# Quick Guide to the Use of **Dorland's Illustrated Medical Dictionary**

For more detailed explanations, see "Notes on the Use of This Dictionary" beginning on page ix.

Word Element — **aden(o)-** [Gr. *adēn,* gen. *adenos* gland] a combining form denoting relationship to a gland or glands.

**ad·e·no·log·a·di·tis** (ad″ə-no-log″ə-di′tis [*adeno-* + Gr. *logades* whites of the eyes + *-itis*] 1. ophthalmia neonatorum. 2. inflammation of the glands of the conjunctiva.

**Des·cartes' law** (da-kahrts′) [René *Descartes,* French mathematician and philosopher, 1596–1650] see under *law.*

**Des·ce·met's membrane** (des-ə-maz′) [Jean *Descemet,* French anatomist, 1732–1810] lamina limitans posterior corneae.

**lam·i·na** (lam′ĭ-nə) gen. and pl. *la′minae* [L.] [TA] layer: a thin flat plate or stratum of a composite structure. The term is often used alone to mean the lamina arcus vertebrae.

**oph·thal·mia** (of-thal′me-ə) [Gr., from *ophthalmos* eye] severe inflammation of the eye or of the conjunctiva or deeper structures of the eye.

**ophthalmia neonato′rum** [MeSH: Ophthalmia Neonatorum], any hyperacute purulent conjunctivitis occurring during the first ten days of life, usually contracted during birth from infected vaginal discharge of the mother; it formerly referred only to gonorrheal infections. An iatrogenic form sometimes occurs after administration of silver nitrate. Called also *neonatal conjunctivitis.*

**seg·men·tum** (seg-men′təm) (pl. *segmen′ta*) [L.] [TA] segment: a general term for a part of an organ or other structure set off by natural or arbitrarily established boundaries.

**segmen′ta medul′lae spina′lis** [TA], segments of spinal cord: the regions of the spinal cord to each of which is attached dorsal and ventral roots of the 31 pairs of spinal nerves, comprising the cervical, thoracic, lumbar, sacral, and coccygeal segments.

**segmen′ta cervica′lia [1–8],** the eight cervical segments; in official terminology the term is considered an alternative to *pars cervicalis medullae spinalis* (q.v.).

**$S_1$** first heart sound; see under *sound.*

**SA** sinoatrial.

**state** (stāt) [L. status] 1. condition or situation; see also *status.* 2. the crisis, or the turning point of an attack of disease.

**dreamy s.,** a state of altered consciousness lasting for a few minutes and accompanied by hallucinations; associated with temporal lobe lesions. See also *temporal lobe epilepsy,* under *epilepsy,* and *petit mal status,* under *status.*

Labels: Word Element; Biographical Information; Eponyms; Pronunciation; Headword; Genitive and Plural; Main entry; Subentry; Subsubentry; Abbreviations; Word Element Used in Etymology; Cross-References to Defined Terms (see entries below); Etymology; Official Terminology; Medical Subject Heading; Synonym; Plural; Definition; Cross-Reference to Subentry; Definitions; Cross-Reference to Related Terms

# Preface

"The aim of the author of this work has been to produce, in a volume of convenient size, an up-to-date Medical Dictionary, sufficiently full for the various requirements of all. . . . The book does not claim to be an encyclopedia; it is a dictionary, a concise and convenient word-book, aiming to furnish full defintions of the terms of medicine and kindred branches. . . . The author has sought a middle course between the large, unwieldy lexicon and the abridged students' dictionary, avoiding the disadvantages of each."

These excerpts from the Preface to the first edition of *The American Illustrated Medical Dictionary,* published in 1900, set forth the principles that have guided a succession of men and women who have worked on this book, both as *The American Illustrated Medical Dictionary* and, following Dr. Dorland's death in 1956, as *Dorland's Illustrated Medical Dictionary.* That *Dorland's* has remained in print for a century is witness to the care taken in ensuring that the essential attributes specified by its originator have been retained. It has, of necessity, grown appreciably over the years, owing to the vast and progressively rapid increase in medical and other scientific knowledge and in the body of vocabulary necessary to describe that knowledge. Balancing the need to include this growing vocabulary against the requirement of keeping the book to a convenient size, all the while updating the existing material, is a challenge that several generations of lexicographers have met successfully through what are now 29 editions.

The vast changes that have occurred in medicine during the 20th century are quickly apparent from a comparison of the original dictionary with the present volume; a handful of examples must suffice here. Immunology was still in its infancy (there is not even an entry for the term in the first edition); antibodies are described simply as "constituents of the blood and tissue-juices of animals rendered immune by inoculation . . ."; blood group antigens were discovered in the same year as the first edition's publication; and the term "allergy" had not yet been coined. A virus is "any animal poison, especially one produced by and capable of transmitting a disease"; filterable viruses would not make their first apearance until the seventh edition. What is now a large body of terms in the specialty of diagnostic imaging is confined primarily to entries for Röntgen rays, discovered only five years before the publication of the book, and skiagraphy ("the art or process of making skiagraphs or photographs by means of the Röntgen rays . . ."). Although entries can be found for aspirin, chloral hydrate, and vaccine, most of the drugs (not to mention entire classes of drugs) used today are absent from the first edition, and many of the drugs listed in the first edition gave only symptomatic relief rather than treating the underlying disease. Other differences between the books reflect changes in the users of the dictionary. In the first edition the etymologies were written with the assumption the user had studied the classical languages and could read Greek words written in Greek characters; this state of affairs continued for over half a century, until in the 23rd edition the Greek was transliterated in recognition of the fact that few people, aside from specialists in classical studies, were still studying ancient Greek.

Turning to the present edition, the most obvious change from the last edition is the addition of a large number of illustrations, bringing the total number of text illustrations and plates to nearly nine hundred. Most of the plates were redrawn for this edition to give them a cleaner, more modern appearance; some of the more crowded ones have been reorganized to improve the clarity of presentation. In all cases the illustrations have been chosen for the practical purpose of aiding the clarity of the definition of an entry and not simply for the sake of having an illustration. The appendices have been updated and reorganized (especially the tables of weights and measures and conversion tables, whose sections have been made easier to find), and a new appendix listing a large number of specific phobias has been added. In the Vocabulary, the format formerly used only for the "Table of Arteries," "Table of Ligaments," and the like, which we felt was easier to read for extremely long blocks of subentries, has been adopted for all long lists of subentries. As always, the entries themselves have been subjected to thorough and merciless revision, and over 8,000 entirely new terms have been added.

In the preparation of this edition, our consultants have performed a great deal of invaluable work in reviewing the entries, and we gratefully acknowledge the generous lending of their expertise. We are indebted to them for their assistance not only in revising existing entries, but also in selecting new terms for inclusion and deleting obsolete terms. The Appendices again include the "Reference Intervals for the Interpretation of Laboratory Tests"; we are grateful to William Z. Borer, M.D., for graciously allowing us to use it once more.

As in past editions, we have used a number of official and standard nomenclatures as guides: for anatomy, the *Terminologia Anatomica* as approved by the Federative Committee on Anatomical Terminology (1998); for enzyme nomenclature, the Recommendations of the Nomenclature Committee of the International Union of Biochemistry and Molecular Biology on the Nomenclature and Classification of Enzymes; for bacteriology, *Bergey's Manual of Systemic Bacteriology* and the ninth edition of *Bergey's Manual of Determinative Bacteriology;* for virology, *Virus Taxonomy: Sixth Report of the International Committee on Taxonomy of Viruses* (1995), together with the proposals approved at the Jerusalem (1996) and Strasburg (1997) ICTV meetings; for psychiatric terms, the *Diagnostic and Statistical Manual of Mental Disorders,* 4th Edition (DSM-IV) (1994), published by the American Psychiatric Association. Drugs are identified as being included in the twenty-fourth edition of the *United States Pharmacopeia (USP 24)* or the nineteenth edition of the *National Formulary (NF 19),* both official from January 1, 2000. The Medical Subject Headings given in the entries are from the 1999 Medical Subject Headings, which are created, maintained, and provided by the U.S. National Library of Medicine. We gratefully acknowledge our indebtedness to the compilers, editors, and publishers of these works, and we emphasize that any inaccuracies that may have arisen from our transcription or interpretation of this material are our sole responsibility.

We also thank the users of this dictionary who, over the years, have provided us with information, opinions, and innumerable suggestions. To them we owe a debt of gratitude; their ongoing interest in the book has helped to maintain *Dorland's* position as the preeminent, most authoritative, and best-selling medical dictionary.

Douglas M. Anderson
Chief Lexicographer

# Consultants

**Thomas E. Andreoli, MD**
Professor and Chairman, Department of Medicine
University of Arkansas for Medical Sciences College of Medicine
Little Rock, Arkansas

**Paul G. Barash, MD**
Professor and Chairman, Department of Anesthesiology
Yale University School of Medicine
New Haven, Connecticut

**Richard E. Behrman, MD**
Clinical Professor of Pediatrics
Stanford University and University of California, San Francisco
Senior Vice President for Medical Affairs
Lucile Packard Foundation for Children's Health

**George L. Blackburn, MD, PhD**
Associate Professor of Surgery
Harvard Medical School
Director, Nutrition Support Service
Chief, Nutrition/Metabolism Laboratory
New England Deaconess Hospital
Boston, Massachusetts

**Neil R. Blacklow, MD**
Chairman, Department of Medicine
Professor of Medicine
University of Massachusetts Medical School
Worcester, Massachusetts

**William Z. Borer, MD**
Professor, Department of Pathology
Thomas Jefferson University
Director, Clinical Chemistry
Thomas Jefferson University Hospital
Philadelphia, Pennsylvania

**George P. Canellos, MD, FACP, FRCP, DSc (hon)**
William Rosenberg Professor of Medicine
Harvard Medical School
Medical Director, Network Development
Dana-Farber/Partners CancerCare
Physician, Brigham and Women's Hospital
Boston, Massachusetts

**Sidney Cohen, MD**
Richard Laylord Evans Professor of Medicine
Chairman, Department of Medicine
Temple University Health Sciences Center
Philadelphia, PA

**M. Wayne Flye, MD, PhD**
Professor of Surgery, Immunology, and Radiology
Washington University School of Medicine
St. Louis, Missouri

**Raymond J. Fonseca, DMD**
Dean, University of Pennsylvania School of Dental Medicine
Professor, Department of Oral and Maxillofacial Surgery
School of Dental Medicine
University of Pennsylvania
Philadelphia, Pennsylvania

**Lester Haddad, MD, FACEP**
Clinical Professor of Family Medicine
Medical University of South Carolina
Charleston, South Carolina
Clinical Professor of Emergency Medicine
Medical College of Georgia
Augusta, Georgia
Staff Physician, Memorial and St. Joseph's Hospital
Savannah, Georgia

**John Bernard Henry, MD**
Professor of Distinguished Service
Director of Pathology 200
Director, Transfusion Medicine
Attending Pathologist
State University of New York Health Science Center at Syracuse
Syracuse, New York

**Donald R. Hoover, MPH, PhD**
Associate Professor, Department of Statistics
Institute for Health Care Policy and Aging Research
Rutgers University
Piscataway, New Jersey

**David T. John, PhD**
Professor of Microbiology and Parasitology
Associate Dean for Basic Sciences and Graduate Studies
Oklahoma State University College of Osteopathic Medicine
Tulsa, Oklahoma

**Jeffrey N. Katz, MD**
Associate Professor of Medicine
Harvard Medical School
Brigham and Women's Hospital
Boston, Massachusetts

**Michael Kienzle, MD**
Associate Professor of Medicine
Office of the Vice President for Research
The University of Iowa
Iowa City, Iowa

**Robert W. Kirk, DVM, Dipl. ACVIM, ADVD**
Professor of Medicine Emeritus
College of Veterinary Medicine
Cornell University
Ithaca, New York

**Juha P. Kokko, MD, PhD**
Asa G. Candler Professor and Chairman of Medicine
Associate Dean for Clinical Research
Emory University School of Medicine
Atlanta, Georgia

**William L. Meyerhoff, MD, PhD**
Professor and Chairman
Arthur E. Meyerhoff Chair in Otolaryngology—Head and Neck Surgery
The University of Texas Southwestern Medical Center at Dallas
Dallas, Texas

**J.P. Mohr, MD**
Sciarra Professor of Clinical Neurology
College of Physicians and Surgeons of Columbia University
The Neurological Institute, Columbia Presbyterian Medical Center
New York, New York

**B. Keith Moore, PhD**
Professor of Dental Materials and Director of the Dental Materials Laboratory
Department of Restorative Dentistry
Indiana University School of Dentistry
Indianapolis, Indiana

**Keith L. Moore, PhD, FIAC, FRSM**
Professor of Anatomy and Cell Biology
Faculty of Medicine, University of Toronto
Toronto, Ontario, Canada
Member of the Federative Committee on Anatomical Terminology of the International Federation of Associations of Anatomists

**Carl E. Ravin, MD**
Professor and Chairman
Department of Radiology
Duke University Medical Center
Durham, North Carolina

**David J. Skorton, MD**
Professor of Medicine, Electrical and Computer Engineering and Biomedical Engineering
Vice President for Research
The University of Iowa
Iowa City, Iowa

**G. Thomas Strickland, MD, PhD**
Professor of Epidemiology and Preventive Medicine, Microbiology and Immunology, and Medicine
Director, International Health Program
University of Maryland School of Medicine
Senior Associate, Department of Immunology and Infectious Diseases
Johns Hopkins School of Public Health
Baltimore, Maryland

**Steven E. Weinberger, MD**
Chief, Pulmonary and Critical Care Division
Associate Chairman for Education, Department of Medicine
Beth Israel Deaconess Medical Center
Harvard Medical School
Boston, Massachusetts

**Sam W. Wiesel, M.D.**
Professor and Chairman, Department of Orthopaedic Surgery
Georgetown University Medical Center
Washington, DC

# CONTENTS

# INDEX TO TABLES

# INDEX TO PLATES

## Main Entries and Subentries

Main entries appear in boldface type, with bullets indicating syllabication. Terms consisting of two or more words are ordinarily given as subentries under the noun, as is traditional in medical dictionaries; subentries are also set in boldface type, and each is set on a new line and followed by a comma. Although this arrangement may be confusing at first to those accustomed to general dictionaries, it has the advantage of allowing related terms to be grouped together (for example, all the *lymphocyte* entries appear under the main entry *lymphocyte*).

According to this scheme, *Howell-Jolly bodies, ketone bodies,* and *pineal body* are all to be found under the main entry *body,* and *carotid pulse, dicrotic pulse,* and *paradoxical pulse* are to be found under the main entry *pulse.* It is important for the user to bear in mind that it is impossible to provide entries for every variation of every term, so that a phrase that is not found under one main entry should be sought under a synonymous main entry. For example, the same entity may be described as a disease or a syndrome (as *Fabry's disease—Fabry's syndrome,* which is to be found under *disease*) or as a sign or a phenomenon (as *Gowers' sign—Gowers' phenomenon,* which appears under *sign*). In such cases, the main entry should be consulted for references to synonymous terms under which the desired phrase may be found.

*Example:*

> **treat·ment** . . . the management and care of a patient for the purpose of combating disease or disorder. See also under *care, maneuver, method, technique, test,* and *therapy.*

In subentries, the main entry word is represented only by the initial letter, e.g., *cogwheel r.* under *respiration,* unless it occurs in the plural form. Regular English plurals are represented by the initial letter followed by *'s,* as *b's* for *bones* under *bone.* Irregular plurals, such as *teeth* under *tooth,* and Latin plurals, as *foramina* under *foramen,* are spelled out in full.

### Chemical Compounds

Exceptions to the use of subentries are made for specific acids and for enzymes and enzyme deficiencies. Names of specific acids will be found as main entries under the first word of the name, e.g., *sulfuric acid* under *S,* as will enzyme names, e.g., *alkaline phosphatase* under *A.* Enzyme deficiencies will be found as main entries immediately following the entry for the enzyme in question, e.g., *carbamoyl phosphate synthetase deficiency* after *carbamoyl phosphate synthetase.*

Chemical compounds embodying the name of an element will be found as subentries under the element; for example, *aluminum acetate, aluminum hydroxide,* and *aluminum sulfate* are all located under *aluminum.* Chemical compounds that begin with the adjectival form denoting valence will be found under the salt or ester, e.g., *ferric citrate* under *citrate.*

### Drug Names

Drugs are to be found under the active moiety, if that is a main entry. For example, *prednisolone acetate, prednisolone hemisuccinate,* and *prednisolone sodium phosphate* all appear under *prednisolone.* If the active moiety is not itself a main entry, then the entire drug name appears as a main entry, e.g., *methadone hydrochloride* under *M.*

## Syllabication

Acceptable word divisions are indicated for main entries by the use of bullets within the entry word; syllabication is based on pronunciation. Not all syllable breaks are given; for example, the separation of a single vowel from the beginning or end of a word is not allowed and is not shown. Likewise, single letters should not be separated from the word elements to which they belong in compound words. In many cases a word may be broken at places other than the ones indicated; for example, different pronunciations imply different sets of breaks, so that *melanocyte* could be divided *mel·a·no·cyte* or *me·lano·cyte,* depending on which syllable, the first or second, is stressed. In any case, breaks that could confuse a reader as to the meaning of a word are to be avoided.

## Sequence of Entries

### Main Entries

Main entries will be found alphabetized on the sequence of letters, regardless of spaces or hyphens that may occur between them. (Special rules govern terms that begin with proper names, which are mainly eponyms; see below.) Thus the following sequences will be found:

| | |
|---|---|
| **formboard** | **heart** |
| **form-class** | **heartbeat** |
| **forme** | **heart block** |
| **form-family** | **heartburn** |

### Subentries

Subentries, like main entries, are alphabetized letter by letter. The main entry word, whether it is represented by the initial letter, the initial plus *'s,* or a spelled-out plural, is ignored in alphabetizing subentries, as are prepositions, conjunctions, and articles. Inflected forms, such as genitives and plurals of Latin words, are treated as if they were nominative singular. (For what is meant by "inflected forms," see "Presentation of Plurals and Other Inflections," page xi.) The following forms, all from *os craniale* "cranial bone," are considered equivalent for purposes of alphabetization: *os craniale, ossis cranialis, ossa cranialia,* and *ossium cranialium.*

In accordance with the above rules, the following sequences of subentries are found under *ganglion* and *prolapse:*

| | |
|---|---|
| **ganglion** | **prolapse** |
| **Andersch's ganglia** | **anal p.** |
| **ganglia aorticorenalia** | **p. of anus** |
| **auditory g.** | **p. of the cord** |
| **Auerbach's g.** | **frank p.** |
| **g. autonomicum** | **p. of the iris** |

A special case is that of what may be called inverted subentries, in which the initial word or words are moved to the end of the entry, set off by a comma. This is done in order to allow related terms to fall together in the subentry list; such inversions are especially common in the anatomical vocabulary for anterior/posterior structures and the like. These terms are alphabetized as usual up to the comma marking the inversion; words following the comma, however, are not counted except within the group of repeated entries:

**lobe**
**inferior l., left**
**inferior l., right**
**inferior l. of lung, left**
**inferior l. of lung, right**

### Proper Names

A number of main entries are included for terms beginning with a proper name, usually eponymic terms; these give information about the term's origin (most often a bit of biographical information) and cross references to entries where definitions may be found. These cross references can be helpful in giving an indication of where to look for an entry that may go by more than one name (such as disease or syndrome). Entries of this sort are alphabetized as entries for the proper name only, following this set of rules:

(1) The *'s*, if one occurs, is never counted for alphabetization. *Addison's planes* precedes *addisonian.*
(2) Words following the name are not counted for alphabetical order unless the names are the same. Thus, *Addison's disease* precedes *Addison's planes.*
(3) Only the first name in a term containing more than one proper name is counted for alphabetization unless the entries are the same in all other respects. *Babinski's reflex, Babinski-Fröhlich syndrome, Babinski-Nageotte syndrome, Babinski-Vaquez* syndrome appear in that order.
(4) Umlauts (*ö, ü*) are ignored for purposes of alphabetization. *Löwe's ring, Lowe's syndrome, Lowe-Terry-MacLachlan syndrome, Löwenberg's canal, Löwenthal's tract, Lower's rings* appear in that order.
(5) Names beginning *Mac* or *Mc* are alphabetized as if spelled *Mac.*

Subentries that begin with a proper name also follow the above rules for sequencing.

Proper nouns (or capitalized entries) appear before common nouns (or lower case entries). Thus *Bacillus* precedes *bacillus.*

### Chemical Terms

In the alphabetization of chemical names, italic prefixes (e.g., *o-*, *p-*, *m-*, *trans-*, *cis-*) are ignored, as are numbers, Greek letters, and the prefixes D-, L-, *d-*, *l-*, (+)-, and (−)-. When a prefix is spelled out, however, the term is to be found under the fully spelled out form, for example, *levodopa* under *L*, *orthocresol* under *O*, and *beta-naphtholsulfonic acid* under *B*.

## Indication of Pronunciation

A phonetic spelling of a term appears in parentheses after the boldface entry word. The pronunciation is given for all main entries; it is generally not given for subentries but does appear in some subentries that are foreign phrases. As a rule, the most common pronunciation is given, with no effort to list the variants, although exceptions to this do occur. The phonetic spelling is kept as simple as possible, with few diacritical marks; the only special character used is ə, the schwa, used to represent the unstressed vowel sound heard at the end of *sofa.* The schwa is also used in combination with *r* to represent the sound heard in *fur* and the second syllable of *other.* This combination may be found in both stressed and unstressed syllables.

There are four basic rules:

(1) An unmarked vowel ending a syllable (an "open" syllable) is long. Thus *ma* represents the pronunciation of *may.*
(2) An unmarked vowel in a syllable ending in a consonant (a "closed" syllable) is short. Thus *not* represents the pronunciation of *knot.*
(3) A long vowel in a closed syllable is indicated by a macron. Thus *māt* represents the pronunciation of *mate.*
(4) A short vowel that ends or itself constitutes a syllable is indicated by a breve. Thus *ĭ-mūn′* represents the pronunciation of *immune.*

Primary (′) and secondary (″) stresses are shown in polysyllabic words, with unstressed syllables followed by hyphens, as in *rep″lĭ-kā′shən.* Monosyllables, even when part of a compound term, have no stress mark, as in *bens jōnz.* Primary stresses are also given as part of the boldface subentries for foreign phrases.

It is impossible with *Dorland's* simplified phonetics to represent the native pronunciations of many foreign words and proper names. These are shown as closely as possible in English phonetics.

### Pronunciation Guide

#### Vowels

(For the use of breves and macrons, see the four rules above.)

| | | | |
|---|---|---|---|
| ə | sof*a* | ŏ | g*o*t |
| ā | m*a*te | ū | f*ue*l |
| ă | b*a*t | ŭ | b*u*t |
| ē | b*ea*m | aw | *a*ll |
| ĕ | m*e*t | oi | b*oi*l |
| ī | b*i*te | o͞o | b*oo*m |
| ĭ | b*i*t | o͝o | b*oo*k |
| ō | h*o*me | ou | f*ow*l |

#### Consonants

| | | | |
|---|---|---|---|
| b | *b*ook | h | *h*eat |
| d | *d*og | j | *j*ewel, *g*em |
| f | *f*og | k | *c*art, pi*ck* |
| g | *g*et | l | *l*ook |

| | | | |
|---|---|---|---|
| m | *m*ouse | ch | *ch*in |
| n | *n*ew | ks | si*x* |
| p | *p*ark | kw | *qu*ote |
| r | *r*at | ng | si*ng* |
| s | *s*igh | sh | *sh*ould |
| t | *t*in | th | *th*in, *th*an |
| w | *w*ood | zh | mea*s*ure |
| z | si*z*e, pha*s*e | | |

## Presentation of Plurals and Other Inflections

In main entries for foreign (nearly always Greek or Latin) nouns, the original and anglicized plurals are given after the phonetic spelling; irregular plurals of English nouns are also given.

*Example:*

**sto·ma** (sto′mə) pl. *stomas* or *sto′mata* . . .

**tooth** (tooth) pl. *teeth* . . .

The original foreign plural is often given a separate boldface listing in its proper alphabetical place in the vocabulary.

*Example:*

**sto·ma·ta** (sto′mə-tə) [Gr.] plural of *stoma.*

Latin is used, especially in anatomy, to form phrases of the type "the X of Y," for example, *arcus aortae,* "the arch of the aorta." The prepositional phrase introduced by "of" corresponds to the Latin genitive case (*aortae* "of the aorta," from *aorta*). For this reason, the genitive case (= English "of") for Latin nouns is also frequently given, introduced by the abbreviation *gen.*

*Examples:*

**pa·pil·la** . . . gen. and pl. *papil′lae* . . .

**os¹** . . . gen. *o′ris,* pl. *o′ra* . . .

**os²** . . . gen. *os′sis,* pl. *os′sa* . . .

Latin and Greek (and a number of other languages, such as German and Russian, for that matter) are said to be inflected, that is, words change form to show how they are related to other words in a sentence. An example of this is the "aortae" phrase given above, where the change in the ending of the word corresponds to the use of the English preposition "of." Other Latin inflected forms are found in subentries; these forms will be the objects in a prepositional phrase. For example, under the main entry *fissura,* there is the subentry *f. in ano; ano* is the object of the preposition *in* and is one of the half dozen or so different inflected forms of *anus,* which is a main entry in the Dictionary and has listed with it the genitive and plural form *ani.* As in all subentries, differences in singular and plural forms do not count for alphabetizing, nor do prepositions or conjunctions (e.g., *et* "and," *in* "in"); thus under the main entry *fissura,* the subentry *f. in ano* precedes *f. antitragohelicina.*

## Etymology

Information on the origin of a word appears in brackets after the phonetic spelling or a plural form of the entry when that is given. The information is necessarily brief, and the reader must often reason from the etymon, the original word from which other words are derived, to the meaning. For example, for the main entry *dualism* the etymological section reads [L. *duo* two]. L. stands for Latin (languages are either abbreviated or spelled out; see "Abbreviations Used in This Dictionary," p. xiii). The word *duo* is the etymon, and "two" is the English translation of the etymon, not of the entry. The reader proceeds from *duo* to *dual* to *dualism.* Furthermore, space limitations preclude the listing of all the stages in the passage from the etymon to the modern derivative (i.e., the entry). For example, the etymological part of the entry for *vein* is simply [L. *vena*]; in full, it would be [Middle English *veine,* from Old Fr., from L. *vena*].

For those foreign words or phrases taken into English entire, only the language is given, with a translation given within quotation marks.

*Example:*

**déjà vu** [Fr. "already seen"] . . .

If the meaning of the foreign word or phrase is the same as that of the entry word, no translation is given.

There are four further additions:

(1) As a guide to related vocabulary, especially for anatomical terms, the main entry may be followed in brackets by its Greek or Latin equivalent (or both).

*Example:*

**kid·ney** . . . [L. *ren;* Gr. *nephros*]

(2) Many technical terms of Greek or Latin derivation are listed twice as main entries (and both times with etymology, meaning, and cross references), first as an independent word, then as a combining form, e.g., *ectomy* and *-ectomy.*
(3) There is an essay, "Fundamentals of Medical Etymology" (see p. xiv), which explains the basic rules for the derivation and composition of Greek, Latin, and Greco-Latin terms in medicine. At the end of the essay there is an analytical word list of Greek and Latin roots, prefixes, and combining forms; the list is an aid for the analysis of existing medical terms and the creation of new ones.
(4) The prefixes (e.g., *hyper-, hypo-*), suffixes (e.g., *-ia, -oid*), and combining forms (e.g., *actino-, -emia*) from the analytical word list are also listed as main entries in the vocabulary.

## Official Publications

Certain terms listed in official publications are identified by an abbreviation in brackets. In main entries, these abbreviations usually appear after the etymology (or after the phonetic spelling if no etymology is given). In subentries, they appear immediately after the boldface subentry word. When a term has more than one meaning, the abbreviation is placed at the beginning of the definition to which it applies. The following abbreviations are used:

| | |
|---|---|
| [DSM-IV] | *Diagnostic and Statistical Manual of Mental Disorders* of the American Psychiatric Association, 4th edition, 1994 |
| [EC] | Enzyme Commission number (e.g., citrate (*si*)-synthase . . . [EC 4.1.3.7]) from the Recommendations of the Nomenclature Committee of the International Union of Biochemistry and Molecular Biology on the Nomenclature and Classification of Enzymes published in *Enzyme Nomenclature* (1992) |
| [TA] | *Terminologia Anatomica* (1998) |
| [NF] | *The National Formulary,* 19th edition (2000) |
| [USP] | *The United States Pharmacopeia,* 24th edition (2000) |

## Medical Subject Headings

Medical Subject Headings (MeSH) and tree numbers are given for a number of terms. In some cases, the Medical Subject Heading is also given on synonyms for such terms; in the interest of conserving space, these are generally confined to MeSH synonyms.

## Placement of Definitions and Cross References

With few exceptions, a definition is given in only one place for two or more synonymous terms. Entries for the synonyms provide cross references to the term where the definition is to be found. Such cross references are in place of a definition and are set in roman type:

**mas·to·plas·ty** (mas′to-plas″te) mammaplasty.

The definition will be found at *mammaplasty.* In many cases, a list of synonyms is given at the end of the entry where the definition appears. This list is introduced by the phrase "called also" and the synonyms are set in italic type.

Cross references from one subentry to another subentry under the same main heading use the abbreviated form of the main entry:

**syndrome**
**hypersomnia-bulimia s.,** Kleine-Levin s.

Cross-referencing has also been used for earlier terms that have been supplanted and for variant spellings of a term. In such instances, the definition is attached to the term that is currently the preferred term. A word of warning is, however, warranted here. In some instances, preference for one term over another may be slight or even nonexistent, while in others, different spellings or terms may be preferred by different authorities, by different specialties, or in different regions. In such cases, the practice of defining words only at one place has been adhered to as a means of keeping down the size of the Dictionary by avoiding duplication of definitions, and the user should remember that the appearance of a cross reference or definition does not always indicate a preference for one form or synonym over another.

### Related Entries

Cross references to related entries or to entries where additional information may be found are also given. They are identified by "see also," "cf.," and "q.v." (or "qq. v."). (For the abbreviations, see "Abbreviations Used in This Dictionary," page xiii). Cross references introduced by "see also" or "cf." are set in italic type.

### Official Terminology

In general, when a term is included in one of the official publications listed in the preceding section ("Official Publications"), its definition appears at the official term. Thus the definition for "pelvic bone" is found at *os coxae;* a cross reference to the official term is found at the subentry under *bone.* Exceptions have been made in a few cases where the nonofficial term is so common or important that it makes the most sense to put the definition on the unofficial term (for example, *heart* is defined, not *cor*).

### Entries Containing a Proper Name

Entries containing a proper name are generally entered twice. The definition for the entity is given in a subentry under the appropriate main entry, as *Down syndrome* under *syndrome.* Biographical, geographical, or other information attached to the proper name is given in a main entry (see "Proper Names" in the section "Sequence of Entries," p. x). A cross reference is given from the main entry for the proper name to the subentry where the term is defined. For example:

**Down syndrome (disease)** (down) [John Langdon Haydon *Down,* English physician, 1828–1896] see under *syndrome.*

## Form of Eponyms

The use of the possessive form ending in *'s* for eponyms is becoming progressively less common, and the entries for eponymic terms in this Dictionary reflect this ongoing change in usage. The Dictionary therefore presents an inconsistent mixture of forms. The user should be aware that although the use of the nonpossessive form is increasingly common, it is by no means universal. (The user should also be aware that some terms, such as *Apgar score,* have never had an *'s* and that for some terms, such as *Christmas disease* and *Down syndrome,* the nonposessive form is actually preferred.) The variation in forms seen in the Dictionary is thus only a reflection of change and *not* a prescription for the use of possessive and nonpossessive forms.

## Symbols and Abbreviations

Symbols, abbreviations, and acronyms are included as main entries; definitions consist of the term for which the symbol or the abbreviation stands, with a translation if the term is in a foreign language. These terms will usually be found at the appropriate places in the vocabulary; some terms, however, are self-explanatory and have no entry, such as the names of organizations and phrases like the following:

**q.h.** abbreviation for L. *qua'que ho'ra,* every hour.

In a few cases, the definition is placed at the abbreviation or acronym instead of at the term for which it stands, e.g., *ELISA;* in such cases, the abbreviation, not the term, is what is actually in use.

Abbreviations appear both with and without periods. This should not be taken to denote proper usage, since abbreviations may appear either way; at the present the trend is away from the use of the period for most abbreviations.

A list of selected abbreviations also appears in Appendix 1.

## Abbreviations Used in This Dictionary

| | |
|---|---|
| a. | artery (L. *arteria*); agar |
| aa. | arteries (L. *arteriae*) |
| ant. | anterior |
| Ar. | Arabic |
| A.S. | Anglo-Saxon |
| c. | about (L. *circa*) |
| cf. | compare (L. *confer*) |
| def. | definition |
| dim. | diminutive |
| EC | Enzyme Commission |
| e.g. | for example (L. *exempli gratia*) |
| Fr. | French |
| gen. | genitive |
| Ger. | German |
| Gr. | Greek |
| i.e. | that is (L. *id est*) |
| inf. | inferior |
| It. | Italian |
| L. | Latin |
| l. | ligament (L. *ligamentum*) |
| ligg. | ligaments (L. *ligamenta*) |
| lat. | lateral |
| m. | muscle (L. *musculus*) |
| med. | medial; median |
| mm. | muscles (L. *musculi*) |
| n. | nerve (L. *nervus*) |
| neg. | negative |
| NF | National Formulary |
| nn. | nerves (L. *nervi*) |
| obs. | obsolete |
| pl. | plural |
| Port. | Portuguese |
| post. | posterior |
| qq. v. | which (things) see (L. *quae vide*) |
| q.v. | which see (L. *quod vide*) |
| sing. | singular |
| Sp. | Spanish |
| sup. | superior |
| TA | Terminologia Anatomica |
| USAN | United States Adopted Names |
| USP | United States Pharmacopeia |
| v. | vein (L. *vena*) |
| vv. | veins (L. *venae*) |

# *Fundamentals of Medical Etymology*

By Joseph M. Patwell, PhD

Twenty-six hundred years ago the Asiatic Greeks of Ionia and the Italian Greeks in Magna Graecia began the speculative and investigational sciences, pushing the then Greek to its limits, pushing beyond those limits, riveting new meanings onto old words, smithing new words for new ideas and discoveries—*philosophia,* "the love of wisdom," was supposedly first used by Pythagoras.

The sciences still go their robust way, iconoclastic but also indebted to and respectful of their ancient tradition. In anatomy, surgery, clinical medicine, and laboratory medicine, Greek, Latin, and Greco-Latin have always formed well over ninety per cent of the technical terms. Knowing the fundamentals of Greek and Latin word formation is immensely helpful in learning the vocabulary of modern medicine or of any modern science and is absolutely necessary for anyone coining a word for a new hypothesis, theory, process, or entity. The purpose of this introduction is to present those fundamentals in as practical and concise a form as possible; any statements contrary to historical and comparative linguistic fact that are made in the following pages are deliberate in keeping with this purpose.

## Alphabet and Pronunciation

The Latin alphabet is a modification of one of the many Greek alphabets. The order and shape of the Latin letters is the same as ours except that the Classical Latin alphabet has no *j*, *u*, or *w*, which are improvements dating from the Middle Ages.

The consonants of the Latin alphabet have about the same values as the English except that *c*, *ch*, *g*, *s*, *t*, and *v* are pronounced as in *c*old, *ch*rome, *g*et, *s*o, *t*in, and *w*ine, and not as in *c*ent, *ch*ill, *g*em, ro*s*e, men*t*ion, and *v*ine. *Ph* and *th* may be pronounced as in *ph*ilosophy and *th*eology.

Latin vowels may be long or short. The short vowels are pronounced very much like the American w*a*nder, b*e*d, *i*t, h*o*pe, and p*u*t; short *y* sounds like the *ü* in German *dünn.* The long vowels are pronounced as in f*a*ther, h*e*y, mar*i*ne, st*o*ve, and r*u*de; long *y* is pronounced like the *ü* in the German *über.*

Words are stressed on the next-to-last syllable, called the penult, if that syllable contains a long vowel or diphthong or is followed by two or more consonants, otherwise on the syllable before the penult.

The Greek alphabet used today is based on that used in Athens by the end of the fifth century B.C. The accompanying table shows one modern English pronunciation of each ancient Greek character in terms of English.

| Capital | Small Letter | Sound | Name | Transcription |
|---|---|---|---|---|
| Α | α | *a*rchaic | alpha | a |
| Β | β | *b*arbarism | beta | b |
| Γ | γ | *g*rammar | gamma | g |
| Δ | δ | *d*ogma | delta | d |
| Ε | ϵ | *e*lephant | epsilon | e |
| Ζ | ζ | *z*oology | zeta | z |
| Η | η | *ai*r | eta | ē |
| Θ | θ, ϑ | *th*eist | theta | th |
| Ι | ι | mach*i*ne | iota | i |
| Κ | κ | s*k*eleton | kappa | c (Latin), k (Dorland's) |
| Λ | λ | *l*ithograph | lambda | l |
| Μ | μ | *m*usic | mu | m |
| Ν | ν | *n*eolithic | nu | n |
| Ξ | ξ | e*x*egesis | xi | x |
| Ο | ο | *o*belisk | omicron | o |
| Π | π | s*p*asm | pi | p |
| Ρ | ρ | a*r*achnid | rho | r |
| Σ | σ, ς | *s*ymbol | sigma | s |
| Τ | τ | s*t*adium | tau | t |
| Υ | υ | ü, über (German) | upsilon | y |
| Φ | ϕ | *ph*oto | phi | ph |
| Χ | χ | Ba*ch* (German) | chi | ch |
| Ψ | ψ | di*ps*omania | psi | ps |
| Ω | ω | *o*cher, Sh*aw* | omega | ō |

The vowels are α, ϵ, η, ι, ο, υ, ω, most of which may be followed by ι or υ to form diphthongs, the most common of which are shown below.

| Diphthong | Sound | Transcription |
|---|---|---|
| αι | *ai*sle | ae, e, or ai |
| αυ | *ou*t | au |
| ϵι | *ei*ght | i or ei |
| ϵυ | *eu*phony | eu |
| οι | p*oi*son | oe, e, or oi |
| ου | gh*ou*l | ou or u |
| υι | s*ui*te | ui, l*ui* (French) |

## Transliteration

The Romans transliterated kappa with *c*, not *k*, and chi with *ch*, not *kh*; thus *ch*ara*c*ter, not *kh*ara*k*ter. This Dictionary transliterates kappa with *k* in its etymologies in order to make immediately clear the nature of the underlying Greek sound: Spelling *cystis* for *kystis,* cyst, could cause doubt whether the sound was "kystis" or "systis." Similar difficulties with chi are less likely, and therefore *Dorland's* retains the traditional *ch*; hence our etymological spelling is *charakter.*

Classical Greek ϵι was pronounced as in *skein,* but by the end of the fourth century B.C. it was pronounced as in *seize;* thus the city that Alexander the Greek founded in Egypt, *Alexandreia,* became Alexandria in Latin. English generally prefers the Latin transliteration, but the use of *ei* for ϵι is growing. This Dictionary transliterates ϵι with *ei* in its etymologies.

The Romans transliterated Greek αι and οι with their own *ae* and *oe*, which had nearly the same pronunciation. By late antiquity the Greek and Latin diphthongs had become simple vowels, having gone through the regular progression *ai*sle to *ai*r to *ai*m, and the spelling wavered between the old diphthongs and the new pronunciation. This vacillation persists in English: the British prefer the diphthongs (*oe*dema, h*ae*morrhage); the Americans, the simple vowel (*e*dema, h*e*morrhage). In official nomenclature, e.g., the *Terminologia Anatom-*

*ica,* the *Index nominum genericorum (plantarum),* and the *International Code of Nomenclature of Bacteria,* the official orthography fluctuates from edition to edition, swinging from *oesophagus* to *esophagus* and *Haemophilus* to *Hemophilus* and back again. In the etymologies of this Dictionary Greek *αι* and *οι* are transliterated by *ai* and *oi,* and Latin *ae* and *oe* retained, for clarity's sake.

The Greeks especially but also the Romans had the same troubles with aitch *(h)* that Cockneys do, dropping it where it belonged and adding it where it did not. In Greek, initial *h-* ordinarily remained in simple words (*haima,* blood) but would either assimilate with or disappear before a prefix. For assimilation, *hypo* and *haima* make *hyphaimos,* suffused with blood (first appearing in Hippocrates); for disappearance, *a-, an-* and *haima* make *anaimia,* anemia (first appearing in Aristotle), not *ahaimia* and *ahemia.*

Latin usually preserved initial *h-* even after prefixes *(homo habilis, habilitas, inhabilitas; honor, honestus, inhonestus),* but very much of our Latin has come through French with inconsistent (to say the least) spellings and pronunciations: *able, ability* and *inability,* not *hable, hability,* and *inhability; honor* and *honest,* not *onor* and *onest.*

Speakers of American English generally have no difficulty with *h-* and treat it as a full consonant when adding prefixes; thus we have *inharmonious,* not *anarmonious; ahaptoglobinemia,* not *anaptoglobinemia;* and *anhydride,* not *anydride* or *ahydride.*

Greek words are written with several accents that now indicate the stressed syllable. Words beginning with a vowel, diphthong, or rho (*ρ*) are written with a so-called breathing mark over the initial vowel or rho or over the second element of the diphthong (*ἑτεροδοξία, heterodoxia; αἰσθητικός, aisthētikos; ῥυθμός, rhythmos*). The *rough* breathing mark (῾) indicates that the syllable begins with an aspiration (aitch) as in *heterodoxia,* above, and words beginning with the rough breathing are usually transcribed into English with an initial *h.* Words beginning with a rho or an upsilon always have a rough breathing (*ὑπέρ, hyper; ῥεῦμα, rheuma*). The smooth breathing (᾿) shows the absence of aspiration and so has no effect on pronunciation (*ἀρωματικός, arōmatikos; αὐτογράφος, autographos*).

The other conventions for transliterations from Greek are as follows: Gamma (*γ*), which before gamma (*γ*), kappa (*κ*), chi (*χ*), or xi (*ξ*) has the sound of *n* as in *finger,* is transcribed as *n.** Initial *rho* and its rough breathing (*ῥ*) are transcribed as *rh* not *hr,* as *rheuma,* above; double *rho* (*ρρ*) is transcribed as *rrh* (*διάρροια, diarrhoea, diarrhea*). *Upsilon* (*υ*) is transcribed as *y* (*ῥυθμός, rhythmos*) except in diphthongs, where it is reproduced by *u* (*ῥεῦμα, rheuma*).

A few Greek words have come into English unchanged (*σκελετόν, skeleton; αὐτόματον, automaton*); most Greek words have passed into English through Latin, undergoing slight change (Greek *στέρνον, sternon;* Latin *sternum*); and some Greek words have passed through a secondary intermediary language, such as French, with still further change (Greek *χειρουργία, cheirourgia;* Latin *chirurgia;* French *cirurgerie;* English *surgery*). Other changes are accounted for by our tendency to drop Greek and Latin inflectional endings (*ἀξίωμα, axioma,* becomes axiom; *dorsalis* becomes dorsal) or replace them with a final mute *e* as if the words had come into English through French (*γονοφόρος, gonophoros,* becomes gonophore; *spina* becomes spine).

* During World War II, *Ancistrodon* (from *ἄγκιστρον,* fishhook, and *ὀδοντ-,* tooth) was reformed to *Agkistrodon,* which is the official spelling. *Ancistrodon* and *Ankistrodon* are both correct, but not *Agkistrodon:* Greek *ἄγγελος* (messenger) becomes *angelus* in Latin and *angel* in English, not *aggelus* and *aggel.*

## Word Formation

The most frequent, the most important, and the seemingly most capricious changes in Greek or Latin words (or in English words, for that matter) arise not when the words pass from Greek or Latin into English, but when these words are first formed in the original language.

Many words in English and nearly all words in the Classical languages are combinations of roots and affixes. The root of a word contains the basic, lexical meaning, and the affixes give the root its shape as a word. (Affixes for the most part are prefixes and suffixes, including the inflections, added before or after the root, respectively.)

For example, in the English *love, loves, lover, lovers, loving, loved, lovingly, unloved,* and *unlovable,* the root is *love,* and the various prefixes *(un-)* and suffixes (*-s, -r, -r-s, -ing, -ing-ly,* etc.) form the foot into a word and modify that word for use in an utterance.

In English a root may very often function as an independent word, as *love, hate, smile, frown, milk;* these "root words" are extremely rare in the Classical languages. Nearly always in Latin and Greek, and usually in English, a word is a complex consisting of a form of a root and one or more affixes, which are not independent words themselves but may be used only to modify the root in some way (as *un-, -er, -ed*); such words are called "derived words."

When the root remains unchanged from derived word to derived word (a "regular" or "weak" root) and the affixes remain unaffected in their surroundings, the entire system of derived words has a transparent, instantly comprehended simplicity, as in *love* and its forms. So in Latin and Greek: there is a systematic clarity to the derivations of the Latin root *laud-* (praise)—the nouns *laudis* and *laudator* (praise, praiser); the principal parts of the regular verb, *laudo* (I praise), *laudare* (to praise); and the adjectives *laudabilis* and *laudatorius* (laudable, laudatory). There is also a regular system in the Greek root *pau-* (stop): the nouns *pausis* (pause) and *paustēr* (reliever, calmer); the regular principal parts of the verb *pauō* (I stop), *pausō* (I shall stop); and the adjectives *pausteon* (to be ended) and *paustērios* (relieving, calming).

Difficulties arise in English, Latin, and Greek with roots that change from word to word ("irregular" or "strong" roots) as in the English *sing, sang, sung, song;* and one says *singer,* not *songer; unsung,* not *unsing;* and *unsingable,* not *unsungable.* One example will suffice. The root *ten-* (stretch) appears in Latin and Greek (and also in English as *thin*). In Latin the root is as regular as the English *talk,* and the derivations are obvious: *ten*do (tendon), *ten*sio (tension), *ten*ius (tenuous, thin), ex*ten*uatus (stretched out, thinned out, weakened). In Greek, however, the same root appears as *ten-, tein-, ton-, ta-, tan-,* and *tain-.* Indeed, the rules for ancient Greek word formation would make a heavy book, and therefore, for efficiency's sake, the analytical word list, which follows this essay, gives examples of which affixes are attached to which forms of the root, for both the methodical Latin and the exuberant Greek.

In the Latin system there is an inconsistency affecting many common Latin and therefore English words: Latin roots with short vowels will have the normal, strong vowel in simple, unprefixed words but a reduced, weakened vowel in prefixed words.

Consider the Latin root *făc-* (do, make). The normal *ă* remains in unprefixed words; hence the principal parts of the verb are:

| | |
|---|---|
| *făcio* | I make |
| *făcere* | to make |
| *făctus* | made |

Other unprefixed derivatives are:

| | |
|---|---|
| *facies* | thing made or formed, face, "facies" |
| *factor* | factor |
| *factura* | as in manu*facture* |
| *faction-* | faction |
| *factiosus* | factious |
| *facil-* | doable, feasible, easy |

From *facil-* are derived in turn:

| | |
|---|---|
| *facultat-* | faculty |
| *facilitat-* | facility |

Now let us add the prefix *ex* to the root *fac-*. *Ex* assimilates to *ef-* before *f* and changes the meaning of *fac-* to "complete." This or any prefix will cause a short *ă* to become a short *ĭ* before one consonant and a short *ĕ* before two consonants. Note the changes in the principal parts of the prefixed verb:

| | | |
|---|---|---|
| *efficio* | from | *exfacio* |
| *efficere* | from | *exfacere* |
| *effectus* | from | *exfactus* |

It is from words like *efficio* that one can most clearly understand the derivations of Latin words. One forms the present participle by dropping the final *-re* from the present active infinitive, which is the form used in the etymologies of *Dorland's,* and adding *-nt* (verbs like *efficio* drop the final *-ere* and add *-ient*). The present participle of *efficio, efficere* is *efficient-* (efficient). And from the present participle is derived the noun *efficientia* (efficiency).

From the last principal part, *effectus,* one forms derivatives by dropping the *-us* and adding other suffixes. Thus from *effect-* one derives

| | |
|---|---|
| *effectum* | effect |
| *effector* | effector |
| *effectivus* | effective |

Occasionally the Romans would recompose a prefixed form according to the unprefixed norm. The most common example, and perfect for medical use, is *calefacio,* I warm, not *caleficio,* and therefore *calefacient-,* not *caleficient-.*

Alas, there are exceptions. *Tenant* comes to English not directly from the Latin *tenēre,* to hold, which would give us *tenent,* but through the French *tenir,* and in French all verbs form their present participles in *-ant,* therefore *tenant;* a *locum tenens* is a *lieu tenant.*

Assimilation may affect the consonants between roots and affixes. In English the *v* in *drive* and *thrive* becomes voiceless and changes to *f* before the voiceless suffix *-t* that forms the nouns *drift* and *thrift.* In Latin, assimilation is usually minimal and obvious: *scribo* ("I write") and *scriba* ("writer, scribe") alternate with *scripsi* ("I wrote") and *scriptura* ("writing, scripture"). Occasionally the assimilation between Latin roots, prefixes, and suffixes may cause enough distortion to result in confusion. Below are listed some common Latin prefixes (most of them are also used as prepositions) showing the assimilation of the prefix to the following element. Note that the prefix *in-* has two sources and hence two uses: as a spatial prefix meaning *in, on,* or *into* (*in*scribe, *im*bibe, *il*luminate, *ir*radiate) and the antonymous prefix (*in*sensitive, *im*mature, *il*legible, *ir*reverent).

| Consonant Changes | | English |
|---|---|---|
| *ad-* | before *c* becomes *ac-* | *ac*celerate |
| *ad-* | before *f* becomes *af-* | *af*finity |
| *ad-* | before *g* becomes *ag-* | *ag*glutinant |
| *ad-* | before *p* becomes *ap-* | *ap*pendix |
| *ad-* | before *s* becomes *as-* | *as*similate |
| *ad-* | before *t* becomes *at-* | *at*trition |
| *ex-* | before *f* becomes *ef-* | *ef*fusion |
| *in-* | before *l* becomes *il-* | *il*linition |
| *in-* | before *m* becomes *im-* | *im*mersion |
| *in-* | before *r* becomes *ir-* | *ir*radiation |
| *ob-* | before *c* becomes *oc-* | *oc*clusion |
| *sub-* | before *f* becomes *suf-* | *suf*focate |
| *sub-* | before *p* becomes *sup-* | *sup*pository |
| *trans-* | before *s* becomes *tran-* | *tran*spiration |

In Greek, assimilation may cause drastic changes to a word, and the phonetic laws governing these assimilations are far beyond the limits of this Dictionary. Fortunately, however, Greek prefixes are fairly regular. Like Latin prefixes, they may also function as prepositions of motion or location. Most Greek prefixes end in a vowel, which is maintained when the following element begins with a consonant and is lost (elided) when that element begins with a vowel: for example, the iota in *epi* ("on, upon") is unchanged in *epi*demic and is elided before *o* in *ep*onychium ("cuticle"). When a Greek prefix ends in a consonant and the following element begins with a consonant, assimilation takes place with results as in Latin: the nu *(n)* of *syn* ("with") changes in *symphatheia* and *syllogismos* (sympathy and syllogism). Note that the prevocalic prefix *an-* has two sources and therefore two uses: it is the spatial preposition *ana* ("up, back"), as in *ana*bolism and *an*ode; and it is the antonymous prefix *a-*, *an-*, as in *a*theist and *an*odyne, coming from the same source as Latin and English antonymous prefixes *in-* and *un-*.

Below are listed some common Greek prefixes with examples of elision and assimilation.

| Preposition | Combining Forms | English |
|---|---|---|
| amphi | amphi- | *amphi*crania |
| | amph- | *amph*eclexis |
| ana | ana- | *ana*bolism |
| | an- | *an*ode |
| anti | anti- | *anti*gen |
| | ant- | *ant*helminthic |
| apo | apo- | *apo*physis |
| | ap- | *ap*andria |
| dia | dia- | *dia*thermy |
| | di- | *di*uretic |
| ek | ek- | *ec*topia |
| ex | ex- | *ex*osmosis |

| | | |
|---|---|---|
| en | en- | *en*ostosis |
| | em- | *em*bolus |
| epi | epi- | *epi*nephrine |
| | ep- | *ep*arterial |
| hyper | hyper- | *hyper*trophy |
| hypo | hypo- | *hypo*dermic |
| | hyp- | *hyp*axial |
| kata | kata- | *cata*lepsy |
| | kat- | *cat*ion |
| meta | meta- | *meta*morphosis |
| | met- | *met*encephalon |
| para | para- | *para*mastoid |
| | par- | *par*otid |
| peri | peri- | *peri*toneum |
| pro | pro- | *pro*gnosis |
| syn | syn- | *syn*thesis |
| | sym- | *sym*physis |
| | syl- | *syl*lepsis |
| | sy- | *sy*stole |

Many Latin suffixes have been naturalized in English for centuries, and little comment is needed on their morphology and use. Some common suffixes of particular use in medicine are listed below with their English derivatives. Note that the suffixes *-abilis* and *-alis*/*-aris* are attached to verb stems of the first conjugation (the infinitives end in *-āre,* as in *laudāre* to praise); and *-ibilis* and *-ilis* are used with the other conjugations *(vidēre, visibilis; legĕre, legibilis; audīre, audibilis).*

| Latin Components | English |
|---|---|
| *avis + -arium* | avi*ary* |
| *dormio (dormitus) + -orium* | dormit*ory* |
| *nutrio (nutritus) + -io* | nutrit*ion* |
| *moveo (motus) + -or* | mot*or* |
| *porosus + -tas* | poros*ity* |
| *frio + -abilis* | fri*able* |
| *edo + -ibilis* | ed*ible* |
| *corpus (corporis) + -alis* | corpor*al* |
| *febris + -ilis* | febr*ile* |
| *oculus + -aris* | ocul*ar* |
| *cilium + -arius* | cili*ary* |
| *sensus + -orius* | sens*ory* |
| *reticulum + -atus* | reticul*ate* |
| *morbus + -idus* | morb*id* |
| *aborior (abortus) + -ivus* | abort*ive* |
| *squama + -osus* | squam*ous* |
| *adeps (adipis) + -osus* | adip*ose* |
| *prae + caveo (cautus) + -io + -arius* | precaut*ionary* |

Greek suffixes in general have not been naturalized in English as the Latin have, with the spectacular exception of the family of suffixes represented by verbs in *-izō* (-ize), agent nouns in *-istēs* (-ist), and verbal nouns in *-ismos* (-ism).

So far we have examined the various forms of roots, root words, and derived words; only compound words remain. A compound word is one formed from two (or more) independent words, the first word modifying, dependent upon, or being object of the next. In English, *housewife, kidney transplant, salesman, schoolboy, store-bought, backbreaking,* and *anteater* are compound words. In English the individual elements undergo little if any change from their basic, lexical forms but remain isolated, as it were, and receive their new meaning solely from juxtaposition (an example is the difference between *house guest* and *guest house*).

The conditions are vastly different in Latin and Greek; in the Classical languages one must use so-called combining forms of substantives (i.e., nouns and adjectives including past participles) that are often considerably different from the lexical forms.

In Latin all native compound words ordinarily will consist of the stem of the first word; then the connecting vowel, usually -i-, sometimes -u-; then the stem of the second word; then the inflection: magn-i-ficient-ia, *magnificientia,* magnificence. In science there are many compounds like *dorsoradial* and *frenosecretory* with Latin words and Greek connecting vowels; the true Latin forms for such compounds would be *dorsiradialis* and *frenisecretorius.*

In Greek the rules for forming compound words are much more complicated. If the first substantive of a Greek compound ends in *-a* (but not *-ma*) or *-ē*, one nearly always changes that vowel to *-o-*:

*glōssa,* tongue + *ptōsis,* fall = glossoptosis

*phōnē,* voice, sound + *logos,* word, reason, study = *phōnologia,* phonology

Substantives ending in *-on*, *-os*, or *-ys* usually drop the final consonant and leave the vowel unchanged:

*osteon,* bone + *arthritis,* gout (first appears in Hippocrates) = osteoarthritis

*myelos,* marrow + *poiēsis,* production = myelopoiesis

*pachys,* thick + *derma,* skin = pachydermia (first appears in Hippocrates)

If the second element begins with a vowel, one merely drops the final *-a* or *-ē* from the first element without adding *-o-*:

*archē,* beginning, chief, rule + *enteron,* intestine = archenteron

*bradys,* slow, dull + *akusis,* hearing = bradyacousia

There are exceptions:

*idea,* idea + *logos* = ideology is regular,

but

*genea,* family, lineage + *logos* = *genealogia,* gene*a*logy is irregular, as are

*architektōn* not *archotektōn,* arch*i*tect

*archetypos* not *archotypos,* arch*e*type

Indeed the regular *archo-* is extremely rare compared with *arche-* and *archi-* and is therefore "irregular."

Forming compounds from other substantives is complicated by the fact that one cannot generally predict the combining form of a substantive from the lexical entry, and in fact one usually predicts the lexical entry from the combining form, not vice versa.

In Greek, substantives ending in *-ma* have a stem or combining form in *-mat-;* so *haima* (blood), *haimat-* and *poiēsis* (making, "poesy") make *haimatopoiēsis,* hematopoiesis. But Hippocrates himself uses *haimorrhagia,* hemorrhage, not *haimatorrhagia.* And no one could predict from the nominative *gynē* (woman), which looks like a regular noun, a combining form *gynaik-,* whence gynecology; or from *gala* (milk), *galakt-,* whence galactophorous.

Latin is not so irregular, but even so *lac* (milk) has a combining stem *lact-* (lactacidemia); *cor* (heart), one in *cord-* (cordial); *miles* (soldier), *milit-* (military); *rex* (king), *reg-* (regicide); *nomen* (name), *nomin-* (nominate). The combining form of *homo* (human being, man) is *homin-* (hominoid ape), but Cicero himself uses *homicida* (murderer, homicide), not *hominicida.*

## Analytical Word List

The following list includes those Greek and Latin words occurring most frequently in this Dictionary, arranged alphabetically under their English combining forms as rubrics. The dash appended to a combining form indicates that it is not a complete word and, if the dash precedes the combining form, that it commonly appears as the terminal element of a compound. Infrequently a combining form is both preceded and followed by a dash, showing that it usually appears between two other elements. Closely related forms are shown in one entry by the use of parentheses: thus carbo(n)-, showing it may be either carbo-, as in *carbo*hydrate, or carbon-, as in *carbon*uria.

Following each combining form the first item of information is the Greek or Latin word, identified by [Gr.] and [L.], from which it is derived. Occasionally both a Greek and a Latin word are given. Presence of a dash before or after such an element indicates that it does not occur as an independent word in the original language. Information necessary to the understanding of the form appears next in parentheses. Then the meaning or meanings of the word are given, followed where appropriate by reference to a synonymous combining form in the other language, that is, on a combining form of Latin derivation, to the synonymous form of Greek derivation, and vice versa. Finally, an example is given to illustrate use of the combining form in a compound English derivative.

If this list is used in close conjunction with the etymological information given in the body of the Dictionary, no confusion should be caused by the similarity of elements in such words as *mel*algia, *mel*ancholia, and *mel*icera, where the similarity is only apparent and the derivation of each word is different.

**a-** *a-* [L.] (*n* is added before words beginning with a vowel) negative prefix. Cf. in-[3]. *a*metria
**ab-** *ab* [L.] away from. Cf. apo-. *ab*ducent
**abdomin-** *abdomen, abdominis* [L.] abdomen. *abdomino*scopy
**ac-** See ad-. *ac*cretion
**acet-** *acetum* [L.] vinegar. *acet*ometer
**acid-** *acidus* [L.] sour. *acid*uric
**acou-** *akouō* [Gr.] hear. *acou*ethesia. (Also spelled acu-)
**acr-** *akron* [Gr.] extremity, peak. *acr*omegaly
**act-** *ago, actus* [L.] do, drive, act. re*act*ion
**actin-** *aktis, aktinos* [Gr.] ray, radius. Cf. radi-. *actino*genesis
**acu-** See acou-. osteo*acu*sis
**ad-** *ad* [L.] (*d* changes to *c*, *f*, *g*, *p*, *s*, or *t* before words beginning with those consonants) to. *ad*renal
**aden-** *adēn* [Gr.] gland. Cf. gland-. *aden*oma
**adip-** *adeps, adipis* [L.] fat. Cf. lip- and stear-. *adip*ocellular
**aer-** *aēr* [Gr.] air. an*aer*obiosis
**aesthe-** See esthe-. *aesthe*sioneurosis
**af-** See ad-. *af*ferent
**ag-** See ad-. *ag*glutinant
**-agogue** *agōgos* [Gr.] leading, inducing. galact*agogue*
**-agra** *agra* [Gr.] catching, seizure. pod*agra*
**alb-** *albus* [L.] white. Cf. leuk-. *alb*ocinereous
**alg-** *algos* [Gr.] pain. neur*alg*ia
**all-** *allos* [Gr.] other, different. *all*ergy
**alve-** *alveus* [L.] trough, channel, cavity. *alve*olar
**amph-** See amphi-. *amph*eclexis
**amphi-** *amphi* [Gr.] (*i* is dropped before words beginning with a vowel) both, doubly. *amphi*celous
**amyl-** *amylon* [Gr.] starch. *amyl*osynthesis
**an-[1]** See ana-. *an*agogic
**an-[2]** See a-. *an*omalous
**ana-** *ana* [Gr.] (final *a* is dropped before words beginning with a vowel) up, positive. *ana*phoresis
**ancyl-** See ankyl-. *ancyl*ostomiasis
**andr-** *anēr, andros* [Gr.] man. gyn*andr*oid
**angi-** *angeion* [Gr.] vessel. Cf. vas-. *angi*emphraxis
**ankyl-** *ankylos* [Gr.] crooked, looped. *ankyl*odactylia. (Also spelled ancyl-)
**ant-** See anti-. *ant*ophthalmic
**anti-** *ante* [L.] before. *ante*flexion
**anti-** *anti* [Gr.] (*i* is dropped before words beginning with a vowel) against, counter. Cf. contra*anti*pyogenic
**antr-** *antron* [Gr.] cavern. *antr*odynia
**ap-[1]** See apo-. *ap*heter
**ap-[2]** See ad-. *append*
**-aph-** *haptō, haph-* [Gr.] touch. dys*aph*ia. (See also hapt-)
**apo-** *apo* [Gr.] (*o* is dropped before words beginning with a vowel) away from, detached. Cf. ab-. *apo*physis
**arachn-** *arachnē* [Gr.] spider. *arachn*odactyly
**arch-** *archē* [Gr.] beginning, origin. *arch*enteron
**arter(i)-** *arteria* [Gr.] windpipe, artery. *arterio*sclerosis, periar*ter*itis
**arthr-** *arthron* [Gr.] joint. Cf. articul-. syn*arthr*osis
**articul-** *articulus* [L.] joint. Cf. arthr-. dis*articul*ation
**as-** See ad-. *as*similation
**at-** See ad-. *at*trition
**aur-** *auris* [L.] ear. Cf. ot-. *aur*inasal
**aux-** *auxō* [Gr.] increase. enter*aux*e
**ax-** *axōn* [Gr.] or *axis* [L.] axis. *ax*ofugal
**axon-** *axōn* [Gr.] axis. *axon*ometer
**ba-** *bainō, ba-* [Gr.] go, walk, stand. hypno*ba*tia
**bacill-** *bacillus* [L.] small staff, rod. Cf. bacter-. actino*bacill*osis
**bacter-** *bactērion* [Gr.] small staff, rod. Cf. bacill-. *bacter*iophage
**ball-** *ballō, bol-* [Gr.] throw. *ball*istics. (See also bol-)
**bar-** *baros* [Gr.] weight. pedo*bar*ometer
**bi-[1]** *bios* [Gr.] life. Cf. vit-. aero*bi*c
**bi-[2]** *bi-* [L.] two (see also di-[1]). *bi*lobate
**bil-** *bilis* [L.] bile. Cf. chol-. *bil*iary
**blast-** *blastos* [Gr.] bud, child, a growing thing in its early stages. Cf. germ-. *blast*oma, zygoto*blast*
**blep-** *blepō* [Gr.] look, see. hemia*blep*sia
**blephar-** *blepharon* [Gr.] (from *blepō;* see blep-) eyelid. Cf. cili-. *blephar*oncus
**bol-** See ball-. em*bol*ism
**brachi-** *brachiōn* [Gr.] arm. *brachi*ocephalic
**brachy-** *brachys* [Gr.] short. *brachy*cephalic
**brady-** *bradys* [Gr.] slow. *brady*cardia
**brom-** *brōmos* [Gr.] stench. podo*brom*idrosis
**bronch-** *bronchos* [Gr.] windpipe. *bronch*oscopy
**bry-** *bryō* [Gr.] be full of life. em*bry*onic
**bucc-** *bucca* [L.] cheek. disto*bucc*al
**cac-** *kakos* [Gr.] bad, abnormal. Cf. mal*cac*odontia, arthro*cac*e. (See also dys-)
**calc-[1]** *calx, calcis* [L.] stone (cf. lith-), limestone, lime. *calci*pexy
**calc-[2]** *calx, calcis* [L.] heel. *calc*aneotibial
**calor-** *calor* [L.] heat. Cf. therm-. *calor*imeter
**cancr-** *cancer, cancri* [L.] crab, cancer. Cf. carcin-. *cancr*ology. (Also spelled chancr-)
**capit-** *caput, capitus* [L.] head. Cf. cephal-. de*capit*ator
**caps-** *capsa* [L.] (from *capio;* see cept-) container. en*caps*ulation
**carbo(n)-** *carbo, carbonis* [L.] coal, charcoal. *carbo*hydrate, *carbon*uria
**carcin-** *karkinos* [Gr.] crab, cancer. Cf. cancr-. *carcin*oma
**cardi-** *kardia* [Gr.] heart. lipo*cardi*ac
**cary-** See kary-. *cary*okinesis
**cat-** See cata-. *cat*hode
**cata-** *kata* [Gr.] (final *a* is dropped before words beginning with a vowel) down, negative. *cata*batic
**caud-** *cauda* [L.] tail. *caud*ad
**cav-** *cavus* [L.] hollow. Cf. coel-. con*cav*e
**cec-** *caecus* [L.] blind. Cf. typhl-. *cec*opexy
**cel-[1]** See coel-. amphi*cel*ous
**cel-[2]** See -cele. *cel*ectome
**-cele** *kēlē* [Gr.] tumor, hernia. gastro*cele*
**cell-** *cella* [L.] room, cell. Cf. cyt-. *cell*iferous
**cen-** *koinos* [Gr.] common. *cen*esthesia
**cent-** *centum* [L.] hundred. Cf. hect-. Indicates fraction in metric system. [This exemplifies the custom in the metric system of identifying fractions of units by stems from the Latin, as centimeter, decimeter, millimeter, and multiples of units by the similar stems from the Greek, as hectometer, decameter, and kilometer.] *cent*imeter, *cent*ipede

**cente-** *kenteō* [Gr.] to puncture. Cf. punct-. entero*centes*is
**centr-** *kentron* [Gr.] or *centrum* [L.] point, center. neuro*centr*al
**cephal-** *kephalē* [Gr.] head. Cf. capit-. en*cephal*itis
**cept-** *capio, -cipientis, -ceptus* [L.] take, receive. re*cept*or
**cer-** *kēros* [Gr.] or *cera* [L.] wax. *cer*oplasty, *cer*omel
**cerat-** See kerat-. a*cerat*osis
**cerebr-** *cerebrum* [L.] brain. *cerebr*ospinal
**cervic-** *cervix, cervicis* [L.] neck. Cf. trachel-. *cervic*itis
**chancr-** See cancr-. *chancr*iform
**cheil-** *cheilos* [Gr.] lip. Cf. labi-. *cheil*oschisis
**cheir-** *cheir* [Gr.] hand. Cf. man-. macro*cheir*ia. (Also spelled chir-)
**chir-** See cheir-. *chir*omegaly
**chlor-** *chlōros* [Gr.] green. a*chlor*opsia
**chol-** *cholē* [Gr.] bile. Cf. bil-. hepato*chol*angeitis
**chondr-** *chondros* [Gr.] cartilage. *chondr*omalacia
**chord-** *chordē* [Gr.] string, cord. peri*chord*al
**chori-** *chorion* [Gr.] protective fetal membrane. endo*chori*on
**chro-** *chrōs* [Gr.] color. poly*chro*matic
**chron-** *chronos* [Gr.] time. syn*chron*ous
**chy-** *cheēo, chy-* [Gr.] pour. ec*chy*mosis
**-cid(e)** *caedo, -cisus* [L.] cut, kill. infanti*cide*, germi*cid*al
**cili-** *cilium* [L.] eyelid. Cf. blephar-. super*cili*ary
**cine-** See kine-. auto*cine*sis
**-cipient** See cept-. in*cipient*
**circum-** *circum* [L.] around. Cf. peri-. *circum*ferential
**-cis-** *caedo, -cisus* [L.] cut, kill. ex*cis*ion
**clas-** *klaō* [Gr.] break. cranio*clas*t
**clin-** *klinō* [Gr.] bend, incline, make lie down. *clin*ometer
**clus-** *claudo, -clusus* [L.] shut. maloc*clus*ion
**co-** See con-. *co*hesion
**cocc-** *kokkos* [Gr.] seed, pill. gono*cocc*us
**coel-** *koilos* [Gr.] hollow. Cf. cav-. *coel*enteron. (Also spelled cel-)
**col-**[1] See colon-. *col*ic
**col-**[2] See con-. *col*lapse
**colon-** *kalon* [Gr.] lower intestine. *colon*ic
**colp-** *kolpos* [Gr.] hollow, vagina. Cf. sin-. endo*colp*itis
**com-** See con-. *com*masculation
**con-** *con-* [L.] (becomes co- before vowels or *h*; col- before *l*; com- before *b*, *m*, or *p*; cor- before *r*) with, together. Cf. syn-. *con*traction
**contra-** *contra* [L.] against, counter. Cf. anti-. *contra*indication
**copr-** *kopros* [Gr.] dung. Cf. sterco-. *copr*oma
**cor-**[1] *korē* [Gr.] doll, little image, pupil. iso*cor*ia
**cor-**[2] See con-. *cor*rugator
**corpor-** *corpus, corporis* [L.] body. Cf. somat-. intra*corpor*al
**cortic-** *cortex, corticis* [L.] bark, find. *cortic*osterone
**cost-** *costa* [L.] rib. Cf. pleur-. inter*cost*al
**crani-** *kranion* [Gr.] or *cranium* [L.] skull. peri*crani*um
**creat-** *kreas, kreato-* [Gr.] meat, flesh. *creat*orrhea
**-crescent** *cresco, crescentis, cretus* [L.] grow. ex*crescent*
**cret-**[1] *cerno, cretus* [L.] distinguish, separate off. Cf. crin-. dis*crete*
**cret-**[2] See -crescent. ac*cret*ion
**crin-** *krinō* [Gr.] distinguish, separate off. Cf. cret-[1]. endo*cri*nology
**crur-** *crus, cruris* [L.] shin, leg. brachio*crur*al
**cry-** *kryos* [Gr.] cold. *cry*esthesia
**crypt-** *kryptō* [Gr.] hide, conceal. *crypt*orchism
**cult-** *colo, cultus* [L.] tend, cultivate. *cult*ure
**cune-** *cuneus* [L.] wedge. Cf. sphen-. *cune*iform
**cut-** *cutis* [L.] skin. Cf. derm(at)-. sub*cut*aneous
**cyan-** *kyanos* [Gr.] blue. antho*cyan*in
**cycl-** *kyklos* [Gr.] circle, cycle. *cycl*ophoria
**cyst-** *kystis* [Gr.] bladder. Cf. vesic-. nephro*cyst*itis
**cyt-** *kytos* [Gr.] cell. Cf. cell-. plasmo*cyt*oma
**dacry-** *dakry* [Gr.] tear. *dacry*ocyst
**dactyl-** *daktylos* [Gr.] finger, toe. Cf. digit-. hexa*dactyl*ism
**de-** *de* [L.] down from. *de*composition
**dec-**[1] *deka* [Gr.] ten. Indicates multiple in metric system. Cf. dec-[2]. *dec*agram
**dec-**[2] *decem* [L.] ten. Indicates fraction in metric system. Cf. dec-[1]. *dec*ipara, *dec*imeter
**dendr-** *dendron* [Gr.] tree. neuro*dendr*ite
**dent-** *dens, dentis* [L.] tooth. Cf. odont-. inter*dent*al
**derm(at)-** *derma, dermatos* [Gr.] skin. Cf. cut-. endo*derm*, *dermat*itis
**desm-** *desmos* [Gr.] band, ligament. syn*desm*opexy
**dextr-** *dexter, dextr-* [L.] right-hand. ambi*dextr*ous
**di-**[1] *di-* [Gr.] two. *di*morphic. (See also bi-[2])
**di-**[2] See dia-. *di*uresis
**di-**[3] See dis-. *di*vergent
**dia-** *dia* [Gr.] (*a* is dropped before words beginning with a vowel) through, apart. Cf. per-. *dia*gnosis
**didym-** *didymos* [Gr.] twin. Cf. gemin-. epi*didym*al
**digit-** *digitus* [L.] finger, toe. Cf. dactyl-. *digit*igrade
**diplo-** *diploos* [Gr.] double. *diplo*myelia
**dis-** *dis-* [L.] (*s* may be dropped before a word beginning with a consonant) apart, away from. *dis*location
**disc-** *diskos* [Gr.] or *discus* [L.] disk. *disc*oplacenta
**dors-** *dorsum* [L.] back. ventro*dors*al
**drom-** *dromos* [Gr.] course. hemo*drom*ometer
**-ducent** See duct-. ad*ducent*
**-duct** *duco, ducentis, ductus* [L.] lead, conduct. ovi*duct*
**dur-** *durus* [L.] hard. Cf. scler-. in*dur*ation.
**dynam(i)-** *dynamis* [Gr.] power. *dynam*oneure, neuro*dynami*c
**dys-** *dys-* [Gr.] bad, improper. Cf. mal-. *dys*trophic. (See also cac-)
**e-** *e* [L.] out from. Cf. ec- and ex-. *e*mission
**ec-** *ek* [Gr.] out of. Cf. e-. *ec*centric
**-ech-** *echō* [Gr.] have, hold, be. syn*ech*otomy
**ect-** *ektos* [Gr.] outside. Cf. extra-. *ect*oplasm
**ede-** *oideō* [Gr.] swell. *ede*matous
**ef-** See ex-. *ef*florescent
**-elc-** *helkos* [Gr.] sore, ulcer. enter*elc*osis. (See also helc-)
**electr-** *ēlectron* [Gr.] amber. *electr*otherapy
**em-** See en-. *em*bolism, *em*pathy, *em*phlysis
**-em-** *haima* [Gr.] blood. an*em*ia. (See also hem(at)-)
**en-** *en* [Gr.] (*n* changes to *m* before *b*, *p*, or *ph*) in, on. Cf. in-[2]. *en*celitis
**end-** *endon* [Gr.] inside. Cf. intra-. *end*angium
**enter-** *enteron* [Gr.] intestine. dys*entery*
**ep-** See epi-. *ep*axial
**epi-** *epi* [Gr.] (*i* is dropped before words beginning with a vowel) upon, after, in addition. *epi*glottis
**erg-** *ergon* [Gr.] work, deed. en*erg*y
**erythr-** *erythros* [Gr.] red. Cf. rub(r)-. *erythr*ochromia
**eso-** *esō* [Gr.] inside. Cf. intra-. *eso*phylactic
**esthe-** *aisthanomai, aisthē-* [Gr.] perceive, feel. Cf. sens-. an*esthe*sia
**eu-** *eu* [Br.] good, normal. *eu*pepsia
**ex-** *ex* [Gr.] or *ex* [L.] out of. Cf. e-. *ex*cretion
**exo-** *exō* [Gr.] outside. Cf. extra-. *exo*pathic
**extra-** *extra* [L.] outside of, beyond. Cf. ect- and exo-. *extra*cellular
**faci-** *facies* [L.] face. Cf. prosop-. brachio*faci*olingual
**-facient** *facio, facientis, factus, -fectus* [L.] make. Cf. poie-. cale*facient*
**-fact-** See -facient. arte*fact*
**fasci-** *fascia* [L.] band. *fasci*orrhaphy
**febr-** *febris* [L.] fever. Cf. pyr-. *febr*icide
**-fect-** See -facient. de*fect*ive
**-ferent** *fero, ferentis, latus* [L.] bear, carry. Cf. phor-. ef*ferent*
**ferr-** *ferrum* [L.] iron. *ferr*oprotein
**fibr-** *fibra* [L.] fiber. Cf. in-[1]. chondro*fibr*oma
**fil-** *filum* [L.] thread. *fil*iform
**fiss-** *findo, fissus* [L.] split. Cf. schis-. *fiss*ion
**flagell-** *flagellum* [L.] whip. *flagell*ation
**flav-** *flavus* [L.] yellow. Cf. xanth-. ribo*flav*in
**-flect-** *flecto, flexus* [L.] bend, divert. de*flect*ion
**-flex-** See -flect-. re*flex*ometer
**flu-** *fluo, fluxus* [L.] flow. Cf. rhe-. *flu*id
**flux-** See flu-. af*flux*ion
**for-** *foris* [L.] door, opening. per*for*ated
**-form** *forma* [L.] shape. Cf. -oid. ossi*form*
**fract-** *frango, fractus* [L.] break. re*fract*ive
**front-** *frons, frontis* [L.] forehead, front. naso*front*al
**-fug(e)** *fugio* [L.] flee, avoid. vermi*fuge*, centri*fug*al
**funct-** *fungor, functus* [L.] perform, serve, function. mal*funct*ion
**fund-** *fundo, fusus* [L.] pour. in*fund*ibulum

**fus-** See fund-. dif*fus*ible

**galact-** *gala, galactos* [Gr.] milk. Cf. lact-. dys*galact*ia

**gam-** *gamos* [Gr.] marriage, reproductive union. a*gam*ont

**gangli-** *ganglion* [Gr.] swelling, plexus. neuro*gangli*itis

**gastr-** *gastēr, gastros* [Gr.] stomach. cholangio*gastr*ostomy

**gelat-** *gelo, gelatus* [L.] freeze, congeal. *gelat*in

**gemin-** *geminus* [L.] twin, double. Cf. didym-. quadri*gemin*al

**gen-** *gignomai, gen-, gon-* [Gr.] become, be produced, originate, or *gennaō* [Gr.] produce, originate. cyto*gen*ic

**germ-** *germen, germinis* [L.] bud, a growing thing in its early stages. Cf. blast-. *germ*inal, ovi*germ*

**gest-** *gero, gerentis, gestus* [L.] bear, carry. con*gest*ion

**gland-** *glans, glandis* [L.] acorn. Cf. aden-. intra*gland*ular

**-glia** *glia* [Gr.] glue. neuro*glia*

**gloss-** *glōssa* [Gr.] tongue. Cf. lingu-. tricho*gloss*ia

**glott-** *glōtta* [Gr.] tongue, language. *glott*ic

**gluc-** See glyc(y)-. *gluc*ophenetidin

**glutin-** *gluten, glutinis* [L.] glue. ag*glutin*ation

**glyc(y)-** *glykys* [Gr.] sweet. *glyc*emia, *glyc*yrrhizin. (Also spelled gluc-)

**gnath-** *gnathos* [Gr.] jaw. ortho*gnath*ous

**gno-** *gignōsiō, gnō-* [Gr.] know, discern. dia*gno*sis

**gon-** See gen-. amphi*gon*y

**grad-** *gradior* [L.] walk, take steps. retro*grad*e

**-gram** *gramma* [Gr.] letter, drawing. cardio*gram*

**gran-** *granum* [L.] grain, particle. lipo*gran*uloma

**graph-** *graphō* [Gr.] scratch, write, record. histo*graph*y

**grav-** *gravis* [L.] heavy. multi*grav*ida

**gyn(ec)-** *gynē, gynaikos* [Gr.] woman, wife, andro*gyn*y, *gyneco*logic

**gyr-** *gyros* [Gr.] ring, circle. *gyr*ospasm

**haem(at)-** See hem(at)-. *haem*orrhagia, *haemat*oxylon

**hapt-** *haptō* [Gr.] touch. *hapt*ometer

**hect-** *hekt-* [Gr.] hundred. Cf. cent-. Indicates multiple in metric system. *hect*ometer

**helc-** *helkos* [Gr.] sore, ulcer. *helc*osis

**hem(at)-** *haima, haimatos* [Gr.] blood. Cf. sanguin-. *hem*angioma, *hemat*ocyturia. (See also -em-)

**hemi-** *hēmi* [Gr.] half. Cf. semi-. *hemi*ageusia

**hen-** *heis, henos* [Gr.] one. Cf. un-. *hen*ogenesis

**hepat-** *hēpar, hēpatos* [Gr.] liver. gastro*hepat*ic

**hept(a)-** *hepta* [Gr.] seven. Cf. sept-$^{2}$. *hept*atomic, *hepta*valent

**hered-** *heres, heredis* [L.] heir. *hered*oimmunity

**hex-$^{1}$** *hex* [Gr.] six. Cf. sex-. *hex*yl-. An *a* is added in some combinations

**hex-$^{2}$** *echō, hech-* [Gr.] (*hech-* added to *s* becomes *hex-*) have, hold, be. ca*chex*ia

**hexa-** See hex-$^{1}$. *hexa*chromic

**hidr-** *hidros* [Gr.] sweat. hyper*hidr*osis

**hist-** *histos* [Gr.] web, tissue. *hist*odialysis

**hod-** *hodos* [Gr.] road, path. *hod*oneuromere. (See also od- and -ode$^{1}$)

**hom-** *homos* [Gr.] common, same. *hom*omorphic

**horm-** *ormē* [Gr.] impetus, impulse. *horm*one

**hydat-** *hydōr, hydatos* [Gr.] water. *hydat*ism

**hydr-** *hydōr, hydr-* [Gr.] water. Cf. lymph-. achlor*hydr*ia

**hyp-** See hypo-. *hyp*axial

**hyper-** *hyper* [Gr.] above, beyond, extreme. Cf. super-. *hyper*trophy

**hypn-** *hypnos* [Gr.] sleep. *hypn*otic

**hypo-** *hypo* [Gr.] (*o* is dropped before words beginning with a vowel) under, below. Cf. sub-. *hypo*metabolism

**hyster-** *hystera* [Gr.] womb. colpo*hyster*opexy

**iatr-** *iatros* [Gr.] physician. ped*iatr*ics

**idi-** *idios* [Gr.] peculiar, separate, distinct. *idi*osyncrasy

**il-** See in-$^{2,3}$. *il*linition (in, on), *il*legible (negative prefix)

**ile-** See ili- [ile- is commonly used to refer to the portion of the intestines known as the ileum]. *ile*ostomy

**ili-** *ilium (ileum)* [L.] lower abdomen, intestines [ili- is commonly used to refer to the flaring part of the hip bone known as the ilium]. *ili*osacral

**im-** See in-$^{2,3}$. *im*mersion (in, on), *im*perforation (negative prefix)

**in-$^{1}$** *is, inos* [Gr.] fiber. Cf. fibr-. *in*osteatoma

**in-$^{2}$** *in* [L.] (*n* changes to *l*, *m*, or *r* before words beginning with those consonants) in, on. Cf. en-. *in*sertion

**in-$^{3}$** *in-* [L.] (*n* changes to *l*, *m*, or *r* before words beginning with those consonants) negative prefix. Cf. a-. *in*valid

**infra-** *infra* [L.] beneath. *infra*orbital

**insul-** *insula* [L.] island. *insul*in

**inter-** *inter* [L.] among, between. *inter*carpal

**intra-** *intra* [L.] inside. Cf. end- and eso-. *intra*venous

**ir-** See in-$^{2,3}$. *ir*radiation (in, on), *ir*reducible (negative prefix)

**irid-** *iris, iridos* [Gr.] rainbow, colored circle. kerato*irid*ocyclitis

**is-** *isos* [Gr.] equal. *is*otope

**ischi-** *ischion* [Gr.] hip, haunch. *ischi*opubic

**jact-** *iacio, iactus* [L.] throw. *jact*itation

**-ject** *iacio, -iectus* [L.] throw. in*ject*ion

**jejun-** *ieiunus* [L.] hungry, not partaking of food. gastro*jejun*ostomy

**jug-** *iugum* [L.] yoke. con*jug*ation

**junct-** *iungo, iunctus* [L.] yoke, join. con*junct*iva

**kary-** *karyon* [Gr.] nut, kernel, nucleus. Cf. nucle-. mega*kary*ocyte. (Also spelled cary-)

**kerat-** *keras, keratos* [Gr.] horn. *kerat*olysis. (Also spelled cerat-)

**kil-** *chilioi* [Gr.] one thousand. Cf. mill-. Indicates multiple in metric system. *kil*ogram

**kine-** *kineō* [Gr.] move. *kine*matograph. (Also spelled cine-)

**labi-** *labium* [L.] lip. Cf. cheil-. gingivo*labi*al

**lact-** *lac, lactis* [L.] milk. Cf. galact-. gluco*lact*one

**lal-** *laleō* [Gr.] talk, babble. glosso*lal*ia

**lapar-** *lapara* [Gr.] flank. *lapar*otomy

**laryng-** *larynx, laryngos* [Gr.] windpipe. *laryng*endoscope

**lat-** *fero, latus* [L.] bear, carry. See -ferent. trans*lat*ion

**later-** *latus, lateris* [L.] side. ventro*later*al

**lent-** *lens, lentis* [L.] lentil. Cf. phac-. *lent*iconus

**lep-** *lambanō, lēp* [Gr.] take, seize. cata*lep*tic

**leuc-** See leuk-. *leuc*inuria

**leuk-** *leukos* [Gr.] white. Cf. alb-. *leuk*orrhea. (Also spelled leuc-)

**lien-** *lien* [L.] spleen. Cf. splen-. *lien*ocele

**lig-** *ligo* [L.] tie, bind. *lig*ate

**lingu-** *lingua* [L.] tongue. Cf. gloss-. sub*lingu*al

**lip-** *lipos* [Gr.] fat. Cf. adip-. glyco*lip*in

**lith-** *lithos* [Gr.] stone. Cf. calc-$^{1}$. nephro*lith*otomy

**loc-** *locus* [L.] place. Cf. top-. *loc*omotion

**log-** *legō, log-* [Gr.] speak, give an account. *log*orrhea, embryo*log*y

**lumb-** *lumbus* [L.] loin. dorso*lumb*ar

**lute-** *luteus* [L.] yellow. Cf. xanth-. *lute*oma

**ly-** *lyō* [Gr.] loose, dissolve. Cf. solut-. kerato*ly*sis

**lymph-** *lympha* [Gr.] water. Cf. hydr-. *lymph*adenosis

**macr-** *makros* [Gr.] long, large, *macr*omyeloblast

**mal-** *malus* [L.] bad, abnormal. Cf. cac- and dys-. *mal*function

**malac-** *malakos* [Gr.] soft. osteo*malac*ia

**mamm-** *mamma* [L.] breast. Cf. mast-. sub*mamm*ary

**man-** *manus* [L.] hand. Cf. cheir-. *man*iphalanx

**mani-** *mania* [Gr.] mental aberration. *mani*graphy, klepto*mani*a

**mast-** *mastos* [Gr.] breast. Cf. mamm-. hyper*mast*ia

**medi-** *medius* [L.] middle. Cf. mes-. *medi*frontal

**mega-** *megas* [Gr.] great, large. Also indicates multiple (1,000,000) in metric system. *mega*colon, *mega*dyne. (See also megal-)

**megal-** *megas, megalou* [Gr.] great, large. acro*megal*y

**mel-** *melos* [Gr.] limb, member. sym*mel*ia

**melan-** *melas, melanos* [Gr.] black. hippo*melan*in

**men-** *mēn* [Gr.] month. dys*men*orrhea

**mening-** *mēninx, mēningos* [Gr.] membrane. encephalo*mening*itis

**ment-** *mens, mentis* [L.] mind. Cf. phren-, psych-, and thym-. de*ment*ia

**mer-** *meros* [Gr.] part. poly*mer*ic

**mes-** *mesos* [Gr.] middle. Cf. med-. *mes*oderm

**met-** See meta-. *met*allergy

**meta-** *meta* [Gr.] (*a* is dropped before words beginning with a vowel) after, beyond, accompanying. *meta*carpal

**metr-$^{1}$** *metron* [Gr.] measure. stereo*metr*y

**metr-**[2] *metra* [Gr.] womb. endo*metr*itis

**micr-** *mikros* [Gr.] small. photo*micr*ograph

**mill-** *mille* [L.] one thousand. Cf. kil-. Indicates fraction in metric system. *milli*gram, *milli*pede

**miss-** See -mittent. intro*miss*ion

**-mittent** *mitto, mittentis, missus* [L.] send. inter*mittent*

**mne-** *mimnēscō, mnē-* [Gr.] remember. pseudo*mne*sia

**mon-** *monos* [Gr.] only, sole. *mono*plegia

**morph-** *morphē* [Gr.] form, shape. poly*morph*onuclear

**mot-** *moveo, motus* [L.] move. vaso*mot*or

**my-** *mys, myos* [Gr.] muscle. leio*my*oma

**-myces** *mykēs, mykētos* [Gr.] fungus. myelo*myces*

**myc(et)-** See -myces. asco*mycet*es, strepto*myc*in

**myel-** *myelos* [Gr.] marrow. polio*myel*itis

**myx-** *myxa* [Gr.] mucus. *myx*edema

**narc-** *narkē* [Gr.] numbness. topo*narc*osis

**nas-** *nasus* [L.] nose. Cf. rhin-. palato*nas*al

**ne-** *neos* [Gr.] new, young. *neo*cyte

**necr-** *nekros* [Gr.] corpse. *necr*ocytosis

**nephr-** *nephros* [Gr.] kidney. Cf. ren-. para*nephr*ic

**neur-** *neuron* [Gr.] nerve. esthesio*neure*

**nod-** *nodus* [L.] knot. *nod*osity

**nom-** *nomos* [Gr.] (from *nemō* deal out, distribute) law, custom. taxo*nomy*

**non-** *nona* [L.] nine. *non*acosane

**nos-** *nosos* [Gr.] disease. *nos*ology

**nucle-** *nucleus* [L.] (from *nux, nucis* nut) kernel. Cf. kary-. *nucle*ide

**nutri-** *nutrio* [L.] nourish. mal*nutri*tion

**ob-** *ob* [L.] (*b* changes to *c* before words beginning with that consonant) against, toward, etc. *ob*tuse

**oc-** See ob-. *oc*clude

**ocul-** *oculus* [L.] eye. Cf. ophthalm-. *ocul*omotor

**-od-** See -ode[1]. peri*od*ic

**-ode**[1] *hodos* [Gr.] road, path. cath*ode*. (See also hod-)

**-ode**[2] See -oid. nemat*ode*

**odont-** *odous, odontos* [Gr.] tooth. Cf. dent-. ortho*dont*ia

**-odyn-** *odynē* [Gr.] pain, distress. gastr*odyn*ia

**-oid** *eidos* [Gr.] form. Cf. -form. hy*oid*

**-ol** See ole-. cholester*ol*

**ole-** *oleum* [L.] oil. *ole*oresin

**olig-** *oligos* [Gr.] few, small. *olig*ospermia

**omphal-** *omphalos* [Gr.] navel. peri*omphal*ic

**onc-** *onkos* [Gr.] bulk, mass. hemat*onc*ometry

**onych-** *onyx, onychos* [Gr.] claw, nail. an*onych*ia

**oo-** *ōon* [Gr.] egg. Cf. ov-. peri*oo*thecitis

**op-** *haraō, op-* [Gr.] see. erythr*op*sia

**ophthalm-** *ophthalmos* [Gr.] eye. Cf. ocul-. ex*ophthalm*ic

**or-** *os, oris* [L.] mouth. Cf. stom(at)-. intra*or*al

**orb-** *orbis* [L.] circle. sub*orb*ital

**orchi-** *orchis* [Gr.] testicle. Cf. test-. *orchi*opathy

**organ-** *organon* [Gr.] implement, instrument. *organ*oleptic

**orth-** *orthos* [Gr.] straight, right, normal. *orth*opedics

**oss-** *os, ossis* [L.] bone. Cf. ost(e)-. *oss*iphone

**ost(e)-** *osteon* [Gr.] bone. Cf. oss-. en*ost*osis, *oste*anaphysis

**ot-** *ous, ōtos* [Gr.] ear. Cf. aur-. par*ot*id

**ov-** *ovum* [L.] egg. Cf. oo-. syn*ov*ia

**oxy-** *oxys* [Gr.] sharp. *oxy*cephalic

**pachy(n)-** *pachynō* [Gr.] thicken. *pachy*derma, myo*pachyn*sis

**pag-** *pēgnymi, pag-* [Gr.] fix, make fast. thoraco*pag*us

**par-**[1] *pario* [L.] bear, give birth to. primi*par*ous

**par-**[2] See para-. *par*epigastric

**para-** *para* [Gr.] (final *a* is dropped before words beginning with a vowel) beside, beyond. *para*mastoid

**part-** *pario, partus* [L.] bear, give birth to. *part*urition

**path-** *pathos* [Gr.] that which one undergoes, sickness. psycho*path*ic

**pec-** *pēgnymi, pēg-* [Gr.] (*pēk-* before *t*) fix, make fast. sym*pec*tothiene. (See also pex-)

**ped-** *pais, paidos* [Gr.] child. ortho*ped*ic

**pell-** *pellis* [L.] skin, hide. *pell*agra

**-pellent** *pello, pellentis, pulsus* [L.] drive. re*pellent*

**pen-** *penomai* [Gr.] need, lack. erythrocyto*pen*ia

**pend-** *pendeo* [L.] hang down. ap*pend*ix

**pent(a)-** *pente* [Gr.] five. Cf. quinque-. *pent*ose, *penta*ploid

**peps-** *peptō, peps-* [Gr.] digest. brady*peps*ia

**pept-** *peptō* [Gr.] digest. dys*pept*ic

**per-** *per* [L.] through. Cf. dia-. *per*nasal

**peri-** *peri* [Gr.] around. Cf. circum-. *peri*phery

**pet-** *peto* [L.] seek, tend toward. centri*pet*al

**pex-** *pēgnumi, pēg-* [Gr.] (*pēg-* added to *s* becomes *pēx-*) fix, make fast. hepato*pexy*

**pha-** *phēmi, pha-* [Gr.] say, speak. dys*pha*sia

**phac-** *phakos* [Gr.] lentil, lens. Cf. lent-. *phac*osclerosis. (Also spelled phak-)

**phag-** *phagein* [Gr.] eat. lipo*phag*ic

**phak-** See phac-. *phak*itis

**phan-** See phen-. dia*phan*oscopy

**pharmac-** *pharmakon* [Gr.] drug. *pharmac*ognosy

**pharyng-** *pharynx, pharyng-* [Gr.] throat. glosso*pharyng*eal

**phen-** *phainō, phan-* [Gr.] show, be seen. phos*phene*

**pher-** *pherō, phor-* [Gr.] bear, support. peri*phery*

**phil-** *phileō* [Gr.] like, have affinity for. eosino*phil*ia

**phleb-** *phleps, phlebos* [Gr.] vein. peri*phleb*itis

**phleg-** *phlogō, phlog-* [Gr.] burn, inflame. adeno*phleg*mon

**phlog-** See phleg-. anti*phlog*istic

**phob-** *phobos* [Gr.] fear, dread. claustro*phob*ia

**phon-** *phōne* [Gr.] sound. echo*phony*

**phor-** See pher-. Cf. -ferent. exo*phor*ia

**phos-** See phot-. *phos*phorus

**phot-** *phōs, phōtos* [Gr.] light. *phot*erythrous

**phrag-** *phrassō, phrag-* [Gr.] fence, wall off, stop up. Cf. sept-[1]. dia*phrag*m

**phrax-** *phrassō, phrag-* [Gr.] (*phrag-* added to *s* becomes *phrax-*) fence, wall off, stop up. em*phrax*is

**phren-** *phrēn* [Gr.] mind, midriff. Cf. ment-. meta*phren*ia, meta*phren*on

**phthi-** *phthinō* [Gr.] decay, waste away. *phthi*sis

**phy-** *phyō* [Gr.] beget, bring forth, produce, be by nature. noso*phy*te

**phyl-** *phylon* [Gr.] tribe, kind. *phyl*ogeny

**-phyll** *phyllon* [Gr.] leaf. xantho*phyll*

**phylac-** *phylax* [Gr.] guard. pro*phylac*tic

**phys(a)-** *physaō* [Gr.] blow, inflate. *phys*ocele, *physa*lis

**physe-** *physaō, physē* [Gr.] blow, inflate. em*physe*ma

**pil-** *pilus* [L.] hair. e*pil*ation

**pituit-** *pituita* [L.] phlegm, rheum. *pituit*ous

**placent-** *placenta* [L.] (from *plakous* [Gr.]) cake. extra*placent*al

**plas-** *plassō* [Gr.] mold, shape. cine*plas*ty

**platy-** *platy-* [Gr.] broad, flat. *platy*rrhine

**pleg-** *plēssō* [Gr.] strike. di*pleg*ia

**plet-** *pleo, -pletus* [L.] fill. de*plet*ion

**pleur-** *pleura* [Gr.] rib, side. Cf. cost-. peri*pleur*al

**plex-** *plēssō, plēg-* [Gr.] (*plēg-* added to *s* becomes *plēx-*) strike. apo*plex*y

**plic-** *plico* [L.] fold. com*plic*ation

**pne-** *pneuma, pneumatos* [Gr.] breathing. traumato*pne*a

**pneum(at)-** *pneuma, pneumatos* [Gr.] breath, air. *pneum*odynamics, *pneumat*othorax

**pneumo(n)-** *pneumōn* [Gr.] lung. Cf. pulmo(n)-. *pneumo*centesis, *pneumon*otomy

**pod-** *pous, podos* [Gr.] foot. *pod*iatry

**poie-** *poieō* [Gr.] make, produce. Cf. -fa-cient. sarco*poie*tic

**pol-** *polos* [Gr.] axis of a sphere. peri*pol*ar

**poly-** *polys* [Gr.] much, many. *poly*spermia

**pont-** *pons, pontis* [L.] bridge. *pont*ocerebellar

**por-**[1] *poros* [Gr.] passage. myelo*pore*

**por-**[2] *pōros* [Gr.] callus. *por*ocele

**posit-** *pono, positus* [L.] put, place. re*posit*or

**post-** *post* [L.] after, behind in time or place. *post*natal, *post*oral

**pre-** *prae* [L.] before in time or place. *pre*natal, *pre*vesical

**press-** *premo, pressus* [L.] press. *press*oreceptive

**pro-** *pro* [Gr.] or *pro* [L.] before in time or place. *pro*gamous, *pro*cheilon, *pro*lapse

**proct-** *prōktos* [Gr.] anus. entero*proct*ia

**prosop-** *prosōpon* [Gr.] face. Cf. faci-. di*prosop*us

**pseud-** *pseudēs* [Gr.] false. *pseud*oparaplegia

**psych-** *psychē* [Gr.] soul, mind. Cf. ment-. *psych*osomatic

**pto-** *piptō, ptō-* [Gr.] fall. nephro*pto*sis

**pub-** *pubes* and *puber, puberis* [L.] adult. ischio*pub*ic. (See also puber-)

**puber-** *puber* [L.] adult. *puber*ty

**pulmo(n)-** *pulmo, pulmonis* [L.] lung. Cf. pneumo(n)-. *pulmo*lith, cardio*pulmo*nary

**puls-** *pello, pellentis, pulsus* [L.] drive. pro*puls*ion

**punct-** *pungo, punctus* [L.] prick, pierce. Cf. cente-. *punct*iform

**pur-** *pus, puris* [L.] pus. Cf. py-. sup*pur*ation

**py-** *pyon* [Gr.] pus. Cf. pur-. nephro*py*osis

**pyel-** *pyelos* [Gr.] trough, basin, pelvis. nephro*pyel*itis

**pyl-** *pylē* [Gr.] door, orifice. *pyl*ephlebitis

**pyr-** *pyr* [Gr.] fire. Cf. febr-. galacto*pyr*a

**quadr-** *quadr-* [L.] four. Cf. tetra-. *quadr*igeminal

**quinque-** *quinque* [L.] five. Cf. pent(a)-. *quinque*cuspid

**rachi-** *rachis* [Gr.] spine. Cf. spin-. encephalo*rachi*dian

**radi-** *radius* [L.] ray. Cf. actin-. ir*radi*ation

**re-** *re-* [L.] back, again. *re*traction

**ren-** *renes* [L.] kidneys. Cf. nephr-. ad*ren*al

**ret-** *rete* [L.] net. *ret*othelium

**retro-** *retro* [L.] backwards. *retro*deviation

**rhag-** *rhēgnymi, rhag-* [Gr.] break, burst. hemor*rhag*ic

**rhaph-** *rhaphē* [Gr.] suture. gastror*rhaph*y

**rhe-** *rheos* [Gr.] flow. Cf. flu-. diar*rhe*al

**rhex-** *rhēgnymi, rhēg-* [Gr.] (*rhēg-* added to *s* becomes *rhēx-*) break, burst. metror*rhex*is

**rhin-** *rhis, rhinos* [Gr.] nose. Cf. nas-. basi*rhin*al

**rot-** *rota* [L.] wheel. *rot*ator

**rub(r)-** *ruber, rubri* [L.] red. Cf. erythr-. bili*rub*in, *rub*rospinal

**salping-** *salpinx, salpingos* [Gr.] tube, trumpet. *salping*itis

**sanguin-** *sanguis, sanguinis* [L.] blood. Cf. hem(at)-. *sanguin*eous

**sarc-** *sarx, sarkos* [Gr.] flesh. *sarc*oma

**schis-** *schizō, schid-* [Gr.] (*schid-* before *t* or added to *s* becomes *schis-*) split. Cf. fiss-. *schis*torachis, rachi*schis*is

**scler-** *sklēros* [Gr.] hard. Cf. dur-. *scler*osis

**scop-** *skopeō* [Gr.] look at, observe. endo*scop*e

**sect-** *seco, sectus* [L.] cut. Cf. tom-. *sect*ile

**semi-** *semi* [L.] half. Cf. hemi-. *semi*flexion

**sens-** *sentio, sensus* [L.] perceive, feel. Cf. esthe-. *sens*ory

**sep-** *sepō* [Gr.] rot, decay. *sep*sis

**sept-**[1] *saepio, saeptus* [L.] fence, wall off, stop up. Cf. phrag-. naso*sept*al

**sept-**[2] *septum* [L.] seven. Cf. hept(a)-. *sept*an

**ser-** *serum* [L.] whey, watery substance. *ser*osynovitis

**sex-** *sex* [L.] six. Cf. hex-[1]. *sex*digitate

**sial-** *sialon* [Gr.] saliva. poly*sial*ia

**sin-** *sinus* [L.] hallow, fold. Cf. colp-. *sin*obronchitis

**sit-** *sitos* [Gr.] food. para*sit*ic

**solut-** *solvo, solventis, solutus* [L.] loose, dissolve, set free. Cf. ly-. dis*solut*ion

**-solvent** See solut-. dis*solvent*

**somat-** *sōma, somatos* [Gr.] body. Cf. corpor-. psycho*somat*ic

**-some** See somat-. dictyo*some*

**spas-** *spaō, spas-* [Gr.] draw, pull. *spas*m, *spas*tic

**spectr-** *spectrum* [L.] appearance, what is seen. micro*spectro*scope

**sperm(at)-** *sperma, spermatos* [Gr.] seed. *sperm*acrasia, *spermato*zoon

**spers-** *spargo, -spersus* [L.] scatter. di*spers*ion

**sphen-** *sphēn* [Gr.] wedge. Cf. cune-. *sphen*oid

**spher-** *sphaira* [Gr.] ball. hemi*spher*e

**sphygm-** *sphygmos* [Gr.] pulsation. *sphygm*omanometer

**spin-** *spina* [L.] spine. Cf. rachi-. cerebro*spin*al

**spirat-** *spiro, spiratus* [L.] breathe. in*spirat*ory

**splanchn-** *splanchna* [Gr.] entrails, viscera. neuro*splanchn*ic

**splen-** *splēn* [Gr.] spleen. Cf. lien-. *splen*omegaly

**spor-** *sporos* [Gr.] seed. *spor*ophyte, zygo*spor*e

**squam-** *squama* [L.] scale. de*squam*ation

**sta-** *histēmi, sta-* [Gr.] make stand, stop. genesi*sta*sis

**stal-** *stellō, stal-* [Gr.] send. peri*stal*sis. (See also stol-)

**staphyl-** *staphylē* [Gr.] bunch of grapes, uvula. *staphyl*ococcus, *staphyl*ectomy

**stear-** *stear, steatos* [Gr.] fat. Cf. adip-. *stear*odermia

**steat-** See stear-. *steat*opygous

**sten-** *stenos* [Gr.] narrow, compressed. *sten*ocardia

**ster-** *sterreos* [Gr.] solid. chole*ster*ol

**sterc-** *stercus* [L.] dung. Cf. copr-. *sterc*oporphyrin

**sthen-** *sthenos* [Gr.] strength. a*sthen*ia

**stol-** *stellō, stol-* [Gr.] send. dia*stol*e

**stom(at)-** *stoma, stomatos* [Gr.] mouth, orifice. Cf. or-. ana*stom*osis, *stomat*ogastric

**strep(h)-** *strephō, strep-* (before *t*) [Gr.] twist. Cf. tors-. *streph*osymbolia, *strep*tomycin. (See also stroph-)

**strict-** *stringo, stringentis, strictus* [L.] draw tight, compress, cause pain. con*strict*ion

**-stringent** See strict-. a*stringent*

**stroph-** *strephō, stroph-* [Gr.] twist. ana*stroph*ic. (See also strep(h)-)

**struct-** *struo, structus* [L.] pile up (against). ob*struct*ion

**sub-** *sub* [L.] (*b* changes to *f* or *p* before words beginning with those consonants) under, below. Cf. hypo-. *sub*lumbar

**suf-** See sub-. *suf*fusion

**sup-** See sub-. *sup*pository

**super-** *super* [L.] above, beyond, extreme. Cf. hyper-. *super*motility

**sy-** See syn-. *sy*stole

**syl-** See syn-. *syl*lepsiology

**sym-** See syn-. *sym*biosis, *sym*metry, *sym*pathetic, *sym*physis

**syn-** *syn* [Gr.] (*n* disappears before *s*, changes to *l* before *l*, and changes to *m* before *b*, *m*, *p*, and *ph*) with, together. Cf. con-. myo*syn*izesis

**ta-** See ton-. ec*ta*sis

**tac-** *tassō, tag-* [Gr.] (*tag-* changes to *tak-* before *t*) order, arrange. a*tac*tic

**tact-** *tango, tactus* [L.] touch. con*tact*

**tax-** *tassō, tag-* [Gr.] (*tag-* added to *s* becomes *tax-*) order, arrange. a*tax*ia

**tect-** See teg-. pro*tect*ive

**teg-** *tego, tectus* [L.] cover. in*teg*ument

**tel-** *telos* [Gr.] end. *tel*osynapsis

**tele-** *taēle* [Gr.] at a distance. *tele*ceptor

**tempor-** *tempus, temporis* [L.] time, timely or fatal spot, temple. *tempor*omalar

**ten(ont)-** *tenōn, tenontos* [Gr.] (from *teinō* stretch) tight stretched band. *ten*odynia, *ten*onitis, *tenont*agra

**tens-** *tendo, tensus* [L.] stretch. Cf. ton-. ex*tens*or

**test-** *testis* [L.] testicle. Cf. orchi-. *test*itis

**tetra-** *tetra-* [Gr.] four. Cf. quadr-. *tetra*genous

**the-** *tithēmi, thē-* [Gr.] put, place. syn*the*sis

**thec-** *thēkē* [Gr.] repository, case. *thec*ostegnosis

**thel-** *thēlē* [Gr.] teat, nipple. *thel*erethism

**therap-** *therapeia* [Gr.] treatment. hydro*therap*y

**therm-** *thermē* [Gr.] heat. Cf. calor-. dia*therm*y

**thi-** *theion* [Gr.] sulfur. *thi*ogenic

**thorac-** *thōrax, thōrakos* [Gr.] chest. *thorac*oplasty

**thromb-** *thrombos* [Gr.] lump, clot. *thromb*openia

**thym-** *thymos* [Gr.] spirit. Cf. ment-. dys*thym*ia

**thyr-** *thyreos* [Gr.] shield (shaped like a door *thyra*). *thyr*oid

**tme-** *temnō, tmē-* [Gr.] cut. axono*tme*sis

**toc-** *tokos* [Gr.] childbirth. dys*toc*ia

**tom-** *temnō, tom-* [Gr.] cut. Cf. sect-. appendec*tom*y

**ton-** *teino, ton-* [Gr.] stretch, put under tension. Cf. tens-. peri*ton*eum

**top-** *topos* [Gr.] place. Cf. loc-. *top*esthesia

**tors-** *torqueo, torsus* [L.] twist. Cf. strep-. ec*tors*ion

**tox-** *toxicon* [Gr.] (from *toxon* bow) arrow poison, poison. *tox*emia

**trache-** *tracheia* [Gr.] windpipe. *trache*otomy

**trachel-** *trachēlos* [Gr.] neck. Cf. cervic-. *trachel*opexy

**tract-** *traho, tractus* [L.] draw, drag. pro*tract*ion

**traumat-** *trauma, traumatos* [Gr.] wound. *traumat*ic

**tri-** *treis, tria* [Gr.] or *tri-* [L.] three. *tri*gonid

**trich-** *thrix, trichos* [Gr.] hair. *trich*oid

**trip-** *tribō* [Gr.] rub. en*trip*sis

**trop-** *trepō, trop-* [Gr.] turn, react. sito*trop*ism

**troph-** *trepō, troph-* [Gr.] nurture. a*troph*y

**tuber-** *tuber* [L.] swelling, node. *tuber*cle

**typ-** *typos* [Gr.] (from *typto* strike) type. a*typ*ical

**typh-** *typhos* [Gr.] fog, stupor. adeno*typh*us

**typhl-** *typhlos* [Gr.] blind. Cf. cec-. *typhl*ectasis

**un-** *unus* [L.] one. Cf. hen-. *un*ioval

**ur-** *ouron* [Gr.] urine. poly*ur*ia

**vacc-** *vacca* [L.] cow. *vacc*ine

**vagin-** *vagina* [L.] sheath. in*vagin*ated
**vas-** *vas* [L.] vessel. Cf. angi-. *vas*cular
**vers-** See vert-. in*vers*ion
**vert-** *verto, versus* [L.] turn. di*vert*iculum
**vesic-** *vesica* [L.] bladder. Cf. cyst-. *vesic*ovaginal
**vit-** *vita* [L.] life. Cf. bi-[1]. de*vit*alize
**vuls-** *vello, vulsus* [L.] pull, twitch. con*vuls*ion

**xanth-** *xanthos* [Gr.] yellow, blond. Cf. flav- and lute-. *xantho*phyll
**-yl-** *hyle* [Gr.] substance. cacod*yl*
**zo-** *zoē* [Gr.] life, *zōon* [Gr.] animal. micro*zo*aria
**zyg-** *zygon* [Gr.] yoke, union. *zyg*odactyly
**zym-** *zymē* [Gr.] ferment. en*zym*e

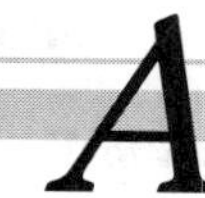

**A** symbol for *accommodation, adenine* or *adenosine, ampere, anode,* and *anterior;* as a subscript, symbol for *alveolar gas.*

**A.** L. *an'num,* year.

***A*** symbol for *absorbance, activity* (def. 3), *admittance, area,* and *mass number.*

**AI** first auditory area; see *auditory areas,* under *area.*

**AII** second auditory area; see *auditory areas,* under *area.*

**$A_2$** symbol for *aortic second sound.*

**Å** symbol for *angstrom.*

**a** symbol for *accommodation* and *atto-;* as a subscript, symbol for *arterial blood.*

**a.** abbreviation for L. *an'num* (year), *a'qua* (water), and *arte'ria* (artery).

**a-**[1] [Gr.] an inseparable prefix denoting want or absence; appears as *an-* before stems beginning with a vowel or with *h.*

**a-**[2] [L.] a prefix denoting separation, or away from.

***a*** symbol for *specific absorptivity, acceleration,* and *activity* (def. 2).

**ā** L. *an'te,* before.

**$\alpha$** alpha, the first letter of the Greek alphabet; symbol for *Bunsen coefficient,* the heavy chain of IgA (see *immunoglobulin*), and the $\alpha$ chain of hemoglobin.

**$\alpha$-** a prefix designating (1) the carbon atom adjacent to the principal functional group, e.g., $\alpha$-amino acids, succeeding letters, $\beta$, $\gamma$, $\delta$, etc., being used to designate succeeding carbon atoms in the chain; (2) the specific rotation of an optically active substance, e.g., $\alpha$-D-glucose; (3) the orientation of an exocyclic atom or group, e.g., 3$\alpha$-hydroxy-5$\alpha$-androstan-17-one (androsterone); (4) a plasma protein migrating with the $\alpha$ band (subdivided into $\alpha_1$ and $\alpha_2$ bands) in protein electrophoresis, e.g., $\alpha$-fetoprotein; (5) one in a series of related chemical compounds, particularly a series of stereoisomeric, isomeric, polymeric or allotropic forms, e.g., $\alpha$-carotene; and (6) one in a group of related entities, e.g., $\alpha$-ray. For compounds prefixed with the symbol $\alpha$-, see the unprefixed form.

**AA** achievement age; Alcoholics Anonymous; amino acid.

**$\overline{AA}$** [Gr. *ana* of each] an abbreviation used in prescription writing, following the names of two or more ingredients and signifying "of each"; also written $\bar{a}\bar{a}$ and *ana.*

**$\overline{aa}$** $\overline{AA}$.

**aa.** abbreviation for L. *arteriae,* arteries.

**AAA** American Association of Anatomists.

**AAAS** American Association for the Advancement of Science.

**AABB** American Association of Blood Banks.

**AACP** American Academy of Child Psychiatry.

**AAD** American Academy of Dermatology.

**AADP** American Academy of Denture Prosthetics.

**AADR** American Academy of Dental Radiology.

**AADS** American Association of Dental Schools.

**AAE** American Association of Endodontists.

**AAFP** American Academy of Family Physicians.

**AAI** American Association of Immunologists.

**AAID** American Academy of Implant Dentistry.

**AAIN** American Association of Industrial Nurses.

**AAMA** American Association of Medical Assistants.

**AAMC** American Association of Medical Colleges.

**AAMD** American Association on Mental Deficiency.

**AAMT** American Association for Medical Transcription.

**AAN** American Academy of Neurology.

**AAO** American Association of Orthodontists; American Academy of Ophthalmology; American Academy of Otolaryngology.

**AAOP** American Academy of Oral Pathology.

**AAOS** American Academy of Orthopaedic Surgeons.

**AAP** American Academy of Pediatrics; American Academy of Pedodontics; American Academy of Periodontology; American Association of Pathologists.

**AAPA** American Academy of Physician Assistants.

**AAPB** American Association of Pathologists and Bacteriologists.

**AAPMR** American Academy of Physical Medicine and Rehabilitation.

**Aar·ane** (ar'ān) trademark for a preparation of cromolyn sodium.

**AARC** American Association for Respiratory Care.

**Aar·on's sign** (ar'ənz) [Charles Dettie *Aaron,* American physician, 1866–1951] see under *sign.*

**Aar·skog syndrome** (ahrs'kog) [Dagfinn Charles *Aarskog,* Norwegian pediatrician, born 1928] see under *syndrome.*

**Aar·skog-Scott syndrome** (ahrs'kog-skot) [D. C. *Aarskog,* Charles I. *Scott,* Jr., American pediatrician, 20th century] Aarskog syndrome; see under *syndrome.*

**Aase syndrome** (ahz) [Jon Morton *Aase,* American pediatrician, born 1936] see under *syndrome.*

**AAV** adeno-associated virus; see *Dependovirus.*

**AB** abbreviation for L. *Artium Baccalaureus,* Bachelor of Arts.

**Ab** abbreviation for antibody.

**ab** Latin preposition meaning *from.*

**ab-** [L. *ab* from] prefix meaning *away from, from.*

**abac·te·ri·al** (a″bak-tēr'e-əl) free from bacteria.

**Aba·die's sign** (ah-bah-dēz') [Joseph Louis Irenée *Abadie,* French neurologist, 1873–1946] see under *sign.*

**abap·tis·ton** (a″bap-tis'tən) pl. *abaptis'ta* [*a-*[1] + Gr. *baptein* to dip] a trephine so shaped that it will not penetrate the brain.

**abar·og·nos·is** (a″bar-əg-no'sis) [*a-*[1] + *baro-* + Gr. *gnosis* knowledge] baragnosis.

**ab·ar·thro·sis** (ab″ahr-thro'sis) [*ab-* + L. *arthrosis*] diarthrosis.

**ab·ar·tic·u·lar** (ab″ahr-tik'u-lər) 1. not affecting a joint. 2. remote from a joint.

**ab·ar·tic·u·la·tion** (ab″ahr-tik″u-la'shən) [*ab-* + L. *articulatio* joint] 1. a dislocation of a joint. 2. junctura synovialis.

**aba·sia** (ə-ba'zhə) [*a-*[1] + Gr. *basis* step + *-ia*] inability to walk.
**a.-asta'sia,** astasia-abasia.
**a. atac'tica,** abasia characterized by uncertainty of movement, due to a defect of coordination.
**choreic a.,** a form due to chorea of the legs.
**paralytic a.,** a form due to paralysis of the leg muscles.
**paroxysmal trepidant a.,** astasia-abasia caused by spastic stiffening of the legs on attempting to stand; called also *spastic a.*
**spastic a.,** paroxysmal trepidant a.
**trembling a., a. tre'pidans,** abasia due to trembling of the legs.

**aba·sic** (ə-bā'sik) pertaining to abasia.

**abate** (ə-bāt') to lessen or decrease.

**abate·ment** (ə-bāt'mənt) a decrease in the severity of a pain or a symptom.

**abat·ic** (ə-bat'ik) abasic.

**ab·bau** (ahp'bou) [Ger. "decomposition," "breakdown"] 1. exergonic breakdown of chemical substances. 2. decomposition of chemical substances. 3. catabolic products.

**Ab·be's condenser** (ah-bəz') [Ernst Karl *Abbe,* German physicist, 1840–1905] see under *condenser.*

**Ab·be's flap, operation** (ab'ēz) [Robert *Abbe,* American surgeon, 1851–1928] see under *flap* and *operation.*

**Ab·be-Zeiss counting chamber (apparatus)** (ah'bə-tsīs) [E. K. *Abbe;* Carl *Zeiss,* German optician, 1816–1888] Thoma-Zeiss counting chamber.

**Ab·bo·cil·lin-DC** (ab″o-sil'in) trademark for preparations of penicillin G procaine.

**Ab·bott's meth·od** (ab'əts) [Edville Gerhardt *Abbott,* American surgeon, 1870–1938] see under *Table of Methods.*

**Ab·bott-Mil·ler tube** (ab'ət-mil'ər) [William Osler *Abbott,* American physician, 1902–1943; T. Grier *Miller,* American physician, 1886–1981] see *Miller-Abbott tube,* under *tube.*

**Ab·bott-Raw·son tube** (ab'ət-raw'sən) [William Osler *Abbott;* Arthur J. *Rawson,* American medical physicist, born 1896] see under *tube.*

**ABC** aspiration biopsy cytology.

**ABCD** a regimen of Adriamycin (doxorubicin), bleomycin, CCNU (lomustine), and dacarbazine, used in cancer chemotherapy.

**ab·cix·i·mab** (ab-sik'sĭ-mab) a human-murine monoclonal antibody Fab fragment that inhibits the aggregation of platelets, used as an antithrombotic in percutaneous transluminal coronary angioplasty; administered by intravenous infusion.

**ab·do·men** (ab′də-mən, ab-do′mən) [L., possibly from *abdere* to hide] [TA] [MeSH: Abdomen] that portion of the body which lies between the thorax and the pelvis; it contains a cavity *(abdominal cavity)* separated by the diaphragm from the thoracic cavity above, and by the plane of the pelvic inlet from the pelvic cavity below, and lined with a serous membrane, the peritoneum. This cavity contains the abdominal viscera (see Plate 56) and is enclosed by a wall *(abdominal wall)* formed by the abdominal muscles, vertebral column, and the ilia. Called also *belly* and *venter.* It is divided into nine regions by four imaginary lines projected onto the anterior wall (see illustration); two of the lines pass horizontally around the body (the upper at the level of the cartilages of the ninth ribs, the lower at the tops of the crests of the ilia), and two extend vertically on each side of the body from the cartilage of the eighth rib to the center of the inguinal ligament. The regions are: three upper—right hypochondriac, epigastric, left hypochondriac; three middle—right lateral, umbilical, left lateral; and three lower—right inguinal, pubic, left inguinal.
**acute a.,** an abdominal condition of abrupt onset usually associated with abdominal pain due to inflammation, perforation, obstruction, infarction, or rupture of intra-abdominal organs. Emergency surgical intervention is usually required. Examples are acute cholecystitis or appendicitis, perforated peptic ulcer, strangulated hernia, superior mesenteric arterial thrombosis, and splenic rupture. Called also *surgical a.*
**boat-shaped a.,** scaphoid a.
**carinate a.,** scaphoid a.
**gridiron a.,** one criss-crossed with scars from multiple surgical procedures, such as may occur in severe forms of Munchausen syndrome.
**navicular a.,** scaphoid a.
**a. obsti′pum,** congenital shortness of the rectus abdominis muscle.
**pendulous a.,** a relaxed condition of the abdominal wall, so that the anterior abdominal wall hangs over the pubis; called also *venter propendens.*
**scaphoid a.,** an abdomen whose anterior wall is hollowed out; seen in children with cerebral disease. Called also *boat-shaped a., carinate a.,* and *navicular a.*
**surgical a.,** acute a.

**ab·dom·i·nal** (ab-dom′ĭ-nəl) [L. *abdominalis*] pertaining to the abdomen. Called also *celiac.*

**abdomin(o)-** [L. *abdomen,* q.v.] a combining form denoting relationship to the abdomen.

**ab·dom·i·no·cen·te·sis** (ab-dom″ĭ-no-sen-te′sis) [*abdomino-* + *-centesis*] paracentesis of the abdominal cavity; called also *celiocentesis* and *celioparacentesis.*

**ab·dom·i·no·cys·tic** (ab-dom″ĭ-no-sis′tik) pertaining to the abdomen and gallbladder. Called also *abdominovesical* and *vesicoabdominal.*

**ab·dom·i·no·gen·i·tal** (ab-dom″ĭ-no-jen′ĭ-təl) pertaining to the abdomen and the reproductive organs.

**ab·dom·i·no·hys·ter·ec·to·my** (ab-dom″ĭ-no-his″tər-ek′tə-me) abdominal hysterectomy.

**ab·dom·i·no·hys·ter·ot·o·my** (ab-dom″ĭ-no-his″tər-ot′ə-me) abdominal hysterotomy.

**ab·dom·i·nos·co·py** (ab-dom″ĭ-nos′kə-pe) [*abdomino-* + *-scopy*] laparoscopy.

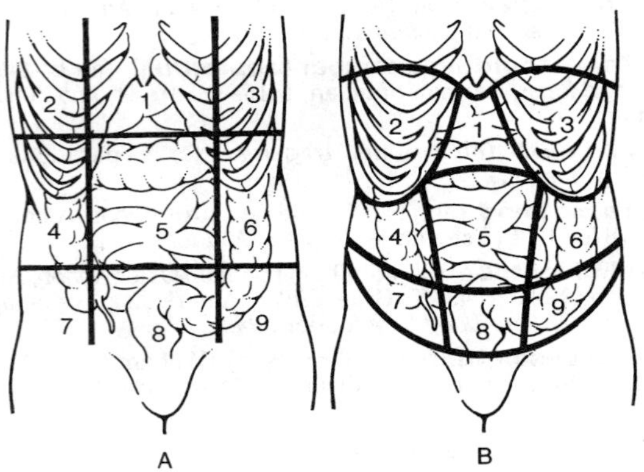


Regions of abdomen bounded according to *(A)* the standard and *(B)* a variant system: *1,* epigastric; *2,* right hypochondriac; *3,* left hypochondriac; *4,* right lateral (or lumbar); *5,* umbilical; *6,* left lateral (or lumbar); *7,* right inguinal (or iliac); *8,* pubic (hypogastric); *9,* left inguinal (or iliac).

**ab·dom·i·no·scro·tal** (ab-dom″ĭ-no-skro′təl) pertaining to the abdomen and scrotum.

**ab·dom·i·no·tho·rac·ic** (ab-dom″ĭ-no-thə-ras′ik) thoracoabdominal.

**ab·dom·i·no·uter·ot·o·my** (ab-dom″mĭ-no-u-tər-ot′ə-me) abdominal hysterotomy.

**ab·dom·i·no·vag·i·nal** (ab-dom″ĭ-no-vaj′ĭ-nəl) pertaining to the abdomen and the vagina.

**ab·dom·i·no·ves·i·cal** (ab-dom″ĭ-no-ves′ĭ-kəl) abdominocystic.

**ab·du·cens** (ab-du′senz) [L. "drawing away"] Latin adjective used in names of structures (e.g., nervus abducens) which serve to abduct a part.

**ab·du·cent** (ab-du′sent) [L. *abducens*] abducting, or effecting a separation, as an abducent nerve.

**ab·duct** (ab-dukt′) [*ab-* + *duct*] to draw away from the median plane or (in the digits) from the axial line of a limb.

**ab·duc·tio** (ab-duk′she-o) [L.] [TA] abduction.

**ab·duc·tion** (ab-duk′shən) the act of abducting or state of being abducted.

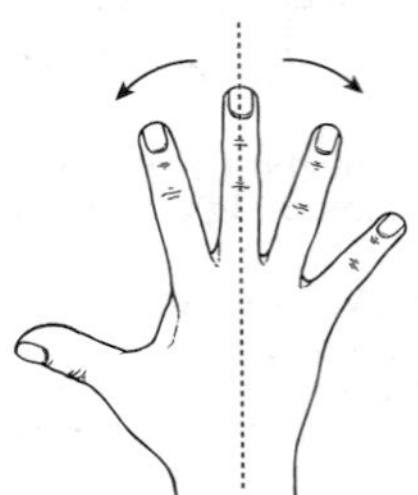

Abduction of the fingers.

**ab·duc·tor** (ab-duk′tər) [L.] that which abducts; see under *musculus.*

**ABE** acute bacterial endocarditis; see *infective endocarditis,* under *endocarditis.*

**Abel·cet** (a′bəl-set) trademark for a preparation of amphotericin B in a lipid complex for injection.

**ab·em·bry·on·ic** (ab″em-bre-on′ik) [*ab-* + *embryonic*] away from the embryo.

**ab·e·quose** (ab′ə-kwōs) an unusual sugar found to be a polysaccharide somatic antigen of *Salmonella* species.

**Ab·er·ne·thy's fascia** (ab′ər-ne″thēz) [John *Abernethy,* British surgeon and anatomist, 1764–1831] see *fascia iliaca.*

**ab·er·ran·cy** (ab-er′ən-se) aberration, def 3.
**acceleration-dependent a.,** aberrancy resulting from the occurrence of impaired intraventricular conduction as the heart attains a specific critical rate.
**bradycardia-dependent a.,** deceleration-dependent a.
**deceleration-dependent a.,** aberrancy resulting from the occurrence of impaired intraventricular conduction after long pauses or slowing of the heart to a critical rate.
**tachycardia-dependent a.,** acceleration-dependent a.

**ab·er·rant** (ab-ar′ənt) wandering or deviating from the usual or normal course.

**ab·er·ra·tio** (ab″ər-a′she-o) [L., from *aberrare* to wander away from] aberration, def. 1.
**a. tes′tis,** situation of the testis in a part distant from the path which it takes in normal descent.

**ab·er·ra·tion** (ab″ər-a′shən) [L. *aberratio,* q.v.] 1. deviation from the usual course or condition. 2. unequal refraction or focalization of light rays by a lens, resulting in degradation of the image they produce. 3. in cardiology, aberrant electrical impulse conduction.
**chromatic a.,** unequal deviation of light rays of different wavelengths passing through a refractive medium, resulting in fringes of color around the image produced; called also *newtonian a.*
**chromatic a., lateral,** difference in magnification due to differences in position of the principal points for light of different wavelengths; also a difference of focal length.
**chromatic a., longitudinal,** difference in position along the axis for the focal points of light, produced by unequal deviation of light rays of different wavelengths by a lens.
**chromosome a.,** an irregularity in the number or structure of chromosomes that may alter the course of development of the embryo, usually in the form of a gain (duplication), loss (deletion), exchange (translocation), or alteration in sequence (inversion) of genetic material. See Plate 1 and see *genetic disease,* under *disease.*

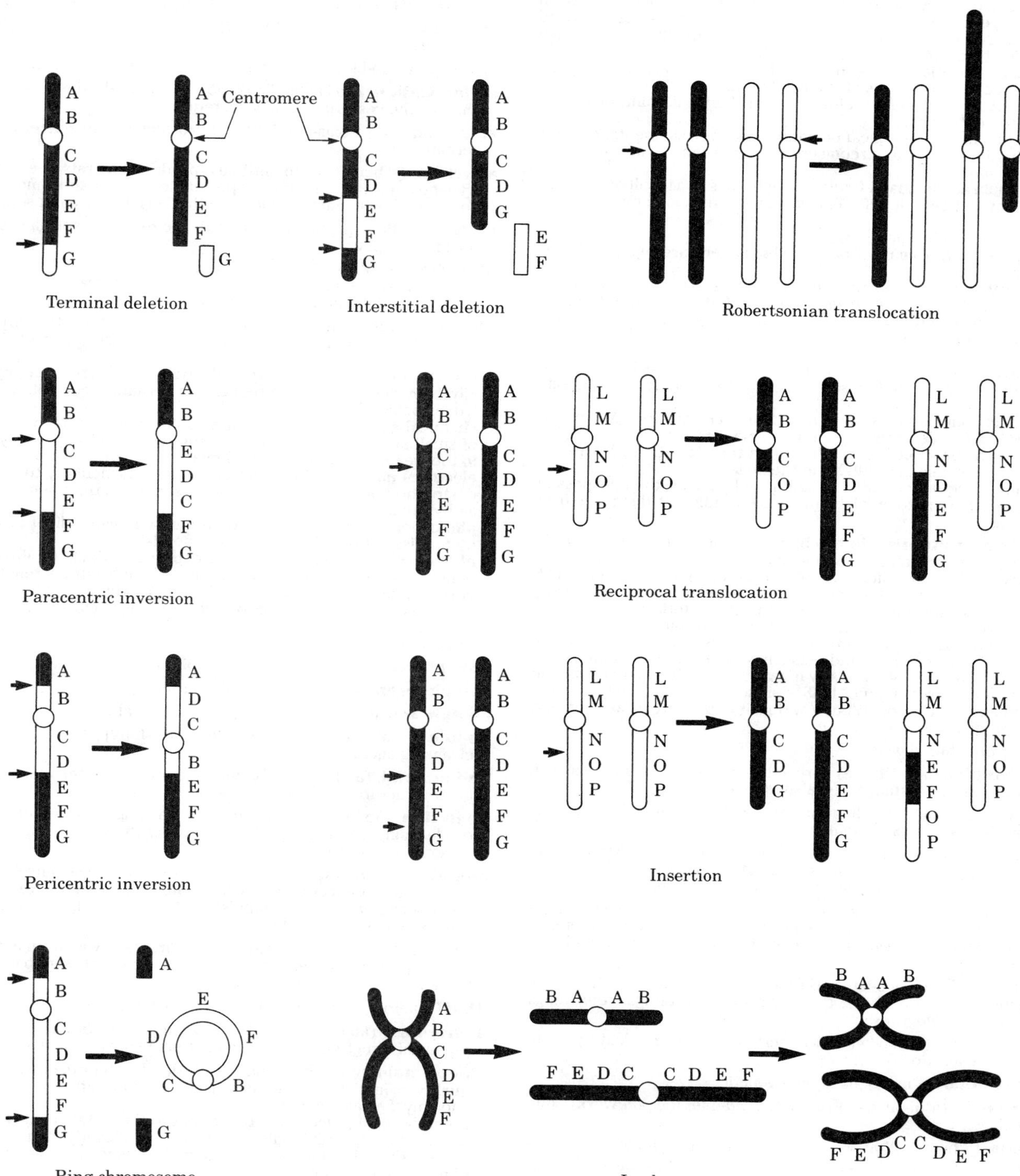


**PLATE 1**—CHROMOSOME ABERRATIONS

Genes are indicated by letters; breaks are indicated by small arrows.

**dioptric a.,** spherical a.
**distantial a.,** a blurring of vision for distant objects.
**intraventricular a.,** aberrant conduction within the ventricles of an impulse generated in the supraventricular region; it is characterized by a bizarre, usually wide QRS complex. Abnormalities due to fixed organic defects in conduction are excluded.
**lateral a.,** deviation of a ray from the focal point, measured on a line perpendicular to the axis at the focal point.
**longitudinal a.,** deviation of a ray from the focal point, measured along the optic axis.
**mental a.,** any pathological deviation from normal mental activity, usually limited to a circumscribed deviation in an otherwise adapted individual.
**meridional a.,** unequal refraction of light rays as a result of variation of refractive power in different portions of the same meridian of a lens.
**newtonian a.,** chromatic a.
**penta-X chromosomal a.,** one in which there are five X chromosomes in a female.
**spherical a.,** zonal aberration in relation to an axial point; see *spherical a., negative,* and *spherical a., positive.* Called also *dioptric a.*
**spherical a., negative,** unequal refraction of light rays by a lens, the peripheral rays being focused farther from the lens than the paraxial rays.
**spherical a., positive,** unequal refraction of light rays by a lens, the peripheral rays being focused closer to the lens than the paraxial rays.
**tetra-X chromosomal a.,** one in which there are four X chromosomes in a female or tetra-XY in the male.
**triple-X chromosomal a.,** one in which there are three X chromosomes in a female or triple-XY in the male.
**zonal a.,** unequal refraction of light rays by a lens, the rays passing through different zones being focused at different distances from the lens.

**abeta·lipo·pro·tein·emia** (a-ba″tə-lip″o-pro″te-ne′me-ə) [MeSH: Abetalipoproteinemia] an autosomal recessive disorder of lipoprotein metabolism in which lipoproteins containing apolipoprotein B (chylomicrons, very low density lipoproteins, and low density lipoproteins) are not synthesized; it is characterized by the presence of acanthocytes in plasma, hypocholesterolemia, progressive ataxic neuropathy, pigmentary retinal degeneration, defective intestinal lipid absorption, and deficiency of fat-soluble vitamins.
**normotriglyceridemic a.,** a variant of abetalipoproteinemia in which apolipoprotein (apo) B-48 is present, but apo B-100 is absent; chylomicrons are formed but low density lipoproteins are not, and some fat absorption may occur.

**ABG** arterial blood gases.

**ab·i·a·tro·phy** (a-bi-ă′trə-fe) premature and endogenous loss of vitality or tissue substance. See also *abiotrophy.*

**ab·i·ent** (ab′e-ənt) avoiding the source of stimulation; said of a response to a stimulus. Cf. *adient.*

**Abi·es** (a′be-ēz) the firs, a genus of evergreens of the family Pinaceae, mainly found in North America. *A. balsa′mea* (L.) Mill. is the balsam fir, which yields Canada balsam.

**abi·et·ic ac·id** (ab″e-et′ik) an acid resin that is the major active component of rosin (q.v.); it is used in the manufacture of soaps and its esters are used in the manufacture of lacquers and varnishes.

**abio·gen·e·sis** (a″bi-o-jen′ə-sis) [*a-*[1] + *bio-* + *-genesis*] the spontaneous generation of life; the origin of living things from things inanimate. Cf. *biogenesis.*

**abio·ge·net·ic** (a″bi-o-jə-net′ik) pertaining to or marked by spontaneous generation.

**abi·og·e·nous** (a″bi-oj′ə-nəs) abiogenetic.

**abi·on·er·gy** (a″bi-on′ər-je) [*a-*[1] + Gr. *bio-* life + *ergon* work] abiotrophy.

**abi·os·is** (a″bi-o′sis) [*a-*[1] + *bio-* + *-osis*] absence of life.

**abi·ot·ic** (a″bi-ot′ik) pertaining to or characterized by absence of life; incapable of living; antagonistic to life.

**abio·troph·ic** (a″bi-o-trof′ik) pertaining to or characterized by abiotrophy.

**abi·ot·ro·phy** (a″bi-ot′rə-fe) [*a-*[1] + *bio-* + *-trophy*] progressive loss of vitality of certain tissues or organs leading to disorders or loss of function; applied especially to degenerative hereditary diseases of late onset, e.g., Huntington's chorea.
**retinal a.,** a general term for a group of degenerative diseases of the retina, such as retinitis pigmentosa and neuronal ceroid-lipofuscinosis.

**ab·ir·ri·tant** (ab-ir′ĭ-tənt) [*ab-* + *irritant*] 1. diminishing or relieving irritation; soothing. 2. an agent that relieves irritation.

**ab·ir·ri·ta·tion** (ab-ir-ĭ-ta′shən) 1. diminished responsiveness to stimulation. 2. atony.

**ab·ir·ri·ta·tive** (ab-ir′ĭ-ta″tiv) reducing irritability; soothing.

**abi·u·ret** (a-bi′u-ret) [*a-*[1] + *biuret*] not giving a positive reaction to the biuret test.

**abi·u·ret·ic** (ə-bi″u-rĕ′tik) not responsive to the biuret test.

**ab·lac·ta·tion** (ab-lac-ta′shən) [*ab-* + *lactation*] the weaning of a child or the cessation of milk secretion.

**ablas·tem·ic** (a″blas-tem′ik) [*a-*[1] + *blastemic*] not concerned with germination.

**ablas·tin** (a″blas′tin) an antibody, produced by rats infected with trypanosomes, that inhibits reproduction of trypanosomes; it has no other known function and is neither a lysin nor an opsonin.

**ab·late** (ab-lāt′) [L. *ablatus* removed] to remove, especially by cutting; to extirpate.

**ab·la·tio** (ab-la′she-o) [L.] ablation.
**a. placen′tae,** premature detachment of a placenta.
**a. re′tinae,** detachment of the retina.

**ab·la·tion** (ab-la′shən) 1. separation or detachment; extirpation; eradication. 2. removal or destruction of a part, especially by cutting.
**catheter-induced a.,** delivery of destructive electrical energy, usually high energy or radiofrequency alternating current, via electrodes on a catheter.
**chemical a.,** destruction of an area of the myocardium by injection of small amounts of alcohol or phenol via a coronary artery; used in the treatment of tachyarrhythmias.
**electrical a.,** fulguration; the term is used particularly to describe destruction of areas of myocardial tissue in the treatment of tachyarrhythmias.
**photochemical a.,** laser ablation of tissue in which light absorbed by the tissue dissociates molecular bonds.
**photomechanical a.,** laser ablation of tissue in which the absorption of light energy causes stress in excess of the tissue's strength.
**photothermal a.,** laser ablation of tissue in which light is absorbed by the tissue and converted to heat, resulting in coagulation, necrosis, and vaporization.
**rotational a.,** rotablation.

**able·pha·ria** (a″blĕ-far′e-ə) cryptophthalmos.

**ableph·a·ron** (a″blef′ə-ron) ablepharia.

**ableph·ar·ous** (a″blef′ə-rəs) pertaining to ablepharia.

**ab·lu·ent** (ab′loo-ənt) [*ab-* + L. *luens* washing] 1. detergent. 2. a cleansing agent.

**ab·lu·mi·nal** (ab-loo′mĭ-nəl) directed away from the lumen of a tubular structure.

**ab·lu·tion** (ab-loo′shən) [L. *ablutio* a washing] the act of washing or cleansing; the application of water by the hand, which may be covered with a bath mitt or towel.

**ab·lu·to·ma·nia** (ab-loo″to-ma′ne-ə) [L. *ablutio* a washing + *-mania*] obsessional preoccupation with cleanliness, washing, or bathing, often accompanied by compulsive rituals, a common symptom in obsessive-compulsive states.

**ab·mor·tal** (ab-mor′təl) situated or directed away from a dead or injured part; applied especially to electric currents set up in injured tissue.

**ABMT** autologous bone marrow transplantation.

**ab·nor·mal** (ab-nor′məl) [*ab-* + *normal*] not normal; contrary to the usual structure, position, condition, behavior, or rule.

**ab·nor·mal·i·ty** (ab″nor-mal′ĭ-te) [MeSH: Abnormalities] 1. the quality or fact of being abnormal. 2. a malformation, deformity, or anomaly. See also *abnormity.*
**potential a. of glucose tolerance (pot AGT),** a statistical classification containing individuals who have a significantly higher than average risk of developing diabetes mellitus, such as identical twins of non-insulin-dependent diabetics.
**previous a. of glucose tolerance (prev AGT),** a statistical classification containing individuals once diagnosed as having diabetes mellitus, gestational diabetes, or impaired glucose tolerance, but who now have normal glucose tolerance.

**ab·nor·mi·ty** (ab-nor′mĭ-te) 1. abnormality; deformity. 2. monstrosity.

**ab·oma·sal** (ab″o-ma′səl) pertaining to the abomasum.

**ab·oma·si·tis** (ab″o-mə-si′tis) inflammation of the abomasum.

**ab·o·ma·so·pexy** (ab″o-ma′so-pek″se) surgical fixation of the abomasum to correct right or left displacement of the abomasum (see under *displacement*).

**ab·o·ma·sot·omy** (ab″o-ma-sot′ə-me) surgical cutting into the abomasum, usually to remove a bezoar or impaction.

**ab·oma·sum** (ab″o-ma′sum) [*ab-* + L. *omasum*] [MeSH: Abomasum] the fourth stomach of a ruminant, comparable in structure and function to the stomach of a nonruminant; it contains gastric glands that secrete gastric juice.

**ab·orad** (ab-or′ad) directed away from the mouth.

**ab·oral** (ab-or′əl) opposite to, away from, or remote from the mouth.

**ab·orig·i·nal** (ab-ə-rij′ĭ-nəl) native to the place inhabited.

**abort** (ə-bort′) [L. *aboriri* to miscarry] 1. to check the usual course of a disease. 2. to miscarry before the fetus is viable. 3. an abortion. 4. to become checked in development.

**abor·tient** (ə-bor′shənt) abortifacient.

**abor·ti·fa·cient** (ə-bor″tĭ-fa′shənt) [L. *abortio* abortion + *-facient*] 1. causing abortion. 2. an agent which causes abortion; called also *abortient.*

**abor·tion** (ə-bor′shən) [L. *abortio*] [MeSH: Abortion] 1. the premature expulsion from the uterus of the products of conception—of the embryo, or of a nonviable fetus. The classic symptoms, usually present in each type of abortion, are uterine contractions, uterine hemorrhage, dilatation of the cervix, and presentation or expulsion of all or part of the products of conception. 2. premature stoppage of a natural or a pathological process.
**accidental a.,** an abortion which is due to an accident.
**ampullar a.,** a variety of tubal abortion occurring from the ampulla of the oviduct.
**artificial a.,** induced a.
**chlamydial a.,** enzootic a. of ewes.
**complete a.,** abortion in which all of the products of conception have been expelled from the uterus and identified.
**contagious a.,** infectious a.
**enzootic a. of cattle,** an infectious abortion caused by organisms of the genus *Chlamydia;* known as *foothill a.* in the western United States. Called also *epidemic* or *epizootic bovine a.*
**enzootic a. of ewes,** abortion in ewes, usually late in the gestation period, caused by *Chlamydia psittaci.*
**epidemic bovine a., epizootic bovine a.,** enzootic a. of cattle.
**equine epizootic a.,** an infectious abortion of horses, caused by the virus of equine rhinopneumonitis.
**equine virus a.,** abortion occurring as part of equine viral rhinopneumonitis.
**foothill a.,** enzootic a. of cattle.
**habitual a.,** the spontaneous expulsion of a dead or nonviable fetus in three or more consecutive pregnancies, at about the same period of development.
**idiopathic a.,** abortion for which no recognized organic cause can be found.
**imminent a.,** impending abortion in which the bleeding is profuse, the cervix softened and dilated, and the uterine contractions approach the character of labor pains.
**incomplete a.,** abortion in which the uterus is not entirely emptied of its contents.
**induced a.,** abortion brought on intentionally; called also *artificial* or *therapeutic a.*
**inevitable a.,** a condition in which vaginal bleeding has been profuse or prolonged and the cervix has become effaced or dilated, and abortion will proceed naturally.
**infected a.,** abortion associated with infection of the genital tract.
**infectious a.,** 1. abortion in cattle caused by *Brucella abortus, Campylobacter* species, or a variety of other bacteria and viruses. Called also *Bang's disease.* See also *enzootic a. of cattle.* 2. abortion in horses caused by *Salmonella abortus equi* or a herpesvirus. See also *equine epizootic a.* and *equine virus a.* 3. abortion in sheep caused by *Campylobacter fetus, Chlamydia* species, or other bacteria. See also *enzootic a. of ewes.*
**missed a.,** retention in the uterus of an abortus that has died, indicated either by cessation of growth and hardening of the uterus or by actual diminution of its size; absence of fetal heart tones after they have been heard is also definitive; more accurate information of fetal death is obtainable by fetal electrocardiography and ultrasonography.
**mycotic a.,** abortion, usually in a cow, due to a fungal infection; common infecting fungi are species of *Absidia, Mortierella, Mucor,* and *Rhizopus.* See also *mucormycosis.*
**a. in progress,** a condition marked by profuse hemorrhage from the uterus and pains resembling those of labor, with softening and dilatation of the cervix, going on to expulsion of the products of conception.
**recurrent a.,** habitual a.
**septic a.,** abortion associated with serious infection of the uterus, leading to generalized infection; more common after illegal abortions.
**spontaneous a.,** abortion occurring naturally; popularly known as miscarriage.
**therapeutic a.,** abortion induced to save the life or health (physical or mental) of a pregnant woman; sometimes performed after rape or incest.
**threatened a.,** a condition in which there is bloody discharge from the uterus but the loss of blood is usually less than in inevitable abortion and there is no dilatation of the cervix; it may proceed to actual abortion or the symptoms may subside and the pregnancy go to full term.
**tubal a.,** extrusion of the conceptus through the open end of the uterine tube into the abdominal cavity, occurring in tubal (ectopic) pregnancy.
**vibrio a.,** an infectious abortion of cattle, sheep, and goats, caused by *Campylobacter (Vibrio) fetus.*

**abor·tion·ist** (ə-bor′shən-ist) one who performs abortions.

**abor·tive** (ə-bor′tiv) [L. *abortivus*] 1. incompletely developed. 2. effecting an abortion; abortifacient. 3. cutting short the course of a disease.

**abor·tus** (ə-bor′təs) [L.] a fetus weighing less than 500 gm. (17 oz.) or being of less than 20 completed weeks' gestational age at the time of expulsion from the uterus, having no chance of survival.

**abouche·ment** (ah-bōōsh-maw′) [Fr.] the termination of a vessel in a larger one.

**abou·lia** (ə-boo′le-ə) abulia.

**ABP** arterial blood pressure.

**abra·chia** (ə-bra′ke-ə) [*a-*[1] + L. *brachia*] congenital absence of the arms.

**abra·chi·a·tism** (ah-bra′ke-ah-tiz″əm) abrachia.

**abra·chio·ceph·a·lia** (ə-brā″ke-o-sĕ-fa′le-ə) [*a-*[1] + *brachio-* + *cephal-* + *-ia*] acephalobrachia.

**abra·chio·ceph·a·lus** (ə-brā″ke-o-sef′ə-lus) acephalobrachius.

**abra·chi·us** (ə-bra′ke-əs) an individual exhibiting abrachia.

**abrad·ant** (ə-bra′dənt) abrasive.

**abrade** (ə-brād′) to rub away the external covering or layer of a part; see also *planing.*

**Abrams' heart reflex** (a′brəmz) [Albert *Abrams,* American physician, 1863–1924] see under *reflex.*

**abra·sio** (ə-bra′se-o) [L.] abrasion.
**a. cor′neae,** a rubbing off of the superficial layers of the cornea.

**abra·sion** (ə-bra′zhən) [L. *abrasio*] 1. the wearing away of a substance or structure (such as the skin or the teeth) through some unusual or abnormal mechanical process; see also *planing.* 2. an area of body surface denuded of skin or mucous membrane by some unusual or abnormal mechanical process.

**abra·sive** (ə-bra′siv) 1. causing abrasion. 2. a substance used for abrading, grinding, or polishing.

**abra·sor** (ə-bra′zor) an instrument used for abrasion.

**ab·re·ac·tion** (ab″re-ak′shən) [*ab-* + *reaction*] [MeSH: Abreaction] the reliving of an experience in such a way that previously repressed emotions associated with it are released, usually also resulting in insight.
**motor a.,** an abreaction achieved through motor or muscular expression.

**ab·reu·og·ra·phy** (ab″roo-og′rə-fe) [Manoel de *Abreu,* Brazilian physician, 1892–1962] *(obs.)* photofluorography.

**Abri·ko·sov's (Abri·kos·soff's) tumor** (ah″bre-kos′ofs) [Aleksei Ivanovich *Abrikosov* (or *Abrikossoff*), Russian pathologist, 1875–1955] see *granular cell tumor,* under *tumor.*

**abrin** (a′brin) [MeSH: Abrin] a powerful phytotoxin or toxalbumin, present in the seeds of *Abrus precatorius* (jequirity bean) and used in the synthesis of immunotoxins; formerly used topically in certain chronic eye disorders.

**abrism** (a′brizm) poisoning by the jequirity bean; see *abrin.*

**ab·rup·tio** (ab-rup′she-o) [L., from *abrumpere* to break off from] a rending asunder.
**a. placen′tae,** premature detachment of a placenta, often attended by maternal systemic reactions in the form of shock, oliguria, and coagulation abnormalities.

**Abrus** (a′brəs) a genus of trees of the family Leguminosae, found in warm regions. *A. precato′rius* L. is found in tropical and subtropical Asia and the Americas; its seed (called *jequirity bean, rosary pea,* or *crab's eye*) is used for rosary beads and jewelry but contains the toxalbumin abrin (q.v.).

**abs-** [L. *abs,* variant of *ab*] a prefix meaning away, from.

**ab·scess** (ab′ses) [L. *abscessus,* from *ab* away + *cedere* to go]

[MeSH: Abscess]a localized collection of pus buried in tissues, organs, or confined spaces. See also *empyema.*
**acute a.,** one which runs a relatively short course, producing some fever and a painful local inflammation.
**alveolar a.,** apical a., def. 2.
**amebic a.,** an abscess cavity of the liver resulting from liquefaction necrosis due to entrance of *Entamoeba histolytica* into the portal circulation in amebiasis; amebic abscesses may also involve lungs, spleen, and brain.
**anorectal a.,** one arising in the anorectum.
**apical a.,** 1. one situated at the apex of an organ. 2. inflammation of tissues surrounding the apical portion of a tooth, associated with the collection of pus, resulting from infection following pulp infection through a carious lesion or as a result of an injury causing pulp necrosis. Called also *alveolar a., dentoalveolar a.,* and *periapical a.*
**apical a., acute,** an apical abscess of a tooth characterized by rapid onset, acute pain, tenderness of the tooth to touch, pus formation, and swelling of tissues in a later stage.
**apical a., chronic,** an apical abscess of a tooth characterized by an intermittent discharge of pus through a sinus tract, with gradual onset, little or no swelling of the affected tissue, and only slight discomfort.
**appendiceal a., appendicular a.,** abscess resulting from perforation of an acutely inflamed appendix.
**arthrifluent a.,** a wandering abscess which has its point of origin in a diseased joint.
**Bartholin's a., bartholinian a.,** abscess of the excretory duct of Bartholin's gland.
**Bezold's a.,** an abscess in the neck resulting from acute mastoiditis *(Bezold's mastoiditis)* in which pus tracts have formed deep to the superior portion of the sternocleidomastoid muscle and along the posterior belly of the digastric muscle.
**bicameral a.,** one which has two chambers or pockets; see *shirt-stud a.*
**bile duct a.,** cholangitic a.
**biliary a.,** abscess of the gallbladder or some part of the biliary tract.
**bone a.,** osteomyelitis; suppurative periostitis.
**brain a.,** one affecting the brain as a result of extension of an infection (e.g., otitis media) from an adjacent area or through blood-borne infection. Called also *pyencephalus* and *pyocephalus.*
**broad ligament a.,** an abscess between the folds of the broad ligament of the uterus; called also *parametric* or *parametrial a.*
**Brodie's a.,** a roughly spherical region of bone destruction, filled with pus or connective tissue, usually found in the metaphyseal region of long bones and caused by *Staphylococcus aureus* or *albus.*
**canalicular a.,** a mammary abscess communicating with a milk duct.
**caseous a.,** one containing cheeselike material, as in pulmonary tuberculosis. Called also *cheesy a.*
**cervical a.,** streptococcal lymphadenitis of swine.
**cheesy a.,** caseous a.
**cholangitic a.,** intrahepatic abscess complicating bacterial cholangitis; called also *bile duct a.*
**chronic a.,** cold a., def. 1.
**circumtonsillar a.,** peritonsillar a.
**cold a.,** 1. an abscess of comparatively slow development with little evidence of inflammation. Called also *chronic a.* 2. tuberculous a.
**collar-button a.,** shirt-stud a.
**dental a.,** an abscess in or about a tooth.
**dentoalveolar a.,** apical a., def. 2.
**diffuse a.,** an uncircumscribed abscess, the pus of which is diffused in the surrounding tissues.
**Douglas' a.,** an abscess in the rectouterine pouch.
**dry a.,** one that disappears without pointing or breaking.
**Dubois' a.,** abscess of the thymus in congenital syphilis; called also *Dubois' disease* and *thymic a.*

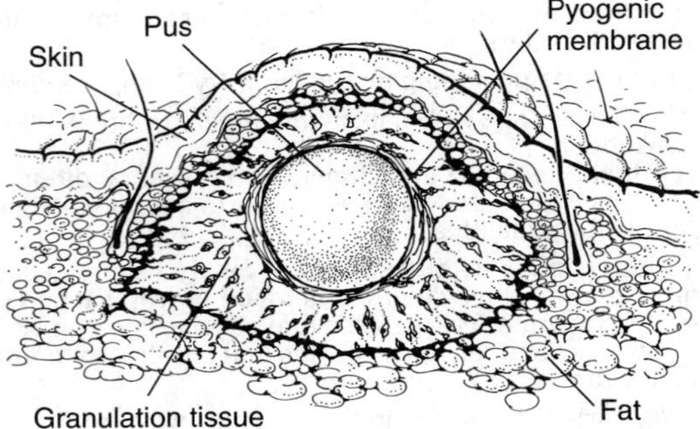

Cross section of abscess.

**epidural a.,** extradural a.
**epiploic a.,** an abscess in the omentum.
**extradural a.,** an abscess of the brain, between the dura and the cranial bone; called also *epidural a.*
**fecal a.,** an abscess, usually pericolic or perirectal, resulting from lower bowel perforation and containing pus and fecal matter; extension to the skin or mucosa leads to a fecal fistula.
**frontal a.,** one in the frontal lobe of the brain.
**gas a.,** a localized collection of seropurulent material containing gas, caused by gas-forming bacteria such as *Clostridium perfringens.* Called also *tympanitic a.* and *Welch's a.*
**gingival a.,** a localized, painful, inflammatory lesion of the gingivae, usually limited to the marginal gingiva or interdental papilla. See also *periodontal a.*
**gravitation a., gravity a.,** one in which the pus migrates or gravitates to a lower or deeper portion of the body.
**heel a.,** abscess of the heel of a sheep with lameness and suppuration at the skin-horn junction, usually as an extension of the infection of interdigital dermatitis. Called also *infectious bulbar necrosis.*
**helminthic a.,** one caused by a worm, such as filaria.
**hot a.,** an acute abscess with symptoms of local inflammation.
**hypostatic a.,** wandering a.
**interlobular a.,** a loculated abscess occurring within the breast stroma between the lobules.
**intersphincteric a.,** an anorectal abscess lying deep to the internal anal sphincter.
**intradural a.,** one within the layers of the dura mater.
**intramastoid a.,** mastoid a.
**ischiorectal a.,** an anorectal abscess located in the ischiorectal fossa.
**jowl a.,** streptococcal lymphadenitis of swine.
**kidney a.,** renal a.
**lacrimal a.,** one in or around the lacrimal sac.
**lacunar a.,** one in the lacunae of the urethra.
**lateral a., lateral alveolar a.,** periodontal a.
**mammary a.,** abscess occurring within the breast, often due to *Staphylococcus aureus* or streptococcal bacteria and usually affecting lactating women; it may be subcutaneous, subareolar, interlobular, central (unicentric or multicentric), or retromammary. See accompanying illustration.
**mammary a., central,** abscess occurring within the deep parenchyma of the breast; it may be unicentric or multicentric. See illustration.
**mammary a., interlobular,** an abscess occurring within the lactiferous ducts of the breast; called also *periductal mammary a.* See illustration.
**mammary a., periductal,** interlobular mammary a.
**mastoid a.,** an abscess within the mastoid process and the air cells, as a complication of mastoiditis. Called also *intramastoid a.* and *mastoid empyema.*

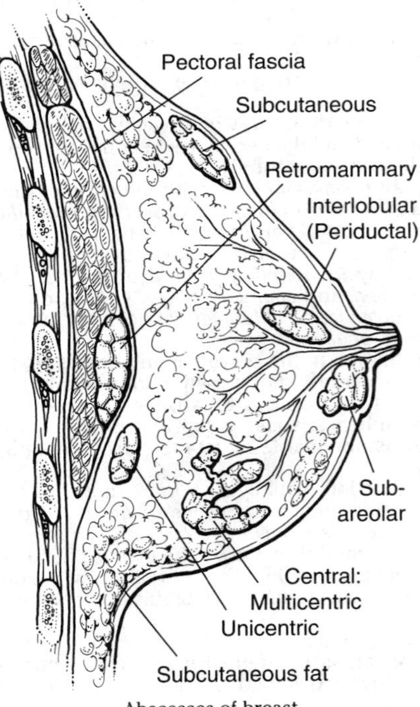

Abscesses of breast.

**metastatic a.**, a secondary abscess, usually of embolic origin, in which organisms are carried by the circulation to a point distant from the primary lesion.
**metastatic tuberculous a.**, tuberculous gumma.
**migrating a.**, wandering a.
**miliary a.**, one of a set of small multiple abscesses.
**Munro a.**, see under *microabscess.*
**orbital a.**, suppuration in the orbit.
**palatal a.**, an apical abscess of a maxillary tooth which erupts or extends toward the palate.
**parafrenal a.**, abscess of the preputial gland.
**parametrial a., parametric a.**, broad ligament a.
**paranephric a.**, one located near the kidney.
**parietal a.**, periodontal a.
**Pautrier's a.**, see under *microabscess.*
**pelvic a.**, abscess of the pelvic peritoneum, usually of the recto-uterine pouch.
**pelvirectal a.**, one lying immediately above the levator ani muscle, in close relation to the wall of the rectum.
**perianal a.**, a superficial anorectal abscess occurring beneath the perianal skin.
**periapical a.**, apical a., def. 2.
**pericoronal a.**, an abscess around the crown of a partially erupted tooth.
**peridental a.**, periodontal a.
**periductal a.**, interlobular a.
**perinephric a.**, one in the tissues immediately around the kidney.
**periodontal a.**, localized collection of purulent material in the periodontal tissue; it may involve the supporting periodontal tissue or the soft tissue wall of a periodontal pocket. Called also *lateral a., lateral alveolar a., parietal a.,* and *peridental a.* See also *gingival a.*
**peritoneal a.**, a confined collection of inflammatory exudate in peritonitis; called also *encysted peritonitis.*
**peritonsillar a.**, an abscess in the peritonsillar tissue extending into the tonsil capsule, resulting from suppuration of the tonsil; called also *quinsy.*
**periureteral a.**, one around the ureter.
**phlegmonous a.**, one associated with acute inflammation of the subcutaneous connective tissues.
**phoenix a.**, an abscess with symptoms identical to those of an acute apical abscess, developing from a chronic apical granuloma and suddenly becoming symptomatic.
**Pott's a.**, one associated with tuberculosis of the spine.
**premammary a.**, abscess occurring in the skin and subcutaneous tissues of the breast.
**psoas a.**, one which arises from disease of the lumbar or lower dorsal vertebrae, the pus descending in the sheath of the psoas muscle.
**pulp a., pulpal a.**, 1. an inflammation of the dental pulp, associated with a circumscribed collection of necrotic tissue and pus arising from breakdown of leukocytes and bacteria, sometimes walled off with connective tissue. 2. an abscess of the tissues of the pulp of a finger; see also *felon.*
**pyemic a.**, one due to pyemia. Called also *septicemic a.*
**renal a.**, a localized renal parenchymal suppuration consequent to bacterial infection.
**residual a.**, one recurring at the site where an incompletely resolved abscess occurred previously.
**retromammary a.**, abscess occurring in the soft tissue behind the breast parenchyma; see illustration.
**retroperitoneal a.**, subperitoneal a.
**retropharyngeal a.**, a suppurative inflammation of the lymph nodes in the posterior and lateral walls of the pharynx.
**retrotonsillar a.**, an abscess behind a tonsil caused by any of the common pyogenic bacteria, usually occurring with or closely following acute tonsillitis or pharyngitis.
**ring a.**, a ring-shaped purulent infiltration at the periphery of the cornea.
**root a.**, a chronic or acute pustular condition affecting the supporting structures of the root of a tooth; when it is of endodontic origin, called *apical a.;* when periodontal in origin, called *periodontal a.*
**satellite a.**, a secondary abscess arising from, and situated near, a primary abscess.
**septicemic a.**, pyemic a.
**serous a.**, periostitis albuminosa.
**shirt-stud a.**, a superficial abscess connected with a deeper one by a passage; called also *collar-button a.*
**spermatic a.**, one in the seminiferous tubules.
**splenic a.**, an abscess of the spleen.
**stercoraceous a., stercoral a.**, fecal a.
**sterile a.**, one from which microorganisms cannot be isolated.
**stitch a.**, one that develops adjacent to a stitch or suture.
**strumous a.**, tuberculous a.
**subaponeurotic a.**, one beneath an aponeurosis or fascia.
**subareolar a.**, a subcutaneous abscess of the breast tissue beneath the areola of the nipple; see illustration.
**subcutaneous a.**, one occurring beneath the skin.
**subdiaphragmatic a.**, one beneath the diaphragm.
**subdural a.**, a brain abscess situated just under the dura mater.
**subfascial a.**, one beneath a fascia.
**subgaleal a.**, one under the galea aponeurotica.
**subhepatic a.**, one situated beneath the liver.
**submammary a.**, one beneath the mammary gland.
**subpectoral a.**, one beneath the pectoral muscles.
**subperiosteal a.**, a bone abscess situated just below the periosteum.
**subperitoneal a.**, one between the parietal peritoneum and the abdominal wall.
**subphrenic a.**, one beneath the diaphragm.
**subscapular a.**, one between the serratus anterior and the posterior thoracic wall.
**sudoriparous a.**, an abscess arising in a sweat gland.
**superficial a.**, one occurring near the surface.
**suprahepatic a.**, one situated in the suspensory ligament between the liver and the diaphragm.
**supralevator a.**, an anorectal abscess occurring above the levator ani muscle and below the pelvic peritoneum.
**sympathetic a.**, one arising some distance from the exciting cause.
**syphilitic a.**, one occurring in the bones during tertiary syphilis.
**thecal a.**, one arising in an enveloping sheath, such as a tendon sheath.
**Thornwaldt's a.**, Tornwaldt's a.
**thymic a.**, Dubois' a.
**toe a.**, abscess of the toe of a sheep with lameness and suppuration at the coronet, usually involving one digit of a front foot.
**Tornwaldt's (Thornwaldt's) a.**, an abscess of the adenoids, usually associated with adenoidism.
**tuberculous a.**, one due to infection with tubercle bacilli *(Mycobacterium tuberculosis);* called also *cold a.* and *strumous a.*
**tubo-ovarian a.**, abscess of the uterine tube and ovary.
**tympanitic a.**, gas a.
**tympanocervical a.**, one arising in the tympanum and extending to the neck. See also *Bezold's a.*
**tympanomastoid a.**, an abscess of the tympanum and mastoid.
**urethral a.**, an abscess of the urethra.
**urinary a.**, one caused by extravasation of infected urine.
**verminous a.**, one which contains insect larvae or other animal parasites.
**vitreous a.**, abscess of the vitreous humor of the eye due to infection, trauma, or foreign body.
**von Bezold's a.**, Bezold's a.
**wandering a.**, one that burrows in the tissues and finally points at a distance from the site of origin; called also *hypostatic a.* and *migrating a.*
**Welch's a.**, gas a.
**worm a.**, one caused by or containing worms; see *helminthic a.* and *verminous a.*

**ab·sces·sus** (ab-ses′us) [L.] abscess.

**ab·scise** (ab-sīz′) excise.

**ab·scis·sa** (ab-sis′ə) [L. *(linea) abscissa* cut-off line, from *abscindere* to cut off] the horizontal coordinate in a two-dimensional coordinate system; the horizontal distance of a point from *y-* (or vertical) axis. Denoted by *x.* Cf. *ordinate.*

**ab·scis·sion** (ab-si′shən) [*ab-* + *scission*] removal by cutting.
**corneal a.**, excision of the prominence of the cornea in staphyloma.

**ab·scon·sio** (ab-skon′se-o) pl. *absconsio′nes* [L.] the cavity of a bone receiving and concealing the head of another bone.

**ab·scop·al** (ab-sko′pəl) pertaining to the effect on nonirradiated tissue resulting from irradiation of other tissue of the organism.

**ab·sence** (ab′sens) 1. absence epilepsy. 2. absence seizure.

**abs. feb.** abbreviation for L. *absen′te feb′re,* while fever is absent. Cf. *adst. feb.*

**Ab·sid·ia** (ab-sid′e-ə) a genus of fungi of the family Mucoraceae. *A. corymbi′fera* (called also *A. ramo′sa, Mucor corymbifer,* and *M. ramosus*) grows on bread and decaying vegetation and sometimes causes mucormycosis and otomycosis in humans, laboratory animals, cattle, and other animals.

**ab·sinthe** (ab′sinth) [MeSH: Absinthe] 1. *Artemisia absinthium.* 2. an extract of *A. absinthium* and other bitter herbs, containing 60 per cent alcohol, formerly used as an alcoholic beverage; its use has been banned because it contains neurotoxins and prolonged ingestion can cause trismus, amblyopia, optic neuritis, and convulsions.

**ab·sin·thi·um** (ab-sin′the-um) 1. *Artemisia absinthium.* 2. the dead leaves and flowering tops of *Artemisia absinthium;* called also *wormwood.*

**ab·so·lute** (ab′sə-lo͞ot) [L. *absolutus,* from *absolvere* to set loose] free from limitations; unlimited; uncombined.

**ab·sorb** (ab-sorb′) [L. *absorbēre*] 1. to take in or assimilate, as to take up substances into or across tissues, e.g., the skin, intestine, or kidney tubules. 2. to react with radiation energy so as to attenuate it. 3. to retain specific wavelengths of radiation incident upon a substance, either increasing its temperature or changing the energy state of its molecules.

**ab·sor·bance** (ab-sor'bəns) 1. in analytical chemistry, the negative logarithm of the transmittance, $-\log_{10}(I/I_0)$, where $I$ is the light intensity transmitted by the solution under analysis and $I_0$ is the intensity transmitted by the pure solvent or other reference solution. Symbol *A*. Formerly referred to as *absorbancy* or *optical density*. 2. in radiation physics, the negative logarithm of the transmittance, defined as the ratio of the radiant energy transmitted by an object $(I)$ to the incident radiant energy $(I_0)$.

**ab·sor·ban·cy** (ab-sor'bən-se) absorbance.

**ab·sor·be·fa·cient** (ab-sor"be-fa'shənt) [L. *absorbere* to absorb + *facient*] 1. causing or promoting absorption. 2. a medicine or an agent that promotes absorption.

**ab·sor·bent** (ab-sor'bənt) [*ab-* + *sorbent*] 1. able to take in, or suck up and incorporate. 2. a tissue structure involved in absorption. 3. a substance that absorbs or acts as an absorbefacient.

**ab·sorp·ti·om·e·ter** (ab-sorp"she-om'ə-tər) [*absorption* + *-meter*] 1. an instrument for measuring the solubility of gas in a liquid. 2. a device for measuring the layer of liquid absorbed between two glass plates; used as a hematoscope.

**ab·sorp·ti·om·e·try** (ab-sorp"she-om'ə-tre) in radiology, the measurement of the degree to which the radiation emitted by a radioisotope is completely dissipated within a tissue.
**dual photon a.**, measurement of the bone mineral content in the axial skeleton, particularly the lumbar spine, by comparing the transmission of the two separate photoelectric energy peaks emitted by gadolinium 153 through both soft and bone tissues.

**ab·sorp·tion** (ab-sorp'shən) [L. *absorptio*] [MeSH: Absorption] 1. the uptake of substances into or across tissues, e.g., skin, intestine, and kidney tubules. 2. in psychology, devotion of thought to one object or activity, with inattention to others. 3. the taking up of energy by matter with which the radiation interacts. Cf. *attenuation*, def. 3. 4. in chemistry, the penetration of a substance within the inner structure of another. Cf. *adsorption*.
**agglutinin a.**, the removal of antibody from an immune serum by treatment with particulate antigen (usually bacteria) homologous to that antibody, followed by separation of the antigen-antibody complex.
**enteral a.**, internal a.
**external a.**, the absorption of foods, poisons, or other agents through the skin or mucous membrane.
**internal a.**, the normal absorption of foods, water, etc., in digestion.
**interstitial a.**, removal of waste matter by the absorbent system.
**intestinal a.**, the uptake from the intestinal lumen of fluids, solutes, proteins, fats, and other nutrients into the intestinal epithelial cells, blood, lymph, or interstitial fluids of the intestine.
**net a.**, the difference between uptake and efflux from a tissue or cell.
**parenteral a.**, absorption otherwise than through the digestive tract.

**ab·sorp·tive** (ab-sorp'tiv) capable of absorbing; absorbent; pertaining to absorption.

**ab·sorp·tiv·i·ty** (ab"sorp-tiv'ĭ-te) a measure of the amount of light absorbed by a solution, defined as the absorbance per unit concentration per unit length of light path. By Beer's law (q.v.) absorptivity is proportional to the concentration of the absorbing solute. Called also *absorbancy index, absorption constant, absorption coefficient,* and *extinction coefficient*.
**molar a.**, absorptivity defined in terms of concentrations expressed in moles per liter. Symbol $\epsilon$.
**specific a.**, absorptivity defined in terms of concentrations expressed in grams per liter. Symbol *a*.

**abst** abstract.

**ab·ster·gent** (ab-ster'jənt) [L. *abstergere* to cleanse] 1. cleansing or purifying. 2. a cleansing application or medicine.

**ab·sti·nence** (ab'sti-nəns) a refraining from the use of or indulgence in food, stimulants, or sexual intercourse. See also *withdrawal* (def. 2).

**abstr** abstract.

**ab·stract** (ab'strakt) [L. *abstractum*, from *abstrahere* to draw off] a summary or epitome of a book, paper, or case history.

**ab·strac·tion** (ab-strak'shən) [L. *abstractus*, past participle of *abstrahere* to draw away] 1. the withdrawal of any ingredient from a compound. 2. a condition in which the teeth or other maxillary and mandibular structures are lower than the normal position, away from the occlusal plane, thereby lengthening the face. Cf. *attraction*, def. 2.

**ab·ter·min·al** (ab-ter'mĭ-nəl) [*ab-* + L. *terminus* end] moving from the end toward the center; said of electric currents in muscle.

**ab·tor·sion** (ab-tor'shən) extorsion.

**Abul·ca·sis** (ah"bool-kas'is) Albucasis.

**abu·lia** (ə-boo'le-ə) [*a-*[1] + Gr. *boulē* will + *-ia*] 1. lack of will or willpower; inability to make decisions. 2. akinetic mutism that is less than total. Called also *aboulia*.

**abu·lic** (ə-boo'lik) affected with or pertaining to abulia.

**Abul·ka·sim** (ah"bool-kas'im) Albucasis.

**abuse** (ə-būs') misuse or wrong use, particularly excessive use of anything.
**child a.**, physical, emotional, or sexual abuse of children, usually by parents, relatives, or caretakers. See also *battered-child syndrome*, under *syndrome*.
**drug a.**, substance a.
**physical a.**, any act resulting in a nonaccidental physical injury, including not only intentional assault but also the result of unreasonable punishment
**psychoactive substance a.**, substance a.
**sexual a.**, any act of a sexual nature performed in a criminal manner, as with a child or with a nonconsenting adult, including rape, incest, sodomy, oral copulation, and penetration of genital or anal opening with a foreign object; also included are lewd and lascivious acts with a child or any sexual act which could be expected to irritate, trouble or offend a child performed by one motivated by an abnormal sexual interest in children, as well as acts related to sexual exploitation of children, including activities related to pornography or prostitution involving minors and coercion of minors to perform obscene acts.
**substance a.** [DSM-IV], a substance use disorder characterized by the use of a mood or behavior-altering substance in a maladaptive pattern resulting in significant impairment or distress, such as failure to fulfill social or occupational obligations or recurrent use in situations in which it is physically dangerous to do so or which end in legal problems, but without fulfilling the criteria for substance dependence (q.v.). Specific disorders are named for their etiology, eg., alcohol abuse, anabolic steroid abuse. DSM-IV includes specific abuse disorders for alcohol, amphetamines or similar substances, cannabis, cocaine, hallucinogens, inhalants, opioids, PCP or similar substances, and sedatives, hypnotics, or anxiolytics.

**abut** (ə-but') to touch, adjoin, or border upon.

**abut·ment** (ə-but'mənt) 1. that on which or at which abutting occurs. 2. a part of a structure that sustains thrust or pressure. 3. a tooth or root used as an anchorage for either a fixed or a removable dental prosthesis, or any other device serving the same purpose. See also under *tooth*.
**auxiliary a.**, secondary a.
**implant a.**, that part of a subperiosteal, intraperiosteal, or intraosseous implant that protrudes into the oral cavity and serves as an abutment for retaining and stabilizing a denture.
**intermediate a.**, a natural tooth or root, without other natural teeth in proximal contact, that is used as an abutment, in addition to two terminal abutments. Called also *pier*.

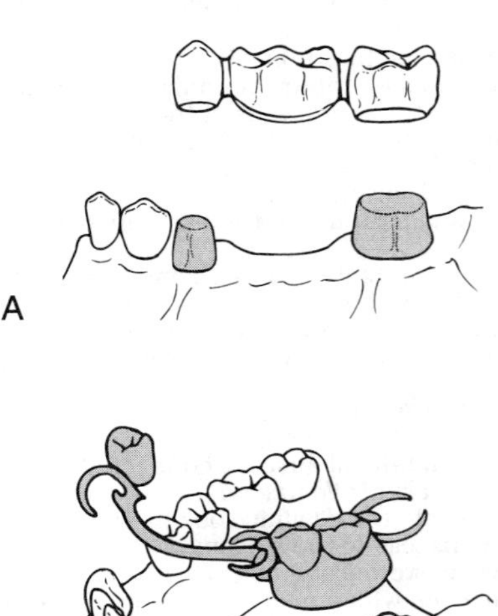

Abutments for fixed bridge *(A)* and removable partial denture *(B)*.

**isolated a.,** an intermediate abutment, particularly one used to support a removable partial denture.
**multiple a.,** one resulting from the fixed splinting of two or more adjacent natural teeth to serve as a unit in the support and retention of a fixed or removable partial denture.
**primary a.,** a tooth used for direct support of a denture.
**secondary a.,** a natural tooth used in addition to the primary abutments to provide support or indirect retention for a removable partial denture; called also *auxiliary a.*
**terminal a.,** a natural tooth located at an extremity of a fixed partial denture and used for the support and retention of the prosthesis.

**ABVD** a regimen consisting of Adriamycin (doxorubicin), bleomycin, vinblastine, and dacarbazine, used in cancer chemotherapy for treatment of Hodgkin's disease.

**AC** 1. air conduction; alternating current; aortic closure; anodal closure; axiocervical; acromioclavicular. 2. a cancer chemotherapy regimen consisting of Adriamycin (doxorubicin) and cyclophosphamide.

**Ac** symbol for *actinium.*

**a.c.** abbreviation for L. *an'te ci'bum,* before meals.

**ACA** American College of Angiology; American College of Apothecaries.

**Aca·cia** (ə-ka'shə) [L.; Gr. *akakia*] [MeSH: Acacia] a genus of shrubs and trees of the family Leguminosae. *A. ca'na* is a selenium accumulator that can cause selenium poisoning in livestock. *A. ca'techu* Willd. is a small tree native to India and Burma that yields catechu. *A. georgi'nae* F. M. Bail. is an Australian tree whose leaves can cause fatal fluoroacetate poisoning to livestock. *A. hor'rida* is a South African species that yields Cape gum. *A. se'negal* is an African tree that yields acacia (gum arabic).

**aca·cia** (ə-ka'shə) [L.; Gr. *akakia*] [MeSH: Acacia] 1. a plant of the genus *Acacia.* 2. the dried, gummy exudate from the stems and branches of *Acacia senegal,* occurring as spheroids, flakes, powder, granules, or spray-dried acacia and prepared as a mucilage or syrup; used as a suspending agent, emollient, and demulcent in pharmaceutical preparations. Called also *gum arabic.*

**acal·cu·lia** (ə-kal-ku'le-ə) [*a-*[1] + L. *calculare* to reckon + *-ia*] inability to do simple arithmetical calculations. Cf. *dyscalculia.*

**acamp·sia** (ə-kamp'se-ə) [*a-*[1] + Gr. *kamptein* to bend + *-ia*] rigidity or inflexibility of a part or of a joint.

**acan·tha** (ə-kan'thə) [Gr. *akantha* thorn] 1. the spine. 2. the spinous process of a vertebra.

**acan·tha·ceous** (ak"an-tha'shəs) bearing prickles or spines.

**acan·tha·me·bi·a·sis** (ə-kan"tha-me-bi'ə-sis) infection with a species of *Acanthamoeba;* the most common manifestations are granulomatous amebic encephalitis and *Acanthamoeba* keratitis.

**Acan·tha·moe·ba** (ə-kan"thə-me'bə) [*acanth-* + *amoeba*] [MeSH: Acanthamoeba] a genus of free-living ameboid protozoa (suborder Acanthopodina, order Amoebida) found usually in fresh water or moist soil. Certain species, such as *A. astronyxis, A. castellanii, A. culbertsoni, A. hatchetti, A. polyphaga,* and *A. rhisodes,* may occur as human pathogens. See also *acanthamebiasis.*

**Acan·thas·ter** (a"kan-thas'tər) a genus of starfish. *A. plan'ci* is the crown-of-thorns starfish, a venomous species.

**acan·thes·the·sia** (ə-kan"thes-the'shə) [*acanth-* + *esthesia*] perverted sensibility with a feeling as of pressure of a sharp point.

**Acan·thia lec·tu·la·ria** (ə-kan'the-ə lek"to͞o-lar'e-ə) *Cimex lectularius.*

**acan·thi·on** (ə-kan'the-on) [Gr. *akanthion* little thorn] a point at the tip of the anterior nasal spine.

**acanth(o)-** [Gr. *akantha,* q.v.] a combining form meaning thorny or spiny, or denoting a relationship to a sharp spine or thorn.

**Acan·tho·bdel·lid·ea** (ə-kan"tho-dĕ-lid'e-ə) an order of leeches of the class Hirudinea, characterized by the presence of spines on the surface of the body.

**Acan·tho·ceph·a·la** (ə-kan"tho-sef'ə-lə) [*acantho-* + Gr. *kephalē* head] [MeSH: Acanthocephala] a phylum of animal parasites, the thorny-headed worms, so called because of the proboscis which projects anteriorly, and is covered with thornlike recurved spines for attachment to the digestive tract of the host. In some systems of classification, they are considered to be a class of the phylum Nemathelminthes.

**acan·tho·ceph·a·lan** (ə-kan"tho-sef'ə-lən) any individual of the phylum Acanthocephala; called also *thorny-headed worm.*

**acan·tho·ceph·a·li·a·sis** (ə-kan"tho-sef"ə-li'ə-sis) infestation of the intestine of a vertebrate with any species of the phylum Acanthocephala.

**acan·tho·ceph·a·lous** (ə-kan"tho-sef'ə-ləs) pertaining to or caused by worms of the phylum Acanthocephala.

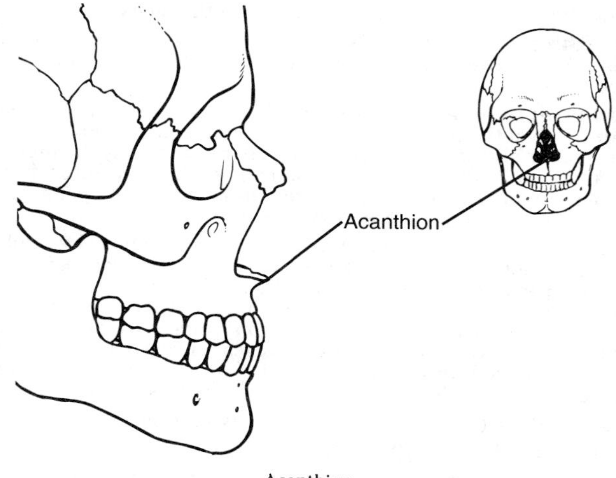

Acanthion.

**Acan·tho·ceph·a·lus** (ə-kan"tho-sef'ə-ləs) a genus of worms of the phylum Acanthocephala; some species are parasitic in fish.

**Acan·tho·chei·lo·ne·ma** (ə-kan"tho-ki"lo-ne'mə) a genus of filarial nematodes.
**A. per'stans,** *Mansonella perstans.*
**A. streptocer'ca,** *Mansonella streptocerca.*

**acan·tho·chei·lo·ne·mi·a·sis** (ə-kan"tho-ki"lo-ne-mi'ə-sis) mansonellosis.

**acan·tho·cyte** (ə-kan'tho-sīt) [*acantho-* + *-cyte*] [MeSH: Acanthocytes] a spiculed erythrocyte with five to ten spiny protoplasmic projections of varying lengths distributed irregularly over its surface; seen in abetalipoproteinemia, malnutrition, liver diseases, and a few other conditions. Called also *acanthrocyte* and *spur cell.*

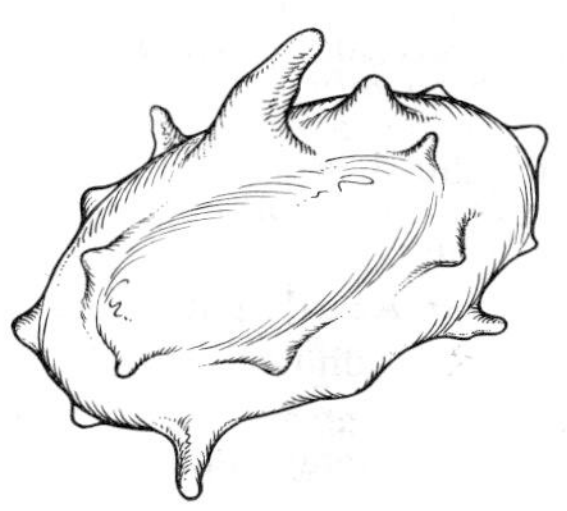
Acanthocyte.

**acan·tho·cy·to·sis** (ah-kan"tho-si-to'sis) [*acanthocyte* + *-osis*] 1. the presence of acanthocytes in the blood. 2. abetalipoproteinemia.

**acan·thoid** (ə-kan'thoid) [*acanth-* + *-oid*] resembling a spine; spinous.

**acan·thol·y·sis** (ak"an-thol'ĭ-sis) [*acantho-* + *-lysis*] [MeSH: Acantholysis] disruption of the intercellular connections between keratinocytes of the epidermis, caused by lysis of intercellular cement substance, resulting in secondary disruption of desmosomes and often in a defined sequence of cellular degenerative events.

**acan·tho·lyt·ic** (ə-kan"tho-lit'ik) pertaining or relating to acantholysis.

**ac·an·tho·ma** (ak"an-tho'mə, a"kan-tho'mə) pl. *acantho'mas* or *acantho'mata* [*acanth-* + *-oma*] a tumor composed of epidermal or squamous cells.
**a. adenoi'des cys'ticum,** multiple trichoepithelioma; see *trichoepithelioma.*
**clear cell a.,** a slightly elevated, erythematous, dome-shaped plaque or papule, with some crusting or scaling, usually occurring on the lower leg in older adults; it is characterized by acanthotic epithelium containing large, pale, glycogen-rich squamous cells.
**Degos a.,** clear cell a.
**pilar sheath a.,** a benign tumor of the hair follicle, usually occurring as an asymptomatic lesion on the upper lip of middle-aged adults; it is characterized by a central keratin-filled cavity lined by stratified squamous epithelium projecting into the connective stroma.

**acan·tho·pel·vis** (ə-kan"tho-pel'vis) [*acantho-* + *pelvis*] a pelvis with a very sharp and prominent pubic crest; called also *acanthopelyx.*

**acan·tho·pel·yx** (ə-kan″tho-pel′iks) acanthopelvis.

**Acan·tho·phis** (ə-kan′tho-fis) a genus of snakes of the family Elapidae. *A. antarc′ticus* is the death adder of Australia and New Guinea. See table at *snake.*

**Acan·tho·po·di·na** (ə-kan″tho-po-di′nə) [*acantho-* + Gr. *pous* foot] [MeSH: Acanthopodina] a suborder of ameboid protozoa (order Amoebida, subclass Gymnamoebia), characterized by the presence of more or less finely tipped, sometimes filiform, often furcate hyaline subpseudopodia produced from a broad hyaline lobe. *Acanthamoeba* is a representative genus.

**ac·an·tho·sis** (ak″an-tho′sis) [*acanth-* + *-osis*] diffuse hyperplasia of the spinous layer of the skin. Called also *hyperacanthosis.*
**a. ni′gricans,** diffuse velvety acanthosis with dark pigmentation, chiefly in axillae, occurring in an adult form, often associated with an internal carcinoma (called *malignant acanthosis nigricans*), and in a benign, nevoid form, more or less generalized. A benign juvenile form associated with obesity, which is sometimes due to endocrine disturbance, is called *pseudoacanthosis nigricans.*

**ac·an·thot·ic** (ak″an-thot′ik) marked by acanthosis.

**acan·thro·cyte** (ə-kan′thro-sīt) acanthocyte.

**acan·thro·cy·to·sis** (ə-kan″thro-si-to′sis) acanthocytosis.

**a ca·pi·te ad cal·cem** (a cap′ĭ-te ad kal′sem) [L.] from head to heel, the classic order for describing symptoms.

**Aca·ra·pis** (a-kar′ə-pis) a genus of mites. *A. woo′di* is a tracheal mite of the honeybee, the cause of Isle of Wight disease.

**acar·bia** (ə-kahr′be-ə) a condition in which the blood bicarbonate is lowered.

**acar·bose** (a′kahr-bōs) an α-glucosidase inhibitor produced by fermentation by *Actinoplanes utahensis,* used as an antihypoglycemic agent in the treatment of non–insulin-dependent diabetes mellitus; administered orally.

**acar·dia** (a-kahr′de-ə) [*a-*[1] + Gr. *kardia* heart] congenital absence of the heart.

**acar·di·ac** (a-kahr′de-ak) having no heart.

**acar·di·a·cus** (a″kahr-di′ə-kus) acardius.

**acar·di·us** (ə-kahr′de-us) [*a-*[1] + *cardia*] an imperfectly formed free twin fetus, lacking a heart and invariably lacking other body parts as well; called also *fetus acardiacus.*
**a. ace′phalus,** holoacardius acephalus.
**a. acor′mus,** holoacardius acormus.
**a. amor′phus,** holoacardius amorphus.
**a. an′ceps,** hemiacardius.

**acari** (ak′ə-ri) [L.] [MeSH: Acari] plural of *acarus.*

**acar·i·an** (ə-kar′e-ən) pertaining to the acarids or mites.

**ac·a·ri·a·sis** (ak″ə-ri′ə-sis) [*acar-* + *-iasis*] infestation with acarids (ticks or mites); see also *mange.* Called also *acaridiasis* and *acarinosis.*
**chorioptic a.,** see under *mange.*
**demodectic a.,** see under *mange.*
**nasal a.,** infestation of the nasal cavity or sinuses of a dog by the nasal mite *Pneumonyssus caninum,* which causes mild rhinitis.

**acar·i·cide** (ə-kar′ĭ-sīd) [*acari* + *-cide*] 1. destructive to mites. 2. an agent that destroys mites.

**ac·a·rid** (ak′ə-rid) 1. a mite or tick of the order Acarina. 2. a mite of the family Acaridae.

**Acar·i·dae** (ə-kar′ĭ-de) a family of small mites of the order Acarina; genera include *Acarus* and *Tyrophagus.* Several species cause skin rashes, such as grocers' itch, copra itch, and vanillism.

**acar·i·dan** (ə-kar′ĭ-dən) acarid.

**acar·i·di·a·sis** (ə-kar″ĭ-di′ə-sis) acariasis.

**Ac·a·ri·na** (ak″ə-ri′nə) an order of the class Arachnida, including the ticks and mites.

**ac·a·rine** (ak′ə-rīn) acarid (def.1).

**acar·i·no·sis** (ə-kar″ĭ-no′sis) acariasis.

**acar·i·o·sis** (ə-kar″e-o′sis) acariasis.

**acar(o)-** [L. *Acarus* a genus of mites, from Gr. *akari*] a combining form denoting relationship to mites.

**ac·a·ro·der·ma·ti·tis** (ak″ə-ro-dər″mə-ti′tis) any skin inflammation caused by mites.
**a. urticarioi′des,** grain itch.

**ac·a·roid** (ak′ə-roid) [Gr. *akari* a mite + *eidos* form] resembling a mite.

**ac·a·rol·o·gist** (ak″ə-rol′ə-jist) a specialist in acarology.

**ac·a·rol·o·gy** (ak″ə-rol′ə-je) [*acaro-* + *-logy*] the scientific study of mites and ticks.

**ac·a·ro·pho·bia** (ak″ə-ro-fo′be-ə) [*acaro-* + *-phobia*] irrational fear of mites or of other minute animate (insects, worms) or inanimate (pins, needles) objects, sometimes accompanied by fear of parasites crawling beneath the skin.

**ac·a·ro·tox·ic** (ak″ə-ro-tok′sik) destructive to mites.

**Acar·to·myia** (ə-kar″to-mi′yə) a genus of culicine mosquitoes.

**Ac·a·rus** (ak′ə-rus) [L.; Gr. *akari* a mite] a genus of small mites of the family Acaridae. They are often ectoparasitic, causing itch, mange, and other skin diseases.
**A. folliculo′rum,** *Demodex folliculorum.*
**A. galli′nae,** *Dermanyssus gallinae.*
**A. hor′dei,** the barley bug, a mite which burrows under the skin of man.
**A. rhyzoglyp′ticus hyacin′thi,** the onion mite which occurs on decaying onions and produces a dermatitis (onion-mite dermatitis) on persons who handle them.
**A. scabie′i,** *Sarcoptes scabiei.*
**A. si′ro,** a mite that causes vanillism in vanilla pod handlers; called also *Tyrophagus siro* and *Tyroglyphus siro.*
**A. tri′tici,** former name for *Pyemotes ventricosus.*

**ac·a·rus** (ak′ə-rus) pl. *a′cari* [L.] mite.

**acar·y·ote** (ə-kăr′e-ōt) akaryocyte.

**ACAT** acyl CoA:cholesterol acyltransferase; see *sterol O-acyltransferase.*

**acat·a·la·se·mia** (a″kat-ə-la-se′me-ə) acatalasia.

**acat·a·la·sia** (a″kat-ə-la′zhə) a rare autosomal recessive disorder due to virtual absence of catalase activity, observed mainly in Japan and Switzerland. It is usually asymptomatic, but in approximately 50 per cent of the Japanese cases it is characterized by a syndrome of oral ulcerations and gangrene and is called also *Takahara's disease.* See also *hypocatalasia.*

**ac·a·thec·tic** (ak″ə-thek′tik) pertaining to or characterized by acathexia.

**ac·a·thex·ia** (ak″ə-thek′se-ə) [*a-*[1] + Gr. *kathexia* a retention] inability to retain bodily secretions.

**ac·a·thex·is** (ak″ə-thek′sis) [*a* neg. + Gr. *kathexis* a retention] a lack of the emotional charge (cathexis) with which an object or idea would normally be invested; detachment of feelings from thoughts and ideas.

**ac·a·this·ia** (ak″ə-thĭ′zhə) akathisia.

**acau·dal** (a-kaw′dəl) acaudate.

**acau·date** (a-kaw′dāt) [*a-*[1] + *caudate*] lacking a tail.

**acau·li·no·sis** (a-kaw″lĭ-no′sis) scopulariopsosis.

**Acau·li·um** (a-kaw′le-əm) former name for *Scopulariopsis.*

**ACC** American College of Cardiology.

**Acc** accommodation.

**ac·cel·er·ant** (ak-sel′ər-ənt) a catalyst.

**ac·cel·er·a·tion** (ak-sel″ər-a′shən) [L. *acceleratio,* from *ad-* intensification + *celerare* to quicken] [MeSH: Acceleration] 1. a quickening, as of the pulse rate or respiration. 2. in physics, the time rate of change of velocity; symbol *a.*
**a. of gravity,** standard gravity.
**negative a.,** a slowing.
**psychomotor a.,** generalized physical and emotional overactivity in response to internal and external stimuli, such as that seen in the manic phase of bipolar disorder.

**ac·cel·er·a·tor** (ak-sel′ər-a″tər) [L. "hastener"] 1. an agent or apparatus that is used to increase the rate at which an object proceeds or a substance acts, or at which some reaction occurs. 2. any nerve or muscle which hastens the performance of a function. 3. any of a group of chemicals used in the vulcanization of rubber or other polymerizations; they frequently cause dermatitis in workers.
**C3b inactivator a.,** former name for *factor H.*
**linear a.,** an accelerator that propels high-energy particles in a linear beam, using energy from an electromagnetic field; its medical use is in radiotherapy to penetrate tissue and minimize the radiation dose at the surface of the body.
**particle a.,** an apparatus that accelerates charged particles to such high speeds that when they bombard a target they cause nuclear reactions.
**serum prothrombin conversion a. (SPCA),** factor VII; see under *coagulation factors,* at *factor.*
**serum thrombotic a.,** a factor in serum that has procoagulant properties and can induce blood coagulation when infused experimentally into locally arrested flow systems.
**a. uri′nae,** musculus bulbospongiosus.

**ac·cel·er·in** (ak-sel′ər-in) factor VI, formerly considered to be one of the coagulation factors (q.v.).

**ac·cel·er·om·e·ter** (ak-sel'ər-om'ĕ-tər) an instrument for measuring the acceleration (rate of change of velocity) of an object.

**ac·cen·tu·a·tion** (ak-sen"choo-a'shən) [L. *accentus* accent] increased loudness or distinctness; intensification.

**ac·cep·tor** (ak-sep'tər) a substance which unites with another substance; specifically a substance which unites with hydrogen or oxygen in an oxidoreduction reaction and so enables the reaction to proceed. Cf. *donor.*
**hydrogen a.,** in oxidation and reduction occurring anaerobically in body tissue, the substance that is reduced.

**ac·cess** (ak'ses) [L. *accessus,* past participle of *accedere* to approach] a means of approaching something.
**arteriovenous a.,** a tube that begins at an artery and ends at a vein, the usual means by which hemodialysis apparatus is connected to blood vessels; see under *fistula* and *shunt.* Called also *angioaccess, hemoaccess, hemodialysis a., hemodialysis vascular a.,* and *vascular a.*
**hemodialysis a., hemodialysis vascular a.,** arteriovenous a.
**vascular a.,** arteriovenous a.
**venovenous a.,** a tube that begins at a vein and ends at a vein, used in hemodialysis and continuous venovenous hemofiltration.

**ac·ces·si·flex·or** (ak-ses'ə-flek"sər) any accessory flexor muscle.

**ac·ces·so·ri·us** (ak"ses-o're-əs) [L. "supplementary"] accessory; used in naming certain structures thought to serve a supplementary function.

**ac·ces·so·ry** (ak-ses'ə-re) [L. *accessorius*] supplementary or affording aid to another similar and generally more important thing; complementary; concomitant.

**ac·ci·dent** (ak'sĭ-dənt) [MeSH: Accidents] an unforeseen occurrence, especially one of an injurious character; an unexpected complicating occurrence in the regular course of a disease.
**cerebrovascular a.,** stroke syndrome.

**ac·ci·den·tal·ism** (ak"sĭ-den'təl-iz-əm) the medical theory that disease is only an accidental change from normal health and can be avoided or cured by changing external conditions; thus one treats only symptoms and ignores etiology and pathology.

**ac·ci·dent prone** (ak'sĭ-dənt prōn) specially susceptible to accidents owing to psychological factors.

**ACCI** anodal closure clonus.

**ac·cli·ma·ta·tion** (ə-kli"mə-ta'shən) acclimation.

**ac·cli·ma·tion** (ak"lĭ-ma'shən) physiological or psychological adjustment to a new environment. Called also *acclimatation* and *acclimatization.*

**ac·cli·ma·ti·za·tion** (ə-kli"mə-tĭ-za'shən) [MeSH: Acclimatization] acclimation.

**Ac·co·late** (ak'ə-lēt) trademark for a preparation of zafirlukast.

**ac·colé** (ah-ko-la') see *appliqué form,* under *form.*

**ac·com·mo·da·tion** (ə-kom"ə-da'shən) [L. *accommodare* to adjust to] 1. adjustment, especially that of the lens of the eye for various distances (see illustration). Symbol A or a. 2. nerve accommodation.
**absolute a.,** the accommodation of either eye separately.
**binocular a.,** accommodation in both eyes in coordination with convergence.
**excessive a.,** accommodation of the eye which is persistently above the normal.
**histologic a.,** a group of changes in the morphology and function of cells following changed conditions.
**negative a.,** adjustment of the eye for long distances by relaxation of the ciliary muscle.

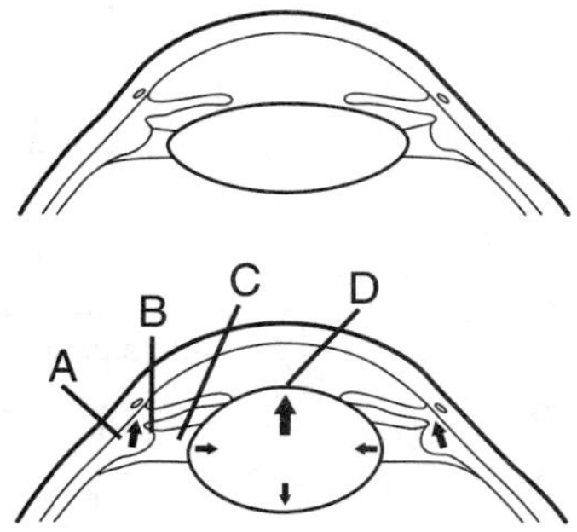


Changes during accommodation: *(A),* contraction of ciliary muscles; *(B),* approximation of ciliary muscles to lens; *(C),* relaxation of suspensory ligament; *(D),* increased curvature of anterior surface of lens.

**nerve a.,** the rise in the threshold during the passage of a constant, direct electric current because of which only the make and break of the current stimulates the nerve.
**positive a.,** adjustment of the eye for short distances by contraction of the ciliary muscle.
**relative a.,** the change in accommodation that is possible with a fixed amount of convergence.
**subnormal a.,** insufficient power of accommodation of the eye.

**ac·com·mo·da·tive** (ə-kom'ə-da"tiv) pertaining to, of the nature of, or affecting accommodation.

**ac·com·mo·dom·e·ter** (ə-kom"ə-dom'ĕ-tər) [*accommodation* + *-meter*] a device for measuring the accommodative capacity of the eye.

**ac·com·plice** (ah-kom-plēs') [Fr.] a bacterium which accompanies the chief infecting agent in a mixed infection and which influences the virulence of the chief organism.

**ac·couche·ment** (ah-ko͞osh-maw') [Fr.] 1. childbirth. 2. delivery.
**a. forcé** (for-sa'), rapid forcible delivery from below by any one of several methods; originally applied to rapid dilatation of the cervix with the hands, followed immediately by version and extraction of the fetus.

**ac·cou·cheur** (ah-koo-shər') [Fr.] obstetrician.

**ac·cou·cheuse** (ah-koo-shooz') [Fr.] midwife.

**ACCP** American College of Chest Physicians.

**ac·cre·men·ti·tion** (ak"rə-men-tish'ən) [L. *ad-* to + *crementum* increase] growth or increase by the addition of similar tissue.

**ac·cre·tio** (ə-kre'she-o) [L.] abnormal adhesion of parts normally separate.
**a. cor'dis, a. pericar'dii,** a form of adhesive pericarditis in which adhesions extend from the pericardium to the pleurae, diaphragm, and chest wall.

**ac·cre·tion** (ə-kre'shən) [L. *ad-* to + *crescere* to grow] 1. growth by addition of material. 2. accumulation. 3. adherence of parts normally separated.

**Ac·cu·pril** (ak'u-pril") trademark for a preparation of quinapril hydrochloride.

**ac·cu·ra·cy** (ak'u-rə-se) the closeness of the expected value to the true value of the measured or estimated quantity; a measure that depends on both precision and bias. Cf. *precision* (def. 1).

**Ac·cu·tane** (ak'u-tān") trademark for a preparation of isotretinoin.

**ACD** acid citrate dextrose.

**ACE** 1. angiotensin-converting enzyme. See *peptidyl-dipeptidase A.* 2. adrenocortical extract.

**ac·e·bu·to·lol** (as"ə-bu'tə-lol) [MeSH: Acebutolol] a cardioselective $\beta_1$-adrenergic blocking agent with intrinsic sympathomimetic activity; its uses are similar to those of propranolol.
**a. hydrochloride** [USP], the hydrochloride salt of acebutolol, used for the treatment of hypertension, anginia pectoris, and arrhythmias; administered orally.

**ac·e·cai·nide hy·dro·chlo·ride** (as"ə-ka'nīd) an antiarrhythmic cardiac depressant.

**acec·li·dine** (ə-sek'lĭ-dēn) a synthetic cholinergic agonist similar to the natural alkaloids arecoline and pilocarpine; used to reduce intraocular pressure in glaucoma.

**ac·e·dap·sone** (as"ə-dap'sōn) [MeSH: Acedapsone] the diacetyl derivative of dapsone, having actions similar to those of the parent compound; used as a leprostatic and antimalarial. Called also *diacetyl diaminodiphenylsulfone (DADDS).*

**Acel-Imune** (a'sel-ĭ-mūn') trademark for a preparation of diphtheria and tetanus toxoids and acellular pertussis vaccine.

**acel·lu·lar** (a-sel'u-lər) not made up of or containing cells.

**ace·lo·mate** (a-se'lə-māt) not having a coelom or body cavity.

**ace·lous** (a-se'ləs) [*a-*[1] + *cel-*[2] + *-ous*] not concave on either surface; said of the vertebral centra of certain animals.

**ace·nes·the·sia** (a-sēn"es-the'zhə) [*a-*[1] + *cenesthesia*] absence of the normal sense of physical existence and well-being and of the regular functioning of the bodily organs.

**ace·no·cou·ma·rin** (ə-se"no-koo'mə-rin) acenocoumarol.

**ace·no·cou·ma·rol** (ə-se"no-koo'mə-rol) [MeSH: Acenocoumarol] One of the synthetic coumarin anticoagulants, occurring as an off-white to light tan powder, having a rapid onset, intermediate duration of action, and little cumulative effect; administered orally.

**acen·tric** (a-sen'trik) [Gr. *akentrikos* not centric] 1. not central; not located in the center. 2. a chromosome lacking a centromere, so that the chromosome will not survive subsequent cell divisions.

**ACEP** American College of Emergency Physicians.

**ace·pha·lia** (a″sĕ-fa′le-ə) [*a-*[1] + *cephal-* + *-ia*] congenital absence of the head.

**Aceph·a·li·na** (a-sef″ə-li′nə) [*a-*[1] + Gr. *kephalē* head] in former systems of classification, a suborder of protozoa (order Eugregarinida) comprising aseptate gregarines, now assigned to the suborders Blastogregarinina and Aseptatina.

**aceph·a·lism** (a-sef′ə-liz-əm) acephalia.

**aceph·a·lo·bra·chia** (a-sef″ə-lo-bra′ke-ə) [*a-*[1] + *cephalo-* + *brachia*] congenital absence of the head and arms.

**aceph·a·lo·bra·chi·us** (a-sef″ə-lo-bra′ke-us) a fetus exhibiting acephalobrachia.

**aceph·a·lo·car·dia** (a-sef″ə-lo-kahr′de-ə) [*a-*[1] + *cephalo-* + *cardia*] congenital absence of the head and heart.

**aceph·a·lo·car·di·us** (a-sef″ə-lo-kahr′de-us) a fetus exhibiting acephalocardia.

**aceph·a·lo·chi·ria** (a-sef″ə-lo-ki′re-ə) [*a-*[1] + *cephalo* + *chir-* + *-ia*] congenital absence of the head and hands.

**aceph·a·lo·chi·rus** (a-sef″ə-lo-ki′rəs) a fetus exhibiting acephalochiria.

**aceph·a·lo·cyst** (a-sef″ə-lo′sist) [*a-*[1] + *cephalo-* + *cyst*] sterile cyst.

**aceph·a·lo·gas·ter** (a-sef″ə-lo-gas′tər) [*a-*[1] + *cephalo-* + *gaster*] a fetus exhibiting acephalogastria.

**aceph·a·lo·gas·tria** (a-sef″ə-lo-gas′tre-ə) congenital absence of the head, thorax, and upper part of the abdomen.

**aceph·a·lo·po·dia** (a-sef″ə-lo-po′de-ə) [*a-*[1] + *cephalo-* + *pod-* + *-ia*] congenital absence of the head and feet.

**aceph·a·lo·po·di·us** (a-sef″ə-lo-po′de-us) a fetus exhibiting acephalopodia.

**aceph·a·lo·rha·chia** (a-sef″ə-lo-ra′ke-ə) [*a-*[1] + *cephalo-* + *rhachi-* + *-ia*] congenital absence of the head and vertebral column.

**aceph·a·lo·sto·mia** (a-sef″ə-lo-sto′me-ə) [*a-*[1] + *cephalo-* + *stom-* + *-ia*] congenital absence of the head, yet with a kind of mouth on the superior aspect.

**aceph·a·los·to·mus** (a-sef″ə-los′tə-məs) a fetus exhibiting acephalostomia.

**aceph·a·lo·tho·ra·cia** (a-sef″ə-lo-tho-ra′se-ə) [*a-*[1] + *cephalo-* + *thorac-* + *-ia*] congenital absence of the head and thorax.

**aceph·a·lo·tho·rus** (a-sef″ə-lo-tho′rəs) a fetus exhibiting acephalothoracia.

**aceph·a·lous** (a-sef′ə-ləs) headless.

**aceph·a·lus** (a-sef′ə-ləs) pl. *aceph′ali* [*a-*[1] + *-cephalus*] a headless fetus.
**a. dibra′chius,** an acephalus with both upper limbs more or less undeveloped.
**a. di′pus,** an acephalus with both lower limbs more or less undeveloped.
**a. monobra′chius,** an acephalus with only one upper limb.
**a. mo′nopus,** an acephalus with only one foot or lower limb.
**a. parace′phalus,** a fetus with a partially formed skull but no brain.
**a. sym′pus,** an acephalus with the two lower limbs fused into one.

**aceph·a·ly** (a-sef′ə-le) acephalia.

**ac·e·pro·ma·zine maleate** (as″ə-pro′mə-zēn) [USP] a tranquilizer used in veterinary medicine to immobilize large animals.

**Acer** (a′sər) the maples, a genus of flowering trees and shrubs of the family Aceraceae. *A. ru′brum* is the red or swamp maple, whose wilted or dry leaves can cause hemolytic anemia in livestock.

**Ace·ra·ria** (as″ə-rar′e-ə) a genus of nematodes. *A. spira′lis* parasitizes the esophagus of fowls.

**acer·in** (ă′ser-in) an extract from the dried fruit of the Norway maple, *Acer plantanoides* L. (Aceraceae); effective against *Escherichia coli* and the vaccinia virus.

**ace·ro·la** (ă-sə-ro′lə) 1. any of various species of trees of the genus *Malpighia,* especially *M. glabra, M. punicifolia,* or *M. urens.* 2. the fruit of these trees, one of the richest natural sources of vitamin C (about 1690 mg. per 100 grams of pitted fruit); it can be used in the diet of individuals allergic to citrus fruits. Called also *Barbados cherry.*

**acer·vu·line** (ə-ser′vu-līn) [L. *acervulus* little heap] aggregated; said of certain glands.

**acer·vu·lus** (ə-ser′vu-lus) pl. *acer′vuli* [L., dim. of *acervus* a heap] in Fungi Imperfecti, a conidioma with a saucer-shaped surface where conidia form underneath a dome of tissue that ruptures at maturity to release the conidia.

**ac·e·tab·u·la** (as″ə-tab′u-lə) plural of *acetabulum.*

**ac·e·tab·u·lar** (as″ə-tab′u-lər) pertaining to the acetabulum.

**Ace·ta·bu·la·ria** (as″ə-tab″u-lar′e-ə) [MeSH: Acetabularia] a genus of large single-celled green algae having a foot, a stalk, and a cap. *A. mediterra′nea* and *A. crenula′ta* have been used in genetic experiments.

**ac·e·tab·u·lec·to·my** (as″ə-tab″u-lek′tə-me) [*acetabulum* + *-ectomy*] excision of the acetabulum.

**ac·e·tab·u·lo·plas·ty** (as″ə-tab′u-lo-plas″te) [*acetabulum* + *-plasty*] plastic reconstruction of the acetabulum.

**ac·e·tab·u·lum** (as″ə-tab′u-ləm) pl. *acetab′ula* [L. "vinegar-cruet," from *acetum* vinegar] [TA] [MeSH: Acetabulum] the large cup-shaped cavity on the lateral surface of the os coxae in which the head of the femur articulates; called also *acetabular bone, cotyloid cavity,* and *os acetabuli.*
**sunken a.,** Otto pelvis.

**ac·e·tal** (as′ə-təl) 1. any of a class of organic compounds of the formula $RCH(OR')_2$, where R and R′ are organic radicals, formed by combination of an aldehyde molecule with two alcohol molecules. 2. $CH_3CH(OC_2H_5)_2$, a colorless volatile liquid used as a solvent and in cosmetics.

**ac·et·al·de·hyde** (as″ə-tal′də-hīd″) [MeSH: Acetaldehyde] a colorless flammable liquid with a pungent odor, used in the manufacture of acetic acid, perfumes, and flavors. It is also an intermediate in the metabolism of alcohol. If ingested, it may cause irritation of mucous membranes, lacrimation, photophobia, conjunctivitis, corneal injury, rhinitis, anosmia, bronchitis, pneumonia, pleurisy, headache, and unconsciousness. Called also *acetic aldehyde, ethanal,* and *ethylaldehyde.*

**ac·et·al·de·hyde de·hy·dro·gen·ase** (as″ə-tal′də-hid de-hi′dro-jen-ās) aldehyde dehydrogenase ($NAD^+$).

**acet·am·ide** (ə-set′ə-mīd) colorless crystals used in organic synthesis and as a general solvent when melted.

**ac·et·am·i·dine** (as″ə-tam′ĭdēn) the imine of acetamide, used in the synthesis of imidazoles and pyrimidines; it is irritating to the skin and mucous membranes.

**ace·ta·min·o·phen** (ə-se″tə-min′o-fen) [USP] [MeSH: Acetaminophen] the amide of acetic acid and *p*-aminophenol; a nonprescription drug having analgesic and antipyretic effects similar to aspirin but only weak anti-inflammatory effects. Administered orally and rectally. Called also *paracetamol.*

**ac·et·an·i·lid** (as″ət-an′ĭ-lid) [*acet-* + *anilid*] the earliest of the *p*-aminophenol derivatives (acetaminophen, phenacetin), produced by combining glacial acetic acid with aniline; it has analgesic and antipyretic actions but has been replaced by other compounds because of its toxicity.

**ac·et·ar·sol** (as″ə-tahr′sol) acetarsone.

**ac·et·ar·sone** (as″ə-tahr′sōn) a pentavalent arsenical used orally in the treatment of intestinal amebiasis, orally and topically in necrotizing ulcerative gingivitis, and topically in trichomonas vaginitis. Also used as an anthelmintic in veterinary medicine. Called also *acetphenarsine.*

**ace·tas** (ə-se′təs) [L.] acetate.

**ac·e·tate** (as′ə-tāt) a salt or ester or the conjugate base of acetic acid.
**cellulose a.,** an acetylated cellulose used as a hemodialyzer membrane; it has a greater permeability and higher ultrafiltration rate than cuprophane.

**ac·e·tate–CoA li·gase** (as′ĕ-tāt ko-a′ li′gās) [EC 6.2.1.1] an en-

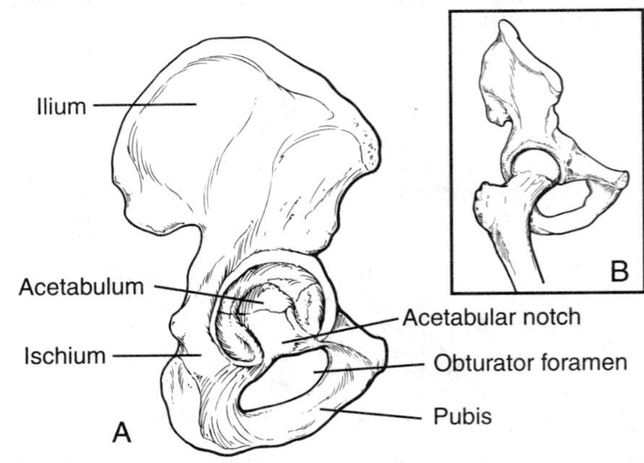


Acetabulum, showing the cup-shaped cavity *(A),* and its articulation with the femur *(B).*

zyme of the ligase class that catalyzes the formation of acetyl coenzyme A from acetate and coenzyme A, as well as analogous reactions linking propionic or acrylic acid to coenzyme A. The enzyme occurs in the mitochondrial membrane and cytosol. Called also *acetyl CoA synthetase.*

**ac·et·a·zol·a·mide** (as″et-ə-zol′ə-mīd) [USP] [MeSH: Acetazolamide] a carbonic anhydrase inhibitor with a wide variety of uses, including adjunctive treatment of glaucoma and epilepsy, treatment of familial periodic paralysis, prophylaxis and treatment of acute mountain sickness, and as a urinary alkalizer in the prophylaxis and treatment of uric acid renal calculi; administered orally, intravenously, and intramuscularly.

**ace·te·nyl** (ə-se′tĕ-nil) ethynyl.

**Ace·test** (as′ə-test) trademark for reagent tablets containing sodium nitroprusside, aminoacetic acid, disodium phosphate, and lactose. A drop of urine is placed on a tablet on a sheet of white paper; if significant quantities of acetone are present the tablet changes from a purple tint (1+), to lavender (2+), to moderate purple (3+), or deep purple (4+).

**ace·tic** (ə-se′tik, ə-set′ik) pertaining to vinegar or its acid; sour.

**ace·tic ac·id** (ə-se′tik) [MeSH: Acetic Acid] the two-carbon carboxylic acid, $CH_3COOH$, which is the characteristic component of vinegar, and, mostly in the form of acetylcoenzyme A, an important biochemical intermediate. In pharmacy, it is used as a solvent and menstruum and as a pharmaceutic necessity in the preparation of aluminum subacetate topical solution; the official preparation [NF] contains 36 to 37 per cent by weight of $C_2H_4O_2$. Systematic name: *ethanoic acid.*
**glacial a. a.,** anhydrous acetic acid, used as a solvent, as a caustic and vesicant, and as a pharmaceutic necessity; the official preparation [USP] contains 99.5–100.5 per cent acetic acid by weight.

**acet·i·fy** (ə-sēt′ĭ-fi, ə-set′ĭ-fi) to turn into acetic acid or vinegar.

**ac·e·tim·e·ter** (as″ə-tim′ə-tər) [*acet-* + *-meter*] an apparatus for determining the amount of acetic acid present in a solution.

**ac·e·tin** (as′ə-tin) a glyceryl acetate, usually containing one acetyl group but sometimes two or three; used in tanning and as a food additive and a solvent for dyes.

**Ace·ti·vib·rio** (ə-se″tĭ-vib′re-ə) [*aceto-* + *vibrio*] a genus of anaerobic, gram-negative, straight or slightly curved rod-shaped bacteria of the family Bacteroidaceae, made up of cells that are motile with flagella and produce acetic acid as the principal acid from carbohydrates. The organisms are found in the intestines of pigs. The type species is *A. cellulolyticus.*

**acet(o)-** a prefix denoting the presence of the acetyl radical or of acetic acid molecules.

**ac·e·to·ac·e·tate** (ə-se″to-as′ə-tāt) a salt or anion of acetoacetic acid.

**ace·to·ace·tic ac·id** (ə-se″to-ə-se′tik) one of the ketone bodies (q.v.) produced in the liver and occurring in excess in the urine and blood in ketosis. Called also *diacetic* or *β-ketobutyric acid.*

**ac·e·to·ac·e·tyl CoA** (as″ə-to-as′ə-til, ə-se′to-as-ə-tēl″) acetoacetyl coenzyme A.

**ac·e·to·ac·e·tyl-CoA re·duc·tase** (as″ə-to-as′ə-təl, ə-se′to-as-ə-tēl″ ko-a′ re-duk-tās) [EC 1.1.1.36] an enzyme of the oxidoreductase class that catalyzes the reduction of 3-ketoacyl coenzyme A to 3-hydroxybutyryl coenzyme A, using NADPH as an electron donor.

**ac·e·to·ac·e·tyl CoA thi·o·lase** (as″ə-to-as′ə-təl, a-se′to-as-ə-tēl″ ko-a′ thi′o-lās) acetyl-CoA *C*-acetyltransferase.

**ac·e·to·ac·e·tyl co·en·zyme A** (as″ə-to-as′ə-təl, a-se′to-as-ə-tēl″ ko-en′zīm) a thioester of acetoacetic acid and coenzyme A. It is an important metabolic intermediate in the oxidation of fatty acids, as a fuel for the citric acid cycle in brain and nervous tissue, and as a precursor of cholesterol. Written also *acetoacetyl CoA.*

**Ace·to·bac·ter** (ə-se″to-bak′tər) [*aceto-* + *-bacter*] [MeSH: Acetobacter] a genus of gram-negative, aerobic, rod-shaped bacteria of the family Acetobacteraceae made up of nonsporogenous organisms that produce acetic acid from ethanol. They are found in fruits, vegetables, souring juices, and alcoholic beverages. The type species is *A. ace′ti.*

**Ace·to·bac·te·ra·ceae** (ə-se″to-bak-tĕ-ra′se-e) [MeSH: Acetobacteraceae] a family of gram-negative, aerobic, ellipsoidal to rod-shaped bacteria that form acetic acid. It includes the genera *Acetobacter* and *Gluconobacter.*

**ace·to·form** (ə-se′to-form) methenamine.

**ac·e·to·hex·a·mide** (as″ə-to-hek′sə-mīd) [USP] [MeSH: Acetohexamide] a sulfonylurea compound used as a hypoglycemic in the treatment of type 2 diabetes mellitus; administered orally.

**ac·e·to·hy·drox·am·ic ac·id** (as″ə-to-hi″droks-am′ik) [USP] an inhibitor of bacterial urease used in the prophylaxis and treatment of struvite renal calculi whose formation is favored by urease-producing bacteria and as an adjunct in the treatment of urinary tract infections caused by urease-producing bacteria; administered orally.

**acet·o·in** (ə-set′o-in) [MeSH: Acetoin] a ketone product formed in the fermentation of glucose by certain bacteria, especially species of Enterobacteriaceae, and detected by the Voges-Proskauer test.

**ac·e·tol·y·sis** (as″-ə-tol′ĭ-sis) the decomposition of an organic compound using acetic acid or acetic anhydride.

**ac·e·tom·e·ter** (as″ə-tom′ə-tər) acetimeter.

**ac·e·to·mor·phine** (as″ə-to-mor′fēn) diacetylmorphine.

**ac·e·to·naph·thone** (as″ə-to-naf′thōn) an acetyl derivative of naphthalene occurring in two isomeric forms. The 2-acetonaphthone isomer is a mosquito repellent; derivatives are used as bactericides and as an antitubercular agent.

**ac·e·to·na·tion** (as″ə-to-na′shən) combination with acetone.

**ac·e·tone** (as′ə-tōn) [MeSH: Acetone] dimethylketone, a flammable colorless, volatile liquid with a pleasant ethereal odor; it is a commonly used solvent and is one of the ketone bodies (q.v.) produced in ketoacidosis. In pharmacy, it is used as a solvent and, in concentrations above 80 per cent, as an antiseptic; the official preparation [NF] contains at least 99 per cent of acetone calculated on an anhydrous basis.

**ac·e·ton·emia** (as″ə-to-ne′me-ə) excessive acetone or ketone bodies in the blood; see *ketonemia.*

**ac·e·to·ni·trile** (as″ə-to-ni′trīl) a colorless liquid with an ethereal odor used as an extractant, solvent, and chemical intermediate; when it is ingested or inhaled one of its metabolic products is inorganic cyanide.

**ac·e·to·num** (as″ə-to′nəm) [L.] acetone.

**ac·e·to·nu·mer·a·tor** (as″ə-to-noo′mər-a″tor) an instrument for estimating the amount of acetone in the urine.

**ac·e·ton·uria** (as″ə-to-nu′re-ə) ketonuria.

**ac·e·to·or·ce·in** (as″ə-to-or′sēn) orcein dissolved in acetic acid, used in making squash preparations of polytene chromosomes.

**ac·e·to·phen·a·zine mal·e·ate** (as″ə-to-fen′ə-zēn) a phenothiazine compound used as an antipsychotic; administered orally.

**ac·e·to·sol·uble** (as″ə-to-sol′u-bəl) soluble in acetic acid.

**ac·e·to·sul·fone so·di·um** (as″ə-to-sul′fōn) an antibacterial derivative of dapsone having actions similar to those of the parent compound; used as leprostatic in lepromatous and tuberculoid leprosy and as a dermatitis herpetiformis suppressant, administered orally.

**ace·tous** (as′ə-təs) pertaining to, producing, or resembling acetic acid.

**ace·to·white** (ə-se′to-hwīt) [*aceto-* + *white*] having a white coloration due to acetowhitening.

**ace·to·whit·en·ing** (ə-se″to-hwi′tən-ing) the process by which certain subclinical lesions of the skin or mucous membranes, especially warts caused by human papillomavirus, change temporarily to a white color when acetic acid is applied topically.

**acet·phe·nar·sine** (as″ət-fen-ahr′sēn) acetarsone.

**acet·py·ro·gall** (as″ət-pi′ro-gəl) used as a topical caustic and keratolytic.

**ac·e·tri·zo·ate** (as″ə-tri-zo′āt) a water-soluble, iodinated radiographic contrast medium, used as *sodium acetrizoate* in hysterosalpingography.

**ace·tum** (ə-se′təm) pl. *ace′ta* [L.] vinegar.

**ac·e·tu·rate** (ə-set′u-rāt) USAN contraction for *N*-acetylglycinate.

**ac·e·tyl** (as′ə-təl, as′ə-tēl″) [*acet-* + *-yl*] the monovalent radical, $CH_3CO$—.
**a. chloride,** a colorless, corrosive, toxic, flammable liquid used as a reagent for forming acetate esters of alcohols.
**a. peroxide,** a highly irritating, flammable, explosive compound used as an initiator and catalyst for resins.
**a. sulfisoxazole,** used as an antimicrobial.

**ac·e·tyl·an·drom·e·dol** (as″ə-təl-, as″ə-tēl-an-drom′ə-dol) andromedotoxin.

**acet·y·lase** (ə-set′ə-lās) an enzyme that catalyzes the addition or removal of an acetyl group; the most common are acetyltransferases.

**acet·y·la·tion** (ə-set″ə-la′shən) [MeSH: Acetylation] the introduction of an acetyl group into the molecule of an organic compound.

**acet·y·la·tor** (ə-set″ə-la′tər) an organism capable of metabolic acetylation; in man, acetylator status (fast or slow) is determined by the rate of acetylation of sulfamethazine.

**ac·e·tyl·cho·line** (as″ə-təl-, as″ə-tēl-ko′lēn) [MeSH: Acetylcholine] a reversible acetic acid ester of choline; it is a cholinergic agonist and serves as a neurotransmitter at the myoneural junctions of striated muscles, at autonomic effector cells innervated by parasympathetic nerves, at the preganglionic synapses of the sympathetic and parasympathetic nervous systems, and at various sites in the central nervous system. ACh has few therapeutic applications owing to its diffuse action and rapid hydrolysis by acetylcholinesterase (AChE); synthetic derivatives are used for more specific, prolonged action. ACh is used as a vasodilator in pharmacoangiography, administered by intra-arterial infusion.
**a. chloride** [USP], a miotic administered by instillation into the anterior chamber of the eye during intraocular surgical procedures.

**ac·e·tyl·cho·lin·es·ter·ase** (as″ə-təl-, as″ə-tēl-ko″lĭ-nes′tə-rās) [EC 3.1.1.7] [MeSH: Acetylcholinesterase] an enzyme of the hydrolase class that catalyzes the cleavage of acetylcholine to choline and acetate; it is found in the central nervous system, particularly in gray matter of nerve tissue, in red blood cells, and in motor endplates of skeletal muscle. Called also *choline esterase I* and *true cholinesterase.* Abbreviated AChE. Cf. *cholinesterase.*

**ac·e·tyl CoA** (as′ə-təl, as″ə-tēl′) acetyl coenzyme A.

**ac·e·tyl-CoA *C*-ac·e·tyl·trans·fer·ase** (as″ə-təl-, as″ə-tēl-ko-a′ as″ə-təl-, as″ə-tēl-trans″fər-ās) [EC 2.3.1.9] an enzyme of the transferase class that catalyzes the synthesis of acetoacetyl coenzyme A from two molecules of acetyl coenzyme A; it can also act as a thiolase, catalyzing the reverse reaction and generating two-carbon units from the four-carbon product of fatty acid oxidation. A mitochondrial form is involved in ketone body synthesis while a cytoplasmic form is involved in the synthesis of cholesterol and other isoprenoids.

**ac·e·tyl-CoA *C*-acyl·trans·fer·ase** (as″ə-təl-, as″ə-tēl-ko-a′ a″səl-trans′fər-ās) [EC 2.3.1.16] any of several enzymes of the transferase class that catalyze the conversion of a 3-ketoacyl CoA to acetyl coenzyme A and an acyl coenzyme A with its chain length shortened by two carbons; the reaction converts fatty acid chains to two-carbon units via beta oxidation. See also individual enzymes, e.g., *α-methylacetoacetyl CoA thiolase.* Called also *β-ketothiolase.*

**ac·e·tyl-CoA car·box·yl·ase** (as″ə-təl-, as″ə-tēl-ko-a′ kahr-bok′sə-lās) [EC 6.4.1.2] [MeSH: Acetyl-CoA Carboxylase] a biotin-containing enzyme of the ligase class that catalyzes the carboxylation of acetyl coenzyme A to form malonyl coenzyme A. The reaction is the key rate-controlling step in the synthesis of fatty acids from acetyl groups, and the enzyme requires citrate or isocitrate for activity.

**ac·e·tyl- CoA:*α*-glu·cos·am·i·nide- *N*-ac·e·tyl·trans·fer·ase** (as′ə-təl, as′ə-tēl ko-a′gloo″kōs-am′ĭ-nīd as″ə-təl-, as″ə-tēl-trans′fər-ās) heparan-*α*-glucosaminide *N*-acetyltransferase.

**ac·e·tyl CoA syn·the·tase** (as′ə-təl, as′ə-tēl ko-a′ sin′thə-tās) acetate–CoA ligase.

**ac·e·tyl co·en·zyme A** (as″ĕ-təl, as-ĕ-tēl″ ko-en′zīm a) [MeSH: Acetyl Coenzyme A] acetyl CoA, a thioester of coenzyme A and acetic acid, the acetyl groups being derived from carbohydrates, fatty acids, and amino acids. Acetyl CoA can enter the tricarboxylic acid cycle, can be used to acetylate numerous compounds, and can be a precursor of steroids and other isoprenoid compounds. Excess acetyl coenzyme A may be converted to fats for storage or may appear as ketone bodies.

**ac·e·tyl·cys·te·ine** (as″ə-təl-, as″ə-tēl-sis′te-ēn) [USP] [MeSH: Acetylcysteine] the *N*-acetyl derivative of L-cysteine used as a mucolytic agent for adjunct therapy in bronchopulmonary disorders to reduce the viscosity of mucus and facilitate its removal, administered by instillation or nebulization; as an antidote for acetaminophen poisoning, administered orally; and to dissolve cystine calculi in cystinuria by pelvicaliceal irrigation.

**ac·e·tyl·dig·i·tox·in** (as″ə-təl-, as″ə-tēl-dij′ĭ-tok″sin) a derivative of digitoxin composed of the aglycone digitoxigenin and three molecules of digitoxose, to one of which an acetyl group is attached, having the same actions and uses as digitalis; administered orally.

**ac·e·tyl·di·hy·dro·lipo·am·ide** (as″ə-təl-, as″ə-tēl″di-hi″dro-lĭ-po-am′īd) acetyl bound to lipoamide, an intermediate in the reaction catalyzed by the pyruvate dehydrogenase complex (q.v.).

**acet·y·lene** (ə-set′ə-lēn) [MeSH: Acetylene] a colorless, volatile, explosive gas; it is the simplest of a class of unsaturated (triple-bonded) hydrocarbons, the alkynes.

**ac·et·yl·eu·ge·nol** (as″ə-təl-u′jə-nol) an essential oil that is a minor constituent of oil of cloves.

***N*-ac·e·tyl·ga·lac·to·sa·mine** (as″ə-təl-, as″ə-tēl-gal″ak-tōs′ə-mēn) the acetyl derivative of galactosamine; it is a component of structural glycosaminoglycans, of glycolipids, and of membrane glycoproteins. Abbreviated GalNAc.

***N*-ac·e·tyl·ga·lac·to·sa·mine-4-sul·fa·tase** (as″ə-təl-, as″ə-tēl″ gal-ak-tōs′ə-mēn sul′fə-tās) [EC 3.1.6.12] a lysosomal enzyme of the hydrolase class that catalyzes the cleavage of sulfate groups from the 4 position of *N*-acetylgalactosamine residues. The reaction is important in the degradation of dermatan sulfate; deficiency of the enzyme, an autosomal recessive trait, results in Maroteaux-Lamy syndrome (mucopolysaccharidosis VI). Called also *arylsulfatase B.*

***N*-ac·e·tyl·ga·lac·to·sa·mine-6-sul·fa·tase** (as″ə-təl-, as″ə-tēl-gal″ak-tōs′ə-mēn sul′fə-tās) [EC 3.1.6.4] a lysosomal enzyme of the hydrolase class that catalyzes the cleavage of the sulfate group from the 6 position of sulfated galactose residues in keratan sulfate or of sulfated *N*-acetylgalactosamine residues in chondroitin 6-sulfate as a step in the degradation of these glycosaminoglycans. Deficiency of the enzyme, an autosomal recessive trait, results in Morquio's syndrome, type A.

***α*-*N*-ac·e·tyl·gal·ac·to·sa·min·i·dase** (as″ə-təl-, as″ə-tēl-gal-ak-tōs″ə-min′ĭ-dās) [EC 3.2.1.49] a lysosomal hexosaminidase specifically catalyzing the cleavage of terminal, *α*-linked, nonreducing *N*-acetylgalactosamine residues from glycoconjugates. Deficiency of the enzyme, an autosomal recessive trait, is a cause of infantile neuroaxonal dystrophy. Called also *α-galactosidase B.*

***β*-*N*-ac·e·tyl·gal·ac·to·sa·min·i·dase** (as″ə-təl-, as″ə-tēl-gal-ak-tōs″ə-min′ĭ-dās) [EC 3.2.1.53] a lysosomal hexosaminidase specifically catalyzing the cleavage of terminal, *β*-linked, nonreducing *N*-acetylgalactosamine residues from gangliosides or other glycosides.

***N*-ac·e·tyl·glu·co·sa·mine** (as″ə-təl-, as″ə-tēl-gloo-kōs′ə-mēn) the acetyl derivative of glucosamine; it is a component of structural glycosaminoglycans, of glycolipids, and of membrane glycoproteins. Abbreviated GlcNAc.

***N*-ac·e·tyl·glu·co·sa·mine-6-sul·fa·tase** (as″ə-təl-, as″ə-tēl-gloo-kōs′ə-mēn sul′fə-tās) [EC 3.1.6.14] a lysosomal enzyme that catalyzes the cleavage of sulfate groups from the 6 position of *N*-acetylglucosamine residues in heparan sulfate and keratan sulfate, a step in the degradation of these glycosaminoglycans. Deficiency of the enzyme, an autosomal recessive trait, results in Sanfilippo's syndrome, type D.

***α*-*N*-ac·e·tyl·glu·co·sa·min·i·dase** (as″ə-təl-, as″ə-tēl-gloo-kōs″ə-min′ĭ-dās) [EC 3.2.1.50] a lysosomal hexosaminidase specifically catalyzing the cleavage of terminal, *α*-linked, nonreducing *N*-acetylglucosamine residues from glycosides; the reaction is necessary for the degradation of heparan sulfate. Deficiency of the enzyme, an autosomal recessive trait, results in Sanfilippo's syndrome, type B.

***β*-D-ac·e·tyl·glu·co·sa·min·i·dase** (as′ə-təl-, as′ə-tēl-gloo-kōs″ə-min′ĭ-dās) [Formerly EC 3.2.1.30] a lysosomal hexosaminidase now recognized as the same enzyme as *β-N*-acetylhexosaminidase (q.v.).

***N*⁴-*β*-*N*-ac·e·tyl·glu·co·sa·min·yl-L-as·par·a·gin·ase** (as″ə-təl-, as″ə-tēl-gloo-kōs″ə-min′əl-as-par″ə-jin′ās) [EC 3.5.1.26] EC nomenclature for *aspartylglucosaminidase.*

***β*-*N*-ac·e·tyl·glu·cos·amin·yl·gly·co·pep·tide *β*-1,4-ga·lac·to·syl·trans·fer·ase** (as″ə-tēl″gloo-kōs″ə-min″əl-gli″ko-pep′tīd gal″ak-tōs″əl-trans′fər-ās) [EC 2.4.1.38] EC nomenclature for *glycoprotein 4-β-galactosyltransferase.*

***N*-ac·e·tyl·glu·cos·am·i·nyl·phos·pho·trans·fer·ase** (as″ə-təl-, as″ə-tēl-gloo-kos″ə-min″əl-fos″fo-trans′fər-ās) UDP-*N*-acetylglucosamine–lysosomal-enzyme *N*-acetylglucosaminephosphotransferase.

***N*-ac·e·tyl·glu·ta·mate** (as″ə-təl-, as″ə-tēl-gloo′tə-māt) *N*-acetylglutamic acid in dissociated form.

***N*-ac·e·tyl·glu·ta·mate syn·the·tase** (as″ə-təl-, as″ə-tēl-gloo′tə-māt sin′thə-tās) amino-acid *N*-acetyltransferase.

***N*-ac·e·tyl·glu·tam·ic ac·id** (as″ə-təl-, as″ə-tēl-gloo-tam′ik) glutamic acid acetylated at its N-terminus, a necessary cofactor in the synthesis of carbamoyl phosphate catalyzed by carbamoyl-phosphate synthase (ammonia). The molecule is an allosteric activator of this enzyme and hence a positive regulator of ureagenesis.

***N*-ac·e·tyl·hex·os·amine** (as″ə-təl-, as″ə-tēl-hek-sōs′ə-mēn) a hexosamine acetylated at its amino group, such as *N*-acetylglucosamine or *N*-acetylgalactosamine.

***β*-*N*-ac·e·tyl·hex·os·amin·i·dase** (as″ə-təl-, as″ə-tēl-hek-sōs″ə-min′ĭ-dās) [EC 3.2.1.52] a lysosomal enzyme of the hydrolase class that catalyzes the cleavage of *N*-acetylhexosamine residues from gangliosides or other glycosides; it is necessary for the degradation of keratan sulfate and also ganglioside $GM_2$ and related compounds. The enzyme comprises two polypeptide chains, $\alpha$ and $\beta$, which are arranged into three isozymes: A ($\alpha\beta$), B ($\beta\beta$), and S ($\alpha\alpha$). Lack of isozyme A activity, due to a defect in the $\alpha$ chain, causes Tay-Sachs disease and other forms of $GM_2$ gangliosidosis, variant B; lack of isozymes A and B, due to a defect in the $\beta$ chain, causes Sandhoff's disease. The enzyme is usually called *hexosaminidase* and has been shown to be identical to *β-D-acetylglucosaminidase.*

**acet·y·li·za·tion** (ə-set″-əl-ĭ-za′shən) acetylation.

***N*-ac·e·tyl·man·no·sa·mine** (as″ə-təl-, as″ə-tēl-mə-nōs′ə-mēn) mannosamine acetylated at its amino group, an intermediate in the biosynthesis and degradation of sialic acids and sialoglycoconjugates.

**N-ac·e·tyl·mu·ram·ate** (as″ə-təl-, as″ə-tēl-mūr′ə-māt) a salt, ester, or anionic form of *N*-acetylmuramic acid.

**N-ac·e·tyl·mu·ram·ic ac·id** (as″ə-təl-, as″ə-tēl-mu-ram′ik) a polysaccharide constituent of bacterial cell walls; it is composed of *N*-acetylglucosamine coupled to lactic acid.

**N-ac·e·tyl·neu·ra·min·ate** (as″ə-təl-, as″ə-tēl-noo-ram′ĭ-nāt) a salt, ester, or anionic form of *N*-acetylneuraminic acid.

**N-ac·e·tyl·neu·ram·i·nate ly·ase** (as″ə-təl-, as″ə-tēl-noo-ram′ĭ-nāt li′ās) [EC 4.1.3.3] a cytoplasmic enzyme of the lyase class that catalyzes the cleavage of a pyruvate residue from *N*-acetylneuraminate to form *N*-acetylmannosamine as a step in the degradation of sialic acids and sialoglycoconjugates.

**N-ac·e·tyl·neu·ra·min·ic ac·id** (as″ə-təl-, as″ə-tēl-noor″ə-min′ik) the acetyl derivative of the amino sugar neuraminic acid; it occurs in many glycoproteins, glycolipids, and polysaccharides.

**ac·e·tyl·sal·i·cyl·ic ac·id** (ə-se′til-sal″ə-sil′ik) chemical name for aspirin. Abbreviated ASA.

**ac·e·tyl·stro·phan·thi·din** (as″ə-təl-, as″ə-tēl-stro-fan′thə-din) a synthetic fast-acting digitalis-like preparation.

**ac·e·tyl·sul·fa·di·a·zine** (as″ə-təl-, as″ə-tēl-sul″fə-di′ə-sēn) the form in which sulfadiazine is excreted in the urine, often occurring in dark green crystalline spheres.

**ac·e·tyl·sul·fa·guan·i·dine** (as″-ə-təl-, as″ə-tēl-sul″fə-gwan′ə-dēn) the form in which sulfaguanidine is excreted in the urine, often occurring in thin oblong crystalline plates.

**ac·e·tyl·sul·fa·thi·a·zole** (as″ə-təl-, as″ə-tēl-sul″fə-thi′ə-zōl) the form in which sulfathiazole is excreted in the urine, often occurring in the form of sheaves-of-wheat crystals.

**ac·e·tyl·trans·fer·ase** (as″ĕ-təl-, as-ə-tēl-trans′fər-ās) an acyltransferase specifically catalyzing the transfer of an acetyl group, often acetyl coenzyme A, to another compound. Those forming esters or amides are also called *acetylases.*

**ac·e·tyl·tri·bu·tyl cit·rate** (as″ĕ-təl-, as-ə-tēl-tri-bu′til) [NF] a compound derived by the esterification and acetylation of citric acid, used as a plasticizer in pharmaceutical preparations.

**ac·e·tyl·tri·eth·yl cit·rate** (as″ĕ-təl-, as-ə-tēl-tri-eth′il) [NF] a compound derived by the esterification and acetylation of citric acid, used as a plasticizer in pharmaceutical preparations.

**ACG** American College of Gastroenterology; angiocardiography; apexcardiogram.

**AcG** [MeSH: Factor V] accelerator globulin (factor V; see under *coagulation factors,* at *factor*).

**ACh** acetylcholine.

**ACHA** American College of Hospital Administrators.

**ach·a·la·sia** (ak″ə-la′zhə) [*a-*[1] + *chalasia*] 1. failure to relax of the smooth muscle fibers of the gastrointestinal tract at any point of junction of one part with another. 2. specifically, failure of the esophagogastric sphincter to relax with swallowing, due to degeneration of ganglion cells in the wall of the organ. The thoracic esophagus also loses its normal peristaltic activity and becomes dilated (megaesophagus). Called also *cardiospasm.*
**cricopharyngeal a.,** achalasia of the cricopharyngeal muscle; see *Asherson's syndrome,* under *syndrome.*
**pelvirectal a.,** congenital megacolon.
**sphincteral a.,** failure of any sphincter of a tubular organ to relax in response to a normal physiological stimulus.

**Achard's syndrome** (ah-shahrz′) [Émile Charles *Achard,* French physician, 1860–1944] see under *syndrome.*

**Achard-Thiers syndrome** (ah-shahr′ tērz) [É. C. *Achard;* Joseph *Thiers,* French physician, born 1885] see under *syndrome.*

**Ach·a·ti·na** (ak″ə-ti′nə) a genus of large land snails of the family Achatinidae, order Stylommatophora, originally native to Africa. *A. fuli′ca* serves as an intermediate host of the lungworm *Angiostrongylus cantonensis.*

**Acha·tin·i·dae** (ak″ə-tin′ĭ-de) a family of African land snails of the suborder Stylommatophora, order Pulmonata; it includes the genus *Achatina.*

**AChE** acetylcholinesterase.

**ache** (āk) 1. to suffer a continuous pain. 2. a continuous, fixed pain, as distinguished from twinges.

**achei·lia** (ə-ki′-le-ə) [*a-*[1] + *cheil-* + *-ia*] congenital absence of one or both lips.

**achei·lous** (ə-ki′lus) lacking lips; exhibiting acheilia.

**achei·ria** (ə-ki′re-ə) [*a-*[1] + *cheir-* + *-ia*] 1. congenital absence of one or both hands. 2. lack of feeling of the hands or a feeling of their absence, sometimes occurring in conversion disorder.

**achei·ro·po·dia** (ə-ki″ro-po′de-ə) [*a-*[1] + *cheir-* + *pod-* + *-ia*] congenital absence of hands and feet.

**achei·rus** (ə-ki′rəs) [L.] an individual exhibiting acheiria.

**Achil·les' bur·sa, jerk (reflex), tendon** (ə-kil′ēz) [Gr. *Achilleus* Greek hero, whose mother held him by the heel to dip him in the Styx] see *bursa tendinis calcanei, triceps surae jerk,* under *jerk,* and *tendo calcaneus.*

**Ach·il·li·ni** (ah″kə-le′ne) Alessandro (1463–1512). A celebrated Bolognese physician and philosopher who wrote on anatomy.

**achil·lo·bur·si·tis** (ə-kil″o-bər-si′tis) [*Achilles* + *bursitis*] inflammation and thickening of the bursae about the Achilles tendon, especially of the bursa in front of it; called also *achillodynia.*

**achil·lo·dy·nia** (ak″ə-lo-din′e-ə) [*Achilles* (tendon) + Gr. *odynē* pain + *-ia*] 1. pain in the Achilles tendon. 2. achillobursitis.

**ach·il·lor·rha·phy** (ak″ə-lor′ə-fe) [*Achilles* (tendon) + Gr. *rhaphē* suture] suture of the Achilles tendon.

**achil·lo·te·not·o·my** (ə-kil″o-tə-not′ə-me) [*Achilles* + Gr. *tenōn* tendon + *tomē* cut] surgical division of the Achilles tendon.
**plastic a.,** elongation of the Achilles tendon by plastic operation.

**achil·lot·o·my** (ak″ə-lot′ə-me) achillotenotomy.

**achi·ria** (ə-ki′re-ə) 1. acheiria. 2. inability to tell which side of the body has been touched; cf. *dyschiria.*

**achi·rus** (ə-ki′rəs) acheirus.

**achlor·hy·dria** (a″klor-hi′dre-ə) [*a-*[1] + *chlorhydria*] [MeSH: Achlorhydria] absence of hydrochloric acid from maximally stimulated gastric secretions; a result of gastric mucosal atrophy. Called also *gastric anacidity.*

**achlor·hy·dric** (a″klor-hi′drik) characterized by achlorhydria.

**Ach·lya** (ak′le-ə) a genus of funguslike organisms of the order Saprolegniales, which form molds on certain fish and insects.

**Acho·le·plas·ma** (a″ko-le-plaz′mə) [*a-*[1] + *chole-* + *plasma*] [MeSH: Acholeplasma] a genus of bacteria of the family Acholeplasmataceae, made up of spherical cells bounded by a triple-layered membrane but lacking a cell wall, and not requiring serum or cholesterol for growth.
**A. granula′rum,** a species found in the nasal cavities of swine and reported to have been isolated from the synovial fluid of arthritic pigs. Called also *Mycoplasma granularum.*
**A. laidlaw′ii,** a species isolated from various human clinical specimens, from the body cavities of cattle, swine, and birds, and from soils. Called also *Mycoplasma laidlawii.*

**Acho·le·plas·ma·ta·ceae** (a-ko″le-plaz″mə-ta′se-e) [MeSH: Acholeplasmataceae] a family of bacteria of the order Mycoplasmatales, class Mollicutes, made up of organisms that do not require sterol for growth. It contains the genus *Acholeplasma.*

**acho·lia** (a-ko′le-ə) [*a-*[1] + *chol-* + *-ia*] absence or failure of secretion of bile.

**acho·lic** (a-ko′lik) free from bile.

**achol·uria** (ak-ol-u′re-ə) [*a-*[1] + Gr. *choluria*] lack of bile pigment in the urine.

**achol·uric** (ak-ol-u′rik) pertaining to or characterized by acholuria, as acholuric jaundice.

**achon·dro·gen·e·sis** (ə-kon″dro-jen′ə-sis) a hereditary disorder characterized by hypoplasia of bone, resulting in markedly shortened limbs; the head and trunk are normal.

**achon·dro·pla·sia** (ə-kon″dro-pla′zhə) [*a-*[1] + *chondroplasia*] [MeSH: Achondroplasia] a hereditary, congenital disturbance of epiphyseal chondroblastic growth and maturation, causing inadequate enchondral bone formation and resulting in a peculiar form of dwarfism with short limbs, normal trunk, small face, normal vault, lordosis, and trident hand. See also *achondroplastic dwarf,* under *dwarf.*

**achon·dro·plas·tic** (ə-kon″dro-plas′tik) pertaining to, or affected with, achondroplasia.

**achon·dro·plas·ty** (ə-kon′dro-plas″te) achondroplasia.

**achor·dal** (a-kor′dəl) achordate.

**achor·date** (a-kor′dāt) without a notochord; used with reference to animals which are not chordates.

**achres·tic** (ə-kres′tik) not using some normal tool or process; see under *anemia.*

**achro·ma·sia** (ak″ro-ma′zhə) [*a-*[1] + *chrom-* + *-asia*] 1. lack of normal pigmentation of the skin. 2. absence of the usual staining reaction in a tissue or cell.

**achro·mat** (ak'ro-mat) [*a-*[1] + *chromat*] 1. an achromatic objective. 2. monochromat.

**achro·mate** (ə-kro'māt) monochromat.

**achro·mat·ic** (ak″ro-mat'ik) [*a-*[1] + *chromatic*] 1. producing no discoloration. 2. staining with difficulty. 3. containing achromatin. 4. refracting light without decomposing it into its component colors. 5. monochromatic, def. 2.

**achro·ma·tin** (ə-kro'mə-tin) [*a-*[1] + *chromatin*] the faintly staining substance forming the karyolymph, linin, and nuclear membrane of the nucleus of a cell.

**achro·ma·tin·ic** (ə-kro″mə-tin'ik) pertaining to or containing achromatin.

**achro·ma·tism** (ə-kro'mə-tiz-əm) 1. the quality or condition of being achromatic. 2. monochromatism.

**achro·ma·tize** (ə-kro'mə-tīz) to render achromatic.

**achro·ma·tol·y·sis** (ə-kro″mə-tol'ə-sis) [*achromatin* + *-lysis*] disorganization of the achromatin of a cell.

**achro·ma·to·phil** (ă″kromat'o-fil) [*a-*[1] + *chromato-* + *-phil*] 1. having no affinity for stains. 2. an organism or tissue element that does not stain easily.

**achro·ma·to·phil·ia** (ə-kro″mə-to-fil'e-ə) the property of resisting the coloring action of stains.

**achro·ma·top·sia** (ə-kro″mə-top'se-ə) monochromatism.

**achro·ma·to·sis** (ə-kro″mə-to'sis) [*a-*[1] + *chromat-* + *-osis*] 1. deficiency of pigmentation in the tissues, as in the skin and the iris. 2. lack of staining power in a cell or tissue.

**achro·ma·tous** (ə-kro'mə-tus) having no color; colorless.

**achro·ma·tu·ria** (ə-kro″mə-tu're-ə) [*a-*[1] + *chromaturia*] the excretion of colorless urine.

**achro·mia** (ə-kro'me-ə) [*a-*[1] + *chrom-* + *-ia*] the lack or absence of normal color or pigmentation, as of the skin.
**cortical a.,** a condition in which an area of the cerebral cortex shows disappearance of ganglion cells.
**a. parasi'tica,** a variant of tinea versicolor occurring in dark-skinned infants, particularly in the tropics, which begins in the diaper region and spreads rapidly, causing marked depigmentation of the skin.

**achro·mic** (ə-kro'mik) pertaining to or characterized by achromia.

**achro·min** (ə-kro'min) achromatin.

**Achro·mo·bac·ter** (ə-kro″mo-bak'tər) [*a-*[1] + *chromo-* + *-bacter*] a genus of gram-negative, nonfermentative, peritrichously flagellated, rod-shaped bacteria of uncertain affiliation, found in water and the human intestinal tract. They have been isolated from various clinical sources, sometimes associated with significant infections. Organisms of this genus are sometimes classified in the genus *Alcaligenes.*

**achro·mo·cyte** (ə-kro'mo-sīt) a crescent-shaped red cell artifact that stains more faintly than intact red cells; cf. *ghost cell.* Called also *demilune body* and *achromic erythrocyte.*

**achro·mo·phil** (ə-kro'mo-fil) [*a-*[1] + *chromo-* + *-phil*] achromatophil.

**achro·moph·i·lous** (a″kro-mof'ĭ-ləs) having no affinity for stains.

**achro·mo·trich·ia** (a-kro″mo-trik'e-ə) loss of pigment in the hair; see also *canities* and *poliosis.* Called also *hypochromotrichia.*

**Achro·my·cin** (ak″ro-mi'sin) trademark for preparations of tetracycline.

**ach·roo·am·y·loid** (a-kro″o-am'ĭ-loid) [*a-*[1] + Gr. *chroa* color + *amyloid*] amyloid in its early nonstainable stage.

**ach·roo·dex·trin** (ə-kro″o-dek'strin) [*a-*[1] + Gr. *chroa* color + *dextrin*] any of the lower-molecular-weight dextrins not colored by iodine.

**Achú·car·ro's stain** (ah-choo'kah-rōz) [Nicolás *Achúcarro,* Spanish histologist, 1881–1918] see under *stain.*

**achy·lia** (ə-ki'le-ə) [Gr. *achylos* juiceless + *-ia*] absence of hydrochloric acid and pepsinogens (pepsin) in the gastric juice *(a. gas'trica).*

**achy·mia** (ə-ki'me-ə) imperfect, insufficient, or absence of formation of chyme.

**achy·mo·sis** (ak″ĭ-mo'sis) achymia.

**acic·u·lar** (ə-sik'u-lər) [L. *acicularis*] shaped like a needle or needle point.

**acic·u·lum** (ə-sik'u-lum) a bent, finger-like spine or bristle found in certain flagellates.

**ac·id** (as'id) [L. *acidum* from *acidus* sharp, sour] any of a large class of chemical substances defined by three chemical concepts of increasing generality. An *Arrhenius acid* is a substance that lowers the pH (increases the hydrogen ion concentration) when added to an aqueous solution; such substances have a sour taste, turn litmus red, and react with alkalis to form salts. A *Bronsted-Lowry acid* is a species that acts as a proton donor in solution; e.g., the ammonium ion ($NH_4^+$) can donate a proton leaving ammonia ($NH_3$); such species are termed conjugate acid-base pairs. A *Lewis acid* is a species that can accept a pair of electrons to form a covalent bond; e.g., $BF_3$ in the reaction $BF_3 + NH_3 \rightarrow BF_3NH_3$. Aqueous solutions of certain compounds that dissociate in solution, e.g., hydrogen chloride, are designated as acids by names beginning with *hydro-,* e.g., hydrochloric acid. Most other common inorganic acids are *oxo acids* (q.v.); common organic acids include carboxylic acids, sulfonic acids, and phenols. The name of the anion formed by the removal of hydrogen from an acid (its conjugate base) and the names of salts and esters of acids are formed by removing the suffix *-ic* and the word *acid* and adding the suffix *-ate,* except for oxo acids ending in *-ous,* when the suffix is *-ite.* For particular acids, see the specific name.
**amino a.,** any organic compound containing an amino and a carboxyl group. See *amino acid.*
**binary a.,** an acid which contains only two elements, e.g., HCl; called also *hydracid.*
**carboxylic a.,** any acid containing the carboxyl (—COOH) group, including amino acids and fatty acids.
**a. citrate dextrose (ACD),** an anticoagulant solution containing citric acid, sodium citrate, and dextrose formerly used for the preservation of stored whole blood but now primarily for plateletpheresis. Called also *anticoagulant citrate dextrose solution* [USP].
**conjugate a.,** a chemical species that is formed from its conjugate base by addition of a proton, e.g., ammonium ($NH_4^+$) is the conjugate acid of ammonia ($NH_3$).
**fatty a.,** see under *F.*
**haloid a.,** an acid which contains no oxygen in the molecule, but is composed of hydrogen and a halogen element.
**hydroxy a.,** an organic acid that contains an additional hydroxyl group.
**inorganic a.,** one containing no carbon atoms.
**monobasic a.,** an acid having but one replaceable hydrogen atom and therefore yielding only one series of salts, e.g., HCl.
**nucleic a.,** see under *N.*
**organic a.,** an acid containing one or more carbon atoms, often specifically a carboxylic acid.
**oxo a.,** 1. oxyacid. 2. keto acid; see under *K.*
**oxygen a.,** an acid that contains oxygen; an oxyacid.
**polybasic a.,** an acid which contains two or more hydrogen atoms which may be neutralized by alkalies and replaced by organic radicals.
**sulfo-a.,** an acid in which oxygen or carbon is replaced by sulfur.
**ternary a.,** an acid which contains three distinct radicals.
**thio a.,** one formed by replacement of an oxygen atom in an oxo acid or carboxylic acid by a sulfur atom, e.g., thiophosphoric acid ($H_3PSO_3$) or thioacetic acid ($CH_3COSH$).
**tribasic a.,** an acid that has three replaceable hydrogen atoms.

**ac·id·al·bu·min** (as″id-al'bu-min) a protein that dissolves in acids and shows an acid reaction.

**Ac·id·ami·no·coc·cus** (as″id-ə-me″no-kok'əs) [*acid* + *amino* + *coccus*] a genus of bacteria of the family Veillonellaceae, found in the intestinal tract of normal humans and pigs, made up of gram-negative anaerobic cocci. The type species is *A. fermentans.*

**ac·id·am·in·uria** (as″id-am″ĭ-nu're-ə) aminoaciduria.

**ac·id–CoA li·gase (GDP-forming)** (as'id ko-a' li'gās) [EC 6.2.1.10] an enzyme of the ligase class that catalyzes the formation of acyl coenzyme A from long chain fatty acids (12 or more carbons) and coenzyme A, using the energy derived from GTP hydrolysis. The enzyme occurs in the mitochondrial matrix and thus can activate any free fatty acids appearing there. Called also *acyl CoA synthetase (GDP-forming).*

**ac·i·de·mia** (as″ĭ-de'me-ə) a decreased pH (increased hydrogen ion concentration) of the blood. For acidemias characterized by increased concentration of a specific acid, see at the acid (e.g., *isovalericacidemia).*
**organic a.,** increased concentration of one or more organic acids in the blood.

**acid-fast** (as'id-fast) not readily decolorized by acid after staining, a characteristic of certain bacteria, particularly *Mycobacterium tuberculosis, Mycobacterium leprae,* and some species of *Nocardia.* See under *stain.*

**acid·ic** (ə-sid'ik) of or pertaining to an acid; acid-forming.

**acid·i·fi·a·ble** (ə-sid'ə-fi″ə-bəl) susceptible of being made acid.

**acid·i·fi·er** (ə-sid″ĭ-fi'ər) an agent that causes acidity; a substance used to increase gastric acidity.

**acid·i·fy** (ə-sid'ĭ-fi) 1. to render acid, as by addition of a strong acid. 2. to become acid.

**ac·i·dim·e·ter** (as″ĭ-dim′ə-tər) [L. *acidum* acid + *-meter*] an instrument used in performing acidimetry.

**ac·i·dim·et·ry** (as″ĭ-dim′ə-tre) the determination of the amount of free acid in a solution.

**ac·id·ism** (as′ĭ-diz-əm) a condition due to introduction into the body of acids from outside; called also *acidismus.*

**ac·i·dis·mus** (as″ĭ-diz′məs) acidism.

**acid·i·ty** (ə-sid′ĭ-te) [L. *aciditas*] the quality of being acid or sour; containing acid (hydrogen ions).

**ac·id li·pase** (as″id li′pās) 1. sterol esterase. 2. a lipase with an acid pH optimum.

**ac·id li·pase de·fi·cien·cy** 1. Wolman's disease. 2. cholesteryl ester storage disease.

**ac·id mal·tase** (as′id mawl′tās) glucan 1,4-α-glucosidase.

**ac·id mal·tase deficiency** glycogen storage disease, type II.

**ac·i·do·gen·ic** (as″ĭ-do-jen′ik) producing acid or acidity, especially acidity of the urine.

**Aci·dol** (a′sĭ-dol) trademark for a preparation of betaine hydrochloride.

**acid·o·phil** (ə-sid′o-fil″) [L. *acidum* acid + Gr. *-phil*] 1. a structure, cell, or other histologic element staining readily with acid dyes. 2. one of the hormone-producing acidophilic cells of the adenohypophysis; types include corticotrophs, lactotrophs, lipotrophs, and somatotrophs. Called also *alpha cell* and *A cell.* 3. an organism that grows well in highly acid media. 4. acidophilic.
**alpha a.,** somatotroph.
**epsilon a.,** lactotroph.

**acid·o·phile** (ə-sid′o-fīl″) 1. acidophil. 2. acidophilic.

**ac·i·do·phil·ic** (as″ĭ-do-fil′ik) 1. readily stained with acid dyes. 2. growing in highly acid media; said of microorganisms. Called also *acidophil, acidophile,* and *oxyphilic.*

**ac·i·do·sic** (as″ĭ-do′sik) acidotic.

**ac·i·do·sis** (as″ĭ-do′sis) [MeSH: Acidosis] 1. the accumulation of acid and hydrogen ions or depletion of the alkaline reserve (bicarbonate content) in the blood and body tissues, resulting in a decrease in pH. 2. the pathologic condition resulting from this process; see also *acidemia..* Cf. *alkalosis.*
**compensated a.,** a condition in which the compensatory mechanisms have returned the pH toward normal; see *metabolic a., compensated,* and *respiratory a., compensated.*
**diabetic a.,** a type of metabolic acidosis produced by accumulation of ketone bodies resulting from uncontrolled diabetes mellitus. Called also *diabetic ketoacidosis.*
**hypercapnic a.,** respiratory a.
**hyperchloremic a.,** metabolic acidosis accompanied by elevated plasma chloride.
**lactic a.,** a metabolic acidosis occurring as a result of excess lactic acid in the blood, due to conditions causing impaired cellular respiration. It occurs most commonly in disorders in which $O_2$ is inadequately delivered to tissues, e.g., shock, septicemia, or extreme hypoxemia, but it can also result from exogenous or endogenous metabolic defects. Initially manifesting as hyperventilation, it progresses to mental confusion and coma.
**metabolic a.,** any of the various kinds of acidosis in which the acid-base status of the body shifts toward the acid side because of loss of base or retention of acids other than carbonic acid (fixed or nonvolatile acids), in contrast to respiratory acidosis. Called also *nonrespiratory a.*
**metabolic a., compensated,** a state of metabolic acidosis in which the pH of the blood has been returned toward normal by respiratory compensatory mechanisms.
**nonrespiratory a.,** metabolic a.
**renal hyperchloremia a.,** renal tubular a.
**renal tubular a. (RTA),** a variety of metabolic acidosis resulting from impairment of renal function; it is usually accompanied by hyperchloremic acidosis, high urinary pH, bicarbonaturia, and lowered excretion of ammonium and titratable acids. Type 1 and Type 2 are distinguished according to whether the primary dysfunction is in the distal or the proximal tubules; see *distal renal tubular a.* and *proximal renal tubular a.*
**renal tubular a., distal,** renal tubular acidosis without the usual lowering of the pH of urine in the distal tubules. Called also *type 1 renal tubular a.*
**renal tubular a., generalized distal,** distal renal tubular acidosis associated with hyporeninemic hypoaldosteronism, most commonly associated with diabetes mellitus. Called also *type 4 renal tubular acidosis.*
**renal tubular a., proximal,** renal tubular acidosis caused by malfunction of the proximal tubules. Mild forms are often accompanied by bicarbonaturia; severe forms such as Fanconi's syndrome may be free of bicarbonaturia but show increased excretion of other solutes. Called also *type 2 renal tubular a.*
**renal tubular a., type 1,** distal renal tubular a.
**renal tubular a., type 2,** proximal renal tubular a.
**renal tubular a., type 4,** generalized distal renal tubular a.
**respiratory a.,** acidosis due to excess retention of carbon dioxide in the body, as opposed to metabolic acidosis; it is seen in chronic obstructive pulmonary disease and other conditions that interfere with normal ventilation. Called also *hypercapnic a.*
**respiratory a., compensated,** respiratory acidosis in which the pH of the blood has been returned toward normal by renal compensatory mechanisms.
**starvation a.,** a type of metabolic acidosis produced by accumulation of ketone bodies which may accompany a caloric deficit. Called also *starvation ketoacidosis.*
**uremic a.,** the condition in chronic renal disease in which the ability to excrete acid is decreased, causing acidosis.

**ac·i·dos·teo·phyte** (as″ĭ-dos′te-o-fīt″) [Gr. *akis* point + *osteo-* + *-phyte*] a sharp-pointed osteophyte.

**ac·i·dot·ic** (as″ĭ-dot′ik) pertaining to or characterized by acidosis.

**ac·id phos·pha·tase** (as′id fos′fə-tās) [EC 3.1.3.2] [MeSH: Acid Phosphatase] an enzyme of the hydrolase class that catalyzes the cleavage of orthophosphate from orthophosphoric monoesters under acid conditions. The enzyme is found in mammalian liver, spleen, bone marrow, plasma and formed blood elements, and prostate gland. The determination of serum acid phosphatase activity is an important diagnostic test. Called also *phosphomonoesterase.*

**acid·u·lat·ed** (ə-sid′u-lāt″ed) rendered acid in reaction.

**Acid·u·lin** (ə-sid′u-lin) trademark for a preparation of glutamic acid hydrochloride.

**acid·u·lous** (ə-sid′u-ləs) somewhat acid.

**ac·id·u·ria** (as″ĭ-du′re-ə) excess of acid in the urine. For acidurias characterized by increased concentration of a specific acid, see at the acid (e.g., *glutaricaciduria).*
**organic a.,** excessive excretion of one or more organic acids in the urine.

**ac·id·uric** (as″ĭ-doo′rik) [L. *acidum* acid + *durare* to endure] acid-tolerant; said of bacteria which are able to withstand a degree of acidity usually fatal to nonsporulating bacteria.

**ac·i·dyl** (as′ĭ-dəl) any acid radical.

**acid·y·la·tion** (ə-sid″ə-la′shən) acylation.

**ac·i·nar** (as′ĭ-nər) pertaining to or affecting an acinus or acini.

**ac·i·ne·sia** (as″ĭ-ne′zhə) akinesia.

**ac·i·net·ic** (as″ĭ-net′ik) akinetic (def. 1).

**Ac·i·net·o·bac·ter** (as″ĭ-net″o-bak′tər) [*a-*[1] + *cineto-* + *-bacter*] [MeSH: Acinetobacter] a genus of bacteria of the family Neisseriaceae, consisting of gram-negative, paired coccobacilli that are aerobic, catalase-positive, and oxidase-negative. The organisms are widely distributed in nature and are part of the normal mammalian flora, but can cause severe primary infections in compromised hosts. The single species is *A. calcoaceticus.*
**A. anitra′tus,** *A. calcoaceticus.*
**A. calcoace′ticus,** the type species of the genus *Acinetobacter;* it can cause fatal pneumonia in immunocompromised patients. See Acinetobacter calcoaceticus *pneumonia,* under *pneumonia.* Called also *A. anitratus, A. lwoffi, Herellea vaginicola, Mima polymorpha,* and *Moraxella lwoffi.*
**A. lwof′fi,** *A. calcoaceticus.*

**ac·i·ni** (as′ĭ-ni) [L.] genitive and plural of *acinus.*

**acin·ic** (ə-sin′ik) pertaining to an acinus.

**acin·i·form** (ə-sin′ĭ-form) [*acini* + *form*] shaped like an acinus, or grape.

**acin·i·tis** (as″ĭ-ni′tis) inflammation of the acini of a gland.

**ac·i·nose** (as′ĭ-nōs) [L. *acinosus* grapelike] 1. made up of acini. 2. acinar.

**ac·i·no·tu·bu·lar** (as″ĭ-no-too′bu-lər) composed of tubular acini or of tubules ending in acini.

**ac·i·nous** (as′ĭ-nəs) 1. resembling a grape. 2. acinar.

**ac·i·nus** (as′ĭ-nəs) pl. *a′cini* [L. "grape"] a general term used in anatomical nomenclature to designate a small saclike dilatation, particularly in the lung or a gland. See also *alveolus.*
**liver a.,** a functional unit of the liver, smaller than a portal lobule, being a diamond-shaped mass of liver parenchyma that is supplied by a terminal branch of the portal vein and of the hepatic artery and drained by a terminal branch of the bile duct.
**pancreatic a.,** one of the secretory units of the exocrine pancreas, where pancreatic juice is produced.
**pulmonary a.,** terminal respiratory unit.

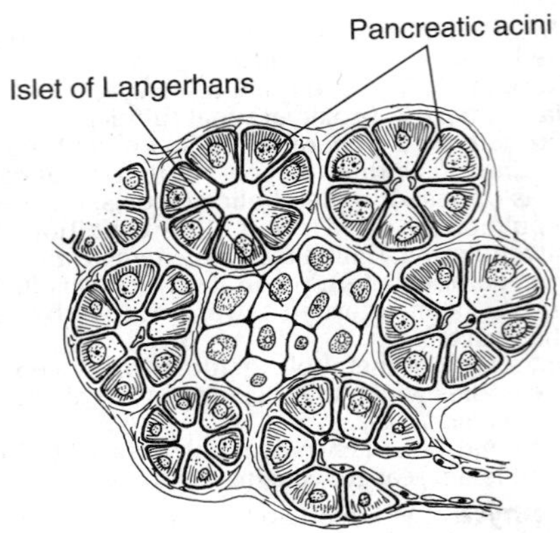

Acini of pancreas.

**a. rena'lis [malpig'hii],** corpuscula renis.
**a. re'nis [malpig'hii],** corpuscula renis.
**thyroid acini,** folliculi glandulae thyroideae.

**ac•i•pen•ser•in** (as″ĭ-pen'sər-in) a toxic substance from the gonads of the sturgeon, *Acipenser.*

**ac•i•tret•in** (as″e-tret'in) a major metabolite of etretinate, used in treatment of severe psoriasis; administered orally.

**ackee** (ă'ke) akee.

**aclad•i•o•sis** (ə-klad″e-o'sis) an ulcerative dermatomycosis that was seen in southern Asia and the Balkans and was caused by a species of *Acladium.*

**Acla•di•um** (ə-kla'de-um) a former genus of Fungi Imperfecti, now reclassified.

**acla•sia** (ə-kla'zhə) aclasis.

**acla•sis** (ak'lə-sis) [*a-*[1] + Gr. *klasis* a breaking] pathologic continuity of structure, as in multiple exostoses.
**diaphyseal a.,** multiple exostoses.
**tarsoepiphyseal a.,** dysplasia epiphysealis hemimelica.

**aclas•tic** (a-klas'tik) 1. pertaining to or characterized by aclasis. 2. not refracting.

**Aclo•vate** (a'klo-vāt″) trademark for preparation of alclometasone dipropionate.

**aclu•sion** (ə-kloo'zhən) [*a-*[1] + *occlusion*] absence of occlusion of the opposing tooth surfaces.

**ac•me** (ak'me) [Gr. *akmē* highest point] the crisis or critical stage of a disease.

**ac•ne** (ak'ne) [possibly a corruption of Greek *akmē* a point or of *achnē* chaff] an inflammatory disease of the pilosebaceous unit, the specific type usually being indicated by a modifying term; frequently used alone to designate common acne, or *a. vulgaris.*
**a. atro'phica,** acne in which, after the disappearance of small papular lesions, there is left a stippling of tiny atrophic pits and scars.
**bromide a.,** an acneiform eruption without comedones, one of the most constant symptoms of brominism.
**chlorine a.,** chloracne.
**common a.,** a. vulgaris.
**a. congloba'ta, conglobate a.,** a severe, chronic form of acne seen almost exclusively in males, beginning during late puberty and often continuing in later life, and characterized by the presence of numerous comedones (often double or triple), large abscesses with interconnecting sinuses, and cysts containing clear or seropurulent material; pronounced and disfiguring scarring remains after healing.
**contact a.,** a. venenata.
**contagious a. of horses, contagious pustular a.,** a contagious disease of the skin in horses caused by infection with *Corynebacterium pseudotuberculosis,* characterized by groups of pustules, especially in areas in contact with the harness; when ruptured, the pustules release greenish pus that dries and forms a crust.
**a. cosme'tica,** a persistent, low-grade type of acne usually involving the chin and cheeks of women who use cosmetics, the lesions of which present as closed comedones and papulopustules, which are thought to be caused by comedogenic substances in the cosmetics.
**cystic a.,** acne with the formation of cysts enclosing a mixture of keratin and sebum in varying proportions.
**a. deter'gicans,** aggravation of the existing lesions of acne by too frequent washing with comedogenic soaps and rough cloths and abrasive pads.
**epidemic a.,** keratosis follicularis contagiosa.
**a. estiva'lis,** a form of acne characterized by the presence of keratotic papules that occurs in the summer or following a vacation in the sun. Called also *Mallorca a.*
**excoriated a., a. excoriée des filles, a. excoriée des jeunes filles,** a superficial type of acne usually seen in girls and young women caused by the compulsive neurotic habit of picking and squeezing minute, trivial, or nonexistent facial lesions, producing secondary lesions that may leave scars. Called also *picker's a.*
**a. fronta'lis,** a. varioliformis.
**a. ful'minans,** a rare form of extremely severe cystic acne occurring primarily in teenage boys, characterized by the presence of highly inflammatory nodules and plaques that undergo suppurative degeneration leaving ulcerations, and by fever, weight loss, anemia, leukocytosis, elevated erythrocyte sedimentation rate, and polyarthritis.
**halogen a.,** an acneiform eruption due to ingestion of the simple salts of bromine and iodine, usually as halogen-containing cold remedies, expectorants, sedatives, analgesics, and vitamins.
**a. indura'ta,** a progression of papular acne, with deep-seated and destructive lesions that may produce severe scarring.
**infantile a.,** a. neonatorum.
**iodide a.,** an eruption caused by the use of iodide compounds.
**a. keloid,** dermatitis papillaris capillitii.
**Mallorca a.,** a. estivalis.
**a. mecha'nica, mechanical a.,** aggravation of the existing lesions of acne by mechanical factors that deform the skin, including friction, rubbing, stretching, pressure, pinching, and pulling, which may be provoked by such factors as chin straps, articles of clothing, orthopedic casts, backpacks, and chair and car or bus seats.
**a. necro'tica milia'ris,** a rare and chronic form of folliculitis of the scalp, occurring principally in adults, with formation of tiny superficial pustules which are destroyed by scratching. See also *a. varioliformis.*
**neonatal a., a. neonato'rum,** acne vulgaris occurring in infants, usually in males before 3 months of age, chiefly characterized by the presence of papules, pustules, and open and closed comedones on the face; the affected child may be predisposed to more severe acne in adolescence. Called also *infantile a.*
**occupational a.,** see *contact a.*
**oil a.,** a follicular acneiform eruption on the dorsa of the hands, on the back of the neck, and on the forearms, face, and thighs caused by contact with water-insoluble cutting oils.
**a. papulo'sa,** a type of acne vulgaris in which the lesions are typically numerous inflammatory papules; this type often progresses into acne indurata.
**picker's a.,** excoriated a.
**pomade a.,** acne vulgaris occurring almost exclusively in blacks who groom their scalp and facial hair with greasy lubricants, and characterized by the presence of closed comedones and occasional papulopustules on the forehead, temples, cheeks, and chin.
**premenstrual a.,** acne of a cyclic nature, appearing shortly before (rarely after) the onset of menses.
**a. pustulo'sa,** acne in which the lesions show central suppuration.
**a. rosa'cea,** rosacea.
**a. scrofuloso'rum,** papulonecrotic tuberculid.
**tropical a., a. tropica'lis,** severe acne vulgaris occurring in hot and moist regions of the tropics, characterized by the presence of large and painful cysts, nodules, and pustules that lead to the formation of conglobate abscesses and frequent scarring, and tend to localize on the back, nape of the neck, buttocks, thighs, and upper arms.
**a. urtica'ta,** an acneiform eruption characterized by edematous papular wheals, resembling acne papules.
**a. variolifor'mis,** a rare condition, with persistent brown papulopustules, usually localized to the brow and scalp; probably a deep

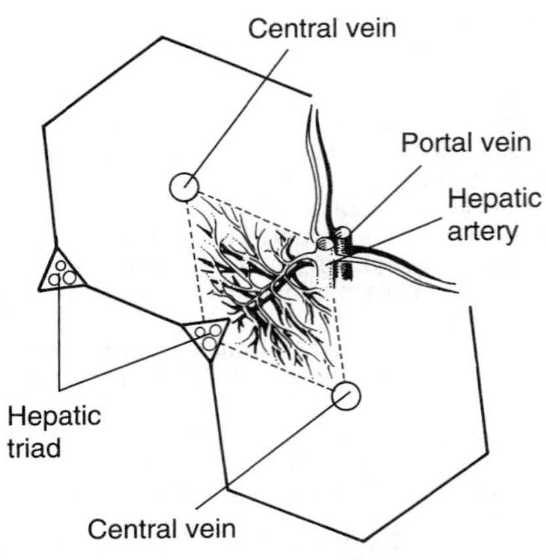

Liver acinus: hepatic lobules are represented by hexagons (solid lines); liver acinus is represented by rhombus (dotted line).

variant of acne necrotica miliaris. Called also *a. frontalis* and *folliculitis varioliformis.*
**a. venena'ta,** acne produced by contact with a great variety of acnegenic chemicals, including those used in cosmetic and grooming agents and industry *(occupational a.)*, including many oils and tars, waxes, and chlorinated hydrocarbons *(chloracne)*. Called also *contact a.*
**a. vulga'ris,** a chronic inflammatory disease of the pilosebaceous apparatus, the lesions occurring most frequently on the face, chest, and back. The inflamed glands may form small pink papules, which sometimes surround comedones so that they have black centers, or form pustules or cysts; the cause is unknown, but it has been suggested that many factors, including stress, hereditary factors, hormones, drugs, and bacteria, especially *Propionibacterium acnes, Staphylococcus albus,* and *Malassezia furfur,* play an etiologic role. Called also *common a.*

**ac·ne·form** (ak'ne-form) acneiform.

**ac·ne·gen** (ak'nə-jen) a substance that causes acne.

**ac·ne·gen·ic** (ak″ne-jen'ĭk) [*acne* + *-genic*] causing or capable of producing acne.

**ac·ne·iform** (ak-ne'ĭ-form″) resembling acne.

**ac·ne·mia** (ak-ne'me-ə) [*a-*[1] + Gr. *knēmē* leg] atrophy of the calves of the legs.

**ac·ni·tis** (ak-ni'tis) [*acne* + *-itis*] a variant of papulonecrotic tuberculid occurring on the face.

**ACNM** American College of Nurse-Midwives; see *nurse-midwife* and *nurse-midwifery.*

**ac·o·as·ma** (ak″o-as'mə) acousma.

**Ac·o·can·the·ra** (ak″o-kan-the'rə) [Gr. *akōkē* a point, edge + *anthēros* blooming] a genus of plants of the family Apocynaceae, native to Africa. *A. schim'peri* (A.D.C.) Schwf. and other species yield the toxic glycoside ouabain (acocantherin).

**ac·o·can·ther·in** (ak″o-kan'thər-in) ouabain.

**acoe·lom·ate** (a-se'lə-māt) 1. lacking a body cavity. 2. an animal lacking a body cavity, as the platyhelminths.

**ACOG** American College of Obstetricians and Gynecologists.

**Ac·o·kan·the·ra** (ak″o-kan-the'rə) *Acocanthera.*

**acol·u·mel·late** (a″kol-u-mel'āt) of certain protozoa and fungi, lacking columellae.

**Acon** (a'kon) trademark for a preparation of vitamin A.

**acon·a·tive** (ə-kon'ə-tiv) without conation; lacking any desire or impulse to act.

**acon·i·tase** (ə-kon'ĭ-tās) aconitate hydratase.

***cis*-acon·i·tate** (ə-kon'ĭ-tāt) an intermediate in the interconversion of citrate and isocitrate in the tricarboxylic acid cycle, formed by dehydration of either compound.

**acon·i·tate hy·dra·tase** (ə-kon'ĭ-tāt hi'drə-tās) [EC 4.2.1.3] [MeSH: Aconitate Hydratase] an enzyme of the lyase class that catalyzes the interconversion of citrate and isocitrate, a reaction of the tricarboxylic acid cycle (q.v.). The enzyme, a nonheme iron protein, is named for the *cis*-aconitate formed as an intermediate in the dehydration and rehydration reaction. Called also *aconitase.*

**ac·o·nite** (ak'ə-nīt) [L *aconitum;* Gr. *akoniton*] [MeSH: Aconite] a poisonous substance from the dried tuberous root of *Aconitum napellus,* which contains aconitine and other related alkaloids; it causes potentially fatal ventricular fibrillation and respiratory paralysis. It was formerly given internally as a febrifuge and gastric anesthetic. Called also *monkshood* and *wolfsbane.*

**acon·i·tine** (ə-kon'ĭ-tin) [L. *aconitina, aconitia*] [MeSH: Aconitine] a poisonous alkaloid, the active principle of aconite.

**Ac·o·ni·tum** (ak″ə-ni'təm) [L.] a genus of poisonous herbs of the family Ranunculaceae. *A. napel'lus* is wolf's bane (or wolfsbane), the source of aconite.

**ac·on·ure·sis** (ak″on-u-re'sis) [Gr. *akōn* unwilling + *uresis*] urinary incontinence.

**acop·ro·sis** (a″kop-ro'sis) [*a-*[1] + *copro-* + *-sis*] absence of fecal matter from the intestine.

**acop·rous** (ə-kop'rəs) having no fecal matter in the intestine.

**aco·rea** (ə-kor'e-ə) [*a-*[1] + Gr. *korē* pupil] absence of the pupil of the eye.

**aco·ria** (ə-kor'e-ə) [*a-*[1] + Gr. *koros* satiety + *-ia*] a form of polyphagia due to loss of the sensation of satiety, a condition in which the patient never feels that he has enough, although the appetite may not be large.

**ac·o·rin** (ak'ə-rin) a bitter glycoside from calamus; it splits into oil of calamus and sugar.

**acorn** (a'korn) the fruit of an oak tree (see *Quercus*). Many types are ground up for food for humans or livestock; because they contain gallic acid and tannic acid, they are poisonous if eaten in large amounts.

**acor·tan** (a-kor'tan) corticotropin (def. 1).

**Ac·o·rus** (ak'ə-rəs) [L.; Gr. *akoros*] a genus of plants of the family Araceae. *A. ca'lamus* L. is calamus, whose rhizome is used as a flavoring agent and insect repellent.

**ACOS** American College of Osteopathic Surgeons.

**Acos·ta's disease** (ah-ko'stahz) [José de *Acosta,* 1539–1600, Spanish Jesuit missionary who first described it after his travels in Peru in 1590] acute mountain sickness.

**acou-** [Gr. *akouein* to hear] a combining form denoting relationship to hearing.

**acous·ma** (ə-ko͞oz'mə) pl. *acous'mata* [Gr. *akousma* a thing heard] a simple auditory hallucination, e.g., buzzing or ringing sounds.

**acous·mat·am·ne·sia** (ə-ko͞oz″mat-am-ne'zhə) [*acousma* hearing + *amnesia*] inability to recall sounds.

**acous·tic** (ə-ko͞os'tik) [Gr. *akoustikos*] [MeSH: Acoustics] pertaining to sound.

**acous·ti·co·pho·bia** (ə-ko͞os″tĭ-ko-fo'be-ə) [*acoustic* + *-phobia*] irrational fear of sounds.

**acous·tics** (ə-ko͞os'tiks) [MeSH: Acoustics] the science of sounds.

**acous·ti·gram** (ə-ko͞os'tĭ-gram) acoustogram.

**acous·to·gram** (ə-ko͞os'to-gram) the graphic tracing of the curves, delineated in frequencies per second and decibel levels, of sounds produced by motion of a joint. Applied to the knee joint, an acoustogram will show the sound of the moving semilunar cartilages, the moving contact between the articular surfaces of the femur and tibia, and the circulation of the synovia.

**ACP** American College of Physicians; acid phosphatase.

**ac·quired** (ə-kwird') [L. *acquirere* to obtain] not genetic, but produced by influences originating outside the organism.

**ac·qui·si·tion** (ă″kwĭ-zĭ'shən) in psychology, the period in learning during which progressive increments in response strength can be measured. Also the process involved in such learning.

**ac·qui·si·tus** (ə-kwis'ĭ-təs) [L.] acquired.

**ACR** American College of Radiology.

**ac·ral** (ak'rəl) [*acr-* + *-al*[1]] pertaining to an extremity or apex; affecting the limbs (extremities).

**acra·nia** (ə-kra'ne-ə) [*a-*[1] + *crani-* + *-ia*] a developmental anomaly characterized by partial or complete absence of the skull (calvaria).

**acra·ni·al** (ə-kra'ne-əl) having no cranium.

**Acra·ni·a·ta** (ə-kra″ne-a'tə) a subphylum of Chordata comprising species without a true skull.

**acra·ni·us** (ə-kra'ne-əs) a fetus exhibiting acrania.

**acrat·ure·sis** (ə-krat″-u-re'sis) dysuria.

**Ac·rel's gan·gli·on** (ahk'relz) [Olof (or Olaf) *Acrel,* Swedish surgeon, 1717–1806] see under *ganglion.*

**Ac·re·mo·ni·el·la** (ak″rə-mo-ne-el'ə) a genus of Fungi Imperfecti of the form-class Hyphomycetes, form-family Dematiaceae; it resembles *Acremonium* and has reportedly been isolated from lung lesions.

**ac·re·mo·ni·o·sis** (ak″rə-mo-ne-o'sis) infection with the fungus *Acremonium,* producing fever and gummalike swellings.

**Ac·re·mo·ni·um** (ak″rə-mo'ne-əm) [MeSH: Acremonium] a genus of Fungi Imperfecti of the form-class Hyphomycetes, form-family Moniliaceae; formerly called *Cephalosporium. A. alabamen'sis* causes opportunistic infections in immunocompromised patients. *A. coenophi'alum* is endophytic in the grass *Festuca arundinacea* and causes fescue foot in cattle and sheep. *A. kilien'se* is an etiologic agent of eumycotic mycetoma. *A. lo'liae* is endophytic in the grass *Lolium perenne* and causes ryegrass staggers in grazing animals.
**A. coenophi'alum,** a species endophytic in the grass *Festuca arundinacea,* causing the disease fescue foot in cattle and sheep.
**A. falcifor'me,** a species that causes eumycotic mycetoma.
**A. kilien'se,** a species that is an etiologic agent of eumycotic mycetoma.
**A. lo'liae,** an endophytic species that infests the grass *Lolium perenne* and causes ryegrass staggers in grazing animals.
**A. reci'fei,** a species that is an etiologic agent of eumycotic mycetoma.

**ac·rid** (ak'rid) [L. *acer, acris* sharp] pungent; producing an irritation.

**ac·ri·dine** (ak'rĭ-dēn) a dibenzopyridine used in the synthesis of

dyes and drugs; its derivatives are mostly fluorescent yellow dyes (acridine dyes), and those used in medicine (as antiseptic agents) are acriflavine hydrochloride, acriflavine base, and proflavine.
**a. orange,** tetramethyl acridine, a fluorescent basic dye; sometimes used for vital staining.

**ac·ri·fla·vine** (ak″rĭ-fla′vēn) [MeSH: Acriflavine] a mixture used in solution as a topical antiseptic for the skin and mucous membranes. Called also *chromoflavine, euflavine, neutral acriflavine,* and *neutroflavine.*

**ac·ri·sor·cin** (ak-rĭ-sor′sin) an acridine derivative with antifungal activity, especially against *Malassezia furfur.* Applied topically to treat tinea versicolor.

**acrit·i·cal** (a-krit′ĭ-kəl) [*a-*[1] + *critical*] having no crisis, said especially of febrile diseases ending by lysis.

**acrit·o·chro·ma·cy** (ə-krit″o-kro′mə-se) monochromatism.

**ACRM** American Congress of Rehabilitation Medicine.

**acr(o)-** [Gr. *akron* extremity, from *akros* extreme] a combining form denoting relation to an extremity, top, or summit, or to an extreme.

**ac·ro·ag·no·sis** (ak″ro-ag-no′sis) [*acro-* + *a-*[1] + Gr. *gnōsis* knowledge] lack of sensory recognition of a limb; lack of acrognosis.

**ac·ro·an·es·the·sia** (ak″ro-an″əs-the′zhə) [*acro-* + *anesthesia*] loss of sensation in the extremities.

**ac·ro·ar·thri·tis** (ak″ro-ahr-thri′tis) [*acro-* + *arthritis*] arthritis affecting the extremities.

**ac·ro·blast** (ak′ro-blast) [*acro-* + *-blast*] Golgi material in the spermatid from which arises the acrosome.

**ac·ro·brachy·ceph·a·ly** (ak″ro-brak″ĭ-sef′ə-le) [*acro-* + *brachycephaly*] a condition resulting from fusion of the coronal suture, causing abnormal shortening of the anteroposterior diameter of the skull.

**ac·ro·bys·tio·lith** (ak″ro-bis′te-o-lith) [Gr. *akrobystia* prepuce + *-lith*] postholith.

**ac·ro·bys·ti·tis** (ak″ro-bis-ti′tis) [Gr. *akrobystia* prepuce + *-itis*] posthitis.

**ac·ro·cen·tric** (ak″ro-sen′trik) [*acro-* + *centric*] a type of chromosome having the centromere near one end of the replicating chromosome, so that one arm is much longer than the other. Cf. *metacentric* and *submetacentric.*

**ac·ro·ce·pha·lia** (ak″ro-sə-fa′le-ə) [*acro-* + *cephal-* + *-ia*] oxycephaly.

**ac·ro·ce·phal·ic** (ak″ro-sə-fal′ik) oxycephalic.

**ac·ro·ceph·a·lo·poly·syn·dac·ty·ly (ACPS)** (ak″ro-sef″ə-lo-pol″e-sin-dak′tĭ-le) [*acrocephaly* + *polysyndactyly*] acrocephalosyndactyly with polydactyly as an additional feature. Four types are known: *type I (ACPS I; Noack's syndrome),* autosomal dominant, is the same as acrocephalosyndactyly type V (Pfeiffer type); *type II (ACPS II; Carpenter syndrome),* with mental retardation and brachydactyly is autosomal recessive; *type III (ACPS with leg hypoplasia; Sakati-Nyhan syndrome),* with hypoplastic tibias and deformed, displaced fibulas, is autosomal dominant; *type IV (ACPS IV; Goodman syndrome),* with congenital heart defects, clinodactyly, camptodactyly, and ulnar deviation, but with unimpaired intelligence, is autosomal recessive.

**ac·ro·ceph·a·lo·syn·dac·tyl·ia** (ak″ro-sef″ə-lo-sin″dak-til′e-ə) [MeSH: Acrocephalosyndactylia] acrocephalosyndactyly.

**ac·ro·ceph·a·lo·syn·dac·ty·lism** (ak″ro-sef″ə-lo-sin-dak′tĭ-liz-əm) acrocephalosyndactyly.

**ac·ro·ceph·a·lo·syn·dac·ty·ly** (ak″ro-sef″ə-lo-sin-dak′tĭ-le) [*acrocephaly* + *syndactyly*] craniostenosis characterized by acrocephaly and syndactyly, probably occurring as an autosomal dominant trait and usually as a new mutation; called also *a. type I, Apert syndrome, Apert-Crouzon disease,* and *Vogt's cephalodactyly.* It also occurs with other anomalies, which have been designated *Chotzen syndrome* (type III) and *Pfeiffer type acrocephalosyndactyly* (type V), which is the same as acrocephalopolysyndactyly type I.

**ac·ro·ceph·a·lous** (ak″ro-sef′ə-ləs) oxycephalic.

**ac·ro·ceph·a·ly** (ak″ro-sef′ə-le) oxycephaly.
**a.-syndactyly,** the characteristic shape of the head seen in acrocephalosyndactyly.

**ac·ro·chor·don** (ak″ro-kor′dən) [*acro-* + *chordo-*] a skin-colored to light brown papillomatous cutaneous lesion usually occurring on the neck, upper chest, or axilla of middle-aged women, characterized by a hyperplastic epidermis enclosing a dermal connective tissue stalk composed of loose, edematous collagen fibers; larger lesions may be pedunculated *(soft fibromas).* Called also *fibroepithelial polyp, cutaneous papilloma* or *tag* and *skin tag.*

**ac·ro·ci·ne·sis** (ak″ro-si-ne′sis) [*acro-* + Gr. *kinēsis* motion] excessive motility; abnormal freedom of movement. Called also *acrokinesia.*

**ac·ro·ci·net·ic** (ak″ro-si-net′ik) affected with acrocinesis.

**ac·ro·con·trac·ture** (ak″ro-kən-trak′chər) [*acro-* + *contracture*] contracture of an extremity; contracture of muscles of the hand or foot.

**ac·ro·cy·a·no·sis** (ak″ro-si″ə-no′sis) [*acro-* + *cyanosis*] a condition marked by symmetrical cyanosis of the extremities, with persistent, uneven blue or red discoloration of the skin of the digits, wrists, and ankles and with profuse sweating and coldness of the digits. Called also *Raynaud's sign.*

**ac·ro·der·ma·ti·tis** (ak″ro-dər″mə-ti′tis) [*acro-* + *dermatitis*] [MeSH: Acrodermatitis] inflammation involving the skin of the extremities, especially the hands and feet.
**a. chro′nica atro′phicans,** a diffuse chronic skin disease usually confined to the extremities, occurring almost exclusively in Northern, Central, and Eastern Europe, most often in women, and characterized initially by an erythematous, edematous, pruritic phase followed by sclerosis and atrophy. It is caused by the spirochete *Borrelia burgdorferi,* the tick *Ixodes ricinus* being the vector. See also *Lyme disease,* under *disease.*
**a. conti′nua,** a variant of pustular psoriasis characterized by a chronic distinctive inflammatory eruption of the digits, palms, and soles, sometimes becoming more generalized, with a thin annular vesiculopustular border that gradually extends and recurs, leaving inflamed mildly exfoliating skin. Called also *a. perstans, Hallopeau's a.,* and *dermatitis repens.*
**a. enteropa′thica,** a severe gastrointestinal and cutaneous disease of early childhood, due to an autosomal recessive disorder of zinc uptake and characterized by a vesiculopustulous dermatitis, preferentially located around the body orifices and on the head, hands, and feet, with diarrhea, true steatorrhea, and loss of hair.
**Hallopeau's a.,** a. continua.
**infantile a.,** Gianotti-Crosti syndrome.
**papular a. of childhood, a. papulo′sa infan′tum,** Gianotti-Crosti syndrome.
**a. per′stans,** a. continua.

**ac·ro·der·ma·to·sis** (ak″ro-dər″mə-to′sis) pl. *acrodermato′ses* [*acro-* + *dermatosis*] any disease involving the skin of the extremities.

**ac·ro·dol·i·cho·me·lia** (ak″ro-dol″ĭ-ko-me′le-ə) [*acro-* + *dolicho-* + *-melia*] abnormal or disproportionate length of hands and feet.

**ac·ro·dyn·ia** (ak″ro-din′e-ə) [*acr-* + *-odynia*] [MeSH: Acrodynia] a disease of early childhood characterized by pink, swollen, painful fingers and toes; listlessness, irritability, failure to thrive, and photophobia; rashes, profuse perspiration, loss of teeth, and sometimes redness of the cheeks and tip of the nose. Most cases are toxic neuropathies caused by mercury poisoning; individual sensitivity may also be a factor. Called also *erythredema polyneuropathy* and *Bilderbeck's, Selter's, Swift's, Swift-Feer,* and *pink disease.*

**ac·ro·dys·pla·sia** (ak″ro-dis-pla′zhə) acrocephalosyndactyly.

**ac·ro·es·the·sia** (ak″ro-es-the′zhə) [*acro-* + *esthesia*] 1. increased sensitiveness. 2. pain in the extremities.

**acrog·e·nous** (ə-kroj′ə-nəs) produced at the apex of a conidiophore; said of conidia.

**ac·rog·no·sis** (ak″rog-no′sis) [*acro-* + Gr. *gnōsis* knowledge] sensory recognition of the limbs and of the different portions of each limb in relation to each other.

**ac·ro·hy·po·ther·my** (ak″ro-hi″po-thər′me) [*acro-* + *hypothermy*] abnormal coldness of the hands and feet.

**ac·ro·ker·a·to·sis** (ak″ro-ker″ə-to′sis) a condition involving the skin of the extremities, with the appearance of horny growths.
**paraneoplastic a.,** Bazex's syndrome.
**a. verrucifor′mis,** a genodermatosis inherited as an autosomal dominant trait, characterized by the occurrence on the dorsal aspects of the hands and feet, elbows, knees, and insteps of numerous closely grouped verrucous papules, and sometimes associated with the presence of diffuse hyperkeratosis of the palms and soles. Acrokeratosis verruciformis and keratosis follicularis frequently occur together.

**ac·ro·ki·ne·sia** (ak″ro-kĭ-ne′zhə) acrocinesis.

**acro·le·in** (ak-ro′le-in) [MeSH: Acrolein] a volatile, acrid, highly toxic liquid from the decomposition of glycerin; it is one of the degradation products of cyclophosphamide and is thought to be the cause of hemorrhagic cystitis and neoplasms of the bladder in patients treated with oral cyclophosphamide.

**ac·ro·mac·ria** (ak″ro-mak′re-ə) arachnodactyly.

**ac·ro·mas·ti·tis** (ak″ro-mas-ti′tis) [*acro-* + *mastitis*] inflammation of the nipple.

**ac·ro·me·ga·lia** (ak″ro-mə-ga′le-ə) acromegaly.

**ac·ro·me·gal·ic** (ak″ro-mə-gal′ik) pertaining to or characterized by acromegaly.

**ac·ro·meg·a·lo·gi·gan·tism** (ak″ro-meg″ə-lo-ji′gan-tiz-əm) gigantism and acromegaly due to hypersecretion of growth hormone beginning before puberty and continuing into maturity.

**ac•ro•meg•a•loid•ism** (ak″ro-meg′ə-loid-iz-əm) a bodily condition resembling acromegaly but not due to pituitary disorder.

**ac•ro•meg•a•ly** (ak″ro-meg′ə-le) [*acro-* + *-megaly*] [MeSH: Acromegaly] a chronic disease of adults caused by hypersecretion of growth hormone, characterized by enlargement of many parts of the skeleton, especially distal portions such as the nose, ears, jaws, fingers, and toes. Joint pain resulting from osteoarthrosis occurs, and the joint spaces are increased because of cartilage proliferation. Complications resulting from increased growth hormone secretion include insulin resistance and glucose intolerance, airway obstruction, hypertension, cardiomyopathy, and abnormalities of calcium and bone metabolism.

**ac•ro•mel•al•gia** (ak″ro-məl-al′jə) erythromelalgia.

**ac•ro•mel•ic** (ak″ro-me′lik) [*acro-* + *mel-* + *-ic*] pertaining to or affecting the end of a limb.

**ac•ro•meta•gen•e•sis** (ak″ro-met″ə-jen′ə-sis) [*acro-* + *meta-* + *-genesis*] undue growth of the extremities.

**acro•mi•al** (ə-kro′me-əl) pertaining to the acromion.

**ac•ro•mic•ria** (ak″ro-mik′re-ə) [*acro-* + *micr-* + *-ia*] hypoplasia of the extremities of the skeleton, including the nose, jaws, fingers, and toes; the converse of acromegaly.

**acromi(o)-** [L. *acromion,* q.v.] a combining form denoting relationship to the acromion.

**acro•mio•cla•vic•u•lar** (ə-kro″me-o-klə-vik′u-lər) pertaining to the acromion and clavicle, especially to the articulation between the acromion and clavicle. See also *articulatio acromioclavicularis.*

**acro•mio•cor•a•coid** (ə-kro″me-o-kor′ə-koid) pertaining to the acromion and the coracoid process; called also *coracoacromial.*

**acro•mio•hu•mer•al** (ə-kro″me-o-hu′mər-əl) pertaining to the acromion and humerus.

**acro•mi•on** (ə-kro′me-on) [*acro-* + Gr. *ōmos* shoulder] [TA] [MeSH: Acromion] the lateral extension of the spine of the scapula, projecting over the shoulder joint and forming the highest point of the shoulder; called also *acromial process* and *acromion scapulae.*

**acro•mio•nec•to•my** (ə-kro″me-o-nek′tə-me) resection of the distal end of the acromion, done in the treatment of acromioclavicular arthritis.

**acro•mio•plas•ty** (ə-kro′me-o-plas″te) surgical removal of the anterior hook of the acromion to relieve mechanical compression of the rotator cuff during movement of the glenohumeral joint; called also *anterior acromioplasty.*

**acro•mio•scap•u•lar** (ə-kro″me-o-skap′u-lər) pertaining to the acromion and scapula.

**acro•mio•tho•rac•ic** (ə-kro″me-o-tho-ras′ik) pertaining to the acromion and thorax.

**acrom•pha•lus** (ə-krom′fə-ləs) [*acr-* + *omphalus*] 1. undue prominence of the navel; sometimes a sign of umbilical hernia. 2. the center of the navel.

**ac•ro•myo•to•nia** (ak″ro-mi-o-to′ne-ə) [*acro-* + *myotonia*] contracture of the hand or foot resulting in spastic deformity.

**ac•ro•my•ot•o•nus** (ak″ro-mi-ot′o-nəs) acromyotonia.

**ac•ro•nar•cot•ic** (ak″ro-nahr-kot′ik) both acrid and narcotic.

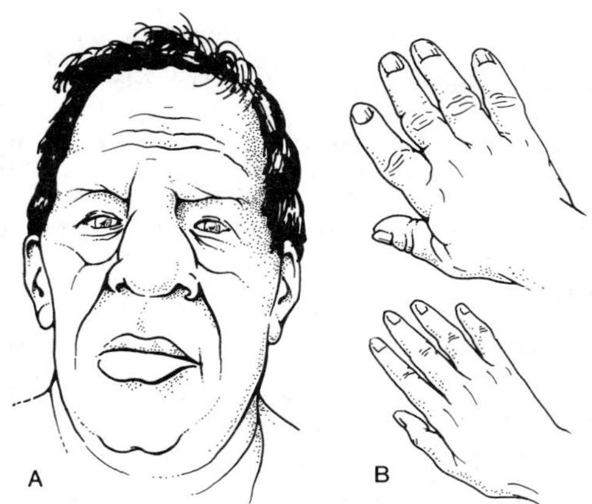


Appearance in acromegaly: *(A),* facial appearance; *(B),* acromegalic hand (upper) and normal hand (lower).

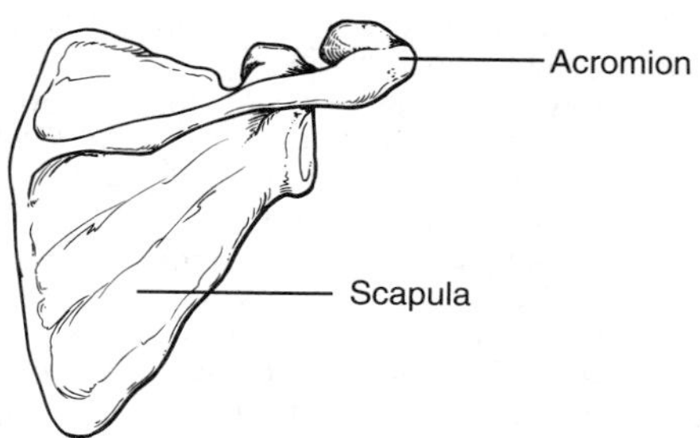


Posterior (dorsal) surface of the scapula, showing the acromion.

**ac•ro•neu•ro•sis** (ak″ro-noo-ro′sis) [*acro-* + *neurosis*] any neuropathy of the extremities.

**ac•ro•nym** (ak′ro-nim) [*acro-* + Gr. *onoma* name] a word formed by the initial letters of the principal components of a compound term, as laser or maser.

**ac•ro•os•te•ol•y•sis** (ak″ro-os″te-ol′ĭ-sis) osteolysis involving the distal phalanges of the fingers and toes.

**ac•ro•pach•ia** (ak″ro-pak′e-ə) [*acro-* + *pachy-* + *-ia*] hypertrophic osteopathy.

**ac•ro•pachy** (ak′ro-pak″e) hypertrophic pulmonary osteoarthropathy.

**ac•ro•pachy•der•ma** (ak″ro-pak″ĭ-der′mə) [*acro-* + *pachy-* + *derma*] thickening of the skin over the extremities, as occurs in acromegaly and pachydermoperiostitis.
**a. with pachyperiostitis,** pachydermoperiostosis.

**ac•ro•pa•ral•y•sis** (ak″ro-pə-ral′ĭ-sis) [*acro-* + *paralysis*] paralysis of the extremities.

**ac•ro•par•es•the•sia** (ak″ro-par″es-the′zhə) [*acro-* + *paresthesia*] 1. paresthesia of the tips of the extremities due to nerve compression at any of several levels, or polyneuritis. 2. a disease marked by attacks of tingling, numbness, and stiffness in the extremities, chiefly the fingers, hands, and forearms, sometimes with pain, pallor of the skin, or slight cyanosis.

**ac•ro•pa•thol•o•gy** (ak″ro-pă-thol′ə-je) [*acro-* + *pathology*] the pathology of diseases affecting the extremities.

**acrop•a•thy** (ă-krop′ə-the) [*acro-* + *-pathy*] any disease of the extremities.
**ulcerative mutilating a.,** hereditary sensory radicular neuropathy.

**ac•ro•pep•tide** (ak″ro-pep′tīd) a protein fraction obtained by heating protein to above 140°C in nonaqueous solvents.

**acrop•e•tal** (ə-krop′ə-təl) [*acro-* + *-petal*] developing from the base toward the summit; pertaining to the production of conidia in fungi.

**ac•ro•pho•bia** (ak″ro-fo′be-ə) [*acro-* + *-phobia*] irrational fear of heights.

**ac•ro•pleu•rog•e•nous** (ak″ro-ploo͝-roj′ə-nəs) produced at the apex and on the sides of a conidiophore; said of conidia.

**ac•ro•pos•thi•tis** (ak″ro-pos-thi′tis) [*acro-* + *posthitis*] posthitis.

**ac•ro•pus•tu•lo•sis** (ak″ro-pus″tu-lo′sis) pustulosis of the extremities.
**infantile a.,** a congenital condition characterized by small pruritic pustules of the hands and feet; episodes last one to two weeks, followed by a remission of a few weeks and another episode. It is usually seen in infants of African descent and resolves completely by age 2 or 3 years.

**ac•ro•scle•ro•der•ma** (ak″ro-sklĕr″o-der′mə) acrosclerosis.

**ac•ro•scle•ro•sis** (ak″ro-sklə-ro′sis) [*acro-* + *sclerosis*] a condition generally regarded as a form of systemic scleroderma that combines the features of Raynaud's disease with scleroderma of the distal parts of the extremities, especially of the digits (sclerodactyly), and of the neck and the face, particularly the nose. Called also *acroscleroderma.*

**ac•ro•some** (ak′ro-sōm) [*acro-* + *-some*] [MeSH: Acrosome] the caplike, membrane-bound structure derived from Golgi elements found at the anterior portion of the nucleus of a spermatozoon; it contains lysosomal enzymes and a proteolytic enzyme, which are believed to facilitate entry of spermatozoa into ova. Called also *acrosomal cap* and *anterior head cap.* See also *acrosome reaction,* under *reaction.*

**ac•ro•sphe•no•syn•dac•tyl•ia** (ak″ro-sfe″no-sin″dak-til′e-ə) acrocephalosyndactyly.

**ac•ro•spi•ro•ma** (ak″ro-spĭ-ro′mə) [*acro-* + *spiroma*] a tumor of the distal portion of a sweat gland.
**eccrine a.,** clear cell hidradenoma.

**ac·ros·te·al·gia** (ak″ros-te-al′jə) [*acr-* + *ostealgia*] a painful apophysitis of the bones of the extremities.

**ac·ro·syn·dac·ty·ly** (ak″ro-sin-dak′tə-le) [*acro-* + *syndactyly*] fusion of the terminal portion of two or more digits, with clefts or sinuses present between their proximal phalanges.

**ac·ro·ter·ic** (ak″ro-ter′ik) pertaining to the tips or outermost parts.

**Ac·ro·the·ca** (ak″ro-the′kə) a former genus of imperfect fungi; *A. pedrosoi* is now called *Fonsecaea pedrosoi.*

**Ac·ro·the·ci·um** (ak″ro-the′se-əm) a former genus of imperfect fungi. *A. flocco′sum* is now called *Epidermophyton floccosum.*

**acrot·ic** (ă-krot′ik) [*a-*[1] + Gr. *krotos* beat] pertaining to absence or weakness of the pulse.

**ac·ro·tism** (ak′ro-tiz-əm) [*a-*[1] + Gr. *krotos* beat + *-ism*] absence or imperceptibility of the pulse.

**ac·ro·tropho·dyn·ia** (ak″ro-trof″o-din′e-ə) [*acro-* + *troph-* + *-odynia*] a trophic disorder with neuritis and paresthesia from exposure of extremities to cold and moisture.

**ac·ro·tropho·neu·ro·sis** (ak″ro-trof″o-noo-ro′sis) trophoneurotic disturbance of the extremities.

**acryl·am·ide** (ə-kril′ə-mīd) a vinyl monomer used in the production of polymers with many industrial uses. The polymers are nontoxic but exposure to acrylamide can cause peripheral neuropathy, polyneuritis, and central nervous system lesions.

**acry·late** (ə-kril′āt) a salt, ester, or conjugate base of acrylic acid.

**acryl·ic** (ə-kril′ik) pertaining to polymers of acrylic acid, methacrylic acid or acrylonitrile, as acrylic fibers or acrylic resins used in dental prostheses, intraocular lenses, ion-exchange resins, and as adsorbents in chromatography.

**acryl·ic ac·id** (ə-kril′ik) a readily polymerizing liquid used as a monomer for acrylic polymers; see also *acrylic.*

**ac·ry·lo·ni·trile** (ak″rə-lo-ni′tril) [MeSH: Acrylonitrile] a colorless halogenated hydrocarbon used in the making of plastics and as a pesticide; its vapors are irritant to the respiratory tract and eyes, may cause systemic poisoning, and are carcinogenic. Called also *2-propenenitrile* and *vinyl cyanide.*

**ACS** American Cancer Society; American Chemical Society; American College of Surgeons.

**ACSM** American College of Sports Medicine.

**act** (akt) a doing, or a thing done; a performance involving motor activity.
**reflex a.,** a relatively fixed action or pattern of response performed as a result of the triggering of a reflex arc and usually without involvement of the higher centers.

**Ac·taea** (ak-te′ə) [L.; Gr. *aktē* elder-tree] a genus of plants of the family Ranunculaceae. *A. odora′ta* (bitter weed) and *A. richardso′ni* (rubber weed) are poisonous to sheep and goats. *A. spica′ta* is the red cohosh, a medicinal plant.

**ac·ta·pla·nin** (ak″tə-pla′nin) any of various glycopeptide antibiotics used as veterinary growth stimulants, derived from species of *Actinoplanes,* containing a chlorophenyl group, glucose, mannose, rhamnose, and other amino acids.

**ACTH** adrenocorticotropic hormone.

**Ac·thar** (ak′thar) trademark for preparations of corticotropin.

**Act·HIB** (akt′hib) trademark from a preparation of *Haemophilus influenzae* b conjugate vaccine.

**Ac·ti·dil** (ak′tĭ-dil) trademark for a preparation of triprolidine hydrochloride.

**Ac·ti·Di·one** (ak″tĭ-di′ōn) trademark for a preparation of cycloheximide.

**Ac·ti·gall** (ak′tĭ-gawl″) trademark for a preparation of ursodiol.

**Ac·tim·mune** (ak′tĭ-mūn) trademark for a preparation of interferon gamma-1b.

**ac·tin** (ak′tin) a protein of the myofibril, localized in the I band; acting along with myosin particles, it is responsible for the contraction and relaxation of muscle. In the absence of salt, it becomes globular *(G-actin),* and in the presence of potassium chloride and adenosine triphosphate it polymerizes, forming long fibers *(F-actin)* Cf. *actomyosin* and *myosin.* See Plate 35.

**act·ing out** (ak′ting out) [MeSH: Acting Out] the expression of unconscious feelings and fantasies in behavior; reacting to present situations as if they were the original situation that gave rise to the feelings and fantasies, i.e., acting out of a transference. Often applied imprecisely to any sort of disapproved impulsive behavior.

**ac·tin·ic** (ak-tin′ik) [*aktin-* + *-ic*] pertaining to those rays of light beyond the violet end of the spectrum that produce chemical effects.

**ac·ti·nic·i·ty** (ak″tĭ-nis′ĭ-te) actinism.

**ac·tin·i·form** (ak-tin′ĭ-form) [*aktin-* + *form*] formed like a ray; radiate.

**α-ac·tin·in** (ak′tə-nin) a protein found in muscle, fibroblasts, and epithelial cells; it is believed to play a role in binding actin molecules together. See also *vinculin.*

**ac·ti·nism** (ak′tĭ-niz-əm) [*aktin-* + *-ism*] that property of radiant energy which produces chemical changes, as in photography or heliotherapy; called also *actinicity.*

**ac·tin·i·um** (ak-tin′e-um) [Gr. *aktis* ray] [MeSH: Actinium] a rare metallic chemical element occurring in the ores of uranium and having radioactive properties; its atomic number is 89, its atomic weight 227, and its symbol Ac.

**actin(o)-** [Gr. *aktis,* gen. *aktinos* a ray] a combining form denoting relation to a ray, as ray-shaped, or pertaining to some form of radiation.

**ac·ti·no·bac·il·lo·sis** (ak″tĭ-no-bas″ĭ-lo′sis) [MeSH: Actinobacillosis] a disease of domestic animals and occasionally humans, resembling actinomycosis but caused by species of *Actinobacillus.* In cattle and sheep the species is *A. lignieresii;* characteristics in cattle include granulomatous lesions in the throat and mouth *(wooden tongue)* and in sheep, suppurative lesions of the skin and lungs. In horses and pigs the species is *A. equuli* and the disease is more commonly known as *equulosis* (q.v.).

**Ac·ti·no·bac·il·lus** (ak″tĭ-no-bə-sil′us) [*actino-* + *bacillus*] [MeSH: Actinobacillus] a genus of gram-negative, fermentative nonmotile, coccoid or rod-shaped bacteria of the family Pasteurellaceae, part of the normal mammalian microflora. They are potentially pathogenic for humans and for cattle, sheep, horses, and pigs, causing granulomatous lesions.
**A. actinoi′des,** a species of uncertain status that is pathogenic for goats and calves, causing lung lesions.
**A. actinomycetemco′mitans,** a species that is found in association with species of *Actinomyces* in actinomycotic lesions and septicemias; the etiologic role is unclear. It has also been isolated from the human gingival crevice.
**A. equu′li,** a species that is found normally on mucous membranes but can also cause equulosis in horses and pigs.
**A. ligniere′sii,** a species that is primarily a commensal and pathogen of domestic animals, although it occasionally infects humans; it causes actinobacillosis.
**A. su′is,** a species isolated from horses, pigs, and cattle. It produces pneumonia and septicemia in pigs. The organisms have also been isolated from human clinical blood and respiratory and wound specimens.

**ac·ti·nob·o·lin** (ak″tĭ-nob′ə-lin) a broad-spectrum antibiotic elaborated by *Streptomyces griseoviridus* var. *atrofaciens,* which exhibits activity against a wide range of bacteria and against various neoplasms, and inhibits cariogenic microorganisms in rats; it is being studied for use in the control of caries in humans.

**ac·ti·no·chem·is·try** (ak″tĭ-no-kem′is-tre) [*actino-* + *chemistry*] photochemistry.

**ac·ti·no·con·ges·tin** (ak″tĭ-no-kən-jes′tin) congestin.

**ac·ti·no·der·ma·ti·tis** (ak″tĭ-no-dər″mə-ti′tis) cutaneous inflammation due to excessive exposure to sunlight or exposure to x-rays.

**ac·tin·o·lyte** (ak-tin′ə-līt) [*actino-* + Gr. *lytos* soluble, from *lyein* to loosen] any substance that is markedly changed by light.

**Ac·ti·no·ma·du·ra** (ak″tĭ-no-mə-dŏŏr′ə) [*actino-* + *Madura* (now *Madurai*), a city in India] a genus of bacteria of the family Nocardiaceae, order Actinomycetales, consisting of non–acid-fast organisms that form nonfragmenting branched filaments.
**A. madu′rae,** a species distributed worldwide in soil, and a common cause of actinomycotic mycetoma; called also *Nocardia madurae.*
**A. pelletie′ri,** a species commonly found in Africa, India, and North and South America; it is the cause of actinomycotic mycetoma.

**ac·ti·nom·e·ter** (ak″tĭ-nom′ə-ter) [*actino-* + *-meter*] an instrument for measuring radiation intensity, particularly that from the sun or other sources capable of causing photochemical reactions.

**ac·ti·nom·e·try** (ak″tĭ-nom′ə-tre) the measurement of the photochemical power of light.

**ac·ti·no·my·ce·li·al** (ak″tĭ-no-mi-se′le-əl) 1. pertaining to the mycelium of an actinomyces. 2. actinomycetic.

**Ac·ti·no·my·ces** (ak″tĭ-no-mi′sēz) [*actino-* + Gr. *mykēs* fungus] [MeSH: Actinomyces] a genus of bacteria of the family Actinomycetaceae, consisting of gram-positive, asporogenous, irregularly staining organisms that form branched filaments. They are non–acid-fast and nonmotile.
**A. asteroi′des,** *Nocardia asteroides.*
**A. bo′vis,** a non–acid-fast, facultatively anaerobic species of serologic group B. It is a normal inhabitant of animal mucous membranes, and the specific etiologic agent of actinomycosis in cattle.

**A. brasilien'sis,** *Nocardia brasiliensis.*
**A. dentocario'sus,** *Rothia dentocariosa.*
**A. epping'ri,** *Nocardia asteroides.*
**A. erikso'nii,** *Bifidobacterium eriksonii.*
**A. gonidiafor'mis,** *Fusobacterium gonidiaformans.*
**A. israe'lii,** a non–acid-fast anaerobic species of serologic group D, parasitic in the mouth and proliferating in necrotic tissue. It is the etiologic agent of human actinomycosis, especially infections associated with the use of intrauterine devices or periodontal disease, and it also can cause actinomycotic mycetoma. Occasionally it is implicated in infections in cattle.
**A. lu'teus,** *Nocardia lutea.*
**A. mu'ris, A. mu'ris-rat'ti,** *Streptobacillus moniliformis.*
**A. naeslun'dii,** an aerobic species of serologic group A. It is a normal inhabitant of the oral cavity and an etiologic agent of human actinomycosis and periodontal disease.
**A. necro'phorus,** *Fusobacterium necrophorum.*
**A. odontoly'ticus,** a facultatively anaerobic species of serologic group E. It is a natural inhabitant of the human oral cavity and has been found in dental caries.
**A. pseudonecro'phorus,** *Fusobacterium necrophorum.*
**A. vina'ceus,** *Streptomyces vinaceus.*
**A. visco'sus,** a facultative anaerobic species of serologic group F. It is found in the oral cavity of man, hamsters, and rats, and is a cause of dental caries in laboratory animals; pathogenicity for humans has not been established.

**ac·ti·no·my·ces** (ak″tĭ-no-mi'sēz) pl. *actinomyce'tes* [MeSH: Actinomyces] A bacterium of the genus *Actinomyces.*

**Ac·ti·no·my·ce·ta·ceae** (ak″tĭ-no-mi″sĕ-ta'se-e) [MeSH: Actinomycetaceae] a family of bacteria, order Actinomycetales, consisting of gram-positive, nonsporulating irregularly shaped rods, which tend to form branched filaments. It contains the genera *Actinomyces, Arachnia, Bacterionema, Bifidobacterium,* and *Rothia.*

**Ac·ti·no·my·ce·ta·les** (ak″tĭ-no-mi″sə-ta'lēz) [MeSH: Actinomycetales] an order of bacteria made up of elongated cells that tend to form branching filaments; it includes the families Actinomycetaceae, Actinoplanaceae, Dermatophilaceae, Frankiaceae, Micromonosporaceae, Mycobacteriaceae, Nocardiaceae, and Streptomycetaceae.

**ac·ti·no·my·cete** (ak″tĭ-no-mi'sēt) any bacterium of the order Actinomycetales.
**nocardioform a's,** a morphological group of actinomycetes characterized by a fugacious mycelium that breaks up into bacillary or coccal forms; all genera in this group are gram-positive and aerobic.

**ac·ti·no·my·ce·tes** (ak″tĭ-no-mi-se'tēz) plural of *actinomyces* and *actinomycete.*

**ac·ti·no·my·cet·ic** (ak″tĭ-no-mi-set'ik) of or caused by actinomyces; of or pertaining to bacteria of the order Actinomycetales or diseases caused by such organisms.

**ac·ti·no·my·ce·tin** (ak″tĭ-no-mi-se'tin) a substance derived from cultures of the actinomycete *Streptomyces albus;* it lyses dead bacteria.

**ac·ti·no·my·ce·to·ma** (ak″tĭ-no-mi″sə-to'mə) [*actino-* + *mycetoma*] actinomycotic mycetoma.

**ac·ti·no·my·cin** (ak″tĭ-no-mi'sin) a large, complex family of antibiotics obtained from cultures of various species of *Streptomyces,* which have antibacterial, antifungal, and cytotoxic properties. Actinomycin D (see *dactinomycin*) is an antineoplastic agent.

**ac·ti·no·my·co·ma** (ak-tĭ-no-mi-ko'mə) [*actinomyces* + *-oma*] a tumor-like reactive lesion due to actinomycetes.

**ac·ti·no·my·co·sis** (ak″tĭ-no-mi-ko'sis) [*actino-* + *mycosis*] [MeSH: Actinomycosis] an infectious disease caused predominantly by *Actinomyces israelii* in humans and by *A. bovis* in cattle. Characteristics include indolent lymphadenitis of the mouth and neck (with the characteristic *lumpy jaw* in cattle); intraperitoneal and pelvic abscesses, including those of the liver; and sometimes lung abscesses due to aspiration. Infection is accompanied by fever and weight loss. Pus from a suppurative lesion may contain yellow clusters called sulfur granules.

**ac·ti·no·my·cot·ic** (ak″tĭ-no-mi-kot'ik) pertaining to or affected with actinomycosis.

**ac·ti·no·my·co·tin** (ak″tĭ-no-mi'kə-tin) a therapeutic preparation of cultures of *Actinomyces,* used in treating actinomycosis.

**ac·ti·no·phage** (ak-tin'o-fāj) a virus that causes the lysis of actinomycetes.

**ac·ti·no·phy·to·sis** (ak″tĭ-no-fi-to'sis) infection with *Actinomyces* or *Nocardia.*

**Ac·ti·no·pla·na·ceae** (ak″tĭ-no-plə-na'se-e) a family of bacteria of the order Actinomycetales, consisting of gram-positive, spore-forming organisms that form a definite mycelium. They occur widely in nature as soil saprophytes.

**Ac·ti·no·pla·nes** (ak″tĭ-no-pla'nēz) [*actino-* + Gr. *planēs* one who wanders] a genus of bacteria of the family Actinoplanaceae, order Actinomycetales, made up of saprophytic forms found on a wide variety of plant material and in soil.
**A. aurantico'lor,** a species that is the source of the antibiotic pluracin.
**A. teichomyce'ticus,** a species that is the source of teicoplanin.
**A. utahen'sis,** a species that produces acarbose.

**ac·tino·qui·nol so·di·um** (ak-tin'o-kwĭ-nōl) an ultraviolet screen.

**ac·ti·no·ther·a·py** (ak″tĭ-no-ther'ə-pe) [*actino-* + *therapy*] phototherapy.

**ac·ti·no·tox·in** (ak″tĭ-no-tok'sin) a crude poison derived from alcoholic extracts of the tentacles of sea anemones.

**ac·tion** (ak'shən) [L. *actio*] any performance of function or movement either of any part or organ or of the whole body.
**ball-valve a.,** the intermittent obstruction caused by a free or partially attached foreign body in a tubular or cavitary structure, as by a foreign body in a bronchus, a stone in a bile duct, or a tumor in the cardiac atrium.
**buffer a.,** an action that tends to stabilize an inanimate system or a body function or state, such as pH, blood pressure, [$Ca^{2+}$], etc.; most commonly used to denote the stabilization of pH by acid-base buffers (tampon a.).
**capillary a.,** the transport of a fluid in a tube, caused by adhesion of the fluid to the tube wall.
**contact a.,** contact catalysis.
**cumulative a.,** action of increased intensity, as may be evidenced after administration of several doses of a drug due to the accumulation of the drug in the body so that the biological effect is greater than after the first dose. Called also *cumulative effect.*
**reflex a.,** a response, often involuntary, resulting from the passage of excitation potential from a receptor to a muscle or gland, over a reflex arc.
**specific a.,** the action of a drug which is exerted on a certain definite pathogenic organism.
**specific dynamic a.,** former name for *obligatory thermogenesis.*
**tampon a.,** buffer a.
**trigger a.,** an action that releases energy whose character has no relation to the process which released it.

**Ac·ti·vase** (ak'tĭ-vās) trademark for a preparation of alteplase.

**ac·ti·vate** (ak'tĭ-vāt) to render active.

**ac·ti·va·tion** (ak″tĭ-va'shən) 1. the act or process of rendering active. 2. the transformation of a proenzyme into an active enzyme by the action of a kinase or another proenzyme. 3. gain in the purifying of sewage by means of activated sludge. 4. the process by which the central nervous system is stimulated into activity through the mediation of the reticular activating system. 5. the deliberate induction of a pattern of electrical activity in the brain in electroencephalography.
**allosteric a.,** increase in enzyme activity by binding of an effector at an allosteric site that causes at the catalytic site either increased binding affinity of the enzyme for the substrate or increased rate of catalytic turnover.
**contact a.,** initiation of the intrinsic pathway of coagulation through interaction of factor XII with various electronegative surfaces, such as collagen fibers, skin, or sebum in vivo, or particulate silicates in vitro.
**lymphocyte a.,** stimulation of lymphocytes by specific antigen or nonspecific mitogens resulting in macromolecular synthesis (RNA, protein, and DNA) and production of lymphokines; it is followed by

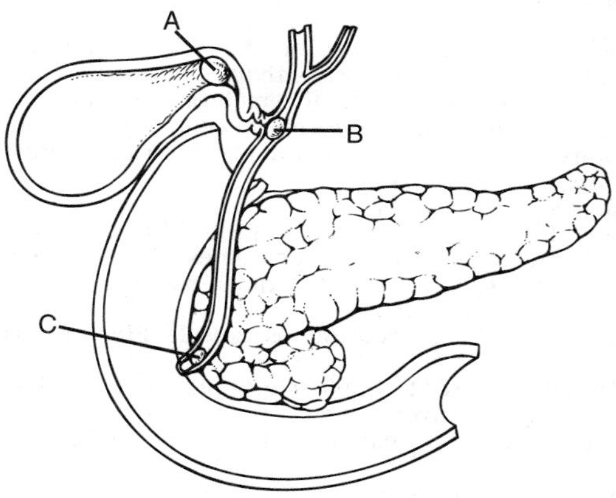

Ball-valve action. Calculi obstructing the cystic duct *(A),* common hepatic duct *(B),* and common bile duct *(C).*

proliferation and differentiation of the progeny into various effector and memory cells.

**ac·ti·va·tor** (ak′tĭ-va″tər) 1. a substance that combines with an enzyme to increase its catalytic activity. 2. a substance that stimulates the development of a particular structure in the embryo. Cf. *inductor* and *organizer.* 3. functional a. 4. a chemical or other form of energy that causes another substance to become reactive or that induces a chemical reaction.
**bow a.,** a functional activator, the halves of which are connected by a wire bow or safety-pin loop; between the halves of the anterior area, a layer of rubber is attached as a shock absorber and to open the bite in front. Called also *Schwarz a.*
**functional a.,** a myofunctional removable orthodontic appliance that acts as a passive transmitter of the force produced by the function of the activated muscle, and applied to the teeth and alveolar processes to effect tooth movement. Called also *Andresen appliance, monoblock a.,* and *monoblock appliance.*
**monoblock a.,** a removable orthodontic appliance utilizing muscle forces to achieve therapeutic correction; called also *Andresen appliance* and *functional a.*
**plasminogen a.,** a general term for a group of substances that have the ability to cleave plasminogen and convert it into plasmin, its active form; see *t-plasminogen a.* and *u-plasminogen a.*
**polyclonal a.,** a mitogen that activates lymphocytes of many antigenic specificities, in contrast to an antigen, which only activates cells specific for the antigen. Some polyclonal activators activate T cells; others activate B cells.
**prothrombin a.,** any of the substances in the intrinsic or extrinsic pathways of coagulation including factors III, VII, X, and XII.
**Schwarz a.,** bow a.
**single chain urokinase-type plasminogen a. (scu-PA),** prourokinase.
**tissue plasminogen a. (TPA, t-PA), t-plasminogen a.** [EC 3.4.21.68], a serine endopeptidase synthesized by endothelial cells, the major physiologic activator of plasminogen; when bound to fibrin clots it catalyzes the conversion of plasminogen to plasmin by hydrolysis of a specific arginine-valine bond. It can be produced by recombinant technology for use in therapeutic thrombolysis.
**u-plasminogen a.** [EC 3.4.21.74], **urinary plasminogen a.,** a serine endopeptidase that acts as a plasminogen activator by catalyzing the preferential cleavage of plasminogen at the same arginine-valine bond where t-plasminogen activator (t-PA) cleaves. It is produced in the kidney and excreted in the urine and has been used to induce therapeutic thrombolysis; unlike t-PA or prourokinase (single chain urokinase-type plasminogen activator) it does not require fibrin for activity. Called also *urokinase.*

**ac·tive** (ak′tiv) characterized by action; not passive; not expectant.
**optically a.,** capable of rotating the plane of polarization of a light wave.

**ac·ti·vin** (ak′tĭ-vin) a nonsteroidal regulator, composed of two covalently linked beta subunits, that is synthesized in the pituitary gland and gonads and stimulates the secretion of follicle-stimulating hormone. The actions of activins are the opposite of those of inhibins.

**ac·tiv·i·ty** (ak-tiv′ĭ-te) [L. *agere* to do, drive] 1. the state of being active; the ability to produce some effect; the extent of some function or action. 2. a thermodynamic quantity that represents the effective concentration of a solute in a nonideal solution; if concentrations are replaced by activities, the equations for equilibrium constants, electrode potentials, osmotic pressure, boiling point elevation, freezing point depression, and vapor pressures of volatile solutes are converted from approximations that hold only for dilute solutions to exact equations that hold for all concentrations. The activity is equal to the product of the concentration and the activity coefficient, a dimensionless number measuring deviation from nonideality. Symbol *a.* 3. for radioactivity, the number of disintegrations per unit time of a radioactive material, measured in curies or becquerels. Symbol *A.* 4. in electroencephalography and electromyography, the presence of recordable electrical energy in a muscle or nerve. 5. optical a.
**alpha a.,** see under *rhythm.*
**background a.,** in measurements of physical or physiological processes, the ongoing generalized, sometimes artifactual, activity from which the more specific activity in question must be distinguished.
**beta a.,** see under *rhythm.*
**continuous muscle a., continuous muscle fiber a.,** Isaacs' syndrome.
**a's of daily living (ADL),** activities routinely performed daily by the average person in a given society; rehabilitation following illness or injury often aims to help patients achieve independence in performing them.
**delta a.,** see under *rhythm.*
**discrete a.,** pathologically reduced electrical activity on a recording from a muscle during maximal voluntary contractions, so that the normal interference pattern (q.v.) is lacking and several discrete motor unit action potentials can be identified.
**electrical a.,** activity (def. 4).
**end-plate a.,** spontaneous activity recorded close to motor end plates in normal muscle. There are two types: *monophasic* (or *end-plate noise*) consists of dense, steady, entirely negative potentials with low amplitude and high frequency, similar to the miniature end-plate potentials of experimental animals; *biphasic* (or *end-plate spikes*) consists of irregular, alternately negative and positive spike potentials that come in short bursts with high frequencies.
**enzyme a.,** the catalytic effect exerted by an enzyme, expressed as units per milligram of enzyme (specific activity) or as molecules of substrate transformed per minute per molecule of enzyme (molecular activity). The conventional unit of enzyme activity is the International Unit (IU), equal to one micromole of substrate transformed per minute. A proposed coherent Système Internationale (SI) unit is the katal (kat), equal to one mole of substrate transformed per second.
**epileptiform a.,** interictal activity on an electroencephalogram, characterized by paroxysmal spike, polyspike, or sharp wave discharges; it may occur in patients who have never had a seizure, and it does not occur in all epileptics. Called also *epileptiform discharges.*
**insertion a., insertional a.,** the electrical activity caused by insertion or movement of a needle electrode; it is prolonged in neuropathies and myopathies and is diminished in some metabolic disorders.
**intermittent rhythmic delta a.,** slow, paroxysmal, relatively constant delta activity seen on the electroencephalogram, associated frequently with metabolic disorders or diffuse encephalopathies and sometimes with subfrontal, deep midline, or posterior fossa lesions; it may be stronger occipitally in children and frontally in adults.
**intrinsic sympathomimetic a. (ISA),** the ability of a $\beta$-blocker to stimulate $\beta$-adrenergic receptors weakly during $\beta$-blockade. Called also *partial agonist a.*
**leukemia-associated inhibitory a. (LIA),** the inhibition of normal marrow cells of donors from forming colonies of granulocytes and macrophages, induced in vitro by the presence of cell extracts, or of culture media conditioned by cells, from the bone marrow, spleen, or blood of patients with acute leukemia.
**nonsuppressible insulin-like a. (NSILA),** insulin-like growth factors.
**optical a.,** the ability of a chemical compound to rotate the plane of polarization of plane-polarized light.
**partial agonist a.,** intrinsic sympathomimetic a.
**plasma renin a.,** a measurement of the enzymatic activity of renin in vitro; angiotensinogen is added to a sample containing renin and the amount of angiotensin I generated is measured.
**polymorphic delta a.,** continuous irregular slow activity that is variable in duration and amplitude and may change little with sleep or other physiological alterations; it may be related to deafferentation of an area of the cortex, to metabolic factors, or to the presence of subcortical cerebral lesions and tumors.
**specific a.,** activity per unit weight of a radioactive material, or the activity of a radioisotope per unit weight of the element (including stable isotopes) present.
**spontaneous a.,** electrical activity recorded from a resting, unstimulated muscle or nerve after insertion activity has ceased.
**theta a.,** see under *rhythm.*
**triggered a.,** triggered automaticity.
**voluntary a.,** electrical and mechanical activity recorded in a muscle during contractions that are under conscious control.

**ac·to·dig·in** (ak″to-dij′in) a cardiac glycoside composed of a steroid nucleus linked to a glucose molecule.

**ac·to·my·o·sin** (ak″to-mi′o-sin) [MeSH: Actomyosin] a complex of the proteins actin and myosin occurring in muscle. Cf. *actin* and *myosin.* See also *myosin ATPase.*

**acu-** [L. *acus* needle] a combining form denoting relationship to a needle.

**Ac·u·a·ria** (ak″u-a′re-ə) a genus of nematodes that infests birds. *A. spira′lis* is found in the proventriculus and esophagus of fowls, causing lesions that may be fatal.

**acu·i·ty** (ə-ku′ĭ-te) [L. *acuitas* sharpness] clarity or clearness, especially of the vision.
**Vernier a.,** displacement threshold; see under *threshold.*
**visual a.,** the ability to discriminate visually between forms, measured by Snellen's test type or, sometimes, by Landolt's rings.

**acu·le·ate** (ə-ku′le-āt) [L. *aculeatus* thorny] covered with sharp points; pointed.

**acu·mi·nate** (ə-ku′mĭ-nāt) [L. *acuminatus*] sharp pointed.

**acu·point** (ak′u-point) [MeSH: Acupuncture Points] a specific site of needle insertion along a body meridian in acupuncture.

**acu·pres·sure** (ak′u-presh″ər) [*acu-* + *pressure*] [MeSH: Acupressure] compression of a bleeding vessel by inserting needles into adjacent tissue.

**acu·punc·ture** (ak′u-punk″chər) [*acu-* + *puncture*] [MeSH: Acupuncture] a traditional Chinese medical practice of insertion of fine needles into specific exterior body locations to relieve pain, to induce surgical anesthesia, and for therapeutic purposes.

**acus** (a′kəs) [L.] a needle or needlelike process.

**acu·sec·tion** (ak′u sek″shən) cutting by means of the electrosurgical needle.

**acu·sec·tor** (ak′u-sek″tər) [*acu-* + *sector*] an electric needle used like a scalpel for incising tissues.

**acute** (ə-kūt′) [L. *acutus* sharp] having a short and relatively severe course.

**acy·a·not·ic** (a-si″ə-not′ik) characterized by absence of cyanosis.

**acy·clic** (a-sik′lik, a-si′klik) 1. in chemistry, having an open-chain structure; aliphatic. 2. occurring independently of a cycle, as of the menstrual cycle.

**acy·clo·vir** (a-si′klo-vir) [USP] [MeSH: Acyclovir] a synthetic acyclic purine nucleoside with selective antiviral activity against herpes simplex virus (types 1 and 2, human herpesvirus 3, Epstein-Barr virus, and cytomegalovirus). It is used in the treatment of genital and mucocutaneous herpesvirus infections in certain patients, both immunocompromised and nonimmunocompromised.
**a. sodium,** the monosodium salt of acyclovir, used intravenously in the treatment of herpes simplex and herpes genitalis in immunocompromised patients and children and severe herpes genitalis in immunocompetent patients.

**acyl** (a′səl) an organic radical derived from an organic acid by removal of the hydroxyl group from the carboxyl group.

**ac·yl·ase** (a′sə-lās) amidase (def. 1).

**ac·yl·a·tion** (a″sə-la′shən) [MeSH: Acylation] the introduction of an acyl radical into the molecule of a chemical compound.

**ac·yl CoA** (a′səl ko-a′) acyl coenzyme A.

**ac·yl CoA:cho·les·ter·ol ac·yl·trans·fer·ase** (a′səl ko-a′ kə-les′tər-ol a″səl-trans′fər-ās) sterol *O*-acyltransferase.

**ac·yl-CoA de·hy·dro·gen·ase** (a′səl ko-a′ de-hi′dro-jən-ās) [EC 1.3.99.3] any of several enzymes of the oxidoreductase class that catalyze the oxidation of acyl coenzyme A thioesters to the enoyl coenzyme A form, using a flavin electron acceptor. The reaction is a step in the degradation of fatty acids and the *trans* isomer of enoyl coenzyme A is formed exclusively. Individual enzymes are specific for certain ranges of acyl chain lengths.
**long-chain a.-C. d. (LCAD) deficiency,** a defect in mitochondrial beta oxidation due to deficiency of the acyl-CoA dehydrogenase acting on long chain length fatty acids. It is clinically similar to MCAD deficiency, but urinary excretion is of long-chain dicarboxylic acids and skeletal muscle weakness and cardiac enlargement may also be present.
**medium-chain a.-C. d. (MCAD) deficiency,** a defect in mitochondrial beta oxidation due to deficiency of the acyl-CoA dehydrogenase acting on medium chain length fatty acids. It is characterized by recurring episodes of hypoglycemia, vomiting, and lethargy, with urinary excretion of medium-chain dicarboxylic acids, minimal ketogenesis, and low plasma and tissue levels of carnitine.
**short-chain a.-C. d. (SCAD) deficiency,** a defect in mitochondrial beta oxidation due to deficiency of the acyl-CoA dehydrogenase acting on short chain length fatty acids. Clinical presentation is variable, but myopathy and abnormalities of carnitine accumulation and excretion are often present.

**acyl-CoA de·sat·ur·ase** (a′səl-ko-a′ de-sach′ə-rās) stearoyl-CoA desaturase.

**ac·yl CoA syn·the·tase** (a′səl-ko-a′ sin′thə-tās) 1. any enzyme of the ligase class that catalyzes the formation of an activated acyl coenzyme A thioester; individual enzymes are specific for a range of fatty acid chain lengths. See also individual enzymes: *acetate–CoA ligase*, *butyrate–CoA ligase*, and *long-chain-fatty-acid–CoA ligase.* 2. long-chain-fatty-acid–CoA ligase.

**ac·yl CoA syn·the·tase (GDP-forming)** (a′səl ko-a′ sin′thə-tās) acid–CoA ligase (GDP-forming).

**ac·yl co·en·zyme A** (a′səl ko-en′zīm) [MeSH: Acyl Coenzyme A] a thiol ester of a carboxylic acid, particularly a long-chain fatty acid, and coenzyme A. Its formation is the first step in fatty acid oxidation, leading to the sequential production of two-carbon groups and progressively shorter acyl coenzyme A compounds until the entire chain is degraded. Also written *acyl CoA.*

**ac·yl·glyc·er·ol** (a″səl-glis′ər-ol) glyceride.

**2-ac·yl·glyc·er·ol *O*-ac·yl·trans·fer·ase** (a″səl-glis′ər-ol a″səl-trans′fər-ās) [EC 2.3.1.22] an enzyme of the transferase class that catalyzes the transfer of the acyl group from palmitoyl coenzyme A or other long chain acyl coenzyme A to a monoglyceride to form a diglyceride. The reaction occurs in the intestinal mucosa, synthesizing triglycerides from monoglycerides produced during digestion. Called also *acylglycerol palmitoyltransferase* and *monoglyceride acyltransferase.*

**ac·yl·glyc·er·ol li·pase** (a″səl-glis′ər-ol li′pās) [EC 3.1.1.23] an enzyme of the hydrolase class that catalyzes the cleavage of the last long-chain fatty acyl group from monoglycerides formed during the digestion of lipids. It occurs in the small intestine.

**ac·yl·glyc·er·ol pal·mi·to·yl·trans·fer·ase** (a″səl-glis′ər-ol pal″mĭ-to″əl-trans′fər-ās) 2-acylglycerol *O*-acyltransferase.

***N*-ac·yl·neu·ra·min·ic ac·id** (a″səl-noor″ə-min′ik) sialic acid.

***N*-ac·yl·neu·ra·min·ate cy·ti·dyl·yl·trans·fer·ase** (a″səl-noo-ram′ĭ-nāt si″tĭ-dəl-əl-trans′fər-ās) [EC 2.7.7.43] an enzyme of the transferase class that catalyzes the transfer of a cytidylyl group from CTP to a sialic acid to form the corresponding CMP-sialic acid, a nucleotide sugar compound that donates sialic acid residues in the biosynthesis of gangliosides.

***N*-ac·yl·sphin·go·sine** (a″səl-sfing′go-sēn) ceramide.

**acyl·sphin·go·sine de·acyl·ase** (a″səl-sfing′go-sēn de-a′səl-ās) ceramidase.

**ac·yl·trans·fer·ase** (a″səl-trans′fər-ās) [EC 2.3] 1. one of a subclass of enzymes of the transferase class that catalyze the transfer of an acyl group from a donor (often the corresponding acyl coenzyme A derivative) to an acceptor compound. Many form esters or amides. 2. a further division of this subclass, a sub-subclass [EC 2.3.1], to distinguish it from the other sub-subclass, aminoacyltransferases. Called also *transacylase.*

**acys·tia** (a-sis′te-ə) [*a-*[1] + *cyst-* + *-ia*] congenital absence of the bladder.

**acys·ti·ner·via** (ə-sis″tĭ-nər′ve-ə) [*a-*[1] + *cysti-* + *nerve* + *-ia*] defective nervous tone in the bladder.

**acys·ti·neu·ria** (ə-sis″tĭ-noo′re-ə) acystinervia.

**AD** anodal duration; alcohol dehydrogenase; [L.] *au′ris dex′tra,* right ear.

**ad** [L. *ad* to] used in writing prescriptions to indicate that a substance (usually a diluent) be added up to a certain amount.

**ad-** [L. *ad* to] a prefix meaning to or toward, addition to, nearness, or intensification.

**-ad**[1] [L. *ad* to] an adverbial suffix meaning toward, as in caudad, cephalad.

**-ad**[2] [Gr. *-as,* gen. *-ados*] a suffix denoting a group, or derivation from or connection with.

**ADA** American Dental Association; American Diabetes Association; American Dietetic Association; adenosine deaminase.

**adac·tyl·ia** (ə-dak-til′e-ə) adactyly.

**adac·ty·lism** (a-dak′tə-lizəm) adactyly.

**adac·ty·lous** (a-dak′tə-ləs) pertaining to adactyly; lacking digits on the hand or foot.

**adac·ty·ly** (a-dak′tə-le) [*a-*[1] + Gr. *daktylos* finger] a developmental anomaly characterized by the absence of digits on the hand or foot.

**Adair Digh·ton's syndrome** (ə-dār′ di′tənz) [Charles Allen *Adair Dighton,* British otolaryngologist, born 1885] osteogenesis imperfecta (type I); see under *osteogenesis.*

**Ad·a·lat** (ad′ə-lat) trademark for a preparation of nifedipine.

**ad·a·man·tine** (ad″ə-man′tin) pertaining to the enamel of the teeth.

**ad·a·man·ti·no·ma** (ad″ə-man″tĭ-no′mə) ameloblastoma.
**a. of long bones,** a rare tumor usually occurring in the tibia and probably of epithelial origin; it resembles an ameloblastoma of the jaw microscopically but is believed to be unrelated to it.
**pituitary a.,** craniopharyngioma.

**ad·a·man·to·blast** (ad″ə-man′to-blast) [Gr. *adamas* a hard substance + *-blast*] ameloblast.

**ad·a·man·to·blas·to·ma** (ad″ə-man″to-blas-to′mə) ameloblastoma.

**ad·a·man·to·ma** (ad″ə-man-to′mə) ameloblastoma.

**ADAMHA** Alcohol, Drug Abuse, and Mental Health Administration, an agency of the United States Public Health Service.

**Adam·kie·wicz's arteries** (ah-dahm-kyĕ′vich-əz) [Albert *Adamkiewicz,* Polish pathologist, 1850–1921] see *rami spinales arteriae vertebralis,* under *ramus.*

**Ad·ams' operation, saw** (ad′əmz) [William *Adams,* English surgeon, 1810–1900] see under *operation* and *saw.*

**Ad·ams-Stokes attack, syndrome (syncope)** (ad′əmz-stōks)

[Robert *Adams,* Irish physician, 1791–1875; William *Stokes,* Irish physician, 1804–1878] see under *attack* and *syndrome.*

**ad·ams·ite** (ad'əmz-īt) diphenylamine chlorarsine.

**Ad·an·so·nia** (ad″an-so'ne-ə) [Michel *Adanson,* French naturalist, 1727–1806] a genus of trees of the family Bombacaceae. *A. digita 'ta* is the baobab, a huge tree of Africa and India. In Africa, the young leaves and seeds are eaten as food and the pulp is used as a diaphoretic.

**ad·an·so·ni·an** (ad″an-so'ne-ən) named for Michel *Adanson;* see *numerical taxonomy,* under *taxonomy.*

**Ada·pin** (ad'ə-pin) trademark for a preparation of doxepin hydrochloride.

**ad·ap·ta·tion** (ad″ap-ta'shən) [L. *adaptare* to fit] 1. the adjustment of an organism to its environment, or the process by which it enhances such fitness. 2. the normal adjustment of the eye to variations in intensity of light. 3. the decline in the frequency of firing of a neuron, particularly of a receptor, under conditions of constant stimulation. 4. in dentistry, *(a)* the proper fitting of a denture, *(b)* the degree of proximity and interlocking of restorative material to a tooth preparation, *(c)* the exact adjustment of bands to teeth. 5. in microbiology, the adjustment of bacterial physiology to a new environment; see *genetic a.* and *phenotypic a.*
**auditory a.,** abnormal decrease in auditory sensitivity as a result of auditory stimulation.
**color a.,** 1. fading of hue and dulling of brightness of visual perceptions with prolonged stimulation. 2. adjustment of vision to degree of brightness or color tone of illumination indoors or out; includes *dark a.*
**dark a.,** the adaptation of the eye to vision in the dark or in reduced illumination (night vision), with build-up of rhodopsin in the retinal rods; called also *scotopic a.*
**genetic a.,** the natural selection of the progeny of a mutant better suited to a new environment; especially seen in the development of bacterial strains resistant to certain antibiotics and drugs.
**light a.,** adaptation of the eye to vision in the sunlight or in bright illumination (photopia), with reduction in the concentration of the photosensitive pigments of the eye; called also *photopic a.*
**phenotypic a.,** a change in the structural and physiological properties of an organism in response to a genetic mutation or to a change in environment.
**photopic a.,** light a.
**retinal a.,** the adjustment of the photoreceptor cell of the eye to the surrounding illumination.
**scotopic a.,** dark a.

**ad·ap·tom·e·ter** (ad″ap-tom'ə-tər) [*adaptation* + *-meter*] an instrument for measuring the time required for retinal adaptation: i.e., for regeneration of the visual purple. It is used to help detect night blindness, vitamin A deficiency, and retinitis pigmentosa.
**color a.,** an instrument using colored and neutral filters and control of illuminant to demonstrate adaptation of eye to color or light.

**ad·ax·i·al** (ad-ak'se-əl) located alongside of, or directed toward, the axis.

**ADCC** antibody-dependent cell-mediated cytotoxicity.

**add.** abbreviation for L. *ad'de,* add, or *adde'tur,* let there be added; used in writing prescriptions.

**adde** (ad'e) [L.] add.

**ad·der** (ad'ər) 1. *Vipera berus.* 2. any of numerous venomous snakes of the family Viperidae; see table at *snake.*
**death a.,** *Acanthophis antarcticus,* an extremely venomous elapid snake of Australia and New Guinea that has a short, stout body and a tail with a spine at the tip.
**puff a.,** *Bitis arrietans,* an extremely venomous, brightly colored, viperine snake found in Africa and Arabia; when annoyed it inflates its stubby body and hisses loudly.

**ad·dict** (ad'ikt) a person who cannot resist a habit, especially the use of drugs or alcohol, for physiological or psychological reasons.

**ad·dic·tion** (ə-dik'shən) 1. the state of being given up to some habit or compulsion. 2. strong physiological and psychological dependence on a drug or other psychoactive substance; see *drug a.*
**alcohol a.,** alcoholism, particularly that in which physiological dependence is present.
**drug a.,** a state of heavy dependence on a drug; sometimes defined as physical dependence but usually also including emotional dependence, i.e., compulsive or pathological drug use. It is often used synonymously with substance dependence.

**Ad·dis count, test** (ad'is) [Thomas *Addis,* American physician, 1881–1949] see under *count* and *test.*

**ad·di·sin** (ad'ĭ-sin) a substance present in the gastric juice that has stimulating power on bone marrow formation; such an extract from the gastric juice of the hog is used in pernicious anemia.

**Ad·di·son's disease** (ad'ĭ-sənz) [Thomas *Addison,* English physician, 1793–1860] [MeSH: Addison's Disease] see under *disease.*

**Ad·di·son's planes, point** (ad'ĭ-sənz) [Christopher *Addison,* English anatomist, 1869–1951] see under *plane* and *point.*

**ad·di·so·ni·an** (ad″ĭ-so'ne-ən) named for Thomas *Addison;* see under *crisis* and *syndrome.*

**ad·di·son·ism** (ad'ĭ-sən-iz″əm) addisonian syndrome.

**ad·di·tive** (ad'ĭ-tiv) 1. characterized by addition; see also under *effect.* 2. a substance, as a flavoring agent, preservative, or vitamin, added to another substance (such as a food or drug) that is to be ingested.
**feed a.,** a chemical, such as a drug or nutritional supplement, that is added to animal feed.

**ad·dress·in** (ə-dres'in) a molecule on the surface of vascular endothelial cells that mediates the attachment of specific leukocytes, particularly lymphocytes, to the endothelium, binding with their homing receptors.

**ad·du·cent** (ə-du'sənt) performing adduction.

**ad·du·cin** (ə-doo'sin) a protein that binds to both actin and spectrin and is thought to play a role in the spectrin-actin complex of the erythrocyte membrane.

**ad·duct**[1] (ə-dukt') [L. *adducere* to draw toward] to draw toward the median plane or (in the digits) toward the axial line of a limb.

**ad·duct**[2] (ă'dukt) inclusion complex.

**ad·duc·tio** (ad-duk'she-o) [L.] [TA] adduction.

**ad·duc·tion** (ə-duk'shən) the act of adducting or the state of being adducted.

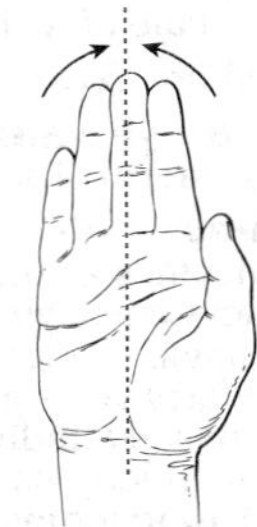

Adduction of fingers.

**ad·duc·tor** (ə-duk'tər) [L.] that which adducts; see under *musculus.*

**Ad·e·le·i·na** (ad″ə-le-i'nə) a suborder of homoxenous or heteroxenous protozoa (order Eucoccidiida, subclass Coccidia) parasitic in the intestinal epithelium and associated glands of invertebrates, characterized by syzygy during development that usually involves a macrogamete and microgamont, with the latter producing one to four sporozoites enclosed in an envelope. Representative genera include *Haemogregarina, Hepatozoon,* and *Klossiella.*

**adelo·mor·phic** (ə-del″o-mor'fik) adelomorphous.

**adelo·mor·phous** (ə-del″o-mor'fəs) [Gr. *adēlos* not evident + *morph-* + *-ous*] not having a clearly defined form; see under *cell.*

**-adelphus** [Gr. *adelphos* brother] a word termination denoting a symmetrical pair of twins conjoined at the site indicated by the stem to which it is affixed; cf. *-pagus.*

**ad·e·nal·gia** (ad″ə-nal'jə) [*aden-* + *-algia*] pain in a gland; called also *adenodynia.*

**aden·dric** (a-den'drik) adendritic.

**aden·drit·ic** (a″den-drit'ik) [*a-*[1] + *dendritic*] lacking dendrites.

**ad·e·nec·to·my** (ad″ə-nek'tə-me) [*aden-* + *-ectomy*] surgical removal of a gland.

**ad·en·ec·to·pia** (ad″ə-nek-to'pe-ə) [*aden-* + *ectopia*] malposition or displacement of a gland.

**ade·nia** (ə-de'ne-ə) chronic great enlargement of the lymphatic glands; see also *lymphoma* and *pseudoleukemia.*

**aden·ic** (ə-de'nik) 1. glandular (def. 1). 2. adenoid (def. 2).

**aden·i·form** (ə-den'ĭ-form) [*aden-* + *form*] resembling a gland, especially in shape.

**ad·e·nine** (ad'ə-nēn) [MeSH: Adenine] 1. a major purine base (see illustration at *base*). In animal and plant cells it usually occurs condensed with ribose or deoxyribose to form the nucleosides adenosine and deoxyadenosine. As such, it is a component of nucleic acids, of certain nucleotides, and of many coenzymes. Symbol A.

2. [USP] a preparation of adenine used to improve the preservation of whole blood.
**a. arabinoside,** vidarabine.
**a. nucleotide,** adenylic acid.

**ad·e·nine phos·pho·ri·bo·syl·trans·fer·ase** (ad′ə-nēn fos″fo-ri′bo-səl-trans′fer-ās) [EC 2.4.2.7] [MeSH: Adenine Phosphoribosyltransferase] an enzyme of the transferase class that catalyzes the transfer of ribose 5-phosphate from phosphoribosylpyrophosphate to adenine to form AMP. The enzyme salvages adenine within the cell.

**ad·e·nine phos·pho·ri·bo·syl·trans·fer·ase de·fi·cien·cy** an autosomal recessive disorder of purine salvage, resulting in accumulation of the insoluble purine 2,8-dihydroxyadenine; clinical signs range from none to urolithiasis (causing colic, hematuria, urinary tract infection, and dysuria) to acute renal failure and permanent kidney damage, with greater severity generally correlated with lower residual enzyme activity.

**ad·e·ni·tis** (ad″ə-ni′tis) inflammation of a gland. Cf. *acinitis.*
**Bartholin's a.,** inflammation of the major vestibular gland (Bartholin's gland) resulting from acute infection of the gland.
**cervical a.,** a condition characterized by enlarged, inflamed, and tender lymph nodes of the neck; seen in certain infectious diseases of children, such as acute infections of the throat. Called also *cervical lymphadenitis.*
**cervical a., tuberculous,** see under *lymphadenitis.*
**mesenteric a.,** mesenteric lymphadenitis.
**phlegmonous a.,** inflammation of a gland and the surrounding connective tissue; called also *adenophlegmon.*
**vestibular a.,** chronic inflammation of the lesser vestibular glands, which produces small, extremely painful ulcerations of the vestibular mucosa.

**Ade·ni·um** (ə-de′ne-um) a genus of African plants of the family Apocynaceae; they contain cardioactive glycosides such as somalin that are close in structure and action to the digitalis glycosides.

**aden(o)-** [Gr. *adēn,* gen. *adenos* gland] a combining form denoting relationship to a gland or glands.

**ad·e·no·ac·an·tho·ma** (ad″ə-no-ak″an-tho′mə) [*adeno-* + *acanth-* + *-oma*] an adenocarcinoma in which some or the majority of the cells exhibit squamous differentiation; called also *adenosquamous* or *adenoid squamous cell carcinoma.*

**ad·e·no·am·e·lo·blas·to·ma** (ad″ə-no-ə-mel″o-blas-to′mə) adenomatoid odontogenic tumor.

**ad·e·no·blast** (ad′ə-no-blast″) [*adeno-* + *-blast*] an embryonic cell that gives rise to glandular tissue.

**ad·e·no·car·ci·no·ma** (ad″ə-no-kahr″sĭ-no′mə) [MeSH: Adenocarcinoma] carcinoma derived from glandular tissue or in which the tumor cells form recognizable glandular structures; adenocarcinomas may be classified according to the predominant pattern of cell arrangement, as papillary, alveolar, etc., or according to a particular product of the cells, as mucinous adenocarcinoma.
**acinar a.,** 1. acinar carcinoma. 2. the most common neoplasm of the prostate, usually arising in the peripheral acini. Histological abnormalities of the acini may include size distortions ranging from giant to tiny, irregular architectural arrangements, and abnormal epithelium that is sometimes cribriform.
**acinic cell a., acinous a.,** see under *carcinoma.*
**alveolar a.,** bronchioloalveolar carcinoma.
**bronchioalveolar a., bronchiolar a.,** bronchioloalveolar carcinoma.
**bronchioloalveolar a., bronchoalveolar a.,** bronchioloalveolar carcinoma.
**bronchogenic a.,** the usual type of adenocarcinoma of the lung, as distinguished from the subtype *bronchioloalveolar carcinoma.*
**clear cell a.,** a rare malignant tumor of the female genital tract, resembling a renal cell carcinoma and containing tubules or small cysts with some cells that are hobnail-shaped and others whose cytoplasm is clear, containing abundant glycogen and inconspicuous stroma. It may occur in the ovary, uterus, cervix, or vagina. One form has been linked to in utero exposure to diethylstilbestrol. Called also *clear cell carcinoma* and *mesonephroma.*
**ductal a. of the prostate,** adenocarcinoma of columnar epithelium in the peripheral prostatic ducts; it may project into the urethra, causing obstruction and hematuria.
**endometrioid a.,** the most common form of endometrial carcinoma, containing tumor cells differentiated into glandular tissue with little or no stroma.
**follicular a.,** see under *carcinoma.*
**gastric a.,** any of a group of common stomach cancers, usually located in the antrum; it may present as a bulky mass with central ulceration invading the wall, a mass that narrows the antral lumen, a polypoid lesion, or a tumor that spreads superficially over the mucosal surface. It is common in Japan, Chile, Iceland, and Finland but the incidence is decreasing in North America and elsewhere. There may be links to certain dietary substances such as nitrosamines and benzpyrene. Called also *gastric carcinoma* and *a. of the stomach.*
**a. of infantile testis,** yolk sac tumor.
**a. of kidney,** renal cell carcinoma.
**a. of the lung,** a type of bronchogenic carcinoma made up of cuboidal or columnar cells in a discrete mass, usually at the periphery of the lungs. Most such tumors form glandular structures containing mucin, although a minority are solid and without mucin. Growth is slow, but there may be early invasion of blood and lymph vessels, giving rise to metastases while the primary lesion is still asymptomatic. Two types are distinguished, *bronchogenic a.* and *bronchioloalveolar carcinoma.*
**mucinous a.,** mucinous carcinoma.
**papillary a., polypoid a.,** an adenocarcinoma in which the tumor elements are arranged as finger-like processes or as a solid spherical nodule projecting from an epithelial surface. See also *papillary carcinoma.*
**polymorphous low-grade a.,** terminal duct carcinoma.
**a. of the prostate,** acinar a. (def. 2).
**renal a.,** renal cell carcinoma.
**a. of the stomach,** gastric a.
**terminal duct a.,** see under *carcinoma.*
**urachal a.,** adenocarcinoma in the urachal region of the dome of the urinary bladder, sometimes extending outwards into the abdomen; the tumor usually has a thick mucous coating, leading to excretion of mucus in the urine.

**ad·e·no·cele** (ad′ə-no-sēl″) [*adeno-* + *-cele*[1]] cystadenoma.

**ad·e·no·cel·lu·li·tis** (ad″ə-no-sel″u-li′tis) inflammation of a gland and the tissue around it.

**ad·e·no·cys·to·ma** (ad″ə-no-sis-to′mə) cystadenoma.
**papillary a. lymphomatosum,** adenolymphoma.

**ad·e·no·cyte** (ad′ə-no-sīt″) [*adeno-* + *-cyte*] a mature secretory cell of a gland.

**ad·e·no·dyn·ia** (ad″ə-no-din′e-ə) [*aden-* + *-odynia*] adenalgia.

**ad·e·no·ep·i·the·li·o·ma** (ad″ə-no-ep″ĭ-the″le-o′mə) [*adeno-* + *epithelioma*] a tumor composed of glandular and epithelial elements.

**ad·e·no·fi·bro·ma** (ad″ə-no-fi-bro′mə) [MeSH: Adenofibroma] a tumor composed of connective tissue containing glandular structures.
**a. edemato′des,** a tumor composed of glandular and connective tissue elements in which there is marked edema of the stroma, as in nasal polyp.

**ad·e·no·fi·bro·sis** (ad″ə-no-fi-bro′sis) fibroid change in a gland.

**ad·e·nog·e·nous** (ad″ə-noj′ə-nəs) [*adeno-* + *-genous*] originating from glandular tissue.

**ad·e·no·graph·ic** (ad″ə-no-graf′ik) pertaining to adenography.

**ad·e·nog·ra·phy** (ad″ə-nog′rə-fe) [*adeno-* + *-graphy*] radiography of a gland or glands.

**ad·e·no·hy·po·phys·e·al** (ad″ə-no-hi-po-fiz′e-əl) adenohypophysial.

**ad·e·no·hy·poph·y·sec·to·my** (ad″ə-no-hi-pof″ĭ-sek′tə-me) excision or ablation of the adenohypophysis.

**ad·e·no·hy·po·phys·i·al** (ad″ə-no-hi-po-fiz′e-əl) pertaining to the adenohypophysis; spelled also *adenohypophyseal.* Called also *prehypophysial.*

**ad·e·no·hy·poph·y·sis** (ad″ə-no-hi-pof′ĭ-sis) [*adeno-* + *hypophysis*] [TA] the anterior lobe of the hypophysis (pituitary gland), the part that secretes growth hormone, fibroblast growth hormone, adrenocorticotropic hormone, β-endorphin, thyrotropin, follicle-stimu-

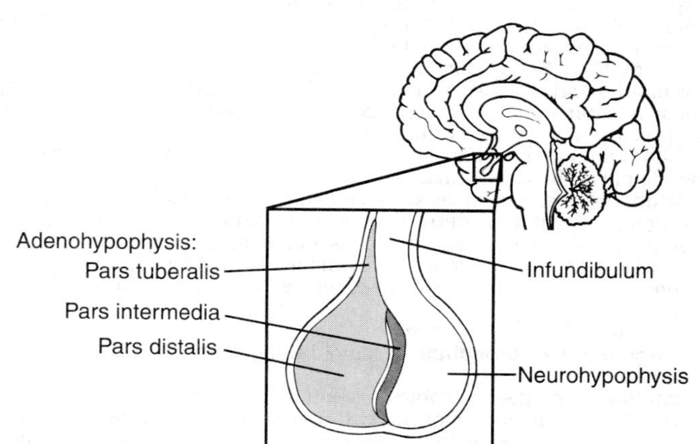

lating hormone, luteinizing hormone, and prolactin; these are released by hypophysiotropic hormones, releasing hormones secreted by the hypothalamus, and they regulate the functioning of the thyroid gland, gonads, adrenal cortex, and other endocrine organs. As a consequence, the hypothalamo-pituitary unit is of vital importance to the growth, maturation, and reproduction of the individual. The adenohypophysis comprises the pars tuberalis; the pars distalis, the main body of the adenohypophysis; and the pars intermedia, which contains cells that secrete β-endorphin, melanotropins, and other regulators but is sometimes considered to be part of the neurohypophysis. The adenohypophysis has its origin in the buccal epithelium of the embryo. Called also *anterior pituitary, anterior lobe of hypophysis, lobus anterior hypophyseos* [TA alternative], and *lobus glandularis hypophyseos.*

**ad•e•noid** (ad'ə-noid) [*aden-* + *-oid*] [MeSH: Adenoids] 1. tonsilla pharyngea. 2. resembling a gland. 3. pertaining to the tonsilla pharyngea.

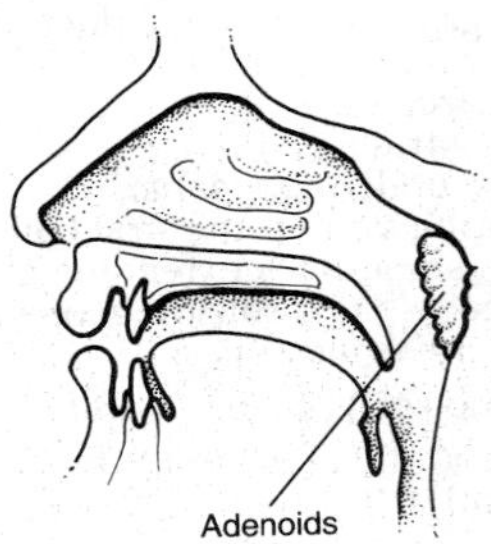


**ad•e•noid•ec•to•my** (ad"ə-noid-ek'tə-me) [*adenoid* + *-ectomy*] [MeSH: Adenoidectomy] excision of the adenoids.

**ad•e•noid•ism** (ad'ə-noid"iz-əm) the syndrome which results from the presence of greatly enlarged adenoids.

**ad•e•noid•i•tis** (ad"ə-noid-i'tis) inflammation of the adenoid tissue of the nasopharynx.

**ad•e•noids** (ad'ə-noidz) [MeSH: Adenoids] popular name for hypertrophy of the pharyngeal tonsils, which occurs primarily in preadolescents and adolescents. See also *adenoidism.*

**ad•e•no•li•po•ma** (ad"ə-no-lĭ-po'mə) a tumor composed of both glandular and fatty tissue elements. Cf. *lipoadenoma.*

**ad•e•no•log•a•di•tis** (ad"ə-no-log"ə-di'tis) [*adeno-* + Gr. *logades* whites of the eyes + *-itis*] 1. ophthalmia neonatorum. 2. inflammation of the glands of the conjunctiva.

**ad•e•no•lym•phi•tis** (ad"ə-no-lim-fi'tis) lymphadenitis.

**ad•e•no•lym•pho•cele** (ad"ə-no-lim'fo-sēl) [*adeno-* + *lymphocele*] lymphadenocele.

**ad•e•no•lym•pho•ma** (ad"ə-no-lim-fo'mə) [*adeno-* + *lymphoma*] [MeSH: Adenolymphoma] a benign tumor of the parotid gland characterized by cystic spaces lined by tall, columnar, eosinophilic epithelial cells, overlying a lymphoid tissue–containing stroma. Called also *Warthin's tumor* and *papillary cystadenoma lymphomatosum.*

**ad•e•no•ma** (ad"ə-no'mə) [*adeno-* + *-oma*] [MeSH: Adenoma] a benign epithelial tumor in which the cells form recognizable glandular structures or in which the cells are clearly derived from glandular epithelium.

## Adenoma

**acidophilic a.,** in a classification system formerly used for pituitary adenomas, an adenoma whose cells stain with acid dyes; most adenomas that secreted excessive amounts of growth hormone were in this group. See *growth hormone–secreting a.*

**acidophil stem-cell a.,** a rapidly growing plurihormonal adenoma; usually a null-cell adenoma, seen in young patients; its single cell type secretes both prolactin and growth hormone and is presumed to be a stem cell for both lactotrophs and somatotrophs.

**ACTH-secreting a.,** corticotroph a.

**a. of the adrenal cortex, adrenocortical a.,** a benign tumor of the adrenal cortex, usually small and unilateral; most types cause endocrine symptoms. See *cortisol-producing a., aldosterone-producing a., feminizing tumor,* and *virilizing tumor.*

**adrenocorticotropic hormone–secreting a.,** corticotroph a.

**aldosterone-producing a., aldosterone-secreting a.,** a benign aldosteronoma, usually small and unilateral.

**alpha subunit a.,** a variant of glycoprotein adenoma that secretes only one subunit of the glycoprotein hormones; most are endocrine-inactive, although a few are endocrine-active.

**a. alveola're,** an adenoma whose cells are arranged like those of an alveolar gland.

**basal cell a.,** a benign, encapsulated, slow-growing, painless salivary gland tumor of intercalated duct or reserve cell origin, occurring mainly in males, in the parotid gland or upper lip; solid, canalicular, trabecular-tubular, and membranous types can be distinguished histologically, but all show little myoepithelial cell participation and little stromal differentiation or metaplasia.

**basophil a., basophilic a.,** in a classification system formerly used for pituitary adenomas, an adenoma whose cells stain with basic dyes; most adenomas that secreted excessive amounts of adrenocorticotrophic hormone were in this group.

**bile duct a.,** a small firm white nodule with multiple bile ducts imbedded in a fibrous stroma.

**bronchial a's,** adenomas situated in the submucosal tissues of large bronchi, thought to be derived from neuroendocrine cells. Sometimes composed of well-differentiated cells and usually circumscribed, they are almost always carcinoid in histologic form. Although termed *adenomas,* these tumors are now recognized as being of low-grade malignancy.

**canalicular a.,** see *basal cell a.*

**carcinoid a. of bronchus,** carcinoid tumor of bronchus; see under *tumor.*

**carcinoma ex pleomorphic a.,** see under *carcinoma.*

**chief cell a.,** adenoma of the parathyroid gland composed of solid masses of small chief cells similar to those seen in the normal gland.

**chromophobe a., chromophobic a.,** a pituitary adenoma composed of cells that lack acidophilic or basophilic granules; this is the same entity as the more precisely named *null-cell a.*

**colloid a.,** macrofollicular a.

**cortical a's,** minute tumors in the cortex of the kidney, arising from the renal tubules; some authorities consider these to be simply small renal cell carcinomas.

**corticotrope a., corticotrope cell a.,** corticotroph a.

**corticotroph a., corticotroph cell a.,** a pituitary adenoma made up predominantly of corticotrophs; excessive corticotropin secretion may cause Cushing's disease or Nelson's syndrome. Called also *ACTH-secreting* or *adrenocorticotropic hormone–secreting a.* and *corticotropinoma.*

**cortisol-producing a.,** the most common adenoma of the adrenal cortex; it secretes cortisol and causes Cushing's syndrome.

**embryonal a.,** trabecular a.

**endocrine-active a.,** a pituitary adenoma that secretes excessive amounts of a hormone; see *prolactinoma, corticotroph a., gonadotroph a., growth hormone–secreting a.,* and *thyrotroph a.* Called also *hyperfunctional a.* and *hyperfunctioning a.*

**endocrine-inactive a.,** a pituitary adenoma that does not secrete excessive amounts of any hormone; many null-cell adenomas are of this type. Called also *nonfunctional a., nonfunctioning a., nonsecreting a.,* and *nonsecretory a.*

**eosinophil a., eosinophilic a.,** growth hormone–secreting a.

**fetal a.,** microfollicular a.

**a. fibro'sum,** fibroadenoma.

**follicular a.,** adenoma of the thyroid in which the cells are arranged in the form of follicles. It is sometimes subclassified as either *macrofollicular a., microfollicular a., trabecular a.,* or *Hürthle cell a.;* however, many adenomas are mixtures of types, and all types have similar clinical characteristics.

**functional a., functioning a.,** endocrine-active a.

**gastric a.,** adenomatous polyp of stomach.

**glycoprotein a., glycoprotein hormone a.,** a pituitary adenoma that causes excessive secretion of one of the three glycoprotein hormones (follicle-stimulating hormone, luteinizing hormone, and thyrotropin); see *gonadotroph a.* and *thyrotroph a.*

**gonadotrope a., gonadotroph a., gonadotroph cell a.,** a rare type of pituitary adenoma made up of gonadotroph-like cells that secrete excessive amounts of follicle-stimulating hormone or luteinizing hormone, or both; it may cause precocious puberty, visual disturbances, or hypogonadism.

**growth hormone cell a.,** growth hormone–secreting a.

**growth hormone–secreting a.,** a pituitary adenoma made up of somatotroph-like cells that secrete excessive amounts of growth hormone; it may cause gigantism in children or acromegaly in adults. Called also *somatotrope a., somatotroph a.,* and *eosinophilic a.*

**hepatocellular a.,** a benign circumscribed tumor of the liver, usually in the right lobe; growth is in a sheetlike fashion and it may be highly vascular with a tendency to hemorrhage and with areas of necrosis. Women are affected more often than men and use of oral contraceptives has been implicated in some cases. Called also *liver cell a.*

**Hürthle cell a.,** a benign Hürthle cell tumor, usually considered a subtype of the follicular adenomas. Called also *oncocytic a., oxyphilic a.,* and *oncocytoma.*

**hyperfunctional a., hyperfunctioning a.,** endocrine-active a.

**islet cell a.,** a benign islet cell tumor.

**a's of kidney,** cortical a's.

**lactotrope a., lactotroph a.,** prolactinoma.

**langerhansian a.,** islet cell a.

**liver cell a.,** hepatocellular a.

**macrofollicular a.,** a follicular adenoma composed of large follicles filled with colloid and lined with flat epithelium. Called also *colloid a.*

**mammosomatotroph a.,** a plurihormonal adenoma composed of mammosomatotrophs, a single cell type secreting both growth hormone and prolactin; cf. *mixed somatotroph-lactotroph a.*

**membranous a.,** see *basal cell a.*

**microfollicular a.,** a follicular adenoma with small closely-packed follicles lined with epithelium; called also *fetal a.*

**mixed-cell a.,** a pituitary adenoma containing more than one cell type, usually making it plurihormonal; see *plurihormonal a.*

**mixed somatotroph-lactotroph a.,** the most common type of mixed-cell adenoma, containing two cell types that produce respectively growth hormone and prolactin. Cf. *mammosomatotroph a.*

**monomorphic a.,** any of a group of benign salivary gland tumors that lack connective tissue changes and are each predominantly composed of a single cell type; included are basal cell adenomas, adenolymphomas, and oxyphilic adenomas. Cf. *pleomorphic a.*

**mucinous a.,** an epithelial tumor whose cells produce mucin.

**nephrogenic a.,** nephrogenic metaplasia.

**nipple a.,** a benign lesion of the breast, clinically resembling Paget's disease of the breast, consisting of ductal and stromal proliferation beneath the nipple, which presents as a mass, ulceration, or erosion, with a serous or bloody discharge. Called also *papillary a., erosive adenomatosis of nipple, florid papillomatosis of nipple,* and *subareolar duct papillomatosis.*

**nonfunctional a., nonfunctioning a.,** endocrine-inactive a.

**nonsecreting a., nonsecretory a.,** endocrine-inactive a.

**null-cell a.,** a pituitary adenoma whose cells give negative results on tests for staining and hormone secretion; although classically they were considered to be composed of sparsely granulated or degranulated (nonfunctioning) cells, some contain functioning cells and may be associated with a hyperpituitary state such as acromegaly or Cushing's syndrome. These tumors are often discovered clinically only when they have grown large and are pressing on surrounding structures. Called also *chromophobic a.*

**oncocytic a.,** 1. oncocytoma. 2. Hürthle cell a.

**a. ova'rii testicula're,** arrhenoblastoma.

**oxyphilic a., oxyphilic granular cell a.,** 1. oncocytoma. 2. Hürthle cell a.

**papillary a.,** nipple a.

**papillary cystic a.,** papillary cystadenoma.

**Pick's testicular a., Pick's tubular a.,** androblastoma, def. 1.

**pituitary a.,** a benign neoplasm of the anterior pituitary gland; some contain hormone-secreting cells *(endocrine-active adenomas)* but some are not secretory *(endocrine-inactive adenomas).*

**pleomorphic a.,** a benign, slow-growing tumor of the salivary gland, occurring as a small, painless, firm nodule, usually of the parotid gland, but also found in any major or accessory salivary gland anywhere in the oral cavity. It is most often seen in women in the fifth decade. Histologically, the tumor presents a variety of cells: cuboidal, columnar, and squamous cells, showing all forms of epithelial growth.

**pleomorphic a., malignant,** any of several malignant epithelial neoplasms arising in a pre-existing pleomorphic adenoma, usually in the salivary glands of an older adult; it occurs in several types, usually divided into *carcinoma ex pleomorphic a.* and *malignant mixed tumor.*

**plurihormonal a.,** an endocrine-active adenoma that secretes two or more hormones, usually growth hormone and one or more of the glycoprotein types, so that its effects are similar to those of a combination of other adenomas such as the growth hormone–secreting adenoma and the glycoprotein hormone adenoma; it may be mixed-cell or a single cell type. Varieties include *acidophil stem-cell a., mammosomatotroph a.,* and some types of *alpha subunit a.*

**prolactin cell a., prolactin-secreting a.,** prolactinoma.

**sebaceous a.,** an uncommon, benign, yellow or flesh-colored, usually solitary, circumscribed nodule occurring on the face or scalp, generally in older men, consisting of incompletely differentiated sebaceous lobules; it may be seen in Muir-Torre syndrome. The term is sometimes used to denote adenoma sebaceum.

**a. seba'ceum,** 1. *Pringle type:* cutaneous angiofibromatous proliferation, usually on the face, occurring in association with tuberous sclerosis; the term is a misnomer since the sebaceous glands are rarely involved. 2. *Balzer type:* nevoid hyperplasia of sebaceous glands, forming multiple yellow papules or nodules of the face.

**somatotrope a., somatotroph a.,** growth hormone–secreting a.

**thyroid stimulating hormone–secreting a.,** thyrotrope a.

**thyrotrope a., thyrotroph a., thyrotroph cell a.,** a rare type of pituitary adenoma made up of thyrotroph-like cells that secrete excess thyrotropin and cause hyperthyroidism; called also *TSH-secreting a.* and *thyroid stimulating hormone–secreting a.*

**toxic a.,** toxic multinodular goiter.

**trabecular a.,** a follicular adenoma whose cells are closely packed to form cords or trabeculae, with only a few small follicles; called also *embryonal a.*

**trabecular-tubular a.,** see *basal cell a.*

**TSH-secreting a.,** thyrotrope a.

**tubular a.,** 1. an adenoma whose cells are arranged in tubules, as occurs with adenomatous polyps of the colon, some fibroadenomas of the breast, and androblastoma. 2. androblastoma (def. 1). 3. the most common type of adenomatous polyp of the colon, usually seen in middle-aged to elderly people; its tubules are highly variable in size and often occur singly, although small and large groups of tubules are also seen. Its potential for malignant transformation is uncertain.

**a. tubula're testicula're ova'rii,** arrhenoblastoma.

**villous a.,** an uncommon type of adenomatous polyp of the colon that is large, soft, and papillary and often premalignant.

---

**ad·e·no·ma·la·cia** (ad″ə-no-mə-la′shə) [*adeno-* + *malacia*] abnormal softening of a gland.

**ad·e·no·ma·toid** (ad″ə-no′mə-toid) resembling adenoma.

**ad·e·no·ma·to·sis** (ad″ə-no-mə-to′tis) a condition characterized by development of numerous adenomatous growths.

**erosive a. of nipple,** nipple adenoma.

**multiple endocrine a.,** multiple endocrine neoplasia.

**a. o'ris,** enlargement of the mucous glands of the lip without secretion or inflammation.

**pluriglandular a., polyendocrine a.,** multiple endocrine neoplasia.

**porcine intestinal a.,** formation of adenomas in the intestines of recently weaned piglets, with anorexia and weight loss; it is seldom fatal, and growths regress within a few weeks. Infection by *Campylobacter sputorum* subspecies *mucosalis* has been implicated.

**pulmonary a.,** 1. bronchioloalveolar carcinoma. 2. a chronic contagious neoplastic lung disease of adult sheep and goats, caused by a retrovirus with adenomatous proliferation in the alveoli and small bronchioles. Called also *jaagsiekte* and *jagziekte.*

**ad·e·no·ma·tous** (ad″ə-nom′ə-təs) 1. pertaining to adenoma. 2. pertaining to nodular hyperplasia of a gland.

**ad·e·no·meg·a·ly** (ad″ə-no-meg′ə-le) enlargement of a gland; called also *adenoncus* and *adenopathy.*

**ad·e·no·mere** (ad′ə-no-mēr″) [*adeno-* + *-mere*] the blind terminal portion of a developing gland, becoming the functional portion of the organ.

**ad·e·no·myo·fi·bro·ma** (ad″ə-no-mi″o-fi-bro′mə) a fibroma containing adenomatous and myomatous tissue.

**ad·e·no·my·o·ma** (ad″ə-no-mi-o′mə) [*adeno-* + *myoma*] [MeSH: Adenomyoma] 1. a benign tumor consisting of smooth muscle and glandular elements. 2. see *adenomyosis.*

**ad·e·no·my·o·ma·to·sis** (ad″ə-no-mi″o-mə-to′sis) the formation of multiple adenomyomatous nodules in the parauterine tissues or in the uterus.

**ad·e·no·my·o·ma·tous** (ad″əno-mi-o′mə-tus) pertaining to or resembling adenomyoma.

**ad·e·no·myo·me·tri·tis** (ad″ə-no-mi″o-mə-tri′tis) an inflammatory lesion of the endometrium, which may lead to adenomyosis.

**ad·e·no·myo·sar·co·ma** (ad″ə-no-mi″o-sahr-ko′mə) a mixed mesodermal tumor in which striated muscle cells are one component.
**embryonal a.,** Wilms' tumor.

**ad·e·no·my·o·sis** (ad″ə-no-mi-o′sis) a benign condition characterized by endometrial glands and stroma within the myometrium, accompanied by hypertrophy of the myometrium. If the lesion forms a circumscribed tumor-like nodule, it is called *adenomyoma.* Called also *endometriosis interna* or *uterina.*
**a. exter′na,** endometriosis.
**stromal a.,** stromatosis.
**a. tu′bae,** 1. an old term for salpingitis isthmica nodosa. 2. the growth of the endometrium into the lumen of the uterine tube from the uterus, replacing the endosalpinx.
**a. u′teri,** adenomyosis.

**ad·e·non·cus** (ad″ə-nong′kəs) adenomegaly.

**ad·e·no·neu·ral** (ad″ə-no-noo͝′rəl) pertaining to a gland and a nerve.

**ad·e·nop·a·thy** (ad″ə-nop′ə-the) [*adeno-* + *-pathy*] 1. adenomegaly. 2. enlargement of a lymph node. 3. lymphadenopathy.

**ad·e·no·phar·yn·gi·tis** (ad″ə-no-far″in-ji′tis) [*adeno-* + *pharyngitis*] inflammation of the adenoids and pharynx, usually involving the tonsils.

**ad·e·no·phleg·mon** (ad″ə-no-fleg′mon) [*adeno-* + *phlegmon*] phlegmonous adenitis.

**ad·e·noph·thal·mia** (ad″ə-nof-thal′me-ə) [*aden-* + *ophthalmia*] inflammation of the meibomian glands.

**ad·e·no·pit·u·i·cyte** (ad″ə-no-pĭ-tu′i-sīt) see *pituicyte.*

**ad·e·no·sar·co·ma** (ad″ə-no-sahr-ko′mə) [MeSH: Adenosarcoma] a mixed tumor composed of sarcomatous and glandular elements, as Wilms' tumor.
**embryonal a.,** Wilms' tumor.

**ad·e·no·scle·ro·sis** (ad″ə-no-sklĕ-ro′sis) [*adeno-* + *sclerosis*] the hardening of a gland.

**aden·o·sine** (ə-den′o-sēn) [USP] [MeSH: Adenosine] 1. a purine nucleoside, adenine linked by its N9 nitrogen to the C1 carbon of ribose. It is a component of ribonucleic acid and its nucleotides play major roles in the reactions and regulation of metabolism. Symbol A. 2. a cardiac depressant of automaticity in the sinus node and conduction in the atrioventricular node; used as an antiarrhythmic.
**cyclic a. monophosphate,** a cyclic nucleotide, adenosine 3′,5′-cyclic monophosphate, that serves as an intracellular and, in some cases, extracellular "second messenger" mediating the action of many peptide or amine hormones. The nucleotide binds to cAMP-dependent kinases and releases free (catalytically active) subunits. Abbreviated 3′,5′-AMP, cAMP, and cyclic AMP.
**a. diphosphate (ADP),** a nucleotide, the 5′-pyrophosphate of adenosine, involved in energy metabolism; it is produced by hydrolysis of ATP and converted back to ATP by the processes of oxidative phosphorylation and substrate-level phosphorylation.
**a. monophosphate (AMP),** a nucleotide, the 5′-phosphate of adenosine, involved in energy metabolism; it is produced by hydrolysis of ATP and converted to ADP by adenylate kinase. Called also *adenylic acid.*
**a. phosphate,** any of the three interconvertible compounds in which adenosine is attached through its ribose group to one *(a. monophosphate),* two *(a. diphosphate),* or three *(a. triphosphate)* phosphoric acid molecules.
**a. triphosphate (ATP),** a nucleotide, the 5′ triphosphate of adenosine, involved in energy metabolism and required for RNA synthesis; it occurs in all cells and is used to store energy in the form of high-energy phosphate bonds. The free energy derived from hydrolysis of ATP is used to drive metabolic reactions including the synthesis of nucleic acids and proteins, to move molecules against concentration gradients (active transport), and to produce mechanical motion (contraction of microfibrils and microtubules).

**aden·o·sine de·am·i·nase** (ə-den′o-sēn de-am′ĭ-nās) [EC 3.5.4.4] [MeSH: Adenosine Deaminase] an enzyme of the hydrolase class that catalyzes the deamination of adenosine to form inosine, a reaction of purine metabolism. Absence of enzyme activity, an autosomal recessive trait, has been found in many individuals with severe combined immunodeficiency syndrome. Abbreviated ADA.

**aden·o·sine ki·nase** (ə-den′o-sēn ki′nās) [EC 2.7.1.20] [MeSH: Adenosine Kinase] an enzyme of the transferase class that catalyzes the phosphorylation of adenosine by ATP to form ADP. The reaction is part of the purine salvage mechanism.

**aden·o·sine·tri·phos·pha·tase** (ə-den″o-sēn-tri-fos′fə-tās) [EC 3.6.1.3] [MeSH: Adenosinetriphosphatase] an enzyme of the hydrolase class that catalyzes the hydrolysis of ATP to ADP. The reaction is a result of the concerted action of proteins using ATP to drive processes such as muscle contraction, maintenance of concentration gradients, membrane transport, and regulation of ion concentrations. Called also *ATPase.* See also *myosin ATPase,* $Na^+,K^+$*-ATPase,* $Ca^{2+}$*-ATPase, dynein ATPase,* and $H^+,K^+$*-ATPase.*

**ad·e·no·sis** (ad″ə-no′sis) 1. any disease of the glands. 2. the abnormal development or formation of gland tissue.
**blunt duct a.,** a form of mammary dysplasia characterized by dominance of the proliferation of the epithelial parenchyma; it is often accompanied by fibrosis and cystic disease of the breast.
**mammary sclerosing a., sclerosing a. of breast,** a form of disease of the breast characterized by multiple firm tender nodules, fibrous tissue, mastodynia, and sometimes small cysts; histologically, it may resemble carcinoma.
**a. vagi′nae,** the presence in the vagina of multiple ectopic areas of glandular (columnar) epithelium.

**aden·o·syl** (ə-den′o-sil″) the radical formed from adenosine on loss of an H or OH group, particularly from the 5′ position.

**aden·o·syl·co·ba·la·min** (ə-den″o-sil-ko-bal′ə-min) a cobalamin derivative in which the substituent is deoxyadenosyl. It is one of two metabolically active forms synthesized upon ingestion of vitamin $B_{12}$ and is the predominant form in the liver; it acts as a coenzyme in the reaction catalyzed by methylmalonyl-CoA mutase. Abbreviated AdoCbl.

**S-aden·o·syl·ho·mo·cys·te·ine** (ə-den″o-sil-ho″mo-sis′tēn) the compound remaining after the methyl group of *S*-adenosylmethionine has been transferred to an acceptor; it is a potent inhibitor of transmethylation reactions and is rapidly hydrolyzed.

**S-aden·o·syl·me·thi·o·nine** (ə-den″o-sil-mə-thi′o-nēn) a reaction product of ATP and methionine in which the sulfur atom of methionine is bound to the ribose of adenosine; it serves as a methyl donor in transmethylation reactions.

**ad·e·no·tome** (ad′ə-no-tōm″) [*adeno-* + *-tome*] an instrument for excision of the adenoids.

**ad·e·no·ton·sil·lec·to·my** (ad″ə-no-ton″sil-ek′tə-me) removal of the adenoids and tonsils.

**ad·e·nous** (ad′ə-nəs) glandular (def. 1).

**ad·e·no·vi·ral** (ad′ə-no-vi″rəl) pertaining to or caused by adenoviruses.

**Ad·e·no·vi·ri·dae** (ad″ə-no-vir′ĭ-de) [MeSH: Adenoviridae] the adenoviruses: a family of DNA viruses having a nonenveloped icosahedral virion 80–110 nm in diameter with 252 capsomers. The genome consists of a single linear molecule of double-stranded DNA (MW 20–30 × $10^6$, size 36–38 kbp). Viruses contain at least ten structural proteins and are ether-resistant and acid-stable; some are heat-sensitive. Replication occurs in the nucleus and structural proteins are synthesized in the cytoplasm; assembly occurs in the nucleus and virions are released by cell destruction. Host range is generally narrow and transmission may be direct or indirect. Genera include *Mastadenovirus* and *Aviadenovirus.*

**ad·e·no·vi·rus** (ad′ə-no-vi″rəs) [MeSH: Adenoviridae] any virus belonging to the family Adenoviridae. For naming of adenovirus species, see *Aviadenovirus* and *Mastadenovirus.*
**a's of birds,** *Aviadenovirus.*
**fowl a.,** a species of viruses of the genus *Aviadenovirus* that is lethal for chicken embryos and induces tumors in newborn hamsters.
**mammalian a's,** *Mastadenovirus.*

**ad·e·nyl** (ad′ə-nəl) 1. the radical of adenine. 2. a term sometimes (incorrectly) used for adenylyl.

**aden·yl·ate** (ə-den′ə-lāt) the dissociated form of adenylic acid.

**aden·yl·ate cy·clase** (ə-den′ə-lāt si′klās) [EC 4.6.1.1] an enzyme of the lyase class that catalyzes the formation of 3′,5′-cyclic adenosine monophosphate (cAMP) from ATP. The enzyme occurs in plasma cell membranes and is activated by certain hormones (epinephrine, vasopressin, glucagon, and adrenocorticotropic hormone). The resultant cyclic AMP serves as an important metabolic regulator. Called also *adenyl cyclase* and *adenylyl cyclase.*

**aden·yl·ate de·am·i·nase** (ə-den′ə-lāt de-am′ĭ-nās) AMP deaminase.

**aden·yl·ate ki·nase** (ə-den′ə-lāt ki′nās) [EC 2.7.4.3] [MeSH: Adenylate Kinase] an enzyme of the transferase class that catalyzes the reaction 2ADP = ATP + AMP. The enzyme occurs predominantly in muscle and provides a means of using both high-energy phosphate bonds from ATP for muscle contraction. The reaction makes AMP concentration a sensitive indicator of depletion of the high-energy phosphate pool and also maintains balance in the nucleotide pool. Called also *AMP kinase.*

**ad·e·nyl cy·clase** (ad′ə-nəl si′klās) [MeSH: Adenyl Cyclase] adenylate cyclase.

**ad·e·nyl·ic ac·id** (ad″ə-nil′ik) phosphorylated adenosine, usually referring to adenosine monophosphate (q.v.).

**ad·e·nylo·suc·ci·nase** (ad″ə-nəl-o-suk′sĭ-nās) adenylosuccinate lyase.

**ad·e·nyl·o·suc·ci·nate** (ad″ə-nəl-o-suk′sĭ-nāt) adenylate with succinate substituted for the C6 amino group, an intermediate in the biosynthesis of adenylate.

**ad·e·nylo·suc·ci·nate ly·ase** (ad″ə-nəl-o-suk′sĭ-nāt li′ās) [EC 4.3.2.2] [MeSH: Adenylosuccinate Lyase] an enzyme of the lyase class that catalyzes the cleavage of adenylosuccinate to form fumarate and AMP. The enzyme occurs in the liver where it catalyzes several steps in purine nucleotide biosynthesis; in muscle it is involved in the utilization of energy. Called also *adenylosuccinase.*

**ad·e·nyl·o·suc·ci·nate syn·thase** (ad″ə-nəl-o-suk′sin-āt sin′thās) [EC 6.3.4.4] an enzyme of the ligase class that catalyzes the substitution of succinate for the carbonyl oxygen of inosine monophosphate, a step in the biosynthesis of adenosine monophosphate.

**aden·yl·yl** (ad′ə-nĭ-lil) the radical formed by removal of OH from the phosphate group of adenosine monophosphate.

**ad·e·nyl·yl cy·clase** (ad′ə-nəl-əl si′klās) adenylate cyclase.

**ad·e·nyl·yl·trans·fer·ase** (ad″ə-nə-ləl-trans′fər-ās) one of the nucleotidyltransferases [EC 2.7.7] that catalyzes the transfer of an adenylyl residue from one compound to another.

**ad·eps** (ad′eps) gen. *ad′ipis* [L.] lard; the purified omental fat of the hog, used in the preparation of ointments.
**a. anseri′nus,** goose grease.
**a. benzoina′tus,** benzoinated lard.
**a. la′nae,** anhydrous lanolin.
**a. la′nae hydro′sus,** lanolin.
**a. ovil′lus,** sheep lard, or tallow.
**a. por′ci,** hog lard.
**a. re′nis,** the fatty capsule of the kidney.
**a. suil′lus,** hog lard.

**ad·e·qua·cy** (ad′ə-kwə-se) the state of being sufficient for a specific purpose.
**velopharyngeal a.,** sufficient velopharyngeal closure so that air and hence sound cannot enter the nasopharyngeal and nasal cavities. Cf. *velopharyngeal insufficiency.*

**ader·mia** (ə-dər′me-ə) [*a-*[1] + *derm-* + *-ia*] congenital defect or absence of the skin.

**ader·mine** (ə-dər′mēn) pyridoxine; vitamin $B_6$.

**ader·mo·gen·e·sis** (ə-dər-mo-jen′ə-sis) [*a-*[1] + *dermo-* + *-genesis*] imperfect development of the skin.

**Ad grat. acid.** abbreviation for L. *ad gra′tum acidita′tem,* to an agreeable sourness, an obsolete instruction in pharmacy.

**ADH** alcohol dehydrogenase; antidiuretic hormone; see *vasopressin.*

**Ad·hat·o·da** (ad-hat′o-də) a genus of plants of the family Acanthaceae. *A. va′sica* is the Malabar nut tree, used in India for its antispasmodic and expectorant properties.

**ad·her·ence** (ad-hēr′əns) the act or quality of sticking to something.
**immune a.,** the adherence of antigen-antibody complexes or cells coated with antibody or complement to cells bearing complement receptors or Fc receptors. The agglutination reaction between antigen-antibody complexes or antibody coated cells and indicator cells, usually human erythrocytes, bearing complement receptors is used as a detector system in complement fixation tests (immune adherence hemagglutination assay).

**ad·he·sin** (ad-he′zin) any of a group of molecular components of the exterior cell wall of bacteria, involved in adhesion processes. See *adhesion* (def. 1).

**ad·he·sio** (ad-he′ze-o) pl. *adhesio′nes* [L. "clinging together"] adhesion.
**a. interthala′mica** [TA], interthalamic adhesion: a mass of gray matter connecting the thalami across the midline of the third ventricle; it develops as a secondary adhesion and is often absent.

**ad·he·sion** (ad-he′zhən) [L. *adhaesio,* from *adhaerere* to stick to] [MeSH: Adhesions] 1. the property of remaining in close proximity, as that resulting from the physical attraction of molecules to a substance, or the molecular attraction existing between the surfaces of contacting bodies. 2. the stable joining of parts to each other, as in wound healing or some abnormal process; called also *conglutination.* 3. a fibrous band or structure by which parts abnormally adhere.
**amniotic a's,** fibrous adhesions from the amnion to the fetus; see *amniotic band,* under *band.*
**interthalamic a.,** adhesio interthalamica.
**primary a.,** healing by first intention.
**secondary a.,** h. by second intention.
**sublabial a.,** abnormal union of the sublabial mucosa of the upper lip to the alveolar process, as seen in cleft lip.
**traumatic uterine a's,** adhesions of the uterus, most often in the cervical canal, frequently in the uterine cavity, and sometimes in both the cervix and the corpus, which are usually caused by trauma or infection; they may cause amenorrhea. See also *Asherman's syndrome,* under *syndrome.*

**ad·he·si·ot·o·my** (ad-he″ze-ot′ə-me) the cutting or division of adhesions.

**ad·he·sive** (ad-he′siv) [MeSH: Adhesives] 1. sticky; tenacious. 2. a substance that causes close adherence of adjoining surfaces.
**cyanoacrylate a.,** any of a group of adhesives and cements containing cyanoacrylate, widely used in surgery and dentistry.
**dental a.,** a chemical capable of forming a mechanical or chemical bond to tooth structures or restorative materials.
**denture a.,** a substance composed of various types of gum, used to help stabilize a denture base on the underlying mucosa.

**ad·he·sive·ness** (ad-he′siv-nəs) [MeSH: Adhesiveness] the property of remaining adherent.
**platelet a.,** the physical property of platelets by which they stick to a variety of materials in vivo and in vitro, particularly as it occurs in the initial formation of a clot and in the maintenance of hemostasis.

**Adhib.** abbreviation for L. *adhiben′dus,* to be administered.

**adi·a·do·cho·ci·ne·sia** (a-di″ə-do″ko-sĭ-ne′zhə) adiadochokinesia.

**adi·a·do·cho·ci·ne·sis** (a-di″ə-do″ko-sĭ-ne′sis) adiadochokinesia.

**adi·a·do·cho·ki·ne·sia** (ə-di″ə-do″ko-kĭ-ne′zhə) [*a-*[1] + *diadochokinesia*] a dyskinesia consisting of inability to perform the rapid alternating movements of diadochokinesia. Called also *adiadochocinesia, adiadochokinesis,* and *adiadokokinesia.*

**adi·a·do·cho·ki·ne·sis** (a-di″ə-ko-kĭ-ne′sis) adiadochokinesia.

**adi·a·do·ko·ki·ne·sia** (a-di″-ə-do″ko-kĭ-ne′zhə) adiadochokinesia.

**adi·a·do·ko·ki·ne·sis** (a-di″-ə-do″ko-kĭ-ne′sis) adiadochokinesia.

**Ad·i·an·tum** (ad″e-an′təm) [*a-*[1] + Gr. *dianein* to moisten] the maidenhair ferns, a genus of the family Polypodiaceae. *A. peda′tum* is a species found in North America and eastern Asia that has been used as an expectorant and demulcent.

**adi·a·pho·ria** (a″-di-ə-fo′re-ə) [Gr. "indifference"] nonresponse to stimuli as a result of previous exposure to similar stimuli; see also *refractory period,* under *period.*

**adi·a·spi·ro·my·co·sis** (ad″e-ə-spi″ro-mi-ko′sis) a pulmonary disease of many species of rodents and occasionally of humans, caused by the inhalation of spores of the fungus *Emmonsia parva* and *E. crescens.* It is marked by huge spherules in the lungs (adiaspores) without endospores, with symptoms ranging from the subclinical to a bilateral pneumonia. The condition is often confused with the tissue phase of *Coccidioides immitis* infection. Called also *adiasporosis* amd *haplomycosis.*

**adi·a·spore** (ad′e-ə-spor″) a spore produced by the soil fungi *Emmonsia parva* and *E. crescens,* which, after inhalation into the lungs, enlarges to form a huge spherule without endospores.

**adi·a·spo·ro·sis** (ad″e-ə-spo-ro′sis) adiaspiromycosis.

**adi·a·ther·man·cy** (a-di″ə-ther′mən-se) [*a-*[1] + *dia-* + *thermansis* heating] the condition of being impervious to heat waves.

**ad·i·cil·lin** (ad″ĭ-sil′in) a cephalosporin that is less active against gram-positive bacteria than penicillin G but more active against gram-negative organisms and is highly active against *Neisseria;* it has been used in the treatment of typhoid fever and gonorrhea. Called also *cephalosporin N* and *penicillin N.*

**Ad·ie's pupil, syndrome** (a′dēz) [William John *Adie,* English neurologist, 1886–1935] see *tonic pupil,* under *pupil,* and see under *syndrome.*

**adi·emor·rhy·sis** (ə-di″ə-mor′ĭ-sis) [*a-*[1] + *dia-* + *hemo-* + *rhysis* flow] stoppage of circulation of blood.

**ad·i·ent** (ad′e-ənt) tending toward the source of stimulation; positive. Cf. *abient.*

**ad·i·pec·to·my** (ad″ĭ-pek′tə-me) [*adip-* + *-ectomy*] lipectomy.

**ad·i·phen·ine hy·dro·chlo·ride** (ad″ĭ-fen′ēn) an antispasmodic anticholinergic, used orally as a smooth muscle relaxant in the treatment of hypermotility and spasm of the genitourinary and gastrointestinal tracts.

**adip·ic** (ə-dip′ik) [L. *adeps* fat] adipose.

**adip(o)-** [L. *adeps,* gen. *adipis* lard, fat] a combining form denoting relationship to fat.

**ad·i·po·cele** (ad′ĭ-po-sēl″) [*adipo-* + *-cele*[1]] a hernia containing fat or fatty tissue, as an epiplocele.

**ad·i·po·cel·lu·lar** (ad″ĭ-po-sel′u-lər) composed of connective tissue and fat.

**ad·i·po·cer·a·tous** (ad″ĭ-po-ser′ə-təs) pertaining to or resembling adipocere.

**ad·i·po·cere** (ad′ĭ-po-sēr″) [*adipo-* + *cera*] a peculiar waxy substance formed during the decomposition of animal bodies, and seen especially in human bodies buried in moist places; it consists principally of insoluble salts of fatty acids. Called also *grave wax* and *corpse* or *grave fat.*

**ad·i·po·cyte** (ad′ĭ-po-sīt″) [MeSH: Adipocytes] a fat cell; see under *cell.*

**ad·i·po·gen·e·sis** (ad″ĭ-po-jen′ə-sis) [*adipo-* + *-genesis*] lipogenesis.

**ad·i·po·gen·ic** (ad″ĭ-po-jen′ik) lipogenic.

**ad·i·pog·e·nous** (ad″ĭ-poj′ə-nəs) lipogenic.

**ad·i·po·he·pat·ic** (ad″ĭ-po-hə-pat′ik) pertaining to or marked by fatty degeneration of the liver.

**ad·i·poid** (ad′ĭ-poid) [*adipo-* + *-oid*] lipoid, def. 1.

**ad·i·po·ki·ne·sis** (ad″ĭ-po-kĭ-ne′sis) the mobilization of fat in the body, often with the liberation of free fatty acids into the blood plasma; see also *lipolytic hormones,* under *hormone.*

**ad·i·po·kin·et·ic** (ad″-ĭ-po-kĭ-net′ik) pertaining to, characterized by, or promoting adipokinesis.

**ad·i·po·ki·nin** (ad″ĭ-po-ki′nin) former name for $\beta$-lipotropin.

**ad·i·pol·y·sis** (ad″ĭ-pol′ĭ-sis) [*adipo-* + *-lysis*] lipolysis.

**ad·i·po·lyt·ic** (ad″ĭ-po-lit′ik) lipolytic.

**ad·i·pom·e·ter** (ad″ĭ-pom′ə-tər) an instrument for measuring the thickness of the skin fold, as a means of determining the presence of obesity.

**ad·i·po·ne·cro·sis** (ad″ĭ-po-nə-kro′sis) necrosis of fatty tissue.
**a. subcuta′nea neonato′rum,** subcutaneous fat induration in newborn and young infants; called also *subcutaneous fat necrosis* and *pseudosclerema.*

**ad·i·po·pec·tic** (ad″ĭ-po-pek′tik) pertaining to, characterized by, or promoting adipopexis.

**ad·i·po·pex·ia** (ad″ĭ-po-pek′se-ə) adipopexis.

**ad·i·po·pex·ic** (ad″ĭ-po-pek′sik) adipopectic.

**ad·i·po·pex·is** (ad″ĭ-po-pek′sis) [*adipo-* + *pexis*] the fixation or storing of fats.

**ad·i·pos·al·gia** (ad″ĭ-pōs-al′jə) [*adipo-* + *-algia*] painful areas of subcutaneous fat.

**ad·i·pose** (ad′ĭ-pōs) [L. *adiposus* fatty] 1. of a fatty nature; fatty; fat. 2. the fat present in the cells of adipose tissue.

**ad·i·po·sis** (ad″ĭ-po′sis) [*adip-* + *-osis*] 1. obesity. 2. fatty change of an organ or tissue.
**a. cerebra′lis,** cerebral adiposity.
**a. doloro′sa,** a disease accompanied by painful localized fatty swellings and by various nerve lesions. The disease is usually seen in women, and may cause death from pulmonary complications. Called also *Dercum's disease.*
**a. hepa′tica,** fatty change of the liver.
**a. tubero′sa sim′plex,** a disorder resembling adiposis dolorosa, marked by development in the subcutaneous tissue of fatty masses which are sometimes painful to pressure; called also *Anders' disease.*
**a. universa′lis,** a deposit of fat generally throughout the body, including the internal organs.

**ad·i·pos·i·tas** (ad″ĭ-pos′ĭ-təs) [L.] obesity.
**a. ex vac′uo,** fatty atrophy.

**ad·i·po·si·tis** (ad″ĭ-po-si′tis) panniculitis.

**ad·i·pos·i·ty** (ad″ĭ-pos′ĭ-te) obesity.
**cerebral a.,** obesity due to a lesion in the brain, especially the hypothalamus, as in adiposogenital dystrophy. Called also *adiposis cerebralis.*
**pituitary a.,** obesity formerly believed to be due to pituitary insufficiency but actually due to a lesion of the diencephalon such as a tumor that impinges on the pituitary gland.

**ad·i·po·su·ria** (ad″ĭ-po-su′re-ə) [*adipo-* + *-uria*] the presence of fat in the urine; lipuria, or lipiduria.

**adip·sia** (ə-dip′se-ə) [*a-*[1] + *dipsia*] absence of thirst, or abnormal avoidance of drinking.

**ad·i·tus** (ad′ĭ-təs) pl. *ad′itus* [L "approach"] [TA] a general term for the entrance or approach to an organ or part.
**a. ad an′trum mastoi′deum** [TA], an opening between the epitympanum and the mastoid antrum.
**a. laryn′gis** [TA], the aperture by which the pharynx communicates with the larynx; called also *aperture of larynx.*
**a. or′bitae, a. orbita′lis** [TA], orbital opening: the opening to the orbit in the cranium; called also *orbital aperture* and *anterior opening of orbital cavity.*
**a. ad pel′vem,** the pelvic inlet (apertura pelvis superior [TA]).
**a. vagi′nae,** ostium vaginae.

**ad·junct** (ad′junkt) an accessory or auxiliary agent or measure.

**ad·just·ment** (ə-just′mənt) 1. the act or process of modification of physical parts made in response to changing conditions. 2. in psychology, the relative degree of harmony between an individual's needs and the requirements of the environment. 3. a modification made in a denture after its completion and insertion in the mouth. 4. the mechanism for raising and lowering the tube of a microscope to bring the object being examined into focus. 5. in chiropractic, manipulation of the spine, said to restore normal nerve function.
**occlusal a.,** selective grinding of occlusal surfaces of the teeth to eliminate premature contacts and occlusal interferences. Called also *occlusal equilibration.* See also *milling-in.*

**ad·ju·vant** (aj′ə-vənt, ă-joo′vənt) [L. *adjuvans* aiding] 1. assisting or aiding. 2. a substance that aids another, such as an auxiliary remedy. 3. in immunology, a nonspecific stimulator of the immune response, such as BCG vaccine.
**A. 65,** trademark for a water-in-oil emulsion containing antigen in peanut oil with Arlacel A and aluminum monostearate as the emulsifying agent.
**aluminum a.,** an aluminum-containing compound, such as aluminum hydroxide or alum, that by combining with soluble antigen forms a precipitate; slow release of the antigen from the precipitate on injection causes prolonged, strong antibody response.
**Freund's a.,** a water-in-oil emulsion incorporating antigen, in the aqueous phase, into lightweight paraffin oil with the aid of an emulsifying agent. On injection, this mixture *(Freund's incomplete a.)* induces strong persistent antibody formation. The addition of killed, dried mycobacteria, e.g., *Mycobacterium butyricum,* to the oil phase *(Freund's complete a.)* elicits cell-mediated immunity (delayed hypersensitivity), as well as humoral antibody formation.
**mycobacterial a.,** Freund's complete a.; see *Freund's a.*

**ad·ju·van·tic·i·ty** (aj″ə-vən-tis′ĭ-te, ă-joo″vən-tis′ĭ-te) the ability to nonspecifically stimulate the immune response.

**ADL** activities of daily living.

**Ad·ler** (ahd′lər) Alfred. Austrian psychiatrist, 1870–1937. A student of Freud who developed his own psychoanalytic theory stating that the need for superiority and power is a more driving force than Freud's postulated unconscious sexual libido. Adler concentrated on overt personality manifestations and was the first to use such terms as inferiority complex and compensation.

**ad lib.** abbreviation for L. *ad lib′itum,* at pleasure.

**ad·me·di·al** (ad-me′de-əl) situated near the median plane.

**ad·me·di·an** (ad-me′de-ən) toward the median plane, or midline of the body.

**ad·mi·nic·u·la** (ad″mĭ-nik′u-lə) [L.] plural of *adminiculum.*

**ad·mi·nic·u·lum** (ad″mĭ-nik′u-ləm) pl. *adminic′ula* [L.] a prop or support.
**a. lin′eae al′bae** [TA], the expansion of fibers extending from the superior pubic ligament to the posterior surface of the linea alba.

**ad·mit·tance** (ad-mit′əns) the measure of how readily an alternating current flows in a circuit; it is the ratio of peak current to peak voltage, the reciprocal of impedance. The unit of admittance is the siemens. Symbol *A.*
**acoustic a.,** the ease of energy flow through the middle ear. See also *acoustic immittance.*

**admov.** abbreviation for L. *ad′move, admovea′tur,* add, let there be added.

**ad nau·se·am** (ad naw′se-əm) [L.] to the extent of producing nausea.

**ad·ner·val** (ad-nər′vəl) 1. situated near a nerve. 2. toward a nerve, said of an electric current which passes through muscle toward the entrance point of a nerve.

**ad·neu·ral** (ad-noor′əl) [*ad-* + *neural*] adnerval.

**ad·nexa** (ad-nek′sə) [L., pl.] appendages or adjunct parts; see also *appendage.*
**a. mastoi′dea,** the structures in the mastoid (posterior) wall of the middle ear, including the mastoid antrum and its aditus and the mastoid air cells.
**a. o′culi,** the eyelids, lacrimal apparatus, and other appendages of the eye.
**a. u′teri,** uterine appendages.

**ad·nex·al** (ad-nek′səl) pertaining to adnexa, especially the adnexa uteri.

**ad·nex·ec·to·my** (ad″nek-sek′tə-me) [*adnexa* + *-ectomy*] excision or removal of the adnexa, especially the adnexa uteri.

**ad·nex·i·tis** (ad″nek-si′tis) [MeSH: Adnexitis] inflammation of the adnexa uteri.

**ad·nex·or·ga·no·gen·ic** (ad-neks″or″gə-no-jen′ik) giving rise to or originating in the adnexa uteri.

**AdoCbl** adenosylcobalamin.

**ad·o·les·cence** (ad″o-les′əns) [L. *adolescentia*] [MeSH: Adolescence] the period of life beginning with the appearance of secondary sex characters and terminating with the cessation of somatic growth, roughly from 11 to 19 years of age; cf. *puberty.*

**ad·o·les·cent** (ad″o-les′ənt) [MeSH: Adolescence] 1. pertaining to adolescence. 2. an individual during the period of adolescence.

**ad·or·al** (ad-o′rəl) [*ad-* + *oral*] toward or near the mouth.

**ADP** adenosine diphosphate; aminohydroxypropylidene diphosphonate (pamidronate, q.v.).

**Ad pond. om.** abbreviation for L. *ad pon′dus om′nium,* to the weight of the whole.

**ad·re·nal** (ə-dre′nəl) [*ad-* + *renal*] 1. pertaining to either of two glands located just above the kidneys; see *glandula suprarenalis.* Called also *suprarenal.* 2. glandula suprarenalis. 3. paranephric (def. 1).
**Marchand's a's,** accessory adrenal bodies in the broad ligament.

**ad·re·nal·ec·to·mize** (ə-dre′nəl-ek′to-mīz) to excise one or both adrenal glands.

**ad·re·nal·ec·to·my** (ə-dre″nəl-ek′to-me) [*adrenal* + *-ectomy*] [MeSH: Adrenalectomy] excision of one *(unilateral adrenalectomy)* or both *(bilateral adrenalectomy)* adrenal glands; called also *suprarenalectomy.*

**Adren·a·lin** (ə-dren′ə-lin) trademark for preparations of epinephrine.

**adren·a·line** (ə-dren′ə-lin) epinephrine.
**a. acid tartrate,** epinephrine bitartrate.

**adren·a·lin·emia** (ə-dren″ə-lin-e′me-ə) the presence of epinephrine in the blood.

**adren·a·lin·uria** (ə-dren″ə-lin-u′re-ə) the presence of epinephrine in the urine.

**adren·al·ism** (ə-dren′əl-iz-əm) any disorder of adrenal function, whether decreased (adrenal or adrenocortical insufficiency) or increased (hyperadrenalism or hyperadrenocorticism). Called also *dysadrenalism* and *suprarenalism.*

**adre·na·li·tis** (ə-dre″nəl-i′tis) inflammation of the adrenal glands; called also *adrenitis.*

**adren·a·lone** (ə-dren′ə-lōn) an adrenergic obtained by oxidation of an epinephrine derivative; it has vasoconstrictor activity.

**adre·nal·op·a·thy** (ə-dre″nəl-op′ə-the) [*adrenal* + *-pathy*] any disease of the adrenal glands. Called also *adrenopathy, suprarenalopathy,* and *suprarenopathy.*

**adren·a·lo·trop·ic** (ə-dren″ə-lo-trop′ik) [*adrenal* + *-tropic*] 1. adrenotropic. 2. pertaining to the developmental stage preceding puberty, during which adrenal androgen secretion increases.

**ad·ren·ar·che** (ad″rən-ahr′ke) [*adren-* + *arche*] augmentation of adrenal cortical secretion, involving especially androgens, a physiologic change that occurs at approximately the age of eight years in both sexes.

**ad·ren·er·gic** (ad″ren-ər′-jik) 1. activated by, characteristic of, or secreting epinephrine or related substances, particularly referring to the sympathetic nerve fibers that liberate norepinephrine at a synapse when a nerve impulse passes. See also under *receptor.* Cf. *cholinergic.* 2. an agent that produces such an effect. Called also *sympathomimetic.*

**adre·nic** (ə-dren′ik) adrenal (def. 1).

**ad·re·ni·tis** (ad″rə-ni′tis) adrenalitis.

**adren(o)-** [*ad-* near + *ren* kidney] a combining form denoting relationship to the adrenal gland.

**adre·no·cep·tive** (ə-dre″no-sep′tiv) pertaining to the sites on effector organs that are acted upon by adrenergic transmitters.

**adre·no·cep·tor** (ə-dre″no-sep′tor) an adrenergic receptor.

**adre·no·chrome** (ə-dre′no-krōm″) [MeSH: Adrenochrome] an oxidation product of epinephrine which has hemostatic properties due to its effect on capillary permeability; it is used in the form of its stable derivative *carbazochrome salicylate.*

**adre·no·cor·ti·cal** (ə-dre″no-kor′tĭ-kəl) pertaining to or arising from the adrenal cortex.

**adre·no·cor·ti·co·hy·per·pla·sia** (ə-dre″no-kor″tĭ-ko-hi″pər-pla′zhə) adrenal cortical hyperplasia.

**adre·no·cor·ti·coid** (ə-dre″no-kor′tĭ-koid″) corticosteroid.

**adre·no·cor·ti·co·mi·met·ic** (ə-dre″no-kor″tĭ-ko-mi-met′ik) producing effects similar to those of the adrenocortical hormones (corticosteroids).

**adre·no·cor·ti·co·troph·ic** (ə-dre″no-kor″tĭ-ko-trof′ik) adrenocorticotropic.

**adre·no·cor·ti·co·troph·in** (ə-dre″no-kor′tĭ-ko-tro″fin) 1. adrenocorticotropic hormone. 2. corticotropin (def. 1).

**adre·no·cor·ti·co·trop·ic** (ə-dre″no-kor″tĭ-ko-trop′ik) having a stimulating effect on the adrenal cortex; called also *adrenocorticotrophic* and *corticotropic.*

**adre·no·cor·ti·co·trop·in** (ə-dre″no-kor″tĭ-ko-tro′pin) 1. corticotropin (def. 1). 2. adrenocorticotropic hormone.

**adre·no·dox·in** (ə-dre″no-dok′sin) [MeSH: Adrenodoxin] an iron-sulfur protein occurring in the mitochondria of the adrenal cortex and serving as an electron carrier in the series of redox reactions by which adrenal steroid hormones are biosynthesized from cholesterol.

**ad·re·no·gen·ic** (ə-dre″no-jen′ik) adrenogenous.

**ad·re·nog·e·nous** (ad″ren-oj′ə-nəs) [*adreno-* + *-genous*] produced or arising in an adrenal gland.

**ad·re·no·gram** (ə-dre′no-gram) a radiograph of the adrenal glands.

**ad·re·no·ki·net·ic** (ə-dre″no-kĭ-net′ik) adrenotropic.

**adre·no·leu·ko·dys·tro·phy** (ə-dre″no-loo″ko-dis′tro-fe) [MeSH: Adrenoleukodystrophy] an X-linked recessive disease of childhood, closely related to Schilder's disease, marked by diffuse abnormality of the cerebral white matter and adrenal atrophy and characterized by mental deterioration progressing to dementia, and by aphasia, apraxia, dysarthria, and loss of vision in about a third of the patients. Almost all show abnormal adrenal functioning when tested.

**adre·no·lyt·ic** (ə-dre″no-lit′ik) [*adreno-* + *-lytic*] inhibiting the action of adrenergic nerves; inhibiting the response to epinephrine. Cf. *adrenergic blocking agent,* under *agent.*

**adre·no·med·ul·lary** (ə-dre″no-med′u-ler″e) pertaining to or originating in the adrenal medulla. Called also *medulloadrenal.*

**adre·no·med·ul·lo·trop·ic** (ə-dre″no-med″u-lo-trop′ik) having a stimulatory influence on the adrenal medulla.

**adre·no·meg·a·ly** (ə-dre″no-meg′ə-le) [*adreno-* + *-megaly*] enlargement of one or both of the adrenal glands.

**adre·no·mi·met·ic** (ə-dre″no-mi-met′ik) sympathomimetic.

**adre·no·my·elo·neu·rop·a·thy** (ə-dre″no-mi″ə-lo-noo͝-rop′ə-the) a hereditary condition related to adrenoleukodystrophy but including spinal cord degeneration and peripheral neuropathy; it affects mainly adults.

**ad·ren·op·a·thy** (ad″rən-op′ə-the) adrenalopathy.

**adre·no·pri·val** (ad-re′no-pri″vəl) pertaining to or characterized by adrenocortical insufficiency.

**adre·no·re·cep·tor** (ə-dre″no-re-sep′tor) an adrenergic receptor.

**Adren·o·sem** (ə-dren′o-sem) trademark for preparations of carbazochrome salicylate.

**adre·no·stat·ic** (ə-dre″no-stat′ik) 1. inhibiting the activity of the adrenal glands. 2. an agent that inhibits the activity of the adrenal glands.

**adre·nos·te·rone** (ă″-drĕ-nos′tər-ōn) an androgenic steroid isolated from the adrenal cortex.

**adre·no·tox·in** (ə-dre″no-tok′sin) any substance that is toxic to the adrenals.

**adre·no·troph·ic** (ə-dre″no-trof′ik) [*adreno-* + *-trophic*] adrenotropic.

**adre·no·tro·phin** (ə-dre′no-tro″fin) 1. adrenocorticotropic hormone. 2. corticotropin (def. 1).

**adre·no·trop·ic** (ə-dre″no-trop′ik) [*adreno-* + *-tropic*] having specific affinity for or growth-promoting or hormonal secretory influence on the adrenal glands; see also *adrenocorticotropic* and *adrenomedullotropic.* Called also *adrenotrophic* and *suprarenotropic.*

**adre·no·tro·pin** (ədre′no-tro″pin) 1. adrenocorticotropic hormone. 2. corticotropin (def. 1).

**Adri·a·my·cin** (a″-dre-ə-mi′sin) trademark for preparations of doxorubicin hydrochloride.

**Adri·an** (a′dre-an) **of Cam·bridge** Baron (Edgar Douglas Adrian). English physiologist, 1889–1977; co-winner, with Sir Charles Scott Sherrington, of the Nobel prize for medicine or physiology in 1932 for their work on the function of the neuron.

**adro·mia** (ə-dro′me-ə) [*a-*[1] + *dromo-* + *-ia*] absence of conduction in nerve of muscle.

**Ad·royd** (ad'roid) trademark for a preparation of oxymetholone.

**Adru·cil** (a'droo-sil) trademark of a preparation of fluorouracil for injection.

**ad·rue** (ad-roo'a) *Cyperus articulatus,* a grasslike plant of the West Indies whose root is aromatic tonic, antiemetic, and anthelmintic.

**ADS** antidiuretic substance; see *vasopressin.*

**Ad·son's maneuver (test)** (ad'sənz) [Alfred Washington *Adson,* American neurosurgeon, 1887–1951] see under *maneuver.*

**ad·sorb** (ad-sorb') to attract and retain other material on the surface; to conduct the process of adsorption.

**ad·sor·bate** (ad-sor'bāt) a substance taken up on a surface by adsorption.

**ad·sor·bent** (ad-sor'bənt) 1. pertaining to or characterized by adsorption. 2. an agent that attracts other materials or particles to its surface by adsorption.

**ad·sorp·tion** (ad-sorp'shən) [L. *ad-* to + *sorption*] [MeSH: Adsorption] the attachment of one substance to the surface of another; the concentration of a gas or a substance in solution in a liquid on a surface in contact with the gas or liquid, resulting in a relatively high concentration of the gas or solution at the surface. Cf. *absorption.*
**agglutinin a.,** the taking up by bacteria suspended in diluted antiserum of those agglutinins specific for that microorganism.
**immune a.,** the use of antigen as a specific adsorbent for antibody or the use of antibody or antiserum as a specific adsorbent for antigen; the antigen-antibody complex is removed by filtration or centrifugation.

**ad·ster·nal** (ad-stər'nəl) toward or near the sternum.

**adst. feb.** abbreviation for L. *adstan'te feb're,* while fever is present; cf. *abs. feb.*

**ad·ter·mi·nal** (ad-tər'mĭ-nəl) [*ad-* + *terminal*] moving from the center toward the end of a muscle; said of an electric current.

**ad·tor·sion** (ad-tor'shən) intorsion.

**adult** (ə-dult') [L. *adultus* grown up] [MeSH: Adult] 1. having attained full growth or maturity. 2. a living organism that has attained full growth or maturity.

**adul·ter·ant** (ə-dul'tər-ənt) a substance used as an addition to another substance for sophistication or adulteration.

**adul·te·ra·tion** (ə-dul"tər-a'shən) addition of an impure, cheap, or unnecessary ingredient to cheat, cheapen, or falsify a preparation; in legal terminology, incorrect labeling, including dosage not in accordance with the label.

**ad·um·bra·tion** (ad"əm-bra'shən) 1. an inherent property of the focal spot which causes the production of double images. 2. in radiology, the giving forth of a shadow.

**Adv.** abbreviation for L. *adver'sum,* against.

**ad·vance** (ad-vans') [Fr. *avancer*] to perform the operation of advancement.

**ad·vance·ment** (ad-vans'mənt) 1. surgical detachment, as of a muscle or tendon, followed by reattachment at an advanced point. 2. orthognathic surgery in which the mandible is moved forward.
**capsular a.,** the artificial attachment of Tenon's capsule in such a way as to draw forward the insertion of an ocular muscle.

**ad·ven·ti·tia** (ad"ven-tish'e-ə) [L. *adventicious* from without] 1. adventitial. 2. tunica adventitia; the outermost connective tissue covering of an organ, vessel, or other structure.

**ad·ven·ti·tial** (ad"ven-tish'əl) pertaining to the tunica adventitia; called also *adventitious.*

**ad·ven·ti·tious** (ad"vent-tish'əs) [*ad-* + *venire* to come] 1. accidental or acquired; not natural or hereditary. 2. found somewhere other than in the normal or usual place. 3. adventitial.

**Ad 2 vic.** abbreviation of L. *ad du'as vi'ces,* at two times, for two doses.

**Ad·vil** (ad'vil) trademark for a preparation of ibuprofen.

**ady·na·mia** (a-di-na'me-ə) [*a-*[1] + *dynam-* + *-ia*] lack or loss of the normal or vital powers; asthenia.
**a. episo'dica heredita'ria,** periodic paralysis II.

**ady·nam·ic** (a-di-nam'ik) characterized by adynamia; asthenic.

**ae-** for words beginning thus, see also those beginning *e-.*

**Ae·by's muscle, plane** (a'bēz) [Christopher Theodore *Aeby,* Swiss anatomist, 1835–1885] see *musculus depressor labii inferioris,* and see under *plane.*

**aec-** for words beginning thus, see also words beginning *ec-.*

**aeci·um** (e'se-əm) pl. *ae'cia* [Gr. *aikia* injury] a cup-shaped fruiting body of a rust fungus; see *rust* (def. 3).

**Ae·des** (a-e'dēz) [Gr. *aēdēs* unpleasant] [MeSH: Aedes] a genus of mosquitoes of the tribe Aedini, subfamily Culicinae, having broad appressed scales on the head and scutellum. The palpi in the female are short and sparsely tufted and have three segments of equal length; in the male, the palpi are long and tufted. In addition to the vectors listed below, the following species are annoying because of their bites: *A. al'drichi, A. commu'nis, A. excru'cians, A. punc'tor, A. sti'mulans,* and *A. vex'ans.* Also written *Aëdes.*
**A. aegyp'ti,** the tiger mosquito, which breeds near houses and transmits urban yellow fever and dengue; it may also transmit filariasis and encephalitis.
**A. africa'nus,** an arboreal mosquito that attacks monkeys and is a vector of the yellow fever virus over much of Central Africa. It also carries the Zika virus.
**A. albopic'tus,** a species that transmits yellow fever, equine encephalomyelitis, and dengue.
**A. atlan'ticus,** a North American species that is a vector of eastern equine encephalitis and of *Dirofilaria immitis.*
**A. canaden'sis,** a North American species that is a vector of eastern equine encephalitis and La Crosse virus.
**A. cine'reus,** a species occurring in certain parts of the United States which transmits equine encephalomyelitis.
**A. flaves'cens,** a species of the Pacific Islands which transmits filariasis.
**A. ingra'mi,** a species found in the pool from which Uganda S virus was isolated in 1947.
**A. leucocelae'nus,** a South American species that transmits jungle yellow fever.
**A. mela'nimon,** a species that is a vector of California encephalitis.
**A. polynesien'sis,** a species of the South Pacific islands which is a vector of filaria and dengue.
**A. pseudoscutella'ris,** a species of the Pacific Islands which is a vector of filaria.
**A. scapula'ris,** a vector of the Cache Valley virus in Trinidad.
**A. serra'tus,** a South American species that is a vector of Oropouche virus.
**A. simp'soni,** a vector of jungle yellow fever in Africa.
**A. sollic'itans,** the common salt-marsh mosquito of the Atlantic and Gulf coasts, a vector of equine encephalomyelitis.
**A. spen'cerii,** a species found on the prairies of western Canada.
**A. taeniorhyn'chus,** a New World species that is the vector of a number of diseases, including equine encephalitis, dengue in Florida, and wuchereriasis.
**A. to'goi,** a species of Japan that serves as a vector of *Brugia malayi,* which causes filariasis malayi.
**A. triseria'tus,** a species that transmits La Crosse encephalitis.
**A. varipal'pus,** a species found along the Pacific coast.

**Ae·di·ni** (a-e-di'ni) a tribe of mosquitoes of the subfamily Culicinae, including the genera *Aedes, Armigeres, Haemagogus,* and *Psorophora.*

**aed·oeo·ceph·a·lus** (ēd"e-o-sef'ə-lus) [Gr. *aidoia* genitals + *-cephalus*] a fetus with no mouth, a nose like a penis, and but one orbit.

**Aeg.** abbreviation for L. *aeger, aegra,* the patient.

**Ae·gyp·ti·a·nel·la** (e-jip"she-ə-nel'ə) [named for *Egypt,* where the organism was first described in 1929] a genus of bacteria of the family Anaplasmataceae, order Rickettsiales, occurring as a parasite in wild and domestic birds.
**A. pullo'rum,** a species found in the blood of fowl. Called also *Balfour's bodies.*

**aelu·ro·pho·bia** (e-loo"ro-fo'be-ə) [Gr. *ailouros* cat + *-phobia*] ailurophobia.

**Aelu·ro·stron·gy·lus** (e-loo"ro-stron'jĭ-lus) a genus of nematodes of the family Angiostrongylidae. *A. abstru'sus* is a lungworm that causes verminous bronchitis or pneumonia in cats.

**-aemia** see *-emia.*

**AEP** auditory evoked potential.

**aequa·tor** (e-kwa'tor) [L. "equalizer"] equator.

**aequor·in** (e-kwor'in) [MeSH: Aequorin] a protein isolated from a species of jellyfish, bioluminescent in proportion to the amount of ionic calcium present; injected into living cells to test for the presence of calcium ions.

**aer·at·ed** (ār'āt"əd) [L. *aeratus*] 1. charged with air. 2. charged with carbon dioxide. 3. oxygenated.

**aer·a·tion** (ār"a'shən) 1. the exchange of carbon dioxide for oxygen by the blood in the lungs. 2. the charging of a liquid with air or gas.

**aer·emia** (ār"e'me-ə) [*aer-* + *-emia*] air embolism.

**aer(o)-** [Gr. *aēr* air] a combining form denoting relationship to air or gas.

**Aero·bac·ter** (ār"o-bak'tər) [*aero-* + *-bacter*] in former systems of

classification, a genus of bacteria of the family Enterobacteriaceae, consisting of gram-negative, facultatively anaerobic, motile rods; individual species have been assigned to the genera *Enterobacter* and *Klebsiella.*
**A. aero'genes,** *Enterobacter aerogenes.*
**A. cloa'cae,** *Enterobacter cloacae.*

**aer·obe** (ār'ōb) [*aero-* + Gr. *bios* life] a microorganism that can live and grow in the presence of free oxygen.
**facultative a's,** microorganisms that are able to live under either aerobic or anaerobic conditions.
**obligate a's,** microorganisms that require molecular oxygen for growth.

**aer·o·bic** (ār-o'bik) 1. having molecular oxygen present. 2. growing, living, or occurring in the presence of molecular oxygen. 3. requiring oxygen for respiration. 4. designed to increase oxygen consumption by the body; see *aerobic exercise,* under *exercise.*

**Aero·Bid** (ār'o-bid") trademark for a preparation of flunisolide.

**aero·bi·ol·o·gy** (ār"o-bi-ol'ə-je) [*aero-* + *biology*] that branch of biology which deals with the distribution of living organisms by the air, either the exterior or outdoor air *(extramural a.)* or the indoor air *(intramural a.).*

**aero·bi·o·sis** (ār"o-bi-o'sis) [*aero-* + *biosis*] [MeSH: Aerobiosis] life in the presence of molecular oxygen.

**aero·bi·ot·ic** (ār"o-bi-ot'ik) pertaining to aerobiosis.

**aero·cele** (ār'o-sēl") [*aero-* + *-cele*[1]] pneumatocele (def. 1).
**epidural a.,** a collection of air between the dura mater and the wall of the spinal column.
**intracranial a.,** pneumocephalus resulting from trauma.

**Aero·coc·cus** (ār"o-kok'əs) a genus of aerobic, gram-positive cocci of the family Streptococcaceae.
**A. vi'ridans,** a species indistinguishable from *Gaffkya homari,* which may be pathogenic for lobsters, and has been found in infections of the urinary tract and in endocarditis in humans.

**aero·col·pos** (ā"ro-kol'pəs) [*aero-* + Gr. *kolpos* bosom or fold] distention of the vagina with gas.

**aero·cys·tog·ra·phy** (ār"o-sis-tog'rə-fe) radiography of the bladder after it has been injected with air; called also *pneumocystography.*

**aero·cys·to·scope** (ār"o-sis'to-skōp) aerourethroscope.

**aero·cys·tos·co·py** (ār"o-sis-tos'ko-pe) [*aero-* + *cysto-* + *-scopy*] aerourethroscopy.

**aero·der·mec·ta·sia** (ār"o-dər"mek-ta'zhə) [*aero-* + *derm-* + *ectasia*] subcutaneous emphysema; it may be spontaneous, traumatic, or surgical in origin.

**aer·o·di·ges·tive** (ār"o-dĭ-jes'tiv) [*aero* + digestive] pertaining to the respiratory and digestive tracts, or parts of them, considered together.

**aer·odon·tal·gia** (ār"o-don-tal'jə) [*aero-* + *odontalgia*] toothache experienced at lowered atmospheric pressures, as in aircraft flight or in a decompression chamber, caused by the expansion of air in the maxillary sinuses. Called also *aero-odontalgia* and *aero-odontodynia.*

**aer·odon·tics** (ār"o-don'tiks) that branch of dentistry which is concerned with effects on the teeth of high altitude flying.

**aero·em·bo·lism** (ār"o-em'bo-liz-əm) air embolism.

**aero·gas·tria** (ār-o-gas'tre-ə) the presence of gas in the stomach; stomach bubble. See also *magenblase.*
**blocked a.,** retention of air in the stomach due to spasm of the esophagus.

**aero·gel** (ār'o-jel") a porous solid formed by replacing the liquid of a gel with a gas, such as rigid plastic foam.

**aero·gen** (ār'-o-jen") an aerogenic, or gas-producing, bacterium.

**aero·gen·e·sis** (ār"o-jen'ə-sis) [*aero-* + *-genesis*] gas production.

**aero·gen·ic** (ār-o-jen'ik) producing gas; said of bacteria that liberate free gaseous products.

**aer·og·e·nous** (ār"oj'ə-nəs) aerogenic.

**aero·med·i·cine** (ār"o-med'ə-sin) aviation medicine.

**Aero·mo·nas** (ār"o-mo'nəs) [*aero-* + Gr. *monas* unit] [MeSH: Aeromonas] a genus of gram-negative, facultatively anaerobic, rod-shaped bacteria of the family Vibrionaceae, consisting of small organisms with polar flagella, found in salt and fresh water, sewage, and soil. They cause disease in humans, amphibians, fish, and reptiles.
**A. ca'viae,** a species found in fresh water and sewage and on fish that causes gastroenteritis and wound infections in humans.
**A. hydro'phila,** a species that causes red leg in frogs. In humans it is a cause of cellulitis, wound infections, acute diarrheal disease, septicemia, and urinary tract infections. Called also *Proteus hydrophilus* and *P. melanovogenes.*
**A. so'bria,** a species found in fresh water, in sewage, and on fish; it causes gastroenteritis and wound infections in humans.

**aero·odon·tal·gia** (ār"o-o"don-tal'jə) aerodontalgia.

**aero·odon·to·dy·nia** (ār"-o-o-don"to-din'e-ə) aerodontalgia.

**aero·oti·tis** (ār"-o-o-ti'tis) [*aero-* + *otitis*] barotitis.

**aer·op·a·thy** (ār"op'ə-the) [*aero-* + *-pathy*] any disease due to change in atmospheric pressure, such as decompression sickness or air sickness.

**aero·peri·to·ne·um** (ār"o-pər"ĭ-to-ne'um) [*aero-* + *peritoneum*] pneumoperitoneum.

**aero·peri·to·nia** (ār"o-per"ĭ-to'ne-ə) pneumoperitoneum.

**aero·pha·gia** (ār"o-fa'jə) [*aero-* + *-phagia*] excessive swallowing of air, usually an unconscious process associated with anxiety, resulting in abdominal distention or belching, often interpreted by the patient as signs of a physical disorder.

**aer·oph·a·gy** (ār"of'ə-je) [MeSH: Aerophagy] aerophagia.

**aero·phil** (ār'o-fil") [*aero-* + *-phil*] an aerophilic organism.

**aero·phil·ic** (ār"o-fil'ik) requiring air for proper growth; aerobic.

**aer·oph·i·lous** (ār-of'-ĭ-lus) aerophilic.

**aero·pho·bia** (ār-o-fo'be-ə) [*aero-* + *-phobia*] irrational fear of drafts or fresh air, often connected with the idea of harmful airborne influences.

**aero·plank·ton** (ār"o-plank'ton) the organisms (bacteria, pollen, etc.) present in the air.

**Aero·plast** (ār'o-plast") trademark for a preparation of vibesate.

**Aero·seb-Dex** (ār'o-seb-deks') trademark for preparations of dexamethasone.

**Aero·seb-HC** (ār'o-seb") trademark for a preparation of hydrocortisone.

**aero·si·a·loph·a·gy** (ār"o-si"ə-lof'ə-je) sialoaerophagy.

**aero·si·nu·si·tis** (ār"o-si"nəs-i'tis) barosinusitis.

**aer·o·sis** (ār"-o'sis) the production of gas in the tissues or organs of the body.

**aer·o·sol** (ār'o-sol) 1. a colloid system, a type of sol, in which the continuous phase (dispersion medium) is a gas, e.g., fog. 2. a liquid stored under pressure along with a propellant so that it can be dispensed as a fine mist, e.g., a bactericidal solution that can be finely atomized for the purpose of sterilizing the air of a room. 3. a solution of a drug that can be atomized into a fine mist for inhalation therapy.

**aero·sol·i·za·tion** (ār"o-sol"ĭ-za'shən) conversion into an aerosol. See also *nebulization.*

**Aero·spo·rin** (ār"o-spor'in) trademark for a preparation of polymyxin B sulfate.

**aero·tax·is** (ār"o-tak'sis) [*aero-* + *-taxis*] a movement of an organism in response to the presence of molecular oxygen.

**aer·oti·tis** (ār"o-ti'tis) barotitis.
**a. me'dia,** barotitis media.

**aero·tol·er·ant** (ār"o-tol'ər-ənt) able to survive or to grow slowly in an aerobic environment; said of certain anaerobic microorganisms.

**aero·to·nom·e·ter** (ār"o-tə-nom'ə-tər) [*aero-* + *tonometer*] an instrument for measuring the partial pressure of the gases in the blood.

**aer·ot·ro·pism** (ār"ot'ro-piz"əm) [*aero-* + *tropism*] movement of an organism toward *(positive a.)* or away from *(negative a.)* a supply of air.

**aero·ure·thro·scope** (ār"o-u-re'thro-skōp") [*aero-* + *urethroscope*] a urethroscope by which the urethra is dilated with air before inspection; called also *aerocystoscope.*

**aero·ure·thros·co·py** (ār"o-u"re-thros̆'kə-pe) examination of the bladder with an aerourethroscope; called also *aerocystoscopy.*

**aes-** for words beginning thus, see also those beginning *es-, et-.*

**aes·cu·la·pi·an** (es"ku-la'pe-ən) pertaining to Aesculapius, the god of medicine, or to the art of medicine.

**Aescu·la·pi·us** (es"ku-la'pe-əs) [L., from Gr. *Asklēpios*] the mythical god or deified hero of healing; also known as *Asclepios.* See also *Asclepiad, asclepion, Hygeia,* and *Panacea,* and under *staff.*

**aes·cu·lin** (es'ku-lin) esculin.

**Aes·cu·lus** (es'ku-ləs) a genus of trees of the family Hippocastanaceae; most species of which contain the coumarin glycoside esculin, which makes them toxic to livestock. *A. hippocasta'num* L. is the horse chestnut, whose bark and seeds were formerly used to treat rheumatism and malaria and as an anticoagulant. *A. glab'ra* is the buckeye.

**aesthesi(o)-** for words beginning thus, see those beginning *esthesi(o)-*.

**aes·thet·ic** (es-thet'ik) esthetic.

**aes·thet·ics** (es-thet'iks) esthetics.

**aet.** abbreviation for L. *ae'tas,* age.

**Aëti·us (Aeti·os) of Ami·da** (a-e'she-əs) [500–575] a Byzantine Greek writer and physician to the Emperor Justinian; his *Tetrabiblion* gives details of the works of Rufus (of Ephesus), Leonides, Soranus, and Philumenus, and accounts of diseases of the eye, ear, nose, and throat, and also of technical procedures (e.g., tonsillectomy, urethrotomy, and the treatment of hemorrhoids). Called also *Aëtius (Aetios) of Antiochenus.*

**AF** atrial fibrillation.

**AFCR** American Federation for Clinical Research.

**afe·brile** (a-feb'ril) without fever; called also *apyretic* and *apyrexial.*

**afe·tal** (a-fe'təl) without a fetus.

**af·fect** (af'ekt) [MeSH: Affect] the external expression of emotion attached to ideas or mental representations of objects; cf. *mood.*
**blunted a.,** severe reduction in the intensity of affect; a common symptom of schizophrenic disorders.
**constricted a.,** restricted a.
**flat a.,** lack of signs expressing affect.
**inappropriate a.,** affect that is incongruent with the situation or with the content of a patient's ideas or speech.
**labile a.,** that characterized by rapid changes in emotion unrelated to external events or stimuli.
**restricted a.,** reduction in the intensity of affect, to a somewhat lesser degree than is characteristic of blunted affect.

**af·fec·tion** (ə-fek'shən) 1. a state of emotion or feeling. 2. an affliction or disease.

**af·fec·tive** (ə-fek'tiv) pertaining to affect.

**af·fec·tiv·i·ty** (af"ek-tiv'ĭ-te) the capacity to feel emotions; the degree of responsiveness or susceptibility to emotional stimuli.

**af·fec·to·mo·tor** (ə-fek"to-mo'tər) [*affect* + *motor*] characterized by mental excitement and muscular hyperactivity, as in the manic phase of bipolar disorder.

**af·fer·ent** (af'ər-ənt) [L. *ad-* to + *ferre* to carry] 1. conveying toward a center; called also *centripetal.* 2. something that so conducts; see under *fiber* and *nerve.* Cf. *corticipetal.*

**af·fil·i·a·tion** (ə-fil"e-a'shən) a social drive to be associated with others in interdependent relationships, involving using others for help or support without making them responsible for problems.

**af·fin·i·ty** (ə-fin'ĭ-te) [L. *affinitas* relationship] 1. a special attraction for a specific element, organ, or structure. 2. chemical a. 3. in immunology, a thermodynamic expression of the strength of interaction between a single antigen-binding site and a single antigenic determinant (and thus of the stereochemical compatibility between them), most accurately applied to interactions among simple, uniform antigenic determinants such as haptens. Expressed as the association constant (K liters mole$^{-1}$), which, owing to the heterogeneity of affinities in a population of antibody molecules of a given specificity, actually represents an average value (mean intrinsic association constant). Cf. *avidity.*
**chemical a.,** the tendency of an atom or compound to combine by chemical reaction with atoms or compounds of unlike composition.
**electron a.,** the energy released when a single electron is combined with an isolated atom; its value is determined by the effective charge on the nucleus and the size and electronic configuration of the atom.

**af·flux** (af'luks) [L. *affluxus, affluxio*] the rush of blood or liquid to a part.

**af·flux·ion** (ə-fluk'shən) afflux.

**af·fri·cate** (af'rĭ-kət) a consonantal speech sound made up of a plosive followed by a fricative, such as *ch* or *j.* Called also *affricative.*

**af·fric·a·tive** (əfrik'ə-tiv) affricate.

**AFib** atrial fibrillation.

**afi·brin·o·gen·emia** (a"fi-brin"o-jə-ne'me-ə) [MeSH: Afibrinogenemia] lack of fibrinogen (coagulation factor I) in the blood; cf. *hypofibrinogenemia.*
**congenital a.,** a rare autosomal recessive hemorrhagic coagulation disorder, characterized by complete incoagulability of the blood; hemorrhagic manifestations vary from mild to serious.

**AFl** atrial flutter.

**af·la·tox·i·co·sis** (af"lə-tok"sĭ-ko'sis) an often fatal type of mycotoxicosis affecting turkeys and other farm animals fed on peanut meal or seedlings of peanut plants *(Arachis hypogaea)* contaminated with the molds *Aspergillus flavus* and related species, which produce aflatoxin. Symptoms include liver necrosis, bile duct proliferation, and cirrhosis, and with prolonged feeding hepatocellular carcinoma and cholangiocarcinoma. Called also *x disease.*

**af·la·tox·in** (af"lə-tok'sin) a toxic factor produced by *Aspergillus flavus* and *A. parasiticus,* molds contaminating seedlings of peanut plants *(Arachis hypogaea).* Domestic fowl and other animals fed with infected peanut meal may die of aflatoxicosis, hepatocellular carcinoma, or cholangiocarcinoma. It has also been implicated as a cause of human hepatic carcinoma.

**AFO** ankle-foot orthosis.

**AFP** alpha fetoprotein.

**Af·rin** (af'rin) trademark for a preparation of oxymetazoline hydrochloride.

**AFS** American Fertility Society.

**af·ter·birth** (af'tər-bərth) the placenta and membranes, delivered from the uterus after the birth of the child. Called also *secundina, secundinae,* and *secundines.*

**af·ter·brain** (af'tər-brān) metencephalon.

**af·ter·care** (af'tər-kār) [MeSH: Aftercare] the care and treatment of a convalescent patient, especially one who has undergone surgery; called also *aftertreatment.*

**af·ter·cat·a·ract** (af"tər-kat'ə-rakt) see under *cataract.*

**af·ter·cur·rent** (af'tər-kər"ənt) a current produced in a muscle and nerve after cessation of an electric current that has been flowing through it.

**af·ter·de·po·lar·iza·tion** (af"tər-de-po"lər-ĭ-za'shən) a depolarizing afterpotential, sometimes occurring in tissues not normally excitable. It is frequently one of a series, failing to reach threshold and self-perpetuating; triggered automaticity may result.
**delayed a. (DAD),** an afterdepolarization occurring after full repolarization, and generally during a period of hyperpolarization, of the cells initially depolarized in the main (spike) potential.
**early a. (EAD),** an afterdepolarization occurring before full repolarization of the cells initially depolarized in the main (spike) potential, thus arising from a low membrane potential.
**late a.,** delayed a.

**af·ter·dis·charge** (af"tər-dis'chahrj) the portion of the response to stimulation in a nerve which persists after the stimulus has ceased.

**af·ter·gil·ding** (af"tər-gild'ing) the histologic application of gold salts to nerve tissue after fixation and hardening.

**af·ter·im·age** (af'tər-im"əj) [MeSH: Afterimage] a visual impression persisting briefly after cessation of the stimuli causing the original image; called also *accidental* or *negative image* and *aftervision.*
**negative a.,** one in which the brights and darks are reversed from, and the colors are complementary to, the original image.
**positive a.,** one in which the bright, dark, and colored areas are the same as in the original image.

**af·ter·im·pres·sion** (af"tər-im-presh'ən) aftersensation.

**af·ter·load** (af'tər-lōd") in cardiac physiology, the force against which cardiac muscle shortens. In isolated muscle it is the force resisting shortening after the muscle is stimulated to contract; in the intact heart it is the pressure against which the ventricle ejects blood, as measured by the stress acting on the ventricular wall following the onset of contraction, determined largely by the peripheral vascular resistance and by the physical characteristics of and blood volume in the arterial system. It is often estimated by determining systolic arterial pressure, from which can be determined the systolic wall stress; see also *Laplace's law,* under *law.*

**af·ter·math** (af'tər-math) mowed second-growth grass, which sometimes causes *fog fever (aftermath disease)* when eaten by ruminants. Called also *fog.*

**af·ter·move·ment** (af"tər-mo͞ov'mənt) spontaneous elevation of the arm by idiomuscular contraction after benumbing it by powerful pressure against a rigid object; called also *Kohnstamm's phenomenon.*

**af·ter·pains** (af'tər-pānz) the cramplike pains felt after the birth of the child, due to the contractions of the uterus.

**af·ter·per·cep·tion** (af"tər-pər-sep'shən) the perception of a sensation after the stimulus producing it has ceased.

**af·ter·po·ten·tial** (af"tər-po-ten'shəl) the small action potential generated following termination of the spike or main potential; it has a negative and a positive phase.
**negative a.,** the period following termination of the spike potential during which there is a lag in the return of the potential of an excitable cell membrane to resting potential.

**positive a.,** the period following termination of the negative afterpotential, during which the potential of an excitable cell membrane is more negative than the resting potential. It is paradoxically called *positive* because it was first detected outside the cell, where the polarity is reversed.

**af·ter·sen·sa·tion** (af″tər-sen-sa′shən) a sensation lasting after the stimulus that produced it has been removed; called also *afterimpression.*

**af·ter·taste** (af′tər-tāst) a taste continuing after the substance producing it has been removed.

**af·ter·treat·ment** (af″tər-trēt′mənt) aftercare.

**af·ter·vi·sion** (af″tər-vizh′ən) afterimage.

**af·to·sa** (af-to′sə) [Sp.] foot-and-mouth disease.

**afunc·tion** (a-funk′shən) loss of function.

**AFX** atypical fibroxanthoma.

**AG** atrial gallop.

**Ag** symbol for *silver* (L. *argentum*); abbreviation for *antigen.*

**AGA** American Gastroenterological Association.

**aga·lac·tia** (a″gə-lak′she-ah) [*a-*[1] + *galacto-* + *-ia*] absence or failure of the secretion of milk; called also *agalactosis.*
**contagious a.,** a contagious disease of goats and sheep in southern Europe and North Africa, usually caused by *Mycoplasma agalactiae;* symptoms include arthritis and eye lesions, with mastitis in females.
**mastitis-metritis-a.,** lactation failure in swine (see under *failure*).

**agal·ac·to·sis** (a-gal″ak-to′sis) agalactia.

**agal·ac·tos·uria** (a-gal″ak-tōs-u′re-ə) [*a-*[1] + *galactose* + *-uria*] absence of galactose from the urine.

**aga·lac·tous** (a″gə-lak′təs) 1. suppressing the secretion of milk. 2. not nursed; artificially fed.

**agal·or·rhea** (a-gal″o-re′ə) [*a-*[1] + Gr. *gala* milk + *rhoia* flow] absence or arrest of the flow of milk.

**agam·ete** (ag′ə-mēt) [*a-*[1] + *gamete*] the product of asexual multiple fission in protozoa.

**agam·ma·glob·u·lin·emia** (a-gam″ə-glob″u-lĭ-ne′me-ə) [*a-*[1] + *gamma globulin* + *-emia*] [MeSH: Agammaglobulinemia] absence of all classes of immunoglobulins in the blood; the term was used before assays sensitive enough to detect very low levels of globulins were developed and consequently most such disorders are really hypogammaglobulinemias (q.v.); see also *dysgammaglobulinemia* and *immunodeficiency.*
**acquired a.,** common variable immunodeficiency.
**Bruton's a.,** X-linked a.
**common variable a.,** see under *immunodeficiency.*
**lymphopenic a.,** severe combined immunodeficiency.
**Swiss-type a.,** former name for *severe combined immunodeficiency.*
**X-linked a., X-linked infantile a.,** a primary X-linked immunodeficiency disorder characterized by absence of circulating B lymphocytes, absence of plasma cells and germinal centers in lymphoid tissues, and very low levels of circulating immunoglobulins. The pathogenic defect appears to be a failure of pre-B cells to differentiate into mature B cells, express surface immunoglobulins, and produce antibody. Patients are unusually prone to bacterial infection and many have symptoms resembling rheumatoid arthritis. Called also *Bruton's a.* or *disease* and *X-linked hypogammaglobulinemia.*

**agam(o)-** [Gr. *agamos* unmarried] a combining form meaning asexual.

**aga·mo·cy·tog·e·ny** (ə-gam″o-si-toj′ə-ne) schizogony.

**Aga·mo·fi·la·ria** (ə-gam″o-fĭ-lar′e-ə) a name given to filarial worms which are known only in immature stages and which cannot be assigned to any known genus or species.

**aga·mo·gen·e·sis** (ag″ə-mo-jen′ə-sis) [*a-*[1] + *gamo-* + *-genesis*] schizogony.

**aga·mo·ge·net·ic** (ag″ə-mo-jə-net′ik) reproducing asexually.

**aga·mog·o·ny** (ag″ə-mog′ə-ne) [*a-*[1] + *gamo-* + *gonos* offspring] schizogony.

**aga·mont** (ag′ə-mont) [*a-*[1] + *gamont*] schizont.

**aga·mous** (ag′ə-məs) 1. asexual. 2. having no recognizable sexual organs.

**agan·gli·on·ic** (a-gang″gle-on′ik) pertaining to or characterized by the absence of ganglion cells.

**agan·gli·on·o·sis** (ə-gang″gle-on-o′sis) [*a-*[1] + *ganglion* + *-osis*] congenital absence of parasympathetic ganglion cells, as in congenital megacolon.

**agar** (ag′ahr) [Malay *agar-agar*] [NF] [MeSH: Agar] a mucilaginous complex sulfated polymer of galactose units, extracted from *Gelidium cartilagineum, Gracilaria confervoides,* and related red algae. It melts at 100°C and solidifies into a gel at 40°C, is not digested by most bacteria, and as a gel is used in the preparation of solid culture media for microorganisms, as a bulk laxative, in making emulsions, as a supporting medium for immunodiffusion and immunoelectrophoresis, and as the principal component in reversible hydrocolloid dental impression material. See under *culture medium* for specific agars.

**agar·ic** (ə-gar′ik, ag′ə-rik) [Gr. *agarikon* a sort of tree fungus] 1. any of various mushrooms, especially any species of *Agaricus.* 2. a preparation of rotten wood mixed with fungi or dried mushrooms.
**fly a.,** a poisonous species, *Amanita muscaria.*
**larch a.,** a preparation obtained from the fungus *Polyporus officinalis;* it contains agaricic acid and was formerly used as an anhidrotic. Called also *purging* or *white a.*
**purging a., white a.,** larch a.

**Agar·i·ca·ceae** (ə-gar″ĭ-ka′se-e) a family of mushrooms (order Agaricales); it includes the genera *Agaricus, Chlorophyllum, Clitocybe, Lepiota,* and *Paxillus.*

**agar·ic ac·id** (ə-gar′ik, ag′ə-rik) agaricic acid.

**Agar·i·ca·les** (ə-gar″ĭ-ka′lēz) [MeSH: Agaricales] the mushrooms, a large order of perfect fungi of the subphylum Basidiomycotina, class Holobasidiomycetes; some are edible, some poisonous, and some hallucinogenic. Families of medical importance include Agaricaceae, Amanitaceae, Coprinaceae, and Strophariaceae.

**ag·a·ri·cic ac·id** (ag″ə-ris′ik) a resinous acid from white agaric, *Polyporus officinalis,* which is responsible for its anhidrotic action.

**Agar·i·cus** (ə-gar′ĭ-kəs) [Gr. *agarikon* a sort of tree fungus] [MeSH: Agaricus]a genus of mushrooms of the family Agaricaceae. *A. campes′tris* is a common edible variety found in fields. *A. musca′rius* has been renamed *Amanita muscaria.* See also *agaric.*

**agas·tria** (a-gas′tre-ə) absence of the stomach.

**agas·tric** (a-gas′trik) [*a-*[1] + *gastric*] having no alimentary canal.

**Ag·a·thi·nus of Spar·ta** (ag″ə-thi′nəs) [1st century A.D.] a Greek physician who was a pupil of Athenaeus and, like his master, a pneumatist.

**Aga·ve** (ə-ga′ve) [L.; Gr. *agauē* noble] a genus of plants of the family Amaryllidaceae; many species have spiny-margined leaves and tall candelabra-shaped inflorescences. Some species serve as a source of a Mexican alcoholic beverage, and others contain saponins.
**A. america′na L.,** the century plant, a species whose juice is purgative and diuretic and has been used as an abortifacient.
**A. lecheguil′la,** a species that grows in the southwestern United States and Mexico; it contains sapotoxins that cause diarrhea and a photodynamic substance that causes lechuguilla fever in sheep and goats. Called also *lechuguilla.*

**AGCT** Army General Classification Test.

**age** (āj) 1. the duration of individual existence measured in units of time. 2. the measure of some individual attribute in terms of the chronological age of an average normal individual showing the same degree of proficiency, e.g., achievement age.
**achievement a.,** a measure of achievement expressed in terms of the chronological age of an average child showing the same degree of attainment.
**anatomical a.,** age expressed in terms of the chronological age of the average individual showing the same body development.
**Binet a.,** mental age as determined by Binet's test.
**bone a.,** osseous development shown radiographically, stated in terms of the chronological age at which the development is ordinarily attained.
**chronological a.,** the age of a person expressed in terms of the period elapsed from the time of birth.
**coital a.,** the age of a conceptus defined by the time elapsed since the coitus that led to fertilization.
**developmental a.,** age estimated from the degree of anatomical development. In psychology, the age of an individual as determined by the degree of his emotional, mental, anatomical, and physiologic maturation.
**emotional a.,** the age of an individual expressed in terms of the chronological age of an average normal individual showing the same degree of emotional maturity.
**fertilization a.,** conceptus age defined by the time elapsed since fertilization.
**functional a.,** the combined expression of the chronological, emotional, mental, and physiological ages of an individual.
**gestational a.,** age of conceptus or pregnancy. In human clinical practice, pregnancy is timed from onset of the last normal menstruation. Elsewhere the onset may be timed from estrus, coitus, artificial insemination, vaginal plug formation, fertilization, or implantation.
**menstrual a.,** conceptus age defined by the time elapsed since the onset of the mother's last normal menstruation.
**mental a.,** the score achieved by a person in an intelligence test,

expressed in terms of the chronological age of an average normal individual showing the same degree of attainment.
**physical a., physiological a.,** the age of an individual expressed in terms of the chronological age of a normal individual showing the same degree of anatomical and physiological development.
**postovulatory a.,** conceptus age defined by the time elapsed since release of the oocyte from the ovary.

**Age•le•ni•dae** a large family of common spiders that build sheetlike or funnel-shaped webs in grass or under rocks or boards; it includes the genus *Tegenaria,* to which the hobo spider (*T. agrestis,* q.v.) belongs.

**agen•e•sia** (a″jə-ne′zhə) agenesis.
**a. cortica′lis,** congenital failure of development of the cortical cells, especially the pyramidal cells, of the brain, resulting in infantile cerebral paralysis and profound mental retardation.

**agen•e•sis** (a-jen′ə-sis) [*a-*[1] + *-genesis*] 1. absence of an organ; frequently used to designate such absence resulting from failure of appearance of the primordium of an organ in embryonic development. Cf. *aplasia.* 2. sterility or impotence.
**callosal a.,** defect of the callosal structures of the brain.
**gonadal a.,** complete failure of gonadal development, as in Turner's syndrome.
**nuclear a.,** Möbius' syndrome.
**ovarian a.,** failure of development of the ovaries, as in Turner's syndrome.
**renal a.,** failure of development of the kidneys.
**sacral a.,** caudal regression syndrome.

**agen•i•tal•ism** (a-jen′ĭ-təl-iz″əm) 1. absence of the genitalia. 2. a condition caused by failure to secrete gonadal hormones. See also *agonadism.*

**ageno•so•mia** (a-jen″o-so′me-ə) congenital absence or rudimentary development of the genitals and eventration of the lower part of the abdomen.

**ageno•so•mus** (a-jen″o-so′məs) [*a-*[1] + *geno-* + *sōma* body] a fetus exhibiting agenosomia.

**agent** (a′jənt) [L. *agens* acting] any power, principle, or substance capable of producing an effect, whether physical, chemical, or biological.
**activating a.,** one of two factors present in adult tissues which, when administered to embryos, interact to induce regional development; when administered alone, this factor induces archencephalic development. Called also *dorsalizing* or *neuralizing a.* Cf. *caudalizing a.*
**adrenergic blocking a.,** a compound that selectively inhibits response to sympathetic impulses and to catecholamines and other adrenergic amines. See *alpha-adrenergic blocking a., beta-adrenergic blocking a.,* and *adrenergic neuron blocking a.*
**adrenergic neuron blocking a.,** one that inhibits the release of norepinephrine from postganglionic adrenergic nerve endings.
**alkylating a.,** a highly reactive compound that can substitute alkyl groups for the hydrogen atoms of certain organic compounds. Such agents are cytotoxic, producing their effects by the scission and cross-linking of DNA chains, and are not cell cycle–specific, but cell killing occurs primarily in rapidly proliferating tissues in which there is not time between mitoses for DNA repair systems to reverse the effects of the agent. Classes of antineoplastic alkylating agents include nitrogen mustards, ethylenimine derivatives, alkyl sulfonates, nitrosoureas, triazenes, and platinum compounds. Hematopoietic, reproductive, and epithelial tissues are particularly sensitive to alkylating agents, and their use may cause depressed blood cell counts, amenorrhea or impaired spermatogenesis, damage to intestinal mucosa, alopecia, and increased risk of malignancy.
**alpha-adrenergic blocking a.,** one that blocks the alpha receptor sites of effector organs to the effects of catecholamines.
**beta-adrenergic blocking a.,** an agent that blocks the beta receptor sites of effector organs to the effects of catecholamines.
**blocking a.,** an agent that inhibits the response of effector organs to neural impulses of the autonomic nervous system; it may be an adrenergic or cholinergic blocking agent.
**caudalizing a.,** one of two factors present in adult tissues which, when administered to embryos, interact to induce regional development; when administered alone, this factor induces only mesodermal development. Called also *mesodermalizing* or *transforming a.* Cf. *activating a.*
**chelating a.,** 1. a compound that combines with metal ions by means of two or more coordinating positions to form stable ring structures, e.g., heme. 2. a substance used to reduce the concentration of free metal ion in solution by complexing it. Called also *metal complexing a.*
**cholinergic blocking a.,** one that blocks or inactivates acetylcholine.
**clearing a.,** an agent used in staining technique for fixed cells, which has the same refractive index as that of protein particles.
**complexing a.,** ligand.
**coupling a.,** a substance used to coat filler particles in a resin matrix composite so that the particles bind to the resin matrix.
**dorsalizing a.,** activating a.
**Eaton a.,** *Mycoplasma pneumoniae.*
**ELB a.,** *Rickettsia felis.*
**emulsifying a.,** emulsifier.
**fixing a's,** agents, such as formalin, alcohol, acids, salts of heavy metals, or mixtures of these, that precipitate the proteins of cells or tissues and render them insoluble.
**ganglionic blocking a.,** one that blocks nerve impulses at autonomic ganglionic synapses.
**inotropic a.,** any of a class of agents affecting the force of muscle contraction, particularly a drug affecting the force of cardiac contraction; positive inotropic agents, such as digitalis glycosides or catecholamines, increase and negative inotropic agents, such as calcium antagonists, decrease the force of cardiac muscle contractions. All such drugs currently used act indirectly, as by affecting sodium pump, calcium transport, or cyclic AMP production, rather than by directly affecting myofibrils or troponin complexes.
**levigating a.,** a material used for moistening a solid before reducing it to a powder.
**luting a.,** lute (def. 1).
**mesodermalizing a.,** caudalizing a.
**metal complexing a.,** chelating a.
**neuromuscular blocking a.,** a compound that causes paralysis of skeletal muscle by blocking neural transmission at the myoneural junction.
**neuromuscular blocking a., depolarizing,** a nicotinic agonist that blocks neural transmission at the myoneural junction by binding to the nicotinic receptors of the motor end plate to produce prolonged depolarization of the postsynaptic membrane.
**neuromuscular blocking a., nondepolarizing,** a compound that blocks neural transmission at the myoneural junction by inhibiting the action of acetylcholine by competitive binding to the nicotinic receptors of the motor end plate without depolarizing the postsynaptic membrane.
**nonsteroidal antiinflammatory a.,** see under *drug.*
**A. Orange,** a herbicide and defoliant containing 2,4-D and 2,4,5-T and the contaminant dioxin which is suspected of being teratogenic and possibly carcinogenic.
**oxidizing a.,** a substance capable of accepting electrons from another substance, thereby oxidizing the second substance and itself becoming reduced.
**phase-specific a.,** a cytotoxic agent that has its maximum effect at a given phase of the cell growth cycle.
**Pittsburgh pneumonia a.,** *Legionella micdadei.*
**progestational a.,** any of a group of hormones secreted by the corpus luteum and placenta and in small amounts by the adrenal cortex, including progesterone; they induce the formation of a secretory endometrium. Many are now also produced synthetically. Called also *gestagen, progestagen, progestin, progestogen,* and *progestational hormone.*
**psychoactive a., psychotropic a.,** see under *substance.*
**reducing a.,** a substance capable of donating electrons to another substance, thereby reducing the second substance and itself becoming oxidized.
**sclerosing a.,** a chemical irritant injected into a vein in sclerotherapy; the most common ones are morrhuate sodium, sodium tetradecyl sulfate, laureth 9, and ethanolamine oleate. Called also *sclerosant.*
**surface-active a.,** a substance that exerts a change on the surface properties of a liquid, especially one that reduces its surface tension, such as a detergent. Called also *surfactant.*
**transforming a.,** a substance that produces transformation in a cell, e.g., a DNA fragment from a bacterial (donor) cell that, when introduced into another bacterial (recipient) cell, is incorporated into the chromosome and produces a permanent, inherited change.
**wetting a's,** substances that lower the surface tension of water and promote wetting.

**AGEPC** acetyl glyceryl ether phosphoryl choline; see *platelet-activating factor,* under *factor.*

**ager•a•sia** (ă-jər-a′zhə) [*a-*[1] + Gr. *gēras* old age] an unusually youthful appearance in a person of advanced years.

**ageu•sia** (ə-goo′zhə) [*a-*[1] + Gr. *geusis* taste] [MeSH: Ageusia] absence of the sense of taste; called also *ageustia* and *gustatory anesthesia.*

**ageu•sic** (ə-goo′zik) pertaining to ageusia.

**ageus•tia** (ə-gōōs′te-ə) ageusia.

**ag•ger** (aj′er) pl. *ag′geres* [L. "mound"] [TA] a general term for an eminence or projection.
**a. na′si** [TA], ridge of nose: a ridgelike elevation midway between the anterior extremity of the middle nasal concha and the inner surface of the dorsum of the nose; called also *nasoturbinal concha.*
**a. perpendicula′ris,** eminentia fossae triangularis auriculae.

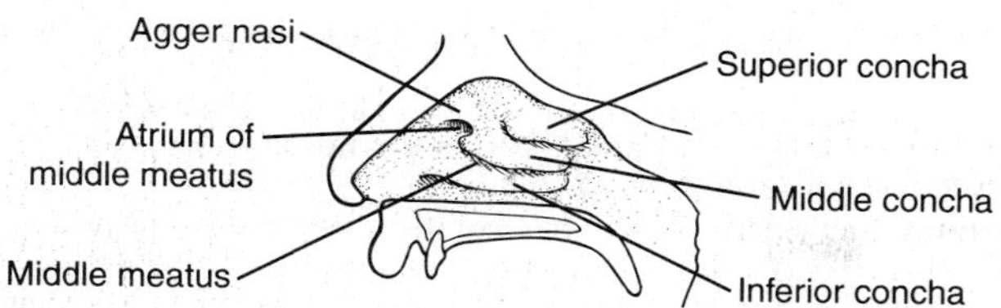


Agger nasi, an elevation anterior to the middle concha on the lateral nasal wall, above the atrium of the middle meatus.

**a. val'vae ve'nae,** an elevation of the wall of a vein over the site of a valve.

**ag·ger·es** (aj'ər-ēz) [L.] plural of *agger.*

**ag·glom·er·at·ed** (ə-glom'ər-āt″əd) [L. *agglomeratus,* from *ad* together + *glomus* mass] crowded into a mass.

**ag·glu·ti·na·ble** (ə-gloo'tĭ-nə-bəl) capable of agglutination.

**ag·glu·ti·nant** (ə-gloo'tĭ-nənt) [L. *agglutinans* gluing] 1. promoting union by adhesion. 2. a tenacious or gluey substance that holds parts together during the process of healing.

**ag·glu·ti·na·tion** (ə-gloo″tĭ-na'shən) [L. *agglutinatio*] [MeSH: Agglutination] 1. the action of an agglutinant substance. 2. the process of union in the healing of a wound. 3. the clumping together in suspension of antigen-bearing cells, microorganisms, or particles in the presence of specific antibodies (agglutinins). Called also *clumping.*

**acid a.,** the nonspecific agglutination of microorganisms at relatively low hydrogen ion concentration; it occurs without participation of antibody.

**bacteriogenic a.,** clumping of cells due to bacterial action. See *T agglutinin,* under *agglutinin.*

**cold a.,** agglutination with cold agglutinins (q.v.), occurring more efficiently below 37°C than at 37°C.

**cross a.,** the agglutination of particulate antigen by antibody raised against a different but related antigen; see also *group a.*

**group a.,** agglutination, usually to a lower titer, of various members of a group of biologically related organisms or corpuscles by an agglutinin specific for one of that group. For instance, the specific agglutinin of typhoid bacilli may agglutinate other members of the colon-typhoid group, such as *Escherichia coli* and *Salmonella enteritidis.*

**H a.,** the agglutination of motile bacteria in the presence of antibody to the heat-labile flagellar antigens.

**intravascular a.,** clumping of particulate elements (usually referring to red blood cells) within the blood vessels, such as after an injury. Called also *sludging of blood.*

**O a.,** the agglutination of bacteria in the presence of antibody to the heat-stable somatic antigen.

**passive a.,** agglutination in antiserum of particles owing to adsorbed specific soluble antigen.

**platelet a.,** the clumping together of platelets under the influence of platelet agglutinins.

**salt a.,** agglutination that occurs in salt solutions of certain concentrations.

**spontaneous a.,** the agglutination of bacteria or other cells in physiologic salt solution due to the lack of sufficient surface polar groups to give stable suspensions in the presence of electrolytes.

**Vi a.,** agglutination of bacteria containing Vi antigen on their surface, in the presence of specific agglutinin.

**ag·glu·ti·na·tive** (ə-gloo'tĭ-na″tiv) promoting adhesion or agglutination.

**ag·glu·ti·na·tor** (ə-gloo'tĭ-na″tər) something which agglutinates; an agglutinin.

**ag·glu·ti·nin** (ə-gloo'tĭ-nin) 1. antibody that aggregates a particulate antigen, e.g., bacteria, following combination with the homologous antigen in vivo or in vitro. 2. any substance other than antibody, e.g., lectin, that is capable of agglutinating particles.

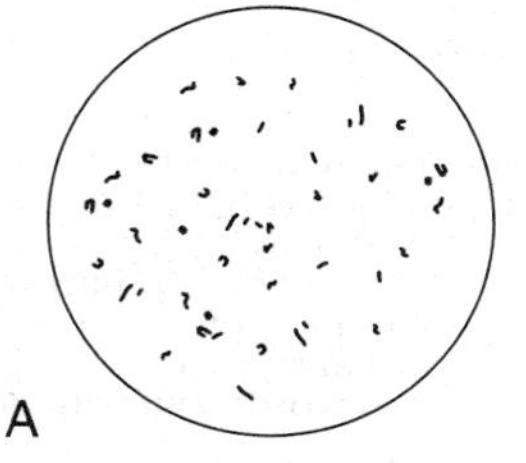


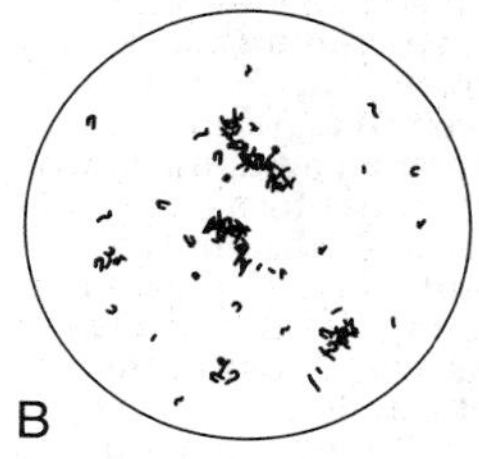


*(A),* Bacteria in suspension; *(B),* agglutinated bacteria.

**anti-Rh a.,** an agglutinin not normally present in human plasma but which may be produced in $Rh^-$ mothers carrying an $Rh^+$ fetus or after transfusion of $Rh^+$ blood into an $Rh^-$ patient. See *blood group.*

**chief a.,** major a.

**cold a.,** antibody that agglutinates erythrocytes or bacteria more efficiently at temperatures below 37°C than at 37°C. Abbreviated CA. See *cold agglutinin syndrome,* under *syndrome,* and *paroxysmal cold hemoglobinuria,* under *hemoglobinuria.*

**complete a.,** see *antibody.*

**cross a., cross-reacting a.,** an agglutinin which, although formed in response to one particulate antigen, also has specific action on a different but related antigen.

**flagellar a.,** an agglutinin specific for the flagella of a microorganism.

**group a.,** an agglutinin that has a specific action on certain organisms or cells but will also agglutinate other closely related species.

**H a.,** see under *antigen.*

**immune a.,** any agglutinating antibody.

**incomplete a.,** see under *antibody.*

**leukocyte a.,** an antibody capable of agglutinating leukocytes; leukocyte autoagglutinins and isoagglutinins are associated with a variety of disorders, both with and without frank leukopenia. Called also *leukoagglutinin.*

**major a.,** the specific agglutinin present at highest titer in an antiserum. Called also *chief a.*

**MG a.,** a specific agglutinin developed against streptococcus MG.

**minor a.,** a specific or cross-reacting agglutinin present in an antiserum at lower titer than the major agglutinin. Called also *partial a.*

**O a.,** see under *antigen.*

**partial a.,** minor a.

**platelet a.,** an antibody capable of agglutinating platelets; platelet autoagglutinins and isoagglutinins are associated with a variety of disorders, both with and without frank thrombocytopenia. Called also *thromboagglutinin.*

**saline a.,** complete antibody.

**somatic a.,** an agglutinin specific for the body of a microorganism.

**T a.,** a natural antibody present in normal human sera that causes agglutination of erythrocytes treated with neuraminidase or incubated with neuraminidase-producing bacteria causing exposure of the T antigen.

**warm a.,** an agglutinin more reactive at 37° C than at lower temperatures.

**ag·glu·tin·o·gen** (ag″loo-tin'o-jen) 1. any substance which, acting as an antigen, stimulates the production of agglutinin. 2. the particulate antigen used in conducting agglutination tests.

**ag·glu·ti·no·gen·ic** (ə-gloo″tĭ-no-jen'ik) pertaining to the production of agglutinin; producing agglutinin.

**ag·glu·ti·no·phil·ic** (ə-gloo″tĭ-no-fil'ik) agglutinating readily.

**ag·glu·to·gen·ic** (ə-gloo″to-jen'ik) agglutinogenic.

**aggred. feb.** abbreviation for L. *aggredien'te feb're,* while the fever is coming on.

**Ag·gre·ga·ta** (ag″rə-ga'tə) [L. *aggregare* to add to] a genus of coccidian protozoa (suborder Eimeriina, order Eucoccidiida), the life cycle of which involves schizogony in a crustacean and sporogony and gametogony in a cephalopod.

**ag·gre·gate** (ag'rə-gāt) [L. *aggregatus,* from *ad* to + *grex* flock] 1. to crowd or cluster together. 2. crowded or clustered together. 3. a mass or assemblage.

**ag·gre·ga·tion** (ag″rə-ga'shən) 1. massing of materials together as in clumping. 2. a clumped mass of material.

**familial a.,** a concentration of cases of a disease in families; the occurrence of more cases of a given disorder in close relatives of a person with the disorder than in control families.

**platelet a.,** a clumping together of platelets, part of a sequential mechanism leading to the initiation and formation of a thrombus or hemostatic plug. It can be induced in vitro, and probably in vivo, by agents such as ADP, thrombin, and collagen.

**ag·gre·gom·e·ter** (ag″rə-gom'ə-tər) an instrument that measures platelet aggregation by detecting changes in optical density of plasma or solution caused by clustering of platelets.

**ag·gre·gom·e·try** (ag″rə-gom'ə-tre) the measurement of platelet aggregation by means of an aggregometer.

**ag·gre·phore** (ag'rə-for) [*aggregate* + *phore*] a cellular organelle that carries water channels as part of its structure and inserts them in cell membranes to cause greater permeability. It has been found in toad urinary bladder cells and is thought to be present in renal tubules of other animals including humans.

**ag·gres·sin** (ə-gres'in) any of a postulated group of nontoxic substances produced by pathogenic bacteria that inhibit the mechanisms of host resistance.

**ag·gres·sion** (ə-gresh'ən) [L. *aggressus,* from *ad* to + *gradi* to step] [MeSH: Aggression] a form of behavior which leads to self-assertion; it may arise from innate drives and/or a response to frustration; it may be manifested by destructive and attacking behavior, by covert attitudes of hostility and obstructionism, or by a healthy self-expressive drive to mastery.

**ag·ing** (āj′ing) [MeSH: Aging] the gradual changes in the structure of any organism that occur with the passage of time, that do not result from disease or other gross accidents, and that eventually lead to the increased probability of death as the individual grows older. Cf. *senescence.*

**ag·i·ta·tion** (aj″ĭ-ta′shən) excessive, purposeless cognitive and motor activity or restlessness, usually associated with a state of tension or anxiety. Called also *psychomotor.*

**ag·i·to·graph·ia** (aj″ĭ-to-graf′e-ə) [L. *agitare* to hurry + *graph-* + *-ia*] a dysgraphia with excessively rapid writing and unconscious omission or distortion of words or parts of words; it is usually associated with logorrhea.

**ag·i·to·la·lia** (aj″ĭ-to-la′le-ə) logorrhea.

**ag·i·to·pha·sia** (aj″ĭ-to-fa′zhə) logorrhea.

**Agit. vas.** abbreviation for L. *agita′to va′se,* the vial being shaken.

**Ag·kis·tro·don** (ag-kis′tro-don) [Gr. *ankistron* fishhook + Gr. *odous* tooth] [MeSH: Agkistrodon] a genus of venomous snakes of the family Crotalidae. *A. contor′trix* is the copperhead of North America and *A. pisci′vorus* is the water moccasin or cottonmouth of North America. The Southeast Asian species *A. rhodosto′ma* has been renamed *Calloselasma rhodostoma.* Called also *Ancistrodon.* See table at *snake.*

**aglo·mer·u·lar** (ă″glo-mər′u-lər) having no glomeruli; said of a kidney in which the glomeruli have been absorbed or in which they have never formed (as in some fishes).

**aglos·sia** (a-glos′e-ə) [*a-*[1] + *gloss-* + *-ia*] congenital absence of the tongue.

**aglos·so·sto·mia** (a″glos-o-sto′me-ə) [*a-*[1] + *glosso-* + *stom-* + *-ia*] a developmental anomaly characterized by a malformed mouth and absence of the tongue.

**aglu·con** (a-gloo′kon) 1. the nonsugar portion of a glucoside. 2. aglycon.

**aglu·cone** (a-gloo′kōn) aglucon.

**aglu·ti·tion** (a-gloo-tish′ən) dysphagia.

**agly·ce·mia** (a″gli-se′me-ə) [*a-*[1] + *glyc-* + *-emia*] virtually total absence of sugar from the blood; see also *hypoglycemia.*

**agly·con** (a-gli′kon) the noncarbohydrate group of a glycoside molecule; called also *genin.*

**agly·cone** (a-gli′kōn) aglycon.

**agly·cos·uric** (a-gli″ko-sur′ik) free from glycosuria.

**ag·min·at·ed** (ag′min-āt″əd) [L. *agmen* a group] clustered.

**ag·na·thia** (ag-na′the-ə) [*a-*[1] + *gnath-* + *-ia*] a developmental anomaly characterized by absence of the lower jaw.

**ag·na·thous** (ag-na′thəs) pertaining to or affected with agnathia.

**ag·na·thus** (ag-na′thəs) a fetus exhibiting agnathia.

**ag·nea** (ag-ne′ə) agnosia.

**ag·no·gen·ic** (ag″no-jen′ik) [Gr. *agnōs* unknown, obscure + *-genesis*] idiopathic.

**ag·no·sia** (ag-no′zhə) [*a-*[1] + *gnosia*] [MeSH: Agnosia] loss of the power to recognize the import of sensory stimuli; the varieties correspond with the several senses and are distinguished as *auditory, visual, olfactory, gustatory,* and *tactile.*
**acoustic a., auditory a.,** inability to recognize the significance of sounds.
**body-image a.,** autotopagnosia.
**face a., facial a.,** prosopagnosia.
**finger a.,** inability to recognize, indicate on command, name, or choose the individual fingers of one's own hand or the hands of others. Also written *fingeragnosia.*
**ideational a.,** loss of the special associations which make up the idea of an object from its component ideas.
**tactile a.,** inability to recognize familiar objects by touch. Cf. *astereognosis* and *stereoanesthesia.*
**time a.,** loss of comprehension of the succession and duration of events.
**visual a.,** inability to recognize familiar objects by sight, usually due to a lesion in one of the visual association areas. Called also *cortical psychic blindness* and *psychic blindness.*
**visual-spatial a., visuospatial a.,** lack of the ability to analyze and orient using visual representations and their spatial relationships.

**-agogue** [Gr. *agōgos* leading, inducing] a word termination meaning an agent that leads or induces.

**ago·nad** (a-go′nad) [*a-*[1] + *gonad*] 1. an individual without gonads; see *agonadism.* 2. agonadal.

**agon·a·dal** (a-gon′ə-dəl) pertaining to or characterized by agonadism.

**ago·na·dism** (a-go′nə-diz″əm) the condition of being without sex glands, as in anorchism and Turner's syndrome. See also *gonadal agenesis,* under *agenesis.*

**ag·o·nal** (ag′ə-nəl) pertaining to or occurring at the time just before death.

**ag·o·nist** (ag′ə-nist) 1. in anatomy, a prime mover. 2. in pharmacology, a drug that has affinity for and stimulates physiologic activity at cell receptors normally stimulated by naturally occurring substances.

**ag·o·ny** (ag′ə-ne) [Gr. *agōnia*] 1. severe pain or extreme suffering. 2. old term for the period just before death occurs, which was thought to be a time of extreme pain.

**ag·o·ra·pho·bia** (ag″ə-rə-fo′be-ə) [Gr. *agora* marketplace + *-phobia*] [MeSH: Agoraphobia] [DSM-IV] intense, irrational fear of open spaces, characterized by marked fear of being alone or of being in public places where escape would be difficult or help might be unavailable. It may be associated with panic attacks (see *panic disorder,* under *disorder*) or may occur independently (called *a. without history of panic disorder* in DSM-IV).
**a. without history of panic disorder** [DSM-IV], agoraphobia with fear of having an attack of one or only a few incapacitating or embarrassing symptoms, which the person may or may not have had in the past, rather than a full panic attack.

**agou·ti** (ə-goo′te) [Fr., from Guarani *acuti*] 1. a rodent of the genus *Dasyprocta,* about the size of a rabbit and with brown and gray fur, found in tropical America; it is a reservoir for the protozoan *Trypanosoma cruzi* and the tapeworm *Echinococcus vogelii.* 2. a term used in genetics to indicate the natural wild color pattern of the hair of certain mammals.

**-agra** [Gr. *agra* a catching, seizure] a word termination denoting a seizure of acute pain.

**agraffe** (ah-grahf′) [Fr.] a clamplike instrument for maintaining the edges of a wound in apposition.

**ag·ram·ma·ti·ca** (ag″ro-mat′ĭ-kə) agrammatism.

**agram·ma·tism** (a-gram′ə-tiz-əm) [Gr. *agrammatos* unlettered] inability to speak grammatically because of brain injury or disease, usually with simplified sentence structure (telegraphic speech) and errors in tense, number, and gender. See also *jargon aphasia* and *syntactical aphasia.* Called also *agrammatologia* and *dysgrammatism.*

**agram·ma·to·lo·gia** (a-gram″ə-to-lo′jə) agrammatism.

**agran·u·lo·cyte** (a-gran′u-lo-sīt″) nongranular leukocyte.

**agran·u·lo·cy·to·sis** (a-gran″u-lo-si-to′sis) [MeSH: Agranulocytosis] 1. any condition involving greatly decreased numbers of granulocytes; see also *leukopenia, neutropenia,* and *granulocytopenia.* 2. more specifically, a symptom complex characterized by marked decrease in the number of circulating granulocytes; severe neutropenia results in lesions of the throat, other mucous membranes, gastrointestinal tract, and skin; in most cases it is caused by sensitization to drugs, chemicals, or radiation affecting the bone marrow and depressing granulopoiesis. Called also *agranulocytic* or *neutropenic angina, malignant* or *pernicious leukopenia, Schultz's angina,* and *Schultz's syndrome.*
**feline a.,** panleukopenia.
**infantile genetic a.,** an autosomal recessive disorder characterized by early onset of recurrent pyogenic infections of the skin and lung, absence of neutrophils in the blood, absolute monocytosis and eosinophilia, and early death. Called also *Kostmann's syndrome.*
**infectious feline a.,** panleukopenia.

**agran·u·lo·plas·tic** (a-gran″u-lo-plas′tik) [*a-*[1] + *granule* + *plastic*] forming nongranular cells only; not forming granular cells.

**agraph·ia** (ə-graf′e-ə) [*a-*[1] + *-graph* + *-ia*] [MeSH: Agraphia] impairment or loss of the ability to write; it takes two forms, one involving poor morphology of written letter forms and the other a reflection of the aphasia also observed in spoken language. See also *dysgraphia.* Called also *graphomotor aphasia.*
**absolute a.,** loss of the power to form even single letters.
**acoustic a.,** loss of the power of writing from dictation.
**a. amnemo′nica,** jargon a.
**a. atac′tica,** absolute a.
**cerebral a.,** mental a.
**jargon a.,** agraphia in which the patient can write correctly formed letters but forms only senseless combinations of letters or words.
**literal a.,** absolute a.
**mental a.,** agraphia due to inability to put thought into phrases.
**motor a.,** inability to write because of lack of motor coordination.
**musical a.,** loss of the power to write musical symbols.
**optic a.,** inability to copy written or printed words, but with ability to write from dictation.

**verbal a.,** ability to write single letters, with loss of ability to combine them into words or sentences.

**agraph·ic** (a-graf'ik) pertaining to, affected with, or of the nature of agraphia.

**Ag·rio·li·max** (ag"re-o-li'maks) a genus of slugs. *A. lae'vis* is a species that serves as an intermediate host for the lungworm *Angiostrongylus cantonensis.*

**Ag·ro·bac·te·ri·um** (ag"ro-bak-te're-əm) [Gr. *agros* field + *bacterium*] [MeSH: Agrobacterium] a genus of bacteria of the family Rhizobiaceae, made up of small, gram-negative, aerobic, flagellated rods, found in soil or in the roots or stems of plants. Most species produce hypertrophy (galls) on plant stems.
**A. radiobac'ter,** a nonpathogenic species isolated occasionally from clinical specimens.

**Ag·ro·stem·ma** (ag"ro-stem'ə) a genus of herbs of the family Caryophyllaceae. *A. githa'go* (called also *Lychnis githago*) is the corn cockle, a flowering plant whose seeds may contaminate human or animal food and cause githagism.

**Agros·tis** (ə-gros'tis) a genus of grasses (family Gramineae). *A. al'ba* is Johnson grass, whose pollen causes hay fever.

**Ag·ry·lin** (ag'rə-lin) trademark for a preparation of anagrelide hydrochloride.

**agryp·node** (ə-grip'nōd) agrypnotic.

**agryp·not·ic** (ă"grip-not'ik) [Gr. *agrypnotikos*] promoting wakefulness.

**AGS** American Geriatrics Society.

**AGT** antiglobulin test.

**AGTH** adrenoglomerulotropin.

**ague** (a'gu) [Fr. *aigu* sharp] 1. old name for malaria, or any other severe recurrent symptom of malarial origin. 2. a chill.
**brassfounder's a.,** see under *fever.*

**AGV** aniline gentian violet.

**agy·ria** (a-ji're-ə) [*a-*[1] + *gyr-* + *-ia*] a malformation in which the convolutions of the cerebral cortex are not fully formed, so that the brain surface is smooth; called also *lissencephaly.*

**agy·ric** (a-ji'rik) 1. pertaining to or characterized by agyria. 2. having no gyri.

**ah** symbol for *hyperopic astigmatism.*

**AHA** American Heart Association; American Hospital Association.

**ahap·to·glo·bin·emia** (a-hap"to-glo"bĭ-ne'me-ə) the presence of little or no haptoglobin in the blood serum; indicative of recent hemolysis.

**AHCPR** Agency for Health Care Policy and Research, an agency of the United States Public Health Service.

**AHF** antihemophilic factor (factor VIII; see *coagulation factors,* under *factor*).

**AHG** [MeSH: Factor VIII] antihemophilic globulin (factor VIII, see under *coagulation factors,* at *factor*).

**AHP** Assistant House Physician.

**AHS** Assistant House Surgeon.

**Ahu·ma·da-del Cas·ti·llo syndrome** (ah-oo-mah'thah dāl kahs-te'yo) [Juan Carlos *Ahumada,* Argentine physician, 20th century; E.B. *del Castillo,* Argentine physician, 20th century] see under *syndrome.*

**A-hy·dro·Cort** (a-hi'dro-kort") trademark for a preparation of hydrocortisone sodium succinate.

**AI** anaphylatoxin inactivator; aortic incompetence; aortic insufficiency; apical impulse; artificial insemination.

**AIC** Association des Infirmières Canadiennes.

**Ai·car·di's syndrome** (ĕ-kahr-dēz') [J. *Aicardi,* French neurologist, 20th century] see under *syndrome.*

**AICD** activation-induced cell death; automatic implantable cardioverter-defibrillator.

**aich·mo·pho·bia** (īk"mo-fo'be-ə) [Gr. *aichmē* spearpoint + phobia] irrational fear of sharp-pointed objects, often connected with the fear that one might use the object to stab someone.

**AID** donor insemination.

**aid** (ād) help or assistance; by extension, applied to any device by which a function can be improved or augmented, as a hearing aid.
**first a.,** the initial emergency care and treatment of an injured or ill person before definitive medical and surgical management can be secured.
**hearing a.,** a device that amplifies sound to help deaf persons hear, often referring specifically to devices worn on the body. See also *assistive listening devices,* under *device.*
**pharmaceutic a., pharmaceutical a.,** see under *necessity.*
**speech a.,** 1. an appliance that improves speech. 2. see under *therapy.*
**speech a., prosthetic,** speech-aid prosthesis.

**AIDS** acquired immunodeficiency syndrome; see under *syndrome.*

**AIH** American Institute of Homeopathy; homologous insemination.

**AIHA** American Industrial Hygiene Association; autoimmune hemolytic anemia.

**AILD** angioimmunoblastic lymphadenopathy with dysproteinemia.

**ail·ment** (āl'mənt) any disease or affection of the body, usually referring to slight or mild disorder.

**ai·lu·ro·pho·bia** (i-loor"o-fo'be-ə) [Gr. *ailouros* cat + *-phobia*] irrational fear of cats.

**ain·hum** (ān'hum, i'num, or [Portuguese] īn-yoom') [Port., from Yoruba *eyun* to saw] [MeSH: Ainhum] a disease affecting the toes, especially the fifth toe, and sometimes the fingers, seen chiefly in black adult males in Africa, in which a linear constriction around the affected digit leads to spontaneous amputation of the distal part of the digit. Called also *dactylolysis spontanea.*

**AIP** acute intermittent porphyria.

**air** (ār) [L. *aer;* from Gr. *aēr*] [MeSH: Air] the gaseous mixture which makes up the earth's atmosphere; it is an odorless, colorless gas, consisting of about 1 part by volume of oxygen and 4 parts of nitrogen, the proportion varying somewhat according to conditions. It also contains small amounts of carbon dioxide, ammonia, argon, nitrites, and organic matter.
**alveolar a.,** see under *gas.*
**liquid a.,** air liquefied by great pressure; on evaporation it produces intense cold. Liquid air has been used to produce local anesthesia and in the treatment of neuralgia and herpes zoster, and as a source of oxygen for medical use.
**residual a.,** see under *volume.*
**tidal a.,** see under *volume.*

**air·borne** (ār'born) suspended in, transported by, or spread by air, as an infectious disease or a pathogen; see under *infection.*

**Air·bra·sive** (ār'bra-siv) trademark for *(a)* an instrument for preparing a cavity in a tooth or removing deposits from teeth by application of silicon carbide or aluminum oxide by air blast; *(b)* the abrasive cutting powder used with the instrument.

**air·flow** (ār'flo) 1. any flowing of air. 2. the flow rate of air through the airways; see *flow* (def. 2).

**air·sac·cu·li·tis** (ār"sak-u-li'tis) inflammation of the air sacs in birds.

**air·way** (ār'wa) 1. the route for passage of air into and out of the lungs; see also *respiratory system,* under *system.* 2. a device for securing unobstructed passage of air into and out of the lungs during general anesthesia or when the patient is not ventilating properly.
**Brain a.,** laryngeal mask a.
**conducting a.,** the lower and upper airways together, from the nares to the terminal bronchioles.
**endotracheal a.,** an endotracheal tube that serves as an airway.
**esophageal obturator a.,** a hollow tube inserted into the esophagus to maintain upper airway patency in unconscious persons and to permit positive-pressure ventilation through the face mask connected to the tube.
**laryngeal mask a.,** a device for maintaining a patent airway without tracheal intubation, consisting of a tube connected to an oval inflatable cuff that seals the larynx. Called also *Brain a.*

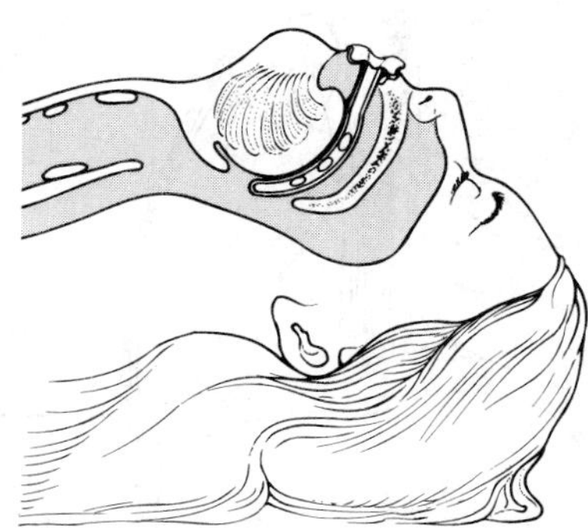

Airway. Oropharyngeal airway in place.

**lower a.,** the airway from the inferior end of the larynx to the ends of the terminal bronchioles.
**nasopharyngeal a.,** a hollow tube inserted into a nostril and directed along the floor of the nose to the nasopharynx to prevent the tongue from blocking off passage of air in unconscious persons.
**oropharyngeal a.,** a hollow tube inserted into the mouth and back of the throat to prevent the tongue from blocking off passage of air in unconscious persons.
**upper a.,** the airway from the nares and lips to the larynx.

**AIUM** American Institute of Ultrasound in Medicine.

**Ajel·lo·my·ces** (a″jə-lo-mi′sēz) a genus of fungi of the family Gymnoascaceae. *A. capsula′tus,* the perfect stage of *Histoplasma capsulatum,* is the etiologic agent of classic histoplasmosis. *A. dermati′tidis,* the perfect stage of *Blastomyces dermatitidis,* is the etiologic agent of North American blastomycosis.

**ak-** for words beginning thus, see also words beginning *ac-*.

**akaryo·cyte** (a-kar′e-o-sīt″) [*a-*[1] + *karyo-* + *-cyte*] a non-nucleated cell, e.g., an erythrocyte.

**akaryo·mas·ti·gont** (a-kar″e-o-mas′tĭ-gont) [*a-*[1] + *karyo-* + *mastigont*] a condition characteristic of certain flagellate protozoa in which the mastigont system is not associated with a nucleus. Cf. *karyomastigont.*

**akar·y·o·ta** (a-kar″e-o′tə) akaryocyte.

**akar·y·ote** (a-kar′e-ōt) [*a-*[1] + Gr. *karyon* kernel] akaryocyte.

**ak·a·this·ia** (ak″ə-thĭ′zhə) [*a-*[1] + Gr. *kathisis* a sitting down + *-ia*] a condition of motor restlessness in which there is a feeling of muscular quivering, an urge to move about constantly, and an inability to sit still, a common extrapyramidal side effect of neuroleptic drugs.

**AK-Dex** (ak′deks) trademark for preparations of dexamethasone sodium phosphate.

**akee** (ăk′ee) 1. *Blighia sapida.* 2. the fruit of *B. sapida;* its whitish, ripe aril is cooked and consumed as a delicacy in the West Indies. The uncooked fruit and aril contain the toxic amino acids hypoglycin A and B, and ingestion without cooking causes Jamaican vomiting sickness. Called also *ackee.*

**Åker·lund deformity** (ek′ər-loond) [Åke Olof *Åkerlund,* Swedish radiologist, 1885–1958] see under *deformity.*

**aki·ne·sia** (a″kĭ-ne′zhə) [*a-*[1] + *kinesi-* + *-ia*] 1. absence, poverty, or lack of control of voluntary muscle movements. 2. the temporary paralysis of a muscle by the injection of procaine.
**a. al′gera,** a condition characterized by generalized pain associated with movement of any kind.
**O'Brien a.,** paralysis of the orbicularis oculi muscle produced by injection of an anesthetic solution directly over the orbital branch of the seventh nerve as it emerges from behind the ear and extends toward the orbital region along the ramus of the jaw, permitting better exposure of the bulb of the eye.

**aki·ne·sis** (a″kĭ-ne′sis) akinesia.

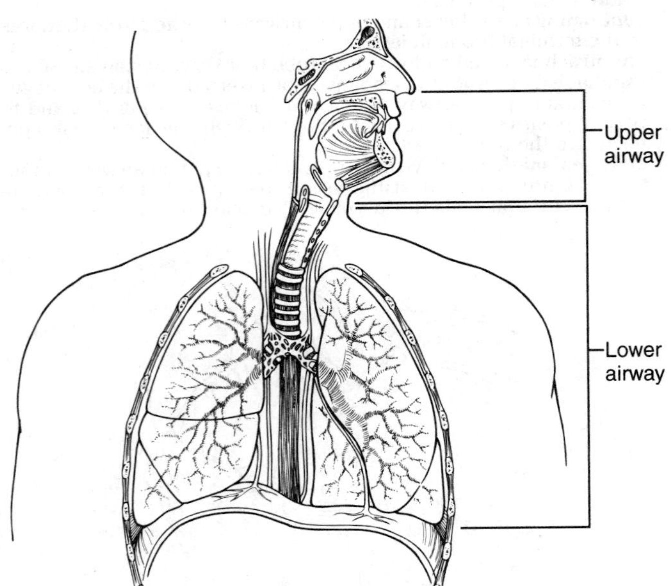

The larynx marks the division between upper and lower airways.

**akin·es·the·sia** (ə-kin″es-the′zhə) absence or loss of movement sense or kinesthesia; called also *kinanesthesia.*

**aki·net·ic** (a-kĭ-net′ik) 1. pertaining to, characterized by, or causing akinesia. 2. amitotic.

**Akin·e·ton** (a-kin′ə-ton) trademark for preparations of biperiden.

**aki·ya·mi** (ah″ke-yah′me) nanukayami.

**ak·lo·mide** (ak′lo-mīd) a coccidiostatic agent used in poultry.

**Ak·o·kan·the·ra** (ak″o-kan-the′rə) *Acocanthera.*

**ako·ria** (ə-ko′re-ə) acoria.

**AK-Pred** (ak′pred) trademark for preparations of prednisolone sodium phosphate.

**Ak·rin·ol** (ak′rin-ol) trademark for a preparation of acrisorcin.

**AK-Tate** (ak′tāt) trademark for preparations of prednisolone.

**Aku·rey·ri disease** (ah-ku′ra-re) [*Akureyri,* town in Iceland where more than 1000 cases occurred in 1948] epidemic neuromyasthenia.

**Al** symbol for *aluminum.*

**-al**[1] [L. *-alis* adjective-forming suffix] an adjective-forming suffix meaning pertaining to or characterized by, as *arterial, diarrheal.*

**-al**[2] [L. *-alia,* neuter plural of *-alis*] a noun-forming suffix denoting an act or process, as *denial.*

**-al** [from *aldehyde*] a suffix used in forming the names of chemical compounds, indicating presence of the aldehyde group, —CHO, as chloral.

**ALA** δ-aminolevulinic acid.

**Ala** alanine.

**ala** (a′lə) pl. *a′lae* [L. "wing"] [TA] wing: a term used in general anatomical nomenclature for a winglike structure or process.
**a. au′ris,** auricula.
**a. of central lobule, a. cerebel′li,** a. lobuli centralis.
**a. cris′tae gal′li** [TA], a small winglike process on the anterior part of the crista galli of the ethmoid bone; called also *frontal hamulus* and *hamulus frontalis.*
**a. i′lii,** a. ossis ilii.
**a′lae lin′gulae cerebel′li,** vincula lingulae cerebelli.
**a. lo′buli centra′lis** [TA], wing of central lobule: the lateral hemispheric extension of the central lobule in the cranial lobe of the cerebellum; called also *a. of central lobule* and *a. cerebelli.*
**a. mag′na os′sis sphenoida′lis, a. ma′jor os′sis sphenoida′lis** [TA], greater wing of sphenoid bone: a large wing-shaped process arising from either side of the body of the sphenoid bone; its cerebral surface forms the anterior part of the floor of the middle cranial fossa, and its orbital surface forms the chief part of the lateral wall of the orbit. Called also *a. temporalis ossis sphenoidalis* and *major* or *temporal wing of sphenoid bone.*
**a. mi′nor os′sis sphenoida′lis** [TA], lesser wing of sphenoid bone: the thin triangular plate of bone that extends horizontally and laterally from either side of the anterior part of the body of the sphenoid bone; it articulates with the frontal bone and helps form the roof of the orbit and the floor of the anterior cranial fossa. Called also *a. orbitalis ossis sphenoidalis* and *minor* or *small wing of sphenoid bone.*
**a. na′si** [TA], wing of nose: the flaring cartilaginous expansion forming the outer side of each naris. See also *cartilago alaris major.*
**a. orbita′lis os′sis sphenoida′lis,** a. minor ossis sphenoidalis.
**a. os′sis i′lii** [TA], **a. os′sis i′lium,** wing of ilium: the expanded superior portion of the ilium which forms the lateral boundary of the greater pelvis.
**a. os′sis sa′cri** [TA], the upper surface of the lateral part of the sacrum.
**a. sacra′lis, a. sa′cri, a. of sacrum,** a. ossis sacri.
**a. tempora′lis os′sis sphenoida′lis,** a. major ossis sphenoidalis.
**a. vespertilio′nis,** ["bat's wing"], mesosalpinx.

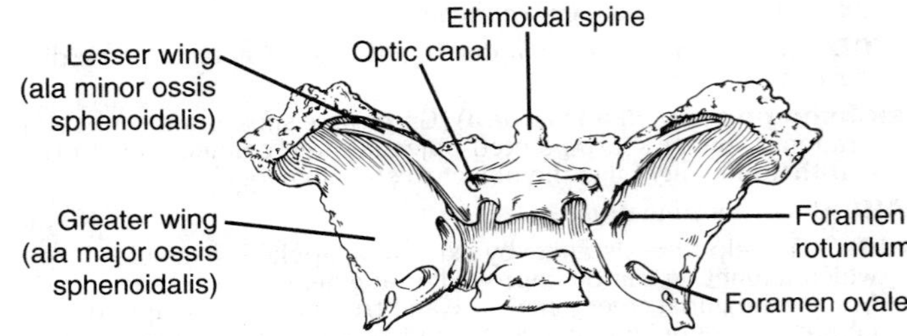

Superior view of ala major ossis sphenoidalis (greater wing of sphenoid bone) and ala minor ossis sphenoidalis (lesser wing of sphenoid bone).

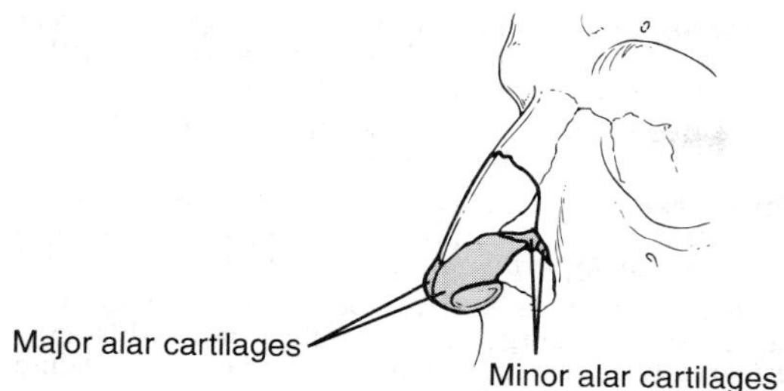

The major and minor alar cartilages of the ala nasi.

**a. of vomer, a. vo′meris** [TA], wing of vomer: one of the two lateral expansions on the superior border of the vomer, coming into contact with the sphenoidal process of the palatine bone and the vaginal process of the medial pterygoid plate.

**alac·ri·ma** (a-lak′rĭ-mə) [*a-*[1] + *lacrima*] deficiency of secretion of tears. The hereditary form is autosomal dominant and is characterized by deficient lacrimation from infancy, punctate corneal epithelial erosions, hypoplasia of the lacrimal gland, and anosmia. Alacrima also occurs in association with dysautonomia, anhidrotic ectodermal dysplasia, and adnexal abnormalities, or as an isolated congenital defect.

**alac·ta·sia** (a″lak-ta′zhə) malabsorption of lactose due to deficiency of lactase; see *lactase deficiency.*

**alae** (a′le) [L.] plural of *ala.*

**Ala·gille syndrome** (ah-lah-zhēl′) [Daniel *Alagille,* French pediatrician, born 1925] [MeSH: Alagille Syndrome] see under *syndrome.*

**Ala·jou·a·nine's syndrome** (ah′lah-zhoo-ah-nēnz′) [Théophile *Alajouanine,* French neurologist, 1890–1980] see under *syndrome.*

**al·a·me·cin** (al-ə-me′sin) an antibiotic substance produced by *Trichoderma viride.*

**Åland eye disease** (ah′lahnt) [Åland Islands, Finnish islands in the Baltic Sea, where it was first observed in the 1960′s] Forsius-Eriksson syndrome.

**Alan·gi·um** (ə-lan′jum) a genus of shrubs and trees of the family Alangiaceae. *A. lamar′ckii* is a species found in Indonesia and Malaysia whose root is emetic, antipyretic, diuretic, and purgative. *A. salviifo′lium* is an Indian species used as an emetic substitute for ipecac.

**al·a·nine** (al′ə-nēn) [MeSH: Alanine] 1. a nonessential amino acid, 2-aminopropanoic acid, occurring in proteins; high levels also occur free in plasma. It is synthesized from pyruvate. Symbols Ala and A. See also table at *amino acid.* 2. [USP] a preparation of alanine used as a dietary supplement.

**β-al·a·nine** (al′ə-nēn) an ω-amino acid, β-aminopropionic acid; it is not found in proteins but occurs both free and in several peptides, is a precursor of acetyl coenzyme A and several related compounds, and is an intermediate in the catabolism of uracil and cytosine.

**al·a·nine ami·no·trans·fer·ase** (al′ə-nēn ə-me″no-trans′fər-ās) [MeSH: Alanine Aminotransferase] alanine transaminase.

**al·a·nine–gly·ox·yl·ate ami·no·trans·fer·ase** (al′ə-nēn gli-ok′səl-āt ə-me″no-trans′fər-ās) alanine–glyoxylate transaminase.

**al·a·nine–gly·ox·y·late trans·am·i·nase** (al′ə-nēn gli-ok′sə-lāt trans-am′ĭ-nās) [EC 2.6.1.44] an enzyme of the transferase class that catalyzes the transamination of glyoxylate to form glycine, using alanine as an amino group donor. Deficiency of the hepatic peroxisomal enzyme, an autosomal recessive trait, causes primary hyperoxaluria, type I.

**β-al·a·nin·emia** (al″ə-nēn-e′me-ə) hyper-β-alaninemia.

**β-al·a·nine–α-ke·to·glu·ta·rate trans·am·i·nase** (al′ə-nēn ke″to-gloo′tə-rāt trans-am′ĭ-nās) an enzyme activity that transfers the amino group from β-alanine to α-ketoglutarate, forming glutamate and malonate semialdehyde as a step in the metabolism of β-alanine. The enzyme can also act on γ-aminobutyrate and *S*-β-aminoisobutyrate; it has been listed as a secondary activity of the enzyme 4-aminobutyrate transaminase but may be a separate enzyme. Deficiency of this enzyme activity causes hyper-β-alaninemia.

**β-al·a·nine–py·ru·vate ami·no·trans·fer·ase** (al′ə-nēn pi′roo-vāt ə-me″no-trans′fər-ās) β-alanine–pyruvate transaminase.

**β-al·a·nine-py·ru·vate trans·am·i·nase** (al′ə-nēn pi′roo-vāt trans-am′ĭ-nās) [EC 2.6.1.18] a mitochondrial enzyme of the transferase class that catalyzes the transfer of the amino group from β-alanine to pyruvate, forming alanine and malonate semialdehyde. The enzyme can also act on *R*-β-aminoisobutyrate.

**al·a·nine trans·am·i·nase** (al′ə-nēn trans-am′ĭ-nās) [EC 2.6.1.2] an enzyme of the transferase class that catalyzes the reversible transfer of an amino group from alanine to α-ketoglutarate to form glutamate and pyruvate, with pyridoxal phosphate as a cofactor. The reaction transfers nitrogen for excretion or for incorporation into other compounds. The enzyme is found in serum and body tissues, especially in the liver. Serum enzyme activity (SGPT) is greatly increased in liver disease and also elevated in infectious mononucleosis. Abbreviated ALT. Called also *alanine aminotransferase* and *glutamic-pyruvic transaminase (GPT).*

**β-al·a·nine trans·am·i·nase** (al′ə-nēn trans-am′ĭ-nās) 1. β-alanine–α-ketoglutarate transaminase. 2. β-alanine–pyruvate transaminase.

**Al·an·son's amputation** (al′ən-sənz) [Edward *Alanson,* English surgeon, 1747–1823] see under *amputation.*

**alan·tin** (ə-lan′tin) inulin.

**al·a·nyl** (al′ə-nəl) the acyl radical of alanine.

**alar** (a′lar) [L. *alaris*] pertaining to an ala, or wing.

**ALARA** as low as reasonably achievable (exposure dose of radiation).

**Ala·ria** (ə-la′re-ə) a genus of trematodes that are intestinal parasites of birds and mammals, occasionally including humans; the animals become infected after eating uncooked or undercooked frogs. Infection is usually subclinical, but a fatal human case has been reported.

**ALAS** 5-aminolevulinate synthase.

**alas·trim** (ə-las′trim) variola minor.

**ALAT** alanine aminotransferase.

**alate** (a′lāt) [L. *alatus* winged] having wings; winged.

**alat·ro·flox·a·cin mes·y·late** (ə-lat″ro-flok′sə-sin) an antibacterial related to the fluoroquinolones, effective against a broad spectrum of gram-positive and gram-negative organisms, used in the treatment of infections due to susceptible organisms. Alatrofloxacin is the prodrug of trovafloxicin; following intravenous infusion, it is rapidly converted to the active drug.

**al·ba** (al′bə) gen. and pl. *al′bae* [L., feminine of *albus*] white; used as an adjective in names of certain anatomical tissues or structures, as substantia alba, and of certain diseases, as pityriasis alba.

**Al·ba·lon** (al′bə-lon) trademark for preparations of naphazoline hydrochloride.

**Al·ba·my·cin** (al′bə-mi″sin) trademark for preparations of novobiocin.

**Al·bar·rán's gland, tubule** (ahl-bah-rahnz′) [Joaquín *Albarrán* y Domínguez, Cuban surgeon in Paris, 1860–1912] see under *gland* and *tubule.*

**al·be·do** (al-be′do) [L.] whiteness.
**a. re′tinae,** edema of the retina.

**Al·bee's operation** (al′bēz) [Fred Houdlett *Albee,* U.S. Army surgeon, 1876–1945] see under *operation.*

**al·ben·da·zole** (al-ben′də-zōl) [USP] [MeSH: Albendazole] a broad-spectrum benzimidazole anthelmintic used against many helminths and in the treatment of hydatid cyst disease and neurocysticercosis and to treat ruminant infestations by either roundworms or flatworms.

**Al·bers-Schön·berg disease** (ahl′berz-shərn′bərg) [Heinrich Ernst *Albers-Schönberg,* German radiologist, 1865–1921] osteopetrosis.

**Al·bert's diphtheria stain** (al′bərts) [Henry *Albert,* American physician, 1878–1930] see under *stain.*

**Al·bert's operation, suture** (ahl′berts) [Eduard *Albert,* Austrian surgeon, 1841–1900] see under *operation* and *suture.*

**al·bi·cans** (al′bĭ-kanz) gen. *albican′tis,* pl. *albican′tia* [L., from *albus* white] white; see *corpus albicans.*

**al·bi·du·ria** (al″bĭ-du′re-ə) [L. *albidus* whitish + *uria*] the discharge of white or pale urine.

**al·bi·dus** (al′bĭ-dəs) [L., from *albus* white] whitish.

**Al·bi·ni's nodules** (ahl-be′nēz) [Giuseppe *Albini,* Italian physiologist, 1827–1911] see under *nodule.*

**al·bi·nism** (al′bĭ-niz-əm) [Port. *albino,* from L. *albus* white + *-ism*] [MeSH: Albinism] 1. the general term for a number of inborn aminoacidopathies affecting the pigment cell (melanocyte) system of the eye and skin and causing hypomelanosis or amelanosis of the eye, skin, and hair. 2. tyrosinase-negative (ty-neg) oculocutaneous a.
**a. I,** tyrosinase-negative (ty-neg) oculocutaneous a.
**a. II,** tyrosinase-positive (ty-pos) oculocutaneous a.

**Amish a.**, yellow mutant oculocutaneous a., so called because first observed among the Amish.
**autosomal dominant oculocutaneous a.**, a form of oculocutaneous albinism characterized by white to red-tinged hair, white to cream-colored skin, and gray to blue-gray irides that are translucent on transillumination, with photophobia, nystagmus, and reduced visual acuity. The number of melanocytes is normal.
**brown a.**, a form of tyrosinase-positive oculocutaneous albinism seen in dark-skinned individuals in which pigmentation is deficient but not absent and photophobia is less severe than in ty-pos OCA. Red reflex and nystagmus are present and visual acuity is moderately reduced.
**complete imperfect a.**, tyrosinase-positive (ty-pos) oculocutaneous a.
**complete perfect a.**, tyrosinase-negative (ty-neg) oculocutaneous a.
**localized a.**, piebaldism.
**ocular a. (OA)**, albinism in which pigment of the hair and skin is normal or only slightly diluted; ocular abnormalities vary with the type of OA, with the X-linked Nettleship type as the classic.
**ocular a., autosomal recessive (AROA)**, a severe form of OA in which both males and females are as severely affected as are hemizygous males with X-linked OA.
**ocular a., Forsius-Eriksson type**, Forsius-Eriksson syndrome.
**ocular a., Nettleship-Falls type**, X-linked (Nettleship) (XOAN) ocular albinism.
**ocular a., X-linked (Nettleship) (XOAN)**, the classic type of OA; hemizygous males are affected with reduced pigmentation of the irides, nystagmus, head nodding and tilting, photophobia, decreased visual acuity of varying degree, and strabismus; the pupillary reflex is present; the fundus is depigmented; and the choroidal vessels stand out. Heterozygous females show translucent irides and a mosaic of pigmentation in the fundus due to lyonization and may also show nystagmus and photophobia. Called also *OA1* and *Nettleship-Falls type ocular a.*
**oculocutaneous a. (OCA)**, a human albinism occurring in ten types all distinguished in their incidence and genetic, biochemical, and clinical characteristics but having in common varying degrees of decreased melanotic pigment of the skin, hair, and eyes, hypoplastic foveas, photophobia, nystagmus, and decreased visual acuity.
**partial a.**, piebaldism.
**red a.**, xanthism.
**rufous a.**, xanthism.
**tyrosinase-negative (ty-neg) oculocutaneous a.**, a recessive disorder characterized by absence of pigment in hair, skin, and eyes. Signs include white hair throughout life, skin that is pink and highly susceptible to neoplasias, absence of pigmented nevi or freckles, gray to blue eyes, prominent red reflexes from the fundi, severe nystagmus, photophobia, and reduced visual acuity (most patients are legally blind). Called also *albinism, a. I,* and *complete perfect a.* Abbreviated ATN.
**tyrosinase-positive (ty-pos) oculocutaneous a.**, a recessive disorder characterized by reduced, but usually visible, pigmentation in hair, skin, and eyes, which varies with race and age. Onset of pigment formation is delayed, pigment accumulates with age, and intensity of accumulation depends on race; hence all ty-pos infants resemble ty-neg infants, and ty-pos adult Blacks may be darker than normal blond Caucasians. The presence of pigmented nevi distinguishes ty-pos and ty-neg Caucasians. Called also *a. II, albinoidism,* and *complete imperfect a.*
**xanthous a.**, yellow mutant oculocutaneous a.
**yellow mutant (ym) oculocutaneous a.**, an autosomal recessive form of oculocutaneous albinism, characterized by yellow hair, fair skin, and severe ocular abnormalities; the hair and skin are white at birth but become pigmented in infancy. The eyes are blue at birth and darken with age; nystagmus persists into adulthood; and from the age of 3 years, transillumination of the iris reveals a cartwheel effect. Pigmentation of the fundus is slight or absent and the macular reflex is absent or minimal. Called also *Amish a.* and *xanthous a.*

**al·bi·nis·mus** (al″bĭ-niz′mus) [L.] albinism.
**a. circumscrip′tus**, piebaldism.

**al·bi·no** (al-bi′no) an individual affected with albinism.

**al·bi·noid·ism** (al-bĭ-noid′iz-əm) [*albinism* + *-oid* + *-ism*] 1. ocular or oculocutaneous hypopigmentation differing from albinism by the absence of hypoplastic foveas, nystagmus, photophobia, and, usually, decreased visual acuity. 2. tyrosinase-positive oculocutaneous albinism.
**oculocutaneous a.**, a dominant hypomelanosis of the skin and hair with rare association of nystagmus, photophobia, and markedly decreased visual acuity. It is a mildly expressed form of tyrosinase-positive oculocutaneous albinism.
**punctate oculocutaneous a.**, a dominant trait marked by blond hair, mildly defective visual acuity (20/30), dilated pupils, and anisocoria.

**al·bi·not·ic** (al″bĭ-not′ik) pertaining to or characterized by albinism.

**al·bin·uria** (al″bĭ-nu′re-ə) albiduria.

**Al·bi·nus' muscle** (ahl-bi′noos) [Bernard Siegfried *Albinus,* German anatomist and surgeon in the Netherlands, 1697–1770] see *musculus risorius* and *musculus scalenus medius.*

**Al·brecht's bone** (ahl′brektz) [Karl Martin Paul *Albrecht,* German anatomist, 1851–1894] basiotic bone.

**Al·bright's hereditary osteodystrophy, syndrome** (awl′brīts) [Fuller *Albright,* American physician and endocrinologist, 1900–1969] see *pseudohyperparathyroidism* and see under *syndrome.*

**Al·bu·cas·is** (al″boo-kas′is) [L., from Ar. Abū-al-Qāsim, 936–1013] an Arabic writer on surgery; the surgical part of his encyclopedic *Altrasrif* greatly influenced medieval European medicine. Known also as *Abulcasis* and *Abulkasim.*

**al·bu·gin·ea** (al″bu-jin′e-ə) [L. from *albus* white] a tough whitish layer of fibrous tissue investing a part, especially a dense white membrane forming the immediate covering of the testicle; called also *tunica albuginea testis* [TA].
**a. o′culi**, the sclera.
**a. ova′rii**, tunica albuginea ovarii.
**a. pe′nis**, the outer envelope of the corpora cavernosa.

**al·bu·gin·e·ot·o·my** (al″bu-jin″e-ot′ə-me) [*albuginea* + *-tomy*] incision of the tunica albuginea of the testis.

**al·bu·gin·e·ous** (al″bu-jin′e-əs) [L. *albugineus*] pertaining to or resembling a tough whitish layer of fibrous tissue (tunica albuginea testis).

**al·bu·gi·ni·tis** (al″bu-jĭ-ni′tis) inflammation of any one of the albugineous tissues or tunics.

**al·bu·men** (al-bu′mən) [L., from *albus* white] 1. egg white. 2. albumin.

**al·bu·mim·e·ter** (al″bu-mim′ə-tər) albuminimeter.

**al·bu·min** (al-bu′min) [*albumen* + *-in*] 1. any protein that is soluble in water and moderately concentrated salt solutions and is coagulable by heat. 2. the major plasma protein, approximately 60 per cent of the total, which is responsible for much of the plasma colloidal osmotic pressure and serves as a transport protein for large organic anions such as fatty acids, bilirubin, and many drugs; it also carries hormones such as cortisol and thyroxine when their specific binding globulins are saturated. It is synthesized in the liver. Decreased serum albumin *(hypoalbuminemia)* occurs in protein malnutrition, active inflammation, and serious hepatic and renal disease. Called also *serum a.* and *seralbumin.*
**a. A**, the normal type of human serum albumin, as opposed to electrophoretic variants.
**acid a.**, albumin altered by the action of an acid.
**aggregated a.**, heat-denatured albumin human; labeled radioactively (technetium 99m), its uses include lung imaging, radionuclide venography, and assessment of peritoneovenous shunt patency. Called also *macroaggregated a. (MAA).* See table at *technetium.*
**alkali a.**, any albumin which has been treated with an alkali.
**blood a.**, albumin (def. 2).
**derived a.**, any albumin denatured by chemical action, as albuminate.
**egg a.**, a glycoprotein that constitutes 20 per cent of the white of hens' eggs; called also *ovalbumin.*
**a. human** [USP], a preparation of serum albumin fractionated from human whole blood, serum, plasma, or placentas; used as a plasma volume expander for emergency treatment of shock or hemorrhage and to increase the binding capacity for bilirubin in the treatment of hyperbilirubinemia and erythroblastosis fetalis; it has also been used to correct hypoalbuminemia of nephrotic syndrome or cirrhosis. Administered intravenously.
**iodinated I 125 a.** [USP], a solution containing normal human albumin adjusted to provide no more than 37 MBq (1 mCi) of radioactivity (from $^{125}$I) per milliliter, used as a diagnostic aid in determining blood or plasma volume and cardiac output.
**iodinated I 131 a.** [USP], a solution containing normal human albumin adjusted to provide no more than 37 MBq (1 mCi) of radioactivity (from $^{131}$I) per milliliter, used as a diagnostic aid in determining blood or plasma volume and cardiac output.
**macroaggregated a.**, MAA; aggregated a.
**native a.**, an albumin in its natural state, i.e., not denatured.
**serum a.**, albumin (def. 2).
**vegetable a.**, any albumin of vegetable origin.

**Al·bu·mi·nar** (al-bu′mĭ-nahr) trademark for preparations of albumin human.

**al·bu·mi·nate** (al-bu′mĭ-nāt″) albumin denatured by a base or an acid, characterized by solubility in dilute acids or alkalis and by being insoluble in dilute salt solutions, water, or alcohol; called also *derived albumin* and *derived protein.*

**al·bu·min·a·tu·ria** (al-bu″mĭ-nă-tu′re-ə) proteinuria in which there is an excess of albuminates in the urine.

**al·bu·min·emia** (al-bu″mĭ-ne′me-ə) the presence of albumin in the blood plasma or serum; proteinemia.

**al·bu·mi·nim·e·ter** (al-bu″mĭ-nim′ə-tər) [*albumin* + *-meter*] an instrument used in determining the proportion of albumin present, as in the urine.

**al·bu·mi·nim·e·try** (al-bu″mĭ-nim′ə-tre) the determination of the proportion of albumin present.

**al·bu·mi·no·cho·lia** (al-bu″mĭ-no-ko′le-ə) [*albumin* + *chol-* + *-ia*] the presence of albumin in the bile.

**al·bu·mi·no·cy·to·log·i·cal** (al-bu″mĭ-no-si″to-loj′ĭ-kəl) pertaining to the level of protein as albumin in relation to number of cells present in cerebrospinal fluid.

**al·bu·mi·noid** (al-bu′mĭ-noid″) [*albumin* + *-oid*] 1. resembling albumin. 2. fibrous protein. 3. a scleroprotein.

**al·bu·mi·nol·y·sis** (al-bu″mĭ-nol′ĭ-sis) the splitting up of albumins.

**al·bu·mi·nom·e·ter** (al-bu″mĭ-nom′ə-tər) albuminimeter.

**al·bu·mi·nop·ty·sis** (al-bu″mĭ-nop′tĭ-sis) [*albumin* + Gr. *ptyein* to spit] presence of albumin in the sputum.

**al·bu·mi·no·re·ac·tion** (al-bu″mĭ-no-re-ak′shən) the reaction of the sputum to tests for albumin; the presence of albumin (positive reaction) is indicative of pulmonary inflammation.

**al·bu·mi·nor·rhea** (al-bu″mĭ-no-re′ə) [*albumin* + *-rrhea*] excessive excretion of albumins.

**al·bu·mi·nous** (al-bu′mĭ-nəs) containing, charged with, or of the nature of an albumin.

**al·bu·min·uret·ic** (al-bu″mĭ-nu-ret′ik) [*albumin* + *uretic*] 1. pertaining to, characterized by, or promoting albuminuria. 2. an agent that promotes albuminuria.

**al·bu·min·uria** (al″bu-mĭ-nu′re-ə) [MeSH: Albuminuria] presence in the urine of serum albumin; see *proteinuria*.

**Al·bu·tein** (al′bu-tēn) trademark for preparations of albumin human.

**al·bu·ter·ol** (al-bu′tər-ol) [USP] [MeSH: Albuterol] a β-adrenergic agent used as a bronchodilator for the treatment and prophylaxis of reversible bronchospasm in obstructive airway disease; administered orally and by inhalation. Called also *salbutamol*.
**a. sulfate** [USP], the sulfate salt of albuterol, having the same actions and uses as the base.

**Al·caine** (al′kān) trademark for a preparation of proparacaine hydrochloride.

**Al·ca·lig·e·nes** (al″kə-lij′ə-nēz) [Arabic *al-qualy* potash + Gr. *gennan* to produce] [MeSH: Alcaligenes] a widespread genus of gram-negative, aerobic, rod-shaped, alkaline-producing bacteria of uncertain affiliation, found in the intestines of vertebrates and as part of the normal skin flora, and occasionally the cause of opportunistic infections.
**A. denitri′ficans**, a species isolated from a variety of clinical specimens.
**A. faeca′lis**, a species isolated from hospital environments and from blood, sputum, and urine specimens. It is a cause of nosocomial septicemia in immunocompromised patients, generally arising from contaminated hemodialysis or intravenous fluids. Called also *A. odorans* and *Bacterium faecalis alcaligenes*.
**A. odo′rans**, *A. faecalis*.

**al·cap·ton·uria** (al-kap″to-nu′re-ə) [MeSH: Alkaptonuria] alkaptonuria.

**al·cap·ton·uric** (al-kap″to-nu′rik) alkaptonuric.

**al·clo·fen·ac** (al-klo′fən-ak) a phenylacetic acid derivative with analgesic, antipyretic, and anti-inflammatory properties, used to treat rheumatoid arthritis.

**al·clo·met·a·sone di·pro·pi·o·nate** (al-klo-met′ə-sōn″) [USP] a synthetic corticosteroid used topically for the relief of inflammation and pruritus in corticosteroid-responsive dermatoses.

**Alc·mae·on of Cro·tona** (alk-me′ən) [c. 500 B.C.] a physician, student of Pythagoras. He described bodily states as an interplay of opposites: health is an *isonomy* of hot and cold, wet and dry, etc.; disease, a *monarchy* of one of these qualities; thus he was one of the precursors of humoralism. Alcmaeon considered the brain to be the seat of sensation and thought, performed the first known human dissections, distinguished veins from arteries, discovered "passages" from the eye to the brain, and was the first observer of the development of a chick embryo. See also *Empedocles*.

**Al·cock's canal** (al′koks) [Benjamin *Alcock*, Irish professor of anatomy; born 1801, date of death unknown] canalis pudendalis.

**al·co·gel** (al′ko-jel) a gel that has alcohol as its dispersion medium.

**al·co·hol** (al′kə-hol) [Arabic *al kuhl* fine powder of antimony or other distilled substance] 1. any of a class of organic compounds formed from the hydrocarbons by substitution of one or more hydroxyl groups for an equal number of hydrogen atoms; the term is extended to various substitution products that are neutral in reaction and that contain one or more of the alcohol groups. 2. ethanol. 3. [USP] the official preparation of ethanol, containing not less than 92.3 per cent and not more than 93.8 per cent of ethanol by weight.
**absolute a.**, dehydrated a.
**amyl a.**, a colorless oily liquid, $C_5H_{11}OH$, with characteristic odor, occurring as several isomers; miscible with alcohol, ether, and chloroform and slightly soluble in water, and used as solvents and in pharmaceutical preparations.
**amyl a., tertiary**, amylene hydrate.
**aromatic a.**, an aromatic compound in which the side chain on the benzene ring contains a hydroxyl group; e.g., phenol.
**azeotropic isopropyl a.** [USP], a preparation containing 91–93 per cent isopropyl alcohol by volume and water.
**benzyl a.** [NF], a clear colorless oily liquid occurring in balsam of Peru, tolu balsam, and styrax; used as a bacteriostatic in solutions for injection and topically as a local anesthetic. Called also *benzenemethanol, phenylcarbinol,* and *phenylmethanol*.
**butyl a.** [NF], a clear, colorless, mobile liquid, $C_4H_9OH$, with a characteristic odor, occurring in four isomeric forms; used as a solvent.
**cetostearyl a.** [NF], a mixture of stearyl alcohol and cetyl alcohol, used as an emulsifier; the official preparation consists of at least 40 per cent stearyl alcohol and at least 90 per cent of stearyl and cetyl alcohols combined.
**cetyl a.** [NF], a solid fatty alcohol prepared by hydrogenation of palmitic acid or by saponification of spermaceti, used as an emulsifying and stiffening agent; the official preparation contains not less than 90 per cent cetyl alcohol, with the remainder consisting mainly of related alcohols.
**dehydrated a.** [USP], an extremely hygroscopic, transparent, colorless, volatile liquid with characteristic odor and burning taste, containing at least 99.5 per cent ethanol by volume; used as a solvent and administered by injection into nerves and ganglia for relief of pain. Called also *absolute a.*
**denatured a.**, ethanol which has been rendered unfit for internal use by addition of an adulterant such as methanol or acetone, but which may still be used for other purposes including industrial processes, as a solvent, on the skin as a cooling agent, and as a skin disinfectant.
**dihydric a.**, an alcohol containing two hydroxyl groups.
**diluted a.** [NF], a mixture of alcohol and water, used as a solvent; the official preparation contains 41 to 42 per cent ethanol by weight, or 48.4 to 49.5 per cent by volume, at 15.56° C.
**ethyl a.**, ethanol.
**fatty a.**, any of a group of high molecular weight primary alcohols, usually straight chain; they may be synthetic or derived from natural oils and are used in pharmacy and as solvents, detergents, and emulsifiers.
**glyceryl a., glycyl a.**, glycerin.
**grain a.**, ethanol.
**isoamyl a.**, one of the isomeric forms of amyl alcohol; used as a solvent and in pharmacy.
**isopropyl a.** [USP], an isomer of propyl alcohol and a homologue of ethyl alcohol, having disinfectant properties similar to those of ethyl alcohol; used as a solvent and disinfectant and applied topically as an antiseptic. Called also *dimethyl carbinol* and *isopropanol*.
**isopropyl rubbing a.** [USP], a preparation containing 68–72 per cent isopropyl alcohol in water, used as a rubefacient.
**lanolin a's** [NF], a mixture of aliphatic alcohols, triterpenoid alcohols, and sterols, obtained by hydrolysis of lanolin; used as an emulsifying agent in the preparation of water-in-oil emulsions. Called also *wool a's*.
**methyl a.**, methanol.
**monohydric a.**, an alcohol containing only one hydroxyl group.
**nicotinyl a.**, a vasodilator with properties similar to those of nicotinic acid, used in peripheral vascular disorders. Called also *nicotinic a.*
**palmityl a.**, cetyl a.
**pantothenyl a.**, 1. panthenol. 2. dexpanthenol.
**phenethyl a.** [USP], a colorless liquid with a roselike odor and a sharp, burning taste, occurring in a number of natural essential oils; used as an antimicrobial agent in pharmaceutical preparations. Called also *benzyl carbinol*.
**polyhydric a.**, polyol.
**polyvinyl a.** [USP], a water-soluble synthetic resin, represented by the formula $(C_2H_4O)_n$, in which *n* varies between 500 and 5000; used as a viscosity-increasing agent in pharmaceutical preparations and as a lubricant and protectant in ophthalmic preparations.
**primary a.**, an alcohol in which the carbon atom attached to the hydroxyl group carries a single alkyl group and two hydrogen groups. See illustration.
***n*-propyl a.**, a clear colorless liquid with an alcohol-like odor, miscible with water and most organic solvents; used as a solvent for resins.
**rubbing a.** [USP], a preparation of acetone, methyl isobutyl ketone, and 68.5 to 71.5 per cent ethanol; used as a rubefacient.
**secondary a.**, an alcohol in which the carbon atom attached to the

Chemical structure of primary *(A)*, secondary *(B)*, and tertiary *(C)* alcohols.

hydroxyl group carries two alkyl groups and one hydrogen group. See illustration.
**stearyl a.,** a solid alcohol prepared from stearic acid by catalytic hydrogenation, used as an ingredient of hydrophilic ointment, hydrophilic petrolatum, and polyethylene glycol ointment; the official preparation [NF] contains at least 90 per cent stearyl alcohol, the remainder consisting mainly of cetyl alcohol.
**sugar a.,** a polyhydric alcohol having no more than one hydroxy group attached to each carbon atom, formed by the reduction of the carbonyl group of a sugar to a hydroxyl group.
**tertiary a.,** an alcohol in which the carbon atom attached to the hydroxyl group carries three alkyl groups. See illustration.
**trihydric a.,** an alcohol containing three hydroxyl groups.
**unsaturated a.,** alcohol that is derived from unsaturated hydrocarbons (alkenes, or olefins).
**wood a.,** methanol.
**wool a's,** lanolin a's.

**al·co·hol de·hy·dro·gen·ase** (al'kə-hol de-hi'dro-jən-ās) [EC 1.1.1.1] [MeSH: Alcohol Dehydrogenase] an enzyme of the oxidoreductase class that catalyzes the reversible oxidation of primary or secondary alcohols to aldehydes using $NAD^+$ as an electron acceptor. The reaction is the first step in the metabolism of alcohols by the liver. Abbreviated AD and ADH.

**al·co·hol de·hy·dro·gen·ase (NADP⁺)** (al'kə-hol de-hi'dro-jən-ās) [EC 1.1.1.2] [MeSH: Alcohol Dehydrogenase] an enzyme of the oxidoreductase class that catalyzes the reversible oxidation of primary (or secondary) alcohols to aldehydes (or ketones), using $NADP^+$ as an electron acceptor.

**al·co·hol de·hy·dro·gen·ase (NAD(P)⁺)** (al'kə-hol de-hi'dro-jən-ās) [EC 1.1.1.71] an enzyme of the oxidoreductase class that catalyzes the reversible oxidation of primary or secondary alcohols to aldehydes or ketones respectively, using $NAD^+$ or $NADP^+$ as an electron acceptor. The enzyme also interconverts retinol and retinal.

**al·co·hol·emia** (al"kə-hol-e'me-ə) the presence of alcohol in the blood.

**al·co·hol·ic** (al"kə-hol'ik) 1. pertaining to or containing alcohol. 2. a person suffering from alcoholism (q.v.).

**al·co·hol·ism** (al'kə-hol-iz-əm) [MeSH: Alcoholism] a disorder characterized by a pathological pattern of alcohol use that causes a serious impairment in social or occupational functioning. In DSM-IV it is covered by alcohol abuse and alcohol dependence.

**al·co·hol·i·za·tion** (al"kə-hol"i-za'shən) treatment by application or injection of alcohol.

**al·co·hol·ize** (al'kə-hol-īz") 1. to treat with alcohol. 2. to transform into alcohol.

**al·co·hol·om·e·ter** (al"kə-hol-om'ə-tər) [*alcohol* + *-meter*] an instrument used in determining the percentage of alcohol in a solution.

**al·co·hol·uria** (al"kə-hol-u're-ə) the presence of alcohol in the urine.

**al·co·hol·y·sis** (al"kə-hol'ĭ-sis) [*alcohol* + *-lysis*] a process analogous to hydrolysis, but in which alcohol takes the place of water.

**al·co·sol** (al'kə-sol) a sol in which the dispersion medium is alcohol.

**al·cu·ro·ni·um chlo·ride** (al-ku-ro'nī-əm) a non-depolarizing skeletal muscle relaxant with effects like those of tubocurarine chloride.

**Al·dac·ta·zide** (al-dak'to-zīd) trademark for a preparation of spironolactone with hydrochlorothiazide.

**Al·dac·tone** (al-dak'tōn) trademark for a preparation of spironolactone.

**al·dar·ic ac·id** (al-dar'ik) a dicarboxylic acid resulting from oxidation of both terminal groups of an aldose to carboxyl groups, e.g., glucaric acid.

**al·de·hyde** (al'də-hīd) [*al*cohol + L. *de* away from + *hyd*rogen] 1. any one of a large class of organic compounds containing the group —CHO, that is, with the carbonyl group, C═O, occurring at the end of the carbon chain. 2. a suffix used to denote a compound occurring in aldehyde conformation. 3. acetaldehyde.
**acetic a.,** acetaldehyde.
**formic a.,** formaldehyde.
**glyceric a.,** glyceraldehyde.

**al·de·hyde de·hy·dro·gen·ase (NAD⁺)** (al'də-hīd de-hi'-dro-jən-ās) [EC 1.2.1.3] [MeSH: Aldehyde Dehydrogenase] an enzyme of the oxidoreductase class that catalyzes the oxidation of various aldehydes, using $NAD^+$ as an electron acceptor, including the oxidation of acetaldehyde to acetate in the metabolism of ethanol. Multiple isozymes exist and deficiencies of the cytosolic or mitochondrial isozymes of liver result in accumulation of acetaldehyde; such deficiencies, particularly prevalent in East Asians, manifest as facial flushing, vasodilation, and tachycardia after ethanol ingestion. Called also *acetaldehyde dehydrogenase.*

**al·de·hyde-ly·ase** (al"də-hīd-li'ās) [EC 4.1.2] any member of a sub-subclass of enzymes of the lyase class that catalyze cleavage of a C—C bond in a molecule containing a hydroxyl group and a carbonyl group to form two smaller molecules, each being an aldehyde or a ketone; chemically, it is the reverse of an aldol condensation. Called also *aldolase.*

**al·de·hyde ox·i·dase** (al'də-hīd ok'sĭ-dās) [EC 1.2.3.1] an enzyme of the oxidoreductase class that catalyzes the oxidation of aldehydes to the corresponding acids, generating a superoxide anion. It is a molybdoflavoprotein found in liver tissue, catalyzing the oxidation of a wide variety of heterocyclic compounds and xenobiotics. Activity of this enzyme is believed to be deficient in molybdenum cofactor deficiency.

**al·de·hyde re·duc·tase** (al'də-hīd re-duk'tās) [EC 1.1.1.21] [MeSH: Aldehyde Reductase] an enzyme of the oxidoreductase class that catalyzes the reduction of aldoses to form alditols, using NADPH as an electron donor. In galactosemia due to galactokinase deficiency, catalysis of the reduction of galactose to galactitol by aldehyde reductase in the lens of the eye results in cataract formation. Called also *aldose reductase.*

**Al·der's anomaly** (ahl'dərz) [Albert von *Alder,* German physician, born 1888] see under *anomaly.*

**Al·der-Reil·ly anomaly, bodies** (ahl'dər ri'le) [A. von *Alder;* William Anthony *Reilly,* American pediatrician, born 1901] see under *anomaly* and *body.*

**al·des·leu·kin** (al"dəs-loo'kin) a recombinant interleukin-2 product used as an antineoplastic and biological response modifier in the treatment of metastatic renal cell carcinoma; administered by intravenous infusion.

**al·di·carb** (al'dĭ-kahrb) [MeSH: Aldicarb] a carbamate pesticide used as an insecticide; in some countries, also used as a rodenticide.

**Al·din·a·mide** (al-din'ə-mīd) trademark for preparations of pyrazinamide.

**al·di·tol** (al'dĭ-tol) the polyhydroxy alcohol produced by reduction of the aldehyde group of an aldose.

**al·do·bi·on·ic ac·id** (al"do-bi-on'ik) 1. an oxidized disaccharide derivative containing an aldose linked to an aldonic acid. 2. more frequently, an incorrectly used term denoting an aldobiuronic acid.

**Al·do·clor** (al'do-klor) trademark for a preparation of methyldopa and chlorothiazide.

**al·do·hex·ose** (al"do-hek'sōs) any aldose containing six carbon atoms, such as glucose or mannose. Cf. *ketohexose.*

**al·do·lase** (al'do-lās) 1. aldehyde-lyase. 2. fructose-bisphosphate aldolase.

**Al·do·met** (al'do-met) trademark for preparations of methyldopa.

**al·don·ic ac·id** (al-don'ik) a carboxylic acid resulting from oxidation of the aldehyde group of an aldose to a carboxyl group, e.g., gluconic acid.

**al·do·pen·tose** (al"do-pen'tōs) any ketose containing five carbon atoms, such as arabinose.

**Al·do·ril** (al'do-ril") trademark for preparations of methyldopa and hydrochlorothiazide.

**al·dose** (al'dōs) one of two subgroups of monosaccharides, being those having a terminal carbonyl (aldehyde) group; it is further subdivided on the basis of the number of carbon atoms in the sugar; see *aldotetrose, aldopentose, aldohexose,* etc. Examples are glucose, galactose, and mannose.

**al·dose 1-epim·er·ase** (al'dōs ə-pim'ər-ās) [EC 5.1.3.3] an enzyme of the isomerase class that catalyzes interconversion of the $\alpha$- and $\beta$- forms of D-glucose, L-arabinose, D-xylose, D-galactose, lactose, and maltose. Commonly called *mutarotase.*

**al·dose re·duc·tase** (al'dōs re-duk'tās) aldehyde reductase.

**al·do·side** (al'do-sīd) a glycoside formed from an aldose; e.g., a glucoside.

**al·dos·ter·one** (al-dos'tər-ōn) [MeSH: Aldosterone] the major mineralocorticoid hormone secreted by the adrenal cortex. It promotes the retention of sodium and bicarbonate, the excretion of potassium and hydrogen ions, and the secondary retention of water. Large excesses can invoke plasma volume expansion, edema, and hypertension. The secretion of aldosterone is stimulated by low plasma potassium concentration and angiotensin II.

**al·dos·ter·on·ism** (al-dos′tə-ro-niz″əm) an abnormality of electrolyte metabolism caused by excessive secretion of aldosterone; called also *hyperaldosteronism.*
**primary a.,** that arising from oversecretion of aldosterone by an adrenal cortical adenoma, characterized typically by hypokalemia, alkalosis, muscular weakness, polyuria, polydipsia, and hypertension. Called also *Conn's syndrome.*
**pseudoprimary a.,** signs and symptoms identical to those of primary aldosteronism but caused by factors other than excessive aldosterone secretion.
**secondary a.,** that due to extra-adrenal stimulation of aldosterone secretion; it is commonly associated with edematous states, such as those accompanying nephrotic syndrome, hepatic cirrhosis, heart failure, or malignant hypertension.

**al·dos·ter·ono·gen·e·sis** (al-dos″tər-o″no-jen′ə-sis) the production of aldosterone by the adrenal cortex.

**al·dos·ter·o·no·ma** (al″do-ster″o-no′mə) a tumor of the adrenal cortex that secretes aldosterone, causing primary aldosteronism; the majority are adenomas, but few are carcinomas. Called also *aldosterone-secreting tumor.*

**al·dos·ter·ono·pe·nia** (al-dos″tər-o″no-pe′ne-ə) hypoaldosteronism.

**al·dos·ter·on·uria** (al-dos″tər-o-nu′re-ə) hyperaldosteronuria.

**al·do·tet·rose** (al″do-tet′rōs) any aldose containing four carbon atoms, such as erythrose.

**al·do·tri·ose** (al″do-tri′ōs) an aldose containing three carbon atoms; see *glyceraldehyde.*

**al·dox·ime** (al-dok′sīm) the —CH═NOH radical formed by the union of an aldehyde with hydroxylamine.

**Al·drich syndrome** (awl′drich) [Robert A. *Aldrich,* American pediatrician, born 1917] Wiskott-Aldrich syndrome; see under *syndrome.*

**Al·drich-Mees lines** (awl′drich-māz) [C.J. *Aldrich,* American physician, early 20th century; *R.A. Mees,* Dutch scientist, 20th century] Mees' lines.

**al·drin** (al′drin) [MeSH: Aldrin] a chlorinated hydrocarbon insecticide, closely related to dieldrin; if ingested or absorbed through the skin by a human or other animal, it causes neurotoxic reactions that can be fatal, including tremors, ataxia, and convulsions.

**alec·i·thal** (a-les′ĭ-thal) [*a-*[1] + *lecith-* + *-al*[1]] without yolk; applied to eggs with very little yolk. See under *ovum.*

**Alec·to·ro·bi·us ta·la·je** (ə-lek″tə-ro′be-əs ta-li′ə) the tick *Ornithodoros talaje.*

**alen·dro·nate sodium** (ə-len′dro-nāt) a bisphosphonate calcium-regulating agent used to inhibit the resorption of bone in the treatment of osteitis deformans, postmenopausal osteoporosis, and hypercalcemia related to malignancy; administered orally.

**aleu·ke·mia** (a″loo-ke′me-ə) 1. leukopenia. 2. aleukemic leukemia.

**aleu·ke·mic** (a″loo-ke′mik) leukopenic.

**aleu·kia** (a-loo′ke-ə) leukopenia.
**alimentary toxic a. (ATA),** a rare form of mycotoxicosis associated with the ingestion of grain that has overwintered in the field and become contaminated with fungi that contain trichothecenes; characteristics include skin inflammation, vomiting, diarrhea, and hemorrhages that can be fatal. Causative fungi include members of the genera *Alternaria, Fusarium, Myrothecium, Piptocephalis, Thamnidium, Trichoderma, Trichothecium, Verticillium,* and others.
**a. hemorrha′gica,** old name for *aplastic anemia.*

**aleu·ko·cyt·ic** (a-loo″ko-sit′ik) leukopenic.

**aleu·ko·cy·to·sis** (a-loo″ko-si-to′sis) [*a-*[1] + *leukocyte* + *-osis*] leukopenia.

**aleu·rio·co·nid·i·um** (ə-lo͞o″re-o-kə-nid′e-əm) [Gr. *aleuron* flour + *conidium*] a terminal or lateral conidium that is released by dissolution of its attachment to the mycelium. Called also *aleuriospore.*

**aleu·rio·spore** (ə-lo͞o′re-o-spor) aleurioconidium.

**al·eu·rone** (ə-lo͞or′ōn, al′yə-rōn″) granules of protein occurring in the endosperm of ripe seeds, particularly those concentrated in the outer layer of the endosperm of cereal grains.

**al·eu·ro·noid** (ə-lu′ro-noid″) resembling flour.

**Al·ex·an·der's deafness (hearing loss)** (al″eg-zan′dərz) [Gustav *Alexander,* Austrian otologist, born 1873] see under *deafness.*

**Al·ex·an·der's disease** (al″eg-zan′dərz) [W. Stewart *Alexander,* English pathologist, 20th century] see under *disease.*

**Al·ex·an·der's operation** (al″eg-zan′dərz) [William *Alexander,* English surgeon, 1844–1919] see under *operation.*

**Al·ex·an·der-Ad·ams operation** (al″eg-zan′dər-ad′əmz) [William *Alexander;* James Alexander *Adams,* Scottish gynecologist, 1857–1930] see *Alexander's operation,* under *operation.*

**Al·ex·an·der of Tral·les** (al″əg-san′dər) [c. 525–605] a Byzantine physician who practiced in Rome; he wrote on pathology and the treatment of internal diseases and described intestinal parasites and vermifuges. Also known as *Alexander Trallianus.*

**alex·ia** (ə-lek′se-ə) [*a-*[1] + Gr. *lexis* word + *-ia*] a form of receptive aphasia in which there is loss of the ability to understand written language as a result of a cerebral lesion; cf. *dyslexia.* Called also *aphemesthesia, optical alexia, visual amnesia, visual aphasia,* and *word blindness.*
**cortical a.,** a form of sensory aphasia due to lesions of the left parietal lobe, especially the gyrus angularis.
**motor a.,** alexia in which the patient understands what he sees written or printed, but cannot read it aloud.
**musical a.,** loss of the ability to read music; called also *music blindness.*
**optical a.,** alexia.
**subcortical a.,** a form due to interruption of the connection between the optic center and the parietal lobe, including the gyrus angularis of the dominant hemisphere.

**alex·ic** (ə-lek′sik) pertaining to alexia.

**alex·i·phar·mac** (ə-lek″sĭ-fahr′mək) antidote.

**alex·i·thy·mia** (ə-lek″sĭ-thi′me-ə) [*a-*[1] + Gr. *lexis* word + *-thymia*] inability to recognize or describe one's emotions.

**aley·dig·ism** (a-li′dig-iz″əm) absence of androgen secretion by Leydig's cells, as occurs in hypogonadotropic hypogonadism.

**Al·ez·zan·dri·ni's syndrome** (ahl″ĕ-tsahn-dre′nēz) [Arturo Alberto *Alezzandrini,* Argentine ophthalmologist, born 1932] see under *syndrome.*

**al·fal·fa** (al-fal′fə) [Sp., from Ar. *al fasfasah*] [MeSH: Alfalfa] *Medicago sativa.*

**Al·fen·ta** (al-fen′tə) trademark for a preparation of alfentanil hydrochloride.

**al·fen·ta·nil hy·dro·chlo·ride** (al-fen′tə-nil) [USP] an opioid analgesic of rapid onset and short duration derived from fentanyl, used as a primary agent for the induction of general anesthesia and as an adjunct in the maintenance of general anesthesia; administered intravenously.

**Al·fer·on N** (al′fēr-on) trademark for a preparation of interferon alfa-n3.

**Al·flo·rone** (al′flo-rōn) trademark for preparations of fludrocortisone.

**ALG** antilymphocyte globulin.

**al·ga** (al′gə) any individual organism of the algae.

**al·gae** (al′je) [L., pl., "seaweeds"] [MeSH: Algae] a group of cryptogamous plants, in which the body is unicellular or consists of a thallus; it includes the seaweed and many unicellular fresh-water plants, most of which contain chlorophyll. Algae account for about 90 per cent of the earth's photosynthetic activity.
**blue-green a.,** *Cyanobacteria.*

**al·gal** (al′gəl) of, pertaining to, or caused by algae.

**al·ga·ro·ba** (al″gə-ro′bə) algarroba.

**al·gar·ro·ba** (al″gə-ro′bə) [Ar. *al kharrubah*] 1. carob (defs. 1 and 2). 2. mesquite.

**alge-** [Gr. *algēsis* sense of pain, from *algos* pain] a combining form denoting relationship to pain.

**al·ge·don·ic** (al″jə-don′ik) [*alge-* + *hedonic*] characterized by or relating to both pleasure and pain.

**al·ge·fa·cient** (al″jə-fa′shənt) [L. *algere* to be cold + *-facient*] cooling; refrigerant.

**al·gel·drate** (al-jel′drāt) nonreactive, powdered, hydrated aluminum hydroxide; an antacid.

**al·ge·sia** (al-je′ze-ə) 1. pain sense. 2. excessive sensitivity to pain, a type of hyperesthesia.

**al·ge·sic** (al-je′zik) 1. painful. 2. pertaining to algesia.

**al·ge·si·chro·nom·e·ter** (al-je″zĭ-kro-nom′ə-tər) [*algesi-* + *chrono-* + *-meter*] an instrument for recording the time required to produce a painful impression.

**al·ge·sim·e·ter** (al′jə-sim′ə-tər) [*algesi-* + *-meter*] an instrument used in measuring the sensitiveness to pain, such as by pricking

with a sharp object or by applying measurable amounts of heat or pressure. Called also *algesiometer* and *algometer*. Cf. *dolorimeter*.
**Björnström's a.,** an apparatus for determining the sensitiveness of the skin.
**Boas' a.,** an instrument for determining the sensitiveness over the epigastrium.

**al·ge·sim·e·try** (al″jə-sim′ə-tre) the measurement of sensitiveness to pain.

**algesi(o)-** [Gr. *algēsis* sense of pain, from *algos* pain] a combining form denoting relationship to pain.

**al·ge·sio·gen·ic** (al-je″ze-o-jen′ik) [*algesio-* + *-genic*] producing pain.

**al·ge·si·om·e·ter** (al-je″ze-om′ə-tər) algesimeter.

**al·ges·the·sia** (al″jes-the′zhə) [*alge-* + *esthesia*] 1. pain sense. 2. any painful sensation.

**al·ges·the·sis** (al″jes-the′sis) algesthesia.

**al·ges·tone ace·to·phen·ide** (al-jes′tōn) [MeSH: Algestone Acetophenide] a progestin with actions similar to those of progesterone.

**al·get·ic** (al-jet′ik) 1. painful. 2. pertaining to algesia.

**-algia** [Gr., from *algos* pain + *-ia*] a word termination denoting a painful condition.

**al·gi·cide** (al′jĭ-sīd) [*algae* + *-cide*] a substance which is destructive to algae.

**al·gid** (al′jid) [L. *algidus*] chilly or cold, def. 1.

**al·gin** (al′jin) sodium alginate, a purified carbohydrate (sodium mannuronate) extracted from brown algae species and used as a stabilizing colloid in numerous pharmaceuticals, cosmetics, and foods.

**al·gi·nate** (al′jĭ-nāt) a salt of alginic acid, which is extracted from marine kelp. Calcium, sodium, and ammonium alginates have been used as foam, clot, or gauze for absorbable surgical dressings. Soluble alginates, such as sodium, potassium, and magnesium alginates, form a viscous sol which can be changed into a gel by a chemical reaction with compounds such as calcium sulfate, a property which makes them useful as materials for taking dental impressions.

**al·gin·ic ac·id** (al-jin′ic) [NF] a hydrophilic colloidal carbohydrate extracted with dilute alkali from species of brown seaweed of the class Phaeophyceae; used as a tablet binder and emulsifying agent.

**al·gin·ure·sis** (al″jin-u-re′sis) [*algi-* + *uresis*] painful urination.

**algi(o)-** [Gr. *algos* pain] a combining form denoting relationship to pain.

**al·gio·mo·tor** (al″je-o-mo′tər) producing painful movements, such as spasm or dysperistalsis.

**al·gio·mus·cu·lar** (al″je-o-mus′ku-lər) algiomotor.

**al·gio·vas·cu·lar** (al″je-o-vas′ku-lər) pertaining to vascular action resulting from painful stimulation. Called also *algovascular*.

**al·glu·cer·ase** (al-gloo′sər-ās″) a modified form of β-glucocerebrosidase, prepared from pooled human placental tissue, used to replace glucocerebrosidase (glucosylceramidase) in the treatment of type 1 Gaucher's disease; administered by intravenous infusion.

**alg(o)-** [Gr. *algos* pain] a combining form denoting relationship to pain.

**al·go·dys·tro·phy** (al″go-dis′tro-fe) [*algo-* + *dystrophy*] reflex sympathetic dystrophy.

**al·go·gen·e·sia** (al″go-jə-ne′zhə) [*algo-* + Gr. *gennan* to produce] the production of pain.

**al·go·gen·e·sis** (al″go-jen′ə-sis) algogenesia.

**al·go·gen·ic** (al-go-jen′ik) algesiogenic.

**al·go·lag·nia** (al″go-lag′ne-ə) [*algo-* + Gr. *lagneia* lust] any psychosexual disorder associated with the derivation of pleasure from experiencing or inflicting physical or psychological pain.
**active a.,** sadism.
**passive a.,** masochism.

**al·gom·e·ter** (al-gom′ə-tər) [*algo-* + *-meter*] algesimeter.
**pressure a.,** an instrument for measuring sensitivity to pressure.

**al·gom·e·try** (al-gom′ə-tre) algesimetry.

**al·go·pho·bia** (al″go-fo′be-ə) [*algo-* + *phobia*] exaggerated, irrational fear of pain.

**al·go·psy·cha·lia** (al″go-si-ka′le-ə) [*algo-* + Gr. *psychē* soul] psychalgia (def. 1).

**al·go·rithm** (al′gə-rith-əm) [MeSH: Algorithms] 1. a step-by-step method of solving a problem or making decisions, as in making a diagnosis. 2. an established mechanical procedure for solving certain mathematical problems.

**al·go·spasm** (al′go-spaz-əm) [*algo-* + *spasm*] painful spasm or cramp.

**al·go·vas·cu·lar** (al″go-vas′ku-lər) algiovascular.

**Ali Ab·bas** (ah′le ah′bahs) [L. *Haly Abbas,* from Ar. *Ali* ibn-al-*Abbās,* al Majūsi, 930–994] a Persian physician whose *Al-Maliki* (*Liber Regius,* "Royal Book") was the leading medical text for 100 years, when it was superseded by Avicenna's *Canon*. Also known as *Haly Abbas*.

**ali·as·ing** (a′le-əs-ing) 1. introduction of an artifact or error in sampling of a periodic signal when the sampling frequency is too low to properly capture the signal. 2. in pulsed Doppler ultrasonography, an artifact occurring when the velocity of the sampled object exceeds the pulse repetition frequency of the sampling system; the system cannot sample rapidly enough for Doppler frequency determination. 3. an artifact appearing in magnetic resonance imaging when a part being examined is larger than the field of view; an image of the area outside the field of view appears as an artifact inside the field of view. Called also *aliasing artifact* and *wraparound artifact*.

**al·i·cy·clic** (al″ĭ-sik′lik) having the properties of both aliphatic and cyclic substances.

**Al·i·dase** (al′ĭ-dās) trademark for a preparation of hyaluronidase for injection.

**alien·a·tion** (āl″e-ən-a′shən) [L. *alienatio,* from *alienus* strange, foreign] 1. estrangement from society; feelings of being an outsider, foreigner, or outcast. 2. estrangement from one's self; feelings of unreality or depersonalization. 3. alienation of affect; isolation of ideas from feelings, avoidance of emotional situations, and other efforts to estrange one's self from one's feelings.

**ali·enia** (a-li-e′ne-ə) [*a-*[1] + *lien-* + *-ia*] asplenia.

**alien·ist** (āl′e-ə-nist) [Fr. *aliéniste,* from *aliéné* insane, from L. *alienatus* estranged] (*obs.*) a psychiatrist.

**al·i·flu·rane** (al″ĭ-floo′rān) an inhalation anesthetic.

**ali·form** (al′ĭ-form) [*ala* + *form*] shaped like a wing.

**align·ment** (ə-līn′mənt) [Fr. *aligner* to put in a straight line] in dentistry, bringing natural or artificial teeth into line, so that they form the two regular parabolic curves of the dental arches and reestablish a harmonious relationship with the supporting structures and with the opposite dentition. Spelled also *alinement*.

**al·i·ment** (al′ə-ment) [L. *alimentum*] food or nutritive material.

**al·i·men·ta·ry** (al″ə-men′tər-e) pertaining to food or nutritive material, or to the organs of digestion.

**al·i·men·ta·tion** (al″ə-men-ta′shən) the act of giving or receiving nutriment.
**artificial a.,** the giving of food or nourishment to persons who cannot take it in the usual way.
**forced a.,** 1. the feeding of a person against his will. 2. the giving of more food to a person than his appetite calls for.
**parenteral a.,** administration of nutriment intravenously.
**rectal a.,** the administration of concentrated nourishment by instillation into the rectum.
**total parenteral a.,** the intravenous administration of the total nutrient requirements of the patient with gastrointestinal dysfunction, accomplished via a central venous catheter, usually inserted in the superior vena cava via a subclavian vein. Called also *parenteral hyperalimentation* and *total parenteral nutrition*.

**ali·na·sal** (al″ĭ-na′səl) pertaining to the ala nasi.

**aline·ment** (ə-līn′mənt) alignment.

**al·i·phat·ic** (al″ĭ-fat′ik) [Gr. *aleiphar, aleiphatos* oil] pertaining to any member of one of the major groups of organic compounds, those having a straight or branched chain structure.

**alipo·gen·ic** (a-lip″o-jen′ik) not lipogenic; not forming fat.

**alipo·trop·ic** (a-lip″o-trop′ik) having no influence on the metabolism of fat.

**al·i·quot** (al′ĭ-kwot) [L. "some, several"] the part of a number which will divide it without a remainder; e.g., 2 is an aliquot of 6. By extension, any portion that bears a known quantitative relationship to a whole or to other portions of the same whole, as an aliquot portion of a solution or specimen, e.g., plasma or serum; a sample of a whole taken to determine the quantitative composition of the whole.

**ali·sphe·noid** (al-ĭ-sfe′noid) [*ala* + *sphenoid*] 1. pertaining to the greater wing of the sphenoid. 2. a cartilage of the fetal chondrocranium on either side of the basisphenoid bone; later in development it forms most of the greater wing of the sphenoid bone. See also *postsphenoidal part of sphenoid bone,* under *part*.

**aliz·a·rin** (ə-liz′ə-rin) [Arabic *ala sara* extract] a red crystalline dye, prepared synthetically or obtained from madder; its compounds are used as indicators.
**a. monosulfonate,** a. red; see under *red*.

**a. No. 6,** purpurin (def. 1).
**a. red,** see under *red.*
**a. yellow, a. yellow g,** see under *yellow.*

**al·i·zar·i·no·pur·pu·rin** (al″ĭ-zar″ĭ-no-pur′pu-rin) purpurin (def. 1).

**al·ka·le·mia** (al″kə-le′me-ə) [*alkali* + *-emia*] increased pH or decreased hydrogen ion concentration of the blood.

**al·ka·les·cence** (al″kə-les′əns) slight or incipient alkalinity.

**al·ka·les·cent** (al″kə-les′ənt) having a tendency to alkalinity.

**al·ka·li** (al′kə-li) [Arabic *al-qalīy* potash] any of a class of compounds which form soluble soaps with fatty acids, turn red litmus blue, have pH values greater than 7.0, and form soluble carbonates. Essentially the hydroxides of cesium, lithium, potassium, rubidium, and sodium, they include also the carbonates of these metals and of ammonia.

**Al·ka·lig·e·nes** (al″kə-lij′ə-nēz) *Alcaligenes.*

**al·ka·lig·e·nous** (al″kə-lij′ə-nəs) yielding an alkali.

**al·ka·lim·e·ter** (al″kə-lim′ə-tər) [*alkali* + *-meter*] an instrument for measuring the alkali contained in any mixture.

**al·ka·lim·e·try** (al″kə-lim′ə-tre) the measurement of the alkalis present in any substance.

**al·ka·line** (al′kə-līn, -lin) 1. having the reactions of an alkali. 2. having a pH greater than 7.0.

**al·ka·line phos·pha·tase** (al′kə-līn, -lin fos′fə-tās) [EC 3.1.3.1] [MeSH: Alkaline Phosphatase] an enzyme of the hydrolase class that catalyzes the cleavage of orthophosphate from orthophosphoric monoesters under alkaline conditions. Differing forms of the enzyme occur in normal and malignant tissues. The activity in serum is useful in the clinical diagnosis of many illnesses. Deficient bone enzyme activity, an autosomal recessive trait, causes hypophosphatasia. Called also *phosphomonoesterase.* Abbreviated ALP.
**leukocyte a. p. (LAP),** the isozyme of alkaline phosphatase occurring in the leukocytes, specifically in the neutrophils; LAP activity is used in the differential diagnosis of neutrophilia, being lowered in chronic myelogenous leukemia but elevated in a variety of other disorders.

**al·ka·lin·i·ty** (al″kə-lin′ĭ-te) the fact, quality, or degree of being alkaline.

**al·ka·lin·i·za·tion** (al″kə-lin″ĭ-za′shən) alkalization.

**al·ka·lin·ize** (al′kə-lin-iz″) alkalize.

**al·ka·lin·uria** (al″kə-lĭ-nu′re-ə) [*alkaline* + *-uria*] an alkaline condition of the urine.

**al·ka·li·za·tion** (al″kə-li-za′shən) the act of making alkaline.

**al·ka·lize** (al′kə-līz) to make alkaline; called also *alkalinize.*

**al·ka·liz·er** (al′kə-li″zər) an agent that neutralizes acids or causes alkalinization.

**al·ka·lo·gen·ic** (al″kə-lo-jen′ik) producing alkalinity.

**al·ka·loid** (al′kə-loid″) [*alkali* + *-oid*] one of a large group of nitrogenous basic substances found in plants. They are usually very bitter and many are pharmacologically active. Examples are atropine, caffeine, coniine, morphine, nicotine, quinine, strychnine. The term is also applied to synthetic substances *(artificial a's)* which have structures similar to plant alkaloids, such as procaine.
**ergot a's,** a group of chemically related alkaloids either derived from ergot or synthesized; some cause ergotism while others are medicinal. Included are ergocornine, ergocristine, ergocryptine, ergonovine, ergotamine, and lysergic acid diethylamide.
**vinca a's,** alkaloids produced by the Madagascar periwinkle, *Vinca rosea;* they are cytotoxic and cell cycle–specific for the M phase of cell division, acting by binding to tabulin, leading to arrest of cells in metaphase. Two, vinblastine and vincristine, are used as antineoplastic agents.

**al·ka·lom·e·try** (al″kə-lom′ə-tre) [*alkaloid* + *-metry*] the dosimetric administration of alkaloids.

**al·ka·lo·sis** (al″kə-lo′sis) [MeSH: Alkalosis] a pathologic condition resulting from accumulation of base, or from loss of acid without comparable loss of base in the body fluids, and characterized by decrease in hydrogen ion concentration (increase in pH). Cf. *acidosis.*
**altitude a.,** increased alkalinity in blood and tissues occurring in mountain sickness.
**compensated a.,** a condition in which compensatory mechanisms have returned the pH toward normal; see *metabolic a., compensated,* and *respiratory a., compensated.*
**hypochloremic a.,** metabolic alkalosis marked by hypochloremia together with hyponatremia and hypokalemia, resulting from the loss of sodium chloride and hydrochloric acid due to prolonged vomiting.
**hypokalemic a.,** a type of metabolic alkalosis associated with a low serum potassium level; retention of alkali or loss of acid occurs in the extracellular (but not intracellular) fluid compartment, although the pH of the intracellular fluid may be below normal. It may be caused by hypertrophy and hypoplasia of the juxtaglomerular cells, as in Bartter's syndrome.
**metabolic a.,** a disturbance in which the acid-base status of the body shifts toward the alkaline side because of retention of base or loss of noncarbonic, or fixed (nonvolatile), acids.
**metabolic a., compensated,** a state of alkalosis in which the pH of the blood has been returned toward normal by respiratory compensation.
**respiratory a.,** a state due to excess loss of carbon dioxide from the body, usually as a result of hyperventilation; hyperventilation may be either psychogenic or physical in nature, with the most common physical problems being disordered regulation in the central nervous system and pulmonary conditions.
**respiratory a., compensated,** a respiratory alkalosis in which the pH of the blood has been returned toward normal through retention of acid or excretion of base by renal mechanisms.

**al·ka·lot·ic** (al″kə-lot′ik) pertaining to or characterized by alkalosis.

**al·kal·uria** (al″kə-lu′re-ə) the presence of an alkali in the urine.

**al·ka·mine** (al′kə-mēn) an alcohol that contains an amine group.

**al·kane** (al′kān) any of a class of saturated hydrocarbons with straight or branched chain structures, with general formula $C_nH_{2n+2}$.

**al·ka·net** (al′kə-net) the reddish dye-containing root of *Alkanna tinctoria* Tausch, Boraginaceae; formerly used as an astringent, but now mainly as a colorant for candies, cosmetics, and wines. It contains alkannin (the dye principle) and tannin.

**al·kan·nin** (al′kə-nin) a red powder, the coloring ingredient of alkanet; used as a colorant and, in the form of alkannin paper as an indicator: alkalis turn the paper blue, acids red.

**al·kap·ton·uria** (al-kap″to-nu′re-ə) [MeSH: Alkaptonuria] an autosomal recessive aminoacidopathy characterized by accumulation of homogentisic acid (HGA), due to a deficiency of homogentisate 1,2-dioxygenase. Manifestations include elevated concentrations of HGA in urine, which darkens on standing or with alkalinization, ochronosis, and arthritis.

**al·kap·ton·uric** (al-kap″to-nu′rik) pertaining to, characterized by, or causing alkaptonuria; by extension, sometimes used as a noun to designate an individual with alkaptonuria.

**al·ka·tri·ene** (al″kə-tri′ēn) an unsaturated aliphatic hydrocarbon containing three double bonds.

**al·ka·ver·vir** (al″kə-vər′vir) a yellow powdery mixture of alkaloids obtained from selective extraction of *Veratrum viride;* it is used orally as a vasodilator in the treatment of hypertension.

**al·kene** (al′kēn) an unsaturated aliphatic hydrocarbon containing one double bond.

**Al·ker·an** (al-ker′ən) trademark for preparations of melphalan.

**al·kyl** (al′kəl) the radical which results when an aliphatic hydrocarbon loses one hydrogen atom.
**a. (C12–15) benzoate** [NF], the esters of a mixture of C12 to C15 alcohols and benzoic acid, used as an oleaginous vehicle and emollient in pharmaceutical preparations.
**a. sulfonate,** a member of a class of alkylating agents comprising a series of symmetrical *bis*-substituted straight chain esters of methanesulfonic acid with a bridge of methylene groups that varies in length; compounds having a methylene bridge of intermediate length (4 or 5 methylene groups) have the highest therapeutic index. Written also *alkylsulfonate.*

**al·kyl·amine** (al′kəl-ə-mēn″) an amine containing an alkyl radical.

**al·kyl·ate** (al′kə-lāt) to cause alkylation; see also *alkylating agent,* under *agent.*

**al·kyl·a·tion** (al″kə-la′shən) [MeSH: Alkylation] the substitution of an alkyl group for an active hydrogen atom in an organic compound.

**al·kyne** (al′kīn) an unsaturated hydrocarbon containing a triple bond between two carbon atoms; the alkynes are members of the acetylene series.

**ALL** acute lymphoblastic leukemia.

**al·la·ches·the·sia** (al″ə-kes-the′zhə) [Gr. *allachē* elsewhere + *esthesia*] allesthesia.
**optical a.,** visual allesthesia.

**al·lan·ti·a·sis** (al″an-ti′ə-sis) [*allanto-* + *-iasis*] a type of sausage poisoning from sausages containing the toxins of *Clostridium botulinum.* See *botulism.*

**allant(o)-** [Gr. *allas,* gen. *allantos* sausage] a combining form denoting relationship to a sausage or to the allantois.

**al·lan·to·cho·ri·on** (ə-lan″to-ko′re-on) a compound membrane formed by fusion of the allantois and chorion.

**al·lan·to·gen·e·sis** (al″an-to-jen′ə-sis) the formation and development of the allantois.

**al·lan·to·ic** (al″an-to′ik) pertaining to the allantois.

**al·lan·toid** (ə-lan′toid) [*allanto-* + Gr. *-oid*] 1. resembling the allantois. 2. sausage-shaped.

**al·lan·toi·de·an** (al″ən-toi′de-ən) 1. pertaining to the allantois. 2. any animal with an allantois during its embryonic development; in the plural, *amniotes* is the more usual term.

**al·lan·toi·do·an·gi·op·a·gous** (al″ən-toi″do-an″je-op′ə-gəs) joined by the vessels of the umbilical cord; see under *twin*.

**al·lan·toi·do·an·gi·op·a·gus** (al″ən-toi″do-an″je-op′ə-gəs) [*allantoid* + *angio-* + *-pagus*] twin fetuses joined by the vessels of the umbilical cord; allantoidoangiopagous twins. Called also *omphaloangiopagus*.

**al·lan·to·in** (ə-lan′to-in) [MeSH: Allantoin] the diureide of glyoxylic acid, found in allantoic fluid, fetal urine, and many plants, and as a urinary excretion product of purine metabolism in most mammals but not in man or the higher apes. It is produced synthetically by the oxidation of uric acid, and was once used to encourage epithelial formation in wounds and ulcers and in osteomyelitis.

**al·lan·to·in·uria** (ə-lan″to-in-u′re-ə) the presence of allantoin in the urine.

**al·lan·to·is** (ə-lan′to-is) [*allanto-* + *eidos* form] [MeSH: Allantois] an initially tubular ventral diverticulum of the hindgut of embryos of reptiles, birds, and mammals. In reptiles and birds, it expands to a large sac for storing urine and, after fusing with the chorion which lines the shell, provides for gas exchange. The allantois is prominent in some mammals (carnivores, ungulates); in others, including humans, it is vestigial except that its blood vessels give rise to those of the umbilical cord. See illustration under *amnion*.

**Al·leg·ra** (ə-leg′rə) trademark for a preparation of fexofenadine hydrochloride.

**al·lel** (ə-lel′) allele.

**al·lele** (ə-lēl′) [Gr. *allēlōn* of one another, from *allos* other] [MeSH: Alleles] any alternative form of a gene that can occupy a particular chromosomal locus. In humans and other diploid organisms there are two alleles, one on each chromosome of a homologous pair. See also *Mendel's laws*, under *law* and *multiple a's*.
**multiple a's**, a series of more than two alleles.
**silent a.**, see under *gene*.

**al·le·lic** (ə-le′lik) pertaining to alleles; produced by alternative genes.

**al·le·lism** (ə-le′liz-əm) the existence of alleles, or their relationship to one another.

**allel(o)-** [Gr. *allēlōn* of one another, from *allos* other] a combining form denoting relationship to another.

**al·le·lo·chem·ics** (ə-le″lo-kem′iks) chemical interactions between species, involving release of active chemical substances, such as scents, pheromones, and toxins.

**al·le·lo·tax·is** (ə-le″lo-tak′sis) [*allelo-* + Gr. *-taxis*] the development of an organ from several embryonic structures.

**al·le·lo·taxy** (ə-le′lo-tak″se) allelotaxis.

**Al·le·mann's syndrome** (ah′lə-mahnz) [Richard *Allemann*, Swiss physician, 1893–1958] see under *syndrome*.

**Al·len's paradoxic law** (al′ənz) [Frederick Madison *Allen*, American physician, 1879–1964] see under *law*.

**Al·len's test** (al′ənz) [Edgar Van Nuys *Allen*, American physician, 1900–1961] see under *test*.

**Al·len-Doi·sy test, unit** (al′ən-doi′se) [Edgar V. *Allen*, American anatomist, 1892–1943; Edward Adelbert *Doisy*, American biochemist, 1893–1986] see under *test* and *unit*.

**al·ler·gen** (al′ər-jen) [*allergy* + *-gen*] an antigenic substance capable of producing immediate-type hypersensitivity (allergy).
**pollen a.**, any protein antigen of weed, tree, or grass pollens capable of causing allergic asthma or rhinitis; pollen allergen extracts are used in skin testing for pollen sensitivity and in immunotherapy (desensitization) for pollen allergy.

**al·ler·gen·ic** (al″ər-jen′ik) acting as an allergen; inducing allergy.

**al·ler·gic** (ə-lər′jik) pertaining to, caused by, affected with, or of the nature of allergy.

**al·ler·gist** (al′ər-jist) a physician who specializes in the diagnosis and treatment of allergic conditions.

**al·ler·gi·za·tion** (al″ər-jĭ-za′shən) active sensitization or the introduction of allergens into the body.

**al·ler·gize** (al′ər-jīz) to subject to sensitization; to make allergic.

**al·ler·goid** (al′ər-goid) an allergen rendered less allergenic but not less antigenic (formation of IgE but not of IgG blocking antibody is decreased) by formalin or glutaraldehyde treatment.

**al·ler·go·log·i·cal** (al″ər-go-loj′ĭ-kəl) pertaining to allergology.

**al·ler·gol·o·gist** (al-ər-gol′ə-jist) one who specializes in allergology.

**al·ler·gol·o·gy** (al″ər-gol′ə-je) the branch of medicine devoted to the study of allergy, its etiology, diagnosis, and treatment.

**al·ler·go·sis** (al″ər-go′sis) any allergic disease.

**al·ler·gy** (al′ər-je) [*all-* + *ergon* work] 1. a state of hypersensitivity induced by exposure to a particular antigen (allergen) resulting in harmful immunologic reactions on subsequent exposures; the term is usually used to refer to hypersensitivity to an environmental antigen (atopic allergy or contact dermatitis) or to drug allergy. 2. The medical specialty dealing with diagnosis and treatment of allergic disorders.
**atopic a.**, atopy.
**bacterial a.**, hypersensitivity to a bacterial antigen, e.g., delayed-type hypersensitivity to *Mycobacterium tuberculosis*.
**bronchial a.**, allergy affecting the bronchi; see *allergic asthma*.
**cold a.**, any condition in which signs and symptoms of allergy are produced by exposure to cold, e.g., cold urticaria.
**contact a.**, see under *dermatitis*.
**delayed a.**, see under *hypersensitivity*.
**drug a.**, an allergic reaction occurring as the result of unusual sensitivity to a drug.
**food a.**, **gastrointestinal a.**, allergy produced by ingested antigens, such as food or drugs; strawberries, milk, and eggs are the most common offenders. The organ affected usually is the skin.
**hereditary a.**, atopy.
**immediate a.**, see under *hypersensitivity*.
**latent a.**, allergy which is not manifested by symptoms but which may be detected by tests.
**physical a.**, any condition in which signs and symptoms of allergy are produced by exposure to cold (cold urticaria or angioedema), heat (cholinergic urticaria), or light (photosensitivity).
**pollen a.**, hay fever.
**polyvalent a.**, a simultaneous allergic response to several allergens.
**spontaneous a.**, atopy.

**Al·les·che·ria** (al″es-ke′re-ə) a former genus of fungi. *A. boy′dii* is now called *Pseudallescheria boydii*.

**al·les·che·ri·a·sis** (al″əs-kə-ri′ə-sis) former name for *pseudallescheriasis*.

**al·les·che·ri·o·sis** (al″əs-ke-re-o′sis) former name for *pseudallescheriasis*.

**al·les·the·sia** (al″es-the′zhə) [*all-* + *esthesia*] a dysesthesia in which a sensation, as of pain or touch, is experienced at a point remote from that at which the stimulus is applied or occurs, as in allochiria. Called also *allachesthesia* and *alloesthesia*.
**visual a.**, a condition in which visual images are transposed from one half of the visual field to the other, either vertically or horizontally; called also *optical allachesthesia*.

**al·le·thrin** (al′ə-thrin) [MeSH: Allethrin] a synthetic analogue of the natural insecticides cinerin, jasmolin, and pyrethrin, used as an insecticide.

**al·li·ance** (ə-li′əns) a union formed for the furtherance of interests of the members; an agreement to cooperate for specific purposes.
**National A. for the Mentally Ill**, NAMI; a self-help and national advocacy group composed of persons with mental illnesses and their family members.
**therapeutic a.**, a conscious contractual relationship between therapist and patient in which each agrees to work together to help the patient with his problems.
**working a.**, therapeutic a.

**al·li·cin** (al′ĭ-sin) an oily substance, extracted from garlic, which has antibacterial activity. See also *Allium*.

**al·li·ga·tion** (al″ĭ-ga′shən) the process of finding the cost of a mixture of known quantities of ingredients, each of known value, or of determining the quantities of solutions of various strengths to be used to form a mixture of a particular strength.

**Al·lis' sign** (al′is) [Oscar Huntington *Allis*, American surgeon, 1836–1921] see under *sign*.

**al·lit·er·a·tion** (ə-lit″ər-a′shən) [*ad-* + *litera* letter] a speech disorder in which the patient uses words containing the same consonant sounds.

**Al·li·um** (al′e-əm) [L. "garlic"] [MeSH: Allium] a genus of flowering plants with bulbous stem bases, of the family Liliaceae. *A. ce′pa* is the onion and *A. sati′vum* is the garlic (q.v.).

**all(o)-** [Gr. *allos* other] a combining form denoting a condition differing from the normal or a reversal, or referring to another.

**al·lo·al·bu·min** (al″o-al-bu′min) any genetic variant of albumin.

**al·lo·an·ti·body** (al″o-an′tĭ-bod″e) isoantibody.

**al·lo·an·ti·gen** (al″o-an′tĭ-jən) an antigen present in allelic forms encoded at the same gene locus in different individuals of the same species.

**al·lo·an·ti·se·rum** (al″o-an″tĭ-se′rəm) an antiserum raised in an individual of a species and directed against antigens of genetically nonidentical members of the same species

**al·lo·bar** (al′o-bahr) [*allo-* + Gr. *baros* weight] a form of a chemical element having an atomic weight different from that of the naturally occurring form.

**al·lo·bar·bi·tal** (al″o-bahr′bĭ-təl) an intermediate to long-acting barbiturate occurring as a white, crystalline powder; used orally as a sedative and hypnotic, and orally in combination with acetaminophen or with acetaminophen and codeine as an analgesic.

**al·lo·bi·o·sis** (al″o-bi-o′sis) [*allo-* + *biosis*] the condition of altered reactivity which an organism manifests under changed environmental or physiologic conditions.

**al·lo·cen·tric** (al″o-sen′trik) focused on the thoughts and feelings of others; not egocentric.

**al·lo·chei·ria** (al″o-ki′re-ə) allochiria.

**al·lo·ches·the·sia** (al″o-kes-the′zhə) allesthesia.

**al·lo·chi·ral** (al″o-ki′rəl) pertaining to allochiria.

**al·lo·chi·ria** (al″o-ki′re-ə) [*allo-* + *chir-* + *-ia*] dyschiria in which, if one extremity is stimulated, the sensation is referred to the opposite side; called also *allocheiria.*

**al·lo·chro·ic** (al″o-kro′ik) pertaining to allochroism.

**al·lo·chro·ism** (al″o-kro′iz-əm) [*allo-* + Gr. *chroa* color + *-ism*] change or variation in color, as in certain minerals.

**al·lo·chro·ma·cy** (al″o-kro′mə-se) the formation of other coloring agents from a dye that is unstable in solution.

**al·lo·chro·ma·sia** (al″o-kro-ma′zhə) change in color of the hair or skin.

**al·lo·cor·tex** (al″o-kor′teks) [*allo-* + *cortex*] [TA] the older, original part of the cerebral cortex, comprising the archicortex and the paleocortex. It does not have the six-layered histologic structure of the larger, phylogenetically newer isocortex. Called also *heterotypical cortex.*

**Al·lo·der·ma·nys·sus** (al″o-der″mə-nis′əs) a genus of blood-sucking mites of the family Dermanyssidae. *A. sangui′neus* parasitizes mice and is a vector of *Rickettsia akari,* the causative agent of rickettsialpox.

**al·lo·dyn·ia** (al″o-din′e-ə) [*all-* + *-odynia*] pain resulting from a non-noxious stimulus to normal skin.

**al·lo·erot·ic** (al″o-ĕ-rot′ik) pertaining to or characterized by alloeroticism.

**al·lo·erot·i·cism** (al″o-ə-rot′ĭ-siz-əm) [*allo-* + *eroticism*] 1. sexual feeling directed to another person. 2. the final stage in the development of object relationships, a state of maturity, characterized both by direction of erotic energies to another and also by the ability to form a love relationship with that other. Cf. *autoeroticism, heteroeroticism.*

**al·lo·er·o·tism** (al″o-er′o-tiz-əm) alloeroticism.

**al·lo·es·the·sia** (al″o-es-the′ze-ah) allesthesia.

**al·log·a·my** (al-og′ə-me) [*allo-* + Gr. *gamos* marriage] cross fertilization.

**al·lo·ge·ne·ic** (al″o-jə-ne′ik) 1. having cell types that are antigenically distinct. 2. in transplantation biology, denoting individuals (or tissues) that are of the same species but antigenically distinct, as opposed to *syngeneic* and *xenogeneic.* Called also *homologous.* See also *allograft* and *allogeneic transplantation.*

**al·lo·gen·ic** (al″o-jen′ik) allogeneic.

**al·lo·graft** (al′o-graft) a graft of tissue between individuals of the same species but of disparate genotype; types of donors are cadaveric, living related, and living unrelated (see under *donor*). Called also *allogeneic graft* and *homograft.*

**al·lo·group** (al′o-gro͞op) an allotype linkage group, especially of allotypes for the four IgG subclasses, which are closely linked and inherited as a unit.

**al·lo·im·mune** (al″o-ĭ-mūn′) specifically immune to an allogeneic antigen.

**al·lo·im·mu·ni·za·tion** (al″o-im″u-nĭ-za′shən) an immune response generated in an individual or strain of one species by an alloantigen from a different individual or strain of the same species, such as that occurring after transplantation of an organ.

**al·lo·isom·er·ism** (al″o-i-som′ər-iz-əm) isomerism which does not appear in the formula.

**al·lo·ker·a·to·plas·ty** (al″o-ker′ə-to-plas″te) [*allo-* + *keratoplasty*] repair of the cornea by the use of foreign material.

**al·lo·ki·ne·sis** (al″o-ki-ne′sis) [*allo-* + *-kinesis*] movement that is not performed voluntarily but is produced passively or occurs by reflex.

**al·lo·ki·net·ic** (al″o-ki-net′ik) pertaining to or characterized by allokinesis.

**al·lo·lac·tose** (al″o-lak′tōs) a derivative of lactose formed in cells of *Escherichia coli;* it is the physiological inducer of β-galactosidase in these cells.

**al·lom·er·ism** (ə-lom′ər-iz-əm) [*allo-* + *merism*] change of chemical constitution without change in the crystalline form. Cf. *allomorphism.*

**al·lo·met·ric** (al″o-met′rik) [*allo-* + *metric*] denoting the change of proportion between organs or parts during the growth of an organism; pertaining to allometry.

**al·lo·met·ron** (al″o-met′ron) [*allo-* + Gr. *metron* measure] an evolutionary change in bodily form or proportion as expressed in measurements and indices.

**al·lom·e·try** (al-om′ə-tre) the measurement of changing shape of an organism with increase in size, i.e., the determination of the relationship of two varying dimensions, usually linear.

**Al·lo·mo·nas** (al″o-mo′nəs) [*allo-* + Gr. *monas* unit, from *monos* single] a proposed genus of facultatively anaerobic, gram-negative, rod-shaped bacteria of uncertain affiliation, found in freshwater reservoirs, sewage, and fecal samples. The type species is *A. ente′rica.*

**al·lo·mor·phism** (al″o-mor′fiz-əm) [*allo-* + *morph-* + *-ism*] change of crystalline form without change in chemical constitution. Cf. *allomerism.*

**al·lon·o·mous** (al″on′ə-məs) [*allo-* + *nom-* + *-ous*] regulated by stimuli from the outside.

**al·lo·path** (al′o-path) a term sometimes applied to a practitioner of allopathy.

**al·lo·path·ic** (al″o-path′ik) pertaining to or characteristic of allopathy.

**al·lop·a·thist** (al-op′ə-thist) allopath.

**al·lop·a·thy** (al-op′ə-the) [*allo-* + *-pathy*] a term applied to that system of therapeutics in which diseases are treated by producing a condition incompatible with or antagonistic to the condition to be cured or alleviated. Called also *heteropathy.* Cf. *homeopathy.*

**al·lo·phan·amide** (al″o-fan-am′īd) biuret.

**al·lo·phan·ate** (al″o-fan′āt) a salt of allophanic acid.

**al·lo·phan·ic ac·id** (al″o-fan′ik) urea carbonic acid which does not occur as the free acid but only in salts or compounds; its amide (allophanamide) is biuret.

**al·lo·phe·nic** (al″o-fe′nik) [*allo-* + *phen-* + *-ic*] 1. of or relating to single individuals originating from more than one conceptus. 2. having orderly coexistence of cells with different phenotypes ascribable to known allelic genotypic differences; mosaic.

**al·lo·phore** (al′o-for) erythrophore.

**al·loph·thal·mia** (al″of-thal′me-ə) heterophthalmia.

**al·lo·pla·sia** (al″o-pla′zhə) [*allo-* + *-plasia*] heteroplasia.

**al·lo·plas·mat·ic** (al″o-plaz-mat′ik) [*allo-* + *plasmatic*] formed by differentiation from the cytoplasm.

**al·lo·plast** (al′o-plast) an inert foreign body used for implantation into tissue.

**al·lo·plas·tic** (al″o-plas′tik) [*allo-* + *plastic*] 1. pertaining to or characterized by alloplasty. 2. pertaining to an alloplast.

**al·lo·plas·ty** (al′o-plas-te) [*allo-* + *-plasty*] in psychoanalytic theory, adaptation by alteration of the external environment (alloplastic change). Cf. *autoplasty* (def. 2).

**al·lo·preg·nane** (al″o-preg′nān) former name for 5α-pregnane.

**al·lo·preg·nane·di·ol** (al″o-preg″nān-di′ol) an isomer of pregnanediol occurring in female urine.

**al·lo·psy·chic** (al″o-si′kik) [*allo-* + *psychic*] pertaining to the mind in its relation to the external world.

**al·lo·pur·i·nol** (al″o-pūr′ĭ-nol) [USP] [MeSH: Allopurinol] an isomer of hypoxanthine; used in the treatment of hyperuricemia of gout and that secondary to blood dyscrasias or cancer chemotherapy, and for prophylaxis of recurrent formation of uric acid and calcium oxalate renal calculi. Both allopurinol and its primary metabolite, oxypurinol, are potent inhibitors of xanthine oxidase and reduce serum levels and urinary excretion of uric acid.

**al·lo·re·ac·tive** (al″o-re-ak′tiv) [*allo-* + *reactive*] pertaining to the immune response in reaction to a transplanted allograft.

**al·lo·rhyth·mia** (al″o-rith′me-ə) [*allo-* + *rhythm* + *-ia*] irregularity in the rhythm of the heart beat or pulse that recurs in a regular fashion.

**al·lo·rhyth·mic** (al″o-rith′mik) affected with or of the nature of allorhythmia.

**all or none** (awl or nun) 1. the principle that the heart muscle, under whatever stimulus, will contract to the fullest extent or not at all; stimulation of any single atrial or ventricular muscle fiber causes the action potential to travel over the entire atrial or ventricular mass, or not to travel at all. 2. in muscles other than cardiac muscle, and in nerves, stimulation of an individual fiber causes an action potential to travel over the entire fiber or not to travel at all. Called also *all-or-none law.*

**al·lor·phine** (al′or-fēn) nalorphine.

**al·lose** (al′ōs) an aldohexose epimeric with glucose at carbon 3.

**al·lo·sen·si·ti·za·tion** (al″o-sen″sĭ-ti-za′shən) sensitization to alloantigens (isoantigens), as to Rh antigens during pregnancy (see *Rh isoimmunization*). Called also *isosensitization.*

**al·lo·some** (al′o-sōm) [*allo-* + *-some*] a foreign constituent of the cytoplasm of a cell which has entered from the outside.
**paired a.**, a diplosome.

**al·lo·ster·ic** (al″o-ster′ik) pertaining to allostery.

**al·lo·ster·ism** (al′o-ster″iz-əm) allostery.

**al·lo·ste·ry** (al″o-ster′e) the condition in which the binding of a substrate, product, or other effector to a subunit of a multi-subunit enzyme or other protein at a site (allosteric site) other than the functional site alters its conformation and functional properties, such as by affecting binding of other ligands at the functional site (cooperativity).

**al·lo·therm** (al′o-thərm″) [*allo-* + *therm*] 1. poikilotherm. 2. heterotherm.

**al·lo·tope** (al′o-tōp) a site on the constant or nonvarying portion of an antibody molecule that can be recognized by a combining site of other antibodies. Cf. *idiotope.*

**al·lo·to·pia** (al″o-to′pe-ə) malposition.

**al·lo·top·ic** (al″o-top′ik) dystopic.

**al·lo·tox·in** (al″o-tok′sin) [*allo-* + *toxin*] any substance formed by tissue change within the body which serves as a defense against toxins by neutralizing their poisonous properties.

**al·lo·trans·plan·ta·tion** (al″o-trans-plan-ta′shən) [*allo-* + *transplantation*] allogeneic transplantation.

**allotri(o)-** [Gr. *allotrios* strange] a combining form meaning strange or foreign.

**al·lot·ri·odon·tia** (ə-lot″re-o-don′shə) [*allotrio-* + *odont-* + *-ia*] 1. the transplantation of teeth from one individual into the mouth of another. 2. the existence of teeth in abnormal places, as in dermoid tumors.

**al·lot·rio·geu·stia** (ə-lot″re-o-goo′ste-ə) [*allotrio-* + Gr. *geusis* taste + *-ia*] abnormal sense of taste or appetite.

**al·lo·tri·os·mia** (al″o-tri-os′me-ə) heterosmia.

**al·lo·trope** (al′o-trōp) an allotropic form.

**al·lo·troph·ic** (al″o-trof′ik) rendered non-nutritious by the process of digestion.

**al·lo·trop·ic** (al″o-trop′ik) 1. exhibiting allotropism. 2. preoccupied with the ideas, actions, and feelings of others; said of a personality that is inclined to be preoccupied by others rather than oneself; not self-centered.

**al·lot·ro·pism** (ə-lot′rə-piz″əm) [*allo-* + *tropism*] the existence of a substance in two or more distinct forms (allotropic forms) with distinct physical properties, e.g., graphite and diamond, allotropic forms of carbon.

**al·lot·ro·py** (ə-lot′rə-pe) 1. allotropism. 2. direction of one's interest more toward others than toward oneself.

**al·lo·type** (al′o-tīp) any of several allelic variants of a protein that are characterized by antigenic differences (allotypic markers), especially allelic variants of immunoglobulin heavy and light chains. Cf. *isotype* and *idiotype.*
**Am a's,** [for alpha chain marker] allotypes of human $\alpha 2$ chains (IgA2 heavy chains); two markers designated A2m(1) and A2m(2) have been identified.
**Gm a's,** [for gamma chain marker] allotypes of human $\gamma$ chains (IgG heavy chains); 25 markers designated Gm(1) through Gm(25) have been identified. Each marker occurs only in certain specific IgG subclasses. A specific allotype (allelic $\gamma$ chain) may have more than one marker.
**Inv a's,** Km a's.
**Km a's,** [for kappa chain marker] allotypes of human $\kappa$ light chains; three markers designated Km(1), Km(2), and Km(3) have been identified. Km(2) always occurs with Km(1), thus the possible serotypes are Km(1), Km(1,2) and Km(3). Called also Inv *a's,* Inv(1)–(3).
**Oz a.,** an allotypic antigenic marker on the lambda chain of human immunoglobulins, equivalent to the Km allotypes on kappa light chains.

**al·lo·typ·ic** (al″o-tip′ik) characterized by allotypes.

**al·lo·ty·py** (al″o-ti′pe) [*allo-* + Gr. *typos* type] the genetically controlled property, in proteins, of existing in antigenically distinguishable forms in different members of the same species, i.e., as serum protein isoantigens (not yet distinguishable by chemical or physiochemical means); the condition of being an allotype.

**al·low·ance** (ə-low′əns) something permitted or allowed.
**recommended daily a.,** popularly used synonym for *recommended dietary a.*
**recommended dietary a.,** RDA; the amount of nutrient and calorie intake per day considered necessary for maintenance of good health, calculated for males and females of various ages and recommended by the Food and Nutrition Board of the National Research Council. Popularly called *recommended daily a.*

**al·lox·an** (ə-lok′san) [MeSH: Alloxan] an oxidized product of uric acid that when administered to experimental animals tends to destroy the islet cells of the pancreas, producing alloxan diabetes. Called also *uroxin.*

**al·lox·an·tin** (al″ok-san′tin) a diabetogenic compound derived from alloxan by reduction.

**al·lox·a·zine** (ə-lok′sə-zēn) a heterocyclic compound that is isomeric with isoalloxazine, which is the parent structure of riboflavin.

**al·loy** (al′oi) [Fr. *aloyer* to mix metals] a mixture of two or more metals or of one or more metals with certain metalloids that are mutually soluble in the molten condition; distinguished as binary, ternary, quaternary, etc., depending on the number of metals in the mixture. An alloy may also be classified on the basis of its behavior when solidified.
**amalgam a.,** an alloy, composed chiefly of silver, tin, and copper, that is mixed with mercury to form dental amalgam; it is prepared by melting its components and casting it in an ingot that is afterward cut into small particles (filings), or it may be produced in the form of spheres.
**solid solution a.,** a type of alloy, commonly used in dentistry, whose molecules are in a solid solution.

**al·loy·age** (ə-loi′əj) the combining of metals into alloys.

**al·lyl** (al′əl) [*allium* + *-yl*] a univalent organic group, $—CH_2=CHCH_2$.
**a. chloride,** a compound derived by the chlorination of propylene, used in the preparation of other allyl compounds, of thermosetting resins, and of pharmaceuticals and insecticides; it is toxic by ingestion, inhalation, and skin absorption and affects the lungs, kidneys, and liver.
**a. isothiocyanate** [USP], a volatile oil derived from sinigrin, which is found in the seeds of black mustard and horseradish; used as a counterirritant in ointments and plasters, in the preparation of flavors, and in the manufacture of war gas. It can cause fatal gastroenteritis in animals consuming the plants.

**al·lyl·am·ine** (al″əl-am′in) [MeSH: Allylamine] a caustic liquid with an ammoniacal odor, used in the manufacture of pharmaceuticals.

**al·lyl·gua·ia·col** (ă″ləl-gwi′ə-kol) eugenol.

**al·ly·sine** (ă-li′sēn) a product of the oxidative deamination of lysine, formed by the action of lysyl oxidase. It is an intermediate in the formation of cross-linkages in collagens.

**al·ma·drate sul·fate** (al′mə-drāt) an antacid.

**Al·mei·da's disease** (ahl-ma′dəz) [Floriano Paulo de *Almeida,* Brazilian physician born 1898] paracoccidioidomycosis.

**al·mond** (ah′mənd) [Fr. *amande,* from L. *amygdala* almond] 1. *Prunus amygdalus.* 2. the fruit or seed of *Prunus amygdalus,* source of almond oil (see under *oil*). Called also *amygdala.*
**bitter a.,** 1. *Prunus amygdalus,* var. *amara.* 2. the fruit or seed of *P. amygdalus,* var. *amara.* The seeds are toxic to humans and animals since they contain amygdalin; they also are the source of bitter almond oil (see under *oil*).

**al·mo·ner** (al′mə-nər) a person who dispenses alms.
**hospital a.,** *Brit.,* a person trained in dispensing the social service funds of a hospital, and in administering social service work.

**alo·chia** (ə-lo′ke-ə) [*a-*[1] + *lochia*] absence of the lochia.

**Alo·cin·ma** (a″lo-sin′mə) a genus of fresh water snails of the family Helicidae. *A. longicor′nis* is a species found in China that can serve as an intermediate host of the liver fluke *Clonorchis sinensis.*

**Al·oe** (al′ə-we) [L. *alöe,* from Gr. *aloē*] [MeSH: Aloe] a large genus of succulent plants of the family Liliaceae, found in southern Africa and elsewhere. Several species, such as *A. barbaden'sis* (called also *A. ve'ra*), *A. fe'rox,* and *A. per'ryi,* have juice that contains the purgative barbaloin. See also *aloe.*

**al·oe** (al'o) [MeSH: Aloe] 1. any plant of the genus *Aloe.* 2. [USP] the dried juice of the leaves of various plants of the genus *Aloe,* which has purgative properties and is used as an ingredient of *compound benzoin tincture.*

**al·oe-em·o·din** (al'o-em'o-din) a compound having cathartic principles, occurring in the free state and as a glycoside in rhubarb, senna leaves, and in various species of *Aloe.*

**alo·et·ic** (al″o-et'ik) [L. *aloeticus*] pertaining to or containing aloe.

**al·o·in** (al'o-in) a mixture of active principles, chiefly barbaloin, extracted from aloes; used as a purgative to relieve temporary constipation and/or atonic chronic constipation.

**Al·o·mide** (al'o-mīd″) trademark for a preparation of lodoxamide tromethamine.

**al·o·pe·cia** (al″o-pe'she-ə) [Gr. *alōpekia* a disease in which the hair falls out] [MeSH: Alopecia] lack or loss of the hair from skin areas where it normally is present. Called also *baldness* and *calvities.*
**androgenetic a., a. androgene'tica,** a progressive, diffuse, symmetric loss of scalp hair. In men it begins in the twenties or early thirties with hair loss from the vertex and the frontoparietal regions, ultimately leaving only a sparse peripheral rim of scalp hair *(male pattern a.* or *male pattern baldness).* In females it begins later, with less severe hair loss in the front area of the scalp. In affected areas, the follicles produce finer and lighter terminal hairs until terminal hair production ceases, with lengthening of the anagen phase and shortening of the telogen phase of hair growth. The etiology is unknown but is believed to be a combination of genetic factors and increased response of hair follicles to androgens.
**a. area'ta,** a microscopically inflammatory, usually reversible, patchy loss of hair, occurring in sharply defined areas and usually involving the beard or scalp. See also *ophiasis.* Called also *a. circumscripta* and *pelade.*
**cicatricial a., a. cicatrisa'ta,** an irreversible loss of hair associated with scarring, usually occurring on the scalp. See also *pseudopelade.*
**a. circumscrip'ta,** a. areata.
**congenital a., a. congenita'lis,** congenital absence of the scalp hair, which may occur alone or be part of a more widespread disorder.
**drug a., drug-induced a.,** transient hair loss caused by administration of certain drugs, such as heparin, antimitotics (e.g., cyclophosphamide, methotrexate, and colchicine), and thallium (formerly used in the treatment of tinea capitis).
**male pattern a.,** see *androgenetic a.*
**moth-eaten a.,** syphilitic alopecia involving the scalp and beard and occurring in small, irregular scattered patches, resulting in a moth-eaten appearance.
**a. mucino'sa,** follicular mucinosis.
**postpartum a.,** telogen effluvium occurring shortly after parturition.
**premature a.,** androgenetic alopecia occurring in young men in their early twenties or before.
**pressure a.,** traumatic alopecia due to persistent pressure on the scalp, as may be seen in babies lying on their backs and in adults after prolonged surgical procedures or in ill persons after prolonged bed rest.
**psychogenic a.,** telogen effluvium due to severe and acute emotional stress, which is believed to be of the alopecia areata type. Called also *stress a.*
**radiation a., radiation-induced a.,** transient hair loss following exposure to ionizing radiation.
**a. seborrhe'ica,** alopecia associated with excessive oiliness of the scalp, dandruff, and other signs of seborrheic dermatitis.
**stress a.,** psychogenic a.

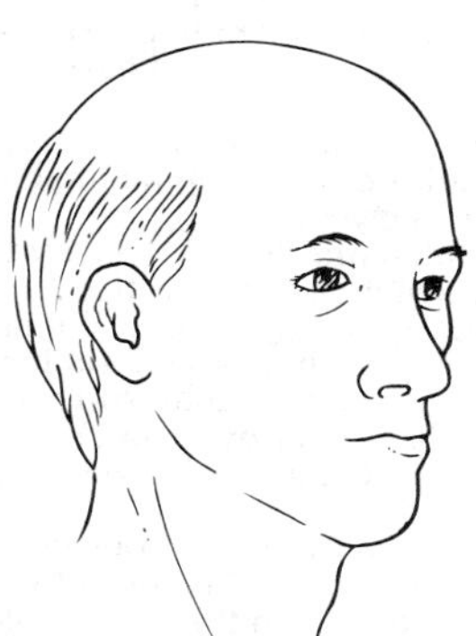

Androgenetic alopecia.

**syphilitic a., a. syphili'tica,** alopecia involving the eyebrows, beard, and scalp in secondary syphilis. See also *moth-eaten a.*
**a. tota'lis,** complete loss of hair from the entire scalp, resulting from progression of alopecia areata.
**traction a.,** traumatic alopecia due to continuous or prolonged traction on the hair, as applied in certain styles of hair dressing or in the habit of twisting the hair.
**traumatic a.,** telogen effluvium due to injury to the hair follicle, as by rubbing, traction, or chemical agent, and limited to the areas thus traumatized.
**traumatic marginal a.,** traction alopecia occurring along the scalp margin.
**a. universa'lis,** loss of hair over the entire body, resulting from progression of alopecia areata.
**x-ray a.,** loss of hair after exposure to x-rays, the extent and permanence of which are dependent on the field and dosage.

**al·o·pe·cic** (al″o-pe'sik) pertaining to or characterized by alopecia.

**al·ox·i·prin** (al-ok'sĭ-prin) a polymeric condensation product of aluminum hydroxide and aspirin, used as an analgesic.

**ALP** alkaline phosphatase.

**Alpers' disease** (al'pərz) [Bernard Jacob *Alpers,* American neurologist, born 1900] see *poliodystrophia cerebri,* under *poliodystrophia.*

**al·pha** (al'fə) [A, $\alpha$] the first letter of the Greek alphabet. See also *$\alpha$-.*

**al·pha$_2$-an·ti·plas·min** (al″fə-an″tĭ-plaz'min) see under *antiplasmin.*

**al·pha$_1$-an·ti·tryp·sin** (al″fə-an″tĭ-trip'sin) a plasma protein (an $\alpha_1$-globulin, $M_r$ 53,000) produced primarily in the liver; it is an acute phase reactant and inhibits the activity of elastase, cathepsin G, trypsin and other proteolytic enzymes. Deficiency of this protein is associated with development of emphysema. Also written *$\alpha_1$-antitrypsin.* Called also *alpha$_1$-proteinase inhibitor.*

**Al·pha Chy·mar** (al'fə ki'mər) trademark for a preparation of chymotrypsin.

**Al·pha·drol** (al'fə-drol) trademark for a preparation of fluprednisolone.

**al·pha fe·to·pro·tein** (al″fə-fe″to-pro'tēn) [MeSH: alpha-Fetoproteins] a plasma protein produced by the fetal liver, yolk sac, and gastrointestinal tract; serum levels decline markedly by the age of one year but are again elevated in many hepatocellular carcinomas and teratocarcinomas and embryonal cell carcinomas; elevated levels may also be seen in benign liver disease, such as cirrhosis and viral hepatitis. Used in monitoring the response of hepatomas and germ cell neoplasms to treatment and in antenatal diagnosis of neural tube defects (indicated by elevated amniotic fluid alpha-fetoprotein levels).

**al·pha glob·u·lin** (al″fə-glob'u-lin) [MeSH: Alpha-Globulins] see under *globulin.*

**al·pha-1,4-glu·co·si·dase de·fi·cien·cy** (al'fə-gloo-kōs'ĭ-dās) glycogen storage disease, type II.

**Al·pha·her·pes·vi·ri·nae** (al″fə-hər″pēz-vir-i'ne) [MeSH: Alphaherpesvirinae] the herpes simplex–like viruses: a subfamily of the Herpesviridae, containing the genera *Simplexvirus* and *Varicellovirus.*

**al·pha·lo·be·line** (al″fə-lōb'ə-len) see *lobeline.*

**al·pha·lyt·ic** (al″fə-lit'ik) blocking the $\alpha$-adrenergic receptors of the sympathetic nervous system; also, an agent that so acts.

**al·pha$_2$-mac·ro·glob·u·lin** (al″fə-mak'ro-glob″u-lin) $\alpha_2$-macroglobulin.

**al·pha·mi·met·ic** (al″fə-mi-met'ik) stimulating or mimicking the stimulation of the $\alpha$-adrenergic receptors of the sympathetic nervous system; also, an agent that so acts.

**al·pha·to·coph·er·ol** (al″fə-to-kof'ər-ol) vitamin E.

**Al·pha·trex** (al″fə-treks′) trademark for preparations of betamethasone maleate.

**Al·pha·vi·rus** (al'fə-vi″rəs) [*alpha* the first letter of the Greek alphabet + *virus*] [MeSH: Alphavirus] a genus of viruses of the family Togaviridae that cause encephalitis or febrile illness with rash or arthralgia, including eastern, western, and Venezuelan equine encephalomyelitis viruses, chikungunya virus, Everglades virus, igbo-ora virus, Mayaro virus, o'nyong-nyong virus, Ross River virus, Semliki Forest virus, and Sindbis virus. Formerly called *group A arboviruses.*

**al·pha·vi·rus** (al'fə-vi″rəs) [MeSH: Alphavirus] any virus belonging to the genus *Alphavirus.*

**Al·port's syndrome** (al'ports) [Arthur Cecil *Alport,* South African-born English physician, 1880–1959] see under *syndrome.*

**al·pra·zo·lam** (al-pra′zo-lam) [USP] [MeSH: Alprazolam] a benzodiazepine used as an anxiolytic in the treatment of anxiety disorders and panic disorders and for short-term relief of anxiety symptoms, administered orally.

**al·pren·o·lol hy·dro·chlo·ride** (al-pren′o-lol) a beta-adrenergic blocking agent, having the same actions as propranolol (q.v.).

**al·pros·ta·dil** (al-pros′tə-dil) [USP] [MeSH: Alprostadil] name for prostaglandin $E_1$ when used pharmaceutically as a vasodilator and platelet aggregation inhibitor; used for the temporary maintenance of patent ductus arteriosus until corrective or palliative surgery can be performed in neonates with congenital heart defects; administered intravenously or intra-arterially. It is also administered by intracavernosal injection to facilitate erection in men with impotence and by intra-arterial infusion to enhance visualization in pharmacoangiography.

**ALS** amyotrophic lateral sclerosis; antilymphocyte serum.

**al·ser·ox·y·lon** (al″sər-ok′sə-lon) a purified extract of *Rauwolfia serpentina,* containing reserpine and other amorphous alkaloids; used orally as an antihypertensive and sedative.

**al·stroe·me·ria** (al-strə-me′re-ə) [Baron Klos von *Alstroemer,* Swedish botanist, 19th century] A genus of flowering South American plants of the family Amaryllidaceae. Several species are popular ornamental plants and are sources of allergic contact dermatitis.

**Al·ström's syndrome** (ahl′stremz) [Carl Henry *Alström,* Swedish geneticist, born 1907] see under *syndrome.*

**Al·tace** (al′tās) trademark for a preparation of ramipril.

**Alt. dieb.** abbreviation for L. *alter′nis die′bus,* every other day.

**al·te·plase** (al′tə-plās) [USP] [MeSH: Alteplase] a tissue plasminogen activator (see *t-plasminogen activator*) produced by recombinant DNA technology; used in fibrinolytic therapy for acute myocardial infarction and as a thrombolytic in the treatment of acute ischemic stroke.

**al·ter** (awl′tər) to castrate, as housepets or livestock.

**al·ter·ego·ism** (awl″tər-e′go-iz-əm) interest and sympathy for persons who are in the same situation as or are otherwise similar to one's self.

**al·ter·nans** (awl-ter′nanz) [L., pres. part. of *alternase* to do by turns] 1. alternating; see *pulsus alternans,* under *pulse.* 2. alternation.
**cardiac a.,** alternation of the heart.
**electrical a.,** alternating variations in the amplitude of specific electrocardiographic waves over successive cardiac cycles.
**mechanical a.,** alternation of the heart, used particularly in contrast with electrical alternans.
**pul′sus a.,** see under *pulsus.*
**total a.,** pulsus alternans in which alternate beats are so weak that they are not detected, causing apparent halving of the pulse rate.

**Al·ter·na·ria** (awl″tər-nar′e-ə) [MeSH: Alternaria] a genus of Fungi Imperfecti of the form-class Hyphomycetes, form-family Dematiaceae; it has dark-colored conidia and somewhat resembles *Trichophyton.* It causes several diseases of plants and is a common allergen in human bronchial asthma; it occasionally causes alternariosis of the skin or lung.

**al·ter·nar·ia·tox·i·co·sis** (awl″tər-nar″e-ə-tok-sĭ-ko′sis) a form of mycotoxicosis in animals caused by members of the genus *Alternaria.*

**al·ter·nar·i·o·sis** (awl″tər-nar-e-o′sis) infection by species of *Alternaria,* usually seen as a cutaneous or lung infection in weak or immunocompromised patients.

**al·ter·nat·ing** (awl′tər-nāt″ing) occurring in regular succession; alternately direct and reversed.

**al·ter·na·tion** (awl″tər-na′shən) [L. *alternare* to do by turns] interrupted occurrence, being interspersed with different or opposite events.
**a. of the heart,** alternating variation in the intensity of the heartbeat or pulse over successive cardiac cycles of regular rhythm. Called also *mechanical alternans.* Cf. *electrical alternans.*
**a. of generations,** metagenesis.

**al·thi·a·zide** (al-thi′ə-zīd) a thiazide diuretic used to treat hypertension.

**Alt. hor.** abbreviation for L. *alter′nis ho′ris,* every other hour.

**Alt·mann's fluid, theory** (ahlt′mahnz) [Richard *Altmann,* German histologist, 1852–1900] see under *fluid* and *theory.*

**Alt·mann-Gersh method** (ahlt′mahn-gersh) [R. *Altmann;* Isidore *Gersh,* American anatomist, born 1907] see under *method.*

**Al·tra·cin** (al-tra′sin) trademark for a preparation of bacitracin zinc.

**al·tret·amine** (al-tret′ə-mēn) [USP] [MeSH: Altretamine] an antineoplastic agent used to treat ovarian carcinoma and other solid tumors. Although structurally related to the alkylating agent triethylenemelamine, it does not act as an alkylating agent; its activity is related to the degree to which it is demethylated by the hepatic microsomal enzyme system, but the exact mechanism is unknown. Formerly called *hexamethylmelamine.*

**al·trose** (al′trōs) an aldohexose isomeric with glucose at carbons 2 and 3.

**al·tru·ism** (al′troo-iz-əm) [MeSH: Altruism] unselfish concern for the needs or interests of others, providing gratification vicariously or from their responses.

**Alu-Cap** (al′u-kap) trademark for a preparation of dried aluminum hydroxide gel.

**Alu·drine** (ə-loo′drin) trademark for a preparation of isoproterenol.

**Alu·drox** (al-u′droks) trademark for a preparation of alumina and magnesia.

**al·um** (al′əm) [L. *alumen*] 1. an odorless, colorless, crystalline substance, with local astringent and styptic properties and sweetish taste, prepared from bauxite (hydrated aluminum oxide) and sulfuric acid, with the addition of ammonium *(ammonium a.)* or potassium *(potassium a.).* It is also used as an adjuvant in adsorbed vaccines and toxoids. 2. a generic term for any member of a class of double sulfates formed on the type of the foregoing compounds. 3. any member of a class of double aluminum-containing compounds.
**ammonium a.** [USP], alum prepared with the addition of ammonium; used topically as an astringent.
**burnt a.,** exsiccated a.
**chrome a.,** chromium and potassium sulfate; a violet pigment.
**dried a.,** exsiccated a.
**exsiccated a.,** ammonium or potassium alum heated to drive off the water of crystallization; used as an astringent. Called also *burnt* or *dried a.*
**iron a.,** iron and potassium sulfate.
**potassium a.** [USP], alum prepared with the addition of potassium; used topically as an astringent.

**alu·men** (ə-loo′men) gen. *alu′minis* [L.] alum.
**a. exsicca′tum,** exsiccated alum.

**alu·mi·na** (ə-loo′mĭ-nə) aluminum oxide.

**alu·mi·nat·ed** (ə-loo′mĭ-nāt″əd) charged with alum.

**al·u·min·i·um** (al″u-min′e-əm) [L.] aluminum.

**Alu·mi·noid** (ə-loo′mĭ-noid) trademark for preparations of aluminum hydroxide gel for use in gastric ulcers and hyperacidity.

**alu·mi·no·sis** (ə-loo′mĭ-no′sis) a form of pneumoconiosis due to the presence of aluminum-bearing dust in the lungs; cf. *bauxite pneumoconiosis.*

**alu·mi·num** (ə-loo′mĭ-nəm) [MeSH: Aluminum] an extremely light, whitish, lustrous, metallic element, obtainable from bauxite or clay: specific gravity, 2.699; atomic weight, 26.982; atomic number, 13; symbol, Al. It is very malleable and ductile, and has many industrial uses. In dentistry it is used for the manufacture of instruments for the fabrication of dentures, obturators, and other prosthetic devices, and as a base for artificial dentures. The aluminum of the pharmacopeia is a fine, free-flowing, silvery powder, free from gritty or discolored particles. Aluminum compounds are used chiefly for their antacid and astringent properties. Excessive amounts in the body have a variety of toxic effects; see *aluminum poisoning,* under *poisoning.*
**a. acetate,** a salt, $C_6H_9AlO_6$, prepared by the reaction of aluminum hydroxide and acetic acid; used in solution as an astringent.
**a. aminoacetate,** dihydroxyaluminum aminoacetate.
**a. ammonium sulfate,** ammonium alum.
**a. carbonate, basic,** an aluminum hydroxide–aluminum carbonate complex, available only in the form of *basic aluminum carbonate gel* (see under *gel*).
**a. chlorhydrex** [USP], a topical astringent, reportedly consisting of a coordination complex of basic aluminum chloride and propylene glycol or polyethylene glycol.
**a. chloride** [USP], aluminum chloride hexahydrate, $AlCl_3 \cdot 6H_2O$, used topically as an astringent and anhidrotic.
**a. chlorohydrate** [USP], the hydrate of aluminum chloride hydroxide, $Al_2Cl(OH)_5$, having astringent and anhidrotic properties; used as an antiperspirant and as an anhidrotic in the treatment of hyperhidrosis. Called also *a. hydroxychloride.*
**a. glycinate,** dihydroxyaluminum aminoacetate.
**a. hydrate,** a. hydroxide.
**a. hydroxide,** a white, bulky, amorphous powder, $Al(OH)_3$, used as an antacid, and as a phosphate binder in the treatment of urolithiasis and hyperphosphatemia in the form of *aluminum hydroxide gel* or *dried aluminum hydroxide gel* (see under *gel*); it is also used as an adjuvant in adsorbed vaccines and toxoids.
**a. hydroxide, colloidal,** aluminum hydroxide gel.

**a. hydroxychloride,** a. chlorohydrate.
**a. monostearate** [NF], a combination of aluminum with variable proportions of stearic acid and palmitic acid; used in preparation of a suspension of penicillin G procaine.
**a. nicotinate,** a complex consisting of aluminum nicotinate, aluminum hydroxide, and nicotinic acid; used chiefly as an anticholesterolemic, antilipoproteinemic, and peripheral vasodilator, administered orally.
**a. oxide,** a compound, occurring naturally as corundum and in hydrated form as bauxite, that is the raw material in aluminum production; impure crystalline forms include emery, ruby, and sapphire. Very fine grains are used in the production of abrasives, refractories, ceramics, catalysts, laboratory wares, and fluxes, to strengthen dental ceramics, and in chromatography.
**a. penicillin,** see under *penicillin.*
**a. phosphate,** a white infusible powder, $AlPO_4$, used as an adjuvant in adsorbed toxoids and vaccines, as a component (with calcium sulfate and sodium silicate) in dental cements, and, in the form of aluminum phosphate gel, as an antacid.
**a. potassium sulfate,** potassium alum.
**a. silicate,** $Al_2SiO_5$, the silicate salt of aluminum. It occurs in several different hydrated forms in nature that have pharmaceutical or dental uses; see *attapulgite, bentonite, fuller's earth, kaolin,* and *zeolite.* See also *silicatosis.*
**a. subacetate,** a basic aluminum acetate, used topically in solution as an astringent.
**a. sulfate** [USP], a powerful astringent, $Al_2(SO_4)_3 \cdot xH_2O$, used topically as a local antiperspirant; also used as a pharmaceutical necessity in the preparation of aluminum subacetate topical solution.

**alun·dum** (ə-lun'dəm) electrically fused aluminum oxide used in making laboratory appliances that must withstand intense heat.

**Al·u·pent** (al'u-pent) trademark for preparations of metaproterenol sulfate.

**Al·ur·ate** (al'ūr-āt) trademark for a preparation of aprobarbital.

**Alu-Tab** (al'u-tab) trademark for a preparation of dried aluminum hydroxide gel.

**al·vei** (al've-i) [L.] genitive and plural of *alveus.*

**al·veo·bron·chi·ol·i·tis** (al″ve-o-brong″ke-o-li'tis) inflammation of the bronchioles and alveoli of the lungs.

**al·veo·lal·gia** (al″ve-o-lal'jə) [*alveolo-* + *-algia*] pain occurring in the dental alveolus, sometimes observed after tooth extraction. See also *dry socket,* under *socket.*

**al·ve·o·lar** (al-ve'ə-lər) [L. *alveolaris*] pertaining to an alveolus.

**al·ve·o·late** (al-ve'ə-lāt) marked by honeycomb-like pits; called also *faveolate.*

**al·ve·o·lec·to·my** (al″ve-o-lek'tə-me) [*alveol-* + *-ectomy*] [MeSH: Alveolectomy] subtotal or complete excision of the alveolar process of the maxilla or mandible.

**al·ve·o·li** (al-ve'o-li) genitive and plural of *alveolus.*

**al·ve·o·li·tis** (al″ve-o-li'tis) 1. inflammation of a pulmonary alveolus. 2. inflammation of a dental alveolus; called also *odontobothritis.*
**allergic a.,** hypersensitivity pneumonitis.
**cryptogenic fibrosing a.,** idiopathic pulmonary fibrosis.
**extrinsic allergic a.,** hypersensitivity pneumonitis.
**fibrosing a.,** idiopathic pulmonary fibrosis.
**a. sic'ca doloro'sa,** dry socket.

**alveol(o)-** [L. *alveolus, q.v.*] a combining form denoting relationship to an alveolus, especially a dental alveolus.

**al·ve·o·lo·cap·il·la·ry** (al-ve″ə-lo-kap'ĭ-lar″e) pertaining to the pulmonary alveoli and capillaries.

**al·ve·o·lo·cla·sia** (al-ve″ə-lo-kla'zhə) [*alveolo-* + Gr. *klasis* breaking] destruction of the dental alveolus; see *marginal periodontitis,* under *periodontitis.*

**al·ve·o·lo·den·tal** (al-ve″ə-lo-den'təl) pertaining to a tooth and its alveolus.

**al·ve·o·lo·la·bi·al** (al-ve″ə-lo-la'be-əl) pertaining to the alveolar processes and the lips.

**al·ve·o·lo·lin·gual** (al-ve″ə-lo-ling'gwəl) pertaining to the alveolar processes and the tongue.

**al·ve·o·lo·me·rot·o·my** (al-ve″ə-lo″mə-rot'ə-me) [*alveolo-* + *mero-*[1] + *-tomy*] excision of part of the alveolar process.

**al·ve·o·lo·na·sal** (al-ve″ə-lo-na'səl) pertaining to the alveolar point and the nasion.

**al·ve·o·lo·pal·a·tal** (al-ve″ə-lo-pal'ə-təl) pertaining to the alveolar process and palate.

**al·ve·o·lo·plas·ty** (al-ve'ə-lo-plas″te) [*alveolo-* + *-plasty*] [MeSH: Alveoloplasty] conservative contouring of the alveolar process, in preparation for immediate or future denture construction.
**interradicular a., intraseptal a.,** the surgical removal of the interradicular bone and collapsing of the cortical plates on each other to achieve an acceptable or more desirable contour.

**al·ve·o·lot·o·my** (al″ve-ə-lot'ə-me) [*alveolo-* + *-tomy*] incision into a dental alveolus; see also *alveolectomy.*

**al·ve·o·lus** (al-ve'ə-ləs) gen. and pl. *alve'oli* [L., dim. of *alveus* hollow] [TA] a general term used in anatomical nomenclature to designate a small saclike structure, especially in the jaws or lungs. Cf. *acinus.*
**dental a., a. denta'lis** [TA], one of the cavities or sockets in the alveolar process of the mandible or maxilla, in which the roots of the teeth are held by fibers of the periodontal ligament. Called also *alveolar cavities* and *tooth sockets.* See also *alveoli dentales mandibulae* and *alveoli dentales maxillae.*
**alve'oli denta'les mandi'bulae** [TA], dental alveoli of the mandible: the cavities or sockets in the alveolar process of the mandible in which the roots of the teeth are held by the periodontal ligament.
**alve'oli denta'les maxil'lae** [TA], dental alveoli of the maxilla: the cavities or sockets in the alveolar process of the maxilla in which the roots of the teeth are held by the periodontal ligament.
**pulmonary alveoli, alve'oli pulmo'nis,** alveoli of lung: small polyhedral outpouchings along the walls of the alveolar sacs and alveolar ducts; through these walls gas exchange takes place between alveolar gas and pulmonary capillary blood.
**alveoli pulmo'num,** alveoli pulmonis.

**al·ve·rine citrate** (al'vĕ-rēn) an anticholinergic used as a smooth muscle relaxant in disorders of the gastrointestinal and genitourinary tracts.

**al·ve·us** (al've-əs) gen. and pl. *al'vei* [L.] a trough or a canal.
**a. hippocam'pi** [TA], **a. of hippocampus,** the thin layer of white matter that covers the ventricular surface of the hippocampus.

**Al·vo·dine** (al'vo-din) trademark for preparations of piminodine esylate.

**alym·phia** (a-lim'fe-ə) [*a-*[1] + *lymph-* + *-ia*] deficiency or absence of the lymph.

**alym·pho·cy·to·sis** (a-lim″fo-si-to'sis) lymphocytopenia.

**alym·pho·pla·sia** (a-lim-fo-pla'zhə) failure of development of lymphoid tissue.
**thymic a.,** former name for *severe combined immunodeficiency.*

**Alz·hei·mer's disease (dementia),** etc. (awltz'hi-mərz) [Alois *Alzheimer,* German neurologist, 1864–1915] see *primary degenerative dementia,* under *dementia,* and see under *cell, disease,* and *stain.*

**AM** abbreviation for L. *artium magister,* Master of Arts.

**Am** 1. symbol for *americium.* 2. see under *allotype.*

**am** symbol for *myopic astigmatism, meter angle,* and *ametropia.*

**AMA** Aerospace Medical Association; American Medical Association; Australian Medical Association.

**am·a·cri·nal** (am″ə-kri'nəl) amacrine.

**am·a·crine** (am'ə-krēn) [*a* neg. + *macro-* + *inos*] 1. having no long processes. 2. amacrine cell; see under *cell.*

**Am·a·dori product** (ah″mah-dor'e) [Mario *Amadori,* Italian chemist, born 1886] see under *product.*

**amal·gam** (ə-mal'gəm) [Gr. *malagma* poultice or soft mass] an alloy in which mercury is one of the components.
**dental a.,** an amalgam containing mercury, silver, tin, copper, and sometimes zinc, which is prepared by mixing mercury with amalgam alloy to form a silvery, soft paste for condensation into the prepared cavity where it hardens to form a dental restoration.
**retrograde a.,** see under *filling.*

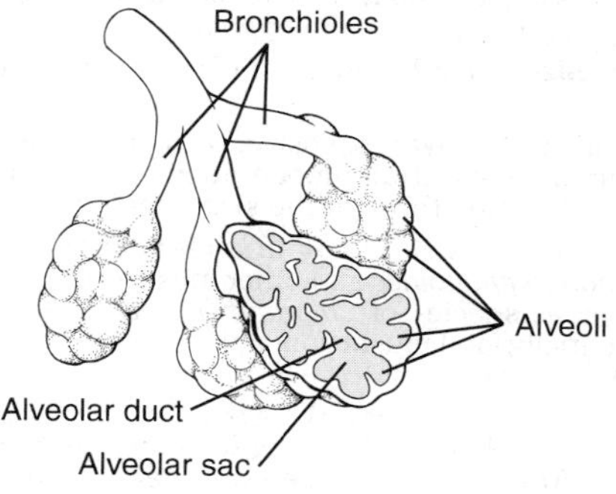


Alveoli pulmonis (pulmonary alveoli), with cross-section showing the alveolar ducts and sacs.

**amal·ga·mate** (ə-mal′gə-māt″) to unite a metal in an alloy with mercury; to form an amalgam. Cf. *triturate*.

**amal·ga·ma·tion** (ə-mal′gə-ma′shən) 1. the formation of an amalgam. 2. trituration (def. 3).

**amal·ga·ma·tor** (ə-mal′gə-māt″ər) triturator.

**Am·a·ni·ta** (am″ə-ni′tə) [Gr. *amanitai* a sort of fungus] [MeSH: Amanita] a genus of mushrooms of the family Amanitaceae, order Agaricales, several of which are poisonous.
**A. musca′ria,** fly agaric, a species that produces muscarine and ibotenic acid; ingestion causes intoxication resembling drunkenness, followed by loss of consciousness.
**A. pantheri′na,** a species that produces muscarine; ingestion causes intoxication followed by loss of consciousness.
**A. phalloi′des,** the destroying angel or death cup, a species that produces a hemolysin and a mixture of amatoxins such as phalloidin, which are protoplasmic poisons; ingestion causes potentially fatal mushroom poisoning (see under *poisoning*).
**A. ver′na,** the death angel, a highly poisonous species that contains peptide toxins similar to those of *A. phalloides.*
**A. viro′sa,** the destroying angel, a highly poisonous species that contains peptide toxins similar to those of *A. phalloides.*

**Am·a·ni·ta·ceae** (am″ə-ni-ta′se-e) a family of mushrooms (order Agaricales), which includes the genus *Amanita.*

**ama·ni·tine** (ə-mă-nĭ′tin) a poisonous glycoside found in the deadly species of *Amanita.*

**aman·i·to·tox·in** (ə-man″ĭ-to-tok′sin) amatoxin.

**aman·ta·dine hy·dro·chlo·ride** (ə-man′tə-dēn) [USP] an antiviral compound used in the prophylaxis and management of type A influenza and, because it augments the release of dopamine, as an antidyskinetic in the treatment of parkinsonism and drug-induced extrapyramidal reactions; administered orally.

**am·a·ranth** (am′ə-ranth) [MeSH: Amaranth] 1. any plant of the genus *Amaranthus.* 2. a red-brown dye, formerly made from amaranth plants but now made synthetically as an azo dye; formerly used as a coloring agent in food, cosmetics, and drugs.

**Am·a·ran·thus** (am″ə-ran′thəs) [L., from Gr. *amarantos* unfading] a genus of herbs of the family Amarantaceae, a source of the dye amaranth. Several species have medical and food uses, and some in the western United States cause hay fever. Some are high in nitrates and oxalates and can cause nitrite or oxalate poisoning in ruminants.
**A. retroflex′us,** pigweed or prince's feather, a species found in pastures that contains oxalates and nitrates and can cause neurologic or kidney disorders in cattle and pigs. See also *oxalate poisoning,* under *poisoning.*

**am·a·rine** (am′ə-rēn) [L. *amarus* bitter] a poisonous crystalline base from oil of bitter almonds, and also prepared artificially.

**am·a·roid** (am′ə-roid) a bitter principle.

**am·a·roi·dal** (am′ə-roi′dəl) somewhat bitter; also resembling a bitter in properties.

**Am·a·ryl** (am′ə-ril) trademark for a preparation of glimepiride.

**am·a·se·sis** (am″ə-se′sis) [*a-*[1] + Gr. *masēsis* chewing] inability to chew food.

**amas·tia** (ə-mas′te-ə) [*a-*[1] + *mast-* + *-ia*] congenital absence of the mammae; sometimes applied to masculine breast characteristics in an adult female. Called also *amazia.*

**amas·ti·gote** (ə-mas′tĭ-gōt) [*a-*[1] + *mastigote*] any of the bodies representing the morphologic (leishmanial) stage in the life cycle of all trypanosomatid protozoa resembling the typical adult form of members of the genus *Leishmania,* in which the oval or round cell has a nucleus, kinetoplast, and basal body but lacks a free-flowing flagellum, the flagellum being either very short or entirely absent. Called also *Leishman-Donovan body.* Cf. *choanomastigote, epimastigote, opisthomastigote, promastigote,* and *trypomastigote.*

**amatho·pho·bia** (ə-math″o-fo′be-ə) [Gr. *amathos* sand + *-phobia*] irrational dread of dust.

**am·a·tol** (am′ə-tol) a war explosive, being a mixture of trinitrotoluene and ammonium nitrate; moderately toxic by ingestion, inhalation, and absorption through the skin; highly irritating.

**am·a·tox·in** (am′ə-tok″sin) any in a class of cyclic hepatotoxins found in *Amanita phalloides* and other mushrooms of the genus *Amanita,* as well as species of *Chlorophyllum* and *Galerina;* ingestion causes potentially fatal mushroom poisoning (see under *poisoning*). Called also *Amanita toxin.*

**am·au·ro·sis** (am″aw-ro′sis) [L. from Gr. *amaurōsis* darkening] blindness, especially that occurring without apparent lesion of the eye, such as from disease of the optic nerve, spine, or brain. Cf. *amblyopia.*
**cat's eye a.,** blindness of one eye, with bright reflection from the pupil, as from the tapetum of a cat; often indicative of retinoblastoma.
**central a.,** amaurosis due to disease of the central nervous system.
**a. centra′lis, cerebral a.,** central a.
**a. conge′nita, a. congenita of Leber, congenital a.,** a type of blindness transmitted as an autosomal recessive trait, occurring at or shortly after birth and associated with an atypical form of diffuse pigmentation and commonly with optic atrophy and attenuation of the retinal vessels.
**diabetic a.,** loss of vision due to diabetes mellitus, such as diabetic retinopathy or diabetic cataracts.
**a. fu′gax,** a transient episode of monocular blindness, or partial blindness, lasting ten minutes or less.
**intoxication a.,** toxic amblyopia.
**Leber's congenital a.,** a. congenita.
**a. partia′lis fu′gax,** sudden transitory partial blindness.
**reflex a.,** that which is caused by the reflex action of a remote irritation.
**saburral a.,** that which occurs in an attack of acute gastritis.
**toxic a.,** toxic amblyopia.
**uremic a.,** loss of vision due to uremia.

**am·au·rot·ic** (am″aw-rot′ik) pertaining to, or of the nature of, amaurosis.

**ama·zia** (ə-ma′zə) [*a-*[1] + *maz-* + *-ia*] amastia.

**amb-** see *ambi-.*

**am·be·no·ni·um chlo·ride** (am″bə-no′ne-əm) [USP] [MeSH: Ambenonium Chloride] a cholinergic used in the treatment of myasthenia gravis to treat the symptoms of muscular weakness and fatigue, administered orally.

**ambi-** [L.] an inseparable prefix meaning on both sides.

**am·bi·dex·ter·i·ty** (am″bĭ-dek-ster′ĭ-te) the ability to perform acts requiring manual skill with either hand, some ordinarily being performed with one and some with the other.

**am·bi·dex·trism** (am″bĭ-dek′striz-əm) ambidexterity.

**am·bi·dex·trous** (am″bĭ-dek′strəs) pertaining to or characterized by ambidexterity.

**Am·bi·en** (am′be-ən) trademark for a preparation of zolpidem tartrate.

**am·bi·ent** (am′be-ənt) [L. *ambire* to surround] surrounding; encompassing; prevailing.

**am·bi·lat·er·al** (am″bĭ-lat′ər-əl) [*ambi-* + *lateral*] pertaining to or affecting both the right and the left side. Cf. *bilateral.*

**am·bi·le·vos·i·ty** (am″bĭ-lə-vos′ĭ-te) the inability to perform acts requiring manual skill with either hand.

**am·bi·le·vous** (am″bĭ-le′vəs) [*ambi-* + *levo-* + *-ous*] pertaining to or characterized by ambilevosity.

**Am·bil·har** (am′bil-hər) trademark for preparations of niridazole.

**am·bi·o·pia** (am″be-o′pe-ə) [L.] diplopia.

**am·bi·sex·u·al** (am″bĭ-sek′shoo-əl) 1. bisexual. 2. hermaphroditic.

**am·bi·sin·is·ter** (am″bĭ-sin′is-tər) [*ambi-* + *sinister*] ambilevous.

**am·bi·si·nis·trous** (am″bĭ-sĭ-nis′trəs) ambilevous.

**am·biv·a·lence** (am-biv′ə-ləns) [*ambi-* + L. *valentia* strength, power] the simultaneous existence of conflicting attitudes, emotions, ideas, or wishes toward the same object.

**am·bi·ver·sion** (am″bĭ-vər′zhən) a balance of introversion and extroversion.

**am·bi·vert** (am′bĭ-vərt) a person who is intermediate between an extrovert and an introvert.

**ambly-** [Gr. *amblys* dull] a combining form denoting dullness.

**am·bly·a·phia** (am-ble-a′fe-ə) [*ambly-* + Gr. *haphē* touch + *-ia*] tactile hypoesthesia.

**am·bly·chro·ma·sia** (am″ble-kro-ma′zhə) the condition of staining faintly or of having little chromatin.

**am·bly·chro·mat·ic** (am″ble-kro-mat′ik) [*ambly-* + *chromatic*] feebly staining.

**am·bly·geu·stia** (am″ble-goo′ste-ə) [*ambly-* + Gr. *geusis* taste + *-ia*] hypogeusia.

**Am·bly·om·ma** (am″ble-om′ə) [*ambly-* + Gr. *omma* eye] a genus of ticks of the family Ixodidae, some of which transmit diseases to humans and other animals.
**A. america′num,** the Lone Star tick of the southern United States, particularly Texas and Louisiana; it is a vector of Rocky Mountain spotted fever and causes tick paralysis in humans and dogs.
**A. cajennen′se,** the Cayenne tick, a species of tropical America that has a particularly vicious bite; it attacks a large variety of mammals and birds and transmits Rocky Mountain spotted fever to humans.

**A. hebrae'um,** the bont tick, an African species that transmits heartwater to sheep, goats, and cattle and boutonneuse fever to humans.
**A. macula'tum,** a species found on the Gulf Coast.
**A. ova'le,** a tropical tick of dogs and tapirs.
**A. tubercula'tum,** a species found in Florida.
**A. variega'tum,** a species which, like *A. hebraeum,* transmits heartwater; it also transmits the virus causing Nairobi sheep disease.

**am·bly·ope** (am'ble-ōp) a person with amblyopia.

**am·bly·o·pia** (am"ble-o'pe-ə) [*ambly-* + *-opia*] [MeSH: Amblyopia] impairment of vision without detectable organic lesion of the eye. Cf. *amaurosis.*
**alcoholic a.,** nutritional amblyopia; toxic amblyopia.
**arsenic a.,** disturbance of vision due to the use of arsenic.
**color a.,** impairment of color vision, caused by toxic or other influences.
**deficiency a.,** nutritional a.
**a. ex anop'sia,** that which results from disuse.
**nocturnal a.,** abnormal dimness of vision at night.
**nutritional a.,** central or cecocentral scotomata due to poor nutrition; seen in alcoholics and patients with severe nutritional deprivation or vitamin $B_{12}$ deficiency, as in pernicious anemia. Complete recovery is possible with good diet and B vitamins; prolonged deficiency results in permanent loss of central vision.
**quinine a.,** amblyopia following large doses of quinine; thought to be due to anemia of the retina.
**reflex a.,** that which results from peripheral irritation.
**strabismic a.,** amblyopia resulting from suppression of vision in one eye to avoid diplopia.
**tobacco a.,** nutritional or toxic amblyopia caused by ingestion of tobacco.
**toxic a.,** amblyopia due to poisoning, as from tobacco or alcohol.
**traumatic a.,** amblyopia due to injury.
**uremic a.,** impairment of vision due to uremia.

**am·blyo·scope** (am'ble-o-skōp") [*amblyopia* + *-scope*] a hand-held reflecting stereoscope that can measure convergence and divergence, measure or train binocular vision, or stimulate vision in an amblyopic eye.
**major a.,** a large, table-mounted amblyoscope that has greater freedom for adjustment than a simple amblyoscope.

**Am·blys·to·ma** (am-blis'to-mə) Ambystoma.

**am·bo** (am'bo) ambon.

**ambo-** [L. *ambo* both] a combining form signifying both, or on both sides.

**am·bo·cep·tor** (am'bo-sep"tər) [*ambo-* + L. *capere* to take] Ehrlich's term for complement-fixing antibody, which he thought had two receptors, one for antigen, one for complement; now used colloquially to denote the anti–sheep red blood cell antibody used in complement fixation tests.

**am·bon** (am'bon) the ring of fibrocartilage forming the edge of the sockets in which the heads of long bones are lodged.

**am·bo·sex·u·al** (am"bo-seks'u-əl) [*ambo-* + *sexual*] 1. bisexual. 2. hermaphroditic.

**Am·bro·sia** (am-bro'zhə) [L. and Gr., from Gr. *ambrotos* immortal] a genus of annual plants of the family Compositae, which produce quantities of windborne pollen and are important causes of hay fever. *A. artemisiaefo'lia* is the common or small ragweed; *A. tri'fida* is the giant ragweed.

**am·bros·te·rol** (am-bros'tə-rol) a phytosterol with a melting point of 147° to 149°C; found in the pollen of ragweed *(Ambrosia).*

**am·bru·ti·cin** (am"broo-ti'sin) an antifungal antibiotic derived from *Polyangium cellulosum* subspecies *fulvum.*

**am·bu·lance** (am'bu-ləns) [Fr.] [MeSH: Ambulances] a vehicle for conveying the sick or injured, and equipped with apparatus for rendering emergency treatment.

**am·bu·lant** (am'bu-lənt) ambulatory.

**am·bu·la·tion** (am"bu-la'shən) walking.

**am·bu·la·to·ry** (am'bu-lə-to"re) [L. *ambulare* to walk] 1. walking or able to walk; not confined to bed. 2. denoting a condition that can be treated without admission to a hospital. 3. pertaining to a procedure perfomed on an outpatient basis, whether in a hospital or a freestanding facility.

**am·bu·phyl·line** (am-bu'fəl-in) a theophylline derivative which has been used as a diuretic and smooth muscle relaxant.

**am·bus·tion** (am-bus'chən) a burn or scald.

**Am·bys·to·ma** (am-bis'to-mə) [MeSH: Ambystoma] a genus of salamanders used for experimental purposes; see *axolotl.* Called also *Amblystoma.*

**am·cin·a·fal** (am-sin'ə-fəl) an anti-inflammatory.

**am·cin·a·fide** (am-sin'ə-fīd) an anti-inflammatory.

**am·cin·o·nide** (am-sin'ə-nīd") [USP] a synthetic corticosteroid used topically for the relief of inflammation and pruritus in corticosteroid-responsive dermatoses.

**am·di·no·cil·lin** (am-de'no-sil"in) [MeSH: Amdinocillin] a semisynthetic penicillin effective against many gram-negative bacteria and used in the treatment of urinary tract infections; administered intravenously or intramuscularly. Called also *mecillinam.*

**ame·ba** (ə-me'bə) pl. *ame'bae* or *amebas* [L., from Gr. *amoibē* change] 1. a type of sarcodine protozoa of the superclass Rhizopoda that move their bodies by cytoplasmic extrusions called *pseudopodia.* Also spelled *amoeba.* 2. any of various other cells or organisms resembling these protozoa.
**a. verruco'sa,** an ameba-like cell having a large knobby nucleus and a deeply staining nucleolus.

**ame·ban** (ə-me'bən) carbarsone.

**ame·bi·a·sis** (am"e-bi'ə-sis) [MeSH: Amebiasis] the state of being infected with amebae, especially with *Entamoeba histolytica.* Although free-living protozoa such as *Acanthamoeba, Hartmannella,* and *Naegleria* are potential human pathogens, the term amebiasis is usually restricted to infection with *E. histolytica.*
**a. cu'tis,** cutaneous manifestation of amebiasis usually manifested as painful ulcers with distinct undermined borders surrounded by erythematous rims, principally seen in patients with active intestinal or hepatic disease, which may occur as a result of direct extension of amebic bowel disease to adjacent skin areas following surgery; direct extension of a hepatic abscess, spontaneously after a surgical procedure; or direct implantation of trophozoites on the skin, with or without preexisting skin lesions.
**hepatic a.,** amebic hepatitis.
**intestinal a.,** amebic dysentery.
**pulmonary a.,** amebic infection in the thoracic space, secondary to intestinal amebiasis and usually associated with amebic liver abscesses; it may affect the pleura, diaphragm, lung, or bronchi.

**ame·bic** (ə-me'bik) pertaining to or of the nature of an ameba.

**ame·bi·ci·dal** (ə-me"bĭ-si'dəl) destructive to amebae.

**ame·bi·cide** (ə-me'bĭ-sīd) [*amebi-* + *-cide*] an agent which is destructive to amebae.

**ame·bi·form** (ə-me'bĭ-form) shaped like or resembling an ameba.

**ameb(i)(o)-** [L., from Gr. *amoibē* change] a combining form denoting a relationship to an ameba. See also words beginning *amoeb(i)(o)-.*

**ame·bi·o·sis** (am"e-bi-o'sis) amebiasis.

**am·e·bism** (am'e-biz-əm) amebiasis.

**ame·bo·cyte** (ə-me'bo-sīt") [*amebo-* + *-cyte*] 1. ameboid cell. 2. old term for *leukocyte.*

**ame·bo·flag·el·late** (ə-me"bo-flag'ə-lāt) [*amebo-* + *flagellate*] a microorganism having both an ameboid and a flagellate stage in its life cycle; said of certain protozoa.

**ame·boid** (ə-me'boid) [*amebo-* + *-oid*] resembling an ameba in form or in movements.

**ame·boid·ism** (ə-me'boid-iz-əm) a type of motility characteristic of amebae and certain other cells, occurring as a result of protrusion of pseudopods.

**am·e·bo·ma** (am"e-bo'mə) a tumor-like mass produced by localized inflammation due to amebiasis.

**ame·bu·la** (ə-me'bu-lə) [dim. of *ameba*] 1. the small ameboid daughter cell occurring following reproduction in certain rhizopod amebae. 2. the motile ameboid stage of a spore prior to aggregation in certain protozoa or on germination of the spore in others. Also written *amoebula.*

**ame·bu·ria** (am"ēb-u're-ə) [*ameb-* + *-uria*] the discharge or presence of amebae in the urine.

**ame·da·lin hy·dro·chlo·ride** (ə-me'də-lin) an antidepressant.

**amei·o·sis** (a"mi-o'sis) aberrant meiosis in which only an equational division occurs, as in parthenogenesis.

**amel·a·no·sis** (ə-mel"ə-no'sis) [*a-*[1] + *melanosis*] complete lack of melanin in the tissues. Cf. *depigmentation, hypomelanosis,* and *hypopigmentation.*

**ame·lia** (ə-me'le-ə) [*a-*[1] + *-melia*] congenital absence of a limb or limbs; cf. *meromelia* and *phocomelia.*

**amel·i·fi·ca·tion** (ə-mel"ĭ-fĭ-ka'shən) [*amel-* + L. *facere* to make] the development of enamel cells into enamel.

**amel·io·ra·tion** (ə-mēl"yə-ra'shən) [L. *ad* to + *melior* better] improvement, as of the condition of a patient.

**amel(o)-** [Middle English *amel* enamel, from Old Fr. *esmal*] a combining form denoting enamel.

**amelo·blast** (ə-mel'o-blast") [*amelo-* + *-blast*[1]] [MeSH: Ameloblasts] a cylindrical epithelial cell in the innermost layer of the enamel organ which takes part in the elaboration of the enamel prism. The ameloblasts cover the dental papilla. Called also *adamantoblast, ganoblast, enamel builder,* and *enameloblast.*

**amelo·blas·to·ma** (ə-mel″o-blas-to′mə) [*ameloblast* + *-oma*] [MeSH: Ameloblastoma] an odontogenic epithelial neoplasm of tissue characteristic of the enamel organ but not differentiated to the point of enamel formation; it usually originates in the mandibular molar-ramus area and is usually benign but locally invasive. Ameloblastomas are often classified on the basis of histologic appearance, the most common subtypes being *follicular, cystic, acanthomatous, plexiform, basal cell,* and *granular cell;* they are also sometimes classified as *multicystic* versus *unicystic.* Called also *adamantinoma.*
**acanthomatous a.**, ameloblastoma in which the cells occupying the position of the stellate reticulum have undergone squamous metaplasia.
**basal cell a.**, a rare form of ameloblastoma microscopically resembling a basal cell carcinoma of the skin.
**cystic a.**, ameloblastoma in which the follicular islands have undergone central cystic degeneration.
**extraosseous a.**, a benign nonaggressive ameloblastoma occurring in the gingiva surrounding the alveolar bone; it resembles the intraosseous form histologically and is believed to originate in surface epithelium or odontogenic remnants.
**follicular a.**, ameloblastoma composed of numerous discrete islands of tumor cells that mimic the normal dental follicle.
**granular cell a.**, ameloblastoma in which the cytoplasm of the central neoplastic cells takes on a coarsely granular eosinophilic appearance.
**malignant a.**, ameloblastoma exhibiting metastases that histologically resemble the primary lesion; cf. *ameloblastic carcinoma.*
**melanotic a.**, melanotic neuroectodermal tumor.
**multicystic a.**, ameloblastoma containing multiple cystic spaces; it may exhibit any or all of the histologic patterns described as subtypes of the lesion and is more aggressive and recurs more frequently than does unicystic ameloblastoma. Cf. *unicystic a.*
**peripheral a.**, extraosseous a.
**pigmented a.**, melanotic neuroectodermal tumor.
**pituitary a.**, craniopharyngioma.
**plexiform a.**, ameloblastoma, often cystic, in which the neoplastic cells have formed an interconnected network of strands.
**plexiform unicystic a.**, a variant of unicystic ameloblastoma in which there is ameloblastic proliferation in an epithelial network on the cyst wall; it occurs in young adults, usually in the mandibular molar area.
**solid a.**, multicystic a.
**unicystic a.**, ameloblastoma containing a single cystic space, characterized by intraluminal or mural growth; it may be a unilocular ameloblastoma or ameloblastic transformation of the epithelial lining of an odontogenic cyst. Cf. *multicystic a.*

**amelo·den·ti·nal** (am″ə-lo-den′tĭ-nəl) pertaining to the enamel and dentin of a tooth.

**amelo·gen·e·sis** (am″ə-lo-jen′ə-sis) [*amelo-* + *genesis*] [MeSH: Amelogenesis] the elaboration of dental enamel by ameloblasts.
**a. imperfec′ta**, an autosomal dominant or X-linked disorder in which there is faulty development of the dental enamel owing to agenesis, hypoplasia, or hypocalcification of the enamel. It is marked by enamel that is very thin and friable and frequently stained in various shades of brown. Called also *hereditary brown enamel.*

**am·e·lo·gen·ic** (am″ə-lo-jen′ik) forming enamel; pertaining to amelogenesis.

**am·e·lo·gen·in** (am″ə-lo-jen′in) any of several proteins secreted by ameloblasts and forming the organic matrix of tooth enamel.

**am·e·lus** (am′ə-ləs) an individual exhibiting amelia.

**Amen** (a′men) trademark for a preparation of medroxyprogesterone acetate.

**ame·nia** (ə-me′ne-ə) [*a-*[1] + *men-* + *-ia*] amenorrhea.

**amen·or·rhea** (ə-men″o-re′ə) [*a-*[1] + *menorrhea*] [MeSH: Amenorrhea] absence or abnormal stoppage of the menses; called also *amenia.*
**dietary a.**, cessation of menstruation accompanying loss of weight due to dietary restriction, the loss of weight and of appetite being less extreme than in anorexia nervosa and unassociated with psychological problems. Called also *nutritional a.*
**dysponderal a.**, amenorrhea associated with disorder of weight, such as obesity or extreme underweight.
**hypothalamic a.**, amenorrhea associated with disorders of the hypothalamus.
**lactation a.**, absence of the menses in association with lactation.
**nutritional a.**, dietary a.
**ovarian a.**, amenorrhea resulting from deficiency of ovarian hormones.
**physiologic a.**, absence of menses not due to organic disorder, such as that occurring in pregnancy.
**pituitary a.**, absence of the menses owing to pituitary deficiency.
**premenopausal a.**, physiologic decrease of menstruation during establishment of the climacterium.
**primary a.**, failure of menstruation to occur at puberty.
**relative a.**, menstrual flow which is less than normal for the individual; called also *oligomenorrhea.*
**secondary a.**, cessation of menstruation after it has once been established at puberty.
**traumatic a.**, amenorrhea due to adhesions, frequently a result of curettage, as in Asherman's syndrome.

**amen·or·rhe·al** (ə-men-o-re′əl) pertaining to amenorrhea.

**amen·sal·ism** (a-men′səl-iz-əm) symbiosis in which one population (or individual) is adversely affected and the other is unaffected.

**amen·tia** (ə-men′shə) [*a-*[2] + *mens* mind + *-ia*] former term for profound mental retardation.

**Amer·i·caine** (ə-mer′ə-kān″) trademark for preparations of benzocaine.

**Amer·i·can Type Cul·ture Col·lec·tion (ATCC)** an organization established in Rockville, MD, as a depository for reference cultures. It maintains and distributes authentic reference strains of algae, bacteria, fungi, and protozoa, bacteriophages and viruses, and cell lines of animal tissues.

**am·er·ic·i·um** (am″ər-is′e-əm) [MeSH: Americium] the chemical element of atomic number 95, atomic weight 243, symbol Am, obtained by cyclotron bombardment of uranium and plutonium.

**am·er·ism** (am′ər-iz-əm) [*a-*[1] + *merism*] the quality of not splitting into segments or fragments.

**am·er·is·tic** (am″ər-is′tik) [*a-*[1] + *meristic*] not split into segments.

**Ames test** (āmz) [Bruce Nathan *Ames,* American biochemist, born 1928] see under *test.*

**ame·tab·o·lon** (am-ə-tab′o-lon) an animal that develops without undergoing metamorphosis.

**ame·tab·o·lous** (a″-mə-tab′ə-ləs) not undergoing metamorphosis.

**ameta·chro·mo·phil** (ə-met″ə-kro′mo-fil) orthochromophil.

**ameta·neu·tro·phil** (ə-met″ə-noo′tro-fil) orthochromophil.

**ameth·o·caine hy·dro·chlo·ride** (ə-meth′o-kān) tetracaine hydrochloride.

**ameth·op·ter·in** (am″əth-op′tə-rin) methotrexate.

**ame·tria** (a-me′tre-ə) [*a-*[1] + *metr-* + *-ia*] congenital absence of the uterus.

**am·e·trom·e·ter** (am″ə-trom′ə-tər) [*ametropia* + *-meter*] an instrument for measuring the degree of ametropia.

**am·e·tro·pia** (am″ə-tro′pe-ə) [Gr. *ametros* disproportionate + *-opia*] discrepancy between the size and refractive powers of the eye, such that images are not brought to a proper focus on the retina; consequently hypermetropia, myopia, or astigmatism are produced. See illustration at *refraction.*
**axial a.**, ametropia due to lengthening of the eyeball along the optic axis.
**curvature a.**, ametropia due to variations in the curvature of the surface of the eye.
**index a.**, ametropia due to alterations in the refractive index media of the eye.
**position a.**, ametropia due to faulty position of the crystalline lens.
**refractive a.**, ametropia due to fault in the dioptric system of the eye.

**am·e·trop·ic** (am″ə-trop′ik) affected with or pertaining to ametropia.

**am·fe·nac so·di·um** (am′fə-nak) an anti-inflammatory.

**am·fo·ne·lic acid** (am-fo-ne′lik) a central nervous system stimulant.

**Amh** mixed astigmatism with myopia predominating over hyperopia.

**AMI** acute myocardial infarction.

**am·i·an·thoid** (am″e-an′thoid) [Gr. *amianthos* asbestos + *-oid*] having the appearance of asbestos; a term applied to certain fibers seen in degenerated costal and laryngeal cartilage.

**am·i·bi·ar·son** (am′ĭ-bi-ahr′son) carbarsone.

**Am·i·car** (am′ĭ-kar) trademark for preparations of aminocaproic acid.

**am·i·chlor·al** (am″ĭ-klor′əl) a compound closely related to glucopyranose, administered as a veterinary feed additive.

**Am·i·ci's disk (line), striae** (ə-me'chēz) [Giovanni Battista *Amici,* Italian physicist, 1786–1863] see *Z band,* under *band,* and see under *stria.*

**ami·cro·scop·ic** (a-mi"kro-skop'ik) submicroscopic.

**amic·u·la** (ə-mik'u-lə) [L.] plural of *amiculum.*

**amic·u·lum** (ə-mik'u-ləm) pl. *amic'ula* [L.] 1. a coat or covering. 2. a. olivare.
**a. oliva're** [TA], **a. of olive,** a capsule of myelinated fibers that surrounds the caudal olivary nucleus; called also *amiculum* and *siliqua olivae.*

**ami·dap·sone** (ă-mĭ-dap'sōn) a member of the dapsone group used as an antiviral in poultry.

**am·i·dase** (am'ĭ-dās) [EC 3.5.1.4] 1. an enzyme of the hydrolase class that catalyzes the formation of a monocarboxylic acid and ammonia by cleavage of the C—N bond of a monocarboxylic acid amide. 2. more generally, a term used in the recommended and trivial names of some amidohydrolases, particularly those acting on linear amides [EC 3.5.1].

**am·ide** (am'īd) [*ammonia* + *-ide*] an organic compound derived from ammonia by substituting an acyl radical for hydrogen, or from an acid by replacing the —OH group by —$NH_2$.
**niacin a., nicotinic acid a.,** niacinamide.

**am·i·dine** (am'ĭ-dēn") any compound containing the amidino group.

**am·i·dine-ly·ase** (am"ĭ-dēn-li'ās) [EC 4.3.2] a sub-subclass of enzymes of the lyase class that catalyze the cleavage of a carbon-nitrogen bond to eliminate the amidino group from an amidine such as adenylosuccinate or argininosuccinate.

**am·i·dino** (am-ĭ-dēn'o) the chemical group —C(=NH)—$NH_2$. As a prefix (amidino-), it indicates the presence in a compound of this group.

**am·i·dino·hy·dro·lase** (am-ĭ-dēn"o-hi'dro-lās) [EC 3.5.3] systematic name for enzymes of the hydrolase class that catalyze the hydrolysis of C—N bonds in linear amidines.

**am·i·dino·trans·fer·ase** (am-ĭ-dēn"o-trans'fər-ās) [EC 2.1.4] a sub-subclass of enzymes of the transferase class that catalyze the transfer of an amidino group from one compound to another. Called also *transaminidase.*

**amido-** a prefix indicating the presence of the radical $NH_2$ along with the radical CO.

**am·i·do·azo·tol·u·ene** (ə-me"do-, am"ĭ-do-a"zo-tol'u-ēn) a reddish brown powder derived from scarlet red; used in an 8 per cent ointment to stimulate the growth of epithelium.

**am·i·do·ben·zene** (ə-me"do-, am"ĭ-do-ben'zēn) aniline.

**am·i·do·gen** (ah-me'do-jen") the hypothetic radical, $NH_2$, found in amido compounds.

**am·i·do·hy·dro·lase** (ə-me"do-, am"ĭ-do-hi'dro-lās) systematic name for enzymes of the hydrolase class that catalyze the cleavage of carbon-nitrogen bonds in linear [EC 3.5.1] or cyclic [EC 3.5.2] amide compounds. Called also *deamidase.*

**am·i·do·li·gase** (ə-me"do-, am"ĭ-do-li'gās) [EC 6.3.5] systematic name for enzymes of the ligase class that catalyze the transfer of the amide nitrogen from glutamine to an acceptor molecule, driven by the concomitant hydrolysis of ATP to ADP or AMP and forming an amide or amidine group on the acceptor.

**am·i·do·phos·pho·ri·bo·syl·trans·fer·ase** (ə-me"do-, am-ĭ"do-fos"fo-ri"bo-səl-trans'fər-ās) [EC 2.4.2.14] an enzyme of the transferase class that catalyzes the first committed step in purine nucleotide biosynthesis, the transfer of an amino group to phosphoribosylpyrophosphate from glutamine, forming phosphoribosylamine as well as glutamate and pyrophosphate. The reaction is inhibited by purine nucleotides.

**Am·i·dos·to·mum** (am"ĭ-dos'to-məm) a genus of nematodes of the superfamily Strongyloides. *A. an'seris* is parasitic in the mucous membrane of the intestinal tract of ducks and geese and may kill young birds by its excessive consumption of their blood.

**am·i·dox·ime** (am-ĭ-dok'sīm) any of a class of compounds formed from the amidines by substituting hydroxyl for a hydrogen atom of the amide group.

**am·i·fos·tine** (am"ĭfos'tēn) [MeSH: Amifostine] a chemoprotectant used to prevent renal toxicity in cisplatin chemotherapy; administered by intravenous infusion. It has also been used investigationally as a radioprotector in radiation therapy.

**Am·i·gen** (am'ĭ-jen) trademark for a protein hydrolysate preparation for intravenous injection.

**am·i·ka·cin** (am"ĭ-ka'sin) [USP] [MeSH: Amikacin] a semisynthetic aminoglycoside antibiotic derived from kanamycin A, effective against a wide range of aerobic gram-negative bacilli and some gram-positive bacteria, including penicillinase- and non–penicillinase-producing staphylococci.
**a. sulfate** [USP], the sulfate salt of amikacin, used in the treatment of a wide variety of serious infections caused by susceptible gram-negative organisms; administered intramuscularly and intravenously.

**Am·i·kin** (am'ĭ-kin) trademark for a preparation of amikacin sulfate.

**amil·o·ride hy·dro·chlo·ride** (ə-mil'ə-rīd) [USP] a potassium-sparing diuretic that inhibits the reabsorption of sodium in the distal and proximal convoluted tubules and the collecting tubule; used in conjunction with a loop or thiazide diuretic for the treatment of congestive heart failure and hypertension and for the prophylaxis and treatment of hypokalemia; administered orally.

**amim·ia** (ə-mim'e-ə) [*a-*[1] + Gr. *mimos* mimic + *-ia*] loss of the power of expression by the use of signs or gestures.

**am·in·a·crine hy·dro·chlo·ride** (am-in-ak'rin) an antiseptic dye which is effective against many gram-negative and gram-positive bacteria; used as a topical anti-infective, mainly in the treatment of infected wounds. Called also *aminoacridine hydrochloride.*

**am·in·ar·sone** (am-in-ahr'sən) carbarsone.

**am·i·na·tion** (am"ĭ-na'shən) [MeSH: Amination] the creation of an amine, either by addition of an amino group to an organic acceptor compound or by reduction of a nitro compound.

**amine** (ə-mēn', am'in) an organic compound containing nitrogen; any member of a group of chemical compounds formed from ammonia by replacement of one or more of the hydrogen atoms by organic (hydrocarbon) radicals. The amines are distinguished as *primary, secondary,* and *tertiary,* according to whether one, two, or three hydrogen atoms are replaced. The amines include allylamine, arylamine, ethylamine, methylamine, phenylamine, propylamine, and many other compounds.
**biogenic a.,** a type of amine synthesized by both plants and animals and frequently involved in signalling; prominent examples are neurotransmitters such as acetylcholine, catecholamines, and serotonin. Others are hormones or components of vitamins, phospholipids, bacteria, and ribosomes and include cadaverine, choline, histamine, muscarine, putrescine, and spermine.
**methyl dimethoxy methyl phenyl ethyl a.,** a long-acting hallucinogenic substance. Abbreviated DMP.
**sympathomimetic a's,** amines that mimic the actions of the sympathetic nervous system, comprising the catecholamines and drugs that mimic their actions.
**vasoactive a's,** amines that cause vasodilation and increase small vessel permeability, e.g., histamine and serotonin.

**amine-ly·ase** (ə-mēn-li'ās) [EC 4.3.3] any member of a sub-subclass of enzymes of the lyase class that catalyze the cleavage of a carbon-nitrogen bond within an amine.

**amine ox·i·dase (cop·per-con·tain·ing)** (ə-mēn', am'in ok'sĭ-dās kop'ər kən-tān'ing) [MeSH: Amine Oxidase (Copper-Containing)] [EC 1.4.3.6] a group of enzymes of the oxidoreductase class that catalyze the oxidative deamination of diamines, including histamine, to form aminoaldehydes, ammonia, and hydrogen peroxide. The enzymes can also convert primary monoamines to aldehydes. They are copper proteins and may contain pyridoxal phosphate. Called also *diamine oxidase.*

**amine ox·i·dase (fla·vin-con·tain·ing)** (ə-mēn' ok'sĭ-dās fla'vin kon-tān'ing) [EC 1.4.3.4] a flavoprotein (FAD) enzyme of the oxidoreductase class that catalyzes the oxidative deamination of primary amines to form aldehydes and hydrogen peroxide. Substrates include serotonin, norepinephrine, epinephrine, dopamine, and also some secondary and tertiary amines. Called also *monoamine oxidase (MAO).* See also *monoamine oxidase inhibitor,* under *inhibitor.*

**am·in·er·gic** (am"ĭ-nər'jik) activated by, characteristic of, or secreting one of the biogenic amines.

**ami·no** (ə-me'no, am'ĭ-no") the monovalent chemical group —$NH_2$. As a prefix (amino-) it indicates the presence in a compound of the group —$NH_2$.

**ami·no·ace·tic ac·id** (ə-me"no-ə-se'tik) former name for *glycine.*

**ami·no ac·id** (ə-me'no) any organic compound containing an amino (—$NH_2$) and a carboxyl (—COOH) group. The 20 $\alpha$-amino acids listed in the accompanying table are the amino acids from which proteins are synthesized by formation of peptide bonds during ribosomal translation of messenger RNA. Other amino acids occurring in proteins, such as hydroxyproline in collagen, are formed by posttranslational enzymatic modification of amino acid residues in polypeptide chains. There are also several important amino acids, such as the neurotransmitter $\gamma$-aminobutyric acid, that have no relation to proteins. Abbreviated AA.

**Amino Acids: The 20 α-Amino Acids Specified by the Genetic Code**

| Name | Symbols* | | Structural Formula |
|---|---|---|---|
| Alanine | Ala | A | $HOOC-CH(NH_2)-CH_3$ |
| Arginine | Arg | R | $HOOC-CH(NH_2)-CH_2-CH_2-CH_2-NH-C(=NH)-NH_2$ |
| Asparagine | Asn | N | $HOOC-CH(NH_2)-CH_2-C(=O)-NH_2$ |
| Aspartic Acid | Asp | D | $HOOC-CH(NH_2)-CH_2-COOH$ |
| Cysteine | Cys | C | $HOOC-CH(NH_2)-CH_2-SH$ |
| Glutamic Acid | Glu | E | $HOOC-CH(NH_2)-CH_2-CH_2-COOH$ |
| Glutamine | Gln | Q | $HOOC-CH(NH_2)-CH_2-CH_2-C(=O)-NH_2$ |
| Glycine | Gly | G | $HOOC-CH(NH_2)-H$ |
| Histidine | His | H | $HOOC-CH(NH_2)-CH_2-$ (imidazolyl) |
| Isoleucine | Ile | I | $HOOC-CH(NH_2)-CH(CH_3)-CH_2-CH_3$ |
| Leucine | Leu | L | $HOOC-CH(NH_2)-CH_2-CH(CH_3)-CH_2$ |
| Lysine | Lys | K | $HOOC-CH(NH_2)-CH_2-CH_2-CH_2-CH_2-NH_2$ |
| Methionine | Met | M | $HOOC-CH(NH_2)-CH_2-CH_2-S-CH_3$ |
| Phenylalanine | Phe | F | $HOOC-CH(NH_2)-CH_2-C_6H_5$ |
| Proline | Pro | P | HOOC– (pyrrolidine ring, N–H) |
| Serine | Ser | S | $HOOC-CH(NH_2)-CH_2-OH$ |
| Threonine | Thr | T | $HOOC-CH(NH_2)-CH(OH)-CH_3$ |
| Tryptophan | Trp | W | $HOOC-CH(NH_2)-CH_2-$ (indolyl) |
| Tyrosine | Tyr | Y | $HOOC-CH(NH_2)-CH_2-C_6H_4-OH$ |
| Valine | Val | V | $HOOC-CH(NH_2)-CH(CH_3)-CH_3$ |

* The three-letter and single-letter symbols that are used in presenting the sequence of a polypeptide or protein, e.g., Gly-Phe-Tyr. By convention, the N-terminal residue is shown at the left, the C-terminal residue at the right. For emphasis, the same formula may be written as H-Gly-Phe-Tyr-OH.

*α*-**a. a.,** one in which the amino and carboxyl groups are both attached to the same carbon atom.
*ω*-**a. a.,** one having the amino and carboxyl groups attached to opposite ends of a carbon chain.
**branched-chain a. a's,** leucine, isoleucine, and valine; they are incorporated into proteins or catabolized for energy.
**essential a. a's,** the nine *α*-amino acids required for protein synthesis that cannot be synthesized by humans and must be obtained in the diet: histidine, isoleucine, leucine, lysine, methionine, phenylalanine, threonine, tryptophan, and valine.
**excitatory a. a's,** a group of nonessential amino acids that act as excitatory neurotransmitters in the central nervous system, including glutamic acid or L-glutamate, aspartic acid or L-aspartate, and the excitotoxins.
**nonessential a. a's,** the eleven *α*-amino acids required for protein synthesis that are synthesized by humans and are not specifically required in the diet.

**ami·no·ac·id *N*-ac·e·tyl·trans·fer·ase** (ə-me′no as′id as″ə-tēl-trans′fər-ās) [EC 2.3.1.1] an enzyme of the transferase class that catalyzes the transfer of an acetyl group from acetyl coenzyme A to the N-terminus of glutamate to form *N*-acetylglutamate. It can also act on aspartate and, slowly, on some other amino acids. Deficiency of the enzyme causes hyperammonemia without orotic aciduria, similar to that seen in carbamoyl phosphate synthetase deficiency. Called also N-*acetylglutamate synthetase.*

**ami·no·ac·id·emia** (ə-me″no-as″ĭ-de′me-ə) an excess of amino acids in the blood.

**ami·no·ac·i·dop·a·thy** (ə-me″no-as″ĭ-dop′ə-the) any of a group of disorders due to a defect in an enzymatic step in the metabolic pathway of one or more amino acids or in a protein mediator necessary for transport of certain amino acids into or out of cells.

**D-ami·no·ac·id ox·i·dase** (ə-me′no as′id ok′sĭ-dās) [EC 1.4.3.3] an enzyme of the oxidoreductase class that catalyzes the oxidative deamination of D-amino acids to form 2-keto acids, producing hydrogen peroxide as a byproduct. The enzyme is a flavoprotein found in the cytoplasm of kidney, brain, and liver; its metabolic role is unclear.

**L-ami·no·ac·id ox·i·dase** (ə-me′no as′id ok′sĭd-ās) [EC 1.4.3.2] an enzyme of the oxidoreductase class that catalyzes the oxidative deamination of L-amino acids to form 2-keto acids, producing hydrogen peroxide as a byproduct. The enzyme is a flavoprotein, present in liver and kidney and found in snake venom. It acts on all naturally occurring monocarboxylic L-amino acids except serine and threonine. The mammalian enzymes also attack 2-hydroxy acids; their function is unclear.

**ami·no·ac·id·u·ria** (ə-me″no-as″ĭ-du′re-ə) an excess of amino acids in the urine; called also *hyperaminoaciduria.*

**ami·no·ac·ri·dine hy·dro·chlo·ride** (ə-me″no-ak′rĭ-din) aminacrine hydrochloride.

**ami·no·acyl** (ə-me″no-a′səl) an acyl radical of an amino acid, e.g., alanyl, glycyl, etc.
**a. adenylate,** an amino acid residue linked via an acid anhydride bond to the 5′ phosphate of adenosine monophosphate; it is a high energy intermediate in the synthesis of aminoacyl-tRNA.
**a.-tRNA,** an amino acid residue joined by an ester linkage to the 2′ or 3′ hydroxyl group of the terminal adenosine residue of a transfer RNA (see also *translation*).

**ami·no·acy·lase** (ə-me″no-a′sə-lās) [EC 3.5.1.14] an enzyme of the hydrolase class that catalyzes the cleavage of the acyl group from acylated L-amino acids. It occurs in the kidney and acts on a variety of substrates, including hippuric acid and benzamide.

**ami·no·acyl-his·ti·dine di·pep·ti·dase** (ə-me″no-a′səl his′tĭ-dēn di-pep′tĭ-dās) X-His dipeptidase.

**ami·no·acyl·trans·fer·ase** (ə-me″no-a″səl-trans′fər-ās) [EC 2.3.2] a sub-subclass of enzymes of the transferase class that catalyze the transfer of an aminoacyl group from one molecule to another with formation of an ester or an amide linkage.

**ami·no·acyl-tRNA syn·the·tase** (ə-me″no-a′səl sin′thə-tās) any of the group of ligases that catalyze the ATP-driven formation of a bond between an amino acid and a tRNA, activating the amino acids as a step in protein synthesis. Individual enzymes are highly specific for one amino acid and for any tRNA corresponding to that amino acid; they are known by the name of the amino acid acted on, e.g., alanyl-tRNA synthetase (formally called alanine–tRNA ligase, EC 6.1.1.7).

**α-ami·no·adip·ate** (ə-me″no-ə-dip′āt) the anionic form of *α*-aminoadipic acid.

**2-ami·no·ad·i·pate trans·am·i·nase** (ə-me″no-ə-dip′āt trans-am′ĭ-nās) [EC 2.6.1.39] an enzyme of the transferase class that catalyzes the oxidative deamination of *α*-ketoglutarate to form glutamate. The reaction is a step in the degradation of lysine and hydroxylysine. Called also *2-aminoadipate aminotransferase.*

**α-ami·no·adip·ic ac·id** (ə-me″no-ə-dip′ik) a dicarboxylic amino acid occurring as an intermediate in the degradation of lysine and hydroxylysine. Written also *2-aminoadipic acid.*

**α-ami·no·adip·ic·ac·id·uria** (ə-me″no-ə-dip″ik-as″ĭ-du′re-ə) excretion of *α*-aminoadipic acid in the urine.

**α-ami·no·adip·ic semi·al·de·hyde syn·thase** (ə-me″no-ə-dip′ik sem″e-al′də-hīd sin′thās) a bifunctional enzyme comprising the two enzyme activities saccharopine dehydrogenase ($NADP^+$, L-lysine-forming) (q.v.) and saccharopine dehydrogenase ($NAD^+$, L-glutamate-forming) (q.v.) and catalyzing the first two steps in the major pathway of lysine degradation. Deficiency of the enzyme, an autosomal recessive trait, causes hyperlysinemia. See also *saccharopinuria.*

**p-ami·no·azo·ben·zene** (ə-me″no-a″zo-ben′zēn) a yellow azo dye; it is carcinogenic.

**o-ami·no·azo·tol·u·ene** (ə-me″no-az″o-tol′u-ēn) a red crystalline azo dye that is actively carcinogenic.

**ami·no·ben·zene** (ə-me″no-ben′zēn) aniline.

**ami·no·ben·zo·ate** (ə-me″no-ben′zo-āt) *p*-aminobenzoate, any salt or ester of *p*-aminobenzoic acid.
**a. potassium,** the potassium salt of *p*-aminobenzoic acid, administered orally as an antifibrotic in the treatment of dermatologic disorders marked by fibrosis or nonsuppurative inflammation; used also in combination with potassium salicylate in an analgesic preparation.
**a. sodium,** the monosodium salt of *p*-aminobenzoic acid, used in combination with sodium salicylate in an analgesic preparation.

**p-ami·no·ben·zo·ic ac·id** (ə-me″no-ben-zo′ik) a substance required for the synthesis of folic acid by many organisms. PABA is included in the B vitamin complex, although it is not an essential nutrient for humans. It also absorbs ultraviolet light and is used as *aminobenzoic acid* [USP] as a topical sunscreen. Abbreviated PAB or PABA.

**p-ami·no·bi·phen·yl** (ə-me″no-bi-fen′əl) a nitrogen-substituted arylamine formerly used in dyemaking and certain other industrial processes; because of its toxicity and carcinogenicity, it is now used mainly to induce cancer in laboratory animals. Written also *4-aminobiphenyl.* Called also p-*aminodiphenyl,* p-*biphenylamine,* and *xenylamine.*

**γ-ami·no·bu·ty·rate** (ə-me″no-bu′tə-rāt) the conjugate base of *γ*-aminobutyric acid.

**4-ami·no·bu·ty·rate trans·am·i·nase** (ə-me″no-bu′-tə-rāt trans-am′ĭ-nās) [EC 2.6.1.19] an enzyme of the transferase class that catalyzes the transfer of an amino group from *γ*-aminobutyrate (GABA) to *α*-ketoglutarate, forming glutamate and succinate semialdehyde. The reaction occurs predominantly in the liver and in the neurons of the brain. The enzyme can also act on *β*-alanine and *β*-aminoisobutyrate. Deficiency of the enzyme, an autosomal recessive trait, causes psychomotor retardation, hypotonia, hyperreflexia, and accelerated linear growth, with high levels of GABA, homocarnosine, and *β*-alanine in the cerebrospinal fluid. See also *β-alanine–α-ketoglutarate transaminase.* Called also *GABA transaminase* and *aminobutyrate aminotransferase.*

**γ-ami·no·bu·tyr·ic ac·id (GABA)** (ə-me″no-bu-tēr′ik) an *ω*-amino acid formed in the metabolism of L-glutamic acid; it is the principal inhibitory neurotransmitter in the brain but is also found in several extraneural tissues, including kidney and pancreatic islet *β* cells. In the brain, it is released from presynaptic cells upon depolarization and via receptor binding it modulates membrane chloride permeability and inhibits postsynaptic cell firing. Called also *4-aminobutyric acid.*

**ε-ami·no·ca·pro·ic ac·id** (ə-me″no-kə-pro′ik) an *ω*-amino acid that inhibits plasminogen activators and, to a lesser degree, plasmin; used orally and intravenously as *aminocaproic acid* [USP] for treatment of acute bleeding syndromes due to excessive fibrinolysis and for the prevention and treatment of postsurgical hemorrhage.

**7-ami·no·ceph·a·lo·spo·ran·ic ac·id** (ə-me″no-sef″ə-lo-spor-an′ik) the active nucleus of the semisynthetic cephalosporins, structurally related to the penicillin nucleus (6-aminopenicillanic acid) and obtained by hydrolysis of cephalosporin C; modification of positions 3 and 7 of this nucleus results in antibiotics with a variety of antibacterial and pharmacologic characteristics.

**ami·no·di·ni·tro·phe·nol** (ə-me″no-di-ni″tro-fe′nol) dinitroaminophenol.

**p-ami·no·di·phen·yl** (ə-me″no-di-fen′əl) *p*-aminobiphenyl.

**ami·no·glu·teth·i·mide** (ə-me″no-gloo-teth′ĭ-mīd) [USP] [MeSH: Aminoglutethimide] an inhibitor of the enzymatic conversion of cholesterol to pregnenolone, thereby reducing corticosteroid synthesis and an aromatase inhibitor which inhibits conversion of androstenedione to estrone in peripheral tissues; used in the treatment of Cushing's syndrome and as an investigational drug in the treatment of breast carcinoma; administered orally. It was formerly used as an anticonvulsant, but this use has been discontinued because of the adrenal suppressant effect.

**ami·no·gly·co·side** (ə-me'no-gli'ko-sīd) any of a group of antibiotics (e.g. amikacin, gentamicin, streptomycin) derived from various species of *Streptomyces* or produced synthetically. Aminoglycosides inhibit protein synthesis by binding with the 30S ribosomal subunit.

**p-ami·no·hip·pu·rate** (ə-me″no-hip'u-rāt) a salt or the conjugate base of *p*-aminohippuric acid.
**p-aminohippurate sodium,** the sodium salt of *p*-aminohippuric acid, used as *aminohippurate sodium injection* [USP] to measure effective renal plasma flow and to determine the functional capacity of the tubular excretory mechanism.

**p-ami·no·hip·pu·ric ac·id** (ə-me″no-hĭ-pūr'ik) PAH, PAHA; the glycine amide of *p*-aminobenzoic acid, which is filtered by the renal glomeruli and secreted into the urine by the proximal tubules. See also *p-aminohippurate sodium.*

**ami·no·hy·dro·lase** (ə-me″no-hi'dro-lās) systematic name for some enzymes of the hydrolase class that catalyze the hydrolysis of an amino group from a cyclic amidine [EC 3.5.4] or a nitrile [EC 3.5.5]. Cf. *deaminase.*

**ami·no·hy·droxy·ben·zo·ic ac·id** (ə-me″no-hi-drok″se-ben-zo'ik) a group of chemotherapeutic agents used in the treatment of infections with acid-fast bacilli.

**ami·no·iso·bu·ty·rate** (ə-me″no-i″so-bu'tər-āt) an anionic form of aminoisobutyric acid.

**β-ami·no·iso·bu·ty·rate–py·ru·vate trans·am·i·nase** (ə-me″no-i″so-bu'tər-āt pi'roo-vāt trans-am'ĭ-nās) an enzyme of the transferase class that catalyzes the oxidative deamination of *R*-β-aminoisobutyrate, transferring the amino group to pyruvate; the reaction is a step in the catabolism of thymine. Deficiency of the enzyme, an autosomal recessive trait, causes β-aminoisobutyricaciduria. In EC nomenclature, called *(R)-3-amino-2-methylpropionate–pyruvate transaminase.* Called also *β-aminoisobutyrate–pyruvate transaminase.*

**ami·no·iso·bu·tyr·ic ac·id** (ə-me″no-i″so-bu-tir'ik) an amino acid not occurring in proteins; the *R*-β- isomer is produced in the degradation of thymine and excreted in excess in β-aminoisobutyricaciduria; the *S*-β-isomer is a metabolite of valine; and the α- form, which does not occur naturally, is used in studies of transport and cytokinin effects.

**β-ami·no·iso·bu·tyr·ic·ac·id·uria** (ə-me″no-i″so-bu-tir″ik-as-ĭ-du're-ə) excessive excretion of *R*-β-aminoisobutyric acid in the urine, occurring as a benign metabolic variant due to deficiency of β-aminoisobutyrate–pyruvate transaminase; it also occurs in certain illnesses in which rapid tissue destruction and deoxyribonucleic acid catabolism occur. Called also *hyper-β-aminoisobutyricaciduria.*

**δ-ami·no·lev·u·lin·ate** (ə-me″no-lev″u-lin'āt) the conjugate base of δ-aminolevulinic acid.

**ami·no·lev·u·lin·ate de·hy·dra·tase** (ə-me″no-lev″u-lin'āt de-hi'drə-tās) porphobilinogen synthase.

**5-ami·no·lev·u·lin·ate syn·thase** (ə-me″no-lev″u-lin'āt sin'thās) [EC 2.3.1.37] an enzyme of the transferase class that catalyzes the condensation of the succinyl group from succinyl coenzyme A with glycine to form δ-aminolevulinate. It is a pyridoxal phosphate protein and the reaction occurs in mitochondria as the first step of the heme biosynthetic pathway. The enzyme is a key regulatory enzyme in heme biosynthesis and, in liver at least, is feedback inhibited by heme. Abbreviated ALAS. Written also *δ-aminolevulinate synthase.*

**δ-ami·no·lev·u·lin·ic ac·id (ALA)** (ə-me″no-lev″u-lin'ik) an intermediate in the synthesis of heme, produced from succinyl-CoA and glycine. Two molecules of ALA are condensed to form porphobilinogen. Blood and urinary ALA levels are increased in lead poisoning, and urinary levels are increased in a variety of porphyrias.

**am·i·nol·y·sis** (am″ə-nol'ə-sis) [*amine* + *-lysis*] reaction with an amine, resulting in the addition of (or substitution by) an imino group, —NH—.

**ami·no·meth·ane** (ə-me″no-meth'ān) methylamine.

**ami·no·meth·yl** (ə-me″no-meth'əl) a methylated amino group, the acyl radical of methylamine (aminomethane).

**(R)-3-ami·no-2-meth·yl·pro·pi·o·nate–py·ru·vate trans·am·i·nase** (ə-me″no-meth″əl-pro'pe-ən-āt pi'roo-vāt trans-am'ĭ-nās) [EC 2.6.1.40] EC nomenclature for *β-aminoisobutyrate–pyruvate.*

**ami·no·met·ra·dine** (ə-me″no-met'rə-dēn) a nonmercurial diuretic, administered orally.

**ami·no·met·ra·mide** (ə-me″no-met'rə-mīd) aminometradine.

**ami·no·ni·tro·thi·a·zole** (ə-me″no-ni″tro-thi'ə-zōl) a green or orange-colored powder used in the treatment and prevention of blackhead in turkeys.

**6-ami·no·pen·i·cil·lan·ic ac·id** (ə-me″no-pen″ĭ-səl-an'ik) the active nucleus common to all penicillins; it may be obtained from cultures of *Penicillium* to which no side-chain precursors have been added. Substitution at the 6-amino position results in semisynthetic penicillins with a variety of antibacterial and pharmacologic characteristics.

**ami·no·pen·ta·mide sul·fate** (ə-me″no-pen'tə-mīd) an anticholinergic with atropine-like action.

**ami·no·pep·ti·dase** (ə-me″-no-pep'tĭ-dās) any member of a sub-subclass of enzymes of the hydrolase class that catalyze the hydrolytic cleavage of the N-terminal amino acid or dipeptide from a peptide chain; they are exopeptidases and occur in plasma and many tissues.

**p-ami·no·phe·nol** (ə-me″no-fe'nol) a dye intermediate and photographic developer and the parent compound of acetaminophen; it is a potent allergen that causes dermatitis as well as asthma and methemoglobinemia on inhalation.

**am·i·noph·yl·line** (am″ĭ-nof'ə-lin) [USP] [MeSH: Aminophylline] a salt of theophylline prepared from theophylline and aqueous ethylenediamine, used as a bronchodilator for the prevention and treatment of symptoms of asthma and of reversible bronchospasm associated with chronic bronchitis or emphysema, administered orally, rectally, or intravenously. Formerly used as an antispasmodic, cardiac stimulant, and diuretic, but now replaced by more effective agents.

**am·i·nop·ter·in** (am″i-nop'tər-in) [MeSH: Aminopterin] a folic acid antagonist formerly used as an antineoplastic, now replaced by methotrexate.

**ami·no·pu·rine** (ə-me″no-pu'ren) a purine that is a component of nucleic acid and the nucleotides; the aminopurines include adenine and guanine.

**ami·no·quin·o·line** (ə-mē″no-kwin'o-lēn) a heterocyclic compound derived from quinoline by the addition of an amino group.
**4-a's,** a group of antimalarial compounds effective against the erythrocytic forms of *Plasmodium* and including amodiaquine, chloroquine, and hydrochloroquine.
**8-a's,** a group of antimalarial compounds effective against the exoerythrocytic forms of *Plasmodium;* of this group, only primaquine is widely used.

**amin·o·rex** (ə-min'o-reks) [MeSH: Aminorex] a sympathomimetic anorexic.

**ami·no·sa·lic·y·late** (ə-me″no-sə-lis'ə-lāt) any salt of *p*-aminosalicylic acid; aminosalicylates are antibacterials effective against mycobacteria and have been used as tuberculostatics.
**a. sodium** [USP], the dihydrated sodium salt of *p*-aminosalicylic acid, an antibacterial effective against mycobacteria; administered orally as a tuberculostatic.

**ami·no·sal·i·cyl·ic ac·id** (ə-me″no-sal-ĭ-sil'ik) [USP] see *p-aminosalicylic acid.*

**5-ami·no·sal·i·cyl·ic ac·id (5-ASA)** (ə-me″no-sal-ĭ-sil'ik) mesalamine.

**p-ami·no·sal·i·cyl·ic ac·id** (ə-me″no-sal-ĭ-sil'ik) an analogue of *p*-aminobenzoic acid (PABA) that inhibits folic acid synthesis in *Mycobacterium tuberculosis* and is bacteriostatic, inhibiting growth and multiplication of the tubercle bacillus; available as *aminosalicylic acid* [USP] and *aminosalicylate sodium* [USP]. Abbreviated PAS and PASA.

**ami·no·si·dine sul·fate** (ə-me″no-si'din) paromomycin sulfate.

**am·i·no·sis** (am″ĭ-no'sis) the pathologic production of amino acids in the body.

**Ami·no·sol** (ə-me'no-sol) trademark for an amino acid preparation for intravenous injection.

**ami·nos·uria** (ə-me″no-su're-ə) [*amine* + *-uria*] an excess of amines in the urine.

**Ami·no·syn** (ə-me'no-sin) trademark for a crystalline amino acid solution for intravenous administration; it contains a mixture of essential and nonessential amino acids but no peptides.

**ami·no·tol·u·ene** (ə-me″no-tol'u-ēn) toluidine.

**ami·no·trans·fer·ase** (ə-me″no-trans'fər-ās) transaminase.

**3-ami·no·tri·az·ole** (ə-me″no-tri'ə-zōl) amitrole.

**am·in·uria** (am″ĭ-nu're-ə) an excess of amines in the urine.

**ami·o·da·rone** (ə-me'o-də-rōn″) [MeSH: Amiodarone] a potassium channel blocker that prolongs the action potential duration and refractory period of all cardiac fibers; administered orally in the treatment of ventricular arrhythmias.

**Am·i·paque** (am'ĭ-pāk) trademark for metrizamide.

**am·i·phen·a·zole hy·dro·chlo·ride** (am″ĭ-fen'ə-zōl) a respiratory stimulant which acts as an antagonist to morphine and other narcotics.

**am·i·quin·sin hy·dro·chlo·ride** (am″ĭ-kwin′sin) an antihypertensive agent.

**am·iso·met·ra·dine** (am″ĭ-so-met′rə-dēn) an oral diuretic.

**ami·to·sis** (am″ĭ-to′sis) [*a-*[1] + *mitosis*] direct cell division; cell division by simple cleavage of the nucleus without the formation of spireme (mitotic) spindle figure or chromosomes. Called also *holoschisis.*

**ami·tot·ic** (am″ĭ-tot′ik) of the nature of amitosis; not occurring by mitosis; called also *akinetic.*

**am·i·traz** (am′ĭ-traz) [USP] a topical acaricide used on cattle, sheep, pigs, and dogs.

**am·i·trip·ty·line hy·dro·chlo·ride** (am″ĭ-trip′tə-lēn) [USP] a tricyclic antidepressant of the dibenzocycloheptadiene group, also having sedative effects; it is also used in the treatment of enuresis, chronic pain, peptic ulcer, and bulimia. Administered orally and intramuscularly.

**am·i·trole** (am′ĭ-trol) [MeSH: Amitrole] an herbicide used on nonfood crops; its use is restricted because it is an epigenetic carcinogen. Called also *3-aminotriazole.*

**AML** acute myelogenous leukemia.

**am·lex·a·nox** (am-lek′sə-noks″) a topical antiulcerative used in the treatment of recurrent aphthous stomatitis.

**am·lo·di·pine bes·yl·ate** (am-lo′dĭ-pēn″) a calcium-channel blocker used in the treatment of hypertension and chronic stable and vasospastic angina; administered orally.

**am·me·ter** (am′me-tər) [*am*pere + *-meter*] an instrument calibrated to read in amperes or subdivisions of amperes the amount of electric current flowing in a circuit.

**Am·mi** (am′e) a genus of plants of the family Umbelliferae, native to Mediterranean countries. *A. ma′jus* and *A. visna′ga* contain psoralens and are toxic in large amounts to poultry and other animals.

**am·mo·ac·id·uria** (am″o-as″ĭ-du′re-ə) an excess of ammonia and amino acids in the urine.

**Am·mon's fissure, operation** (ah′mənz) [Friedrich August von *Ammon,* German ophthalmologist and pathologist, 1799–1861] see under *fissure* and *operation.*

**Am·mon's horn** (am′ənz) [*Ammon,* a ram-headed god of the Egyptians] hippocampus.

**am·mo·ne·mia** (ă-mo-ne′me-ə) hyperammonemia.

**am·mo·nia** (ə-mōn′yə) [named from Jupiter *Ammon,* near whose temple in Libya it was formerly obtained] [MeSH: Ammonia] a colorless alkaline gas, $NH_3$, having a penetrating odor; it is soluble in water, forming *ammonia water.*
**a. hemate,** a compound of ammonia and hematein, used as a violet-black stain for microscopic specimens.
**a. N 13** [USP], ammonia in which a portion of the molecules are labeled with $^{13}N$; used in positron emission tomography of the heart and liver.

**am·mo·ni·a·cal** (am″o-ni′ə-kəl) containing ammonia or treated with excess ammonia.

**am·mo·nia-ly·ase** (ə-mōn′yə-li′ās) [EC 4.3.1] a sub-subclass of enzymes of the lyase class that catalyze the formation of a C═C bond in a molecule by liberation of ammonia, e.g., histidine ammonia-lyase.

**am·mo·ni·ate** (ə-mo′ne-āt) 1. to treat or to combine with ammonia. 2. the product of combination with ammonia.

**am·mo·ni·emia** (ə-mo″ne-e′me-ə) hyperammonemia.

**am·mo·ni·fi·ca·tion** (ə-mo″nĭ-fĭ-ka′shən) the formation of ammonia by the action of bacteria on proteins.

**am·mo·ni·um** (ə-mo′ne-əm) the hypothetical radical, $NH_4$; it forms salts analogous to those of the alkaline metals.
**a. alum,** see under *alum.*
**a. bromide,** a sedative, $NH_4Br$, occurring as colorless crystals or a yellowish white crystalline powder; used occasionally in treatment of grand mal seizures. See also *bromide.*
**a. carbonate** [NF], a mixture of ammonium bicarbonate and ammonium carbamate in varying proportions, used as an ingredient of aromatic ammonia spirit and as a source of ammonia in smelling salts. It has also been used as an expectorant. Called also *hartshorn* and *sal volatile.*
**a. chloride** [USP], a systemic and urinary acidifying agent and diuretic administered orally or by intravenous infusion. It is also administered orally as an expectorant. Called also *a. muriate* and *sal ammoniac.*
**a. lactate,** lactic acid neutralized with ammonium hydroxide, applied topically as a humectant in ichthyosis vulgaris and xerosis.
**a. mandelate,** the ammonium salt of mandelic acid, used orally as a urinary anti-infective.
**a. molybdate** [USP], the hexaammonium salt of molybdic acid, used as a supplement in parenteral feeding solutions and as a reagent.
**a. muriate,** a. chloride.
**a. nitrate,** $NH_4NO_3$; a chemical used in fertilizers, in matches, and in the manufacture of nitrous oxide gas and freezing compounds; it may accumulate in plants and lead to nitrite poisoning in livestock.
**a. oxalate,** $NH_4OOCCOONH_4$; used as a test solution.
**a. phosphate** [NF], the diammonium salt of phosphoric acid, $(NH_4)_2HPO_4$, used as a buffering agent in pharmaceutical preparations; formerly used as a urinary acidifier in the treatment of gout and rheumatism.
**a. purpurate,** murexide.
**a. tartrate,** a white crystalline compound soluble in water and alcohol; used in Cohn's solution.

**am·mo·ni·uria** (ə-mo″ne-u′re-ə) an excess of ammonia in the urine.

**am·mo·nol·y·sis** (am″o-nol′ĭ-sis) a process analogous to hydrolysis, but in which ammonia takes the place of water, resulting in attachment of (or replacement by) an amino group, $NH_2$.

**am·mo·no·tel·ic** (ə-mo″no-tel′ik) [*ammonia* + Gr. *telikos* belonging to the completion, or end] having ammonia as the chief excretory product of nitrogen metabolism, as in fresh-water fishes.

**Am·mo·sper·moph·i·lus** (am″o-spər-mof′ĭ-ləs) the antelope squirrels, a genus found in the deserts of western North America. *A. leucu′rus* is a natural host of a plague-transmitting flea.

**am·ne·sia** (am-ne′zhə) [Gr. *amnēsia* forgetfulness] [MeSH: Amnesia] lack or loss of memory; inability to remember past experiences.
**anterograde a.,** impairment of memory for events occurring after the onset of amnesia; inability to form new memories. Cf. *retrograde a.*
**circumscribed a.,** loss of memory for all events during a discrete, specific period of time. Called also *localized a.*
**continuous a.,** loss of memory for all events after a certain time, continuing up to and including the present.
**dissociative a.,** [DSM-IV], a dissociative disorder characterized by a sudden loss of memory for important personal information, usually circumscribed or selective amnesia, rarely generalized or continuous amnesia, and which is not due to the direct effects of a psychogenic substance or a general medical condition; the amnesia may follow severe psychological stress or may be an unconscious response to internal conflicts or an intolerable life situation; complete recovery of memory almost always occurs.
**episodic a.,** amnesia for a particular episode or a small area of experience.
**generalized a.,** loss of memory encompassing the individual's entire life.
**infantile a.,** the usual inability to recall the events of infancy and early childhood.
**lacunar a.,** partial loss of memory; amnesia for certain isolated experiences.
**localized a.,** 1. circumscribed a. 2. lacunar a.
**neurological a.,** that caused by disease of or injury to the nervous system.
**postconcussional a.,** amnesia resulting from a concussion of the brain.
**posthypnotic a.,** a directed forgetfulness of the subject for experiences undergone while in the hypnotic state.
**post-traumatic a.,** amnesia resulting from concussion or other head trauma. Called also *traumatic a.* See *amnestic syndrome,* under *syndrome.*
**psychogenic a.,** dissociative a.
**retrograde a.,** inability to recall events that occurred before the actual onset of amnesia; loss of memories of past events. Cf. *anterograde a.*
**selective a.,** loss of memory for a group of related events but not for other events occurring during the same period of time.
**tactile a.,** astereognosis.
**transient global a.,** an episode of short-term memory loss, usually nonrecurrent, and lasting a few hours, without other signs or symptoms of neurological impairment; the cause is usually unknown but may occasionally be an ischemic or epileptic attack.
**traumatic a.,** post-traumatic a.
**visual a.,** alexia.

**am·ne·si·ac** (am-ne′se-ak) a person affected with amnesia.

**am·ne·sic** (am-ne′sik) affected with or characterized by amnesia.

**am·nes·tic** (am-nes′tik) 1. amnesic. 2. causing amnesia.

**Am·nes·tro·gen** (am-nes′tro-jen) trademark for a preparation of esterified estrogens.

**amni(o)-** [*amnion,* q.v.] a combining form denoting relationship to the amnion.

**am·nio·cele** (am′ne-o-sēl) omphalocele.

**am·nio·cen·te·sis** (am″ne-o-sen-te′sis) [MeSH: Amniocentesis] percutaneous transabdominal puncture of the uterus to obtain amniotic fluid.

**am·nio·cho·ri·al** (am″ne-o-kor′e-əl) pertaining to the amnion and chorion.

**am·nio·cyte** (am′ne-o-sīt) a cell of fetal origin obtained in an amniotic fluid specimen.

**am·nio·gen·e·sis** (am″ne-o-jen′ə-sis) [*amnio-* + *-genesis*] the development of the amnion.

**am·ni·og·ra·phy** (am″ne-og′rə-fe) [*amnio-* + *-graphy*] radiography of the gravid uterus after injection of opaque media into the amniotic fluid, outlining the amniotic cavity and fetus.

**am·nio·in·fu·sion** (am″ne-o-in-fu′zhən) introduction of solutions into the amnion, such as to induce abortion, to counteract the late decelerations caused by cord compression, or to dilute thick meconium.

**am·ni·on** (am′ne-on) [Gr. "bowl"; "membrane enveloping the fetus"] [MeSH: Amnion] the thin but tough extraembryonic membrane of reptiles, birds, and mammals that lines the chorion and contains the embryo and later the fetus, with the amniotic fluid around it; in mammals it is derived from trophoblast by folding or splitting. See also *amniotic sac,* under *sac.*

**a. nodo′sum,** multiple focal lesions of the amnion, consisting of masses of adherent amniotic squamae partially invaded by amniotic mesoderm; a nodular condition of the fetal surface of the amniotic membrane.

**am·ni·on·ic** (am″ne-on′ik) amniotic.

**am·ni·o·ni·tis** (am″ne-o-ni′tis) inflammation of the amnion.

**Am·ni·o·plas·tin** (am-ne-o-plas′tin) trademark for the dried and sterilized amnionic membrane applied to prevent adhesions after craniotomy.

**am·ni·or·rhea** (am″ne-o-re′ə) [*amnio-* + *-rrhea*] the escape of the amniotic fluid.

**am·ni·or·rhex·is** (am″ne-o-rek′sis) [*amnio-* + *-rrhexis*] rupture of the amnion.

**am·nio·scope** (am′ne-o-skōp″) an endoscope used in amnioscopy.

**am·ni·os·co·py** (am″ne-os′kə-pe) [MeSH: Amnioscopy] direct observation of the fetus and the color and amount of the amniotic fluid by means of a specially designed endoscope inserted through the uterine cervix.

**Am·ni·o·ta** (am-ne-o′tə) a major group of vertebrates comprising those which develop an amnion, including reptiles, birds, and mammals; opposed to Anamniota.

**am·ni·ote** (am′ne-ōt) any animal or group belonging to the Amniota.

**am·ni·ot·ic** (am″ne-ot′ik) pertaining to or developing an amnion.

**Am·ni·o·tin** (am-ni′o-tin) trademark for estrogens derived from the urine of pregnant mares.

**am·ni·o·tome** (am′ne-ə-tōm″) [*amnio-* + *-tome*] an instrument for cutting the fetal membranes.

**am·ni·ot·o·my** (am″ne-ot′ə-me) [*amnio-* + *-tomy*] deliberate rupture of the fetal membranes to induce labor.

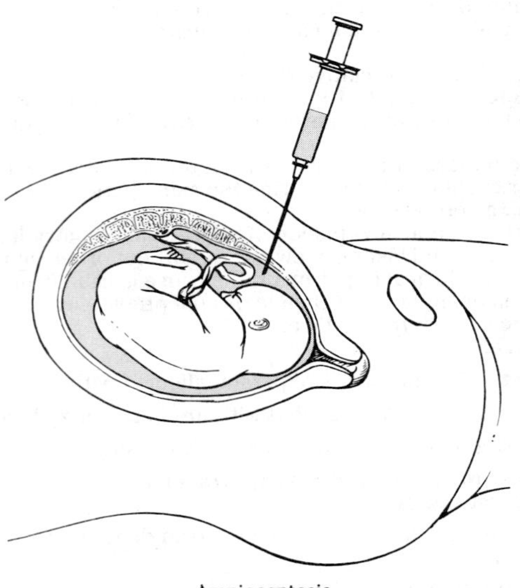

Amniocentesis.

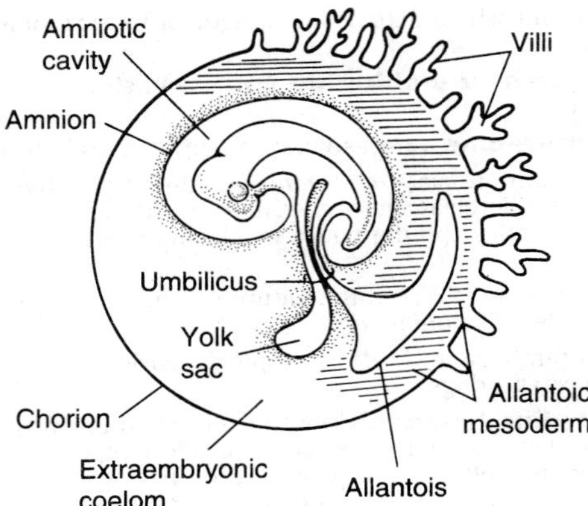


Amnion, chorion, and other embryonic membranes surrounding the embryo of a placental mammal.

**amo·bar·bi·tal** (am″o-bahr′bĭ-təl) [MeSH: Amobarbital] an intermediate-acting barbiturate used orally as a sedative and hypnotic; called also *amylobarbitone.*

**a. sodium** [USP], the monosodium salt of amobarbital, administered orally, intravenously, and intramuscularly as a hypnotic and sedative and intravenously in macroanalysis.

**a. hydrochloride** [USP], the dihydrated dihydrochloride salt of amodiaquine, having the same actions and uses as the base; administered orally.

**am·o·di·a·quine** (am″o-di′ə-kwin) [USP] [MeSH: Amodiaquine] a 4-aminoquinoline compound with anti-inflammatory properties, used for the suppression and treatment of malaria, for the treatment of giardiasis and extraintestinal amebiasis, for suppression of lupus erythematosus, and as an anti-inflammatory in the treatment of rheumatoid arthritis; administered orally.

**amoeb-** [L., from Gr. *amoibē* change] a combining form denoting relationship to an ameba. See also words beginning *ameb(i)(o)-.*

**Amoe·ba** (ə-me′bə) [L. from Gr. *amoibē* change] [MeSH: Amoeba] a genus of ameboid protozoa (suborder Tubulina, order Amoebida), characterized by the presence of a vesicular nucleus, usually one contractile vacuole, and lobopodia. Most are free living. Those parasitic in humans and once included in this genus have been assigned to other genera.

**A. pro′teus,** a species found in fresh water and widely studied in the laboratory.

**amoe·ba** (ə-me′bə) [MeSH: Amoeba] ameba.

**Amoe·bi·da** (ə-me′bid-ə) [MeSH: Amoebida] an order of ameboid, largely freshwater protozoa (subclass Gymnamoebia, class Lobosea) containing all of the amebae parasitic in animals, including humans, most of which are nonpathogenic or only mildly so. They are typically uninucleate and have mitochondria but no flagellate stage. It comprises five suborders: Tubulina, Thecina, Flabellina, Conopodina, and Acanthopodina.

**Amoe·bo·tae·nia** (ə-me″bo-te′ne-ə) a genus of tapeworms of the family Dipylidiidae. *A. cunea′ta* is found in the intestines of fowls and causes hemorrhagic enteritis.

**amoe·bu·la** (ə-me′bu-lə) [dim. of *amoeba*] amebula.

**amok** (ə-mok′) [Malay "furious attack"] a culture-specific syndrome first reported in the Malay people, almost always male, consisting of a sudden outburst of indiscriminate aggressive or homicidal fury provoked by a perceived slight or insult or possibly unprovoked (running amuck). Spelled also *amuck.*

**am·o·py·ro·quin hy·dro·chlo·ride** (am-o-pi′ro-kwin) an antimalarial drug.

**amorph** (a′morf) see *silent gene,* under *gene.*

**amor·phia** (ə-mor′fe-ə) [*a-*[1] + *morph-* + *-ia*] the fact or quality of being amorphous.

**amor·phism** (ə-mor′fiz-əm) amorphia.

**amor·pho·syn·the·sis** (a-mor″fo-sin′thə-sis) [*a-*[1] + *morpho-* + *synthesis*] defective perception of somatic sensations from one side of the body, such as astereognosis or lack of position sense on one side. It may be accompanied by a generalized faulty awareness of spatial relationships and is often a sign of a parietal lobe lesion. Cf. *asomatognosia.*

**amor·phous** (ə-mor′fəs) [*a-*[1] + *morph-* + *-ous*] 1. having no definite form; shapeless. 2. having no specific orientation of atoms. 3. in pharmacy, not crystallized.

**amor·phus** (ə-mor′fəs) [*a* neg. + Gr. *morphē* form] a shapeless malformed fetus. See also *holoacardius amorphus.*

**am·o·site** (a′mə-sīt″) a mineral in the amphibole class of asbestos, used industrially but now restricted because it causes asbestosis and certain forms of cancer such as mesotheliomas. Called also *brown asbestos.*

**Amoss' sign** (a′məs) [Harold Lindsay *Amoss,* American physician, 1886–1956] see under *sign.*

**amo·tio** (ə-mo′she-o) gen. *amotio′nis,* pl. *amotio′nes* [L., from *amovēre* to move away from] a removing.
**a. re′tinae,** detachment of the retina.

**amox·a·pine** (ə-moks′ə-pēn) [USP] [MeSH: Amoxapine] a tricyclic antidepressant of the dibenzoxazepine class used for the treatment of symptoms of depression in neurotic and psychotic depressive disorders and endogenous and reactive depression; administered orally.

**amox·i·cil·lin** (ə-mok″sĭ-sil′in) [USP] [MeSH: Amoxicillin] a semi-synthetic derivative of ampicillin effective against a broad spectrum of gram-positive and gram-negative bacteria; used especially in the treatment of infections due to susceptible strains of *Haemophilus influenzae, Escherichia coli, Proteus mirabilis, Neisseria gonorrhoeae,* streptococci (including *Streptococcus faecalis* and *S. pneumoniae*), and nonpenicillinase-producing staphylococci. It is administered orally.

**Amox·il** (ə-mok′sil) trademark for preparations of amoxicillin.

**AMP** adenosine monophosphate.
**3′,5′-AMP, cyclic AMP,** cyclic adenosine monophosphate.

**amp** former abbreviation for *ampere.*

**AMP de·am·i·nase** (de-am′ĭ-nās) [EC 3.5.4.6] [MeSH: AMP Deaminase] an enzyme of the hydrolase class that catalyzes the deamination of AMP to form inosine monophosphate. Isoenzyme A (myoadenylate deaminase) is present in large amounts in muscle tissue and is a major source of ammonium ions during muscle contraction. Deficiency of this isoenzyme, an autosomal recessive trait, is characterized by muscle fatigue following exercise. Two additional isoenzymes have been identified: isoenzyme B, found in liver, kidney, and testes, and isoenzyme C, found in heart muscle. Called also *adenylate deaminase.*

**am·per·age** (am′pər-əj) the amount of electric current expressed in amperes or milliamperes.

**am·pere** (am′pēr) [André M. *Ampère,* 1775–1836] the SI unit of electric current, defined as the constant current that if maintained in two parallel straight conductors (of infinite length and negligible circular cross section) separated by a distance of 1 meter in a vacuum, produces a force between the wires of $2 \times 10^{-7}$ neutrons per meter of length; it is equivalent to one coulomb per second. Symbol A. Formerly abbreviated amp.

**Am·phe·drox·yn** (am″fə-drok′sin) trademark for a preparation of methamphetamine.

**am·phet·a·mine** (am-fet′ə-mēn″) [MeSH: Amphetamine] 1. racemic amphetamine, (±)-α-methylphenethylamine, a sympathomimetic amine that has a stimulating effect on both the central and peripheral nervous systems. It relaxes both systolic and diastolic blood pressure and bronchial muscle, contracts the sphincter of the urinary bladder, and depresses the appetite. Abuse of this drug and its salts may lead to dependence, characterized by strong psychic dependence, to marked tolerance. Abrupt withdrawal can cause severe fatigue, mental depression, and abnormalities in the electroencephalogram. 2. [pl.] a group of closely related compounds having similar actions, including amphetamine and its salts, dextroamphetamine, and methamphetamine.
**a. aspartate,** the aspartate salt of amphetamine, having the same actions and uses as the sulfate salt; administered orally.
**a. sulfate** [USP], the sulfate salt of amphetamine, having the same actions as the base, used orally in the treatment of narcolepsy and attention-deficit/hyperactivity disorder; it has been used as an anorexiant in the treatment of obesity but is no longer recommended for this purpose.

**amph(i)-** [Gr. *amphi* on both sides] a prefix meaning on both sides; around or about; double.

**am·phi·ar·thro·di·al** (am″fe-ahr-thro′de-əl) pertaining to amphiarthrosis.

**am·phi·ar·thro·sis** (am″fe-ahr-thro′sis) [*amphi-* + *arthrosis*] junctura cartilaginea.

**am·phi·as·ter** (am′fe-as″tər) [*amphi-* + *aster*] the figure of achromatin fibers formed in karyokinesis, consisting of two asters joined by a spindle; called also *diaster.*

**Am·phib·ia** (am-fib′e-ə) [*amphi-* + Gr. *bios* life] [MeSH: Amphibia] a class of vertebrate animals that breathe by means of gills in the larval state, but after metamorphosis generally breathe by means of lungs; orders include Anura (frogs and toads) and Caudata (salamanders).

**am·phib·i·ous** (am-fib′e-əs) capable of living both on land and in water.

**am·phi·blas·tic** (am″fe-blas′tik) [*amphi-* + *blast-* + *-ic*] denoting the complete but unequal cleavage of a telolecithal egg.

**am·phi·blas·tu·la** (am″fĭ-blas′tu-lə) [*amphi-* + *blastula*] a blastula with unequal blastomeres.

**am·phi·bol·ic** (am″fĭ-bol′ik) 1. uncertain; vacillating; of doubtful prognosis. See under *stage.* 2. See under *pathway.*

**am·phi·ce·lous** (am″fe-se′lus) [*amphi-* + Gr. *koilos* hollow] concave on both sides; said of the vertebral centra of certain cold-blooded vertebrates. Called also *dicelous.*

**am·phi·cen·tric** (am″fĭ-sen′trik) [*amphi-* + *centric*] beginning and ending in the same vessel, as a branch of a rete mirabile.

**am·phi·chro·ic** (am″fĭ-kro′ik) [*amphi-* + Gr. *chrōma* color] exhibiting two colors; affecting both red and blue litmus.

**am·phi·chro·mat·ic** (am″fĭ-kro-mat′ik) amphichroic.

**am·phi·cre·at·i·nine** (am″fĭ-kre-at′ĭ-nin) [*amphi-* + *creatinine*] a poisonous leukomaine, $C_9H_{19}N_7O_4$, from muscle.

**am·phi·cro·ic** (am″fĭ-kro′ik) [*amphi-* + Gr. *krouein* to test] amphichroic.

**am·phi·cyte** (am′fĭ-sīt) [*amphi-* + *-cyte*] a satellite cell, def. 1.

**am·phi·cyt·u·la** (am″fĭ-sit′u-lə) [*amphi-* + *cytula*] a fertilized telolecithal ovum.

**am·phi·di·ar·thro·sis** (am″fĭ-di″ahr-thro′sis) [*amphi-* + *diarthrosis*] a joint having the nature of both a ginglymus and articulatio plana (arthrodia), as the articulation of the mandible.

**am·phi·gas·tru·la** (am″fĭ-gas′troo-lə) [*amphi-* + *gastrula*] a gastrula composed of cells unequal in size in its upper and lower hemispheres.

**am·phi·ge·net·ic** (am″fĭ-jə-net′ik) produced by means of both sexes, as amphigenetic reproduction.

**am·phi·gon·a·dism** (am″fĭ-gon′ə-diz-əm) 1. possession of both ovarian and testicular tissue by the same animal. 2. true hermaphroditism.

**am·phig·o·ny** (am-fig′o-ne) sexual reproduction.

**am·phi·kar·y·on** (am″fĭ-kar′e-on) [*amphi-* + *karyon*] a diploid nucleus.

**am·phi·leu·ke·mic** (am″fĭ-loo-ke′mik) [*amphi-* + *leukemic*] showing leukemic changes which vary in degree with the changes in the organ.

**Am·phim·er·us** (am-fim′ər-əs) a genus of trematodes. *A. nover′ca* is a biliary-duct parasite of dogs and foxes and occasionally of hogs and man. *A. pseudofeli′neus* infects cats and coyotes in the central United States.

**am·phi·mor·u·la** (am″fĭ-mor′u-lə) [*amphi-* + *morula*] the morula resulting from unequal cleavage, the cells of the two hemispheres being of unequal size.

**am·phi·nu·cle·us** (am″fĭ-noo′kle-əs) [*amphi-* + *nucleus*] a nucleus that consists of a single body made of spindle fibers and centrosome, around which the chromatin is massed; it is the ordinary form of protozoan nucleus. Called also *centronucleus.*

**am·phi·path** (am′fĭ-path) a molecule showing amphipathic properties.

**am·phi·path·ic** (am″fĭ-path′ik) of or relating to molecules containing groups with characteristically different properties, e.g., both hydrophilic and hydrophobic properties.

**am·phi·py·re·nin** (am″fĭ-pi′rə-nin) [*amphi-* + Gr. *pyrēn* stone of a fruit] the substance of the nuclear membrane of a cell.

**am·phi·reg·u·lin** (am″fe-reg′u-lin) a 78–amino acid glycoprotein,

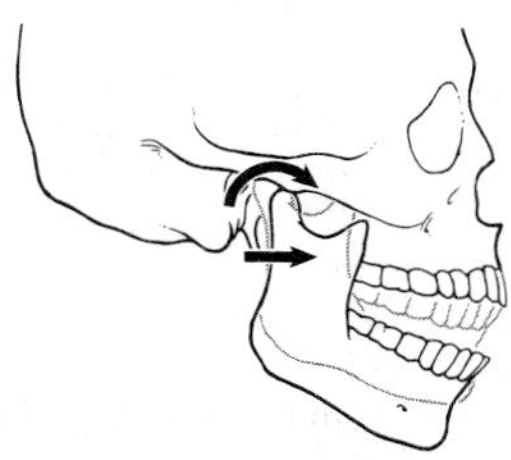

Amphidiarthrosis, exemplified by the temporomandibular joint. Arrows show the gliding component (arthrodia or articulatio plana) and hinge component (ginglymus) of movement.

originally identified in cultures from human breast carcinoma cells; it is 38 per cent identical with epidermal growth factor and can inhibit the growth of several carcinoma cell lines while stimulating the proliferation of normal cells.

**Am·phis·to·ma** (am-fis'tə-mə) [*amphi-* + *stoma*] a genus of parasitic trematode worms, many species of which have been reassigned to other genera.
**A. co'nicum,** *Paramphistomum cervi.*
**A. ho'minis,** *Gastrodiscoides hominis.*
**A. watso'ni,** *Watsonius watsoni.*

**am·phis·tome** (am-fis'tōm) paramphistome.

**am·phi·sto·mi·a·sis** (am″fĭ-sto-mi'ə-sis) paramphistomiasis.

**am·phi·tene** (am'fĭ-tēn) zygotene.

**am·phi·the·a·ter** (am″fĭ-the'ə-tər) an operating room or lecture room with seats arranged in tiers for students or spectators.

**am·phit·ri·chous** (am-fit'rĭ-kəs) [*amphi-* + *trich-* + *-ous*] having a single flagellum, or a single tuft of flagella, at each end; said of a bacterial cell. See *flagellum.*

**am·phit·y·py** (am-fit'ĭ-pe) the condition of showing both types.

**ampho-** [Gr. *amphō* both] a prefix meaning both.

**am·pho·chro·ma·to·phil** (am″fo-kro'mə-tə-fil) 1. amphophilic cell. 2. amphophilic.

**am·pho·chro·mo·phil** (am″fo-kro'mə-fil) [*ampho-* + *chromophil*] 1. amphophilic cell. 2. amphophilic.

**am·pho·cyte** (am'fo-sīt) amphophilic cell.

**am·pho·di·plo·pia** (am″fo-dĭ-plo'pe-ə) [*ampho-* + *diplopia*] double vision in both eyes.

**am·pho·gen·ic** (am″fo-jen'ik) [*ampho-* + *-genic*] producing offspring of both sexes.

**Am·pho·jel** (am'fo-jəl) trademark for preparations of aluminum hydroxide gel.

**am·pho·lyte** (am'fo-līt) [*ampho-* + *electrolyte*] an amphoteric electrolyte.

**am·pho·my·cin** (am-fo-mi'sin) an antibiotic substance produced by *Streptomyces canus.*

**am·pho·phil** (am'fo-fil) 1. amphophilic cell. 2. amphophilic.

**am·pho·phile** (am'fo-fīl″) 1. amphophil. 2. amphophilic cell.

**am·pho·phil·ic** (am-fo-fil'ik) [*ampho-* + *-philic*] stainable with either acid or basic dyes; see also *amphophilic cell,* under *cell.* Called also *amphophil, amphophile,* and *amphophilous.*
**a.-basophil,** staining with both acid and basic stains, but having a greater affinity for basic ones.
**gram-a.,** tending to stain both positive and negative with Gram stain.
**a.-oxyphil,** staining with both acid and basic dyes, but having a greater affinity for the acid ones.

**am·phoph·i·lous** (am-fof'ĭ-ləs) amphophilic.

**am·phor·ic** (am-for'ik) [L. *amphoricus,* from L. *amphora,* Gr. *amphoreus* jar] 1. pertaining to a bottle. 2. said of certain high-pitched auscultatory sounds resembling the sound made by blowing across the mouth of a bottle.

**am·pho·ric·i·ty** (am″fə-ris'ĭ-te) the quality of being amphoric; see *cavernous voice,* under *voice.*

**am·pho·ril·o·quy** (am″fə-ril'o-kwe) [L. *amphora* jar + *loqui* to speak] cavernous voice.

**am·pho·roph·o·ny** (am″fə-rof'ə-ne) [Gr. *amphoreus* jar + *phonē* voice] cavernous voice.

**am·pho·ter·ic** (am-fə-ter'ik) [Gr. *amphoteros* pertaining to both] having opposite characters; capable of acting either as an acid or as a base; combining with both acids and bases; affecting both red and blue litmus.

**am·pho·ter·i·cin B** (am″fə-ter'ĭ-sin) [USP] [MeSH: Amphotericin B] one of two antifungal antibiotics, the other designated amphotericin A (not used clinically), derived from a strain of *Streptomyces nodosus* and effective against a wide range of fungi and against some species of *Leishmania.* It is used intravenously in the treatment of progressive, potentially fatal fungal infections and as a secondary drug in the treatment of mucocutaneous leishmaniasis and topically in the treatment of superficial candidiasis.

**am·pho·ter·ic·i·ty** (am″fə-tər-is'ĭ-te) amphoterism.

**am·pho·ter·ism** (am-fo'tər-iz-əm) the condition or quality of possessing both basic and acid properties.

**am·phot·ero·di·plo·pia** (am-fot″ər-o-dĭ-plŏ'pe-ə) [Gr. *amphoteros* both + *diplopia*] amphodiplopia.

**am·phot·er·ous** (am-fot'ər-əs) amphoteric.

**am·phot·o·ny** (am-fot'ə-ne) [*ampho-* + Gr. *tonos* tension] a condition in which both sympathicotonia and vagotony is said to exist; hypertonia of the entire sympathetic nervous system.

**amp·i·cil·lin** (amp″ĭ-sil'in) [USP] [MeSH: Ampicillin] a semisynthetic, acid-resistant, penicillinase-sensitive penicillin, effective against a broad spectrum of gram-positive and gram-negative bacteria, used in the treatment of infections caused by susceptible organisms; administered orally.
**a. sodium** [USP], the monosodium salt of ampicillin, having the same actions and uses as the base; administered intramuscularly or intravenously.

**AMP ki·nase** (ki'nās) adenylate kinase.

**am·plex·a·tion** (am″plek-sa'shən) [L. *amplexus* embrace] treatment of fractured clavicle by an apparatus which fixes the shoulder and embraces the chest and neck.

**am·plex·us** (am-plek'səs) [L.] an embrace, as in the sexual clasping of the female by the male frog; see *pseudocopulation.*

**am·pli·fi·ca·tion** (am″plĭ-fĭ-ka'shən) [L. *amplifica'tio*] the process of making larger, as the increase of an auditory or visual stimulus, as a means of improving its perception.
**gene a.,** a process by which the number of copies of a gene is increased in certain cells because extra copies of DNA are made in response to certain signals of cell development or of stress from the environment. In humans this process is seen most often in malignant cells.
**image a.,** amplification of an image by means of an electron-image or electron multiplier tube.

**am·pli·fi·er** (am'plĭ-fi″ər) [MeSH: Amplifiers] an electronic device that increases the strength of an input signal, or an apparatus for increasing the magnification of a microscope.

**am·pli·tude** (am'plə-to̅o̅d) [L. *amplus* full] 1. largeness or fullness; wideness or breadth of range or extent. 2. in a phenomenon that occurs in waves, the maximal deviation of a wave from the baseline, measured as either *peak a.* or *peak-to-peak a.*
**a. of accommodation,** range of accommodation; see under *range.*
**a. of convergence,** the difference in the power required to turn the eyes from their far point to their near point of convergence.
**peak a.,** the maximal deviation of a wave in just one direction from the baseline.
**peak-to-peak a.,** the sum of the peak amplitude in a positive direction and that in a negative direction from the baseline.

**am·poule** (am'pūl) ampule.

**Am·prol** (am'prol) trademark for a preparation of amprolium.

**am·pro·li·um** (am-pro'le-əm) [USP] [MeSH: Amprolium] a thiamine analogue used in veterinary medicine for the prevention and treatment of coccidiosis.

**Am·pro·vine** (am'pro-vēn) trademark for a preparation of amprolium.

**am·pul** (am'pūl) ampule.

**am·pule** (am'pūl) [Fr. *ampoule*] a small glass or plastic container capable of being sealed so as to preserve its contents in a sterile condition; used principally for containing sterile parenteral solutions.

**am·pul·la** (am-pul'ə) gen. and pl. *ampul'lae* [L. "a jug"] [TA] a general term used in anatomical nomenclature to designate a flasklike dilatation of a tubular structure.
**biliaropancreatic a.,** ampulla hepatopancreatica.
**a. biliaropancrea'tica,** TA alternative for ampulla hepatopancreatica.
**a. canali'culi lacrima'lis** [TA], ampulla of lacrimal canaliculus: a dilatation of a lacrimal canaliculus just before it opens into the lacrimal sac; called also *a. ductus lacrimalis.*
**a. chy'li,** cisterna chyli.
**a. duc'tus deferen'tis** [TA], the enlarged and tortuous distal end of the ductus deferens; called also *Henle's a.* and *a. of vas deferens.*
**a. duc'tus lacrima'lis,** a. canaliculi lacrimalis.
**duodenal a., a. duode'ni** [TA], duodenal cap: the superior part of the duodenum, as seen radiographically after a barium meal. A true duodenal ampulla is seen in some domestic mammals.
**Henle's a.,** a. ductus deferentis.
**hepatopancreatic a., a. hepatopancrea'tica** [TA], the dilatation formed by junction of the common bile and the pancreatic ducts proximal to their opening into the lumen of the duodenum; called also *biliaropancreatic a., ampulla biliaropancreatica* [TA alternative], and *a. of Vater.*
**a. of lacrimal canaliculus,** a. canaliculi lacrimalis.
**ampul'lae lacti'ferae,** sinus lactiferi.
**Lieberkühn's a.,** the termination of a lacteal in an intestinal villus.
**ampul'lae membrana'ceae,** membranous ampullae: the dilatations at one end of each of the three membranous semicircular ducts, each named according to the duct of which it forms a part.
**a. membrana'cea ante'rior** [TA], anterior membranous ampulla:

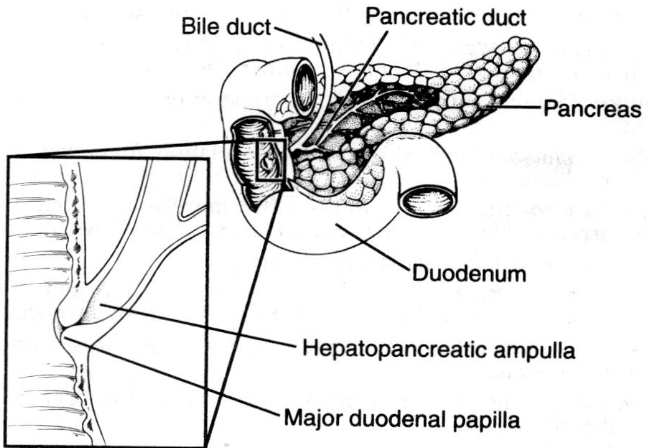


Ampulla hepatopancreatica (hepatopancreatic ampulla), receiving the common bile and pancreatic ducts and entering the duodenum at the major duodenal papilla.

the dilatation at the end of the anterior membranous semicircular duct.
**a. membrana'cea latera'lis** [TA], lateral membranous ampulla: the dilatation at the end of the lateral membranous semicircular duct.
**a. membrana'cea poste'rior** [TA], posterior membranous ampulla: the dilatation at the end of the posterior membranous semicircular duct.
**membranous a., anterior,** a. membranacea anterior.
**membranous a., lateral,** a. membranacea lateralis.
**membranous a., posterior,** a. membranacea posterior.
**ampul'lae os'seae,** osseous ampullae: the dilatations at one of the ends of the bony semicircular canals, each named according to the canal of which it forms a part, and lodging the correspondingly named ampulla of a semicircular duct.
**a. os'sea ante'rior** [TA], the dilatation at one end of the anterior semicircular canal; see *ampullae osseae.*
**a. os'sea latera'lis** [TA], the dilatation at one end of the lateral semicircular canal; see *ampullae osseae.*
**a. os'sea poste'rior** [TA], the dilatation at one end of the posterior semicircular canal; see *ampullae osseae.*
**phrenic a.,** the dilatation at the lower end of the esophagus.
**rectal a., a. rec'ti** [TA], the dilated portion of the rectum just proximal to the anal canal.
**a. of Thoma,** one of the small terminal expansions of an interlobar artery in the pulp of the spleen.
**a. tu'bae uteri'nae** [TA], ampulla of uterine tube: the thin-walled, almost muscle-free, midregion of the uterine tube; its mucosa is greatly plicated.
**a. of vas deferens,** a. ductus deferentis.
**a. of Vater,** a. hepatopancreatica.

**am·pul·lae** (am-pul'e) [L.] genitive and plural of *ampulla.*

**am·pul·lar** (am-pul'ər) pertaining to an ampulla, especially to the ampulla hepatopancreatica.

**am·pul·la·ry** (am'pu-la"re) ampullar.

**am·pul·late** (am-pul'āt) flask-shaped.

**am·pul·li·tis** (am"pul-li'tis) inflammation of an ampulla, especially of the ampulla ductus deferentis.

**am·pul·lu·la** (am-pul'oo-lə) [L.] any minute ampulla, like many of those of the lymphatic and lacteal vessels.

**am·pu·ta·tion** (am"pu-ta'shən) [L. *amputare* to cut off, or to prune] [MeSH: Amputation] the removal of a limb or other appendage or outgrowth of the body.
**above-elbow a.,** amputation of the upper limb between the elbow and the shoulder.
**above-knee (A-K) a.,** amputation of the leg between the knee and the hip; the femur may be divided in the supracondylar region *(long above-knee amputation),* at midthigh, or high on the thigh. Called also *transfemoral a.*
**Alanson's a.,** circular amputation, the stump being shaped like a hollow cone.
**Alouette's a.,** amputation at the hip, with a semicircular outer flap to the great trochanter and a large internal flap from within outward; called also *Alouette's operation.*
**aperiosteal a.,** amputation with complete removal of the periosteum from the end of the stump of the bone; called also *Bunge's a.*
**Béclard's a.,** hip disarticulation with cutting of the posterior flap first.
**below-elbow a.,** amputation of the upper limb between the wrist and the elbow.
**below-knee (B-K) a.,** amputation of the lower leg between the ankle and the knee; called *long below-knee* when in the distal third of the tibia and *short below-knee* when in the proximal third of the tibia. Called also *transtibial a.*
**Bier's a.,** osteoplastic amputation of the leg with a bone flap cut out of the tibia and fibula above the stump; called also *Bier's operation.*
**Bunge's a.,** aperiosteal a.
**Callander's a.,** a tenoplastic knee disarticulation with long anterior and posterior flaps, the patella being removed to leave a fossa for the end of the divided femur.
**Carden's a.,** a single flap above-knee amputation done just above the knee.
**central a.,** one in which the scar is situated at or near the center of the stump.
**chop a.,** guillotine a.
**Chopart's a.,** amputation of the foot, with the calcaneus, talus, and other parts of the tarsus being retained; called also *mediotarsal a.*
**cinematic a., cineplastic a.,** kineplasty.
**circular a.,** one performed by means of a single flap and by a circular cut in a direction vertical to the long axis of a limb.
**closed a.,** one in which flaps are made from the skin and subcutaneous tissue and sutured over the end of the bone; called also *flap a.*
**coat-sleeve a.,** a circular amputation, with a single skin flap made very long, the end being closed with a tape.
**a. in contiguity,** an amputation at a joint.
**a. in continuity,** an amputation elsewhere than at a joint.
**cutaneous a.,** amputation in which the flaps are composed entirely of skin.
**Dieffenbach's a.,** see under *operation,* def. 1.
**double-flap a.,** one in which two flaps are formed.
**Dupuytren's a.,** shoulder disarticulation.
**eccentric a.,** one in which the scar is not at the center of the stump.
**elliptic a.,** one in which the cut has an elliptic outline on account of the oblique direction of the incision.
**Farabeuf's a.,** amputation of the leg, with a large external flap.
**flap a.,** closed a.
**flapless a.,** guillotine a.
**forequarter a.,** interscapulothoracic a.
**Gritti's a.,** knee disarticulation using the patella as an osteoplastic flap over the end of the femur. Called also *Gritti's operation.*
**Gritti-Stokes a.,** a modification of Gritti's amputation, using an oval anterior flap; called also *Stokes' a.* or *operation.*
**guillotine a.,** rapid amputation of a limb by a circular sweep of the knife and a cut of the saw, the entire cross-section being left open for dressing; done when primary closure of the stump is contraindicated, owing to the possibility of recurrent or developing infection. Called also *chop a., flapless a.,* and *open a.*
**Guyon's a.,** below-knee amputation just above the malleoli.
**Hancock's a.,** a modification of Pirogoff's amputation, a part of the astragalus (talus) being retained in the flap, the lower surface being sawed off, and the cut surface of the calcaneus being brought into contact with it; called also *Hancock's operation.*
**Hey's a.,** disarticulation of the tarsus from the metatarsus with removal of a part of the medial cuneiform bone. Called also *Hey's operation.* Cf. *Lisfranc's a.*
**hindquarter a.,** hemipelvectomy.
**interilioabdominal a., interinnominoabdominal a.,** amputation of an entire lower limb, including the whole or part of the hip bone; called also *hindquarter a.*
**interpelviabdominal a.,** hemipelvectomy.
**interscapulothoracic a.,** amputation of the upper extremity, including the scapula and the clavicle; called also *forequarter a.*
**Jaboulay's a.,** hemipelvectomy.
**kineplastic a.,** kineplasty.
**Kirk's a.,** a tenoplastic above-knee amputation done just above the femoral condyles, with the tendon of the quadriceps femoris muscle sutured over the end of the divided femur.
**Langenbeck's a.,** amputation in which the flaps are cut from without inward.
**Larrey's a.,** shoulder disarticulation with an incision extending from the acromion about three inches down the arm, splitting the deltoid muscle, and from this point going around the arm to the center of the axilla; called also *Larrey's operation.*
**Le Fort's a.,** a modification of Pirogoff's amputation in which the calcaneus is sawed through horizontally instead of vertically.
**linear a.,** amputation by a simple straight division of all the tissues.
**Lisfranc's a.,** 1. amputation of the foot between the tarsus and the metatarsus. 2. shoulder disarticulation. Called also *Lisfranc's operation.*
**Mackenzie's a.,** amputation like that of Syme except that the flap is taken from the inner side of the ankle.
**Maisonneuve's a.,** amputation by breaking the bone, followed by cutting of the soft parts.
**major a.,** amputation of a leg above the ankle or of an arm above the wrist.
**Malgaigne's a.,** subastragalar a.
**mediotarsal a.,** Chopart's a.

**minor a.**, amputation of a small part, as of a finger or toe.
**mixed a.**, that which is performed by a combination of the circular and flap methods.
**musculocutaneous a.**, one in which the flap consists of muscle and skin.
**oblique a.**, oval a.
**open a.**, guillotine a.
**osteoplastic a.**, one in which the two severed surfaces of bone are brought into contact so as to unite.
**oval a.**, one in which the incision consists of two reversed spirals; called also *oblique a.* and *loxotomy.*
**periosteoplastic a.**, subperiosteal a.
**phalangophalangeal a.**, amputation of a digit at a phalangeal joint.
**Pirogoff's a.**, amputation of the foot at the ankle, part of the calcaneus being left in the lower end of the stump.
**pulp a.**, pulpotomy.
**ray a.**, amputation of a metacarpal or metatarsal and all the phalangeal segments distal to it.
**racket a.**, one in which there is a single longitudinal incision continuous below with a spiral incision on each side of the limb.
**rectangular a.**, one with a long and a short rectangular skin flap, as in Teale's amputation.
**Ricard's a.**, amputation of the foot with disarticulation of the tibia from the calcaneus, astragalectomy, and the placing of the calcaneus in the mortise between the tibia and fibula.
**root a.**, excision of the root of a tooth; amputation of the root of a single-rooted tooth is called *apicoectomy,* and that of one root of a two-rooted mandibular tooth is *hemisectomy.* Called also *radiectomy* and *radisectomy.*
**spontaneous a.**, loss of a part which occurs without surgical intervention, as in leprosy, diabetes mellitus, and Buerger's disease.
**Stokes' a.**, Gritti-Stokes a.
**subastragalar a.**, amputation of the foot, leaving the astragalus (talus) in the lower end of the stump; called also *Malgaigne's a.*
**subperiosteal a.**, one in which the cut end of the bone is covered with a flap of periosteum; called also *periosteoplastic a.*
**Syme's a.**, ankle disarticulation with removal of both malleoli; called also *Syme's operation.*
**Teale's a.**, amputation with preservation of a long rectangular flap of muscle and integument on one side of the limb and a short rectangular flap on the other.
**transfemoral a.**, above-knee a.
**a. by transfixion**, one performed by thrusting a long knife through the limb and cutting the flaps from within outward.
**transmetatarsal a.**, amputation of the anterior part of the foot across the metatarsal bones.
**transtibial a.**, below-knee a.
**traumatic a.**, amputation of a part by accidental injury.
**Tripier's a.**, one like Chopart's, except that a part of the tarsus is removed.
**Vladimiroff-Mikulicz a.**, a type of osteoplastic amputation (q.v.) of the foot with incision of the calcaneus and talus.

**am·pu·tee** (am″pu-te′) [MeSH: Amputees] a person who has had one or more limbs amputated.

**am·ri·none** (am′rĭ-nōn) [USP] [MeSH: Amrinone] a phosphodiesterase inhibitor that prevents enzymatic breakdown of cyclic AMP by phosphodiesterase, having positive inotropic and vasodilator effects; used as a cardiotonic.
**a. lactate**, the lactate salt of amrinone, used for the short-term management of congestive heart failure in patients unresponsive to digitalis, diuretics, or vasodilators; administered intravenously.

**AMRL** Aerospace Medical Research Laboratories.

**AMS** American Meteorological Society.

**ams.** *a*mount of a *s*ubstance.

**AMSA** American Medical Student Association.

**am·sa·crine** (am′sə-krēn) [MeSH: Amsacrine] an antineoplastic drug that inhibits DNA synthesis, used to treat some forms of leukemia; administered intravenously.

**Am·sler's charts, marker** (ahm′zlərz) [Marc *Amsler,* Swiss ophthalmologist, 1891–1968] see under *chart* and *marker.*

**Am·sus·tain** (am′səs-tān) trademark for a preparation of dextroamphetamine.

**amu** atomic mass unit.

**amuck** (ə-muk′) [Malay *amok*] 1. amok. 2. *(colloq.)* wild, frenzied, or uncontrollable.

**amu·sia** (ə-mu′ze-ə) [Gr. *amousia* want of harmony] a form of auditory agnosia in which a person has lost the ability to recognize or produce music; cf. *paramusia.*
**instrumental a.**, that in which the patient has lost the power of playing a musical instrument.
**sensory a.**, loss of the ability to comprehend musical sounds; called also *tone deafness.*
**vocal motor a.**, that in which the patient cannot sing in tune.

**Amus·sat's operation** (ah″mu-sahz′) [Jean Zuléma *Amussat,* French surgeon, 1796–1856] see under *operation.*

**Am·visc** (am′visk) trademark for a preparation of sodium hyaluronate.

**AMWA** American Medical Women's Association; American Medical Writers' Association.

**amy·cho·pho·bia** (ə-mi″ko-fo′be-ə) [Gr. *amychē* a scratch + *-phobia*] irrational fear of being scratched, as by the claws of a cat.

**amyc·tic** (ə-mik′tik) caustic or irritating.

**amy·el·en·ce·pha·lia** (ə-mi″əl-en-sə-fa′le-ə) [*a-*[1] + *myelo-* + *encephal-* + *-ia*] congenital absence of the brain and spinal cord.

**amy·el·en·ceph·a·lus** (ə-mi″əl-en-sef′ə-ləs) a fetus exhibiting amyelencephalia.

**amy·e·lia** (a″mi-e′le-ə) [*a-*[1] + *myel-* + *-ia*] congenital absence of the spinal cord.

**amy·el·ic** (a″mi-el′ik) having no spinal cord.

**amy·e·lin·ic** (a-mi″ə-lin′ik) unmyelinated.

**amy·e·lon·ic** (a-mi″ə-lon′ik) [*a* neg. + Gr. *myelos* marrow] 1. amyelic. 2. having no bone marrow.

**amy·e·lus** (a-mi′ə-ləs) [*a-*[1] + Gr. *myelos* marrow] a fetus exhibiting amyelia.

**amyg·da·la** (ə-mig′də-lə) [Gr. *amygdalē* almond] 1. almond. 2. a term used in anatomical nomenclature to designate an almond-shaped structure. 3. corpus amygdaloideum.
**a. ama′ra**, bitter almond.

**amyg·da·lic ac·id** (ə-mig′də-lik) mandelic acid.

**amyg·da·lin** (ə-mig′də-lin) [MeSH: Amygdalin] 1. a cyanogenetic glycoside found in seeds and other plant parts of the bitter almond and other members of the family Rosaceae, often the cause of cyanide poisoning in animals eating them in large amounts. It is split by enzymatic hydrolysis into glucose, benzaldehyde, and hydrocyanic acid. 2. Laetrile.

**amyg·da·line** (ə-mig′də-lēn″) [L. *amygdalinus*] 1. like an almond. 2. tonsillar.

**amygdal(o)-** [Gr. *amygdalē* almond] a combining form denoting relationship to an almond-shaped structure or to the tonsil.

**amyg·da·lo·hip·po·cam·pec·to·my** (ə-mig″də-lo-hip″o-cam-pek′tə-me) [*amygdalo-* + *hippocampus* + *-ectomy*] surgical removal of all or part of the amygdala, hippocampus, and parahippocampal gyrus; done for the treatment of temporal lobe epilepsy resistant to medical treatment.

**amyg·da·loid** (ə-mig′də-loid) [*amygdalo-* + *-oid*] resembling an almond, or tonsil.

**am·yl** (am′əl) [Gr. *amylon* starch] the univalent radical, $—C_5H_{11}$.
**a. acetate**, a colorless limpid liquid, the acetic acid ester of amyl alcohol, $CH_3{\cdot}CO{\cdot}OC_5H_{11}$; it has the odor of bananas and is also called *banana oil.*
**a. nitrite** [USP], a mixture of the nitrite esters of 3-methyl-1-butanol and 2-methyl-1-butanol, a flammable clear liquid with an ethereal odor, volatile at low temperatures and administered by inhalation. It is a vasodilator and is used as a diagnostic aid in tests of reserve cardiac function; it has also been used in the treatment of acute angina pectoris, although it has largely been replaced by other agents. It is also used in treatment of a cyanide poisoning to promote formation of methemoglobin, which combines with the cyanide ion to form nontoxic cyanmethemoglobin. It is abused to produce euphoria and as a sexual stimulant and may cause methemoglobinemia, hemolytic anemia, and immunologic disorders.

**am·y·la·ceous** (am″ə-la′shəs) [L. *amylaceus*] starchy; containing starch; of the nature of starch.

**am·y·lase** (am′ə-lās) an enzyme of the hydrolase class that catalyzes the hydrolysis of $\alpha$-1,4-glucosidic linkages in polysaccharides.
**$\alpha$-a.** [EC 3.2.1.1], an endoamylase catalyzing the hydrolysis of internal $\alpha$-1,4-glucosidic linkages in polysaccharides that contain three or more glucose residues, yielding a mixture of linear and branched oligosaccharides. The enzyme is secreted by the salivary glands and pancreas of mammals.
**$\beta$-a.** [EC 3.2.1.2], an exoamylase occurring in plants and bacteria; it cleaves alternate glucosidic bonds to remove maltose units from the polysaccharide chains.

**am·y·las·uria** (am″ə-lās-u′re-ə) an excess of amylase in the urine, a sign of pancreatitis.

**am·y·le·mia** (am″ə-le′me-ə) [*amyl-* + *-emia*] an excess of starch in the blood.

**am·y·lene** (am′ə-lēn) a flammable liquid hydrocarbon of five isomeric forms.

**a. hydrate,** [NF], a clear, colorless liquid with a camphoraceous odor, miscible with alcohol, chloroform, ether, and glycerin; used as a solvent in pharmaceutical preparations. See also *amylism.*

**amyl·ic** (ə-mil'ik) [L. *amylicus*] pertaining to amyl.

**am·yl·in** (am'ə-lin) a 37–amino acid polypeptide with over 40 per cent homology with calcitonin gene–related peptide, occurring packaged with insulin in the beta cell secretory granules in normal pancreatic islets; it is also a major component of islet amyloid in patients with type 2 diabetes. Amylin inhibits insulin-stimulated glycogen synthesis in isolated skeletal muscle and inhibits insulin-induced glucose utilization *in vivo*. Called also *islet amyloid polypeptide.*

**am·y·lism** (am'ə-liz-əm) poisoning by amylene hydrate.

**amyl(o)-** [Gr. *amylon* starch] a combining form denoting relationship to starch.

**am·y·lo·bar·bi·tone** (am″ə-lo-bahr'bĭ-tōn) amobarbital.

**am·y·lo·dex·trin** (am″ə-lo-dek'strin) any of the class of water-soluble dextrins staining blue with iodine and formed in the early stages of hydrolysis of starch.

**am·y·lo·dys·pep·sia** (am″ə-lo-dis-pep'se-ə) [*amylo-* + *dyspepsia*] inability to digest starch-containing foods.

**am·y·lo·gen·e·sis** (am″ə-lo-jen'ə-sis) [*amylo-* + *-genesis*] the biosynthesis of starch.

**am·y·lo·gen·ic** (am″ə-lo-jen'ik) 1. producing starch. 2. of or pertaining to amylogenesis.

**am·y·lo-1,6-glu·co·si·dase** (am″ə-lo-gloo-ko'sĭ-dās, gloo-kosīd'ās) [EC 3.2.1.33] an enzyme of the hydrolase class that catalyzes the cleavage of terminal $\alpha$-1,6-glucoside linkages, releasing free glucose residues. In mammals, the enzyme also has a transferase activity on the same polypeptide chain (see *oligo-1,4-1,4-glucantransferase*) and can hydrolyze such linkages occurring at points of branching in glycogen molecules by first transferring to nearby chains those triglucosides adjacent to branch points, thereby exposing the $\alpha$-1,6-linked branch points to the glucosidase activity. In concert with glycogen phosphorylase, the enzyme can thus degrade glycogen to free glucose and glucose 1-phosphate. It is found in liver and muscle. Deficiency of the enzyme, an autosomal recessive trait, results in glycogen storage disease type III. Called also *debranching enzyme (of glycogen).*

**am·y·loid** (am'ə-loid) [*amylo-* + *-oid*] [MeSH: Amyloid] 1. resembling starch; characterized by starchlike staining properties. 2. a substance produced by the action of sulfuric acid on cellulose, which gives a blue color when treated with iodine. 3. the pathologic extracellular proteinaceous substance deposited in amyloidosis; it is a waxy eosinophilic material that exhibits a green birefringence under polarized light when stained with Congo red. Amyloid deposits are composed primarily of straight, nonbranching fibrils 7.5–10 nm in diameter and of indefinite length, arranged either in bundles or in a feltlike meshwork; each fibril is composed of identical polypeptide chains arranged in stacked antiparallel $\beta$-pleated sheets. There are two major biochemical types of amyloid protein: *amyloid light chain protein* and *amyloid A protein* (see under *protein*), as well as less common types.
**a. A,** see under *protein.*
**a. L,** amyloid light chain protein; see under *protein.*

**am·y·loi·do·sis** (am″ə-loi-do'sis) [*amyloid-* + *-osis*] [MeSH: Amyloidosis] a group of conditions of diverse etiologies characterized by the accumulation of insoluble fibrillar proteins (amyloid) in various organs and tissues of the body such that vital function is compromised. The associated disease states may be inflammatory, hereditary, or neoplastic, and the deposition can be local or generalized or systemic. The most widely used classification is based on the chemistry of the amyloid fibrils and includes primary or *immunocyte-derived* and secondary or *reactive systemic* forms. Amyloidosis associated with multiple myeloma or familial Mediterranean fever has been considered to be in a separate category because the pattern of tissue involvement resembles that of the primary type but the amyloidosis is secondary to a known cause. Also, since the hereditary forms of amyloidosis have their own distinctive pattern of organ involvement, they may constitute a separate, heterogenetic group.
**AA a.,** reactive systemic a.
**a. of aging,** senile a.
**AL a.,** immunocyte-derived a.
**cutaneous a.,** amyloidosis localized to the skin and usually associated with pruritus, which may be a characteristic of primary disease or occur in secondary amyloidosis. See *lichen a., macular a.,* and *nodular a.*
**dialysis a.,** hemodialysis-associated a.
**familial a.,** hereditary a.
**hemodialysis-associated a.,** that occurring in patients on long-term hemodialysis, caused by the deposition of beta$_2$-microglobulin, which cannot be removed from the blood by dialysis, in the joints, synovial membranes, and tendon sheaths. Manifestations include carpal tunnel syndrome and arthritis. Called also *dialysis a.*
**hereditary a.,** a group of amyloidoses, usually found in limited geographic areas, and characterized by widespread tissue involvement indistinguishable from the reactive systemic form and by the presence of fibrillar proteins of the AA type. Most have autosomal dominant inheritance, the exception being familial Mediterranean fever, which is autosomal recessive. Based on the principal sites of amyloid deposition, it is classified in the following major subtypes: neuropathies, nephropathies, cardiopathies, and miscellaneous. Called also *familial a.* and *heredofamilial a.*; see also *familial amyloid polyneuropathy,* under *polyneuropathy.*
**hereditary neuropathic a.,** familial amyloid polyneuropathy.
**heredofamilial a.,** hereditary a.
**idiopathic a.,** primary a.
**immunocyte-derived a.,** that in which the deposited fibrillar material is usually of the AL type and is most often systemic or generalized in distribution. It is a primary type of amyloidosis, usually involving the heart, tongue, carpal ligaments, peripheral nerves, gastrointestinal tract, and skin. Called also *AL a., light chain–related a.,* and *primary a.*
**immunocytic a.,** systemic amyloidosis in which the amyloid is composed of the AL protein derived from immunoglobulin light chains; this category includes amyloidosis associated with multiple myeloma and other plasma cell dyscrasias and primary amyloidosis.
**lichen a.,** the most common form of cutaneous amyloidosis, characterized by the symmetrical distribution over the extensor surfaces of the lower extremities, thighs, dorsal feet, and lower back of translucent, yellow to brown, dome-shaped, discrete pruritic papules; the chest, shoulders, and skin of the abdominal walls may be involved later. Called also *lichen amyloidosus.*
**light chain–related a.,** immunocyte-derived a.
**macular a.,** cutaneous amyloidosis manifested by ill-defined, sometimes pruritic grayish brown macules distributed on the upper back, breasts, buttocks, arms, ankles, and thighs.
**nodular a.,** a form of localized amyloidosis in which single or multiple, amyloid-containing nodular or tumefactive masses are found most often in the lung, urinary bladder, larynx, tongue, conjunctiva, and skin, especially that of the extremities, trunk, genitals, and face.
**primary a.,** that in which no obvious predisposing condition is associated. The term is sometimes used synonymously with *immunocyte-derived a.* (q.v.). Called also *idiopathic a.*
**reactive systemic a.,** that in which the deposited fibrillar material is of the AA type, and occurs secondary to a chronic infectious process (e.g., tuberculosis and osteomyelitis) or a chronic noninfectious inflammatory disease (e.g., rheumatoid arthritis). It may also occur in association with certain nonlymphoid tumors and some nonimmunoglobulin-producing lymphomas, the two most common being renal cell carcinoma and Hodgkin's disease. Called also *secondary a.*
**renal a.,** amyloid deposits in the kidneys; in the primary type the fibrils are mainly of AL amyloid, and in secondary types they are of AA amyloid. Secondary types may accompany inflammatory disorders such as rheumatoid arthritis and paraplegias, chronic infectious diseases such as tuberculosis and leprosy, and neoplastic diseases such as multiple myeloma. Called also *amyloid nephrosis.*
**secondary a.,** reactive systemic a.
**senile a.,** that seen in the elderly and usually involving the heart, brain, pancreas, or spleen. Called also *a. of aging.*

**am·y·lol·y·sis** (am″ə-lol'ə-sis) [*amylo-* + *-lysis*] the degradation of starch to water-soluble dextrins and sugars, particularly that catalyzed by enzymes.

**am·y·lo·lyt·ic** (am'ə-lo-lit'ik) pertaining to, characterized by, or promoting amylolysis.

**am·y·lo·pec·tin** (am″ə-lo-pek'tin) [MeSH: Amylopectin] a highly branched, water-insoluble glucan, the more prevalent of the two constituents of starch (see also *amylose* ); it consists of a chain of glucose residues in $\alpha$-(1,4) linkage to which branches are formed by $\alpha$-(1,6) linkages. It stains violet to red-violet with iodine.

**am·y·lo·pec·ti·no·sis** (am″ə-lo-pek″tĭ-no'sis) glycogen storage disease, type IV.

**am·y·lo·pha·gia** (am″ə-lo-fa'jə) [*amylo-* + *-phagia*] starch eating; an abnormal craving for starch.

**am·y·lo·plas·tic** (am″ə-lo-plas'tik) [*amylo-* + *-plastic*] forming starch.

**am·y·lor·rhea** (am″ə-lo-re'ə) [*amylo-* + *rrhea*] the presence of an abnormal amount of starch in the stools.

**am·y·lose** (am'ə-lōs) [MeSH: Amylose] a linear, water-soluble glucan, a lesser constituent of starch (see also *amylopectin*); it consists of a chain of glucose residues in $\alpha$-(1,4) linkage and it stains blue with iodine.

**am·y·lo·su·ria** (am″ə-lo-sur'e-ə) the presence of amylose in the urine.

**am·y·lo-1:4,1:6-trans·glu·co·si·dase** (am″ə-lo-trans″gloo-kōs′ə-dās) 1,4-α-glucan branching enzyme.

**Am·yl·sine Hy·dro·chlo·ride** (am′əl-sin) trademark for a preparation of naepaine.

**am·y·lum** (am′ə-ləm) [L.; Gr. *amylon*] starch.

**am·y·lu·ria** (am″əl-u′re-ə) [*amylo-* + *uria*] an excess of starch in the urine.

**amyo·es·the·sia** (a-mi″o-es-the′zhə) [*a-*[1] + *myo-* + *esthesia*] muscular anesthesia.

**amyo·es·the·sis** (a-mi″o-es-the′sis) [*a-*[1] + *myo-* + Gr. *aisthēsis* sensation] muscular anesthesia.

**amyo·pla·sia** (a-mi″o-pla′zhə) [*a-*[1] + *myo-* + *-plasia*] lack of muscle formation.
**a. conge′nita,** a generalized lack of muscular development and growth, with contracture and deformity at most of the joints; called *congenital multiple arthrogryposis* and *arthrogryposis multiplex congenita.*

**amyo·sta·sia** (a-mi″o-sta′zhə) [*a-*[1] + *myo-* + *stasis*] a tremor of the muscles, seen especially in locomotor ataxia.

**amyo·stat·ic** (a-mi″o-stat′ik) marked by amyostasia or muscular tremors.

**amyo·to·nia** (a″mi-o-to′ne-ə) [*a-*[1] + *myotonia*] atonic condition of the musculature of the body; called also *myatonia* and *myatony.*

**amyo·tro·phia** (a-mi″o-tro′fe-ə) [*a-*[1] + *myotrophia*] amyotrophy.
**neuralgic a.,** neuralgic amyotrophy.
**a. spina′lis progressi′va,** progressive muscular atrophy.

**amyo·troph·ic** (a-mi″o-trof′ik) pertaining to or characterized by amyotrophy.

**amy·ot·ro·phy** (a″mi-ot′rə-fe) atrophy of muscle tissue.
**diabetic a.,** progressive asymmetrical weakening and wasting of muscles accompanied by aching or stabbing pain, usually limited to the muscles of the pelvic girdle and thigh, and associated with uncontrolled diabetes.
**neuralgic a.,** a condition characterized by pain across the shoulder and upper arm, with atrophy and paralysis of the muscles of the shoulder girdle.

**am·y·ous** (am′e-əs) [*a-*[1] + *myo-* + *-ous*] deficient in muscular tissue.

**Am·y·tal** (am′ĭ-təl) trademark for preparations of amobarbital.

**amyx·ia** (ə-mik′se-ə) [*a-*[1] + *myx-* + *-ia*] absence of mucus.

**amyx·or·rhea** (ə-mik″sə-re′ə) [*a-*[1] + *myxo-* + *rrhea*] absence of mucus secretion.

**An** anode; anodal.

**an-**[1] the form of *a-* neg. used before a vowel or *h;* see *a-*[1].

**an-**[2] the form of the prefix *ana-* used before a vowel or *h;* see *ana-.*

**ANA** American Nurses' Association, antinuclear antibodies.

**ana** (an′ah) [Gr.] so much of each; usually written āā.

**ana-** [Gr. *ana* up, back, again] a prefix meaning upward, excessive, or again.

**Anab·aena** (an″ə-be′nə) [MeSH: Anabaena] a genus of cyanobacteria that sometimes contaminates water, giving it an offensive odor and danger of cyanobacteria poisoning.

**anab·a·sine** (ə-nab′ə-sēn) [MeSH: Anabasine] an alkaloid, from the plant *Anabasis aphylla,* which closely resembles nicotine; it is used as an insecticide.

**Anab·e·na** (an″ə-be′nə) Anabaena.

**ana·bi·o·sis** (an″ə-bi-o′sis) [Gr. *anabiōsis* a reviving] restoration of vital processes after their apparent cessation.

**ana·bi·ot·ic** (an″ə-bi-ot′ik) apparently lifeless, but still capable of living.

**an·a·bol·ic** (an″ə-bol′ik) pertaining to or serving to promote anabolism.

**anab·o·lism** (ə-nab′ə-liz″-əm) [Gr. *anabolē* a throwing up] any constructive metabolic process by which organisms convert substances into other components of the organism's chemical architecture.

**anab·o·lite** (ə-nab′ə-līt″) any product of anabolism or of a constructive metabolic process.

**ana·cata·did·y·mus** (an″ə-kat″ə-did′ə-məs) anakatadidymus.

**ana·cat·es·the·sia** (an″ə-kat″es-the′zhə) [*ana-* + *cata-* + *esthesia*] a hovering feeling or perception.

**an·acid·i·ty** (an″ə-sid′ĭ-te) [*an-* neg. + *acidity*] lack of normal acidity.
**gastric a.,** achlorhydria.

**anac·la·sis** (ə-nak′lə-sis) [Gr. *anaklasis* reflection] reflection or refraction of light.

**an·a·cli·sis** (an″ə-kli′sis) [*ana-* + Gr. *klinein* to lean] physical and emotional dependence on another for protection and gratification; used to refer to the normal dependence of an infant on its mother or to excessive leaning on others for emotional support in an older individual.

**an·a·clit·ic** (an″ə-klit′ik) pertaining to anaclisis; exhibiting excessive emotional dependency.

**ana·co·bra** (an″ə-ko′brə) cobra venom treated with formaldehyde and heat.

**an·acou·sia** (an″ə-koo′zhə) anakusis.

**an·a·crot·ic** (an″ə-krot′ik) 1. pertaining to the ascending limb of a pulse tracing. 2. said of an ascending limb of a pulse tracing that has a notch, i.e. has two waveforms. Called also *anadicrotic.*

**anac·ro·tism** (ə-nak′rə-tiz-əm) [*ana-* + Gr. *krotos* beat + *-ism*] presence of an anacrotic pulse.

**an·acu·sis** (an″ə-koo′sis) anakusis.

**Ana·cys·tis** (an″ə-sis′tis) *Microcystis.*

**an·a·di·crot·ic** (an″ə-di-krot′ik) anacrotic (def. 2).

**an·a·did·y·mus** (an″ə-did′ĭ-məs) [*ana-* + *didymus*] conjoined twins that are divided below but single toward the cephalic pole; called also *duplicitas inferior* and *duplicitas posterior.*

**an·a·dip·sia** (an″ə-dip′shə) [*ana-* + *dipsia*] intense thirst.

**an·ad·re·nal·ism** (an″ə-dre′nəl-iz-əm) absence or failure of adrenal function.

**an·ad·re·nia** (an″ə-dre′ne-ə) anadrenalism.

**An·a·drol** (an′ə-drol) trademark for a preparation of oxymetholone.

**an·aer·obe** (an′ə-rōb) [*an-* neg. + *aerobe*] a microorganism that lives and grows in the complete, or almost complete, absence of molecular oxygen.
**facultative a's,** microorganisms which are able to grow under either anaerobic or aerobic conditions.
**obligate a's,** microorganisms that can grow only in the complete absence of molecular oxygen; some are killed by oxygen.
**spore-forming a.,** see *Clostridium* and *Desulfotomaculum.*

**an·aer·o·bic** (an″ə-ro′bik) 1. lacking molecular oxygen. 2. growing, living, or occurring in the absence of molecular oxygen; pertaining to an anaerobe.

**an·aer·o·bi·o·sis** (an-ār″o-bi-o′sis) [*an-* neg. + *aero* + *biosis*] [MeSH: Anaerobiosis] metabolic processes occurring in the absence of molecular oxygen.

**an·aero·gen·ic** (an-ār″o-jen′ik) [*an-* neg. + *aero-* + *-genic*] 1. producing little or no gas. 2. suppressing the formation of gas by the gas-producing bacteria.

**An·af·ra·nil** (ə-naf′rə-nil) trademark for a preparation of clomipramine hydrochloride.

**an·a·gen** (an′ə-jen) the phase of the hair cycle during which synthesis of hair takes place.

**Anag·nos·ta·kis' operation** (ah-nahg″no-stah′kēs) [Andreas *Anagnostakis,* Greek ophthalmologist, 1826–1897] see under *operation.*

**an·a·go·ge** (an″ə-go′je) anagogy.

**an·a·gog·ic** (an″ə-goj′ik) [*ana-* + Gr. *agogē* leading] pertaining to the moral, uplifting, progressive strivings of the unconscious.

**an·a·go·gy** (an″ə-go′je) psychic material that has an idealistic quality.

**an·ag·o·tox·ic** (an-ag″o-tok′sik) acting antagonistically to toxin; counteracting toxic action.

**an·ag·re·lide hy·dro·chlo·ride** (an-ag′rə-līd) an agent used to reduce elevated platelet counts and the risk of thrombosis in the treatment of hemorrhagic thrombocythemia; administered orally.

**ana·kata·did·y·mus** (an″ə-kat″ə-did′ĭ-məs) [*ana-* + *cata-* + *didymus*] conjoined twins that are separate above and below, but united in the middle.

**ana·khré** (ah-nah-kra′) [Fr., from native West African name] goundou.

**an·ak·me·sis** (an-ak′me-sis) [*an-* neg. + Gr. *akmēnos* full grown] arrest of maturation; specifically, increase of granulocyte precursors in the marrow with lack of further maturation, as seen in agranulocytosis.

**an·aku·sis** (an″ə-koo′sis) [*an* neg. + Gr. *akouein* to hear] total deafness. Called also *anacusis* and *anacousia.*

**anal** (a'nəl) [L. *analis*] pertaining to the anus.

**an·al·bu·min·emia** (an"al-bu"mĭ-ne'me-ə) a state characterized by deficiency or absence of albumins in the blood serum.

**an·a·lep·tic** (an"ə-lep'tik) [Gr. *analepsis* a repairing] a drug which acts as a restorative, such as caffeine, amphetamine, pentylenetetrazol, etc.

**an·al·ge·sia** (an"əl-je'ze-ə) [*an-* neg. + *algesia*] [MeSH: Analgesia] 1. absence of sensibility to pain; absence of pain on noxious stimulation. 2. the relief of pain without loss of consciousness.
**a. al'gera,** spontaneous pain in a denervated part; pain in an area or region that is anesthetic; called also *anesthesia dolorosa.*
**audio a.,** audioanalgesia.
**continuous epidural a.,** a method of pain relief consisting of continuous bathing of lumbar or thoracic nerve roots within the epidural space with an injected anesthetic solution; used during labor and childbirth, in general surgery for blockage of pain pathways below the umbilicus, and postoperatively. Called also *continuous epidural anesthesia.*
**epidural a.,** see under *anesthesia.*
**infiltration a.,** see under *anesthesia.*
**paretic a.,** loss of the sense of pain accompanied by partial paralysis.
**patient controlled a.,** a technique for pain control using an infusion pump so that small doses of a narcotic can be administered intravenously by the patient; it includes safeguards against overdose.
**patient controlled epidural a.,** patient controlled analgesia in which a narcotic or local anesthetic is administered into the epidural space via a catheter.
**relative a.,** in dental anesthesia, a maintained level of conscious-sedation, short of general anesthesia, in which the pain threshold is elevated, usually induced in inhalation of nitrous oxide and oxygen.
**spinal a.,** analgesia produced by injection of an opioid into the subarachnoid space around the spinal cord; cf. *spinal anesthesia.*

**an·al·ge·sic** (an"əl-je'zik) 1. relieving pain. 2. not sensitive to pain. 3. an agent that alleviates pain without causing loss of consciousness.
**narcotic a.,** opioid a.
**nonsteroidal antiinflammatory a.,** NSAIA; see under *drug.*
**opiate a.,** opioid a.
**opioid a.,** any of a class of compounds that bind with a number of closely related specific receptors (opioid receptors) in the central nervous system to block the perception of pain or affect the emotional response to pain; such compounds include opium and its derivatives, as well as a number of synthetic compounds, and are used for moderate to severe pain. Chronic administration or abuse may lead to dependence.

**an·al·get·ic** (an"əl-jet'ik) analgesic.

**an·al·gia** (an-al'jə) [*an-* + Gr. *-algia*] analgesia (def. 1).

**an·al·gic** (an-al'jik) analgesic (def. 2).

**anal·i·ty** (a-nal'ĭ-te) the psychic organization of all the sensations, impulses, and personality traits derived from the anal stage (q.v.) of psychosexual development.

**an·al·ler·gic** (an"ə-lər'jik) not allergic; not causing anaphylaxis or hypersensitivity.

**an·a·log** (an'ə-log) [shortening of *analogue*] 1. pertaining to electronic equipment in which data are represented by electrical signals or physical magnitudes having continuously varying values. Cf. *digital,* def. 3. 2. analogue.

**anal·o·gous** (ə-nal'ə-gəs) [Gr. *analogos* according to a due ratio, conformable, proportionate] resembling or similar in some respects, as in function or appearance, but not in origin or development; cf. *homologous,* def. 1.

**an·a·logue** (an'ə-log) 1. a part or organ having the same function as another, but of a different evolutionary origin; cf. *homologue* (def. 1). 2. a chemical compound with a structure similar to that of another but differing from it in respect to a certain component; it may have a similar or opposite action metabolically. Cf. *homologue* (def. 2).
**folic acid a.,** a structural analogue of folic acid; see *folic acid antagonist,* under *antagonist.*
**homologous a.,** a part that is similar to another in both function and structure.
**metabolic a.,** a closely similar compound which tends to replace an essential metabolite.
**purine a.,** a structural analogue of one of the purine bases (purine, adenine, or guanine): 6-mercaptopurine and 6-thioguanine are used as antineoplastics, azathioprine as an immunosuppressive; the antiviral agent vidarabine (adenine arabinoside) is an analogue of the adenine nucleoside adenosine.
**pyrimidine a.,** a structural analogue of one of the pyrimidine bases (cytosine, thymine, or uracil): 5-fluorouracil and cytarabine (cytosine arabinoside), analogues of the cytosine nucleotide deoxycytidine, are important antineoplastic agents.
**substrate a.,** a substance with a structure similar to the natural substrate of an enzyme and which, because of this similarity, in some cases inhibits the action of the enzyme, as in competitive inhibition.

**anal·o·gy** (ə-nal'ə-je) [Gr. *analogia* equality of ratios, proportion] the quality of being analogous; resemblance or similarity in function or appearance, but not in origin or development.

**an·al·pha·li·po·pro·tein·emia** (an-al"fə-lip"o-pro"te-ne'me-ə) 1. absence of high-density (alpha) lipoproteins in the blood. 2. Tangier disease.

**anal·y·sand** (ə-nal'ĭ-sand) one who is being psychoanalyzed.

**anal·y·sis** (ə-nal'ĭ-sis) pl. *anal'yses* [*ana-* + *-lysis*] 1. separation into component parts or elements; the act of determining the component parts of a substance. 2. psychoanalysis.
**activation a.,** a quantitative or qualitative determination of trace levels of atoms possessing certain types of nuclei in a sample by bombarding it with radioactivity and analyzing the emanating radiation.
**behavior a.,** Skinner's model for examination and prediction of the behavior of individuals in the environment based on theories of operant and respondent conditioning and social learning and depending on observation.
**bite a.,** occlusal a.
**bivariate a.,** any of various statistical methods for analysis of the association between one independent and one dependent variable.
**blood gas a.,** the determination of oxygen and carbon dioxide concentrations and pressures with the pH of the blood by laboratory tests; the following measurements may be made: $PO_2$, partial pressure of oxygen in arterial blood; $PCO_2$, partial pressure of carbon dioxide in arterial blood; $SO_2$, percent saturation of hemoglobin with oxygen in arterial blood; the total $CO_2$ content of (venous) plasma; and the pH.
**bradykinetic a.,** cineradiographic study of motor activity.
**cephalometric a.,** measurement of the head, using the vector quantities distance and direction, based on the tracing of the radiograph of the living head, usually in the lateral view.
**character a.,** psychoanalysis of the personality traits and character defenses particular to an individual.
**chromatographic a.,** chromatography.
**cluster a.,** in epidemiology, statistical techniques used to analyze observations that are clustered in subgroups.
**colorimetric a.,** analysis based on the principle that in certain instances the color intensity of a solution is proportional to the concentration of a specific substance in that solution.
**a. of covariance (ANCOVA),** a statistical procedure used with one dependent variable and multiple independent variables of both categorical (ordinal, dichotomous, or nominal) and continuous types; it is a variation of analysis of variance that adjusts for confounding by continuous variables; see also *a. of variance.*
**decision a.,** a statistical method used for delineating the probabilities of various outcomes by determining the probabilities of each option available at each point where a decision can be made; often graphed as a decision tree to display the array of choices and outcomes as nodes and branches.
**densimetric a.,** analysis by ascertaining the specific gravity of a solution and estimating the amount of matter dissolved.
**discriminant function a.,** a form of multivariate analysis useful when the dependent variable is nominal or dichotomous and the independent variables are continuous; used to find the combination of variables that maximizes the separation between categories for the dependent variable. In recent years it has largely been replaced by logistic regression.
**Downs' a.,** radiographic cephalometric criteria developed by Downs as an aid in orthodontic diagnosis.
**ego a.,** in a psychoanalytic treatment, the analysis of the strengths and weaknesses of the ego, especially its defense mechanisms against unacceptable unconscious impulses.
**end-group a.,** evaluation of the degree of linearity and branching of polysaccharide by determination of the number of end groups; determination of the amino- and carboxyl-terminal amino acids of a protein permitting an evaluation of the number of peptide chains per molecule as well as the state of purity of the protein.
**gasometric a.,** the measurement of the different components of a gaseous mixture.
**gravimetric a.,** a form of quantitative analysis in which the sample is purified by precipitation or combustion before being dried, weighed, and analyzed.
**group a.,** group therapy in which interpretation is given to the patients and insight is evoked on the basis of the communication and interactions occurring within the group.
**log-linear a.,** a form of multivariate analysis useful for examining the effects of multiple independent variables, at least some of which

are categorical, on a nominal dependent variable; it is used to construct models for the evaluation of relationships between categorical variables.
**multivariate a.,** any of various statistical methods for analyzing more than two variables simultaneously.
**Northern blot a.,** see under *technique.*
**occlusal a.,** an analysis of the contact of the teeth in centric relation and during excursions of the mandible to determine if occlusal dysfunction is present. Called also *bite a.*
**organic a.,** the analysis of animal and vegetable tissues.
**proximate a.,** quantitative analysis separating and identifying categories of compounds in a mixture.
**pulse-chase a.,** a method for examining a cellular process occurring over time: organisms, cells, or organelles are briefly exposed to a radioactive compound (pulse) and washed; then they are exposed to the same compound, but in a nonradioactive form, for varying lengths of time (chase), and their characteristics over time are observed.
**qualitative a., qualitive a.,** the determination of the nature of the constituents of a compound or a mixture of compounds.
**quantitative a., quantitive a.,** the determination of the proportionate quantities of the constituents of a compound.
**radiochemical a.,** direct or indirect identification or determination of the content of specific elements in a substance through measurement of the disintegration rates of radionuclides.
**regression a.,** interpretation of a finite population of data by exploring the relationship between several variables using the principle of regression; see *regression* (def. 5).
**sequential a.,** a statistical technique in which the sample size is not fixed in advance, rather, sampling is stopped as soon as significant results are observed. The criteria for stopping the trials at each sample size are set so that the overall probability (for all sample sizes) of falsely rejecting the null hypothesis at any step is held to a preset level. Cf. *hypothesis test.*
**Southern blot a.,** see under *technique.*
**Southwestern blot a.,** see under *technique.*
**spectroscopic a., spectrum a.,** analysis by means of determining the wave length(s) at which electromagnetic energy is absorbed by a sample.
**survival a.,** statistical analysis that evaluates the timing of events, particularly survival but also by extension other nonrecurrent events occurring in a cohort over time, such as relapse, death, or marriage. It involves following the cohort, plotting the occurrence of events, and calculating their probabilities for each time interval. See also *Kaplan-Meier survival curve,* under *curve.*
**transactional a.,** a type of psychotherapy based on an understanding of the interactions (transactions) between patient and therapist and between patient and others in the environment. It focuses primarily on ego states, principally the Parent, Adult, and Child.
**ultimate a.,** the determination of the proportions of elements in a chemical compound.
**a. of variance (ANOVA),** a statistical method for analyzing the effects of each of one or more categorical (nominal, ordinal, or dichotomous) independent variables on a continuous dependent variable as well as on each other, examining more than two groups simultaneously; if the null hypothesis that the variables' effects do not differ and all outcomes are drawn from the same population is true, then the means of all outcome groups approximate each other. To test the hypothesis, the variability between group means is compared to that within groups using the *F*-test; if their ratio approximates 1.0 then the null hypothesis cannot be rejected. When a single independent variable is tested the method is sometimes called *one-way ANOVA;* when multiple independent variables are tested, N-*way ANOVA.*
**vector a.,** analysis of a directed quantity to determine both its magnitude and its direction, e.g., analysis of the scalar electrocardiogram to determine the magnitude and direction of the electromotive force for one complete cycle of the heart.
**volumetric a.,** quantitative analysis of solutions of known volume but unknown strength: reagents of known concentration are added by volume to the solution until a reaction endpoint is reached; the most common method is by titration.
**Western blot a.,** see under *technique.*

**an·a·lyst** (an'ə-list) 1. one who performs analysis. 2. psychoanalyst.

**an·a·lyte** (an'ə-līt) a substance undergoing analysis.

**an·a·lyt·ic** (an"ə-lit'ik) pertaining to analysis.

**an·a·ly·zer** (an'ə-li"zer) 1. a Nicol prism attached to a polarizing apparatus which extinguishes the ray of polarized light. 2. Pavlov's name for a specialized part of the nervous system which controls the reactions of the organism to changing external conditions. 3. a nervous receptor together with its central connections, by means of which sensitivity to stimulations is differentiated.
**amino acid a.,** an analytical instrument that separates, identifies, and measures quantities of amino acids and related compounds.
**blood gas a.,** an instrument for measuring partial pressures of oxygen, carbon dioxide, carbon monoxide, and nitrogen in blood.
**breath a.,** an instrument for determining the volume and composition of respired gases; some types are specifically designed for detecting alcohol in the breath.
**image a.,** an instrument that counts, measures, and classifies cells and images viewed on microscopes, photographs, transparencies, etc.
**oxygen gas a.,** an instrument for measuring the oxygen content of a gaseous mixture, or dissolved oxygen in a liquid, or saturation of blood hemoglobin with $O_2$ or partial pressure of $O_2$ in blood.
**pulse height a.,** an electronic circuit designed to respond to voltage pulses only within a certain range, or window, of amplitudes.
**voice a.,** an electronic instrument that prints out waveforms corresponding to vocal characteristics; used for analysis of voice and speech problems or identification of a particular speaker.

**An·a·me** (an'ə-me) a genus of spiders of the family Theraphosidae, including the venomous bird spiders.

**Ana·mir·ta** (an"ə-mir'tə) a genus of East Indian flowering vines of the family Menispermaceae. *A. coc'culus* L. Wight & Arn is cocculus indicus, a poisonous variety whose seeds yield picrotoxin.

**an·am·ne·sis** (an"am-ne'sis) [Gr. *anamnēsis* a recalling] 1. recollection. 2. a medical or psychiatric patient case history, particularly using the patient's recollections; cf. *catamnesis.* 3. immunologic memory.

**an·am·nes·tic** (an"am-nes'tik) 1. pertaining to anamnesis. 2. aiding the memory.

**An·am·ni·o·ta** (an"am-ne-o'tə) [*an-* neg. + Gr. *amnion*] a major group of vertebrates comprising those which develop no amnion, including fishes and amphibians; opposed to Amniota.

**an·am·ni·ote** (an-am'ne-ōt") any animal or group belonging to the Anamniota.

**an·am·ni·ot·ic** (an"am-ne-ot'ik) [*an-* neg. + *amnion*] having no amnion.

**an·a·morph** (an'ə-morf") [*ana-* + *-morph*] the stage of a fungus where reproduction results from mitosis of a parent cell by means of condidia only (asexual spores), as opposed to a teleomorph. See also *imperfect fungus,* under *fungus.* Called also *asexual stage* or *state* and *imperfect stage* or *state.*

**ana·mor·pho·sis** (an"ə-mor-fo'sis) [*ana-* + *morphosis*] an ascending progression or change of form in the evolution of a group of animals or plants.

**An·a·nase** (an'ə-nās) trademark for a preparation of bromelains.

**an·an·cas·tic** (an"an-kas'tik) [Gr. *anankastos* forced] obsessive-compulsive; see under *personality.*

**an·an·gi·oid** (an-an'je-oid) [*an-* neg. + *angioid*] seemingly without blood vessels.

**an·a·pep·sia** (an"ə-pep'se-ə) complete absence of pepsin from the stomach secretion.

**ana·phase** (an'ə-fāz) [*ana-* + *phase*] [MeSH: Anaphase] that stage in meiosis and mitosis, following the metaphase, in which the centromeres divide and the chromatids lined up on the spindle begin to move apart toward the poles of the spindle to form the daughter chromosomes. See also *meiosis* and *mitosis.*
**flabby a.,** a mitotic phase in which the gel is disoriented and separation of the doubled chromosomes fails to occur, owing to interference with spindle formation caused by cell poisoning.

**an·a·phia** (an-a'fe-ə) [*an-* + Gr. *haphē* touch + *-ia*] tactile anesthesia.

**an·a·pho·re·sis** (anə-fə-re'sis) the passage of charged particles toward the positive pole (anode) in electrophoresis.

**an·a·pho·ria** (an"ə-fo're-ə) [*ana-* + Gr. *phoros* carrying + *-ia*] a tendency for the visual axes of both eyes to divert above the horizontal plane.

**an·aph·ro·dis·iac** (an"af-ro-diz'e-ak) 1. repressing sexual desire. 2. a drug or medicine that allays sexual desire.

**ana·phy·lac·tic** (an"ə-fə-lak'tik) pertaining to anaphylaxis.

**ana·phy·lac·to·gen** (an"ə-fə-lak'to-jen) an antigen capable of inducing anaphylaxis.

**ana·phy·lac·to·gen·e·sis** (an"ə-fə-lak"to-jen'ə-sis) the production of anaphylaxis.

**ana·phy·lac·to·gen·ic** (an"-ə-fə-lak"to-jen'ik) producing anaphylaxis.

**ana·phy·lac·toid** (an"ə-fə-lak'toid) resembling anaphylaxis.

**ana·phyl·a·tox·in** (an"ə-fil"ə-tok'sin) a substance produced by complement activation that causes the release of histamine and other mediators of immediate hypersensitivity from basophils and mast cells, thereby producing signs and symptoms of immediate hypersensitivity (anaphylaxis) without involvement of IgE. The anaphylatoxins are low-molecular-weight complement cleavage products, C3a, C4a, and C5a, which bind to specific receptors on mast cells and basophils; C4a has comparatively weak anaphylatoxin activity; C5a is also a chemotactic factor for granulocytes and macrophages.

**ana·phy·lax·is** (an″ə-fə-lak′sis) [*ana-* + *phylaxis*] [MeSH: Anaphylaxis] 1. systemic or generalized anaphylaxis, anaphylactic shock; a type I hypersensitivity reaction (see under *hypersenstivity reaction*) in which exposure of a sensitized individual to a specific antigen or hapten results in urticaria, pruritus, and angioedema, followed by vascular collapse and shock and often accompanied by life-threatening respiratory distress. Common agents causing anaphylaxis include Hymenoptera venom, pollen extracts, certain foods, horse and rabbit sera, heterologous enzymes and hormones, and certain drugs, such as penicillin and lidocaine. 2. a general term originally applied to the situation in which exposure to a toxin resulted not in development of immunity (prophylaxis) but in hypersensitivity. The term was extended to include all cases of systemic anaphylaxis in response to foreign antigens and also to include a variety of experimental models, e.g., passive cutaneous anaphylaxis. Anaphylaxis has now been subsumed under the more general concept of type I (immediate) hypersensitivity.
**active a.,** the anaphylactic state produced in an individual by the injection of a foreign immunogen; distinguished from *passive anaphylaxis.*
**aggregate a.,** an anaphylactic reaction initiated by the formation of large amounts of antigen-antibody complexes upon injection of the antigen. The complexes activate complement, producing anaphylatoxins (C3a and C5a) that trigger the release of mediators of immediate hypersensitivity from basophils and mast cells.
**antiserum a.,** passive a.
**generalized a.,** see *anaphylaxis.*
**inverse a.,** 1. anaphylaxis in which the shocking agent is antibody rather than antigen. 2. anaphylactic shock produced by a single intravenous injection into guinea pigs of Forssman antibody which interacts with Forssman antigen in their tissues. Called also *reverse a.*
**local a.,** anaphylaxis confined to a limited area, e.g., passive cutaneous anaphylaxis.
**passive a.,** anaphylaxis occurring in a normal individual as a result of the injection of the serum of a previously sensitized individual; called also *antiserum a.*
**passive cutaneous a. (PCA),** a passively transferred local anaphylactic reaction used in the study of reaginic antibodies; the skin of an animal is sensitized by intradermal injection of serum from a sensitized animal, and after a 24- to 72-hour latent period the antigen and Evans blue dye are injected intravenously. Reaction of the antigen with skin-fixed antibody causes the release of histamine, which increases vascular permeability, permits leakage of the albumin-bound dye, and produces a blue spot at the site of the intradermal injection.
**reverse a.,** anaphylaxis following the injection of antigen succeeded by the injection of antiserum; also local reactions from the union of circulating antibodies with antigen fixed by tissue cells.
**systemic a.,** see *anaphylaxis.*

**ana·phy·lo·tox·in** (an″ə-fi″lo-tok′sin) anaphylatoxin.

**an·a·pla·sia** (an″ə-pla′zhə) [*ana-* + *-plasia*] [MeSH: Anaplasia] a loss of differentiation of cells and of their orientation to one another and to their axial framework and blood vessels, a characteristic of tumor tissue; called also *dedifferentiation.*

**An·a·plas·ma** (an″ə-plaz′mə) [Gr. *anaplasma* something without form] [MeSH: Anaplasma] a genus of bacteria of the family Anaplasmataceae, order Rickettsiales. *A. margina′le* causes anaplasmosis in cattle and deer, and *A. o′vis* causes anaplasmosis in sheep.

**An·a·plas·ma·ta·ce·ae** (an″ə-plaz″mə-ta′se-e) [MeSH: Anaplasmataceae] a family of bacteria of the order Rickettsiales, made up of microorganisms parasitic in red blood cells or free in the plasma of various vertebrates, in which they appear as reddish violet bodies when stained with Giemsa stain. They are naturally parasitic in ruminants and transmitted by arthropods, causing disease in cattle, deer, birds, and cats but not in humans. The family includes the genera *Aegyptianella, Anaplasma, Eperythrozoon,* and *Haemobartonella.*

**an·a·plas·mo·da·stat** (an″ə-plaz-mo′də-stat″) any of a group of chemical agents for control of anaplasmosis in animals.

**an·a·plas·mo·sis** (an″ə-plaz-mo′sis) [MeSH: Anaplasmosis] a disease of cattle and related ruminants marked by fever, anemia, and icterus; caused by *Anaplasma marginale* or *Anaplasma ovis,* which is transmitted by ticks and other blood-sucking arthropods. Called also *gallsickness* or *gall sickness.*

**an·a·plas·tic** (an″ə-plas′tik) [*ana-* + *plastic*] undifferentiated; characterized by anaplasia or reversed development; said of cells.

**an·a·ple·ro·sis** (an″ə-plĕ-ro′sis) [Gr. "filling up, restoration"] the repair or replacement of lost or defective parts.

**an·a·ple·rot·ic** (an″ə-plĕ-rot′ik) [*anaplerosis*] pertaining to a filling up or restoration; see under *reaction.*

**an·apoph·y·sis** (an″ə-pof′ĭ-sis) [*ana-* + *apophysis*] an accessory vertebral process, especially an accessory process of a thoracic or lumbar vertebra.

**An·a·prox** (an′ə-proks) trademark for preparations of naproxen sodium.

**an·ap·tic** (an-ap′tik) marked by anaphia (tactile anesthesia).

**an·a·rith·mia** (an″ə-rith′me-ə) [*an-* + Gr. *arithmos* number] acalculia.

**an·ar·rhex·is** (an″ə-rek′sis) [*ana-* + *-rrhexis*] the operation of refracturing a bone.

**an·ar·thria** (an-ahr′thre-ə) [*an-* + *arthr-*[2] + *-ia*] severe dysarthria (q.v.) resulting in speechlessness.

**an·a·sar·ca** (an″ə-sahr′kə) [*ana-* + *sarco*] generalized massive edema.

**an·a·sar·cous** (an″ə-sahr′kəs) affected with or of the nature of anasarca.

**an·a·scit·ic** (an″ə-sit′ik) without ascites.

**an·a·stig·mat·ic** (an″ə-stig-mat′ik) not astigmatic; corrected for astigmatism.

**anas·to·mose** (ə-nas′tə-mōs) 1. to connect with one another by anastomosis, as arteries and veins. 2. to create a connection between two formerly separate structures.

**an·as·to·mo·sis** (ə-nas″tə-mo′sis) pl. *anastomo′ses* [Gr. *anastomōsis* opening, outlet] 1. a connection between two vessels. 2. an opening created by surgical, traumatic, or pathological means between two normally separate spaces or organs. Cf. *shunt.*
**antiperistaltic a.,** enterostomy in which the intestinal segments are so joined that the directions of the peristaltic waves in the two conjoined portions are opposed.
**arteriolovenular a., glomeriform,** a. arteriovenosa glomeriformis.
**arteriolovenular a., simple,** a. arteriovenosa simplex.
**a. arteriolovenula′ris** [TA], arteriolovenular anastomosis: a vessel that directly interconnects an arteriole and a venule and that acts as a shunt to bypass the capillary bed. Called also *a. arteriovenosa* [TA alternative].
**a. arteriolovenula′ris glomerifor′mis,** a. arteriovenosa glomeriformis.
**a. arteriolovenula′ris sim′plex,** TA alternative for *a. arteriovenosa simplex.*
**a. arterioveno′sa,** TA alternative for *a. arteriolovenularis.*
**a. arterioveno′sa glomerifor′mis,** glomeriform arteriovenous anastomosis: a specialized type of arteriovenous shunt that helps regulate blood flow and is also concerned with maintenance or regulation of temperature; these are found most abundantly in the skin of the hands and feet (especially the digital pads and nail beds), the skin of the nose and ears, and along certain nerves and blood vessels. See also *glomus tumor,* under *tumor.* Called also *a. arteriolovenularis glomeriformis, glomiform gland, glomeriform arteriolovenular a., glomus,* and *glomus body.*
**a. arterioveno′sa sim′plex,** simple arteriovenous anastomosis: a vessel that directly interconnects an artery and a vein, acting as a shunt to bypass the capillary bed. Called also *a. arteriolovenularis simplex* and *simple arteriolovenular a.*
**arteriovenous a.,** 1. a. arteriolovenularis. 2. see under *shunt.*
**arteriovenous a., glomeriform,** a. arteriovenosa glomeriformis.
**arteriovenous a., simple,** a. arteriovenosa simplex.
**Braun's a.,** formation of an anastomosis between the afferent and

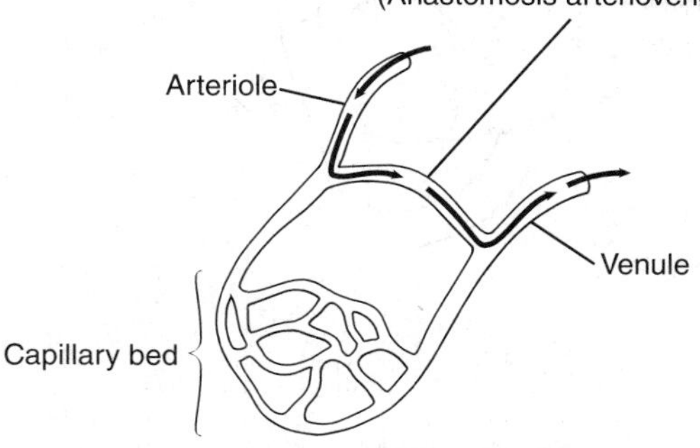

Anastomosis arteriovenosa simplex

efferent intestinal loops just distal to a gastroenteric stoma to prevent vicious cycling of gastric and duodenal contents.
**Clado's a.,** the anastomosis between the appendicular and ovarian arteries in the appendiculo-ovarian ligament.
**crucial a., cruciate a.,** an arterial anastomosis in the proximal part of the thigh, formed by the anastomotic branch of the sciatic, the internal circumflex, the first perforating, and the transverse portion of the external circumflex.
**end-to-end a.,** 1. an anastomosis connecting the end of an artery and that of some other vessel, either directly or with a synthetic graft. 2. anastomosis of two sections of colon, such as with partial colectomy or when an ileostomy is closed.
**end-to-side a.,** an anastomosis connecting the end of one vessel with the side of a larger one.
**Galen's a.,** ramus communicans nervi laryngei superioris cum nervo laryngeo inferiore.
**Glenn a.,** see under *operation.*
**heterocladic a.,** one between branches of different arteries.
**homocladic a.,** one between two branches of the same artery.
**Hyrtl's a.,** see *Hyrtl's loop,* under *loop.*
**ileoanal a.,** anastomosis of the terminal ileum and anus following colectomy, often in conjunction with creation of a reservoir from terminal ileum; performed in the management of ulcerative colitis.
**ileoanal pull-through a.,** anastomosis of an ileoanal reservoir to the anal canal by means of a short conduit of ileum pulled through the rectal cuff and sutured to the anus; done to allow continent elimination of feces following colectomy in the management of ulcerative colitis. See also *Duhamel operation, Soave operation,* and *Swenson's operation,* under *operation.* Called also *ileoanal pull-through procedure.*
**ileorectal a.,** surgical anastomosis of the ileum and rectum after total colectomy, as is often done in treatment of ulcerative colitis.
**intestinal a.,** the establishment of a communication between two portions of the intestinal tract.
**isoperistaltic a.,** enterostomy in which the intestinal segments are so joined that the peristaltic waves in the two conjoined portions progress in the same direction.
**portal-systemic a., portosystemic a.,** 1. a naturally-occurring anastomosis between the portal and systemic venous circulations. 2. see under *shunt.*
**postcostal a.,** a longitudinal linkage of the seven highest intersegmental arteries in the embryo that gives rise to the vertebral artery.
**Potts a.,** see under *operation.*
**precapillary a.,** anastomosis between small arteries just before they become capillaries.
**precostal a.,** a longitudinal anastomosis of intersegmental arteries in the embryo that gives rise to the thyrocervical and costocervical trunks.
**pyeloileocutaneous a.,** direct connection of the renal pelvis to an isolated loop of the ileum, which is then anchored to the abdominal wall at the stoma, to drain exteriorly.
**a. of Riolan,** the part of the marginal artery of the colon that is an anastomosis of the superior and inferior mesenteric arteries.
**Roux-en-Y a.,** any Y-shaped anastomosis in which the small intestine is included; after division of the small intestine segment, the distal end is implanted into another organ, such as the stomach or esophagus, and the proximal end into the small intestine below the anastomosis to provide drainage without reflux.
**stirrup a.,** an arterial branch sometimes seen connecting the dorsalis pedis and external plantar arteries.

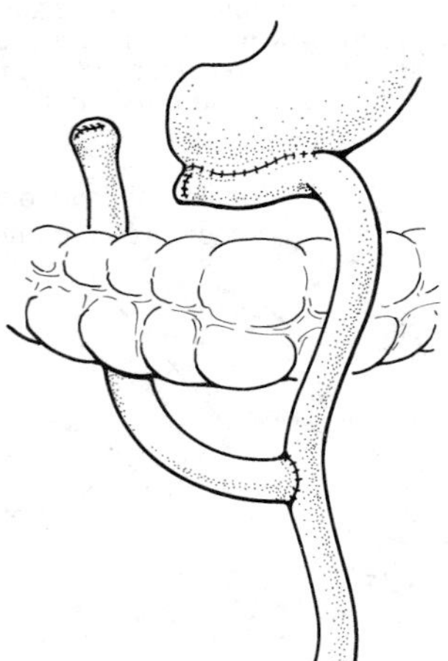

Roux-en-Y anastomosis

**Sucquet-Hoyer a.,** segmentum arteriale anastomosis arteriovenosae glomeriformis.
**terminoterminal a.,** surgical anastomosis between the distal end of an artery and the proximal end of the corresponding vein and between the proximal end of the artery and the distal end of the vein.
**transureteroureteral a.,** the operation of connecting one ureter to the ureter on the opposite side.
**ureteroileocutaneous a.,** connection of the transected ureter to an isolated loop of the ileum, which is then anchored to the abdominal wall at the stoma, to drain exteriorly.
**ureteroureteral a.,** the operation of joining portions of the same ureter.
**Waterston a.,** see under *operation.*

**an·as·to·mot·ic** (ə-nas″tə-mot′ik) pertaining to or of the nature of an anastomosis.

**an·as·tral** (an-as′trəl) [*an-* neg. + *astral*] lacking, or pertaining to the lack of, an aster; used in reference to a mitotic figure.

**an·as·tro·zole** (an-as′trə-zōl) a nonsteroidal aromatase inhibitor that lowers levels of serum estradiol and is used in chemotherapy for carcinoma of the breast, especially in postmenopausal women; administered orally.

**anat.** anatomy; anatomical.

**an·a·tom·ic** (an″ə-tom′ik) anatomical.

**an·a·tom·i·cal** (an″ə-tom′ĭ-kəl) pertaining to anatomy, or to the structure of an organism.

**an·a·tom·i·co·med·i·cal** (an-ə-tom″ĭ-ko-med′ĭ-kəl) pertaining to anatomy and medicine or to medical anatomy.

**an·a·tom·i·co·path·o·log·i·cal** (an″ə-tom″ĭ-ko-path″o-loj′ĭ-kəl) pertaining to anatomic pathology.

**an·a·tom·i·co·phys·i·o·log·i·cal** (an-ə-tom″ĭ-ko-fiz″e-o-loj′ĭ-kəl) pertaining to anatomy and physiology.

**an·a·tom·i·co·sur·gi·cal** (an-ə-tom″ĭ-ko-sər′jĭ-kəl) pertaining to anatomy and surgery.

**anat·o·mist** (ə-nat′ə-mist) a person skilled or learned in anatomy; a specialist in the science of anatomy.

**anat·o·my** (ə-nat′ə-me) [*ana-* + *-tomy*] [MeSH: Anatomy] 1. the science of the structure of the body and the relation of its parts; it is largely based on dissection, from which it obtains its name. 2. dissection of an organized body.
**applied a.,** anatomy as applied to diagnosis and treatment.
**artificial a.,** the study of anatomical structure by use of models or other artificial means.
**artistic a.,** the study of anatomy as applied to drawing, painting, and sculpture.
**clastic a.,** anatomy studied by the aid of models in which various layers can be removed to show the position of organs and parts underneath.
**clinical a.,** anatomy as applied to clinical practice.
**comparative a.,** a comparison of the structure of different animals and plants, one with another.
**corrosion a.,** anatomy studied by means of corrosive agents that remove the tissues not intended to be observed.
**dental a.,** the study of the structure of the teeth and their correlated parts.
**descriptive a.,** the study or description of individual parts of the body; called also *systematic a.*
**developmental a.,** the field of embryology concerned with the changes that cells, tissues, organs, and the body as a whole undergo from a germ cell of each parent to the resulting offspring; it includes both prenatal and postnatal development.
**general a.,** the study of the structure and composition of the body, and its tissues and fluids in general.
**gross a.,** that which deals with structures that can be distinguished with the unaided eye; called also *macroscopic a.*
**histologic a.,** histology.
**homologic a.,** the study of the correlated parts of the body in different animals.
**macroscopic a.,** gross a.
**medical a.,** anatomy concerned with the study of points connected with the physical examination and localization of internal abnormalities.
**microscopic a., minute a.,** histology.
**morbid a., pathological a.,** anatomic pathology.
**physiognomonic a.,** the study of the external expression of the body surface, especially of the face.
**physiological a.,** the study of the organs with respect to their normal functions.
**plastic a.,** the study of anatomy by the aid of models and manikins, especially those that can be taken apart.
**practical a.,** anatomy studied by means of demonstration and dissection.

**radiological a.,** the study of the anatomy of organs and tissues using radiological techniques.
**regional a.,** descriptive anatomy arranged according to the regions of the body. The study of limited portions or regions of the body, and the relationships of their parts.
**special a.,** the study of particular organs or parts.
**surface a.,** the study of the form and markings of the surface of the body, especially in relation to deeper parts.
**surgical a.,** the study of limited portions or regions of the body, with a view to the diagnosis and treatment of surgical conditions.
**systematic a.,** descriptive a.
**topographic a.,** the study of parts in their relation to surrounding parts.
**transcendental a.,** the study of the general design and morphology of the body and the analogies and homologies of its parts.
**veterinary a.,** the anatomy of domestic animals.
**x-ray a.,** radiological a.

**ana·tox·ic** (an″ə-tok′sik) pertaining to anatoxin.

**ana·tox·in** (an″ə-tok′sin) [*ana-* + *toxin*] toxoid.
**diphtheria a., a.-Ramon,** diphtheria toxoid.

**ana·tri·crot·ic** (an″ə-tri-krot′ik) on a pulse tracing, having two notches, i.e. three waveforms, on the ascending limb.

**ana·troph·ic** (an″ə-trof′ik) 1. correcting or preventing atrophy. 2. a remedy that prevents waste of the tissues.

**ana·tro·pia** (an″ə-tro′pe-ə) [*ana-* + Gr. *trepein* to turn] upward deviation of the visual axis of one eye when the other eye is fixing.

**ana·trop·ic** (an″ə-trop′ik) pertaining to anatropia; deviating upward.

**ana·ven·in** (an″ə-ven′in) a venom which has become inactivated by the addition of formaldehyde but which retains its antigenic properties.

**an·az·o·lene so·di·um** (an-az′o-lēn) a diagnostic aid in the determination of blood volume and cardiac output.

**ANCA** antineutrophil cytoplasmic autoantibody (or antibody).

**An·cef** (an′sef) trademark for a preparation of cefazolin sodium.

**an·chor** (ang′kər) a means by which something is held securely.
**endosteal implant a.,** a metal implant in the shape of a ship's anchor, usually made of a chromium-cobalt alloy, which is placed deep into the bone to provide retention for an implant denture.

**an·chor·age** (ang′kər-ij) 1. surgical fixation of a displaced viscus. 2. in operative dentistry, the fixation of fillings or of artificial crowns or bridges. 3. in orthodontics, the nature and degree of resistance to displacement offered by an anatomical unit when used for the purpose of effecting tooth movement. 4. in tissue cell culture, the attachment of proliferating cells to a solid surface.
**cervical a.,** an orthodontic anchorage in which the back of the neck is used for resistance through a strap fitted around the neck.
**compound a.,** an orthodontic anchorage in which the resistance is obtained from two or more teeth.
**extramaxillary a.,** extraoral a.
**extraoral a.,** an orthodontic anchorage in which the resistance unit is outside of the oral cavity, the force being transmitted to the teeth by means of headgear attached to the teeth. Called also *extramaxillary a.*
**intermaxillary a.,** an orthodontic anchorage in which the resistance units situated in one jaw are used to effect tooth movement in the other jaw. Called also *maxillomandibular a.*
**intraoral a.,** an orthodontic anchorage in which the resistance units are all located within the oral cavity.
**maxillomandibular a.,** intermaxillary a.
**multiple a.,** an orthodontic anchorage in which more than one type of resistance unit is utilized. Called also *reinforced a.*
**occipital a.,** an orthodontic anchorage in which the resistance is borne by the top and back of the head, and the force transmitted to the teeth by means of the headgear and heavy elastics connected with attachment on the teeth.
**precision a.,** see under *attachment.*
**reciprocal a.,** anchorage in which the movement of one or more dental units is balanced against the movement of one or more opposing dental units. Cf. *reciprocal force.*
**reinforced a.,** multiple a.
**simple a.,** an orthodontic anchorage in which larger teeth or groups of teeth and their location are used to move teeth of lesser size; the resistance to the movement comes solely from resistance to tipping movement of the anchored unit.
**stationary a.,** an orthodontic anchorage in which the resistance to the movement of one or more dental units comes from the resistance to bodily movement of the anchorage unit; a questionable concept of anchorage implying that selected teeth remain stable.

**anchyl(o)-** for words beginning thus, see those beginning *ankyl(o)-.*

**an·cil·la·ry** (an′sĭ-lar″e) [L. *ancillaris* relating to a maid servant] assisting in the performance of a service or the achievement of a result.

**an·cip·i·tal** (an-sip′ĭ-təl) [L. *an′ceps* two headed] having two heads or two edges.

**An·cis·tro·don** (an-sis′tro-don) *Agkistrodon.*

**an·cis·troid** (an-sis′troid) [Gr. *ankistron* fishhook + *-oid*] hook shaped.

**An·co·bon** (an′ko-bon) trademark for a preparation of flucytosine.

**an·co·nad** (ang′ko-nad) [Gr. *ankōn* elbow + L. *ad* toward] toward the elbow or olecranon.

**an·con·ag·ra** (ang″kon-ag′rə) [Gr. *ankōn* elbow + *agra* seizure] gout of the elbow.

**an·co·nal** (ang′kə-nəl) cubital.

**an·co·ne·al** (ang-ko′ne-əl) cubital.

**an·co·ni·tis** (ang″ko-ni′tis) inflammation of the elbow joint.

**an·co·noid** (ang′ko-noid) resembling the elbow.

**ANCOVA** analysis of covariance.

**an·crod** (an′krod) [MeSH: Ancrod] a proteinase obtained from the venom of the Malayan pit viper *Agkistrodon rhodostoma,* acting specifically on fibrinogen; used as an anticoagulant in the treatment of retinal vein occlusion and deep vein thrombosis and to prevent postoperative rethrombosis.

**ancyl(o)-** for words beginning thus, see also words beginning *ankyl(o)-.*

**An·cy·los·to·ma** (ang″kĭ-los′tə-mə, an″sĭ-los′tə-mə) [*ancylo-* + *stoma*] [MeSH: Ancylostoma] a genus of nematode parasites of the family Ancylostomatidae, the Old World hookworms.
**A. america′num,** *Necator americanus.*
**A. brazilien′se,** a hookworm found in cats and dogs in the southeastern United States, Brazil, and other tropical countries; its larvae may cause cutaneous larva migrans (q.v.) in humans.
**A. cani′num,** the most common hookworm of dogs; it also infects cats, and its larvae may cause cutaneous larva migrans (q.v.) in humans.
**A. ceylo′nicum,** *A. braziliense.*
**A. duodena′le,** the common European or Old World hookworm, which inhabits the small intestine of humans and other animals and causes ancylostomiasis. Males are 10 to 12 mm long and females are somewhat larger.
**A. tubaefor′mis,** a common hookworm of cats.

**an·cy·lo·sto·mat·ic** (an″kĭ-lo-stə-mat′ik, an″sĭ-lo-stə-mat′ik) caused by *Ancylostoma.*

**An·cy·lo·sto·ma·ti·dae** (ang″kĭ-lo-, an″sĭ-lo-sto-mat′ĭ-de) the hookworms, a family of often parasitic phasmid nematodes that includes the genera *Ancylostoma, Bunostomum, Gaigeria, Necator,* and *Uncinaria.* See also *hookworm disease,* under *disease.*

**an·cy·lo·stome** (an-kil′ə-stōm, an-sil′ə-stōm) 1. an individual of the genus *Ancylostoma.* 2. an individual of the family Ancylostomidae; a hookworm.

**an·cy·los·to·mi·a·sis** (an″kĭ-los″to-mi′ə-sis) [MeSH: Ancylostomiasis] 1. hookworm disease in carnivores caused by members of the genus *Ancylostoma.* 2. cutaneous larva migrans (def. 1).

**An·cy·lo·sto·mi·dae** (ang″kĭ-lo-, an″sĭ-lo-sto′mĭ-de) Ancylostomatidae.

**An·cy·los·to·mum** (an″kĭ-los-to′məm, an″sĭ-los-to′məm) *Ancylostoma.*

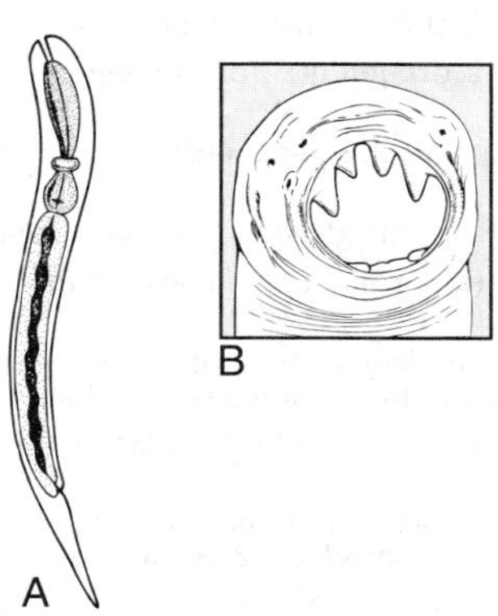

*Ancylostoma duodenale. (A),* Larval form; *(B),* mouth of adult, showing the two pairs of teeth.

**an·cy·roid** (an'sə-roid) [Gr. *ankyra* anchor + *oid*] shaped like an anchor or hook.

**An·der·nach's ossicles** (ahn'der-nahks) [Johann Winther von *Andernach,* German physician, 1487–1574] see *os suturale.*

**An·ders' disease** (an'dərs) [James Meschter *Anders,* American physician, 1854–1936] adiposis tuberosa simplex.

**An·dersch's ganglion, nerve** (ahn'dərsh-əz) [Carolus Samuel *Andersch,* German anatomist, 1732–1777] see *ganglion inferius nervi glossopharyngei* and *nervus tympanicus.*

**An·der·sen's disease, syndrome (triad)** (an'dər-sənz) [Dorothy Hansine *Andersen,* American pathologist, 1901–1963] see under *disease* and *syndrome.*

**An·der·son splint** (An'dər-son) [Roger *Anderson,* American orthopedic surgeon, 1891–1971] see under *splint.*

**An·des disease** (an'dēz) [*Andes* Mountains in Peru, where it was first observed] chronic mountain sickness.

**An·di·ra** (an-di'rə) a genus of tropical trees of the family Leguminosae. *A. araro'ba* is a Brazilian species that is a source of Goa powder and chrysarobin. Many species are poisonous, and several are anthelmintic.

**An·dra·de type familial amyloid polyneuropathy (syndrome)** (ahn-drah'da) [Corino M. *Andrade,* Portuguese physician, 20th century] Portuguese type familial amyloid polyneuropathy; see under *polyneuropathy.*

**An·dral's decubitus (sign)** (ahn-drahlz') [Gabriel *Andral,* French physician, 1797–1876] see under *decubitus.*

**An·dre·sen appliance** (ahn'drə-sən) [Viggo *Andresen,* Norwegian orthodontist, 1870–1950] see *functional activator,* under *activator.*

**An·dré Tho·mas sign** (ahn-dra' to-mahs') [*André* Antoine Henri *Thomas,* French neurologist, 1867–1963] see under *sign.*

**andr(o)-** [Gr. *anēr, andros* man] a combining form denoting relationship to the male.

**an·dro·blas·to·ma** (an″dro-blas-to'mə) [MeSH: Androblastoma] 1. a rare, benign tumor of the testis that histologically resembles the fetal testis; there are three varieties: diffuse stromal, mixed (stromal and epithelial), and tubular (epithelial). Sertoli cells in the epithelial elements may produce estrogen and cause feminization. Called also *gonadal stromal tumor, Pick's testicular* or *tubular adenoma, tubular adenoma,* and *Sertoli cell tumor.* 2. a rare tumor of the ovary, usually occurring in young women; both Sertoli cells (sex cord origin) and Leydig cells (stromal origin) are present. The tumor may cause masculinization and hirsutism, although occasionally estrogenic activity results. Called also *Sertoli-Leydig cell tumor* and *arrhenoblastoma.*

**an·dro·cyte** (an'dro-sīt) [*andro-* + *-cyte*] male sex cell, especially an immature stage.

**an·dro·de·do·tox·in** (an″dro-de″do-tok'sin) a poisonous principle from the leaves of rhododendrons.

**an·droe·ci·um** (an-dre'she-əm) stamen.

**an·dro·ga·lac·to·ze·mia** (an″dro-gə-lak″to-ze'me-ə) [*andro-* + *galacto-* + Gr. *zēmia* loss] lactation from the male breast.

**an·dro·gen** (an'dro-jən) [*andro-* + *-gen*] any substance that promotes masculinization; see *adrenal a's* and *testosterone.*
**adrenal a's,** any of the 19-carbon steroids synthesized by the adrenal cortex that function as weak steroids or steroid precursors, including dehydroepiandrosterone, dehydroepiandrosterone sulfate, and androstenedione.

**an·dro·gen·e·sis** (an″dro-jen'ə-sis) [*andro-* + *-genesis*] development of a zygote that contains only paternal chromosomes.

**an·dro·gen·ic** (an″dro-jen'ik) producing masculine characteristics.

**an·dro·ge·nic·i·ty** (an″dro-jə-nis'ĭ-te) the quality of exerting a masculinizing effect.

**an·dro·gen·i·za·tion** (an″dro-jen-ĭ-za'shən) masculinization.

**an·drog·e·nized** (an-droj'ə-nīzd) showing the effects of a response to androgens.

**an·drog·e·nous** (an-droj'ə-nəs) [*andro-* + *-genous*] pertaining or tending to the production of male rather than female offspring.

**an·dro·gone** (an'dro-gōn) [*andro-* + Gr. *gonos* seed] spermatogenic cell.

**an·dro·gyne** (an'dro-jīn) 1. a person characterized by androgyny; see also *pseudohermaphrodite.* 2. female pseudohermaphrodite.

**an·drog·y·nism** (an-droj'ĭ-niz″əm) 1. androgyny. 2. pseudohermaphroditism.

**an·drog·y·noid** (an-droj'ĭ-noid) 1. pseudohermaphrodite. 2. androgynous.

**an·drog·y·nous** (an-droj'ĭ-nəs) pertaining to or characterized by androgyny; see also *pseudohermaphrodite.* Called also *androgynoid, bisexual,* and *intersexual.*

**an·drog·y·ny** (an-droj'ĭ-ne) 1. sexual ambiguity, either physical or psychological; called also *androgynism* and *bisexuality.* 2. female pseudohermaphroditism.

**an·droid** (an'droid) [*andr-* + *-oid*] resembling a man; see *male.* Called also *androidal* and *andromorphous.*

**an·droi·dal** (an-droi'dəl) android.

**an·drol·o·gy** (an-drol'ə-je) [*andro-* + *-logy*] scientific study of the masculine constitution and of the diseases of the male sex; especially the study of diseases of the male organs of generation.

**An·drom·e·da** (an-drom'ə-də) [L.] a genus of shrubs and trees of the family Ericaceae; some species contain andromedotoxin.

**an·drom·e·do·tox·in** (an-drom″ə-do-tok'sin) [*Andromeda* + *toxin*] a crystalline principle, poisonous to humans and other animals, found in various ericaceous plants, such as species of *Andromeda, Azalea, Kalmia,* and *Rhododendron.* In sheep and other livestock that graze on the plants, it causes salivation, nasal discharge, emesis, and central nervous system symptoms that may include paralysis, coma, and death. Called also *acetylandromedol* and *grayanotoxin.*

**an·dro·mer·o·gon** (an″dro-mer'ə-gon) [*andro-* + *mero-*[1] + *gonē* seed] an organism developed from an oocyte containing the male pronucleus only; as a result, the cells contain only the paternal set of chromosomes.

**an·dro·mer·o·gone** (an″dro-mer'ə-gōn) andromerogon.

**an·dro·me·rog·o·ny** (an″dro-mə-rog'o-ne) [*andro-* + *merogony*] development of a portion of an oocyte containing the male pronucleus only, the nucleus of the ovum having been removed before fusion of the male and female pronuclei occurred. Cf. *gynomerogony* and *merogony.*

**an·dro·mi·met·ic** (an″dro-mĭ-met'ik) [*andro-* + *mimetic*] exerting influences of the sort promoted by testosterone and other androgens. See also *masculinization.*

**an·dro·mor·phous** (an″dro-mor'fəs) [*andro-* + *morph-* + *-ous*] android.

**an·drop·a·thy** (an-drop'ə-the) [*andro-* + *-pathy*] any disease peculiar to males.

**an·dro·phile** (an'dro-fīl) anthropophilic.

**an·droph·i·lous** (an-drof'ĭ-ləs) anthropophilic.

**an·dro·stane** (an'dro-stān) the 19-carbon tetracyclic hydrocarbon nucleus, $C_{19}H_{32}$, that is the parent structure of the androgens; used in steroid nomenclature.

**an·dro·stane·di·ol** (an″dro-stān'de-ol) an androgen, $C_{19}H_{32}O_2$, implicated as a regulator of gonadotropin secretion.
**a. glucuronide,** a metabolite of dihydrotestosterone formed in the peripheral tissues; plasma and urinary concentrations are used to estimate peripheral androgen activity.

**an·dro·stene** (an'dro-stēn) a cyclic hydrocarbon nucleus, $C_{19}H_{30}$, with one double bond; used in androgen nomenclature.

**an·dro·stene·di·ol** (an″dro-stēn'de-ol) a testosterone metabolite, $C_{19}H_{30}O_2$, occurring in two isomeric forms, 3-*trans,*17-dihydroxy $\Delta^5$-androstene and 3-*cis,*17-dihydroxy $\Delta^5$-androstene, that may contribute to gonadotropin secretion.

**an·dro·stene·di·one** (an″dro-stēn'de-ōn) [MeSH: Androstenedione] an androgenic steroid produced by the testis, adrenal cortex, and ovary, occurring as two types, $\Delta^4$-androstenedione and $\Delta^5$-androstenedione. Androstenediones can be converted metabolically to testosterone and other androgens.

**an·dros·ter·one** (an-dros'tər-ōn) [MeSH: Androsterone] an androgen degradation product, 3$\alpha$-hydroxy-5$\alpha$-androstan-17-one, $C_{19}H_{30}O_2$; in some species it exerts weak androgen-like effects.

**AN-DTPA** trademark for a kit for the preparation of technetium Tc 99m pentetate.

**-ane** a word termination denoting a saturated open-chain hydrocarbon, $C_nH_{2n+2}$.

**an·ec·do·tal** (an″ek-do'təl) [Gr. *anekdotos* not published] based on descriptions of unmatched individual cases rather than on controlled studies.

**an·ec·dy·sis** (an-ek'dĭ-sis) [*an-* neg. + *ecdysis*] a long period during the molting cycle of arthropods when there are no signs of either recovery from a molt or preparations for the next molt.

**an·echo·ic** (an-ə-ko'ik) [*an-* neg. + *echo* + *-ic*] 1. without echoes, as an anechoic chamber. 2. sonolucent.

**an·ec·ta·sis** (an-ek'tə-sis) [*an-* neg. + *ectasis*] primary atelectasis.

**An•ec•tine** (an-ek′tin) trademark for preparations of succinylcholine chloride.

**Anel's probe, syringe** (ah-nelz′) [Dominique *Anel,* French surgeon, 1679–1730] see under *probe* and *syringe.*

**an•elec•tro•ton•ic** (an″ə-lek″tro-ton′ik) pertaining to anelectrotonus.

**an•elec•trot•o•nus** (an″ə-lek-trot′ə-nəs) [*ana-* + *electrotonus*] lessened irritability of a nerve in the region of the positive pole or anode during the passage of an electric current.

**ane•mia** (ə-ne′me-ə) [*an-* neg. + *-emia*] [MeSH: Anemia] a reduction below normal in the concentration of erythrocytes or hemoglobin in the blood, measured per cu mm or by volume of packed red cells per 100 mL of blood; it occurs when the equilibrium is disturbed between blood loss (through bleeding or destruction) and blood production.

## Anemia

**achrestic a.,** any of various types of megaloblastic anemia that resemble pernicious anemia but are unresponsive to therapy with vitamin $B_{12}$.

**achylic a.,** iron deficiency a.

**anhematopoietic a.,** aplastic a.

**aplastic a.,** any of a diverse group of anemias characterized by bone marrow failure with reduction of hematopoietic cells and their replacement by fat, resulting in pancytopenia, often accompanied by granulocytopenia and thrombocytopenia. It may be hereditary; it may be secondary to causes such as toxic, radiant, or immunologic injury to bone marrow stem cells or their microenvironment; it may be associated with various diseases; or it may be idiopathic.

**Arctic a.,** polar a.

**aregenerative a.,** an anemia characterized by bone marrow failure, so that functional marrow cells are regenerated slowly or not at all; the term has been used to denote specific disorders with this characteristic, including aplastic anemia and pure red cell anemia.

**aregenerative a., congenital,** congenital hypoplastic anemia (def. 1).

***Bartonella* a.,** Oroya fever.

**Blackfan-Diamond a.,** congenital hypoplastic a. (def. 1).

**cameloid a.,** hereditary elliptocytosis.

**a. of chronic disease, a. of chronic disorders,** mild to moderate anemia secondary to any of numerous chronic diseases lasting more than two months, such as infections, inflammatory conditions, or malignancies, characterized by hypoferrinemia in combination with siderosis of the reticuloendothelial system.

**congenital a. of newborn,** erythroblastosis fetalis.

**Cooley's a.,** thalassemia major.

**cow's milk a.,** milk anemia in infants fed exclusively on cow's milk.

**deficiency a.,** anemia caused by lack of a specific substance required for normal hemoglobin synthesis and erythrocytic maturation and arising by several means, such as malabsorption or poor dietary intake. See *folic acid deficiency a., iron deficiency a.,* and *scorbutic a.* Called also *nutritional a.*

**Diamond-Blackfan a.,** congenital hypoplastic a., def. 1.

**dilution a.,** hydremia.

**dimorphic a.,** anemia with erythrocytes of two different sizes, such as with combined deficiencies of vitamin $B_{12}$ and iron or after a blood transfusion.

**dyserythropoietic a., congenital,** any of several rare hereditary anemias, mostly types of macrocytic anemia, characterized by nuclear anomalies of the erythrocytes, such as multinuclearity, karyorrhexis, or macrocytosis. The most common type (called also HEMPAS) is an autosomal recessive condition characterized by multinuclear erythrocytes and a positive acidified serum test.

**elliptocytary a., elliptocytic a., elliptocytotic a.,** hereditary elliptocytosis.

**equine infectious a.,** a disease of equines caused by a lentivirus and spread through the blood by inoculation, especially by blood-sucking insects; characteristics include abrupt fevers and recurring attacks of malaise. Called also *infectious a. of horses* and *swamp fever.*

**Fanconi's a.,** Fanconi's syndrome (def. 1).

**feline infectious a.,** a cyclic type of hemolytic anemia in domestic cats caused by infection of red blood cells with the rickettsia *Haemobartonella felis,* which may be spread from cat to cat during fights; acute cases are characterized by fever, jaundice, anorexia, and splenomegaly and can be fatal. Called also *haemobartonellosis.*

**folic acid deficiency a.,** macrocytic anemia due to deficiency of folic acid. Called also *nutritional macrocytic a.*

**goat's milk a.,** milk anemia in infants fed exclusively on goat's milk.

**ground itch a.,** hookworm a.

**Heinz body a's,** a group of hemolytic anemias of diverse etiology with the common morphologic characteristic of having Heinz bodies within affected erythrocytes.

**hemolytic a.,** any of a group of acute or chronic anemias characterized by shortened survival of mature erythrocytes and inability of bone marrow to compensate for the decreased life span. They are classified as either *inherited* (generally due to intrinsic cell defects such as in the erythrocyte membrane, glycolytic pathway, glutathione metabolism, or hemoglobin molecule; see *congenital* and *congenital nonspherocytic hemolytic a.*), or *acquired* (due to the actions of extrinsic agents such as infectious agents, poisons, physical trauma, or antibodies; see *autoimmune, immune, infectious, microangiopathic,* and *toxic hemolytic a.*).

**hemolytic a., autoimmune (AIHA),** any of a large group of anemias involving autoantibodies against red cell antigens. Those due to warm-reactive antibodies, usually IgG but occasionally IgM or IgA, may be idiopathic or secondary to autoimmune diseases, hematologic neoplasms, viral infections, or immunodeficiency diseases, and usually involve sequestration of sensitized erythrocytes by the spleen. Those due to cold-reactive antibodies, usually IgM but occasionally IgG, include cold agglutinin syndrome and paroxysmal cold hemoglobinuria and usually involve complement-dependent intravascular hemolysis or sequestration of erythrocytes by the liver.

**hemolytic a., congenital,** 1. a general term for hemolytic anemia that is present from birth and in which the lifespan of red blood cells is diminished, such as occurs in hereditary spherocytosis. 2. hereditary spherocytosis.

**hemolytic a., congenital nonspherocytic,** any of a heterogeneous group of inherited anemias characterized by shortened red cell survival, lack of spherocytosis, and normal osmotic fragility associated with erythrocyte membrane defects, multiple intracellular enzyme deficiencies or other defects, or unstable hemoglobins. The most common enzyme defects are in glucose-6-phosphate dehydrogenase or pyruvate kinase.

**hemolytic a., drug-induced immune,** immune hemolytic anemia induced by drugs, classified by mechanism as *penicillin type,* in which the drug, acting as a hapten bound to the red cell membrane, induces the formation of specific antibodies; *methyldopa type,* in which the drug, possibly by inhibition of suppressor T cells, induces the formation of anti-Rh antibodies; or *stibophen* or *"innocent bystander" type,* in which circulating drug-antibody immune complexes bind nonspecifically to red cells. The first two types usually involve warm-reactive antibodies and accelerated sequestration of red cells by the reticuloendothelial system; the third usually involves cold-reactive antibodies and complement-dependent intravascular hemolysis.

**hemolytic a., immune,** an acquired hemolytic anemia in which a hemolytic response is caused by isoantibodies or autoantibodies produced on exposure to drugs, toxins, or other antigens. See also *autoimmune hemolytic a., drug-induced immune hemolytic a.,* and *erythroblastosis fetalis.*

**hemolytic a., infectious,** that due to an incompletely compensated decrease in red blood cell survival secondary to infectious agents, including protozoa (e.g., *Plasmodium* in malaria), bacteria, and certain viruses.

**hemolytic a., microangiopathic,** thrombotic thrombocytopenic purpura.

**hemolytic a., nonspherocytic,** see *congenital nonspherocytic hemolytic a.*

**hemolytic a., toxic,** that due to toxic agents, including drugs, bacterial lysins, and snake venoms.

**hemolytic a. of newborn,** erythroblastosis fetalis.

**hemorrhagic a.,** anemia caused by the sudden and acute loss of blood; called also *acute posthemorrhagic a.*

**hereditary iron-loading a.,** hereditary sideroblastic a.

**hookworm a.,** hypochromic microcytic anemia in humans or other animals occurring as part of hookworm disease (q.v.). Called also *ground itch a.*

**hypochromic a.,** anemia characterized by a disproportionate reduction of red cell hemoglobin and an increased area of central pallor in the red cells. It may be hereditary (e.g., hereditary sideroblastic anemia, thalassemia minor) or acquired (e.g., iron deficiency anemia). Called also *Faber's syndrome.*

**hypochromic microcytic a.,** any anemia with microcytes that are hypochromic (reduced in size and in hemoglobin content); the most common type is iron deficiency anemia.

**a. hypochro'mica sideroachres'tica heredita'ria,** hereditary sideroblastic a.

**hypoplastic a.,** a general term indicating a form of anemia due to varying degrees of erythrocytic hypoplasia without leukopenia or thrombocytopenia; it sometimes develops into aplastic anemia.

**hypoplastic a., congenital,** 1. a progressive anemia of unknown etiology encountered in the first year of life, characterized by deficiency of red cell precursors in an otherwise normally cellular bone marrow; it is unresponsive to hematinics and often requires multiple blood transfusions. Called also *Blackfan-Diamond a.* or *syndrome, Diamond-Blackfan a.* or *syndrome, congenital pure red cell a.* or *aplasia, congenital aregenerative a.,* and *erythrogenesis imperfecta.* 2. Fanconi's syndrome (def. 1).

**immunohemolytic a.,** immune hemolytic a.

**infectious a. of horses,** equine infectious a.

**iron deficiency a.,** a type of hypochromic microcytic anemia caused by low or absent iron stores and serum iron concentration; there is elevated free erythrocyte porphyrin, low transferrin saturation, elevated transferrin, low serum ferritin, and low hemoglobin concentration. Symptoms may include pallor, angular stomatitis and other oral lesions, gastrointestinal complaints, retinal hemorrhages and exudates, and thinning and brittleness of the nails, occasionally leading to spoon nails (koilonychia).

**leukoerythroblastic a.,** leukoerythroblastosis.

**macrocytic a.,** any of various anemias of diverse etiologies that are characterized by macrocytes (larger than normal red cells) lacking the usual central area of pallor; there is also increased mean corpuscular volume and mean corpuscular hemoglobin.

**macrocytic a., nutritional,** folic acid deficiency a.

**macrocytic a., tropical,** a type of nutritional macrocytic anemia seen in impoverished tropical regions, resembling pernicious anemia but without achlorhydria and only erratically responsive to vitamin $B_{12}$. The etiology is often related to folate deficiency and administration of folic acid usually produces marked improvement.

**Mediterranean a.,** thalassemia major.

**megaloblastic a.,** any anemia characterized by the presence of megaloblasts in the bone marrow, such as pernicious anemia.

**megalocytic a.,** macrocytic a.

**microangiopathic a.,** thrombotic thrombocytopenic purpura.

**microcytic a.,** any anemia characterized by microcytes (erythrocytes smaller than normal), such as iron deficiency anemia or β-thalassemia. See also *hypochromic microcytic a.*

**milk a.,** iron deficiency anemia in infants fed a diet of only milk; see *cow's milk a.* and *goat's milk a.*

**miners' a.,** hookworm anemia in humans.

**mountain a.,** a misnomer for *mountain sickness.*

**myelopathic a., myelophthisic a.,** leukoerythroblastosis.

**a. neonato'rum,** erythroblastosis fetalis.

**normoblastic a., refractory,** refractory sideroblastic a.

**normochromic a.,** anemia in which the hemoglobin content of the red cells as measured by the MCHC is in the normal range.

**normocytic a.,** anemia with erythrocytes of normal size but a proportionate decrease in hemoglobin content, packed red cell volume, and number of erythrocytes per cubic millimeter of blood.

**nutritional a.,** deficiency a.

**osteosclerotic a.,** anemia due to bone marrow failure associated with osteosclerosis, as a result of the effect on bone marrow of changes in the bones.

**pernicious a.,** a type of megaloblastic anemia usually seen in older adults, caused by impaired intestinal absorption of vitamin $B_{12}$ due to lack of availability of intrinsic factor; it is often characterized by pallor, achlorhydria, glossitis, gastric mucosal atrophy, weakness, antibodies against gastric parietal cells or intrinsic factor, and neurologic manifestations.

**pernicious a., congenital, pernicious a., juvenile,** a rare disorder occurring in children, clinically very similar to the adult form but differing in that gastric acid secretion is normal, the gastric mucosa is not atrophied, and development is delayed.

**physiologic a.,** the normocytic, normochromic anemia that occurs in infants at the age of two or three months, owing to normal depression of erythropoiesis and hemoglobin synthesis, probably resulting as an adjustment to the changeover from placental to pulmonary oxygenation.

**polar a.,** an anemic condition that occurs during exposure to low temperature; it is initially microcytic but later becomes normocytic. Called also *Arctic a.*

**posthemorrhagic a., acute,** hemorrhagic a.

**posthemorrhagic a. of newborn,** anemia of the newborn due to hemorrhage, such as into the placenta or from umbilical vessels; it may range from mild to severe.

**pure red cell a.,** anemia characterized by absence of red cell precursors in the bone marrow. It may be acquired or congenital; the latter is called *congenital hypoplastic a.*

**pyridoxine-responsive a.,** a form of sideroblastic anemia in which there is a therapeutic response to pyridoxine; it affects predominately young or middle-aged males.

**a. refracto'ria sideroblas'tica,** refractory sideroblastic a.

**refractory a.,** anemia unresponsive to hematinics.

**scorbutic a.,** anemia due to deficiency of ascorbic acid (vitamin C); in naturally occurring human scurvy the anemia is generally normocytic, although in experimentally induced vitamin C deficiency the anemia is of the megaloblastic type.

**sickle cell a.,** an autosomal dominant type of hemolytic anemia, seen primarily in West Africa and in people of West African descent, and less often in the Mediterranean basin and a few other areas; it is caused by the presence of hemoglobin S with abnormal sickle-shaped erythrocytes *(sickle cells).* Homozygous individuals have 85 to 95 per cent sickle cells and have the full-blown syndrome with accelerated hemolysis, increased blood viscosity and vaso-occlusion, arthralgias, acute attacks of abdominal pain, ulcerations of the lower extremities, and periodic attacks of any of the conditions called *sickle cell crises* (see under *crisis*). The heterozygous condition is called *sickle cell trait* and is usually asymptomatic. See also *sickle cell disease,* under *disease.* Called also *sicklemia.*

**sideroachrestic a.,** sideroblastic a.

**sideroachrestic a., acquired,** refractory sideroblastic a.

**sideroachrestic a., congenital,** hereditary sideroblastic a.

**sideroachrestic a., hereditary,** hereditary sideroblastic a.

**sideroblastic a.,** any of a heterogenous group of acquired and hereditary anemias with diverse clinical manifestations; commonly characterized by large numbers of ringed sideroblasts in the bone marrow, ineffective erythropoiesis, variable proportions of hypochromic erythrocytes in the peripheral blood, and usually increased levels of tissue iron.

**sideroblastic a., acquired,** refractory sideroblastic a.

**sideroblastic a., hereditary,** an X-linked anemia, usually detected in childhood or early adulthood, characterized by an abundance of ringed sideroblasts, hypochromic, microcytic erythrocytes, poikilocytosis, weakness, and iron overload in later years. Called also *Rundles-Falls syndrome.*

**sideroblastic a., primary acquired,** refractory sideroblastic a.

**sideroblastic a., refractory,** a sideroblastic anemia clinically similar to the hereditary sideroblastic form but occurring in adults and often only slowly progressive. It is unresponsive to hematinics or withdrawal of toxic agents or drugs and can be a preleukemic disorder.

**sideroblastic a., X-linked,** hereditary sideroblastic a.

**sideropenic a.,** any of a group of anemias characterized by low levels of iron in the plasma; it includes iron deficiency anemia and the anemias of chronic disorders.

**slaty a.,** a term applied to a grayish color of the face in poisoning by acetanilid or silver.

**spherocytic a.,** hereditary spherocytosis.

**splenic a.,** congestive splenomegaly.

**spur cell a.,** anemia in which the red cells have a bizarre spiculated shape and are destroyed prematurely, primarily in the spleen; it is an acquired form occurring in severe liver disease and represents an abnormality in the cholesterol content of the red-cell membrane.

---

**ane·mic** (ə-ne'mik) pertaining to or characterized by anemia.

**an·e·mom·e·try** (an″ə-mom'ə-tre) velocimetry.

**Anem·o·ne** (ə-nem'o-ne) a large genus of plants of the family Ranunculaceae with divided leaves and conspicuous flowers of sepals. Most species contain ranunculin, which converts enzymatically to protoanemonin, an irritant toxin that can cause poisoning *(anemonism)* in humans and livestock. *A. pulsatil'la* and certain other species contain anemonin rather than its precursors, and have been used medicinally.

**anem·o·nin** (ə-nem'o-nin) a substituted diacrylic acid dilactone that has been used as a sedative and hypnotic; formed as a breakdown product from protoanemonin (q.v.).

**anem·o·nism** (ə-nem'o-niz-əm) poisoning of humans or other animals by plants of the genus *Anemone.*

**anem·o·nol** (ə-nem'o-nol) a highly toxic volatile oil from various species of *Anemone* and from other ranunculaceous plants.

**Anem·o·nop·sis** (ə-nem″ə-nop'sis) a genus of herbs. *A. califor'nica* Hook and Arn., a species found in the southwestern United States and northern Mexico, is the source of mansa.

**an·e·mo·pho·bia** (an″ə-mo-fo′be-ə) [Gr. *anemos* wind + *-phobia*] irrational fear of wind or of drafts.

**an·en·ce·pha·lia** (an″ən-sə-fa′le-ə) anencephaly.

**an·en·ceph·a·lic** (an″ən-sə-fal′ik) exhibiting anencephaly; having no brain.

**an·en·ceph·a·lous** (an″ən-sef′ə-ləs) anencephalic.

**an·en·ceph·a·lus** (an″ən-sef′ə-ləs) an infant exhibiting anencephaly.

**an·en·ceph·a·ly** (an″ən-sef′ə-le) [*an-* neg. + Gr. *enkephalos* brain] [MeSH: Anencephaly] congenital absence of the calvaria, with cerebral hemispheres missing or reduced to small masses attached to the base of the skull; complete absence of the brain is rare. Cf. *meroanencephaly.*

**an·en·ter·ous** (an-en′tər-əs) [*an-* neg. + *entero-* + *-ous*] lacking intestines.

**aneph·ric** (a-nef′rik) without kidneys.

**aneph·ro·gen·e·sis** (a″nef-ro-jen′ə-sis) [*a-*[1] + *nephrogenesis*] congenital absence of kidney tissue.

**an·ep·i·plo·ic** (an-ep″ĭ-plo′ik) devoid of omentum.

**an·er·gia** (an-ər′je-ə) anergy.

**an·er·gic** (an-ər′jik) [*an-* neg. + Gr. *ergon* work] 1. characterized by abnormal inactivity; inactive. 2. marked by lack of energy. 3. pertaining to anergy.

**an·er·gy** (an′ər-je) 1. lack of energy, extreme passivity. 2. diminished reactivity to all antigens; it may take the form of diminished immediate hypersensitivity or diminished delayed hypersensitivity, or both. Cf. *immunologic tolerance.*
**negative a.,** transient reduction in reactivity to allergens in a sensitized individual, occurring as a result of intervening events, such as cachexia.
**positive a.,** reduction in reactivity to allergens in a sensitized individual, owing to alterations in the immune response in the course of disease, as in tuberculosis.

**an·er·oid** (an′ər-oid) [*a-*[1] + Gr. *nēros* liquid + *-oid*] not containing liquid.

**an·eryth·ro·pla·sia** (an″ə-rith″ro-pla′zhə) [*an-* neg. + *erythro-* + *-plasia*] anerythropoiesis.

**an·eryth·ro·plas·tic** (an″ə-rith″ro-plas′-tik) pertaining to or characterized by anerythropoiesis.

**an·eryth·ro·poi·e·sis** (an″ə-rith″ro-poi-e′sis) [*an-* neg. + *erythropoiesis*] deficient or absent erythropoiesis; see also *erythropenia.* Called also *anerythroplasia.*

**an·eryth·ro·re·gen·er·a·tive** (an″ə-rith″ro-re-jen′ər-a″tiv) characterized by lack of regeneration of erythrocytes; see also *aregenerative.*

**anes·the·ci·ne·sia** (an-es″the-sĭ-ne′zhə) [*an-* neg. + *esthesi-* + *cinesi-* + *-ia*] loss of sensibility and motor power.

**anes·the·ki·ne·sia** (an-es″the-kĭ-ne′zhə) anesthecinesia.

**an·es·the·sia** (an″es-the′zhə) [*an-* neg. + *esthesia*] [MeSH: Anesthesia] 1. loss of sensation, usually by damage to a nerve or receptor; called also *numbness.* 2. loss of the ability to feel pain, caused by administration of a drug or by other medical interventions; cf. *anesthetic* (def. 2).
**acupuncture a.,** regional anesthesia using the principles of acupuncture.
**ambulatory a.,** anesthesia performed on an outpatient basis for ambulatory surgery.
**angiospastic a.,** loss of sensibility dependent on spasm of the blood vessels.
**balanced a.,** anesthesia that uses a combination of drugs, each in an amount sufficient to produce its major or desired effect to the optimum degree and keep its undesirable or unnecessary effects to a minimum.
**basal a.,** anesthesia which acts as a basis for further and deeper anesthesia; a state of narcosis produced by preliminary medication so profound that the added inhalation anesthetic necessary to produce surgical anesthesia is greatly reduced.
**Bier's local a.,** Bier block.
**block a.,** regional a.
**brachial plexus a.,** see under *block.*
**bulbar a.,** lack of sensation caused by a lesion of the pons.
**caudal a.,** see under *block.*
**closed circuit a.,** inhalation anesthesia maintained by the continuous rebreathing of a relatively small amount of anesthetic gas and a basal amount of oxygen, normally used with an absorption apparatus for the removal of carbon dioxide.
**compression a.,** loss of sensation resulting from pressure on a nerve.
**conduction a.,** regional a.
**continuous epidural a.,** see under *analgesia.*
**crossed a.,** hemianesthesia cruciata.
**dissociated a., dissociation a.,** loss of sensitivity to pain, heat, and cold without loss of other tactile senses; seen in syringomyelia.
**a. doloro′sa,** analgesia algera.
**electric a.,** anesthesia induced by passage of an electric current.
**endotracheal a.,** anesthesia produced by introduction of a gaseous mixture through a wide-bore tube inserted into the trachea through either the mouth or the nose.
**epidural a.,** regional anesthesia produced by injection of the anesthetic agent between the vertebral spines and beneath the ligamentum flavum into the epidural space; see also *continuous epidural analgesia.* Called also *epidural block* and *peridural a.*
**facial a.,** loss of sensation caused by a lesion of the facial nerve.
**frost a.,** former name for *cryoanesthesia.*
**gauntlet a.,** loss of sensation in the hand and wrist; called also *glove a.*
**general a.,** a reversible state of unconsciousness, produced by anesthetic agents, with absence of pain sensation over the entire body and a greater or lesser degree of muscular relaxation; the drugs producing this state can be administered by inhalation, intravenously, intramuscularly, or rectally.
**girdle a.,** loss of sensation in a zone encircling the hips.
**glove a.,** gauntlet a.
**gustatory a.,** ageusia.
**high pressure a.,** anesthesia produced by controlled application of pressure to a nerve trunk or its branches.
**hypnosis a.,** production of insensibility to pain during surgical procedures by means of hypnotism.
**hypotensive a.,** anesthesia accompanied by deliberate lowering of blood pressure to reduce blood loss and improve usability of the surgical field.
**hypothermic a.,** anesthesia accompanied by the deliberate lowering of the body temperature. See also *cryoanesthesia.*
**hysterical a.,** loss of tactile sensation occurring as a symptom of conversion disorder, often recognizable by its lack of correspondence with nerve distributions.
**infiltration a.,** the production of local anesthesia by deposition of anesthetic solution into a superficial area.
**inhalation a.,** anesthesia produced by the inhalation of vapors of a volatile liquid or gaseous anesthetic agent.
**insufflation a.,** anesthesia produced by blowing a mixture of gases or vapors through a tube introduced into the respiratory tract.
**intercostal a.,** see under *block.*
**intrapulpal a.,** a local anesthetic effect produced by the administration of an anesthetic agent directly into the dental pulp.
**intraspinal a.,** spinal a. (def. 1).
**intravenous a.,** 1. anesthesia produced by introduction of an anesthetic agent into a vein, usually in a limb to which a pneumatic tourniquet has been applied. 2. Bier block.
**intravenous regional a.,** Bier block.
**local a.,** anesthesia confined to one area of the body; see also *regional a.*
**lumbar epidural a.,** anesthesia produced by injection of the anesthetic agent into the epidural space at the second or third lumbar interspace.
**muscular a.,** loss or lack of muscle sense; called also *amyoesthesia* and *amyoesthesis.*
**nausea a.,** loss of the sensation of nausea that is normally stimulated by noxious and disgusting substances.
**olfactory a.,** anosmia.
**open a.,** general inhalation anesthesia utilizing a cone or ether mask; there is no significant rebreathing of expired gases.
**paraneural a.,** perineural block.
**paravertebral a.,** see under *block.*
**peridural a.,** epidural a.
**perineural a.,** see under *block.*
**peripheral a.,** loss of sensation which is due to changes in the peripheral nerves.
**plexus a.,** anesthesia produced by the injection of a local anesthetic around a nerve plexus.
**pressure a.,** anesthesia caused by pressure on a nerve.
**rectal a.,** anesthesia induced by introduction of an anesthetic agent into the rectum.
**refrigeration a.,** former name for *cryoanesthesia.*
**regional a.,** the production of insensibility of a part by interrupting the sensory nerve conductivity from that region of the body. It may be produced by (1) *field block,* that is, the creation of walls of anesthesia encircling the operative field by means of injections of a local anesthetic; or (2) *nerve block,* that is, injection of the anesthetic agent close to the nerves whose conductivity is to be cut off. Called also *block, blockade, block a.,* and *conduction a.*
**sacral a.,** regional anesthesia produced by injection of a local anesthetic into the extradural space of the sacral canal. Called also *transsacral a.* or *block.*
**saddle block a.,** see under *block.*
**segmental a.,** loss of sensation caused by lesions of nerve roots.

**semiclosed a.,** general inhalation anesthesia in which there is partial rebreathing of the expired gases, with a carbon dioxide absorber in the circuit.
**semiopen a.,** general inhalation anesthesia administered by use of a partially open circuit; there is partial rebreathing of the expired gases without a carbon dioxide absorber in the circuit.
**spinal a.,** 1. regional anesthesia produced by injection of a local anesthetic into the subarachnoid space around the spinal cord; cf. *epidural a.* Called also *intraspinal a.* or *block* and *subarachnoid a.* or *block.* 2. loss of sensation due to a spinal lesion.
**subarachnoid a.,** spinal a. (def. 1).
**surgical a.,** that degree of anesthesia at which surgery may safely be performed; ordinarily used to designate such depth of general anesthesia.
**tactile a.,** loss or impairment of the sense of touch; called also *anaphia.* Cf. *paraphia.*
**thalamic hyperesthetic a.,** thalamic syndrome; see under *syndrome.*
**thermal a.,** thermoanesthesia.
**topical a.,** anesthesia produced by application of a local anesthetic directly to the area involved, as to the oral mucosa or the cornea.
**transsacral a.,** sacral a.
**traumatic a.,** loss of sensation caused by injury to a nerve.
**unilateral a.,** hemianesthesia.
**visceral a.,** loss or lack of the visceral sense.

**an·es·the·si·ol·o·gist** (an″əs-the″ze-ol′ə-jist) a physician or dentist specializing in anesthesiology. Cf. *anesthetist.*

**an·es·the·si·ol·o·gy** (an″əs-the″ze-ol′ə-je) [*anesthesia* + *-logy*] [MeSH: Anesthesiology] that branch of medicine which studies anesthesia and anesthetics.

**an·es·the·si·o·phore** (an″əs-the′ze-o-for″) [*anesthesia* + *-phore*] the portion of the molecule of a chemical compound which is responsible for its anesthetic action.

**an·es·thet·ic** (an″əs-thet′ik) 1. characterized by anesthesia (def. 1); called also *numb.* 2. producing anesthesia (defs. 1 and 2). 3. a drug or agent that is used to abolish the sensation of pain.
**general a.,** an agent that produces general anesthesia.
**local a.,** an agent whose anesthetic action is limited to an area of the body determined by the site of its application; it produces its effect by blocking nerve conduction.
**topical a.,** a local anesthetic applied directly to the area to be anesthetized, usually the mucous membranes or the skin.

**anes·the·tist** (ə-nes′thə-tist) a nurse or technician trained to administer anesthetics. Cf. *anesthesiologist.*

**anes·the·ti·za·tion** (ə-nes″thə-tĭ-za′shən) the production of insensibility to pain.

**anes·the·tize** (ə-nes′thə-tīz) to put under the influence of anesthetics.

**an·es·trum** (an-es′trəm) anestrus.

**an·es·trus** (an-es′trəs) [MeSH: Anestrus] 1. abnormal lack of ovarian activity in a female mammal; the term is sometimes extended to include any prolonged lack of sexual responsiveness. 2. a period of the estrous cycle during which there is no ovarian activity; in cats, horses, sheep, goats, and certain other species this occurs annually for periods of weeks to months. Called also *diestrus.*

**an·e·thole** (an′ə-thōl) [NF] a flavoring agent for drugs, obtained from anise and fennel oils and other sources, or prepared synthetically. Called also *anise camphor.*

**Ane·thum** (ə-ne′thəm) [L.; Gr. *anēthon*] a genus of plants of the family Umbelliferae, originally native to Asia. *A. graveo′lens* is dill, the source of oil of dill, whose fruit is carminative and stimulant.

**anet·ic** (ə-net′ik) sedative.

**an·e·to·der·ma** (an″ə-to-dər′mə) [Gr. *anetos* slack + *derma*] localized elastolysis producing circumscribed areas of soft, thin, wrinkled skin that often protrude as small outpouchings. It may be primary and may be associated with inflammatory lesions, or it may be secondary to syphilis, leprosy, or tuberculosis. Called also *atrophia cutis, atrophia maculosa, atrophoderma maculatum,* and *macular atrophy.* See also *atrophoderma.*
**Jadassohn's a., Jadassohn-Pellizari a.,** primary anetoderma occurring after an inflammatory or urticarial eruption; the lesions are round or oval erythematous macules that become atrophic, wrinkled, and pale protrusions. It is usually seen in women in the second to fourth decade. Cf. *Schweninger-Buzzi a.*
**perifollicular a.,** anetoderma occurring around hair follicles not preceded by folliculitis; it may be caused by an elastase-producing strain of *Staphylococcus epidermidis,* it may be drug induced, or endocrine factors may be involved. Called also *perifollicular elastolysis.*
**postinflammatory a.,** a condition usually occurring during infancy, characterized by the development of erythematous papules that enlarge to form oval plaques with a cordlike border and a scaly collarette at the inner margin. All areas of the body except the palms and soles may be affected, with the face, ears, and neck always being involved; it is followed by laxity of the skin clinically resembling cutis laxa. Called also *postinflammatory elastolysis.*
**Schweninger-Buzzi a.,** progressive primary anetoderma without any preceding inflammatory condition, characterized by the abrupt appearance of many bluish white macules, some of which are protuberant; usually seen in women. Cf. *Jadassohn's a.*

**an·eu·ga·my** (an-u′gə-me) [*an-* neg. + *eugamy*] union of gametes in one or both of which the chromosomes have not been reduced to the normal haploid number, resulting in an abnormal number of chromosomes (aneuploidy) in the zygote.

**an·eu·ploid** (an′u-ploid) [*an-* neg. + *euploid*] 1. a chromosome number that is not an exact multiple of the normal diploid number. 2. an individual or cell having an aneuploid number of chromosomes.

**an·eu·ploi·dy** (an″u-ploi′de) [MeSH: Aneuploidy] any deviation from an exact multiple of the haploid number of chromosomes, whether fewer (hypoploidy, as in Turner's syndrome) or more (hyperploidy, as in Down syndrome).

**aneu·rine** (an-u′rin) [*an-* neg. + Gr. *neuron* nerve] thiamine.
**a. hydrochloride,** thiamine hydrochloride.

**aneu·ro·gen·ic** (a″noo͡-ro-jen′ik) pertaining to or characterized by absence of formation of nerve fibers.

**an·eu·rysm** (an′u-rizm) [Gr. *aneurysma* a widening] [MeSH: Aneurysm] a sac formed by the dilatation of the wall of an artery, a vein, or the heart; it is filled with fluid or clotted blood, often forming a pulsating tumor.
**abdominal a., abdominal aortic a.,** a common type of aneurysm, found in the abdominal aorta, usually in an area of severe atherosclerosis.
**ampullary a.,** sacculated a.
**aortic a.,** aneurysm of the aorta.
**aortic sinusal a.,** aneurysm arising in the aortic sinuses of Valsalva; it is a rare, usually congenital lesion that begins as finger-like projections in the right or noncoronary sinuses and can progress to rupture, usually into the right ventricle or atrium, causing volume overload and congestive heart failure.
**arterial a.,** aneurysm in the wall of an artery; the chief signs are formation of a pulsating tumor, often a bruit *(aneurysmal bruit)* heard over the swelling, and sometimes symptoms from pressure on contiguous parts.
**arteriosclerotic a.,** an aneurysm arising in a large artery, most commonly the abdominal aorta, as a result of weakening of the wall in severe atherosclerosis; called also *atherosclerotic a.*
**arteriovenous a.,** a communication, either congenital or traumatic, between an artery and a vein; arterial blood may flow directly into the vein *(aneurysmal varix)* or be carried into it by a connecting sac *(varicose aneurysm).*
**arteriovenous pulmonary a.,** pulmonary arteriovenous fistula.
**atherosclerotic a.,** arteriosclerotic a.
**axillary a.,** aneurysm of the axillary artery.
**bacterial a.,** see *infected a.*
**berry a.,** a saccular aneurysm of a cerebral artery, usually at the

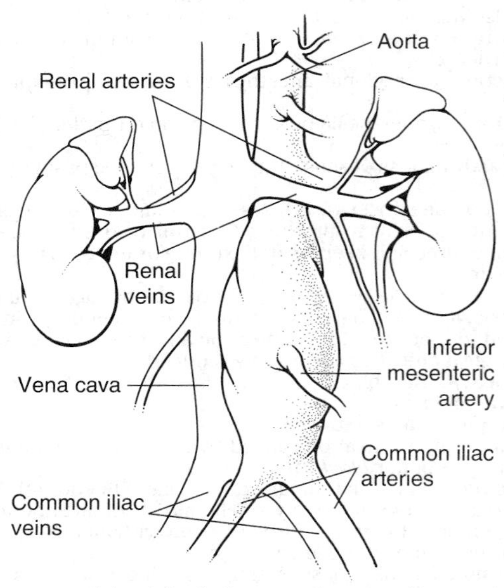


Aneurysm of the abdominal aorta and common iliac arteries.

junction of vessels in the circle of Willis; its narrow neck of origin and larger dome resemble those of a berry. Called also *cerebral a.*
**brain a.,** berry a.
**cardiac a.,** ventricular a.
**cerebral a.,** berry a.
**Charcot-Bouchard a.,** a type of miliary aneurysm found in the small vessels affected by hypertension; not thought to be a cause of bleeding.
**cirsoid a.,** racemose a.
**compound a.,** one in which some of the coats are ruptured and others merely dilated; called also *mixed a.*
**congenital cerebral a.,** berry a.
**cylindroid a.,** the uniform dilatation of a considerable part of an artery; called also *tubular a.*
**dissecting a.,** longitudinal splitting of the arterial wall resulting from hemorrhage, producing a tear in the intima and establishing communication with the lumen; it usually affects the aorta *(aortic dissection)* but may also affect other large arteries.
**ectatic a.,** one formed by distention of a section of an artery without rupture of any of its coats.
**embolic a.,** an infected aneurysm caused by a septic embolus from infective endocarditis; it was formerly the most common form of mycotic aneurysm.
**false a.,** 1. one in which the entire wall is injured and the blood is contained by the surrounding tissues, with eventual formation of a sac communicating with the artery (or heart); called also *aneurysmal hematoma.* 2. pseudoaneurysm.
**fusiform a.,** a spindle-shaped arterial aneurysm in which the stretching process affects the entire circumference of the artery, as opposed to a *saccular aneurysm.* Called also *Richet's a.*
**hernial a.,** one in which the sac is formed by an inner coat projecting through the outer.
**infected a.,** aneurysm produced by growth of bacteria *(bacterial a.)* or fungi *(mycotic a.)* in the vessel wall, or infection arising within a preexisting arteriosclerotic aneurysm.
**innominate a.,** aneurysm of the innominate artery (brachiocephalic trunk).
**intracranial a.,** any aneurysm situated within the cranium.
**lateral a.,** one that projects from one side of an artery.
**luetic a.,** syphilitic a.
**miliary a.,** aneurysm of a minute artery, chiefly intracranial or retinal.
**mixed a.,** compound a.
**mycotic a.,** see *infected a.*
**Park's a.,** an arteriovenous aneurysm occurring at the elbow and establishing communication between the brachial artery and the brachial and median basilic veins.
**Pott's a.,** aneurysmal varix (def. 2).
**racemose a.,** a condition in which the blood vessels become dilated, lengthened, and tortuous; called also *cirsoid a., cirsoid varix,* and *diffuse arterial ectasia.*
**Rasmussen's a.,** dilatation of an artery in a tuberculous cavity; its rupture produces hemorrhage.
**renal a.,** an aneurysm within the kidney.
**Richet's a.,** fusiform a.
**saccular a., sacculated a.,** an eccentric, localized distended sac affecting only a part of the circumference of the arterial wall, as opposed to a *fusiform aneurysm.* Called also *ampullary a.*
**serpentine a.,** an elongated and varicose senile condition of certain arteries, such as the splenic, iliac, and temporal.
**spurious a.,** 1. false a. (def. 1). 2. pseudoaneurysm.
**suprasellar a.,** aneurysm of the internal carotid artery above the sella turcica.
**syphilitic a.,** an aortic aneurysm, usually of the ascending aorta, occurring in cases of cardiovascular syphilis; called also *luetic a.*
**traumatic a.,** an aneurysm due to injury.
**true a.,** an aneurysm in which the sac is formed by the arterial walls, at least one of which is unbroken.
**tubular a.,** cylindroid a.
**varicose a.,** an aneurysm in which the artery communicates with contiguous veins by means of an intervening sac.
**venous a.,** aneurysm of a vein; called also *phlebangioma.*
**ventricular a.,** an aneurysmal dilatation of a portion of the wall of a ventricle, usually the left, or, rarely, a saccular protrusion through it *(false a.* of the heart). It is usually consequent to myocardial infarction but other causes, such as bacterial endocarditis or trauma, have been described.
**verminous a., worm a.,** an aneurysm of equines caused by the nematode *Strongylus vulgaris,* usually in the anterior mesenteric artery. Called also *verminous mesenteric arteritis.*

**an·eu·rys·mal** (an″u-riz′məl) pertaining to or resembling an aneurysm.

**an·eu·rys·mat·ic** (an″u-riz-mat′ik) aneurysmal.

**an·eu·rys·mec·to·my** (an″u-riz-mek′to-me) [*aneurysm* + *-ectomy*] extirpation of an aneurysm by removal of the sac.

**an·eu·rys·mo·plas·ty** (an″u-riz′mo-plas″te) [*aneurysm* + *-plasty*] plastic reconstruction of an aneurysmal artery.

**an·eu·rys·mor·rha·phy** (an″u-riz-mor′ə-fe) [*aneurysm* + *-rrhaphy*] the operation of suturing an aneurysm.

**an·eu·rys·mot·o·my** (an″u-riz-mot′ə-me) [*aneurysm* + *-tomy*] the operation of incising the sac of an aneurysm.

**ANF** antinuclear factor; see *antinuclear antibodies (ANA),* under *antibody.*

**angei-** for words beginning thus, see those beginning *angi-.*

**An·gel·i·ca** (an-jel′ĭ-kəh) [L., from Gr. *angelikos* angelic] a genus of plants of the family Umbelliferae. *A. archange′lica* is the garden angelica, which has carminative, diaphoretic, and diuretic properties; its roots and fruit were formerly used as a source for various medicinal substances.

**An·gel·man's syndrome** (ān′jəl-mənz) [Harry *Angelman,* British physician, 20th century] see under *syndrome.*

**An·ge·luc·ci's syndrome** (ahn″jə-loo′chēz) [Arnaldo *Angelucci,* Italian ophthalmologist, 1854–1934] see under *syndrome.*

**An·ger camera** (ang′gər) [Hal Oscar *Anger,* American electrical engineer, born 1920] see under *camera.*

**An·ghe·les·cu's sign** (ahn-jə-les′ko͞oz) [Constantin *Anghelescu,* Romanian surgeon, 1869–1948] see under *sign.*

**an·gi·al·gia** (an″je-al′jə) [*angi-* + Gr. *algos* pain + *-ia*] pain in a blood vessel; called also *angiodynia* and *vasalgia.*

**an·gi·as·the·nia** (an″je-əs-the′ne-ə) [*angi-* + *asthenia*] instability or loss of tone in the vascular system.

**an·gi·ec·ta·sis** (an″je-ek′tə-sis) [*angi-* + *ectasis*] abnormal, usually gross dilatation and often lengthening of a blood or lymphatic vessel; see also *lymphangiectasis* and *vasodilation.* Called also *hemangiectasia.*

**an·gi·ec·tat·ic** (an″je-ek-tat′ik) pertaining to or characterized by angiectasis.

**an·gi·ec·to·my** (an″je-ek′tə-me) [*angi-* + *-ectomy*] the excision or resection of a vessel.

**an·gi·ec·to·pia** (an″je-ek-to′pe-ə) [*angi-* + *ectopia*] abnormal position or course of a vessel.

**an·gi·i·tis** (an″je-i′tis) pl. *angii′tides* [*angi-* + *-itis*] vasculitis.
**allergic granulomatous a.,** Churg-Strauss syndrome.
**granulomatous a. of central nervous system, isolated a. of central nervous system,** 1. isolated vasculitis of central nervous system. 2. hypersensitivity vasculitis.
**hypersensitivity a., leukocytoclastic a.,** hypersensitivity vasculitis.
**necrotizing a.,** systemic necrotizing vasculitis.

**an·gi·na** (an-ji′nə, an′jə-nə) [L.] 1. a. pectoris. 2. any spasmodic, choking, or suffocative pain. 3. old term for sore throat.
**abdominal a., a. abdomina′lis, a. abdo′minis,** intestinal a.
**agranulocytic a.,** old name for *agranulocytosis.*
**a. cor′dis,** a. pectoris.
**crescendo a.,** former term for unstable angina pectoris.
**a. cru′ris,** intermittent claudication.
**a. decu′bitus,** cardiac pain occurring in a recumbent position.
**a. dyspep′tica,** a condition resembling angina pectoris but due to distention of the stomach with gas.
**herpes a., a. herpe′tica,** herpangina.
**intestinal a.,** cramping postprandial abdominal pain caused by ischemia of the smooth muscle of the bowel in patients with mesenteric vascular insufficiency.
**a. inver′sa,** Prinzmetal's a.
**Ludwig's a.,** a severe form of cellulitis of the submaxillary space and secondary involvement of the sublingual and submental spaces, usually resulting from an infection in the mandibular molar area or a penetrating injury of the floor of the mouth. Elevation of the tongue, difficulty in eating and swallowing, edema of the glottis, fever, rapid breathing, and moderate leukocytosis are the most common symptoms.
**microvascular a.,** angina pectoris resulting from ischemia caused by microvascular dysfunction.
**neutropenic a.,** old name for *agranulocytosis.*
**a. pec′toris,** a paroxysmal thoracic pain, often radiating to the arms, particularly the left, sometimes accompanied by a feeling of suffocation and impending death; it is most often due to ischemia of the myocardium and precipitated by effort or excitement. It is subdivided into *stable* and *unstable a. pectoris.* Called also *a. cordis, angor pectoris, Heberden's disease,* and *Rougnon-Heberden disease.*
**a. pectoris, stable,** angina pectoris occurring in attacks of predictable frequency and duration after provocation by circumstances that increase myocardial oxygen demands, such as exercise, emotional stress, or excitement, the precipitating circumstances tending to remain constant across episodes. Cf. *unstable a.*

**a. pectoris, unstable,** angina pectoris occurring unpredictably or suddenly increasing in severity or frequency; attacks may occur without provocation, such as during sleep or rest, may not respond to nitroglycerin, and may be of unusually long duration. Prinzmetal's (variant) angina is often included in this category. Cf. *stable a. pectoris.*
**a. pectoris, variant,** Prinzmetal's a.
**a. pec'toris elec'trica,** pain and tightness in the chest on effort, without specific electrocardiographic changes, persisting for several weeks following electrical injury.
**preinfarction a.,** 1. angina pectoris preceding a myocardial infarction. 2. unstable a. pectoris.
**Prinzmetal's a.,** a variant of angina pectoris, often considered a form of unstable angina, in which the attacks occur during rest, exercise capacity is often well preserved, and attacks are associated electrocardiographically with elevation of the ST segment. Focal spasm of an epicardial coronary artery causes transient abrupt reduction of arterial diameter, resulting in myocardial ischemia. Called also *variant a. pectoris.*
**pseudomembranous a.,** necrotizing ulcerative gingivostomatitis.
**Schultz's a.,** old name for *agranulocytosis.*
**silent a., a. sine dolo're,** an episode of coronary insufficiency in which no pain is experienced.
**stable a., typical a.,** stable a. pectoris.
**unstable a.,** unstable a. pectoris.
**variant a.,** variant a. pectoris.
**Vincent's a.,** a type of membranous pharyngitis consisting of painful ulceration with edema and hyperemic patches; it represents spread of acute necrotizing ulcerative gingivitis to the oropharynx.

**an·gi·nal** (an-ji'nəl, an'jə-nəl) pertaining to or characteristic of angina.

**an·gin·i·form** (an-jin'ĭ-form) resembling angina.

**an·gi·noid** (an'jĭ-noid) anginiform.

**an·gino·pho·bia** (an″jin-o-fo'be-ə) [*angina* + *-phobia*] irrational dread of choking.

**an·gi·nous** (an'jĭ-nəs) anginal.

**angi(o)-** [Gr. *angeion* vessel] a combining form denoting relationship to a vessel, usually a blood vessel.

**an·gio·ac·cess** (an″je-o-ak'ses) arteriovenous access.

**an·gio·atax·ia** (an″je-o-ə-tak'se-ə) [*angio-* + *ataxia*] irregular tension of the blood vessels.

**an·gio·blast** (an'je-o-blast″) [*angio-* + *-blast*[1]] 1. the mesenchymal tissue of the embryo from which the blood cells and blood vessels differentiate; called also *angioderm.* 2. an individual vessel-forming cell; called also *vasofactive* or *vasoformative cell.*

**an·gio·blas·tic** (an″je-o-blas'tik) pertaining to angioblast.

**an·gio·blas·to·ma** (an″je-o-blas-to'mə) 1. hemangioblastoma. 2. angioblastic meningioma.

**an·gio·car·dio·gram** (an″je-o-kahr'de-o-gram) the film produced by angiocardiography.

**an·gio·car·di·og·ra·phy** (an″je-o-kahr″de-og'rə-fe) [*angio-* + *cardiography*] [MeSH: Angiocardiography] angiography of the heart and great vessels; contrast material may be injected into a blood vessel or one of the cardiac chambers. Images obtained can be analyzed to determine parameters of ventricular function, including ventricular ejection fractions, cardiac output, ejection rates, stroke volume, end-diastolic volume, and end-systolic volume, as well as to test the effects of exercise. Called also *cardioangiography.*
**equilibrium radionuclide a.,** a form of radionuclide angiocardiography in which images are taken at specific phases of the cardiac cycle over a series of several hundred cycles. Timing of image recording is set, or gated, by the occurrence of specific electrocardiographic waveforms, and the data can be used to determine average activity during specific cardiac cycle phases or can be accumulated and displayed in rapid sequence, as a movie. Called also *multiple gated acquisition* or *MUGA scanning* and *gated cardiac blood pool imaging.*
**first pass radionuclide a.,** a form of radionuclide angiocardiography in which a rapid sequence of images is taken immediately after administration of a bolus of radionuclide, recording only the initial transit of the isotope through the central circulation.
**gated equilibrium radionuclide a.,** equilibrium radionuclide a.
**radionuclide a.,** a form in which the contrast material is a radionuclide, usually a compound of technetium Tc 99m such as Tc 99m pyrophosphate or Tc 99m–labeled red blood cells, and images are obtained using a gamma camera.

**an·gio·car·dio·ki·net·ic** (an″je-o-kahr″de-o-kĭ-net'ik) [*angio-* + *cardiokinetic*] 1. affecting the motions or movements of the heart and blood vessels. 2. any agent that affects the movements of the heart and vessels.

**an·gio·car·di·tis** (an″je-o-kahr-di'tis) [*angio-* + *carditis*] inflammation of the heart and great blood vessels.

**an·gio·cen·tric** (an″je-o-sen'trik) angiogenic (def. 1).

**an·gio·chei·lo·scope** (an″je-o-ki'lo-skōp″) [*angio-* + *cheilo-* + *-scope*] an instrument for observing blood circulation of the lips under magnification.

**An·gio-Con·ray** (an″je-o-kon'ra) trademark for a preparation of iothalamate sodium.

**an·gio·crine** (an'je-o-krīn) [*angio-* + *endocrine*] denoting vasomotor disorders of endocrine origin.

**an·gio·cri·no·sis** (an″je-o-krĭ-no'sis) a vasomotor disorder of endocrine origin.

**an·gio·cyst** (an'je-o-sist″) [*angio-* + *cyst*] angioblastic cyst.

**an·gio·derm** (an'je-o-dərm) angioblast, def. 1.

**an·gio·der·ma·ti·tis** (an″je-o-dər-mə-ti'tis) [*angio-* + *dermatitis*] inflammation of the vessels of the skin. Angiodermatitis occurring in association with arteriovenous fistula is known as *pseudo–Kaposi sarcoma.*
**disseminated pruritic a.,** itching purpura.

**an·gio·di·as·co·py** (an″je-o-di-as'kə-pe) [*angio-* + *diascopy*] direct visual inspection of blood vessels of the extremities, a light being held behind the part.

**an·gi·odyn·ia** (an″je-o-din'e-ə) [*angi-* + *-odynia*] angialgia.

**an·gio·dys·pla·sia** (an″je-o-dis-pla'zhə) [MeSH: Angiodysplasia] small vascular abnormalities, such as of the intestinal tract.
**papular a.,** small superficial papular lesions occurring around the face, considered by some to be a variant of angiolymphoid hyperplasia with eosinophilia but lacking the lymphocytic response and eosinophils.

**an·gio·dys·tro·phia** (an″je-o-dis-tro'fe-ah) [*angio-* + *dystrophy*] any disorder of blood vessels caused by a defective supply of nutrients.

**an·gio·dys·tro·phy** (an″je-o-dis'tro-fe) angiodystrophia.

**an·gio·ec·tat·ic** (an″je-o-ek-tat'ik) angiectatic.

**an·gio·ede·ma** (an″je-o-ə-de'mə) [*angio-* +*edema*] a vascular reaction involving the deep dermis or subcutaneous or submucosal tissues, representing localized edema caused by dilatation and increased permeability of capillaries, and characterized by development of giant wheals. *Urticaria* is the same physiologic reaction occurring in the superficial portions of the dermis. Called also *angioneurotic, circumscribed,* or *giant edema; Quincke's disease* or *edema;* and *giant urticaria.*
**hereditary a.,** inherited C1 inhibitor (C1 INH) deficiency, an autosomal dominant disorder manifested as recurrent episodes of edema of the skin, upper respiratory tract, and gastrointestinal tract with increased levels of several vasoactive mediators of anaphylaxis. It may be mediated by such factors as minor trauma, sudden changes in environmental temperature, and sudden emotional stress. There are two variants: one in which no C1 INH is produced, and another in which there are normal serum levels of a nonfunctional C1 INH. The lack of C1 INH causes uncontrolled activation of the classical complement pathway and the production of a kininlike substance (C2 kinin) derived from the attack of C1 on C2 and C4.
**vibratory a.,** angioedema due to vibratory stimuli to the skin, occurring as a dominant disorder, with cholinergic urticaria, or after prolonged occupational exposure to vibration.

**an·gio·ede·ma·tous** (an″je-o″ə-de'mə-təs) pertaining to or characterized by angioedema.

**an·gio·el·e·phan·ti·a·sis** (an″je-o-el″ə-fən-ti'ə-sis) [*angio-* + *elephantiasis*] extensive angiomatosis of the subcutaneous tissues.

**an·gio·en·do·the·li·o·ma** (an″je-o-en″do-the″le-o'mə) hemangioendothelioma.

**an·gio·en·do·the·lio·ma·to·sis** (an″je-o-en″do-the″le-o-mə-to'sis) [*angio-* + *endotheliomatosis*] intravascular proliferation of tumors derived from endothelial cells.
**systemic proliferating a.,** cutaneous and visceral intravascular proliferation of tumor cells believed to be of endothelial origin, with obstruction of vascular lumina and thromboses; it occurs in a benign, self-limited form in which involvement is limited to the cutaneous vasculature and in a malignant, systemic, usually fatal form in which various organs as well as cutaneous and central nervous system vessels may be involved, with variable clinical manifestations. The malignant form has been noted to frequently follow or precede lymphoma.

**an·gio·fi·bro·ma** (an″je-o-fi-bro'mə) [*angioma* + *fibroma*] [MeSH: Angiofibroma] a lesion characterized by fibrous tissue and vascular proliferation; it often occurs as one or more small, flesh-colored papules, particularly on the face.

**juvenile nasopharyngeal a., nasopharyngeal a.,** a benign tumor of the nasopharynx composed of fibrous connective tissue with abundant endothelium-lined vascular spaces, usually occurring during puberty, most commonly in boys. It is characterized by nasal obstruction which may become total, hyponasality, discomfort in swallowing, auditory tube obstruction and massive epistaxis. Called also *juvenile arrhythmia*

**an·gio·fol·lic·u·lar** (an″je-o-fŏ-lik′u-lər) pertaining to a lymphoid follicle and its blood vessels.

**an·gio·gen·e·sis** (an″je-o-jen′ə-sis) [*angio-* + *genesis*] 1. development of blood vessels in the embryo. 2. any formation of new blood vessels; see also *neovascularization* (def. 2) and *revascularization.* Called also *angiopoiesis* and *vasculogenesis.*
**tumor a.,** the induction of the growth of blood vessels from surrounding tissue into a tumor by a diffusible protein factor released by the tumor cells.

**an·gio·gen·ic** (an″je-o-jen′ik) 1. pertaining to angiogenesis; called also *angiopoietic* and *vasculogenic.* 2. arising in the circulatory system.

**an·gio·gram** (an′je-o-gram″) a radiograph of blood vessels taken during angiography.

**an·gio·gran·u·lo·ma** (an″je-o-gran″u-lo′mə) [*angio-* + *granuloma*] an angioma containing granulation tissue, which represents a vasoproliferative inflammatory response. When the epithelial surface is ulcerated and suppuration is evident, the lesion is referred to as pyogenic granuloma.

**an·gio·graph** (an′je-o-graf″) angiogram.

**an·gi·og·ra·phy** (an″je-og′rə-fe) [*angio-* + *-graphy*] [MeSH: Angiography] the radiographic visualization of blood vessels following introduction of contrast material; used as a diagnostic aid in such conditions as stroke syndrome and myocardial infarction. See also *arteriography* and *phlebography.* Called also *vasography.*
**cerebral a.,** angiography of the vascular system of the brain.
**coronary a.,** angiography of the coronary arteries.
**digital subtraction a., intra-arterial,** arteriography that uses electronic circuitry to subtract the background of bone and soft tissue to provide a useful image of the arteries injected with contrast medium.
**digital subtraction a., intravenous,** phlebography that uses electronic circuitry to subtract the background of bone and soft tissue to provide a useful image of vessels injected with contrast medium.
**magnetic resonance a. (MRA),** a form of magnetic resonance imaging used to study blood vessels and blood flow, particularly for detection of abnormalities in the vessels of the head and neck and for evaluation of the peripheral vasculature of the lower extremities.
**pulmonary a.,** angiography of the pulmonary vessels, used to detect pulmonary embolism or less frequently to delineate pulmonary arteriovenous malformations, pulmonary varices, or pulmonary vessel anatomy.
**retinal a.,** examination of the ophthalmic vasculature after injection of a contrast medium, such as fluorescein sodium.

**an·gio·he·mo·phil·ia** (an″je-o-he′mo-fil′e-ə) von Willebrand's disease.

**an·gio·hy·a·li·no·sis** (an″je-o-hi″ə-lĭ-no′sis) [*angio-* + *hyalinosis*] hyaline degeneration of the walls of blood vessels.

**an·gi·oid** (an′je-oid) [*angi-* + *-oid*] resembling a blood vessel.

**an·gio·in·va·sive** (an″je-o-in-va′siv) tending to invade the walls of blood vessels.

**an·gio·ker·a·to·ma** (an″je-o-ker″ə-to′mə) [*angio-* + *keratoma*] [MeSH: Angiokeratoma] a discrete, pink to red telangiectasia having a tendency to undergo secondary epithelial changes, including acanthosis and hyperkeratosis. An underlying vascular abnormality is present in many cases. Called also *angiokeratosis* and *telangiectatic wart.*
**a. circumscrip′tum,** a condition mainly occurring in infancy or early childhood, chiefly in females, characterized by the usually unilateral development of papules and small nodules that may coalesce to form plaques, which are generally localized in a small patch, often with a linear configuration.
**a. cor′poris diffu′sum, diffuse a.,** Fabry disease.
**a. of Fordyce,** the existence of small vascular papules, which become keratotic, along the superficial veins of the scrotum and rarely over the penis, inguinal area, or upper thigh; seen in older men, usually with a history of venous obstruction. Similar lesions may occur on the vulva in women. Called also *a. of scrotum.*
**a. of Mibelli,** symmetrical development on the dorsum of the fingers, toes, elbows, and knees of discrete, aggregated, or confluent, soft red to purple vascular papules that later become hyperkeratotic. Most cases are seen in children or young adults, often with a history of chilblains, cold sensitivity, or frost bite.
**a. of scrotum,** a. of Fordyce.
**solitary a.,** angiokeratoma manifested as a small, bluish black warty papule that occurs most frequently on the lower extremities, usually singly, in childhood and adolescence.

**an·gio·ker·a·to·sis** (an″je-o-ker″ə-to′sis) angiokeratoma.

**an·gio·ki·ne·sis** (an″je-o-kĭ-ne′sis) vasomotion.

**an·gio·ki·net·ic** (an″je-o-kĭ-net′ik) vasomotor.

**an·gio·leio·my·o·ma** (an″je-o-li″o-mi-o′mə) [*angio-* + *leiomyoma*] a leiomyoma arising from vascular smooth muscle, usually occurring as a solitary nodular, sometimes painful, subcutaneous tumor on the lower extremity, more deeply situated than ordinary leiomyoma; usually seen in middle-aged women. Called also *angiomyoma* and *vascular leiomyoma.*

**an·gio·leu·ci·tis** (an″je-o-loo-si′tis) [*angio-* + *leucitis*] lymphangitis.

**an·gio·leu·ki·tis** (an″je-o-loo-ki′tis) lymphangitis.

**an·gio·lipo·leio·my·o·ma** (an″je-o-lip″o-li-o-mi-o′mə) [*angio-* + *lipo-* + *leiomyoma*] a benign tumor composed of blood vessel, adipose tissue, and smooth muscle elements, such as occurs in the kidney in association with tuberous sclerosis, where it is usually called *angiomyolipoma.*

**an·gio·li·po·ma** (an″je-o-lĭ-po′mə) [*angio-* + *lipoma*] [MeSH: Angiolipoma] a lipoma containing clusters of thin-walled proliferating blood vessels; it is frequently painful.

**an·gio·lo·gia** (an″je-o-lo′jə) 1. angiology. 2. a term used in anatomic terminology to encompass the nomenclature relating to the heart, arteries, veins, lymphatic system, and spleen.

**an·gi·ol·o·gy** (an″je-ol′ə-je) [*angio-* + *-logy*] 1. the study of the blood and lymph vessels of the body. 2. the sum of knowledge about the blood and lymph vessels.

**an·gio·lu·poid** (an″je-o-loo′poid) [*angio-* + *lupoid*] a rare manifestation of cutaneous sarcoidosis localized to the malar region, bridge of the nose, or around the eyes, and consisting of livid nodular lesions that coalesce to form plaques.

**an·gio·lym·phan·gi·o·ma** (an″je-o-lim-fan″je-o′mə) a mixed angioma in which lymph vessels and blood vessels are involved.

**an·gio·lym·phi·tis** (an″je-o-lim-fi′tis) lymphangitis.

**an·gi·ol·y·sis** (an″je-ol′ĭ-sis) [*angio-* + *-lysis*] retrogression or obliteration of blood vessels, such as occurs during embryonic development.

**an·gi·o·ma** (an″je-o′mə) [*angio-* + *-oma*] a tumor whose cells tend to form blood vessels *(hemangioma)* or lymph vessels *(lymphangioma);* a tumor made up of blood vessels or lymph vessels. Called also *endothelioma angiomatosum* and *vascular tumor.*
**a. arteria′le racemo′sum,** a dilatation and complex intertwining of many new-formed and altered vessels of small caliber with subsequent involvement of normal vessels.
**arteriovenous a. of brain,** cerebral arteriovenous malformation.
**capillary a's,** cherry a's.
**a. caverno′sum, cavernous a.,** cavernous hemangioma.
**cherry a's,** bright red to purple, smooth, dome-shaped lesions representing a telangiectatic vascular disturbance, usually found on the trunk and proximal extremities; they occur in most of the elderly, but the onset may be in early adult life. Called also *capillary a's, De Morgan's spots,* and *senile a's.*
**a. cu′tis,** vascular nevus.
**fissural a.,** a hemangioma occurring in embryonal fissures (clefts) of the face, neck, or lips.
**hypertrophic a.,** angioma characterized by proliferation of endothelial tissue.
**a. lympha′ticum,** lymphangioma.
**senile a's,** cherry a's.
**a. serpigino′sum,** generalized essential telangiectasia characterized by groups of tiny, copper-colored to bright red angiomatous puncta that enlarge by forming new puncta at the periphery with central clearing, which produces annular or serpiginous patterns. The eruption usually occurs on the lower extremities. Called also *Hutchinson's disease.*
**spider a.,** vascular spider.
**a. veno′sum racemo′sum,** the swellings caused by severe varicosity of superficial veins.
**venous a. of brain,** congenital angioma of the brain, composed of abnormal branches of veins, usually with a common center, found most often near the ventricular wall; it is often asymptomatic.

**an·gi·o·ma·toid** (an″je-o′mə-toid) 1. resembling an angioma. 2. a mass of dilated, twisted vessels that resembles an angioma.

**an·gi·o·ma·to·sis** (an″je-o-mə-to′sis) [MeSH: Angiomatosis] a diseased state of the vessels with the formation of multiple angiomas.
**bacillary a.,** a condition seen in immunocompromised patients, caused by *Bartonella henselae* and *B. quintana;* characteristics range

from raised erythematous angiomatous skin lesions to more widespread disease including hepatitis, osteomyelitis, or obstruction of the lungs.
**cerebroretinal a.,** von Hippel-Lindau disease.
**encephalofacial a., encephalotrigeminal a.,** Sturge-Weber syndrome.
**hepatic a.,** peliosis hepatis.
**a. of retina,** von Hippel's disease.
**retinocerebral a.,** von Hippel-Lindau disease.

**an·gi·om·a·tous** (an″je-om′ə-təs) of the nature of angioma.

**an·gio·meg·a·ly** (an″je-o-meg′ə-le) [*angio-* + *-megaly*] enlargement of blood vessels, causing swelling, such as of the eyelids.

**an·gio·myo·li·po·ma** (an″je-o-mi″o-lĭ-po′mə) [*angio-* + *myo-* + *lipoma*] [MeSH: Angiomyolipoma] a benign tumor containing vascular, adipose, and muscle elements; it occurs most often as a renal tumor with smooth muscle elements (more correctly called *angiolipoleiomyoma*) usually in association with tuberous sclerosis, and is considered to be a hamartoma.

**an·gio·my·o·ma** (an″je-o-mi-o′mə) [*angio-* + *myoma*] [MeSH: Angiomyoma] angioleiomyoma.

**an·gio·myo·sar·co·ma** (an″je-o-mi″o-sahr-ko′mə) a tumor made up of elements of angioma, myoma, and sarcoma.

**an·gio·myx·o·ma** (an″je-o-mik-so′mə) a chorioangioma containing capillary-like blood vessels; it may extend into the umbilical cord and often contains myxomatous tissue resembling that in the normal cord.

**an·gio·ne·cro·sis** (an″je-o-nə-kro′sis) [*angio-* + *necrosis*] necrosis of the walls of blood vessels.

**an·gio·neu·ral·gia** (an″je-o-noo͡-ral′jə) [*angio-* + *neuralgia*] burning pain in an extremity with edema and redness.

**an·gio·neu·rec·to·my** (an″je-o-noo͡-rek′to-me) [*angio-* + *neurectomy*] excision of vessels and nerves.

**an·gio·neu·ro·path·ic** (an″je-o-noo͡r″o-path′ik) pertaining to or of the nature of an angioneuropathy.

**an·gio·neu·rop·a·thy** (an″je-o-noo-rop′ə-the) [*angio-* + *neuropathy*] 1. angiopathic neuropathy. 2. any neuropathy affecting primarily the blood vessels; a disorder of the vasomotor system, as angiospasm, angioparalysis, or vasomotor paralysis.

**an·gio·neu·rot·ic** (an″je-o-noo͡-rot′ik) angioneuropathic.

**an·gio·neu·rot·o·my** (an″je-o-noo͡-rot′o-me) [*angio-* + *neurotomy*] the operation of cutting vessels and nerves.

**an·gio·no·ma** (an″je-o-no′mə) [*angio-* + *noma*] ulceration of a blood vessel.

**an·gio·pa·ral·y·sis** (an″je-o-pə-ral′ə-sis) [*angio-* + *paralysis*] vasomotor paralysis.

**an·gio·pa·re·sis** (an″je-o-pə-re′sis) [*angio-* + *paresis*] vasoparesis.

**an·gio·path·ol·o·gy** (an″je-o-pə-thol′ə-je) the pathology of, or the changes seen in, diseases of the blood vessels.

**an·gi·op·a·thy** (an-je-op′ə-the) [*angio-* + *-pathy*] any disease of the blood vessels or lymphatics.
**cerebral amyloid a., congophilic a.,** vascular amyloidosis affecting small and medium-sized arteries of the leptomeninges and cerebral cortex, resulting in microinfarcts or in hemorrhage; it may be asymptomatic or may result in hemorrhagic stroke or dementia. Most cases are sporadic and occur most often in the elderly. A hereditary form with autosomal dominant inheritance also exists.

**an·gio·phak·o·ma·to·sis** (an″je-o-fak″o-mə-to′sis) [*angio-* + *phakomatosis*] von Hippel-Lindau disease.

**an·gio·plas·ty** (an′je-o-plas″te) [*angio-* + *-plasty*] [MeSH: Angioplasty] an angiographic procedure for elimination of areas of narrowing in blood vessels.

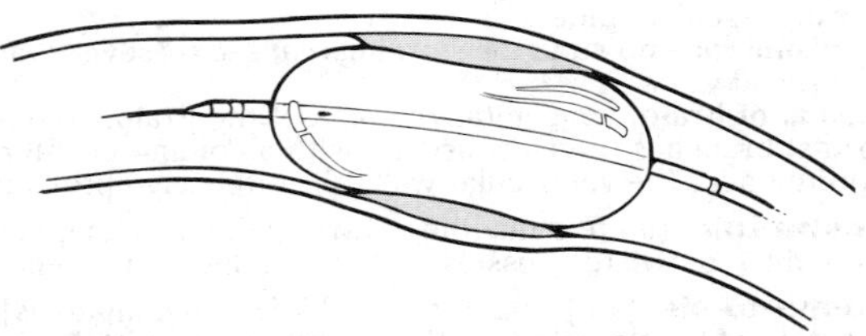
Balloon angioplasty, the expanded balloon pressing against a stenotic site in an artery.

**balloon a.,** angioplasty using a balloon-tip catheter that is inflated inside an artery, stretching the intima and leaving a ragged interior surface after deflation, which triggers a healing response and breaking up of plaque. See also *percutaneous transluminal a.* and *transluminal coronary a.*
**laser a., laser thermal a.,** the recanalization of an occluded artery by vaporizing the occlusion using laser energy delivered by a fiberoptic probe with a metal tip that converts light energy to heat energy.
**percutaneous transluminal a.,** a type of balloon angioplasty in which the catheter is inserted through the skin and through the lumen of the vessel to the site of the narrowing.
**transluminal coronary a.,** PTCA; percutaneous transluminal angioplasty to enlarge the lumen of a sclerotic coronary artery, an alternative to bypass cardiac surgery for selected patients with ischemic heart disease.

**an·gio·poi·e·sis** (an″je-o-poi-e′sis) [*angio-* + *-poiesis*] angiogenesis.

**an·gio·poi·et·ic** (an″je-o-poi-et′ik) angiogenic (def. 1).

**an·gio·pres·sure** (an′je-o-presh″ər) the application of pressure to a blood vessel to control hemorrhage.

**an·gio·re·tic·u·lo·en·do·the·li·o·ma** (an″je-o-rĕ-tik″u-lo-en″do-the-le-o′mə) Kaposi's sarcoma.

**an·gio·re·tic·u·lo·ma** (an″je-o-re-tik″u-lo′mə) hemangioblastoma.

**an·gi·or·rha·phy** (an″je-or′ə-fe) [*angio-* + *rrhaphy*] suture of a vessel or vessels.
**arteriovenous a.,** the suturing of an artery to a vein, so as to divert the arterial current into the vein.

**an·gio·sar·co·ma** (an″je-o-sahr-ko′mə) [*angio-* + *sarcoma*] a malignant neoplasm arising from vascular endothelial cells; the term may be used generally or may denote a specific histologic subtype, usually hemangiosarcoma but also others such as lymphangiosarcoma or hemangiopericytoma.
**hepatic a.,** a malignant tumor of the liver characterized by dilated sinusoids with hypertrophied or necrotic hepatocytes that leave vascular channels lined by malignant cells. It usually affects older men and has been linked to exposure to toxins such as vinyl chloride gas, inorganic arsenic compounds, and thorium dioxide. Called also *Kupffer cell sarcoma.*

**an·gio·scle·ro·sis** (an″je-o-sklĕ-ro′sis) [*angio-* + *sclerosis*] hardening of walls of blood vessels; see *arteriosclerosis* and *phlebosclerosis.*

**an·gio·scope** (an′je-o-skōp″) [*angio-* + *-scope*] 1. a fiberoptic catheter for viewing the inside of a blood vessel. 2. a microscope for observing capillary blood vessels.

**an·gi·os·co·py** (an″ge-os′kə-pe) [MeSH: Angioscopy] 1. use of a fiberoptic angioscope to visualize the lumen of a blood vessel. 2. visualization of capillary blood vessels with a special microscope (angioscope).

**an·gio·sco·to·ma** (an″je-o-sko-to′mə) [*angio-* + *scotoma*] a cecocentral scotoma caused by shadows of the retinal blood vessels.

**an·gio·sco·tom·e·try** (an″je-o-sko-tom′ə-tre) [*angio-* + *scotoma* + *-metry*] the plotting or mapping of the scotoma caused by the shadow of retinal blood vessels; used particularly in the diagnosis of glaucoma.

**an·gio·spasm** (an′je-o-spaz″əm) [*angio-* + *spasm*] vasospasm.

**an·gio·spas·tic** (an″je-o-spas′tik) vasospastic.

**an·gio·sperm** (an′je-o-spərm″) [*angio-* + *sperm*] a true flowering plant; a plant having its seeds in an enclosed ovary.

**an·gio·ste·no·sis** (an″je-o-stə-no′sis) [*angio-* + *stenosis*] narrowing of the caliber of a vessel.

**an·gi·os·te·o·sis** (an″je-os″te-o′sis) [*angi-* + *osteosis*] ossification or calcification of a vessel.

**an·gi·os·the·nia** (an″je-os-the′ne-ə) [*angio-* + *sthenia*] arterial pressure.

**an·gi·os·to·my** (an″je-os′tə-me) [*angio-* + *-stomy*] 1. the making of an opening into a blood vessel. 2. the opening so made.

**an·gio·stron·gy·li·a·sis** (an″je-o-stron″jĭ-li′ə-sis) infection by a species of *Angiostrongylus.* In humans the usual species is *A. cantonensis,* and infection comes after eating contaminated raw snails, slugs, or paratenic hosts such as prawns or crabs. The larval worms migrate to the central nervous system and cause eosinophilic meningitis. In dogs the most common infecting species is *A. vasorum* and the worms are found in the pulmonary arteries.

**An·gio·stron·gy·li·dae** (an″je-o-stron-jil′ĭ-de) a family of nematodes that includes the genera *Aelurostrongylus* and *Angiostrongylus.* Several species are lungworms in mammals.

**an·gio·stron·gy·lo·sis** (an″je-o-stron″jĭ-lo′sis) angiostrongyliasis.

**An·gio·stron·gy·lus** (an″je-o-stron′jĭ-ləs) [*angio-* + *strongylos* round] [MeSH: Angiostrongylus] a genus of parasitic nematodes of the family Angiostrongylidae.
**A. cantonen′sis,** a lungworm that parasitizes the domestic rat in Australia and many Pacific islands, including Hawaii. Larval development occurs in snails, slugs, and planarians; in rats, the adult worms are found in the bronchioles. Human infection is caused by ingestion of larvae in raw seafood; see *angiostrongyliasis*.
**A. costaricen′sis,** a species that normally inhabits the mesenteric arteries of rodents but has been found in the mesenteric and nearby arteries of humans in Central America and Brazil.
**A. vaso′rum,** a species parasitic in dogs; see *angiostrongyliasis*.

**an·gi·os·tro·phe** (an″je-os′trə-fe) [*angio-* + Gr. *strophē* a twist] the twisting of a vessel to arrest hemorrhage.

**an·gi·os·tro·phy** (an″je-os′trə-fe) angiostrophe.

**an·gio·te·lec·ta·sis** (an″je-o-tə-lek′tə-sis) pl. *angiotelec′tases* [*angio-* + *tel-* + *ectasis*] dilatation of the minute arteries and veins.

**an·gio·ten·sin** (an″je-o-ten′sin) any of a family of polypeptide vasopressor hormones formed by the catalytic action of renin on angiotensinogen. Called also *angiotonin*.
**a. I,** a decapeptide cleaved from angiotensinogen by renin; it has some biological activity but serves mainly as a precursor to a. II.
**a. II,** an octapeptide hormone formed by the action of angiotensin-converting enzyme (peptidyl-dipeptidase A) on a. I, chiefly in the lungs but also at other sites, including the blood vessel walls, uterus, and brain. It is a powerful vasopressor and stimulator of aldosterone secretion by the adrenal cortex, and it also functions as a neurotransmitter. Its vasopressor action raises blood pressure and diminishes fluid loss in the kidney by restricting blood flow.
**a. III,** a heptapeptide degradation product of a. II, having less vasopressor activity than the parent compound.
**a. amide,** an amide derivative of angiotensin and a powerful vasoconstrictor and vasopressor, used in the treatment of certain hypotensive states; usually administered by slow intravenous infusion, and sometimes intramuscularly or subcutaneously.

**an·gio·ten·sin·ase** (an″je-o-ten′sin-ās) any of a group of plasma or tissue peptidases that cleave and inactivate angiotensin.

**an·gio·ten·sin-con·vert·ing en·zyme** (an″je-o-ten′sin kən-vərt′ing en′zīm) peptidyl-dipeptidase A.

**an·gio·ten·sin·o·gen** (an″je-o-ten-sin′o-jen) [MeSH: Angiotensinogen] a serum $\alpha_2$-globulin secreted in the liver and produced in many organs, which is cleaved by renin to give rise to angiotensin I. Called also *renin substrate*.

**an·gio·tome** (an′je-o-tōm″) [*angio-* + *-tome*] any one of the segments of the vascular system of the embryo.

**an·gi·ot·o·my** (an″je-ot′ə-me) [*angio-* + *-tomy*] the cutting or severing of a blood or lymph vessel.

**an·gio·to·nia** (an″je-o-to′ne-ə) vasotonia.

**an·gio·ton·ic** (an″je-o-ton′ik) [*angio-* + *tonic*] vasotonic.

**an·gio·to·nin** (an″je-o-to′nin) angiotensin.

**an·gio·tribe** (an′je-o-trīb″) [*angio-* + Gr. *tribein* to crush] an exceedingly strong forceps in which pressure is applied by means of a screw; the instrument is used to crush tissue containing an artery in order to control hemorrhage from the vessel. Called also *vasotribe*.

**an·gio·trip·sy** (an′je-o-trip″se) production of hemostasis by use of the angiotribe; called also *vasotripsy*.

**an·gio·troph·ic** (an″je-o-trof′ik) [*angio-* + *-trophic*] vasotrophic.

**an·gi·tis** (an-ji′tis) angiitis.

**An·gle's classification, splint** (ang′gəlz) [Edward Hartley *Angle*, American orthodontist, 1855–1930] see under *classification* and *splint;* see also *malocclusion*.

**an·gle** (ang′gəl) [L. *angulus*] 1. the area or point of junction of two intersecting borders or surfaces. 2. the degree of divergence of two intersecting lines or planes. Symbol $\theta$.

## Angle

For specific anatomic structures not found here, see under *angulus*.

**a. of aberration,** a. of deviation.
**acromial a.,** angulus acromii.
**acromial a. of scapula,** angulus lateralis scapulae.
**alpha a.,** that formed by the intersection of the visual axis with the optic axis at the nodal point. It is *positive* when the visual axis crosses the cornea on the nasal side of the optic axis, as in most individuals; *negative* when the visual axis crosses the cornea on the temporal side of the optic axis; and *nil* when the visual axis and the optic axis coincide.
**Alsberg's a.,** see under *triangle*.
**alveolar a.,** the angle between a line running through a point beneath the nasal spine and the most prominent point of the lower border of the alveolar process of the superior maxilla and the cephalic horizontal (glabella to opisthocranion).
**a. of anterior chamber of eye,** the angle formed at the border of the anterior chamber by the trabecular reticulum, the ciliary body, and the part of the iris attached to the ciliary body.
**anterior a. of petrous portion of temporal bone,** angulus anterior pyramidis ossis temporalis.
**a. of aperture,** the angle between two lines from the focus of a lens to the ends of its diameter.
**auriculo-occipital a.,** the angle between lines from the auricular point to the lambda and opisthion.
**axial a.,** any angle the formation of which is partially dependent on the axial wall of a tooth cavity preparation, as the axiodistal angle or buccoaxial angle. See table of *cavity a's* and illustration of *tooth a's*.
**axial line a.,** any line angle which is parallel with the long axis of a tooth. For names of various angles see table of *cavity a's* and illustration of *tooth a's*.
**Baumann's a.,** on an anteroposterior radiograph of the distal humerus, the angle formed by a line perpendicular to the long axis of the humerus and a line tangential to the straight epiphyseal border of the distal lateral metaphysis, normally 70°–75°; a larger angle indicates cubitus varus and a smaller, cubitus valgus.
**Bennett a.,** the angle formed by the sagittal plane and the path of the advancing condyle during lateral movement of the mandible, as viewed in the horizontal plane. See also *Bennett movement,* under *movement*.

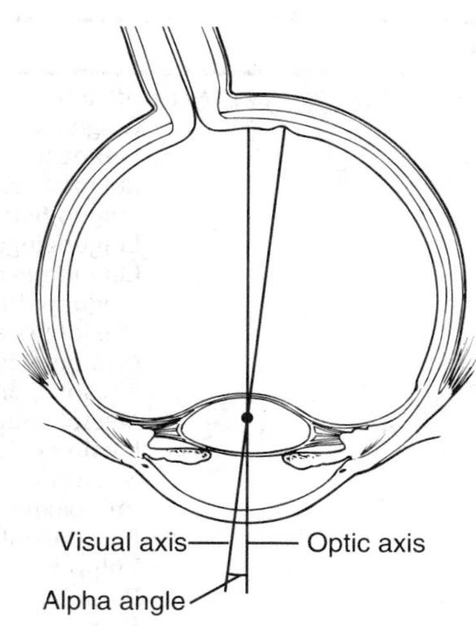

Positive alpha angle.

**beta a.,** the angle between the radius fixus and a line joining the bregma and hormion.
**biorbital a.,** the angle formed by intersection of a posterior extension of the axes of the two orbits.
**Broca's a.,** ophryospinal a.
**buccal a's,** the angles formed between the buccal surface and the other surfaces of a posterior tooth, or between the buccal wall of a tooth cavity and other walls, named according to the surfaces which participate in their formation. See table of *cavity a's* and illustration of *tooth a's*.
**cardiodiaphragmatic a.,** the angle formed by the junction of the

shadows of the heart and diaphragm in posteroanterior radiographs of the chest; called also *cardiophrenic a.*

**cardiohepatic a.,** the angle formed by the horizontal limit of hepatic dullness with the upright line of cardiac dullness in the fifth right intercostal space, close to the sternal border; called also *Ebstein's a.*

**cardiophrenic a.,** cardiodiaphragmatic a.

**carrying a.,** the angle formed laterally by the axes of the arm and forearm when the forearm is extended in the anatomical position.

**cavity a's,** the angles formed by the junction of two or more walls of a tooth cavity, named according to the walls participating in their formation. See accompanying table.

**cavosurface a.,** the angle formed by the junction of a wall of a tooth cavity preparation and a surface of the crown of the tooth.

**cephalic a's,** various angles of the skull or face.

**cephalic-medullary a.,** the angle at which the brain stem meets the base of the brain.

**cephalometric a.,** measurement of intersecting anthropometric lines on tracings made of oriented head films in radiologic orthodontic diagnosis.

**cerebellopontine a.,** that between the cerebellum and the pons.

**chi a.,** the angle between two lines from the hormion to the staphylion and to the basion, respectively.

**Cobb a.,** an angle measuring scoliosis as seen on a radiograph: for a given group of vertebrae, lines are drawn across the vertebral column on the upper surface of the upper vertebra and the lower surface of the lower vertebra. The angle measured may be either that between these two lines or that between lines drawn perpendicular to them.

**collodiaphyseal a.,** the angle formed by the intersection of the long axes of the neck and shaft of the femur.

**condylar a.,** the angle between the planes of the basilar clivus and the foramen magnum.

**a. of convergence,** that between the visual axis and the median line when an object is looked at.

**a. of convexity,** a radiographic cephalometric measurement formed by connecting the nasion, point A, and pogonion (NAP), which reflects the convexity or concavity of the facial profile.

**coronary a.,** angulus frontalis ossis parietalis.

**costal a.,** angulus costae.

**costophrenic a.,** the angle formed at the junction of the costal and diaphragmatic pleurae. See also *recessus costodiaphragmaticus pleuralis.*

**costovertebral a.,** the angle formed on either side of the vertebral column, between the last rib and the lumbar vertebrae.

**Cavity Angles**

*Line Angles (Formed by the Junction of Two Walls)*

| | |
|---|---|
| Axiodistal | Gingivoaxial |
| Axiogingival | Labiogingival |
| Axioincisal | Linguoaxial |
| Axiolabial | Linguodistal |
| Axiolingual | Linguogingival |
| Axiomesial | Linguomesial |
| Axio-occlusal | Linguopulpal |
| Axiopulpal | Mesiobuccal |
| Buccoaxial | Mesiogingival |
| Buccodistal | Mesiolabial |
| Buccogingival | Mesiolingual |
| Buccomesial | Mesio-occlusal |
| Buccopulpal | Mesiopulpal |
| Distobuccal | Pulpoaxial |
| Distogingival | Pulpodistal |
| Distolabial | Pulpolabial |
| Distolingual | Pulpolingual |
| Disto-occlusal | Pulpomesial |
| Distopulpal | |

*Point Angles (Formed by the Junction of Three Walls)*

| | |
|---|---|
| Axiodistogingival | Distopulpolingual |
| Axiodisto-occlusal | Gingivobuccoaxial |
| Axiolabiogingival | Gingivolinguoaxial |
| Axiolinguogingival | Mesiobuccopulpal |
| Axiomesiogingival | Mesiolinguopulpal |
| Axiomesio-occlusal | Mesiopulpolabial |
| Distobuccopulpal | Mesiopulpolingual |
| Distolinguopulpal | Pulpobuccoaxial |
| Distopulpolabial | Pulpolinguoaxial |

**craniofacial a.,** the angle between the basifacial and basicranial axes at the middle of the ethmoidosphenoid suture.

**critical a.,** the angle of incidence at which a ray of light passing from one medium to another of different density changes from refraction to total reflection; called also *limiting a.*

**cusp a.,** 1. the angle made by the slopes of a cusp of a tooth with the plane that passes through the tip of the cusp and that is perpendicular to a line bisecting the cusp, measured mesiodistally or buccolingually. 2. the angle made by the slopes of a cusp with a perpendicular line bisecting the cusp, measured mesiodistally or buccolingually. 3. one half of the included angle between the buccal and lingual or mesial and distal cusp inclines.

**cusp plane a.,** the incline of the cusp plane in relation to the plane of occlusion.

**Daubenton's a.,** an angle formed by junction of the opisthiobasial and opisthionasial lines; called also *occipital a.*

**a. of declination,** Mikulicz's a.

**a. of deviation,** the angle between a refracted ray and the incident ray prolonged; called also *a. of aberration.*

**a. of direction,** the angle through which the eye must move to bring the image onto the fovea.

**distal a's,** the angles formed between the distal surface and other surfaces of a tooth, or between the distal wall of a tooth cavity and other walls; named according to the surfaces which participate in their formation. See table of *cavity a's* and illustration of *tooth a's.*

**Ebstein's a.,** cardiohepatic a.

**elevation a.,** 1. the angle made by the visual plane when moved upward or downward with its normal position. 2. Alsberg's triangle; see under *triangle.*

**epigastric a.,** the angle made by the xiphoid process with the body of the sternum.

**ethmocranial a.,** the angle formed by the plane of the cribriform plate of the ethmoid bone prolonged to meet the basicranial axis; called also *ethmoid a.*

**ethmoid a.,** ethmocranial a.

**external a. of border of tibia,** margo interosseus tibiae.

**external a. of scapula,** angulus lateralis scapulae.

**facial a.,** the angle formed by the junction of the Frankfort horizontal plane and the nasion-pogonion line in the lateral radiographic cephalometric tracing. Used to express the degree of retrusion or protrusion of the chin. See also *prognathism* and *retrognathia.*

**filtration a.,** angulus iridocornealis.

**frontal a. of parietal bone,** angulus frontalis ossis parietalis.

**gamma a.,** the angle formed by junction of the line of fixation and the optic axis at the center of rotation of the eye.

**gonial a.,** the angle formed by the intersection of the body of the mandible and the ascending mandibular ramus; an important consideration in prognathic procedures. Called also *angulus mandibulae* [TA].

**horizontal a.,** in dental radiology the angle, measured within a horizontal plane, at which the central ray of the useful beam is projected relative to a vertical plane of reference.

**a. of incidence,** the angle made with the perpendicular by a ray of light which strikes a denser or a rarer medium; see *refraction.*

**incisal a.,** one of the angles formed by the junction of the incisal and the mesial or distal surfaces of an anterior tooth; called the *mesial* and the *distal incisal angle,* respectively.

**incisal guide a.,** the angle formed with the horizontal plane by drawing a line in the sagittal plane between incisal edges of the maxillary and mandibular central incisors when the teeth are in centric occlusion.

**incisal mandibular plane a.,** one of the three angles composing the Tweed triangle, designating the axial inclination of the lower incisor to the mandibular plane in the lateral cephalometric radiograph.

**a. of inclination,** inclinatio pelvis.

**inferior a. of duodenum,** flexura duodeni inferior.

**inferior a. of parietal bone, anterior,** angulus sphenoidalis ossis parietalis.

**inferior a. of parietal bone, posterior,** angulus mastoideus ossis parietalis.

**inferior a. of scapula,** angulus inferior scapulae.

**infrasternal a. of thorax,** angulus infrasternalis.

**inner a. of humerus,** margo medialis humeri.

**internal a. of tibia,** margo medialis tibiae.

**iridial a., iridocorneal a., a. of iris,** angulus iridocornealis.

**Jacquart's a.,** ophryospinal a.

**a. of jaw,** angulus mandibulae.

**kappa a.,** the angle between the pupillary axes.

**kyphotic a.,** the superior angle formed by intersection of two lines drawn on the lateral chest radiogram, tangential to the anterior borders of the second and eleventh intervertebral spaces; an index of the degree of deformity in thoracic kyphosis.

**labial a's,** the angles formed between the labial surface and other surfaces of an anterior tooth, or between the labial wall of a tooth cavity and other walls; named according to the surfaces participating in their formation. See table of *cavity a's* and illustration of *tooth a's.*

**lambda a.,** the angle between the pupillary axis and the line of sight.

**lateral a. of border of tibia,** margo interosseus tibiae.

**lateral a. of eye,** see *angulus oculi lateralis.*

**lateral a. of humerus,** margo lateralis humeri.

**lateral a. of scapula,** angulus lateralis scapulae.

**limiting a.,** critical a.

**line a.,** an angle formed by the junction of two planes; used to designate the junction of two surfaces of a tooth, or of two walls of a tooth cavity preparation. Line angles of the posterior teeth include the mesio-occlusal, linguo-occlusal, mesiolingual, distolingual, mesiobuccal, distobuccal, bucco-occlusal, and disto-occlusal angles. Those of the anterior teeth include the labioincisal, linguoincisal, mesiolabial, distolabial, mesiolingual, and distolingual angles. See table of *cavity a's* and illustration of *tooth a's.*

**lingual a's,** the angles formed between the lingual and other surfaces of a tooth, or between the lingual wall of a tooth cavity preparation and other walls; named according to the surfaces which participate in their formation, e.g., the linguopulpal angle is formed at the junction of the lingual and pulpal walls of a cavity preparation. See table of *cavity a's* and illustration of *tooth a's.*

**Louis' a., Ludwig's a.,** angulus sterni.

**lumbosacral a.,** sacrovertebral a.

**a. of mandible, mandibular a.,** angulus mandibulae.

**mastoid a. of parietal bone,** angulus mastoideus ossis parietalis.

**maxillary a.,** the angle between two lines extending from the point of contact of the upper and lower central incisors to the ophryon and the most prominent point of the lower jaw (pogonion).

**medial a. of eye,** see *angulus oculi medialis.*

**medial a. of humerus,** margo medialis humeri.

**medial a. of scapula,** angulus superior scapulae.

**medial a. of tibia,** margo medialis tibiae.

**mesial a's,** the angles formed between the mesial surface and other surfaces of a tooth, or between the mesial wall of a tooth cavity and other walls, named according to the surfaces participating with the mesial in their formation. See table of *cavity a's* and illustration of *tooth a's.*

**metafacial a.,** the angle between the base of the skull and the pterygoid process; called also *Serres' a.*

**meter a.,** a unit of convergence of the eye: that amount of convergence required for binocular fixation of an object at 1 meter and using 1 diopter of accommodation.

**Mikulicz's a.,** an angle formed by two planes, one passing through the long axis of the epiphysis of the femur and the other through the long axis of the diaphysis; it is normally 130 degrees. Called also *a. of declination.*

**minimum separabile a., minimum separable a.,** 1. the smallest angle of separation at which the eye recognizes two points, lines, or objects as being separate. 2. minimum visible a.

**minimum visible a., minimum visual a.,** the angle which the minimum separabile subtends at the eye; 60 seconds of arc is usually taken as standard for a normal eye.

**a. of mouth,** angulus oris.

**a. of Mulder,** the angle formed by the intersection of the facial line of Camper and a line from the root of the nose to the spheno-occipital suture.

**nu a.,** the angle between the radius fixus and a line joining the hormion and nasion.

**occipital a.,** Daubenton's a.

**occipital a. of parietal bone,** angulus occipitalis ossis parietalis.

**olfactive a.,** the angle formed by the line of the olfactory fossa and the os planum of the sphenoid bone; called also *olfactory a.*

**olfactory a.,** olfactive a.

**ophryospinal a.,** the angle at the anterior nasal spine between lines from the auricular point and the glabella; called also *Jacquart's a., Topinard's a.,* and *Broca's a.*

**optic a.,** visual a.

**orofacial a.,** one of the facial angles formed by the junction of the Frankfort horizontal plane with the nasion-pogonion plane.

**parietal a.,** the angle formed by junction of lines passing through the extremities of the transverse bizygomatic diameter and the maximum transverse frontal diameter; called also *Quatrefages' a.*

**parietal a. of sphenoid bone,** margo parietalis alae majoris.

**a. of pelvis,** inclinatio pelvis.

**pelvivertebral a.,** inclinatio pelvis.

**phrenopericardial a.,** the space or angle between the pericardium and the diaphragm.

**Pirogoff's a.,** venous a.

**point a.,** any angle formed by the junction of three surfaces of a tooth crown, or three walls of a tooth cavity preparation, named according to the tooth surfaces or the cavity walls participating in its formation. Point angles on the posterior teeth include the mesiolinguo-occlusal, mesiobucco-occlusal, distolinguo-occlusal, and distobucco-occlusal angles. Point angles on the anterior teeth include the mesiolabioincisal, mesiolinguoincisal, distolabioincisal, and distolinguoincisal angles. See table of *cavity a's* and illustration of *tooth a's.*

**a. of polarization,** the angle at which light reflected from a surface is most completely polarized.

**posterior a. of petrous portion of temporal bone,** angulus posterior pyramidis ossis temporalis.

**principal a.,** refracting a.

**a. of pubis,** angulus subpubicus.

**Q a.,** the angle formed by the intersection of a line connecting the center of the patella and the anterior iliac spine (representing the line of pull of the quadriceps tendon) and a line connecting the center of the patella and the center of the tibial tuberosity; in a normal knee it is 15 degrees.

**Quatrefages' a.,** parietal a.

**Ranke's a.,** the angle between the horizontal plane of the skull and a line through the center of the maxillary alveolar margin and the center of the nasofrontal suture.

**a. of reflection,** that which a reflected ray makes with a line perpendicular to the reflecting surface.

**refracting a.,** that between the two refracting faces of a prism; called also *principal a.*

**a. of refraction,** the angle between a refracted ray and a line perpendicular to the refracting surface; see *refraction.*

**a. of rib,** angulus costae.

**rolandic a., a. of Rolando,** the angle formed by junction of the median plane and the central sulcus (fissure of Rolando).

**sacrovertebral a.,** the angle formed at the junction of the sacrum with the lowest lumbar vertebra; called also *lumbosacral a.*

**Serres' a.,** metafacial a.

**sigma a.,** the angle between the radius fixus and a line from the staphylion to the hormion.

**somatosplanchnic a.,** the angle formed by junction of the somatic and splanchnic layers of the mesoblast in the embryo.

**sphenoid a., sphenoidal a.,** 1. an angle at the top of the sella turcica between lines from the nasal point and from the tip of the rostrum of the sphenoid. 2. angulus sphenoidalis ossis parietalis.

**sphenoidal a. of parietal bone,** angulus sphenoidalis ossis parietalis.

**squint a.,** the angle by which the visual line of the squinting eye deviates from a line drawn to the object which should be fixed; called also *squint deviation.*

**sternal a.,** angulus sterni.

**sternoclavicular a.,** the angle formed by junction of the sternum and clavicle.

**a. of sternum,** angulus sterni.

**subcostal a.,** angulus infrasternalis.

**subpubic a.,** angulus subpubicus.

**subscapular a.,** a transverse depression on the costal or ventral surface of the scapula, where the bone appears bent on itself perpendicular to and passing through the glenoid cavity.

**substernal a.,** angulus infrasternalis.

**superior a. of duodenum,** flexura duodeni superior.

**superior a. of parietal bone, anterior,** angulus frontalis ossis parietalis.

**superior a. of parietal bone, posterior,** angulus occipitalis ossis parietalis.

**superior a. of petrous portion of temporal bone,** angulus superior pyramidis ossis temporalis.

**superior a. of scapula,** angulus superior scapulae.

**a. of Sylvius,** the angle formed by junction of the lateral sulcus (fissure of Sylvius) and a line perpendicular to the horizontal plane tangential to the highest point of the hemisphere.

**tentorial a.,** the angle between the basicranial axis and the plane of the tentorium.

**tooth a's,** the angles formed by the junction of two or more surfaces of a tooth, named according to the surfaces participating in their formation (see illustration).

**Topinard's a.,** ophryospinal a.

**a. of torsion,** the angle between the axes of any two different portions of long bones.

**tuber a.,** the angle formed by junction of two lines, one parallel with the superior surface of the tuber calcanei and the other joining the anterior and posterior articular facets; normally about 30 degrees.

**venous a.,** the angle formed by junction of the internal jugular and subclavian veins; called also *angulus venosus* and *Pirogoff's a.*

**vertical a.,** in dental radiology, the angle measured within a vertical plane at which the central ray of the useful beam is projected relative to a horizontal plane of reference.

**Angle** *Continued*

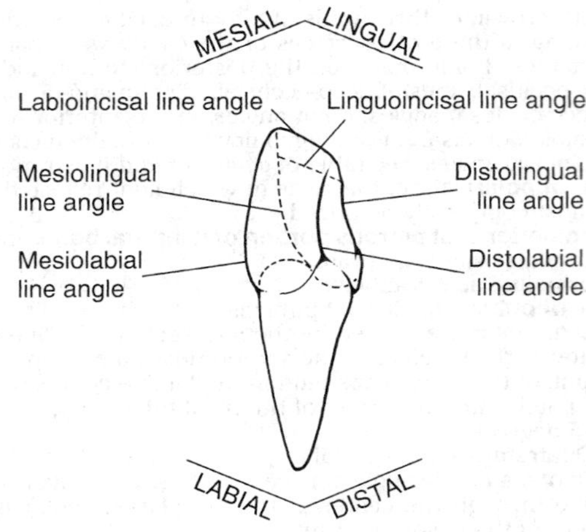


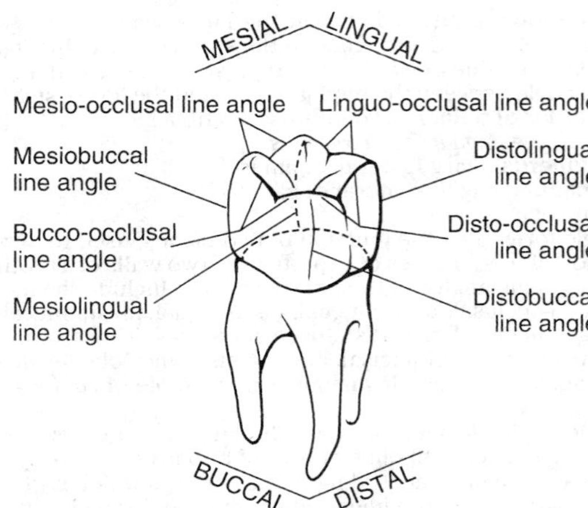


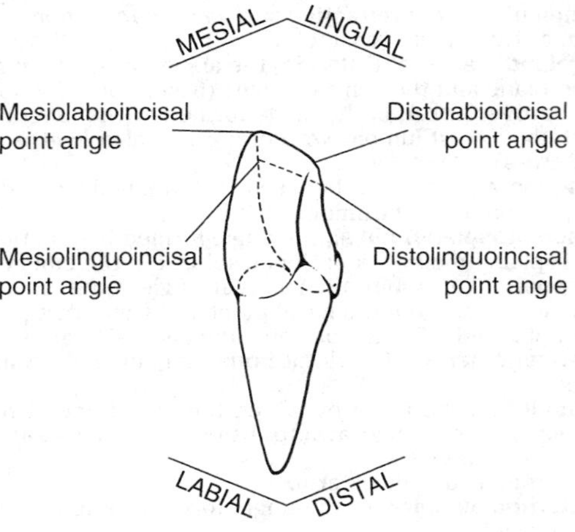


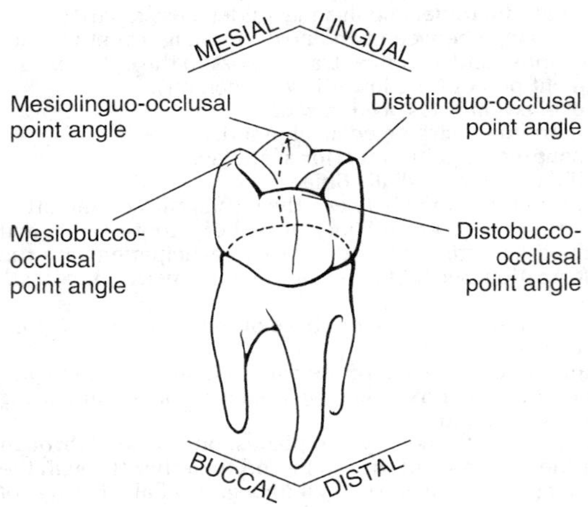


Tooth angles: *Top,* line angles; *Bottom,* point angles.

**vesicourethral a.,** the angle formed by junction of the bladder wall and the urethra.

**vesicourethral a., anterior,** the angle formed by junction of the anterior wall of the bladder and the urethra.

**vesicourethral a., posterior,** the angle formed by junction of the posterior wall of the bladder and the urethra.

**a. of Virchow,** the angle between the nasobasilar line and the nasosubnasal line.

**visual a.,** the angle formed between two lines extending from the nodal point of the eye to the extremities of the object seen; called also *optic a.*

**Vogt's a.,** the angle between the nasobasilar and alveolonasal lines.

**Weisbach's a.,** the angle at the alveolar point between lines passing from the basion and from the middle of the frontonasal suture.

**Welcker's a.,** angulus sphenoidalis ossis parietalis.

**xiphoid a's,** the angles formed by the borders of the xiphoid notch.

**Y a.,** the angle between the radius fixus and a line joining the lambda and the inion.

**ang·li·cus su·dor** (ang′glĭ-kəs soo′dor) the English sweating fever; a deadly pestilential fever which several times ravaged England during the Middle Ages.

**an·gor** (ang′gor) [L. "a strangling"] angina.
**a. a′nimi,** a feeling of life slipping away and impending death.
**a. ocula′ris,** a condition marked by fear of imminent blindness and by sudden attacks of mist before the eyes, possibly due to angiospasm of ocular vessels.
**a. pec′toris,** angina pectoris.

**Ång·ström's law, unit** (ang′strəm) [Anders Jonas *Ångström,* Swedish physicist, 1814–1874] see under *law,* and see *angstrom.*

**ang·strom** (ang′strəm) a unit of length used for atomic dimensions and light wavelengths; it is defined in terms of the wavelength of the red line of cadmium but is nominally equivalent to $10^{-10}$ meter. Symbol Å. Called also *Angström unit.*

**An·guil·lu·la** (ang-gwil′u-lə) [L. "little eel"] a genus of nematode parasites, many species of which have been reassigned to other genera.
**A. ace′ti,** *Turbatrix aceti.*
**A. intestina′lis, A. stercora′lis,** *Strongyloides stercoralis.*

**An·guil·lu·li·na pu·tre·fa·ci·ens** (ang-gwil″u-li′nə pu″trə-fa′she-ənz) *Ditylenchus dipsaci.*

**an·gu·lar** (ang′gu-lər) [L. *angula′ris*] sharply bent; having corners or angles.

**an·gu·la·tion** (ang″gu-la′shən) [L. *angulatus* bent] 1. the formation of a sharp obstructive angle, as in the intestine, the ureter, or similar tubes. 2. deviation from a straight line, as in a poorly set bone.

**an·gu·li** (ang′gu-li) [L.] genitive and plural of *angulus.*

**an·gu·lus** (ang′gu-ləs) gen. and pl. *an′guli* [L.] [TA] angle: term used in general anatomical nomenclature to designate a triangular area or the angle of a particular structure or part of the body.
**a. acromia′lis, a. acro′mii** [TA], acromial angle: the easily palpable subcutaneous bony point where the lateral border of the acromion becomes continuous with the spine of the scapula.
**a. ante′rior pyra′midis os′sis tempora′lis,** a short area on the petrous part of the temporal bone consisting of two parts: one, adjoined to the squamous part of the bone at the petrosquamous suture; the other, a free part articulating with the great wing of the sphenoid; called also *anterior angle of petrous portion of temporal bone.*
**a. cos′tae** [TA], costal angle: a prominent line on the external surface of a rib, slightly anterior to the tubercle, where the rib is bent in two directions and at the same time twisted on its long axis; called also *angle of rib.*
**a. fronta′lis os′sis parieta′lis** [TA], frontal angle of parietal bone: the anterosuperior angle of the parietal bone, which is membranous at birth and forms part of the anterior fontanelle; called also *anterior superior angle of parietal bone* and *coronary angle.*
**a. infectio′sus,** perlèche.
**a. infe′rior sca′pulae** [TA], inferior angle of scapula: the angle formed by the junction of the medial and lateral borders of the scapula.
**a. infrasterna′lis** [TA], infrasternal angle of thorax: the angle on the anteroinferior surface of the thorax, the apex of which is the sternoxiphoid junction, and the sides of which are the seventh, eighth, and ninth costal cartilages; it partially delimits two sides of the triangular epigastric region on the ventral body surface; called also *subcostal* or *substernal angle.*
**a. i′ridis, a. iridocornea′lis** [TA], iridocorneal angle: a narrow recess between the sclerocorneal junction and the attached margin of the iris, marking the periphery of the anterior chamber of the eye; it is the principal exit site for the aqueous fluid. Called also *filtration angle, iridial angle,* and *angle of iris.*
**a. latera′lis sca′pulae** [TA], lateral angle of scapula: the head of the scapula, which bears the glenoid cavity and articulates with the head of the humerus; called also *acromial* or *external angle of scapula* and *condyle of scapula.*
**a. latera′lis ti′biae,** margo interosseus tibiae.
**a. Ludovi′ci,** a. sterni.
**a. mandi′bulae** [TA], angle of mandible: the angle created at the junction of the posterior edge of the ramus and the lower edge of the mandible; called also *angle of jaw, gonial angle,* and *mandibular angle.*
**a. mastoi′deus os′sis parieta′lis** [TA], mastoid angle of parietal bone: the posteroinferior angle of the parietal bone, which articulates with the posterior part of the temporal bone and the occipital bone; called also *posterior inferior angle of parietal bone.*
**a. media′lis sca′pulae,** a. superior scapulae.
**a. media′lis ti′biae,** margo medialis tibiae.
**a. occipita′lis os′sis parieta′lis** [TA], occipital angle of parietal bone: the posterosuperior angle of the parietal bone, which during fetal life participates in the formation of the posterior fontanelle; called also *posterior superior angle of parietal bone.*
**a. o′culi latera′lis** [TA], lateral angle of eye: the angle formed by the lateral junction of the superior and inferior eyelids.
**a. o′culi media′lis** [TA], medial angle of eye: the angle formed by the medial junction of the superior and inferior eyelids.
**a. o′ris** [TA], angle of mouth: the angle formed at either side of the mouth by junction of the upper and the lower lip.

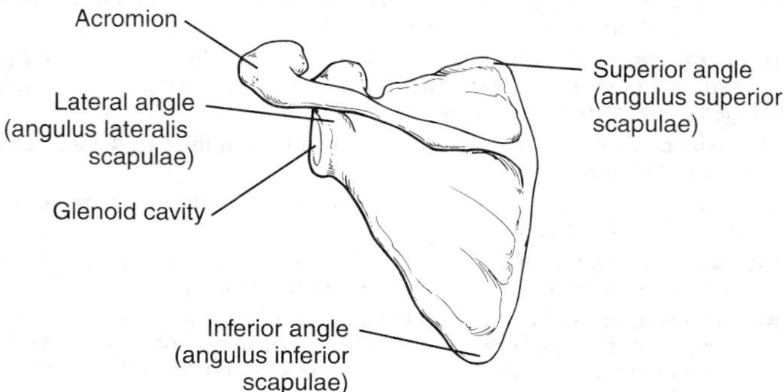

Scapula, showing the lateral, superior, and inferior angles.

**a. poste′rior pyra′midis os′sis tempora′lis,** the angle on the petrous portion of the temporal bone that separates the posterior from the inferior surface; called also *posterior angle* or *order of petrous portion of temporal bone.*
**a. pu′bis,** a. subpubicus.
**a. sphenoida′lis os′sis parieta′lis** [TA], sphenoid angle of parietal bone: the anteroinferior angle of the parietal bone, which articulates with the greater wing of the sphenoid bone and the frontal bone; called also *anterior inferior angle of parietal bone* and *Welcker's angle.*
**a. sterna′lis, a. ster′ni** [TA], sternal angle: the angle formed on the anterior surface of the sternum at the junction of its body and manubrium; called also *a. Ludovici* and *Louis'* or *Ludwig's angle.*
**a. of stomach,** incisura angularis gastris.
**a. subpu′bicus** [TA], subpubic angle: the apex of the pubic arch; the angle formed at the point of meeting of the conjoined rami of the ischial and pubic bones of the two sides of the body. Called also *a. pubis, subpubic arch,* and *arch of pelvis.*
**a. supe′rior pyra′midis os′sis tempora′lis,** the angle on the internal surface of the petrous portion of the temporal bone that separates its posterior and anterior surfaces. Called also *superior angle of petrous portion of temporal bone* and *superior border of petrous portion of temporal bone.*
**a. supe′rior sca′pulae** [TA], superior angle of scapula: the angle made by the superior and medial borders of the scapula; called also *medial angle of scapula* and *a. medialis scapulae.*
**a. veno′sus,** venous angle.

**an·hal·o·nine** (an″hə-lo′nēn) a crystalline alkaloid from *Lophophora williamsii,* with the pharmacological properties of mescaline.

**An·ha·lo·ni·um le·win·ii** (an-″hə-lo′ne-əm loo-win′e-e) *Lophophora williamsii.*

**an·ha·phia** (an-ha′fe-ə) anaphia.

**an·he·do·nia** (an″he-do′ne-ə) [*an*[1] + Gr. *hēdonē* pleasure + *-ia*] total loss of feeling of pleasure in acts that normally give pleasure.

**an·hi·dro·sis** (an″hĭ-dro′sis) [*an-*[1] + *hidro-* + *-osis*] 1. absence or severe deficiency of sweating; in humans this is usually due to absence or paralysis of the sweat glands or to obstruction of the sweat ducts. See also *hypohidrosis.* 2. absence of sweating in horses, a condition more noticeable in hot climates; affected animals develop severe dyspnea and cannot work. Called also *dry coat* and *puff disease.* Defs. 1 and 2 called also *anidrosis* and *hidroschesis.*
**thermogenic a.,** tropical anhidrotic asthenia.

**an·hi·drot·ic** (an″hĭ-drot′ik) 1. pertaining to or characterized by anhidrosis. 2. antiperspirant.

**an·hy·drase** (an-hi′drās) an older, common term used in naming some enzymes of the hydro-lyase (q.v.) sub-subclass.

**an·hy·dre·mia** (an″hi-dre′me-ə) [*an-*[1] + *hydremia*] deficiency of water in the blood. See also *dehydration* and *hypovolemia.*

**an·hy·dride** (an-hi′drīd) [*an-*[1] + *hydride*] a chemical compound derived from a substance, especially an acid, by the abstraction of a molecule of water. The anhydrides of bases are oxides; those of alcohols are ethers.
**acetic a.,** a colorless mobile liquid of a pungent acetic odor, the anhydride of acetic acid.
**acid a.,** an anhydride formed by dehydration of an acid or one that forms an acid upon hydration; if bimolecular, it can be composed of two molecules of the same acid (e.g., acetic anhydride or pyrophosphate), or it can be a mixed anhydride.
**arsenous a.,** arsenic trioxide.
**chromic a.,** chromic acid.
**mixed a.,** an acid anhydride composed of two different acids, e.g., adenosine triphosphate or an aminoacyl adenylate.
**perosmic a.,** osmium tetroxide.
**phthalic a.,** a reactive, low-molecular-weight compound with a wide variety of industrial uses, including the manufacture of dyes, pharmaceuticals, and insecticides, and as a hardener for resins. It is an allergen that causes skin irritation, and if its fumes are inhaled it can cause *epoxy resin lung,* a form of hypersensitivity pneumonitis.
**silicic a.,** silica.
**sorbitol a.,** sorbitan.
**sulfurous a.,** sulfur dioxide.
**trimellitic a.,** TMA; a low-molecular-weight reactive chemical used in the manufacture of plastics, epoxy resin, coatings, and paints; inhalation of its dust or fumes produces a variety of respiratory symptoms. See under *flu* and *pneumonitis.*

**an·hy·dro·chlo·ric** (an″hi-dro-klor′ik) achlorhydric.

**an·hy·dro·hy·droxy·pro·ges·ter·one** (an-hi″dro-hi-drok′se-pro-jes′tər-ōn) ethisterone.

**An·hy·dron** (an-hi′dron) trademark for a preparation of cyclothiazide.

**an·hy·dro·sug·ar** (an-hi″dro-shoog′ər) a sugar from which one or more molecules of water have been removed, resulting in the formation of an internal acetal structure.

**an·hy·drous** (an-hi'drəs) [*an-*[1] + *hydrous*] deprived or destitute of water.

**ani·a·cin·am·i·do·sis** (ə-ni-ə-sin-am″ĭ-do'sis) any disorder due to niacinamide deficiency; see *pellagra.*

**ani·a·ci·no·sis** (ə-ni″ə-sĭ-no'sis) pellagra.

**Anich·kov's (Anitsch·kow's) myocyte (cell)** (ah-nich'kofs) [Nikolai Nikolaevich *Anichkov* (or *Anitschkow*), Russian pathologist, 1885–1964] see under *myocyte.*

**an·ic·ter·ic** (an″ik-ter'ik) without icterus; not associated with jaundice.

**anid·e·an** (ə-nid'e-ən) pertaining to anideus.

**anid·e·us** (ə-nid'e-əs) [*an-*[1] + *idea*] holoacardius amorphus.
**embryonic a.,** a blastoderm in which no embryonic axis develops.

**an·idro·sis** (an-ĭ-dro'sis) anhidrosis.

**an·idrot·ic** (an″ĭ-drot'ik) 1. anhidrotic (def. 1). 2. antiperspirant.

**an·ile** (a'nīl) [L. *anus* old woman] 1. like an old woman. 2. senile; in one's dotage.

**an·i·ler·i·dine** (an″ĭ-ler'ĭ-dēn) [USP] a synthetic narcotic analgesic used as the phosphate salt for premedication for general anesthesia in surgery, as a postoperative sedative, and as an obstetric analgesic; administered subcutaneously or intramuscularly. Abuse of this drug may lead to dependence.
**a. hydrochloride** [USP], the hydrochloride salt of leritine, used as an analgesic for the relief of moderate to severe pain and as an obstetric analgesic.

**an·i·lid** (an'ĭ-lid) anilide.

**an·i·lide** (an'ĭ-līd) any compound formed from aromatic amines by substitution of an acyl group for the hydrogen of $NH_2$.

**an·i·line** (an'ĭ-lin) [Arabic *an-nil* indigo plant] a colorless oily liquid arylamine derived from coal tar or indigo, made commercially by reducing nitrobenzene. It is slightly soluble in water and freely so in ether and alcohol. Combined with other substances, especially chlorine and the chlorates, it forms the aniline colors or dyes. It is an important cause of serious industrial poisoning *(anilinism),* and high doses or long exposure may be carcinogenic. Called also *amidobenzene* and *aminobenzene.*

**ani·lin·gus** (a″nĭ-ling'gəs) [L. *anus* q.v. + *lingere* to lick] sexual stimulation of the anus with the lips or tongue.

**an·i·lin·ism** (an'ĭ-lin-iz-əm) a condition produced by exposure to aniline, and marked by methemoglobinemia and aplastic anemia, vertigo, muscular weakness, cyanosis, and digestive derangement.

**an·i·lism** (an'ĭ-liz-əm) anilinism.

**anil·i·ty** (ə-nil'ĭ-te) [L. *anus* old woman] 1. the state of existing as or like an old woman. 2. senility; dotage.

**an·il·o·pam hy·dro·chlo·ride** (an'il-o-pam″) an analgesic.

**an·il·quin·o·line** (an″il-kwin'o-lin) synthetic quinoline prepared from aniline.

**an·i·ma** (an'ĭ-mə) [L., the animating spirit present in any animal] 1. the soul. 2. the active principle of a drug. 3. in jungian psychology, the soul or inner being of a person, as opposed to the *persona,* the social role or facade presented to the world; because the inner and outer facades are often opposing, Jung also used the term to refer to the feminine aspect of a man's soul, the analogous masculine aspect of a woman's soul being termed the *animus.*

**an·i·mal** (an'ĭ-məl) [L. *animalis,* from *anima* life, breath] [MeSH: Animal] 1. a living organism having sensation and the power of voluntary movement and requiring for its existence oxygen and organic food. 2. pertaining to such an organism. 3. any animal organism other than a human being.
**control a.,** see *control,* def. 2.
**conventional a.,** an experimental animal that has not been reared under gnotobiotic conditions.
**decerebrate a.,** an experimental animal that has been subjected to decerebration; such an animal exhibits rigid extension of the legs, with strong tonic contraction of the extensor muscles and to some extent the flexor muscles. See also *decerebrate,* and see *decerebrate rigidity,* under *rigidity.*
**experimental a.,** an animal which is used as a subject of experimental procedures in the laboratory.
**Houssay a.,** an experimental animal deprived of both pituitary gland and pancreas; see *Houssay phenomenon,* under *phenomenon.*
**hyperphagic a.,** an experimental animal in which the cells of the ventromedial nucleus of the hypothalamus have been destroyed, abolishing its awareness of the point at which it should stop eating; excessive eating and savageness characterize such an animal.
**Long-Lukens a.,** an experimental animal which has been deprived of the pancreas and adrenal glands.
**nuclein a.,** an animal into which a certain amount of nuclein has been injected.
**spinal a.,** an animal whose spinal cord has been severed, thus cutting off communication with the brain.
**thalamic a.,** an animal in which the brain stem has been transected just above the thalamus.

**an·i·mal·cu·list** (an″ĭ-mal'ku-list) a believer in the theory that the undeveloped embryo exists preformed in the spermatozoon; cf. *ovist.*

**an·i·ma·tion** (an″ĭ-ma'shən) 1. the state of being alive. 2. liveliness of spirits.
**suspended a.,** a temporary state of apparent death.

**an·i·mism** (an'ĭ-miz-əm) [L. *anima* soul] 1. the obsolete doctrine that the soul is the source of all organic development. 2. the belief that nonliving objects and phenomena (such as clouds) are inhabited and motivated by a nonphysical agent; it is a characteristic of the thinking of early childhood. 3. the theory that behavior is controlled by an immaterial mind or soul.

**an·i·mus** (an'ĭ-məs) [L., the rational part of the mind; intellect or motivations] 1. disposition. 2. ill will or hostility; animosity. 3. in jungian psychology, the masculine aspect of a woman's soul or inner being; see *anima.*

**an·ion** (an'i-on) [*ana-* + *ion*] an ion carrying a negative charge owing to a surplus of electrons; in an electrolytic cell anions migrate toward the anode, the positively charged electrode.

**an·ion·ic** (an″i-on'ik) pertaining to or containing an anion.

**an·ion·ot·ro·py** (an″e-on-ot'rə-pe) [*anion* + Gr. *tropos* a turning] a type of tautomerism in which the migrating group is a negative ion rather than the more usual hydrogen ion. Cf. *prototropy.*

**an·irid·ia** (an″ĭ-rid'e-ə) [*an-*[1] + *irid-* + *-ia*] [MeSH: Aniridia] absence of the iris; a usually bilateral, hereditary anomaly that is rarely complete, a rudimentary stump usually being visible on gonioscopy.

**an·i·sa·ki·a·sis** (an″i-sə-ki'ə-sis) [MeSH: Anisakiasis] infection of humans or other animals with any nematode of the family Anisakidae. Human infection is usually caused by third-stage larvae of *Anisakis marina* eaten in undercooked infected marine fish (e.g., herring); the larvae then burrow into the stomach wall, producing an eosinophilic granulomatous mass. Called also *eosinophilic granuloma.*

**An·i·sa·ki·dae** (an″ĭ-sak'ĭ-de) a family of nematodes, many of which cause anisakiasis in humans and other animals that eat raw fish. Genera include *Anisakis* and *Phocanema.*

**An·i·sa·kis** (an″ĭ-sa'kis) [MeSH: Anisakis] a genus of nematodes of the family Anisakidae; the usual infecting species is *A. mari'na.* It parasitizes the stomachs of marine mammals and birds, where it reaches the adult stage. Infective third-stage larvae occur in various marine fishes, and humans may become infected by ingestion of such fish raw. See also *anisakiasis.*

**an·i·sate** (an'ĭ-sāt) a salt of anisic acid.

**an·ise** (an'is) [L. *anisum*] 1. *Pimpinella anisum.* 2. the fruit of *P. anisum,* used as a carminative and expectorant. 3. any of several other similar fruits.
**Chinese a., Indian a.,** the dried ripe fruit of *Illicium verum;* it yields anise oil and is used as a stimulant and carminative.
**star a.,** 1. *Illicium religiosum.* 2. the poisonous fruit of *I. religiosum.*

**an·is·ei·ko·nia** (an″is-i-ko'ne-ə) [*anis-* + *eikōn* image + *-ia*] [MeSH: Aniseikonia] a condition in which the ocular image of an object as seen by one eye differs in size and shape from that seen by the other.

**an·is·ei·kon·ic** (an″is-i-kon'ik) pertaining to or correcting aniseikonia.

**anis·ic acid** (ə-nis'ik) *p*-methoxybenzoic acid, an antiseptic compound obtained from anise and fennel.

***o*-an·is·i·dine** (ə-nis'ĭ-dēn) a yellow to red oily aromatic amine used as a chemical intermediate in the manufacture of azo dyes; it is a strong irritant and carcinogen.

**an·is·in·di·one** (an″is-in-di'ōn) an orally administered indanedione anticoagulant.

**anis(o)-** [Gr. *anisos* unequal, uneven] a combining form meaning unequal or dissimilar.

**an·iso·ac·com·mo·da·tion** (an-i″so-ə-kom″ə-da'shən) a difference in the accommodative capacity of the two eyes.

**an·iso·chro·ma·sia** (an-ĭ″so-kro-ma'zhə) [*aniso-* + Gr. *chrōma* color] a condition in which only the peripheral zone of an erythrocyte is colored; seen in some forms of anemia. Called also *anisochromia.*

**an·iso·chro·mat·ic** (an-i″so-kro-mat'ik) [*aniso-* + *chromatic* color] 1. not of the same color throughout. 2. pertaining to solutions used for testing color blindness, containing two pigments which are distinguished by both the normal and the color blind eye. Cf. *pseudoisochromatic.*

**an·iso·chro·mia** (an″i-so-kro′me-ə) [*aniso-* + *chrom-* + *-ia*] anisochromasia.

**an·iso·co·ria** (an-i″so-ko′re-ə) [*aniso-* + *cor-* + *-ia*] [MeSH: Anisocoria] inequality in diameter of the pupils.

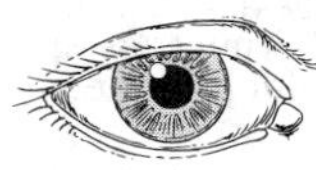
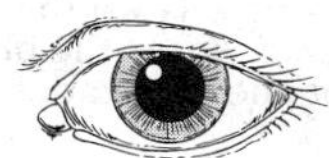

Anisocoria.

**an·iso·cy·to·sis** (an-i″so-si-to′sis) [*aniso-* + *cyt-* + *-osis*] presence in the blood of erythrocytes with excessive variation in size; see also *macrocythemia* and *microcythemia.* Called also *anisopoikilocytosis.*

**an·iso·dac·ty·lous** (an″i-so-dak′tə-ləs) [*aniso-* + *dactylo-* + *-ous*] having corresponding digits of unequal length.

**an·iso·dac·ty·ly** (an-i-so-dak′tə-le) a condition characterized by having corresponding digits of unequal length.

**an·iso·di·a·met·ric** (an-i″so-di″ə-met′rik) characterized by different dimensions in different diameters.

**an·iso·dont** (an-i′so-dont) [*anis-* + Gr. *odous* tooth] 1. one who has unequal, asymmetric teeth. 2. an animal having irregular, asymmetric teeth, as in certain reptiles.

**an·iso·gam·ete** (an″i-so-gam′ēt) a gamete of different size and structure from the one with which it unites. See *macrogamete* and *microgamete.*

**an·iso·ga·met·ic** (an″i-so-gə-met′ik) characterized by the production of gametes of different size and structure.

**an·isog·a·mous** (an″i-sog′ə-məs) having conjugating elements (gametes) that differ in size and structure.

**an·isog·a·my** (an″i-sog′ə-me) [*aniso-* + Gr. *gamos* marriage] sexual conjugation in which the gametes differ in structure and size.

**an·iso·ico·nia** (an-i″so-i-ko′ne-ə) aniseikonia.

**an·iso·kary·o·sis** (an-i″so-kar″e-o′sis) [*aniso-* + *kary-* + *-osis*] inequality in the size of the nuclei of cells.

**An·iso·lo·bis** (an-i″so-lo′bis) a genus of beetles, the earwigs. Nymphs and adults of *A. euborel′lia* (Lucas) are intermediate hosts of helminth parasites of humans and other animals.

**an·iso·mas·tia** (an-i″so-mas′te-ə) [*aniso-* + *mast-* + *-ia*] inequality in the size of the breasts.

**an·iso·me·lia** (an-i″so-me′le-ə) [*aniso-* + *-melia*] inequality between paired limbs.

**an·iso·mer·ic** (an-i″so-mer′ik) not isomeric.

**an·iso·met·rope** (an-i″so-met′rōp) a person with anisometropia.

**an·iso·me·tro·pia** (an-i″so-mə-tro′pe-ə) [*aniso-* + Gr. *metron* measure + *-opia*] [MeSH: Anisometropia] a difference in the refractive power of the two eyes.

**an·iso·me·trop·ic** (an-i″so-mĕ-trop′ik) pertaining to or characterized by anisometropia.

**An·iso·mor·pha** (an-i″so-mor′fə) a genus of insects.
**A. buprestoi′des,** the walking stick; a species of orthopterous insects capable of discharging an irritating fluid.

**an·iso·pho·ria** (an″i-so-for′e-ə) [*aniso-* + *phoria*] a condition in which the balance of the vertical muscles of one eye differs from that of the other eye, so that the visual lines do not lie in the same horizontal plane.

**an·iso·pia** (an″i-so′pe-ə) [*aniso-* + *-opia*] inequality of vision in the two eyes.

**an·iso·pi·esis** (an-i″so-pi-e′sis) [*aniso-* + *-piesis*] variation or inequality in the blood pressure as registered in different parts of the body.

**an·iso·poi·ki·lo·cy·to·sis** (an-i″so-poi″kĭ-lo-si-to′sis) presence in the blood of erythrocytes of abnormal sizes and shapes; anisocytosis with poikilocytosis.

**an·i·sos·mot·ic** (an″i-sos-mot′ik) not having the same osmotic pressure or not containing the same effective concentration of osmotically active components.

**an·iso·spore** (an-i′so-spor″) [*aniso-* + *spore*] 1. a sexual spore, the male and female differing in size or shape. 2. an asexual spore produced by a heterosporous organism. See *isospore.*

**an·isos·po·rous** (an″ĭ-sos′pə-rəs) having anisospores.

**an·isos·then·ic** (an-i″sos-then′ik) [*aniso-* + *sthenic*] not having equal strength; said of paired muscles.

**an·iso·ton·ic** (an-i″so-ton′ik) 1. showing a variation in tonicity or tension. 2. having an osmotic pressure differing from that of a solution with which it is compared.

**an·isot·ro·pal** (an″i-sot′ro-pəl) anisotropic.

**an·iso·trop·ic** (an-i″so-trop′ik) [*aniso-* + *tropic*] 1. having unlike properties in different directions, as in any unit lacking spherical symmetry. 2. doubly refracting or having a double polarizing power.

**an·i·so·tro·pine meth·yl·bro·mide** (an-i″so-tro′pēn) an orally administered anticholinergic that produces relaxation of visceral smooth muscle and is used as a spasmolytic in various gastrointestinal disorders.

**an·isot·ro·py** (an″i-sot′rə-pe) [MeSH: Anisotropy] the quality or condition of being anisotropic.

**an·is·trep·lase** (an-is-trep′lās) [MeSH: Anistreplase] a thrombolytic agent, primarily used to clear coronary vessel occlusions after myocardial infarction; administered intravenously.

**an·i·su·ria** (an″i-su′re-ə) [*anis-* + *-uria*] a condition marked by alternating oliguria and polyuria.

**ani·trog·e·nous** (a″ni-troj′ə-nəs) not nitrogenous.

**Anitsch·kow** (ah-nich′kov) see *Anichkov.*

**Anix·i·op·sis** (ə-nik″se-op′sis) *Aphanoascus.*

**an·kle** (ang′kəl) [A.S. *anclēow*] [MeSH: Ankle] 1. articulatio talocruralis. 2. the region of the ankle joint (articulatio talocruralis). 3. talus. 4. hock.
**tailors′ a.,** an abnormal bursa over the lower end of the fibula in tailors, from pressure caused by sitting on the floor with the legs crossed in front.

**ankyl(o)-** [Gr. *ankylos* bent or crooked] a combining form meaning bent, or denoting fusion or adhesion.

**an·ky·lo·bleph·a·ron** (ang″kə-lo-blef′ə-ron) [*ankylo-* + Gr. *blepharon* eyelid] the adhesion of the ciliary edges of the eyelid to each other.
**a. filifor′me adna′tum,** congenital adhesion of the margins of the upper and lower lids by filamentous bands.

**an·ky·lo·chei·lia** (ang″kə-lo-ki′le-ə) [*ankylo-* + *cheilo-* + *-ia*] adhesion of the lips to each other.

**an·ky·lo·col·pos** (ang-kə-lo-kol′pos) [*ankylo-* + Gr. *kolpos* vagina] atresia or imperforation of the vagina.

**an·ky·lo·dac·ty·ly** (ang″kə-lo-dak′tə-le) [*ankylo-* + Gr. *daktylos* finger] fusion or adhesion of fingers or toes to one another.

**an·ky·lo·glos·sia** (ang″kə-lo-glos′e-ə) [*ankylo-* + *glossa* + *-ia*] restricted movement of the tongue, resulting in speech difficulty. Called also *adherent tongue, lingua frenata,* and *tongue-tie.* See also *complete a.* and *partial a.*
**complete a.,** ankyloglossia resulting from fusion between the tongue and the floor of the mouth.
**partial a.,** ankyloglossia resulting from a short lingual frenum or one which is attached too near the tip of the tongue.
**a. supe′rior,** an unusual association of an extensive adhesion of the tongue to the palate, sometimes with deformities of the extremities.

**an·ky·lo·poi·et·ic** (ang″kə-lo-poi-et′ik) [*ankylo-* + Gr. *poiein* to make] producing or characterized by ankylosis.

**An·ky·lo·pro·glypha** (ang″kə-lo-pro-glif′ə) Proteroglypha.

**an·ky·losed** (ang′kə-lōzd) fused or obliterated, as a joint.

**an·ky·lo·ses** (ang″kə-lo′sēz) [MeSH: Ankylosis] plural of *ankylosis.*

**an·ky·lo·sis** (ang″kə-lo′sis) pl. *ankylo′ses* [Gr. *ankylōsis*] [MeSH: Ankylosis] immobility and consolidation of a joint due to disease, injury, or surgical procedure. Called also *arthrokleisis.*
**artificial a.,** arthrodesis.
**bony a.,** the union of the bones of a joint by proliferation of bone cells, resulting in complete immobility; called also *true a.*
**cricoarytenoid joint a.,** fixation of the cricoarytenoid joint due to inflammation; characterized by hoarseness, cough, and difficulty in expectoration.
**extracapsular a.,** ankylosis due to rigidity of structures exterior to the joint capsule.
**false a.,** fibrous a.
**fibrous a.,** reduced mobility of a joint due to proliferation of fibrous tissue; called also *false a.* and *spurious a.*
**intracapsular a.,** obliteration of joint motion due to disease, injury, or surgical procedure within the joint capsule.
**spurious a.,** fibrous a.
**stapedial a.,** fixation of the footplate of the stapes in otosclerosis, causing a conductive hearing loss.
**true a.,** bony a.

**An·ky·los·to·ma** (ang″kə-los′to-mə) *Ancylostoma.*

**an·ky·lo·sto·mi·a·sis** (ang″kə-lo-sto-mi′ə-sis) ancylostomiasis.

**an·ky·lot·ic** (ang″kə-lot′ik) pertaining to or marked by ankylosis.

**an·ky·lot·o·my** (ang″kə-lot′ə-me) [*ankylo-* + *-tomy*] frenotomy for relieving ankyloglossia.

**an·kyl·ure·thria** (ang″kəl-u-re′thre-ə) [*ankylo-* + *urethra* + *-ia*] stricture of the urethra.

**an·ky·rin** (ang′kə-rin) a membrane protein of erythrocytes and brain that anchors spectrin to the plasma membrane at the sites of anion channels.

**an·ky·roid** (ang′kĭ-roid) ancyroid.

**an·lage** (ahn-lah′-gə, an′lāj) pl. *anla′gen* [Ger. "a laying on"] primordium.

**AN-MAA** trademark for a kit for the preparation of technetium Tc 99m albumin aggregated.

**AN-MDP** trademark for a kit for the preparation of technetium Tc 99m medronate.

**an·neal** (ə-nēl′) 1. to heat a material, such as glass or metal, followed by controlled cooling to remove internal stresses and induce a desired degree of toughness, temper, or softness of the material. 2. to homogenize an amalgam alloy ingot by heating it in an oven. 3. to degas; see *degassing,* def. 2. 4. in molecular biology, to cause the association or reassociation of single-stranded nucleic acids so that double-stranded molecules are formed, often by heating followed by cooling.

**an·nec·tent** (ə-nek′tənt) [L. *annectens*] connecting or joining; spelled also *annectant.*

**an·ne·lid** (an′ə-lid) 1. any member of the phylum Annelida. 2. of or pertaining to the phylum Annelida.

**An·ne·li·da** (ə-nel′ĭ-də) [Fr. *anneler* to arrange in rings, from L. *anellus* a little ring] [MeSH: Annelida] a phylum of metazoan invertebrates comprising the segmented worms, and including marine annelids, freshwater annelids and earthworms, and leeches (class Hirudinea); only the latter are of medical interest.

**an·nel·lide** (an′ə-līd) a type of conidiogenous cell formed in blastic conidiogenesis, having multiple ringlike scars around its tip resulting from release of successive conidia.

**an·nex·in** (ə-nek′sin) any of a family of $Ca^{2+}$/phospholipid-dependent proteins, thought to mediate intracellular calcium signals and inhibit activation of phospholipase $A_2$, which means also inhibiting synthesis of prostaglandins and other arachidonic acid derivatives. Called also *lipocortin.*

**An·no·na** (ə-no′nə) a genus of trees and shrubs of the family Annonaceae, found in tropical regions of the Americas. *A. murica′ta* L. is the soursop, source of a popular edible fruit. The bark, fruit, and leaves of various species are used in native medicine, and the seeds of some have emetic properties and are poisonous for fish and insects.

**an·nu·lar** (an′u-lər) [L. *annularis*] shaped like a ring. See also *circular.*

**an·nu·li** (an′u-li) [L.] genitive and plural of *annulus.*

**an·nu·lo·aor·tic** (an″u-lo-a-or′tĭk) [*annulus* + *aortic*] pertaining to the aorta and aortic annulus.

**an·nu·lo·plas·ty** (an″u-lo-plas′te) [*annulus* + *-plasty*] plastic repair of a cardiac valve.
**DeVega a.,** a method for repair of an incompetent tricuspid valve by placing a series of purse-string sutures around the valve annulus to reduce it to the size of the obturator.
**Kay a.,** a method for repairing a tricuspid valve with a dilated annulus but little prolapse: by placing several sutures at the commissures, the posterior leaflet is drawn forward toward the anterior leaflet and their surface area of approximation is increased.

**an·nu·lor·rha·phy** (an″u-lor′ə-fe) [*annulus* + *-rrhaphy*] closure of a hernial ring or defect by sutures.

**an·nu·lus** (an′u-ləs) gen. and pl. *an′nuli* [L., from *anus* ring] a ring or ringlike structure; in official anatomical terminology, spelled *anulus* [TA], q.v. for terms not found here.
**a. cilia′ris,** orbiculus ciliaris.
**a. of nuclear pore,** a filamentous, circular structure at the edge of the nuclear pore of a cell nucleus and extending into the pore as a lining layer; the pore and its annulus together form the pore complex.
**a. ova′lis,** limbus fossae ovalis.
**an′nuli tra′cheae,** cartilagines tracheales.
**a. urethra′lis,** a thickening around the urethral opening of the bladder formed by a thickening of the middle muscular coat.
**Vieussens′ a.,** 1. limbus fossae ovalis. 2. ansa subclavia.

**Ano·cen·tor** (a″no-sen′tər) a genus of ticks of the family Ixodidae.
**A. ni′tens,** a species of yellow-brown ticks parasitizing horses, found first in the West Indies and later in the southern United States; it transmits *Babesia caballi,* an etiologic agent of equine babesiosis. Called also *Dermacentor nitens* and *Otocentor nitens.*

**ano·chro·ma·sia** (an″o-kro-ma′zhə) 1. absence of the usual staining reaction from a tissue or cell. 2. a condition in which the erythrocytes show a piling up of hemoglobin at the periphery so that the center is pale.

**ano·ci·as·so·ci·a·tion** (ə-no″se-ə-so″se-a′shən) [*a-*[1] + L. *nocere* to injure + *association*] the blunting of harmful association impulses; a method of anesthesia designed to minimize the effect of surgical shock.

**ano·ci·ated** (ə-no′se-āt″əd) in a condition of anociassociation.

**ano·ci·a·tion** (ə-no″se-a′shən) anociassociation.

**ano·coc·cy·ge·al** (a″no-kok-sij′e-əl) pertaining to the anus and coccyx.

**an·o·dal** (an′o-dəl) pertaining to the anode.

**an·ode** (an′ōd) [Gr. *ana-* up + *hodos* way] 1. in an electrochemical cell, the electrode at which oxidation occurs, i.e., the positive electrode in an electrolytic cell or a storage battery. It is the negative electrode in a voltaic cell that is delivering current. 2. the positive electrode of devices such as electron tubes, x-ray tubes, and electrophoresis cells. Symbol A. Cf. *cathode.*
**hooded a.,** in radiology, an anode incorporating a copper shield to overcome problems of secondary ray emission.
**rotating a.,** in radiology, an anode in the form of a disk with the target material annealed to its rim; the anode is continuously rotated so that the electron stream strikes only a small part of the target at one time, thus allowing heat dissipation.

**ano·derm** (a′no-dərm) the epithelial lining of the anal canal.

**an·od·mia** (an-od′me-ə) [*an-*[1] + Gr. *odmē* smell + *-ia*] anosmia.

**an·odon·tia** (an″o-don′shə) [*an-*[1] + *odont-* + *-ia*] [MeSH: Anodontia] congenital absence of the teeth; it may involve all *(total a.)* or only some of the teeth *(partial a., hypodontia),* and both the deciduous and the permanent dentition, or only teeth of the permanent dentition. See also *Kennedy classification* and *Skinner classification,* under *classification.* Called also *anodontism* and *edentia.*
**partial a.,** hypodontia.
**total a.,** a rare condition characterized by congenital absence of all teeth, both deciduous and permanent.
**true a., a. ve′ra,** total or partial (hypodontia) congenital absence of the teeth.

**an·odon·tism** (an″o-don′tiz-əm) anodontia.

**an·o·dyne** (an′o-dīn) [*an-*[1] + Gr. *odynē* pain] 1. relieving pain. 2. a medicine that relieves pain; the anodynes include opium, morphine, codeine, aspirin, and others. Called also *acesodyne.*

**Ano·geis·sus** (a″no-ji′səs) a genus of trees of the family Combretaceae, found in southern Asia. *A. latifo′lia* is the dhava, source of ghatti gum.

***p*-anol** (a′nol) an intermediate in the production of estrogens; it is readily polymerized to form active carcinogenic and estrogenic substances.

**anom·a·lad** (ə-nom′ə-lad) sequence, def. 2.
**amniotic band a.,** see under *sequence.*
**Robin's a.,** Pierre Robin syndrome.

**anomal(o)-** [Gr. *anōmalos* irregular] a combining form meaning irregular or uneven.

**anom·a·lo·scope** (ə-nom′ə-lo-skōp″) [*anomalo-* + *-scope*] an instrument used in testing for anomalies of color vision by having the subject match mixed spectral lines.

**anom·al·ot·ro·phy** (ə-nom″əl-ot′ro-fe) [*anomalo-* + *-trophy*] abnormality of nutrition.

**anom·a·lous** (ə-nom′ə-ləs) [Gr. *anōmalos*] irregular; marked by deviation from the natural order. Applied particularly to congenital and hereditary defects.

**anom·a·ly** (ə-nom′ə-le) [Gr. *anōmalia*] marked deviation from the normal standard, especially as a result of congenital defects.
**Alder's a., Alder's constitutional granulation a., Alder-Reilly a.,** an autosomal dominant condition in which leukocytes of the myelocytic series, and sometimes all leukocytes, contain coarse azurophil granules (Alder-Reilly bodies); it is usually clinically unimportant but is sometimes associated with Hurler's syndrome or other pathological conditions.
**Aristotle's a.,** if the first and second fingers are crossed and a pencil is placed between them, the person feels two pencils.
**Axenfeld's a.,** a developmental anomaly consisting of posterior embryotoxon and iris processes to Schwalbe's ring. Called also *arcus juvenilis, posterior embryotoxon,* and *posterior embryotoxon of Axenfeld.* See also *anterior chamber cleavage syndrome,* under *syndrome.*

**Chédiak-Higashi a., Chédiak-Steinbrinck-Higashi a.,** see under *syndrome.*
**chromosomal a., chromosome a.,** see under *aberration.*
**collie eye a.,** an autosomal recessive ocular defect seen in collies and a few other breeds of dog, characterized by an area of choroidal hyperplasia lateral to the optic disk, sometimes with colobomas, retinal detachment, and intraocular hemorrhaging.
**developmental a.,** 1. a structural abnormality of any type. 2. a defect resulting from imperfect development of the embryo.
**Ebstein's a.,** a malformation of the tricuspid valve, the septal and posterior leaflets being adherent to the wall of the right ventricle to a varying degree, producing tricuspid deficiency, and the anterior leaflet being normally attached to the annulus fibrosus; usually associated with an atrial septal defect. Called also *Ebstein's disease.*
**Freund's a.,** stenosis of the upper thoracic aperture from shortening of the first rib, resulting in deficient expansion of the apex of the lung.
**Hegglin's a.,** May-Hegglin a.
**Jordans' a.,** presence of lipid vacuoles in the cytoplasm of granulocytes, monocytes, and occasionally plasma cells and lymphocytes; some affected persons develop muscular dystrophy while others develop ichthyosis.
**May-Hegglin a.,** an autosomal dominant disorder of blood cell morphology, characterized by blue, RNA-containing cytoplasmic inclusions similar to Döhle's bodies in most of the granulocytes, accompanied by abnormally large, poorly granulated platelets and sometimes thrombocytopenia, usually without other distinguishing features. Called also *Hegglin's a.*
**Pelger's nuclear a., Pelger-Huët a.,** Pelger-Huët nuclear a., def. 1.
**Pelger-Huët nuclear a.,** 1. an autosomal dominant defect of neutrophils and eosinophils in which their nuclei are bilobed or dumbbell-shaped and have a coarse and lumpy structure. Called also *Pelger's nuclear a.* and *Pelger-Huët a.* 2. an acquired condition with changes similar to those observed in the genetically determined abnormality, occurring in certain types of anemia and leukemia.
**Peters' a.,** a developmental defect in structures around the anterior chamber of the eye, characterized by corneal clouding and sometimes adhesions of the iris, lens, and cornea; it is often accompanied by other defects such as dwarfism and mental retardation.
**Poland's a.,** see under *syndrome.*
**Rieger's a.,** a developmental anomaly consisting of posterior embryotoxon, hypoplasia of iris stroma, and usually glaucoma. See also *anterior chamber cleavage syndrome,* under *syndrome.*
**Uhl's a.,** congenital hypoplasia of the myocardium of the right ventricle, resulting in decreased output of the right side of the heart.

**an·o·mer** (an'o-mər) [*ana-* + *-mere*] either of a pair of cyclic diastereoisomers of a sugar or glycoside, differing only in the configuration at the reducing carbon atom and resulting from the new point of symmetry created by ring formation; they are designated $\alpha$- and $\beta$- to denote position of the hydroxyl group below and above the plane of the ring, respectively.

**an·o·mer·ic** (an″o-mer'ik) pertaining to an anomer; denoting the reducing carbon atom in an anomer.

**ano·mia** (ə-no'me-ə) [MeSH: Anomia] anomic aphasia.

**an·onych·ia** (an″o-nik'e-ə) [*an-*[1] + *onych-* + *-ia*] absence of the nail(s).

**anon·y·mous** (ə-non'ĭ-məs) nameless; innominate.

**ano·per·i·ne·al** (a″no-per-ĭ-ne'əl) pertaining to the anus and perineum.

**Anoph·e·les** (ə-nof'ə-lēz) [Gr. *anōphelēs* hurtful] [MeSH: Anopheles] a large genus of mosquitoes of the tribe Anophelini, subfamily Anophelinae, characterized by long slender palpi, nearly as long as the proboscis, and by holding the body at an angle with the surface on which it rests while the head and proboscis are in line with the body. Many species are vectors of malaria, and some are vectors of *Wuchereria bancrofti.* It has been subdivided into several subgenera, including *Cellia, Kerteszia, Nyssorhynchus,* and one called *Anopheles.* 1. a subgenus of genus *Anopheles.*

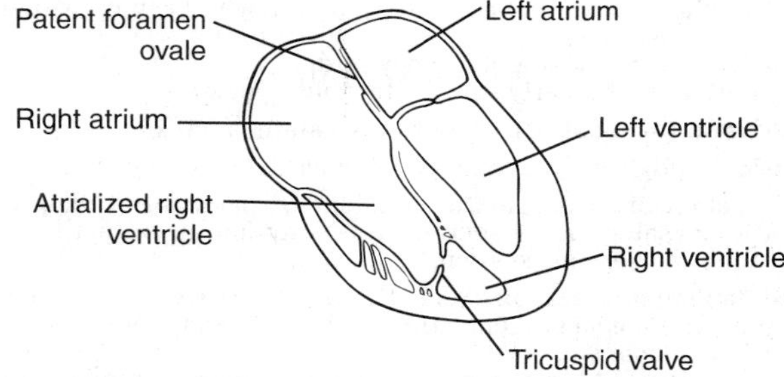

Ebstein's anomaly, showing displacement of the septal and posterior leaflets of the tricuspid valve into the right ventricle and accompanied by a patent foramen ovale.

The $\alpha$- and $\beta$- anomers of glucose: *(A)* $\alpha$-D-glucopyranose; *(B)* $\beta$-D-glycopyranose. The hydroxyl group of interest is indicated by the arrows.

**anoph·e·li·cide** (ə-nof'ə-lĭ-sīd) [*anopheles* + *-cide*] destructive to anopheline mosquitoes.

**anoph·e·li·fuge** (ə-nof'ə-lĭ-fūj) [*anopheles* + *-fuge*] preventing the bite or attack of anopheline mosquitoes.

**anoph·e·line** (ə-nof'ə-lēn) pertaining to or caused by mosquitoes of the tribe Anophelini.

**Anoph·e·li·nae** (ə-nof″ə-li'ne) a subfamily of mosquitoes of the family Culicidae. It includes one tribe, Anophelini, which contains the genera *Anopheles* and *Chagasia.*

**Anoph·e·li·ni** a tribe of mosquitoes of the subfamily Anophelinae; genera of medical interest include *Anopheles* and *Chagasia.*

**anoph·e·lism** (ə-nof'ə-liz-əm) infestation of a district with anopheline mosquitoes.

**Malaria-Carrying Anopheles Species**

| Malaria-Carrying Anopheles Species |
|---|
| Subgenus *Anopheles* |
| *A. (A.) anthropophagus* |
| *A. (A.) atroparvus* |
| *A. (A.) aztecus* |
| *A. (A.) bancroftii* |
| *A. (A.) campestris* |
| *A. (A.) claviger* |
| *A. (A.) donaldi* |
| *A. (A.) freeborni* |
| *A. (A.) labranchiae* |
| *A. (A.) letifer* |
| *A. (A.) messeae* |
| *A. (A.) nigerrimus* |
| *A. (A.) pseudopunctipennis* |
| *A. (A.) punctimacula* |
| *A. (A.) quadrimaculatus* |
| *A. (A.) sacharovi* |
| *A. (A.) sinensis* |
| *A. (A.) whartoni* |
| Subgenus *Cellia* |
| *A. (C.) aconitus* |
| *A. (C.) annularis* |
| *A. (C.) arabiensis* |
| *A. (C.) balabacensis* |
| *A. (C.) culicifacies* |
| *A. (C.) dirus* |
| *A. (C.) farauti* |
| *A. (C.) flavirostris* |
| *A. (C.) fluviatilis* |
| *A. (C.) funestus* |
| *A. (C.) gambiae* |
| *A. (C.) hilli* |
| *A. (C.) karwari* |
| *A. (C.) koliensis* |
| *A. (C.) leucosphyrus* |
| *A. (C.) ludlowae* |
| *A. (C.) maculatus* |
| *A. (C.) melas* |
| *A. (C.) merus* |
| *A. (C.) minimus* |
| *A. (C.) moucheti* |
| *A. (C.) multicolor* |
| *A. (C.) nili* |
| *A. (C.) pattoni* |
| *A. (C.) pharoensis* |
| *A. (C.) philippinensis* |
| *A. (C.) pulcherrimus* |
| *A. (C.) punctulatus* |
| *A. (C.) sergentii* |
| *A. (C.) stephensi* |
| *A. (C.) subpictus* |
| *A. (C.) sundaicus* |
| *A. (C.) superpictus* |
| *A. (C.) tessellatus* |
| Subgenus *Nyssorhynchus* |
| *A. (N.) albimanus* |
| *A. (N.) albitarsis* |
| *A. (N.) aquasalis* |
| *A. (N.) argyritarsis* |
| *A. (N.) darlingi* |
| *A. (N.) nuneztovari* |
| *A. (N.) triannulatus* |
| Subgenus *Kerteszia* |
| *A. (K.) bellator* |
| *A. (K.) cruzii* |

**an·o·pho·ria** (an-o-for'e-ə) [Gr. *anō* upward + Gr. *pherein* to bear] hyperphoria.

**an·oph·thal·mia** (an″of-thal'me-ə) [*an-*[1] + *ophthalm-* + *-ia*] a developmental defect characterized by complete absence of the eyes (rare) or by the presence of vestigial eyes.

**an·oph·thal·mos** (an″of-thal'mos) [MeSH: Anophthalmos] anophthalmia.

**ano·plas·ty** (a'no-plas″te) [*anus* + *-plasty*] a plastic or restorative operation on the anus.

**An·op·lo·ceph·a·la** (an″op-lo-sef'ə-lə) [Gr. *anoplos* unarmed + Gr. *kephalē* head] a genus of tapeworms of the family Anoplocephalidae, found in horses.

**An·op·lo·ce·phal·i·dae** (an″op-lo-sə-fal'ĭ-de) a family of medium-sized or large tapeworms of the order Cyclophyllidea, subclass Cestoda, commonly parasitic in various herbivorous animals and man. Genera of medical and veterinary importance are *Anoplocephala, Bertiella, Moniezia, Paranoplocephala,* and *Thysanosoma.*

**An·o·plu·ra** (an″o-ploo'rə) [Gr. *anoplos* unarmed + *oura* tail] [MeSH: Anoplura] an order of insects, the sucking lice, characterized by claws and sucking mouth parts; genera of medical or veterinary interest include *Haematopinus, Linognathus, Pediculus, Phthirus, Polyplax,* and *Solenopotes.*

**an·or·chia** (an-or'ke-ə) anorchism.

**an·or·chid** (an-or'kid) [*an-*[1] + *orchis*] 1. a male who lacks testes. 2. a male whose testes are not in the scrotum.

**an·or·chid·ic** (an″or-kid'ik) 1. pertaining to or characterized by anorchism. 2. having no testes in the scrotum.

**an·or·chi·dism** (an-or'kĭ-diz″əm) anorchism.

**an·or·chism** (an-or'kiz-əm) congenital absence of the testis in a male; it may be either unilateral or bilateral. See also *hypogonadism* and *vanishing testes syndrome.* Called also *anorchia* and *anorchidism.*

**ano·rec·tal** (a″no-rek'təl) pertaining to the anus and rectum or to the junction region between the two.

**ano·rec·tic** (an″o-rek'tik) [Gr. *anorektos* without appetite for] 1. pertaining to anorexia; having no appetite. 2. a substance that diminishes the appetite. Called also *anoretic, anorexic, anorexiant,* and *anorexigenic.*

**ano·rec·ti·tis** (a″no-rek-ti'tĭs) inflammation of the anorectum.

**ano·rec·to·co·lon·ic** (a″no-rek″to-ko-lon'ik) pertaining to the anus, rectum, and colon.

**ano·rec·tum** (a″no-rek'təm) [*anus* + *rectum*] the anus and rectum considered together as a single unit.

**ano·ret·ic** (an″o-ret'ik) anorectic.

**an·orex·ia** (an″o-rek'se-ə) [Gr. "want of appetite"] [MeSH: Anorexia] lack or loss of the appetite for food.
**a. nervo'sa,** [DSM-IV], an eating disorder primarily affecting females, usually with onset in adolescence, characterized by refusal to maintain a normal minimal body weight, intense fear of gaining weight or becoming obese, and a disturbance of body image resulting in a feeling of being fat or having fat in certain areas even when extremely emaciated, undue reliance on body weight or shape for self-evaluation, and amenorrhea. Associated features often include denial of the illness and resistance to psychotherapy, depressive symptoms, markedly decreased libido, and obsessions or peculiar behavior regarding food, such as hoarding. The disorder is divided into two subtypes, a *restricting* type, in which weight loss is achieved primarily through diet or exercise, and a *binge-eating/purging* type, in which binge eating or purging behavior also occur regularly; the latter type resembles *bulimia nervosa*, which is not diagnosed in the presence of anorexia nervosa.

**ano·rex·i·ant** (an″o-rek'se-ənt) anorectic (def. 2).

**ano·rex·ic** (an″o-rek'sik) anorectic.

**ano·rex·i·gen·ic** (an″o-rek″sĭ-jen'ik) [*anorexia* + *-genic*] 1. producing anorexia, or diminishing the appetite. 2. anorectic (def. 2).

**an·or·gan·ic** (an″or-gan'ik) denoting tissue (e.g., bone) from which the organic material has been removed.

**an·or·gas·mia** (an″or-gaz'me-ə) anorgasmy.

**an·or·gas·my** (an-or-gaz'me) [*an-*[1] + *orgasm*] inability or failure to experience orgasm.

**an·or·thog·ra·phy** (an″or-thog'rə-fe) [*an-*[1] + *ortho-* + *-graphy*] agraphia.

**an·or·tho·pia** (an″or-tho'pe-ə) [*an-*[1] + *ortho-* + *-opia*] 1. distorted vision in which straight lines appear as curves or angles, and symmetry is incorrectly perceived. 2. strabismus.

**an·or·tho·scope** (an-or'thə-skōp″) [*an-*[1] + *ortho* + *-scope*] an instrument for combining two disconnected pictures in one perfect visual image.

**ano·scope** (a'nə-skōp) [*anus* + *-scope*] a speculum for examining the anus and lower rectum.

**anos·co·py** (a-nos'kə-pe) examination of the anus and lower rectum by means of an anoscope.

**ano·sig·moi·do·scop·ic** (a″no-sig-moi″do-skop'ik) pertaining to anosigmoidoscopy.

**ano·sig·moi·dos·co·py** (a″no-sig″moi-dos'kə-pe) [*anus* + *sigmoid* + *-scopy*] endoscopic examination of the anus, rectum, and sigmoid colon.

**an·os·mat·ic** (an″oz-mat'ik) [*an-* + *osmastic*] anosmic.

**an·os·mia** (an-oz'me-ə) [*an-*[1] + *osm-*[1] + *-ia*] [MeSH: Anosmia] absence of the sense of smell; called also *anosphresia* and *olfactory anesthesia.*
**a. gustato'ria,** the loss of the power to smell foods.
**preferential a.,** lack of ability to sense certain odors only.
**a. respirato'ria,** loss of smell due to nasal obstruction.

**an·os·mic** (an-oz'mik) pertaining to or characterized by anosmia; called also *anosmatic.*

**ano·sog·no·sia** (an-o″so-no'zhə) [*a-*[1] + *noso-* + *gnosia*] unawareness or denial of a neurological deficit such as hemiplegia; see also *Anton's syndrome,* under *syndrome,* and *asomatognosia.*

**an·os·phre·sia** (an″os-fre'zhə) [*an-*[1] + *osphresi-* + *-ia*] anosmia.

**ano·spi·nal** (a″no-spi'nəl) pertaining to the anus and the spinal cord.

**an·os·teo·pla·sia** (an-os″te-o-pla'zhə) [*an-*[1] + *osteo-* + *-plasia*] defective bone formation.

**an·os·to·sis** (an″os-to'sis) [*an-*[1] + *osteo-* + *-osis*] defective development of bone.

**an·otia** (an-o'shə) [*an-*[1] + *ot-* + *-ia*] congenital absence of the external ear(s).

**ano·tro·pia** (an″o-tro'pe-ə) [*ano-* + *trepein* to turn] a condition in which the visual axes tend to rise above the object looked at.

**an·otus** (an-o'təs) [*an-*[1] + *ot-* + *-ous*] an earless fetus.

**ANOVA** analysis of variance.

**ano·vag·i·nal** (a″no-vaj'ĭ-nəl) pertaining to the anus and vagina, or communicating with the anal canal and vagina, as an anovaginal fistula.

**an·ova·ria** (an″o-var'e-ə) anovarism.

**an·ovar·i·an·ism** (an″o-var'e-ən-iz-əm) anovarism.

**an·ovar·ism** (an-o'vər-iz-əm) [*an-*[1] + *ovary*] absence of the ovaries; see also *hypogonadism* and *Turner's syndrome.* Called also *anovarianism.*

**ano·ves·i·cal** (a″no-ves'ĭ-kəl) [L. *anus* fundament + *vesica*] pertaining to the anus and urinary bladder.

**an·ov·u·lar** (an-ov'u-lər) not accompanied with the discharge of an ovum.

**an·ov·u·la·tion** (an″ov-u-la'shən) [MeSH: Anovulation] absence of ovulation.

**an·ov·u·la·to·ry** (an-ov'u-lə-to″re) anovular.

**an·ov·u·lo·men·or·rhea** (an-ov″u-lo-men″o-re'ə) anovular menstruation.

**anox·ia** (ə-nok'se-ə) [MeSH: Anoxia] a total lack of oxygen; often used interchangeably with *hypoxia* to mean a reduced supply of oxygen to the tissues.
**altitude a.,** see under *sickness.*
**anemic a.,** anoxia resulting from a decrease in amount of hemoglobin or number of erythrocytes in the blood. Cf. *anemic hypoxia.*
**anoxic a.,** anoxia resulting from interference with the source of oxygen. Cf. *hypoxic hypoxia.*
**histotoxic a.,** particularly severe histotoxic hypoxia.
**myocardial a.,** failure of coronary blood flow to keep up with myocardial needs.
**a. neonato'rum,** anoxia of the newborn.
**stagnant a.,** particularly severe stagnant hypoxia.

**anox·i·ate** (ə-nok'se-āt) to put into a state of anoxia.

**anox·ic** (ə-nok'sik) pertaining to or characterized by anoxia.

**ANS** 1. anterior nasal spine, a cephalometric landmark; the tip of the anterior nasal spine as seen on the x-ray film in norma lateralis. 2. autonomic nervous system.

**an·sa** (an'sə) gen. and pl. *an'sae* [L. "handle"] [TA] a general term used in anatomical nomenclature to designate a looplike structure; called also *loop.*
**a. cervica'lis** [TA], a nerve loop in the neck that supplies the infrahyoid muscles and that presents an anterior (superior) root, which connects with the hypoglossal nerve (and actually consists of fibers of the second or first cervical nerve), and an inferior root

(nervus descendens cervicalis), which connects with the second and third cervical nerves. Called also *a. hypoglossi* and *loop of hypoglossal nerve.*
**a. lenticula'ris** [TA], a small fiber tract arising in the globus pallidus of the lenticular nucleus and extending around the medial border of the internal capsule to join and mingle with the fibers of the fasciculus lenticularis, some of which synapse with cells in the subthalamic nucleus, nucleus of the prerubral field (field H of Forel), and the zona incerta, and others of which continue to the ventral nuclei of the thalamus.
**a. nephro'ni,** a long, U-shaped part of the renal tubule, extending through the medulla from the end of the proximal convoluted tubule to the beginning of the distal convoluted tubule. It begins with a *descending limb* having a thick-walled segment called the *proximal straight tubule,* followed by a thin-walled segment called the *thin* or *attenuated tubule;* this is followed by the *ascending limb,* which sometimes includes the distal end of the attenuated tubule and always ends with a long thick-walled segment called the *distal straight tubule.* The loops vary in the lengths of their segments according to their locations in the kidney. Called also *loop of Henle.*
**an'sae nervo'rum spina'lium,** loops of spinal nerves: loops of nerve fibers joining the ventral roots of the spinal nerves.
**a. peduncula'ris** [TA], peduncular loop: a complex grouping of fibers connecting the amygdaloid nucleus, the piriform area, and the anterior part of the hypothalamus, and various thalamic nuclei. The fiber bundles pass below the internal capsule, a principal bundle being the inferior peduncle of the thalamus.
**a. subcla'via** [TA], subclavian loop: nerve filaments that pass anterior and posterior to the subclavian artery to form a loop interconnecting the middle and inferior cervical ganglia; called also *a. of Vieussens* and *annulus of Vieussens.*
**a. of Vieussens,** a. subclavia.
**a. vitelli'na,** an embryonic vein from the yolk sac to the umbilical vein.

**an·sae** (an'se) [L.] genitive and plural of *ansa.*

**An·said** (an'sād) trademark for a preparation of flurbiprofen.

**an·sate** (an'sāt) [L. *ansatus,* from *ansa* handle] having a handle; loop-shaped.

**Ans·bach·er unit** (ahns'bahk-ər) [Stefan *Ansbacher,* German-American biologist, born 1905] see under *unit.*

**an·ser·ine** [L. *anser* goose] [MeSH: Anserine] 1. (an'sər-īn) pertaining to or like a goose. 2. (an'sər-ēn) a dipeptide related to carnosine, composed of *β*-alanine and methylated histidine; it was first identified in goose muscle and occurs in the skeletal muscle of birds and some mammals, excluding humans.

**an·se·ri·nus** (an"sə-ri'nəs) [L.] anserine, def. 1.

**an·si·form** (an'sĭ-form) loop-shaped.

**An·so·ly·sen** (an"so-li'sən) trademark for preparations of pentolinium tartrate.

**An·spor** (an'spor) trademark for a preparation of cephradine.

**AN-Sul·fur Col·loid** trademark for a kit or the preparation of technetium Tc 99m sulfur colloid.

**ant.** anterior.

**ant-** see *anti-.*

**ant** (ant) [MeSH: Ants] any of several crawling insects of the family Formicoidae. See *Formica* and *Solenopsis.*
**fire a.,** 1. any ant of the genus *Solenopsis.* 2. any ant with a fierce sting.

**An·ta·buse** (an'tə-būs") trademark for a preparation of disulfiram.

**ant·ac·id** (ant-as'id) [*ant-* + *acid*] 1. counteracting acidity. 2. a substance that counteracts or neutralizes acidity, usually of the stomach.

**an·tag·o·nism** (an-tag'ə-niz"əm) [Gr. *antagōnisma* struggle] opposition or contrariety between similar things, as between muscles, medicines, or organisms; cf. *antibiosis.*
**bacterial a.,** the antagonistic (inhibiting) effect of one bacterial organism on another by reason of its production of an antibiotic (antibiosis) or by its superior competitive ability to absorb nutrients.
**metabolic a.,** interference with the metabolism or function of a given chemical compound by another bearing a close structural resemblance, the similarity in structure being the basis of the interference. For the various forms of such interference, see under *inhibition.*
**salt a.,** the antagonistic action of different salts in maintaining normal permeability of the plasma membrane.

**an·tag·o·nist** (an-tag'ə-nist) [Gr. *antagōnistēs* an opponent] 1. a muscle whose action is the direct opposite of that of another muscle. 2. a substance that tends to nullify the action of another, as a drug that binds to a cell receptor without eliciting a biological response, blocking binding of substances that could elicit such responses. 3. a tooth in one jaw that articulates with a tooth in the other jaw.
**aldosterone a.,** a compound that blocks the action of aldosterone. A class of potassium-sparing diuretics, typified by spironolactone, competes with aldosterone for receptor sites, thus blocking the aldosterone-dependent exchange of sodium and potassium in the distal tubule.
***α*-adrenergic a.,** *α*-blocker.
***β*-adrenergic a.,** *β*-blocker.
**competitive a.,** a substance that competes with a substrate or with an enzyme which ordinarily attacks the substrate, thus interfering with usual metabolic activity. The antagonist is usually a substrate analogue. See *antimetabolite.*
**enzyme a.,** an antimetabolite that interferes with the normal action of an enzyme. See *enzyme inhibition,* under *inhibition.*
**folic acid a.,** an antimetabolite of folic acid; those used as chemotherapeutic agents are competitive inhibitors of dihydrofolate reductase: trimethoprim is used as an antibacterial, pyrimethamine as an antimalarial, and methotrexate as an antineoplastic. Called also *antifol* and *antifolate.*
**$H_1$ receptor a.,** any of a large number of agents that block the action of histamine by competitive binding to the $H_1$ receptor. Such agents also have sedative, anticholinergic, and antiemetic effects, the exact effect varying from drug to drug, and are used for the relief of allergic symptoms and as antiemetics, antivertigo agents, sedatives, and antidyskinetics in parkinsonism.
**$H_2$ receptor a.,** an agent that blocks the action of histamine by competitive binding to the $H_2$ receptor; used to inhibit gastric secretion in the treatment of peptic ulcer.
**insulin a's,** hormones, antibodies, and other factors that block the action of insulin, such as epinephrine, somatotropin, glucocorticoids, and glucagon.
**metabolic a.,** an antimetabolite that interferes with the utilization of a substance essential in metabolism.
**narcotic a.,** an agent that opposes the action of narcotics on the nervous system.
**sulfonamide a.,** *p*-aminobenzoic acid.

**ant·al·gic** (ant-al'jik) analgesic.

**ant·al·ka·line** (ant-al'kə-līn") [*ant-* + *alkali*] 1. neutralizing alkalinity. 2. an agent that neutralizes alkalis.

**ant·aph·ro·di·si·ac** (ant"af-ro-diz'e-ak) 1. abrogating the sexual instinct. 2. an agent that allays sexual impulses; called also *anterotic.*

**ant·ap·o·plec·tic** (ant"ap-o-plek'tik) [*ant-* + *apoplectic*] an agent for alleviating stroke.

**ant·arth·rit·ic** (ant"ahr-thrit'ik) [*ant-* + *arthritic*] 1. alleviating arthritis. 2. an agent that alleviates arthritis.

**ant·as·then·ic** (ant"as-then'ik) [*ant-* + *asthenic*] 1. alleviating weakness, or restoring strength. 2. an agent that alleviates weakness and restores strength.

**ant·asth·mat·ic** (ant"az-mat'ik) [*ant-* + *asthmatic*] 1. affording relief in asthma. 2. an agent that relieves the spasm of asthma.

**ant·atroph·ic** (ant"ə-trof'ik) correcting or opposing the progress of atrophy.

**an·taz·o·line** (an-taz'o-lēn) [MeSH: Antazoline] an ethylenediamine derivative used as an antihistaminic.
**a. hydrochloride,** the hydrochloride salt of antazoline, used to relieve allergic symptoms and to treat allergic manifestations; administered orally.
**a. phosphate** [USP], the phosphate salt of antazoline, used in a 0.5 per cent solution, applied topically to the eyes in the treatment of allergic conjunctivitis.

**ante-** [L. *ante* before] a prefix meaning prior to or in front of.

**an·te·bra·chi·um** (an"te-bra'ke-əm) [*ante-* + L. *brachium* arm] [TA]

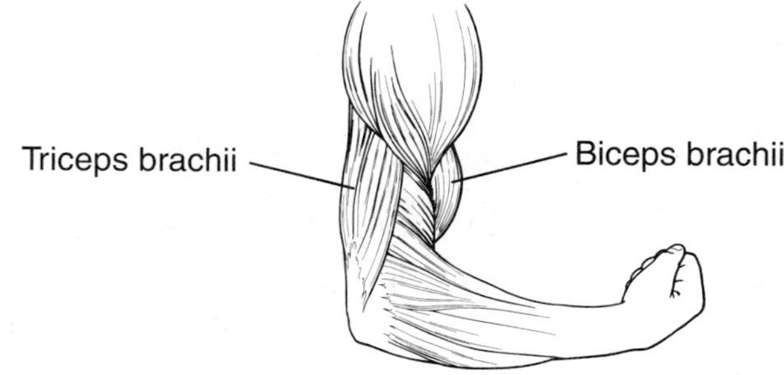


Antagonist. The triceps brachii extends the forearm at the elbow while the biceps brachii, its antagonist, flexes the elbow.

the part of the upper limb of the body between the elbow and the wrist; called also *forearm.*

**an·te·car·di·um** (an″te-kahr′de-əm) [*ante-* + Gr. *kardia* heart] epigastrium.

**an·te·ce·dent** (an″te-se′dənt) [L. *antecedere* to go before, precede] a precursor.
**plasma thromboplastin a. (PTA),** factor XI; see under *coagulation factors,* at *factor.*

**an·te ci·bum** (an′te si′bəm) [L.] before meals, usually abbreviated *a.c.* in prescriptions, etc.

**an·te·cu·bi·tal** (an″te-ku′bĭ-təl) situated anterior to the cubitus, or elbow.

**an·te·cur·va·ture** (an″te-kər′və-chər) [*ante-* + *curvature*] a slight anteflexion.

**an·te·flect** (an′te-flekt) to bend anteriorly.

**an·te·flexed** (an′te-flekst) in a condition of anteflexion.

**an·te·flex·ion** (an-te-flek′shən) [*ante-* + *flexion*] forward curvature of an organ or part, so that its top is turned anteriorly; particularly, the normal forward curvature of the uterus.

**an·te·grade** (an′te-grād) anterograde.

**an·te·lo·ca·tion** (an″te-lo-ka′shən) [*ante-* + L. *locatio* placement] the forward displacement of an organ.

**an·te mor·tem** (an′te mor′təm) [L.] before death.

**an·te·mor·tem** (an″te-mor′tem) [L.] occurring before death.

**an·te·na·tal** (an″te-na′təl) [*ante-* + *natal*] prenatal.

**an·ten·na** (an-ten′ə) pl. *anten′nae.* a feeler of an arthropod; one of the two lateral appendages on the anterior segment of the head of arthropods.

**An·te·par** (an′te-par) trademark for a preparation of piperazine citrate and piperazine phosphate.

**an·te·par·tal** (an″te-pahr′təl) antepartum.

**an·te·par·tum** (an″te-pahr′təm) [L.] occurring before parturition, or childbirth, with reference to the mother. Cf. *prenatal.* Spelled also *ante partum.* Called also *antepartal* and *prepartal.*

**an·te·phase** (an′te-fāz) the portion of interphase immediately preceding mitosis (or meiosis) when energy is being produced and stored for mitosis (or meiosis) and chromosome reproduction is taking place.

**ant·ephi·al·tic** (ant″ef-e-al′tik) [*ant-* + Gr. *ephialtēs* nightmare] alleviating or preventing nightmare.

**an·te·po·si·tion** (an″te-pə-zish′ən) forward displacement, as of the uterus.

**an·te·pros·tate** (an″te-pros′tāt) [*ante-* + *prostate*] glandula bulbourethralis.

**an·te·pros·ta·ti·tis** (an″te-pros-tə-ti′tis) inflammation of glandula bulbourethralis.

**an·te·py·ret·ic** (an″te-pi-ret′ik) [*ante-* + *pyretic*] occurring before the stage of fever.

**an·te·ri·ad** (an-tēr′e-ad) toward the anterior surface of the body.

**an·te·ri·or** (an-tēr′e-ər) [L. "before"; neut. *anterius*] 1. situated in front of or in the forward part of an organ. 2. [TA] in humans and other bipeds, toward the belly surface of the body; called also *ventral.* 3. in quadruped anatomy, a term sometimes used as a synonym for *cranial.*

**antero-** [L. *anterior* before] a prefix signifying before.

**an·tero·clu·sion** (an″tər-o-kloo′zhən) mesioclusion.

**an·tero·ex·ter·nal** (an″tər-o-eks-ter′nəl) anterolateral.

**an·tero·grade** (an′tər-o-grād″) [*antero-* + L. *gredi* to go] moving or extending anteriorly; called also *antegrade.*

**an·tero·in·fe·ri·or** (an″tər-o-in-fēr′e-ər) situated anteriorly and inferiorly.

**an·tero·in·ter·nal** (an″tər-o-in-ter′nəl) anteromedial.

**an·tero·lat·er·al** (an″tər-o-lat′ər-əl) situated anteriorly and to one side; preferred to *anteroexternal.*

**an·tero·me·di·al** (an″tər-o-me′de-əl) situated anteriorly and to the medial side; preferred to *anterointernal.*

**an·tero·me·di·an** (an″tər-o-me′de-ən) situated anteriorly and toward the median plane.

**an·tero·pos·te·ri·or** (an″tər-o-pos-tēr′e-ər) from front to back of the body, such as the direction of a radiographic projection.

**an·tero·sep·tal** (an″tər-o-sep′təl) situated in front of a septum, particularly the atrioventricular septum.

**an·tero·su·pe·ri·or** (an″tər-o-soo-pēr′e-ər) situated anteriorly and superiorly.

**ant·erot·ic** (ant″ə-rot′ik) antaphrodisiac.

**an·tero·ven·tral** (an″tər-o-ven′trəl) situated anteriorly and toward the ventral surface.

**an·te·ver·sion** (an″te-vər′zhən) [*ante-* + *version*] the forward tipping or tilting of an organ; displacement in which the entire organ or part is tipped forward, but is not bent at an angle (cf. *anteflexion*); particularly, the normal tipping forward of the entire uterus relative to the pelvic axis.

**ant·he·lix** (ant′he-liks) [*ant-* + Gr. *helix* coil] antihelix.

**ant·hel·min·thic** (ant″həl-min′thik) anthelmintic.

**ant·hel·min·tic** (ant″həl-min′tik) [*ant-* + Gr. *helmins* worm] 1. destructive to parasitic worms; called also *anthelminthic, vermicidal,* and *vermifugal.* 2. an agent that is destructive to parasitic worms. Called also *helminthagogue, helminthicide, vermicide,* and *vermifuge.*

**an·thel·my·cin** (an-thəl-mi′sin) an antibiotic substance produced by *Streptomyces longissimus,* which has anthelmintic activity.

**an·the·lot·ic** (ant″he-lot′ik) [*ant-* +Gr. *hēlos* nail] 1. effective against corns. 2. a remedy for corns.

**An·the·mis** (an′thə-mis) [L.; Gr. *anthemis*] a genus of composite-flowered plants (family Compositae). *A. cotu′la,* or mayweed, is a contact allergen that has been associated with severe contact dermatitis with bullous lesions; it also contains cyanogenetic compounds that can cause cyanide poisoning in livestock. *A. no′bilis* is one of two plants called chamomile, whose flowering tops are used medicinally.

**ant·hem·or·rhag·ic** (ant″hem-ə-raj′ik) [*ant-* + *hemorrhage*] antihemorrhagic.

**an·ther** (an′thər) [Gr. *anthēros* blooming] the portion of the stamen of flowering plants containing the microsporangia (pollen sacs) in which haploid microspores (pollen grains) are formed.

**an·ther·id·i·um** (an″thər-id′e-um) pl. *antherid′ia* [*anther-* +Gr. *idion* a diminutive ending] male organ of a cryptogamic plant or fungus in which microgametes are produced. Cf. *archegonium.*

**an·thero·zoid** (an′thər-o-zoid″) the motile fertilizing cell of certain fungi.

**ant·her·pet·ic** (ant″hər-pet′ik) curing or preventing herpes.

**An·tho·my·ia** (an″tho-mi′yə) a genus of small black houseflies. Two species of medical importance were formerly assigned to this genus; see *Fannia canicularis* and *F. scalaris.*

**An·tho·my·ii·dae** (an″tho-mi′ə-de) [Gr. *anthos* flower + *myia* fly] in some systems of classification, a family of the order Diptera; the only genus of medical importance is *Fannia.*

**An·tho·xan·thum** (an″tho-zan′thəm) a genus of grasses (family Gramineae). *A. odora′tum* is sweet vernal grass, whose pollen causes hay fever.

**An·thox·i·um** (an-thok′se-um) a genus of grasses. *A. odora′tum* is

Rectum
Uterus
Bladder
Vagina

Anteflexion of uterus.

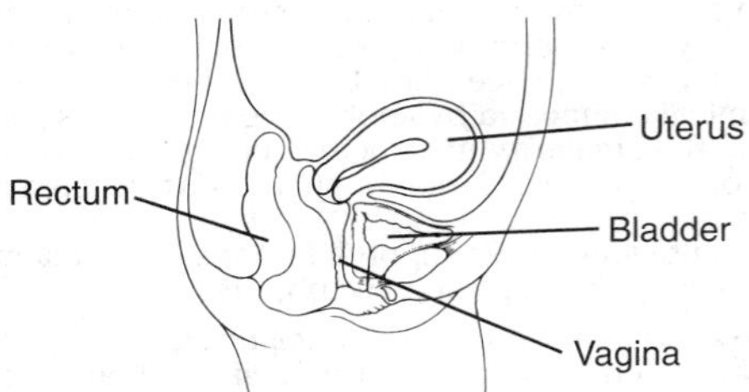


Anteversion of uterus.

sweet vernal grass, a species used as fodder for horses and cattle in the British Isles; since it contains dicumarol, animals consuming excessive amounts of it can suffer fatal hemorrhaging. It causes hay fever in susceptible humans.

**An·tho·zoa** (an″tho-zo′ə) [Gr. *anthos* flower + *zoia* animal] a class of coelenterates with large polyps and no medusa stage; it includes corals.

**an·thra·cene** (an′thrə-sēn) a colorless crystalline hydrocarbon derived from coal tar and used in the manufacture of anthracene dyes.

**an·thra·cene·di·one** (an″thrə-sēn-di′ōn) any of a class of derivatives of anthraquinone; some have antineoplastic properties. Cf. *mitoxantrone hydrochloride.*

**an·thrac·ic** (an-thras′ik) pertaining to or resembling anthrax.

**anthrac(o)-** [Gr. *anthrax* charcoal, carbuncle] a combining form denoting relationship to coal or carbon, or to a carbuncle.

**an·thra·coid** (an′thrə-koid) [*anthrac-* + *-oid*] resembling anthrax or a carbuncle.

**an·thra·com·e·ter** (an″thrə-kom′ə-tər) [*anthraco-* + *-meter*] an instrument for measuring the carbon dioxide of the air.

**an·thra·co·ne·cro·sis** (an″thrə-ko-nə-kro′sis) [*anthraco-* + *necrosis*] necrotic transformation of a tissue into a black dry mass.

**an·thra·co·sil·i·co·sis** (an″thrə-ko-sil″ĭ-ko′sis) [*anthraco-* + *silicon*] [MeSH: Anthracosilicosis] a type of mixed dust pneumoconiosis consisting of both anthracosis and silicosis, caused by coal with a high silica content. Called also *silicoanthracosis.*

**an·thra·co·sis** (an-thrə-ko′sis) [*anthraco-* + *-osis*] a usually asymptomatic form of pneumoconiosis caused by deposition of anthracite coal dust in the lungs. When the dust accumulates in large amounts, it may result in coal workers' pneumoconiosis.
**a. lin′guae,** black tongue.

**an·thra·co·ther·a·py** (an″thrə-ko-ther′ə-pe) [*anthraco-* + *therapy*] treatment with charcoal.

**an·thra·cot·ic** (an″thrə-kot′ik) pertaining to or affected with anthracosis.

**an·thra·cy·cline** (an″thrə-si′klēn) any of a class of antineoplastic antibiotics, including daunorubicin and doxorubicin, produced by *Streptomyces peucetius* or *S. coeruleorubidus* and having a four-ring system to which a daunosamine molecule is attached by glycoside linkage (see illustration). Although the precise mechanism of action is unknown, anthracyclines can damage DNA by intercalation, metal ion chelation, and the generation of free radicals and can inhibit enzyme activity critical to DNA function. The use of these drugs is limited by dose-related cardiotoxicity.

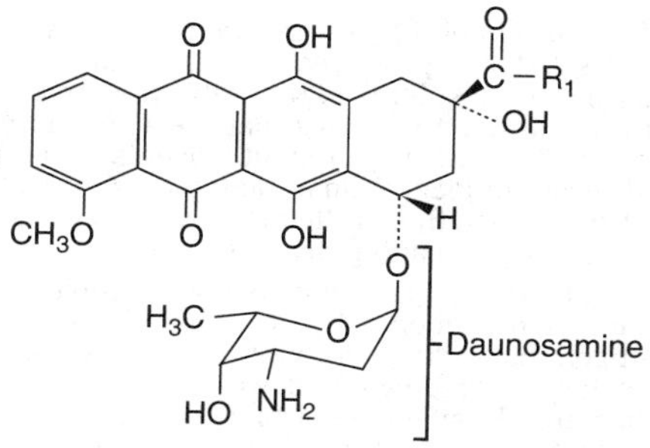

Anthracycline. For daunorubicin, $R_1$ = —$CH_3$; for doxorubicin, $R_1$ = —CHOH.

**An·thra-Derm** (an′thrə-dərm) trademark for a preparation of anthralin.

**an·thra·lin** (an′thrə-lin) [USP] [MeSH: Anthralin] an anthraquinone derivative that reduces DNA synthesis and mitotic activity in hyperplastic epidermis, restoring the normal rate of epidermal cell proliferation and keratinization; used topically in the treatment of psoriasis. Called also *dithranol.*

**an·thra·nil·ate** (an″thrə-nil′āt) a salt, anion, or ester of anthranilic acid.

**an·thra·nil·ic ac·id** (an″thrə-nil′ik) a cyclic aromatic compound, the *ortho* form of aminobenzoic acid; it is a product of tryptophan catabolism.

**an·thra·quin·one** (an″thrə-kwin′ōn) 1. the 9, 10 quinone derivative of anthracene, used in dye manufacture. 2. more commonly, any of the usually highly colored derivatives, yellow, orange, red, red-brown, or violet, of this compound, some of which are used as dyes. Anthraquinones occur in aloe, cascara sagrada, senna, and rhubarb, and have cathartic properties. The antineoplastic mitoxantrone is a synthetic derivative.

**an·thra·ro·bin** (an″thrə-ro′bin) [*anthracene* + *araroba*] a derivative of alizarin used to treat psoriasis and various skin diseases in 10 to 20 per cent ointment, and as a parasiticide.

**an·thrax** (an′thraks) [Gr. "coal," "carbuncle"] [MeSH: Anthrax] an infectious bacterial zoonotic disease usually acquired by ingestion of *Bacillus anthracis* or its spores from infected pastures by herbivores or indirectly from infected carcasses by carnivores. It is transmitted to humans usually by contact with infected animals or their discharges *(agricultural a.)* or with contaminated animal products *(industrial a.).* Anthrax is classified by primary routes of inoculation as *cutaneous, gastrointestinal,* or *inhalational.*
**agricultural a.,** see *anthrax.*
**cerebral a.,** meningeal a.
**cutaneous a.,** the most common type of anthrax in humans, due to inoculation of *Bacillus anthracis* into superficial wounds or abrasions. It occurs in two forms manifested by: (1) a small, painless, pruritic papular lesion (which has been called malignant carbuncle or pustule even though no liquefactive necrosis or pus formation occurs) at the site of inoculation, often with one or more satellite lesions, that enlarges, ulcerates, and becomes crusted with an adherent dense black eschar, which often heals spontaneously, but may progress to a systemic condition and may involve the meninges; and (2) bullae at the site of inoculation that break down to form a necrotic eschar surrounded by massive spreading edema *(malignant edema)* associated with induration, high fever, and severe toxemia.
**gastrointestinal a.,** anthrax due to ingestion of poorly cooked meat contaminated with *Bacillus anthracis,* with deposition of spores in the submucosa of the intestinal tract, where they germinate, multiply, and produce toxin, resulting in massive edema that may obstruct the bowel, with hemorrhage and necrosis. Called also *intestinal a.*
**industrial a.,** see *anthrax.*
**inhalational a.,** a highly fatal form of anthrax due to inhalation of dust containing anthrax spores, which are transported by the alveolar pneumocytes to the regional lymph nodes, where they germinate, multiply, and produce toxin, and characterized by hemorrhagic edematous mediastinitis, pleural effusions, dyspnea, cyanosis, stridor, and shock. It is usually an occupational disease, most often affecting those who handle and sort contaminated wools and fleeces. Called also *pulmonary a.; ragpicker's, ragsorter's,* or *woolsorter's disease; anthrax pneumonia;* and *woolsorter's pneumonia.*
**intestinal a.,** gastrointestinal a.
**malignant a.,** anthrax.
**meningeal a.,** a rare, highly fatal form of anthrax resembling typical hemorrhagic meningitis due to hematogenous spread of the anthrax bacillus from a primary focus of infection, and manifested by hemorrhagic cerebrospinal fluid and accompanying neurological signs and symptoms. Called also *cerebral a.*
**pulmonary a.,** inhalational a.
**symptomatic a.,** blackleg.

**anthrop(o)-** [Gr. *anthrōpos* man, human being] a combining form denoting a relationship to man, or to a human being.

**an·thro·po·bi·ol·o·gy** (an″thrə-po-bi-ol′ə-je) the biological study of human beings and the anthropoid apes.

**an·thro·po·cen·tric** (an″thrə-po-sen′trik) [*anthropo-* + *centric*] with a human bias; considering humans the center of the universe.

**an·thro·pog·e·ny** (an″thrə-poj′ə-ne) [*anthropo-* + *-geny*] the evolution and development of human beings.

**an·thro·pog·ra·phy** (an″thrə-pog′rə-fe) [*anthropo-* + *-graphy*] that branch of anthropology that deals with the distribution of the varieties of humans, as distinguished by factors such as physical character, institutions, or customs. Cf. *ethnography.*

**an·thro·poid** (an′thrə-poid) [*anthropo-* + *-oid*] [MeSH: Haplorhini] 1. resembling that of a man, as an anthropoid pelvis. 2. resembling a human being, as an anthropoid ape.

**An·thro·poi·dea** (an″thrə-poi′de-ə) a suborder of Primates characterized by well-developed brains and walking with an upright stance; it includes human beings (family Hominidae) and the anthropoid apes (family Pongidae). Cf. *Hominoidea.*

**an·thro·po·ki·net·ics** (an″thrə-po-kĭ-net′iks) [*anthropo-* + *kinetics*] the study of the total human being in action, with integrated applications from the special fields of the biological and physical sciences, psychology, and sociology.

**an·thro·pol·o·gy** (an″thrə-pol′ə-je) [*anthropo-* + *-ology*] [MeSH: Anthropology] the science that treats of humans, their origins, historical and cultural development, and races.
**criminal a.,** that branch of anthropology which treats of criminals and crimes.

**cultural a.,** that branch of anthropology which treats of humans in relation to their fellows and to their environment.
**physical a.,** that branch of anthropology which treats of the physical characteristics of humans.

**an·thro·pom·e·ter** (an″thrə-pom′ə-tər) an instrument especially designed for measuring various dimensions of the body.

**an·thro·po·met·ric** (an″thrə-po-met′rik) pertaining to or connected with anthropometry.

**an·thro·pom·e·trist** (an″thrə-pom′ə-trist) a person skilled in anthropometry.

**an·thro·pom·e·try** (an″thrə-pom′ə-tre) [*anthropo-* + *-metry*] [MeSH: Anthropometry] the science which deals with the measurement of the size, weight, and proportions of the human body.

**an·thro·po·mor·phism** (an″thrə-po-mor′fiz-əm) [*anthropo-* + *morph-* + *-ism*] the attribution of human form or character to nonhuman objects.

**an·thro·pon·o·my** (an″thrə-pon′ə-me) [*anthropo-* + Gr. *nomos* law] the science that deals with the laws of human development in relation to environment and to other organisms.

**an·thro·po·no·sis** (an″thrə-pə-no′sis) [*anthropo-* + Gr. *nosos* disease] a disease that is spread from humans to humans; said of diseases with some varieties that spread from animals to humans *(zoonoses)* and others that spread from humans to humans, particularly in reference to parasitic disease such as dry cutaneous leishmaniasis in which the disease can be spread from one human to another by an appropriate vector.

**an·thro·po·not·ic** (an″thrə-pə-not′ik) pertaining to or constituting an anthroponosis.

**an·thro·pop·a·thy** (an″thrə-pop′ə-the) [*anthropo-* + *-pathy*] the ascription of human emotions to nonhuman subjects.

**an·thro·po·phil·ic** (an″thrə-po-fil′ik) [*anthropo-* + *-philic*] preferring human beings to other animals, such as a mosquito or a dermatophyte. Cf. *anthropozoophilic* and *zoophilic.*

**an·thro·po·pho·bia** (an″thrə-po-fo′be-ə) [*anthropo-* + *-phobia*] irrational dread of human society.

**an·thro·pos·co·py** (an″thrə-pos′kə-pe) [*anthropo-* + *-scopy*] the judging of the type of body build by inspection rather than by anthropometry.

**an·thro·po·zoo·phil·ic** (an″thrə-po-zo″o-fil′ik) [*anthropo-* + *zoophilic*] attracted to both human beings and animals, such as certain mosquitoes and fungi. Cf. *anthropophilic* and *zoophilic.*

**ant·hys·ter·ic** (ant″his-ter′ik) antihysteric.

**anti-** [Gr. *anti* against] a prefix signifying counteracting, effective against, opposing, or opposite; sometimes shortened to *ant-.*

**an·ti·abor·ti·fa·cient** (an″te-ə-bor″tĭ-fa′shənt) an agent that prevents abortion or promotes successful gestation.

**an·ti·ad·re·ner·gic** (an″te-ad″-rə-nər′jik) 1. opposing the effects of impulses conveyed by adrenergic postganglionic fibers of the sympathetic nervous system. 2. an agent that so acts. Called also *sympatholytic.* Cf. *anticholinergic.*

**an·ti·ag·glu·ti·nin** (an″te-ə-gloo′tĭ-nin) a substance that opposes the action of an agglutinin.

**an·ti·al·bu·min** (an″te-al-bu′min) a precipitin for albumin.

**an·ti·ame·bic** (an″te-ə-me′bik) 1. destroying or suppressing the growth of amebas. 2. an agent that destroys or suppresses the growth of amebas.

**an·ti·ana·phy·lax·is** (an″te-an-ə-fə-lak′sis) a condition in which the anaphylaxis reaction is not obtained because of the presence of free antibodies in the blood; the state of desensitization to antigens.

**an·ti·an·dro·gen** (an″te-an′drə-jən) any substance capable of inhibiting the biological effects of androgens.

**an·ti·ane·mic** (an″te-ə-ne′mik) 1. counteracting or preventing anemia. 2. an agent that counteracts or prevents anemia.

**an·ti·an·gi·nal** (an″te-an-ji′nəl) 1. preventing or alleviating angina. 2. an agent that prevents or alleviates angina.

**an·ti·anoph·e·line** (an″te-ə-nof′ə-lēn) directed against anopheline mosquitoes or their larvae.

**an·ti·an·ti·body** (an″te-an′tĭ-bod″e) an antibody directed against antigenic determinants on other antibody (immunoglobulin) molecules.

**an·ti·an·ti·tox·in** (an″te-an″tĭ-tok′sin) an antibody, formed in immunization with an antitoxin, which counteracts the effect of the latter.

**an·ti·an·xi·e·ty** (an″te-ang-zi′ə-te) reducing anxiety. Called also *anxiolytic.*

**an·ti·ap·o·plec·tic** (an″te-ap″o-plek′tik) affording relief in or preventing stroke (apoplexy).

**an·ti·a·rin** (an-te′ə-rin) a poisonous principle from the upas tree, *Antiaris toxicaria;* formerly used as a heart depressant.

**An·ti·a·ris** (an″te-ă′rĭs) [Javanese *antiar*] a genus of plants of the family Moraceae, having fleshy fruit and milky juice. *A. toxica′ria* is the Bohun upas or upas tree, an Indonesian species that yields a latex used as an arrow poison. The major toxic principle is a digitalis-like cardioactive glycoside, $\alpha$-antiarin.

**an·ti·ar·rhyth·mic** (an″te-ə-rith′mik) 1. preventing or alleviating cardiac arrhythmia. 2. an agent that prevents or alleviates cardiac arrhythmia.

**an·ti·ar·thrit·ic** (an″te-ahr-thrit′ik) antarthritic.

**an·ti·asth·mat·ic** (an″te-az-mat′ik) antasthmatic.

**an·ti·ath·ero·gen·ic** (an″te-ath″ər-o-jen′ik) combating the formation of atheromatous lesions in arterial walls.

**an·ti·au·tol·y·sin** (an″te-aw-tol′ĭ-sin) a substance which opposes the action of autolysin.

**an·ti·bac·te·ri·al** (an″tĭ-bak-te′re-əl) 1. destroying or suppressing the growth or reproduction of bacteria. 2. a substance that destroys bacteria or suppresses their growth or reproduction.

**an·ti·bech·ic** (an″tĭ-bek′ik) antitussive.

**an·ti·bi·o·sis** (an″tĭ-bi-o′sis) [*anti-* + *biosis*] [MeSH: Antibiosis] an association between two organisms that is detrimental to one of them, or between one organism and an antibiotic produced by another.

**an·ti·bi·ot·ic** (an″tĭ-bi-ot′ik) [*anti-* + *biotic*] 1. destructive of life. 2. a chemical substance produced by a microorganism which has the capacity, in dilute solutions, to inhibit the growth of or to kill other microorganisms. Antibiotics that are sufficiently nontoxic to the host are used as chemotherapeutic agents in the treatment of infectious diseases of man, animals, and plants.
**broad-spectrum a.,** one that is effective against a wide range of bacteria, both gram-positive and gram-negative.

**an·ti·body** (an′tĭ-bod″e) an immunoglobulin molecule that has a specific amino acid sequence by virtue of which it interacts only with the antigen that induced its synthesis in cells of the lymphoid series (especially plasma cells), or with antigen closely related to it. Antibodies are classified according to their mode of action as agglutinins, bacteriolysins, hemolysins, opsonins, precipitins, etc. See *immunoglobulin.*

## Antibody

**acetylcholine receptor a's,** anti–acetylcholine receptor a's.
**anaphylactic a.,** IgE antibody causing anaphylaxis.
**anti–acetylcholine receptor (anti-AChR) a's,** circulating autoantibodies against the acetylcholine receptors of the myoneural junction. High titers are demonstrable in about 85 per cent of myasthenia gravis patients; false positives are rare. Called also *acetylcholine receptor a's.*
**anticardiolipin a.,** an antibody directed against cardiolipin, seen with increased frequency in systemic lupus erythematosus; its presence correlates with increased risk for thrombotic events.
**anti-D a.,** antibody directed against the "$Rh_0$" or "D" antigen of the Rh blood group.
**anti-DNA a.,** see *antinuclear a's.*
**antigliadin a's,** circulating IgA and IgG antibodies to gliadin occurring in the serum of patients with celiac disease; measurement of antigliadin antibodies is used in the diagnosis of celiac disease.
**anti–glomerular basement membrane (anti-GBM) a's,** see *anti–glomerular basement membrane antibody disease,* under *disease.*
**anti-idiotype a.,** antibody that binds selectively to a specific idiotope.
**anti-La a.,** anti–SS-B a.
**antimicrosomal a's,** organ-specific autoantibodies directed against a thyroid microsomal antigen, demonstrable in almost all patients with Hashimoto's thyroiditis.
**antimitochondrial a's,** circulating antibodies directed against inner

mitochondrial membrane antigens seen in almost all patients with primary biliary cirrhosis and rarely in other liver diseases. Called also *mitochondrial a's.*

**antineutrophil cytoplasmic a.,** see under *autoantibody.*

**antinuclear a's (ANA),** antibodies directed against nuclear antigens; ANA against a variety of different antigens are almost invariably found in systemic lupus erythematosus and are frequently found in rheumatoid arthritis, scleroderma (systemic sclerosis), Sjögren's syndrome, and mixed connective tissue disease. ANA may be detected by immunofluorescent staining. Serologic tests are also used to determine antibody titers against specific antigens.

**antiphospholipid a's,** a group of antibodies against phosphorylated polysaccharide esters of fatty acids, thought to be markers of a hypercoagulable state of the blood; included are anticardiolipin antibodies and lupus anticoagulant.

**antireceptor a's,** autoantibodies against cell-surface receptors, e.g., those directed against acetylcholine receptors in myasthenia gravis, against TSH receptors in Graves' disease, against insulin receptors in type B insulin resistance with acanthosis nigricans, and against $\beta_2$-adrenergic receptors in some patients with allergic disorders.

**anti-Ro a.,** anti–SS-A a.

**anti–SS-A a.,** an antinuclear antibody that occurs in Sjögren's syndrome and systemic lupus erythematosus. Called also *anti-Ro a.*

**anti–SS-B a.,** an antinuclear antibody that occurs in Sjögren's syndrome and systemic lupus erythematosus. Called also *anti-La a.*

**antithyroglobulin a's,** autoantibodies directed against thyroglobulin, demonstrable in about 50 to 75 per cent of patients with Hashimoto's thyroiditis and in about one-third of patients with other types of thyroiditis, Graves' disease, and thyroid carcinoma.

**antithyroid a's,** see *antimicrosomal a's* and *antithyroglobulin a's.*

**auto–anti-idiotypic a's,** autologous anti-idiotype antibodies that suppress the immune response in many experimental situations; auto–anti-idiotypic antibodies occur in certain autoimmune disorders.

**autologous a.,** self-derived antibody; autoantibody.

**bispecific a.,** antibody in which each of two antigen-binding sites is specific for separate antigenic determinants. It is an artificial antibody produced in the laboratory, formed by reassociating half molecules of two different antibody specificities to form a hybrid or bispecific antibody with antigen-binding sites of separate specificities. Called also *hybrid a.*

**blocking a.,** any antibody that by combining with an antigen blocks another immunologic reaction with the antigen. In most patients, immunotherapy (hyposensitization or desensitization) for allergic disorders induces IgG blocking antibodies that can bind the allergen and prevent it from binding to cell-fixed IgE, triggering immediate hypersensitivity; it can thus induce partial immunologic tolerance. Blocking antibodies directed against tumor-specific antigens have been suggested as one mechanism allowing tumors to escape immune surveillance. Blocking antibodies can prevent agglutination in serologic tests (see *incomplete a.*)

**cell-bound a., cell-fixed a.,** any antibody bound to a cell surface either by its antigen combining sites to cell-surface antigenic determinants or by other sites to specific cell-surface receptors (Fc receptors, IgE receptors).

**cold a., cold-reactive a.,** antibody, usually IgM but occasionally IgG, that reacts less efficiently with antigen at 37°C than at lower temperatures.

**complement-fixing a.,** antibody that activates complement when reacted with antigen; IgM and IgG (the usual complement-fixing antibodies) fix complement by the classic pathway, whereas IgA fixes complement by the alternative pathway.

**complete a.,** antibody capable of agglutinating cells in physiologic saline solution. Called also *saline agglutinin.* Cf. *incomplete a.*

**cross-reacting a.,** one that combines with an antigen other than the one that induced its production.

**cytophilic a.,** cytotropic a.

**cytotoxic a.,** any specific antibody directed against cellular antigens, which when bound to the antigen, activates the complement pathway or activates killer cells, resulting in cell lysis.

**cytotropic a.,** antibody that binds to mast cells and basophils at specific receptors; subsequent binding of antigen to the cell-fixed antibody triggers release of mediators of immediate hypersensitivity. Such antibodies produced by the animal itself in response to antigenic challenge or transferred from another animal of the same species (*homocytotropic* or *reaginic antibodies* or *reagin*) are always of the IgE class. In some cases IgG, IgA, or IgM from one species (heterocytotropic antibodies) can sensitize tissues of another species; e.g., rabbit IgG can sensitize guinea pig skin for passive cutaneous anaphylaxis.

**Donath-Landsteiner a.,** an IgG antibody directed against the P blood group antigen, first noted in cases of syphilis, that binds to red cells at low temperatures and induces complement-mediated lysis on warming; it is responsible for hemolysis in paroxysmal hemoglobinuria.

**duck virus hepatitis yolk a.,** yolk antibody derived from chicken eggs, used for treatment of duck virus hepatitis.

**Forssman a.,** heterophile antibody directed against the Forssman antigen.

**heteroclitic a.,** antibody produced in response to immunization with one antigen but having a higher affinity for a second antigen that was not present during immunization.

**heterocytotropic a.,** see *cytotropic a.*

**heterogenetic a., heterophil a., heterophile a.,** antibody directed against heterophile antigens. Heterophile sheep erythrocyte agglutinins appear in the serum of patients with infectious mononucleosis (see *Paul-Bunnell test* under *tests*).

**homocytotropic a.,** see *cytotropic a.*

**hybrid a.,** bispecific a.

**immune a.,** antibody induced by immunization or by transfusion incompatibility, in contrast to the natural antibodies.

**incomplete a.,** 1. antibody that binds to erythrocytes or bacteria but does not produce agglutination; the nonagglutinating antibody is detectable with the antiglobulin (Coombs) test. For example, IgG anti-Rh antibodies do not agglutinate erythrocytes in physiologic saline whereas IgM antibodies do (the large IgM molecule can cross-link the erythrocytes at a wider separation so that there is less electrostatic repulsion due to the zeta potential). 2. a univalent antibody fragment, e.g., Fab fragment.

**indium-111 antimyosin a.,** a monoclonal antibody against myosin, labeled with indium 111; it binds selectively to irreversibly damaged myocytes and is used in infarct avid scintigraphy.

**isophil a.,** antibody against red blood cell antigens produced in members of the species from which the red cells originated.

**mitochondrial a's,** antimitochondrial a's.

**monoclonal a's,** chemically and immunologically homogeneous antibodies produced by hybridomas, used as laboratory reagents in radioimmunoassays, ELISA, and immunofluorescence assays; also used experimentally in cancer immunotherapy.

**natural a's,** antibodies present in the serum of normal individuals in the apparent absence of any contact with the specific antigen, probably induced by exposure to cross-reacting antigens. They may result from unknown exposure to naturally occurring antigens, e.g., food or bacterial flora.

**neutralizing a.,** see *viral neutralization,* under *neutralization.*

**OKT3 monoclonal a.,** a mouse monoclonal antibody directed against T3 lymphocytes and used to prevent or treat rejection after organ transplantation.

**panel-reactive a. (PRA),** 1. the pre-existing anti-HLA antibody in the serum of a potential allograft recipient that reacts with specific antigen in a panel of leukocytes (see *antibody screening,* under *screening*). A higher percentage of PRA indicates a higher risk of a positive crossmatch. 2. the percentage of such antibody in the recipient's serum.

**P-K a's,** Prausnitz-Küstner a's.

**polyclonal a.,** antibody produced by more than one clone of antibody-synthesizing plasma cells (B-lymphocytes); antibody that is not monoclonal, e.g., that produced by immunizing an animal.

**Prausnitz-Küstner a's,** cytotropic IgE antibodies responsible for cutaneous anaphylaxis; see *Prausnitz-Küstner reaction,* under *reaction.*

**protective a.,** antibody responsible for immunity to an infectious agent observed in passive immunity.

**reaginic a.,** reagin.

**Rh a's,** those directed against Rh antigen(s) of human erythrocytes. Not normally present, but may be produced when Rh-negative persons receive Rh-positive blood by transfusion or when an Rh-negative person is pregnant with an Rh-positive fetus.

**saline a.,** complete a.

**sensitizing a.,** a loosely used term, applied to antibodies that are attached to body cells and that "sensitize" the cells or render them susceptible to destruction by body defenses.

**thyroid colloidal a's,** antibodies to antigens in the thyroid colloid such as thyroglobulin or $CA_2$, seen in Hashimoto's disease.

**TSH-displacing a. (TDA),** TSH-binding inhibitory immunoglobulins.

**warm a., warm-reactive a.,** antibody, usually IgG but occasionally IgM or IgA, that reacts more efficiently with antigen at 37°C than at lower temperatures.

**an·ti·bra·chi·um** (an″tĭ-bra′ke-əm) incorrect spelling of *antebrachium.*

**an·ti·bro·mic** (an″tĭ-bro′mik) [*anti-* + Gr. *brōmos* smell] deodorant.

**an·ti·ca·chec·tic** (an″tĭ-kə-kek′tik) 1. preventing or relieving cachexia. 2. an agent that prevents or relieves cachexia.

**an·ti·cal·cu·lous** (an″tĭ-kal′ku-ləs) preventing or alleviating calculus.

**an·ti·car·cin·o·gen** (an″tĭ-kahr-sin′ə-jen) an agent that counteracts the effect of a carcinogen.

**an·ti·car·ci·no·gen·ic** (an″tĭ-kahr-sin″o-jen′ik) inhibiting or preventing the development of carcinoma.

**an·ti·car·di·um** (an″tĭ-kahr′de-um) [*anti-* + Gr. *kardia* heart] epigastrium.

**an·ti·car·io·gen·ic** (an″tĭ-kār″e-o-jen′ik) suppressing the development of caries; anticarious.

**an·ti·car·i·ous** (an″tĭ-kar′e-əs) anticariogenic.

**an·ti·cat·a·lyst** (an″tĭ-kat′ə-list) a substance that retards the action of a catalyzer by acting on the catalyzer itself.

**an·ti·cat·a·lyz·er** (an″tĭ-kat′ə-līz″ər) anticatalyst.

**an·ti·ca·thex·is** (an″tĭ-kə-thek′sis) [*anti-* + *cathexis*] in psychoanalytic theory, the energy required for the ego to maintain repression of unacceptable ideas and impulses.

**an·ti·ceph·a·lal·gic** (an″tĭ-sef-ə-lal′jik) curing or preventing headache.

**an·ti·cho·le·litho·gen·ic** (an″tĭ-ko″le-lith″o-jen′ik) 1. serving to prevent the formation of gallstones. 2. an agent that so acts.

**an·ti·cho·les·ter·emic** (an″tĭ-kə-les″tər-e′mik) 1. promoting a reduction of cholesterol levels in the blood. 2. any agent that promotes a reduction of blood cholesterol levels, e.g., the sitosterols and clofibrate. Called also *anticholesterolemic.*

**an·ti·cho·les·te·rol·emic** (an″tĭ-kə-les″tĕ-rə-le′mik) anticholesteremic.

**an·ti·cho·lin·er·gic** (an″tĭ-ko″lin-ər′jik) [*anti-* + *cholinergic*] 1. blocking the passage of impulses through the parasympathetic nerves. 2. an agent that blocks the parasympathetic nerves. Called also *parasympatholytic.* Cf. *antiadrenergic.*

**an·ti·cho·lin·es·ter·ase** (an″tĭ-ko″lin-es′tər-ās) [*anti-* + *cholinesterase*] cholinesterase inhibitor.

**an·ti·chy·mo·sin** (an″tĭ-ki′mo-sin) an antibody that prevents the action of rennin on milk.

**an·ti·ci·pate** (an-tis′ĭ-pāt) [*ante-* + L. *capere* to take] to occur or recur before the regular time; said of a disease or of symptoms. See *anticipation.*

**an·ti·ci·pa·tion** (an-tis″ĭ-pa′shən) 1. the apparent occurrence of a hereditary disease at a progressively earlier age in successive generations; now considered by most authorities to be an artifact arising from the ease of identification of succeeding cases or because cases of later onset are more likely to be fertile. 2. looking forward to future events, experiences, or emotions, preexperiencing them; it can be used as a defense mechanism.

**an·ti·clin·al** (an″tĭ-kli′nəl) [*anti-* + Gr. *klinein* to slope] sloping in opposite directions, as opposite sides of triangular structures.

**an·tic·ne·mi·on** (an″tik-ne′me-on) [*anti-* + Gr. *knēmē* leg] the shin.

**an·ti·co·ag·u·lant** (an″tĭ-ko-ag′u-lənt) 1. preventing blood clotting. 2. any substance that prevents blood clotting. Those used in anticoagulant therapy (q.v.) are heparin, administered parenterally, and the oral anticoagulants warfarin, dicumarol, and their congeners. Anticoagulant solutions used for the preservation of stored whole blood and blood fractions are acid citrate dextrose (ACD), citrate phosphate dextrose (CPD), citrate phosphate dextrose-adenine (cPDA-l), and heparin. Anticoagulants used to prevent clotting of blood specimens for laboratory analysis are heparin ethylenediaminetetraacetic acid (EDTA), citrate, oxalate, and fluoride.
**circulating a.,** a substance present in the blood that inhibits normal clotting and thus may cause a hemorrhagic syndrome; it may be directed against a specific coagulation factor and may accompany various hematologic and nonhematologic diseases.
**lupus a.,** a circulating anticoagulant that inhibits the conversion of prothrombin to thrombin, found in 5–10 per cent of patients with systemic lupus erythematosus, but also seen in other disorders. Although associated with a prolonged partial thromboplastin time, it rarely causes abnormal bleeding and, paradoxically, increases the risk of thromboembolism. Called also *lupus inhibitor.*

**an·ti·co·ag·u·la·tion** (an″tĭ-ko-ag″u-la′shən) 1. the prevention of coagulation. 2. anticoagulant therapy.

**an·ti·co·ag·u·la·tive** (an″tĭ-ko-ag′u-la″tiv) anticoagulant (def. 1).

**an·ti·coc·cid·i·al** (an″tĭ-kok-sid′e-əl) coccidiostatic.

**an·ti·co·don** (an″tĭ-ko′don) [MeSH: Anticodon] a triplet of nucleotides in transfer RNA that is complementary to the codon in messenger RNA which specifies the amino acid.

**an·ti·com·ple·ment** (an″tĭ-kom′plə-mənt) a substance that opposes or counteracts the action of a complement.

**an·ti·com·ple·men·ta·ry** (an″tĭ-kom″plə-men′tə-re) capable of reducing or destroying the power of a complement.

**an·ti·con·cep·tive** (an″tĭ-kən-sep′tiv) contraceptive.

**an·ti·con·vul·sant** (an″tĭ-kən-vul′sənt) 1. preventing or relieving convulsions. 2. an agent that prevents or relieves convulsions.

**an·ti·con·vul·sive** (an″tĭ-kən-vul′siv) anticonvulsant.

**an·ti·cro·tin** (an″tĭ-kro′tin) the antitoxin of crotin.

**an·ti·cu·ra·re** (an″tĭ-koo-rah′re) an agent that counteracts the action of curare on skeletal muscle.

**an·ti·cus** (an-ti′kəs) [L.] anterior.

**an·ti·cy·tol·y·sin** (an″tĭ-si-tol′ĭ-sin) a substance opposing the action of cytolysin.

**an·ti·cy·to·tox·in** (an″tĭ-si″to-tok′sin) a substance that opposes the action of a cytotoxin.

**an·ti-D** antibody against the "D" or "$Rh_0$" Rh blood group antigen; see *$Rh_0(D)$ immune globulin,* under *globulin.*

**an·ti·de·pres·sant** (an″tĭ-de-pres′ənt) 1. preventing or relieving depression. 2. an agent that stimulates the mood of a depressed patient, including tricyclic antidepressants and monoamine oxidase inhibitors.
**tetracyclic a.,** an antidepressant drug that includes four fused rings in its chemical structure.
**tricyclic a.,** any of a group of antidepressant drugs that contain three fused rings in their chemical structure and that potentiate the action of catecholamines; the tricyclic antidepressants include a number of compounds, which may be grouped into four classes on the basis of chemical structure: dibenzazepines, dibenzocycloheptadienes, dibenzoxazepines, and dibenzoxepines.

**an·ti·di·a·bet·ic** (an″tĭ-di″ə-bet′ik) 1. preventing or alleviating diabetes. 2. an agent that prevents or alleviates diabetes.

**an·ti·di·a·be·to·gen·ic** (an″tĭ-di″ə-be″to-jen′ik) 1. preventing the development of diabetes. 2. an agent that prevents the development of diabetes.

**an·ti·di·ar·rhe·al** (an″tĭ-di″ə-re′əl) 1. counteracting diarrhea. 2. an agent that is effective in combating diarrhea.

**an·ti·di·ar·rhe·ic** (an″tĭ-di″ə-re′ik) antidiarrheal.

**an·ti·di·u·re·sis** (an″tĭ-di″u-re′sis) suppression of urinary excretion.

**an·ti·di·uret·ic** (an″tĭ-di″u-ret′ik) 1. suppressing the rate of urine formation. 2. an agent that suppresses urine formation.

**an·ti·do·tal** (an″tĭ-do′təl) serving as an antidote.

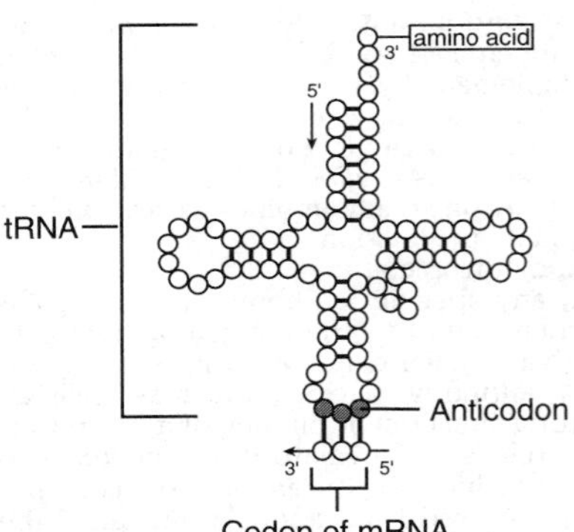


Anticodon. The three nucleotides *(shaded)* on a transfer RNA bind to a complementary messenger RNA codon.

**an·ti·dote** (an'tĭ-dōt) [L. *antidotum,* from Gr. *anti* against + *didonai* to give] a remedy for counteracting a poison.
**chemical a.,** an antidote that reacts chemically with a poison to form a harmless compound.
**mechanical a.,** an antidote that prevents the absorption of a poison.
**physiologic a.,** an antidote that counteracts the effects of a poison by producing opposing physiologic effects.
**"universal" a.,** a mixture of 2 parts activated charcoal, 1 part magnesium oxide, and 1 part tannic acid; given when the exact poison is not known. There is no true "universal" antidote and this mixture is no longer recommended by most authorities; activated charcoal alone is preferred.

**an·ti·dot·ic** (an"tĭ-dot'ik) antidotal.

**an·ti·drom·ic** (an"tĭ-drom'ik) [Gr. *antidromein* to run in a contrary direction] conducting impulses in a direction opposite to the normal; see under *conduction.* Cf. *orthodromic.*

**an·ti·dys·en·ter·ic** (an"tĭ-dis"ən-ter'ik) 1. preventing, alleviating, or curing dysentery. 2. an agent that prevents, alleviates, or cures dysentery.

**an·ti·dys·ki·net·ic** (an"tĭ-dis"kĭ-net'ik) 1. relieving or preventing dyskinesia. 2. an agent that relieves or prevents dyskinesia.

**an·ti·ec·ze·mat·ic** (an"tĭ-ek"-zə-mat'ik) 1. alleviating eczema. 2. an agent that alleviates eczema.

**an·ti·edem·a·tous** (an"te-e-dem'ə-təs) antiedemic.

**an·ti·edem·ic** (an"te-ə-dem'ik) 1. preventing or alleviating edema. 2. an agent that prevents or alleviates edema.

**an·ti·emet·ic** (an"te-ə-met'ik) [*anti-* + *emetic*] 1. preventing or alleviating nausea and vomiting. 2. an agent that prevents or alleviates nausea and vomiting. See also *antinauseant.*

**an·ti·en·zyme** (an"te-en'zīm) [*anti-* + *enzyme*] an agent that prevents or retards the action of an enzyme, such as a protease inhibitor or an antibody.

**an·ti·ep·i·lep·tic** (an"te-ep"ĭ-lep'tik) 1. combating epilepsy. 2. an agent that combats epilepsy.

**an·ti·ep·i·the·li·al** (an"te-ep"ĭ-the'le-əl) destructive to epithelial cells.

**an·ti·es·tro·gen** (an"te-es'trə-jen) any substance capable of inhibiting the biological effects of estrogens.

**an·ti·es·tro·gen·ic** (an"te-es-trə-jen'ik) counteracting or suppressing estrogenic activity.

**an·ti·fe·brile** (an"tĭ-feb'ril) antipyretic (def. 1).

**an·ti·fib·ril·la·tory** (an"tĭ-fib'rĭ-lə-tor"e) 1. preventing or stopping fibrillation of the heart. 2. an agent that prevents or stops fibrillation of the heart.

**an·ti·fi·bri·nol·y·sin** (an"tĭ-fi"brĭ-nol'ĭ-sin) antiplasmin.

**an·ti·fi·bri·no·lyt·ic** (an"tĭ-fi"brĭ-no-lit'ik) 1. inhibiting fibrinolysis. 2. a substance that prevents fibrinolysis.

**an·ti·fi·brot·ic** (an"tĭ-fi-brot'ik) 1. causing regression of fibrosis. 2. an agent that causes the regression of fibrosis.

**an·ti·fi·lar·i·al** (an"tĭ-fĭ-lar'e-əl) 1. effective against filaria. 2. an agent that is effective against filaria.

**an·ti·flat·u·lent** (an"tĭ-flat'u-lənt) 1. relieving or preventing flatulence. 2. an agent that relieves or prevents flatulence.

**an·ti·flux** (an"tĭ-fluks') a substance that prevents the attachment of solder.

**an·ti·fol** (an'tĭ-fōl) folic acid antagonist.

**an·ti·fo·late** (an"tĭ-fo'lāt) folic acid antagonist.

**an·ti·fun·gal** (an"tĭ-fung'gəl) antimycotic.

**an·ti·ga·lac·tic** (an"tĭ-gə-lak'tik) [*anti-* + *galactic*] 1. diminishing the secretion of milk. 2. an agent that tends to suppress milk secretion.

**an·ti·gen** (an'tĭ-jən) [*antibody* + *-gen*] any substance which is capable, under appropriate conditions, of inducing a specific immune response and of reacting with the products of that response, that is, with specific antibody or specifically sensitized T-lymphocytes, or both. Antigens may be soluble substances, such as toxins and foreign proteins, or particulate, such as bacteria and tissue cells; however, only the portion of the protein or polysaccharide molecule known as the antigenic determinant (q.v.) combines with antibody or a specific receptor on a lymphocyte. Abbreviated Ag.

## Antigen

**allogeneic a.,** one occurring in some but not all individuals of the same species, e.g., histocompatibility antigens and human blood group antigens; isoantigen.
**Am a's,** see under *allotype.*
**Au a., Australia a.,** former name for *hepatitis B surface a.*
**blood group a's,** the antigens responsible for specificities of blood groups; those of the ABO and Lewis blood groups were the first to be characterized. They are formed by sequential addition of monosaccharide moieties to any of several different types of precursor substances; addition of one moiety produces the Lewis antigen, addition of a second produces the H antigen, and addition of a third produces either the A or the B antigen. Secreted blood group antigens (in individuals with the secretor phenotype) are glycoproteins, and red cell antigens are glycosphingolipids; the oligosaccharide chains determining blood group specificity are the same in both.
**cancer a. 125 (CA 125),** a surface glycoprotein associated with müllerian epithelial tissue; elevated serum levels are often associated with epithelial ovarian carcinomas, particularly with nonmucinous tumors, but are also seen in some other malignant and various benign pelvic disorders. See also *cancer antigen 125 (CA 125) assay,* under *assay.*
**capsular a.,** K a.
**carcinoembryonic a. (CEA),** a glycoprotein, mol. wt. 200,000, secreted into the glycocalyx coating the luminal surface of gastrointestinal epithelia. Originally thought to be a specific antigen of the fetal digestive tract and adenocarcinoma of the colon, CEA is now known to occur normally in feces and pancreaticobiliary secretions and to appear in the plasma in a diverse group of neoplastic and non-neoplastic conditions, including cancers of the colon, pancreas, stomach, lung, and breast, alcoholic cirrhosis and pancreatitis, inflammatory bowel disease, rectal polyps, and cigarette smoking. The primary use of CEA is in monitoring response to treatment of colorectal cancer.
**CD a.,** any of a number of cell surface markers expressed by leukocytes and used to distinguish cell lineages, developmental stages, and functional subsets; such markers can be identified by specific monoclonal antibodies and are numbered CD1, CD2, CD3, etc. Markers used to identify T lymphocyte subsets were formerly called *T antigens.* See also *CD system,* under *system.*
**class I a's,** major histocompatibility antigens found on virtually every cell, human erythrocytes being the only notable exception; they are found on molecules consisting of two noncovalently bound chains. One, a 44,000-dalton polymorphic glycoprotein partially embedded in the cell membrane, is determined by an MHC gene (HLA-A, -B, or -C in humans); the other, $\beta_2$-microglobulin, a 12,000-dalton nonpolymorphic protein, is determined by a non-MHC gene. Class I antigens are the classic histocompatibility antigens recognized during graft rejection and are also the antigens involved in MHC restriction (q.v.).
**class II a's,** major histocompatibility antigens found only on immunocompetent cells, primarily B lymphocytes and macrophages; they are found on molecules consisting of two noncovalently bound chains, the 34,000-dalton $\alpha$ chain and the 29,000-dalton $\beta$ chain, both glycoproteins partially embedded in the cell membrane and both determined by MHC genes. The human HLA-D, -DR, -DQ, -DT, -MB, -MT, and -Te loci are all associated with antigenic determinants on class II antigen molecules.
**class III a's,** a term used to refer to nonhistocompatibility antigens mapping in the major histocompatibility complex, e.g., the complement components C2, C4, and factor B.
**common a.,** an antigenic determinant group (epitope) that is present in two or more different antigen molecules and frequently leads to cross-reactions among them.
**common acute lymphoblastic leukemia a. (CALLA),** a tumor-associated antigen, CD10, occurring on lymphoblasts in about 80 per cent of patients with acute lymphoblastic leukemia (ALL) and also in 40–50 per cent of patients with blastic phase chronic myelogenous leukemia (CML). It does not occur on normal lymphoid cells except during fetal development.
**common leukocyte a's,** a group of glycoproteins, antigenically similar but of different molecular weights, found on B cells, T cells, thymocytes, and leukopoietic cells.
**complete a.,** an antigen which both stimulates the immune response and reacts with the products (e.g., antibody) of that response.

**conjugated a.,** antigen produced by coupling a hapten to a protein carrier molecule through covalent bonds; when it induces immunization, the resultant immune response is directed against both the hapten and the carrier.

**cross-reacting a.,** 1. one that combines with antibody produced in response to a different but related antigen, owing to similarity of antigenic determinants. 2. identical antigens in two bacterial strains, so that antibody produced against one strain will react with the other.

**D a.,** one of the Rh factors, an antigen of the Rh blood group, important in the development of isoimmunization in Rh-negative persons exposed to the blood of Rh-positive persons.

**delta a.,** a 32- to 37-nm RNA particle coated with hepatitis B surface antigen.

**E a.,** one of the Rh factors, an antigen of the Rh blood group system.

**epithelial membrane a.,** a protein specific to the epithelial membrane; used as an immunohistochemical marker for epithelium.

**extractable nuclear a's,** ENA; protein antigens, not containing DNA, that are extractable from cell nuclei in phosphate-buffered saline; anti-ENA antibodies are a component of the antinuclear antibodies occurring in systemic lupus erythematosus and other connective tissue diseases.

**febrile a's,** a standard panel of serologic antigens (*Salmonella, Proteus, Francisella tularensis,* and *Brucella*) used in screening patients with unexplained fever.

**flagellar a.,** H a. (def. 1).

**Forssman a.,** a heterogenetic antigen inducing the production of antisheep hemolysin, occurring in various unrelated animals, mainly in the organs but not in the erythrocytes (guinea pig, horse), but sometimes only in the erythrocytes (sheep), and occasionally in both (chicken). In the original and strict sense, the antigen is typified by that found in the guinea pig kidney and characterized by heat stability and solubility in alcohol; the antigenic determinant is polysaccharide in nature. Its antibody is absorbed by tissues containing the antigen and contains no lysin for bovine cells and little or no agglutinin for sheep cells. The term is also used loosely to refer to any antigen producing sheep hemolysin, but antibodies to it are not identical, as they are in the case of the true Forssman (or F) antigen.

**Frei a.,** antigen for the Frei test, material prepared from lymphogranuloma venereum organisms grown in chick embryo yolk sacs.

**Gm a's,** see under *allotype.*

**H a.** [*Hauch,* q.v.], 1. the precursor of the A and B blood group antigens. Normal type O individuals lack enzymes to convert H antigen to A or B antigens. Those individuals having the rare *Bombay phenotype* lack the ability to make H antigen and thus are phenotypically type O whether or not they possess A or B genes. Called also *H substance.* 2. one of the bacterial flagellar antigens important in the serological classification of enteric bacilli, especially *Salmonella.* Cf. *O a.*

**H-2 a's,** the major histocompatibility antigens in mice.

**hepatitis a., hepatitis-associated a. (HAA),** former name for *hepatitis B surface a.*

**hepatitis B core a. (HBcAg),** a core protein antigen of the hepatitis B virus present inside complete virions (Dane particles) and in the nuclei of infected hepatocytes, indicating the presence of replicating hepatitis B virus; the antigen is not present in the blood of infected individuals, but anti-HBc antibodies appear during the acute infection; they do not protect against reinfection.

**hepatitis B e a. (HBeAg),** an antigen of hepatitis B virus sometimes present in the blood during acute infection, usually disappearing afterward but sometimes persisting in chronic disease. Anti-HBe antibodies appear transiently during convalescence; they do not protect against reinfection.

**hepatitis B surface a. (HBsAg),** a coat protein antigen of the hepatitis B virus present on complete virions (Dane particles) and smaller spherical and filamentous particles circulating in the blood of individuals with active or chronic infections, being first detectable several weeks prior to clinical disease and peaking with the appearance of symptoms. Anti-HBs antibodies appear in the blood in late convalescence and are protective against reinfection. Originally called *Australia* or *Au antigen* because it was first found in an Australian aborigine; also formerly called *hepatitis-associated a. (HAA)* and *serum hepatitis (SH) a.* See *hepatitis B vaccine,* under *vaccine.*

**heterogeneic a.,** xenogeneic a.

**heterogenetic a.,** heterophile a.

**heterologous a.,** an antigen that reacts with an antibody that is not the one (the homologous antigen) that induced its formation.

**heterophil a., heterophile a.,** any of a group of cross-reacting antigens occurring in several species and having a species distribution that does not correspond to phylogenetic relationships, e.g., Forssman antigen. Called also *heterogenetic a.*

**high frequency a's, high incidence a's,** public a's (def. 1).

**histocompatibility a's,** systems of allelic alloantigens that can stimulate an immune response that leads to transplant rejection when the donor and recipient are mismatched. Called also *transplantation a's.* See *HLA a's.*

**histocompatibility a's, major,** those in the major histocompatibility complex; HLA antigens in humans and H-2 antigens in mice.

**histocompatibility a's, minor,** systems of allelic alloantigens that can cause transplant rejection, but with a long delay (up to 100 days); about 15–30 such systems have been found in mice.

**HLA a's** [*H*uman *L*eukocyte *A*ntigens], histocompatibility antigens governed by genes of the HLA complex (the human major histocompatibility complex), a region on the short arm of chromosome 6 containing several genetic loci, each having multiple alleles. Loci are designated by letters, HLA-A, -B, -C, -DP, -DQ, -DR (there are at least three subloci in the D region), -MB, -MT, and -Te, and alleles at each locus by numbers, e.g., HLA-A1, provisional designations being indicated by "w" (for "workshop"), e.g., HLA-DRw10. The A, B, C, DR, MB, MT, and Te antigens are defined and typed by serologic reactions. The D antigens are defined and typed by one-way mixed lymphocyte culture (MLC) using panels of HLA-D-homozygous typing cells. The SB (for "secondary B cell") antigens are defined and typed by primed lymphocyte typing. See *class I, class II,* and *class III a's.*

**homologous a.,** 1. the antigen that induces the formation of an antibody. 2. isoantigen.

**H-Y a.,** a minor histocompatibility antigen present in all tissues of normal males and coded for by a structural gene on the short arm of the Y chromosome; it is thought to promote the differentiation of indifferent gonads into testes, thus determining male sex.

**I a.,** see *cold agglutinin syndrome,* under *syndrome.*

**i a.,** see *cold agglutinin syndrome,* under *syndrome.*

**Ia a's** [*I* region–*a*ssociated], class II histocompatibility antigens found on the surface of mouse B cells, macrophages, and accessory cells. They are also found on granulocyte precursors but disappear during maturation. Ia antigens are governed by the Ia genes of the H-2 complex (q.v.).

**Inv group a.,** see *Km allotypes,* under *allotype.*

**isogeneic a.,** isoantigen.

**isophile a.,** isoantigen.

**K a.** [Ger. *Kapsel* capsule], a bacterial capsular antigen, a surface antigen external to the cell wall, such as the *Salmonella* Vi antigens and pneumococcal capsular antigens.

**Km a's,** see under *allotype.*

**Kveim a.,** a saline suspension of human sarcoid tissue prepared from the spleen or lymph nodes of a patient with active sarcoidosis.

**La a.,** SS-B a.

**LD a's,** lymphocyte-defined a's.

**leukocyte function–associated a. 1 (LFA-1),** a $\beta_2$ integrin expressed on most lymphocytes, granulocytes, and monocytes that mediates leukocyte adhesion; it also plays a role in antibody-dependent cellular cytotoxicity.

**leukocyte function–associated a. 2 (LFA-2),** a cell membrane glycoprotein, perhaps related to the immunoglobulins, expressed on thymocytes and NK cells that mediates leukocyte adhesion.

**leukocyte function–associated a. 3 (LFA-3),** a cell surface glycoprotein expressed on a wide variety of cells that serves as a ligand for LFA-2.

**leu-M1 a.,** an antigen present on granulocytes and Reed-Sternberg cells in Hodgkin's disease, except in the lymphocyte-predominant diffuse subtype.

**low frequency a's, low incidence a's,** private antigens (def. 1).

**Ly a's,** cell-surface markers differentiating subpopulations of murine T lymphocytes: Ly 1, Ly 2, and Ly 3. Most thymocytes and undifferentiated peripheral T cells are Ly $1^+2^+3^+$; helper cells are Ly $1^+2^-3^-$; cytotoxic T cells and suppressor cells are Ly $1^-2^+3^+$.

**Lyb a's,** cell-surface markers on murine B lymphocytes: Lyb 1,2,3,4, and 5. Lyb 1,2, and 4 are found on all B cells, Lyb 3 and 5 on a subset of mature B cells.

**lymphocyte-defined (LD) a's,** major histocompatibility antigens defined and typed by the mixed lymphocyte reaction (MLR), e.g., HLA-D antigens.

**Lyt a's,** Ly a's.

**M a.,** M protein (def. 1).

**Mitsuda a.,** lepromin.

**mumps skin test a.** [USP], a preparation of killed mumps virus, used in the mumps skin test (q.v.).

**nuclear a's,** the components of cell nuclei with which antinuclear antibodies (see under *antibody*) react.

**O a.** [*ohne Hauch,* q.v.], the lipopolysaccharide-protein somatic antigens of gram-negative bacteria, important in the serological classification of enteric bacilli. See *lipopolysaccharide.* Cf. *H a.*

**oncofetal a.,** an antigenic gene product that is expressed during fetal development, partially or completely repressed in adult tissues, and derepressed in some tissues that have undergone neoplastic transformation; oncofetal antigens, e.g., alpha-fetoprotein, carcinoembryonic antigen, and pancreatic oncofetal antigen, are thus useful tumor markers.

**organ-specific a.,** any antigen that occurs exclusively in a particular organ and serves to distinguish it from other organs. Two types of organ specificity have been proposed: (1) first-order or tissue specificity is attributed to the presence of an antigen characteristic of a particular organ in a single species; (2) second-order organ specificity is attributed to an antigen characteristic of the same organ in many, even unrelated species. Called also *tissue-specific a.*

**Oz a.,** an antigenic marker on the lambda chain of human immunoglobulins, equivalent to Km allotypes on kappa light chains. Together with Kern markers, they delineate three types of human lambda chain.

**pancreatic oncofetal a.,** POA; a glycoprotein, mol. wt. 800,000, found in fetal and neoplastic pancreatic tissue but not in that of normal adults; it also occurs at lower levels in the serum of patients with cancer at other sites and some normal adults.

**partial a.,** hapten.

**Pl(A1) a.,** the most commonly expressed antigen of platelets; patients not expressing this isoantigen are at risk for transfusion-induced hematologic disorders of platelets, such as thrombocytopenic purpura.

**platelet a.,** any of several isoantigens expressed by platelets.

**pollen a.,** see under *allergen.*

**Pr a.,** see *cold agglutinin syndrome,* under *syndrome.*

**private a's,** 1. blood group antigens that occur in only a few kindreds *(low frequency blood groups).* Called also *low frequency a's.* 2. HLA antigens found only on the gene product of a single allele. 3. a tumor antigen expressed only on a particular type of chemically induced tumor. Cf. *public a's.*

**proliferating cell nuclear a. (PCNA),** a 36 kd nuclear acidic protein whose levels in the body correlate with the rates of DNA synthesis and cellular proliferation in transformed cells of certain tumors. Called also *cyclin.*

**prostate-specific a. (PSA),** a serine endopeptidase secreted by the epithelial cells of the prostate gland; serum levels are elevated in benign prostatic hyperplasia and prostate cancer. Measurement of PSA serum levels is sometimes used as a screening test for prostate cancer.

**prostate-specific membrane a. (PSMA),** a substance often expressed by the most aggressive clones of prostate cancer cells; monoclonal antibody tests for PSMA appear to be more sensitive than those using prostate-specific antigen alone in finding circulating prostate cancer cells and may be useful in identifying patients with a high risk of advanced disease.

**public a's,** 1. blood group antigens that occur in the general population at high frequencies; see *high frequency blood group,* under *blood group.* Called also *high frequency a's.* 2. HLA antigens occurring on the products of several allelic genes. Cf. *private a's.*

**recall a.,** an antigen to which an individual has previously been sensitized and which is subsequently administered as a challenging dose to elicit a hypersensitivity reaction.

**Rh a.,** see under *factor.*

**RNP a.** [*ribo*nucleo*p*rotein], one of the extractable nuclear antigens.

**Ro a.,** SS-A a.

**SD a's,** serologically defined a's.

**self-a.,** autoantigen.

**sequestered a's,** the cellular constituents of tissue (e.g., lens of the eye) sequestered anatomically from the lymphoreticular system during embryonic development and thus thought not to be recognized as "self." Should such tissue be exposed to the lymphoreticular system during adult life, an autoimmune response would be elicited.

**sero-defined (SD) a's, serologically defined (SD) a's,** major histocompatibility antigens defined by serologic reactions, e.g., HLA-A, HLA-B, and HLA-C antigens.

**serum hepatitis a., SH a.,** former name for *hepatitis B surface a.*

**shock a.,** an antigen capable of eliciting anaphylactic shock in a sensitized animal.

**Sm a.** [after a patient, *Smith*], an uncharacterized nuclear antigen that is a nonhistone acidic protein not complexed with DNA or RNA; anti-Sm antibodies make up a part of the antinuclear antibodies in about one-third of patients with systemic lupus erythematosus, but do not occur in other connective tissue diseases, except mixed connective tissue disease.

**somatic a's,** antigens, usually cell surface antigens, of the body of a bacterial cell, in contrast to flagellar or capsular antigens. See *O a.*

**species-specific a's,** antigens that are restricted to a single species but occur in all members of that species.

**SS-A a.,** a ribonucleoprotein extractable nuclear antigen; see also *anti–SS-A antibody,* under *antibody.*

**SS-B a.,** a ribonucleoprotein extractable nuclear antigen; see also *anti–SS-B antibody,* under *antibody.*

**T a.,** 1. tumor antigen; any of several antigens, coded for by the viral genome, associated with transformation of infected cells by certain DNA tumor viruses, e.g., SV 40. 2. an antigen present on human erythrocytes that is exposed by treatment with neuraminidase or contact with certain bacteria. See *T agglutinin* under *agglutinin.* 3. see *CD a.*

**$\theta$ a.,** Thy 1 a.

**Tac a.,** the receptor for interleukin 2.

**T-dependent a.,** one that requires the presence of helper T cells to stimulate antibody production by B cells; most antigens are T-dependent.

**theta a., Thy 1 a.,** a cell-surface marker occurring on all murine T lymphocytes.

**T-independent a.,** an antigen that can trigger B cells to produce antibodies without the participation of T cells; most are polymers with a simple repeating pattern and are B cell mitogens; only IgM is produced and few memory cells are formed.

**tissue-specific a.,** organ-specific a.

**TL a.** [*t*hymus *l*eukemia], a differentiation antigen, first discovered on thymic leukemia cells, that occurs on thymocytes but not peripheral T cells in some strains of mice.

**transplantation a's,** histocompatibility a's.

**tumor a.,** 1. T a. (def. 1). 2. tumor-specific a.

**tumor-associated a.,** a new antigen acquired by a tumor cell line in the process of neoplastic transformation, such as a tumor-specific antigen, a tissue specific antigen, or an oncofetal antigen.

**tumor-specific a. (TSA),** any cell-surface antigen of a tumor that does not occur on normal cells of the same origin.

**tumor-specific transplantation a. (TSTA),** any of the cell surface histocompatibility antigens of any given tumor that evoke a specific immune response on transplantation to a syngeneic host.

**VDRL a.,** an alcohol solution containing 0.03 per cent cardiolipin, 0.99 per cent cholesterol, and enough lecithin to produce standard reactivity. See *VDRL test,* under *test.*

**very late activation (VLA) a.,** $\beta_1$ integrin.

**Vi a.,** a K antigen of *Salmonella typhi* originally thought to be responsible for virulence.

**xenogeneic a.,** an antigen common to members of one species but not to members of other species; called also *heterogeneic a.*

---

**an·ti·gen·emia** (an″tĭ-jə-ne′me-ə) [*antigen* + *-emia*] the presence of antigen (e.g., hepatitis B antigen) in the blood.

**an·ti·gen·emic** (an″tĭ-jen-e′mik) exhibiting antigenemia.

**an·ti·gen·ic** (an-tĭ-jen′ik) having the properties of an antigen.

**an·ti·ge·nic·i·ty** (an″tĭ-jə-nis′ĭ-te) the property of being able to induce a specific immune response or the degree to which a substance is able to stimulate an immune response. Called also *immunogenicity.*

**an·ti·glob·u·lin** (an′tĭ-glob″u-lin) an antibody directed against gamma globulin; see also under *test.*

**an·ti·goit·ro·gen·ic** (an″tĭ-goi″tro-jen′ik) preventing or inhibiting the development of goiter.

**an·ti·go·nado·trop·ic** (an″tĭ-go″nad-o-tro′pik) inhibiting the secretion or actions of the gonadotropins.

**an·ti·grav·i·ty** (an″tĭ-grav′ə-te) counteracting the pull of gravity.

**an·ti·hal·lu·cin·a·to·ry** (an″tĭ-hə-loo′sĭ-nə-to″re) counteracting hallucinogenesis; suppressing hallucinations.

**an·ti-HBc** antibody to hepatitis B core antigen ($HB_cAg$).

**an·ti-HBs** antibody to hepatitis B surface antigen ($HB_sAg$).

**an·ti·he·lix** (an″te-he′liks) [TA] the prominent semicircular ridge seen on the lateral aspect of the auricle of the external ear, anteroinferior to the helix; called also *anthelix.*

**an·ti·hel·min·tic** (an″tĭ-hel-min′tik) anthelmintic.

**an·ti·he·mag·glu·ti·nin** (an″tĭ-he″mə-gloo′tĭ-nin) a substance whose action is antagonistic to hemagglutinin.

**an·ti·he·mol·y·sin** (an″tĭ-he-mol′ə-sin) any agent that opposes the action of a hemolysin.

**an·ti·he·mo·lyt·ic** (an″tĭ-he″mo-lit′ik) preventing hemolysis.

**an·ti·he·mo·phil·ic** (an″tĭ-he″mo-fil′ik) 1. counteracting hemophilia. 2. an agent that acts to counteract hemophilia.

**an·ti·hem·or·rhag·ic** (an″tĭ-hem″o-raj′ik) 1. stopping hemorrhage. 2. an agent that prevents or stops hemorrhage.

**an·ti·het·er·ol·y·sin** (an″tĭ-het″ər-ol′ĭ-sin) a substance that counteracts heterolysin.

**an·ti·his·ta·mine** (an″tĭ-his′tə-mēn) a drug that counteracts the action of histamine. The antihistamines are of two types. The conventional ones, as those used in allergies, block the $H_1$ histamine receptors, whereas the others block the $H_2$ receptors. See *histamine*. Called also *antihistaminic*.

**an·ti·his·ta·min·ic** (an″tĭ-his-tə-min′ik) 1. counteracting the effect of histamine. 2. antihistamine.

**an·ti·hor·mone** (an″tĭ-hor′mōn) any substance that opposes the action of a hormone.

**an·ti·hy·per·cho·les·ter·ol·emic** (an″tĭ-hi″pər-kə-les″tər-ol-e′mik) effective in decreasing or preventing an excessively high level of cholesterol in the blood. By extension, sometimes used to designate an agent that exerts such an effect.

**an·ti·hy·per·gly·ce·mic** (an″tĭ-hi″pər-gli-se′mik) 1. counteracting high levels of glucose in the blood. 2. an agent that counteracts high levels of glucose in the blood.

**an·ti·hy·per·lipo·pro·tein·emic** (an″tĭ-hi″pər-lip″o-pro″tēn-e′mik) 1. promoting a reduction of lipoprotein levels in the blood. 2. an agent that so acts.

**an·ti·hy·per·ten·sive** (an″tĭ-hi″pər-ten′siv) 1. counteracting high blood pressure. 2. an agent that reduces high blood pressure.

**an·ti·hyp·not·ic** (an″tĭ-hip-not′ik) 1. preventing or hindering sleep. 2. an agent that prevents or hinders sleep.

**an·ti·hy·po·ten·sive** (an″tĭ-hi″po-ten′siv) 1. counteracting low blood pressure. 2. an agent that so acts.

**an·ti·hy·ster·ic** (an″tĭ-his-ter′ik) 1. preventing or relieving hysteria. 2. an agent that counteracts hysteria.

**an·ti·ic·ter·ic** (an″te-ik-ter′ik) relieving icterus or jaundice.

**an·ti·id·io·type** (an″te-id′e-o-tīp) an antibody directed against an idiotypic determinant of another antibody. See *idiotype–anti-idiotype network,* under *network.*

**an·ti·in·fec·tive** (an″te-in-fek′tiv) 1. capable of killing infectious agents or of preventing them from spreading and causing infection. 2. an agent that so acts.

**an·ti·in·flam·ma·to·ry** (an″te-in-flam′ə-to″re) 1. counteracting or suppressing inflammation. 2. an agent that counteracts or suppresses the inflammatory process.

**an·ti·in·su·lin** (an″te-in′su-lin) a substance that counteracts the action of insulin; see also *insulin antagonists,* under *antagonist.*

**an·ti·isol·y·sin** (an″te-i-sol′ĭ-sin) a substance that counteracts an isolysin.

**an·ti·ke·to·gen** (an″tĭ-ke′to-jen) a substance that inhibits the formation of ketone bodies.

**an·ti·ke·to·gen·e·sis** (an″tĭ-ke″to-jen′ə-sis) inhibition of the formation of ketone bodies.

**an·ti·ke·to·ge·net·ic** (an″tĭ-ke″to-jə-net′ik) antiketogenic.

**an·ti·ke·to·gen·ic** (an″tĭ-ke″to-jen′ik) preventing or inhibiting the formation of ketone bodies.

**an·ti·ke·to·plas·tic** (an″tĭ-ke″to-plas′tik) antiketogenic.

**an·ti·leish·ma·ni·al** (an″tĭ-līsh-ma′ne-əl) 1. effective against leishmania. 2. an agent that is effective against leishmania.

**an·ti·lep·rot·ic** (an″tĭ-lep-rot′ik) 1. therapeutically effective against leprosy. 2. an agent that is therapeutically effective against leprosy.

**an·ti·leu·ko·ci·din** (an″tĭ-loo-ko′sĭ-din) a substance that counteracts leukocidin; called also *antileukotoxin.*

**an·ti·leu·ko·cyt·ic** (an″tĭ-loo″ko-sit′ik) leukocytolytic.

**an·ti·leu·ko·tox·in** (an″tĭ-loo″ko-tok′sin) antileukocidin.

**an·ti·lew·is·ite** (an″tĭ-loo′ĭ-sīt) dimercaprol; also called *British antilewisite,* or *BAL.*

**an·ti·li·pe·mic** (an″tĭ-lĭ-pe′mik) 1. counteracting high levels of lipids in the blood. 2. an agent that counteracts high levels of lipids in the blood.

**an·ti·lipo·trop·ic** (an″tĭ-lip″o-trop′ik) interfering with the mobilization of fat in the liver.

**an·ti·lip·ot·rop·ism** (an″tĭ-lip-ət′rə-piz-əm) interference with the mobilization of fat in the liver.

**An·ti·lir·i·um** (an″tĭ-lir′e-əm) trademark for a preparation of physostigmine salicylate.

**an·ti·lith·ic** (an″tĭ-lith′ik) [*anti-* + *lithic*] 1. preventing the formation of stone or calculus. 2. an agent that prevents the formation of stone or calculus.

**an·ti·ly·sin** (an″tĭ-li′sin) [*anti-* + *lysin*] a substance that opposes the action of a lysin.

**an·ti·ly·sis** (an″tĭ-li′sis) the inhibition or suppression of lysis.

**an·ti·lyt·ic** (an″tĭ-lit′ik) pertaining to antilysis; inhibiting or suppressing lysis.

**an·ti·ma·lar·i·al** (an″tĭ-mə-lar′e-əl) 1. therapeutically effective against malaria. 2. an agent that is therapeutically effective against malaria.

**an·ti·me·phit·ic** (an″tĭ-mə-fit′ik) preventing or neutralizing mephitic substances.

**an·ti·mere** (an′tĭ-mēr) [*anti-* + *-mere*] one of the opposite corresponding parts of an organism which are symmetrical with respect to the longitudinal axis of its body; cf. *metamere.*

**an·ti·mes·en·ter·ic** (an″tĭ-mes′ən-ter″ik) designating that part of the intestine which is opposite to the site of attachment of the mesentery.

**an·ti·me·tab·o·lite** (an″tĭ-mə-tab′o-līt) a substance bearing a close structural resemblance to one required for normal physiological functioning, and exerting its effect by interfering with the utilization of the essential metabolite. For various ways in which antimetabolites inhibit metabolic processes, see under *inhibition.*

**an·ti·met·he·mo·glo·bin·emic** (an″tĭ-met-he″mo-glo″bĭ-ne′mik) 1. effective in reducing the production of methemoglobin; effective in the treatment of methemoglobinemia. 2. an agent that produces such effects.

**an·ti·me·tro·pia** (an″tĭ-mə-tro′pe-ə) [*anti-* + *metr-* + *-opia*] difference in the refractive error of the two eyes, e.g., hyperopia in one eye with myopia in the other.

**an·ti·mi·cro·bi·al** (an″tĭ-mi-kro′be-əl) 1. killing microorganisms, or suppressing their multiplication or growth. 2. an agent that kills microorganisms or suppresses their multiplication or growth. Cf. *antibiotic.*

**an·ti·min·er·alo·cor·ti·coid** (an″tĭ-min″ər-əl-o-kor′tĭ-koid) a substance that suppresses the secretion or opposes the action of mineralocorticoids.

**An·ti·minth** (an′tĭ-minth) trademark for a preparation of pyrantel pamoate.

**an·ti·mi·tot·ic** (an″tĭ-mi-tot′ik) inhibiting or preventing mitosis.

**an·ti·mon·go·lism** (an″tĭ-mon′go-liz-əm) a term applied to the syndromes associated with group chromosome 21 deletions or chromosome 21 monosomy, characterized by antimongoloid obliquity of the palpebral fissures, hypertonia, high-arched palate, micrognathia, and microcephaly, and by mental and growth retardation.

**an·ti·mon·go·loid** (an″tĭ-mon′go-loid) denoting a feature opposite to one characteristic of mongolism, as antimongoloid slant of the palpebral fissures.

**an·ti·mo·ni·al** (an″tĭ-mo′ne-əl) pertaining to or containing antimony.

**an·ti·mon·ic** (an″tĭ-mon′ik) containing antimony in its pentad valency.

**an·ti·mon·ic ac·id** (an″tĭ-mon′ik) antimony pentoxide.

**an·ti·mo·nid** (an″tĭ-mo′nīd) any binary compound of antimony.

**an·ti·mo·ni·ous** (an″tĭ-mo′ne-əs) containing antimony in its triad valency.

**an·ti·mo·ni·um** (an″tĭ-mo′ne-əm) gen. *antimo′nii* [L.] antimony.

**an·ti·mo·ny** (an′tĭ-mo″ne) [L. *antimonium* or *stibium*] [MeSH: Antimony] a crystalline metallic element with a bluish luster, symbol Sb, atomic number 51, atomic weight 121.75, forming various medicinal and poisonous salts. See also *antimony poisoning* and *antimony pneumoconiosis.*

**a. pentoxide,** a white or yellowish powder, $Sb_2O_5$, used in preparation of antimony compounds; called also *antimonic acid.*

**a. potassium tartrate** [USP], a trivalent antimony compound used as an antischistosomal, especially for treatment of *Schistosoma japonicum* infections, administered intravenously; now rarely used because of its toxicity. It was formerly used in other tropical diseases and as a nauseant emetic.

**a. sodium dimercaptosuccinate,** stibocaptate.

**a. sodium tartrate** [USP], a trivalent antimony compound having the same actions and uses as the potassium tartrate but more water-soluble and less irritant when injected; now rarely used because of its toxicity.

**tartrated a.,** a. potassium tartrate.

**a. trioxide,** a white odorless crystalline powder, $Sb_2O_3$, used in the preparation of tartar emetic (antimony potassium tartrate).

**an·ti·mo·nyl** (an-tim′o-nil″) the univalent radical SbO—.

**an·ti·mül·le·ri·an** (an″tĭ-mu-le′re-ən) inhibiting the development of müllerian ducts, such as an antimüllerian hormone.

**an·ti·mus·ca·rin·ic** (an″tĭ-mus′kə-rin′ik) 1. effective against the toxic effects of muscarine. 2. blocking the muscarinic receptors. 3. an agent that counteracts the effects of muscarine or blocks the muscarinic receptors.

**an·ti·mu·ta·gen** (an″tĭ-mu′tə-jen) a substance that antagonizes the mutagenic effects of other substances.

**an·ti·my·as·then·ic** (an″tĭ-mi″əs-then′ik) 1. counteracting or relieving muscular weakness in myasthenia gravis. 2. an agent that counteracts or relieves muscular weakness in myasthenia gravis.

**an·ti·my·co·bac·te·ri·al** (an″tĭ-mi″ko-bak-te′re-əl) 1. effective against mycobacteria. 2. an agent that is effective against mycobacteria.

**an·ti·my·cot·ic** (an″tĭ-mi-kot′ik) 1. destructive to fungi, or suppressing their reproduction or growth; effective against fungal infections. 2. an agent that is destructive to fungi, suppresses the growth or reproduction of fungi, or is effective against fungal infections. Called also *antifungal.*

**an·ti·nar·cot·ic** (an″tĭ-nahr-kot′ik) counteracting narcotic depression.

**an·ti·na·tri·ure·sis** (an″tĭ-na″tre-u-re′sis) any condition characterized by low excretion of sodium in the urine.

**an·ti·nau·se·ant** (an″tĭ-naw′ze-ənt) 1. preventing or relieving nausea. 2. an agent that prevents or relieves nausea. See also *antiemetic.*

**an·ti·neo·plas·tic** (an″tĭ-ne″o-plas′tik) 1. inhibiting or preventing the development of neoplasms; checking the maturation and proliferation of malignant cells. 2. an agent having such properties.

**an·ti·ne·phrit·ic** (an″tĭ-nə-frit′ik) counteracting inflammation of the kidneys.

**an·ti·neu·ral·gic** (an″tĭ-noo͞-ral′jik) counteracting neuralgia.

**an·ti·neu·rit·ic** (an″tĭ-noo͞-rit′ik) counteracting neuritis.

**an·ti·neu·ro·tox·in** (an″ti-noo͞″ro-tok′sin) a substance that counteracts a neurotoxin.

**an·ti·neu·tri·no** (an″tĭ-noo-tre′no) the antiparticle of the neutrino.

**an·ti·neu·tron** (an″tĭ-noo′tron) an elementary particle without a charge and with a mass and spin equal to that of a neutron, but with magnetic moment opposite to that of a neutron; the antiparticle of a neutron.

**an·tin·i·ad** (an-tin′e-ad) toward the antinion.

**an·tin·i·al** (an-tin′e-əl) pertaining to the antinion.

**an·tin·ion** (an-tin′e-on) [*anti-* + *inion*] the frontal pole of the head; the median frontal point farthest from the inion.

**an·ti·no·ci·cep·tive** (an″tĭ-no″sĭ-sep′tiv) having an analgesic effect; reducing sensitivity to painful stimuli.

**an·ti·nu·cle·ar** (an″tĭ-noo′kle-ər) destructive to or reactive with components of the cell nucleus, as antinuclear antibody.

**an·ti·odon·tal·gic** (an″tĭ-o″don-tal′jik) relieving toothache.

**an·ti·on·co·gene** (an″te-ong′ko-jēn″) [MeSH: Genes, Suppressor, Tumor] tumor suppressor gene.

**an·ti·op·so·nin** (an″te-op′so-nin) a substance that has an inhibitory influence on opsonins; called also *antitropin.*

**an·ti·ov·u·la·to·ry** (an″te-ov′u-lə-to″re) suppressing ovulation.

**an·ti·ox·i·dant** (an″te-ok′sĭ-dənt) one of many widely used synthetic or natural substances added to a product to prevent or delay its deterioration by action of oxygen in the air. Rubber, paints, vegetable oils, and prepared foods commonly contain antioxidants.

**an·ti·ox·i·da·tion** (an″te-ok-sĭ-da′shən) the prevention of oxidation.

**an·ti·oxy·gen** (an″te-ok′sĭ-jen) antioxidant.

**an·ti·par·al·lel** (an″tĭ-par′ə-lel) denoting molecules that are arranged side by side, but in opposite directions. For example, the strands of deoxyribonucleic acid are antiparallel with their 5′ to 3′ linkages running in opposite directions.

**an·ti·par·a·lyt·ic** (an″tĭ-par″ə-lit′ik) [*anti-* + *paralysis*] relieving paralysis.

**an·ti·par·a·sit·ic** (an″tĭ-par″ə-sit ′ik) 1. destructive to parasites. 2. an agent destructive to parasites.

**an·ti·pa·ras·ta·ta** (an″tĭ-pə-ras′tə-tə) [*anti-* + Gr. *parastatēs* testis] glandula bulbourethralis.

**an·ti·para·sym·patho·mi·met·ic** (an″tĭ-par″ə-sim″pə-tho-mĭ-met′ik) opposing or blocking a parasympathomimetic agent or effect.

**an·ti·par·kin·so·ni·an** (an″tĭ-pahr″kin-so′ne-ən) 1. effective in the treatment of parkinsonism. 2. an agent effective in the treatment of parkinsonism.

**an·ti·par·ti·cle** (an′tĭ-pahr″tĭ-kəl) either of a pair of particles, as an electron and a positron, that are identical in mass and spin but opposite in charge and magnetic moment; the collision of two antiparticles results in annihilation.

**an·ti·pe·dic·u·lar** (an″tĭ-pĕ-dik′u-lər) effective against *Pediculus* (sucking lice), or in the treatment of pediculosis; antipediculotic.

**an·ti·ped·i·cu·lot·ic** (an″tĭ-pĕ-dik″u-lot′ik) 1. effective against lice. 2. an agent effective against lice.

**an·ti·pe·ri·od·ic** (an″tĭ-pe″re-od′ik) preventing periodic recurrence of symptoms, as in malaria.

**an·ti·per·i·stal·sis** (an″tĭ-per″ĭ-stal′sis) reversed peristalsis.

**an·ti·per·i·stal·tic** (an″tĭ-per′ĭ-stal′tik) 1. pertaining to or causing antiperistalsis. 2. diminishing peristaltic action. 3. an agent that diminishes peristaltic action.

**an·ti·per·spir·ant** (an″tĭ-pər′spər-ant″) 1. inhibiting or preventing perspiration. 2. an agent that inhibits or prevents perspiration.

**an·ti·phago·cyt·ic** (an″tĭ-fag-o-sit′ik) counteracting or opposing phagocytosis.

**an·ti·phlo·gis·tic** (an″tĭ-flo-jis′tik) 1. counteracting inflammation and fever. 2. an agent that counteracts inflammation and fever.

**an·ti·phry·nol·y·sin** (an″tĭ-frĭ-nol′ĭ-sin) the antivenin for the toxin of toad venom.

**an·ti·phthi·ri·ac** (an″tĭ-thĕr′e-ak) effective against lice.

**an·ti·plas·min** (an″tĭ-plaz′min) [MeSH: Antiplasmin] a substance in the blood that inhibits plasmin.

**$\alpha_2$-a.,** the most important inhibitor of fibrinolysis, an $\alpha_2$-globulin, $M_r$ 53,000, found in large quantities in normal blood; it is synthesized predominantly in the liver and functions by forming stable complexes with free plasmin. It is also cross-linked to fibrin by the action of coagulation factor XIII and inhibits the binding of plasminogen to fibrin. Deficiency of this protein, an autosomal recessive trait, is associated with severe bleeding, including hemarthrosis.

**an·ti·plas·mo·di·al** (an″tĭ-plaz-mo′de-əl) having a destructive action on plasmodia.

**an·ti·plas·tic** (an″tĭ-plas′tik) [*anti-* + *plastic*] 1. unfavorable to the healing process. 2. suppressing cell formation. 3. myelosuppressive.

**an·ti·plate·let** (an″tĭ-plāt′lət) directed against or destructive to blood platelets. See also *platelet inhibitor,* under *inhibitor.*

**an·ti·pneu·mo·coc·cal** (an″tĭ-noo″mo-kok′əl) destroying or inhibiting the growth of *Streptococcus pneumoniae.*

**an·ti·pneu·mo·coc·cic** (an″tĭ-noo″mo-kok′sik) antipneumococcal.

**an·ti·po·dag·ric** (an″tĭ-po-dag′rik) effective against gout.

**an·tip·o·dal** (an-tip′ə-dəl) occupying opposite positions, as of a cell or body; diametrically opposed.

**an·ti·pode** (an′tĭ-pōd) something occupying a directly opposed position. In chemistry, a molecule whose atoms are arranged in a directly opposite manner.

**an·ti·poly·cy·the·mic** (an″tĭ-pol″e-si-the′mik) 1. effective against polycythemia. 2. an agent effective against polycythemia.

**an·ti·port** (an′tĭ-port) a mechanism of coupling the transport of two compounds across a membrane in opposite directions. Cf. *countertransport* and *symport.*

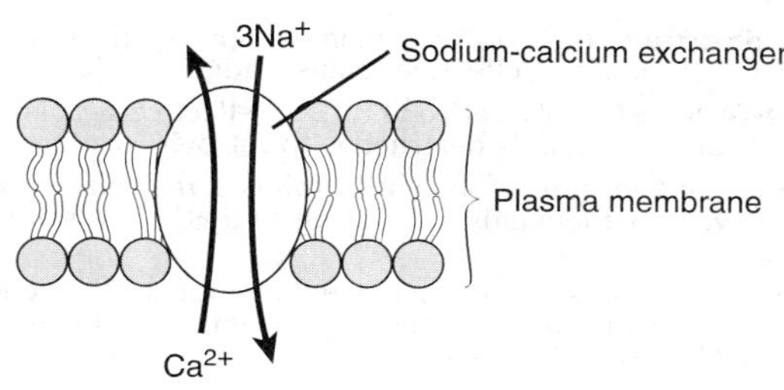


Antiport: sodium-calcium exchanger. The electrochemical gradient of $Na^+$ is used to pump $Ca^{2+}$ out of the cell and thereby regulate the cytosolic $Ca^{2+}$ level.

**an·ti·po·sia** (an″tĭ-po′zhə) antipathy to drinking.

**an·ti·pre·ci·pi·tin** (an″tĭ-pre-sip′ĭ-tin) a substance antagonistic in its action to precipitin.

**an·ti·pro·ges·tin** (an″tĭ-pro-jes′tin) a substance that inhibits the formation of progestational agents; the most common example is mifepristone.

**an·ti·pros·tate** (an″tĭ-pros′tāt) glandula bulbourethralis.

**an·ti·pro·throm·bin** (an″tĭ-pro-throm′bin) 1. directed against prothrombin. 2. any of a diverse group of anticoagulants that retard the conversion of prothrombin to thrombin by any means.

**an·ti·pro·to·zo·al** (an″tĭ-pro-tə-zo′əl) 1. destroying protozoa, or checking their growth or reproduction. 2. an agent that destroys protozoa, or checks their growth or reproduction.

**an·ti·pro·to·zo·an** (an″tĭ-pro-tə-zo′ən) antiprotozoal.

**an·ti·pru·rit·ic** (an″tĭ-proo-rit′ik) 1. relieving or preventing itching. 2. an agent, usually a topical application, that relieves or prevents itching.

**an·ti·pso·ri·at·ic** (an″tĭ-so″re-at′ik) 1. effective against psoriasis. 2. an agent effective against psoriasis.

**an·ti·psy·cho·mo·tor** (an″tĭ-si′ko-mo′tor) suppressing or inhibiting hyperactivity or hyperkinesis.

**an·ti·psy·chot·ic** (an″tĭ-si-kot′ik) effective in the treatment of psychosis, or an agent that so acts. Antipsychotic agents (called also *neuroleptic* agents) are a chemically diverse (including phenothiazines, thioxanthenes, butyrophenones, dibenzoxazepines, dibenzodiazepines, dihydroindolones, and diphenylbutylpiperidines) but pharmacologically similar class of drugs used to treat schizophrenic, paranoid, schizoaffective, and other psychotic disorders; acute delirium and dementia and manic episodes (during induction of lithium therapy); to control the movement disorders associated with Huntington's chorea, Gilles de la Tourette's syndrome, and ballismus; and to treat intractable hiccups and severe nausea and vomiting. Antipsychotic agents bind to dopamine, histamine, muscarinic cholinergic, $\alpha$-adrenergic, and serotonin receptors. Blockade of dopaminergic transmission in various areas is thought to be responsible for their major effects: antipsychotic action by blockade in the mesolimbic and mesocortical areas; extrapyramidal side effects (dystonia, akathisia, parkinsonism, and tardive dyskinesia) by blockade in the basal ganglia; and antiemetic effects by blockade in the chemoreceptor trigger zone of the medulla. Sedation and autonomic side effects (orthostatic hypotension, blurred vision, dry mouth, nasal congestion, and constipation) are caused by blockade of histamine, cholinergic, and adrenergic receptors.

**an·ti·pu·tre·fac·tive** (an″tĭ-pu″trə-fak′tiv) counteracting putrefaction.

**an·ti·pyo·gen·ic** (an″tĭ-pi″o-jen′ik) [*anti-* + *pyogenic*] preventing or hindering the development of pus.

**an·ti·py·re·sis** (an″tĭ-pi-re′sis) [*anti-* + Gr. *pyressein* to have a fever] the therapeutic use of antipyretics.

**an·ti·py·ret·ic** (an″tĭ-pi-ret′ik) [*anti-* + *pyretic*] 1. relieving or reducing fever. Called also *antifebrile, antithermic,* and *febrifugal.* 2. an agent that relieves or reduces fever. Called also *febricide* and *febrifuge.*

**an·ti·py·rine** (an″tĭ-pi′rēn) [USP] [MeSH: Antipyrine] phenazone; a pyrazolone analgesic and antipyretic. Because it can cause agranulocytosis, it has been replaced by safer and more effective agents. Now used as a component of antipyrine and benzocaine otic solution; as a component of antipyrine, benzocaine, and phenylephrine otic solution; and complexed with chloral hydrate in dichloralphenazone.

**an·ti·py·rot·ic** (an″tĭ-pi-rot′ik) [*anti-* + *pyrotic*] 1. therapeutically effective against burns. 2. an agent that is effective in the treatment of burns.

**an·ti·ra·di·a·tion** (an″tĭ-ra″de-a′shən) capable of counteracting the effects of radiation; effective against radiation injury.

**an·ti·ret·ro·vi·ral** (an″tĭ-ret′ro-vi″rəl) 1. effective against retroviruses. 2. an agent that is destructive to retroviruses.

**an·ti·rheu·mat·ic** (an″tĭ-roo-mat′ik) [*anti-* + *rheumatic*] 1. relieving or preventing rheumatism. 2. an agent that relieves or prevents rheumatism.

**an·ti·ri·cin** (an″tĭ-ri′sin) a substance that opposes the action of ricin (e.g., antitoxin produced following the introduction of ricin into the animal body).

**an·ti·rick·ett·si·al** (an″tĭ-rĭ-ket′se-əl) 1. effective against rickettsiae. 2. an agent that is effective against rickettsiae.

**an·ti·ro·bin** (an″tĭ-ro′bin) the antitoxin of robin, a poison of the locust tree.

**an·ti·sal·ure·sis** (an″tĭ-sal″u-re′sis) antinatriuresis.

**an·ti·schis·to·so·mal** (an″tĭ-shis″to-so′məl) 1. effective against schistosomes. 2. an agent that is destructive to schistosomes.

**an·ti·scor·bu·tic** (an″tĭ-skor-bu′tik) [*anti-* + *scorbutus*] effective in the prevention or relief of scurvy.

**an·ti·se·cre·to·ry** (an″tĭ-sə-kre′to-re) 1. inhibiting or diminishing secretion; called also *secretoinhibitory.* 2. an agent that so acts, as certain drugs that inhibit or diminish gastric secretions.

**an·ti·sense** (an″tĭ-sens′) pertaining to the antisense strand of a nucleic acid; see under *strand* and *RNA.*

**an·ti·sep·sis** (an″tĭ-sep′sis) [*anti-* + *sepsis*] [MeSH: Antisepsis] 1. the prevention of sepsis by antiseptic means. 2. any procedure that reduces to a significant degree the microbial flora of skin or mucous membranes.
**physiologic a.,** the combination of methods by which the body excludes germs; called also *autoantisepsis.*

**an·ti·sep·tic** (an″tĭ-sep′tik) 1. pertaining to antisepsis. 2. preventing decay or putrefaction. 3. a substance that inhibits the growth and development of microorganisms without necessarily killing them. Cf. *disinfectant* and *germicide.*

**an·ti·se·rum** (an″tĭ-se′rəm) a serum that contains antibody or antibodies; it may be obtained from an animal that has been immunized either by injection of antigen into the body or by infection with microorganisms containing the antigen. Antisera may be monovalent (specific for one antigen) or polyvalent (specific for more than one antigen).
***Erysipelothrix rhusiopathiae* a.,** an antiserum prepared by hyperimmunization of horses with *Erysipelothrix rhusiopathiae,* used for prevention and treatment of swine erysipelas.

**an·ti·si·al·a·gogue** (an″tĭ-si-al′ə-agog) 1. counteracting the formation of saliva. 2. an agent that counteracts any influence that promotes the flow of saliva.

**an·ti·si·al·ic** (an″tĭ-si-al′ik) [*anti-* + *sialic*] 1. checking the flow of saliva. 2. an agent that checks the secretion of saliva.

**an·ti·sid·er·ic** (an″tĭ-sĭ-der′ik) [*anti-* + *sider-* + *-ic*] incompatible with iron.

**an·ti·so·cial** (an″tĭ-so′shəl) 1. denoting behavior that violates the rights of others, societal mores, or the law. 2. denoting the specific personality traits seen in *antisocial personality disorder* (see under *personality*).

**an·ti·spas·mod·ic** (an″tĭ-spaz-mod′ik) 1. relieving spasm, usually of smooth muscle, as in arteries, bronchi, intestine, bile duct, ureters or sphincters, but also of voluntary muscle. Cf. *antispastic.* 2. an agent that relieves spasm.
**biliary a.,** an agent that relieves spasm of the biliary duct and sphincter.
**bronchial a.,** an agent that relieves bronchial spasm.

**an·ti·spas·tic** (an″tĭ-spas′tik) antispasmodic with specific reference to skeletal muscle.

**an·ti·staph·y·lo·coc·cic** (an″tĭ-staf″ə-lo-kok′sik) killing or suppressing staphylococci.

**an·ti·staph·y·lo·he·mol·y·sin** (an″tĭ-staf″ə-lo-he-mol′ĭ-sin) antistaphylolysin.

**an·ti·staph·y·lol·y·sin** (an″tĭ-staf-ə-lol′ĭ-sin) an antibody that opposes the action of staphylolysin.

**an·ti·ste·ril·i·ty** (an″tĭ-stĕ-ril′ĭ-te) combating sterility.

**An·tis·tine** (an-tis′tin) trademark for preparations of antazoline.

**an·ti·strep·to·coc·cic** (an″tĭ-strep″to-kok′sik) 1. effective against streptococci. 2. an agent that is effective against streptococci.

**an·ti·strep·to·ki·nase** (an″tĭ-strep″to-ki-nās) an antibody that inhibits streptokinase.

**an·ti·strep·tol·y·sin** (an″tĭ-strep-tol′ĭ-sin) [MeSH: Antistreptolysin] an antibody that inhibits streptolysin.

**an·ti·su·do·ral** (an″tĭ-soo′də-rəl) antisudorific.

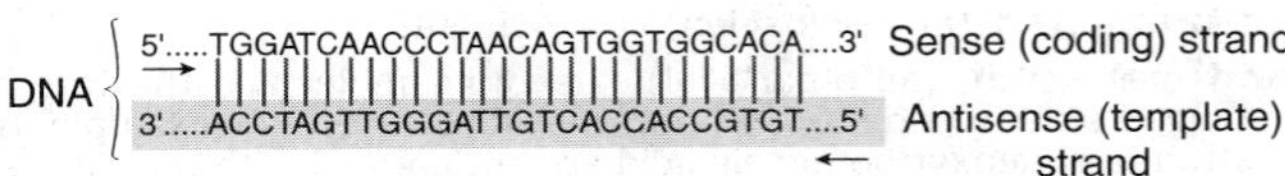


Antisense strand of DNA, complementary to the sense (coding) strand and serving as a template for RNA synthesis.

**an·ti·su·dor·if·ic** (an″tĭ-soo″dor-if′ik) [*anti-* + *sudorific*] 1. inhibiting perspiration. 2. an agent that inhibits perspiration.

**an·ti·sym·pa·thet·ic** (an″tĭ-sim″pə-thet′ik) sympatholytic.

**an·ti·tem·plate** (an″tĭ-tem′plāt) a hypothetical substance said to inhibit mitosis of normal cells and, on injury to cells, to diffuse out of the cells to initiate mitosis.

**an·ti·te·tan·ic** (an″tĭ-tə-tan′ik) preventing or curing tetanus.

**an·ti·the·nar** (an″tĭ-the′nar) [*anti-* + *thenar*] situated opposite to the palm or the sole.

**an·ti·ther·mic** (an″tĭ-thər′mik) [*anti-* + *thermic*] antipyretic (def. 1).

**an·ti·throm·bin** (an″tĭ-throm′bin) [*anti-* + *thrombin*] any naturally occurring or therapeutically administered substance that neutralizes the action of thrombin and thus limits or restricts blood coagulation. Six naturally occurring antithrombins have been designated by Roman numerals I to VI; antithrombins I and III are the most common and significant ones. Heparin is also considered an antithrombin.
**a. I,** fibrin; referring to the capacity of fibrin to adsorb large amounts of thrombin and thus neutralize (but not inactivate) it.
**a. III,** an $\alpha_2$-globulin of the serpin family synthesized in the liver and found in plasma and various extravascular sites, which inactivates thrombin in a time-dependent irreversible reaction. It also inhibits certain other proteinases with serine active sites, including coagulation factors Xa, XIIa, XIa, and IXa, and kallikrein. Inherited deficiency of the protein, a rare autosomal dominant disorder, is associated with recurrent deep vein thrombosis and pulmonary emboli.

**an·ti·throm·bo·plas·tin** (an″tĭ-throm″bo-plas′tin) any agent or substance that prevents or interferes with the interaction of the blood coagulation factors as they generate prothrombinase.

**an·ti·throm·bot·ic** (an″tĭ-throm-bot′ik) 1. preventing or interfering with the formation of thrombi. 2. an agent that so acts; see also *anticoagulant* and *thrombolytic.*

**an·ti·thy·roid** (an″tĭ-thi′roid) counteracting the functioning of the thyroid, especially in its synthesis of thyroid hormones.

**an·ti·thy·ro·tox·ic** (an″tĭ-thi″ro-tok′sik) counteracting the toxic effects of excessive amounts of thyroid hormones.

**an·ti·thy·ro·trop·ic** (an″tĭ-thi″ro-trop′ik) inhibiting the secretion or actions of thyrotropin.

**an·ti·ton·ic** (an″tĭ-ton′ik) reducing tone or tonicity.

**an·ti·tox·ic** (an″tĭ-tok′sik) 1. effective against a poison. 2. pertaining to antitoxin.

**an·ti·tox·i·gen** (an″tĭ-tok′sĭ-jən) antitoxinogen.

**an·ti·tox·in** (an″tĭ-tok′sin) 1. antibody against a toxin. 2. a purified antiserum from animals (usually horses) immunized by injections of a toxin or toxoid, administered as a passive immunizing agent to neutralize a specific bacterial toxin, e.g., botulinus, tetanus, or diphtheria.
**botulinal a., botulinum a., botulinus a.,** botulism a.
**botulism a.** [USP], an equine antitoxin against the toxins produced by the type A, B, or E strain of *Clostridium botulinum.* Generally trivalent (ABE) antitoxin is used. Called also *botulinal a., botulinum a.,* and *botulinus a.*
**bovine a.,** antitoxin containing antibodies derived from the cow instead of from the horse, for use on persons who are hypersensitive to horse serum.
***Clostridium perfringens* types C and D a.,** an antitoxin prepared from serum of animals hyperimmunized with toxins of *C. perfringens* types C and D, administered immediately after birth for prevention of enterotoxemia in calves, lambs, and suckling pigs.
**diphtheria a.** [USP], equine antitoxin against the toxin of *Corynebacterium diphtheriae,* used for treatment of diphtheria.
**equine a.,** an antitoxin derived from the blood of healthy horses that have been immunized against a specific bacterial toxin.
**gas gangrene a.,** a polyvalent equine antitoxin against toxins of *Clostridium* species causing gas gangrene, formerly administered for prevention or treatment of gas gangrene.
**tetanus a.** [USP], equine antitoxin against the toxins of *Clostridium tetani;* used for the passive prevention and treatment of tetanus. It is rarely used, tetanus immune globulin being preferred if available.
**tetanus and gas gangrene a's,** a combination of tetanus and gas gangrene antitoxins.

**an·ti·tox·in·o·gen** (an″tĭ-tok-sin′o-jen) [*antitoxin* + *-gen*] an antigen that stimulates the production of antitoxin, i.e., a toxin or toxoid.

**an·ti·tox·i·num** (an″tĭ-tok-si′nəm) [L.] antitoxin.

**an·ti·trag·i·cus** (an″tĭ-traj′ĭ-kəs) see under *musculus.*

**an·ti·tra·gus** (an″tĭ-tra′gəs) [*anti-* + *tragus*] [TA] a projection opposite the tragus, bounding the cavitas conchae posteroinferiorly and continuous above with the anthelix.

**an·ti·trep·o·ne·mal** (an″tĭ-trep″o-ne′məl) 1. effective against *Treponema.* 2. an agent that is effective against *Treponema.*

**an·ti·trich·o·mo·nal** (an″tĭ-trik″o-mo′nəl) 1. effective against *Trichomonas.* 2. an agent that is destructive to *Trichomonas.*

**an·ti·tris·mus** (an″tĭ-triz′məs) a spasm that prevents the closure of the mouth.

**an·ti·trope** (an′tĭ-trōp) [*anti-* + Gr. *trepein* to turn] any organ that forms a symmetrical pair with another.

**an·ti·trop·ic** (an″tĭ-trop′ik) corresponding, but oppositely oriented, as a right and a left glove.

**an·ti·tro·pin** (an″tĭ-tro′pin) antiopsonin.

**an·ti·try·pan·o·so·mal** (an″tĭ-trĭ-pan″ə-so′məl) 1. effective against trypanosomes. 2. a drug for combating trypanosomiasis.

**$\alpha_1$-an·ti·tryp·sin** (an″tĭ-trip′sin) alpha$_1$-antitrypsin.

**an·ti·tu·ber·cu·lin** (an″tĭ-too-bər′ku-lin) an antibody developed following the injection of tuberculin.

**an·ti·tu·ber·cu·lot·ic** (an″tĭ-too-bər″ku-lot′ik) 1. therapeutically effective against tuberculosis; called also *antituberculous.* 2. an agent that is therapeutically effective against tuberculosis.

**an·ti·tu·ber·cu·lous** (an″tĭ-too-bər′ku-ləs) therapeutically effective against tuberculosis.

**an·ti·tu·bu·lin** (an″tĭ-too′bu-lin) an agent that prevents the polymerization of tubulin, and thus the formation of microtubules in a cell.

**an·ti·tu·mor·i·gen·ic** (an″tĭ-too″mər-ĭ-jen′ik) counteracting tumor formation.

**an·ti·tus·sive** (an″tĭ-tus′iv) 1. relieving or preventing cough. 2. an agent that relieves or prevents cough.

**an·ti·ty·phoid** (an″tĭ-ti′foid) counteracting or preventing typhoid.

**an·ti·ul·cer·a·tive** (an″te-ul′sər-ə″tiv) 1. preventing or promoting the healing of ulcers. 2. an agent that so acts.

**an·ti·urat·ic** (an″tĭ-u-rat′ik) preventing the deposit of urates.

**an·ti·uro·lith·ic** (an″tĭ-u″ro-lith′ik) 1. preventing the formation of urinary calculi. 2. an agent that prevents the formation of urinary calculi.

**an·ti·vac·ci·na·tion·ist** (an″tĭ-vak″sĭ-na′shən-ist) a person who is opposed to vaccination.

**an·ti·ven·ene** (an″tĭ-vĕ-nēn′) [*anti-* + L. *venenum* poison] antivenin.

**an·ti·ven·in** (an″tĭ-ven′in) [*anti-* + L. *venenum* poison] a proteinaceous material used in the treatment of poisoning by animal venom. See also *antivenomous serum,* under *serum.*
**black widow spider a.,** a. *(Latrodectus mactans).*
**a. (Crotalidae) polyvalent** [USP], a lyophilized preparation containing specific venom-neutralizing globulins obtained from the serum of horses immunized with the venoms of *Crotalus atrox* (western diamondback rattlesnake), *C. adamanteus* (eastern diamondback rattlesnake), *C. durissus terrificus* (tropical rattlesnake), and *Bothrops atrox* (fer-de-lance); used to neutralize the effects of envenomation by pit vipers native to North, Central, and South America.
**a. *(Latrodectus mactans)*** [USP], a lyophilized preparation containing specific venom-neutralizing globulins obtained from the serum of horses immunized with the venom of *Latrodectus mactans* (the black widow spider); occasionally used to treat the symptoms of black widow spider bites. Called also *black widow spider a.*
**a. *(Micrurus fulvius)*** [USP], a lyophilized preparation containing specific venom-neutralizing globulins obtained from the serum of horses immunized with the venom of *Micrurus fulvius* (the eastern coral snake); used to neutralize the effects of envenomation by the eastern coral snake *(M. fulvius fulvius)* and the Texas coral snake *(M. fulvius tenere).* Called also *North American coral snake a.*
**North American coral snake a.,** a. *(Micrurus fulvius).*
**polyvalent crotaline a.,** a. (Crotalidae) polyvalent.

**an·ti·ven·om** (an″tĭ-ven′om) antivenin.

**an·ti·ven·om·ous** (an″tĭ-ven′ə-məs) counteracting venom.

**An·ti·vert** (an′tĭ-vert″) trademark for a preparation of meclizine hydrochloride.

**an·ti·vi·ral** (an″tĭ-vi′rəl) 1. destroying viruses or suppressing their replication. 2. an agent that destroys viruses or suppresses their replication.

**an·ti·vi·rot·ic** (an″tĭ-vi-rot′ik) antiviral.

**an·ti·vi·ta·min** (an″tĭ-vi′tə-min) a substance that interferes with the synthesis or metabolism of a vitamin.

**an·ti·vivi·sec·tion** (an″tĭ-viv″ĭ-sek′shən) opposition to vivisection.

**an·ti·vivi·sec·tion·ist** (an″tĭ-viv″ĭ-sek′shən-ist) an individual opposed to vivisection.

**an·ti·xen·ic** (an″tĭ-ze′nik) [*anti-* + Gr. *xenos* strange or foreign] pertaining to the reaction of living tissue to any foreign substance.

**an·ti·xe·roph·thal·mic** (an″tĭ-ze″rof-thal′mik) counteracting xerophthalmia.

**an·ti·xe·rot·ic** (an″tĭ-ze-rot′ik) counteracting or preventing xerosis.

**ant·odon·tal·gic** (ant″-o-don-tal′jik) antiodontalgic.

**An·ton's syndrome (symptom)** (ahn′tonz) [Gabriel *Anton,* German neuropsychiatrist, 1858–1933] see under *syndrome.*

**An·ton-Ba·bin·ski syndrome** (ahn′ton-bə-bin′ske) [G. *Anton;* Joseph François Félix *Babinski,* French physician, 1857–1932] Anton's syndrome.

**ant·oph·thal·mic** (ant″of-thal′mik) relieving ophthalmia.

**ant·or·phine** (ant-or′fēn) nalorphine.

**an·tra** (an′trə) [L.] plural of *antrum.*

**an·tral** (an′trəl) of or pertaining to an antrum.

**an·trec·to·my** (an-trek′tə-me) [*antr-* + *-ectomy*] surgical excision of an antrum, as resection of the pyloric antrum of the stomach.

**An·tre·nyl** (an′trə-nəl) trademark for a preparation of oxyphenonium.

**An·tri·co·la** (an-trik′ə-lə) a genus of ticks of the family Argasidae; they infest birds and bats.

**an·tri·tis** (an-tri′tis) 1. inflammation of an antrum. 2. maxillary sinusitis.

**antr(o)-** [L. *antrum,* q.v.] a combining form denoting relationship to an antrum, or sinus; often used with specific reference to the maxillary antrum, or sinus.

**an·tro·at·ti·cot·o·my** (an″tro-at″ĭ-kot′ə-me) atticoantrotomy.

**an·tro·buc·cal** (an″tro-buk′əl) pertaining to or communicating with the maxillary antrum (sinus) and (oral) buccal cavity, as an antrobuccal fistula.

**an·tro·cele** (an′tro-sēl) [*antro-* + *-cele*[1]] a cystic accumulation of fluid in the maxillary antrum (sinus).

**an·tro·du·o·de·nal** (an″tro-doo″o-de′nəl) [*antro-* + *duodenal*] pertaining to the antrum of the stomach and the duodenum.

**an·tro·du·o·de·nec·to·my** (an″tro-doo″o-de-nek′tə-me) surgical removal of the pyloric antrum and adjacent portion of the duodenum, formerly done in the treatment of duodenal ulcer.

**an·tro·dyn·ia** (an″tro-din′e-ə) [*antro-* + *-odynia*] pain in an antrum.

**an·tro·na·sal** (an″tro-na′zəl) pertaining to the maxillary antrum and the nose.

**an·tro·phore** (an′tro-for) [*antro-* + Gr. *pherein* to bear] a form of soluble medicated bougie.

**an·tro·phose** (an′tro-fōz) [*antro-* + *phose*] a phose originating in the central ocular mechanism.

**an·tro·py·lo·ric** (an″tro-pi-lor′ik) pertaining to or affecting the pyloric part of the stomach, including its antrum.

**an·tro·scope** (an′trə-skōp″) [*antro-* + *-scope*] an instrument for illuminating and examining the maxillary antrum.

**an·tros·co·py** (an-tros′kə-pe) inspection of an antrum using an antroscope.

**an·tros·to·my** (an-tros′tə-me) [*antro-* + *-stomy*] the operation of making an opening into an antrum for purposes of drainage.

**an·trot·o·my** (an-trot′ə-me) [*antro-* + *-tomy*] antrostomy.

**an·tro·tym·pan·ic** (an″tro-tim-pan′ik) pertaining to the mastoid antrum and the tympanic cavity.

**an·trum** (an′trəm) pl. *an′trums* or *an′tra* [L.; Gr. *antron* cave] [TA] general term used in anatomical nomenclature for a cavity or chamber, especially within a bone.
**a. au′ris,** meatus acusticus externus.
**cardiac a., a. cardi′acum,** the short conical portion of the esophagus below the diaphragm, its base being continuous with the cardiac orifice of the stomach.
**ethmoid a., a. ethmoida′le,** bulla ethmoidalis ossis ethmoidalis.
**frontal a.,** sinus frontalis.
**gastric a.,** a. pylori.
**a. of Highmore, a. highmo′ri,** sinus maxillaris.
**a. mastoi′deum** [TA], mastoid antrum: an air space in the mastoid portion of the temporal bone, communicating with the tympanic cavity and the mastoid cells; called also *a. tympanicum, tympanic a.,* and *mastoid cavity.*
**a. maxilla′re, maxillary a.,** sinus maxillaris.
**a. pylo′ri, a. pylor′icum** [TA], pyloric antrum: the dilated portion of the pyloric part of the stomach, between the body of the stomach and the pyloric canal; called also *a. of Willis* and *gastric a.*

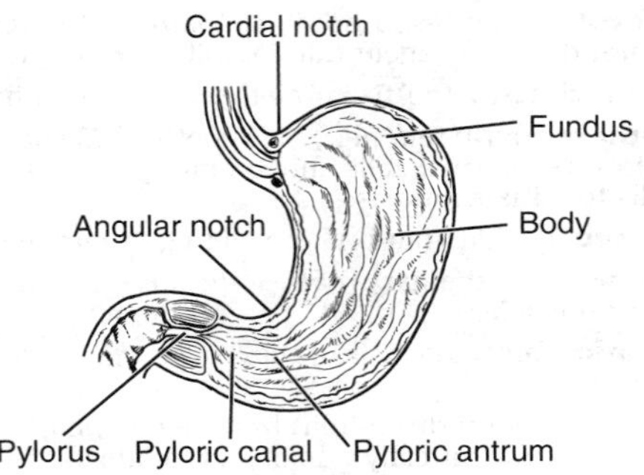

Antrum pyloricum (pyloric antrum).

**tympanic a., a. tympa′nicum,** a. mastoideum.
**a. of Willis,** a. pyloricum.

**An·try·pol** (an′trə-pol) trademark for a preparation of suramin sodium.

**ANTU** alphanaphthyl thiourea, a compound used as a rodenticide; it produces massive pulmonary edema and pleural effusion in rats and many other mammals.

**An·tu·rane** (an′choo-rān) trademark for a preparation of sulfinpyrazone.

**An·tyl·lus** (an-til′əs) (2nd or 3rd century A.D.) a noted Greek surgeon of antiquity, a Pneumatist, whose treatment of aneurysms by ligation above and below remained standard practice until the time of John Hunter (18th century). He also made contributions to plastic surgery, ophthalmology, and public health. His writings remain only in fragments, and in the works of others (particularly Oribasius).

**a·nu·cle·ar** (a-noo′kle-ər) having no nuclei; said of cells, such as erythrocytes, which have lost their nuclei.

**a·nu·cle·at·ed** (a-noo′kle-āt″əd) denucleated.

**ANUG** acute necrotizing ulcerative gingivitis.

**anu·lo·plas·ty** (an″u-lo-plas′te) annuloplasty.

**anu·lus** (an′u-ləs) gen. and pl. *a′nuli* [L., from *anus* ring] [TA] ring: general anatomic nomenclature for a circular or ringlike structure; written also *annulus.* See also *circle* and *circulus.*
**a. abdomina′lis, a. abdomina′lis abdo′minis,** anulus inguinalis profundus.
**atrioventricular anuli, atrioventricular valve anuli,** see *anulus fibrosus dexter/sinister cordis.*
**a. conjunc′tivae** [TA], conjunctival ring: a ring at the junction of the conjunctiva and cornea.
**a. femora′lis** [TA], femoral ring: the abdominal opening of the femoral canal, normally closed by the crural septum and peritoneum; called also *crural* or *femoral fossa, inferior digital fossa, crural* or *femoral fovea* and *hiatus femoralis.*
**a. fibrocartilagi′neus membra′nae tym′pani** [TA], fibrocartilaginous ring of tympanic membrane: the margin of the pars tensa of the tympanic membrane, which attaches to the sulcus tympanicus.
**a. fibro′sus dex′ter/sinis′ter cor′dis** [TA], right/left fibrous ring of heart: one of the dense fibrous rings that surround the right and left atrioventricular orifices. To these rings, either directly or indirectly, are attached the atrial and ventricular muscle fibers. The rings form part of the cardiac skeleton. Called also *Lower's rings.*
**a. fibro′sus dis′ci intervertebra′lis** [TA], fibrous ring of intervertebral disk: the circumferential ringlike portion of an intervertebral disk, composed of fibrocartilage and fibrous tissue.
**a. inguina′lis profun′dus** [TA], deep inguinal ring: an aperture in the fascia transversalis for the spermatic cord or for the round ligament; called also *a. abdominalis abdominis, a. inguinalis abdominalis, deep* or *internal abdominal ring,* and *internal inguinal ring.*
**a. inguina′lis superficia′lis** [TA], superficial inguinal ring: an opening in the aponeurosis of the external oblique muscle for the spermatic cord or for the round ligament; called also *anulus inguinalis subcutaneus, external abdominal ring,* and *superficial* or *external inguinal ring.*
**a. i′ridis ma′jor** [TA], greater ring of iris: the less coarsely striated outer concentric circle on the anterior surface of the iris; called also *greater circle of iris.*
**a. i′ridis mi′nor** [TA], lesser ring of iris: the more coarsely striated inner concentric circle on the anterior surface of the iris; called also *lesser circle of iris.*
**a. lympha′ticus car′diae** [TA], cardiac lymphatic ring: a chain of lymph nodes (paracardial lymph nodes) around the cardiac opening of the stomach.

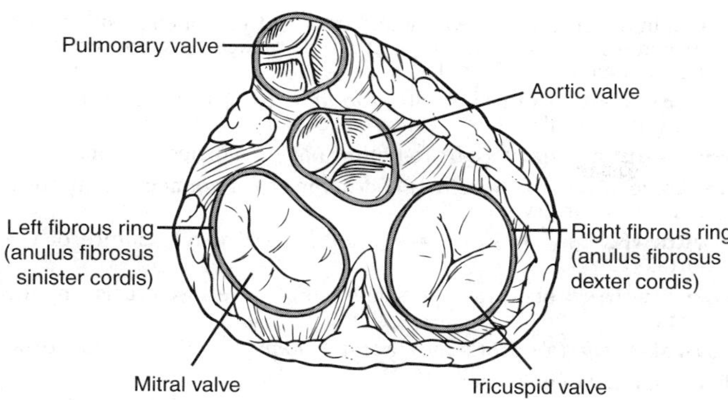


Anuli fibrosi cordis (fibrous rings of heart), one surrounding each of the two atrioventricular valves.

**mitral a., mitral valve a.,** see *anulus fibrosus dexter/sinister cordis.*
**a. of spermatozoon,** ring centriole.
**a. tendi'neus commu'nis** [TA], **a. tendi'neus commu'nis [Zin'ni],** common tendinous ring: the annular ligament of origin common to the recti muscles of the eye, attached to the edge of the optic canal and the inner part of the superior orbital fissure; called also *anulus of Zinn, Zinn's ligament* or *ring,* and *common annular tendon.*
**tricuspid a., tricuspid valve a.,** see *anulus fibrosus dexter/sinister cordis.*
**a. tympa'nicus** [TA], tympanic anulus or ring: the bony ring forming part of the temporal bone at the time of birth and developing into the pars tympanica of the bone.
**a. umbilica'lis** [TA], umbilical ring: the aperture in the abdominal wall through which the umbilical cord communicates with the fetus. After birth it is felt for some time as a distinct fibrous ring surrounding the umbilicus; these fibers later shrink progressively. Called also *umbilical canal.*
**a. of Zinn,** *a. tendineus communis.*

**Anu•ra** (ə-nu'rə) [MeSH: Anura] an order of amphibians, including the frogs and toads.

**an•u•ran** (ə-nu'rən) any member of Anura.

**an•ure•sis** (an″u-re'sis) 1. retention of urine in the bladder. 2. anuria.

**an•uret•ic** (an-u-ret'ik) pertaining to or characterized by anuresis.

**an•uria** (an-u're-ə) [*an-*[1] + *-uria*] [MeSH: Anuria] complete suppression of urinary secretion by the kidneys; called also *anuresis.*
**angioneurotic a.,** anuria occurring in cortical necrosis of the kidney.
**calculous a.,** anuria caused by a renal calculus.
**obstructive a.,** failure of urinary excretion due to a blockage, as by a calculus, in the urinary passages.
**postrenal a.,** anuria resulting from obstruction of the ureters or urethra.
**prerenal a.,** cessation of renal secretion of urine resulting from fall of blood pressure below the level necessary to maintain adequate filtration pressure in the glomeruli.
**renal a.,** failure of urinary secretion by the kidney in the presence of adequate filtration pressure in the glomeruli and patency of the ureters.
**suppressive a.,** failure of secretion of urine in the kidneys.

**an•uric** (an-u'rik) pertaining to or characterized by anuria.

**an•u•rous** (an-u'rəs) [*an-*[1] +Gr. *oura* tail] acaudate.

**anus** (a'nəs) gen. *a'ni,* pl. *a'nus* [L. "ring, circle"] [TA] [MeSH: Anus] the distal or terminal orifice of the alimentary canal.
**artificial a.,** an opening from the bowel formed by the creation of a colostomy.
**ectopic a.,** imperforate a.
**imperforate a.,** persistence of the anal membrane, so that the anus is closed. The defect is not always complete; sometimes a narrow opening permits the passage of the bowel contents. When the anus is completely imperforate, there is simply a dimple in the skin of the perineum; this condition is often associated with atresia of the lower rectum. Called also *anal atresia, atresia ani,* and *proctatresia.*
**preternatural a.,** an anus situated at some unusual or abnormal place.
**a. of Rusconi,** the blastopore.
**a. vesica'lis,** anomalous opening of the rectum into the bladder, the anus being imperforate.
**a. vestibula'ris,** anomalous opening of the rectum on the vulva, the anus being imperforate.
**vulvovaginal a.,** a. vestibularis.

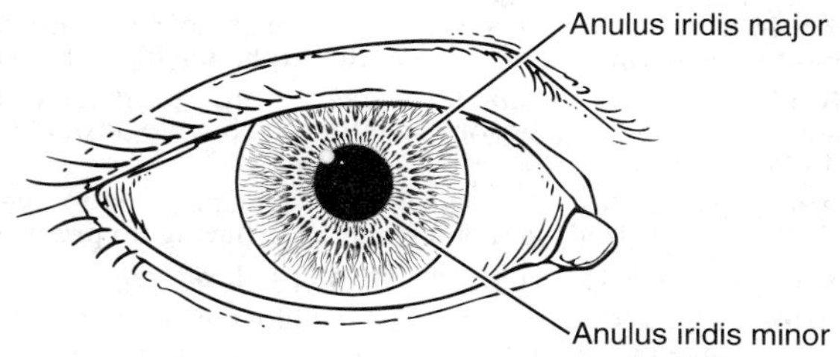


Anulus iridis major and anulus iridis minor.

**anus•i•tis** (a-nəs-i'tis) inflammation of the anus.

**an•vil** (an'vil) incus.

**an•xi•e•ty** (ang-zi'ə-te) [MeSH: Anxiety] the unpleasant emotional state consisting of psychophysiological responses to anticipation of unreal or imagined danger, ostensibly resulting from unrecognized intrapsychic conflict. Physiological concomitants include increased heart rate, altered respiration rate, sweating, trembling, weakness, and fatigue; psychological concomitants include feelings of impending danger, powerlessness, apprehension, and tension. Cf. *fear.*
**castration a.,** see under *complex.*
**free-floating a.,** severe, generalized anxiety having no apparent connection to any specific object, situation, or idea.
**performance a.,** a social phobia characterized by extreme anxiety and episodes of panic when performance, particularly public performance, is required.
**separation a.,** apprehension due to removal of significant persons or familiar surroundings, common in infants 12 to 24 months old; see also under *disorder.*
**situational a.,** that occurring specifically in relation to a situation or object.

**anx•io•lyt•ic** (ang″zi-o-lit'ik) 1. antianxiety. 2. an agent that reduces anxiety; the group includes the benzodiazepines (diazepam and congeners) and a few less widely used nonbenzodiazepines (meprobamate, hydroxyzine). Called also *minor tranquilizer.*

**An•ze•met** trademark for preparations of dolasetron mesylate.

**AO** opening of the atrioventricular valves.

**AOA** American Optometric Association; American Orthopsychiatric Association; American Osteopathic Association.

**AOMA** American Occupational Medical Association.

**aor•ta** (a-or'tə) pl. *aor'tas, aor'tae* [L. from Gr. *aortē*] [TA] [MeSH: Aorta] the main trunk from which the systemic arterial system proceeds. It arises from the left ventricle of the heart; passes upward *(pars ascendens aortae* or *ascending aorta),* bends over *(arcus aortae* or *aortic arch),* and then proceeds downward *(pars descendens aortae* or *descending aorta);* the latter is divided into an upper, thoracic part *(pars thoracica aortae)* and a lower, abdominal part *(pars abdominalis aortae).* At about the level of the fourth lumbar vertebra it divides into the two common iliac arteries.
**abdominal a.,** pars abdominalis aortae.
**a. abdomina'lis,** TA alternative for *pars abdominalis aortae.*
**a. ascen'dens,** TA alternative for *pars ascendens aortae.*
**ascending a.,** pars ascendens aortae.
**a. descen'dens,** TA alternative for *pars descendens aortae.*
**descending a.,** pars descendens aortae.

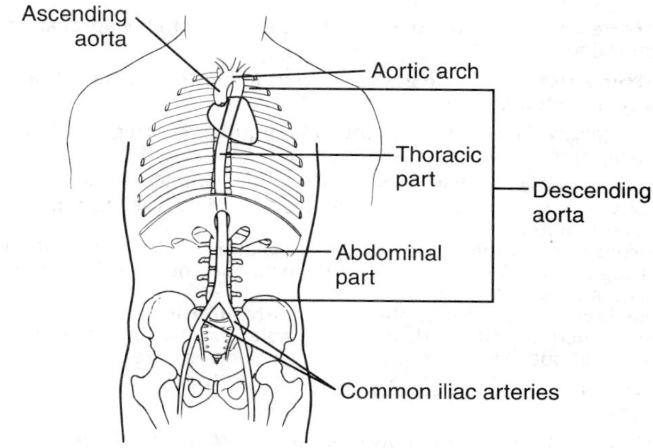


Aorta, arising from the left ventricle, ascending, arching, then descending through the thorax to the abdomen, where it divides into the common iliac arteries.

**dextropositioned a.**, overriding a.
**overriding a.**, a congenital anomaly occurring in tetralogy of Fallot, in which the aorta is displaced to the right so that it appears to arise from both ventricles and straddles the ventricular septal defect.
**palpable a.**, one that is easily palpable, on account of a thin retracted abdominal wall.
**paravisceral a.**, thoracoabdominal a.
**primitive a., primordial a.**, either of two main vascular trunks before fusion into a single aorta in the early embryo.
**a. thoraca'lis, thoracic a.**, pars thoracica aortae.
**a. thora'cica**, TA alternative for *pars thoracica aortae.*
**thoracoabdominal a.**, the lower part of the thoracic aorta and the upper part of the abdominal aorta, where the visceral branches originate.
**ventral a.**, a single short vascular segment that, in fishes, in some amphibians, and in the embryo of higher vertebrates, connects the heart with the aortic arches. In mammalian development, it becomes continuous with the aortic arch.

**aor·tae** (a-or'te) [L.] genitive and plural of *aorta.*

**aor·tal** (a-or'təl) aortic.

**aor·tal·gia** (a″or-tal'jə) [*aorta* + *-algia*] pain in the region of the aorta.

**aor·tec·to·my** (a″or-tek'tə-me) [*aorta* + *-ectomy*] excision of part of the aorta.

**aor·tic** (a-or'tik) of or pertaining to the aorta.

**aor·ti·co·me·di·as·ti·nal** (a-or″tĭ-ko-me″de-ə-sti'nəl) pertaining to the aorta and mediastinum.

**aor·ti·co·pul·mo·nary** (a-or″tĭ-ko-pul'mo-nar″e) pertaining to or lying between the aorta and pulmonary artery. Called also *pulmoaortic.*

**aor·ti·co·re·nal** (a-or″tĭ-ko-re'nəl) pertaining to the aorta and the kidneys.

**aor·ti·tis** (a″or-ti'tis) [*aorta* + *-itis*] [MeSH: Aortitis] inflammation of the aorta.
**Döhle-Heller a.**, syphilitic a.
**luetic a.**, syphilitic a.
**nummular a.**, aortitis with white circular patches on the inner coat of the vessel.
**rheumatic a.**, inflammation of the aorta due to rheumatism, which may progress to patchy fibrosis.
**syphilitic a., a. syphili'tica**, aortitis caused by syphilis; its complications include insufficiency of the aortic valve, stenosis or occlusion of the coronary orifices, and aortic aneurysm. Called also *Döhle-Heller a., Heller-Döhle disease,* and *luetic a.*

**aor·to·bi·fem·o·ral** (a-or″to-bi-fem'ə-rəl) pertaining to the aorta and both femoral arteries.

**aor·to·ca·val** (a-or″to-ka'vəl) pertaining to or connecting the aorta and vena cava.

**aor·to·cor·o·nary** ( a-or″to-kor'ə-nar-e) pertaining to or communicating with the aorta and coronary arteries.

**aor·to·du·o·de·nal** (a-or″to-doo″o-de'nəl) pertaining to or connecting the aorta and duodenum.

**aor·to·en·ter·ic** (a-or″to-en-ter'ik) pertaining to or connecting the aorta and gastrointestinal tract.

**aor·to·esoph·a·ge·al** (a-or″to-e-sof″ə-je'əl) pertaining to or connecting the aorta and esophagus.

**aor·to·fem·o·ral** (a-or″to-fem'ə-rəl) pertaining to the aorta and the femoral artery.

**aor·to·gas·tric** (a-or″to-gas'trik) pertaining to or connecting the aorta and stomach.

**aor·to·gram** (a-or'to-gram) the radiographic record resulting from aortography.

**aor·tog·ra·phy** (a″or-tog'rə-fe) [*aorta* + *-graphy*] [MeSH: Aortography] radiography of the aorta after the intravascular injection of an opaque medium.
**retrograde a.**, radiography of the aorta after passage of a catheter through a peripheral artery to the aorta and the rapid injection of a radiopaque substance.
**translumbar a.**, radiography of the aorta after injection of a radiopaque medium into it through a needle inserted into the lumbar area at about the level of the 12th thoracic vertebra.

**aor·to·il·i·ac** (a-or″to-il'e-ak) pertaining to the aorta and the iliac artery.

**aor·top·a·thy** (a″or-top'ə-the) [*aorta* + *-pathy*] any disease of the aorta.

**aor·to·pexy** (a-or'to-pek″se) [*aorta* + *-pexy*] suturing of the anterior walls of the aortic arch and right subclavian artery to the sternum in order to pull the attached trachea to an open position; performed for relief of airway obstruction caused by compression of the trachea in tracheomalacia.

**aor·to·plas·ty** (a″or-to-plas'te) [*aorta* + *-plasty*] surgical repair of the aorta; see also *aortic reconstruction.*

**aor·to·pul·mo·nary** (a-or″to-pul'mə-nar″e) aorticopulmonary.

**aor·to·re·nal** (a-or″to-re'nəl) pertaining to or connecting the aorta and a renal artery.

**aor·tor·rha·phy** (a″or-tor'ə-fe) [*aorta* + *-rrhaphy*] suture of the aorta.

**aor·to·scle·ro·sis** (a-or″to-sklə-ro'sis) arteriosclerosis in the aorta.

**aor·tot·o·my** (a″or-tot'ə-me) [*aorta* + *-tomy*] incision of the aorta.

**AOS** anodal opening sound.

**AOTA** American Occupational Therapy Association.

**AP** action potential; angina pectoris; anterior pituitary (gland); anteroposterior; arterial pressure.

**ap-** see *apo-.*

**APA** American Pharmaceutical Association; American Podiatric Association; American Psychiatric Association; American Psychological Association.

**ap·a·con·i·tine** (ap″ə-kon'ĭ-tēn) [*ap-* + *aconitine*] a poisonous base derived from aconitine.

**apal·les·the·sia** (ə-pal″əs-the'zhə) pallanesthesia.

**Ap·a·mide** (ap'ə-mīd) trademark for a preparation of acetaminophen.

**apan·crea** (a-pan'kre-ə) absence of the pancreas.

**apan·cre·at·ic** (a-pan″kre-at'ik) due to absence of the pancreas.

**Apan·sporo·blas·ti·na** (a″pan-spor″o-blas-ti'nə) [*a-*[1] + *pansporoblast*] [MeSH: Apansporoblastina] a suborder of parasitic protozoa (order Microsporida, class Microsporea) in which a pansporoblastic membrane is usually absent, being vestigial when present, and never persisting as a sporophorous vesicle; the sporoblast is most often dinucleate. Representative genera include *Encephalitozoon, Glugea,* and *Nosema.*

**apar·a·lyt·ic** (a-par″ə-lit'ik) without paralysis.

**apar·a·thy·roid·ism** (a-par″ə-thi'roid-iz-əm) aparathyrosis.

**apar·a·thy·ro·sis** (a-par″ə-thi-ro'sis) absence or deficiency of the parathyroid glands; see also *hypoparathyroidism.* Called also *aparathyroidism.*

**ap·ar·thro·sis** (ap″ahr-thro'sis) [Gr. *aparthrōsis*] junctura synovialis.

**ap·a·thet·ic** (ap″ə-thet'ik) indifferent; undemonstrative.

**ap·a·thy** (ap'ə-the) [Gr. *apatheia*] lack of feeling or emotion; indifference.

**ap·a·tite** (ap'ə-tīt) [Gr. *apatan* to deceive] any of a group of minerals with the general formula $10Ca^{2+}$: $6PO_4^{3-}$: $X^-$ where X is a monovalent anion such as a chloride, carbonate, fluoride, or hydroxyl ion; when it contains a hydroxyl ion the compound is hydroxyapatite (q.v.), an important inorganic constituent of teeth and bones.

**ap·a·zone** (ap'ə-zōn) [MeSH: Apazone] a pyrazolone derivative having anti-inflammatory, analgesic, antipyretic, uricosuric effects; used for treatment of rheumatoid arthritis and osteoarthritis. Called also *azapropazone.*

**APB** atrial premature beat; see *atrial premature complex,* under *complex.*

**APC** atrial premature complex; activated protein C (see *protein C*).

**APD** atrial premature depolarization; see *atrial premature complex,* under *complex.*

**APE** anterior pituitary extract.

**ape** (āp) [MeSH: Pongidae] an imprecise term used to refer to most of the larger Old World monkeys.
**anthropoid a.**, any member of the family Pongidae; some are used in laboratory experiments because of their relationship to humans.

**ap·ei·do·sis** (ap″i-do'sis) [*ap-* + Gr. *eidos* form] progressive disappearance of characteristic form in either the histologic or clinical aspect of a disease.

**apel·lous** (a-pel'əs) [*a-*[1] + L. *pellis* skin] 1. skinless; not covered with skin; not cicatrized; said of a wound. 2. having no prepuce.

**ape·ri·ent** (ə-pe're-ənt) [L. *aperiens* opening] laxative.

**ape·ri·od·ic** (a″pēr-e-od'ik) having no definite period; said of membranes that have no definite periods of vibration of their own, but are free to take up any vibrations imparted to them.

**aper·i·stal·sis** (a-per-ĭ-stal′sis) [*a-*[1] + *peristalsis*] absence of peristaltic action.

**aper·i·tive** (ə-per′ĭ-tiv) 1. stimulating the appetite. 2. laxative.

**Ap·ert's disease** (ah-pārz′) [Eugène *Apert,* French pediatrician, 1868–1940] acrocephalosyndactyly.

**Ap·ert-Crou·zon disease** (ah-pār′kroo-zaw′) [E. *Apert;* Octave *Crouzon,* French neurologist, 1874–1938] see under *disease.*

**ap·er·tog·na·thia** (ə-per″tog-na′the-ə) open bite.

**ap·er·tom·e·ter** (ap″ər-tom′ə-tər) an apparatus for measuring the angle of aperture of microscopical objectives.

**ap·er·tu·ra** (ap″ər-too′rə) gen. and pl. *apertu′rae* [L., from *aperire* to open] [TA] aperture: term used in general anatomical nomenclature to designate an opening in the body.
**a. exter′na aqueduc′tus vestib′uli** [TA], external aperture of aqueduct of vestibule: the external opening for the aqueduct of the vestibule, located on the posterior surface of the petrous part of the temporal bone, lateral to the opening for the internal acoustic meatus; called also *fissure of aqueduct of vestibule.*
**a. exter′na canalic′uli coch′leae** [TA], external aperture of canaliculus of cochlea: the external opening of the cochlear canaliculus on the margin of the jugular foramen in the temporal bone.
**a. infe′rior canali′culi tympa′nici,** inferior aperture of tympanic canaliculus: the lower opening of the tympanic canaliculus on the inferior surface of the petrous portion of the temporal bone; called also *external aperture of tympanic canaliculus.*
**a. latera′lis ventri′culi quar′ti** [TA], lateral aperture of fourth ventricle: an opening at the end of each lateral recess of the fourth ventricle by which the ventricular cavity communicates with the subarachnoid space; called also *foramen of Luschka* and *foramen of Key and Retzius.*
**a. media′na ventri′culi quar′ti** [TA], median aperture of fourth ventricle: a deficiency in the lower portion of the roof of the fourth ventricle through which the ventricular cavity communicates with the subarachnoid space; called also *foramen of Magendie.*
**a. nasa′lis ante′rior,** a. piriformis.
**a. pel′vica infe′rior,** a. pelvis inferior.
**a. pel′vica supe′rior,** a. pelvis superior.
**a. pel′vis infe′rior** [TA], inferior aperture of pelvis: the inferior, very irregular aperture of the minor pelvis, bounded by the coccyx, the sacrotuberous ligaments, part of the ischium, the sides of the pubic arch, and the pubic symphysis; called also *a. pelvica inferior, exitus pelvis, pelvic outlet,* and *inferior aperture of minor pelvis.*
**a. pel′vis supe′rior** [TA], superior aperture of pelvis: the superior aperture of the minor pelvis, bounded by the crest and pecten of the pubic bones, the arcuate lines of the ilia, and the anterior margin of the base of the sacrum; called also *aditus ad pelvem, apertura pelvica superior, pelvic brim, pelvic inlet,* and *superior aperture of minor pelvis.*
**a. pirifor′mis** [TA], piriform aperture: the anterior end of the bony nasal opening, connecting the external nose with the skull; called also *anterior nasal aperture, a. nasalis anterior,* and *base of nose.*
**a. si′nus fronta′lis** [TA], aperture of frontal sinus: the external opening of the frontal sinus into the nasal cavity; its structure is variable, but it usually drains into the middle meatus. Called also *frontal ostium, frontal sinus ostium,* and *ostium of frontal sinus.*
**a. si′nus sphenoida′lis** [TA], aperture of sphenoid sinus: a round opening just above the superior nasal concha, connecting the sphenoid sinus and the nasal cavity. Called also *sphenoid ostium, sphenoid sinus ostium,* and *ostium of sphenoid sinus.*
**a. supe′rior canali′culi tympa′nici,** superior aperture of tympanic canaliculus: the upper opening of the tympanic canaliculus in the temporal bone, leading to the tympanum; called also *internal aperture of tympanic canaliculus.*
**apertu′rae supe′rior et infe′rior fos′sae axilla′ris,** superior and inferior apertures of axillary fossa: the openings of the axillary fossa into the axillary region; the superior is between the clavicle, scapula, and first rib and the inferior is covered by the axillary fascia.
**a. thora′cis infe′rior** [TA], inferior aperture of thorax: the irregular opening at the inferior part of the thorax bounded by the twelfth thoracic vertebra, the twelfth ribs, and the curving edge of the costal cartilages as they meet the sternum; called also *thoracic outlet* and *inferior thoracic aperture* or *opening.*
**a. thora′cis supe′rior** [TA], superior aperture of thorax: the elliptical opening at the summit of the thorax, bounded by the first thoracic vertebra, the first ribs and cartilage, and the upper margin of the manubrium sterni. Called also *thoracic inlet* and *superior thoracic aperture* or *opening.* NOTE: In clinical usage, the term "thoracic outlet syndrome" refers to this, not to the apertura thoracis inferior.
**a. tympa′nica canali′culi chor′dae tym′pani** [TA], tympanic aperture of canaliculus of chorda tympani: the opening in the posterior part of the middle ear through which the chorda tympani nerve enters the tympanic cavity. Called also *iter chordae posterius.*

**ap·er·tu·rae** (ap″ər-too′re) [L.] genitive and plural of *apertura.*

**ap·er·ture** (ap′ər-chər) [L. *apertura,* q.v.] 1. an opening, or orifice; see also *apertura.* 2. the diameter of a microscope objective lens or the (adjustable) diameter of the iris diaphragm of a camera lens.
**angle of a., angular a.,** the angle formed at a luminous point between the most divergent rays that are capable of passing through the objective of a microscope; called also *a. of lens.*
**cloacal a.,** the posterior opening on the body surface of the cloaca in vertebrates such as birds, reptiles, fish, and amphibians. Called also *vent.*
**external a. of aqueduct of vestibule,** apertura externa aqueductus vestibuli.
**external a. of canaliculus of cochlea, external a. of cochlear aqueduct,** apertura externa canaliculi cochleae.
**external a. of tympanic canaliculus,** apertura inferior canaliculi tympanici.
**a. of frontal sinus,** apertura sinus frontalis.
**a. of glottis,** rima glottidis.
**inferior a. of minor pelvis, inferior a. of pelvis,** apertura pelvis inferior.
**inferior thoracic a., inferior a. of thorax,** apertura thoracis inferior.
**inferior a. of tympanic canaliculus,** apertura inferior canaliculi tympanici.
**internal a. of tympanic canaliculus,** apertura superior canaliculi tympanici.
**a. of larynx,** aditus laryngis.
**lateral a. of fourth ventricle,** apertura lateralis ventriculi quarti.
**a. of lens,** angle of a.
**median a. of fourth ventricle,** apertura mediana ventriculi quarti.
**nasal a., anterior,** apertura piriformis.
**nasal a's, posterior,** choanae; see *choana,* def. 2.
**numerical a.,** a measure of the efficiency of a microscope objective, being the product of the sine of one-half the angle of the aperture times the lowest refractive index of any medium between the objective and the specimen; usually abbreviated N.A.
**orbital a.,** aditus orbitalis.
**piriform a.,** apertura piriformis.
**a. of sphenoid sinus,** apertura sinus sphenoidalis.
**spinal a.,** foramen vertebrale.
**superior and inferior a's of axillary fossa,** aperturae superior et inferior fossae axillaris.
**superior a. of minor pelvis, superior a. of pelvis,** apertura pelvis superior.
**superior thoracic a., superior a. of thorax,** apertura thoracis superior.
**superior a. of tympanic canaliculus,** apertura superior canaliculi tympanici.
**thoracic a., inferior,** apertura thoracis inferior.
**thoracic a., superior,** apertura thoracis superior.
**tympanic a. of canaliculus of chorda tympani,** apertura tympanica canaliculi chordae tympani.

**apex** (a′peks) pl. *apexes* or *a′pices* [L.] 1. [TA] a general term used in anatomical nomenclature to designate the superior aspect of a body, organ, or part, or the pointed extremity of a conical structure such as the heart or lung; called also *tip.* 2. the point of greatest activity, or the point of greatest response to any type of stimulation, such as electrical stimulation of a muscle.
**a. of arytenoid cartilage,** a. cartilaginis arytenoideae.
**a. auri′culae** [TA], **a. auricula′re,** a point sometimes present on the posterior superior part of the helix of the ear. Cf. *tuberculum auriculare.*
**a. of bladder,** a. vesicae.
**a. ca′pitis fi′bulae** [TA], apex of head of fibula: a process pointing upward on the posterior surface of the head of the fibula, giving attachment to the arcuate popliteal ligament of the knee joint and part of the biceps tendon.
**cardiac a.,** a. cordis.
**a. cartila′ginis arytenoi′deae** [TA], apex of arytenoid cartilage: the upper part of the arytenoid cartilage, which bends posteriorly and medially and connects with the corniculate cartilage.
**a. cor′dis** [TA], apex of heart: the blunt rounded extremity of the heart formed by the left ventricle; it is directed ventrally, inferiorly, and to the left.
**a. cor′nus dorsa′lis medul′lae spina′lis,** a. cornus posterioris medullae spinalis.
**a. cor′nus posterio′ris medul′lae spina′lis** [TA], apex of posterior horn of spinal cord: the extremity of the posterior horn, or column, of the spinal cord, which is capped by the substantia gelatinosa. Called also *a. cornus dorsalis medullae spinalis* and *a. of dorsal horn of spinal cord.*
**a. cus′pidis den′tis** [TA], the apex of the cusp of a tooth.
**darwinian a.,** tuberculum auriculare.
**a. den′tis** [TA], apex of dens: the tip of the dens of the axis.
**a. of dorsal horn of spinal cord,** a. cornus posterioris medullae spinalis.
**a. of head of fibula,** a. capitis fibulae.
**a. of heart,** a. cordis.

**a. lin'guae** [TA], **a. lingua'lis,** tip of tongue: the most distal portion of the tongue.
**a. of lung,** a. pulmonis.
**a. na'si** [TA], tip of nose: the most distal portion of the nose.
**a. os'sis sacra'lis,** TA alternative for *a. ossis sacri.*
**a. os'sis sa'cri** [TA], apex of the sacrum: the caudal end of the body of the fifth sacral vertebra, which articulates with the coccyx.
**a. par'tis petro'sae os'sis tempora'lis** [TA], apex of petrous part of temporal bone: the truncated portion of the petrous part of the temporal bone that is directed anteriorly and medially and ends at the medial opening of the carotid canal.
**a. patel'lae** [TA], apex of patella: the inferiorly directed blunt point of the patella, to which the patellar ligament is attached.
**a. of petrous part of temporal bone,** a. partis petrosae ossis temporalis.
**a. of posterior horn of spinal cord,** a. cornus posterioris medullae spinalis.
**a. prosta'tae** [TA], **a. of prostate gland,** the lower portion of the prostate, located just above the urogenital diaphragm.
**a. pulmo'nis** [TA], **a. pulmona'lis,** apex of the lung: the rounded upper extremity of either lung, extending upward as high as the first thoracic vertebra. Called also *a. pulmonalis* [TA alternative].
**a. ra'dicis den'tis** [TA], **root a.,** apex of root of tooth: the terminal end of the root of a tooth.
**a. of sacrum,** a. ossis sacri.
**a. of tongue,** a. linguae.
**a. vesi'cae** [TA], **a. vesica'lis,** apex of bladder: the site of junction of the superior and inferolateral surfaces of the urinary bladder, from which the middle umbilical ligament (urachus) extends to the umbilicus; called also *fundus of bladder, vertex vesicae urinariae,* and *fundus* or *vertex of urinary bladder.*

**apex·car·dio·gram** (a″peks-kahr'de-o-gram) a graphic record, in the form of a simple displacement curve, of the thrust of the apex of the heart as manifested on the surface of the body. Abbreviated ACG.

**apex·car·di·og·ra·phy** (a″peks-kahr″de-og'rə-fe) a method of graphically recording the pulsations of the anterior chest wall over the apex of the heart.

**apex·i·fi·ca·tion** (a-pek″sĭ-fĭ-ka'shən) treatment of an immature tooth whose pulp has died by creating an environment that encourages a calcified barrier to form over the open apex; done by cleaning the tooth and applying a paste.

**Ap·gar score (scale)** (ap'gahr) [Virginia *Apgar,* American anesthesiologist, 1909–1974] see under *score.*

**APHA** American Public Health Association.

**APhA** American Pharmaceutical Association.

**apha·cia** (ə-fa'shə) aphakia.

**apha·cic** (ə-fa'sik) aphakic.

**apha·gia** (ə-fa'jə) [*a-*[1] + *-phagia*] refusal or inability to swallow. See also *dysphagia.*
**a. al'gera,** refusal of a person to take food because it gives pain.

**apha·go·prax·ia** (ə-fa″go-prak'se-ə) dysphagia.

**apha·kia** (ə-fa'ke-ə) [*a-*[1] + *phak-* + *-ia*] [MeSH: Aphakia] absence of the lens of the eye; it may occur congenitally or from trauma, but is most commonly caused by extraction of a cataract.

**apha·kic** (ə-fa'kik) pertaining to aphakia.

**apha·lan·gia** (a-fə-lan'jə) [*a-*[1] + *phalang-* + *-ia*] a developmental anomaly characterized by absence of a digit or of one or more phalanges of a finger or toe.

**Aphan·i·zo·men·on** (ə-fan″ĭ-zo-men'on) a genus of cyanobacteria that sometimes contaminates water and can cause cyanobacteria poisoning.

**Aphan·o·as·cus** (ə-fan″o-as'kəs) a genus of fungi of the family Gymnoascaceae; called also *Anixiopsis. A. fulves'cens* and *A. steroca'ria* are keratinophilic soil fungi that occasionally cause hyalohyphomycosis in humans and other animals.

**apha·sia** (ə-fa'zhə) [*a-*[1] + Gr. *phasis* speech] [MeSH: Aphasia] any of a large group of speech disorders involving defect or loss of the power of expression by speech, writing, or signs, or of comprehending spoken or written language, due to injury or disease of the brain or to psychogenic causes. Less severe forms are known as *dysphasia.* For types of aphasia not given below, see *agrammatism, anomia, dysphasia, paragrammatism,* and *paraphasia.*
**acoustic a.,** auditory a.
**acquired epileptic a.,** Landau-Kleffner syndrome.
**amnesic a., amnestic a.,** anomic a.
**anomic a.,** defective recall of names of objects or words, with intact abilities of comprehension and repetition. Called also *amnesic a., amnestic a., nominal a.,* and *anomia.*
**associative a.,** conduction a.
**auditory a.,** a form of receptive aphasia in which sounds are heard but convey no meaning to the person affected, due to disease of the subcortical pathways leading to the main auditory center of the brain, or disease of the center itself; called also *acoustic a.* and *word deafness.*
**Broca's a.,** motor a.
**central a.,** a term that has been used as a synonym for various aphasias that involve disturbance in word selection, grammar, and sentence structure apart from elementary auditory or visual comprehension and the ability to write legible characters and speak aloud. Many are presumed to be due to lesions of brain centers *(motor speech areas).* See *global a., motor a.,* and *receptive a.*
**combined a.,** aphasia of two or more forms occurring concomitantly in the same person.
**commissural a.,** conduction a.
**complete a.,** global a.
**conduction a.,** a type of aphasia characterized by normal comprehension but inability to repeat words correctly; said to be caused by lesions in the pathways connecting Broca's motor speech area and Wernicke's area. Called also *associative a.* and *commissural a.*
**expressive a.,** motor a.
**expressive-receptive a.,** global a.
**fluent a.,** a type of receptive aphasia in which speech is well articulated with satisfactory melodic intonation, syllable stress, and phrasing but has gross errors in grammatical structure and is lacking in content.
**frontocortical a.,** motor a.
**functional a.,** aphasia associated with a psychogenic disorder.
**gibberish a.,** jargon a.
**global a.,** aphasia involving all the functions of spoken or written language and comprehension; called also *central a., complete a., expressive-receptive a.,* and *total a.*
**graphomotor a.,** agraphia.
**impressive a.,** receptive a.
**intellectual a.,** true a.
**jargon a.,** utterance of meaningless phrases, either neologisms or incoherently arranged known words (see *agrammatism*); it is sometimes a symptom of certain types of schizophrenia. Written also *jargonaphasia.*
**mixed a.,** global a.
**motor a.,** aphasia in which there is impairment of the ability to speak and write, owing to a lesion in the insula and surrounding operculum, including Broca's motor speech area. The patient understands many written and spoken words but has difficulty uttering the words. Cf. *receptive a.* Called also *Broca's a., expressive a., frontocortical a., nonfluent a.,* and *logaphasia.*
**nominal a.,** anomic a.
**nonfluent a.,** motor a.
**receptive a.,** inability to understand written, spoken, or tactile speech symbols, due to disease of the auditory and visual word centers. Cf. *motor a.* Called also *impressive a., sensory a.,* and *Wernicke's a.*
**semantic a.,** aphasia characterized by a lack of recognition of the full significance of words and phrases, or faulty use of words, phrases, or sentences; words heard, seen, spoken, or written are misunderstood or used incorrectly in place of other words in the same class.
**sensory a.,** receptive a.
**syntactical a.,** a type of agrammatism in which some necessary elements for coherent sentences are lacking.
**tactile a.,** anomic aphasia characterized by inability to name objects that are touched. Cf. *tactile agnosia.*
**total a.,** global a.
**transcortical a.,** a type of conduction aphasia believed to be caused by a lesion of a pathway between the speech center and other cortical centers, but often reflecting large lesions in brain areas other than the perisylvian region of the hemisphere dominant for speech and language. The patient may repeat words *(echolalia)* but cannot speak independently.
**true a.,** aphasia due to a lesion of any one of the speech centers; called also *intellectual a.*
**visual a.,** alexia.
**Wernicke's a.,** receptive a.

**apha·si·ac** (ə-fa'ze-ak) aphasic, def. 2.

**apha·sic** (ə-fa'zik) 1. pertaining to or affected with aphasia. 2. a person affected with aphasia.

**apha·si·ol·o·gy** (ə-fa″ze-ol'ə-je) the scientific study of aphasia and the specific neurologic lesions producing it.

**aphas·mid** (a-faz'mid) [*a-*[1] + *phasmid*] a nematode belonging to the subclass Aphasmidia. Cf. *phasmid.*

**Aphas·mid·ia** (a-faz-mid'e-ə) a subclass of Nematoda comprising those organisms which do not possess phasmids, and including the superfamilies Trichuroidea, Mermithoidea, and Dioctophymoidea.

**ap·he·li·ot·ro·pism** (ap″he-le-ot'rə-piz-əm) negative heliotropism.

**aphe·mes·the·sia** (ə-fe-mes-the′zhə) [*a-*[1] + Gr. *phēmē* voice + *esthesia*] alexia.

**aphe·mia** (ə-fe′me-ə) [*a-*[1] + *-phemia*] a term formerly used to describe a type of motor aphasia and more recently proposed as a synonym for *apraxia of speech.*

**aphe·pho·bia** (af″ə-fo′be-ə) [Gr. *haphē* touch + *-phobia*] haphephobia.

**aph·e·re·sis** (af-ə-re′sis) [Gr. *aphairesis* removal] any procedure in which blood is withdrawn from a donor, a fluid or solid portion (plasma, leukocytes, platelets, etc.) is separated and retained, and the remainder is retransfused into the donor. Types include erythrocytapheresis, leukapheresis, lymphocytapheresis, plasmapheresis, and plateletpheresis. Called also *hemapheresis* and *pheresis.*

**apho·nia** (a-fo′ne-ə) [*a-*[1] + *phon-* + *-ia*] [MeSH: Aphonia] loss of voice. Cf. *dysphonia.*
**hysteric a.,** loss of speech due to emotional conflicts in conversion disorder.
**spastic a.,** see under *dysphonia.*

**aphon·ic** (a-fon′ik) 1. pertaining to or affected with aphonia. 2. without audible voice.

**apho·no·ge·lia** (a″fo-no-je′le-ə) [*a-*[1] + *phono-* + *gelōs* laughter] inability to laugh aloud.

**aphose** (ā′fōz) [*a-*[1] + *phose*] any phose or subjective visual sensation due to absence or interruption of light.

**aphos·pha·gen·ic** (a-fos″fə-jen′ik) due to deficiency of phosphorus.

**aphos·pho·ro·sis** (a-fos″fə-ro′sis) a deficiency of dietary phosphorus in animals, particularly grazing cattle, characterized by inappetence, lameness, osteomalacia, bone fragility, decline in milk production, and lowered fertility.

**aphot·es·the·sia** (a″fōt-es-the′zhə) [*a-*[1] + *phot-* + *esthesia*] reduced sensitivity of the retina to light resulting from excessive exposure to rays of the sun.

**aphot·ic** (a-fot′ik) without light; totally dark.

**aphra·sia** (ə-fra′zhə) [*a-*[1] + Gr. *phrasis* utterance] inability to speak or to understand phrases. See also *aphasia* and *mute.*

**aph·ro·dis·ia** (af″ro-diz′e-ə) [Gr. *aphrodisia* sexual pleasures] sexual excitement.

**aph·ro·dis·iac** (af″ro-diz′e-ak) 1. exciting the libido. 2. any drug that arouses the sexual instinct.

**aph·tha** (af′thə) pl. *aph′thae* [L.; Gr. "thrush"] a small ulcer, such as the round lesion with a grayish exudate surrounded by a red halo characteristic of recurrent aphthous stomatitis.
**Bednar's aphthae,** symmetric excoriation of the hard palate over the pterygoid plates in infants; thought to be due to pressure of the nipple against the palate during nursing, or to sucking of the tongue or foreign objects.
**contagious aphthae,** foot-and-mouth disease of cattle.
**epizootic aphthae,** foot-and-mouth disease.
**Mikulicz's aphthae,** periadenitis mucosa necrotica recurrens.
**recurring scarring aphthae,** periadenitis mucosa necrotica recurrens.

**aph·thae** (af′the) [L.] 1. plural of *aphtha.* 2. recurrent aphthous stomatitis.

**Aph·tha·sol** (af′thə-sol) trademark for a preparation of amlexanox.

**aph·thoid** (af′thoid) [*aphtha* + *-oid*] 1. resembling thrush; thrush-like. 2. an exanthema resembling that of thrush.

**aph·thon·gia** (af-thon′jə) [*a-*[1] + Gr. *phthongos* sound] aphasia due to spasm of the speech muscles.

**aph·tho·sis** (af-tho′sis) any condition marked by aphthae.

**aph·thous** (af′thəs) pertaining to, characterized by, or affected with aphthae.

**Aph·tho·vi·rus** (af′tho-vi″rəs) [*aphtha* + *virus*] [MeSH: Aphthovirus] foot-and-mouth disease viruses; a genus of viruses of the family Picornaviridae that cause foot-and-mouth disease.

**aphy·lac·tic** (a″fə-lak′tik) pertaining to or characterized by aphylaxis.

**aphy·lax·is** (a″fə-lak′sis) absence of phylaxis.

**Aphyl·lo·pho·ra·les** (ə-fil″ə-fə-ra′lēz) an order of perfect fungi of the subphylum Basidiomycotina, class Holobasidiomycetes; it includes the family Polyporaceae. Called also *Polyporales.*

**ap·i·cal** (ap′ĭ-kəl) pertaining to or located at the apex.

**ap·i·ca·lis** (ă″pĭ-ka′lis) [L., from *apex,* gen. *apicis,* top] 1. apical. 2. [TA] a general term denoting relationship to or location at an apex.

**api·cec·to·my** (a″pĭ-sek′tə-me) [*apic-* + *-ectomy*] excision of the apex of the petrous portion of the temporal bone.

**ap·i·ces** (ap′ĭ-sēz) [L.] plural of *apex.*

**api·ci·tis** (a″pĭ-si′tis) [*apic-* + *-itis*] inflammation of an apex, as the apex of a tooth, of the lung, or of the petrous portion of the temporal bone (petrositis).

**apic(o)-** [L. *apex* top, summit] a prefix denoting a relationship to the top, as of an organ or other structure.

**api·co·ec·to·my** (a″pĭ-ko-ek′to-me) [*apico-* + *-ectomy*] [MeSH: Apicoectomy] excision of the apical portion of a tooth through an opening made in the overlying labial, buccal, or palatal alveolar bone; see also *root amputation.* Called also *root resection.*

**Ap·i·com·plexa** (ap″ĭ-kəm-plek′sə) [*apico-* + *complex*] [MeSH: Apicomplexa] a phylum of uninucleate, parasitic tissue-dwelling protozoa characterized by the presence of an apical complex; one or more micropores are generally present at some stage of development. Flagella and cilia are absent in the adult stage; many mature apicomplexans glide by means of ultrastructural ridges and fibers on the body surface. They typically reproduce asexually by means of multiple fission, forming merozoites or schizoites, or by endodyogeny, or sexually by syngamy. It comprises two classes: Perkinsea and Sporozoea. Called also *Sporozoa.*

**ap·i·com·plex·an** (ap″ĭ-kom-plek′san) 1. any protozoan of the subphylum Apicomplexa. 2. pertaining or relating to protozoa of the subphylum Apicomplexa.

**api·cos·to·my** (a″pĭ-kos′to-me) dental trephination.

**api·cot·o·my** (a″pĭ-kot′ə-me) puncture of the apex of the petrous portion of the temporal bone.

**apic·u·late** (ə-pik′u-lāt) having an apiculus.

**apic·u·lus** (ə-pik′u-ləs) a short pointed projection at or near the end of a conidium or spore.

**Api·dae** (ap′ĭ-de) the bees, a family of flying insects with relatively large bodies, of the order Hymenoptera; many species can sting. Genera include *Apis* and *Bombus.*

**APIM** abbreviation for *Association Professionnelle Internationale des Médecins,* an international body which deals with the conduct of medical practice from the economic point of view.

**apio·ther·a·py** (a″pe-o-ther′ə-pe) treatment with bee venom.

**api·pho·bia** (a″pĭ-fo′be-ə) [L. *apis* bee + *-phobia*] irrational fear of bees.

**Apis** (a′pis) a genus of bees of the family Apidae, smaller than the bumblebees (genus *Bombus*). *A. melli′fera* is the most common type of honeybee, which can sting if bothered.

**apis·i·na·tion** (a″pis-ĭ-na′shən) [L. *apis* bee] poisoning by the sting of bees.

**api·tox·in** (a″pĭ-tok′sin) the toxic protein constituent of bee venom.

**api·tu·i·tar·ism** (a″pĭ-too′ĭ-tər-iz″əm) 1. lack of pituitary tissue; it may be congenital, as with anencephaly, or acquired, as by hypophysectomy. 2. hypopituitarism.

**APL** trademark for a preparation of human chorionic gonadotropin.

**apla·cen·tal** (a-plə-sen′təl) [*a-*[1] + *placenta*] having no placenta.

**ap·la·nat·ic** (ap″lə-nat′ik) [*a-*[1] + Gr. *planan* to wander] pertaining to aplanatism.

**aplan·a·tism** (ə-plan′ə-tiz-əm) freedom from spherical aberration and coma; said of a lens.

**apla·sia** (ə-pla′zhə) [*a-*[1] + *-plasia*] lack of development of an organ or tissue. Cf. *agenesis* and *hypoplasia.*
**a. axia′lis extracortica′lis conge′nita,** Pelizaeus-Merzbacher disease.
**a. cu′tis conge′nita,** a usually lethal congenital condition consisting of localized failure of development of skin, usually of the scalp but sometimes of the trunk or limbs. The defects are usually covered by a thin translucent membrane or scar tissue, or may be raw, ulcerated, or covered by granulation tissue. Called also *epitheliogenesis imperfecta.*
**hereditary retinal a.,** amaurosis congenita.
**Michel's a.,** lack of development of the inner ear, which causes Michel's deafness.
**nuclear a.,** Möbius' syndrome.
**pure red cell a.,** severe normochromic, normocytic anemia, reticulocytosis, and erythroblastopenia in bone marrow that produces the other cellular elements in a normal way. It occurs as either a primary chronic form *(congenital hypoplastic anemia),* in chronic forms secondary to immune disorders, or in an acute form that is self-limited and associated with drugs or infection.
**retinal a.,** retinal dysplasia, defs. 1 and 2.

**Scheibe's a.,** partial aplasia of the saccule and cochlear duct, which causes Scheibe's deafness.
**thymic a.,** absence of the thymus gland, as in DiGeorge's syndrome.
**thymic-parathyroid a.,** DiGeorge's syndrome.

**aplas·tic** (a-plas'tik) [*a-*[1] + *plastic*] pertaining to or characterized by aplasia; anatomically undeveloped from the primordium or from the stem cell.

**Aplec·ta·na** (ə-plek'tə-nə) a genus of nematodes parasitic in the intestinal tract of amphibians and reptiles.

**apleu·ria** (a-ploor'e-ə) [*a-*[1] + *pleur-* + *-ia*] absence of ribs.

**ap·nea** (ap'ne-ə) [*a-*[1] + *-pnea*] [MeSH: Apnea] cessation of breathing.
**central a.,** central sleep a.
**deglutition a.,** a temporary arrest of the activity of the respiratory nerve center during an act of swallowing.
**initial a.,** a condition in which an infant fails to establish sustained respiration within two minutes of delivery.
**late a.,** cessation of respiration in an infant for more than 45 seconds after spontaneous breathing has been established and sustained.
**a. neonato'rum,** failure of the newborn infant to initiate pulmonary ventilation.
**obstructive a.,** obstructive sleep a.
**sleep a.,** transient periods of cessation of breathing during sleep. It may result in hypoxemia and vasoconstriction of pulmonary arterioles, producing pulmonary arterial hypertension. The two primary types are *central sleep a.* and *obstructive sleep a.*
**sleep a., central,** sleep apnea resulting from failure of stimulation by the respiratory centers in the medulla; both hereditary varieties and varieties accompanying other brain stem disorders have been observed.
**sleep a., obstructive,** sleep apnea resulting from collapse or obstruction of the airway with the inhibition of muscle tone that occurs during REM sleep. In adults it is seen primarily in middle-aged obese individuals, with a male predominance; in children it is often seen accompanying conditions such as adenotonsillar hypertrophy, Down syndrome, or morbid obesity.
**traumatic a.,** cessation of pulmonary ventilation following physical injury. See also *traumatic asphyxia,* under *asphyxia.*

**ap·ne·ic** (ap'ne-ik) pertaining to apnea or affected with apnea.

**ap·neu·ma·to·sis** (ap″noo-mə-to'sis) [*a-*[1] + *pneumat-* + *-osis*] congenital atelectasis.

**ap·neu·mia** (ap-noo'me-ə) [*a-*[1] + *pneum-* + *-ia*] congenital absence of the lungs.

**ap·neu·sis** (ap-noo'sis) [*a-*[1] + *pneusis*] a condition marked by maintained inspiratory activity unrelieved by expiration, each inspiration being long and cramplike; it follows excision of the pneumotaxic center in the upper part of the pons.

**ap·neus·tic** (ap-noo͞s'tik) pertaining to or characterized by apneusis.

**apo-** [Gr. *apo* from] a prefix denoting separation or derivation from. Also, *ap-*.

**apo·at·ro·pine** (ap″o-ă'tro-pēn) An antispasmodic alkaloid derived from belladonna.

**ap·o·cam·no·sis** (ap″o-kam-no'sis) apokamnosis.

**apo·chro·mat** (ap″o-kro'mat) [*apo-* + *chromatic aberration*] an apochromatic objective; see under *objective.*

**apo·chro·mat·ic** (ap″o-kro-mat'ik) free from chromatic and spherical aberration; see under *objective.*

**apoc·o·pe** (ə-pok'o-pe) [Gr. *apokopē*] a cutting off; amputation.

**ap·o·cop·tic** (ap″o-kop'tik) resulting from or pertaining to an amputation.

**apo·crine** (ap'o-krin) [Gr. *apokrinesthai* to be secreted] denoting that type of glandular secretion in which the free end or apical portion of the secreting cell is cast off along with the secretory products that have accumulated therein.

**apo·crin·i·tis** (ap″o-krin-i'tis) [*apo-* + Gr. *krinein* to separate] hidradenitis suppurativa.

**ap·o·crus·tic** (ap″o-krus'tik) 1. astringent and repellent. 2. an astringent and repellent agent.

**apoc·y·nin** (ə-pos'ĭ-nin) a cardiotonic found in species of *Apocynum,* formerly used like digitalis but now considered poisonous; animals consuming the plants may develop an increased pulse rate with fever that can be fatal.

**Apoc·y·num** (ə-pos'ĭ-nəm) the dogbanes, a genus of poisonous North American plants of the family Apocynaceae, noted for their digitalis-like cardioactive principles. *A. cannabi'num* L. (Canadian or Indian hemp) and *A. androsaemifo'lium* L. contain apocynin.

**apo·dal** (ə-po'dəl) having no feet; see also *symmelia.*

**Ap·o·de·mus** (ap″o-de'məs) a genus of Old World field mice that are reservoirs of infectious disease. Species include *A. sylva'ticus,* the wood mouse, *A. agra'rius,* the Manchurian striped field mouse, and *A. flavicollis,* the yellow-necked field mouse.

**apo·dia** (a-po'de-ə) [*a-*[1] + *pod-* + *-ia*] 1. a developmental anomaly characterized by absence of one foot or both feet. 2. apodal symmelia.

**apo·en·zyme** (ap″o-en'zīm) the protein component of an enzyme that is separable from the prosthetic group (cofactor or coenzyme) but that requires the presence of the prosthetic group to form the functioning compound (holoenzyme).

**ap·o·fer·ri·tin** (ap″o-fer'ĭ-tin) [MeSH: Apoferritin] a colorless protein closely related to transferrin, of molecular weight 460,000, produced in the mucosal cells of the small intestine; it binds iron and forms ferritin.

**apo·gam·ia** (ap″o-gam'e-ə) apogamy.

**apog·a·my** (ə-pog'ə-me) [*apo-* + Gr. *gamein* to wed] 1. reproduction without conjugation of gametes and usually without meiosis, as in certain seed plants. 2. parthenogenesis.

**apo·kam·no·sis** (ap″o-kam-no'sis) abnormal liability to fatigue in myasthenia; a feeling of tiredness, numbness, and heaviness in a limb motion.

**apo·lar** (a-po'lər) [*a-*[1] + *polar*] not having poles or processes.

**apo·le·gam·ic** (ap″o-lə-gam'ik) [Gr. *apolegein* to pick out + *gamic*] pertaining to selection, especially sexual selection.

**apo·leg·a·my** (ap″ə-leg'ə-me) selection, especially sexual selection in breeding.

**apo·lipo·pro·tein** (ap″o-lip″o-pro'tēn) any of the protein constituents of lipoproteins; grouped by function in four classes A, B, C, and E (the former apo D is now apo A-III).
**a. A,** a class of apolipoproteins, apo A-I, -II, -III, and -IV, that occur primarily in HDL and in lesser amounts in chylomicrons; apo A-I is the activator of lecithin-cholesterol acyltransferase (LCAT), which forms cholesteryl esters in HDL.
**a. B,** a class of apolipoproteins recognized by specific cell-surface receptors that mediate endocytosis of lipoprotein particles; apo B-100 on VLDL, IDL, and LDL is recognized by LDL receptors on liver and extrahepatic cells; apo B-48 on chylomicrons is recognized by chylomicron remnant receptors on liver cells.
**a. C,** a class of apolipoproteins, apo C-I, -II, and -III, that occur in VLDL, HDL, and chylomicrons; apo C-II activates lipoprotein lipase, which hydrolyzes triglycerides for transfer from VLDL and chylomicrons to tissues.
**a. D,** a. A-III.
**a. E,** an apolipoprotein, apo E, that occurs in all classes of lipoproteins; it may be involved in the conversion of VLDL to IDL and its clearance from the circulation.

**Ap·ol·lo·nia** (ap″ə-lo'ne-ə) a Christian martyr and the patron saint of dentistry; her teeth were knocked out, and then she was burned alive in 249. Her feast day is February 9.

**ap·o·mix·ia** (ap″o-mik'se-ə) apomixis.

**ap·o·mix·is** (ap″o-mik'sis) [*apo-* + Gr. *mixis* a mingling] 1. asexual reproduction in a species normally reproducing sexually, as in certain seed plants. 2. apogamy.

**apo·mor·phine hy·dro·chlo·ride** (ap″o-mor'fēn) [USP] a derivative of morphine used as a central emetic in the treatment of drug overdose and accidental poisoning; administered subcutaneously.

**ap·o·neu·rec·to·my** (ap″o-noo͞-rek'to-me) [*aponeurosis* + *-ectomy*] excision of the aponeurosis of a muscle.

**ap·o·neu·rol·o·gy** (ap″o-noo͞-rol'ə-je) [*aponeurosis* + *-logy*] the sum of knowledge regarding aponeuroses and fasciae.

**ap·o·neu·ror·rha·phy** (ap″o-noo͞-ror'ə-fe) [*aponeurosis* + *-rrhaphy*] suture of an aponeurosis; fasciorrhaphy.

**ap·o·neu·ro·ses** (ap″o-noo͞-ro'sēz) plural of *aponeurosis.*

**ap·o·neu·ro·sis** (ap″o-noo͞-ro'sis) pl. *aponeuro'ses* [Gr. *aponeurōsis*] [TA] 1. a white, flattened or ribbon-like tendinous expansion, serving mainly to connect a muscle with the parts that it moves. 2. a term formerly applied to certain fasciae.
**abdominal a.,** the conjoined tendons of the oblique and transverse muscles on the abdomen.
**a. of biceps muscle of arm, bicipital a.,** a. musculi bicipitis brachii.
**bicipital a.,** a. musculi bicipitis brachii.
**a. bicipita'lis,** TA alternative for *a. musculi bicipitis brachii.*
**clavicoracoaxillary a.,** fascia clavipectoralis.
**crural a.,** fascia cruris.
**Denonvilliers' a.,** septum rectovesicale.
**epicranial a.,** galea aponeurotica.
**a. epicrania'lis,** TA alternative for *galea aponeurotica.*

**falciform a. of rectus abdominis muscle,** falx inguinalis.
**femoral a.,** fascia lata.
**a. glutea'lis** [TA], gluteal aponeurosis: that part of the fasciculata femoris which lies between the iliac crest and the superior border of the gluteus maximus; from it arises a part of the gluteus medius muscle.
**a. of insertion,** the connection of a muscle with the part or parts that it moves.
**intercostal a's, external,** see *membrana intercostalis externa.*
**intercostal a's, internal,** see *membrana intercostalis interna.*
**ischiorectal a.,** fascia inferior diaphragmatis pelvis.
**a. lin'guae** [TA], **lingual a.,** the connective tissue framework of the tongue, supporting and giving attachment to the intrinsic and extrinsic muscles; composed of the connective tissue layer of the tunica mucosa, the lingual septum, and the posterior transverse expansion of the septum which attaches to the hyoid bone.
**a. mus'culi bici'pitis bra'chii** [TA], aponeurosis of biceps muscle of arm: an expansion of the tendon of the biceps brachii muscle by which it is attached to the fascia of the forearm and to the ulna; called also *bicipital a., a. bicipitalis* [TA alternative], *lacertus fibrosus musculi bicipitis brachii* [TA alternative], *bicipital fascia, semilunar fascia,* and *fibrous fasciculus of biceps muscle.*
**a. of occipitofrontal muscle,** galea aponeurotica.
**a. palati'na** [TA], palatine aponeurosis: a fibrous sheet in the anterior part of the soft palate, derived mainly from the tendons of the two tensor muscles, giving attachment to the musculus uvulae and to the palatopharyngeus and levator veli palatini muscles.
**a. palma'ris** [TA], palmar aponeurosis: bundles of fibrous tissue radiating toward the bases of the fingers from the tendon of the palmaris longus muscle; called also *Dupuytren's fascia* and *volar fascia.*
**pharyngeal a., a. pharyn'gis, pharyngobasilar a., a. pharyngobasila'ris,** fascia pharyngobasilaris.
**a. planta'ris** [TA], plantar aponeurosis: bands of fibrous tissue radiating toward the bases of the toes from the medial process of the tuber calcanei; called also *plantar fascia.*
**Sibson's a.,** membrana suprapleuralis.
**subscapular a.,** a fascia attached to the circumference of the subscapular fossa.
**a. of superior surface of levator ani muscle,** fascia superior diaphragmatis pelvis.
**supraspinous a.,** a dense fascia that partly envelops the supraspinous muscle.
**temporal a.,** fascia temporalis.
**vertebral a.,** fascia thoracolumbalis.
**a. of Zinn,** see *fibrae zonulares.*

**ap·o·neu·ro·si·tis** (ap″o-no͞o-ro-si'tis) [*aponeurosis* + *-itis*] inflammation of an aponeurosis.

**ap·o·neu·rot·ic** (ap″o-no͞o-rot'ik) pertaining to or of the nature of an aponeurosis.

**ap·o·neu·ro·tome** (ap″o-no͞o'ro-tōm) a knife for cutting aponeuroses.

**ap·o·neu·rot·o·my** (ap″o-no͞o-rot'ə-me) [*aponeurosis* + *-tomy*] surgical cutting of an aponeurosis.

**Ap·o·nom·ma** (ap″o-nom'ə) a genus of ticks of the family Ixodidae; they infest tropical reptiles of the Old World.

**ap·o·phleg·mat·ic** (ap″o-fleg-mat'ik) causing a discharge of mucus; expectorant.

**apoph·y·sa·ry** (ə-pof'ə-ză-re) apophyseal.

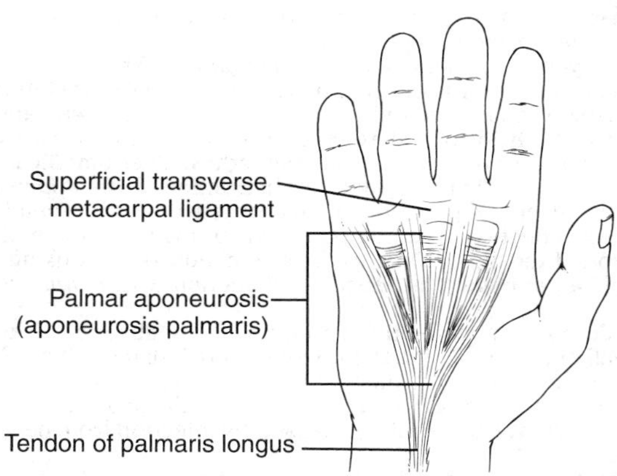


Palmar aponeurosis. A fifth longitudinal band, radiating toward the base of the thumb, is sometimes present.

**apoph·y·se·al** (ə-pof'ə-se″əl, ap″o-fiz'e-əl) pertaining to or of the nature of an apophysis.

**apoph·y·se·op·a·thy** (ap″o-fiz-e-op'ə-the) [*apophysis* + *-pathy*] disease of an apophysis, particularly Osgood-Schlatter disease.

**apoph·y·ses** (ə-pof'ə-sēz) plural of *apophysis.*

**apoph·y·si·al** (ə-pof'ə-se″əl, ap″o-fiz'e-əl) apophyseal.

**ap·o·phys·i·ary** (ap″o-fiz'e-ar″e) apophyseal.

**apoph·y·sis** (ə-pof'ə-sis) pl. *apoph'yses* [Gr. "an offshoot"] 1. [TA] any outgrowth or swelling, especially a bony outgrowth that has never been entirely separated from the bone of which it forms a part, such as a process, tubercle, or tuberosity. 2. in fungi, a V-shaped swelling of the sporangiophore just below the columella. See Plate 29.
**a. anula'ris,** annular apophysis: a raised ring of compact bone on the periphery of the superior and inferior surfaces of the vertebral body, giving attachment to the anulus fibrosus and the longitudinal ligaments.
**basilar a.,** pars basilaris ossis occipitalis.
**cerebral a., a. ce'rebri,** glandula pinealis.
**genial a.,** spina mentalis.
**a. of Ingrassia,** ala minor ossis sphenoidalis.
**a. lenticula'ris incu'dis,** processus lenticularis incudis.
**odontoid a.,** dens axis.
**a. os'sium,** epiphysis.
**pterygoid a.,** processus pterygoideus ossis sphenoidalis.
**a. of Rau,** processus anterior mallei.

**apoph·y·si·tis** (ə-pof″ə-zi'tis) inflammation of an apophysis, especially a disorder of the foot caused by disease of the epiphysis of the calcaneus.
**a. tibia'lis adolescen'tium,** Osgood-Schlatter disease.

**Apo·phy·so·my·ces** (ap″o-fiz″o-mi'sēz) [*apophysis* (def. 2) + Gr. *mykēs* fungus] a genus of fungi of the family Mucoraceae. *A. e'legans* is a soil saprobe that occasionally causes mucormycosis in humans.

**apo·plas·mat·ic** (ap″o-plaz-mat'ik) pertaining to substances that are produced by cells and form a constituent part of the tissues of an organism, such as fibers of connective tissue or the matrix of bone and cartilage.

**ap·o·plec·tic** (ap″o-plek'tik) [Gr. *apoplēktikos*] pertaining to, caused by, or affected with apoplexy.

**ap·o·plec·ti·form** (ap″o-plek'tĭ-form) resembling apoplexy.

**ap·o·plec·toid** (ap″o-plek'toid) resembling apoplexy.

**ap·o·plex·ia** (ap″o-plek'se-ə) [Gr. *apoplēxia*] apoplexy.
**a. u'teri,** sudden uterine hemorrhage.

**ap·o·plexy** (ap'o-plek″se) [Gr. *apoplēxia*] 1. old name for *stroke syndrome.* 2. hemorrhage into an organ.
**abdominal a.,** spontaneous intraperitoneal hemorrhage due to rupture of an intra-abdominal blood vessel, independent of any trauma to the abdomen.
**adrenal a.,** massive hemorrhage into the adrenal glands, as seen in Waterhouse-Friderichsen syndrome.
**bulbar a.,** stroke syndrome affecting the substance of the pons; called also *pontile* or *pontine a.*
**cerebellar a.,** stroke syndrome affecting the cerebellum.
**cerebral a.,** stroke syndrome affecting the cerebrum.
**embolic a.,** see under *stroke.*
**heat a.,** old term for *heat stroke.*
**ovarian a.,** hemorrhage into the ovary.
**pancreatic a.,** extensive hemorrhage of the pancreas; seen in cardiac failure and portal hypertension.
**pituitary a.,** sudden massive degeneration with hemorrhagic necrosis of the pituitary gland, associated with a pituitary tumor; it is signaled by abrupt headache followed by loss of sight, diplopia, drowsiness, confusion or other mentally deranged states, and coma.
**placental a.,** hemorrhage into a separated placenta with formation of a hematoma between the placenta and the uterine wall.
**pontile a., pontine a.,** bulbar a.
**Raymond's a.,** a type of stroke in evolution marked by paresthesia of the hand on the side which later becomes paralyzed.
**renal a.,** hemorrhage from a ruptured intrarenal blood vessel.
**spinal a.,** hematomyelia.
**thrombotic a.,** see under *stroke.*
**uteroplacental a.,** Couvelaire's term for a severe uterine condition seen in some cases of separation of the placenta, in which the uterine musculature is disrupted and infiltrated with blood.

**apo·pro·tein** (ap″o-pro'tēn) the protein moiety of a conjugated protein or protein complex. See also *apolipoprotein.*

**ap·op·to·sis** (ap″op-to'sis) [Gr. "a falling off," from *apo* off + *ptosis* fall] [MeSH: Apoptosis] a morphologic pattern of cell death affecting single cells, marked by shrinkage of the cell, condensation of chromatin, formation of cytoplasmic blebs, and fragmentation of the cell into membrane-bound apoptotic bodies that are eliminated by phagocytosis. It is a mechanism for cell deletion in the regulation of cell populations, as of B and T lymphocytes following cytokine depletion. Often used synonymously with *programmed cell death.*

**ap•op•tot•ic** (ap″op-tot′ic) pertaining to apoptosis.

**apo•re•pres•sor** (ap″o-re-pres′ər) in genetic theory, a product of regulator genes, of unknown structure, which combines with low-molecular weight corepressor to form the complete repressor, which specifically represses the activity of certain structural genes.

**ap•o•some** (ap′o-sōm) [*apo-* + *-some*] an inclusion within the cytoplasm that has been made by the activity of the cell itself.

**apos•ta•sis** (ə-pos′tə-sis) [Gr.] the end or crisis of an attack of disease.

**apos•thia** (ə-pos′the-ə) [*a-*[1] + Gr. *posthē* foreskin + *-ia*] congenital absence of the prepuce.

**apoth•e•cary** (ə-poth′ĕ-kar″e) [Gr. *apothēke* storehouse] pharmacist.

**ap•o•the•ci•um** (ap″o-the′se-əm) an open or expanded fruiting body seen in lichens and actinomycetous fungi (see *ascocarp*), having asci contained on its exposed surface.

**ap•pa•ra•tus** (ap″-ə-ră′təs) pl. *apparatus* or *apparatuses* [L., from *ad-* to + *parare* to make ready] an arrangement of a number of parts acting together in the performance of some special function; used in anatomical nomenclature to designate a number of structures or organs which act together in serving some particular function.
**Abbe-Zeiss a.,** Thoma-Zeiss counting chamber.
**biliary a.,** the parts concerned in the formation, conduction, and storage of bile, including the secreting cells of the liver, bile ducts, and gallbladder.
**branchial a.,** pharyngeal a.
**Brown-Roberts-Wells a.,** the equipment used in the Brown-Roberts-Wells technique of stereotactic surgery; see under *technique.*
**central a.,** the dynamic organ of the cell that participates in mitosis; it consists of a centrosome, a centrosphere, and an astrosphere.
**Charnley's a.,** see under *prosthesis.*
**chromidial a.,** the chromatin staining material of the cytoplasm of a cell, occurring in the form of granules, rods, strands, and networks.
**ciliary a.,** corpus ciliare.
**cytopharyngeal a.,** a cytopharynx with walls supported by nematodesmata; see *cyrtos* and *rhabdos.*
**Desault's a.,** see under *bandage.*
**Golgi a.,** see under *complex.*
**Haldane a.,** see under *chamber.*
**Hodgen's a.,** see under *splint.*
**Jaquet's a.,** a recording apparatus for venous and cardiac impulses.
**juxtaglomerular a.,** a complex comprising the juxtaglomerular cells, the macula densa, and the lacis cells of the polkissen that acts as a feedback mechanism in the autoregulation of the glomerular filtration rate; called also *juxtaglomerular complex.*
**Kirschner's a.,** see under *wire.*
**a. lacrima′lis** [TA], lacrimal apparatus: the system concerned with the secretion and circulation of the tears and the normal fluid of the conjunctival sac; it consists of the lacrimal gland and ducts, and associated structures. See Plate 17.
**Leksell a.,** the equipment used in the Leksell technique of stereotactic surgery; see under *technique.*
**a. ligamento′sus col′li,** membrana tectoria.
**masticatory a.,** the organs and structures involved in mastication, including the teeth and jaws and their supporting structures, temporomandibular joints, mandibular muscles, accessory facial muscles, tongue, lips, cheeks, and oral mucosa together with their innervation. Called also *organs of mastication* and *masticatory system.*
**mucociliary a.,** on the inner surface of the respiratory tract, a layer of columnar epithelial cells covered by a thin mucous layer and many projecting cilia that beat in a rhythmic manner to bring about mucociliary clearance (see under *clearance*).
**parabasal a.,** the structure comprising the parabasal body and the fibril or thread that connects it to the basal body.
**a. of Perroncito,** a mass of fibrils in the form of spirals and networks with newly formed axons which develop in the cut stump of a nerve during regeneration; called also *Perroncito's spirals.*
**pharyngeal a.,** the branchial (pharyngeal) arches and clefts considered as a unit; called also *branchial a.*
**pilosebaceous a.,** the complex consisting of a hair follicle and its sebaceous gland, and the erector pili muscle.
**a. respirato′rius, respiratory a.,** the organs and structures by means of which pulmonary ventilation and gas exchange are brought about between ambient air and the blood. See *respiratory system,* under *system.*
**Riechert-Mundinger a.,** the equipment used in the Riechert-Mundinger technique of stereotactic surgery; see under *technique.*
**Sayre's a.,** an apparatus for suspending a patient during the application of a plaster-of-Paris jacket.
**Soxhlet's a.,** an apparatus by which fatty or lipid constituents can be extracted from solid matter by repeated treatment with distilled solvent.
**spindle a.,** see *spindle,* def. 1.
**subneural a.,** see under *cleft.*
**sucker a.,** pericapillary end foot.
**a. suspenso′rius len′tis,** zonula ciliaris.
**Taylor's a.,** see under *brace.*
**Tiselius a.,** an apparatus for the electrophoretic separation of the proteins of blood serum, plasma, and other body fluids.
**Todd-Wells a.,** the equipment used in the Todd-Wells technique of stereotactic surgery; see under *technique.*
**a. urogenita′lis,** urogenital system; see under *system.*
**vasomotor a.,** the neuromuscular mechanism controlling the constriction and dilation of blood vessels and thus the amount of blood supplied to a part.
**vestibular a.,** the structures in the inner ear concerned with reception and transduction of stimuli of equilibrium; they include the semicircular canals, the utricle, and the saccule.
**Wangensteen's a.,** see under *tube.*
**Warburg a.,** a device for measuring the quantity of gas liberated or consumed by respiring tissue slices enclosed in a chamber which is attached to a manometer and immersed in water at constant temperature.

**ap•pen•dage** (ə-pen′dəj) a thing or part appended; limb. See also *adnexa* and *appendix.*
**atrial a., auricular a.,** auricula atrialis.
**cecal a.,** appendix vermiformis.
**a. of epididymis,** appendix epididymidis.
**epiploic a's,** appendices epiploicae.
**a's of the eye,** the lids, eyebrows, lacrimal apparatus, and conjunctiva; called also *adnexa oculi.*
**a's of the fetus,** the trophoblast derivatives and extraembryonic or fetal membranes, including the umbilical cord, amnion, and chorion (placenta).
**fibrous a. of liver,** appendix fibrosa hepatis.
**ovarian a.,** the parovarium.
**a's of the skin,** the hair, nails, sebaceous glands, sweat glands, and mammary glands.
**testicular a., a. of the testis,** appendix testis.
**uterine a's,** the ligaments of the uterus, and the oviducts and the ovaries; called also *adnexa uteri.*
**a. of ventricle of larynx,** sacculus laryngis.
**vermicular a.,** appendix vermiformis.
**vesicular a's of epoöphoron,** appendices vesiculosae epoophori.

**ap•pen•da•gi•tis** (ə-pen″də-ji′tis) inflammation of an appendage, particularly of the epiploic appendages.
**epiploic a.,** inflammation of one or more of the epiploic appendages of the colon, characterized by pain and tenderness over the affected area.

**ap•pen•dec•to•my** (ap″en-dek′tə-me) [MeSH: Appendectomy] surgical removal of the vermiform appendix.
**auricular a.,** excision of the auricula atrii.

**ap•pen•di•cal** (ə-pen′dĭ-kəl) appendiceal.

**ap•pen•dic•e•al** (ap-en-dis′e-əl) pertaining to an appendix.

**ap•pen•di•cec•to•my** (ə-pen″dĭ-sek′to-me) [*appendix* + *-ectomy*] appendectomy.

**ap•pen•di•ces** (ə-pen′dĭ-sēz) [L.] [MeSH: Appendix] plural of *appendix.*

**ap•pen•di•ci•tis** (ə-pen″dĭ-si′tis) [MeSH: Appendicitis] inflammation of the vermiform appendix.
**actinomycotic a.,** that caused by *Actinomyces israelii.*
**acute a.,** appendicitis of acute onset requiring surgical intervention and usually characterized by pain in the right lower abdominal quadrant with local and referred rebound tenderness, overlying muscle spasm, and cutaneous hyperesthesia. Periumbilical, colicky pain at the onset may be due to obstruction of the appendix by a fecalith. Fever and polymorphonuclear leukocytosis result from the localized infection. Symptoms and signs may be modified by the location of the appendix, by adhesive bands, or by kinking.
**amebic a.,** appendicitis caused by infection with *Entamoeba histolytica.*
**chronic a.,** 1. appendicitis characterized by fibrotic thickening of the wall of the organ due to previous acute inflammation. 2. a term formerly applied to chronic or recurrent pain in the appendiceal area in the absence of evidence of acute inflammation.
**a. by contiguity,** appendicitis caused by infection from neighboring tissues.
**foreign-body a.,** appendicitis, usually obstructive, due to a foreign body in the lumen.
**fulminating a.,** appendicitis marked by sudden onset and rapid, fatal termination.

**gangrenous a.,** appendicitis complicated by gangrene of the organ, owing to interference with the blood supply.
**helminthic a.,** verminous a.
**left-sided a.,** 1. diverticulitis; so called because the symptoms resemble those of appendicitis, and the descending (or left) colon is the usual site of involvement. 2. left-sided appendicitis associated with situs inversus.
**lumbar a.,** a type of appendicitis in which the appendix is posterior, lying against the peritoneum behind or below the cecum.
**a. obli'terans,** appendicitis with sclerosis and shrinking of the submucous tissue and plastic peritonitis, causing obliteration of the lumen of the appendix; called also *protective a.*
**obstructive a.,** a common form of appendicitis attended by obstruction of the lumen of the appendix, usually by a fecalith.
**perforating a., perforative a.,** appendicitis with perforation of the organ.
**protective a.,** a. obliterans.
**purulent a.,** suppurative a.
**recurrent a.,** that characterized by recurrent attacks of acute appendicitis.
**relapsing a.,** recurrence of appendiceal inflammation after improvement; recurrent appendicitis.
**segmental a.,** inflammation confined to a segment of the appendix; it may be proximal, central, or distal.
**skip a.,** appendicitis in which two or more areas of focal inflammation are separated by normal appendiceal tissue.
**stercoral a.,** appendicitis in which a fecal concretion is the assumed cause.
**subperitoneal a.,** appendicitis in which the appendix is buried under the peritoneum instead of being free in the peritoneal cavity.
**suppurative a.,** purulent infiltration of the walls of the appendix; called also *purulent a.*
**traumatic a.,** appendicitis caused by external trauma.
**verminous a.,** appendicitis due to the presence of a worm in the appendix.

**appendic(o)-** [L. *appendix,* q.v., gen. *appendicis*] a combining form denoting relation to an appendix, especially to the vermiform appendix.

**ap·pen·di·co·ce·cos·to·my** (ə-pen″dĭ-ko-se-kos'tə-me) the formation of an abnormal opening between the appendix and cecum, usually by surgical means; also, the orifice so established.

**ap·pen·di·co·cele** (ə-pen'dĭ-ko-sēl) hernia containing the vermiform appendix.

**ap·pen·di·co·en·ter·os·to·my** (ə-pen″dĭ-ko″en-tər-os'tə-me) the formation of an anastomosis between the vermiform appendix and the intestine.

**ap·pen·di·co·li·thi·a·sis** (ə-pen″dĭ-ko″lĭ-thi'ə-sis) [*appendix* + *lithiasis*] a condition in which the lumen of the vermiform appendix becomes obstructed with calculi; it is said to run in families, and to be akin to gout and rheumatism. Called also *appendicular lithiasis.*

**ap·pen·di·col·y·sis** (əpen″dĭ-kol'ĭ-sis) [*appendix* + *-lysis*] the surgical division of adhesions about the appendix.

**ap·pen·di·cop·a·thy** (ə-pen″dĭ-kop'ə-the) [*appendix* + *-pathy*] any diseased condition of the vermiform appendix.

**ap·pen·di·cos·to·my** (ə-pen″dĭ-kos'tə-me) [*appendix* + *-stomy*] surgical creation of an opening from the surface of the abdominal wall into the vermiform appendix for the purpose of irrigating or draining the large bowel.

**ap·pen·dic·u·lar** (ap″en-dik'u-lər) 1. pertaining to the vermiform appendix. 2. pertaining to an appendage.

**ap·pen·dix** (ə-pen'diks) pl. *appendixes, appen'dices* [L. from *appendere* to hang upon] [TA] [MeSH: Appendix] a general term used in anatomical nomenclature to designate a supplementary, accessory, or dependent part attached to a main structure; called also *appendage.* Frequently used alone to refer to the *vermiform appendix* (*a. vermiformis* [TA]) of the colon.
**auricular a.,** auricula atrii.
**cecal a.,** a. vermiformis.
**ensiform a.,** processus xiphoideus.
**a. epidi'dymidis** [TA], appendix of epididymis: a remnant of the mesonephros sometimes situated on the head of the epididymis; called also *appendage of epididymis.*
**appen'dices epiplo'icae** [TA], epiploic appendices: peritoneum-covered tabs of fat, 2 to 10 cm long, attached in rows along the tenia of the colon; called also *appendices omentales* [TA alternative] and *omental appendices.*
**a. fibro'sa he'patis** [TA], fibrous appendix of liver: a fibrous band at the left extremity of the liver, being the atrophied remnant of formerly more extensive liver tissue.
**Morgagni's a.,** see *a. testis* and *appendices vesiculosae epoöphorontis.*
**omental appendices,** appendices epiploicae.
**appen'dices omenta'les,** TA alternative for *appendices epiploicae.*
**a. tes'tis** [TA], the remnant of the müllerian duct (ductus paramesonephricus) on the upper end of the testis; called also *hydatid of Morgagni, morgagnian cyst, sessile hydatid,* and *testicular appendage.*
**a. of ventricle of larynx, a. ventri'culi laryn'gis,** sacculus laryngis.
**a. vermicula'ris,** a. vermiformis.
**a. vermifor'mis** [TA], vermiform appendix: a wormlike diverticulum of the cecum, varying in length from 7 to 15 cm, and measuring about 1 cm in diameter.
**appen'dices vesiculo'sae epooph'ori** [TA], vesicular appendages of epoophoron: small pedunculated structures attached to the uterine tubes near their fimbriated end, being remnants of the mesonephric ducts; called also *a. morgagnii, hydatids of Morgagni, Morgagni's a.,* and *morgagnian cyst.*
**appen'dices vesiculo'sae epoophoron'tis,** appendices vesiculosae epoophori.
**xiphoid a.,** processus xiphoideus.

**ap·pen·do·li·thi·a·sis** (ə-pen″do-lĭ-thi'ə-sis) appendicolithiasis.

**ap·per·cep·tion** (ap″ər-sep'shən) [L. *ad* to + *percipere* to perceive] conscious perception and appreciation; the power of receiving, appreciating, and interpreting sensory impressions.

**ap·per·cep·tive** (ap″ər-sep'tiv) pertaining to apperception.

**ap·per·son·a·tion** (ə-pər″so-na'shən) appersonification.

**ap·per·son·i·fi·ca·tion** (ap″ər-son-ĭ-fĭ-ka'shən) unconscious identification with another person or delusional belief that one is another person; it may be associated with various mental disorders, particularly schizophrenia.

**ap·pe·stat** (ap'ə-stat) [*appe*tite + *stat*] the brain center (probably in the hypothalamus) concerned with controlling the amount of food intake.

**ap·pe·tite** (ap'ə-tīt) [L. *appetere* to desire] [MeSH: Appetite] a natural longing or desire, especially the natural and recurring desire for food.

**ap·pe·ti·tion** (ap″ə-tish'ən) [L. *ad* toward + *petere* to seek] the directing of desire toward a definite purpose or object.

**ap·pet·i·tive** (ə-pet'ĭ-tiv″) characterized by approach, or exciting approach behavior; said of stimuli or behavior. Cf. *aversive.*

**ap·pla·na·tion** (ap″lə-na'shən) [L. *applanatio*] undue flatness, as of the cornea.

**ap·pla·nom·e·ter** (ap″lə-nom'ĕ-tər) applanation tonometer.

**ap·ple** (ap'əl) 1. *Malus sylvestris.* L. 2. the edible fruit of *M. sylvestris.* In dried and powdered form it is used as an antidiarrheal; its seeds are cyanogenetic, and ingestion of large quantities can cause cyanide poisoning. 3. Something that resembles this fruit.
**Adam's a.,** prominentia laryngea.
**bitter a.,** colocynth.
**Indian a., May a.,** podophyllum.
**thorn a.,** 1. *Datura stramonium.* 2. stramonium, def. 2.

**ap·pli·ance** (ə-pli'əns) in dentistry, a general term referring to various devices used to provide a function or therapeutic effect, e.g., dental prostheses, obturators, or orthodontic appliances.
**Andresen a.,** functional activator.
**Begg a.,** an orthodontic appliance consisting of a light wire and brackets permitting the tipping of tooth crowns, horizontal buccal tubes on the anchor molars to prevent their tipping, and elastics. See also *Begg technique,* under *technique.*
**Bimler a.,** a removable orthodontic appliance believed to stimulate reflex muscle activity, which in turn produces the desired tooth movement. Called also *Bimler stimulator.*
**craniofacial a.,** a device used to immobilize and/or reduce mandibular or midfacial fractures.

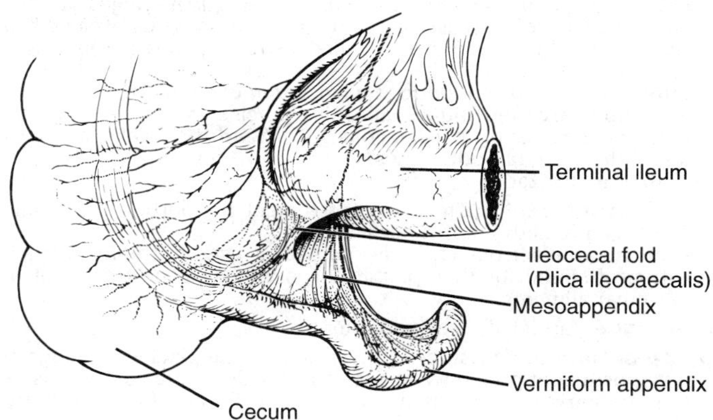

Vermiform appendix and adjacent structures.

**Crozat a.**, a removable orthodontic appliance, usually made of a precious metal, used to align teeth during orthodontic therapy. Called also *crozat* and *Walker a.*
**Denholz a.**, an orthodontic appliance consisting of a wire assembly containing a vestibular acrylic screen and open coil spring segments that fit over the wire arch.
**edgewise a.**, a fixed, multiunit orthodontic appliance using a rectangular labial arch wire ligated to brackets cemented to individual teeth or to bands encircling the teeth. So called because the bracket is machined so that the rectangular arch wire is inserted with its long cross section horizontal instead of vertical as in the ribbon arch bracket. Called also *edgewise attachment.*
**expansion plate a.**, any orthodontic appliance equipped with an expansion plate. Called also *split plate a.*
**extraoral a.**, an orthodontic appliance using a resistance unit outside of the oral cavity; see under *anchorage.*
**fixed a.**, an appliance that is cemented to the teeth or attached by means of an adhesive material. Called also *permanent a.*
**Fränkel a.**, function corrector.
**habit-breaking a.**, an orthodontic appliance designed to correct faulty habits, such as finger-sucking, tongue-thrusting, infantile swallowing.
**Hawley a.**, see under *retainer.*
**Jackson a.**, a removable orthodontic appliance retained in position by crib-shaped wires, bent to follow the outline of the buccal and lingual contours of the bicuspid and molar teeth, and united by cross wires lying in the occlusal embrasures. Called also *Jackson crib.*
**Johnston twin wire a.**, twin wire a.
**jumping-the-bite a.**, Kingsley a.
**Kesling a.**, an occlusal splint made of soft acrylic resin or latex rubber that fits over the occlusal and incisal surfaces of the teeth; it is designed to hold the mandible in a certain relationship to the maxilla to treat bruxism.
**Kingsley a.**, an active plate appliance having a bite plate with an inclined anterior plane to move the mandible forward by jumping the bite. Called also *jumping-the-bite a., jumping-the-bite plate,* and *Kingsley plate.*
**labiolingual a.**, an orthodontic appliance for intermaxillary therapy, consisting of a maxillary labial arch introduced into horizontal buccal tubes attached to the anchor bands and lingual arches of the same diameter fitted into vertical or horizontal tubes fastened to the lingual side of the anchor bands.
**monoblock a.**, functional activator.
**orthodontic a.**, a device, either fixed to the teeth or removable, that applies force to the teeth and their supporting structures to produce changes in their relationship to each other and to control their growth and development. Used in orthodontic therapy to move the teeth into esthetically or physiologically better positions, such as better alignment within the dental arch or with the opposing dentition; also used in the treatment of fractures or other injuries to the maxilla, to stabilize or immobilize the teeth and jaws. Called also *braces.*
**permanent a.**, fixed a.
**prosthetic a.**, a device affixed to or implanted in the body, designed to take the place, or perform the function, of a missing body part, such as an artificial arm or leg, or a complete or partial denture.
**removable a.**, any orthodontic appliance that the patient is able to insert and remove from the mouth.
**ribbon arch a.**, an orthodontic appliance consisting of a flattened wire inserted into a special bracket against the labial and buccal surfaces of the teeth; usually done to move the teeth laterally. Called also *ribbon arch.*
**Schwarz a.**, a removable orthodontic appliance with a tissue-borne anchorage and appurtenances of wire for tooth movement.
**split plate a.**, expansion plate a.
**twin wire a.**, an orthodontic appliance using fixed lingual arches and a labial arch consisting of a pair of round wires attached to brackets on the anterior teeth. Called also *Johnston twin wire a.* and *twin wire.*
**universal a.**, an orthodontic appliance that combines the edgewise and ribbon arch techniques, affording precise control of individual teeth in all planes of space; it consists of bands or brackets or both for all the teeth in both arches.
**Walker a.**, Crozat a.

**ap·pli·ca·tor** (ap′lĭ-ka″tər) an instrument for putting something (such as a remedy) onto a surface.
**sonic a.**, an electromechanical transducer used in the local application of sound for therapeutic purposes, as in the treatment of muscular ailments.

**ap·pli·qué** (ap″lĭ-ka′) see under *form.*

**ap·po·si·tion** (ap″ə-zish′ən) [L. *appositio*] the placing of things in juxtaposition or proximity; specifically, the deposition of successive layers upon those already present, as in cell walls. Called also *juxtaposition.*

**ap·pre·hen·sion** (ap″re-hen′shən) 1. perception and understanding. 2. anticipatory fear or anxiety.

**ap·proach** (ə-prōch′) the specific anatomic dissection by which an organ or part is exposed in surgery.
**Risdon a.**, a surgical method of exposing the ascending ramus of the mandible by means of an incision made below and behind the angle of the mandible, for treatment of fractures, e.g., condylar fractures, or for reconstructive surgery.

**ap·prox·i·mal** (ə-prok′sĭ-məl) situated close together.

**ap·prox·i·mate** (ə-prok′sĭ-māt″) 1. to bring close together, or into apposition. 2. approximal.

**ap·prox·i·ma·tion** (ə-prok″sĭ-ma′shən) the act or process of bringing closer together or into apposition.
**successive a.**, shaping.

**ap·ro·clon·i·dine hy·dro·chlo·ride** (ap″rə-klon′ĭ-dēn) [USP] an $\alpha_2$-adrenergic receptor agonist used to reduce intraocular pressure in the treatment of open-angle glaucoma and ocular hypertension; administered topically.

**aprac·tag·no·sia** (ə-prak″tag-no′zhə) [*apractic* + *agnosia*] a type of agnosia marked by inability to use objects or perform skilled motor activities, due to lesions in the lower occipital or parietal lobes; subtypes include *ideomotor apraxia* and *sensory apraxia.*

**aprac·tic** (ə-prak′tik) pertaining to or characterized by apraxia.

**ap·ra·my·cin** (ap″rə-mi′sin) an aminoglycoside antibiotic, part of the nebramycin complex, effective against a wide variety of aerobic gram-negative bacilli; used as the sulfate salt in the treatment of enteric colibacillosis in swine.

**aprax·ia** (ə-prak′se-ə) [Gr. "a not acting," "want of success"] [MeSH: Apraxia] loss of ability to carry out familiar, purposeful movements in the absence of paralysis or other motor or sensory impairment. Cf. *dyspraxia.*
**akinetic a.**, loss of ability to carry out spontaneous movement.
**amnestic a.**, loss of ability to carry out a movement on command as a result of inability to remember the command, although ability to perform the movement is present.
**Bruns' a. of gait**, Bruns' frontal ataxia.
**buccofacial a.**, facial a.
**classic a.**, ideokinetic a.
**Cogan's oculomotor a., congenital oculomotor a.**, an absence or defect of horizontal eye movements, so that when the patient tries to look at an object off to one side, the head must turn to bring the eyes into line with the object and the eyes exhibit nystagmus; the cause is probably a brain lesion. Called also *Cogan's syndrome.*
**constructional a.**, a type of deficit in motor skills characterized by lack of ability to copy simple drawings or to reproduce patterns created with building blocks or matchsticks.
**dressing a.**, inability to dress oneself properly, often on just one side, as a result of a lesion in the parietal lobe, usually on the nondominant side. See also *unilateral neglect,* under *neglect.*
**facial a.**, apraxia of the facial muscles with inability to carry out movements for expression, articulation, and other functions; caused by a lesion in either the supramarginal gyrus or the motor association area on the dominant side. It may be associated with ideokinetic apraxia. Called also *buccofacial a.*
**ideational a.**, sensory a.
**ideokinetic a., ideomotor a.**, inability to carry out movements that are part of normal activities when requested, in imitation of a demonstration, or even when the person spontaneously wishes to do them. The name is derived from the older concept that ideas were not linked to movements. Called also *transcortical a.*
**innervatory a.**, motor a.
**Liepmann's a.**, apraxia.
**motor a.**, impairment of skilled movements that is greater than or different in form from that caused by weakness of the affected parts; the patient appears clumsy rather than weak. Called also *innervatory a.*
**sensory a.**, loss of ability to make proper use of an object, due to lack of perception of its proper nature and purpose or to gross disorganization of a plan of usage. Called also *ideational a.*
**a. of speech**, a speech disorder similar to motor aphasia, due to apraxia of mouth and neck muscles because of a lesion interfering with coordination of impulses from Broca's motor speech area. Called also *aphemia.*
**transcortical a.**, ideokinetic a.

**aprax·ic** (ə-prak′sik) apractic.

**Apres·a·zide** (ə-pres′ə-zīd) trademark for preparations of hydralazine hydrochloride with hydrochlorothiazide.

**Apres·o·line** (ə-pres′o-lēn) trademark for preparations of hydralazine hydrochloride.

**ap·ro·bar·bi·tal** (ap″ro-bahr′bĭ-təl) an intermediate-acting barbiturate, used as a sedative and hypnotic; administered orally. Abuse of this drug may lead to dependence.

**aproc·tia** (ə-prok'she-ə) [*a-*[1] + *procto-* + *-ia*] congenital absence or imperforation of the anus.

**apro·so·dia** (a″pro-so'de-ə) aprosody.

**apros·o·dy** (a-pros'ə-de) severe dysprosody.

**apro·so·pia** (ap″ro-so'pe-ə) [*a-*[1] + *prosopo-* + *-ia*] partial or complete congenital absence of structures of the face.

**apro·so·pus** (ə-pro'sə-pəs) a fetus exhibiting aprosopia.

**apro·tic** (a-pro'tik) denoting a substance that neither accepts nor donates protons.

**apro·ti·nin** (ap″ro-ti'nin) [MeSH: Aprotinin] a polypeptide inhibitor of proteolytic enzymes, used as an antihemorrhagic and to reduce perioperative blood loss during cardiopulmonary bypass; administered intravenously. It has also been used in the treatment of acute pancreatitis.

**APS** American Physiological Society.

**APTA** American Physical Therapy Association.

**ap·ter·ous** (ap'tər-əs) [*a-*[1] + Gr. *pteron* wing] wingless.

**ap·ti·tude** (ap'tĭ-to͞od) [MeSH: Aptitude] natural ability and skill in certain lines of endeavor.

**APTT, aPTT** activated partial thromboplastin time.

**ap·ty·a·lia** (ap″ti-a'le-ə) aptyalism.

**ap·ty·a·lism** (ap-ti'ə-liz-əm) deficiency or absence of the saliva.

**APUD** [*a*mine *p*recursor *u*ptake (and) *d*ecarboxylation] see under *cell.*

**apud·o·ma** (a″pəd-o'mə) [MeSH: Apudoma] any tumor composed of cells with APUD properties.

**apul·mo·nism** (a-pul'mo-niz-əm) [*a-*[1] + *pulmon-* + *-ism*] apneumia.

**apus** (a'pəs) [*a-*[1] + Gr. *pous* foot] sirenomelus.

**apy·e·tous** (a-pi'ə-təs) [*a-*[1] + Gr. *pyon* pus] showing no pus; nonpurulent.

**apyk·no·mor·phous** (ə-pik″no-mor'fəs) [*a-*[1] + *pyknomorphous*] not pyknomorphous; not having the stainable cell elements compactly placed; said of certain nerve cells.

**apy·o·gen·ic** (a″pi-o-jen'ik) not caused by pus.

**apy·ous** (a-pi'əs) [*a-*[1] + Gr. *pyon* pus] having no pus; nonpurulent.

**apy·rene** (a'pi-rēn) [*a-*[1] + Gr. *pyrēn* fruit stone, nucleus] having no nucleus or nuclear material.

**apy·ret·ic** (a″pi-ret'ik) [*a-*[1] + *pyretic*] afebrile.

**apy·rex·ia** (a″pi-rek'se-ə) [*a-*[1] + *pyrexia*] 1. absence of fever. 2. the intermission of fever.

**apy·rex·i·al** (a″pi-rek'se-əl) afebrile.

**apy·ro·gen·ic** (a-pi″ro-jen'ik) [*a-*[1] + *pyrogenic*] not producing fever.

**AQ** achievement quotient.

**Aq.** Abbreviation for L. *a'qua,* water.

**Aq. dest.** [L. *a'qua destilla'ta*] distilled water.

**Aq. pur.** [L. *a'qua pu'ra*] pure water.

**Aq. tep.** [L. *a'qua tep'ida*] tepid water.

**aq·ua** (ah'kwə, ak'wə, ā'kwə) gen. and pl. *a'quae* [L.] water. See also *aromatic water* and various other forms listed under *water.*
**a. am'nii,** amniotic fluid.
**a. aromat'ica,** aromatic water.
**a. cinnamo'mi,** cinnamon water.
**a. destilla'ta,** distilled water.
**a. for'tis,** a solution of nitric acid.
**a. men'thae piperi'tae,** peppermint water.
**a. o'culi,** the aqueous humor or fluid of the eye.
**a. re'gia,** a mixture of one part concentrated nitric acid to three or four parts concentrated hydrochloric acid; it is able to dissolve gold and platinum.
**a. ro'sae,** rose water.
**a. ro'sae for'tior,** stronger rose water.

**Aqua·bir·na·vi·rus** (ah″kwə-bər'nə-vi″rəs) [L. *aqua* water + *bi*segmented *RNA* + *virus*] a genus of viruses of the family Birnaviridae that infect fish, mollusks, and crustaceans; it includes a single species, infectious pancreatic necrosis virus, which is the cause of infectious pancreatic necrosis of fish.

**Aq·ua·care** (ak'wə-kār) trademark for preparations of urea.

**aq·uae** (ah'kwe, ak'we, a'kwe) [L.] genitive and plural of *aqua.*

**aq·uae·duc·tus** (ak″we-duk'təs) [L.] aqueductus.

**aq·ua·gen·ic** (ak″wə-jen'ik) caused by water or by contact with water.

**Aq·ua·MEPH·Y·TON** (ak″wə-mef'ĭtən) trademark for a preparation of phytonadione.

**aq·ua·pho·bia** (ak″wə-fo'be-ə) [*aqua-* + *-phobia*] irrational fear of water, i.e., of swimming or of being near water where one might fall in and drown.

**aq·ua·punc·ture** (ak'wə-pungk″chər) [*aqua* + *puncture*] the subcutaneous injection of water.

**Aq·ua·reo·vi·rus** (ak″wə-re'o-vi″rəs) [L. *aqua* water + *reovirus*] a genus of viruses of the family Reoviridae that infect fresh- and saltwater fish and invertebrates; some species cause economically important diseases of fish.

**Aq·ua·ten·sen** (ak″wə-ten'sən) trademark for a preparation of methyclothiazide.

**aquat·ic** (ə-kwat'ik) inhabiting or frequenting water.

**aq·ue·duct** (ak'wə-dukt″) a passage or channel in a body structure or organ; see also *aqueductus.*
**cerebral a.,** aqueductus mesencephali.
**a. of cochlea, cochlear a.,** aqueductus cochleae.
**a. of Cotunnius,** 1. aqueductus vestibuli. 2. canaliculus cochleae.
**fallopian a., a. of Fallopius,** canalis nervi facialis.
**a. of mesencephalon,** aqueductus mesencephali.
**a. of midbrain,** aqueductus mesencephali.
**a. of Sylvius,** aqueductus mesencephali.
**ventricular a.,** aqueductus mesencephali.
**vestibular a., a. of vestibule,** aqueductus vestibuli.

**aq·ue·duc·tus** (ak″wə-duk'təs) gen. and pl. *aqueduc'tus* [L., from *aqua* water + *ductus* canal] [TA] a passage or channel in a body structure or organ, especially a channel for the conduction of fluid; called also *aqueduct* and *aquaeductus.*
**a. ce'rebri,** TA alternative for *a. mesencephali.*
**a. coch'leae** [TA], aqueduct of cochlea: a small channel that connects the scala tympani with the subarachnoid space; called also *cochlear aqueduct, ductus perilymphatici, ductus perilymphaticus,* and *perilymphatic duct.*
**a. mesence'phali** [TA], aqueduct of mesencephalon: the narrow channel in the mesencephalon that connects the third and fourth ventricles; called also *aqueduct of Sylvius, a. cerebri* [TA alternative], *cerebral aqueduct,* and *iter of Sylvius.*
**a. vesti'buli** [TA], aqueduct of vestibule: a small canal extending from the vestibule of the inner ear to open onto the posterior surface of the petrous part of the temporal bone. It lodges the endolymphatic duct and an arteriole and a venule. Called also *vestibular aqueduct* and *aqueduct of Cotunnius.*

**aque·ous** (a'kwe-əs) 1. watery; prepared with water. 2. the aqueous humor of the eye; see under *humor.*

**Aq·uex** trademark for a preparation of clopamide.

**aq·uip·a·rous** (ak-wip'ə-rəs) [*aqua* + *parere* to produce] producing water or a watery secretion.

**AR** alarm reaction; aortic regurgitation; artificial respiration.

**Ar** symbol for *argon.*

**ara-A** adenine arabinoside; see *vidarabine.*

**ar·a·ban** (ar-ə-ban) any of a group of pentosans composed of L-arabinose residues; they are major constituents of gums and pectins.

**ar·a·bic ac·id** (ar'ə-bik) arabin.

**ar·a·bin** (ar'ə-bin) an amorphous carbohydrate gum composed of residues of arabinose, rhamnose, galactose, and an aldobionic acid composed of glucuronic acid and galactose; its salts with calcium, potassium, and magnesium are the main constituents of gum arabic (acacia). Called also *arabic acid.*

**arab·i·nose** (ə-rab'ĭ-nōs) [MeSH: Arabinose] an aldopentose epimeric with ribose at the 2 carbon, occurring naturally in both D- and L-forms, widely distributed in plants in the form of complex polysaccharides, glycosides, and mucilages and also occurring in some bacteria.

**ar·a·bin·o·side** (ar″ə-bin'o-sīd) a glycoside of arabinose.

**arab·in·o·sis** (ə-rab″ĭ-no'sis) poisoning by arabinose, which may produce nephrosis.

**arab·i·no·su·ria** (ə-rab″ĭ-nōs-u're-ə) the presence of arabinose in the urine.

**arab·i·no·syl·cy·to·sine** (ə-rab″ĭ-no-səl-si'to-sēn) cytarabine.

**arab·i·tol** (ə-rab'ĭ-tol) a sugar alcohol formed by the reduction of the carbonyl group of arabinose.

**ara-C** cytarabine.

**arach·ic ac·id** (ə-rak'ik) arachidic acid.

**arach·i·date** (ə-rak′ĭ-dāt) a salt (soap), ester, or anionic form of arachidic acid.

**ar·a·chid·ic** (ar″ə-kid′ik) [L. *arachis* peanut] pertaining to or caused by peanuts or other members of the genus *Arachis*; see under *bronchitis*.

**ar·a·chid·ic ac·id** (ar″ə-kid′ik) a saturated 20-carbon fatty acid found in vegetable (e.g. peanut) oils and fish oils. Called also *eicosanoic acid*. See table accompanying *fatty acid*.

**arach·i·don·ate** (ə-rak″ĭ-don′āt) a salt, ester, or anion of arachidonic acid.

**arach·i·don·ate 5-lip·oxy·gen·ase** (ə-rak″ĭ-don′āt lĭ-pok′sə-jən-ās) [EC 1.13.11.34] [MeSH: Arachidonate 5-Lipoxygenase] an enzyme of the oxidoreductase class that catalyzes the oxidation of arachidonate at the 5 position to form 5-hydroperoxyeicosatetraenoic acid (5-HPETE). The reaction occurs in leukocytes, particularly neutrophils, as the first step of the lipoxygenase pathway for conversion of arachidonic acid to leukotrienes.

**arach·i·don·ate 12-lip·oxy·gen·ase** (ə-rak′ĭ-don″āt lĭ-pok′sə-jən-ās) [EC 1.13.11.31] [MeSH: Arachidonate 12-Lipoxygenase] an enzyme of the oxidoreductase class that catalyzes the oxidation of arachidonate at the 12 position to form 12-hydroperoxyeicosatetraenoic acid (12-HPETE). The reaction occurs primarily in platelets and is the first step of the lipoxygenase pathway for conversion of arachidonic acid to the leukotriene 12-hydroxyeicosatetraenoic acid (12-HETE).

**arach·i·don·ate 15-lip·oxy·ge·nase** (ə-rak′ĭ-don′āt lĭ-pok′sə-jən-ās) [EC 1.13.11.33] [MeSH: Arachidonate 15-Lipoxygenase] an enzyme of the oxidoreductase class that catalyzes the oxidation of arachidonate at the 15 position to form 15-hydroperoxyeicosatetraenoic acid (15-HPETE). The reaction occurs primarily in vascular endothelium and is the first step in the conversion of arachidonic acid to 15-hydroxyeicosatetraenoic acid (15-HETE) and to lipoxins.

**arach·i·don·ic acid** (ə-rak″ĭ-don′ik) [MeSH: Arachidonic Acid] a polyunsaturated 20-carbon essential fatty acid (see table at *fatty acid*) occurring in animal fats and also formed by biosynthesis from dietary linoleic acid. It is a precursor in the biosynthesis of leukotrienes, prostaglandins, and thromboxanes.

**ara·chis** (ar′ə-kis) a genus of herbs of the family Leguminosae, having yellow flowers, originally native to southern Brazil. *A. hypogae′a* is the peanut, source of peanut oil. See also *arachidic* and *aflatoxin*.

**arach·ne·pho·bia** (ə-rak″nə-fo′be-ə) arachnophobia.

**Arach·nia** (ə-rak′ne-ə) [Gr. *arachnion* a cobweb] a genus of bacteria of the family Actinomycetaceae, order Actinomycetales. The organisms are gram-positive, anaerobic or microaerophilic, nonsporulating, branched, diphtheroid rods that form thin branching filaments but no mycelia.
**A. propio′nica,** a species that is a normal inhabitant of the body cavities and skin of humans and other mammals. It causes human actinomycosis and periodontal disease and infections in cattle. Called also *Propionibacterium propionicum*.

**arach·nid** (ə-rak′nid) [MeSH: Arachnida] any member of the class Arachnida.

**Arach·ni·da** (ə-rak′nĭ-də) [Gr. *arachnē* spider] [MeSH: Arachnida] a class of the Arthropoda; orders include Araneae (the spiders), Acarina (the ticks and mites), and Scorpionida (the scorpions).

**arach·nid·ism** (ə-rak′nĭ-diz-əm) [MeSH: Arachnidism] the condition produced by the bite of a venomous spider; envenomation by a spider. Called also *araneism* and *arachnoidism*.
**necrotic a.,** spider envenomation marked by necrosis at the site of the bite, resulting in slow-healing, ulcerating lesions.

**arach·ni·tis** (ar″ak-ni′tis) [*arachno-* + *-itis*] arachnoiditis.

**arachn(o)-** [Gr. *arachnē* spider] a combining form denoting relationship to the arachnoid membrane or to a spider.

**arach·no·dac·tyl·ia** (ə-rak″no-dak-til′e-ə) arachnodactyly.

**arach·no·dac·ty·ly** (ə-rak″no-dak′tə-le) [*arachno-* + Gr. *daktylos* finger] a condition characterized by abnormal length and slenderness of the fingers and toes; called also *acromacria, dolichostenomelia,* and *spider finger*. Sometimes used in the past as a synonym for *Marfan's syndrome*.
**contractural a., congenital (CCA),** a form of hereditary bone dysplasia; see under *dysplasia*.

**arach·no·gas·tria** (ə-rak″no-gas′tre-ə) [*arachno-* + *gastr-* + *-ia*] the prominent network of veins on the protuberant abdomen caused by ascites, especially in hepatic cirrhosis.

**arach·noid** (ə-rak′noid) [MeSH: Arachnoid] 1. resembling a spider's web. 2. arachnoidea mater.
**a. of brain, cranial a.,** arachnoidea mater encephali.
**spinal a., a. of spinal cord,** arachnoidea mater spinalis.

**arach·noi·dal** (ar″ak-noi′dəl) or of pertaining to the arachnoid.

**arach·noi·dea** (ar″ak-noi′de-ə) pl. *arachnoi′deae* [Gr. *arachnoidēs* like a cobweb] arachnoidea mater.
**a. ence′phali,** arachnoidea mater encephali; see under *arachnoidea mater*.
**a. spina′lis,** arachnoidea mater spinalis; see under *arachnoidea mater*.

**arach·noi·dea ma·ter** (ar″ak-noi′de-ə ma′tər, mah′ter) [TA] a delicate membrane interposed between the dura mater and the pia mater, separated from the pia mater by the subarachnoid space.
**a. m. crania′lis** [TA], the arachnoidea covering the brain; called also *arachnoid of brain, cranial arachnoid,* and *a.m. encephali* [TA alternative].
**a. m. ence′phali,** TA alternative for *a. m. cranialis*.
**a. m. et pi′a ma′ter,** TA alternative for *leptomeninx*.
**a. m. spina′lis** [TA], spinal arachnoid: the arachnoidea covering the spinal cord; called also *arachnoid of spinal cord*.

**arach·noid·ism** (ə-rak′noid-iz″əm) arachnidism.

**arach·noid·i·tis** (ə-rak″noid-i′tis) [*arachnoid* + *-itis*] [MeSH: Arachnoiditis] inflammation of the arachnoidea; called also *arachnitis*.
**chronic adhesive a.,** thickening and adhesions of the leptomeninges in the brain or spinal cord, resulting from previous meningitis, other disease processes, or trauma; it is sometimes secondary to therapeutic or diagnostic injection of substances into the subarachnoid space. The signs and symptoms vary with extent and location. See also *spinal a.*
**spinal a.,** chronic adhesive arachnoiditis in the spinal arachnoid, with root and spinal cord symptoms similar to those caused by pressure from a tumor.

**arach·noid ma·ter** (ə-rak′noid ma′tər, mah′ter) arachnoidea mater.
**cranial a. m.,** arachnoidea mater cranialis.
**spinal a. m.,** arachnoidea mater spinalis.

**arach·nol·y·sin** (ar″ak-nol′ə-sin) [*arachno-* + *lysin*] the active hemolytic principle of spider venom.

**arach·no·me·lia** (ə-rak″no-me′le-ə) [*arachno-* + *-melia*] an autosomal recessive skeletal defect in calves and lambs in which the limbs are long, thin, and fragile, resembling the legs of a spider.

**arach·no·pho·bia** (ə-rak″no-fo′be-ə) [*arachno-* + *-phobia*] irrational fear of spiders.

**Ar·a·len** (ār′ə-len) trademark for preparations of chloroquine.

**aral·kyl** (ə-ral′kəl) an organic group in which an aryl group has replaced an alkyl hydrogen.

**Ar·a·mine** (ar′ə-min) trademark for a preparation of metaraminol.

**Ar·an's law** (ah-rahnz′) [François Amilcar *Aran,* French physician, 1817–1861] see under *law*.

**Ar·an-Du·chenne muscular atrophy (disease)** (ah-rahn′du-shen′) [F. A. *Aran;* Guillaume Benjamin Amand *Duchenne,* French neurologist, 1806–1875] spinal muscular atrophy; see under *atrophy*.

**Aran·e·ae** (ə-rān′e-e) an order of the Arachnida comprising the spiders; it is divided into the suborders Labidognatha and Orthognatha.

**Ar·a·ne·i·da** (ar″ə-ne′ĭ-də) Araneae.

**ara·ne·ism** (ə-ra′ne-iz-əm) arachnidism.

**Aran·ti·us' bodies, etc.** (ə-ran′shəs) [Julius Caesar *Arantius* (Italian *Aranzi*), Italian anatomist and physician, 1530–1589] see under *body, canal, duct, ligament, nodule,* and *ventricle*.

**Aran·zi** (ah-rahn′tse) Arantius.

**ara·phia** (ə-ra′fe-ə) dysraphia.

**ar·a·ro·ba** (ahr″ə-ro′bə) [Brazilian] 1. *Andira.* 2. Goa powder.

**ar·ba·pros·til** (ahr′bə-pros′til) [MeSH: Arbaprostil] a synthetic 15-methyl analogue of dinoprostone, a prostaglandin of the E type; its esters have been used orally to reduce gastric secretion in the treatment of gastric ulcer and intramuscularly for termination of pregnancy.

**Ar·ber** (ahr′bər) Werner. Swiss microbiologist, born 1929; co-winner, with Daniel Nathans and Hamilton Othanel Smith, of the Nobel prize for medicine or physiology in 1978 for his work on restriction enzymes.

**ar·bor** (ahr′bər) pl. *ar′bores* [L.] a treelike structure or part; a structure or system resembling a tree with its branches.
**a. bronchia′lis** [TA], bronchial tree: the bronchi and their branching structures.
**dendritic a.,** see under *tree*.
**a. vi′tae,** 1. *Thuja occidentalis.* 2. a. vitae cerebelli.
**a. vi′tae cerebel′li** [TA], the treelike outline of white substance seen in a median section of the cerebellum; called also *medullary body of vermis* and *arborescent white substance of cerebellum*.
**a. vi′tae u′teri,** plicae palmatae.

**ar·bo·re·al** (ahr-bo′re-əl) pertaining to trees; inhabiting or attached to trees.

**ar·bo·res** (ahr-bor′ēz) [L.] plural of *arbor.*

**ar·bo·res·cent** (ahr″bo-res′ənt) [L. *arborescens*] branching like a tree.

**ar·bo·ri·za·tion** (ahr″bə-rĭ-za′shən) 1. the branching termination of certain nerve cell processes. 2. a form of the termination of a nerve fiber when in contact with a muscle fiber. 3. the treelike appearance of capillary vessels in inflamed conditions.

**ar·bo·roid** (ahr′bə-roid) [*arbor* + *-oid*] branching like a tree.

**ar·bor·vi·rus** (ahr′bor-vi″rəs) former term for *arbovirus.*

**ar·bo·vi·ral** (ahr″bo-vi′rəl) pertaining to or caused by arboviruses.

**ar·bo·vi·rus** (ahr′bo-vi″rəs) [from *ar*thropod-*bo*rne + virus] [MeSH: Arboviruses] any member of an epidemiologic class of viruses (the arboviruses) that replicate in blood-feeding arthropods and are transmitted by bite to the host. Arboviruses can be grouped serologically; the original groups were designated A, B, and C, but new groups are named from the first member of the group to be discovered. Arboviruses are contained in the families Arenaviridae, Bunyaviridae, Flaviviridae, Reoviridae, Rhabdoviridae, and Togaviridae; a few are unclassified. "Arbovirus" has no relationship to viral chemistry, morphology, or replication and so has no standing as a legitimate taxonomic term.
**group A a's,** *Alphavirus.*
**group B a's,** *Flavivirus.*

**ARC** American Red Cross; anomalous retinal correspondence; AIDS-related complex.

**arc** (ahrk) [*arcus*] 1. a structure or projected path having a curved or bowlike outline. 2. a visible electrical discharge generally taking the outline of an arc. 3. in neurophysiology, the pathway of neural reactions.
**auricular a., binauricular a.,** a measurement from the center of one auditory meatus to that of the other.
**bregmatolambdoid a.,** the arc extending along the course of the sagittal suture from the bregma to the lambda.
**carbon a.,** an electrical discharge between carbon electrodes that gives off an intense white light.
**mercury a.,** an electric discharge between electrodes in mercury vapor in a vacuum tube which gives off light rich in ultraviolet rays.
**nasobregmatic a.,** the arc extending from the nasion to the bregma.
**naso-occipital a.,** the arc extending from the nasion to the most inferior part of the external occipital protuberance.
**neural a.,** a series of two or more neurons connecting certain receptors and effectors, and constituting the pathway for neural reactions and reflexes; called also *sensorimotor a.*
**nuclear a.,** vortex lentis.
**reflex a.,** the neural arc used in a reflex action; an impulse travels to a nerve center over afferent fibers and the response travels outward from the center to an effector organ or part over efferent fibers. See illustration.
**sensorimotor a.,** neural a.

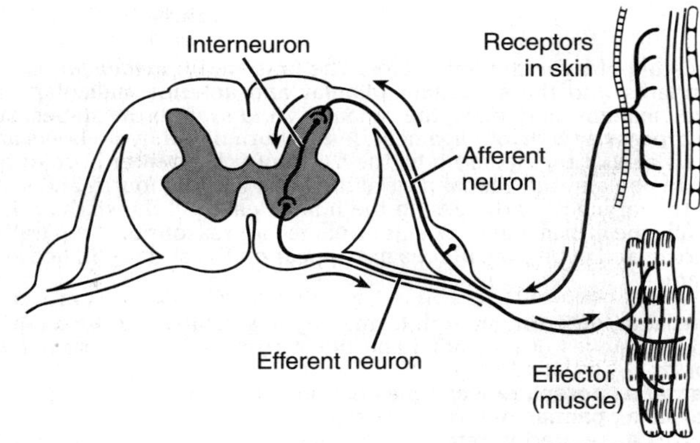

Three-neuron reflex arc.

**ar·cade** (ahr-kād′) an anatomical structure composed of a series of arches.
**arterial a's,** a series of anastomosing arterial arches as in the intestinal branches of the superior mesenteric artery.
**Flint's a.,** a series of arteriovenous arches at the base of the renal pyramids.
**dental a., lower,** arcus dentalis mandibularis.
**dental a., mandibular,** arcus dentalis mandibularis.
**dental a., maxillary,** arcus dentalis, maxillaris.
**dental a., upper,** arcus dentalis, maxillaris.

**Ar·ca·no·bac·te·ri·um** (ahr-ka″no-bak-tēr′e-əm) [L. *arcanus* secret + *bacterium*] a genus of irregular, rod-shaped, non–spore-forming, gram-positive bacteria. Organisms are non-motile, facultatively anaerobic, and catalase-negative.
**A. haemoly′ticum,** a genus, formerly *Corynebacterium haemolyticum,* that can cause infections in both humans and animals. In adolescents, infection is manifested by pharyngitis and a scarlatiniform rash similar to those seen in streptococcal infection.

**ar·cate** (ahr′kāt) arcuate.

**Ar·cel·la** (ahr-sel′ə) [L., dim. of *arca* box, chest] a genus of ameboid protozoa (order Arcellinida, subclass Testacealobosia) characterized by the presence of a few slender lobopodia and a transparent test to which the body of the organism is attached by numerous strands of ectoplasm.

**Ar·cel·lin·i·da** (ahr″sə-lin′ĭ-də) an order of free-living protozoa (subclass Testacealobosia, class Lobosiea) comprising those amebas enclosed in a test, tectum, or other external membrane that is composed of either organic or inorganic material or both and has a definite aperture through which pseudopodia (lobopodia or filopodia) can be extruded. Representative genera include *Arcella* and *Difflugia.* Called also *Testacea* and *Testacida.*

**arch** (arch) [L. *arcus* bow] a structure with a curved or bowlike outline.

## Arch

For specific anatomic structures not listed here, see under *arcus.*

**abdominothoracic a.,** the lower boundary of the anterior aspect of the thorax.
**alveolar a.,** an arch formed by the ridge of the alveolar process of the mandible or maxilla; see *arcus alveolaris mandibulae* and *arcus alveolaris maxillae.*
**anterior a. of atlas,** arcus anterior atlantis.
**a. of aorta, aortic a.,** arcus aortae.
**aortic a's,** paired vessels arching from the ventral to the dorsal aorta through the branchial arches of fishes and amniote embryos. In mammalian development, arches 1 and 2 disappear; arch 3 joins the common to the internal carotid; the left arch 4 remains as the arch of the definitive aorta while the right arch 4 joins the aorta to the subclavian artery; arch 5 is absent or disappears; and the ventral halves of arch 6 form the pulmonary arteries while the connections to the dorsal aorta are lost, although the left half, or ductus arteriosus, serves until birth.
**aortic a., cervical,** a rare, usually asymptomatic, congenital anomaly in which the aortic arch has an abnormally superior location, occasionally extending to the thoracic inlet or into the neck.
**aortic a., double,** a congenital anomaly in which the aorta divides into two branches which embrace the trachea and esophagus and reunite to form the descending aorta.
**arterial a's of kidney,** arteriae arcuatae renis.
**axillary a.,** a muscular slip occasionally arising from the cranial border of the latissimus dorsi muscle, crossing the axilla ventral to the axillary vessels and nerves, and joining the under surface of the tendon of the pectoralis major, the coracobrachialis, or the fascia of the biceps brachii muscle.
**a. of azygos vein,** arcus venae azygou.
**basal a.,** apical base.
**branchial a's,** paired arched columns that bear the gills in lower aquatic vertebrates and that, in the embryos of higher vertebrates, appear in comparable form before subsequent modification into structures of the head and neck. In humans they are also called *pharyngeal arches* because gills do not develop. Each contains a cartilaginous bar,

consisting of right and left halves. The first arch *(mandibular a.)* differentiates into the sphenomandibular and anterior malleolar ligaments, malleus, and incus; the second *(hyoid a.)* into the stapes, styloid process, stylohyoid ligament, lesser horn of the hyoid bone, and cranial part of the hyoid body; the third into the greater horn of the hyoid bone and the caudal part of its body; and the fourth and sixth into the laryngeal cartilages. In the human embryo, the sixth arch is actually the fifth in number but is so named for reasons of comparative anatomy and evolution; it does not appear on the surface. Called also *visceral a's.*

**carpal a., anterior,** an arch formed by anastomosis of the anterior carpal branches of the radial and ulnar arteries. Called also *palmar carpal a.*
**carpal a., dorsal,** rete carpale dorsale.
**carpal a., palmar,** anterior carpal a.
**carpal a., posterior,** rete carpale dorsale.
**a's of Corti,** a series of arches in the organ of Corti formed by inner and outer pillar cells.
**costal a.,** arcus costalis.
**a. of cricoid cartilage,** arcus cartilaginis cricoideae.
**crural a.,** ligamentum inguinale.
**crural a., deep,** tractus iliopubicus.
**dental a.,** the curving structure formed by a line described by the buccal surfaces or through the central grooves of the molars and bicuspids of the teeth in their normal position, viewed from the incisal and occlusal aspects. See also *arcus dentalis mandibularis* and *arcus dentalis maxillaris.*
**dental a., inferior,** arcus dentalis mandibularis.
**dental a., superior,** arcus dentalis maxillaris.
**diaphragmatic a., external,** ligamentum arcuatum laterale.
**diaphragmatic a., internal,** ligamentum arcuatum mediale.
**digital venous a's,** arcus venosi digitales.
**dorsal venous a. of foot,** arcus venosus dorsalis pedis.
**epiphyseal a.,** the embryonic structure in the roof of the third ventricle from which the pineal body develops.
**femoral a., superficial,** ligamentum inguinale.
**fibrous a. of soleus muscle,** arcus tendineus musculi solei.
**a's of foot,** see *arcus pedis longitudinalis* and *arcus pedis transversalis.*
**glossopalatine a.,** arcus palatoglossus.
**Haller's a's,** see *ligamentum arcuatum laterale* and *ligamentum arcuatum mediale.*
**hemal a.,** one of the cartilaginous structures surrounding the caudal vein in the tail of the vertebrate embryo, formed by the ventrad growth of the ventrolateral arcualia. In fish, the arches are also present in the thoracic region. Cf. *neural a.*
**hyoid a.,** the second pharyngeal (branchial) arch; see *branchial a's.*
**inguinal a.,** ligamentum inguinale.
**jugular venous a.,** arcus venosus jugularis.
**Langer's axillary a.,** axillary a.
**lateral a.,** lateral longitudinal arch.
**lingual a.,** a wire appliance made to conform to the lingual aspect of the dental arch; used to promote or to prevent movement of the teeth in orthodontic therapy.
**lingual a., fixed,** a space-retaining appliance consisting of an arch wire designed to fit the lingual surface of the teeth, and soldered to metal crowns or orthodontic bands. Called also *stationary lingual a.*

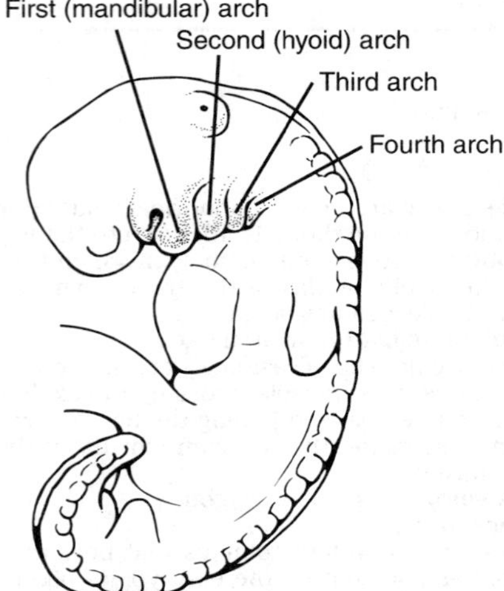

Branchial arches.

**lingual a., passive,** an orthodontic appliance for maintaining space and preserving arch length when bilateral primary molars are prematurely lost.
**lingual a., stationary,** fixed lingual a.
**longitudinal a.,** arcus pedis longitudinalis.
**longitudinal a., lateral,** pars lateralis arcus pedis longitudinalis.
**longitudinal a., medial,** pars medialis arcus pedis longitudinalis.
**longitudinal a. of foot,** arcus pedis longitudinalis.
**lumbocostal a. of diaphragm, external,** ligamentum arcuatum laterale.
**lumbocostal a. of diaphragm, internal,** ligamentum arcuatum mediale.
**lumbocostal a. of Haller, lateral,** ligamentum arcuatum laterale.
**lumbocostal a. of Haller, medial,** ligamentum arcuatum mediale.
**malar a.,** arcus zygomaticus.
**mandibular a.,** 1. the first pharyngeal (branchial) arch; see *branchial a's.* 2. arcus dentalis mandibularis.
**maxillary a.,** 1. palatal a. 2. arcus dentalis maxillaris.
**medial a.,** medial longitudinal arch.
**metatarsal a.,** arcus pedis transversalis.
**nasal a.,** the arch formed in the embryo by the nasal bones and by the nasal processes of the maxilla.
**neural a.,** one of the cartilaginous structures surrounding the embryonic spinal cord, formed by the dorsad growth of the dorsolateral arcualia; it is the primordium of the vertebral arch. Cf. *hemal a.*
**neural a. of vertebra,** arcus vertebrae.
**open pubic a.,** a congenital anomaly in which the pubic arch is not fused, the bodies of the pubic bones being spread apart.
**oral a.,** see *palatal a.*
**orbital a. of frontal bone,** margo supraorbitalis ossis frontalis.
**palatal a.,** the arch formed by the roof of the mouth from the teeth on one side of the maxilla to the teeth on the other or, if the teeth are missing, from the residual dental arch on one side to that on the other. Called also *maxillary a., palatomaxillary a.,* and *oral a.*
**palatine a., anterior,** arcus palatoglossus.
**palatine a., posterior,** arcus palatopharyngeus.
**palatoglossal a.,** arcus palatoglossus.
**palatomaxillary a.,** palatal a.
**palatopharyngeal a.,** arcus palatopharyngeus.
**palmar arterial a., deep,** arcus palmaris profundus.
**palmar arterial a., superficial,** arcus palmaris superficialis.
**palmar venous a., deep,** arcus venosus palmaris profundus.
**palmar venous a., superficial,** arcus venosus palmaris superficialis.
**palpebral a., inferior,** arcus palpebralis inferior.
**palpebral a., superior,** arcus palpebralis superior.
**paraphyseal a.,** the embryonic structure in the roof of the third ventricle of vertebrates from which the paraphysis develops.
**a. of pelvis,** angulus subpubicus.
**pharyngeal a's,** see *branchial a's.*
**pharyngoepiglottic a.,** arcus palatopharyngeus.
**pharyngopalatine a.,** arcus palatopharyngeus.
**plantar a., deep, plantar arterial a.,** arcus plantaris profundus.
**plantar venous a.,** arcus venosus plantaris.
**popliteal a.,** ligamentum popliteum arcuatum.
**postaural a's,** branchial a's.
**posterior a. of atlas,** arcus posterior atlantis.
**pubic a.,** arcus pubicus.
**pulmonary a's,** the most caudal of the aortic arches, which become the pulmonary arteries.
**residual a., residual dental a.,** the curved contour of the ridge remaining after tooth removal.
**ribbon a.,** see under *appliance.*
**a. of ribs,** arcus costalis.
**right aortic a.,** a congenital anomaly in which the aorta is displaced to the right and passes behind the esophagus, thus forming a vascular ring that may cause compression of the trachea and esophagus.
**Riolan's a.,** the arch formed by the mesentery of the transverse colon.
**Shenton's a.,** Shenton's line.
**subpubic a.,** angulus subpubicus.
**superciliary a.,** arcus superciliaris.
**supraorbital a. of frontal bone,** margo supraorbitalis ossis frontalis.
**tarsal a's,** see *arcus palpebralis inferior* and *arcus palpebralis superior.*
**tendinous a.,** arcus tendineus.
**tendinous a. of diaphragm, external,** ligamentum arcuatum laterale.
**tendinous a. of diaphragm, internal,** ligamentum arcuatum mediale.
**tendinous a. of levator ani muscle,** arcus tendineus musculi levatoris ani.

**tendinous a. of lumbodorsal fascia,** ligamentum lumbocostale.
**tendinous a. of pelvic fascia,** arcus tendineus fasciae pelvis.
**tendinous a. of soleus muscle,** arcus tendineus musculi solei.
**a. of thoracic duct,** see *ductus thoracicus.*
**thyrohyoid a.,** the third pharyngeal (branchial) arch, which becomes represented by the greater horn of the hyoid bone.
**transverse a. of foot,** arcus pedis transversalis.
**Treitz's a.,** an arch sometimes found in the paraduodenal fold, composed of the left superior colic artery and the inferior mesenteric vein.
**venous a's of kidney,** venae arcuatae renis.
**a. of vertebra, vertebral a.,** arcus vertebrae.
**visceral a's,** branchial a's.
**volar venous a., deep,** arcus venosus palmaris profundus.
**volar venous a., superficial,** arcus venosus palmaris superficialis.
**V-shaped a.,** a dental arch which narrows and comes to a point at the lingual junction of the maxillary central incisors.
**Zimmermann's a.,** an inconstant, rudimentary arch of the embryo, supposed to explain the origin of certain occasionally occurring vessels between the fourth aortic and the pulmonary arch.
**zygomatic a.,** arcus zygomaticus.

**arch-** See *archi-.*

**archae(o)-** for words beginning thus, see also those beginning *arche(o)-.*

**ar·chaeo·cer·e·bel·lum** (ahr″ke-o-ser″ə-bel′əm) [*archaeo-* + *cerebellum*] archicerebellum.

**ar·chaeo·cor·tex** (ahr″ke-o-kor′teks) [*archaeo-* + *cortex*] archicortex.

**ar·chae·us** (ahr-ke′-əs) Paracelsus' term for the vital principle, the living force in the body or the animate universe.

**Arch·ag·a·thus** (ahrk-ag′ə-thəs) the first Greek physician to practice in Rome (219 B.C.), according to Pliny. At first known as "the wound-curer" *(Vulnerarius),* because of his surgical exploits he was later termed "the executioner" *(Carnifex).*

**ar·cha·ic** (ahr-ka′ik) [Gr. *archaios* ancient] very ancient; pertaining to early evolutionary stages.

**arch·am·phi·as·ter** (ahrk-am′fe-as″tər) [*arch-* + *amphiaster*] the primitive amphiaster associated with the formation of polar bodies.

**ar·che·go·nium** (ahr″kə-go′ne-əm) [*arche-* + Gr. *gonos* offspring] the female organ of a cryptogamic plant taking part in the formation of sexually produced spores; cf. *antheridium.*

**arch·en·ceph·a·lon** (ahrk″ən-sef′ə-lon) [*arche-* + *encephalon*] the primordial brain, anterior to the end of the notochord, from which the midbrain and the forebrain are developed.

**arch·en·ter·on** (ahrk-en′tər-on) [*arche-* + *enteron*] the primordial digestive cavity of those embryonic forms whose blastula becomes a gastrula by invagination; called also *coelenteron, gastrocoele,* and *primitive gut.*

**arche(o)-** [Gr. *archaios* ancient, from *archē* beginning, from *archein* to begin] a combining from meaning first, beginning, original, primitive. Written also *archae(o)-.*

**ar·cheo·cer·e·bel·lum** (ahr″ke-o-ser″ə-bel′əm) [*archeo-* + *cerebellum*] archicerebellum.

**ar·cheo·cor·tex** (ahr″ke-o-kor′teks) [*archeo-* + *cortex*] archicortex.

**ar·che·spore** (ahr′kə-spor) [*arche-* + *-spore*] the mass of cells that give rise to spore mother cells; called also *archesporium* and *archispore.*

**ar·che·spo·ri·um** (ahr″kə-spo′re-əm) archespore.

**ar·che·type** (ahr′kə-tīp) [*arche-* + *type*] an ideal, original, or standard type or form.

**archi-** [Gr., from *archein* to begin, to rule] a prefix meaning (1) chief or principal, (2) beginning, original, or primitive. Written *arch-* before a vowel.

**ar·chi·blast** (ahr′kĭ-blast) [*archi-* + *-blast*] 1. the components of an ovum that actively form the embryo, as distinguished from the yolk. 2. His' term for the fundamental part of the blastodermic layers as distinguished from the parablast or peripheral portion of the mesoderm.

**ar·chi·blas·tic** (ahr″kĭ-blas′tik) derived from or pertaining to the archiblast.

**ar·chi·carp** (ahr′kĭ-kahrp) 1. the group of cells, including the ascogonium, that give rise to the fruiting body of ascomycetous fungi. Cf. *ascocarp.* 2. archegonium.

**ar·chi·cer·e·bel·lum** (ahr″kĭ-ser″ə-bel′əm) [*archi-* + *cerebellum*] [TA] the phylogenetically oldest part of the cerebellum; namely, the flocculonodular lobe. Because this lobe is the site of termination of most of the projections of vestibular afferents, the term is sometimes equated with *vestibulocerebellum.* Called also *archaeocerebellum* and *archeocerebellum.* Cf. *neocerebellum* and *paleocerebellum.*

**ar·chi·cor·tex** (ahr″kĭ-kor′teks) [TA] that portion of the cerebral cortex that, with the palaeocortex, develops in association with the olfactory system, and which is phylogenetically older than the neocortex and lacks its layered structure. The embryonic archaeocortex corresponds to the cortex of the dentate gyrus and hippocampus in mature mammals. Called also *archaeocortex* or *archeocortex, archipallium,* and *olfactory cortex.*

**ar·chi·gas·tru·la** (ahr″kĭ-gas′troo-lə) [*archi-* + *gastrula*] the gastrula in its most primordial form of development.

**Ar·chi·ge·nes of Apa·mea** (ar-kij′ĕ-nēz) [c. 53–c. 117] a Greek physician, a pupil of Agathinus, an Eclectic influenced by Pneumatist theories. He practiced at Rome and wrote several works, including observations on amputation and ligation, some portions of which are preserved. Galen's theory of pulse was taken from Archigenes'.

**ar·chi·kary·on** (ahr-kĭ-kar′e-on) [*archi-* + *karyon*] the nucleus of a zygote.

**ar·chil** (ahr′kil) 1. the lichen *Roccella tinctoria.* 2. a violet coloring from this and other lichens, employed as an indicator dye for litmus paper: alkalies give a blue color, and acids a red color.

**ar·chi·mor·u·la** (ahr-kĭ-mor′u-lə) [*archi-* + *morula*] a mass of cells arising from the division of the archicytula and preceding the archigastrula.

**ar·chi·neph·ron** (ahr″kĭ-nef′ron) [*archi-* + *nephron*] a unit of the pronephros.

**arch·i·pal·li·al** (ahr″kĭ-pal′e-əl) pertaining to the archipallium.

**ar·chi·pal·li·um** (ahr″kĭ-pal′e-əm) [*archi-* + *pallium*] archicortex.

**ar·chi·spore** (ahr′kĭ-spor) archespore.

**ar·chi·stome** (ahr′kĭ-stōm) [*archi-* + *-stome*] blastopore.

**ar·chi·stri·a·tum** (ahr″kĭ-stri-a′təm) [*archi-* + *striatum*] the primordial corpus striatum, represented in humans by the amygdaloid body.

**ar·chi·tec·ton·ic** (ahr″kĭ-tek-ton′ik) 1. pertaining to architectural pattern. 2. the structure or construction of, as architectonic structure of the brain.

**ar·ci·form** (ahr′sĭ-form) [L. *arcus* bow + *form*] bow-shaped; arcuate.

**arc-quad·rant** (ahrk-kwod′rənt) an arc guidance system that has a 90° arc.

**arc·ta·tion** (ahrk-ta′shən) [L. *arctare* to draw together] stenosis.

**Arc·to·mys** (ahrk′tə-mis) Marmota.

**Arc·to·staph·y·los** (ahrk″to-staf′ə-lōs) a genus of North American evergreen plants of the family Ericaceae. *A. uva-ur′si* L. is the bearberry or uva ursi, a shrub whose leaves are used medicinally (see *uva ursi,* under *uva*). *A. manzani′ta* Parry is manzanita, a small shrub or tree of the western United States whose leaves are used as a medicinal tea, astringent, tonic, and diuretic.

**ar·cu·al** (ahr′ku-əl) [L. *arcualis*] pertaining to an arch.

**ar·cu·al·ia** (ahr″ku-a′le-ə) nodules of cartilage in the continuous mesenchymal sheath in close apposition to the external surface of the notochord in vertebrate embryos, typically occurring in double pairs, one pair dorsolateral and one pair ventrolateral to the notochord; the dorsolateral pairs give rise to the neural arches, while the ventrolateral pairs give rise to the rudiments of the ribs and the hemal arches.

**ar·cu·ate** (ahr'ku-āt) [L. *arcuatus* bow shaped] shaped like an arc; arranged in arches.

**ar·cu·a·tion** (ahr-ku-a'shən) [L. *arcuatio*] curvature; especially an abnormal curvature.

**ar·cus** (ahr'kəs) pl. *ar'cus* [L. "a bow"] [TA] arch: a general term used in anatomical nomenclature to designate any structure having a curved or bowlike outline.

**a. adipo'sus,** a. corneae.

**a. alveola'ris mandi'bulae** [TA], alveolar arch of mandible: the superior free border of the alveolar process of the mandible. Called also *alveolar border* or *alveolar limbus of mandible,* and *limbus alveolaris mandibulae.*

**a. alveola'ris maxil'lae** [TA], alveolar arch of maxilla: the inferior free border of the alveolar process of the maxilla; called also *alveolar border* or *alveolar limbus of maxilla,* and *limbus alveolaris maxillae.*

**a. ante'rior atlan'tis** [TA], anterior arch of atlas: the more slender portion joining the lateral masses of the atlas ventrally, constituting about one-fifth of the entire circumference of the atlas.

**a. aor'tae** [TA], arch of aorta: the continuation of the ascending aorta, giving rise to the brachiocephalic trunk, and the left common carotid and left subclavian arteries; it continues as the thoracic aorta. Called also *aortic arch.*

**a. cartila'ginis cricoi'deae** [TA], arch of cricoid cartilage: the slender anterior portion of the cricoid cartilage.

**a. cor'neae, a. cornea'lis,** a white or gray opaque ring in the corneal margin, present at birth, or appearing later in life, and becoming quite frequent in those over 50; it results from cholesterol deposits in or hyalinosis of the corneal stroma and may be associated with ocular defects or with familial hyperlipidemia. Called also *a. adiposus, a. juvenilis, a. lipoides corneae,* and *a. senilis.*

**a. costa'lis** [TA], **a. costa'rum,** costal arch: the anterior portion of the apertura thoracis inferior, consisting of the costal cartilages of ribs 7 to 10, inclusive; called also *arch of ribs.*

**a. denta'lis infe'rior** [TA], TA alternative for *a. dentalis mandibularis.*

**a. denta'lis mandibula'ris** [TA], mandibular dental arch: the portion of the dental arch formed by the teeth of the mandible. Called also *arcus dentalis inferior* [TA alternative] and *inferior dental arch.*

**a. denta'lis maxilla'ris** [TA], maxillary dental arch: the portion of the dental arch formed by the teeth of the maxilla. Called also *arcus dentalis superior* [TA alternative] and *superior dental arch.*

**a. denta'lis supe'rior** [TA], TA alternative for *a. dentalis maxillaris.*

**a. duc'tus thora'cici** [TA], the arch of the thoracic duct; see *ductus thoracicus.*

**a. glossopalati'nus,** a. palatoglossus.

**a. iliopecti'neus** [TA], the fascial partition that separates the lacuna musculorum and the lacuna vasorum; called also *fascia iliopectinea.*

**a. inguina'lis,** TA alternative for *ligamentum inguinale.*

**a. juveni'lis,** 1. a. corneae. 2. Axenfeld's anomaly.

**a. lipoi'des cor'neae,** a. corneae.

**a. lumbocosta'lis latera'lis,** ligamentum arcuatum laterale.

**a. lumbocosta'lis media'lis,** ligamentum arcuatum mediale.

**a. palati'ni,** see *a. palatoglossus* and *a. palatopharyngeus.*

**a. palatoglos'sus** [TA], palatoglossal arch: the anterior of the two folds of mucous membrane on either side of the oropharynx, connected with the soft palate and enclosing the palatoglossal muscle; called also *a. glossopalatinus, glossopalatine arch, anterior palatine arch,* and *anterior column* or *pillar of fauces.*

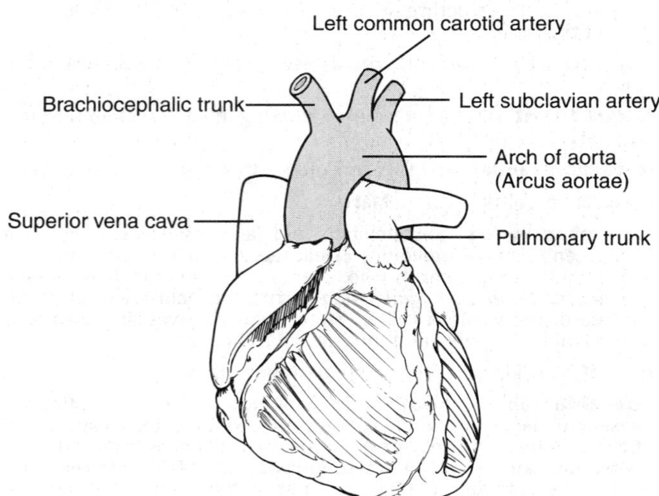


Arcus aortae (arch of aorta).

**a. palatopharyn'geus** [TA], palatopharyngeal arch: the posterior of the two folds of mucous membrane on each side of the oropharynx, connected with the soft palate and enclosing the palatopharyngeal muscle; called also *a. pharyngopalatinus, pharyngopalatine* or *pharyngoepiglottic arch, posterior palatine arch,* and *posterior column* or *pillar of fauces.*

**a. palma'ris profun'dus** [TA], deep palmar arch: an arterial arch formed by the terminal part of the radial artery and its anastomosis with the deep branch of the ulnar, and extending from the base of the metacarpal bone of the little finger to the proximal end of the first interosseous space; it gives off palmar metacarpal arteries and perforating branches. Called also *a. volaris profundus.*

**a. palma'ris superficia'lis** [TA], superficial palmar arch: an arterial arch formed by the terminal part of the ulnar artery and its anastomosis with the superficial palmar branch of the radial, giving rise to the palmar digital arteries and supplying blood to the palmar aspect of the hands and fingers. Called also *a. volaris superficialis.*

**a. palpebra'lis infe'rior** [TA], inferior palpebral arch: an arch derived from the medial palpebral artery, supplying the lower lid of the eye.

**a. palpebra'lis supe'rior** [TA], superior palpebral arch: an arch derived from the medial palpebral artery, supplying the upper lid of the eye.

**a. parieto-occipita'lis,** the curved convolution formed by the backward continuation into the occipital lobe of the superior postcentral sulcus.

**a. pe'dis longitudina'lis** [TA], longitudinal arch of foot: the arch running longitudinally along the sole of the foot, consisting of lateral and medial parts (see *pars lateralis arcus pedis longitudinalis* and *pars medialis arcus pedis longitudinalis*).

**a. pe'dis transversa'lis,** transverse arch of foot: an arch formed by the navicular, cuneiform, cuboid, and five metatarsal bones; called also *metatarsal arch.*

**a. pharyngopalati'nus,** a. palatopharyngeus.

**a. planta'ris,** a. plantaris profundus.

**a. planta'ris profun'dus** [TA], deep plantar arch: the deep arterial arch in the foot, formed by the anastomosis of the lateral plantar artery with the deep plantar branch of the dorsal artery of the foot, and giving off the plantar metatarsal arteries. Called also *plantar arch, plantar arterial arch,* and *a. plantaris.*

**a. poste'rior atlan'tis** [TA], posterior arch of atlas: the slender portion joining the lateral masses of the atlas dorsally, constituting about two-fifths of the entire circumference of the atlas.

**a. pu'bicus** [TA], **a. pu'bis,** pubic arch: the arch formed by the conjoined rami of the ischial and pubic bones of the two sides of the body.

**a. seni'lis,** a. corneae.

**a. supercilia'ris** [TA], superciliary arch: a smooth elevation arching superolaterally from the glabella, slightly superior to the margin of the orbit.

**a. tendi'neus** [TA], tendinous arch: a linear thickening of fascia over some part of a muscle, such as that over the soleus or the obturator internus.

**a. tendi'neus fas'ciae pel'vis** [TA], tendinous arch of pelvic fascia: a thickening of the superior fascia, extending from the ischial spine to the posterior part of the body of the pubis.

**a. tendi'neus mus'culi levato'ris a'ni** [TA], tendinous arch of levator ani muscle: a linear thickening of the fascia over the levator ani muscle.

**a. tendi'neus mus'culi so'lei** [TA], tendinous arch of soleus muscle: an aponeurotic band in the front part of the soleus muscle, extending from a tubercle on the neck of the fibula to the soleal line of the tibia.

**a. ve'nae azy'gou** [TA], arch of azygos vein: an arch formed by the azygos vein above the root of the right lung.

**a. veno'si digita'les,** digital venous arches: communicating branches of veins across the backs of the fingers at their bases.

**a. veno'sus dorsa'lis pe'dis** [TA], dorsal venous arch of foot: a transverse venous arch across the dorsum of the foot near the bases of the metatarsal bones.

**a. veno'sus jugula'ris** [TA], jugular venous arch: a transverse connecting trunk between the anterior jugular veins of either side.

**a. veno'sus palma'ris profun'dus** [TA], deep palmar venous arch: a venous arch accompanying the deep palmar arterial arch; called also *a. volaris venosus profundus.*

**a. veno'sus palma'ris superficia'lis** [TA], superficial palmar venous arch: a venous arch accompanying the superficial palmar arterial arch; called also *a. volaris venosus superficialis.*

**a. veno'sus planta'ris** [TA], plantar venous arch: the deep venous arch that accompanies the plantar arterial arch.

**a. ver'tebrae** [TA], **a. vertebra'lis,** vertebral arch: the bony arch on the dorsal aspect of a vertebra, composed of the laminae and pedicles; called also *arch of vertebra,* and *neural arch of vertebra.*
**a. vola'ris profun'dus,** a. palmaris profundus.
**a. vola'ris superficia'lis,** a. palmaris superficialis.
**a. vola'ris veno'sus profun'dus,** a. venosus palmaris profundus.
**a. vola'ris veno'sus superficia'lis,** a. venosus palmaris superficialis.
**a. zygoma'ticus** [TA], zygomatic arch: the arch formed by the articulation of the broad temporal process of the zygomatic bone and the slender zygomatic process of the temporal bone, giving attachment to the masseter muscle and serving as a line of demarcation between the temporal and infratemporal fossae; called also *malar arch.*

**ARD** acute respiratory disease (of any undefined form).

**ar·dor** (ahr'dor) [L.] intense heat.
**a. uri'nae,** a scalding sensation during the passage of urine.

**ARDS** acute respiratory distress syndrome; adult respiratory distress syndrome.

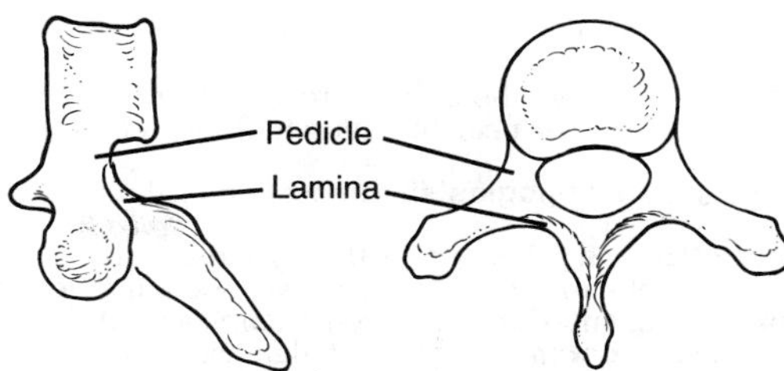

Arcus vertebrae (vertebral arch). The vertebral arch consists anteriorly of a pair of pedicles and posteriorly of a pair of laminae.

**ar·ea** (ar'e-ə) pl. *a'reae* or *areas* [L.] [TA] a limited space; a general term used in anatomical nomenclature to designate a specific surface or functional region.

## Area

See also entries under *region.*

**AI a.,** see *auditory a's.*
**AII a.,** see *auditory a's.*
**acoustic a's, a. acus'tica,** auditory a's.
**a. amygdaloi'dea ante'rior** [TA], anterior amygdaloid area: a poorly differentiated transition zone in the corticomedial part of the amygdaloid body, through which the nuclei are continuous with adjacent areas.
**anterior amygdaloid a.,** a. amygdaloidea anterior.
**aortic a.,** the area on the thorax over the medial end of the right second costal cartilage.
**association a's,** areas of the cerebral cortex (excluding the primary areas) that are connected with each other and with the neothalamus by numerous fibers passing through the corpus callosum and the white matter of the hemispheres; these areas are responsible for the higher mental and emotional processes, such as memory, learning, speech, and the interpretation of sensations.
**auditory a's,** two contiguous areas of the temporal lobe in the region of the anterior transverse temporal gyrus (Brodmann's areas 41 and 42); designated AI *(first* or *primary auditory area)* and AII *(second* or *secondary auditory area).*
**auditory association a.,** a sensory association area for auditory stimuli.
**auditory receiving a's,** auditory a's.
**Bamberger's a.,** an area of cardiac dullness in the left intercostal region, suggestive of pericardial effusion.
**bare a. of liver,** a. nuda hepatis.
**basal seat a.,** denture-bearing a.
**B-dependent a.,** thymus-independent a.
**Betz cell a.,** primary somatomotor a.
**brain a.,** cortical a.
**Broca's motor speech a.,** an area comprising parts of the opercular portion of the inferior frontal gyrus; injury to this area may result in a minor form of motor aphasia.
**Broca's parolfactory a.,** a. subcallosa.
**Brodmann's a's,** areas of the cerebral cortex distinguished by hypothesized differences in the arrangement of their six cellular layers and identified by numbers; although the histologic basis is in dispute, the topographic numbering is widely used as a descriptor for mapping cortical locations that control different functions of the nervous system and the body.
**catchment a.,** the geographical area that a specialized health care facility is responsible for serving.
**a. centra'lis,** macula luteae.
**a. cerebrovasculo'sa,** a membrane-covered, reddish, spongy mass, consisting of thin-walled blood vessels and variable amounts of ependyma, choroid plexus, and glial tissue, that replaces the forebrain in anencephaly.
**cingulate a.,** the area comprising the cingulate gyrus and isthmus, an important component of the limbic system.
**a. coch'leae** [TA], the anterior part of the inferior portion of the fundus of the internal acoustic meatus, near the base of the cochlea; called also *cochlear a. of internal acoustic meatus.*
**cochlear a. of internal acoustic meatus,** a. cochleae.

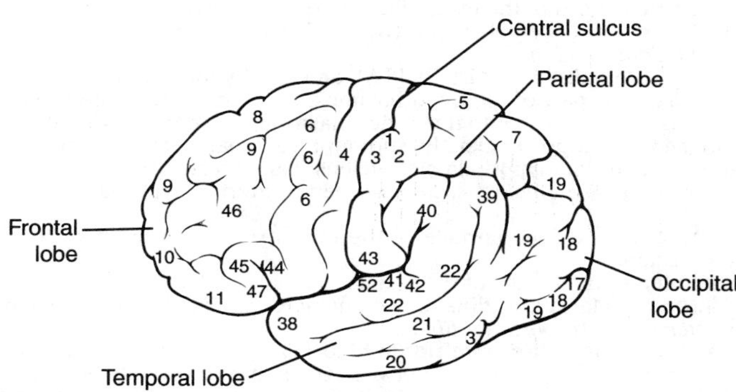

Lateral view of the cerebral hemisphere, showing some of Brodmann's areas.

**Cohnheim's a's,** dark, polygonal areas of myofibrils seen on cross-section of a poorly fixed muscle fiber.
**contact a.,** 1. any area at which two bodies or materials touch. Called also *contact surface.* See also *proximal surface,* def. 2, under *surface.* 2. a. contingens dentis.
**a. contin'gens den'tis** [TA], contact area: the area of the mesial or distal surface of a tooth that touches the adjoining tooth.
**cortical a.,** any portion of the cerebral cortex that can be differentiated functionally from its neighbors; see names of specific areas and see also *cortex, field,* and *zone.*
**cribriform a. of renal papilla,** a. cribrosa papillae renalis.
**a. cribro'sa papil'lae rena'lis** [TA], cribriform area of renal papilla: the tip of a pyramid of a kidney, which is perforated by 10–25 openings for the papillary ducts.
**a. of critical definition,** that part of an optic image within which the detail is clear.
**denture-bearing a., denture foundation a., denture-supporting a.,** the surface of the oral tissues (residual alveolar ridge) that supports a denture. Called also *basal seat a.* and *stress-bearing a.*
**dermatomic a.,** dermatome.
**embryonic a.,** see under *disc.*
**entorhinal a.,** Brodmann's area 28, the inferior and posterior parts of the piriform area, including the caudal part of the parahippocampal gyrus.
**eye a.,** see *frontal eye field* and *occipital eye field.*
**a. of facial nerve,** a. nervi facialis.
**a's of Forel,** see under *field.*
**fusion a.,** Panum's a.
**a'reae gas'tricae** [TA], gastric areas: small patches of gastric mucosa, 1 to 5 mm in diameter, separated by the plicae villosae and containing the foveolae (gastric pits); they present a reticular pattern on endoscopy and double-contrast radiography.
**germinal a.,** embryonic disc.

**gustatory receiving a.,** the primary receiving area for taste sensations; thought to be in or near the opercular part of the postcentral gyrus.

**hypoglossal a., a. hypoglos'si,** the portion of the mouth beneath the tongue.

**hypophysiotropic a.,** the part of the hypothalamus that contains neurons that secrete hormones that regulate adenohypophysial cells.

**hypothalamic a., anterior,** area hypothalamica rostralis.

**hypothalamic a., dorsal,** area hypothalamica dorsalis.

**hypothalamic a., intermediate,** area hypothalamica intermedia.

**hypothalamic a., lateral,** area hypothalamica lateralis.

**hypothalamic a., posterior,** area hypothalamica posterior.

**a. hypothala'mica dorsa'lis** [TA], dorsal hypothalamic area: the most dorsal part of the hypothalamus, comprising the entopeduncular nucleus and the nucleus of the ansa lenticularis. Called also *regio hypothalamica dorsalis* and *dorsal hypothalamic region.*

**a. hypothala'mica interme'dia** [TA], intermediate hypothalamic area: the part of the hypothalamus comprising the lateral hypothalamic region and the following nuclei: arcuate, tuberal, ventromedial hypothalamic, dorsomedial hypothalamic, dorsal hypothalamic, posterior periventricular, and infundibular. Called also *regio hypothalamica intermedia* and *intermediate hypothalamic region.*

**a. hypothala'mica latera'lis** [TA], lateral hypothalamic area: a part of the intermediate hypothalamic area lateral to the fornix and the mammillothalamic fasciculus; called also *regio hypothalamica lateralis* and *lateral hypothalamic region.*

**a. hypothala'mica poste'rior** [TA], posterior hypothalamic area: the most posterior part of the hypothalamus, consisting of the lateral and medial nuclei of the mammillary body and the posterior hypothalamic nucleus. Called also *regio hypothalamica posterior* and *posterior hypothalamic region.*

**a. hypothala'mica rostra'lis** [TA], anterior hypothalamic area: the most anterior part of the hypothalamus, lying adjacent to the lamina terminalis and superior to the optic chiasm, and comprising the lateral and medial preoptic nuclei, the supraoptic and paraventricular nuclei; and the anterior hypothalamic nucleus; called also *preoptic area* or *region, regio hypothalamica anterior,* and anterior hypothalamic region.

**impression a.,** the surface of the oral structures recorded in an impression.

**insular a.,** the cortex of the insula.

**intercondylar a's of tibia,** see *a. intercondylaris anterior tibiae* and *a. intercondylaris posterior tibiae.*

**a. intercondyla'ris ante'rior ti'biae** [TA], anterior intercondylar area of tibia: the broad area between the superior articular surfaces of the tibia; called also *fossa intercondyloidea anterior tibiae, anterior intercondylar fossa of tibia,* and *patellar fossa of tibia.*

**a. intercondyla'ris poste'rior ti'biae** [TA], posterior intercondylar area of tibia: a deep notch separating the condyles on the posterior surface of the tibia; called also *posterior intercondylar a., fossa intercondyloidea posterior tibiae, posterior intercondylar fossa of tibia,* and *popliteal fossa of tibia.*

**Kiesselbach's a.,** an area on the anterior part of the nasal septum above the intermaxillary bone, which is richly supplied with blood vessels and is a common site of nosebleed; called also *Little's a.*

**Laimer-Haeckerman a.,** a triangular area of sparse musculature just below the pharyngoesophageal junction, where Zenker's diverticulum most frequently develops.

**language a.,** any center of the cortex, usually in the dominant hemisphere, controlling the understanding or use of language.

**Little's a.,** Kiesselbach's a.

**a. martegia'ni,** a slightly enlarged space at the optic disk, marking the beginning of the hyaloid canal.

**a. medullovasculo'sa,** a median elongated area of vascular granulation-like tissue in rachischisis.

**mesobranchial a.,** the pharyngeal floor in the embryo, between the pharyngeal arches and pouches of each side.

**midarm muscle a.,** a value used to estimate lean body mass, calculated by the formula where $n$ is 10 for males and 6.5 for females.

**mirror a.,** the reflecting surface of the cornea and lens when illuminated through the slit lamp.

**motor a.,** any area of the cerebral cortex primarily involved in stimulating muscle contractions; often used alone to refer to the primary somatomotor area. See also *premotor a., sensorimotor a.,* and *Broca's motor speech a.*

**motor speech a.,** see *Broca's motor speech a.* and *Wernicke's second motor speech a.*

**a. ner'vi facia'lis** [TA], area of facial nerve: the part of the fundus of the internal acoustic meatus where the facial nerve enters the facial canal.

**a. nu'da he'patis** [TA], bare area of liver: the superior surface of the liver, adjacent to the diaphragm, that lacks a peritoneal covering; its boundaries are formed by the hepatic coronary ligament proper and the triangular ligaments.

**olfactory a.,** 1. a general area, including the olfactory bulb, tract, and trigone, the anterior portion of the gyrus cinguli, and the uncus. 2. substantia perforata rostralis.

**a. opa'ca,** the outer part of the embryonic disc, as seen in the bird egg.

**Panum's a.,** the area on the retina of one eye over which a point-sized image can range and still provide a stereoscopic image with a specific point of stimulus on the retina of the other eye. Called also *fusion a.*

**parastriate a.,** Brodmann's area 18, an area of the occipital cortex partly surrounding the striate cortex and having some of the functions of an association area for visual sensations.

**a. pellu'cida,** the central clear part of the embryonic disc, as seen in the bird egg.

**periamygdaloid a.,** the intermediate part of the piriform area, between the piriform area and the entorhinal area; it covers the amygdaloid body.

**peristriate a.,** Brodmann's area 19, an area of the occipital cortex partly surrounding the striate cortex and having some functions of an association area for visual sensations.

**piriform a.,** an area in the rhinencephalon, pear-shaped in some species but not in humans; it includes the lateral olfactory process or gyrus, the limen insulae, the uncus, and part of the parahippocampal gyrus; subdivided into the prepiriform area, the periamygdaloid area, and the entorhinal area. Called also *piriform lobe.*

**postcentral a.,** the sensory area just posterior to the central sulcus of the cerebral hemisphere, the primary receptive area for general sensations; called also *postrolandic a.* and *somesthetic cortex.*

**post dam a.,** posterior palatal seal a.

**posterior palatal seal a.,** the soft tissues along the junction of the hard and soft palates on which pressure can be applied by a denture to aid in its retention; called also *post dam a.*

**a. postre'ma,** a small tongue-shaped area on the lateral wall of the fourth ventricle, between the funiculus separans and the tuberculum gracile, in which the blood-brain barrier may be modified. See also *circumventricular organs,* under *organ.*

**postrolandic a.,** postcentral a.

**precentral a.,** primary somatomotor a.

**prefrontal a.,** the cortex of the frontal lobe immediately in front of the premotor cortex, concerned chiefly with associative functions.

**premotor a.,** the motor cortex of the frontal lobe immediately in front of the precentral gyrus.

**preoptic a.,** 1. a. preoptica. 2. area hypothalamica rostralis.

**a. preop'tica** [TA], preoptic area: several groups of cells in the median plane immediately below the rostral commissure of the telencephalon that are functionally related to the hypothalamus; called also *preoptic region.*

**prepiriform a.,** the anterior part of the piriform area, consisting primarily of the lateral olfactory gyrus.

**pressure a.,** an area subjected to excessive pressure with consequent displacement of tissue or fluid.

**pretectal a., a. pretecta'lis** [TA], an area at the junction of the mesencephalon and diencephalon, extending from a position dorsolateral to the commissure of the epithalamus toward the cranial colliculus, within which is situated the pretectal nucleus; called also *pretectal region.*

**primary a's,** areas of the cerebral cortex comprising the motor and sensory regions. Cf. *association a's.*

**primary receiving a's, primary receptive a's,** the areas of the cerebral cortex that receive the thalamic projections of the primary sensory modalities.

**primary somatomotor a.,** an area in the posterior part of the frontal lobe just anterior to the central sulcus, corresponding to Brodmann's area 4; different regions control motor activity of specific parts of the body. Called also *Betz cell a., motor a., precentral a., rolandic a.,* and *Rolando's zone.*

**projection a's,** those areas of the cerebral cortex that receive the most direct projection of the sensory systems of the body.

**pyriform a.,** piriform a.

**receptive a's,** primary receptive a's.

**relief a.,** the portion of the surface of the mouth upon which pressures or forces are reduced or eliminated in prosthodontic therapy. See also *relief,* def. 3.

**rest a.,** the prepared surface of a tooth or fixed restoration into which the rest fits, giving support to a removable partial denture. Called also *rest seat.*

**a. retrooliva'ris** [TA], **retroolivary a.,** the most caudal part of the lateral region of the medulla oblongata, towards the posterolateral sulcus.

**rolandic a.,** primary somatomotor a.

**rugae a.,** the portion of the mouth in which rugae are found; called also *rugae zone.*

**SI a.,** first somatosensory a.

**SII a.,** second somatosensory a.

**saddle a.**, the edentulous portion of the dental arch upon which a fixed or removable prosthesis rests.

**sensorimotor a.**, the cortex of the pre- and postcentral gyri—the motor area and the primary receptive area for general sensations, respectively.

**sensory a's**, primary receptive a's.

**sensory association a.**, an association area around the borders of a primary receptive area, where sensory stimuli are interpreted.

**septal a.**, the area on either cerebral hemisphere comprising the area subcallosa and the corresponding half of the septum pellucidum; the area has olfactory, hypothalamic, and hippocampal connections.

**silent a.**, 1. an area of the brain in which pathologic conditions may occur without producing symptoms obvious to the clinician. 2. association a.

**somatic sensory a., somatosensory a.**, either of the two cortical regions where conscious perception of somatic sensations occurs, called the *first* or *primary somatosensory area* and the *second* or *secondary somatosensory area.*

**somatosensory a., first, somatosensory a., primary,** the cortical projection area in the postcentral gyrus for receiving into consciousness somatosensory information initiated by stimulation of receptors in the skin, joints, muscles, and viscera. Called also *SI a.*

**somatosensory a., second, somatosensory a., secondary,** a cortical projection area lateral and posterior to the primary somatosensory area; it receives somatic sensations mainly from the skin, particularly sensations of pain and of movement across the skin. Called also *SII a.*

**somesthetic a.**, somatosensory a.

**stress-bearing a.**, 1. the portion of the mouth capable of providing support for a denture. 2. surfaces of oral structures which resist forces, strains, or pressures brought upon them during function. 3. denture-bearing a.

**striate a.**, striate cortex.

**strip a.**, a strip of cortex between the motor and premotor areas thought to be suppressor in function.

**a. subcallo'sa** [TA], **subcallosal a.**, a small area of cortex on the medial surface of each cerebral hemisphere, between the anterior and posterior parolfactory sulci..

**a. of superficial cardiac dullness**, a triangular area of dullness observed on percussion of the chest, corresponding to that area of the heart not covered by lung tissue.

**supplementary a's**, small motor and sensory areas of the cerebral cortex in addition to the primary areas.

**supplementary motor a.**, an area in the gyrus frontalis medius just above the cingulate gyrus and anterior to the part of the first somatomotor area that mediates movements of the lower extremity.

**supporting a.**, 1. the surface of the mouth available for support of a denture. 2. those areas of the maxillary and mandibular edentulous ridges which are considered best suited to carry the forces of mastication when the dentures are in function.

**suppressor a's**, cortical areas whose activation is thought to suppress or prevent movement; see also *strip a.*.

**taste receiving a.**, gustatory receiving a.

**T-dependent a.**, thymus-dependent a.

**thymus-dependent a.**, any of the areas of the peripheral lymphoid organs populated by T lymphocytes, e.g., the periarteriolar lymphatic sheath in the spleen, the paracortex in lymph nodes, and the parafollicular areas of gut-associated lymphoid tissue. Called also *paracortex, T- dependent a.,* and *tertiary cortex.*

**thymus-independent a.**, any of the areas of the peripheral lymphoid organs populated by B lymphocytes, e.g., the lymph nodules (lymphoid follicles) of the spleen, lymph nodes, and gut-associated lymphoid tissue. Called also *B-dependent a.* and *T-independent a.*

**T-independent a.**, thymus-independent a.

**trigger a.**, see under *zone.*

**a. under the curve (AUC),** the area enclosed between a probability curve with nonnegative values and the axis of the quality being measured; of the total area under a curve, the proportion that falls between two given points on the curve defines a probability density function (see under *function*).

**vagus a.**, trigonum nervi vagi.

**a. vasculo'sa**, that part of the area opaca where the blood vessels are first seen, as in the bird egg.

**vestibular a.**, a rounded triangular elevation lateral to foveae of the fourth ventricle over which pass the striae medullares; it extends into the lateral recess, where it forms the *auditory,* or *acoustic, tubercle.*

**vestibular a. of internal acoustic meatus, inferior,** a. vestibularis inferior meatus acustici interni.

**vestibular a. of internal acoustic meatus, superior,** a. vestibularis superior meatus acustici interni.

**a. vestibula'ris infe'rior mea'tus acus'tici inter'ni** [TA], inferior vestibular area of internal acoustic meatus: the lower portion of the fundus of the internal acoustic meatus, transmitting fibers of the saccular nerve.

**a. vestibula'ris supe'rior mea'tus acus'tici inter'ni** [TA], superior vestibular area of internal acoustic meatus: the upper portion of the fundus of the internal acoustic meatus, transmitting fibers of the utricular and superior ampullary nerves.

**visual a.**, see under *cortex.*

**visual a., first,** striate cortex.

**visual a., second,** parastriate a.

**visual a., third,** peristriate a.

**visual association a's**, the peristriate and parastriate areas considered together.

**visual receiving a.**, visual cortex.

**visuopsychic a's**, visual association a's.

**visuosensory a.**, striate cortex.

**a. vitelli'na**, the yolk area beyond the area vasculosa in meroblastic eggs.

**vocal a.**, rima glottidis.

**watershed a.**, any of several areas over the convexities of the cerebral or cerebellar hemispheres, distant from the circle of Willis, where the vascular beds of two cerebral arteries meet and form anastomoses. At times of prolonged systemic hypotension, these are particularly susceptible to infarction, with those fed by the largest arterial branches being the first affected. See also *watershed infarction,* under *infarction.*

**Wernicke's a., Wernicke's second motor speech a.**, originally a term denoting a speech center thought to be confined to the posterior part of the superior temporal gyrus adjacent to the transverse temporal gyri; the term now includes a wider zone that encompasses the supramarginal and angular gyri as well; called also *Wernicke's field* or *zone.*

---

**ar·e·a·ta** (ar″e-a′tə) occurring in patches, as alopecia areata.

**ar·e·a·tus** (ar″e-a′tus) areata.

**Ar·e·ca** (ar′ə-kə) [from Malayalam *atekka*] [MeSH: Areca] a genus of palm trees (family Palmae), native to southern Asia and nearby islands. *A. ca'techu* L. is the betel palm, an East Indian species that is the source of areca and betel.

**ar·e·ca** (ar′ə-kə) [MeSH: Areca] 1. any palm tree of the genus *Areca.* 2. the dried ripe seed of *Areca catechu,* a common masticatory in India and elsewhere in Asia. It contains the alkaloid arecoline and astringent tannins and has parasympathomimetic and anthelmintic properties. Called also *areca nut* and *betel nut.*

**arec·o·line** (ə-rek′o-lēn) [MeSH: Arecoline] a cholinomimetic alkaloid obtained from areca (betel nut) having both muscarinic and nicotinic effects, used as an ingredient of the veterinary anthelmintic *drocarbil.*

**Are·dia** (ə-re′de-ə) trademark for a preparation of pamidronate disodium.

**are·flex·ia** (a″re-flek′se-ə) [*a-*[1] + *reflex* + *-ia*] absence of reflexes.

**are·gen·er·a·tive** (a″re-jen′ər-ə-tiv) characterized by absence of regeneration; applied especially to blood cells in aplastic anemia.

**ar·e·na·ceous** (ar″ə-na′shəs) sandy; gritty.

**Are·na·vi·ri·dae** (ə-re″nə-vir′ĭ-de) [MeSH: Arenaviridae] the arenaviruses: a family of RNA viruses having a pleomorphic virion 50–300 nm in diameter consisting of a lipid bilayer envelope, with large peplomers, surrounding a coiled nucleocapsid with two members and a variable number of ribosomes. The genome consists of two circular molecules of ambisense single-stranded RNA, designated L (MW $1.1\times10^6$) and S (MW $2.2–2.8\times10^6$) (size of total genome 10–14 kb). Viruses contain three major polypeptides, including a transcriptase, and are ultraviolet- and gamma radiation–sensitive. Replication and assembly occur in the cytoplasm; virions are released by budding through the plasma membrane. Host ranges are narrow. There is a single genus, *Arenavirus.*

**Are·na·vi·rus** (ə-re′nə-vi″rəs) [L. *arena* sand + *virus* (from the granules that give the virions a sandy appearance)] [MeSH: Arenavirus] arenaviruses; a genus of viruses of the family Arenaviridae that includes lymphocytic choriomeningitis (LCM) virus, Lassa virus, and viruses of the Tacaribe complex (Amapari, Flexal, Guanarito, Junin, Machupo, Parana, Pichinde, Tacaribe, and Tamiami viruses, some of which cause hemorrhagic fever). Rodents are common hosts.

**are·na·vi·rus** (ə-re′nə-vi″rəs) [MeSH: Arenavirus] any virus belonging to the family Arenaviridae.

**ar·e·noid** (ar′ə-noid) [L. *arena* sand + *-oid*] resembling sand.

**are·o·la** (ə-re′o-lə) pl. *are′olae* [L., dim. of *area* space] 1. any minute space or interstice in a tissue; see *areolar tissue,* under *tissue.* 2. a circular area of a different color, surrounding a central point, as such an area surrounding a pustule or vesicle, or the part of the iris surrounding the pupil of the eye, or the area surrounding the nipple of the breast.
**a. mam′mae** [TA], **a. of mammary gland,** the darkened ring surrounding the nipple of a breast.
**a. of nipple,** a. mammae.
**a. papilla′ris,** a. mammae.
**second a.,** a ring which, during pregnancy, surrounds the areola mammae.
**umbilical a.,** a pigmented patch that sometimes surrounds the navel.

**are·o·lae** (ə-re′o-le) [L.] genitive and plural of *areola.*

**are·o·lar** (ə-re′o-lər) pertaining to or containing areolae.

**are·o·li·tis** (ar″e-o-li′tis) inflammation of the areola of the breast.

**ar·e·om·e·ter** (ar″e-om′ə-tər) [Gr. *araios* thin + *-meter*] a hydrometer.

**Ar·e·tae·us of Cap·pa·do·cia** (ar-ə-te′us) [c. 81–c. 138] a Greek physician, contemporary of Galen; he was an Eclectic, but influenced by Pneumatist theories. Aretaeus wrote works on acute and chronic diseases. His clinical descriptions (e.g., of diabetes, pleurisy, tetanus) are outstanding and firmly established upon Archigenes' work.

**Ar·ey's rule** (ār′ēz) [Leslie Brainerd *Arey,* American anatomist, 1891–1988] see under *rule.*

**Ar·fon·ad** (ahr′fon-ad) trademark for a preparation of trimethaphan camsylate.

**Arg** arginine.

**arg.** abbreviation for L. *argen′tum,* silver.

**ar·gam·bly·opia** (ahr″gam-ble-o′pe-ə) [Gr. *argos* idle + *amblyopia*] amblyopia due to long disuse of the eye.

**Ar·gand burner** (ahr-gah′) [Aimé *Argand,* Swiss physicist, 1755–1803] see under *burner.*

**Ar·gas** (ahr′gəs) a genus of ticks of the family Argasidae, some of which transmit diseases to humans and other animals.
**A. america′nus,** *A. persicus.*
**A. brump′ti,** a species found in Africa whose bite causes local inflammation in man.
**A. minia′tus,** *A. persicus.*
**A. per′sicus,** the tampan tick, one of the most important blood-sucking parasites of poultry, which produces a weak condition of flocks, with great economic losses. In Iran, Egypt, India, Australia, and Brazil, it acts as the carrier of fowl spirochetosis. Called also *A. americanus* or *A. miniatus, tampan, miana bug,* and *Mianeh bug.*
**A. reflex′us,** an ectoparasite of pigeons and other roosting birds, which frequently attacks man and may cause a cutaneous inflammatory lesion.

**ar·ga·sid** (ahr′gə-sid) 1. pertaining to ticks of the family Argasidae. 2. a tick of the family Argasidae; called also *soft tick* and *soft-bodied tick.* 3. pertaining to ticks of the genus *Argas.*

**Ar·gas·i·dae** (ahr-gas′ĭ-de) the soft ticks, a family of the superfamily Ixodoidea, distinguished from the hard ticks (Ixodidae) by absence of the scutum. The genera are *Argas, Otobius, Antricola,* and *Ornithodoros.*

**ar·ge·ma** (ahr′jə-mə) a white ulcer of the cornea.

**Ar·gem·o·ne** (ahr-jem′ə-ne) a genus of herbs of the family Papaveraceae, originally native to the Americas, having prickly leaves and yellow or white flowers. *A. mexica′na* is the prickly poppy, which contains argemone oil and can cause epidemic dropsy.

**ar·gen·taf·fin** (ahr-jen′tə-fin) [L. *argentum* silver + *affinis* having affinity for] having an affinity for silver and chromium salts; said of tissues. See also under *cell.*

**ar·gen·taf·fi·no·ma** (ahr″jən-taf″ĭ-no′mə) a carcinoid tumor of the gastroenteric tract formed from the argentaffin cells (Kulchitzky's cells) found in the enteric canal; such tumors elaborate a variety of catecholamines that produce the symptom complex called carcinoid syndrome.
**a. of bronchus,** carcinoid tumor of bronchus.

**ar·gen·ta·tion** (ahr″jen-ta′shən) [L. *argentum* silver] staining with a silver salt.

**ar·gen·tic** (ahr-jen′tik) containing silver.

**ar·gen·tum** (ahr-jen′təm) gen. *argen′ti.* [L.] silver.

**ar·gil·la** (ahr-jil′ə) kaolin (def. 1).

**ar·gil·la·ceous** (ahr″jĭ-la′shəs) composed of clay.

**ar·gi·nase** (ahr′jĭ-nās) [EC 3.5.3.1] [MeSH: Arginase] an enzyme of the hydrolase class that catalyzes the hydrolysis of arginine to form ornithine and urea. The reaction occurs in the liver as part of the urea cycle.

**ar·gi·nase de·fi·cien·cy** an autosomal recessive aminoacidopathy involving the biosynthesis of urea; arginine is elevated in blood and urine and may cause secondary cystinuria; oroticaciduria is common, but hyperammonemia is rare. Clinical signs include psychomotor retardation, hepatomegaly, and scalp discoloration. Called also *argininemia* and *hyperargininemia.*

**ar·gi·nine** (ahr′jĭ-nēn) [MeSH: Arginine] 1. a nonessential amino acid, 2-amino-5-guanidinovaleric acid, produced by the hydrolysis or digestion of proteins. It is one of the hexone bases and supplies the amidine group for the synthesis of creatine. Arginine is also formed by the transfer of a nitrogen atom from aspartate to citrulline in the urea cycle. It then gives off urea, to form ornithine. Symbols Arg and R. See table at *amino acid.* 2. [USP] a preparation of L-arginine used in the treatment of hyperammonemia and as a diagnostic aid in the assessment of pituitary function.
**a. glutamate,** a salt composed of L-arginine and L-glutamic acid, used as an adjunct in the treatment of hyperammonemia; administered intravenously.
**a. hydrochloride** [USP], the monohydrochloride salt of L-arginine, used as an adjunct in the treatment of hyperammonemia and as a stimulant of growth hormone release by the pituitary in tests of pituitary function; administered intravenously.
**a. monohydrochloride,** a salt of arginine sometimes used in place of ammonium chloride to potentiate mercurial diuretics in refractory heart failure.

**ar·gi·nine car·boxy·pep·ti·dase** (ahr′jĭ-nēn kahr-bok″se-pep′tĭ-dās) lysine carboxypeptidase.

**ar·gi·ni·ne·mia** (ahr′jĭ-nĭ-ne′me-ə) arginase deficiency.

**ar·gi·ni·no·suc·cin·ase** (ahr″jĭ-ne″no-suk′sĭ-nās) argininosuccinate lyase.

**ar·gi·ni·no·suc·cin·ase de·fi·cien·cy** argininosuccinicaciduria.

**ar·gi·ni·no·suc·cin·ate** (ahr″jĭ-ne″no-suk′sĭ-nāt) the anionic form of argininosuccinic acid.

**ar·gi·ni·no·suc·cin·ate ly·ase** (ahr″jĭ-ne″no-suk′sĭ-nāt li′ās) [EC 4.3.2.1] [MeSH: Argininosuccinate Lyase] an enzyme of the lyase class that catalyzes the cleavage of argininosuccinate to form fumarate and arginine. The reaction is part of the urea cycle in the liver (see illustration at *urea cycle,* under *cycle*). Deficiency of the enzyme, an autosomal recessive trait, results in argininosuccinicaciduria. Called also *argininosuccinase.*

**ar·gi·ni·no·suc·cin·ate syn·thase** (ahr″jĭ-ne″no-suk′sĭ-nāt sin′thās) [EC 6.3.4.5] an enzyme of the ligase class that catalyzes the condensation of citrulline and aspartate to form argininosuccinate. The reaction is a part of the urea cycle in the liver (see illustration at *urea cycle,* under *cycle*). Written also *argininosuccinate synthetase.*

**ar·gi·ni·no·suc·ci·nate syn·thase de·fi·cien·cy** an autosomal recessive aminoacidopathy characterized by marked elevation in plasma and urine levels of citrulline, with hyperammonemia and sometimes secondary oroticaciduria. Neonatal and late onset forms exist and clinical findings, which vary widely in severity, include mental retardation and neurologic abnormalities. Called also *citrullinemia* and *citrullinuria.*

**ar·gi·ni·no·suc·cin·ic ac·id** (ahr″jĭ-ne″no-suk-sin′ik) a compound formed by the condensation of aspartic acid and citrulline as a step in the urea cycle (q.v.).

**ar·gi·ni·no·suc·cin·ic·ac·i·de·mia** (ahr″jĭ-ne″no-suk-sin″ik-as″ĭ-de′me-ə) the presence in the blood of argininosuccinic acid.

**ar·gi·ni·no·suc·cin·ic·ac·id·uria** (ahr″jĭ-ne″no-suk-sin″ik-as″ĭ-du′re-ə) 1. an autosomal recessive aminoacidopathy characterized by urinary excretion of argininosuccinic acid, due to a deficiency of argininosuccinate lyase, with hyperammonemia, argininosuccinicacidemia, and citrullinemia. Neonatal and late onset forms exist, and clinical findings, which vary widely in severity, include mental retardation, seizures, ataxia, hepatomegaly, and friable hair (trichorrhexis nodosa). Called also *argininosuccinase* or *argininosuccinate lyase deficiency.* 2. excretion of argininosuccinic acid in the urine.

**ar·gi·nyl** (ahr′jĭ-nəl) the acyl radical of arginine.

**ar·gi·pres·sin** (ahr″jĭ-pres′in) [MeSH: Argipressin] arginine vasopressin.

**ar·gon** (ahr′gon) [Gr. *argos* inert] [MeSH: Argon] a chemical element, atomic number 18, discovered in the atmosphere in 1895. One of the inert gases, its symbol is Ar and its atomic weight 39.948.

**Ar·gyll Rob·ert·son pupil (pupil sign)** (ahr-gil′rob′ərt-son) [Douglas Moray Cooper Lamb *Argyll Robertson,* Scottish physician, 1837–1909] see under *pupil.*

**ar·gyr·emia** (ahr″jə-re′me-ə) [Gr. *argyros* silver + *-emia*] the presence of silver or silver salts in the blood.

**ar·gyr·ia** (ahr-jir′e-ə) [MeSH: Argyria] a permanent ashen-gray discoloration of the skin, conjunctiva, and internal organs that results from long-continued use of silver salts. Called also *argyrosis.*
**a. nasa′lis,** argyric discoloration of the nasal mucosa.

**ar·gyr·i·a·sis** (ahr″jə-ri′ə-sis) argyria.

**ar·gyr·ic** (ahr-jir′ik) 1. pertaining to or caused by silver. 2. pertaining to argyria.

**ar·gyr·ism** (ahr′jə-riz-əm) argyria.

**Ar·gyr·ol** (ahr′jə-rol) trademark for mild silver protein; see under *silver.*

**ar·gy·ro·phil** (ahr′jə-ro-fil) [Gr. *argyros* silver + *-phil*] capable of binding silver salts, which may subsequently be reduced by light or by a reducing agent to give a black deposit of silver; said of tissues.

**ar·gy·ro·sis** (ahr″jə-ro′sis) [Gr. *argyros* silver] argyria.

**arhin·en·ceph·a·lia** (a″rin-en″sə-fa′le-ə) [*a-*[1] + *rhinencephalon*] arrhinencephalia.

**arhin·ia** (ə-rin′e-ə) [*a-*[1] + *rhin-* + *-ia*] arrhinia.

**Arias-Stel·la reaction** (ahr′yahs-stel′ə) [Javier *Arias-Stella,* Peruvian pathologist, born 1924] see under *reaction.*

**ari·bo·fla·vin·o·sis** (a-ri″bo-fla″vĭ-no′sis) [*a-*[1] + *riboflavin* + *-osis*] deficiency of riboflavin in the diet. It produces a syndrome chiefly marked by cheilosis or cheilitis, angular stomatitis, glossitis associated with a purplish red or magenta-colored tongue that may show fissures, corneal vascularization, dyssebacia, and anemia.

**Ar·i·cept** (ar′ĭ-sept) trademark for a preparation of donepezil hydrochloride.

**ar·il** (ar′il) [L. *arillus* dried grape] an accessory covering or appendage of seeds.

**ar·il·lode** (ar′ĭ-lōd) an appendage of certain seeds attached to the micropyle or raphe.

**Arim·i·dex** (ə-rim′ĭ-deks) trademark for a preparation of anastrozole.

**aris·tin** (ə-ris′tin) a crystalline compound found in various species of *Aristolochia.*

**Aris·to·cort** (ə-ris′to-cort) trademark for preparations of triamcinolone.

**Aris·to·lo·chia** (ə-ris″to-lo′ke-ə) [L.; Gr. *aristos* best + *lochia* lochia] a large genus of shrubs and herbs of the family Aristolochiaceae; many species contain aristolochic acid and are actively medicinal, although high doses are toxic to livestock, causing diarrhea and limb weakness.

**aris·to·lo·chic acid** (ə-ris″to-lo′kik) a phenanthrene-carboxylic acid derivative, the major bitter aromatic principle of herbs of the genus *Aristolochia* and related species; high doses cause cardiac and respiratory arrest in experimental animals and diarrhea with limb weakness in livestock. Called also *aristolochine.*

**aris·tol·o·chine** (ə-ris-tol′o-chēn) aristolochic acid.

**Aris·to·span** (ə-ris′to-span) trademark for preparations of triamcinolone hexacetonide.

**Ar·is·tot·le** (ar′is-tot″əl) [384–322 B.C.] Greek philosopher, student of Plato. As a physical scientist, Aristotle stressed direct observation and induction; in biology his teleology is still accepted by vitalists. His studies included comparative anatomy and physiology, embryology, and ethology. Unfortunately, Aristotle adopted Empedocles' theory of the heart's being the center of intelligence, and also the theory of the four elements and the four qualities (cf. *humoralism*).

**Ar·is·tot·le's anomaly** (ar′is-tot″əlz) [*Aristotle*] see under *anomaly.*

**arith·mo·ma·nia** (ə-rith″mo-ma′ne-ə) [Gr. *arithmos* number + *mania*] compulsive counting, as paces when walking, steps in a staircase, etc., a common symptom in obsessive-compulsive disorder.

**Ar·i·zo·na** (ar″ĭ-zo′nə) [MeSH: Arizona] see *Salmonella arizona.*

**Ar·li·din** (ahr′lĭ-din) trademark for preparations of nylidrin hydrochloride.

**Arlt's recess, sinus, trachoma** (ahrlts) [Carl Ferdinand Ritter von *Arlt,* Austrian ophthalmologist, 1812–1887] see under *trachoma* and see *sinus of Maier.*

**arm** (ahrm) [A.S. *earm*] [MeSH: Arm] 1. brachium (def. 1). 2. in common usage, the entire upper limb (*membrum superius* [TA]). 3. a slender part or extension, usually having mobility and independent function, that projects from a main structure. 4. an extension or projection by which a removable partial denture is retained in position in the mouth.
**bar clasp a.,** a clasp arm that serves as an extracoronal retainer, originating from the denture base, a major or minor connector, or the framework of a denture, traverses soft tissue, approaches the tooth undercut area from a gingival direction, and terminates in a retentive undercut lying gingival to the height of contour.
**bird a.,** a wasted condition of the forearm due to atrophy of the muscles.
**chromosome a.,** either of the two segments of the chromosome separated by the centromere; the symbol p indicates the short arm and q the long arm.

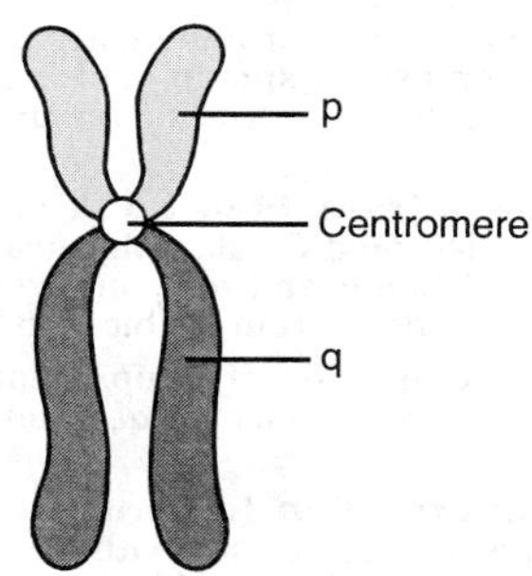


Chromosome arms.

**circumferential clasp a.,** a clasp arm that originates above the height of contour, traverses part of the suprabulge portion of the tooth, approaches the tooth undercut from an occlusal direction, and terminates in a retentive undercut lying gingival to the height of contour.
**clasp a.,** an extension or projection of the clasp of a partial denture, helping to stabilize and retain it in the mouth.
**glass a.,** a painful condition of the upper arm due to an injury to the long tendon of the biceps muscle or to the tendon of the supraspinatus muscle, at times resulting in subdeltoid bursitis.
**golf a.,** a form of neuritis seen in golf players after excessive exercise.
**reciprocal a.,** a clasp arm located in such a manner as to reciprocate any force arising from an opposing clasp arm on the same tooth.
**retention a., retentive a.,** a rigid clasp that engages the infrabulge area at the terminal end of the arm.
**stabilizing a.,** a rigid clasp arm that contacts the tooth at or occlusal to the surveyed height of contour.

**ar·ma·dil·lo** (ahr″mə-dil′o) [Sp. "little armored thing"] [MeSH: Armadillos] one of a group of burrowing mammals of the order Edentata, family Dasypodidae, that have horny shields on the dorsal surface of the body; one species in South America is a reservoir for *Trypanosoma cruzi.*

**ar·ma·men·tar·i·um** (ahr″mə-men-tar′e-əm) [L.] the equipment of a practitioner or institution, including books, instruments, medicines, and surgical appliances.

**Ar·man·ni-Eb·stein cells, kidney, lesion (degeneration)** (ahr-mah′ne eb′shtīn) [Luciano *Armanni,* Italian pathologist, 1839–1903; Wilhelm *Ebstein,* German internist, 1836–1912] see under *cell, kidney,* and *lesion.*

**ar·mar·i·um** (ahr-mar′e-əm) [L.] armamentarium.

**ar·ma·ture** (ahr′mə-choor) [L. *armatura* a defensive apparatus] 1. the iron bar or keeper across the open end of a horseshoe magnet. 2. a protective organ or structure.

**Ar·mig·er·es** (ahr-mij′ər-ēz) a genus of mosquitoes of the tribe Aedini, subfamily Culicinae. A. obtur′bans transmits dengue in Japan.

**Ar·mil·li·fer** (ahr-mil′ĭ-fər) a genus of endoparasitic degenerate arthropods of the family Porocephalidae.
**A. armilla′tus,** a species whose adults are found in the lungs and trachea of the python and whose larvae are found in the internal organs of monkeys, lions, and occasionally humans in Africa. Called also *Porocephalus armillatus* and *P. constrictus.*
**A. monilifor′mis,** a species whose larvae are parasitic in man in China, the Philippines, and other Asian islands.

**Ar·mo·ra·cia** (ahr″mo-ra′shə) a genus of flowering herbs of the family Cruciferae. *A. lapathifo'lia* is the horseradish plant, whose root yields the condiment horseradish; it can cause fatal gastroenteritis in livestock. Formerly called *Cochlearia armoracia.*

**arm·pit** (ahrm'pit) the externally visible portion of the axilla.

**Ar·nal·dus de Vil·la·no·va** see *Arnold of Villanova.*

**Arndt's law** (ahrnts) [Rudolf *Arndt,* German psychiatrist, 1835–1900] see under *law.*

**Arndt-Schulz law** (ahrnt-shoolts) [R. *Arndt;* Hugo *Schulz,* German pharmacologist, 1853–1932] Arndt's law.

**Ar·neth classification, count, formula, index** (ahr-net') [Joseph *Arneth,* German physician, 1873–1955] see under *classification, count, formula,* and *index.*

**Ar·ni·ca** (ahr'nĭ-kə) [L.] [MeSH: Arnica] a genus of composite-flowered plants (family Compositae), known also as *leopard's bane, wolf's bane,* and *mountain tobacco.* The dried flowerheads of *A. monta'na* are called *arnica* and are used medicinally.

**ar·ni·ca** (ahr'nĭ-kə) [MeSH: Arnica] 1. any plant of the genus *Arnica.* 2. the dried flowerheads of *Arnica montana;* they contain arnicin, arnisterol, anthoxanthins, tannin, and resins and are used topically in tincture form for contusions, sprains, and superficial wounds, and as a counterirritant. Called also *wolf's bane* or *wolfsbane* and *leopard's bane.*

**Ar·nold of Vil·la·no·va (Ar·nal·dus de Vil·la·no·va)** (ahr'nəld) [c. 1235–1312] a celebrated Catalan physician who wrote extensively on medicine, alchemy, and religion and who translated Avicenna's writings on the heart from Arabic into Latin.

**Ar·nold's canal,** etc. (ahr'nəldz) [Philipp Friedrich *Arnold,* German anatomist, 1803–1890] see under *canal, ligament, nerve,* and *syndrome.*

**Ar·nold-Chi·ari malformation (deformity, syndrome)** (ahr'nəld-ke-ahr'e) [Julius *Arnold,* German pathologist, 1835–1915; Hans *Chiari,* Austrian pathologist, 1851–1916] see under *malformation.*

**AROA** autosomal recessive ocular albinism.

**aro·ma** (ə-ro'mə) [Gr. *arōma* spice] fragrance or odor, especially that of a spice or medicine or of articles of food or drink.

**aro·ma·tase** (ə-ro'mə-tās) [MeSH: Aromatase] an enzyme activity occurring in the endoplasmic reticulum and catalyzing the conversion of testosterone to the aromatic compound estradiol, proceeding via three successive hydroxylations, loss of a carbon atom, and rearrangement.

**ar·o·mat·ic** (ar"o-mat'ik) [L. *aromaticus;* Gr. *arōmatikos*] 1. having a spicy odor. 2. in organic chemistry, denoting a compound containing a ring system stabilized by a closed circle of conjugated double bonds or nonbonding electron pairs, such as benzene, naphthalene, or the arylamines.

**ar·o·mat·ic-L-ami·no-ac·id de·car·box·y·lase** (ar"o-mat'ik ə-me'no as'id de"kahr-bok'sə-lās) [EC 4.1.1.28] an enzyme of the lyase class that catalyzes the decarboxylation of aromatic amino acids, notably converting dopa to dopamine, tryptophan to tryptamine, and hydroxytryptophan to serotonin. The enzyme is bound to a pyridoxal phosphate cofactor and occurs particularly in liver, kidney, brain, and vas deferens; the reaction is important in the biosynthesis of catecholamines and of melanin.

**aro·ma·ti·za·tion** (ə-ro"mə-tĭ-za'shən) chemical conversion to an aromatic form.

**arous·al** (ə-rou'zəl) [MeSH: Arousal] 1. a state of responsiveness to sensory stimulation or excitability. 2. the act or state of waking from or as if from sleep. 3. the act of stimulating to readiness or to action.
**sexual a.,** physical and psychological responses to mental or physical erotic stimulation, including altered respiration, muscular tension, pulse, and blood flow to the genitals as well as increased interest in sexual activity.

**ar·pri·no·cid** (ahr-pri'no-sid) a coccidiostat used in poultry.

**ar·rache·ment** (ahr"ahsh-mahwn') [Fr. "extraction"] extraction of a membranous cataract by pulling out the capsule through a corneal incision.

**ar·range·ment** (ə-rānj'mənt) the disposal or positioning of parts.
**anterior tooth a.,** the arrangement of anterior teeth for esthetic or phonetic effects.
**tooth a.,** 1. the positioning of teeth on a denture for specific purposes. 2. the setting of teeth on temporary bases.

**ar·rec·tor** (ə-rek'tər) pl. *arrecto'res* [L.] raising, or that which raises.
**a. pi'li,** pl. **arrecto'res pilo'rum,** [L. "raisers of the hair"], minute smooth muscles of the skin, attached to the connective tissue sheath of the hair follicles, the contraction of which causes the hair to stand erect and produces the appearance called cutis anserina, or goose flesh.

**ar·rec·to·res** (ar"ek-to'res) [L.] plural of *arrector.*

**ar·rest** (ə-rest') stoppage; the act of stopping.
**cardiac a.,** sudden cessation of the pumping function of the heart, with disappearance of arterial blood pressure, connoting either ventricular fibrillation or ventricular standstill; it usually leads to death unless corrected but may be temporary or paroxysmal.
**deep transverse a.,** the condition during delivery in which the occiput of the fetus turns and stops in the transverse diameter of the pelvis.
**developmental a.,** a temporary or permanent cessation of the process of development.
**epiphyseal a.,** interruption of growth at the epiphysis of a bone by diaphyseal-epiphyseal fusion.
**heart a.,** cardiac a.
**maturation a.,** interruption of the process of development before it is complete; applied especially to failure of maturation of granulocytes, with myeloblasts and promyelocytes predominating, as seen in certain forms of leukemia.
**sinus a.,** a halt, usually transient, in the normal cardiac (sinus) rhythm due to a slowing or cessation of impulse initiation by the sinus node, lasting for an interval that is not an exact multiple of the normal cardiac cycle; either ectopic pacemakers assume control of the rhythm or periods of ventricular asystole occur. See also *sinus pause,* under *pause.*

**ar·rest·ed** (ə-rest'əd) detained; stopped. In obstetrics, the head of the child is said to be arrested when it is *detained,* but not *impacted,* in the pelvic cavity.

**ar·res·tin** (ə-res'tin) [MeSH: Arrestin] a protein of the retina that binds activated phosphorylated rhodopsin and prevents it from binding transducin; it deactivates rhodopsin as part of the visual cycle.

**ar·rha·phia** (ə-ra'fe-ə) [*a-*[1] + *-rhaphy*] status dysraphicus.

**Ar·rhe·ni·us' equation, formula, theory (doctrine)** (ə-re'ne-əs) [Svante August *Arrhenius,* Swedish chemist, 1859–1927] see under *equation, formula,* and *theory.*

**arrheno-** [Gr. *arrhēn* male] a combining form meaning male.

**ar·rhe·no·blas·to·ma** (ə-re"no-blas-to'mə) [*arrheno-* + *blast-* + *-oma*] androblastoma (def. 2)

**ar·rhi·go·sis** (a"rĭ-go'sis) [*a-*[1] + *rhigosis*] inability to perceive cold; absence of the cold sense.

**ar·rhin·en·ce·pha·lia** (ə-rin"ən-sə-fa'le-ə) [*a-*[1] + *rhinencephalon*] congenital absence of the rhinencephalon.

**ar·rhin·ia** (ə-rin'e-ə) [*a* neg. + *rhin-* + *-ia*] congenital absence of the nose.

**ar·rhyth·mia** (ə-rith'me-ə) [*a-*[1] + *rhythm* + *-ia*] [MeSH: Arrhythmia] any variation from the normal rhythm of the heartbeat; it may be an abnormality of either the rate, regularity, or site of impulse origin or the sequence of activation. The term encompasses abnormal regular and irregular rhythms as well as loss of rhythm. Cf. *dysrhythmia* and see also entries under *rhythm.*
**chronic a.,** continuous a.
**compound a.,** one with multiple disturbances in rhythm.
**continuous a.,** irregularity in the force, quality, and sequence of the pulse beat, continuing as a permanent phenomenon; called also *chronic* or *perpetual a.*
**juvenile a.,** sinus arrhythmia occurring in children.
**nodal a.,** arrhythmia occurring when the atrioventricular node or surrounding junctional tissue is acting as pacemaker.
**nonphasic a.,** a form of sinus arrhythmia in which the irregularity is not linked to the phases of respiration. Cf. *phasic a.*
**perpetual a.,** continuous a.
**phasic a.,** a form of sinus arrhythmia linked to the phases of respiration, the heart rate increasing with inspiration and decreasing with expiration. Cf. *nonphasic a.*
**sinus a.,** the physiologic cyclic variation in heart rate related to vagal impulses to the sinoatrial node, which can be linked to or independent of the phases of respiration (see *phasic a.* and *nonphasic a.*). It is common, particularly in children, and is not considered abnormal.
**sinus a., nonrespiratory,** nonphasic a.
**sinus a., respiratory,** phasic a.
**supraventricular a.,** an arrhythmia originating in the atria, including the atrioventricular node; it may be a bradyarrhythmia or a tachyarrhythmia.
**ventricular a.,** an arrhythmia originating in the ventricles.

**ar·rhyth·mic** (ə-rith'mik) [*a-*[1] + Gr. *rhythmos* rhythm] 1. characterized by absence of rhythm. 2. pertaining to or characterized by arrhythmia.

**ar·rhyth·mo·gen·esis** (ə-rith"mo-jen'ə-sis) [*arrhythmia* + *genesis*] the development of an arrhythmia.

**ar·rhyth·mo·gen·ic** (ə-rith"mo-jen'ik) [*arrhythmia* + *-genic*] producing or promoting arrhythmia.

**ar·rhyth·mo·ki·ne·sis** (ə-rith″mo-kĭ-ne′sis) [*arrhythmia* + *kinesis*] a dyskinesia consisting of defective ability to perform voluntary successive movements of a definite rhythm. Cf. *adiadochokinesia.*

**Ar·ro·yo's sign** (ah-ro′yōz) [Carlos F. *Arroyo,* American physician, 1892–1928] asthenocoria.

**ARRS** American Roentgen Ray Society.

**ar·sam·bide** (ahr-sam′bīd) carbarsone.

**ar·sa·nil·ic ac·id** (ahr″sə-nil′ik) [USP] [MeSH: Arsanilic Acid] an arsenical antibacterial used in veterinary practice for the prevention and treatment of swine dysentery.

**ar·se·ni·a·sis** (ahr″sə-ni′ə-sis) chronic arsenic poisoning.

**ar·se·nic**[1] (ahr′sə-nik) [L. *arsenicum, arsenium,* or *arsenum;* from Gr. *arsēn* strong] a nonmetallic element, occurring as a brittle, lustrous, grayish solid, with a garlicky odor. Symbol, As; atomic number, 33; atomic weight, 74.922; specific gravity, 5.73; it is toxic by inhalation and ingestion and is carcinogenic. Although arsenic and its compounds have been widely employed in medicine, it is now rarely used and is important only in the treatment of certain tropical parasitic diseases. See also arsenic poisoning, under *poisoning.*
**a. chloride,** a. trichloride.
**a. disulfide,** a poisonous compound, used as a pigment, in fireworks, in shot manufacture, and in the leather industry; called also *red a. sulfide* and *realgar.*
**fuming liquid a.,** a. trichloride.
**red a. sulfide,** a. disulfide.
**a. trichloride,** a very poisonous fuming liquid, $AsCl_3$, which readily liberates highly irritant hydrochloric acid; it is used in war gas and as an intermediate for organic chemicals.
**a. trioxide,** white arsenic, a white or glassy compound, with a sweetish taste and erythropoietic effect; taken in repeated small doses in Alpine countries to increase hemoglobin, resulting in increased working capacity and a ruddy complexion. Formerly used in treatment of skin and hematologic disorders. Called also *arsenous acid, arsenous anhydride,* and *flowers of arsenic.*
**a. trisulfide,** a poisonous substance, occurring in nature as the mineral orpiment; used as a pigment and sometimes as a medicine. Called also *a. yellow* and *auripigment.*
**white a.,** a. trioxide.
**a. yellow,** a. trisulfide.

**ar·sen·ic**[2] (ahr-sen′ik) pertaining to or containing arsenic in a pentavalent state.

**ar·sen·ic ac·id** (ahr-sen′ik) the hydrate, $H_3AsO_4$, of arsenic pentoxide, which is itself also referred to as arsenic acid.

**ar·sen·i·cal** (ahr-sen′ĭ-kəl) [L. *arsenicalis*] 1. pertaining to or containing arsenic. 2. a drug or other compound (such as a pesticide) containing arsenic; all arsenicals are toxic to humans and some are carcinogenic.

**ar·sen·i·cal·ism** (ahr-sen′ĭ-kəl-iz″əm) chronic arsenic poisoning.

**ar·se·nide** (ahr′sə-nīd) any compound of arsenic with another element, in which arsenic is the negative element.

**ar·sen·i·ous** (ahr-sen′e-əs) arsenous.

**ar·se·nism** (ahr′sə-niz″əm) chronic arsenic poisoning.

**ar·se·nite** (ahr′sə-nīt) any salt of arsenous acid.

**arseno-** a prefix indicating the chemical group —As:As—.

**ar·se·no·ther·a·py** (ahr″sə-no-ther′ə-pe) [*arsenic* + *therapy*] treatment of disease by the use of arsenic and arsenical preparations.

**ar·se·nous** (ahr′sə-nəs) containing arsenic in its lower or triad valency.

**ar·se·nous ac·id** (ahr′sə-nəs) the hydrate, $H_3AsO_3$, of arsenic trioxide, which is itself also referred to as arsenous acid.

**ar·sine** (ahr′sēn) any member of a peculiar group of volatile arsenical bases, formed when arsenous acid is brought in contact with albuminous substances. The typical arsine is $AsH_3$, arsenous hydride or arseniuretted hydrogen, a very poisonous gas, and some of its compounds have been used in warfare. A major industrial use is in the production of microelectronic components. It is carcinogenic and also causes hemolysis, jaundice, gastroenteritis, and nephritis.

**ar·sin·ic ac·id** (ahr-sin′ik) an organic compound containing the $—AsO_2H$ functional group.

**ar·son·ic ac·id** (ahr-son′ik) an organic compound containing the $—AsO(OH)_2$ functional group.

**ar·so·ni·um** (ahr-so′ne-əm) the univalent radical or ion, $AsH_4$, which acts in combination like the ammonium ion, $NH_4$.

**ars·phen·a·mine** (ahrs-fen′ə-mēn) [MeSH: Arsphenamine] the first medicine specific for the treatment of syphilis, yaws, and other spirillum infections, later replaced by oxophenarsine and then by penicillin. Called also *salvarsan.*

**ars·thi·nol** (ahrs′thĭ-nol) an antiprotozoal agent, effective in amebiasis and yaws; administered orally.

**ART** [MeSH: Art] Accredited Record Technician; assisted reproductive technology; automated reagin test.

**Ar·tane** (ahr′tān) trademark for preparations of trihexyphenidyl.

**ar·te·fact** (ahr′tə-fakt) [MeSH: Artifacts] artifact.

**Ar·te·mi·sia** (ahr″tə-mis′e-ə) [L.; Gr. *artemisia* from *Artemis* Diana] [MeSH: Artemisia] a genus of composite-flowered plants (family Compositae). *A. abro′tanum* is southernwood; *A. absin′thium* is wormwood or absinthe (q.v.); and *A. mari′tima* (or *A. pauciflo′ra*) is santonica, the source of santonin.

**ar·te·ral·gia** (ahr″tər-al′jə) pain emanating from an artery, such as headache from an inflamed temporal artery.

**ar·ter·ec·to·my** (ahr″tər-ek′to-me) arteriectomy.

**ar·te·re·nol** (ahr″tə-re′nol) norepinephrine hydrochloride.

**ar·te·ria** (ahr-te′re-ə) pl. *arte′riae* [L. *arteria;* from Gr. *artēria,* possibly from *aēr* air + *tērein* to keep, because the arteries were thought to contain air, or from *aeirein* to lift or attach] [TA] artery.

## Arteria

**a. aceta′buli,** 1. ramus acetabularis arteriae obturatoriae. 2. ramus acetabularis arteriae circumflexae femoris medialis.

**a. adrena′lis me′dia,** a. suprarenalis media.

**a. alveola′ris infe′rior** [TA], inferior alveolar artery: *origin,* maxillary artery; *branches,* dental, peridental, mental, and mylohyoid rami; *distribution,* lower jaw, lower lip, and chin. Called also *inferior dental artery* and *mandibular artery.*

**arte′riae alveola′res superio′res anterio′res** [TA], anterior superior alveolar arteries: *origin,* infraorbital artery; *branches,* dental and peridental rami; *distribution,* incisors and canine regions of upper jaw, maxillary sinus. Called also *anterior dental arteries.*

**a. alveola′ris supe′rior poste′rior** [TA], posterior superior alveolar artery: *origin,* maxillary artery; *branches,* dental and peridental rami; *distribution,* molar and premolar regions of upper jaw, maxillary sinus. Called also *posterior dental artery.*

**a. angula′ris** [TA], angular artery: *origin,* facial artery; *branches,* none; *distribution,* lacrimal sac, lower eyelid, nose.

**a. aor′ta,** aorta.

**a. appendicula′ris** [TA], appendicular artery: *origin,* ileocolic artery; *branches,* none; *distribution,* vermiform appendix. Called also *vermiform artery.*

**arte′riae arcifor′mes re′nis,** arteriae arcuatae renis.

**a. arcua′ta pe′dis** [TA], arcuate artery of foot: *origin,* dorsal artery of foot; *branches,* deep plantar branch and dorsal metatarsal artery; *distribution,* foot, toes.

**arte′riae arcua′tae re′nis** [TA], arcuate arteries of kidney: *origin,* interlobar artery; *branches,* interlobular artery and arteriolae rectae; *distribution,* parenchyma of kidney. Called also *arteriae arciformes renis* and *arterial arches of kidney.*

**a. ascen′dens ileoco′lica,** ramus colicus arteriae ileocolicae.

**a. auditi′va inter′na,** a. labyrinthina.

**arte′riae auricula′res anterio′res,** rami auriculares anteriores arteriae temporalis superficialis.

**a. auricula′ris poste′rior** [TA], posterior auricular artery: *origin,* external carotid; *branches,* auricular and occipital rami, stylomastoid artery; *distribution,* middle ear, mastoid cells, auricle, parotid gland, digastric and other muscles.

**a. auricula′ris profun′da** [TA], deep auricular artery: *origin,* maxillary artery; *branches,* none; *distribution,* skin of auditory canal, tympanic membrane, temporomandibular joint.

**a. axilla′ris** [TA], axillary artery: *origin,* continuation of subclavian artery; *branches,* subscapular rami, and superior thoracic, thoracoacromial, lateral thoracic, subscapular, and anterior and posterior circumflex humeral arteries; *distribution,* upper limb, axilla, chest, shoulder.

**arte'riae azy'goi vagi'nae,** rami vaginales arteriae uterinae.

**a. basila'ris** [TA], basilar artery: *origin,* from junction of right and left vertebral arteries; *branches,* pontine branches, and anterior inferior cerebellar, labyrinthine, superior cerebellar, and posterior cerebral arteries; *distribution,* brain stem, internal ear, cerebellum, posterior cerebrum.

**a. brachia'lis** [TA], brachial artery: *origin,* continuation of axillary artery; *branches,* superficial brachial, deep brachial, nutrient of humerus, superior ulnar collateral, inferior ulnar collateral, radial, and ulnar arteries; *distribution,* shoulder, arm, forearm, hand.

**a. brachia'lis superficia'lis** [TA], superficial brachial artery: an occasional vessel that arises from high bifurcation of the brachial artery and assumes a more superficial course than usual.

**arte'riae bronchia'les,** rami bronchiales partis thoracicae aortae.

**a. bucca'lis** [TA], buccal artery: *origin,* maxillary artery; *branches,* none; *distribution,* buccinator muscle, mucous membrane of mouth. Called also *a. buccinatoria* and *buccinator artery.*

**a. buccinato'ria,** a. buccalis.

**a. bul'bi pe'nis** [TA], artery of bulb of penis: *origin,* internal pudendal artery; *branches,* none; *distribution,* bulbourethral gland, bulb of penis. Called also *a. bulbi urethrae* and *bulbourethral artery.*

**a. bul'bi ure'thrae,** a. bulbi penis.

**a. bul'bi vesti'buli** [TA], artery of bulb of vestibule: *origin,* internal pudendal artery; *branches,* none; *distribution,* vestibular bulb, greater vestibular glands.

**a. caeca'lis ante'rior** [TA], anterior cecal artery: *origin,* ileocolic; *branches,* none; *distribution,* cecum. Spelled also *a. cecalis anterior.*

**a. caeca'lis poste'rior** [TA], posterior cecal artery: *origin,* ileocolic; *branches,* none; *distribution,* cecum. Spelled also *a. cecalis posterior.*

**a. callosomargina'lis** [TA], callosomarginal artery: *origin,* postcommunical part of anterior cerebral artery; *branches,* anteromedial frontal, mediomedial frontal, posteromedial frontal, and singular branches; *distribution,* medial and superolateral surfaces of cerebral hemisphere.

**a. cana'lis pterygoi'dei** [TA], artery of pterygoid canal: *origin,* maxillary artery; *branches,* pterygoid; *distribution,* roof of pharynx, auditory tube. Called also *vidian artery.*

**arte'riae capsula'res,** capsular arteries: *origin,* renal artery; *branches,* none; *distribution,* renal capsule. Called also *arteriae perirenales* [TA alternative], and *perirenal arteries.*

**arte'riae caroticotympa'nicae** [TA], caroticotympanic arteries: branches of the petrous part of the internal carotid artery that supply the tympanic cavity; called also *rami caroticotympanici arteriae carotidis internae.*

**a. caro'tis commu'nis** [TA], common carotid artery: *origin,* brachiocephalic trunk (right), aortic arch (left); *branches,* external and internal carotids; *distribution,* see *a. carotis externa* and *a. carotis interna.*

**a. caro'tis exter'na** [TA], external carotid artery: *origin,* common carotid; *branches,* superior thyroid, ascending pharyngeal, lingual, facial, sternocleidomastoid, occipital, posterior auricular, superficial temporal, maxillary; *distribution,* neck, face, skull.

**a. caro'tis inter'na** [TA], internal carotid artery: *origin,* common carotid; *branches,* caroticotympanic, ophthalmic, posterior communicating, anterior choroid, anterior cerebral, and middle cerebral arteries; *distribution,* middle ear, brain, pituitary gland, orbit, choroid plexus. It is divided into four parts: cervical, petrous, cavernous, and cerebral.

**a. cau'dae pancre'atis** [TA], artery of tail of pancreas: *origin,* splenic; *branches and distribution,* supplies branches to tail of pancreas, and accessory spleen (if present).

**a. ceca'lis ante'rior,** a. caecalis anterior.

**a. ceca'lis poste'rior,** a. caecalis posterior.

**arte'riae centra'les anterolatera'les** [TA], anterolateral central arteries: *origin,* sphenoidal part of middle cerebral artery; *branches,* two sets of branches, medial and lateral; *distribution,* anterior lenticular and caudate nuclei and internal capsule of brain. Called also *arteriae thalamostriatae anterolaterales, anterolateral thalamostriate arteries,* and *striate arteries.*

**arte'riae centra'les anteromedia'les arte'riae ce'rebri anterio'ris** [TA], anteromedial central arteries of anterior cerebral artery: *origin,* precommunical part of anterior cerebral artery; *branches,* none; *distribution,* anterior and medial corpus striatum. Called also *arteriae thalamostriatae anteromediales* and *anteromedial thalamostriate arteries.*

**arte'riae centra'les anteromedia'les arte'riae communican'tis anterio'ris** [TA], anteromedial central arteries of anterior communicating artery: *origin,* anterior communicating artery; *branches,* none; *distribution,* corpus callosum, septum pellucidum, lentiform and caudate nuclei.

**a. centra'lis bre'vis,** short central artery: a branch from the precommunical part of the anterior cerebral artery.

**a. centra'lis lon'ga,** long central artery: a branch of the precommunical part of the anterior cerebral artery; called also *a. recurrens.*

**arte'riae centra'les posterolatera'les** [TA], posterolateral central arteries: *origin,* postcommunical part of posterior cerebral artery; *branches,* none; *distribution,* cerebral peduncle, posterior thalamus, colliculi, pineal and medial geniculate bodies.

**arte'riae centra'les posteromedia'les arte'riae ce'rebri posterio'ris** [TA], posteromedial central arteries of posterior cerebral artery: *origin,* precommunical part of posterior cerebral artery; *branches,* none; *distribution,* anterior thalamus, lateral wall of third ventricle, and globus pallidus of lentiform nucleus. Called also *paramedian arteries.*

**arte'riae centra'les posteromedia'les arte'riae communican'tis posterio'ris** [TA], posteromedial central arteries of posterior communicating artery: *origin,* posterior communicating artery; *branches,* none; *distribution,* medial thalamic surface and walls of third ventricle.

**a. centra'lis re'tinae** [TA], central artery of retina: *origin,* ophthalmic artery; *branches,* none; *distribution,* retina. Called also *artery of Zinn.*

**a. cerebel'li infe'rior ante'rior,** a. inferior anterior cerebelli.

**a. cerebel'li infe'rior poste'rior,** a. inferior posterior cerebelli.

**a. cerebel'li supe'rior,** a. superior cerebelli.

**a. ce'rebri ante'rior** [TA], anterior cerebral artery: *origin,* internal carotid artery; *branches* (precommunical part) anteromedial central arteries, long and short central arteries, anterior communicating artery, and (postcommunical part) medial frontobasal, callosomarginal (anteromedial, interomedial, posteromedial, and cingular branches), paracentral, precuneal, and parieto-occipital arteries; *distribution,* orbital, frontal, and parietal cortex, corpus callosum, diencephalon, corpus striatum, internal capsule, and choroid plexus of lateral ventricle.

**a. ce'rebri me'dia** [TA], middle cerebral artery: *origin,* internal carotid; *branches* sphenoidal part: anterolateral central artery (with medial and lateral branches); insular part: insular artery, lateral frontobasal artery, and anterior, intermediate, and posterior temporal arteries; terminal or cortical part: arteries of central, precentral, and postcentral sulcus, anterior and posterior parietal arteries, artery of angular gyri; *distribution,* orbital, frontal, parietal, and temporal cortex, corpus striatum, internal capsule. Called also *sylvian artery.*

**a. ce'rebri poste'rior** [TA], posterior cerebral artery: *origin,* terminal bifurcation of basilar artery; *branches* (precommunical part) posteromedial central arteries, (postcommunical part) posterolateral central arteries, and thalamic, medial and lateral posterior choroidal, and peduncular branches, and (terminal, or cortical, part) lateral occipital artery (anterior, medial intermediate and posterior temporal branches) and medial occipital artery (dorsal corpus callosum, parietal, parieto-occipital, calcarine, and occipitotemporal branches); *distribution,* occipital and temporal cortex, diencephalon, midbrain, choroid plexus of lateral and third ventricles, and visual area of cerebral cortex and other structures associated with the visual pathway.

**a. cervica'lis ascen'dens** [TA], ascending cervical artery: *origin,* inferior thyroid artery; *branches,* spinal rami; *distribution,* muscles of neck, vertebrae, vertebral canal.

**a. cervica'lis profun'da** [TA], deep cervical artery: *origin,* costocervical trunk; *branches,* none; *distribution,* deep neck muscles.

**a. cervica'lis superficia'lis,** ramus superficialis arteriae transversae cervicis.

**arte'riae cervicovagina'les,** cervicovaginal arteries: several large branches of the uterine artery given off at the side of the uterus at the level of the cervix, to supply the vagina.

**a. choroi'dea ante'rior** [TA], anterior choroidal artery: *origin,* internal carotid or middle cerebral artery; *branches,* many small branches; *distribution,* interior of brain, including choroid plexus of lateral ventricle and adjacent parts.

**arte'riae cilia'res anterio'res** [TA], anterior ciliary arteries: *origin,* ophthalmic and lacrimal arteries; *branches,* episcleral and anterior conjunctival arteries; *distribution,* iris, conjunctiva.

**arte'riae cilia'res posterio'res bre'ves** [TA], short posterior ciliary arteries: *origin,* ophthalmic artery; *branches,* none; *distribution,* choroid coat of eye. Called also *short ciliary arteries.*

**arte'riae cilia'res posterio'res lon'gae** [TA], long posterior ciliary arteries: *origin,* ophthalmic artery; *branches,* none; *distribution,* iris, ciliary process. Called also *long ciliary arteries.*

**a. circumflex'a ante'rior hu'meri,** a. circumflexa humeri anterior.

**a. circumflex'a fe'moris latera'lis** [TA], lateral circumflex femoral artery: *origin,* deep femoral artery; *branches,* ascending, descending, and transverse branches; *distribution,* hip joint, thigh muscles.

**a. circumflex'a fe'moris media'lis** [TA], medial circumflex femoral artery: *origin,* deep femoral artery; *branches,* deep, superficial, ascending, transverse, and acetabular branches; *distribution,* hip joint, thigh muscles.

**a. circumflex'a hu'meri ante'rior** [TA], anterior circumflex humeral artery: *origin,* axillary artery; *branches,* none; *distribution,* shoulder joint and head of humerus, long tendon of biceps, tendon of pectoralis major muscle. Called also *a. circumflexa anterior humeri.*

**a. circumflex'a hu'meri poste'rior** [TA], posterior circumflex humeral artery: *origin,* axillary artery; *branches;* none; *distribution,* deltoideus, shoulder joint, teres minor and triceps muscles. Called also *a. circumflexa posterior humeri.*

**a. circumflex'a i'lium profun'da** [TA], deep circumflex iliac artery: *origin,* external iliac artery; *branches,* ascending branches; *distribution,* iliac region, abdominal wall, groin.

**a. circumflex'a i'lium superficia'lis** [TA], superficial circumflex iliac artery: *origin,* femoral artery; *branches,* none; *distribution,* groin, abdominal wall.

**a. circumflex'a poste'rior hu'meri,** a. circumflexa humeri posterior.

**a. circumflex'a sca'pulae** [TA], circumflex artery of scapula: *origin,* subscapular artery; *branches,* none; *distribution,* inferolateral muscles of the scapula.

**a. co'lica dex'tra** [TA], right colic artery: *origin,* superior mesenteric artery; *branches,* none; *distribution,* ascending colon.

**a. co'lica me'dia** [TA], middle colic artery: *origin,* superior mesenteric artery; *branches,* none; *distribution,* transverse colon. Called also *accessory superior colic artery.*

**a. co'lica sinis'tra** [TA], left colic artery: *origin,* inferior mesenteric; *branches,* none; *distribution,* descending colon.

**a. collatera'lis me'dia** [TA], middle collateral artery: *origin,* deep brachial artery; *branches,* none; *distribution,* triceps muscle, elbow joint.

**a. collatera'lis radia'lis** [TA], radial collateral artery: *origin,* deep brachial artery; *branches,* none; *distribution,* brachioradialis and brachialis muscles.

**a. collatera'lis ulna'ris infe'rior** [TA], inferior ulnar collateral artery: *origin,* brachial artery; *branches,* none; *distribution,* arm muscles at back of elbow.

**a. collatera'lis ulna'ris supe'rior** [TA], superior ulnar collateral artery: *origin,* brachial artery; *branches,* none; *distribution,* elbow joint, triceps muscle.

**a. co'mitans ner'vi ischia'dici** [TA], accompanying artery of ischiadic nerve: *origin,* inferior gluteal artery; *branches,* none; *distribution,* accompanies sciatic nerve. Called also *a. comitans nervi sciatici, artery to sciatic nerve,* and *sciatic artery.*

**a. co'mitans ner'vi media'ni** [TA], accompanying artery of median nerve: *origin,* anterior interosseous artery; *branches,* none; *distribution,* median nerve, muscles of front of forearm. Called also *a. mediana* and *median artery.*

**a. co'mitans ner'vi scia'tici,** a. comitans nervi ischiadici.

**a. commu'nicans ante'rior** [TA], anterior communicating artery: *origin,* precommunical part of anterior cerebral artery; *branches,* none; *distribution,* establishes connection between the anterior cerebral arteries.

**a. commu'nicans poste'rior** [TA], posterior communicating artery: establishes connection between internal carotid and posterior cerebral arteries; *branches,* to the optic chiasm, oculomotor nerve, thalamus, hypothalamus, and tail of caudate nucleus.

**arte'riae conjunctiva'les anterio'res** [TA], anterior conjunctival arteries: *origin,* anterior ciliary; *branches,* none; *distribution,* conjunctiva.

**arte'riae conjunctiva'les posterio'res** [TA], posterior conjunctival arteries: *origin,* medial palpebral artery; *branches,* none; *distribution,* caruncula lacrimalis, conjunctiva.

**a. corona'ria [cor'dis] dex'tra,** a. coronaria dextra.

**a. corona'ria dex'tra** [TA], right coronary artery of heart: *origin,* right aortic sinus; *branches,* conus artery and atrial, atrioventricular node, intermediate atrial, posterior interventricular right marginal, and sinoatrial node rami; *distribution,* right ventricle, right atrium. Formerly called *right auricular artery.*

**a. corona'ria [cor'dis] sinis'tra,** a. coronaria sinistra.

**a. corona'ria sinis'tra** [TA], left coronary artery of heart: *origin,* left aortic sinus; *branches,* anterior interventricular and circumflex rami; *distribution,* left ventricle, left atrium. Formerly called *left auricular artery.*

**a. cremaste'rica** [TA], cremasteric artery: *origin,* inferior epigastric; *branches,* none; *distribution,* cremaster muscle, coverings of spermatic cord. Called also *a. spermatica externa* and *external spermatic artery.*

**a. cys'tica** [TA], cystic artery: *origin,* right branch of proper hepatic artery; *branches,* none; *distribution,* gallbladder.

**a. deferentia'lis,** a. ductus deferentis.

**a. descen'dens genicula'ris,** a. descendens genus.

**a. descen'dens ge'nus** [TA], descending genicular artery: *origin,* femoral artery; *branches,* saphenous, articular; *distribution,* knee joint, upper and medial leg. Called also *a. descendens genicularis.*

**arte'riae digita'les dorsa'les ma'nus** [TA], dorsal digital arteries of hand: *origin,* dorsal metacarpal arteries; *branches,* none; *distribution,* dorsum of fingers.

**arte'riae digita'les dorsa'les pe'dis** [TA], dorsal digital arteries of foot: *origin,* dorsal metatarsal arteries; *branches,* none; *distribution,* dorsum of toes.

**arte'riae digita'les palma'res commu'nes** [TA], common palmar digital arteries: *origin,* superficial volar arch; *branches,* proper palmar digital arteries; *distribution,* fingers. Called also *arteriae digitales volares communes, common volar digital arteries,* and *ulnar metacarpal arteries.*

**arte'riae digita'les palma'res pro'priae** [TA], proper palmar digital arteries: *origin,* common palmar digital arteries; *branches,* none; *distribution,* fingers. Called also *arteriae digitales volares propriae, collateral digital arteries,* and *proper volar digital arteries.*

**arte'riae digita'les planta'res commu'nes** [TA], common plantar digital arteries: *origin,* plantar metatarsal arteries; *branches,* proper plantar digital arteries; *distribution,* toes.

**arte'riae digita'les planta'res pro'priae** [TA], proper plantar digital arteries: *origin,* common plantar digital arteries; *branches,* none; *distribution,* toes.

**arte'riae digita'les vola'res commu'nes,** arteriae digitales palmares communes.

**arte'riae digita'les vola'res pro'priae,** arteriae digitales palmares propriae.

**a. dorsa'lis clito'ridis** [TA], dorsal artery of clitoris: *origin,* internal pudendal artery; *branches,* none; *distribution,* clitoris.

**a. dorsa'lis na'si** [TA], dorsal artery of nose: *origin,* ophthalmic artery; *branches,* lacrimal; *distribution,* dorsum of nose. Called also *a. nasi externa.*

**a. dorsa'lis pe'dis** [TA], dorsal artery of foot: *origin,* continuation of anterior tibial; *branches,* lateral and medial tarsal, arcuate, and deep plantar arteries; *distribution,* foot, toes.

**a. dorsa'lis pe'nis** [TA], dorsal artery of penis: *origin,* internal pudendal artery; *branches,* none; *distribution,* glans, corona, prepuce.

**a. dorsa'lis sca'pulae** [TA], dorsal scapular artery: *origin,* second or third part of subclavian artery, or may be the deep branch of transverse cervical artery *(ramus profundus arteriae transversae cervicis)*; *branches,* none; *distribution,* rhomboid, latissimus dorsi, and trapezius muscles. Called also *a. scapularis dorsalis.*

**a. duc'tus deferen'tis** [TA], artery of ductus deferens: *origin,* umbilical artery; *branches,* ureteral artery; *distribution,* ureter, ductus deferens, seminal vesicles, testes. Called also *a. deferentialis* and *deferential artery.*

**a. epigas'trica infe'rior** [TA], inferior epigastric artery: *origin,* external iliac; *branches,* pubic branch, cremasteric artery, a. of round ligament of uterus; *distribution,* abdominal wall.

**a. epigas'trica superficia'lis** [TA], superficial epigastric artery: *origin,* femoral; *branches,* none; *distribution,* abdominal wall, groin.

**a. epigas'trica supe'rior** [TA], superior epigastric artery: *origin,* internal thoracic artery; *branches,* none; *distribution,* abdominal wall, diaphragm.

**arte'riae episclera'les** [TA], episcleral arteries: *origin,* anterior ciliary artery; *branches,* none; *distribution,* iris, ciliary process.

**a. ethmoida'lis ante'rior** [TA], anterior ethmoidal artery: *origin,* ophthalmic artery; *branches,* anterior meningeal, anterior septal, and anterior lateral nasal rami; *distribution,* dura mater, nose, frontal sinus, anterior ethmoidal cells.

**a. ethmoida'lis poste'rior** [TA], posterior ethmoidal artery: *origin,* ophthalmic artery; *branches,* none; *distribution,* posterior ethmoidal cells, dura mater, nose.

**a. facia'lis** [TA], facial artery: *origin,* external carotid; *branches,* ascending palatine, tonsillar, submental, inferior labial, superior labial, septal, lateral nasal, angular, glandular; *distribution,* face, tonsil, palate, submandibular gland. Called also *a. maxillaris externa* or *external maxillary artery.*

**a. femora'lis** [TA], femoral artery: *origin,* continuation of external iliac; *branches,* superficial epigastric, superficial circumflex iliac, external pudendal, deep femoral, descending geniculate; *distribution,* lower abdominal wall, external genitalia, lower extremity. NOTE: Vascular surgeons refer to the portion of the femoral artery proximal to the branching of the deep femoral as the *common femoral a.,* and to its continuation as the *superficial femoral a.* In this classification, the descending geniculate artery is a branch of the superficial femoral artery.

**a. fibula'ris** [TA], fibular artery: *origin,* posterior tibial artery; *branches,* perforating, communicating, calcaneal, and lateral and medial malleolar branches, and calcaneal rete; *distribution,* outside and back of ankle, deep calf muscles. Called also *a. peronea* and *peroneal artery.*

**a. fronta'lis,** a. supratrochlearis.

**a. frontobasa'lis latera'lis** [TA], lateral frontobasal artery: *origin,* insular part of middle cerebral artery: *branches,* none; *distribution,* cortex of lateroinferior frontal lobe.

**a. frontobasa'lis media'lis** [TA], medial frontobasal artery: *origin,* postcommunical part of anterior cerebral artery; *branches,* none; *distribution,* medioinferior cortex of frontal lobe. Called also *ramus orbitofrontalis medialis arteriae cerebri anterioris* [TA alternative].

**arte'riae gas'tricae bre'ves** [TA], short gastric arteries: *origin,* splenic; *branches,* none; *distribution,* upper part of stomach.

**a. gas'trica dex'tra** [TA], right gastric artery: *origin,* common hepatic artery; *branches,* none; *distribution,* lesser curvature of stomach. Called also *pyloric artery.*

**a. gas'trica poste'rior** [TA], posterior gastric artery: *origin,* splenic artery; *branches,* none; *distribution,* posterior gastric wall.

**a. gas'trica sinis'tra** [TA], left gastric artery: *origin,* celiac; *branches,* esophageal; *distribution,* esophagus, lesser curvature of stomach. Called also *left coronary artery of stomach.*

**a. gastroduodena'lis** [TA], gastroduodenal artery: *origin,* common hepatic artery; *branches,* supraduodenal and posterior superior pancreaticoduodenal arteries; *distribution,* stomach, duodenum, pancreas, greater omentum.

**a. gastroepiplo'ica dex'tra,** a. gastro-omentalis dextra.

**a. gastroepiplo'ica sinis'tra,** a. gastro-omentalis sinistra.

**a. gastroomenta'lis dex'tra** [TA], right gastro-omental artery: *origin,* gastroduodenal artery; *branches,* gastric, omental; *distribution,* stomach, greater omentum. Called also *a. gastroepiploica dextra* and *right inferior gastric artery.*

**a. gastroomenta'lis sinis'tra** [TA], left gastro-omental artery: *origin,* splenic artery; *branches,* gastric, omental; *distribution,* stomach, greater omentum. Called also *a. gastroepiploica sinistra* and *left inferior gastric artery.*

**a. ge'nus infe'rior latera'lis,** a. inferior lateralis genus.

**a. ge'nus infe'rior media'lis,** a. inferior medialis genus.

**a. ge'nus me'dia,** a. media genus.

**a. ge'nus supe'rior latera'lis,** a. superior lateralis genus.

**a. ge'nus supe'rior media'lis,** a. superior medialis genus.

**a. glu'tea infe'rior** [TA], inferior gluteal artery: *origin,* internal iliac; *branches,* sciatic; *distribution,* buttock, back of thigh. Called also *a. glutealis inferior.*

**a. glu'tea supe'rior** [TA], superior gluteal artery: *origin,* internal iliac artery; *branches,* superficial and deep branches; *distribution,* buttocks. Called also *a. glutealis superior.*

**a. glutea'lis infe'rior,** a. glutea inferior.

**a. glutea'lis supe'rior,** a. glutea superior.

**a. gy'ri angula'ris,** artery of angular gyrus: *origin,* terminal part of middle cerebral artery; *branches,* none; *distribution,* temporal, parietal, and occipital lobes.

**a. haemorrhoida'lis infe'rior,** a. rectalis inferior.

**a. haemorrhoida'lis me'dia,** a. rectalis media.

**a. haemorrhoida'lis supe'rior,** a. rectalis superior.

**arte'riae helici'nae pe'nis** [TA], helicine arteries of penis: helicine arteries arising from the vessels of the penis, whose engorgement causes erection of the organ. Called also *arteries of Mueller.*

**a. hepa'tica,** a. hepatica communis.

**a. hepa'tica commu'nis** [TA], common hepatic artery: *origin,* celiac trunk; *branches,* right gastric, gastroduodenal, hepatic proper; *distribution,* stomach, pancreas, duodenum, liver, gallbladder, greater omentum. Called also *a. hepatica.*

**a. hepa'tica pro'pria** [TA], hepatic artery proper: *origin,* common hepatic artery; *branches,* right and left branches; *distribution,* liver, gallbladder.

**a. hyaloi'dea** [TA], hyaloid artery: a fetal vessel that continues forward from the central retinal artery through the vitreous body to supply the lens; it normally is not present after birth.

**a. hypogas'trica,** a. iliaca interna.

**a. hypophysia'lis infe'rior** [TA], inferior hypophyseal artery: a small branch from the cerebral part of the internal carotid artery that supplies the pituitary gland.

**a. hypophysia'lis supe'rior** [TA], superior hypophyseal artery: a small branch from the cerebral part of the internal carotid artery that supplies the pituitary gland.

**arte'riae i'leae, arte'riae ilea'les** [TA], ileal arteries: *origin,* superior mesenteric; *branches,* none; *distribution,* ileum. Called also *arteriae ilei* and *arteries of ileum.*

**arte'riae i'lei,** arteriae ileales.

**a. ileoco'lica** [TA], ileocolic artery: *origin,* superior mesenteric; *branches,* anterior and posterior cecal and appendicular arteries and colic (ascending) and ileal rami; *distribution,* ileum, cecum, vermiform appendix, ascending colon. Called also *inferior right colic artery.*

**a. ili'aca commu'nis** [TA], common iliac artery: *origin,* abdominal aorta; *branches,* internal and external iliac; *distribution,* pelvis, abdominal wall, lower limb.

**a. ili'aca exter'na** [TA], external iliac artery: *origin,* common iliac; *branches,* inferior epigastric, deep circumflex iliac; *distribution,* abdominal wall, external genitalia, lower limb. Called also *anterior iliac artery.*

**a. ili'aca inter'na** [TA], internal iliac artery: *origin,* continuation of common iliac; *branches,* iliolumbar, obturator, superior gluteal, inferior gluteal, umbilical, inferior vesical, uterine, middle rectal, and internal pudendal arteries; *distribution,* wall and viscera of pelvis, buttock, reproductive organs, medial aspect of thigh. Called also *a. hypogastrica, hypogastric artery,* and *posterior pelvic artery.*

**a. iliolumba'lis** [TA], iliolumbar artery: *origin,* internal iliac; *branches,* iliac and lumbar branches, lateral sacral arteries; *distribution,* pelvic muscles and bones, fifth lumbar segment, sacrum. Called also *small iliac artery.*

**a. infe'rior ante'rior cerebel'li** [TA], anterior inferior cerebellar artery: *origin,* basilar artery; *branches,* posterior, spinal (usually) and labyrinthine (usually) arteries; *distribution,* anteroinferior part of cerebellum, lower and lateral parts of pons and sometimes upper part of medulla oblongata. Called also *a. cerebelli inferior anterior.*

**a. infe'rior latera'lis ge'nus** [TA], lateral inferior artery of knee: *origin,* popliteal artery; *branches,* none; *distribution,* knee joint. Called also *lateral inferior genicular artery* and *a. genus inferior lateralis.*

**a. infe'rior media'lis ge'nus** [TA], medial inferior artery of knee: *origin,* popliteal artery; *branches,* none; *distribution,* knee joint. Called also *medial inferior genicular artery* and *a. genus inferior medialis.*

**a. infe'rior poste'rior cerebel'li** [TA], posterior inferior cerebellar artery: *origin,* vertebral artery; *branches,* medial and lateral; *distribution,* lower cerebellum, medulla, choroid plexus of fourth ventricle. Called also *a. cerebelli inferior posterior.*

**a. infraorbita'lis** [TA], infraorbital artery: *origin,* maxillary artery; *branches,* anterior superior alveolar; *distribution,* maxilla, maxillary sinus, upper teeth, lower lid, cheek, nose.

**a. innomina'ta,** truncus brachiocephalicus.

**arte'riae insula'res** [TA], insular arteries: *origin,* insular part of middle cerebral artery; *branches,* none; *distribution,* cortex of insula.

**arte'riae intercosta'les posterio'res** [TA], posterior intercostal arteries: for the first two, see *a. intercostalis posterior prima* and *a. intercostalis posterior secunda;* there are nine other pairs (III–XI): *origin,* thoracic aorta; *branches,* dorsal, spinal, lateral and medial cutaneous, collateral, and lateral mammary; *distribution,* thoracic wall.

**a. intercosta'lis poste'rior pri'ma** [TA], first posterior intercostal artery: *origin,* highest intercostal artery; *branches,* dorsal and spinal branches; *distribution,* upper thoracic wall.

**a. intercosta'lis poste'rior secun'da** [TA], second posterior intercostal artery: *origin,* highest intercostal artery; *branches,* dorsal and spinal branches; *distribution,* upper thoracic wall.

**a. intercosta'lis supre'ma** [TA], highest intercostal artery: *origin,* costocervical trunk; *branches,* first and second posterior intercostal arteries; *distribution,* upper thoracic wall. Called also *superior intercostal artery.*

**arte'riae interloba'res re'nis** [TA], interlobar arteries of kidney: *origin,* lobar branches of segmental arteries; *branches,* arcuate arteries; *distribution,* parenchyma of kidney.

**arte'riae interlobula'res he'patis** [TA], interlobular arteries of liver: arteries originating from the right or left branch of the proper hepatic artery, and passing between the lobules of the liver.

**arte'riae interlobula'res re'nis** [TA], interlobular arteries of kidney: arteries originating from the arcuate arteries of the kidney and distributed to the renal glomeruli. Called also *radiate arteries of kidney.*

**a. interos'sea ante'rior** [TA], anterior interosseous artery: *origin,* posterior or common interosseous artery; *branches,* median artery; *distribution,* deep parts of front of forearm. Called also *a. interossea volaris* or *volar interosseous artery.*

**a. interos'sea commu'nis** [TA], common interosseous artery: *origin,* ulnar artery; *branches,* anterior and posterior interosseous arteries; *distribution,* antecubital fossa.

**a. interos'sea dorsa'lis,** a. interossea posterior.

**a. interos'sea poste'rior** [TA], posterior interosseous artery: *origin,* common interosseous artery; *branches,* recurrent interosseous; *distribution,* deep parts of back of forearm. Called also *a. interossea dorsalis* and *dorsal* or *posterior interosseous artery.*

**a. interos'sea recur'rens** [TA], recurrent interosseous artery: *origin,* posterior interosseous or common interosseous artery; *branches,* none; *distribution,* back of elbow joint.

**a. interos'sea vola'ris,** a. interossea anterior.

**arte'riae intestina'les,** intestinal arteries: the arteries arising from the superior mesenteric, and supplying the intestines, including the pancreaticoduodenal, jejunal, ileal, ileocolic, and colic arteries.

**arte'riae intrarena'les** [TA], intrarenal arteries: the arteries of the kidney, including the interlobar, arcuate, and interlobular arteries, and the arteriolae rectae.

**arte'riae jejuna'les** [TA], jejunal arteries: *origin,* superior mesenteric; *branches,* none; *distribution,* jejunum.

**arte'riae labia'les anterio'res vul'vae,** rami labiales anteriores arteriae pudendae externae profundae.

**a. labia'lis infe'rior** [TA], inferior labial artery: *origin,* facial artery; *branches,* none; *distribution,* lower lip.

**arte'riae labia'les posterio'res vul'vae,** rami labiales posteriores arteriae pudendae internae.

**a. labia'lis supe'rior** [TA], superior labial artery: *origin,* facial artery; *branches,* septal and alar; *distribution,* upper lip, nose.

**a. labyrin'thi** [TA], **a. labyrinthi'na,** labyrinthine artery: *origin,* basilar or anterior inferior cerebellar artery; *branches,* vestibular and cochlear rami; *distribution,* through the internal acoustic meatus to the internal ear. Called also *a. auditiva interna, internal auditory artery, artery of labyrinth,* and *ramus meatus acustici interni arteriae basilaris* [TA alternative].

**a. lacrima'lis** [TA], lacrimal artery: *origin,* ophthalmic artery; *branches,* lateral palpebral arteries and recurrent meningeal; *distribution,* lacrimal gland, upper and lower eyelids, conjunctiva.

**a. laryn'gea infe'rior** [TA], inferior laryngeal artery: *origin,* inferior thyroid artery; *branches,* none; *distribution,* larynx, trachea, esophagus.

**a. laryn'gea supe'rior** [TA], superior laryngeal artery: *origin,* superior thyroid artery; *branches,* none; *distribution,* larynx.

**a. liena'lis,** TA alternative for *a. splenica.*

**a. ligamen'ti te'retis u'teri** [TA], artery of round ligament of uterus: *origin,* inferior epigastric artery; *branches,* none; *distribution,* round ligament of uterus.

**a. lingua'lis** [TA], lingual artery: *origin,* external carotid; *branches,* suprahyoid, sublingual, dorsal lingual, deep lingual; *distribution,* tongue, sublingual gland, tonsil, epiglottis.

**a. lingula'ris** [TA], lingular artery: a branch of the left pulmonary artery to the superior lobe, consisting almost entirely of the superior and inferior lingular arteries and supplying the lingular segments. Called also *lingular segmental artery.*

**a. lingula'ris infe'rior** [TA], inferior lingular artery: a branch of the left pulmonary artery to the superior lobe, supplying the inferior lingular segment. Called also *inferior lingular segmental artery.*

**a. lingula'ris supe'rior** [TA], superior lingular artery: a branch of the left pulmonary artery to the superior lobe, supplying the superior lingular segment. Called also *superior lingular segmental artery.*

**arte'riae loba'res inferio'res pulmo'nis dex'tri** [TA], inferior lobar arteries of right lung: the branches of the right pulmonary artery that supply the inferior lobe of the right lung, consisting of the superior, anterior basal, lateral basal, medial basal, and posterior basal segmental arteries.

**arte'riae loba'res inferio'res pulmo'nis sinis'tri** [TA], inferior lobar arteries of left lung: the branches of the left pulmonary artery that supply the inferior lobe of the left lung, consisting of the superior, anterior basal, lateral basal, medial basal, and posterior basal segmental arteries.

**a. loba'ris me'dia pulmo'nis dex'tri** [TA], middle lobar artery of right lung: the branch of the right pulmonary artery that carries blood to the middle lobe of the right lung, giving rise to the lateral and medial lobar arteries.

**arte'riae loba'res superio'res pulmo'nis dex'tri** [TA], superior lobar arteries of right lung: the branches of the right pulmonary artery that carry blood to the superior lobe of the right lung, consisting of the apical, anterior, and posterior segmental arteries.

**arte'riae loba'res superio'res pulmo'nis sinis'tri** [TA], superior lobar arteries of left lung: the branches of the left pulmonary artery that carry blood to the superior lobe of the left lung, consisting of the apical, anterior, and posterior segmental arteries.

**a. lo'bi cauda'ti** [TA], artery of caudate lobe: either of two branches, one from the right and one from the left hepatic artery, supplying twigs to the caudate lobe of the liver.

**arte'riae lumba'les** [TA], lumbar arteries: *origin,* abdominal aorta; *branches,* dorsal and spinal branches; *distribution,* posterior abdominal wall, renal capsule.

**arte'riae lumba'les i'mae** [TA], lowest lumbar arteries: *origin,* middle sacral; *branches,* none; *distribution,* sacrum, gluteus maximus muscle. Called also *fifth lumbar arteries.*

**a. luso'ria,** an abnormally situated retroesophageal vessel, usually the subclavian artery from the aortic arch, which may cause symptoms by compression of the esophagus, the trachea, or a nerve.

**a. malleola'ris ante'rior latera'lis** [TA], lateral anterior malleolar artery: *origin,* anterior tibial artery; *branches,* none; *distribution,* ankle joint.

**a. malleola'ris ante'rior media'lis** [TA], medial anterior malleolar artery: *origin,* anterior tibial artery; *branches,* none; *distribution,* ankle joint.

**a. mamma'ria inter'na,** a. thoracica interna.

**a. margina'lis co'li** [TA], marginal artery of colon; a continuous vessel running along the inner perimeter of the large intestine from the ileocolic junction to the rectum, formed by branches from the superior and inferior mesenteric arteries and giving rise to straight arteries that supply the intestinal wall. Called also *marginal artery of Drummond.*

**a. massete'rica** [TA], masseteric artery: *origin,* maxillary artery; *branches,* none; *distribution,* masseter muscle.

**a. maxilla'ris** [TA], maxillary artery: *origin,* external carotid artery; *branches,* pterygoid rami, and deep auricular, anterior tympanic, inferior alveolar, middle meningeal, masseteric, deep temporal, buccal, posterior superior alveolar, infraorbital, descending palatine, sphenopalatine, and the artery of the pterygoid canal; *distribution,* both jaws, teeth, muscles of mastication, ear, meninges, nose, nasal sinus, palate. Called also *a. maxillaris interna* and *internal maxillary artery.*

**a. maxilla'ris exter'na,** a. facialis.

**a. maxilla'ris inter'na,** a. maxillaris.

**a. me'dia ge'nus** [TA], middle artery of knee: *origin,* popliteal artery; *branches,* none; *distribution,* knee joint, cruciate ligaments, patellar synovial and alar folds. Called also *middle genicular artery* and *a. genus media.*

**a. media'na,** a. comitans nervi mediani.

**arte'riae mediastina'les anterior'res,** rami mediastinales arteriae thoracicae internae.

**arte'riae mem'bri inferio'ris** [TA], arteries of lower limb: the arteries supplying the thigh, leg, and foot, including the external iliac, femoral, deep femoral, popliteal, anterior and posterior tibial, dorsalis pedis, medial and lateral plantar, and fibular arteries.

**arte'riae mem'bri superio'ris** [TA], arteries of upper limb: the arteries supplying the arm, forearm, and hand, including the axillary, brachial, radial, and ulnar arteries.

**a. menin'gea ante'rior,** ramus meningeus anterior arteriae ethmoidalis anterioris.

**a. menin'gea me'dia** [TA], middle meningeal artery: *origin,* maxillary artery; *branches,* frontal, parietal, and lacrimal anastomotic, accessory meningeal, and petrosal rami, and the superior tympanic artery; *distribution,* cranial bones, dura mater.

**a. menin'gea poste'rior** [TA], posterior meningeal artery: *origin,* ascending pharyngeal; *branches,* none; *distribution,* bones, dura mater of posterior cranial fossa.

**a. menta'lis,** ramus mentalis arteriae alveolaris inferioris.

**arte'riae mesencepha'licae** [TA], mesencephalic arteries: *origin,* basilar artery; *branches,* none; *distribution:* cerebral peduncle.

**a. mesente'rica infe'rior** [TA], inferior mesenteric artery: *origin,* abdominal aorta; *branches,* left colic, sigmoid, and superior rectal arteries; *distribution,* descending colon, rectum.

**a. mesente'rica supe'rior** [TA], superior mesenteric artery: *origin,* abdominal aorta; *branches,* inferior pancreaticoduodenal, jejunal, ileal, ileocolic, right colic, and middle colic arteries; *distribution,* small intestine, proximal half of colon.

**arte'riae metacarpa'les dorsa'les** [TA], dorsal metacarpal arteries: *origin,* dorsal carpal rete and radial artery; *branches,* dorsal digital arteries; *distribution,* dorsum of fingers. Called also *arteriae metacarpeae dorsales.*

**arte'riae metacarpa'les palma'res** [TA], palmar metacarpal arteries: *origin,* deep palmar arch; *branches,* none; *distribution,* deep parts of metatarsus. Called also *arteriae metacarpeae palmares, arteriae metacarpeae volares, volar metacarpal arteries,* and *palmar intermetacarpal arteries.*

**arte'riae metacar'peae dorsa'les,** arteriae metacarpales dorsales.

**arte'riae metacar'peae palma'res, arte'riae metacar'peae vola'res,** arteriae metacarpales palmares.

**arte'riae metatarsa'les dorsa'les** [TA], dorsal metatarsal arteries: *origin,* arcuate artery of foot; *branches,* dorsal digital arteries; *distribution,* foot, toes. Called also *arteriae metatarseae dorsales.*

**arte'riae metatarsa'les planta'res** [TA], plantar metatarsal arteries: *origin,* plantar arch; *branches,* perforating branches, common and proper plantar digital arteries; *distribution,* toes. Called also *arteriae metatarseae plantares* and *common digital arteries of foot.*

**arte'riae metatar'seae dorsa'les,** arteriae metatarsales dorsales.

**arte'riae metatar'seae planta'res,** arteriae metatarsales plantares.

**arte'riae muscula'res** [TA], muscular arteries: branches of the ophthalmic artery consisting of a superior group and an inferior group; the inferior group gives origin to the anterior ciliary arteries.

**a. musculophre'nica** [TA], musculophrenic artery: *origin,* internal thoracic artery; *branches,* none; *distribution,* diaphragm, abdominal and thoracic walls.

**arte'riae nasa'les posterio'res latera'les** [TA], posterior lateral nasal arteries: *origin,* sphenopalatine artery; *branches,* none; *distribution,* frontal, maxillary, ethmoidal, and sphenoidal sinuses.

**a. na'si exter'na,** a. dorsalis nasi.

**a. nutri'cia** [TA], nutrient artery: any artery that supplies the marrow of a long bone; called also *a. nutriens* [TA alternative] and *medullary artery.* See also *nutrient vessels,* under *vessel.*

**arte'riae nutri'ciae fe'moris** [TA], nutrient arteries of femur: *origin,* third perforating artery; *branches,* none; *distribution,* femur. Called also *arteriae nutrientes femoris.*

**a. nutri'cia fi'bulae** [TA], nutrient artery of fibula: *origin,* fibular artery; *branches,* none; *distribution,* fibula. Called also *a. nutriens fibulae* [TA alternative].

**arte'riae nutri'ciae hu'meri** [TA], nutrient arteries of humerus: *origin,* brachial and deep brachial arteries; *branches,* none; *distribution,* humerus. Called also *arteriae nutrientes humeri* [TA alternative].

**a. nutri'cia ti'biae** [TA], **a. nutri'cia tibia'lis,** nutrient tibial artery: *origin,* posterior tibial artery; *branches,* none; *distribution,* tibia. Called also *nutrient artery of tibia, a. nutriens tibiae* [TA alternative], and *a. nutriens tibialis.*

**a. nu'triens,** TA alternative for *a. nutricia.*

**arte'riae nutrien'tes fe'moris,** TA alternative for *arteriae nutriciae femoris.*

**a. nu'triens fi'bulae,** TA alternative for *a. nutricia fibulae.*

**arte'riae nutrien'tes hu'meri,** TA alternative for *arteriae nutriciae humeri.*

**a. nu'triens ti'biae,** TA alternative for *a. nutricia tibiae.*

**a. nu'triens tibia'lis,** a. nutricia tibiae.

**a. obturato'ria** [TA], obturator artery: *origin,* internal iliac; *branches,* pubic, acetabular, anterior, and posterior branches; *distribution,* pelvic muscles, hip joint.

**a. obturato'ria accesso'ria** [TA], accessory obturator artery: a name given to the obturator artery when it arises from the inferior epigastric instead of the internal iliac artery.

**a. occipita'lis** [TA], occipital artery: *origin,* external carotid; *branches,* auricular, meningeal, mastoid, descending, occipital, and sternocleidomastoid rami; *distribution,* muscles of neck and scalp, meninges, mastoid cells.

**a. occipita'lis latera'lis** [TA], lateral occipital artery: *origin,* terminal, or cortical, part of posterior cerebral artery; *branches,* lateral occipital artery and anterior temporal, middle intermediate temporal and posterior temporal branches; *distribution,* anterior, medial, intermediate, and posterior parts of temporal lobe.

**a. occipita'lis media'lis** [TA], middle occipital artery: *origin,* terminal, or cortical, part of posterior cerebral artery; *branches,* dorsal corpus callosum, parietal, parieto-occipital, calcarine, and occipitotemporal branches; *distribution,* dorsum of corpus callosum, precuneus, cuneus, lingual gyrus, and posterior part of lateral surface of occipital lobe.

**a. ophthal'mica** [TA], ophthalmic artery: *origin,* internal carotid; *branches,* lacrimal, supraorbital, central artery of retina, ciliary, posterior and anterior ethmoidal, palpebral, supratrochlear, dorsal nasal; *distribution,* eye, orbit, adjacent facial structures.

**a. ova'rica** [TA], ovarian artery: *origin,* abdominal aorta; *branches,* ureteral, tubal; *distribution,* ureter, ovary, uterine tube. Called also *tubo-ovarian artery* or *aortic uterine artery.*

**a. palati'na ascen'dens** [TA], ascending palatine artery: *origin,* facial artery; *branches,* none; *distribution,* soft palate, wall of pharynx, tonsil, auditory tube.

**a. palati'na descen'dens** [TA], descending palatine artery: *origin,* maxillary artery; *branches,* greater and lesser palatine arteries; *distribution,* soft palate, hard palate, tonsil.

**a. palati'na ma'jor** [TA], greater palatine artery: *origin,* descending palatine; *branches,* none; *distribution,* hard palate.

**arte'riae palati'nae mino'res** [TA], lesser palatine arteries: *origin,* descending palatine; *branches,* none; *distribution,* soft palate, tonsil.

**arte'riae palpebra'les latera'les** [TA], lateral palpebral arteries: *origin,* lacrimal artery; *branches,* none; *distribution,* eyelids, conjunctiva.

**arte'riae palpebra'les media'les** [TA], medial palpebral arteries: *origin,* ophthalmic artery; *branches,* posterior conjunctival; *distribution,* eyelids.

**a. pancrea'tica dorsa'lis** [TA], dorsal pancreatic artery: *origin,* splenic; *branches,* inferior pancreatic; *distribution,* neck and body of pancreas.

**a. pancrea'tica infe'rior** [TA], inferior pancreatic artery: *origin,* dorsal pancreatic; *branches,* none; *distribution,* body and tail of pancreas.

**a. pancrea'tica mag'na** [TA], great pancreatic artery: *origin,* splenic artery; *branches and distribution,* right and left branches anastomose with other pancreatic arteries.

**arte'riae pancreaticoduodena'les infe'riores** [TA], inferior pancreaticoduodenal arteries: *origin,* superior mesenteric artery; *branches,* anterior, posterior; *distribution,* pancreas, duodenum.

**a. pancreaticoduodena'lis supe'rior ante'rior** [TA], anterior superior pancreaticoduodenal artery: *origin,* gastroduodenal artery; *branches,* pancreatic and duodenal; *distribution,* pancreas and duodenum.

**a. pancreaticoduodena'lis supe'rior poste'rior** [TA], posterior superior pancreaticoduodenal artery: *origin,* gastroduodenal artery; *branches,* pancreatic and duodenal; *distribution,* pancreas, duodenum.

**a. paracentra'lis,** paracentral artery: *origin,* postcommunical part of anterior cerebral artery; *branches,* none; *distribution,* cerebral cortex and medial central sulcus.

**arte'riae parieta'les ante'rior et poste'rior** [TA], anterior and posterior parietal arteries: *origin,* terminal part of middle cerebral artery; *branches,* anterior and posterior branches; *distribution,* anterior parietal lobe and posterior temporal lobe.

**arteriae parietooccipita'les,** see *rami parietooccipitalis arteriae cerebri anterioris* and *ramus parietooccipitalis arteriae occipitalis medialis.*

**arte'riae perforan'tes** [TA], perforating arteries: *origin,* branches (usually three) of the deep femoral artery that perforate the insertion of the adductor magnus to reach the back of the thigh; *branches,* nutrient arteries; *distribution,* adductor, hamstring, and gluteal muscles, and femur.

**a. pericallo'sa,** pars postcommunicalis arteriae cerebri anterioris.

**a. pericardiacophre'nica** [TA], pericardiacophrenic artery: *origin,* internal thoracic artery; *branches,* none; *distribution,* pericardium, diaphragm, pleura. Called also *superior phrenic artery.*

**a. perinea'lis** [TA], perineal artery: *origin,* internal pudendal artery; *branches,* none; *distribution,* perineum, skin of external genitalia. Called also *a. perinei.*

**a. perine'i,** a. perinealis.

**arte'riae perirena'les,** arteriae capsulares.

**a. perone'a,** TA alternative for a. fibularis.

**a. pharyn'gea ascen'dens** [TA], ascending pharyngeal artery: *origin,* external carotid; *branches,* posterior meningeal, pharyngeal, and inferior tympanic; *distribution,* pharynx, soft palate, ear, meninges.

**a. phre'nica infe'rior** [TA], inferior phrenic artery: *origin,* abdominal aorta; *branches,* superior suprarenal; *distribution,* diaphragm, suprarenal gland. Called also *great phrenic artery* and *diaphragmatic artery.*

**arte'riae phre'nicae superio'res** [TA], superior phrenic arteries: *origin,* thoracic aorta; *branches,* none; *distribution,* upper surface of vertebral portion of diaphragm. Called also *superior diaphragmatic arteries.*

**a. planta'ris latera'lis** [TA], lateral plantar artery: *origin,* posterior tibial artery; *branches,* plantar arch, and plantar metatarsal arteries; *distribution,* sole of foot and toes. Called also *external plantar artery.*

**a. planta'ris media'lis** [TA], medial plantar artery: *origin,* posterior tibial artery; *branches,* deep and superficial branches; *distribution,* sole of the foot and toes.

**a. planta'ris profun'da** [TA], deep plantar artery: *origin,* dorsal artery of foot; *branches,* none; *distribution,* sole of foot to help form plantar arch. Called also *ramus plantaris profundus arteriae dorsalis pedis.*

**arte'riae pon'tis** [TA], pontine arteries: *origin,* basilar artery; *branches,* none; *distribution,* pons and adjacent areas of brain. Called also *rami ad pontem arteriae basilaris.*

**a. popli'tea** [TA], popliteal artery: *origin,* continuation of femoral artery; *branches,* lateral and medial superior genicular, middle genicular, sural, lateral and medial inferior genicular, anterior and posterior tibial arteries, and the genicular articular and the patellar rete; *distribution,* knee, calf.

**a. precunea'lis,** precuneal artery: *origin,* postcommunical part of the anterior cerebral artery; *branches,* none; *distribution,* inferior precuneus.

**a. prepancrea'tica** [TA], prepancreatic artery: an arterial arch between the neck and uncinate process of the pancreas, formed by the right branch of the dorsal ramus of the splenic artery and a branch from the anterior superior pancreaticoduodenal artery.

**a. prin'ceps pol'licis** [TA], principal artery of thumb: *origin,* radial artery; *branches,* radial of index finger; *distribution,* each side and palmar aspect of thumb.

**a. profun'da bra'chii** [TA], deep brachial artery: *origin,* brachial artery; *branches,* deltoid ramus, nutrient artery, medial and radial collateral arteries; *distribution,* humerus, muscles and skin of arm.

**a. profun'da clito'ridis** [TA], deep artery of clitoris: *origin,* internal pudendal artery; *branches,* none; *distribution,* clitoris.

**a. profun'da fe'moris** [TA], deep femoral artery: *origin,* femoral artery; *branches,* medial and lateral circumflex arteries of thigh, perforating arteries; *distribution,* thigh muscles, hip joint, gluteal muscles, femur.

**a. profun'da lin'guae** [TA], deep lingual artery: *origin,* lingual artery; *branches,* none; *distribution,* tongue. Called also *ranine artery.*

**a. profun'da pe'nis** [TA], deep artery of penis: *origin,* internal pudendal artery; *branches,* none; *distribution,* corpus cavernosum penis.

**a. puden'da exter'na profun'da** [TA], deep external pudendal artery: *origin,* femoral artery; *branches,* anterior scrotal or anterior labial and inguinal branches; *distribution,* external genitalia, upper medial thigh.

**a. puden'da exter'na superficia'lis** [TA], superficial external pudendal artery: *origin,* femoral artery; *branches,* none; *distribution,* external genitalia.

**a. puden'da inter'na** [TA], internal pudendal artery: *origin,* internal iliac artery; *branches,* posterior scrotal or posterior labial branches and inferior rectal, perineal, urethral arteries, artery of bulb of penis or vestibule, deep artery of penis or clitoris, dorsal artery of penis or clitoris; *distribution,* external genitalia, anal canal, perineum.

**a. pulmona'lis,** truncus pulmonalis.

**a. pulmona'lis dex'tra** [TA], right pulmonary artery: *origin,* pulmonary trunk; *branches, of superior lobe:* apical, anterior ascending and descending, posterior ascending and descending, *of medial lobe:* medial and lateral, *of inferior lobe:* anterior basal, lateral basal, medial basal; posterior basal; *distribution,* right lung.

**a. pulmona'lis sinis'tra** [TA], left pulmonary artery: *origin,* pulmonary trunk; *branches, of superior lobe:* apical, ascending and descending, posterior, lingular (inferior and superior), *of inferior lobe:* superior, anterior basal, lateral basal, medial basal, posterior basal; *distribution,* left lung.

**a. radia'lis** [TA], radial artery: *origin,* brachial artery; *branches,* palmar carpal, superficial palmar and dorsal carpal rami, recurrent radial artery, principal artery of thumb, deep palmar arch; *distribution,* forearm, wrist, hand.

**a. radia'lis in'dicis** [TA], radial artery of index finger: *origin,* principal artery of thumb; *branches,* none; *distribution,* index finger. Called also *volar radial artery of index finger.*

**a. recta'lis infe'rior** [TA], inferior rectal artery: *origin,* internal pudendal artery; *branches,* none; *distribution,* rectum, anal canal. Called also *a. haemorrhoidalis inferior* and *inferior hemorrhoidal artery.*

**a. recta'lis me'dia** [TA], middle rectal artery: *origin,* internal iliac artery; *branches,* vaginal; *distribution,* rectum, prostate, seminal vesicles, vagina. Called also *a. haemorrhoidalis media* and *middle hemorrhoidal artery.*

**a. recta'lis supe'rior** [TA], superior rectal artery: *origin,* inferior mesenteric artery; *branches,* none; *distribution,* rectum. Called also *a. haemorrhoidalis superior* and *superior hemorrhoidal artery.*

**a. recur'rens,** a. centralis longa.

**a. recur'rens radia'lis** [TA], radial recurrent artery: *origin,* radial artery; *branches,* none; *distribution,* brachioradialis, brachialis, elbow region.

**a. recur'rens tibia'lis ante'rior** [TA], anterior tibial recurrent artery: *origin,* anterior tibial artery; *branches,* none; *distribution,* tibialis anterior, extensor digitorum longus, knee joint, contiguous fascia and skin.

**a. recur'rens tibia'lis poste'rior** [TA], posterior tibial recurrent artery: *origin,* anterior tibial artery; *branches,* none; *distribution,* knee.

**a. recur'rens ulna'ris** [TA], ulnar recurrent artery: *origin,* ulnar artery; *branches,* anterior and posterior; *distribution,* elbow joint region.

**arte'riae recurren'tes ulna'res,** see *a. recurrens ulnaris.*

**a. rena'lis** [TA], renal artery: *origin,* abdominal aorta; *branches,* ureteral branches, inferior suprarenal artery; *distribution,* kidney, suprarenal gland, ureter.

**arte'riae retroduodena'les** [TA], retroduodenal arteries: *origin,* first branch of gastroduodenal; *branches,* none; *distribution,* bile duct, duodenum, head of pancreas.

**arte'riae sacra'les latera'les** [TA], lateral sacral arteries: *origin,* iliolumbar artery; *branches,* spinal branches; *distribution,* structures about coccyx and sacrum.

**a. sacra'lis media'na** [TA], median sacral artery: *origin,* continuation of abdominal aorta; *branches,* lowest lumbar artery; *distribution,* sacrum, coccyx, rectum. Called also *caudal, coccygeal,* or *sacrococcygeal artery.*

**a. scapula'ris descen'dens,** ramus profundus arteriae transversae cervicis.

**a. scapula'ris dorsa'lis,** 1. a. dorsalis scapulae. 2. ramus profundus arteriae transversae colli.

**arte'riae scrota'les anterio'res,** rami scrotales anteriores arteriae pudendae externae profundae.

**arte'riae scrota'les posterio'res,** rami scrotales posteriores arteriae pudendae internae.

**a. segmenta'lis ante'rior pulmo'nis dex'tri** [TA], anterior segmental artery of right lung: one of the branches of the right pulmonary artery to the superior lobe of the right lung, supplying its anterior segment; it gives rise to ascending and descending branches.

**a. segmenta'lis ante'rior pulmo'nis sinis'tri** [TA], anterior segmental artery of left lung: one of the branches of the left pulmonary artery to the superior lobe of the left lung, supplying its anterior segment; it gives rise to ascending and descending branches.

**a. segmenta'lis apica'lis pulmo'nis dex'tri** [TA], apical segmental artery of right lung: one of the branches to the superior lobe, supplying its apical segment.

**a. segmenta'lis apica'lis pulmo'nis sinis'tri** [TA], apical segmental artery of left lung: one of the branches to the superior lobe, supplying its apical segment.

**a. segmenta'lis basa'lis ante'rior pulmo'nis dex'tri** [TA], anterior basal segmental artery of right lung: one of the branches to the inferior lobe, supplying the anterior basal segment.

**a. segmenta'lis basa'lis ante'rior pulmo'nis sinis'tri** [TA], anterior basal segmental artery of left lung: one of the branches to the inferior lobe, supplying its anterior basal segment.

**a. segmenta'lis basa'lis latera'lis pulmo'nis dex'tri** [TA], lateral basal segmental artery of right lung: one of the branches to the inferior lobe, supplying the lateral basal segment.

**a. segmenta'lis basa'lis latera'lis pulmo'nis sinis'tri** [TA], lateral basal segmental artery of left lung: one of the branches to the inferior lobe, supplying its lateral basal segment.

**a. segmenta'lis basa'lis media'lis pulmo'nis dex'tri** [TA], medial basal segmental artery of right lung: one of the branches to the inferior lobe, supplying the medial basal segment.

**a. segmenta'lis basa'lis media'lis pulmo'nis sinis'tri** [TA], medial basal segmental artery of left lung: one of the branches to the inferior lobe, supplying its medial basal segment.

**a. segmenta'lis basa'lis poste'rior pulmo'nis dex'tri** [TA], posterior basal segmental artery of right lung: one of the branches to the inferior lobe, supplying the posterior basal segment.

**a. segmenta'lis basa'lis poste'rior pulmo'nis sinis'tri** [TA], posterior basal segmental artery of left lung: one of the branches to the inferior lobe, supplying its posterior basal segment.

**a. segmenta'lis latera'lis pulmo'nis dex'tri** [TA], lateral segmental artery of right lung: one of the two branches to the middle lobe, supplying its lateral segment.

**a. segmenta'lis media'lis pulmo'nis dex'tri** [TA], medial segmental artery of right lung: one of the two branches to the middle lobe, supplying its medial segment.

**a. segmenta'lis poste'rior pulmo'nis dex'tri** [TA], posterior segmental artery of right lung: one of the branches of the right pulmonary artery to the superior lobe of the right lung, supplying its posterior segment; it gives rise to ascending and descending branches.

**a. segmenta'lis poste'rior pulmo'nis sinis'tri** [TA], posterior segmental artery of left lung: one of the branches of the left pulmonary artery to the superior lobe of the left lung, supplying its posterior segment; it gives rise to ascending and descending branches.

**a. segmenta'lis supe'rior pulmo'nis dex'tri** [TA], superior segmental artery of right lung: one of the branches of the right pulmonary artery to the inferior lobe, supplying its superior segment.

**a. segmenta'lis supe'rior pulmo'nis sinis'tri** [TA], superior segmental artery of left lung: one of the branches of the left pulmonary artery to the inferior lobe, supplying its superior segment.

**a. segmen'ti anterio'ris hepa'tici** [TA], anterior segmental artery of liver: *origin,* right hepatic; *branches,* none; *distribution,* anterior segment of right lobe of liver.

**a. segmen'ti anterio'ris inferio'ris rena'lis** [TA], anterior inferior segmental artery of kidney: *origin,* anterior branch of renal artery; *branches,* none; *distribution,* anterior inferior segment of kidney.

**a. segmen'ti anterio'ris superio'ris rena'lis** [TA], anterior superior segmental artery of kidney: *origin,* anterior branch of renal artery; *branches,* none; *distribution,* anterior superior segment of kidney.

**a. segmen'ti inferio'ris rena'lis** [TA], inferior segmental artery of kidney: *origin,* anterior branch of renal artery; *branches,* none; *distribution,* inferior segment of kidney.

**a. segmen'ti latera'lis hepa'tici** [TA], lateral segmental artery of liver: *origin,* left branch of common hepatic artery; *branches,* none; *distribution,* lateral segment of left lobe of liver.

**a. segmen'ti media'lis hepa'tici** [TA], medial segmental artery of liver: *origin,* left branch of common hepatic artery; *branches,* none; *distribution,* medial segment of left lobe of liver.

**a. segmen'ti posterio'ris hepa'tici** [TA], posterior segmental artery of liver: *origin,* right hepatic; *branches,* none; *distribution,* posterior segment of right lobe of liver.

**a. segmen'ti posterio'ris rena'lis** [TA], posterior segmental artery of kidney: *origin,* posterior branch of renal artery; *branches,* none; *distribution,* posterior segment of kidney.

**a. segmen'ti superio'ris rena'lis** [TA], superior segmental artery of kidney: *origin,* anterior branch of renal artery; *branches,* none; *distribution,* superior segment of kidney.

**arte'riae sigmoi'deae** [TA], sigmoid arteries: *origin,* inferior mesenteric artery; *branches,* none; *distribution,* sigmoid colon.

**a. sperma'tica exter'na,** a. cremasterica.

**a. sphenopalati'na** [TA], sphenopalatine artery: *origin,* maxillary artery; *branches,* posterior lateral nasal artery and posterior septal rami; *distribution,* structures adjoining nasal cavity, the nasopharynx. Called also *nasopalatine artery.*

**a. spina'lis ante'rior** [TA], anterior spinal artery: *origin,* intracranial part of vertebral artery; *branches,* none; *distribution,* spinal cord.

**a. spina'lis poste'rior** [TA], posterior spinal artery: *origin,* anterior inferior cerebellar artery (usually); *branches,* none; *distribution,* spinal cord.

**a. sple'nica** [TA], splenic artery: *origin,* celiac trunk; *branches,* pancreatic and splenic branches, prepancreatic, left gastro-omental, and short gastric arteries; *distribution,* spleen, pancreas, stomach, greater omentum. Called also *a. lienalis* [TA alternative].

**arte'riae sternocleidomastoi'deae,** see *rami sternocleidomastoidei arteriae occipitalis.*

**a. stylomastoi'dea** [TA], stylomastoid artery: *origin,* posterior auricular; *branches,* mastoid and stapedial rami, posterior tympanic artery; *distribution,* tympanic cavity walls, mastoid cells, stapedius muscle.

**a. subcla'via** [TA], subclavian artery: *origin,* brachiocephalic trunk (right), arch of aorta (left); *branches,* vertebral, internal thoracic arteries, thyrocervical and costocervical trunks; *distribution,* neck, thoracic wall, spinal cord, brain, meninges, upper limb.

**a. subcosta'lis** [TA], subcostal artery: *origin,* thoracic aorta; *branches,* dorsal and spinal branches; *distribution,* upper posterior abdominal wall.

**a. sublingua'lis** [TA], sublingual artery: *origin,* lingual artery; *branches,* none; *distribution,* sublingual gland.

**a. submenta'lis** [TA], submental artery: *origin,* facial artery; *branches,* none; *distribution,* tissues under chin.

**a. subscapula'ris** [TA], subscapular artery: *origin,* axillary artery; *branches,* thoracodorsal and circumflex scapular arteries; *distribution,* scapular and shoulder region.

**a. sul'ci centra'lis** [TA], artery of central sulcus: *origin,* terminal part of middle cerebral artery; *branches,* none: *distribution,* cortex on either side of central sulcus.

**a. sul'ci postcentra'lis** [TA], artery of postcentral sulcus: *origin,* terminal part of middle cerebral artery; *branches,* none; *distribution,* cortex on either side of postcentral sulcus.

**a. sul'ci precentra'lis** [TA], artery of precentral sulcus: *origin,* terminal part of middle cerebral artery; *branches,* none; *distribution,* cortex on either side of precentral sulcus.

**a. supe'rior cerebel'li** [TA], superior artery of cerebellum: *origin,* basilar artery; *branches,* none; *distribution,* upper cerebellum, midbrain, pineal body, choroid plexus of third ventricle. Called also *superior cerebellar artery* and *a. cerebelli superior.*

**a. supe'rior latera'lis ge'nus** [TA], lateral superior artery of knee: *origin,* popliteal artery; *branches,* none; *distribution,* knee joint, femur, patella, contiguous muscles. Called also *lateral superior genicular artery* and *a. genus superior lateralis.*

**a. supe'rior media'lis ge'nus** [TA], medial superior artery of knee: *origin,* popliteal artery; *branches,* none; *distribution,* knee joint, femur, patella, contiguous muscles. Called also *medial superior genicular artery* and *a. genus superior medialis.*

**a. supraduodena'lis** [TA], supraduodenal artery: *origin,* gastroduodenal; *branches,* duodenal; *distribution,* superior first part of duodenum.

**a. supraorbita'lis** [TA], supraorbital artery: *origin,* ophthalmic artery; *branches,* superficial, deep, diploic; *distribution,* forehead, upper muscles of orbit, upper eyelid, frontal sinus.

**a. suprarena'lis infe'rior** [TA], inferior suprarenal artery: *origin,* renal artery; *branches,* none; *distribution,* suprarenal gland. Called also *inferior capsular artery.*

**a. suprarena'lis me'dia** [TA], middle suprarenal artery: *origin,* abdominal aorta; *branches,* none; *distribution,* suprarenal gland. Called also *a. adrenalis media, middle capsular artery,* and *aortic suprarenal artery.*

**arte'riae suprarena'les superio'res** [TA], superior suprarenal arteries: *origin,* inferior phrenic artery; *branches,* none; *distribution,* suprarenal gland.

**a. suprascapula'ris** [TA], suprascapular artery: *origin,* thyrocervical trunk; *branches,* acromial branch; *distribution,* clavicular, deltoid, and scapular regions. Called also *a. transversa scapulae* and *transverse scapular artery.*

**a. supratrochlea'ris** [TA], supratrochlear artery: *origin,* ophthalmic artery; *branches,* none; *distribution,* anterior scalp. Called also *a. frontalis* and *frontal artery.*

**arte'riae sura'les** [TA], sural arteries: *origin,* popliteal artery; *branches,* none; *distribution,* popliteal space, calf.

**a. tarsa'lis latera'lis** [TA], lateral tarsal artery: *origin,* dorsal artery of foot; *branches,* none; *distribution,* tarsus. Called also *a. tarsea lateralis.*

**arte'riae tarsa'les media'les** [TA], medial tarsal arteries: *origin,* dorsal artery of foot; *branches,* none; *distribution,* side of foot. Called also *arteriae tarseae mediales.*

**a. tar'sea latera'lis,** a. tarsalis lateralis.

**arte'riae tar'seae media'les,** arteriae tarsales mediales.

**a. tempora'lis ante'rior** [TA], anterior temporal artery: *origin,* insular part of middle cerebral artery; *branches,* none; *distribution,* cortex of anterior temporal lobe.

**a. tempora'lis me'dia** [TA], 1. middle temporal artery: *origin,* superficial temporal artery; *branches,* none; *distribution* temporal region. 2. intermediate temporal artery: *origin,* insular part of middle cerebral artery; *branches,* none; *distribution,* cortex of temporal lobe between anterior and posterior arteries. Called also *middle temporal artery.*

**a. tempora'lis poste'rior,** posterior temporal artery: *origin,* insular part of middle cerebral artery; *branches,* none; *distribution,* cortex of posterior temporal lobe.

**a. tempora'lis profun'da ante'rior** [TA], anterior deep temporal artery: *origin,* maxillary artery; *branches,* to zygomatic bone and greater wing of sphenoid bone; *distribution,* temporal muscle, and anastomoses with middle temporal artery.

**a. tempora'lis profun'da poste'rior** [TA], posterior deep temporal artery: *origin,* maxillary artery; *branches,* none; *distribution,* temporal muscle, and anastomoses with middle temporal artery.

**a. tempora'lis superficia'lis** [TA], superficial temporal artery: *origin,* external carotid; *branches,* parotid, auricular, and occipital rami, transverse facial, zygomatico-orbital, and middle temporal arteries; *distribution,* parotid and temporal regions.

**a. testicula'ris** [TA], testicular artery: *origin,* abdominal aorta; *branches,* ureteral, epididymal; *distribution,* ureter, epididymis, testis. Called also *funicular artery.*

**arte'riae thalamostria'tae anterolatera'les,** arteriae centrales anterolaterales arteriae cerebri anterioris.

**arte'riae thalamostria'tae anteromedia'les,** arteriae centrales anteromediales.

**a. thora'cica inter'na** [TA], internal thoracic artery: *origin,* subclavian artery; *branches,* mediastinal, thymic, bronchial, tracheal, sternal, perforating, medial mammary, lateral costal, and anterior intercostal branches, pericardiacophrenic, musculophrenic, and superior epigastric arteries; *distribution,* anterior thoracic wall, mediastinal structures, diaphragm. Called also *a. mammaria interna* and *internal mammary artery.*

**a. thora'cica latera'lis** [TA], lateral thoracic artery: *origin,* axillary artery; *branches,* mammary branches; *distribution,* pectoral muscles, mammary gland. Called also *external mammary artery.*

**a. thora'cica supe'rior** [TA], superior thoracic artery: *origin,* axillary artery; *branches,* none; *distribution,* axillary aspect of chest wall. Called also *a. thoracica suprema* and *highest thoracic artery.*

**a. thora'cica supre'ma,** a. thoracica superior.

**a. thoracoacromia'lis** [TA], thoracoacromial artery: *origin,* axillary artery; *branches,* clavicular, pectoral, deltoid, acromial rami; *distribution,* deltoid, clavicular, and thoracic regions. Called also *acromiothoracic artery, thoracicoacromial artery,* and *thoracic axis.*

**a. thoracodorsa'lis** [TA], thoracodorsal artery: *origin,* subscapular artery; *branches,* none; *distribution,* subscapular and teretes muscles.

**arte'riae thy'micae,** rami thymici arteriae thoracicae internae.

**a. thyroi'dea i'ma** [TA], lowest thyroid artery: *origin,* arch of aorta, brachiocephalic trunk or right common carotid; *branches,* none; *distribution,* thyroid gland. Called also *Neubauer's artery.*

**a. thyroi'dea infe'rior** [TA], inferior thyroid artery: *origin,* thyrocervical trunk; *branches,* pharyngeal, esophageal, and tracheal rami, inferior laryngeal and ascending cervical arteries; *distribution,* thyroid gland and adjacent structures.

**a. thyroi'dea supe'rior** [TA], superior thyroid artery: *origin,* external carotid artery; *branches,* hyoid, sternocleidomastoid, superior laryngeal, cricothyroid, muscular, and anterior, posterior, and lateral glandular branches; *distribution,* thyroid gland and adjacent structures.

**a. tibia'lis ante'rior** [TA], anterior tibial artery: *origin,* popliteal artery; *branches,* posterior and anterior tibial recurrent, and lateral and medial anterior malleolar arteries, lateral and medial malleolar retes; *distribution,* leg, ankle, foot.

**a. tibia'lis poste'rior** [TA], posterior tibial artery: *origin,* popliteal artery; *branches,* fibular circumflex branch, peroneal, medial plantar, and lateral plantar arteries; *distribution,* leg, foot.

**a. transver'sa cer'vicis** [TA], transverse artery of neck: *origin,* subclavian artery; *branches,* deep and superficial rami; *distribution,* root of neck, muscles of scapula. Called also *transverse cervical artery* and *a. transversa colli* [TA alternative].

**a. transver'sa col'li,** TA alternative for *a. transversa cervicis.*

**a. transver'sa facia'lis,** a. transversa faciei.

**a. transver'sa facie'i** [TA], transverse facial artery: *origin,* superficial temporal artery; *branches,* none; *distribution,* parotid region.

**a. transver'sa sca'pulae,** a. suprascapularis.

**a. tympa'nica ante'rior** [TA], anterior tympanic artery: *origin,* maxillary artery; *branches,* none; *distribution,* tympanic cavity.

**a. tympa'nica infe'rior** [TA], inferior tympanic artery: *origin,* ascending pharyngeal; *branches,* none; *distribution,* tympanic cavity.

**a. tympa'nica poste'rior** [TA], posterior tympanic artery: *origin,* stylomastoid artery; *branches,* none; *distribution,* tympanic cavity.

**a. tympa'nica supe'rior** [TA], superior tympanic artery: *origin,* middle meningeal artery; *branches,* none; *distribution,* tympanic cavity.

**a. ulna'ris** [TA], ulnar artery: *origin,* brachial artery; *branches,* palmar carpal, dorsal carpal, and deep palmar rami, ulnar recurrent and common interosseous arteries, superficial palmar arch; *distribution,* forearm, wrist, hand.

**a. umbilica'lis** [TA], umbilical artery: *origin,* internal iliac artery; *branches,* deferential, superior vesical arteries; *distribution,* ductus deferens, seminal vesicles, testes, urinary bladder, ureter.

**a. urethra'lis** [TA], urethral artery: *origin,* internal pudendal artery; *branches,* none; *distribution,* urethra.

**a. uteri'na** [TA], uterine artery: *origin,* internal iliac artery; *branches,* ovarian and tubal rami, vaginal artery; *distribution,* uterus, vagina, round ligament of uterus, uterine tube, ovary. Called also *fallopian artery.*

**a. vagina'lis** [TA], vaginal artery: *origin,* uterine artery; *branches,* none; *distribution,* vagina, fundus of bladder.

**a. vertebra'lis** [TA], vertebral artery: divided into four parts: the *first* or *prevertebral part (pars prevertebralis),* the *second* or *atlantal part (pars atlantica),* the *third* or *transverse part (pars transversaria),* and the *fourth* or *intracranial part (pars intracranialis); origin,* subclavian artery; *branches, transverse part:* spinal and muscular rami; *intracranial part:* anterior spinal artery and posterior inferior cerebellar artery and its branches; *distribution,* muscles of neck, vertebrae, spinal cord, cerebellum, interior of cerebrum.

**a. vesica'lis infe'rior** [TA], inferior vesical artery: *origin,* internal iliac; *branches,* prostatic; *distribution,* bladder, prostate, seminal vesicles, lower ureter.

**arte'riae vesica'les superio'res** [TA], superior vesical arteries: *origin,* umbilical artery; *branches,* none; *distribution,* bladder, urachus, ureter.

**a. zygomaticoorbita'lis** [TA], zygomatico-orbital artery: *origin,* superficial temporal; *branches,* none; *distribution,* lateral side of orbit.

---

**ar•te•ri•ae** (ahr-te're-e) [L.] plural of *arteria.*

**ar•te•ri•al** (ahr-tēr'e-əl) pertaining to an artery or to the arteries.

**ar•te•ri•al•i•za•tion** (ahr-te"re-əl-ĭ-za'shən) surgical alteration of a vein so that it functions as an artery.

**ar•te•ri•ec•ta•sia** (ahr"tə-re-ek-ta'zhə) arteriectasis.

**ar•te•ri•ec•ta•sis** (ahr-tēr"e-ek'tə-sis) [*arteri-* + *ectasis*] dilatation and, usually, lengthening of an artery.

**ar•te•ri•ec•to•my** (ahr-tēr"e-ek'tə-me) [*arteri-* + *-ectomy*] excision of a portion of an artery.

**ar•te•ri•ec•to•pia** (ahr-tēr"e-ek-to'pe-ə) [*arteri-* + *ectopia*] displacement of an artery from its normal location.

**arteri(o)-** [L. *arteria,* q.v.] a combining form denoting relationship to an artery or arteries.

**ar•te•rio•cap•il•lary** (ahr-tēr"e-o-kap'ĭ-lar"e) pertaining to the arteries and the capillaries.

**ar•te•rio•di•lat•ing** (ahr-tēr"e-o-di'lāt-ing) increasing the caliber of the arteries, particularly of arterioles.

**ar•te•rio•gen•e•sis** (ahr-tēr"e-o-jen'ə-sis) the formation of arteries. Cf. *vascularization.*

**ar•te•rio•gram** (ahr-tēr'e-o-gram) [*arterio-* + *-gram*] a radiograph of an artery taken during arteriography.

**ar•te•rio•graph** (ahr-tēr'e-o-graf) a film produced by arteriography.

**ar•te•ri•og•ra•phy** (ahr"tēr-e-og'rə-fe) [*arterio-* + *-graphy*] angiography of arteries.

**catheter a.,** radiography of vessels after introduction of contrast material through a catheter inserted into an artery.

**coronary a.,** angiography of the coronary arteries, in which a cardiac catheter is inserted into an artery, usually the femoral or brachial artery, advanced under fluoroscopic guidance, and used to inject contrast medium directly into the coronary orifices. It is most often used in evaluations of patients with angina pectoris, prior to coronary artery surgery or percutaneous transluminal coronary angioplasty.

**selective a.,** radiography of a specific vessel which is opacified by a medium introduced directly into it, usually via a catheter.

**ar•te•ri•o•la** (ahr-tēr"e-o'lə) pl. *arterio'lae* [L., dim. of *arteria*] [TA] arteriole: a minute arterial branch, especially one just proximal to a capillary.

**a. glomerula'ris af'ferens** [TA], afferent glomerular arteriole: a branch of an interlobular artery that goes to a renal glomerulus; called also *afferent artery of glomerulus, afferent vessel of glomerulus,* and *vas afferens glomeruli.*

**a. glomerula'ris ef'ferens** [TA], efferent glomerular arteriole: an arteriole that arises from a renal glomerulus and breaks up into capillaries to supply renal tubules. Called also *efferent artery of glomerulus, efferent vessel of glomerulus,* and *vas efferens glomeruli.*

**a. macula'ris infe'rior** [TA], inferior macular arteriole: the inferior arteriole supplying the macula retinae.

**a. macula'ris me'dia** [TA], medial arteriole of retina: the small branch supplying blood to the central region of the retina.

**a. macula'ris supe'rior** [TA], superior macular arteriole: the superior arteriole supplying the macula retinae.

**a. nasa'lis re'tinae infe'rior** [TA], inferior nasal arteriole of retina: a small branch of the central artery of the retina supplying the inferior nasal region of the retina.

**a. nasa'lis re'tinae supe'rior** [TA], superior nasal arteriole of retina: a small branch of the central artery of the retina, supplying the superior nasal region of the retina.

**arterio'lae rec'tae re'nis** [TA], straight arterioles of kidney: branches of the arcuate arteries of the kidney arising from the efferent glomerular arterioles, and passing down to the renal pyramids; called also *straight arteries of kidney* and *vasa recta renis* [TA alternative]. Also sometimes called *arteriolae rectae spuriae* or *false straight arterioles of the kidney* to distinguish them from straight direct branches from the arcuate and interlobular arteries that are called *arteriolae rectae verae* or *true straight arterioles of the kidney.*

**arterio'lae rec'tae spu'riae,** see *arteriolae rectae renis.*

**arterio'lae rec'tae ve'rae,** see *arteriolae rectae renis.*

**a. tempora'lis re'tinae infe'rior** [TA], inferior temporal arteriole of retina: a branch of the central artery of the retina, supplying the inferior temporal region of the retina.

**a. tempora'lis re'tinae supe'rior** [TA], superior temporal arteriole of retina: a branch of the central artery of the retina, supplying the superior temporal region of the retina.

**ar•te•ri•o•lae** (ahr-tēr"e-o'le) [L.] genitive and plural of *arteriola.*

**ar•te•ri•o•lar** (ahr-tēr"e-o'lər) pertaining to or resembling arterioles.

**ar•te•ri•ole** (ahr-tēr'e-ōl) [L. *arteriola*] [MeSH: Arterioles] arteriola.

**afferent glomerular a.,** arteriola glomerularis afferens.

**efferent glomerular a.,** arteriola glomerularis efferens.

**ellipsoid a's,** sheathed arteries.

**Isaacs-Ludwig a.,** an arteriolar twig that sometimes branches from the afferent glomerular arteriole of the kidney to communicate directly with the tubular capillary plexus.

**macular a., inferior,** arteriola macularis inferior.

**macular a., superior,** arteriola macularis superior.

**medial a. of retina,** arteriola medialis retinae.

**nasal a. of retina, inferior,** arteriola nasalis retinae inferior.

**nasal a. of retina, superior,** arteriola nasalis retinae superior.

**postglomerular a.,** efferent glomerular a.

**precapillary a.,** arterial capillaries.

**preglomerular a.,** afferent glomerular a.

**sheathed a's,** see under *artery.*

**straight a's of kidney,** arteriolae rectae renis.

**straight a's of kidney, false,** see *arteriolae rectae renis.*

**straight a's of kidney, true,** see *arteriolae rectae renis.*

**temporal a. of retina, inferior,** arteriola temporalis retinae inferior.

**temporal a. of retina, superior,** arteriola temporalis retinae superior.

**ar•te•rio•lith** (ahr-tēr'e-o-lith") [*arterio-* + *-lith*] a chalky concretion in an artery.

**ar•te•rio•li•tis** (ahr-tēr"e-o-li'tis) inflammation of the arterioles.

**hyperplastic a.,** onionskin lesion.

**necrotizing a.,** fibrinoid necrosis.

**arteriol(o)-** [L. *arteriola,* dim. of *arteria* artery] a combining form denoting relationship to one or more arterioles.

**ar•te•ri•ol•o•gy** (ahr-tēr"e-ol'ə-je) [*arterio-* + *-logy*] the sum of what is known regarding the arteries; the science or study of the arteries.

**ar•te•rio•lo•ne•cro•sis** (ahr-tēr"e-o"lo-nə-kro'sis) necrosis of arterioles, as may be seen in nephrosclerosis; called also *arteriolar necrosis.*

**ar•te•ri•o•lop•a•thy** (ahr-tēr"e-o-lop'ə-the) any disease of the arterioles.

**ar•te•rio•lo•scle•ro•sis** (ahr-tēr"e-o"lo-sklə-ro'sis) sclerosis and thickening of the walls of the smaller arteries (arterioles). *Hyaline arteriolosclerosis,* in which there is homogeneous pink hyaline thickening of the arteriolar walls, is associated with benign nephrosclerosis. *Hyperplastic arteriolosclerosis,* in which there is a concentric thickening with progressive narrowing of the lumina, may be associated with malignant hypertension, nephrosclerosis, and scleroderma.

**hyaline a.,** a variety with homogeneous pink hyaline thickening of vessel walls, associated with benign nephrosclerosis.

**hyperplastic a.,** a variety characterized by concentrated thickening with progressive narrowing of the lumina, sometimes associated with malignant hypertension, nephrosclerosis, and scleroderma.

**ar•te•rio•lo•scle•rot•ic** (ahr-tēr"e-o"lo-sklə-rot'ik) pertaining to or characterized by arteriolosclerosis.

**ar•te•rio•mo•tor** (ahr-tēr"e-o-mo'tər) pertaining to or causing change in the caliber of an artery.

**ar·te·rio·ne·cro·sis** (ahr-tēr″e-o-nə-kro′sis) necrosis of an artery or of arteries.

**ar·te·ri·op·a·thy** (ahr-tēr″e-op′ə-the) [*arterio-* + *-pathy*] any arterial disease.
**cyclosporine-associated a.**, a manifestation of chronic cyclosporine-induced nephrotoxicity, consisting of hyaline degeneration of the tunica media and mucoid thickening of the intima of the arterioles of the peripheral vascular tree.
**hypertensive a.**, widespread involvement, chiefly of arterioles and small arteries, associated with arterial hypertension and characterized primarily by hypertrophy and thickening of the media.
**plexogenic a., plexogenic pulmonary a.**, hypertrophy of arterial walls in part of the pulmonary vasculature, which may become obstructed, leading to plexiform thin-walled vessels distally; seen in some cases of pulmonary hypertension. Cf. *Ayerza's syndrome.*

**ar·te·rio·plas·ty** (ahr-tēr″e-o-plas′te) [*arterio-* + *-plasty*] surgical repair or reconstruction of an artery.

**ar·te·rio·pres·sor** (ahr-tēr″e-o-pres′ər) hypertensive (def. 2).

**ar·te·rio·re·nal** (ahr-tēr″e-o-re′nəl) pertaining to the arteries of the kidney.

**ar·te·ri·or·rha·phy** (ahr-tēr″e-or′ə-fe) [*arterio-* + *-rrhaphy*] suture of an artery.

**ar·te·ri·or·rhex·is** (ahr-tēr″e-o-rek′sis) [*arterio-* + *-rrhexis*] rupture of an artery.

**ar·te·rio·scle·ro·sis** (ahr-tēr″e-o-sklə-ro′sis) [*arterio-* + *sclerosis*] [MeSH: Arteriosclerosis] any of a group of diseases characterized by thickening and loss of elasticity of arterial walls; there are three distinct forms: *atherosclerosis, Mönckeberg's a.,* and *arteriolosclerosis.* Called also *arterial sclerosis* and *vascular sclerosis.*
**cerebral a.**, arteriosclerosis of the arteries of the brain.
**coronary a.**, arteriosclerosis or atherosclerosis of the coronary arteries.
**hyaline a.**, a homogeneous hyaline thickening of the walls of arterioles with consequent narrowing of the lumina.
**hypertensive a.**, arteriosclerosis intensified by hypertension.
**infantile a.**, see *infantile arteritis,* under *arteritis.*
**intimal a.**, arteriosclerosis in which the major changes affect the intima of the arteries.
**medial a.**, 1. a condition of large and medium-sized arteries, with primary destruction of the muscle and elastic fibers of the medial coat, which are replaced by fibrous tissue; when there are deposits of calcium it is called *Mönckeberg's arteriosclerosis.* 2. Mönckeberg's a.
**Mönckeberg's a.**, medial arteriosclerosis with extensive deposits of calcium in the media of the artery; called also *Mönckeberg's calcification, degeneration, mesarteritis,* or *sclerosis; medial a.;* and *medial calcific sclerosis.*
**a. obli′terans**, arteriosclerosis in which proliferation of the intima of small vessels has caused obliteration of the lumen. See also *endarteritis obliterans.*
**peripheral a.**, arteriosclerosis of the extremities.
**presenile a.**, a type of unknown cause occurring at an unusually early age.
**senile a.**, arteriosclerosis occurring in old age.

**ar·te·rio·scle·rot·ic** (ahr-tēr″e-o-sklə-rot′ik) pertaining to or affected with arteriosclerosis.

**ar·te·rio·spasm** (ahr-tēr′e-o-spaz″əm) spasm of an artery.

**ar·te·rio·spas·tic** (ahr-ter″e-o-spas′tik) pertaining to, characterized by, or causing arteriospasm.

**ar·te·rio·ste·no·sis** (ahr-tēr″e-o-stə-no′sis) [*arterio-* + *stenosis*] the narrowing or diminution of the caliber of an artery.

**ar·te·ri·os·teo·gen·e·sis** (ahr-tēr″e-os′te-o-jen′ə-sis) [*arteri-* + *osteogenesis*] calcification of an artery.

**ar·te·ri·os·to·sis** (ahr-tēr″e-os-to′sis) [*arteri-* + *ostosis*] arteriosteogenesis.

**ar·te·ri·ot·o·my** (ahr-tēr″e-ot′ə-me) [*arterio-* + *-tomy*] incision of an artery.

**ar·te·ri·ot·o·ny** (ahr-tēr″e-ot′ə-ne) [*artery* + *-tony*] blood pressure.

**ar·te·rio·ve·nous** (ahr-tēr″e-o-ve′nəs) both arterial and venous; pertaining to or affecting an artery and a vein.

**ar·te·rit·i·des** (ahr″tə-rit′ĭ-dēz) [MeSH: Arteritis] plural of *arteritis.*

**ar·te·ri·tis** (ahr″tə-ri′tis) pl. *arterit′ides* [*arteri-* + *-itis*] [MeSH: Arteritis] inflammation of an artery.
**aortic arch a.**, Takayasu's a.
**brachiocephalic a., a. brachiocepha′lica,** Takayasu's a.
**coronary a.**, inflammation of the coronary arteries.
**cranial a.**, temporal a.
**equine viral a.**, a frequently fatal disease of horses, caused by the equine arteritis virus, affecting especially the smaller arteries, with hemorrhagic enteritis, abdominal pain and diarrhea, and pulmonary edema. Abortion is common in affected mares.
**giant cell a.**, a chronic vascular disease of unknown origin in the elderly, often associated with polymyalgia rheumatica, seen usually in the external carotid arteries but sometimes in other arteries. Characteristics include proliferative inflammation, often with giant cells and granulomas; headache, pain with chewing, weight loss, fever, and sometimes ocular symptoms; and increased erythrocyte sedimentation rate. Called also *cranial, granulomatous,* or *temporal a.* and *Horton's a., disease,* or *syndrome.*
**granulomatous a., Horton's a.**, giant cell a.
**infantile a.**, diffuse arteritis in infants and children, rarely with atherosclerotic processes.
**infectious a.**, arteritis secondary to an infectious disorder, caused by direct invasion by or, less commonly, hematogenous spread of infectious organisms.
**localized visceral a.**, hypersensitivity vasculitis.
**necrotizing a.**, polyarteritis nodosa
**a. obli′terans**, endarteritis obliterans.
**rheumatic a.**, generalized inflammation of arterioles and arterial capillaries occurring in rheumatic fever.
**syphilitic a.**, a late manifestation of syphilis characterized by intimal proliferation and degeneration of the medial coat, usually involving the ascending aorta, aortic arch, and pulmonary artery, which may lead to aneurysm.
**Takayasu's a.**, progressive obliteration of the brachiocephalic trunk and the subclavian and common carotid arteries above their origin in the aortic arch, leading to loss of pulse in both arms and carotids. This may be followed by symptoms associated with ischemia of the brain (such as syncope or transient hemiplegia), of the eyes (such as transient blindness or retinal atrophy), of the face (such as muscular atrophy), of the arms (such as claudication), or of the kidneys. Called also *aortic arch a., brachiocephalic a.* or *ischemia, Martorell's syndrome, pulseless disease, reversed coarctation,* and *Takayasu's disease* or *syndrome.*
**temporal a.**, giant cell a.
**tuberculous a.**, endarteritis obliterans in those arteries intimately involved in a tubercular focus.
**a. umbilica′lis**, septic inflammation of the umbilical artery in newborn infants.
**verminous mesenteric a.**, verminous aneurysm.

**Ar·te·ri·vi·ri·dae** (ahr-tēr″ĭ-vir′ĭ-de) the arteriviruses; a family of RNA viruses having a virion 60 nm in diameter consisting of a lipid envelope with 12–15 ringlike surface structures surrounding an isometric nucleocapsid about 35 nm in diameter. The genome consists of a single molecule of linear positive-sense RNA (size about 13 kb). Viruses contain at least four major structural proteins. Replication is similar to that of the Coronaviridae. Host range is narrow and transmission is horizontal. There is a single genus, *Arterivirus.*

**Ar·te·ri·vi·rus** (ahr-tēr′ĭ-vi″rəs) [*arteritis* + *virus*] [MeSH: Arterivirus] a genus of viruses of the family Arteriviridae. Species include equine arteritis virus and swine infertility and respiratory syndrome virus.

**ar·te·ri·vi·rus** (ahr-tēr′ĭ-vi″rəs) [MeSH: Arterivirus] any virus belonging to the family Arteriviridae.

**ar·te·ry** (ahr′tər-e) [Gr. *artēria* q.v.] [MeSH: Arteries] a vessel through which the blood passes away from the heart to the various parts of the body. The wall of an artery consists typically of an outer coat (tunica externa), a middle coat (tunica media), and an inner coat (tunica intima). Called also *arteria* [TA].

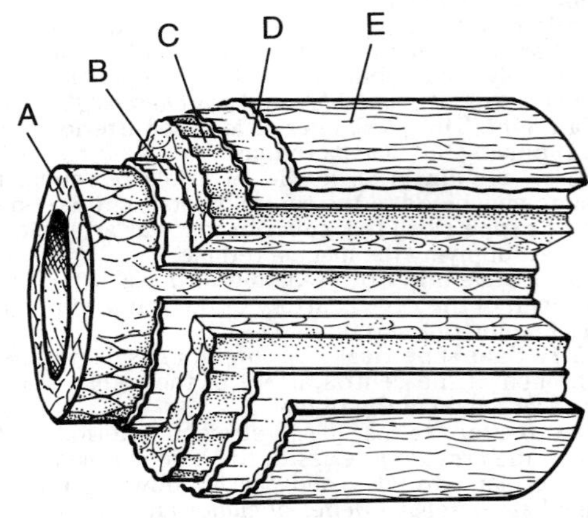

Representation of arterial coats: *(A),* tunica intima; *(B),* internal elastic lamina; *(C),* tunica media; *(D),* external elastic lamina; *(E),* tunica externa.

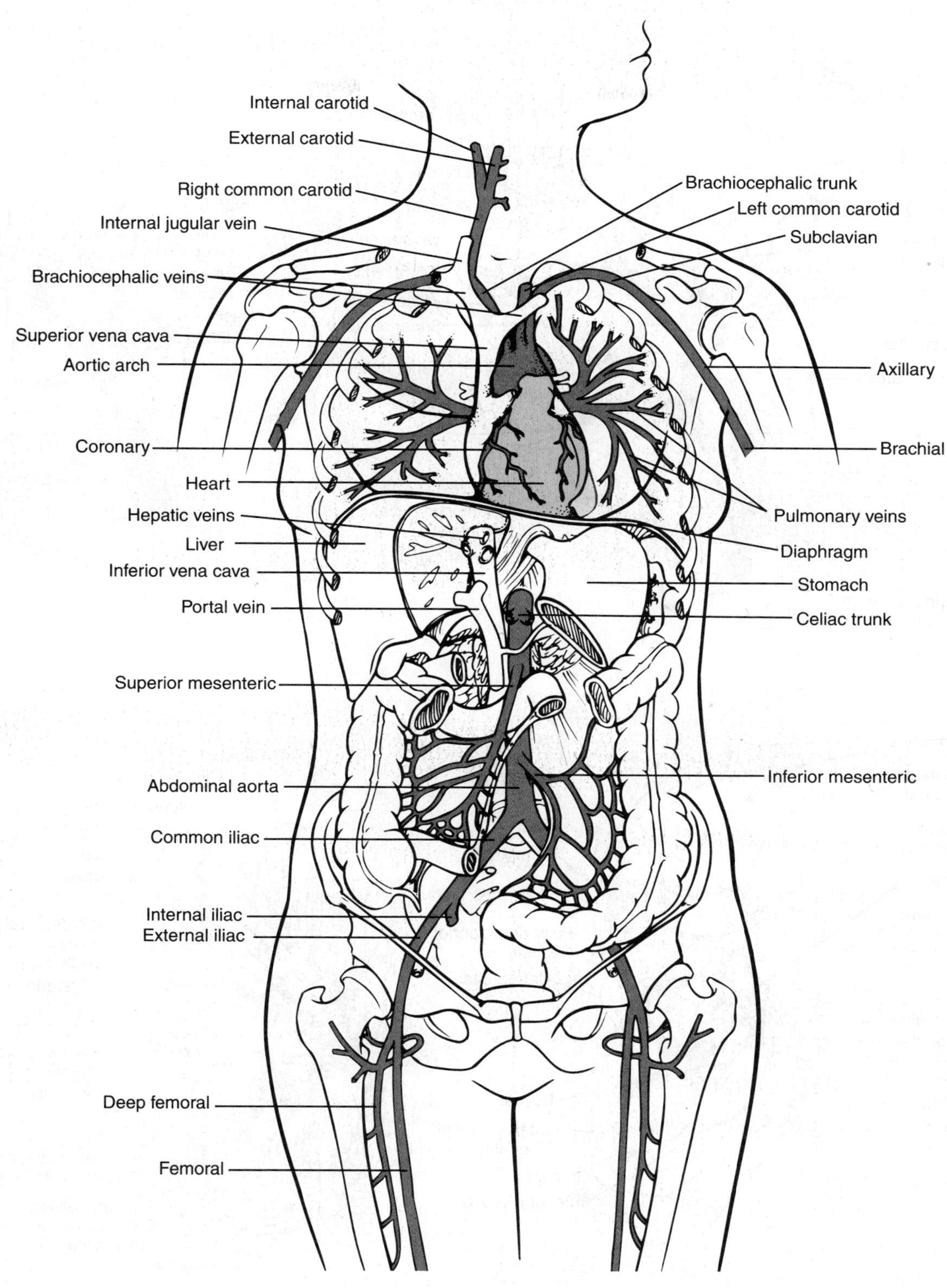


**PLATE 2**—PRINCIPAL ARTERIES OF THE BODY AND THE PULMONARY VEINS

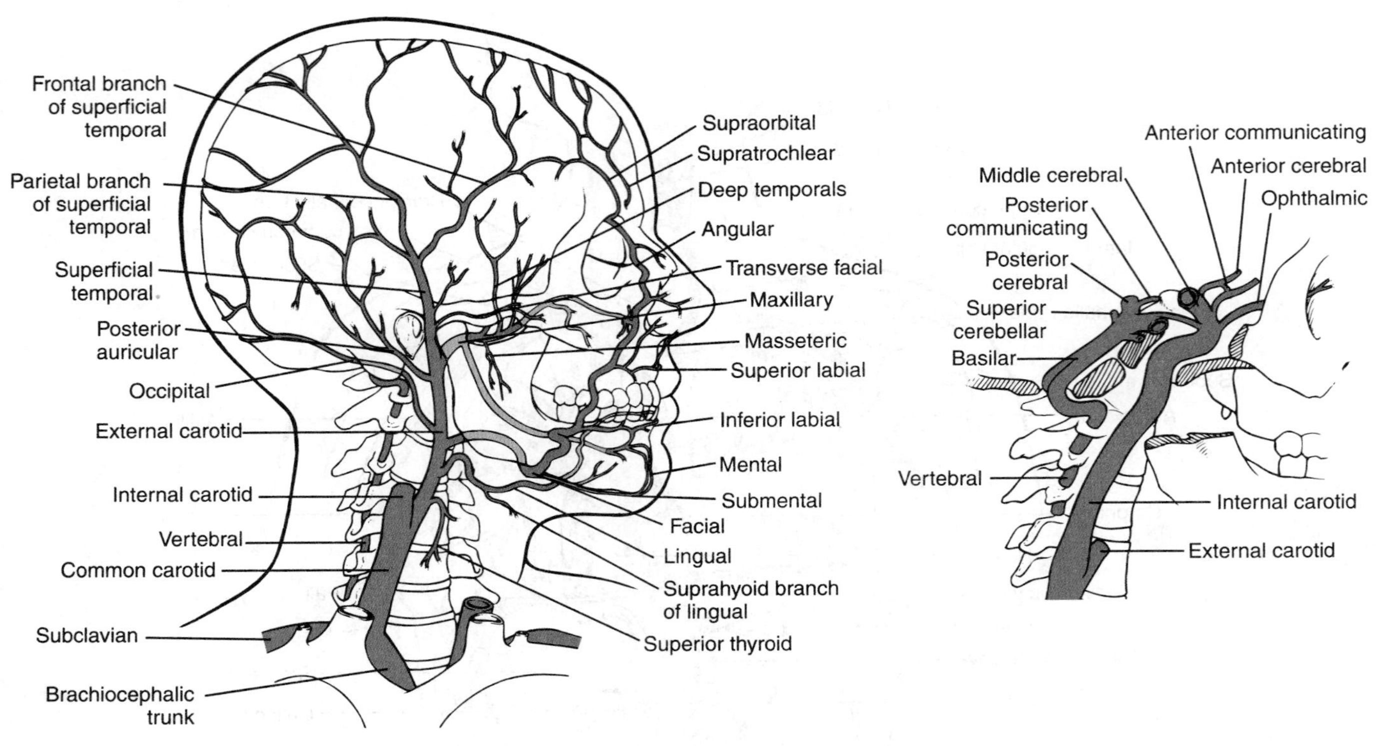


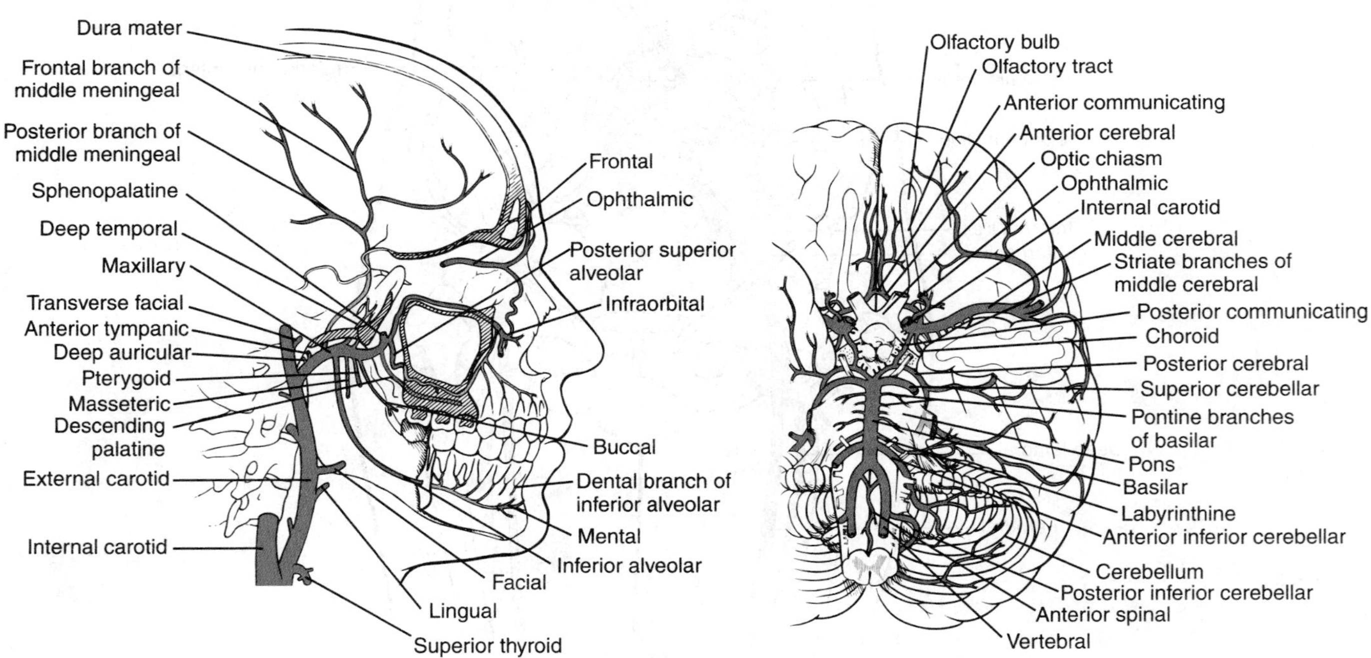


**PLATE 3**—ARTERIES OF THE HEAD, NECK, AND BASE OF THE BRAIN

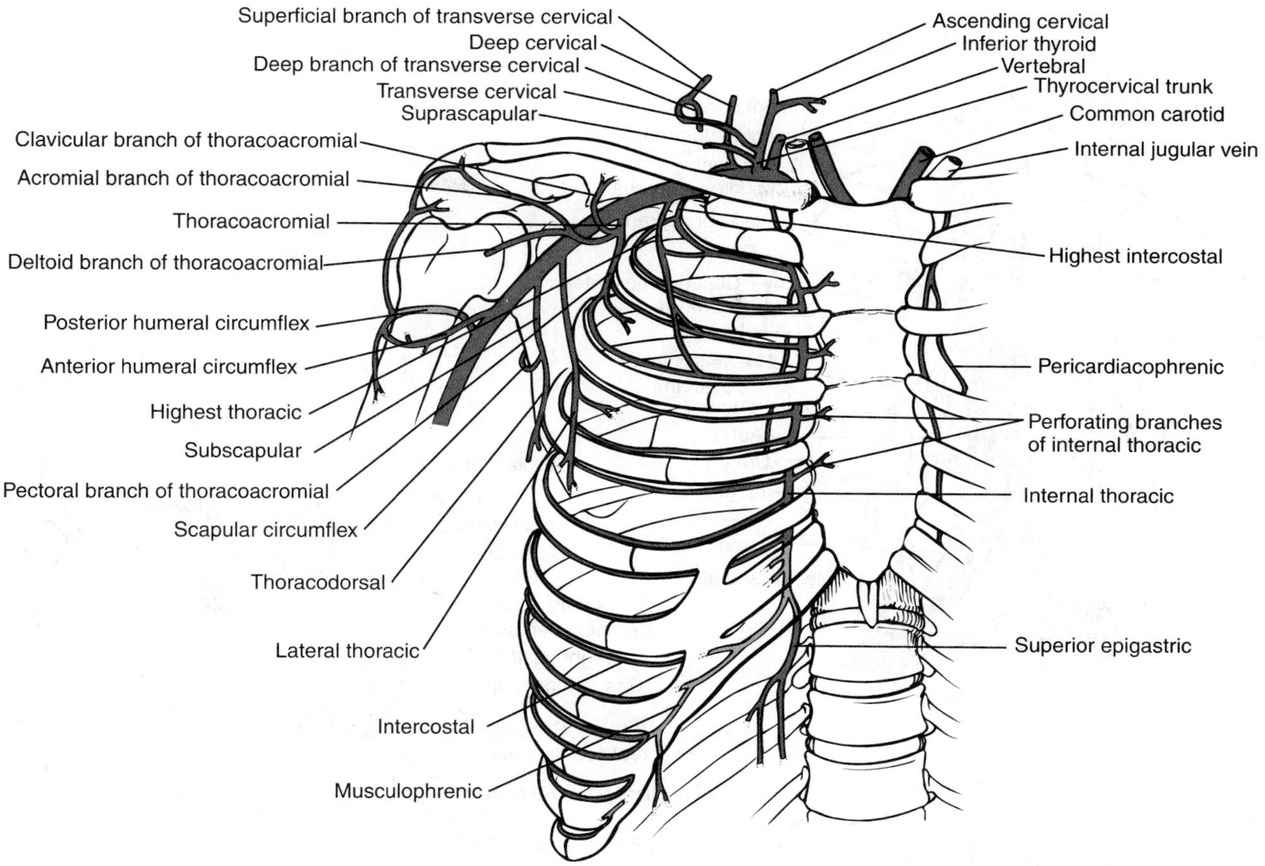

Superficial branch of transverse cervical
Deep cervical
Deep branch of transverse cervical
Transverse cervical
Suprascapular
Clavicular branch of thoracoacromial
Acromial branch of thoracoacromial
Thoracoacromial
Deltoid branch of thoracoacromial
Posterior humeral circumflex
Anterior humeral circumflex
Highest thoracic
Subscapular
Pectoral branch of thoracoacromial
Scapular circumflex
Thoracodorsal
Lateral thoracic
Intercostal
Musculophrenic
Ascending cervical
Inferior thyroid
Vertebral
Thyrocervical trunk
Common carotid
Internal jugular vein
Highest intercostal
Pericardiacophrenic
Perforating branches of internal thoracic
Internal thoracic
Superior epigastric

Ascending cervical
Inferior thyroid
Thyrocervical trunk
Vertebral
Common carotids
Internal jugular vein
Subclavian
Brachiocephalic
Internal thoracic
Brachiocephalic veins
Superior vena cava
Pulmonary
Right coronary
Left coronary
Heart
Aorta
Inferior vena cava
Deep cervical
Suprascapular
Transverse cervical
Deep branch of transverse cervical
Subclavian
Highest intercostal
Thoracoacromial
Highest thoracic
Lateral thoracic
Axillary
Subscapular
Anterior circumflex humeral
Posterior circumflex humeral
Scapular circumflex
Brachial
Intercostal

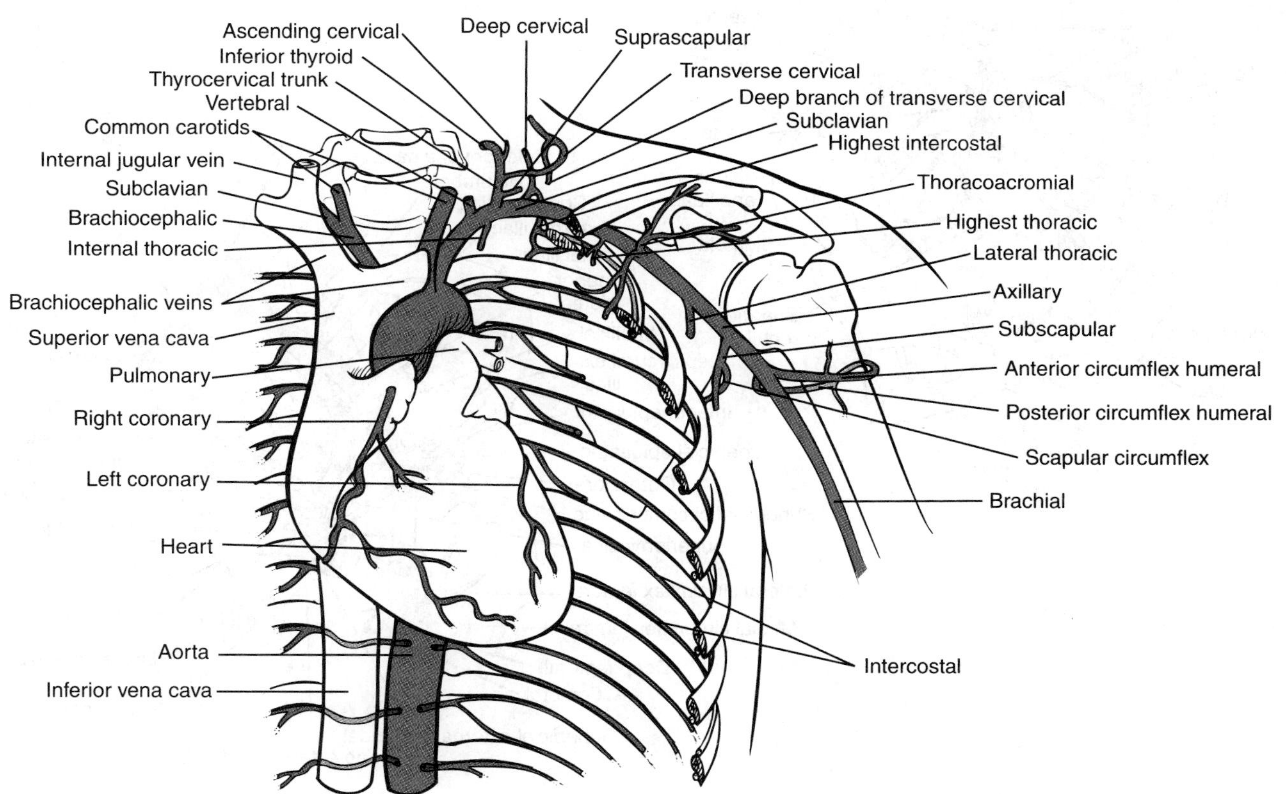

**PLATE 4—**ARTERIES OF THE THORAX AND AXILLA

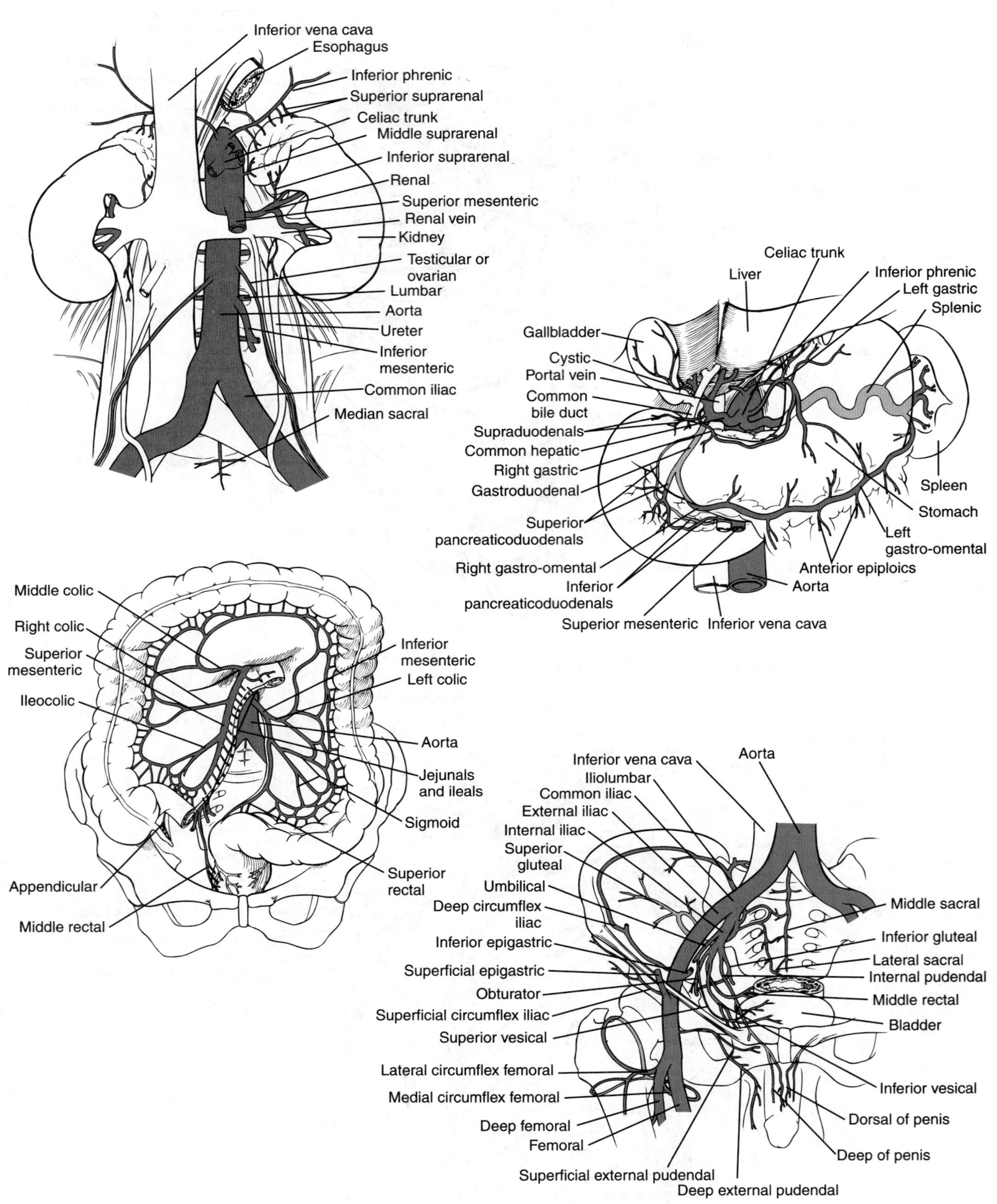


**PLATE 5**—ARTERIES OF THE ABDOMEN AND PELVIS

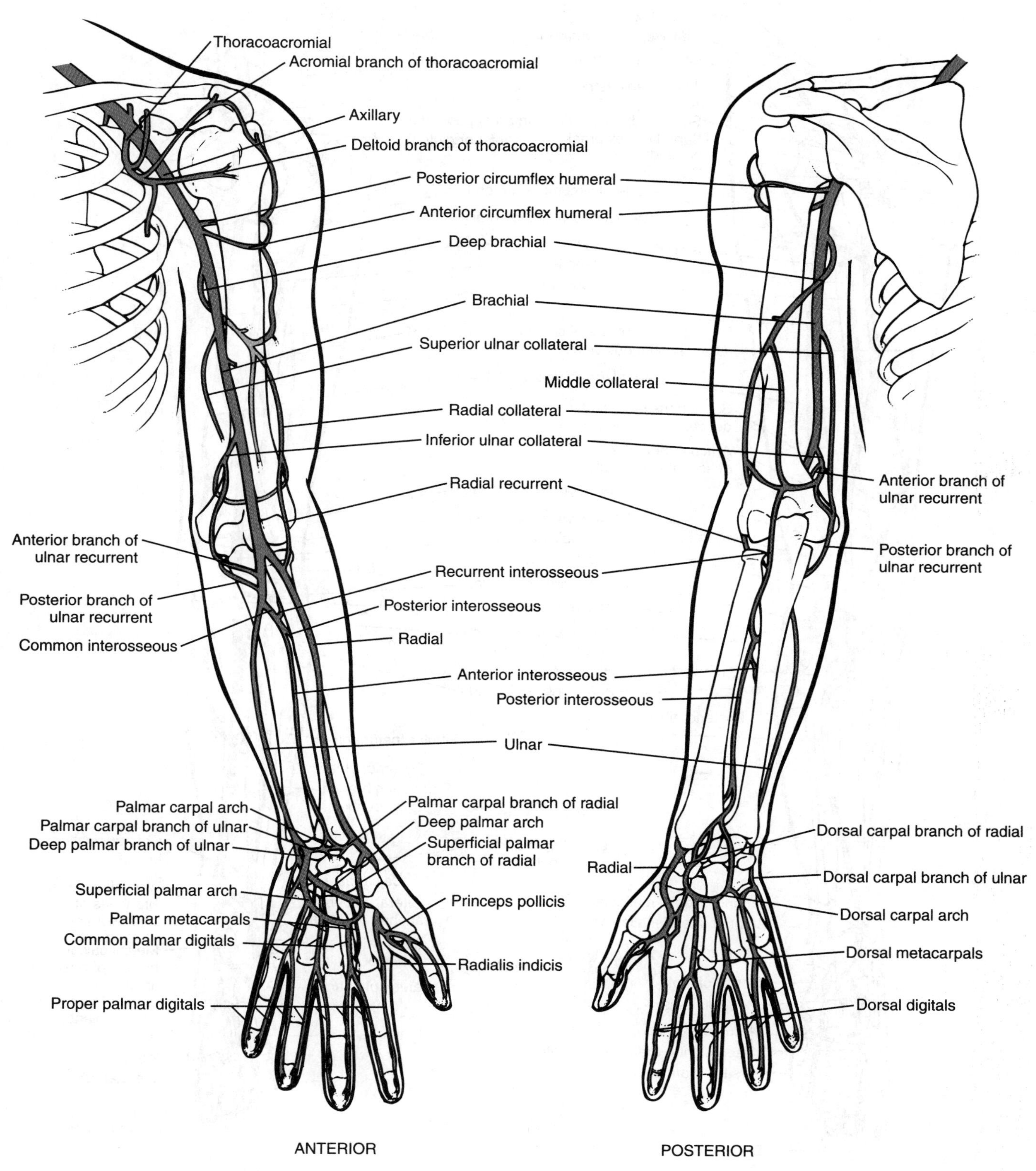


**PLATE 6**—ARTERIES OF THE UPPER LIMB

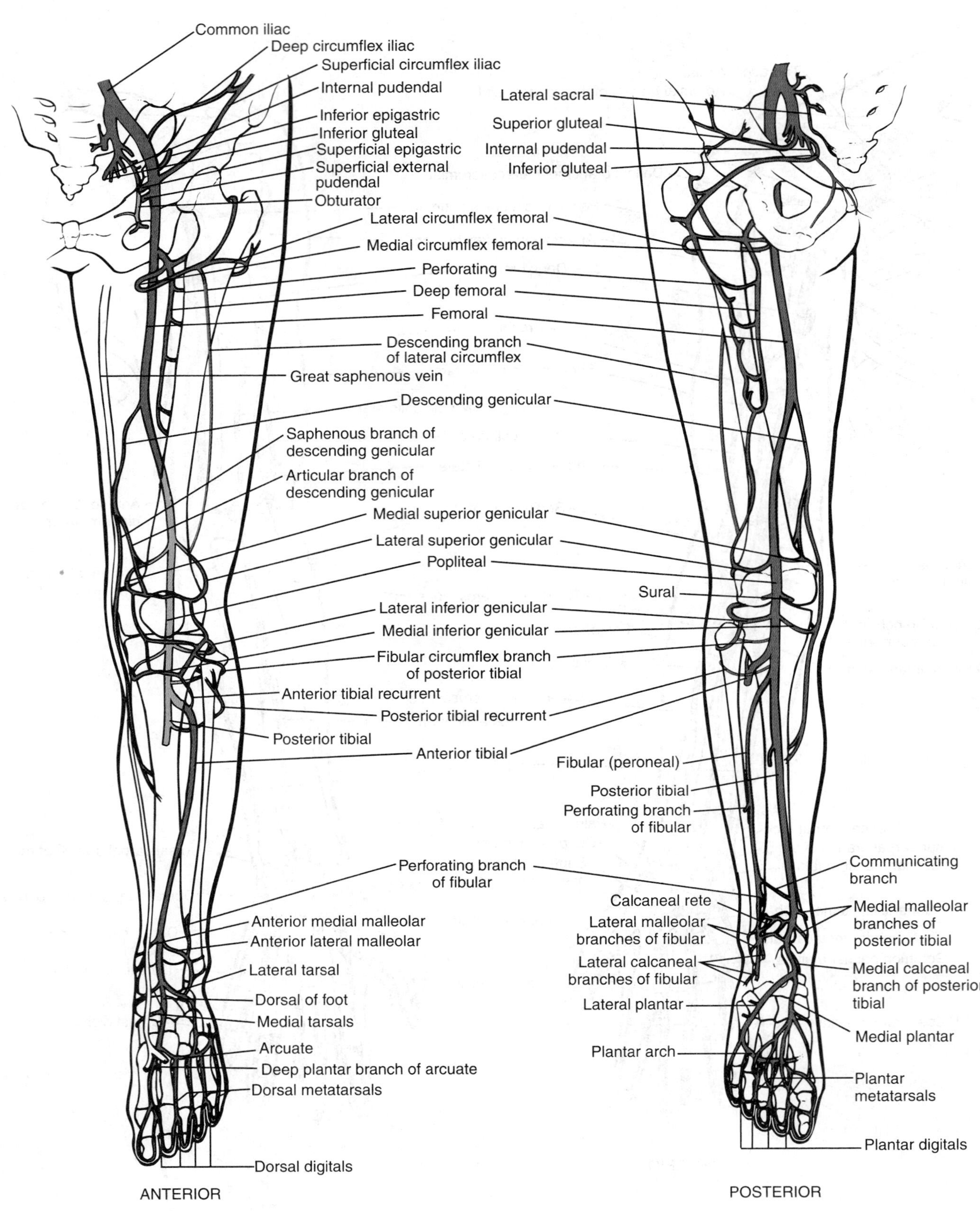


**PLATE 7**—ARTERIES OF THE LOWER LIMB

## Artery

For names and descriptions of specific arteries, see under *arteria.*

**accompanying a. of ischiadic nerve,** arteria comitans nervi ischiadici.
**accompanying a. of median nerve,** arteria comitans nervi mediani.
**acetabular a.,** 1. ramus acetabularis arteriae circumflexae femoris medialis. 2. ramus acetabularis arteriae obturatoriae.
**acromiothoracic a.,** arteria thoracoacromialis.
**a's of Adamkiewicz,** rami spinales arteriae vertebralis.
**adipose a's of kidney,** rami capsulares arteriae renalis.
**adrenal a., middle,** arteria suprarenalis media.
**afferent a. of glomerulus,** arteriola glomerularis afferens.
**alveolar a's, anterior superior,** arteriae alveolares superiores anteriores.
**alveolar a., inferior,** arteria alveolaris inferior.
**alveolar a., posterior superior,** arteria alveolaris superior posterior.
**anastomotic atrial a.,** ramus atria'lis anastomo'ticus ra'mi circumflex'i arte'riae corona'riae sinis'trae
**angular a.,** arteria angularis.
**a. of angular gyrus,** arteria gyri angularis.
**appendicular a.,** arteria appendicularis.
**arcuate a. of foot,** arteria arcuata pedis.
**arcuate a's of kidney,** arteriae arcuatae renis.
**atrial anastomotic a.,** ramus atria'lis anastomo'ticus ra'mi circumflex'i arte'riae corona'riae sinis'trae
**atrioventricular nodal a.,** ramus nodi atrioventricularis arteriae coronariae dextrae.
**auditory a., internal,** arteria labyrinthina.
**auricular a's, anterior,** rami auriculares anteriores arteriae temporalis superficialis.
**auricular a., deep,** arteria auricularis profunda.
**auricular a., left,** arteria coronaria sinistra.
**auricular a., posterior,** arteria auricularis posterior.
**auricular a., right,** arteria coronaria dextra.
**axillary a.,** arteria axillaris.
**azygos a's of vagina,** rami vaginales arteriae uterinae.
**basilar a.,** arteria basilaris.
**brachial a.,** arteria brachialis.
**brachial a., deep,** arteria profunda brachii.
**brachial a., superficial,** arteria brachialis superficialis.
**brachiocephalic a.,** truncus brachiocephalicus.
**bronchial a's,** rami bronchiales partis thoracicae aortae.
**bronchial a's, anterior,** rami bronchiales arteriae thoracicae internae.
**buccal a., buccinator a.,** arteria buccalis.
**a. of bulb of penis,** arteria bulbi penis.
**a. of bulb of vestibule,** arteria bulbi vestibuli.
**bulbourethral a.,** arteria bulbi penis.
**capsular a., inferior,** arteria suprarenalis inferior.
**capsular a., middle,** arteria suprarenalis media.
**caroticotympanic a's,** arteriae caroticotympanicae.
**carotid a., common,** arteria carotis communis.
**carotid a., external,** arteria carotis externa.
**carotid a., internal,** arteria carotis interna.
**caudal a.,** arteria sacralis mediana.
**cecal a., anterior,** arteria caecalis anterior.
**cecal a., posterior,** arteria caecalis posterior.
**central a's, anterolateral,** arteriae centrales anterolaterales arteriae cerebri anterioris.
**central a's, anteromedial, of anterior cerebral a.,** arteriae centrales anteromediales arteriae cerebri anterioris.
**central a's, anteromedial, of anterior communicating a.,** arteriae centrales anteromediales arteriae communicantis anterioris.
**central a., long,** arteria centralis longa.
**central a's, posterolateral,** arteriae centrales posterolaterales.
**central a's, posteromedial, of posterior cerebral a.,** arteriae centrales posteromediales arteriae cerebri posterioris.
**central a's, posteromedial, of posterior communicating a.,** arteriae centrales posteromediales arteriae communicantis posterioris.
**central a., short,** arteria centralis brevis.
**central a. of retina,** arteria centralis retinae.
**central a's of spleen,** branches of the splenic artery after they leave the trabeculae; their tunica adventitia is replaced by a cylindrical lymphoid sheath and they pass through the aggregations of lymphatic nodules and branch out to terminate as splenic penicilli.
**a. of central sulcus,** arteria sulci centralis.
**cerebellar a., anterior inferior,** arteria inferior anterior cerebelli.
**cerebellar a., posterior inferior,** arteria inferior posterior cerebelli.
**cerebellar a., superior,** arteria cerebelli superior.
**cerebral a's,** the arteries supplying the cerebral hemispheres, derived from the internal carotid artery (anterior choroid, anterior cerebral, middle cerebral, and posterior communicating arteries and the circle of Willis) or from the basilar artery (posterior cerebral artery).
**cerebral a., anterior,** arteria cerebri anterior.
**cerebral a., middle,** arteria cerebri media.
**cerebral a., posterior,** arteria cerebri posterior.
**a. of cerebral hemorrhage,** any of various medial or lateral striate arteries that are common sites of cerebral hemorrhage; called also *lenticulostriate a.*
**a's of cerebrum,** cerebral a's.
**cervical a., ascending,** arteria cervicalis ascendens.
**cervical a., deep,** arteria cervicalis profunda.
**cervical a., deep descending,** the deep branch of the descending branch of the occipital artery; see *ramus descendens arteriae occipitalis.*
**cervical a., superficial,** ramus superficialis arteriae transversae colli.
**cervical a., transverse,** arteria transversa cervicis.
**cervicovaginal a's,** arteriae cervicovaginales.
**choroid a., anterior, choroidal a., anterior,** arteria choroidea anterior.
**ciliary a's, anterior,** arteriae ciliares anteriores.
**ciliary a's, long,** arteriae ciliares posteriores longae.
**ciliary a's, long posterior,** arteriae ciliares posteriores longae.
**ciliary a's, short,** arteriae ciliares posteriores breves.
**ciliary a's, short posterior,** arteriae ciliares posteriores breves.
**circumflex a.,** ramus circumflexus arteriae coronariae sinistrae.
**circumflex a., internal deep,** ramus profundus arteriae circumflexae femoris medialis.
**circumflex femoral a., lateral ,** arteria circumflexa femoris lateralis.
**circumflex femoral a., medial,** arteria circumflexa femoris medialis.
**circumflex humeral a., anterior,** arteria circumflexa anterior humeri.
**circumflex humeral a., posterior,** arteria circumflexa posterior humeri.
**circumflex iliac a., deep,** arteria circumflexa ilium profunda.
**circumflex iliac a., superficial,** arteria circumflexa ilium superficialis.
**circumflex a. of scapula,** arteria circumflexa scapulae.
**coccygeal a.,** arteria sacralis mediana.
**cochlear a.,** ramus cochlearis arteriae vestibulocochlearis.
**colic a., accessory superior,** arteria colica media.
**colic a., inferior right,** arteria ileocolica.
**colic a., left,** arteria colica sinistra.
**colic a., middle,** arteria colica media.
**colic a., right,** arteria colica dextra.
**collateral a., inferior ulnar,** arteria collateralis ulnaris inferior.
**collateral a., middle,** arteria collateralis media.
**collateral a., radial,** arteria collateralis radialis.
**collateral a., superior ulnar,** arteria collateralis ulnaris superior.
**communicating a., anterior,** arteria communicans anterior.
**communicating a., posterior,** arteria communicans posterior.
**conal a.,** 1. ramus coni arteriosi arteriae coronariae dextrae. 2. ramus coni arteriosi arteriae coronariae sinistrae.
**conducting a's,** arterial trunks characterized by large size and elasticity, such as the aorta, subclavian artery, common carotid artery, brachiocephalic trunk, and pulmonary trunk. Called also *elastic a's.*
**conjunctival a's, anterior,** arteriae conjunctivales anteriores.
**conjunctival a's, posterior,** arteriae conjunctivales posteriores.
**conus a., left,** ramus coni arteriosi arteriae coronariae sinistrae.
**conus a., right, conus a., third,** ramus coni arteriosi arteriae coronariae dextrae.
**copper-wire a's,** retinal arteries on which the bright line of reflex is exaggerated; seen in arteriosclerosis.
**corkscrew a's,** small arteries in the macular region of the eye that appear markedly tortuous.
**coronary a., left,** arteria coronaria sinistra.
**coronary a., left anterior descending,** ramus interventricularis anterior arteriae coronariae sinistrae.
**coronary a., posterior descending,** ramus interventricularis posterior arteriae coronariae dextrae.
**coronary a., right,** arteria coronaria dextra.
**coronary a. of stomach, left,** arteria gastrica sinistra.
**cremasteric a.,** arteria cremasterica.
**cricothyroid a.,** ramus cricothyroideus arteriae thyroideae superioris.
**cystic a.,** arteria cystica.
**deep a. of clitoris,** arteria profunda clitoridis.
**deep a. of penis,** arteria profunda penis.
**deferential a.,** arteria ductus deferentis.
**deltoid a.,** see *ramus deltoideus arteriae profundae brachii* and *ramus deltoideus arteriae thoracoacromialis.*
**dental a's, anterior,** arteriae alveolares superiores anteriores.
**dental a., inferior,** arteria alveolaris inferior.
**dental a., posterior,** arteria alveolaris superior posterior.
**diaphragmatic a.,** arteria phrenica inferior.
**diaphragmatic a's, superior,** arteriae phrenicae superiores.

**digital a's, collateral,** arteriae digitales palmares propriae.
**digital a's, common palmar,** arteriae digitales palmares communes.
**digital a's, common plantar,** arteriae digitales plantares communes.
**digital a's, common volar,** arteriae digitales palmares communes.
**digital a's, proper palmar,** arteriae digitales palmares propriae.
**digital a's, proper plantar,** arteriae digitales plantares propriae.
**digital a's, proper volar,** arteriae digitales palmares propriae.
**digital a's of foot, common,** arteriae metatarsales plantares.
**digital a's of foot, dorsal,** arteriae digitales dorsales pedis.
**digital a's of hand, dorsal,** arteriae digitales dorsales manus.
**distributing a's,** most of the arteries except the conducting arteries; of muscular type, they extend from the large vessels to the arterioles. Called also *muscular a's.*
**dorsal a. of clitoris,** arteria dorsalis clitoridis.
**dorsal a. of foot,** arteria dorsalis pedis.
**dorsal a. of nose,** arteria dorsalis nasi.
**dorsal a. of penis,** arteria dorsalis penis.
**dorsal a. of tongue,** see *rami dorsales linguae arteriae lingualis.*
**a. of ductus deferens,** arteria ductus deferentis.
**efferent a. of glomerulus,** arteriola glomerularis efferens.
**elastic a's,** conducting a's.
**end a.,** one which undergoes progressive branching without development of channels connecting with other arteries, so that if occluded it cannot supply sufficient blood to the tissue depending on it.
**epigastric a., inferior,** arteria epigastrica inferior.
**epigastric a., superficial,** arteria epigastrica superficialis.
**epigastric a., superior,** arteria epigastrica superior.
**episcleral a's,** arteriae episclerales.
**esophageal a.,** the esophageal branch of an artery; see terms starting with *rami oesophageales,* under *ramus.*
**esophageal a's, inferior,** rami oesophageales arteriae gastricae sinistrae.
**ethmoidal a., anterior,** arteria ethmoidalis anterior.
**ethmoidal a., posterior,** arteria ethmoidalis posterior.
**facial a.,** arteria facialis.
**facial a., transverse,** arteria transversa faciei.
**fallopian a.,** arteria uterina.
**femoral a.,** arteria femoralis.
**femoral a., common,** see *arteria femoralis.*
**femoral a., deep,** arteria profunda femoris.
**femoral a., superficial,** see *arteria femoralis.*
**fibular a.,** arteria fibularis.
**frontal a.,** arteria supratrochlearis.
**frontobasal a., lateral,** arteria frontobasalis lateralis.
**frontobasal a., medial,** arteria frontobasalis medialis.
**funicular a.,** arteria testicularis.
**gastric a., left,** arteria gastrica sinistra.
**gastric a., left inferior,** arteria gastro-omentalis sinistra.
**gastric a., posterior,** arteria gastrica posterior.
**gastric a., right,** arteria gastrica dextra.
**gastric a., right inferior,** arteria gastro-omentalis dextra.
**gastric a's, short,** arteriae gastricae breves.
**gastroduodenal a.,** arteria gastroduodenalis.
**gastroepiploic a., left,** arteria gastro-omentalis sinistra.
**gastroepiploic a., right,** arteria gastro-omentalis dextra.
**gastro-omental a., left,** arteria gastro-omentalis sinistra.
**gastro-omental a., right,** arteria gastro-omentalis dextra.
**genicular a., descending,** arteria descendens genicularis.
**genicular a., lateral inferior,** arteria inferior lateralis genus.
**genicular a., lateral superior,** arteria superior lateralis genus.
**genicular a., medial inferior,** arteria inferior medialis genus.
**genicular a., medial superior,** arteria superior medialis genus.
**genicular a., middle,** arteria media genus.
**gluteal a., inferior,** arteria glutea inferior.
**gluteal a., superior,** arteria glutea superior.
**gonadal a's,** the ovarian arteries or the testicular arteries.
**helicine a's,** 1. small arteries that for their entire length have a band of thickened intima on one side, in which longitudinal muscle fibers are embedded. They follow a convoluted or curled course and open directly into cavernous sinuses instead of capillaries; they play a dominant role in erection of erectile tissue. 2. arteriae helicinae penis. 3. rami helicinae arteriae uterinae.
**hemorrhoidal a., inferior,** arteria rectalis inferior.
**hemorrhoidal a., middle,** arteria rectalis media.
**hemorrhoidal a., superior,** arteria rectalis superior.
**hepatic a., common,** arteria hepatica communis.
**hepatic a., proper,** arteria hepatica propria.
**hyaloid a.,** arteria hyaloidea.
**a's of hybrid type,** a term denoting the short transitional regions where arteries of the mixed or elastic (conducting) type pass into arteries of the muscular (distributing) type.
**hypogastric a.,** arteria iliaca interna.
**hypophysial a., inferior,** arteria hypophysialis inferior.
**hypophysial a., superior,** arteria hypophysialis superior.
**ileal a's,** arteriae ileales.
**ileocolic a.,** arteria ileocolica.
**ileocolic a., ascending,** ramus colicus arteriae ileocolicae.
**a's of ileum,** arteriae ileales.
**iliac a., anterior,** arteria iliaca externa.
**iliac a., common,** arteria iliaca communis.
**iliac a., external,** arteria iliaca externa.
**iliac a., internal,** arteria iliaca interna.
**iliac a., small,** arteria iliolumbalis.
**iliolumbar a.,** arteria iliolumbalis.
**infracostal a.,** ramus costalis lateralis arteriae thoracicae internae.
**infraorbital a.,** arteria infraorbitalis.
**inguinal a's,** rami inguinales arteriae pudendae externae profundae.
**innominate a.,** truncus brachiocephalicus.
**insular a's,** arteriae insulares.
**intercostal a's, anterior,** rami intercostales anteriores arteriae thoracicae internae.
**intercostal a., first posterior,** arteria intercostalis posterior prima.
**intercostal a., highest,** arteria intercostalis suprema.
**intercostal a's, posterior,** arteriae intercostales posteriores.
**intercostal a., second posterior,** arteria intercostalis posterior secunda.
**intercostal a., superior,** arteria intercostalis suprema.
**interlobar a's of kidney,** arteriae interlobares renis.
**interlobular a's of kidney,** arteriae interlobulares renis.
**interlobular a's of liver,** arteriae interlobulares hepatis.
**intermediate atrial a., left,** ramus atrialis intermedius rami circumflexi arteriae coronariae sinistrae.
**intermediate atrial a., right,** ramus atrialis intermedius arteriae coronariae dextrae.
**intermetacarpal a's, palmar,** arteriae metacarpales palmares.
**interosseous a., anterior,** arteria interossea anterior.
**interosseous a., common,** arteria interossea communis.
**interosseous a., dorsal,** arteria interossea posterior.
**interosseous a., posterior,** arteria interossea posterior.
**interosseous a., recurrent,** arteria interossea recurrens.
**interosseous a., volar,** arteria interossea anterior.
**intersegmental a's,** paired dorsal branches of the embryonic aorta, originally going to the spinal cord but later mainly to the neck, back, and body wall.
**interventricular a., anterior,** ramus interventricularis anterior arteriae coronariae sinistrae.
**interventricular septal a's, anterior,** rami interventriculares septales arteriae coronariae sinistrae.
**interventricular septal a's, posterior,** rami interventriculares septales arteriae coronariae dextrae.
**intestinal a's,** arteriae intestinales.
**intrarenal a's,** arteriae intrarenales.
**jejunal a's,** arteriae jejunales.
**a's of kidney,** arteriae intrarenales.
**labial a., inferior,** arteria labialis inferior.
**labial a., superior,** arteria labialis superior.
**labial a's of vulva, anterior,** rami labiales anteriores arteriae pudendae externae profundae.
**labial a's of vulva, posterior,** rami labiales posteriores arteriae pudendae internae.
**a. of labyrinth, labyrinthine a.,** arteria labyrinthina.
**lacrimal a.,** arteria lacrimalis.
**laryngeal a., inferior,** arteria laryngea inferior.
**laryngeal a., superior,** arteria laryngea superior.
**lateral inferior a. of knee,** arteria inferior lateralis genus.
**lateral superior a. of knee,** arteria superior lateralis genus.
**lenticulostriate a.,** a. of cerebral hemorrhage.
**lingual a.,** arteria lingualis.
**lingual a., deep,** arteria profunda linguae.
**lingular a.,** arteria lingularis.
**lingular a., inferior,** arteria lingularis inferior.
**lingular a., superior,** arteria lingularis superior.
**lobar a's of left lung, inferior,** arteriae lobares inferiores pulmonis sinistri.
**lobar a's of left lung, superior,** arteriae lobares superiores pulmonis sinistri.
**lobar a's of right lung, inferior,** arteriae lobares pulmonis dextri.
**lobar a. of right lung, middle,** arteria lobaris media pulmonis dextri.
**lobar a's of right lung, superior,** arteriae lobares superiores pulmonis dextri.
**a's of lower limb,** arteriae membri inferioris.
**lumbar a's,** arteriae lumbales.
**lumbar a's, fifth, lumbar a's, lowest,** arteriae lumbales imae.
**malleolar a., lateral anterior,** arteria malleolaris anterior lateralis.
**malleolar a., lateral posterior,** see *rami malleolares laterales arteriae fibularis.*
**malleolar a., medial anterior,** arteria malleolaris anterior medialis.

**mammary a., external,** 1. arteria thoracica lateralis. 2. see *rami mammarii laterales arteriae thoracicae lateralis.*
**mammary a., internal,** arteria thoracica interna.
**mandibular a.,** arteria alveolaris inferior.
**marginal a., left,** ramus marginalis sinister rami circumflexi arteriae coronariae sinistrae.
**marginal a., right,** ramus marginalis dexter arteriae coronariae dextrae.
**marginal a. of colon, marginal a. of Drummond,** arteria marginalis coli.
**masseteric a.,** arteria masseterica.
**mastoid a.,** ramus mastoideus arteriae occipitalis.
**maxillary a.,** arteria maxillaris.
**maxillary a., external,** arteria facialis.
**maxillary a., internal,** arteria maxillaris.
**medial a. of foot, superficial,** ramus superficialis arteriae plantaris medialis.
**medial inferior a. of knee,** arteria inferior medialis genus.
**medial superior a. of knee,** arteria superior medialis genus.
**median a.,** arteria comitans nervi mediani.
**mediastinal a's, anterior,** rami mediastinales arteriae thoracicae internae.
**mediastinal a's, posterior,** rami mediastinales aortae thoracicae.
**medullary a.,** arteria nutricia.
**meningeal a., accessory,** ramus meningeus accessorius arteriae meningeae mediae.
**meningeal a., anterior,** ramus meningeus anterior arteriae ethmoidalis anterioris.
**meningeal a., middle,** arteria meningea media.
**meningeal a., posterior,** arteria meningea posterior.
**mental a.,** ramus mentalis arteriae alveolaris inferioris.
**mesencephalic a's,** arteriae mesencephalicae.
**mesenteric a., inferior,** arteria mesenterica inferior.
**mesenteric a., superior,** arteria mesenterica superior.
**metacarpal a., deep volar,** ramus palmaris profundus arteriae ulnaris.
**metacarpal a's, dorsal,** arteriae metacarpales dorsales.
**metacarpal a's, palmar,** arteriae metacarpales palmares.
**metacarpal a's, ulnar,** arteriae digitales palmares communes.
**metacarpal a's, volar,** arteriae metacarpales palmares.
**metatarsal a's, dorsal,** arteriae metatarsales dorsales.
**metatarsal a's, plantar,** arteriae metatarsales plantares.
**a's of mixed type,** arteries having both elastic (conducting) and muscular (distributing) elements.
**a's of Mueller,** arteriae helicinae penis.
**muscular a's,** 1. distributing a's. 2. arteriae musculares.
**musculophrenic a.,** arteria musculophrenica.
**mylohyoid a.,** ramus mylohyoideus arteriae alveolaris inferioris.
**myomastoid a.,** ramus occipitalis arteriae auricularis posterioris.
**nasal a., dorsal, nasal a., external,** arteria dorsalis nasi.
**nasal a's, lateral posterior,** arteriae nasales posteriores laterales.
**nasopalatine a.,** arteria sphenopalatina.
**Neubauer's a.,** arteria thyroidea ima.
**nodal a.,** see *ramus nodi atrioventricularis arteriae coronariae dextrae* and *ramus nodi sinuatrialis arteriae coronariae dextrae.*
**nutrient a.,** arteria nutricia.
**nutrient a's of femur,** arteriae nutriciae femoris.
**nutrient a. of fibula,** arteria nutricia fibulae.
**nutrient a's of humerus,** arteriae nutriciae humeri.
**nutrient a. of tibia,** arteria nutricia tibiae.
**obturator a.,** arteria obturatoria.
**obturator a., accessory,** arteria obturatoria accessoria.
**occipital a.,** arteria occipitalis.
**occipital a., lateral,** arteria occipitalis lateralis.
**occipital a., middle,** arteria occipitalis medialis.
**ophthalmic a.,** arteria ophthalmica.
**ovarian a.,** arteria ovarica.
**palatine a., ascending,** arteria palatina ascendens.
**palatine a., descending,** arteria palatina descendens.
**palatine a., greater,** arteria palatina major.
**palatine a's, lesser,** arteriae palatinae minores.
**palpebral a's, lateral,** arteriae palpebrales laterales.
**palpebral a's, medial,** arteriae palpebrales mediales.
**pancreatic a., dorsal,** arteria pancreatica dorsalis.
**pancreatic a., great,** arteria pancreatica magna.
**pancreatic a., inferior,** arteria pancreatica inferior.
**pancreaticoduodenal a., anterior superior,** arteria pancreaticoduodenalis superior anterior.
**pancreaticoduodenal a's, inferior,** arteriae pancreaticoduodenales inferiores.
**pancreaticoduodenal a., posterior superior,** arteria pancreaticoduodenalis superior posterior.
**paracentral a.,** arteria paracentralis.
**paramedian a's,** arteriae centrales posteromediales arteriae cerebri posterioris.
**parietal a's, anterior and posterior,** arteriae parietales anterior et posterior.
**pelvic a., posterior,** arteria iliaca interna.
**perforating a's,** arteriae perforantes.
**pericallosal a.,** pars postcommunicalis arteriae cerebri anterioris.
**pericardiac a's, posterior,** rami pericardiaci partis thoracicae aortae.
**pericardiacophrenic a.,** arteria pericardiacophrenica.
**perineal a.,** arteria perinealis.
**perirenal a's,** arteriae capsulares.
**peroneal a.,** arteria fibularis.
**peroneal a., perforating,** ramus perforans arteriae fibularis.
**pharyngeal a., ascending,** arteria pharyngea ascendens.
**phrenic a., great, phrenic a., inferior,** arteria phrenica inferior.
**phrenic a., superior,** 1. arteria pericardiacophrenica. 2. see *arteriae phrenicae superiores.*
**plantar a., deep,** arteria plantaris profunda.
**plantar a., external,** arteria plantaris lateralis.
**plantar a., lateral,** arteria plantaris lateralis.
**plantar a., medial,** arteria plantaris medialis.
**pontine a's,** arteriae pontis.
**popliteal a.,** arteria poplitea.
**a. of postcentral sulcus,** arteria sulci postcentralis.
**a. of precentral sulcus,** arteria sulci precentralis.
**precuneal a.,** arteria precunealis.
**prepancreatic a.,** arteria prepancreatica.
**principal a. of thumb,** arteria princeps pollicis.
**pterygoid a's,** rami pterygoidei arteriae maxillaris.
**a. of pterygoid canal,** arteria canalis pterygoidei.
**pubic a.,** ramus pubicus arteriae epigastricae inferioris.
**pudendal a., deep external,** arteria pudenda externa profunda.
**pudendal a., internal,** arteria pudenda interna.
**pudendal a., superficial external,** arteria pudenda externa superficialis.
**pulmonary a.,** truncus pulmonalis.
**pulmonary a., left,** arteria pulmonalis sinistra.
**pulmonary a., right,** arteria pulmonalis dextra.
**a. of the pulp,** a name given the first portion of one of the penicilli arteriae splenicae (see under *penicillus*).
**pyloric a.,** arteria gastrica dextra.
**quadriceps a. of femur,** ramus descendens arteriae circumflexae femoris lateralis.
**radial a.,** arteria radialis.
**radial a., collateral,** arteria collateralis radialis.
**radial a. of index finger,** arteria radialis indicis.
**radial a. of index finger, volar,** arteria radialis indicis.
**radiate a's of kidney,** arteriae interlobulares renis.
**ranine a.,** arteria profunda linguae.
**rectal a., inferior,** arteria rectalis inferior.
**rectal a., middle,** arteria rectalis media.
**rectal a., superior,** arteria rectalis superior.
**recurrent a.,** arteria centralis longa.
**recurrent a., anterior tibial,** arteria recurrens tibialis anterior.
**recurrent a., posterior tibial,** arteria recurrens tibialis posterior.
**recurrent a., radial,** arteria recurrens radialis.
**recurrent a., ulnar,** arteria recurrens ulnaris.
**renal a.,** arteria renalis.
**retrocostal a.,** ramus costalis lateralis arteriae thoracicae internae.
**retroduodenal a's,** arteriae retroduodenales.
**revehent a.,** arteriola glomerularis efferens.
**a. of round ligament of uterus,** arteria ligamenti teretis uteri.
**sacral a's, lateral,** arteriae sacrales laterales.
**sacral a., median,** arteria sacralis mediana.
**sacrococcygeal a.,** arteria sacralis mediana.
**scapular a., descending,** ramus profundus arteriae transversae cervicis.
**scapular a., dorsal,** 1. arteria dorsalis scapulae. 2. ramus profundus arteriae transversae cervicis.
**scapular a., transverse,** arteria suprascapularis.
**sciatic a., a. to sciatic nerve,** arteria comitans nervi ischiadici.
**scrotal a's, anterior,** rami scrotales anteriores arteriae pudendae externae profundae.
**scrotal a's, posterior,** rami scrotales posteriores arteriae pudendae internae.
**segmental a., inferior lingular,** ramus lingularis inferior arteriae pulmonalis sinistrae.
**segmental a., lingular,** arteria lingularis.
**segmental a. of kidney, anterior inferior,** arteria segmenti anterioris inferioris renalis.
**segmental a. of kidney, anterior superior,** arteria segmenti anterioris superioris renalis.
**segmental a. of kidney, inferior,** arteria segmenti inferioris renalis.

**segmental a. of kidney, posterior,** arteria segmenti posterioris renalis.
**segmental a. of liver, anterior,** arteria segmenti anterioris hepatici.
**segmental a. of liver, lateral,** arteria segmenti lateralis hepatici.
**segmental a. of liver, medial,** arteria segmenti medialis of liver.
**segmental a. of liver, posterior,** arteria segmenti posterioris hepatici.
**segmental a. of kidney, superior,** arteria segmenti superioris renalis.
**segmental a., superior lingular,** ramus lingularis superior arteriae pulmonalis sinistrae.
**segmental a. to inferior lobe of right lung, superior,** ramus superior lobi inferioris arteriae pulmonalis dextrae.
**segmental a. of left lung, anterior,** arteria segmentalis anterior pulmonis sinistri.
**segmental a. of left lung, anterior ascending,** ramus ascendens arteriae segmentalis anterioris pulmonis sinistri.
**segmental a. of left lung, anterior basal,** arteria segmentalis basalis anterior pulmonis sinistri.
**segmental a. of left lung, anterior descending,** ramus descendens arteriae segmentalis anterioris pulmonis sinistri.
**segmental a. of left lung, apical,** arteria segmentalis apicalis pulmonis sinistri.
**segmental a. of left lung, lateral basal,** 1. ramus basalis lateralis arteriae pulmonalis sinistrae. 2. arteria segmentalis basalis lateralis pulmonis sinistri.
**segmental a. of left lung, medial basal,** arteria segmentalis basalis medialis pulmonis sinistri.
**segmental a. of left lung, posterior,** arteria segmentalis posterior pulmonis sinistri.
**segmental a. of left lung, posterior ascending,** ramus ascendens arteriae segmentalis posterioris pulmonis sinistri.
**segmental a. of left lung, posterior basal,** arteria segmentalis basalis posterior pulmonis sinistri.
**segmental a. of left lung, posterior descending,** ramus descendens arteriae segmentalis posterioris pulmonis sinistri.
**segmental a. of left lung, superior,** arteria segmentalis superior pulmonis sinistri.
**segmental a. of right lung, anterior,** arteria segmentalis anterior pulmonis dextri.
**segmental a. of right lung, anterior ascending,** ramus ascendens arteriae segmentalis anterioris pulmonis dextri.
**segmental a. of right lung, anterior basal,** arteria segmentalis basalis anterior pulmonis dextri.
**segmental a. of right lung, anterior descending,** ramus descendens arteriae segmentalis anterioris pulmonis dextri.
**segmental a. of right lung, apical,** arteria segmentalis apicalis pulmonis dextri.
**segmental a. of right lung, lateral,** arteria segmentalis lateralis pulmonis dextri.
**segmental a. of right lung, lateral basal,** arteria segmentalis basalis lateralis pulmonis dextri.
**segmental a. of right lung, medial,** arteria segmentalis medialis pulmonis dextri.
**segmental a. of right lung, medial basal,** arteria segmentalis basalis medialis pulmonis dextri.
**segmental a. of right lung, posterior,** arteria segmentalis posterior pulmonis dextri.
**segmental a. of right lung, posterior ascending,** ramus posterior ascendens arteriae pulmonalis dextrae.
**segmental a. of right lung, posterior basal,** arteria segmentalis basalis posterior pulmonis dextri.
**segmental a. of right lung, posterior descending,** ramus descendens arteriae segmentalis posterioris pulmonis dextri.
**segmental a. of right lung, superior,** arteria segmentalis superior pulmonis dextri.
**septal a's, anterior,** rami interventriculares septales arteriae coronariae sinistrae.
**septal a's, posterior,** rami interventriculares septales arteriae coronariae dextrae.
**sheathed a's,** arterial branches having spindle-shaped thickenings in their walls (Schweigger-Seidel sheaths) and forming the penicilli of the spleen; called also *ellipsoid* or *sheathed arterioles.*
**sigmoid a's,** arteriae sigmoideae.
**sinoatrial nodal a., sinuatrial nodal a., sinus node a.,** ramus nodi sinuatrialis arteriae coronariae dextrae.
**spermatic a., external,** arteria cremasterica.
**spermatic a., internal,** arteria testicularis.
**sphenopalatine a.,** arteria sphenopalatina.
**spinal a's,** rami spinales arteriae vertebralis.
**spinal a., anterior,** arteria spinalis anterior.
**spinal a., posterior,** arteria spinalis posterior.
**splenic a.,** arteria splenica.
**sternal a's, posterior,** rami sternales arteriae thoracicae internae.
**sternocleidomastoid a's,** see *rami sternocleidomastoidei arteriae occipitalis.*
**sternocleidomastoid a., superior,** ramus sternocleidomastoideus arteriae thyroideae superioris.
**straight a's of kidney,** arteriolae rectae renis.
**striate a's,** arteriae centrales anterolaterales arteriae cerebri anterioris.
**striate a's, lateral,** rami laterales arteriarum centralium anterolateralium.
**striate a's, medial,** rami mediales arteriarum centralium anterolateralium.
**stylomastoid a.,** arteria stylomastoidea.
**subclavian a.,** arteria subclavia.
**subcostal a.,** arteria subcostalis.
**sublingual a.,** arteria sublingualis.
**submental a.,** arteria submentalis.
**subscapular a.,** arteria subscapularis.
**superior a. of cerebellum,** arteria superior cerebelli.
**supraduodenal a.,** arteria supraduodenalis.
**suprahyoid a.,** ramus suprahyoideus arteriae lingualis.
**supraorbital a.,** arteria supraorbitalis.
**suprarenal a., aortic,** arteria suprarenalis media.
**suprarenal a., inferior,** arteria suprarenalis inferior.
**suprarenal a., middle,** arteria suprarenalis media.
**suprarenal a's, superior,** arteriae suprarenales superiores.
**suprascapular a.,** arteria suprascapularis.
**supratrochlear a.,** arteria supratrochlearis.
**sural a's,** arteriae surales.
**sylvian a.,** arteria cerebri media.
**tarsal a., lateral,** arteria tarsalis lateralis.
**tarsal a's, medial,** arteriae tarsales mediales.
**temporal a., anterior,** arteria temporalis anterior.
**temporal a., anterior deep,** arteria temporalis profunda anterior.
**temporal a's, deep,** see *arteria temporalis profunda anterior* and *arteria temporalis profunda posterior.*
**temporal a., intermediate,** arteria temporalis media (def. 2).
**temporal a., middle,** 1. arteria temporalis media (def. 1). 2. arteria temporalis media (def. 2).
**temporal a., posterior,** arteria temporalis posterior.
**temporal a., posterior deep,** arteria temporalis profunda posterior.
**temporal a., superficial,** arteria temporalis superficialis.
**terminal a.,** 1. end a. 2. an artery that does not divide into branches, but is directly continuous with capillaries. Called also *telangion.*
**testicular a.,** arteria testicularis.
**thalamostriate a's, anterolateral,** arteriae centrales anterolaterales arteriae cerebri anterioris.
**thalamostriate a's, anteromedial,** arteriae centrales anteromediales arteriae cerebri anterioris.
**thoracic a., highest,** arteria thoracica superior.
**thoracic a., internal,** arteria thoracica interna.
**thoracic a., lateral,** arteria thoracica lateralis.
**thoracic a., superior,** arteria thoracica superior.
**thoracicoacromial a., thoracoacromial a.,** arteria thoracoacromialis.
**thoracodorsal a.,** arteria thoracodorsalis.
**thymic a's,** rami thymici arteriae thoracicae internae.
**thyroid a., inferior,** arteria thyroidea.
**thyroid a. of Cruveilhier, inferior,** ramus cricothyroideus arteriae thyroideae superioris.
**thyroid a., lowest,** arteria thyroidea ima.
**thyroid a., superior,** arteria thyroidea superior.
**tibial a., anterior,** arteria tibialis anterior.
**tibial a., posterior,** arteria tibialis posterior.
**tonsillar a.,** ramus tonsillaris arteriae facialis.
**transverse cervical a.,** arteria transversa cervicis.
**transverse a. of face,** arteria transversa faciei.
**transverse a. of neck,** arteria transversa cervicis.
**tubo-ovarian a.,** arteria ovarica.
**tympanic a., anterior,** arteria tympanica anterior.
**tympanic a., inferior,** arteria tympanica inferior.
**tympanic a., posterior,** arteria tympanica posterior.
**tympanic a., superior,** arteria tympanica superior.
**ulnar a.,** arteria ulnaris.
**ulnar collateral a., inferior,** arteria collateralis ulnaris inferior.
**ulnar collateral a., superior,** arteria collateralis ulnaris superior.
**umbilical a.,** arteria umbilicalis.
**a's of upper limb,** arteriae membri superioris.
**urethral a.,** arteria urethralis.
**uterine a.,** arteria uterina.
**uterine a., aortic,** arteria ovarica.
**vaginal a.,** arteria vaginalis.
**venous a's,** venae pulmonales.

**vermiform a.**, arteria appendicularis.
**vertebral a.**, arteria vertebralis.
**vesical a., inferior**, arteria vesicalis inferior.
**vesical a's, superior**, arteriae vesicales superiores.
**vestibular a's,** rami vestibulares arteriae labyrinthi.
**vidian a.**, arteria canalis pterygoidei.
**a. of Zinn**, arteria centralis retinae.
**zygomatico-orbital a.**, arteria zygomatico-orbitalis.

**ar·thral** (ahr'thrəl) pertaining to a joint.

**ar·thral·gia** (ahr-thral'jə) [*arthr-* + *-algia*] [MeSH: Arthralgia] pain in a joint; called also *arthrodynia*.
**a. saturni'na**, arthralgia of lead poisoning.

**ar·thral·gic** (ahr-thral'jik) pertaining to arthralgia; affected with arthralgia.

**ar·threc·to·my** (ahr-threk'to-me) [*arthr-* + *-ectomy*] the excision of a joint.

**ar·threm·py·e·sis** (ahr"threm-pi-e'sis) [*arthr-* + *empyesis*] arthropyosis.

**ar·thres·the·sia** (ahr"thres-the'zhə) [*arthr-* + *esthesia*] joint sensibility; the perception of joint motions.

**ar·thrit·ic** (ahr-thrit'ik) 1. pertaining to or affected with arthritis. 2. a person affected with arthritis.

**ar·thri·tide** (ahr'thrĭ-tīd) any skin eruption of arthritic or gouty origin.

**ar·thrit·i·des** (ahr-thrit'ĭ-dēz) [MeSH: Arthritis] plural of *arthritis*.

**ar·thri·tis** (ahr-thri'tis) pl. *arthrit'ides* [*arthr-* + *-itis*] [MeSH: Arthritis] inflammation of joints; see also *rheumatism*.
**acute a.**, arthritis marked by pain, heat, redness, and swelling, due to inflammation, infection, or trauma.
**acute rheumatic a.**, joint tenderness and swelling due to rheumatic fever.
**acute suppurative a.**, septic a.
**bacterial a.**, septic a.
**Bekhterev's (Bechterew's) a.**, ankylosing spondylitis.
**caprine a.-encephalitis**, see under *encephalitis*.
**chronic inflammatory a.**, inflammation of joints in chronic disorders such as rheumatoid arthritis.
**climacteric a.**, menopausal a.
**cricoarytenoid a.**, inflammation of the cricoarytenoid joint in rheumatoid arthritis; it may cause laryngeal dysfunction and rarely stridor.
**crystal-induced a.**, that due to the deposition of inorganic crystalline material within the joints; see *gout* and see *calcium pyrophosphate deposition disease*, under *disease*.
**a. defor'mans**, severe destruction of joints, seen in disorders such as rheumatoid arthritis.
**degenerative a.**, osteoarthritis.
**enteropathic a.**, arthritis associated with inflammatory bowel disease or following bacterial infection of the bowel.
**exudative a.**, arthritis with exudate into or about the joint.
**fungal a., a. fungo'sa**, mycotic a.
**gonococcal a., gonorrheal a.**, bacterial arthritis occurring secondary to gonorrhea, often characterized by migratory polyarthritis that usually involves one and sometimes two joints, and commonly associated with erythematous skin lesions and tenosynovitis.
**gouty a.**, arthritis due to gout.
**hemophilic a.**, bleeding into the joint cavities.
**hypertrophic a.**, osteoarthritis.
**infectious a.**, arthritis caused by bacteria, rickettsiae, mycoplasmas, viruses, fungi, or parasites.
**Jaccoud's a.**, see under *syndrome*.
**juvenile a., juvenile chronic a.**, juvenile rheumatoid a.
**Lyme a.**, see under *disease*.
**menopausal a.**, a condition sometimes seen in women at menopause, due to ovarian hormonal deficiency and marked by pain in the small joints, shoulders, elbows, or knees; called also *arthropathia ovaripriva* and *climacteric a.*
**a. mu'tilans**, a severe deforming polyarthritis with gross bone and cartilage destruction, usually an atypical variant of rheumatoid arthritis.
**mycoplasmal a.**, see under *polyarthritis*.
**mycotic a.**, infectious arthritis secondary to any invasive mycosis, such as coccidioidomycosis, blastomycosis, histoplasmosis, actinomycosis, candidiasis, and sporotrichosis, usually by extension from adjacent bone, and having manifestations similar to those of tuberculous arthritis. Called also *fungal a.* and *a. fungosa*.
**navicular a.**, inflammation of the navicular bursa and the cartilage covering the navicular bone of the foot of a horse.
**neuropathic a.**, neuropathic arthropathy.
**proliferative a.**, inflammation of joints with proliferation of the synovium, seen in rheumatoid arthritis.
**psoriatic a.**, a syndrome of psoriasis in association with inflammatory arthritis; rheumatoid factor is usually not present in the sera of affected individuals. Called also *arthritic psoriasis, psoriasis arthropathica*, and *psoriatic arthropathy*.
**pyogenic a.**, septic a.
**reactive a.**, arthritis after an infection, such as urethritis caused by *Chlamydia trachomatis* or enteritis caused by *Campylobacter, Salmonella, Shigella*, or *Yersinia*. Cf. *Reiter's syndrome*.
**rheumatoid a.**, a chronic systemic disease primarily of the joints, usually polyarticular, marked by inflammatory changes in the synovial membranes and articular structures and by muscle atrophy and rarefaction of the bones. In late stages deformity and ankylosis develop. The cause is unknown, but autoimmune mechanisms and virus infection have been postulated.
**rheumatoid a., juvenile**, rheumatoid arthritis of children, with swelling, tenderness, and pain in one or more joints, which may lead to impaired growth and development, limitation of movement, ankylosis, and flexion contractures. It is often accompanied by systemic manifestations such as spiking fever, transient rash on the trunk and extremities, hepatosplenomegaly, generalized lymphadenopathy, and anemia. The form with systemic features is also called *Still's disease*.
**rheumatoid a., seronegative**, any of various rare types of rheumatoid arthritis in which patients are seronegative for rheumatoid factor.
**septic a.**, infectious a., usually acute, characterized by inflammation of synovial membranes with purulent effusion into a joint or joints, most often due to *Staphylococcus aureus, Streptococcus pyogenes, S. pneumoniae*, or *Neisseria gonorrhoeae*, usually caused by hematogenous spread from a primary site of infection although joints may also become infected by direct inoculation or local extension. Called also *bacterial, pyogenic*, or *suppurative a.*
**suppurative a.**, septic a.
**syphilitic a.**, a rare form of bacterial arthritis occurring as a manifestation of primary, secondary, or tertiary syphilis; types include *neuropathic arthropathy, Clutton's joint*, and *Parrot's pseudoparalysis*.
**tuberculous a.**, bacterial arthritis occurring secondary to tuberculosis; it usually affects a single joint and is characterized by chronic inflammation with effusion and destruction of contiguous bone.
**a. urethri'tica, venereal a.**, Reiter's syndrome.
**vertebral a.**, inflammation involving the intervertebral disks.
**viral a.**, infectious arthritis, usually polyarticular and self-limited, associated with a viral disease, such as rubella, mumps, infectious mononucleosis, varicella, hepatitis B, and arboviral or adenoviral infection.

**arthr(o)-** [Gr. *arthron* joint] a combining form denoting some relationship to a joint or joints.

**Ar·thro·bo·trys** (ahr"thro-bo'trəs) a genus of Fungi Imperfecti of the form-family Moniliaceae, some of which infect and destroy nematodes.

**ar·thro·cele** (ahr'thro-sēl) [*arthro-* + *-cele*] a swollen joint.

**ar·thro·cen·te·sis** (ahr"thro-sen-te'sis) puncture and aspiration of a joint.

**ar·thro·cha·la·sis** (ahr"thro-kal'ə-sis) [*arthro-* + Gr. *chalasis* relaxation] abnormal relaxation or flaccidity of a joint.
**a. multiplex congenita**, Ehlers-Danlos syndrome, type VII.

**ar·thro·chon·dri·tis** (ahr"thro-kon-dri'tis) [*arthro-* + *chondritis*] inflammation of the cartilage of a joint.

**ar·thro·cla·sia** (ahr"thro-kla'zhə) [*arthro-* + Gr. *klaein* to break] the surgical breaking down of an ankylosis in order to secure free movement in a joint.

**ar·thro·cli·sis** (ahr"thro-kli'sis) ankylosis.

**ar·thro·co·nid·ium** (ahr"thro-kə-nid'e-əm) arthrospore.

**Ar·thro·der·ma** (ahr"thro-dər'mə) a genus of fungi of the family Gymnoascaceae; the hyphae around the gymnothecium are dichotomously branched, and cells have deep constrictions to give them a dumbbell shape. It has been found to be identical to the former genus *Nannizzia*. This genus contains the perfect (sexual) stages of fungi of genera *Microsporum* and *Trichophyton*. *A. cajeta'ni* is the sexual stage of *M. cookei* and *A. persi'color* is the sexual stage of *M. persicolor*.

**ar·thro·de·sia** (ahr″thro-de′zhə) arthrodesis.

**ar·thro·de·sis** (ahr-thro-de′sis) [*arthro-* + *-desis*] [MeSH: Arthrodesis] the surgical fixation of a joint by a procedure designed to accomplish fusion of the joint surfaces by promoting the proliferation of bone cells; called also *artificial ankylosis*.
**Moberg a.,** fusion of a finger joint with a small squared bone peg.
**triple a.,** fusion of the subtalar, calcaneocuboid, and talonavicular joints, to provide lateral stability to the paralyzed foot.

**ar·thro·dia** (ahr-thro′de-ə) [Gr. *arthrōdia* a particular kind of articulation] articulatio plana.

**ar·thro·di·al** (ahr-thro′de-əl) of the nature of an arthrodia.

**ar·thro·dyn·ia** (ahr″thro-din′e-ə) [*arthro-* + *-odynia*] arthralgia.

**ar·thro·dys·pla·sia** (ahr″thro-dis-pla′zhə) [*arthro-* + *dysplasia*] a hereditary condition marked by deformity of various joints.

**ar·thro·em·py·e·sis** (ahr″thro-em″pi-e′sis) [*arthro-* + *empyesis*] arthropyosis.

**ar·thro·en·dos·co·py** (ahr″thro-en-dos′ko-pe) arthroscopy.

**ar·thro·erei·sis** (ahr″thro-ə-ri′sis) [*arthro-* + Gr. *ereisis* a raising up] operative limiting of the motion in a joint that is abnormally mobile from paralysis.

**ar·throg·e·nous** (ahr-troj′ə-nəs) [*arthro-* + *-genous*] formed as a separate joint, as arthrogenous spore.

**ar·thro·gram** (ahr′thro-gram) a radiographic record after introduction of opaque contrast material into a joint.

**Ar·thro·graph·is** (ahr″thro-graf′is) a genus of Fungi Imperfecti of the form-class Hyphomycetes, form-family Dematiaceae. Some species cause dermatomycosis, and *A. kal'rae* has been found chronically in the sputum of patients with lung disease.

**ar·throg·ra·phy** (ahr-throg′rə-fe) [*arthro-* + *-graphy*] [MeSH: Arthrography] radiography of a joint after injection of opaque contrast material.
**air a.,** pneumoarthrography.

**ar·thro·gry·po·sis** (ahr″thro-grə-po′sis) [*arthro-* + *gryposis*] [MeSH: Arthrogryposis] 1. persistent flexure or contracture of a joint. 2. tetanoid spasm.
**congenital a.,** congenital articular rigidity.
**congenital multiple a., a. mul'tiplex conge'nita,** a syndrome characterized by congenital immobility of most of the joints, fixed in various postures, with lack of muscle development and growth.

**ar·thro·ka·tad·y·sis** (ahr″thro-kə-tad′ə-sis) [*arthro-* + Gr. *katadysis* a falling down] a sinking in or subsidence of the floor of the acetabulum with protrusion of the femoral head through it (intrapelvic protrusion) resulting in limitation of movement of the hip joint; called also *Otto's disease* and *protrusio acetabuli*.

**ar·thro·klei·sis** (ahr″thro-kli′sis) [*arthro-* + Gr. *kleisis* closure] ankylosis.

**ar·thro·lith** (ahr′thro-lith) [*arthro-* + *-lith*] a calculous deposit in a joint; cf. *arthrophyte* and *joint mouse*.

**ar·thro·li·thi·a·sis** (ahr″thro-lĭ-thi′ə-sis) gout.

**ar·thro·lo·gia** (ahr″thro-lo′jə) arthrology; in anatomic terminology, the nomenclature relating to the articulations (joints) and ligaments. Called also *syndesmologia*.

**ar·throl·o·gy** (ahr-throl′ə-je) [*arthro-* + *-logy*] the scientific study of the joints and ligaments; also applied to the body of knowledge relating thereto. Called also *syndesmology*.

**ar·throl·y·sis** (ahr-throl′ə-sis) [*arthro-* + *-lysis*] the operative loosening of adhesions in an ankylosed joint.

**ar·thro·men·in·gi·tis** (ahr″thro-men″in-ji′tis) [*arthro-* + *mening-* + *-itis*] synovitis.

**ar·throm·e·ter** (ahr-throm′ə-tər) [*arthro-* + *-meter*] goniometer.

**ar·throm·e·try** (ahr-throm′ə-tre) goniometry.

**ar·thron·cus** (ahr-throng′kəs) [*arthro-* + Gr. *onkos* mass] swelling of a joint.

**ar·thro·neu·ral·gia** (ahr″thro-noo͝-ral′jə) [*arthro-* + *neuralgia*] pain arising in or around a joint.

**ar·thro-ony·cho·dys·pla·sia** (ahr″thro-on″ə-ko-dis-pla′zhə) onycho-osteodysplasia.

**ar·thro-oph·thal·mop·a·thy** (ahr″thro-of-thəl-mop′ə-the) an association of degenerative joint disease and eye disease.
**hereditary progressive a.-o.,** an autosomal dominant disorder consisting of myopia progressing to retinal detachment and blindness, and premature degenerative changes in the joints; sensorineural deafness may also occur. Called also *Stickler's syndrome*.

**Ar·thro·pan** (ahr′thro-pan) trademark for a preparation of choline salicylate.

**ar·thro·path·ia** (ahr″thro-path′e-ə) [L.] arthropathy.
**a. ovaripri'va,** menopausal arthritis.
**a. psoria'tica,** a disease of the joints seen in persons suffering from psoriasis; it resembles rheumatoid arthritis.

**ar·thro·path·ic** (ahr″thro-path′ik) pertaining to or characterized by arthropathy.

**ar·thro·pa·thol·o·gy** (ahr″thro-pə-thol′ə-je) [*arthro-* + *pathology*] the study of the structural and functional changes produced in the joints by disease.

**ar·throp·a·thy** (ahr-throp′ə-the) [*arthro-* + *-pathy*] any joint disease.
**Charcot's a.,** neuropathic a.
**chondrocalcific a.,** progressive polyarthritis with joint swelling and bony enlargement, most commonly in the small joints of the hand but also affecting other joints, characterized radiographically by narrowing of the joint space with subchondral erosions and sclerosis and frequently chondrocalcinosis.
**crystal a.,** crystal-induced arthritis.
**hemophilic a.,** chronic arthropathy in hemophiliacs due to bleeding into a joint followed by inflammation and thickening of the synovial membrane.
**inflammatory a.,** a disease of a joint of inflammatory origin.
**neurogenic a.,** neuropathic a.
**neuropathic a.,** chronic progressive degeneration of the stress-bearing portion of a joint, with bizarre hypertrophic changes at the periphery; it is usually a complication of a neurologic disorder such as tabes dorsalis, syringomyelia, or diabetic neuropathy. Loss of sensation leads to relaxation of supporting structures and chronic instability of the joint. Called also *Charcot's a., neurogenic a., Charcot's disease* or *joint,* and *neuropathic arthritis*.
**osteopulmonary a.,** clubbing of the fingers and toes, enlargement and swelling of the ends of the long bones associated with cardiac and pulmonary disease.
**psoriatic a.,** see under *arthritis*.
**pyrophosphate a.,** calcium pyrophosphate deposition disease (q.v.), particularly the structural joint changes that occur in the disease.
**static a.,** a disturbance in a joint of the extremity secondary to a disturbance in some other joint of the same extremity, as one in the knee joint secondary to one in the hip joint.
**syphilitic a.,** see under *arthritis*.
**tabetic a.,** neuropathic arthropathy (q.v.) occurring in patients with tabes dorsalis.

**ar·thro·phy·ma** (ahr″thro-fi′mə) [*arthro-* + *phyma*] the swelling of a joint.

**ar·thro·phyte** (ahr′thro-fīt) [*arthro-* + *-phyte*] an abnormal growth in a joint cavity; cf. *arthrolith* and *joint mouse*.

**ar·thro·plas·tic** (ahr″thro-plas′tik) pertaining to arthroplasty.

**ar·thro·plas·ty** (ahr′thro-plas″te) [*arthro-* + *-plasty*] [MeSH: Arthroplasty] plastic surgery of a joint or of joints; the formation of movable joints. Called also *joint replacement*.
**Austin Moore a.,** hip reconstruction surgery using an Austin Moore prosthesis.
**capsular a.,** correction of dislocation or deformation of the hip by soft tissue manipulation, curetting of the acetabulum, and muscle transfer but without osteotomy.
**Charnley's hip a.,** a hip replacement operation involving insertion of Charnley's prosthesis to form a low-friction joint.
**interposition a.,** surgical correction of ankylosis of the temporomandibular joint by separating the immobile fragment from the mobilized fragment and interposing a substance, such as fascia, cartilage, metal, or plastic, between them.
**intracapsular temporomandibular joint a.,** operative recontouring of the articular surface of the mandibular condyle without the removal of the articular disk.
**Thompson a.,** hip reconstruction surgery using a Thompson prosthesis.
**total joint a.,** arthroplasty in which both sides of a joint are removed and replaced by artificial implants anchored to the bones. Called also *total joint replacement*.
**total knee a.,** arthroplasty of both sides of the knee joint.

**ar·thro·pneu·mog·ra·phy** (ahr″thro-noo-mog′rə-fe) arthropneumoradiography.

**ar·thro·pneu·mo·ra·di·og·ra·phy** (ahr′thro-noo″mo-ra″de-og′rə-fe) [*arthro-* + *pneumo-* + *radiography*] radiography of a joint after injection into it of air, oxygen, or carbon dioxide.

**ar·thro·pod** (ahr′thro-pod) [MeSH: Arthropods] an animal belonging to the Arthropoda.

**Ar·throp·o·da** (ahr-throp′ə-də) [*arthro-* + Gr. *pous* foot] a phylum of the animal kingdom composed of organisms having a hard, jointed exoskeleton and paired, jointed legs, and including, among other classes, the Arachnida and Insecta, many species of which are important medically as parasites or as vectors of organisms capable of causing disease in man.

**ar·throp·o·dan** (ahr-throp′ə-dən) arthropodous.

**ar·thro·po·dic** (ahr″thro-po′dic) arthropodous.

**ar·throp·o·dous** (ahr-throp′ə-dəs) pertaining to or caused by arthropods.

**ar·thro·py·o·sis** (ahr″thro-pi-o′sis) [*arthro-* + *pyo-* + *-sis*] the formation of pus in a joint cavity. Called also *arthrempyesis* and *arthroempyesis.*

**ar·thro·ri·sis** (ahr″thro-ri′sis) arthroereisis.

**ar·thro·scle·ro·sis** (ahr″thro-sklə-ro′sis) [*arthro-* + *sclerosis* hardening] stiffening or hardening of the joints.

**ar·thro·scope** (ahr′thro-skōp) [*arthro-* + *-scope*] an endoscope for examining the interior of a joint and for carrying out diagnostic and therapeutic procedures within the joint.

**ar·thros·copy** (ahr-thros′kə-pe) [MeSH: Arthroscopy] examination of the interior of a joint with an arthroscope.

**ar·thro·sis** (ahr-thro′sis) 1. [Gr. *arthrōsis* a jointing] a joint or articulation. 2. [*arthr-* + *-osis*] arthropathy.

**ar·thro·spore** (ahr′thro-spor) [*arthro-* + *spore*] an asexual fungal spore formed by hyphal segmentation. Called also *arthroconidium.*

**ar·thros·to·my** (ahr-thros′tə-me) [*arthro-* + *-stomy*] surgical creation of an opening into a joint, as for the purpose of drainage.

**ar·thro·syn·o·vi·tis** (ahr″thro-sin″o-vi′tis) [*arthro-* + *synovitis*] inflammation of the synovial membrane of a joint.

**Ar·thro·tec** (ahr′thro-tek) trademark for a preparation of diclofenac sodium and misoprostol.

**ar·thro·tome** (ahr′thro-tōm) [*arthro-* + *-tome*] a knife for incising a joint.

**ar·throt·o·my** (ahr-throt′ə-me) [*arthro-* + *-tomy*] surgical incision of a joint.

**ar·thro·trop·ic** (ahr″thro-trop′ik) [*arthro-* + *-tropic*] having an affinity for or tending to settle in the joints.

**ar·throx·e·sis** (ahr-throk′sə-sis) [*arthro-* + Gr. *xesis* scraping] the scraping of diseased tissue from an articular surface.

**Ar·thus reaction (phenomenon), Arthus-type reaction** (ahr-tūs′) [Nicolas-Maurice *Arthus,* French physiologist, 1862–1945] see under *reaction.*

**ar·ti·cle** (ahr′tĭ-kəl) [L. *articulus* a little joint] an interarticular segment; one of the portions or segments forming a jointed series.

**ar·tic·u·lar** (ahr-tik′u-lər) [L. *articularis*] of or pertaining to a joint.

**ar·tic·u·la·re** (ahr-tik″u-lăr′e) a craniometric landmark used in radiographic cephalometry, being the point of intersection of the posterior margin of the ascending ramus of the mandible and the shadow of the cranial base, as seen on the lateral x-ray of the head. Called also *point Ar.*

**ar·tic·u·late**[1] (ahr-tik′u-lāt) [L. *articulatus* jointed] 1. to pronounce clearly and distinctly. 2. to make speech sounds by manipulation of the vocal organs. 3. to express in coherent verbal form. 4. to divide into or to unite so as to form a joint. 5. in dentistry, to adjust or place the teeth in their proper relation to each other in making an artificial denture.

**ar·tic·u·late**[2] (ahr-tik′u-lət) 1. divided into distinct, meaningful syllables or words. 2. endowed with the power of speech. 3. characterized by the use of clear, meaningful language. 4. divided into or united by joints.

**ar·tic·u·lat·ed** (ahr-tik′u-lāt″əd) connected by movable joints; consisting of separate segments so joined as to be movable on each other.

**ar·tic·u·la·tio** (ahr-tik″u-la′she-o) pl. *articulatio′nes* [L.] 1. articulation: any place of junction between two different parts or objects. 2. TA alternative for *junctura synovialis.*

## Articulatio

Descriptions of articulations are given on TA terms, and include anglicized names of specific articulations.

**a. acromioclavicula′ris** [TA], acromioclavicular articulation: the joint formed by the acromion of the scapula and the acromial extremity of the clavicle; called also *scapuloclavicular articulation* or *joint.*

**a. atlantoaxia′lis latera′lis** [TA], lateral atlantoaxial articulation: one of a pair of joints, one on either side of the body, formed by the inferior articular surface of the atlas and the superior surface of the axis.

**a. atlantoaxia′lis media′na** [TA], medial atlantoaxial articulation: a single joint formed by the two articular facets of the dens of the axis, one in relation with the articular facet on the anterior arch of the atlas, the other in relation with the transverse ligament of the atlas.

**a. atlantoepistro′phica,** see *a. atlantoaxialis lateralis* and *a. atlantoaxialis mediana.*

**a. atlantooccipita′lis** [TA], atlantooccipital articulation: one of two joints, each formed by a superior articular pit of the atlas and a condyle of the occipital bone; called also *craniovertebral articulation* or *junction, occipital* or *occipito-atlantal articulation,* and *Cruveilhier's* or *atlantooccipital joint.*

**a. bicondyla′ris** [TA], bicondylar articulation: a condylar joint with a meniscus between the articular surfaces, as in the temporomandibular joint; called also *bicondylar joint.*

**a. calcaneocuboi′dea** [TA], calcaneocuboid articulation: one formed between the cuboidal articular surface of the calcaneus and the cuboid bone.

**a. ca′pitis cos′tae** [TA], articulation of head of rib: the articulation of the head of the rib with the bodies of two vertebrae, one of the two types of articulations between ribs and vertebrae. Called also *articulation of head of rib,* and *capitular* or *costocentral articulation.* Cf. *a. costotransversaria.*

**a. ca′pitis hu′meri,** a. humeri.

**articulatio′nes capitulo′rum costa′rum,** see *a. capitis costae.*

**articulatio′nes car′pi** [TA], carpal articulations: any of the joints that connect the carpal bones together, comprising: the joints between each row, distal and proximal *(articulationes intercarpales)*; the joint between the distal and proximal rows *(a. mediocarpalis)*; and the joint formed by the pisiform and triquetral bones *(a. ossis pisiformis).* Called also *carpal joints.*

**articulatio′nes carpometacarpa′les** [TA], **articulatio′nes carpometacar′peae,** carpometacarpal articulations: joints formed by the trapezial, trapezoid, capitate, and hamate bones together with the bases of the four medial metacarpal bones; called also *metacarpocarpal articulations.*

**a. carpometacarpa′lis pol′licis** [TA], **a. carpometacar′pea pol′licis,** carpometacarpal articulation of thumb: the joint formed by the first metacarpal and the trapezial bones; called also *carpometacarpal joint of thumb* and *first carpometacarpal articulation.*

**a. cartilagi′nea,** junctura cartilaginea.

**articulatio′nes cin′guli mem′bri inferio′ris,** juncturae cinguli pelvici.

**articulatio′nes cin′guli mem′bri superio′ris,** juncturae cinguli pectoralis.

**articulatio′nes cin′guli pectora′lis,** juncturae membri pectoralis.

**articulatio′nes cin′guli pel′vici,** juncturae cinguli pelvici.

**a. cochlea′ris,** a form of hinge joint that permits some lateral motion.

**articulatio′nes colum′nae vertebra′lis** [TA], synovial joints of vertebral column: the articulations of the vertebrae, including zygapophyseal, lumbosacral, sacrococcygeal, and lateral and medial atlantoaxial joints.

**a. complex′a, a. compo′sita** [TA], composite joint: a type of synovial joint in which more than two bones are involved; called also *compound articulation* or *joint.*

**a. condyla′ris,** a. ellipsoidea.

**a. condyla′ris inver′sa,** a. sellaris.

**articulatio′nes costochondra′les** [TA], costochondral articulations: articulations between the lateral extremity of each costal cartilage and the sternal ends of the ribs.

**a. costotransversa′ria** [TA], costotransverse articulation: one of the two types of articulations between ribs and vertebrae: the articulation of the tubercle of the rib with the transverse process of a vertebra. This is lacking for the eleventh and twelfth ribs. Called also *articulation of tubercle of rib.* Cf. *a. capitis costae.*

**articulatio′nes costovertebra′les** [TA], costovertebral articulations: the articulations between the ribs and vertebrae, of which there are two types: a. capitis costae and a. costotransversaria.

**a. coty'lica** [TA], a type of ball and socket joint.

**a. cox'ae** [TA], articulation of hip: the joint formed between the head of the femur and the acetabulum of the hip bone; called also *a. coxofemoralis* [TA alternative], *coxofemoral articulation of Buisson, femoral* or *iliofemoral articulation,* and *coxal* or *hip joint;* loosely called *hip* or *coxa.*

**a. coxofemora'lis,** TA alternative for *a. coxae.*

**articulatio'nes cra'nii** [TA], cranial synovial joints: the temporomandibular joint and the atlanto-occipital joint.

**a. cricoarytenoi'dea** [TA], cricoarytenoid articulation: the synovial joint between the upper border of the cricoid cartilage and the base of the arytenoid cartilage.

**a. cricothyroi'dea** [TA], cricothyroid articulation: the articulation between the lateral aspect of the cricoid cartilage and the inferior horn of the thyroid cartilage.

**a. crurotala'ris,** a. talocruralis.

**a. cubita'lis,** a. cubiti.

**a. cu'biti** [TA], cubital articulation: the joint between the arm and forearm, comprising the humeroulnar, humeroradial, and proximal radioulnar articulations; called also *a. cubitalis, articulation of elbow,* and *cubital* or *elbow joint.*

**a. cuneocuboi'dea,** cuneocuboid articulation: the synovial joint between the lateral cuneiform bone and the cuboid bone.

**a. cuneonavicula'ris** [TA], cuneonavicular articulation: the joint between the anterior surface of the navicular bone and the proximal ends of the three cuneiform bones.

**a. ellipsoi'dea** [TA], ellipsoidal joint: a modification of the ball-and-socket type of synovial joint in which the articular surfaces are ellipsoid rather than spheroid; owing to the arrangement of the muscles and ligaments around the joint, all movements are permitted except rotation about a vertical axis. Called also *a. condylaris, condylar articulation,* and *condylar* or *condyloid joint.*

**a. fibro'sa,** junctura fibrosa.

**a. genua'lis,** a. genus.

**a. ge'nus** [TA], articulation of knee: the compound joint formed between the articular surface of the patella, the condyles and patellar surface of the femur, and the superior articular surface of the tibia; called also *a. genualis* and *knee joint.*

**a. glenohumera'lis,** TA alternative for *a. humeri.*

**a. hu'meri** [TA], articulation of shoulder: the joint formed by the head of the humerus and the glenoid cavity of the scapula; called also *a. capitis humeri, a. glenohumeralis* [TA alternative], *glenohumeral articulation, articulation of head of humerus, articulation of humerus,* and *humeral* or *shoulder joint.*

**a. humeroradia'lis** [TA], humeroradial articulation: the joint between the humerus and the radius; called also *brachioradial articulation.*

**a. humeroulna'ris** [TA], humeroulnar articulation: the joint between the humerus and the ulna; called also *brachioulnar articulation.*

**a. iliofemora'lis,** a. coxae.

**a. incudomallea'ris** [TA], **a. incudomalleola'ris,** incudomalleolar articulation: the junction of the incus and the malleus.

**a. incudostapedia'lis** [TA], incudostapedial articulation: the junction of the incus and the stapes.

**articulatio'nes intercarpa'les** [TA], **articulatio'nes intercar'peae,** intercarpal articulations: the joints between the bones, within each row, distal and proximal, of carpal bones. Called also *intercarpal joints.* See also *articulationes carpi.*

**articulatio'nes interchondra'les** [TA], interchondral articulations: the unions, on either side, between the costal cartilages of the upper false ribs, usually ribs seven through ten; called also *intercostal articulations.*

**articulatio'nes intercuneifor'mes** [TA], intercuneiform articulations: the synovial joints between the cuneiform bones.

**articulatio'nes intermetacarpa'les** [TA], **articulatio'nes intermetacar'peae,** intermetacarpal articulations: the joints formed between the adjoining bases of the second, third, fourth, and fifth metacarpal bones; called also *articulations of metacarpal bones.*

**articulatio'nes intermetatarsa'les** [TA], **articulatio'nes intermetatar'seae,** intermetatarsal articulations: the joints formed between the adjoining bases of the five metatarsal bones; called also *articulations of metatarsal bones.*

**articulatio'nes interphalan'geae ma'nus** [TA], **articulatio'nes interphalangea'les ma'nus,** interphalangeal articulations of hand: the hinge joints between the phalangeal articulations of the hand. Called also *digital joints of hand, phalangeal articulations or joints of hand,* and *interphalangeal articulations* or *joints of fingers.*

**articulatio'nes interphalan'geae pe'dis** [TA], **articulatio'nes interphalangea'les pe'dis,** interphalangeal articulations of foot: the hinge joints between the phalangeal articulations of the foot. Called also *digital joints of foot, phalangeal articulations* or *joints of foot,* and *interphalangeal articulations* or *joints of toes.*

**articulatio'nes intertarsa'les,** intertarsal articulations: the articulations between the various tarsal bones.

**a. lumbosacra'lis** [TA], lumbosacral articulation: the articulation between the sacrum and the lumbar vertebrae; called also *junctura lumbosacralis.*

**a. mandibula'ris,** a. temporomandibularis.

**articulatio'nes ma'nus** [TA], articulations of hand: the joints of the hand, including those of the wrist and the intercarpal, carpometacarpal, intermetacarpal, metacarpophalangeal, and interphalangeal articulations.

**a. mediocarpa'lis** [TA], **a. mediocar'pea,** mediocarpal articulation: the joint between the two rows, distal and proximal, of carpal bones. Called also *midcarpal joint.* See also *articulationes carpi.*

**articulatio'nes mem'bri inferio'ris li'beri** [TA], synovial joints of free lower limb: the synovial joints of the thigh, leg, and foot.

**articulatio'nes mem'bri superio'ris li'beri** [TA], synovial joints of free upper limb: the synovial joints of the arm, forearm, and hand.

**articulatio'nes metacarpophalan'geae** [TA], **articulatio'nes metacarpophalangea'les,** metacarpophalangeal articulations: joints formed between the heads of the five metacarpal bones and the bases of the corresponding proximal phalanges.

**articulatio'nes metatarsophalan'geae** [TA], **articulatio'nes metatarsophalangea'les,** metatarsophalangeal articulations: the joints formed between the heads of the five metatarsal bones and the bases of the corresponding proximal phalanges.

**articulatio'nes ossiculo'rum audi'tus** [TA], articulations of auditory ossicles, including *a. incudomallearis* and *a. incudostapedialis.*

**articulatio'nes ossiculo'rum auditorio'rum,** TA alternative for *articulationes ossiculorum auditus.*

**a. os'sis pisifor'mis** [TA], articulation of pisiform bone: the carpal joint formed by the pisiform and triquetral bones. Called also *pisotriquetral joint.*

**a. ovoida'lis,** a. sellaris.

**articulatio'nes pe'dis** [TA], articulations of foot: the joints of the foot, including the talocrural, intertarsal, tarsometatarsal, metatarsophalangeal, and interphalangeal articulations.

**a. pla'na** [TA], plane articulation: a type of synovial joint in which the opposed surfaces are flat or only slightly curved; it permits only simple gliding movement, in any direction, within narrow limits imposed by ligaments. Called also *arthrodia, gliding articulation, plane* or *gliding joint,* and *arthrodial joint.*

**a. radiocarpa'lis** [TA], **a. radiocar'pea,** radiocarpal articulation: a condylar joint formed by the radius and the articular disk with the scaphoid, lunate, and triquetral bones; called also *brachiocarpal articulation, radiocarpal joint, wrist,* and *wrist joint.*

**a. radioulna'ris,** syndesmosis radioulnaris.

**a. radioulna'ris dista'lis** [TA], distal radioulnar articulation: the joint formed by the head of the ulna and the ulnar notch of the radius; called also *inferior radioulnar articulation, inferior cubitoradial articulation,* and *distal radioulnar joint.*

**a. radioulna'ris proxima'lis** [TA], proximal radioulnar articulation: the proximal of the two joints between the radius and the ulna; it enters into pronation and supination of the forearm. Called also *superior radioulnar articulation, superior cubitoradial articulation,* and *proximal radioulnar joint.*

**a. sacrococcy'gea** [TA], sacrococcygeal articulation: the articulation between the coccyx and sacrum; called also *junctura sacrococcygea, sacrococcygeal symphysis,* and *symphysis sacrococcygea.*

**a. sacroili'aca** [TA], sacroiliac articulation: the joint formed between the auricular surfaces of the sacrum and ilium; called also *sacroiliac symphysis,* and *iliosacral articulation.*

**a. sella'ris** [TA], sellar or saddle joint: a type of synovial joint in which the articular surface of one bone is concave in one direction and convex in the direction at right angles to the first (concavoconvex), and the articular surface of the second bone is reciprocally convexoconcave; movement is possible along two main axes at right angles to each other. Called also *a. condylaris inversa, a. ovoidalis, ovoid articulation,* and *saddle articulation.*

**a. sim'plex** [TA], simple joint: a type of synovial joint in which only two bones are involved.

**a. spheroi'dea** [TA], spheroidal joint: a type of synovial joint in which a spheroidal surface on one bone ("ball") moves within a concavity ("socket") on the other bone; it is the most movable type of joint. Called also *ball-and-socket articulation* or *joint, spheroidal articulation, multiaxial* or *polyaxial joint,* and *enarthrodial joint.*

**a. sternoclavicula'ris** [TA], sternoclavicular articulation: the joint formed by the sternal extremity of the clavicle, the clavicular notch of the manubrium of the sternum, and the first costal cartilage.

**articulatio'nes sternocosta'les** [TA], sternocostal articulations: the joints between the costal notches of the sternum and the medial ends of the costal cartilages of the upper seven ribs; called also *costosternal* or *chondrosternal articulations.*

**a. subtala'ris** [TA], subtalar articulation: the joint formed between the posterior calcaneal articular surface of the talus and the posterior articular surface of the calcaneus; called also *a. talocalcanea, subtalar joint,* and *talocalcaneal joint.*

**a. synovia'lis,** junctura synovialis.

**articulatio'nes cra'nii** [TA], **articulatio'nes synovia'les cra'nii,** synovial articulations of cranium: the temporomandibular and atlanto-occipital articulations.

**a. talocalca'nea,** TA alternative for *a. subtalaris.*

**a. talocalcaneonavicula'ris** [TA], talocalcaneonavicular articulation: a joint formed by the head of the talus, the anterior articular surface of the calcaneus, the plantar calcaneonavicular ligament, and the posterior surface of the navicular bone.

**a. talocrura'lis** [TA], talocrural articulation: the ankle joint, formed by the inferior articular and malleolar articular surfaces of the tibia, the malleolar articular surface of the fibula, and the medial malleolar, lateral malleolar, and superior surfaces of the talus; called also *ankle, ankle joint, a. crurotalaris, crurotalar articulation,* and *talocrural joint.*

**a. talonavicula'ris,** talonavicular articulation: the junction between the talus and navicular bone.

**a. tar'si transver'sa** [TA], **a. tar'si transver'sa [Choparti],** transverse tarsal articulation: a joint comprising the articulation of the calcaneus and the cuboid bone and the articulation of the talus and the navicular bone. Called also *a. tarsi transversa* [*Choparti*], *transverse tarsal joint,* and *Chopart's articulation* or *joint.*

**articulatio'nes tarsometatarsa'les** [TA], **articulatio'nes tarsometatar'seae,** tarsometatarsal articulations: joints formed by the cuneiform and cuboid bones together with the bases of the metatarsal bones; called also *Lisfranc's joints* and *tarsometatarsal joints.*

**a. temporomandibula'ris** [TA], temporomandibular joint: a bicondylar joint formed by the head of the mandible and the mandibular fossa, and the articular tubercle of the temporal bone; called also *a. mandibularis, temporomandibular* or *temporomaxillary articulation,* and *mandibular articulation* or *joint.*

**articulatio'nes tho'racis** [TA], thoracic synovial joints: the costovertebral, costotransverse, sternocostal, costochondral, and interchondral articulations and the joints of the heads of ribs.

**a. tibiofibula'ris** [TA], 1. tibiofibular articulation: a plane joint between the lateral condyle of the tibia and the head of the fibula. Called also *proximal tibiofibular joint* and *superior tibiofibular articulation* or *joint* 2. syndesmosis tibiofibularis.

**a. trochoi'dea** [TA], trochoidal joint: a type of synovial joint that allows a rotary motion in but one plane; a pivot-like process turns within a ring, or a ring turns on a pivot. Called also *pivot articulation* or *joint.*

**articulatio'nes vertebra'les,** articulationes columnae vertebralis.

**articulatio'nes zygapophysia'les** [TA], zygapophyseal articulations: the articulations between the articular processes of the vertebrae (zygapophyses); called also *zygapophyseal joints* and *juncturae zygapophyseales.*

---

**ar·tic·u·la·tion** (ahr-tik″u-la'shən) [L. *articulatio*] 1. articulatio. 2. the forming of speech sounds. 3. in dentistry: *(a)* the contact relationship of the occlusal surfaces of the teeth while in action; *(b)* the arrangement of artificial teeth so as to accommodate the various positions of the mouth and to serve the purpose of the natural teeth which they are to replace.

**acromioclavicular a.,** articulatio acromioclavicularis.

**articulator a.,** the use of a mechanical device that simulates the movements of the temporomandibular joint, permitting the orientation of casts in a manner duplicating or simulating various positions or movements of the mandible.

**atlantoaxial a., lateral,** articulatio atlantoaxialis lateralis.

**atlantoaxial a., medial,** articulatio atlantoaxialis mediana.

**atlantoepistrophic a.,** see *articulatio atlantoaxialis lateralis* and *articulatio atlantoaxialis mediana.*

**atlantooccipital a.,** articulatio atlantooccipitalis.

**a's of auditory ossicles,** articulationes ossiculorum auditoriorum.

**balanced a.,** the simultaneous contact between the upper and lower teeth as they glide over each other when the mandible is moved from centric relation to the various eccentric relations and back to centric relation again.

**ball-and-socket a.,** articulatio spheroidea.

**bicondylar a.,** articulatio bicondylaris.

**brachiocarpal a.,** articulatio radiocarpalis.

**brachioradial a.,** articulatio humeroradialis.

**brachioulnar a.,** articulatio humero-ulnaris.

**calcaneocuboid a.,** articulatio calcaneocuboidea.

**capitular a.,** articulatio capitis costae.

**carpal a's,** 1. articulationes carpi. 2. see *articulationes intercarpales.*

**carpometacarpal a's,** articulationes carpometacarpales.

**carpometacarpal a., first, carpometacarpal a. of thumb,** articulatio carpometacarpalis pollicis.

**chondrosternal a's,** articulationes sternocostales.

**Chopart's a.,** articulatio tarsi transversa.

**composite a.,** articulatio composita.

**compound a.,** articulatio composita.

**condylar a.,** articulatio ellipsoidea.

**confluent a.,** a manner of speaking in which the syllables are run together.

**costocentral a.,** articulatio capitis costae.

**costosternal a's,** articulationes sternocostales.

**costotransverse a.,** articulatio costotransversaria.

**costovertebral a's,** articulationes costovertebrales.

**coxofemoral a. of Buisson,** articulatio coxae.

**craniovertebral a.,** articulatio atlanto-occipitalis.

**cricoarytenoid a.,** articulatio crico-arytenoidea.

**cricothyroid a.,** articulatio cricothyroidea.

**crurotalar a.,** articulatio crurotalaris.

**cubital a.,** articulatio cubiti.

**cubitoradial a., inferior,** articulatio radioulnaris distalis.

**cubitoradial a., superior,** articulatio radioulnaris proximalis.

**cuneocuboid a.,** articulatio cuneocuboidea.

**cuneonavicular a.,** articulatio cuneonavicularis.

**dentoalveolar a.,** syndesmosis dentoalveolaris.

**a's of digits of foot,** articulationes interphalangeae pedis.

**a's of digits of hand,** articulationes interphalangeae manus.

**a. of elbow,** articulatio cubiti.

**ellipsoidal a.,** articulatio ellipsoidea.

**femoral a.,** articulatio coxae.

**fibrous a.,** junctura fibrosa.

**glenohumeral a.,** articulatio humeri.

**gliding a.,** articulatio plana.

**a's of hand,** articulationes manus.

**a. of head of humerus,** articulatio humeri.

**a. of head of rib,** articulatio capitis costae.

**a. of hip,** articulatio coxae.

**humeroradial a.,** articulatio humeroradialis.

**humeroulnar a.,** articulatio humeroulnaris.

**a. of humerus,** articulatio humeri.

**iliofemoral a.,** articulatio coxae.

**iliosacral a.,** articulatio sacroiliaca.

**incudomalleolar a.,** articulatio incudomallearis.

**incudostapedial a.,** articulatio incudostapedialis.

**intercarpal a's,** 1. articulationes intercarpales. 2. See *articulationes carpi.*

**interchondral a's,** articulationes interchondrales.

**intercostal a's,** articulationes interchondrales.

**intercuneiform a's,** articulationes intercuneiformes.

**intermetacarpal a's,** articulationes intermetacarpales.

**intermetatarsal a's,** articulationes intermetatarsales.

**interphalangeal a's of fingers,** articulationes interphalangeales manus.

**interphalangeal a's of foot,** articulationes interphalangeales pedis.

**interphalangeal a's of hand,** articulationes interphalangeales manus.

**interphalangeal a's of toes,** articulationes interphalangeales pedis.

**intertarsal a's,** articulationes intertarsales.

**a. of knee,** articulatio genus.

**laryngeal a's,** see *cartilagines et articulationes laryngeales.*

**lumbosacral a.,** articulatio lumbosacralis.

**mandibular a.,** articulatio temporomandibularis.

**manubriosternal a.,** see *symphysis manubriosternalis* and *synchondrosis manubriosternalis.*

**maxillary a.,** articulatio temporomandibularis.

**mediocarpal a.,** articulatio mediocarpalis.

**a's of metacarpal bones,** articulationes intermetacarpales.

**metacarpocarpal a's,** articulationes carpometacarpales.

**metacarpophalangeal a's,** articulationes metacarpophalangeales.

**a's of metatarsal bones,** articulationes intermetatarsales.

**metatarsophalangeal a's,** articulationes metatarsophalangeales.

**occipital a., occipitoatlantal a.,** articulatio atlantooccipitalis.

**ovoid a.,** articulatio sellaris.

**patellofemoral a.,** the joint between the articular surface of the patella and the patellar surface of the femur.

**petrooccipital a.,** synchondrosis petrooccipitalis.

**phalangeal a's,** see *articulationes interphalangeales manus* and *articulationes interphalangeales pedis.*
**a. of pisiform bone,** articulatio ossis pisiformis.
**pisocuneiform a.,** articulatio ossis pisiformis.
**pivot a.,** articulatio trochoidea.
**plane a.,** articulatio plana.
**a. of pubis,** symphysis pubica.
**radiocarpal a.,** articulatio radiocarpalis.
**radioulnar a.,** syndesmosis radioulnaris.
**radioulnar a., distal, radioulnar a., inferior,** articulatio radioulnaris distalis.
**radioulnar a., proximal, radioulnar a., superior,** articulatio radioulnaris proximalis.
**sacrococcygeal a.,** articulatio sacrococcygea.
**sacroiliac a.,** articulatio sacroiliaca.
**saddle a.,** articulatio sellaris.
**scapuloclavicular a.,** articulatio acromioclavicularis.
**a. of shoulder,** articulatio humeri.
**simple a.,** articulatio simplex.
**spheroidal a.,** articulatio spheroidea.
**sternoclavicular a.,** articulatio sternoclavicularis.
**sternocostal a's,** articulationes sternocostales.
**subtalar a.,** articulatio subtalaris.
**synovial a.,** junctura synovialis.
**synovial a's of cranium,** articulationes synoviales cranii.
**talocalcaneonavicular a.,** articulatio talocalcaneonavicularis.
**talocrural a.,** articulatio talocruralis.
**talonavicular a.,** articulatio talonavicularis.
**tarsometatarsal a's,** articulationes tarsometatarsales.
**temporomandibular a., temporomaxillary a.,** articulatio temporomandibularis.
**a's of thorax,** articulationes thoracis.
**tibiofibular a.,** 1. articulatio tibiofibularis (def. 1). 2. syndesmosis tibiofibularis
**tibiofibular a., inferior,** syndesmosis tibiofibularis.
**tibiofibular a., superior,** articulatio tibiofibularis (def. 1).
**a's of toes,** articulationes interphalangeae pedis.
**transverse tarsal a.,** articulatio tarsi transversa.
**trochoidal a.,** articulatio trochoidea.
**a. of tubercle of rib,** articulatio costotransversaria.
**zygapophyseal a's,** articulationes zygapophysiales.

**ar·tic·u·la·ti·o·nes** (ahr-tik″u-la″she-o′nēz) [L.] plural of *articulatio.*

**ar·tic·u·la·tor** (ahr-tik′u-la″tər) [MeSH: Dental Articulators] 1. a device for effecting a jointlike union. 2. dental a.
**adjustable a.,** 1. a dental articulator that can be adjusted to permit movement of the casts into recorded eccentric relationships. 2. a dental articulator capable of adjustment to more than one eccentric position.
**dental a.,** a mechanical device that represents the temporomandibular joint and jaws and simulates jaw movements, and to which maxillary and mandibular dental casts may be attached. It is used for the mounting of dental casts for diagnosis, treatment planning, and patient presentation; fabrications of occlusal surfaces for dental restorations; and arrangement of teeth for complete and partial dentures. There are four groups or classes: those of *Class I* accept a single interocclusal record and vertical motion may or may not be possible; those of *Class II* permit horizontal and vertical motion but do not orient the motion to the temporomandibular joint through a face-bow transfer; those of *Class III* simulate condylar pathways by using an average or mechanical equivalent for all or part of the motion and allow orientation of the casts to the temporomandibular joint through a face-bow transfer; and those of *Class IV* accept three-dimensional dynamic registrations and allow orientation of the casts to the temporomandibular joint through a face-bow transfer.
**semiadjustable a.,** a dental articulator that can be adjusted so that one movement conforms with a mandibular movement.

**ar·tic·u·la·to·ry** (ahr-tik′u-lə″to-re) pertaining to utterance.

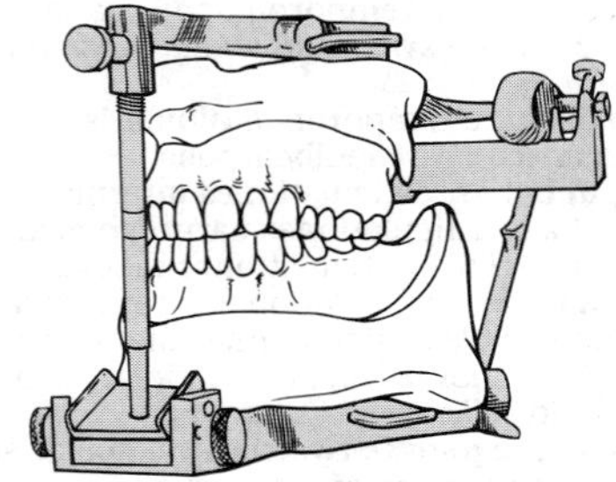

Dental articulator with wax-up of dentures.

**ar·tic·u·lo** (ahr-tik′u-lo) [L., ablative of *articulus,* q.v.] at the moment or crisis of.
**a. mor′tis,** at the moment or point of death.

**ar·tic·u·lus** (ahr-tik′u-ləs) pl. *articuli* [L.] a joint.

**ar·ti·fact** (ahr′tĭ-fakt″) [L. *ars* art + *factum* made] [MeSH: Artifacts] any artificial product. In histology or microscopy, any structure or feature that has been introduced by processing a tissue. In radiology, a substance or structure not naturally present in living tissue, but of which an authentic image appears in a radiograph.
**aliasing a.,** aliasing, def. 3.
**wraparound a.,** aliasing, def. 3.

**ar·ti·fac·ti·tious** (ahr′tĭ-fak-tish′əs) having the character of an artifact.

**ar·ti·fi·cial** (ahr″tĭ-fish′əl) [L. *ars* art + *facere* to make] made by art; not natural or pathological.

**Ar·tio·dac·ty·la** (ahr″te-o-dak′tə-lə) [Gr. *artios* even + *daktylos* finger] [MeSH: Artiodactyla] an order of mammals, the ungulates with an even number of toes, including ruminants, pigs, deer, and antelopes. Cf. *Perissodactyla.*

**ar·tio·dac·ty·lous** (ahr″te-o-dak′tə-ləs) 1. having an even number of digits on the hands or feet. 2. pertaining to Artiodactyla.

**Ar·ty·fech·i·nos·to·mum** (ahr-tə-fek″ĭ-nos′tə-məm) *Paryphostomum.*

**ARVO** Association for Research in Vision and Ophthalmology.

**ary·ep·i·glot·tic** (ar″e-ep″ĭ-glot′ik) arytenoepiglottic.

**ary·ep·i·glot·ti·cus** (ar″e-ep″ĭ-glot′ĭ-kəs) see under *musculus.*

**ary·ep·i·glot·tid·e·an** (ar″e-ep″ĭ-glo-tid′e-ən) arytenoepiglottic.

**aryl-** a chemical prefix indicating a radical derived from an aromatic compound by removal of a hydrogen atom.

**ar·yl·amine** (ar″əl-ə-mēn′) any of a group of amines in which one or more of the hydrogen atoms are replaced by aromatic groups. Some are poisonous or carcinogenic, such as *p*-aminobiphenyl, the anilines, benzidine, and naphthylamine.

**ar·yl·ar·son·ic ac·id** (ar″il-ahr-son′ik) an arsonic acid in which the —$AsO(OH)_2$ functional group is bonded to an aryl radical.

**ar·yl·es·ter·ase** (ar″əl-es′tər-ās) [EC 3.1.1.2] an enzyme of the hydrolase class that catalyzes the hydrolytic cleavage of the ester group from a variety of esterified phenols. The enzyme occurs in normal serum.

**ar·yl·for·mam·i·dase** (ar″əl-for-mam′ĭ-dās) [EC 3.5.1.9] [MeSH: Arylformamidase] an enzyme of the hydrolase class that catalyzes the cleavage of formylkynurenine to formate and kynurenine, a step in the catabolism of tryptophan. The enzyme also acts on other formyl aromatic amines.

**ar·yl·sul·fa·tase** (ar″əl-sul′fə-tās) [EC 3.1.6.1] any of a group of enzymes of the hydrolase class that catalyze the cleavage of sulfate residues from sulfate esters; physiological substrates are generally sulfolipids or sulfated polysaccharides, while in vitro substrates include aryl or alkyl sulfates. Called also *sulfatase.*
**a. A,** cerebroside-sulfatase.
**a. B,** *N*-acetylgalactosamine-4-sulfatase.
**a. C,** an arylsulfatase believed to be identical to steryl-sulfatase.

**ar·yl·sul·fa·tase A de·fi·cien·cy** metachromatic leukodystrophy.

**ar·yl·sul·fa·tase B deficiency** (ar″əl-sul′fə-tās) Maroteaux-Lamy syndrome.

**ar·y·te·no·ep·i·glot·tic** (ar-it″ə-no-ep″ĭ-glot′ik) [Gr. *arytaina* ladle + *epiglottis*] pertaining to the arytenoid cartilage and to the epiglottis.

**ar·y·te·noid** (ar″ə-te′noid) [Gr. *arytaina* ladle + *-oid*] shaped like a jug or pitcher, as arytenoid cartilage.

**ar·y·te·noid·ec·to·my** (ar″ə-te″noid-ek′tə-me) [*arytenoid* + *-ectomy*] surgical removal of an arytenoid cartilage.

**ar·y·te·noi·de·us** (ar″ə-te-noi′de-əs) [L.] see *musculus arytenoideus obliquus* and *transversus.*

**ar·y·te·noi·di·tis** (ar-ə-te″-noi-di′tis) inflammation of the arytenoid cartilage or muscles.

**ar·y·te·noi·do·pexy** (ar″ə-te-noi′do-pek″se) [*arytenoid* + *-pexy*] surgical fixation of arytenoid cartilage or muscle.

**AS** aortic stenosis; arteriosclerosis; [L.] *au′ris sinis′tra,* left ear.

**As** symbol for *arsenic;* abbreviation for *astigmatism.*

**ASA** American Society of Anesthesiologists; American Standards Association; American Surgical Association; acetylsalicylic acid; argininosuccinic acid.

**asa·cria** (ə-sa′kre-ə) congenital absence of the sacrum.

**as·a·fet·i·da** (as″ə-fet′ĭ-də) the oleo-gum-resin obtained from the roots of *Ferula asafoetida* L. and other related species of Umbelliferae; the main odorous principle is isobutylpropanyldisulfide. Used in India, Iran, and elsewhere as a condiment and food flavoring, and formerly used as an animal repellent in veterinary medicine to prevent bandage chewing, and as a carminative, expectorant, and antispasmodic both in humans and animals.

**as•a•ron** (as'ə-ron) a camphorlike aromatic principle found in *Asarum europaeum*.

**As•a•rum** (as'ə-rəm) [Gr. *asaron*] the snakeroots, a genus of herbs found in temperate regions. *A. europae'um* L. yields asaron. *A. canaden'se* L. (Canadian snakeroot or wild ginger) yields from its dried roots and rhizomes an acrid resin, methyl eugenol, and an aromatic volatile oil.

**ASAS** American Society of Abdominal Surgeons.

**ASAT** aspartate aminotransferase; see *aspartate transaminase*.

**ASB** American Society of Bacteriologists.

**as•bes•ti•form** (as-bes'tĭ-form) having a fibrous structure like asbestos.

**as•bes•tos** (as-bes'təs) [Gr. *asbestos* unquenchable] [MeSH: Asbestos] any of several fibrous, incombustible materials, forms of magnesium and calcium silicate, used as thermal insulation; the two major types are *amphibole a.* and *serpentine a.* Its dust causes asbestosis and acts as an epigenetic carcinogen for pleural mesothelioma and possibly bronchogenic carcinoma.
**amphibole a.,** one of the two major classes of asbestos, characterized by fibers too brittle to be spun but more resistant to chemicals and heat than the serpentine form. It is less widely used than serpentine asbestos and is thought to be much more carcinogenic. The group includes amosite and crocidolite.
**blue a.,** crocidolite.
**brown a.,** amosite.
**chrysotile a.,** chrysotile.
**crocidolite a.,** crocidolite.
**serpentine a.,** one of the two major classes of asbestos, characterized by strong, flexible fibers that can be spun; it includes chrysotile.
**white a.,** chrysotile.

**as•bes•to•sis** (as″bes-to'sis) [*asbestos* + *-osis*] [MeSH: Asbestosis] a form of pneumoconiosis (silicatosis) caused by inhaling fibers of asbestos, marked by interstitial fibrosis of the lung varying in extent from minor involvement of the basal areas to extensive scarring; it is associated with pleural mesothelioma and bronchogenic carcinoma.

**As•bron G** (az'bron) trademark for a preparation of theophylline sodium glycinate and guaifenesin.

**A-scan** see under *scan*.

**as•ca•ri•a•sis** (as″kə-ri'ə-sis) [*ascaris* + *-iasis*] [MeSH: Ascariasis] 1. human infection by the roundworm *Ascaris lumbricoides*, which is found in the small intestine, causing colicky pains and diarrhea, especially in children. On ingestion, the larvae migrate from the intestine to the lungs, where they cause a pneumonitis, and then to the trachea, esophagus, and intestine, where they mature. If adult worms are present in sufficient number, they may cause intestinal obstruction. 2. infection of humans or other animals, usually in the intestine, liver, or lungs, by any member of the family Ascarididae.
**pulmonary a.,** *Ascaris* pneumonitis.

**as•car•i•cid•al** (as-kar″ĭ-si'dəl) destructive to intestinal parasites of the genus *Ascaris*.

**as•car•i•cide** (as-kar'ĭ-sīd″) [*ascaris* + *-cide*] an agent that destroys worms of the genus *Ascaris*.

**as•ca•rid** (as'kə-rid) any member of the superfamily Ascaridoidea.

**as•car•i•des** (as-kar'ĭ-dēz) plural of *ascaris*.

**As•ca•rid•ia** (as″kə-rid'e-ə) [MeSH: Ascaridia] a genus of nematode parasites of the superfamily Ascaridoidea. *A. gal'li* is parasitic in the large intestines of chickens and other birds, causing enteritis and diarrhea. *A. linea'ta* is a common roundworm parasitizing the small intestines of birds in the United States.

**as•ca•ri•di•a•sis** (as″kə-rĭ-di'ə-sis) [MeSH: Ascaridiasis] ascariasis.

**As•ca•ri•di•dae** (as-kə-rid'ĭ-de) a family of nematodes that includes the genera *Ascaris, Parascaris, Toxascaris,* and *Toxocara*. Many species are intestinal parasites in mammals, including humans.

**As•ca•ri•doi•dea** (as″kə-rĭ-doi'de-ə) [MeSH: Ascaridoidea] a superfamily of phasmid nematodes, including the families Ascarididae and Heterakidae.

**as•ca•ri•do•sis** (as″kə-rĭ-do'sis) ascariasis.

**As•ca•ris** (as'kə-ris) [L.; Gr. *askaris*] [MeSH: Ascaris] a genus of large intestinal nematode parasites of the family Ascarididae.
**A. e'qui, A. equo'rum,** *Parascaris equorum*.
**A. lumbricoi'des,** a species parasitic in humans and occasionally pigs; it is found in the small intestine and lungs. See also *ascariasis* and *Ascaris pneumonitis*.

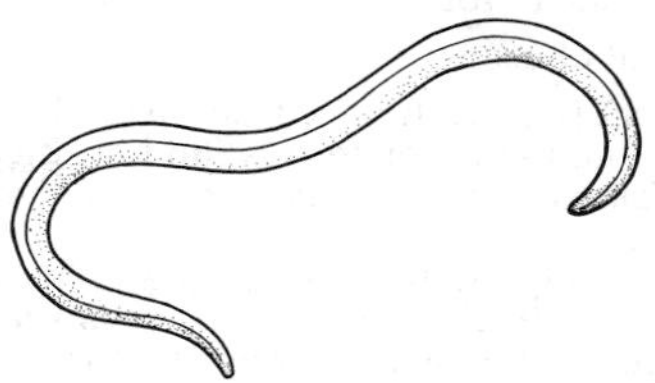

*Ascaris lumbricoides.*

**A. megaloce'phala,** *Parascaris equorum*.
**A. o'vis,** A. lumbricoides.
**A. su'is, A. suil'la, A. su'um,** a species closely related to *A. lumbricoides*, usually found in pigs although it has also been reported in humans.
**A. vermicula'ris,** see *Enterobius vermicularis*.
**A. vitulo'rum,** a species found in cattle and the Indian buffalo.

**as•ca•ris** (as'kə-ris) pl. *ascar'ides* [MeSH: Ascaris] a worm of the genus *Ascaris*.

**As•ca•rops** (as'kə-rops) a genus of parasitic nematodes of the superfamily Spiruroidea. *A. strongyli'na* is a small red blood-sucking species found in the stomachs of pigs.

**as•cend•ing** (ə-send'ing) having an upward course.

**as•cer•tain•ment** (ă″sər-tān'mənt) in genetic studies, the method by which persons with a trait or disease are selected or found by an investigator.
**complete a.,** the method in which families for study are selected through affected parents, and all their offspring are included.
**incomplete a.,** ascertainment in which only those sibships with at least one affected sib are identified; this is far more common than complete ascertainment.
**multiple a.,** a type of incomplete ascertainment in which some sibships are counted more than once because they have more than one affected member; multiplex families (those with more than one affected member) have a higher chance of being ascertained than simplex families.
**single a.,** a type of incomplete ascertainment in which there is no chance that any one sibship will be ascertained more than once; thus there is only one proband in each sibship, and the change that a sibship will be ascertained is proportional to the number of its affected members.
**truncate a.,** a type of incomplete ascertainment in which any sibship in which there is no affected member is not ascertained.

**as•cet•i•cism** (ə-set'ĭ-siz-əm) a way of life or character trait described by the elimination of pleasurable effects associated with experiences and characterized by renunciation, self-denial, withdrawal from society, and sometimes dedication to an unattainable ideal or to eradication of some specific evil.

**ASCH** American Society of Clinical Hypnosis.

**Asch's forceps, operation, splint** (ash'əs) [Morris Joseph *Asch*, American laryngologist, 1833–1902] see under *forceps, operation,* and *splint*.

**asc•hel•minth** (ask'həl-minth) any worm of the phylum Aschelminthes.

**Asc•hel•min•thes** (ask″həl-minth'ēz) a phylum of unsegmented, bilaterally symmetrical, pseudocoelomate, mostly vermiform animals whose bodies are almost entirely covered with a cuticle, and possess a complete digestive tract lacking definite muscular walls. It includes the classes Gastrotricha, Kinorhyncha, Nematoda, Nematomorpha, and Rotifera.

**Asch•er's negative glass-rod phenomenon, positive glass-rod phenomenon, syndrome** (ahsh'ərz) [Karl Wolfgang *Ascher*, Czech-born American ophthalmologist, 1887–1971] see *blood-influx phenomenon* and *aqueous-influx phenomenon*, under *phenomenon*, and see under *syndrome*.

**Asch•er•son's membrane** (ahsh'ər-sənz) [Ferdinand Moritz *Ascherson*, German physician, 1798–1879] see under *membrane*.

**Asch•heim-Zon•dek test** (ahsh'hīm tson'dək) [Selmar *Aschheim*, German gynecologist, 1878–1965; Bernhardt *Zondek*, German gynecologist, 1891–1966] see under *test*.

**Asch•ner's reflex (phenomenon)** (ahsh'nərz) [Bernhard *Aschner*, Austrian gynecologist, 1883–1960] oculocardiac reflex.

**Asch•off's bodies (nodules), cell, node** (ahsh'ofs) [Karl Albert Ludwig *Aschoff*, German pathologist, 1866–1942] see under *body* and *cell*, and see *nodus atrioventricularis*.

**Asch•off-Ta•wa•ra node** (ahsh'of tah-wah'rah) [K. A. L. *Aschoff*; K.

Sunao *Tawara,* Japanese pathologist, 1873–1938] nodus atrioventricularis.

**ASCI** American Society for Clinical Investigation.

**as·ci** (as'i) plural of *ascus.*

**as·ci·tes** (ə-si'tēz) [L.; Gr. *askitēs,* from *askos* bag] [MeSH: Ascites] effusion and accumulation of serous fluid in the abdominal cavity; called also *abdominal* or *peritoneal dropsy, hydroperitonia,* and *hydrops abdominis.*
**a. adipo'sus,** a variety characterized by a milky appearance of the contained fluid, due to the presence of cells that have undergone fatty degeneration; called also *fatty* or *milky a.*
**bile a.,** choleperitoneum.
**bloody a.,** hemorrhagic a.
**chyliform a., a. chylo'sus, chylous a.,** the presence of chyle in the peritoneal cavity as a result of anomalies, injuries, or obstruction of the thoracic duct.
**exudative a.,** ascites in which the fluid in the peritoneal cavity is an exudate.
**fatty a.,** a. adiposus.
**hemorrhagic a.,** that in which the fluid is mixed with blood.
**hydremic a.,** that which is associated with, or due to, a watery state of the blood, as in severe malnutrition.
**milky a.,** a. adiposus.
**a. prae'cox,** ascites that develops prior to edema in constrictive pericarditis.
**preagonal a.,** a flow of serum into the peritoneal cavity just before death.
**pseudochylous a.,** ascites in which the contained fluid resembles chyle in appearance but does not contain fatty matter.
**transudative a.,** ascites in which the fluid in the peritoneal cavity is a transudate.

**as·cit·ic** (ə-sit'ik) pertaining to or characterized by ascites.

**as·ci·tog·e·nous** (as"ī-toj'ə-nəs) causing ascites.

**As·cle·pi·a·des of Bithynia** (as"klə-pi'ə-dēz) [124–c. 40 B.C.] a Greek physician born in Prusa in Bithynia (southwest coast of the Black Sea), who studied at Alexandria and taught and practiced in Rome after 91 B.C. An Epicurean, he opposed humoralism and introduced into medicine Democritus' atomic theory, according to which inharmonious or irregular movement of atoms causes disease, which one cures by restoring harmony. Asclepiades' methods included diet, friction, bathing, exercise, emetics, and blood-letting. His influence continued (through the Methodical School, founded by his students) until Galen began to practice in A.D. 164. Asclepiades established humane treatment for the mentally ill and made Greek medicine honorable in Rome through his own good character. See also *Democritus.*

**as·cle·pi·a·din** (as"klə-pi'ə-din) a toxic bitter principle found in species of *Asclepias.*

**As·cle·pi·as** (as-kle'pe-əs) [L.] the milkweeds or swallow-worts, a genus of herbs of the family Umbelliferae. Most species are poisonous to animals, containing asclepiadin, volatile oils, cardiac glycosides, or toxic resins. Some species, such as *A. tubero'sa* (pleurisy root), have medicinal qualities.

**as·cle·pi·on** (as-kle'pe-on) pl. *asclepia* [Gr. *Asklēpieion* temple of Asklepios (Æsculapius)] one of the early Greek temples of healing, the most celebrated of which were at Cos, Epidaurus, Cnidus, and Pergamos. See also *Aesculapius.*

**As·clep·i·os** (as-klep'e-os) Aesculapius.

**ASCLT** American Society of Clinical Laboratory Technicians.

**ASCO** American Society of Clinical Oncology; American Society of Contemporary Ophthalmology.

**As·co·bo·la·ceae** (as"ko-bo-la'se-e) a family of coprophilic fungi of the order Pezizales; it includes the genus *Ascobolus.*

**As·cob·o·lus** (as-kob'ə-lus) [*ascus* + *bolus*] a genus of fungi of the family Ascobolaceae that eject their sporangia forcefully; used in genetic studies of crossing over.

**as·co·carp** (as'ko-kahrp) [Gr. *askos* bag + *carp*] the fruiting body of an ascomycetous fungus, including the asci and ascospores. Types include *apothecium, cleistothecium, gymnothecium,* and *perithecium.* Called also *ascoma.*

**as·co·gen·ous** (as-koj'ə-nəs) producing asci; said of hyphae.

**as·co·go·ni·um** (as"ko-go'ne-əm) the receiving (female) organ in ascomycetous fungi which, after fertilization, gives rise to ascogenous hyphae and later to asci and ascospores. Called also *carpogonium* and, in British usage, *archicarp.*

**as·co·ma** (as-ko'mə) pl. *asco'mata* [Gr. *askōma* the leather padding that protected the opening for the oar] ascocarp.

**as·co·my·cete** (as"ko-mi'sə-te) any individual fungus of the Ascomycotina.

**As·co·my·ce·tes** (as"ko-mi-se'tēz) [MeSH: Ascomycetes] name given to Ascomycotina when it is considered a class and placed within the phylum Eumycota.

**as·co·my·ce·tous** (as"ko-mi-se'təs) of or pertaining to the Ascomycotina.

**As·co·my·co·ta** (as"ko-mi-ko'tə) name given to Ascomycotina when it is considered a separate phylum.

**As·co·my·co·ti·na** (as"ko-mi"ko-ti'nə) [Gr. *askos* bag + *mykēs* fungus] the sac fungi, a subphylum of perfect fungi variously grouped under either Dikaryomycota or Eumycota, characterized by the formation of an ascus in which sexual spores (ascospores) are produced; it includes the yeasts, mildews, and cheese, jelly, and fruit molds. Some authorities consider this group a class and call it Ascomycetes, whereas others consider it a separate phylum and call it Ascomycota. A number of different classifications of fungi within this group have been proposed.

**ascor·bate** (ə-skor'bāt) a compound or derivative of ascorbic acid.

**as·cor·be·mia** (as"kor-be'me-ə) the presence of ascorbic acid in the blood.

**ascor·bic ac·id** (ə-skor'bik) [MeSH: Ascorbic Acid] 1. vitamin C; a water-soluble vitamin found in many fruits and vegetables. Ascorbic acid is required for the optimal function of a number of enzymes; deficiency causes scurvy and poor wound repair. Called also *cevitamic acid.* 2. [USP] a preparation of ascorbic acid used as an antiscorbutic and nutritional supplement, as an adjunct to improve absorption in the treatment of iron deficiency anemia and to improve chelation during deferoxamine therapy for chronic iron toxicity, and for the treatment of methemoglobinemia; administered orally or by intravenous or intramuscular injection. Ascorbic acid is also used as an adjunct in the sodium chromate Cr 51 labeling of red blood cells.

**as·corb·uria** (as"korb-u're-ə) the presence of ascorbic acid in the urine.

**ascor·byl pal·mi·tate** (ə-skor'bəl) [NF] an antioxidant used as a preservative in pharmaceutical preparations.

**as·co·spore** (as'ko-spor) [Gr. *askos* bag + *spore*] a sexual spore formed within a special sac, or ascus, as in ascomycetous fungi.

**ASCP** American Society of Clinical Pathologists.

**as·cus** (as'kəs) pl. *as'ci* [Gr. *askos* bag] the sporangium or spore case of certain lichens and fungi, consisting of a single terminal cell. See *Ascomycotina.*
**bitunicate a.,** a cylindrical ascus whose wall has two layers; at maturity, the outer layer splits and the inner layer expands during expulsion of spores. See also *Bitunicatae.*
**prototunicate a.,** a type of ascus that is more or less spherical (as opposed to cylindrical) and has a thin wall that ruptures or disintegrates at maturity to release spores. See also *Prototunicatae.*
**unitunicate a.,** a cylindrical ascus whose wall has a single layer. There are two types: the *operculate* type has a small cap at the end of the ascus,which pops open when the mature organism is ready to eject its spores; and the *inoperculate* type has no cap and ejects its spores through a pore or slit that momentarily opens. See also *Unitunicatae.*

**ASCVD** arteriosclerotic cardiovascular disease.

**-ase** a word termination used in forming the names of enzymes, ordinarily affixed to a stem that indicates the substrate, the type of reaction catalyzed, or a combination of these factors.

**ase·cre·to·ry** (a-se'krə-to"re) without secretion.

**Asel·li's pancreas (glands)** (ə-sel'ēz) [Gasparo *Aselli* (or Gaspare Asellio, or Gaspar Asellius), Italian anatomist, 1581–1626] see under *pancreas.*

**Asel·lio** (ə-sel'e-o), **Asel·li·us** (ə-sel'e-us) see *Aselli.*

**as·e·ma·sia** (as"ə-ma'zhə) [*a-*[1] + Gr. *sēmasia* the giving of a signal] asemia.

**ase·mia** (a-se'me-ə) [*a-*[1] + Gr. *sēma* sign + *-ia*] aphasia with inability to employ or to understand either speech or signs. Called also *asemasia* and *asymbolia.*

**Asen·din** (ə-sen'din) trademark for a preparation of amoxapine.

**asep·sis** (a-sep'sis) [*a-*[1] + *sepsis*] [MeSH: Asepsis] 1. freedom from infection. 2. prevention of contact with microorganisms; see also *aseptic techniques,* under *technique.* Defs. 1 and 2 called also *sterility.*

**asep·tic** (a-sep'tik) [*a-*[1] + Gr. *sēpsis* decay] free from infection or septic material; called also *sterile.*
**a.-antiseptic,** both aseptic and antiseptic.

**asep·ti·cism** (a-sep'tĭ-siz-əm) the principles and practices of aseptic techniques.

**as·e·ta·ke** (as"e-tak'e) any of various poisonous Japanese mushrooms of the genus *Hebeloma.*

**asex·u·al** (a-sek'shoo-əl) having no sex; not sexual; not pertaining to sex. Called also *agamic* or *agamous.*

**asex·u·al·i·ty** (a″seks-u-al'ĭ-te) the state of being asexual; absence of sexual interests.

**ASF** a synthetic resin composed of aniline, formaldehyde, and sulfur, used for mounting microscopic objects.

**ASGE** American Society for Gastrointestinal Endoscopy.

**ASH** American Society of Hematology; asymmetrical septal hypertrophy.

**ash** (ash) 1. the incombustible residue remaining after any process of incineration. 2. any tree of the genus *Fraxinus.*

**ASHA** American School Health Association; American Speech and Hearing Association.

**ASHD** arteriosclerotic heart disease; see *ischemic heart disease,* under *disease.*

**Ash·er·man's syndrome** (ash'ər-mənz) [Joseph G. *Asherman,* Czechoslovakian-born physician in Israel, born 1889] see under *syndrome.*

**Ash·er·son's syndrome** (ash'ər-sənz) [Nehemiah *Asherson,* English physician, born 1897] see under *syndrome.*

**ASHP** American Society of Hospital Pharmacists.

**ASI** Addiction Severity Index.

**ASIA** American Spinal Injury Association.

**asi·a·lia** (a″si-a'le-ə) [*a-*[1] + Gr. *scialon* spittle] aptyalism.

**asi·a·lo** (a-si″ə-lo) [*a-*[1] + *sialo*] lacking a sialic acid group, as do certain sphingolipids.

**asi·at·i·co·side** (a″zhe-at'ĭ-ko-sīd″) the active principle of the umbelliferous plant *Centella asiatica* L., which has been used for various dermatological conditions, including wounds and burns.

**asid·er·o·sis** (a″sid-ər-o'sis) [*a-*[1] + *sider-* + *-sis*] abnormal decrease of the iron reserve of the body.

**ASII** American Science Information Institute.

**ASIM** American Society of Internal Medicine.

**Asim·i·na** (ə-sim'ĭ-nə) [L., from Algonquian] a genus of North American trees and shrubs of the family Annonaceae. *A. trilo'ba* (L.) Dunal is the papaw or pawpaw.

**asim·i·nine** (ə-sim'ĭ-nin) an alkaloid from the seeds of *Asimina triloba.*

**-asis** [Gr.] a word termination denoting an action, process or condition; see also *-sis.*

**asit·ia** (ə-sish'e-ə) [*a-*[1] + *sit-* + *-ia*] anorexia.

**As·ka·na·zy cells** (as'kə-nah″ze) [Max *Askanazy,* German pathologist, 1865–1940] see under *cell.*

**As·kin's tumor** (as'kinz) [Frederic Barton *Askin,* American pathologist, 20th century] see under *tumor.*

**As·kle·pi·os** (as-kle'pe-əs) [Gr. *Asklēpios* son of Apollo and Coronis, tutelary god of medicine] see *Æsculapius.*

**ASL** antistreptolysin.

**ASM** American Society for Microbiology.

**ASN** American Society of Nephrology.

**Asn** asparagine.

**ASO** arteriosclerosis obliterans.

**aso·ma** (a-so'mə) pl. *aso'mata* [*a-*[1] + *soma*] a fetus with an imperfect head and the merest rudiments of a trunk.

**aso·ma·tog·no·sia** (ə-so″mə-tog-no'zhə) lack of awareness of the condition of all or part of one's body; lack of somatognosis. Cf. *amorphosynthesis* and *anosognosia.*

**aso·ma·to·phyte** (a-so'mə-to-fīt″) [*a* neg. + *somato-* + *-phyte*] a plant in which there is no distinction between body and reproductive cells.

**Aso·pia** (ə-so'pe-ə) a genus of pyralid moths. *A. farina'lis* is a meal moth that acts as the intermediate host of the tapeworm *Hymenolepis diminuta.*

**ASP** American Society of Parasitologists.

**Asp** aspartic acid.

**as·pal·a·so·ma** (as″pal-ə-so'mə) [Gr. *aspalax* mole + *soma*] a fetus with lateral or median abdominal eventration and other deformities.

**as·par·a·gin·ase** (as-par'ə-jin-ās″) [EC 3.5.1.1] [MeSH: Asparaginase] 1. an enzyme of the hydrolase class that catalyzes the hydrolytic deamination of asparagine to form aspartate, a step in the degradation of asparagine. 2. a preparation of this enzyme isolated from *Escherichia coli* and used in the treatment of childhood acute lymphoblastic leukemia to reduce availability of asparagine to tumor cells; administered intravenously or intramuscularly.

**as·par·a·gine** (as-par'ə-jēn, as-par'ə-jin) [Gr. *asparagos* asparagus] [MeSH: Asparagine] a nonessential amino acid that is the β-amide of aspartic acid. It is found in most plants, and has diuretic properties. It is used as a culture medium for certain bacteria. Symbols Asn and N. See also table at *amino acid.*

**as·par·a·gin·yl** (as-par'ə-jin″əl) the acyl radical of asparagine.

**as·par·tame** (ə-spahr'tām, as'pahr-tām″) [NF] [MeSH: Aspartame] an artificial sweetener about 200 times as sweet as sucrose and used as a low-calorie sweetener.

**as·par·tate** (ə-spahr'tāt) a salt of aspartic acid, or aspartic acid in dissociated form.

**as·par·tate ami·no·trans·fer·ase** (ə-spahr'tāt ə-me″no-trans'fər-ās) [MeSH: Aspartate Aminotransferase] aspartate transaminase.

**as·par·tate car·bam·o·yl·trans·fer·ase** (ə-spahr'tāt kahr-bam″o-əl-trans'fər-ās) [EC 2.1.3.2] [MeSH: Aspartate Carbamoyltransferase] an enzyme activity of the trifunctional CAD protein; it is a transferase that catalyzes the formation of carbamoylaspartate from carbamoyl phosphate and aspartate in the first committed step in pyrimidine biosynthesis. Called also *aspartate transcarbamoylase.*

**as·par·tate trans·am·i·nase** (ə-spahr'tāt trans-am'ĭ-nās) [EC 2.6.1.1] an enzyme of the transferase class that catalyzes the reversible transfer of an amino group from aspartate to α-ketoglutarate to form glutamate and oxaloacetate, with pyridoxal phosphate required as a cofactor. The enzyme is present in most eukaryotic cells, occurring as distinct isozymes in mitochondria and cytosol. Both isozymes participate in the malate-aspartate shuttle, and in the liver the reaction transfers excess metabolic nitrogen into aspartate for disposal via the urea cycle. The serum level of aspartate transaminase (SGOT) and that of other transaminases are frequently elevated in a variety of disorders causing tissue damage (e.g., myocardial infarction). Abbreviated AST and ASAT. Called also *aspartate aminotransferase* and *glutamic-oxaloacetic transaminase (GOT).*

**as·par·tate trans·car·bam·oyl·ase** (ə-spahr'tāt trans″kahr-bam'o-əl-ās) aspartate carbamoyltransferase.

**as·par·thi·one** (ə-spahr'thi-ōn″) a tripeptide analogous to glutathione but containing aspartic acid in place of glutamic acid.

**as·par·tic ac·id** (ə-spahr'tik) [MeSH: Aspartic Acid] a nonessential amino acid, aminosuccinic acid, occurring in proteins; it is also an excitatory neurotransmitter in the central nervous system. Symbols Asp and D. See also table at *amino acid.*

**as·par·tic en·do·pep·ti·dase** (ə-spahr'tik en″do-pep'tĭ-dās) [EC 3.4.23] any member of the group of endopeptidases that have an acidic residue involved in the catalytic process and so have a pH optimum below 5.

**as·par·to·cin** (ə-spahr'to-sin) an antibacterial substance produced by *Streptomyces griseus.*

**as·par·tyl** (ə-spahr'təl) the acyl radical of aspartic acid.

**as·par·tyl·glu·co·sa·mine** (ə-spahr″təl-gloo-kōs'ə-mēn) *N*-acetylglucosamine in *N*-glycosidic linkage with the amino group of asparagine; it is an intermediate in the degradation of glycoproteins and accumulates abnormally in aspartylglycosaminuria.

**as·par·tyl·glu·co·sa·min·i·dase** (ə-spahr″təl-gloo-kōs″ə-min'ĭ-dās) a lysosomal enzyme of the hydrolase class that catalyzes the cleavage of *N*-glycosidic linkages between *N*-acetylglucosamine and asparagine in glycoproteins, a step in the degradation of glycoproteins. Deficiency of the enzyme, an autosomal recessive trait, causes aspartylglycosaminuria. In EC nomenclature, called $N^4$-(*β-N-acetylglucosaminyl*)-L-*asparaginase.*

**as·par·tyl·glu·co·sa·min·uria** (ə-spahr″təl-gloo″kōs-am″in-u're-ə) aspartylglycosaminuria.

**as·par·tyl·gly·cos·amin·i·dase** (ə-spahr″təl-gli-kōs″ə-min'ĭ-dās) $N^4$-(β-*N*-acetylglucosaminyl)-L-asparaginase; see *aspartylglucosaminidase.*

**as·par·tyl·gly·cos·a·mi·nu·ria** (ə-spahr'təl-gli'kōs-ə-min-u're-ə) an autosomal recessive lysosomal storage disease caused by deficiency of aspartylglucosaminidase. The disorder is preceded by diarrhea and frequent infections in infancy, with later onset of severe mental retardation, coarsening of features, lens opacity, and skeletal dysplasia, as well as storage and urinary excretion of abnormal levels of aspartylglucosamine and related glycopeptides. Called also *aspartylglucosaminuria.*

**aspe·cif·ic** (a″spə-sif'ik) nonspecific; not caused by a specific organism.

**as·pect** (as'pekt) [L. *aspectus,* from *aspicere* to look toward] 1. that part of a surface facing in any designated direction. 2. the look or appearance.

**anterior a. of cranium,** norma facialis.
**dorsal a.,** the surface of a body as viewed from a posterior direction (human anatomy) or, for quadrupeds, from a superior direction (veterinary anatomy).
**facial a. of cranium, frontal a. of cranium,** norma facialis.
**inferior a. of cranium,** norma inferior.
**lateral a. of cranium,** norma lateralis.
**occipital a. of cranium,** norma occipitalis.
**sagittal a. of cranium,** norma sagittalis.
**superior a. of cranium,** norma superior.
**temporal a. of cranium,** norma lateralis.
**ventral a.,** the surface of a body as viewed from an anterior direction (human anatomy) or, for quadrupeds, from an inferior direction (veterinary anatomy).
**vertical a. of cranium,** norma superior.

**As·per·ger's syndrome** (ahs'pər-gərz) [Hans *Asperger,* Austrian psychiatrist, 20th century] see under *syndrome.*

**as·per·gil·lar** (as"pər-jil'ər) pertaining to or caused by *Aspergillus.*

**as·per·gil·li** (as"pər-jil'i) plural of *aspergillus.*

**as·per·gil·lic acid** (as"pər-jil'ik) an antibiotic substance isolated from *Aspergillus flavus.*

**as·per·gil·lin** (as"pər-jil'in) a black antibiotic substance, from the spore of various species of *Aspergillus;* formerly called *vegetable hematin.*

**as·per·gil·lo·ma** (as"pər-jil-o'mə) the most common kind of fungus ball, formed by colonization of *Aspergillus* in a bronchus or lung cavity.

**as·per·gil·lo·my·co·sis** (as"pər-jil"o-mi-ko'sis) aspergillosis.

**as·per·gil·lo·sis** (as"pər-jil-o'sis) [MeSH: Aspergillosis] infection of humans or other animals by species of *Aspergillus,* marked by inflammatory granulomatous lesions in the skin, ear, orbit, nasal sinuses, lungs, and sometimes the bones and meninges; called also *aspergillomycosis.*
**allergic a.,** an allergic reaction to *Aspergillus* in body passages or orifices, such as the bronchi and lungs in atopic asthma. Species commonly implicated include *A. clava'tus, A. fla'vus, A. fumiga'tus, A. ni'dulans, A. ni'ger,* and *A. ter'reus.* See also *malt worker's lung,* under *lung.*
**aural a.,** *Aspergillus* otomycosis.
**bronchopneumonic a., bronchopulmonary a.,** infection of the bronchi and lungs by species of *Aspergillus*; subtypes include *allergic bronchopulmonary a., chronic necrotizing a., invasive a.,* and *aspergilloma.* Called also *bronchoaspergillosis.*
**bronchopulmonary a., allergic,** bronchopulmonary a. accompanied by allergic (immunologic) symptoms in the bronchi, often with expectoration of yellow or brown bronchial plugs composed of eosinophils and fungal hyphae. It is frequently seen in patients with asthma or cystic fibrosis and may progress to bronchiectasis or bronchocentric granulomatosis.
**chronic necrotizing a.,** a slowly progressive invasive type of aspergillosis seen in patients with severe lung disease such as chronic obstructive pulmonary disease, often in diabetics or the immunocompromised. Characteristics include cavitary infiltration that may extend into the pleura and sometimes fungus balls in the cavities.
**invasive a.,** a frequently fatal type of bronchopulmonary a. seen in immunocompromised or debilitated patients, characterized by fungal invasion of the tissues. In lung involvement, there is pneumonia with dyspnea, coughing, and hemoptysis. Invasion of blood vessels can lead to infarction of tissues supplied by the vessels. Less often, the fungus invades the central nervous system and may cause seizures.
**pulmonary a.,** infection of the lungs with *Aspergillus*; an acute invasive form is sometimes seen in immunocompromised patients, characterized by pulmonary infiltration and often pulmonary vascular involvement, necrosis, cavitation, areas of hemorrhagic pulmonary infarction, and sometimes aspergillomas that may impede air flow. Cf. Aspergillus *pneumonia.*

**as·per·gil·lo·tox·i·co·sis** (as"pər-jil"o-tok"sĭ-ko'sis) any mycotoxicosis caused by *Aspergillus* species, such as those containing aflatoxin, citrinin, ochratoxin A, patulin, or sterigmatocystin. Called also *aspergillustoxicosis.*

**As·per·gil·lus** (as"pər-jil'əs) [L. *aspergere* to scatter] [MeSH: Aspergillus] a genus of Fungi Imperfecti of the form-class Hyphomycetes, form-family Moniliaceae. When found, the perfect, or sexual, stage is classified with the ascomycetous fungi in the family Trichocomaceae. This genus includes several common molds and some that are opportunistic pathogens and is characterized by elongated conidiophores thickly set with chains of basipetally formed conidia. See Plate 29.
**A. amsteloda'mi,** a species with blue to green conidial heads, found in nasal and occasionally cerebral infections.
**A. clava'tus,** a species with blue or green conidial heads, found in soils and manure; inhalation of its spores in contaminated barley dust causes malt worker's lung. Its cultures produce the toxic antibacterial substance patulin.
**A. fishe'rii,** a thermophilic soil fungus.
**A. fla'vus,** a species with yellow or yellow-green conidial heads, usually found on corn, peanuts, or grain; it contains aflatoxin and causes aflatoxicosis. It also can cause allergic aspergillosis, eumycotic mycetoma, and pulmonary disease in humans, and in weak or immunocompromised patients it can cause disseminated forms of aspergillosis.
**A. fumiga'tus,** a thermotolerant species with blue or green conidial heads, usually found growing in soils and manure. It has also been found in infections of the ear, nose, lungs and other organs of humans and animals and is a primary pathogen of birds, causing brooder pneumonia. Inhalation of its spores in contaminated barley dust causes malt worker's lung. Its cultures produce various antibiotics, such as fumagillin and gliotoxin.
**A. gigan'teus,** a species that contains the carcinogenic mycotoxin patulin.
**A. glau'cus,** a group of species of bluish molds common on dry and decaying vegetation and sometimes found in otomycosis, nasal and pulmonary infections, and other human infectious processes.
**A. ni'dulans,** a species common in soil and sometimes isolated from onychomycosis, maduromycosis, eumycotic mycetoma, and other disease processes.
**A. ni'ger,** a species common in soil, which can cause severe or persistent otomycosis; it has also been implicated in allergic aspergillosis.
**A. ni'veus,** a species that contains the mycotoxin citrinin and sometimes contaminates grain, causing fatal renal failure in rats and possibly Balkan nephritis in humans.
**A. ochra'ceus,** a species with yellow conidial heads, important economically because it ferments the coffee berry and produces the characteristic and desirable odor; it contains ochratoxin and sometimes contaminates cereals, causing ochratoxicosis in animals. In humans it has been implicated in nasal and orbital infections and allergic aspergillosis.
**A. ory'zae,** a species with yellow-green conidial heads that change to brown with age, closely related to *A. flavus;* it is commonly found in soil and manure and can cause aspergillosis.
**A. parasi'ticus,** a mold found on peanut seedlings that elaborates aflatoxin.
**A. re'pens,** a species that is the perfect stage of *Eurotium repens* and is sometimes found in the human external auditory canal or lungs.
**A. restric'tus,** a species with blue to green conidial heads, found in pulmonary and occasionally disseminated infections.
**A. ter'reus,** a species associated with infection of the bronchi and lungs in humans (see *aspergilloma* and *allergic aspergillosis*), and occasionally with other infections such as of the orbit or central nervous system. It also contains the mycotoxin patulin.
**A. versi'color,** a species with yellow to green conidial heads, common soil saprobes that have been found in human infections of the lungs, bronchi, and occasionally the central nervous system.

**as·per·gil·lus** (as"pər-jil'əs) pl. *aspergil'li* [MeSH: Aspergillus] An individual of the genus *Aspergillus.*

**as·per·gil·lus·tox·i·co·sis** (as"pər-jil"əs-tok"sĭ-ko'sis) aspergillotoxicosis.

**asper·ma·tism** (ə-spər'mə-tiz-əm) aspermia.

**as·per·ma·to·gen·e·sis** (a-spər"mə-to-jen'ə-sis) absence of development of spermatozoa.

**asper·mia** (ə-spər'me-ə) [*a-*[1] + *sperm-* + *-ia*] failure of formation or emission of semen.

**ASPET** American Society for Pharmacology and Experimental Therapeutics.

**as·phyg·mia** (as-fig'me-ə) temporary disappearance of the pulse.

**as·phyx·ia** (as-fik'se-ə) [Gr. "a stopping of the pulse"] [MeSH: Asphyxia] pathological changes caused by lack of oxygen in respired air, resulting in hypoxia and hypercapnia; see also *respiration.*
**birth a.,** perinatal a.
**blue a., a. cyano'tica,** a. livida.
**fetal a.,** asphyxia in utero due to hypoxia; see also *fetal hypoxia,* under *hypoxia.*
**a. li'vida,** perinatal asphyxia in which the skin is cyanotic from the lack of oxygen in the blood. Called also *blue a.* and *a. cyanotica.*
**a. neonato'rum,** perinatal asphyxia in the newborn.
**a. pal'lida,** perinatal asphyxia attended with paleness of the skin; called also *white a.*
**perinatal a.,** asphyxia in the infant during labor, delivery, or the immediate postnatal period, a common cause of hypoxic-ischemic encephalopathy. See also *respiratory distress syndrome of the newborn,* under *syndrome.* Called also *birth a.*
**secondary a.,** asphyxia recurring after apparent recovery from suffocation.
**traumatic a.,** asphyxia occurring as a result of sudden or severe

compression of the thorax or upper abdomen, or both. See also *traumatic apnea,* under *apnea.*
**white a.,** a. pallida.

**as·phyx·i·al** (as-fik′se-əl) characterized by or pertaining to asphyxia.

**as·phyx·i·ant** (as-fik′se-ənt) a substance capable of producing asphyxia.

**as·phyx·i·ate** (as-fik′se-āt) to put into a state of asphyxia.

**as·phyx·i·a·tion** (as-fik″se-a′shən) the causing of or state of asphyxia. Called also *suffocation.*

**As·pid·i·um** (as-pid′e-əm) [L.; Gr. *aspidion* little shield] *Dryopteris.*

**as·pid·i·um** (as-pid′e-əm) 1. any fern of the genus *Aspidium.* 2. the rhizome and stipes of ferns of the genus *Aspidium,* yielding not less than 1.5 per cent of crude filicin. It is a violent poison and is highly irritant to the gastrointestinal tract when taken internally. It is also the source of the anthelmintic aspidium oleoresin (see under *oleoresin*).

**as·pi·rate** (as′pĭ-rāt) 1. to treat by aspiration. 2. the substance or material obtained by aspiration. 3. a consonantal speech sound in which part of the respiratory tract is constricted, the nasal cavity shut off, and the breath makes a whistling noise; an example is *h.*

**as·pi·ra·tion** (as″pĭ-ra′shən) [L. *ad-* to + *spirare* to breathe] [MeSH: Aspiration] 1. inhalation. 2. removal by suction; used to remove excess fluid or gas from a body cavity and to obtain biopsy specimens.
**fine-needle a.,** see under *biopsy.*
**meconium a.,** aspiration of meconium by the fetus or newborn, which may result in atelectasis, emphysema, pneumothorax, or pneumonia.
**vacuum a.,** removal of the uterine contents by application of a vacuum using a hollow curet or a cannula introduced into the uterus.

**as·pi·ra·tor** (as″pĭ-ra′tər) an apparatus used for removal by suction of fluids or gases contained within a cavity.

**as·pi·rin** (as′pĭ-rin) [USP] [MeSH: Aspirin] acetylsalicylic acid, a drug having anti-inflammatory, analgesic, and antipyretic effects; it is the prototype of the nonsteroidal anti-inflammatory agents whose mechanism of action is inhibition of prostaglandin synthesis; used for relief of pain and fever and for treatment of rheumatoid arthritis and osteoarthritis. Because it is a platelet inhibitor, it is also used to reduce the risk of recurrent transient ischemic attacks or of cerebrovascular accident.

**asple·nia** (a-sple′ne-ə) [*a-*[1] + *splenia*] absence of the spleen.
**functional a.,** impaired reticuloendothelial function of the spleen, as in children with sickle-cell anemia.

**asplen·ic** (a-splen′ik) pertaining to asplenia; caused by absence of the spleen.

**aspo·ro·gen·ic** (as″po-ro-jen′ik) [*a-*[1] + *sporogenic*] not producing spores; not reproduced by spores.

**as·po·rog·e·nous** (as″po-roj′ə-nəs) asporogenic.

**aspor·ous** (ə-spor′əs) [*a-*[1] + Gr. *sporos* seed] having no true spores; applied to microorganisms.

**ASRT** American Society of Radiologic Technologists.

**ASS** anterior superior spine.

**as·say** (as′a) determination of the amount of a particular constituent of a mixture, or determination of the biological or pharmacological potency of a drug.
**antigen capture a.,** one used to identify minute quantities of antigen in solution: large quantities of antibody against the desired antigen are fixed to a solid support matrix, over which the solution is passed. The antigen is retained by the matrix and can be identified by reaction with labeled antibody.
**biological a.,** bioassay.
**blastogenesis a.,** see *lymphocyte proliferation test,* under *tests.*
**cancer antigen 125 (CA 125) a.,** determination of the level of CA 125 in serum by radioimmunoassay after reaction with a specific murine monoclonal antibody; it is used in the evaluation of women with suspected, diagnosed, or treated primary epithelial ovarian cancer to aid diagnosis, assess prognosis, or predict recurrence.
**cell-mediated lympholysis (CML) a.,** see under *lympholysis.*
**CH50 a.,** a functional assay of total complement activity that measures the capacity of serial dilutions of serum to lyse a standard preparation of sheep red blood cells coated with anti–sheep erythrocyte antibody. The reciprocal of the dilution of serum that lyses 50 per cent of the erythrocytes is reported as the whole complement titer in CH50 units per milliliter of serum. Called also *hemolytic, total,* or *whole complement a.*
**Clauss a.,** see under *method.*
**competitive protein-binding a.,** a radioimmunoassay in which labeled and unlabeled ligands compete for sites on a carrier that has the same avidity for both; the concentration of unlabeled ligand is inversely proportional to the amount of labeled ligand bound.
**D-dimer a.,** an immunoassay for the fibrin degradation product D dimer. Levels are elevated in deep venous thrombosis, acute myocardial infarction, pulmonary embolism, unstable angina, and disseminated intravascular coagulation (DIC). Called also *D-dimer test.*
**EAC rosette a.,** an assay for human B lymphocytes using complement receptors, a B cell marker. Peripheral blood cells are mixed with ox red blood cells, IgM antierythrocyte antibody, and complement deficient in C5 (to prevent red cell lysis). The antibody-and-complement-coated erythrocytes (EAC) form rosettes with B cells, which are counted using a hemocytometer.
**electrophoretic mobility shift a.,** gel retardation a.
**enzyme-linked immunosorbent a.,** see *ELISA.*
**E rosette a.,** an assay for human T lymphocytes based on the existence of a specific receptor on T cells for a sheep red blood cell membrane antigen. Peripheral blood lymphocytes are incubated with sheep red cells. T cells are surrounded by a ring of red cells—an E (erythrocyte) rosette—and are counted using a hemacytometer.
**fibrinogen a.,** an assay for the level of fibrinogen in a plasma sample; a thrombin reagent is added to the diluted sample and the time needed to form clots is compared with that for a reference containing a known amount of fibrinogen.
**four-point a.,** an assay based on a mixture of two doses of test material and two doses of standard material.
**gel retardation a.,** an assay used to determine whether a specific protein binds to DNA or to determine some characteristics of such binding; protein is incubated with or without nucleic acid under various conditions and the electrophoretic mobilities of the samples are compared. In a nondenaturing type of gel electrophoresis, a decreased rate of migration relative to an unbound control is indicative of binding.
**hemagglutination inhibition (HI, HAI) a.,** see under *test.*
**hemolytic complement a.,** CH50 a.
**hemolytic plaque a.,** a quantitative assay that counts antibody-producing cells. Lymphocytes sensitized against sheep erythrocytes (SRBCs) are plated in agar with SRBCs. After incubation complement is added; this lyses SRBCs, leaving a clear circular plaque around each cell that produced antibody against SRBC. The plaques are counted and reported as the number of plaque-forming cells (PFCs, pfcs). Called also *Jerne plaque a.*
**immune a.,** immunoassay.
**immune adherence hemagglutination a. (IAHA),** see *immune adherence,* under *adherence.*
**immunofluorescence a. (IFA),** fluorescence immunoassay.
**immunoradiometric a. (IRMA),** a variant of radioimmunoassay in which the antigen being measured reacts directly with radiolabeled antibody.
**Jerne plaque a.,** hemolytic plaque a.
**lymphocyte proliferation a.,** see under *test.*
**microbiological a.,** assay by the use of microorganisms.
**microcytotoxicity a.,** the standard method of typing serologically defined HLA antigens (HLA-A, -B, and -C antigens). Multiple typing sera are placed in wells of a microtiter plate, and peripheral blood lymphocytes and complement are added to each well. The pattern of lysed cells indicates the HLA phenotype.
**microhemagglutination a.–*Treponema pallidum* (MHA-TP),** a *Treponema pallidum* hemagglutination assay using microtechniques; used in the detection of syphilis.
**mixed lymphocyte culture a., MLC a.,** see under *culture.*
**radioimmunoprecipitation a. (RIPA),** immunoprecipitation conducted with radiolabeled antibody or antigen.
**radioligand a.,** any assay procedure that uses radioisotopic labeling and biologically specific binding of reagents, such as a radioimmunoassay, competitive protein-binding assay, or radioreceptor assay.
**radioreceptor a.,** a radioligand assay in which a radiolabeled hormone is used to measure the concentration of specific cellular receptors for the hormone in tissue specimens, an example being radioassay of estrogen receptors in breast tissue.
**Raji cell a.,** an assay for immune complexes using the Raji lymphoblastoid cell line (see *Raji cell,* under *cell*).
**stem cell a.,** a test for determining the effectiveness of particular drugs against human cancer, in which human tumor cell suspensions are first incubated with various drugs and then suspended in agar and plated over a layer of agar at the bottom of the plate. Effectiveness of the drugs is determined by counting the number of colonies that grow in comparison with the number of colonies on control plates.
**total complement a.,** CH50 a.
***Treponema pallidum* hemagglutination a. (TPHA),** a treponemal antigen serologic test for syphilis using tanned sheep red blood cells coated with antigen from the Nichol's strain of *Treponema pallidum* and patient serum absorbed with an extract of Reiter treponemes to remove nonspecific antibodies. It is similar in sensitivity and specificity to the FTA-ABS test except that it is less sensitive in detecting primary syphilis.
**whole complement a.,** CH50 a.

**as·sess·ment** (ə-ses'mənt) an evaluation or appraisal.
**Fugl-Meyer a.,** a standardized assessment of motor function of a part after neurological damage.
**functional a.,** an objective evaluation of a patient's functional level, including ability to perform activities of daily living, done to prescribe or evaluate rehabilitation measures.

**As·sé·zat's triangle** (ah-sa-zahz') [Jules *Assézat,* French anthropologist, 1832–1876] facial triangle.

**as·si·dent** (as'ĭ-dənt) generally but not always accompanying a disease.

**as·sim·i·la·ble** (ə-sim'ĭ-lə-bəl) capable of being assimilated.

**as·sim·i·la·tion** (ə-sim"ĭ-la'shən) [L. *assimilatio,* from *ad* to + *similare* to make like] 1. the transformation of food into living tissue; anabolism. 2. in psychology, the absorption of new experiences into the existing psychological make-up.

**as·sis·tant** (ə-sis'tənt) one who aids or helps another; an auxiliary.
**physician a., physician's a.,** see under *physician.*

**Ass·mann's focus (tuberculous infiltrate)** (ahs'mahnz) [Herbert *Assmann,* German internist, 1882–1950] see under *focus.*

**as·so·ci·a·tion** (ə-so"se-a'shən) [L. *associatio,* from *ad* to + *socius* a fellow] [MeSH: Association] 1. a state in which two attributes occur together either more or less often than expected by chance. 2. in neurology, a term applied to those regions of the brain that link the primary motor and sensory cortices; see *association areas,* under *area.* 3. in genetics, the occurrence together of two or more phenotypic characteristics more often than would be expected by chance. To be distinguished from linkage (q.v.). 4. in psychiatry, a connection between ideas or feelings, especially between conscious thoughts and elements of the unconscious, or the formation of such a connection.
**CHARGE a.,** a syndrome of associated defects, including *c*oloboma of the eye, *h*eart anomaly, choanal *a*tresia, *r*etardation, and *g*enital and *e*ar anomalies. Facial palsy, cleft palate, and dysphagia are often present, and familial transmission has been postulated.
**clang a.,** see *clanging.*
**dream a's,** emotions or thoughts associated with previous dreams, as developed by the patient in psychoanalysis.
**free a.,** a psychoanalytical method in which the patient is encouraged to describe the association of thoughts and emotions as they arise spontaneously during the analysis.

**as·sort·ment** (ə-sort'mənt) the random distribution of different combinations of the parental chromosomes to the gametes. As a result, each gamete normally possesses one genome (set of 23 chromosomes) that includes one chromosome of each type. The genes on the chromosome also assort independently unless they are linked. Called also *independent a.*

**AST** aspartate transaminase.

**Ast.** astigmatism.

**asta·sia** (as-ta'zhə) [*a-*[1] + Gr. *stasis* stand] motor incoordination with inability to stand; cf. *dysstasia* and *posture.*
**a.-aba'sia,** motor incoordination with an inability to stand or walk despite normal ability to move the legs when sitting or lying down, a form of hysterical ataxia. Called also *abasia-astasia.*

**astat·ic** (as-tat'ik) pertaining to astasia.

**as·ta·tine** (as'tə-tēn) [Gr. *astatos* unstable] [MeSH: Astatine] the radioactive element of atomic number 85, atomic weight 210, symbol At. It is prepared by alpha particle bombardment of bismuth on the cyclotron. It has a half-life of 75 hours and may be of use in the treatment of hyperthyroidism.

**aste·a·to·des** (as"te-ə-to'dēz) asteatosis.

**aste·a·to·sis** (as"te-ə-to'sis) [*a-*[1] + *stear-* + *-osis*] any disease characterized by such persistent fine dry scaling of the skin surface as to suggest scantiness or absence of the sebaceous secretion. Called also *asteatodes.* See also *chapping; winter itch,* under *itch;* and *xerotic eczema,* under *eczema.*

**as·tem·i·zole** (ə-stem'ĭ-zōl) [USP] [MeSH: Astemizole] an $H_1$-receptor antagonist used in the treatment of chronic urticaria and seasonal allergic rhinitis (hay fever).

**as·ter** (as'tər) [L.; Gr. *astēr* star] a structure seen in a cell during the prophase of mitosis, composed of a system of microtubules arranged in astral rays around the centrosome; called also *astrosphere, cytaster,* and *kinosphere.*
**sperm a.,** the centriole, with astral rays, that precedes the male pronucleus during fertilization.

**As·ter·a·ce·ae** (as"tər-a'se-e) Compositae.

**aste·reo·cog·no·sy** (ə-ste"re-o-kog'nə-se) astereognosis.

**aste·re·og·no·sis** (ə-ster"e-og-no'sis) [*a-*[1] + Gr. *stereo-* + *gnōsis*] loss or lack of the ability to understand the form and nature of objects that are touched (stereognosis), a form of tactile agnosia; called also *astereocognosy, stereoagnosis,* and *tactile amnesia.*

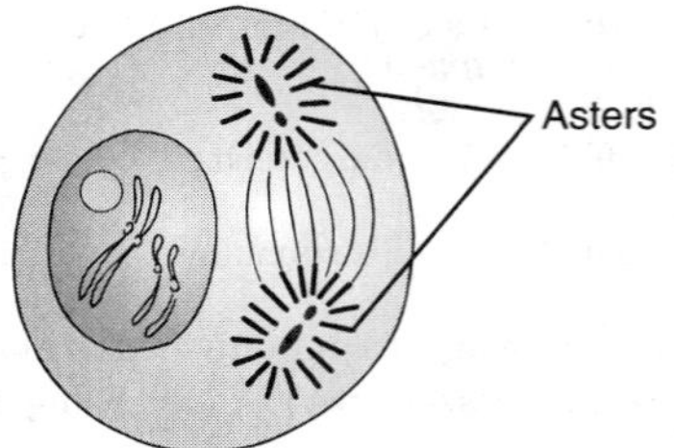

Asters separating in prophase of mitosis.

**as·te·ri·on** (as-te're-on) pl. *aste'ria* [Gr. "starred"] [TA] the point on the surface of the skull where the lambdoid, parietomastoid, and occipitomastoid sutures meet.

**as·ter·ix·is** (as"tər-ik'sis) [*a-*[1] + Gr. *stērixis* a fixed position] a motor disturbance marked by intermittent lapse of an assumed posture, as a result of intermittency of the sustained contraction of groups of muscles, a characteristic of hepatic coma but observed also in numerous other conditions; called also *liver flap* and *flapping tremor.*

**aster·nal** (a-stər'nəl) 1. not joined to the sternum. 2. pertaining to asternia; lacking a sternum.

**aster·nia** (a-stər'ne-ə) [*a-*[1] + *stern-* + *-ia*] congenital absence of the sternum.

**as·ter·oid** (as'tər-oid) [*aster* + *-oid*] star-shaped; resembling the aster.

**As·ter·ol** (as'tər-ol) trademark for preparations of diamthazole dihydrochloride.

**Asth.** asthenopia.

**as·the·nia** (as-the'ne-ə) [*asthen-* + *-ia*] [MeSH: Asthenia] lack or loss of strength and energy; weakness.
**cutaneous a.,** 1. a disease of cattle and sheep, similar to human Ehlers-Danlos syndrome; the skin is fragile and easily torn. It is due to an abnormally low activity of procollagen N-endopeptidase. Called also *dermatosparaxis* and *Ehlers-Danlos syndrome.* 2. Ehlers-Danlos syndrome (def. 1).
**myalgic a.,** any condition characterized by a sensation of general fatigue and muscular pains.
**neurocirculatory a.,** a syndrome characterized by palpitations, dyspnea, a sense of fatigue, fear of effort, and discomfort brought on by exercise or even slight effort; considered by most authorities to be a particular presentation of an anxiety disorder, the physical symptoms being attributed to autonomic responses to anxiety or to hyperventilation. Called also *DaCosta's syndrome, effort syndrome,* and *irritable* or *soldier's heart.*
**periodic a.,** a condition marked by periodically recurring attacks of marked asthenia.
**tropical anhidrotic a.,** a rare condition seen under conditions of heat stress, in which miliaria profunda causes extensive occlusion of the sweat ducts, producing anhidrosis and heat retention that may lead to heat exhaustion with weakness, dyspnea, tachycardia, elevation of body temperature, and collapse. Called also *sweat retention syndrome* and *thermogenic anhidrosis.*

**as·then·ic** (as-then'ik) pertaining to or characterized by asthenia.

**asthen(o)-** [Gr. *asthenēs* weak, from *a-*[1] + *sthenos* strength] a combining form denoting lack of strength or weakness.

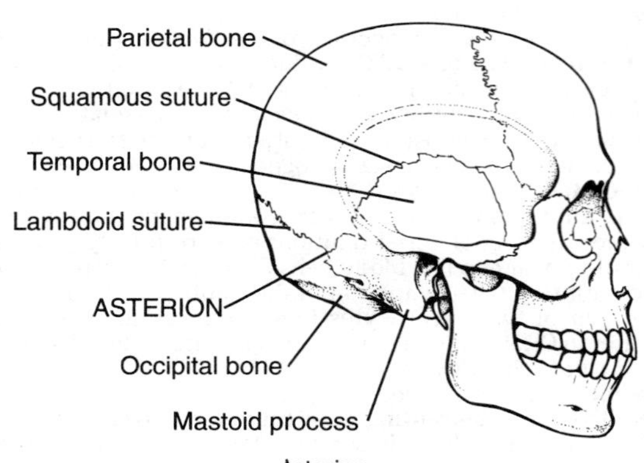

Asterion.

**as·the·no·bi·o·sis** (as-the″no-bi-o′sis) [*asthen-* + *biosis*] a condition of reduced biologic activity resembling hibernation or estivation but not directly related to or dependent on temperature or humidity.

**as·the·no·co·ria** (as-the″no-kor′e-ə) [*astheno-* + *cor-* + *-ia*] sluggishness of the pupillary reflex, as seen in hypoadrenalism. Called also *Arroyo's sign.*

**as·the·nope** (as′then-ōp) a person affected with asthenopia.

**as·the·no·pia** (as″thə-no′pe-ə) [*asthen-* + *-opia*] [MeSH: Asthenopia] weakness or easy fatigue of the visual organs, attended by pain in the eyes, headache, dimness of vision, etc. Previously a diagnostic term; now used mainly as a descriptive term.
**accommodative a.,** asthenopia due to strain of the ciliary muscle.
**muscular a.,** that which is due to weakness of the external ocular muscles.
**nervous a.,** 1. that due to a functional disorder. 2. that due to organic nervous disease.
**tarsal a.,** asthenopia due to irregular astigmatism produced by the pressure of the lids on the cornea.

**as·the·nop·ic** (as″thə-nop′ik) characterized by asthenopia.

**as·the·no·sper·mia** (as″thə-no-spər′me-ə) [*astheno-* + *sperm-* + *-ia*] reduction in the vitality of spermatozoa.

**as·the·nox·ia** (as″then-ok′shə) [*astheno-* + *oxygen*] lack of power to oxidize waste products.

**as·thma** (az′mə) [Gr. *asthma* panting] [MeSH: Asthma] recurrent attacks of paroxysmal dyspnea, with airway inflammation and wheezing due to spasmodic contraction of the bronchi. Some cases are allergic manifestations in sensitized persons *(allergic a.)*; others are provoked by factors such as vigorous exercise, irritant particles, psychologic stresses, and others. Called also *bronchial a.* and *spasmodic a.*
**allergic a.,** atopic a.
**atopic a.,** asthma due to atopy (atopic allergy). Called also *allergic a.* and *extrinsic a.*
**bakers' a.,** a usually mild form of occupational asthma seen in bakery workers, caused by the inhalation of flour; some cases are due to contaminants such as mites in the flour.
**bronchial a.,** asthma.
**bronchitic a.,** asthmatic disorder accompanying bronchitis; see also *asthmatic bronchitis,* under *bronchitis.*
**cardiac a.,** paroxysmal nocturnal dyspnea that occurs in association with heart disease, such as left ventricular failure.
**cat a.,** atopic asthma brought on by inhalation of cat dander by a sensitized person.
**catarrhal a.,** bronchitic a.
**colophony a.,** a type of occupational asthma in workers in electronics industries caused by inhalation of fumes of colophony (rosin), which is used to solder parts together.
**cotton-dust a.,** byssinosis.
**cough variant a.,** asthma characterized by minimal wheezing and a nonproductive, often severe cough lasting from a few hours to days.
**cryptogenic a.,** intrinsic a.
**diisocyanate a.,** isocyanate a.
**dust a.,** atopic asthma caused by inhalation of dust; many cases are caused by presence in the dust of the house dust mite (*Dermatophagoides pteronyssinus*), and some other cases are caused by allergies to animal dander.
**exercise-induced a.,** asthma due to a narrowing of the airways occurring in moderate to heavy exercise.
**extrinsic a.,** 1. asthma caused by some factor in the environment, usually atopic asthma. Onset is usually in childhood and almost always before age 30. Cf. *intrinsic a.* 2. atopic a.
**food a.,** atopic asthma brought on by ingestion of certain foods to which the person is allergic.
**horse a.,** atopic asthma caused by an allergy to horses or horse products.
**intrinsic a.,** asthma attributed to pathophysiologic disturbances and not to environmental factors; usually seen in adults. Called also *cryptogenic a.*
**isocyanate a.,** asthma, usually occupational, caused by allergy to toluene diisocyanate and similar materials.
**millers' a.,** occupational asthma in millers, caused by the inhalation of cereal dusts.
**nasal a.,** asthma caused by a disease of the nose.
**occupational a.,** asthma, sometimes atopic in nature, caused by inhalation of an irritant in the workplace.
**reflex a.,** asthma attributed to a reflex reaction to another condition.
**Rostan's a.,** cardiac a.
**spasmodic a.,** asthma.
**steam-fitters' a.,** occupational asthma in steam-fitters, associated with asbestosis.
**stripper's a.,** byssinosis.
**western red cedar a.,** occupational asthma in sawmill workers, carpenters, and other susceptible persons who work with the wood of *Thuja plicata,* the western red cedar; the causative agent is probably the plicatic acid in the wood.

**asth·mat·ic** (az-mat′ik) [L. *asthmaticus*] pertaining to or affected with asthma.

**asth·mat·i·form** (az-mat′ĭ-form) resembling asthma.

**asth·mo·gen·ic** (az″mo-jen′ik) causing asthma.

**As·ti·ban** (as′tĭ-ban) trademark for preparations of stibocaptate.

**astig·ma·graph** (ə-stig′mə-graf) [*astigma*tism + *-graph*] an instrument for demonstrating astigmatism.

**astig·mat·ic** (as″tig-mat′ik) pertaining to or affected with astigmatism.

**astig·ma·tism** (ə-stig′mə-tiz -əm) [*a-*[1] + Gr. *stigma* point] [MeSH: Astigmatism] unequal curvature of the refractive surfaces of the eye; hence a point source of light cannot be brought to a point focus on the retina but is spread over a more or less diffuse area. This results from the radius of curvature in one plane being longer or shorter than the radius at right angles to it.
**acquired a.,** that due to some disease or injury of the eye.
**a. against the rule,** that in which the greatest refraction takes place along the horizontal meridian; called also *inverse a.*
**compound a.,** that which is complicated in all meridians by hypermetropia or myopia.
**congenital a.,** that which exists at birth.
**corneal a.,** that due to irregularity in the curvature or refracting power of the cornea.
**direct a.,** a. with the rule.
**hypermetropic a., compound, hyperopic a., compound,** astigmatism in which all meridians are hyperopic, both principal meridians having their foci behind the retina.
**hypermetropic a., hyperopic a.,** that which complicates hyperopia.
**hyperopic a., simple,** astigmatism in which one meridian, usually the vertical, is emmetropic and the horizontal meridian is hyperopic. The focus of the vertical meridian is not in the retina; that of the horizontal is behind the retina; horizontal lines appear distinct.
**inverse a.,** a. against the rule.
**irregular a.,** astigmatism in which the curvature in different parts of the same meridian of the eye varies or in which successive meridians differ irregularly in refraction, the image produced being an irregular area.
**lenticular a.,** that which is due to some irregularity or abnormality of the lens.
**mixed a.,** that in which one principal meridian is myopic and the other hyperopic.
**myopic a.,** that which complicates myopia.
**myopic a., compound,** astigmatism in which all meridians are myopic, both principal meridians having their foci in front of the retina; vertical lines are usually more distinct.
**myopic a., simple,** astigmatism in which the focus of one meridian is situated on the retina, while that of the other lies in front of the retina; vertical lines appear distinct.
**oblique a.,** astigmatism in which the direction of the principal meridians approaches 45° and 135°.
**physiological a.,** the slight astigmatism possessed by nearly all eyes and causing the twinkling sensation when distant points of light are viewed.
**regular a.,** astigmatism in which the refractive power of the eye shows a uniform increase or decrease from one meridian to the other, being practically constant in each meridian; the image produced is regular in shape, either a line, an oval, or a circle. See also *Sturm's conoid,* under *conoid.*
**a. with the rule,** that wherein the meridian in which the greatest refraction takes place is vertical or nearly so; called also *direct a.*

**astig·ma·tom·e·ter** (ə-stig″mə-tom′ə-tər) [*astigmatism* + *-meter*] an instrument used in measuring astigmatism.

**astig·ma·tom·e·try** (ə-stig″mə-tom′ə-tre) [*astigmatism* + *-metry*] the measurement of astigmatism; the use of the astigmatometer. Called also *astigmometry.*

**as·tig·mato·scope** (as″tig-mat′ə-skōp) [*astigmatism* + *-scope*] an instrument for discovering and measuring astigmatism.

**as·tig·ma·tos·co·py** (ə-stig″mə-tos′kə-pe) the use of the astigmatoscope.

Astigmatism: the appearance of lines as seen by *(A)* the normal eye and *(B)* the astigmatic eye.

**astig·mia** (ə-stig′me-ə) [*a-*[1] + Gr. *stigma* a point + *ia*] astigmatism.

**as·tig·mic** (ə-stig′mik) astigmatic.

**as·tig·mom·e·ter** (as″tig-mom′ə-tər) astigmatometer.

**as·tig·mom·e·try** (as″tig-mom′ə-tre) astigmatometry.

**as·tig·mo·scope** (ə-stig′mo-skōp) astigmatoscope.

**as·tig·mos·co·py** (as″tig-mos′kə-pe) astigmatoscopy.

**astom·a·tous** (ə-stom′ə-təs) [*a-*[1] + *stomat-* + *-ous*] having no mouth, as certain ciliates.

**asto·mia** (ə-sto′me-ə) [*a* neg. + *stom-* + *-ia*] congenital absence of the mouth.

**asto·mus** (ə-sto′məs) a fetus without a mouth opening.

**As·tra·fer** (as′trə-fər) trademark for a preparation of dextriferron.

**as·trag·a·lar** (as-trag′ə-lər) pertaining to the astragalus (talus).

**as·trag·a·lec·to·my** (as″trag-ə-lek′to-me) [*astragalus* + *-ectomy*] excision of the astragalus (talus).

**as·trag·a·lo·cal·ca·ne·an** (as-trag″ə-lo-kal-ka′ne-ən) pertaining to the astragalus (talus) and the calcaneus.

**as·trag·a·lo·cru·ral** (as-trag″ə-lo-kro̅o̅r′əl) relating to the astragalus (talus) and the leg.

**as·trag·a·lo·scaph·oid** (as-trag″ə-lo-skaf′oid) pertaining to the astragalus (talus) and the scaphoid (navicular) bone.

**as·trag·a·lo·tib·i·al** (as-trag″ə-lo-tib′e-əl) pertaining to the astragalus (talus) and the tibia.

**As·trag·a·lus** (as-trag′ə-ləs) a genus of plants of the family Leguminosae, having many species, some poisonous and others medicinal. *A. gum′mifer* and other Asian species are sources of tragacanth. *A. mollis′simus* and at least seven other North American species are types of *locoweed* and have a mydriatic active principle. Six other species grow preferentially in seleniferous soil and may accumulate large quantities of selenium, causing selenium poisoning in livestock.

**as·trag·a·lus** (as-trag′ə-ləs) [L.; Gr. *astragalos* ball of the ankle joint or dice] the talus, def. 1.

**as·tral** (as′trəl) of or relating to an aster.

**as·tra·pho·bia** (as″trə-fo′be-ə) [Gr. *astrapē* lightning + *-phobia*] irrational fear of thunder and lightning.

**as·tra·po·pho·bia** (as″trə-po-fo′be-ə) astraphobia.

**astric·tion** (ə-strik′shən) [L. *astringere* to constrict] the action of an astringent.

**astringe** (ə-strinj′) to act as an astringent.

**astrin·gent** (ə-strin′jənt) [L. *astringens,* from *ad* to + *stringere* to bind] 1. causing contraction, usually locally after topical application. 2. an agent which has an astringent action.

**astro-** [Gr. *astron* star] a combining form denoting relationship to a star, or to an aster.

**as·tro·blast** (as′tro-blast) [*astro-* + *-blast*] an embryonic cell that develops into an astrocyte.

**as·tro·blas·to·ma** (as″tro-blas-to′mə) an astrocytoma of Grade II; its cells resemble astroblasts, with abundant cytoplasm and two or three nuclei.

**as·tro·cele** (as′tro-sēl) astrocoele.

**as·tro·ci·net·ic** (as″tro-si-net′ik) astrokinetic.

**as·tro·coele** (as′tro-sēl) [*astro-* + *-coele*] the clear space within the astrosphere of a cell in which the centrosome lies.

**as·tro·cyte** (as′tro-sīt) [*astro-* + *-cyte*] [MeSH: Astrocytes] a neuroglial cell of ectodermal origin, characterized by fibrous, protoplasmic, or plasmatofibrous processes. Collectively, such cells are called *astroglia.*
**fibrillary a's, fibrous a's,** astrocytes found mainly in the white matter of the brain, having long, thin, infrequently branched cytoplasmic processes containing numerous fibrillar structures.
**gemistocytic a.,** gemistocyte.
**plasmatofibrous a's,** astrocytes found at the junction of the gray and white matter of the brain; the cytoplasmic processes extending into the white matter are fibrous and those extending into the gray matter are protoplasmic.
**protoplasmic a's,** astrocytes found mainly in the gray matter of the brain, having many branching, thick cytoplasmic processes.

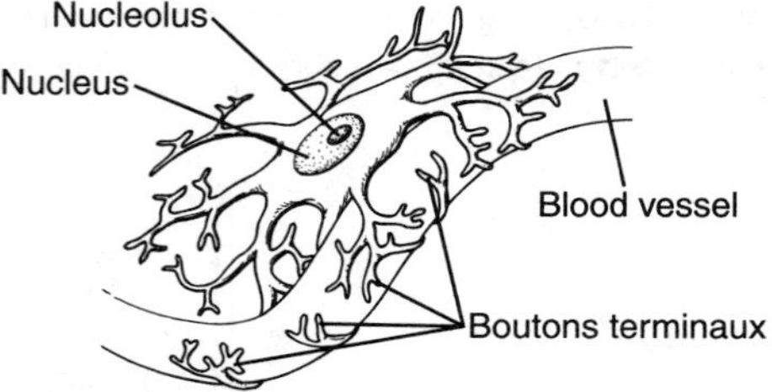

Astrocyte in association with a blood vessel.

**as·tro·cy·to·ma** (as″tro-si-to′mə) [MeSH: Astrocytoma] a tumor composed of astrocytes; it is the most common type of primary brain tumor and is also found throughout the central nervous system. One classification groups astrocytomas according to their histologic appearance and distinguishes *pilocytic, protoplasmic, gemistocytic,* and *fibrillary* types. Another classification groups them in order of increasing malignancy as *Grade I, Grade II, Grade III,* and *Grade IV* types. Called also *astrocytic glioma.*
**anaplastic a.,** a malignant to highly malignant form of astrocytoma that often degenerates into a glioblastoma multiforme; variously classified as a Grade II or a Grade III astrocytoma.
**cerebellar a.,** an astrocytoma in the cerebellum; the most common kind, the *juvenile pilocytic a.,* has a low grade of malignancy, but a second variety, the *diffuse cerebellar a.,* is of a higher grade.
**diffuse cerebellar a.,** a cerebellar astrocytoma that is solid, dense, and infiltrative and resembles a fibrillary astrocytoma; it occurs more frequently in adults and has a higher grade of malignant potential than a pilocytic astrocytoma.
**a. fibrilla′re, fibrillary a.,** an astrocytoma whose cells resemble fibrous astrocytes, usually a Grade I or Grade II astrocytoma found in the cerebrum of an adult, but occasionally occurring in the brain stem or cerebellum. A minority are malignant and undergo anaplastic changes.
**gemistocytic a.,** an astrocytoma whose cells resemble gemistocytes; their cytoplasm is swollen, homogeneously hyaline, and acidophilic in appearance. Their tendency to undergo malignant transformation is variable.
**Grade I a's,** a group of generally slow-growing astrocytomas, including most fibrillary and pilocytic astrocytomas.
**Grade II a's,** astrocytomas with slightly more malignant potential than those of Grade I, including astroblastomas and some fibrillary and pilocytic astrocytomas. One classification system includes some anaplastic astrocytomas in this group.
**Grade III a's,** moderately malignant astrocytomas, including most anaplastic astrocytomas and sometimes including the less malignant of the glioblastoma multiforme group.
**Grade IV a's,** astrocytomas that are highly malignant; this group includes only the glioblastoma multiforme type, although some less malignant glioblastomas are sometimes classified as Grade III.
**juvenile pilocytic a.,** a pilocytic astrocytoma found in the cerebellum in children, one of the most common juvenile brain tumors; it grows slowly and has a low grade of malignancy.
**malignant a.,** an astrocytoma of Grade III or Grade IV; see *anaplastic a.* and *glioblastoma multiforme.*
**pilocytic a.,** an astrocytoma resembling the fibrillary type but with its fibrils arranged in parallel rows; its grade of malignancy is low. The most common kind is the cerebellar *juvenile pilocytic a.* In adults the pilocytic type is usually found in the cerebrum.
**piloid a.,** 1. pilocytic a. 2. polar spongioblastoma.
**protoplasmic a., a. protoplasma′ticum,** a tumor composed of protoplasmic astrocytes. The distinction between this type and fibrillary astrocytoma has been questioned.
**subependymal giant cell a.,** a rare, usually slow-growing astrocytoma found in the wall of the lateral ventricle; it is sometimes associated with tuberous sclerosis.

**as·tro·cy·to·sis** (as″tro-si-to′sis) the proliferation of astrocytes owing to the destruction of nearby neurons during a hypoxic or hypoglycemic episode.

**as·trog·lia** (as-trog′le-ə) [*astro-* + *neuroglia*] 1. astrocytes. 2. the astrocytes considered as tissue; see *macroglia.*

**as·tro·ki·net·ic** (as″tro-kī-net′ik) [*astro-* + *kinetic*] pertaining to the movements of the centrosome.

**as·tro·phor·ous** (as″trof′ə-rəs) [*astro-* + Gr. *phoros* bearing] having star-shaped processes.

**as·tro·pyle** (as″tro-pīl) [*astro-* + *pyle*] the main opening in the capsular membrane of certain marine planktonic protozoa. See also *parapyle.*

**as·tro·sphere** (as′tro-sfēr) [*astro-* + *sphere*] 1. the central mass of an aster, exclusive of the rays. 2. aster.

**as·tro·stat·ic** (as″tro-stat′ik) [*astro-* + *static*] pertaining to the centrosome in its resting condition.

**As·tro·vi·ri·dae** (as″-tro-vir′ĭ-de) the astroviruses; a family of RNA viruses having a nonenveloped spherical virion 28–30 nm in diameter with a characteristic star-shaped outline. The genome consists of a single molecule of polyadenylated positive-sense single-stranded RNA (size 6.8–7.9 kb). Viruses contain four structural proteins and are chloroform-resistant. Infection is host restricted and transmission is by the fecal-oral route. There is a single genus, *Astrovirus.*

**As·tro·vi·rus** (as'tro-vi″rəs) [*astro-* + *virus*] [MeSH: Astrovirus] the sole genus of the family Astroviridae. At least seven serotypes of human viruses have been identified. Infection causes gastroenteritis in humans and many animals and hepatitis in ducklings.

**as·tro·vi·rus** (as'tro-vi″rəs) [MeSH: Astrovirus] any virus belonging to the family *Astroviridae.*

**asul·fu·ro·sis** (a-sul″fu-ro'sis) a condition due to lack of sulfur in the body.

**asyl·la·bia** (ă″sə-la'be-ə) a type of alexia in which the patient recognizes letters but is unable to form them into syllables.

**asy·lum** (ə-si'ləm) [L.] a place of refuge and shelter, as an institution of the past for the support and care of helpless and deprived individuals, such as the mentally deficient, emotionally disturbed, or the blind.

**asym·bo·lia** (ă-sim-bo'le-ə) [*a-*[1] + *symbolia*] 1. loss of power to comprehend the symbolic meaning of things such as words, figures, gestures, and signs; cf. *dyssymbolia.* 2. asemia.
**pain a.,** absence of psychic reaction to pain sensations; it may be congenital or result from brain lesion, particularly of the supramarginal gyrus of the dominant parietal lobe.

**asym·bo·ly** (ə-sim'bo-le) 1. asymbolia, def. 1. 2. asemia.

**asym·met·ri·cal** (a-sim-et'rĭ-kəl) characterized by or pertaining to asymmetry.

**asym·me·try** (a-sim'ə-tre) [*a-*[1] + *symmetry*] lack or absence of symmetry; dissimilarity in corresponding parts or organs on opposite sides of the body which are normally alike. In chemistry, lack of symmetry in the special arrangements of the atoms and radicals within the molecule or crystal.
**chromatic a.,** difference in color in the irides of the two eyes.
**encephalic a.,** a condition in which the two sides of the brain are not the same size.

**asym·phy·tous** (ə-sim'fə-təs) separate or distinct; not grown together.

**asymp·to·mat·ic** (a″simp-to-mat'ik) showing or causing no symptoms.

**asyn·ap·sis** (a-sĭ-nap'sis) [*a-*[1] + *synapsis*] the failure of homologous chromosomes to pair during meiosis.

**asyn·chro·nism** (a-sin'krə-niz-əm) [*a-*[1] + *synchronism*] the occurrence at distinct times of events normally synchronous; disturbance of coordination. See also *heterochronism* and *metachronous.*

**asyn·chro·ny** (a-sin'krə-ne) asynchronism.

**asyn·cli·tism** (ə-sin'klĭ-tiz-əm) [*a-*[1] + *synclitism*] 1. lateral deflection of the fetal head in labor so that the sagittal suture is deflected anteriorly toward the symphysis or posteriorly toward the sacrum. 2. dyserythropoiesis.
**anterior a.,** Nägele's obliquity.
**posterior a.,** Litzmann's obliquity.

**asyn·de·sis** (ə-sin'də-sis) [*a-*[1] + *syn-* + *-desis*] a pattern of language in which words and phrases are juxtaposed without grammatical linkage; seen in schizophrenic and other mental disorders.

**asyn·ech·ia** (a″sin-ek'e-ə) [*a-*[1] + Gr. *synecheia* continuity] absence of continuity of structure.

**asyn·er·gia** (a″sin-ər'je-ə) asynergy.

**asyn·er·gic** (a″sin-ər'jik) marked by asynergy.

**asyn·er·gy** (a-sin'ər-je) [*a-*[1] + *synergy*] lack of coordination among parts or organs normally acting in harmony. See also *ataxia* and *dyssynergia.*

**asy·no·via** (as″ə-no've-ə) deficiency of the synovial secretion.

**asyn·tax·ia** (a″sin-tak'se-ə) [Gr. "want of arrangement"] lack of proper and orderly embryonic development.
**a. dorsa'lis,** failure of the neural groove to close in the developing embryo.

**asys·to·le** (a-sis'to-le) [*a-*[1] + *systole*] absence of a heartbeat; see *cardiac arrest,* under *arrest.*

**asys·to·lia** (a″sis-to'le-ə) asystole.

**asys·tol·ic** (a″sis-tol'ik) characterized by asystole.

**AT** atrial tachycardia.

**At** symbol for *astatine.*

**ATA** alimentary toxic aleukia; see under *aleukia.*

**Ata·brine** (at'ə-brēn) trademark for a preparation of quinacrine hydrochloride.

**At·a·cand** (at'ə-kand) trademark for a preparation of candesartan cilexetil.

**atac·tic** (ə-tak'tik) [Gr. *ataktos* irregular] lacking coordination; irregular; pertaining to or characterized by ataxia.

**atac·ti·form** (ə-tak'tĭ-form) resembling ataxia.

**at·a·rac·tic** (at″ə-rak'tik) [Gr. *ataraktos* without disturbance; quiet] 1. pertaining to or capable of producing ataraxia. 2. tranquilizer.

**At·a·rax** (at'əraks) trademark for preparations of hydroxyzine hydrochloride.

**at·a·rax·ia** (at″ə-rak'se-ə) [Gr. "impassiveness," "calmness"] serenity, calmness, peace of mind.

**at·a·rax·ic** (at″ə-rak'sik) ataractic.

**at·a·raxy** (at″ə-rak'se) ataraxia.

**at·a·vic** (at'ə-vik) atavistic.

**at·a·vism** (at'ə-viz-əm) [L. *atavus* grandfather] the apparent inheritance of a characteristic from remote rather than from immediate ancestors, due to a chance recombination of genes or to unusual environmental conditions favorable to their expression in the embryo. Called also *reversion.*

**at·a·vis·tic** (at″ə-vis'tik) characterized by atavism.

**atax·ia** (ə-tak'se-ə) [Gr., from *a-*[1] + *taxis* order] [MeSH: Ataxia] failure of muscular coordination; irregularity of muscular action. Cf. *asynergy* and *dystaxia.*
**acute a.,** ataxia of sudden onset.
**acute cerebellar a.,** cerebellar ataxia, usually unilateral, associated with infectious disease, tumor, or trauma, resulting in marked hypotonia of muscles on the affected side, asynergy, and assumption of a characteristic posture.
**Bruns' frontal a.,** a disturbance of equilibrium and gait due to a lesion in the frontal lobe; the patient walks with a broad-based gait, taking short steps with feet flat on the ground and a tendency to retropulsion. Called also *Bruns' apraxia of gait* and *frontal a.*
**cerebellar a.,** ataxia due to disease of the cerebellum. See also *acute cerebellar a.* and *spinocerebellar a.*
**cerebral a.,** ataxia due to disease of the cerebrum.
**enzootic a.,** congenital ataxia of lambs, with cerebral demyelination, sometimes proceeding to paralysis, blindness, and death; the cause is thought to be a copper deficiency. Called also *swayback.*
**equine sensory a.,** wobbler syndrome (def. 2).
**feline a.,** panleukopenia.
**Ferguson-Critchley a.,** a rare hereditary ataxia resembling multiple sclerosis, with onset between ages 30 and 45.
**Friedreich's a.,** an autosomal recessive disease, usually beginning in childhood or youth, with sclerosis of the dorsal and lateral columns of the spinal cord. It is attended by ataxia, speech impairment, lateral curvature of the spinal column, and peculiar swaying and irregular movements, with paralysis of the muscles, especially of the lower extremities, and a high-arched foot. It is often associated with hypertrophic cardiomyopathy. Called also *hereditary a.* and *Friedreich's tabes.*
**frontal a.,** Bruns' frontal a.
**hereditary a.,** 1. Friedreich's a. 2. an autosomal recessive disease of fox terrier and Jack Russell terrier dogs in which demyelination of the ventromedial and dorsolateral columns of the spinal cord begins before age 6 months and progresses at varying rates until the animals cannot walk.
**hysterical a.,** ataxia recognizable as a conversion symptom; see also *astasia-abasia,* under *astasia.*
**intrapsychic a.,** the separation of ideas and affect seen in schizophrenic disorders; inappropriateness of affect.
**kinetic a.,** motor a.
**locomotor a.,** tabes dorsalis.
**Menzel's a.,** former name for an adult-onset form of olivopontocerebellar atrophy, now considered to be a type of Friedreich's ataxia.
**motor a.,** inability to coordinate the movements of the muscles; called also *kinetic a.*
**ocular a.,** nystagmus.
**Sanger Brown a.,** former name for a type of olivopontocerebellar atrophy, now considered to be a type of Friedreich's ataxia.
**sensory a.,** ataxia due to loss of proprioception (joint position sensation) between the motor cortex and peripheral nerves, resulting in poorly judged movements, the incoordination becoming aggravated when the eyes are closed.
**spinal a.,** that which is due to disease of the spinal cord.
**spinocerebellar a.,** any hereditary ataxia with cerebellar malfunction resulting in clinical manifestation.
**a.-telangiectasia,** an autosomal recessive disorder characterized by cerebellar ataxia and nystagmus, oculocutaneous telangiectasia, variable degrees of humoral and cellular immunodeficiency, recur-

rent bacterial infections of the respiratory tract from sinuses to lungs, and an increased incidence of lymphoreticular malignancies. There is an increased sensitivity to ionizing radiation caused by a defect in DNA repair. Gonadal hypoplasia, insulin resistance and hyperglycemia, liver function abnormalities, and elevated levels of alpha-fetoprotein and carcinoembryonic antigen are also seen in some patients. Called also *Louis-Bar's syndrome.*
**thermal a.,** a condition characterized by great and paradoxic fluctuations of the temperature of the body.
**truncal a.,** ataxia affecting the muscles of the trunk.

**atax·ia·gram** (ə-tak'se-ə-gram") a tracing drawn by an ataxic patient; also the record made by an ataxiagraph.

**atax·ia·graph** (ə-tak'se-ə-graf") [*ataxia* + *-graph*] an apparatus used to assess the extent of ataxia by measuring the amount of swaying of the body when standing erect with eyes closed.

**atax·i·am·e·ter** (ə-tak"se-am'ə-tər) [*ataxia* + *-meter*] ataxiagraph.

**ataxi·apha·sia** (ə-tak"se-ə-fa'zhə) [*ataxia* + *aphasia*] syntactical aphasia.

**atax·ic** (ə-tak'sik) atactic.

**atax·io·phe·mia** (ə-tak"se-o-fe'me-ə) dysarthria.

**atax·io·pho·bia** (ə-tak"se-o-fo'be-ə) ataxophobia.

**ataxo·phe·mia** (ə-tak"so-fe'me-ə) dysarthria.

**ataxo·pho·bia** (ə-tak"so-fo'be-ə) [Gr. *ataxia* disorder + *-phobia*] irrational dread of disorder or untidiness.

**ataxy** (ə-tak'se) ataxia.

**ATCC** American Type Culture Collection.

**-ate** [L. *-atus,* past participial ending of verbs ending in *-are*] a word termination forming a participial noun, as the object of the process indicated by the root to which it is affixed, e.g., *hemolysate,* something hemolyzed; *homogenate,* something homogenized; *injectate,* something injected. Also forming adjectives, signifying possession of the quality indicated by the root, e.g., *dentate* and *corticate;* and verbs, signifying performance of the action indicated by the root, e.g., *decussate* and *pulsate.*

**-ate** [L. *-atus,* past participial ending of verbs ending in *-are*] in chemistry, a suffix replacing the suffix *-ic* and the word *acid* in forming the names of anions, salts, and esters, e.g., acetate ion, sodium acetate, methyl acetate from acetic acid. Cf. *-ite.*

**at·e·lec·ta·sis** (at"ə-lek'tə-sis) [*atel-* + *-ectasis*] [MeSH: Atelectasis] 1. incomplete expansion of a lung or a portion of a lung; it may be a primary (congenital), secondary, or otherwise acquired condition. 2. airlessness or collapse of a lung that had once been expanded. 3. absence of air in a normally air-filled space such as the middle ear.
**absorption a., acquired a.,** produced by any factor, e.g., secretions, foreign body, tumor, or abnormal external pressure, that completely obstructs the airway, preventing intake of air into the alveolar sacs and permitting absorption of air into the bloodstream. Called also *obstructive a., resorption a.,* and *secondary a.*
**adhesive a.,** alveolar collapse with patent airways, often related to absence or inactivation of surfactant, such as in respiratory distress syndrome of the newborn or radiation pneumonitis.
**cicatrization a.,** loss of lung volume due to fibrosis and the resultant cicatrization.
**compression a.,** acquired atelectasis due to abnormal external pressure on the lung, such as from a large pleural effusion.
**congenital a.,** that present at birth or shortly thereafter; it may occur as a primary condition (see *primary a.*) or secondary to some other congenital disorder (see *secondary a.*).
**initial a.,** primary a.
**lobar a.,** that affecting one lobe of the lung; see also *middle lobe syndrome,* under *syndrome.*
**lobular a.,** that affecting a lobule of the lung; called also *patchy a.*
**obstructive a.,** absorption a.
**passive a.,** relaxation a.
**patchy a.,** lobular a.
**platelike a.,** subsegmental a.
**primary a.,** congenital atelectasis, common among premature infants, in which there is failure of initial alveolar expansion, due to pulmonary immaturity or to inadequacy of respiratory effort that may be a result of weakness of respiratory muscles, severe illness, softness of thoracic cage, brain damage with injury to the respiratory center, or oversedation. Called also *anectasis* and *initial a.*
**relaxation a.,** atelectasis occurring because of large amounts of air or fluid in the pleural cavity, as in pneumothorax or pleural effusion. Called also *passive a.*
**resorption a.,** absorption a.
**round a., rounded a.,** a localized, reversible form in subjacent peripheral tissue, often following resorption of a pleural effusion and characterized by focal pleural scarring. Called also *folded lung syndrome.*
**secondary a.,** 1. absorption atelectasis occurring at birth or in the newborn period, in which the pulmonary alveoli collapse after initial expansion by air; it is due to obstruction of the airway which prevents further entrance of air or to prevention of air from remaining in the alveoli by increased surfaces forces, occurring as a result of inhalation of amniotic debris or mucous plugs, deficiency of pulmonary surfactant (see *respiratory distress syndrome of newborn,* under *syndrome*), obstruction by congenital abnormalities, or abnormal external pressure upon the lung. 2. absorption a.
**segmental a.,** atelectasis affecting one segment of a lung.
**subsegmental a.,** that affecting only the part of a lung distal to an occluded segmental bronchus; called also *platelike a.*
**tympanic membrane a.,** a complication of chronic serous otitis media in which the middle ear contains a viscous fluid and the tympanic membrane has become thin, atrophic, retracted, and adherent to middle ear structures; there is usually conductive hearing loss. Called also *adhesive* or *atelectatic otitis media.*

**at·e·lec·tat·ic** (at"ə-lek-tat'ik) pertaining to or characterized by atelectasis.

**atel·en·ce·pha·lia** (ə-tel"en-sə-fa'le-ə) [*atel-* + *encephal-* + *-ia*] congenital imperfect development of the brain.

**ate·lia** (ə-te'le-ə) [Gr. *ateleia* incompleteness] imperfect or incomplete development.

**ate·li·ot·ic** (ə-te"le-ot'ik) pertaining to or characterized by atelia.

**atel(o)-** [Gr. *atelēs* incomplete] a combining form meaning imperfect or incomplete.

**at·e·lo·car·dia** (at"ə-lo-kahr'de-ə) [*atelo-* + Gr. *kardia* heart] congenitally incomplete development of the heart.

**at·e·lo·ceph·a·lous** (at"ə-lo-sef'ə-ləs) [*atelo-* + Gr. *kephalē* head] having an incomplete head.

**at·e·lo·ceph·a·ly** (at"ə-lo-sef'ə-le) congenitally incomplete development of the skull.

**at·e·lo·chei·lia** (at"ə-lo-ki'le-ə) [*atelo-* + *cheil-* + *-ia*] congenitally incomplete development of a lip.

**at·e·lo·chei·ria** (at"ə-lo-ki're-ə) [*atelo-* + *cheir-* + *-ia*] congenitally incomplete development of the hand.

**at·e·lo·en·ce·pha·lia** (at"ə-lo-en"sə-fa'le-ə) atelencephalia.

**at·e·lo·glos·sia** (at"ə-lo-glos'e-ə) [*atelo-* + *gloss-* + *-ia*] congenitally incomplete development of the tongue.

**at·e·log·na·thia** (at"ə-log-na'the-ə) [*atelo-* + *gnath-* + *-ia*] congenitally incomplete development of the jaw.

**at·e·lo·my·e·lia** (at"ə-lo-mi-e'le-ə) [*atelo-* + *myel-* + *-ia*] congenitally incomplete development of the spinal cord.

**atel·op·id·tox·in** (a-təl-op"id-tok'sin) a potent dialyzable toxin derived from the skin of frogs of the genus *Atelopus,* of Central and South America. The $LD_{50}$ in mice is 16 $\mu$g/kg. Its chemical and pharmacological nature has not been fully defined.

**at·e·lo·po·dia** (at"ə-lo-po'de-ə) [*atelo-* + *pod-* + *-ia*] congenitally incomplete development of the foot.

**at·e·lo·pro·so·pia** (at"ə-lo-pro-so'pe-ə) [*atelo-* + *prosop-* + *-ia*] congenitally incomplete development of the face.

**at·e·lo·ra·chid·ia** (at"ə-lo-ra-kid'e-ə) [*atelo-* + *rhachi-* + *-ia*] congenitally incomplete development of the vertebral column.

**at·e·lo·sto·mia** (at"ə-lo-sto'me-ə) [*atelo-* + *stom-* + *-ia*] congenitally incomplete development of the mouth.

**aten·o·lol** (ə-ten'ə-lol) [USP] [MeSH: Atenolol] a cardioselective $\beta_1$-adrenergic receptor blocking agent used in the treatment of hypertension and chronic angina pectoris.

**ATG** antithymocyte globulin.

**At·gam** trademark for preparations of lymphocyte immune globulin and antithymocyte globulin (equine).

**athe·lia** (ə-the'le-ə) [*a-*[1] + *thel-* + *-ia*] congenital absence of the nipple(s).

**Ath·e·nae·us** (ath"ə-ne'əs) a Greek physician, born in Asia Minor, who practiced in Rome under the Emperors Claudius and Nero (A.D. 41–68). He considered medicine part of general education, followed Aristotle's physiology, added pneuma ("breath," "spirit") to the four elements as the fifth, and founded the Pneumatist School. His school, speculative, not practical or empirical, explained health and sickness in terms of good and bad temperaments.

**ath·er·ec·to·my** (ath"ər-ek'tə-me) [*ather-* + *ectomy*] [MeSH: Atherectomy] the removal of atherosclerotic plaque from an artery using a rotary cutter inside a special catheter guided radiographically; it does not extend to the tunica intima as endarterectomy does.
**directional a.,** that done using a directional atherectomy catheter.
**rotational a.,** rotablation.
**transluminal a.,** see under *endarterectomy.*

**ather·man·cy** (ə-thər′mən-se) the state of being athermanous.

**ather·ma·nous** (ə-thər′mə-nəs) [*a-*[1] + *thermic*] absorbing heat rays and not permitting them to pass.

**ather·mic** (a-thər′mik) afebrile.

**ather·mo·sys·tal·tic** (ə-thər″mə-sis-tal′tik) [*a-*[1] + *thermo-* + *systaltic*] not contracting under the action of cold or heat; said of skeletal muscle.

**ather(o)-** [Gr. *athērē* gruel] a combining form denoting fatty degeneration, or relationship to an atheroma.

**ath·ero·em·bo·lism** (ath″ər-o-em′bo-liz-əm) [*athero-* + *embolism*] embolism due to blockage of a blood vessel by an atheroembolus.

**ath·ero·em·bo·lus** (ath″ər-o-em′bo-ləs) pl. *atheroem′boli* [*athero-* + *embolus*] an embolus composed of cholesterol or its esters or of fragments of atheromatous plaques, typically lodging in small arteries.

**ath·ero·gen·e·sis** (ath″ər-o-jen′ə-sis) [*athero-* + *genesis*] the formation of atheromatous lesions in the arterial intima.

**ath·ero·gen·ic** (ath″ər-o-jen′ik) conducive to or causing atherogenesis.

**ath·er·o·ma** (ath″ər-o′mə) [Gr. *athērōma* a tumor filled with gruel-like matter, from *athērē* gruel] a mass of plaque of degenerated, thickened arterial intima occurring in atherosclerosis; called also *atherosis* and *atheromatous degeneration.*

**ath·er·o·ma·to·sis** (ath″ər-o″mə-to′sis) a diffuse atheromatous disease of the arteries.

**ath·er·o·ma·tous** (ath″ər-o′mə-təs) affected with or of the nature of atheroma.

**ath·ero·scle·ro·sis** (ath″ər-o-sklə-ro′sis) [*athero-* + *sclerosis*] [MeSH: Atherosclerosis] a common form of arteriosclerosis in which deposits of yellowish plaques (atheromas) containing cholesterol, lipoid material, and lipophages are formed within the intima and inner media of large and medium-sized arteries.
**a. obli′terans,** arteriosclerosis obliterans.

**ath·er·o·sis** (ath″ər-o′sis) atheroma.

**ath·e·toid** (ath′ə-toid) [Gr. *athetos* not fixed + *-oid*] resembling or affected with athetosis.

**ath·e·to·sic** (ath″ə-to′sik) athetotic.

**ath·e·to·sis** (ath″ə-to′sis) [Gr. *athetos* not fixed + *-osis*] [MeSH: Athetosis] a form of dyskinesia marked by ceaseless occurrence of slow, sinuous, writhing movements, especially severe in the hands, and performed involuntarily; it may occur after hemiplegia, and is then known as *posthemiplegic chorea.* Called also *mobile spasm.*
**double a., double congenital a.,** congenital bilateral athetosis due to birth trauma, which may occur in association with spastic paraplegia, as in *Vogt's syndrome* and *Little's disease.*
**pupillary a.,** hippus.

**ath·e·tot·ic** (ath″ə-tot′ik) pertaining to athetosis.

**athi·a·mi·no·sis** (a-thi″ə-mĭ-no′sis) thiamine deficiency.

**athrep·sia** (ə-threp′se-ə) [*a-*[1] + Gr. *threpsis* nutrition] 1. marasmus. 2. Ehrlich's term for immunity to tumor inoculation due to a supposed lack of the special nutritive material necessary for tumor growth.

**ath·rep·sy** (ə-threp′se) athrepsia.

**athrep·tic** (ə-threp′tik) pertaining to or characterized by athrepsia.

**ath·ro·cy·to·sis** (ath″ro-si-to′sis) absorption of macromolecules from the lumen of the renal tubules by renal tubular cells by means of a process similar to phagocytosis.

**ath·ro·phago·cy·to·sis** (ath″ro-fag″o-si-to′sis) non-nutritive phagocytosis; phagocytosis of inert particles, as the removal of injected carbon particles.

**athym·ia** (ə-thīm′e-ə) 1. [*a-*[1] + *thymus*] athymism. 2. [Gr. "lack of spirit"] name formerly given to absence of feeling or emotion, as seen in depression or the dysthymic disorder.

**athym·ism** (ə-thīm′iz-əm) 1. absence of the thymus. 2. the condition resulting from absence of the thymus; if it is congenital or the result of neonatal thymectomy, it will be accompanied by a lack of T lymphocytes with some degree of immunodeficiency. Called also *athymia.*

**athy·rea** (ə-thi′re-ə) 1. hypothyroidism. 2. athyria (def. 2).

**athy·re·o·sis** (ə-thi″re-o′sis) 1. hypothyroidism. 2. athyria (def. 2).

**athy·re·ot·ic** (ə-thi″re-ot′ik) 1. hypothyroid. 2. athyrotic (def. 2).

**athy·ria** (ə-thi′re-ə) 1. hypothyroidism. 2. complete absence of thyroid function; the concept has largely been replaced by severe hypothyroidism.

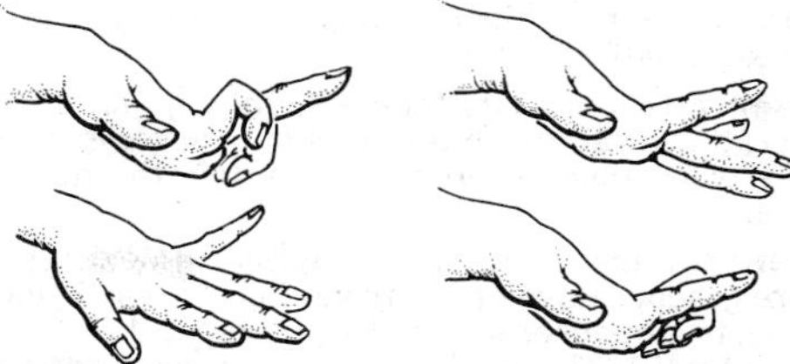
Positions of fingers in movements of athetosis.

**athy·roid·emia** (a-thi″roi-de′me-ə) [*a-*[1] + *thyroid* + *-emia*] absence of thyroid hormone from the blood.

**athy·roid·ism** (a-thi′roid-iz-əm) 1. hypothyroidism. 2. athyria (def. 2).

**athy·roi·do·sis** (a-thi″roi-do′sis) 1. hypothyroidism. 2. athyria (def. 2).

**athy·ro·sis** (a″thi-ro′sis) 1. hypothyroidism. 2. athyria (def. 2).

**athy·rot·ic** (a″thi-rot′ik) 1. hypothyroid. 2. pertaining to or characterized by athyria.

**Athys·a·nus** (ə-this′ə-nəs) a genus of blood-sucking flies of Algeria.

**At·i·van** (at′ĭ-van) trademark for preparations of lorazepam.

**ATL** adult T-cell leukemia/lymphoma; see under *leukemia.*

**atlant(o)-** [Gr. *atlas,* q.v., gen. *atlantos*] a combining form denoting relationship to the atlas.

**at·lan·tad** (at-lan′tad) toward the atlas.

**at·lan·tal** (at-lan′təl) pertaining to the atlas.

**at·lan·to·ax·i·al** (at-lan″to-ak′se-əl) pertaining to the atlas and the axis.

**at·lan·to·did·y·mus** (at-lan″to-did′ə-məs) dicephalus.

**at·lan·to·mas·toid** (at-lan″to-mas′toid) pertaining to the atlas and the mastoid process.

**at·lan·to·odon·toid** (at-lan″to-o-don′toid) pertaining to the atlas and the odontoid process of the axis.

**at·las** (at′ləs) [Gr. *Atlas* the Greek god who bears up the pillars of Heaven] [MeSH: Atlas] 1. [TA] the first cervical vertebra, which articulates above with the occipital bone and below with the axis. 2. a collection of illustrations on one subject, such as anatomy, blood and bone marrow, brain, cardiac disease.
**stereotactic a.,** a group of maps of the areas of the cerebrum, usually stressing physiologic functions, for use in stereotactic surgery.

**at·lo·ax·oid** (at″lo-ak′soid) pertaining to the atlas and the axis.

**at·lo·did·y·mus** (at″lo-did′ə-mus) [*atlas* + Gr. *didymos* twin] dicephalus.

**at·loi·do·oc·cip·i·tal** (at-loi″do-ok-sip′ĭ-təl) pertaining to the atlas and the occiput.

**atm** atmosphere.

**atm(o)-** [Gr. *atmos* steam or vapor] a combining form denoting relationship to steam or vapor.

**at·mol·y·sis** (at-mol′ə-sis) [*atmo-* + *-lysis*] 1. the separation of mixed gases by passing through a porous plate, the more diffusible

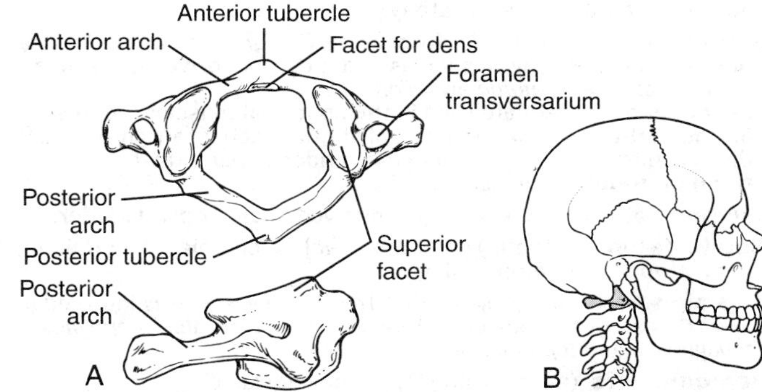

Atlas. *(A), (Top)* superior aspect; *(bottom)* transverse aspect. Note the absence of the body and spinous process. *(B),* Position.

passing through first. 2. the disintegration of organic tissue by the fumes of toxic volatile fluids.

**at·mom·e·ter** (at-mom'ə-tər) [*atmo-* + *-meter*] an instrument for measuring exhaled vapors, or the amount of water exhaled by evaporation in a given time, in order to ascertain the humidity of the atmosphere.

**at·mos·phere** (at'məs-fēr) [*atmo-* + *sphere*] [MeSH: Atmosphere] 1. the entire gaseous envelope surrounding the earth, including the troposphere, tropopause, and stratosphere. 2. the unit of pressure equal to exactly 101325 pascals, the pressure exerted by the earth's atmosphere at sea level, approximately 760 mm Hg. Symbol, atm.

**at·mos·pher·ic** (at″məs-fer'ik) of or pertaining to the atmosphere.

**ATN** tyrosinase-negative (ty-neg) oculocutaneous albinism.

**at no** atomic number.

**ato·cia** (a-to'shə) [*a-*[1] + *toc-* + *-ia*] 1. nulliparity. 2. sterility in the female.

**at·om** (at'əm) [Gr. *atomos* indivisible] any one of the ultimate particles of a molecule or of any matter. An atom is the smallest particle of an element that is capable of entering into a chemical reaction. The atom consists of a minute central nucleus, in which practically all of the mass of the atom is concentrated, and of surrounding electrons. The nucleus is positively charged; the amount of the charge corresponds to the atomic number of the atom. See *Table of Elements,* at *element.* In a neutral atom the surrounding negative electrons are equal in number to the positive charges on the nucleus. The number and arrangement of these electrons determine all the properties of the atom except its atomic weight and its radioactivity.
**activated a.,** 1. an ionized atom. 2. an atom in which some of the orbital electrons have been driven out into larger and less stable orbits; the atom is thus prepared to release its stored energy as these electrons return to their normal and stable orbits. Called also *excited a.*
**asymmetric carbon a.,** a carbon atom with four different substituents. Such a molecule does not have a mirror plane passing through the asymmetric atom, and thus may be optically active.
**Bohr a.,** the conception of a nuclear atom in which the orbital electrons are able to occupy only certain orbits, these orbits being determined by quantum limitations.
**excited a.,** activated a.
**ionized a.,** an atom from which one or more of the outer or valence electrons have been removed, or to which one or more electrons have been added (hence positive and negative ions).
**nuclear a.,** the conception or theory of the atom as composed of a small central nucleus surrounded by orbital electrons; called also *Rutherford a.*
**recoil a., rest a.,** the portion of an atom from which an alpha particle or other subatomic particle has been given off; this remaining part recoils with a velocity inversely proportional to its mass.
**Rutherford a.,** nuclear a.
**stripped a.,** an atom from which the orbital electrons have been more or less completely removed.
**tagged a.,** one which has been made radioactive, so that its course in the body may be checked; see *radioactive tracer,* under *tracer.*

**atom·ic** (ə-tom'ik) of or pertaining to an atom.

**at·om·i·za·tion** (at″əm-ĭ-za'shən) nebulization.

**at·om·iz·er** (at'əm-īz″ər) [MeSH: Nebulizers and Vaporizers] nebulizer.

**ato·nia** (ə-to'ne-ə) atony.
**choreatic a.,** deficient muscular tonicity often seen in chorea.

**aton·ic** (ə-ton'ik) lacking normal tone or strength; pertaining to or characterized by atony.

**at·o·nic·i·ty** (at″ə-nis'ĭ-te) atony.

**at·o·ny** (at'ə-ne) [L. *atonia,* from *a-*[1] + Gr. *tonos* tension] lack of normal tone or strength, such as in a muscle deprived of its innervation. Called also *atonia* and *atonicity.*
**abomasal a.,** inadequate tone in the abomasal muscles, often seen in postparturient cows and a contributing factor to right and left displacement of the abomasum (see under *displacement*).
**primary ureteral a.,** megaloureter.

**at·o·pen** (at'ə-pen) the allergen involved in an atopic disorder.

**atop·ic** (a-top'ik, ə-top'ik) [*a-*[1] + *top-* + *-ic*] 1. ectopic. 2. pertaining to an atopen or to atopy; allergic.

**atop·og·no·sia** (ə-top″og-no'zhə) [*a-*[1] + *topo-* + *gnōsis* knowledge + *-ia*] loss of the power of topesthesia; called also *atopognosis, topagnosia,* and *topoanesthesia.*

**atop·og·no·sis** (ə-top″og-no'sis) atopognosia.

**at·o·py** (at'ə-pe) [Gr. *atopos* out of place] a genetic predisposition toward the development of immediate (type I) hypersensitivity reactions against common environmental antigens (atopic allergy). The most common clinical manifestation is allergic rhinitis; bronchial asthma, atopic dermatitis, and food allergy occur less frequently.

**ator·va·stat·in cal·ci·um** (a-tor″və-sta'tin) an antihyperlipidemic agent that acts by inhibiting cholesterol synthesis, used in the treatment of primary hypercholesterolemia and dyslipidemia; administered orally.

**atox·ic** (a-tok'sik) [*a-*[1] + *toxic*] not poisonous; not due to a poison.

**atox·i·gen·ic** (a-tok″sĭ-jen'ik) not producing or elaborating toxins.

**ATP** adenosine triphosphate.

**ATPase** adenosinetriphosphatase.

**ATP cit·rate ly·ase** (sit'rāt li'ās) [MeSH: ATP Citrate Lyase] an enzyme of the lyase class that catalyzes the ATP-dependent cleavage of citrate to form oxaloacetate and acetate, the latter then condensing with coenzyme A to form acetyl coenzyme A. The reaction is part of the mechanism by which acetyl coenzyme A produced in the mitochondria from pyruvate can be transported to the cytosol to be used in fatty acid synthesis. In EC nomenclature, called *ATP citrate* (pro-S) *lyase* [EC 4.1.3.8]. Called also *citrate cleavage enzyme.*

**ATP syn·thase** (sin'thās) $H^+$-transporting ATP synthase.

**Atrac·tas·pis** (ə-trak-tas'pis) a genus of African vipers whose bite is toxic to humans.

**atra·cu·rium bes·y·late** (at″rə-kūr'e-əm) a nondepolarizing neuromuscular blocking agent of intermediate duration, administered intravenously as an adjunct to general anesthesia to facilitate endotracheal intubation, induce skeletal muscle relaxation during surgery, and facilitate mechanical ventilation.

**atrans·fer·ri·ne·mia** (a-trans″fər-ĭ-ne'me-ə) absence from the circulating blood of iron-binding protein (transferrin).

**atrau·mat·ic** (a″traw-mat'ik) [*a-*[1] + *traumatic*] not inflicting or causing damage or injury.

**Atrax** (a'traks) the funnel-web spiders, a tarantulalike genus found in Australia, of the family Dipluridae. *A. formida'bilis* is the tree funnel-web spider. This and other species have a venomous bite. *A. robus'tus* has caused human deaths.

**at·rep·sy** (at'rep-se) [*a-*[1] + Gr. *threpsis* nutrition] athrepsia (def. 1).

**atrep·tic** (ə-trep'tik) athreptic.

**atre·sia** (ə-tre'zhə) [*a-*[1] + Gr. *trēsis* a hole + *-ia*] congenital absence or closure of a normal body orifice or tubular organ; called also *clausura.*
**anal a., a. a'ni,** imperforate anus.
**aortic a.,** absence or closure of the aortic root orifice, a rare congenital anomaly in which the left ventricle is hypoplastic, oxygenated blood passing from the left into the right atrium through a septal defect, and the mixed venous and arterial blood passing from the pulmonary artery to the aorta by way of a patent ductus.
**aural a.,** obstruction of the external acoustic meatus; it may be either congenital or acquired through trauma or disease.
**biliary a.,** obliteration or hypoplasia of one or more components of the bile ducts due to arrested fetal development, resulting in persistent jaundice and liver damage ranging from biliary stasis to biliary cirrhosis, with splenomegaly as portal hypertension progresses.
**bronchial a.,** atresia of a lobar or segmental bronchus, usually in the left upper lobe; the affected lung segment is often hyperinflated due to leakage of air through the alveolar pores.
**choanal a.,** congenital bony or membranous occlusion of one or both choanae, due to failure of the embryonic bucconasal membrane to rupture. Cf. *atretorrhinia.*
**duodenal a.,** congenital absence or occlusion of a portion of the duodenum, characterized by vomiting a few hours after birth, cessation of bowel movements after one to three days, and usually distention of the epigastrium. It is often associated with Down syndrome.
**esophageal a.,** congenital lack of continuity of the esophagus, commonly associated with tracheosophageal fistula and characterized by excessive salivation, gagging, vomiting when fed, cyanosis, and dyspnea.
**follicular a., a. folli'culi,** the degeneration and resorption of an ovarian follicle before it reaches maturity and ruptures.
**intestinal a.,** congenital obstruction of the intestine at any level, most commonly of the ileum, due to lack of continuity of the lumen; symptoms vary with the site of obstruction.
**a. i'ridis,** closure of the pupillary opening.
**lacrimal duct a.,** blockage of a lacrimal duct, as in congenital imperforation or with scar tissue. Called also *dacryagogatresia.*
**laryngeal a.,** congenital lack of the normal opening into the larynx. See also *laryngeal web.*
**mitral a.,** congenital obliteration of the mitral valve orifice; it is associated with hypoplastic left-heart syndrome or transposition of the great vessels.

**prepyloric a.,** congenital obstruction of the gastric outlet by an antral or pyloric membrane, characterized by vomiting of gastric contents only. Called also *pyloric a.*
**pulmonary a.,** congenital severe narrowing or obstruction of the opening between the pulmonary artery and the right ventricle, characterized by cardiomegaly, reduced pulmonary vascularity, and right ventricular atrophy. It is usually associated with tetralogy of Fallot, transposition of the great vessels, or other cardiovascular anomalies.
**pyloric a.,** prepyloric a.
**tricuspid a.,** absence of the orifice between the right atrium and ventricle, circulation being made possible by the presence of an atrial septal defect, blood passing from the right to the left atrium and thence to the left ventricle and aorta. Classification by type is made according to the presence or absence of pulmonary stenosis and of transposition of the great vessels.

**atre·sic** (ə-tre′zik) atretic.

**atret·ic** (ə-tret′ik) [*atret-* + *-ic*] without an opening; pertaining to or characterized by atresia.

**atret(o)-** [Gr. *atrētos* not perforated] a combining form denoting absence of a normal opening; imperforate or closed.

**atre·to·ble·pha·ria** (ə-tre″to-blə-far′e-ə) [*atreto-* + *blepharo-* + *-ia*] symblepharon.

**atre·to·ceph·a·lus** (ə-tre″to-sef′ə-ləs) [*atreto-* + Gr. *-cephalus*] a fetus lacking the orifices normally present in the head.

**atre·to·cor·mus** (ə-tre″to-kor′məs) [*atreto-* + Gr. *kormos* trunk] a fetus or infant having one of the body openings imperforate.

**atre·to·cys·tia** (ə-tre″to-sis′te-ə) [*atreto-* + *cyst-* + *-ia*] lack of the normal opening from the bladder.

**atre·to·gas·tria** (ə-tre″to-gas′tre-ə) [*atreto-* + *gastr-* + *-ia*] lack of the normal opening into the stomach.

**atre·to·le·mia** (ə-tre″to-le′me-ə) [*atreto-* + Gr. *laimos* gullet + *-ia*] laryngeal atresia.

**atre·to·me·tria** (ə-tre″to-me′tre-ə) [*atreto-* + *metr-* + *-ia*] hysteratresia.

**atre·top·sia** (ă″tre-top′se-ə) atresia iridis; see under *atresia.*

**atre·tor·rhi·nia** (ə-tre″to-ri′ne-ə) [*atreto-* + *rhin-* + *-ia*] absence of the external opening into the nose. Cf. *choanal atresia,* under *atresia.*

**atre·to·sto·mia** (ə-tre″to-sto′me-ə) [*atreto-* + *stom-* + *-ia*] lack of the normal opening into the oral cavity.

**atre·ture·thria** (ah-tre″tu-re′thre-ah) [*atret-* + *urethr-* + *-ia*] urethratresia.

**atria** (a′tre-ə) [L.] plural of *atrium.*

**atri·al** (a′tre-əl) pertaining to an atrium.

**at·ri·cho·sis** (at″rĭ-ko′sis) alopecia.

**atrich·ous** (ə-trik′əs) [*a-*[1] + *trich-* + *-ous*] 1. having no flagella; said of bacteria. 2. having no hair.

**atri(o)-** [L. *atrium,* q.v.] a combining form denoting relationship to an atrium of the heart.

**atrio·com·mis·su·ro·pexy** (a″tre-o-kom″ĭ-su′ro-pek″se) [*atrio-* + *commissure* + *-pexy*] repair of the mitral valve with sutures passed from the ventricle through the valve leaflets and the atrial wall, for correction of mitral insufficiency.

**atrio·his·i·an** (a″tre-o-his′e-ən) connecting the atrium and the bundle of His.

**atrio·meg·a·ly** (a″tre-o-meg′ə-le) [*atrio-* + *-megaly*] abnormal dilatation or enlargement of an atrium of the heart.

**atri·o·pep·tin** (a″tre-o-pep′tin) atrial natriuretic peptide.

**atrio·sep·to·pexy** (a″tre-o-sep′to-pek″se) [*atrio-* + *septo-* + *-pexy*] a closed technique for surgical repair of a defect in the interatrial septum by suturing together part of the atrial wall to obstruct the defect.

**atrio·sep·to·plas·ty** (a″tre-o-sep′to-plas″te) [*atrio-* + *septo-* + *-plasty*] plastic repair of the interatrial septum.

**atri·ot·o·my** (a″tre-ot′ə-me) [*atrio-* + *-tomy*] surgical incision of an atrium of the heart.

**atrio·ven·tric·u·lar** (a″tre-o-ven-trik′u-lər) pertaining to both an atrium and a ventricle of the heart.

**atri·o·ven·tric·u·la·ris com·mu·nis** (a″tre-o-ven-trik″u-la′ris kə-mu′nis) a congenital cardiac anomaly in which the endocardial cushions fail to fuse, the ostium primum persists (producing a low-lying atrial septal defect), sometimes a single atrioventricular valve occurs which has anterior and posterior cusps, and there is commonly a defect of the membranous interventricular septum. Called also *persistent common atrioventricular canal.*

**Atrip·lex** (ə-trip′leks) a genus of herbs and shrubs. *A. littora′lis* and other species are commonly fed to livestock, but in selenium-rich soils they may absorb large amounts of selenium and be a cause of atriplicism, a form of selenium poisoning.

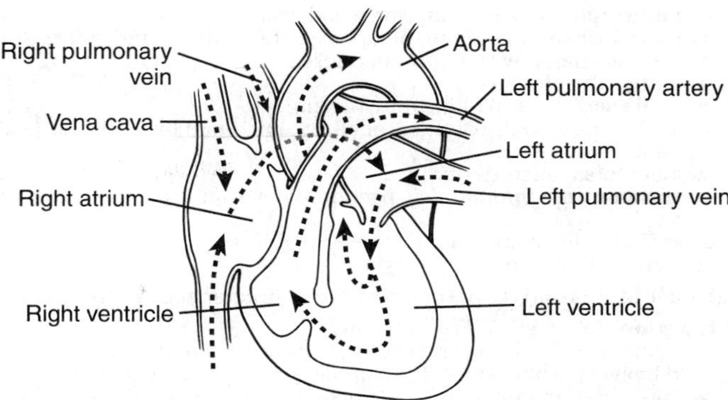


Tricuspid atresia, here displaying a ventricular septal defect and normally related great arteries, the arrows showing the altered flow of blood through the heart.

**atrip·li·cism** (ə-trip′lĭ-siz-əm) selenium poisoning in livestock produced by eating *Atriplex littoralis* or other species grown in selenium-rich soil.

**atri·um** (a′tre-əm) pl. *a′tria* [L.; Gr. *atrion* hall] [TA] a chamber; used in anatomical nomenclature to designate a chamber affording entrance to another structure or organ. Usually used alone to designate an atrium of the heart *(a. cordis).*
**common a.,** the single atrium found in a form of three-chambered heart.
**a. dex′trum** [TA], right atrium: the atrium of the right side of the heart; it receives blood from the superior and the inferior venae cavae and delivers it to the right ventricle.
**a. of glottis,** vestibulum laryngis.
**left a.,** a. sinistrum.
**a. mea′tus me′dii** [TA], atrium of middle meatus: a depression in front of the middle nasal meatus, between the agger nasi and the middle nasal concha.
**right a.,** a. dextrum.
**a. sinis′trum** [TA], left atrium: the atrium of the left side of the heart; it receives blood from the pulmonary veins, and delivers it to the left ventricle.
**a. vagi′nae,** vestibulum vaginae.

**At·ro·mid-S** (at′ro-mid) trademark for a preparation of clofibrate.

**At·ro·pa** (at′ro-pə) [Gr. *Atropos* "undeviating," one of the Fates] a genus of plants of the family Solanaceae, many of which contain alkaloids such as atropine, hyoscyamine, and scopolamine. *A. belladon′na* is deadly nightshade or belladonna (q.v.).

**atroph·e·de·ma** (ə-trof″ə-de′mə) angioedema.

**atro·phia** (ə-tro′fe-ə) [L.; Gr., from *a-*[1] + Gr. *trophē* nourishment] atrophy.

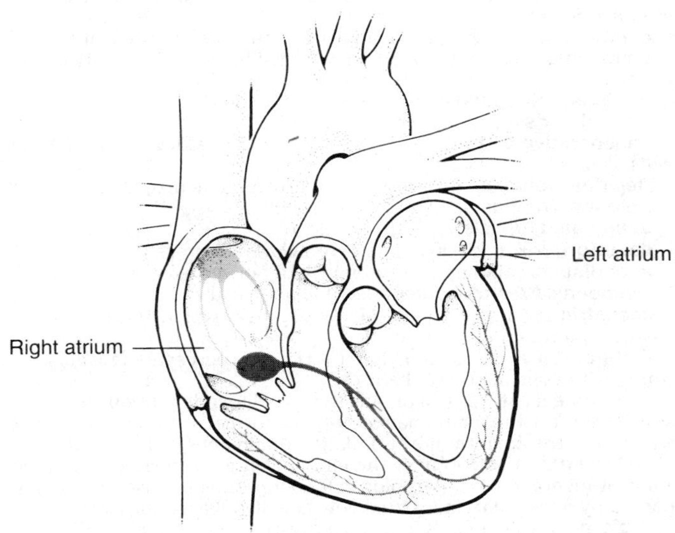


Atria of the heart.

**a. bulbo'rum heredita'ria,** Norrie's disease.
**a. choroi'deae et re'tinae,** atrophy of the choroid and retina, formerly associated with night blindness.
**a. cu'tis,** atrophoderma.
**a. cu'tis seni'lis,** senile atrophy of skin.
**a. doloro'sa,** atrophy of the eyeball accompanied by violent attacks of pain.
**a. maculo'sa,** anetoderma.
**a. musculo'rum lipomato'sa,** pseudohypertrophic muscular dystrophy.
**a. seni'lis,** senile atrophy.
**a. testic'uli,** wasting of the testis.

**atroph·ic** (a-trof'ik) pertaining to or characterized by atrophy.

**atro·phie** (ah-tro-fe') [Fr.] atrophy.
**a. blanche** (blahnsh) [Fr. "white atrophy"], a condition characterized by ivory-white, smooth, atrophic scar tissue with telangiectasia within a hyperpigmented areola, usually occurring on the ankles of middle-aged women.
**a. noire** (nwahr) [Fr. "black atrophy"], a condition characterized by ulcers surrounded by areas of blue-black pigmentation on the ankles, the pigmentation occurring after recurrent attacks of dermatitis with ulceration.

**at·ro·phied** (at'ro-fēd) marked by atrophy; shrunken.

**atroph(o)-** [Gr. *atrophia* want of nourishment] a combining form pertaining to atrophy.

**at·ro·pho·der·ma** (at″ro-fo-dər'mə) [*atropho-* + *derma*] atrophy of the skin or of any part of it. Called also *atrophia cutis* and *atrophodermia.* See also *anetoderma.*
**a. biotrip'ticum,** senile atrophy of skin.
**idiopathic a. of Pasini and Pierini,** see *a. of Pasini and Pierini.*
**a. macula'tum,** anetoderma.
**a. neuri'ticum,** glossy skin.
**a. of Pasini and Pierini,** a condition most commonly occurring on the trunk, especially the back, of young women, characterized by the development of soft, bluish-brown to violaceous atrophic plaques with central induration that resemble the lesions of the late stages of morphea. The etiology is unknown, and it usually resolves spontaneously after months or years. Two types have been suggested: one idiopathic and one closely related to or the same as morphea.
**a. reticula'tum symme'tricum facie'i,** folliculitis ulerythematosa reticulata.
**a. seni'le,** senile atrophy of skin.
**a. vermicula'ris,** atrophodermia vermiculata.

**at·ro·pho·der·ma·to·sis** (at-ro″fo-dər″mə-to'sis) any skin disease having cutaneous atrophy as a prominent symptom.

**at·ro·pho·der·mia** (at″ro-fo-dər'me-ə) atrophoderma.
**a. vermicula'ta,** a group of genodermatoses chiefly characterized by inflammation and later by a reticulated honeycomb- or wormlike follicular atrophy, often accompanied by erythema and follicular plugging, which are transmitted as an autosomal recessive trait and are usually seen in children and young adults. The lesions are usually confined to the cheeks *(folliculitis ulerythematosa reticulata)* but they may primarily involve the forehead and eyebrow region *(ulerythema ophryogenes)* and from there may spread to the scalp. Called also *atrophoderma vermicularis.*

**at·ro·phy** (at'rə-fe) [L., Gr. *atrophia*] [MeSH: Atrophy] 1. a wasting away; a diminution in the size of a cell, tissue, organ, or part. See also *atrophia* and *atrophie.* 2. to undergo this process.

## Atrophy

**acute yellow a.,** massive hepatic necrosis.
**Aran-Duchenne muscular a.,** spinal muscular a.
**arthritic a.,** wasting of the muscles and bone that surround a joint, due to injury or to constitutional disease.
**black a.,** atrophie noire.
**blue a.,** a blue pigmentation that sometimes follows self-injection of drugs by individuals addicted to their use.
**bone a.,** resorption of bone evident both in external form and in internal density. Cf. *osteoporosis.*
**brown a.,** atrophy in which the affected viscus assumes a brownish hue, due to intracellular accumulation of lipofuscin; it is seen chiefly in the heart, liver, and spleen of the elderly.
**Charcot-Marie a., Charcot-Marie-Tooth a.,** Charcot-Marie-Tooth disease.
**circumscribed cerebral a.,** Pick's disease (def. 1).
**compensatory a.,** atrophy, particularly of an endocrine organ, caused by negative feedback mechanisms when its paired organ or another structure releases large amounts of a regulator similar to or identical with the gland's product.
**compression a.,** atrophy of a part due to constant pressure.
**concentric a.,** atrophy of a hollow organ in which its cavity is contracted.
**corticostriatospinal a.,** Creutzfeldt-Jakob disease.
**Cruveilhier's a.,** spinal muscular a.
**degenerative a.,** the wasting of a part due to a degeneration of its cells.
**Dejerine-Sottas a.,** progressive hypertrophic neuropathy.
**Dejerine-Thomas a.,** olivopontocerebellar a.
**denervated muscle a.,** neuropathic a.
**dentatorubral a.,** dyssynergia cerebellaris progressiva.
**a. of disuse,** wasting caused by lack of normal exercise of a part.
**Duchenne-Aran muscular a.,** spinal muscular a.
**eccentric a.,** atrophy of a hollow organ in which the size of the cavity is increased.
**Eichhorst's a.,** the femorotibial form of progressive muscular atrophy with contraction of the toes.
**endocrine a.,** atrophy in organs that are dependent upon endocrine stimulation for the maintenance of their normal structure, occurring when their tropic hormone stimulation diminishes or is absent.
**endometrial a.,** atrophy of the endometrium, occurring physiologically at menopause or pathologically before menopause and accompanied by absence of menstrual flow and shrinkage of the uterus.
**Erb's a.,** 1. Duchenne's muscular dystrophy. 2. limb-girdle muscular dystrophy.
**exhaustion a.,** atrophy of an endocrine organ, presumably caused by prolonged overwork of that organ.
**facial a.,** facial hemiatrophy.
**facioscapulohumeral muscular a.,** see under *dystrophy.*
**fatty a.,** fatty infiltration following atrophy of a tissue or organ; called also *adipositas ex vacuo.*
**Fazio-Londe a.,** progressive bulbar palsy of childhood.
**gastric a.,** a condition in which the thickness of the mucosa of the stomach is greatly reduced, with complete or almost complete disappearance of the gastric and pyloric glands and their replacement by simple mucus-secreting epithelium and by extensive intestinal metaplasia.
**granular a. of kidney,** chronic interstitial inflammation of the kidney producing compression and atrophy of the parenchyma.
**gray a.,** secondary optic a.
**gyrate a. of choroid and retina,** an autosomal recessive form of tapetoretinal degeneration marked by ring-shaped areas of thinning in the periphery of the fundus which enlarge and become confluent, resulting in tunnel vision; night blindness and other disturbances of vision follow. It is characterized by hyperornithinemia and caused by a deficiency of the enzyme ornithine aminotransferase.
**healed yellow a.,** macronodular cirrhosis.
**hemifacial a.,** facial hemiatrophy.
**hemilingual a.,** atrophy of one side of the tongue.
**Hoffmann's a.,** Werdnig-Hoffmann spinal muscular a.
**Hunt's a.,** neuropathic atrophy of the small muscles of the hand unattended by sensory disturbance.
**idiopathic muscular a.,** spinal muscular a.
**infantile a.,** marasmus.
**inflammatory a.,** atrophy of the functioning part of an organ caused by overgrowth of the fibrous elements from inflammation.
**interstitial a.,** absorption of the mineral matter of bones, so that only the reticulated portion remains.
**a. of iris, essential,** a progressive disease of unknown etiology, marked by patchy degeneration and disappearance of the iris stroma followed by loss of epithelium and formation of holes in the iris; it is associated with severe glaucoma.
**ischemic muscular a.,** Volkmann's contracture.
**juvenile muscular a.,** Kugelberg-Welander syndrome.
**lactation a.,** hyperinvolution of the uterus which may follow prolonged lactation.
**Landouzy-Dejerine a.,** facioscapulohumeral muscular dystrophy.
**leaping a.,** progressive muscular atrophy beginning in the hand and extending to the shoulder without affecting the muscles of the arm.
**Leber's hereditary optic a.,** see under *neuropathy.*

**linear a.,** striae atrophicae.
**lobar a.,** Pick's disease (def. 1).
**macular a.,** anetoderma.
**multiple system a.,** a name grouping the cerebral degenerative diseases olivopontocerebellar atrophy, Shy-Drager syndrome, striatonigral degeneration, and one form of parkinsonism as different forms of the same disease process.
**muscular a.,** a wasting of muscle tissue; there are many kinds and causes. See also *spinal muscular a.*
**myelopathic muscular a.,** muscular atrophy due to lesion of the spinal cord, as in spinal muscular atrophy.
**myopathic a.,** muscular atrophy due to disease of the muscle tissue.
**neural a.,** neuropathic a.
**neuritic muscular a.,** neuropathic a.
**neuropathic a.,** atrophy of muscular tissue due to disease of the peripheral nervous system; called also *neural a.*
**neurotrophic a.,** atrophy attributed to destruction of the peripheral neurons that maintain the nutrition of a tissue.
**numeric a.,** atrophy due to diminution in the number of the constituent elements of a tissue, as well as shrinkage of those that remain.
**olivopontocerebellar a.,** any of a group of progressive hereditary disorders involving degeneration of the cerebellar cortex, middle peduncles, ventral pontine surface, and olivary nuclei. They occur in the young to middle-aged and are characterized by ataxia, dysarthria, and tremors similar to those of parkinsonism. Both autosomal dominant and autosomal recessive types have been distinguished. Called also *olivopontocerebellar degeneration* and *Dejerine-Thomas syndrome.*
**optic a.,** atrophy of the optic disk resulting from degeneration of the nerve fibers of the optic nerve and optic tract.
**optic a., hereditary,** Leber's hereditary optic neuropathy.
**optic a., Leber's,** see under *neuropathy.*
**optic a., primary,** a form in which the optic disk is characterized by sharp margins, enlarged physiologic cup, enhanced visibility of the lamina cribrosa, and a white color.
**optic a., secondary,** a form in which the optic disk is characterized by blurred margins, poor visibility of the lamina cribrosa, filling-in of the physiologic cup, and gray-white glial tissue on its surface and along its blood vessels; called also *gray a.*
**pallidal a.,** juvenile paralysis agitans (of Hunt); see under *paralysis.*
**Parrot's a. of the newborn,** primary marasmus.
**pathologic a.,** a decrease in the size of tissues or organs beyond the range of normal variability.
**periodontal a.,** reduction of the size of the alveolar process, associated with recession of the gingiva with subsequent exposure of the root surface.
**peroneal a., peroneal muscular a.,** Charcot-Marie-Tooth disease.
**physiologic a.,** atrophy which affects certain organs in all individuals as part of the normal aging process.
**pigmentary a.,** wasting marked by the deposit of pigment in the atrophied cells, as in brown a.
**postmenopausal a.,** atrophy of various tissues, such as the genital mucosa, occurring after menopause.
**post-traumatic a. of bone,** post-traumatic osteoporosis.
**pressure a.,** decrease in the size of a tissue cell caused by excessive pressure.
**progressive choroidal a.,** choroideremia.
**progressive hemifacial a.,** facial hemiatrophy.
**progressive muscular a.,** spinal muscular a.
**progressive neural muscular a., progressive neuromuscular a.,** Charcot-Marie-Tooth disease.
**progressive retinal a.,** any of a group of hereditary retinal diseases of dogs characterized by progressive dysplasia or degeneration of the retinal rods or cones. Affected animals first have night blindness and then increasingly lose their daytime vision; some develop cataracts.
**pseudohypertrophic muscular a.,** pseudohypertrophic muscular dystrophy.
**pulp a.,** a degenerative process of the dental pulp, characterized by a diminution in size and wasting away of pulpal cells, usually associated with an interference with nutrition. Called also *atrophic pulp degeneration.*
**red a.,** congestive atrophy, mainly of the liver, due to right heart failure.
**rheumatic a.,** atrophy of muscles after an attack of rheumatism.
**segmental sensory dissociation with brachial muscular a.,** see *syringomyelia.*
**senile a.,** the natural atrophy of tissues and organs occurring with advancing age. Called also *atrophia senilis.* Cf. *senile degeneration.*
**senile a. of skin,** the mild atrophic changes in the epidermis and dermis that occur naturally with aging. Called also *atrophia cutis senilis, atrophoderma biotripticum,* and *atrophoderma senile.* See also *actinic elastosis,* under *elastosis.*
**serous a.,** atrophy with the effusion of a serous fluid into the wasted tissues; wasting of fat.
**simple a.,** atrophy due to a shrinkage in size of individual cells.
**spinal muscular a.,** a progressive degenerative disease of the motor cells of the spinal cord. Beginning usually in the small muscles of the hands, but in some cases (scapulohumeral type) in those of the upper arm and shoulder, the atrophy progresses slowly to the muscles of the lower extremity. Called also *Aran-Duchenne disease* or *muscular a., Duchenne-Aran disease* or *muscular a., Cruveilhier's a.* or *paralysis, progressive spinal muscular a.,* and *wasting paralysis.*
**spinal muscular a., infantile,** Werdnig-Hoffmann spinal muscular a.
**spinal muscular a., juvenile,** Kugelberg-Welander syndrome.
**spinal muscular a., progressive,** spinal muscular a.
**spinal muscular a., proximal,** Kugelberg-Welander syndrome.
**spinal muscular a., Werdnig-Hoffmann,** a progressive, infantile, autosomal recessive form of muscular dystrophy, usually occurring in siblings rather than in successive generations, and resulting from degeneration of the anterior horn cells of the spinal cord. It is marked by early onset (usually at about six months of age, but sometimes prenatally), hypotonia and wasting of the muscles, complete flaccid paralysis, and death, usually in early life. Called also *Hoffmann's a., infantile spinal muscular a.,* and *Werdnig-Hoffmann disease.*
**subacute a. of liver, subchronic a. of liver,** subacute hepatic necrosis.
**Sudeck's a.,** post-traumatic osteoporosis.
**Tooth's a.,** Charcot-Marie-Tooth disease.
**toxic a.,** atrophy of an organ in the course of infectious disease.
**trophoneurotic a.,** atrophy due to disease of the nerves or of a center supplying a part.
**vascular a.,** progressive loss of substance in cells and organs when the blood supply to that organ or tissue becomes reduced below a critical level.
**Vulpian's a.,** scapulohumeral type of spinal muscular atrophy.
**white a.,** 1. atrophy of a nerve, leaving only white connective tissue. 2. atrophie blanche.
**yellow a.,** acute yellow a.
**Zimmerlin's a.,** Duchenne's muscular dystrophy.

---

**at•ro•pine** (at'ro-pēn) [USP] [MeSH: Atropine] an alkaloid derived from species of belladonna, hyoscyamus, or stramonium, or produced synthetically. It is an anticholinergic and antispasmodic and is used to relax smooth muscles; to relieve the tremor and rigidity of parkinsonism, and to increase the heart rate by blocking the vagus nerve; as an antidote for various toxic and anticholinesterase agents; and as an antisecretory, mydriatic, and cycloplegic. Ingestion of excessive amounts causes atropinism.
**a. methonitrate, a. methylnitrate,** methylatropine nitrate.
**a. oxide hydrochloride,** a salt of atropine, having the same actions as atropine.
**a. sulfate** [USP], the sulfate salt of atropine, having the same actions as the base; administered parenterally and orally as an anticholinergic, intravenously as a cholinesterase inhibitor, and applied topically to the conjunctiva as a cycloplegic and mydriatic.

**at•ro•pin•ic** (at″ro-pin'ik) having actions similar to atropine, that is, antagonizing the muscarinic effects of acetylcholine.

**at•ro•pin•ism** (at'ro-pin-iz-əm) poisoning caused by ingestion of atropine or belladonna or parts or preparations of any of the plants from which the drugs are derived; the symptoms include excessive dryness of the mouth and throat, dilation of the pupils, fever, rapid pulse, flushing of the face, confusion, mania, and hallucinations, and sometimes a rash.

**at•ro•pin•i•za•tion** (at-ro″pin-ĭ-za'shən) subjection to the influence of atropine.

**at•ro•pism** (at'ro-piz-əm) atropinism.

**At•ro•pi•sol** (at'ro-pĭ-sol″) trademark for preparations of atropine sulfate.

**ATS** American Thoracic Society; antitetanic serum.

**ATSDR** Agency for Toxic Substances and Diseases Registry, an agency of the United States Public Health Service.

**at·tach·ment** (ə-tach'mənt) 1. a connection by which one thing is fixed to another. 2. a device for retention and stabilization of a dental prosthesis.
**edgewise a.,** see under *appliance.*
**epithelial a. (of Gottlieb),** a band or wedge of epithelium whose external surface adheres to the tooth crown and whose internal surface adheres to the lamina propria of the free gingiva, forming a peripheral cuff that seals the periodontal tissue and protects it from foreign material in the oral cavity.
**extracoronal a.,** a precision attachment in which the retaining mechanism is outside the crown of an abutment tooth or restoration.
**friction a., internal a.,** intracoronal a.
**intracoronal a., key-and-keyway a.,** a precision attachment with a slotlike unit (female part) built entirely into the crown and an insert or flange (male part) extending from the prosthesis proper and fitting into the slot when the denture is attached to the crown; the flange may be retained by friction alone or by augmenting mechanical locks, screws, or adjustable latches. Called also *friction a., internal a., parallel a., precision a.,* and *slotted a.*
**orthodontic a.,** see *bracket* (def. 2).
**parallel a.,** intracoronal a.
**precision a.,** 1. a device using a precision rest (q.v.) to attach fixed or removable partial dentures to the crown of an abutment tooth or a restoration; the two primary types are the intracoronal attachment and the extracoronal attachment. Called also *precision anchorage.* See also *extracoronal a., intracoronal a.,* and *semiprecision a.* 2. intracoronal a.
**semiprecision a.,** attachment of a denture to an abutment tooth or a restoration by a semiprecision rest, (q.v.), sometimes supplemented by a spring-loaded plunger or clip, fitting into a rest seat on the lateral surface of a crown, which is especially deepened to provide added retention.
**slotted a.,** intracoronal a.

**at·tack** (ə-tak') an episode or onset of illness.
**Adams-Stokes a.,** an episode of syncope in Adams-Stokes syndrome.
**anxiety a.,** panic a.
**drop a.,** sudden loss of balance without loss of consciousness, usually seen in elderly women; various causes are hypothesized.
**heart a.,** 1. popular term for myocardial infarction. 2. any of various types of acute episodes of ischemic heart disease.
**panic a.** [DSM-IV], an episode of acute intense anxiety, with symptoms such as racing or pounding heart, sweating, trembling, chest pains, nausea, dizziness, faintness, chills or hot flashes, and feelings of choking or smothering. It is the essential feature of panic disorder (q.v.) but may also occur in agoraphobia and other anxiety disorders, as well as in other psychiatric disorders such as schizophrenic disorders or mood disorders. Called also *anxiety a.*
**Stokes-Adams a.,** Adams-Stokes a.
**transient ischemic a. (TIA),** a brief attack (from a few minutes to an hour) of cerebral dysfunction of vascular origin, with no persistent neurological deficit; TIAs are most commonly associated with occlusive vascular disease, especially in the distribution of the carotid and vertebral-basilar systems.
**vagal a.,** vasovagal a.
**vasovagal a.,** a transient vascular and neurogenic reaction marked by pallor, nausea, sweating, bradycardia, and rapid fall in arterial blood pressure which, when below a critical level, results in loss of consciousness and characteristic electroencephalographic changes. It is most often evoked by emotional stress associated with fear or pain. Called also *vasovagal* or *vasodepressor syncope* and *Gowers' syndrome.*

**at·ta·pul·gite** (at"ə-pul'jīt) [*Attapulgus,* a town in Georgia near which it is found] a hydrated aluminum silicate containing magnesium, which is the chief ingredient of fuller's earth (q.v.).
**activated a.** [USP], attapulgite that has been heat treated to increase its adsorbency; used as an adjunct to adsorb bacteria and toxins in the treatment of diarrhea; administered orally.

**at·tar** (at'ar) [Persian "essence"] any essential or volatile oil of vegetable origin.
**a. of roses,** rose oil.

**at·ten·tion** (ə-ten'shən) [MeSH: Attention] 1. selective awareness of a part or aspect of the environment. 2. selective responsiveness to one class of stimuli.

**at·ten·u·ant** (ə-ten'u-ənt) 1. causing thinness, as of the blood. 2. a medicine that thins the blood.

**at·ten·u·ate** (ə-ten'u-āt) [L. *attenuare* to thin] 1. to render thin. 2. to render less virulent; see *attenuation,* def. 2.

**at·ten·u·a·tion** (ə-ten"u-a'shən) [L. *attenuatio,* from *ad-* to + *tenuis* thin] 1. the act of thinning or weakening. 2. the reduction of the virulence of a pathogenic organism, usually by adaptation to another host or to a different culture medium. 3. the process by which a beam of radiation is reduced in energy when passed through tissue or other material. Cf. *adsorption,* def. 3.

**At·ten·u·vax** (ə-ten'u-vaks) trademark for a preparation of live attenuated measles virus vaccine.

**at·tic** (at'ik) [L. *atticus*] recessus epitympanicus.

**at·ti·co·an·trot·o·my** (at"ĭ-ko-an-trot'ə-me) the operation of opening the mastoid antrum and the attic of the middle ear; called also *antroatticotomy.*

**at·ti·co·mas·toid** (at"ĭ-ko-mas'toid) pertaining to the recessus epitympanicus (attic) and the mastoid process of the temporal bone.

**at·ti·cot·o·my** (at"ĭ-kot'ə-me) [*attic* + *-tomy*] the surgical opening of the attic.
**transmeatal a.,** removal through the external auditory meatus of the outer wall of the attic.

**at·ti·tude** (at'ĭ-to͞od) [L. *attitudo* posture] [MeSH: Attitude] 1. a posture or position of the body. In obstetrics, the relation of the various parts of the fetal body to one another, the normal attitude being one of moderate flexion of all the joints, with the back curved forward, the head slightly bent on the chest, and the arms and legs free to move in all natural directions (habitus). 2. a tendency to respond positively or negatively to other individuals, institutions, or programs of activity.
**a. of combat** [Fr. *attitude de combat*], the stiff defensive position with flexion of the elbows, knees, fingers, and neck, like those of a boxer, seen in burned corpses.
**discobolus a.,** a position resembling that of a discus thrower, caused by stimulation of the semicircular canals.
**forced a.,** an abnormal position or attitude due to some disease, such as is seen in meningitis or as the result of contractures.
**military a.,** the condition early in labor in which the fetal neck is deflexed and the cervical spine is in extension.

**atto-** [Danish *atten* eighteen] a combining form used in naming units of measurement to indicate one-quintillionth ($10^{-18}$) of the unit designated by the root with which it is combined. Symbol, a.

**at·trac·tant** (ə-trak'tənt) [L. *attrahere* to draw toward] a substance that exerts an attracting influence, such as one used to attract insect or animal pests to traps or to poisons.

**at·trac·tion** (ə-trak'shən) [L. *attractus* past participle of *attrahere* to draw together] 1. the process of drawing one body toward another. 2. a condition in which the teeth or other maxillary and mandibular structures are higher than normal position, thereby causing shortening of the face. Cf. *abstraction,* def. 2.
**a. of affinity,** chemical a.
**capillary a.,** the force that attracts the particles of a fluid into and along the caliber of a very narrow tube.
**chemical a.,** the tendency of atoms of one element to unite with those of another; called also *a. of affinity.*
**electric a.,** the tendency of bodies bearing opposite electric charges to move toward each other.
**magnetic a.,** the tendency of bodies possessing circulating electric currents to move toward each other.

**at·tri·tion** (ə-trish'ən) [L. *attritio* a rubbing against] the physiologic wearing away of a substance or structure (such as the teeth) in the course of normal use.

**at vol** atomic volume.

**at wt** atomic weight.

**atyp·ia** (a-tip'e-ə) the condition of being irregular or not conforming to type.
**koilocytotic a.,** an abnormal condition of cells of the stratified squamous epithelium of the uterine cervix, characterized by vacuolization and nuclear abnormalities; it may be a premalignant condition.

**atyp·i·cal** (a-tip'ĭ-kəl) [*a-*[1] + *typical*] irregular; not conformable to the type; in microbiology, applied specifically to strains of unusual type.

**atyp·ism** (a-tip'iz-əm) atypia.

**AU** L. *au'res uni'tas* (both ears together) or *au'ris uter'que* (each ear).

**Au** symbol for *gold* (L. *au'rum*); abbreviation for Australia antigen (see *hepatitis B surface antigen,* under *antigen*).

**AUA** American Urological Association.

**Au-an·ti·gen·emia** (an"tĭ-jə-ne'me-ə) hepatitis B antigenemia.

**Aub-Du·bois table** (awb doo-bois') [Joseph Charles *Aub,* American physician, 1890–1973; Eugene Floyd *Dubois,* American physician, 1882–1959] see under *table.*

**Au·ber·ger blood group** (o-bār-zhā') [from the name of the French propositus first reported on in 1961] see under *blood group.*

**Au·bert's phenomenon** (ou-berts') [Hermann *Aubert,* German physiologist, 1826–1892] see under *phenomenon.*

**AUC** area under the curve.

**Auch·mero·my·ia** (awk″mər-o-mi′yə) a genus of flies of the family Calliphoridae. *A. lute′ola* has a larva called the Congo floor maggot that parasitizes humans and pigs in Nigeria and Central Africa.

**au·dile** (aw′dīl) pertaining to hearing; understanding or recalling most readily what has been heard. Cf. *visile.*

**audi(o)-** [L. *audire* to hear] a combining form denoting relationship to hearing.

**au·dio·an·al·ge·sia** (aw″de-o-an″al-je′ze-ə) [MeSH: Audioanalgesia] reduction or abolition of the perception of pain by listening through a head set to recorded music to which a background of "white noise" has been added.

**au·dio·gen·ic** (aw″de-o-jen′ik) produced by sound.

**au·dio·gram** (aw′de-o-gram″) [*audio-* + *-gram*] a record of the thresholds of hearing of an individual for various sound frequencies.
**cortical a.,** a graphic representation of the result of cortical audiometry.

**au·di·ol·o·gist** (aw″de-ol′ə-jist) a person skilled in audiology, including diagnostic testing and the rehabilitation of those whose impaired hearing cannot be improved by medical or surgical means.

**au·di·ol·o·gy** (aw″de-ol′ə-je) [*audio-* + *-logy*] [MeSH: Audiology] the science of hearing, particularly diagnostic testing and the study of impaired hearing that cannot be improved by medication or surgical therapy.

**au·di·om·e·ter** (aw″de-om′ə-tər) [*audio-* + *-meter*] an electronic device that produces acoustic stimuli of known frequency and intensity for the measurement of hearing.
**evoked potential a.,** an instrument that detects response to sound stimuli by changes in the electroencephalogram.

**au·dio·met·ric** (aw″de-o-met′rik) pertaining to the measurement of hearing, as by means of an audiometer.

**au·dio·me·tri·cian** (aw″de-o-mə-trish′ən) a technician specializing in the measurement of hearing ability (audiometry).

**au·di·om·e·try** (aw″de-om′ə-tre) [MeSH: Audiometry] measurement of hearing, as by means of an audiometer.
**Békésy a.,** audiometry in which the patient, by pressing a signal button, traces monaural thresholds for pure tones: the intensity of the tone decreases as long as the button is depressed and increases when it is released. Both continuous and interrupted tones are used.
**cortical a.,** a method of determining auditory acuity by recording and averaging auditory evoked potentials from the cortex of the brain in response to pure tones.
**electrocochleographic a.,** electrocochleography.
**electrodermal a.,** audiometry in which the subject is conditioned to pure tones by harmless electric shock; thereafter when a pure tone is heard a shock is anticipated, resulting in a brief electrodermal response, which is recorded. The lowest intensity at which the response is elicited is taken to be the subject's hearing threshold.
**localization a.,** a technique for measuring the capacity to locate the source of a pure tone received binaurally in a sound field.
**pure tone a.,** audiometry utilizing pure tones that are relatively free of noise and overtones.
**speech a.,** audiometry that measures speech reception threshold in decibels and speech discrimination (ability to understand).

**au·dio·scope** an instrument for the detection of hearing impairment, consisting of an otoscope combined with an audiometer.

**au·di·tion** (aw-dish′ən) [L. *auditio*] 1. hearing. 2. the act of hearing.
**chromatic a.,** color hearing.
**gustatory a.,** a synesthesia in which certain sounds call up a sensation of taste.

**au·di·tive** (aw′dĭ-tiv) a person in whom the prime sense is hearing.

**au·di·tog·no·sis** (aw″dĭ-tog-no′sis) [L. *auditio* hearing + Gr. *gnōsis* knowledge] the sense by which sounds are understood and interpreted.

**au·di·to·ry** (aw′dĭ-tor″e) [L. *auditorius*] pertaining to the sense of hearing; called also *aural.*

**Au·en·brug·ger's sign** (ou-en-broog′ərz) [Leopold Joseph Elder von *Auenbrugger,* Austrian physician, 1722–1809] see under *sign.*

**Au·er bodies (rods)** (ou′ər) [John *Auer,* American physician, 1875–1948] see under *body.*

**Au·er·bach's ganglion, plexus** (ou′ər-bahks) [Leopold *Auerbach,* German anatomist, 1828–1897] see under *ganglion,* and see *plexus myentericus.*

**aug·men·ta·tion** (awg″men-ta′shən) an adding on.
**bladder a.,** augmentation cystoplasty .
**breast a.,** popular name for augmentation mammaplasty.

**Aug·men·tin** (awg-men′tin) trademark for a preparation of amoxicillin and clavulanate potassium.

**aug·men·tor** (awg-men′tor) 1. increasing; a term applied to nerves or nerve cells concerned in increasing the size and force of heart contractions. 2. a substance supposed to increase the action of an auxetic.

**aug·na·thus** (awg-na′thəs) [Gr. *au* again + *gnathos* jaw] dignathus.

**Au·jesz·ky's disease** (ou-yes′kēz) [Aladár *Aujeszky,* Hungarian physician, 1869–1933] pseudorabies.

**AUL** acute undifferentiated leukemia.

**au·la** (aw′lə) [L.; Gr. *aulē* hall] the red erythematous areola formed about the periphery of the vesicle of the vaccination lesion.

**au·ra** (aw′rə) pl. *auras* or *au′rae* [L. "breath"] a subjective sensation or motor phenomenon that precedes and marks the onset of an episode of a neurological condition, particularly an epileptic seizure *(epileptic a.)* or a migraine *(migraine a.).* Cf. *prodrome.*
**a. asthma′tica,** premonitory symptoms preceding an attack of asthma.
**auditory a.,** a simple partial seizure marked by auditory sensations.
**electric a.,** the tingling sensation experienced on the receipt of a discharge of static electricity through the air.
**epigastric a.,** a simple partial seizure with autonomic manifestations, causing an uncomfortable sensation in the epigastrium.
**epileptic a.,** a subjective sensation or motor phenomenon that sometimes gives warning of an approaching generalized or complex partial seizure. Formerly considered part of the prodrome of a seizure, it is now known to be itself a type of simple partial seizure and may occur without progression to a more serious attack.
**a. hyste′rica,** an aura like that preceding an epileptic attack, sometimes experienced by hysterical patients.
**intellectual a.,** a simple partial seizure with psychic manifestations, causing a dreamy mental condition; called also *reminiscent a.*
**kinesthetic a.,** 1. a sensation of movement of some part of the body, with or without such actual movement. 2. focal motor seizure.
**migraine a.,** visual, motor, or psychic disturbances, paresthesias, and other neurologic abnormalities that accompany a migraine; see also *migraine with aura, migraine without aura,* and *migraine a. without headache.*
**migraine a. without headache,** symptoms such as teichopsia that fit the definition of migraine aura but occur without headache or brain lesions; called also *migraine equivalent.*
**motor a.,** an epileptic aura that is a focal motor seizure.
**reminiscent a.,** intellectual a.
**vertiginous a.,** a sensory seizure affecting the vestibular sense, causing a feeling of vertigo. See also *vertiginous epilepsy.*

**Au·ra·fair** (aw″rə-fār″) trademark for a preparation of antipyrine and benzocaine otic solution.

**au·ral**[1] (aw′rəl) [L. *auris* ear] 1. auditory. 2. otic.

**au·ral**[2] (aw′rəl) [L. *aura*] pertaining to or of the nature of an aura.

**Au·ral·gan** (aw-ral′gan) trademark for a preparation of antipyrine and benzocaine otic solution.

**au·ra·mine O** (aw′rə-mēn o) a yellow fluorescent dye used to stain acid-fast bacteria and DNA and as a component of the Truant auramine-rhodamine stain for tubercle bacilli.

**au·ran·o·fin** (aw-ran′ə-fin) [MeSH: Auranofin] a gold-containing compound used in the treatment of active rheumatoid arthritis not adequately controlled by nonsteroidal antiinflammatory drugs, or in combination with nonsteroidal antiinflammatory agents or nondrug therapy such as physical therapy; administered orally.

**au·ran·tia** (aw-ran′shə) an orange coal tar stain, the ammonium salt of hexanitrodiphenylamine; used in staining mitochondria.

**Au·re·lia** (aw-rel′e-ə) a genus of large discophorous jellyfish found in oceans throughout the world; nematocysts of many of the larger forms can penetrate the human skin and produce intense pain.

**Au·reo·ba·sid·i·um** (aw″re-o-bə-sid′e-əm) a genus of Fungi Imperfecti of the form-class Hyphomycetes, form-family Dematiaceae, which produce black yeastlike cells; inhalation of sawdust contaminated with the spores causes sequoiosis. *A. pul′lulans* is a common soil organism and contaminant. Called also *Pullularia.*

**au·re·o·lin** (aw-re′o-lin) a yellow dye.

**Au·reo·my·cin** (aw″re-o-mi′sin) trademark for preparations of crystalline chlortetracycline hydrochloride.

**au·res** (aw′rēz) [L.] plural of *auris.*

**auri-** [L. *auris* ear] a combining form denoting relationship to the ear.

**au·ri·a·sis** (aw-ri′ə-sis) chrysiasis (def. 1).

**au·ric** (aw′rik) pertaining to or containing gold.

**au·ri·cle** (aw′rĭ-kəl) [L. *auricula,* q.v.] 1. auricula. 2. auricula atrialis. 3. formerly, the atrium of the heart (atrium cordis).
**cervical a.,** a flap of skin and yellow cartilage sometimes seen on

the side of the neck at the external opening of a persistent branchial cleft.
**left a. of heart,** auricula sinistra.
**right a. of heart,** auricula dextra.

**au·ric·u·la** (aw-rik′u-lə) pl. *auri′culae* [L., dim of *auris*] [TA] 1. auricle: the portion of the external ear not contained within the head; the flap of the ear. Called also *ala auris* and *pinna.* 2. auricula atrialis. 3. formerly, the atrium of the heart *(atrium cordis).*
**atrial a., a. atria′lis,** the ear-shaped appendage of either atrium of the heart; called also *atrial appendage.*
**a. a′trii dex′tri,** a. dextra.
**a. a′trii sinis′tri,** a. sinistra.
**a. dex′tra** [TA], right auricle: the ear-shaped appendage of the right atrium of the heart.
**a. sinis′tra** [TA], left auricle: the ear-shaped appendage of the left atrium of the heart.

**au·ric·u·lar** (aw-rik′u-lər) 1. pertaining to an auricle. 2. pertaining to the ear.

**au·ric·u·la·re** (aw-rik″u-lă′re) [L. *auricularis* pertaining to the ear] a craniometric point at the top of the opening of the external auditory meatus.

**au·ric·u·la·ris** (aw-rik″u-lă′ris) [L.] pertaining to the ear; auricular.

**au·ric·u·lo·cra·ni·al** (aw-rik″u-lo-kra′ne-əl) pertaining to an ear and the cranium.

**au·ric·u·lo·tem·po·ral** (aw-rik″u-lo-tem′pŏ-rəl) pertaining to an ear and the temporal region.

**au·ric·u·lo·ther·a·py** (aw-rik″u-lo-ther′ə-pe) electrical stimulation of the outer ear for the relief of pain.

**au·ric·u·lo·ven·tric·u·lar** (aw-rik″u-lo-ven-trik′u-lər) a former term for *atrioventricular.*

**au·rid** (aw′rid) [L. *aurum* gold] a skin eruption produced by the systemic administration of gold salts.

**au·ri·form** (aw′rĭ-form) ear-shaped.

**au·rin** (aw′rin) a triphenylmethane derivative occurring as deep red masses with a greenish metallic luster; used as an indicator and dye intermediate. Called also *corallin.*

**auri·na·ri·um** (aw″ri-nar′e-əm) a medicated suppository for insertion into the external auditory meatus.

**au·ri·na·sal** (aw″rĭ-na′zəl) pertaining to the ear and the nose.

**au·ri·pig·ment** (aw″rĭ-pig′mənt) arsenic trisulfide.

**au·ris** (aw′ris) pl. *au′res* [L.] [TA] the ear; the organ of hearing. See Plate 16.
**a. exter′na** [TA], external ear: the portion of the auditory organ comprising the auricle and the external acoustic meatus.
**a. inter′na** [TA], internal ear: the labyrinth, comprising the vestibule, cochlea, and semicircular canals; called also *inner ear.*
**a. me′dia** [TA], middle ear: the cavity in the temporal bone comprising the cavitas tympani, adnexa mastoidea, and tuba auditiva.

**au·ri·scope** (aw′rĭ-skōp) [*auri-* + *-scope*] otoscope.

**au·ro·chro·mo·der·ma** (aw″ro-kro″mo-der′mə) [*aurum* + *chromo-* + *derma*] a permanent greenish-blue staining of the skin due to injection of certain gold compounds.

**au·ro·ther·a·py** (aw″ro-ther′ə-pe) chrysotherapy.

**au·ro·thio·glu·cose** (aw″ro-thi″o-gloo′kōs) [USP] [MeSH: Aurothioglucose] a monovalent gold salt used in the treatment of early active rheumatoid arthritis (both adult and juvenile types) not controlled by nonsteroidal antiinflammatory agents, rest, and physical therapy; administered intramuscularly.

**au·ro·thio·ma·late di·so·di·um** (aw″ro-thi″o-ma′lāt) gold sodium thiomalate.

**au·rum** (aw′rəm) [L.] gold.

**aus·cult** (aws-kult′) auscultate.

**aus·cul·tate** (aws′kəl-tāt) [L. *auscultare* to listen to] to examine by listening, usually to the sounds of the thoracic or abdominal viscera, with or without a stethoscope.

**aus·cul·ta·tion** (aws″kəl-ta′shən) [MeSH: Auscultation] the act of listening for sounds within the body, chiefly for ascertaining the condition of the lungs, heart, pleura, abdomen and other organs, and for the detection of pregnancy.
**direct a., immediate a.,** auscultation performed without the stethoscope.
**Korányi's a.,** auscultatory percussion done by tapping with one forefinger the second joint of the other forefinger applied perpendicularly to the part; called also *Korányi's percussion.*
**mediate a.,** auscultation performed by the aid of an instrument (stethoscope) interposed between the ear and the part being examined.
**obstetric a.,** auscultation in pregnancy for the study of the sounds of the fetal heart.

**aus·cul·ta·to·ry** (aws-kul″tə-tore) of or pertaining to auscultation.

**aus·cul·to·plec·trum** (aws-kul″to-plek′trəm) an instrument for use both in auscultation and percussion.

**aus·cul·to·scope** (aws-kul′tə-skōp) phonendoscope.

**Aus·spitz sign** (ou′spitz) [Heinrich *Auspitz,* Austrian dermatologist, 1835–1886] see under *sign.*

**Aus·tin Flint murmur, respiration** (aw′stin flint) [*Austin Flint,* American physiologist, 1812–1886] see *Flint's murmur,* under *murmur.*

**Aus·tin Moore arthroplasty, prosthesis** (aw′stin mo͞or) [*Austin* Talley *Moore,* American orthopedic surgeon, 1899–1963] see under *arthroplasty* and *prosthesis.*

**Aus·tra·lor·bis** (aws″trə-lor′bis) *Biomphalaria.*

**au·ta·coid** (aw′tə-koid) [*aut-* +Gr. *akos* remedy] local hormone.

**au·techo·scope** (aw-tek′o-skōp) [*aut-* + *echo* + *-scope*] an instrument for auscultating one's own body.

**au·te·cic** (aw-te′sik) autoecious.

**au·te·cious** (aw-te′shəs) autoecious.

**au·te·col·o·gy** (aw″tə-kol′ə-je) [*aut-* + *ecology*] the ecology of an organism as an individual; cf. *synecology.*

**au·te·me·sia** (aw″tə-me′shə) [*aut-* + *emesia*] functional or idiopathic vomiting.

**au·tism** (aw′tiz-əm) [*aut-* + *-ism*] [MeSH: Autism] 1. autistic disorder. 2. autistic thinking.
**infantile a.,** autistic disorder.

**au·tis·tic** (aw-tis′tik) characterized by or pertaining to autism.

**aut(o)-** [Gr. *autos* self] a prefix denoting relationship to self.

**au·to·ac·ti·va·tion** (aw″to-ak″tĭ-va′shən) the activation of a cell by its own secretory products.

**au·to·ag·glu·ti·na·tion** (aw″to-ə-gloo″tĭ-na′shən) 1. clumping or agglutination of an individual's cells by his own serum, as in autohemagglutination. 2. nonspecific clumping or agglutination of particulate antigens (e.g., bacteria) that does not involve antibody; an important cause of error in bacterial agglutination tests.

**au·to·ag·glu·ti·nin** (aw″to-ə-gloo′tĭ-nin) an autologous serum factor with the property of agglutinating the individual's own cellular elements.

**au·to·al·ler·gic** (aw′to-ə-lər′jik) pertaining to or characterized by autoallergy.

**au·to·al·ler·gy** (aw′to-al′ər-je) autoimmunity.

**au·to·am·pu·ta·tion** (aw″to-am″pu-ta′shən) the spontaneous detachment from the body and elimination of an appendage or of an abnormal growth, such as a polyp.

**au·to·anal·y·sis** (aw″to-ə-nal′ə-sis) [MeSH: Autoanalysis] self-analysis.

**au·to·an·ti·body** (aw″to-an′tĭ-bod″e) an antibody directed against a self antigen, i.e., against a normal tissue constituent. An antibody (immunoglobulin) formed in response to, and reacting against, one of the individual's own normal antigenic endogenous body constituents.
**antineutrophil cytoplasmic a. (ANCA),** an autoantibody to cytoplasmic constituents of monocytes and neutrophils, found in increased amounts in some types of vasculitis. There are several different subtypes, each characterized serologically by reactivity against particular cellular antigens; some are specific to given disease states. Called also *antineutrophil cytoplasmic antibody.*

**au·to·an·ti·com·ple·ment** (aw″to-an″ti-kom′plə-mənt) an anticomplement formed in the body against its own complement.

**au·to·an·ti·gen** (aw″to-an′tĭ-jen) an antigen that, despite being a normal tissue constituent, is the target of a humoral or cell-mediated immune response, as in autoimmune disease. Called also *self antigen.*

**au·to·an·ti·sep·sis** (aw″to-an″tĭ-sep′sis) physiological antisepsis.

**au·to·an·ti·tox·in** (aw″to-an″tĭ-tok′sin) [*auto-* + *antitoxin*] antitoxin produced by the animal itself, as opposed to exogenous antitoxin.

**au·to·bi·ot·ic** (aw″to-bi-ot′ik) any of a group of substances produced by cells and controlling the behavior of the producing cells.

**au·to·body** (aw′to-bod″e) an antibody that both carries an idiotypic determinant that is stereochemically similar to the epitope on the antigen against which the antibody was originally directed and at the same time expresses a binding site for the antigen; autobodies therefore have the potential for self-aggregation.

**au·to·ca·tal·y·sis** (aw″to-kə-tal′ə-sis) a catalytic reaction that gradually accelerates in velocity because some of the products of the reaction themselves act as catalytic agents.

**au·to·cat·a·lyst** (aw″to-kat′ə-list) an element participating in autocatalysis.

**au·to·cat·a·lyt·ic** (aw″to-kat-ə-lit′ik) pertaining to, characterized by, or producing autocatalysis.

**au·to·ca·thar·sis** (aw″to-kə-thahr′sis) a form of psychiatric treatment in which the patient writes down thoughts, feelings, and experiences in order to release disturbing emotions associated with them.

**au·to·cath·e·ter·ism** (aw″to-kath′ə-tər-iz-əm) [*auto-* + *catheterism*] self-insertion of a urinary catheter by the patient.

**au·to·cho·le·cys·tec·to·my** (aw″to-ko″le-sis-tek′tə-me) [*auto-* + *cholecystectomy*] invagination of the gallbladder into the intestine, with final separation and expulsion of the organ.

**au·toch·tho·nous** (aw-tok′thə-nəs) [Gr. *autochthōn* sprung from the land itself] 1. found in the place of formation; not removed to a new site. 2. denoting a tissue graft to a new site on the same individual.

**au·to·ci·ne·sis** (aw″to-si-ne′sis) [*auto-* + Gr. *kinēsis* motion] autokinesis.

**au·toc·la·sis** (aw-tok′lə-sis) [*auto-* + Gr. *klasis* breaking] destruction of a part due to conditions within the part.

**au·to·clave** (aw′to-klāv) [*auto-* + L. *clavis* key] an apparatus for effecting sterilization by steam under pressure; it is fitted with a gauge that automatically regulates the pressure and therefore the degree of heat to which the contents are subjected.

**Au·to·clip** (aw′to-klip) trademark for a stainless steel surgical clip for wound closing, inserted by means of a mechanical applicator that automatically feeds a series of clips.

**au·to·coid** (aw′to-koid) local hormone.

**au·to·crine** (aw′to-krin) denoting a mode of hormone action in which a hormone binds to receptors on and affects the function of the cell type that produced it.

**au·to·cys·to·plas·ty** (aw″to-sis′tə-plas″te) a plastic operation on the bladder using grafts from the patient's body.

**au·to·cy·tol·y·sin** (aw″to-si-tol′ĭ-sin) autolysin.

**au·to·cy·tol·y·sis** (aw″to-si-tol′ĭ-sis) autolysis.

**au·to·cy·to·lyt·ic** (aw″to-si″to-lit′ik) autolytic.

**au·to·cy·to·tox·in** (aw″to-si″to-tok′sin) a cytotoxin for the cells of the body in which it is formed.

**au·to·der·mic** (aw″to-dər′mik) [*auto-* + *derma*] of the patient's own skin; a term applied to skin grafts. See *dermatoautoplasty* and *autograft.*

**au·to·di·ges·tion** (aw″to-di-jes′chən) self-digestion; autolysis; applied especially to the digestion of the walls of the stomach and contiguous structures after death.

**au·to·drain·age** (aw″to-drān′əj) drainage of an abscess or cavity by diversion of the fluid into a different channel or viscus within the patient's own body; this may be accomplished by surgery or may occur spontaneously.

**au·to·echo·la·lia** (aw″to-ek″o-la′le-ə) [*auto-* + *echolalia*] parrot-like repetition of words and phrases initially uttered by the patient himself; seen in catatonic schizophrenia and in certain cerebral degenerative disorders.

**au·toe·cic** (aw-te′sik) [*auto-* + Gr. *oikos* house] autoecious.

**au·toe·cious** (aw-te′shəs) [*auto-* + Gr. *oikos* house] term describing parasitic fungi that pass through their entire developmental cycle upon the same host, as opposed to *heteroecious.* Called also *autecious* and *autoecic.*

**au·to·ec·zem·a·ti·za·tion** (aw″to-ek-zem″ə-tĭ-za′shən) the spread, at first locally, and later more generally, of lesions from an originally circumscribed focus of eczema.

**au·to·erot·ic** (aw″to-e-rot′ik) pertaining to autoeroticism.

**au·to·erot·i·cism** (aw″to-ə-rot′ĭ-siz-əm) 1. sexual self-gratification or arousal without the participation of another person, such as masturbation. 2. in psychoanalytic theory, the most primitive stage in the development of object relations, preceding the narcissistic stage. Cf. *heteroeroticism, alloeroticism.*

**au·to·er·o·tism** (aw″to-ər′o-tiz-əm) autoeroticism.

**au·to·eryth·ro·phago·cy·to·sis** (aw″to-ə-rith″ro-fa″go-si-to′sis) [*auto* + *erythro*cyte + *phagocytosis*] phagocytosis of erythrocytes by autologous neutrophils or monocytes.

**au·to·flu·o·res·cence** (aw″to-floo″-res′ens) fluorescence in tissues produced by substances normally present in the tissues. Cf. *secondary fluorescence,* under *fluorescence.*

**au·to·flu·o·ro·scope** (aw″to-floor′-o-skōp″) a type of scintillation camera that utilizes in its detector sodium iodide crystals packed in an array, each connected to specific photomultiplier tubes by individual light pipes.

**au·to·fun·do·scope** (aw″to-fun′do-skōp) [*auto-* + *fundus* + *-scope*] an instrument that makes use of the fact that by observing an illuminated blank space through a pin-perforated card, one can see faint images of the retinal vessels of one's own eyes.

**au·to·fun·dos·co·py** (aw″to-fən-dos′kə-pe) examination with the autofundoscope.

**au·tog·a·mous** (aw-tog′ə-məs) characterized by self-fertilization.

**au·tog·a·my** (aw-tog′ə-me) [*auto-* + Gr. *gamos* marriage] 1. self-fertilization; fertilization within a cell itself by union of two chromatin masses derived from the same primary nucleus; called also *automixis* and *syngamic nuclear union.* Cf. *endogamy* (def. 1) and *exogamy.* 2. a special case of syngamy in which the gametes are sister cells, resulting from the division of a single mother cell.

**au·to·gen·e·ic** (aw″to-jen-e′ik) autologous.

**au·to·gen·e·sis** (aw″to-jen′ə-sis) [*auto-* + *-genesis*] self-generation; origination within the organism.

**au·to·ge·net·ic** (aw″to-jə-net′ik) pertaining to autogenesis.

**au·tog·e·nous** (aw-toj′ə-nəs) [*auto-* + *-genous*] autologous.

**au·to·graft** (aw′to-graft) a graft of tissue derived from another site in or on the body of the organism receiving it; called also *autologous* or *autochthonous graft.*

**au·to·graft·ing** (aw″to-graft′ing) autotransplantation.

**au·to·gram** (aw′to-gram) [*auto-* + *-gram*] a mark forming on the skin following pressure by a blunt instrument.

**au·to·he·mag·glu·ti·na·tion** (aw″to-hem″ə-gloo″tĭ-na′shən) hemagglutination of the subject's own erythrocytes.

**au·to·he·mag·glu·ti·nin** (aw″to-hem-ə-gloo′tĭ-nin) a hemagglutinin that causes the clumping or agglutination of the subject's own erythrocytes.

**au·to·he·mol·y·sin** (aw″to-he-mol′ĭ-sin) a hemolysin that causes complement-dependent hemolysis of the patient's own erythrocytes.

**au·to·he·mol·y·sis** (aw″to-he-mol′ĭ-sis) hemolysis of the blood cells of a person by his own serum.

**au·to·he·mo·lyt·ic** (aw″to-he″mo-lit′ik) pertaining to autohemolysis.

**au·to·he·mo·ther·a·py** (aw″to-he″mo-ther′ə-pe) [*auto-* + *hemo-* + *therapy*] therapy using an autotransfusion.

**au·to·he·mo·trans·fu·sion** (aw″to-he″mo-trans-fu′zhən) autotransfusion.

**au·to·his·to·ra·dio·graph** (aw″to-his″to-ra′de-o-graf) autoradiograph.

**au·to·hyp·no·sis** (aw″to-hip-no′sis) the act or process of hypnotizing oneself.

**au·to·hyp·not·ic** (aw″to-hip-not′ik) pertaining to autohypnosis.

**au·to·im·mune** (aw″to-ĭ-mūn′) pertaining to autoimmunity.

**au·to·im·mu·ni·ty** (aw″to-ĭ-mun′ĭ-te) [MeSH: Autoimmunity] a condition characterized by a specific humoral or cell-mediated immune response against constituents of the body's own tissues (self antigens or autoantigens). See also *autoimmune disease,* under *disease.*

**au·to·im·mu·ni·za·tion** (aw″to-im″u-nĭ-za′shən) the induction in an individual of an immune response to its own tissue constituents, which may lead to pathological sequelae, i.e., to autoimmune disease. Called also *autosensitization.* See also *autoantibody.*

**au·to·in·fec·tion** (aw″to-in-fek′shən) [*auto-* + *infection*] infection by an agent already present in the body, such as the transferral of a microbe or other organism from one part of the body to another.

**au·to·in·fu·sion** (aw″to-in-fu′zhən) [*auto-* + *infusion*] the forcing of the blood toward the heart by bandaging the extremities, compression of the abdominal aorta, etc.

**au·to·in·oc·u·la·ble** (aw″to-in-ok′u-lə-bəl) [*auto-* + *inoculable*] susceptible of being inoculated with microorganisms from one's own body.

**au·to·in·oc·u·la·tion** (aw″to-in-ok′u-la″shən) [*auto-* + *inoculation*] inoculation with microorganisms from one's own body.

**au·to·in·ter·fer·ence** (aw″to-in″tər-fēr′əns) interference with the replication of a virus by an intact, attenuated, or inactivated virus of the same kind.

**au·to·isol·y·sin** (aw″to-i-sol′ĭ-sin) autoantibody that causes complement-dependent lysis of cells in the individual from which it was obtained, as well as those of other animals of the same species.

**au·to·ker·a·to·plas·ty** (aw″to-ker′ə-to-plas″te) [*auto-* + *keratoplasty*] corneal grafting with tissue from the patient's other eye.

**au·to·ki·ne·sis** (aw″to-kĭ-ne′sis) [*auto-* + *-kinesis*] voluntary motion.
**visible light a.**, see *autokinetic visible light phenomenon,* under *phenomenon.*

**au·to·ki·net·ic** (aw″to-kĭ-net′ik) having the power of voluntary motion.

**au·to·la·vage** (aw″to-lah-vahj′) [*auto-* + *lavage*] lavage performed on one's self or on one's own stomach.

**au·to·le·sion** (aw″to-le′zhən) a self-inflicted injury.

**au·to·leu·ko·ag·glu·ti·nin** (aw″to-loo″ko-ə-gloo′tĭ-nin) an antibody capable of agglutinating leukocytes of the same individual in which it is generated.

**au·tol·o·gous** (aw-tol′ə-gəs) [*auto-* + *log-* + *-ous*] related to self; originating within an organism itself, as an autograft or autotransfusion. Called also *autogeneic* and *autogenous.*

**au·tol·y·sate** (aw-tol′ĭ-sāt) a substance or substances produced by autolysis.

**au·tol·y·sin** (aw-tol′ĭ-sin) autoantibody causing complement-dependent lysis of autologous cells; called also *autocytolysin.*

**au·tol·y·sis** (aw-tol′ĭ-sis) [*auto-* + *-lysis*] [MeSH: Autolysis] digestion of cellular components by endogenous hydrolases released from lysosomes following cell death, seen as a postmortem change and in certain pathological conditions.
**postmortem a.**, enzymatic self-digestion of cells or tissues after death.

**au·to·ly·so·some** (aw″to-li′so-sōm) a vacuolar element of the lysosome system of cells to which hydrolases have been added by fusion with lysosomes.

**au·to·lyt·ic** (aw-to-lit′ik) pertaining to or causing autolysis; autocytolytic.

**au·to·lyze** (aw′to-līz) to undergo or to cause to undergo autolysis.

**au·to·mat·ic** (aw″to-mat′ik) [Gr. *automatos* self-acting] 1. spontaneous or involuntary; done by no act of the will. 2. self-moving; self-regulating.

**au·to·ma·ti·ci·ty** (aw″to-mə-tis′ĭ-te) 1. the state or quality of being automatic. 2. the capacity of a cell to initiate an impulse, such as depolarization, without an external stimulus.
**triggered a.**, pacemaker activity occurring as a result of a propagated or stimulated action potential, such as an afterdepolarization, in cells or tissues not normally displaying a spontaneous automaticity.

**au·tom·a·tism** (aw-tom′ə-tiz-əm) [Gr. *automatismos* self-action] [MeSH: Automatism] aimless and apparently undirected behavior that is not under conscious control and is performed without conscious knowledge; seen in psychomotor epilepsy, catatonic schizophrenia, dissociative fugue, and other conditions. Called also *automatic behavior.*
**ambulatory a.**, a condition in which the patient walks about and performs acts mechanically and without consciousness of what he is doing.
**command a.**, the performance of suggested acts without exercise of critical judgment; seen in catatonic schizophrenia and in the hypnotic state.

**au·to·mato·graph** (aw″to-mat′o-graf) [Gr. *automatismos* self-action + *-graph*] an instrument for recording involuntary movements.

**Au·tom·eris io** (aw-tom′ə-ris i′o) a genus of moths. *A. io* is the io moth, whose larva has irritant hairs that produce moth dermatitis.

**au·to·mix·is** (aw″to-mik′sis) [*auto-* + Gr. *mixis* mixture] autogamy, def. 1.

**au·to·my·so·pho·bia** (aw″to-mi″so-fo′be-ə) [*auto-* + *mysophobia*] irrational fear of being unclean or smelling bad.

**au·to·ne·phrec·to·my** (aw″to-nə-frek′to-me) [*auto-* + *nephr-* + *-ectomy*] obliteration of a kidney as the result of disease.

**au·to·neph·ro·tox·in** (aw″to-nef″ro-tok′sin) a substance toxic to the cells of the kidney of the body in which it is formed.

**au·to·nom·ic** (aw″to-nom′ik) self-controlling; functionally independent. See *autonomic nervous system,* under *system.*

**au·to·nomo·trop·ic** (aw″to-nom-o-trop′ik) [*autonomic* + *-tropic*] having an affinity for the autonomic nervous system.

**au·ton·o·mous** (aw-ton′ə-məs) pertaining to or characterized by autonomy.

**au·ton·o·my** (aw-ton′ə-me) [*auto-* + Gr. *nomos* law] the state of functioning independently, without extraneous influence.

**au·to·oph·thal·mo·scope** (aw″to-of-thal′mə-skōp) [*auto-* + *ophthalmoscope*] an ophthalmoscope for examining one's own eyes.

**au·to·oph·thal·mos·co·py** (aw″to-of-thəl-mos′kə-pe) the use of the auto-ophthalmoscope.

**au·to·ox·i·da·tion** (aw″to-ok″sĭ-da′shən) spontaneous direct combination, at ordinary temperatures, of a substance with molecular oxygen.

**auto-ox·i·di·za·ble** (aw″to-ok″sĭ-di′zə-bəl) capable of spontaneous combination with oxygen.

**au·to·pa·thog·ra·phy** (aw″to-pə-thog′rə-fe) [*auto-* + *patho-* + *-graphy*] a written description of one's own disease.

**au·to·pha·gia** (aw″to-fa′jə) [*auto-* + *-phagia*] 1. the biting or eating of one's own flesh. 2. nutrition of the body by the consumption of its own tissues. 3. autophagy.

**au·to·phago·ly·so·some** (aw″to-fag″ə-li′sə-sōm) an organelle, formed by the fusion of an autophagosome with a primary lysosome, in which digestion of intracellular elements occurs in autophagy.

**au·to·phago·some** (aw″to-fag′ə-sōm) [*auto-* + *phagosome*] an intracytoplasmic vacuole containing elements of the cell's own cytoplasm; it fuses with a lysosome to form an autophagolysosome, subjecting its contents to enzymatic digestion. Called also *autosome* and *cytolysosome.*

**au·toph·a·gy** (aw-tof′ə-je) 1. the segregation of part of the cell's own cytoplasmic material within a membrane and its digestion after fusion of the segregated vacuole with a lysosome. Cf. *heterophagy.* 2. autophagia.

**au·to·phar·ma·co·log·ic** (aw″to-fahr″mə-kə-loj′ik) pertaining to or of the nature of autopharmacology.

**au·to·phar·ma·col·o·gy** (aw″to-fahr″mə-kol′ə-je) the chemical regulation of bodily function by the natural constituents of the body tissues, sucvh as hormones.

**au·to·pho·bia** (aw″to-fo′be-ə) [*auto-* + *-phobia*] irrational dread of oneself, of being alone.

**au·to·pho·nom·e·try** (aw″to-fo-nom′ə-tre) [*auto-* + *phono-* + *-metry*] the application of a vibrating tuning fork to the body of a patient for the purpose of having him describe the sensations that it produces.

**au·toph·o·ny** (aw-tof′ə-ne) [*auto-* + Gr. *phōnē* voice] abnormal hearing of one's own voice and respiratory sounds, usually as a result of a patulous eustachian tube.

**au·toph·thal·mo·scope** (aw″tof-thal′mə-skōp) auto-ophthalmoscope.

**au·to·phyte** (aw′to-fīt) [*auto-* + *-phyte*] a plant that does not depend on organized food material, but derives its nourishment directly from inorganic matter. Cf. *saprophyte.*

**au·to·plast** (aw′to-plast) autograft.

**au·to·plas·tic** (aw″to-plas′tik) 1. autologous. 2. pertaining to autoplasty.

**au·to·plas·ty** (aw′to-plas″te) [*auto-* + *-plasty*] 1. autotransplantation. 2. in psychoanalytic theory, adaptation by changing one self (autoplastic change) rather than changing the external environment. Cf. *alloplasty.*
**peritoneal a.**, peritonization.

**au·to·po·di·um** (aw″to-po′de-əm) see *limb* (def. 1).

**au·to·poi·son·ous** (aw″to-poi′zən-əs) poisonous to the organism by which it is formed.

**au·to·pol·y·mer** (aw″to-pol′i-mər) a material that polymerizes without the use of heat, but on the addition of an activator and a catalyst.

**au·to·pol·y·mer·i·za·tion** (aw″to-pol″ĭ-mər″ĭ-za′shən) polymerization occurring without the use of heat but as a chemical reaction following the addition of an activator and a catalyst.

**au·to·pro·te·ol·y·sis** (aw″to-pro-te-ol′ĭ-sis) autolysis.

**au·to·pro·throm·bin** (aw″to-pro-throm′bin) older term for certain coagulation factors.
**a. II**, factor IX; see under *coagulation factors,* at *factor.*
**a. C**, factor X; see under *coagulation factors,* at *factor.*

**au·to·pro·tol·y·sis** (aw″to-pro-tol′ĭ-sis) proton transfer from one molecule to another of the same substance.

**au·top·sy** (aw′top-se) [*auto-* + Gr. *opsis* view] [MeSH: Autopsy] the postmortem examination of a body, including the internal organs and structures after dissection, so as to determine the cause of death or the nature of pathological changes. Called also *necropsy.*

**au·to·psy·chic** (aw″to-si′kik) [*auto-* + *psychic*] pertaining to one's own mind or to self-consciousness.

**au·to·ra·dio·gram** (aw″to-ra′de-o-gram) an autoradiograph.

**au·to·ra·dio·graph** (aw″to-ra′de-o-graf) a radiograph of an object or tissue made by recording the radiation emitted by radioactive material within it, especially after the purposeful introduction of radioactive material.

**au·to·ra·di·og·ra·phy** (aw″to-ra″de-og′rə-fe) [MeSH: Autoradiography] the making of a radiograph of an object or tissue by recording on a photographic plate the radiation emitted by radioactive material within the object, such as in studying DNA synthesis and location within cells, using radioactive isotopes which have been incorporated into the DNA.

**au·to·reg·u·la·tion** (aw″to-reg″u-la′shən) 1. the process occurring when some mechanism within a biological system detects and adjusts for changes within the system; exercised by negative feedback. 2. in circulatory physiology, the intrinsic tendency of an organ or tissue to maintain constant blood flow despite changes in arterial pressure, or the adjustment of blood flow through an organ in order to provide for its metabolic needs.
**heterometric a.**, those intrinsic mechanisms controlling the strength of ventricular contractions that depend on the length of myocardial fibers at the end of diastole.
**homeometric a.**, 1. those intrinsic mechanisms controlling the strength of ventricular contractions that are independent of the length of myocardial fibers at the end of diastole. 2. Anrep effect.

**au·to·re·in·fu·sion** (aw″to-re″in-fu′zhən) intravenous infusion of a patient's own blood or serum which has escaped into the pleural or peritoneal cavities, usually because of trauma or spontaneous rupture of a major vessel.

**au·to·sen·si·ti·za·tion** (aw″to-sen″sĭ-tĭ-za′shən) sensitization toward one's own tissues; see *autoimmunization*.
**erythrocyte a.**, painful bruising syndrome.

**au·to·sen·si·tized** (aw″to-sen′sĭ-tīzd) rendered hypersensitive to one's own serum or tissues; see *autoimmunization*.

**au·to·sep·ti·ce·mia** (aw″to-sep″tĭ-se′me-ə) septicemia arising from microorganisms within the body; endosepsis.

**au·to·se·rous** (aw″to-sēr′əs) pertaining to autoserum.

**au·to·se·rum** (aw″to-sēr′əm) [*auto-* + *serum*] a serum administered to the patient from whom it was derived.

**au·to·sex·ing** (aw″to-seks′ing) in avian genetics, the deliberate breeding of an early-appearing sex-linked phenotype to distinguish male from female chicks.

**au·to·site** (aw′to-sīt) [*auto-* + *site*] the larger, more nearly normal component of asymmetrical conjoined twins, to which the parasite is attached as a dependent growth.

**au·to·sit·ic** (aw″to-sit′ik) pertaining to or of the nature of an autosite.

**au·tos·mia** (aw-tos′me-ə) [*auto-* + *osm-*[1] + *-ia*] the smelling of one's own bodily odor.

**au·to·so·mal** (aw-to-so′məl) pertaining to an autosome.

**au·to·so·ma·tog·no·sis** (aw″to-so″mə-tog-no′sis) [*auto-* + *somato-* + *gnōsis* recognition] the feeling that a part of the body that has been removed, as by amputation, is still present. See *phantom limb*, under *limb*.

**au·to·so·ma·tog·nos·tic** (aw″to-so″mə-tog-nos′tik) pertaining to autosomatognosis.

**au·to·some** (aw′to-sōm) [*auto-* + *-some*] 1. any ordinary paired chromosome that is alike in males and females, as distinguished from sex chromosomes; in humans there are 22 pairs. 2. autophagosome.

**au·to·sper·mo·tox·in** (aw″to-spər″mo-tok′sin) a substance capable of agglutinating the spermatozoa of the animal in which they are formed.

**au·to·sple·nec·to·my** (aw″to-sple-nek′tə-me) the almost complete disappearance of the spleen through progressive fibrosis and shrinkage, such as may occur in sickle cell anemia.

**au·to·spray** (aw′to-spra) an apparatus for spraying, to be used by the patient.

**au·to·stim·u·la·tion** (aw″to-stim″u-la′shən) stimulation of an animal with antigenic material originating from its own tissues.

**au·to·sug·ges·ti·bil·i·ty** (aw″to-səg-jes″tĭ-bil′ĭ-te) the state of being readily amenable to autosuggestion.

**au·to·sug·ges·tion** (aw″to-səg-jes′chən) [*auto-* + *suggestion*] [MeSH: Autosuggestion] self-suggestion; the process by which a person induces in himself an uncritical acceptance of an idea, belief, or opinion, such as by self-hypnosis.

**au·to·syn·the·sis** (aw″to-sin′thə-sis) self-reproduction.

**au·to·tem·nous** (aw″to-tem′nəs) [*auto-* + Gr. *temnein* to cut] capable of spontaneous division.

**au·to·ther·a·py** (aw″to-ther′ə-pe) [*auto-* + *therapy*] 1. the spontaneous cure of disease. 2. self-cure. 3. treatment of disease by filtrates from the patient's own secretions.

**au·to·throm·bo·ag·glu·ti·nin** (aw″to-throm″bo-ə-gloo′tĭ-nin) a platelet autoagglutinin.

**au·to·tomo·graph·ic** (aw″to-tom″o-graf′ik) pertaining to autotomography.

**au·to·to·mog·ra·phy** (aw″to-to-mog′rə-fe) a method of tomography involving movement of the patient instead of the x-ray tube.

**au·tot·o·my** (aw-tot′ə-me) [*auto-* + *-tomy*] 1. self-division; fission. 2. the spontaneous shedding of an appendage, as in some invertebrates.

**au·to·top·ag·no·sia** (aw″to-top″ag-no′zhə) [*auto-* + *topo-* + *agnosia*] agnosia affecting the posture sense, characterized by inability to localize or orient correctly different parts of the body; the cause is usually a lesion in the parietal part of the posterior thalamic radiations. Called also *body-image agnosia* and *somatotopagnosia*.

**au·to·trans·fu·sion** (aw″to-trans-fu′zhən) reinfusion of blood or blood products derived from the patient's own circulation. Called also *autologous transfusion*.
**intraoperative a.**, the collection, processing, and reinfusion of a patient's blood shed from a wound or body cavity during surgery.
**postoperative a.**, the collection, processing, and reinfusion of the patient's blood shed from the mediastinum following open heart or chest surgery or from the chest following traumatic hemothorax.

**au·to·trans·plant** (aw″to-trans′plant) autograft.

**au·to·trans·plan·ta·tion** (aw″to-trans″plan-ta′shən) transplantation of an autograft.

**au·to·trep·a·na·tion** (aw″to-trep″ə-na′shən) erosion of the skull by a brain tumor.

**au·to·troph** (aw′to-trōf) an autotrophic organism.
**facultative a.**, an organism, especially a bacterium, having a metabolism that is either autotrophic or heterotrophic and thus is capable of growth on either inorganic or organic media.
**obligate a.**, a microorganism that can exist only by autotrophic means.

**au·to·troph·ic** (aw″to-trof′ik) [*auto-* + *-trophic*] self-sustaining; said of a type of nutrition in which organisms are capable of synthesizing organic molecules as nutritive substances. Cf. *heterotrophic*.

**au·tot·ro·phy** (aw-tot′rə-fe) the state of being autotrophic; autotrophic nutrition.

**au·to·vac·ci·na·tion** (aw″to-vak″sĭ-na′shən) 1. treatment of a patient with autovaccine. 2. treatment of a patient by causing liberation of antigenic products from some invading microorganism or diseased tissue and thus bringing about the formation of antibodies.

**au·to·vac·cine** (aw″to-vak′sēn) a bacterial vaccine prepared from cultures of organisms isolated from the patient's own secretions or tissues.

**au·to·vac·cin·ia** (aw″to-vak-sin′e-ə) [*auto-* + *vaccinia*] a vaccinial reaction appearing on an area of the body other than at the primary site of smallpox vaccination as a result of transference of vaccinia virus by scratching.

**au·to·vac·ci·no·ther·a·py** (aw″to-vak″sĭ-no-ther′ə-pe) autovaccination.

**au·tox·i·da·tion** (aw″tok-sĭ-da′shən) auto-oxidation.

**au·to·zy·gous** (aw″to-zi′gəs) homozygous by virtue of parental descent from a common ancestor.

**aux·ano·gram** (awk-san′ə-gram) the plate culture in auxanography.

**aux·ano·graph·ic** (awk″san-ə-graf′ik) pertaining to auxanography.

**aux·an·og·ra·phy** (awk″san-og′rə-fe) [Gr. *auxanein* to increase + *-graphy*] determination of the most suitable medium for a microbe by placing drops of various solutions on a plate containing a poor medium; the microbe will develop the strongest colonies on the spot that contains the best medium.

**aux·e·sis** (awk-se′sis) [Gr. *auxēsis*] increase in the size of an organism; often used specifically to designate increase in volume of an organism as a result of growth of its individual cells, without increase in their number.

**aux·et·ic** (awk-set′ik) [Gr. *auxētikos* growing] 1. pertaining to auxesis. 2. a substance that stimulates auxesis.

**aux·il·i·a·ry** (awg-zil′yə-re) [L. *auxiliaris*] 1. affording aid. 2. that which affords aid.

**torquing a.**, an accessory arch wire used to apply torsion on a tooth in any of the three planes of space; used in orthodontic therapy.

**aux·il·io·mo·tor** (awk-sil″e-o-mo′tor) aiding or stimulating motion.

**aux·i·lyt·ic** (awk-sĭ-lit′ik) [Gr. *auxein* to increase + *-lytic*] increasing the lytic or destructive power.

**aux·in** (awk′sin) [Gr. *auxē* increase] a phytohormone from sprouts of plants and from human urine that promotes growth in plant cells and tissues by elongation rather than by multiplication of cells. Examples are the gibberellins and indoleacetic acid.

**aux·in B** (awk′sin) indoleacetic acid.

**aux·i·om·e·ter** (awk″se-om′ə-tər) [Gr. *auxein* to increase + *-meter*] an apparatus for measuring the magnifying powers of lenses; called also *auxometer.*

**aux(o)-** [Gr. *auxē* increase] a combining form denoting relationship to growth, or to stimulation or acceleration.

**auxo·chrome** (awk′so-krōm) [*auxo-* + *-chrome*] a chemical group which, if introduced into a chromogen, will convert the latter into a dye.

**auxo·chro·mous** (awk″so-kro′məs) pertaining to an auxochrome.

**auxo·cyte** (awk′so-sīt) [*auxo-* + *-cyte*] an oocyte, spermatocyte, or sporocyte in the early stages of its development; called also *gonotokont.*

**auxo·drome** (awk′so-drōm) [*auxo-* + Gr. *dromos* a course] the course of growth as plotted on a Wetzel grid.

**auxo·flore** (awk′so-flor) an atom or group that increases the intensity of fluorescence of a compound in which it occurs; cf. *bathoflore.*

**auxo·gluc** (awk′so-glo͞ok) [*auxo-* + Gr. *glykys* sweet] a tasteless atom with which a glucophore combines to form a compound that has a sweet taste.

**aux·om·e·ter** (awk-som′ə-tər) auxiometer.

**auxo·met·ric** (awk″so-met′rik) pertaining or relating to auxometry.

**aux·om·e·try** (awk-som′ə-tre) [*auxo-* + *-metry*] measurement of rate of growth.

**auxo·spi·reme** (awk″so-spi′rēm) the spireme of an auxocyte during the growth cycle.

**auxo·ton·ic** (awk″so-ton′ik) [*auxo-* + *tonic*] contracting against increasing resistance.

**auxo·tox** (awk′so-toks) a chemical group that causes a compound to be toxic.

**auxo·troph** (awk′so-trōf) an auxotrophic organism.

**auxo·troph·ic** (awk″so-trof′ik) [*auxo-* + *-trophic*] 1. requiring a growth factor that is not required by the parental or prototype strain; said of microbial mutants. 2. requiring specific organic growth factors in addition to the carbon source present in a minimal medium.

**auxo·type** (awk′so-tīp) [*auxo-* + *type*] the type of an individual strain of *Neisseria gonorrhoeae* as determined by its nutritional requirements.

**AV, A-V** atrioventricular; arteriovenous.

**Av** average; avoirdupois.

**aval·vu·lar** (a-val′vu-lər) having no valves.

**avas·cu·lar** (a-vas′ku-lər) [*a-*[1] + *vascular*] not supplied with blood vessels.

**avas·cu·lar·i·za·tion** (a-vas″ku-lər-i-za′shən) the diversion of blood from tissues; it may be accomplished by ligating vessels or by applying tight elastic bandages.

**Av·el·lis' syndrome (paralysis)** (ah-vel′is) [Georg *Avellis,* German laryngologist, 1864–1916] see under *syndrome.*

**Ave·na** (ə-ve′nə) [L.] a genus of grasses (family Gramineae). *A. sati′va* is the oat plant, whose seeds are the edible cereal called *oats.*

**ave·nin** (ə-ve′nin) an albuminoid present in oats *(Avena sativa),* which may be harmful to patients with celiac disease.

**ave·no·lith** (ə-ve′no-lith) [L. *avena* oats + *-lith*] an intestinal calculus or enterolith formed around a grain of oats.

**Aven·tyl** (ə-ven′təl) trademark for a preparation of nortriptyline hydrochloride.

**Av·en·zo·ar** (av″ən-zo′ər) [from Ar. Abū Marwan Abdal-Malīk *ibn* Abū al-Ala *Zuhr,* c. 1091 to c. 1162] an Arab physician born in Seville, Spain; he was the teacher of Averroes. His surviving works deal with therapeutics, hygiene, and diet. Also known as *Abumeron* and *Ibn Zuhr.*

**av·er·ag·ing** (av′ər-əj-ing) 1. the finding of a mean value in a population. 2. reducing to or taking a typical example of the group under consideration.

**signal a.**, a method for minimizing noise interference in a periodic signal; the relative constancy of the signal intensity over time versus the randomness of noise is exploited by averaging the waveforms over a number of periods.

**av·er·mec·tin** (av″ər-mek′tin) any of a group of lactones that are potent anthelmintics and insecticides for domestic animals and sometimes humans; the one most widely used is ivermectin.

**Av·er·ro·es** (av-er′o-ēz) [L., from Ar. Abul-Walīd Muhammad ibn-Ahmad Ibn-Muhammad *ibn-Rushd,* 1126–1198] the last and greatest of the Arab physicians and philosophers of the West, born in Cordova, Spain. His *Kitab-al-Kullyat* or *Colliget* ("Book of Universals") tried to establish a system of medicine on neo-Platonic modifications of Aristotle. Also known as *Ibn Rushd.*

**aver·sive** (ə-vər′siv) characterized by or giving rise to avoidance; noxious. Cf. *appetitive.*

**Aver·tin** (ə-vər′tin) trademark for a preparation of tribromoethanol.

**Avi·ad·e·no·vi·rus** (a″vĭ-ad′ə-no-vir″əs) [L. *avis* bird + *adenovirus*] [MeSH: Aviadenovirus] adenoviruses of birds; a genus of viruses of the family Adenoviridae that infect many bird species, causing a wide variety of diseases; infection by some viral species is asymptomatic. Species names are abbreviated by a prefix derived from the host genus and a number designating the serotype, e.g., DAdV-2 for duck adenovirus 2.

**avi·an** (a′ve-ən) [L. *avis* bird] of or pertaining to birds. Cf. *gallid.*

**Avi·bir·na·vi·rus** (a″vĭ-bər′nə-vi″rəs) [L. *avis* bird + *bi*segmented *RNA* + *virus*] a genus of viruses of the family Birnaviridae that infect birds, containing a single species, infectious bursal disease virus, which causes infectious bursal disease of chickens.

**Av·i·cen·na** (av″ĭ-sen′ə) [L., from Ar. Abū Ali al-Husayn ibn Abdallah *ibn Sinā,* 979–1037] the greatest physician and philosopher of the Eastern Arab world, born in Persia. His *Canon* is one of the most famous medical books ever written and was the standard text in Europe through the 17th century. He completely expounded the entire corpus of speculative and practical medicine according to Hippocrates, Aristotle, and Galen and systematically compiled all of Greco-Arabic medicine. Called also *Ibn Sina.*

**av·i·din** (av′ĭ-din) [MeSH: Avidin] a protein from egg whites that binds biotin, rendering it unavailable for absorption and resulting in biotin deficiency if large quantities of raw egg whites are ingested. Because binding is strong and specific, it has been used in biochemical assays (see *biotinylation*).

**avid·i·ty** (ə-vid′ĭ-te) 1. the strength of an acid or a base. 2. the strength of binding between antibody and a complex antigen. Since the antigen has more than one determinant and many of the determinants differ from one another, avidity expresses the overall interaction between antigen and antibody; it is, however, greater than the sum of the affinities for the single determinants, since the effective multivalency of the antigen gives rise to a cooperative "bonus" effect. Often represented by constant $K_a$ (the value of the association constant for the reaction Ab + Ag $\rightleftarrows$ AbAg). Avidity is a function of the techniques used in its measurement and can be expressed only in arbitrary units. Cf. *affinity.*

**avi·fau·na** (a″vĭ-faw′nə) the bird life present in or characteristic of a given region or locality.

**Avi·hep·ad·na·vi·rus** (a′vĭ-hep-ad′nə-vi″rəs) [L. *avis* bird + *hepadnavirus*] a genus of viruses of the family Hepadnaviridae containing hepatitis B viruses that infect birds.

**Avi·pox·vi·rus** (a′vĭ-poks″vi-rəs) [L. *avis* bird + *poxvirus*] [MeSH: Avipoxvirus] avipoxviruses; a genus of viruses of the subfamily Chordopoxvirinae (family Poxviridae) with antigenic cross-reactivity, comprising the fowlpox and related viruses.

**avi·pox·vi·rus** (a′vĭ-poks″vi-rəs) [MeSH: Avipoxvirus] any virus of the genus *Avipoxvirus.*

**avir·u·lence** (a-vir′u-ləns) lack of virulence; lack of competence of an infectious agent to produce pathologic effects.

**avir·u·lent** (a-vir′u-lənt) not virulent.

**avi·ta·min·o·sis** (a-vi″tə-mĭ-no′sis) [MeSH: Avitaminosis] hypovitaminosis.

**avi·ta·min·ot·ic** (a-vi″tə-mĭ-not′ik) pertaining to or characterized by avitaminosis.

**avive·ment** (ah-vēv-mon′) [Fr.] the refreshing of the edges of a wound by surgical procedure.

**Av·lo·sul·fon** (av-lo-sul′fon) trademark for a preparation of dapsone.

**AVMA** American Veterinary Medical Association.

**AVN** atrioventricular node.

**av•o•ben•zone** (av″o-ben′zōn) [USP] a sunscreen that absorbs light in the UVA range.

**Avo•gad•ro's law, number (constant)** (ah-vo-gahd′rōz) [Amedeo *Avogadro,* Italian physicist, 1776–1856] see under *law* and *number.*

**avo•gram** (av′o-gram) one septillionth ($10^{-24}$) of a gram, or one picopicogram (ppg); so named from Avogadro's number, 6.0233 × $10^{23}$. The mass of a molecule in avograms is therefore 1.66 times its conventional molecular weight.

**avoid•ance** (ə-void′əns) a conscious or unconscious defense mechanism consisting of refusal to encounter situations, activities, or objects that would produce anxiety or conflict.

**avoid•ant** (ə-void′ənt) moving away from; negatively oriented.

**av•oir•du•pois** (av″ər-də-poiz′, av-wahr″doo-pwah′) see under *weight.*

**av•o•par•cin** (av-o-pah′sin) a glycopeptide antibiotic derived from *Streptomyces candidus;* an antibacterial.

**AVP** arginine vasopressin.

**AVRT** atrioventricular reciprocating tachycardia; see *atrioventricular nodal reentrant tachycardia,* under *tachycardia.*

**avul•sion** (ə-vul′shən) [L. *avulsio,* from *a-*[2] + *vellere* to pull] the ripping or tearing away of a part either accidentally or surgically.
**nerve a.,** the operation of tearing a nerve by traction.

**awu** atomic weight unit; see *atomic mass unit,* under *unit.*

**ax.** axis.

**Ax•el•rod** (ak′səl-rod) Julius. American biochemist and pharmacologist, born 1912; co-winner, with Ulf Svante von Euler and Sir Bernard Katz, of the Nobel prize for medicine or physiology in 1970 for research on the chemical aspects of nerve impulse transmission.

**Ax•en•feld's anomaly, syndrome** (ahk′sən-felts″) [Theodor *Axenfeld,* German ophthalmologist, 1867–1930] see under *anomaly* and *syndrome.*

**axen•ic** (a-zen′ik) [*a-*[1] + *xen-* + *-ic*] not contaminated by or associated with any foreign organisms; used in reference to pure cultures of microorganisms or to germ-free animals. Cf. *gnotobiotic.*

**ax•es** (ak′sēz) [L.] plural of *axis.*

**ax•i•al** (ak′se-əl) of or pertaining to the axis of a structure or part, as the long axis of a tooth.

**ax•i•a•lis** (ak″se-a′lis) [L., from *axis,* q.v.] [TA] axial; a general term denoting relationship to an axis or location near the long axis or central part of the body.

**ax•i•a•tion** (ak″se-a′shən) the establishment of an axis, or the development of polarity, in an ovum, embryo, organ, or other body structure.

**Ax•id** (ak′sid) trademark for a preparation of nizatidine.

**ax•if•u•gal** (ak-sif′u-gəl) [*axi-* + *-fugal*] directed away from an axon or axis.

**ax•i•lem•ma** (ak″sĭ-lem′ə) [*axi-* + *-lemma*] axolemma.

**ax•il•la** (ak-sil′ə) gen. and pl. *axil′lae* [L.] [TA] [MeSH: Axilla] the pyramidal region between the upper thoracic wall and the arm, its base formed by the skin and apex bounded by the approximation of the clavicle, coracoid process, and first rib; it contains axillary vessels, the brachial plexus of nerves, many lymph nodes and vessels, and loose areolar tissue.

**ax•il•lary** (ak′sĭ-lar″e) pertaining to the axilla.

**ax•il•lo•bi•fem•o•ral** (ak-sil″o-bi-fem′ə-rəl) pertaining to the axillary artery and both femoral arteries.

**ax•il•lo•fem•o•ral** (ak-sil″o-fem′ə-rəl) pertaining to the axillary and femoral arteries.

**ax•il•lo•pop•lit•e•al** (ak-sil″o-pop-lit′e-əl) pertaining to the axillary and popliteal arteries.

**axi(o)-** [L. *axis,* q.v.] a combining form denoting relationship to an axis. In dentistry, it is used in special reference to the long axis of a tooth, as in the names of cavity angles. See specific terms.

**ax•io•buc•cal** (ak″se-o-buk′əl) pertaining to or formed by the axial and buccal walls of a tooth cavity.

**ax•io•buc•co•cer•vi•cal** (ak″se-o-buk″o-sər′vĭ-kəl) pertaining to or formed by the axial, buccal, and cervical walls of a tooth cavity.

**ax•io•buc•co•gin•gi•val** (ak″se-o-buk″o-jin′jĭ-vəl) pertaining to or formed by the axial, buccal, and gingival walls of a tooth cavity.

**ax•io•buc•co•lin•gual** (ak″se-o-buk″o-ling′gwəl) pertaining to the long axis and the buccal and lingual surfaces of a posterior tooth.

**ax•io•cer•vi•cal** (ak″se-o-sər′vĭ-kəl) pertaining to or formed by the axial and cervical walls of a tooth cavity.

**ax•io•dis•tal** (ak″se-o-dis′təl) pertaining to or formed by the axial and distal walls of a tooth cavity.

**ax•io•dis•to•cer•vi•cal** (ak″se-o-dis″to-ser′vĭ-kəl) pertaining to or formed by the axial, distal, and cervical walls of a tooth cavity.

**ax•io•dis•to•gin•gi•val** (ak″se-o-dis″to-jin′jĭ-vəl) pertaining to or formed by the axial, distal, and gingival walls of a tooth cavity.

**ax•io•dis•to•in•ci•sal** (ak″se-o-dis″to-in-si′zəl) pertaining to or formed by the axial, distal, and incisal walls of a tooth cavity.

**ax•io•dis•to•oc•clu•sal** (ak″se-o-dis″to-ə-kloo′zəl) pertaining to or formed by the axial, distal, and occlusal walls of a tooth cavity.

**ax•io•gin•gi•val** (ak″se-o-jin′jĭ-vəl) pertaining to or formed by the axial and gingival walls of a tooth cavity.

**ax•io•in•ci•sal** (ak″se-o-in-si′zəl) pertaining to or formed by the axial and incisal walls of a tooth cavity.

**ax•io•la•bi•al** (ak″se-o-la′be-əl) pertaining to or formed by the axial and labial walls of a tooth cavity.

**ax•io•la•bio•gin•gi•val** (ak″se-o-la″be-o-jin′jĭ-vəl) pertaining to or formed by the axial, labial, and gingival walls of a tooth cavity.

**ax•io•la•bio•lin•gual** (ax″se-o-la″be-o-ling′gwəl) pertaining to the long axis and the labial and lingual surfaces of an anterior tooth.

**ax•io•lin•gual** (ak″se-o-ling′gwəl) pertaining to or formed by the axial and lingual walls of a tooth cavity.

**ax•io•lin•guo•cer•vi•cal** (ak″se-o-ling″gwo-sər′vĭ-kəl) pertaining to or formed by the axial, lingual, and cervical walls of a tooth cavity.

**ax•io•lin•guo•gin•gi•val** (ak″se-o-ling″gwo-jin′jĭ-vəl) pertaining to or formed by the axial, lingual, and gingival walls of a tooth cavity.

**ax•io•lin•guo•oc•clu•sal** (ak″se-o-ling″gwo-ə-kloo′zəl) pertaining to or formed by the axial, lingual, and occlusal walls of a tooth cavity.

**ax•io•me•si•al** (ak″se-o-me′zhəl) pertaining to or formed by the axial and mesial walls of a tooth cavity.

**ax•io•me•sio•cer•vi•cal** (ak″se-o-me″ze-o-sər′vĭ-kəl) pertaining to or formed by the axial, mesial, and cervical walls of a tooth cavity.

**ax•io•me•sio•dis•tal** (ak″se-o-me″ze-o-dis′təl) pertaining to the long axis and the mesial and distal surfaces of a tooth.

**ax•io•me•sio•gin•gi•val** (ak″se-o-me″ze-o-jin′jĭ-vəl) pertaining to or formed by the axial, mesial, and gingival walls of a tooth cavity.

**ax•io•me•sio•in•ci•sal** (ak″se-o-me″ze-o-in-si′zəl) pertaining to or formed by the axial, mesial, and incisal walls of a tooth cavity.

**ax•io•me•sio•oc•clu•sal** (ak″se-o-me″ze-o-ə-kloo′zəl) pertaining to or formed by the axial, mesial, and occlusal walls of a tooth cavity.

**ax•io•oc•clu•sal** (ak″se-o-ə-kloo′zəl) pertaining to or formed by the axial and occlusal walls of a tooth cavity.

**ax•io•po•di•um** (ak″se-o-po′de-əm) axopodium.

**ax•io•pul•pal** (ak″se-o-pul′pəl) pertaining to or formed by the axial and pulpal walls of a tooth cavity.

**ax•ip•e•tal** (ak-sip′ə-təl) [*axi-* + *-petal*] directed toward an axon or axis.

**ax•is** (ak′sis) pl. *ax′es* [L.; Gr. *axōn* axle] [MeSH: Axis] 1. a line about which a revolving body turns or about which a structure would turn if it did revolve. 2. a line around which specified parts of the body are arranged. Used as a general term in TA terminology. 3. [TA] the second cervical vertebra; called also *epistropheus, odontoid vertebra,* and *vertebra dentata.* 4. one of the reference lines in a coordinate system. In a two-dimensional coordinate system there are two axes, one horizontal (designated the *x*-axis), and the other intersecting it (designated the *y*-axis). Cf. *abscissa* and *ordinate.*
**basibregmatic a.,** a vertical line from the basion to the bregma; the maximum height of the cranium.
**basicranial a.,** a line from the basion to the gonion.
**basifacial a.,** a line joining the gonion and the subnasal point; called also *facial a.*
**binauricular a.,** a line joining the two auricular points.
**a. bul′bi exter′nus** [TA], external axis of eye: an imaginary line that passes from the anterior to the posterior pole of the eyeball.
**a. bul′bi inter′nus** [TA], internal axis of eye: an imaginary line in the eyeball, passing from the anterior pole to a point on the anterior surface of the retina just deep to the posterior pole.
**celiac a.,** truncus celiacus.
**cell a.,** an imaginary line connecting the proximal and distal sides of a cell or passing through the centrosome and nucleus of a cell.
**cephalocaudal a.,** the long axis of the body.
**condylar a.,** an imaginary line passing through the two mandibular

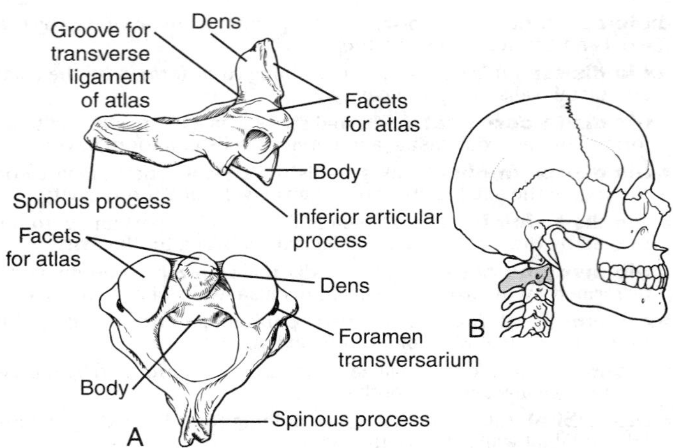


Axis. *(A), (Top)* transverse aspect; *(bottom)* superior aspect. *(B),* Position.

condyles around which the mandible may rotate during a part of the opening movement of the jaw; called also *condyle chord.*
**costocervical arterial a.,** truncus costocervicalis.
**craniofacial a.,** the axis of the bones at the base of the skull, including the mesethmoid, presphenoid, basisphenoid, and basioccipital bones.
**dorsoventral a.,** any line in the median plane at right angles to the long axis of the body.
**Downs Y a.,** Y a.
**electrical a. of heart,** the resultant of the electromotive forces within the heart at any instant. See also *axis deviation,* under *deviation.*
**embryonic a.,** an imaginary line from the head end to the tail end of an embryo or, before that, the line of elongation of the primitive streak and groove.
**external a. of eye,** a. bulbi externus.
**facial a.,** basifacial a.
**frontal a.,** an imaginary line running from right to left through the center of the eyeball.
**a. of heart,** an imaginary line passing through the center of the base of the heart and the apex.
**hinge a.,** the imaginary line connecting the mandibular condyles around which the mandible can rotate without translatory movement; called also *mandibular a.*
**hypothalamic-pituitary a.,** the interrelationships between the hypothalamus and the adenohypophysis, both endocrine and neural, including stimulation of the adenohypophysis by neurosecretory neurons, production of releasing and inhibiting hormones in the hypothalamus, reception of the hormones at sites on pituitary acidophils and basophils, production of hormones by acidophils and basophils, and negative feedback mechanisms by which high levels of circulating hormones act on the hypothalamus and adenohypophysis to inhibit secretion of anterior pituitary hormones.
**hypothalamic-pituitary-adrenal a.,** the interrelationships between the endocrine structures and functions of the hypothalamus and adenohypophysis (the *hypothalamic-pituitary axis*) and the adrenal cortex, including production of adrenocorticotropic hormone, its reception at sites in the adrenal cortex, and negative feedback mechanisms by which high levels of circulating glucocorticoids such as cortisol act on the hypothalamus and adenohypophysis to inhibit secretion of adrenocorticotropic hormone.
**hypothalamic-pituitary-gonadal a.,** the interrelationships between the hypothalamic-pituitary axis and the gonads, including production of gonadotropins, their reception at sites in the testis or ovary, and negative feedback mechanisms by which high levels of circulating estrogens or androgens act on the hypothalamus and adenohypophysis to inhibit secretion of gonadotropins.
**hypothalamic-pituitary-thyroid a.,** the interrelationships between the hypothalamic pituitary axis and the thyroid gland, including production of thyrotropin, its reception at sites in the thyroid gland, and negative feedback mechanisms by which high levels of circulating thyroid hormones act on the hypothalamus and adenohypophysis to inhibit secretion of thyrotropin.
**internal a. of eye,** a. bulbi internus.
**a. len'tis** [TA], axis of lens: an imaginary line joining the anterior and posterior poles of the lens of the eye.
**long a. of body,** the imaginary straight line projected on the median plane through the neck, thorax, abdomen, and pelvis about which the weights of the torso are most symmetrically distributed.
**mandibular a.,** hinge a.
**opening a.,** an imaginary line passing through the mandibular condyles around which the condyles may rotate during opening and closing movements of the mandible.
**optic a., optical a.,** 1. a. opticus. 2. the straight line that passes through the centers of the surfaces and the centers of curvature of a lens system. In a spherical system, it is the axis of symmetry, in the eye being the line passing through the center of the cornea and of the lens of the eye; in a simple lens system it is the line perpendicular to both surfaces of the lens, the lens being regarded as a spherical segment.
**a. op'ticus** [TA], optic axis: a line connecting the center of the anterior curvature of the cornea (anterior pole) with that of the posterior curvature of the sclera (posterior pole).
**a. pel'vis** [TA], axis of pelvis: an imaginary curved line through the minor pelvis at right angles to the plane of the superior aperture, the plane of the cavity, and the plane of the inferior aperture at their central points.
**a. of preparation,** the path taken by a dental restoration as it slides on or off the preparation.
**principal a.,** optic a.
**pupillary a.,** the imaginary line perpendicular to the cornea that passes through the center of the pupil of entrance.
**renal a.,** an imaginary straight line extending through the upper and lower poles of the kidney or, radiographically, through the most inferior and superior calices of the kidney; when projected superiorly, it intersects the thoracic spine.
**renin-aldosterone a., renin-angiotensin a.,** renin-angiotensin-aldosterone system.
**secondary a.,** an imaginary line passing through the optical center of a lens.
**thoracic a.,** arteria thoracoacromialis.
**thyroid a.,** truncus thyrocervicalis.
**vertical a. of eye,** an imaginary line connecting the extreme upper and lower points of the eyeball.
**visual a.,** the line between the fovea centralis retinae and the point of fixation, intersecting the optic axis as it passes through the nodal point; it is sometimes defined as the line extending from the fovea to the nodal point and then continuing anteriorly through the cornea.
**Y a.,** the angle of an imaginary line connecting the sella turcica and the gnathion related to the Frankfort horizontal plane; it is an indicator of downward and forward growth of the mandible.

**ax(o)-** [Gr. *axōn* axle, axis] a combining form denoting relationship to an axis, or to an axon.

**axo·ax·on·ic** (ak″so-ak-son′ik) [*axo-* + *axon*] referring to a synapse between the axon of one neuron and the axon of another.

**axo·den·drit·ic** (ak″so-den-drit′ik) [*axo-* + *dendritic*] referring to a synapse between the axon of one neuron and dendrites of another; see *synapse.*

**ax·of·u·gal** (ak-sof′u-gəl) axifugal.

**ax·o·graph** (ak′so-graf) an apparatus for recording axes in kymographic tracings.

**ax·oid** (ak′soid) pertaining to the axis or second cervical vertebra.

**ax·oi·de·an** (ak-soi′de-ən) axoid.

**axo·lem·ma** (ak-so-lem′ə) [*axo-* + *lemma*] the plasma membrane of an axon; called also *Mauthner's membrane* or *sheath.*

**ax·o·lotl** (ak′so-lot-əl) [Nahuatl] a larval salamander of the genus *Ambystoma;* used in experiments with thyroid feeding.

**ax·ol·ysis** (ak-sol′ĭ-sis) [*axo-* + *-lysis*] degeneration and breaking up of the axon of a nerve cell.

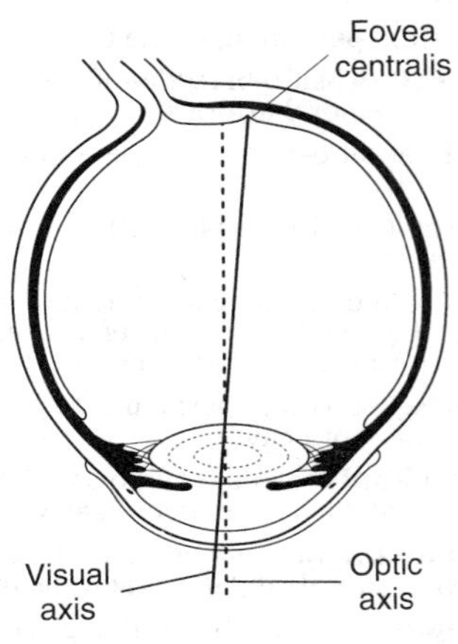


Axes of the eye.

**ax·om·e·ter** (ak-som′ə-tər) [*axo-* + *-meter*] an instrument for measuring an axis, especially an instrument for adjusting a pair of spectacles with respect to the optic axes of the eyes.

**ax·on** (ak′son) [Gr. *axōn* axle, axis] [MeSH: Axons] 1. that process of a neuron by which impulses travel away from the cell body; at the terminal arborization of the axon, the impulses are transmitted to other nerve cells or to effector organs. The larger axons are surrounded by a myelin sheath (see under *sheath* ). Called also *axone.* See also *neurofibra.* 2. columna vertebralis.
**fusimotor a.,** see under *fiber.*
**giant a.,** an axon of certain invertebrates, e.g., the squid, whose size (500 to 700 microns) has facilitated physiological studies of cell membrane excitation.
**myelinated a.,** an axon with a myelin sheath.
**naked a.,** an axon which has no myelin sheath.
**unmyelinated a.,** naked a.

**ax·o·nal** (ak′so-nəl) pertaining to or affecting an axon.

**ax·on·aprax·ia** (ak″son-ə-prak′shə) neurapraxia.

**ax·one** (ak′sōn) axon (def. 1).

**ax·o·neme** (ak′so-nēm) [*axo-* + Gr. *nēma* thread] 1. the axial thread of the chromosome in which is located the axial combination of genes. 2. the central core of a cilium or flagellum, consisting of a central pair of filaments surrounded by nine other pairs; called also *axial filament.*

**ax·o·nom·e·ter** (ak″so-nom′ə-tər) axometer.

**axo·nop·a·thy** (ak″sə-nop′ə-the) [*axon* + *-pathy*] a disorder disrupting the normal functioning of the axons.
**distal a.,** the more common kind of axonopathy, in which the disease process starts centrally and proceeds towards the periphery; cf. *wallerian degeneration.*
**proximal a.,** axonopathy in which the disease process starts at the periphery and proceeds towards the center; cf. *dying-back.*

**ax·on·ot·me·sis** (ak″son-ot-me′sis) [*axo-* + Gr. *tmēsis* a cutting apart] nerve injury characterized by disruption of the axon and myelin sheath but with preservation of the connective tissue fragments, resulting in degeneration of the axon distal to the injury site; regeneration of the axon is spontaneous and of good quality. Cf. *neurapraxia* and *neurotmesis.*

**ax·op·e·tal** (ak-sop′ə-təl) axipetal.

**axo·phage** (ak′so-fāj) [*axo-* + *-phage*] a neuroglial cell occurring in excavations in the myelin in myelitis.

**axo·plasm** (ak′so-plaz-əm) [*axo-* + *plasma*] the cytoplasm of an axon.

**axo·plas·mic** (ak″so-plas′mik) pertaining to the axoplasm.

**axo·po·di·um** (ak″so-po′de-əm) pl. *axopo′dia* [*axo-* + Gr. *pous* foot] a long and slender, semipermanent type of locomotor pseudopodium that has a central axial filament composed of a bundle of microtubules; cf. *filopodium, lobopodium,* and *reticulopodium.* Called also *axiopodium.*

**axo·so·mat·ic** (ak′so-so-mat′ik) [*axo-* + *somatic*] referring to a synapse between the axon of one neuron and the cell body of another.

**axo·style** (ak′so-stīl) [*axo-* + Gr. *stylos* pillar] a filamentous or hyaline-supporting structure passing through the longitudinal axis of certain flagellate protozoa, such as trichomonads, and sometimes extending beyond the posterior end of the organism. Its enlarged capitulum may give rise to or be covered by a pelta.

**ax·ot·o·my** (ak-sot′ə-me) transection or severing of an axon.

**aya·pa·na** (ah″yah-pah′nah) 1. *Eupatorium ayapana.* 2. the leaves of *E. ayapana,* which are used in South America as an aromatic, stomachic, diaphoretic, stimulant, and household remedy for many conditions.

**Ayer's test** (a′yər) [James Bourne *Ayer,* American neurologist, 1882–1963] see under *test.*

**Ayer-To·bey test** (a′ər-to′be) [J. B. *Ayer;* George L. *Tobey,* Jr., American otolaryngologist, 1881–1947] Tobey-Ayer test.

**Ayer·za's disease, syndrome** (ah-yār′sahz) [Abel *Ayerza,* Argentine physician, 1861–1918] see under *disease* and *syndrome.*

**Az** azote, French for nitrogen.

**aza·ci·ti·dine** (a″zə-si′tĭ-dēn) [MeSH: Azacitidine] USAN for 5-azacytidine.

**aza·cos·ter·ol hy·dro·chlo·ride** (a″zə-kos′tər-ol) a hypocholesterolemic agent and avian chemosterilant.

**Azac·tam** (a-zak′-tam) trademark for a preparation of aztreonam.

**aza·cy·clo·nol** (a″zə-si′klo-nol) the gamma isomer of pipradrol, used in the hydrochloride form as a tranquilizer in the treatment of schizophrenia. Called also *gamma-pipradrol.*

**5-aza·cy·ti·dine** (a″zə-si′tĭ-dēn) a cytidine analogue that can be incorporated into RNA and DNA; unlike cytidine it cannot be 5-methylated, a process that is important in gene regulation and post-transcriptional processing of RNA; 5-azacytidine is an investigational antineoplastic agent.

**az·a·guan·ine** (az″ə-gwahn′ēn) [MeSH: Azaguanine] a mitotic poison that resembles the purine guanine but is actually incorporated into nucleic acids and acts to block nucleic acid synthesis by competitive inhibition.

**Aza·lea** (ə-za′le-ə) a former genus of shrubs and trees now classified as part of the genus *Rhododendron;* they contain andromedotoxin and have caused poisoning in sheep.

**az·a·lide** (az′ə-līd) a subclass of the macrolide antibiotics to which the antibacterial azithromycin belongs.

**aza·per·one** (a″zəper′ōn) [USP] [MeSH: Azaperone] a butyrophenone antipsychotic used as a tranquillizer in veterinary medicine.

**aza·pet·ine phos·phate** (a″zə-pet′ēn) an $\alpha$-adrenergic blocking agent used as a vasodilator in peripheral vascular disease in which vasospasm is prominent, administered orally.

**aza·pro·pa·zone** (a″zə-pro′pə-zōn) apazone.

**aza·ri·bine** (a″zə-ri′bēn) the prodrug of the uridine metabolite 6-azauridine (AzU), which is metabolically activated to the monophosphate nucleotide (AzUMP), an inhibitor of de novo pyrimidine synthesis. Azaribine is investigational; potential indications are treatment of severe, disabling psoriasis, mycosis fungoides, and polycythemia vera.

**azat·a·dine mal·e·ate** (ə-zat′ə-dēn) [USP] an antihistamine used in the treatment of perennial and seasonal allergic rhinitis and chronic urticaria, administered orally.

**aza·thio·prine** (az′ə-thi′o-prēn) [USP] [MeSH: Azathioprine] the imidazolyl derivative of 6-mercaptopurine, its active metabolite; used as an immunosuppressive agent for prevention of transplant rejection in organ transplantation and for the treatment of severe, progressive rheumatoid arthritis unresponsive to other agents; also used (investigationally) to prevent transplant rejection in cardiac, hepatic, and pancreatic transplantation and in the treatment of a number of autoimmune disorders, such as systemic lupus erythematosus and autoimmune hemolytic anemia; administered orally.
**a. sodium** [USP], the sodium salt of azathioprine, used to prevent transplant rejection in organ transplantation; administered intravenously.

**azed·a·rach** (ə-zed′ə-rak″) *Melia azedarach.*

**az·e·la·ic ac·id** (az″ə-la′ik) a dicarboxylic acid occurring in whole grains and animal products; it has a cytotoxic effect on malignant or hyperactive melanocytes, apparently affecting their mitochondria; applied topically in the treatment of acne vulgaris.

**Az·e·lex** (az′ə-leks) trademark for a preparation of azelaic acid.

**azeo·trope** (a′ze-o-trōp″) [*a-*[1] + Gr. *zein* to boil + *tropē* a turn, or turning] a mixture of two substances that has a constant boiling point and cannot be separated by fractional distillation.

**azeo·trop·ic** (a″ze-o-trop′ik) pertaining to or having the characteristics of an azeotrope.

**aze·ot·ro·py** (a″ze-ot′rə-pe) having the characteristics of an azeotrope; the absence of any change in the composition of a mixture of substances when it is boiled under a given pressure, the vapor having the same characteristics as the liquid.

**az·ide** (az′īd) a compound that contains the group $—N_3$.

**3′-az·i·do-3′-de·oxy·thy·mi·dine** (az″ĭ-do″de-ok″se-thi′mĭ-dēn) zidovudine.

**az·i·do·thy·mi·dine** (az″ĭ-do-thi′mĭ-dēn) zidovudine.

**azir·i·dine** (ə-zir′ĭ-dēn) ethylenimine.

**az·ith·ro·my·cin** (az-ith″ro-mi′sin) [USP] [MeSH: Azithromycin] an azalide antibiotic, derived from erythromycin, that inhibits bacterial protein synthesis, effective against a wide range of gram-positive, gram-negative, and anaerobic bacteria; used in the treatment of mild to moderate infections caused by susceptible organisms, administered orally and intravenously.

**Az·lin** (az′lin) trademark for a preparation of azlocillin sodium.

**az·lo·cil·lin** (az″lo-sil′in) [MeSH: Azlocillin] a broad-spectrum penicillin antibiotic effective against a wide variety of gram-positive and gram-negative organisms but used primarily in the treatment of *Pseudomonas aeruginosa* infections; its bactericidal activity results from interference with cell wall synthesis.
**a. sodium,** the monosodium salt of azlocillin, administered intravenously by infusion or injection.

**Az·ma·cort** (az′mə-kort) trademark for a preparation of triamcinolone acetonide.

**azo-** a prefix indicating the presence of the group —N=N—, as in azobenzene.

**azo·ben·zene** (az″o-ben′zēn) [*azo-* + *benzene*] an orange-red crystalline product, of the reduction of nitrobenzene; it is the parent substance of azo dyes and some pH indicators and is carcinogenic. Called also *diphenyldiimide.*

**azo·bil·i·ru·bin** (a″zo-bil′ĭ-roo″bin) bilirubin that has been diazotized by exposure to Ehrlich's diazo reagent during the Jendrassik-Grof method of bilirubin measurement.

**azo·car·mine** (az″o-kahr′min) either azocarmine G or azocarmine B, red basic dyes used in certain staining procedures.

**azo·ic** (a-zo′ik) [*a-*[1] + Gr. *zōe* life] 1. devoid of living organisms. 2. a protoplasmic poison, hydrazoic acid, $N_3H$, resembling hydrocyanic acid in its action, made by heating hydrogen chloride with sodium nitrate. It is highly explosive. Called also *triazoic acid* and *hydronitric acid.*

**az·ole** (az′ōl) 1. a derivative of a five-membered ring containing nitrogen and either oxygen, sulfur, or an additional nitrogen atom, as well as carbon atoms. 2. pyrrole.

**Az·o·lid** (az′o-lid) trademark for preparations of phenylbutazone.

**azo·lit·min** (az″o-lit′min) a coloring principle, from litmus; it is used as a pH indicator, being red at a pH of 4.5 and blue at 8.3.

**Azo·mo·nas** (a″zo-mo′nəs) [*azo-* + Gr. *monas* unit] a genus of gram-negative, aerobic, ovoid to coccoid bacteria of the family Azotobacteraceae, found in soil and water, made up of sometimes capsulated cells that fix nitrogen. The type species is *A. a′gilis.*

**azo·my·cin** (a″zo-mi′sin) an antibiotic produced by a species of *Streptomyces.*

**azoo·sper·ma·tism** (a-zo″ə-spər′mə-tiz-əm) azoospermia.

**azoo·sper·mia** (a-zo″ə-spər′me-ə) [*a-*[1] + *zoospermia*] absence of spermatozoa in the semen, or failure of formation of spermatozoa.

**azo·pig·ment** (a″zo-pig′mənt) a purple derivative of bile pigment containing an azo (—N=N—) linkage; formed by reacting bile pigments with diazotizing agents.

**azo·pro·tein** (az″o-pro′tēn) a protein some constituents of which have been diazotized.

**Azor·e·an disease** (a-zor′e-ən) [*Azores* Islands, because it occurs in families of Portuguese-Azorean descent] see under *disease.*

**azo·sul·fa·mide** (az″o-sul′fə-mīd) an antibacterial compound; it was one of the forerunners of the sulfonamide drugs.

**az·ote** (az′ōt) [Fr., from *a-*[1] + Gr. *zōe* life] nitrogen; used only in France. It is the basis of the prefix *azo-* and occurs as a stem in such words as *azotemia.*

**az·o·te·mia** (az″o-te′me-ə) [*azote* + *-emia*] an excess of urea or other nitrogenous compounds in the blood; called also *uremia.*
**extrarenal a.,** that due to a condition or process outside the kidney; see *prerenal a.* and *postrenal a.*
**postrenal a.,** azotemia due to obstruction of the urinary tract.
**prerenal a.,** azotemia resulting from inadequate perfusion of the kidneys, as in hypovolemic shock or congestive heart failure.
**renal a.,** azotemia due to reduced glomerular filtration resulting from acute or chronic renal disease.

**az·o·te·mic** (az″o-te′mik) pertaining to or characterized by azotemia.

**az·o·tom·e·ter** (az″o-tom′ə-tər) [*azote* + *-meter*] an instrument for measuring the proportion of nitrogen compounds in a solution.

**azo·to·my·cin** (ə-zo″to-mi′sin) an antibiotic substance with antineoplastic properties produced by *Streptomyces ambofaciens.*

**az·o·tor·rhea** (az″o-tə-re′ə) [*azote* + *-rrhea*] excessive loss of nitrogen in the feces.

**az·o·tu·ria** (az″o-tu′re-ə) [*azote* + *-uria*] 1. an excess of urea or other nitrogen compounds in the urine. 2. a type of exertional rhabdomyolysis in horses marked by sudden perspiration and paralysis of the hind quarters and by the passing of light red to dark brown urine. It occurs in animals that, after being engaged in continuous work, are given a long rest (such as a weekend for work horses) with continuation of the high-protein diet and then return to work. Called also *cording-up, set- fast, tying up, tying-up syndrome, Monday morning disease,* and *paralytic myoglobinuria.*

**az·o·tu·ric** (az″o-tu′rik) pertaining to azoturia or the urinary excretion of nitrogen.

**az·oxy** (az-ok′se) the group:

N—
O
N—

**az·oxy·ben·zene** (az-ok″se-ben′zēn) a pale yellow product, $C_6H_5 \cdot N \cdot (\cdot O)N \cdot C_6H_5$, of the reduction of nitrobenzene.

**AZQ** diaziquone.

**AZT** zidovudine.

**az·tre·o·nam** (az′tre-o-nam″) [USP] [MeSH: Aztreonam] a monobactam antibiotic effective against a wide range of gram-negative bacteria; used for the treatment of infections caused by susceptible organisms. Administered intravenously or intramuscularly.

**Azul·fi·dine** (a-zul′fĭ-dēn) trademark for a preparation of sulfasalazine.

**az·ure** (azh′ər) any of the partially methylated homologues of the series of basic dyes extending from thionine to methylene blue or to certain mixtures of members of this series. They are metachromatic and are used in many important staining procedures.
**a. I,** a. B.
**a. II,** a mixture of equal parts of azure I and methylene blue.
**a. A,** asymmetrical dimethylthionine, $(CH_3)_2N \cdot C_6H_3(SN)C_6H_3 \cdot NH_2 \cdot Cl$.
**a. B,** trimethylthionine chloride; a dye used as a biological stain; it is a component of polychrome methylene blue.
**a. C,** monomethylthionine chloride, $(CH_3)N \cdot C_6H_3(SN)C_6H_3NH_2 \cdot Cl$.
**methylene a.,** a. B.

**az·u·res·in** (azh″u-rez′in) a complex combination of azure A dye and carbacrylic cationic exchange resin, used as a diagnostic aid in detection of gastric secretion.

**az·u·ro·phil** (azh-u′ro-fil) [*azure* + *-phil*] 1. an element or cell that stains well with blue aniline dyes. 2. azurophilic.

**az·u·ro·phile** (azh′u-ro-fīl) 1. azurophil. 2. azurophilic.

**az·u·ro·phil·ia** (azh″u-ro-fil′e-ə) 1. the quality of staining well with blue aniline dyes. 2. the presence of azurophil granules, as in many lymphocytes.

**az·u·ro·phil·ic** (azh″u-ro-fil′ik) 1. easily stained with blue aniline dyes. 2. pertaining to or characterized by azurophilia. Called also *azurophil* and *azurophile.*

**azyg(o)-** [Gr. *azygos* unpaired, from *a-*[1] + *zygon* yoke] 1. combining form denoting something unpaired. 2. combining form denoting relationship to the azygous vein.

**az·y·go·esoph·a·ge·al** (az″ĭ-go-e-sof″ə-je′əl) pertaining to or located between the azygos vein and esophagus.

**az·y·go·gram** (az′ĭ-go-gram) the radiographic record obtained by azygography.

**az·y·gog·raphy** (az″ĭ-gog′rə-fe) radiography of the azygos venous system following its opacification with contrast material; usually employed for evaluation of abnormal tumor masses in the mediastinum, as evidenced by extrinsic pressure upon, or complete obstruction of, the visualized azygos vein.

**az·y·go·me·di·as·ti·nal** (az″ĭ-go-me″de-ə-sti′nəl) pertaining to or located between the azygos vein and mediastinum.

**az·y·gos** (az′ĭ-gəs) [Gr., from *a-*[1] + Gr. *zygon* yoke] 1. unpaired. 2. any unpaired part, such as the azygos vein.

**azy·go·sperm** (ə-zi′go-sperm″) [*a-*[1] + *zygosperm*] azygospore.

**azy·go·spore** (ə-zi′go-spōr) [*a-*[1] + *zygospore*] a spore developed directly from a gamete without conjugation; called also *azygosperm.*

**az·y·gous** (az′ĭ-gəs) [Gr. *azygos,* q.v.] having no fellow; unpaired.

# B

**B** symbol for *bel, boron,* and *magnetic flux density.*

***B*** symbol for *magnetic flux density.*

**b** symbol for *barn, born,* and *base* (def. 6), used in designating lengths of nucleic acid sequence, e.g., 50 b, a sequence of 50 bases (50 nucleotides long).

***β*** beta, the second letter of the Greek alphabet; symbol for the *β* chain of hemoglobin.

***β*-** a prefix designating (1) the second carbon atom of a chain starting with that adjacent to the principal functional group, e.g., *β*-hydroxybutyric acid (see *α*-); (2) the specific rotation of an optically active substance, e.g., *β*-D-glucose; (3) the orientation of an exocyclic atom or group, e.g., cholest-5-en-3-*β*-ol (cholesterol); (4) a plasma protein migrating with the *β* band (subdivided into $\beta_1$ and $\beta_2$ bands) in protein electrophoresis, e.g., *β*-lipoprotein; (5) one in a series of related chemical compounds, particularly a series of stereoisomeric, isomeric, polymeric, or allotropic forms, e.g., *β*-carotene; and (6) one in a group of related entities, e.g., *β*-ray. For compounds prefixed with the symbol *β*-, see the unprefixed form.

**BA** Bachelor of Arts.

**Ba** symbol for *barium.*

**Baas·trup's disease (syndrome)** (bah'stroops) [Christian Ingerslev *Baastrup,* Danish physician, 1885–1950] kissing spines; see under *spine.*

**Bab·cock's operation** (bab'koks) [William Wayne *Babcock,* American surgeon, 1872–1963] see under *operation.*

**Ba·bès' nodules (nodes, tubercles)** (bah'besh) [Victor *Babeş,* Romanian bacteriologist, 1854–1926] see under *nodule.*

**Ba·bès-Ernst granule (body)** (bah'besh ārnst) [Victor *Babeş;* Paul *Ernst,* Swiss pathologist, 1859–1937] metachromatic granule.

**Ba·be·sia** (bə-be'ze-ə) [Victor *Babeş*] [MeSH: Babesia] a genus of protozoa of the order Piroplasmida, occurring as single or paired parasites within the erythrocytes of various vertebrates, causing babesiosis and other diseases in domestic and wild animals and humans and transmitted by ticks, in which a sexual multiplicative cycle occurs. Certain species have been reported to cause a malarialike disease in both healthy and splenectomized individuals. Formerly called *Babesiella* and *Piroplasma.*
**B. argenti'na,** an etiologic agent of bovine babesiosis in Central and South America, transmitted by *Boophilus microplus,* and in Australia, transmitted by *B. microplus* and *B. australis.*
**B. bige'mina,** an etiologic agent of bovine babesiosis in Central and South America, certain regions in Europe, North, Central, and South Africa, the Middle East, the West Indies, and formerly the southern United States, which is transmitted by various ticks, especially *Boophilus annulatus* and *B. microplus.*
**B. bo'vis,** a species found in some of the same regions but not always together with *B. bigemina,* being the major cause of bovine babesiosis in Europe and the former Soviet Union; ticks of *Boophilus* spp. are the chief vectors but in some areas *Ixodes* ticks are vectors.
**B. cabal'li,** a species causing equine babesiosis in Africa and the former Soviet Union, transmitted by ticks of the genera *Anocentor, Dermacentor, Hyalomma,* and *Rhipicephalus.*
**B. ca'nis,** an etiologic agent of canine babesiosis in the domestic dog, wolf, and certain jackals, transmitted by *Rhipicephalus sanguineus, Haemophilus leachi, Hyalomma plumbeum,* and *Dermacentor* spp., and occurring worldwide.
**B. ca'ti,** an etiologic agent of feline babesiosis in the domestic cat and Indian wildcat, occurring in India; the vector is unknown.
**B. diver'gens,** an etiologic agent of bovine babesiosis in temperate regions of northern, western, and central Europe and perhaps Asia, transmitted chiefly by the ticks *Ixodes ricinus* and *Haemaphysalis punctata.*
**B. e'qui,** a species causing equine babesiosis in eastern Russia, Italy, Africa, India, and Brazil, transmitted by ticks of the genera *Dermacentor, Rhipicephalus,* and *Hyalomma.*
**B. fe'lis,** an etiologic agent of feline babesiosis in the domestic cat, Sudanese wildcat, puma, and leopard in the Sudan and South Africa; the vector is unknown.
**B. gibso'ni,** an etiologic agent of canine babesiosis in the domestic dog, jackal, wolf, and fox, and also infecting the mongoose, ferret, and badger, transmitted by the ticks *Haemaphysalis bispinosa* and *Rhipicephalus sanguineus,* and occurring in India, Sri Lanka, Malaysia, Korea, Egypt, Japan, and the United States.
**B. herpailu'ri,** an etiologic agent of feline babesiosis in the jaguarundi in South America and Africa; the vector is unknown.
**B. ma'jor,** an etiologic agent of bovine babesiosis, transmitted by the tick *Boophilus calcaratus,* and occurring in North Africa, Europe, and the former Soviet Union.
**B. micro'ti,** a parasite of rodents causing babesiosis in both healthy and splenectomized humans in North America; usually transmitted by the tick *Ixodes scapularis* but transmission by means of blood transfusion has been reported.
**B. mota'si,** a species infecting sheep and goats in parts of Europe, the Middle East, Southeast Asia, Northern Africa, and the former Soviet Union, transmitted by the ticks *Rhipicephalus bursa, Dermacentor sylvarum,* and *Haemaphysalis punctata.*
**B. o'vis,** a species infecting sheep and goats in the tropics and in southern Europe, the former Soviet Union, and the Middle East, transmitted by the ticks *Rhipicephalus bursa* and *Ixodes persulcatus.*
**B. panthe'rae,** an etiologic agent of feline babesiosis in the leopard in Kenya; the vector is unknown.
**B. perronci'toi,** a species causing swine babesiosis in Africa; the vector is unknown.
**B. trautman'ni,** a species causing swine babesiosis in Europe, Asia, Africa, and Central and South America; transmitted by the tick *Rhipicephalus sanguineus.*
**B. voge'li,** an etiologic agent of canine babesiosis in the domestic dog, transmitted by the tick *Rhipicephalus sanguineus,* and occurring in Asia and Africa.

**ba·be·si·a·sis** (bă"be-zi'ə-sis) 1. the chronic, asymptomatic form of infection with protozoa of the genus *Babesia;* cf. *babesiosis.* 2. babesiosis.

**Ba·be·si·el·la** (bə-be"ze-el'ah) former name for *Babesia.*

**ba·be·si·o·sis** (bə-be"ze-o'sis) [MeSH: Babesiosis] 1. any of various tickborne diseases due to infection with protozoa of the genus *Babesia,* occurring in wild animals, in domestic animals including cattle, horses, sheep, goats, pigs, cats, and dogs, and in humans as a zoonosis. 2. human infection with species of *Babesia,* particularly *B. divergens* and *B. microti,* a classic type of zoonosis occurring after exposure to infected animals, manifesting as anemia, hemoglobinemia, hemoglobinuria, and a malarialike fever with chills, sweats, myalgia, nausea and vomiting, hemolytic anemia, and splenomegaly. Called also *babesiasis* and *piroplasmosis.*
**bovine b.,** infection of cattle by *Babesia;* the acute phase is manifested by fever, hemoglobinuria, anemia, icterus, and splenomegaly. The variety that was once endemic in the southern United States, infection with *B. bigemina,* has been largely eliminated by eradicating its tick vector, *Boophilus annulatus. B. bovis, B. divergens, B. argentina,* and other *Babesia* spp. still cause the disease in various parts of the world, each employing one or more tick vectors, e.g., *B. microplus, Haemaphysalis* spp., and *Rhipicephalus* spp. Called also *redwater, redwater fever, Texas fever,* and *Texas cattle fever.*
**canine b.,** infection of dogs or other canines with *Babesia canis, B. felis, B. gibsoni,* or *B. vogeli,* transmitted by various ticks, the most common being *Rhipicephalus sanguineus.* The acute phase, which may be fatal, is characterized by depression, weakness, loss of appetite, pallor of the mucous membranes, icterus, fever, and splenomegaly. Called also *biliary fever of dogs* and *malignant jaundice of dogs.*
**equine b.,** infection of horses or other equines with *Babesia caballi* or *B. equi,* transmitted by ticks of the genera *Dermacentor, Hyalomma,* or *Rhipicephalus;* characteristics include high fever, immobility, icterus, gastrointestinal disturbances, rapid emaciation, and dependent edema. Called also *biliary fever of horses* and *equine biliary fever.*
**feline b.,** infection of cats and other felines with *Babesia cati, B. felis, B. herpailuri,* or *B. pantherae,* the vectors of which are unknown. It is characterized by loss of appetite, lethargy, weakness, rough coat, and pale mucous membranes.
**human b.,** babesiosis (def. 2).
**ovine b.,** infection in sheep and goats with *Babesia motasi* or *B. ovis,* transmitted to mammals by tick vectors. Symptoms include jaundice and hematuria; the *B. motasi* form is usually more severe than the *B. ovis* form.
**porcine b.,** swine b.
**swine b.,** infection of swine with *Babesia trautmanni* or *B. perroncitoi;* the former occurs in Europe, Asia, Africa, and Central and South America and is transmitted by *Rhipicephalus sanguineus,* and the latter occurs in Africa but its vector is unknown. Called also *porcine b.*

**Ba·bin·ski's reflex, sign, syndrome** (bə-bin'skēz) [Joseph François Félix *Babinski,* French physician, 1857–1932] see under *reflex, sign,* and *syndrome.*

**Ba·bin·ski-Fröh·lich syndrome** (bə-bin'ske-frer'lik) [J.F.F. *Babinski;* Alfred *Fröhlich,* Austrian-born neurologist in United States, 1871–1953] adiposogenital dystrophy.

**Ba·bin·ski-Na·geotte syndrome** (bə-bin'ske-nahzh-ot') [J.F.F. *Babinski;* Jean *Nageotte,* French pathologist, 1866–1948] see under *syndrome.*

**Ba·bin·ski-Va·quez syndrome** (bə-bin'ske-vah-ka') [J.F.F. *Babin-*

*ski;* Louis Henri *Vaquez,* French physician, 1860–1936] Babinski syndrome.

**ba·by** (ba'be) infant.
**blue b.**, an infant born with cyanosis due to a congenital heart lesion.
**collodion b.**, an infant born encased in a tight membrane resembling collodion or parchment, which is subsequently shed, occasionally leaving normal-appearing skin *(lamellar exfoliation of newborn* or *lamellar desquamation of newborn).* It is usually a primary manifestation of various forms of ichthyosis, most often the lamellar type.

**ba·cam·pi·cil·lin hy·dro·chlo·ride** (bə-kam"pĭ-sil'in) [USP] a semisynthetic penicillin of the ampicillin class, for oral administration; it is hydrolyzed to ampicillin during absorption from the gastrointestinal tract and has the same actions and uses as ampicillin.

**bac·cate** (bak'āt) resembling a berry.

**Bac·cel·li's sign** (bə-chel'ēz) [Guido *Baccelli,* Italian physician, 1832–1916] aphonic pectoriloquy.

**bac·ci·form** (bak'sĭ-form) [L. *bacca* berry + *form*] berry-shaped.

**Bach·mann's bundle** (bahk'mənz) [Jean George *Bachmann,* American physiologist, 1877–1959] see under *bundle.*

**Bac·i·guent** (bas'ĭ-gwənt) trademark for preparations of bacitracin.

**Bac·il·la·ceae** (bas"ĭ-la'se-e) [MeSH: Bacillaceae] a family of bacteria made up of endospore-forming rods and cocci. The mostly gram-positive organisms are usually soil saprophytes, but a few are insect or animal parasites and may produce disease. It includes five genera: *Bacillus, Clostridium, Desulfotomaculum, Sporolactobacillus,* and *Sporosarcina;* the first two contain important human pathogens.

**bac·il·la·ry** (bas'ĭ-lar"e) pertaining to bacilli or to rodlike forms.

**bacille** (bah-sēl') [Fr.] bacillus.
**b. Calmette-Guérin (BCG),** an organism of the strain *Mycobacterium bovis,* rendered completely avirulent by cultivation for many years on bile-glycerol-potato medium. The strain, commonly called BCG, is used for immunization of humans against tuberculosis and in cancer chemotherapy. See also *BCG vaccine,* under *vaccine.*

**bac·il·le·mia** (bas"ĭ-le'me-ə) [*bacill-* + *-emia*] the presence of bacilli in the blood.

**ba·cil·li** (bə-sil'i) [L.] plural of *bacillus.*

**bacilli-** [L. *bacillus,* q.v.] a combining form denoting relationship to a bacillus or to bacilli. Also *bacill(o)-.*

**ba·cil·lif·er·ous** (bă"sĭ-lif'ər-əs) bearing or carrying bacilli.

**ba·cil·li·form** (bə-sil'ĭ-form) [*bacilli-* + *form*] having the appearance of a bacillus; rod-shaped.

**ba·cil·lin** (bə-sil'in) an antibiotic substance isolated from strains of *Bacillus subtilis.*

**bacill(o)-** see *bacilli-.*

**ba·cil·lu·ria** (bas"ĭ-lu're-ə) [*bacill-* + *-uria*] the presence of bacilli in the urine.

**Ba·cil·lus** (bə-sil'əs) [L. "little rod"] [MeSH: Bacillus] a genus of bacteria of the family Bacillaceae, including large aerobic or facultatively anaerobic, spore-forming, rod-shaped cells, the great majority of which are gram-positive and motile. The genus is separated into 48 species, of which three are pathogenic, or potentially pathogenic, and the remainder are saprophytic soil forms. Many organisms historically called *Bacillus* are now classified in other genera.
**B. aero'genes capsula'tus,** *Clostridium perfringens.*
**B. al'vei,** the etiologic agent of European foulbrood of honeybees.
**B. an'thracis,** the causative agent of anthrax in lower animals and humans. Virulence is associated with the production of capsules and a potent exotoxin.
**B. botuli'nus,** *Clostridium botulinum.*
**B. bre'vis,** an organism that is the source of the antibiotics gramicidin and tyrocidin.
**B. bronchisep'ticus,** *Bordetella bronchiseptica.*
**B. ce'reus,** a sometimes motile, aerobic or facultatively anaerobic spore-forming species that is a common soil saprophyte. It causes food poisoning by the formation of an enterotoxin in contaminated foods.
**B. co'li,** *Escherichia coli.*
**B. dysente'riae,** *Shigella dysenteriae.*
**B. enteri'tidis,** *Salmonella enteritidis.*
**B. faeca'lis alcali'genes,** *Alcaligenes faecalis.*
**B. fra'gilis,** *Bacteroides fragilis.*
**B. fusifor'mis,** *Fusobacterium nucleatum.*
**B. lar'vae,** the specific etiologic agent of American foulbrood of honeybees, not pathogenic for humans.
**B. lep'rae,** *Mycobacterium leprae.*
**B. megate'rium,** a widely distributed saprophytic soil form, commonly occurring as a laboratory contaminant.
**B. necro'phorus,** *Fusobacterium necrophorum.*
**B. oedema'tiens,** *Clostridium novyi.*
**B. oede'matis malig'ni No. II,** *Clostridium novyi.*
**B. pilifor'mis,** a species that is the etiologic agent of Tyzzer's disease.
**B. pneumo'niae,** *Klebsiella pneumoniae.*
**B. polymyx'a,** a saprophytic soil and water microorganism that produces the antibiotic polymyxin.
**B. pyocya'neus,** *Pseudomonas aeruginosa.*
**B. stearothermo'philus,** a thermophilic species that produces very resistant spores and is capable of growth at 65°C. It is used to test for autoclave quality control.
**B. sub'tilis,** a common saprophytic soil and water form, often occurring as a laboratory contaminant and occasionally causing conjunctivitis in humans. It produces the antibiotic bacitracin.
**B. te'tani,** *Clostridium tetani.*
**B. ty'phi, B. typho'sus,** *Salmonella typhi.*
**B. wel'chii,** *Clostridium perfringens.*

**ba·cil·lus** (bə-sil'us) pl. *bacil'li* [L.] [MeSH: Bacillus] 1. an organism of the genus *Bacillus.* 2. any rod-shaped bacterium.
**anthrax b.,** *Bacillus anthracis.*
**Bang's b.,** *Brucella abortus.*
**Battey b.,** *Mycobacterium intracellulare.*
**Boas-Oppler b.,** a microorganism, probably a species of *Lactobacillus,* first found in the gastric juice of patients with stomach carcinoma. Called also *lactobacillus of Boas-Oppler.*
**Bordet-Gengou b.,** *Bordetella pertussis.*
**butter b.,** *Clostridium butyricum.*
**Calmette-Guérin b.,** bacille Calmette-Guérin.
**coliform bacilli,** gram-negative bacilli found in the intestinal tract that resemble *Escherichia coli,* particularly in the fermentation of lactose with gas. The term generally is used to refer to the genera *Citrobacter, Escherichia, Edwardsiella, Enterobacter, Klebsiella,* and *Serratia.*
**colon b.,** *Escherichia coli.*
**DF-2 b.,** *Capnocytophaga canimorsus.*
**diphtheria b.,** *Corynebacterium diphtheriae.*
**Döderlein's b.,** one of the gram-positive rods commonly found in vaginal secretions that may consist of mixtures of *Lactobacillus acidophilus, L. casei, L. cellobiosisus, L. fermentum,* or *Leuconostoc mesenteroides.* Said by some to be identical with *L. acidophilus.*
**Ducrey's b.,** *Haemophilus ducreyi.*
**dysentery bacilli,** gram-negative, non–spore-forming rods causing dysentery in humans; see *Shigella.*
**enteric b.,** a bacillus belonging to the family Enterobacteriaceae.
**Escherich's b.,** *Escherichia coli.*
**Flexner's b.,** *Shigella flexneri.*
**Friedländer's b.,** *Klebsiella pneumoniae.*
**Frisch b.,** *Klebsiella pneumoniae rhinoscleromatis.*
**fusiform b.,** fusobacterium.
**Gärtner's b.,** *Salmonella enteritidis.*
**Ghon-Sachs b.,** *Clostridium septicum.*
**glanders b.,** *Pseudomonas mallei.*
**Hansen's b.,** *Mycobacterium leprae.*
**Hofmann's b.,** *Corynebacterium pseudodiphtheriticum.*
**hog cholera b.,** *Salmonella choleraesuis.*
**Johne's b.,** *Mycobacterium paratuberculosis.*
**Klebs-Löffler b.,** *Corynebacterium diphtheriae.*
**Koch's b.,** *Mycobacterium tuberculosis.*
**Koch-Weeks b.,** *Haemophilus aegyptius.*
**legionnaire's b.,** *Legionella pneumophila.*
**lepra b., leprosy b.,** *Mycobacterium leprae.*
**Morax-Axenfeld b.,** *Moraxella (Moraxella) lacunata.*
**Morgan's b.,** *Morganella morganii.*
**Newcastle-Manchester b.,** *Shigella flexneri* type 6, Boyd 88.
**paracolon bacilli,** microorganisms commonly found in the intestinal flora, distinguished by delayed (5–21 days) fermentation of lactose. Organisms of this type belong to the genera *Escherichia, Citrobacter,* or *Klebsiella.*
**Pfeiffer's b.,** *Haemophilus influenzae.*
**Preisz-Nocard b.,** *Corynebacterium pseudotuberculosis.*
**rhinoscleroma b.,** *Klebsiella pneumoniae rhinoscleromatis.*
**Schmitz's b.,** *Shigella dysenteriae* type 2.
**Schmorl's b.,** *Fusobacterium necrophorum.*
**Shiga b.,** *Shigella dysenteriae* type 1.
**smegma b.,** *Mycobacterium smegmatis.*
**Sonne-Duval b.,** *Shigella sonnei.*
**Stanley b.,** a serotype of *Salmonella enteritidis* isolated from patients with food poisoning in Stanley, England.
**Strong's b.,** *Shigella flexneri.*
**swine rotlauf b.,** *Erysipelothrix rhusiopathiae.*
**tetanus b.,** *Clostridium tetani.*
**timothy b.,** *Mycobacterium phlei.*
**tubercle b.,** *Mycobacterium tuberculosis.*
**typhoid b.,** *Salmonella typhi.*
**vole b.,** *Mycobacterium microti.*

**Weeks' b.**, *Haemophilus aegyptius.*
**Welch's b.**, *Clostridium perfringens.*

**bac·i·tra·cin** (bas″ĭ-tra′sin) [USP] [MeSH: Bacitracin] an antibacterial polypeptide produced by the growth of a gram-positive, spore-forming organism belonging to the *licheniformin* group of *Bacillus subtilis,* which acts by interfering with bacterial cell wall synthesis. It is effective against many gram-positive bacteria, such as staphylococci, streptococci, and pneumococci, and some gram-negative bacteria, such as gonococci and meningococci. It is applied topically to the skin or conjunctiva or administered by intramuscular injection in the treatment of infections caused by susceptible organisms.
**b. zinc** [USP], the zinc salt of bacitracin, used for topical application to the skin and administered orally in the treatment of antibiotic-associated pseudomembranous enterocolitis caused by *Clostridium difficile* toxins A and B.

**back** (bak) [MeSH: Back] the posterior part of the trunk from the neck to the pelvis; called also *dorsum* [TA].
**angry b.**, excited skin syndrome.
**flat b.**, a back that appears flat as a result of a decrease of normal lumbar lordosis and normal thoracic kyphosis.
**functional b.**, a condition of fatigue and defective balance marked by more or less continuous lumbar or dorsal pain.
**hollow b.**, see *lordosis.*
**hump b., hunch b.**, kyphosis.
**kinky b.**, a type of developmental spondylolisthesis in chickens in which the sixth thoracic vertebra is deformed and downwardly rotated; pressure on the spinal cord can cause posterior paralysis.
**poker b.**, ankylosing spondylitis.
**saddle b.**, see *lordosis.*

**back·bone** (bak′bōn) columna vertebralis.

**back-cal·cu·la·tion** (bak-kal″ku-la′shən) a statistical method that uses the current incidence and the length of incubation of a disease to estimate the cumulative incidence of the disease and project the number of cases that will occur in the future.

**back·cross** (bak′kros) in experimental genetics, a mating between a heterozygote and a homozygote.
**double b.**, the mating between a double heterozygote and a homozygote.

**back·flow** (bak′flo) the flowing of a current in a direction the reverse of that normally taken; regurgitation.
**pyelovenous b.**, the drainage of fluid from the pelvis of the kidney into the venous system under certain conditions of back pressure.

**back·ing** (bak′ing) in dentistry, the piece of metal that supports a porcelain or resin facing on a fixed or removable partial denture.

**back·knee** (bak′ne) genu recurvatum.

**back-rak·ing** (bak-rāk′ing) see under *raking.*

**back·scat·ter** (bak′skat-ər) in radiology, radiation deflected by scattering processes at angles greater than 90 degrees to the original direction of the beam of radiation; see *scatter,* and see also *scattered rays,* under *ray.*

**bac·lo·fen** (bak′lo-fen″) [USP] [MeSH: Baclofen] an analogue of $\gamma$-aminobutyric acid used as a muscle relaxant and antispastic in the treatment of multiple sclerosis, spinal cord diseases, and spinal cord injury; administered orally.

**BACOP** a regimen of bleomycin, Adriamycin (doxorubicin), cyclophosphamide, Oncovin (vincristine), and prednisone, used in cancer chemotherapy.

**Bact.** *Bacterium.*

**-bacter** [L. *bacterium,* q.v.] a word termination denoting a bacterium.

**bac·ter·as·ci·tes** (bak″tər-əsi′tēz) [*bacterium* + *ascites*] bacterial infection of ascitic fluid.
**monomicrobial non-neutrocytic b.**, spontaneous bacterial peritonitis caused by a single organism; the ascitic fluid neutrophil count is less than 250 cells/mm$^3$.
**polymicrobial b.**, an iatrogenic infection of ascitic fluid caused by needle perforation of the bowel during paracentesis and characterized by the presence of several species of bacteria.

**bac·ter·e·mia** (bak″tər-e′me-ə) [*bacteri-* + *-emia*] [MeSH: Bacteremia] the presence of bacteria in the blood.

**Bac·te·ria** (bak-tēr′e-ə) [MeSH: Bacteria] in former systems of classification, a division of the kingdom Procaryotae, including all prokaryotic organisms except the blue-green algae (Cyanobacteria). See also *Procaryotae.*

**bac·te·ria** (bak-tēr′e-ah) [L.] [MeSH: Bacteria] plural of *bacterium.*

**Bac·te·ri·a·ceae** (bak″te-re-a′se-e) in former systems of classification, a name given to a family of bacteria.

**bac·te·ri·al** (bak-te′re-əl) pertaining to or caused by bacteria.

**bac·te·ri·ci·dal** (bak-ter″ĭ-si′dəl) [*bacteri-* + L. *caedere* to kill] destructive to bacteria.

**bac·te·ri·cide** (bak-tēr′ĭ-sīd) an agent that destroys bacteria.
**specific b.**, bacteriolysin.

**bac·te·ri·ci·din** (bak-tēr″ĭ-si′din) a substance that leads to the death of bacteria; such substances include both antibody and certain nonantibody components in the serum.

**bac·ter·id** (bak′tər-id) [*bacteri-* + *-id*] an id reaction associated with a bacterial infection.
**pustular b.**, a chronic relapsing cutaneous eruption consisting of vesicles or pustules frequently localized to the palms and soles, which generally occurs in association with a focal infection elsewhere in the body.

**bac·ter·i·form** (bak-tēr′ĭ-form) resembling a bacterium in form.

**bac·ter·in** (bak′tər-in) bacterial vaccine.
***Bordetella bronchiseptica* b.**, a suspension of inactivated and adsorbed *Bordetella bronchiseptica,* used for prevention of atrophic rhinitis of swine.
***Clostridium chauvoei-septicum* b.**, see under *bacterin-toxoid.*
***Clostridium haemolyticum* b.**, a chemically killed culture of *Clostridium haemolyticum,* used for prevention of bacillary hemoglobinuria in cattle, sheep, and goats.
***Erysipelothrix rhusiopathiae* b.**, a formalin-killed, adsorbed culture of *Erysipelothrix rhusiopathiae,* used for immunization of swine against erysipelas.
***Haemophilus paragallinarum* b.**, a chemically inactivated and adsorbed suspension of *Haemophilus paragallinarum,* used for immunization of chickens against infectious coryza.
***Leptospira canicola-grippotyphosa-hardjo-icterohaemorrhagiae-pomona* b.**, chemically inactivated, adsorbed whole cultures of *Leptospira canicola, L. grippotyphosa, L. hardjo, L. icterohaemorrhagiae,* and *L. pomona,* used for immunization of cattle against leptospirosis.
***Pasteurella haemolytica-multocida* b.**, an inactivated and adsorbed whole culture of *Pasteurella haemolytica* and *P. multocida,* used for prevention of pasteurellosis in cattle and sheep.
***Pasteurella multocida* b.**, 1. chemically killed, adsorbed whole culture of *Pasteurella multocida* bovine and porcine isolates, used for prevention of pasteurellosis in cattle, sheep, goats, and swine. 2. chemically killed, emulsified whole culture of *Pasteurella multocida* avian isolates, used for prevention of fowl cholera in chickens and turkeys.
***Salmonella dublin-typhimurium* b.**, a formalin-inactivated, adsorbed suspension of *Salmonella dublin* and *S. typhimurium,* used for prevention of salmonellosis in cattle.
***Staphylococcus aureus* b.**, a formalin-inactivated, adsorbed lysed culture of *Staphylococcus aureus,* used for prevention of *S. aureus* infection in cattle.
***Streptococcus equi* b.**, a chemically killed, adsorbed suspension of *Streptococcus equi,* used for prevention of strangles in horses.
***Vibrio fetus* b.**, a chemically inactivated, adsorbed whole culture of *Campylobacter (Vibrio) fetus,* used for immunization of cows *(C. fetus* subspecies *fetus)* or of ewes *(C. fetus* subspecies *intestinalis* or *jejuni)* for prevention of bovine or ovine genital campylobacteriosis.

**bac·ter·in-tox·oid** (bak′tər-in-tok′soid) an active immunizing agent prepared from chemically inactivated bacterial cultures containing both killed bacteria and inactivated toxin.
***Clostridium botulinum* type C b.-t.**, a chemically killed, alum-adsorbed culture of *Clostridium botulinum,* type C, used for prevention of type C botulism in mink.
***Clostridium chauvoei-septicum* b.-t.**, a chemically killed culture of *Clostridium chauvoei* and *C. septicum,* used for prevention of blackleg and malignant edema in cattle, horses, sheep, and goats.
***Clostridium novyi-sordelli* b.-t.**, a chemically inactivated suspension of *Clostridium novyi* and *C. sordelli,* used for immunization of cattle and sheep against diseases caused by these organisms (e.g., black disease, bighead).
***Clostridium perfringens* b.-t.**, a chemically killed culture of *Clostridium perfringens* type C and/or type D organisms, used for prevention of enterotoxemia caused by these strains in sheep and cattle.

**bacteri(o)-** [L. *bacterium,* q.v.] a combining form denoting relationship to bacteria.

**bac·te·rio·chlo·ro·phyll** (bak-tēr″e-o-klor′ə-fil) any of a group of pigments (designated bacteriochlorophyll *a, b, c, d,* or *e* ) occurring in bacteria and functioning in anaerobic photosynthesis.

**bac·te·rio·ci·din** (bak-tēr″e-o-si′din) bactericidin.

**bac·te·rio·cin** (bak-tēr′e-o″sin) a protein substance, e.g., colicin or staphylococcin, released by certain bacteria that kills but does not lyse closely related strains of bacteria. Specific bacteriocins attach to specific receptors on cell walls and induce specific metabolic block, e.g., cessation of nucleic acid or protein synthesis of oxidative phosphorylation.

**bac·te·ri·o·cin·o·gen** (bak-tēr″e-o-sin′o-jen) a bacterial plasmid that controls the synthesis of bacteriocin.

**bac·te·ri·o·cin·o·gen·ic** (bak-tēr″e-o-sin″o-jen′ik) giving rise to bacteriocin.

**bac·te·rio·cla·sis** (bak-tēr″e-ok′lə-sis) [*bacterio-* + Gr. *klasis* breaking] bacteriolysis.

**bac·te·rio·flu·o·res·cin** (bak-tēr″e-o-floo-res′in) a fluorescent dye produced by *Pseudomonas aeruginosa.*

**bac·te·ri·o·gen·ic** (bak-tēr″e-o-jen′ik) caused by bacteria.

**bac·te·ri·og·e·nous** (bak-tēr″e-oj′ə-nəs) bacteriogenic.

**bac·te·ri·oid** (bak-tēr′e-oid) [*bacteri-* + *-oid*] 1. resembling the bacteria. 2. a structure resembling a bacterium.

**bac·te·rio·log·ic** (bak-tēr″e-o-loj′ik) pertaining to bacteriology.

**bac·te·rio·log·i·cal** (bak-tēr″e-o-loj′ĭ-kəl) bacteriologic.

**bac·te·ri·ol·o·gist** (bak-tēr″e-ol′ə-jist) an expert in bacteriology.

**bac·te·ri·ol·o·gy** (bak-tēr″e-ol′ə-je) [*bacterio-* + *-logy*] [MeSH: Bacteriology] the science that treats of bacteria. Cf. *microbiology.*
**clinical diagnostic b.,** the science and practice of collecting specimens from persons or the environment, examining them for bacteria or evidence of bacterial infection, and evaluating the results.
**medical b.,** that branch of bacteriology that deals chiefly with bacteria causing human disease.
**pathological b.,** that branch of bacteriology which treats chiefly of the effects produced upon the animal body by the presence of bacteria and their toxins.
**public health b.,** that branch of bacteriology that deals with the spread and prevention of bacterial disease.
**sanitary b.,** bacteriology that deals chiefly with disease prevention based upon sanitation in food and water supplies and distribution, and upon disposal of sewage.
**systematic b.,** that branch of bacteriology that studies the classification and relationship of bacteria (taxonomy).

**bac·te·ri·ol·y·sin** (bak-tēr″e-ol′ĭ-sin) an antibacterial antibody that produces lysis of bacterial cells.

**bac·te·ri·ol·y·sis** (bak-tēr″e-ol′ĭ-sis) [*bacterio-* + *-lysis*] [MeSH: Bacteriolysis] disruption of the structural integrity of a bacterial cell resulting in release of the cell contents.

**bac·te·rio·lyt·ic** (bak-tēr″e-o-lit′ik) pertaining to, characterized by, or promoting the dissolution or destruction of bacteria.

**Bac·te·rio·ne·ma** (bak-tēr″e-o-ne′mə) [*bacterio-* + Gr. *nēma* thread] a genus of bacteria of the family Actinomycetaceae, order Actinomycetales, occurring as facultative anaerobic, gram-positive, pleomorphic organisms, comprising nonseptate and septate filaments and bacilli.
**B. matrucho′tii,** a species found in the oral cavity of humans and other primates, particularly in dental calculus and plaque.

**bac·te·ri·o·op·so·nin** (bak-tēr″e-o-op-so′nin) an opsonin that acts on bacteria.

**bac·te·rio·phage** (bak-tēr′e-o-fāj″) [*bacterio-* + *-phage*] [MeSH: Bacteriophages] a virus that lyses bacteria; see *bacterial virus,* under *virus.*
**temperate b.,** a bacteriophage whose genetic material (prophage) becomes an intimate part of the bacterial cell, persisting through many cell division cycles. The affected bacterial cell is known as a *lysogenic bacterium* (q.v.).

**bac·te·rio·pha·gia** (bak-tēr″e-o-fa′jə) lysis of bacteria by a bacteriophage.

**bac·te·rio·phag·ic** (bak-tēr″e-o-faj′ik) [*bacterio-* + *phag-* + *-ic*] pertaining to, characterized by, or producing bacteriophagia.

**bac·te·rio·pha·gol·o·gy** (bak-tēr″e-o-fə-gol′ə-je) the study of bacteriophage.

**bac·te·ri·oph·a·gy** (bak-tēr″e-of′ə-je) bacteriophagia.

**bac·te·rio·phy·to·ma** (bak-tēr″e-o-fi-to′mə) a tumorlike, reactive lesion caused by bacteria.

**bac·te·rio·plas·min** (bak-tēr″e-o-plaz′min) plasmin produced by bacteria.

**bac·te·rio·pre·cip·i·tin** (bak-tēr″e-o-pre-sip′ĭ-tin) a precipitin formed in the body in response to bacterial antigens.

**bac·te·rio·pro·tein** (bak-tēr″e-o-pro′tēn) any protein of bacterial origin.

**bac·te·ri·op·son·ic** (bak-tēr″e-op-son′ik) exerting an opsonic effect on bacteria.

**bac·te·ri·op·so·nin** (bak-tēr″e-op′so-nin) an antibody that interacts with bacteria to render them more susceptible to ingestion by phagocytic cells than they otherwise would be.

**bac·te·rio·pur·pu·rin** (bak-tēr″e-o-pur′pu-rin) [*bacterio-* + L. *purpur* purple] a light purple pigment produced by certain bacteria.

**bac·te·rio·rho·dop·sin** (bak-tēr″e-o-ro-dop′sin) [*bacterio-* + *rhodo-* + *opsin*] [MeSH: Bacteriorhodopsin] a purple pigment, similar to rhodopsin, occurring in the cell membrane of bacteria of the genus *Halobacterium,* which converts sunlight directly into electrochemical energy.

**bac·te·ri·o·sis** (bak-tēr″e-o′sis) any bacterial disease.

**bac·te·rio·sper·mia** (bak-tēr″e-o-spər′me-ə) the presence of bacteria in the semen.

**bac·te·rio·sta·sis** (bak-tēr″e-o-sta′sis) [*bacterio-* + *stasis*] the inhibition of growth, but not the killing, of bacteria by chemicals or biologic materials.

**bac·te·rio·stat** (bak-tēr′e-o-stat″) an agent that inhibits the growth of bacteria.

**bac·te·rio·stat·ic** (bak-tēr″e-o-stat′ik) 1. inhibiting the growth or multiplication of bacteria. 2. an agent that inhibits the growth or multiplication of bacteria.

**bac·te·rio·ther·a·py** (bak-tēr″e-o-ther′ə-pe) [*bacterio-* + *therapy*] treatment of disease by the introduction of bacteria into the system.

**bac·te·rio·tox·emia** (bak-tēr″e-o-tok-se′me-ə) the presence of bacterial toxins in the blood.

**bac·te·rio·tox·ic** (bak-tēr″e-o-tok′sik) toxic to bacteria.

**bac·te·rio·tox·in** (bak-tēr″e-o-tok′sin) [*bacterio-* + *toxin*] any toxin produced by or toxic to bacteria.

**bac·te·ri·o·trop·ic** (bak-tēr″e-o-trop′ik) [*bacterio-* + *-tropic*] turning toward or changing bacteria; bacteriopsonic.

**bac·te·ri·ot·ro·pin** (bak-tēr″e-ot′ro-pin) bacteriopsonin.

**bac·ter·it·ic** (bak″tər-it′ik) caused by or characterized by bacteria.

**Bac·te·ri·um** (bak-tēr′e-əm) [L.; Gr. *baktērion* little rod] in former systems of classification, a genus of bacteria made up of non–spore-forming, rod-shaped bacteria, not necessarily closely related, that were not fitted into other formally defined genera.
**B. actinomyce′tem co′mitans,** *Actinobacillus actinomycetemcomitans.*
**B. aero′genes,** *Enterobacter aerogenes.*
**B. aerugino′sum,** *Pseudomonas aeruginosa.*
**B. cho′lerae su′is,** *Salmonella choleraesuis.*
**B. cloa′cae,** *Enterobacter cloacae.*
**B. co′li, B. co′li commu′ne,** *Escherichia coli.*
**B. dysente′riae,** *Shigella dysenteriae.*
**B. pes′tis,** *Yersinia pestis.*
**B. son′nei,** *Shigella sonnei.*
**B. tularen′se,** *Francisella tularensis.*

**bac·te·ri·um** (bak-tēr′e-əm) pl. *bacte′ria* [L.; Gr. *baktērion* little rod] in general, any of the unicellular prokaryotic microorganisms that commonly multiply by cell division (fission) and whose cell is typically contained within a cell wall. They may be aerobic or anaerobic, motile or nonmotile, and may be free-living, saprophytic, parasitic, or even pathogenic, the last causing disease in plants or animals. See also *Bacteria.*
**acid-fast b.,** one that retains stains by dyes (e.g., carbolfuchsin or auramine) so tenaciously that it is not decolorized by 5 per cent mineral acids, especially *Mycobacterium* species and *Nocardia.*
**autotrophic b.,** one that has no organic nutritional requirements; none are pathogenic.
**beaded b.,** one having deeply staining granules equally spaced along the rod.
**bifid b.,** one that has a branched rod- or cleft-shaped cell, especially *Bifidobacterium.*
**blue-green b.,** see *Cyanobacteria.*
**chemoautotrophic b.,** one that is autotrophic and obtains energy by the oxidation of inorganic compounds of iron, nitrogen, sulfur, or hydrogen; none is pathogenic.
**chemoheterotrophic b.,** one that is heterotrophic and obtains energy by the oxidation of organic compounds by mechanisms closely similar to those existing in higher animals.
**chromo b., chromogenic b.,** one that produces pigment.
**coliform b.,** one of the facultative gram-negative, rod-shaped bacteria that are normal inhabitants of the intestinal tract of humans and animals. See *Citrobacter, Edwardsiella, Enterobacter, Escherichia, Klebsiella,* and *Serratia.*
**coryneform bacteria,** a group of bacteria that are morphologically similar to the organisms of the genus *Corynebacterium;* corynebacteria. Called also *coryneform group.*
**Dar es Salaam b.,** *Salmonella salamae.*
**denitrifying b.,** one that is able to reduce nitrates to nitrites, ammonia, or nitrogen gas.
**gram-negative b.,** see *gram-negative,* under *G.*
**gram-positive b.,** see *gram-positive,* under *G.*
**hemophilic b.,** one that has a nutritional affinity for constituents of blood or whose growth is stimulated by blood-enriched media.
**heterotrophic b.,** one that requires organic compounds of carbon and nitrogen as sources of energy or as essential parts of the cell.

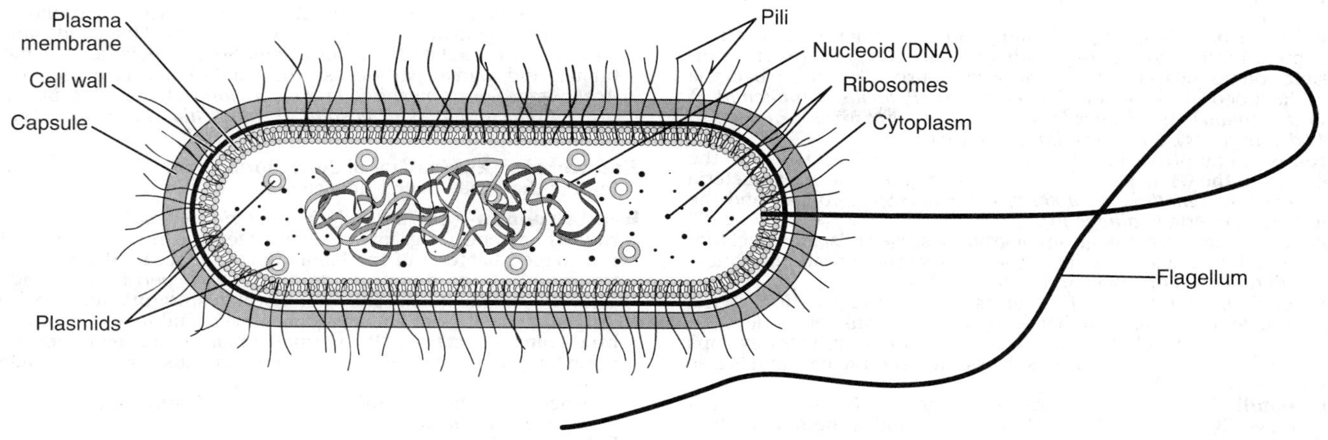


Generalized structure of a monotrichous bacterium (Not all structures occur in all cells)

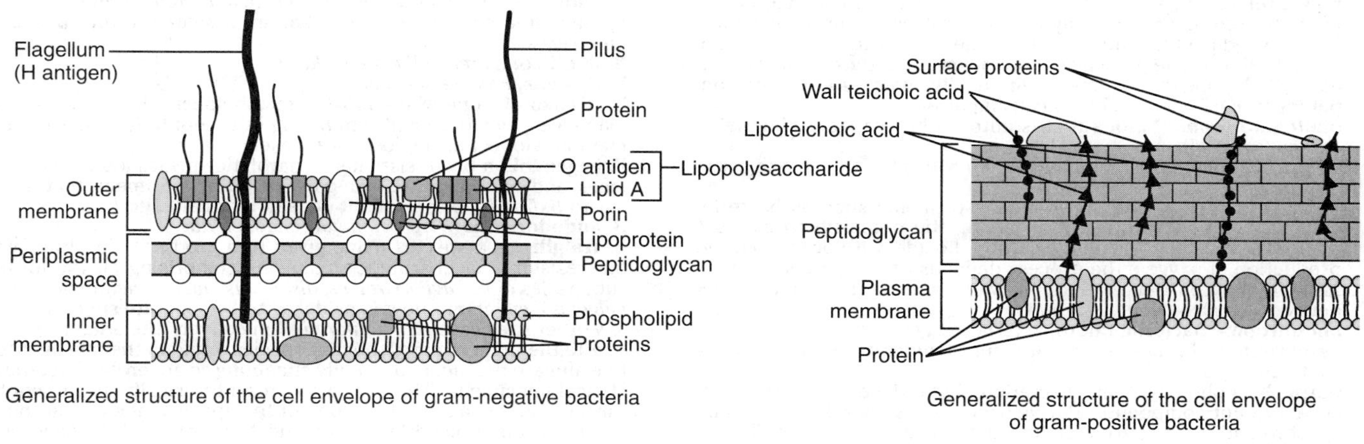


Generalized structure of the cell envelope of gram-negative bacteria

Generalized structure of the cell envelope of gram-positive bacteria

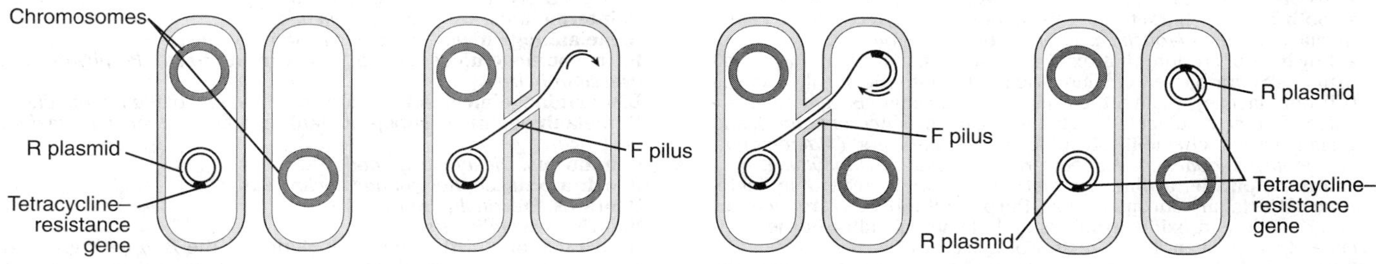


Transfer of drug resistance, in this case to tetracycline, between bacteria by transfer of the R plasmid during conjugation

**PLATE 8**—GENERALIZED STRUCTURES OF TYPICAL BACTERIAL CELLS AND TRANSFER OF A PLASMID BETWEEN BACTERIAL CELLS VIA CONJUGATION

**higher bacteria,** a term used to denote filamentous bacteria (e.g., Actinomycetales) that seem to be intermediate between bacteria and fungi.
**hydrogen b.,** a facultative chemoautotrophic microorganism that respires by the oxidation of hydrogen to water, using various organic compounds as carbon and energy sources. Hydrogen bacteria are included in the genera *Pseudomonas (P. facilis, P. ruhlandii, P. saccharophila), Alcaligenes (A. eutrophus, A. paradoxus), Paracoccus (P. denitrificans),* and *Nocardia (N. opaca).*
**iron b.,** an autotrophic microorganism that oxidizes iron from the ferrous to the ferric state, including some of the sheathed bacteria *(Clonothrix, Aenothrix, Leptothrix, Lieskeela, Sphaerotilus)* and the budding bacteria *(Gallionella).*
**lactic acid bacteria,** the group of gram-positive rods and cocci that produce lactic acid as an endproduct of carbohydrate formation; included are streptococci and lactobacilli.
**lysogenic b.,** one that harbors in its genome the genetic material (prophage) of a temperate bacteriophage and thus reproduces the bacteriophage in cell division; occasionally the prophage develops into the mature form, replicates, lyses the bacterial cell, and is free to infect other cells.
**mesophilic b.,** one whose optimal temperature for growth is in a midrange (30° to 45°C, 86° to 113°F) that includes the temperature of the human body.
**nitrifying b.,** a soil bacterium of the family Nitrobacteraceae that oxidizes ammonia to nitrites *(Nitrobacter, Nitrococcus, Nitrospina)* or nitrites to nitrates *(Nitrosococcus, Nitrosolobus, Nitrosomonas).*
**nodule bacteria,** bacteria which by their growth in specific nodules on the roots of plants (legumes) tend to bring about fixation of atmospheric nitrogen.
**nonsulfur b., purple,** a photosynthetic, heterotrophic, microaerophilic bacterium of the family Rhodospirillaceae. Purple nonsulfur bacteria reduce $CO_2$ and oxidize sulfide or thiosulfate but not elemental sulfur in the presence of the pigment bacteriochlorophyll *a.*
**parasitic b.,** one that is dependent on a living host for its nutrition.
**pathogenic b.,** one capable of causing disease.
**photoautotrophic b.,** one that is autotrophic, capable of deriving energy from light.
**photoheterotrophic b.,** one that is heterotrophic, capable of deriving energy from light.
**photosynthetic b.,** one that contains pigments such as bacteriochlorophylls and carotenoids enabling the organism to conduct photosynthesis and assimilate carbon dioxide, with or without the production of oxygen; the process depends on the presence of oxidizable electron donors such as water and reduced sulfur compounds. See also *Cyanobacteria.*
**phototrophic bacteria,** Photobacteria.
**psychrophilic b.,** one whose optimum temperature for growth is 15° to 20°C (59° to 68°F).
**purple b.,** a photosynthetic bacterium that reduces $CO_2$ in the presence of sulfur compounds. Purple bacteria are classified in the family Chromatiaceae (purple sulfur bacteria) and Rhodospirillaceae (purple nonsulfur bacteria).
**pyogenic b.,** one that produces suppuration when it infects an organism.
**pyrogenetic b.,** one that produces fever when it infects an organism.
**rough b.,** a variant form of a bacterium characterized by dry, wrinkled colonies on solid media. See *smooth-rough variation,* under *variation.*
**saprophytic b.,** one that lives in decaying organic matter.
**smooth b.,** one characterized by smooth, glossy colonies on solid media. See *smooth-rough variation,* under *variation.*
**sulfur b.,** a bacterium that oxidizes hydrogen sulfide, sulfur, or thiosulfate. Sulfur bacteria include the photosynthetic purple bacteria (Chromatiaceae), filamentous gliding organisms *(Beggiatoa, Thioploca, Thiothrix),* unicellular gliding organisms *(Achromatium),* and gram-negative chemolithotrophic sulfur oxidizers *(Macromonas, Sulfolobus, Thiobacillus, Thiobacterium, Thiospira, Thiovulum).*
**sulfur b., purple,** a photosynthetic autotrophic anaerobic bacterium of the family Chromatiaceae. Purple sulfur bacteria reduce carbon dioxide and oxidize sulfides and elemental sulfur in the presence of the pigment bacteriochlorophyll *a* or *b.*
**thermophilic b.,** one that grows best at temperatures above 40°C (104°F) with an optimal range of 50° to 70°C (122° to 158°F).
**toxigenic b., toxinogenic b.,** one that produces a toxin.
**water b.,** a gram-negative bacterium capable of rapid growth in all types of water and producing pyrogenic infections, especially in immunocompromised hospital patients, occurring as a contaminant in hemodialysis fluids and in flood waters. The most common water bacteria are species of *Achromobacter, Acinetobacter, Aeromonas, Flavobacterium,* and *Pseudomonas.*

**bac·te·ri·uria** (bak-tēr″e-u′re-ə) [*bacteri-* + *-uria*] [MeSH: Bacteriuria] the presence of bacteria in the urine.

**bac·te·ri·uric** (bak-tēr″e-u′rik) pertaining to bacteriuria.

**bac·ter·oid** (bak′tər-oid) [*bacteria* + Gr. *eidos* form] 1. resembling a bacterium. 2. a structurally modified bacterium.

**Bac·te·roi·da·ceae** (bak″tər-oi-da′se-e) [MeSH: Bacteroidaceae] a family of gram-negative, obligately anaerobic bacteria, occurring as nonsporogenous rods, nonmotile or motile with peritrichous flagella. The organisms occur naturally in cavities of man and animals, and have been isolated from infections. Some species are significant human and animal pathogens. The family consists of the genera *Acetivibrio, Angerobiospirillum, Angerovibrio, Bacteroides, Butyrivibrio, Fusobacterium, Lachnospira, Leptotrichia, Pectinatus, Selenomonas, Succinimonas, Succinivibrio,* and *Wolinella.*

**Bac·te·roi·deae** (bak″tər-oi′de-e) former name for a tribe of bacteria of the family Bacteroidaceae.

**Bac·te·roi·des** (bak″tər-oi′dēz) [*bacterio-* + *-oid*] [MeSH: Bacteroides] a genus of gram-negative, anaerobic, non–spore-forming, rod-shaped bacteria of the family Bacteroidaceae, made up of organisms that are nonmotile or motile with peritrichous flagella. They are normal inhabitants of the oral, respiratory, intestinal, and urogenital cavities of humans and animals, and may constitute the predominant bacteria of the normal human colon. Some species are potential pathogens, causing possibly fatal abscesses and bacteremias.
**B. asaccharoly′ticus,** *Porphyromonas asaccharolytica.*
**B. bi′vius,** *Prevotella bivia.*
**B. buc′cae,** *Prevotella buccae.*
**B. capillo′sus,** a weakly fermentative, bile-sensitive, nonpigmented species isolated from cysts, wounds, and feces of humans and the intestinal tract of animals.
**B. clostridiifor′mis,** *Clostridium clostridioforme.*
**B. cor′poris,** *Prevotella corporis.*
**B. corro′dens,** a former species including facultative organisms that are now assigned to the species *Eikenella corrodens* and microaerophilic, urease-positive strains that are assigned to the species *B. ureolyticus.*
**B. denti′cola,** *Prevotella denticola.*
**B. di′siens,** *Prevotella disiens.*
**B. distaso′nis,** one of the most common species isolated from human feces, which is similar to *B. fragilis* except that it does not ferment amylopectin, amylose, or fucose.
**B. egger′thii,** a bile-resistant saccharolytic species found in human feces, and occasionally isolated from clinical specimens, that is similar to *B. fragilis* except that it does not ferment sucrose.
**B. endodonta′lis,** *Porphyromonas endodontalis.*
**B. fra′gilis,** 1. a species name given to a group of closely related bile-resistant, saccharolytic organisms comprising all the former subspecies of *B. fragilis (fragilis, distasonis, ovatus, thetaiotaomicron, vulgatus),* which are now considered to be separate species, and a few other species, e.g., *B. uniformis.* Collectively, the organisms constitute the numerically dominant species found in the human intestine and are the most commonly encountered anaerobic bacteria in clinical specimens. They are also present normally in the mouth, throat, and vaginal tract. 2. one of the species included in the *B. fragilis* group of bacteria. It is the most important of the anaerobic bacteria causing human infection, being most frequently implicated in intra-abdominal infections, but is also found in bacteremias, abscesses, and other lesions throughout the body. Organisms in this species are more resistant to antibiotics than any other anaerobe. Called also *Bacillus fragilis.*
**B. fundulifor′mis,** *Fusobacterium necrophorum.*
**B. gingiva′lis,** *Porphyromonas gingivalis.*
**B. heparinoly′ticus,** *Prevotella heparinolytica.*
**B. interme′dius,** *Prevotella intermedia.*
**B. melaninoge′nicus,** *Prevotella melaninogenica.*
**B. melaninoge′nicus** subsp. **asaccharoly′ticus,** *Porphyromonas asaccharolytica.*
**B. melaninoge′nicus** subsp. **interme′dius,** *Prevotella intermedia.*
**B. melaninoge′nicus** subsp. **melaninoge′nicus,** *Prevotella melaninogenica.*
**B. nodo′sus,** *Dichelobacter nodosus.*
**B. ochra′ceus,** *Capnocytophaga ochraceus.*
**B. ora′lis,** *Prevotella oralis.*
**B. o′ris,** *Prevotella oris.*
**B. ova′tus,** one of the species included in the *B. fragilis* group of bacteria, isolated from normal human feces and occasionally from clinical specimens.
**B. pneumosin′tes,** a species isolated from the nasopharynx, blood, and abscesses of the lung and brain.
**B. praeacu′tus,** *Tissierella praeacutus.*
**B. putre′dinis,** a bile-sensitive, nonpigmented, nonfermentative species isolated from abdominal and rectal abscesses and from feces of humans, from soil, and from sheep foot rot.
**B. rumini′cola,** *Prevotella ruminicola.*
**B. splanch′nicus,** a bile-resistant, saccharolytic species isolated from human feces, the vagina, and occasionally from abdominal infections, which is similar to *B. fragilis* except that it does not ferment sucrose.
**B. thetaiotao′micron,** one of the species included in the *B. fragilis* group of bacteria. Except for *B. fragilis,* it is the most important

anaerobe causing human infection. *B. thetaiotaomicron,* with *B. vulgatus,* is the organism most frequently isolated from fecal specimens, and it is frequently found in other human clinical specimens.
**B. unifor'mis,** one of the species included in the *B. fragilis* group of bacteria, occurring as part of the normal flora in human and swine feces, and isolated from various human clinical specimens.
**B. ureoly'ticus,** a bile-sensitive, nonpigmented, microaerophilic, nonfermentative species that is urease positive, isolated from infections of the respiratory and intestinal tracts and from various clinical specimens. See also *B. corrodens.*
**B. vulga'tus,** one of the species included in the *B. fragilis* group of bacteria. *B. vulgatus,* with *B. thetaiotaomicron,* is the organism most frequently isolated from fecal specimens, and it has occasionally been isolated from human infections.

**bac·te·roi·des** (bak″tər-oi'dēz) [MeSH: Bacteroides] any bacterium of the genus *Bacteroides.*

**bac·te·roi·do·sis** (bak″tər-oi-do'sis) infection with organisms of the genus *Bacteroides.*

**bac·ter·uria** (bak″tēr-u're-ə) bacteriuria.

**Bac·to·cill** (bak'to-sil) trademark for a preparation of oxacillin sodium.

**Bac·trim** (bak'trim) trademark for preparations of trimethoprim and sulfamethoxazole.

**Bac·tro·ban** (bak'tro-ban″) trademark for preparations of mupirocin.

**bac·u·lum** (bak'u-ləm) [L. "a stick, staff"] a heterotopic bone developed in the fibrous septum between the corpora cavernosa and above the urethra, forming the skeleton of the penis in all insectivores, bats, rodents, carnivores, and pinnipeds, and in nonhuman primates. Called also *os penis* and *os priapi.*

**badge** (baj) see *film badge.*

**Baelz's disease** (bāltz'əz) [Erwin von *Baelz,* German physician, 1849–1913] see *cheilitis glandularis.*

**BAEP** brain stem auditory evoked potential.

**Baer's cavity, law** (bārz) [Karl Ernst von *Baer* (Ber), Estonian anatomist, 1792–1876] see under *cavity* and *law.*

**Bä·fver·stedt's syndrome** (ba'fər-shtets) [Bo Erik *Bäfverstedt,* Swedish physician, born 1905] lymphocytoma cutis.

**bag** (bag) a sac or pouch.
**Bunyan b.,** a bag of light waterproof material for covering wet dressings.
**colostomy b.,** a receptacle worn over the stoma to receive the fecal discharge from a colostomy.
**Douglas b.,** a receptacle for the collection of expired air, permitting measurement of respiratory gases.
**Hagner b.,** an inflatable rubber bag to be used by traction through the urethra to prevent hemorrhage following prostatectomy.
**ice b.,** a bag filled with ice, for applying cold to the body.
**ileostomy b.,** any of various plastic or latex bags for the collection of urine or fecal material following ileostomy or the establishment of an ileal bladder; a flange or similar device fits closely about the ileal stoma and the bag is cemented to the skin or strapped to the body.
**micturition b.,** a receptacle for urine used by ambulatory patients with urinary incontinence.
**nuclear b.,** the central portion of the central or equatorial segment of intrafusal fibers of muscle; it is usually devoid of obvious cross striations and contains an accumulation of 40 to 50 spherical nuclei, which completely fill and often slightly distend the fiber.
**Perry b.,** an ileostomy bag with a small latex cuff reinforced by a plastic disk which fits snugly around a protruding stoma; the cuff is held down by a large plastic ring to which a belt is attached.
**Petersen's b.,** an inflatable rubber bag inserted into the rectum so as to elevate the bladder in the operation of suprapubic cystotomy.
**Pilcher b.,** a modification of the Hagner bag which provides urethral drainage as well as hemostasis.
**Politzer's b.,** a soft bag of rubber for inflating the middle ear.
**testicular b.,** scrotum.
**b. of waters,** popular name for the amniotic sac.
**Whitmore b.,** an ileostomy bag with a malleable flange and a valvular device for urine drainage at the lower end of the bag.

**bag·as·so·sis** (bag″ə-so'sis) a type of hypersensitivity pneumonitis caused by inhalation of the dust of bagasse, the waste of sugar cane after the sugar has been extracted.

**Bail·lar·ger's bands,** etc. (bi-yahr-zhāz') [Jules Gabriel François *Baillarger,* French psychiatrist, 1809–1890] see *stria laminae granularis internae* and *stria laminae pyramidalis internae,* and see under *sign.*

**Bain·bridge reflex** (bān'brij) [Francis Arthur *Bainbridge,* English physiologist, 1874–1921] see under *reflex.*

**bake** (bāk) to expose to high temperature at low humidity, as in the processing of porcelain.

**Ba·ker's cyst** (ba'kərz) [William Morrant *Baker,* British surgeon, 1839–1896] see under *cyst.*

**BAL** [*British antilewisite*] dimercaprol.

**Bal·a·mu·thia** (bal″ə-moo'the-ə) a genus of amoebae of the order Leptomyxida. *B. mandrilla'ris* is the cause of primary amebic meningoencephalitis in both immunocompromised and previously healthy patients; some cases are fatal.

**bal·ance** (bal'əns) [L. *bilanx*] 1. an instrument for weighing. 2. the harmonious adjustment of parts; the harmonious performance of functions. 3. equilibrium.
**acid-base b.,** a condition in which the net rate of acid or alkali production by the body is balanced by the net rate of acid or alkali excretion from the body, resulting in a stable concentration of $H^+$ (hydrogen ions) in the body fluids.
**analytical b.,** a laboratory balance sensitive to variations of the order of 0.05 to 0.1 mg.
**calcium b.,** the balance between the calcium intake and its output through the body excretions.
**fluid b.,** the state of the body in relation to ingestion and excretion of water and electrolytes; called also *water b.*
**genic b.,** the ratio of male-determining to female-determining genes in the chromosome assortment as the determiner of sex.
**microchemical b.,** a laboratory balance sensitive to variations of the order of 0.001 mg.
**nitrogen b.,** the state of the body in regard to ingestion and excretion of nitrogen. In *negative nitrogen balance* the amount of nitrogen excreted is greater than the quantity ingested; in *positive nitrogen balance* the amount excreted is smaller than the amount ingested.
**occlusal b.,** balanced occlusion.
**semimicro b.,** a balance sensitive to variations of 0.01 mg.
**torsion b.,** 1. a weighing balance in which the scale beam is supported by metallic ribbons that act by torsion. 2. an electrometer that acts by the twisting of a single fiber of the web of a silkworm.
**water b.,** fluid b.

**ba·lan·ic** (bə-lan'ik) pertaining to the glans penis or glans clitoridis.

**bal·a·ni·tis** (bal″ə-ni'tis) [*balano-* + *-itis*] [MeSH: Balanitis] inflammation of the glans penis; it is usually associated with phimosis.
**amebic b.,** a variety caused by *Entamoeba histolytica.*
**b. circina'ta,** a variety attributed to the presence of spirochetes.
**b. circumscrip'ta plasmacellula'ris,** a benign erythroplasia histologically characterized by plasma cell infiltration of the dermis, and clinically by persistent inflammation, usually involving the inner surface of the prepuce and glans penis and associated with the development of a single erythematous, moist, shiny lesion. Called also *b. plasmocellularis, balanoposthitis circumscripta plasmocellularis, chronic circumscribed plasmocytic balanoposthitis, plasma cell b.,* and *Zoon's erythroplasia.* Cf. *plasma cell vulvitis.*
**b. diabet'ica,** a variety caused by the irritation of the urine in diabetes.
**erosive b.,** balanitis due to mixed microbial infection that progresses to gangrenous ulcerations of the penis similar to the lesions seen in noma of oral tissues.
**Follmann's b.,** a serous balanitis and posthitis without induration.
**b. gangraeno'sa, gangrenous b.,** a rapidly destructive infection producing erosion of the glans penis and often destruction of the entire external genitals; the infection is believed to be due to a spirochete. Called also *balanoposthomycosis* and *Corbus' disease.*
**phagedenic b.,** gangrenous b.
**plasma cell b., b. plasmacellula'ris,** b. circumscripta plasmacellularis.
**b. xero'tica obli'terans,** lichen sclerosus in males; see under *lichen.*

**balan(o)-** [Gr. *balanos* acorn] a combining form indicating relationship to the glans penis or to the glans clitoridis.

**bal·a·no·cele** (bal'ə-no-sēl) [*balano-* + *-cele*[1]] protrusion of the glans penis through a rupture of the prepuce.

**bal·a·no·plas·ty** (bal'ə-no-plas″te) [*balano-* + *-plasty*] plastic surgery of the glans penis.

**bal·a·no·pos·thi·tis** (bal'ə-no-pos-thi'tis) [*balano-* + Gr. *posthē* prepuce + *-itis*] inflammation of the glans penis and prepuce.
**chronic circumscribed plasmocytic b., b. chro'nica circumscrip'ta plasmocellula'ris,** balanitis circumscripta plasmacellularis.
**enzootic b.,** a disease of castrated male sheep in Australia and New Zealand, marked by spreading ulceration of the glans penis and prepuce and severe swelling and distention of the sheath; the cause is infection by *Corynebacterium renale* of animals fed a high protein diet so that their urine is high in urea. Called also *enzootic posthitis, pizzle rot,* and *sheath rot.*
**infectious pustular b.,** a venereal infection of bulls, caused by bovine herpesvirus 1 and characterized by small pustules on the penis and prepuce; it can also be spread through artificial insemination. It is the male counterpart of infectious pustular vulvovaginitis.

**specific gangrenous and ulcerative b.,** an acute inflammatory disease of the glans penis and opposed surface of the prepuce, marked by ulcerations and sometimes by gangrene, with a flow of odorous pus, and caused by a spirochete; called also *fourth venereal disease.*

**bal·a·no·pos·tho·my·co·sis** (bal″ə-no-pos″tho-mi-ko′sis) gangrenous balanitis.

**bal·a·no·pre·pu·ti·al** (bal″ə-no-pre-poo′shəl) pertaining to the glans penis and the prepuce.

**bal·a·nor·rha·gia** (bal″ə-no-ra′jə) [*balano-* + *-rrhagia*] balanitis with free discharge of pus.

**bal·an·ti·di·a·sis** (bal″an-tĭ-di′ə-sis) [MeSH: Balantidiasis] infection by protozoa of the genus *Balantidium;* in humans and many other vertebrates, *Bacillus coli* may cause diarrhea and dysentery, with ulceration of the colon mucosa.

**bal·an·tid·i·o·sis** (bal″an-tid-e-o′sis) balantidiasis.

**Bal·an·tid·i·um** (bal″an-tid′e-əm) [Gr. *balantidion* little bag] [MeSH: Balantidium] a genus of ciliate protozoa of the order Trichostomatida, suborder Trichostomatina, including many species found in the intestines of vertebrates and invertebrates.
**B. co′li,** the largest protozoan and the only ciliate parasite of humans (see *balantidiasis*), which is also found in pigs and monkeys; it may measure 30 to 150 μm long by 25 to 120 μm wide.
**B. su′is,** a nonpathogenic species found in pigs considered by some to be identical with *B. coli* and by others to be a separate species.

**bal·an·ti·do·sis** (bal″an-tĭ-do′sis) balantidiasis.

**bal·a·nus** (bal′ə-nəs) the glans penis.

**Bal·bi·a·ni's nucleus (body)** (bahl-be-ah′nēz) [Edouard Gérard *Balbiani,* French embryologist, 1823–1899] yolk nucleus.

**bald·ness** (bawld′nəs) alopecia, especially of the scalp.
**common b.,** androgenetic alopecia; in men called *common male b.* and in women called *common female b.*
**male pattern b.,** see *androgenetic alopecia,* under *alopecia.*

**Bal·dy's operation** (bawl′dēz) [John Montgomery *Baldy,* American gynecologist, 1860–1934] see *Webster's operation,* under *operation.*

**Bal·dy-Web·ster operation** (bawl′de-web′stər) [J. M. *Baldy;* John Clarence *Webster,* American gynecologist, 1863–1950] see *Webster's operation,* under *operation.*

**Bal·int syndrome** (bah-lēnt′) [Rezsoe *Balint,* Hungarian neurologist and psychiatrist, 1874–1929] see under *syndrome.*

**Bal·kan frame, splint** (bawl′kən) [*Balkan* countries, where first used] see under *frame* and *splint.*

**Ball's valve** (bawlz) [Sir Charles Bent *Ball,* Irish surgeon, 1851–1916] valvulae anales.

**ball** (bawl) a more or less spherical mass. Cf. *sphere.*
**chondrin b.,** one of the ball-like masses in hyaline cartilage, consisting of cells surrounded by a capsule of basophilic matrix.
**food b.,** phytobezoar.
**fungus b.,** a tumorlike mass formed by colonization of a fungus in a body cavity, usually a bronchus or pulmonary cavity but occasionally a nasal cavity; the organism may disseminate through the bloodstream to the brain, heart, and kidneys. The most common type is the aspergilloma. Called also *fungoma.*
**hair b.,** trichobezoar.
**Marchi b's,** ellipsoid or ovoid segments of myelin produced by degeneration, staining brown by Marchi methods.
**oat hair b.,** a trichobezoar formed in the stomach of the horse from the fine hairs within the outer husk of the oat grain and other materials.
**pleural fibrin b's,** fibrin bodies of pleura.
**wool b.,** a trichobezoar containing wool fibers and other substances.

**Bal·lance's sign** (bal′ən-səz) [Sir Charles Alfred *Ballance,* English surgeon, 1857–1936] see under *sign.*

**Bal·ler-Ger·old syndrome** (bah′lər ga′rōlt) [Friedrich *Baller,* German physician, 20th century; M. *Gerold,* German physician, 20th century] see under *syndrome.*

**Bal·let's sign** (bah-lāz′) [Louis Gilbert *Ballet,* French neurologist, 1853–1916] see under *sign.*

**bal·lism** (bal′iz-əm) ballismus.

**bal·lis·mus** (bə-liz′məs) [Gr. *ballismos* a jumping about, dancing] violent flinging dyskinetic movements caused by contractions of the proximal limb muscles as a result of destruction of the subthalamic nucleus or its fiber connections, sometimes affecting only one side of the body (hemiballismus). Called also *ballism.*

**bal·lis·tic** (bə-lis′tik) 1. jerking or twitching; pertaining to or characterized by ballismus. 2. pertaining to or caused by projectiles.

**bal·lis·tics** (bə-lis′tiks) [Gr. *ballein* to throw] the scientific study of the motion of projectiles in flight.
**wound b.,** the scientific study of the speed and direction of missiles (bullets and other projectiles) in relation to the injuries they produce.

**bal·lis·to·car·dio·gram** (bə-lis″to-kahr′de-o-gram″) the tracing made by a ballistocardiograph; abbreviated BCG.

**bal·lis·to·car·di·o·graph** (bə-lis″to-kahr′de-o-graf″) an apparatus for recording the movements of the body caused by cardiac contractions and associated blood flow; it has been used to determine cardiac output and other aspects of cardiac function.

**bal·lis·to·car·di·og·ra·phy** (bə-lis″to-kahr″de-og′rə-fe) [MeSH: Ballistocardiography] the graphic recording, by means of a ballistocardiograph, of the recoil movements of the body which result from motion of the heart and blood.

**bal·lis·to·spore** (bə-lis′to-spor) a fungal spore that is forcibly discharged upon maturity; seen in some basidiomycetes.

**bal·loon** (bə-lo͞on′) 1. a sac that can be inserted into a body cavity or tube and distended with air or gas. 2. to distend with air or gas; to inflate.
**Shea-Anthony antral b.,** sinus b.
**sinus b.,** a balloon expandable with liquid or air to support depressed fractures of the walls of the maxillary sinus; a Foley catheter may also be used. Called also *Shea-Anthony antral b.*

**bal·loon·ing** (bə-lo͞on′ing) distending any cavity of the body with air or gas for therapeutic purposes.

**bal·lot·a·ble** (bə-lot′ə-bəl) capable of showing ballottement.

**bal·lotte·ment** (bə-lot′mənt) [Fr. "a tossing about"] a palpatory maneuver to test for a floating object. The term is applied especially to a maneuver for detecting the existence of pregnancy by pushing up the head or breech of a fetus by fingers inserted into the vagina, so as to cause the fetus to rise and fall again like a heavy body in water.
**abdominal b., indirect b.,** that which is effected by the finger applied to the abdominal wall.
**renal b.,** palpation of the kidney by pressing one hand into the abdominal wall while the other hand makes quick thrusts forward from behind so as to throw the kidney against the anterior hand.

**balm** (bahm) [Fr. *baume*] 1. a healing or soothing medicine. 2. a plant of the genus *Melissa,* especially *M. officinalis;* it is carminative and aromatic. 3. b. of Gilead. 4. balsam.
**blue b.,** *Melissa.*
**b. of Gilead,** 1. any of various trees of the genus *Commiphora,* especially *C. opobalsamum.* 2. Mecca balsam. 3. Canada balsam. 4. the buds of the poplar tree *Populus candicans,* which contain volatile oils and resins and are used as a stimulating expectorant in cough syrups. Called also *balsam of Gilead.*
**lemon b.,** *Melissa.*
**mountain b.,** *Eriodictyon.*
**sweet b.,** *Melissa.*

**Balme's cough** (bahlmz) [Paul Jean *Balme,* French physician, born 1857] see under *cough.*

**bal·neo·ther·a·py** (bal″ne-o-ther′ə-pe) [L. *balneum* bath + *therapy*] the treatment of disease by baths.

**Bal·ne·tar** (bal′nə-tahr) trademark for a preparation of coal tar.

**Ba·ló's disease (concentric sclerosis)** (bah-lōz′) [Jozsef Matthius *Baló,* Hungarian physician, born 1895] see under *disease.*

**bal·sam** (bawl′səm) [L. *balsamum;* Gr. *balsamon*] 1. a semifluid, resinous, and fragrant liquid of vegetable origin, usually trees, which is often composed chiefly of resins, volatile oils, and various esters. 2. balm.

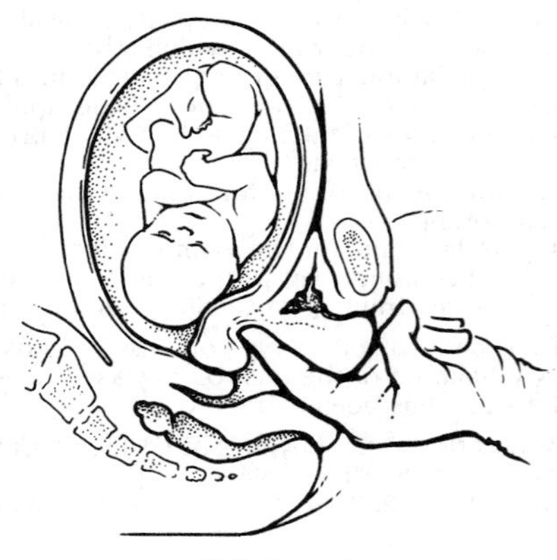

Ballottement.

**Canada b.**, a liquid oleoresin from *Abies balsamea,* which contains volatile oils, chiefly *l*-pinene, and over 70 per cent resins; a microscopic medium that was formerly used medicinally. Called also *balm* or *b. of Gilead.*
**b. of Gilead,** 1. Mecca b. 2. Canada b. 3. balm of Gilead (def. 4).
**Holland b.,** juniper tar.
**Mecca b.,** the resinous juice of *Commiphora opobalsamum,* a light colored viscid liquid with an aromatic aroma used in medicines and cosmetics in northeastern Africa and southern and southwestern Asia. Called also *balm* or *b. of Gilead.*
**b. of Peru, peruvian b.,** a dark brown viscid liquid obtained from *Myroxylon pereirae* Klotzsch (Leguminosae) used as a local protectant and as a rubefacient; applied topically.
**silver b.,** juniper tar.
**tolu b.** [USP], a balsam obtained from *Myroxylon balsamum,* used as an ingredient of compound benzoin tincture and as an expectorant.
**Turlington's b., Wade's b.,** compound benzoin tincture.

**Bal·ser's fatty necrosis** (bahl'zərz) [Wilhelm August *Balser,* German physician, died 1892] see under *necrosis.*

**Bal·ti·more** (bawl'tĭ-mor) [MeSH: Baltimore] David. American biologist, born 1938; co-winner, with Renato Dulbecco and Howard Temin, of the Nobel prize in medicine and physiology for 1975, for discoveries concerning the interaction between tumor viruses and the genetic material of host cells and the role of reverse transcriptase.

**Bam·ber·ger's disease, sign** (bahm'bər-gərz) [Heinrich von *Bamberger,* Austrian physician, 1822–1888] see under *disease* and *sign.*

**Bam·ber·ger-Ma·rie disease** (bahm'bər-gər mah-re') [Eugen *Bamberger,* Austrian physician, 1858–1921; Pierre *Marie,* French physician, 1853–1940] hypertrophic pulmonary osteoarthropathy.

**bam·ber·my·cins** (bam"bər-mi'sinz) [MeSH: Bambermycins] an antibacterial antibiotic complex containing at least four components, with two (the A and C components) predominating; produced by various species of *Streptomyces,* as well as synthetically; used as a feed additive or food supplement for pigs, poultry, and calves. Called also *moenomycins.*

**bam·nid·a·zole** (bam-nid'ə-zōl) an antiprotozoal effective against *Trichomonas.*

**BAN** British Approved Name, an official nonproprietary name approved by the British Pharmacopoeia Commission.

**ban·crof·ti·an** (bang-krof'te-ən) named for Joseph *Bancroft,* English physician in Australia, 1836–1894.

**ban·crof·to·sis** (ban"krof-to'sis) infection with *Wuchereria bancrofti.*

**band** (band) 1. an object or appliance that confines or restricts while allowing a limited or desired degree of movement. 2. in dentistry, a thin metal hoop that horizontally encircles the crown or root of a natural tooth. 3. a strip that holds together or binds two or more separate objects or parts; for anatomical structures, see *frenulum, taenia, trabecula,* and *vinculum.* 4. an elongated area with parallel or roughly parallel borders that is distinct from the surrounding surface by its color, texture, or other characteristics, such as a chromosome band. See also *layer, stria,* and *stripe.*
**A b.,** the dark-staining zone of a sarcomere, whose center is traversed by the paler H band, which in turn contains the darker M band; called also *A disk, Q disk, anisotropic disk,* and *transverse disk.*
**absorption b's,** dark bands in the spectrum due to absorption of light by the medium (a solid, a liquid, or a gas) through which the light has passed. Cf. *absorption lines,* under *line.*
**amniotic b.,** a fibrous band passing from fetus to amnion. See also *amniotic band sequence,* under *sequence.*
**anchor b.,** orthodontic b.
**anogenital b.,** the primordium of the embryonic perineum.
**anterior b. of colon,** taenia libera.
**atrioventricular b.,** bundle of His.

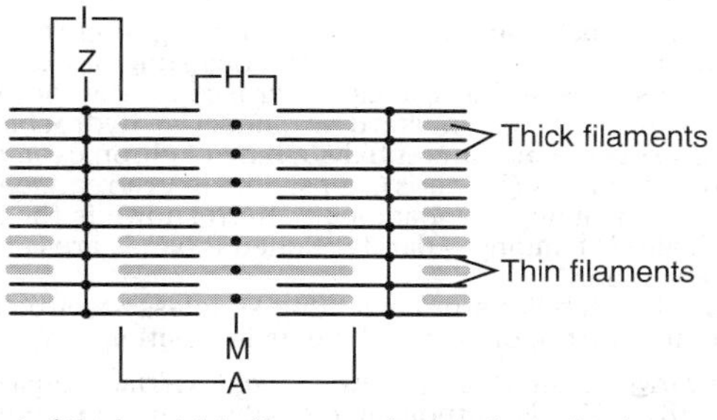

Arrangement of thick and thin filaments of striated muscle, showing the A, H, I, M, and Z bands.

**axis b.,** primitive streak.
**Baillarger's external b.,** stria laminae granularis internae.
**Baillarger's inner b., Baillarger's internal b.,** stria laminae pyramidalis internae.
**Baillarger's outer b.,** stria laminae granularis internae.
**b. of Broca, Broca's diagonal b.,** stria diagonalis (Broca).
**Büngner's b's,** bands of syncytium formed by the union of sheath cells during the regeneration of peripheral nerves; called also *Ledbänder.*
**C b., C-b.,** see *chromosome b.,* and *C banding,* under *banding.*
**chromosome b.,** any of the alternating dark and light or fluorescent transverse bands produced on chromosomes by differential staining; named according to the procedure used, i.e., C band, G band, Q band, and R band. See *chromosome banding,* under *banding.*
**Clado's b.,** the suspensory ligament of the ovary covered with peritoneum.
**clamp b.,** an orthodontic band held in place with a screw nut.
**b's of colon, longitudinal,** taeniae coli.
**contoured b.,** an orthodontic band shaped to the contour of the tooth.
**contraction b.,** one of the bands seen by light microscopy in fully contracted muscle on either side of the Z band, caused by distortion of the ends of the myosin filaments by the Z band.
**coronary b.,** a band of vascular tissue at the upper edge of the wall of the hoof, which is concerned in the secretion of the wall; called also *coronary cushion, coronary ring, coronet,* and *cutidure.*
**dentate b.,** gyrus dentatus, def. 1.
**diagonal b., diagonal b. of Broca,** stria diagonalis.
**elastic b.,** see *elastic,* def. 2.
**external b. of Baillarger,** stria laminae granularis internae.
**free b. of colon,** taenia libera.
**furrowed b.,** a strip of cortex that connects the tonsil of the hemisphere of the cerebellum to the uvula of the vermis.
**G b., G-b.,** see *chromosome b.,* and *chromosome banding,* under *banding.*
**b. of Gennari,** see under *line.*
**Giacomini's b.,** the grayish band constituting the anterior extension of the gyrus dentatus of the hippocampus over the inferior surface of the uncus.
**H b.,** a relatively pale zone sometimes seen traversing the center of the A band of fibrils of striated muscle; called also *Hensen's* or *Engelmann's disk.*
**Harris' b.,** anomalous peritoneal folds which extend from the gallbladder to the inferior surface of the liver to the proximal duodenum, sometimes traversing the mesocolon near the hepatic flexure.
**Henle's b.,** fibers from the anterior aponeurosis of the transversus abdominis muscle extending posterior to the rectus abdominis muscle and inferior to the arcuate line.
**His' b.,** see under *bundle.*
**Hunter-Schreger b's, b's of Hunter and Schreger,** lines of Schreger.
**I b.,** the band or disk within a striated muscle fibril that appears as a light region under the light microscope and as a dark region under polarized light; it contains the proteins actin, troponin, and tropomyosin. Called also *isotropic disk* and *J disk.*
**iliotibial b.,** tractus iliotibialis.
**inner b. of Baillarger, internal b. of Baillarger,** stria laminae pyramidalis internae.
**Ladd's b's,** bands of peritoneum that attach the cecum to the right lateral abdominal wall. See also *Ladd's syndrome,* under *syndrome.*
**Lane's b's,** adhesions between tight loops of the terminal ileum which may extend as ligamentous bands to the right iliac fossa.
**limbic b's,** a superior and an inferior muscular band developed in the right atrium of the fetal heart that become the basis of Lower's tubercle and the sinus septum.
**M b.,** the narrow dark band in the center of the H band of the sarcomere; called also *M disk, Hensen's line,* and *mesophragma.* Cf. *Z b.*
**Maissiat's b.,** tractus iliotibialis.
**matrix b.,** a cylindrical stainless steel or copper band or short tube with a special clamp or holder; it is filled with a softened impression compound and seated over a tooth, so that the compound flows into the prepared cavity and an impression of a single tooth can be obtained. Also used in the placement and contouring of restorative materials such as resin or glass ionomer cement, and to form the fourth wall of a class II cavity preparation during the condensation of an amalgam restoration.
**Meckel's b.,** a part of the anterior ligament fastening the malleus to the wall of the tympanum. Called also *Meckel's ligament.*
**mesocolic b.,** taenia mesocolica.
**moderator b.,** trabecula septomarginalis.
**molar b.,** an orthodontic band applied to a molar tooth; a bracket is attached to the band to hold the arch wire of the appliance.
**oligoclonal b's,** discrete bands of immunoglobulins with decreased electrophoretic mobility; their appearance in electrophoretograms of cerebrospinal fluid is a sign of possible multiple sclerosis or other diseases of the central nervous system.
**omental b.,** taenia omentalis.

**orthodontic b.**, a band fitted over a tooth to anchor a fixed orthodontic appliance. Called also *anchor b.*
**outer b. of Baillarger,** stria laminae granularis internae.
**Parham b.**, a metallic ribbon used to fix a fractured long bone by encircling the bone at the site of the fracture.
**perioplic b.**, the band of secretor cells at the upper border of the hoof of animals; it secretes the periople.
**periosteal b.**, see under *collar.*
**Q b., Q-b.**, see *chromosome b.*, and *chromosome banding,* under *banding.*
**R b., R-b.**, see *chromosome b.*, and *chromosome banding,* under *banding.*
**b. of Reil,** trabecula septomarginalis.
**retention b.**, musculus suspensorius duodeni.
**Schreger's b's, b's of Schreger,** see under *line.*
**Simonart's b.**, 1. Simonart's thread. 2. a weblike band of tissue that sometimes joins the medial and lateral parts of a cleft lip.
**Soret b.**, the absorption band of porphyrins at 400–410 nm.
**Vicq d'Azyr's b.**, Kaes-Bekhterev layer.
**Z b.**, a thin membrane seen on longitudinal section as a dark line in the center of the I band; the distance between successive Z bands serves to delimit the sarcomeres of striated muscle. Called also *Z disk* or *line, Amici's disk, Dobie's line* or *layer, intermediate disk, Krause's membrane, telophragma,* and *thin disk.* See also *inophragma* and *M b.*
**zonular b.**, zona orbicularis articulationis coxae.

**ban·dage** (ban'dəj) [MeSH: Bandages] 1. a strip or roll of gauze or other material for wrapping or binding any part of the body. 2. to cover by wrapping with a strip of gauze or other material. See also *dressing* and *strapping.*
**Ace b.**, trademark for a bandage of woven elastic material.
**adhesive b.** [USP], a sterile compress of four layers of Type I absorbent gauze affixed to a fabric or film coated with a pressure-sensitive adhesive.
**Barton's b.**, a figure-of-8 bandage supporting the lower jaw below and in front. See Plate 9.
**Borsch's b.**, an eye bandage covering both the diseased and the healthy eye.
**Buller's b.**, see under *shield.*
**capeline b.**, a bandage applied like a cap or hood to the head or shoulder or to an amputation stump.
**circular b.**, a bandage applied in circular turns, usually about a limb.
**compression b.**, a bandage by which pressure is applied to a limb to prevent edema.
**crucial b.**, T b.
**demigauntlet b.**, a bandage that covers the hand but leaves the fingers exposed.
**Desault's b.**, a bandage binding the elbow to the side, with a pad in the axilla, for fractured clavicle; called also *Desault's apparatus.*
**elastic b.**, a bandage of elastic material applied to an area to exert continuous pressure upon it.
**Esmarch's b.**, a rubber bandage applied around a part from distal to proximal in order to expel blood from it; the limb is often elevated as the elastic pressure is applied. Called also *Esmarch tourniquet.*
**figure-of-eight b.**, a bandage in which the turns cross each other like the figure eight (8). See Plate 9.
**four-tailed b.**, one with each end cut into two strips of equal width, which are used to secure the center portion under or over the jaw or other prominence. See Plate 9.
**gauntlet b.**, a bandage that covers the hand and fingers like a glove.
**gauze b.** [USP], Type I absorbent gauze containing no dyes or additives; it may be sterilized.
**Gibney b.**, strips of $\frac{1}{2}$-inch adhesive overlapped along the sides and back of the foot and leg to hold the foot in slight varus position and leave the dorsum of the foot and anterior aspect of the leg exposed; called also *Gibney's strapping.*
**hammock b.**, a bandage for retaining dressings on the head; it consists of a broad strip placed over the dressing, brought down over the ears, and held in place by a circular bandage around the head.
**immobilizing b.**, a bandage for partially immobilizing a part.
**many-tailed b.**, a wide bandage with each end cut into several strips of equal width which may be overlapped as the bandage is applied, usually to the abdomen or chest. See *Scultetus b.*
**Martin's b.**, a roller bandage of thin elastic rubber.
**oblique b.**, a bandage applied obliquely up a limb without reverses. Cf. *reversed b.*
**plaster b.**, a bandage stiffened with a paste of plaster of Paris, which sets and becomes very hard.
**pressure b.**, a bandage for applying pressure.
**recurrent b.**, one used on a distal stump, such as a finger, toe, or amputation stump, that is turned lengthwise to cover the end of the stump and is secured in place by circular turns. See Plate 9.
**reversed b.**, one applied to a limb in such a way that the roll is inverted or half-turned at each revolution, so as to make it fit smoothly the varying dimensions of the limb.
**roller b.**, a tightly rolled, circular bandage of varying widths and materials, often commercially prepared.
**Scultetus b.**, a many-tailed b. applied with the tails overlapping each other and held in position by safety pins; see Plate 9. Called also *scultetus.*
**spica b.**, a figure-of-eight bandage with turns that cross one another regularly like the letter V, usually applied to anatomical areas of quite different dimensions, as the pelvis and thigh or the thorax and arm. See Plate 9.
**spiral b.**, a roller bandage applied spirally around a limb.
**spiral reverse b.**, a spiral bandage applied with reverse turns in order to fit more snugly the varying contours and dimensions of a limb. See Plate 9.
**suspensory b.**, a bandage for supporting the scrotum.
**T b.**, a bandage shaped like the letter T; called also *crucial b.*
**triangular b.**, a triangle of cloth used as a sling or bandage.
**Velpeau's b.**, a bandage to support the arm and provide immobilization of the elbow and shoulder; it is useful in supporting the upper extremity in severe injuries involving the shoulder girdle and upper end of humerus.
**Y b.**, a bandage shaped like the letter Y.

**ban·da·let·ta** (ban″də-let'ə) [L., from Fr. *bandelette* (q.v.)] 1. a small band. 2. a small bandlike anatomical structure.
**b. diagona'lis (Broca),** stria diagonalis (Broca).

**ban·de·lette** (ban″də-let') [Fr., dim. of *bande* band] a small band.

**ban·di·coot** (ban'dĭ-ko͞ot) [Teluga *bantikoku*] an Indian rodent, *Nesokia bengalensis,* which is a reservoir of *Spirillum minus,* the causative organism of rat-bite fever; it also harbors *Coxiella burnetii,* which may be transmitted by the bandicoot tick, *Haemaphysalis humerosa.*

**band·ing** (band'ing) 1. the act of encircling and binding with a thin strip of material. 2. any of several techniques of staining chromosomes so that a characteristic pattern of transverse dark and light bands becomes visible; see *chromosome b.*
**C b., C-b., centromeric b.**, differential staining of chromosomes to elicit chromosome bands, using a method that specifically stains the regions of the chromosomes that contain constitutive heterochromatin (C bands), particularly the pericentromeric areas, secondary constrictions of chromosomes 1, 9, and 16, and the distal segment of the long arm of the Y chromosome; the method consists of a denaturation and renaturation technique involving treatment of the chromosomes with acid, alkali, or heat before Giemsa staining.
**chromosome b.**, the use of various physical and cytochemical preparations with differential staining techniques, which allows visualization of differentially stained regions of a chromosome as a continuous series of light and dark bands specific for the chromosome and species, thus permitting definitive identification and delineation of all the chromosomes and chromosomal segments of humans and many other organisms. Named according to the staining technique used, see *C b., G b., Q b.*, and *R b.*
**G b., G-b., Giemsa b.**, differential staining of chromosomes to elicit chromosome bands (G bands), consisting of pretreatment with a salt solution or with proteolytic enzymes (usually trypsin or pronase) before staining with Giemsa solution. The same banding pattern may be obtained with other agents.
**high-resolution b.**, a banding technique in which cultured cells are blocked in the S phase of the cell cycle; the block is then released, and the culture is harvested when the greatest number of cells are in late prophase or prometaphase, revealing 800–1400 bands rather than the 400–600 seen in metaphase preparations. Used to detect precise breakpoints or small structural alterations. Called also *prophase b.*
**prophase b.**, high-resolution b.
**pulmonary artery b.**, an operation to provide constriction of the pulmonary artery with a band to reduce pulmonary blood flow and relieve congestive heart failure in children with congenital heart defects that produce left to right shunts between ventricles or the great arteries.
**Q b., Q-b., quinacrine b.**, differential staining of chromosomes to elicit chromosome bands (Q bands), consisting of examination of the chromosomes by fluorescence microscopy after they have been stained with quinacrine mustard or quinacrine hydrochloride.
**R b., R-b., reverse b.**, differential staining of chromosomes to elicit chromosome bands (R bands), consisting of pretreatment with hot alkali before staining; the banding pattern shown is the reverse of that of G and Q banding—darkly stained R bands are G and Q light and vice versa.
**tooth b.**, the technique of cementing stainless steel bands to the teeth to hold orthodontic attachments in position.

**Ban·dl's ring** (bahn'dəlz) [Ludwig *Bandl,* German obstetrician in Austria, 1842–1892] pathologic retraction ring; see *retraction ring,* under *ring.*

**band·pass** (band'pas) the range of frequencies passed by a filter,

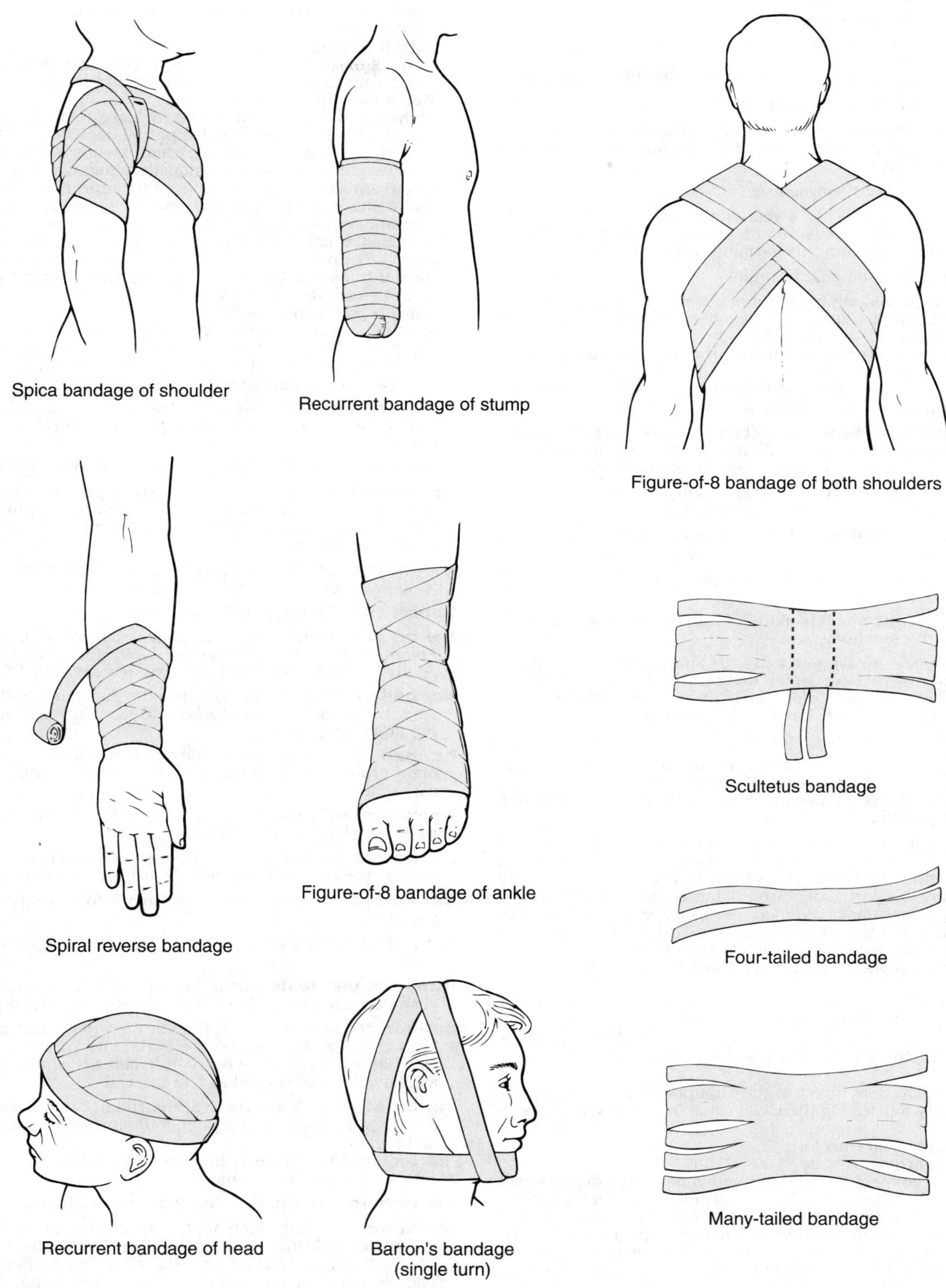


**PLATE 9**—VARIOUS TYPES OF BANDAGES

or the range of wavelengths used by a spectrophotometer or colorimeter; equal to the range in which the transmittance is equal to or greater than one-half the peak transmittance.

**band·width** (band'width) bandpass.

**bane** (bān) old term for *poison*.
**leopard's b.,** 1. *Arnica.* 2. arnica.
**wolf's b.,** 1. *Arnica.* 2. arnica. 3. *Aconitum napellus.* 4. aconite.

**bane·wort** (bān'wort) belladonna (def. 1).

**Bang's bacillus, disease, test** (bahngz) [Bernhard Laurits Frederik *Bang,* Danish physician, 1848–1932] see *Brucella abortus,* and under *disease* and *test.*

**ban·ian** (ban'yən) *Ficus bengalensis.*

**Ban·is·te·ria** (ban″is-te're-ə) a genus of plants of the family Malpighiaceae. *B. caa'pi* Spruce is a South American woody vine whose seeds contain the hallucinogens harmine and harmaline.

**ban·is·ter·ine** (ban-is'tər-ēn) harmine.

**bank** (bangk) a stored supply of human material or tissues for future use by other individuals, such as a *blood bank, bone bank, eye bank, human-milk bank,* or *skin bank.*
**blood b.,** an organization that collects, processes, and stores blood in preparation for transfusions.
**eye b.,** an agency that collects and stores eye tissue and then prepares it and supplies it for transplantation.

**Ban·na·yan-Zo·na·na syndrome** (ban'ə-yən zo-nă'nə) [George A. *Bannayan,* American physician, 20th century; Jonathan *Zonana,* American physician, 20th century] see under *syndrome.*

**Ban·nis·ter's disease** (ban'is-tərz) [Henry Martyn *Bannister,* American physician, 1844–1920] angioedema.

**Bann·warth's syndrome** (bahn'vahrts) [Alfred *Bannwarth,* German neurologist, 1903–1970] see under *syndrome.*

**Ban·thine** (ban'thēn) trademark for preparations of methantheline bromide.

**Ban·ti's disease** (bahn'tēz) [Guido *Banti,* Italian pathologist, 1852–1925] congestive splenomegaly.

**Ban·ting** (ban'ting) Sir Frederick Grant. Canadian physician, 1891–1941; co-winner, with John James Richard Macleod, of the Nobel prize for medicine or physiology in 1923 for their isolation, with Charles Herbert Best, of insulin from the pancreas.

**ban·yan** (ban'yən) *Ficus bengalensis.*

**Bap·tis·ia** (bap-tiz'e-ə) [L.; Gr. *baptizein* to dip in or under water] a genus of plants of the family Leguminosae. *B. leucan'tha* is the wild indigo, which contains quinolizidine alkaloids and may cause poisoning of horses and cattle.

**bar** (bahr) 1. a unit of pressure, being a pressure of $10^6$ dyne/cm$^2$; 1 bar = 0.987 atm or $10^5$ Pa; called also *barye.* 2. a metal segment of greater length than width that serves to connect two or more parts of a removable partial denture. 3. tarsal coalition; for this and its various types, see under *coalition.* 4. the upper part of the gums of a horse, between the grinders and the tusks, which bears no teeth. 5. that portion of the wall of a horse's hoof reflected posteriorly at an acute angle. Called also *pars inflexa, spine, stay,* and *frog stay.*
**arch b.,** any of several types of heavy wire bars shaped to the outer circumference of the dental arch and extending from one side to the other so that intervening teeth may be attached to it; used for treatment of fractures of the jaws and for stabilization of injured teeth.
**Bill's b.,** a vertical bony crest in the superior half of the internal acoustic meatus, separating the facial canal from the superior vestibular nerve.
**b. of bladder,** plica interureterica.
**chromatoid b.,** bromatid body.
**connector b.,** a connector unit of a removable partial denture that is fabricated as parallel-, round-, or oval-sided bars and serves to connect parts of dentures, splint or connect abutments, connect and splint crowns, or splint teeth that have received root therapy. Called also *connecting b.* and *minor connector.* Cf. *major connector.*
**Dolder b.,** an attachment designed to secure and stabilize an overlay denture; it consists of a bar transected by several screw holes, which are used to attach it to the jaw, and is ovoid to allow some rotational movement of the denture.
**Erich arch b.,** an arch bar made of soft, readily contoured metal, used for intermaxillary fixation.
**hyoid b's,** a pair of cartilaginous plates forming the second pharyngeal (branchial) arch, from which a part of the hyoid bone is developed.
**Kazanjian T b.,** an appliance useful in reconstruction of the lip and jaw; it is fixed with an acrylic prosthesis to provide soft tissue support during reconstruction.
**Kennedy b.,** 1. a metal bar, usually resting on the lingual surfaces of teeth, that aids in their stabilization and acts as an indirect retainer. 2. continuous clasp.
**labial b.,** a major connector located labial to the dental arch, and joining two or more bilateral parts of a mandibular removable partial denture.
**lingual b.,** continuous clasp.
**median b.,** a fibrotic formation across the neck of the prostate gland, causing obstruction of the urethra.
**Mercier's b.,** plica interureterica.
**occlusal rest b.,** a minor connector used to attach an occlusal rest to a major part of a removable partial denture.
**palatal b.,** a major connector that extends across the palate and joins two or more parts of a maxillary removable partial denture.
**Passavant's b.,** a horizontal ridge that appears on the posterior wall of the pharynx during swallowing, produced by contraction of the palatopharyngeal sphincter; it also occurs during speech in persons with cleft palate. Called also *pharyngeal ridge* and *Passavant's cushion, pad,* or *ridge.*
**sternal b.,** one of the paired cartilaginous bars in the embryo that unite to form the sternum.
**tarsal b.,** see under *coalition.*
**terminal b's,** zones where epithelial cells contact one another, once thought to represent an accumulation of dense cementing substance, but with the electron microscope shown to be a junctional complex (see under *complex*).

**bar·ag·no·sis** (bar″ag-no'sis) [*bar-* + *a-*[1] + Gr. *gnosis* knowledge] lack or loss of the faculty of barognosis; called also *abarognosis* and *baroagnosis.*

**Ba·ra·lyme** (bar'ə-līm″) trademark for barium hydroxide lime.

**Bá·rá·ny** (bah'rah-ne) Robert. Austrian physician in Sweden, 1876–1936; winner of the Nobel prize for medicine or physiology in 1914 for his work on the physiology and pathology of the vestibular apparatus of the ear.

**Bá·rá·ny's symptom (sign, test), pointing test** (bah'rah-nēz) [Robert *Bárány*] see under *symptom* and *test.*

**bar·ba** (bahr'bə) [L.] [TA] the beard.

**bar·ba ama·ri·lla** (bahr'bah ah-mah-re'yah) [Sp. "yellow beard"] *Bothrops atrox,* a large venomous pit viper found in Central and South America; it is sometimes erroneously called *fer-de-lance.*

**bar·ba·loin** (bahr'bə-lo-īn) an anthraquinone pentoside that occurs in various species of *Aloe* and is mainly responsible for their purgative properties.

**bar·ban** (bahr'ban) an herbicide chemically related to the carbamate group, which in heavy doses causes a condition similar to carbamate poisoning.

**bar·bar·a·la·lia** (bahr″bər-ə-la'le-ə) a form of dyslalia that is shown when speaking a foreign language.

**bar·bas·co** (bahr-bas'ko) either of two tropical plants, *Jacquinia paramensis* and *Paullinia pinnata,* used as fish poisons.

**Bar·ba·sed** (bahr'bə-sed″) trademark for a preparation of butabarbital sodium.

**bar·bei·ro** (bahr-ba'ro) [Port.] Brazilian name for *Panstrongylus megistus.*

**Bar·ber's psoriasis** (bahr'bərz) [Harold Wordsworth *Barber,* English dermatologist, 1886–1955] localized pustular psoriasis.

**bar·ber·ry** (bahr'bər-e) 1. the shrub *Berberis vulgaris,* which contains resins and berberine; the bark of its stems and roots is used as a bitter tonic. 2. the berry of *B. vulgaris,* which is the source of a yellow dye and is used as a preservative.

**bar·bi·tal** (bahr'bĭ-tawl) [MeSH: Barbital] the oldest of the barbiturates, a long-acting compound administered orally as a sedative and hypnotic.
**b. sodium,** the soluble monosodium salt of barbital, having the same actions and uses as the base.

**bar·bi·tone** (bahr'bĭ-tōn) British name for barbital.

**bar·bi·tur·ate** (bahr-bich'ər-ət) any of a class of sedative-hypnotic agents derived from barbituric acid or thiobarbituric acid and classified into long-, intermediate-, short-, and ultrashort-acting classes. The ultrashort-acting barbiturates, e.g., thiopental, are used as intravenous anesthetics. The long-acting barbiturate phenobarbital is an important anticonvulsant used in the treatment of epilepsy. Many other barbiturates were widely used as sedatives or hypnotics, but benzodiazepines have replaced them in most uses. Some of these have a high potential for abuse and are Schedule II controlled substances.

**bar·bi·tur·ic ac·id** (bahr-bĭ-tūr'ik) the parent compound of the barbiturates, 2,4,6-trioxohexahydropyrimidine. It is not itself a central nervous system depressant; the presence of alkyl or aryl groups at position 5 gives its derivatives their sedative and hypnotic effects.

**bar·bo·tage** (bahr″bo-tahzh′) [Fr. *barboter* to dabble] repeated injection and withdrawal of fluid, as in the administration of an anesthetic into the subarachnoid space by alternate injection of a small amount of the anesthetic and withdrawal of a small quantity of cerebrospinal fluid into the syringe, until the anesthetic is completely administered.

**bar·bu·la** (bahr′bu-lə) [L.] a little beard.
**b. hir′ci,** 1. hirci. 2. tufts of hair in the ears.

**Bar·coo disease (rot), vomit** (bahr-koo′) [*Barcoo* River in South Australia] see *desert sore,* under *sore* and see under *vomit.*

**Bard's sign** (bahrdz′) [Louis *Bard,* French physician, 1857–1930] see under *sign.*

**Bar·det-Biedl syndrome** (bahr-da′ be′dəl) [Georges *Bardet,* French physician, born 1885; Artur *Biedl,* Austrian physician, 1869–1933] see under *syndrome.*

**bar·es·the·sia** (bar″es-the′zhə) [*bar-* + *esthesia*] pressure sense.

**bar·es·the·si·om·e·ter** (bar″əs-the″ze-om′ə-tər) [*bar-* + *esthesio-* + *-meter*] an instrument for determining sensitivity to weight or pressure.

**bar·iat·rics** (bar″e-at′riks) [*bar-* + *-iatrics*] the study of overweight, its causes, prevention, and treatment.

**bar·ite** (bar′īt) 1. barium oxide. 2. barium sulfate.

**bar·i·to·sis** (bar-ĭ-to′sis) a benign pneumoconiosis due to inhalation of the dust of barium or barite. Called also *barytosis.*

**bar·ium** (bar′e-əm) gen. *ba′rii* [L.; Gr. *baros* weight] [MeSH: Barium] a pale yellowish, metallic element belonging to the alkaline earths; its atomic number is 56; atomic weight 137.34; symbol, Ba. Its acid-soluble salts are poisonous; see *barium poisoning,* under *poisoning.*
**b. hydrate, b. hydroxide,** $Ba(OH)_2$, a crystalline soluble base employed as a test for sulfates.
**b. oxide,** $BaO_2$, a white or light yellow powder used for drying gases; called also *barite, baryta,* and *baryte.*
**b. sulfate** [USP], $BaSO_4$, an odorless fine white powder used as a contrast medium in radiography of the digestive tract. Called also *barite, baryta,* and *baryte.*

**bark** (bahrk) [L. *cortex*] the rind or outer cortical cover of the woody parts of a plant, tree, or shrub; called also *cascara.*
**buckthorn b.,** the dried bark of *Rhamnus frangula,* a purgative.
**calisaya b.,** cinchona (def. 2).
**casca b.,** the bark of *Erythrophloeum guineense,* an ordeal poison used in western Africa; called also *Mancona b.*
**chittem b.,** cascara sagrada.
**cinchona b.,** cinchona (def. 2).
**cramp b.,** the dried bark of *Viburnum opulus,* the high bush or cranberry tree; it has been used as an antispasmodic, uterine sedative, and antiscorbutic.
**cuprea b.,** the bark of *Remijia pedunculata,* which contains cupreine and has been used as an antimalarial.
**elm b.,** slippery elm b.
**Jesuit's b.,** cinchona (def. 2).
**Mancona b.,** casca b.
**Peruvian b.,** cinchona (def. 2).
**Purshiana b.,** cascara sagrada.
**quillay b.,** quillaia.
**sacred b.,** cascara sagrada.
**slippery elm b.,** the dried inner bark of the slippery elm, *Ulmus rubra,* which is mucilaginous and demulcent; the official preparation [USP] is *elm.* Called also *elm b.*
**soap b., soap tree b.,** quillaia.
**white oak b.,** the dried inner bark of *Quercus alba,* used as an astringent.
**wild black cherry b.,** wild cherry; see under *cherry.*

**Bar·kan's operation** (bahr′kənz) [Otto *Barkan,* American ophthalmologist, 1887–1958] goniotomy.

**bark·er** (bahr′kər) a foal with neonatal maladjustment syndrome.

**Bar·low's disease** (bahr′lōz) [Sir Thomas *Barlow,* British physician, 1845–1945] infantile scurvy; see under *scurvy.*

**Bar·low syndrome** (bahr′lo) [John Brereton *Barlow,* South African cardiologist, born 1924] mitral valve prolapse syndrome; see under *syndrome.*

**barn** (bahrn) [jocular "big as a barn"] a unit of area equal to $10^{-24}$ square centimeter, used in measuring nuclear scattering cross sections. Symbol b.

**Barnes' curve** (bahrnz) [Robert *Barnes,* English obstetrician, 1817–1907] see under *curve.*

**bar(o)-** [Gr. *baros* weight] a combining form denoting relationship to weight or pressure.

**baro·ag·no·sis** (bar″o-ag-no′sis) baragnosis.

**baro·cep·tor** (bar″o-sep′tər) baroreceptor.

**bar·og·no·sis** (bar″og-no′sis) [*baro-* + Gr. *gnosis* knowledge] conscious perception of weight; the faculty by which weight is recognized, such as when an object is placed in the hand. Cf. *baragnosis.*

**baro·oti·tis** (bar″o-o-ti′tis) barotitis.
**b.-o. me′dia,** barotitis media.

**baro·pac·er** (bar′o-pās″ər) an electronic unit implanted in the necks of dogs for continuous stimulation of the carotid sinuses.

**baro·phil·ic** (bar″o-fil′ik) [*baro-* + *-philic*] growing best under high atmospheric pressure; said of bacterial cells.

**baro·re·cep·tor** (bar″o-re-sep′tər) [MeSH: Pressoreceptors] a type of interoceptor that is stimulated by changes in pressure, particularly those in the walls of blood vessels; see also under *reflex.* Called also *baroceptor* and *pressoreceptor.*

**baro·re·flex** (bar′o-re″fleks) [MeSH: Baroreflex] baroreceptor reflex.

**baro·si·nus·itis** (bar″o-si″nəs-i′tis) inflammation and pain of one or more paranasal sinuses (usually the frontal sinus) due to difference in pressure between the surrounding atmosphere and the air within the sinus cavity; it occurs on ascent to or descent from a high altitude, such as in an airplane, when the opening into the sinus is obstructed. Called also *aerosinusitis* and *sinus barotrauma.*

**baro·tax·is** (bar″o-tak′sis) [*baro-* + *taxis*] stimulation of living matter by change of the pressure relations under which it exists; see also *barotropism.*

**bar·oti·tis** (bar″o-ti′tis) a morbid condition of the ear produced by exposure to differing atmospheric pressures. Called also *aerotitis.*
**b. me′dia,** traumatic inflammation of the middle ear caused by a difference in pressure between the surrounding atmosphere and the air in the middle ear space, marked by otalgia, tinnitus, hearing loss, and sometimes vertigo. It occurs in rapid descent in altitude, such as in an aircraft or in diving. Called also *aerotitis media, aviator's ear, aviation otitis,* and *otitic barotrauma.*

**baro·trau·ma** (bar″o-traw′mə) [*baro-* + *trauma*] [MeSH: Barotrauma] injury caused by pressure, especially to enclosed cavities of the body such as the eustachian tube, middle ear, paranasal sinuses, or lung. See also *barotitis media.*
**pulmonary b.,** traumatic damage to the lung as a result of pressure changes, such as in divers, usually characterized by peribronchial rupture and pneumomediastinum.
**otitic b.,** barotitis media.
**sinus b.,** barosinusitis.

**bar·ot·ro·pism** (bar-ot′rə-piz-əm) [*baro-* + *tropism*] a relatively stereotyped response, often a movement, to pressure stimuli.

**Barr body** (bahr) [Murray Llewellyn *Barr,* Canadian anatomist, 1908–1995] [MeSH: Sex Chromatin] sex chromatin.

**Bar·ra·quer's disease** (bah-rah-kārz′) [José Luis Antonio Roviralta *Barraquer,* Spanish physician, 1855–1928] partial lipodystrophy; see under *lipodystrophy.*

**Bar·ra·quer's method, operation** (bah-rah-kārz′) [Ignacio *Barraquer,* Spanish ophthalmologist, 1884–1965] phacoerysis.

**Bar·ra·quer-Si·mons syndrome** (bah-rah-kār′ se′monz) [J.L.A.R. *Barraquer;* Arthur *Simons,* German physician, born 1879] partial lipodystrophy; see under *lipodystrophy.*

**Bar·ré's sign** (bah-rāz′) [Jean Alexandre *Barré,* French neurologist, 1880–1971] see under *sign.*

**Bar·ré-Guil·lain syndrome** (bah-ra′ ge-ă′) [J. A. *Barré;* Georges *Guillain,* French neurologist, 1876–1951] acute idiopathic polyneuritis.

**bar·ren** (bar′ən) sterile (def. 1).

**Bar·rett's epithelium, syndrome (esophagus), ulcer** (bar′əts) [Norman Rupert *Barrett,* English surgeon, 1903–1979] see under *epithelium, syndrome,* and *ulcer.*

**bar·ri·er** (bar′e-ər) an obstruction.
**alveolar b., alveolar-capillary b., alveolocapillary b.,** alveolocapillary membrane.
**blood-air b.,** alveolocapillary membrane.
**blood-aqueous b.,** the anatomical mechanism that prevents exchange of materials between the chambers of the eye and the blood.
**blood-brain b., blood-cerebral b.,** the barrier system separating the blood from the parenchyma of the central nervous system. Its anatomical component consists of unique endothelial cells in the brain capillaries, having tight junctions without fenestrations and with few microvilli and few vesicles for fluid transport. Its physiologic component in part consists of enzymes unique to the brain endothelia and of active transport via carrier proteins.
**blood–cerebrospinal fluid b.,** blood-brain b.
**blood-gas b.,** alveolocapillary membrane.
**blood-testis b.,** a barrier separating the blood from the seminiferous tubules, consisting of special junctional complexes between adjacent Sertoli cells near the base of the seminiferous epithelium.

**blood-thymus b.**, a barrier in the thymus which excludes certain substances, possibly constituted by the interposition of a sheet of epithelial cell processes around the periphery of the lobules and between the lymphocytes and the perivascular connective tissue.
**filtration b.**, the structures separating the blood in the glomerular capillaries and capsular space of the renal corpuscle, consisting of the fenestrated epithelium, the basal lamina, and the slit pores between the pedicels of the podocytes.
**gastric mucosal b.**, a physiological property of the gastric mucosa rendering the epithelium relatively impermeable to ions. Its function is impaired by aspirin, organic acids, and bile salts, and in patients subjected to severe trauma or shock. Back diffusion of acid from the gastric lumen may cause mucosal erosion or ulceration.
**hematoencephalic b.**, blood-brain b.
**histohematic connective tissue b.**, the barrier between the blood and the dependent parenchymal tissue through which diffusion of nutrients and gases takes place.
**placental b.**, the placental separation of fetal from maternal blood and bloodborne materials of greater than molecular size; in humans this is the placental membrane.
**protective b.**, an intervening shield of radiation-absorbing material such as lead, concrete, or plastic whose atomic number and thickness are specifically sufficient to give adequate body protection against ionizing radiation of various types.
**protective b's, primary,** barriers sufficient to reduce a primary beam of radiation to a permissible exposure rate.
**protective b's, secondary,** barriers sufficient to reduce stray or scattered radiation to a permissible exposure rate.
**radiation b.**, protective b.

**bar·sati** (bahr-saht'e) [Hindi "of the rainy season"] 1. cutaneous habronemiasis. 2. pythiosis.

**Bart's syndrome** (bahrtz) [Bruce Joseph *Bart,* American dermatologist, born 1936] see under *syndrome.*

**Barth's hernia** (bahrts) [Jean Baptiste Philippe *Barth,* French physician, 1806–1877] see under *hernia.*

**Bar·thel index** (bahr-tel') [D.W. *Barthel,* American physiatrist, 20th century] see under *index.*

**Bar·tho·lin's abscess, adenitis, cyst, duct, gland** (bahr'to-linz) [Caspar Thomèson *Bartholin,* Jr., Danish anatomist, 1655–1738] see under *abscess, adenitis,* and *cyst,* and see *ductus sublingualis major* and *glandula vestibularis major.*

**bar·tho·lin·i·an** (bahr″to-lin'e-ən) [C. T. *Bartholin,* Jr.] pertaining to Bartholin's duct or gland (glandula vestibularis major).

**bar·tho·lin·itis** (bahr″to-lin-i'tis) inflammation of Bartholin's ducts.

**Bar·ton's bandage, fracture, operation** (bahr'tənz) [John Rhea *Barton,* American surgeon, 1794–1871] see under *bandage, fracture,* and *operation.*

**Bar·to·nel·la** (bahr″tə-nel'ə) [A. L. *Barton,* Peruvian physician, 1871–1950] [MeSH: Bartonella] a genus of bacteria of the family Bartonellaceae, order Rickettsiales, made up of gram-negative cells in chains found in fixed tissue cells and in or on erythrocytes. The organism occurs in humans, sometimes asymptomatically, and in arthropod vectors. The genus includes organisms formerly classified in the genus *Rochalimaea.*
**B. bacillifor'mis**, a species transmitted to humans by the sandfly *Phlebotomus verrucarum;* it is the etiologic agent of Carrión's disease.
**B. elizabe'thae**, a species that is a cause of bacterial endocarditis.
**B. hen'selae**, a species that is the etiologic agent of cat-scratch disease and is the primary cause of bacillary angiomatosis and bacillary peliosis; it also is a cause of bacteremia in immunocompromised patients and of bacterial endocarditis. Cats are the reservoir and transmission is by a cat bite or scratch.
**B. quinta'na**, the etiologic agent of trench fever, transmitted by the body louse *Pediculus humanus.* It is also a cause of bacterial endocarditis and of bacillary angiomatosis and peliosis. Formerly called *Rochalimaea quintana, Rickettsia quintana,* and *Rickettsia wolhynica.*
**B. vinso'nii**, a species that is a cause of bacterial endocarditis.

**Bar·to·nel·la·ceae** (bahr″tə-nel-a'se-e) [MeSH: Bartonellaceae] a family of bacteria of the order Rickettsiales, made up of small rod-shaped, coccoid, or ring- or disk-shaped, filamentous and beaded organisms, usually measuring less than 3$\mu$, occurring as pathogenic parasites in the erythrocytes of humans and other animals. It includes the genera *Bartonella* and *Grahamella.*

**bar·to·nel·li·a·sis** (bahr″to-nel-i'ə-sis) bartonellosis.

**bar·to·nel·lo·sis** (bahr-tə-nel-o'sis) 1. infection with organisms of the genus *Bartonella.* 2. infection by *Bartonella bacilliformis,* transmitted by sandflies of the genus *Phlebotomus,* especially *P. verrucarum,* found only in certain Andean valleys in Peru, Ecuador, and Colombia; besides humans, it also affects dogs and rodents, especially after splenectomy. It occurs in two distinct stages: the first or acute stage is *Oroya fever,* a highly fatal febrile illness associated with severe hemolytic anemia (*Bartonella* anemia); the second or chronic stage in humans is *verruga peruana,* manifested by a benign skin eruption of hemangioma-like macules surrounded by hyperpigmented borders. Called also *Carrión's disease* and *bartonelliasis.*

**Bart·ter's syndrome** (bahr'tərz) [Frederic Crosby *Bartter,* American internist, 1914–1983] see under *syndrome.*

**bar·u·ria** (bar-u're-ə) [*bar-* + *uria*] the passage of urine of a high specific gravity.

**bary-** [Gr. *barys* heavy] a combining form meaning heavy or difficult.

**bar·ye** (bar'e) bar, def. 1.

**bary·es·the·sia** (bar″e-es-the'zhə) baresthesia.

**bary·la·lia** (bar″ĭ-la'le-ə) [*bary-* + *lal-* + *-ia*] thick, indistinct speech due to imperfect articulation.

**ba·ry·ta** (bə-ri'tə) 1. barium oxide. 2. barium sulfate.

**bar·yte** (bar'īt) 1. barium oxide. 2. barium sulfate.

**bar·y·to·sis** (bar″ĭ-to'sis) baritosis.

**ba·sad** (ba'sad) toward a base or basal aspect.

**ba·sal** (ba'səl) pertaining to or situated near a base.

**ba·sa·lis** (ba-sa'lis) [L., from Gr. *basis* base] [TA] basal; a general term denoting relationship to or location near a base.

**Ba·sal·jel** (ba'səl-jel″) trademark for basic aluminum carbonate gel.

**ba·sa·loid** (ba'sə-loid) resembling basal cells of the skin; see under *carcinoma.*

**ba·sa·lo·ma** (ba″sə-lo'mə) basal cell carcinoma.

**bas·cule** (bas'kūl) [Fr. "seesaw"] a device working on the principle of the seesaw, so that when one end is lowered the other is raised.
**cecal b.**, a form of cecal volvulus in which the cecum becomes folded anteriorly and medially over bands or adhesions that run across the ascending colon.

**base** (bās) [L., Gr., *basis*] 1. the lowest part or foundation of anything; see also *basis.* 2. the main ingredient of a compound. 3. in chemistry, the nonacid part of a salt; a substance that combines with acids to form salts; a substance that dissociates to give hydroxide ions in aqueous solutions; a substance whose molecule or ion can combine with a proton (hydrogen ion); a substance capable of donating a pair of electrons (to an acid) for the formation of a coordinate covalent bond. 4. a unit of a removable prosthesis that supports the supplied tooth and any intermediary material and in turn receives support from the tissue of the basal seat. 5. in genetics, a nucleotide, particularly one in a nucleic acid sequence. 6. See also *base pair,* under *pair.*
**acidifiable b.**, a chemical substance that will unite with water to form an acid.
**acrylic resin b.**, a denture base made of an acrylic resin.
**apical b.**, that portion of the jaws giving support to the teeth; called also *basal arch.*
**b. of brain,** facies inferior cerebri.
**buffer b.**, the sum of all the buffer anions in the blood (bicarbonate, hemoglobin, proteins, and phosphate), determined by titrating the blood with a strong acid; it is used as an index of the degree of metabolic disturbance in the acid-base balance.
**cement b.**, a layer of insulating, sometimes medicated dental cement placed in the deep portions of a cavity preparation to protect the pulp or eliminate undercuts in tapered preparation.
**conjugate b.**, a chemical species that is formed from its conjugate acid by removal of a proton; e.g., acetate ($CH_3COO^-$) is the conjugate base of acetic acid ($CH_3COOH$).
**b. of cranium,** see *basis cranii externa* and *basis cranii interna.*
**denture b.**, that part of a denture, made either of metal or resin or a combination of both materials, that supports the supplied teeth and receives support from the abutment teeth, the residual alveolar ridge, or both. See also *denture base saddle,* under *saddle.*
**denture b., tinted,** a denture base which simulates the coloring and shading of natural oral tissues.
**b. of dorsal horn of spinal cord,** basis cornus posterioris medullae spinalis.
**external b. of skull,** basis cranii externa.
**film b.**, a thin, flexible, transparent sheet of cellulose acetate or similar material which carries the radiation and light-sensitive emulsion of x-ray or photographic films.
**b. of heart,** basis cordis.
**Lewis b.**, an electron-pair donor, e.g., ammonia and halide ion.
**b. of lung,** basis pulmonis.
**metal b.**, a metallic portion of a denture base forming a part or all of the basal surface of the denture, which serves as the attachment for the plastic (resin) part of the denture base and the teeth.
**nitrogenous b.**, an aromatic, nitrogen-containing molecule that serves as a proton acceptor, e.g., purine or pyrimidine.
**b. of nose,** apertura piriformis.

**ointment b.,** a vehicle for medicinal substances intended for external application to the body.
**plastic b.,** a denture or baseplate made of a plastic material.
**b. of posterior horn of spinal cord,** basis cornus posterioris medullae spinalis.
**b. of prostate,** basis prostatae.
**purine b's,** a group of chemical compounds of which purine is the base, including 6-oxypurine (hypoxanthine); 2,6-dioxypurine (xanthine); 6-aminopurine (adenine); 2-amino-6-oxypurine (guanine); 2,6,8-trioxypurine (uric acid); and 3,7-dimethyl xanthine (theobromine). Called also *xanthine b's.* See illustration.
**pyrimidine b's,** a group of chemical compounds of which pyrimidine is the base, including 2,4-dioxypyrimidine (uracil), 2,4-dioxy-5-methylpyrimidine (thymine), and 2-oxy-4-aminopyrimidine (cytosine), which are common constituents of nucleic acids. See illustration.
**record b.,** baseplate.
**Schiff b.,** any of a class of compounds having the general formula R—CH═N—R′, formed by condensation of primary amines with ketones or aldehydes.
**shellac b's,** resinous materials adapted to maxillary or mandibular edentulous casts to form baseplates for the construction of dentures.
**b. of skull,** see *basis cranii externa* and *basis cranii interna.*
**b. of stapes,** basis stapedis.
**temporary b.,** baseplate.
**tinted denture b.,** a denture base which simulates the coloring and shading of natural oral tissues.
**tooth-borne b.,** the base of a partial denture which is supported by the abutment teeth and not by the tissues beneath it.
**trial b.,** baseplate.
**xanthine b's,** purine b's.

**bas·e·doid** (baz′ə-doid) a condition resembling Graves' (Basedow's) disease, but without thyrotoxicosis.

**Bas·e·dow's disease** (bah′zə-dōz) [Karl Adolf von *Basedow,* German physician, 1799–1854] see *Graves' disease,* under *disease.*

**bas·e·dow·i·form** (baz″ə-do′ĭ-form) resembling Graves' (Basedow's) disease.

**base·line** (bās′līn″) an observation or value that represents the normal background level, or an initial level, of a measurable quantity; used for comparison with values representing response to experimental intervention or an environmental stimulus, usually implying that the baseline and response values refer to the same individual or system.

**base·plate** (bās′plāt″) 1. a temporary preformed shape made of shellac, wax, or acrylic resin, representing the base of a denture and used for making maxillomandibular relation records, for arranging artificial teeth, or for trial placement in the mouth. Called also *record base, temporary base,* and *trial base.* Written also *base plate.* 2. Hutch's term for the tissue circumferential to and somewhat eccentric to the urethral orifice which, it is postulated, may act as a floor during the filling of the bladder and assume a cone shape during micturition to allow the proximal urethra to fill.
**stabilized b.,** a baseplate lined with a plastic or other suitable material to improve its adaptation and stability.

**ba·ses** (ba′sēz) [L.] plural of *basis.*

**bas-fond** (bah-fawn′) [Fr.] a fundus, especially that of the urinary bladder.

**ba·si·al** (ba′se-əl) pertaining to the basion.

**ba·si·a·lis** (ba″se-a′lis) [L.] basial; denoting relationship to a base or to the basion.

**ba·si·al·ve·o·lar** (ba″se-al-ve′ə-lər) extending from the basion to the alveolar point.

**ba·sic** (ba′sik) 1. pertaining to or having the properties of a base. 2. capable of neutralizing acids.

**ba·si·caryo·plas·tin** (ba″sĭ-kar′e-o-plas″tin) [*basi-* + *caryo-* + *plastin*] the basophil paraplastin of the cell nucleus.

**ba·si·chro·ma·tin** (ba″sĭ-kro′mə-tin) the basophil portion of the chromatin of the cell nucleus.

**ba·si·chro·mi·ole** (ba-sĭ-kro′me-ōl) [*basophil* + *chromiole*] one of the basophil particles forming the chromatin of the cell nucleus.

**ba·sic·i·ty** (bə-sis′ĭ-te) 1. the quality of being a base, or basic. 2. the combining power of an acid; it is measured by the number of hydrogen atoms replaceable by a base.

**ba·si·cra·ni·al** (ba″sĭ-kra′ne-əl) [*basi-* + *cranial*] pertaining to the base of the skull.

**ba·si·cy·to·para·plas·tin** (ba″sĭ-si″to-par″ə-plas′tin) the basophil paraplastin of the cytoplasm.

**ba·sid·ia** (bə-sid′e-ə) plural of *basidium.*

**Ba·sid·i·ob·o·la·ceae** (bə-sid″e-ob″o-la′se-e) a family of fungi of

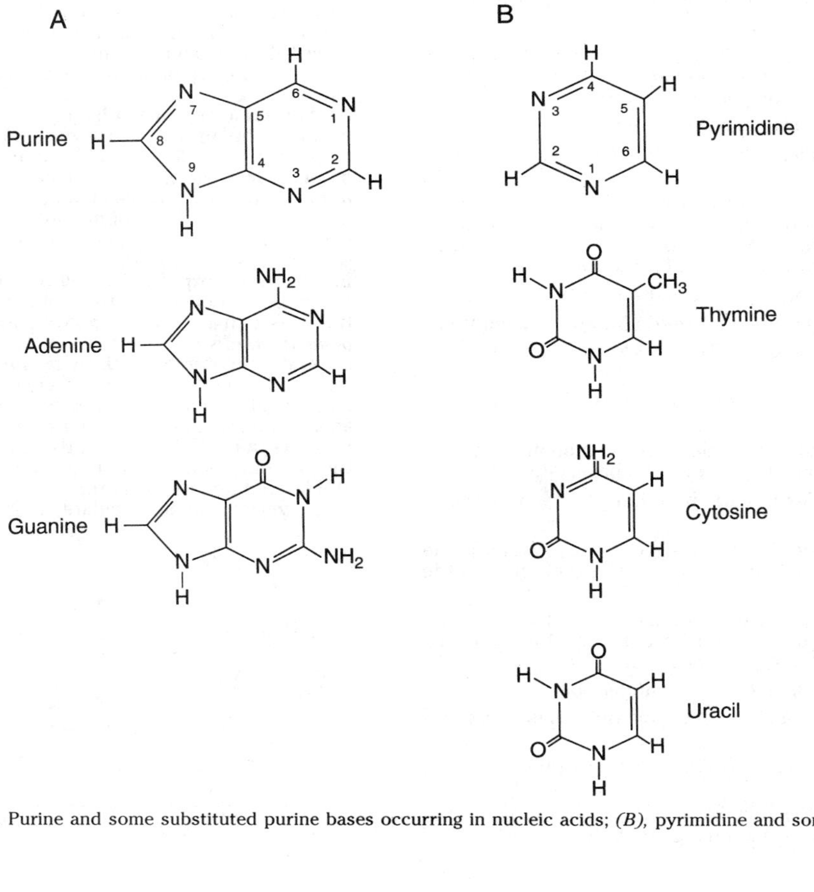

Purine and pyrimidine bases. *(A),* Purine and some substituted purine bases occurring in nucleic acids; *(B),* pyrimidine and some substituted pyrimidine bases occurring in nucleic acids.

the order Entomophthorales, consisting of widespread saprobes; one genus, *Basidiobolus,* contains organisms pathogenic for humans and horses.

**ba·sid·i·ob·o·lo·my·co·sis** (bə-sid″e-ob″ə-lo-mi-ko′sis) entomophthoromycosis basidiobolae.

**Ba·sid·i·ob·o·lus** (bə-sid″e-ob′ə-ləs) [*basidium,* def. 2 + Gr. *bolos* a throw] a mainly saprobic genus of fungi of the family Basidiobolaceae, which produces zygospores, chlamydospores, and conidia that carry along a piece of the conidiophore when they are ejected. *B. rana′rum* (called also *B. haptospo′rus* or *B. meristospo′rus*) causes entomophthoromycosis in humans and horses.

**ba·sid·io·carp** (bə-sid′e-o-kahrp″) [*basidium* + *carp*] the large fruiting body characteristic of the majority of fungi of the subphylum Basidiomycotina; it is composed of masses of intertwined hyphal elements and produces basidia. Mushrooms and toadstools are common examples.

**ba·sid·io·my·cete** (bə-sid″e-o-mi′sēt) an individual fungus of the Basidiomycotina.

**Ba·sid·io·my·ce·tes** (bə-sid″e-o-mi-se′tēz) [MeSH: Basidiomycetes] name given to Basidiomycotina when it is considered a class and placed within the phylum Eumycota.

**ba·sid·io·my·ce·tous** (bə-sid″e-o-mi-se′təs) of or pertaining to fungi of the class Basidiomycotina.

**Ba·sid·i·o·my·co·ta** (bə-sid″e-o-mi-ko′tə) name given to Basidiomycotina when it is considered a separate phylum.

**Ba·sid·io·my·co·ti·na** (bə-sid″e-o-mi″ko-ti′nə) [*basidium* + Gr. *mykēs* fungus] the club fungi, a subphylum of perfect fungi variously grouped under either Dikaryomycota or Eumycota. Spores (basidiospores) are borne on club-shaped organs (basidia). Some authorities consider this group a class and call it Basidiomycetes, whereas others consider it a separate phylum and call it Basidiomycota. Several different systems have been proposed for classifying the taxa above family within this group.

**ba·sid·io·spore** (bə-sid′e-o-spor) a type of sexual spore that forms on a basidium.

**ba·sid·i·um** (bə-sid′e-əm) pl. *basid′ia* [Gr. *basis* base] 1. the club-like organ of the fungal class Basidiomycotina which, following karyogamy and meiosis, bears the basidiospore. 2. *(obs.)* conidiophore or phialide.

**ba·si·fa·cial** (ba-sĭ-fa′shəl) [*basi-* + *facial*] pertaining to the inferior part of the face.

**ba·sig·e·nous** (bə-sij′ə-nəs) capable of forming a chemical base.

**ba·si·hy·al** (ba″sĭ-hi′əl) basihyoid.

**ba·si·hy·oid** (ba″sĭ-hi′oid) the body of the hyoid bone (corpus ossis hyoidei [TA]); in certain of the lower animals, either of the two lateral bones that are its homologues.

**bas·i·lad** (bas′ĭ-ləd) toward the basilar aspect.

**bas·i·lar** (bas′ĭ-lər) [L. *basilaris,* from *basis* base] pertaining to a base or basal part.

**bas·i·la·ris** (bas″ĭ-la′ris) [L., from Gr. *basis* base] [TA] basilar; a general term denoting relationship to a base or location at a base.
**b. cra′nii,** a composite of the numerous bones which serve the brain as a supportive floor and form the axis of the whole skull.

**ba·si·lat·er·al** (ba″sĭ-lat′ər-əl) both basilar and lateral.

**ba·si·lem·ma** (ba″sĭ-lem′ə) [*basi-* + *lemma*] basement membrane.

**ba·sil·ic** (bə-sil′ik) [L. *basilicus;* Gr. *basilikos* royal] important or prominent.

**ba·si·na·si·al** (ba″sĭ-na′ze-əl) pertaining to the basion and the nasion.

**basi(o)-** [Gr. *basis*] a combining form denoting relationship to a base or foundation, to the basion, or to a chemical base.

**ba·si·oc·cip·i·tal** (ba″se-ok-sip′ĭ-təl) pertaining to the basilar process of the occipital bone.

**ba·sio·glos·sus** (ba″se-o-glos′əs) [*basio-* + Gr. *glōssa* tongue] the part of the hyoglossus muscle that is attached to the base of the hyoid bone.

**ba·si·on** (ba′se-on) [Gr. *basis* base] [TA] a craniometric landmark located at the midpoint of the anterior border of the foramen magnum in the median plane. Called also *point Ba.*

**ba·si·ot·ic** (ba″se-ot′ik) [*basi-* + *otic*] see under *bone.*

**ba·si·para·chro·ma·tin** (ba″sĭ-par″ə-kro′mə-tin) basicaryoplastin.

**ba·si·para·plas·tin** (ba″sĭ-par″ə-plas′tin) the basophil portion of the paraplastin.

**ba·sip·e·tal** (bə-sip′ə-təl) [*basi-* + *-petal*] descending toward the base; developing in the direction of the base, as a spore.

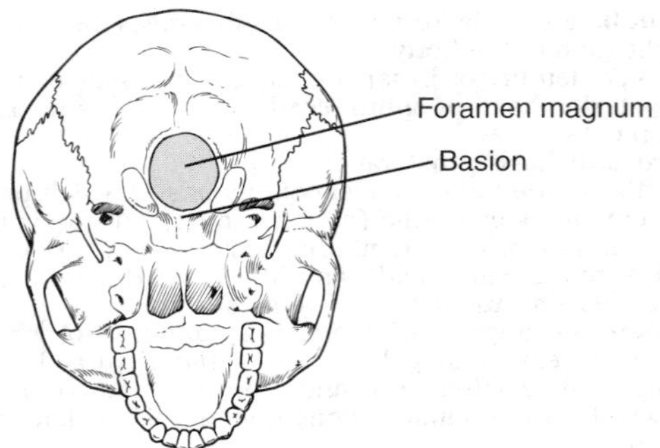


Basion, visible on the inferior view of the skull.

**ba·si·phil·ic** (ba″sĭ-fil′ik) basophilic.

**ba·si·rhi·nal** (ba″sĭ-ri′nəl) [*basi-* + *rhinal*] pertaining to the base of the brain and to the nose.

**ba·sis** (ba′sis) pl. *ba′ses* [L.; Gr.] [TA] base: a general anatomical term designating the lowest or fundamental part of a structure or organ, or the part opposite to or distinguished from the apex.
**b. cartila′ginis arytenoi′deae** [TA], base of arytenoid cartilage: the triangular inferior part of the arytenoid cartilage, which bears the articular surface.
**b. ce′rebri,** facies inferior cerebri.
**b. coch′leae** [TA], base of cochlea: the posterior of the cochlea, which rests upon the internal acoustic meatus.
**b. cor′dis** [TA], base of heart: a poorly delimited region of the heart, formed, in general, by the atria and the area occupied by the roots of the great vessels. It lies opposite the middle thoracic vertebrae, its exact position varying with heart action, and is directed superiorly, posteriorly, and to the right.
**b. cor′nus dorsa′lis medul′lae spina′lis,** b. cornus posterioris medullae spinalis.
**b. cor′nus posterio′ris medul′lae spina′lis** [TA], base of posterior horn of spinal cord: the portion of the posterior horn of gray substance in the spinal cord that is continuous with the lateral horn. Called also *b. cornus dorsalis medullae spinalis* and *base of dorsal horn of spinal cord.*
**b. cra′nii exter′na** [TA], external surface of cranial base: the outer surface of the inferior aspect of the skull; called also *norma ventralis, external base of skull,* and *scaphion.*
**b. cra′nii inter′na** [TA], internal base of cranium: the inner surface of the inferior region of the skull, constituting the floor of the cranial cavity.
**b. glan′dulae suprarena′lis,** facies renalis glandulae suprarenalis.
**b. mandi′bulae** [TA], base of mandible: the lower margin of the body of the mandible; called also *inferior border of mandible.*
**b. metacarpa′lis,** b. ossis metacarpi.
**b. metatarsa′lis,** b. ossis metatarsi.
**b. modi′oli** [TA], base of modiolus: the broad part of the modiolus situated near the lateral part of the internal acoustic meatus.
**b. na′si,** apertura piriformis.
**b. os′sis metacarpa′lis, b. os′sis metacar′pi** [TA], the base of a metacarpal bone, being the proximal end of each metacarpal, which articulates with a carpal(s) and with adjacent metacarpals. Called also *b. metacarpalis.*
**b. os′sis metatarsa′lis, b. os′sis metatar′si** [TA], the base of the metatarsal bone, being the wedge-shaped proximal end of each metatarsal, which articulates with bone(s) of the tarsus and with adjacent metatarsals. Called also *b. metatarsalis.*
**b. os′sis sa′cri** [TA], base of the sacral bone: the cranial surface of the sacrum; its lateral portions consist of the alae of the sacrum, and its middle portion is the upper surface of the body of the first sacral vertebra that articulates with the fifth lumbar vertebra.

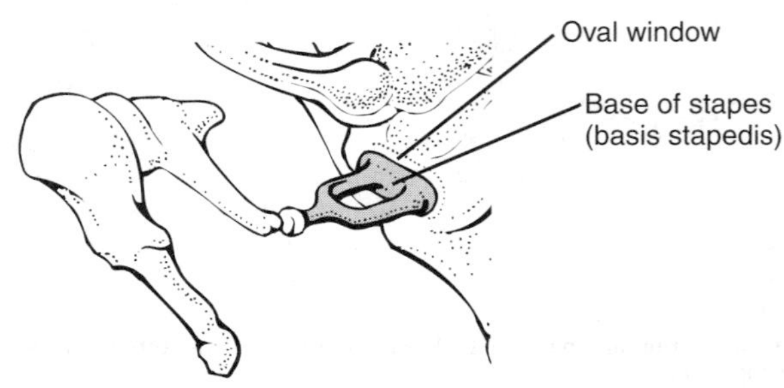

**b. patel'lae** [TA], base of patella: the superior border of the patella, to which the tendon of the quadriceps femoris muscle is attached; called also *superior border of patella.*
**b. pedun'culi ce'rebri** [TA], base of cerebral peduncle: the large bundle of nerve fiber tracts forming the anterior part of the cerebral peduncles, which consists of corticospinal, corticonuclear, corticopontine, parietotemporopontine, and frontopontine fibers descending from the cerebral cortex and terminating in the pons and spinal cord. Called also *crus cerebri.*
**b. phalan'gis digito'rum ma'nus** [TA], base of phalanx of fingers: the proximal end of each phalanx of the fingers; called also *proximal extremity of phalanx of finger.*
**b. phalan'gis digito'rum pe'dis** [TA], base of phalanx of toes: the proximal end of each phalanx of the toes; called also *proximal extremity of phalanx of toe.*
**b. prosta'tae** [TA], base of prostate: the broad upper part of the prostate, in contact with the lower surface of the urinary bladder.
**b. pulmo'nis** [TA], **b. pulmona'lis,** base of lung: the portion of each lung that is directed toward the diaphragm.
**b. pyra'midis rena'lis,** base of renal pyramid: the part of a renal pyramid that is directed away from the renal sinus.
**b. sca'pulae,** a name applied to both the vertebral and the axillary borders of the scapula (margo medialis and margo lateralis).
**b. stape'dis** [TA], base of stapes: the flat oval plate of bone on the stapes that fits into the fenestra vestibuli (oval window) on the medial wall of the middle ear. Called also *footplate* and *stapedial footplate.*

**ba·si·sphe·noid** (ba″sĭ-sfe′noid) 1. postsphenoid. 2. basisphenoid bone.

**ba·si·tem·po·ral** (ba″sĭ-tem′pə-rəl) [*basi-* + *temporal*] pertaining to the lower part of the temporal bone.

**ba·si·ver·te·bral** (ba″sĭ-ver′tə-brəl) [*basi-* + *vertebral*] pertaining to the body of a vertebra.

**bas·ket** (bas′kət) 1. a container made of material woven together. 2. something resembling such a container. 3. basket cell.
**cytopharyngeal b.,** cyrtos.
**Dormia b.,** a tiny apparatus consisting of four wires that can be advanced through an endoscope into a body cavity or tube, manipulated to trap a calculus or other object, and withdrawn.
**fiber b's,** fine fibers extending from the external limiting membrane of the retina to surround the adjacent portions of the rods and cones.

**Basle No·mi·na Ana·to·mi·ca** (bah′zəl no′mĭ-nə an-ə-tom′ĭ-kə) the official body of anatomical nomenclature prepared by a group of German anatomists with some help from anatomists in other countries, and presented for final criticism at the annual meeting of the German Anatomic Society held in Basle, Switzerland in 1895. Abbreviated BNA. It has been superseded by *Terminologia Anatomica* (TA) (1998).

**bas(o)-** see *basi(o)-.*

**ba·so·ca·ten·u·late** (ba″so-kə-ten′u-lāt) [*baso-* + *catenulate*] said of a chain of conidia in which the youngest cells are at the base away from the apex. Cf. *blastocatenulate.*

**ba·so·graph** (ba′so-graf) [*baso-* + *-graph*] an instrument for recording abnormalities of gait.

**ba·so·lat·er·al** (ba″so-lat′ər-əl) pertaining to the base and sides.

**ba·so·meta·chro·mo·phil** (ba″so-met″ə-kro′mo-fil) [*baso-* + *metachromophil*] staining with basic dyes to a color different from that of surrounding substances.

**Ba·som·ma·toph·o·ra** (ba″som-ə-tof′o-rə) a suborder of snails of the order Pulmonata, including mostly fresh water snails; two families of medical importance are Planorbidae and Lymnaeidae.

**ba·so·phil** (ba′so-fil) [*baso-* + *-phil*] [MeSH: Basophils] 1. a structure, cell, or other histologic element that stains readily with basic dyes. 2. a granular leukocyte with an irregularly shaped, pale-staining nucleus that is partially constricted into two lobes, and with cytoplasm that contains coarse, bluish-black granules of variable size. Basophils contain vasoactive amines such as histamine and serotonin, which are released on appropriate stimulation. Called also *basophilic leukocyte.* 3. one of the hormone-producing basophilic cells of the adenohypophysis; types include *gonadotrophs* and *thyrotrophs.* Called also *beta cell* and *B cell.* 4. basophilic.
**beta b.,** thyrotroph.
**Crooke-Russell b's,** the basophils in Crooke's hyaline degeneration; see under *degeneration.*
**delta b.,** gonadotroph, def. 1.

**ba·so·phile** (ba′so-fīl) 1. basophilic. 2. basophil (def. 3).

**ba·so·phil·ia** (ba″so-fil′e-ə) 1. an abnormal increase of basophils in the blood, as seen in myxedema, hypothyroid conditions, ulcerative colitis, certain types of anemia, and other conditions. Called also *basophilism* and *basophilic leukocytosis.* 2. the reaction of immature erythrocytes to basic dyes so that they become stippled; there are two varieties, *diffuse b.* and *punctate b.*
**diffuse b.,** basophilia in which erythrocytes are blue-gray and not stippled.
**punctate b.,** basophilia in which erythrocytes are blue and stippled; seen in poisoning with lead and certain other heavy metals.

**ba·so·phil·ic** (ba-so-fil′ik) 1. pertaining to basophils. 2. staining readily with basic dyes; called also *basophil, basophile,* and *basophilous.*

**ba·soph·i·lism** (ba-sof′ĭ-liz-əm) basophilia (def. 1).
**Cushing's b., pituitary b.,** Cushing's syndrome (def. 1); see under *syndrome.*

**ba·so·phil·o·pe·nia** (ba″so-fil″o-pe′ne-ə) abnormal reduction in the number of basophils in the blood; seen in hypothyroidism, stress, and a few other conditions. Called also *basophilic leukopenia.*

**ba·soph·i·lous** (ba-sof′ĭ-ləs) basophilic.

**ba·so·plasm** (ba′so-plaz″əm) cytoplasm that stains with basic dyes.

**Bas·sen-Korn·zweig syndrome** (bas′ən korn′zwīg) [Frank Albert *Bassen,* American physician, born 1903; Abraham Leon *Kornzweig,* American physician, born 1900] abetalipoproteinemia; see *familial lipoprotein deficiency,* under *deficiency.*

**Bas·set's operation** (bah-sāz′) [Antoine *Basset,* French surgeon, 1882–1951] see under *operation.*

**Bas·si·ni's operation** (bə-se′nēz) [Edoardo *Bassini,* Italian surgeon, 1847–1924] see under *operation.*

**bas·so·rin** (bas′ə-rin) a principal constituent of tragacanth gum, made up of a complex of polymethoxylated acids (bassoric acid) which swell in water to form an irreversible gel; used as a pharmaceutical adjuvant.

**bass·wood** (bas′wood) linden.

**bas·tard** (bas′tərd) [Old Fr.] 1. a person born out of wedlock. 2. born out of wedlock. 3. of inferior quality; not genuine.

**Bas·te·do's rule** (bas-te′dōz) [Walter Arthur *Bastedo,* American physician, 1873–1952] see under *rule.*

**Bas·ti·an-Bruns law (sign)** (bas′chən-broonz) [Henry Charlton *Bastian,* English neurologist, 1837–1915; Ludwig *Bruns,* German neurologist, 1858–1916] see under *law.*

**bat** (bat) [MeSH: Chiroptera] any member of the order *Chiroptera,* small flying mammals.
**vampire b.,** a member of either of the genera *Desmodus* or *Diphylla,* found in South America, Central America, Mexico, and the West Indies, which subsist on the blood of warm-blooded animals; some are reservoirs of rabies virus while others are reservoirs of *Trypanosoma cruzi.*

**bath** (bath) [MeSH: Baths] 1. a conductive or convective medium, as water, vapor, sand, or mud, with which the body is laved or in which the body is wholly or partly immersed for therapeutic or cleansing purposes; called also *balneum.* 2. the application of a conductive or convective medium to the body for therapeutic or cleansing purposes. 3. a piece of equipment or scientific apparatus in which a body or object may be immersed.
**acid b.,** one of water medicated with a mineral acid.
**air b.,** the therapeutic exposure of the body to air, which is usually warm.
**alcohol b.,** the laving of the body with dilute alcohol; it is defervescent and stimulant.
**alkaline b.,** the washing of a patient in a weak solution of an alkaline carbonate; useful in skin diseases.
**bubble b.,** a bath in which the water has been filled with bubbles produced by mechanical or chemical means.
**cabinet b.,** a hot-air bath or a radiant heat bath in which the patient is enclosed in a special cabinet.
**cold b.,** one in which cold water is used at a temperature of less than 65°F.
**colloid b.,** a bath containing gelatin, oatmeal, starch, or similar substances, used for its soothing or antipruritic effects.
**continuous b.,** a method of calming agitated or delirious patients by immersing them in a tub of warm water that has continuous inflow and outflow and is at approximately body temperature.
**contrast b.,** immersion of a part of the body alternately in hot and in cold water.
**cool b.,** one in water from 65° to 75°F.
**douche b.,** the application of water to the body from a jet spray.
**drip-sheet b.,** see *drip sheet,* under *sheet.*
**emollient b.,** a bath in a solution of an emollient substance, used in the treatment of pruritic conditions and other dermatoses.
**foam b.,** a bath of foam produced by blowing air or oxygen through the water to which a foam-forming substance (saponin) has been added.

**full b.**, one in which the patient's body is fully immersed in the water.
**half b.**, a bath of the hips and lower part of the body.
**hip b.**, sitz b.
**hot b.**, one in water from 98° to 104°F.
**hot-air b.**, one in air or vapor from 100° to 130°F.
**hyperthermal b.**, a hot bath in which the water is above 104°F.
**immersion b.**, one in which the body of the patient is immersed.
**kinetotherapeutic b.**, a bath providing facilities for underwater exercise.
**light b.**, exposure of all or part of the body to light rays, either of the sun or from an apparatus.
**lukewarm b.**, a neutral bath in which the water is between 92° and 97°F.
**medicated b.**, a bath containing medicinal substances.
**needle b.**, a shower bath in which the water is projected in a fine, needle-like spray.
**oatmeal b.**, a colloid bath containing oatmeal, used for its soothing or antipruritic effects in some dermatoses.
**paraffin b.**, wax b.
**sand b.**, the immersion of the body in dry, heated sand.
**sauna b.**, a sweat bath given in an enclosed room, usually followed by a cold shower.
**sedative b.**, a warm bath in which the patient's body is immersed, usually for several hours, to reduce agitated behavior.
**sheet b.**, the application of wet sheets to the body as an antipyretic measure.
**sitz b.**, a bath in which the patient sits in the tub, the hips and buttocks being immersed; called also *hip b.*
**sponge b.**, one in which the patient's body is not immersed in water but is rubbed with a wet cloth or sponge.
**sweat b.**, any bath given to promote sweating.
**tepid b.**, one in water from 75° to 92°F.
**vapor b.**, exposure of the body to steam.
**warm b.**, one taken in water from 92° to 97°F.
**water b.**, a vessel containing water for immersing bodies or for immersing liquid-containing vessels that are to be heated or cooled, or are to be held at a given temperature.
**wax b.**, the application of heated liquid wax to a part of the body, the wax being permitted to solidify; also the immersion of a part of the body in heated liquid wax maintained at a constant temperature. Called also *paraffin b.*
**whirlpool b.**, a variously sized tank in which the body or an extremity can be submerged as the heated water is mechanically agitated.

**bath·es·the·sia** (bath″es-the′zhə) [*bath-* + *esthesia*] deep sensibility.

**bath·mo·trop·ic** (bath″mo-trop′ik) [*bathmo-* + *-tropic*] influencing the response of muscle tissue to stimuli.
**negatively b.**, lessening response of muscle tissue to stimuli.
**positively b.**, increasing response of muscle tissue to stimuli.

**bath·mot·ro·pism** (bath-mot′ro-piz-əm) influence on the excitability of muscular tissue.

**bath(o)-** see *bathy-*.

**batho·chrome** (bath′o-krōm) an atom or group whose introduction into a compound shifts the compound's absorption peak to a longer wavelength; cf. *hypsochrome.*

**batho·chro·my** (bath″o-kro′me) a shift of the absorption band toward lower frequencies (longer wavelengths) with deepening of color from yellow to red to black.

**batho·flore** (bath′o-flor) [*batho-* + *fluorescence*] an atom or group that decreases the intensity of fluorescence of a compound in which it occurs; cf. *auxoflore.*

**batho·mor·phic** (bath″o-mor′fik) having a deep or myopic eye.

**batho·rho·dop·sin** (bath″o-ro-dop′sin) a transient intermediate produced upon irradiation of rhodopsin in the visual cycle; see illustration at *visual cycle.*

**bath·ro·ceph·a·ly** (bath″ro-sef′ə-le) [Gr. *bathron* a step + *-cephaly*] a developmental anomaly characterized by a steplike posterior projection of the skull, caused by excessive bone formation at the lambdoid suture.

**bathy-** [Gr. *bathys* deep, *bathos* depth] a combining form meaning deep or denoting relationship to depth. Also *bath(o)-*.

**bathy·an·es·the·sia** (bath″e-an″es-the′zhə) [*bathy-* + *anesthesia*] loss of deep sensibility (bathyesthesia).

**bathy·car·dia** (bath″ĭ-kahr′de-ə) [*bathy-* + Gr. *kardia* heart] a fixed low position of the heart due to anatomical conditions and not to disease.

**bathy·es·the·sia** (bath″e-əs-the′zhə) [*bathy-* + *esthesia*] deep sensibility.

**bathy·hy·per·es·the·sia** (bath″e-hi″pər-əs-the′zhə) [*bathy-* + *hyperesthesia*] increased sensitiveness of deep structures of the body. Cf. *deep sensibility,* under *sensibility.*

**bathy·hyp·es·the·sia** (bath″e-hip″əs-the′zhə) [*bathy-* + *hypesthesia*] decreased deep sensibility.

**bathy·pnea** (bath″ĭp-ne′ə) [*bathy-* + *-pnea*] deep breathing.

**BATO** a boronic acid adduct of a technetium oxime; as a class they are neutral lipid-soluble agents some of which have been used as radioactive tracers for diagnostic imaging, including siboroxime and teboroxime.

**ba·to·net** (ba-to-net′) pseudochromosome.

**Bat·son's plexus** (bat′sənz) [Oscar Vivian *Batson,* American otolaryngologist, 1894–1979] see under *plexus.*

**Bat·ten disease** (bat′ən) [Frederick Eustace *Batten,* English ophthalmologist, 1865–1918] see under *disease.*

**Bat·ten-Ma·you disease** (bat′ən-ma-yoo′) [F.E. *Batten;* Marmaduke Stephen *Mayou,* English ophthalmologist, 1876–1934] Batten disease; see under *disease.*

**bat·te·ry** (bat′ər-e) 1. a set or series of cells which afford an electric current. 2. any set, series, or grouping of similar things, as a battery of tests.

**Bat·tey ba·cil·li** (bat′e) [*Battey,* a tuberculosis hospital in Rome, Georgia, where many strains of these mycobacteria were first recognized] see under *bacillus.*

**bat·tey·in** (bat′e-in) [*Battey* bacillus] a product prepared from Battey bacilli (Group III of the unclassified mycobacteria), comparable to tuberculin, used in a cutaneous test of hypersensitivity.

**Bat·tle's incision, operation, sign** (bat′əlz) [William Henry *Battle,* English surgeon, 1855–1936] see under *operation* and *sign,* and see *Kammerer-Battle incision,* under *incision.*

**Bat·tle-Ja·la·guier-Kam·mer·er incision** (bat′əl-zhah-lah-ge-a′-kam′ər-ər) [W. H. *Battle;* Adolphe *Jalaguier,* French surgeon, 1853–1924; Frederic *Kammerer,* American surgeon, 1856–1928] see *Kammerer-Battle incision,* under *incision.*

**Bau·de·locque's diameter (line)** (bo-də-lōks′) [Jean Louis *Baudelocque,* French obstetrician, 1746–1810] conjugata externa pelvis.

**Bau·hin's gland, valve** (bo-az′) [Gaspard (Caspar) *Bauhin,* Swiss anatomist, 1560–1624] see *glandulae linguales anteriores* and *valva ileocaecalis.*

**Bau·mé's scale** (bo-māz′) [Antoine *Baumé,* French chemist, 1728–1804] see under *scale.*

**baux·ite** (bawk′sīt) [Les *Baux,* France, site of the first bauxite mines] an impure mixture of aluminum hydroxides, clay, and other metal oxides, the primary natural source of aluminum. See also *bauxite pneumoconiosis.*

**bay** (ba) a recess or inlet.
**lacrimal b.**, lacus lacrimalis.

**Bayes' theorem** (bāz) [Thomas *Bayes,* English mathematician, 1702–1761] see under *theorem.*

**bayes·ian statistics** (ba′ze-ən) [T. *Bayes*] see under *statistics.*

**Bayle's disease** (bālz) [Antoine Laurent Jesse *Bayle,* French physician, 1799–1858] paralytic dementia.

**Bay·lis·as·car·is** (ba″lis-as′kə-ris) a genus of nematodes of the family Ascaridae. *B. columna′ris* infests the central nervous system of dogs. *B. procy′onis* is usually found in raccoons and rodents, but fecal contamination from those animals can cause spread to domestic animals and humans, resulting in nervous system infection or larva migrans.

**Bay·liss effect** (ba′lis) [Sir William Maddock *Bayliss,* British physician, 1860–1924] see under *effect.*

**Ba·zex's syndrome** (bah-zeks′əz) [J. *Bazex,* French dermatologist, 20th century] see under *syndrome.*

**Ba·zin's disease** (bah-zaz′) [Antoine Pierre Ernest *Bazin,* French dermatologist, 1807–1878] see *erythema induratum.*

**BBB** 1. blood-brain barrier; see under *barrier.* 2. bundle branch block.

**BBBB** bilateral bundle branch block.

**BBT** basal body temperature.

**BC** bone conduction.

**$\beta$1C** former name for complement factor *C3;* see under *complement.*

**BCAA** branched-chain amino acids.

**B-CAVe** a regimen of bleomycin, CCNU (lomustine), Adriamycin (doxorubicin), and vinblastine, used in cancer chemotherapy.

**BCDF** B cell differentiation factors.

**BCF** basophil chemotactic factor.

**BCG** bacille Calmette-Guérin; bicolor guaiac test (see under *tests*); ballistocardiogram.

**BCGF** B cell growth factors.

**BCNU** carmustine.

**b.d.** abbreviation for L. *bis di'e,* twice a day.

**BDA** British Dental Association.

**Bdel·la** (del'ə) [Gr. "leech"] a genus of mites. *B. cardina'lis* is parasitic on other insects.

**bdel·li·um** (del'e-əm) [L.; Gr. *bdellion*] the fragrant gum-resin of several species of *Commiphora* trees; used as an adulterant of myrrh because of its similar appearance and aromatic properties.

**Bdel·lo·vib·rio** (del"o-vib're-o) [*bdella* + *vibrio*] [MeSH: Bdellovibrio] a genus of small, aerobic, motile, vibrioid, gram-negative bacteria that are obligate parasites on other gram-negative bacteria, replicating between the cell wall and the plasma membrane of the host bacterium; they are found worldwide in soil and fresh and marine waters. The type species is *B. bacteriovorus.*

**bdel·lo·vib·rio** (del"o-vib're-o) [MeSH: Bdellovibrio] any microorganism of the genus *Bdellovibrio.*

**B-DNA** see under *DNA.*

**BDS** Bachelor of Dental Surgery.

**BDSc** Bachelor of Dental Science.

**Be** symbol for *beryllium.*

**$\beta$1E** former name for complement factor *C4;* see under *complement.*

**bead** (bēd) a small spherical structure or mass.
**rachitic b's,** a series of palpable or visible prominences at the points where the ribs join their cartilages; seen in certain cases of rickets.
**scorbutic b's,** a series of visible prominences at the costochondral joints, sometimes seen in children with scurvy.

**bead·ed** (bēd'əd) having the appearance of a string of beads.

**bead·ing** (bēd'ing) alternate local constriction and dilatation of a blood vessel so that on an angiograph it resembles a string of beads.

**Bea·dle** (be'dəl) George Wells. American biochemist, 1903–1989; co-winner, with Edward Lawrie Tatum and Joshua Lederberg, of the Nobel prize for medicine or physiology in 1958 for work on the bread mold *Neurospora crassa,* showing that genes control a cell's production of enzymes and therefore the chemistry of the cell.

**beak** (bēk) [Fr. *bec*] [MeSH: Beak] 1. the forward-projecting jaws of a bird, along with their leathery or horny covering. 2. something shaped like the beak of a bird. See also *rostrum.*

**beak·er** (bēk'ər) a form of glass cup, usually with a lip for pouring, used by chemists and pharmacists.

**Beale's ganglion cells** (bēlz) [Lionel Smith *Beale,* British physician, 1828–1906] see under *cell.*

**Beals' syndrome** (bēlz) [Rodney Kenneth *Beals,* American orthopedic surgeon, born 1931] congenital contractural arachnodactyly; see under *arachnodactyly.*

**beam** (bēm) 1. a unidirectional, or approximately unidirectional, emission of electromagnetic radiation or particles. 2. any slender structure of a denture or orthodontic appliance designed to provide support to the structure and subjected to lateral stresses, such as a dental bar or an orthodontic arch wire whose curvature changes under load.
**cantilever b.,** a beam that is supported by one fixed support at only one of its ends.
**continuous b.,** a beam that continues over three or more supports, those supports not at the beam ends being equally free supports.
**primary b.,** useful b.
**restrained b.,** one that has two or more supports, at least one of which permits some freedom of rotation to the point of support.
**simple b.,** a straight beam that has two supports, one at either end.
**useful b.,** in radiology, that part of the primary radiation which is permitted to emerge from the tubehead assembly of an x-ray machine, as limited by the tubehead aperture or port and accessory collimating devices.

**bean** (bēn) [MeSH: Legumes] 1. any of various leguminous plants of the pea family. 2. the seed of such a plant.
**broad b.,** 1. *Vicia faba.* 2. the seed of *Vicia faba.*
**cacao b's,** cacao, def. 2.
**Calabar b.,** 1. *Physostigma venenosum.* 2. the poisonous seed of *P. venenosum,* which contains physostigmine and has been used by natives in ordeal trials. Called also *ordeal b.*
**carob b.,** 1. *Ceratonia siliqua.* 2. carob (def. 2).
**castor b.,** 1. *Ricinus communis.* 2. the seed of *Ricinus communis,* which yields castor oil but is also toxic to humans and other animals.
**cocoa b's,** cacao, def. 2.
**djenkol b.,** 1. *Pithecolobium lobatum.* 2. the seed of *P. lobatum,* a broad round reddish bean eaten as a delicacy in Indonesia and nearby areas, sometimes causing djenkol bean poisoning. Called also *jering b.*
**fava b.,** 1. *Vicia faba.* 2. the seed of *Vicia faba.*
**jack b.,** any of various beans of the genus *Canavalia,* used as food for humans and livestock.
**jequirity b.,** 1. *Abrus precatorius.* 2. the toxic seed of *A. precatorius,* which is used as a decorative bead but contains abrin. Called also *crab's eye* and *rosary pea.*
**jering b.,** djenkol b.
**locust b.,** 1. *Ceratonia siliqua.* 2. carob (def. 2).
**mescal b.,** *Sophora secundiflora.*
**ordeal b.,** Calabar b.
**St. Ignatius' b.,** the poisonous seed of the tropical tree *Strychnos ignatii;* it contains strychnine and brucine.
**tonka b.,** 1. *Dipteryx odorata.* 2. the seed of *D. odorata,* which has been used as a flavoring agent and contains coumarin.
**vanilla b.,** vanilla (def. 2).

**bear·ber·ry** (ber'ber-e) *Arctostaphylos uva-ursi.*

**beard** (bērd) the heavy hair growing on the lower part of a man's face, normally appearing after puberty as a secondary sex characteristic; called also *barba* [TA].

**bear·ing** (bar'ing) a supporting surface or point.
**central b.,** application of forces between the maxillae and mandible at a single point as near as possible to the center of the supporting areas of the upper and lower jaws, for the purpose of distributing closing forces evenly throughout the areas of the supporting structures during the registration and recording of maxillomandibular (jaw) relations and during the correction of occlusal errors.

**bear·ing down** (bār'ing down) 1. a feeling of weight in the pelvis occurring in certain diseases. 2. the expulsive effort of a woman in labor.

**Bearn-Kun·kel syndrome** (bərn-kung'kəl) [Alexander Gordon *Bearn,* English-born American physician, 1923–1983; Henry George *Kunkel,* American physician, born 1916] lupoid hepatitis; see under *hepatitis.*

**Bearn-Kun·kel-Sla·ter syndrome** (bərn-kung'kəl-sla'tər) [A. G. *Bearn;* H. G. *Kunkel;* Robert James *Slater,* Canadian-born American pediatrician, born 1923] lupoid hepatitis.

**bear·wood** (bār'wood) cascara sagrada.

**beat** (bēt) a throb or pulsation, as of the heart or of an artery; see also *pulse.*
**apex b.,** the most inferolateral point of visible or palpable pulsation of the chest wall due to movement of the apex of the heart, normally medial and superior to the intersection of the left midclavicular line and the fifth left intercostal space. Generally it corresponds roughly to the position of the apex of the heart and is often the point of maximal impulse.
**atrial escape b.,** an ectopic beat originating within the atria; it occurs when the sinus node does not fire or fires ineffectively.
**atrial premature b. (APB),** see under *complex.*
**atrioventricular (AV) junctional escape b.,** a depolarization initiated in the atrioventricular junction when one or more impulses from the sinus node are nonexistent or ineffective.
**atrioventricular (AV) junctional premature b.,** see under *complex.*
**capture b's,** in atrioventricular dissociation, occasional ventricular responses to a sinus impulse that reaches the atrioventricular node in a nonrefractory phase.
**ciliary b.,** the rhythmic, coordinated contraction of cilia of cells in a two-step process involving intraciliary excitation followed by interciliary conduction. The beat may be divided into two parts, the *effective stroke* and the *recovery stroke.* The rhythm may be either *isochronous* (all cilia beating simultaneously) or *metachronous* (beats moving along the cilia in waves).
**dropped b.,** absence of a single ventricular contraction.
**echo b.,** reciprocal b.
**ectopic b.,** a heart beat originating at some point other than the sinus node.
**escape b., escaped b.,** an ectopic beat that follows an abnormally long pause between impulses propagated by the sinoatrial node; name for the escape of impulse propagation from normal control.
**forced b.,** an extrasystole produced by artificial stimulation of the heart.
**fusion b.,** in electrocardiography, the complex resulting when an ectopic ventricular beat coincides with normal conduction to the ventricle; the complex has features of both the normal and the ectopic beat.
**heart b.,** heartbeat.
**interpolated b.,** a contraction occurring exactly between two normal beats without altering the sinus rhythm.
**interpolated ventricular premature b.,** see under *complex.*
**junctional escape b.,** atrioventricular junctional escape b.
**junctional premature b.,** atrioventricular junctional complex.

**nodal b.**, atrioventricular junctional escape b.
**postectopic b.**, the normal beat following an ectopic beat.
**premature b.**, extrasystole.
**pseudofusion b.**, an ineffective pacing stimulus delivered during the absolute refractory period following a spontaneous depolarization but before sufficient charge accumulates to prevent pacemaker discharge; on the electrocardiogram the pacemaker impulse spike is superimposed on the QRS complex of the spontaneous complex.
**reciprocal b.**, a cardiac impulse that in one cycle causes ventricular contraction, travels back toward the atria, then reexcites the ventricles; a series of such beats constitutes a reciprocal rhythm.
**reentrant b.**, any of the characteristic beats of a reentrant circuit.
**retrograde b.**, a beat occurring as a result of impulse conduction backward relative to the normal atrioventricular direction.
**sinus b.**, a natural pulsation of the heart, originating in the sinus node.
**ventricular escape b.**, an ectopic beat of ventricular origin occurring in the absence of supraventricular impulse generation or conduction; it is characterized by a bizarre, usually wide QRS complex and lack of an ectopic P wave.
**ventricular premature b. (VPB)**, see under *complex*.

**Beau's lines** (bōz) [Joseph Honoré Simon *Beau,* French physician, 1806–1865] see under *line*.

**Beau·ver·ia** (bo-vēr′e-ə) a genus of Fungi Imperfecti of the form-class Hyphomycetes, form-family Moniliaceae. *B. bassia′na* causes muscardine in silkworms, and *B. tenel′la* causes a disease of the larvae of beetles; formerly called *Botrytis bassiana* and *B. tenella,* respectively.

**bech·ic** (bek′ik) [L. *bechicus,* from Gr. *bēx* cough] tussive.

**Bech·te·rew** see *Bekhterev*.

**Beck's disease** (beks) [E.V. *Beck* (or *Bek*), Russian physician, early 20th century] Kashin-Bek disease.

**Beck's gastrostomy** (beks) [Carl *Beck,* American surgeon, 1856–1911] see under *gastrostomy*.

**Beck's triad** (beks) [Claude Schaeffer *Beck,* American surgeon, 1894–1971] see under *triad*.

**Beck·er's nevus** (bek′ərz) [Samuel William *Becker,* American physician, born 1924] see under *nevus*.

**Beck·er's phenomenon (sign), test** (bek′ərz) [Otto Heinrich Enoch *Becker,* German oculist, 1828–1890] see under *phenomenon* and *test*.

**Beck·with's syndrome** (bek′withs) [John Bruce *Beckwith,* American pediatric pathologist, born 1933] Beckwith-Wiedemann syndrome; see under *syndrome*.

**Beck·with-Wie·de·mann syndrome** (bek′with-ve′də-mahn) [J. B. *Beckwith;* Hans Rudolf *Wiedemann,* German pediatrician, born 1915] [MeSH: Beckwith-Wiedemann Syndrome] see under *syndrome*.

**Bé·clard's amputation,** etc. (ba-klahrz′) [Pierre Augustin *Béclard,* French anatomist, 1785–1825] see under *amputation, hernia, nucleus, sign,* and *triangle*.

**bec·lo·meth·a·sone di·pro·pi·o·nate** (bek″lo-meth′ə-sōn) [USP] a synthetic glucocorticoid administered by inhalation for the chronic treatment of bronchial asthma and intranasally for the treatment of perennial and seasonal rhinitis and to prevent the recurrence of nasal polyps following surgical removal; also used topically for the relief of inflammation and pruritus in corticosteroid-responsive dermatoses.

**Bec·lo·vent** (bek′lo-vent″) trademark for a preparation of beclomethasone dipropionate.

**Bec·on·ase** (bek′ə-nāz″) trademark for a preparation of beclomethasone dipropionate.

**bec·que·rel** (bek-ə-rel′) [Antoine Henri *Becquerel,* French physicist, 1852–1908; co-winner, with M. S. Curie and P. Curie, of the Nobel Prize in physics for 1903 for studies in spontaneous radioactivity] a unit of radioactivity, defined as that of quantity of a radioactive nuclide whose rate of spontaneous nuclear transformation is one decay per second ($1\ s^{-1}$); 1 curie equals $3.7 \times 10^{10}$ becquerels; 1 microcurie equals 37 kilobecquerels. Abbreviated Bq.

**bed** (bed) [MeSH: Beds] 1. a supporting structure or tissue. 2. a couch or support for the body during sleep.
**air b.**, an airtight, inflatable mattress.
**capillary b.**, the total combined mass of capillaries forming a large reservoir which may be more or less completely filled with blood. See illustration at *capillary*.
**CircOlectric b.**, trademark for a revolving circular bed which induces constant pressure alteration.
**fracture b.**, a bed for the use of patients with broken bones.
**Gatch b.**, a bed fitted with joints beneath the hips and knees of the patient, allowing him to be raised to a half-sitting position and be so maintained by elevating his knees to prevent his sliding toward the footboard.
**hydrostatic b.**, water b.
**metabolic b.**, a bed so arranged that all the feces and urine of the patient are saved; the amount of excreta compared with the intake gives an indication of the metabolism in the body.
**nail b.**, matrix unguis.
**rocking b.**, a bed mounted on a rocking apparatus, moving between the head up and head down positions to promote movement of the diaphragm and thus breathing, particularly for patients who are quadriplegic or have paralysis of the diaphragm.
**Sanders b.**, a rocking bed used to improve circulation in the treatment of chronic occlusive arterial disease.
**sawdust b.**, a bed made from sawdust, used to prevent bed sores.
**vascular b.**, the sum of the blood vessels supplying an organ or region.
**water b.**, a plastic or rubber mattress filled with water; used to prevent bed sores by distributing the patient's weight. Called also *hydrostatic b.*

**bed·bug** (bed′bug) [MeSH: Bedbugs] 1. any bug of the genus *Cimex*. 2. any of various other biting insects that infest human bedding.
**Mexican b.**, any of various biting reduviid bugs of the genus *Triatoma* found in the southern United States and Mexico.

**Bed·nar's aphthae** (bed′nahrz) [Alois *Bednar,* Austrian physician, 1816–1888] see under *aphtha*.

**bed·pan** (bed′pan) a vessel for receiving the urinary and fecal discharges of a patient unable to leave his bed.

**Bed·so·nia** (bed-so′ne-ə) *Chlamydia*.

**bed·sore** (bed′sor″) decubitus ulcer.

**bee** [MeSH: Bees] any of several flying insects of the family Apidae. See *Apis* and *Bombus*.

**Beer's law** (bārz) [August *Beer,* German physicist, 1825–1863] see under *law*.

**Beer's operation** (bārz) [Georg Joseph *Beer,* Austrian ophthalmologist, 1763–1821] see under *operation*.

**beer·wort** (bēr′wərt) an infusion of malt in water intended to be converted into beer; it is sometimes used for the cultivation of yeasts and molds.

**bees·wax** (bēz′waks) wax derived from the honeycomb of *Apis mellifera;* see *yellow wax,* under *wax*.
**bleached b.**, see *white wax,* under *wax*.
**unbleached b.**, see *yellow wax,* under *wax*.

**beet** (bēt) 1. any plant of the genus *Beta*. 2. the enlarged root of such a plant.

**bee·tle** (be′təl) [MeSH: Beetles] an insect of the order Coleoptera.
**blister b.**, any beetle of the family Meloidae; their dried bodies raise blisters when rubbed on human skin and are sometimes used as counterirritants.
**coconut b.**, any beetle of the genus *Sessinia*.
**grain b.**, a beetle of the genus *Tenebrio;* its larva is the mealworm.
**rove b.**, any beetle of the family Staphylinidae.

**Bee·vor's sign** (be′vərz) [Charles Edward *Beevor,* British neurologist, 1854–1908] see under *sign*.

**Begg's appliance, technique** (begz) [Peter Raymond *Begg,* Australian orthodontist, born 1898] see under *appliance* and *technique*.

**beg·ma** (beg′mə) [Gr.] phlegm.

**Bé·guez Cé·sar disease** (ba′gās sa′sahr) [Antonio *Béguez César,* Cuban pediatrician, 20th century] Chédiak-Higashi syndrome.

**be·hav·ior** (be-hāv′yər) [MeSH: Behavior] deportment or conduct; any or all of a person's total activity, especially that which can be externally observed.
**automatic b.**, automatism.
**invariable b.**, activity whose character is determined by innate structure, such as reflex action.
**operant b.**, see under *conditioning*.
**respondent b.**, see *conditioning*.
**variable b.**, behavior that is modifiable by individual experience.

**be·hav·ior·ism** (be-hāv′yər-iz-əm) [MeSH: Behaviorism] a school of psychology founded by John B. Watson that regards as the subject matter of psychology only overt actions capable of direct observation and measurement and ignores unobservable mental events such as ideas and emotions.

**be·hav·ior·ist** (be-hāv′yər-ist) a psychologist who is a disciple of behaviorism.

**Beh·çet's syndrome** (beh-chets′) [Hulûsi *Behçet,* Turkish dermatologist, 1889–1948] see under *syndrome*.

**be·hen·ate** (bə-hen′āt) a salt (soap), ester, or anionic form of behenic acid.

**be·hen·ic acid** (bə-hen'ik) a saturated 22-carbon fatty acid present in oil of mustard and other plant seed oils. See table accompanying *fatty acid.*

**Behr's disease, pupil** (bārz) [Carl *Behr,* German ophthalmologist, 1874–1943] see under *disease* and *pupil.*

**Beh·ring** (ba'ring) Emil Adolf von. German physician and bacteriologist, 1854–1917; winner of the first Nobel prize for medicine or physiology in 1901 for his demonstration of immunization against diphtheria and tetanus by injections of antitoxins.

**Beh·ring's law** (ba'ringz) [Emil Adolf von *Behring*] see under *law.*

**Bei·gel's disease** (bi'gəlz) [Hermann *Beigel,* German physician, 1830–1879] piedra.

**bej·el** (bej'əl) [Ar. *bajlah*] endemic syphilis.

**Bé·ké·sy** (ba'ka-she) Georg von. Hungarian-born American physicist, 1899–1972; winner of the Nobel prize for medicine or physiology in 1961 for his discoveries concerning the physical mechanisms of stimulation within the cochlea.

**Bé·ké·sy audiometry** (ba'ka-she) [Georg von *Békésy*] see under *audiometry.*

**Bekh·te·rev's (Bech·te·rew's) layer, nucleus, reaction,** etc. (bek-ter'yevz) [Vladimir Mikhailovich *Bekhterev* (or *Bechterew*), Russian neurologist, 1857–1927] see under *nucleus, reaction, reflex, sign,* and *test*; see *rheumatoid spondylitis* under *spondylitis;* and see *Kaes-Bekhterev layer,* under *layer.*

**Bekh·te·rev-Men·del reflex** (bek-ter'yev-men'dəl) [V. M. *Bekhterev;* Kurt *Mendel,* German neurologist, 1874–1946] Mendel-Bekhterev reflex.

**bel** (bel) [Alexander Graham *Bell,* American inventor, 1847–1922] a unit of relative power intensity used for acoustic or electric power, defined as the base 10 logarithm of the ratio of the measured power to some reference power level. A change of one bel is a tenfold power increase. Measurements are usually expressed in decibels (q.v.). Symbol B.

**belch·ing** (belch'ing) eructation.

**be·lem·noid** (bə-lem'noid) [Gr. *belemnon* dart + *-oid*] 1. dart-shaped. 2. the styloid process of the ulna or of the temporal bone.

**Bell's muscle** (belz) [John *Bell,* Scottish surgeon and anatomist, 1763–1820] see under *muscle.*

**Bell's nerve, palsy (paralysis), phenomenon** (belz) [Sir Charles *Bell,* Scottish physiologist in London, 1774–1842] see *nervus thoracicus longus,* and see under *palsy* and *phenomenon.*

**bel·la·don·na** (bel"ə-don'ə) [Ital. "fair lady"] [MeSH: Belladonna] 1. *Atropa belladonna,* a perennial plant indigenous to central and southern Europe and cultivated in North America; it contains various anticholinergic alkaloids, including atropine, hyoscyamine, and scopolamine, which are used medicinally. Ingestion of belladonna or its alkaloids can cause anticholinergic poisoning (q.v.). Called also *banewort, deadly nightshade, death's herb,* and *dwale.* 2. belladonna leaf.

**bel·la·don·nine** (bel"ə-don'ēn) an alkaloid derived from belladonna and related solanaceous plants, produced during the process of extraction.

**Bel·li·ni's duct (tubule), ligament** (bel-e'nēz) [Lorenzo *Bellini,* Italian anatomist, 1643–1704] see *ductus papillaris,* and see under *ligament.*

**bel·ly** (bel'e) 1. abdomen. 2. the fleshy contractile part of a muscle (venter [TA]).
**anterior b. of digastric muscle,** venter anterior musculi digastrici.
**drum b.,** tympanitic abdomen.
**frontal b. of occipitofrontal muscle,** venter frontalis musculi occipitofrontalis.
**inferior b. of omohyoid muscle,** venter inferior musculi omohyoidei.
**occipital b. of occipitofrontal muscle,** venter occipitalis musculi occipitofrontalis.
**posterior b. of digastric muscle,** venter posterior musculi digastrici.
**prune b.,** see under *syndrome.*
**superior b. of omohyoid muscle,** venter superior musculi omohyoidei.
**wooden b.,** abdominal rigidity.

**bel·o·ne·pho·bia** (bel"o-nə-fo'be-ə) [Gr. *belonē* needle + *-phobia*] irrational fear of pins, needles, and other sharp objects.

**bel·o·noid** (bel'o-noid) [Gr. *belonē* needle + *-oid*] needle-shaped; styloid.

**bel·o·no·ski·as·co·py** (bel"ə-no-ski-as'kə-pe) [Gr. *belonē* needle + *skia-* + *-scopy*] a subjective type of retinoscopy in which refractive error is determined by eliminating the perceived shadow of a needle passing in front of the eye fixating on a distant point of light; called also *velonoskiascopy.*

**Bel·sey Mark IV operation** (bel'se) [Ronald Herbert Robert *Belsey,* English surgeon, 20th century] see under *operation.*

**Be·na·cer·raf** (ba-nə-sə-rahf') Baruj. Venezuelan-born American pathologist, born 1920; co-winner, with Jean Baptiste Gabriel Dausset and George Davis Snell, of the Nobel prize for medicine or physiology in 1980 for their work on the major histocompatibility complex and the genetic control of immune responses.

**ben·ac·ty·zine hy·dro·chlo·ride** (ben-ak'tĭ-zēn) an anticholinergic which has the ability to increase the emotional threshold of outside influences and to block the thought processes; used as a tranquilizer, administered orally.

**Ben·a·dryl** (ben'ə-dril) trademark for preparations of diphenhydramine hydrochloride.

**ben·a·ze·pril hy·dro·chlo·ride** (ben-a'zə-pril) an angiotensin-converting enzyme inhibitor administered orally for treatment of hypertension.

**Bence Jones protein,** etc. (bens-jōnz) [Henry *Bence Jones,* English physician, 1814–1873] see under *cylinder, protein, proteinuria,* and *reaction.*

**bend** (bend) a flexure or curve; a flexed or curved part.
**first order b's,** adjustments made in a labial arch wire, incorporating offsets in the horizontal plane, which are usually made in the areas of the cuspids and premolar and molar teeth, accommodating differences in thickness in the labiolingual or buccolingual diameters of the teeth.
**head b., neck b.,** cervical flexure.
**second order b's,** bends in the vertical plane of an arch wire.
**third order b's,** bends in an arch wire to maintain or produce torsion of a tooth.
**V b's,** V-shaped bends incorporated in an arch wire, usually placed mesial or distal to the cuspids to improve the axial relationship of teeth.
**varolian b.,** the third cerebral flexure in the developing fetus.

**ben·da·zac** (ben'də-zak) a nonsteroidal antiinflammatory drug structurally related to indomethacin, applied topically in the treatment of inflammatory skin disorders.

**Ben·der Vis·u·al-Mo·tor Ges·talt test** (ben'dər) [Lauretta *Bender,* American psychiatrist, 1897–1987] see under *test.*

**ben·dro·flu·a·zide** (ben"dro-floo'ə-zīd) bendroflumethiazide.

**ben·dro·flu·me·thi·a·zide** (ben"dro-floo"mə-thi'ə-zīd) [USP] [MeSH: Bendroflumethiazide] a thiazide diuretic used for treatment of hypertension and edema; administered orally.

**bends** (bendz) pain in the limbs and abdomen occurring as a result of rapid reduction of air pressure; see *decompression sickness,* under *sickness.*

**Ben·dy·late** (ben'də-lāt) trademark for preparations of diphenhydramine hydrochloride.

**be·ne** (ben'a) [L.] well.

**bene·cep·tor** (ben'ə-sep-tər) [*bene* + *-ceptor*] a rarely used term for a receptor that transmits stimuli of a beneficial character. Cf. *nociceptor.*

**Be·neck·ea** (be-nek'e-ə) in former systems of classification, a genus of bacteria, species of which have now been assigned to the genus *Vibrio.*

**Ben·e·dict's solution, test** (ben'ə-dikts) [Stanley Rossiter *Benedict,* American physiological chemist, 1884–1936] see under *solution* and *test.*

**Ben·e·dikt's syndrome** (ben'ə-dikts) [Moritz *Benedikt,* Austrian physician, 1835–1920] see under *syndrome.*

**Ben·e·mid** (ben'ə-mid) trademark for probenecid.

**be·nign** (bə-nīn') [L. *benignus*] not malignant; not recurrent; favorable for recovery.

**Ben·i·sone** (ben'ĭ-sōn) trademark for preparations of betamethasone benzoate.

**ben·ja·min** (ben'jə-min) benzoin, def. 1.

**Ben·nett's fracture** (ben'əts) [Edward Hallaran *Bennett,* Irish surgeon, 1837–1907] see under *fracture.*

**Ben·o·quin** (ben'o-kwin) trademark for preparations of monobenzone.

**ben·ox·i·nate hy·dro·chlo·ride** (ben-ok'sĭ-nāt) [USP] a benzoic acid ester related to procaine, used as a local anesthetic in ophthalmology; applied topically to the conjunctiva to produce anesthesia of short duration for tonometry, goniometry, foreign object removal, and short operative procedures on the conjunctiva and cornea.

**Ben·ox·yl** (ben-ok′səl) trademark for preparations of benzoyl peroxide.

**ben·ser·a·zide** (ben-ser′ə-zīd) [MeSH: Benserazide] an inhibitor of the decarboxylation of peripheral levodopa to dopamine, having actions similar to those of carbidopa. When given with levodopa, carbidopa produces higher brain concentrations of dopamine with lower doses of levodopa, thus lessening the side effects seen with higher doses. It is used orally, in conjunction with levodopa, as an antiparkinsonian agent.

**Ben·son's disease** (ben′sənz) [Alfred Hugh *Benson,* Irish ophthalmologist, 1852–1912] asteroid hyalosis.

**ben·taz·e·pam** (ben-taz′ə-pam) a benzodiazepine tranquilizer, with properties similar to those of diazepam, used as an antianxiety agent; administered orally.

**ben·thos** (ben′thos) [Gr. *benthos* bottom of the sea] the flora and fauna of the bottom of oceans.

**ben·tir·o·mide** (ben-tēr′o-mīd) a compound containing *p*-aminobenzoic acid used in a noninvasive screening test for pancreatic exocrine insufficiency and to monitor therapy with pancreatic supplements.

**ben·ton·ite** (ben′ton-īt) [Fort *Benton,* Montana, after which the geological formation where it was found was named] [NF] [MeSH: Bentonite] a colloidal hydrated aluminum silicate, which on the addition of water swells to produce a slippery paste; its chief pharmaceutical use is as a suspending agent, and it has also been used as a bulk laxative.

**Ben·tyl** (ben′til) trademark for preparations of dicyclomine hydrochloride.

**ben·zal·de·hyde** (ben-zal′də-hīd) [NF] artificial essential oil of almond; used as a flavoring agent in orally administered medicaments.

**ben·za·lin** (ben′zə-lin) nigrosin.

**ben·zal·ko·ni·um chlo·ride** (ben″zal-ko′ne-əm) [NF] a mixture of alkylbenzyl dimethylammonium chlorides; a rapidly acting surface disinfectant and detergent active against both gram-negative and gram-positive bacteria and certain viruses, fungi, yeasts, and protozoa; applied topically to the skin and mucous membranes. It is also used as an antimicrobial preservative in ophthalmic solutions.

**ben·za·mine** (ben′zə-mēn) eucaine.

**ben·zan·thra·cene** (ben-zan′thrə-sēn) one of a group of aromatic hydrocarbons consisting of anthracene with one benzene substitution; some of them have carcinogenic properties.

**ben·zaz·o·line hy·dro·chlo·ride** (ben-zaz′o-lēn) tolazoline hydrochloride.

**benz·bro·ma·rone** (benz-bro′mə-rōn) [MeSH: Benzbromarone] a potent uricosuric agent that blocks tubular reabsorption of uric acid; used in the treatment of hyperuricemia of gout.

**benz·cu·rine io·dide** (benz′ku-rēn) gallamine triethiodide.

**Ben·ze·drex** (ben′zə-dreks) trademark for a propylhexedrine inhaler.

**ben·zene** (ben′zēn) [MeSH: Benzene] a colorless volatile liquid hydrocarbon, $C_6H_6$, obtained mainly as a by-product in the destructive distillation of coal, along with coal tar, etc. It has an aromatic odor, and burns with a light-giving flame. It dissolves sulfur, phosphorus, iodine, and organic compounds. It is harmful by transdermal absorption and acutely toxic by ingestion or inhalation, causing mucous membrane irritation, neurological symptoms, and death due to respiratory failure; chronic exposure may result in bone marrow depression and aplasia and leukemia. Benzene is a known carcinogen. See illustration under *ring.* Called also *benzol.*
**dimethyl b.,** xylene.
**b. hexachloride,** a compound prepared by chlorination of benzene in actinic light, consisting of five isomers; the gamma isomer (see *lindane*) is a powerful insecticide. Called also *hexachlorocyclohexane.*
**methyl b.,** toluene.

**1,2-ben·zene·di·car·box·yl·ic ac·id** (ben″zēn-di-kahr″bok-sil′ik) see *phthalic acid.*

**ben·zene·meth·a·nol** (ben″zēn-meth′ə-nol) benzyl alcohol.

**ben·ze·noid** (ben′zə-noid) a compound having a structure related to benzene or other compounds of aromatic character.

**ben·zes·tro·fol** (ben-zes′trə-fōl) estradiol benzoate.

**ben·ze·tho·ni·um chlo·ride** (ben″zə-tho′ne-əm) [USP] a synthetic quaternary ammonium compound used as a local anti-infective applied topically as a solution and as a preservative in pharmaceutical preparations. It is also used in various concentrations for cleaning eating and cooking utensils, as a disinfectant in laundering, to control algal growth in swimming pools, and as an environmental deodorant.

**benz·hex·ol hy·dro·chlo·ride** (benz-hek′sol) trihexyphenidyl hydrochloride.

**benz·hy·dra·mine hy·dro·chlo·ride** (benz-hi′drə-mēn) diphenhydramine hydrochloride.

**ben·zi·dine** (ben′zĭ-dēn) a colorless, crystalline arylamine compound formed by the action of acids on hydrazobenzene; once widely used in testing for occult blood, its use is now limited because it is a carcinogen and is toxic if absorbed through the skin, ingested, or inhaled. Called also *p-diaminodiphenyl.*

**ben·zil·o·ni·um bro·mide** (ben″zil-o′ne-əm) an anticholinergic used in the treatment of peptic ulcer and functional gastrointestinal disorders.

**ben·zi·mid·a·zole** (ben″zĭ-mid′ə-zol) a dicyclic compound comprising a benzene ring and an imidazole ring, occurring as part of the nucleotide portion of vitamin $B_{12}$. Substituted benzimidazoles inhibit the action of $H^+/K^+$-ATPase at the secretory surface of the parietal cells, thus blocking the final step of gastric acid production, and are used as inhibitors of gastric acid secretion. Several benzimidazoles are used as anthelmintics.

**ben·zin** (ben′zin) petroleum benzin.
**petroleum b.,** see under *petroleum.*

**ben·zine** (ben′zēn) petroleum benzin.

**ben·zo·ate** (ben′zo-āt) a salt of benzoic acid.

**ben·zo·at·ed** (ben′zo-āt-əd) containing or combined with benzoic acid.

**ben·zo·caine** (ben′zo-kān) [USP] [MeSH: Benzocaine] an insoluble ester that is a local anesthetic, applied topically to the skin and mucous membranes; used to suppress the gag reflex in dental procedures, endoscopy, and intubation.

**ben·zo·di·az·e·pine** (ben″zo-di-az′ə-pēn) any of a group of minor tranquilizers, having a common molecular structure and similar pharmacological activity, including antianxiety, sedative, hypnotic, amnestic, anticonvulsant, and muscle relaxing effects.

**ben·zo·di·ox·an** (ben″zo-di-ok′san) a class of $\alpha$-adrenergic blocking agents, the most important member of which is piperoxan.

**ben·zo·gy·nes·tryl** (ben″zo-gi-nes′trəl) estradiol benzoate.

**ben·zo·ic ac·id** (ben-zo′ik) [USP] benzenecarboxylic acid, a fungistatic compound widely used as a food preservative; it is conjugated to glycine in the liver and excreted as hippuric acid. See also *benzoic and salicylic acids ointment,* under *ointment.*

**ben·zo·ic al·de·hyde** (ben-zo′ik) benzaldehyde.

**ben·zo·in** (ben′zo-in) [MeSH: Benzoin] 1. [USP] a balsamic resin with an aromatic odor and taste, obtained from certain species of *Styrax;* it is used as a topical protectant, topical antiseptic, irritant expectorant, and inhalant in respiratory tract inflammation. Called also *benjamin, gum benjamin,* and *gum benzoinoil.* 2. a highly toxic crystalline compound, $C_{14}H_{12}O_2$, prepared by the condensation of benzaldehyde in an alkaline cyanide solution, used in organic synthesis and as a catalyst in photopolymerization.

**ben·zol** (ben′zol) benzene.

**ben·zo·na·tate** (ben-zo′nə-tāt) [USP] a peripherally acting antitussive that reduces the cough reflex by anesthetizing the stretch receptors in the respiratory passages, lungs, and pleura; administered orally.

**ben·zo·no·na·tine** (ben-zo″no-na′tēn) benzonatate.

**ben·zo·pur·pu·rine** (ben′zo-pur′pu-rin) any one of a series of azo-dyes of a scarlet color, used especially as a contrast stain with hematoxylin and other blue stains.
**b. 4B,** a compound used as an analytical reagent, as a biological stain, and as an indicator with a pH range of 1.2 (violet) to 4.0 (red).

**1,2-ben·zo·pyr·an** (ben″zo-pir′an) 1,2-chromene.

**ben·zo[*a*]py·rene** (ben″zo-pi′rēn) 3,4-benzpyrene; a highly carcinogenic polycyclic aromatic hydrocarbon occurring as a product of incomplete combustion of carbonaceous materials. It is a procarcinogen that requires metabolic activation to exert a mutagenic effect.

**ben·zo·qui·none** (ben″zo-kwin′ōn) 1. a substituted benzene ring containing two carbonyl groups, usually in the *para* (1,4) position. *p*-Benzoquinone is used in the manufacture of dyes and hydroquinone, and in fungicides; it is toxic by inhalation and is an irritant to skin and mucous membranes. Called also *quinone.* 2. any of a subclass of quinones that are derived from or contain this structure, such as those involved in the electron transport chain of respiration.

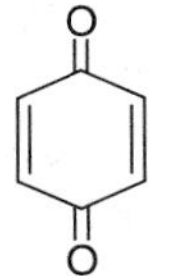

*p*-Benzoquinone.

**ben·zo·thi·a·di·a·zide** (ben″zo-thi″ə-di′ə-zīd) thiazide.

**ben·zo·thi·a·di·a·zine** (ben″zo-thi″ə-di′ə-zēn) thiazide.

**benz·ox·i·quine** (ben-zok′sĭ-kwin″) the benzoate ester of oxyquinoline, used as a disinfectant.

**ben·zo·yl** (ben′zo-il) the radical, $C_6H_5CO$—, of benzoic acid and of an extensive series of compounds.
**b. peroxide, hydrous b. peroxide** [USP], a crystalline substance formed by the action of sodium peroxide on benzoyl chloride, used as a topical antibacterial and to initiate free radical reactions and to induce skin peeling so as to promote evacuation of comedones in acne vulgaris.

**ben·zo·yl·ec·go·nine** (ben″zo-il-ek′go-nēn) the major metabolite of cocaine, produced by hydrolysis of the drug by plasma esterases and detectable in the blood by laboratory testing.

**ben·zo·yl·gly·cine** (ben″zo-il-gli′sēn) hippuric acid.

**ben·zo·yl·pas cal·ci·um** (ben″zo-il′paz) a derivative of aminosalicylic acid used as a tuberculostatic; administered orally. Called also *calcium benzamidosalicylate.*

**ben·zo·yl·phen·yl·car·bi·nol** (ben″zo-il-fen″əl-kahr′bĭ-nol) benzoin, def. 2.

**benz·phet·amine hy·dro·chlo·ride** (benz-fet′ə-mēn) a sympathomimetic amine, related to amphetamine, used as an oral anorexiant in the control of exogenous obesity.

**3,4-benz·py·rene** (benz-pi′rēn) benzo[*a*]pyrene.

**benz·py·rin·i·um bro·mide** (benz″pi-rin′e-əm) a cholinergic having anticholinesterase actions similar to those of neostigmine.

**benz·quin·amide hy·dro·chlo·ride** (benz-kwin′ə-mīd) an antiemetic compound with antihistaminic, mild anticholinergic, and sedative properties; used to prevent and treat nausea and vomiting associated with anesthesia and surgery and also that associated with cancer chemotherapy. Administered intramuscularly or intravenously.

**benz·thi·a·zide** (benz-thi′ə-zīd) a thiazide diuretic, used for the treatment of hypertension and edema; administered orally.

**benz·tro·pine mes·y·late** (benz′tro-pēn) [USP] a synthetic compound combining the active moieties of atropine and diphenylhydramine, and having anticholinergic, antihistaminic, and local anesthetic effects, used as an antidyskinetic in the treatment of parkinsonism and for the control of extrapyramidal reactions (except tardive dyskinesia) to neuroleptic drugs; administered orally, intramuscularly, and intravenously.

**ben·zyd·ro·flu·me·thi·a·zide** (ben-zid″ro-floo-mə-thi′ə-zīd) bendroflumethiazide.

**ben·zyl** (ben′zəl) the hydrocarbon radical, $C_7H_7$ or $C_6H_5CH_2$—, of benzyl alcohol and various other compounds.
**b. benzoate** [USP], a clear, colorless, oily liquid, one of the active substances in peruvian balsam and produced synthetically; applied topically as a scabicide.
**b. bromide,** a war gas causing lacrimation and irritation of the skin; called also *cylite.*
**b. carbinol,** phenylethyl alcohol.

**ben·zyl·i·dene** (ben-zil′ĭ-dēn) a hydrocarbon radical, $C_6H_5CH$=.

***p*-ben·zyl·oxy·phe·nol** (ben″zəl-ok″se-fe′nol) monobenzone.

**ben·zyl·pen·i·cil·lin** (ben″zəl-pen″ĭ-sil′in) penicillin G; see under *penicillin.*
**b. potassium,** penicillin G potassium; see under *penicillin.*
**b. procaine,** penicillin G procaine; see under *penicillin.*
**b. sodium,** penicillin G sodium; see under *penicillin.*

**ben·zyl·pen·i·cil·lo·yl poly·ly·sine** (ben″zəl-pen″ĭ-sil′o-əl pol″e-li′sēn) a skin test antigen composed of a benzylpenicilloyl moiety (a major antigenic determinant of benzylpenicillin) conjugated to poly-L-lysine as a carrier, used in assessing hypersensitivity to penicillin by scratch test or intradermal test. Available as *benzylpenicilloyl polylysine concentrate* [USP] and *benzylpenicilloyl polylysine injection* [USP].

**be·phe·ni·um hy·droxy·naph·tho·ate** (bə-fe′ne-əm hi-drok″se-naf′tho-āt) an anthelmintic effective against intestinal nematodes, especially hookworms *(Ancylostoma duodenale* and *Necator americanus)* and some other roundworms *(Ascaris lumbricoides* and *Strongyloides stercoralis);* it is a cholinergic agonist that causes the worms to relax and be expelled.

**ber·ac·tant** (bər-ak′tənt) a modified bovine lung extract containing chiefly phospholipids that mimics the action of pulmonary surfactant, used in the prevention and treatment of respiratory distress syndrome of the newborn; administered by endotracheal instillation.

**Be·rar·di·nel·li-Seip syndrome** (bər-ahr″dĭ-nel′e sīp) [Waldemar *Berardinelli,* Argentine physician, 1903–1956; Martin Fredrik *Seip,* Norwegian pediatrician, born 1921] total lipodystrophy.

**Bé·rard's ligament** (ba-rahrz′) [Auguste *Bérard,* French surgeon, 1802–1846] see under *ligament.*

**Bé·raud's valve** (ba-rōz′) [Bruno Jean Jacques *Béraud,* French surgeon, 1823–1865] see under *valve.*

**Ber·ber·i·da·ceae** (bər″bər-ĭ-da′se-e) a family of herbs and shrubs, many of which have berries. Genera include *Berberis, Jeffersonia,* and *Podophyllum.*

**ber·ber·ine** (bər′bər-ēn) [MeSH: Berberine] an alkaloid obtained from species of *Berberis* and other plants of the family Berberidaceae, as well as from *Hydrastis canadensis;* used as an antimalarial, carminative, and febrifuge, and externally in dressings for indolent ulcers.

**Ber·ber·is** (bər′bər-is) [L.] a genus of shrubs of the family Berberidaceae that contain berberine. *B. vulga′ris* is the barberry (q.v.).

**be·reave·ment** (bə-rēv′mənt) [MeSH: Bereavement] a deprivation causing grief and desolation, especially the death or loss of a loved one. The period of grief and mourning following a bereavement often resembles clinical depression. See also *mourning.*

**Be·reit·schafts·po·ten·tial** (bə-rīt″shahfts-pə-ten′shəl) [Ger] readiness potential.

**ber·ga·mot** (bər′gə-mot) [L. *bergamium*] 1. *Citrus bergamia.* 2. the orangelike fruit of *C. bergamia,* whose rind is a source of bergamot oil. 3. any of various fragrant labiate plants, such as *Mentha citrata* and *Monarda fistulosa.*

**Ber·ger's disease** (bār-zhārz′) [Jean *Berger,* French nephrologist, 20th century] IgA nephropathy.

**Ber·ger's operation** (bār′zhārz) [Paul *Berger,* French surgeon, 1845–1908] see under *operation.*

**Ber·ger rhythm** (ber′gər) [Hans *Berger,* German neurologist, 1873–1941] alpha rhythm; see under *rhythm.*

**Ber·ger's sign** (ber′gərz) [Emil *Berger,* Austrian ophthalmologist, 1855–1926] see under *sign.*

**Ber·gey's classification** (bər′gēz) [David Hendricks *Bergey,* American bacteriologist, 1860–1937] see under *classification.*

**Berg·man's sign** (bərg′mənz) [Harry *Bergman,* American urologist, born 1912] see under *sign.*

**Berg·mann's cells, cords, fibers** (berg′mahnz) [Gottlieb Heinrich *Bergmann,* German physician, 1781–1861] see *striae acusticae,* and see under *cell* and *fiber.*

**Ber·go·nié-Tri·bon·deau law** (bār-go-nya′ tre-bon-do′) [Jean Alban *Bergonié,* French physician, 1857–1925; Louis *Tribondeau,* French naval physician, 1872–1918] see under *law.*

**Berg·ström** (berk′strəm) Sune. Swedish biochemist, born 1916; co-winner, with Bengt Ingemar Samuelsson and John Robert Vane, of the Nobel prize for medicine or physiology in 1982, for their discoveries of prostaglandins and related substances.

**beri·beri** (ber″e-ber′e) [Singhalese, "I cannot," signifying that the person is too ill to do anything] [MeSH: Beriberi] a disease caused by a deficiency of thiamine (vitamin $B_1$) and characterized by polyneuritis, cardiac pathology, and edema. The epidemic form is found primarily in areas in which white (polished) rice is the staple food, as in Japan, China, the Philippines, India, and other countries of Southeast Asia. Called also *rice disease, dietetic neuritis, neuritis multiplex endemica,* and *endemic polyneuritis.* See also *nutritional polyneuropathy.*
**atrophic b.,** dry b.
**cerebral b.,** Wernicke-Korsakoff syndrome.
**dry b.,** a form of beriberi in which flaccid paralysis, muscular atrophy, and areflexia are the prominent signs; cardiac enlargement and tachycardia may be present. Called also *atrophic b.* and *paralytic b.*
**infantile b.,** a disease of breast-fed infants whose mothers have thiamine deficiency; it is characterized by diminished urine secretion, progressive edema, and often by acute cardiac failure, which may

terminate in sudden death. Vomiting, aphonia, opisthotonos, and convulsions may occur.
**paralytic b.**, dry b.
**wet b.**, a form marked by cardiac failure and edema, but without extensive nervous system involvement.

**beri·ber·ic** (ber″e-ber′ik) pertaining to or of the nature of beriberi.

**Berke operation** (bərk) [Raynold N. *Berke,* American ophthalmologist, born 1901] see under *operation.*

**berke·li·um** (bərk′le-əm) [named for *Berkeley,* California, where it was produced] [MeSH: Berkelium] an element of atomic number 97, atomic weight 247, symbol Bk, produced by bombardment of the isotope of americium of atomic weight 241 by helium ions; half-life $4\frac{1}{2}$ hours.

**Ber·lin's edema** (bər-linz′) [Rudolf *Berlin,* German oculist, 1833–1897] commotio retinae.

**Ber·nard's duct,** etc. (bār-nahrz′) [Claude *Bernard,* French physiologist, 1813–1878] see under *duct, layer, puncture,* and *syndrome.*

**Ber·nard-Hor·ner syndrome** (bār-nahr′ hor′nər) [C. *Bernard;* Johann Friedrich *Horner,* Swiss ophthalmologist, 1831–1886] Horner's syndrome; see under *syndrome.*

**Ber·nard-Sou·li·er syndrome** (bār-nahr′ so͞ol-ya′) [Jean Alfred *Bernard,* French hematologist, born 1907; Jean-Pierre *Soulier,* French hematologist, born 1915] [MeSH: Bernard-Soulier Syndrome] see under *syndrome.*

**Ber·nays' sponge** (bər′nāz) [Augustus Charles *Bernays,* American surgeon, 1854–1907] see under *sponge.*

**Bern·hardt's disease, paresthesia** (bern′hahrts) [Martin *Bernhardt,* German neurologist, 1844–1915] meralgia paresthetica.

**Bern·hardt-Roth disease, syndrome** (bern′hahrt-rōt) [M. *Bernhardt;* Vladimir Karlovich *Roth,* Russian neurologist, 1848–1916] meralgia paresthetica.

**Bern·heim's syndrome** (bārn′hīmz) [P. *Bernheim,* French physician, early 20th century] see under *syndrome.*

**Ber·noul·li distribution, theorem, trial** (bər-noo′le, bār-noo-e′) [Jakob *Bernoulli,* Swiss mathematician, 1654–1705] see under *distribution, theorem,* and *trial.*

**Ber·o·tec** (ber′o-tek) trademark for a preparation of fenoterol hydrobromide.

**Ber·ry's ligament** (ber′ēz) [Sir James *Berry,* Canadian surgeon, 1860–1946] ligamentum thyroideum laterale.

**ber·ry** (ber′e) [MeSH: Fruit] a small fruit with a succulent pericarp.
**bear b.**, 1. *Arctostaphylos uva-ursi.* 2. the fruit of *A. uva-ursi.*
**buckthorn b.**, *Rhamnus cathartica.*
**horse nettle b.**, *Solanum carolinense.*

**Ber·the·lot reaction (reagent)** (bār-tə-lo′) [Pierre Eugène Marcellin *Berthelot,* French chemist, 1827–1907] see under *reaction.*

**Ber·ti·el·la** (bər″te-el′ə) a genus of tapeworms of the family Anoplocephalidae. *B. sa′tyri* (or *B. stu′deri*) is found in humans and other primates in India, Africa, the West Indies, the Philippines, and various islands in the Indian Ocean.

**ber·ti·el·li·a·sis** (bər″te-ə-li′ə-sis) infection with *Bertiella.*

**Ber·tin's bone (ossicles), column, ligament** (bār-taz′) [Exupère Joseph *Bertin,* French anatomist, 1712–1781] see *concha sphenoidalis, columnae renales,* and *ligamentum iliofemorale.*

**Ber·to·lot·ti's syndrome** (bār-to-lot′ēz) [Mario *Bertolotti,* Italian physician, born 1876] see under *syndrome.*

**Be·ru·bi·gen** (bə-roo′bĭ-jen) trademark for preparations of cyanocobalamin.

**ber·yl·li·o·sis** (bər-il″e-o′sis) [*beryllium* + *-osis*] [MeSH: Berylliosis] a hypersensitivity response to beryllium, usually involving the lungs and less often the skin, subcutaneous tissues, lymph nodes, liver, or other structures. Beryllium fumes, its oxide and salts, and finely divided dust all may cause a tissue reaction when inhaled or implanted in the skin. Two varieties are distinguished: *acute b.* and *chronic b.* Called also *beryllium poisoning.*
**acute b.**, an often fulminating reaction to inhalation of beryllium, characterized by a toxic or allergic pneumonitis, sometimes with rhinitis, pharyngitis, and tracheobronchitis. Symptoms may last for weeks, and serious cases can be fatal.
**chronic b.**, the usual form of berylliosis, characterized by beryllium granulomas (q.v.), a diffuse inflammatory reaction that may be indistinguishable from sarcoidosis, and sometimes dyspnea and hypertrophic pulmonary osteoarthropathy. In time the granulomas may combine to form pulmonary nodules with fibrosis.

**ber·yl·li·um** (bər-il′e-əm) [Gr. *bēryllos* beryl] [MeSH: Beryllium] a metallic element of atomic number 4, atomic weight 9.012, symbol Be. It is often found mixed with coal, and has many uses both in alloys and in pure form. Inhalation of its fumes causes berylliosis.

**bes·i·clom·e·ter** (bes″i-klom′ə-tər) [Fr. *besides* spectacles + *-meter*] an instrument for measuring the forehead to ascertain the proper width of spectacle frames.

**Bes·nier's prurigo** (ba-nyāz′) [Ernest *Besnier,* French dermatologist, 1831–1909] see *atopic dermatitis,* under *dermatitis,* and *prurigo gestationis of Besnier.*

**Bes·nier-Boeck disease** (ba-nya′ bek) [E. *Besnier;* Caesar P. M. *Boeck,* Norwegian dermatologist and syphilologist, 1845–1917] sarcoidosis.

**Bes·noi·tia** (bes-noi′te-ə) a genus of coccidian protozoa (suborder Eimeriina, order Eucoccidiida) whose oocysts resemble those of *Toxoplasma;* various species cause besnoitiosis in mammals. *B. bennet′ti* infects horses; *B. besnoi′ti* infects cattle; and *B. jelliso′ni* and *B. walla′cei* infect rodents.

**bes·noi·ti·o·sis** (bes-noi″te-o′sis) infection of cattle, horses, sheep, goats, or other herbivores with protozoa of the genus *Besnoitia,* transmitted mechanically by certain biting flies or by ingestion of oocysts shed in the feces of the cat, the definitive host. The organisms localize in the skin, blood vessels, mucous membranes of the upper respiratory tract, and subcutaneous and other tissues, where they eventually form characteristic thick-walled cysts. Other symptoms include fever, anasarca, loss of appetite, photophobia, rhinitis, sclerodermatitis, and alopecia of varying severity. Formerly called *globidiosis.*

**Best** (best) Charles Herbert. Canadian physiologist, born in the United States; he discovered histaminase and was associated with Sir Frederick Banting and John James Macleod in the discovery of insulin in 1922.

**Best's disease** (bests) [Franz *Best,* German ophthalmologist, 1878–1920] congenital macular degeneration; see under *degeneration.*

**bes·ti·al·i·ty** (bes-te-al′ĭ-te) [L. *bestia* beast] sexual connection with an animal. See also *zoophilia.*

**bes·y·late** (bes′ə-lāt) USAN contraction for benzenesulfonate.

**Be·ta** (be′tə) [L.] the beets, a genus of herbaceous plants of the family Chenopodiaceae. *B. vulga′ris* L. is the sugar beet, a commercial source of sucrose. The leafy tops of beets are rich in oxalates and can cause oxalate poisoning in animals that eat them in large amounts.

**be·ta** (ba′tə) [B, $\beta$] the second letter of the Greek alphabet. See also *$\beta$-.*

**Be·ta·bac·te·ri·um** (be″tə-bak-tēr′e-əm) [L. *beta* beet + Gr. *baktērion* little rod] in former systems of classification, a genus of bacteria made up of organisms now assigned to the genus *Lactobacillus.*

**be·ta·car·o·tene** (ba″tə-kar′ə-tēn) see under *carotene.*

**Be·ta-Chlor** (ba′tə-klōr) trademark for a preparation of chloral betaine.

**be·ta·cho·les·ta·nol** (ba″tə-ko-les′tə-nol) see under *cholestanol.*

**be·ta·cism** (ba′tə-siz-əm) [*beta*] a speech disorder involving excessive use of the *b* sound.

**be·ta·dex** (ba′tə-deks) [NF] $\beta$-cyclodextrin, a sequestrant used as a pharmaceutic aid; it has also been used as a carrier molecule for drug delivery. Called also *beta cyclodextrin.*

**Be·ta·dine** (ba′tə-dīn) trademark for preparations of povidone-iodine.

**be·ta glob·u·lin** (ba″tə-glob′u-lin) [MeSH: Beta-Globulins] see under *globulin.*
**pregnancy-specific b. g.**, a beta globulin secreted by the placenta; its function is unknown.

**Be·ta·her·pes·vi·ri·nae** (ba″tə-hər″pēz-vir-i′ne) [MeSH: Betaherpesvirinae] the cytomegalovirus group: a subfamily of viruses of the family Herpesviridae, containing the genera *Cytomegalovirus, Muromegalovirus,* and *Roseolovirus,* along with a number of species not yet assigned to a genus. See *cytomegalovirus.*

**be·ta·his·tine hy·dro·chlo·ride** (ba″tə-his′tēn) a histamine analogue used as a vasodilator to reduce the frequency of attacks of vertigo in Meniere's disease, especially in patients having a high frequency of such attacks; administered orally.

**be·ta·ine** (be′tə-ēn) [MeSH: Betaine] an oxidation product of choline which is a transmethylating intermediate in metabolism, and has been shown to have lipotropic activity. Betaine was first found in the sugar beet and was later shown to be present in many other plants and in animals. It is produced synthetically, and has been used in the treatment of muscular weakness and degeneration. The term has also been used to designate any of a class of trimethyl derivatives of amino acids, e.g., carnitine, or, more generally, the internal salts of quaternary ammonium bases. Called also *lycine* and *oxyneurine.*
**b. hydrochloride** [USP], the hydrochloride salt of betaine, which on hydrolysis yields hydrochloric acid; used as a gastric acidifier.

It has been used as a lipotropic agent in the treatment of fatty infiltration of the liver.

**Be·ta·lin** (ba'tə-lin) trademark for preparations containing components of the vitamin B complex. *Betalin Complex* is a sterile solution of synthetic B complex factors in sterile distilled water. *Betalin Complex F.C.* consists of synthetic vitamin B factors and synthetic ascorbic acid in sterile distilled water. *Betalin S* is a synthetic preparation of thiamine hydrochloride. *Betalin 12 crystalline* is a sterile isotonic solution of crystalline cyanocobalamin.

**be·ta·ly·sin** (ba″tə-li'sin) [so-called to distinguish it from antibodies, "alpha lysins"] a heat-stable cationic protein released by platelets during coagulation that is bactericidal for gram-positive bacteria with the exception of streptococci. Written also *beta lysin.*

**be·ta·meth·a·sone** (ba″tə-meth'ə-sōn) [USP] [MeSH: Betamethasone] a synthetic glucocorticoid, the most active of the anti-inflammatory steroids; used topically as an anti-inflammatory and administered orally in replacement therapy for adrenal insufficiency and as an anti-inflammatory and immunosuppressant in a wide variety of disorders.
**b. acetate** [USP], an ester of betamethasone, having the same actions as the base; used in combination with betamethasone sodium phosphate for intramuscular, intra-articular, intrasynovial, or intralesional injection.
**b. benzoate** [USP], the 17-benzoate ester of betamethasone, having the same actions as the base; used topically for the relief of inflammation and pruritus in corticosteroid-responsive dermatoses.
**b. dipropionate** [USP], the 17,21-dipropionate ester of betamethasone, having the same uses as the base; used topically for the relief of inflammation and pruritus in corticosteroid-responsive dermatoses.
**b. sodium phosphate** [USP], the disodium salt of the 21-phosphate ester of betamethasone, having the same actions as the base; used in combination with betamethasone acetate for intramuscular, intra-articular, intrasynovial, or intralesional injection.
**b. valerate** [USP], the 17-valerate ester of betamethasone, used topically for the relief of inflammation and pruritus in corticosteroid-responsive dermatoses.

**be·ta$_2$-mi·cro·glob·u·lin** (ba″tə-mi″kro-glob'u-lin) a small (mol. wt. 12,000), nonpolymorphic protein, homologous to the C3 domain of IgG, that is one subunit of class I major histocompatibility antigens.

**be·ta·naph·thol** (ba″tə-naf'thol) a form of naphthol, formerly used locally as a counterirritant in alopecia and as an anthelmintic; now used as a topical antiseptic, especially in fungal infections. Called also *isonaphthol.*

**be·ta·naph·thol·sul·fon·ic ac·id** (ba″tə-naf″thol-sul-fon'ik) white pearly scales tinged with red, $OH{\cdot}C_{10}H_6SO_2{\cdot}OH$, used as a test for albumin in the urine; it is a toxic drug that causes profound narcotism and symptoms resembling diabetic coma and is not used as a medication.

**be·ta·nin** (be'tə-nin) the red pigment of the root of the beet.

**Be·ta·pace** (ba'tə-pās″) trademark for a preparation of sotalol hydrochloride.

**Be·ta·par** (ba'tə-pahr) trademark for a preparation of meprednisone.

**Be·ta·pen-VK** (ba'tə-pen) trademark for a preparation of penicillin V potassium.

**Be·ta·prone** (ba'tə-prōn) trademark for a preparation of propiolactone.

**be·ta·pro·pio·lac·tone** (ba″tə-pro″pe-o-lak'tōn) propiolactone.

**be·ta·qui·nine** (ba″tə-kwi'nīn) quinidine.

**Be·ta·trex** (ba″tə-treks') trademark for preparations of betamethasone valerate.

**be·ta·tron** (ba'tə-tron) [MeSH: Particle Accelerators] an apparatus for accelerating electrons to millions of electron volts by means of magnetic induction.

**Beta-Val** (ba'tə-val″) trademark for preparations of betamethasone valerate.

**Be·tax·in** (be-tak'sin) trademark for preparations of thiamine hydrochloride.

**be·tax·o·lol hy·dro·chlo·ride** (ba-tak'sə-lol) [USP] a cardioselective beta-blocker that acts at *β*-adrenergic receptors; used as an antihypertensive and antianginal and also as an ophthalmic preparation to treat ocular hypertension and open-angle glaucoma.

**be·ta·zole hy·dro·chlo·ride** (ba'tə-zōl) an isomer of histamine that stimulates gastric secretion of hydrochloric acid; formerly used intramuscularly or subcutaneously in tests of gastric secretion.

**bête** (bet) [Fr.] beast.
**b. rouge,** (ro͞ozh) [Fr. "red beast"], chigger.

**be·tel** (be'təl) [Tamil *vettilei*] 1. *Piper betle.* 2. a masticatory used in India and Southeast Asia, consisting of a piece of areca (betel nut) rolled up with lime in a leaf of *P. betle* (betel leaf); it is tonic, astringent, and stimulant.

**be·than·e·chol chlo·ride** (bə-than'ə-kol) [USP] a cholinergic agonist having primarily muscarinic effects; used to stimulate smooth muscle contraction of the urinary bladder and gastrointestinal tract in the treatment of postoperative, postpartum, or neurogenic atony of the bladder with retention, postoperative atony of the gastrointestinal tract, congenital megacolon, and gastrointestinal reflux. Administered orally or subcutaneously.

**be·than·i·dine sul·fate** (bə-than'ĭ-dēn) an adrenergic neuron-blocking agent used in the treatment of essential hypertension, particularly in the malignant phase.

**Be·thea's sign (method)** (bə-tha'əz) [Oscar Walter *Bethea,* American physician, 1878–1963] see under *sign.*

**Be·thes·da Sys·tem** (bə-thez'də) [*Bethesda,* Maryland, location of the National Cancer Institute, which sponsored its development] see under *system.*

**Be·top·tic** (ba-top'tik) trademark for a preparation of betaxolol hydrochloride.

**Bet·u·la** (bet'u-lə) [L.] the birches, a genus of deciduous trees of the family Betulaceae, native to the Northern Hemisphere. *B. al'ba* L. is the white birch, whose bark yields rectified birch tar oil. *B. len'ta* is the black birch, whose bark is an important commercial source of methyl salicylate.

**Betz's cells, cell area** (bet'zəs) [Vladimir Aleksandrovich *Betz,* Russian anatomist, 1834–1894] see under *cell,* and see *primary somatomotor area,* under *area.*

**BeV, Bev** billion electron volts, now largely replaced by the term *gigaelectron volt* (GeV).

**Bev·an's incision, operation** (bev'ənz) [Arthur Dean *Bevan,* American surgeon, 1861–1943] see under *incision* and *operation.*

**bev·el** (bev'əl) 1. a slanting edge. 2. to produce a slanting of the enamel margins of a tooth cavity.

**Bev·i·dox** (bev'ĭ-doks) trademark for a solution of vitamin $B_{12}$; see *cyanocobalamin.*

**be·zoar** (be'zor) [Farsi *pādzohr* antidote to poison] [MeSH: Bezoars] a concretion of foreign material found in the stomach or intestines of humans or other animals; there are three types: trichobezoar (hair), phytobezoar (fruit and vegetable fibers), and trichophytobezoar (a mixture of hair and fruit and vegetable fibers).

**Be·zold's abscess,** etc. (bāt'solts) [Friedrich *Bezold,* German otologist, 1842–1908] see under *abscess, mastoiditis, perforation, sign,* and *triad.*

**Be·zold's ganglion, reflex** (bāt'sōlts) [Albert von *Bezold,* German physiologist, 1836–1868] see under *ganglion* and *reflex.*

**Be·zold-Jar·isch reflex** (bāt'sōlt-yah'rish) [A. von *Bezold;* Adolf *Jarisch,* Austrian dermatologist, 1850–1902] Bezold reflex.

**BF** blastogenic factor; see *lymphocyte mitogenic factor,* under *factor.*

**β1F** former name for complement factor *C5;* see under *complement.*

**BFP** biologic false-positive; see under *false-positive.*

**BFU-E** burst-forming unit–erythroid.

**β1H** former name for complement *factor H;* see under *complement.*

**BHA** butylated hydroxyanisole.

**BHCDA** Bureau of Health Care Delivery and Assistance, an agency of the Health Resources and Services Administration.

**BHPR** Bureau of Health Professions, an agency of the Health Resources and Services Administration.

**BHRD** Bureau of Health Resources Development, an agency of the Health Resources and Services Administration.

**BHT** butylated hydroxytoluene.

**Bi** symbol for *bismuth.*

**bi-** [L. *bi-,* from *bis* twice] a prefix meaning two, twice, or double. In chemistry, it denotes the presence of a component in twice the proportion of the other component or in twice the usual proportion, or a double radical, except that in bicarbonate, bisulfate, and bitartrate, the prefix *di-* is preferred. Before vowels it appears as *bin-.*

**bi·acro·mi·al** (bi-ə-kro'me-əl) between the two acromia.

**Bi·al's reagent, test** (be'əlz) [Manfred *Bial,* German physician, 1870–1908] see under *reagent* and *test.*

**bi·al·lyl·am·i·col** (bi-al″əl-am'ĭ-kol) former name for bialamicol hydrochloride.

**Bi·an·chi's nodules, valve** (be-ahng'kēz) [Giovanni Battista *Bian-*

*chi,* Italian anatomist, 1681–1761] see *noduli valvularum semilunarium valvae aortae,* and see under *valve.*

**bi·ar·tic·u·lar** (bi″ahr-tik′u-lər) pertaining to two joints.

**bi·ar·tic·u·late** (bi″ahr-tik′u-lāt) having two joints.

**bi·as** (bi′əs) 1. (in a measurement process) systematic error. 2. (of a statistical estimator) the difference between the expected value of the estimator and the true parameter value.
**conservative b.,** a bias in study design that makes it less likely to find a true difference than it would be with an unbiased study.
**lead-time b.,** systematic error introduced when monitoring of all groups or individuals does not begin at precisely the same time, such as an illusion of longer survival that is really due to earlier diagnosis of the disease.
**measurement b.,** that due to systematic error in measurement during data collection.
**misclassification b.,** see *misclassification.*
**recall b.,** systematic error due to differential recall across subjects, particularly a tendency for cases to remember more events from the study period than do controls.
**selection b.,** systematic error in the manner in which cases and controls are chosen for a study or for allocation to groups.
**surveillance b.,** increased detection of signs or symptoms, many of which would otherwise go unnoticed, caused by increased frequency and intensity of surveillance, as that of subjects under treatment in a study.

**bi·as·ter·ic** (bi″əs-ter′ik) pertaining to the two asteria, especially to the shortest distance between them (biasteric width).

**bi·au·ric·u·lar** (bi″aw-rik′u-lər) [*bi-* + *auricular*] pertaining to the two auricles of the ears. Called also *binauricular.*

**Bi·ax·in** (bi-ak′sin) trademark for a preparation of clarithromycin.

**Bib.** abbreviation for L. *bi′be,* drink.

**bib** (bib) the remaining fragment of an erythrocyte in which the crescentic gametocyte of *Plasmodium falciparum* is developing in malaria.

**bi·ba·sic** (bi-ba′sik) doubly basic; having two hydrogen atoms that may react with bases. Cf. *dibasic.*

**bi·bev·eled** (bi-bev′əld) having a slanting surface on two sides, as some dental instruments; hatchet-edged.

**bib·lio·ther·a·py** (bib″le-o-ther′ə-pe) [Gr. *biblion* book + *therapy*] [MeSH: Bibliotherapy] the reading of selected books as part of the treatment of mental disorders or for mental health.

**bib·u·lous** (bib′u-ləs) [L. *bibulus,* from *bibere* to drink] 1. absorbent or spongy. 2. having the property of absorbing moisture. Cf. *hygroscopic.*

**bi·ca·lu·ta·mide** (bi″kə-loo′tə-mīd) an androgen antagonist used as a treatment adjunct, in combination with a luteinizing hormone–releasing hormone analogue, in the treatment of prostatic carcinoma; administered orally.

**bi·cam·er·al** (bi-kam′ər-əl) [*bi-* + *camera*] having two chambers.

**bi·cap·su·lar** (bi-kap′su-lər) [*bi-* + *capsular*] having two capsules, as an articular capsule.

**bi·car·bo·nate** (bi-kahr′bə-nāt) any salt containing the $HCO_3^-$ anion.
**blood b., plasma b.,** the bicarbonate of the blood, an index of the alkali reserve.
**b. of soda,** sodium bicarbonate.
**standard b.,** the plasma bicarbonate concentration in blood equilibrated with a gas mixture having a $P_{CO_2}$ of 40 mm Hg and a $P_{O_2}$ over 100 mm Hg at 37°C.

**bi·cau·dal** (bi-kaw′dəl) [*bi-* + *caudal*] having two tails.

**bi·cau·date** (bi-kaw′dāt) bicaudal.

**bi·cel·lu·lar** (bi-sel′u-lər) made up of two cells, or having two cells.

**bi·ceph·a·lus** (bi-sef′ə-ləs) dicephalus.

**bi·ceps** (bi′seps) [*bi-* + L. *caput* head] a muscle having two heads.
**b. bra′chii,** see under *musculus.*
**b. fem′oris,** see under *musculus.*

**Bi·chat's fissure, ligament,** etc. (be-shahz′) [Marie François Xavier *Bichat,* French anatomist and physiologist, 1771–1802, founder of scientific histology and pathological anatomy] see under *ligament,* see *fenestrated membrane* under *membrane,* and see *fissura transversa cerebri* and *tunica intima vasorum.*

**bi·chlo·ride** (bi-klor′īd) any chloride that contains two equivalents of chlorine.

**bi·chro·mate** (bi-kro′māt) dichromate.

**Bi·cil·lin** (bi′sĭ-lin) trademark for a preparation of penicillin G benzathine.

**bi·cip·i·tal** (bi-sip′ĭ-təl) 1. having two heads. 2. pertaining to a biceps muscle.

**bi·cir·o·mab** (bi-sir′o-mab) mouse anti-human monoclonal antibody to fibrin; used in the radioactive form (complexed with technetium 99m) in the diagnosis of deep vein thrombosis. See table at *technetium.*

**bi·cis·ate** (bi-sis′āt) ECD; ethyl cysteinate dimer, a lipophilic amine having the ability to cross the blood-brain barrier and localize in the brain; complexed with technetium 99m, it is used in imaging of the cerebrovascular system, giving a static image of regional cerebral blood flow. See table at *technetium.*

**Bic·ker·staff's migraine** (bik′ər-stafs) [Edwin Robert *Bickerstaff,* British physician, born 1920] basilar migraine.

**BiCNU** (bik′noo) trademark for preparations of carmustine.

**bi·col·lis** (bi-kol′is) [L., from *bi-* + *collum*] having a double cervix; see *uterus bicornis bicollis,* under *uterus.*

**bi·con·cave** (bi″kon-kāv′) [*bi-* + *concave*] having two concave surfaces, as the opposite sides of a structure.

**bi·con·vex** (bi″kon-veks′) having two convex surfaces, as the opposite sides of a structure.

**bi·cor·nate** (bi-kor′nāt) bicornuate.

**bi·cor·nu·ate** (bi-kor′nu-āt) [*bi-* + *cornuate*] having two horns or horn-shaped branches, as the uterus of humans and most other mammals.

**bi·co·ro·nal** (bi-kə-ro′nəl) 1. pertaining to the two coronae radiatae, one radiating from each internal capsule of the brain. 2. pertaining to or performed through both coronal sutures.

**bi·cor·po·rate** (bi-kor′pə-rət) [*bi-* + *corpora* + *-ate*] having two bodies.

**bi·cu·cul·line** (bi-koo′kə-lēn″) [MeSH: Bicuculline] an alkaloid neurotoxin found in species of *Corydalis, Dicentra,* and other plants; it is a convulsant and acts as an antagonist to the inhibitory neurotransmitter $\gamma$-aminobutyric acid.

**bi·cus·pid** (bi-kus′pid) [*bi-* + *cuspid*] [MeSH: Bicuspid] 1. having two cusps or points. 2. pertaining to a bicuspid valve of the heart. 3. premolar tooth.

**bi·cus·pi·dal** (bi-kus′pĭ-dəl) 1. pertaining to a bicuspid tooth (premolar tooth). 2. having two cusps.

**bi·cus·pi·date** (bi-kus′pĭ-dāt) having two cusps.

**bi·cus·poid** (bi-kus′poid) a figure in space resembling a bicuspid tooth (premolar tooth) and representing the space traversed in all its movements by a point in one jaw in relation to the other jaw.

**b.i.d.** abbreviation for L. *bis in di′e,* twice a day.

**Bid·der's ganglia, organ** (bid′ərz) [Heinrich Friedrich *Bidder,* Estonian anatomist, 1810–1894] see under *ganglion* and *organ.*

**bi·den·tal** (bi-den′təl) [*bi-* + *dental*] having, pertaining to, or affecting two teeth.

**bi·den·tate** (bi-den′tāt) having two teeth or toothlike structures.

**bi·der·mo·ma** (bi″dər-mo′mə) didermoma.

**Bie·der·man's sign** (be′dər-mənz) [Joseph Bear *Biederman,* American physician, born 1907] see under *sign.*

**Biedl's disease, syndrome** (be′dəlz) [Artur *Biedl,* Austrian physician, 1869–1933] Bardet-Biedl syndrome.

**Biels·chow·sky's head tilting test** (byels-chov′skēz) [Alfred *Bielschowsky,* German ophthalmologist, 1871–1940] see under *test.*

**Biels·chow·sky's method** (byels-chov′skēz) [Max *Bielschowsky,* German neuropathologist, 1869–1940] see under *stain.*

**Biels·chow·sky-Jan·ský disease** (byels-chov′ske yahn′ske) [A. *Bielschowsky;* Jan *Janský,* Czech psychiatrist, 1873–1921] Janský-Bielschowsky disease; see under *disease.*

**Bie·mond syndrome** (be-maw′) [A. *Biemond,* French physician, born 1902] see under *syndrome.*

**Bier's amputation, anesthesia** (bērz) [August Karl Gustav *Bier,* German surgeon, 1861–1949] see under *amputation* and *block.*

**Bier·nac·ki's sign** (byer-naht′skēz) [Edmund Adolfevich *Biernacki,* Polish physician, 1866–1912] see under *sign.*

**Bie·sia·dec·ki's fossa** (byĕ-syah-det′skēz) [Alfred von *Biesiadecki,* Polish physician, 1839–1888] fossa iliacosubfascialis.

**Biette's collarette** (byets) [Laurent Théodore *Biette,* French dermatologist, 1781–1840] see under *collarette.*

**bi·fe·ri·ens** (bi-fer′e-ənz) [L.] bisferious.

**bi·fer·i·ous** (bi-fer′e-əs) [*bi-* + L. *ferire* to beat] bisferious.

**bi•fid** (bi'fid) [L. *bifidus* divided into two parts] cleft into two parts or branches.

**Bi•fid•o•bac•te•ri•um** (bi"fid-o-bak-tēr'e-əm) [*bifidus* + *bacterium*] [MeSH: Bifidobacterium] a genus of gram-positive, anaerobic bacteria of the family Actinomycetaceae, occurring as irregularly staining rods of bifurcated Y and V forms and club or spatulate shapes.
**B. adolescen'tis,** a species isolated from human feces, the appendix, the vagina, dental caries, and abscesses.
**B. bi'fidum,** a species found in the alimentary tract and in the stools of breast- and bottle-fed infants and in human adults. Called also *Lactobacillus bifidum.*
**B. cornu'tum,** *Eubacterium lentum.*
**B. erikso'nii,** a species that has been isolated from the feces and from subcutaneous and pulmonary lesions of humans. Called also *Actinomyces eriksonii.*
**B. infan'tis,** a species that is the predominant bifidobacterium found in the feces of breast-fed infants.

**bi•fid•o•bac•te•ri•um** (bi"fid-o-bak-tēr'e-əm) pl. *bifidobacte'ria* [MeSH: Bifidobacterium] any bacterium of the genus *Bifidobacterium.*

**bif•i•dus** (bif'ĭ-dəs) bifid.

**bi•fo•cal** (bi'fo-kəl) 1. having two foci. 2. pertaining to the compound spectacle, which contains a smaller lens for near vision placed below the center of the larger lens, which is for distant vision. 3. (pl.) bifocal glasses.

**bi•fo•rate** (bi-for'āt) [*bi-* + L. *fora* opening] having two foramina or openings.

**bi•for•myl** (bi-for'məl) glyoxal.

**bi•fur•cate** (bi-fər'kāt) [L. *bifurcatus,* from *bi-* + *furca* fork] forked; divided into two branches.

**bi•fur•ca•tio** (bi"fər-ka'she-o) pl. *bifurcatio'nes* [L.] [TA] bifurcation; the site where a single structure divides into two, as in blood vessels or teeth.
**b. aor'tae** [TA], **b. aor'tica,** bifurcation of aorta: the site on the left side of the body of the fourth lumbar vertebra, where the abdominal aorta divides into the right and left common iliac arteries.
**b. caro'tidis** [TA], carotid bifurcation: the site where the common carotid artery divides into the external carotid artery and internal carotid artery, usually marked by a dilatation, the carotid sinus.
**b. tra'cheae** [TA], bifurcation of trachea: the site of division of the trachea into the right and left main bronchi.
**b. trun'ci pulmona'lis** [TA], bifurcation of pulmonary trunk: the site of the division of the pulmonary trunk into right and left pulmonary arteries.

**bi•fur•ca•tion** (bi"fər-ka'shən) [L. *bifurcatio,* from *bi-* + *furca* fork] 1. division into two branches. 2. bifurcatio.
**b. of aorta,** bifurcatio aortae.
**carotid b.,** bifurcatio carotidis.
**b. of pulmonary trunk,** bifurcatio trunci pulmonalis.
**b. of trachea,** bifurcatio tracheae.

**bi•fur•ca•ti•o•nes** (bi"fər-ka"she-o'nēz) [L.] plural of *bifurcatio.*

**Big•e•low's ligament, operation, septum** (big'ə-lōz) [Henry Jacob *Bigelow,* American surgeon, 1818–1890] see *ligamentum iliofemorale,* see *litholapaxy,* and see under *septum.*

**bi•gem•i•na** (bi-jem'ĭ-nə) 1. plural of *bigeminum.* 2. bigeminal pulse.

**bi•gem•i•nal** (bi-jem'ĭ-nəl) 1. twin. 2. pertaining to bigeminy.

**bi•gem•i•num** (bi-jem'ĭ-nəm) pl. *bigem'ina* [L. "twin"] either of the corpora bigemina; see under *corpus.*

**bi•gem•i•ny** (bi-jem'ĭ-ne) [*bi-* + *geminus*] 1. occurring in pairs. 2. the occurrence of a bigeminal pulse.
**atrial b.,** an arrhythmia consisting of the repetitive sequence of one atrial premature complex followed by one normal sinus impulse.

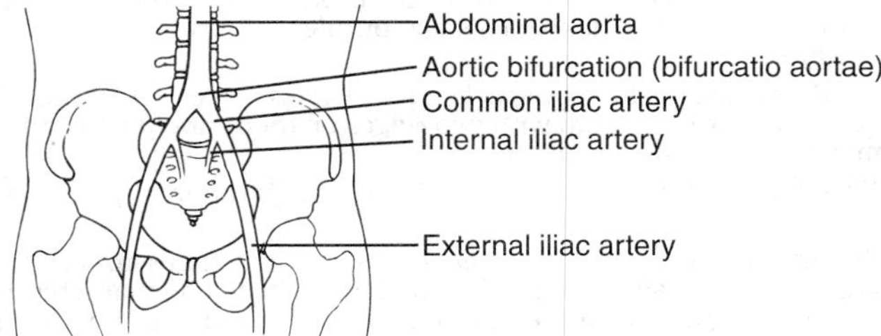


Bifurcatio aortae (aortic bifurcation), showing the branching of the abdominal aorta into the common iliac arteries, and from there to the internal and external iliac arteries.

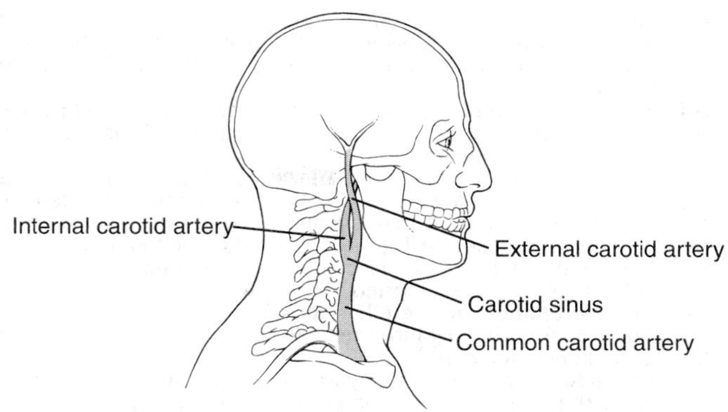


Bifurcatio carotidis (carotid bifurcation).

**atrioventricular nodal b.,** an arrhythmia in which an atrioventricular extrasystole is followed by a normal sinus impulse in repetitive sequence.
**nodal b.,** atrioventricular nodal b.
**ventricular b.,** an arrhythmia consisting of the repeated sequence of one ventricular premature complex followed by one normal beat.

**bi•ger•mi•nal** (bi-jər'mĭ-nəl) pertaining to two germs or ova.

**big•head** (big'hed) 1. bulging of the skull bones of an animal, due to osteomalacia. 2. acute infection of young rams by *Clostridium novyi,* which enters the tissues through head wounds acquired in fighting; it is characterized by intense edematous swelling of the head, face, and neck. Called also *swellhead* and *swelled head.* 3. photosensitization in white-faced sheep after ingestion of certain plants, characterized by thickening and pendulous swelling of the face and ears. 4. hydrocephalus in mink. 5. nutritional secondary hyperparathyroidism.

**bi•go•ni•al** (bi-go'ne-əl) connecting the two gonions.

**bi•labe** (bi'lāb) [*bi-* + *labium*] an instrument for taking small calculi from the bladder through the urethra.

**bi•la•bi•al** (bi-la'be-əl) a consonantal speech sound produced using the two lips, such as *b, p,* or *m.* Called also *labial.*

**bi•lam•i•nar** (bi-lam'ĭ-nər) [*bi-* + *laminar*] having or pertaining to two layers, as the basement membrane that comprises the basal lamina and the reticular lamina.

**Bil•ar•cil** (bil-ahr'sil) trademark for preparations of metrifonate.

**bi•lat•er•al** (bi-lat'ər-əl) [*bi-* + *lateral*] having two sides, or pertaining to both sides.

**bi•lat•er•al•ism** (bi-lat'ər-əl-iz-əm) bilateral symmetry.

**bi•lay•er** (bi'la-ər) a membrane consisting of two molecular layers, such as the cell membrane or the envelope of some viruses.

**bile** (bīl) [L. *bilis*] [MeSH: Bile] a fluid secreted by the liver and poured into the small intestine via the bile ducts. Important constituents are conjugated bile salts, cholesterol, phospholipid, bilirubin diglucuronide, and electrolytes. Bile is alkaline due to its bicarbonate content, is golden brown to greenish yellow in color, and has a bitter taste. Bile secreted by the liver (see *A b.*) is concentrated in the gallbladder. Its formation depends on active secretion by liver cells into the bile canaliculi. Excretion of bile salts by liver cells and secretion of bicarbonate rich fluid by ductular cells in response to secretin are the major factors which normally determine the volume of secretion. Conjugated bile salts and phospholipid normally dissolve cholesterol in a mixed micellar solution. In the upper small intestine, bile is in part responsible for alkalinizing

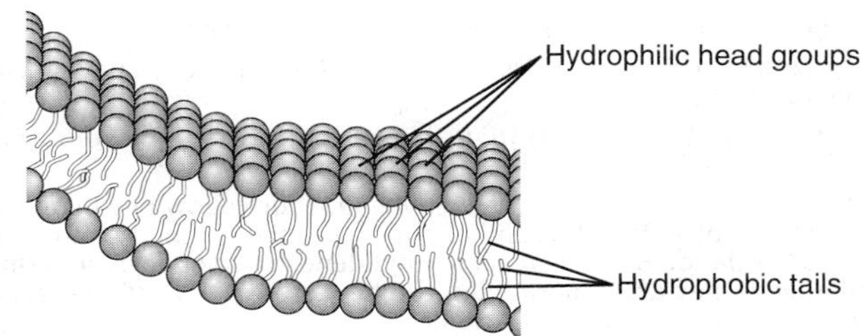


Lipid bilayer, a fluid barrier to permeability, with polar head groups exposed and hydrophobic tails sequestered.

the intestinal content, and conjugated bile salts play an essential role in fat absorption by dissolving the products of fat digestion (fatty acids and monoglycerides) in water soluble micelles. Called also *fel* and *gall.*

**A b.,** bile from the common bile duct; samples are obtained by use of a duodenal tube before gallbladder stimulation. It usually contains 20–200 mg. of bilirubin per 100 mL.

**B b.,** bile from the gallbladder; samples are obtained by use of a duodenal tube after gallbladder contraction stimulation, usually with magnesium sulfate. It may occur despite absence of the gallbladder and contains up to 1 gram of bilirubin per 100 mL.

**C b.,** hepatic bile; it is obtained from a duodenal drainage tube after the gallbladder has been emptied.

**cystic b., gallbladder b.,** the bile that is held for some time in the gallbladder before moving into the intestine.

**limy b.,** milk of calcium b.

**milk of calcium b.,** bile containing an increased amount of calcium, usually as the carbonate but sometimes as the phosphate or bilirubinate. It varies in consistency from a thick, milky fluid to a putty, gel, or solid. It is usually suspended in a thin, more watery bile. Called also *limy b.*

**ox b.,** the fresh bile of the ox, a brownish green to dark green viscous fluid; the extract is used as a choleretic. Called also *fel bovis* and *oxgall.*

**white b.,** the colorless liquid containing mucoproteins and calcium salts sometimes found in the gallbladder in obstructions above the entrance of the cystic duct. Its accumulation in the distended biliary tract is called *hydrops.*

**bile ac·id** (bīl) any of the steroid carboxylic acids derived from cholesterol. The *primary bile acids,* cholic and chenodeoxycholic acids, are formed in the liver and conjugated to glycine or taurine forming bile salts (e.g., cholylglycine), which are secreted in the bile and aid in the digestion of fats. *Secondary bile acids,* deoxycholic, lithocholic, and ursodeoxycholic acids, are formed from the primary bile acids by the action of intestinal bacteria, either as bile salts or as deconjugated bile acids. Most of the bile acids are reabsorbed and returned to the liver via enterohepatic circulation, where, after free acids are reconjugated, they are again excreted. Because the lithocolyl conjugates are relatively insoluble they are excreted mostly in the form of sulfate esters (e.g., sulfolithocholylglycine) produced by the liver.

**Bil·har·zia** (bil-hahr'ze-ə) [Theodor Maximilian *Bilharz,* German physician, 1825–1862] *Schistosoma.*

**bil·har·zi·al** (bil-hahr'ze-əl) schistosomal.

**bil·har·zi·a·sis** (bil″hahr-zi'ə-sis) schistosomiasis.

**bil·har·zic** (bil-hahr'zik) schistosomal.

**bil·har·zi·o·ma** (bil-hahr″ze-o'mə) a tumor in the skin or mucous membrane caused by a schistosome. Cf. *schistosomal bladder carcinoma.*

**bil·har·zi·o·sis** (bil-hahr″ze-o'sis) schistosomiasis.

**bili-** [L. *bilis* bile] a combining form denoting relationship to the bile.

**bil·i·a·ry** (bil'e-ar-e) pertaining to the bile, to the bile ducts, or to the gallbladder. See also *bilious.*

**bil·i·cy·a·nin** (bil″ĭ-si'ə-nin) [*bili-* + L. *cyaneus* blue] a blue pigment derivable from biliverdin by oxidation; called also *cholecyanin* and *cholocyanin.*

**bil·i·fla·vin** (bil″ĭ-fla'vin) [*bili-* + L. *flavus* yellow] a yellow pigment obtainable from biliverdin.

**bil·i·ful·vin** (bil″ĭ-ful'vin) [*bili-* + L. *fulvus* tawny] an impure bilirubin of a tawny color; also a tawny pigment from extract of ox bile; not normally found in healthy human bile.

**bil·i·fus·cin** (bil″ĭ-fus'in) [*bili-* + L. *fuscus* brown] a pigment from human bile and gallstones.

**bil·i·gen·e·sis** (bil″ĭ-jen'ə-sis) the production or formation of bile.

**bil·i·ge·net·ic** (bil″ĭ-jə-net'ik) 1. pertaining to biligenesis. 2. biligenic.

**bil·i·gen·ic** (bil″ĭ-jen'ik) [*bili-* + *-genic*] producing bile.

**bi·lig·u·late** (bi-lig'u-lāt) [*bi-* + L. *ligula* little tongue] having two tonguelike structures.

**bil·i·hu·min** (bil″ĭ-hu'min) [*bili-* + L. *humus* earth] an insoluble ingredient of gallstones.

**bi·lin** (bi'lin) [L. *bilis* bile] collective name for yellow bile pigments including i-urobilin, stercobilin, and d-urobilin, formed by spontaneous oxidation of the central methylidene group of corresponding bilinogen; they are generated in the final steps of bilirubin catabolism.

**bil·ious** (bil'yəs) [L. *biliosus*] characterized by bile, by excess of bile, or by biliousness. See also *biliary.*

**bil·ious·ness** (bil'yəs-nəs) a symptom complex comprising nausea, abdominal discomfort, headache, and constipation, formerly attributed to excessive secretion of bile.

**bil·i·pra·sin** (bil″ĭ-pra'sin) [*bili-* + Gr. *prasinos* green] a green pigment from gallstones.

**bil·i·ra·chia** (bil″ĭ-ra'ke-ə) [*bili-* + *rachi-* + *-ia*] the presence of bile pigments in the spinal fluid.

**bil·i·ru·bin** (bil″ĭ-roo'bin) [*bili-* + *ruber*] [MeSH: Bilirubin] a bile pigment; it is a breakdown product of heme mainly formed from the degradation of erythrocyte hemoglobin in reticuloendothelial cells, but also formed by breakdown of other heme pigments, e.g., cytochromes. Bilirubin normally circulates in plasma as a complex with albumin, and is taken up by the liver cells and conjugated to form bilirubin diglucuronide, which is the water-soluble pigment excreted in bile. In patients with cholestasis conjugated bilirubin (bilirubin diglucuronide) accumulates in the blood and tissues and is excreted in the urine; unconjugated bilirubin is not excreted in the urine. High concentrations of bilirubin may result in jaundice.

**conjugated b., direct b.,** bilirubin that has been taken up by the liver cells and conjugated to form the water-soluble bilirubin diglucuronide.

**indirect b.,** unconjugated b.

**unconjugated b.,** the lipid-soluble form of bilirubin that circulates in loose association with the plasma proteins; called also *indirect b.*

**bil·i·ru·bi·nate** (bil″ĭ-roo'bĭ-nāt) a salt of bilirubin.

**bil·i·ru·bin·emia** (bil″ĭ-roo″bĭ-ne'me-ə) the presence of bilirubin in the blood; see *hyperbilirubinemia.*

**bil·i·ru·bin·ic** (bil″ĭ-roo-bin'ik) pertaining to bilirubin.

**bil·i·ru·bin UDPglu·cu·ron·yl·trans·fer·ase** (bil″ĭ-roo'bin gloo-ku'ron-əl-trans″fər-ās) former name for an enzyme of the glucuronosyltransferase family.

**bil·i·ru·bin·uria** (bil″ĭ-roo″bĭ-nu're-ə) presence of bilirubin in the urine.

**bi·lis** (bi'lis) [L.] bile.

**b. bovi'na, b. buba'ta,** ox bile extract; see under *extract.*

**bil·i·uria** (bil″ĭ-u're-ə) [*bili-* + *-uria*] the presence of bile pigments in the urine.

**bil·i·ver·din** (bil″ĭ-vər'din) [*bili-* + L. *viridis* green] a green pigment, the initial bile pigment from catabolism of hemoglobin, converted to bilirubin by reduction of a methene bridge; it may arise from air oxidation of bilirubin. Called also *dehydrobilirubin.*

**bil·i·ver·di·nate** (bil″ĭ-vər'dĭ-nāt) a salt of biliverdin.

**bil·i·ver·din re·duc·tase** (bil″ĭ-vər'din re-duk'tās) [EC 1.3.1.24] an enzyme of the oxidoreductase class that catalyzes the reduction of biliverdin to bilirubin, using NADH or NADPH as an electron donor; the reaction is a step in heme catabolism.

**bil·i·xan·thin, bil·i·xan·thine** (bil″ĭ-zan'thin, bil″ĭ-zan'thēn) [*bili-* + Gr. *xanthos* yellow] choletelin.

**Bill·roth's cords, disease,** etc. (bil'rōts) [Christian Albert Theodor *Billroth,* German surgeon in Austria, 1829–1894] see under *cord, disease, operation,* and *strand.*

**bi·lo·bate** (bi-lo'bāt) [*bi-* + *lobate*] having two lobes.

**bi·lob·u·lar** (bi-lob'u-lər) having two lobules.

**bi·lob·u·late** (bi-lob'u-lāt) bilobular.

**bi·loc·u·lar** (bi-lok'u-lər) [*bi-* + *locular*] having two compartments.

**bi·loc·u·late** (bi-lok'u-lāt) bilocular.

**bi·lo·ma** (bi'lo-mə) an encapsulated collection of bile in the peritoneal cavity.

**Bi·lo·phi·la** (bi-lof'ĭ-lə) [L. *bilis* bile + Gr. *philos* loving] a genus of gram-negative, anaerobic, bile-tolerant, nonmotile, rod-shaped bacteria, originally isolated from infections of the vermiform appendix and from human feces.

**B. wadswor'thia,** a $\beta$-lactamase species that causes intra-abdominal infections; it has also been isolated in other infections, including pericarditis, empyema, bacteremia, purulent arthritis, and soft tissue infection.

**bi·loph·odont** (bi-lof'ə-dont) [*bi-* + Gr. *lophos* ridge + *odous* tooth] having molariform teeth with two ridges on them; applied to certain mammals, e.g., the kangaroo.

**Bil·tri·cide** (bil'trĭ-sīd) trademark for a preparation of praziquantel.

**Bim·a·na** (bim'ə-nə) [*bi-* + *manus*] a name sometimes applied to a group of mammals distinguished by having hands of character different from that of the feet; humans are the only species in the group.

**bi·man·u·al** (bi-man'u-əl) [*bi-* + *manual*] with both hands; performed by both hands.

**bi·mas·toid** (bi-mas'toid) pertaining to both mastoid processes.

**bi•max•il•lary** (bi-mak'sĭ-lar"e) pertaining to or affecting both jaws.

**Bim•ler's appliance** (bim'lerz) [H.P. *Bimler,* German orthodontist, 20th century] see under *appliance.*

**bi•mo•dal** (bi-mo'dəl) having two modes; of a graph, having two maxima.

**bi•mo•lec•u•lar** (bi"mo-lek'u-lər) relating to or formed from two molecules.

**bin-** see *bi-.*

**bin•an•gle** (bin'ang-gəl) having two angles; a dental instrument having two angulations in the shank connecting the handle, or shaft, with the working portion of the instrument, known as the blade, or nib.

**bi•na•ry** (bi'nar-e) [L. *binarius* of two] 1. made up of two elements. 2. denoting a number system with a base of two.

**bi•nau•ral** (bi-naw'rəl) [*bin-* + *aural*] pertaining to both ears; called also *binotic.*

**bi•nau•ric•u•lar** (bi"naw-rik'u-lər) [*bin-* + *auricular*] biauricular.

**bind** (bīnd) 1. to wrap with a binder or bandage. 2. to form a weak, reversible chemical bond, e.g., antigen to antibody or hormone to receptor. 3. a predicament or dilemma.
**double b.,** a situation in which one person receives conflicting messages from another and in which response to either message, recognition of the conflict, or withdrawal is met with rejection or disapproval; thought to be a characteristic mode of interaction in some families of schizophrenics and in other dysfunctional families.
**nail b.,** foot pain and lameness in a horse due to a horseshoe nail having been driven close to, but not into, the soft tissue. If a nail penetrates soft tissue, the condition is called *pricked foot* or *nail prick.*

**bind•er** (bīnd'ər) an abdominal girdle or bandage, especially one applied after childbirth to support the relaxed abdominal walls.

**bi•neg•a•tive** (bi-neg'ə-tiv) having two negative charges, especially in ions such as $SO_4^{2-}$.

**binge** (binj') 1. a period of uncontrolled or excessive self-indulgent activity, particularly of eating or drinking. 2. to engage in such activity. See also under *eating.*

**binge•ing** (binj'ing) engaging in a binge, particularly of eating; see also *binge eating,* under *eating.*

**Bi•net's test** (be-nāz') [Alfred *Binet,* French psychologist, 1857–1911] see under *test.*

**Bi•net-Si•mon test** (be-na'-se-maw') [A. *Binet;* Théodore *Simon,* French physician, 1873–1961] Binet's test.

**Bing's test** (bingz) [Albert *Bing,* German otologist, 1844–1922] see under *test.*

**Bing-Neel syndrome** (bing-nāl) [Jens *Bing,* Danish physician, born 1906; Axel Valdemar *Neel,* Danish physician, 1878–1952] see under *syndrome.*

**bin•ir•a•my•cin** (bĭ-nēr"ə-mi'sin) an antibacterial substance produced by a variant of *Streptomyces bikiniensis.*

**bin•oc•u•lar** (bĭ-nok'u-lər) [*bin-* + *ocular*] 1. pertaining to both eyes. 2. having two eyepieces, as in a microscope.

**bi•no•mi•al** (bi-nōm'e-əl) [*bi-* + L. *nomen* name] 1. composed of two names, as the scientific names of organisms formed by combination of genus and species names (binomial nomenclature). 2. a mathematical expression obtained by taking powers of the sums or differences of two terms; see *binomial coefficient* and *distribution,* under *coefficient* and *distribution.*

**bin•oph•thal•mo•scope** (bin"of-thal'mə-skōp) [*bin-* + *ophthalmoscope*] an ophthalmoscope for examining both fundi of the patient at one time.

**bino•scope** (bin'o-skōp) [L. *bini* two + *-scope*] an instrument for inducing binocular vision in squint by presenting one object in the central part of the field of vision, the peripheral parts of the field being screened out.

**bin•ot•ic** (bin-ot'ik) [*bin-* + *otic*] binaural.

**bin•ov•u•lar** (bin-ov'u-lər) [*bin-* + *ovular*] pertaining to or derived from two distinct ova.

**Bins•wang•er's disease (dementia, encephalitis)** (bin' swahng-ər) [Otto *Binswanger,* German neurologist, 1852–1929] see under *disease.*

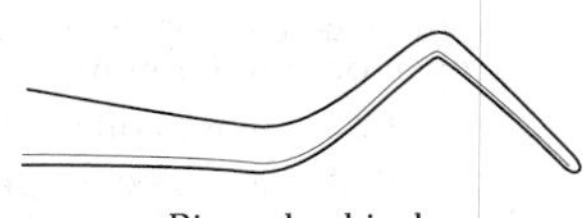
Binangle chisel.

**bi•nu•cle•ar** (bi-noo'kle-ər) [*bi-* + *nuclear*] having two nuclei.

**bi•nu•cle•ate** (bi-noo'kle-āt) binuclear.

**bi•nu•cle•a•tion** (bi"noo-kle-a'shən) the formation of two nuclei within a cell through division of the nucleus without division of the cytoplasm.

**bi•nu•cleo•late** (bi-noo-kle'o-lāt) [*bi-* + L. *nucleolus*] having two nucleoli.

**bio-** [Gr. *bios* life] combining form denoting relationship to life, or to living organisms.

**bio•acous•tics** (bi"o-ə-koo'stiks) the science dealing with the communicating sounds made by animals.

**bio•ac•tive** (bi"o-ak'tiv) having an effect on or eliciting a response from living tissue.

**bio•aer•a•tion** (bi"o-ār-a'shən) a modification of the activated sludge method of purifying sewage.

**bio•amine** (bi'o-ə-mēn") biogenic amine.

**bio•am•in•er•gic** (bi"o-am"in-ər'jik) of or pertaining to neurons that secrete biogenic amines.

**bio•as•say** (bi"o-as'a) [*bio-* + *assay*] determination of the active power of a sample of a drug by noting its effect on a live animal or an isolated organ preparation, as compared with the effect of a standard preparation; called also *biological assay.*

**bio•as•tro•nau•tics** (bi"o-as"trə-nawt'iks) the science concerned with study of the effects of space and interplanetary travel on living organisms.

**bio•avail•a•bil•i•ty** (bi"o-ə-vāl"ə-bil'ĭ-te) the degree to which a drug or other substance becomes available to the target tissue after administration.

**bio•cat•a•lyst** (bi"o-kat'ə-list) enzyme.

**bio•ce•no•sis** (bi"o-se-no'sis) [*bio-* + *ceno-*[3] + *-sis*] the relation of diverse organisms that live in association.

**bio•ce•not•ic** (bi"o-se-not'ik) characterized by biocenosis.

**bio•chem•is•try** (bi"o-kem'is-tre) [*bio-* + *chemistry*] [MeSH: Biochemistry] the chemistry of living organisms and of vital processes; physiological chemistry.

**bio•che•mor•phic** (bi"o-ke-mor'fik) pertaining to biochemorphology.

**bio•che•mor•phol•o•gy** (bi"o-ke-mor-fol'ə-je) the study of the relationship between chemical constitution and biological action.

**bio•ci•dal** (bi"o-si'dəl) pertaining to that which kills living organisms.

**bio•cide** (bi'o-sīd) an agent that kills living organisms.

**bio•cli•mat•ics** (bi"o-kli-mat'iks) bioclimatology.

**bio•cli•ma•tol•o•gist** (bi"o-kli"mə-tol'ə-jist) an individual skilled in bioclimatology.

**bio•cli•ma•tol•o•gy** (bi"o-kli"mə-tol'ə-je) [*bio-* + *climatology*] the science devoted to the study of effects on living organisms of conditions of the natural environment (rainfall, daylight, temperature, humidity, air movement) prevailing in specific regions of the earth. See also *biometeorology.*

**bio•coe•no•sis** (bi"o-se-no'sis) biocenosis.

**bio•col•loid** (bi"o-kol'oid) [*bio-* + *colloid*] a colloid from animal, plant, or microbial tissue.

**bio•com•pat•i•bil•i•ty** (bi"o-kom-pat"ĭ-bil'ĭ-te) the quality of being biocompatible.

**bio•com•pat•i•ble** (bi"o-kom-pat'ĭ-bəl) being harmonious with life; not having toxic or injurious effects on biological function.

**bio•cy•ber•net•ics** (bi"o-si"bər-net'iks) the science of communications and control in animals.

**bio•cy•cle** (bi"o-si'kəl) [*bio-* + *cycle*] the rhythmic repetition of certain phenomena observed in living organisms.

**bio•cy•tin** (bi"o-si'tin) biotin in amide linkage with the ϵ-amino group of lysine, as occurs in the holoenzymes for which biotin is the coenzyme.

**bio•de•grad•a•ble** (bi"o-de-grād'ə-bəl) susceptible of decomposition by natural biological processes, as by the action of bacteria, plants, animals, etc.

**bio•deg•ra•da•tion** (bi"o-deg"rə-da'shən) [MeSH: Biodegradation] the series of processes by which living systems render chemicals less noxious to the environment.

**bio•de•tri•tus** (bi"o-de-tri'təs) detritus derived from the disintegration and decomposition of once-living organisms; further designated as phytodetritus or zoodetritus, depending on whether the original organism was vegetal or animal.

**bio·dy·nam·ics** (bi″o-di-nam′iks) [*bio-* + *dynamics*] the scientific study of the nature and determinants of all organismic (including human) behavior.

**bio·elec·tric·i·ty** (bi″o-e″lek-tris′ĭ-te) the electrical phenomena that appear in living tissues, as that generated by muscle and nerve tissue.

**bio·elec·tron·ics** (bi″o-e″lek-tron′iks) the study of the role of intermolecular transfer of electrons in biological regulation and defense.

**bio·el·e·ment** (bi″o-el′ə-mənt) any chemical element that is a component of living tissue.

**bio·en·er·get·ics** (bi″o-en″ər-jet′iks) the study of the energy transformations in living organisms.

**bio·en·gi·neer·ing** (bi″o-en″jĭ-nēr′ing) biomedical engineering.

**bio·equiv·a·lence** (bi″o-e-kwiv′ə-ləns) the quality of being bioequivalent.

**bio·equiv·a·lent** (bi″o-e-kwiv′ə-lənt) having the same strength and similar bioavailability in the same dosage form as another specimen of a given drug substance.

**bio·eth·ics** (bi″o-eth′iks) [MeSH: Bioethics] obligations of a moral nature relating to biological research and its applications.

**bio·feed·back** (bi″o-fēd′bak) the process of furnishing an individual information, usually in an auditory or visual mode, on the state of one or more physiological variables such as heart rate, blood pressure, or skin temperature; such a procedure often enables the individual to gain some voluntary control over the physiological variable being sampled.
**alpha b.**, a procedure in which a person is presented with continuous information, usually auditory, on the state of his brain-wave pattern, with the intent of increasing the percentage of alpha activity; this is done with the expectation that it will be associated with a state of relaxation and peaceful wakefulness. Called also *alpha feedback*.
**electromyographic b.**, a method of muscle retraining for patients with neurological deficits; electrical activity of the muscle is recorded by electromyography and displayed on a video screen in front of the patient, accompanied by a variable audible signal, in order to monitor muscle movements.

**biofilm** (bi′o-film″) a thin layer of microorganisms adhering to the surface of a structure, which may be organic or inorganic, together with the polymers that they secrete.

**bio·fla·vo·noid** (bi″o-fla′və-noid) any of the flavonoids (q.v.) with biological activity in mammals; despite being reported to decrease capillary fragility, they have not been shown to be essential or to have any medical or nutritional value.

**bio·gen·e·sis** (bi″o-jen′ə-sis) [*bio-* + *-genesis*] [MeSH: Biogenesis] 1. Thomas Huxley's theory, opposed to spontaneous generation, that living matter always arises by the agency of preexisting living matter; see also *panspermy*. 2. recapitulation; see under *theory*.

**bio·ge·net·ic** (bi″o-jə-net′ik) pertaining to biogenesis.

**bi·o·gen·ic** (bi″o-jen′ik) having origins in biological processes, as a biogenic amine.

**bi·og·e·nous** (bi-oj′ə-nəs) originating from life or producing life.

**bio·ge·og·ra·phy** (bi″o-je-og′rə-fe) the scientific study of geographic distribution of living organisms.

**bio·haz·ard** (bi′o-haz″ərd) a potentially dangerous infectious agent such as may be found in a clinical microbiology laboratory or used in experimental studies on genetic recombination.

**bio·hy·drau·lic** (bi″o-hi-draw′lik) [*bio-* + Gr. *hydōr* water] pertaining to the action of water and solutions in living tissue.

**bio·im·plant** (bi″o-im′plant) denoting a prosthesis made of biosynthetic material.

**bio·in·com·pat·i·ble** (bi″o-in″kəm-pat′ə-bəl) being inharmonious with life; having toxic or injurious effects on biological function.

**bio·in·for·mat·ics** (bi″o-in″for-mat′iks) the organization and use of biological information, particularly computer-driven processing and analysis of data and databases in the fields of molecular biology and genetics.

**bio·ki·net·ics** (bi″o-kĭ-net′iks) [*bio-* + Gr. *kinētikos* of or for putting in motion] the science of the movements within developing organisms.

**bi·o·log·ic, bi·o·log·i·cal** (bi-o-loj′ik, bi-o-loj′ĭ-kəl) pertaining to biology.

**bi·o·log·i·cals** (bi-o-loj′ĭ-kəls) medicinal preparations made from living organisms and their products, including serums, vaccines, antigens, antitoxins, etc.

**bi·ol·o·gist** (bi-ol′ə-jist) an expert in biology.

**bi·ol·o·gy** (bi-ol′ə-je) [*bio-* + *-logy*] [MeSH: Biology] the science that deals with the phenomena of life and living organisms in general.
**molecular b.**, the study of molecular structures and events underlying biological processes, including the relation between genes and the functional characteristics they determine.
**radiation b.**, the scientific study of effects of ionizing radiation on living organisms.

**bio·lu·mi·nes·cence** (bi″o-loo″mĭ-nes′əns) chemoluminescence occurring in living cells, especially the emission of light as a result of cellular oxidation of a heat-stable substrate (luciferin) in the presence of a heat-sensitive enzyme (luciferase).

**bi·ol·y·sis** (bi-ol′ĭ-sis) chemical decomposition of organic matter by the action of living organisms.

**bio·lyt·ic** (bi-o-lit′ik) [*bio-* + *-lytic*] 1. pertaining to or characterized by biolysis. 2. destructive to life.

**bio·mark·er** (bi′o-mahr″kər) 1. a biological molecule used as a marker for the substance or process of interest. 2. tumor marker.

**bio·mass** (bi′o-mas) [MeSH: Biomass] the entire assemblage of living organisms, both animal and vegetable, of a particular region, considered collectively.

**bio·ma·te·ri·al** (bi″o-mə-tēr-e-əl) any substance (other than a drug), synthetic or natural, that can be used as a system or part of a system that treats, augments, or replaces any tissue, organ, or function of the body.

**bio·math·e·mat·ics** (bi″o-math″ə-mat′iks) [*bio-* + *mathematics*] the application of mathematics to biology and medicine.

**bi·ome** (bi′ōm) [Gr. *bios* life + *-ome* (-oma) mass] the recognizable community unit of a given region, produced by interaction of climatic factors, biota, and substrate, usually designated according to the characteristic adult or climax vegetation, as tundra, coniferous forest or taiga, deciduous forest, grassland, and the like.

**bio·me·chan·ics** (bi″o-mə-kan′iks) [*bio-* + *mechanics*] [MeSH: Biomechanics] the application of mechanical laws to living structures, as to a locomotor system. See also *kinesiology* and *bionics*.
**dental b.**, the relationship between the biologic behavior of oral structures and the physical influence of a dental restoration or appliance. Called also *dental biophysics*.

**bio·med·i·cal** (bi″o-med′i-kəl) biological and medical; pertaining to the application of the natural sciences (biology, biochemistry, biophysics, etc.) to the study of medicine.

**bio·med·i·cine** (bi″o-med′ĭ-sin) clinical medicine based on the principles of the natural sciences (biology, biochemistry, biophysics, etc.).

**bio·mem·brane** (bi″o-mem′brān) any membrane, e.g., cell membrane, of an organism.

**bio·mem·bra·nous** (bi″o-mem′brə-nəs) of or pertaining to a biomembrane.

**bio·me·te·or·ol·o·gist** (bi″o-me″te-or-ol′ə-jist) an individual skilled in biometeorology.

**bio·me·te·or·ol·o·gy** (bi″o-me″te-or-ol′ə-je) [*bio-* + *meteorology*] that branch of ecology which deals with the effects on living organisms of the extraorganic aspects of the physical environment (such as temperature, humidity, barometric pressure, rate of air flow, and air ionization). It considers not only the natural atmosphere but also artificially created atmospheres such as those to be found in buildings and shelters, and in closed ecological systems, such as satellites and submarines.

**bi·om·e·ter** (bi-om′ə-tər) [*bio-* + *-meter*] an apparatus by which extremely minute quantities of carbon dioxide can be measured; used in measuring the carbon dioxide given off from functioning tissue.

**bio·me·tri·cian** (bi″o-mə-trish′ən) a specialist in biometry.

**bio·met·rics** (bi″o-met′riks) biometry.

**bi·om·e·try** (bi-om′ə-tre) [*bio-* + *-metry*] [MeSH: Biometry] 1. the science of the application of statistics in biology and medicine. 2. in life insurance, the calculation of the expectation of life.

**bio·mi·cro·scope** (bi″o-mi′krə-skōp) a microscope for examining living tissue in the body.
**slit-lamp b.**, see *slit lamp*, under *lamp*.

**bio·mi·cros·co·py** (bi″o-mi-kros′kə-pe) [*bio-* + *microscopy*] 1. microscopic examination of living tissue in the body. 2. examination of the cornea or the lens by a combination of slit lamp and corneal microscope.

**bio·mod·u·la·tion** (bi″o-mod″u-la′shən) reactive or associative adjustment of the biochemical or cellular status of an organism.

**bio·mod·u·la·tor** (bi″o-mod′u-la″tər) biologic response modifier.

**bio·mol·e·cule** (bi″o-mol′ə-kūl) a molecule produced by a living cell, as a protein, carbohydrate, or lipid.

**Bi·om·pha·la·ria** (bi-om″fə-lar′e-ə) [MeSH: Biomphalaria] a genus of snails of the family Planorbidae; some species are intermediate hosts of *Schistosoma mansoni.* Called also *Australorbis.*

**bi·on** (bi′on) [Gr. *bioun* a living being] an individual living organism.

**bio·ne·cro·sis** (bi″o-nə-kro′sis) necrobiosis.

**bi·on·ics** (bi-on′iks) [MeSH: Bionics] the science concerned with study of the functions, characteristics, and phenomena found in the living world and application of the knowledge gained to new devices and techniques in the world of machines. See also *biomechanics.*

**bi·o·nom·ics** (bi″o-nom′iks) [*bio-* + Gr. *nomos* law] the study of the relations of organisms to their environment; ecology.

**bi·on·o·my** (bi-on′ə-me) [*bio-* + Gr. *nomos* law] the sum of knowledge regarding the laws of life.

**bio·nu·cle·on·ics** (bi″o-noo″kle-on′iks) the study of the biological applications of radioactive and rare stable isotopes.

**bio·os·mot·ic** (bi″o-oz-mot′ik) [*bio-* + *osmotic*] a term applied to osmotic pressure phenomena in living organisms.

**bi·oph·a·gism** (bi-of′ə-jiz-əm) [*bio-* + *phag-* + *-ism*] the eating or absorption of living matter.

**bi·oph·a·gous** (bi-of′ə-gəs) feeding on living matter.

**bi·oph·a·gy** (bi-of′ə-je) biophagism.

**bio·phys·i·cal** (bi″o-fiz′ĭ-kəl) pertaining to biophysics.

**bio·phys·ics** (bi-o-fiz′iks) [*bio-* + *physics*] [MeSH: Biophysics] the science dealing with the application of physical methods and theories to biological problems.
**dental b.**, see under *biomechanics.*

**bio·phys·i·og·ra·phy** (bi″o-fiz-e-og′rə-fe) [*bio-* + *physiography*] structural or descriptive biology.

**bio·phys·i·ol·o·gy** (bi″o-fiz-e-ol′ə-je) [*bio-* + *physiology*] that part of biology which includes organogeny, morphology, and physiology.

**bio·pla·sia** (bi″o-pla′zhə) [*bio-* + *-plasia*] the storing up of food energy in the form of growth.

**bio·plasm** (bi′o-plaz-əm) [*bio-* + *-plasm*] 1. protoplasm. 2. the more essential or vital part of cytoplasm, contrasted with the *hyaloplasm.* Called also *plasmogen.*

**bio·plas·mic** (bi-o-plaz′mik) of or pertaining to bioplasm.

**bio·poi·e·sis** (bi″o-poi-e′sis) [*bio-* + *-poiesis*] the origin of life from inorganic matter.

**bio·poly·mer** (bi″o-pol′ĭ-mər) a polymer formed in a living organism, as a polypeptide formed from amino acids (monomers).

**bio·pros·the·sis** (bi″o-pros-the′sis) [*bio-* + *prosthesis*] [MeSH: Bioprosthesis] a prosthesis that contains biological material.

**bi·o·pros·thet·ic** (bi″o-pros-thet′ik) pertaining to a bioprosthesis; see under *valve.*

**bi·op·sy** (bi′ŏp-se) [*bio-* + Gr. *opsis* vision] [MeSH: Biopsy] the removal and examination, usually microscopic, of tissue from the living body, performed to establish precise diagnosis.
**aspiration b.**, biopsy in which the tissue is obtained by the application of suction through a needle attached to a syringe.
**bite b.**, the instrumental removal of a fragment of tissue.
**brush b.**, biopsy in which cells or tissue is obtained by manipulating tiny brushes against the tissue or lesion in question (e.g., through a bronchoscope) at the desired site.
**chorionic villus b.**, see under *sampling.*
**cone b.**, biopsy in which an inverted cone of tissue is excised, as from the uterine cervix.
**core b., core needle b.**, needle biopsy with a large hollow needle that extracts a core of tissue; used in diagnosis of prostate and kidney conditions.
**cytological b.**, a procedure in which cells are obtained by various methods for pathological examinations, as by irrigation of hollow viscera.
**endomyocardial b.**, sampling of the endomyocardial tissue with a bioptome inserted percutaneously and advanced via the femoral or internal jugular vein to the right heart or via the femoral artery to the left heart; used to assess cardiac transplant rejection or anthracycline-induced cardiotoxicity, and sometimes in diagnosing myocarditis, cardiomyopathy, or infiltrative diseases.
**endoscopic b.**, removal of tissue by appropriate instruments introduced through an endoscope.
**excisional b.**, biopsy of tissue removed by excision; biopsy of an entire lesion, including a significant margin of contiguous normal-appearing tissue. Cf. *lumpectomy.*
**exploratory b.**, exploration combined with biopsy to determine the type and extent of neoplasms, both deep and superficial.
**fine-needle aspiration b.**, aspiration biopsy using a fine needle; for superficial tissue such as the thyroid, breast, or prostate the needle is unguided but for deep tissue it must be guided radiologically.
**incisional b.**, biopsy of a selected portion of a lesion and, if possible, of adjacent normal-appearing tissue.
**needle b.**, biopsy in which tissue from deep within the body is obtained by insertion through the skin of a specifically designed needle that detaches tissue with an inner needle so that the tissue can be brought to the surface in the needle's lumen.
**percutaneous b.**, needle b.
**punch b.**, biopsy in which tissue is obtained by a punch.
**shave b.**, biopsy of a skin lesion in which the sample is excised using a cut parallel to the surface of the surrounding skin.
**stereotactic b.**, biopsy of the brain using a stereotactic technique to locate the biopsy site.
**sternal b.**, biopsy of bone marrow of the sternum; done by puncture or trephining.
**surface b.**, biopsy of cells scraped from the surface of suspicious or obvious lesions, most commonly employed in examination for cancer of the cervix.
**transbronchial lung b.**, biopsy of the lung through a bronchofiberscope (or rigid bronchoscope in small children) positioned under fluoroscopic guidance.

**bio·psy·chic** (bi″o-si′kik) pertaining to mental phenomena in their relation to the living organism.

**bio·psy·chol·o·gy** (bi″o-si-kol′ə-je) psychobiology (def. 1).

**bi·op·ter·in** (bi-op′tər-in) [MeSH: Biopterin] an oxidized degradation product of tetrahydrobiopterin; the term is also used to denote the class of related compounds.

**bi·op·tic** (bi-op′tik) pertaining to or dependent on biopsy.

**bi·op·tome** (bi′op-tōm″) a cutting instrument for taking biopsy specimens.

**bio·pyo·cul·ture** (bi″o-pi″o-kul′chər) [*bio-* + *pyo-* + *culture*] a culture made from pus whose cells are alive.

**bio·ra·tion·al** (bi″o-rash′ə-nəl) based on biological principles; having an effect by natural means; said, for example, of such pesticidal agents as viruses, bacteria, protozoa, fungi, or naturally occurring biochemicals.

**bi·or·bi·tal** (bi-or′bĭ-təl) pertaining to both orbits.

**bio·re·ver·si·ble** (bi″o-re-vər′sĭ-bəl) capable of being changed back to the original biologically active chemical form by processes within the organism; said of drugs.

**bi·or·gan** (bi′or-gən) a physiological organ, as distinguished from a morphological organ, or *idorgan.*

**bio·rhe·ol·o·gy** (bi″o-re-ol′ə-je) the study of the deformation and flow of matter in living systems and in materials directly derived from them.

**bio·rhythm** (bi′o-rith-əm) [MeSH: Periodicity] the cyclic occurrence of physiological events, as a circadian rhythm.

**bio·sci·ence** (bi″o-si′ens) the study of biology wherein all the sciences (physics, chemistry, etc.) are applied.

**bi·o·sis** (bi-o′sis) [Gr. *bios* life] vitality, or life.

**bi·os·mo·sis** (bi″os-mo′sis) osmosis through a living membrane.

**bio·spec·trom·e·try** (bi″o-spek-trom′ə-tre) measurement by a spectroscope of the quantity of a substance in living tissue.

**bio·spec·tros·co·py** (bi″o-spek-tros′kə-pe) examination of living tissue with the spectroscope.

**bio·sphere** (bi′ŏ-sfēr) 1. that part of the universe in which living organisms are known to exist, comprising the atmosphere, hydrosphere, and lithosphere. 2. the sphere of action between an organism and its environment.

**bio·stat·ics** (bi″o-stat′iks) [*bio-* + *statics*] the science of the structure of organisms in relation to their function.

**bio·stat·is·ti·cian** (bi″o-stat″is-tish′ən) a specialist in biostatistics.

**bio·sta·tis·tics** (bi″o-stə-tis′tiks) biometry.

**bio·ste·reo·met·rics** (bi″o-ster-e-o-met′riks) analysis of the spatial and spatial-temporal characteristics of biological form and function by means of three-dimensional mapping of the body.

**bio·syn·the·sis** (bi″o-sin′thə-sis) the building up of a chemical compound in the physiologic processes of a living organism.

**bio·syn·thet·ic** (bi″o-sin-thet′ik) pertaining to or characterized by biosynthesis.

**Bi·ot's respiration (breathing, sign)** (be-ōz′) [Camille *Biot,* French physician, born 1878] see under *respiration.*

**bi·o·ta** (bi-o′tə) [Gr. *bios* life] all the living organisms of a particular area; the combined flora and fauna of a region.

**bio·tax·is** (bi″o-tak′sis) [*bio-* + *taxis*] the selecting and arranging powers of living cells.

**bio·taxy** (bi″o-tak′se) 1. biotaxis. 2. taxonomy.

**bio·tel·em·e·try** (bi″o-təl-em′ə-tre) the use of telemetry to record and measure certain vital phenomena of living organisms.

**bio·ther·a·py** (bi″o-ther′ə-pe) [*bio-* + *-therapy*] biological therapy.

**bio·the·si·om·e·ter** (bi″o-the″ze-om′ə-tər) an instrument for measuring the vibratory-perception threshold.

**bio·tic** (bi-ot′ik) 1. pertaining to life or living matter. 2. pertaining to the biota.

**bio·tics** (bi-ot′iks) [Gr. *biōtikos* living] the functions and qualities peculiar to living organisms, or the sum of knowledge regarding these qualities.

**bio·tin** (bi′o-tin) [MeSH: Biotin] 1. a water-soluble dicyclic monocarboxylic acid considered to be part of the vitamin B complex; it is an essential cofactor for several carboxylases, plays a role in the metabolism of fatty acids and the deamination of certain amino acids, and is also used in vitro in biochemical assays based on biotinylation (q.v.) of various molecules. Deficiencies in humans have occurred only after prolonged total parenteral nutrition not supplemented with biotin or on ingestion of large quantities of raw egg whites (see *avidin*); manifestations have included dermatologic, neurologic, and ocular disorders. In some animals, deficiency has resulted in graying and loss of hair. 2. [USP] a preparation of biotin used as a nutritional supplement.

**bi·o·tin·i·dase** (bi″o-tin′ĭ-dās) [EC 3.5.1.12] an enzyme of the hydrolase class essential for the recycling of biotin; it catalyzes the cleavage of biocytin or of biotin in amide linkage with peptide fragments, freeing biotin for reuse. Deficiency of the enzyme, an autosomal recessive trait, results in multiple carboxylase deficiency.

**bi·o·tin·yl** (bi″o-tin′əl) the acyl radical of biotin.

**bi·o·tin·yl·a·tion** (bi″o-tin″ə-la′shən) the incorporation of biotinyl groups into molecules, either that catalyzed by holocarboxylase synthetase during enzyme biosynthesis or that undertaken *in vitro* to visualize specific substrates by incubating them with biotin-labeled probes and avidin that has been linked to any of a variety of substances amenable to biochemical assay.

**bi·ot·o·my** (bi-ot′ə-me) [*bio-* + *-tomy*] 1. the study of animal and plant structure by dissection. 2. vivisection.

**bio·tox·i·ca·tion** (bi″o-tok″sĭ-ka′shən) an intoxication resulting from a plant or animal poison (biotoxin).

**bio·tox·i·col·o·gy** (bi″o-tok″sĭ-kol′ə-je) [*bio-* + *toxicology*] the science of poisons produced by living things, their cause, detection, and their effects, and of the treatment of conditions produced by them.

**bio·tox·in** (bi″o-tok′sin) any poisonous substance produced by and derived from a living organism, either plant or animal.

**bio·trans·for·ma·tion** (bi″-trans″for-ma′shən) [MeSH: Biotransformation] the series of chemical alterations of a compound (e.g., a drug) which occur within the body, as by enzymatic activity.

**bi·ot·re·py** (bi-ot′rə-pe) the study of the body by means of its reactions to chemical substances.

**bio·type** (bi′o-tīp) 1. a group of individuals possessing the same genotype. 2. a variant strain of a bacterial species, differing in identifiable physiologic characteristics.

**bio·ty·pol·o·gy** (bi″o-ti-pol′ə-je) the study of anthropological types with their constitutional variations, inadequacies, etc.

**bi·ov·u·lar** (bi-ov′u-lər) binovular.

**bi·para·sit·ic** (bi″par-ə-sit′ik) living parasitically upon a parasite; hyperparasitic.

**bi·par·en·tal** (bi″pə-ren′təl) derived from two parents, male and female.

**bi·pa·ri·e·tal** (bi″pə-ri′ə-təl) pertaining to the two parietal eminences or bones.

**bip·a·rous** (bip′ə-rəs) [*bi-* + *-parous*] producing two ova or offspring at one time.

**bi·par·tite** (bi-pahr′tīt) [L. *bipartitus*] having two parts or divisions.

**bi·ped** (bi′ped) [*bi-* + L. *pes* foot] 1. having two feet. 2. an animal with two feet.

**bip·e·dal** (bip′ə-dəl) [*bi-* + *pedal*] having or pertaining to both feet.

**bi·pen·ni·form** (bi-pen′ĭ-form) doubly feather-shaped; said of muscles whose fibers are arranged on each side of a tendon, like the barbs on the shaft of a feather.

**bi·per·fo·rate** (bi-pər′fə-rāt) [*bi-* + L. *perforatus* bored through] having two perforations.

**bi·per·i·den** (bi-per′ĭ-den) [USP] [MeSH: Biperiden] a synthetic anticholinergic agent having antisecretory, spasmolytic, and mydriatic activity, used in the form of its salts as an antidyskinetic.
**b. hydrochloride** [USP], the hydrochloride of biperiden, used in the treatment of parkinsonism and drug-induced antipyramidal reactions; administered orally.
**b. lactate,** the lactate salt of biperiden, available as biperiden lactate injection [USP], used in the treatment of parkinsonism and drug-induced extrapyramidal reactions; administered intramuscularly or intravenously.

**bi·phen·amine hy·dro·chlo·ride** (bi-fen′ə-mēn) an antibacterial, antifungal, and topical anesthetic.

**bi·phen·yl** (bi-fen′əl) diphenyl.
**polychlorinated b. (PCB),** any of a group of substances in which chlorine replaces hydrogen in biphenyls, used as heat-transfer agents and as insulators in electrical equipment. They are chemically very stable and accumulate in animal tissues, causing a variety of toxic effects including carcinogenesis.

***p*-bi·phen·yl·amine** (bi-fen″əl-am′ēn) *p*-aminobiphenyl.

**bi·po·lar** (bi-po′lər) 1. having two poles or pertaining to both poles. 2. describing neurons that have processes at both ends. 3. denoting bacterial staining confined to the poles (ends) of the organism. 4. pertaining to mood disorders in which both depressive episodes and manic or hypomanic episodes occur.

**Bi·po·la·ris** (bi-po-la′ris) a genus of Fungi Imperfecti of the form-class Hyphomycetes, form-family Dematiaceae, closely related to *Drechslera* and *Exserohilum*. *B. australien′sis, B. hawaiien′sis,* and *B. spici′fera* have occasionally been isolated from humans with fatal encephalitis or meningoencephalitis, as well as nasal polyps and sinusitis. The perfect (sexual) stage of *Bipolaris* species is in genus *Cochliobolus*.

**bi·pos·i·tive** (bi-poz′ĭ-tiv) having two positive charges, as in $Ca^{2+}$.

**bi·po·ten·tial** (bi″po-ten′shəl) pertaining to or characterized by bipotentiality.

**bi·po·ten·ti·al·i·ty** (bi″po-ten″she-al′ĭ-te) [*bi-* + L. *potentia* power] possession of the power of developing or acting in either of two possible ways.
**b. of the gonad,** the capability of an undifferentiated gonad to develop into either an ovary or a testis.

**bi·pus** (bi′pəs) [*bi-* + Gr. *pous* foot] having two feet.

**bi·ra·mous** (bi-ra′məs) [*bi-* + L. *ramus* branch] consisting of or possessing two branches.

**birch** (bərch) any tree of the genus *Betula*.

**Bird's sign** (bərdz) [Samuel Dougan *Bird,* Australian physician, 1832–1904] see under *sign*.

**bi·re·frac·tive** (bi″re-frak′tiv) doubly refractive.

**bi·re·frin·gence** (bi″re-frin′jəns) [MeSH: Birefringence] the quality of transmitting light unequally in different directions; double refraction. In biological materials, it indicates an ordering of the molecules, e.g., they may be oriented to one another much as in a crystal.
**crystalline b.,** birefringence occurring in systems in which the bonds between molecules or ions have a regular asymmetrical arrangement; it is independent of the refractive index of the medium.
**flow b.,** that exhibited only when the substance is in solution and flowing; e.g., it is seen in solutions of long thin molecules, such as nucleoproteins.
**form b.,** that produced by regular orientation of submicroscopic asymmetrical particles in a substance or object, differing in refractive index from the surrounding medium; it is the most common form occurring in organisms.
**intrinsic b.,** crystalline b.
**strain b.,** birefringence observed occasionally in isotropic structures when subjected to tension or pressure; it occurs in muscle and in embryonic tissues.
**streaming b.,** flow b.

**bi·re·frin·gent** (bi″re-frin′jənt) [*bi-* + *refringent*] doubly refractive.

**Bir·kett's hernia** (bər′kets) [John *Birkett,* English surgeon, 1815–1904] synovial hernia.

**Bir·na·vi·ri·dae** (bər′nə-vir″ĭ-de) [*bi*segmented *RNA* + *virus*] [MeSH: Birnaviridae] the two-segmented double-stranded RNA viruses: a family of RNA viruses having a nonenveloped icosahedral virion 60 nm in diameter with 92 capsomers in a T = 9 arrangement. The genome consists of two segments of linear double-stranded RNA (MW 2.2–2.5 × $10^6$ and 2.4–2.6 × $10^6$, size of total genome about 6 kbp). Viruses contain five major structural polypeptides and are resistant to light and ultraviolet radiation, heat, lipid solvents, and trypsin. Replication and assembly occur in the cytoplasm; *Aquabirnavirus* (infecting fish, mollusks, and crustaceans), *Avibirnavirus* (infecting birds), and *Entomobirnavirus* (infecting insects).

**Bir·na·vi·rus** (bər′nə-vi″rəs) [*bi*segmented *RNA* + *virus*] a former genus of viruses of the family Birnaviridae; see *Aquabirnavirus* and *Avibirnavirus*.

**bir·na·vi·rus** (bər′nə-vi″rəs) any virus belonging to the family Birnaviridae.

**birth** (bərth) the act or process of being born.
**complete b.,** the complete separation of the infant from the maternal body (after cutting of the umbilical cord).
**cross b.,** labor with the fetus lying transversely in the uterus.
**dead b.,** birth of a fetus which, during or before birth, has lost all signs of antenatal life, including heart beat, pulsation, and movement.
**head b.,** a birth in which the head presents.
**multiple b.,** the birth of two or more offspring produced in the same gestation period, the frequency of birth of viable offspring after such multiple pregnancy having been computed as follows: twins, 1 in 80; triplets, 1 in 6400 (80 × 80); quadruplets, 1 in 512,000 (80 × 80 × 80); etc. (Hellin's law).
**post-term b.,** birth of a post-mature, or over-term, infant.
**premature b.,** birth of a premature infant.

**birth·mark** (bərth′mahrk) any congenital blemish or spot on the skin, usually visible at birth or shortly after, such as a nevus or mole.

**bis-** [L. *bis* twice] a prefix meaning two or twice.

**bis·ac·o·dyl** (bis-ak′ə-dil; bis″ə-ko′dil) [USP] [MeSH: Bisacodyl] a contact laxative used for short-term relief of constipation and for bowel evacuation prior to radiography, endoscopy, and elective colon surgery; administered orally or by rectal suppository.
**b. tannex,** a water-soluble complex of bisacodyl and tannic acid; a cathartic.

**bis·acro·mi·al** (bis-ə-kro′me-əl) pertaining to the two acromial processes.

**bis·ax·il·lary** (bis-ak′sĭ-lar″e) pertaining to both axillae.

**bis(chlo·ro·meth·yl)ether** (bis-klor″o-meth′əl-e′thər) an alkylating agent used as a chemical intermediate in industry; it is irritating to eyes and mucous membranes and carcinogenic. Called also *sym-dichloromethyl ether*.

**Bis·chof's myelotomy** (bish′ofs) [W. *Bischof*, German neurosurgeon, 20th century] see under *myelotomy*.

**bis·cuit** (bis′kət) dental porcelain that has undergone the first firing and has assumed a surface texture like that of a cookie. Called also *bisque*.

**bis·cuit·ing** (bis′kət-ing) the first baking of porcelain paste, by which biscuit is formed.

**bi·sec·tion** (bi-sek′shən) [*bi-* + *section*] division into two parts by cutting.

**bi·seg·men·tec·to·my** (bi″seg-men-tek′tə-me) resection of two segments (i.e., one lobe) of the liver; hepatic lobectomy.

**bi·sep·tate** (bi-sep′tāt) [*bi-* + *septate*] divided into two parts by a septum.

**bi·sex·u·al** (bi-sek′shoo-əl) [*bi-* + *sexual*] [MeSH: Bisexuality] 1. of or pertaining to bisexuality. 2. an individual exhibiting bisexuality. Called also *ambisexual*. 3. hermaphroditic. 4. androgynous.

**bi·sex·u·al·i·ty** (bi-sek″shoo-al′ĭ-te) [MeSH: Bisexuality] 1. true hermaphroditism. 2. sexual attraction to persons of both sexes; exhibition of both homosexual and heterosexual behavior. 3. androgyny (def. 2).

**bis·fe·ri·ens** (bis-fēr′e-ənz) [L.] bisferious.

**bis·fe·ri·ous** (bis-fe′re-əs) [*bis-* + L. *ferire* to beat] having two beats; usually refers to a widely notched arterial pulse, sometimes palpable. Called also *biferiens* and *biferious*.

**BIS-GMA** dimethacrylate.

**Bish·op** (bish′əp) John Michael. American microbiologist and immunologist, born 1936. Co-winner with Harold Eliot Varmus of the Nobel prize for medicine or physiology in 1989 for their discovery that oncogenes of animal tumor viruses are derived from cellular genes called proto-oncogenes.

**Bish·op's sphygmoscope** (bish′əps) [Louis Faugères *Bishop*, American physician, 1864–1941] see under *sphygmoscope*.

**bis·hy·droxy·cou·ma·rin** (bis″hi-drok″se-koo′mə-rin) dicumarol (def. 1).

**bis·il·i·ac** (bis-il′e-ak) [*bis* + *iliac*] pertaining to both iliac bones or to any two corresponding points on the two iliac bones.

**bis in die** (bis in de′a) [L.] twice a day; abbreviated b.d. or b.i.d.

**bis·muth** (biz′məth) [L. *bismuthum*] [MeSH: Bismuth] a silver-white metal; atomic number 83; atomic weight 208.980; symbol Bi. Its salts have astringent, antacid, and mildly germicidal properties and are used to treat diarrhea, nausea, indigestion, and other gastrointestinal conditions; they were formerly used in the treatment of syphilis but have been superseded by antibiotics. Excessive ingestion can cause bismuth poisoning; see under *poisoning*.
**b. carbonate, basic,** b. subcarbonate.
**b. glycoloylarsanilate,** glycobiarsol.
**b. magma,** milk of bismuth; see under *milk*.
**b. oxyiodide,** a brownish-red powder, BiOI, formerly used as a local antiseptic.
**b. subcarbonate** [USP], a topical protectant to relieve skin irritations; it has been used internally as an antacid and astringent. Called also *basic bismuth carbonate*.
**b. subgallate** [USP], a basic salt, which on drying yields 52 to 57 per cent bismuth trioxide; it has been used in the treatment of peptic ulcer disease.
**b. subnitrate** [USP], a basic salt, used as a pharmaceutic necessity in the preparation of milk of bismuth; the official preparation contains at least 79 per cent bismuth trioxide, calculated on the dried basis.
**b. subsalicylate** [USP], a basic salt, $C_7H_5BiO_4$, which on ignition yields 62 to 66 per cent bismuth trioxide; it has been given orally in the treatment of enteritis and intramuscularly in the treatment of syphilis, lupus erythematosus, and necrotizing ulcerative gingivitis.

**bis·mu·thia** (biz-mu′the-ə) blue discoloration of the skin and mucous membranes from excessive ingestion of bismuth compounds; see *bismuth poisoning*, under *poisoning*.

**bis·muth·ism** (biz′məth-iz-əm) bismuth poisoning.

**bis·mu·tho·sis** (biz″mə-tho′sis) bismuth poisoning.

**bis·o·pro·lol fu·ma·rate** (bis″ə-pro′lol) a synthetic beta-adrenergic blocking agent used in the treatment of hypertension; administered orally.

**1,3-bis·phos·pho·glyc·er·ate** (bis″fos-fo-glis′ər-āt) an anion of the form of bisphosphoglyceric acid phosphorylated at the 1 and 3 carbons; it is an intermediate in gluconeogenesis and glycolysis, and a precursor to 2,3-bisphosphoglycerate.

**2,3-bis·phos·pho·glyc·er·ate** (bis-fos″fo-glis′ər-āt) a salt or ester of bisphosphoglyceric acid; it is contained in red blood cells, where it plays a role in liberating oxygen from hemoglobin in the peripheral circulation. It is also an intermediate in the conversion of 3-phosphoglycerate to 2-phosphoglycerate. Called also *2,3-diphosphoglycerate*.

**bis·phos·pho·glyc·er·ate mu·tase** (bis-fos″fo-glis′ər-āt mu′tās) [EC 5.4.2.4] [MeSH: Bisphosphoglycerate Mutase] an enzyme of the isomerase class that catalyzes the interconversion of 1,3-bisphosphoglycerate and 2,3-bisphosphoglycerate; it requires $Mg^{2+}$ as a cofactor and is more active in the presence of 3-phosphoglycerate. The reaction produces 2,3-bisphosphoglycerate necessary for glucose catabolism and for erythrocytic regulation of hemoglobin oxygen affinity. Deficient enzyme activity, an autosomal recessive trait, results in a form of hemolytic anemia.

**bis·phos·pho·glyc·er·ate phos·pha·tase** (bis-fos″fo-glis′ər-āt fos′fə-tās) [EC 3.1.3.13] an enzyme of the hydrolase class that catalyzes the hydrolysis of 2,3-bisphosphoglycerate to form 3-phosphoglycerate. The reaction is one of the control mechanisms regulating the affinity of hemoglobin for oxygen.

**bis·phos·pho·gly·cer·ic ac·id** (bis″fos-fo-glĭ-sēr′ik) glyceric acid esterified with phosphate at two positions.

**bis·phos·pho·glyc·ero·mu·tase** (bis-fos″fo-glis″ər-o-mu′tās) bisphosphoglycerate mutase.

**bis·phos·pho·nate** (bis-fos′fo-nāt) diphosphonate.

**bi·spore** (bi′spor) one of two asexual spores produced by the red algae.

**bisque** (bisk) [Fr.] biscuit.

**bi·ste·phan·ic** (bi-stə-fan′ik) pertaining to the two stephanions, especially to the shortest distance between them (bistephanic width).

**Bis·ton** (bis′tən) a genus of moths. *B. betula′ria* is the peppered moth, a species used in the study of industrial melanism.

**bis·tou·ry** (bis′tə-re) [Fr. *bistouri*] a long, narrow surgical knife, straight or curved, used for incising abscesses and enlarging sinuses, fistulas, etc.

**bi·stra·tal** (bi-stra′təl) [*bi-* + *stratum*] disposed in two layers.

**bi·sul·fate** (bi-sul′fāt) an acid sulfate (not to be confused with *disulfate*).

**bi·sul·fide** (bi-sul′fīd) disulfide.

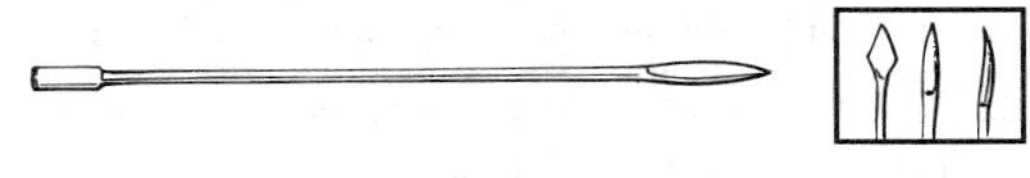

Bistoury.

**bi·sul·fite** (bi-sul'fīt) an acid sulfite.

**bi·tar·trate** (bi-tahr'trāt) any salt containing the anion $C_4H_5O_6^-$ derived from the diacid tartaric acid ($C_4H_6O_6$).

**bite** (bīt) [MeSH: Bites and Stings] 1. the forcible closure of the lower against the upper teeth. 2. the measure of force exerted in the closure of the teeth. 3. a record of the relationship of upper and lower teeth, in occlusion, obtained by biting into a mass of modeling substance. 4. the part of an artificial tooth on the lingual side between the shoulder and the incisal edge of the tooth. 5. a wound or puncture made by the teeth or other parts of the mouth. 6. a morsel of food.
**balanced b.,** balanced occlusion.
**check b.,** a thin sheet of wax or a modeling compound placed between the teeth in centric, eccentric, lateral, or protrusive occlusion, and pressed to their buccal or labial surfaces after the jaws have been closed; used to check dental occlusion in the articulator in properly aligning study models. Written also *check-bite.*
**closed b.,** malocclusion with decreased occlusal vertical dimension and an abnormal overbite in which the mandible protrudes. Called also *deep b., closed-bite malocclusion,* and *deep overbite.*
**cross b.,** crossbite.
**deep b.,** closed b.
**edge-to-edge b., end-to-end b.,** see under *occlusion.*
**open b.,** a condition marked by failure of certain opposing teeth to establish occlusal contact when the jaws are closed. Called also *apertognathia* and *nonocclusion.*
**over b.,** vertical overlap (def. 1).
**overshot b.,** veterinary term for *retrognathia.*
**scissors b.,** total lingual crossbite of the mandible, with the mandibular teeth completely contained within the maxillary dental arch in habitual occlusion.
**underhung b.,** a characteristic of mandibular prognathism in which the incisal edges of the mandibular anterior teeth extend labially to the incisal edges of the maxillary anterior teeth when the jaws are in habitual occlusion.
**undershot b.,** veterinary term for *prognathism;* it is normal in animals such as boxers and bulldogs.
**wax b.,** a simultaneous impression of both the upper and the lower jaw, made by having the subject bite on a double layer of soft baseplate wax.
**X-b.,** crossbite.

**bite-block** (bīt'blok) occlusion rim.

**bite·gage** (bīt'gāj) a device used in prosthetic dentistry as an aid in securing proper occlusion of the maxillary and mandibular teeth.

**bite·lock** (bīt'lok) occlusion rim.

**bi·tem·po·ral** (bi-tem'pə-rəl) pertaining to both temples or temporal bones.

**bite·plane** (bīt'plān) an orthodontic removable appliance, made of acrylic resin, covering all the maxillary teeth, and kept in place by orthodontic wrought wire clasps and labial wires; used in the diagnosis and treatment of pain of the temporomandibular joint and adjacent muscles. Written also *bite plane.*

**bite·plate** (bīt'plāt) bite plate; see under *plate.*

**bi·ter·mi·nal** (bi-tər'min-al) performed by using two terminals of an alternating current.

**bite-wing** (bīt'wing) a central tab or wing of a dental x-ray film, which is held between the upper and lower teeth during radiography of oral structures. See also under *film* and *radiograph.*

**bi·thi·o·nol** (bĭ-thi'ə-nol) [MeSH: Bithionol] A bacteriostatic agent especially effective against gram-positive cocci; formerly used in the formulation of surgical soap compositions. Called also *TBP.*

**Bi·thyn·ia** (bĭ-thin'e-ə) *Bulimus.*

**Bi·tis** (bi'tis) a genus of venomous snakes of the family Viperidae. *B. arrie'tans* is the puff adder; *B. gabo'nica* is the Gaboon viper; and *B. nasicor'nis* is the rhinoceros viper. See table at *snake.*

**bi·tol·ter·ol mes·y·late** (bi-tol'tər-ol) a beta-adrenergic bronchodilator administered as an aerosol in the treatment of asthma; bitolterol is an inactive prodrug that is hydrolyzed to the active drug colterol by blood and tissue esterases.

**Bi·tot's spots (patches)** (be-tōz') [Pierre A. *Bitot,* French physician, 1822–1888] see under *spot.*

**bi·tro·chan·ter·ic** (bi″tro-kan-ter'ik) pertaining to both trochanters on one femur or to both greater trochanters.

**bit·ter** (bit'ər) 1. having an austere and unpalatable taste, like that of quinine. 2. [pl.] a medicinal agent that has a bitter taste; used as a tonic, alterative, or appetizer. Called also *amara.*
**aromatic b's,** bitter vegetable drugs that have an aromatic quality.

**bit·ters** (bit'ərz) see under *bitter.*

**bit·ter·wood** (bit'ər-wood) *Picrasma excelsa.*

**Bitt·ner virus** (bit'nər) [John Joseph *Bittner,* American pathologist, 1904–1961] see *mouse mammary tumor virus,* under *virus.*

**Bit·torf's reaction** (bit'orfs) [Alexander *Bittorf,* German physician, 1876–1949] see under *reaction.*

**bi·tu·mi·no·sis** (bi″tu-mĭ-no'sis) coal workers' pneumoconiosis caused by inhalation of the dust from soft (bituminous) coal.

**Bi·tu·ni·ca·tae** (bi-too″nĭ-ka'te) in fungal taxonomy, a series of the subphylum Ascomycotina, consisting of those having a bitunicate ascus. It includes the orders Dothideales and Erysiphales.

**bi·urate** (bi'u-rāt) an acid urate; a monobasic salt of uric acid.

**bi·u·ret** (bi'u-rət) [*bis-* + *urea*] [MeSH: Biuret] a derivative of urea, equivalent to two molecules of urea less one of ammonia; see also under *reaction.* Called also *allophanamide.*

**bi·va·lence** (bi-va'ləns) [*bi-* + L. *valens* powerful] the property of an atom of certain chemical elements of forming chemical bonds with two other atoms or groups.

**bi·va·lent** (bi-va'lənt) 1. divalent. 2. the structure formed by a pair of homologous chromosomes joined by synapsis along their length during the zygotene and pachytene stages of the first meiotic prophase. After each of the paired chromosomes separates into two sister chromatids during the pachytene stage, this structure is then called a *tetrad.*

**bi·valve** (bi'valv) [*bi-* + *valve*] having two valves, as the shells of such mollusks as clams.

**Bi·val·via** (bi-val've-ə) [*bi-* + *valva* + *-ia*] Pelecypoda.

**Bi·val·vu·li·da** (bi″val-vu'lĭ-də) [*bi-* + *valve*] an order of parasitic protozoa (class Myxosporea, phylum Myxozoa), the spores of which have two valves.

**bi·ven·ter** (bi-ven'tər) [*bi-* + *venter*] a part or organ (as a muscle) with two bellies.
**b. cer'vicis,** musculus spinalis capitis.

**bi·ven·tral** (bi-ven'trəl) 1. having two bellies. 2. musculus digastricus.

**bi·ven·tric·u·lar** (bi″ven-trik'u-lər) pertaining to or affecting both ventricles of the heart.

**bi·vi·tel·line** (bi″vĭ-tel'in) having two yolks.

**bi·zy·go·mat·ic** (bi″zi-go-mat'ik) [*bi-* + *zygoma*] pertaining to the two most prominent points on the two zygomatic arches. See also *bizygomatic breadth,* under *breadth.*

**Bjer·rum's scotoma (sign)** (byer'oomz) [Jannik Petersen *Bjerrum,* Danish ophthalmologist, 1851–1920] see under *scotoma.*

**Bjer·rum's screen** (byer'oomz) [J. *Bjerrum,* Danish ophthalmologist, 1827–1892] tangent screen.

**Björn·stad's syndrome** (byorn'stahdz) [R. *Björnstad,* Swedish dermatologist, 20th century] see under *syndrome.*

**Bk** symbol for *berkelium.*

**BKV** BK virus.

**Black** (blak) Sir James Whyte. British pharmacologist, born 1924. Co-winner, with Gertrude B. Elion and George H. Hitchings, of the Nobel prize for medicine or physiology in 1988 for his pioneering work developing rational principles of drug research and development.

**Black's classification** (blaks) [Greene Vardiman *Black,* American dentist, 1836–1915] see under *classification.*

**black** (blak) reflecting no light or true color; of the darkest hue.
**animal b., bone-b.,** animal charcoal.
**fat b. HB,** Sudan black B.
**indulin b.,** nigrosin.
**ivory b.,** animal charcoal.
**lamp b.,** finely divided carbon deposited from the smoky flame of burning oils, rosin, and other substances.
**Paris b.,** animal charcoal.
**solvent b. 3,** Sudan black B.

**black·ber·ry** (blak'ber-e) 1. any of various plants of the genus *Rubus;* some have medicinal root bark. 2. the fruit of one of these plants.

**Black·fan-Di·a·mond anemia (syndrome)** (blak'fan-di'mənd) [Kenneth D. *Blackfan,* American pediatrician, 1883–1941; Louis Klein *Diamond,* American pediatrician, born 1902] see *hypoplastic anemia, congenital,* under *anemia.*

**black haw** (blak haw) *Viburnum prunifolium.*

**black·head** (blak'hed) 1. open comedo. 2. histomoniasis.

**black·leg** (blak'leg) an acute anaerobic bacterial disease of cattle and sheep caused by *Clostridium chauvoei;* symptoms include crepitant swelling in the musculature and a high fever, often leading to death within a day. Called also *symptomatic anthrax, blackquarter,* and *quarter evil* or *ill.* Spelled also *black leg.*

**black·out** (blak'out) a condition characterized by failure of vision and momentary unconsciousness, due to diminished circulation to the brain.
**alcoholic b.,** anterograde amnesia experienced by alcoholics during episodes of drinking, even when not fully intoxicated; indicative of early but still reversible brain damage.

**black·quar·ter** (blak-kwor'tər) blackleg.

**black·snake** (blak'snāk) 1. *Pseudechis porphyriacus,* a large venomous semiaquatic Australian snake whose body is black on top and red underneath. 2. *Coluber constrictor,* a nonvenomous snake found in North America; called also *black racer.* See table at *snake.*

**black·tongue** (blak'tung") black tongue, def. 2.

**blad·der** (blad'ər) [L. *vesica, cystis;* Gr. *kystis*] [MeSH: Bladder] 1. a membranous sac, such as one serving as receptacle for a secretion; see also *vesica* and *cyst.* 2. urinary b.; see *vesica urinaria.*
**allantoic b.,** a membranous sac formed in amphibians as an outgrowth of the cloaca for the storage of urine.
**areflexic b.,** autonomous b.
**atonic b.,** a condition marked by a dilated, poorly contracting urinary bladder without evidence of a lesion of the central nervous system.
**atonic neurogenic b.,** neurogenic bladder due to destruction of the sensory nerve fibers from the bladder to the spinal cord, marked by the absence of control of bladder functions and of the desire to void, overdistention of the bladder, and an abnormal amount of residual urine; it is most frequently associated with tabes dorsalis *(tabetic b.)* and pernicious anemia, but may be seen in association with other diseases. Called also *paralytic b.* and *sensory paralytic b.*
**automatic b.,** neurogenic bladder due to complete transection of the spinal cord above the sacral segments, marked by complete loss of micturition reflexes and bladder sensation, violent involuntary voiding, and an abnormal amount of residual urine. Called also *cord b., reflex b.,* and *spastic b.*
**autonomic b.,** autonomous b.
**autonomous b.,** neurogenic bladder due to a lesion in the sacral portion of the spinal cord that interrupts the reflex arc which controls the bladder. The lesion may be in the cauda equina, conus medullaris, sacral roots, or pelvic nerve. It is marked by loss of normal bladder sensation and reflex activity, inability to initiate urination normally, and incontinence. Called also *denervated b.* and *nonreflex b.*
**chyle b.,** cisterna chyli.
**cord b.,** automatic b.
**denervated b.,** autonomous b.
**double b.,** reduplication of the bladder.
**fasciculated b.,** a bladder ridged on its inner surface due to hypertrophy of the muscular coat.
**gall b.,** vesica biliaris.
**irritable b.,** a state of the bladder marked by increased frequency of contraction with associated desire to urinate.
**motor paralytic b.,** neurogenic bladder due to impairment of the motor neurons or nerves controlling the bladder. The *acute* form is marked by painful distention and inability to initiate micturition, the *chronic* form by difficulty in initiating micturition, straining, decrease in size and force of stream, interrupted stream, and recurrent infection of the urinary tract.
**nervous b.,** a colloquial term for a functional condition characterized by a constant desire to urinate without the power to do so completely.
**neurogenic b.,** any condition of dysfunction of the urinary bladder caused by a lesion of the central or peripheral nervous system, as *atonic neurogenic b., automatic b., autonomous b., motor paralytic b.,* and *uninhibited neurogenic b.*
**nonneurogenic neurogenic b.,** Hinman syndrome.
**nonreflex b.,** autonomous b.
**paralytic b.,** atonic neurogenic b.
**reflex b.,** automatic b.
**sacculated b.,** a bladder with pouches between the hypertrophied muscular fibers.
**sensory paralytic b.,** atonic neurogenic b.
**spastic b.,** automatic b.
**string b.,** a term sometimes erroneously used as a synonym for cord bladder; see *automatic b.*
**tabetic b.,** see *atonic neurogenic b.*
**uninhibited neurogenic b.,** neurogenic bladder due to a lesion in the region of the upper motor neurons with subtotal interruption of the corticospinal pathways, marked by urgency, frequent involuntary voiding, and small-volume threshold of activity.
**urinary b.,** vesica urinaria.

**Blain·ville's ears** (blă-vēlz') [Henri Marie Ducrotay de *Blainville,* French zoologist, 1777–1850] see under *ear.*

**Blake's disk** (blāks) [Clarence John *Blake,* American otologist, 1843–1919] see under *disk.*

**Bla·lock-Han·lon operation** (bla'lok-han'lən) [Alfred *Blalock,* American surgeon, 1899–1964; C. Rollins *Hanlon,* American surgeon, born 1915] see under *operation.*

**Bla·lock-Taus·sig operation (shunt)** (bla'lok-taw'sig) [A. *Blalock;* Helen Brooke *Taussig,* American pediatrician, 1898–1986] see under *operation.*

**Blanc·o·phor** (blank'o-for) trademark for optical whitening agents (blankophores), chemically related to the sulfonamides, which produce brightness by absorbing invisible ultraviolet light and reflecting it as visible blue light. They are added to detergents, paper, and textiles, and may produce phototoxic effects, e.g., phototoxic dermatitis; they may also produce allergic contact sensitization.

**bland** (bland) [L. *blandus*] mild or soothing.

**Blan·din's glands** (blah-daz') [Philippe Frédéric *Blandin,* French surgeon, 1798–1849] see *glandulae linguales anteriores.*

**Blan·din and Nuhn's glands** (blah-dă', nōōnz) [P.F. *Blandin;* Anton *Nuhn,* German anatomist, 1814–1889] glandulae linguales anteriores.

**blank·o·phore** (blank'o-for) see *Blancophor.*

**Bla·si·us' duct** (blah'se-ooz) [Gerhard *Blasius* (Blaes), Dutch anatomist, 1625–1692] ductus parotideus.

**Blas·ko·vics operation** (blahs'ko-vitz) [Laszlo de Blaskovics, Hungarian ophthalmologist, 1869–1938] see under *operation.*

**blast**[1] (blast) [Gr. *blastos* germ] 1. an immature stage in cellular development before appearance of the definitive characteristics of the cell; used also as a word termination (see *-blast*). 2. blast cell (def. 2).

**blast**[2] (blast) [A.S. *blaest,* blast] the wave of air pressure *(air concussion)* produced by the detonation of a high-explosive bomb shell or other explosion. A wave of high-pressure velocity (shock wave) is created and this is followed by one of negative decreased velocity, exerting a suction-like action. Blast causes pulmonary concussion and hemorrhage *(lung blast, blast chest),* laceration of other thoracic and abdominal viscera, ruptured ear drums, and minor effects in the central nervous system.

**-blast** [Gr. *blastos* germ] a word termination denoting a type of blast[1]. See also *blast(o)-.*

**blas·te·ma** (blas-te'mə) [Gr. *blastēma* shoot] a group of cells that give rise to a new individual, in asexual reproduction, or to an organ or part, in either normal development or in regeneration.

**blas·tem·ic** (blas-tem'ik) pertaining to the blastema.

**blas·tic** (blas'tik) said of conidiogenesis in which new growth of a conidium takes place by a process of enlargement before delimitation by a septa.

**blas·tid** (blas'tid) the site indicative of an organizing nucleus in a fertilized ovum.

**blas·tide** (blas'tīd) blastid.

**blas·tin** (blas'tin) a substance that stimulates or increases cell proliferation; a substance providing alimentation for cells.

**blast(o)-** [Gr. *blastos* shoot, germ] a combining form denoting relationship to a bud or budding, particularly to an early embryonic stage, as to a primitive or formative element, cell, or layer.

**blas·to·cat·e·nate** [*blasto-* + L. *catena* chain] said of a chain of conidia in which the youngest cells are at the apex. Cf. *basocatenulate.*

**blas·to·cele** (blas'to-sēl) blastocoele.

**blas·to·ce·lic** (blas"to-se'lik) blastocoelic.

**blas·to·chyle** (blas'to-kīl) [*blasto-* + Gr. *chylos* juice] the fluid contained in the blastocoele.

**blas·to·coele** (blas'to-sēl) [*blasto-* + *-coele*] the fluid-filled cavity of the mass of cells (blastula) produced by cleavage of a fertilized ovum. Sometimes spelled *blastocoel.* Called also *cleavage,* or *segmentation, cavity.*

**blas·to·coel·ic** (blas"to-se'lik) pertaining to the blastocoele.

**blas·to·co·nid·i·um** (blas"to-kə-nid'e-əm) blastospore.

**Blas·to·cri·thid·ia** (blas"to-krĭ-thid'e-ə) [*blasto-* + Gr. *krithē* barleycorn] a genus of protozoa (suborder Trypanosomatina, order Kinetoplastida) parasitic in arthropods and other invertebrates, which pass through epimastigote, amastigote, and presumably promastigote developmental stages in their life cycle.

**blas·to·cyst** (blas'to-sist) [*blasto-* + Gr. *kystis* bladder] [MeSH: Blastocyst] the mammalian conceptus in the post-morula stage; it is like a blastula in having a fluid-filled cavity, unlike it in having the surface layer not exclusively embryoblast but mainly or entirely trophoblast, in having an eccentric embryoblast, and in not being limited to one germ layer.

**Blas·to·cys·tis** (blas"to-sis'tis) [MeSH: Blastocystis] a genus of

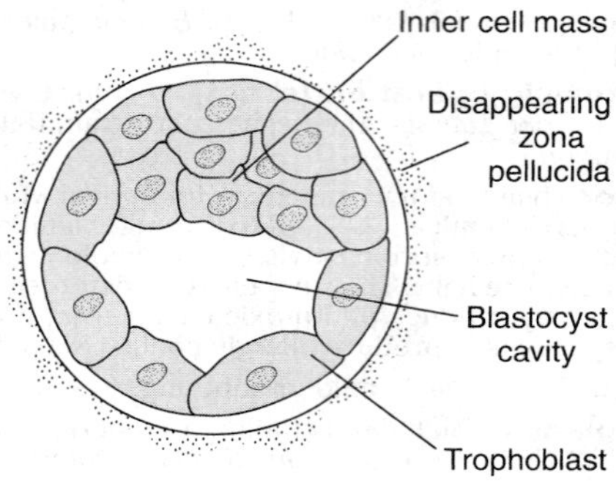

Early blastocyst.

yeasts of the family Entomophthoraceae. *B. ho'minis* is a nonpathogenic species frequently found in human feces.

**blas·to·cyte** (blas'to-sīt) [*blasto-* + *-cyte*] [MeSH: Blastomeres] an undifferentiated embryonic cell.

**blas·to·derm** (blas'to-dərm) [*blasto-* + *-derm*] [MeSH: Blastoderm] collectively, the mass of cells produced by cleavage of a fertilized ovum, forming the hollow sphere of the blastula, or the cellular cap above a floor of segmented yolk in the discoblastula of telolecithal eggs. Called also *germinal membrane,* or *membrana germinativa.*
**bilaminar b.,** the stage of development in which the embryo is represented by two primary layers: the ectoderm and the endoderm. See *gastrula.*
**embryonic b.,** the region of the blastoderm forming the embryo proper.
**extraembryonic b.,** the region of the blastoderm forming membranes rather than the embryo proper.
**trilaminar b.,** the stage of development in which the embryo is represented by the three primary layers: the ectoderm, the mesoderm, and the endoderm.

**blas·to·der·mal** (blas″to-dər'məl) pertaining to or derived from the blastoderm.

**blas·to·der·mic** (blas″to-dər'mik) blastodermal.

**blas·to·disc** (blas'to-disk) [*blasto-* + Gr. *diskos* disk] the convex structure formed by the blastomeres at the animal pole of an ovum undergoing incomplete cleavage.

**blas·to·gen·e·sis** (blas″to-jen'ə-sis) 1. the development of an individual from a blastema, that is, by asexual reproduction. 2. transmission of inherited characters by the germ plasm. 3. the morphological transformation of small lymphocytes into larger cells resembling blast cells, occurring on exposure to phytohemagglutinin or to antigens to which the donor is immunized.

**blas·to·ge·net·ic** (blas″to-jə-net'ik) blastogenic.

**blas·to·gen·ic** (blas″to-jen'ik) originating in the germ or germ cell; pertaining to or characterized by blastogenesis.

**blas·tog·e·ny** (blas-toj'ə-ne) [*blasto-* + *-geny*] the germ history of an organism or species.

**blas·to·ki·nin** (blas″to-ki'nin) a globulin found in the uterine lumen of some mammals near the time of blastocyst implantation; called also *uteroglobulin.*

**blas·tol·y·sis** (blas-tol'ĭ-sis) [*blasto-* + *-lysis*] destruction or splitting up of germ substance.

**blas·to·lyt·ic** (blas″to-lit'ik) pertaining to, characterized by, or producing blastolysis.

**blas·to·ma** (blas-to'mə) pl. *blasto'mas* or *blasto'mata* [*blast-* + *-oma*] a neoplasm composed of embryonic cells derived from the blastema of an organ or tissue.
**pulmonary b.,** a rare malignant pulmonary neoplasm whose cells resemble those of the fetal pulmonary blastema; it is usually large, develops in the peripheral portions of the lungs, and may invade the bronchi.

**blas·to·ma·toid** (blas-to'mə-toid) [*blastoma* + *-oid*] resembling blastomas.

**blas·to·ma·tous** (blas-to'mə-təs) pertaining to or of the nature of blastoma.

**blas·to·mere** (blas'to-mēr) [*blasto-* + *-mere*] [MeSH: Blastomeres] one of the cells produced by cleavage of a zygote; called also *segmentation sphere* and *cleavage cell.*

**blas·to·mer·ot·o·my** (blas″to-mēr-ot'o-me) [*blastomere* + *-tomy*] destruction of a blastomere or of blastomeres; called also *blastotomy.*

**blas·to·mo·gen·ic** (blas″to-mo-jen'ik) producing or tending to produce blastomas.

**blas·to·mog·e·nous** (blas″to-moj'ə-nəs) blastomogenic.

**Blas·to·my·ces** (blas″to-mi'sēz) [*blasto-* + Gr. *mykēs* fungus] [MeSH: Blastomyces] a genus of thermal dimorphic Fungi Imperfecti of the form-class Hyphomycetes; species grow as mycelial forms at room temperature and as yeastlike forms at body temperature. It includes several yeasts pathogenic for humans and other animals.
**B. brasilien'sis,** *Paracoccidioides brasiliensis.*
**B. dermati'tidis,** a species endemic in the midwestern United States and adjacent parts of Canada, the etiologic agent of North American blastomycosis; its perfect (sexual) stage is *Ajellomyces dermatitidis.*

**blas·to·my·ces** (blas″to-mi'sēz) pl. *blastomyce'tes* [MeSH: Blastomyces] a fungus of the genus *Blastomyces.* Called also *blastomycete.*

**blas·to·my·cete** (blas″to-mi'sēt) 1. blastomyces. 2. any yeastlike organism.

**Blas·to·my·ce·tes** (blas″to-mi-se'tēz) a form-class of Fungi Imperfecti (subphylum Deuteromycotina), comprising the yeasts. Most members of the group do not have known teleomorphs; those that do are classified under Ascomycotina or Basidiomycotina. The form-family Cryptococcaceae is sometimes classified here and sometimes in Hyphomycetes.

**blas·to·my·cin** (blas″to-mi'sin) a skin test antigen prepared from *Blastomyces dermatitidis* organisms, formerly used in diagnosis of blastomycosis but found to be unreliable.

**blas·to·my·co·sis** (blas″to-mi-ko'sis) [MeSH: Blastomycosis] 1. an infection usually acquired through the pulmonary route, caused by *Blastomyces dermatitidis.* There may be suppurating tumors in the skin *(cutaneous b.)* or lesions in the lungs, bones, subcutaneous tissues, liver, spleen, and kidneys *(systemic b.).* It runs a fulminant, sometimes fatal, course in immunocompromised patients. Called also *North American b., Gilchrist's disease* or *mycosis,* and *Chicago disease.* 2. a general term for any infection caused by a yeastlike organism.
**Brazilian b.,** paracoccidioidomycosis.
**cutaneous b.,** see *blastomycosis* (def. 1).
**European b.,** cutaneous cryptococcosis.
**keloidal b.,** an infection caused by *Loboa loboi,* characterized by the appearance of red, smooth, hard cutaneous nodules which have the histologic appearance of a keloid. Called also *Lobo's disease* and *lobomycosis.*
**North American b.,** blastomycosis (def. 1).
**pulmonary b.,** blastomycosis affecting primarily the lungs and bronchi; it often resolves with fibrosis or takes an indolent course, sometimes with cavitation and eventual spread to other organs. In some patients there is an acute onset of symptoms with acute respiratory distress syndrome that can be fatal. Called also bronchoblastomycosis.
**South American b.,** paracoccidioidomycosis.
**systemic b.,** see *blastomycosis* (def. 1).

**blas·to·neu·ro·pore** (blas″to-no͞o'ro-pōr) [*blasto-* + *neuro-* + *pore*] in certain embryos, a temporary aperture formed by the coalescence of the blastopore and neuropore.

**blas·toph·tho·ria** (blas″tof-thor'e-ə) [*blasto-* + Gr. *phthora* corruption] degeneration of the germ cells.

**blas·toph·tho·ric** (blas″tof-thor'ik) pertaining to, characterized by, or producing blastophthoria.

**blas·to·phyl·lum** (blas″to-fil'əm) [*blasto-* + Gr. *phyllon* leaf] a primordial germ layer.

**blas·toph·y·ly** (blas-tof'ə-le) [*blasto-* + Gr. *phylē* tribe] the tribal history, or arrangement, of organisms.

**blas·to·pore** (blas'to-por) [*blasto-* + *pore*] the opening of the archenteron to the exterior of the embryo, at the gastrula stage; called also *archistome, protostoma,* and *anus of Rusconi.*

**Blas·to·schiz·o·my·ces** (blas″to-skiz″o-mi'sēz) a genus of Fungi Imperfecti of the form-class Hyphomycetes. *B. capita'tus* (formerly called *Trichosporon capitatum*) has caused fatal opportunistic infections.

**blas·to·sphere** (blas'to-sfēr) [*blasto-* + *sphere*] blastula.

**blas·to·spore** (blas'to-spor) [*blasto-* + *spore*] a spore formed by budding, as in yeast. Called also *blastoconidium.*

**blas·to·stro·ma** (blas″to-stro'mə) that part of the egg which takes an active part in the formation of the blastoderm.

**blas·tot·o·my** (blas-tot'ə-me) blastomerotomy.

**blas·to·zo·oid** (blas″to-zo'oid) [*blasto-* + *zooid*] an individual developed as a result of asexual reproduction. Cf. *oozooid.*

**blas·tu·la** (blas'tu-lə) pl. *blas'tulae* [L.] the usually spherical structure produced by cleavage of a zygote, consisting of a single layer of cells (blastoderm) surrounding a fluid-filled cavity (blastocoele); called also *blastosphere.* See also *discoblastula.*

**blas·tu·lae** (blas'tu-le) [L.] plural of *blastula.*

**blas·tu·lar** (blas'tu-lər) pertaining to the blastula.

**blas·tu·la·tion** (blas"tu-la'shən) conversion of a morula to a blastula by the development of a central cavity (the blastocoele, blastocyst, or cleavage cavity).

**Bla·tin's sign, syndrome** (blah-taz') [Marc *Blatin,* French physician, 1878–1943] see under *sign* and see *hydatid thrill,* under *thrill.*

**Blat·ta** (blat'ə) [L.] a genus of cockroaches of the family Blattidae. Their dried, crushed bodies were formerly administered medically as diuretics. They may act as intermediate hosts of *Raillietina madagascariensis* and *Gongylonema pulchrum. B. orienta'lis* is the Oriental cockroach.

**Blat·tar·ia** (blă-tar'e-ə) the cockroaches, an order of crawling winged insects with flat oval bodies; many are household pests or reservoirs of disease. See also *cockroach.*

**Blat·tel·la** (blă-tel'ə) a genus of cockroaches of the family Blattidae. *B. germa'nica* is the German cockroach.

**Blat·ti·dae** (blat'ĭ-de) a family of cockroaches (order Blattaria); genera include *Blatta* and *Blattella.*

**BLB mask** [Walter Meredith *Boothby,* American medical researcher, 1880–1953; William R. *Lovelace,* American surgeon, 1907–1965; Arthur H. *Bulbulian,* Turkish-born American medical researcher, born 1900] see under *mask.*

**bleach·ing** (blēch'ing) the act or process of removing stains or color by chemical means.
**coronal b.,** the use of a chemical agent, usually but not necessarily in combination with heat, to remove discolorations from the crown of a pulpless tooth.

**bleb** (bleb) bulla.

**bleed·er** (blēd'ər) 1. popular term for a person who tends to bleed too easily, usually because of a deficiency of one of the coagulation factors, such as in hemophilia. 2. any blood vessel cut during a surgical procedure that requires clamping, cautery, or ligature.

**bleed·ing** (blēd'ing) 1. the escape of blood from an injured vessel; see also *hemorrhage.* 2. phlebotomy.
**dysfunctional uterine b.,** bleeding from the uterus when no organic uterine lesions are present.
**implantation b.,** bleeding occurring at the time of implantation of the fertilized ovum in the decidua, being due to leakage of blood into the uterine lumen from disrupted blood vessels about the implantation site.
**occult b.,** escape of such a small amount of blood that it can be detected only by chemical test or by examination with the microscope or spectroscope.
**summer b.,** dermatorrhagia parasitica.

**blen·nad·e·ni·tis** (blen"ad-ə-ni'tis) [*blenn-* + *adeno-* + *-itis*] inflammation of mucous glands.

**blen·nem·e·sis** (blen-em'ə-sis) [*blenn-* + *emesis*] the vomiting of mucus.

**blenn(o)-** [Gr. *blenna* mucus] a combining form denoting relationship to mucus.

**blen·no·gen·ic** (blen-o-jen'ik) [*blenno-* + *-genic*] muciparous.

**blen·nog·e·nous** (blen-oj'ə-nəs) muciparous.

**blen·noid** (blen'oid) [*blenn-* + *-oid*] mucoid, def. 1.

**blen·nor·rha·gia** (blen"o-ra'jə) [*blenno-* + *-rrhagia*] 1. blennorrhea. 2. former name for *gonorrhea.*

**blen·nor·rhag·ic** (blen"o-raj'ik) blennorrheal.

**blen·nor·rhea** (blen"o-re'ə) [*blenno-* + *-rrhea*] 1. a free discharge from the mucous surfaces, especially a gonorrheal discharge from the urethra or vagina. Called also *blennorrhagia* and *myxorrhea.* 2. former name for *gonorrhea.*
**inclusion b.,** see under *conjunctivitis.*
**b. neonato'rum,** ophthalmia neonatorum.
**Stoerk's b.,** blennorrhea with profuse chronic suppuration producing hypertrophy of the mucosa of the nose, pharynx, and larynx.

**blen·nor·rhe·al** (blen"o-re'əl) pertaining to or of the nature of blennorrhea.

**blen·no·sta·sis** (blen-os'tə-sis) [*blenno-* + *-stasis*] the suppression of an abnormal mucous discharge, or the correction of an excessive one.

**blen·no·stat·ic** (blen"o-stat'ik) [*blenno-* + *-static*] 1. pertaining to blennostasis. 2. mucostatic, def. 1.

**blen·no·tho·rax** (blen"o-thor'aks) [*blenno-* + *thorax*] a pleural effusion consisting of mucus.

**blen·nu·ria** (blen-u're-ə) [*blenn-* + *-uria*] the existence of mucus in the urine.

**Blen·ox·ane** (blen-oks'ān) trademark for a preparation of bleomycin sulfate.

**ble·o·my·cin** (ble"o-mi'sin) [MeSH: Bleomycin] any of a mixture of glycopeptide antibiotics produced by a strain of *Streptomyces verticillus,* designated $A_1$ to $A_6$, $A_2'$, and $B_1$ to $B_6$, that bind to DNA causing chain scission and removal of purine and pyrimidine bases, resulting in inhibition of DNA synthesis and, to a lesser extent, RNA and protein synthesis and also accumulation of cells in the $G_2$ phase of the cell cycle. The drug used clinically is a mixture consisting primarily of bleomycins $A_2$ and $B_2$; it is used in the form of bleomycin sulfate as an antineoplastic.
**b. sulfate** [USP], a mixture of the sulfate salts of the components of bleomycin, especially that of bleomycin $A_2$, used alone or in conjunction with other chemotherapeutic agents in the palliative treatment of squamous cell carcinoma of the head and neck, Hodgkin's disease and other lymphomas, and testicular tumors; administered intravenously, intramuscularly, intra-arterially, or subcutaneously.

**Bleph** (blef) trademark for preparations of sulfacetamide sodium.

**bleph·ar·ad·e·ni·tis** (blef"ər-ad"ə-ni'tis) [*blephar-* + *aden-* + *-itis*] inflammation of the meibomian glands; called also *blepharoadenitis.*

**bleph·a·ral** (blef'ə-ral) pertaining to the eyelids.

**bleph·a·rec·to·my** (blef"ə-rek'to-me) [*blephar-* + *ectomy*] excision of a lesion of the eyelids.

**bleph·a·rel·o·sis** (blef"ə-rel-o'sis) [*blephar-* + Gr. *eilein* to roll] entropion.

**bleph·a·rism** (blef'ə-riz"əm) [L. *blepharismus,* from Gr. *blepharizein* to wink] spasm of the eyelids; continuous blinking.

**bleph·a·ri·tis** (blef"ə-ri'tis) [*blephar-* + *-itis*] [MeSH: Blepharitis] inflammation of the eyelids.
**b. angula'ris,** blepharitis ulcerosa affecting the medial commissure (angle) and blocking the punctum lacrimalis.
**b. cilia'ris, marginal b., b. margina'lis,** a chronic inflammation of the hair follicles and sebaceous gland openings of the margins of the eyelids; called also *blear eye, lippa,* and *lippitude.*
**nonulcerative b.,** blepharitis often associated with seborrhea of the scalp, brows, and skin behind the ears, marked by greasy scaling of the margins of the lids, scales around the lashes, hyperemia, and thickening; called also *seborrheic b.* and *squamous seborrheic b.*
**seborrheic b.,** nonulcerative b.
**squamous b.,** nonulcerative b.
**b. ulcero'sa,** an ulcerous form of marginal blepharitis.

**blephar(o)-** [Gr. *blepharon* eyelid] a combining form denoting relationship to an eyelid.

**bleph·a·ro·ad·e·ni·tis** (blef"ə-ro-ad"ə-ni'tis) blepharadenitis.

**bleph·a·ro·ad·e·no·ma** (blef"ə-ro-ad"ə-no'mə) adenoma of the eyelid.

**bleph·a·ro·ath·er·o·ma** (blef"ə-ro-ath"ər-o'mə) an encysted tumor or sebaceous cyst of an eyelid.

**bleph·a·ro·chal·a·sis** (blef"ə-ro-kal'ə-sis) [*blepharo-* + Gr. *chalasis* relaxation] relaxation of the skin of the eyelid, due to atrophy of the intercellular tissue; called also *dermatolysis palpebrarum.*

**bleph·a·ro·chro·mi·dro·sis** (blef"ə-ro-kro-mĭ-dro'sis) [*blepharo-* + *chrom-* + *hidr-* + *-osis*] excretion of a sweat containing pigment from the eyelids, usually of a bluish shade.

**bleph·a·roc·lo·nus** (blef"ə-rok'lə-nəs) [*blepharo-* + *clonus*] clonic spasm of the orbicularis oculi muscle, appearing as an increased winking of the eye.

**bleph·a·ro·con·junc·ti·vi·tis** (blef"ə-ro-kən-junk"-tĭ-vi'tis) inflammation of the eyelids and conjunctiva.

**Bleph·a·ro·co·ryn·thi·na** (blef"ə-ro-ko"rin-thi'nə) [*blepharo-* + Gr. *koryntheus* basket] a suborder of ciliate protozoa (order Trichostomatida, subclass Vestibuliferia) found in herbivorous mammals, especially horses, and characterized by a marked reduction in somatic ciliature and apically by a retractable oral area, prominent frontal lobe, and a distinctive corkscrew-like process.

**bleph·a·ro·di·as·ta·sis** (blef"ə-ro-di-as'tə-sis) [*blepharo-* + *diastasis*] excessive separation of the eyelids, or inability to close them completely, causing the fissure to be very wide.

**bleph·a·ron·cus** (blef"ə-rong'kəs) [*blepharo-* + Gr. *onkos* bulk, mass] a tumor on the eyelid.

**bleph·a·ro·pach·yn·sis** (blef"ə-ro-pak-in'sis) [*blepharo-* + *pachynsis*] abnormal thickening of an eyelid.

**bleph·a·ro·phi·mo·sis** (blef"ə-ro-fĭ-mo'sis) [*blepharo-* + Gr. *phimōsis* a muzzling] [MeSH: Blepharophimosis] abnormal narrowness of the palpebral fissures in the horizontal direction, caused by lateral displacement of the inner canthi.

**bleph·a·ro·plast** (blef′ə-ro-plast) [*blepharo-* + *-plast*] basal body.

**bleph·a·ro·plas·ty** (blef′ə-ro-plas″te) plastic surgery of the eyelids.

**bleph·a·ro·ple·gia** (blef″ə-ro-ple′jə) [*blepharo-* + *-plegia*] paralysis of an eyelid or of both muscles of the eyelid.

**bleph·a·rop·to·sis** (blef″ə-rop-to′sis) [*blepharo-* + *-ptosis*] [MeSH: Blepharoptosis] drooping of an upper eyelid due to paralysis; ptosis.

**bleph·a·ro·py·or·rhea** (blef″ə-ro-pi″ə-re′ə) [*blepharo-* + *pyo-* + *-rrhea*] purulent ophthalmia.

**bleph·a·ror·rha·phy** (blef″ə-ror′ə-fe) [*blepharo-* + *-rrhaphy*] tarsorrhaphy.

**bleph·a·ro·spasm** (blef′ə-ro-spaz″əm) [*blepharo-* + *spasm*] [MeSH: Blepharospasm] tonic spasm of the orbicularis oculi muscle, producing more or less complete closure of the eyelids.
**essential b.,** blepharospasm that is present when there is no abnormality of the eye, or trigeminal (fifth cranial) nerve.
**symptomatic b.,** blepharospasm occurring in association with a lesion of the eye or of the trigeminal (fifth cranial) nerve.

**bleph·a·ro·sphinc·ter·ec·to·my** (blef″ə-ro-sfingk″tər-ek′tə-me) [*blepharo-* + *sphincter* + *ectomy*] excision of some of the fibers of the orbicularis muscle, together with overlying skin, to relieve pressure of the eyelid on the cornea in blepharospasm.

**bleph·a·ro·stat** (blef′ə-ro-stat″) [*blepharo-* + *-stat*] an instrument for holding the eyelids and keeping them apart during surgical operations on the eye.

**bleph·a·ro·ste·no·sis** (blef″ə-ro-stə-no′sis) blepharophimosis.

**bleph·a·ro·syn·ech·ia** (blef″ə-ro-sĭ-nek′e-ə) [*blepharo-* + *synechia*] the growing together or adhesion of the eyelids.

**bleph·a·rot·o·my** (blef″ə-rot′ə-me) [*blepharo-* + *-tomy*] surgical incision of an eyelid; tarsotomy.

**Bles·sig's cysts (spaces, lacunae), groove** (bles′igz) [Robert *Blessig,* German physician, 1830–1878] see under *cyst* and *groove.*

**Blighia** (bli′yə) a genus of evergreen trees of the family Sapindaceae, native to West Africa. *B. sa′pida* Kon. is the akee or ackee, whose aril is cooked and considered a delicacy in the West Indies but is poisonous if eaten raw. See *Jamaican vomiting sickness,* under *sickness.*

**blind** (blīnd) [A.S. *blind*] 1. not having the sense of sight; see *blindness.* 2. pertaining to a clinical trial or other experiment (blind study) in which one or more of the groups receiving, administering, and evaluating the treatment are unaware of which treatment any particular subject is receiving; sometimes referred to as masked to avoid confusion. See *single blind, double blind,* and *triple blind.* Cf. *open.*

**blind·gut** (blīnd′gut″) caecum (def. 2).

**blind·ness** (blīnd′nəs) [MeSH: Blindness] lack or loss of ability to see; lack of perception of visual stimuli, due to disorder of the organs of sight or to lesions in certain areas of the brain; see also *amaurosis.*
**amnesic color b.,** a form of aphasia in which the patient sees a color correctly but cannot name it, due to a brain lesion.
**blue b.,** imperfect perception of the blue spectrum; see *tetartanopia* (def. 2) and *tritanopia.*
**blue-yellow b.,** imperfect perception of blue and yellow tints; see *tetartanopia* (def. 2.) and *tritanopia.*
**Bright's b.,** former term for dimness or complete loss of sight occurring in uremia, without lesion of the retina or optic disk.
**color b.,** a term colloquially and incorrectly applied to any deviation from normal perception of hues; see *deuteranopia, monochromatism, protanopia, quadrantanopia,* and *tritanopia.*
**color b., complete, color b., total,** monochromatism.
**concussion b.,** functional blindness due to violent explosions, as by high explosive shells, bombs, etc.
**cortical b.,** blindness due to a lesion of the cortical visual center.
**cortical psychic b.,** visual agnosia.
**day b.,** hemeralopia.
**eclipse b.,** partial or total loss of central vision caused by a burn on the macula from direct fixation on the sun or from viewing a partial solar eclipse without proper protective lenses.

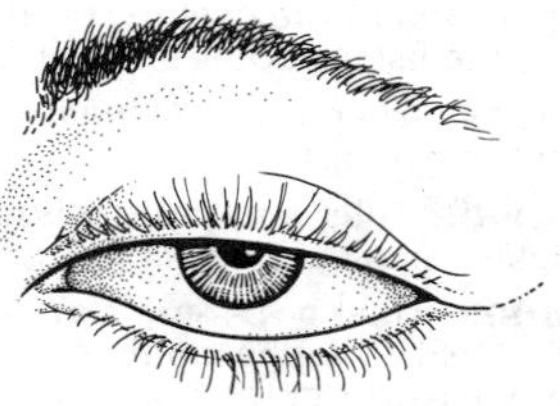
Blepharoptosis.

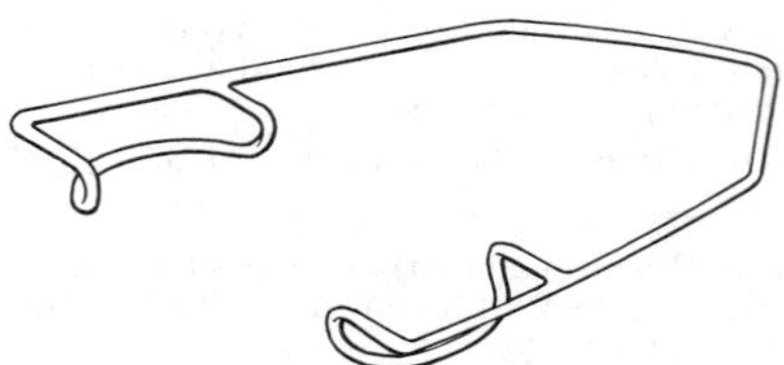
Blepharostat.

**electric-light b.,** temporary impairment of vision due to exposure to ultraviolet rays. Photophobia, blepharospasm, redness of the eye, and swelling of the conjunctiva are the symptoms, which usually occur several hours after exposure.
**flight b.,** amaurosis fugax caused by high centrifugal forces encountered in aviation.
**functional b.,** inability to see because of conversion hysteria; it occurs without disorder of the organs of sight.
**green b.,** imperfect perception of green tints; see *deuteranopia* and *protanopia.*
**heather b.,** infectious ovine keratoconjunctivitis.
**hysterical b.,** functional b.
**legal b.,** blindness as defined by law; in most states of the United States, maximal visual acuity of the better eye, after correction, of 20/200 or less, with a total diameter of the visual field in that eye of 20 degrees or less.
**letter b.,** alexia characterized by inability to recognize individual letters.
**moon b.,** periodic ophthalmia.
**music b.,** musical alexia.
**night b.,** nyctalopia.
**object b.,** visual agnosia.
**psychic b.,** visual agnosia.
**red b.,** imperfect perception of red tints; see *deuteranopia* and *protanopia.*
**red-green b.,** imperfect perception of red and green tints; see *deuteranopia* and *protanopia.*
**river b.,** blindness caused by onchocerciasis.
**snow b.,** dimness of vision, usually temporary, due to the glare of the sun upon snow.
**taste b.,** partial ageusia, with only some substances producing no sensation of taste.
**text b.,** alexia.
**total b.,** complete absence of light perception.
**twilight b.,** aknephascopia.
**word b.,** alexia.
**yellow b.,** imperfect perception of yellow tints; see *tetartanopia* and *tritanopia.*

**blis·ter** (blis′tər) [L. *vesicula*] [MeSH: Blister] 1. bulla (def. 1). 2. vesicle (def. 2).
**blood b.,** a blister containing blood; it may be caused by a pinch, a bruise, or persistent friction.
**fever b.,** herpes febrilis.
**water b.,** one with clear watery contents.

**bloat** (blōt) 1. indigestion with excessive formation of gas in one or more of the stomachs of a ruminant. 2. ruminal tympany. 3. enteritis in young rabbits, accompanied by gaseous distention of the abdomen.
**abomasal b.,** bloat in calves or lambs on milk replacement diets, seen especially when the milk replacer is warm or contains insoluble ingredients or if the animals have not been fed for a few hours and drink too much. The distended abomasum may compress adjacent organs and vessels, resulting in fatal asphyxia or heart failure.
**free gas b.,** bloat in ruminants caused by an esophageal obstruction that prevents eructation; called also *secondary ruminal tympany.*
**frothy b.,** primary ruminal tympany.
**leguminous b.,** primary ruminal tympany caused by a diet excessively high in legumes such as alfalfa or clover.

**Blo·ca·dren** (blo′kə-dren) trademark for a preparation of timolol maleate.

**Bloch** (blok) Konrad Emil. German-born American biochemist born 1912; co-winner, with Feodor Lynen, of the Nobel prize for medicine or physiology in 1964, for investigations in biosynthesis and metabolism of cholesterol and fatty acids.

**Bloch-Sulz·ber·ger syndrome** (blok-sulz′berg-ər) [Bruno *Bloch,* Swiss dermatologist, 1878–1933; Marion Baldur *Sulzberger,* American dermatologist, 1895–1983] incontinentia pigmenti.

**block** (blok) 1. obstruction. 2. to obstruct. 3. regional anesthesia; see under *anesthesia.*

**adrenergic b.**, see under *blockade*.
**air b.**, interference with the normal inflation and deflation of the lungs and with the pulmonary blood flow, produced by the leakage of air from the pulmonary alveoli into the interstitial tissue of the lung (interstitial emphysema) and into the mediastinum (mediastinal emphysema).
**alveolar-capillary b.**, interference in the normal diffusion of gases across the membrane between the alveolar spaces and the pulmonary capillaries.
**ankle b.**, regional anesthesia of the foot by the injection of a local anesthetic around the anterior and posterior tibial nerves at the level of the ankle.
**anodal b.**, a conduction block resulting from hyperpolarization of the nerve cell membrane by an electric stimulus.
**anterior fascicular b.**, left anterior hemiblock; see *hemiblock*. See also *fascicular b.*
**atrioventricular b., AV b.**, impairment of conduction of cardiac impulses from the atria to the ventricles, usually due to a block in the atrioventricular junctional tissue (atrioventricular node, bundle of His, or bundle branches). It is generally subclassified as first, second, or third degree atrioventricular block. Cf. *heart b.*
**2:1 AV b.**, second degree atrioventricular block in which conduction of every other impulse through the atrioventricular conduction system is prevented, resulting in a 2:1 ratio of atrial to ventricular depolarizations.
**Bier b.**, regional anesthesia by intravenous injection, used for surgical procedures on the arm below the elbow or the leg below the knee; performed in a bloodless field maintained by a pneumatic tourniquet that also prevents the anesthetic from entering the systemic circulation. Called also *Bier's local anestheia, intravenous regional anesthesia,* and *intravenous b.*
**bifascicular b.**, impairment of conduction in two of the three fascicles of the bundle branches (see *fascicular b.*), i.e., in the left bundle branch or in the right bundle branch plus either the anterior or posterior limb of the left bundle branch.
**bilateral bundle branch b. (BBBB),** interruption of conduction of cardiac impulses through both bundle branches, clinically indistinguishable from complete atrioventricular block.
**brachial plexus b.**, regional anesthesia of the shoulder, arm, and hand by injection of a local anesthetic into the brachial plexus; called also *brachial plexus anesthesia.*
**bundle branch b. (BBB),** interruption of conduction in one of the main bundle branches, left or right; the sequence of ventricular depolarization is altered since the impulse reaches one ventricle and then travels to the other.
**caudal b.**, regional anesthesia produced by injection of a local anesthetic into the caudal or sacral canal. Called also *caudal anesthesia.*
**cervical plexus b.**, regional anesthesia of the neck by injection of a local anesthetic into the cervical plexus.
**comparator b.**, see *comparator.*
**complete atrioventricular b.**, third degree atrioventricular b.
**complete heart b.**, third degree heart b.
**conduction b.**, a blockage in a nerve that prevents impulses from being conducted across a given segment although the nerve is viable beyond that segment. Cf. *neurapraxia.*
**congenital complete heart b.**, third degree atrioventricular block that presents in the fetal or neonatal period and is caused by defective development of the atrioventricular junctional tissue; it may be associated with other cardiac anomalies.
**cryogenic b.**, local cooling of tissue.
**depolarization b.**, failure of an excitable cell to respond to a stimulus, because the membrane is depolarized.
**dynamic b.**, spinal subarachnoid b.
**elbow b.**, regional anesthesia of the forearm and hand by injection of local anesthetic around the median, radial, and ulnar nerves at the elbow.
**entrance b.**, in cardiology, a unidirectional impasse to conduction that prevents an impulse from entering a specific region of excitable tissue; it is part of the mechanism underlying parasystole.
**epidural b.**, see under *anesthesia.*
**exit b.**, in cardiology, delay or failure of an impulse to be conducted from a specific region to surrounding tissues; the region may be either a physiologic or artificial cardiac pacemaker.
**fascicular b.**, any of a group of disorders of conduction localized within the bundle branches or their ramifications. The block may occur in any combination of the three fascicles of the bundle branches: the right bundle branch or the anterior or posterior limb of the left bundle branch. See also *unifascicular b., bifascicular b.,* and *trifascicular b.*
**femoral b.**, regional anesthesia of the posterior thigh and the leg below the knee by injection of a local anesthetic around the femoral nerve just below the inguinal ligament at the lateral border of the fossa ovalis.

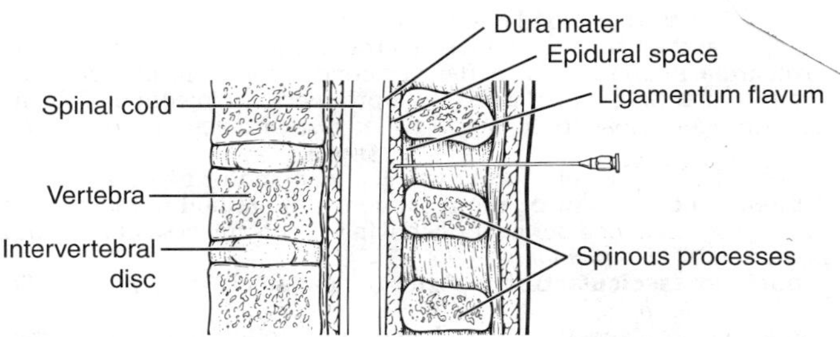

Production of epidural block by injection through the ligamentum flavum into the epidural space, the needle stopping just short of the dura mater.

**field b.**, regional anesthesia obtained by blocking conduction in nerves with chemical or physical agents.
**first degree atrioventricular b.**, a first degree heart block due to a block in the atrioventricular junctional tissue; the rate of conduction of impulses from the atria to the ventricles is slowed, resulting in regular electrocardiographic P–R intervals of greater than 0.21 second.
**first degree heart b.**, the mildest form of heart block, in which conduction time is prolonged but all impulses are conducted; often used specifically for first degree atrioventricular block.
**heart b.**, impairment of conduction of an impulse in heart excitation, either permanent or transient and due to anatomical or functional impairment. It is subclassified as first, second, or third degree heart block and is frequently used specifically to denote atrioventricular block.
**high grade atrioventricular b.**, either second or third degree atrioventricular b.
**incomplete heart b.**, heart block in which at least some impulses are conducted, i.e., first or second degree heart block.
**intercostal b., intercostal nerve b.**, regional anesthesia produced by blocking intercostal nerves with a local anesthetic.
**interventricular b.**, bundle branch b.
**intra-Hisian b., intrahisian b.**, atrioventricular block located within the bundle of His.
**intranasal b.**, local anesthesia produced by insertion into the nasal fossae of pledgets soaked in a solution of local anesthetic.
**intraspinal b.**, spinal anesthesia (def. 1).
**intravenous (IV) b.**, Bier b.
**intraventricular b.**, impaired conduction within the ventricles due to absence of conduction within the bundle branches, their ramifications, or the ventricles.
**left anterior fascicular b.**, left anterior hemiblock; see *hemiblock.* See also *fascicular b.*
**left bundle branch b. (LBBB),** see *bundle branch b.*
**left posterior fascicular b.**, left posterior hemiblock; see *hemiblock.* See also *fascicular b.*
**lumbar plexus b.**, regional anesthesia of the anterior and medial aspects of the leg by injection of a local anesthetic into the lumbar plexus.
**mental b.**, *blocking* (def. 2).
**metabolic b.**, the blockade of a biosynthetic pathway caused by a genetic enzyme deficiency or by inhibition of an enzyme by a drug or other substance.
**methadone b.**, see *narcotic blockade,* under *blockade.*
**Mobitz type I b.**, Wenckebach b.
**Mobitz type II b.**, a type of second degree atrioventricular block in which dropped beats occur periodically without previous lengthening of the P–R interval (cf. *Wenckebach b.*); it is due to a block within or below the bundle of His.
**motor point b.**, interruption of impulses, by anesthesia or destruction of the nerve, at a motor point in order to relieve spasticity; a common method is *phenol motor point b.* Called also *intramuscular neurolysis.*
**nerve b.**, 1. regional anesthesia secured by making extraneural or paraneural injections of anesthetics in close proximity to the nerve whose conductivity is to be cut off. 2. neurolysis (def. 4).
**neurolytic b.**, neurolysis (def. 4).
**paracervical b.**, regional anesthesia of the inferior hypogastric plexus and ganglia produced by injection of the local anesthetic into the lateral fornices of the vagina; called also *uterosacral b.*
**paraneural b.**, perineural b.
**parasacral b.**, regional anesthesia produced by injection of a local anesthetic around the sacral nerves as they emerge from the sacral foramina.
**paravertebral b.**, regional anesthesia produced by injection of a local anesthetic around the spinal nerves at their exit from the spinal column, usually to cause anesthesia of the sympathetic trunk at a given level. Called also *paravertebral anesthesia.*

**partial heart b.**, second degree heart b.
**periinfarction b.**, disturbance of intraventricular conduction after a myocardial infarction, due to delayed conduction in the infarct region.
**perineural b.**, regional anesthesia produced by injection of the anesthetic agent close to the nerve; called also *paraneural b.* or *anesthesia.*
**phenol b.**, 1. phenol neurolysis. 2. phenol motor point b.
**phenol motor point b.**, the most common method of motor point block; a solution of 5 per cent phenol in water is injected at the motor point. Called also *phenol b.*
**posterior fascicular b.**, left posterior hemiblock; see *hemiblock.* See also *fascicular b.*
**presacral b.**, anesthesia produced by injection of the local anesthetic into the sacral nerves on the anterior aspect of the sacrum.
**pudendal b.**, anesthesia produced by blocking the pudendal nerves, accomplished by injection of the local anesthetic into the region of the tuberosity of the ischium.
**right bundle branch b. (RBBB)**, see *bundle branch b.*
**sacral b.**, see under *anesthesia.*
**saddle b.**, the production of spinal anesthesia in a region corresponding roughly with the areas of the buttocks, perineum, and inner aspects of the thighs which impinge on the saddle in riding, by introducing the anesthetic agent low in the dural sac.
**sciatic b.**, regional anesthesia of the lower leg and foot by injection of a local anesthetic around the sciatic nerve.
**second degree atrioventricular b.**, a second degree heart block due to partial impairment of impulse conduction through the atrioventricular junctional tissue; impulses intermittently fail to reach the ventricles (dropped beats). It occurs as two types: *type I* is Wenckebach or Mobitz type I block and *type II* is Mobitz type II block.
**second degree heart b.**, the partial form of heart block, in which some impulses are not conducted; often used specifically for second degree atrioventricular block. Called also *partial heart b.*
**sinoatrial b., sinoatrial exit b.**, a disturbance in which the atrial response is delayed or omitted because of partial or complete interference with the propagation of impulses from the sinoatrial node to the atria.
**sinus b.**, sinoatrial b.
**sinus exit b.**, sinoatrial exit b.
**spinal b.**, spinal anesthesia.
**spinal subarachnoid b.**, a condition in which the flow of cerebrospinal fluid is interfered with by an obstruction in the spinal canal; called also *dynamic b.*
**splanchnic b.**, regional anesthesia produced by blocking the splanchnic nerves and the celiac ganglia; it is accomplished by injection of the anesthetic agent into the retroperitoneal tissues in the immediate vicinity of the celiac plexuses.
**stellate b., stellate ganglion b.**, regional anesthesia produced by blocking of the stellate (cervicothoracic) ganglion.
**subarachnoid b.**, spinal anesthesia (def. 1).
**sympathetic b.**, blocking of the sympathetic trunk by paravertebral infiltration with an anesthetic agent.
**third degree atrioventricular b.**, a third degree heart block due to total cessation of impulse conduction through the atrioventricular junctional tissue; no correspondence exists between atrial and ventricular activity, and ventricular asystole and death occur unless a ventricular pacemaker is activated.
**third degree heart b.**, the complete form of heart block, in which no impulses are conducted; often used specifically for third degree atrioventricular block. Called also *complete heart b.*
**transsacral b.**, sacral anesthesia.
**trifascicular b.**, impairment of conduction in all three fascicles of the bundle branches, i.e., the right bundle branch and both anterior and posterior limbs of the left bundle branch. It is a form of complete heart block. See also *fascicular b.*
**unifascicular b.**, impairment of conduction in the right bundle branch or in either the anterior or posterior limb of the left bundle branch. See also *fascicular b.*
**uterosacral b.**, paracervical b.
**vagal b., vagus nerve b.**, regional anesthesia produced by blocking of vagal impulses by injection of a local anesthetic into the vagus nerve at its exit from the skull.
**ventricular b.**, obstruction to the flow of cerebrospinal fluid within the ventricular system or through the exit foramina (foramina of Magendie and Luschka) by which the ventricles communicate with the subarachnoid space; it results in obstructive hydrocephalus.
**Wenckebach b.**, a type of second degree atrioventricular block in which one or more dropped beats occur periodically after a series of steadily increasing P–R intervals (cf. *Mobitz type II b.*); it is usually due to a block within the atrioventricular node. Called also *Mobitz type I b.*
**wrist b.**, regional anesthesia of the hand by injection of a local anesthetic around the median, radial, and ulnar nerves at the wrist.

**block·ade** (blok-ād′) 1. receptor blockade, the blocking of the effect of a hormone or neurotransmitter at a cell-surface receptor by a pharmacologic antagonist bound to the receptor. 2. in histochemistry, a chemical reaction that by modifying certain chemical groups blocks a specific staining method. 3. regional anesthesia.
**adrenergic b.**, selective inhibition of the response to sympathetic impulses and to catecholamines and other adrenergic amines at either the alpha or beta receptor sites of the effector organ or at the postganglionic adrenergic neuron.
**adrenergic neuron b.**, see *adrenergic b.*
**alpha-adrenergic b., alpha-b.**, see *adrenergic b.*
**beta-adrenergic b., beta-b.**, see *adrenergic b.*
**cholinergic b.**, selective inhibition of cholinergic nerve impulses at autonomic ganglionic synapses, at postganglionic parasympathetic effectors, or at the neuromuscular junction.
**combined androgen b.**, treatment of prostate cancer by blocking both testicular and adrenal androgens, usually through orchiectomy followed by administration of an agent that blocks adrenal androgens.
**narcotic b.**, inhibition of the euphoric effects of narcotic drugs by the use of other drugs, such as methadone, in the treatment of addiction.
**neuromuscular b.**, a failure in neuromuscular transmission that can be induced pharmacologically or may result from pathological disturbance at the myoneural junction.
**renal b.**, obstructive uropathy with involvement of the genitourinary system distal to the collecting tubules; blockade of individual nephrons or nephron groups and the resultant anuria.
**virus b.**, interference by a virus with the action of another virus; attenuated virus of a disease has been used to inhibit the multiplication of an active virus.

**block·age** (blok′əj) obstruction.
**tendon b.**, fixation of a tendon by a Kirschner wire to bone or tendon sheath to relieve tension and prevent retraction.

**Block·ain** (blok′ān) trademark for a preparation of propoxycaine hydrochloride.

**block·er** (blok′ər) something that obstructs passage or activity. See also *blocking agent*, under *agent.*
**α-b.**, a drug that induces adrenergic blockade at α-adrenergic receptors.
**β-b.**, a drug that induces adrenergic blockade at either $\beta_1$- or $\beta_2$-adrenergic receptors or at both.
**calcium channel b.**, one of a group of drugs that inhibit the entry of calcium into cells or inhibit the mobilization of calcium from intracellular stores, resulting in slowing of atrioventricular and sinoatrial conduction and relaxation of arterial smooth and cardiac muscle; used in the treatment of angina, cardiac arrhythmias, and hypertension.
**calcium entry b.**, calcium channel b.
**potassium channel b.**, any of a class of drugs that inhibit the movement of potassium ions through the potassium channels, thus prolonging repolarization of the cell membrane; such drugs are used as antiarrhythmic agents.
**sodium channel b.**, any of a class of antiarrhythmic agents that prevent ectopic beats by acting on partially inactivated sodium channels to inhibit abnormal depolarizations.

**block·ing** (blok′ing) 1. interfering with afferent nerve impulses; see *regional anesthesia,* under *anesthesia.* 2. sudden cessation of the train of thought or speech, such as may occur in a period of extreme emotion or when a repressed painful thought is approached. Called also *thought b.* or *deprivation.* 3. casting of tissue blocks in an embedding medium such as paraffin wax so that sections can be cut with a microtome.

**adrenergic b.,** see under *blockade.*

**thought b.,** *blocking* (def. 2).

**block·out** (blok′out) elimination in a master cast of undesirable undercut areas, including all areas that would offer interference to the placement of the denture framework and those not crossed by a rigid part of the denture, accomplished by filling in areas to be blocked out with suitable materials. See also *relief,* def. 4.

**Blocq's disease** (bloks) [Paul Oscar *Blocq,* French physician, 1860–1896] astasia-abasia.

**Blom-Sing·er puncture** (blom sing′ər) [Eric D. *Blom,* American speech pathologist, 20th century; Mark Irwin *Singer,* American otolaryngologist, born 1945] see *tracheoesophageal puncture,* under *puncture.*

**blood** (blud) [L. *sanguis, cruor;* Gr. *haima*] [MeSH: Blood] the fluid that circulates through the heart, arteries, capillaries, and veins, carrying nutriment and oxygen to the body cells. It consists of the *plasma,* a pale yellow liquid containing the microscopically visible formed elements of the blood: the *erythrocytes,* or red blood corpuscles; the *leukocytes,* or white blood corpuscles; and the *platelets,* or thrombocytes. Called also *haema* [TA], *hema,* and *sanguis* [TA alternative].

**arterial b.,** oxygenated blood, found in the pulmonary veins, the left chambers of the heart, and the systemic arteries; it is bright red in color.

**citrated b.,** blood treated with sodium citrate or citric acid to prevent its coagulation.

**cord b.,** blood contained within the umbilical vessels at the time of delivery of the infant.

**defibrinated b.,** whole blood from which fibrin was separated during the clotting process.

**laky b.,** blood that has undergone laking and contains at least some lysed erythrocytes.

**occult b.,** blood present in such small quantities that, while it is not visible to the naked eye, it can be detected only by chemical tests of suspected material, e.g., feces.

**peripheral b.,** blood obtained from acral areas, or from the circulation remote from the heart, as from earlobe, fingertip, or heel pad (in a child), or from the antecubital vein; the blood in the systemic circulation.

**sludged b.,** blood in which the red cells have become aggregated into masses; see *intravascular agglutination,* under *agglutination.*

**venous b.,** deoxygenated blood, found in the systemic veins, the right chambers of the heart, and the pulmonary arteries; it is dark red in color.

**whole b.,** 1. blood from which none of the elements have been removed. 2. [USP] blood that has been drawn from a selected donor under strict aseptic conditions, containing citrate ion or heparin as an anticoagulant; used as a blood replenisher. Called also *whole human b.*

**blood group** (blud gro͞op) [MeSH: Blood Groups] 1. an allotype (or phenotype) of erythrocytes defined by one or more cell surface antigens that are under the control of allelic genes. Antigenic determinants irregularly incite allotypic and sometimes xenotypic immune responses. Human blood groups are identified by agglutination supported by specific human or animal antisera and by lectins extracted from certain plants. An abbreviated classification of human blood groups is given in the accompanying table. 2. any of certain other characteristics or traits of a cellular or fluid component of blood, considered as the expression (phenotype or allotype) of the actions and interactions of dominant genes; used in medicolegal and other studies of human inheritance. Such characteristics include the antigenic groupings of erythrocytes, leukocytes, platelets, and plasma proteins. Called also *blood type.*

**ABO b. g.,** the major human blood group system, dependent on the presence or absence of A and B antigens, which are largely glycolipids on the cell membrane. The gene for A is responsible for synthesis of *N*-acetyl-α-D-galactosaminyl transferase, whereas that for B is responsible for α-D-galactosyl transferase. Either A or B is created when one of these hexasaccharides is positioned by a specific transferase in 1→3 linkage to the β-D-galactose of an H-active oligosaccharide. Type O occurs when neither transferase is present or, very rarely *(Bombay phenotype),* when H antigen does not exist. When both transferases are present, type AB results. Differences in degree of transferase activity are determined at the same locus: weak transferase gives rise to weak antigens ($A_2$, $A_3A_x$, $B_3B_x$). Similar oligosaccharides, especially in bacterial cell walls, immunize persons lacking A or B so that their serum contains anti-A or anti-B activity. A and B antigens are on the mucopolysaccharides of secretors; persons with dominant genes have H-active mucoids.

**Auberger b. g.,** a blood group consisting of the erythrocytic antigen $Au^a$, related to the Lutheran blood group.

**Bg b. g.,** a blood group consisting of the erythrocytic HLA antigens $Bg^a$, $Bg^b$, $Bg^c$, DBG, Ho, Ho-like, Ot, and Sto.

**Cartwright b. g.,** Yt b. g.

**Chido-Rodgers b. g.,** a blood group consisting of antigens $Ch^a$ and $Rg^a$, antigenic determinants of fragments of the C4 component of complement.

**Colton b. g.,** a blood group consisting of erythrocytic antigens $Co^a$ and $Co^b$.

**Cromer b. g.,** a blood group consisting of erythrocytic antigens $Cr^a$, $Tc^a$, $Tc^{ab}$, $Dr^a$, $Es^a$, $WES^b$, UMC, and IFC, which are located on the membrane protein called *decay accelerating factor.*

**Diego b. g.,** a blood group consisting of the erythrocytic antigens $Di^a$ and $Di^b$, determined by allelic genes. $Di^a$ is most frequent in South American Indians, Japanese, and Chinese.

**Dombrock b. g.,** a blood group consisting of the erythrocytic antigens $Do^a$ and $Do^b$, most common in people of European descent.

**Duffy b. g.,** a blood group consisting principally of the erythrocytic antigens $Fy^a$ and $Fy^b$, determined by allelic genes. Amorphic genes are common in individuals of African descent.

**Gerbich b. g.,** a blood group consisting of the erythrocytic antigens Ge 1, Ge 2, and Ge 3; although rare in most parts of the world, it has been found often in Papua New Guinea.

**H b. g.,** a blood group consisting of antigen H; see also *Bombay phenotype.*

**high frequency b. g.,** a group containing over 99 per cent of individuals, who have a type of erythrocyte antigens called *public antigens.*

**Ii b. g.,** a high frequency blood group involving receptors of most cold reactive hemagglutinins; it is expressed most strongly on cord blood cells.

**Kell b. g.,** a blood group consisting of multiple erythrocytic antigens, especially three pairs of alternates, determined by complex genes at one locus, including an amorph; also regulated by the X chromosome, it is associated with sex-linked chronic granulomatous disease. One antigen, K6, is more frequent in people of African descent.

**Kidd b. g.,** a blood group consisting principally of $Jk^a$ and $Jk^b$ antigens, determined by allelic genes; amorphic genes are most common in those of East Asian descent.

**Knops b. g.,** a blood group consisting of antigens $Kn^a$, $Kn^b$, $McC^a$, $Sl^a$, and $Yk^a$, which are located on complement receptor type 1.

**Lan b. g.,** a blood group consisting of the erythrocytic antigen Lan.

**Lewis b. g.,** a blood group determined by plasma glycolipids that adhere to erythrocytic surfaces. It is based on dominant independent *Le* genes, but interacts with the H precursor oligosaccharides of A and B. Whereas *le/le* provides the "double negative" blood type Le(a−b−), *Le* without H gives rise to $Le^a$, i.e., blood type Le(a+b−), and that with H gives rise to $Le^bH$, i.e., blood type Le(a−b+).

**low frequency b. g.,** any small group that has erythrocytic antigens found in fewer than 1 per cent of the population *(private antigens).*

**Lutheran b. g.,** a complex blood group system consisting of antigens $Lu^a$ and $Lu^b$; it somewhat resembles the Kell group in having pairs of alternative antigens and amorphic genes, but is also subject to a dominant independently segregating repressor.

**MNSs b. g.,** a complex blood group system consisting principally of two pairs of antigens determined by closely linked genes (crossovers have been observed, but rarely). M and N, determined by allelic genes, depend on sialic (neuraminic) acid residues. S and s are also determined by allelic genes, and an amorphic gene is common in blacks when another antigen (U) is missing. The system also includes numerous low frequency antigens.

**P b. g.,** a blood group system originally consisting of only P (now P1) antigen, but later found to include P2 ($Tj^a$), a very high frequency antigen, and P3 ($P^k$), a very low frequency antigen. P1 is most common in people of African descent (90 per cent), less so in those of European descent (75 per cent), and least in those of East Asian descent (30 per cent).

**Rh b. g.,** the most complex of all human blood groups because the genes differ by determining different numbers of antigens *(Rh factors)* and do so with remarkably different quality; over 40 antigens have been described to date. People of African descent show the greatest degree of diversity and East Asians the least. The major antigen, *Rh1* (*$Rh_0$, D,* or *$Rh_0D$*), is highly immunogenic and before the development of passive immunization prophylaxis it was responsible for serious hemolytic disease of the newborn. Two other pairs of alternative antigens are inherited with or without Rh1; these are *Rh21* (*$rh^G$* or *$C^G$*) and *Rh4* (*hr′* or *c*), and *Rh3* (*rh′* or *E*) and *Rh5* (*hr′* or *e*). The most common groups of antigens are $R^{-1,-3,-21}$ (in Caucasians), $R^{1,-3,-21}$ (in blacks), $R^{1,-3,21}$ (in East Asians and Caucasians), and $R^{1,3,-21}$ (in East Asians and Caucasians). Another antigen Rh10 ($hr^v$, V) is common in blacks.

**Scianna b. g.,** a blood group consisting of erythrocytic antigens Sc1 (formerly Sm) and Sc2 (formerly $Bu^a$).

**Sid b. g.,** a blood group consisting of those with extra amounts of the public erythrocytic antigen $Sd^a$, referred to as Sd(a++).

**Human Blood Group Systems and Erythrocytic Antigenic Determinants**

| Blood Group System | Antigenic Determinants* |
|---|---|
| ABO | A [Subgroups $A_1$, $A_2$, $A_3$, $A_m$, $A_o$, $A_x$, $A_{int}$, $A_{end}$, $A_{finn}$, $A_{el}$, $A_{bantu}$], B [Subgroups $B_3$, $B_x$, $B_{el}$] |
| Auberger | Au$^a$ |
| Bg | Bg$^a$, Bg$^b$, Bg$^c$, DBG, Ho, Ho-like, Ot, Sto |
| Cartwright | Yt$^a$, Yt$^b$ |
| Colton | Co$^a$, Co$^b$ |
| Cost-Sterling | Cs$^a$, Yk$^a$ |
| Diego | Di$^a$, Di$^b$ |
| Dombrock | Do$^a$, Do$^b$ |
| Duffy | Fy$^a$ (Fy1), Fy$^b$ (Fy2), Fy$^{ab}$ (Fy3), Fy4, Fy5 |
| Gerbich | Ge 1, Ge 2, Ge 3 |
| H | H |
| Ii | I, I$^D$, I$^F$, I$^T$, i |
| Kell | K1 (K), K2 (k), K3 (Kp$^a$), K4 (Kp$^b$), K5 (Ku), K6 (Js$^a$), K7 (Js$^b$), K8 (kw), K9 (K1) K10 (U1$^a$), K11 (Côté), K12 (Bøk), K13 (Sgro), K14 (San), K15 (Kx), K16 (K-like), K17 (Wk$^a$), K18, K19, Kp$^c$ |
| Kidd | Jk$^a$ (Jk1), Jk$^b$ (Jk2), Jk$^{ab}$ (Jk3) |
| Lewis | Le$^a$ (Le1), Le$^b$ (Le2), Le$^c$ (Le5), Le$^d$, Le$^x$ (L$^{ab}$, Le3), Mag (Le4) |
| Lutheran | Lu$^a$ (Lu1), Lu$^b$ (Lu2), Lu$^{ab}$ (Lu3), Lu4, Lu5, Lu6, Lu7, Lu8, Lu9, Lu10, Lu11, Lu12, Lu13, Lu14 (Sw$^a$) |
| MNSs | Cl$^a$, Far, He, Hill, Hu, M, $M_1$, M$^A$, M$^c$, M$^e$, M$^g$, M$^k$, M$^r$, M$^v$, M$^z$, Mi$^a$, Mt$^a$, Mur, N, N$^A$, N$^a$, $N_2$, Ny$^a$, Ri$^a$, S, $S_2$, S$^B$, s, Sj, St$^a$, Sul, Tm, U, U$^B$, Vr, Vw, Z |
| P | P1, P2 (Tj$^a$), P3 (P$^k$) |
| Rh | Rh1 (D, $Rh_0$), Rh2 (C, rh′) Rh3 (E, rh′), Rh4 (c, hr′), Rh5 (e, hr′), Rh6 (ce, f, hr), Rh7 (Ce, $Rh_i$), Rh8 (C$^w$, rh$^{wI}$), Rh9 (C$^x$, rh$^x$), Rh10 (V, ce$^S$, hr$^v$), Rh11 (E$^w$, rh$^{w2}$), Rh12 (G, rh$^G$), Rh13 (Rh$^A$), Rh14 (Rh$^B$), Rh15 (Rh$^C$), Rh16 (Rh$^D$), Rh17 ($Hr_0$), Rh18 (Hr), Rh19 (Hr$^S$), Rh20 (VS, e$^s$), Rh21 (C$^G$), Rh22 (CE), Rh23 (D$^w$), Rh24 (E$^T$), Rh25 (L$^W$), Rh26 (c-like), Rh27 (cE), Rh28 (hr$^H$), Rh29 (RH), Rh30 (D$^{cor}$), Rh31 (hr$^B$), Rh32, Rh33, Rh34 (Hr$^B$), Rh35, Rh36, Rh37, Rh38, Rh39, Rh40, Rh41, Rh42 (Ce$^s$) |
| Scianna | Sm (Sc1), Bu$^a$ (Sc2) |
| Stoltzfus | Sf$^a$ |
| Vel | Vel 1, Vel 2 |
| Wright | Wr$^a$, Wr$^b$ |
| Xg | Xg$^a$ |

*Antigenic Determinants that Depend on Gene Interactions*

| | | | |
|---|---|---|---|
| ABO/I | P/ABO | IP1, IP2 (IT$^a_j$), I$^T$P1, iP1 | Fy5 |
| P/I | Xor/Duffy | ILe$^{bh}$ | Rh25 (L$^W$) |
| Lewis/I | Rh/L$^W$ | $A_1$Le$^b$(Seidler) | |
| Lewis/ABO | Ih, IA, IB, iH | Luke | |

*Selected Antigenic Determinants Not Thus Far Associated with a Blood Group System*

754, An$^a$, At$^a$, Be$^a$, Bec, Bi, Big Charles, Bp*a*, Bra, Bx*a*, By, Cad, Car, Chido (Gursha), Chr$^a$, Cip, Coates, Craig, Dahl, Donaviesky, Dp, Driver, Duch, E1, En$^a$, Evans, Evelyn, Fin, Fuerhart, Fuj, Gf$^a$, Gilbraith, Gn$^a$, Go$^b$, Good, Green, Gy$^a$, Hands, Hen, Heibel, Hill, Ht$^a$, Hy, Je$^a$, Jn$^a$, Jo$^a$, Job, Jr, Kam, Kelly, Ken, Knops (Kn$^a$), Kosis, Lan, Lev, Lw$^a$, McCall, McCoy (McC$^a$), Man, Mar, Mo$^a$, MZ443, Nij, Ola, Orr, Pea, Pt$^a$, Rd$^a$, Reid, Rogers (Rg$^a$), Savior, Sch, Sd$^a$, Simon, Skjelbred, Ters, Th$^a$, To$^a$, Todd, Tr$^a$, Ven, Vennera, Wb, Weeks, Wil, Winbourne, Wu, Yh$^a$, York (Yk$^a$), Za

*Symbols within parentheses are those of alternative nomenclatures. Antigenic determinants are systematized according to observed and assumed independent assortment of their responsible genes. Within many systems, alleles are responsible for differing combinations of antigenic determinants.

**Vel b. g.,** a blood group consisting of the erythrocytic antigens Vel 1 and Vel 2.

**Wright b. g.,** a blood group consisting of the erythrocytic antigens Wr$^a$ and Wr$^b$.

**Xg b. g.,** a blood group consisting of erythrocytic antigen Xg$^a$, which is determined by a gene on the long arm of the X chromosome.

**Yt b. g.,** a blood group consisting of the erythrocytic antigens Yt$^a$ and Yt$^b$. Called also *Cartwright b. g.*

**blood·less** (blud′ləs) 1. deprived of blood; cf.*anemic.* Called also *exsanguinate.* 2. performed with little or no loss of blood.

**blood·root** (blud′ro͞ot) sanguinaria.

**blood stream, blood·stream** (blud′strēm) the blood flowing through the circulatory system in the living body.

**Bloom's syndrome** (blo͞omz) [David *Bloom,* American dermatologist, born 1892] see under *syndrome.*

**bloom** (blo͞om) 1. a surface texture on a colony of microorganisms that appears velvety or powdery owing to aerial projections of hyphae. 2. a film of cyanobacteria on the surface of water, often containing substances toxic to humans and other animals.

**blot** (blot) a technique for transferring ionic solutes separated by electrophoresis onto a nitrocellulose membrane, filter, or treated paper for analysis; also used to describe the substrate containing the transferred material. For specific techniques, see under *technique.*

**blotch** (bloch) a blemish or spot.

**blot·ting** (blot′ing) soaking up with or transferring to absorbent material.

**Blount brace, disease** (blunt) [Walter Putnam *Blount,* American orthopedic surgeon, born 1900] see under *brace* and see *tibia vara.*

**blow·fly** (blo′fli) blow fly.

**blow·pipe** (blo′pīp) a tube through which a current of air or other gas is forced upon a flame to concentrate and intensify the heat.

**blue** (bloo) 1. one of the principal colors of the spectrum, the color of the sky. 2. having the color of the clear sky. 3. a dye that is blue in color.

**alcian b.,** a copper-containing dye for staining acid mucopolysaccharides; it may be combined with periodic acid–Schiff reagent.

**alizarin b.,** a blue dyestuff derived from anthracene.

**alkali b.,** a dye, sodium triphenylrosaniline monosulfate; called also *isamine b.*

**aniline b.,** a mixture of the trisulfonates of triphenylrosaniline and of diphenylrosaniline; also known variously as *anthracene b., China b., marine b., soluble b. (3M* or *2R),* and *water b.*

**aniline b., W. S.,** a mixture of the sulfonation products of mixtures of phenylated rosaniline and pararosaniline, soluble in water.

**anthracene b.,** alizarin b.

**azidine b., 3 B.,** trypan b.

**benzamine b., 3 B.,** trypan b.

**benzo b.,** trypan b.

**Berlin b.,** Prussian b.

**Borrel's b.,** a silver oxide stain for spirochetes.

**brilliant b., C.,** brilliant cresyl b.

**brilliant cresyl b.,** an oxazin dye, usually $C_{15}H_{16}N_3OCl$, used in staining blood; called also *C. brilliant b.* and *cresyl b., 2R.N* or *B.B.S.*

**bromchlorphenol b.,** an indicator, dibromodichlorophenolsulfonphthalein, used in the determination of hydrogen ion concentration;

yellow at pH 3.2 and blue at pH 4.8. Written also *bromochlorphenol b.*
**bromphenol b.**, an indicator, tetrabromophenolsulfonphthalein, used in determining hydrogen ion concentration, being yellow at pH 3.0 and blue at pH 4.6. Written also *bromophenol b.*
**bromthymol b.**, a dye, dibromothymolsulfonphthalein, used as an indicator in determining hydrogen ion concentration, being yellow at pH 6.0 and blue at pH 7.6. Written also *bromothymol b.*
**china b.**, aniline b.
**chlorazol b., 3 B.**, trypan b.
**Congo b., 3 B.**, trypan b.
**cresyl b., 2 R. N.** or **B. B. S.**, brilliant cresyl b.
**cyanol b.**, a bright blue acid coal tar color related to triphenylmethane.
**diamine b.**, trypan b.
**dianil b., H. 3 G.**, trypan b.
**Evans b.**, a dye in the form of a green, blue green, or brown powder, $C_{34}H_{24}N_6Na_4O_{14}S_4$, injected intravenously to determine blood volume and movement. Called also *T-1824.*
**Helvetia b.**, methyl benzene
**indigo b.**, indigotin.
**indigo b., soluble,** indigotindisulfonate sodium.
**indophenol b.**, the blue pigment produced in the Nadi reaction and in the indophenol test; it is $(CH_3)_2N{\cdot}C_6H_4{\cdot}N{:}C_{10}H_6{:}O$.
**isamine b.**, alkali b.
**Kühne's methylene b.**, a mixture of methylene blue and dehydrated alcohol in phenol solution.
**leukomethylene b.**, see *methylene b.*
**Löffler's methylene b.**, a mixture of methylene blue and alcohol in aqueous solution of potassium hydroxide.
**Luxol fast b. MBS**, an alcohol soluble dye used to stain myelinated nerve fibers. Called also *solvent b. 38.*
**marine b.**, aniline b.
**methylene b.** [USP], methylthionine chloride; dark green crystals or crystalline powder having a bronze-like luster, readily reduced to colorless leukomethylene blue, which in turn is readily oxidized to methylene blue. Administered orally or intravenously in the treatment of congenital methemoglobinemia and intravenously in the treatment of toxic methemoglobinemia, and used as a bacteriological and pathological stain and as a diagnostic aid in the detection of the premature rupture of fetal membranes and to identify separate amniotic sacs in multiple pregnancies. Called also *Swiss b.*
**methylene b. O,** toluidine blue O.
**naphthamine b., 3 B. X.**, trypan b.
**Niagara b., 3 B.**, trypan b.
**Nile b., A., Nile b. sulfate,** an oxazin dye which stains fatty acids blue; it is $(C_2H_5)_2N{\cdot}C_6H_3(ON)C_{10}H_5{\cdot}NH_2{\cdot}(SO_4)_{\frac{1}{2}}$.
**polychrome methylene b.**, a mixture of methylene green, methylene azure, methylene violet, and methylene blue.
**Prussian b.**, an amorphous blue powder, $Fe_4[Fe(CN)_6]_3$; called also *Berlin b.*
**pyrrole b.**, $C_4H_4N{\cdot}C[C_6H_4{\cdot}N(CH_3)_2]_2$.
**quinaldine b.**, chemical name: 1-ethyl-2-[3-(1-ethyl-2(1*H*)quinolylidene)propenyl]quinolinium chloride. A bright blue-green stain, $C_{25}H_{25}ClN_2$, used in the cytodiagnosis of ruptured fetal membranes.
**soluble b., 3 M., soluble b., 2 R.**, aniline b.
**solvent b. 38,** Luxol b. MBS.
**spirit b.**, a mixture of diphenylrosaniline and triphenylrosaniline; cf. *rosaniline.*
**Swiss b.**, methylene b.
**thymol b.**, an indicator, thymolsulfonphthalein, with an acid pH range of 1.2 to 2.8, being red at 1.2 and yellow at 2.8, and an alkaline pH range of 8.0 to 9.6, being yellow at 8.0 and blue at 9.6.
**toluidine b., toluidine b. O,** the chloride salt or zinc chloride double salt of aminodimethylaminotoluphenazthionium chloride; useful as a stain for demonstrating basophilic and metachromatic substances. Called also *methylene b. O.*
**trypan b.**, an acid, azo dye that has been used in vital staining and as a remedy in protozoan infections; it is the sodium salt of toluidin-diazo-diamino-naphthol-disulfonic acid. Variously known as *azidine b., 3 B; benzamine b., 3 B; benzo b.; chlorazol b.; Congo b., 3 B; diamine b.; dianil b., H. 3G.; naphthamine b., 3 B. X.;* and *Niagara b., 3 B. X.*
**Unna's alkaline methylene b.**, see under *stain.*
**Victoria b.**, a triphenylmethane dye with bacteriostatic properties.
**b. vitriol,** cupric sulfate.
**water b.**, aniline b.

**blue·grass** (bloo'gras) any of various species of grasses of the genus *Poa* that have bluegreen leaves. Some are commonly used as fodder for horses and cattle and cause hay fever in susceptible humans.

**blue·nose** (bloo'nōz) photosensitization in horses in Great Britain, with cyanosis around the muzzle, after they eat fresh spring grass; in some cases edema becomes so severe that the condition resembles purpura hemorrhagica.

**blu·en·so·my·cin** (bloo″ən-so-mi'sin) an antibiotic substance, originally obtained from cultures of *Streptomyces bluensis.*

**blue·stone** (bloo'stōn) cupric sulfate.

**blue·tongue** (bloo'tung″) [MeSH: Bluetongue] a viral disease of sheep, cattle, goats, and wild ruminants, transmitted by biting flies of the genus *Culicoides;* the etiologic agent is an orbivirus. Characteristics include inflammation, ulceration, and necrosis of the tongue, lips, and dental pads, and fever.

**Blum·berg** (blum'bərg) Baruch Samuel. American physician, born 1925; co-winner, with Daniel Carleton Gajdusek, of the Nobel prize for medicine or physiology in 1976 for their discoveries of new mechanisms for the origin and dissemination of infectious diseases, specifically hepatitis B virus.

**Blum·berg's sign** (blum'bərgz) [Jacob Moritz *Blumberg,* surgeon and gynecologist in Berlin, and later in London, 1873–1955] see under *sign.*

**Blu·men·au's nucleus** (bloo'mən-ouz) [Leonid Wassiljewitsch *Blumenau,* Russian neurologist, 1862–1932] see under *nucleus.*

**Blu·men·bach's clivus, plane** (bloo'mən-bahks) [Johann Friederich *Blumenbach,* German physiologist, 1752–1840] see under *plane.*

**blunt·hook** (blunt'hook) an instrument used mainly in embryotomy.

**blur** (blər) indistinctness, clouding, or fogging.
**spectacle b.**, the indistinct vision with spectacles occurring after removal of hard contact lenses, particularly non–gas permeable lenses; it is thought to result from chronic hypoxia of the cornea and attendant corneal edema.

**blush** (blush) sudden, brief erythema of the face and neck, resulting from vascular dilatation due to emotion or heat.

**BMA** British Medical Association.

**BMI** body mass index.

**BMR** basal metabolic rate.

**BMS** Bachelor of Medical Science.

**BMT** behavioral marital therapy; bone marrow transplantation.

**BNA** abbreviation for *Basle Nomina Anatomica.*

**BOA** British Orthopaedic Association.

**board** (bord) 1. a long flat piece of wood or other material. 2. a group of administrators or experts serving a special function.
**angle b.**, in dental radiology, a device used to facilitate the establishment of reproducible angular relationships between a patient's head and the plane of an x-ray film.
**bed b.**, a rigid board put under the mattress of a bed for firm support of the patient.
**Institutional Review B.**, an official group associated with an institution performing medical research. The group reviews research studies being planned within the institution to ensure that the research is legal and ethical and safeguard the safety, well-being, and rights of study subjects.

**Bo·a·ri flap** (bo-ah're) [Achille *Boari,* Italian surgeon, late 19th century] see under *flap.*

**Bo·as' algesimeter, point** (bo'ahs) [Ismar Isidor *Boas,* German physician, 1858–1938] see under *algesimeter* and *point.*

**Bo·as-Op·pler bacillus (lactobacillus)** (bo'ahs-op'lər) [I. I. *Boas;* Bruno *Oppler,* German physician, 19th century] see under *bacillus.*

**Bo·bath method** (bo'baht) [Berta and Karel *Bobath,* German physical therapists in England, 20th century] see under *method.*

**bob·bing** (bob'ing) a quick, jerky, up-and-down movement.
**ocular b.**, a jerky downward deviation of the eyes with slow return to the middle position, seen in comatose patients and thought to be due to a pontine lesion.

**Boch·da·lek's duct,** etc. (bok'dəl-əks) [Vincent Alexander *Bochdalek,* Czech anatomist, 1801–1883] see *ductus thyroglossalis, hiatus pleuroperitonealis,* and *plexus dentalis superior,* and see under *hernia* and *valve.*

**Bock's ganglion, nerve** (boks) [August Carl *Bock,* German anatomist, 1782–1833] see *carotid ganglion,* under *ganglion,* and see *ramus pharyngeus nervi vagi.*

**Bock·hart's impetigo** (bok'hahrts) [Max *Bockhart,* German physician, 1883–1921] see under *impetigo.*

**Bo·dan·sky unit** (bo-dan'ske) [Aaron *Bodansky,* American biochemist, 1887–1961] see under *unit.*

**bo·den·plat·te** (bo″dən-plah'tə) [Ger.] floor plate.

**body** (bod'e) 1. corpus. 2. any mass or collection of material. 3. a cadaver or corpse. 4. the trunk, or animal frame, with its organs.

## Body

For descriptions of specific anatomic structures not found here, see under *corpus.*

**acetone b's,** ketone b's.
**adrenal b.,** glandula suprarenalis.
**Alder-Reilly b's,** coarse azurophil granules found in leukocytes in the Alder-Reilly anomaly.
**Amato b's,** Döhle's b's.
**amygdaloid b.,** corpus amygdaloideum.
**amylaceous b's, amyloid b's,** corpora amylacea.
**anococcygeal b.,** corpus anococcygeum.
**aortic b's,** corpora para-aortica.
**apical b.,** acrosome.
**apoptotic b's,** the membrane-bound cell fragments produced during apoptosis, containing organelles and, sometimes, fragments of the nucleus.
**b's of Arantius,** noduli valvularum semilunarium valvae aortae.
**asbestos b's, asbestosis b's,** golden yellow ferruginous bodies whose central core is asbestos.
**Aschoff b's,** submiliary collections of cells and leukocytes in the interstitial tissues of the heart in rheumatic myocarditis; called also *Aschoff's nodules.*
**asteroid b.,** an irregularly star-shaped inclusion body found in the giant cells in sarcoidosis and also found in numerous other diseases.
**Auer b's,** finely granular lamellar bodies having acid phosphatase activity; they are found in the cytoplasm of myeloblasts, myelocytes, monoblasts, granular histiocytes, and occasionally plasma cells, but never lymphoblasts or lymphocytes; their presence is virtually pathognomonic of leukemia. Called also *Auer rods.*
**Babès-Ernst b.,** metachromatic granule.
**Balbiani's b.,** yolk nucleus.
**Balfour b's,** *Aegyptianella pullorum.*
**Barr b.,** sex chromatin.
**basal b.,** one of the cylindrical cytoplasmic bodies structurally resembling the centriole, from which it originates, located on the subsurface of flagellate protozoa and giving rise to the axoneme. Basal bodies are connected together in longitudinal rows by bundles of fibrils called kinetodesmata. Called also *basal granule, blepharoplast,* and *kinetosome.* See also *kinetoplast* and *parabasal b.*
**Bollinger's b's,** inclusion bodies found in all tissue cells in fowlpox; they contain the fowlpox virus. Called also *Bollinger's granules.* Cf. *Borrel b's.*
**Borrel b's,** minute virus-containing granules that aggregate to form Bollinger bodies.
**Bracht-Wächter b's,** nonspecific inflammatory foci of lymphocytic and mononuclear cells in the myocardium, observed in bacterial endocarditis.
**brassy b.,** a dark, shrunken blood corpuscle seen in malaria.
**bull's eye b.,** dense b. (def. 2).
**Cabot's ring b's,** lines in the form of loops or figures of eight, possibly remnants of the nuclear membrane, seen in stained erythrocytes in severe anemias. Called also *Cabot's rings.*
**Call-Exner b's,** the accumulations of densely staining material that appear among granulosa cells in maturing ovarian follicles and that may be intracellular precursors of follicular fluid; also seen in ovarian tumors of granulosal origin.
**cancer b's,** Plimmer's b's.
**carotid b.,** glomus caroticum.
**b. of caudate nucleus,** corpus nuclei caudati.
**cavernous b. of clitoris,** corpus cavernosum clitoridis.
**cavernous b. of penis,** corpus cavernosum penis.
**cell b.,** that portion of a cell which contains the nucleus, independent of any such projections as an axon or dendrites which the cell may have.
**central b.,** the structures at the center of the aster during mitosis.
**central fibrous b. of heart,** trigonum fibrosum dextrum cordis.
**b. of cerebellum,** corpus cerebelli.
**chromaffin b.,** paraganglion.
**chromatin b., chromatinic b.,** the genetic material of bacteria. See nucleoid (def. 3).
**chromatoid b.,** 1. one of the dense accumulations of RNA found in the cysts of certain amebae (e.g., *Entamoeba* species), manifested as a deeply staining rodlike body. Called also *chromatoid bar.* 2. a dense chromatoid mass near the distal centriole of a spermatozoon, from which the so-called ring centriole seemingly arises.
**chromophilous b's,** Nissl b's.
**ciliary b.,** corpus ciliare.
**Civatte b's,** an anuclear keratinocyte that has become incorporated into the papillary dermis, seen in lichen planus. Called also *colloid b's.*
**coccoid x b's,** minute bodies found in the blood in psittacosis.
**coccygeal b.,** glomus coccygeum.
**colloid b's,** Civatte b's.
**colostrum b's,** colostrum corpuscles.
**conchoid b's,** Schaumann's b's.
**Councilman's b's,** apoptotic bodies of hepatocellular origin seen in viral hepatitis, yellow fever, and other hepatic diseases; called also *Councilman's lesions.*
**Cowdry type I inclusion b's,** eosinophilic nuclear inclusions composed of nucleic acid and protein seen in cells infected with herpes simplex or varicella-zoster virus.
**crystalloid b.,** a body seen near the nuclei of the cells of the seminiferous tubules.
**cytoid b's,** globular, shiny white structures resembling cell nuclei in size and shape, appearing in degenerated retinal nerve fibers; seen histologically in cotton-wool spots.
**Deetjen's b.,** old term for *platelet.*
**demilune b.,** achromocyte.
**dense b.,** 1. any of the small regions of increased density in the sarcoplasm of skeletal muscles to which myofilaments seem to attach; cf. *attachment plaques,* under *plaque.* 2. an electron-dense granule occurring in blood platelets that stores and secretes adenosine nucleotides and serotonin. Called also *bull's eye b.* or *granule, dense granule,* and *platelet dense b.*
**Döhle's b's, Döhle's inclusion b's,** round to oval blue-staining inclusions seen in the periphery of the cytoplasm of neutrophils, consisting mainly of RNA derived from rough endoplasmic reticulum; they are found in association with many infections, burns, aplastic anemia, uncomplicated pregnancy, and after administration of toxic agents. Similar structures, usually larger and more prominent, are present in granulocytes other than neutrophils in the May-Hegglin anomaly. Called also *Amato b's* and *leukocyte inclusions.*
**Donné's b's,** colostrum corpuscles.
**Donovan's b.,** *Calymmatobacterium granulomatis.*
**Dutcher b.,** an intranuclear invagination of immunoglobulin-containing cytoplasm found in neoplastic plasmacytoid lymphocytes and plasma cells in both benign and malignant conditions.
**elementary b.,** 1. old term for *platelet.* 2. an inclusion body. 3. the infectious extracellular form of *Chlamydia,* consisting of electron-dense nuclear material and a few ribosomes surrounded by a rigid trilaminar wall. Elementary bodies are taken up into cells where they reorganize into reticulate bodies (q.v.); following reproduction, chlamydiae are released from the cell as elementary bodies.
**Elschnig b's,** clear grapelike clusters formed by proliferation of epithelial cells after extracapsular extraction of a cataractous lens; called also *Elschnig's pearls.*
**embryoid b's,** structures resembling embryos, occurring in several types of germ cell tumors.
**b. of epididymis,** corpus epididymidis.
**epithelial b's,** parathyroid glands.
**fat b. of ischioanal fossa,** corpus adiposum fossae ischioanalis.
**ferruginous b's,** small masses of mineral matter of various shapes found in the lungs as a result of deposition of calcium salts, iron salts, and protein around a central core of foreign matter. See also *asbestos b's.*
**fibrin b's of pleura,** movable or adherent, round, homogeneous, sharply demarcated opacities near the base of the pleural cavity, which may occur secondary to pleural effusion, pneumothorax, or hemopneumothorax; called also *pleural fibrin balls.*
**foreign b.,** a mass or particle of material that is not normal to the place where it is found.
**b. of fornix,** corpus fornicis.
**fruiting b.,** a specialized structure that produces spores; see Plate 29 and see also *carp.*
**fuchsin b's,** Russell b's.
**b. of gallbladder,** corpus vesicae biliaris.
**Gamna-Favre b's,** small intracytoplasmic inclusion bodies found in lymphogranuloma venereum.
**gastric b.,** corpus gastricum.
**geniculate b., lateral,** corpus geniculatum laterale.
**geniculate b., medial,** corpus geniculatum mediale.
**Giannuzzi's b's,** crescents of Giannuzzi.
**glomus b.,** anastomosis arteriovenosa glomeriformis.
**Golgi b.,** see under *complex.*
**Guarnieri's b's,** inclusion bodies in the cells of the affected tissues in smallpox and vaccinia, regarded as caused by the reaction of the cell to the virus of the disease; called also *Guarnieri's corpuscles.*
**habenular b.,** habenula, def. 2.
**Halberstaedter-Prowazek b's,** trachoma b's.
**Harting b's,** deposits of calcium (calcospherites) in the cerebral capillaries.
**Hassall's b's,** Hassall's corpuscles.
**Hassall-Henle b's,** see under *wart.*
**Heinz b's, Heinz-Ehrlich b's,** coccoid inclusion bodies resulting from oxidative injury to and precipitation of hemoglobin, seen in the presence of abnormal hemoglobins such as Hb H, Hb Köln, etc. and

in erythrocytes with enzyme deficiencies. Refractile in fresh blood smears, they are not visible when stained with Romanowsky dyes but may be stained supravitally. See also *Heinz body anemias,* under *anemia.* Called also *Heinz granules.*

**hematoxylin b.,** a dense, homogeneous, cyanophilous particle consisting of the denatured nuclear material of an injured cell together with a small amount of cytoplasm, occurring in systemic lupus erythematosus; lymphocytes that ingest such particles are known as LE cells. Called also *LE b.*

**Henderson-Paterson b's,** molluscum b's.

**Hensen's b.,** a rounded modified Golgi net under the cuticle of an outer hair cell of the organum spirale.

**Herring b's,** hyaline or colloid masses scattered throughout the pars nervosa of the pituitary gland.

**b. of Highmore,** mediastinum testis.

**Hirano b's,** glassy, eosinophilic, rod-shaped inclusions, composed primarily of actin, seen in the cytoplasm of neurons of the central nervous system, chiefly the hippocampus, particularly in older persons; although they may occur in the absence of disease, they are more prevalent in patients with neurodegenerative disorders such as Alzheimer's disease.

**Howell's b's, Howell-Jolly b's,** smooth, round remnants of nuclear chromatin seen in erythrocytes in megaloblastic anemia, hemolytic anemia, and after splenectomy. Called also *Jolly's b's.*

**HX b's,** Birbeck granules.

**hyaline b's,** drusen.

**hyaloid b.,** corpus vitreum.

**b. of ilium,** corpus ossis ilii.

**immune b.,** antibody.

**inclusion b's,** round, oval, or irregular-shaped bodies occurring in the cytoplasm and nuclei of cells of the body, as in disease caused by filtrable virus infection such as rabies, smallpox, herpes, etc.; called also *elementary b's* and *intranuclear inclusions.*

**b. of incus,** corpus incudis.

**infrapatellar fatty b.,** corpus adiposum infrapatellare.

**infundibular b.,** neurohypophysis.

**intermediate b. of Flemming,** a small bridge of acidophil material connecting the two daughter cells for a time at the end of mitosis.

**interrenal b.,** an elongated organ that lies between the kidneys in elasmobranch fishes and that corresponds to the adrenal medulla in mammals.

**b. of ischium,** corpus ossis ischii.

**Jaworski b's,** see under *corpuscle.*

**Joest's b's,** intranuclear inclusion bodies found in the brain of animals with Borna disease.

**Jolly's b's,** Howell-Jolly b's.

**jugulotympanic b.,** tympanic b.

**juxtarestiform b.,** a structure connecting the lateral vestibular nucleus with the nucleus fastigii and conveying vestibular impulses.

**ketone b's,** the substances $\beta$-hydroxybutyric acid, acetoacetic acid, and acetone, which are produced by fatty acid and carbohydrate metabolism in the liver in approximately a 78:20:2 ratio. Acetoacetate is produced from acetyl-CoA; most is enzymatically converted to $\beta$-ketobutyrate, but a small amount is spontaneously decarboxylated to acetone. The ketone bodies can be used as fuels by muscle and brain tissue. In starvation and uncontrolled diabetes mellitus, large quantities are produced causing metabolic acidosis and elevated blood and urine levels of all three ketone bodies.

**Kurloff's (Kurlov's) b's,** bodies seen in the large mononuclear leukocytes of guinea pigs and related rodents. Observations with the electron microscope indicate that they probably result from intracellular secretion or from a sequestering and concentration of a serum molecular component.

**Lafora's b's,** intracytoplasmic inclusions consisting of a complex of glycoprotein and acid mucopolysaccharide; widespread deposits of these bodies are found in Lafora's myoclonus epilepsy.

**Lallemand's b's, Lallemand-Trousseau b's,** Bence Jones cylinders.

**lamellar b.,** keratinosome.

**b. of lateral ventricle,** pars centralis ventriculi lateralis.

**L.C.L. b's,** minute coccoid bodies found in tissue infected with psittacosis; called also *Levinthal-Coles-Lillie b's.*

**LE b.,** hematoxylin b.

**Leishman-Donovan b.,** amastigote.

**Levinthal-Coles-Lillie b's,** L.C.L. b's.

**Lewy b's,** concentrically laminated, round bodies found in vacuoles in the cytoplasm of some of the neurons of the midbrain in paralysis agitans.

**Lieutaud's b.,** trigonum vesicae.

**Lindner's initial b's,** cytoplasmic elementary bodies, resembling those in trachomatous epithelia, found in inclusion conjunctivitis of newborns.

**Lipschütz b's,** intranuclear inclusion bodies found in the lesions of herpes simplex, both in the epithelial cells of the primary skin lesion (skin or cornea) and in the affected nerve cells.

**Lostorfer's b's,** Lostorfer's corpuscles.

**Luschka's b.,** glomus coccygeum.

**Luys' b.,** nucleus subthalamicus.

**lyssa b's,** red staining masses somewhat resembling Negri bodies but less sharply defined and with less internal structure.

**Mallory's b's,** hyaline cytoplasmic inclusions of cytokeratin within hepatocytes in alcoholic cirrhosis and other hepatic disorders.

**malpighian b's of kidney,** corpuscula renis.

**malpighian b's of spleen,** noduli lymphoidei splenici; see under *nodulus.*

**mamillary b., mammillary b.,** corpus mammillare.

**Marchal b's,** cell inclusion bodies observed in infectious ectromelia.

**Masson b's,** the cellular components that fill the pulmonary alveoli and alveolar ducts in rheumatic pneumonia, thought to be modified Aschoff bodies.

**medullary b. of cerebellum,** corpus medullare cerebelli.

**medullary b. of vermis,** arbor vitae cerebelli.

**melon-seed b.,** any of a class of small fibrous masses sometimes occurring in the joints and in cysts of the tendon sheaths.

**metachromatic b's,** metachromatic granules.

**Michaelis-Gutmann b's,** bodies found in the lesion of malacoplakia of the urinary tract or kidney.

**mitochondrial b.,** a fused colony of mitochondria found in the spermatids of insects.

**molluscum b's,** large homogeneous intracytoplasmic inclusions found in the stratum granulosum and stratum corneum in molluscum contagiosum, which contain replicating virions and cellular debris.

**Mooser b's,** bodies resembling rickettsiae, seen in the epithelial cells of the tunica vaginalis exudate in some forms of typhus.

**Mott b's,** clear globules found in the cytoplasm of plasma cells *(Mott cells)* in multiple myeloma and certain other conditions.

**multilamellar b.,** any of the osmiophilic, lipid-rich, layered bodies found in the type II alveolar cells of the lung; called also *cytosome.*

**multivesicular b.,** a secondary lysosome manifested as a spherical, membrane-bound vacuole, containing numerous small vesicles in a matrix that exhibits acid phosphatase activity.

**b. of nail,** corpus unguis.

**Negri b's,** oval or round inclusion bodies, seen in the cytoplasm and sometimes in the processes of nerve cells of rabid animals or patients with rabies after death; their presence is considered conclusive proof of rabies.

**Neill-Mooser b's,** large mononuclear cells filled with rickettsiae, seen in the inflammatory exudate of the scrotal swelling of laboratory animals infected with murine typhus (Neill-Mooser reaction).

**nemaline b's,** small threadlike or rod-shaped bodies found scattered through muscle fibers in nemaline myopathy.

**nigroid b.,** granula iridica.

**Nissl b's,** large granular basophilic bodies found in the cytoplasm of neurons, composed of rough endoplasmic reticulum and free polyribosomes; called also *chromophilous b's, chromophilic* or *chromatic granules, tigroid bodies* or *substance,* and *Nissl's granules* or *substance.*

**Nothnagel's b's,** oval or round bodies, plain or striated, from 15 to 60 $\mu$m in diameter, sometimes found in the stools of persons who eat meat.

**no-threshold b's,** no-threshold substances.

**Odland b.,** keratinosome.

**Oken's b.,** mesonephros.

**olivary b.,** oliva.

**oryzoid b's,** rice b's.

**pacchionian b's,** granulationes arachnoideae.

**pampiniform b.,** epoöphoron.

**orbital fat b.,** corpus adiposum orbitae.

**b. of pancreas,** corpus pancreatis.

**Pappenheimer b's,** basophilic iron-containing granules observed in erythrocytes in sideroblastic anemia, sickle cell anemia, and certain other conditions.

**para-aortic b's,** corpora para-aortica.

**parabasal b.,** a cytoplasmic body of varying appearance, structure, and function closely associated with the nucleus, kinetoplast, and basal body in certain parasitic flagellate protozoa; it is usually connected to the basal body by a fibril or thread, which together are known as the *parabasal apparatus.* More than one such structure may be present in each organism. Some authorities consider the parabasal body to be the Golgi complex of these cells.

**paranephric b.,** corpus adiposum pararenale.

**paranuclear b.,** centrosphere, def. 1.

**paraphyseal b.,** paraphysis (def. 1).

**pararenal fat b.,** corpus adiposum pararenale.

**paraterminal b.,** gyrus paraterminalis.

**parathyroid b's,** parathyroid glands.

**parietal b.,** epiphyseal eye.

**parolivary b's,** accessory olivary nuclei; see *nucleus olivaris accessorius posterior* and *nucleus olivaris accessorius medialis.*

**Paschen b's,** inclusion bodies in the cells of the tissues in variola and vaccinia; they are infective but whether they are the infective agents or mechanical carriers of the invisible virus is not known. Called also *Paschen's corpuscles* or *granules*.

**pearly b's,** epithelial pearls.

**perineal b.,** corpus perineale.

**pheochrome b.,** paraganglion.

**Pick b's,** filamentous intracytoplasmic inclusions seen in neurons in Pick's disease (def. 1).

**pineal b.,** 1. glandula pinealis. 2. the posterior eyelike structure arising from the median of the dorsal wall of the thalamus in some lower vertebrates. See also *epiphyseal eye,* under *eye.*

**pituitary b.,** hypophysis.

**platelet dense b.,** dense b. (def. 2).

**Plimmer's b's,** small round capsulated bodies found in cancer, and thought by the discoverer to be the parasite causing the disease but now considered to be cell necrosis products. Called also *cancer b's.*

**polar b's,** 1. the small nonfunctional cells with a haploid chromosome complement, consisting of a small amount of cytoplasm and a nucleus, resulting from unequal division of the primary oocyte *(first polar b.)* and, if fertilization occurs, of the secondary oocyte *(second polar b.)*; the polar body appears as a speck at the animal pole of the egg. 2. metachromatic granules located at one or both ends of a bacterial cell.

**polyglucosan b's,** corpora amylacea.

**postbranchial b's,** ultimobranchial b's.

**preepiglottic fat b.,** corpus adiposum pre-epiglotticum.

**presegmenting b's,** malarial parasites *(Plasmodium)* before they undergo segmentation.

**Prowazek's b's,** 1. trachoma b's. 2. extremely small inclusion bodies found in the material from smallpox pustules and in cowpox vaccine and regarded by Prowazek as the cause of the disease.

**Prowazek-Greeff b's,** trachoma b's.

**psammoma b.,** a spherical, concentrically laminated mass of calcareous material, usually of microscopic size; such bodies occur in both benign and malignant epithelial and connective-tissue tumors, and are sometimes associated with chronic inflammation.

**purine b's,** purine bases.

**pyknotic b's,** bodies in the mucus of stools in amebiasis; they are the nuclear remains of tissue cells and leukocytes.

**quadrigeminal b's,** corpora quadrigemina.

**Reilly b's,** large, coarse granulations found in the leukocytes in Hurler's syndrome.

**Renaut's b's,** pale granules in the degenerating nerve fibers in muscular dystrophy.

**residual b.,** 1. a secondary lysosome that has completed its digestive processes but retains indigestible or very slowly digestible material. 2. residuum, def. 2.

**residual b. of Regnaud,** an anucleate mass consisting of fine granules, lipid droplets, and degenerating organelles, cast off after the completion of regional differentiation of the tail during spermiogenesis.

**restiform b.,** pedunculus cerebellaris inferior.

**reticulate b.,** the noninfectious intracellular form of *Chlamydia,* consisting of fibrillar nuclear material and more ribosomes that occur in elementary bodies (q.v.), surrounded by a thin trilaminar wall. Reticulate bodies reproduce within vacuoles in the host cell; following the reproductive cycle, reticulate bodies condense into elementary bodies, which are released from the cell.

**b. of Retzius,** a protoplasmic mass containing pigment granules at the lower end of a hair cell of the organum spirale.

**b. of rib,** corpus costae.

**rice b's,** small bodies resembling grains of rice which form in the tendons of joints and in the fluid of hygroma; called also *oryzoid b's* and *corpora oryzoidea.*

**Ross's b's,** spherical copper-colored bodies showing dark granulations and sometimes having ameboid movements; seen in the blood and tissue fluids in syphilis.

**Russell b's,** globular plasma cell inclusions, mucoprotein in nature, containing surface gamma globulin, and representing aggregates of immunoglobulins synthesized by the cell; they are seen in both chronic inflammatory and malignant disorders. Called also *fuchsin b's.*

**sand b's,** the mass of gritty matter lying in or near the pineal body, the choroid plexus, and other parts of the brain; called also *acervulus* and *brain sand.*

**Sandström's b's,** parathyroid glands.

**Schaumann's b's,** iron- and calcium-containing, red to brown, laminated inclusion bodies found in the cytoplasm of giant cells in sarcoidosis and other granulomatoses; called also *conchoid b's.*

**Schiller-Duval b.,** a structure resembling a glomerulus seen in yolk sac tumors, composed of germ cells surrounding a central blood vessel and occurring within a space lined by germ cells.

**Schmorl b.,** a portion of the nucleus pulposus that has protruded into an adjoining vertebra.

**sclerotic b's,** a type of rounded cells surrounded by thick walls, characteristic of the dematiaceous fungi that cause chromoblastomycosis. Called also *muriform* or *sclerotic cells.*

**semilunar b's,** crescents of Giannuzzi.

**spongy b. of male urethra,** corpus spongiosum penis.

**spongy b. of penis,** corpus cavernosum penis.

**Stieda b.,** an ultrastructural organelle located at the polar region of the sporocyst of certain coccidia, appearing as a knoblike structure or representing a plug occluding a hole in the sporocyst, the breakdown of which allows excystation of the sporozoites.

**b. of stomach,** corpus gastricum.

**striate b.,** corpus striatum.

**suprarenal b.,** glandula suprarenalis.

**Symington's b.,** corpus anococcygeum.

**telobranchial b's,** ultimobranchial b's.

**threshold b's,** threshold substances.

**thyroid b.,** glandula thyroidea.

**tigroid b's,** Nissl b's.

**Todd b's,** eosinophilic structures formed in the cytoplasm of the red cells of certain amphibians.

**Torres-Teixeira b's,** inclusion bodies found in the cells in variola minor.

**trachoma b's,** inclusion bodies found in clusters in the cytoplasm of the epithelial cells from the conjunctiva of a trachomatous eye; called also *Halberstaedter-Prowazek b's, Prowazek's b's,* and *Prowazek-Greeff b's.*

**trapezoid b.,** corpus trapezoideum.

**Trousseau-Lallemand b's,** Bence Jones cylinders.

**tympanic b.,** an ovoid body found in the adventitia of the upper part of the superior bulb of the internal jugular vein; its structure and presumably its function are similar to those of the glomus caroticum (carotid body). Called also *glomus jugulare, jugular glomus,* and *jugulotympanic b.* See also *glomus jugulare tumor,* under *tumor.*

**ultimobranchial b's,** embryonic derivatives of the fifth pharyngeal pouches, which migrate along with the parathyroid glands and are incorporated in the thyroid gland. In submammalian vertebrates they remain as discrete masses in the neck or mediastinum throughout adult life. The parafollicular cells of these bodies produce calcitonin. Called also *postbranchial b's* and *telobranchial b's.*

**b. of uterus,** corpus uteri.

**vagal b's,** corpora para-aortica.

**vermiform b's,** peculiar sinuous invaginations of the plasma membrane of Kupffer cells of the liver, having a central linear density between parallel membranes and a faint transverse striation; similar structures are seen in macrophages of certain organs and in the Langerhans cells of the epidermis.

**Verocay b's,** small groups of fibrils surrounded by rows of palisaded nuclei, seen in schwannomas.

**vertebral b.,** corpus vertebrae.

**vitelline b.,** yolk nucleus.

**vitreous b.,** corpus vitreum.

**Weibel-Palade b's,** rod-shaped intracytoplasmic bundles of microtubules, believed derived from the Golgi complex; they are specific for vascular endothelial cells and are used as markers for benign or malignant endothelial cell neoplasms in electron microscopy.

**Winkler's b's,** spherical bodies seen in the lesions of syphilis.

**wolffian b.,** mesonephros.

**yellow b. of ovary,** corpus luteum.

**zebra b.,** concentric, laminated, cytoplasmic inclusions of Schwann cells, occurring singly or in clusters as a result of degeneration phenomena.

**Zuckerkandl's b's,** corpora para-aortica.

**body rock·ing** (bod'e rok'ing) a rhythmic backward and forward motion in a sitting position.

**body snatch·ing** (bod'e snach'ing) the illegal procural of dead bodies, especially the robbing of a grave of a recently buried corpse.

**Boeck's disease, sarcoid** (bərks) [Caesar P. M. *Boeck,* Norwegian dermatologist and syphilologist, 1845–1917] sarcoidosis.

**Boer·haa·ve's syndrome** (boor'hah-vēz) [Hermann *Boerhaave,* Dutch physician, 1668–1738] see under *syndrome.*

**Boet·tcher** (bərt'shər) see *Böttcher.*

**Bo·gros' space** (bōg-rōz') [Annet Jean *Bogros,* French anatomist, 1786–1823] see under *space.*

**Bohr effect** (bor) [Christian *Bohr,* Danish physiologist, 1855–1911] see under *effect.*

**Bo·hun upas** (bo'hən u'pəs) *Antiaris toxicaria.*

**boil** (boil) furuncle.
**Aleppo b., Bagdad b., Biskra b.,** Old World cutaneous leishmaniasis.
**blind b.,** a boil that does not develop a white or yellow "head" at its apex through which pus may be discharged; an abscess.
**Delhi b.,** Old World cutaneous leishmaniasis.
**gum b.,** parulis.
**Jericho b., Oriental b.,** Old World cutaneous leishmaniasis.
**shoe b.,** capped elbow in the horse.

**Bol.** abbreviation for L. *bo'lus,* pill.

**bol·de·none un·dec·y·len·ate** (bōl'də-nōn) an anabolic steroid used in veterinary practice.

**bol·dine** (bol-dēn') an alkaloid from *Peumus (Boldu) boldus* Molina (Monimiaceae), which possesses diuretic properties.

**bol·do** (bol'do) [L. *boldus, boldoa*] the leaves and stems of *Peumus (Boldu) boldus* Molina (Monimiaceae), a Chilean evergreen shrub. Once official in the U.S. National Formulary (1936) and still common in numerous over-the-counter remedies in Canada and other countries, it contains over 15 alkaloids and is used variously as a choleretic, diuretic, stomachic, sedative, and anthelmintic.

**bol·doa** (bol'do-ə) [L.] boldo.

**Bo·le·tus** (bo-le'təs) [L.; Gr. *bōlitēs*] a genus of fungi of the subphylum Basidiomycotina; some species are edible and others poisonous. *B. sata'nas* causes mycetismus gastrointestinalis.

**Bolk's retardation theory** (bōlks) [Louis *Bolk,* Dutch anatomist, 1866–1930] see under *theory.*

**Bol·lin·ger's bodies, granules** (bol'in-gərz) [Otto *Bollinger,* German pathologist, 1843–1909] see under *body* and *granule.*

**bo·lom·e·ter** (bo-lom'ə-tər) [Gr. *bolē* a throw, a ray + *-meter*] an instrument for measuring minute changes in heat radiated by an object, such as a portion of the human body.

**bo·lus** (bo'ləs) [L. from Gr. *bōlos* lump] 1. a rounded mass of food or a pharmaceutical preparation ready to swallow, or such a mass passing through the gastrointestinal tract. 2. a concentrated mass of pharmaceutical preparation given intravenously for diagnostic purposes, e.g., an opaque contrast medium or radioactive isotope. 3. a mass of scattering material, such as wax, paraffin, bags of water, or a rice-flour mixture, placed between the radiation source and the skin so as to achieve precalculated isodose pattern in the tissue irradiated.
**b. al'ba,** kaolin.
**alimentary b.,** the mass of food in the oropharynx or the esophagus, comprising one swallow.

**bomb** (bom) a heavy metal-shielded apparatus containing a quantity of radium or other radioactive element for use in clinical teleradiation therapy.

**bom·bard** (bom-bahrd') to expose the whole body or a specific tissue target to the action of ionizing radiation.

**Bom·bay phenotype** (bom-ba') [*Bombay,* India, where it was first reported on in 1952] see under *phenotype.*

**bom·be·sin** (bom'bə-sin) [MeSH: Bombesin] a tetradecapeptide neurohormone and pressor substance with paracrine and autocrine effects, found in small amounts in brain and intestinal tissue in humans under normal conditions and in increased amounts in certain pulmonary and thyroid tumors. It was first isolated from the skin of frogs and is an important amphibian hormone. It is a potent mitogen, and its effects on gastrin and other hormones are attributed to increased cell numbers.

**Bom·bi·na** (bom-bi'nə) a genus of toads. *B. bombi'na* (the fire-bellied toad) and *B. variega'ta* are European species with colored bellies; their skin is toxic and contains serotonin with various amino acids.

**Bom·bi·na·tor** (bom'bĭ-na"tər) a genus of toads. *B. ig'neus* is the fire toad, whose venom contains the toxin phrynolysin.

**Bom·bus** (bom'bəs) a genus of bees of the family Apidae; the bumblebees. They are larger than honeybees (genus *Apis*), produce smaller amounts of honey, and can sting when bothered.

**bom·by·kol** (bom'bĭ-kol) a pheromone secreted by silkworms that serves as a sex attractant; it is a 16-carbon alcohol with two double bonds.

**Bom·byx** (bom'biks) a genus of moths of the family Bombycidae. *B. mo'ri* is the silkworm moth, a species native to Asia whose larva is the commercial silkworm and which is used extensively in experimental genetics.

**bond** (bond) 1. the linkage between two atoms or radicals of a chemical compound. 2. a mark used to indicate the number and attachment of the valences of an atom in constitutional formulas; it is represented by a pair of dots or a line between the atoms, e.g., H—O—H, H—C≡C—H or H:O:H, H:C:::C:H.
**coordinate covalent b.,** a covalent bond in which one of the bonded atoms furnishes both of the shared electrons.
**covalent b.,** a chemical bond between two atoms or radicals formed by the sharing of a pair (single bond), two pairs (double bond), or three pairs of electrons (triple bond).
**disulfide b.,** a strong covalent bond, —S—S—, important in linking polypeptide chains in proteins, the linkage arising as a result of the oxidation of the sulfhydryl (SH) groups of two molecules of cysteine; called also *disulfide bridge.*
**energy rich b.,** high energy b.
**glycosidic b's,** the bonds between the monosaccharide components of a polysaccharide.
**high energy b.,** a chemical bond the hydrolysis of which yields high levels of free energy; such bonds involve phosphate *(high energy phosphate b.)* or sulfur *(high energy sulfur b.)* or other mixed anhydride types of chemical structures.
**high energy phosphate b.,** a high energy bond containing phosphate, occurring in ATP, phosphocreatine, phospho*enol*pyruvate, and other phosphate-containing high energy compounds; see *high energy compounds,* under *compound.* The energy released on hydrolysis of the bond can be transferred, stored, or used to drive metabolic processes such as the synthesis of glycogen from glucose.
**high energy sulfur b.,** a high energy bond containing sulfur, occurring particularly in a variety of thioesters that are high energy compounds (q.v.); the most important such bond is that of the metabolic intermediate acetyl coenzyme A. The energy released by hydrolysis of a high energy sulfur bond can be transferred, stored, or used to drive metabolic processes such as the biosynthesis of fatty acids.
**hydrogen b.,** a relatively weak, primarily electrostatic, bond between a hydrogen atom bound to a highly electronegative element (such as oxygen or nitrogen) in a given molecule, or part of a molecule, and a second highly electronegative atom in another molecule or in a different part of the same molecule. The hydrogen bond is generally represented by three dots, e.g., X—H···Y, where X and Y are electronegative atoms.
**hydrophobic b.,** a linkage resulting from the tendency of nonpolar molecules (or their side chains) to aggregate in an aqueous environment because of their mutual repulsion of solvent.
**ionic b.,** a chemical bond in which electrons are transferred from one atom (e.g., sodium) to another (e.g., chlorine) so that one bears a positive and the other a negative charge, the attraction between these opposite charges forming the bond.
**pair b.,** in ethology, the more or less permanent relationship between a male and a female for the purposes of mating and rearing the young.
**peptide b.,** the —CO—NH— bond formed between the carboxyl group of one amino acid and the amino group of another; it is an amide linkage joining amino acids to form peptides.
**van der Waals b.,** a weak electrostatic attraction arising from a nonspecific attractive force originating when two molecules are close to one another and the distribution of electrons is uneven, the locations lacking electrons attracting the locations with surplus electrons.

**bond·ing** (bond'ing) joining together securely with an adhesive substance, such as glue or cement.
**tooth b.,** the technique of fixing orthodontic brackets and other attachments directly to the enamel surface with orthodontic adhesives.

**Bon·dy's mastoidectomy** (bon'dēz) [G. *Bondy,* German otologist, early 20th century] modified radical mastoidectomy.

**bone** (bōn) [L. *os;* Gr. *osteon*] [MeSH: Bone and Bones] 1. the hard form of connective tissue that constitutes the majority of the skeleton of most vertebrates; it consists of an organic component (the cells and matrix) and an inorganic, or mineral, component; the matrix contains a framework of collagenous fibers and is impregnated with the mineral component, chiefly calcium phosphate (85 per cent) and calcium carbonate (10 per cent), which imparts the quality of rigidity to bone. Called also *osseous tissue.* 2. any distinct piece of the osseous framework, or skeleton, of the body; called also *os* [TA]. See Plates 10 and 45.

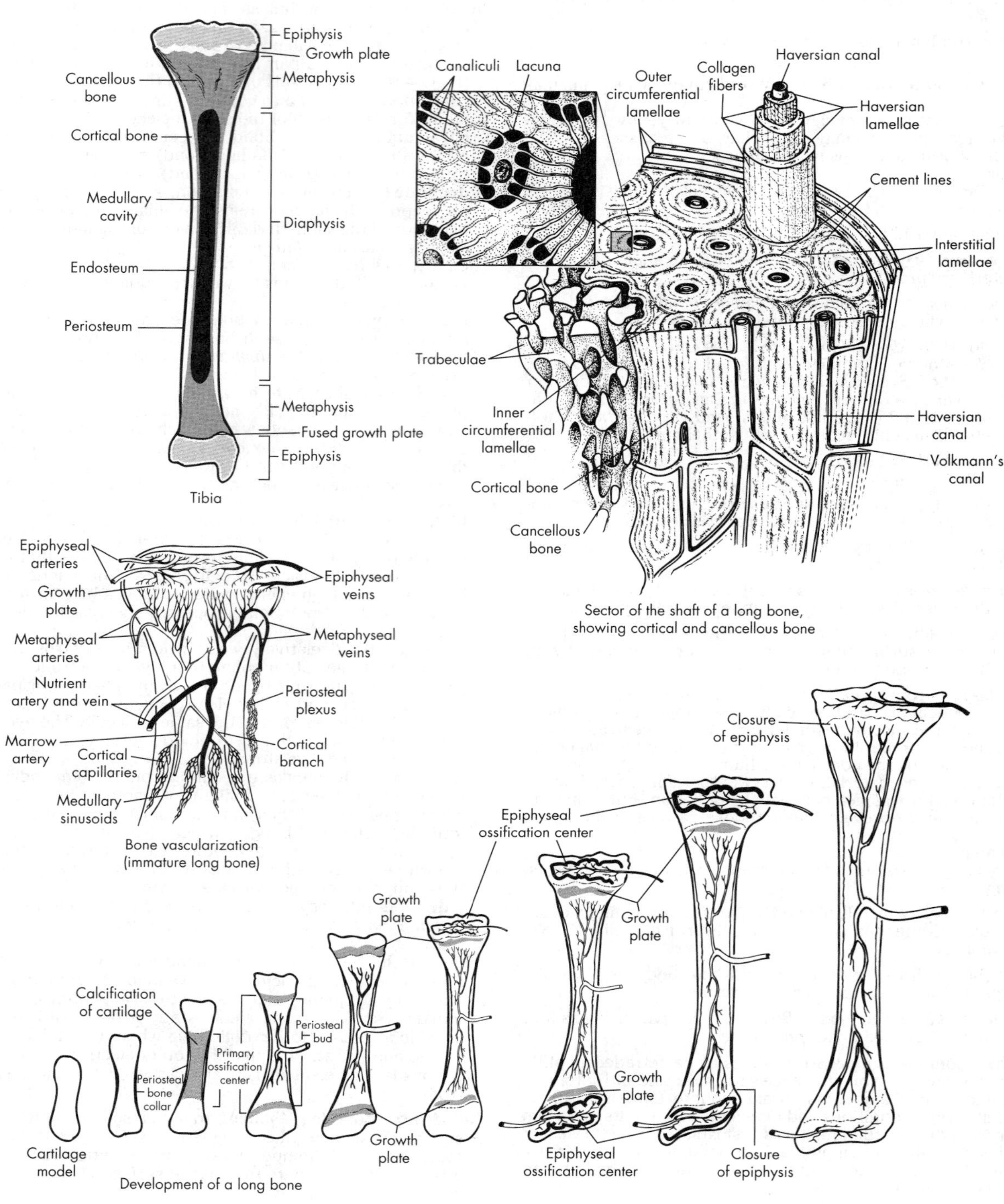


**PLATE 10**—STRUCTURE, VASCULARIZATION, AND DEVELOPMENT OF BONE

**accessory b.,** an occasionally occurring bone or ossicle adjoining one of the bones of the carpus or of the tarsus; recognized in the radiograph.

**acetabular b.,** acetabulum.

**acromial b.,** acromion.

**alar b.,** os sphenoidale.

**Albers-Schönberg marble b's,** osteopetrosis.

**Albrecht's b.,** basiotic b.

**alisphenoid b.,** ala major ossis sphenoidalis.

**alveolar b.,** the thin layer of bone making up the bony processes of the maxilla and mandible, and surrounding and containing the teeth; it is pierced by many small openings through which blood vessels, lymphatics, and nerve fibers pass. See also *alveolar process.*

**ankle b.,** talus.

**astragaloid b.,** talus.

**astragaloscaphoid b.,** Pirie's b.

**back b.,** columna vertebralis.

**basal b.,** the relatively fixed and unchangeable framework of the mandible and maxilla, which limits the extent to which teeth can be moved in the alveolar or supporting bone if the occlusion is to remain stable.

**basihyal b.,** corpus ossis hyoidei.

**basilar b., basioccipital b.,** a bone developing from a separate ossification center in the fetus, which becomes the basilar part of the occipital bone.

**basiotic b.,** a small bone of the fetus between the basisphenoid and the basioccipital bones; called also *Albrecht's b.*

**basisphenoid b.,** a bone in the floor of the skull of the human embryo and many animal species. In humans, before birth it becomes part of the postsphenoidal part of the sphenoid bone (see under *part*); in most animals it persists as a separate bone between the basioccipital bone and the presphenoidal bone.

**Bertin's b.,** concha sphenoidalis.

**breast b.,** sternum.

**bregmatic b.,** os parietale.

**brittle b's,** osteogenesis imperfecta.

**bundle b.,** one of the two types of bones composing the alveolar bone, so called because of the continuation into it of the principal fibers of the periodontal ligament. Large amounts of more calcified cementing substance render bundle bone more resistant to x-rays than surrounding bones; therefore it appears on dental radiographs as a thin radiopaque line (hence the synonym *lamina dura*). Called also *lamellated b.*

**calcaneal b.,** calcaneus.

**calf b.,** fibula.

**cancellated b., cancellous b.,** substantia spongiosa ossium.

**cannon b.,** a bone in the limb of hoofed animals, extending from the fetlock to the hock joint in the hind leg or the fetlock to the carpus in the foreleg; equivalent to a metacarpal or metatarsal in humans.

**capitate b.,** os capitatum.

**carpal b's,** ossa carpi; see under *os.*

**carpal b., central,** os centrale.

**carpal b., first,** os trapezium.

**carpal b., fourth,** os hamatum.

**carpal b., great,** os capitatum.

**carpal b., intermediate,** os lunatum.

**carpal b., radial,** os scaphoideum.

**carpal b., second,** os trapezoideum.

**carpal b., third,** os capitatum.

**carpal b., ulnar,** os triquetrum.

**cartilage b.,** any bone that develops within cartilage, in contrast to membrane bone, ossification taking place within a cartilage model; called also *endochondral b., replacement b.,* and *substitution b.*

**cavalry b.,** rider's b.

**central b.,** os centrale.

**chalky b's,** osteopetrosis.

**cheek b.,** os zygomaticum.

**chevron b.,** the V-shaped hemal arches of the third, fourth, and fifth coccygeal vertebrae of a dog.

**coccygeal b.,** os coccygis.

**coffin b.,** the third or distal phalanx of the foot of a horse; called also *pedal b.* and *os pedis.*

**collar b.,** clavicula.

**compact b.,** substantia compacta ossium.

**coronary b.,** small pastern bone; see *pastern b.*

**cortical b.,** the compact bone of the shaft of a bone that surrounds the medullary cavity.

**costal b.,** os costale.

**cranial b's, b's of cranium,** ossa cranii.

**cribriform b.,** os ethmoidale.

**cuboid b.,** os cuboideum.

**cuneiform b., external,** os cuneiforme laterale.

**cuneiform b., first,** os cuneiforme mediale.

**cuneiform b., intermediate,** os cuneiforme intermedium.

**cuneiform b., internal,** os cuneiforme mediale.

**cuneiform b., lateral,** os cuneiforme laterale.

**cuneiform b., medial,** os cuneiforme mediale.

**cuneiform b., middle, cuneiform b., second,** os cuneiforme intermedium.

**cuneiform b., third,** os cuneiforme laterale.

**cuneiform b. of carpus,** os triquetrum.

**dermal b.,** a bone developed by ossification in the skin.

**b's of digits of foot,** ossa digitorum pedis.

**b's of digits of hand,** ossa digitorum manus.

**ear b's,** ossicula auditus.

**ectethmoid b.,** labyrinthus ethmoidalis.

**ectocuneiform b.,** os cuneiforme laterale.

**endochondral b.,** cartilage b.

**entocuneiform b.,** os cuneiforme mediale.

**epactal b.,** os suturale.

**epactal b., proper,** os interparietale.

**ethmoid b.,** os ethmoidale.

**exercise b.,** a bone developed in a muscle, tendon, or fascia, as a result of excessive exercise.

**exoccipital b.,** one of the two lateral portions of the occipital bone, developing, from separate centers of ossification, into the portions that bear the condyles.

**b's of face, facial b's,** the bones that constitute the facial part of the skull, including the hyoid, palatine, and zygomatic bones, the mandible, and the maxilla; many authorities also include the lacrimal and nasal bones, the inferior nasal concha, and the vomer, and exclude the hyoid bone. Called also *ossa faciei* and *ossa facialia.*

**femoral b.,** femur (def. 1).

**fibular b.,** fibula.

**b's of fingers,** ossa digitorum manus.

**flank b.,** os ilium.

**flat b.,** os planum.

**frontal b.,** os frontale.

**funny b.,** the region of the median condyle of the humerus where it is crossed by the ulnar nerve.

**hamate b.,** os hamatum.

**haunch b.,** os coxae.

**heel b.,** calcaneus.

**hip b.,** os coxae.

**humeral b.,** humerus.

**hyoid b.,** os hyoideum.

**iliac b.,** os ilium.

**incarial b.,** os interparietale.

**incisive b.,** os incisivum.

**innominate b.,** os coxae.

**intermediate b.,** os lunatum.

**interparietal b.,** os interparietale.

**intrachondrial b.,** osseous tissue occurring in cartilage matrix which has undergone calcification; found particularly in patches within the middle layer of the otic capsule. Called also *globuli ossei.*

**irregular b.,** os irregulare.

**ischial b.,** os ischii.

**ivory b's,** osteopetrosis.

**jaw b., lower,** mandibula.

**jaw b., upper,** maxilla.

**jugal b.,** os zygomaticum.

**lacrimal b.,** os lacrimale.

**lacrimal b., lesser,** the lacrimal hamulus when it exists as a part separated from the rest of the lacrimal bone.

**lamellar b.,** the normal type of adult bone, organized in layers (lamellae), which may be parallel (cancellous bone) or concentrically arranged (compact bone).

**lamellated b.,** one of the two types of bone composing the alveolar bone, with some lamellae roughly parallel with the marrow spaces and others forming haversian systems. Cf. *bundle b.*

**lenticular b. of hand, lentiform b.,** os pisiforme.

**lingual b.,** os hyoideum.

**long b.,** os longum.

**lunate b.,** os lunatum.

**malar b.,** os zygomaticum.

**marble b's,** osteopetrosis.

**mastoid b.,** mastoid part of temporal bone.

**maxillary b.,** maxilla.

**maxilloturbinal b.,** concha nasalis inferior.

**membrane b.,** any bone that develops within a connective tissue membrane, in contrast to cartilage bone.

**mesethmoid b.,** a cranial bone present in some vertebrates, forming the most anterior part of the internal base of the cranium.

**mesocuneiform b.,** os cuneiforme intermedium.

**metacarpal b's,** ossa metacarpi.

**metacarpal b., middle, metacarpal b., third,** os metacarpi tertium.

**metatarsal b's,** ossa metatarsi.
**multangular b., accessory,** os centrale.
**multangular b., larger,** os trapezium.
**multangular b., smaller,** os trapezoideum.
**nasal b.,** os nasale.
**navicular b. of foot,** os naviculare.
**navicular b. of hand,** os scaphoideum.
**nonlamellated b.,** woven b.
**occipital b.,** os occipitale.
**odontoid b.,** dens axis.
**orbitosphenoidal b.,** ala minor ossis sphenoidalis.
**palate b., palatine b.,** os palatinum.
**parietal b.,** os parietale.
**pastern b.,** either of two bones of the horse's foot just proximal to the hoof: the *large pastern bone* is the first phalanx and the *small pastern bone* (called also *coronary b.*) is the second phalanx.
**pedal b.,** coffin b.
**pelvic b.,** os coxae.
**periosteal b.,** bone that is developed directly from and beneath the periosteum.
**petrosal b., petrous b.,** pars petrosa ossis temporalis.
**phalangeal b's of foot,** ossa digitorum pedis.
**phalangeal b's of hand,** ossa digitorum manus.
**Pirie's b.,** an occasionally occurring ossicle found above the head of the talus; called also *astragaloscaphoid b.*
**pisiform b.,** os pisiforme.
**plowshare b.,** pygostyle.
**pneumatic b.,** os pneumaticum.
**postsphenoid b., postsphenoidal b.,** see under *part.*
**postulnar b.,** os pisiforme.
**prefrontal b.,** pars nasalis ossis frontalis.
**preinterparietal b.,** a wormian bone sometimes observed, detached from the anterior part of the interparietal bone.
**premaxillary b.,** premaxilla.
**presphenoid b., presphenoidal b.,** see under *part.*
**primitive b.,** woven b.
**pterygoid b.,** processus pterygoideus ossis sphenoidalis.
**pubic b.,** os pubis.
**pyramidal b.,** os triquetrum.
**radial b.,** radius (def. 2).
**replacement b.,** cartilage b.
**resurrection b.,** os sacrum.
**rider's b.,** a localized ossification of the inner aspect of the lower end of the tendon of the adductor muscle of the thigh (adductor tubercle), sometimes seen in horseback riders; called also *cavalry b.*
**Riolan's b's,** small bones resembling wormian (sutural) bones, sometimes found in the suture between the occipital bone and the petrous portion of the temporal bone.
**rostral b.,** a bone supporting the apex of the nose in cattle or of the snout in pigs.
**rudimentary b.,** a bone that has only partially developed.
**sacral b.,** os sacrum.
**scaphoid b.,** os scaphoideum.
**scaphoid b. of foot,** os naviculare.
**scaphoid b. of hand,** os scaphoideum.
**scapular b.,** scapula.
**semilunar b.,** os lunatum.
**sesamoid b's,** numerous ovoid nodular bones, often small, usually found embedded within a tendon or joint capsule, principally in the hands and feet (*ossa sesamoidea manus* and *ossa sesamoidea pedis,* respectively); two sesamoid bones, the fabella and patella, are associated with the knee.
**sesamoid b's of foot,** ossa sesamoidea pedis.
**sesamoid b's of hand,** ossa sesamoidea manus.
**shin b.,** tibia.
**short b.,** os breve.
**b's of skull,** ossa cranii.
**solid b.,** substantia compacta ossium.
**sphenoid b.,** os sphenoidale.
**sphenoturbinal b.,** concha sphenoidalis.
**splint b's,** the reduced second and fourth metacarpal and metatarsal bones of equines.
**spoke b.,** radius (def. 2).
**spongy b.,** substantia spongiosa ossium.
**spongy b., inferior,** concha nasalis inferior.
**spongy b., superior,** concha nasalis superior.
**squamo-occipital b.,** the squamous portion of the fetal occipital bone, including the supraoccipital and interparietal bones.
**squamous b.,** pars squamosa ossis temporalis.
**stifle b.,** the patella of the horse.
**stirrup b.,** stapes.
**substitution b.,** cartilage b.
**supernumerary b.,** a bone occurring in addition to the normal one, as a vertebra or a rib (cervical or lumbar rib).
**suprainterparietal b.,** a wormian (sutural) bone sometimes occurring at the posterior part of the sagittal suture.
**supraoccipital b.,** a bone developing from a separate ossification center in the fetus, which becomes the squamous part of the occipital bone below the superior nuchal line.
**suprasternal b's,** ossa suprasternalia.
**sutural b.,** os suturale.
**tail b.,** os coccygis.
**tarsal b's,** ossa tarsi.
**tarsal b., first,** os cuneiforme mediale.
**tarsal b., second,** os cuneiforme intermedium.
**tarsal b., third,** os cuneiforme laterale.
**temporal b.,** os temporale.
**thigh b.,** femur (def. 1).
**thoracic b's,** ossa thoracis.
**b's of toes,** ossa digitorum pedis.
**tongue b.,** os hyoideum.
**trapezium b.,** os trapezium.
**trapezium b., lesser, trapezium b. of Lyser,** os trapezoideum.
**trapezoid b.,** os trapezoideum.
**trapezoid b. of Henle,** processus pterygoideus ossis sphenoidalis.
**trapezoid b. of Lyser,** os trapezium.
**triangular b.,** os triquetrum.
**triquetral b.,** os triquetrum.
**turbinate b., highest,** concha nasalis suprema.
**turbinate b., inferior,** concha nasalis inferior.
**turbinate b., middle,** concha nasalis media.
**turbinate b., superior,** concha nasalis superior.
**turbinate b., supreme,** concha nasalis suprema.
**tympanic b.,** pars tympanica ossis temporalis.
**ulnar b.,** ulna.
**unciform b., uncinate b.,** os hamatum.
**vesalian b.,** os vesalianum pedis.
**vomer b.,** vomer.
**whettle b's,** vertebrae thoracicae.
**wormian b.,** os suturale.
**woven b.,** bony tissue found in the embryo and young children and in various pathologic conditions in adults, in which the bone fails to show the oriented arrangement of collagen fibers characteristic of lamellated bone; called also *nonlamellated b.* and *primitive b.*
**xiphoid b.,** processus xiphoideus.
**zygomatic b.,** os zygomaticum.

**bone·let** (bōn'lət) a small bone, or ossicle.

**Bon·hoef·fer's symptom** (bon'hərf-ərz) [Karl *Bonhoeffer,* German psychiatrist, 1868–1948] see under *symptom.*

**Bo·nine** (bo'nēn) trademark for preparations of meclizine hydrochloride.

**Bon·net's capsule, sign** (bo-nāz') [Amédée *Bonnet,* French surgeon, 1802–1858] see *vagina bulbi* and see under *sign.*

**Bon·will crown, triangle** (bon'wil) [William Gibson Arlington *Bonwill,* American dentist, 1833–1899] see under *crown* and *triangle.*

**book·lung** (book'lung") see under *lung.*

**Böök's syndrome** (bo'oks) [Jan Arvid *Böök,* Swedish geneticist, born 1915] PHC syndrome.

**boom·slang** (bōōm'slang) *Dispholidus typus,* a venomous, green to brownish black, arboreal snake found in southern Africa. See table at *snake.*

**BOOP** bronchiolitis obliterans with organizing pneumonia.

**Bo·oph·i·lus** (bo-of'ĭ-ləs) [Gr. *bous* ox + *philein* to love] a genus of blood-sucking ixodid cattle ticks comprising many species that are vectors of bovine anaplasmosis and babesiosis. *B. annula'tus* is a vector of *Babesia bigemina; B. mi'croplus* is a vector of *B. bovis; B. calcara'tus* is a vector of *B. major;* and *B. decolora'tus* is a vector of *Anaplasma marginale.*

**Bo·op·o·nus** (bo-op′ə-nəs) [Gr. *bous* ox + *ponos* pain] a genus of flies of the family Calliphoridae, found in the Philippines; the larvae of *B. inton′sus* (foot maggots) cause lameness in cattle and goats.

**boost·er** (bōōst′ər) see under *dose.*

**boot** (bōōt) an encasement for the foot; a protective casing or sheath.
**De Lorme b.,** quadriceps b.
**Gibney's b.,** an adhesive tape support used in treatment of sprains and other painful conditions of the ankle, the tape being applied in a basketweave fashion with strips placed alternately under the sole of the foot and around the back of the leg.
**quadriceps b.,** a metal plate that fits over the sole of a shoe and can be fitted with weights of various sizes for therapeutic exercise of the quadriceps muscles. Called also *De Lorme b.*
**Unna's b., Unna's paste b.,** a dressing for varicose ulcers, consisting of a paste made from gelatin, zinc oxide, and glycerin, which is applied to the entire leg, then covered with a spiral bandage, this in turn being given a coat of the paste; the process is repeated until satisfactory rigidity is attained.

**boot·strap** (bōōt′strap) in statistics, a method for computing the distribution of values based on random resampling from the observed data.

**bo·rate** (bor′āt) any salt of boric acid.

**bo·rat·ed** (bor′at-əd) combined with or containing borax or boric acid.

**bo·rax** (bor′aks) gen. *bora′cis* [L. from Arabic; Farsi *būrah*] sodium borate.

**bor·bo·ryg·mus** (bor″bə-rig′məs) pl. *borboryg′mi* [L.] a rumbling noise caused by the propulsion of gas through the intestines.

**bor·der** (bor′dər) a bounding line or edge; called also *margin* and *margo* [TA].
**b. of acetabulum,** limbus acetabuli.
**alveolar b. of mandible,** arcus alveolaris mandibulae.
**alveolar b. of maxilla,** arcus alveolaris maxillae.
**anterior b. of body of pancreas,** margo anterior corporis pancreatis.
**anterior b. of lung,** margo anterior pulmonis.
**anterior b. of pancreas,** margo anterior corporis pancreatis.
**brush b.,** a specialization of the free surface of a cell, consisting of minute cylindrical processes (microvilli) that greatly increase the surface area; noted especially on the cells of the proximal convolution in a renal tubule and on the intestinal epithelium of vertebrates. Called also *striated b.*
**denture b.,** 1. the limit, boundary, or circumferential margin of a denture base. 2. the margin of the denture base at the junction of the polished surface with the impression (tissue) surface. 3. the extreme edges of a denture base at the buccolabial, lingual, and posterior limits. 4. the extreme margins of a denture base. Called also *denture edge.*
**external b. of tibia,** facies lateralis tibiae.
**fibular b. of foot,** margo lateralis pedis.
**frontal b. of parietal bone,** margo frontalis ossis parietalis.
**inferior b. of body of pancreas,** margo inferior corporis pancreatis.
**inferior b. of heart,** margo dexter cordis.
**inferior b. of liver,** margo inferior hepatis.
**inferior b. of lung,** margo inferior pulmonis.
**inferior b. of mandible,** basis mandibulae.
**inferior b. of pancreas,** margo inferior corporis pancreatis.
**lateral b. of foot,** margo lateralis pedis.
**lateral b. of forearm,** margo radialis antebrachii.
**medial b. of adrenal gland, medial b. of suprarenal gland,** margo medialis glandulae suprarenalis.
**medial b. of foot,** margo medialis pedis.
**medial b. of forearm,** margo ulnaris antebrachii.
**orbital b. of sphenoid bone,** facies orbitalis alae majoris.
**b. of oval fossa,** limbus fossae ovalis.

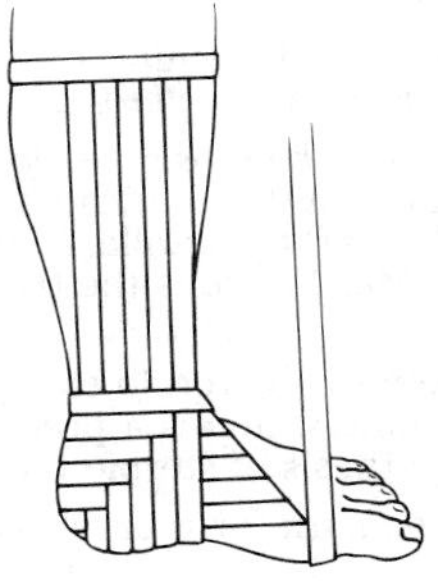
Gibney's boot.

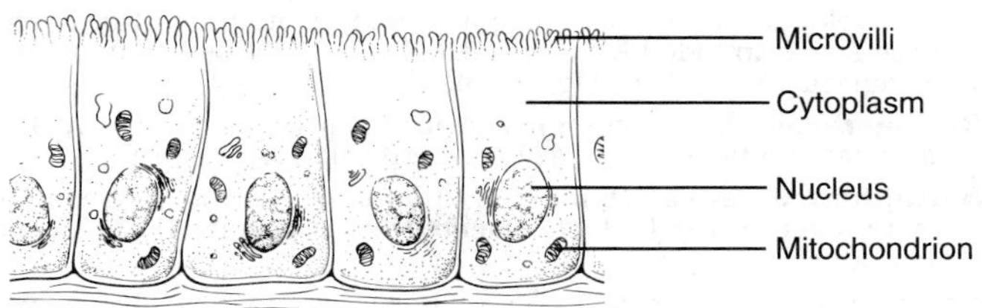

Brush border, characterized by closely packed microvilli.

**parietal b. of squamous part of temporal bone,** margo parietalis partis squamosae ossis temporalis.
**peroneal b. of foot,** margo lateralis pedis.
**posterior b. of petrous part of temporal bone,** margo posterior partis petrosae ossis temporalis.
**posterior b. of petrous portion of temporal bone,** angulus posterior pyramidis ossis temporalis.
**posterointernal b. of fibula,** crista medialis fibulae.
**radial b. of forearm,** margo radialis antebrachii.
**right b. of heart,** margo dexter cordis.
**sagittal b. of parietal bone,** margo sagittalis ossis parietalis.
**squamous b. of parietal bone,** margo squamosus ossis parietalis.
**striated b.,** brush b.
**superior b. of adrenal gland,** margo superior glandulae suprarenalis.
**superior b. of body of pancreas, superior b. of pancreas,** margo superior corporis pancreatis.
**superior b. of patella,** basis patellae.
**superior b. of petrous part of temporal bone,** margo superior partis petrosae ossis temporalis.
**superior b. of petrous portion of temporal bone,** angulus superior pyramidis ossis temporalis.
**superior b. of suprarenal gland,** margo superior glandulae suprarenalis.
**tibial b. of foot,** margo medialis pedis.
**ulnar b. of forearm,** margo ulnaris antebrachii.
**vermilion b.,** the exposed red portion of the upper and lower lips.

**bor·der·line** (bor′dər-līn) of a phenomenon, straddling the dividing line between two categories; see also under *personality.*

**Bor·det** (bor-da′) Jules Jean Baptíste Vincent. Belgian bacteriologist and serologist, 1870–1961; winner of the Nobel prize for medicine or physiology in 1919 for his work in immunology.

**Bor·det-Gen·gou agar (culture medium), bacillus, phenomenon (reaction)** (bor-da′zhahn-goo′) [J.J.B.V. *Bordet;* Octave *Gengou,* French bacteriologist, 1875–1957] see under *culture medium,* and see *Bordetella pertussis* and *complement fixation.*

**Bor·de·tel·la** (bor″də-tel′ə) [J.J.B.V. *Bordet*] [MeSH: Bordetella] a genus of gram-negative aerobic, minute coccobacilli of uncertain affiliation. It is made up of organisms that are parasites and pathogens of the respiratory tract of humans and lower animals and produce a dermonecrotic toxin.
**B. bronchisep′tica,** a species resembling *B. pertussis* morphologically, culturally, and antigenically except that *B. bronchiseptica* is motile and grows sparsely on nutrient agar; it is a frequent cause of bronchopneumonia in guinea pigs and other rodents, swine, dogs, and lower primates, and of canine infectious tracheobronchitis. Called also *Bacillus bronchisepticus, Brucella bronchiseptica,* and *Haemophilus bronchisepticus.*
**B. parapertus′sis,** a species immunologically related to *B. pertussis,* from which it can be distinguished by the readiness with which it grows on simple culture media. It causes parapertussis and occasionally classic pertussis. Called also *Haemophilus parapertussis.*
**B. pertus′sis,** the usual causative agent of pertussis (whooping cough) in humans, found only in the human respiratory tract. Virulent strains are encapsulated with smooth colonies (Phase I); prolonged laboratory culture produces loss of surface K antigens and altered colonial morphology (Phases II, III, and IV) progressing to obviously rough strains that are avirulent. Called also *Bordet-Gengou bacillus, Haemophilus pertussis,* and *Pseudomonas pertucinogena* (Phase IV).

**bo·ric ac·id** (bor′ik) [NF] a mild acid used as an acidifying agent and in buffer solutions; it is also a weak germicide used on intact skin, mucous membranes, and cornea. Accidental ingestion may cause fatal poisoning in humans or other animals; see *boron poisoning,* under *poisoning.*

**Bör·je·son's syndrome** (bor′yə-sunz) [Mats Gunnar *Börjeson,* Swedish physician, born 1922] see under *syndrome.*

**Bor·na disease** (bor′nə) [*Borna,* a district in Germany where an epidemic occurred] [MeSH: Borna Disease] see under *disease.*

**Bor·na·vir·i·dae** (bor″nə-vir′ĭ-de) a family of RNA viruses having an enveloped virion containing a genome consisting of negative-sense single-stranded RNA (size 8.9 kb). Replication occurs within the nucleus. There is a single genus, *Bornavirus.*

**Bor·na·vi·rus** (bor'nə-vi″rəs) a genus of viruses of the family Bornaviridae, containing a single species, Borna disease virus.

**Born·holm disease** (born'hōm) [*Bornholm,* island in Denmark where some of the first documented cases occurred] epidemic pleurodynia.

**bo·ron** (bor'on) [L. *borium*] [MeSH: Boron] a nonmetallic element occurring in the form of crystals and as a powder. It is the base of borax and boric acid: symbol B, atomic number 5, specific gravity 2.54, atomic weight 10.811. See also *boron poisoning,* under *poisoning.*
**b. carbide,** a compound, $B_4C$, slightly harder than silicon carbide (q.v.), obtained by heating boron at very high temperature to effect its union with carbon; used as a neutron absorber in nuclear reactors, and as an abrasive agent in industry and dentistry.

**Bor·rel bo·dies** (bo-rel') [Amédée *Borrel,* French bacteriologist, 1867–1936] see under *body.*

**Bor·rel·ia** (bə-rel'e-ə) [after A. *Borrel*] [MeSH: Borrelia] a genus of bacteria of the family Spirochaetaceae, order Spirochaetales, made up of gram-negative, anaerobic, helical cells up to 1$\mu$ wide by 20$\mu$ long, with coarse, shallow, irregular coils surrounding a central fibrillar substance. The organisms are parasitic, living on mucous membranes, and are the cause of relapsing fever in humans and animals.
**B. afze'lii,** a genospecies, formerly classed as group 3 of *B. burgdorferi,* that is an agent of Lyme borreliosis in Europe.
**B. anseri'na,** the etiologic agent of fowl spirochetosis, transmitted by species of the tick *Argas,* which occurs worldwide in wild and domestic fowl. It is not pathogenic for humans.
**B. ber'bera,** *B. recurrentis.*
**B. bucca'lis,** *Treponema buccale.*
**B. burgdor'feri,** the causative agent of acrodermatitis chronica atrophicans, erythema chronicum migrans, and Lyme disease, transmitted by ixodid ticks. See also *B. afzelii* and *B. garinii.*
**B. car'teri,** *B. recurrentis.*
**B. cauca'sica,** an etiologic agent of relapsing fever in the Caucasus, transmitted by the tick *Ornithodoros verrucosus* from a reservoir of infection in field mice.
**B. crocidu'rae,** an etiologic agent of relapsing fever in humans in North Africa, transmitted by the tick *Ornithodoros erraticus sonrai,* which is carried by small rodents.
**B. dipodil'li,** a species of uncertain status that is an etiologic agent of North African tickborne relapsing fever, transmitted by the tick *Ornithodoros erraticus sonrai,* which is carried by small rodents.
**B. dutto'nii,** an etiologic agent of endemic relapsing fever in Central and South Africa, carried by the tick *Ornithodoros moubata,* which transmits the microorganism from human to human in its saliva. Called also *B. hochii* and *Dutton's spirochete.*
**B. gari'nii,** a genospecies, formerly classed as group 2 of *B. burgdorferi,* that is an agent of Lyme borreliosis in Europe.
**B. herm'sii,** an etiologic agent of endemic relapsing fever in western North America, transmitted by the tick *Ornithodoros hermsii,* which is transported by chipmunks and tree squirrels.
**B. hispa'nica,** the etiologic agent of endemic relapsing fever in the Iberian peninsula and Northwest Africa, transmitted by the large tick *Ornithodoros erraticus,* which lives on rodents, reptiles, and amphibians; the organism is transmitted as the tick is feeding.
**B. ko'chii,** *B. duttonii.*
**B. latysche'wii,** the etiologic agent of a type of relapsing fever in Iran and Central Asia, transmitted by the tick *Ornithodoros tartakovskyi,* which is carried by rodents and reptiles.
**B. mazzot'tii,** the etiologic agent of relapsing fever in the southern United States, Mexico, and Central and South America, transmitted by the tick *Ornithodoros talaje,* which is carried by rodents, armadillos, and monkeys.
**B. merione'si,** a species of uncertain status that is an etiologic agent of North African tickborne relapsing fever and is transmitted by *Ornithodoros erraticus sonrai,* which is carried by small rodents.
**B. micro'ti,** a species that causes North African tickborne relapsing fever. It is transmitted by *Ornithodoros erraticus sonrai,* which is carried by small rodents.
**B. neotropica'lis,** *B. venezuelensis.*
**B. no'vyi,** *B. recurrentis.*
**B. obermey'eri,** *B. recurrentis.*
**B. par'keri,** an etiologic agent of endemic relapsing fever in the western United States. Burrowing rodents, such as ground squirrels, carry the tick vector, *Ornithodoros parkeri,* which transmits the organism in its bite.
**B. per'sica,** an etiologic agent of endemic relapsing fever in Asia and Africa. The organism is transmitted in the bite of the tick vector *Ornithodoros tholozani,* which is carried by rodents living in caves, stables, and burrows.
**B. recurren'tis,** the causative agent of worldwide epidemic louse-borne relapsing fever, transmitted by the human body louse, *Pediculus humanus.* The organism is spread by rubbing infected hemolymph of lice into the skin, as in scratching. The organism produces successive antigenic mutants that cause the clinical relapses. Called also *B. berbera, B. carteri, B. novyi,* and *B. obermeyeri.*
**B. theile'ri,** an etiologic agent of tickborne spirochetosis in cattle, horses, and sheep in South Africa and Australia, transmitted by species of *Rhipicephalus* and *Boophilus.*
**B. turica'tae,** an etiologic agent of endemic relapsing fever in southwestern United States and Mexico. The organism is transmitted by the bite of the tick *Ornithodoros turicata,* which is carried by rodents and reptiles.
**B. venezuelen'sis,** an etiologic agent of relapsing fever in Central and South America, transmitted by the tick *Ornithodoros rudis,* which is carried by monkeys and rodents. Called also *B. neotropicalis.*
**B. vincen'tii,** *Treponema vincentii.*

**bor·rel·i·o·sis** (bə-rel″e-o'sis) infection with spirochetes of the genus *Borrelia.*
**Lyme b.,** a general term encompassing a number of diseases that are caused by *Borrelia burgdorferi* and have similar manifestations, including Lyme disease, acrodermatitis chronica atrophicans, Bannwarth's syndrome, and erythema chronicum migrans.

**Borr·mann's classification** (bor'mahnz) [R. *Borrmann,* German, 20th century] see under *classification.*

**Bor·si·eri's sign (line)** (bor″se-er'ēz) [Giovanni Battista *Borsieri* de Kanilfeld, Italian physician, 1725–1785] see under *sign.*

**boss** (bos) a rounded eminence, as on the surface of a bone or tumor.
**parietal b's,** sharp prominences on each side of the parietal bones.

**Bos·ker implant** (bos'kər) [Hans *Bosker,* Dutch surgeon, 20th century] see under *implant.*

**bos·se·lat·ed** (bos'ə-lāt-əd) [Fr. *bosseler*] marked or covered with bosses.

**bos·se·la·tion** (bos″ə-la'shən) 1. a small eminence; one of a set of bosses. 2. the condition or fact of being bosselated; the process of becoming bosselated.

**Bos·ton's sign** (bos'tənz) [L. Napoleon *Boston,* American physician, 1871–1931] see under *sign.*

**bot** (bot) the larva of a botfly, which may be parasitic in the stomach of animals or sometimes of humans.
**sheep nose b.,** the larva of *Oestrus ovis,* which is frequently found in the nasal passages of sheep.

**Bo·tal·lo's duct, foramen, ligament** (bo-tah'lōz) [Leonardo *Botallo,* Italian surgeon in Paris, 1530–1600] see *ductus arteriosus, foramen ovale cordis,* and *ligamentum arteriosum.*

**bo·tan·ic** (bo-tan'ik) 1. pertaining to or derived from plants; of the vegetable kingdom. 2. pertaining to botany.

**bot·a·ny** (bot'ə-ne) [L. *botanica* from Gr. *botanē* herb] [MeSH: Botany] the science of plants or of the vegetable kingdom.
**medical b.,** the botany of plants used in medicine.

**bot·fly** (bot'fli) an insect of the family Oestridae whose larvae (called *bots*) are parasitic, especially in horses and sheep. Genera include *Cuterebra, Dermatobia, Gasterophilus,* and *Oestrus.*

**both·rid·i·um** (both-rid'e-əm) one of the four leaf-like suckers symmetrically placed around the anterior end of the scolex of a tetraphyllidean cestode; called also *phyllidea.*

**both·rio·ceph·a·li·a·sis** (both″re-o-sef″ə-li'ə-sis) diphyllobothriasis.

**Both·rio·ceph·a·lus** (both″re-o-sef'ə-ləs) [Gr. *bothrion* pit + *-cephalus*] *Diphyllobothrium.*

**both·ri·um** (both're-əm) [Gr. *bothrion* pit] a sucker in the form of a groove such as is seen on either side of the head of *Diphyllobothrium latum.*

**both·rop·ic** (both-rop'ik) pertaining to, characteristic of, or derived from snakes of the genus *Bothrops.*

**Both·rops** (both'rops) [Gr. *bothros* pit + *ōps* eye] [MeSH: Bothrops] a genus of tropical and South American snakes of the family Crotalidae. *B. atrox'* is the barba amarilla, *B. jarara'ca* is the jararaca, and *B. lanceola'tus* of Martinique is the true fer-de-lance. See table at *snake.*

**bot·o·ge·nin** (bot-o-je'nin) a steroid sapogenin, $C_{27}H_{40}O_4$, derived from *Dioscorea mexicana,* which is a precursor in a patented process for the partial synthesis of steroid hormones.

**Bo·tox** (bo'toks) trademark for a preparation of botulinum toxin type A.

**bot·ry·oid** (bot're-oid) [Gr. *botrys* bunch of grapes + *-oid*] resembling a bunch of grapes.

**bot·ryo·my·co·sis** (bot″re-o-mi-ko'sis) [Gr. *botrys* bunch of grapes + *myco-* + *-osis*] a chronic purulent granulomatous bacterial infection usually caused by *Staphylococcus aureus,* originally thought to be due to fungi called "botryomycetes," characterized by lesions containing sulfur granules composed of a central mass of bacteria surrounded by a capsule, and histologically resembling actinomycosis or mycetoma. Human infection is usually localized to the skin but may involve other organs such as the viscera and lymph nodes, especially in debilitated patients; infection in domestic animals most often occurs as chronic, localized or spreading abscesses of the skin.

**bot·ryo·my·cot·ic** (bot″re-o-mi-kot'ik) pertaining to or affected with botryomycosis.

**Bo·try·tis** (bo-tri'tis) a genus of Fungi Imperfecti of the form-class Hyphomycetes, form-family Moniliaceae; it includes the common gray mold and plant pathogens such as those that cause onion rot, peony blight, and turnip fire. *B. bassia'na* and *B. tenel'la* have been reclassified in genus *Beauveria.*

**Böt·tcher's space** (bərt'shərz) [Arthur *Böttcher,* German anatomist, 1831–1889] saccus endolymphaticus.

**bot·tle** (bot'əl) a hollow narrow-necked vessel of glass or other material, used in laboratory procedures or for other purposes.
**Castaneda b.,** a biphasic bottle containing both broth and a solid agar slant; used in the cultivation of fastidious organisms from blood.
**Spritz b.,** a wash bottle for laboratory use.
**wash b.,** 1. a flexible squeeze-bottle with delivery tube, or a bottle having two tubes through the cork, so arranged that blowing into one will force a stream of liquid from the other; used in washing chemical materials. 2. a bottle containing some washing fluid, through which gases are passed for the purpose of freeing them from impurities.
**Woulfe's b.,** a three-necked bottle used for washing gases or for saturating liquids with a gas.

**bot·u·li·form** (boch'u-lĭ-form) [L. *botulus* sausage + *form*] sausage-shaped.

**bot·u·lin** (boch'u-lin) [L. *botulus* sausage] botulinum toxin.

**bot·u·li·nal** (boch″u-li'nəl) 1. pertaining to *Clostridium botulinum.* 2. pertaining to botulinum toxin.

**bot·u·lin·o·gen·ic** (boch'u-lin″o-jen'ik) [*botulin* + *-genic*] producing or containing botulinum toxin.

**bot·u·lism** (boch'u-liz-əm) [L. *botulus* sausage] [MeSH: Botulism] 1. in humans, food poisoning with neurotoxicity resulting from eating spoiled food contaminated with *Clostridium botulinum,* which produces botulinum toxin (q.v.). Characteristics include central nervous system symptoms with motor disturbances; visual and oculomotor difficulties; and disturbances of secretion such as dryness of the mouth and pharynx with coughing. In adults it is usually due to ingestion of preformed toxin, although sometimes toxins can be produced in the gastrointestinal tract by ingested organisms. See also *infant b.* and *allantiasis.* 2. any of various neurotoxic syndromes in animals caused by ingestion of feed contaminated with *Clostridium botulinum,* such as moldy hay, grain, or silage. See *lamziekte, limberneck,* and *shaker foal syndrome.*
**infant b.,** that affecting infants, typically 4 to 26 weeks of age, marked by constipation, lethargy, hypotonia, and feeding difficulty; it may lead to respiratory insufficiency. It results from toxin produced in the gut by ingested organisms, rather than from preformed toxins.
**wound b.,** botulism resulting from infection of a wound with *Clostridium botulinum;* it is marked by the same symptoms as the food-borne form except for the absence of gastrointestinal symptoms.

**bot·u·lis·mo·tox·in** (boch'u-liz″mo-tok'sin) botulinum toxin.

**bou·fée dé·li·rante** (boo-fa' da-le-rahnt') [Fr. "delirious outburst"] a reactive psychosis resembling schizophrenia but having a duration of less than three months and a favorable prognosis. It is roughly the French counterpart to schizophreniform disorder.

**Bou·chard's disease, nodes (nodules)** (boo-shahrz') [Charles Jacques *Bouchard,* French physician, 1837–1915] see under *disease* and *node.*

**Bou·chardat's test, treatment** (boo-shahr-dahz') [Apollinaire *Bouchardat,* French chemist, 1806–1886] see under *treatment.*

**Bou·chut's respiration, tubes** (boo-shūz') [Jean Antoine Eugène *Bouchut,* French physician, 1818–1891] see under *tube.*

**bou·gie** (boo-zhe') [Fr. "wax candle"] a slender, flexible, hollow or solid, cylindrical instrument for introduction into the urethra or other tubular organ, usually for the purpose of calibrating or dilating constricted areas.

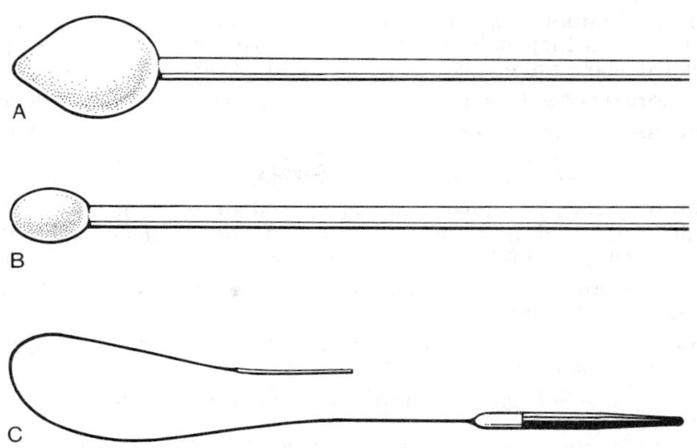

Bougies: *(A),* Otis bougie à boule; *(B),* olive-tipped bougie; *(C),* filiform bougie.

**b. à boule,** (ah-bo͞ol') [Fr.], bulbous b.
**acorn-tipped b.,** a bulbous bougie with a tip shaped like an acorn.
**bulbous b.,** one with a bulb-shaped tip; called also *b. à boule.*
**caustic b.,** one that has a piece of silver nitrate or other caustic agent attached to its end; used as a portcaustic.
**conic b.,** one with a cone-shaped tip.
**cylindrical b.,** one with a round or circular section.
**dilating b.,** a bougie whose diameter can be increased by turning a screw; commonly used for dilating a stricture of the urethra.
**elastic b.,** one made of rubber or other elastic material.
**elbowed b.,** one with an elbow or sharp bend near the tip.
**filiform b.,** one of very slender caliber; often used for the gentle exploration of strictures or sinus tracts of small diameter with multiple false passages.
**fusiform b.,** one with a belly or expansion in its shaft.
**Hurst's b's,** a series of mercury-filled tubes of graded diameter for dilating the cardioesophageal region.
**Maloney b's,** a series similar to Hurst's bougies but having cone-shaped tips.
**olive-tipped b.,** a bulbous bougie with a tip shaped like an olive.
**rosary b.,** a beaded bougie for use in a strictured urethra.
**wax-tipped b.,** a long, slender, flexible bougie with a wax tip for passage into the ureter through the cystoscope to confirm the diagnosis of ureteral calculus.
**whip b.,** one with a filiform point and a stem of gradually increasing caliber.

**bou·gie·nage** (boo″zhe-nahzh') the passage of a bougie through a tubular structure or organ, to increase its caliber, as in the treatment of stricture of the esophagus.

**boug·i·nage** (boo-zhe-nahzh') bougienage.

**Bouil·laud's disease, sign, syndrome** (boo-e-yōz') [Jean Baptiste *Bouillaud,* French physician, 1796–1881] see *rheumatic endocarditis,* under *endocarditis,* and see under *sign* and *syndrome.*

**bouil·lon** (boo-yaw') [Fr.] a broth or soup prepared from the flesh of animals; used in food preparations and as a bacteriological culture medium. In the latter use, it is generally called *broth;* see under *culture medium* for specific broths.

**Bou·in's fluid (solution)** (boo-az') [Pol André *Bouin,* French anatomist, 1870–1962] see under *fluid.*

**bound** (bound) 1. restrained or confined; not free. 2. held in chemical combination.

**bou·quet** (boo-ka') [Fr.] a structure suggesting resemblance to a bunch of flowers, as a cluster of vessels, nerves, or fibers, or the polarized stage of synapsis at the start of meiosis.

**Bour·gery's ligament** (bo͞or-zhə-rēz') [Marc Jean *Bourgery,* French anatomist and surgeon, 1797–1849] ligamentum popliteum obliquum.

**Bourne·ville's disease** (bo͞orn-vēlz') [Désiré-Magloire *Bourneville,* French neurologist, 1840–1909] tuberous sclerosis.

**Bourne·ville-Prin·gle syndrome** (bo͞orn-vēl' pring'gəl) [D.-M. *Bourneville;* John James *Pringle,* British dermatologist, 1855–1922] tuberous sclerosis.

**bout** (bout) an attack or episode of illness.

**bou·ton** (boo-tahn') [Fr. "button"] a button-like swelling on an axon where it has a synapse with another neuron.
**b. de passage, b. en passant,** a button-like swelling on an axon at a synapse that is not at the end of the axon. See also *en passant synapse.*
**synaptic b.,** b. terminal.

**b. terminal** **boutons' terminaux'**, a button-like terminal enlargement of an axon that ends in relation to another neuron at a synapse; called also *terminal button, end-foot,* and *synaptic knob.*

**bou·ton·neuse** (boo-tə-nooz') [Fr. "pimply"] boutonneuse fever.

**Bou·ve·ret's syndrome** (boo-və-rāz') [Léon *Bouveret,* French physician, 1850–1929] see *paroxysmal supraventricular tachycardia,* under *tachycardia,* and see under *syndrome.*

**Bo·vet** (bo-va') Daniele. Swiss-born Italian pharmacologist, born 1907; winner of the Nobel prize for medicine or physiology in 1957 for developing antihistamines and muscle relaxants.

**Bo·vi·my·ces pleu·ro·pneu·mo·niae** (bo"vĭ-mi'sēz ploor"o-noo-mo'ne-e) *Mycoplasma mycoides.*

**bo·vine** (bo'vīn) [L. *bos, bovis* ox, bullock, cow] pertaining to, characteristic of, or derived from cattle.

**bow** (bo) [A.S. *boga* bow, arch] an arched or curved appliance or device.
**Logan b.,** an appliance used to prevent tension on sutures after surgical repair of cleft lip.

**Bow·ditch's law, staircase phenomenon** (bo'dich-əz) [Henry Pickering *Bowditch,* American physiologist, 1840–1911] see *all or none,* under *A,* and see *treppe.*

**bow·el** (bou'əl) [Fr. *boyau*] intestinum.

**Bo·wen's disease (precancerous dermatosis)** (bo'ənz) [John Templeton *Bowen,* American dermatologist, 1857–1941] see under *disease.*

**bow·en·oid** (bo'ən-oid) pertaining to or resembling the lesions of Bowen's disease.

**bow·ie** (bo'e) a disease resembling rickets that affects unweaned lambs in New Zealand.

**bowl** (bōl) [A.S. *bolla*] a rounded, more or less hemispherical open container, or a structure resembling such a container.
**mastoid b., mastoidectomy b.,** the hollow bony defect in the temporal bone created by open mastoidectomy.

**bow·leg** (bo'leg) genu varum.
**nonrachitic b.,** tibia vara.

**Bow·man's capsule,** etc. (bo'mənz) [Sir William *Bowman,* English physician, 1816–1892] see under *probe* and *tube* and see *capsula glomeruli, lamina limitans anterior corneae, musculus ciliaris,* and *glandulae olfactoriae.*

**box** (boks) a rectangular structure.
**anatomical snuff-b.,** a triangular depression on the dorsum of the wrist at its radial border formed between the tendon of the extensor pollicis longus medially and the tendons of the extensor pollicis brevis and abductor pollicis longus laterally, formed when the thumb is abducted and extended.
**brain b.,** neurocranium.
**CAAT b.,** a conserved noncoding DNA sequence approximating the consensus sequence 5'-GGCCAATCT-3'; it is located approximately 40 to 110 base pairs upstream from the site of transcription initiation in some eukaryotic genes and serves a promoter function.
**GC b.,** a conserved noncoding DNA sequence approximating the consensus sequence 5'-GGGCGG-3'; it is located approximately 40 to 110 base pairs upstream from the site of transcription in some eukaryotic genes, particularly constitutively expressed housekeeping genes, and serves a promoter function.
**Goldberg-Hogness b., Hogness b.,** TATA b.
**Skinner b.,** an experimental enclosure for testing animal conditioning, in which the subject animal performs (e.g., presses a bar or lever) to obtain a reward.
**TATA b.,** a conserved noncoding DNA sequence approximating the consensus sequence 5'-TATAAAA-3'; it occurs approximately 25 base pairs upstream from the site of transcription initiation in most eukaryotic genes and serves a promoter function. See also *CAAT b.* Called also *Goldberg-Hogness b.* and *Hogness b.*
**Yerkes discrimination b.,** a maze with a series of doors, used in the laboratory in studies of visual discrimination in animals; opening of the proper door produces a reward, but opening of the wrong door produces an electric stimulus.

**box·ing** (bok'sing) [MeSH: Boxing] in the fabrication of dental restorations and appliances, the building up of vertical walls of wax or other suitable material to form a box around a dental impression into which the freshly mixed plaster or stone is poured; done to produce the desired size and form of the base of the cast and to preserve certain landmarks of the impression.

**box-note** (boks'nōt) a hollow percussion sound heard in the chest of a person with emphysema.

**Boyce's sign** (boi'səz) [Frederick Fitzherbert *Boyce,* American physician, born 1903] see under *sign.*

**Boy·er's bursa, cyst** (bwah-yāz') [Alexis de *Boyer,* French surgeon, 1757–1833] see under *cyst* and see *retrohyoid bursa* under *bursa.*

**Boyle's law** (boilz) [Robert *Boyle,* English physicist, 1627–1691] see under *law.*

**Boze·man's operation, position, speculum** (bōz'mənz) [Nathan *Bozeman,* American surgeon, 1825–1905] see under *position* and *speculum,* and see *hysterocystocleisis.*

**Boz·zo·lo's sign** (bot-so'lōz) [Camillo *Bozzolo,* Italian physician, 1845–1920] see under *sign.*

**BP** 1. blood pressure. 2. British Pharmacopoeia, a publication of the General Medical Council, describing and establishing standards for medicines, preparations, materials, and articles used in the practice of medicine, surgery, or midwifery.

**bp** base pair; boiling point.

**BPA** British Paediatric Association.

**BPI** bactericidal permeability increasing protein.

**B Ph** British Pharmacopoeia.

**BPIG** bacterial polysaccharide immune globulin.

**BPRS** Brief Psychiatric Rating Scale.

**Bq** abbreviation for *becquerel.*

**Br** symbol for *bromine.*

**Braasch bulb catheter** (brahsh) [William F. *Braasch,* American urologist, 1878–1975] see under *catheter.*

**brace** (brās) [MeSH: Braces] 1. a device that holds parts together or in place. 2. an orthopedic appliance (orthosis) used to support, align, or hold parts of the body in correct position. 3. (pl.) orthodontic appliance; see under *appliance.*
**back b.,** spinal orthosis.
**Blount b.,** a spinal orthosis consisting of a molded pelvic band with anterior and posterior metal bars connecting to chin or throat piece and occipital hold; used in scoliosis.
**chairback b.,** any of a number of thoracolumbosacral orthoses that have a pelvic band passing between the iliac crest and the greater trochanter and a thoracic band passing just below the angle of the scapula; steel upright bars connect the bands and provide rigidity.
**collar b.,** cervical orthosis.
**Fisher b.,** a thoracolumbar orthosis with axillary holds and a corset front.
**Goldthwait b.,** a thoracolumbar orthosis consisting of three padded, leather-covered metal strips, the uppermost fitting above the nipple line and the lowest encircling the pelvis.
**Jewett b.,** a hyperextension orthosis with pads as corrective pressure points at the sternal notch, above the pubis, and in the lumbar lordosis.
**Jones b.,** a thoracolumbosacral orthosis consisting of two vertical parallel bars that join a wider horizontal bar at the bottom, held in place by shoulder straps, an abdominal support, and groin straps, leaving the chest free.
**Knight b.,** one of the oldest kinds of chairback brace; the upper and lower bands and the upright bars are made of aluminum.
**leg b.,** knee-ankle-foot orthosis.
**long leg b.,** hip-knee-ankle-foot orthosis.
**McKee b.,** a lumbosacral orthosis with a lumbar pad; used to support the lumbar spine and prevent flexion.
**Milwaukee b.,** a spinal orthosis with a molded pelvic belt that fits above the upper edge of the iliac crest, joined to a turnbuckle that extends the length of the spine to an occipital hold with a throat mold; used in scoliosis and ankylosing spondylitis.
**neck b.,** cervical orthosis.
**Taylor b.,** a. thoracolumbosacral orthosis with steel rods that support the spine; used in cases of disease or mechanical derangement. Called also *Taylor's apparatus* and *Taylor splint.*

**brace·let** (brās'let) a small encircling band, denoting, in the plural, transverse markings across the palmar surface of the skin of the wrists.
**Nageotte's b's,** bands covered with circular spines on the axons at the level of the nodes of Ranvier.

**bra·chia** (bra'ke-ə) [L.] plural of *brachium.*

**bra·chi·al** (bra'ke-əl) [L. *brachialis,* from *brachium* arm] pertaining to the arm.

**bra·chi·al·gia** (bra"ke-al'jə) [*brachi-* + *-algia*] pain in the arm or arms.
**b. sta'tica paresthe'tica,** painful paresthesias in the arm and hand during sleep due to compression of the blood vessels.

**bra·chi·a·tion** (bra"ke-a'shən) [*brachi-* + *-ation* suffix implying action] locomotion in a position of suspension by means of the hands and arms, as exhibited by monkeys when swinging from branch to branch.

**brachi(o)-** [L. *brachium,* q.v.] a combining form denoting arm.

**bra·chio·ce·phal·ic** (brak"e-o-sə-fal'ik) [*brachio-* + *cephalic*] pertaining to the arm and head.

**bra·chio·cru·ral** (brak″e-o-kroo′rəl) [*brachio-* + *crural*] pertaining to the arm and leg.

**bra·chio·cu·bi·tal** (brak″e-o-ku′bĭ-təl) [*brachio-* + *cubital*] pertaining to the arm and elbow or forearm.

**bra·chio·cyl·lo·sis** (brak″e-o-sə-lo′sis) [*brachio-* + Gr. *kyllōsis* a crooking] brachiocyrtosis.

**bra·chio·cyr·to·sis** (brak″e-o-sər-to′sis) [*brachio-* + *cyrtosis*] crookedness of the arm.

**bra·chio·fa·cio·lin·gual** (brak″e-o-fa″she-o-ling′gwəl) pertaining to or affecting the arm, face, and tongue.

**bra·chio·tho·ra·co·om·pha·lo·is·chi·op·a·gus** (bra″ke-o-thor″ə-ko-om″fə-lo-is″ke-op′ə-gəs) conjoined twins joined from the forearms and shoulder to the pelvis.
**b. bi′pus,** conjoined twins joined from the forearms and shoulder to the pelvis and having two feet.

**bra·chi·um** (bra′ke-əm) pl. *bra′chia* [L.; Gr. *brachiōn*] [TA] 1. arm: the part of the upper limb from shoulder to elbow. 2. a general term used to designate an armlike process or structure.
**b. of caudal colliculus, b. coll′iculi cauda′lis,** b. colliculi inferioris.
**b. colli′culi inferio′ris** [TA], brachium of inferior colliculus: fibers from the lateral lemniscus that pass deep to the inferior colliculus and run forward to terminate in the medial geniculate body; called also *b. of caudal colliculus* and *b. colliculi caudalis.*
**b. colli′culi rostra′lis,** b. colliculi superioris.
**b. colli′culi superio′ris** [TA], brachium of superior colliculus: fibers ascending ventrolaterally from the lateral aspect of the superior colliculus of the mesencephalon, conveying fibers from the retina and the optic radiation to the superior colliculus; called also *b. colliculi rostralis, b. of rostral colliculus,* and *b. opticum.*
**b. of inferior colliculus,** b. colliculi inferioris.
**b. op′ticum,** b. colliculi superioris.
**b. pon′tis,** pedunculus cerebellaris medius.
**b. of rostral colliculus,** b. colliculi superioris.
**b. of superior colliculus,** b. colliculi superioris.

**Brach·mann-de·Lange syndrome** (brahk′mahn-da-lahng′ə) [W. *Brachmann,* German physician, early 20th century; Cornelia *de Lange,* Dutch pediatrician, 1871–1950] de Lange's syndrome.

**Bracht's maneuver** (brokts) [Erich Franz Eugen *Bracht,* German gynecologist and obstetrician, born 1882] see under *maneuver.*

**Bracht-Wäch·ter lesion** (brokt-vek′tər) [E. F. E. *Bracht;* Hermann Julius Gustav *Wächter,* German physician, born 1878] see under *lesion.*

**brachy-** [Gr. *brachys* short] a combining form meaning short.

**brachy·ba·sia** (brak″e-ba′zhə) [*brachy-* + Gr. *basis* walking] a slow, shuffling, short-stepped gait, as seen in double hemiplegia.

**brachy·ce·pha·lia** (brak″e-sə-fă′le-ə) brachycephaly.

**brachy·ce·phal·ic** (brak″e-sə-fal′ik) pertaining to or characterized by brachycephaly. Called also *brachycephalous* and *eurycephalic.* See also *brachycranic.*

**brachy·ceph·a·lism** (brak″e-sef′əl-iz-əm) brachycephaly.

**brachy·ceph·a·lous** (brak″e-sef′ə-ləs) brachycephalic.

**brachy·ceph·a·ly** (brak″e-sef′ə-le) [*brachy-* + Gr. *-cephaly*] having a comparatively short head, with a cephalic index of 81.0 to 85.4, a characteristic of American Indians, Malayans, and Burmese.

**brachy·chei·lia** (brak″e-ki′le-ə) [*brachy-* + *cheil-* + *-ia*] abnormal shortness of the lip.

**brach·ych·i·ly** (brak-ik′ĭ-le) brachycheilia.

**brachy·chron·ic** (brak″e-kron′ik) acute.

**brachy·cne·mic** (brak″e-ne′mik) brachyknemic.

**brachy·cra·ni·al** (brak″e-kra′ne-əl) brachycranic.

**brachy·cra·nic** (brak″e-kra′nik) [*brachy-* + Gr. *kranion* skull] having a comparatively short head, with a cranial index of 80.0 to 84.9. Called also *brachycranial* and *eurycranic.* See also *brachycephalic.*

**brachy·dac·ty·ly** (brak″e-dak′tə-le) [*brachy-* + Gr. *daktylos* finger] abnormal shortness of the fingers and toes.

**brachy·esoph·a·gus** (brak″e-ə-sof′ə-gəs) [*brachy-* + *esophagus*] abnormal shortness of the esophagus.

**brachy·fa·cial** (brak″e-fa′shəl) [*brachy-* + *facial*] having a comparatively low, broad face, with a facial index of 90 or less.

**brach·yg·na·thia** (brak″ig-na′the-ə) [*brachy-* + *gnath-* + *-ia*] micrognathia (def. 1).

**brach·yg·na·thous** (brak-yg′nə-thəs) having an unusually short mandible; see *micrognathia.*

**brachy·ker·kic** (brak″e-kər′kik) [*brachy-* + Gr. *kerkis* radius] having a short radius, with a radiohumeral index less than 75.

**brachy·kne·mic** (brak″e-ne′mik) [*brachy-* + Gr. *knēmē* shin] having short legs, with a tibiofemoral index of 82 or less; also spelled *brachycnemic.*

**brachy·meta·car·pal·ism** (brak″e-met″ə-kahr′pəl-iz-əm) brachymetacarpia.

**brachy·meta·car·pia** (brak″e-met″ə-kahr′pe-ə) [*brachy-* + *metacarpus* + *-ia*] abnormal shortness of the metacarpal bones.

**brachy·me·tap·o·dy** (brak″e-mə-tap′o-de) [*brachy-* + *meta-* (2) + *pod-* + *-ia*] abnormal shortness of some of the metacarpal or metatarsal bones.

**brachy·meta·tar·sia** (brak″e-met″ə-tahr′se-ə) [*brachy-* + *metatarsus* + *-ia*] abnormal shortness of the metatarsal bones.

**brachy·mor·phic** (brak″e-mor′fik) [*brachy-* + *morph-* + *-ic*] built along lines that are shorter and broader than those of the normal figure; called also *brachytypical* and *brevilineal.*

**brachy·pha·lan·gia** (brak″e-fə-lan′jə) [*brachy-* + *phalanx*] abnormal shortness of one or more of the phalanges of a finger or toe.

**brachy·ske·lous** (brak″e-ske′ləs) [*brachy-* + Gr. *skelos* leg] abnormal shortness of one or both legs.

**brachy·staph·y·line** (brak″e-staf′ĭ-lēn) [*brachy-* + *staphyline*] pertaining to or characterized by a short, wide palate, with a palatal index of 85.0 or more.

**brach·ys·ta·sis** (brak-is′tə-sis) [*brachy-* + *stasis*] a state in which a muscle fiber is relatively decreased in length, and resists stretch; it contracts and relaxes, manifesting the same tension after contraction as before.

**brachy·ther·a·py** (brak″e-ther′ə-pe) [MeSH: Brachytherapy] in radiotherapy, treatment with ionizing radiation whose source is applied to the surface of the body or is located a short distance from the body area being treated; cf. *teletherapy.*

**brachy·typ·i·cal** (brak″e-tip′ĭ-kəl) brachymorphic.

**brachy·uran·ic** (brak″e-u-ran′ik) having a narrow maxilla, with a maxilloalveolar index of 115.0 or more.

**brac·ing** (brās′ing) 1. holding parts together or in place. 2. making something rigid or steady. 3. resistance to horizontal components of masticatory force.

**brack·en** (brak′ən) *Pteridium aquilinum,* a fern of worldwide distribution that causes bracken poisoning (q.v.) in many species of animals. Called also *bracken fern.*

**brack·et** (brak′ət) 1. a support projecting from the main structure. 2. orthodontic b., a small metal attachment soldered or welded to an orthodontic band or cemented directly to the teeth, serving to fasten the arch wire to the band or tooth. Called also *orthodontic attachment.* See also *orthodontic appliance,* under *appliance.*

**bract** (brakt) a small modified leaf in a flower cluster.

**Brad·bury-Eg·gle·ston syndrome** (brad′bə-re-eg′əl-stən) [Samuel *Bradbury,* American physician, 1883–1947; Cary *Eggleston,* American physician, 1884–1966] see under *syndrome.*

**Brad·ford frame** (brad′fərd) [Edward Hickling *Bradford,* American orthopedic surgeon, 1848–1926] see under *frame.*

**Brad·ley's disease** (brad′lēz) [W.H. *Bradley,* British physician, 20th century] see under *disease.*

**brad·shot** (brad′shot) braxy.

**brad·sot** (brad′sot) braxy.

**brady-** [Gr. *bradys* slow] a combining form meaning slow.

**brady·acu·sia** (brad″e-ə-ku′se-ə) [*brady-* + Gr. *akouein* to hear] dullness of hearing.

**brady·ar·rhyth·mia** (brad″e-ə-rith′me-ə) [*brady-* + *arrhythmia*] any disturbance in the heart rhythm in which the heart rate is abnormally slowed, usually to less than 60 beats per minute in an adult.

**brady·ar·thria** (brad″e-ahr′thre-ə) [*brady-* + *arthr-*[2] + *-ia*] bradylalia.

**brady·aux·e·sis** (brad″e-awk-se′sis) [*brady-* + *auxesis*] a form of heterauxesis in which the part grows more slowly than the whole.

**Brady·bae·na** (brad″e-be′nə) a genus of land snails; they serve as hosts to the liver fluke *Dicrocoelium dentriticum* in Malaysia.

**brady·car·dia** (brad″e-kahr′de-ə) [*brady-* + Gr. *kardia* heart] [MeSH: Bradycardia] slowness of the heartbeat, as evidenced by slowing of the pulse rate to less than 60.
**Branham's b.,** see under *sign.*
**central b.,** bradycardia dependent on disease of the central nervous system.
**essential b.,** bradycardia occurring without discoverable cause.
**fetal b.,** a fetal heart rate of less than 120 beats per minute, generally associated with hypoxia; it is usually due to placental insufficiency; it may also result from placental transfer of local anesthetics or

beta-adrenergic blocking agents, and rarely from heart block associated with congenital heart disease or maternal collagen vascular disease.
**nodal b.,** bradycardia in which the stimulus of the heart's contraction arises in the atrioventricular node or common bundle.
**postinfective b.,** bradycardia occurring after infectious disease.
**sinoatrial b.,** sinus b.
**sinus b. (SB),** a slow sinus rhythm, with a heart rate of less than 60 beats per minute in an adult; it is common in young adults and in athletes but is also a manifestation of some disorders.
**vagal b.,** bradycardia due to increased vagal tone.

**brady·car·di·ac** (brad″e-kahr′de-ak) 1. pertaining to, characterized by, or causing bradycardia. 2. an agent that acts to slow the pulse.

**brady·car·dic** (brad″e-kahr′dik) bradycardiac.

**brady·ci·ne·sia** (brad″e-sĭ-ne′zhə) bradykinesia.

**brady·crot·ic** (brad″e-krot′ik) [*brady-* + Gr. *krotos* pulsation] pertaining to, characterized by, or inducing slowness of pulse.

**brady·dys·rhyth·mia** (brad″e-dis-rith′me-ə) [*brady-* + *dysrhythmia*] an abnormal heart rhythm with rate less than 60 beats per minute in an adult; the term *bradyarrhythmia* is usually used instead.

**brady·es·the·sia** (brad″e-es-the′zhə) [*brady-* + *esthesia*] slowness or dullness of perception; cf. *hypesthesia.*

**brady·gen·e·sis** (brad″e-gen′ə-sis) [*brady-* + *-genesis*] the lengthening of certain stages in embryonic development.

**brady·glos·sia** (brad″e-glos′e-ə) [*brady-* + *gloss-* + *-ia*] slowness of speech due to impaired mobility of the tongue; cf. *bradylalia.*

**brady·ki·ne·sia** (brad″e-kĭ-ne′zhə) [*brady-* + *kinesi-* + *-ia*] abnormal slowness of muscular movement. Called also *bradycinesia* and *bradypragia.* Cf. *hypokinesia.*

**brady·ki·net·ic** (brad″e-kĭ-net′ik) [*brady-* + *kinetic*] 1. characterized by or performed by slow movement. 2. denoting a method of showing the details of motor action by motion pictures taken very rapidly and shown very slowly.

**brady·ki·nin** (brad″e-ki′nin) [*brady-* + Gr. *kinein* to move] [MeSH: Bradykinin] a nonapeptide (Arg-Pro-Pro-Gly-Phe-Ser-Pro-Phe-Arg) produced by activation of the kinin system in a variety of inflammatory conditions. It is a potent vasodilator and also increases vascular permeability, stimulates pain receptors, and causes contraction of a variety of extravascular smooth muscles. The name refers to the slowly developing contraction produced in isolated guinea pig ileum. It is produced by the action of plasma kallikrein, trypsin, or plasmin on high-molecular-weight kininogen, a plasma $\alpha_2$-globulin, and is destroyed by several kininases in the lungs and other tissues.
**lysyl-b.,** older name for *kallidin.*

**brady·la·lia** (brad″e-la′le-ə) [*brady-* + *lal-* + *-ia*] abnormally slow utterance of words due to a brain lesion or mental disorder; called also *bradyarthria* and *bradyphasia.*

**brady·lex·ia** (brad″e-lek′se-ə) [*brady-* + Gr. *lexis* word] abnormal slowness in reading, due neither to defect of intelligence or of vision nor to ignorance of the alphabet.

**brady·lo·gia** (brad″e-lo′jə) [*brady* + *log-* + *-ia*] bradylalia.

**brady·pha·gia** (brad″ĭ-fa′jə) [*brady-* + *-phagia*] abnormal slowness in eating.

**brady·pha·sia** (brad″ĭ-fa′zhə) [*brady-* + *-phasia*] bradylalia.

**brady·phra·sia** (brad″e-fra′zhə) [*brady-* + Gr. *phrasis* utterance + *-ia*] 1. bradylalia. 2. bradyphrenia.

**brady·phre·nia** (brad″e-fre′ne-ə) [*brady-* + *phren-* + *-ia*] slowness of thought or fatigability of initiative, resulting from depression or central nervous system disease; called also *bradyphrasia.*

**brady·pnea** (brad″e-ne′ə, brad-ip-ne′ə) [*brady-* + *-pnea*] abnormal slowness of breathing. Cf. *hypopnea* and *hypoventilation.*

**brady·pra·gia** (brad″e-pra′je-ə) [*brady-* + Gr. *prattein* to act] bradykinesia.

**brady·rhyth·mia** (brad″e-rith′me-ə) [*brady-* + *rhythm* + *-ia*] bradycardia.

**brady·sper·ma·tism** (brad″e-spər′mə-tiz-əm) [*brady-* + *spermatism*] abnormally slow ejaculation of semen.

**brady·sphyg·mia** (brad″e-sfig′me-ə) [*brady-* + *sphygm-* + *-ia*] abnormal slowness of the pulse, usually linked to bradycardia.

**brady·tachy·car·dia** (brad″e-tak″ĭ-kahr′de-ə) [*brady-* + *tachy-* + Gr. *kardia* heart] alternating attacks of bradycardia and tachycardia, as may occur in sick sinus syndrome.

**brady·tel·eo·ci·ne·sia** (brad″e-tel″e-o-si-ne′zə) bradyteleokinesis.

**brady·tel·eo·ki·ne·sis** (brad″e-tel″e-o-kĭ-ne′sis) [*brady-* + *teleo-* + *-kinesis*] a dyskinesia in which a movement is slowed or stopped prior to reaching its goal; called also *bradyteleocinesia.*

**brady·to·cia** (brad″e-to′se-ə) [*brady-* + *toc-* + *-ia*] lingering or slow parturition.

**brady·tro·phia** (brad″e-tro′fe-ə) a condition characterized by slow-acting nutritive processes.

**brady·troph·ic** (brad″e-trof′ik) [*brady-* + *-trophic*] having slow-acting nutritive processes.

**brady·uria** (brad″e-u′re-ə) [*brady-* + *-uria*] abnormally slow passage of urine.

**brady·zo·ite** (brad″e-zo′īt) [*brady-* + *zōon* animal] a small, comma-shaped form of *Toxoplasma gondii,* found in clusters enclosed by an irregular wall (pseudocyst) in the tissues, chiefly muscles and the brain, in chronic (latent) toxoplasmosis; considered to be the slow-growing form. Cf. *tachyzoite.*

**Bra·gard's sign** (brah′gahrts) [Karl *Bragard,* German orthopedist, 20th century] see under *sign.*

**braid·ism** (brād′iz-əm) [after James *Braid,* who coined the word *hypnosis*] obsolete term for hypnotism.

**braille** (brāl) [Louis *Braille,* a French teacher of the blind, 1809–1852] a system of writing and printing for the blind by means of tangible points or dots.

**Brain airway** (brān) [A. I. *Brain,* British anesthesiologist, 20th century] see under *airway.*

**Brain's reflex** (brānz) [Walter Russell *Brain,* English neurologist, 1895–1966] see under *reflex.*

**brain** (brān) [Anglo-Saxon *braegen*] [MeSH: Brain] that part of the central nervous system contained within the cranium, comprising the prosencephalon (forebrain: telencephalon plus diencephalon), mesencephalon (midbrain), and rhombencephalon (hindbrain: metencephalon plus myelencephalon). It is derived (developed) from the anterior part of the embryonic neural tube. Functions include muscle control and coordination, sensory reception and integration, speech production, memory storage, and the elaboration of thought and emotion. See also *cerebrum.* Called also *encephalon* [TA]. See Plates 11 and 12.
**olfactory b.,** rhinencephalon, def. 1.
**respirator b.,** the congested, swollen brain of a patient who has been on a respirator longer than one day after suffering cerebral anoxia and ischemia; necrotic and autolytic changes begin to occur and the patient is comatose or brain dead.
**split b.,** a brain in which connections between the hemispheres, mainly the corpus callosum, have been severed or otherwise disrupted; done surgically on experimental laboratory animals and in humans to provide access to the third ventricle or to control epilepsy. See also *split-brain syndrome,* under *syndrome,* and *corpuscallosotomy.*
**smell b.,** rhinencephalon, def. 1.
**wet b.,** cerebral edema.

**brainstem** (brān′stem″) [MeSH: Brain Stem] the stalklike portion of the brain connecting the cerebral hemispheres with the spinal cord and comprising the mesencephalon, pons, and medulla oblongata; the diencephalon is considered part of the brain stem by some. Called also *truncus encephalicus* [TA]. Also written *brain stem.*

**brain·wash·ing** (brān′wahsh″ing) any systematic effort aimed at instilling certain attitudes and beliefs in a person against his will, usually beliefs in conflict with his prior beliefs and knowledge. It initially referred to political indoctrination of prisoners of war and political prisoners.

**bran** (bran) the meal derived from the epidermis or outer covering of a cereal grain. It is a source of dietary fiber, which may be soluble (e.g., oats) or insoluble (e.g., wheat) depending on the type of grain.
**wheat b.** [USP], the outer covering of the cereal grain derived from various species of *Triticum.*

**branch** (branch) a division or offshoot from a main stem, especially of blood vessels, nerves, or lymphatics; for specific anatomical structures not found here, see under *ramus.*
**anterior b. of axillary nerve,** a branch that winds around the humeral neck beneath the deltoid muscle and innervates both the muscle and the overlying skin.
**anterior b's of thoracic nerves,** nervi intercostales.
**articular b. of deep fibular nerve,** a twig that innervates the ankle joint.
**bundle b.,** a branch of the bundle of His.
**communicating b. with ciliary ganglion, communicating b. with nasociliary nerve, communicating b. of nasociliary nerve with ciliary ganglion,** radix sensoria ganglii ciliaris.
**b. to coracobrachialis,** a branch of the musculocutaneous nerve that innervates the coracobrachialis muscle.

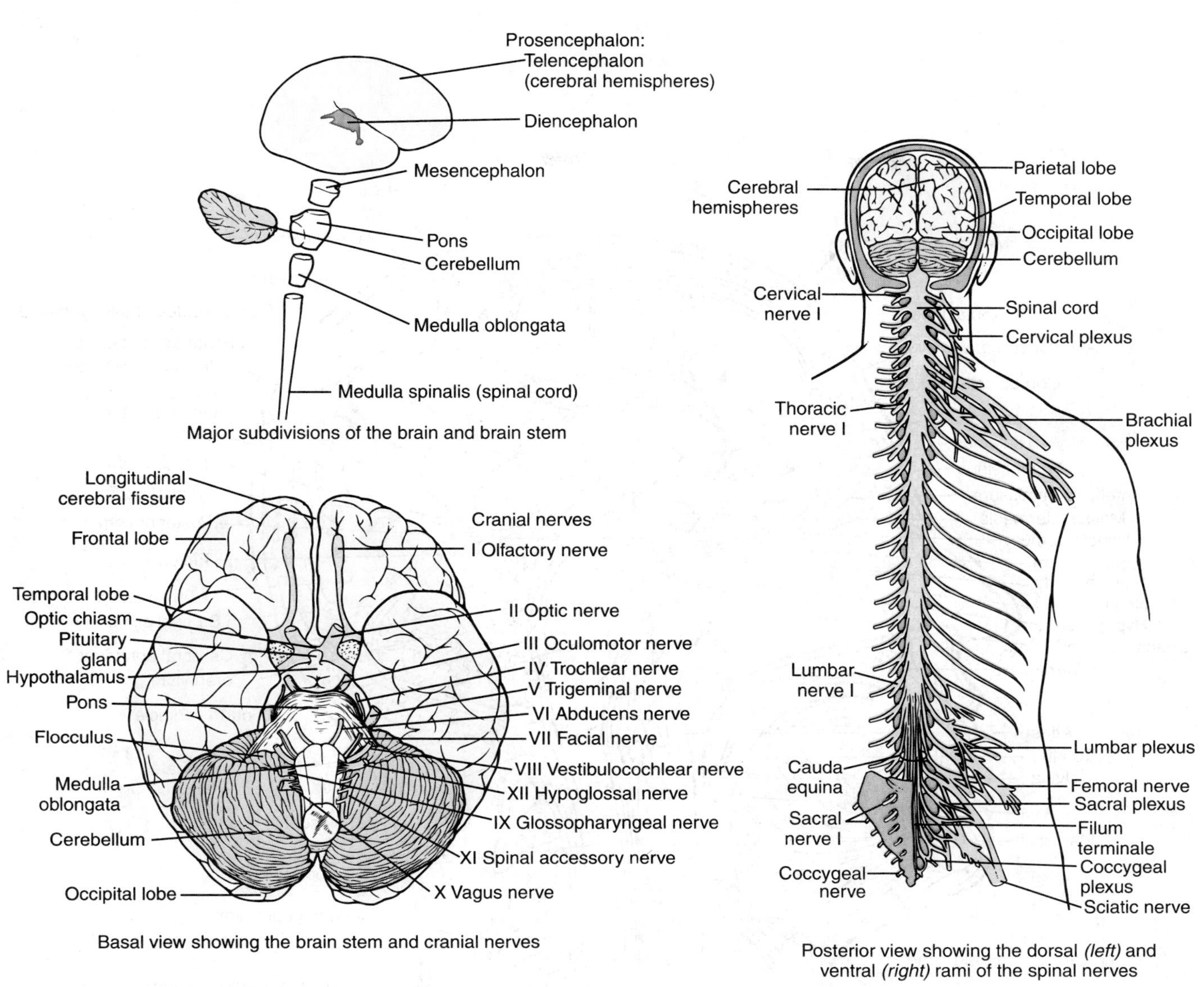


Major subdivisions of the brain and brain stem

Basal view showing the brain stem and cranial nerves

Posterior view showing the dorsal *(left)* and ventral *(right)* rami of the spinal nerves

Central sucus
Postcentral gyrus
Precentral gyrus
Parietal lobe
Lateral sulcus (sylvian fissure)
Occipital lobe
Cerebellum
Lateral ventricle
Frontal lobe
Thalamus
Temporal lobe
Pons
Medulla oblongata

Lateral view showing cortical lobes

Interventricular foramen
Frontal (anterior) horn of lateral ventricle
Lateral ventricle
Collateral trigone
Third ventricle
Occipital (posterior) horn of lateral ventricle
Temporal (inferior) horn of lateral ventricle
Fourth ventricle
Cerebral aqueduct
Median aperture of fourth ventricle
Lateral aperture of fourth ventricle

Lateral view of ventricles

**PLATE 11**—VARIOUS ASPECTS OF BRAIN AND SPINAL CORD

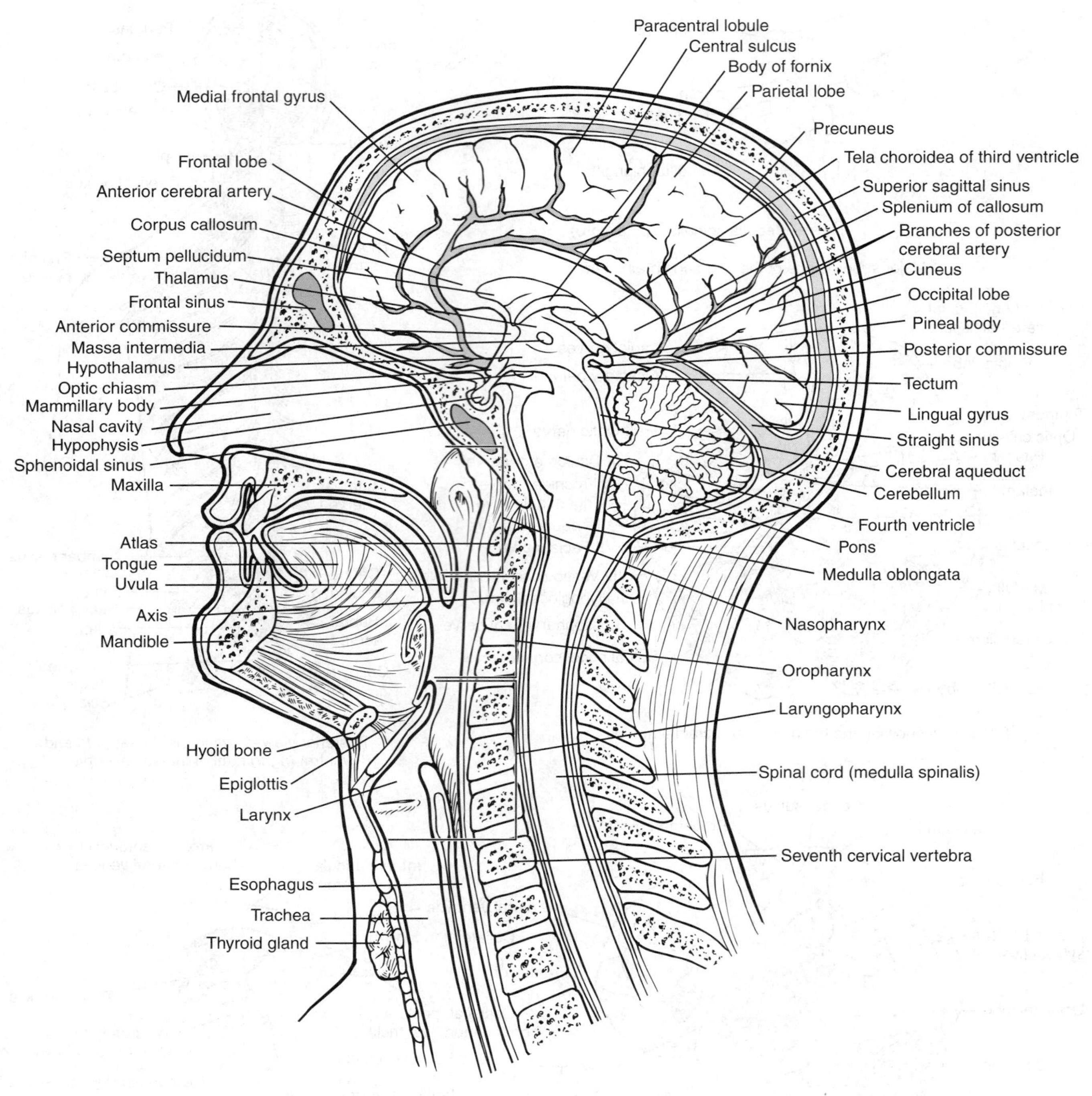


**PLATE 12**—HEMISECTION OF THE HEAD AND NECK, SHOWING VARIOUS PARTS OF THE BRAIN IN RELATION TO OTHER STRUCTURES

**interosseous b's of lateral terminal b. of deep fibular nerve,** twigs of the lateral terminal branch that innervate the metatarsophalangeal joints of the second, third, and fourth toes.
**interosseous b. of medial terminal b. of deep fibular nerve,** a small branch of the medial terminal branch that innervates the metatarsophalangeal joint of the great toe and the first dorsal interosseous space.
**left b. of atrioventricular bundle, left bundle b.,** crus sinistrum fasciculi atrioventricularis.
**muscular b's of deep fibular nerve,** branches innervating the tibialis anterior, extensor hallucis longus, extensor digitorum longus, and third peroneal muscles.
**b. of oculomotor nerve to ciliary ganglion,** ramus parasympathica ganglii ciliaris.
**posterior b's of axillary nerve,** rami musculares nervi axillaris.
**pulmonary b's of vagus nerve, anterior,** anterior bronchial branches of vagus nerve; see *rami bronchiales nervi vagi,* under *ramus.*
**pulmonary b's of vagus nerve, posterior,** posterior bronchial branches of vagus nerve; see *rami bronchiales nervi vagi,* under *ramus.*
**right b. of atrioventricular bundle, right bundle b.,** crus dextrum fasciculi atrioventricularis.
**b's to sternocleidomastoid,** deep branches of the cervical plexus that are proprioceptive sensory connectors to the sternocleidomastoid muscle.
**terminal b. of deep fibular nerve, lateral,** a branch beginning deep within the ankle and supplying the extensor digitorum brevis muscles.
**terminal b. of deep fibular nerve, medial,** a branch beginning in the ankle and running along the dorsum of the foot to the first interosseous space, where it combines with the medial dorsal cutaneous nerve and then subdivides into the dorsal digital nerves of the great and second toes.
**ventral b's of thoracic nerves,** nervi intercostales.
**zygomaticofacial b. of zygomatic nerve,** ramus zygomaticofacialis nervi zygomatici.
**zygomaticotemporal b. of zygomatic nerve,** ramus zygomaticotemporalis nervi zygomatici.

**branched-chain-ami·no-ac·id trans·am·i·nase** (brancht-chān-ə-me′no-as′id trans-am′ĭ-nās) [EC 2.6.1.42] an enzyme of the transferase class that catalyzes the removal of the α-amino group of leucine, isoleucine, or valine to form the corresponding keto acid, transferring the amino group to α-ketoglutarate or a similar acceptor. The reaction is the first step in the catabolism of branched-chain amino acids. In humans, the enzyme for leucine and isoleucine may be separate from the one for valine. Called also *branched-chain-amino-acid aminotransferase.*

**branched-chain α-ke·to ac·id de·hy·dro·gen·ase** (brancht chān ke′to as′id de-hi′dro-jən-ās) see under *complex.*

**branch·er en·zyme** (branch′ər en′zīm) 1,4-α-glucan branching enzyme.

**branch·er en·zyme de·fi·cien·cy** glycogen storage disease, type IV.

**bran·chia** (brang′ke-ə) [Gr. *branchia* gills] the gills of fishes and of others of the lower vertebrates; represented in the human fetus by the pharyngeal (branchial) arches, separated by clefts.

**bran·chi·al** (brang′ke-əl) pertaining to or resembling the gills of a fish or the derivatives of homologous parts in higher forms.

**branch·ing en·zyme** (branch′ing en′zīm) 1,4-α-glucan branching enzyme.

**bran·chi·o·gen·ic** (brang″ke-o-jen′ik) gill-forming; forming a branchial arch.

**bran·chi·og·e·nous** (brang″ke-oj′ə-nəs) [*branchia* + *-genous*] formed from a branchial cleft or arch.

**bran·chi·o·ma** (brang″ke-o′mə) [MeSH: Branchioma] a tumor derived from branchial epithelium or branchial rests.

**bran·chio·mere** (brang′ke-o-mēr″) a segment of the splanchnic mesoderm from which the branchial arches are developed.

**bran·chio·mer·ic** (brang″ke-o-mer′ik) pertaining to the branchiomeres or branchial arches.

**bran·chi·om·er·ism** (brang″ke-om′ər-iz-əm) [*branchia-* + *merism*] metamerism based on the serial repetition of the branchial arches.

**Brandt-An·drews maneuver** (brahnt-an′dro͞oz) [Thure *Brandt,* Swedish obstetrician and gynecologist, 1819–1895; Henry Russell *Andrews,* English obstetrician and gynecologist, 1871–1942] see under *maneuver.*

**Brâ·ne·mark implant** (brā̆′nə-mahrk) [Per-Ingmar *Brånemark,* Swedish physician, 20th century] see under *implant.*

**Bran·ham's sign (bradycardia)** (bran′həmz) [H. H. *Branham,* American surgeon, 19th century] see under *sign.*

**Bran·ha·mel·la** (bran″hə-mel′ə) [Sara Elizabeth *Branham,* American bacteriologist, 1888–1962] *Moraxella (Branhamella).*
**B. catarrha′lis,** *Moraxella (Branhamella) catarrhalis.*

**brash** (brash) heartburn.
**water b.,** heartburn with regurgitation of sour fluid or almost tasteless saliva into the mouth.

**Bras·si·ca** (bras′ĭ-kə) [L.] [MeSH: Brassica] a genus of plants of the family Cruciferae, including cabbage, turnip, mustard, rape, and others. Species of medical interest are *B. na′pus,* the rape (q.v.) plant; *B. al′ba* (L.) Rabenh., white mustard; and *B. ni′gra* (L.) Koch., black mustard (see under *mustard*).

**Braun's anastomosis** (brounz) [Heinrich *Braun,* German surgeon, 1847–1911] see under *anastomosis.*

**Braun's canal** (brounz) [Carl Ritter *Braun* von Fernwald, Austrian obstetrician, 1822–1891] neurenteric canal; see under *canal.*

**Brau·ne's muscle** (brow′nəz) [Christian Wilhelm *Braune,* German anatomist, 1831–1892] musculus puborectalis.

**Braun·wald sign** (broun′wahldz) [Eugene *Braunwald,* American cardiologist, born 1929] see under *sign.*

**Bra·vais-jack·so·ni·an epilepsy** (brah-va′jak-so′ne-ən) [Louis François *Bravais,* French physician, early 19th century; John Hughlings *Jackson,* English neurologist, 1835–1911] jacksonian epilepsy.

**Brax·ton Hicks contraction (sign), version** (brak′stən hiks) [John *Braxton Hicks,* English gynecologist, 1823–1897] see under *contraction* and *version.*

**braxy** (brak′se) a disease of sheep caused by *Clostridium septicum,* and marked by hemorrhagic abomasitis, with hemorrhage into the peritoneal cavity, by abdominal pain, and, usually, by diarrhea and high fever. Called also *bradshot, bradsot,* and *malignant edema.*

**bra·ye·ra** (bra-ye′rə) the dried panicles of the pistillate flowers of *Hagenia abyssinica* J. F. Gmel., used as a vermifuge.

**braze** (brāz) in dentistry, to solder with a relatively infusible alloy.

**bra·zil·in** (brə-zil′in) a yellow crystalline substance obtained from the bark of *Biancea sappan* and other redwood trees; it is very similar to hematoxylin and oxidizes to a bright red dye, brazilein.

**breadth** (bredth) the distance measured horizontally from side to side; see also under *diameter.*
**b. of accommodation,** range of accommodation.
**bizygomatic b.,** the distance between the most laterally situated points (zygia) on the zygomatic arches.

**break** (brāk) 1. to interrupt the continuity, or an interruption in the continuity of a structure, especially a bone. See *fracture.* 2. the interruption of an electric circuit, as distinguished from the make.
**chromatid b.,** interruption of the continuity of a chromatid; the portions immediately proximal and distal to the site may then become out of alignment.

**break·down** (brāk′doun) 1. the act or process of ceasing to function, or the resulting condition. 2. an often sudden collapse in health, physical or mental. 3. loss of self-control.
**nervous b.,** a nonspecific, popular name for any type of mental disorder that interferes with the affected individual's normal activities, often implying a severe episode with sudden onset.

**breast** (brest) [MeSH: Breast] 1. the anterior aspect of the thorax. 2. mamma.
**caked b.,** stagnation mastitis.
**chicken b.,** pectus carinatum.
**Cooper's irritable b.,** neuralgia of the breast.
**funnel b.,** pectus excavatum.
**pigeon b.,** pectus carinatum.
**proemial b.,** that condition of the female breast which is a prelude to pathologic changes.
**shoemakers' b.,** sinking in of the sternum as in shoemakers, produced by the pressure of tools against the lower part of the sternum and the xiphoid cartilage.
**shotty b.,** cystic disease of the breast; see under *disease.*
**thrush b.,** the speckled appearance of the myocardium under the endocardium in fatty degeneration of the heart.

**breast-feed·ing** (brest′ fēd′ing) the nursing of an infant at the mother's breast.

**breath** (breth) [L. *spiritus halitus*] the air taken in and expelled during ventilation (q.v.).
**bad b.,** halitosis.
**lead b.,** the metallic odor of the breath in lead poisoning.
**liver b.,** fetor hepaticus (hepatic fetor).

**breath·ing** (brēth′ing) ventilation (def. 2).
**Biot's b.,** see under *respiration.*
**bronchial b.,** bronchial breath sounds; see under *sound.*
**Cheyne-Stokes b.,** see under *respiration.*
**frog b., glossopharyngeal b.,** respiration unaided by the primary or ordinary accessory muscles of respiration, the air being "swal-

lowed" rapidly into the lungs by use of the tongue and muscles of the pharynx; used by patients with chronic muscle paralysis to augment their breathing.
**intermittent positive pressure b.**, IPPB: the active inflation of the lungs during inspiration under positive pressure from a cycling valve. Called also *intermittent positive pressure ventilation.*
**mouth b.**, breathing through the mouth instead of the nose, usually because of some obstruction of the nasal passages.
**periodic b.**, Cheyne-Stokes respiration.
**pursed lip b.**, an abnormal breathing style in which the lips are pursed during expiration, usually due to dyspnea in an effort to reduce respiratory muscle effort.

**bre•douille•ment** (brĕ″dwe-maw′) a speech defect in which only part of the word is pronounced, due to extreme rapidity of utterance.

**breech** (brēch) buttocks (nates [TA]).

**breg•ma** (breg′mə) [Gr. "front of the head"] [TA] the point on the surface of the skull at the junction of the coronal and sagittal sutures; used as a craniometric landmark.

**breg•mat•ic** (breg-mat′ik) pertaining to the bregma.

**breg•ma•to•dym•ia** (breg″mə-to-dim′e-ə) [*bregma* + Gr. *didymos* twin + *-ia*] the state of conjoined twins fused at the bregmas.

**brei** (bri) [Ger. "pulp"] tissue that has been ground to a pulp; a homogenate.

**Brei•sky's disease** (bri′skēz) [August *Breisky,* Czechoslovakian gynecologist, 1832–1889] lichen sclerosus in females; see under *lichen.*

**brems•strah•lung** (brem′strah-loong) [Ger. "braking radiation"] 1. the continuous spectrum of electromagnetic radiation produced by the rapid deceleration of a fast-moving charged particle (such as an electron or beta particle) in the electric field of another charged particle (usually a nucleus). Called also *braking radiation, white radiation* (by analogy to the continuous optical spectrum obtained from white light), and *continuous x-ray spectrum.* 2. the deceleration of a charged particle that produces this radiation.

**Bren•ne•mann's syndrome** (bren′ə-mənz) [Joseph *Brennemann,* American pediatrician, 1872–1944] see under *syndrome.*

**Bren•ner tumor** (bren′ər) [Fritz *Brenner,* German pathologist, born 1877] [MeSH: Brenner Tumor] see under *tumor.*

**breph•ic** (bref′ik) [*breph-* + *-ic*] pertaining to an early stage of development.

**breph(o)-** [Gr. *brephos* embryo, newborn infant] a combining form denoting relationship to the embryo, fetus, or newborn infant.

**brepho•plas•tic** (bref″o-plas′tik) [*brepho-* + *plastic*] formed from embryonic tissue or during embryonic life.

**brepho•troph•ic** (bref″o-trof′ik) [*brepho-* + *-trophic*] pertaining to the nourishment of infants.

**Bres•chet's canals, hiatus, sinus, veins** (brə-shāz′) [Gilbert *Breschet,* French anatomist, 1783-1845] see *canales diploici, helicotrema, sinus sphenoparietalis,* and *venae diploicae.*

**Bres•cia-Ci•mi•no fistula** (bresh′-e-ə sĭ-me′no) [Michael J. *Brescia,* American nephrologist, born 1933; James E. *Cimino,* American nephrologist, born 1928] see under *fistula.*

**Breth•aire** (breth′ār) trademark for a preparation of terbutaline sulfate.

**Breth•ine** (breth′ēn) trademark for preparations of terbutaline sulfate.

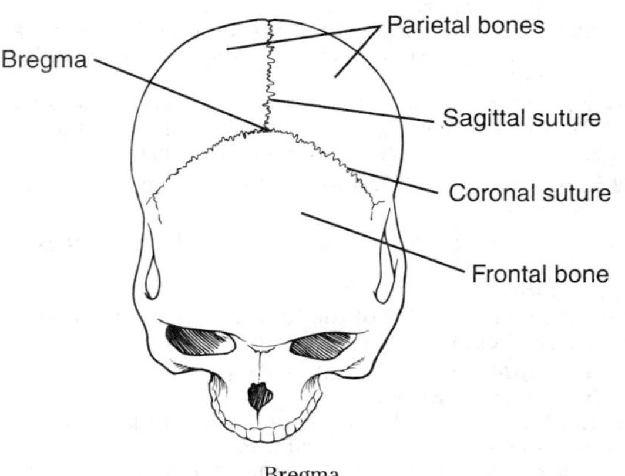


Bregma.

**Bre•ty•late** (brĕ′tə-lāt) trademark for a preparation of bretylium tosylate.

**bre•tyl•i•um to•sy•late** (brə-til′e-əm) [USP] [MeSH: Bretylium Tosylate] an adrenergic blocking agent originally used as an antihypertensive agent; it is now used as an antiarrhythmic in certain cases of ventricular tachycardia or fibrillation.

**Bre•ty•lol** (brĕ′tə-lol) trademark for a preparation of bretylium tosylate.

**Breus' mole** (brois) [Karl *Breus,* Austrian obstetrician, 1852–1914] see under *mole.*

**brevi-** [L. *brevis* short] a combining form meaning short.

**Brev•i•bac•te•ri•um** (brev″ĭ-bak-tēr′e-əm) [*brevi-* + *bacterium*] [MeSH: Brevibacterium] a genus of coryneform bacteria of uncertain status, consisting of short, unbranched rods found in salt and fresh water, dairy products, and decomposing material of many types. Many are of industrial importance.

**Brevi•bloc** (brev′ĭ-blok″) trademark for a preparation of esmolol hydrochloride.

**brev•i•col•lis** (brev″ĭ-kol′is) [*brevi-* + *collum*] shortness of the neck; see *dystrophia brevicollis.*

**brev•i•flex•or** (brev″ĭ-flek′sər) [*brevi-* + *flexor*] a short flexor muscle.

**brevi•lin•e•al** (brev″ĭ-lin′e-əl) brachymorphic.

**brevi•ra•di•ate** (brev″ĭ-ra′de-āt) having short processes; a term applied to one type of neuroglia cells.

**Brev•i•tal** (brev′ĭ-təl) trademark for a preparation of methohexital sodium.

**Brew•er's infarcts, point** (broo′ərz) [George Emerson *Brewer,* American surgeon, 1861–1939] see under *infarct* and *point.*

**Bric•a•nyl** (brik′ə-nəl) trademark for preparations of terbutaline sulfate.

**Brick•er's operation** (brik′ərz) [Eugene M. *Bricker,* American surgeon, born 1908] see under *operation.*

**BrIDA** mebrofenin.

**bridge** (brij) 1. a structure that connects two distant points, including parts of an organ. Called also *pons.* 2. fixed partial denture. 3. tarsal coalition. 4. intercellular b.
**arteriolovenular b.**, the main and largest capillary connecting an arteriole and a venule; it retains some muscle elements and is rarely completely collapsed.
**cantilever b.**, a fixed partial denture in which the pontic is cantilevered, i.e., retained only on one side by the abutment tooth. Called also *extension b.*
**cell b's**, see *intercellular b.* and *protoplasmic b.*
**conjugative b.**, in bacterial conjugation, a connection formed between two bacterial cells by the attachment of an F pilus from an $F^+$ cell to an $F^-$ cell.
**cytoplasmic b.**, 1. protoplasmic b. 2. see *intercellular b.*
**dentin b.**, a scarlike deposit of reparative dentin or other calcific substance which reseals exposed pulp or which forms across the excised surface of pulp after pulpotomy.
**disulfide b.**, see under *bond.*
**extension b.**, cantilever b.
**fixed b.**, fixed partial denture.
**fixed-fixed b.**, fixed b. with rigid connectors.
**fixed-movable b.**, fixed b. with rigid and nonrigid connectors.
**fixed b. with rigid connectors**, a fixed partial denture in which all components are rigidly soldered or cast in one piece. Called also *fixed-fixed b.*
**fixed b. with rigid and nonrigid connectors**, a fixed partial denture consisting of a major retainer attached to a pontic and supplied with a dovetail, and a minor retainer supplied with a slot into which the dovetail of the pontic fits; it provides some stress-breaking by allowing some movement. Called also *fixed-movable b.*
**intercellular b.**, a structure seen especially in the prickle cell layer of the epidermis, formed by the meeting of short cytoplasmic projections from the cell surface of adjacent cells. The structure was formerly thought to constitute a bridge for cytoplasmic continuity between cells, but it has been demonstrated to be an artifact caused by dehydration during fixation and represents a desmosome in which are terminated the projections from each cell.
**b. of the nose**, the upper portion of the external nose formed by the junction of the nasal bones.
**protoplasmic b.**, a strand of protoplasm connecting two secondary spermatocytes, occurring as a result of incomplete cytokinesis; called also *cytoplasmic b.*
**removable b.**, partial removable denture.
**salt b.**, 1. an inverted-U–shaped tube filled with a gel, usually composed of agar, water, and potassium chloride, used to separate two chemically incompatible solutions in an electrochemical cell. 2. a

chemical bond between a nitrogen atom, carrying a positive charge, and an oxygen atom, carrying a negative charge.
**stationary b.,** fixed partial denture.
**tarsal b.,** see under *coalition.*
**ureteric b.,** Bell's muscle.

**bridge·work** (brij'wərk) partial denture.
**fixed b.,** fixed partial denture.
**removable b.,** removable partial denture.

**bri·dle** (bri'dəl) 1. a frenum. 2. a loop or filament that crosses the lumen of a passage or the surface of an ulcer.

**bri·dou** (bre-doo') perlèche.

**Bright's disease** (brīts) [Richard *Bright,* English physician, 1789–1858] see under *disease.*

**bright·ic** (bri'tik) 1. affected with glomerulonephritis (Bright's disease). 2. a person with glomerulonephritis.

**bright·ism** (brīt'iz-əm) acute or chronic nephritis.

**Brill's disease** (brilz) [Nathan Edwin *Brill,* American physician, 1860–1925] Brill-Zinsser disease.

**Brill-Sym·mers disease** (brill-sim'ərz) [N. E. *Brill;* Douglas *Symmers,* American physician, 1879–1952] nodular lymphoma.

**Brill-Zins·ser disease** (brill-zin'sər) [N. E. *Brill;* Hans *Zinsser,* American bacteriologist, 1878–1940] see under *disease.*

**brim** (brim) the upper edge of a basin.
**pelvic b.,** apertura pelvis superior.

**Bri·nell hardness number** (brĭ-nel') [Johann August *Brinell,* Swedish engineer, 1849–1925] see under *number.*

**bri·no·lase** (bri'no-lās) [MeSH: Brinolase] a fibrinolytic enzyme produced by the fungus *Aspergillus oryzae.*

**Brin·ton's disease** (brin'tonz) [William *Brinton,* English physician, 1823–1867] linitis plastica.

**Bri·on-Kay·ser disease** (bre-on'ki'zer) [Albert *Brion,* German physician, born 1874; Heinrich *Kayser,* German physician, 1876–1940] paratyphoid.

**Bri·quet's syndrome** (bre-kāz') [Paul *Briquet,* French physician, 1796–1881] see under *syndrome.*

**brise·ment** (brēz-maw') [Fr. "crushing"] the breaking up or tearing of anything, as of an ankylosis.
**b. forcé,** the forcible breaking up or tearing of a bony ankylosis.

**bris·ket** (bris'kət) the connective tissue and fat over the sternum of a ruminant, hanging down between the front legs.

**Bris·saud's dwarf, infantilism, reflex, scoliosis** (bre-sōz') [Edouard *Brissaud,* French physician, 1852–1909] see under *dwarf* and *reflex;* see *cretinism;* and see *sciatic scoliosis,* under *scoliosis.*

**Bris·saud-Si·card syndrome** (bre-so'-se-kahr') [E. *Brissaud;* Jean Athanase *Sicard,* French neurologist, 1872–1929] see under *syndrome.*

**Bris·towe's syndrome** (bris'tōz) [John Syer *Bristowe,* British physician, 1827–1895] see under *syndrome.*

**BRM** biologic response modifier.

**broach** (brōch) 1. an elongated, tapered, and serrated cutting tool for shaping and enlarging holes. 2. barbed b.; root canal b.
**barbed b.,** a thin, flexible, hand-operated or engine-driven endodontic instrument, usually tapered, with a series of sharply pointed barbs along the operative head; used for engaging and removing the dental pulp and other substances intact from the root canal or pulp chamber.
**pathfinder b.,** root canal probe.
**root canal b.,** a broach, usually barbed, used for removing the soft tissue contents of the root canal; see *barbed b.*
**smooth b.,** root canal probe.

**Broad·bent's sign** (brod'bentz) [Sir William Henry *Broadbent,* English physician, 1835–1907] see under *sign.*

**Bro·ca's amnesia, motor speech area,** etc. (bro-kahz') [Pierre Paul *Broca,* French anatomist, anthropologist, and surgeon, 1824–1880] see under *area, convolution,* and *fissure,* and see *expressive aphasia,* under *aphasia, visual plane,* under *plane,* and *stria diagonalis (Broca),* under *stria.*

**Brock's infundibulectomy, operation, syndrome** (broks) [Sir Russell Claude *Brock,* British surgeon, born 1903] see under *infundibulectomy;* see *transventricular closed valvotomy,* under *valvotomy;* and see *middle lobe syndrome,* under *syndrome.*

**Brock·en·brough's sign** (brok'en-brōz) [Edwin C. *Brockenbrough,* American surgeon, born 1930] see under *sign.*

**Brö·del's white line** (brər'delz) [Max *Brödel,* American medical artist, 1870–1941] see under *line.*

**Bro·ders' index (classification)** (bro'dərz) [Albert Compton *Broders,* American pathologist, 1885–1964] see under *index.*

**Bro·die's abscess,** etc. (bro'dēz) [Sir Benjamin Collins *Brodie,* English surgeon, 1783–1862] see under *abscess, disease, knee,* and *sign.*

**Bro·die's ligament** (bro'dēz) [C. Gordon *Brodie,* British anatomist, 1786–1818] transverse humeral ligament.

**bro·di·fa·coum** (bro'dĭ-fə-ko͞om) a long-acting anticoagulant rodenticide.

**Brod·mann's areas** (brod'mahnz) [Korbinian *Brodmann,* German neurologist, 1868–1918] see under *area.*

**Broe·si·ke's fossa** (brər'ze-kəz) [Gustav *Broesike,* German anatomist, late 19th century] parajejunal fossa.

**bro·mat·ed** (bro'māt-əd) brominated.

**bro·ma·ther·a·py** (bro"mə-ther'ə-pe) diet therapy.

**bro·ma·tol·o·gy** (bro"mə-tol'ə-je) [Gr. *brōma* food + *-logy*] dietetics.

**bro·ma·to·ther·a·py** (bro"mə-to-ther'ə-pe) [Gr. *brōma* food + *therapy*] diet therapy.

**bro·ma·to·tox·in, bro·ma·to·tox·is·mus** (bro"mə-to-tok'sin) [Gr. *brōma* food + *toxin*] a poison formed in food by fermentation.

**bro·maz·e·pam** (bro-maz'ə-pam") [MeSH: Bromazepam] a benzodiazepine used as an anxiolytic in the treatment of anxiety disorders; administered orally.

**bro·me·lain** (bro'mə-lān) any of several cysteine endopeptidases that catalyze the cleavage of proteins on the carboxyl side of alanine, glycine, lysine, and tyrosine bonds. Differing forms are derived from the fruit (fruit bromelain) and stem (stem bromelain) of the pineapple plant, *Ananas comosus.* The enzyme is administered orally as an anti-inflammatory agent and is also used in immunology to render red cells agglutinable by incomplete antibody. Called also *bromelin.*

**bro·mel·in** (bro-mel'in) bromelain.

**brom·hex·ine hy·dro·chlo·ride** (brom-hek'sēn) an expectorant and mucolytic agent, administered orally and by inhalation in the treatment of respiratory disorders characterized by the production of excess or viscous mucus, and orally in the treatment of keratoconjunctivitis sicca in Sjögren's syndrome.

**brom·hi·dro·sis** (bro"mĭ-dro'sis) [*brom-* (1) + *hidro-* + *-sis*] axillary (apocrine) sweat which has become foul-smelling as a result of its bacterial decomposition.

**bro·mic** (bro'mik) pertaining to or containing pentavalent bromine, as in bromic acid, $HBrO_3$.

**bro·mide** (bro'mīd) any binary compound of bromine in which the bromine carries a negative charge ($Br^-$); specifically a salt (or organic ester) of hydrobromic acid ($H^+Br^-$). Bromides produce depression of the central nervous system, and were once widely used for their sedative effect. Because overdosage causes serious mental disturbances they are now seldom used, except occasionally in grand mal seizures. See also *bromism.*

**bro·mi·dro·sis** (bro"mĭ-dro'sis) bromhidrosis.

**bro·mi·nat·ed** (bro'mĭ-nāt"əd) combined with or containing bromine; called also *bromated* and *brominized.*

**bro·mine** (bro'mēn, bro'min) [L. *bromium, brominium, bromum;* Gr. *brōmos* stench] [MeSH: Bromine] a reddish-brown liquid element, symbol Br, giving off suffocating vapors. Its atomic number is 35; atomic weight, 79.909. See also *bromide* and *brominism.*

**bro·min·ism** (bro'min-iz-əm) bromism.

**bro·min·ized** (bro'min-īzd) brominated.

**bro·mism** (bro'miz-əm) [*brom-* (2) + *-ism*] chronic bromide intoxication, once a common problem, now rare, caused by chronic ingestion of proprietary bromide preparations; it is characterized by mental dullness, deficient memory, slurred speech, drowsiness, tremors, and ataxia. Skin eruptions of various forms are common. In most cases bromism also produces a mental disorder, which may be a delirium, a hallucinosis, or a transitory psychotic state resembling paranoid schizophrenia. Called also *brominism.*

**bro·mi·za·tion** (bro"mĭ-za'shən) impregnation with bromides or bromine; the administration of large doses of bromides.

**bro·mized** (bro'mīzd) under the influence of bromides.

**brom(o)-** [Gr. *brōmos* stench] 1. a combining form meaning foul-smelling. 2. in chemical terms, indicating the presence of bromine.

**bro·mo·chlo·ro·tri·flu·o·ro·eth·ane** (bro"mo-klor"o-tri-flo͞or"o-eth'ān) halothane.

**bro·mo·crip·tine mes·y·late** (bro"mo-krip'tēn) [USP] an ergot alkaloid that acts as a dopamine agonist, used to suppress prolactin secretion and thereby to inhibit lactation and stimulate ovulation in galactorrhea-amenorrhea syndrome and hypogonadism; it is also used in the treatment of Parkinson's disease. It raises serum growth hormone levels in normal persons, but lowers them in those with acromegaly.

**5-bro·mo·de·oxy·uri·dine** (bro″mo-de-ok-se-u′rĭ-din) a thymidine analogue causing breakage in chromosomal regions rich in heterochromatin.

**bro·mo·der·ma** (bro″mo-dər′mə) [*brom-* (2) + *derma*] a skin eruption due to the use of bromides.

**bro·mo·di·phen·hy·dra·mine hy·dro·chlo·ride** (bro″mo-di″fen-hi′drə-mēn) [USP] a derivative of monoethanolamine, closely related to diphenhydramine, used as an antihistaminic; administered orally.

**bro·mo·men·or·rhea** (bro″mo-men-o-re′ə) [*bromo-* (1) + *menorrhea*] the discharge of menses characterized by an offensive odor.

**bro·mop·nea** (bro-mop′ne-ə, bro″mo-ne′ə) [*bromo-* (1) + *-pnea*] halitosis.

**5-bro·mo·ura·cil** (bro″mo-u′rə-sil) a pyrimidine analogue with mutagenic properties.

**brom·per·i·dol** (brom-per′ĭ-dōl) an antipsychotic of the butyrophenone group, having properties similar to those of haloperidol, used in the treatment of schizophrenia and other psychoses; administered orally, and by intramuscular or intravenous injection.

**brom·phen·ir·amine** (brōm″fən-ir′ə-mēn) [MeSH: Brompheniramine] the bromine analogue of chlorpheniramine, an antihistaminic agent having anticholinergic and sedative effects.
**b. maleate** [USP], the maleate salt of brompheniramine, used for therapy and prophylaxis of conditions in which antihistamines may be effective; administered orally or by intramuscular, intravenous, or subcutaneous injection.

**brom·phe·nol** (brōm-fe′nol) one of a series of brominized phenols, sometimes found in the precipitates of tested urine.

**brom·sa·lans** (brom′sə-lanz) the brominated salicylanilides, a group of disinfectants; see *dibromsalan, metabromsalan,* and *tribromsalan.*

**Brom·sul·pha·lein** (brōm-sul′fə-lēn) trademark for a preparation of sulfobromophthalein sodium. Abbreviated BSP.

**bro·mum** (bro′məm) [L.] bromine.

**brom·u·rat·ed** (brōm′u-rāt″əd) containing bromine or bromine salts.

**brom·u·ret** (brōm′u-rət) a bromide.

**bronch·ad·e·ni·tis** (brong″kad-ə-ni′tis) [*bronch-* + *adenitis*] inflammation of the bronchial glands. Called also *bronchoadenitis.*

**bron·chi** (brong′ki) [L.] [MeSH: Bronchi] genitive and plural of *bronchus.*

**bron·chia** (brong′ke-ə) [L.] plural of *bronchium.*

**bron·chi·al** (brong′ke-əl) pertaining to a bronchus.

**bron·chi·ec·ta·sia** (brong″ke-ek-ta′zhə) bronchiectasis.

**bron·chi·ec·ta·sic** (brong″ke-ek-ta′zik) bronchiectatic.

**bron·chi·ec·ta·sis** (brong″ke-ek′tə-sis) [*bronchi-* + *ectasis*] [MeSH: Bronchiectasis] chronic dilatation of the bronchi marked by fetid breath and paroxysmal coughing, with the expectoration of mucopurulent matter. Types are distinguished according to the nature of the dilatations. Called also *bronchiectasia.*
**capillary b.,** bronchiolectasis.
**cylindrical b.,** a type in which whole sections of the bronchi are uniformly widened.
**cystic b.,** saccular b.
**dry b.,** a rare type with usually a nonproductive cough but episodes of infection that may be attended by hemoptysis.
**follicular b.,** bronchiectasis in which the lymphoid tissue in the affected regions becomes greatly enlarged and, by projecting into the bronchial lumen, may seriously distort and partially obstruct the bronchus.
**fusiform b.,** a type in which the dilated tubes have terminal bulbous enlargements.
**saccular b., sacculated b.,** a type in which the bronchi terminate in enlarged blind sacs; called also *cystic b.*
**varicose b.,** a type resembling cylindrical bronchiectasis but with local constrictions that result in an irregular varicose shape.

**bron·chi·ec·tat·ic** (brong″ke-ek-tat′ik) pertaining to or characterized by bronchiectasis.

**bron·chil·o·quy** (brong-kil′ə-kwe) [*bronchi-* + L. *loqui* to speak] bronchophony (def. 2).

**bronchi(o)-** a combining form denoting relationship to a bronchus. See also *bronch(o)-.*

**bron·chio·cele** (brong′ke-o-sēl) [*bronchio-* + *-cele*] bronchocele.

**bron·chio·gen·ic** (brong″ke-o-jen′ik) bronchogenic.

**bron·chi·ole** (brong′ke-ōl) [MeSH: Bronchi] bronchiolus.
**alveolar b's,** bronchioli respiratorii.
**lobular b.,** terminal b.
**respiratory b's,** bronchioli respiratorii.
**terminal b.,** the last portion of a bronchiole that does not contain alveoli, i.e., whose sole function is gas conduction; it subdivides into respiratory bronchioles. Called also *lobular b.*

**bron·chio·lec·ta·sis** (brong″ke-o-lek′tə-sis) [*bronchiole* + *ectasis*] dilatation of the bronchioles. Called also *capillary bronchiectasis.*

**bron·chi·o·li** (brong-ki′o-li) [L.] genitive and plural of *bronchiolus.*

**bron·chi·o·li·tis** (brong″ke-o-li′tis) [MeSH: Bronchiolitis] inflammation of the bronchioles, usually occurring in children less than 2 years old and resulting from a viral infection, particularly with respiratory syncytial virus. See also *bronchopneumonia.*
**constrictive b.,** bronchiolitis fibrosa obliterans in which the fibrous tissue is between the muscularis mucosa layer and the epithelium.
**b. exudati′va, exudative b.,** bronchiolitis accompanied by exudation of Curschmann's spirals and grayish, tenacious sputum; often associated with asthma.
**b. fibro′sa obli′terans,** a usually chronic bronchiolitis with ingrowth of connective tissue from the wall of the terminal bronchi and occlusion of their lumina; it may be a complication of connective tissue disease or heart-lung transplant, and in children it may follow an acute attack of bronchiolitis or pneumonia. An acute form occurs in silo workers (silo filler's lung). Called also *b. obliterans* and *obliterative b.*
**b. obli′terans,** b. fibrosa obliterans.
**b. obliterans with organizing pneumonia (BOOP),** an idiopathic disease combining organizing pneumonia with a condition resembling bronchiolitis fibrosa obliterans; terminal bronchioles and alveoli become occluded with masses of inflammatory cells and fibrotic tissue. Called also *cryptogenic organizing pneumonia.*
**obliterative b.,** b. fibrosa obliterans.
**proliferative b.,** that in which the lumen of the bronchioles is obliterated by epithelial proliferation and exudate.
**respiratory b.,** fibrosis in the respiratory bronchioles, seen mainly in cigarette smokers; see also *respiratory bronchiolitis–associated interstitial lung disease.*

**bron·chi·o·lus** (brong-ki′o-ləs) pl. *bronchi′oli* [L.] [TA] bronchiole: one of the finer subdivisions of the branched bronchial tree, 1 mm or less in diameter, differing from the bronchi in having no cartilage plates and having cuboidal epithelial cells.
**bronchi′oli respirato′rii,** respiratory bronchioles: the final branches of bronchioles, subdivisions of the terminal bronchioles that have alveolar outcroppings and divide further into several alveolar ducts. Called also *alveolar bronchioles.*
**b. termina′lis,** terminal bronchiole.

**bron·chio·spasm** (brong′ke-o-spaz″əm) bronchospasm.

**bron·chio·ste·no·sis** (brong″ke-o-stə-no′sis) bronchostenosis.

**bron·chis·mus** (brong-kis′məs) bronchospasm.

**bron·chit·ic** (brong-kit′ik) [L. *bronchiticus*] pertaining to, affected with, or of the nature of bronchitis.

**bron·chi·tis** (brong-ki′tis) [*bronch-* + *-itis*] [MeSH: Bronchitis] inflammation of a bronchus or bronchi; there are both acute and chronic varieties. Symptoms usually include fever, coughing, and expectoration. Chronic forms may involve secondary changes to lung tissue. See also *chronic obstructive pulmonary disease,* under *disease.*
**acute b.,** a bronchitic attack with a short and more or less severe

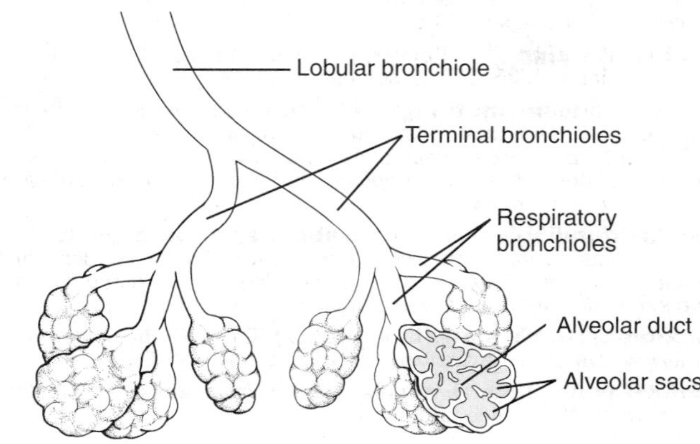

course; symptoms include fever and a productive cough. Repeated attacks may indicate chronic bronchitis.
**arachidic b.,** bronchitis caused by the presence of a peanut kernel in a bronchus.
**asthmatic b.,** bronchitis accompanying or just preceding asthma; see also *bronchitic asthma,* under *asthma.*
**capillary b.,** bronchopneumonia.
**Castellani's b.,** hemorrhagic b.
**chronic b.,** a type of chronic obstructive pulmonary disease in which there is bronchial irritation with increased secretions and a productive cough for at least three months, two years in succession; it is usually accompanied by pulmonary emphysema. The most common cause is long-term inhalation of irritants.
**equine infectious b.,** equine influenza.
**exudative b., fibrinous b.,** bronchitis with a violent cough, paroxysmal dyspnea, and expectoration of casts of the bronchi containing Charcot-Leyden crystals. Called also *fibrobronchitis, membranous b., plastic b.,* and *pseudomembranous b.*
**hemorrhagic b.,** chronic bronchitis with hemoptysis caused by a spirochetal infection. Called also *bronchospirochetosis, Castellani's bronchitis* or *disease* and *bronchopulmonary spirochetosis.*
**infectious avian b.,** an acute, highly contagious, respiratory disease of chickens, caused by a coronavirus and characterized by tracheal rales, coughing, sneezing, nasal discharge, and a drop in egg production.
**laryngotracheal b.,** laryngotracheobronchitis.
**membranous b.,** fibrinous b.
**b. obli'terans,** a form in which the smaller bronchi become filled with nodules made up of fibrinous exudate.
**parasitic b.,** verminous b.
**plastic b., pseudomembranous b.,** fibrinous b.
**putrid b.,** chronic bronchitis in which the sputum has an offensive smell; see also *Dittrich's plugs,* under *plug.*
**secondary b.,** bronchitis secondary to some other condition.
**vanadium b.,** irritation of the bronchi in workers inhaling excessive amounts of vanadium pentoxide dust, usually accompanied by a green to black discoloration of the tongue. See also *vanadiumism.*
**verminous b.,** hoose; a coughing and dyspnea in domestic animals due to presence in the bronchial tubes of nematode lungworms. In sheep, cattle, goats, and pigs it is called *hoose*; it also occurs in horses, donkeys, dogs, and cats. Called also *parasitic b.*

**bron·chi·um** (brong'ke-əm) pl. *bron'chia* [L.] a term sometimes used for one of the subdivisions of a bronchus larger than a bronchiole.

**bronch(o)-** [L. *bronchus,* q.v.] a combining form denoting relationship to a bronchus.

**bron·cho·ad·e·ni·tis** (brong"ko-ad"ə-ni'tis) bronchadenitis.

**bron·cho·al·ve·o·lar** (brong"ko-al-ve'ə-lər) pertaining to a bronchus and alveoli; called also *bronchovesicular.*

**bron·cho·as·per·gil·lo·sis** (brong"ko-as"pər-jil-o'sis) bronchopulmonary aspergillosis.

**bron·cho·blas·to·my·co·sis** (brong"ko-blas"to-mi-ko'sis) pulmonary blastomycosis.

**bron·cho·can·di·di·a·sis** (brong"ko-kan"dĭ-di'ə-sis) bronchopulmonary candidiasis.

**bron·cho·cav·ern·ous** (brong"ko-kav'ər-nəs) having both bronchial and cavernous qualities, such as abnormal respiration.

**bron·cho·cav·i·ta·ry** (brong"ko-kav'ĭ-ter-e) pertaining to or communicating between a bronchus and a cavity.

**bron·cho·cele** (brong'ko-sēl) [*broncho-* + *cele*[1]] a localized dilatation of a bronchus.

**bron·cho·con·stric·tion** (bron"ko-kən-strik'shən) [MeSH: Bronchoconstriction] constriction or narrowing the lumina of the air passages of the lungs, typically as a result of bronchial smooth muscle contraction.

**bron·cho·con·stric·tor** (bron"ko-kən-strik'tər) 1. constricting or narrowing the lumina of the air passages of the lungs. 2. an agent that causes narrowing of the lumina of the air passages of the lungs.

**bron·cho·di·la·ta·tion** (brong"ko-di-lə-ta'shən) 1. a dilated state of a bronchus. 2. a dilated area of a bronchus.

**bron·cho·di·la·tion** (brong"ko-di-la'shən) the act or process of increasing the caliber of a bronchus.

**bron·cho·di·la·tor** (brong"ko-di'la-tor) 1. dilating or expanding the lumina of air passages of the lungs. 2. an agent that causes expansion of the lumina of the air passages of the lungs.

**bron·cho·egoph·o·ny** (brong"ko-e-gof'ə-ne) egophony.

**bron·cho·esoph·a·ge·al** (brong"ko-ə-sof"ə-je'əl) pertaining to or communicating with a bronchus and the esophagus; called also *esophagobronchial.*

**bron·cho·esoph·a·gol·o·gy** (brong"ko-ə-sof"ə-gol'ə-je) that branch of medicine which deals with the tracheobronchial tree and the esophagus.

**bron·cho·esoph·a·gos·co·py** (brong"ko-ə-sof"-ə-gos'kə-pe) the instrumental examination of the bronchi and esophagus.

**bron·cho·fi·ber·scope** (brong"ko-fi'bər-skōp) a flexible bronchoscope that uses fiberoptics. Called also *fiberoptic bronchoscope.*

**bron·cho·fi·ber·sco·py** (brong"ko-fi-bər'skə-pe) bronchofibroscopy.

**bron·cho·fi·bros·co·py** (brong"ko-fi-bros'kə-pe) examination of the bronchi through a bronchofiberscope. Called also *bronchofiberscopy* and *fiberoptic bronchoscopy.*

**bron·cho·gen·ic** (brong-ko-jen'ik) originating in a bronchus.

**bron·cho·gram** (brong'ko-gram) the radiogram obtained by bronchography.
**air b.,** a radiographic shadow of an air-filled bronchus running through an airless lung; applied also to any tapering, branching radiolucency in an opacified lung that corresponds in size and distribution to (and is assumed to be) a part of the bronchial tree.

**bron·cho·graph·ic** (brong"ko-graf'ik) pertaining to or obtained by bronchography.

**bron·chog·ra·phy** (brong-kog'rə-fe) [*broncho-* + *-graphy*] [MeSH: Bronchography] radiography of the lung after the instillation of an opaque medium in a bronchus.

**bron·cho·lith** (brong'ko-lith) [*broncho-* + *-lith*] a concretion in the bronchi, formed by accretion about an inorganic nucleus, or from calcified portions of lung tissue or adjacent lymph nodes; called also *bronchial calculus.*

**bron·cho·li·thi·a·sis** (brong"ko-lĭ-thi'ə-sis) the presence of broncholiths in the lumen of the tracheobronchial tree.

**bron·cho·log·ic** (brong"ko-loj'ik) pertaining to bronchology.

**bron·chol·o·gy** (brong-kol'ə-je) the study and treatment of diseases of the tracheobronchial tree.

**bron·cho·ma·la·cia** (brong"ko-mə-la'shə) a deficiency in the cartilaginous wall of a bronchus, often accompanied by some degree of tracheomalacia, which may lead to atelectasis or obstructive emphysema; it may be congenital or acquired.

**bron·cho·mo·tor** (brong"ko-mo'tər) affecting the caliber of the bronchi.

**bron·cho·mu·co·trop·ic** (brong"ko-mu"ko-trop'ik) augmenting secretion by the respiratory mucosa.

**bron·cho·my·co·sis** (brong"ko-mi-ko'sis) [*broncho-* + *mycosis*] any infection of the bronchi or lungs by a fungus, particularly *Candida albicans;* see also *bronchopulmonary candidiasis.*

**bron·cho·no·car·di·o·sis** (brong"ko-no-kahr"de-o'sis) nocardiosis in the bronchi.

**bron·cho·pan·cre·at·ic** (brong"ko-pan"kre-at'ik) communicating with a bronchus and the pancreas, as a bronchopancreatic fistula.

**bron·chop·a·thy** (brong-kop'ə-the) [*broncho-* + *-pathy*] any disease of a bronchus.

**bron·choph·o·ny** (brong-kof'ə-ne) [*broncho-* + Gr. *phōnē* voice] 1. the normal voice sounds heard over a healthy large bronchus. 2. abnormal voice sounds heard over the lung, with the voice transmitted unusually clearly and with a high pitch; it is a type of pectoriloquy, indicating solidification of the lung tissue. Called also *bronchiloquy.*
**whispered b.,** see under *pectoriloquy.*

**bron·cho·plas·ty** (brong'ko-plas"te) [*broncho-* + *-plasty*] plastic surgery of a bronchus.

**bron·cho·ple·gia** (brong"ko-ple'jə) paralysis of the muscles of the walls of the bronchial tubes.

**bron·cho·pleu·ral** (brong"ko-ploor'əl) 1. pertaining to a bronchus and the pleura. 2. communicating with a bronchus and the pleural cavity, as a bronchopleural fistula.

**bron·cho·pleu·ro·pneu·mo·nia** (brong"ko-ploor"o-noo͞-mo'ne-ə) bronchopneumonia with pleurisy.

**bron·cho·pneu·mo·nia** (brong"ko-noo͞-mo'ne-ə) [*broncho-* + *pneumonia*] [MeSH: Bronchopneumonia] an inflammation of the lungs that begins in the terminal bronchioles, which become clogged with a mucopurulent exudate forming consolidated patches in adjacent lobules. Called also *bronchial* or *lobular pneumonia, capillary bronchitis,* and *bronchopneumonitis.*
**postoperative b.,** bronchopneumonia following surgical operations, particularly those on the abdomen. It may be due to the inhalation of irritant anesthesia or of infected material from the mouth or nose during the temporary depression of the cough reflex.

**bron·cho·pneu·mon·ic** (brong"ko-noo͞-mon'ik) pertaining to, affected with, or caused by bronchopneumonia.

**bron·cho·pneu·mo·ni·tis** (brong″ko-noo″mə-ni′tis) bronchopneumonia.

**bron·cho·pneu·mop·a·thy** (brong″ko-noo͝-mop′ə-the) disease of the bronchi and lung tissue.

**bron·cho·prov·o·ca·tion** (brong″ko-prov″ə-ka′shən) bronchial challenge.

**bron·cho·pul·mo·nary** (brong″ko-pul′mə-nar″e) pertaining to the lungs and their air passages; both bronchial and pulmonary.

**bron·cho·ra·di·og·ra·phy** (brong″ko-ra-de-og′rə-fe) radiographic visualization of the bronchial tree.

**bron·chor·rha·gia** (brong″ko-ra′jə) [*broncho-* + *-rrhagia*] hemorrhage from the bronchi.

**bron·chor·rha·phy** (brong-kor′ə-fe) [*broncho-* + *-rrhaphy*] suture of a bronchus.

**bron·chor·rhea** (brong-ko-re′ə) [*broncho-* + *-rrhea*] excessive discharge of mucus from the bronchi.

**bron·cho·scope** (brong′ko-skōp) an instrument for inspecting the interior of the tracheobronchial tree and carrying out endobronchial diagnostic and therapeutic maneuvers, such as taking specimens for culture and biopsy and removing foreign bodies.
**fiberoptic b.,** bronchofiberscope.

**bron·cho·scop·ic** (brong″ko-skop′ik) pertaining to bronchoscopy or to the bronchoscope.

**bron·chos·co·py** (brong-kos′kə-pe) [*broncho-* + *-scopy*] [MeSH: Bronchoscopy] examination of the bronchi through a bronchoscope.
**fiberoptic b.,** bronchofibroscopy.

**bron·cho·si·nus·itis** (brong″ko-si″nəs-i′tis) coexisting infection of the paranasal sinuses and the lower respiratory passages.

**bron·cho·spasm** (brong′ko-spaz″əm) spasmodic contraction of the smooth muscle of the bronchi, as occurs in asthma. Called also *bronchial spasm.*

**bron·cho·spi·ro·che·to·sis** (brong″ko-spi″ro-ke-to′sis) hemorrhagic bronchitis.

**bron·cho·spi·rog·ra·phy** (brong″ko-spi-rog′rə-fe) the recording of bronchospirometry results.

**bron·cho·spi·rom·e·ter** (brong″ko-spi-rom′ə-tər) an instrument used in bronchospirometry.

**bron·cho·spi·rom·e·try** (brong″ko-spi-rom′ə-tre) [MeSH: Bronchospirometry] determination of the vital capacity, oxygen intake, and carbon dioxide excretion of a single lung, or simultaneous measurements of the function of each lung separately. Called also *bronchoscopic spirometry.*
**differential b.,** measurement of the function of each lung separately.

**bron·cho·stax·is** (brong″ko-stak′sis) bronchorrhagia.

**bron·cho·ste·no·sis** (brong″ko-stə-no′sis) [*broncho-* + *stenosis*] stricture or cicatricial diminution of the caliber of a bronchial tube.

**bron·chos·to·my** (brong-kos′tə-me) [*broncho-* + *-stomy*] the surgical creation of an opening into a bronchus.

**bron·cho·tome** (brong′ko-tōm) a cutting instrument used in performing bronchotomy.

**bron·chot·o·my** (brong-kot′ə-me) [*broncho-* + *-tomy*] surgical incision of a bronchus.

**bron·cho·tra·che·al** (brong″ko-tra′ke-əl) tracheobronchial.

**bron·cho·ve·sic·u·lar** (brong″ko-vĕ-sik′u-lər) 1. bronchoalveolar. 2. vesiculobronchial.

**bron·chus** (brong′kəs) pl. *bron′chi* [L.; Gr. *bronchos* windpipe] [TA] [MeSH: Bronchi] any of the larger air passages of the lungs, having an outer fibrous coat with irregularly placed plates of hyaline cartilage, an interlacing network of smooth muscle, and a mucous membrane of columnar ciliated epithelial cells.
**apical b.,** 1. b. segmentalis apicalis. 2. b. segmentalis superioris. See table and illustration.
**cardiac b.,** b. segmentalis basalis medialis; see table and illustration.
**eparterial b.,** a name sometimes given to the superior lobar bronchus on the right, which arises above the level of the pulmonary artery; see table and illustration. Called also *ramus bronchialis eparterialis.*
**hyparterial bronchi,** a name sometimes given to the middle and inferior lobar bronchi on the right and the lobar bronchi on the left, all of which arise below the level of the pulmonary artery. See table and illustration. Called also *rami bronchiales hyparteriales.*
**lingular b., inferior,** b. lingularis inferior; see table and illustration.
**lingular b., superior,** b. lingularis superior; see table and illustration.
**bron′chi loba′res** [TA], lobar bronchi: passages arising from the primary bronchi and passing to the lobes of the right and left lungs. There are three right and two left lobar bronchi, which divide into the segmental bronchi. See table and illustration, and see plate at *lung.*
**main bronchi, right and left, primary bronchi, right and left,** bronchi principales dexter/sinister.
**bron′chi principa′les dexter/sinis′ter** [TA], right and left primary bronchi: the two main branches into which the trachea divides, each passing to the respective lung. Called also *right and left main bronchi.*
**secondary bronchi,** subdivisions of the primary bronchi; see *bronchi lobares* and *bronchi segmentales.*
**segmental bronchi,** bronchi segmentales.
**segmental b., anteromedial basal,** the bronchus segmentalis basalis anterior and bronchus segmentalis basalis medialis of the left lung considered as a unit. See table and illustration.
**segmental b., apical,** 1. b. segmentalis apicalis. 2. b. segmentalis superior. See table and illustration.
**bron′chi segmenta′les** [TA], segmental bronchi: air passages arising from the lobar bronchi and passing to the different segments of the two lungs, where they further subdivide into smaller and smaller passages (bronchioles). The segmental bronchi are designated by roman numerals, with the three right lobar bronchi divided into ten segmental bronchi and the two left lobar bronchi into eight or nine, depending on the system of classification. See accompanying table and illustration; see also table at *segmenta bronchopulmonalia* and plate at *lung.*
**stem b.,** the continuation of the primary bronchus of the embryo, from which branches are given off to the lobes of the lungs.
**tracheal b.,** an ectopic or supernumerary bronchus, extending directly from the trachea to the apical segment of the upper lobe of the right lung, occurring normally in some animals but as a congenital anomaly in man.

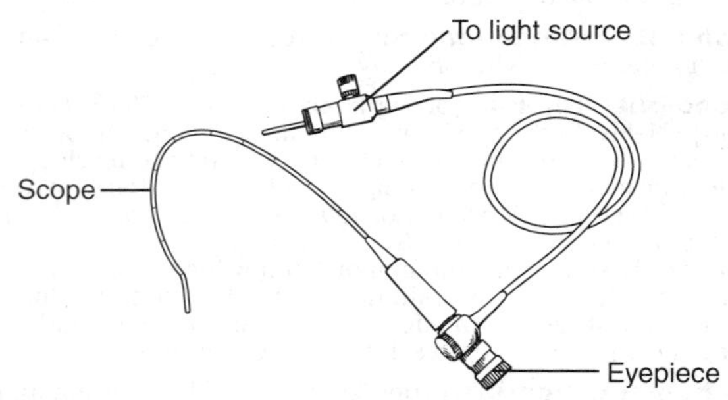

Bronchoscope.

**bron·to·pho·bia** (bron″to-fo′be-ə) [Gr. *brontē* thunder + *phobia*] irrational fear of thunder; astraphobia.

**Brooke's disease, tumor** (brooks) [Henry Ambrose Grundy *Brooke,* English dermatologist, 1854–1919] see *keratosis follicularis multiplex,* and *trichoepithelioma papillosum multiplex.*

**broom** (bro͞om) any of various shrubs with long slender branches, such as *Cytisus scoparius;* see also *broom poisoning,* under *poisoning.*

**brosse** (bros) [Fr. *brush*] a brushlike organelle of cilia seen on the anterodorsal surface of certain ciliate protozoa, such as those of the suborder Prorodontina; its function is unknown.

**broth** (broth) 1. a thin soup prepared by boiling meat or vegetables. 2. a liquid culture medium for the cultivation of microorganisms; see under *culture medium* for specific broths.

**Bro·vi·ac catheter** (bro′ve-ak) [J. W. *Broviac,* American surgeon, 20th century] see under *catheter.*

**brow** (brou) 1. frons. 2. either of the halves of the frons (forehead).
**olympian b., olympic b.,** the prominent forehead seen in congenital syphilis.

**Brown** (broun) Michael Stuart. American physician, born 1941; co-winner, with Joseph Leonard Goldstein, of the Nobel prize for medicine or physiology in 1985 for their discoveries about the regulation of cholesterol metabolism and the treatment of diseases caused by abnormally high levels of cholesterol in the blood.

**brown** (broun) a dusky, reddish yellow color.
**aniline b., Bismarck b.,** a basic aniline dye, phenylene-diazo-meta-phenylene-diamine, $C_6H_4[N_2C_6H_3(NH)_2]_2$, much used as a stain and counterstain in histology; called also *Manchester b.* and *phenylene b.*
**Manchester b., phenylene b.,** aniline b.
**Bismark b. R,** a dark brown solid, synthetically prepared, used as a leather and textile dye and as a biological stain.

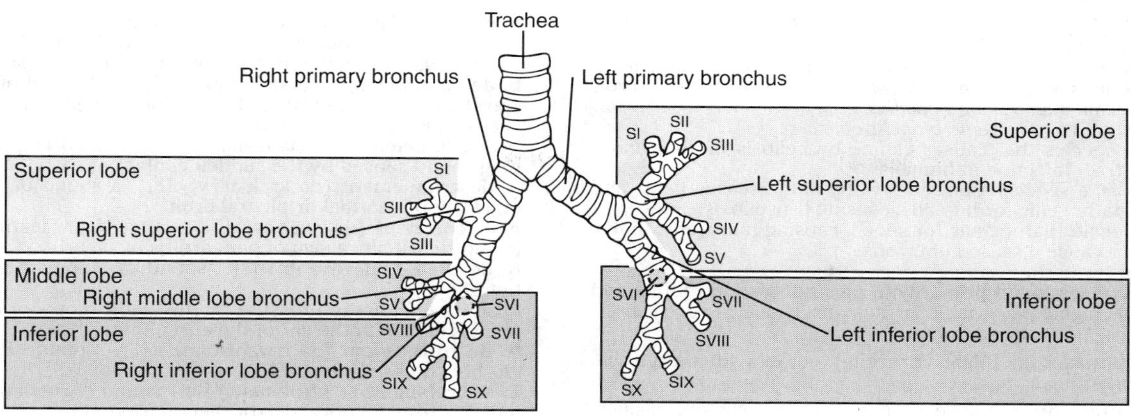


Bronchi, showing primary, lobar, and segmental (S I–X) bronchi of the right and left lungs. For correlation of the segmental bronchi with subdivisions of the lungs, see Plate 20.

**Bismark b. Y,** a blackish brown powder, synthetically prepared, used as a textile dye and as a stain for demonstrating mucus in intestinal goblet cells and cartilage in the trachea and in embryonic tissue.

**Brown-Rob·erts-Wells apparatus, technique** (broun-rob'ərts-welz) [R.A. *Brown,* American neurosurgeon, 20th century; T.S. *Roberts,* American neurosurgeon, 20th century; T.H. *Wells,* Jr., American neurosurgeon, 20th century] see under *apparatus* and *technique.*

**Brown-Sym·mers disease** (broun-sim'ərz) [Charles Leonard *Brown,* American physician, 1899–1959; Douglas *Symmers,* American physician, 1879–1952] see under *disease.*

**Brown-Vi·a·let·to-van Laere syndrome** (broun ve-ah-lĕ'to vahn-lĕr') [C.H. *Brown,* American physician, late 19th century; E. *Vialetto,* Italian physician, 20th century; J. *van Laere,* Belgian physician, 20th century] see under *syndrome.*

**Browne operation** (broun) [Sir Denis John *Browne,* Australian-born English pediatric surgeon,1892–1967] see under *operation.*

**brown·i·an move·ment** (broun'e-ən) [Robert *Brown,* English botanist, 1773–1858] see under *movement.*

**Brown·ing's vein** (broun'ingz) [William *Browning,* American anatomist, 1855–1941] vena anastomotica inferior.

**Brown-Sé·quard's syndrome, treatment** (brōōn'sa-kahrz') [Charles Edouard *Brown-Séquard,* French physiologist, 1817–1894] see under *syndrome* and *treatment.*

**Brox·o·lin** (brok'sə-lin) trademark for a preparation of glycobiarsol.

**B.R.S.** British Roentgen Society.

**Bruce's tract** (brōōs'əz) [Alexander *Bruce,* Scottish anatomist, 1854–1911] fasciculus septomarginalis.

**Bru·cea** (broo'se-ə) a genus of evergreen shrubs of the family Simaroubaceae, found from Southeast Asia to Australia. *B. sumatra'na* Roxb. is the medicinal plant called *kosam.*

**Bru·cel·la** (broo-sel'ə) [Sir David *Bruce,* English physician, 1855–1931] [MeSH: Brucella] a genus of gram-negative, aerobic coccobacilli of uncertain affiliation, made up of nonmotile cells that require biotin, niacin, thiamine, and sometimes serum for growth; they are animal parasites and pathogens, causing brucellosis, and

**Bronchi Segmentales (Segmental Bronchi)**

| Terminologia Anatomica | Common Name |
|---|---|
| *Bronchus lobaris superior dexter* | *Right superior lobar bronchus* |
| Bronchus segmentalis apicalis [B I] | Apical segmental bronchus |
| Bronchus segmentalis posterior [B II] | Posterior segmental bronchus |
| Bronchus segmentalis anterior [B III] | Anterior segmental bronchus |
| *Bronchus lobaris medius* | *Middle lobar bronchus* |
| Bronchus segmentalis lateralis [B IV] | Lateral segmental bronchus |
| Bronchus segmentalis medialis [B V] | Medial segmental bronchus |
| *Bronchus lobaris inferior dexter* | *Right inferior lobe bronchus* |
| Bronchus segmentalis superior [B VI] | Superior segmental bronchus |
| Bronchus segmentalis basalis medialis [B VII] [B. cardiacus]* | Medial basal segmental bronchus (Cardiac bronchus) |
| Bronchus segmentalis basalis anterior [B VIII] | Anterior basal segmental bronchus |
| Bronchus segmentalis basalis lateralis [B IX] | Lateral basal segmental bronchus |
| Bronchus segmentalis basalis posterior [B X] | Posterior basal segmental bronchus |
| *Bronchus lobaris superior sinister* | *Left superior lobar bronchus* |
| Bronchus segmentalis apicoposterior [B I + II] | Apicoposterior segmental bronchus |
| Bronchus segmentalis anterior [B III] | Anterior segmental bronchus |
| Bronchus lingularis superior [B IV] | Superior lingular bronchus |
| Bronchus lingularis inferior [B V] | Inferior lingular bronchus |
| *Bronchus lobaris inferior sinister* | *Left inferior lobar bronchus* |
| Bronchus segmentalis superior [B VI] | Superior segmental bronchus |
| Bronchus segmentalis basalis medialis [B VII] [B. cardiacus]* | Medial basal segmental bronchus† (Cardiac bronchus) |
| Bronchus segmentalis basalis anterior [B VIII] | Anterior basal segmental bronchus† |
| Bronchus segmentalis basalis lateralis [B IX] | Lateral basal segmental bronchus |
| Bronchus segmentalis basalis posterior [B X] | Posterior basal segmental bronchus |

*TA alternative.
†The anterior basal and medial basal segmental bronchi of the left inferior lobe are often described collectively as the anteromedial basal segmental bronchus.

are transmissible to humans through contact with infected tissue or dairy products.
**B. abor'tus,** the most common cause of brucellosis in humans; it causes infectious abortion in cattle, which are the animal reservoir of infection; called also *Bang's bacillus.*
**B. bronchisep'tica,** *Bordetella bronchiseptica.*
**B. ca'nis,** a species that causes canine brucellosis in dogs and a respiratory tract infection in humans.
**B. meliten'sis,** a species found in healthy and diseased goats and sheep; it is pathogenic for humans, causing brucellosis.
**B. o'vis,** a species pathogenic for sheep, causing ram epididymitis; not known to cause disease in humans.
**B. rangi'feri taran'di,** *B. suis.*
**B. su'is,** a species found primarily in pigs but also in rabbits and reindeer; it is highly pathogenic for humans, causing brucellosis.
**B. tularen'sis,** *Francisella tularensis.*

**bru·cel·la** (broo-sel'ah) [MeSH: Brucella] an individual organism of the genus *Brucella.*

**Bru·cel·la·ceae** (broo″sə-la'se-e) in former systems of classification, a family of gram-negative aerobic cocci and rod-shaped bacteria. It included the genera *Actinobacillus, Bordetella, Brucella, Calymmatobacterium, Haemophilus, Moraxella, Noguchia,* and *Pasteurella.*

**bru·cel·lar** (broo-sel'ər) pertaining to or caused by *Brucella.*

**bru·cel·lin** (broo-sel'in) a preparation from pooled cultures of the three species of *Brucella,* used in the diagnosis of brucellosis.

**bru·cel·lo·sis** (broo″sə-lo'sis) [MeSH: Brucellosis] 1. in humans, a generalized infection caused by species of *Brucella,* transmitted by contact with the natural animal reservoirs, including cattle, sheep, goats, swine, deer, and rabbits, or their infected products or tissue. It involves primarily the reticuloendothelial system and is characterized by fever, sweating, weakness, malaise, and weight loss. Called also *Malta fever, Mediterranean fever,* and *undulant fever.* 2. in livestock, infection by species of *Brucella,* characterized primarily by infertility or abortion.
**canine b.,** infection of dogs by *Brucella canis,* characterized by lymphadenitis, splenitis, and infertility; fetal death or abortion in pregnant females; and epididymitis, scrotal dermatitis, and testicular atrophy in males.

**Bruch's glands, layer (membrane)** (brooks) [Karl Wilhelm Ludwig *Bruch,* German anatomist, 1819–1884] see under *gland,* and see *lamina basalis choroideae.*

**bru·cine** (broo'sēn) [from *Brucea,* a genus of shrubs named for J. *Bruce,* Scottish explorer, 1730–1794] a poisonous alkaloid, from *Strychnos ignatii* and *S. nux-vomica,* which resembles strychnine in its action, but is less poisonous. One of the principal constituents of nux vomica and ignatia, it was formerly used in the same manner as strychnine (q.v.).

**Bruck's disease** (brooks) [Alfred *Bruck,* German physician, late 19th century] see under *disease.*

**Brü·cke's lines, muscle, tunic** (bre'kez) [Ernst Wilhelm von *Brücke,* Austrian physiologist, 1819–1892] see under *line* and *muscle,* and see *tunica nervea of Brücke.*

**Bru·dzin·ski's sign (reflex)** (broo-jin'skēz) [Józef *Brudzinski,* Polish physician, 1874–1917] see under *sign.*

**Brue·ghel's syndrome** (broi'gəlz) [Pieter *Brueghel* the Elder, Flemish painter, 1525–1569, whose painting *De Gaper* shows a person with this syndrome] Meige's syndrome (def. 2).

**Brug's filaria** (broogz) [S.L. *Brug,* Dutch parasitologist in Indonesia, 1879–1946] *Brugia malayi.*

**Brug·ia** (bruj'ə) [S.L. *Brug*] [MeSH: Brugia] a genus of filarial worms of the superfamily Filarioidea, which parasitize humans and other mammals.
**B. ma'layi,** a species causing human filariasis and elephantiasis throughout Southeast Asia, the China Sea, and eastern India; it is similar to, and often found in association with, *Wuchereria bancrofti.* Called also *W. malayi* and *Brug's filaria.*
**B. pahan'gi,** a species found in humans, cats, tigers, and other wild and domestic animals in Malaya; in humans, it may produce the symptoms of tropical eosinophilia.
**B. ti'mori,** a species causing filariasis and elephantiasis among the inhabitants of Timor and the small islands of southeastern Indonesia.

**brug·i·an** (brooj'e-ən) named for S. L. *Brug.*

**bruise** (bro͞oz) contusion.
**stone b.,** a painful bruise, especially of the bare feet of children.

**bruisse·ment** (brwēs-ə-maw') [Fr.] a purring tremor; see under *tremor.*

**bruit** (brwe, bro͞ot) [Fr.] sound (def. 4).
**aneurysmal b.,** a blowing sound heard over an aneurysm.
**b. de canon** (də kah-naw') [Fr. "sound of cannon"], an abnormally loud first heart sound, heard intermittently in complete heart block when atrial contraction just precedes ventricular contraction.
**b. de clapotement** (də klah-pōt-maw') [Fr. "sound of rippling"], a splashing sound indicative of dilatation of the stomach when pressure is put on the wall of the abdomen.
**b. de claquement** (də klahk-maw') [Fr. "sound of clapping"], a snapping sound caused by the sudden contact of parts.
**b. de craquement** (də krak-maw') [Fr. "a sound of crackling"], a crackling pericardial or pleural bruit.
**b. de cuir neuf** (də kwĕr nəf) [Fr. "sound of new leather"], a creaking noise; usually a sign of pericarditis or pleurisy.
**b. de diable** (də dyahbl) [Fr. "sound of humming top"], venous hum.
**false b.,** one due to pressure by the stethoscope, or derived from the circulation in the ear of the auscultator.
**b. de froissement** (də frwahs-maw') [Fr. "sound of clashing"], a clashing noise of varying origin.
**b. de frolement** (də frōl-maw') [Fr. "sound of rustling"], a rustling murmur from a pericardial or pleural friction rub.
**b. de galop** (də gah-lop') [Fr.], gallop rhythm.
**b. de lime** (də lēm) [Fr. "sound of a file"], a cardiac sound resembling filing.
**b. de moulin** (də moo-lă') [Fr. "sound of a mill"], a splashing or waterwheel sound synchronous with systole, sometimes audible at some distance from the patient, variously attributed to cardiac, pericardiac, or mediastinal causes.
**b. de parchemin** (də parsh-mă') [Fr. "sound of parchment"], a sound as of two pieces of parchment rubbed together, of valvular cardiac origin.
**b. de piaulement** (də pyōl-maw') [Fr. "sound of whining"], a cardiac murmur like the mewing of a cat.
**b. placentaire** (plah″sawn-tār') [Fr. "placental sound"], placental souffle.
**b. de pot fêlé** (də po fĕ-la') [Fr.], cracked-pot resonance.
**b. de rape** (də rahp) [Fr. "sound of a grater"], a rasping, cardiac, valvular murmur.
**b. de rappel** (də rah-pel') [Fr. "sound of a drum beating to arms"], a double sound as of two beats of a drum, describing splitting of the second heart sound or a second sound followed by an opening snap.
**Roger's b., b. de Roger** (də ro-zha'), a loud, long systolic murmur heard in the third interspace to the left of the sternum, characteristic of a small ventricular septal defect. Called also *Roger's murmur.*
**b. de scie** (də se) [Fr. "sound of a saw"], a cardiac murmur resembling the sound of a saw.
**b. de soufflet** (də soo-fla') [Fr. "sound of a bellows"], see *souffle.*
**systolic b.,** see under *murmur.*
**b. de tabourka** (də tah-bo͞or'kah) [Fr. "sound of drum"], timbre métallique.
**b. de tambour** (də tahm-bo͞or') [Fr. "sound of drum"], a ringing sound heard in syphilitic aortic regurgitation.
**Verstraeten's b.,** an abnormal sound heard in auscultation over the lower border of the liver in cachectic patients.

**Bru·na·ti's sign** (broo-nah'tēz) [M. *Brunati,* Italian physician, 20th century] see under *sign.*

**Brunn's membrane, epithelial nests** (broonz) [Albert von *Brunn,* German anatomist, 1849–1895] see under *membrane* and *nest.*

**Brun·ner's glands** (broon'ərz) [Johann Conrad *Brunner,* Swiss anatomist, 1653–1727] [MeSH: Brunner's Glands] glandulae duodenales.

**Brunn·strom meth·od** (brun'strəm) [Signe *Brunstrom,* American physical therapist, 20th century] see under *method.*

**Bruns' frontal ataxia, syndrome (sign)** (broonz) [Ludwig *Bruns,* German neurologist, 1858–1916] see under *ataxia* and *syndrome.*

**Brun·schwig's operation** (broon'shwigz) [Alexander *Brunschwig,* American surgeon, 1901–1969] pancreatoduodenectomy.

**Brun·sting's syndrome** (broon'stings) [Louis A. *Brunsting,* Sr., American dermatologist, born 1900] see under *syndrome.*

**brush** (brush) tufts of bristles, hair, or other flexible materials set into a handle.
**Haidinger's b.,** two conical brushlike images with apexes touching, seen on looking through a Nicol prism; used in determining visual function.
**Ruffini's b.,** see under *corpuscle.*
**stomach b.,** a brush used to cleanse and stimulate the mucous lining of the stomach.

**Brush·field's spots** (brush'fēldz) [Thomas *Brushfield,* English physician, 1858–1937] see under *spot.*

**Brush·field-Wy·att syndrome** (brush'fēld-wi'ət) [T. *Brushfield;* W. *Wyatt,* British physician, 20th century] see under *syndrome.*

**brush·ite** (brush'īt) a nearly colorless type of acid calcium phosphate, found in rock phosphates and sometimes as a component of human dental or renal calculi.

**Bru·ton's agammaglobulinemia, disease** (broo'tənz) [Ogden C. *Bruton,* American pediatrician, born 1908] see *X-linked agammaglobulinemia,* under *agammaglobulinemia.*

**brux** (bruks) to grind the teeth rhythmically or spasmodically; cf. *bruxism.*

**brux·ism** (bruk'siz-əm) [Gr. *brychein* to gnash the teeth] [MeSH: Bruxism] involuntary, nonfunctional, rhythmic or spasmodic gnashing, grinding, and clenching of teeth (not including chewing movements of the mandible), usually during sleep, sometimes leading to occlusal trauma. Causes may be related to repressed aggression, emotional tension, anger, fear, and frustration. See also *bruxomania* and *clenching.*
**centric b.,** bruxism characterized by clenching in centric occlusion. Called also *clamping habit* and *clenching habit.*

**bruxo·ma·nia** (bruk"so-ma'ne-ə) [Gr. *brychein* +*mania*] bruxism occurring in the daytime, usually performed unconsciously.

**Bry·ant's line, sign, traction, triangle** (bri'ənts) [Sir Thomas *Bryant,* English surgeon, 1828–1914] see under *line, sign,* and *traction* and see *iliofemoral triangle* under *triangle.*

**Bryce-Teach·er ovum** (brīs-te'chər) [Thomas Hastie *Bryce,* Scottish anatomist, 1862–1946; John Hammond *Teacher,* Scottish pathologist, 1869–1930] see under *ovum.*

**Bry·o·bia** (bri-o'be-ə) a genus of spider mites. *B. praetio'sa* is the clover mite or spinning mite, a species found on clover and sometimes greatly annoying humans.

**Bry·o·nia** (bri-o'ne-ə) a genus of plants of the family Cucurbitaceae, all called *bryony.* They are poisonous to humans and other animals, containing bryonidin, bryonin, and other glycosides that cause diarrhea and sometimes convulsions. They were formerly used medicinally as drastic purgatives.

**bry·o·nia** (bri-o'ne-ə) [L.; Gr. *bryōnia*] the air-dried root of *Bryonia alba* or related species, which was formerly used as a drastic purgative for humans and other animals; toxic alkaloids causing diarrhea include bryonidin and bryonin.

**bry·o·ni·din** (bri-o'nĭ-din) a toxic glycoside found in species of *Bryonia,* partially responsible for their purgative effects.

**bry·o·nin** (bri'o-nin) a toxic glycoside found in species of *Bryonia,* partially responsible for their purgative effects.

**BS** Bachelor of Surgery; Bachelor of Science; breath sounds; blood sugar.

**BSA** body surface area.

**B-scan** see under *scan.*

**BSP** Bromsulphalein.

**BSS** Bernard-Soulier syndrome.

**BThU, BTU** British thermal unit.

**bu·bo** (bu'bo) [L. from Gr. *boubōn* groin] a tender, enlarged, and inflamed lymph node, particularly in the axilla or groin, due to such infections as plague, syphilis, gonorrhea, chancroid, lymphogranuloma venereum, and tuberculosis.
**bullet b.,** the characteristic hard bubo of primary syphilis.
**chancroidal b.,** a suppurating form accompanying or following chancroid; called also *virulent b.*
**climatic b.,** lymphogranuloma venereum.
**malignant b.,** the bubo of bubonic plague.
**primary b.,** a bubo which is due to venereal exposure but which is not preceded by any visible lesion; called also *bubon d'emblée.*
**syphilitic b.,** nontender, nonfluctuant, firm regional lymphadenopathy that follows the chancre of syphilis.
**tropical b.,** lymphogranuloma venereum.
**virulent b.,** chancroidal b.

**bu·bon** (bu-baw') [Fr.] bubo.
**b. d'emblée,** (dahm-bla') [Fr. "at the first onset"], primary bubo.

**bu·bon·ic** (bu-bon'ik) [L. *bubonicus*] characterized by or pertaining to buboes; see also under *plague.*

**bu·bono·cele** (bu-bon'o-sēl) [Gr. *boubōn* groin + *-cele*[1]] inguinal or femoral hernia forming a swelling in the groin.

**bu·bon·u·lus** (bu-bon'u-ləs) [L. "a small bubo"] a nodule or abscess along a lymphatic vessel, especially one on the dorsum of the penis.

**bu·cai·nide mal·e·ate** (bu-ka'nīd) a cardiac depressant with antiarrhythmic action.

**buc·ca** (buk'ə) [L.] [TA] cheek: the fleshy portion of the side of the face, constituting the lateral wall of the oral cavity. Called also *mala.*

**buc·cal** (buk'əl) [L. *buccalis,* from *bucca* cheek] pertaining to or directed toward the cheek. In dental anatomy, used to refer to the buccal surface of a tooth; see *buccal surface,* under *surface.* Cf. *labial.*

**buc·cal·ly** (buk'ə-le) toward the cheek.

**buc·ci·na·tor** (buk'sĭ-na"tor) [L. "trumpeter"] see under *musculus.*

**bucc(o)-** [L. *bucca* cheek] a combining form denoting relationship to the cheek.

**buc·co·ax·i·al** (buk"o-ak'se-əl) pertaining to or formed by the buccal and axial walls of a tooth cavity preparation.

**buc·co·ax·io·cer·vi·cal** (buk"o-ak"se-o-sər'vĭ-kəl) buccoaxiogingival.

**buc·co·ax·io·gin·gi·val** (buk"o-ak"se-o-jin'jĭ-vəl) pertaining to or formed by the buccal, axial, and gingival walls of a tooth cavity; called also *buccoaxiocervical.*

**buc·co·cer·vi·cal** (buk"o-sər'vi-kəl) 1. pertaining to the cheek and neck. 2. pertaining to the buccal surface of the neck of a posterior tooth. 3. buccogingival.

**buc·co·clu·sal** (buk"o-kloo'zəl) 1. pertaining to buccoclusion. 2. bucco-occlusal.

**buc·co·clu·sion** (buk"o-kloo'zhən) malocclusion in which the dental arch or a quadrant or group of teeth is buccal to the normal.

**buc·co·dis·tal** (buk"o-dis'təl) distobuccal.

**buc·co·gin·gi·val** (buk"o-jin'jĭ-vəl) 1. pertaining to the cheek and gingiva. 2. pertaining to or formed by the buccal and gingival walls of a tooth cavity preparation.

**buc·co·glos·so·phar·yn·gi·tis** (buk"o-glos'o-far"in-ji'tis) inflammation involving the cheek, tongue, and pharynx.
**b. sic'ca,** inflammation and dryness of the buccal mucosa, tongue, and pharynx. Cf. *Sjögren's syndrome,* under *syndrome.*

**buc·co·la·bi·al** (buk"o-la'be-əl) pertaining to the cheek and lip.

**buc·co·lin·gual** (buk"o-ling'gwəl) 1. pertaining to the cheek and tongue. 2. pertaining to the buccal and lingual surfaces of a posterior tooth.

**buc·co·lin·gual·ly** (buk"o-ling'gwə-le) from the cheek toward the tongue.

**buc·co·max·il·lary** (buk"o-mak'sĭ-lar"e) 1. pertaining to the cheek and maxilla. 2. communicating with the buccal cavity and the maxillary sinus, as a buccomaxillary fistula.

**buc·co·me·si·al** (buk"o-me'ze-əl) pertaining to or formed by the buccal and mesial surfaces of a tooth, or the buccal and mesial walls of a tooth cavity.

**buc·co-oc·clu·sal** (buk"o-ə-kloo'zəl) pertaining to or formed by the buccal and occlusal surfaces of a tooth.

**buc·co·pha·ryn·ge·al** (buk"o-fə-rin'je-əl) pertaining to the mouth and pharynx.

**buc·co·place·ment** (buk'o-plās"ment) displacement of a tooth toward the cheek.

**buc·co·pul·pal** (buk"o-pul'pəl) pertaining to or formed by the buccal and pulpal walls of a tooth cavity.

**buc·cos·to·my** (buk-os'tə-me) an old method of treating cribbing in horses, consisting of the surgical creation of permanent buccal fistulae.

**buc·co·ver·sion** (buk"o-vər'zhən) the position of a tooth which lies buccally to the line of occlusion.

**Bu·ceph·a·lus** (bu-sef'ə-ləs) a genus of trematodes. *B. papillo'sus* is parasitic in the stomach and intestines of freshwater fish.

**Buck's extension, fascia, operation** (buks) [Gurdon *Buck,* American surgeon, 1807–1877] see under *extension, fascia,* and *operation.*

**buck·eye** (buk'i) *Aesculus glabra* or any of several other plants of the same genus, whose fruit and seeds are toxic to livestock.

**Buck·ley's syndrome** (buk'lēz) [Rebecca H. *Buckley,* American physician, born 1933] hyperimmunoglobulinemia E syndrome.

**buck·ling** (buk'ling) the process or an instance of becoming crumpled or warped.
**scleral b.,** a technique for repair of detachment of the retina, in which indentations or infoldings of the sclera are made over the tears in the retina so as to promote adherence of the retina to the choroid.

**buck·thorn** (buk'thorn) 1. any of various trees and shrubs of the genus *Rhamnus.* 2. *Karwinskia humboldtiana;* see also under *poisoning.*

**buck·wheat** (buk'hwēt) *Fagopyrum esculentum.* See also *fagopyrism.*

**bu·cli·zine hy·dro·chlo·ride** (bu'klĭ-zēn) an antihistamine, used mainly as an antinauseant in the management of motion sickness; administered orally.

**bu·cry·late** (bu'krə-lāt) [MeSH: Bucrylate] a compound, isobutyl 2-cyanoacrylate, used as a tissue adhesive.

**bud** (bud) any small part of the embryo or adult metazoon more or less resembling the bud of a plant and presumed to have potential for growth and differentiation.
**bronchial b.,** an outgrowth from the stem bronchus giving rise to the air passages of its respective pulmonary lobe.
**end b.,** the remnant of the primitive knot, from which arises the caudal portion of the trunk; called also *tail b.*
**farcy b's,** small tubercular nodules on the skin seen in some cases of farcy.
**gustatory b.,** caliculus gustatorius.
**limb b.,** a swelling on the trunk of the embryo that becomes a limb.
**liver b.,** a diverticulum from the foregut that gives rise to the liver and its ducts.
**lung b.,** an outgrowth from the foregut that gives rise to the trachea, bronchi, and all the branchings that form a tracheobronchial tree.
**metanephric b.,** ureteric b.
**periosteal b.,** vascular connective tissue from the periosteum growing through apertures in the periosteal bone collar into the cartilaginous matrix of the primary center of ossification.
**tail b.,** 1. the primordium of the caudal appendage. 2. end b.
**taste b.,** caliculus gustatorius.
**tongue b., distal,** either of the two oval swellings, one on each side of the median tongue bud in the embryo; they grow over the median tongue bud and converge to form the anterior part of the tongue. Called also *lingual swelling* and *lateral lingual swelling.*
**tongue b., median,** tuberculum impar.
**tooth b.,** a knoblike tooth primordium developing into an enamel organ surrounded by a dental sac and encasing the dental papilla. See also *tooth germ,* under *germ.*
**ureteric b.,** an outgrowth of the mesonephric duct that gives rise to all but the nephrons of the permanent kidney; called also *metanephric b.* or *diverticulum.*
**b. of urethra,** bulbus penis.
**vascular b.,** an outgrowth of an existing vessel from which a new blood vessel arises.
**wing b.,** a swelling on the trunk of an avian embryo that gives rise to a wing.

**Budd-Chi·a·ri syndrome (disease)** (bud'ke-ah're) [George *Budd,* English physician, 1808–1882; Hans *Chiari,* Austrian pathologist, 1851–1916] see under *syndrome.*

**bud·ding** (bud'ing) 1. gemmation; a form of asexual reproduction in which the body divides into two unequal parts, the larger part being considered the parent and the smaller one the bud. 2. the process by which a new blood vessel arises from a preexisting vessel.

**bu·des·o·nide** (bu-des'ə-nīd) an anti-inflammatory glucocorticoid used to treat rhinitis and asthma, administered orally in powdered form or intranasally by inhalation of a mist.

**Bud·ge's center** (bood'gēz) [Julius Ludwig *Budge,* German physiologist, 1811–1888] 1. the ciliospinal center. 2. the genital center.

**bud·ger·i·gar** (buj'ər-ĭ-gahr") [Australian aboriginal *gijirrigaa*] [MeSH: Parrots] a species of parakeet, *Melopsittacus undulatus,* native to Australia, popular as a cage pet and used for experimental work in psittacosis. Called also *budgie.*

**bud·gie** (buj'e) budgerigar.

**Bu·din's joint, rule** (boo-daz') [Pierre-Constant *Budin,* French gynecologist, 1846–1907] see under *joint* and *rule.*

**BUDR** 5-bromodeoxyuridine.

**Buer·ger's disease, symptom** (bər'gərz) [Leo *Buerger,* American physician, 1879–1943] see *thromboangiitis obliterans* and under *symptom.*

**Buer·gi's theory** (būr'gēz) [Emil *Buergi,* Swiss pharmacologist, born 1872] see under *theory.*

**buf·fer** (buf'ər) 1. a chemical system that prevents change in the concentration of another chemical substance, e.g., proton donor and acceptor systems that prevent marked changes in hydrogen ion concentration (pH). 2. a physical or physiological system that tends to maintain constancy, e.g., reflexes regulating blood pressure.
**bicarbonate b.,** a buffer system composed of bicarbonate ions and dissolved carbon dioxide; in the body, this system is an important factor in determining the pH of the blood as the concentration of bicarbonate ions is regulated by the kidneys and of carbon dioxide by the respiratory system.
**cacodylate b.,** one containing an organic arsenical salt, used in preparing fixatives for electron microscopy.
**phosphate b.,** a buffer system composed of acid phosphate and sodium or potassium salts, e.g., monosodium and disodium acid phosphate; in the body, it is important in regulating the pH of the renal tubular fluids.
**protein b.,** a buffer system involving proton donor and proton acceptor groups of the amino acid residues of proteins.
**TRIS b.,** see *tromethamine.*
**veronal b.,** a barbital buffer commonly used in the preparation of fixatives for electron microscopy.

**buf·fer·ing** (buf'ər-ing) the action produced by a buffer.
**secondary b.,** chloride shift.

**bu·fil·con A** (bu-fil'kon) a contact lens material (hydrophobic).

**bu·fin** (bu'fin) a white secretion obtained by stimulating the parotid gland of certain species of toads by electricity; it has a physiologic action similar to that of digitalis but is not used in Western medicine.

**Bu·fo** (bu'fo) [L. "toad"] a genus of toads, species of which have been extensively studied by population geneticists. Several species have alkaloids in their skins or secretions; see *bufotoxin* and *bufotherapy. B. bu'fo bu'fo* contains bufotenin; *B. mari'nus* contains the cardiac poison marinobufagin; *B. val'liceps* contains the cardiac poison vallicepobufagin; and *B. vulga'ris* contains the toxin bufotalin.

**bu·for·min** (bu-for'min) [MeSH: Buformin] an antihyperglycemic agent related to metformin that potentiates the action of insulin, used in the treatment of type 2 diabetes mellitus; administered orally.

**bu·fo·tal·in** (bu"fo-tal'in) a poisonous principle, $C_{26}H_{36}O_6$, present in the skin and saliva of the common European toad, *Bufo vulgaris.*

**bu·fo·te·nin** (bu-fo'tə-nin) [MeSH: Bufotenin] a specific basic pressor principle, prepared from the skin glands of the toad, *Bufo bufo bufo.* It is used as a hallucinogenic in experimental medicine.

**bu·fo·ther·a·py** (bu"fo-ther'ə-pe) [L. *bufo* toad + *therapy*] the use of toad toxins in the treatment of disease.

**bu·fo·tox·in** (bu"fo-tok'sin) any toxin derived from the skin of toads, such as bufotalin, bufotenin, marinobufagin, or vallicepobufagin. See also *bufotherapy.*

**bug** (bug) an insect of the order Hemiptera.
**assassin b.,** any of various species of reduviids that attack and kill other insects; some also inflict poisonous bites on humans and other mammals.
**barley b.,** *Acarus hordei.*
**blister b.,** *Lytta vesicatoria.*
**blue b.,** *Argas persicus.*
**cone-nose b.,** any of various species of reduviid bugs; some have poisonous bites and others (such as those of genus *Triatoma*) spread disease.
**Croton b.,** German cockroach.
**great black b.,** *Triatoma infestans.*
**harvest b.,** chigger.
**hematophagous b.,** a bug that lives on blood, such as the bedbug.
**kissing b.,** any of various species of reduviids that bite humans around the mouth.
**Malay b.,** see *Reduviidae.*
**miana b., Mianeh b.,** *Argas persicus.*
**red b.,** chigger.
**wheat b.,** *Pyemotes.*

**Buhl's disease, desquamative pneumonia** (bo͞olz) [Ludwig von *Buhl,* German pathologist, 1816–1880] see under *disease.*

**bu·iat·rics** (bu"e-at'riks) [Gr. *bous* ox, cow + *-iatrics*] the treatment of diseases of cattle.

**bulb** (bulb) [L. *bul'bus;* Gr. *bolbos*] 1. a rounded mass, or enlargement. See also *bulbus.* 2. myelencephalon; see *medulla oblongata.*
**b. of aorta,** bulbus aortae.
**b. of corpus spongiosum,** bulbus penis.
**duodenal b.,** pars superior duodeni.
**end b.,** corpusculum nervosum terminale.
**end b. of Held,** an enlarged process at the end of an axon of a primary neuron of the cochlear nerve, synapsing with the body of a secondary neuron in the ventral cochlear nucleus.
**end b. of Krause,** corpusculum bulboideum.
**b. of eye,** bulbus oculi.
**b. of hair,** bulbus pili.
**b. of heart,** bulbus cordis.
**b. of jugular vein, inferior,** bulbus inferior venae jugularis.
**b. of jugular vein, superior,** bulbus superior venae jugularis.
**b. of Krause, Krause's end b.,** corpusculum bulboideum.
**b. of occipital horn of lateral ventricle,** bulbus cornus posterioris ventriculi lateralis.
**olfactory b.,** bulbus olfactorius.
**onion b.,** in neuropathology, a collection of overlapping Schwann cells resembling the bulb of an onion, encircling an axon that has become demyelinated; seen in progressive hypertrophic neuropathy and similar conditions that are characterized by repeated demyelination and remyelination.
**b. of ovary,** a bulb formed by the interweaving of veins with the

bundles of involuntary muscle within the mesovarium; called also *Rouget's b.*
**b. of penis,** bulbus penis.
**b. of posterior horn of lateral ventricle,** bulbus cornus posterioris ventriculi lateralis.
**Rouget's b.,** b. of ovary.
**sinovaginal b.,** one of the pair of endodermal outgrowths of the urogenital sinus, which later fuse to form the lower part of the vagina.
**terminal b. of Krause,** corpusculum bulboideum.
**b. of urethra,** bulbus penis.
**vaginal b.,** sinovaginal b.
**b. of vestibule of vagina, vestibulovaginal b.,** bulbus vestibuli vaginae.

**bul•bar** (bul'bər) 1. bulbous (def. 1). 2. pertaining to or involving the medulla oblongata.

**bul•bi** (bul'bi) [L.] genitive and plural of *bulbus.*

**bul•bi•form** (bul'bĭ-form) bulb-shaped.

**bul•bi•tis** (bul-bi'tis) inflammation of the bulb of the penis.

**bul•bo•atri•al** (bul"bo-a'tre-əl) pertaining to the bulbus cordis and atrium.

**bul•bo•cap•nine** (bul"bo-kap'nin) an alkaloid derived from various species of *Corydalis* and *Dicentra,* which inhibits the reflex and motor activities of striated muscle. It has been used in the treatment of muscular tremors and vestibular nystagmus. Ruminants eating such plants suffer neurotoxic effects with agitation, convulsions, and sometimes death (see also *bulbocapnine experiment,* under *experiment*).

**bul•bo•cav•er•no•sus** (bul"bo-kav"ər-no'səs) musculus bulbospongiosus.

**bul•bo•gas•trone** (bul"bo-gas'trōn) a polypeptide secreted by the duodenal bulb when the bulb is acidified; it inhibits gastric acid secretion in dogs.

**bul•boid** (bul'boid) bulb-shaped.

**bul•bo•pon•tine** (bul"bo-pon'tīn) pertaining to the pons and the region of the medulla oblongata situated dorsad to it.

**bul•bo•spi•ral** (bul"bo-spi'rəl) pertaining to the root of the aorta (bulbus aortae) and having a spiral course; said of certain bundles of cardiac muscle fibers. See also under *fiber.*

**bul•bo•spon•gi•o•sus** (bul"bo-spon"je-o'səs) see under *musculus.*

**bul•bo•ure•thral** (bul"bo-u-re'thrəl) pertaining to the bulb of the penis.

**bul•bous** (bul'bəs) 1. having the form or nature of a bulb; called also *bulbar* and *bulboid.* 2. bearing or arising from a bulb.

**bul•bus** (bul'bəs) gen. and pl. *bul'bi* [L.] 1. [TA] bulb: a general term for a rounded mass or enlargement. 2. b. encephali.
**b. aor'tae** [TA], bulb of aorta: the enlargement of the aorta at its point of origin from the heart, where the bulges of the aortic sinuses occur.
**b. arterio'sus,** b. cordis.
**b. caro'ticus,** carotid sinus.
**b. cor'dis,** the foremost of the three parts of the primordial heart of the embryo; called also *bulb of heart* and *b. arteriosus.*
**b. cor'nus occipita'lis ventri'culi latera'lis, b. cor'nus posterio'ris ventri'culi latera'lis** [TA], bulb of occipital horn of lateral ventricle: an eminence in the upper part of the medial wall of the occipital horn of the lateral ventricle, above the calcar avis, produced by the splenial fibers of the forceps frontalis as they pass posteriorly into the occipital lobe; called also *bulb of posterior horn of lateral ventricle.*
**b. cor'poris spongio'si,** b. penis.
**b. ence'phali,** TA alternative for *myelencephalon;* see *medulla oblongata.*
**b. infe'rior ve'nae jugula'ris** [TA], inferior bulb of jugular vein: a dilatation of the internal jugular vein just before it joins the brachiocephalic vein; called also *b. venae jugularis inferior.*
**b. o'culi** [TA], the eyeball or bulb of the eye; see illustration at *eye.* Called also *globe.*
**b. olfacto'rius** [TA], olfactory bulb; the bulblike expansion of the olfactory tract on the undersurface of the frontal lobe of each cerebral hemisphere; the olfactory nerves enter it. Called also *Morgagni's tubercle.*
**b. pe'nis** [TA], bulb of penis: the enlarged proximal part of the corpus spongiosum found between the two crura of the penis; called also *b. corporis spongiosi* and *b. urethrae.*
**b. pi'li,** bulb of hair: the bulbous expansion at the proximal end of a hair, in which the hair shaft is generated.
**b. supe'rior ve'nae jugula'ris** [TA], superior bulb of jugular vein: a dilatation at the beginning of the internal jugular vein; called also *b. venae jugularis superior* and *Heister's diverticulum.*
**b. ure'thrae,** b. penis.
**b. ve'nae jugula'ris infe'rior,** b. inferior venae jugularis.
**b. ve'nae jugula'ris supe'rior,** b. superior venae jugularis.
**b. vesti'buli vagi'nae** [TA], bulb of vestibule of vagina: a body consisting of paired elongated masses of erectile tissue, one on either side of the vaginal opening, united anteriorly by a narrow median band, which then expands slightly to form the glans clitoridis.

**bu•le•sis** (bu-le'sis) [Gr. *boulēsis*] the will, or an act of the will.

**bu•lim•ia** (bu-lim'e-ə) [L.; Gr. *bous* ox + *limos* hunger] [MeSH: Bulimia] episodic binge eating usually followed by behavior designed to negate the excessive caloric intake, most commonly purging behaviors such as self-induced vomiting or laxative abuse but sometimes other methods such as excessive exercise or fasting. While it is usually associated with *b. nervosa,* it may also occur in other disorders, such as *anorexia nervosa.*
**b. nervo'sa,** [DSM-IV], an eating disorder occurring predominantly in females, with onset usually in adolescence or early adulthood and characterized by episodic binge eating followed by behaviors designed to prevent weight gain, including purging, fasting, and excessive exercise. Episodes of binge eating involve intake of quantifiably excessive quantities of food within a short, discrete period as well as a sense of loss of control over food intake during these periods. The person with bulimia nervosa has a preoccupying pathological fear of becoming overweight, feels an unusually strong tie between self-worth and body shape and size, is aware that the eating pattern is abnormal, and frequently experiences feelings of self-recrimination. In contrast to persons with anorexia nervosa, patients with bulimia nervosa tend to be somewhat older, more socially inclined, have less obsessive characteristics, and do not exhibit extreme weight loss; it is not diagnosed in the presence of anorexia nervosa.

**bu•lim•ic** (bu-lim'ik) pertaining to or affected with bulimia.

**Bu•lim•i•dae** (bu-lim'ĭ-de) a family of fresh water snails of the subclass Streptoneura, order Mesogastropoda. It includes the genera *Bulimus, Oncomelania, Parafossarulus,* and *Pomatiopsis.*

**Bu•lim•i•nae** (bu-lim'ĭ-ne) a subfamily of snails of the family Hydrobiidae; medically important genera include *Bulimus* and *Parafossarulus.*

**Bu•li•mus** (bu-li'məs) a genus of small fresh water snails of the family Bulimidae; formerly called *Bithynia.*
**B. fuchsia'nus,** the chief intermediate host of the human liver flukes *Clonorchis* and *Opisthorchis;* it is commonly found in southern China.
**B. lea'chii,** a species found in northern Europe and the northwestern United States, which ingests the eggs of the liver fluke *Opisthorchis felineus* and in whose body the eggs hatch.

**Bu•li•nus** (bu-li'nəs) [MeSH: Bulinus] a genus of snails of the family Planorbidae. Several species are intermediate hosts of *Schistosoma haematobium* and *Opisthorchis.*

**bulk•age** (bulk'əj) material that will increase the bulk of the intestinal contents and consequently stimulate peristalsis.

**Bull.** abbreviation for L. *bul'liat,* let it boil.

**bul•la** (bul'ə) pl. *bul'lae* [L.] 1. a large elevation on the skin, containing serous or seropurulent fluid. Cf. *vesicle* (def. 1). Called also *bleb* and *blister.* 2. a rounded, projecting anatomical structure.
**emphysematous b.,** any space in a distended area of an emphysematous lung, ranging in size from one centimeter to most of a hemithorax.
**ethmoid b.,** see *b. ethmoidalis cavi nasi* and *b. ethmoidalis ossis ethmoidalis.*
**b. ethmoida'lis ca'vi na'si** [TA], ethmoidal bulla of nasal cavity: the large ethmoid air cell lodged in the bulla ethmoidalis ossis ethmoidalis.
**b. ethmoida'lis os'sis ethmoida'lis** [TA], ethmoidal bulla of ethmoidal bone: a rounded projection of the ethmoid bone into the lateral wall of the middle nasal meatus just below the middle nasal concha, enclosing a large ethmoid air cell; called also *antrum ethmoidale* and *ethmoid antrum.*
**b. mastoi'dea,** a large air cell in the mastoid of certain animals.
**b. os'sea,** the dilated part of the bony external meatus of the ear.

**bul•lae** (bul'e) plural of *bulla.*

**bul•late** (bul'āt) [L. *bullatus*] 1. bullous (def. 2). 2. inflated.

**bul•la•tion** (bə-la'-shən) [L. *bullatio*] 1. the presence of bullae. 2. the state of being inflated.

**bul•lec•to•my** (bə-lek'tə-me) [*bulla* + *-ectomy*] excision of a bulla, especially one of the giant ones seen in bullous emphysema in order to improve pulmonary function. See also *reduction pneumoplasty.*

**Bul•ler's shield (bandage)** (bul'ərz) [Frank *Buller,* Canadian ophthalmologic surgeon, 1844–1905] see under *shield.*

**bull•neck** (bool'nek) bull neck; see under *neck.*

**bull•nose** (bool'nōz) necrotic rhinitis.

**bul·lo·sis** (bul-o'sis) the production of, or a condition characterized by, bullous lesions.
**diabetic b.,** a condition in which bullae appear spontaneously, usually on the ankles and feet, in some uncontrolled diabetics.

**bul·lous** (bul'əs) 1. pertaining to bullae. 2. characterized by bullae; called also *bullate.*

**bum·ble·foot** (bum'bəl-foot) inflammation of the ball of the foot of fowls, usually caused by staphylococcus.

**bu·met·a·nide** (bu-met'ə-nīd) [USP] [MeSH: Bumetanide] a loop diuretic used in the treatment of edema associated with congestive heart failure or hepatic or renal disease; administered orally, intramuscularly, or intravenously.

**Bu·mex** (bu'meks) trademark for preparations of bumetanide.

**Bu·mi·nate** (bu'mĭ-nāt) trademark for a preparation of albumin human.

**Bum·ke's pupil** (boom'kez) [Oswald Conrad Edward *Bumke,* German neurologist, 1877–1950] see under *pupil.*

**bumps** (bumps) erythema nodosum sometimes seen in cases of primary coccidioidomycosis; called also *desert bumps* and *valley bumps.*

**BUN** blood urea nitrogen; see *urea nitrogen.*

**bu·nam·i·dine hy·dro·chlo·ride** (bu-nam'ĭ-dēn) an anthelmintic used in cats and dogs.

**bun·dle** (bun'dəl) a collection of muscle or nerve fibers; see also *fasciculus, fiber, lemniscus, tract,* and *tractus.*
**aberrant b's,** collections of pyramidal fibers leaving the corticonuclear tract at successive levels of the brain stem, and giving off fibers to the motor nuclei of the cranial nerves.
**atrioventricular b., AV b.,** b. of His.
**Bachmann's b.,** a group of fibers of the anterior internodal tract that penetrate the interatrial septum and diverge in the left atrium, connecting the atria.
**comb b.,** nigrostriate tract.
**common b.,** truncus fasciculi atrioventricularis.
**hair b.,** the organelle that contains the receptors for hearing and equilibrium, found at the apex of a hair cell; it consists of about 100 stereocilia and usually a kinocilium.
**Helweg's b.,** olivospinal tract.
**b. of His,** a small band of atypical cardiac muscle fibers that originates in the atrioventricular node in the interatrial septum, passes through the atrioventricular junction, and then runs beneath the endocardium of the right ventricle on the membranous part of the interventricular septum. It divides at the upper end of the muscular part of the interventricular septum into right and left bundle branches which descend in the septal wall of the right and left ventricle, respectively, to be distributed to those two chambers. This bundle propagates the atrial contraction rhythm to the ventricles, and its interruption produces heart block. The term is often used to refer specifically to the trunk of the bundle *(truncus fasciculi atrioventricularis)* rather than the entire bundle. Called also *fasciculus atrioventricularis* [TA], *atrioventricular b., AV b., Kent-His b.,* and *His' band.* See illustration.
**Kent's b.,** a muscular bundle in the heart of several mammalian species forming a direct connection between the atrial and ventricular walls; it occasionally occurs in the human heart, where it can form an accessory conducting pathway allowing the preexcitation of the ventricle that occurs in the Wolff-Parkinson-White syndrome. Called also *atrioventricular pathway.*
**Kent-His b.,** b. of His.
**longitudinal medial b.,** fasciculus longitudinalis medialis.
**medial forebrain b.,** fasciculus medialis telencephali.
**Meynert's b.,** tractus habenulointerpeduncularis.
**Monakow's b.,** tractus rubrospinalis.
**muscle b.,** one of the primary longitudinal subdivisions of a muscle, made up of muscle fibers and separated from other bundles by fascial septa or perimysium.
**olivocochlear b. of Rasmussen,** tractus olivocochlearis.
**b. of Oort,** tractus olivocochlearis.
**papillomacular b's,** an oval shaped arrangement of ganglion cell axons extending from the macula lutea to the optic disk, then entering the optic nerve as discrete bundles.
**posterior longitudinal b.,** fasciculus longitudinalis medialis.
**b. of Rasmussen,** tractus olivocochlearis.
**Schütz's b.,** fasciculus longitudinalis posterior.
**solitary b.,** tractus solitarius medullae oblongatae.
**thalamomammillary b.,** fasciculus mammillothalamicus.
**Thorel's b.,** a bundle of muscle fibers in the human heart, connecting the sinoatrial and atrioventricular nodes, and passing around the mouth of the inferior vena cava.
**transverse b's of palmar aponeurosis,** fasciculi transversi aponeurosis palmaris; see under *fasciculus.*

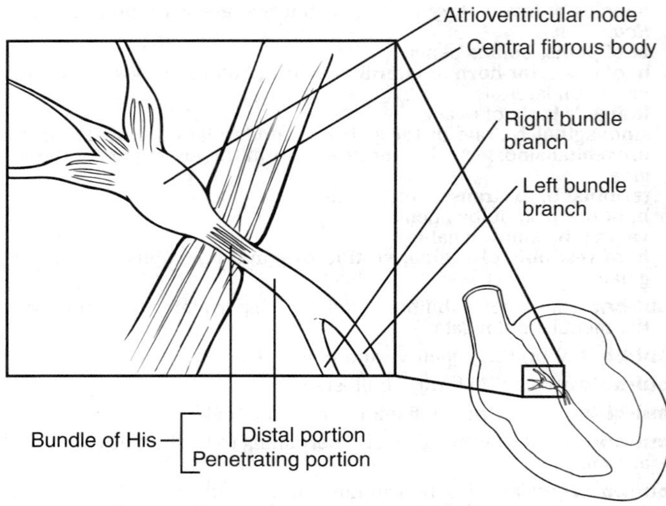

Bundle of His considered as the trunk of the bundle and excluding the bundle branches.

**Türck's b.,** fibrae thalamopontinae.
**Weissmann's b.,** the bundle of striated muscle fibers of a neuromuscular spindle.

**bun·dle branch** (bun'dəl branch) see under *branch.*

**bun·ga·ro·tox·in** (bung″gə-ro-tok'sin) a strong neurotoxin from the venom of kraits *(Bungarus);* three electrophoretic fractions, α-, β-, and γ-bungarotoxin, have been identified. α-Bungarotoxin, the chief fraction, binds irreversibly with acetylcholine receptors, producing neuromuscular block.

**Bun·ga·rus** (bung'gə-rəs) [MeSH: Bungarus] the kraits, a genus of venomous snakes of the family Elapidae, found in the Indian subcontinent, Southeast Asia, and China. See table at *snake.*

**Bun·ge's amputation** (boon'gəz) [Richard *Bunge,* German surgeon, born 1870] aperiosteal amputation.

**bung·eye** (bung'i) cutaneous habronemiasis around the eye.

**Büng·ner's bands** (bēng'nərz) [Otto von *Büngner,* German neurologist, 1858–1905] see under *band.*

**bun·ion** (bun'yən) [L. *bunio;* Gr. *bounion* turnip] abnormal prominence of the inner aspect of the first metatarsal head, accompanied by bursal formation and resulting in a lateral or valgus displacement of the great toe.
**tailor's b.,** bunionette.

**bun·ion·ec·to·my** (bun″yən-ek'tə-me) [*bunion* + *ectomy*] excision of an abnormal prominence on the mesial aspect of the first metatarsal head.

**bun·ion·ette** (bun″yən-et') enlargement of the lateral aspect of the fifth metatarsal head; called also *tailor's bunion.*

**Bun·nell's suture** (bə-nelz') [Sterling *Bunnell,* American surgeon, 1882–1957] see under *suture.*

**bu·no·dont** (bu'no-dont) [Gr. *bounos* hill + *odous* tooth] having cheek teeth with low rounded cusps on the occlusal surface of the

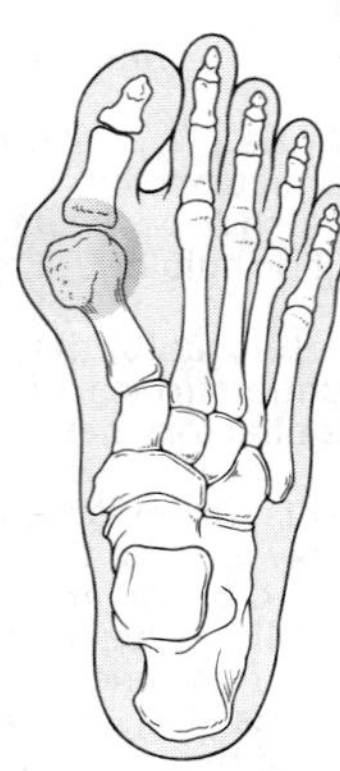
Bunion.

crown, as in mammals with mixed diet, such as swine, many rodents, and humans.

**bu·no·lol hy·dro·chlo·ride** (bu'no-lol) a beta-adrenergic blocking agent, having the same actions as propranolol (q.v.).

**bu·no·lo·pho·dont** (bu″no-lo'fə-dont) [Gr. *bounos* hill + *lophodont*] having cheek teeth with both rounded cusps and transverse ridges on the occlusal surface of the crown, as in some kangaroos.

**bu·no·se·le·no·dont** (bu″no-sə-le'no-dont) [Gr. *bounos* hill + *selenodont*] having cheek teeth with both rounded cusps and crescentic ridges on the occlusal surface of the crown.

**bu·no·sto·mi·a·sis** (bu″no-stə-mi'ə-sis) hookworm disease in ruminants caused by species of *Bunostomum.*

**Bu·no·sto·mum** (bu″no-sto'məm) a genus of hookworms of the family Ancylostomatidae that parasitize cattle, sheep, and other ruminants; called also *Monodontus.*

**Bun·sen burner, coefficient** (bun'sən) [Robert Wilhelm Eberhard *Bunsen,* German chemist, 1811–1899] see under *burner* and *coefficient.*

**Bun·ya·vi·ri·dae** (bun″yə-vir'ĭ-de) [MeSH: Bunyaviridae] the bunyaviruses: a family of RNA viruses having a spherical or oval virion 80–120 nm in diameter consisting of a lipid bilayer envelope, with glycoprotein surface projections 5–10 nm long and 10–12 nm across in hexagonal arrangement, surrounding three loosely helical nucleocapsids. The genome consists of three molecules of circular negative-sense or ambisense single-stranded RNA, designated L, M, and S (total MW $4.8–8 \times 10^6$, size of total genome 11–20 kb). Viruses contain four major structural polypeptides, including a transcriptase, and are sensitive to lipid solvents and detergents. Replication occurs in the cytoplasm and assembly is by budding through the smooth membrane of the Golgi apparatus. Host ranges vary; transmission is generally by arthropod vectors, although transmission by aerosols and avian vectors sometimes occurs. Genera include *Bunyavirus, Hantavirus, Nairovirus, Phlebovirus,* and *Tospovirus.*

**Bun·ya·vi·rus** (bun'yə-vi″rəs) [*Bunyamwera,* town in Uganda where the type species was isolated] [MeSH: Bunyavirus] the Bunyamwera supergroup of viruses; a widespread genus of viruses of the family Bunyaviridae, containing at least 161 species in 18 serogroups and 4 unclassified species; human pathogens of this genus cause febrile disease and encephalitis. Important pathogenic species include Bunyamwera, Bwamba, California encephalitis, Guama, Jamestown Canyon, LaCrosse, Oropouche, and Tahyna viruses. The usual mode of transmission is by the bite of infected mosquitoes, although a few species are tick-borne.

**bun·ya·vi·rus** (bun'yə-vi″rəs) [MeSH: Bunyavirus] any virus belonging to the family Bunyaviridae.

**buph·thal·mia** (bŭf-thal'me-ə) buphthalmos; hydrophthalmos.

**buph·thal·mos** (bŭf-thal'mos) [Gr. *bous* ox + *ophthalmos* eye] enlargement and distention of the fibrous coats of the eye; hydrophthalmos; congenital glaucoma. Called also *megophthalmos.*

**buph·thal·mus** (bŭf-thal'məs) buphthalmos; hydrophthalmos.

**bu·piv·a·caine hy·dro·chlo·ride** (bu-piv'ə-kān) [USP] a homologue of mepivacaine, chemically related to lidocaine, used as a local anesthetic for local infiltration, peripheral nerve block, retrobulbar block, sympathetic block, and caudal and epidural anesthesia.

**bu·pre·nor·phine hy·dro·chlo·ride** (bu″prə-nor'fēn) [USP] a synthetic opioid agonist-antagonist derived from thebaine, used as an analgesic for moderate to severe pain and as an anesthesia adjunct; administered sublingually or by intramuscular or intravenous injection.

**bu·pro·pi·on hy·dro·chlo·ride** (bu-pro'pe-on) a monocyclic compound structurally similar to amphetamine, used as an antidepressant and as an aid in smoking cessation to reduce the symptoms of nicotine withdrawal; administered orally.

**bur** (bər) 1. a metal rotary dental instrument with cutting heads of various shapes, held and revolved in a handpiece; used to remove carious material from within decayed teeth, reduce decayed or fractured hard tissues, form the design of the cavity preparation, and finish and polish the teeth and restorations. Called also *drill.* 2. a type of surgical drill for making holes in bones. In both senses, also spelled *burr.*

**bur·bu·lence** (bər'bu-ləns″) gaseousness; a group of symptoms of intestinal origin, including a feeling of fullness, bloating or distention, borborygmus, and flatulence.

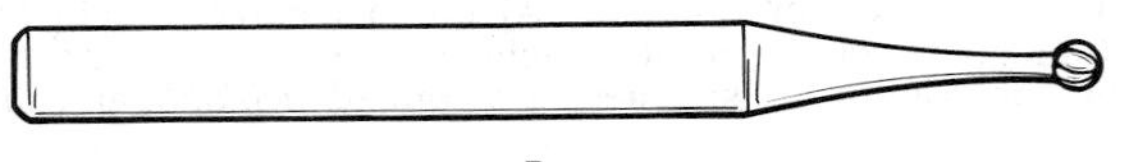

Bur.

**Bur·dach's cuneate fasciculus (bundle, columns, fibers, tract),** etc. (bo͞or'dahks) [Karl Friedrich *Burdach,* German physiologist, 1776–1847] see under *fissure;* see *fasciculus cuneatus medullae spinalis* and *fasciculus longitudinalis superior cerebri,* under *fasciculus;* and see *nucleus cuneatus,* under *nucleus.*

**bu·ret, bu·rette** (bu-ret') a graduated glass tube used in volumetric chemistry to deliver a measured amount of liquid.

**Bür·ger-Grütz syndrome** (bĕr'gər-grĕtz) [Max *Bürger,* German physician, born 1885; Otto *Grütz,* German physician, 20th century] familial hyperlipoproteinemia, type I; see under *hyperlipoproteinemia.*

**bu·rim·amide** (bu-rim'ə-mīd) [MeSH: Burimamide] an antagonist to histamine, competing for the $histamine_2$ receptor site on cells.

**Burk·hol·de·ria** (bərk″hol-der'e-ə) [MeSH: Burkholderia] a genus of gram-negative, rod-shaped bacteria of the family Pseudomonadaceae, comprising animal and plant pathogens formerly classified in group II of the genus *Pseudomonas.*
**B. cepa'cia,** the type species; a widespread species isolated from clinical specimens and hospital equipment and supplies that is an opportunistic pathogen and causes various nosocomial infections. It appears to be an important respiratory pathogen in children with cystic fibrosis. Formerly classified as *Pseudomonas cepacia.*
**B. mal'lei,** a nonmotile species that is pathogenic chiefly for horses, causing glanders; it may also infect other animals and humans. Formerly classified as *Pseudomonas mallei.*
**B. picket'tii,** former name for *Ralstonia pickettii.*
**B. pseudomal'lei,** the species that causes melioidosis in humans and animals; it has been isolated from soil and water in tropical regions. Formerly classified as *Pseudomonas pseudomallei.*

**Bur·kitt's lymphoma** (bər'kits) [Denis Parsons *Burkitt,* Irish surgeon in Uganda, 1911–1993] [MeSH: Burkitt's Lymphoma] see under *lymphoma.*

**burn** (bərn) [MeSH: Burns] injury to tissues caused by contact with dry heat (fire), moist heat (steam or hot liquid), chemicals (e.g., corrosive substances), electricity (current or lightning), friction, or radiant and electromagnetic energy. Burns of the *first degree* show redness; of the *second degree,* vesication; of the *third degree,* necrosis through the entire skin. Burns of the first and second degree are known as *partial-thickness* burns, those of the third degree as *full-thickness* burns.
**brush b.,** a wound caused by violent rubbing or friction, as by a rope pulled through the hands; called also *friction b.*
**chemical b.,** irritant dermatitis caused by various caustic substances, such as acids, disinfectants, and alkalis.
**contact b.,** a burn produced by contact with electric current.
**electric b., electrical b.,** see *flash b.* and *contact b.*
**flash b.,** a thermal lesion produced by a very brief exposure to radiant heat of high intensity, as in an explosion or a sudden discharge of electricity.
**friction b.,** brush b.
**radiation b.,** a burn caused by exposure to x-ray, radium, sunlight, atomic, or any other type of radiant energy.
**sun b.,** sunburn.
**thermal b.,** injury due to contact with flame, hot objects, or hot liquids, as distinguished from chemical and electric burns.
**x-ray b.,** a lesion caused by exposure to x-rays.

**burn·er** (bər'nər) the part of a lamp, stove, or furnace from which the flame issues.
**Argand b.,** a burner for oil or gas, with an inner tube for supplying air to the flame.
**Bunsen b.,** a gas burner in which the gas is mixed with air before ignition, in order to give complete oxidation.

**Bur·net** (bər-net') Sir Frank Macfarlane. Australian physician and virologist, 1899–1985; co-winner, with Peter B. Medawar, of the Nobel prize in medicine and physiology for 1960, for the discovery of acquired immunological tolerance and for the conceptual framework of immunology in the clonal selection theory.

**Bur·nett's disinfecting fluid** (bər-nets') [Sir William *Burnett,* Scottish surgeon, 1779–1861] see under *fluid.*

**Bur·nett's syndrome** (bər-nets') [Charles Hoyt *Burnett,* American physician, 1913–1967] milk alkali syndrome.

**bur·nish·er** (bər'nish-ər) a dental instrument with a blade or nib with a beveled edge used for smoothing out roughness at the margin of a restoration and the enamel.

**bur·nish·ing** (bər'nish-ing) 1. condensation and polishing under the sliding pressure of a smooth hard instrument, as in finishing the surface of a gold filling. 2. adaptation of a thin, annealed sheet metal by means of a burnisher, as in forming a band about a tooth root or in fitting a matrix for porcelain.

**Burns' ligament, space** (bərnz) [Allan *Burns,* Scottish anatomist, 1781–1813] see *margo falciformis hiatus saphenus* and *fossa jugularis,* def. 1.

**Bur·ow's operation, solution, vein** (bo͞or'ovz) [Karl August *Burow,* German surgeon, 1809–1874] see under *operation* and *vein,* and see *aluminum acetate topical solution,* under *solution.*

**burr** (bər) bur.

**bur·sa** (bər'sə) pl. *bur'sae* [L.; Gr. "a wine skin"] [TA] a sac or saclike cavity filled with a viscid fluid and situated at places in the tissues at which friction would otherwise develop.

## Bursa

Descriptions are given on TA terms, and include anglicized names of specific bursae.

**b. of Achilles, b. of Achilles tendon,** b. tendinis calcanei.
**acromial b.,** b. subdeltoidea.
**adventitious b.,** an abnormal cyst due to friction or some other mechanical cause, and containing synovial fluid; called also *supernumerary b.*
**anconeal b.,** b. subcutanea olecrani.
**anconeal b. of triceps muscle,** b. subtendinea musculi tricipitis brachii.
**b. anseri'na** [TA], **anserine b.,** a bursa between the tendons of the sartorius, gracilis, and semitendinosus muscles, and the tibial collateral ligament; called also *anterior genual b.*
**bicipital b.,** 1. b. subtendinea musculi bicipitalis femoris inferior. 2. intertubercular b., def. 2.
**bicipitofibular b.,** b. subtendinea musculi bicipitalis femoris inferior.
**bicipitoradial b., b. bicipitoradia'lis** [TA], a bursa between the radial tuberosity and the biceps tendon.
**Boyer's b.,** b. retrohyoidea.
**Brodie's b.,** b. subtendinea musculi gastrocnemii medialis.
**calcaneal b.,** b. tendinis calcanei.
**calcaneal b., subcutaneous,** b. subcutanea calcanea.
**b. of calcaneal tendon,** b. tendinis calcanei.
**Calori's b.,** a bursa situated between the trachea and the arch of the aorta.
**b. copula'trix,** an appendage at the posterior end of the male of certain nematodes.
**coracobrachial b.,** b. musculi coracobrachialis.
**coracoid b.,** b. subtendinea musculi subscapularis.
**b. cubita'lis interos'sea** [TA], **cubitoradial b.,** interosseous cubital bursa: a bursa between the ulna, the biceps tendon, and nearby muscles; called also *ulnoradial b.*
**deltoid b.,** b. subacromialis.
**b.-equivalent,** analogous to the bursa of Fabricius; see *B lymphocyte,* under *lymphocyte,* and *bursa-equivalent tissue,* under *tissue.*
**b. of Fabricius,** a lymphoid organ of birds that, like the thymus, develops as an epithelial outpouching of the gut but near the cloaca rather than the foregut; it atrophies at 5 or 6 months of age, persisting as a fibrous remnant in sexually mature birds; before involution it is the site of maturation of B lymphocytes (q.v.).
**fibular b.,** b. subtendinea musculi bicipitis femoris inferior.
**Fleischmann's b.,** one beneath the tongue.
**b. of flexor carpi radialis muscle,** vagina synovialis tendinis musculi flexoris carpi radialis.
**gastrocnemiosemimembranous b.,** b. musculi semimembranosi.
**genual b., anterior,** b. anserina.
**genual b., external inferior,** b. subtendinea musculi bicipitis femoris inferior.
**genual bursae, internal superior,** bursae subtendineae musculi sartorii.
**genual b., posterior,** b. musculi semimembranosi.
**bur'sae glutaeofemora'les,** bursae intermusculares musculorum gluteorum.
**gluteal b.,** one situated beneath the gluteus maximus muscle.
**gluteal intermuscular bursae,** bursae intermusculares musculorum gluteorum.
**gluteofascial bursae,** bursae intermusculares musculorum gluteorum.
**gluteofemoral bursae,** bursae intermusculares musculorum gluteorum.
**gluteotuberosal b.,** b. ischiadica musculi glutei maximi.
**His' b.,** the dilatation at the end of the archenteron.
**humeral b.,** 1. b. subacromialis. 2. b. subtendinea musculi gastrocnemii lateralis.
**hyoid b.,** b. subcutanea prominentiae laryngeae.
**iliac b., subtendinous, b. ili'aca subtendi'nea,** b. subtendinea iliaca.
**b. iliopecti'nea** [TA], **iliopectineal b.,** a bursa between the iliopsoas tendon and the iliopectineal eminence; called also *subiliac b.* and *iliopubic vesicular b.*
**b. of iliopsoas muscle,** b. subtendinea iliaca.
**inferior b. of biceps femoris muscle,** b. subtendinea musculi bicipitis femoris inferior.
**infracardiac b.,** the cranial end of a coelomic recess of the embryo, extending upward between the esophagus and right lung bud; frequently persisting in the adult.
**infracondyloid b., external,** recessus subpopliteus.
**infragenual b.,** b. infrapatellaris profunda.
**infrahyoid b., b. infrahyoi'dea** [TA], a bursa sometimes present below the hyoid bone at the attachment of the sternohyoid muscle.
**infrapatellar b.,** b. subtendinea prepatellaris.
**infrapatellar b., deep,** b. infrapatellaris profunda.
**infrapatellar b., subcutaneous,** b. subcutanea infrapatellaris.
**infrapatellar b., superficial inferior,** b. subcutanea tuberositatis tibiae.
**b. infrapatella'ris profun'da** [TA], deep infrapatellar bursa: a bursa between the patellar ligament and the tibia; called also *infragenual b., subpatellar b.,* and *subligamentous b.*
**b. infrapatella'ris subcuta'nea,** b. subcutanea infrapatellaris.
**bur'sae intermuscula'res musculo'rum gluteo'rum** [TA], intermuscular gluteal bursae: several sacs that surround the tendon attaching the gluteus maximus to the femur; called also *bursae glutaeofemorales, gluteofascial bursae,* and *gluteofemoral bursae.*
**interosseous cubital b.,** b. cubitalis interossea.
**intertubercular b.,** 1. vagina synovialis intertubercularis. 2. on a quadruped, a bursa between the tendon of the biceps brachii muscle and the intertubercular groove of the humerus. Called also *bicipital b.*
**b. intratendi'nea olecra'ni** [TA], intratendinous bursa of olecranon: a bursa within the triceps tendon near its insertion; called also *intratendinous supra-anconeal b.* and *Monro's b.*
**ischiadic b.,** b. ischiadica musculi obturatorii interni.
**b. ischia'dica mus'culi glu'tei max'imi** [TA], ischial bursa of gluteus maximus muscle: a bursa between the ischial tuberosity and the gluteus maximus; called also *b. sciatica musculi glutei maximi* [TA alternative], *gluteotuberosal b.,* and *sciatic b. of gluteus maximus muscle.*
**b. ischia'dica mus'culi obturato'rii inter'ni** [TA], sciatic bursa of obturator internus muscle: a bursa between the tendon of the obturator internus muscle and the lesser sciatic notch; called also *b. sciatica musculi obturatorii interni, ischiadic b., ischial b. of obturator internus muscle,* and *tuberoischiadic b.*
**ischial b. of gluteus maximus muscle,** b. ischiadica musculi glutei maximi.
**ischial b. of obturator internus muscle,** b. ischiadica musculi obturatorii interni.
**lateral b. of gastrocnemius muscle,** b. subtendinea musculi gastrocnemii lateralis.
**b. of latissimus dorsi muscle,** subtendinea musculi latissimi dorsi.
**Luschka's b.,** b. pharyngealis.
**medial b. of gastrocnemius muscle,** b. subtendinea musculi gastrocnemii medialis.
**Monro's b.,** b. intratendinea olecrani.
**b. muco'sa,** b. synovialis.
**b. muco'sa submuscula'ris,** b. synovialis submuscularis.
**mucous b.,** b. synovialis.
**multilocular b.,** one which is subdivided into several compartments.
**b. mus'culi bici'pitis fe'moris infe'rior,** b. subtendinea musculi bicipitis femoris inferior.
**b. mus'culi bici'pitis fe'moris supe'rior** [TA], superior bursa of biceps femoris muscle: a bursa between the long head of the biceps, the semitendinosus, the tendon of the semimembranosus, and the ischial tuberosity; called also *subtendinous b.*
**b. mus'culi coracobrachia'lis** [TA], bursa of coracobrachialis muscle: a bursa between the coracobrachialis and subscapularis muscles and the coracoid process; called also *coracobrachial b.* and *subcoracoid b.*
**b. mus'culi extenso'ris car'pi radia'lis bre'vis,** a bursa between the tendon and the base of the third metacarpal bone.

**b. mus′culi gastrocne′mii latera′lis,** b. subtendinea musculi gastrocnemii lateralis.
**b. mus′culi gastrocne′mii media′lis,** b. subtendinea musculi gastrocnemii medialis.
**b. mus′culi infraspina′ti,** b. subtendinea musculi infraspinati.
**b. mus′culi latis′simi dor′si,** b. subtendinea musculi latissimi dorsi.
**b. mus′culi obturato′ris inter′ni,** see *b. ischiadica musculi obturatorii interni* and *b. subtendinea musculi obturatorii interni.*
**b. mus′culi pirifor′mis** [TA], bursa of piriform muscle: a bursa between the piriformis tendon, the superior gemellus muscle, and the femur; called also *piriform b.*
**b. mus′culi popli′tei,** recessus subpopliteus.
**b. mus′culi sarto′rii pro′pria,** see *bursae subtendineae musculi sartorii.*
**b. mus′culi semimembrano′si** [TA], bursa of semimembranosus muscle: a bursa between the semimembranosus muscle and the medial head of the gastrocnemius. Called also *gastrocnemiosemimembranous b., posterior genual b., retrocondyloid b., semimembranosogastrocnemial b.,* and *semimembranous b.*
**b. mus′culi sternohyoi′dei,** see *b. infrahyoidea* and *b. retrohyoidea.*
**b. mus′culi subscapula′ris,** b. subtendinea musculi subscapularis.
**b. mus′culi tenso′ris ve′li palati′ni** [TA], bursa of tensor veli palatini muscle: a bursa between the hamular process of the sphenoid bone and the tendon of the tensor veli palatini.
**b. mus′culi te′retis majo′ris,** b. subtendinea musculi teretis majoris.
**b. mus′culi thyrohyoi′dei,** a bursa under the thyrohyoid muscle.
**b. of olecranon,** b. subcutanea olecrani.
**omental b., b. omenta′lis** [TA], a serous peritoneal cavity situated behind the stomach, the lesser omentum, and part of the liver and in front of the pancreas and duodenum. It communicates with the general peritoneal cavity (greater sac) through the epiploic foramen and sometimes is continuous with the cavity of the greater omentum. Called also *lesser peritoneal cavity.*
**ovarian b., b. ova′rica,** the peritoneal fossa in which the ovary is situated.
**patellar b., deep,** b. subtendinea prepatellaris.
**patellar b., middle,** b. subfascialis prepatellaris.
**patellar b., prespinous,** b. subcutanea tuberositatis tibiae.
**patellar b., subcutaneous,** b. subcutanea prepatellaris.
**peroneal b., common,** vagina synovialis musculorum peroneorum communis.
**b. pharyn′gea, pharyngeal b., b. pharyngea′lis** [TA], an inconstant blind sac located above the pharyngeal tonsil in the midline of the posterior wall of the nasopharynx; it represents persistence of an embryonic communication between the anterior tip of the notochord and the roof of the pharynx. Called also *Luschka's b., Tornwaldt's b.,* and *Tornwaldt's cyst.*
**b. of piriform muscle,** b. musculi piriformis.
**popliteal b., b. of popliteal muscle,** recessus subpopliteus.
**postcalcaneal b.,** b. subcutanea calcanea.
**postcalcaneal b., deep,** b. tendinis calcanei.
**postgenual b., external,** b. subtendinea musculi gastrocnemii lateralis.
**b. praepatella′ris subcuta′nea,** b. subcutanea prepatellaris.
**b. praepatella′ris subfascia′lis,** b. subfascialis prepatellaris.
**b. praepatella′ris subtendin′ea,** b. subtendinea prepatellaris.
**prepatellar b., middle,** b. subfascialis prepatellaris.
**prepatellar b., subcutaneous,** b. subcutanea prepatellaris.
**prepatellar b., subfascial,** b. subfascialis prepatellaris.
**prepatellar b., subtendinous,** b. subtendinea prepatellaris.
**bur′sae prepatella′res,** see *b. subcutanea prepatellaris, b. subfascialis prepatellaris,* and *b. subtendinea prepatellaris.*
**b. prepatella′ris profun′da, b. prepatella′ris subaponeuro′tica,** b. subtendinea prepatellaris.
**pretibial b.,** b. subcutanea tuberositatis tibiae.
**bur′sae pro′priae mus′culi sarto′rii,** bursae subtendineae musculi sartorii.
**pyriform b.,** b. musculi piriformis.
**b. of quadratus femoris muscle,** b. subtendinea iliaca.
**retrocalcaneal b.,** b. tendinis calcanei.
**retrocondyloid b.,** b. musculi semimembranosi.
**retroepicondyloid b., lateral, deep,** b. subtendinea musculi gastrocnemii lateralis.
**retrohyoid b., b. retrohyoi′dea** [TA], a bursa sometimes present behind the hyoid bone at the attachment of the sternohyoid muscle.
**retromammary b.,** a well-defined loose areolar tissue between the deep layer of superficial fascia on the posterior aspect of the breast, and the deep fascia covering the pectoralis major and other muscles of the chest wall.
**sciatic b. of gluteus maximus muscle,** b. ischiadica musculi glutei maximi.
**sciatic b. of obturator internus muscle,** b. ischiadica musculi obturatorii interni.
**b. scia′tica mus′culi glu′tei max′imi,** b. ischiadica musculi glutei maximi.
**b. scia′tica mus′culi obturato′rii inter′ni,** b. ischiadica musculi obturatorii interni.
**semimembranosogastrocnemial b., semimembranous b.,** b. of semimembranosus muscle.
**semitendinous b.,** b. musculi bicipitis femoris superior.
**sternohyoid b., b. sternohyoi′dea,** either of two bursae located where the sternohyoid muscle attaches to the hyoid bone; see *b. infrahyoidea* and *b. retrohyoidea.*
**subachilleal b.,** b. tendinis calcanei.
**subacromial b., b. subacromia′lis** [TA], one between the acromion and the insertion of the supraspinatus muscle, extending between the deltoid and the greater tubercle of the humerus; called also *deltoid b.* and *humeral b.*
**subcalcaneal b.,** b. subcutanea calcanea.
**subclavian b.,** an inconstant bursa between the fibers of the rhomboid ligament.
**subcoracoid b.,** 1. b. musculi coracobrachialis. 2. b. subtendinea musculi subscapularis.
**subcrural b.,** b. suprapatellaris.
**b. subcuta′nea** [TA], subcutaneous bursa: a synovial sac found beneath the skin; called also *b. synovialis subcutanea* and *subcutaneous synovial b.*
**b. subcuta′nea acromia′lis** [TA], subcutaneous acromial bursa: a bursa between the acromion and the overlying skin.
**b. subcuta′nea calca′nea** [TA], subcutaneous calcaneal bursa: a bursa between the calcaneus and the skin on the sole of the foot; called also *postcalcaneal b.,* and *subcalcaneal b.*
**b. subcuta′nea infrapatella′ris** [TA], subcutaneous infrapatellar bursa: a bursa between the upper end of the patellar ligament and the skin; called also *b. infrapatellaris subcutanea, subpatellar b.,* and *superficial b. of knee.*
**b. subcuta′nea malle′oli latera′lis** [TA], subcutaneous bursa of lateral malleolus: a bursa between the lateral malleolus and the skin.
**b. subcuta′nea malle′oli media′lis** [TA], subcutaneous bursa of medial malleolus: a bursa between the medial malleolus and the skin.
**b. subcuta′nea olecra′ni** [TA], subcutaneous bursa of olecranon: a bursa between the olecranon process and the skin; called also *anconeal b.* and *superficial b. of olecranon.*
**b. subcuta′nea prepatella′ris** [TA], subcutaneous prepatellar bursa: a bursa between the patella and the skin; called also *b. praepatellaris subcutanea.*
**b. subcuta′nea prominen′tiae laryn′geae** [TA], **b. subcuta′nea prominen′tiae laryngea′lis,** subcutaneous bursa of laryngeal prominence: a bursa anterior to the laryngeal prominence of the thyroid cartilage, under the skin; called also *hyoid b., subhyoid b.,* and *thyrohyoid b.*
**b. subcuta′nea tuberosita′tis ti′biae** [TA], subcutaneous bursa of tuberosity of tibia: a bursa between the tibial tuberosity and the skin; called also *patellar b., prespinous, pretibial b.,* and *superficial inferior infrapatellar b.*
**subcutaneous b.,** b. subcutanea.
**subcutaneous acromial b.,** b. subcutanea acromialis.
**subcutaneous b. of laryngeal prominence,** b. subcutanea promentiae laryngealis.
**subcutaneous b. of lateral malleolus,** b. subcutanea malleoli lateralis.
**subcutaneous b. of medial malleolus,** b. subcutanea malleoli medialis.
**subcutaneous b. of olecranon,** b. subcutanea olecrani.
**subcutaneous synovial b.,** b. subcutanea.
**subcutaneous b. of tuberosity of tibia,** b. subcutanea tuberositatis tibiae.

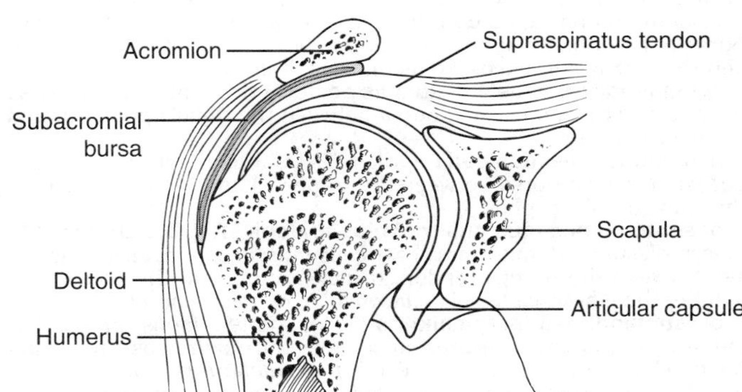


Bursa subacromialis (subacromial bursa), lying between the acromion and supraspinatus tendon and extending between the deltoid and greater tubercle.

**subdeltoid b., b. subdeltoi'dea** [TA], a bursa between the deltoid and the shoulder joint capsule, usually connected to the subacromial bursa; called also *acromial b.*

**b. subfascia'lis** [TA], **subfascial synovial b.,** subfascial bursa: synovial sac found beneath a fascial layer; called also *b. synovialis subfascialis.*

**b. subfascia'lis prepatella'ris** [TA], subfascial prepatellar bursa: a bursa between the front of the patella and the investing fascia of the knee; called also *b. praepatellaris subfascialis, middle patellar,* or *middle prepatellar b.*

**subhyoid b.,** b. subcutanea prominentiae laryngeae.

**subiliac b.,** 1. b. iliopectinea. 2. b. subtendinea iliaca.

**subligamentous b.,** b. infrapatellaris profunda.

**b. submuscula'ris** [TA], **submuscular synovial b.,** submuscular bursa: a synovial sac found beneath a muscle; called also *b. synovialis.*

**subpatellar b.,** 1. b. infrapatellaris profunda. 2. b. subcutanea infrapatellaris.

**b. subtendi'nea** [TA], subtendinous bursa: a synovial sac found between tendons and bone, tendons and ligaments, and one tendon and another. Called also *b. synovialis subtendinea* and *subtendinous synovial b.*

**b. subtendi'nea ili'aca** [TA], subtendinous iliac bursa: a bursa between the iliopsoas tendon and the lesser trochanter; called also *b. iliaca subtendinea, b. of quadratus femoris muscle, b. of iliopsoas muscle,* and *subiliac b.*

**b. subtendi'nea mus'culi bici'pitis fe'moris infe'rior** [TA], inferior subtendinous bursa of bicipitis femoris muscle: a bursa between the tendon of the biceps femoris muscle and the fibular collateral ligament of the knee joint; called also *bicipital b., bicipitofibular b., fibular b., external inferior genual b.,* and *b. musculi bicipitis femoris inferior.*

**b. subtendi'nea mus'culi gastrocne'mii latera'lis** [TA], lateral subtendinous bursa of gastrocnemius muscle: a bursa between the tendon of the lateral head of the gastrocnemius muscle and the joint capsule; called also *b. musculi gastrocnemii lateralis, humeral b., lateral b. of gastrocnemius muscle, external postgenual b.,* and *deep lateral retroepicondyloid b.*

**b. subtendi'nea mus'culi gastrocne'mii media'lis** [TA], medial subtendinous b. of gastrocnemius muscle: a bursa between the tendon of the medial head of the gastrocnemius, the condyle of the femur, and the joint capsule; called also *b. musculi gastrocnemii medialis, Brodie's b., internal supracondyloid b., medial b. of gastrocnemius muscle,* and *medial supracondyloid b.*

**b. subtendi'nea mus'culi infraspina'ti** [TA], subtendinous bursa of infraspinatus muscle: a bursa between the tendon of the infraspinatus and the joint capsule or the greater tubercle; called also *b. musculi infraspinati.*

**b. subtendi'nea mus'culi latis'simi dor'si** [TA], subtendinous bursa of latissimus dorsi muscle: a bursa between the tendons of the latissimus dorsi and teres major muscles; called also *b. musculi latissimi dorsi* and *b. of latissimus dorsi muscle.*

**b. subtendi'nea mus'culi obturato'rii inter'ni** [TA], subtendinous bursa of internal obturator muscle: a bursa beneath the tendon of the obturator internus muscle; called also *b. musculi obturatoris interni.*

**bur'sae subtendi'neae mus'culi sarto'rii** [TA], subtendinous bursae of sartorius muscle: bursae between the tendons of the sartorius, semitendinosus, and gracilis muscles; called also *internal superior genual bursae, b. musculi sartorii propria,* and *bursae propriae musculi sartorii.*

**b. subtendi'nea mus'culi subscapula'ris** [TA], subtendinous bursa of subscapularis muscle: a bursa between the tendon of the subscapularis muscle and the glenoid border of the scapula; called also *b. musculi subscapularis, coracoid b.,* and *subcoracoid b.*

**b. subtendi'nea mus'culi te'retis majo'ris** [TA], subtendinous bursa of teres major muscle: a bursa deep to the tendon of insertion of the teres major muscle; called also *b. musculi teretis majoris.*

**b. subtendi'nea mus'culi tibia'lis anterio'ris** [TA], subtendinous bursa of anterior tibial muscle: a bursa between the tibialis anterior and the medial surface of the medial cuneiform bone.

**b. subtendi'nea mus'culi tibia'lis posterio'ris,** subtendinous bursa of posterior tibial muscle: a bursa between the tibialis posterior and the navicular bone.

**b. subtendi'nea mus'culi trape'zii** [TA], subtendinous bursa of trapezius muscle: a bursa between the trapezius and the medial end of the spine of the scapula.

**b. subtendi'nea mus'culi trici'pitis bra'chii** [TA], **b. subtendi'nea olecra'ni,** subtendinous bursa of triceps muscle of arm: an inconstant sac between the triceps tendon, the olecranon, and the dorsal ligament of the elbow; called also *anconeal b. of triceps muscle.*

**b. subtendi'nea prepatella'ris** [TA], subtendinous prepatellar bursa: a bursa sometimes present between the quadriceps tendon and the patellar periosteum; called also *b. praepatellaris subtendinea, deep patellar b., infrapatellar b., b. prepatellaris profunda* or *subaponeurotica,* and *subcutaneous patellar b.*

**subtendinous b.,** b. subtendinea.

**subtendinous b. of anterior tibial muscle,** b. subtendinea musculi tibialis anterioris.

**subtendinous b. of biceps femoris muscle, inferior,** b. subtendinea musculi bicipitis femoris inferior.

**subtendinous b. of gastrocnemius muscle, lateral,** b. subtendinea musculi gastrocnemii lateralis.

**subtendinous b. of gastrocnemius muscle, medial,** b. subtendinea musculi gastrocnemii medialis.

**subtendinous b. of infraspinatus muscle,** b. subtendinea musculi infraspinati.

**subtendinous b. of internal obturator muscle,** b. subtendinea musculi obturatorii interni.

**subtendinous b. of lateral head of gastrocnemius muscle,** b. subtendinea musculi gastrocnemii lateralis.

**subtendinous b. of latissimus dorsi muscle,** b. subtendinea musculi latissimi dorsi.

**subtendinous b. of medial head of gastrocnemius muscle,** b. subtendinea musculi gastrocnemii medialis.

**subtendinous b. of obturator internus muscle,** b. subtendinea musculi obturatorii interni.

**subtendinous b. of posterior tibial muscle,** b. subtendinea musculi tibialis posterioris.

**subtendinous bursae of sartorius muscle,** bursae subtendineae musculi sartorii.

**subtendinous b. of subscapularis muscle,** b. subtendinea musculi subscapularis.

**subtendinous synovial b.,** b. subtendinea.

**subtendinous b. of teres major muscle,** b. subtendinea musculi teretis majoris.

**subtendinous b. of trapezius muscle,** b. subtendinea musculi trapezii.

**subtendinous b. of triceps muscle of arm,** b. subtendinea musculi tricipitis brachii.

**superficial b. of knee,** b. subcutanea infrapatellaris.

**superficial b. of olecranon,** b. subcutanea olecrani.

**superior b. of biceps femoris muscle,** b. musculi bicipitis femoris superior.

**supernumerary b.,** adventitious b.

**supra-anconeal b., intratendinous,** b. intratendinea olecrani.

**supracondyloid b., internal, supracondyloid b., medial,** b. subtendinea musculi gastrocnemii medialis.

**supragenual b., suprapatellar b.,** b. suprapatellaris.

**b. suprapatella'ris** [TA], suprapatellar bursa: a bursa between the distal end of the femur and the quadriceps tendon; called also *supragenual b.* and *subcrural b.*

**synovial b.,** b. synovialis.

**synovial b. of trochlea,** vagina tendinis musculi obliqui superioris.

**b. synovia'lis** [TA], synovial bursa: a closed synovial sac interposed between surfaces which glide upon each other; it may be simple or multilocular in structure, and subcutaneous, submuscular, subfascial, or subtendinous in location; called also *b. mucosa* and *mucous b.*

**b. synovia'lis subcuta'nea,** b. subcutanea.

**b. synovia'lis subfascia'lis,** b. subfascialis.

**b. synovia'lis submuscula'ris,** b. submuscularis.

**b. synovia'lis subtendi'nea,** b. subtendinea.

**b. ten'dinis Achil'lis,** b. tendinis calcanei.

**b. ten'dinis calca'nei** [TA], b. of calcaneal tendon: a bursa between the calcaneal tendon and the back of the calcaneus; called also *b. of Achilles, b. of Achilles tendon, b. tendinis Achillis,* and *calcaneal, deep postcalcaneal, retrocalcaneal,* and *subachilleal b.*

**b. of tendon of Achilles,** b. tendinis calcanei.

**b. of tensor veli palatini muscle,** b. musculi tensoris veli palatini.

**b. of testes,** scrotum.

**Thornwaldt's b.,** b. pharyngealis.

**thyrohyoid b.,** b. subcutanea prominentiae laryngeae.

**thyrohyoid b., anterior,** either of two bursae found below or behind the hyoid bone; see *b. infrahyoidea* and *b. retrohyoidea.*

**Tornwaldt's (Thornwaldt's) b.,** b. pharyngealis.

**trochanteric b., subcutaneous,** b. trochanterica subcutanea.

**trochanteric b. of gluteus maximus muscle,** b. trochanterica musculi glutei maximi.

**trochanteric bursae of gluteus medius muscle,** bursae trochantericae musculi glutei medii.

**trochanteric b. of gluteus minimus muscle,** b. trochanterica musculi glutei minimi.

**b. trochanter'ica mus'culi glu'tei max'imi** [TA], trochanteric bursa of gluteus maximus muscle: a bursa between the fascial tendon of the gluteus maximus, the posterolateral surface of the greater trochanter, and the vastus lateralis muscle.

**bur'sae trochanter'icae mus'culi glu'tei me'dii** [TA], trochanteric bursae of gluteus medius muscle: bursae between the gluteus medius and the lateral surface of the greater trochanter, and sometimes between the tendons of the gluteus medius and the piriformis.

**b. trochanter'ica mus'culi glu'tei min'imi** [TA], trochanteric bursa

of gluteus minimus muscle: a bursa between the edge of the gluteus minimus and the greater trochanter.
**b. trochanter'ica subcuta'nea** [TA], subcutaneous trochanteric bursa: a bursa between the greater trochanter of the femur and the skin.
**trochlear synovial b.**, vagina synovialis musculi obliqui superioris.
**tuberoischiadic b.**, b. ischiadica musculi obturatorii interni.
**ulnoradial b.**, b. cubitalis interossea.
**vesicular b., iliopubic**, b. iliopectinea.
**vesicular b. of sternohyoid muscle**, either of two bursae located where the sternohyoid muscle attaches to the hyoid bone; see *b. infrahyoidea* and *b. retrohyoidea.*

**bur·sae** (bər'se) [L.] genitive and plural of *bursa.*

**bur·sal** (bər'səl) [L. *bursalis*] of or pertaining to a bursa.

**bur·sal·o·gy** (bər-sal'ə-je) [*bursa* + *-logy*] the sum of knowledge regarding the bursae.

**Bur·sa·ta** (bər-sa'tə) a term sometimes used to designate those Nematoda which have a bursa copulatrix.

**bur·sat·ti, bur·saut·ee** (bər-sat'e, bər-sawt'e) [Hindi *barsati* of the rainy season] 1. pythiosis. 2. cutaneous habronemiasis. Spelled also *bursatti, bursattee,* and *bursautee.*

**bur·sec·to·my** (bər-sek'to-me) [*bursa* + *-ectomy*] excision of a bursa.

**bur·si·tis** (bər-si'tis) [MeSH: Bursitis] inflammation of a bursa, occasionally accompanied by a calcific deposit in the underlying tendon; the most common site is the subdeltoid bursa.
**Achilles b.**, achillobursitis.
**adhesive b.**, see under *capsulitis.*
**anserine b.**, inflammation of the anserine bursa with pain on the medial side of the knee, sometimes seen after jogging or other heavy knee exercise and in heavy individuals with genu valgum.
**bicipital b.**, inflammation of the intertubercular bursa in the forelimb of a horse, usually caused by trauma and resulting in lameness and stumbling. Called also *intertubercular b.*
**calcific b.**, see under *tendinitis.*
**intertubercular b.**, bicipital b.
**ischiogluteal b.**, inflammation of the bursa over the ischial tuberosity, characterized by sudden onset of excruciating pain over the center of the buttock and down the back of the leg.
**olecranon b.**, inflammation and enlargement of the bursa over the olecranon; called also *miners' elbow.*
**omental b.**, peritonitis localized to the omental bursa (lesser sac).
**pharyngeal b.**, Tornwaldt's b.
**popliteal b.**, a swelling behind the knee, caused by escape of synovial fluid which then becomes enclosed in a sac or membrane; called also *Baker's cyst.*
**prepatellar b.**, inflammation of the bursa in front of the patella, with fluid accumulating within it; called also *housemaid's knee.*
**radiohumeral b.**, tennis elbow.
**retrocalcaneal b.**, achillodynia.
**scapulohumeral b.**, calcific tendinitis.
**septic b.**, that caused by infection, usually the result of bacterial inoculation due to trauma.
**subacromial b.**, see *calcific tendinitis,* under *tendinitis.*
**subdeltoid b.**, see *calcific tendinitis,* under *tendinitis.*
**superficial calcaneal b.**, achillobursitis.
**Tornwaldt's (Thornwaldt's) b.**, chronic inflammation of the pharyngeal bursa, with formation of a pus-containing cyst, and nasopharyngeal stenosis; called also *pharyngeal b.* and *Tornwaldt's disease.*
**trochanteric b.**, inflammation of a trochanteric bursa with pain on the lateral part of the hip and thigh.

**bur·so·lith** (bər'so-lith) [*bursa* + *-lith*] a calculus or concretion in a bursa.

**bur·sop·a·thy** (bər-sop'ə-the) [*bursa* + *-pathy*] any disease of a bursa.

**bur·sot·o·my** (bər-sot'ə-me) [*bursa* + *-tomy*] incision of a bursa.

**burst** (bərst) 1. a sudden, intense increase in activity. 2. a small explosion. 3. on an electroencephalogram, any short waveform that has an abrupt onset and termination and differs from background activity.
**metabolic b.**, respiratory b.
**respiratory b.**, a sequence of four metabolic events that occur during oxidative killing of ingested microorganisms by granulocytes and mononuclear phagocytes, consisting of (1) an increase in oxygen consumption, (2) formation of superoxide anion, (3) formation of hydrogen peroxide, and (4) activation of the hexose monophosphate shunt. Molecular oxygen is converted to superoxide by NADPH oxidase and NADH oxidase. Superoxide is converted to hydrogen peroxide by superoxide dismutase. Hydrogen peroxide is utilized in myeloperoxidase-dependent bacterial killing, and both superoxide and hydrogen peroxide are spontaneously converted to other toxic metabolites, e.g., singlet oxygen and hydroxyl radicals. The hexose monophosphate shunt regenerates NADPH.
**spider b.**, radiating lines of capillaries on the leg caused by venous dilatation but without distinct varicosity.

**Bur·ton's line (sign)** (bər'tənz) [Henry *Burton,* British physician, 1799–1849] see *lead line,* under *line.*

**Bu·ru·li ulcer** (boo'rə-le) [*Buruli* district in Uganda, where a large number of cases have occurred] see under *ulcer.*

**Busch·ke's disease, scleredema** (boosh'kəz) [Abraham *Buschke,* German dermatologist, 1868–1943] see *cryptococcosis.*

**Busch·ke-Lö·wen·stein tumor** (boosh'kə-ler'ven-shtīn) [A. *Buschke;* Ludwig W. *Löwenstein,* German-born American physician, 1885–1959] see under *tumor.*

**Busch·ke-Ol·len·dorff syndrome** (boosh'kə-o'len-dorf) [A. *Buschke;* Helene *Ollendorff,* German dermatologist, 20th century] dermatofibrosis lenticularis disseminata.

**Bu·sel·mei·er shunt** (boo͝'səl-mi"ər) [T.J. *Buselmeier,* American nephrologist, 20th century] see under *shunt.*

**bu·se·rel·in ace·tate** (bu"sə-rel'in) a synthetic analogue of luteinizing hormone–releasing hormone, used in the palliative treatment of advanced prostatic carcinoma; administered intranasally.

**bush·mas·ter** (bush'mas-tər) *Lachesis mutus,* a large venomous pit viper of the Amazon region of South America. See table at *snake.* Called also *suruçucu.*

**Bu·Spar** (bu'spar) trademark for a preparation of buspirone hydrochloride.

**bu·spi·rone hy·dro·chlo·ride** (bu-spi'rōn) [USP] an anxiolytic drug used in the treatment of anxiety disorders and for short-term relief of anxiety symptoms; it is not related chemically or pharmacologically to the benzodiazepines, barbiturates, or other sedative/anxiolytic agents.

**Bus·quet's disease** (boo͝s-kāz') [Paul *Busquet,* French physician, 1866–1930] see under *disease.*

**Buss disease** (bus) [*Buss,* name of farmer whose animals were first observed with the disease] see under *disease.*

**Bus·se-Busch·ke disease** (boo͝'sə-boosh'kə) [Otto Emil Franz Ulrich *Busse,* German physician, 1867–1922; Abraham *Buschke,* German dermatologist, 1868–1943] cryptococcosis.

**bu·sul·fan** (bu-sul'fan) [USP] [MeSH: Busulfan] a bifunctional cytotoxic alkylating agent, an antineoplastic agent unrelated to the nitrogen mustards; used primarily for the palliative treatment of chronic granulocytic leukemia and also for the treatment of myeloproliferative syndromes, polycythemia vera, and myeloid metaplasia; administered orally. It is also used at high doses in lieu of whole body irradiation in bone marrow transplantation.

**But.** abbreviation for L. *bu'tyrum,* butter.

**bu·ta·bar·bi·tal** (bu-tə-bahr'bĭ-təl) [USP] an intermediate-acting barbiturate used as a sedative and hypnotic; administered orally.
**b. sodium** [USP], the monosodium salt of butabarbital having the same actions and uses as the base.

**bu·ta·caine sul·fate** (bu'tə-kān") a local anesthetic applied topically for the relief of pain associated with dental appliances.

**Bu·ta·lan** (bu'tə-lan") trademark for a preparation of butabarbital sodium.

**bu·tal·bi·tal** (bu-tal'bĭ-təl) [USP] a short- to intermediate-acting barbiturate, used as a sedative in combination with an analgesic in the treatment of tension headache; administered orally.

**bu·tam·ben** (bu-tam'bən) [USP] a local anesthetic applied topically to relieve pain and pruritus. Called also *butyl aminobenzoate.*

**b. picrate,** a local anesthetic applied topically for temporary relief of pain due to minor burns.

**bu·tam·i·sole hy·dro·chlo·ride** (bu-tam'ĭ-sōl) a veterinary anthelmintic used to treat whipworm and hookworm infestations; administered parenterally or by subcutaneous injection.

**bu·tane** (bu'tān) [NF] *n*-butane; an aliphatic hydrocarbon of the methane series, $C_4H_{10}$, from petroleum, occurring as a colorless flammable gas with a characteristic odor, used in pharmacy as an aerosol propellant.
**normal b.,** butane in straight line configuration, $CH_3(CH_2)_2CH_3$, cf. *isobutane* and see illustration at *isomerism.*

**bu·ta·no·ic ac·id** (bu"tə-no'ik) systematic name for *n-butyric acid.* See also table at *fatty acid.*

**bu·ta·per·a·zine** (bu-tə-per'ə-zēn) a phenothiazine derivative, used as an antipsychotic drug in the treatment of acute and chronic schizophrenia; administered orally.
**b. maleate,** the maleate ester of butaperazine, having the same actions and uses as the base.

**Bu·ta·zol·i·din** (bu"tə-zol'ĭ-din) trademark for preparations of phenylbutazone.

**Butch·er's saw** (booch'ərz) [Richard George Herbert *Butcher,* Irish surgeon, 1819–1891] see under *saw.*

**Bu·te·sin** (bu'tə-sin) trademark for a preparation of butamben.

**bu·te·thal** (bu'tə-thal") an intermediate-acting barbiturate, used as a sedative; administered orally.

**bu·teth·amine hy·dro·chlo·ride** (bu-teth'ə-mēn) a local anesthetic, used for nerve block anesthesia in dentistry.

**Bu·thus** (bu'thəs) a genus of scorpions. *B. carolinia'nus* is found in the southern United States and *B. quinquestria'tus* is a dangerous Egyptian species.

**Bu·ti·caps** (bu'tĭ-kaps") trademark for a preparation of butabarbital sodium.

**bu·tir·o·sin sul·fate** (bu-tir'o-sin) [MeSH: Butirosin Sulfate] an aminoglycoside antibiotic complex obtained from certain strains of *Bacillus circulans,* consisting of butirosins A and B; an antibacterial.

**Bu·ti·sol so·di·um** (bu'tĭ-sol) trademark for preparations of butabarbital sodium.

**bu·to·con·az·ole ni·trate** (bu"to-kon'ə-zōl) an imidazole derivative used as a topical antifungal, applied intravaginally in the treatment of vulvovaginal candidiasis.

**bu·to·nate** (bu'tə-nāt) an insecticide and anthelmintic that is a potent cholinesterase inhibitor.

**bu·to·py·ro·nox·yl** (bu"to-pi"ro-nok'səl) an insect repellent effective against ticks.

**bu·tor·pha·nol** (bu-tor'fə-nol) [MeSH: Butorphanol] a synthetic opioid, having analgesic and antitussive properties.
**b. tartrate** [USP], the tartrate salt of butorphanol, administered intramuscularly, intravenously, or intranasally as an analgesic.

**bu·tox·amine hy·dro·chlo·ride** (bu-tok'sə-mēn) a beta-adrenergic blocking agent.

**bu·trip·ty·line hy·dro·chlo·ride** (bu-trip'tə-lēn) an antidepressant.

**Bütsch·li's nuclear spindle** (būtsh'lēz) [Otto *Bütschli,* German zoologist, 1848–1920] spindle (def. 1).

**butt** (but) to bring the surfaces of two distinct objects squarely or directly into contact with each other.

**but·ter** (but'ər) [L. *butyrum;* Gr. *boutyron*] [MeSH: Butter] the oily mass procured by churning cream.
**b. of arsenic,** arsenic trichloride.
**cacao b., cocoa b.** [NF], the fat obtained from the roasted seed of *Theobroma cacao;* used as a suppository base, for its emollient properties in cosmetics, and sometimes for softening and protecting the skin. Called also *theobroma oil.*
**b. of tin,** stannic chloride.
**b. of zinc,** zinc chloride.

**but·ter·fat** (but'ər-fat") the fat content of milk and the major component of butter; it is composed largely of glycerides of stearic, oleic, and palmitic acids and has high levels of saturated fats and cholesterol.

**but·ter·fly** (but'ər-fli) [MeSH: Butterflies] 1. any of numerous flying insects of the order Lepidoptera, or something resembling this insect. 2. a small piece of adhesive tape with broad, wing-shaped ends by means of which the edges of a superficial wound may be approximated. 3. a pattern formed by a skin eruption across the nose and adjacent areas of the cheeks, as in systemic lupus erythematosus, seborrheic dermatitis, and rosacea. Called also *butterfly rash.*

**But·ti·aux·el·la** (but"e-awk-sel'ə) a genus of gram-negative, facultatively anaerobic, rod-shaped bacteria of the family Enterobacteriaceae. The organisms belong to Enteric Groups 63 and 64, and are sucrose negative. The type species is *B. agres'tis.*

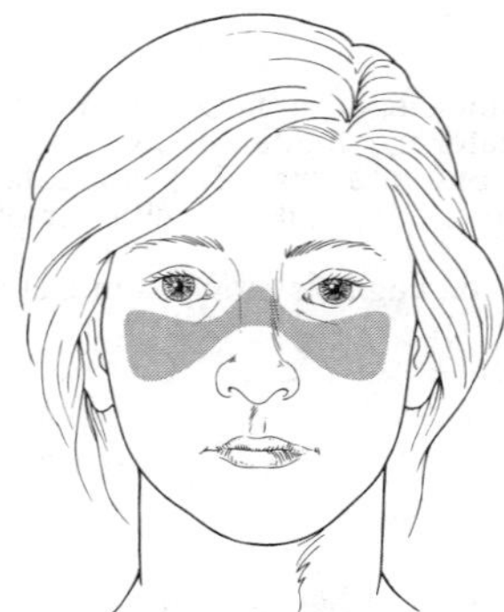

Butterfly.

**but·tocks** (but'əks) [MeSH: Buttocks] nates.

**but·ton** (but'ən) 1. a knoblike elevation or structure. 2. a small appliance shaped like a spool or disk and used in surgery for the construction of intestinal anastomosis.
**bromide b.,** a verrucous cutaneous lesion occurring as a result of sensitivity to bromides.
**dog b.,** nux vomica.
**iodide b.,** a verrucous cutaneous lesion occurring as a result of sensitivity to iodides.
**Jaboulay b.,** a device for performing lateral intestinal anastomosis without the aid of sutures, consisting of two buttonlike cylinders of metal that are fitted together on the screw and key-ring principle through a small intestinal opening.
**mescal b's,** transverse slices of the flowering heads of the Mexican dumpling cactus, *Lophophora williamsii,* whose major active principle is mescaline; used in divinatory and religious ceremonies in some North American Indian cultures.
**Murphy's b.,** a device for joining the ends of a divided intestine so that union may take place. It consists of two short metal cylinders of different diameter, each having a collar at one end; the collars are sutured to the divided ends, and the narrower cylinder is locked into its mate.
**peritoneal b.,** a short flanged glass tube for insertion between the peritoneal cavity and a subcutaneous pocket through which peritoneal transudate may be drained.
**quaker b.,** nux vomica.
**skin b.,** a connector or stretch of tubing covered with dacron velour fabric, designed to encourage tissue ingrowth where it passes through the skin.
**terminal b.,** bouton terminal; see under *bouton.*

**but·ton·hole** (but'ən-hōl) 1. a short straight incision into a cavity or organ. 2. an abnormal narrowing of the caliber of a structure.
**mitral b.,** an advanced state of stenosis of the mitral orifice of the heart, adhesion and shortening of the cusps having produced a narrow slitlike orifice.

**bu·tyl** (bu'təl) a hydrocarbon radical, $C_4H_9$, being $CH_3(CH_2)_2CH_2$—, $(CH_3)_2CHCH_2$—, $CH_3CH_2CHCH_3$—, or $(CH_3)_3C$—.
**b. acetate,** a liquid compound, used in the manufacture of lacquer, artificial leather, photographic film, plastics, and safety glass; it is an irritant which may cause conjunctivitis, and is narcotic in high concentrations.
**b. aminobenzoate,** butamben.
**b. formate,** an industrial solvent, the vapors of which are powerfully lacrimatory and suffocating.

**bu·ty·lat·ed hy·droxy·an·isole (BHA)** (bu'tə-la"təd hi-drok"se-an'ĭ-sōl) [MeSH: Butylated Hydroxyanisole] a white or slightly yellow waxy solid with a faint characteristic odor; used as an antioxidant in foods, cosmetics, and pharmaceuticals that contain fats or oils.

**bu·ty·lat·ed hy·droxy·tol·u·ene (BHT)** (bu'tə-la"təd hi-drok"se-tol'u-ēn) [MeSH: Butylated Hydroxytoluene] an antioxidant, occurring as white, tasteless crystals with a faint odor, used in foods, cosmetics, pharmaceuticals, and petroleum products.

**bu·ty·lene** (bu'tə-lēn) a gaseous hydrocarbon, $C_4H_8$.

**bu·tyl·par·a·ben** (bu"təl-par'ə-ben) [NF] an antifungal compound, closely related to ethylparaben and methylparaben, used as a preservative in pharmaceutic preparations.

**Bu·tyn** (bu'tin) trademark for a preparation of butacaine sulfate.

**bu·ty·ra·ceous** (bu″tə-ra′shəs) of a buttery consistency.

**bu·ty·rate** (bu′tə-rāt) a salt, ester, or anionic form of butyric acid.

**bu·ty·rate–CoA li·gase** (bu′tə-rāt ko-a′ li′gās) [EC 6.2.1.2] an enzyme of the ligase class that catalyzes the formation of acyl coenzyme A from medium chain length fatty acids (4 to 12 carbons) and coenzyme A, using energy derived from ATP hydrolysis. The enzyme occurs in the mitochondrial matrix and acts on saturated and unsaturated fatty acids as well as on some hydroxy acids.

**bu·tyr·ic ac·id** (bu-tēr′ik as′id) 1. any four-carbon carboxylic acid, either *n*-butyric acid or isobutyric acid. 2. *n*-butyric acid, a saturated four-carbon fatty acid occurring in butter, particularly rancid butter, and in much animal fat. Systematic name: *butanoic acid.*

**bu·ty·rin** (bu′tər-in) tributyrin.

**bu·ty·rine** (bu′tə-rēn) an amino acid derivative of butyric acid; it is $\alpha$-amino butyric acid.

**Bu·ty·ri·vib·rio** (bu-tir″ĭ-vib′re-o) [L. *butyricus* butyric + *vibrio*] a genus of gram-negative, non–spore-forming, anaerobic bacteria of the family Bacteroidaceae, found in the rumen contents of animals, and consisting of motile curved rods that may be in chains or filaments. The type species is *B. fibrosol′vens.*

**butyr(o)-** [L. *butyrum* butter] a combining form denoting relationship to butter, or to butyric acid.

**bu·ty·roid** (bu′tə-roid) [*butyr-* + *-oid*] resembling or having the consistency of butter.

**bu·tyr·o·mel** (bu-tir′o-məl) fresh, unsalted butter, 2 parts, and honey, 1 part: a substitute for cod liver oil.

**bu·ty·ro·phe·none** (bu″tə-ro-fe′nōn) any of a class of structurally related antipsychotic agents; the prototype is haloperidol.

**bu·ty·rous** (bu′tə-rəs) like butter; having a butterlike appearance.

**bu·ty·ryl** (bu′tə-rəl) the radical of *n*-butyric acid.

**bu·ty·ryl CoA syn·the·tase** (bu′tə-rəl ko-a′ sin′thə-tās) butyrate–CoA ligase.

**BVAD** biventricular assist device.

**by·pass** (bi′pas) an auxiliary flow, such as in the circulatory system or alimentary tract; see also *shunt* (def. 2).
**aortobifemoral b.**, aortofemoral bypass involving both femoral arteries.
**aortocoronary b.**, coronary artery b.
**aortofemoral b.**, insertion of a vascular prosthesis from the aorta to the femoral artery as a passage around atherosclerotic occlusions in the aorta and the iliac artery.
**aortofemoral b., thoracic**, insertion of a vascular prosthesis from the thoracic aorta to the femoral artery, with femorofemoral bypass, as a passage around aortoiliac occlusion in patients in whom the abdominal aorta is unsuitable for grafting.
**aortoiliac b.**, insertion of a vascular prosthesis from the abdominal aorta to the iliac artery as a passage around intervening atherosclerotic segments.
**aortorenal b.**, insertion of a section of saphenous vein, hypogastric artery, or suitable substitute between the aorta and renal artery as a passage around occluded or stenotic segments.
**aortosubclavian b.**, insertion of a vascular prosthesis from the aorta to a subclavian artery, serving as a passage around an occluded segment in or around their junction.
**axillary-axillary b.**, insertion of a vascular prosthesis between the axillary arteries, passing over the sternum, serving as a passage around occluded or stenosed segments.
**axillobifemoral b.**, an axillofemoral bypass combined with a femorofemoral bypass.

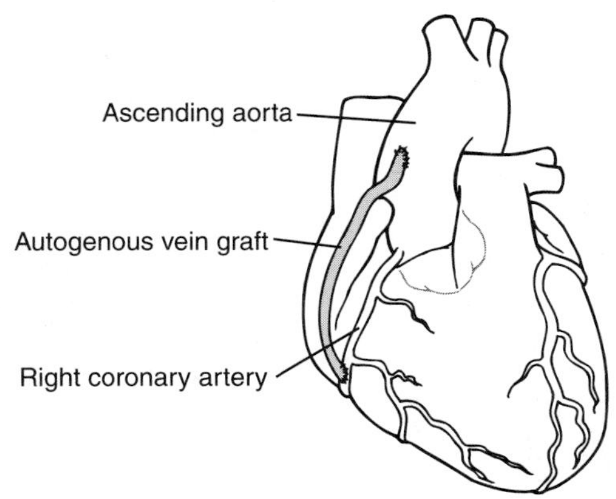

Single coronary artery bypass of an occluded right coronary artery (RCA).

**axillofemoral b.**, an extra-anatomic bypass consisting of a vascular prosthesis or section of saphenous vein extending from the axillary artery to the ipsilateral femoral artery to relieve lower limb ischemia in patients in whom normal anatomic placement of a graft is contraindicated, as by abdominal infection or aortic aneurysm.
**axillopopliteal b.**, an extra-anatomic bypass consisting of a vascular prosthesis extending from the axillary artery to the popliteal artery to relieve lower limb ischemia in patients in whom the femoral artery is unsuitable for axillofemoral bypass.
**cardiopulmonary b.**, diversion of the flow of blood to the heart directly to the aorta, via a pump oxygenator, avoiding both the heart and the lungs; a form of extracorporeal circulation used in heart surgery.
**carotid-carotid b.**, insertion of a vascular prosthesis from the left carotid to the right carotid artery, serving as a passage around an occluded or stenosed portion of the brachiocephalic trunk.
**carotid-subclavian b.**, insertion of a vascular prosthesis from the subclavian artery to the common carotid artery as a passage around occluded or stenotic segments of either artery.
**coronary b., coronary artery b.**, a section of vein or other conduit grafted between the aorta and a coronary artery distal to an obstructive lesion in the latter.
**extra-anatomic b.**, an arterial bypass that does not follow the normal anatomic pathway, such as an axillofemoral or axillopopliteal bypass.
**extracranial/intracranial (EC/IC) b.**, anastomosis of the superficial temporal artery to a branch of the middle cerebral artery on the brain surface to improve collateral blood flow that has been reduced by occlusion or stenosis of the internal carotid or middle cerebral artery.
**femorofemoral b.**, insertion of a vascular prosthesis between the femoral arteries as a passage around an occluded or injured iliac artery.
**femorofemoropopliteal b.**, insertion of a vascular prosthesis, or of a vascular prosthesis anastomosed to a section of saphenous vein, between the popliteal artery and the contralateral femoral artery as a passage around occluded, stenotic, or injured iliac and femoral arteries.
**femoropopliteal b.**, insertion of a vascular prosthesis from the femoral to the popliteal artery as a passage around occluded, narrowed, or injured segments.
**gastric b.**, gastrojejunostomy in which the stomach is transected high on the body, the proximal remnant being joined to a loop of jejunum in end-to-side anastomosis.
**hepatorenal b.**, insertion of a vascular prosthesis between the common hepatic artery and the renal artery, serving as a passage around an occluded segment in or near their junction.
**iliofemoral b.**, insertion of a vascular prosthesis from the iliac artery to the femoral artery, serving as a passage around an occluded or stenosed segment.
**infrainguinal b.**, any of the bypass procedures connecting arteries of the lower limb, including femorofemoral, femoropopliteal, iliofemoral, and inframalleolar bypasses.
**inframalleolar b.**, insertion of a vascular prosthesis in arteries of the foot to serve as a passage around an occluded or stenotic segment.
**infrapopliteal b.**, a bypass procedure connecting arteries below the knee.
**intestinal b.**, resection of the intestine, with anastomosis of the proximal to the distal portion, as in jejunoileostomy.
**jejunal b., jejunoileal b.**, surgical anastomosis of the proximal part of the jejunum to the distal part of the ileum so as to circumvent much of the small intestine and reduce intestinal absorption.
**left heart b.**, diversion of the flow of blood from the pulmonary veins directly to the aorta, avoiding the left atrium and the left ventricle.
**obturator b., obturator foramen b.**, an extra-anatomic type of iliofemoral bypass in which the graft passes through the obturator foramen; used when trauma or infection makes it necessary to avoid the femoral triangle.
**partial b.**, the deviation of only a portion of blood flowing through an artery.
**partial ileal b.**, anastomosis of the proximal end of the transected ileum to the cecum, the bypass of the portion of the small intestine resulting in decreased intestinal absorption of and increased fecal excretion of cholesterol; sometimes used in treatment of hyperlipidemia and in weight reduction.
**right heart b.**, diversion of the flow of blood from the entrance of the right atrium directly to the pulmonary arteries, avoiding the right atrium and right ventricle.

**by·prod·uct** (by′prod′əkt) a secondary product obtained during the manufacture of a primary product.

**bys·sa·ceous** (bĭ-sa′shəs) [Gr. *byssos* flax] composed of fine flax-like threads.

**bys·si·no·sis** (bis″ĭ-no′sis) [Gr. *byssos* flax + *-osis*] [MeSH: Byssinosis] a pulmonary disease seen in cotton textile workers and preparers of flax and soft hemp, due to inhalation of textile dust. Two forms are distinguished, *acute* and *chronic b.* Called also *brown lung, cotton-dust asthma,* and *stripper's asthma.*

**acute b.,** a form occurring in those who return to work after a weekend or other time away, marked by tightness of the chest, wheezing, and cough. See also *mill fever,* under *fever.*

**chronic b.,** byssinosis in workers who have had years of exposure to textile dust, marked by permanent dyspnea, probably due to smooth muscle contraction after histamine release induced by chemicals in the dust.

**bys·si·not·ic** (bis″ĭ-not′ik) 1. pertaining to byssinosis. 2. one affected with byssinosis.

**bys·so·cau·sis** (bis″o-kaw′sis) [Gr. *byssos* flax + *kausis* burning] moxibustion.

**bys·soid** (bis′oid) [Gr. *byssos* flax + *-oid*] made up of a fringe, the filaments of which are unequal in length.

**bys·sus** (bis′əs) pl. *bys′suses* or *bys′si* [L., from Gr. *byssos* flax] lint, charpie, or cotton.

**by·stand·er** (bi′stan-dər) that which is only incidentally involved in a process.

**innocent b.,** a tissue cell that is lysed because it is in close proximity to the actual target of lysis, rather than itself being a target.

**Byth·nia** (bith′ne-ah) *Bithynia.*

**By·wa·ters' syndrome** (bi′wah-tərz) [Eric George Lapthorne *Bywaters,* British physician, born 1910] see under *syndrome.*

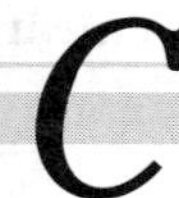

**C** symbol for *canine* (see under *tooth*), *carbon* (molecular carbon atoms are frequently designated C1, C2, C3, etc., or α-C, β-C, etc., beginning from one end or other standard reference point), *large calorie, cathode* (or *cathodal*), *cervical vertebrae* (C1 through C7), *clonus, closure, color sense, complement* (numbered C1 through C9; see *complement* for additional symbols), *compliance* (subscripts denote the structure, e.g., $C_L$ lung compliance), *contraction, coulomb, cylinder, cytidine* or *cytosine,* and *cylindrical lens.*

**C.** symbol for L. *con'gius,* gallon.

***C*** symbol for *capacitance, clearance* (subscripts denote the substance, e.g., $C_I$ or $C_{In}$ inulin clearance), and *heat capacity.*

**$C_H$** see *constant region,* under *region.*

**$C_L$** see *constant region,* under *region.*

**°C** symbol for degree Celsius.

**c** symbol for *small calorie, contact,* and *centi-.*

**c.** symbol for L. *ci'bus* (food) and *cum* (with).

***c*** symbol for *molar concentration, specific heat capacity* (see *specific heat,* under *heat*), and the velocity of light in a vacuum.

**c̄** symbol for L. *cum,* with.

**χ** chi, the twenty-second letter of the Greek alphabet.

**$\chi^2$** chi-square; see under *distribution* and *test.*

**CA** cardiac arrest; chronological age; cold agglutinin; coronary artery; croup-associated (virus).

**CA 125** cancer antigen 125.

**Ca** symbol for *calcium.*

**ca** abbreviation for L. *circa,* about.

**$CA_2$** a colloid antigen lacking iodine, the second most common antigen in thyroid colloid (the first being thyroglobulin); the presence in serum of antibodies against $CA_2$ is a sign of autoimmune disorders such as Hashimoto's disease.

**$Ca^{2+}$-ATP·ase** (a-te-pe'ās) a membrane-bound enzyme that hydrolyzes ATP to provide the energy necessary to drive the cellular calcium pump (q.v.). See also *adenosinetriphosphatase.* In EC nomenclature, called *$Ca^{2+}$-transporting ATPase.*

**CABG** coronary artery bypass graft; see under *bypass.*

**Cab·ot's ring bodies** (kab'əts) [Richard Clarke *Cabot,* American physician, 1868–1939] see under *body.*

**cab·u·fo·con** (kab″u-fo'kon) chemical name: cellulose acetate butanoate; either of two hydrophobic contact lens materials, designated A or B.

**ca·cao** (kə-ka'o) [Nahuatl *cacahuatl*] [MeSH: Cacao] 1. *Theobroma cacao.* 2. the seeds of *T. cacao;* called also *cocoa beans* and *cacao beans.* 3. cocoa, def. 1.

**cac·a·tion** (kak-a'shən) defecation.

**cac·a·to·ry** (kak'ə-tor″-e) marked by severe diarrhea.

**Cac·chi-Ric·ci disease** (kah'ke-re'che) [Roberto *Cacchi,* Italian physician, 20th century; Vincenzo *Ricci,* Italian physician, 20th century] sponge kidney; see under *kidney.*

**ca·chec·tic** (kə-kek'tik) pertaining to or characterized by cachexia.

**ca·chec·tin** (kə-kek'tin) tumor necrosis factor.

**ca·chet** (kă-sha') [Fr.] a disk-shaped wafer or capsule for enclosing a dose of medicine.

**ca·chex·ia** (kə-kek'se-ə) [*cac-* + Gr. *hexis* habit + *-ia*] [MeSH: Cachexia] a profound and marked state of constitutional disorder; general ill health and malnutrition.
**cancerous c.,** the weak, emaciated condition seen in cases of malignant tumor.
**cardiac c.,** emaciation due to heart disease, usually caused by a combination of increased caloric expenditure and decreased caloric intake or utilization.
**fluoric c.,** that seen in fluorosis.
**hypophysial c.,** see *panhypopituitarism.*
**c. hypophysiopri'va,** the train of symptoms resulting from total deprivation of function of the pituitary gland, including phthisis, loss of sexual function, atrophy of the pituitary target glands, bradycardia, hypothermia, apathy, and coma.
**malarial c.,** a group of physical signs of a chronic nature that result from antecedent attacks of severe malaria; the principal signs are anemia, sallow skin, yellow sclera, splenomegaly, hepatomegaly, and, in children, retardation of body growth and puberty.
**c. mercuria'lis,** that seen in chronic mercury poisoning.
**pituitary c.,** see *panhypopituitarism.*
**saturnine c.,** that seen in chronic lead poisoning.
**c. suprarena'lis,** Addison's disease.
**uremic c.,** cachexia associated with other systemic symptoms of advanced renal failure.

**ca·chexy** (kə-kek'se) cachexia.

**cach·in·na·tion** (kak″ĭ-na'shən) [L. *cachinnare* to laugh aloud] immoderate, loud, and inappropriate laughter; commonly seen in disorganized schizophrenia.

**cac(o)-** [Gr. *kakos* bad] a combining form meaning bad, or ill.

**caco·de·mono·ma·nia** (kak″o-de″mon-o-ma'ne-ə) a condition marked by delusions of being possessed by evil spirits.

**cac·o·dyl** (kak'o-dəl) [*caco-* + Gr. *ozein* to smell + *hylē* matter] tetramethylbiarsine, a colorless liquid arsenic-containing compound, $(CH_3)_2As—As(CH_3)_2$, with an offensive odor; it gives off a poisonous vapor and is inflammable when exposed to air.
**c. cyanide,** a white powder, $(CH_3)_2AsCN$, which, when exposed to air, gives off an extremely poisonous vapor.
**c. hydride,** a colorless liquid, $(CH_3)_2AsH$, with a strong, garlicky odor; on exposure to air, it gives off a poisonous vapor and ignites spontaneously. Symptoms of poisoning are the same as those of arsenic poisoning.

**cac·o·dyl·ate** (kak'o-dəl-āt) a salt of cacodylic acid; the cacodylates were formerly used medicinally but release arsenic compounds when they metabolize, causing symptoms of arsenic poisoning.

**cac·o·dyl·ic ac·id** (kak″o-dil'ik) [MeSH: Cacodylic Acid] dimethylarsinic acid, a highly toxic herbicide.

**caco·ethic** (kak″o-e'thik) [*caco-* + Gr. *ēthos* the manners and habits of an individual or a group] ill-conditioned; malignant.

**caco·gen·e·sis** (kak″o-jen'ə-sis) [*caco-* + *-genesis*] dysgenesis.

**caco·geu·sia** (kak″o-goo'zhə) [*caco-* + Gr. *geusis* taste + *-ia*] a parageusia consisting of bad taste not related to the ingestion of specific substances, or associated with gustatory stimuli usually considered to be pleasant.

**caco·me·lia** (kak″o-me'le-ə) [*caco-* + *-melia*] dysmelia.

**cac·os·mia** (kak-oz'me-ə) [*caco-* + *osm-*[1] + *-ia*] a parosmia consisting of bad smell not related to exposure to a specific odor, or associated with olfactory stimuli usually considered to be pleasant.

**caco·then·ic** (kak″o-then'ik) pertaining to cacothenics.

**caco·then·ics** (kak″o-then'iks) [Gr. *kakothēnein* to be in a bad state] deterioration of a race resulting from deleterious influences in the environment.

**cac·ot·ro·phy** (kak-ot'rə-fe) [*caco-* + *-trophy*] malnutrition.

**CAD** coronary artery disease.

**ca·dav·er** (kə-dav'ər) [L., from *cadere* to fall, to perish] [MeSH: Cadaver] a dead body; generally applied to a human body preserved for anatomical study. Cf. *corpse.*

**ca·dav·er·ic** (kə-dav'ər-ik) of or pertaining to a cadaver.

**ca·dav·er·ine** (kə-dav'ər-in) [L. *cadaver* corpse] [MeSH: Cadaverine] a foul-smelling nitrogenous base, pentamethylenediamine, produced by decarboxylation of lysine. It is produced in decaying protein material by the action of bacteria, particularly species of *Vibrio.*

**ca·dav·er·ous** (kə-dav'ər-əs) resembling a cadaver.

**cad·dis** (kad'is) see under *fly.*

**cad·her·in** (kad-hēr'in) any of a family of calcium-dependent cell adhesion molecules.

**cad·mi·o·sis** (kad″me-o'sis) pneumoconiosis due to inhalation of and tissue reaction to cadmium dust. Cf. *cadmium lung.*

**cad·mi·um** (kad'me-əm) [Gr. *kadmia* earth] [MeSH: Cadmium] a bivalent metal, similar to tin in appearance and properties; symbol, Cd; atomic number, 48; atomic weight, 112.40. Cadmium and its salts are poisonous; see *cadmium poisoning, cadmiosis,* and *cadmium lung.*
**c. bromide,** $CdBr_2$, a compound used in photography, process engraving, and lithography; when swallowed it causes cadmium poisoning.

**ca·du·ca** (kə-doo'kə) the decidua.

**ca·du·ce·us** (kə-doo'shəs) [L., from Doric Gr. *karykeion,* herald's staff] the winged staff of Hermes or Mercury, the messenger of the gods, with two snakes winding around it. Used as a medical symbol and as the emblem of the Medical Corps, U.S. Army. The official symbol of the medical profession is the staff of Aesculapius.

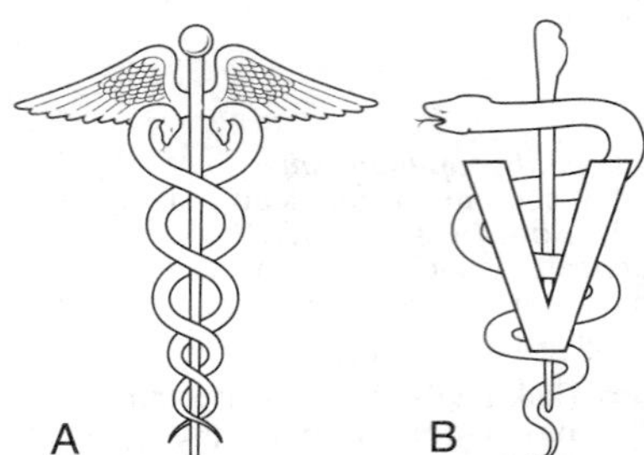


Caduceus. *(A),* United States Army Medical Corps; *(B),* American Veterinary Medicine Association.

**ca·du·cous** (kə-doo'kəs) [L. *cadere* to fall] falling off; deciduous.

**cae-** for words beginning thus, see also those beginning *ce-*.

**caec(o)-** for words beginning thus, see also those beginning *cec(o)-*.

**cae·cum** (se'kəm) [L.] 1. a blind pouch or cul-de-sac. 2. [TA] the first part of the large intestine, forming a dilated pouch into which open the ileum, colon, and appendix vermiformis; spelled also *cecum.* Called also *blindgut, blind intestine,* and *intestinum caecum.*
**c. cupula're duc'tus cochlea'ris** [TA], cupular caecum of cochlear duct: the closed blind apical end of the cochlear duct.
**c. vestibula're duc'tus cochlea'ris** [TA], vestibular caecum of cochlear duct: a small blind outpouching at the vestibular end of the cochlear duct.

**cae·cus** (se'kəs) [L. "blind"] a blind pouch.
**c. mi'nor ventric'uli,** cardia.

**Cae·di·bac·ter** (se"dī-bak'tər) [L. *caedes* slaughter + *-bacter*] a genus of bacteria of uncertain affiliation that are parasites of paramecia.

**caen(o)-** see *cen(o)-* (def. 1).

**cae·ru·le·us** (sə-roo'le-əs) [L. "dark blue," "azure," probably from *caelum* sky] blue; azure; cerulean. Written also *ceruleus* and *coeruleus* (q.v.).

**cae·sa·re·an** (sə-za're-ən) cesarean.

**cae·si·um** (se'ze-əm) cesium.

**caf·feine** (kă-fēn', kaf'ēn) [Ger. *Kaffein,* from *Kaffee* coffee] [USP] [MeSH: Caffeine] one of the methylxanthines (q.v.), soluble in water and alcohol, and obtainable from coffee, tea, guarana, and maté. It stimulates the central nervous system, especially the cerebrum; has a diuretic effect on the kidneys; stimulates striated muscle; and has a group of effects on the cardiovascular system. It is used as a central and respiratory stimulant, in combination with ergotamine in the treatment of vascular headache, and as an adjunct to enhance pain relief in combination with analgesics; administered orally. Ingestion of excessive amounts can cause caffeinism (q.v.). Called also *guaranine* and *methyltheobromine.*
**c. benzoate,** a salt used as an accelerator for the conversion of unconjugated bilirubin to azobilirubin in the Jendrassik-Grof method for determining total bilirubin.
**c. citrate, citrated c.,** a preparation of equal parts of caffeine and citric acid, used for the same purposes as caffeine; administered orally.
**c. and sodium benzoate,** see under *injection.*

**caf·fein·ism** (kaf'ēn-iz-əm, kaf'e-in-iz"əm) a morbid condition resulting from ingestion of excessive amounts of caffeine. The manifestations include insomnia, restlessness, excitement, tachycardia, tremors, and diuresis.

**Caf·fey's disease** (kaf'ēz) [John *Caffey,* American pediatrician, 1895–1978] infantile cortical hyperostosis.

**cage** (kāj) a box or enclosure.
**population c.,** an enclosure in which populations of *Drosophila* can be isolated through many generations.
**rib c., thoracic c.,** skeleton thoracis.

**Ca·got ear** (kah-go') [*Cagot,* region in the Pyrenees Mountains where this deformity frequently occurs] see under *ear.*

**CAH** congenital adrenal hyperplasia.

**cain(o)-** see *cen(o)-* (def. 1).

**Ca·jal** see *Ramón y Cajal.*

**Ca·jal's cells, interstitial nucleus, stain** (kah-hahlz') [Santiago Ramón y *Cajal,* Spanish physician and histologist, 1852–1934] see under *cell,* see *nucleus interstitialis,* and see *stain.*

**caj·e·put** (kaj'ə-poot) [Malay *kayu puteh* white tree] *Melaleuca leucadendron.*

**caj·e·pu·tol** (kaj'e-pu-tol) eucalyptol.

**caj·u·put** (kaj'ə-poot) *Melaleuca leucadendron.*

**Cal** large calorie (kilocalorie).

**cal** calorie.

**Cal·a·bar bean, edema (swellings)** (kal'ə-bahr) [*Calabar* River and region in southeastern Nigeria] see under *bean* and *edema.*

**ca·lage** (kah-lahzh') [Fr.] propping with pillows to immobilize the viscera and thus relieve seasickness.

**cal·a·mine** (kal'ə-mīn) 1. [USP] a mild astringent and protectant, consisting of zinc oxide with a small proportion of ferric oxide, and occurring as a fine, pink powder; applied topically in the treatment of skin diseases. 2. a similar preparation containing zinc carbonate instead of zinc oxide.

**cal·a·mus** (kal'ə-məs) [L.] 1. a reedlike structure. 2. *Acorus calamus.* 3. the aromatic rhizome of *A. calamus,* used as a flavoring agent and insect repellent, and formerly as a carminative and vermifuge.
**c. scripto'rius,** the lowest portion of the floor of the fourth ventricle, shaped like a pen when viewed from the dorsal side and situated between the restiform bodies.

**Cal·an** (kal'an) trademark for preparations of verapamil hydrochloride.

**cal·ca·ne·al** (kal-ka'ne-əl) pertaining to the calcaneus.

**cal·ca·ne·an** (kal-ka'ne-ən) calcaneal.

**cal·ca·ne·itis** (kal-ka"ne-i'tis) inflammation of the calcaneus.

**calcane(o)-** [L. *calcaneus,* q.v.] a combining form denoting relationship to the calcaneus.

**cal·ca·neo·apoph·y·si·tis** (kal-ka"ne-o-ə-pof"ə-zi'tis) an affection of the posterior part of the calcaneus marked by pain at the point of insertion of the Achilles tendon, with swelling of the soft parts.

**cal·ca·neo·as·trag·a·loid** (kal-ka"ne-o-ə-strag'ə-loid) pertaining to the calcaneus and astragalus.

**cal·ca·neo·ca·vus** (kal-ka"ne-o-ka'vəs) see under *talipes.*

**cal·ca·neo·cu·boid** (kal-ka"ne-o-ku'boid) pertaining to the calcaneus and cuboid bone.

**cal·ca·ne·odyn·ia** (kal-ka"ne-o-din'e-ə) pain in the heel, or calcaneus.

**cal·ca·neo·fib·u·lar** (kal-ka"ne-o-fib'u-lər) pertaining to the calcaneus and the fibula.

**cal·ca·neo·na·vic·u·lar** (kal-ka"ne-o-nə-vik'u-lər) pertaining to the calcaneus and navicular bone.

**cal·ca·neo·plan·tar** (kal-ka"ne-o-plan'tər) pertaining to the calcaneus and the sole of the foot.

**cal·ca·neo·scaph·oid** (kal-ka"ne-o-skaf'oid) calcaneonavicular.

**cal·ca·neo·tib·i·al** (kal-ka"ne-o-tib'e-əl) pertaining to the calcaneus and the tibia.

**cal·ca·neo·val·go·ca·vus** (kal-ka"ne-o-val"go-ka'vəs) clubfoot in which talipes calcaneus, talipes valgus, and talipes cavus are combined.

**cal·ca·ne·um** (kal-ka'ne-əm) pl. *calca'nea* [L.] calcaneus.

**cal·ca·ne·us** (kal-ka'ne-əs) pl. *calca'nei* [L.] [MeSH: Calcaneus] 1. [TA] the irregular quadrangular bone at the back of the tarsus; called also *calcaneal bone, calcaneum, heel bone, os calcis,* and *os tarsi fibulare.* 2. talipes calcaneus.

**cal·ca·no·dyn·ia** (kal"kə-no-din'e-ə) calcaneodynia.

**cal·car** (kal'kər) [L. "spur"] 1. spur. 2. a structure resembling a spur.
**c. a'vis** [TA], calcarine spur: an eminence on the medial wall of the occipital horn of the lateral ventricle, below the bulb of the occipital horn, produced by lateral extension of the calcarine sulcus.
**c. femora'le,** the plate of strong tissue which strengthens the neck of the femur.
**c. pe'dis,** the heel.

**cal·car·ea** (kal-kar'e-ə) [L.] calcium oxide or hydroxide.
**c. chlora'ta,** chlorinated lime, a disinfectant and bleaching agent.
**c. hy'drica,** calcium hydroxide topical solution.
**c. phospho'rica,** precipitated calcium phosphate.
**c. us'ta,** calcium oxide.

**cal·car·e·ous** (kal-kar'e-əs) [L. *calcarius*] pertaining to or containing lime or calcium; chalky.

**cal·ca·rine** (kal'kə-rīn) [L. *calcarinus* spur-shaped] 1. spur-shaped. 2. pertaining to a calcar.

**cal·ca·ri·uria** (kal-ka"re-u're-ə) [L. *calcarius* containing lime + *-uria*] the presence of lime salts in the urine.

**cal·ca·roid** (kal'kə-roid) resembling calcium; a term given to certain deposits in cerebral tissue which resemble calcification but do not give a specific reaction for calcium.

**cal·ce·mia** (kal-se′me-ə) [*calci-* + *-emia*] hypercalcemia.

**calci-** [L. *calx,* gen. *calcis* lime] a combining form denoting relationship to calcium or calcium salts.

**cal·ci·bil·ia** (kal″sĭ-bil′e-ə) the presence of calcium in the bile.

**Cal·ci·bind** (kal′sĭ-bīnd) trademark for a preparation of cellulose sodium phosphate.

**cal·cic** (kal′sik) of or pertaining to lime or to calcium.

**cal·ci·co·sil·i·co·sis** (kal″sĭ-ko-sil″ĭ-ko′sis) a type of mixed dust pneumoconiosis due to the inhalation of mineral dust containing silica and calcium-containing minerals such as lime, limestone, or marble.

**cal·ci·co·sis** (kal″sĭ-ko′sis) [*calci-* + *-osis*] pneumoconiosis resulting from the inhalation of dust containing calcium, such as from lime, limestone, or marble.

**cal·ci·di·ol** (kal″sĭ-di′ol) 25-hydroxycholecalciferol.

**cal·cif·e·di·ol** (kal″sif-ə-di′ol) [MeSH: Calcifediol] 1. 25-hydroxycholecalciferol. 2. [USP] a preparation of this compound, used to treat renal osteodystrophy or hypocalcemia associated with chronic renal failure, as well as a variety of disorders of vitamin D nutrition or metabolism.

**Cal·cif·er·ol** (kal-sif′ər-ol) trademark for a preparation of ergocalciferol.

**cal·cif·er·ol** (kal-sif′ər-ol) 1. a compound having vitamin D activity, e.g., cholecalciferol or ergocalciferol. 2. ergocalciferol.

**cal·cif·ic** (kal-sif′ik) forming lime.

**cal·ci·fi·ca·tion** (kal″sĭ-fĭ-ka′shən) [*calci-* + L. *facere* to make] the process by which organic tissue becomes hardened by a deposit of calcium salts within its substance.
**dystrophic c.,** the deposition of calcium in abnormal tissue, such as scar tissue or atherosclerotic plaques, but without abnormalities of blood calcium.
**eggshell c.,** deposition of a thin layer of calcium around a thoracic lymph node, often seen in silicosis.
**metastatic c.,** the deposition of calcium in vital tissues as a result of elevations in calcium and phosphate levels in the blood and tissue fluids.
**Mönckeberg's c.,** see under *arteriosclerosis.*

**cal·cig·er·ous** (kal-sij′ər-əs) [*calci-* + L. *gerere* to bear] producing or carrying calcium salts.

**Cal·ci·jex** (kal′sĭ-jeks) trademark for a preparation of calcitriol.

**Cal·ci·mar** (kal′sĭ-mar) trademark for a preparation of calcitonin.

**cal·ci·na·tion** (kal″sĭ-na′shən) [L. *calcinare* to char] the process of reducing to a dry powder by heat.

**cal·cine** (kal′sin) to reduce to a dry powder by heat.

**cal·ci·no·sis** (kal″sĭ-no′sis) [MeSH: Calcinosis] a condition marked by the deposition of calcium salts in various tissues of the body.
**c. circumscrip′ta,** localized deposition of calcium in small nodules in subcutaneous tissues or muscle, usually in systemic scleroderma or dermatomyositis.
**c. cu′tis,** a condition marked by deposits of calcium salts in the skin in the form of nodules or plaques.
**enzootic c.,** a chronic condition in ruminants caused by plant poisoning or mineral imbalance; symptoms include calcification of soft tissues, joint inflammation, diarrhea, and emaciation. Plants causing it include *Cestrum diurnum;* several species of *Solanum,* especially *S. malacoxylon;* and *Trisetum flavescens.* Called also *enteque* and *Manchester wasting disease.*
**c. intervertebra′lis,** deposit of calcium in one or more intervertebral disks; called also *chondritis intervertebralis calcanea* and *Verse's disease.*
**tumoral c.,** development of large periarticular masses about the shoulder, elbow, and hip, marked by symptoms such as sciatica due to pressure on adjacent nerves. It is of unknown etiology, with onset usually in the first or second decade of life.
**c. universa′lis,** widespread deposition of calcium salts in the dermis, panniculus, and muscles, in the form of nodules or plaques, most often in children, principally girls, with dermatomyositis.

**cal·cio·ki·ne·sis** (kal″se-o-kĭ-ne′sis) mobilization of calcium stored in the body.

**cal·cio·ki·net·ic** (kal″se-o-kĭ-net′ik) pertaining to or causing calciokinesis.

**cal·ci·or·rha·chia** (kal″se-o-ra′ke-ə) [*calcio-* + *rhachi-* + *-ia*] the presence of calcium in the spinal fluid.

**cal·ci·pec·tic** (kal″sĭ-pek′tik) pertaining to, characterized by, or causing calcipexy.

**cal·ci·pe·nia** (kal″sĭ-pe′ne-ə) [*calci-* + *-penia*] deficiency of calcium; called also *hypocalcia.* See also *hypocalcemia.*

**cal·ci·pe·nic** (kal″sĭ-pe′nik) pertaining to or characterized by calcipenia.

**cal·ci·pex·ic** (kal″sĭ-pek′sik) calcipectic.

**cal·ci·pex·is** (kal″sĭ-pek′sis) calcipexy.

**cal·ci·pexy** (kal′sĭ-pek″se) [*calci-* + *-pexy*] fixation of calcium in the tissues of the organism.

**cal·ci·phil·ia** (kal″sĭ-fil′e-ə) [*calci-* + *-philia*] a tendency to absorb calcium salts from the blood and thus to become calcified.

**cal·ci·phy·lac·tic** (kal″sĭ-fə-lak′tik) pertaining to or characterized by calciphylaxis.

**cal·ci·phy·lax·is** (kal″sĭ-fə-lak′sis) [MeSH: Calciphylaxis] the formation of calcified tissue in response to administration of a challenging agent subsequent to induction of a hypersensitive state.
**systemic c.,** the generalized appearance of calcifications in internal organs or tissues, occurring in response to intravenous or intraperitoneal injection of the challenging agent.
**topical c.,** the formation of a circumscribed area of calcification in response to subcutaneous injection of the challenging agent.

**cal·ci·po·tri·ene** (kal″sĭ-po-tri′ēn) a synthetic derivative of vitamin $D_3$ (cholecalciferol), applied topically as an antipsoriatic.

**cal·ci·priv·ia** (kal″sĭ-priv′e-ə) [*calci-* + L. *privus* without + *-ia*] deprivation or loss of calcium; see also *hypocalcemia.*

**cal·ci·priv·ic** (kal″sĭ-priv′ik) pertaining to or characterized by calciprivia.

**cal·ci·py·eli·tis** (kal″sĭ-pi-ə-li′tis) calculous pyelitis.

**Calcitite** (kal′sĭ-tīt) trademark for hydroxylapatite.

**cal·ci·to·nin** (kal″sĭ-to′nin) [MeSH: Calcitonin] a 32-amino-acid polypeptide hormone elaborated by the parafollicular cells of the thyroid gland in response to hypercalcemia; it lowers plasma calcium and phosphate levels, inhibits bone resorption, and acts as an antagonist to parathyroid hormone. It is secreted in lower vertebrates by the ultimobranchial bodies. It is used in the treatment of severe hypercalcemia and Paget's disease of bone. Called also *thyrocalcitonin.*
**c.-salmon, c. (salmon), salmon c.,** a form of calcitonin originally obtained from salmon but now also prepared synthetically; administered by subcutaneous or intramuscular injection.

**cal·ci·tri·ol** (kal″sĭ-tri′ol) [MeSH: Calcitriol] 1. 1,25-dihydroxycholecalciferol. 2. a preparation of this compound, used in the treatment of hypocalcemia, hypophosphatemia, rickets, and osteodystrophy associated with a variety of disorders, particularly chronic renal failure and hypoparathyroidism. It is also used in the prophylaxis and treatment of tetany in premature infants, and of vitamin D deficiencies due to metabolic or nutritional inadequacies.

**cal·ci·um** (kal′se-əm) [L. *calx* lime] [MeSH: Calcium] a silvery yellow metal, the basic element of lime. Symbol, Ca; atomic number, 20; atomic weight, 40.08. It is found in nearly all organized tissues, being the most abundant mineral in the body. In combination with phosphorus it forms calcium phosphate, the dense, hard material of the teeth and bones. It is an essential dietary element, a constant blood calcium level being essential for the maintenance of the normal heartbeat, and for the normal functioning of nerves and muscles. It also plays a role in multiple phases of blood coagulation (in which it is called *coagulation factor IV*) and in many enzymatic processes.
**c. 45,** see *radiocalcium.*
**c. 47,** see *radiocalcium.*
**c. acetate** [USP], the calcium salt of acetic acid; administered orally as a source of calcium for hemodialysis patients and others.
**c. ascorbate** [USP], ascorbic acid calcium salt, used as a source of vitamin C (ascorbic acid) in nutritional supplements.
**c. benzamidosalicylate,** benzoylpas calcium.
**c. carbimide,** 1. c. cyanamide. 2. c. carbimide, citrated.
**c. carbimide, citrated,** a mixture containing calcium cyanamide and citric acid; an antialcoholic. See also *c. cyanamide.*
**c. carbonate** [USP], a compound, $CaCO_3$, occurring naturally in a variety of sources, including bones, shells, and limestone. It is used chiefly as an antacid in its native form, in a prepared form (see *prepared chalk,* under *chalk*), and in a precipitated form.
**c. caseinate,** a nutrient preparation of casein and calcium.
**c. chloride** [USP], a salt, $CaCl_2 2H_2O$, occurring as white, hard fragments or granules. It is used as a calcium replenisher, administered intravenously, and has been used as an acid-producing diuretic and urinary acidifier and to control bleeding in such conditions as purpura, intestinal bleeding, and small multiple hemorrhages. It is also a specific antidote for magnesium poisoning, administered intravenously.
**c. cyanamide,** a compound, $CaCN_2$, obtained by the interaction of nitrogen and calcium carbide in an electric furnace, which inhibits

one or more of the enzymes required for oxidation of acetaldehyde formed from alcohol; used as a fertilizer, defoliant, herbicide, and pesticide. Drinking of alcohol after inhalation or ingestion of calcium cyanamide causes unpleasant symptoms (see *mal rouge*); thus it has been used to treat alcoholism in a mixture with citric acid *(citrated c. carbimide)*. Called also *c. carbimide* and *cyanamide.*
**c. cyclamate,** cyclamate calcium.
**c. disodium edathamil, c. disodium edetate,** edetate calcium disodium.
**C. Disodium Versenate,** trademark for edetate calcium disodium.
**c. EDTA,** edetate calcium disodium.
**c. fluoride,** a compound, $CaF_2$, occurring in the bones and teeth.
**c. glubionate,** a calcium replenisher, used as a nutritional supplement and for the treatment of hypocalcemia; administered orally.
**c. gluconate** [USP], a calcium salt of gluconic acid, used as a calcium replenisher, administered intravenously or orally. It is an oral antidote for fluoride or oxalic acid poisoning.
**c. hydroxide** [USP], a salt, $Ca(OH)_2$, occurring as a white powder; used in solution as a topical astringent.
**c. lactate** [USP], a calcium replenisher, administered orally in the treatment of calcium deficiency.
**c. levulinate** [USP], a calcium replenisher, administered parenterally in the treatment of calcium deficiency.
**c. oxalate,** $CaC_2O_4$, a salt of oxalic acid which, when formed in high concentrations in the urine, may lead to formation of an oxalate calculus (see under *calculus*).
**c. oxide,** a corrosively alkaline and caustic earth, CaO, used for absorbing carbon dioxide from air, and industrially as a cheap alkali and as a base for mortar; called also *calcarea usta, calx, lime,* and *quicklime.*
**c. pantothenate** [USP], the calcium salt of the dextrorotatory isomer of pantothenic acid, the B-complex vitamin; used, usually in combination with other B vitamins, as a nutritional supplement. See also *racemic c. pantothenate.*
**c. pantothenate, racemic** [USP], a mixture of the calcium salts of the dextrorotatory and levorotatory isomers of pantothenic acid, with a physiological activity about half that of calcium pantothenate.
**c. phosphate,** any of three salts containing calcium and the phosphate radical $(PO_4)$.
**c. phosphate, dibasic** [USP], an odorless, tasteless, white powder, $CaHPO_4 \cdot 2H_2O$, used as a calcium supplement and as a base in preparation of tablets; called also *dicalcium phosphate.*
**c. phosphate, tribasic,** 1. the compound $Ca_3(PO_4)_2$, true tribasic calcium phosphate, a rarely occurring form. 2. [NF] an amorphous variable mixture of calcium phosphates with approximate formula $(Ca_3(PO_4)_2)_3 \cdot Ca(OH)_2$ (see *hydroxyapatite*), used as a calcium supplement; it is also used as an antacid and as a laxative.
**c. polycarbophil** [USP], a calcium salt of a loosely cross-linked, hydrophilic resin of the polycarboxylic type; a cathartic.
**c. propionate,** the calcium salt of propionic acid, which has antifungal properties; used alone or in combination with sodium propionate or other agents as a preservative to inhibit mold production in bakery and milk products, other foods, tobacco, and pharmaceuticals and as a topical antifungal in the treatment of various mycoses.
**c. pyrophosphate,** the pyrophosphate salt of calcium, $Ca_2O_7P_2$, used as a polishing agent in dentifrices. Crystals of the dihydrate form occur in the joints in calcium pyrophosphate deposition disease.
**c. stearate** [NF], a compound of calcium with organic acids obtained from fats, used as a tablet lubricant.
**c. sulfate** [NF], the sulfate salt of calcium, $CaSO_4$, found commonly in nature as anhydrite and in a hydrated form known as *gypsum;* when gypsum is calcined it forms *plaster of Paris.* Dried calcium sulfate dihydrate is used as a tablet diluent.
**c. trisodium pentetate,** pentetate calcium trisodium.
**c. undecylenate** [USP], the calcium salt of undecylenic acid, applied topically in the treatment of infection by *Epidermophyton, Microsporum,* and *Trichophyton.*

**cal·ci·um·ed·e·tate so·di·um** (kal″se-əm-ed′ə-tāt) edetate calcium disodium.

**cal·ci·uria** (kal″se-u′re-ə) the presence of calcium in the urine.

**calc(o)-** see *calci-.*

**cal·co·glob·u·lin** (kal″ko-glob′u-lin) the form of globulin that occurs in calcifying tissue.

**cal·co·spher·ite** (kal″ko-sfēr′it) one of the small globular bodies formed during the process of calcification, by chemical union between the calcium particles and the albuminous organic matter of the intercellular substance. These particles coalesce to form calcoglobulin.

**cal·cu·li** (kal′ku-li) [MeSH: Calculi] plural of *calculus.*

**cal·cu·lo·gen·e·sis** (kal″ku-lo-jen′ə-sis) lithogenesis.

**cal·cu·lo·sis** (kal″ku-lo′sis) lithiasis.

**cal·cu·lous** (kal′ku-ləs) pertaining to, of the nature of, or affected with a calculus or calculi.

**cal·cu·lus** (kal′ku-ləs) pl. *cal′culi* [L. "pebble"] [MeSH: Calculi] an abnormal concretion occurring within the body and usually composed of mineral salts. Called also *stone.*
**alternating c.,** a urinary calculus made up of successive layers of different composition; called also *combination c.*
**apatite c.,** a urinary calculus composed of apatite.
**articular c.,** a deposit in a joint; it is usually composed of sodium urate, sometimes of calcium urate. Called also *joint c., calculous concretion,* and *chalk stone.*
**bile duct c.,** choledocholith.
**biliary c.,** gallstone.
**bronchial c.,** broncholith.
**brushite c.,** a hard, light-colored urinary calculus composed of brushite.
**calcium oxalate c.,** oxalate c.
**cholesterol c.,** a calculus formed of cholesterol; see also under *gallstone.*
**combination c.,** alternating c.
**cystine c.,** a soft variety of urinary calculus composed of cystine.
**decubitus c.,** a calculus formed in the urinary tract as a result of long immobilization.
**dental c.,** a hard, stonelike concretion, varying in color from creamy yellow to black, that forms on the teeth or dental prostheses through calcification of dental plaque. According to location, there are two general types: *supragingival c.* and *subgingival c.* Called also *odontolith, tartar,* and *dental tophus.*
**encysted c.,** a urinary calculus enclosed in a sac developed from the wall of the bladder; called also *pocketed c.*
**fibrin c.,** a urinary calculus formed largely from fibrinogen in blood.
**fusible c.,** a calculus formed of a mixture of calcium phosphate and triple phosphates which fuses to a black, enamel-like mass when submitted to high heat.
**gastric c.,** gastrolith.
**gonecystic c.,** spermatic c.
**hemic c.,** a calculus developed from a blood clot.
**hemp seed c.,** a small, smooth, oxalate calculus the size and shape of a hemp seed.
**hepatic c.,** a gallstone formed in the intrahepatic bile ducts.
**indigo c.,** calculus formed by oxidation of the indican of the urine.
**intestinal c.,** enterolith.
**joint c.,** articular c.
**lacrimal c.,** one in a lacrimal gland or duct; dacryolith.
**lacteal c.,** mammary c.
**lung c.,** 1. pneumolith. 2. broncholith.
**mammary c.,** a concretion in one of the lactiferous ducts; called also *lacteal c.*
**matrix c.,** a yellowish white to light tan urinary calculus with the consistency of putty, containing calcium salts but composed chiefly of an organic matrix consisting of a mucoprotein and a sulfated mucopolysaccharide.
**mulberry c.,** a hard, smooth oxalate calculus shaped like a mulberry.
**nasal c.,** rhinolith.
**nephritic c.,** renal c.
**oxalate c.,** a hard urinary calculus of calcium oxalate, often in the form of weddellite or whewellite; some are covered with minute sharp spines that may abrade the renal pelvic epithelium, and others (such as *hemp seed* and *mulberry calculi*) are smooth. Called also *calcium oxalate c.*
**pancreatic c.,** a concretion formed in the pancreatic duct from calcium carbonate with other salts and organic materials. Called also *pancreatolith.*
**phosphate c., phosphatic c.,** a urinary calculus composed of a phosphate such as brushite, struvite, or whitlockite along with calcium oxalate; it may be hard, soft, or friable, and so large that it may fill the renal pelvis and calices.
**pocketed c.,** encysted c.
**preputial c.,** postholith.
**prostatic c.,** a concretion formed in the prostate, chiefly of calcium carbonate and phosphate.
**renal c.,** a calculus occurring in the kidney; cf. *urinary c.* Called also *nephritic c., nephrolith,* and *kidney stone.*
**renal c., primary,** one formed in an apparently healthy urinary tract, usually composed of oxalates or urates.
**renal c., secondary,** one associated with infection and obstruction, usually composed of ammonium magnesium phosphate.
**salivary c.,** 1. sialolith. 2. supragingival c.
**serumal c.,** subgingival c., so called because it is supposed to result from exudation of serum.
**shellac c.,** a gastrolith caused by drinking shellac varnish.
**spermatic c.,** a concretion in a seminal vesicle. Called also *gonecystic c.*
**staghorn c.,** a calculus of the renal pelvis usually extending into multiple calices.

**stomachic c.,** gastrolith.
**struvite c.,** a urinary calculus composed of struvite, seen when the renal pelvis is infected with urea-splitting bacteria such as *Proteus.* Called also *infection stone.*
**subgingival c.,** calculus located below the crest of the marginal gingiva, usually in periodontal pockets. Called also *serumal c.*
**submorphous c.,** a calculus made up of molecules of a crystalline salt, together with molecules of the colloid matter in which the salt is contained.
**supragingival c.,** calculus covering the coronal surface of the tooth to the crest of the gingival margin. Called also *salivary c.*
**tonsillar c.,** tonsillolith.
**triple phosphate c.,** struvite c.
**urate c.,** a calculus composed of urates, usually smooth, round, and yellow-brown, occurring chiefly in newborn or young infants.
**urethral c.,** calculus of the urethra with symptoms varying according to sex and the site of lodgment.
**uric acid c.,** a hard, yellow or reddish-yellow urinary calculus formed from uric acid.
**urinary c.,** a calculus in any part of the urinary tract; *vesical calculi* are those lodged in the bladder and *renal calculi* are those in the pelvis of the kidney. Common types named for their primary components are *oxalate calculi, phosphate calculi,* and *uric acid calculi.* Called also *urolith.*
**urostealith c.,** a urinary calculus formed of fatty matter.
**uterine c.,** an intrauterine concretion formed mainly by the calcification of a tumor; called also *womb stone.*
**vesical c.,** a calculus found in the urinary bladder; cf. *urinary c.* Called also *bladder stone* and *cystolith.*
**vesicoprostatic c.,** a prostatic calculus extending into the urinary bladder.
**weddellite c.,** a common type of oxalate calculus, containing weddellite.
**whewellite c.,** a common type of oxalate calculus, containing whewellite.
**whitlockite c.,** a urinary calculus composed of whitlockite.
**xanthic c.,** a urinary calculus composed mainly of xanthine.

**Cal·da·ni's ligament** (kal-dah'nēz) [Leopoldo Marcantonio *Caldani,* Italian anatomist, 1725–1813] see under *ligament.*

**cal·des·mon** (kal-dez'mən) a protein that exists in two isoforms: a high molecular weight form found in smooth muscles that can bind to actin and tropomyosin, prevent actin-myosin linkage, and inhibit muscle contraction, and a low molecular weight form found in nonmuscle tissue and cells that plays a role in regulating the microfilament network.

**Cald·well's position, projection** (kawld'welz) [Eugene Wilson *Caldwell,* American radiologist, 1870–1918] see under *position* and *projection.*

**Cald·well-Luc operation** (kawld'wel lūk) [George W. *Caldwell,* American physician, 1834–1918; Henri *Luc,* French laryngologist, 1855–1925] see under *operation.*

**Cald·well-Mo·loy classification** (kawld'wel-mə-loi') [William Edgar *Caldwell,* American obstetrician, 1880–1943; Howard Carman *Moloy,* Canadian obstetrician, 1903–1953] see under *classification.*

**Calef.** abbreviation for L. *calefactus,* warmed, or for L. *calefac,* make warm.

**cal·e·fa·cient** (kal"ə-fa'shənt) [L. *calidus* warm + *-facient*] 1. warming; causing a sensation of warmth. 2. an agent that causes a sensation of warmth.

**Ca·len·du·la** (kə-len'du-lə) [L.] a genus of composite-flowered plants (family Compositae). The dried florets of *C. officina'lis,* the pot marigold, are stimulant and resolvent, and were once used externally for inflammatory lesions of the skin and mucous membranes.

**calf** (kaf) [L. *sura*] 1. sura. 2. the young of a bovine. 3. the young of any of several other mammalian species.
**baldy c.,** a calf with a lethal inherited condition characterized by alopecia, cracked and ulcerated skin, elongated feet, and hypersalivation.
**bulldog c.,** a calf born with lethal skeletal defects including short limbs, a swollen cranium, and a cleft palate.

**cal·i·ber** (kal'ĭ-bər) [Fr. *calibre* the bore of a gun] the diameter of a canal or tube.

**cal·i·bra·tion** (kal"ĭ-bra'shən) [MeSH: Calibration] 1. determination of the accuracy of an instrument, usually by measurement of its variation from a standard, to ascertain necessary correction factors. 2. measurement of the caliber of a tube.

**cal·i·ce·al** (kal"ĭ-se'əl) pertaining to or affecting a calix.

**cal·i·cec·ta·sis** (kal"ĭ-sek'tə-sis) dilatation of a calix of a kidney.

**cal·i·cec·to·my** (kal"ĭ-sek'tə-me) excision of a calix of a kidney.

**ca·li·ces** (ka'lĭ-sēz) [L.] plural of *calix.* In TA nomenclature, this plural is used with the singular *calyx.*

**cal·i·cine** (kal'ĭ-sēn) related to or resembling a calix.

**ca·li·ci·vi·ral** (kə-lis"-ĭ-vi'rəl) pertaining to or caused by caliciviruses.

**Ca·li·ci·vi·ri·dae** (kə-lis"ĭ-vir'ĭ-de) [MeSH: Caliciviridae] the caliciviruses: a family of RNA viruses having a nonenveloped virion 27–40 nm in diameter with 32 cuplike depressions in a $t = 3$ arrangement. The genome consists of a single molecule of positive-sense single-stranded polyadenylated RNA (MW $2.6–2.7 \times 10^6$, size 7.4–7.7 kb). Viruses contain one major and two minor polypeptides and are resistant to chloroform, ether, mild detergents, and lipid solvents; some are inactivated by trypsin. Replication and assembly occur in the cytoplasm; virions are released by cell destruction. Host range is narrow and transmission is via infested food, by contact, or by airborne particles. There is a single genus, *Calicivirus.*

**Ca·li·ci·vi·rus** (kə-lis'ĭ-vi"rəs) [L. *calix,* gen. *calicis* cup + *virus*] [MeSH: Calicivirus] caliciviruses; a genus of the family Caliciviridae that includes vesicular exanthema of swine virus, human calicivirus, feline calicivirus, Norwalk virus and other Norwalk-like viruses, hepatitis E virus, rabbit hemorrhagic fever virus, and other viruses infecting animals.

**ca·li·ci·vi·rus** (kə-lis'ĭ-vi"rəs) [MeSH: Calicivirus] a member of the family Caliciviridae.
**feline c.,** a virus of the genus *Calicivirus,* transmitted by aerosol droplets and fomites, that causes respiratory disease in cats.
**human c's,** a group of viruses of the genus *Calicivirus* that includes Norwalk virus and a number of other strains that cause acute, self-limited gastroenteritis in humans.

**Cal·i·coph·o·ron** (kal"ĭ-kof'ə-ron) a genus of trematodes of the family Paramphistomatidae that infest the rumen and intestines of ruminants, causing paramphistomiasis.

**ca·lic·u·li** (kə-lik'u-li) genitive and plural of *caliculus.*

**ca·lic·u·lus** (kə-lik'u-ləs) pl. *cali'culi* [L., dim. of *calix*] a bud-shaped or cup-shaped structure.
**c. gustato'rius** [TA], taste bud: one of the minute, barrel-shaped terminal organs of the gustatory nerve, situated around the bases of the vallate, fungiform, and foliate papillae of the tongue. It contains several types of cells, including basal cells, taste cells, supporting cells, and some that are both supporting and taste cells. Called also *gustatory bud, Schwalbe's corpuscle,* and *gemma gustatoria* [TA alternative].
**c. ophthal'micus,** ophthalmic cup: an indentation of the distal wall of the optic vesicle, brought about by rapid marginal growth and producing a double-layered cup, attached to the diencephalon by a tubular stalk. Called also *ocular cup* and *optic cup.*

**ca·li·ec·ta·sis** (ka"le-ek'tə-sis) [*calix* + *ectasis*] calicectasis.

**ca·li·ec·to·my** (ka"le-ek'to-me) [*calix* + *-ectomy*] calicectomy.

**cal·i·for·ni·um** (kal"ĭ-for'ne-əm) [named from *California* (University and state), where it was first produced] [MeSH: Californium] chemical element of atomic number 98, atomic weight 249, symbol Cf, produced by irradiation of the isotope of curium of atomic weight 242 with helium ions; half-life 45 minutes.

**cal·i·pers** (kal'ĭ-pərz) [from *caliber*] compasses with bent or curved legs used for measuring the thickness or diameter of a solid.
**skinfold c.,** calipers designed for measuring skinfolds (q.v.).

**cal·is·then·ics** (kal"is-then'iks) [Gr. *kalos* beautiful + *sthenic*] a system of light gymnastics for promoting strength and grace of carriage.

**ca·lix** (ka'liks) pl. *cal'ices* [L. "drinking cup"] calyx.
**renal calices,** calices renales.
**renal calices, greater,** calices renales majores.
**renal calices, major,** calices renales majores.
**renal calices, minor,** calices renales minores.
**ca'lices rena'les,** renal calices: the recesses of the pelvis of the kidney which enclose the pyramids; called also *calyces renales* and *infundibula of kidney.*
**ca'lices rena'les majo'res** [TA], major renal calices: the two or more larger subdivisions of the renal pelvis, into which the minor calices open; called also *calyces renales majores* and *greater renal calices.*
**ca'lices rena'les mino'res** [TA], minor renal calices: a varying number of smaller subdivisions of the renal pelvis which enclose the pyramids, and open into the major calices; called also *calyces renales minores.*

**Call-Ex·ner bodies** (kahl-eks'nər) [Friedrich von *Call,* Austrian physician, 1844–1917; Siegmund *Exner,* Austrian physiologist, 1846–1926] see under *body.*

**CALLA** common acute lymphoblastic leukemia antigen.

**Cal·lan·der's amputation** (kal'ən-dərz) [C. Latimer *Callander,* American surgeon, 1892–1947] see under *amputation.*

**Cal·le·ja's islands (islets)** (kahl-ya'hahz) [Julián *Calleja* y Sánchez, Spanish anatomist, 1836–1913] see under *island.*

**Cal·liph·o·ra** (kə-lif'o-rə) [Gr. *kallos* beauty + *phoros* bearing] a genus of scavenger flies of the family Calliphoridae, including the blow flies and bluebottle flies, which deposit their eggs in decaying matter, on wounds, or in the openings of the body. Several species lay eggs on wounds or wool, causing cutaneous myiasis. Species include *C. azu'rea, C. erythroce'phala, C. lionen'sis,* and *C. vomito'ria.*
**C. vomito'ria,** the common bluebottle fly, whose larvae may invade the nasal fossae or produce intestinal myiasis.

**cal·liph·o·rid** (kə-lif'ə-rid) a member of the family Calliphoridae.

**Cal·li·phor·i·dae** (kal"ĭ-for'ĭ-de) a family of medium-sized to large flies of the order Diptera, including the genera *Auchmeromyia, Booponus, Calliphora* (type genus), *Cordylobia, Cochliomyia, Chrysomyia, Lucilia, Phaenicia,* and *Phormia;* all species may serve as vectors of pathogens and may also produce myiasis in humans; several are causes of cutaneous myiasis in domestic animals.

**Cal·li·son's fluid** (kal'ĭ-sənz) [James S. *Callison,* American physician, born 1873] see under *fluid.*

**Cal·lis·ta** (kə-lis'tə) a genus of shellfish. *C. brevisphona'ta* was the cause of callistin shellfish poisoning in Japan.

**Cal·li·tro·ga** (kal"ĭ-tro'gə) *Cochliomyia.*

**cal·lo·sal** (kə-lo'səl) pertaining to the corpus callosum.

**Cal·lo·se·las·ma** (kə-lo"sə-laz'mə) a genus of venomous snakes of the family Crotalidae. *C. rhodosto'ma* (formerly called *Agkistrodon rhodostoma*) is the Malayan pit viper, found in Southeast Asia, Malaysia, and Indonesia, whose bite can be fatal to humans.

**cal·los·i·tas** (kə-los'ĭ-təs) [L.] callus.

**cal·los·i·ty** (kə-los'ĭ-te) [L. *callositas,* from *callus*] [MeSH: Callosities] callus.

**cal·lo·so·mar·gin·al** (kə-lo"so-mahr'jĭ-nəl) pertaining to the callosal and marginal gyri.

**cal·lo·sot·o·my** (kal"ə-sot'ə-me) corpuscallosotomy.

**cal·lo·sum** (kə-lo'səm) corpus callosum.

**cal·lous** (kal'əs) hard; like callus.

**cal·lus** (kal'əs) [L.] [MeSH: Callus] 1. localized hyperplasia of the horny layer of the epidermis due to pressure or friction. Called also *callosity, keratoma,* and *tyloma.* See also *hyperkeratosis* (def. 1) and *keratoderma.* 2. an unorganized meshwork of woven bone developed on the pattern of the original fibrin clot, which is formed following fracture of a bone and is normally ultimately replaced by hard adult bone; called also *bony c.* 3. a mass of plant tissue formed over a wound or at the base of a cutting.
**bony c.,** see *callus* (def. 2).
**central c.,** a provisional callus formed within the medullary cavity of a fractured bone; it arises from the cells covering the endosteal and trabecular surfaces near the fracture. Called also *inner c., medullary c.,* and *myelogenous c.*
**definitive c.,** the exudate formed between the fractured ends of the bone, which is permanent and becomes changed into true bone; called also *intermediate c.* and *permanent c.*
**ensheathing c.,** provisional callus forming a sheath about the ends of the fragments of a fractured bone.
**external c.,** the collar of callus formed by the periosteum in a long bone.
**inner c.,** central c.
**intermediate c.,** definitive c.
**internal c., medullary c., myelogenous c.,** central c.
**permanent c.,** definitive c.
**provisional c., temporary c.,** callus formed within the medullary cavity and about the ends of a broken bone, and which is absorbed as the repair is completed.

**cal·ma·tive** (kal'mə-tiv, kahm'ə-tiv) sedative.

**Cal·mette's test, vaccine** (kahl-mets') [Albert Léon Charles *Calmette,* French bacteriologist, 1863–1933] see *BCG vaccine,* under *vaccine.*

**Cal·mette-Gué·rin bacillus** (kahl-met'-ga-ră') [A.L.C. *Calmette;* Camille *Guérin,* French bacteriologist, 1872–1961] see *bacille Calmette-Guérin.*

**cal·mod·u·lin** (kal-mod'u-lin) [MeSH: Calmodulin] a ubiquitous calcium-binding protein of eukaryotic cells that mediates a variety of cellular responses to calcium. The calcium-calmodulin complex acts as a messenger, affecting the activity of many enzymes and nonenzyme proteins, including the calcium pump, numerous specific protein kinases and cyclic nucleotide phosphodiesterases, spectrin, histones, and tubulin.

**Ca·lo·ba·ta** (kə-lo'bə-tə) a genus of South American flies whose larvae sometimes occur in the human intestine.

**cal·o·mel** (kal'o-məl) [L. *calomelas;* Gr. *kalos* fair + *melas* black] chemical name: mercurous chloride. A heavy, white, odorless, impalpable powder, HgCl, insoluble in water, alcohol, ether, and cold dilute acids; rarely used today as a cathartic.
**vegetable c.,** podophyllum.

**ca·lor** (ka'lor) [L.] heat; one of the cardinal signs of inflammation.
**c. febri'lis,** the heat of fever.
**c. fer'vens,** an intense heat.
**c. inna'tus,** the normal or natural heat of the body.
**c. inter'nus,** the heat of the interior of the body.
**c. mor'dax, c. mor'dicans,** 1. biting or stinging heat. 2. the hot, burning, reddish-colored skin occurring in scarlet fever.

**cal·o·ra·di·ance** (kal"ə-ra'de-əns) the radiation or rays which lie between 250 and 55,000 millimicrons, such as the rays from the sun, carbon arcs, incandescent rods and filaments, and hot black bodies.

**cal·o·res·cence** (kal"ə-res'əns) the conversion of nonluminous into luminous heat rays.

**Ca·lo·ri's bursa** (kah-lo'rēz) [Luigi *Calori,* Italian anatomist, 1807–1896] see under *bursa.*

**calori-** [L. *calor,* gen. *caloris* heat] a combining form denoting relationship to heat.

**ca·lo·ric** (kə-lor'ik) pertaining to heat or to calories.

**cal·o·ric·i·ty** (kal"ə-ris'ĭ-te) the power of the animal body of developing and maintaining heat.

**cal·o·rie** (kal'ə-re) [Fr.; L. *calor* heat] any of several units of heat defined as the amount of heat required to raise the temperature of 1 kilogram of water 1 degree Celsius at a specified temperature. The calorie used in chemistry and biochemistry is equal to exactly 4.184 joules. Symbol cal. NOTE: There was formerly a distinction made between the "small calorie," defined above, and the "large calorie," written Calorie with a capital "C" and abbreviated Cal, which was equal to 1000 small calories or one kilocalorie. The use of the large calorie survives only in nutrition, where calorie, now usually written with a small "c," means kilocalorie when specifying the energy content of foods.
**gram c.,** small c.
**IT c., International Table c.,** a unit of heat, equivalent to 4.1868 joules.
**large c.,** the calorie used in metabolic studies, being the amount of heat required to raise the temperature of 1 kilogram of water 1 degree Celsius, specifically from 14.5° to 15.5°C at a pressure of 1 atmosphere; abbreviated kg-cal. Called also *kilocalorie.* Also used to express the fuel or energy value of food.
**mean c.,** one one-hundredth of the amount of heat required to raise the temperature of 1 gram of water from 0° to 100°C.
**small c.,** the amount of heat required to raise the temperature of 1 gram of water 1 degree Celsius, specifically from 14.5° to 15.5°C at a pressure of 1 atmosphere; abbreviated g-cal. Called also *gram c.* and *standard c.*
**standard c.,** small c.
**thermochemical c.,** a unit of heat, equivalent to 4.184 joules.

**cal·or·i·fa·cient** (kə-lor"ĭ-fa'shənt) [*calori-* + *-facient*] producing heat; said of certain foods.

**cal·o·rif·ic** (kal"ə-rif'ik) [*calori-* + L. *facere* to make] producing heat.

**ca·lor·i·ge·net·ic** (kə-lor"ĭ-jə-net'ik) calorigenic.

**ca·lor·i·gen·ic** (kə-lor"ĭ-jen'ik) [*calori-* + *-genic*] producing heat or energy; increasing heat or energy production; increasing the consumption of oxygen.

**cal·o·rim·e·ter** (kal"o-rim'ə-tər) [*calori-* + *-meter*] an instrument for measuring the amount of heat exchanged in any system. In physiology, an apparatus for measuring the amount of heat produced by an individual.
**bomb c.,** an apparatus for measuring the potential energy of food, a weighed amount of the food being placed on a platinum dish inside a hollow steel container (bomb) filled with pure oxygen. The heat produced by its combustion is absorbed by a known quantity of water in which the container is immersed, permitting its measurement.
**compensating c.,** an apparatus in which the object to be tested, such as a developing chick in an egg, is placed at one junction of a thermocouple and an electrical resistance at the other. From the amount of current that must pass through the resistance to keep both junctions at the same temperature (as shown by lack of current in the thermocouple circuit), it is possible to calculate the amount of heat generated in the object being tested.

**ca·lor·i·met·ric** (kah-lor"ĭ-met'rik) pertaining to or performed by calorimetry.

**cal·o·rim·e·try** (kal"ə-rim'ə-tre) [*calori-* + *-metry*] [MeSH: Calorimetry] measurement of the amounts of heat absorbed or given out.
**direct c.,** measurement of the amount of heat produced by a subject enclosed within a small chamber.

**indirect c.,** measurement of the amount of heat produced by a subject by determination of the amount of oxygen consumed and the quantity of nitrogen and carbon dioxide eliminated.

**ca·lor·i·scope** (kə-lor'ĭ-skōp) an instrument for showing the caloric values of mixtures for infant feedings.

**ca·lor·i·trop·ic** (kə-lor"ĭ-trop'ik) [*calori-* + *-tropic*] thermotropic.

**cal·o·ry** (kal'o-re) calorie.

**Ca·lot's triangle** (kah-lōz') [Jean-François *Calot,* French surgeon, 1861–1944] see under *triangle.*

**ca·lotte** (kə-lot') [Fr. "cap"] 1. a part shaped like a skull cap. 2. in ophthalmology, a cap-shaped specimen removed from the eyeball for histopathologic examination. 3. in anatomy, the superior part of the calvaria.

**cal·pain** (kal'pān) [MeSH: Calpain] a calcium-activated proteinase of eukaryotic cells that itself activates several cellular enzymes. In erythrocytes, it affects several proteins important for the determination of cellular shape and deformability.

**cal·re·tic·u·lin** (kal"rə-tik'u-lin) a 55–65 kDa high-affinity calcium-binding protein found in the sarcoplasmic reticulum and also in the endoplasmic reticulum of nonmuscle cells; its many functions include roles in calcium homeostasis, control of viral RNA replication, lymphocyte activation, and cytotoxicity.

**cal·se·ques·trin** (kal"sə-kwes'trin) [MeSH: Calsequestrin] a calcium-binding protein rich in carboxylate side chains, occurring on the inner membrane surface of the sarcoplasmic reticulum; it serves to chelate and store calcium ions.

**cal·va·ria** (kal-var'e-ə) [L.] the domelike superior portion of the cranium, derived from the membranous neurocranium and consisting of the frontal and parietal bones and the squamous parts of the occipital and temporal bones. Called also *concha of cranium* and *skull cap.*

**cal·var·i·al** (kal-var'e-əl) pertaining to the calvaria.

**cal·va·ri·um** (kal-va're-əm) incorrect term for *calvaria.*

**Cal·vé-Per·thes disease** (kahl-va'per'təz) [Jacques *Calvé,* French orthopedist, 1875–1954; Georg Clemens *Perthes,* German surgeon, 1869–1927] osteochondrosis of the capitular epiphysis of the femur.

**Cal·vin cycle** (kal'vin) [Melvin *Calvin,* American chemist, born 1911; winner of the Nobel prize in chemistry for 1961 for development of techniques to determine the chemical reactions of plant carbon dioxide assimilation] see under *cycle.*

**cal·vi·ti·es** (kal-vish'e-ēz) [L.] alopecia.

**calx** (kalks) [L.] 1. [TA] heel: the hindmost projection of the foot. 2. any residue obtained by calcination. 3. lime or calcium oxide, CaO; quicklime: alkaline, caustic, and escharotic.
**c. chlora'ta, c. chlorina'ta,** chlorinated lime.

**cal·y·ce·al** (kal"ĭ-se'əl) caliceal.

**cal·y·cec·ta·sis** (kal"ĭ-sek'tə-sis) calicectasis.

**cal·y·cec·to·my** (kal"ĭ-sek'tə-me) calicectomy.

**cal·y·ces** (kal'ĭ-sēz) plural of *calyx.*

**cal·y·cine** (kal'ĭ-sĭn) calicine.

**cal·y·cle** (kal'ĭ-kəl) a caliculus.

**ca·lyc·u·lus** (kə-lik'u-ləs) gen. and pl. *caly'culi* [L., dim. of Gr. *kalyx* cup of a flower] caliculus.

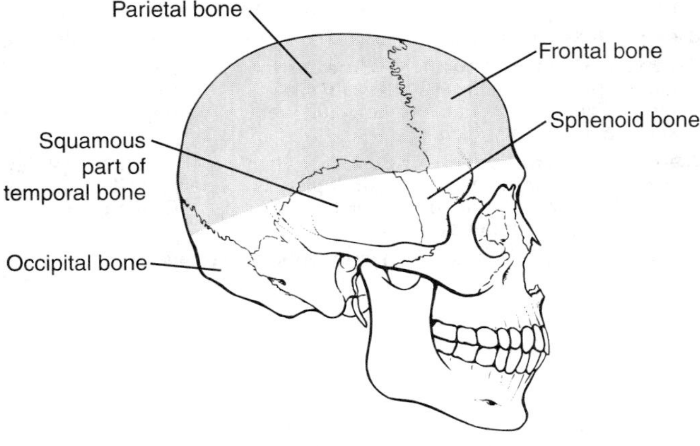


Calvaria.

**Ca·lym·ma·to·bac·te·ri·um** (kə-lim"ə-to-bak-tēr'e-əm) [Gr. *kalymma* a hood or veil + *bacterium*] [MeSH: Calymmatobacterium] a genus of facultatively anaerobic, gram-negative, rod-shaped, capsulated bacteria, characteristically found as intracellular organisms in the cytoplasm of large mononuclear phagocytes; all are human pathogens.
**C. granulo'matis,** a species that is not viable on ordinary media but cultivable on fresh egg-yolk medium. It is serologically related to *Klebsiella pneumoniae* and is the causative agent of human granuloma inguinale. Called also *Donovan's body* and *Donovania granulomatis.*

**ca·lyx** (ka'liks) pl. *cal'yces* [Gr. *kalyx* cup of a flower] [TA] a general term in anatomical nomenclature for a cup-shaped organ or cavity. Called also *calix.*
**cal'yces rena'les,** calices renales; see under *calix.*
**cal'yces rena'les majo'res,** calices renales majores; see under *calix.*
**cal'yces rena'les mino'res,** calices renales minores; see under *calix.*

**CAM** cell adhesion molecules.

**Cam·al·la·nus** (kam"ə-la'nəs) a genus of nematodes of the superfamily Spiruroidea, species of which are parasites in the intestines of fishes, reptiles, and amphibians.

**Cam·ba·roi·des** (kam"bə-roi'dēz) a genus of crayfish which harbor the metacercariae of *Paragonimus.*

**cam·ben·da·zole** (kam-ben'də-zōl) [MeSH: Cambendazole] a benzimidazole used as an anthelmintic in humans and farm animals.

**cam·bi·um** (kam'be-əm) [L. "exchange"] 1. the loose cellular inner layer of the periosteal tissue in the intramembranous ossification of bone. 2. a layer of cells beneath the bark of woody plants.

**Ca·mel·lia** (kə-mel'e-ə) a genus of flowering evergreen trees and shrubs of the family Theaceae, native to hot regions of Asia. *C. sinen'sis* (L.) Kuntze is the tea plant, whose leaves are dried to make the most common type of tea.

**cam·el·pox** (kam'əl-poks) an eruptive disease of camels due to a poxvirus.

**cam·era** (kam'ə-rə) pl. *cameras* or *cam'erae* [L. "chamber"] 1. a box or compartment. 2. [TA] chamber: general anatomical nomenclature for an enclosed space or ventricle. 3. a device for converting light or other energy from an object into a visible image.
**Anger c.,** a device used to form an image of the distribution of a gamma ray–emitting radionuclide in a patient. The radiation is passed through a collimator to reduce scatter and interacts with a sodium iodide crystal, resulting in the production of pulses of light, which are detected and converted to amplified electrical signals by an array of photomultiplier tubes behind the crystal. A pulse height analyzer then discards all but those signals arising from the photopeak of the nuclide being imaged, and the remaining signals are used to form an image of the distribution of the radionuclide on a cathode ray tube. It was the original, and is by far the most commonly used, form of scintillation (or gamma) camera, and the terms are often used interchangeably.
**c. ante'rior bul'bi** [TA], anterior chamber of eye: that portion of the aqueous-containing space between the cornea and the lens which is bounded in front by the cornea and part of the sclera, and behind by the iris, part of the ciliary body, and that part of the lens which presents through the pupil. Called also *c. oculi anterior.* See figure at *chamber.*
**gamma c.,** scintillation c.; see also *Anger c.*
**c. lu'cida,** an optical device utilizing a prism or mirrors so arranged as to throw the reflected image of an object upon paper, thus permitting its outlines to be traced with a pencil.
**c. obscu'ra,** a combined box, lens, and screen, used for viewing, tracing, or making photographs.
**c. o'culi,** any of the chambers of the eye; see figure at *chamber.*
**c. o'culi ante'rior,** c. anterior bulbi.
**c. o'culi poste'rior,** c. posterior bulbi.
**c. poste'rior bul'bi** [TA], posterior chamber of eye: that portion of the aqueous-containing space between the cornea and the lens which is bounded in front by the iris, and behind by the lens and ciliary zonule; called also *c. oculi posterior.* See figure at *chamber.*
**recording c.,** photokymograph.
**scintillation c.,** an electronic instrument that produces photographs or cathode-ray tube images of the gamma ray emissions from organs containing tracer compounds; the original and most commonly used type is the Anger camera (q.v.), with which the term is often equated, although other types, such as multicrystal versions, have also been used.
**c. vi'trea bul'bi** [TA], vitreous chamber of eye: the space in the eyeball enclosing the vitreous humor, bounded anteriorly by the lens and ciliary body and posteriorly by the posterior wall of the eyeball. See figure at *chamber.*

**cam·erae** (kam'ə-re) [L.] plural of *camera.*

**Cam·er·er's law** (kahm'ər-ərz) [Johann Friedrich Wilhelm *Camerer,* German pediatrician, 1842–1910] see under *law.*

**cam·i·sole** (kam′ĭ-sōl) [Fr. "dressing gown"] a device for restraining the limbs, especially the arms, of a violently disturbed person; it consists of a canvas jacket with long sleeves that can be fastened behind the back of the patient. Called also *straitjacket.*

**Cam·mann's stethoscope** (kam′ənz) [George Philip *Cammann,* American physician, 1804–1863] a binaural stethoscope.

**Cam·o·quin** (kam′o-kwin) trademark for a preparation of amodiaquine hydrochloride.

**cAMP** cyclic AMP; see *cyclic adenosine monophosphate.*

**Camp·bell's ligament** (kam′bəlz) [William Francis *Campbell,* American surgeon, 1867–1926] the suspensory ligament of the axilla.

**cAMP-de·pen·dent pro·tein ki·nase** (de-pen′dənt pro′tēn ki′nās) any of a group of closely related protein kinases that are activated by cyclic adenosine monophosphate and catalyze the activity of a variety of intracellular proteins via phosphorylation of specific serine and threonine moieties of other proteins. Called also *protein kinase A* and *cyclic AMP–dependent protein kinase*

**cam·pea·chy** (kam-pe′che) *Haematoxylon campechianum.*

**cam·pe·chy** (kam-pe′che) [*Campeche* state in southeastern Mexico] *Haematoxylon campechianum.*

**Cam·per's fascia, ligament** (kahm′pərz) [Pieter *Camper,* Dutch physician, 1722–1789] see *diaphragma urogenitale,* and see under *fascia.*

**cam·phe·chlor** (kam′fə-klor) toxaphene.

**cam·phene** (kam-fēn′) a terpene found in many essential oils or prepared synthetically from pinene in the process of producing synthetic camphor; it is toxic by ingestion.

**cam·phor** (kam′for, kam′fer) [L. *camphora;* Gr. *kamphora*] [MeSH: Camphor] 1. [USP] a ketone with a characteristic penetrating odor and a pungent taste, obtained from the wood of *Cinnamomum camphora* or produced synthetically. It is applied topically to the skin as an antipruritic and anti-infective and is also used as a pharmaceutic necessity. Called also *gum camphor.* 2. any compound having characteristics similar to those of camphor.
**anise c.,** anethole.
**peppermint c.,** natural menthol.
**synthetic c.,** a camphor produced from pinene, the principal constituent of turpentine.
**thyme c.,** thymol.

**cam·pho·ra** (kam-fo′rə) [L.] camphor.

**cam·pho·ra·ceous** (kam″fə-ra′shəs) having characteristics resembling those of camphor.

**cam·pho·rat·ed** (kam″fə-rāt′əd) [L. *camphoratus*] containing or tinctured with camphor.

**cam·phor·ism** (kam′for-iz-əm) poisoning by camphor; the condition is marked by convulsions, coma, and gastritis.

**cam·pim·e·ter** (kam-pim′ə-tər) [L. *campus* field + *-meter*] an apparatus for mapping the central portion of the visual field on a flat surface.

**cam·pim·e·try** (kam-pim′ə-tre) the determination of the presence of defects in the central portion of the visual field by use of the campimeter.

**cam·po·spasm** (kam′po-spaz-əm) [Gr. *kampē* a bending + *spasm*] camptocormia.

**cam·pot·o·my** (kam-pot′ə-me) [L. *campi* fields (of Forel) + *-tomy*] the stereotaxic surgical technique of producing a lesion in Forel's fields, beneath the thalamus, for correction of tremor in Parkinson's disease.

**camp·to·cor·mia** (kamp″to-kor′me-ə) [Gr. *kamptos* bent + *kormos* trunk + *-ia*] a static deformity consisting of forward flexion of the trunk; called also *camptospasm.*

**camp·to·cor·my** (kamp″to-kor′me) camptocormia.

**camp·to·dac·tyl·ia** (kamp″to-dak-til′e-ə) camptodactyly.

**camp·to·dac·tyl·ism** (kamp″to-dak′tə-liz-əm) camptodactyly.

**camp·to·dac·ty·ly** (kamp″to-dak′tə-le) [Gr. *kamptos* bent + *daktylos* finger] permanent and irreducible flexion of one or more fingers.

**camp·to·me·lia** (kamp″to-me′le-ə) [Gr. *kamptos* bent + *-melia*] bending of the limbs, producing permanent bowing or curving of the affected part; see also *camptomelic syndrome,* under *syndrome.*

**camp·to·me·lic** (kamp″to-me′lik) pertaining to camptomelia.

**Camp·to·sar** (kamp′to-sahr) trademark for a preparation of irinotecan hydrochloride.

**camp·to·spasm** (kamp′to-spaz-əm) camptocormia.

**Cam·py·lo·bac·ter** (kam″pə-lo-bak′tər) [Gr. *kampylos* curved + *-bacter*] [MeSH: Campylobacter] a genus of curved or spiral rod-shaped bacteria made up of gram-negative microaerophilic to anaerobic cells that are motile with polar flagella. The organisms are found in the oral cavity, intestinal tract, and reproductive organs of humans and animals. Some species are pathogenic, causing enteritis and systemic disease in humans and abortion in cattle and sheep.
**C. cinae′di,** *Helicobacter cinaedi.*
**C. co′li,** a species that causes diarrhea in humans.
**C. feca′lis,** a nonpathogenic species isolated from sheep feces and the reproductive organs of cattle.
**C. fennel′liae,** a species that causes proctitis and diarrhea in homosexual men.
**C. fe′tus,** a microaerophilic species occurring as several subspecies. Called also *Vibrio fetus.*
**C. fe′tus** subsp. **fe′tus,** a subspecies that causes abortion and infertility in cattle (bovine genital campylobacteriosis). It is an occasional human pathogen, capable of causing systemic infection in immunocompromised hosts.
**C. fe′tus** subsp. **intestina′lis,** *C. fetus* subsp. *fetus.*
**C. fe′tus** subsp. **jeju′ni,** *C. jejuni.*
**C. fe′tus** subsp. **venera′lis,** a subspecies that causes abortion and infertility in cattle.
**C. hyointestina′lis,** a species that causes porcine proliferative enteritis.
**C. jeju′ni,** a subspecies that is a common cause of acute bacterial gastroenteritis in humans, infectious abortion in sheep, and avian vibrionic hepatitis in fowls; it is also found as a commensal in swine, cattle, cats, and chickens. Called also *Vibrio coli* and *V. jejuni.*
**C. pylo′ri,** *Helicobacter pylori.*
**C. rec′tus,** a species associated with periodontal disease and isolated from dental root canal infections; called also *Wolinella recta.*
**C. sputo′rum,** a usually nonpathogenic, microaerophilic to anaerobic species occurring as three subspecies.
**C. sputo′rum** subsp. **bu′bulus,** a subspecies found in the genital tracts of sheep and cattle.
**C. sputo′rum** subsp. **mucosa′lis,** a subspecies commonly found in the intestinal mucosa and oral cavity of pigs, which sometimes causes porcine proliferative enteritis.
**C. sputo′rum** subsp. **sputo′rum,** a subspecies found in the human oral cavity.

**cam·py·lo·bac·ter** (kam″pə-lo-bak′tər) [MeSH: Campylobacter] a bacterium of the genus *Campylobacter.*

**cam·py·lo·bac·te·ri·o·sis** (kam″pə-lo-bak-tēr″e-o′sis) infection with organisms of the genus *Camylobacter.*
**avian c.,** infection of chickens and other birds by *Campylobacter jejuni,* with hepatitis of varying severity; symptoms range from the subclinical or a simple drop in egg production to weight loss, hemorrhage, depression, and death. Called also *vibrionic, avian vibrionic,* or *avian infectious hepatitis.*
**bovine genital c.,** a venereal disease of cattle caused by *Campylobacter fetus* subspecies *fetus;* characterized by infertility and early embryonic death. Called also *bovine genital vibriosis.*
**enteric c.,** intestinal infection with a species of *Campylobacter;* it occurs in many mammals, including humans.
**ovine genital c.,** an infectious disease of sheep caused by *Campylobacter fetus* subspecies *fetus* and *C. jejuni,* characterized by abortion, and transmitted orally. Called also *ovine genital vibriosis.*

**cam·sy·late** (kam′sə-lāt) USAN contraction for camphorsulfonate.

**Cam·u·ra·ti-En·gel·mann disease** (kah-moo-rah′te-eng′gəl-mahn) [Mario *Camurati,* Italian physician, 1896–1948; Guido *Engelmann,* Czechoslovakian surgeon, 20th century] diaphyseal dysplasia; see under *dysplasia.*

**Can·a·da-Cronk·hite syndrome** (kan′ə-də-krong′kīt) [Wilma Jeanne *Canada,* American radiologist, 20th century; Leonard W. *Cronkhite,* Jr., American internist, born 1919] Cronkhite-Canada syndrome; see under *syndrome.*

**ca·nal** (kə-nal′) a relatively narrow tubular passage or channel; see also *canalis.*

## Canal

For descriptions of specific anatomic structures not found here, see under *canalis.*

**abdominal c.**, canalis inguinalis.
**adductor c.**, canalis adductorius.
**Alcock's c.**, canalis pudendalis.
**alimentary c.**, digestive tract.
**alisphenoid c.**, a canal through the greater wing of the sphenoid bone of various animals, which transmits the internal carotid artery.
**alveolar c's**, see *canalis mandibulae* and *canales alveolares maxillae.*
**alveolar c., anterior**, an alveolar canal of the maxilla located anteriorly; see *canales alveolares maxillae.*
**alveolar c., posterior**, an alveolar canal of the maxilla located posteriorly; see *canales alveolares maxillae.*
**alveolar c's of maxilla**, canales alveolares maxillae.
**anal c.**, canalis analis.
**c. of Arantius**, ductus venosus.
**archenteric c.**, neurenteric c.
**archinephric c.**, pronephric duct.
**Arnold's c.**, 1. canaliculus mastoideus. 2. sulcus nervi petrosi minoris.
**arterial c.**, ductus arteriosus.
**atrioventricular c.**, the common canal connecting the primordial atrium and ventricle; it sometimes persists as a congenital anomaly as a result of failure of closure of the gap between the interatrial and interventricular septa due to arrest in development of the endocardial cushions.
**atrioventricular c., persistent common**, atrioventricularis communis.
**auditory c., external**, meatus acusticus externus.
**auditory c., internal**, meatus acusticus internus.
**basipharyngeal c.**, canalis vomerovaginalis.
**biliary c's, interlobular**, ductuli interlobulares.
**biliary c's, intralobular**, ductuli biliferi.
**birth c.**, the canal through which the fetus passes in birth, comprising the cervix uteri, vagina, and vulva; called also *obstetric c.* and *parturient c.*
**blastoporic c.**, neurenteric c.
**bony c's of ear**, canales semicirculares ossei.
**Braun's c.**, neurenteric c.
**Breschet's c's**, canales diploici.
**calciferous c's**, canals containing lime salts in cartilage that is undergoing calcification.
**caroticotympanic c's**, canaliculi caroticotympanici.
**carotid c.**, canalis caroticus.
**carpal c.**, canalis carpi.
**c's of cartilage**, canals in an ossifying cartilage during its stage of vascularization.
**central c. of modiolus**, see *canales longitudinales modioli.*
**central c. of spinal cord**, canalis centralis medullae spinalis.
**central c. of Stilling, central c. of vitreous**, canalis hyaloideus.
**cerebrospinal c.**, the primordial cavity of the brain and spinal cord.
**cervical c. of uterus**, canalis cervicis uteri.
**chordal c.**, notochordal c.
**c. of chorda tympani**, canaliculus chordae tympani.
**ciliary c's**, spatia anguli iridocornealis.
**Civinini's c.**, canaliculus chordae tympani.
**Cloquet's c.**, canalis hyaloideus.
**cochlear c.**, 1. ductus cochlearis. 2. canalis spiralis cochleae.
**common atrioventricular c.**, atrioventricularis communis.
**condylar c., condyloid c.**, canalis condylaris.
**condyloid c., anterior**, canalis nervi hypoglossi.
**connecting c.**, tubulus renalis arcuatus.
**c. of Corti**, inner tunnel.
**c. of Cotunnius**, the aqueductus vestibuli and canaliculus cochleae considered as a continuous passage.
**craniopharyngeal c.**, an occasional passage through the sphenoid bone, opening into the sella turcica. Some authorities consider it a remnant of Rathke's pouch.
**crural c.**, canalis femoralis.
**crural c. of Henle**, canalis adductorius.
**c. of Cuvier**, ductus venosus.
**dental c., inferior**, canalis mandibulae.
**dental c's, posterior**, 1. canales alveolares maxillae. 2. foramina alveolaria maxillae.
**dentinal c's**, canaliculi dentales.
**digestive c.**, see under *tract.*
**diploic c's**, canales diploici.
**Dorello's c.**, an opening sometimes found in the temporal bone through which the abducens nerve and inferior petrosal sinus together enter the cavernous sinus.
**entodermal c.**, the primordial gut; see *gut* (def. 2).
**c. of epididymis**, ductus epididymidis.
**ethmoidal c., anterior**, foramen ethmoidale anterius.
**ethmoidal c., posterior**, foramen ethmoidale posterius.
**eustachian c.**, tuba auditiva.
**facial c., c. for facial nerve**, canalis nervi facialis.
**fallopian c.**, canalis nervi facialis.
**femoral c.**, canalis femoralis.
**Ferrein's c.**, rivus lacrimalis.
**flexor c.**, canalis carpi.
**Gartner's c.**, ductus longitudinalis epoöphori.
**gastric c.**, canalis gastricus.
**genital c.**, any canal for the passage of ova or for copulatory use; called also *genital duct.*
**gubernacular c's**, four small openings in young crania, one behind each incisor tooth.
**c. of Guidi**, canalis pterygoideus.
**Guyon's c.**, a small superficial canal at the base of the hypothenar bounded by the retinaculum flexorum manus and the musculus flexor carpi ulnaris, which transmits blood vessels and the ulnar nerve from the forearm to the hand. Called also *loge de Guyon.*
**gynecophoral c., gynecophorous c.**, the ventral slot in which the male schistosome carries the female.
**hair c.**, an epidermal canal through which a hair grows in order to erupt.
**Hannover's c.**, a potential space existing between the anterior and posterior portions of the suspensory ligament of the lens.
**haversian c.**, canalis nutricius.
**hemal c.**, the space within the hemal arch.
**Henle's c.**, ansa nephroni.
**Hensen's c.**, ductus reuniens.
**c's of Hering**, openings through which the bile canaliculi communicate with the terminal branches of the bile duct system, the cholangioles; distinguished by their walls, which consist of parenchymal liver cells on one side and cells of the ductules (cholangioles) on the other.
**hernial c.**, that through which a hernia passes.
**Hirschfeld's c's**, interdental c's.
**His' c.**, ductus thyroglossalis.
**Holmgren-Golgi c's**, minute canals in the cytoplasm of cells, particularly of nerve cells, forming a complex apparatus throughout the cytoplasm; called also *intracytoplasmic c's.*
**c. of Hovius**, one of a series of connections between the venae vorticosae in certain mammals.
**Huguier's c.**, iter chordae anterius.
**Hunter's c.**, canalis adductorius.
**Huschke's c.**, see under *foramen.*
**hyaloid c.**, canalis hyaloideus.
**hypoglossal c.**, canalis nervi hypoglossi.
**iliac c.**, lacuna musculorum.
**incisive c's**, canales incisivi.
**incisive c. of mandible**, an extension of the mandibular canal, leading forward to the symphysis inferiorly to the incisor teeth.
**infraorbital c.**, canalis infraorbitalis.
**inguinal c.**, canalis inguinalis.
**intercellular c's**, interfacial c's.
**interdental c's**, channels in the alveolar process of the mandible, between the roots of the medial and lateral incisors, for the passage of anastomosing blood vessels between the sublingual and inferior dental arteries; called also *Hirschfeld's c's.*
**interfacial c's**, a labyrinthine system of expanded intercellular spaces between desmosomes; called also *intercellular c's.*
**intersacral c's**, foramina intervertebralia ossis sacri.
**intestinal c.**, the intestine; that part of the alimentary canal which lies between the pylorus and the anus.
**intracytoplasmic c's**, Holmgren-Golgi c's.
**Jacobson's c., c. for Jacobson's nerve**, canaliculus tympanicus.
**Kovalevsky's c.**, neurenteric c.
**lacrimal c.**, canalis nasolacrimalis.
**Laurer's c.**, a passage in trematode worms extending from the ovarian duct to the dorsal surface of the body.
**longitudinal c's of modiolus**, canales longitudinales modioli.
**Löwenberg's c.**, ductus cochlearis.
**mandibular c.**, canalis mandibulae.
**maxillary c., superior**, foramen rotundum ossis sphenoidalis.
**medullary c.**, 1. cavitas medullaris. 2. canalis vertebralis.
**mental c.**, an extension of the mandibular canal, leading superiorly to connect with the mental foramen.
**c's of modiolus**, see *canalis spiralis modioli* and *canales longitudinales modioli.*
**Müller's c.**, ductus paramesonephricus.
**musculotubal c.**, canalis musculotubarius.
**nasal c., nasolacrimal c.**, canalis nasolacrimalis.
**nasopalatine c's**, canales incisivi.
**neural c.**, canalis vertebralis.
**neurenteric c. (of Kovalevsky)**, a passage, in the embryo, from the

posterior part of the neural tube into the archenteron; called also *Braun's c., archenteric c.,* and *blastoporic c.*

**notochordal c.,** a tunnel extending from the primitive pit into the notochordal process of the embryo; called also *chordal c.*

**c. of Nuck,** processus vaginalis peritonei.

**nutrient c.,** canalis nutricius.

**obstetric c.,** birth c.

**obturator c.,** canalis obturatorius.

**obturator c. of pubic bone,** sulcus obturatorius ossis pubis.

**c. of Oken,** ductus mesonephricus.

**olfactory c.,** the nasal fossae at an early stage of their embryonic development.

**omphalomesenteric c.,** yolk stalk.

**optic c.,** canalis opticus.

**orbital c., anterior internal,** foramen ethmoidale anterius.

**orbital c., posterior internal,** foramen ethmoidale posterius.

**palatine c's, accessory,** canales palatini minores.

**palatine c., greater,** canalis palatinus major.

**palatine c's, lesser,** canales palatini minores.

**palatomaxillary c.,** canalis palatinus major.

**palatovaginal c.,** canalis palatovaginalis.

**paraurethral c's of male urethra,** ductus paraurethrales urethrae masculinae.

**parturient c.,** birth c.

**pelvic c.,** the passage from the superior to the inferior aperture of the pelvis.

**perivascular c.,** a lymph space about a blood vessel.

**Petit's c.,** spatia zonularia.

**pharyngeal c.,** canalis palatovaginalis.

**plasmatic c.,** canalis nutricius.

**pleural c's,** a pair of passages in the embryo, connecting the primordial pericardial and peritoneal cavities.

**portal c.,** a space within the capsule of Glisson and liver substance, containing branches of the portal vein, of the hepatic artery, and of the hepatic duct.

**pterygoid c.,** canalis pterygoideus.

**pterygopalatine c.,** 1. canalis palatinus major. 2. canalis palatovaginalis.

**pudendal c.,** canalis pudendalis.

**pulmoaortic c.,** ductus arteriosus.

**pulp c.,** canalis radicis dentis.

**pyloric c.,** canalis pyloricus.

**c's of Recklinghausen,** small lymph spaces in the connective tissue.

**recurrent c.,** canalis pterygoideus.

**Reichert's c.,** ductus reuniens.

**c's of Rivinus,** ductus sublinguales minores.

**root c.,** canalis radicis dentis.

**root c., accessory,** a lateral branching of the main root canal, usually occurring in the apical third of the root.

**root c. of tooth,** canalis radicis dentis.

**Rosenthal's c.,** canalis spiralis modioli.

**sacculocochlear c.,** ductus reuniens.

**sacculoutricular c.,** ductus utriculosaccularis.

**sacral c.,** canalis sacralis.

**Santorini's c.,** ductus pancreaticus accessorius.

**Schlemm's c.,** a branching, circumferential vessel lying in the internal scleral sulcus, a major component of the drainage pathway for aqueous humor; called also *sinus venosus sclerae* [TA].

**scleral c., scleroticochoroidal c.,** the channel in the choroid and sclera of the eye through which the optic nerve passes; see also *lamina cribrosa sclerae.*

**semicircular c's,** canales semicirculares ossei.

**semicircular c., anterior,** canalis semicircularis anterior.

**semicircular c's, bony,** canales semicirculares ossei.

**semicircular c., horizontal,** canalis semicircularis lateralis.

**semicircular c., lateral,** canalis semicircularis lateralis.

**semicircular c's, membranous,** ductus semicirculares.

**semicircular c., posterior,** canalis semicircularis posterior.

**semicircular c., superior,** canalis semicircularis anterior.

**seminal c.,** a passage for the transmission of semen, or of spermatozoa.

**serous c.,** a minute lymph space.

**sheathing c.,** the passage from the peritoneal cavity to the tunica vaginalis testis.

**singular c.,** foramen singulare.

**Sondermann's c's,** conical extensions of the lumen of Schlemm's canal sometimes observed in the inner wall of the canal.

**spermatic c.,** the canalis inguinalis in the male, providing for passage of the spermatic cord.

**sphenopalatine c.,** 1. canalis palatovaginalis. 2. canalis palatinus major.

**sphenopharyngeal c.,** canalis palatovaginalis.

**spinal c.,** canalis vertebralis.

**spiral c. of cochlea,** canalis spiralis cochleae.

**spiral c. of modiolus,** canalis spiralis modioli.

**c. of Steno, Stensen's c.,** ductus parotideus.

**c. of Stilling,** canalis hyaloideus.

**c. of stomach,** canalis gastricus.

**streak c.,** teat c.

**subsartorial c.,** canalis adductorius.

**Sucquet-Hoyer c.,** segmentum arteriale anastomosis arteriovenosae glomeriformis.

**supraciliary c.,** a small opening sometimes present near the supraorbital notch, which transmits a nutrient artery and a branch of the supraorbital nerve to the frontal sinus.

**supraoptic c.,** a minute canal which is the anterior continuation of the optic recess above the optic chiasma.

**supraorbital c.,** incisura frontalis.

**tarsal c.,** sinus tarsi.

**teat c.,** the canal leading from the lactiferous sinus to the exterior of the udder of an animal. Called also *streak c.*

**c. for tensor tympani muscle,** semicanalis musculi tensoris tympani.

**Theile's c.,** sinus transversus pericardii.

**tubal c.,** semicanalis tubae auditoriae.

**tubotympanic c.,** the inner division of the first pharyngeal (branchial) cleft in the embryo, from which the auditory tube and middle ear cavity are derived.

**tympanic c. of cochlea,** scala tympani.

**umbilical c.,** anulus umbilicalis.

**urogenital c's,** that portion of the urogenital sinus used jointly by the müllerian and mesonephric ducts.

**uterine c.,** cavitas uteri.

**uterocervical c.,** canalis cervicis uteri.

**utriculosaccular c.,** ductus utriculosaccularis.

**vaginal c.,** the space within the vagina; called also *vulvouterine c.*

**Van Hoorne's c.,** ductus thoracicus.

**Velpeau's c.,** canalis inguinalis.

**ventricular c.,** canalis gastricus.

**Verneuil's c's,** collateral vessels of a venous trunk.

**vertebral c.,** canalis vertebralis.

**vestibular c.,** scala vestibuli.

**vidian c.,** canalis pterygoideus.

**Volkmann's c's,** passages other than haversian canals, for the passage of blood vessels through bone.

**vomerine c.,** canalis vomerovaginalis.

**vomerobasilar c., lateral inferior,** canalis palatovaginalis.

**vomerobasilar c., lateral superior,** canalis vomerovaginalis.

**vomerorostral c.,** canalis vomerorostralis.

**vomerovaginal c.,** canalis vomerovaginalis.

**vulvar c.,** vestibulum vaginae.

**vulvouterine c.,** vaginal c.

**c. of Wirsung,** ductus pancreaticus.

**zygomaticotemporal c.,** foramen zygomaticotemporale.

**ca·na·les** (kə-na'lēz) [L.] plural of *canalis.*

**can·a·lic·u·lar** (kan"ə-lik'u-lər) resembling or pertaining to a canaliculus.

**can·a·lic·u·li** (kan"ə-lik'u-li) [L.] plural of *canaliculus.*

**can·a·lic·u·li·tis** (kan"ə-lik"u-li'tis) [L. *canaliculus,* from *canalis* channel + *-itis* inflammation] inflammation of the lacrimal ducts.

**can·a·lic·u·li·za·tion** (kan"ə-lik"u-lĭ-za'shən) the development of canaliculi, as in bone.

**can·a·lic·u·lo·rhi·nos·to·my** (kan"ə-lik"u-lo-ri-nos'tə-me) dacryocystorhinostomy.

**can·a·lic·u·lus** (kan"ə-lik'u-ləs) pl. *canalic'uli* [L. dim. of *canalis*] [TA] an extremely narrow tubular passage or channel; used as a general term in anatomical nomenclature for various small channels.

**apical c.,** any of the numerous tubular invaginations arising from the clefts between the microvilli of the proximal convoluted tubule of the kidney and extending downward into the apical cytoplasm.

**bile canaliculi, biliary canaliculi,** fine tubular canals running between liver cells, throughout the parenchyma, usually occurring singly between each adjacent pair of cells, and forming a three-dimensional network of polyhedral meshes, with a single cell in each mesh. Called also *bile capillaries.*
**bone canaliculi,** branching tubular passages radiating like wheel spokes from each bone lacuna to connect with the canaliculi of adjacent lacunae, and with the haversian canal.
**canali'culi caroticotympan'ici** [TA], caroticotympanic canaliculi: tiny passages in the temporal bone interconnecting the carotid canal and the tympanic cavity, and carrying communicating twigs between the internal carotid and tympanic plexuses; called also *caroticotympanic foramina.*
**c. chor'dae tym'pani** [TA], canaliculus of chorda tympani: a small canal that opens off the facial canal just before its termination, transmitting the chorda tympani nerve into the tympanic cavity; called also *canal of chorda tympani, canalis chordae tympani,* and *Civinini's canal.*
**c. coch'leae** [TA], **cochlear c.,** canaliculus of cochlea: a small canal in the petrous part of the temporal bone that interconnects the scala tympani of the inner ear with the subarachnoid cavity; it houses the perilymphatic duct and a small vein. Called also *aqueduct of Cotunnius.*
**canali'culi denta'les,** dental canaliculi: minute channels in dentin, extending from the pulp cavity to the cementum and enamel. Called also *dental* or *dentinal tubules.*
**haversian c.,** any one of a system of minute channels in compact bone connected with each haversian canal.
**incisor c.,** ductus incisivus.
**innominate c., c. innomina'tus,** 1. sulcus nervi petrosi minoris. 2. foramen petrosum.
**intercellular c.,** one located between adjacent cells, such as one of the secretory capillaries (secretory canaliculi) of the gastric parietal cells.
**intracellular canaliculi of parietal cells,** a system of canaliculi that seem to be intracellular, but are formed by deep invaginations of the surface of the gastric parietal cells rather than extending into the cytoplasm of the cell.
**c. lacrima'lis** [TA], lacrimal canaliculus: the short passage in an eyelid, beginning at the punctum, that leads from the lacrimal lake to the lacrimal sac; called also *lacrimal duct* and *ductus lacrimalis.*

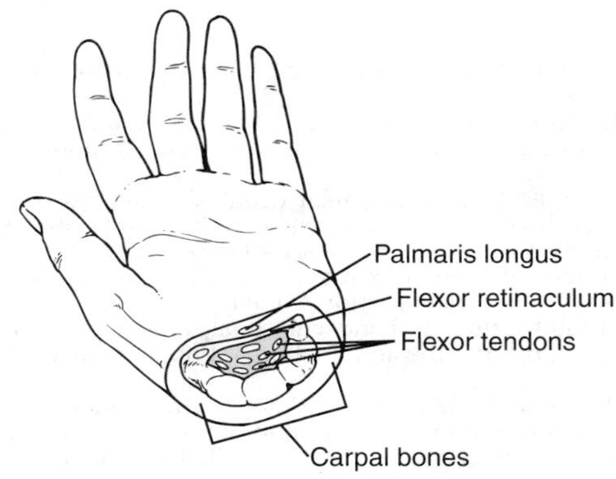

Canalis carpi (carpal tunnel), carrying the tendons of the flexor muscles.

**mastoid c., mastoid c. for Arnold's nerve,** c. mastoideus.
**c. mastoi'deus** [TA], mastoid canaliculus: a minute passage beginning in the lateral wall of the jugular fossa of the temporal bone and passing into the temporal bone. The auricular branch of the vagus nerve passes through it to exit via the tympanomastoid fissure. Called also *mastoid c. for Arnold's nerve.*
**c. petro'sus, petrous c.,** sulcus nervi petrosi minoris.
**pseudobile c.,** one of the dark-staining columns of cells from the bile ducts seen in the portal area of the liver in cirrhosis.
**secretory c.,** see under *capillary.*
**tympanic c. for Jacobson's nerve,** c. tympanicus.
**c. tympa'nicus** [TA], tympanic canaliculus: a small opening on the inferior surface of the petrous part of the temporal bone in the floor of the petrosal fossa; it transmits the tympanic branch of the glossopharyngeal nerve and a small artery. Called also *Jacobson's canal, canal for Jacobson's nerve,* and *tympanic c. for Jacobson's nerve.*

**ca•na•lis** (kə-na'lis) pl. *cana'les* [L.] [TA] canal: a general term for a relatively narrow tubular passage or channel. Cf. *channel, tube,* and *tunnel.*

## Canalis

Descriptions are given on TA terms, and include anglicized names of specific canals.

**c. adducto'rius** [TA], adductor canal: an intramuscular interval on the medial aspect of the middle third of the thigh, which contains the femoral vessels and the saphenous nerve. The lateral wall is formed by the vastus medialis, the posterior wall by the adductor longus and adductor magnus, the roof by a layer of fascia, and it is covered by the sartorius. Called also *crural canal of Henle, Hunter's canal, subsartorial canal,* and *c. subsartorialis.*
**c. alimenta'rius,** digestive tract.
**cana'les alveola'res,** see *canales alveolares maxillae* and *c. mandibulae.*
**cana'les alveola'res maxil'lae** [TA], alveolar canals of maxilla: several canals in the maxilla for the passage of the posterior superior alveolar vessels and nerves, each canal beginning on the infratemporal surface of the maxilla at an alveolar foramen; called also *posterior dental canals.*
**c. ana'lis** [TA], anal canal: the terminal portion of the alimentary canal, extending from the rectum to the anus; called also *pars analis recti.*
**c. caro'ticus** [TA], carotid canal: a passage in the petrous portion of the temporal bone, beginning on the inferior surface just anterior to the jugular foramen, and running anteromedially for about 2 cm.; it is seen interiorly in the floor of the middle cranial fossa, where it meets the carotid sulcus on the body of the sphenoid bone. It houses the internal carotid artery.
**c. car'pi** [TA], carpal canal: an osseofibrous tunnel for passage of the tendons of the flexor muscles of the hand and digits, formed by the flexor retinaculum as it roofs over the concavity of the carpus on the palmar surface; called also *carpal tunnel* and *flexor canal.*
**c. centra'lis medul'lae spina'lis** [TA], central canal of spinal cord: a small canal extending throughout the length of the spinal cord, lined by ependymal cells. Above, it continues into the medulla oblongata, where it opens into the fourth ventricle.
**c. cer'vicis u'teri** [TA], cervical canal of uterus: the part of the uterine cavity that lies within the cervix.
**c. chor'dae tym'pani,** canaliculus chordae tympani.
**c. condyla'ris** [TA], condylar canal: an opening sometimes present in the floor of the condylar fossa for the transmission of a vein from the transverse sinus; called also *condyloid canal* and *posterior condyloid foramen.*
**cana'les diplo'ici** [TA], diploic canals: bony canals in the cranial bones, located in the spongy bone between the compact tables and providing for passage of the veins of the diploë; called also *Breschet's canals.*
**c. facia'lis, c. facia'lis [Fallo'pii],** canalis nervi facialis.
**c. femora'lis** [TA], femoral canal: the cone-shaped medial part of the femoral sheath lateral to the base of the lacunar ligament; called also *crural canal.*
**c. gas'tricus** [TA], gastric canal: the longitudinal grooved channel formed by the more or less regular ridges along the lesser curvature of the stomach; called also *canal of stomach, magenstrasse, ventricular canal, c. ventricularis,* and *c. ventriculi.*
**c. hyaloi'deus** [TA], hyaloid canal: a passage running from in front of the optic disk to the lens of the eye; in the fetus it transmits the hyaloid artery. Called also *central canal of Stilling, central canal of vitreous,* and *Cloquet's canal.*
**c. hypoglossa'lis,** c. nervi hypoglossi.
**canales incisi'vi** [TA], incisive canals: the small canals opening into the incisive fossa of the hard palate, and transmitting small vessels and nerves from the floor of the nose into the front part of the roof of the mouth; called also *nasopalatine canals* and *foramina of Stensen.* See also *foramen incisivum.*
**c. infraorbita'lis** [TA], infraorbital canal: a passage beneath the orbital surface of the maxilla, continuous posteriorly with the infraorbital sulcus, and opening anteriorly on the anterior surface of the body of the maxilla in the infraorbital foramen. It contains the infraorbital vessels and nerve.
**c. inguina'lis** [TA], inguinal canal: the passage superficial to the deep inguinal ring for transmission of the spermatic cord in the male

and the round ligament in the female; called also *abdominal canal* and *Velpeau's canal.*

**cana'les longitudina'les modi'oli** [TA], longitudinal canals of modiolus: short tunnels in the modiolus that transmit blood vessels and nerves.

**c. mandi'bulae** [TA], mandibular canal: a canal that traverses the ramus and body of the mandible between the mandibular and mental foramina, transmitting the inferior alveolar vessels and nerve; beneath the first or second premolars it splits into the mental canal and the incisive canal. Called also *inferior dental canal.*

**c. musculotuba'rius** [TA], musculotubal canal: the combined semicanals of the auditory tube and the tensor tympani muscle in the temporal bone.

**c. nasolacrima'lis** [TA], nasolacrimal canal: a canal formed by the lacrimal sulcus of the maxilla, lacrimal bone, and inferior nasal concha; it contains the nasolacrimal duct. Called also *lacrimal canal* and *nasal canal.*

**c. ner'vi facia'lis** [TA], facial canal: a canal in the temporal bone for the facial nerve, beginning in the internal acoustic meatus and passing anterolaterally dorsal to the vestibule of the inner ear for about 2 mm. Turning sharply backward at the genu of the facial canal, it runs along the medial wall of the tympanic cavity, then turns inferiorly and reaches the exterior of the petrous part of the bone at the stylomastoid foramen. Called also *canal for facial nerve, fallopian aqueduct* or *canal,* and *aqueduct of Fallopius.*

**c. ner'vi hypoglos'si** [TA], hypoglossal canal: an opening in the lateral part of the occipital bone at the base of the condyle, which transmits the hypoglossal nerve and a branch of the posterior meningeal artery; called also *anterior condyloid canal, canalis hypoglossalis,* and *anterior condyloid foramen.*

**c. nutri'cius** [TA], nutrient canal of bone: one of the freely anastomosing channels of the haversian system of compact bone, which contain blood vessels, lymph vessels, and nerves; called also *c. nutriens* [TA alternative], *haversian canal,* and *haversian space.*

**c. nu'triens,** TA alternative for *c. nutricius.*

**c. obturato'rius** [TA], obturator canal: an opening within the obturator membrane for the passage of the obturator vessels and nerve; its boundaries are the edge of the obturator membrane, together with the obturator groove of the pubic bone.

**c. op'ticus** [TA], optic canal: one of the paired openings in the sphenoid bone where the small wings are attached to the body of the bone at the apex of the orbit; each canal transmits one of the optic nerves and the ophthalmic artery of that side. Called also *foramen opticum ossis sphenoidalis* and *optic foramen of sphenoid bone.*

**c. palati'nus ma'jor** [TA], greater palatine canal: a passage in the sphenoid and palatine bones for the greater palatine vessels and nerve; it ends at the foramen palatinum majus. Called also *c. pterygopalatinus, palatomaxillary canal, pterygopalatine canal,* and *sphenopalatine canal.*

**cana'les palati'ni mino'res** [TA], lesser palatine canals: openings in the palatine bone that branch off the great palatine canal to carry the lesser and middle palatine nerves and vessels to the roof of the mouth; they end at the foramina palatina minora. Called also *accessory palatine canals.*

**c. palatovagina'lis** [TA], palatovaginal canal: a narrow canal located in the roof of the nasal cavity between the inferior surface of the body of the sphenoid bone and the sphenoidal process of the palatine bone; it opens posteriorly into the nasal cavity and anteriorly into the pterygopalatine fossa. Called also *c. pharyngeus, pharyngeal canal, pterygopalatine canal, sphenopalatine canal, sphenopharyngeal canal,* and *lateral inferior vomerobasilar canal.*

**cana'les paraurethra'les ure'thrae masculi'nae,** ductus paraurethrales urethrae masculinae.

**c. pharyn'geus,** c. palatovaginalis.

**c. pterygoi'deus** [TA], pterygoid canal: a horizontally running canal that passes forward through the base of the medial pterygoid plate of the sphenoid bone to open into the posterior wall of the pterygopalatine fossa just medial and inferior to the foramen rotundum; it transmits the pterygoid vessels and nerves. Called also *canal of Guidi, recurrent canal,* and *vidian canal.*

**c. pterygopalati'nus,** c. palatinus major.

**c. pudenda'lis** [TA], pudendal canal: the tunnel in the special fascial sheath through which the pudendal vessels and nerve pass; it is intimately related to the obturator fascia. Called also *Alcock's canal.*

**c. pylo'ricus** [TA], pyloric canal: the short, narrow part of the stomach extending from the gastroduodenal junction to the pyloric antrum.

**c. ra'dicis den'tis** [TA], root canal: the portion of the dental pulp cavity in the root of a tooth, extending from the pulp chamber to the apical foramen; more than one canal may be present in a single root, two commonly being present in the mesial root of the mandibular first molar. Called also *pulp canal.*

**c. reu'niens,** ductus reuniens.

**c. sacra'lis** [TA], sacral canal: the continuation of the vertebral canal through the sacrum.

**c. semicircula'ris ante'rior** [TA], anterior semicircular canal: the anterior of the osseous semicircular canals, lodging the ductus semicircularis anterior of the membranous labyrinth. Called also *c. semicircularis superior* and *superior semicircular canal.*

**c. semicircula'ris latera'lis** [TA], lateral semicircular canal: the lateral of the osseous semicircular canals, lodging the ductus semicircularis lateralis of the membranous labyrinth; called also *horizontal semicircular canal.*

**cana'les semicircula'res os'sei** [TA], bony semicircular canals: three long canals of the bony labyrinth of the ear, forming loops and opening into the vestibule by five openings; they lodge the semicircular ducts. See *c. semicircularis anterior, c. semicircularis lateralis,* and *c. semicircularis posterior.* Called also *semicircular canals.*

**c. semicircula'ris poste'rior** [TA], posterior semicircular canal: the posterior of the semicircular canals, lodging the ductus semicircularis posterior of the membranous labyrinth.

**c. semicircula'ris supe'rior,** c. semicircularis anterior.

**c. spina'lis,** c. vertebralis.

**c. spira'lis coch'leae** [TA], spiral canal of cochlea: a winding tube that makes two and one-half turns about the modiolus of the cochlea; it is divided into two compartments, scala tympani and scala vestibuli, by the lamina spiralis.

**c. spira'lis modi'oli** [TA], spiral canal of modiolus: a canal following the course of the bony spiral lamina of the cochlea and containing the spiral ganglion of the cochlear division of the vestibulocochlear nerve. Called also *Rosenthal's canal.*

**c. subsartoria'lis,** c. adductorius.

**c. ventricula'ris, c. ventri'culi,** c. gastricus.

**c. vertebra'lis** [TA], vertebral canal: the canal formed by the foramina in the successive vertebrae, which encloses the spinal cord and meninges; called also *c. spinalis, medullary canal, neural canal,* and *spinal canal.*

**c. vomerorostra'lis** [TA], vomerorostral canal: a canal located between the vomer and sphenoidal rostrum.

**c. vomerovagina'lis** [TA], vomerovaginal canal: an inconstant opening formed by the articulating margins of the ala of the vomer and the body of the sphenoid bone; called also *basipharyngeal canal, lateral superior vomerobasilar canal,* and *vomerine canal.*

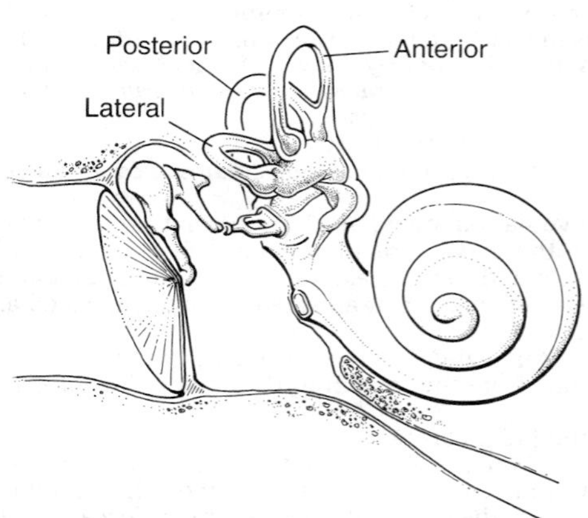


Semicircular canals (canales semicirculares ossei).

**can·a·li·za·tion** (kan″əl-i-za′shən) 1. formation of canals, natural or pathologic. 2. surgical establishment of canals for drainage. 3. recanalization. 4. in psychology, formation in the central nervous system of new pathways by repeated passage of nerve impulses.

**ca·nalo·plas·ty** (kan′ə-lo-plas″te) plastic reconstruction of a passage, as of the external auditory meatus.

**ca·nal·plas·ty** (kə-nal′plas-te) canaloplasty.

**ca·na·ry·pox** (kə-na′re-poks) a type of fowlpox seen in canaries.

**Can·a·val·ia** (kan″ə-val′yə) the jack bean, a genus of West Indian plants of the family Leguminosae, widely used as food for humans and livestock. *C. ensifor′mis* D.C. and other species are the source of canavalin, canavanine, and concanavalin.

**can·a·val·in** (kan″ə-val′in) an antibacterial substance isolated from the meal of the jack bean.

**Can·a·van's disease** (kan′ə-vanz) [Myrtelle May *Canavan,* American neurologist, 1879–1953] spongy degeneration of the central nervous system; see under *degeneration.*

**Can·a·van-van Bo·gaert-Ber·trand disease** (kan′ə-van-vahn bo′gert-bār-trahn′) [M.M. *Canavan;* Ludo *van Bogaert,* Belgian neurologist, born 1897; Ivan Georges *Bertrand,* French neurologist, 1863–1965] spongy degeneration of the central nervous system; see under *degeneration.*

**can·av·a·nine** (kə-nav′ə-nēn) [MeSH: Canavanine] an analogue of arginine found in alfalfa seeds and the jack bean; used in experimental medicine to study enzymes that usually act on arginine.

**can·cel·lat·ed** (kan′sə-lāt″əd) having a lattice-like structure; cancellous.

**can·cel·li** (kan-sel′i) [L.] plural of *cancellus.*

**can·cel·lous** (kan-səl′əs) of a reticular, spongy, or lattice-like structure; said mainly of bony tissue.

**can·cel·lus** (kan-səl′əs) pl. *cancel′li* [L. "a lattice"] any structure arranged like a lattice.

**can·cer** (kan′sər) [L. "crab, malignant tumor"] a neoplastic disease the natural course of which is fatal. Cancer cells, unlike benign tumor cells, exhibit the properties of invasion and metastasis and are highly anaplastic. Cancer includes the two broad categories of carcinoma and sarcoma, but in normal usage it is often used synonymously with carcinoma.
**aniline c.**, cancer usually of the urinary bladder, occurring among those who work with aniline dyes; called also *dye workers' c.*
**betel c.**, squamous cell carcinoma of the cheek mucous membranes, seen in India and other Asian countries where betel nut, often mixed with tobacco, is held in the buccal vestibule for prolonged periods.
**buyo cheek c.**, [Philippine *buyo,* betel], betel c.
**cerebriform c.**, medullary carcinoma.
**chimney-sweeps' c.**, squamous cell carcinoma of the skin of the scrotum due to soot poisoning; called also *soot c.*
**clay pipe c.**, squamous cell carcinoma of the lip due to irritation caused by a pipe stem.
**colloid c.**, mucinous carcinoma.
**contact c.**, cancer developing in a part of the body in contact with a previously existing cancer.
**cystic c.**, see under *tumor.*
**dendritic c.**, papillary carcinoma.
**c. à deux,** [Fr. "cancer in two"], cancer attacking simultaneously or consecutively two persons who live together.
**duct c.**, see under *carcinoma.*
**dye workers' c.**, aniline c.
**encephaloid c.**, medullary carcinoma.
**c. en cuirasse**, see under *carcinoma.*
**endometrial c.**, see under *carcinoma.*
**endothelial c.**, endothelioma.
**epithelial c.**, carcinoma.
**glandular c.**, adenocarcinoma.
**c. in si′tu,** carcinoma in situ.
**kang c., kangri c.**, squamous cell carcinoma in the thigh or abdomen affecting Indian and Chinese natives, and attributed to irritation from the kang (heated brick oven) or from the kangri (fire basket).
**latent c.**, cancer discovered, in the absence of any clinical manifestations, in the course of histological examination; cf. *occult c.*
**medullary c.**, see under *carcinoma.*
**melanotic c.**, malignant melanoma.
**mule-spinners' c.**, a form of squamous cell carcinoma affecting mule spinners in the cotton-spinning industry, due to continued soaking of the clothes and abdomen by arsenic, tar, and carcinogenic oils; it is now rare.
**non–small cell lung c.**, see under *carcinoma.*
**occult c.**, a small cancer that may give rise to clinically evident distant metastases before it is itself clinically detectable; cf. *latent c.*
**paraffin c.**, carcinoma of the skin occurring in those who work in paraffin.
**pitch workers' c.**, carcinoma of the skin of the face, neck, and scrotum seen in workers frequently exposed to pitch.
**scar c.**, see under *carcinoma.*
**schistosomal bladder c.**, see under *carcinoma.*
**scirrhous c.**, see under *carcinoma.*
**small cell lung c.**, see under *carcinoma.*
**soft c.**, medullary carcinoma.
**soot c.**, chimney-sweeps' c.
**spindle cell c.**, see under *carcinoma.*
**swamp c.**, 1. pythiosis. 2. a general term for several syndromes in horses consisting of skin or mucosal lesions with ulcers and granulomatous tissue on the head, trunk, or lower extremities. See *cutaneous habronemiasis, entomophthoromycosis,* and *pythiosis.*
**tar c.**, squamous cell carcinoma caused by inflammatory irritation of fumes of tar or by the irritating effect of tar on the skin.
**tubular c.**, tubular carcinoma (def. 1).

**can·cer·emia** (kan″sər-e′me-ə) the presence of cancer cells in the blood.

**can·cer·i·ci·dal** (kan″sər-ĭ-si′dəl) [*cancer* + L. *caedere* to kill] destructive to cancer or malignant cells; cf. *carcinolytic.*

**can·cer·i·gen·ic** (kan″sər-ĭ-jen′ik) giving rise to a malignant tumor; cf. *carcinogenic* and *sarcomagenic.* Called also *cancerogenic.*

**can·cero·ci·dal** (kan″sər-o-si′dəl) cancericidal.

**can·cer·o·gen·ic** (kan″sər-o-jen′ik) cancerigenic.

**can·cero·pho·bia** (kan″ser-o-fo′be-ə) cancerphobia.

**can·cer·ous** (kan′sər-əs) of the nature of or pertaining to cancer.

**can·cer·pho·bia** (kan″sər-fo′be-ə) [*cancer* + *-phobia*] irrational fear of cancer.

**can·cri·form** (kang′krĭ-form) resembling a cancer.

**can·croid** (kang′kroid) [L. *cancer,* gen. *cancri,* crab, malignant tumor + *-oid*] resembling cancer.

**can·crum** (kang′krəm) [L.] canker.
**c. na′si,** gangrenous rhinitis of children.
**c. o′ris,** noma (def. 1).
**c. puden′di,** gangrenous erosion of the genitalia; see *erosive balanitis,* under *balanitis,* and *erosive vulvitis,* under *vulvitis.*

**can·dela** (kan-del′ə) [L. *candēla* candle] the SI unit of luminous intensity equal to one-sixtieth of the luminous intensity per square centimeter of a blackbody radiating at the temperature of the freezing point of platinum. Called also *candle, new candle,* and *standard candle.* Abbreviated cd.

**can·de·lil·la** (kan″də-lil′ə) [Sp. "little candle"] *Euphorbia antisyphilitica,* the source of candelilla wax.

**Can·dep·tin** (kan-dep′tin) trademark for preparations of candicidin.

**can·de·sar·tan ci·lex·e·til** (kan″də-sahr′tan) an angiotensin II receptor antagonist, used in the treatment of hypertension; administered orally.

**can·di·ci·din** (kan″dĭ-si′din) [MeSH: Candicidin] an antifungal antibiotic produced by a strain of *Streptomyces griseus;* it is especially effective against *Candida albicans,* and is administered intravaginally in the treatment of vaginal candidiasis.

**Can·di·da** (kan′dĭ-də) [L. *candidus* glowing white] [MeSH: Candida] a genus of yeastlike Fungi Imperfecti of the form-family Cryptococcaceae, characterized by producing yeast cells, mycelia, pseudomycelia, and blastospores. Some species are part of the normal flora of human skin and mucous membranes but can also cause various infections. Formerly called *Monilia, Mycotoruloides,* and *Oidium.*
**C. al′bicans,** a species that is part of the normal flora of human skin and mucous membranes and is the most frequent cause of candidiasis.
**C. glabra′ta,** *Torulopsis glabrata.*
**C. guilliermon′dii,** a species that sometimes causes cutaneous candidiasis, onychomycosis, meningitis, and endocarditis.
**C. kru′sei,** a species occasionally associated with candidiasis, esophagitis, endocarditis, and vaginitis.
**C. lusita′niae,** a species that causes opportunistic infections in humans; its perfect (sexual) stage is *Clavispora lusitaniae.*
**C. mesente′rica,** a species which causes fermentation in fruit acids; called also *Saccharomyces mesentericus.*
**C. parapsilo′sis,** a species that sometimes causes endocarditis, paronychia, or otitis externa.
**C. pseudotropica′lis,** a species that sometimes causes *Candida* vaginitis.
**C. stellatoi′dea,** a species that sometimes causes *Candida* vaginitis or endocarditis. Some authorities consider it a variant of *C. albicans.*
**C. tropica′lis,** a species that sometimes causes *Candida* vaginitis, meningitis, onychomycosis, or bronchopulmonary infection.

**C. vi'ni,** a species found in fermenting liquors and diabetic urine. Called also *Saccharomyces mycoderma.*

**can·di·dal** (kan'dĭ-dəl) pertaining to or caused by *Candida.*

**can·di·de·mia** (kan″dĭ-de'me-ə) the presence in the blood of fungi of the genus *Candida,* usually resulting from *Candida* endocarditis or systemic candidiasis.

**can·di·di·a·sis** (kan″dĭ-di'ə-sis) [MeSH: Candidiasis] infection with a fungus of the genus *Candida,* especially *C. albicans.* It is usually a superficial infection of the skin or mucous membranes, although sometimes it manifests as a systemic infection or endocarditis; any form can become more severe in immunocompromised patients. Called also *moniliasis* and *candidosis.*
**acute pseudomembranous c.,** thrush, def. 1.
**atrophic c.,** a type of oral c. (thrush) marked by erythematous, pebbled patches on the hard or soft palate, buccal mucosa, and dorsal surface of the tongue, a complication of numerous different conditions such as vitamin deficiency, diabetes mellitus, or poorly-fitting dentures. There are acute forms and a chronic form called *denture stomatitis.*
**bronchopulmonary c.,** candidiasis of the respiratory tract, either from colonization of the tracheobronchial tree in immunocompromised patients or those on antibiotics, or associated with pneumonia in the immunocompromised. It ranges from mild to severe and life-threatening. Called also *bronchocandidiasis.*
**chronic mucocutaneous c.,** any of a diverse group of candidal infections of the oral mucosa, skin, nails, and vaginal mucosa; they are usually resistant to treatment, may be localized or diffuse, are sometimes familial, and may be associated with endocrinopathy or immunosuppression.
**cutaneous c.,** candidiasis of the skin, which may be manifested as eczemalike lesions of the interdigital spaces, perlèche, or chronic paronychia.
**endocardial c.,** *Candida* endocarditis.
**oral c.,** thrush (def. 1).
**pulmonary c.,** a type of fungal pneumonia caused by infection with *Candida* species, seen especially in immunocompromised patients or those with malignancies. Called also Candida *pneumonia.*
**vaginal c.,** *Candida* vaginitis.
**vulvovaginal c.,** *Candida* vulvovaginitis.

**can·di·did** (kan'dĭ-did) a secondary skin eruption that is the expression of hypersensitivity to infection with *Candida* elsewhere on the body; called also *moniliid.*

**can·di·din** (kan'dĭ-din) a skin test antigen derived from *Candida albicans,* used in testing for the development of delayed-type hypersensitivity to constituents of the microorganism.

**can·di·do·sis** (kan-dĭ-do'sis) candidiasis.

**can·did·uria** (kan″did-u're-ə) the presence of *Candida* organisms in the urine.

**can·dle** (kan'dəl) 1. a mass of wax or similar substance, usually cylindrical in shape, with a wick for burning, to furnish illumination or heat. 2. a cylindrical mass of material used as a filter in microbiology. 3. candela.
**foot c.,** see under *F.*
**meter c.,** see *lux.*
**new c., standard c.,** candela.

**cane** (kān) [MeSH: Canes] a wooden stick or metal rod used for support in walking.
**adjustable c.,** a cane whose length can be easily altered.
**English c.,** forearm crutch.
**quadripod c.,** one adapted for increased stability by forking to provide a four-legged rectangular base of support.
**quadruped c.,** quadripod c.
**tripod c.,** one similar to a quadripod cane except that it forks to provide a three-legged, triangular base of support.

**ca·nes·cent** (kə-nes'ənt) [L. *canus* gray] 1. becoming white or grayish. 2. in biology, having grayish or whitish hairs or down; hoary.

**ca·nine** (ka'nīn) [L. *canis* a dog, hound] 1. of, pertaining to, or like that which belongs to a dog. 2. canine tooth.

**ca·ni·nus** (ka-ni'nəs) musculus levator anguli oris.

**ca·ni·ti·es** (kə-nish'e-ēz) [L.] diffuse grayness or whiteness of the scalp hair, especially as associated with aging. Cf. *achromotrichia, leukotrichia,* and *poliosis.*

**can·ker** (kang'kər) 1. ulceration, chiefly of the mouth and lips. 2. a disease of the keratogenous membrane in horses, usually in the hindlimb, with loss of function of horn-secreting cells and discharge of a serous exudate in place of the normal horny hoof; it begins at the frog and extends to the sole and wall. 3. otitis externa in a dog or cat.

**can·na·bi·di·ol** (kan″ə-bĭ-di'ol) [MeSH: Cannabidiol] a nonpsychoactive diphenol isolated from cannabis.

**can·nab·i·noid** (kə-nab'ĭ-noid) any of the principles of cannabis, including tetrahydrocannabinol, cannabinol, and cannabidiol.

**can·nab·i·nol** (kə-nab'ĭ-nol) [MeSH: Cannabinol] a nonpsychoactive constituent of resinous exudates of *Cannabis sativa* L.; its tetrahydro derivatives are active principles.

**Can·na·bis** (kan'ə-bis) [MeSH: Cannabis] a genus of flowering herbs. *C. sati'va* L. (Cannabaceae) is the hemp plant, widely used for fiber and rope; its dried leaves and flowers are called marijuana (q.v.) and contain tetrahydrocannabinol and other cannabinoids.

**can·na·bis** (kan'ə-bis) [Gr. *kannabis* hemp] [MeSH: Cannabis] the dried flowering tops of *Cannabis sativa,* which contain the euphoric principles $\Delta^1$-3,4-*trans* and $\Delta^6$-3,4-*trans* tetrahydrocannabinol, as well as cannabinol and cannabidiol. It is classified as hallucinogenic and is most commonly prepared as hashish or marijuana.

**Can·niz·za·ro's reaction** (kahn″e-tsah'rōz) [Stanislao *Cannizzaro,* Italian chemist, 1826–1910] see under *reaction.*

**Can·non's ring (point), theory** (kan'ənz) [Walter Bradford *Cannon,* American physiologist, 1871–1945] see under *ring* and see *emergency theory,* under *theory.*

**Can·non-Bard theory** (kan'ən bahrd) [W.B. *Cannon;* Philip *Bard,* American psychologist, 1898–1977] emergency theory.

**can·nu·la** (kan'u-lə) [L. dim. of *canna* "reed"] a tube for insertion into a vessel, duct, or cavity; during insertion its lumen is usually occupied by a trocar. Cf. *catheter.*
**nasal c.,** a cannula that fits into the nostrils for delivery of oxygen therapy. Called also *nasal prongs.*
**perfusion c.,** a double tube for running a continuous flow of liquid into and out of an organ.
**washout c.,** a cannula attached to a manometer and inserted into a blood vessel so that the connection between the artery and the manometer can be irrigated in long observations.

**can·nu·late** (kan'u-lāt) to introduce a cannula, which may be left in place.

**can·nu·la·tion** (kan″u-la'shən) the insertion of a cannula.

**can·nu·li·za·tion** (kan″u-lĭ-za'shən) cannulation.

**can·on** (kan'ən) [L. "rule"] a working rule or formula for use in scientific procedure.

**can·ren·o·ate po·tas·si·um** (kan-ren'o-āt) [MeSH: Canrenoate Potassium] a potassium sparing diuretic with actions and uses similar to those of spironolactone.

**can·ren·one** (kan-ren'ōn) [MeSH: Canrenone] an aldosterone antagonist, the active metabolite of canrenoate potassium and spironolactone, used as a potassium sparing diuretic; administered orally.

**cant** (kant) an inclination or slope.
**c. of mandible,** the angle formed by the intersection of the mandibular (gonion-gnathion) plane with the sella-nasion or Frankfort plane.

**can·thal** (kan'thəl) pertaining to a canthus.

**can·tha·ri·a·sis** (kan″thə-ri'ə-sis) [Gr. *kantharos* beetle] infection by beetles as endoparasites in the body of a mammal, following ingestion of larval or adult forms.

**can·thar·i·dal** (kan-thar'ĭ-dəl) containing or pertaining to cantharides.

**can·thar·i·date** (kan-thar'ĭ-dāt) any salt of cantharidic acid.

**can·thar·i·des** (kan-thar'ĭ-dēz) [L.] the dried body of *Lytta (Cantharis) vesicatoria,* containing the toxic active principle cantharidin (q.v.); it was formerly applied externally as a powerful rubefacient and blistering agent and given internally as a diuretic and aphrodisiac. Called also *Spanish fly.*

**can·tha·rid·ic acid** (kan″thə-rid'ik) a dibasic acid formed when cantharidin dissolves in water.

**can·thar·i·din** (kan-thar'ĭ-din) [MeSH: Cantharidin] a bitter-tasting crystalline substance, the lactone of cantharidic acid and the most important active principle of cantharides; it is also found in the bodies of other beetles such as *Epicauta.* On human skin it produces blistering; consumption of the dead bodies of the beetles in hay or other feed can be lethal to farm animals.

**can·thar·i·dism** (kan-thar'ĭ-diz-əm) 1. a toxic reaction in humans from the misuse of cantharides. 2. cantharidin poisoning.

**Can·tha·ris** (kan'thə-ris) [L.; Gr. *kantharos* beetle] *Lytta.*
**C. vesicato'ria,** *Lytta vesicatoria.*

**can·thec·to·my** (kan-thek'tə-me) [*canth-* + *ectomy*] surgical removal of a canthus.

**can·thi** (kan'thi) [L.] plural of *canthus.*

**can·thi·tis** (kan-thi'tis) inflammation of a canthus or of the canthi.

**canth(o)-** [Gr. *kanthos*] a combining form denoting relationship to the canthus.

**can·thol·y·sis** (kan-thol'ĭ-sis) [*cantho-* + *-lysis*] surgical division of the canthus of an eye or of a canthal ligament.

**can·tho·plas·ty** (kan'tho-plas″te) [*cantho-* + *-plasty*] plastic surgery of the medial and/or lateral canthus, especially section of the lateral canthus to lengthen the palpebral fissure; also the surgical restoration of a defective canthus.

**can·thor·rha·phy** (kan-thor'ə-fe) [*cantho-* + *-rrhaphy*] the suturing of the palpebral fissure at either canthus.

**can·thot·o·my** (kan-thot'ə-me) [*cantho-* + *-tomy*] surgical division of the outer canthus.

**can·thus** (kan'thəs) pl. *can'thi* [L.; Gr. *kanthos*] the angle at either end of the fissure between the eyelids; see *angulus oculi lateralis* and *angulus oculi medialis.*
**inner c., nasal c.,** angulus oculi medialis.
**outer c., temporal c.,** angulus oculi lateralis.

**Can·til** (kan'til) trademark for a preparation of mepenzolate bromide.

**Can·tor tube** (kan'tor) [Meyer O. *Cantor,* American physician, born 1907] see under *tube.*

**Can·trell's pentalogy** (kan-trelz') [James R. *Cantrell,* American physician, 20th century] see under *pentalogy.*

**can·u·la** (kan'u-lə) cannula.

**CAP** College of American Pathologists.

**Cap.** abbreviation for L. *ca'piat,* let him take.

**cap** (kap) 1. a protective covering for the head or for a similar structure. 2. colloquial term for an artificial crown.
**acrosomal c.,** acrosome.
**bishop's c.,** pars superior duodeni.
**5′ c.,** a structure consisting of a 7-methylguanosine ($m^7G$) residue attached backwards (i.e., 5′ to 5′) by a triphosphate linkage to the 5′ end of primary mRNA transcripts in eukaryotes: In addition, the first and, in some cases, second nucleotide of the mRNA are methylated at the 2′ position of the ribose residue. The 5′ cap protects the mRNA from attack by 5′ exonucleases and also functions in the recognition of the mRNA by ribosomes.
**cradle c.,** crusta lactea.
**duodenal c.,** see under *ampulla.*
**dutch c.,** a contraceptive cervical diaphragm.
**enamel c.,** a caplike structure of the enamel organ, developed during the third month of fetal development, and composed of an outer layer and an inner enamel layer; between the two layers are looser ectodermal cells that become the stellate reticulum. Called also *germinal c.*
**germinal c.,** enamel c.
**head c.,** the double-layered caplike structure over the upper two-thirds of the acrosome of a spermatozoon, consisting of the collapsed acrosomal vesicle.
**head c., anterior,** acrosome.
**ink c., inky c.,** any mushroom of the genus *Coprinus.*
**knee c.,** patella.
**metanephric c's,** masses of metanephric mesoderm (blastema) that adhere to the primordial pelvis of the kidney and to its ampullary dilatations.
**phrygian c.,** the cholecystographic appearance of the gallbladder showing kinking between the body and the fundus, in which the fundus is fixed and folded.
**polar c.,** a chromophilic, saclike organelle occurring beneath the spore wall in the polar region of microsporidian protozoa. Called also *polar capsule.*
**postnuclear c.,** a broad band encircling the postacrosomal region of the nucleus of a spermatozoon.
**pyloric c.,** pars superior duodeni.
**root c.,** a thimble-shaped group of cells forming a protective covering over the apical meristem in the tip of a plant root.
**skull c.,** calvaria.
**c. of Zinn,** a prominence of the pulmonary arc in the left upper portion of the cardiac silhouette, usually seen in posteroanterior radiograms in cases of patent ductus arteriosus, and representing the dilated pulmonary artery.

**ca·pac·i·tance** (kə-pas'ĭ-təns) 1. the property of being able to store an electric charge. 2. the ratio of the charge stored by a capacitor to the voltage across the capacitor. Symbol *C.* Formerly called *capacity.* The SI unit of capacitance is the farad.
**membrane c.,** the electrical capacitance of a cell membrane, as of an axon or muscle fiber.

**ca·pac·i·ta·tion** (kə-pas″ĭ-ta'shən) the process by which spermatozoa become capable of fertilizing an oocyte (ovum) after it reaches the ampullary portion of the uterine tube.

**ca·pac·i·tor** (kə-pas'ĭ-tər) a device for holding and storing charges of electricity.

**ca·pac·i·ty** (kə-pas'ĭ-te) [L. *capacitas,* from *capere* to take] 1. power or ability to hold, retain, or contain, or the ability to absorb. 2. the volume or potential volume of material (solid, liquid, or gas) that can be held or contained. 3. capacitance. 4. mental ability to receive, accomplish, endure, or understand.
**closing c.,** the volume of gas in the lungs at the time the airways close during respiration; the closing volume added to the residual volume, usually expressed as a percentage of total lung capacity.
**cranial c.,** an expression of the amount of space within the cranium.
**diffusing c., diffusion c.,** the ability of the alveolocapillary membrane to transfer gas: a reflection of the thinness and area of the alveolocapillary membrane. It is the amount of gas transferred per minute from the alveolar gas to the pulmonary capillary blood divided by the mean pressure gradient of the gas between the alveolar gas and the capillary blood; unit, mL/min/torr (or mm Hg). Symbol D.
**forced vital c. (FVC),** vital capacity measured when the patient is exhaling with maximum speed and effort.
**functional residual c.,** the volume of gas remaining at the end of a normal quiet exhalation; abbreviated FRC. See illustration.
**heat c.,** the amount of heat required to raise the temperature of a specific quantity of a substance by one degree Celsius. Symbol *C* ($C_p$ at constant pressure, $C_v$ at constant volume).
**inspiratory c.,** the volume of gas that can be taken into the lungs on a full inspiration, starting from the functional residual capacity; it is equal to the tidal volume plus the inspiratory reserve volume. Abbreviated IC. See illustration.
**iron-binding c. (IBC),** the extent to which transferrin in the serum of a given patient can bind serum iron; see also *total iron-binding c.*
**maximal breathing c.,** maximum voluntary ventilation.
**maximal tubular excretory c.,** see *tubular maximum,* under *maximum.*
**molar heat c.,** heat capacity when the amount of the substance is expressed in moles.
**specific heat c.,** specific heat. Symbol *c.*
**thermal c.,** heat c.
**total iron-binding c. (TIBC),** a measure of the total amount of iron that can be bound by the transferrin in a serum sample, determined by saturating the transferrin with iron, then removing the unbound iron with an absorbent and measuring the iron in the filtrate; used in the evaluation of patients with iron deficiency or overload. See also *transferrin saturation,* under *saturation.*
**total lung c.,** the volume of gas contained in the lungs at the end of a maximal inspiration; abbreviated TLC. See illustration.
**virus neutralizing c.,** the ability of a serum to inhibit the infectivity of a virus.
**vital c.,** VC; the volume of gas that can be expelled from the lungs from a position of full inspiration, with no limit to the duration of expiration; it is equal to the inspiratory capacity plus the expiratory reserve volume. See illustration.

**Cap·a·stat** (kap'ə-stat) trademark for a preparation of capreomycin sulfate.

**CAPD** continuous ambulatory peritoneal dialysis.

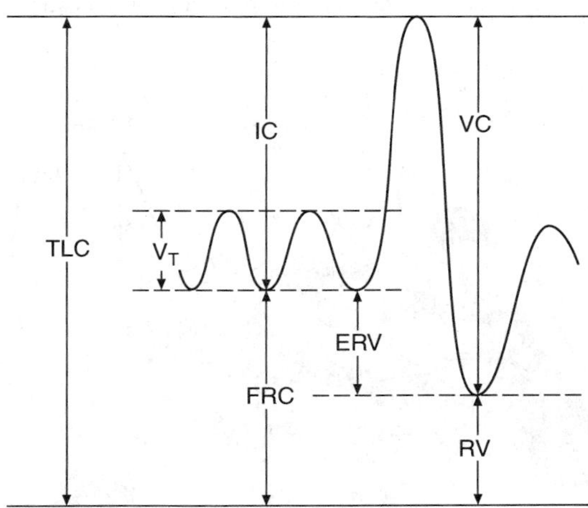


Subdivisions of total lung capacity: *TLC,* total lung capacity; $V_T$, tidal volume; *IC,* inspiratory capacity; *FRC,* functional residual capacity; *ERV,* expiratory reserve volume; *VC,* vital capacity; *RV,* residual volume.

**Cape gum** (kāp) [*Cape* of Good Hope, South Africa, where the trees are found] see under *gum.*

**cap·e·line** (kap'ə-līn) [Fr.] a cap-shaped bandage for the head or for the stump of an amputated limb.

**Cap·gras syndrome** (kahp-grah) [Jean Marie Joseph *Capgras,* French psychiatrist, 1873–1950] see under *syndrome.*

**cap·il·lar·ec·ta·sia** (kap″ĭ-lar″ək-ta'zhə) [*capillary* + *ectasia*] dilatation of capillaries.

**Ca·pil·la·ria** (kap″ĭ-lar'e-ə) [MeSH: Capillaria] a genus of nematodes of the family Trichuridae, superfamily Trichuroidea; called also *Hepaticola* and *Trichosoma.*
**C. contor'ta,** a roundworm parasitic in domestic fowls; called also *Trichosoma contortum.*
**C. hepa'tica,** a species parasitic in the liver of rats and many other mammals; a few human infections have been reported.
**C. philippinen'sis,** a parasite of the human intestine in the Philippines, causing severe diarrhea, malabsorption, and high mortality.

**cap·il·la·ri·a·sis** (kap″ĭ-lə-ri'ə-sis) infection with nematodes of the genus *Capillaria.* In birds the species is *C. contorta;* in many mammals it is *C. hepatica;* and in humans it is often *C. philippinensis.*

**cap·il·lar·io·mo·tor** (kap″ĭ-lar″e-o-mo'tər) pertaining to the functional activity of the capillaries.

**cap·il·lar·i·os·co·py** (kap″ĭ-lar″e-os'kə-pe) capillaroscopy.

**cap·il·lar·itis** (kap″ĭ-lər-i'tis) inflammation of the capillaries; called also *telangiitis.*

**cap·il·lar·i·ty** (kap″ĭ-lar'ĭ-te) [MeSH: Capillarity] the action by which the surface of a liquid where it is in contact with a solid, as in capillary tubes, is elevated or depressed.

**cap·il·la·rop·a·thy** (kap″ĭ-lə-rop'ə-the) [*capillary* + *-pathy*] any disease of the capillaries; called also *telangiosis.*

**cap·il·la·ros·co·py** (kap″ĭ-lər-os'kə-pe) [*capillary* + *-scope*] diagnostic examination of the capillaries with the microscope. Called also *capillarioscopy* and *microangioscopy.*

**cap·il·lary** (kap'ĭ-lar″e) [L. *capillaris* hair-like] [MeSH: Capillaries] 1. pertaining to or resembling a hair. 2. any of the minute vessels that connect the arterioles and venules, forming a network in nearly all parts of the body. Their walls act as semipermeable membranes for the interchange of various substances, including fluids, between the blood and tissue fluid. The two principal types are *continuous* and *fenestrated capillaries.* Called also *vas capillare* [TA]. 3. vas lymphocapillare.
**arterial c.,** a type of minute vessel lacking a continuous muscular coat, intermediate in structure and location between an arteriole and a capillary; called also *precapillary, precapillary arteriole,* and *metarteriole.*
**bile c's,** 1. bile canaliculi. 2. a term sometimes used to designate the cholangioles.
**continuous c's,** one of the two major types of capillaries, found in muscle, skin, lung, central nervous system, and other tissues, and characterized by an uninterrupted endothelium, a continuous basal lamina, fine filaments, and numerous pinocytotic vesicles. Cf. *fenestrated c's.*
**erythrocytic c's,** capillaries of the bone marrow of early life which seem to produce erythrocytes.
**fenestrated c's,** one of the two major types of capillaries, found in the intestinal mucosa, renal glomeruli, pancreas, endocrine glands, and other tissues, and characterized by circular fenestrae or pores that penetrate the endothelium and may be closed by a very thin diaphragm. Cf. *continuous c's.*
**glomerular c.,** any of the capillaries of a renal glomerulus.
**lymph c., lymphatic c.,** vas lymphocapillare.
**Meigs' c's,** capillaries in the myocardium.
**secretory c.,** any of the extremely fine intercellular canaliculi situated between adjacent gland cells, such as the gastric parietal cells, being formed by the apposition of grooves in the surfaces of the cells, and opening into the gland's lumen.
**sheathed c's,** see under *artery.*
**sinusoidal c.,** vas sinusoideum.
**venous c.,** a type of minute vessel lacking a muscular coat, intermediate in structure and location between a venule and a capillary. Called also *postcapillary* and *postcapillary venule.*

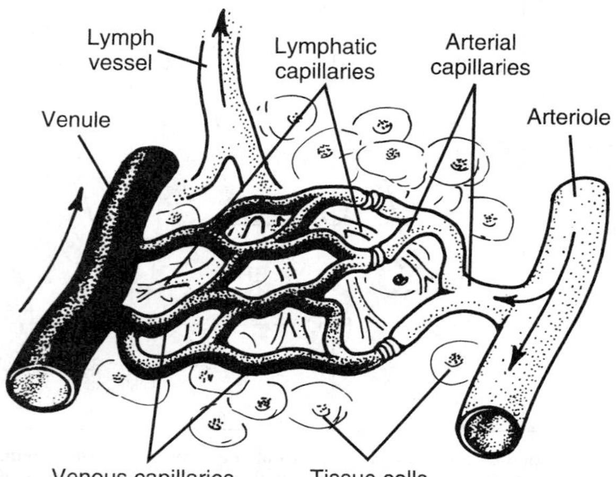

Capillary bed. Lighter areas indicate oxygenated blood.

**cap·il·li** (kə-pil'i) sing. *capillus* [L.] [TA] the aggregate of hair on the scalp.

**cap·il·li·ti·um** (kap″ĭ-lish'e-əm) [L. "head of hair"] a filamentous structure that interlaces among the spores in the fruiting bodies of certain bacteria (Myxobacterales), protozoa (Eumycetozoa), and fungi (Gasteromycetes).

**cap·il·lus** (kə-pil'əs) pl. *capil'li* [L.] a hair; see *capilli.*

**cap·i·stra·tion** (cap″ĭ-stra'shən) [L. *capistratus* masked] phimosis.

**cap·i·ta** (kap'ĭ-tə) [L.] plural of *caput.*

**cap·i·tal** (kap'ĭ-təl) 1. of the highest importance; involving danger to life. 2. of or pertaining to the head of the femur.

**cap·i·tate** (kap'ĭ-tāt) [L. *caput* head] head-shaped.

**cap·i·ta·tion** (kap″ĭ-ta'shən) the annual fee paid to a physician or group of physicians by each participant in a health plan.

**cap·i·ta·tum** (kap″ĭ-ta'təm) [L. "having a head"] the capitate bone, or os capitatum [TA].

**cap·i·tel·lum** (kap″ĭ-tel'əm) [L. dim. of *caput* head] capitulum humeri.

**cap·i·ton·nage** (kap″ĭ-to-nahzh') [Fr.] the surgical closure of a cyst cavity by applying sutures in such a way as to cause approximation of the opposing surfaces.

**cap·i·to·ped·al** (kap″ĭ-to-ped'əl) pertaining to the head and foot.

**Cap·i·trol** (kap'ĭ-trol) trademark for a preparation of chloroxine.

**ca·pit·u·la** (kə-pit'u-lə) [L.] plural of *capitulum.*

**ca·pit·u·lar** (kə-pit'u-lər) pertaining to a capitulum or head of a bone.

**ca·pit·u·lum** (kə-pit'u-ləm) pl. *capit'ula* [L. dim. of *caput*] 1. [TA] a little head, or a small eminence on a bone by which it articulates with another bone. 2. c. humeri. 3. a bulbous, knoblike, or enlarged terminal protuberance of a body or part, such as: *(a)* the movable head zone bearing the mouth parts of a tick or mite (called also *gnathosoma*); *(b)* the calcareous framework enclosing the mantle and body of a barnacle; *(c)* the end of an insect's antennae; *(d)* the proximal ends of the nematodesmata of certain ciliate protozoa of the superclass Hyperstomatia, which may be prominent and toothlike; or *(e)* the anterior end of the axostyle of certain zooflagellates, containing the nucleus of the organism.
**c. cos'tae,** caput costae.
**c. fi'bulae,** caput fibulae.
**c. hu'meri** [TA], **c. of humerus,** an eminence on the distal end of the lateral epicondyle of the humerus for articulation with the head of the radius; called also *capitellum* and *little* or *radial head of humerus.*
**c. mal'lei,** caput mallei.
**c. [proces'sus condyloi'dei] mandib'ulae,** caput mandibulae.
**c. ra'dii,** caput radii.
**c. stape'dis,** caput stapedis.
**c. ul'nae,** caput ulnae.

**Cap·la** (kap'lə) trademark for a preparation of mebutamate.

**Cap·lan's syndrome** (kap'lənz) [Anthony *Caplan,* British physician, 1907–1976] [MeSH: Caplan's Syndrome] see under *syndrome.*

**cap·ne·ic** (kap'ne-ik) [*capno-* + *-ic*] under conditions of increased carbon dioxide in the atmosphere; said of the incubation of bacterial cultures.

**capn(o)-** [Gr. *kapnos* smoke] a combining form signifying a sooty or smoky appearance, or the presence of carbon dioxide.

**Cap·no·cy·toph·a·ga** (kap″no-si-tof'ə-gə) [*capno-* + Gr. *kytos* cell + *phagein* to eat] [MeSH: Capnocytophaga] a genus of gram-negative, facultatively anaerobic, rod-shaped or fusiform bacteria of uncertain affiliation, which occur in normal and diseased sites of the human oral cavity. It has also been associated with systemic disease in debilitated persons. It includes the species *C. gingiva'lis, C. ochra'ceus* (called also *Bacteroides ochraceus*), and *C. sputi'gena.*
**C. canimor'sus,** a species that is part of the normal oral flora of dogs and cats; when a human is bitten by an infected animal, an

infection may follow that can be fatal, characterized by cellulitis, bacteremia, purulent meningitis, endocarditis, peripheral gangrene, malar purpura, and Waterhouse-Friderichsen syndrome. Infection is more severe in persons with asplenia, alcoholism, or a hematologic malignancy. Formerly called *DF-2 bacillus.*

**cap·no·gram** (kap'no-gram") a real-time waveform record of the concentration of carbon dioxide in the respiratory gases.

**cap·no·graph** (kap'no-graf") [*capno-* + *-graph*] a system for monitoring the concentration of exhaled carbon dioxide, consisting of a sensor placed in the breathing circuit or a tube that carries part of the exhaled gases to the analyzing device, a mass spectrometer or an infrared spectrometer, and devices to provide continuous visual (cathode ray tube) and graphic (printer) displays.

**cap·nog·ra·phy** (kap-nog'rə-fe) [*capno-* + *-graphy*] [MeSH: Capnography] monitoring of the concentration of exhaled carbon dioxide in order to assess the physiologic status of patients with acute respiratory problems or who are receiving mechanical ventilation and to determine the adequacy of ventilation in anesthetized patients.

**cap·no·hep·a·tog·ra·phy** (kap"no-hep"ə-tog'rə-fe) radiography of the liver after intravenous injection of carbon dioxide gas.

**cap·nom·e·ter** (kap-nom'ə-tər) a device for measuring the end-tidal partial pressure of carbon dioxide.

**cap·nom·e·try** (kap-nom'ə-tre) the determination of the end-tidal partial pressure of carbon dioxide.

**cap·no·phil·ic** (kap-no-fil'ik) [*capno-* + *-philic*] growing best in the presence of carbon dioxide; said of bacteria.

**cap·o·ben·ate so·di·um** (kap-o-ben'āt) the monosodium salt of capobenic acid, having cardiac depressant activity; used as an antiarrhythmic.

**cap·o·ben·ic ac·id** (kap-o-ben'ik) a vasodilator used in the treatment and prevention of myocardial infarction.

**ca·pon** (ka'pon) a castrated domestic fowl.

**ca·pon·ize** (ka'pon-īz) to castrate, especially male domestic fowl.

**ca·pote·ment** (kah-pōt-maw') [Fr.] a splashing sound heard in the dilated stomach.

**Cap·o·ten** (kap'o-ten) trademark for a preparation of captopril.

**Cap·o·zide** (kap'o-zīd") trademark for a combination preparation of captopril and hydrochlorothiazide.

**capped** (kapt) said of joints, especially of the legs of horses or cattle, that are swollen with hygromas or fibrous degeneration due to prolonged pressure or repeated minor injuries.

**cap·pie** (kap'e) double scalp.

**cap·ping** (kap'ing) 1. the provision of a protective or obstructive covering. 2. the movement of cell surface antigens into a small region (cap) on the cell surface owing to the cross linking of antigens by specific antibody. 3. in restorative dental procedures: *(a)* covering of tooth cusps weakened by caries with a protective metal overlay; see *cusp restoration,* under *restoration; (b)* colloquial term for replacement of the crown of a natural tooth with an artificial crown (cap).
**pulp c.,** covering of an exposed or nearly exposed pulp with a dressing or cement to protect the pulp against further injury and to provide an environment for healing and repair processes. In *direct capping,* the dressing is placed directly over the pulp at the site of exposure. In *indirect capping,* it is placed over a thin partition of remaining dentin, which if removed, might expose the dental pulp.

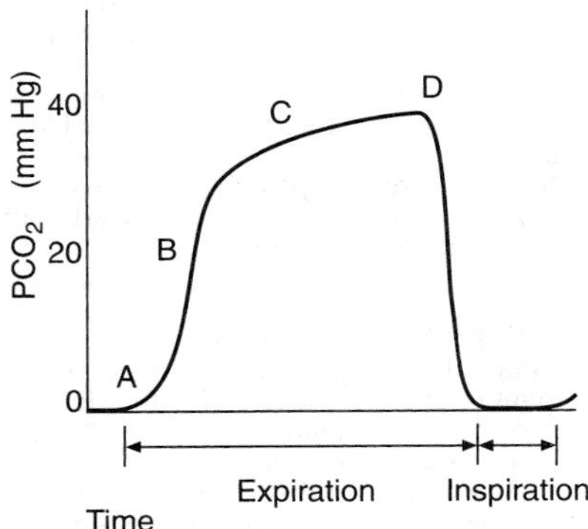


Normal capnogram. *(A),* Carbon dioxide cleared from the anatomic dead space; *(B),* dead space and alveolar carbon dioxide; *(C),* alveolar plateau; *(D),* end-tidal carbon dioxide tension ($P_{ET}CO_2$).

**cap·rate** (kap'rāt) any salt, ester, or anionic form of capric acid.

**cap·reo·lary** (kap're-o-lar"e) capreolate.

**cap·reo·late** (kap're-o-lāt) tendril shaped, like the spermatic vessels.

**cap·reo·my·cin** (kap"re-o-mi'sin) a polypeptide antibiotic produced by *Streptomyces capreolus,* which is active against human strains of *Mycobacterium tuberculosis* and has four microbiologically active components.
**c. sulfate** [USP], the disulfate salt of capreomycin, occurring as a white to practically white, amorphous powder; used as a tuberculostatic, administered intramuscularly.

**cap·ric ac·id** (kap'rik) a saturated ten-carbon fatty acid occurring as a minor constituent of numerous fats and oils. See also table accompanying *fatty acid.*

**ca·pril·o·quism** (kə-pril'o-kwiz"əm) [L. *caper* goat + *loqui* to speak] egophony.

**cap·rine** (kap'rin) [L. *caper* goat] [MeSH: Goats] 1. pertaining to or derived from a goat. 2. norleucine.

**Cap·ri·pox·vi·rus** (kap'rĭ-poks"vi-rəs) [L. *caper,* gen. *capri* goat + *poxvirus*] [MeSH: Capripoxvirus] a genus of viruses of the subfamily Chordopoxvirinae (family Poxviridae) with serologic cross-reactivity, comprising the sheeppox, goatpox, and lumpy skin disease viruses.

**cap·ri·zant** (kap'rĭ-zənt) [L. *caprizans,* from *caper* a goat] bounding (like a goat); old term used to describe a strong pulse.

**cap·ro·ate** (kap'ro-āt) 1. any salt of caproic acid. 2. USAN contraction for *hexanoate.*

**ca·pro·ic ac·id** (kə-pro'ik) a saturated six-carbon fatty acid occurring in butterfat and coconut and palm oils. Called also *hexanoic acid.* See also table accompanying *fatty acid.*

**cap·ro·yl** (kap-ro'əl) the acyl radical of caproic acid.

**cap·ry·late** (kap'rə-lāt) any salt, ester, or anionic form of caprylic acid.

**ca·pryl·ic ac·id** (kə-pril'ik) an eight-carbon saturated fatty acid occurring in butterfat and palm and coconut oils. Called also *octanoic acid.* See also table accompanying *fatty acid.*

**cap·sa·i·cin** (kap-sa'ĭ-sin) [USP] [MeSH: Capsaicin] an alkaloid irritating to the skin and mucous membranes, the pungent active principle in capsicum, used as the active ingredient in a cream as a counterirritant and topical analgesic.

**Cap·se·bon** (kap'sə-bon) trademark for a suspension of cadmium sulfide.

**Cap·si·cum** (kap'sĭ-kəm) [L.] [MeSH: Capsicum] a genus of plants of the family Solanaceae, including types of hot peppers. *C. frutes'cens* is the African chili; *C. an'num* var. *conoi'dis* is the tabasco pepper; and *C. an'num* var. *lon'gum* is the Louisiana long pepper. See also *capsicum.*

**cap·si·cum** (kap'sĭ-kəm) [MeSH: Capsicum] 1. any plant of the genus *Capsicum;* oleoresin extracts are used in pepper spray. Called also *cayenne pepper.* 2. [USP] the dried fruit of certain species of *Capsicum,* used as an irritant and carminative.

**cap·sid** (kap'sid) [L. *capsa* a box] [MeSH: Capsid] the shell of protein that protects the nucleic acid of a virus; it may have helical or icosahedral symmetry and is composed of structural units, or capsomers. According to the number of subunits possessed by capsomers, they are called dimers (2), trimers (3), pentamers (5), or hexamers (6).

**cap·si·tis** (kap-si'tis) inflammation of the capsule of the crystalline lens.

**cap·so·mer** (kap'so-mər) [L. *capsa* a box + Gr. *meros* part] the morphological unit of the capsid of a virus.

**cap·so·mere** (kap'so-mēr) capsomer.

**cap·sot·o·my** (kap-sot'ə-me) capsulotomy.

**Capsul.** abbreviation for L. *cap'sula,* capsule.

**cap·su·la** (kap'su-lə) pl. *cap'sulae* [L. "a small box"] [TA] capsule: a general term for a cartilaginous, fatty, fibrous, or membranous structure enveloping another structure, organ, or part.

## Capsula

Descriptions are given on TA terms, and include anglicized names of specific capsules.

**c. adipo'sa,** a capsule consisting principally of fat.

**c. adipo'sa re'nis** [TA], adipose capsule of kidney: the investment of fat surrounding the fibrous capsule of the kidney and continuous at the hilum with the fat in the renal sinus; called also *fatty capsule of kidney* and *perinephric* or *perirenal fat.*

**c. articula'ris** [TA], articular capsule: the sac-like envelope which encloses the cavity of a synovial joint by attaching to the circumference of the articular end of each involved bone; it consists of a fibrous membrane and a synovial membrane. Called also *joint capsule* and *synovial capsule.*

**c. articula'ris acromioclavicula'ris,** acromioclavicular articular capsule: a ligamentous sac surrounding the acromioclavicular joint.

**c. articula'ris articulatio'nis tar'si transver'sae,** a ligamentous sac surrounding the transverse tarsal joint.

**c. articula'ris articulatio'nis temporomandibula'ris,** a ligamentous sac surrounding the temporomandibular joint; called also *c. articularis mandibulae* and *capsule of temporomandibular joint.*

**c. articula'ris articulatio'num vertebra'rum,** capsule of vertebral articulations: one of the bands of tissue, partly white fibrous and partly yellow elastic, that unite the articular processes of adjacent vertebrae.

**c. articula'ris atlantoaxia'lis latera'lis,** atlantoaxial articular capsule: a ligamentous sac surrounding the lateral atlantoaxial joint; called also *c. articularis atlantoepistrophica.*

**c. articula'ris atlantoepistro'phica,** c. articularis atlantoaxialis lateralis.

**c. articula'ris atlantooccipita'lis,** capsule of atlantooccipital articulation: one of a pair of distinct ligamentous bands, each of which is attached at one end to the lateral mass of the atlas and at the other end to the margins of an occipital condyle.

**c. articula'ris calcaneocuboi'dea,** capsule of calcaneocuboid joint: a ligamentous sac surrounding the calcaneocuboid joint.

**c. articula'ris ca'pitis cos'tae,** articular capsule of head of rib: a ligamentous sac surrounding the articulation of the head of a rib.

**cap'sulae articula'res carpometacar'peae,** capsules of carpometacarpal joints: ligamentous sacs surrounding the carpometacarpal joints; they are continuous with the capsules of the intercarpal joints.

**c. articula'ris carpometacar'pea pol'licis,** capsule of carpometacarpal articulation of thumb: a ligamentous sac surrounding the carpometacarpal joint of the thumb.

**c. articula'ris costotransversa'ria,** capsule of costotransverse joint: a ligamentous sac surrounding the costotransverse articulation.

**c. articula'ris cox'ae,** capsule of hip joint: a large, strong ligamentous sac surrounding the hip joint.

**c. articula'ris cricoarytenoi'dea,** capsule of cricoarytenoid joint: the fibrous and synovial layers enclosing the cricoarytenoid joint.

**c. articula'ris cricothyroi'dea,** the capsule of the cricothyroid joint.

**c. articula'ris cu'biti,** articular capsule of elbow: the capsule formed around the cubital articulation by its various ligaments.

**cap'sulae articula'res digito'rum man'us,** capsulae articulares interphalangearum manus.

**cap'sulae articula'res digito'rum pe'dis,** capsulae articulares interphalangearum pedis.

**c. articula'ris ge'nus,** capsule of knee joint: the loose, thin, but strong sac enclosing the knee joint.

**c. articula'ris hu'meri,** articular capsule of humerus: a ligamentous sac surrounding the shoulder joint.

**cap'sulae articula'res intermetacar'peae,** capsules of intermetacarpal joints: ligamentous sacs that surround the intermetacarpal joints; they are continuous with the capsules of the carpometacarpal joints.

**cap'sulae articula'res intermetatar'seae,** capsules of intermetatarsal joints: the capsules around the four joints between the bases of the metatarsal bones.

**cap'sulae articula'res interphalangea'rum ma'nus,** capsules of interphalangeal joints of hand: incomplete ligamentous sacs surrounding the interphalangeal joints of the hand; called also *capsulae articulares digitorum manus.*

**cap'sulae articula'res interphalangea'rum pe'dis,** capsules of interphalangeal joints of foot: the capsules surrounding the interphalangeal articulations of the toes; called also *capsulae articulares digitorum pedis.*

**c. articula'ris mandi'bulae,** c. articularis articulationis temporomandibularis.

**c. articula'ris ma'nus,** a loose ligamentous sac surrounding the radiocarpal joint and the intercarpal joints together; called also *capsule of radiocarpal joint.*

**cap'sulae articula'res metacarpophalan'geae,** capsules of metacarpophalangeal joints: ligamentous sacs that surround the metacarpophalangeal joints.

**cap'sulae articula'res metatarsophalan'geae,** capsules of metatarsophalangeal joints: the five capsules surrounding the metatarsophalangeal articulations.

**c. articula'ris os'sis pisifor'mis,** articular capsule of pisiform bone: a thin, loose ligamentous sac surrounding the joint of the pisiform bone.

**c. articula'ris radioulna'ris dista'lis,** distal radioulnar articular capsule: a loose ligamentous sac surrounding the distal radioulnar joint.

**c. articula'ris sternoclavicula'ris,** capsule of sternoclavicular joint: a ligamentous sac surrounding the sternoclavicular joint.

**c. articula'ris sternocosta'lis,** sternocostal articular capsule: the ligamentous sac that surrounds a sternocostal joint.

**c. articula'ris talocalca'nea,** a loose ligamentous sac surrounding the subtalar joint; called also *capsule of subtalar joint.*

**c. articula'ris talocrura'lis,** a thin ligamentous sac surrounding the ankle joint; called also *capsule of ankle joint.*

**c. articula'ris talonavicula'ris,** a capsule surrounding the talonavicular joint.

**cap'sulae articula'res tarsometatar'seae,** capsules of tarsometatarsal joints: the three capsules that surround the joints between the metatarsal and cuneiform bones.

**c. articula'ris tibiofibula'ris,** capsule of tibiofibular joint: a fibrous sac enclosing the tibiofibular articulation.

**c. bul'bi,** vagina bulbi.

**c. exter'na** [TA], external capsule: the thin layer of white substance that separates the lateral part of the lentiform nucleus (putamen) from the claustrum.

**c. extre'ma** [TA], extreme capsule: the white matter between the claustrum and the cortex of the insula.

**c. fibro'sa,** a capsule consisting largely of fibrous elements.

**c. fibro'sa glan'dulae thyroi'deae** [TA], fibrous capsule of thyroid gland: a connective tissue coat intimately adherent to the underlying gland; called also *c. glandulae thyroideae.*

**c. fibro'sa [Glisso'ni], c. fibro'sa he'patis,** c. fibrosa perivascularis.

**c. fibro'sa perivascula'ris** [TA], perivascular fibrous capsule: the connective tissue sheath that accompanies the vessels and ducts through the hepatic portal. It is continuous with the fibrous coat. Called also *c. fibrosa hepatis, fibrous capsule of liver, Glisson's capsule, hepatobiliary capsule,* and *c. fibrosa* [*Glissoni*].

**c. fibro'sa re'nis** [TA], fibrous capsule of kidney: the connective tissue investment of the kidney, which continues through the hilus to line the renal sinus; called also *tunica fibrosa renis.*

**c. gan'glii** [TA], capsule of ganglion: the laminated connective tissue capsule surrounding a neural ganglion and continuous with epineurium of its associated nerve root.

**c. glan'dulae thyroi'deae,** c. fibrosa glandulae thyroideae.

**c. glome'ruli,** capsule of glomerulus: the double-walled globular dilatation that forms the beginning of a uriniferous tubule of the kidney and surrounds the glomerulus; it consists of an inner, or visceral, layer *(capsular epithelium)* and an outer, or parietal, layer *(glomerular epithelium)*; called also *Bowman's, glomerular, malpighian,* and *müllerian capsule.*

**c. inter'na** [TA], internal capsule: a fanlike mass of white fibers that separates the lentiform nucleus laterally from the head of the caudate nucleus, the dorsal thalamus, and the tail of the caudate nucleus medially; it consists of an anterior limb, a genu, and a posterior limb consisting of three parts, thalamolenticular, sublenticular, and retrolenticular. The internal capsule is known to carry corticofugal (efferent) fibers from the cerebral cortex; its exact role in carrying afferent fibers to the cortex remains uncertain.

**c. len'tis** [TA], capsule of lens: the elastic envelope covering the lens of the eye and fusing with the fibers of the ciliary zonule; called also *crystalline capsule.*

**c. no'di lympha'tici, c. no'di lymphoi'dei** [TA], capsule of lymph node: the outer layer of a lymph node, composed mainly of collagen fibers with a few fibroblasts and elastin fibers.

**c. nu'clei denta'ti,** a layer formed by fibers passing to and from the dentate nucleus.

**cap'sulae nu'clei lentifor'mis,** see *c. externa* and *c. interna.*

**c. pancre'atis,** capsule of pancreas: a thin sheath of areolar tissue that invests the pancreas (but does not form a definite capsule), the septa of which extend into the gland and divide it into lobules.

**c. prosta'tica** [TA], capsule of prostate: the fibroelastic capsule that surrounds the prostate and contains an extensive plexus of veins.

**cap'sulae re'nis,** see *c. adiposa renis* and *c. fibrosa renis.*

**c. sero'sa lie'nis,** tunica serosa splenis.

**c. sple'nis** [TA], capsule of spleen: the fibroelastic coat of the spleen; called also *tunica fibrosa lienis* and *tunica fibrosa splenis* [TA alternatives].

**c. tonsilla'ris** [TA], tonsillar capsule: a fibrous capsule covering the lateral surface of the palatine tonsils and separating them from the underlying connective tissue.

**cap·su·lae** (kap′su-le) [L.] plural of *capsula.*

**cap·su·lar** (kap′su-lər) pertaining to a capsule.

**cap·su·la·tion** (kap″su-la′shən) the enclosure of a medicine in a capsule.

**cap·sule** (cap′səl) [L. *capsula* a little box] 1. a structure in which something is enclosed, such as a hard or a soft, soluble container of a suitable substance, for enclosing a dose of medicine. 2. an anatomical structure enclosing an organ or body part; see *capsula.*
**adherent c.,** an investing structure that is not readily separated from the organ or substance contained within it.
**adipose c.,** one consisting largely of fat.
**adipose c. of kidney,** capsula adiposa renis.
**adrenal c.,** glandula suprarenalis.
**c. of ankle joint,** capsula articularis talocruralis.
**articular c.,** capsula articularis.
**articular c., fibrous,** membrana fibrosa capsulae articularis.
**auditory c.,** the cartilaginous capsule of the embryo that develops into the bony labyrinth of the inner ear.
**bacterial c.,** an envelope of gel surrounding a bacterial cell, usually polysaccharide but sometimes polypeptide in nature, which is associated with the virulence of pathogenic bacteria.
**biopsy c.,** a device which may be passed into the intestine for the purpose of securing specimens of the mucosa for examination under the microscope.
**Bonnet's c.,** vagina bulbi.
**Bowman's c.,** capsula glomeruli.
**brood c's,** capsular projections from the internal membrane of hydatid cysts, from which the scoleces arise.
**cartilage c.,** a basophilic zone of cartilage matrix bordering on a lacuna and its enclosed cartilage cell.
**central c.,** a structure seen in certain protozoa of the superclass Actinopoda, such as radiolarians, that encloses the central nucleated core of cytoplasm and is surrounded by a membrane perforated to permit communication with the outer cortex *(calymma).*
**Crosby c.,** an instrument used to obtain intestinal material for biopsy, consisting of a cylindrical capsule containing a knife which is spring-activated and triggered by suction.
**crystalline c.,** capsula lentis.
**external c.,** capsula externa.
**extreme c.,** capsula extrema.
**fatty c. of kidney,** capsula adiposa renis.
**fibrous c.,** capsula fibrosa.
**fibrous c. of corpora cavernosa of penis,** tunica albuginea corporum cavernosorum penis.
**fibrous c. of graafian follicle,** tunica externa thecae folliculi.
**fibrous c. of kidney,** capsula fibrosa renis.
**fibrous c. of liver,** capsula fibrosa perivascularis.
**fibrous c. of spleen,** capsula splenis.
**fibrous c. of testis,** tunica albuginea testis.
**fibrous c. of thyroid gland,** capsula fibrosa glandulae thyroideae.
**c. of ganglion,** capsula ganglii.
**Gerota's c.,** fascia renalis.
**Glisson's c.,** capsula fibrosa perivascularis.
**glomerular c., c. of glomerulus,** capsula glomeruli.
**c. of heart,** pericardium.
**hepatobiliary c.,** capsula fibrosa perivascularis.
**internal c.,** capsula interna.
**joint c.,** capsula articularis.
**c. of lens,** capsula lentis.
**c. of lymph node,** capsula nodi lymphoidei.
**malpighian c.,** capsula glomeruli.
**Müller c., müllerian c.,** capsula glomeruli.
**ocular c.,** vagina bulbi.
**optic c.,** the embryonic structure from which the sclera is developed.
**otic c.,** the skeletal element enclosing the inner ear mechanism. In the human embryo, it develops as cartilage at various ossification centers and becomes completely bony and unified at about the twenty-third week of fetal life.
**c. of pancreas,** capsula pancreatis.
**pelvioprostatic c.,** fascia prostatae.
**perinephric c.,** see *capsula adiposa renis* and *capsula fibrosa renis.*
**periotic c.,** the tissue surrounding the otic sac in the embryo.
**perirenal fat c.,** capsula adiposa renis.
**polar c.,** 1. any of the thick-walled vesicles seen in the spores of

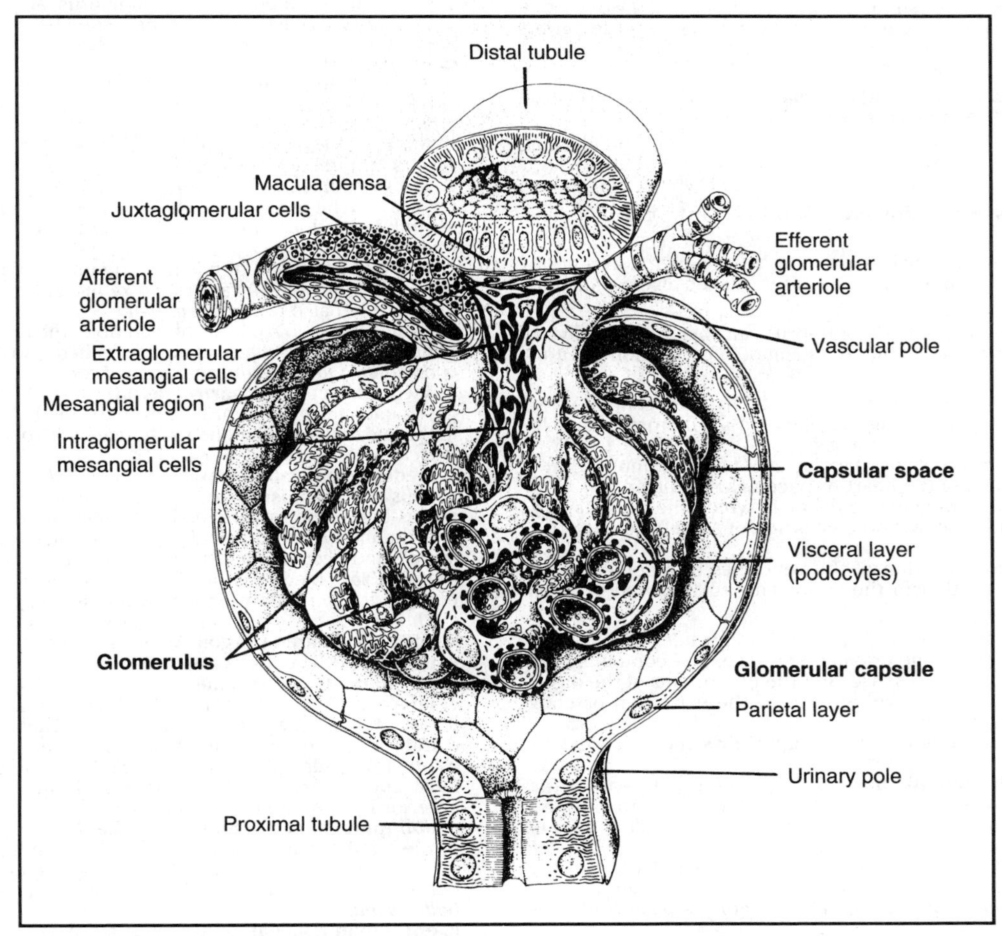


Capsula glomeruli (glomerular capsule), showing the double-walled cup shape invaginated by the glomerulus, which is closely approximated by the podocytes of the visceral layer of the capsule.

certain protozoa and containing the polar filament. 2. see under *cap.*
**c. of prostate,** capsula prostatica.
**c. of radiocarpal joint,** capsula articularis manus.
**radiotelemetering c.,** telemetering c.
**renal c.,** see *capsula adiposa renis* and *capsula fibrosa renis.*
**serous c. of spleen,** tunica serosa splenis.
**c. of spleen,** capsula splenis.
**c. of subtalar joint,** capsula articularis talocalcanea.
**suprarenal c.,** glandula suprarenalis.
**synovial c.,** capsula articularis.
**telemetering c.,** a small radio transmitter encased in a capsule the size of an ordinary drug capsule that can be swallowed or otherwise inserted in the body to give information about conditions (pressure, temperature, pH, etc.) within an organ; called also *radio pill.*
**Tenon's c.,** vagina bulbi.
**tonsillar c.,** capsula tonsillaris.
**triasyn B c's,** capsules containing thiamine, riboflavin, and nicotinamide, used as a vitamin supplement.

**cap·su·lec·to·my** (kap″su-lek′tə-me) [*capsule* + *-ectomy*] excision of a capsule, especially a joint capsule or the capsule of the lens; called also *decapsulation.*
**renal c.,** renal decapsulation.

**cap·su·li·tis** (kap″su-li′tis) the inflammation of a capsule, as that of the lens, joint, liver, or labyrinth.
**adhesive c.,** adhesive inflammation between the joint capsule and the peripheral articular cartilage of the shoulder with obliteration of the subdeltoid bursa, characterized by painful shoulder of gradual onset, with increasing pain, stiffness, and limitation of motion. Called also *adhesive bursitis* and *frozen shoulder.*
**hepatic c.,** perihepatitis.

**cap·su·lo·len·tic·u·lar** (kap″su-lo-len-tik′u-lər) pertaining to the lens of the eye and its capsule.

**cap·su·lo·plas·ty** (kap′su-lo-plas″te) [*capsule* + *-plasty*] a plastic operation on a joint capsule.

**cap·su·lor·rha·phy** (kap″su-lor′ə-fe) [*capsule* + *-rrhaphy*] suturing of a capsule, especially a joint capsule.

**cap·su·lor·rhex·is** (kap″su-lo-rek′sis) [*capsule* + *-rrhexis*] the making of a continuous circular tear in the anterior capsule during cataract surgery in order to allow expression or phacoemulsification of the nucleus of the lens.

**cap·su·lo·tome** (kap-su′lo-tōm) [*capsule* + *-tome*] a cutting instrument used for incising the capsules of the lens.

**cap·su·lot·o·my** (kap″su-lot′ə-me) [*capsule* + *-tomy*] the incision of a capsule, such as of the lens, the kidney, or a joint.
**renal c.,** incision of a renal capsule.

**cap·to·di·ame hy·dro·chlo·ride** (kap″to-di′ām) captodiamine hydrochloride.

**cap·to·di·amine hy·dro·chlo·ride** (kap″to -di′ə-mēn) a tranquilizer and muscle relaxant used as a sedative. Called also *captodiame hydrochloride.*

**cap·to·pril** (kap′to-pril) [MeSH: Captopril] an angiotensin-converting enzyme inhibitor used in the treatment of hypertension and congestive heart failure.

**cap·ture** (kap′chər) 1. to seize or catch; to take control over. 2. the coalescence of an atomic nucleus and a subatomic particle, usually resulting in an unstable mass.
**atrial c.,** depolarization of the atria in response to stimulus either originating elsewhere in the heart or pacemaker induced.
**electron c.,** a type of radioactive decay in which the nucleus captures an orbital electron, with the emission of a neutrino and characteristic rays.
**ventricular c.,** depolarization of the ventricles in response to an impulse originating either in the supraventricular region or in an artificial pacemaker.

**cap·ut** (kap′ət) pl. *cap′ita* [L.] [TA] 1. head: the superior extremity of the body, comprising the cranium and face, and containing the brain, the organs of special sense, and the first organs of the digestive system. 2. a general term applied to the expanded or chief extremity of an organ or part.
**c. angula′re mus′culi quadra′ti la′bii superio′ris,** musculus levator labii superioris alaeque nasi.
**c. bre′ve mus′culi bicip′itis bra′chii** [TA], the short head of the biceps brachii muscle, arising from the apex of the coracoid process; called also *medial head of biceps brachii muscle, short head of coracoradialis muscle,* and *coracoradialis.*
**c. bre′ve mus′culi bicip′itis fem′oris** [TA], the short head of the biceps femoris muscle, arising from the linea aspera femoris.
**c. cor′nus dorsa′lis medul′lae spina′lis,** c. cornus posterioris medullae spinalis.
**c. cor′nus posterio′ris medul′lae spina′lis** [TA], head of posterior horn of spinal cord: the oval or fusiform portion of the dorsal horn of gray substance in the spinal cord between the constricted portion (neck) and the apex of the horn. Called also *c. cornus dorsalis medullae spinalis* and *head of dorsal horn of spinal cord.*
**c. cos′tae** [TA], head of rib: the posterior end of a rib, which articulates with the body of a vertebra; called also *capitulum costae.*
**c. distor′tum,** torticollis.
**c. epididy′midis** [TA], head of epididymis: the upper part of the epididymis, in which are found the straight and coiled portions of the efferent ductules of the testis; called also *globus major epididymidis.*
**c. fe′moris** [TA], the main part or shaft of the femur.
**c. fi′bulae** [TA], **c. fibula′re,** head of fibula: the proximal extremity of the fibula; called also *capitulum fibulae.*
**c. gallina′ginis,** [L. "woodcock's head"], colliculus seminalis.
**c. humera′le,** c. humeri.
**c. humera′le mus′culi flexo′ris car′pi ulna′ris** [TA], the humeral head of the flexor carpi ulnaris muscle, arising from the medial epicondyle of the humerus.
**c. humera′le mus′culi flexo′ris digito′rum subli′mis,** c. humeroulnare musculi flexoris digitorum superficialis.
**c. humera′le mus′culi pronato′ris tere′tis** [TA], the humeral head of the pronator teres muscle arising from the medial epicondyle of the humerus.
**c. hu′meri** [TA], head of humerus: the proximal end of the humerus, which articulates with the glenoid cavity of the scapula; called also *c. humerale.*
**c. humeroulna′re mus′culi flexo′ris digito′rum superficia′lis** [TA], the humeroulnar head of the flexor digitorum superficialis muscle, arising from the medial epicondyle of the humerus and coronoid process of ulna; called also *c. humerale musculi flexoris digitorum sublimis* and *humeral head of flexor digitorum sublimis muscle.*
**c. infraorbita′le mus′culi quadra′ti la′bii superio′ris,** musculus levator labii superioris.
**c. latera′le mus′culi gastrocne′mii** [TA], the lateral head of the gastrocnemius muscle, arising from the lateral condyle and posterior surface of the femur, and the capsule of the knee joint; called also *lateral gastrocnemius muscle.*
**c. latera′le mus′culi tricip′itis bra′chii** [TA], the lateral head of the triceps brachii muscle, arising from the posterior surface of the humerus, the lateral border of the humerus, and the lateral intermuscular septum; called also *great* or *second head of triceps brachii muscle,* and *lateral* or *short anconeus muscle.*
**c. lie′nis,** extremitas posterior lienis.
**c. lon′gum mus′culi bicip′itis bra′chii** [TA], the long head of the biceps brachii muscle, arising from the upper border of the glenoid cavity; called also *interarticular ligament of articulation of humerus.*
**c. lon′gum mus′culi bicip′itis fem′oris** [TA], the long head of the biceps femoris muscle, arising from the ischial tuberosity.
**c. lon′gum musculi tricip′itis bra′chii** [TA], the long head of the triceps brachii muscle, arising from the infraglenoid tubercle of the scapula; called also *first, middle,* or *scapular head of triceps brachii muscle.*
**c. mal′lei** [TA], head of malleus: the upper portion of the malleus, which includes the surface *(facet for incus)* that articulates with the incus; called also *capitulum mallei.*
**c. mandi′bulae** [TA], head of mandible: the articular surface of the condyloid process of the mandible; called also *capitulum [processus condyloidei] mandibulae* and *head of condyloid process of mandible.*
**c. media′le mus′culi gastrocne′mii** [TA], the medial head of the gastrocnemius muscle, arising from the medial condyle of the femur and the capsule of the knee joint; called also *medial gastrocnemius muscle.*
**c. media′le mus′culi tricip′itis bra′chii** [TA], the medial head of the triceps brachii muscle, arising from the posterior surface of the humerus below the radial groove, the medial border of the humerus, and the medial intermuscular septum; called also *medial anconeus muscle* and *deep* or *short head of triceps brachii muscle.*
**c. medu′sae,** Medusa's head: dilated cutaneous veins around the umbilicus, seen mainly in the newborn and in patients suffering with cirrhosis of the liver; so called because the veins resemble the head of the snake-haired Gorgon, Medusa. Called also *cirsomphalos.*
**c. metacarpa′le,** c. ossis metacarpi.
**c. metatarsa′le,** c. ossis metatarsi.
**c. mus′culi** [TA], head of muscle: the end of a muscle at the site of its attachment to a bone or other fixed structure (origin).
**c. natifor′me,** former name for *c. quadratum.*
**c. nu′clei cauda′ti** [TA], head of caudate nucleus: the largest and most anterior part of the caudate nucleus, which bulges into the anterior horn of the lateral ventricle.
**c. obli′quum mus′culi adducto′ris hal′lucis** [TA], the oblique head of the adductor hallucis muscle, originating from the bases of the second, third, and fourth metatarsal bones, and the sheath of the peroneus longus muscle; called also *great* or *long head of adductor hallucis muscle.*
**c. obli′quum mus′culi adducto′ris pol′licis** [TA], the oblique head of the adductor pollicis muscle, arising from the capitate and trapezoid bones and the base of the second metacarpals.

**c. os'sis metacarpa'lis, c. os'sis metacar'pi** [TA], head of metacarpal bone: the distal extremity of a metacarpal bone, which articulates with the base of a proximal digit. Called also *c. metacarpalis.*
**c. os'sis metatarsa'lis, c. os'sis metatar'si** [TA], head of metatarsal bone: the distal extremity of a metatarsal bone, which articulates with the base of a digit. Called also *c. metatarsalis.*
**c. pancre'atis** [TA], head of pancreas: the discoidal mass forming the enlarged right extremity of the pancreas, lying in a flexure of the duodenum.
**c. pe'nis,** glans penis.
**c. phalan'gis ma'nus** [TA], head of phalanx of hand: the distal articular surface of each of the proximal and middle phalanges of the fingers.
**c. phalan'gis pe'dis** [TA], head of phalanx of foot: the distal articular extremity of each of the proximal and middle phalanges of the toes.
**c. pla'num,** a flattened head occurring with osteochondritis deformans juvenilis.
**c. proge'neum,** prognathism.
**c. quadra'tum,** a head deformity seen in rickets in which the eminences of the frontal and parietal bones form elevations separated by depressions marking the lines of the cranial sutures.
**c. radia'le,** c. radii.
**c. radia'le mus'culi flexo'ris digito'rum superficia'lis** [TA], the radial head of the flexor digitorum superficialis muscle, arising from the oblique line and anterior border of the radius.
**c. ra'dii** [TA], head of radius: the disk on the proximal end of the radius that articulates with the capitulum of the humerus and the radial notch of the ulna; called also *capitulum radii* and *c. radiale.*
**c. rec'tum mus'culi rec'ti fe'moris** [TA], straight head of rectus femoris muscle: the head of the rectus femoris that arises from anteroinferior iliac spine, which fuses with the reflected or posterior head and continues down into the belly of the muscle. Called also *anterior head of rectus femoris muscle.*
**c. reflex'um mus'culi rec'ti fe'moris** [TA], reflected head of rectus femoris muscle: the head of the rectus femoris that arises from a groove above the rim of the acetabulum, which fuses with the straight or anterior head and continues down into the belly of the muscle. Called also *posterior head of rectus femoris muscle.*
**c. stape'dis** [TA], head of stapes: the part that articulates with the incus; called also *capitulum stapedis.*
**c. succeda'neum,** edema occurring in and under the fetal scalp during labor.
**c. tala're,** c. tali.
**c. ta'li** [TA], head of talus: the rounded anterior end of the talus; called also *head of astragalus.*
**c. transver'sum mus'culi adducto'ris hal'lucis** [TA], the transverse head of the adductor hallucis muscle, arising from the capsules of the metatarso-phalangeal joints of the third, fourth, and fifth toes.
**c. transver'sum mus'culi adducto'ris pol'licis** [TA], the transverse head of the adductor pollicis muscle arising from the lower two thirds of the anterior surface of the third metacarpal.
**c. ul'nae** [TA], head of ulna: the articular surface of the distal extremity of the ulna; called also *capitulum ulnae.*
**c. ulna're mus'culi flexo'ris car'pi ulna'ris** [TA], the ulnar head of the flexor carpi ulnaris muscle, arising from the olecranon, and the adjacent part of the ulna.
**c. ulna're mus'culi pronato'ris ter'etis** [TA], the ulnar head of the pronator teres muscle, arising from the coronoid process of the ulna; called also *coronoid head of pronator teres muscle.*
**c. zygomat'icum mus'culi quadra'ti la'bii superio'ris,** musculus zygomaticus minor.

**CAR** Canadian Association of Radiologists.

**Ca·ra·bel·li cusp (sign, tubercle)** (kah-rə-bel'e) [Georg *Carabelli,* Hungarian dentist in Vienna, 1787–1842] see under *cusp.*

**Car·a·fate** (kar'ə-fāt) trademark for a preparation of sucralfate.

**car·a·mel** (kar'ə-məl, kahr'məl) [NF] a concentrated solution of the product obtained by heating sugar or glucose until the sweet taste is destroyed and a uniform dark brown mass results; used as a coloring agent for pharmaceuticals and foods.

**ca·ram·i·phen** (kə-ram'ĭ-fen) an anticholinergic with actions similar to but weaker than those of atropine (q.v.).
**c. edisylate, c. ethanedisulfonate,** an ester of caramiphen, with the anticholinergic effects of the base; used as an antitussive, administered orally.
**c. hydrochloride,** an ester of caramiphen with the anticholinergic effects of the base; used mainly in the treatment of Parkinson's disease and parkinsonism, administered orally.

**car·at** (kar'ət) 1. a measure of the fineness of gold, pure gold being 24 carats. 2. a unit of weight of precious stones, being 205.5 milligrams or $3\frac{1}{6}$ grains troy.

**car·a·way** (kar'ə-wa) [Ar. *karawyā,* from Gr. *karon*] 1. *Carum carvi.* 2. the dried ripe fruit of *C. carvi;* its brown mericarps have an aromatic odor and taste and are used as a flavoring agent.

**car·ba·ceph·em** (kahr"bə-sef'əm) any of a class of $\beta$-lactam antibiotics closely related to the cephalosporins, having a methylene group substituted for the sulfur atom in the 7-aminocephalosporanic acid nucleus; carbacephems are chemically more stable than cephalosporins.

**car·ba·chol** (kahr'bə-kol) [USP] [MeSH: Carbachol] a cholinergic agonist, carbamylcholine chloride, that is not hydrolyzed by acetylcholinesterase or pseudocholinesterase; used as a miotic and to lower intraocular pressure in the treatment of glaucoma and following cataract surgery.

**car·ba·dox** (kahr'bə-doks) [MeSH: Carbadox] an antibacterial used in veterinary medicine.

**car·ba·mate** (kahr'bə-māt) 1. any ester of carbamic acid. 2. any of a group of insecticides and parasiticides that act by inhibiting cholinesterase; heavy exposure to some of them can cause carbamate poisoning (q.v.) in humans or livestock. See table.

**car·ba·maz·e·pine** (kahr"bə-maz'ə-pēn) [USP] [MeSH: Carbamazepine] an anticonvulsant and antineuralgic, used in the treatment of pain associated with trigeminal neuralgia and in epilepsy manifested by tonic-clonic and partial seizures, administered orally.

**car·bam·ic ac·id** (kahr-bam'ik) a compound, $H_2NCOOH$, that exists only in the form of salts or esters (carbamates), amides (carbamides), and other derivatives (its acyl radical, $H_2NCO$—, is carbamoyl).
**c. a. peroxide** [USP], an equimolecular compound of urea and hydrogen peroxide used topically as a cerumen-softening agent and as a dental cleanser, bleaching agent, and anti-inflammatory.

**car·ba·mide** (kahr'bə-mīd) urea.

**car·bam·i·no·he·mo·glo·bin** (kahr-bam"ĭ-no-he"mo-glo'bin) a chemical combination of carbon dioxide with hemoglobin, $CO_2HHb$, being one of the forms in which carbon dioxide exists in the blood. Called also *carbhemoglobin* and *carbohemoglobin.*

**car·bam·o·yl** (kahr-bam'o-əl) the radical $NH_2CO$—. Called also *carbamyl.*

**car·bam·o·yl·as·par·tate** (kahr-bam"o-əl-as-pahr'tāt) aspartate linked at the amino end to a carbamoyl moiety; it is an intermediate in pyrimidine biosynthesis.

**car·bam·o·y·la·tion** (kahr-bam"o-ə-la'-shən) the transfer of a carbamoyl moiety to the amino group of an acceptor compound.

**car·bam·o·yl-phos·phate syn·thase (am·mo·nia)** (kahr-bam'o-əl fos'fāt sin'thās ə-mo'ne-ə) [EC 6.3.4.16] an enzyme of the ligase class that catalyzes the synthesis of carbamoyl phosphate from ammonia and carbon dioxide, the first committed step in the urea cycle (see illustration at *urea cycle,* under *cycle*). The reaction occurs predominantly in liver mitochondria, requires *N*-acetylglutamate as a cofactor, and hydrolyzes two molecules of ATP. Decreased enzyme activity, an autosomal recessive trait, causes carbamoyl phosphate synthetase deficiency.

**car·bam·o·yl-phos·phate syn·thase (glu·ta·mine-hy·dro·lyz·ing)** (kahr-bam'o-əl fos'fāt sin'thās gloo'tə-mēn hi'dro-li-zing) [EC 6.3.5.5] an enzyme activity of the trifunctional CAD protein (q.v.); it is a ligase that catalyzes the formation of carbamoyl phosphate as the first step in the biosynthesis of pyrimidine nucleotides. Glutamine is the nitrogen donor in the reaction, which is cytosolic and is inhibited by UTP.

**car·bam·o·yl phos·phate syn·the·tase (CPS)** (kahr-bam'o-əl fos'fāt sin'thə-tās) 1. carbamoyl-phosphate synthase (ammonia); written also *carbamoyl phosphate synthetase I* (CPSI). 2. carbamoyl-phosphate synthase (glutamine hydrolyzing); written also *carbamoyl phosphate synthetase II* (CPSII).

**car·bam·o·yl phos·phate syn·the·tase de·fi·cien·cy** a genetic aminoacidopathy due to a deficiency of carbamoyl phosphate synthase (ammonia); characteristic symptoms include pronounced hyperammonemia without orotic aciduria, protein intolerance, and neurologic disorders. Symptoms may begin in the neonatal period or appear later in infancy, with varying degrees of severity. Written also *carbamoyl phosphate synthetase I (CPSI) deficiency.*

**car·bam·o·yl·trans·fer·ase** (kahr-bam'o-əl-trans'fər-ās) a term

| Carbamate Insecticides |
|---|
| Aldicarb |
| Aminocarb |
| Carbaril |
| Carbofuran |
| Dimetilan |
| Methomyl |
| Propoxur |

used in the names of some of the enzymes of the sub-subclass carbamoyltransferases and carboxyltransferases [EC 2.1.3] to denote those that catalyze the transfer of a carbamoyl group from a donor compound to an acceptor compound. Called also *transcarbamoylase.*

**car·ba·myl** (kahr'bə-məl) carbamoyl.

**car·bam·y·la·tion** (kahr-bam"əl-a'shən) carbamoylation.

**car·ba·myl·cho·line chlo·ride** (kahr"bə-məl-ko'lēn klor'īd) carbachol.

**car·ba·ril** (kahr'bə-ril) a carbamate compound with cholinesterase-inhibiting activity, used as an insecticide and parasiticide in shampoos and lotions for humans and domestic animals. Excessive exposure can cause mild carbamate poisoning. Called also *carbaryl.*

**car·bar·sone** (kahr-bahr'sōn) a pentavalent organic arsenical used as an antiamebic in the treatment of intestinal amebiasis; administered orally or by retention enema. Because of its toxicity, it has largely been replaced by other agents.

**car·ba·ryl** (kahr'bə-rəl) [MeSH: Carbaryl] carbaril.

**car·ba·zide** (kahr'bə-zīd) a urea derivative, carbodihydrazide, $CO(NHNH_2)_2$, in which both the amide groups of urea have been replaced by hydrazine residues.

**car·baz·o·chrome sal·i·cyl·ate** (kahr-baz'ə-krōm) a complex of adrenochrome monosemicarbazone with sodium salicylate, used as a hemostatic to control capillary bleeding and to prevent capillary permeability, administered orally or intramuscularly.

**car·baz·o·tate** (kahr-baz'o-tāt) any salt of picric acid; a picrate.

**car·ben·i·cil·lin** (kahr"bən-ĭ-sil'in) [MeSH: Carbenicillin] a semisynthetic penicillin, effective against gram-negative bacteria, such as susceptible strains of *Pseudomonas aeruginosa,* indole-positive *Proteus* species, certain strains of *Escherichia coli,* and *Haemophilus influenzae;* it also inhibits the growth of some gram-positive pathogens. Called also *carfecillin.*
**c. disodium** [USP], the disodium salt of carbenicillin, having the same actions as the base; administered intramuscularly or intravenously in severe systemic infections and septicemia, urinary and genitourinary tract infections, acute and chronic respiratory infections, and soft tissue infections.
**c. indanyl sodium** [USP], the sodium salt of the indanyl ester of carbenicillin disodium, having the same actions as the base; administered orally in the treatment of upper and lower urinary tract infections due to susceptible strains of *Pseudomonas* species, *Proteus* species, *Escherichia coli, Enterobacter,* and enterococci. Called also *carindacillin sodium.*
**c. phenyl sodium,** the sodium salt of the phenyl ester of carbenicillin disodium, which has been used for the same purposes as carbenicillin indanyl sodium. Called also *carfecillin sodium.*
**c. potassium,** the potassium salt of carbenicillin.
**c. sodium,** c. disodium.

**car·ben·ox·o·lone so·di·um** (kahr"bən-ok'sə-lōn) a derivative of glycyrrhizin having marked anti-inflammatory actions and aldosterone-like activity; used in the treatment of gastric ulcer.

**car·be·ta·pen·tane** (kahr-ba"tə-pen'tān) an antitussive agent with mild atropine-like antisecretory activity; used in the treatment of cough associated with upper respiratory infections, administered orally; available as *carbetapentane citrate* and *carbetapentane tannate.*

**carb·he·mo·glo·bin** (kahrb"he-mo-glo'bin) carbaminohemoglobin.

**car·bide** (kahr'bīd) a compound of carbon with an element or radical.
**metallic c.,** a compound of carbon with a transition metal, as in $Fe_3C$ (as distinguished from a salt-like carbide, such as $CaC_2$).

**car·bi·do·pa** (kahr"bĭ-do'pə) [USP] [MeSH: Carbidopa] an inhibitor of the decarboxylation of peripheral levodopa to dopamine, which does not penetrate the central nervous system. When given with levodopa, carbidopa produces higher brain concentrations of dopamine with lower doses of levodopa, thus lessening the side effects seen with higher doses. It is used orally, in conjunction with levodopa, as an antiparkinsonian agent, and has been used in the treatment of Lesch-Nyhan syndrome and Gilles de la Tourette syndrome.

**car·bim·a·zole** (kahr-bim'ə-zōl) [MeSH: Carbimazole] an inhibitor of thyroid hormone synthesis, administered orally in the treatment of hyperthyroidism.

**car·bi·nol** (kahr'bĭ-nol) 1. methanol. 2. any aromatic or fatty alcohol formed by substituting one, two, or three hydrocarbon groups for hydrogen in methanol.
**acetylmethyl c.,** a keto-isomer of aldol, $CH_3{\cdot}CHOH{\cdot}CO{\cdot}CH_3$, which is formed from glucose by certain bacteria and which is detected in a broth culture of bacteria by the Voges-Proskauer reaction.
**dimethyl c.,** isopropyl alcohol.

**car·bi·nox·amine** (kahr"bin-ok'sə-mēn) an ethanolamine derivative with $H_1$ antihistaminic, antimuscarinic, and sedative properties.
**c. maleate** [USP], the maleate salt of carbinoxamine, used as an antihistaminic; administered orally.

**car·bo** (kahr'bo) [L.] charcoal.
**c. activa'tus,** activated charcoal.
**c. anima'lis,** a variety prepared from bones and other animal matter; a decolorizing agent.
**c. anima'lis purifica'tus,** purified animal charcoal.

**Car·bo·caine** (kahr'bo-kān) trademark for preparations of mepivacaine hydrochloride.

**car·bo·cho·line** (kahr"bo-ko'lēn) carbachol.

**car·bo·cy·clic** (kahr"bo-sik'lik) having or pertaining to a closed chain or ring formation which includes only carbon atoms; said of chemical compounds.

**car·bo·cys·te·ine** (kahr"bo-sis'tēn) [MeSH: Carbocysteine] a mucolytic agent, administered orally and by inhalation in the treatment of respiratory disorders characterized by the production of excess or viscous mucus.

**car·bo·di·im·ide** (kahr"bo-di-im'id) a derivative of urea, NH:C:NH.

**car·bo·gas·e·ous** (kahr"bo-gas'e-əs) charged with carbon dioxide gas.

**car·bo·gen** (kahr'bo-jen) a mixture of oxygen with 5 per cent carbon dioxide.

**car·bo·he·mo·glo·bin** (kahr"bo-he"mo-glo'bin) carbaminohemoglobin.

**car·bo·hy·drate** (kahr"bo-hi'drāt) any of a class of aldehyde or ketone derivatives of polyhydric alcohols, particularly of the pentahydric and hexahydric alcohols. They are so named because the hydrogen and oxygen are usually in the proportion to form water, $C_n(H_2O)_n$; the most important include the small sugars as well as the large starches, glycogens, celluloses, and gums. See also *saccharide.*
**reserve c's,** carbohydrates that can be stored in the plant or animal in the form of high molecular weight, hydrolyzable compounds such as starch or glycogen.

**car·bo·hy·dra·tu·ria** (kahr"bo-hi"drət-u're-ə) excess of carbohydrates in the urine.

**car·bo·hy·dro·gen·ic** (kahr"bo-hi"dro-jen'ik) producing carbohydrates.

**car·bo·late** (kahr'bo-lāt) 1. phenolate. 2. to charge with carbolic acid.

**car·bol·fuch·sin** (kahr"bol-fūk'sin) see under *stain,* and *solution.*

**car·bol·ic ac·id** (kahr-bol'ik) trivial name for *phenol* (def. 1).

**car·bol·ism** (kahr'bol-iz-əm) phenol poisoning.

**car·bol·ize** (kahr'bəl-īz) to treat with phenol.

**car·bol·uria** (kahr"bol-u're-ə) [*carbolic* acid + *-uria*] the presence of phenol in the urine.

**car·bol·xy·lene** (kahr"bol-zi'lēn) a mixture of 1 part carbolic acid and 3 parts xylene, used for clearing microscopical sections.

**car·bo·mer** (kahr'bo-mər) a polymer of acrylic acid, cross-linked with a polyfunctional agent; used as an emulsifying agent and as a suspending agent in pharmaceutical preparations.

**car·bon** (kahr'bon) [*carbo*] [MeSH: Carbon] 1. a nonmetallic tetrad element, found nearly pure in the diamond, and approximately pure in charcoal, graphite, and anthracite; symbol C; atomic number, 6; atomic weight, 12.011. The two naturally occurring, stable isotopes are $^{12}C$ (98.89 per cent) and $^{13}C$ (1.11 per cent). 2. an electrode made of carbon shell in which medicaments may be enclosed.
**c. 11,** a radioactive isotope of carbon, atomic mass 11, having a half-life of 20.39 minutes; it decays by positron emission, with energy of 0.961 MeV, and is used as a tracer in positron emission tomography.
**c. 14,** a radioactive isotope of carbon, atomic mass 14, having a half-life of 5730 years; it decays by beta emission, with energy of 0.156 MeV, and is used as a tracer in cancer and metabolic research.
**c. dioxide,** 1. an odorless, colorless gas, $CO_2$, resulting from the oxidation of carbon. It is formed in the tissues and eliminated by the lungs. $CO_2$ and the carbonates assist in maintaining the neutrality of the tissues and fluids of the body. Solid carbon dioxide *(Dry Ice* or *carbon dioxide snow)* has been used as an escharotic to destroy certain skin lesions. 2. [USP] a preparation of not less than 99 per cent carbon dioxide by volume, used for inhalation to stimulate respiration.
**c. disulfide,** a colorless, flammable, poisonous liquid, $CS_2$, used as a solvent, as a fruit preservative, and for numerous other industrial purposes. Excessive inhalation of its fumes causes carbon disulfide poisoning (q.v.).
**c. monoxide,** a colorless poisonous gas, CO, formed by burning car-

bon or organic fuels with a scanty supply of oxygen; it causes asphyxiation by combining irreversibly with the blood hemoglobin. See also *carbon monoxide poisoning,* under *poisoning.*
**c. monoxide C 11** [USP], carbon monoxide in which a portion of the molecules are labeled with [11]C; used to label erythrocytes for measurement of blood volume.
**c. oxysulfide,** a colorless gas, COS, uniting with air to form an explosive mixture.
**c. tetrachloride,** a clear, colorless, volatile liquid, $CCl_4$, used as a solvent in pharmaceutical preparations. Inhalation of its vapors can depress central nervous system activity and cause degeneration of the liver and kidneys. Called also *perchlormethane* and *tetrachlormethane.*

**car·bon·ate** (kahr′bə-nāt) any salt of carbonic acid.

**car·bon·ate de·hy·dra·tase** (kahr′bə-nāt de-hi′drə-tās) [EC 4.2.1.1] [MeSH: Carbonate Dehydratase] an enzyme of the lyase class that catalyzes the equilibration of dissolved carbon dioxide and carbonic acid, speeding the movement of carbon dioxide from tissues to blood to alveolar air. It is a zinc protein found in kidney tubule cells and red blood cells. Called also *carbonic anhydrase.*

**car·bon·ic ac·id** (kahr-bon′ik) [MeSH: Carbonic Acid] the chemical species $H_2CO_3$, which exists in chemical equilibrium with dissolved carbon dioxide in water; its dissociated forms are the bicarbonate ($HCO_3^-$) and carbonate ($CO_3^{2-}$) ions. In the blood the predominant species are $HCO_3$ and dissolved $CO_2$ in approximately a 20:1 ratio. The conversion of $CO_2$ to $H_2CO_3$ is catalyzed by the enzyme carbonic anhydrase.

**car·bon·ic an·hy·drase** (kahr-bon′ik an-hi′drās) carbonate dehydratase.

**car·bon·ize** (kahr′bon-īz) to char or to convert into charcoal.

**car·bon·uria** (kahr″bə-nu′re-ə) [*carbon* + *-uria*] the presence of carbon dioxide or other carbon compounds in the urine.

**car·bon·yl** (kahr′bə-nəl) [*carbon* + Gr. *hylē* matter] the divalent group C═O, occurring in compounds such as aldehydes, ketones, carboxylic acids, and esters.

**car·bo·pla·tin** (kahr′bo-plat″in) [USP] [MeSH: Carboplatin] a platinum coordination compound having the same mechanism of action as cisplatin, although its rate of action is slower and its spectrum of toxicity is different. Used in the treatment of ovarian carcinoma refractory to standard chemotherapy or in patients who cannot be safely treated with cisplatin; also used experimentally in the treatment of small and non–small cell lung carcinoma, head and neck carcinoma, testicular carcinoma, and seminoma. Administered intravenously.

**car·bo·prost** (kar′bo-prost) [MeSH: Carboprost] a synthetic 15-methyl analogue of dinoprost, a prostaglandin of the F type; it has been used as an oxytocic for termination of pregnancy and missed abortion, administered intramuscularly.
**c. methyl,** the methyl ester of carboprost, having the same actions and similar uses as the base; administered in vaginal suppositories or in an intravaginal device.
**c. tromethamine,** an oxytocic compound of carboprost and 2-amino-2-(hydroxymethyl)-1,3-propanediol (1:1).

**Car·bo·run·dum** (kahr″bo-run′dəm) trademark for a preparation of silicon carbide.

**Car·bo·wax** (kar′bo-waks) trademark for a series of polyethylene glycols; used in compounding water-soluble ointment vehicles.

**γ-car·boxy·glu·ta·mate** (kahr-bok″se-gloo′tə-māt) a salt or dissociated form of γ-carboxyglutamic acid.

**γ-car·boxy·glu·ta·mic ac·id** (kahr-bok″se-gloo-tam′ik) an amino acid occurring in biologically active prothrombin and in noncollagen bone proteins; it is formed in the liver in the presence of vitamin K by carboxylation of glutamic acid residues.

**car·boxy·he·mo·glo·bin** (kahr-bok″se-he′mo-glo″bin) [MeSH: Carboxyhemoglobin] hemoglobin in which the sites usually bound to oxygen are bound to carbon monoxide, which has an affinity for hemoglobin over 200 times that of oxygen. See *carbon monoxide poisoning,* under *poisoning.*

**car·box·y·he·mo·glo·bin·e·mia** (kahr-bok″se-he″mo-glo″bin-e′me-ə) the presence of carboxyhemoglobin in the blood; see *carbon monoxide poisoning,* under *poisoning.*

**car·box·yl** (kahr-bok′səl) the monovalent radical, —COOH, occurring in those organic acids termed carboxylic acids.

**car·box·y·lase** (kahr-bok′sə-lās) an enzyme that catalyzes the addition of a molecule of carbon dioxide to another compound to form a carboxyl group. The carboxylases include some carboxy-lyases [EC 4.1.1] and those ligases, usually biotinyl-proteins, that cleave ATP to drive the reaction [EC 6.4.1].
**amino acid c.,** an enzyme in many bacteria that catalyzes the removal of $CO_2$ from amino acids, thus producing amines.
**multiple c. deficiency,** an inherited aminoacidopathy correctable by biotin therapy and due to deficiency of either holocarboxylase synthetase or biotinidase, which causes deficiency of activity of the biotin-containing carboxylases (acetyl-CoA carboxylase, methylcrotonoyl-CoA carboxylase, propionyl-CoA carboxylase, and pyruvate carboxylase); it is characterized by metabolic ketoacidosis, organic aciduria, hyperammonemia, and variable manifestation of breathing difficulties, hypotonia, seizures, ataxia, alopecia, skin rash, and developmental delay. Urine contains organic acids characteristic of each individual carboxylase deficiency, particularly 3-hydroxyisovaleric acid. The *neonatal* form, due to deficiency of holocarboxylase synthetase, is apparently an autosomal recessive trait, often of earlier onset, and may progress rapidly to coma; the *juvenile* form, due to deficiency of biotinidase, is an autosomal recessive trait and is characterized additionally by sensorineural deafness and optic atrophy. See also the individual enzymes and *propionicacidemia.*

**car·box·y·late** (kahr-bok′sə-lāt) any salt, ester, or conjugate base of a carboxylic acid.

**car·box·y·la·tion** (kahr-bok″sə-la′shən) the addition of a carboxyl group, as to pyruvate to form oxaloacetate.

**car·box·yl·es·ter·ase** (kahr-bok″səl-es′tər-ās) [EC 3.1.1.1] an enzyme of the hydrolase class that catalyzes the cleavage of the ester bond in a carboxylic ester to form an alcohol and a carboxylic acid. It has a wide specificity, usually acting on short-chain acids linked to monohydric alcohols, and also hydrolyzes esters of vitamin A.

**car·box·yl·trans·fer·ase** (kahr-bok″səl-trans′fər-ās) a term used in the names of some of the enzymes of the sub-subclass carbamoyltransferases and carboxyltransferases [EC 2.1.3] to denote those that catalyze the transfer of a carboxyl group from a donor compound to an acceptor compound. Called also *transcarboxylase.*

**car·box·y·ly·ase** (kahr-bok′se-li′ās) [EC 4.1.1] any member of a sub-subclass of enzymes of the lyase class that catalyze the nonhydrolytic addition or removal of a carboxyl group to or from a compound; it includes the carboxylases and decarboxylases.

**car·boxy·meth·yl·cel·lu·lose so·di·um** (kahr-bok″se-meth″əl-sel′u-lōs) [USP] the sodium salt of a polycarboxymethyl ether of cellulose; used as a suspending agent, tablet excipient, and viscosity-increasing agent in pharmaceutical preparations, and administered orally as a cathartic.

**car·boxy·myo·glo·bin** (kahr-bok″se-mi″o-glo′bin) a compound formed from myoglobin on exposure to carbon monoxide, with formation of a covalent bond with oxygen and without change of the charge of the ferrous state.

**car·boxy·pep·ti·dase** (kahr-bok″se-pep′tĭ-dās) [EC 3.4.15–18] any exopeptidase that catalyzes the hydrolytic cleavage of the terminal or penultimate peptide bond at the C-terminal end of a peptide or polypeptide.

**car·boxy·pep·ti·dase A** (kahr-bok″se-pep′tĭ-dās) [EC 3.4.17.1] an enzyme of the hydrolase class that catalyzes the cleavage from aminopolypeptides of C-terminal acid residues other than arginine, lysine, or proline. It is a zinc metalloenzyme found in pancreatic juice.

**car·boxy·pep·ti·dase B** (kahr-bok″se-pep′tĭ-dās) [EC 3.4.17.2] an enzyme of the hydrolase class that catalyzes the cleavage of C-terminal arginine or lysine residues from polypeptides. It is a zinc metalloenzyme found in pancreatic juice.
**lysosomal c. B,** cysteine-type carboxypeptidase, def. 2.

**car·bro·mal** (kahr-bro′məl) a sedative with weak hypnotic activity, administered orally.

**car·bun·cle** (kahr′bəng-kəl) [L. *carbunculus* little coal] [MeSH: Carbuncle] a necrotizing infection of skin and subcutaneous tissue composed of a cluster of boils (furuncles), usually due to *Staphylococcus aureus,* with multiple formed or incipient drainage sinuses.
**malignant c.,** see *cutaneous anthrax,* under *anthrax.*
**renal c.,** a massive localized parenchymal suppuration consequent to bacterial metastasis, following localized vascular thrombosis or infarction of the kidney.

**car·bun·cu·lar** (kahr-bung′ku-lər) resembling or of the nature of a carbuncle.

**car·bun·cu·loid** (kahr-bung′ku-loid) resembling a carbuncle.

**car·bun·cu·lo·sis** (kahr-bung″ku-lo′sis) a condition marked by the development of carbuncles.

**car·bu·ta·mide** (kahr-bu′tə-mīd) [MeSH: Carbutamide] a sulfonylurea compound used as a hypoglycemic in the treatment of type 2 diabetes mellitus; administered orally.

**car·bu·ter·ol hy·dro·chlo·ride** (kahr-bu′tər-ol) an adrenergic, which has been used as a bronchodilator, administered by inhalation.

**car·cass** (kahr′kəs) [Fr. *carcasse*] a dead body; generally applied to other than a human body.

**Car·cas·sonne's ligament, perineal ligament** (kahr-kah-sunz′)

[Bernard Gauderic *Carcassonne,* French surgeon, 18th century] see *ligamentum puboprostaticum* and *ligamentum transversum perinei.*

**car•cin•emia** (kahr″sin-e′me-ə) [*carcin-* + *-emia*] canceremia.

**carcin(o)-** [Gk. *karkinos* a crab] a combining form meaning relationship to carcinoma.

**car•ci•no•cy•the•mia** (kahr″sĭ-no″si-the′me-ə) canceremia.

**car•ci•no•em•bry•on•ic** (kahr″sĭ-no-em″bre-on′ik) [*carcino-* + *embryonic*] occurring both in carcinoma and in embryonic tissue; see under *antigen.*

**car•cin•o•gen** (kahr-sin′ə-jen) any cancer-producing substance; often a distinction is made between *epigenetic* and *genotoxic carcinogens.*

**epigenetic c.,** an agent that does not itself damage DNA but causes alterations such as hormonal derangements, immunosuppression, or chronic tissue injury that in turn predispose to cancer.

**genotoxic c.,** a carcinogen that reacts directly with DNA or with macromolecules that then react with DNA.

**car•ci•no•gen•e•sis** (kahr″sĭ-no-jen′ə-sis) [*carcino-* + *-genesis*] the production of carcinoma.

**car•cin•o•gen•ic** (kahr″sin-o-jen′ik) 1. producing carcinoma; cf. *cancerigenic.* 2. pertaining to a carcinogen.

**car•ci•no•ge•nic•i•ty** (kahr″sĭ-no-jə-nis′ĭ-te) the ability or tendency to produce carcinoma; the quality of being carcinogenic.

**car•ci•noid** (kahr′sĭ-noid) a yellow circumscribed tumor arising from enterochromaffin cells, usually in the small intestine, appendix, stomach, or colon and less commonly in the bronchus. The term is sometimes used alone to refer to the gastrointestinal tumor (called also *argentaffinoma*). See also *carcinoid tumor of bronchus* and *carcinoid syndrome.* Called also *carcinoid tumor.*

**bronchial c., c. of bronchus,** carcinoid tumor of bronchus; see under *tumor.*

**car•ci•nol•y•sin** (kahr″si-nol′ə-sin) [*carcino-* + *lysin*] a ferment derived from a Chinese variety of pine called "haisung." It has been given subcutaneously or intramuscularly for cancer.

**car•ci•nol•y•sis** (kahr″sĭ-nol′ə-sis) destruction of carcinoma cells, as by perfusion of an antineoplastic agent through the vessels of the body segment in which the growth occurs.

**car•ci•no•lyt•ic** (kahr-sĭ-no-lit′ik) [*carcino-* + *-lytic*] pertaining to, characterized by, or causing carcinolysis.

**car•ci•no•ma** (kahr″sĭ-no′mə) pl. *carcinomas* or *carcino′mata* [Gr. *karkinōma* from *karkinos* crab, cancer] [MeSH: Carcinoma] a malignant new growth made up of epithelial cells tending to infiltrate the surrounding tissues and give rise to metastases.

## Carcinoma

**acinar c., acinic cell c., acinous c.,** a slow-growing malignant tumor characterized by acinic cells arranged in small glandlike structures, usually occurring in the pancreas or salivary glands, particularly in females. Called also *acinar, acinic cell,* or *acinous adenocarcinoma* and *acinar cell* or *acinic cell tumor.*

**adenocystic c.,** adenoid cystic c.

**adenoid cystic c.,** carcinoma characterized by bands or cylinders of hyalinized or mucinous stroma separating or surrounded by nests or cords of small epithelial cells. It appears as one or more of three patterns: cribriform, solid, and tubular. The usual site is the salivary glands, but histologically similar tumors appear elsewhere. Malignant and invasive but slow growing, it spreads by infiltrating the bloodstream and perineural spaces. Called also *adenocystic c., cribriform c.,* and *cylindroma.* NOTE: Certain unrelated tumors may have a cylindromatous or adenoid cystic pattern, e.g., ameloblastoma.

**adenoid squamous cell c.,** adenoacanthoma.

**c. adenomato′sum,** adenocarcinoma.

**adenosquamous c.,** 1. adenoacanthoma. 2. a diverse category of bronchogenic carcinoma with areas of glandular, squamous, and large-cell differentiation; in some cases inclusion of a tumor in this category rather than in one of the more specific categories of bronchogenic carcinoma has been questioned.

**adnexal c.,** carcinoma arising from, or forming structures resembling, the cutaneous appendages, particularly the sweat or sebaceous glands.

**c. of adrenal cortex, adrenocortical c.,** a malignant adrenal cortical tumor that can cause endocrine disorders such as Cushing's syndrome or adrenogenital syndrome.

**aldosterone-producing c., aldosterone-secreting c.,** a rare malignant form of aldosteronoma; it is larger than an aldosterone-producing adenoma.

**alveolar c., alveolar cell c.,** bronchioloalveolar c.

**ameloblastic c.,** a type of ameloblastoma in which malignant epithelial transformation has occurred; the metastatic lesions do not resemble the primary tumor histologically, instead usually resembling squamous cell carcinoma. Cf. *malignant ameloblastoma.*

**ampullary c.,** a subset of periampullary carcinoma that comprises tumors arising in the immediate vicinity of the sphincter of Oddi.

**anaplastic c. of thyroid gland,** a type of thyroid gland carcinoma with atypical cells of various types and patterns; it may be silent for years but then become highly malignant and locally invasive. It affects mainly the elderly and somewhat more women than men. Called also *anaplastic thyroid c.* and *undifferentiated c. of thyroid gland.*

**apocrine c.,** 1. carcinoma of an apocrine gland. 2. a rare breast malignancy with a ductal or acinar growth pattern and apocrine secretions.

**basal cell c.,** the most common form of skin cancer, consisting of an epithelial tumor of the skin originating from neoplastic differentiation of basal cells, rarely metastatic but locally invasive and aggressive; it usually occurs as one or several small, pearly nodules or plaques with central depressions on the face of an older adult, particularly on a sun-exposed area of persons with fair skin. It has been divided into numerous and variable subtypes on the basis of clinical and histological characteristics; the more constant subtypes include *nodulo-ulcerative, morphea-like, cystic,* and *superficial.*

**basal cell c., alveolar,** cystic basal cell c.

**basal cell c., comedo,** a form in which the cores of the basal cell masses are necrotic.

**basal cell c., cystic,** an uncommon subtype occurring as a cystic lesion formed by central degeneration, characterized histologically by edematous stroma rimmed by neoplastic cells.

**basal cell c., morphea-like,** a form usually occurring on the face or neck as scar-like, telangiectatic, ivory lesions with poorly defined borders, characterized histologically by strands of basal cells surrounded by dense hyalinized stroma, and usually spreading laterally.

**basal cell c., multicentric,** superficial basal cell c.

**basal cell c., nodulo-ulcerative,** the most common form of basal cell carcinoma, usually occurring on the face as one or several small, waxy, translucent nodules with rolled edges around a central depression, which may be ulcerated, crusted, or bleeding. It may spread laterally or invade deeply.

**basal cell c., pigmented,** a form in which the lesions contain brown or black pigment; it is frequently associated with long term ingestion of arsenic. It grows slowly and occurs more often in darker complexioned individuals.

**basal cell c., sclerosing,** morphea-like basal cell c.

**basal cell c., superficial,** a form usually occurring on the trunk as one or several superficial, slowly spreading, erythematous, scaly plaques with thread-like raised borders; it is frequently associated with long-term exposure to arsenic.

**basaloid c.,** 1. a nonspecific term used to refer to any of numerous carcinomas that resemble basal cell carcinoma. 2. a rare transitional cell carcinoma of the anus, resembling basal cell carcinoma of the skin. Called also *cloacogenic anal c.*

**basosquamous cell c.,** carcinoma that histologically exhibits both basal and squamous elements.

**bile duct c.,** 1. cholangiocarcinoma. 2. cholangiocellular c.

**bile duct c., extrahepatic,** cholangiocellular c.

**bile duct c., intrahepatic,** cholangiocarcinoma (def. 1).

**bilharzial c.,** schistosomal bladder c.

**bronchioalveolar c., bronchiolar c., bronchioloalveolar c.,** a variant type of adenocarcinoma of the lung, with columnar to cuboidal epithelial cells lining the alveolar septa and projecting into alveolar spaces in branching papillary formations. Called also *alveolar c.* or *adenocarcinoma, alveolar cell c.* or *tumor, bronchiolar c.* or *adenocarcinoma, bronchoalveolar c.* or *adenocarcinoma,* and *bronchioalveolar adenocarcinoma.*

**bronchoalveolar c., bronchoalveolar cell c.,** bronchioloalveolar c.

**bronchogenic c.,** any of a large group of carcinomas of the lung, so called because they arise from the epithelium of the bronchial tree. Four primary subtypes are distinguished: *adenocarcinoma of the lung, large cell carcinoma, small cell carcinoma,* and *squamous cell carcinoma.*

**cerebriform c.,** medullary c.

**cholangiocellular c.,** a rare hepatocellular carcinoma arising from the cholangioles, composed of tumor cells resembling the epithelial cells of the cholangioles arranged in cords consisting of two layers of cells surrounding a minute lumen. Called also *bile duct c., extrahepatic bile duct c.,* and *cholangiocarcinoma.*

**chorionic c.,** choriocarcinoma.

**choroid plexus c.,** an aggressive anaplastic tumor representing malignant transformation of a choroid plexus papilloma.

**clear cell c.,** 1. see under *adenocarcinoma.* 2. renal cell c.

**cloacogenic anal c.,** basaloid c. (def. 2).

**colloid c.,** mucinous c.

**comedo c.,** comedocarcinoma.

**corpus c., c. of corpus uteri,** uterine corpus c.

**cortisol-producing c.,** a type of carcinoma of the adrenal cortex that secretes cortisol, causing Cushing's syndrome.

**cribriform c.,** 1. adenoid cystic c. 2. an adenoid cystic carcinoma of the lactiferous ducts, one of the subtypes of ductal carcinoma in situ; many tumors have combined cribriform and micropapillary patterns.

**cylindrical c., cylindrical cell c.,** carcinoma in which the cells are cylindrical or nearly so.

**duct c., ductal c.,** carcinoma of a duct, such as of the pancreas or breast; see also *ductal c. in situ.*

**ductal c. of the prostate,** see under *adenocarcinoma.*

**ductal c. in situ (DCIS),** any of a large group of in situ carcinomas of the lactiferous ducts; subtypes distinguished by histology include comedocarcinoma, cribriform carcinoma, and micropapillary carcinoma, but many tumors include areas of more than one type. Called also *intraductal c.*

**eccrine c.,** carcinoma of the eccrine sweat glands.

**embryonal c.,** a highly malignant germ cell tumor that is a primitive form of carcinoma, probably of primitive embryonal cell derivation; it may be found either in pure form or as part of a mixed germ cell tumor and has a histological appearance similar to that of a yolk sac tumor. In females, there is a median age of 15; in males the majority of patients are adolescents or older.

**c. en cuirasse,** carcinoma of the skin manifest as thickening and induration over large areas of the thorax, frequently as a result of metastasis from a primary breast lesion. Called also *cancer en cuirasse.*

**endometrial c., c. of endometrium,** carcinoma of the endometrium of the corpus uteri, one of the most common gynecological cancers, mainly affecting postmenopausal women; a common symptom is abnormal vaginal bleeding. It includes types ranging in malignancy from locally invasive to metastasizing.

**endometrioid c.,** carcinoma characterized by glandular patterns that resemble those of the endometrium, occurring in the uterine fundus and in the ovaries; see also under *adenocarcinoma.*

**epidermoid c.,** squamous cell c.

**c. ex mixed tumor,** c. ex pleomorphic adenoma.

**c. ex pleomorphic adenoma,** a type of malignant pleomorphic adenoma that usually occurs in the salivary glands of older adults; an epithelial malignancy arises in a preexisting mixed tumor, with metastasis only of the malignant epithelial component. The term is sometimes used synonymously with *malignant mixed tumor.*

**exophytic c.,** a malignant epithelial neoplasm with marked outward growth like a wart or papilloma.

**fibrolamellar c.,** a rare variant of hepatocellular carcinoma in which there is a solitary mass, no evidence of cirrhosis, and no male predominance. It is characterized histologically by eosinophilic polygonal hepatocytes that contain swollen mitochondria, cytoplasmic bodies, and hyaline bodies and have prominent nucleoli; the cells are surrounded by a stroma of thin parallel collagen bands. Called also *fibrolamellar hepatoma.*

**c. fibro'sum,** scirrhous c.

**follicular c. of thyroid gland,** a type of thyroid gland carcinoma with many follicles, although it may have areas without follicles; it is more common in women and is more malignant than papillary carcinoma of thyroid gland. Called also *follicular thyroid carcinoma.*

**gastric c.,** see under *adenocarcinoma.*

**gelatiniform c., gelatinous c.,** mucinous c.

**giant cell c.,** a poorly differentiated, highly malignant, epithelial neoplasm containing numerous very large, multinucleated tumor cells, such as occurs in the lungs.

**giant cell c. of thyroid gland,** a type of anaplastic carcinoma of the thyroid gland, containing numerous giant cells, some with multiple nuclei.

**c. gigantocellula're,** giant cell c.

**glandular c.,** adenocarcinoma.

**granulosa cell c.,** a granulosa cell tumor that has undergone malignant transformation.

**hepatocellular c.,** primary carcinoma of the liver cells; symptoms include hepatomegaly, abdominal pain, weight loss, jaundice, hemoperitoneum, and other symptoms of the presence of an abdominal mass. It is rare in North America and Western Europe but is one of the most common malignancies in parts of sub-Saharan Africa, Southeast Asia, East Asia, and elsewhere. A strong association seems to exist with chronic hepatitis B virus infection, and definite but less strong associations with some types of cirrhosis and hepatitis C virus infection. Called also *hepatoma, malignant hepatoma,* and *hepatocarcinoma.*

**Hürthle cell c.,** a malignant Hürthle cell tumor.

**hypernephroid c.,** renal cell c.

**infantile embryonal c.,** yolk sac tumor.

**inflammatory c. of the breast,** a highly malignant carcinoma of the breast, presenting with pink to red skin discoloration, tenderness, edema, and rapid enlargement of the breast; it usually invades dermal lymphatic vessels.

**c. in si'tu,** a neoplastic entity wherein the tumor cells are confined to the epithelium of origin, without invasion of the basement membrane; the likelihood of subsequent invasive growth is presumed to be high. See also *ductal c. in situ* and *lobular c. in situ.* Called also *cancer in situ* and *preinvasive c.*

**intraductal c.,** 1. any carcinoma of the epithelium of a duct. 2. ductal c. in situ.

**intraepidermal c.,** carcinoma confined within the epidermis, the basal layer of the epidermis not being penetrated by the proliferating cells, e.g., Bowen's disease.

**intraepithelial c.,** c. in situ.

**juvenile embryonal c.,** yolk sac tumor.

**Kulchitzky cell c.,** carcinoid tumor of the small or large intestine.

**large cell c.,** a bronchogenic tumor of undifferentiated (anaplastic) cells of large size; it may be a variety of squamous cell carcinoma of the lung that has undergone further dedifferentiation.

**leptomeningeal c.,** meningeal c.

**lobular c.,** 1. terminal duct c. 2. see *lobular c. in situ.*

**lobular c., infiltrating,** invasive lobular c.

**lobular c., invasive,** an invasive type of carcinoma of the breast characterized by linear growth into desmoplastic stroma around the terminal part of the lobules of mammary glands; most cases develop from lobular carcinoma in situ. Called also *infiltrating lobular c.*

**lobular c. in situ (LCIS),** a type of precancerous neoplasia found in the lobules of mammary glands, usually small and widely dispersed so that it is not palpable physically and is identified only on microscopic examination. It progresses slowly, sometimes developing into invasive lobular carcinoma 10 to 15 years after first being observed. Called also *lobular neoplasia.*

**lymphoepithelial c.,** lymphoepithelioma.

**c. medulla're, medullary c.,** carcinoma composed mainly of epithelial elements with little or no stroma; sites where this is commonly found are the breast and thyroid gland. Called also *encephaloid, medullary,* or *soft cancer; cerebriform cancer* or *carcinoma; c. molle;* and *c. spongiosum.*

**medullary c. of thyroid gland, medullary thyroid c.,** a type of thyroid gland carcinoma that contains amyloid deposits and parafollicular cells and secretes calcitonin. It occurs in both an autosomal dominant form as a component of multiple endocrine neoplasia, types II and III, and in a nonfamilial form. Called also *medullary thyroid c.*

**melanotic c.,** malignant melanoma.

**meningeal c.,** carcinomatous infiltration of the meninges, particularly the pia and arachnoid; it may be primary or secondary, especially metastatic from small-cell lung carcinoma or breast cancer. Called also *leptomeningeal c.* and *leptomeningeal* or *meningeal carcinomatosis.*

**Merkel cell c.,** a rapidly growing malignant dermal or subcutaneous tumor occurring on sun-exposed areas in middle-aged or older adults and containing irregular anastomosing trabeculae and small dense granules typical of Merkel cells; whether these are the cells of origin is still under debate. Called also *neuroendocrine* or *trabecular c. of the skin* and *Merkel cell tumor.*

**metatypical cell c.,** basosquamous c.

**micropapillary c.,** a type of ductal carcinoma in situ characterized by a regular pattern of small bulbous papillae; many tumors have combined micropapillary and cribriform patterns.

**c. mol'le,** medullary c.

**mucinous c.,** an adenocarcinoma that produces mucin in significant amounts. Called also *colloid cancer* or *c., gelatinous c., mucinous adenocarcinoma, c. mucosum,* and *mucous c.*

**c. muci'parum,** mucinous c.

**c. mucocellula're,** Krukenberg's tumor.

**mucoepidermoid c.,** a malignant epithelial tumor of glandular tissue, especially the salivary glands, characterized by acini with mucus-producing cells and by the presence of malignant squamous elements; it may occur as a low, intermediate, or high grade malignancy.

**c. muco'sum, mucous c.,** mucinous c.

**nasopharyngeal c.,** a malignant tumor arising in the epithelial lining of the space behind the nose (the nasopharynx) and occurring with a high frequency in people of Chinese ancestry. The Epstein-Barr virus has been implicated as a causative agent.

**neuroendocrine c. of the skin,** Merkel cell c.

**noninfiltrating c.,** c. in situ.

**non–small cell c., non–small cell lung c. (NSCLC),** a general term comprising all lung carcinomas except small cell carcinoma, and including adenocarcinoma of the lung, large cell carcinoma, and squamous cell carcinoma. Called also *non–small cell lung cancer.*
**oat cell c.,** a form of small cell carcinoma in which the cells are round or elongated and slightly larger than lymphocytes; they have scanty cytoplasm and clump poorly.
**c. ossi'ficans, osteoid c.,** carcinoma in which there is osteoid or osseous metaplasia of the stroma.
**Paget's c.,** Paget's disease (def. 1).
**papillary c.,** carcinoma in which there are papillary excrescences.
**papillary c. of thyroid gland,** the most common thyroid gland carcinoma, often occurring before age 40 and much more common in women than in men. It usually has both papillary and follicular elements, grows slowly, and may remain localized for years. Called also *papillary thyroid c.*
**periampullary c.,** carcinoma arising in the immediate vicinity of the ampulla of Vater.
**preinvasive c.,** c. in situ.
**prickle cell c.,** squamous cell c.
**primary intraosseous c.,** a rare epithelial odontogenic malignancy occurring in the mandible and maxilla, particularly of male adults, and believed to arise from odontogenic epithelial remnants.
**renal cell c.,** carcinoma of the renal parenchyma usually occurring in middle age or later and composed of tubular cells in varying arrangements; symptoms depend on extent of invasion. Called also *adenocarcinoma of kidney, renal adenocarcinoma, hypernephroid c., clear cell c., hypernephroma,* and *Grawitz's tumor.*
**scar c.,** carcinoma associated with scarring, usually an adenocarcinoma of the lung; the scar may either precede the carcinoma or be a fibrotic response to it. Called also *scar cancer.*
**schistosomal bladder c.,** carcinoma of the wall of the urinary bladder, usually a squamous cell carcinoma, caused by chronic infection and irritation by *Schistosoma haematobium;* called also *bilharzial c.* and *schistosomal bladder cancer.*
**schneiderian c.,** a neoplasm of the mucosa of the nose and the paranasal sinuses.
**scirrhous c.,** carcinoma with a hard structure owing to the formation of dense connective tissue in the stroma. Called also *fibrocarcinoma, carcinoma fibrosum,* and *scirrhous cancer.*
**sebaceous c.,** carcinoma of the sebaceous glands, usually occurring as a slow-growing hard yellow nodule on the eyelid.
**signet-ring cell c.,** a highly malignant, mucus-secreting tumor in which the mucus-secreting cells are anaplastic and appear rounded, with the nucleus displaced to one side by a globule of mucus in the cytoplasm.
**c. sim'plex,** an undifferentiated carcinoma.
**small cell c., small cell lung c. (SCLC),** a common, highly malignant form of bronchogenic carcinoma in the wall of a major bronchus, occurring mainly in middle-aged individuals with a history of tobacco smoking; it is radiosensitive and has small oval undifferentiated cells that are intensely hematoxyphilic. Metastasis to the hilum and to mediastinal lymph nodes is common. Called also *small cell lung cancer.*
**spindle cell c.,** carcinoma, usually of the squamous cell type, marked by fusiform development of rapidly proliferating cells.
**c. spongio'sum,** medullary c.
**squamous c., squamous cell c.,** 1. carcinoma developed from squamous epithelium, having cuboid cells and characterized by keratinization and often by preservation of intercellular bridges. Initially local and superficial, the lesion may later invade and metastasize. 2. the form occurring in the skin, usually originating in sun-damaged areas or preexisting lesions. 3. in the lung, one of the most common types of bronchogenic carcinoma, generally forming polypoid or sessile masses that obstruct the airways of the bronchi. It usually occurs in middle-aged individuals with a history of smoking. There is frequent invasion of blood and lymphatic vessels with metastasis to regional lymph nodes and other sites. Called also *epidermoid c.* and *prickle cell c.*
**terminal duct c.,** a slow-growing, locally invasive malignant neoplasm composed of myoepithelial and ductal elements, occurring in the minor salivary glands, particularly in the palate.
**thyroid c., anaplastic,** anaplastic c. of thyroid gland.
**thyroid c., follicular,** follicular c. of thyroid gland.
**thyroid c., medullary,** medullary c. of thyroid gland.
**thyroid c., papillary,** papillary c. of thyroid gland.
**trabecular c. of the skin,** Merkel cell c.
**transitional cell c.,** a malignant tumor arising from a transitional type of stratified epithelium, usually affecting the urinary bladder.
**tubular c.,** 1. an adenocarcinoma in which the cells are arranged in the form of tubules; called also *tubular cancer.* 2. a type of breast cancer in which small glandlike structures are formed and infiltrate the stroma; it usually develops from an earlier ductal carcinoma in situ and is rarely metastatic.
**undifferentiated c. of thyroid gland,** anaplastic c. of thyroid gland.
**uterine corpus c.,** carcinoma of the corpus uteri, usually endometrial carcinoma, one of the most common gynecological cancers; it ranges in malignancy from locally invasive to metastatic. Called also *corpus c.*
**verrucous c.,** 1. a variety of squamous cell carcinoma that has a predilection for the buccal mucosa but also affects other oral soft tissue and the larynx. It is a slow-growing, somewhat invasive, exophytic neoplasm, either papillary or verrucous in appearance. 2. Buschke-Löwenstein tumor, so called because it is histologically similar to the oral lesion.
**villous c., c. villo'sum,** carcinoma in which the cells are arranged in a villous pattern, as papillary projections which are covered with neoplastic epithelium; usually seen in the gastrointestinal tract.
**yolk sac c.,** see under *tumor.*

**car·ci·no·ma·ta** (kahr″sĭ-no'mə-tə) plural of *carcinoma.*

**car·ci·nom·a·toid** (kahr″sĭ-nom'ə-toid) resembling carcinoma.

**car·ci·no·ma·to·pho·bia** (kahr″sĭ-no″mə-to-fo'be-ə) cancerphobia.

**car·ci·no·ma·to·sis** (kahr″sĭ-no-mə-to'sis) the condition of widespread dissemination of cancer throughout the body; called also *carcinosis.*
**leptomeningeal c.,** meningeal carcinoma.
**meningeal c.,** see under *carcinoma.*

**car·ci·nom·a·tous** (kahr″sĭ-nom'ə-təs) pertaining to or of the nature of cancer; cf. *malignant.*

**car·ci·no·pho·bia** (kahr″sĭ-no-fo'be-ə) [*carcino-* + *phobia*] cancerphobia.

**car·ci·no·sar·co·ma** (kahr″sĭ-no-sahr-ko'mə) [*carcino-* + *sarcoma*] [MeSH: Carcinosarcoma] a malignant tumor composed of carcinomatous and sarcomatous tissues.
**embryonal c.,** Wilms' tumor.

**car·ci·no·stat·ic** (kahr″sĭ-no-stat'ik) tending to check the growth of carcinoma.

**car·da·mom** (kahr'də-məm) [L. *cardamomum;* Gr. *kardamōmon*] 1. *Elettaria cardamomum.* 2. any of various other closely related plants that yield seeds similar to those of *E. cardamomum.* 3. the dried ripe seeds of *E. cardamomum* or related plants, used as a flavoring agent and formerly as a carminative; see also *cardamom oil,* under *oil.* Called also *cardamom seed.*

**car·del·my·cin** (kahr″dəl-mi'sin) novobiocin.

**Car·den's amputation** (kahr'dənz) [Henry Douglas *Carden,* English surgeon, died 1872] see under *amputation.*

**Car·dene** (kahr'dēn) trademark for a preparation of nicardipine hydrochloride.

**car·dia** (kahr'de-ə) [Gr. *kardia* heart] [TA] [MeSH: Cardia] the part of the stomach immediately adjacent to and surrounding the cardiac opening of the esophagus, distinguished only by the presence of the cardiac glands, and lacking acid (parietal) and pepsin (chief) cells. Called also *pars cardiaca gastris* [TA alternative] and *cardiac* or *cardial part of stomach.*

**car·di·ac** (kahr'de-ak) [L. *cardiacus,* from Gr. *kardiakos*] 1. pertaining to the heart. 2. a cordial, or restorative medicine. 3. a person with a heart disorder. 4. pertaining to the orifice *(ostium cardiacum)* between the esophagus and the part of the stomach immediately adjacent to and surrounding the orifice *(pars cardiaca gastris).*

**car·di·al·gia** (kahr″de-al'jə) [*cardi-*(1) + *-algia*] cardiodynia.

**car·di·ec·ta·sis** (kahr″de-ek'tə-sis) [*cardi-*(1) + *ectasis*] dilatation of the heart.

**car·di·ec·to·mized** (kahr″de-ek'tə-mīzd) having the heart removed, as a cardiectomized animal.

**car·di·ec·to·my** (kahr″de-ek'tə-me) [*cardi-*(2) + *-ectomy*] excision of the cardiac portion of the stomach.

**Car·di·late** (kahr'dĭ-lāt) trademark for a preparation of erythrityl tetranitrate.

**car·di·nal** (kahr'dĭ-nəl) [L. *cardinalis,* from *cardo* a hinge] of primary or preeminent importance.

**cardi(o)-** [Gr. *kardia* heart] a combining form denoting relationship (1) to the heart or (2) to the cardiac orifice or portion of the stomach.

**car·dio·ac·cel·er·a·tor** (kahr"de-o-ak-sel'ər-a-tər) 1. quickening the heart action. 2. an agent that accelerates the heart action.

**car·dio·ac·tive** (kahr"de-o-ak'tiv) having an effect upon the heart.

**car·dio·an·gi·og·ra·phy** (kahr"de-o-an"je-og'rə-fe) angiocardiography.

**car·dio·an·gi·ol·o·gy** (kahr"de-o-an"je-ol'ə-je) [*cardio-*(1) + *angio-* + *-logy*] the medical specialty which deals with the heart and blood vessels.

**Car·dio·bac·te·ri·um** (kahr"de-o-bak-tēr'e-əm) [*cardio-*(1) + *bacterium*] a genus of gram-negative, facultatively anaerobic, fermentative, rod-shaped bacteria, part of the normal flora of the nose and throat, and also isolated from blood.
**C. ho'minis,** a species that is part of the normal flora of the nose and pharynx, and also an etiologic agent of endocarditis.

**car·dio·cai·ro·graph** (kahr"de-o-ki'ro-graf) [*cardio-*(1) + Gr. *kairos* time + *-graph*] a technique by means of which radiographs of the heart can be made at any chosen phase of its cycle.

**car·dio·cele** (kahr'de-o-sēl") [*cardio-*(1) + *-cele*[1]] protrusion of the heart through a fissure of the diaphragm or through a wound.

**car·dio·cen·te·sis** (kahr"de-o-sən-te'sis) [*cardio-*(1) + *centesis*] surgical puncture or incision of the heart.

**car·dio·cha·la·sia** (kahr"de-o-kə-la'zhə) [*cardio-*(2) + *chalasia*] relaxation or incompetence of sphincter action of the cardiac orifice of the stomach.

**car·dio·ci·net·ic** (kahr"de-o-sĭ-net'ik) cardiokinetic.

**car·dio·cir·rho·sis** (kahr"de-o-sĭ-ro'sis) cardiac cirrhosis.

**car·dio·cyte** (kahr'de-o-sīt") [*cardio-*(1) + *-cyte*] myocyte.

**car·dio·di·la·tin** (kahr"de-o-di'lə-tin) [*cardio-*(1) + *dilation*] former name for the prohormone form of atrial natriuretic peptide.

**car·dio·di·la·tor** (kahr"de-o-di'la-tər) an instrument for dilating the pars cardiaca gastris (cardia) in cardiospasm or stricture.

**car·dio·di·o·sis** (kahr"de-o-di-o'sis) the dilatation of the cardiac end of the stomach.

**car·dio·dy·nam·ics** (kahr"de-o-di-nam'iks) [*cardio-*(1) + *dynamics*] the science of the motions and forces involved in the heart's action.

**car·di·odyn·ia** (kahr"de-o-din'e-ə) [*cardio-*(1) + *-odynia*] pain in the heart.

**car·dio·esoph·a·ge·al** (kahr"de-o-ə-sof"ə-je'əl) pertaining to the cardia of the stomach and the esophagus, as the cardioesophageal junction or sphincter.

**car·dio·gen·e·sis** (kahr"de-o-jen'ə-sis) [*cardio-*(1) + *genesis*] the development of the heart in the embryo.

**car·dio·gen·ic** (kahr"de-o-jen'ik) [*cardio-*(1) + *-genic*] 1. originating in the heart; caused by normal or abnormal function of the heart. 2. pertaining to cardiogenesis.

**Car·dio·gra·fin** (kahr"de-o-gra'fin) trademark for meglumine diatrizoate.

**car·dio·gram** (kahr'de-o-gram") [*cardio-*(1) + *-gram*] a tracing of a cardiac event made by means of the cardiograph.
**apex c.,** apexcardiogram.
**esophageal c.,** a tracing of the contractions of the left atrium made by registering the pulsations in the esophagus.
**precordial c.,** kinetocardiogram.
**vector c.,** vectorcardiogram.

**car·dio·graph** (kahr'de-o-graf") [*cardio-*(1) + -graph] an instrument designed to record some element of the heartbeat.

**car·dio·graph·ic** (kahr"de-o-graf'ik) pertaining to cardiography.

**car·di·og·ra·phy** (kahr"de-og'rə-fe) [*cardio-*(1) + *-graphy*] the technique of graphically recording some physical or functional aspects of the heart. See also *apexcardiography, cardiokymography, echocardiography, electrocardiography, kinetocardiography, phonocardiography, telecardiography, vectorcardiography,* etc.
**ultrasonic c.,** echocardiography.

**car·dio·he·pat·ic** (kahr"de-o-hə-pat'ik) pertaining to the heart and the liver.

**car·dio·hep·a·to·meg·a·ly** (kahr"de-o-hep"ə-to-meg'ə-le) enlargement of the heart and liver.

**car·di·oid** (kahr'de-oid) heartlike; resembling a heart.

**car·dio·in·hib·i·tor** (kahr"de-o-in-hib'ĭ-tər) an agent which restrains the heart's action.

**car·dio·in·hib·i·to·ry** (kahr"de-o-in-hib'ĭ-tor-e) restraining or inhibiting the movements of the heart.

**car·dio·ki·net·ic** (kahr"de-o-kĭ-net'ik) 1. stimulating the action of the heart. 2. an agent that stimulates action of the heart.

**car·dio·ky·mo·graph·ic** (kahr"de-o-ki"mo-graf'ik) pertaining to cardiokymography.

**car·dio·ky·mog·ra·phy** (kahr"de-o-ki-mog'rə-fe) the recording of the motion of the heart by means of the electrokymograph.

**car·dio·lip·in** (kahr"de-o-lip'in) [*cardio-*(1) + Gr. *lipos* fat] 1,3-diphosphatidylglycerol, a phospholipid occurring primarily in mitochondrial inner membranes and in bacterial plasma membranes. Cardiolipin is the main antigenic component of Wassermann-type antigens used in nontreponemal serologic tests for syphilis.

**Car·dio·lite** (kahr'de-o-līt") trademark for a kit for the preparation of technetium Tc 99m sestamibi.

**car·di·ol·o·gist** (kahr"de-ol'ə-jist) a physician skilled in the prevention, diagnosis, and treatment of heart disease.

**car·di·ol·o·gy** (kahr"de-ol'ə-je) [*cardio-*(1) + *-logy*] [MeSH: Cardiology] the study of the heart and its functions.
**invasive c.,** the theory and practice of diagnostic and therapeutic cardiac procedures that involve entry into the heart or central circulation, such as cardiac catheterization, coronary angioplasty, or electrophysiologic studies.

**car·di·ol·y·sis** (kahr"de-ol'ə-sis) [*cardio-*(1) + *lysis*] an operation of freeing the heart and pericardium in adhesive mediastinopericarditis; it is done by resecting the ribs and the sternum over the pericardium.

**car·dio·ma·la·cia** (kahr"di-o-mə-la'shə) [*cardio-*(1) + *malacia*] morbid softening of the muscular substance of the heart.

**car·dio·me·ga·lia** (kahr"di-o-mə-ga'le-ə) cardiomegaly.
**c. glycoge'nica diffu'sa,** glycogen storage disease, type II; see under *disease.*

**car·dio·meg·a·ly** (kahr"de-o-meg'ə-le) [*cardio-*(1) + *-megaly*] hypertrophy of the heart.

**car·dio·mel·a·no·sis** (kahr"de-o-mel"ə-no'sis) melanosis of the heart.

**car·di·om·e·ter** (kahr"de-om'ə-tər) [*cardio-*(1) + *-meter*] an instrument used in estimating the size of the heart or the force of its action.

**car·di·om·e·try** (kahr"de-om'ə-try) [*cardio-*(1) + *-metry*] the estimation of the size of the heart or the force of its action.

**car·dio·mo·til·i·ty** (kahr"de-o-mo-til'ĭ-te) [*cardio-*(1) + *motility*] the movements of the heart; the motility of the heart.

**car·dio·myo·li·po·sis** (kahr"de-o-mi"o-lĭ-po'sis) [*cardio-*(1) + *myo-* + *lipo-* + *-osis*] fatty degeneration of the heart muscle.

**car·dio·my·op·a·thy** (kahr"de-o-mi-op'ə-the) [*cardio-*(1) + *myopathy*] [MeSH: Myocardial Diseases] 1. a general diagnostic term designating primary noninflammatory disease of the heart muscle, often of obscure or unknown etiology and not the result of ischemic, hypertensive, congenital, valvular, or pericardial disease. It is usually subdivided into *dilated, hypertrophic,* and *restrictive c.* 2. In World Health Organization nomenclature, only those disorders in which the pathological process involves solely the myocardium and in which the cause is unknown and not part of a disease affecting other organs; called also *primary c.* Cf. *secondary c.*
**alcoholic c.,** dilated cardiomyopathy occurring in patients with a history of chronic alcohol abuse; it is believed to be due to a direct toxic effect of alcohol or its metabolites.
**beer-drinkers' c.,** cardiac dilatation and hypertrophy due to excessive beer consumption; in at least some cases it has been caused by addition of cobalt to the beer during manufacturing. See also *alcoholic c.*
**congestive c.,** dilated c.
**dilated c.,** a syndrome of ventricular dilatation, systolic contractile dysfunction, and often congestive heart failure; the course is usually progressive with a poor prognosis. It is believed to be an expression of myocardial damage caused by a variety of factors, such as alcohol, pregnancy, systemic hypertension, or certain infections.
**hypertrophic c. (HCM),** a cardiomyopathy, possibly of autosomal dominant inheritance, marked by ventricular hypertrophy, particularly of the left ventricle and often involving the interventricular septum, with diastolic dysfunction manifest as impaired ventricular filling. See also *idiopathic hypertrophic subaortic stenosis,* under *stenosis.*
**hypertrophic obstructive c. (HOCM),** a form of hypertrophic cardiomyopathy in which the location of the septal hypertrophy causes obstructive interference to left ventricular outflow. Cf. *asymmetrical septal hypertrophy.*

**idiopathic c.**, primary c.
**infectious c.**, chronic myocardial disease following infection.
**infiltrative c.**, restrictive cardiomyopathy characterized by deposition in the heart tissue of abnormal substances, as may occur in amyloidosis, hemochromatosis, etc.
**ischemic c.**, heart failure with left ventricular dilatation resulting from ischemic heart disease; it does not meet the strict definition of a cardiomyopathy.
**obliterative c.**, restrictive c.
**obstructive hypertrophic c.**, hypertrophic obstructive c.
**peripartum c.**, cardiac enlargement and congestive heart failure of unknown cause beginning in the last month of gestation or the first few months after delivery.
**postpartum c.**, peripartum c.
**primary c.**, cardiomyopathy, def. 2.
**restrictive c.**, a form in which the ventricular walls are excessively rigid, impeding ventricular filling; it is marked by abnormal diastolic function sometimes with normal or nearly normal systolic function.
**right ventricular c.**, a right-sided cardiomyopathy occurring predominantly in young males, characterized by dilatation of the right ventricle with partial to total replacement of its muscle by fibrous or adipose tissue, palpitations, syncope, and sometimes sudden death.
**secondary c.**, any form that is due to another cardiovascular disorder (e.g., hypertension) or is a manifestation of systemic disease (e.g., sarcoidosis). See also *cardiomyopathy.*
**toxic c.**, that due to agents causing toxic damage to the myocardium, such as alcohol, certain antitumor agents, catecholamines, snake venom, and some metals.

**car·dio·my·ot·o·my** (kahr″de-o-mi-ot′ə-me) [*cardio-*(1) + *myo-* + *-tomy*] esophagocardiomyotomy.
**Heller's c.**, esophagocardiomyotomy.

**car·dio·na·trin** (kahr″de-o-na′trin) [*cardio-*(1) + *natrium*] former name for *atrial natriuretic peptide.*

**car·dio·neph·ric** (kahr″de-o-nef′rik) pertaining to the heart and the kidney.

**car·dio·neu·ral** (kahr″de-o-noo͝′rəl) pertaining to the heart and nervous system.

**car·dio·path·ic** (kahr″de-o-path′ik) pertaining to or marked by disease of the heart.

**car·di·op·a·thy** (kahr″de-op′ə-the) [*cardio-*(1) + *-pathy*] any disorder or disease of the heart.
**infarctoid c.**, a heart condition with symptoms resembling those of myocardial infarction.

**car·dio·peri·car·dio·pexy** (kahr″de-o-per″ĭ-kahr′de-o-pek″se) [*cardio-*(1) + *pericardium* + *-pexy*] the operative establishment of adhesive pericarditis; formerly used to increase blood flow to the heart.

**car·dio·peri·car·di·tis** (kahr″de-o-per″ĭ-kahr-di′tis) [*cardio-*(1) + *pericarditis*] inflammation of both the heart and the pericardium.

**car·dio·pho·bia** (kahr″de-o-fo′be-ə) [*cardio-*(1) + *-phobia*] irrational dread of heart disease.

**car·dio·plas·ty** (kahr′de-o-plas″te) [*cardio-*(2) + *-plasty*] esophagogastroplasty.

**car·dio·ple·gia** (kahr″de-o-ple′jə) [*cardio-*(1) + Gr. *plēgē* stroke + *-ia*] arrest of contraction of the myocardium, as may be induced by the use of chemical compounds or of cold (cryocardioplegia) in the performance of surgery upon the heart.

**car·dio·ple·gic** (kahr″de-o-plej′ik) pertaining to or inducing cardioplegia.

**car·dio·pneu·mat·ic** (kahr″de-o-noo-mat′ik) [*cardio-*(1) + *pneumatic*] of or pertaining to the heart and respiration.

**car·dio·pro·tec·tant** (kahr″de-o-pro-tek′tənt) 1. counteracting cardiotoxicity. 2. an agent that counteracts cardiotoxicity.

**car·dio·pro·tec·tive** (kahr-de-o-pro-tek′tiv) cardioprotectant.

**car·di·op·to·sia** (kahr″de-op-to′se-ə) cardioptosis.

**car·di·op·to·sis** (kahr″de-op′tə-sis) [*cardio-*(1) + *-ptosis*] downward displacement of the heart.

**car·dio·pul·mo·nary** (kahr″de-o-pul′mə-nar-e) pertaining to the heart and lungs. Called also *cardiorespiratory* and *pneumocardial.*

**car·dio·py·lo·ric** (kahr″de-o-pi-lor′ik) pertaining to the cardia (ostium cardiacum [TA]) and the pylorus.

**Car·dio·quin** (kahr′de-o-kwin″) trademark for a preparation of quinidine polygalacturonate.

**car·dio·re·nal** (kahr″de-o-re′nəl) pertaining to the heart and the kidney. Called also *nephrocardiac.*

**car·dio·res·pi·ra·to·ry** (kahr″de-o-res′pĭ-rə-to″re) cardiopulmonary.

**car·di·or·rha·phy** (kahr″de-or′ə-fe) [*cardio-*(1) + *-rrhaphy*] the operation of suturing the heart muscle.

**car·di·or·rhex·is** (kahr″de-o-rek′sis) [*cardio-*(1) + *-rrhexis*] rupture of the heart.

**car·dio·scle·ro·sis** (kahr″de-o-sklə-ro′sis) [*cardio-*(1) + *sclerosis*] fibrous induration of the heart.

**car·dio·se·lec·tive** (kahr″de-o-sə-lek′tiv) having greater activity on heart tissue than on other tissue.

**car·dio·spasm** (kahr′de-o-spaz″əm) achalasia of the esophagus; see under *achalasia.*

**car·dio·ta·chom·e·ter** (kahr″de-o-tə-kom′ə-tər) [*cardio-*(1) + *tacho-* + *-meter*] the instrument used in cardiotachometry.

**car·dio·ta·chom·e·try** (kahr″de-o-tə-kom′ə-tre) [*cardio-*(1) + *tacho-* + *-metry*] continuous recording of the heart rate for long periods of time.

**Car·dio·Tec** (kahr′de-o-tek″) trademark for a kit for the preparation of technetium Tc 99m teboroxime.

**car·dio·ther·a·py** (kahr″de-o-ther′ə-pe) [*cardio-*(1) + *therapy*] the treatment of heart diseases.

**car·dio·thy·ro·tox·i·co·sis** (kahr″de-o-thi″ro-tok″sĭ-ko′sis) hyperthyroidism with cardiac involvement.

**car·dio·to·co·graph** (kahr″de-o-to′ko-graf) the instrument used in cardiotocography.

**car·dio·to·cog·ra·phy** (kahr″de-o-to-kog′rə-fe) [*cardio-*(1) + *toco-* + *-graphy*] [MeSH: Cardiotocography] the monitoring of the fetal heart rate, as during delivery. Also spelled *cardiotokography.* See also *contraction stress test* and *nonstress test,* under *test.*

**car·dio·to·kog·ra·phy** (kahr″de-o-to-kog′rə-fe) cardiotocography.

**car·di·ot·o·my** (kahr″de-ot′ə-me) [*cardio-* + *-tomy*] 1. surgical incision of the heart for repair of cardiac defects. 2. incision into the cardiac end of the stomach or the cardiac orifice.

**car·dio·ton·ic** (kahr″de-o-ton′ik) 1. having a tonic effect on the heart. 2. an agent that has a tonic effect on the heart.

**car·dio·to·pom·e·try** (kahr″de-ə-tə-pom′ə-tre) [*cardio-*(1) + *topo-* + *-metry*] measurement of the area of superficial cardiac dullness observed in percussion of the chest.

**car·dio·tox·ic** (kahr″de-o-tok′sik) having a poisonous or deleterious effect upon the heart.

**car·dio·tox·ic·i·ty** (kahr″de-o-tok-sis′ĭ-te) the quality of being cardiotoxic.

**car·dio·val·vu·lar** (kahr″de-o-val′vu-lər) pertaining to the valves of the heart.

**car·dio·val·vu·li·tis** (kahr″de-o-val″vu-li′tis) [*cardio-*(1) + *valvulitis*] inflammation of the valves of the heart.

**car·dio·val·vu·lo·tome** (kahr″de-o-val′vu-lə-tōm″) [*cardio-*(1) + *valvula* + *-tome*] an instrument for performing cardiovalvulotomy.

**car·di·o·val·vu·lot·o·my** (kahr″de-o-val″vu-lot′ə-me) [*cardio-*(1) + *valvula* + *-tomy*] the operation of incising a cardiac valve, or of excising a portion of it, done for the relief of stenosis.

**car·dio·vas·cu·lar** (kahr″de-o-vas′ku-lər) pertaining to the heart and blood vessels.

**car·dio·vas·cu·lar·re·nal** (kahr″-de-o-vas′ku-lər-re′nəl) pertaining to the heart, blood vessels, and kidney.

**car·dio·ver·sion** (kahr′de-o-vər″zhən) the restoration of normal rhythm of the heart by electrical shock.

**car·dio·ver·ter** (kahr′de-o-vər″tər) an energy-storage capacitor-discharge type of condenser which is discharged with an inductance; it delivers a direct-current shock which restores normal rhythm of the heart.
**automatic implantable c.-defibrillator,** an implantable device that detects sustained ventricular tachycardia or fibrillation and terminates it by a shock or shocks delivered directly to the myocardium.

**Car·dio·vi·rus** (kahr′de-o-vi″rəs) [*cardio-*(1) + *virus*] [MeSH: Cardiovirus] EMC-like viruses; a genus of viruses of the family Picornaviridae that cause encephalomyelitis and myocarditis, comprising two groups, the encephalomyocarditis (EMC) viruses and the murine encephalomyelitis viruses.

**car·dio·vi·rus** (kahr′de-o-vi″rus) [MeSH: Cardiovirus] any member of the genus *Cardiovirus.*

**car·di·tis** (kahr-di′tis) [*cardi-*(1) + *-itis*] inflammation of the heart.
**Lyme c.**, cardiac involvement, generally transient, in Lyme disease; it usually manifests as some degree of atrioventricular block but ventricular tachycardia and left ventricular dysfunction may occur.
**rheumatic c.**, cardiac involvement in rheumatic fever, which when severe may be manifested by congestive heart failure, progressive

cardiac enlargement, pericarditis, and significant murmurs due to valvular dysfunction.
**streptococcal c.**, carditis occurring as a result of streptococcal sore throat.
**verrucous c.**, a nonbacterial endocarditis marked by a continuous chain of wartlike vegetations near the line of closure of the cusps of the mitral and tricuspid valves; seen in lupus erythematosus and occasionally in scleroderma, thrombotic purpura, and other collagen diseases.

**Car·di·zem** (kahr′dĭ-zem) trademark for preparations of diltiazem hydrochloride.

**Car·dura** (kahr-du′rə) trademark for a preparation of doxazosin mesylate.

**care** (kār) [A.S. *caru* anxiety] the services rendered by members of the health professions for the benefit of a patient. Called also *treatment*.
**coronary c.**, see under *unit*.
**critical c.**, intensive c.; see under *unit*.
**intensive c.**, see under *unit*.
**palliative c.**, see under *treatment*.
**primary c.**, the care a patient receives at first contact with the health care system, usually involving coordination of care and continuity over time.
**respiratory c.**, 1. the health care profession providing, under a physician's supervision, diagnostic evaluation, therapy, monitoring, and rehabilitation of patients with cardiopulmonary disorders. 2. a general term for the type of medical care provided by the members of this profession. Defs. 1 and 2 called also *respiratory therapy*. 3. the diagnostic and therapeutic use of medical gases and their administering apparatus, environmental control systems, humidification, aerosols, medications, ventilatory support, bronchopulmonary drainage, pulmonary rehabilitation, cardiopulmonary resuscitation, and airway management. Called also *inhalation therapy* and *respiratory therapy*.
**secondary c.**, treatment by specialists to whom a patient has been referred by primary care providers.
**tertiary c.**, treatment given in a health care center that includes highly trained specialists and often advanced technology.

**car·fe·cil·lin so·di·um** (kahr″fə-sil′in) carbenicillin phenyl sodium.

**Car·i·ca** (kar′ĭ-kə) a genus of trees of the family Caricaceae, native to tropical regions of the Americas. *C. papa′ya* L. is the papaya or papaw tree, source of the fruit called papaya and of the enzyme papain.

**car·i·cous** (kar′ĭ-kəs) [L. *carica* fig] shaped like or resembling a fig.

**car·ies** (kar′e-ēz, kar′ēz) [L. "rottenness"] 1. the molecular decay or death of a bone, in which it becomes softened, discolored, and porous. It produces a chronic inflammation of the periosteum and surrounding tissues, and forms a cold abscess filled with a cheesy, fetid, puslike liquid, which generally burrows through the soft parts until it opens externally by a sinus or fistula. 2. dental c.
**backward c.**, dental caries that progresses backward from the dentinoenamel junction into the enamel; called also *internal c.*
**cemental c.**, dental caries that involves the cementum of a tooth.
**central c.**, a chronic abscess in the interior of a bone.
**dental c.**, localized destruction of calcified tissue initiated on the tooth surface by decalcification of the enamel of the teeth, followed by enzymatic lysis of organic structures, leading to cavity formation that, if left unchecked, penetrates the enamel and dentin and may reach the pulp. There are several theories on etiology: see *acidogenic theory, proteolytic theory,* and *proteolysis-chelation theory,* under *theory*. Classified by Black into five groups on the basis of similarity of treatment required; a sixth group is sometimes added. (See table.) See also *cavity*. Called also *tooth decay*.
**dental c., primary,** dental caries in which the lesion constitutes the initial attack on the tooth surface.
**dental c., rampant,** dental caries that involve several teeth, appear suddenly, and often progress rapidly.
**dental c., secondary,** dental caries occurring around the edges and under restorations.
**dentinal c.**, dental caries that spreads along the dentinoenamel junction and involves dentinal tubules, eventually reaching the pulp.
**dry c.**, a form of tuberculous caries of the joints and ends of bones; called also *c. sicca*.
**enamel c.**, dental caries that involves the enamel of a tooth.
**internal c.**, backward c.
**lateral c.**, dental caries that extends laterally at the dentinoenamel junction.
**necrotic c.**, a disease in which pieces of bone lie in a suppurating cavity.

**Black's Classification of Dental Caries**

| | |
|---|---|
| Class I | Cavities occurring in pit and fissure defects in occlusal surfaces of bicuspids and molars, lingual surfaces of upper incisors, and facial and lingual grooves sometimes found on occlusal surfaces of molar teeth. |
| Class II | Cavities in proximal surfaces of bicuspids and molars. |
| Class III | Cavities in proximal surfaces of incisors and cuspids not requiring removal of incisal angle. |
| Class IV | Cavities in proximal surfaces of incisors and cuspids that require removal of incisal angle. |
| Class V | Cavities in gingival third of labial, lingual, or buccal surfaces. |
| Class VI (not a true Black classification) | Cavities in incisal edges and smooth surfaces of teeth above the height of contour. |

**pit c.**, dental caries originating in pits or fissures, usually of the occlusal surfaces of molars and premolars or on the lingual surfaces of the maxillary incisors, typically occurring as a deep cavity with a narrow point of penetration.
**rampant c.**, rampant dental c.
**c. sic′ca**, dry c.
**spinal c.**, tuberculotic osteitis of the vertebrae and of the intervertebral cartilages.

**ca·ri·na** (kə-ri′nə) pl. *cari′nae* [L. "keel"] a ridge or ridgelike structure.
**c. for′nicis,** carina of fornix: a ridge on the under surface of the fornix.
**c. tra′cheae** [TA], carina of trachea: a projection of the lowest tracheal cartilage, forming a prominent semilunar ridge running anteroposteriorly between the orifices of the two bronchi.
**c. urethra′lis vagi′nae** [TA], urethral carina of vagina: the column of rugae in the lower part of the anterior wall of the vagina, immediately beneath the urethra.

**ca·ri·nae** (kə-ri′ne) [L.] genitive and plural of *carina*.

**car·i·nate** (kar′ĭ-nāt) [L. *carina* a keel] keel shaped; having a keellike process.

**car·i·na·tion** (kar″ĭ-na′shən) a ridged condition of a part.

**car·in·da·cil·lin so·di·um** (kar″in-də-sil′in) carbenicillin indanyl sodium.

**car·io·gen·e·sis** (kar″e-o-jen′ə-sis) development of caries.

**car·io·gen·ic** (kar″e-o-jen′ik) [*caries* + *-genic*] conducive to the production of caries.

**car·io·ge·nic·i·ty** (kar″e-o-jə-nis′ĭ-te) the quality of being conducive to the production of caries.

**car·i·ol·o·gy** (kar″e-ol′ə-je) [*caries-* + *-logy*] the study of cariogenesis and its prevention.

**car·i·os·i·ty** (kar″e-os′ĭ-te) the quality of being carious.

**ca·ri·ous** (kar′e-əs) [L. *cariosus*] affected with or of the nature of caries.

**car·iso·pro·dol** (kar″i-so-pro′dol) [MeSH: Carisoprodol] a centrally acting skeletal muscle relaxant, for the symptomatic management of acute, painful musculoskeletal disorders, administered orally. Called also *isopropyl meprobamate*.

**Car·lens' tube** (kahr′lənz) [Eric *Carlens,* Swedish physician, born 1908] see under *tube*.

**Carle·ton's spots** (kahrl′tənz) [Bukk G. *Carleton,* American physician, 1856–1914] see under *spot*.

**car·mal·um** (kahr-mal′əm) a stain composed of carmine, alum, and water.

**Carman's sign** (kahr′mənz) [Russell Daniel *Carman,* American physician, 1875–1926] meniscus sign; see under *sign*.

**Car·man-Kirk·lin sign (meniscus sign)** (kahr′mən-kərk′lin) [R.D. *Carman;* Byrl Raymond *Kirklin,* American radiologist, 1888–1957] meniscus sign.

**car·min·a·tive** (kahr-min′ə-tiv) [L. *carminare* to card, to cleanse, from *carmen,* a card for wool] 1. relieving flatulence. 2. a medicine that relieves flatulence and assuages pain.

**car·mine** (kahr′min) [MeSH: Carmine] a red coloring matter de-

rived from cochineal by the addition of alum and used as a histologic stain; called also *carminum* and *coccinellin.*
**alizarin c.,** alizarin red.
**indigo c.,** indigotindisulfonate sodium.
**lithium c.,** vital stain for macrophages.
**Schneider's c.,** a saturated solution of carmine in concentrated acetic acid.

**car·min·ic acid** (kahr-min'ik) an aromatic acid that is the essential constituent of the dye carmine.

**car·min·o·phil** (kahr-min'o-fil) [*carmine* + *-phil*] 1. easily stainable with carmine. 2. a cell or other element that readily takes a stain from carmine. 3. lactotroph.

**car·mi·num** (kahr-mi'nəm) carmine.

**car·mus·tine** (kahr-mus'tēn) [MeSH: Carmustine] a cytotoxic alkylating agent of the nitrosourea (q.v.) group, used as an antineoplastic primarily against brain tumors, multiple myeloma, colorectal carcinoma, and Hodgkin's disease and non-Hodgkin's lymphomas; administered intravenously. Called also *BCNU.*

**car·nas·si·al** (kahr-nas'e-əl) 1. adapted for shearing and tearing. 2. carnassial tooth.

**car·nau·ba** (kahr-naw'bə) *Copernicia cerifera,* the source of carnauba wax.

**car·ne·ous** (kahr'ne-əs) [L. *carneus,* from *caro* flesh] fleshy.

**Car·nett's sign** (kahr-nets') [J.B. *Carnett,* American physician, 20th century] see under *sign.*

**Car·ney's complex (syndrome, triad)** (kahr'nēz) [J.A. *Carney,* American physician, 20th century] see under *complex.*

**car·ni·fi·ca·tion** (kahr"nĭ-fĭ-ka'shən) [L. *caro,* gen. *carnis* flesh + *facere* to make] the change of tissue, such as that of the lungs, into a fleshy substance.

**car·ni·tine** (kahr'nĭ-tēn) [MeSH: Carnitine] a betaine derivative found in skeletal muscle and liver; it is required for mitochondrial beta oxidation of fatty acids, carrying the acyl groups (fatty acids) across the mitochondrial membrane to the matrix, where they are transferred back to coenzyme A prior to oxidation. It has been used as an investigational antithyroid and antiangina agent.

**car·ni·tine ac·yl·trans·fer·ase** (kahr'nĭ-tēn a"səl-trans'fər-ās) carnitine *O*-palmitoyltransferase.

**car·ni·tine *O*-pal·mi·to·yl·trans·fer·ase** (kahr'nĭ-tēn pahl"mĭ-to"əl-trans'fər-ās) [EC 2.3.1.21] an enzyme of the transferase class that catalyzes the transfer between coenzyme A and carnitine of long chain fatty acids. *Carnitine palmitoyltransferase I* transfers the fatty acid to carnitine; the acyl carnitine can then traverse the inner mitochondrial membrane. Once in the matrix, the fatty acid is transferred from carnitine back to coenzyme A by *carnitine palmitoyltransferase II;* the resultant acyl coenzyme A is a substrate for oxidation. Deficiency of the enzyme is a cause of defective fatty acid oxidation. Written also *carnitine palmityltransferase.*

**car·ni·tine pal·mi·tyl·trans·fer·ase de·fi·cien·cy** (kahr'nĭ-tēn pahl"mĭ-til-trans'fər-ās) a disorder of lipid metabolism in which the altered enzyme is abnormally regulated, resulting in muscle aches, fatigability, and myoglobinuria, but without lipid accumulation, in the wake of prolonged exercise, particularly in the cold or after fasting. It is an autosomal recessive trait with reduced penetrance in women.

**Car·ni·tor** (kahr'nĭ-tor) trademark for preparations of levocarnitine.

**Car·niv·o·ra** (kahr-niv'ə-rə) [L. *caro* flesh + *vorare* to devour] [MeSH: Carnivora] an order of mammals that are primarily carnivorous, with teeth adapted for flesh eating, a simple stomach, and a short intestine. Included are the dog family, the cat family, bears, walruses, raccoons, and numerous others.

**car·ni·vore** (kahr'nĭ-vor) an animal that eats flesh, especially members of the order Carnivora.

**car·niv·o·rous** (kahr-niv'ə-rəs) eating or subsisting on flesh.

**car·no·sin·ase** (kahr'no-sĭ-nās") X-His dipeptidase.
**serum c. deficiency,** an autosomal recessive aminoacidopathy of carnosine metabolism, due to deficiency of the serum isozyme of X-His dipeptidase; it is characterized by urinary excretion of carnosine and accumulation of homocarnosine in the cerebrospinal fluid and may cause myoclonic seizures, severe mental retardation, and spasticity. See also *homocarnosinosis.*

**car·no·sine** (kahr'no-sēn) [MeSH: Carnosine] a dipeptide composed of β-alanine and histidine, in humans found in skeletal muscle and in the brain, particularly in the primary olfactory pathways. It may play a role as a neurotransmitter.

**car·no·si·ne·mia** (kahr"no-sĭ-ne'me-ə) 1. accumulation of carnosine in the blood. 2. former name for *serum carnosinase deficiency.*

**car·no·sin·u·ria** (kahr"no-sĭ-nu're-ə) urinary excretion of high levels of carnosine, such as occurs after ingestion of meat or fowl or in serum carnosinase deficiency.

**car·nos·i·ty** (kahr-nos'ĭ-te) [L. *carnositas* fleshiness] any abnormal fleshy excrescence.

**car·ob** (kar'əb) [Ar. *al kharrubah*] 1. *Ceratonia siliqua.* 2. the finely pulverized meal of the dried ripe fruit of *Ceratonia siliqua;* it contains albuminous proteins, carbohydrates, and small amounts of fat and crude fiber, and is used in pharmaceutical formulations as an adsorbent and demulcent in treatment of diarrhea. Called also *algaroba* or *algarroba, carob bean,* and *locust bean.*

**Ca·ro·li's disease** (kah-ro-lēz') [Jacques *Caroli,* French physician, born 1902] [MeSH: Caroli's Disease] see under *disease.*

**car·o·tene** (kar'ə-tēn) [L. *carota* carrot] [MeSH: Carotene] one of four isomeric pigments (α-, β-, γ-, and δ-carotene), having colors from violet to red-yellow to yellow, found in many dark green, leafy, and yellow vegetables (e.g., collards, turnips, carrots, sweet potatoes, and squash), and yellow fruit (e.g., apricots, oranges, peaches, and cantaloupes). They are fat-soluble, unsaturated aliphatic hydrocarbons that are converted to vitamin A in animals by an enzyme in the intestinal wall and the liver. β-Carotene is the major precursor (provitamin) of vitamin A in humans, although it is less well absorbed than is retinol. See also *retinol equivalent,* under *equivalent.*
**beta c.,** 1. the β isomer of carotene (q.v.), usually written *β-carotene* or *beta-carotene.* 2. [USP] a preparation of β-carotene (see *carotene*) administered orally to reduce the severity of photosensitivity in patients with erythropoietic protoporphyria. Written also *beta-carotene.*

**β-car·o·tene 15,15'-di·oxy·gen·ase** (kar'o-tēn di-ok'sĭ-jən-ās) [EC 1.13.11.21] an enzyme of the oxidoreductase class that catalyzes the oxidative cleavage of β-carotene in the intestinal mucosa, forming two molecules of all-*trans* retinal.

**car·o·ten·emia** (kar"ə-tə-ne'me-ə) hypercarotenemia.

**ca·rot·e·noid** (kə-rot'ə-noid) 1. any group of pigments, yellow to deep red in color, chemically consisting of tetraterpene (polyisoprene) hydrocarbons. Carotenoids are synthesized by prokaryotes and higher plants, and they concentrate in animal fat when eaten (where they are called *lipochromes).* Examples are β-carotene, cryptoxanthin, lycopene, and xanthophyll. 2. marked by a yellow color.
**provitamin A c's,** carotenoids, particularly the carotenes and cryptoxanthin, that can be converted to vitamin A in the body; they are a major source of vitamin A in a normal diet.

**car·o·te·no·sis** (kar"o-tə-no'sis) the yellow discoloration of the skin occurring in hypercarotenemia. The palms, soles, and area behind the ears are most heavily pigmented, while the sclerae remain white.

**ca·rot·i·co·tym·pan·ic** (kə-rot"ĭ-ko-tim-pan'ik) pertaining to the carotid canal and the tympanum.

**ca·rot·i·co·ver·te·bral** (kə-rot"ĭ-ko-vər'tə-brəl) pertaining to or affecting the carotid and vertebral arteries.

**ca·rot·id** (kə-rot'id) [Gr. *karōtis* from *karos* deep sleep] pertaining to the principal artery of the neck (arteria carotis communis).

**ca·rot·i·dyn·ia** (kə-rot"ĭ-din'e-ə) [contracted form from *carotid* + *-odynia*] episodic, usually unilateral neck pain with tenderness along the course of the common carotid artery.

**ca·rot·o·dyn·ia** (kə-rot"o-din'e-ə) carotidynia.

**carp** (kahrp) [Gr. *karpos* fruit] a fruiting body of a fungus; see also *ascocarp* and *basidiocarp.*

**car·pal** (kahr'pəl) [L. *carpalis*] of or pertaining to the carpus, or wrist.

**car·pa·le** (kahr-pa'le) a carpal bone.

**car·pec·to·my** (kahr-pek'tə-me) [*carpus* + Gr. *ektomē* excision] excision of a carpal bone.

**car·pel** (kahr'pəl) a one-celled pistil, or one of the members composing a compound pistil or seed vessel.

**Car·pen·ter's syndrome** (kahr'pən-tərz) [George *Carpenter,* British physician, 1859–1910] acrocephalopolysyndactyly, type II.

**car·phen·a·zine mal·e·ate** (kahr-fen'ə-zēn) a phenothiazine antipsychotic agent used in the treatment of acute or chronic schizophrenic reactions in hospitalized patients, administered orally.

**car·pho·lo·gia** (kahr"fo-lo'jə) floccillation.

**car·phol·o·gy** (kahr-fol'ə-je) [Gr. *karphologein* to pick bits of wool off a person's coat] floccillation.

**car·pi·tis** (kahr-pi'tis) inflammation of the synovial membranes of the knee (carpal joint) of the horse, with swelling, pain, and lameness. Called also *popped knee.*

**car·po·car·pal** (kahr″po-kahr′pəl) pertaining to two parts of the carpus, especially to the articulations between carpal bones.

**Car·po·gly·phus** (kahr″po-gli′fəs) a genus of mites of the family Acaridae. Some species infest dried fruit and cause dermatitis in those who handle the fruit.

**car·po·go·ni·um** (kahr″po-go′ne-əm) 1. the female sex organ (ascogonium) of members of the order Erysiphales. 2. the female sex organ of any of various algae. 3. ascogonium.

**car·po·meta·car·pal** (kahr″po-met″ə-kahr′pəl) pertaining to the carpus and metacarpus.

**car·po·ped·al** (kahr″po-ped′əl) [*carpus* + *pedal*] pertaining to or affecting the carpus and the foot, as carpopedal spasm.

**car·po·pha·lan·ge·al** (kahr″po-fə-lan′je-əl) pertaining to the carpus and the phalanges.

**car·pop·to·sis** (kahr″pop-to′sis) [*carpus* + *ptosis*] wristdrop.

**car·po·spore** (kahr′po-spor) a diploid spore in the red algae which, by germination, produces tetraspores.

**Car·pue's operation, rhinoplasty** (kahr′pūz) [Joseph Constantine *Carpue,* English surgeon, 1764–1846] Indian rhinoplasty.

**Car·pule** (kahr′pūl) trademark for a glass, rubber-stoppered cartridge containing local anesthetic solutions, fitted in a special syringe for hypodermic injection.

**car·pus** (kahr′pəs) [L., from Gr. *karpos*] 1. [TA] wrist: the joint between the arm and hand, made up of eight bones (see *ossa carpi,* under *os*). See also *articulatio radiocarpalis.* 2. the region of the hand between the forearm and metacarpus. 3. the part of the forelimb of a quadruped that corresponds to this part in the human; called also *knee* and *wrist.*
**c. cur′vus,** Madelung's deformity.

**car·ra·geen** (kar′ə-gēn) 1. *Chondrus crispus.* 2. chondrus (def. 2).

**car·ra·gee·nan** (kar″ə-ge′nən) [*Carragheen,* village in southeastern Ireland] [NF] [MeSH: Carrageenan] a colloidal extractive derived from certain red marine algae, such as of the genera *Chondrus, Eucheuma,* and *Gigartina,* composed of a mixture of sodium, potassium, calcium, and magnesium salts of an acid sulfate of a galactose-containing polysaccharide. Used chiefly as a suspending agent in foods, pharmaceuticals, and cosmetics. Spelled also *carrageenin, carragheenan,* and *carragheenin.*

**car·ra·gee·nin** (a kar″ə-gee′nən) carrageenan.

**car·ra·gheen** (kar′ə-gēn) 1. *Chondrus crispus.* 2. chondrus (def. 2).

**car·ra·ghee·nan** (kar″ə-gee′nən) carrageenan.

**car·ra·ghee·nin** (kar″ə-gee′nən) carrageenan.

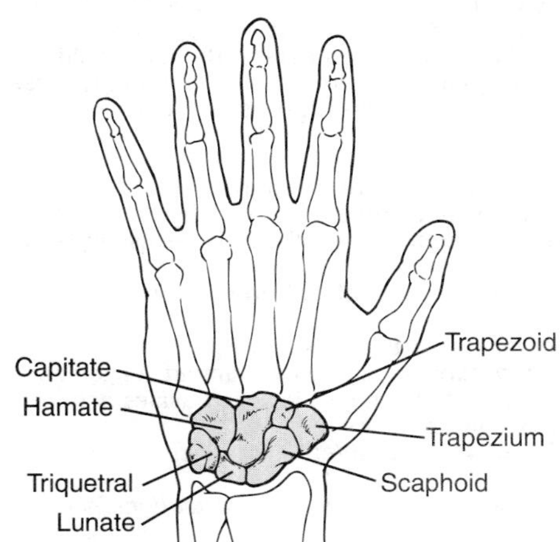


Carpus, viewed from the dorsal aspect. The eighth bone, the pisiform, is palmar to the triquetral bone.

**Car·rel** (kah-rel′) Alexis. French surgeon in the United States, 1873–1944; winner of the Nobel prize for medicine or physiology in 1912 for his work in suturing blood vessels, transfusion, and organ transplants.

**Car·rel's method, treatment** (kah-relz′) [A. *Carrel*] see under *method* and *treatment.*

**Car·rel-Da·kin fluid, treatment** (kah-rel′ da′kin) [A. *Carrel;* Henry Drysdale *Dakin,* English chemist in United States, 1880–1952] see *diluted sodium hypochlorite solution,* under *solution,*

**car·ri·er** (kar′e-ər) 1. an instrument or apparatus for carrying something. 2. an individual who harbors the specific organisms of a disease without manifest symptoms and is capable of transmitting the infection; the condition of such an individual is referred to as the *carrier state.* 3. a chemical substance that can accept one or more electrons and then donate them to another substance (being reduced and then reoxidized). Called also *electron carrier.* 4. [MeSH: Heterozygote] in genetics, an individual who is heterozygous for a recessive gene and thus does not express the recessive phenotype but can transmit it to offspring. Only females can be carriers of X-linked recessive traits. 5. a substance that carries a radioisotopic or other label, as in a tracer study. A second isotope mixed with a particular isotope is also referred to as a carrier; see *carrier-free.* 6. a transport protein that attaches to and carries a specific substance, particularly one that transports the substance across the cell membrane. 7. in immunology, a macromolecular substance to which a hapten is coupled in order to produce an immune response against the hapten, immune responses being usually produced only against large molecules capable of simultaneously binding both B cells and helper T cells. Called also *Schlepper.*
**amalgam c.,** an instrument for carrying freshly mixed amalgam to the prepared cavity.
**electron c.,** carrier (def. 3).
**foil c.,** see under passer.
**gametocyte c.,** in malaria, a person who has gametocytes in his blood stream and so can infect *Anopheles* mosquitoes that feed on him and thus transmit malaria.
**lentulo paste c.,** lentulo.
**paste c.,** lentulo.

**car·ri·er-free** (kar′e-ər-fre) a term denoting a radioisotope of an element in pure form, i.e., essentially undiluted with a stable isotope carrier.

**Car·rión's disease** (kah-re-ōnz′) [Daniel A. *Carrión,* 1850–1885, Peruvian physician who inoculated himself and died of the disease] bartonellosis.

**car·rot** (kar′ət) [L. *carota*] [MeSH: Carrots] 1. *Daucus carota.* 2. the orange or yellow root of *D. carota,* a food rich in vitamin A whose seed is diuretic and stimulant.

**cart** (kahrt) a wheeled vehicle for conveying patients or equipment and supplies in a hospital.
**crash c.,** resuscitation c.
**dressing c.,** one containing all the supplies and equipment that may be necessary for changing dressings of surgical or injured patients.
**resuscitation c.,** one containing all the equipment necessary for initiating emergency resuscitation.

**car·te·o·lol hy·dro·chlo·ride** (kahr′te-ə-lol) [USP] a beta-adrenergic blocking agent with intrinsic sympathetic activity, administered orally in the treatment of hypertension and angina pectoris and applied topically to the conjunctiva in the treatment of glaucoma.

**Car·tha·mus** (kahr-tha′məs) a genus of herbs of the family Compositae, native to Europe and Asia, having brightly colored flowers. *C. tincto′rius* is the safflower, source of safflower oil.

**car·ti·lage** (kahr′tĭ-ləj) [L. *cartilago*] [MeSH: Cartilage] a specialized, fibrous connective tissue, forming most of the temporary skeleton of the embryo, providing a model in which most of the bones develop, and constituting an important part of the growth mechanism of the organism. It exists in several types, the most important of which are hyaline cartilage, elastic cartilage, and fibrocartilage. Also used as a general term to designate a mass of such tissue in a particular site in the body. See *cartilago.*

**accessory c's of nose,** cartilagines nasales accessoriae.
**c. of acoustic meatus,** cartilago meatus acustici.
**alar c., greater,** cartilago alaris major.
**alar c's, lesser,** cartilagines alares minores.
**annular c.,** cartilago cricoidea.
**aortic c.,** the second costal cartilage on the right side.
**arthrodial c.,** articular c.
**articular c.,** a thin layer of cartilage, usually hyaline, on the articular surface of bones in synovial joints. Called also *cartilago articularis* [TA], *arthrodial c., diarthrodial c., investing c.,* and *obducent c.*
**arytenoid c.,** cartilago arytenoidea.
**c. of auditory tube,** cartilago tubae auditivae.
**c. of auricle, auricular c.,** cartilago auricularis.
**branchial c.,** one of the rods of cartilage in the branchial arches of the embryo; called also *pharyngeal c.*
**calcified c.,** cartilage in which granules of calcium phosphate and calcium carbonate have been deposited in the interstitial substance.
**cariniform c.,** the cartilaginous prolongation at the anterior end of the sternum of a horse.
**cellular c.,** a variety composed almost entirely of cells, with little interstitial substance; called also *parenchymatous c.*
**ciliary c's,** palpebral c's.
**circumferential c.,** labrum glenoidale.
**conchal c.,** the part of the auricular cartilage that is in the concha.
**connecting c.,** cartilage connecting the surfaces of an immovable joint; called also *interosseous c.*
**corniculate c.,** cartilago corniculata.
**costal c.,** cartilago costalis.
**costal c., interarticular,** ligamentum sternocostale intraarticulare.
**cricoid c.,** cartilago cricoidea.
**cuneiform c.,** cartilago cuneiformis.
**dentinal c.,** the substance remaining after the lime salts of dentin have been dissolved in an acid.
**diarthrodial c.,** articular c.
**elastic c.,** a substance that is more opaque, flexible, and elastic than hyaline cartilage, and is further distinguished by its yellow color. The interstitial substance is penetrated in all directions by frequently branching fibers which give all the reactions for elastin. Called also *reticular c.* and *yellow c.*
**ensiform c.,** processus xiphoideus.
**epiglottic c.,** cartilago epiglottica.
**epiphyseal c.,** cartilago epiphysialis.
**eustachian c.,** cartilago tubae auditivae.
**falciform c's,** see *meniscus lateralis articulationis genus* and *meniscus medialis articulationis genus.*
**first arch c.,** Meckel's c.
**floating c.,** a detached piece of cartilage, usually from the articular surface of the medial condyle and femur, but also from the patella or lateral condyle of the femur.
**gingival c.,** the tissue covering the loculus which contains an unerupted tooth.
**hyaline c.,** a flexible, somewhat elastic, semitransparent substance with an opalescent bluish tint, composed of a basophilic, fibril-containing interstitial substance with cavities in which the chondrocytes occur; called also *chondroid.*
**inferior c. of nose,** cartilago alaris major.
**innominate c.,** cartilago cricoidea.
**interarticular c.,** 1. ligamentum longitudinale posterius. 2. an interarticular disk.

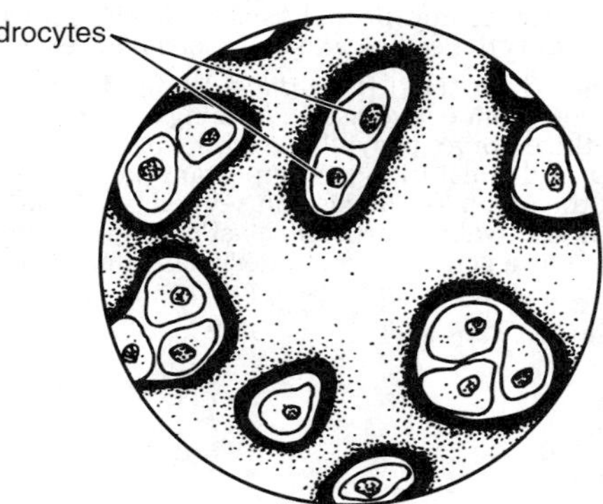

Hyaline cartilage. The matrix nearest the chondrocytes is intensely staining; although the matrix appears homogeneous, collagen fibrils may be visualized by polarized light or electron microscopy.

**interarticular c. of little head of rib,** ligamentum capitis costae intraarticulare.
**interosseous c.,** connecting c.
**intervertebral c's,** disci intervertebrales.
**intrathyroid c.,** a cartilage connecting the alae of the thyroid cartilage in early life.
**investing c.,** articular c.
**Jacobson's c.,** cartilago vomeronasalis.
**laryngeal c's,** see *cartilagines et articulationes laryngeales.*
**laryngeal c. of Luschka,** cartilago sesamoidea ligamenti vocalis.
**lateral c's,** in the horse, the cartilages from the end of the third phalanx to the heel of the hoof.
**lateral c. of nose,** cartilago nasi lateralis.
**lower lateral c.,** cartilago alaris major.
**Luschka's c.,** cartilago sesamoidea ligamenti vocalis.
**mandibular c.,** Meckel's c.
**meatal c.,** cartilago meatus acustici.
**Meckel's c.,** the cartilaginous bar (in the embryo) into which the mesenchymal core of the mandibular process of the first mandibular arch is converted; from it or its sheath, the sphenomandibular ligament, the anterior malleolar ligament, the malleus, and the incus develop. Called also *first arch c., mandibular c., tympanomandibular c.,* and *Meckel's rod.*
**mucronate c.,** processus xiphoideus.
**nasal c's,** cartilagines nasi.
**nasal c's, accessory,** 1. cartilagines nasales accessoriae. 2. cartilagines alares minores.
**nasal c., inferior, nasal c., inferior lateral,** cartilago alaris major.
**nasal c., lateral,** cartilago nasi lateralis.
**nasal c., lower lateral,** cartilago alaris major.
**nasal c., superior, nasal c., superior lateral,** cartilago nasi lateralis.
**nasal c., upper lateral,** cartilago nasi lateralis.
**c. of nasal septum,** cartilago septi nasi.
**c's of nose,** cartilagines nasi.
**obducent c.,** articular c.
**ossifying c.,** temporary c.
**palpebral c's,** the firm cartilaginous framework that gives shape to the eyelids; see *tarsus superior palpebrae* and *tarsus inferior palpebrae.*
**parachordal c's,** the two cartilages at the sides of the occipital part of the notochord of the embryo.
**parenchymatous c.,** cellular c.
**periotic c.,** an oval mass on the upper surface of the fetal chondrocranium investing the inner ear.
**permanent c.,** cartilage that does not normally become ossified.
**pharyngeal c.,** branchial c.
**precursory c.,** temporary c.
**pulmonary c.,** the third costal cartilage on the left side.
**quadrilateral c.,** cartilago nasi lateralis.
**Reichert's c's,** cartilaginous bars in the lateral side of the embryonic tympanum from which develop the styloid processes, the stylohyoid ligaments, and the lesser horns of the hyoid bone. Called also *second arch c's.*
**reticular c.,** elastic c.
**Santorini's c.,** cartilago corniculata.
**second arch c's,** Reichert's c's.
**semilunar c. of knee joint, external,** meniscus lateralis articulationis genus.
**semilunar c. of knee joint, internal,** meniscus medialis articulationis genus.
**septal c. of nose,** cartilago septi nasi.
**sesamoid c. of larynx,** cartilago sesamoidea ligamenti vocalis.
**sesamoid c's of nose,** 1. cartilagines nasales accessoriae. 2. cartilagines alares minores.
**sesamoid c. of vocal ligament,** cartilago sesamoidea ligamenti vocalis.
**sigmoid c's,** see *meniscus lateralis articulationis genus* and *meniscus medialis articulationis genus.*
**slipping rib c.,** loosening and deformity of the costal cartilages, causing painful symptoms.
**sternal c.,** cartilago costalis.
**stratified c.,** fibrocartilage.
**subvomerine c.,** cartilago vomeronasalis.
**supra-arytenoid c.,** cartilago corniculata.
**tarsal c's,** palpebral c's.
**temporary c.,** any cartilage that is being replaced by bone or that is normally destined to be replaced by bone; called also *ossifying c.* and *precursory c.*
**tendon c.,** a form of embryonic cartilage by which tendons and bones are united.
**thyroid c.,** cartilago thyroidea.

**tip c.,** cartilago alaris major.
**tracheal c's,** cartilagines tracheales.
**triangular c. of nose,** cartilago nasi lateralis.
**triquetral c., triquetrous c.,** 1. cartilago arytenoidea. 2. discus articularis articulationis radioulnaris distalis.
**triticeal c., triticeous c.,** cartilago triticea.
**tubal c.,** cartilago tubae auditivae.
**tympanomandibular c.,** Meckel's c.
**upper lateral c.,** cartilago nasi lateralis.
**vomeronasal c.,** cartilago vomeronasalis.
**Weitbrecht's c.,** discus articularis articulationis acromioclavicularis.
**Wrisberg's c.,** cartilago cuneiformis.
**xiphoid c.,** processus xiphoideus.
**Y c.,** a Y-shaped cartilage in the acetabulum, joining the ilium, ischium, and pubes.
**yellow c.,** elastic c.

---

**car·ti·lag·in** (kahr'tĭ-laj″in) a protein found in cartilage, which is changed by boiling into chondrin; called also *chondrigen.*

**car·ti·lag·i·nes** (kahr″tĭ-laj'ĭ-nēz) [L.] plural of *cartilago.*

**car·ti·la·gin·i·fi·ca·tion** (kahr″tĭ-lə-jin'ĭ-fĭ-ka'shən) conversion into cartilage.

**car·ti·la·gin·i·form** (kahr″tĭ-lə-jin'ĭ-form) resembling cartilage; called also *cartilaginoid.*

**car·ti·lag·i·noid** (kahr″tĭ-laj'ĭ-noid) cartilaginiform.

**car·ti·lag·i·nous** (kahr″tĭ-laj'ĭ-nəs) consisting of or of the nature of cartilage.

**car·ti·la·go** (kahr″tĭ-lah'go) pl. *cartilag'ines* [L.] [TA] cartilage: general anatomical nomenclature for a mass of specialized fibrous connective tissue at a particular site in the body.

**c. ala'ris ma'jor** [TA], greater alar cartilage: either of two thin, curved cartilages, one on either side at the apex of the nose, each of which possesses a lateral and a medial crus; called also *inferior cartilage of nose, inferior lateral* or *lower lateral nasal cartilage,* and *tip cartilage.*

**cartila'gines ala'res mino'res** [TA], lesser alar cartilages: various small cartilages located in the fibrous tissue of the alae nasi posterior to a cartilago alaris major; called also *accessory cartilages of nose* and *sesamoid cartilages.*

**c. articula'ris,** articular cartilage: a thin layer of cartilage, usually hyaline, on the articular surface of bones in synovial joints; called also *arthrodial, diarthrodial, investing,* and *obducent cartilage.*

**cartila'gines et articulatio'nes laryngea'les, cartila'gines et articulatio'nes laryn'gis** [TA], laryngeal cartilages and articulations: cartilages of the larynx, including the cricoid, thyroid, and epiglottic, and two each of the arytenoid, corniculate, and cuneiform, together with the articulations between them.

**c. arytenoi'dea** [TA], arytenoid cartilage: one of the paired, pitcher-shaped cartilages of the back of the larynx at the upper border of the cricoid cartilage; called also *c. arytaenoidea, triquetral cartilage,* and *triquetrous cartilage.*

**c. auri'culae** [TA], **c. auricula'ris,** auricular cartilage: the internal plate of elastic cartilage which is found in the external ear; called also *cartilage of auricle.*

**c. cornicula'ta** [TA], **c. cornicula'ta [Santori'ni],** corniculate cartilage: a small nodule of cartilage at the apex of each arytenoid cartilage; called also *Santorini's* and *supra-arytenoid cartilage, corniculum,* and *corpus santorianum.*

**c. costa'lis** [TA], costal cartilage: a bar of hyaline cartilage by which the ventral extremity of a rib is attached to the sternum in the case of the true ribs, or to the superiorly adjacent ribs in the case of the upper false ribs; called also *sternal cartilage.*

**c. cricoi'dea** [TA], cricoid cartilage: a ringlike cartilage forming the lower and back part of the larynx; called also *annular* or *innominate cartilage.*

**c. cuneifor'mis** [TA], cuneiform cartilage: either of the paired cartilages, one on either side in the aryepiglottic fold; called also *Wrisberg's cartilage.*

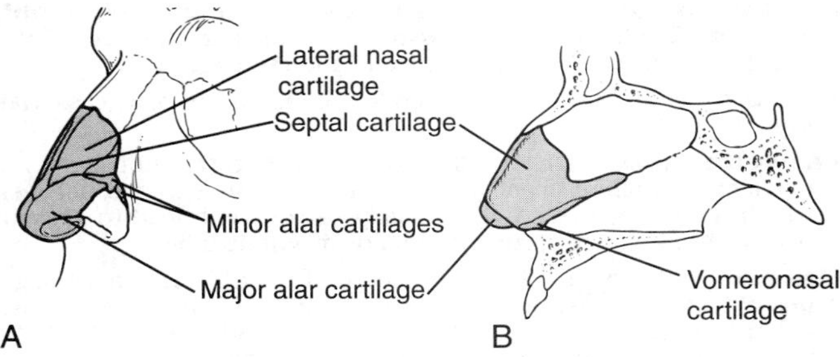


Cartilagines nasi (nasal cartilages). *(A)* Lateral view; *(B)* median section.

**c. ensifor'mis,** processus xiphoideus.

**c. epiglot'tica** [TA], epiglottic cartilage: the plate of cartilage that constitutes the central part of the epiglottis.

**c. epiphysia'lis** [TA], epiphyseal cartilage: the disk or plate of cartilage interposed between the epiphysis and the shaft of the bone during the period of growth; by its growth the bone increases in length. Called also *epiphyseal disk* or *plate* and *growth disk* or *plate.*

**cartila'gines falca'tae,** see *meniscus lateralis articulationis genus* and *meniscus medialis articulationis genus.*

**cartila'gines laryngea'les,** see *cartilagines et articulationes laryngeales.*

**c. mea'tus acus'tici** [TA], cartilage of acoustic meatus: the trough-shaped cartilage of the cartilaginous part of the external acoustic meatus; called also *meatal cartilage.*

**cartila'gines nasa'les,** cartilagines nasi.

**cartila'gines nasa'les accesso'riae,** cartilagines nasi accessoriae.

**cartila'gines na'si** [TA], cartilages of nose: see *c. nasi lateralis, c. alaris major, cartilagines alares minores, c. septi nasi, c. vomeronasalis* and *cartilagines nasales accessoriae.*

**cartila'gines na'si accesso'riae** [TA], accessory nasal cartilages: one or more small cartilages on either side of the nose between the greater alar and lateral nasal cartilages; called also *accessory* or *sesamoid cartilages of nose.*

**c. na'si latera'lis,** lateral nasal cartilage: either of a pair of triangular cartilages extending laterally from the septal cartilages on either side of the nose, attached superiorly to the nasal bone and the frontal process of the maxilla. Called also *superior lateral* or *upper lateral nasal cartilage* and *triangular cartilage of nose.*

**c. sep'ti na'si** [TA], cartilage of nasal septum: the hyaline cartilage forming the framework of the cartilaginous part of the nasal septum, adjacent to and partly fused with the lateral nasal cartilages; called also *septal cartilage of nose* and *quadrilateral cartilage.*

**c. sesamoi'dea ligamen'ti voca'lis** [TA], sesamoid cartilage of vocal ligament: a small cartilage occasionally found within the vocal ligaments; called also *laryngeal cartilage of Luschka,* and *Luschka's cartilage.*

**c. thyroi'dea** [TA], thyroid cartilage: the largest cartilage of the larynx, with two broad, posteriorly diverging laminae and two pairs of horns, superior and inferior, that extend from the posterior borders of the laminae; called also *c. thyreoidea.*

**cartila'gines trachea'les** [TA], tracheal cartilages: the 16 to 20 incomplete rings which, held together and enclosed by a strong, elastic, fibrous membrane, constitute the wall of the trachea. Called also *annuli tracheae* and *tracheal rings.*

**c. triti'cea** [TA], triticeal cartilage: a small cartilage in the thyrohyoid ligament. Called also *corpusculum triticeum* and *corpus triticeum.*

**c. tu'bae auditi'vae** [TA], cartilage of auditory tube: the cartilage on the inferomedial surface of the temporal bone that supports the walls of the cartilaginous portion of the auditory tube; called also *tubal* or *eustachian cartilage* and *c. tubae auditoriae* [TA alternative].

**c. tu'bae audito'riae,** TA alternative for *c. tubae auditivae.*

**c. vomeronasa'lis** [TA], **c. vomeronasa'lis [Jacobso'ni],** vomeronasal cartilage: either of the two narrow, longitudinal strips of cartilage, one lying on either side of the anterior portion of the lower margin of the septal cartilage; called also *Jacobson's* or *subvomerine cartilage.*

**car·ti·la·go·trop·ic** (kahr″tĭ-la″go-trop'ik) [*cartilago* + *-tropic*] having affinity for cartilage.

**Car·trol** (kar'trol) trademark for a preparation of carteolol hydrochloride.

**Cart·wright blood group** (kahrt'rīt) [from the name of the propositus first observed in 1956] Yt blood group.

**ca·ru·bi·cin hy·dro·chlo·ride** (kə-roo'bĭ-sin) an anthracycline antibiotic isolated from *Actinomadura carminata;* it has antineoplastic activity and has been used experimentally in the treatment of acute leukemias and some solid tumors.

**Ca·ru·kia** (kə-roo'ke-ə) a genus of jellyfish. *C. barne'si* Southcott is an Australian species whose sting causes Irukandji syndrome.

**Ca·rum** (kar'əm) a genus of plants of the family Umbelliferae. *C. car'vi* is caraway, a species native to Europe, the Middle East, and Central Asia whose fruit is used as a flavoring.

**car·un·cle** (kar'əng-kəl) caruncula.
**amniotic c's,** small epithelial amniotic growths occasionally found at the placental insertion of the umbilical cord, the fold of amnion, or Schultze's fold, carrying the vitelline duct.
**hymenal c's,** carunculae hymenales.
**lacrimal c.,** caruncula lacrimalis.
**major c. of Santorini,** papilla duodeni major.
**Morgagni's c., morgagnian c.,** lobus medius prostatae.
**myrtiform c's,** carunculae hymenales.
**sublingual c.,** caruncula sublingualis.
**urethral c.,** a small, polypoid, deep red growth on the mucous membrane of the urinary meatus in women.

**ca·run·cu·la** (kə-rung'ku-lə) pl. *carun'culae* [L. dim. of *caro* flesh] [TA] caruncle: a small fleshy eminence, which may be normal or abnormal.
**carun'culae hymena'les** [TA], hymenal caruncles: small elevations of the mucous membrane encircling the vaginal orifice, being relics of the torn hymen; called also *carunculae myrtiformes.*
**c. lacrima'lis** [TA], lacrimal caruncle: the red eminence at the medial angle of the eye.
**carun'culae myrtifor'mes,** carunculae hymenales.
**c. saliva'ris,** c. sublingualis.
**c. sublingua'lis** [TA], sublingual caruncle: an eminence on each side of the frenulum of the tongue, at the apex of which are the openings of the major sublingual duct and the submandibular duct. Called also *c. salivaris.*

**ca·run·cu·lae** (kə-rung'ku-le) [L.] plural of *caruncula.*

**Ca·rus' curve (circle)** (kah'rəs) [Karl Gustav *Carus,* German obstetrician, 1789–1869] see under *curve.*

**Car·val·lo's sign** (kahr-vah'yōz) [J.M. Rivero *Carvallo,* Mexican cardiologist, 20th century] see under *sign.*

**car·ver** (kahr'vər) a knife or other instrument used for carving or fashioning an object by cutting, such as one used for shaping artificial teeth and dental restorations.

**car·vone** (kahr'vōn) a terpene ketone found in many volatile oils, such as caraway oil, oil of dill, and spearmint oil.

**cary(o)-** [Gr. *karyon* nucleus, or nut] a combining form denoting relationship to a nucleus; see also words beginning *karyo-.*

**caryo·chrome** (kar'e-o-krōm") [*caryo-* + *-chrome*] karyochrome.

**Caryo·pha·non** (kar"e-o'fə-non) [*caryo-* + Gr. *phanus* bright] a genus of bacteria of uncertain affiliation, consisting of gram-positive, asporogenous, rod-shaped organisms found in cow dung.

**caryo·phil** (kar'e-o-fil) staining easily with thiazinammonium stains.

**Car·y·so·my·ia** (kar"ī-so-mi'yə) *Chrysomyia.*

**Ca·sal's necklace (collar)** (kah-sahlz') [Gaspar *Casal,* Spanish physician, 1679–1759] see under *necklace.*

**ca·san·thra·nol** (kə-san'thrə-nōl) [USP] a purified mixture of the anthranol glycosides derived from *Cascara sagrada;* used as a contact laxative.

**cas·ca·bel** (kahs-kah-bel') [Sp. "little round bell"] *Crotalus duris'sus terri'ficus,* a highly venomous rattlesnake found in South and Central America.

**cas·cade** (kas-kād') a series of steps or stages (as of a physiological process) that once initiated continues to the final step by virtue of each step being triggered by the preceding one, sometimes with cumulative effect.
**coagulation c.,** the series of steps beginning with activation of the intrinsic or extrinsic pathways of coagulation, or of one of the related alternative pathways, and proceeding through the common pathway of coagulation to the formation of the fibrin clot; each step involves zymogen activation, the activated zymogen catalyzing activation of the following step.
**electron c.,** the electron transport chain (q.v.), emphasizing the passage of electrons from a large negative (reducing) potential to a positive (oxidizing) potential.

**cas·cara** (kas-kār'ə) [Sp.] [MeSH: Cascara] bark.
**c. amar'ga,** [Sp. "bitter bark"], the bark of *Sweetia panamensis* Benth. (Leguminosae), a tree of tropical America; it is alterative and tonic.
**c. sagra'da** [USP] [Sp. "sacred bark"], the dried bark of *Rhamnus purshiana,* used as a cathartic; its laxative principles are glycosidal anthraquinones such as emodin and barbaloin. Called also *bearberry bark, bearwood, chittem bark, dogwood bark, Persian bark, Purshiana bark,* and *sacred bark.*

**case** (kās) 1. a particular instance of disease, as a *case* of leukemia; sometimes used incorrectly to designate the patient with the disease. 2. a term sometimes used incorrectly in dentistry to designate a flask, denture, casting, or the like.
**borderline c.,** an instance of a disease in which the symptoms resemble those of a recognized condition but are not typical of it.
**index c.,** 1. the case of the original patient *(proband)* that provides the stimulus for study of other members of a family to investigate for possible genetic factors in causation of the presenting condition. 2. in epidemiology of contagious disease, the first case of a disease, as opposed to subsequent cases.
**trial c.,** a box containing convex and concave spherical, and convex and concave cylindrical lenses, arranged in pairs, a trial spectacle frame, and various other devices used in testing vision.

**ca·se·a·tion** (ka"se-a'shən) [L. *caseus* cheese] 1. the precipitation of casein. 2. necrosis in which the tissue becomes a soft, dry, crumbly mass resembling cheese, usually caused by mycobacterial infection. Called also *caseous* or *cheesy necrosis.*

**case·book** (kās'book") a book in which a physician enters records of cases.

**case his·to·ry** (kās his'ta-re) the collected data concerning an individual, his family, and environment, including his medical history and any other information that may be useful in analyzing and diagnosing his condition or for instructional purposes.

**ca·sein** (ka'sēn, ka-sēn') [L. *caseus* cheese] a phosphoprotein, the principal protein of milk, the basis of curd and of cheese. It is precipitated from milk as a white amorphous substance by dilute acids, and redissolves on the addition of alkalis or of excess acid. Rennin (and other milk-clotting enzymes) influence the hydrolysis of casein to soluble paracasein, which in the presence of calcium ($Ca^{2+}$) is converted to an insoluble curd (insoluble paracasein or calcium paracaseinate). Casein, usually in the form of its calcium, potassium, or sodium salts, is added to other ingredients of the diet to increase its protein content. NOTE: In British nomenclature, casein is called *caseinogen,* and paracasein is called *casein.*
**c.-calcium,** calcium caseinate.
**c.-sodium,** a nutrient preparation of casein and sodium hydroxide.

**ca·sei·nate** (ka'se-ə-nāt", ka-se'nāt) 1. any salt of casein. 2. a combination of casein and a metal.

**ca·sein·o·gen** (ka-sēn'o-jen) [*casein* + *-gen*] the British term for casein.

**ca·sein·og·e·nate** (ka"se-noj'ə-nāt) a salt of caseinogen.

**ca·se·og·e·nous** (ka"se-oj'ə-nəs) producing caseation; conversion into cheese (casein).

**ca·se·ous** (ka'se-əs) resembling cheese or curd; cheesy.

**ca·se·um** (ka'se-əm) [L. "cheese"] cellular debris of a cheeselike consistency, produced as a result of caseation.

**case·worm** (kās'wərm) echinococcus.

**Cas·o·dex** (kas'o-deks) trademark for a preparation of bicalutamide.

**Ca·so·ni's intradermal test (reaction)** (kə-so'nēz) [Tommaso *Casoni,* Italian physician, 1880–1933] see under *test.*

**cas·sa·va** (kə-sah'və) [Sp., from Taino *casavi*] [MeSH: Cassava] 1. a shrub of the genus *Manihot,* especially *M. esculenta.* 2. a starchy substance from the root of *Manihot,* used in many tropical regions in soups, breads, tapioca, and other foods, as well as in glue. The root contains hydrogen cyanide, which is removed during processing; if eaten raw, it causes cyanide poisoning in humans and domestic animals. Called also *manioc.*

**Cas·sel·ber·ry's position** (kas'əl-ber"ēz) [William Evans *Casselberry,* American laryngologist, 1858–1916] see under *position.*

**Cas·ser's (Cas·se·rio's, Cas·se·ri·us') fontanelle, ligament, muscle** (kah'sərz) [Giulio *Casserio,* Italian anatomist, c. 1552–1616] see under *fontanelle, ligament,* and *muscle.*

**cas·se·ri·an** (kə-se're-ən) named for Giulio Casserio, as casserian fontanelle.

**cas·sette** (kə-set') [Fr. "a little box"] 1. a lightproof housing for x-ray film, containing front and back intensifying screens between which the film is placed; it is usually backed with lead to prevent backscatter. 2. a magazine for film or magnetic tape.

**Cas·sia** (kash'e-ə) [L.; Gr. *kasia*] [MeSH: Cassia] the sennas, a genus of tropical trees, shrubs, and herbs of the family Leguminosae.
**C. acutifo'lia** Del., a species native to Africa and cultivated in India that is the source of Alexandria senna; see *senna.*
**C. angustifo'lia** Vahl., a species native to Arabia that is the source of India or Tinnevelly senna; see *senna.*

**C. obtusifo'lia,** *C. occidentalis.*
**C. occidenta'lis,** coffee senna, a species whose seeds are often found as a contaminant in feed corn or soybeans; when eaten in excess by domestic animals, they cause muscle degeneration that can lead to fatal cardiomyopathy.

**cast** (kast) 1. a solid reproduction of an enclosed space such as a hollow organ (e.g., a renal tubule or bronchiole), formed of effused proteinaceous matter and extruded from the body. 2. an accurate reproduction of an object or part, made of plastic that has taken form in an impression or mold. 3. to form an object in a mold. 4. a rigid dressing, molded to the body while pliable, and hardening as it dries, to give firm support. 5. a positive reproduction of all or part of the maxillary or mandibular arch, made from an impression. Called also *model* and *dental c.* 6. strabismus.
**bacterial c.,** a urinary cast made up of bacteria or containing a large number of bacteria.
**blood c.,** a urinary cast that bears blood cells on its surface.
**bronchial c.,** a cylindrical solid or semisolid plug that blocks a bronchus and is sometimes expectorated.
**coma c.,** a urinary cast containing strongly refracting granules; said to indicate oncoming coma in diabetes. Called also *Külz's c.* or *cylinder.*
**decidual c.,** the mass of degenerating or necrotic decidua discharged from the uterus at the time of rupture of an ectopic pregnancy.
**dental c.,** cast, def. 5.
**diagnostic c.,** a positive reproduction of the maxillary and/or mandibular arches, usually made from gypsum, and used for study and treatment planning. Called also *preextraction c., preoperative c.,* and *study c.*
**epithelial c.,** a urinary cast made up of columnar renal epithelium or of round cells.
**false c.,** pseudocast.
**fatty c.,** any cast made up of material loaded with fat globules and indicating renal tubular damage, the fat being derived from the tubular cells.
**fibrinous c.,** a cast resembling a waxy cast, but having a distinctly yellow color like beeswax; often seen in acute nephritis.
**gnathostatic c.,** a cast of the teeth trimmed so that the occlusal plane is in its normal position in the mouth when the cast is set on a plane surface; used in orthodontic diagnosis.
**granular c.,** a dark colored urinary cast of a granular or cell-like substance, it being a degenerated form of a hyaline or waxy cast.
**hair c.,** 1. trichobezoar. 2. (usually pl.) a hair disorder marked by the presence of discrete, white, shiny, freely movable keratinous tubular structures, about 3 to 5 mm. long, encircling the hair shafts within 1 to 3 cm. of the scalp surface, which are formed by retention and desquamation of segments of the internal root sheath. They may be mistaken for nits.
**hanging c.,** one applied to the arm in fracture of the shaft of the humerus and suspended by a sling looped around the neck.
**hemoglobin c.,** an irregular, dark, granular cast composed of disintegrated red blood corpuscles.
**hyaline c.,** a nearly transparent urinary cast made up of homogeneous protein, but slightly refractive.
**investment c.,** refractory c.
**Külz's c.,** coma c.
**leukocyte c.,** a hyaline cast in which leukocytes are incorporated; called also *pus c.*
**master c.,** a facsimile of oral structures, including the prepared tooth surfaces, residual ridge areas, and/or other parts of the dental arch, reproduced from an impression from which a prosthesis is to be fabricated.
**mucous c.,** cylindroid, def. 2.
**preextraction c., preoperative c.,** diagnostic c.
**pus c.,** leukocyte c.
**red cell c.,** hyaline cast in which red cells are incorporated.
**refractory c.,** one made of heat-resistant materials that will withstand high temperatures without disintegrating and that, when used in partial denture casting, has expansion to compensate for metal shrinkage. Called also *investment c.*
**renal c.,** urinary c.
**spiral c.,** a urinary cast having a spiral or twisted shape.
**spurious c., spurious tube c.,** cylindroid, def. 2.
**study c.,** diagnostic c.
**tube c.,** urinary c.
**urate c.,** an agglomeration of urates on a shred of fibrin or other substance.
**urinary c.,** a cast formed from gelled protein precipitated in the renal tubules and molded to the tubular lumen; pieces of these casts break off and are washed out with the urine. There are various different types, including *granular, hyaline,* and *epithelial.* Called also *renal c., tube c.,* and *urinary cylinder.*
**waxy c.,** a urinary cast made up of a highly refractive, translucent, amyloid substance.

**Cas·ta·nea** (kas-ta'ne-ə) [L.; Gr. *kastanea*] the chestnuts, a genus of trees of the family Fagaceae. *C. denta'ta* (Marsh.) Borkh. is the American chestnut, which has an edible nut. Its wood and leaves contain tannin, and it has been used as an astringent and in pertussis. Its leaves and buds may be poisonous to livestock if consumed in large quantities.

**Cas·tel·la·ni's bronchitis (disease), paint** (kahs-tə-lah'nēz) [Marquis Aldo *Castellani,* Italian physican, 1879–1971] see *bronchospirochetosis,* and see under *paint.*

**Cas·tel·la·ni-Low symptom** (kahs-tə-lah'ne lo) [A. *Castellani;* George Carmichael *Low,* British physician, 1872–1952] see under *symptom.*

**cast·ing** (kast'ing) 1. any object formed by the solidification of plastic material, such as a gypsum product or molten metal, poured into an impression or mold. 2. the act of forming such an object, e.g., the fabrication of a metallic dental restoration or appliance, 3. a metallic dental restoration or appliance fabricated by this process. 4. a metallic dental restoration made to fit a cavity preparation and retained to or luted into it with a cementing medium.
**centrifugal c.,** the use of centrifugal force to cause a plastic material to flow into an impression or mold, a process commonly used in dental casting.
**vacuum c.,** the pouring of plastic material into an impression or mold, under conditions of lowered atmospheric pressure, the end of the mold distal to the sprue is subjected to a vacuum, allowing atmospheric pressure to force the casting material into the mold.

**Cas·tle's intrinsic factor** (kas'əlz) [William Bosworth *Castle,* American physician, 1897–1990] intrinsic factor.

**Cas·tle·man's disease** (kas'əl-mənz) [Benjamin *Castleman,* American pathologist, 1906–1982] see under *disease.*

**cas·trate** (kas'trāt) 1. to deprive of the gonads, rendering the individual incapable of reproduction. Called *geld* for male horses; *emasculate* for any male; *spay* for female animals; and *oophorectomize* (if bilateral) for any female. Called also *neuter* (in veterinary medicine), *desexualize,* and *unsex.* 2. an individual that has been castrated, such as a *eunuch* (human being), or an *ox* or *gelding* (farm animals).

**cas·tra·tion** (kas-tra'shən) [L. *castratio*] [MeSH: Castration] 1. removal of the gonads; bilateral orchiectomy or bilateral oophorectomy. 2. destruction of the gonads, as by radiation.
**female c.,** bilateral oophorectomy.
**male c.,** bilateral orchiectomy; called also *emasculation.*

**cas·troid** (kas'troid) eunuchoid.

**ca·su·al·ty** (kazh'oo-əl-te) 1. an accident; an accidental wound; death or disablement from an accident; also the person so injured or killed. 2. in the armed forces, one missing from his unit as a result of death, injury, illness, capture, because his whereabouts are unknown, or other reasons.

**cas·u·is·tics** (kaz"u-is'tiks) the recording and study of cases of disease.

**CAT** computerized axial tomography.

**cat** (kat) [MeSH: Cats] any member of the family Felidae (lions, leopards, wildcats, etc.), especially the domesticated cat, *Felis catus.*

**cata-** [Gr. *kata* down] a prefix signifying down, lower, under, against, along with, very; see also words beginning *kata-.*

**cata·ba·si·al** (kat"ə-ba'zhəl) [*cata-* + *basial*] having the basion lower than the opisthion; said of certain skulls.

**catab·a·sis** (kə-tab'ə-sis) [*cata-* + Gr. *bainein* to go] the stage of decline of a disease.

**cata·bat·ic** (kat"ə-bat'ik) pertaining to the decline of a disease; abating.

**cata·bi·o·sis** (kat"ə-bi-o'sis) [Gr. *katabiōsis* a passing life] the normal senescence of cells.

**cata·bi·ot·ic** (kat"ə-bi-ot'ik) 1. pertaining to or characterized by catabiosis. 2. dissipated or used up in the performance of function; said of the energy obtained from food.

**cat·a·bol·ic** (kat"ə-bol'ik) pertaining to or of the nature of catabolism.

**ca·tab·o·lism** (kə-tab'o-liz-əm) [Gr. *katabolē* a throwing down] any destructive metabolic process by which organisms convert substances into excreted compounds.
**antibody c.,** the rapid degradation (shortened half-life) of foreign gamma globulin in the body.

**ca·tab·o·lite** (kə-tab'o-līt) any product of catabolism.

**ca·tab·o·lize** (kə-tab'o-līz) to subject to catabolism; to undergo catabolism.

**cata·crot·ic** (kat"ə-krot'ik) 1. pertaining to the descending limb of a pulse tracing. 2. said of a descending limb of a pulse tracing that has a notch, i.e., has two waveforms.

**ca·tac·ro·tism** (kə-tak′ro-tiz-əm) [*cata-* + Gr. *krotos* beat] an anomaly of the pulse evidenced by appearance of a small additional wave or notch in the descending limb of the pulse tracing.

**cata·di·crot·ic** (kat″ə-di-krot′ik) on a pulse tracing, having two waveforms on the descending limb; see under *pulse.*

**cata·di·cro·tism** (kat″ə-di′kro-tiz-əm) [*cata-* + *di-* + *krotos* beat] presence of a catadicrotic pulse.

**cata·did·y·mus** (kat″ə-did′ĭ-məs) katadidymus.

**cata·di·op·tric** (kat″ə-di-op′trik) deflecting and reflecting light at the same time.

**cat·a·gen** (kat′ə-jən) the brief portion of the hair growth cycle in which growth (anagen) stops and resting (telogen) starts.

**cata·gen·e·sis** (kat″ə-jen′ə-sis) [*cata-* + *-genesis*] involution or retrogression.

**cata·ge·net·ic** (kat″ə-jə-net′ik) pertaining to catagenesis.

**cat·ag·mat·ic** (kat″ag-mat′ik) [Gr. *katagma* fracture] having the power of consolidating a broken bone.

**cat·a·lase** (kat′ə-lās) [EC 1.11.1.6] [MeSH: Catalase] a hemoprotein enzyme of the oxidoreductase class that catalyzes the conversion of hydrogen peroxide to water and oxygen, protecting cells. It is found in almost all animal cells except certain obligate anaerobic bacteria. Deficiency of the enzyme, an autosomal recessive trait, results in acatalasia.

**cat·a·lep·sy** (kat′ə-lep″se) [Gr. *katalēpsis*] [MeSH: Catalepsy] indefinitely prolonged maintenance of a fixed body posture; seen in severe cases of catatonic schizophrenia. The term is sometimes used to denote *cerea flexibilitas.*

**cat·a·lep·tic** (kat″ə-lep′tik) 1. pertaining to, characterized by, or inducing catalepsy. 2. a person affected with catalepsy.

**cat·a·lep·ti·form** (kat″ə-lep′tĭ-form) resembling catalepsy.

**cat·a·lep·toid** (kat″ə-lep′toid) cataleptiform.

**cat·a·lo·gia** (kat″ə-lo′jə) verbigeration.

**ca·tal·y·sis** (kə-tal′ə-sis) [Gr. *katalysis* dissolution] [MeSH: Catalysis] increase in the velocity of a chemical reaction or process produced by the presence of a substance that is not consumed in the net chemical reaction or process; *negative catalysis* denotes the slowing down or inhibition of a reaction or process by the presence of such a substance.
**contact c., heterogeneous c.,** catalysis produced by the adsorbing power of contact surfaces; e.g., catalysis caused by colloidal platinum.
**surface c.,** catalysis in which the reacting substances are adsorbed onto the surface of the catalyst and there react. Cf. *contact c.*

**cat·a·lyst** (kat′ə-list) any substance that brings about catalysis; called also *accelerant.*
**negative c.,** a catalyst that retards the velocity of a reaction.

**cat·a·lyt·ic** (kat″ə-lit′ik) [Gr. *katalyein* to dissolve] causing or pertaining to an alterative effect; causing catalysis.

**cat·a·ly·za·tor** (kat″ə-lə-za′tor) catalyst.

**cat·a·lyze** (kat′ə-līz) to cause or produce catalysis.

**cat·a·lyz·er** (kat′ə-līz″ər) catalyst.

**cat·a·me·nia** (kat″ə-me′ne-ə) [Gr. *katamēnia*] 1. menses. 2. menstruation.

**cat·a·me·ni·al** (kat″ə-me′ne-əl) menstrual.

**cat·a·men·o·gen·ic** (kat″ə-men″o-jen′ik) emmenagogic.

**cat·am·ne·sis** (kat″am-ne′sis) 1. the follow-up medical or psychiatric history of a patient after he is discharged from treatment or a hospital. 2. the history of a patient after the onset of medical or mental illness.

**cat·am·nes·tic** (kat″am-nes′tik) pertaining to catamnesis.

**cat·a·pasm** (kat′ə-paz-əm) [Gr. *katapasma*] a dusting powder applied to an injured surface.

**cata·pha·sia** (kat″ə-fa′zhə) [*cata-* + *-phasia*] verbigeration.

**cata·pho·re·sis** (kat″ə-fo-re′sis) [*cata-* + *-phoresis*] the passage of charged particles toward the negative pole (cathode) in electrophoresis.

**cata·pho·ret·ic** (kat″ə-fo-ret′ik) of, or pertaining to, cataphoresis.

**cata·pho·ria** (kat″ə-for′e-ə) [*cata-* + Gr. *pherein* to bear] a permanent downward turning of the visual axes of both eyes after the visual fusional stimuli have been eliminated.

**cata·phor·ic** (kat″ə-for′ik) cataphoretic.

**cata·phy·lax·is** (kat″ə-fə-lak′sis) [*cata-* + *phylaxis*] a breaking down of the body's natural defense to infection.

**cat·a·plasm** (kat′ə-plaz″əm) [L. *cataplasma;* Gr. *kataplasma*] a poultice or soft external application, often medicated.
**kaolin c.,** a poultice prepared with kaolin, boric acid, and glycerin; called also *cataplasma kaolini.*

**cat·a·plas·ma** (kat′ə-plaz′mə) [L.; Gr. *kataplasma*] cataplasm.
**c. fermen′ti,** a poultice containing yeast.
**c. kaoli′ni,** kaolin cataplasm.

**cat·a·plec·tic** (kat″ə-plek′tik) 1. pertaining to or characterized by cataplexy. 2. coming on suddenly and overwhelmingly.

**cat·a·plex·is** (kat′ə-plek″sis) [Gr.] cataplexy.

**cat·a·plexy** (kat′ə-plek″se) [MeSH: Cataplexy] a condition in which there are abrupt attacks of muscular weakness and hypotonia triggered by an emotional stimulus such as mirth, anger, fear, or surprise. It is often associated with narcolepsy.

**cat·a·poph·y·sis** (kat″ə-pof′ə-sis) a process, or projection, of bone or of brain matter.

**Cat·a·pres** (kat′ə-pres) trademark for a preparation of clonidine hydrochloride.

**cat·a·ract** (kat′ə-rakt) [L. *cataracta,* from Gr. *katarraktēs* waterfall, portcullis (perhaps because an ocular opacity and a portcullis are obstructions)] [MeSH: Cataract] a partial or complete opacity on or in the lens or lens capsule of the eye, especially one impairing vision or causing blindness. Cataracts are classified by their morphology (size, shape, location) or etiology (cause or time of occurrence).

## Cataract

**after-c.,** a recurrent capsular cataract; any membrane in the pupillary area after performance of a procedure for extraction or absorption of the lens.

**aminoaciduria c.,** capsular thickening occurring in aminoaciduria, homocystinuria, and oculocerebrorenal syndrome.

**atopic c.,** cataract sometimes occurring in the third decade or later in those with longstanding atopic dermatitis.

**axial fusiform c.,** anterior and posterior polar cataracts joined with threadlike opacities extending axially through the lens; called also *spindle c.*

**black c.,** black or dark-colored opacity occurring in senile nuclear sclerotic cataract.

**blue c., blue dot c.,** 1. a small, round developmental opacity that appears white, brown, or blue; it is common in the periphery of the cortex and occasionally moves into the axial zone of the lens; it rarely affects vision. Called also *cerulean c., punctate c.,* and *cataracta caerulea.* 2. coronary c..

**brown c., brunescent c.,** senile cataract appearing as a brown opacity.

**calcareous c.,** dystrophic calcium salt deposits in the subcapsular and cortical areas of the lens.

**capsular c.,** capsular thickening occurring in heat cataracts and oculocerebrorenal syndrome.

**cerulean c.,** 1. blue c. 2. coronary c.

**complete c.,** total c.

**complicated c.,** secondary c.

**congenital c.,** 1. any of various usually bilateral opacities present at birth; they may be mild or severe and may or may not impair vision, depending upon their size, location, and density. Some have a hereditary, usually autosomal dominant cause; others result from intrauterine infection, drug-induced toxicity, ionizing radiation, trauma, prematurity, or chromosomal, endocrine, metabolic, or systemic disorders.; and a sizable percentage are of unknown cause. Congenital cataracts are often associated with low birth weight, central nervous system abnormalities, mental retardation, convulsions, and cerebral palsy. 2. developmental c..

**contusion c.,** one due to shock or to injury of the eyeball.

**coralliform c.,** a developmental, sutural opacity radiating axially forward and outward from the lens and ending in ampullae behind the capsule.

**coronary c.,** 1. a white punctate or flakelike opacity around the periphery of the lens, forming a ring or crown. Coronary cataracts are transmitted by dominant inheritance and may be present in 25 per cent of the general population. 2. blue c..

**cortical c.,** 1. developmental punctate opacity common in the cortex and present in most lenses. The cataract is white or cerulean, increases in number with age, but rarely affects vision. 2. cuneiform c..

**cuneiform c.,** the most common senile cataract, consisting of white, wedgelike opacities distributed like spokes around the periphery of the cortex.

**cupuliform c.,** a posterior subcapsular cortical opacity seen as brown, saucer-shaped granules or cysts. It is centrally located and therefore seriously impairs vision very quickly. Cupuliform cataracts occur between the ages of 60 and 80, but earlier appearance may be an inherited trait.

**dermatogenic c.,** syndermatotic c.

**developmental c.,** a small, common opacity occurring in youth as a result of a congenitally caused defect such as heredity, malnutrition, toxicity, or inflammation. The number of developmental cataracts increases with age, but they rarely impair vision. Called also *evolutionary c.*

**diabetic c.,** a rare, usually bilateral, opacity shaped like a snowflake, affecting the anterior and posterior cortices of young diabetics. Sometimes it can be reversed when the blood glucose is brought under control, but in most cases it progresses rapidly to a mature cataract.

**duplication c.,** a disk-shaped cortical opacity forming in layers under capsular cataracts with clear zones between the layers.

**electric c.,** a cataract occurring after an electric shock, especially to the head. Anterior subcapsular cataracts may form and develop within days after a severe shock; slowly developing or stationary opacities may follow a shock not on the head.

**embryonal nuclear c.,** an opacity confined to the embryonic nucleus of the lens. It is an autosomal dominant trait, is often bilateral, has a powdery appearance, and seldom affects vision. Called also *cataracta centralis pulverulenta.*

**embryopathic c.,** a congenital opacity caused by intrauterine infection, e.g., rubella, syphilis, or toxoplasmosis.

**evolutionary c.,** developmental c.

**galactosemic c.,** a cataract commonly observed in infants with galactosemia. The opacities look like oil droplets, are bilateral, and are zonular or nuclear.

**glassblowers' c.,** heat c.

**glaucomatous c.,** a patchy anterior subcapsular opacity following an attack of acute glaucoma; called also *glaukomflecken.*

**heat c.,** posterior subcapsular opacity caused by chronic exposure to infrared radiation.

**heterochromic c.,** a secondary, posterior cortical cataract symptomatic of heterochromic cyclitis; failing vision is often the first symptom.

**hypermature c.,** a cataract with a swollen, milky cortex, the result of autolysis of the lens fibers of a mature cataract.

**hypocalcemic c.,** punctate, sometimes cerulean, opacities, initially subcapsular, becoming lamellar, occurring with infantile tetany, hypoparathyroidism, or rickets.

**immature c., incipient c.,** an incomplete cataract; the lens is only slightly opaque and the cortex clear.

**intumescent c.,** a mature cataract that progresses; the lens becomes swollen from the osmotic effect of degenerated lens protein, and this may lead to secondary angle closure (acute) glaucoma.

**juvenile c.,** a cataract in a child under nine years old; such cataracts are usually congenital or traumatic.

**lamellar c.,** a concentric opacity, broad or narrow, usually consisting of powdery white dots, affecting one lamella or zonule of an otherwise clear lens. This is the most common type of congenital cataract, and causes include hypocalcemia, hypoglycemia, galactosemia, and rubella. Called also *zonular c.*

**mature c.,** a cataract that produces swelling and opacity of the entire lens. Most cataracts are removed before maturity.

**membranous c.,** a cataract formed of a collapsed, flattened capsule with little or no cortex or epithelium.

**metabolic c.,** an opacity due to an endocrine or biochemical disorder.

**morgagnian c.,** a mature cataract in which most of the cortex has become opaque and liquefied, so that the nucleus moves freely within the lens.

**nuclear c.,** 1. embryonal nuclear c. 2. senile nuclear sclerotic c.

**nutritional deficiency c.,** subcapsular opacity observed in patients with anorexia nervosa and in alcoholics.

**overripe c.,** hypermature c.

**polar c.,** an anterior or posterior subcapsular opacity, usually disk-shaped; the anterior cataract is the more common; the posterior reduces visual acuity more often.

**postinflammatory c.,** a secondary cataract due to inflammation.

**c's of prematurity,** clusters of vacuoles of unknown cause in the Y-shaped sutures of the lens in a premature infant; the condition usually disappears spontaneously within a month.

**presenile c.,** a subcapsular senile cataract in a person under 40.

**primary c.,** a cataract developing independently of any other disease.

**punctate c.,** 1. blue c. 2. coronary c.

**pyramidal c.,** a conoid anterior polar cataract with its apex pointing forward.

**radiation c.,** a subcapsular opacity caused by ionizing radiation such as x-rays, gamma rays, and neutrons, and by nonionizing radiation such as infrared (heat) rays, ultraviolet waves, microwaves, and laser radiation.

**ringform congenital c.,** a very rare opacity in which the lens nucleus is absent, and only a doughnut-shaped remnant of lens is left.

**ripe c.,** mature c..

**rubella c.,** a congenital nuclear cataract caused by maternal rubella during the first trimester of pregnancy.

**secondary c.,** a cataract, usually posterior subcapsular, secondary to some other condition, such as disease (especially iridocyclitis), degeneration (such as chronic glaucoma or retinal detachment), or surgery (particularly glaucoma filtering or retinal reattachment). Called also *complicated c.*

**senile c.,** the most common kind of cataract, painless and of unknown cause, developing without any traumatic, ocular, systemic, or congenital disorder. Senile cataracts are associated solely with aging, some degree of cataract being normal in persons over 50. Most form in the cortical area of the lens, but some form in the nuclear area and a few in the subcapsular area.

**senile nuclear sclerotic c.,** an increasing hardening of the nucleus, with the opacity appearing brown or black and the lens becoming inelastic and unable to accommodate; the opacity is usually bilateral, begins between ages 50 and 60, and progresses slowly.

**snowflake c., snowstorm c.,** the most common type of diabetic cataract, having the appearance of gray to bluish-white flaky opacities.

**Soemmering's ring c.,** see under *ring.*

**spindle c.,** axial fusiform c.

**subcapsular c.,** an opacity beneath the anterior or posterior capsule of the lens.

**sunflower c.,** a brightly colored, usually red anterior capsular opacity with a sunflower pattern that occurs in patients with Wilson's disease and hypercupremia; it has little effect on vision and clears after treatment with penicillamine.

**supranuclear c.,** an opacity in the deep cortex of the lens, just above the nucleus.

**sutural c.,** a congenital opacity of the lens affecting the Y-shaped sutures of the fetal membrane; it usually does not affect vision.

**syndermatotic c.,** an inherited, usually bilateral opacity associated with cutaneous disease and occurring in youth; called also *dermatogenic c.*

**thermal c.,** heat c.

**total c.,** an opacity of all the fibers of the lens; called also *complete c.*

**toxic c.,** an opacity caused by exposure to a drug or other toxic substance, such as a miotic, antimiotic, corticosteroid, metal, nitro compound, or substituted hydrocarbon.

**traumatic c.,** a cataract resulting from injury to the eye, either immediately after injury (e.g., from perforation of the capsule) or years later (e.g., from concussion of the lens without a rupture of the capsule).

**zonular c.,** lamellar c.

---

**cat·a·rac·ta** (kat″ə-rak′tə) [L.] cataract.

**c. brunes′cens,** brown cataract.

**c. caeru′lea,** blue c..

**c. centralis pulverulen′ta,** embryonal nuclear cataract.

**c. complica′ta,** secondary cataract.

**c. ni′gra,** black cataract.

**cat·a·rac·to·gen·ic** (kat″ə-rak″to-jen′ik) tending to induce the formation of cataracts.

**cat·a·rac·tous** (kat″ə-rak′təs) of the nature of or affected with cataract.

**ca·ta·ria** (kə-tar′e-ə) [L. "catnip"] the leaves and tops of *Nepeta cataria* (catnip); used as a carminative and mild nerve stimulant.

**ca·tarrh** (kə-tahr′) [L. *catarrhus,* from Gr. *katarrhein* to flow down] inflammation of a mucous membrane, especially in the air passages of the head and throat, with a free discharge of mucus.
**bovine malignant c.,** malignant catarrhal fever.
**malignant c. of cattle, malignant head c.,** malignant catarrhal fever.
**postnasal c.,** chronic rhinopharyngitis.
**sinus c.,** a disorder of the lymph nodes characterized by dilatation of the sinuses accompanied by some proliferation of the littoral cells, which become swollen and detach themselves from the wall of the sinuses to lie free in the lumen.
**vernal c.,** see under *conjunctivitis.*

**ca·tar·rhal** (kə-tahr′əl) of the nature of or pertaining to catarrh.

**Cat·ar·rhi·na** (kat″ə-ri′nə) [*cata-* + Gr. *rhis* nose] Cercopithecoidea.

**cat·ar·rhine** (kat′ə-rīn) 1. pertaining to the superfamily Catarrhina. 2. characterized by nostrils that are close together and directed downward.

**cat·a·stal·tic** (kat″ə-stal′tik) [Gr. *katastaltikos*] 1. inhibitory; restraining. 2. an agent that tends to restrain or check any process.

**cata·ther·mom·e·ter** (kat″ə-thər-mom′ə-tər) katathermometer.

**cata·thy·mia** (kat″ə-thi′me-ə) the existence in the unconscious of elements sufficiently affect-laden to produce effects in consciousness.

**cata·thy·mic** (kat″ə-thi′mik) pertaining to catathymia.

**cata·to·nia** (kat″ə-to′ne-ə) [*cata-* + *ton-* + *-ia*] [MeSH: Catatonia] a wide group of motor abnormalities, most involving extreme under- or overactivity, occurring primarily in catatonic schizophrenia but also in other disorders; included are catalepsy, catatonic excitement, catatonic stupor, catatonic rigidity, bizarre posturing, unusual mannerisms, stereotypy, waxy flexibility, and negativism.

**cata·ton·ic** (kat″ə-ton′ik) 1. pertaining to catatonia or to catatonic schizophrenia. 2. an individual affected with catatonia or catatonic schizophrenia.

**cata·tri·crot·ic** (kat″ə-tri-krot′ik) on a pulse tracing, having three waveforms on the descending limb; see under *pulse.*

**cata·tri·cro·tism** (kat″ə-tri′kro-tiz-əm) [*cata-* + *tricrotism*] presence of a catatricrotic pulse.

**cat·e·chin** (kat′ə-kin) [MeSH: Catechin] a crystalline astringent principle from catechu. Called also *catechol* and *catechuic acid.*

**cat·e·chol** (kat′ə-kol) 1. catechin. 2. pyrocatechol.

**cat·e·chol·amine** (kat″ə-kol′ə-mēn) one of a group of biogenic amines having a sympathomimetic action, the aromatic portion of whose molecule is catechol, and the aliphatic portion an amine; examples are dopamine, norepinephrine, and epinephrine.

**cat·e·chol·am·in·er·gic** (kat″ə-kol-əm″in-ər′jik) activated by or secreting catecholamines.

**cat·e·chol *O*-meth·yl·trans·fer·ase** (kat′ə-kol meth″əl-trans′fər-ās) [EC 2.1.1.6] an enzyme of the transferase class that catalyzes the transfer of a methyl group from *S*-adenosylmethionine to a catechol or catecholamine such as dopa, dopamine, epinephrine, or norepinephrine. The enzyme occurs in the cytoplasm, particularly in the kidney, liver, and central nervous system.

**cat·e·chol ox·i·dase** (kat′ə-kol ok′sĭ-dās) [EC 1.10.3.1] [MeSH: Catechol Oxidase] any of a group of enzymes of the oxidoreductase class that catalyze the oxidation of catechols to 1,2-benzoquinones. They are copper-containing proteins that act also upon substituted catechols and many catalyze the reaction of monophenol monooxygenase. The group includes enzymes called also *diphenol oxidase* or *polyphenol oxidase,* based on their substrates. Cf. *monophenol monooxygenase.*

**cat·e·chu** (kat′ə-ku) 1. a powerfully astringent extract from the heartwood of *Acacia catechu;* its chief constituents are catechin, quercetin, and catechutannic acid; formerly used as an antidiarrheal agent. Called also *black c.* 2. gambir.
**black c.,** catechu.
**pale c.,** gambir.

**cat·e·chu·ic acid** (kat″ə-ku′ik) catechin.

**cat·elec·trot·o·nus** (kat″ə-lek-trot′ə-nəs) [*cata-* + *electrotonus*] increase of irritability of a nerve or muscle near the cathode during passage of an electric current.

**Cat·e·na·bac·te·ri·um** (kat″ə-nə-bak-tēr′e-əm) [L. *catena* chain +*bacterium*] in former systems of classification, a genus of bacteria of the family Lactobacillaceae, made up of nonsporulating, anaerobic, gram-positive, rod-shaped organisms. These organisms are now assigned to the genera *Eubacterium* and *Lactobacillus.*

**cat·e·nat·ing** (kat′ə-nāt′ing) [L. *catena* a chain] forming part of a chain or complex of symptoms.

**cat·e·noid** (kat′ə-noid) [L. *catena* chain] 1. resembling a chain. 2. arranged in a chain; called also *catenulate.*

**ca·ten·u·late** (kə-ten′u-lāt) catenoid, def. 2.

**cat·er·pil·lar** (kat′ər-pil″ər) the larva of an insect of the order Lepidoptera. Certain species have hairs that cause insect dermatitis (q.v.) in humans.

**cat·gut** (kat′gut″) [MeSH: Catgut] surgical gut.
**chromic c., chromicized c.,** see *chromic gut,* under *gut.*

**Cath.** abbreviation for L. *cathar′ticus,* cathartic.

**Ca·tha** (kath′ə) a genus of evergreen shrubs and trees of the family Celastracheae, native to East Africa. *C. e′dulis* Forsk. is a species whose leaves contain the central nervous system stimulant D-norpseudoephedrine and are chewed or made into a tea.

**ca·thaer·e·sis** (kə-thĕr′ə-sis) catheresis.

**cath·a·rom·e·ter** (kath″ə-rom′ə-tər) an instrument for measuring the thermal conductivity of air by the rate of heat loss from a heated platinum wire.

**ca·thar·sis** (kə-thahr′sis) [Gr. *katharsis* a cleansing] [MeSH: Catharsis] 1. purgation. 2. in psychiatry, release of ideas, thoughts, and repressed material from the unconscious, accompanied by an emotional response and relief.

**ca·thar·tic** (kə-thahr′tik) 1. causing emptying of the bowels. 2. an agent that causes emptying of the bowels, such as by increasing bulk or stimulating peristaltic action. Called also *evacuant* and *purgative.* 3. producing emotional catharsis.
**bulk c.,** one that stimulates evacuation of the bowel by increasing the bulk of the feces.
**lubricant c.,** one that acts by softening the feces and reducing friction between them and the intestinal wall.
**saline c.,** one that increases fluidity of the intestinal contents by retention of water by osmotic forces, and indirectly increases motor activity.
**stimulant c.,** one that directly increases motor activity of the intestinal tract.

**ca·thec·tic** (kə-thek′tik) pertaining to cathexis.

**ca·the·mo·glo·bin** (kə-the-mo-glo′bin) a substance produced by oxidizing hemochromogen; it consists of oxidized heme and denatured globin.

**ca·thep·sin** (kə-thep′sin) one of a number of enzymes of the hydrolase class that catalyze the hydrolysis of peptide bonds. Most cathepsins are lysosomal endopeptidases with an acidic optimum pH.
**c. B** [EC 3.4.22.1], a cysteine endopeptidase with specificity similar to that of papain; it occurs predominantly in lysosomes.
**c. B1,** c. B.
**c. $B_2$,** cysteine-type carboxypeptidase, def. 2.
**c. C,** dipeptidyl peptidase I.
**c. D** [EC 3.4.23.5], an aspartic endopeptidase of the hydrolase class with specificity resembling, but narrower than, that of pepsin A. The enzyme is optimally active at acidic pH and occurs in lysosomes.
**c. G** [EC 3.4.21.20], a serine endopeptidase with specificity similar to that of chymotrypsin; it is found in polymorphonuclear leukocyte lysosomes.
**c. H** [EC 3.4.22.16], a cysteine endopeptidase that also catalyzes the removal of amino acids from the N-terminus of peptides with that end free; it is present in the lysosomes of most mammalian tissues.
**c. L** [EC 3.4.22.15], a cysteine endopeptidase of the lysosomes, structurally related to papain.

**ca·ther·e·sis** (kə-thĕr′ə-sis) [Gr. *kathairesis* a reduction] 1. weakness caused by medicine. 2. a mild action.

**cath·e·ret·ic** (kath″ə-ret′ik) 1. mildly caustic. 2. weakening or prostrating.

**cath·e·ter** (kath′ə-tər) [Gr. *kathetēr*] 1. a tubular, flexible, surgical instrument that is inserted into a cavity of the body to withdraw or introduce fluid. See also *cannula.* 2. urethral c.

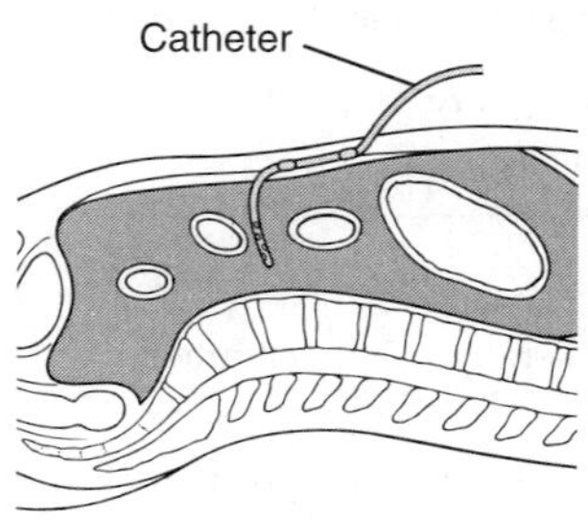

Catheter inserted into the abdomen.

**acorn-tipped c.,** one used in ureteropyelography to occlude the ureteral orifice and prevent backflow from the ureter during and following the injection of an opaque medium.
**Amplatz coronary c.,** a preformed J-shaped angiographic catheter used as an alternative to a Judkins coronary catheter in coronary arteriography.
**angiographic c.,** a catheter through which a contrast medium is injected for visualization of the vascular system of an organ; it may have a preformed end to facilitate selective locating (as in a renal or coronary vessel) from a remote entry site. Different types may be named according to the site of entry and destination, such as *femoral-renal* or *brachial-coronary*.
**atherectomy c.,** a catheter containing a rotating cutter and a collecting chamber for debris, used for atherectomy and endarterectomy; it is inserted percutaneously under radiographic guidance.
**balloon c., balloon-tip c.,** a catheter whose tip is provided with an inflatable balloon that holds the catheter in place or is used to dilate the lumen of a vessel, such as in balloon angioplasty; common types are the *Gruentzig balloon c.* and the *Swan-Ganz c.*
**bicoudate c., c. bicoudé,** an elbowed catheter with two bends.
**Braasch bulb c.,** a bulb-tipped ureteral catheter used for dilation and determination of the inner diameter of the ureter.
**Brockenbrough transseptal c.,** a specialized cardiac catheter with a curved steel inner needle that can puncture the interatrial septum; used to catheterize the left ventricle when the aortic valve cannot be crossed in a retrograde approach.
**Broviac c.,** a type of central venous catheter similar to a Hickman catheter but with a smaller lumen.
**cardiac c.,** a long, fine catheter especially designed for passage, usually through a peripheral blood vessel, into the chambers of the heart under radiologic control; used to obtain blood samples and intracardiac pressures, in diagnosing cardiac abnormalities, and in therapeutic intervention.
**cardiac c.-microphone,** phonocatheter.
**Castillo c.,** a cardiac catheter similar to an Amplatz catheter in shape and use, but shorter and introduced via the brachial artery.
**central venous c.,** a catheter introduced via a large vein, such as the jugular or subclavian, into the superior vena cava or right atrium to administer parenteral fluids (as in hyperalimentation) or medications or to measure central venous pressure.
**closed end-hole c.,** one lacking a hole in its tip; used for rapid injection of large volumes of contrast solution. Cf. *end-hole c.*
**conical c.,** a ureteral catheter that has a cone-shaped tip designed to dilate the lumen.
**c. coudé,** an elbowed catheter.
**Cournand c.,** a cardiac catheter with a single end hole; used for pressure measurement, usually in the right heart.
**DeLee c.,** a catheter used to suction meconium and amniotic debris from the nasopharynx and oropharynx of neonates.
**c. à demeure,** indwelling c.
**de Pezzer c.,** a self-retaining urethral catheter having a bulbous extremity.
**directional atherectomy c.,** a type of atherectomy catheter whose direction can be shifted to shave off additional plaque.
**double-current c., double-lumen c.,** a catheter having two channels, one for injection and one for removal of fluid. Called also *two-way c.*
**Drew-Smythe c.,** an instrument used for the artificial rupture of the amniotic membranes to induce labor.
**elbowed c.,** a urethral catheter with a sharp bend near the beak; used principally in cases of enlarged prostate. Called also *c. coudé*.
**electrode c.,** a cardiac catheter containing one or more electrodes; it may be used to pace the heart or to deliver high-energy shocks.
**end-hole c.,** a cardiac catheter with a hole in the tip, through which a guidewire may be passed or pressure monitored.
**eustachian c.,** an instrument for inflating the eustachian tube for treatment of diseases of the middle ear.
**female c.,** a short urethral catheter for passage through the female urethra.
**filiform-tipped c.,** a catheter used to dilate tight urethral strictures and to bypass obstructions due to angulations or calculi in the ureter.
**fluid-filled c.,** an intravascular catheter connected by a saline-filled tube to an external pressure transducer; used to measure intravascular pressure.
**Fogarty c.,** a type of balloon-tip catheter used to remove thrombi and emboli from blood vessels.
**Foley c.,** an indwelling urethral catheter retained in the bladder by a balloon inflated with air or liquid.
**Garceau c.,** conical c.
**Gensini coronary c.,** a nonpreformed catheter used for coronary arteriography; it has an end-hole to accommodate a guidewire or monitor pressure as well as side holes for rapid injection of large volumes of contrast material.
**Gouley's c.,** a solid, curved steel instrument, grooved on its inferior surface so that it can be passed over a guide through a urethral stricture.
**Gruentzig balloon c.,** a flexible balloon catheter with a short guidewire fixed to the tip, used for dilation of arterial stenoses; the balloon is made of low-compliance plastic to reduce the risk of arterial rupture.
**Hickman c.,** a type of central venous catheter used for the long term administration of substances via the venous system, such as antibiotics, total parenteral nutrition, or chemotherapeutic agents; it can be used for continuous or intermittent administration and may have either a single or a double lumen.
**indwelling c.,** a urethral catheter that is held in position in the urethra.
**Judkins coronary c.,** a preformed J-shaped angiographic catheter used in coronary arteriography to cannulate and deliver contrast material to one of the coronary arteries via a percutaneous femoral route. It is composed of polyurethane or polyethylene with a fine wire braid within its walls; right and left catheters are shaped specifically for use in the respective coronary arteries.
**Judkins pigtail left ventriculography c.,** a specialized pigtail catheter used for left ventriculography.
**left coronary c.,** one designed for coronary arteriography of the left coronary artery.
**Malecot c.,** a two- or four-winged female catheter.
**manometer-tipped c.,** one with a small pressure transducer on its tip; used in measuring intravascular or intracardiac pressure.
**multipurpose c.,** 1. a catheter with several functions or applications. 2. a catheter for coronary angiography that is shaped so that it can be used in either coronary artery.
**Nélaton's c.,** a type of flexible rubber urethral catheter.
**NIH c.,** a nonpreformed catheter used for coronary arteriography; it has a closed end and several side holes for rapid injection of large volumes of contrast material.
**olive-tip c.,** a ureteral catheter with an olive-shaped end, used to dilate a constricted ureteral orifice; larger sizes are also utilized for dilating urethral strictures or for calibrating the diameter of such strictures.
**pacing c.,** a cardiac catheter containing one or more electrodes on pacing wires; used as a temporary cardiac pacing lead.
**Pezzer's c.,** see *de Pezzer c.*
**Phillips' c.,** a urethral catheter with a woven filiform guide.
**pigtail c.,** an angiographic catheter ending in a tightly curled tip that resembles the tail of a pig.
**preformed c.,** a preshaped catheter designed to require less operator manipulation but usually restricted to a single function.
**prostatic c.,** a urethral catheter having a short angular tip for passing an enlarged prostate.
**right coronary c.,** one designed for coronary arteriography of the right coronary artery.
**Robinson c.,** a straight urethral catheter with two to six openings to allow drainage, especially useful in the presence of blood clots which may occlude one or more openings.
**self-retaining c.,** a urethral catheter constructed to be retained in the bladder and urethra.
**snare c.,** one designed to remove intracardiac catheter fragments introduced iatrogenically.
**Sones coronary c.,** a woven Dacron or polyurethane catheter used in coronary arteriography to cannulate and deliver contrast material to the coronary arteries via the brachial artery. It is not preformed and may be used for several tasks or approaches.
**spiral-tip c.,** a catheter with an off-center filiform tip.
**Swan-Ganz c.,** a soft, flow-directed cardiac catheter with a balloon at the tip for measuring pulmonary arterial pressures; it is introduced into the venous system (via the basilic, internal jugular, or subclavian vein) and is guided by blood flow into the superior vena cava, the right atrium and ventricle, and into the pulmonary artery.
**Tenckhoff c.,** any of several types of catheter commonly used in peritoneal dialysis, consisting of a flexible silicone rubber tube with end and side holes and one or two extraperitoneal Dacron felt cuffs that help provide a bacteria-tight seal.
**thermodilution c.,** a catheter used in thermodilution for introduction of the cold liquid indicator into the cardiovascular system.
**toposcopic c.,** a miniature catheter that can pass through narrow, tortuous vessels to convey chemotherapy directly to brain tumors.
**tracheal c.,** an instrument for removing mucus from the trachea by application of suction.
**transluminal endarterectomy c.,** a type of atherectomy catheter

with a conical cutting window, inserted through the lumen of the vessel; debris is collected in a special vacuum bottle.
**transtracheal c., transtracheal oxygen c.,** a catheter inserted into the trachea through a tracheostomy for patients who cannot tolerate a nasal or oral cannula.
**two-way c.,** double-lumen c.
**ureteral c.,** a catheter inserted into the ureter, either through the urethra and bladder or posteriorly via the kidney.
**urethral c.,** a catheter for insertion through the urethra into the urinary bladder.
**vertebrated c.,** a catheter made in small sections fitted together so as to be flexible.
**whistle-tip c.,** a urethral catheter with a terminal opening as well as a lateral one.
**winged c.,** a urethral catheter that has winglike projections on the end to retain it in the bladder.

**cath·e·ter·iza·tion** (kath″ə-tər-ī-za′shən) [MeSH: Catheterization] 1. the insertion of a catheter. 2. the use of a catheter.
**cardiac c.,** passage of a small catheter through a vein in an arm or leg or the neck and into the heart, permitting the securing of blood samples, determination of intracardiac pressure, detection of cardiac anomalies, planning of operative approaches, and determination, implementation, or evaluation of appropriate therapy.
**hepatic vein c.,** passage of a cardiac catheter through an arm vein, right atrium, inferior vena cava, and hepatic vein, into a small hepatic venule, for recording of intrahepatic venous pressures.
**retrograde c.,** passage of a cardiac catheter along an artery, usually the femoral artery, against the direction of blood flow and into the heart.
**retrourethral c.,** passage through the urethra of a catheter first introduced through an incision into the bladder, and then passed through the internal urethral orifice.
**transseptal c.,** passage of a cardiac catheter through the right atrium and across the interatrial septum into the left atrium; used in cases of valve obstruction and in techniques such as balloon mitral valvuloplasty.

**cath·e·ter·ize** (kath′ə-tər-īz) to introduce a catheter within a body cavity; usually used to designate the passage of a catheter into the bladder for the drainage of urine.

**cath·e·tero·stat** (kath-e′tər-o-stat″) a holder for containing and sterilizing catheters.

**cath·e·tom·e·ter** (kath″ə-tom′ə-tər) an instrument for aiding in the reading of thermometers, burets, and other equipment.

**ca·thex·is** (kə-thek′sis) [Gr. *kathexis*] [MeSH: Cathexis] in psychiatry, conscious or unconscious investment of psychic energy in a person, idea, or any other object.

**cath·iso·pho·bia** (kath″ĭ-so-fo′be-ə) [Gr. *kathizein* to sit down + *-phobia*] kathisophobia.

**cath·ode** (kath′ōd) [*cata-* + *hodos* way] 1. in an electrochemical cell, the electrode at which reduction occurs, i.e., the negative electrode in an electrolytic cell or a storage battery and the positive electrode in a voltaic cell that delivers current. 2. the negative electrode of devices such as electron tubes, x-ray tubes, and electrophoresis cells. Symbol C. Cf. *anode.*

**ca·thod·ic** (kə-thod′ik) pertaining to or emanating from a cathode.

**cath·o·lyte** (kath′o-līt) that portion of an electrolyte that adjoins the cathode.

**Cath·o·my·cin** (kath′o-mi″sin) trademark for preparations of novobiocin.

**cat·ion** (kat′i-on) [*cata-* + *ion*] an ion carrying a positive charge owing to a deficiency of electrons; in an electrolytic cell cations migrate toward the cathode, which is negatively charged.

**cat·ion·ic** (kat″i-on′ik) pertaining to or containing a cation.

**cat·i·on·o·gen** (kat″i-on′ə-jən) a compound that may become or may liberate a cation in the body.

**cat·lin** (kat′lin) a long, straight, sharp-pointed, double-edged knife used in amputations.

**cat·ling** (kat′ling) catlin.

**cat·nip** (kat′nip) *Nepeta cataria.*

**ca·top·tric** (kə-top′trik) [Gr. *katoptrikos* in a mirror] pertaining to a reflected image, or to reflected light.

**ca·top·trics** (kə-top′triks) that branch of physics which treats of reflected light.

**ca·top·tro·scope** (kə-top′trə-skōp) [Gr. *katoptron* mirror + *-scope*] an instrument for examining objects by reflected light.

**$Ca^{2+}$-trans·port·ing ATP·ase** (trans-por′ting a-te-pe′ās) [EC 3.6.1.38] EC nomenclature for *$Ca^{2+}$-ATPase.*

**cau·da** (kaw′də) pl. *cau′dae* [L.] [TA] a tail, or taillike appendage; in anatomical nomenclature, a general term for a structure resembling such an appendage.
**c. epididy′midis** [TA], tail of epididymis: the lower part of the epididymis, where the ductus epididymidis is continuous with the ductus deferens; called also *globus minor epididymidis.*
**c. equi′na** [TA], the collection of spinal roots that descend from the lower part of the spinal cord and occupy the vertebral canal below the cord; their appearance resembles the tail of a horse.
**c. he′licis** [TA], tail of helix: the termination of the posterior margin of the cartilage of the helix.
**c. nu′clei cauda′ti** [TA], tail of caudate nucleus: the part of the caudate nucleus that tapers off from the body, curves around in the roof of the inferior horn of the lateral ventricle, and extends rostrally as far as the amygdaloid nucleus.
**c. pancre′atis** [TA], tail of pancreas: the left extremity of the pancreas, usually in contact with the medial aspect of the spleen and the junction of the transverse and descending colon.

**cau·dad** (kaw′dad) directed toward the tail or the inferior end of the trunk, as opposed to *cephalad.* Called also *cephalocaudad.*

**cau·dae** (kaw′de) [L.] genitive and plural of *cauda.*

**cau·dal** (kaw′dəl) 1. pertaining to a cauda or tail. 2. in embryology and nonhuman anatomy, denoting a position more toward the cauda or tail; see also *posterior,* def. 2. 3. in human anatomy, a synonym of *inferior.*

**cau·da·lis** (kaw-da′lis) [TA] caudal.

**cau·dal·ward** (kaw′dəl-wərd) caudad.

**Cau·da·ta** (kaw-da′tə) an order of amphibians, including the salamanders (q.v.).

**cau·date** (kaw′dāt) [L. *caudatus*] having a tail.

**cau·da·to·len·tic·u·lar** (kaw-da″-to-len-tik′u-lər) pertaining to the caudate and lenticular nuclei of the striatum.

**cau·dec·to·my** (kaw-dek′tə-me) the surgical removal of all or part of the tail; see also *dock.*

**cau·do·ceph·a·lad** (kaw″do-sef′ə-ləd) [*cauda* + *cephalad*] 1. proceeding in a direction from the tail toward the head. 2. cephalad. 3. in both a caudal and a cephalic direction.

**caul** (kawl) a piece of amnion that sometimes envelops a child's head at birth; called also *cowl, pileus,* and *veil.*

**Cau·lo·bac·ter** (kaw″lo-bak′tər) [Gr. *kaulos* stalk + *-bacter*] [MeSH: Caulobacter] a genus of appendaged bacteria found in soil and fresh water containing organic matter, made up of rod-shaped, fusiform, or vibrioid cells that typically produce a stalk extending

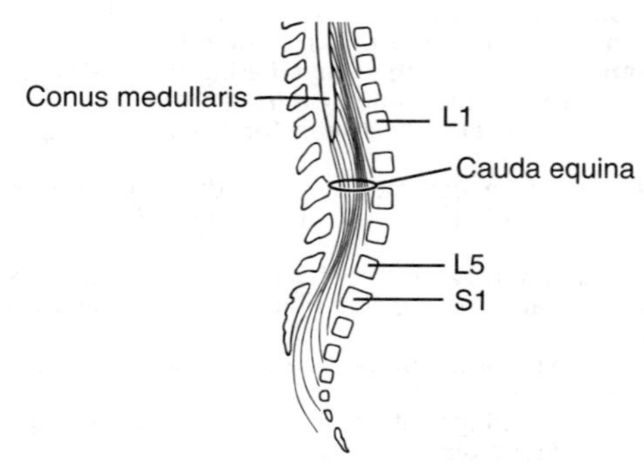


Cauda equina, descending from the conus medullaris of the spinal cord.

from one pole and reproduce by asymmetrical cell fission. The type species is *C. vibrioi'des.*

**cau·mes·the·sia** (kaw"məs-the'zhə) [Gr. *kauma* burn + *esthesia*] a condition in which, with a low temperature, the patient experiences a sense of burning heat.

**cau·sal** (kaw'zəl) pertaining to a cause; directed against a cause.

**cau·sal·gia** (kaw-zal'jə) [Gr. *kausos* heat + *-algia*] [MeSH: Causalgia] a burning pain, often accompanied by trophic skin changes, due to injury of a peripheral nerve, particularly the median nerve.

**caus·a·tive** (kawz'ə-tiv) effective or responsible as a cause or agent.

**cause** (kawz) [L. *causa*] that which brings about any condition or produces any effect.
**constitutional c.,** one acting within the body that is not restricted to a specific site, but is systemic or has a genetic basis.
**c. of death,** the injury or disease responsible for a death; cf. *manner of death,* under *manner.*
**exciting c.,** one that leads directly to a specific condition.
**immediate c.,** a cause that is operative at the beginning of the specific effect; called also *precipitating c.*
**local c.,** one that is not general or constitutional, but is confined to the site where the effect is produced.
**precipitating c.,** immediate c.
**predisposing c.,** anything that renders a person more liable to a specific condition without actually producing it.
**primary c.,** the principal factor contributing to the production of a specific result.
**proximate c.,** that which immediately precedes and produces an effect.
**remote c.,** any cause that does not immediately precede and produce a specific condition; a predisposing, secondary, or ultimate cause.
**secondary c.,** one that is supplemental to the primary cause.
**specific c.,** one that produces a special or specific effect.
**ultimate c.,** the earliest factor, in point of time, that has contributed to production of a specific result.

**caus·tic** (kaws'tik) [L. *causticus;* Gr. *kaustikos*] 1. burning or corrosive; destructive to living tissues. 2. having a burning taste. 3. an escharotic or corrosive agent. Called also *cauterant.*
**Churchill's iodine c.,** a caustic solution of iodine and potassium iodide in water.
**Filhos's c.,** 5 parts of potassium hydroxide and 1 part of calcium oxide.
**Landolfi's c.,** a compound containing chlorides of antimony, bromine, gold, and zinc.
**Lugol's c.,** 1 part each of iodine and potassium iodide dissolved in 2 parts of water.
**lunar c.,** toughened silver nitrate.
**mitigated c.,** silver nitrate diluted with potassium nitrate.
**Plunket's c.,** a caustic paste made of 60 parts of arsenic, 100 of sulfur, and 480 each of *Ranunculus acris* and *R. flammula.*
**Rousselot's c.,** a caustic containing red mercuric sulfide, burnt sponge, and arsenic trioxide.
**Vienna c.,** caustic potash with lime.
**zinc c.,** a mixture of 1 part of zinc chloride and 3 parts of flour.

**caus·ti·cize** (kaws'tĭ-sīz) to render caustic.

**cau·ter·ant** (kaw'tər-ənt) 1. any caustic material or application. 2. caustic.

**cau·ter·iza·tion** (kaw"tər-ĭ-za'shən) the destruction of tissue with a hot instrument, an electric current, a caustic substance, or some other agent. Called also *cautery.*

**cau·tery** (kaw'tər-e) [L. *cauterium;* Gr. *kautērion*] [MeSH: Cautery] 1. a caustic substance or hot instrument used in cauterization. 2. cauterization.
**actual c.,** the application of an agent that actually burns tissue.
**chemical c.,** chemocautery.
**cold c.,** cryocautery.
**electric c., galvanic c.,** electrocautery.
**gas c.,** cauterization by means of a specially controlled jet of burning gas.
**potential c.,** cauterization by an escharotic without applying heat; called also *virtual c.*
**virtual c.,** potential c.

**ca·va** (ka'və) [L.] 1. plural of *cavum.* 2. a vena cava.

**ca·val** (kā'-vəl) pertaining to a vena cava; called also *venacaval* or *vena caval.*

**cav·a·scope** (kav'ə-skōp) [*cavum* + *-scope*] an instrument for illuminating and examining a cavity.

**CAVB** complete atrioventricular block.

**cave** (kāv) [L. *cavum*] cavum.
**Meckel's c.,** cavum trigeminale.
**c. of septum pellucidum,** cavum septi pellucidi.
**trigeminal c.,** cavum trigeminale.

**ca·ve·o·la** (ka-ve-o'lə) pl. *caveo'lae* [L.] a small pit, depression, or invagination, such as any of the minute pits or incuppings of the cell membrane formed during pinocytosis, which close and then pinch off to form small, free, fluid-filled vesicles (pinosomes) in the cytoplasm. Called also *c. intracellularis* and *plasmalemmal vesicle.*

**Cav·er·ject** (kav'ər-jekt") trademark for a preparation of alprostadil.

**cav·ern** (kav'ərn) caverna.
**c's of corpora cavernosa of penis,** cavernae corporum cavernosorum penis.
**c's of corpus spongiosum,** cavernae corporis spongiosi.
**Schnabel's c's,** glaucomatous optic atrophy with elevated intraocular pressure.

**ca·ver·na** (ka-vər'nə) pl. *caver'nae* [L.] [TA] cavern: a type of cavity.
**caver'nae cor'poris spongio'si** [TA], caverns of corpus spongiosum: the dilatable spaces within the corpus spongiosum of the penis, which fill with blood and become distended with erection.
**caver'nae cor'porum cavernoso'rum pe'nis** [TA], caverns of corpora cavernosa of penis: the dilatable spaces within the corpora cavernosa of the penis, which fill with blood and become distended with erection.

**cav·er·nil·o·quy** (kav"ər-nil'ə-kwe) [*caverna* + *loqui* to speak] cavernous voice.

**cav·er·ni·tis** (kav"ər-ni'tis) inflammation of the corpora cavernosa or corpus spongiosum of the penis.
**fibrous c.,** Peyronie's d..

**cav·er·no·sal** (kav"ər-no'səl) 1. pertaining to a corpus cavernosum. 2. cavernous.

**cav·er·no·scope** (kav'ər-nə-skōp) an instrument for viewing any cavity, as one inserted through an intercostal space into the pleural cavity.

**cav·er·nos·co·py** (kav"ər-nos'kə-pe) the inspection of a cavity with the aid of a cavernoscope.

**cav·er·no·si·tis** (kav"ər-no-si'tis) cavernitis.

**cav·er·no·sog·ra·phy** (kav"ər-no-sog'rah-fe) radiographic visualization of the corpus cavernosum of the penis.
**dynamic infusion c.,** radiographic imaging of the corporal bodies and associated vasculature following infusion of contrast medium or saline solution directly into the corpus cavernosum; used for detection of venous leaks.

**cav·er·no·som·e·try** (kav"ər-no-som'ə-tre) measurement of the vascular pressure in the corpus cavernosum.
**dynamic infusion c.,** a graphic representation of intracorporal vascular pressure as a function of infused volume.

**cav·er·nos·to·my** (kav"ər-nos'tə-me) operative incision into a cavity.

**cav·er·nous** (kav'ər-nəs) [L. *cavernosus*] 1. containing caverns or hollow spaces. 2. said of certain low-pitched auscultatory sounds due to having a cavitary resonating chamber.

**Ca·via** (ka've-ə) a genus of small South American rodents of the family Caviidae. *C. coba'ya* is the guinea pig.

**cav·i·ta·ry** (kav'ĭ-tar"e) 1. characterized by the presence of a cavity or cavities. 2. any entozoon with a body space or alimentary canal.

**cav·i·tas** (kav'ĭ-təs) pl. *cavita'tes* [L., from *cavus* hollow] [TA] cavity: a hollow space or depression within the body. Called also *cavum.*
**c. abdomina'lis,** TA alternative for *c. abdominis.*
**c. abdo'minis** [TA], abdominal cavity: the body cavity located inferior to the diaphragm and superior to the pelvis, forming the superior and major part of the abdominopelvic cavity.
**c. abdo'minis et pel'vis** [TA], abdominopelvic cavity: the space within the trunk between the diaphragm and the inferior boundary of the lesser pelvis; it is divided into the abdominal and pelvic cavities.
**c. articula'ris** [TA], articular cavity: the minute space of a synovial joint, enclosed by the synovial membrane and articular cartilages.
**c. con'chae** [TA], **c. concha'lis,** cavity of concha: the inferior part of the concha of the auricle, which leads into the external acoustic meatus; called also *cavum conchae* [TA alternative] and *innominate fossa of auricle.*
**c. coro'nae** [TA], **c. corona'lis,** pulp chamber: the portion of the dental (pulp) cavity located in the tooth crown, occupied by the dental pulp.
**c. cra'nii** [TA], cranial cavity: the space enclosed by the bones of the cranium.
**c. den'tis** [TA], dental cavity: the natural cavity in the central por-

tion of a tooth occupied by the dental pulp, which is divided into the pulp chamber *(c. coronalis)* and the root canal *(canalis radicis dentis)*; called also *c. pulparis* [TA alternative], *nerve cavity,* and *pulp cavity.*

**c. epidura'lis,** spatium epidurale.

**c. glenoida'lis** [TA], glenoid cavity: a depression in the lateral angle of the scapula for articulation with the humerus; called also *glenoid fossa of scapula.*

**c. infraglot'tica** [TA], infraglottic cavity: the most inferior part of the laryngeal cavity, extending from the rima glottidis above to the cavity of the trachea below. Called also *subglottis.*

**c. laryn'gea interme'dia,** intermediate laryngeal cavity: the smallest part of the laryngeal cavity, extending from the rima vestibuli to the rima glottidis.

**c. laryn'gis** [TA], laryngeal cavity: the space enclosed by the walls of the larynx.

**c. medulla'ris** [TA], medullary cavity: the space in the diaphysis of a long bone containing the marrow; called also *marrow cavity, medullary canal,* and *medullary space.*

**c. nasa'lis,** cavitas nasi.

**c. na'si** [TA], nasal cavity: the portion of the passages of the respiratory system extending from the nares to the pharynx. It is divided into left and right halves by the nasal septum; its floor is the hard palate, which separates it from the oral cavity; and its lateral walls contain the nasal conchae and nasal meatus.

**c. o'ris** [TA], oral cavity: the cavity of the mouth and associated structures, including the cheek, palate, oral mucosa, the glands whose ducts open into the cavity, the teeth, and the tongue.

**c. o'ris exter'na,** vestibulum oris.

**c. o'ris pro'pria** [TA], oral cavity proper: the part of the oral cavity internal to the teeth.

**c. pel'vica,** c. pelvis.

**c. pelvi'na,** TA alternative for *c. pelvis.*

**c. pel'vis** [TA], pelvic cavity: the space within the walls of the pelvis, forming the inferior and lesser part of the abdominopelvic cavity. Called also *c. pelvica* and *c. pelvina* [TA alternative].

**c. pericardi'aca** [TA], **c. pericardia'lis,** pericardial cavity: the potential space between the parietal layer and the visceral layer (epicardium) of the serous pericardium.

**c. peritonea'lis** [TA], peritoneal cavity: the potential space of capillary thinness between the parietal and the visceral peritoneum, which is normally empty except for a thin serous fluid that keeps the surfaces moist. Called also *greater peritoneal cavity.*

**c. pharyn'gis** [TA], pharyngeal cavity: the space enclosed by the walls of the pharynx.

**c. pleura'lis** [TA], pleural cavity: the potential space between the parietal and visceral pleurae. Called also *pleural space.*

**c. pulpa'ris,** TA alternative for *c. dentis.*

**c. sep'ti pellu'cidi,** cavum septi pellucidi.

**c. subarachnoi'dea, c. subarachnoidea'lis,** spatium subarachnoideum.

**c. thora'cica,** TA alternative for *c. thoracis.*

**c. thora'cis** [TA], thoracic cavity: the portion of the body cavity situated between the neck and the diaphragm; called also *c. thoracica* [TA alternative], *pectoral cavity,* and *thorax.*

**c. trigemina'le, c. trigemina'lis,** cavum trigeminale.

**c. tympa'nica, c. tym'pani** [TA], tympanic cavity: the major portion of the middle ear (auris media), consisting of a narrow air-filled cavity in the temporal bone that contains the auditory ossicles. It communicates with the mastoid air cells and the mastoid antrum via the aditus and with the nasopharynx via the auditory tube. The middle ear and the tympanic cavity were formerly regarded as being synonymous. Called also *tympanum.*

**c. u'teri** [TA], uterine cavity: the flattened space within the uterus, communicating on either side at the cornu with the uterine tubes and below with the vagina.

**cav·i·ta·tes** (kav″ĭ-ta'tēz) [L.] plural of *cavitas.*

**cav·i·ta·tion** (kav″ĭ-ta'shən) 1. the formation of pathological cavities, as in pulmonary tuberculosis. 2. a pathological cavity.

**ca·vi·tis** (ka-vi'tis) inflammation of the vena cava; called also *celophlebitis.*

**cav·i·ty** (kav'ĭ-te) [L. *cavitas*] 1. a hollow place or space, or a potential space, within the body or in one of its organs; it may be normal (called *cavitas* in anatomical nomenclature) or pathological (see *cavitation*). See also *pocket, pouch,* and *recess.* Called also *cave, cavern, caverna,* and *cavum.* 2. the lesion, or area of destruction in a tooth, produced by dental caries; classified as simple, compound, or complex, according to the number of surfaces involved. See also *dental caries,* under *caries.* 3. prepared c.

**abdominal c.,** cavitas abdominis.

**abdominopelvic c.,** *cavitas abdominis et pelvis.*

**absorption c's,** cavities in developing compact bone due to osteoclastic erosion, usually occurring in the areas laid down first.

**alveolar c's,** dental alveoli.

**amniotic c.,** the closed sac between the embryo and the amnion, containing the amniotic fluid.

**articular c.,** cavitas articulare.

**Baer's c.,** the cleavage cavity beneath the blastoderm.

**body c.,** a visceral cavity, such as the thoracic, abdominal, or pelvic cavity.

**buccal c.,** 1. that portion of the oral cavity bounded on one side by the teeth and gingivae (or the residual alveolar ridges), and on the other by the cheeks. 2. a carious lesion beginning on the buccal surface of a posterior tooth. 3. cavitas oris. 4. a preoral chamber seen in higher ciliate protozoa, manifested as an indentation or pouch containing compound ciliary organelles and leading to the cytostomal-cytopharyngeal complex. Called also *peristome.*

**cleavage c.,** the cavity of the blastula; blastocoele.

**complex c.,** a carious lesion that involves three or more surfaces of a tooth in its prepared state.

**compound c.,** a carious lesion that involves two surfaces of a tooth.

**c. of concha,** cavitas conchae.

**cotyloid c.,** acetabulum.

**cranial c.,** cavitas cranii.

**dental c.,** 1. see *cavity* (def. 2), and see under *caries.* 2. cavitas dentis.

**distal c.,** a carious lesion beginning on the distal surface of a tooth.

**epidural c.,** spatium epidurale.

**fibrotic c's,** cavities of the lung composed of granulation tissue surrounded by scar tissue, as in idiopathic pulmonary fibrosis or tuberculosis; in tuberculosis they may be the source from which the disease spreads to other pulmonary segments.

**fissure c.,** a carious lesion beginning in a fissure of a tooth. See *pit caries,* under *caries.*

**gastrovascular c.,** the body cavity of a coelenterate, which opens to the outside at one end to form a mouth; called also *coelenteron.*

**glandular c.,** a hollow sac formed by invagination of the epithelial sheath in the developing multicellular gland.

**glenoid c.,** cavitas glenoidalis.

**head c.,** modified somites that in lower vertebrates give rise to the extrinsic eye muscles.

**hemal c.,** hemocoelom.

**incisal c.,** a carious lesion beginning on the incisal surface of an anterior tooth.

**infraglottic c.,** cavitas infraglottica.

**ischioanal c., ischiorectal c.,** fossa ischioanalis.

**labial c.,** a carious lesion beginning on the labial surface of an anterior tooth.

**laryngeal c.,** cavitas laryngis.

**laryngeal c., intermediate,** cavitas laryngealis intermedia.

**laryngopharyngeal c.,** pars laryngea pharyngis.

**lingual c.,** a carious lesion beginning on the lingual surface of a tooth.

**lymph c's,** the larger lymph spaces and cisterns of the body.

**marrow c.,** cavitas medullaris.

**mastoid c.,** antrum mastoideum.

**mediastinal c., anterior,** mediastinum anterius.

**mediastinal c., middle,** mediastinum medium.

**mediastinal c., posterior,** mediastinum posterius.

**mediastinal c., superior,** mediastinum superius.

**medullary c.,** cavitas medullaris.

**mesial c.,** a carious lesion beginning on the mesial surface of a tooth.

**nasal c.,** cavitas nasi.

**nerve c.,** cavitas dentis.

**occlusal c.,** a carious iesion beginning on the occlusal surface of a posterior tooth.

**oral c.,** cavitas oris.

**oral c., external,** vestibulum oris.

**oral c., proper,** cavitas oris propria.

**orbital c.,** orbita.

**pectoral c.,** thoracic cavity; see *cavitas thoracis.*

**pelvic c.,** cavitas pelvis.

**pericardial c.,** cavitas pericardialis.

**peritoneal c., peritoneal c., greater,** cavitas peritonealis.

**peritoneal c., lesser,** bursa omentalis.

**pharyngeal c.,** cavitas pharyngis.

**pharyngolaryngeal c.,** pars laryngea pharyngis.

**pharyngonasal c.,** pars nasalis pharyngis.

**pharyngo-oral c.,** pars oralis pharyngis.

**pit c.,** see *pit caries,* under *caries.*

**pleural c.,** cavitas pleuralis.

**pleuroperitoneal c.,** the temporarily continuous coelomic cavity in the embryo, which will later be partitioned by the developing diaphragm to become the pleural and peritoneal cavities.

**popliteal c.,** fossa poplitea.

**prepared c.,** one that is produced in a tooth to support and retain the filling material and protect the tooth structure remaining after removal of all carious tissue. See also *cavity preparation,* under *preparation.*

**proximal c.,** a carious lesion beginning on a proximal (the mesial or distal) surface of a tooth.

**pulp c.**, cavitas dentis.
**rectoischiadic c.**, fossa ischioanalis.
**resorption c.**, the area excavated by the osteoclasts in the process of bone turnover.
**Retzius' c.**, spatium retropubicum.
**Rosenmüller's c.**, recessus pharyngeus.
**segmentation c.**, the blastocoele.
**c. of septum pellucidum**, cavitas septi pellucidi.
**serous c.**, a coelomic cavity, like that enclosed by the pericardium, peritoneum, or pleura, not communicating with the outside of the body, and whose lining membrane secretes a serous fluid.
**sigmoid c. of radius**, incisura ulnaris radii.
**sigmoid c. of ulna, greater**, incisura trochlearis ulnae.
**sigmoid c. of ulna, lesser**, incisura radialis ulnae.
**simple c.**, a carious lesion that involves only one surface of a tooth in its preparation, designated according to the surface involved as buccal, distal, incisal, labial, lingual, mesial, or occlusal.
**somatic c.**, the intraembryonic portion of the coelom.
**somite c.**, myocoele.
**splanchnic c.**, visceral c.
**subarachnoid c.**, spatium subarachnoideum.
**subdural c.**, spatium subdurale.
**tension c's**, cavities of the lung in which the air pressure is greater than that of the atmosphere, as in tension pneumothorax. Radiologically, they appear as large, spherical, thin-walled defects indicative of productive inflammatory reaction in the bronchus that drains the cavity or of partial stenosis due to peribronchial fibrosis.
**thoracic c.**, cavitas thoracis.
**trigeminal c.**, cavum trigeminale.
**tympanic c.**, cavitas tympanicum.
**uterine c.**, cavitas uteri.
**visceral c.**, one of the cavities of the body containing organs, such as the thoracic, abdominal, or pelvic cavity; called also *splanchnic c.*
**yolk c.**, the space between the embryonic disc and the yolk of the developing ovum of some animals.

**ca·vog·ra·phy** (ka-vog'rə-fe) venacavography.

**ca·vo·sur·face** (ka'vo-sər"fis) the surface of a cavity, as of a tooth.

**ca·vo·val·gus** (ka"vo-val'gəs) see *talipes cavovalgus.*

**ca·vo·va·rus** (ka"vo-va'rəs) see under *talipes.*

**ca·vum** (ka'vəm) pl. *ca'va* [L.] [TA] cave: a type of cavity.
**c. con'chae**, TA alternative for *cavitas conchae.*
**c. epidurale**, spatium epidurale.
**c. o'ris exter'num**, vestibulum oris.
**c. psalte'rii**, Verga's ventricle.
**c. rectoischia'dicum**, fossa ischioanalis.
**c. sep'ti pellu'cidi** [TA], cave of septum pellucidum: the median cleft between the two laminae of the septum pellucidum; called also *pseudocele* or *pseudocoele, pseudoventricle, cavity of septum pellucidum, Duncan's ventricle, fifth ventricle, ventricle of Sylvius,* or *Vieussens' ventricle.*
**c. subarachnoi'deum**, spatium subarachnoideum.
**c. trigemina'le** [TA], trigeminal cave: the small outpocketing of the dura mater surrounding the ganglion and divisions of the trigeminal nerve at the end of the petrous portion of the temporal bone; it contains the trigeminal ganglion. Called also *Meckel's space, trigeminal cavity, cavitas trigeminale,* and *cavitas trigeminalis.*

**ca·vus** (ka'vəs) [L. "hollow"] see under *talipes.*

**ca·vy** (ka've) guinea pig.

**Cay·tine** (ka'tēn) trademark for a preparation of protokylol hydrochloride.

**CB** abbreviation for L. *Chirur'giae Baccalau'reus,* Bachelor of Surgery.

**cbc** complete blood count.

**CBF** cerebral blood flow.

**CBG** corticosteroid-binding globulin; see *transcortin.*

**C3b INA** C3b inactivator, former name for complement *factor I.*

**Cbl** cobalamin. A variety of defects in the intracellular utilization of cobalamin (vitamin $B_{12}$) and the synthesis of its coenzyme forms have been denoted *CblA–CblG.*

**CBS** chronic brain syndrome.

**CC** chief complaint.

**CC 914** a thioarsenite, *p*-carbamido-phenyl-bis (carboxymethylmercapto) arsine, used in treatment of intestinal amebiasis.

**CC 1037** a thioarsenite, *p*-carbamido-phenyl-bis (2-carboxyphenylmercapto) arsine, used in intestinal amebiasis.

**cc** symbol for *cubic centimeter.*

**CCA** congenital contractural arachnodactyly; see *hereditary bone dysplasia,* under *dysplasia.*

**CCAT** conglutinating complement absorption test.

**CCF** crystal-induced chemotactic factor.

**CCK** cholecystokinin.

**CCK-179** the methanesulfonate salts of equal parts of dihydroergocornine, dihydroergocristine, and dihydroergocryptine, used as an antihypertensive and as a vasodilator in the treatment of peripheral vascular diseases.

**c cm** symbol for *cubic centimeter.*

**CCNU** lomustine.

**CCP** complement control protein.

**CCPD** continuous cycling peritoneal dialysis.

**CCU** critical care unit.

**CD** cadaveric donor; conjugata diagonalis; curative dose; cluster designation (see under *antigen* and *system*).

**$CD_{50}$** median curative dose; a dose that abolishes symptoms in 50 per cent of the test subjects.

**Cd** 1. chemical symbol for *cadmium.* 2. abbreviation for *caudal* or *coccygeal;* used in vertebral formulas.

**cd** candela.

**2-CdA** cladribine.

**CDC** Centers for Disease Control and Prevention.

**CDC/AIDS** see *acquired immunodeficiency syndrome,* under *syndrome.*

**CDDP** cisplatin (*cis*-diamminedichloroplatinum).

**cdf** cumulative distribution function.

**cDNA** complementary DNA or copy DNA.

**CDP** cytidine diphosphate.

**CDP·di·ac·yl·glyc·er·ol** (di-a"səl-glis'ər-ol) cytidine diphosphate carrying a diacylglycerol moiety; it is a key intermediate in the synthesis and resynthesis of phospholipids.

**CDP·di·ac·yl·glyc·er·ol–ino·si·tol 3-phos·pha·ti·dyl·trans·fer·ase** (di-a"səl-glis'ər-ol in-o'sĭ-tol fos"fə-ti"dəl-trans'fər-ās) [EC 2.7.8.11] an enzyme of the transferase class that catalyzes the formation of phosphatidylinositol from *myo*-inositol and the diacylglycerol moiety of CDPdiacylglycerol.

**Ce** symbol for *cerium.*

**CEA** carcinoembryonic antigen.

**ce·as·mic** (se-as'mik) [Gr. *keasma* chip] characterized by the persistence after birth of embryonic fissures.

**ce·bo·ceph·a·lus** (se"bo-sef'ə-ləs) a fetus exhibiting cebocephaly.

**ce·bo·ceph·a·ly** (se"bo-sef'ə-le) [Gr. *kebos* monkey + *-cephaly*] a developmental anomaly characterized by a monkey-like head, the nose being defective and the eyes close together.

**ce·ca** (se'kə) [L.] plural of *cecum.*

**ce·cal** (se'kəl) [L. *caecalis*] 1. ending in a blind passage. 2. pertaining to the cecum.

**ce·cec·to·my** (se-sek'tə-me) [*ceco-* + *-ectomy*] surgical removal of the cecum.

**Ce·cil's operation** (se'səlz) [Arthur Bond *Cecil,* American surgeon, 1885–1967] see under *operation.*

**ce·ci·tis** (se-si'tis) inflammation of the cecum; called also *typhlitis.*

**Cec·lor** (se'klor) trademark for preparations of .cefaclor

**cec(o)-** [L. *cecum,* q.v.] a combining form denoting relation to the cecum.

**ce·co·cele** (se'ko-sēl) a hernia containing part of the cecum.

**ce·co·cen·tral** (se"ko-sen'trəl) centrocecal.

**ce·co·col·ic** (se"ko-kol'ik) pertaining to the cecum and the colon.

**ce·co·co·lon** (se"ko-ko'lən) the cecum and colon considered as a unit.

**ce·co·co·lo·pexy** (se"ko-ko'lə-pek"se) an operation for fixing the cecum and ascending colon to the abdominal wall.

**ce·co·co·los·to·my** (se"ko-kə-los'tə-me) the surgical creation of an anastomosis between the cecum and the colon; also, the anastomosis so constructed. Called also *colocecostomy.*

**ce·co·fix·a·tion** (se"ko-fik-sa'shən) cecopexy.

**ce·co·il·e·ost·o·my** (se"ko-il"e-os'tə-me) [*ceco-* + *ileostomy*] ileocecostomy.

**Ce·con** (se'kon) trademark for preparations of ascorbic acid.

**ce·co·pexy** (se'ko-pek'se) [*ceco-* + *-pexy*] fixation or suspension of the cecum to correct excessive mobility of the organ; called also *cecofixation.*

**ce·co·pli·ca·tion** (se″ko-plĭ-ka′shən) [*ceco-* + *plication*] plication of the cecal wall to correct ptosis or dilatation of the organ.

**ce·cor·rha·phy** (se-kor′ə-fe) [*ceco-* + *-rrhaphy*] suture or repair of the cecum.

**ce·co·sig·moid·os·to·my** (se″ko-sig″moi-dos′tə-me) formation of an artificial opening between the cecum and sigmoid, usually by surgical procedure; also, the opening so constructed.

**ce·cos·to·my** (se-kos′tə-me) [*ceco-* + *-stomy*] [MeSH: Cecostomy] the surgical creation of an artificial opening or fistula into the cecum; also, the opening so constructed.

**ce·cot·o·my** (se-kot′ə-me) [*ceco-* + *-tomy*] the operation of cutting into the cecum.

**ce·cum** (se′kəm) [L. *caecum* blind, blind gut] [MeSH: Cecum] 1. any blind pouch or cul-de-sac. 2. *caecum*.
**gastric ceca,** outpocketings of the midgut, of uncertain function, seen in many insects.
**high c.,** a cecum situated higher up in the abdomen than normal.
**mobile c., c. mo′bile,** abnormal mobility of the cecum and lower portion of the ascending colon, caused by incomplete rotation or faulty fixation of the cecum in embryonic development.

**ce·dar** (se′dər) 1. one of the true cedars, evergreen trees of the genus *Cedrus*. 2. any of numerous coniferous evergreen trees resembling those of the genus *Cedrus*, especially from the genera *Juniperus* and *Thuja*.
**red c.,** *Juniperus virginiana*.
**western red c.,** *Thuja plicata*.
**white c.,** *Thuja occidentalis*.

**Ce·dax** (se′daks) trademark for a preparation of ceftibuten.

**Ce·de·cea** (se-de′se-ə) [named for *Ce*nters for *D*isease *C*ontrol, Atlanta, Georgia] a genus of gram-negative, facultatively anaerobic, rod-shaped bacteria of the family Enterobacteriaceae, isolated primarily from clinical specimens of the human respiratory tract, and a possible opportunistic pathogen. The type species is *C. da′visae*.

**Ce·di·lan·id** (se″dĭ-lan′id) trademark for a preparation of lanatoside C.

**Ce·di·lan·id-D** (se″dĭ-lan′id) trademark for a preparation of deslanoside.

**Ce·dio·psyl·la** (se″de-o-sil′ə) a genus of fleas, including some of the rabbit fleas.

**CeeNU** trademark for preparations of lomustine.

**cef·a·clor** (sef′ə-klor) [MeSH: Cefaclor] a semisynthetic, second-generation cephalosporin effective against a wide range of gram-positive and gram-negative bacteria, used in the treatment of infections of the urinary and respiratory tracts and of the skin and soft tissues; administered orally.

**cef·a·drox·il** (sef″ə-droks′il) [USP] [MeSH: Cefadroxil] a semisynthetic cephalosporin antibiotic.

**Cef·a·dyl** (sef′ə-dəl) trademark for a preparation of cephapirin sodium.

**cef·a·man·dole** (sef″ə-man′dōl) [MeSH: Cefamandole] a semisynthetic cephalosporin antibiotic.
**c. nafate** [USP], the monosodium salt of cefamandole.

**cef·a·pa·role** (sef′ə-pə-rōl″) a semisynthetic cephalosporin antibiotic.

**cef·a·tri·zine** (sef″ə-tri′zēn) [MeSH: Cefatrizine] a semisynthetic cephalosporin antibiotic.

**ce·faz·a·flur so·di·um** (sə-faz′ə-flər) a semisynthetic cephalosporin antibiotic.

**ce·faz·o·lin** (sə-faz′o-lin) [MeSH: Cefazolin] a semisynthetic analogue of the natural antibiotic cephalosporin C, effective against a wide range of gram-negative and gram-positive bacteria.
**c. sodium** [USP], the monosodium salt of cefazolin, having the same actions as the base; used in the treatment of infections of the respiratory tract, genitourinary tract, skin, soft tissues, bones, joints, and blood due to sensitive pathogens; administered intramuscularly and intravenously.

**ce·fix·ime** (sə-fik′sēm) [USP] a third-generation, semisynthetic cephalosporin effective against a wide range of bacteria, used in the treatment of otitis media and bronchitis; administered orally.

**Cef·i·zox** (sef′ĭ-zoks) trademark for a preparation of ceftizoxime sodium.

**cef·men·ox·ime hy·dro·chlo·ride** (sef″men-ok′sēm) [USP] a third-generation cephalosporin structurally related to cefotaxime and ceftizoxime, and having actions and uses similar to those of cefotaxime sodium; administered intramuscularly and intravenously.

**cef·met·a·zole** (sef-met′ə-zōl) [USP] [MeSH: Cefmetazole] a cephamycin antibiotic derived from cephamycin C and generally classified with the second-generation cephalosporins, having activity and uses similar to those of cefoxitin.
**c. sodium** [USP], the monosodium salt of cefmetazole, having the same actions and uses as the base.

**Cef·o·bid** (sef′o-bid) trademark for preparations of cefoperazone sodium.

**ce·fon·i·cid so·di·um** (sə-fon′ĭ-sid) [USP] a semisynthetic, broad-spectrum, $\beta$-lactamase–resistant cephalosporin effective against a wide range of gram-positive and gram-negative bacteria; administered parenterally.

**cef·o·per·a·zone so·di·um** (sef″o-per′ə-zōn) [USP] a semisynthetic, broad-spectrum, $\beta$-lactamase–resistant cephalosporin antibiotic effective against a wide range of aerobic and anaerobic gram-positive and gram-negative bacteria.

**ce·for·a·nide** (sə-for′ə-nīd) [USP] a semisynthetic cephalosporin antibiotic with actions and uses similar to those of cefamandole; administered intramuscularly or intravenously.

**Cef·o·tan** (sef′o-tan) trademark for preparations of cefotetan disodium.

**cef·o·tax·ime** (sef″o-tak′sēm) [MeSH: Cefotaxime] a semisynthetic broad-spectrum cephalosporin antibiotic effective against many organisms that have become resistant to penicillin, cephalosporin, and aminoglycoside antibiotics.
**c. sodium** [USP], the sodium salt of cefotaxime, having the same actions as the base.

**cef·o·te·tan** (sef′o-te″tən) [USP] [MeSH: Cefotetan] a semisynthetic cephamycin derived from cephamycin C and generally classified with the second-generation cephalosporins, effective against a wide range of gram-positive, gram-negative, and anaerobic bacteria.
**c. disodium** [USP], the disodium salt of cefotetan, used for the treatment of a wide variety of infections caused by susceptible organisms; administered intravenously or intramuscularly.

**cef·o·ti·am hy·dro·chlo·ride** (sef″o-ti′əm) [USP] a cephalosporin antibiotic having actions and uses similar to those of cefamandole; administered intramuscularly and intravenously.

**ce·fox·i·tin** (sə-fok′sĭ-tin) [MeSH: Cefoxitin] a cephamycin antibiotic derived from cephamycin C and generally classified with the second-generation cephalosporins, effective against a wide range of gram-positive and gram-negative organisms, with strong resistance to $\beta$-lactamase.
**c. sodium** [USP], the monosodium salt of cefoxitin, used to treat infections caused by susceptible organisms; administered intramuscularly or intravenously.

**cef·pir·a·mide** (sef-pir′ə-mīd) [USP] a third-generation cephalosporin structurally related to cefoperazone, effective against *Pseudomonas aeruginosa*, staphylococci, and streptococci; administered by injection.

**cef·po·dox·ime prox·e·til** (sef″po-dok′sēm prok′sə-til) a broad-spectrum $\beta$-lactamase–resistant cephalosporin, effective against a wide range of gram-positive and gram-negative bacteria; administered orally.

**cef·pro·zil** (sef-pro′zil) [USP] a semisynthetic broad-spectrum cephalosporin effective against a wide range of gram-negative and gram-positive organisms, used in the treatment of infections of the respiratory tract and skin; administered orally.

**cef·ta·zi·dime** (sef′ta-zĭ-dēm″) [USP] [MeSH: Ceftazidime] a semisynthetic, broad-spectrum, $\beta$-lactam antibiotic, which acts by inhibiting enzymes responsible for cell-wall synthesis; effective against gram-positive and gram-negative bacteria.

**cef·ti·bu·ten** (sef-ti′bu-tən) an antibacterial compound used in the treatment of bronchitis, pharyngitis, tonsillitis, and acute otitis media; administered orally.

**Cef·tin** (sef′tin) trademark for a preparation of cefuroxime axetil.

**cef·ti·o·fur so·di·um** (sef-ti′o-foor) a semisynthetic cephalosporin used in cattle.

**cef·ti·zox·ime so·di·um** (sef″tĭ-zok′sēm) [USP] a semisynthetic, broad-spectrum, $\beta$-lactamase–resistant cephalosporin antibiotic effective against a wide range of aerobic and anaerobic gram-positive and gram-negative bacteria.

**cef·tri·ax·one so·di·um** (sef″tri-ak′sōn) [USP] a semisynthetic, $\beta$-lactamase–resistant, broad-spectrum cephalosporin antibiotic effective against a wide range of gram-positive and gram-negative bacteria.

**cef·u·rox·ime** (sef″u-rok′sēm) [MeSH: Cefuroxime] a semisynthetic, broad-spectrum, $\beta$-lactamase–resistant cephalosporin effective against a wide range of gram-positive and gram-negative bacteria.
**c. axetil** [USP], an ester of cefuroxime with increased lipid solubility and better gastrointestinal absorption, for oral administration.

**c. sodium** [USP], the monosodium salt of cefuroxime, used in the treatment of infections by susceptible organisms.

**Cef•zil** (sef'zil) trademark for a preparation of cefprozil.

**Ceg•ka's sign** (cheg'kahz) [Josephus Joannes *Cegka*, Czech physician, 1812–1862] see under *sign*.

**Cel** Celsius (thermometric scale).

**cel** (sel) a unit of velocity, being the velocity of 1 cm. per second.

**ce•la•ri•um** (sə-lar'e-əm) mesothelium.

**Cel•be•nin** (sel'bə-nin) trademark for preparations of methicillin sodium.

**-cele**[1] [Gr. *kēlē* hernia] a word termination denoting relationship to a tumor or swelling.

**-cele**[2] [Gr. *koilia* cavity] a word termination denoting relationship to a cavity; see also words spelled *-coele*.

**Cel•e•brex** (sel'ə-breks) trademark for a preparation of celecoxib.

**cel•e•cox•ib** (sel"ə-kok'sib) a nonsteroidal antiinflammatory drug that inhibits cyclooxygenase-1 activity, used for the symptomatic treatment of osteoarthritis and rheumatoid arthritis; administered orally.

**ce•len•ter•on** (sə-len'tər-on) 1. archenteron. 2. gastrovascular cavity.

**Ce•les•tone** (sə-les'tōn) trademark for preparations of betamethasone.

**Ce•lex•a** (sə-lek'sə) trademark for a preparation of citalopram hydrobromide.

**ce•li•ac** (se'le-ak) abdominal.

**ce•li•ec•to•my** (se"le-ek'tə-me) [*celi-* + *-ectomy*] surgical removal of an abdominal organ.

**celi(o)-** [Gr. *koilia* belly] a combining form denoting relationship to the abdomen. For words beginning thus, see also words beginning *cel(o)-* and *coel(o)-*.

**ce•lio•cen•te•sis** (se"le-o-sen-te'sis) [*celio-* + *-centesis*] abdominocentesis.

**ce•lio•col•pot•o•my** (se"le-o-kol-pot'ə-me) [*celio-* + *colpo-* + *-tomy*] incision into the abdomen through the vaginal wall.

**ce•lio•en•ter•ot•o•my** (se"le-o-en"tər-ot'ə-me) [*celio-* + *enterotomy*] incision through the abdominal wall into the intestine.

**ce•lio•gas•trot•o•my** (se"le-o-gas-trot'ə-me) [*celio-* + *gastrotomy*] laparogastrotomy.

**ce•lio•hys•ter•ec•to•my** (se"le-o-his"tə-rek'tə-me) [*celio-* + *hysterectomy*] abdominal hysterectomy.

**ce•li•o•ma** (se"le-o'mə) [*celio-* + *-oma*] a tumor of the abdomen, especially mesothelioma of the peritoneum.

**ce•lio•myo•mec•to•my** (se"le-o-mi"o-mek'tə-me) [*celio-* + *myomectomy*] abdominal myomectomy.

**ce•lio•myo•mot•o•my** (se"le-o-mi"o-mot'ə-me) [*celio-* + *myomotomy*] incision into a muscular organ or tumor through the abdominal wall.

**ce•lio•myo•si•tis** (se"le-o-mi"o-si'tis) [*celio-* + *myositis*] inflammation of the abdominal muscles.

**ce•lio•para•cen•te•sis** (se"le-o-par"ə-sen-te'sis) [*celio-* + *paracentesis*] abdominocentesis.

**ce•li•op•a•thy** (se"le-op'ə-the) [*celio-* + *-pathy*] any abdominal disease.

**ce•li•or•rha•phy** (se"le-or'ə-fe) [*celio-* + *-rrhaphy*] laparorrhaphy.

**ce•lio•sal•pin•gec•to•my** (se"le-o-sal"pin-jek'tə-me) [*celio-* + *salpingectomy*] laparosalpingectomy.

**ce•lio•sal•pin•got•o•my** (se"le-o-sal"pin-got'ə-me) laparosalpingotomy.

**ce•lio•scope** (se'le-o-skōp") laparoscope.

**ce•li•os•co•py** (se"le-os'kə-pe) laparoscopy.

**ce•li•ot•o•my** (se"le-ot'ə-me) [*celio-* + *-tomy*] surgical incision into the abdominal cavity. Called also *laparotomy* and *peritoneotomy*.
**vaginal c.,** incision into the abdominal cavity through the vagina.
**ventral c.,** incision into the abdominal cavity through the abdominal wall.

**ce•li•tis** (se-li'tis) any abdominal inflammation.

**cell** (sel) [L. *cella* compartment] [MeSH: Cells] 1. any of the minute protoplasmic masses that make up organized tissue, consisting of a nucleus which is surrounded by cytoplasm which contains the various organelles and is enclosed in the cell or plasma membrane. A cell is the fundamental, structural, and functional unit of living organisms. See Plates 13 and 14. In some of the lower forms of life, e.g., bacteria, a morphological nucleus is absent, although nucleoproteins (and genes) are present. 2. a small, more or less enclosed space.

## Cell

**A c.,** 1. alpha cell (def. 1). 2. acidophil. 3. (in plural) amacrine cells.
**absorptive c., intestinal,** one of the cells of the intestinal epithelium, having a brush border made up of many closely packed parallel microvilli, and believed to be associated with absorption, particularly of macromolecules.
**accessory c's,** cells, predominantly of the monocyte-macrophage lineage, that cooperate with B and T lymphocytes in the generation of the immune response.
**acid c's,** parietal c's.
**acinar c., acinic c., acinous c.,** any of the cells lining an acinus, especially applied to the zymogen-secreting cells of the pancreatic acini.
**acoustic hair c.,** any one of the cells provided with cilia that serve as sensory receptors in the organ of Corti; called also *auditory c.*
**adipose c.,** a fat cell.
**adventitial c.,** pericyte.
**agger nasi c's,** the cells of the anterior part of the ethmoid crest, constituting the pneumatized portion of the lacrimal bone.
**air c.,** 1. any minute bodily chamber filled with air, such as an alveolus of the lung. 2. a cavity containing air and surrounded by a bodily structure, usually one of the bones of the head, such as an ethmoidal air cell, mastoid air cell, or tubal air cell.
**air c's, anterior ethmoidal,** sinus ethmoidales anteriores.
**air c's, mastoid,** cellulae mastoideae.
**air c's, middle ethmoidal,** sinus ethmoidales medii.
**air c's, posterior ethmoidal,** sinus ethmoidales posteriores.
**air c's, tubal,** cellulae pneumaticae tubae auditivae.
**air c's of auditory tube,** cellulae pneumaticae tubae auditivae.
**albuminous c.,** serous c.
**algoid c's,** cells resembling algae, seen in cases of chronic diarrhea.
**alpha c.,** 1. one of the cells in the periphery of the pancreatic islets that secrete somatostatin (alpha$_1$ cells) and glucagon (alpha$_2$ cells). 2. acidophil (def. 2).
**alveolar c.,** any cell of the walls of the pulmonary alveoli; the term is often limited to alveolar epithelial cells (type I and type II alveolar cells) and alveolar macrophages. Called also *pneumocyte* and *pneumonocyte*.
**alveolar c's, great,** type II alveolar c's.
**alveolar c's, large,** type II alveolar c's.
**alveolar c's, small,** type I alveolar c's.
**alveolar c's, squamous,** type I alveolar c's.
**alveolar c's, type I,** the flattened cells of the alveolar epithelium, distinguished by their greatly attenuated cytoplasm and paucity of organelles; called also *membranous pneumonocytes* and *squamous* or *small alveolar cells*.
**alveolar c's, type II,** pleomorphic cells of the pulmonary alveolar epithelium that secrete surfactant and are distinguished by abundant cytoplasm containing numerous lipid-rich multilamellar bodies; called also *granular pneumonocytes* and *great* or *large alveolar cells*.
**alveolar epithelial c's,** the cells of the alveolar epithelium; see *type I alveolar c's* and *type II alveolar c's*.
**Alzheimer's c's,** 1. giant astrocytes with large, prominent nuclei found in the brain in hepatolenticular degeneration and hepatic coma. 2. degenerated astrocytes.
**amacrine c's,** five types of retinal neurons that seem to lack large axons, having only processes that resemble dendrites. Called also *A c's*.
**ameboid c.,** any cell that is able to change its form and move about; called also *amebocyte, migratory c., wandering c.,* and *planocyte*.
**amine precursor uptake and decarboxylation c's,** APUD c's.
**amphophilic c.,** one that stains readily with either acid or basic dyes; called also *amphocyte, amphophil, amphochromatophil,* and *amphochromophil*.

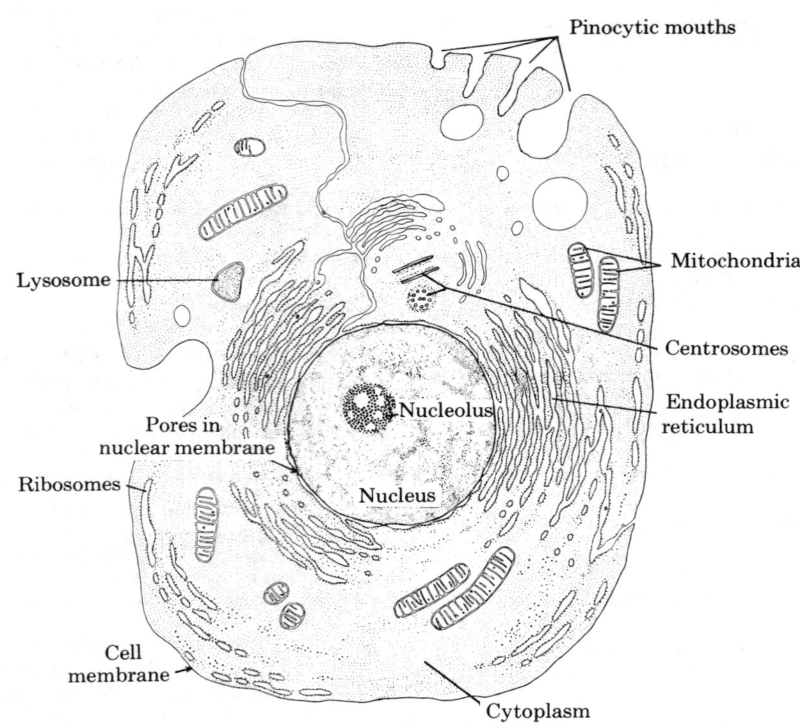


TYPICAL ANIMAL CELL

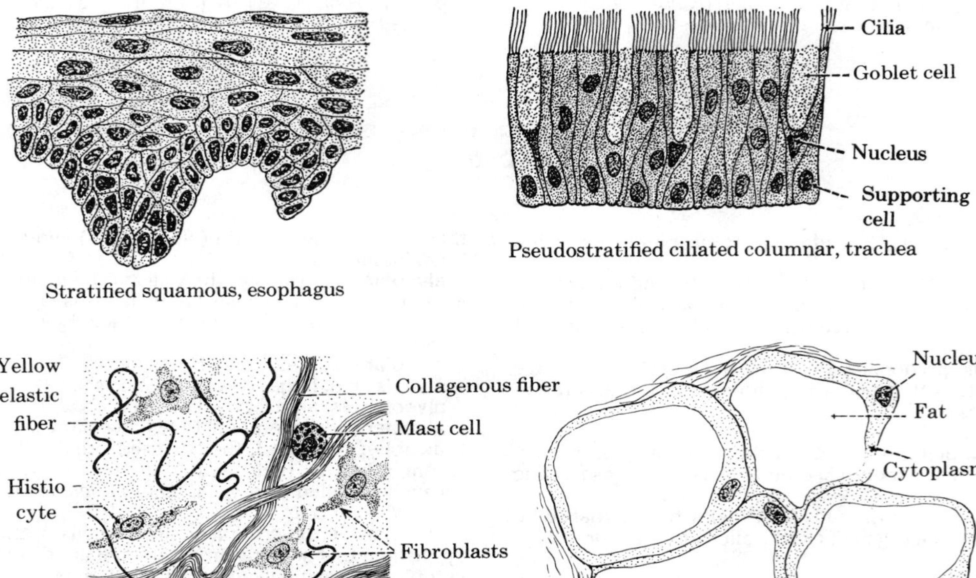


VARIOUS TYPES OF EPITHELIAL CELL

**PLATE 13**—THE CELL: CELL STRUCTURES AND EPITHELIAL CELL TYPES

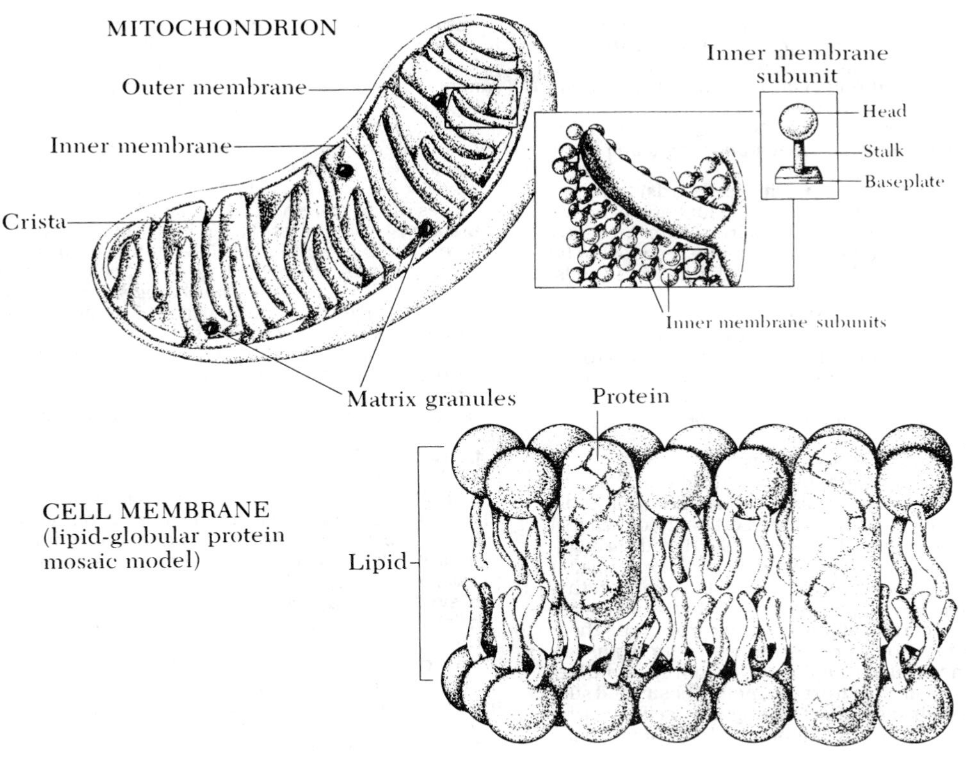


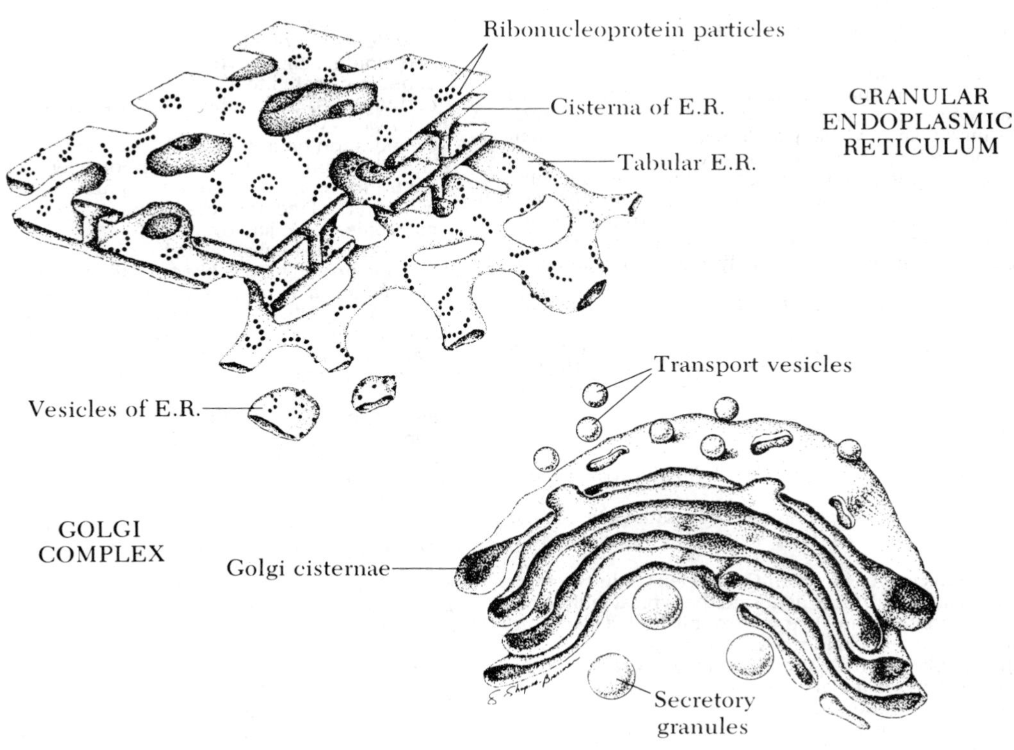


**PLATE 14**—CELL ORGANELLES AND CELL MEMBRANE

**Anichkov's (Anitschkow's) c.,** a plump modified macrophage found in the Aschoff bodies, inflammatory lesions of the heart characteristic of rheumatic fever; they contain round to ovoid nuclei with a central, slender, caterpillar-like ribbon of chromatin. Called also *Anichkov's myocyte, cardiac histiocyte,* and *caterpillar c.*

**anterior horn c's,** motoneurons whose cell bodies are in the anterior horn of the spinal cord; see *alpha motoneuron* and *gamma motoneuron.*

**antigen-presenting c's,** a group of dendritic cells arising in the bone marrow and migrating to other body sites, the function of which seems to be the retention of antigens on their surfaces for presentation to the lymphocytes, thereby inducing an immune response. The group includes follicular dendritic cells, interdigitating cells, veil cells, and Langerhans cells.

**antigen-reactive c's,** 1. T lymphocytes that rapidly proliferate in response to challenge by antigen. 2. antigen-sensitive c's.

**antigen-sensitive c's,** small lymphocytes that when exposed to antigen can differentiate into antibody-producing cells. Called also *antigen-reactive c's.*

**antipodal c's,** a group of four cells in the early embryo.

**apocrine c's,** see *apocrine.*

**apolar c.,** a neuron with no processes or poles.

**APUD c's** [*a*mine *p*recursor *u*ptake and *d*ecarboxylation], amine precursor uptake and decarboxylation cells: a diffuse group of cells, many originating in the neural crest, that share certain cytochemical and ultrastructural characteristics and are found scattered throughout the body; types include melanocytes, the cells of the chromaffin system, and cells in the hypothalamus, hypophysis, thyroid, parathyroids, lungs, gastrointestinal tract, and pancreas. They concentrate the amino acid precursors of certain amines and decarboxylate them to form the amines, which function as regulators and neurotransmitters. They produce substances such as epinephrine, norepinephrine, dopamine, serotonin, enkephalin, somatostatin, neurotensin, and substance P, the actions of which may affect contiguous cells, nearby groups of cells, or distant cells, thus functioning as local or systemic hormones. See also *basal granular c's.*

**argentaffin c's,** enterochromaffin cells (q.v.) whose granules stain readily with chromium and silver salts, located in the basilar portions of the glands of the gastrointestinal tract. Based upon their staining reactions with silver, these cells have been divided into two groups: those that reduce silver without pretreatment *(argentaffin c's),* and those that require prior exposure to a reducing substance *(argyrophilic c's).* See also *argentaffinoma.*

**argyrophilic c's,** enterochromaffin cells that require exposure to a reducing substance before their granules will react with silver; they are located in the fundic and pyloric glands between the basement lamina and zymogenic cells. See also *argentaffin c's.*

**Arias-Stella c's,** cells in the endometrial epithelium which have hyperchromatic enlarged nuclei; they appear to be hypersecretory and associated with chorionic tissue in an intrauterine or extrauterine site.

**Armanni-Ebstein c's,** vacuolated epithelial cells in the proximal straight renal tubule containing deposits of glycogen; see also under *lesion.*

**Aschoff c.,** Anichkov's cell, particularly in the larger, multinucleate giant cell form.

**Askanazy c's,** large granular eosinophilic cells, rich in mitochondria, found in the thyroid gland in autoimmune thyroiditis and Hürthle cell tumors. Called also *Hürthle c's, interfollicular c's, oxyphil c's,* and *oxyphils.*

**auditory c.,** acoustic hair c.

**automatic c.,** pacemaker c.

**B c.,** 1. beta c. (def. 1). 2. basophil (def. 3). 3. (in plural) see under *lymphocyte.*

**balloon c's,** unusual swollen degenerated cells with pale, almost clear, abundant cytoplasm, such as those seen in the vesicles of herpes zoster or varicella.

**band c.,** a late metamyelocyte in which the nucleus is in the form of a curved or coiled band, not having acquired the typical multilobar shape of the mature polymorphonuclear neutrophil. Called also *band form* or *neutrophil, rod neutrophil,* and *stab c.* or *neutrophil.*

**basal c.,** the name applied to the early keratinocyte, present in the basal layer of the epidermis; called also *foot cell.*

**basal granular c's,** enteroendocrine c's.

**basket c.,** 1. a cell of the cerebellar cortex whose axon gives off brushes of fibrils, forming a basket-like nest in which the body of each Purkinje cell rests. 2. myoepithelial c.

**beaker c.,** goblet c.

**Beale's ganglion c's,** bipolar cells with one process coiled around the other; found in cardiac ganglia.

**Bergmann's c's,** peculiar glial cells in the molecular layer of the cerebellar cortex having dendrites that extend outward through that layer; called also *Bergmann's glia.*

**berry c.,** Mott c.

**beta c.,** 1. one of the cells that compose the bulk of the islets of Langerhans and secrete insulin. 2. basophil (def. 3).

**Betz's c's,** large pyramidal ganglion cells found in the internal pyramidal layer of the cerebral cortex; called also *giant pyramidal c's.*

**bipolar c.,** a nerve cell with two processes.

**bipolar retinal c's,** various types of bipolar neurons that are the second, intermediate, neurons in the vertical linkage of the retina and are analogous to the spinal ganglia. See also *visual c's.*

**bladder c's,** swollen cells in the epidermis of the tips of the fingers and toes of the embryo. Called also *Zander's c's.*

**blast c.,** 1. blast[1] (def. 1). 2. in the monophyletic theory, the least differentiated, totipotential blood cell without commitment as to its particular series, from which all blood cells are derived, preceding a *stem cell.* Called also *blast, hematoblast, hematocytoblast, hemoblast,* and *hemocytoblast.* Formerly used terms include *hematogone, hematohistioblast,* and *hemohistioblast.*

**blood c.,** one of the formed elements of the blood; a leukocyte, erythrocyte, or platelet. Called also *blood corpuscle, hemacyte, hematocyte,* and *hemocyte.*

**bone c.,** a nucleated cell occupying a lacuna of bone; called also *osseous c.* and *bone corpuscle.*

**border c's,** 1. a row of columnar supporting cells that delimit the inner boundary of the organ of Corti. 2. parietal c's.

**Böttcher's c's,** small groups of polyhedral cells interposed between Claudius' cells and the basilar membrane of the cochlea.

**bowenoid c's,** neoplastic cells derived from the epidermis, which constitute lesions of intraepidermal squamous cell carcinoma (Bowen's disease).

**breviradiate c's,** neuroglial cells that have short processes.

**bristle c's,** the hair cells associated with the cochlear nerve.

**brood c.,** mother c.

**burr c.,** a spiculed erythrocyte that has multiple small projections evenly spaced over the cell circumference; observed in azotemia, gastric carcinoma, and bleeding peptic ulcer. Called also *burr erythrocyte, crenated erythrocyte, crenocyte,* and *echinocyte.*

**C c's,** 1. parafollicular c's. 2. a type of cells that lack granules, found especially in the pancreatic islets in guinea pigs. 3. chromophobe c's.

**Cajal c.,** 1. astrocyte. 2. one of the neuroglial cells arranged horizontally in the molecular layer of the cerebral cortex; called also *horizontal c. of Cajal.*

**caliciform c.,** goblet c.

**cameloid c.,** elliptocyte.

**capsule c.,** satellite c., def. 1.

**cartilage c's,** cells embedded in the lacunae of the cartilages; called also *chondrocyte.*

**Caspersson type B c's,** cells rich in nucleolar ribonucleic acid and relatively poor in nuclear deoxyribonucleic acid.

**castration c's,** vacuolated basophil cells that develop in the anterior pituitary gland after castration.

**caterpillar c.,** Anichkov's c.

**caudate c's,** neuroglial cells of the gray matter having several streaming prolongations like the tail of a comet.

**caveolated c's,** epithelial cells with thick, short, apical microvilli containing bundles of filaments extending down into the cytoplasm and with irregular tubules (caveolae) passing as invaginations from the apical surface between microvilli; occasionally found in the small intestine and respiratory tract and thought to function as chemoreceptors.

**cement c.,** cementocyte.

**central c.,** chief c's (def. 1).

**centroacinar c's,** the beginnings of the intralobular duct system of the pancreas within the pancreatic acini.

**chalice c.,** goblet c.

**chief c's,** 1. epithelial cells, either columnar or cuboidal, that line the lower portions of the gastric glands and secrete pepsin; called also *central c's, Heidenhain's c's, peptic c's,* and *zymogenic c's.* 2. pinealocytes. 3. the most abundant cells of the parathyroid glands, being polygonal epithelial cells rich in glycogen, having granular cytoplasm and vesicular nuclei, and arranged in plates or cords.They are sometimes divided between the more numerous *clear cells* that have clear cytoplasm, large nuclei, and few granules, and *dark cells* that have cytoplasm with smaller, darker nuclei and many fine granules; intermediate forms also exist. Called also *principal c's.* 4. the principal chromaffin cells of the paraganglia, each of which is surrounded by supporting cells. 5. chromophobe c's.

**Chinese hamster ovary c's, CHO c's,** an established line of fibroblasts isolated from the ovary of a spontaneous aneuploid mutant Chinese hamster; used in a variety of biomedical applications.

**chromaffin c's,** a type of APUD cells that stain readily with chromium salts, their cytoplasmic granules taking on a characteristic brown color; they are found especially in cells of the adrenal medulla and in paraganglia of the coccygeal gland and carotid gland, along the sympathetic nerves, and in various organs. They contain chromaffin granules. See also *enterochromaffin c's* and *argentaffin c's.* Called also *pheochrome cells* and *pheochromocytes.*

**chromophobe c's, chromophobic c's,** small, faintly staining cells with scanty cytoplasm found often in clusters in the center of the cell cords in the adenohypophysis; their cytoplasm was formerly thought to be nongranular, but the granules are now known to be simply small and sparse. These cells are increased in chromophobic or null-cell adenomas. Called also *C c's, chief c's,* and *gamma c's of hypophysis.*

**ciliated c.,** any cell with cilia.

**Clara c's,** unciliated cells found in the epithelium of the respiratory and terminal bronchioles.

**Clarke's c's,** pigmented cells in the thoracic column of the spinal cord.

**Claudius' c's,** cuboidal cells found in the floor of the external spiral sulcus, external to the organ of Corti.

**clear c's,** cells with empty-appearing cytoplasm.

**cleavage c.,** any one of the cells derived from the zygote by mitosis; a blastomere.

**cleaved c.,** see *follicular center c., small cleaved* and *follicular center c., large cleaved.*

**clump c's,** round, thick, pigmented cells seen in the sphincter muscle of the iris.

**collenchyma c's,** elongated living cells with walls thickened in the corners, which compose the collenchyma of plants. Cf. *sclerenchyma c's.*

**columnar c.,** an elongate epithelial cell.

**commissural c's,** heteromeral c's.

**committed c.,** a lymphocyte which, after contact with antigen, is obligated to follow an individual course of development. In the bone marrow, these arise from pluripotential stem cells and themselves form precursor lines for various blood cells.

**compound granule c.,** gitter c.

**cone c.,** retinal cone.

**conidiogenous c.,** a fungal cell that produces a conidium; see also *conidiogenesis.*

**connective tissue c's,** a general name for the cellular elements of the fibrous and nonfibrous components of the various forms of connective tissue.

**contractile fiber c's,** the spindle-shaped and nucleated cells which, collected into bundles, make up unstriated or smooth muscle.

**contrasuppressor c's,** cells that augment the immune response by suppressing the activity of other suppressor cells, or by rendering the reactive cell unresponsive to suppression.

**corneal c.,** a modified connective tissue cell occupying each corneal space.

**c. of Corti,** acoustic hair c.

**corticotrope c., corticotroph c.,** corticotroph.

**corticotroph-lipotroph c.,** corticotroph.

**corticotropic c.,** corticotroph.

**counting c.,** hemacytometer.

**cover c.,** any cell that covers and protects other cells, especially any long epithelial cell of the outer layer of the taste buds; called also *encasing c.* and *incasing c.*

**crescent c's,** crescents of Giannuzzi.

**cribrate c.,** a cell whose walls are perforated with numerous sieve-like pores.

**Crooke's c's,** the pituitary corticotrophs seen in Crooke's hyalinization.

**cuboid c.,** an epithelial cell of which the transverse and vertical diameters are approximately equal.

**Custer c's,** cells with long delicate protoplasmic processes replacing the lymphoid tissue of lymph nodes in reticuloendothelial disease.

**cylindric c.,** columnar c.

**cytotoxic T c's,** cytotoxic T lymphocytes.

**cytotrophoblastic c's,** polygonal, mononucleate cells resembling the cells of the cytotrophoblast, having prominent nucleoli and clear, eosinophilic or cyanophilous cytoplasm; one of the two cell types that compose a choriocarcinoma. Cf. *syncytiotrophoblastic c's.*

**D c.,** delta cell (def. 1).

**daughter c.,** any cell formed by the division of a mother cell.

**Davidoff's (Davidov's) c's,** Paneth's c's.

**decidual c's,** cells of the uterine endometrium that become modified and specialized during pregnancy.

**Deiters' c's,** the outer phalangeal cells of the organ of Corti.

**delta c.,** 1. a type of cell in the pancreatic islets that secretes somatostatin. 2. gonadotroph.

**demilune c's,** crescents of Giannuzzi.

**dendritic c's,** 1. a heterogeneous group of nonphagocytic lymph node constituents comprising follicular dendritic cells of the germinal centers, interdigitating cells of the deep cortex, and veil cells of the afferent lymph and lymphatic sinuses, all of which have an irregular shape with numerous branching processes and an inconspicuous complement of cell organelles. 2. follicular dendritic c's.

**dendritic c's, follicular,** antigen-presenting cells found in the germinal centers of the lymph nodes, and having the property of retaining for long periods of time antigen-antibody complexes in the labyrinth of clefts bounded by their surface processes. Called also *dendritic c's.*

**dentin c.,** odontoblast.

**dome c's,** the large cells that compose the epitrichium of the fetus.

**Dorothy Reed c's,** Reed-Sternberg c's.

**Downey c's,** atypical lymphocytes of three types invariably present in infectious mononucleosis. Type I is a mature cell with a kidney-shaped or lobulated nucleus with vacuolated, basophilic foamy cytoplasm; type II cells contain plasmacytoid nuclei with less vacuolated and basophilic cytoplasm; type III has a finer chromatin pattern and one or two nucleoli.

**dust c.,** alveolar macrophage.

**effector c.,** 1. a cell that becomes active in response to stimulation. 2. in immunology, a differentiated lymphocyte that carries out some part of the immune response, e.g., antibody production, lymphokine production, or helper, suppressor, or killer function. Cf. *memory c.*

**electrochemical c.,** an apparatus consisting of two half-cells, each containing a solution in which an electrode is placed, connected by a salt bridge or semipermeable membrane. A voltaic cell is one in which chemical reactions occurring at the electrodes supply a voltage to an external circuit; an electrolytic cell is one in which an applied voltage drives the reactions occurring at the electrodes in the opposite direction from that in which they proceed spontaneously.

**electrolytic c.,** an electrochemical cell (q.v.) to which voltage is applied to drive chemical reactions.

**elementary c., embryonic c.,** blastomere.

**emigrated c.,** a leukocyte that has undergone diapedesis through the wall of a blood vessel and is in the neighboring tissue.

**enamel c.,** ameloblast.

**encasing c.,** cover c.

**endocrine c's of the gut,** enteroendocrine c's.

**endothelioid c's,** large protoplasmic cells frequently seen in disease of the blood-making organs and believed by some to be derived from the endothelial lining of the blood vessels and lymph vessels.

**enterochromaffin c's,** a group of enteroendocrine cells whose granules stain readily with silver and chromium salts, and which are sites of synthesis and storage of serotonin. Based upon their staining reactions with silver, these cells have been divided between those that reduce silver without pretreatment *(argentaffin cells)* and those that require prior exposure to a reducing substance *(argyrophilic cells).*

**enteroendocrine c's,** a group of APUD cells, which may be divided into a number of populations on the basis of polypeptide hormone and biogenic amine production, found scattered throughout the gastrointestinal epithelium, mainly at the base of the epithelium; their numerous small secretory granules are concentrated chiefly between the nucleus and the cell base. Their secretions affect gastrointestinal motility, pancreatic and biliary secretions, and gastrointestinal epithelial growth, as well as being regulators of other enteroendocrine products. Called also *basal granular c's* and *endocrine c's of the gut.*

**ependymal c's,** the cells of the ependyma; called also *ependymocytes.*

**epidermic c's,** the cells of the epidermis.

**epithelial c's,** cells that cover the surface of the body and line its cavities.

**epithelioid c's,** 1. large polyhedral cells of connective tissue origin. 2. highly phagocytic, modified macrophages, resembling epithelial cells, having large, pale and vesicular nuclei with abundant, eosinophilic cytoplasm, which are characteristic of granulomatous inflammation; they may coalesce to form multinucleate giant cells. 3. pinealocytes.

**erythroid c's,** blood cells of the erythrocytic series.

**ethmoidal c's,** 1. sinus ethmoidales. 2. any of the ethmoidal air cells; see *sinus ethmoidales anteriores, medii,* and *posteriores.*

**eukaryotic c.,** a cell with a true nucleus; see *eukaryote.*

**excitable c.,** a cell that can generate an action potential at its membrane in response to depolarization and may transmit an impulse along the membrane; most are nerve cells or muscle cells, although other kinds of cells have also been shown to be excitable.

**F c.,** 1. in bacterial genetics, a cell with an inheritable mating type. The $F^+$ cell (male donor) carries the F (fertility) plasmid, while the $F^-$ cell (female recipient) lacks this factor. 2. (in plural) PP cells.

**Fañanás' c.,** a type of neuroglial cell found in the molecular layer of the cerebellar cortex; called also *glia of Fañanás.*

**fat c.,** a connective tissue cell specialized for the synthesis and storage of fat; such cells are bloated with globules of triglycerides, the nucleus being displaced to one side and the cytoplasm seen as a thin line around the fat droplet. Called also *adipose c., adipocyte,* and *lipocyte.*

**fat-storing c's of liver,** lipid-accumulating, stellate cells located in the perisinusoidal space of the liver.

**fatty granule c.,** gitter c.

**Ferrata's c.,** old name for *blast cell* (def. 2).

**fiber c.,** any elongated and linear cell.

**flagellate c.,** any cell having a flagellum, usually motile.
**foam c's,** 1. abnormal histiocytes with a peculiar vacuolated appearance due to the presence of complex lipids, seen in storage diseases, xanthomas, and certain other conditions. 2. a specific type of these cells found in xanthomas; called also *xanthoma cells.* 3. Mikulicz's c's.
**follicle c's, follicular c's,** cells located in the epithelium of follicles, e.g., the cells of the thyroid follicles and ovarian follicles. Called also *follicular epithelial c's.*
**follicular center c.,** any of a series of B lymphocytes occurring normally in the germinal center and pathologically in the neoplastic nodules of follicular cell lymphoma; they are regarded as intermediate stages in the development of lymphoblasts and plasma cells from activated lymphocytes and are distinguished according to size (large vs. small) and presence or absence of folds or clefts on the nucleus (cleaved or uncleaved). Follicular center cells are thought to be the B memory cells.
**follicular center c., large cleaved,** a follicular center cell considered to be intermediate between the small cleaved and small noncleaved stages; it has a diameter of about 12 μm, a nucleus with deep folds or clefts and clumped chromatin, and cytoplasm that is not pyroninophilic but may have immunoglobulin inclusions.
**follicular center c., large noncleaved,** a follicular center cell considered to be the stage immediately preceding the development of the B lymphoblast and migration out of the follicle; it has a diameter of 15–20 μm, a nucleus without clefts that contains finely dispersed chromatin, and cytoplasm that is abundant and pyroninophilic.
**follicular center c., small cleaved,** a follicular center cell considered to be the precursor of the other stages; it has a diameter of about 8 μm, a nucleus with a deep fold or cleft and clumped chromatin, and cytoplasm that is not pyroninophilic.
**follicular center c., small noncleaved,** a follicular center cell considered to be intermediate between the large cleaved and the large noncleaved stages; it has a diameter of about 12 μm, a nucleus without folds or clefts that contains finely dispersed chromatin, and cytoplasm that is pyroninophilic and basophilic.
**follicular epithelial c's,** follicle c's.
**foot c's,** 1. basal cells. 2. Sertoli's c's.
**foreign body giant c's,** giant cells, resembling Langhans' giant cells, having clusters of nuclei scattered in an irregular pattern throughout the cytoplasm, formed by coalescence and fusion of macrophages, with only a rare internal nuclear division, characteristic of inflammation induced by inoculation or implantation of exogenous materials resistant to degradation in dermis or subcutaneous tissue.
**formative c.,** a cell of the inner cell mass of the conceptus, a blastomere destined to form a part of the embryo, as distinct from a trophoblast cell.
**fusiform c.,** spindle c.
**G c's,** granular enterochromaffin cells in the mucosa of the pyloric part of the stomach that are the source of gastrin.
**galvanic c.,** voltaic c.
**gametoid c's,** carcinoma cells resembling reproductive cells (gametes).
**gamma c's of hypophysis,** chromophobic c's.
**ganglion c.,** 1. a form of large nerve cell characteristic of ganglia; called also *gangliocyte.* 2. any of those retinal cells that are the third, last, neurons in the vertical linkage of the retina and are analogous to the relays in the spinal cord and brain stem. At least six types of ganglion cells have been classified according to their dendritic patterns. See also *visual cone*
**Gaucher's c.,** a large and distinctive cell characteristic of Gaucher's disease, with one or more eccentrically placed nuclei and with fine wavy kerasin fibrils running parallel to the long axis of the cell, imparting a wrinkled, tissue-paper appearance to the gray or bluish opaque cytoplasm.
**Gegenbaur's c.,** osteoblast.
**germ c's,** the cells of an organism whose function it is to reproduce the kind, i.e., oocytes and spermatozoa and their immature stages. See also *gamete.* Called also *initial c's, sex c's,* and *sexual c's.*
**germ c., primordial,** the earliest recognizable precursor in the embryo of an oocyte or spermatozoon.
**germinal c.,** a cell capable of dividing and differentiating.
**ghost c.,** 1. a keratinized denucleated cell with an unstained, shadowy center where the nucleus had been. Called also *shadow c.* 2. a degenerating or fragmented erythrocyte with no hemoglobin; cf. *achromocyte.* Called also *erythroclast* and *shadow cell.*
**c's of Giannuzzi,** see under *crescent.*
**giant c.,** 1. any very large cell, such as the megakaryocyte of bone marrow. 2. any of the very large, multinucleate, modified macrophages that may be formed by coalescence of epithelioid cells or by nuclear division without cytoplasmic division of monocytes, such as those characteristic of granulomatous inflammation *(Langhans' giant c's)* and those that form around large foreign bodies *(foreign body giant c's).* 3. any very large tumor cell.
**giant pyramidal c's,** Betz's c's.
**Gierke's c's,** small, deeply staining Golgi type II neurons that constitute the chief cells of Rolando's gelatinous substance; cf. *Rolando's c's.*
**gitter c.,** a microglial cell that is globular and swollen after having phagocytized debris from cells destroyed pathologically in the central nervous system; called also *compound granule c.* and *compound granular corpuscle.*
**Gley's c's,** large glandular cells in the interstitial tissue of the testicle.
**glial c's,** neuroglial c's.
**glitter c's,** polymorphonuclear leukocytes that stain a pale blue with gentian-violet-safranin and contain granules in the cytoplasm that exhibit brownian movement; their presence in urine may indicate pyelonephritis.
**globoid c.,** an abnormal large histiocyte found in large numbers in intracranial tissues in Krabbe's disease.
**glomerular c.,** glomus c., def. 1.
**glomus c.,** 1. any of the moderately large specific epithelioid cells (type I) of the carotid body (see *glomus caroticum*) containing abundant cytoplasm and membrane-bound, electron-dense granules and having a few dendritic processes; they are richly supplied with nerve endings and are surrounded by cells without cytoplasmic granules (type II). Called also *glomerular c.* 2. any of the modified smooth muscle cells with uniform nuclei, pale-staining cytoplasm, and indistinct margins that surround the arterial segment of a glomeriform arteriovenous anastomosis, which are richly innervated by fibers of the autonomic nervous system.
**goblet c.,** a unicellular mucous gland found in the epithelium of various mucous membranes, especially that of the respiratory passages and intestines. Droplets of mucigen collect in the upper part of the cell and distend it, while the basal end remains slender, and the cell assumes the shape of a goblet. Called also *beaker c., caliciform c.,* and *chalice c.* See also *ptyocrinous.*
**Golgi's c's,** Golgi type I neurons or Golgi type II neurons; see under *neuron.*
**gonadotrope c., gonadotroph c., gonadotropic c.,** gonadotroph.
**Goormaghtigh c's,** lacis c's.
**granular c.,** the name applied to a keratinocyte in the stratum granulosum of the epidermis, when it has become flattened and rhomboidal in shape and contains a dense collection of variously sized darkly staining granules, before it dies and desquamates.
**granule c's,** 1. diminutive stellate cells found chiefly in the granular layers of the cerebral and cerebellar cortices. 2. small nerve cells without axons, whose bodies are in the granular layer of the olfactory bulb; they have many dendrites that synapse with dendrites of mitral and tufted cells and probably act as dampers.
**granulosa c's,** cells surrounding the vesicular ovarian follicle and forming the stratum granulosum and cumulus oophorus; after ovulation they are transformed into lutein cells.
**granulosa c's, primitive, granulosa c's, primordial,** prefollicle c's.
**granulosa-lutein c's,** lutein cells of the corpus luteum derived from granulosa cells.
**grape c.,** Mott c.
**ground-glass c.,** a hepatocyte having finely granular, eosinophilic cytoplasm and staining positively for hepatitis B surface antigen, characteristic of chronic hepatitis B.
**gustatory c's,** taste c's.
**H c.,** horizontal c.
**hair c's,** neuroepithelial cells with hairlike processes (kinocilia or stereocilia, or both) found in the organ of Corti, ampullar crest, and utricle and saccule of the inner ear; the hair cells receive afferent and efferent fibers of the cochlear nerve (organ of Corti) or the vestibular nerve. See also *acoustic hair c.*

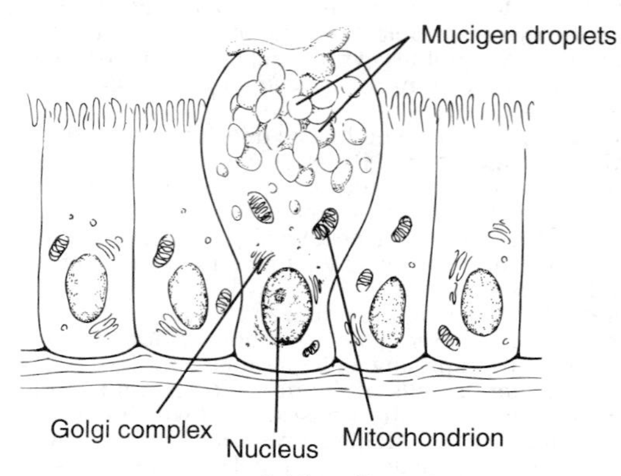

Goblet cell.

**hairy c.,** a type of abnormal large leukocyte, probably in the B lymphocyte lineage, found in the blood in hairy cell leukemia; it has numerous irregular cytoplasmic villi that give it a flagellated or hairy appearance, a round or oval nucleus, gray-blue cytoplasm, moderately clumped nuclear chromatin, and small to imperceptible nucleoli. Called also *tricholeukocyte.*

**Hammar's myoid c's,** myoid c's (def. 2).

**heart-disease c's, heart-failure c's, heart-lesion c's,** macrophages containing granules of iron, found in the pulmonary alveoli and sputum in congestive heart failure.

**hecatomeral c's,** cells of gray matter of the spinal cord whose axis cylinder processes divide and send one branch into the white substance of the same side of the cord and another into the anterolateral columns of the other side.

**heckle c.,** prickle c.

**Heidenhain's c's,** 1. chief c's (def. 1). 2. parietal c's.

**HeLa c's,** cells of the first continuously cultured carcinoma strain, descended from a human cervical carcinoma; used in the study of life processes, including viruses, at the cell level.

**helmet c.,** schistocyte.

**helper c's,** differentiated T lymphocytes whose cooperation (help) is required for the production of antibody against most (T-dependent) antigens. B cell activation requires recognition of the antigenic determinant against which specific antibody is produced by antigen receptors on a B cell, recognition of some other antigenic determinant by antigen receptors on a helper cell, and a signal passed from the helper cell to the B cell, probably requiring direct cell-to-cell contact. Murine helper cells are marked by the Ly-1 antigen, human helper cells by the CD4 antigen. See *lymphocyte.*

**Hensen's c's,** tall supporting cells arranged in rows adjacent to the last row of outer phalangeal cells, constituting the outer border of the organ of Corti.

**hepatic c's,** the polyhedral epithelial cells that constitute the substance of an acinus of the liver; called also *liver c's.*

**heteromeral c's, heteromeric c's,** nerve cells of the gray matter of the spinal cord whose axon processes pass to the white matter of the opposite side; called also *commissural c's.*

**hilus c's,** groups of large epithelioid cells closely associated with vascular spaces and unmyelinated nerve fibers in the hilus of the ovary and the adjacent mesovarium.

**Hodgkin's c's,** Reed-Sternberg c's.

**Hofbauer c's,** large, globular cells filled with vacuoles and large spherical nuclei, which are found in the connective tissue core of the chorionic villi of the placenta; they are probably macrophages.

**homozygous typing c's (HTC),** cells homozygous for a known HLA-D specificity; panels of HTC of all established HLA-D types are used to determine the HLA-D type of unknown cells using one-way mixed lymphocyte reactions.

**horizontal c.,** a retinal neuron; there are two types, and their functions are unclear. Each cell has a multipolar soma in the internal nuclear layer and one long neurite and several short ones. All the neurites serve as both axons and dendrites, extending along and ramifying within the internal nuclear layer. The long neurites synapse in the outer plexiform layer with both pedicles and spherules; the short neurites synapse either with pedicles or with spherules. Called also *H c.*

**horizontal c. of Cajal,** Cajal's c., def. 2.

**horizontal c. of retina,** horizontal c.

**horn c's,** 1. epithelial cells that have lost their protoplasm, have sharp edges, and look horny. 2. any ganglion cell of the horns of the spinal cord.

**Hortega c.,** microglial c.

**Hürthle c's,** Askanazy c's.

**hyperchromatic c.,** one that stains more intensely than is typical of its cell type.

**I-c.,** an abnormal fibroblast containing a large number of dark inclusions that fill the central part of the cytoplasm except for the juxtanuclear zone; seen in mucolipidosis II.

**immunologically competent c.,** immunocyte.

**incasing c.,** cover c.

**indifferent c.,** a cell that has no characteristic structure, or that is not an essential part of the tissue in which it is found.

**inflammatory c.,** a cell (neutrophil, macrophage, etc.) participating in the inflammatory response to a foreign substance.

**initial c's,** germ c's.

**integrator c.,** interneuron.

**intercalary c's,** dark, rodlike structures between the other (secretory and nonsecretory) cells of the endosalpinx, which may be emptied secretory cells; called also *peg c's.*

**intercalated c's,** dark-colored cells in the renal collecting tubules that are responsible for acidification of the urine.

**intercapillary c's,** mesangial c's.

**interdental c's,** cells found in the spiral limbus between the dentes acustici, which secrete the tectorial membrane of the cochlear duct.

**interdigitating c's,** antigen-presenting cells found in the thymus-dependent (parafollicular) areas of the deep cortex of lymph nodes and spleen and having numerous surface processes that interdigitate with adjacent lymphocytes; the surface of these cells contains an Ia antigen of the major histocompatibility complex that causes T cells to cluster.

**interfollicular c's,** Askanazy c's.

**interstitial c's,** 1. Leydig's c's. 2. masses of large epithelioid, lipid-containing cells in the ovarian stroma, believed to have a secretory function, derived from the theca interna of atretic ovarian follicles, and thus, in humans, more numerous during the first year of life when atresia proceeds rapidly. In women, they are either absent or poorly represented, but in some other mammals, especially rabbits, they are more prominent; see also *interstitial gland* (def. 2), under *gland.* 3. cells with elongated nuclei and long cytoplasmic processes, found in the perivascular areas and between the cords of pinealocytes in the pineal body, and regarded by some to be glial elements. 4. fat-storing c's of liver.

**interstitial c's of Cajal,** pleomorphic cells having an oval nucleus and long, branching cytoplasmic processes that interlace with processes of adjacent cells, interspersed between the circular and longitudinal muscle layers of the gastrointestinal tract and in the smooth muscle of the esophagus; they are thought to act as pacemakers.

**interstitial c's of Leydig,** Leydig's c's.

**islet c's,** cells composing the islets of Langerhans, including the *alpha cells, beta cells, delta cells,* and *PP cells.*

**Ito c's,** stellate lipocytes in the space of Disse that are the major site of vitamin A storage in the body; they also synthesize collagen and may be involved in hepatic tissue repair and be responsible for the excess collagen produced in cirrhosis.

**juvenile c.,** metamyelocyte.

**juxtaglomerular c's,** specialized smooth muscle cells, located in the tunica media of the afferent glomerular arterioles and containing secretory granules. They are the major structural component responsible for the release of renin and play a major role in renal autoregulation.

**K c's,** 1. killer cells; cells mediating antibody-dependent cell-mediated cytotoxicity (ADCC). They are small lymphocytes without T or B cell surface markers. K cells recognize IgG antibody coating the target cell by means of Fc receptors. Lysis of the target cell is extracellular, requires direct cell-to-cell contact, and does not involve complement. 2. cells located predominantly in the midzone of the duodenal and jejunal mucosa that synthesize gastric inhibitory polypeptide.

**karyochrome c.,** karyochrome.

**killer c's,** 1. K c's. 2. cytotoxic T lymphocytes; see under *lymphocyte.*

**killer T c's,** cytotoxic T lymphocytes; see under *lymphocyte.*

**Kulchitsky's c's,** argentaffin cells situated between the cells that line the glands of Lieberkühn of the intestine.

**Kupffer's c's,** large star-shaped or pyramidal cells with a large oval nucleus and a small prominent nucleolus. These intensely phagocytic cells line the walls of the sinusoids of the liver and form a part of the reticuloendothelial system (q.v.). Called also *stellate c's of liver* and *von Kupffer's c's.*

**L c's,** 1. cells from a strain (C3H) of mouse fibroblasts grown in tissue culture for many years; employed for their ability to support replication of many types of viruses. 2. a type of argyrophilic cells with large cytoplasmic granules in the mucosa of the upper intestine; their ultrastructure resembles that of the alpha cells of the islets of Langerhans, and they secrete glicentin; called also *large granule c's.* 3. Langerhans' c's. 4. Langhans' c's. 5. null cells with natural killer or killer properties.

**lacis c's,** lacelike cells with pale-staining of the polkissen, having numerous processes and connecting gap junctions; thought to provide electrical coupling among themselves and to the mesangium and

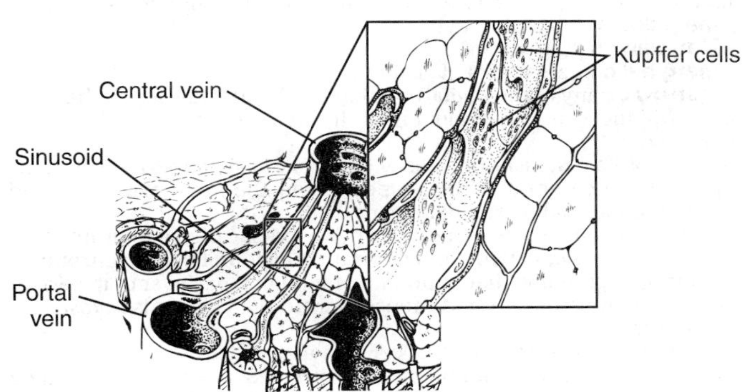


Kupffer cells lining a hepatic sinusoid.

glomerular arterioles. Called also *Goormaghtigh c's* and *extraglomerular mesangium.*

**lacrimoethmoid c's,** the ethmoidal cells situated under the lacrimal bone.

**lactotrope c., lactotroph c., lactotropic c.,** lactotroph.

**lacunar c.,** a variant of the Reed-Sternberg cell, typically having a single nucleus surrounded by an ample, pale-staining cytoplasm enclosed in a sharply defined cell membrane; it is primarily associated with the nodular sclerosis type of Hodgkin's disease.

**LAK c's,** lymphokine-activated killer c's.

**Langerhans' c's,** stellate dendritic cells, derived from precursors in the bone marrow, that appear clear on light microscopy and have a dark-staining, indented nucleus and characteristic inclusions *(Birbeck granules)* in the cytoplasm; they lack tonofilaments, desmosomes, and melanosomes. Langerhans' cells are found principally in the stratum spinosum of the epidermis, but they also occur in other stratified epithelia and have been identified in the lung, lymph nodes, spleen, and thymus. They have surface markers characteristic of macrophages and are believed to be antigen-presenting cells involved in contact allergic responses and other cell-mediated immune reactions in the skin.

**Langhans' c's,** 1. polyhedral epithelial cells constituting cytotrophoblast (Langhans' layer). 2. Langhans' giant c's.

**Langhans' giant c's,** giant cells, resembling foreign body giant cells but having their nuclei arranged in a complete circle or in a horseshoe-shaped pattern at the periphery of the cells, characteristically seen in granulomatous inflammations, as occur in tuberculosis, syphilis, sarcoidosis, and deep fungal infections.

**large cleaved c.,** see *follicular center c., large cleaved.*

**large granule c's,** L c's (def. 2).

**large noncleaved c., large uncleaved c.,** see *follicular center c., large noncleaved.*

**LE c.,** a neutrophil or macrophage that has phagocytized the denatured nuclear material of an injured cell (LE or hematoxylin body); a characteristic of systemic lupus erythematosus, but also found in analogous disorders of connective tissue.

**Leishman's chrome c's,** basophil granular leukocytes occurring in black water fever.

**lepra c.,** a histiocyte in a leprous nodule that has been converted by the action of lepra bacilli into a sac containing degenerated protoplasm and bacilli; called also *Virchow's c.*

**Leydig's c's,** 1. clusters of epithelioid cells constituting the endocrine tissue of the testis, which elaborate androgens, chiefly testosterone; called also *interstitial c's* or *interstitial c's of Leydig,* and *interstitial glands.* 2. mucous cells that do not pour their secretion out over the surface of the epithelium.

**light c's,** parafollicular c's.

**littoral c's,** flattened cells lining the walls of lymph or blood sinuses. Called also *rod* or *stave c's.*

**liver c's,** hepatic c's.

**luteal c's, lutein c's,** the plump, pale-staining, polyhedral cells of the corpus luteum; they include the granulosa lutein cells and the theca lutein cells.

**lymph c.,** lymphocyte.

**lymphoid c's,** cells of the immune system that react specifically with antigen and elaborate specific cell products; they comprise the lymphocytes and plasma cells.

**lymphokine-activated killer c's,** killer cells activated by interleukin-2 that have specificity towards tumors refractory to NK cells; they may represent a further activation state of the NK cell. Called also *LAK c's.*

**M c's,** specialized cells of the epithelium overlying the lymphoid nodules of the intestines that bind antigens and transport them to the underlying lymphocytes; it is believed that they may provide a continuous sampling of the intestinal contents to the immune system.

**malpighian c.,** keratinocyte.

**Marchand's c.,** pericyte.

**marginal c's,** crescents of Giannuzzi.

**marrow c.,** any of the immature blood cells that develop in the bone marrow, such as those involved in hematopoiesis. Called also *myeloid c.*

**Martinotti's c's,** fusiform cells with ascending axon processes in the layers of the cerebral cortex, especially in the multiform layer and also in the internal pyramidal layer.

**mast c.,** a connective tissue cell whose specific physiologic function remains unknown; capable of elaborating basophilic, metachromatic cytoplasmic granules that contain histamine, heparin, and, in certain species, such as the rat and mouse, serotonin; called also *mastocyte* and *labrocyte.*

**mastoid c's, mastoid air c's,** cellulae mastoideae.

**matrix c's,** flat cells found in the lobules of sebaceous glands; they undergo a rather abrupt transformation into the pale, foamy-looking, fat-containing cells of the alveoli.

**Mauthner's c.,** a large cell in the metencephalon of fishes and amphibians that gives rise to Mauthner's fiber.

**megaspore mother c.,** any of the diploid cells developed in the megasporangium of plants which divide by meiosis to produce four haploid daughter cells (megaspores), usually only one of which survives to become a megagametophyte, or female gametophyte.

**memory c's,** T and B lymphocytes that mediate immunologic memory (q.v.); believed to retain information that permits a subsequent challenge to be followed by a more rapid efficient immunologic reaction on subsequent exposures to an antigen than occurred on first exposure.

**Merkel c.,** a specialized cell at or near the epithelial–dermal junction, characterized by numerous membrane-bound granules with dense cores, some desmosomes, cytoplasmic microfilaments, intranuclear filaments bundled in parallel to form rodlets, and spikelike processes that interdigitate with keratinocytes. They are believed to act as touch receptors by association with flat, disklike endings of nerve fibers (tactile menisci).

**Merkel-Ranvier c's,** clear cells in the basal layer of the epidermis that contain catecholamine granules and resemble melanocytes.

**Merkel tactile c.,** Merkel c.

**mesangial c's,** cells found in the mesangium, the connective tissue stalk in the glomerular capsule of the kidney.

**mesenchymal c's,** the pluripotential cells constituting the mesenchyme.

**mesothelial c's,** flattened epithelial cells of mesenchymal origin that line the serous cavities.

**metallophil c's,** cells in which the cytoplasm has a great affinity for metal salts; these are cells of the reticuloendothelial system, and also a series of related cells that are not selectively stained by vital staining.

**Mexican hat c.,** target c.

**Meynert's c's,** large solitary pyramidal cells in the cerebral cortex, found in a single row near the calcarine fissure; called also *solitary c's of Meynert.*

**microglia c., microglial c.,** one of the small interstitial phagocytic cells of the microglia; see also *gitter c.* Called also *microgliocyte* and *Hortega c.*

**microspore mother c.,** any of the diploid cells with large nuclei developed in the microsporangium of plants which divide by meiosis to produce four haploid microspores.

**migratory c.,** ameboid c.

**Mikulicz's c's,** the cells in rhinoscleroma that contain the bacillus of the disease; called also *foam c's.*

**mitral c's,** neurons with pyramidal bodies located in the olfactory bulb, being the second stage in the pathway to the cortex; they receive impulses in the olfactory glomeruli from the olfactory cells and transmit impulses through the olfactory tracts to various areas of the cortex.

**Mooser c.,** a large mononuclear (serosal) cell with numerous rickettsiae in the cytoplasm, observed in inflammatory exudate in murine typhus; called also *Neill-Mooser bodies.*

**morular c.,** Mott c.

**mossy c.,** 1. protoplasmic astrocyte. 2. any of the cells of the oligodendroglia or of the microglia.

**mother c.,** a cell that divides so as to form new or daughter cells; called also *brood c.* and *parent c.*

**motor c.,** motoneuron.

**Mott c.,** an abnormal plasma cell that contains Mott bodies or Russell bodies, seen in multiple myeloma and in the brain in late stages of African trypanosomiasis. Called also *berry, grape,* or *morular c.*

**mouth c's,** squamous cells detached from the epithelium lining the oropharynx, found in the sputum.

**mucoalbuminous c's, mucoserous c's,** trophochrome c's.

**mucous c's,** cells that secrete mucus or mucin.

**mucous neck c's,** cells found in the necks of gastric glands; they fill the spaces between the parietal cells and are filled with pale transparent granules.

**mulberry c.,** 1. Mott c. 2. a round cell with centrally placed nuclei and coarse cytoplasmic vacuoles near the outer border, developing at the periphery of a retrogressing corpus luteum.

**c's of Müller,** see under *fiber.*

**muriform c's,** sclerotic bodies.

**muscle c.,** any contractile cell peculiar to muscle. Smooth muscle cells are elongated spindle-shaped cells containing a single nucleus and longitudinally arranged myofibrils. For cardiac and skeletal muscle cells, see *muscle fiber,* under *fiber.*

**myeloid c.,** marrow c.

**myeloma c.,** a cell found in bone marrow and occasionally in peripheral blood of patients with multiple myeloma. In the more anaplastic forms, the cell is large, has abundant blue-staining cytoplasm with no perinuclear pallor, and has one or more moderately large and vesicular nuclei that may be centrally or eccentrically placed and may contain nucleoli. In better differentiated tumors, the cell is smaller and, except for the finer chromatic structure, greatly resembles a plasmacyte.

**myoepithelial c's,** modified smooth muscle cells, contractile in nature, believed to be of ectodermal origin, located around the secretory units of certain glands (salivary, mammary, sweat, and lacrimal glands) between the gland cells and basement membrane, having long dendritic interweaving cytoplasmic processes, and containing myofilaments. It is assumed that contraction of these cells functions to help express secretion from the gland. Called also *basket c's.*

**myoepithelioid c's,** juxtaglomerular c's; so called because they appear to be highly modified smooth muscle cells.

**myoid c's,** 1. cells found in the seminiferous tubules of common laboratory rodents, which cytologically resemble smooth muscle and are presumed to be contractile and to be responsible for the rhythmic shallow contractions of the seminiferous tubules of these species; called also *peritubular contractile c's.* 2. striated muscle cells found in the thymus of nonmammalian vertebrates, especially reptiles and birds, and rarely in mammals; called also *Hammar's myoid c's.*

**myointimal c.,** a smooth muscle cell found in the intima of an artery.

**Nageotte's c's,** cells of the cerebrospinal fluid that become greatly increased in number in disease.

**naive c.,** a lymphocyte that has not yet undergone activation (q.v.).

**natural killer c's,** NK c's.

**nerve c.,** neuron.

**neuroendocrine c's,** the specialized neurons that secrete neurohormones.

**neuroepithelial c's,** cells of the neuroepithelium.

**neuroglia c's, neuroglial c's,** the cells of the supportive tissue of the central nervous system (neuroglia); these non-neural cells are of three kinds: astrocytes, oligodendrocytes (collectively termed macroglia) and microglia. See Plate 36.

**neuromuscular c.,** a form of cell chiefly or always seen in the lower animals, of which the outer part receives stimuli and the inner part is contractile.

**neurosecretory c.,** any cell with neuron-like properties that secretes a biologically active substance acting on another structure, often at a distant site; examples are the paraganglia and cells in the hypothalamus. See also *neuroendocrine c's.*

**neutrophilic c.,** a cell, particularly a leukocyte, stainable by neutral dyes; called also *neutrophil.*

**nevus c.,** a polymorphic, melanin-containing cell variously postulated to be a normal mature melanocyte or a modified one, or to be derived from a Schwann cell or an embryonal nevoblast. Such cells occur in aggregations, or nests *(theques),* in the epidermis and reach the dermis by a kind of centripetal extrusion *(abtropfung),* and are the main constituents of nevocytic nevi. Called also *nevocyte.*

**Niemann-Pick c's,** round, oval, or polyhedral cells present in the bone marrow and spleen in Niemann-Pick disease; they have foamy, lipid-containing cytoplasm, in the form of sphingomyelin, which gives a positive reaction with Sudan III and other fat stains. Called also *Pick's c's.*

**NK c's,** natural killer cells; cells capable of mediating cytotoxic reactions without prior sensitization against the target. NK cells are small lymphocytes without B or T cell surface markers that originate in the bone marrow and develop fully in the absence of the thymus; their cytotoxic activity is not antibody-dependent. They can lyse a wide variety of tumor cells and other cell types and are probably important in natural resistance to tumors. Interferon augments their activity. See *lymphocyte.*

**noble c's,** the differentiated cells of the organs and tissues of the body.

**nodal c's,** P c's.

**noncleaved c.,** see *follicular center c., small noncleaved* and *follicular center c., large noncleaved.*

**normal c.,** any cell found naturally in any part or organ free from disease.

**nucleated c.,** any cell having a nucleus.

**null c's,** lymphocytes that lack the surface markers for B or T cells; see *K c's* and *NK c's.*

**nurse c's, nursing c's,** Sertoli's c's.

**oat c's, oat-shaped c's,** small round cells with little cytoplasm, resembling oat grains, seen in small cell lung carcinoma.

**olfactory c's, olfactory receptor c's,** a set of specialized, fusiform nerve cells with large nuclei, embedded among the epithelial cells in the mucous membrane of the nose; they carry impulses from the olfactory receptors to the glomeruli in the olfactory bulb. Called also *Schultze's c's.*

**osseous c.,** a bone cell.

**osteoprogenitor c's,** relatively undifferentiated cells found on or near all of the free surfaces of bone, which, under certain circumstances, undergo division and transform into osteoblasts or coalesce to give rise to osteoclasts.

**owl's eye c's,** desquamated renal epithelial cells.

**oxyntic c's,** parietal c's.

**oxyphil c's, oxyphilic c's,** 1. acidophilic cells found, along with the more numerous chief cells, in the parathyroid glands; they increase in number with age, have small dark nuclei and abundant finely granular cytoplasm, and are larger and have many more mitochondria than the chief cells. 2. any of various pathological acidophilic cells found in the thyroid gland. 3. Askanazy cells.

**P c's,** poorly staining, pale, small cells almost devoid of myofibrils, mitochondria, or other organelles; they are clustered in the center of the sinoatrial node, where they are thought to be the source of impulse formation, and also in the atrioventricular node.

**pacemaker c.,** a myocardial cell demonstrating automaticity; i.e., one that initiates electrical activity in the absence of external stimuli. Called also *automatic c.*

**packed red blood c's,** red blood cells [USP].

**Paget's c., pagetoid c.,** a large, irregularly shaped, pale anaplastic tumor cell with vacuolated cytoplasm and a vesicular nucleus that is usually hyperchromatic and surrounded by a clear zone; cells occur singly or in small clusters in the epidermis in Paget's disease of the breast and extramammary Paget's disease.

**palatine c's,** those parts of ethmoid cells that are extended into the palatine bone.

**palisade c's,** a compact layer of cylindrical chloroplast-bearing cells located in the mesophyll layer of a leaf, and so arranged that their long axes are at right angles to the epidermal surface of the leaf.

**Paneth's c's,** narrow, pyramidal, or columnar epithelial cells with a round or oval nucleus close to the base of the cell, occurring in the fundus of the crypts of Lieberkühn; they contain large secretory granules that may contain peptidase. Called also *Davidoff's c's.*

**parafollicular c's,** ovoid cells with an irregular nucleus and many brown or black cytoplasmic granules, located in the follicular epithelium and interfollicular spaces along with the principal cells of the thyroid follicles, in the follicular epithelium and interfollicular spaces, and which elaborate calcitonin. They arise during embryonic life from the fifth pharyngeal pouches and are incorporated in the thyroid gland in mammals, but form discrete epithelial cell masses *(ultimobranchial bodies)* in submammalian vertebrates. Called also *C c's* and *light c's.*

**paraluteal c's, paralutein c's,** theca-lutein c's.

**parenchymal hepatic c's, parenchymal liver c's,** hepatic c's.

**parent c.,** mother c.

**parietal c's,** large spheroidal or pyramidal cells that are the source of gastric hydrochloric acid and are the site of intrinsic factor production; they are found scattered along the walls of the gastric glands, with their tapered ends pushed between the chief cells. Called also *acid c's, border c's, Heidenhain's c's, and oxyntic c's.*

**pathologic c.,** any cell that results from a disease process or that belongs to or arises from a pathogenic microorganism.

**pavement c's,** the flat cells composing pavement epithelium.

**peg c's,** intercalary c's.

**peptic c's,** a name sometimes given to the chief cells of the stomach.

**pericapillary c.,** pericyte.

**periglomerular c's,** nerve cells in the olfactory bulb that have synaptic connections with glomeruli, mitral cells, and tufted cells, and are thought to act as dampers.

**perithelial c.,** pericyte.

**peritubular contractile c's,** myoid c's, def. 1.

**perivascular c.,** pericyte.

**pessary c.,** a hypochromic erythrocyte with the hemoglobin in a narrow circumferential rim; cf. *achromocyte.* Called also *pessary corpuscle.*

**phalangeal c's,** elongated supporting cells of the organ of Corti with bases that rest on the basilar membrane adjacent to the pillar cells; the *inner* ones are arranged in a row on the inner surface of the inner pillar cells and surround the inner hair cells; the *outer* ones *(c's of Deiters)* support the outer hair cells.

**pheochrome c's,** chromaffin c's.

**photoautotrophic c's,** green plant cells.

**photoreceptor c's,** visual c's.

**physaliferous c's, physaliphorous c's,** spheroidal nucleated cells, containing glycogen or mucin, causing them to appear vacuolated; they are characteristic of chordoma.

**Pick's c's,** Niemann-Pick c's.

**pigment c.,** any cell containing pigment granules.

**pillar c's,** elongated supporting cells in a double row *(inner* and *outer pillar c's)* in the organ of Corti, having their heads joined and their bases resting on the basilar membrane widely separated so as to form a tunnel *(inner tunnel* or *canal of Corti)* that extends the length of the cochlea. Called also *Corti's rods.*

**pineal c.,** pinealocyte.

**plasma c.,** a terminally differentiated cell of the B lymphocyte lineage that produces antibodies; plasma cells are oval or round with extensive rough endoplasmic reticulum, a well-developed Golgi apparatus, and a round nucleus having a characteristic "cartwheel" heterochromatin pattern. Called also *plasmacyte.*

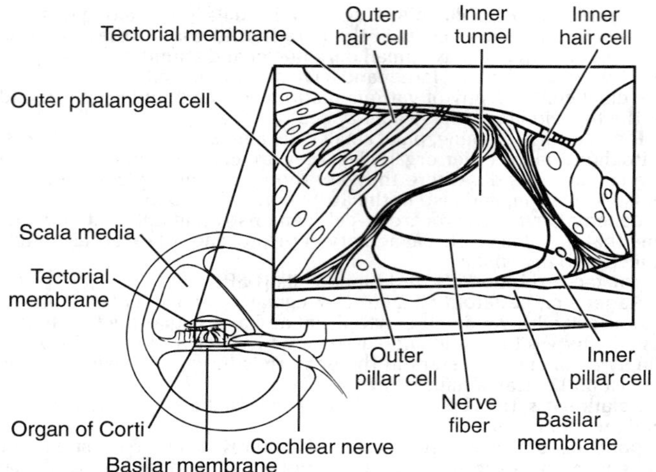

Pillar cells forming the inner tunnel in the organ of Corti in the inner ear.

**plasma c., flaming,** an abnormal plasma cell that stains red to violet, probably because it contains immunoglobulins with a high carbohydrate content; it may be related to a thesaurocyte.

**pneumatic c.,** air c. (def. 2).

**PNH c's,** abnormal erythrocytes seen in paroxysmal nocturnal hemoglobinuria (PNH); they are classified in three groups: *PNH I cells,* which have normal or nearly normal sensitivity to complement; *PNH II cells,* which require about one fourth as much complement as normal cells for an equal amount of lysis; and *PNH III cells,* which have about one fifteenth the normal sensitivity to complement.

**polar c's,** polar bodies (def. 1).

**polychromatic c's, polychromatophil c's,** immature erythrocytes staining with both acid and basic stains so that their color is a diffuse mixture of blue-gray and pink.

**polyhedral c.,** a cell that is many-sided in form.

**polyplastic c.,** a cell made up of various structural elements; also one that passes through various modifications of form.

**popcorn c.,** a variant of the Reed-Sternberg cell, having a multilobed nucleus that resembles an exploded popcorn kernel.

**PP c's,** cells in the pancreatic islets, exocrine pancreas, and intestine that secrete pancreatic polypeptide. Called also *F c's.*

**pre-B c's,** the earliest identifiable precursors of B lymphocytes: large, rapidly dividing cells found in the fetal liver and adult bone marrow that lack surface immunoglobulin but contain diffuse cytoplasmic immunoglobulin of the IgM type.

**prefollicle c's,** cells encapsulating the germ cells in the fetal ovary. Called also *primitive* or *primordial granulosa c's.*

**pregnancy c.,** an altered chromophobe cell found in the adenohypophysis in pregnant women.

**pre-T c.,** a T lymphocyte precursor before undergoing induction of the maturation process in the thymus; it lacks the characteristics of a mature T lymphocyte.

**prickle c.,** a cell with delicate radiating processes that connect with similar cells; the name applied to one of the dividing keratinocytes present in the stratum germinativum of the epidermis. Called also *heckle c.*

**primary c.,** an irreversible (non-rechargeable) electromotive force cell.

**primordial germ c's,** the earliest germ cells, originating extragonadally but migrating early in embryonic development to the gonads.

**principal c's,** 1. chief c's, def. 3. 2. the fundamental cells of an organ, which usually have a specific function. 3. light-staining cells of the renal collecting tubules that transport water in response to antidiuretic hormone and sodium in response to aldosterone.

**progenitor c.,** stem c.

**progenitor c., hematopoietic,** stem c. (def. 2).

**progenitor c's, peripheral blood (PBPC),** stem cells found in the peripheral blood rather than the bone marrow; their numbers can be artificially increased by exposure to hematopoietic growth factors so that they can be extracted before myeloablative chemotherapy and later infused as an autologous bone marrow transplantation.

**prokaryotic c.,** a cell without a true nucleus; see *prokaryote.*

**prolactin c.,** lactotroph.

**pulmonary epithelial c's,** alveolar epithelial c's.

**pulpar c's,** the typical cells of the spleen substance.

**Purkinje c's,** 1. large neurons in the cerebellar cortex that have piriform cell bodies in the Purkinje layer (the *stratum purkinjense cerebelli*) and large branching dendrite trees going through the outer (molecular) layer towards the surface. 2. cells of the Purkinje fibers of the heart; they are large, clear, tightly packed cells with many gap junctions between them and thus conduct impulses rapidly.

**pus c's,** polymorphonuclear leukocytes, chiefly neutrophils, occurring in pus.

**pyramidal c.,** one of the large multipolar pyramid-shaped cells of the cerebral cortex, having a single apical dendrite extending outward toward the surface and several dendrites extending inward; a few are inverted so that their apical dendrites extend inward. They vary in size from small to the giant Betz's cells. Called also *pyramidal neuron.*

**RA c.,** ragocyte.

**racket c.,** one shaped like a tennis racket, with a swollen outer end, found in the racket hyphae of various dermatophytes.

**radial c's of Müller,** Müller's fibers.

**Raji c's,** cells from a cultured human lymphoblastoid cell line, derived from a patient with Burkitt's lymphoma, that have receptors for the C1q, C3b, and C3d complement components and can be used for detection of immune complexes.

**red c., red blood c.,** erythrocyte.

**red blood c's** [USP], the remaining red blood cells of whole blood from which plasma has been removed; used therapeutically in blood transfusions. Called also *packed red blood c's.*

**Reed c's, Reed-Sternberg c's,** giant histiocytic cells, typically multinucleate, most often binucleate with the two halves of the cell appearing as mirror-images of each other; the nuclei are enclosed in abundant amphophilic cytoplasm and contain prominent nucleoli. The presence of the cells is the common histiologic characteristic of Hodgkin's disease. A variant form is the lacunar cell (q.v.). Called also *Dorothy Reed c's, Sternberg-Reed c's, Hodgkin's c's,* and *Sternberg's giant c's.*

**Renshaw c's,** interneurons in the ventromedial region of the spinal cord that make inhibitory connections with the motoneurons.

**reserve c's,** cells of the basal or germinal layer of the bronchial epithelium.

**residential c.,** a cell that does not wander, especially one of the cells of the substantia propria of the cornea.

**resting c.,** a cell that is not undergoing karyokinesis.

**resting wandering c.,** a fixed macrophage.

**reticular c's,** the cells forming the reticular fibers of connective tissue; those forming the framework of lymph nodes, bone marrow, and spleen are part of the reticuloendothelial system and under appropriate stimulation may differentiate into macrophages.

**reticuloendothelial c.,** any of the cells of the reticuloendothelial system.

**reticulum c's,** reticular cells.

**rhagiocrine c.,** macrophage.

**Rieder's c.,** a myeloblast seen in a type of acute myelogenous leukemia *(Rieder's cell leukemia)* and chronic lymphocytic leukemia; it has a nucleus with wide and deep indentations suggesting lobulation, which may represent asynchronism of nuclear and cytoplasmic maturation. Called also *Rieder's lymphocyte.*

**rod c's,** 1. retinal rods. 2. microglia as observed in chronic diseases of the cerebral cortex and in dementia paralytica, in which the cells are markedly attenuated in form, their processes being confined mainly to the two extremities. 3. littoral c's.

**Rohon-Beard c's,** giant ganglion cells in the spinal cord of some vertebrates.

**Rolando's c's,** the ganglion cells of Rolando's gelatinous substance; cf. *Gierke's c's.*

**root c's,** neurons whose axons form nerve roots.

**Rouget c.,** pericyte.

**round c.,** any cell having a spherical shape, especially a lymphocyte.

**RS c's,** Reed-Sternberg c's.

**S c's,** 1. mucoid cells of the adenohypophysis that contain a cysteine-rich protein. 2. enteroendocrine cells found predominantly in the duodenum, which have cytoplasmic granules that store and release secretin; called also *small granule c's.*

**Sala's c's,** star-shaped cells of connective tissue in the fibers that form the sensory nerve endings situated in the pericardium.

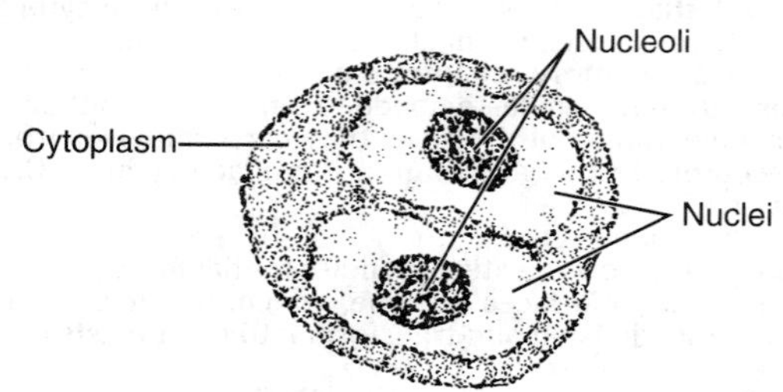

Binucleate Reed-Sternberg cell.

**sarcogenic c's,** the cells that are developed into muscle fiber.

**satellite c's,** 1. glial cells that cluster about a neuron. 2. free nuclei that accumulate around cells in certain diseases. 3. elongated cells that are closely associated with a muscle fiber; they either are flattened against the fiber or occupy shallow depressions in its surface.

**scavenger c.,** a cell which absorbs and removes irritant products.

**Schultze's c's,** olfactory c's.

**Schwann c.,** any of the large nucleated cells whose cell membrane spirally enwraps the axons of myelinated peripheral neurons and is the source of myelin; a single Schwann cell supplies the myelin sheath between two nodes of Ranvier.

**sclerenchyma c's,** thick-walled, lignified, usually dead cells, which compose the sclerenchyma of plants. Cf. *collenchyma c's.*

**sclerotic c's,** see under *body.*

**segmented c.,** a mature granulocyte in which the nucleus is divided into definite lobes joined by a filamentous connection, as distinguished from a band cell.

**seminal c's,** epithelial cells within the tubuli seminiferi.

**sensitized c.,** 1. a cell that has been immunologically activated by an antigen (primed). 2. an antibody-coated cell used in complement fixation tests.

**sensory c.,** primary sensory neuron.

**septal c's,** type II alveolar c's.

**serous c.,** a cell concerned in the secretion of a watery fluid rich in protein, like the secretory cells of the parotid gland; called also *albuminous c.*

**Sertoli's c's,** elongated cells in the seminiferous tubules, to which the spermatids become attached; they provide support, protection, and, apparently, nutrition until the spermatids become transformed into mature spermatozoa; called also *sustentacular c's, nurse* or *nursing c's, foot c's,* and *trophocytes.*

**sex c's, sexual c's,** germ c's.

**Sézary c.,** an abnormal mononuclear cell with a hyperchromic infolded cribriform nucleus and a narrow rim of cytoplasm that may contain vacuoles, occurring in small and large cell variants; it is a characteristic finding in cutaneous T-cell lymphoma and its variants.

**shadow c.,** ghost c..

**sickle c.,** an erythrocyte shaped like a sickle or crescent owing to the presence of hemoglobin S; seen in sickle cell anemia and other sickle cell diseases (see under *disease*). Called also *drepanocyte* and *meniscocyte.*

**signet-ring c.,** one in which the nucleus has been pressed to one side by an accumulation of intracytoplasmic mucin; see *Krukenberg's tumor,* under *tumor.*

**skeletogenous c.,** an osteoblast.

**small cleaved c.,** see *follicular center c., small cleaved.*

**small granule c's,** S c's, def. 2.

**small noncleaved c., small uncleaved c.,** see *follicular center c., small noncleaved.*

**smudge c.,** a disrupted leukocyte appearing during preparation of a peripheral blood smear.

**solitary c's of Meynert,** Meynert's c's.

**somatic c's,** the cells of the somatoplasm; undifferentiated body cells.

**somatostatin c's,** endocrine cells that secrete somatostatin, found in oxyntic and pyloric glands.

**somatotrope c., somatotroph c., somatotropic c.,** somatotroph.

**sperm c.,** spermatozoon.

**spermatogenic c.,** a cell that produces sperm; called also *androgone.*

**spermatogonial c.,** spermatogonium.

**sphenoid c.,** *sinus sphenoidalis.*

**spider c.,** 1. astrocyte. 2. a cell occurring in rhabdomyosarcoma; its nucleus, with a narrow rim of cytoplasm, is located in what appears to be a large vacuole, with thread-like processes radiating to the outer cell wall.

**spindle c.,** a spindle-shaped cell; called also *fusiform c.*

**spur c.,** acanthocyte.

**squamous c.,** a flat, scalelike epithelial cell.

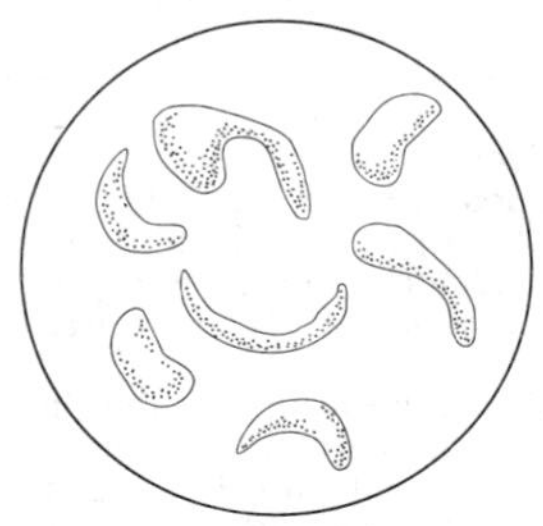

Sickle cells.

**stab c., staff c.,** band c.

**star c's,** cells with large vacuoles in their cytoplasm and cytoplasmic bridges; seen in ameloblastoma.

**stave c's.,** littoral c's.

**stellate c.,** any cell having a star-shaped appearance produced by numerous processes that extend in different directions, such as the Kupffer cells in the liver, astrocytes, and granule cells in the granular layers of the cerebral and cerebellar cortices.

**stem c.,** 1. any precursor cell. 2. a blood cell progenitor or mother cell representing a slightly later stage than the blast cell; it has the capacity for both replication and differentiation, and has pluripotentiality, giving rise to precursors of various different blood cell lines, such as the proerythrocyte and myeloblast, which cannot self-replicate and must differentiate into more mature daughter cells. Called also *progenitor c., hematopoietic stem c.,* and *colony-forming unit–spleen.*

**stem c., hematopoietic,** stem c. (def. 2).

**stem c's, peripheral blood,** peripheral blood progenitor c's.

**Sternberg's giant c's, Sternberg-Reed c's,** Reed-Sternberg c's.

**stippled c.,** an erythrocyte containing granules of varying size and shape, taking a basic or bluish stain with Wright's stain, as in punctate basophilia.

**supporting c's,** cells that serve to provide support and protection and perhaps contribute to the nutrition of principal or other cells of certain organs; such cells are found in the labyrinth of the inner ear, organ of Corti, olfactory epithelium, taste buds, and seminiferous tubules (Sertoli's cells). Called also *sustentacular c's.*

**suppressor c's,** differentiated T lymphocytes that suppress antibody synthesis or cell-mediated immunity. They may be activated in response to antigen or to idiotypic determinants present on antibodies and T and B cell antigen receptors and may act either by suppressing the activity of helper cells or by inhibiting the differentiation of activated lymphocytes into effector cells. Murine suppressor cells are marked by the Ly-2 and Ly-3 antigens, human suppressor cells by the T5 and T8 antigens. Cf. *contrasuppressor c's.*

**sustentacular c's,** supporting c's.

**sympathicotrophic c's,** large epithelioid cells occurring in groups and connected with bundles of nonmyelinated nerve fibers in the hilus of the ovary.

**sympathochromaffin c's,** small round cells in the fetal suprarenal gland, the forerunners of the sympathetic and medullary cells.

**syncytial c.,** a cell whose cytoplasm is confluent with that of an adjacent cell.

**syncytiotrophoblastic c's,** large, multinucleate cells resembling the syncytiotrophoblast, having hyperchromatic nuclei and abundant eosinophilic, sometimes vacuolated cytoplasm; one of the cell types that compose a choriocarcinoma. Cf. *cytotrophoblastic c's.*

**synovial c's,** fibroblasts lying between the cartilaginous fibers in the synovial membrane of joints.

**T c's,** T lymphocytes; see under *lymphocyte.*

**$T_{DTH}$ c's,** activated T cells producing lymphokines mediating the delayed-type hypersensitivity reaction; most are in the population exhibiting the same surface markers as helper cells.

**tactile c.,** 1. corpuscula tactus. 2. an epithelial cell that contains a tactile corpuscle.

**tadpole c's,** cells with an elongated cytoplasmic tail.

**target c.,** 1. an abnormally thin erythrocyte that when stained shows a dark center and a peripheral ring of hemoglobin, separated by a pale unstained ring containing less hemoglobin; seen in certain congenital and acquired anemias, thalassemia, certain hemoglobinopathies, liver disease, especially obstructive jaundice, and other disorders, and the postsplenectomy state. Called also *codocyte, leptocyte, Mexican hat c.* or *erythrocyte,* and *target erythrocyte.* 2. any cell selectively affected by a particular agent, such as a hormone or drug.

**tart c.,** a macrophage or monocytoid reticuloendothelial cell that contains a phagocytized nucleus with well preserved nuclear structure; the phagocytized nucleus, as distinguished from an LE cell inclusion, shows an intact chromatin pattern, chromatin that is more dense and tends to become vacuolated, and is frequently smaller than that in a true LE cell.

**taste c's,** the cells in a taste bud that have gustatory receptors and are thus directly involved in taste; they undergo degeneration and replacement every few days. Called also *gustatory c's.*

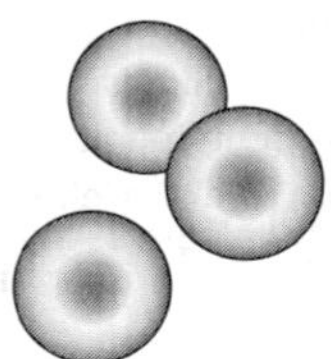

Target cells.

**tautomeral c's,** cells of the gray matter of the spinal cord whose axons pass into the white substance of the same side of the cord.
**teardrop c.,** dacryocyte.
**tegmental c's,** cells that cover any delicate structure.
**tendon c's,** flattened tissue cells of connective tissue occurring in rows between the primary bundles of the tendons.
**T$\gamma$ c's,** T lymphocytes bearing Fc receptors for IgG; they exhibit suppressor cell function.
**theca c's,** theca-lutein c's.
**theca-lutein c's,** lutein cells derived from the theca interna; called also *paraluteal* or *paralutein c's.*
**Thoma-Zeiss counting c.,** see under *chamber.*
**thyroidectomy c's,** hypertrophied thyrotrophs found in the adenohypophysis after thyroidectomy and in severe thyroid hormone deficiency.
**thyrotrope c., thyrotroph c., thyrotropic c.,** thyrotroph.
**T$\mu$ c's,** lymphocytes bearing Fc receptors for IgM; they exhibit helper cell function.
**totipotential c.,** an embryonic cell that is capable of developing into any variety of body cells.
**touch c.,** 1. corpusculum tactus. 2. tactile c. (def. 2).
**Touton giant c.,** a large vacuolated cell with numerous nuclei surrounding a peripheral rim of foamy cytoplasm; characteristic of such diseases as xanthomas, juvenile xanthogranuloma, and histiocytosis X.
**transitional c's,** 1. cells in the process of changing from one type to another. 2. in the sinoatrial and atrioventricular nodes, small, slow-conducting, heterogeneous cells interposed between the P cells and Purkinje cells; they are thought to link the impulses generated by the P cells with the rest of the myocardium.
**trophochrome c's,** serous cells whose secretory granules give a staining reaction for mucus with mucicarmine; called also *mucoalbuminous c's* and *mucoserous c's.*
**tufted c.,** a type of cell in the olfactory bulb, smaller, more numerous, and more superficially located than a mitral cell but with similar functions and connections.
**Türk's c.,** a nongranular, mononuclear cell displaying morphologic characteristics of both an atypical lymphocyte and a plasma cell, observed in the peripheral blood during severe anemias, chronic infections, and leukemoid reactions; called also *Türk's irritation leukocyte.*
**tympanic c's,** cellulae tympanicae.
**type I c's,** alveolar c's, type I.
**type II c's,** alveolar c's, type II.
**Tzanck c.,** a degenerated epithelial cell caused by acantholysis, and found especially in pemphigus.
**ultimobranchial c's,** parafollicular c's.
**vacuolated c.,** a cell whose protoplasm contains vacuoles.
**vasofactive c., vasoformative c.,** angioblast (def. 2).
**veil c's, veiled c's,** antigen-presenting cells with numerous surface ruffles or veil-like processes found in the afferent lymph and lymphatic sinuses; they may contain inclusions similar to those characteristic of the Langerhans' cells of the epidermis (Birbeck granules).
**ventricular c.,** any of the columnar epithelial cells of the neural tube.
**Vero c's,** a cell line derived from African green monkey kidney cells, used in the isolation of viruses.
**veto c's,** a subset of suppressor cells that are passively recognized by autoreactive cytotoxic T cells that recognize major histocompatibility antigens on the veto cells; this one-way recognition results in the elimination of the autoreactive cytotoxic T cells.
**Vignal's c's,** embryonic connective tissue cells secreting myelin and associated with the formation of the axons of nerves in the fetus.
**Virchow c's,** lepra c's.
**visual c's,** the neuroepithelial photoreceptor portion of the retina, the first neurons of the vertical linkage of the retina, consisting of two kinds of cells: the *retinal cones* and *retinal rods* (see under *cone* and *rod*). Each rod or cone has an inner, axonal, process synapsing with one or more horizontal or bipolar retinal cells, has a soma in the outer nuclear layer, and has a photosensitive outer dendritic process that extends toward the pigment epithelium. See also *ganglion c.* Called also *photoreceptor c's.*
**voltaic c.,** an electrochemical cell (q.v.) that serves as a voltage source. Called also *galvanic c.*
**von Hansemann c's,** macrophages containing Michaelis-Gutmann bodies, occurring as sheets of cells in malacoplakia of the urinary tract or kidney.
**von Kupffer's c's,** Kupffer's c's.
**wandering c.,** ameboid c.
**wandering c., primitive, wandering c., primordial,** a small mononuclear cell of the embryo that arises from the mesoderm and subsequently by differentiation gives rise to wandering cells of the body.
**Warthin-Finkeldey c's,** multinucleate giant cells with intranuclear inclusions, of lymphoreticular origin, seen in various organs, including lymph nodes, tonsil, appendix, and thymus, just prior to or during the prodromal phase of measles.
**wasserhelle c., water-clear c.,** a large clear cell found in the parathyroid gland; these cells have a ballooned appearance and are especially numerous in adenoma of the gland.
**Wedl c's,** large swollen cells (bladder cells) formed by the capsular epithelium in cataract development.
**white c., white blood c.,** leukocyte.
**wing c's,** cells in the corneal epithelium with convex anterior surfaces and concave posterior surfaces.
**xanthoma c's,** foam c's (def. 2).
**Zander's c's,** bladder c's.
**zymogenic c's,** chief c's, def. 1.

---

**cel·lac·e·fate** (sel-as'ə-fāt) [NF] a reduction product of phthalic anhydride and a partial acetate ester of cellulose; it is a free-flowing white powder used as a tablet-coating agent. Called also *cellulose acetate phthalate.*

**Cel·lase 1000** (sel'ās) trademark for a preparation of cellulase, used as a digestant adjunct.

**Cell·Cept** (sel'sept) trademark for a preparation of mycophenolate mofetil.

**Cell·fal·cic·u·la** (sel"fəl-sik'u-lə) a genus of bacteria of uncertain status, which have been assigned conditionally to the genus *Pseudomonas.*

**Cel·lia** (sel'e-ə) [Angelo *Celli,* Italian physician, 1857–1914] a subgenus of mosquitoes of the genus *Anopheles,* vectors of malaria in Africa and Asia.

**cel·lic·o·lous** (sə-lik'ə-ləs) [*cella* + *colere* to dwell] inhabiting cells.

**cel·lif·er·ous** (sə-lif'ər-əs) producing or bearing cells.

**cel·li·form** (sel'ĭ-form) cell-like.

**cel·lif·u·gal** (sə-lif'u-gəl) cellulifugal.

**cel·lip·e·tal** (sə-lip'ə-təl) cellulipetal.

**cel·lo·bi·ose** (sel"lo-bi'ōs) [MeSH: Cellobiose] a disaccharide, two glucose moieties in $\beta$-(1,4) linkage, forming the basic repeating unit of cellulose and obtained by partial hydrolysis of the polysaccharide.

**cel·lo·bi·uron·ic ac·id** (sel"o-bi"u-ron'ik) a disaccharide consisting of glucose and glucuronic acid linked at positions 1 and 4, found in the capsular polysaccharides of *Streptococcus pneumoniae.* See also *pneumococcus polysaccharide,* under *polysaccharide.*

**cel·loi·din** (sə-loi'din) a concentrated preparation of pyroxylin, employed in microscopy for embedding specimens for section cutting.

**cel·lo·phane** (sel'o-fān) [MeSH: Cellophane] a transparent tissue of regenerated cellulose used as a dialysis membrane and for bandages, compresses, etc.

**cel·lu·la** (sel'u-lə) pl. *cel'lulae* [L., dim. of *cella*] 1. [TA] a general term for a small, more or less enclosed space. 2. in histology, a cell.
**cel'lulae ethmoida'les** [TA], ethmoidal cells: collective name for a type of paranasal sinus occurring in groups within the ethmoid bone and communicating with the ethmoidal infundibulum and bulla and the superior and highest meatuses. They are often subdivided into *cellulae ethmoidales anteriores, medii,* and *posteriores,* named according to the location of their openings into the nasal meatus. Called also *sinus ethmoidales.*
**cel'lulae ethmoida'les anterio'res** [TA], anterior ethmoidal cells: ethmoidal air cells that open into the middle nasal meatus; they are often grouped with adjacent middle and posterior ethmoidal cells and called simply *ethmoidal cells* or *sinuses.*Called also *sinus ethmoidales anteriores.*
**cel'lulae ethmoida'les me'diae** [TA], middle ethmoidal cells: ethmoidal air cells that open into the middle nasal meatus; they are often grouped with adjacent anterior and posterior ethmoidal sinuses and called simply *ethmoidal cells.* Called also *sinus ethmoidales medii.*

**cel'lulae ethmoida'les posterio'res** [TA], posterior ethmoidal cells: ethmoidal air cells that open into the superior nasal meatus; they are often grouped with adjacent middle and anterior ethmoidal sinuses and called simply *ethmoidal cells.* Called also *sinus ethmoidales posteriores.*
**cel'lulae len'tis,** fibrae lentis.
**cel'lulae mastoi'deae** [TA], mastoid cells: the air cells in the mastoid process of the temporal bone.
**cel'lulae pneuma'ticae tu'bae auditi'vae** [TA], air cells of auditory tube: air cells in the floor of the auditory tube close to the carotid canal, being similar to the air cells of the mastoid part of the temporal bone; called also *cellulae pneumaticae tubae auditoriae* [TA alternative], *cellulae pneumaticae tubariae,* and *tubal air cells.*
**cel'lulae pneuma'ticae tu'bae audito'riae,** TA alternative for *cellulae pneumaticae tubae auditivae.*
**cel'lulae pneuma'ticae tuba'riae,** cellulae pneumaticae tubae auditivae.
**cel'lulae tympa'nicae** [TA], tympanic cells: spaces in the tympanic cavity between the bony projections from the floor, or jugular wall.

**cel·lu·lae** (sel'u-le) [L.] plural of *cellula.*

**cel·lu·lar** (sel'u-lər) pertaining to, or made up of, cells.

**cel·lu·lar·i·ty** (sel″u-lar'ĭ-te) the state of a tissue or other mass as regards the number of constituent cells.

**cel·lu·lase** (sel'u-lās) [EC 3.2.1.4] [MeSH: Cellulase] an enzyme of the hydrolase class that catalyzes the cleavage of internal $\beta$-(1,4) glycosidic linkages, such as occur in cellulose. It occurs in various bacteria, fungi, plants, and lower animals but is absent from higher animals.

**cel·lule** (sel'ūl) [L. *cellula*] a small cell; see also *cellula.*
**c. claire,** clear cell.

**cel·lu·lic·i·dal** (sel″u-lis'ĭ-dəl) [*cellula* + *-cide* + *-al*[1]] cytocidal.

**cel·lu·lif·u·gal** (sel″u-lif'ə-gəl) [*cellula* + *-fugal*] directed away from a cell body.

**cel·lu·lip·e·tal** (cel″u-lip'ə-təl) [*cellula* + *-petal*] directed toward a cell body.

**cel·lu·li·tis** (sel″u-li'tis) [*cellule* + *-itis*] [MeSH: Cellulitis] an acute, diffuse, spreading, edematous, suppurative inflammation of the deep subcutaneous tissues and sometimes muscle, sometimes with abscess formation; the skin is warm and tender. It is usually caused by infection of a wound, burn, or other cutaneous lesion by bacteria, especially group A streptococci and *Staphylococcus aureus,* but it may also occur in immunocompromised hosts or following erysipelas. It tends to spread to tissue spaces and cleavage planes owing to bacterial elaboration of large amounts of hyaluronidases that break down polysaccharide ground substance, fibrinolysins that digest fibrin barriers, and lecithinases that destroy cell membranes. Cf. *erysipelas* and *phlegmon,* def. 1.
**anaerobic c.,** see *clostridial anaerobic c.* and *nonclostridial anaerobic c.*
**clostridial anaerobic c.,** cellulitis due to a necrotizing clostridial infection, especially one caused by *Clostridium perfringens,* usually arising in devitalized tissue in a contaminated wound or in otherwise compromised tissues, and characterized by a foul-smelling discharge, widespread gas formation, and frank crepitus. The clinical findings are relatively milder than those seen in true gas gangrene.
**dissecting c. of scalp,** perifolliculitis capitis abscedens et suffodiens.
**eosinophilic c.,** Wells' syndrome.
**facial c.,** acute cellulitis involving the face, especially the cheek or periorbital or orbital tissues, although other areas such as the neck may be affected, which may be produced by spread of an infection from nearby or distant foci. It is characterized by a bluish or purplish red, tender, poorly demarcated area of indurated cellulitis with an edematous border, and often accompanied by fever, local pain, and bacteremia. *Haemophilus influenzae* type b is the etiologic agent in children under 5 years of age. Group B streptococci and *Streptococcus pneumoniae* have also been shown to cause a clinically similar condition in children. In adults and older children, *Staphylococcus aureus* and group A streptococci are the predominant etiologic agents.
**finger c.,** felon.
**gangrenous c.,** 1. necrotizing fasciitis. 2. necrotic dermatitis.
**indurated c.,** a hard, brawny induration of the skin of the lower leg, sometimes painful and disabling, caused by a low-grade inflammation in association with chronic venous insufficiency (see *postphlebitic syndrome,* under *syndrome*); it is seen most often proximal to the internal malleolus but can affect other areas and even the entire circumference of the leg. Called also *phlebitic induration.*
**intermandibular c.,** pharyngeal phlegmon.
**juvenile c.,** see under *pyoderma.*
**necrotizing c.,** see under *fasciitis.*
**nonclostridial anaerobic c.,** cellulitis usually occurring as a result of microbial synergism between different aerobic and anaerobic bacteria, generally characterized by progressive tissue destruction, which eventually leads to a fatal septicemia caused by the aerobic component, with or without an associated anaerobic bacteremia.
**orbital c.,** facial cellulitis usually secondary to sinusitis in children, characterized by proptosis, lid swelling, chemosis, and impaired ocular motility; it occasionally can cause blindness and death.
**pelvic c.,** parametritis.
**periurethral c.,** see under *phlegmon.*
**phlegmonous c.,** phlegmon, def. 1.
**preseptal c.,** facial cellulitis affecting the anterior part of the orbital septum, with edema of the eyelids; it may be caused by spread of infection from some other area or by trauma to the periorbital tissue.
**ulcerative c.,** see under *lymphangitis.*

**cel·lu·lo·fi·brous** (sel″u-lo-fi'brəs) partly cellular and partly fibrous.

**cel·lu·lose** (sel'u-lōs) [MeSH: Cellulose] the most abundant polysaccharide in nature, a rigid, colorless, unbranched, insoluble, long chain polymer, consisting of 3000 to 5000 glucose residues in $\beta$-(1,4) linkage and forming the skeleton of most plant structures and of plant cells; it can be enzymatically hydrolyzed to the disaccharide cellobiose, although man lacks the necessary enzyme, cellulase.
**absorbable c.,** oxidized c.
**c. acetate phthalate,** cellacefate.
**hydroxyethyl c.** [NF], a partially substituted, nonionic, water-soluble cellulose ether available in several grades that vary in viscosity and degree of substitution and some of which are modified to improve their dispersion in water; it may contain suitable anticaking agents. Used as a pharmaceutic aid (suspending agent and viscosity-increasing agent).
**hydroxypropyl c.** [NF], a partially substituted, water-soluble cellulose ether, which may contain suitable anticaking agents, used as a pharmaceutic aid (emulsifying agent and tablet-coating agent) and as an ophthalmic protectant and lubricant, applied topically.
**microcrystalline c.** [NF], purified, partially depolymerized cellulose prepared by treating alpha cellulose, obtained as a pulp from fibrous plant material with mineral acids; used as a tablet and capsule diluent.
**oxidized c.** [USP], cellulose partially oxidized and with a varying content of carboxylic acid groups, which confers some solubility in dilute alkali; it is insoluble in water. Dried in a vacuum over phosphorus pentoxide, it is used as a local hemostatic. Called also *absorbable c.* and *absorbable cotton.*
**c. sodium phosphate** [USP], an insoluble, nonabsorbable ion-exchange resin prepared by phosphorylation of cellulose; it exchanges sodium for calcium and when taken orally binds calcium, which is then excreted in the feces. Used to reduce urinary calcium in the treatment of hyperabsorptive hypercalciuria.
**tetranitrate c.,** $(C_{12}H_{16}N_4O_{18})_n$, the principal constituent of pyroxylin.

**cel·lu·lo·sic ac·id** (sel″u-lo'sik) oxidized cellulose.

**cel·lu·los·i·ty** (sel″u-los'ĭ-te) the condition of being composed of cells.

**cel·lu·lo·tox·ic** (sel″u-lo-tok'sik) toxic to cells.

**cel·lu·lous** (sel'u-ləs) made up of cells.

**cel(o)-**[1] [Gr. *kēlē* tumor] a combining form denoting relationship to a tumor or swelling.

**cel(o)-**[2] [Gr. *koilos* hollow] see *coel(o)-.*

**cel(o)-** [Gr. *koilia* belly] see *celi(o)-.*

**ce·lom** (se'ləm) coelom.

**ce·lom·ic** (se-lom'ik) coelomic.

**Ce·lon·tin** (se-lon'tin) trademark for a preparation of methsuximide.

**ce·lo·phle·bi·tis** (se″lo-flə-bi'tis) [*celo-*[2] + *phlebitis*] cavitis.

**ce·los·chi·sis** (se-los'kĭ-sis) [*celo-*[3] + *-schisis*] abdominal fissure.

**celo·scope** (sel'o-skōp) celioscope.

**ce·los·co·py** (sə-los'kə-pe) celioscopy.

**ce·lo·so·mia** (se″lo-so'me-ə) [*celo-*[3] + *soma*] a developmental anomaly characterized by fissure or absence of the sternum and hernial protrusion of the viscera. Cf. *thoracoceloschisis.*

**ce·lo·so·mus** (se″lo-so'məs) a fetus exhibiting celosomia; called also *kelosomus.*

**ce·lo·thel** (se'lo-thəl) mesothelium.

**ce·lo·the·li·um** (se″lo-the'le-əm) mesothelium.

**ce·lot·o·my** (se-lot'ə-me) herniotomy.

**ce·lo·zo·ic** (se″lo-zo'ik) [*celo-*[2] + *zoic*] inhabiting the intestinal cavities of the body; said of parasites.

**Cel·si·us scale, thermometer** (sel'se-əs) [Anders *Celsius,* Swedish astronomer, 1701–1744] see under *scale* and *thermometer.*

**Cel·sus** (sel'səs) Aulus Cornelius (1st century A.D.) a Roman encyclopedist. Of his many writings, only his *De re medicina* (in eight books) survives; the four classical signs (Celsus' quadrilateral) of inflammation—*calor* (heat), *dolor* (pain), *rubor* (redness), and *tumor* (swelling)—are mentioned in the third book of this work. Celsus was a layman writing for other laymen; his outline of the history of medicine is very important.

**CEM** contagious equine metritis.

**ce·ment** (sə-ment') [L. *cemen'tum*] 1. a substance that serves to produce solid union between two surfaces. 2. a filling material, such as zinc phosphate, used in dentistry to assist in retaining gold castings in prepared teeth and to insulate the tooth pulp from metallic and other fillings. 3. cementum.
**calcium hydroxide c.**, a dental cement that promotes the formation of a protective layer of secondary dentin, which is particularly beneficial in aiding healing of the pulp; used principally for pulp capping, as a thermal insulating base, and for protection from chemical insult.
**dental c.**, any of several bonding substances that are placed in the mouth as a viscous liquid and set to a hard mass; used in restorative and orthodontic dental procedures as luting (cementing) agents, as bases, and as restorative materials. Resins and polymers used as restorative materials are usually called restorative resins rather than cements.
**glass ionomer c.**, a dental cement produced by mixing a powder prepared from a calcium fluoroaluminosilicate glass and a liquid prepared from an aqueous solution of polyacrylic acid; used for small restorations on the proximal surfaces of anterior teeth, for restoration of eroded areas at the gingival margin, and as a luting agent for restorations and orthodontic bands.
**glass ionomer c., hybrid,** resin-modified glass ionomer c.
**glass ionomer c., resin-modified,** a type of glass ionomer cement with pendant methacrylate groups attached to polycarboxylic acid; it also may contain other water-soluble methacrylate monomers and complex vinyl-carboxylate monomers. Hardening occurs by acid-base reaction plus addition polymerization. Called also *hybrid glass ionomer c.*
**intercellular c.**, a mucilaginous substance that holds cells, and especially epithelial cells, together.
**muscle c.**, myoglia.
**polycarboxylate c.**, a dental cement made by mixing a powder consisting chiefly of zinc oxide and an aqueous solution of polyacrylic acid; used as a luting agent for cementing restorations and as a cavity lining.
**resin c.**, one of several polymer or monomer/polymer systems, usually containing finely divided inorganic filler particles, used as an insoluble dental luting agent in the cementation of orthodontic brackets, ceramic, resin, and metal restorations, and etched based metal extracoronal retainers to etched enamel.
**root canal c.**, see under *sealer.*
**silicate c.**, a dental cement that is translucent and porcelainlike when set; formerly used for esthetic temporary and semipermanent restorations of anterior teeth.
**silicophosphate c.**, a mixture of silicate and zinc phosphate cements, formerly used as temporary filling material and for cementation of orthodontic bands, cast restorations, and porcelain jacket crowns; it has been replaced by resin cements and glass ionomer cements.
**zinc oxide–eugenol c.**, a dental cement made by mixing zinc oxide powder with eugenol liquid and a small amount of water; used chiefly in temporary restorations, thermal insulating bases, and root canal fillings and as a temporary luting agent.
**zinc phosphate c.**, a dental cement made by mixing a powder that consists chiefly of zinc oxide and magnesium oxide as a modifier with a liquid that is a mixture of phosphoric acid, water, and metallic salts that act as buffering agents; used primarily as a luting agent for fabricated restorations and secondarily in temporary restorations and as a thermal insulating agent.

**ce·men·ta·tion** (se″mən-ta'shən) [MeSH: Cementation] the attachment of anything by the means of cement, such as the use of cement in attaching restorative material to a natural tooth, or the use of an adhesive material to attach bands to the tooth.

**ce·men·ti·cle** (sə-men'tĭ-kəl) a small, discrete focus of calcified tissue that may or may not represent true cementum, found in the periodontal ligament.
**adherent c., attached c.,** one that is firmly connected with the cementum.
**free c., interstitial c.,** one that is completely surrounded by connective tissue of the periodontal ligament.

**ce·men·ti·fi·ca·tion** (sə-men″tĭ-fĭ-ka'shən) cementogenesis.

**ce·men·tin** (sə-men'tin) the material that sometimes unites the margins of squamous endothelial cells.

**ce·men·ti·tis** (se″mən-ti'tis) inflammation of the cementum of a tooth.

**cement(o)-** [L. *cementum,* q.v.] a combining form denoting relationship to the cementum.

**ce·men·to·blast** (sə-men'to-blast) [*cemento-* + *-blast*] a large cell ranging in shape from cuboidal to squamous with a large central nucleus and usually a single nucleolus, which is active in the formation of cementum (cementogenesis).

**ce·men·to·blas·to·ma** (sə-men″to-blas-to'mə) a rare, benign odontogenic tumor arising from the cementum and presenting as a proliferating mass contiguous with a tooth root, particularly that of a mandibular molar. Patients are generally asymptomatic, although cortical expansion and pain can occur.

**ce·men·to·cla·sia** (sə-men″to-kla'zhə) [*cemento-* + Gr. *klasis* breaking + *-ia*] dissolution and resorption of the cementum of a tooth; usually a complication of trauma or pathologic conditions.

**ce·men·to·clast** (sə-men'to-klast″) [*cemento-* + *clast*] a cell, cytomorphologically the same as an osteoclast, involved in cementum resorption; the cavities produced by resorption are known as *resorption lacunae.* Called also *odontoclast.*

**ce·men·to·cyte** (sə-men'to-sīt) [*cemento-* + *-cyte*] a cell in the lacunae of cellular cementum, ranging in shape from round to oval or flattened, and exhibiting numerous protoplasmic processes extending from its free surface. Called also *cement cell.*

**ce·men·to·gen·e·sis** (sə-men″to-jen'ə-sis) [*cemento-* + *-genesis*] the development of the cementum on the root dentin of a tooth; called also *cementification.*

**ce·men·toid** (sə-men'toid) [*cement* + *-oid*] the surface uncalcified layer of the cementum in areas of intact periodontal tissue. Called also *precementum* and *uncalcified cementum.*

**ce·men·to·ma** (se″mən-to'mə) [MeSH: Cementoma] any of a variety of benign cementum-producing tumors including cementoblastoma, cementifying fibroma, florid osseous dysplasia, and periapical cemental dysplasia, particularly the last.
**gigantiform c.**, florid osseous dysplasia.
**true c.**, cementoblastoma.

**ce·men·to·path·ia** (sə-men'to-path'e-ə) periodontitis or periodontosis resulting from disease or defect of the cementum.

**ce·men·to·peri·os·ti·tis** (sə-men″to-pər″e-os-ti'tis) periodontitis.

**ce·men·to·sis** (se″mən-to'sis) hypercementosis.

**ce·men·tum** (sə-men'təm) [L.] [TA] the bonelike rigid connective tissue covering the root of a tooth from the cementoenamel junction to the apex and lining the apex of the root canal; it also serves as an attachment structure for the periodontal ligament, thus assisting in tooth support. Called also *substantia ossea dentis.*
**acellular c.**, the cementum without cellular components that covers one-third to one-half of the tooth root adjacent to the cementoenamel junction; it is usually apposed by a layer of cellular cementum.
**afibrillar c.**, a layer of cementum, containing acid mucopolysaccharides and possibly nonfibrillar collagen, that sometimes extends onto the enamel of a tooth at the cementoenamel junction.
**cellular c.**, the cementum covering the apical one-half to two-thirds of the tooth root, which contains cementocytes embedded in the calcified matrix; it is usually apposed by a layer of acellular cementum.
**uncalcified c.**, cementoid.

**ce·na·del·phus** (se″nə-del'fəs) [*ceno-*[3] + *-adelphus*] symmetrical conjoined twins.

**ce·nes·the·sia** (se″nes-the'zhə) [*ceno-*[3] + *esthesia*] somatognosis.

**ce·nes·the·sic** (se″nəs-the'sik) pertaining to cenesthesia.

**ce·nes·the·si·op·a·thy** (se″nəs-the″ze-op'ə-the) [*cenesthesia* + *-pathy*] cenesthopathy.

**ce·nes·thet·ic** (se″nəs-thet'ik) cenesthesic.

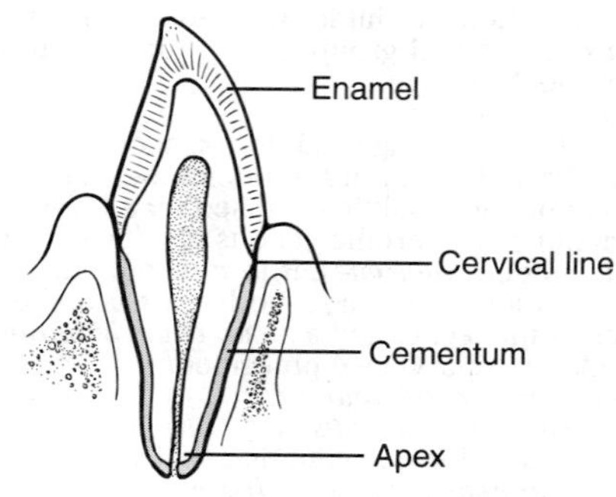


Cementum covering the anatomical root of an anterior tooth.

**ce·nes·thop·a·thy** (se″nəs-thop′ə-the) a general feeling of discomfort, unease, and lack of wellness not referable to any particular part of the body.

**cen(o)-**[1] [Gr. *kainos* new, fresh] a combining form meaning new; written also *cain(o)-* and *kain(o)-*.

**cen(o)-**[2] [Gr. *kenos* empty] a combining form meaning empty; written also *caen(o)-* and *ken(o)-*.

**cen(o)-**[3] [Gr. *koinos* shared in common] a combining form denoting relationship to a common feature or characteristic; written also *coen(o)-*, *coin(o)-*, and *koin(o)-*.

**ce·no·bi·um** (sə-no′be-əm) [Gr. *koinobios* living in communion with others] a colony of independent cells or organisms held together by a common investment.

**ce·no·cyte** (se′no-sīt) coenocyte.

**ce·no·gen·e·sis** (se″no-jen′ə-sis) [*ceno-*[1] + *-genesis*] the appearance of new features in development, in adaptive response to environmental conditions. Cf. *palingenesis*, def. 2.

**ce·no·psych·ic** (se″no-si′kik) [*ceno-*[1] + *psychic*] of recent appearance in mental development.

**ce·no·site** (se′no-sīt) coinosite.

**ce·no·type** (se′no-tīp) [*ceno-*[3] + *type*] the original type from which all forms have arisen.

**cen·sor** (sen′sər) a term used by Freud to refer to the mental faculty that guards the border between the unconscious and preconscious, preventing unconscious thoughts and wishes from coming into consciousness unless disguised, as in dreams. In Freud's later theory, the actions of the censor (displacement, condensation, symbolism, and repression) are considered defense mechanisms of the ego and superego.

**cen·sor·ship** (sen′sər-ship) the operation of the censor.

**Cen·tau·rea** (sen-taw′re-ə) a genus of plants with yellow flowers, found mainly in the western United States and Australia; when eaten by horses they cause nigropallidal encephalomalacia. *C. re′pens* is the Russian knapweed and *C. solstitia′lis* is the yellow star thistle.

**cen·ter** (sen′tər) [Gr. *kentron;* L. *centrum*] 1. the middle point of a body. 2. a collection of neurons in the central nervous system concerned with performance of a particular function; see also *area.*

## Center

**accelerating c.**, the part of the vasomotor center involved in acceleration of the heart; called also *cardioaccelerating c.*

**anospinal c's**, the centers for contracting the sphincter ani, for relaxing it (defecation center), and for the anal reflex; all are in the lumbar enlargement.

**apneustic c.**, the neurons in the brain stem that control normal respiration; not a true center.

**auditopsychic c.**, auditory association area.

**Broca's c.**, Broca's motor speech area.

**Budge's c.**, erection c.

**cardioaccelerating c.**, accelerating c.

**cardioinhibitory c.**, the part of the vasomotor center that exerts an inhibitory influence on the heart by way of the vagus. Called also *Kronecker's c.*.

**cardiovascular control c's**, vasomotor c's.

**cell c.**, centrosome.

**chiral c.**, the center of dyssymmetry in a molecule, usually an atom with four different substituents (e.g., a carbon with four single bonds or the nitrogen of a quaternary amine).

**c's of chondrification**, dense aggregations of embryonic mesenchymal cells at sites of future cartilage formation; called also *protochondral tissue.*

**ciliospinal c.**, a center in the lower cervical and upper thoracic portions of the spinal cord, connected with the dilatation of the pupil.

**community mental health c. (CMHC)**, a mental health facility or group of affiliated agencies that provide various psychotherapeutic services to a designated catchment area.

**coordination c.**, a nerve center serving the function of coordination.

**coughing c.**, a center in the medulla oblongata, situated above the respiratory center, which controls the act of coughing.

**defecation c.**, see *anospinal c's.*

**deglutition c.**, a nerve center in the medulla oblongata that controls the function of swallowing.

**dentary c.**, an ossification center of the mandible, giving origin to the lower border and outer plate.

**C's for Disease Control and Prevention (CDC)**, an agency of the U.S. Department of Health and Human Services, with headquarters in Atlanta, Georgia, concerned with all phases of control of communicable, vector-borne, and occupational diseases and with the prevention of disease, injury, and disability. The CDC's responsibilities include epidemiology, surveillance, detection, laboratory science, ecologic investigations, training, disease control methods, chronic disease prevention, health promotion, and injury prevention and control. Formerly called *Communicable Disease Center* (1946), *Center for Disease Control* (1970), and *Centers for Disease Control* (1980).

**ejaculation c.**, the reflex center in the lumbar spinal cord that regulates ejaculation of semen during sexual stimulation.

**epiotic c.**, the center of ossification that forms the mastoid process.

**erection c.**, a reflex center in the sacral spinal cord that regulates erection of the penis or clitoris. Called also *Budge's c.* or *genital c.*

**eupraxic c.**, premotor area.

**feeding c.**, a group of cells in the lateral hypothalamus that when stimulated cause a sensation of hunger; called also *hunger c.*

**Flemming c.**, germinal c.

**genital c., genitospinal c.**, erection c.

**germinal c.**, the area in the center of a lymph nodule containing aggregations of actively proliferating lymphocytes (antibody-forming B cells); it appears as a spherical mass surrounded by a capsule of elongated cells that is partially invested by a crescentic cap of small lymphocytes. Called also *Flemming c.* and *secondary nodule.*

**glossokinesthetic c.**, motor speech area.

**health c.**, 1. a community health organization for creating health work and coordinating the efforts of all health agencies. 2. an educational complex consisting of a medical school and various allied health professional schools.

**heat-regulating c's**, thermoregulatory c's.

**hunger c.**, feeding c.

**Kerckring's (Kerkring's) c.**, an ossification center sometimes present in the posterior margin of the foramen magnum at about the sixteenth week of fetal life, which unites with the other squamous parts prior to birth. Called also *Kerckring's ossicle.*

**kinetic c.**, the centrospheres of a fertilized ovum.

**Kronecker's c.**, cardioinhibitory c.

**Lumsden's c.**, pneumotaxic c.

**medullary c.**, 1. medullary c. of cerebellum. 2. medullary respiratory c.

**medullary c. of cerebellum**, corpus medullare cerebelli.

**medullary respiratory c.**, the part of the respiratory centers that is in the medulla oblongata, divided between the *dorsal respiratory group* and the *ventral respiratory group.*

**micturition c.**, a center controlling the bladder and inhibiting the tension of the vesical sphincter, situated in the lumbar enlargement.

**nerve c.**, center (def. 2).

**optic c.**, that point in a lens, or combination of lenses, where all rays that help to form a clear image cross the principal axis; in the eye, about 2 mm. behind the cornea.

**ossification c.**, centrum ossificationis.

**ossification c., primary**, centrum ossificationis primarium.

**ossification c., secondary**, centrum ossificationis secundarium.

**panting c.**, polypneic c.

**phrenic c.**, centrum tendineum diaphragmatis.

**pneumotaxic c.**, a center in the upper part of the pons that rhythmically inhibits inspiration independently of the vagi; called also *Lumsden's c.*

**polypneic c.**, a center in the tuber cinereum that accelerates the rate of breathing.

**pteriotic c.**, a center of ossification in the fetus and infant, from which are developed the tegmen tympani and the covering of the lateral semicircular canal.

**reaction c.**, germinal c.

**rectovesical c.**, a cord reflex center for the rectum and bladder.

**reflex c.**, any center in the brain or spinal cord in which a sensory impression is changed into a motor impulse.

**respiratory c's**, a series of centers in the medulla and pons which coordinate respiratory movements; they include the pneumotaxic center, the apneustic center, and the dorsal and ventral respiratory groups.

**rotation c.**, the point or axis about which a body rotates.

**satiety c.**, a group of cells in the ventromedial hypothalamus that when stimulated suppress the desire for food.

**semioval c.**, centrum semiovale.

**sensory c's**, primary receptive areas.

## Center *Continued*

**sex-behavior c.**, ventromedial nucleus of hypothalamus.
**sphenotic c.**, a center of ossification in the fetal sphenoid bone for the lingula.
**splenial c.**, one of the ossification centers of the mandible, forming a part of its inner plate.
**sudorific c.**, 1. a center in the anterior hypothalamus controlling diaphoresis. 2. any of several centers in the medulla oblongata or spinal cord that exercise parasympathetic control over diaphoresis.
**swallowing c.**, deglutition c.
**sweat c.**, sudorific c.
**thermoregulatory c's**, hypothalamic centers regulating the conservation and dissipation of heat.
**thirst c.**, a group of cells in the lateral hypothalamus that when stimulated cause a sensation of thirst.
**vasoconstrictor c.**, a center in the medulla oblongata and lower pons that controls contraction of the blood vessels.
**vasodilator c.**, a center in the medulla oblongata that causes dilation of blood vessels by repressing the activity of the vasoconstrictor center.
**vasomotor c's**, centers in the medulla oblongata and the lower pons that regulate the caliber of the blood vessels and increase or decrease the heart rate and contractility. See also *vasoconstrictor c.* and *vasodilator c.;* called also *cardiovascular control c's.*
**vesical c., vesicospinal c.**, micturition c.
**vomiting c.**, a center in the lower central region of the medulla oblongata; its stimulation causes vomiting. See also *chemoreceptor trigger zone,* under *zone.*
**word c., auditory**, Wernicke's area.

**cen·tes·i·mal** (sen-tes'ĭ-məl) [L. *centesimus* hundredth] divided into hundredths or based upon divisions into hundredths.

**cen·te·sis** (sen-te'sis) [Gr. *kentēsis*] perforation or tapping, as with an aspirator, trocar, or needle.

**-centesis** a word termination used to denote a perforation or tapping operation, with the part on which it is performed indicated by the root to which the suffix is affixed, e.g., *abdominocentesis* or *thoracocentesis.*

**centi-** [L. *centum* one hundred] a combining form denoting (1) one hundredth ($10^{-2}$) of the unit designated by the root with which it is combined (symbol, c) as in centimeter (cm) or (2) one hundred, as in centipede.

**cen·ti·grade** (sen'tĭ-grād) [*centi-* + L. *gradus* a step] consisting of or having 100 gradations (steps or degrees); abbreviated C. See *Celsius (centigrade) scale,* under *scale.*

**cen·ti·gray** (sen'tĭ-grā") a unit of absorbed radiation dose equal to one hundredth of a gray, or 1 rad; abbreviated cGy.

**cen·ti·li·ter** (sen'tĭ-le"tər) one one-hundredth of a liter ($10^{-2}$ L), or the equivalent of 0.33815 of a fluid ounce; abbreviated cL or cl.

**cen·ti·me·ter** (sen'tĭ-me"tər) [Fr. *centimètre*] a unit of length equal to one one-hundredth of a meter ($10^{-2}$ m); abbreviated cm.
**cubic c.**, a unit of volume equal to that of a cube one centimeter on a side, equal to 1 mL or $10^{-6}$ $m^3$. Symbol $cm^3$. Abbreviated cc or cu cm.

**cen·ti·mor·gan** (sen"tĭ-mor'gən) one one-hundredth of a morgan; the unit of distance on a linkage map. The map distance between adjacent loci, expressed in centimorgans, is equal to the recombination frequency, expressed as a percentage. For nonadjacent loci the map distance can be greater than the recombination frequency, because recombination frequencies are not always additive. Symbol, cM. Called also *map unit.*

**cen·ti·pede** (sen'tĭ-pēd) any arthropod of the class Chilopoda.

**cen·ti·poise** (sen'tĭ-poiz) one one-hundredth of a poise.

**cen·ti·stoke** (sen'tĭ-stōk) one one-hundredth of a stoke.

**cen·ti·u·nit** (sen"tĭ-u'nit) one one-hundredth of the conventional unit.

**cen·tra** (sen'trə) [L.] plural of *centrum.*

**cen·trad** (sen'trad) 1. [*centr-* + *-ad*] toward the center or a center, especially toward the center of the body. 2. [L. *centum* hundred + *radian*] a measure of an angle of deviation, being 0.57 degree, or one one-hundredth part of a radian; its symbol is $\triangle$; called also *prism degree.*

**cen·trage** (sen'trāj) the condition in which the centers of the various refracting surfaces of the eye are in the same straight line.

**cen·tral** (sen'trəl) situated at or pertaining to a center; not peripheral.

**cen·tra·lis** (sən-tra'lis) [L.] [TA] a general term denoting a centrally located structure.

**cen·tra·phose** (sen'trə-fōz) any aphose, or sensation of darkness, originating in the optic or visual centers.

**cen·tra·tion** (sən-tra'shən) the inability to pay attention to more than one salient feature at a time; it is a normal stage in human intellectual development.

**Cen·trax** (sen'traks) trademark for a preparation of prazepam.

**cen·trax·o·ni·al** (sen"trak-so'ne-əl) having the axis in a central median line.

**cen·tre** (sen'tər) center.

**cen·tren·ce·phal·ic** (sen"trən-sə-fal'ik) pertaining to the center of the encephalon; see under *system.*

**centri-** [L. *centrum* center, from Gr. *kentron* sharp point] a combining form denoting relationship to a center, or to a central location. Also, *centr(o)-.*

**cen·tric** (sen'trik) 1. pertaining to or situated at the center; central. 2. a term sometimes used as a noun to refer to *centric occlusion, centric relation,* or *power c.*
**power c.**, the position of the mandible during a forceful bite.
**true c.**, centric relation.

**cen·tric·i·put** (sən-tris'ĭ-pət) [*centri-* + *caput*] the central part of the upper surface of the head, located between the occiput and sinciput.

**cen·trif·u·gal** (sen-trif'ə-gəl) [*centri-* + *-fugal*] moving away from a center, moving away from the cerebral cortex; efferent.

**cen·trif·u·gate** (sən-trif'u-gāt) material subjected to centrifugation.

**cen·trif·u·ga·tion** (sen-trif"u-ga'shən) [MeSH: Centrifugation] the process of separating the lighter portions of a solution, mixture, or suspension from the heavier portions by centrifugal force.
**density gradient c.**, ultracentrifugation in a liquid, such as cesium chloride solution, the density of which increases along the lines of centrifugal force, the substances under test or preparation seeking their level of density.
**differential c.**, that based on the sedimentation coefficient of the substances under investigation; applied to homogenates to derive various subcellular fractions.
**isopyknic c.**, that in which the solvent is of the same density as the substance to be isolated.

**cen·tri·fuge** (sen'trĭ-fūj) [*centri-* + *-fuge*] 1. a machine by which centrifugation is effected. 2. to subject to centrifugation.
**microscope c.**, a high-speed centrifuge with a built-in microscope, permitting a specimen to be viewed under centrifugal force.

**cen·tri·lob·u·lar** (sen"trĭ-lob'u-lər) pertaining to the central portion of a lobule.

**cen·tri·ole** (sen'tre-ōl) [MeSH: Centrioles] either of the two cylindrical organelles located in the centrosome and containing nine triplets of microtubules arrayed around their edges; centrioles migrate to opposite poles of the cell during cell division and serve to organize the spindles. They are capable of independent replication and of migrating to form basal bodies.
**anterior c.**, proximal c.
**distal c.**, that centriole of a spermatozoon which, after migrating to the cell surface and giving rise to a slender flagellum, returns to a position just caudal to the proximal centriole; called also *posterior c.*
**posterior c.**, distal c.
**proximal c.**, that centriole of a spermatozoon which migrates to a position in a depression in the wall of the posterior portion of the nucleus, with its axis at right angles to the main axis of the spermatozoon, and from which the axoneme extends; called also *anterior c.*
**ring c.**, a dark annular structure at the posterior end of the middle piece of a spermatozoon; it is not a true centriole. Called also *anulus of spermatozoon.*

**cen·trip·e·tal** (sən-trip′ə-təl) [*centri-* + *-petal*] moving toward a center; moving toward the cerebral cortex; afferent.

**centr(o)-** see *centri-*.

**cen·tro·blast** (sen′tro-blast″) [*centro-* + *-blast*] a general term encompassing both large and small noncleaved follicular center cells.

**cen·tro·ce·cal** (sen″tro-se′kəl) pertaining to the central macular area and the blind spot; called also *cecocentral*.

**Cen·tro·ces·tus** (sen″tro-ses′təs) a genus of flukes.
**C. cuspida′tus,** a fluke occurring in the Egyptian kite. *C. cuspidatus* var. *canina* is reported from dogs in Taiwan; it may be the same as *Stamnosoma formosanum*.

**cen·tro·cyte** (sen′tro-sīt″) [*centro-* + *-cyte*] a general term encompassing both large and small cleaved follicular center cells.

**cen·tro·des·mose** (sen″tro-des′mōs) the connection between intranuclear centrioles during mitosis in certain protozoa; see *desmose*. Called also *centrodesmus*.

**cen·tro·des·mus** (sen″tro-des′məs) centrodesmose.

**cen·tro·lec·i·thal** (sen″tro-les′ĭ-thəl) [*centro-* + *lecithal*] having the yolk centrally located; see under *ovum*.

**cen·tro·lob·u·lar** (sen″tro-lob′u-lər) centrilobular.

**cen·tro·mere** (sen′tro-mēr) [*centro-* + *-mere*] [MeSH: Centromere] the constricted portion of the chromosome at which the chromatids are joined and by which the chromosome is attached to the spindle during cell division. According to its location, a centromere is said to be metacentric (central), submetacentric (off center), acrocentric (near one end), or telocentric (at one end). The last type does not occur in human chromosomes. Called also *kinetochore* and *primary constriction*.

**cen·tro·mer·ic** (sen″tro-mer′ik) pertaining to or resembling a centromere.

**cen·tro·nu·cle·us** (sen″tro-noo′kle-əs) amphinucleus.

**cen·tro·os·teo·scle·ro·sis** (sen″tro-os″te-o-sklə-ro′sis) centrosclerosis.

**cen·tro·phen·ox·ine** (sen″tro-fən-ok′sēn) meclofenoxate.

**cen·tro·phose** (sen′tro-fōz) any phose, or sensation of light, originating in the visual centers.

**cen·tro·plasm** (sen′tro-plaz-əm) the substance of the centrosome.

**cen·tro·plast** (sen′tro-plast) a central granule from which the axial filaments of the axopodia of certain heliozoa arise.

**cen·tro·scle·ro·sis** (sen″tro-sklə-ro′sis) [*centro-* + osteo*sclerosis*] the filling of the marrow cavity of a bone with osseous material.

**cen·tro·some** (sen′tro-sōm) [*centro-* + *-some*] [MeSH: Centrosome] the cell center; the centrosphere together with the two centrioles.

**cen·tro·sphere** (sen′tro-sfēr) [*centro-* + *sphere*] 1. a specialized area of condensed cytoplasm that contains the centrioles and plays an important part in mitosis; called also *cytocentrum, microcentrum, attraction sphere,* and *paranuclear body*. 2. centrosome.

**cen·trum** (sen′trəm) pl. *cen′tra* [L.; Gr. *kentron*] 1. [TA] a center. 2. the large, central portion of the body of a vertebra, formed from the cranial and caudal portions of adjacent sclerotomes and ossified from a single center.
**c. ossificatio′nis** [TA], ossification center: any point at which the process of ossification begins in bones; in a long bone there is a primary center for the diaphysis and a secondary center for the epiphysis. Called also *ossification point* and *punctum ossificationis*.
**c. ossificatio′nis prima′rium,** primary ossification center: the first point at which a bone begins to ossify. Called also *primary ossification point* and *punctum ossificationis primarium*.
**c. ossificatio′nis secunda′rium,** secondary ossification center: a point from which ossification proceeds that arises after a primary ossification center; it is concerned with progressive ossification toward the end of a bone. Called also *secondary ossification point* and *punctum ossificationis secundarium*.
**c. perine′i,** TA alternative for *corpus perineale*.
**c. semiova′le,** semioval center: the white matter of the cerebral hemispheres which underlies the cerebral cortex and which, in horizontal sections superior to the corpus callosum, has a semioval shape; it contains projection, commissural, and association fibers.
**c. tendi′neum diaphrag′matis** [TA], central tendon of diaphragm: the cloverleaf-shaped aponeurosis, immediately below the pericardium, onto which the diaphragmatic fibers converge to insert; called also *trefoil tendon, cordiform ligament of diaphragm,* and *phrenic center*.
**c. tendi′neum perine′i,** corpus perineale.
**c. of vertebra, vertebral c.,** centrum, def. 2.

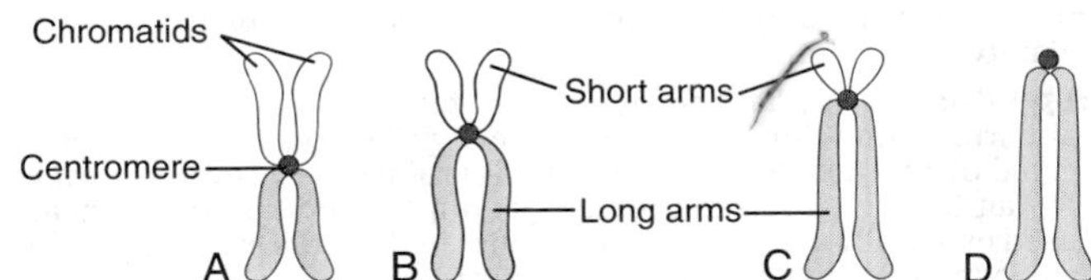

Position of the centromere in *(A)* metacentric, *(B)* submetacentric, *(C)* acrocentric, and *(D)* telocentric chromosomes.

**Cen·tru·roi·des** (sen″troo-roi′dēz) a genus of tropical and subtropical American scorpions, including several called bark scorpions. *C. suffu′sus* is a dangerous Mexican species.

**Cen·u·rus** (sən-u′rəs) *Coenurus*.

**CEP** congenital erythropoietic porphyria.

**ceph·a·ce·trile so·di·um** (sef′ə-sə-trīl″) an antibiotic effective against a wide range of gram-positive and gram-negative bacteria.

**Ceph·a·elis** (sef″ə-e′lis) a genus of tropical shrubs and trees of the family Rubiaceae. *C. acumina′ta* and *C. ipecacua′nha* are sources of ipecac.

**ceph·a·lad** (sef′ə-lad) [*cephal-* + *-ad*] proceeding toward the head, as opposed to *caudad*. Called also *caudocephalad* and *craniad*.

**ceph·a·lal·gia** (sef″ə-lal′jə) [Gr. *kephalalgia*] headache.
**histamine c.,** cluster headache.
**pharyngotympanic c.,** glossopharyngeal neuralgia.
**quadrantal c.,** headache affecting one quadrant of the head.

**ceph·al·ede·ma** (sef″əl-ə-de′mə) [*cephal-* + *edema*] edema of the head.

**ceph·a·lex·in** (sef″ə-lek′sin) [USP] [MeSH: Cephalexin] a semisynthetic analogue of the natural antibiotic cephalosporin C, effective against a wide range of gram-negative and gram-positive bacteria; used in the treatment of infections of the urinary and respiratory tracts and of skin and soft tissues due to sensitive pathogens, administered orally.
**c. hydrochloride** [USP], the hydrochloride salt of cephalexin, having the same actions and uses as the base; administered orally.

**ce·phal·gia** (sə-fal′jə) headache.

**ceph·al·he·mat·o·cele** (sef″əl-he-mat′o-sēl) [*cephal-* + *hemato-* + *-cele*[1]] a bloody tumor under the pericranium, communicating with one or more sinuses of the dura through the cranial bones.
**Stromeyer's c.,** a subperiosteal cephalhematocele which communicates with veins and becomes filled with blood during strong expiratory efforts.

**ceph·al·he·ma·to·ma** (sef″əl-he″mə-to′mə) [*cephal-* + *hematoma*] a subperiosteal hemorrhage limited to the surface of one cranial bone, a usually benign condition seen frequently in the newborn as a result of bone trauma. Called also *cephalohematoma*.
**c. defor′mans,** a bulging of the anterior part of the skull due to hyperostosis, osteoporosis, and cavity formation in the bone.

**ceph·al·hy·dro·cele** (sef″əl-hi′dro-sēl) [*cephal-* + *hydrocele*] a serous or watery accumulation under the pericranium.
**c. trauma′tica,** traumatic meningocele.

**ce·phal·ic** (sə-fal′ik) [Gr. *kephalikos*] 1. pertaining to the head. 2. cranial, def. 2.

**ceph·a·li·za·tion** (sef″ə-lĭ-za′shən) [Gr. *kephalē* head] 1. the concentration or initiation of the growth tendency at the head end of the embryo. 2. the development of a head; the concentration of nervous tissue and sense organs at the anterior end of the organism.

**cephal(o)-** [Gr. *kephalē* head] a combining form denoting relationship to the head.

**ceph·a·lo·ca·thar·tic** (sef″ə-lo-kə-thahr′tik) [*cephalo-* + *cathartic* (3)] cleansing or clearing the head.

**ceph·a·lo·cau·dad** (sef″ə-lo-kaw′dəd) 1. proceeding from the head toward the tail. 2. caudad. 3. in both a cephalic and caudal direction.

**ceph·a·lo·cau·dal** (sef″ə-lo-kaw′dəl) [*cephalo-* + *caudal*] pertaining to the long axis of the body, in a direction from head to tail.

**ceph·a·lo·cele** (sef′ə-lo-sēl″) [*cephalo-* + *-cele*[1]] encephalocele.
**orbital c.,** protrusion of the cranial contents through a defect in the orbital wall, named according to its contents as meningocele, encephalocele, etc.

**ceph·a·lo·cen·te·sis** (sef″ə-lo-sən-te′sis) [*cephalo-* + *-centesis*] the surgical puncture of the skull.

**ceph·a·lo·chord** (sef′ə-lo-kord″) [*cephalo-* + *chord*] the intracranial portion of the embryonic notochord.

**Ceph·a·lo·chor·da·ta** (sef″ə-lo-kor-da′tə) a subphylum of primitive, small, fishlike chordates in which the notochord extends the entire length of the body; it includes the genus *Amphioxus*.

**ceph·a·lo·chor·date** (sef″ə-lo-kor′dāt) any member of the Cephalochordata.

**ceph·a·lo·cyst** (sef′ə-lo-sist″) a larval cestode, such as a hydatid cyst.

**ceph·a·lo·dac·ty·ly** (sef″ə-lo-dak′tə-le) [*cephalo-* + Gr. *daktylos* a finger or toe] malformation of the head and digits.
**Vogt's c.,** acrocephalosyndactyly.

**ceph·a·lo·di·pros·o·pus** (sef″ə-lo-di-pros′o-pəs) [*cephalo-* + *di-* + Gr. *prosopus* face] a fetus with a partially incomplete head attached to the head proper.

**ceph·a·lo·dym·ia** (sef″ə-lo-dim′e-ə) the condition of a cephalodymus.

**ceph·a·lod·y·mus** (sef″ə-lod′ə-məs) [*cephalo-* + *didymus* (2)] conjoined twins with a single or united head.

**ceph·al·odyn·ia** (sef″ə-lo-din′e-ə) [*cephal-* + *-odynia*] headache.

**ceph·a·lo·gen·e·sis** (sef″ə-lo-jen′ə-sis) [*cephalo-* + *-genesis*] the development of the head in the embryo.

**ceph·a·lo·gly·cin** (sef″ə-lo-gli′sin) [MeSH: Cephaloglycin] a semisynthetic analogue of the natural antibiotic cephalosporin C, effective against a wide range of gram-negative and gram-positive bacteria; used in the treatment of acute and chronic urinary infections due to sensitive pathogens; administered orally.

**ceph·a·lo·gram** (sef′ə-lo-gram) [*cephalo-* + *-gram*] cephalometric radiograph.

**ceph·a·log·ra·phy** (sef″ə-log′rə-fe) [*cephalo* + *-graphy*] radiography of the head.

**ceph·a·lo·gy·ric** (sef″ə-lo-ji′rik) [*cephalo-* + *gyr-* + *-ic*] pertaining to turning motions of the head.

**ceph·a·lo·hem·a·to·cele** (sef″ə-lo-he-mat′o-sēl) cephalhematocele.

**ceph·a·lo·he·ma·to·ma** (sef″ə-lo-he″mə-to′mə) cephalhematoma.

**ceph·a·lom·e·lus** (sef″ə-lom′ə-ləs) [*cephalo-* + Gr. *melos* limb] a fetus with an accessory limb growing from the head.

**ceph·a·lo·me·nia** (sef″ə-lo-me′ne-ə) [*cephalo-* + *men-* + *-ia*] vicarious menstruation from the head, as in a nasal discharge at the menstrual period.

**ceph·a·lom·e·ter** (sef″ə-lom′ə-tər) [*cephalo-* + *-meter*] an instrument for measuring the head; an orienting device for positioning the head for radiographic examination and measurement.

**ceph·a·lom·e·try** (sef″ə-lom′ə-tre) [MeSH: Cephalometry] scientific measurement of the dimensions of the head. In dentistry, certain combinations of linear and angular measurements developed from tracing the oriented lateral and frontal radiographic head film are used to assess craniofacial growth and development on a longitudinal basis and to determine the nature of orthodontic treatment response.
**fetal c.,** measurement of the fetal skull *in utero* by means of x-ray films or by interpreting the echoes of ultrasonic radiation received from each side of the skull.

**ceph·a·lo·mo·tor** (sef″ə-lo-mo′tər) [*cephalo-* + *motor*] moving the head; pertaining to motions of the head.

**Ceph·a·lo·my·ia** (sef″ə-lo-mi′yə) *Oestrus.*

**ceph·a·lo·nia** (sef″ə-lo′ne-ə) a condition in which the head is abnormally large with sclerotic hyperplasia of the brain.

**ceph·a·lop·a·gus** (sef″ə-lop′ə-gəs) craniopagus.

**ceph·a·lop·a·thy** (sef″ə-lop′ə-the) [*cephalo-* + *-pathy*] any disease of the head.

**ceph·a·lo·pel·vic** (sef″ə-lo-pəl′vik) pertaining to the relationship of the fetal head to the maternal pelvis.

**ceph·a·lo·pel·vim·e·try** (sef″ə-lo-pəl-vim′ə-tre) pelvicephalometry.

**ceph·a·lo·pha·ryn·ge·us** (sef″ə-lo-fə-rin′je-əs) musculus constrictor pharyngis superior.

**ceph·a·lo·ple·gia** (sef″ə-lo-ple′jə) [*cephalo-* + *-plegia*] paralysis of the muscles about the head and face.

**Ceph·a·lop·o·da** (sef″ə-lop′ə-də) [*cephalo-* + Gr. *pous* foot] a class of large mollusks with elongated muscular arms; it includes the octopus, squid, cuttlefish, and nautilus.

**ceph·a·lo·rha·chid·i·an** (sef″ə-lo-rə-kid′e-ən) pertaining to the head and the spinal column. Spelled also *cephalorachidian.*

**ceph·a·lor·i·dine** (sef″ə-lor′ĭ-dēn) [MeSH: Cephaloridine] a first-generation, semisynthetic cephalosporin effective against a wide range of gram-positive and some gram-negative bacteria and having uses similar to those of cephalothin sodium; administered intramuscularly and intravenously. Its use is severely limited by its nephrotoxicity and it is no longer available in the United States.

**ceph·a·lo·spo·rin** (sef″ə-lo-spor′in) any of a group of broad-spectrum, relatively penicillinase-resistant antibiotics originally derived from a species of the fungus *Emericellopsis minimum,* a teleomorph of *Acremonium* (formerly called *Cephalosporium*). They are related to the penicillins in both structure and mode of action; their antibacterial activity results from inhibition of the cross-linking of peptidoglycan units in the cell wall. The cephalosporins available for medicinal use are semisynthetic derivatives of the natural antibiotic *c. C.* (The cephamycins cefotetan and cefoxitin and the β-lactam moxalactam are included with the cephalosporins because of their close relationship to them.)
**c. C,** a cephalosporin that is the parent compound of a number of semisynthetic antibiotics, including cefazolin sodium, cephalexin, cephaloridine, cephaloglycin, cephalothin, cephapirin, and cephradine, used in the treatment of a wide variety of infections due to sensitive gram-positive and gram-negative bacteria.
**first-generation c's,** a group containing the first cephalosporins developed, comprising agents with a broad range of activity against gram-positive organisms but a narrow range of activity against gram-negative organisms and including cephalothin, cefazolin, cephaloridine, cephapirin, cephadrine, cephalexin, and cefadroxil.
**c. N,** adicillin.
**c. P,** an antibacterial steroid; the crude form contains at least five components ($P_1$, $P_2$, $P_3$, $P_4$, $P_5$), $P_1$ being the major active substance.
**second-generation c's,** a group containing cephalosporins that are more active against gram-negative organisms but less active against gram-positive organisms than first-generation agents; it includes cefamandole, cefoxitin, cefaclor, and cefuroxime.
**third-generation c's,** a group of β-lactamase–resistant cephalosporins that are more active against gram-negative organisms but less active against gram-positive organisms than second-generation agents; it includes cefoperazone, cefotaxime, ceftriaxone, ceftazidime, ceftizoxime, and moxalactam.

**ceph·a·lo·spo·rin·ase** (sef″ə-lo-spor′in-ās) [MeSH: Cephalosporinase] a β-lactamase (q.v.) preferentially cleaving cephalosporins.

**ceph·a·lo·spo·ri·o·sis** (sef″ə-lo-spor″e-o′sis) acremoniosis.

**Ceph·a·lo·spo·ri·um** (sef″ə-lo-spor′e-əm) [*cephalo-* + Gr. *sporos* seed] former name for *Acremonium.*

**ceph·a·lo·stat** (sef′ə-lo-stat″) a head-positioning device used in dental radiology, facial photography, cephalometry, and other procedures requiring exact positioning of the head. See also *gnathostat.*

**ceph·a·lo·style** (sef′ə-lo-stīl″) the cranial end of the notochord.

**ceph·a·lo·tet·a·nus** (sef″ə-lo-tet′ə-nəs) [*cephalo-* + *tetanus*] cephalic tetanus.

**ceph·a·lo·thin** (sə-fal′o-thin) [MeSH: Cephalothin] a semisynthetic analogue, of the natural antibiotic cephalosporin C, effective against a wide range of gram-positive and gram-negative bacteria.
**c. sodium** [USP], the monosodium salt of cephalothin, used in the treatment of infections of the major organ and tissue systems due to sensitive pathogens; administered parenterally.

**ceph·a·lo·tho·rac·ic** (sef″ə-lo-thə-ras′ik) pertaining to the head and thorax.

**ceph·a·lo·tho·ra·cop·a·gus** (sef″ə-lo-thor″ə-kop′ə-gəs) conjoined twins united at the head, neck, and thorax.
**c. disym′metros,** a cephalothoracopagus fused squarely in the frontal plane and presenting two broad anterior surfaces and two narrow posterior ones, with a common head bearing two faces, each being formed by the right and left halves of the different components.
**c. monosym′metros,** a cephalothoracopagus with one complete face formed by a right and a left half of the two components, the other face being only rudimentary.

**ceph·a·lo·tome** (sef′ə-lo-tōm″) an instrument for cutting the fetal head.

**ceph·a·lot·o·my** (sef″ə-lot′ə-me) [*cephalo-* + *-tomy*] 1. the cutting up of the fetal head to facilitate delivery. 2. dissection of the fetal head.

**ceph·a·lo·trop·ic** (sef″ə-lo-trop′ik) [*cephalo-* + *-tropic*] having an affinity for brain tissue.

**-cephalus** [Gr. *kephalē* head] a word termination denoting *(a)* an abnormal condition of the head, the specific condition being indicated by the stem to which the ending is affixed, e.g., *hydrocephalus; (b)* an individual affected by an abnormal condition of the head, used especially of congenital anomalies in the fetus, e.g., *dicephalus; (c)* in taxonomy, having a head of a certain type.

**-cephaly** [Gr. *kephalē* head] a word termination denoting an abnormal condition of the head, the specific condition being indicated by the stem to which the ending is attached.

**ceph·a·my·cin** (sef″ə-mi′sin) any of a family of naturally occurring antibacterial antibiotics derived from various species of *Streptomyces* or produced semisynthetically, which are resistant to degradation by $\beta$-lactamase. Cephamycins A, B, and C have been isolated.
**c. sodium** [USP], the sodium salt of cephamycin, used in the prophylaxis and treatment of anaerobic and mixed bacterial infections, especially intra-abdominal and pelvic infections; administered intravenously.

**ceph·a·pi·rin** (sef-ə-pi′rin) [MeSH: Cephapirin] a semisynthetic analogue of the natural antibiotic cephalosporin C, effective against a wide range of gram-negative and gram-positive bacteria.
**c. benzathine** [USP], administered by intramammary infusion.
**c. sodium** [USP], the monosodium salt of cephapirin, used in the treatment of infections of the respiratory and genitourinary tracts, skin, soft tissues, bones, joints, and blood due to sensitive pathogens; administered intramuscularly and intravenously.

**ceph·ra·dine** (sef′rə-dēn) [USP] [MeSH: Cephradine] a semisynthetic analogue of the natural antibiotic cephalosporin C, effective against a wide range of gram-positive and gram-negative bacteria; used in the treatment of infections of the urinary tract, skin, and soft tissues due to sensitive pathogens, administered orally or by intramuscular or intravenous injection.

**-ceptor** [shortened from *receptor*] a word termination denoting a receptor, with the root preceding it specifying the type.

**cera** (se′rə) [L.] wax.
**c. al′ba,** white wax.
**c. fla′va,** yellow wax.

**ce·ra·ceous** (sə-ra′shəs) [L. *cera* wax] waxlike in appearance.

**ce·ram·ic** (sə-ram′ik) [MeSH: Ceramics] 1. of or pertaining to ceramics. 2. a product, such as porcelain, produced by the action of heat on earthy materials, in which silicon and silicates occupy a predominant position. 3. a metal oxide.
**castable c.,** a glass ceramic having a high compressive strength and hardness with translucency, and wear characteristics that approximate those of enamel; used in the casting of dental restorations.
**glass c.,** any of a number of forms of partially crystallized glass having a variety of properties and uses, including the manufacture of dental restorations, formed by heating to the point of crystallization an amorphous glass matrix to which impurities have been added to provide nuclei for crystal formation.
**metal c.,** a composite material made by mixing powdered metal with powdered ceramic and sintering the mixture. See also *cermet.*
**metal-c.,** a dental restoration consisting of a cast metal substructure covered with an external fused ceramic veneer.

**ce·ram·ics** (sə-ram′iks) [Gr. *keramos* potters' clay] [MeSH: Ceramics] 1. the modeling and processing of objects made of clay or similar material. 2. objects made of ceramic material.
**dental c.,** the employment of porcelain and similar materials in restorative dentistry.

**cer·am·i·dase** (sər-am′ĭ-dās) [EC 3.5.1.23] an enzyme of the hydrolase class that catalyzes the cleavage of a ceramide (*N*-acylsphingosine) to form sphingosine and a fatty acid anion, a step in the degradation of sphingolipids. Acid, neutral, and alkaline isozymes occur; deficiency of the acid (lysosomal) enzyme, an autosomal recessive trait, results in accumulation of ceramides and gangliosides in Farber's disease. Called also *acylsphingosine deacylase.*

**cer·am·i·dase deficiency** Farber's disease.

**cer·a·mide** (ser′ə-mīd) the basic unit of the sphingolipids; it is sphingosine, or a related base, attached via its amino group to a long chain fatty acyl group. Ceramides are accumulated abnormally in Farber's disease. Called also N-*acylsphingosine.*
**c. trihexoside,** any of a specific family of glycosphingolipids of composition galactose-galactose-glucose-ceramide; due to deficiency of $\alpha$-galactosidase A activity, they accumulate abnormally in plasma and tissues in Fabry's disease.

**cer·a·mide cho·line·phos·pho·trans·fer·ase** (ser′ə-mīd ko″lēn-fos″fo-trans′fər-ās) [EC 2.7.8.3] an enzyme of the transferase class that catalyzes the transfer of a phosphorylated choline group from CDPcholine to ceramide to form sphingomyelin.

**cer·a·mide tri·hex·o·si·dase** (ser′ə-mīd tri″hek-so′sĭ-dās) [MeSH: Ceramide Trihexosidase] $\alpha$-galactosidase A.

**cer·a·mide tri·hex·o·si·dase deficiency** Fabry's disease.

**cer·a·sine** (ser′ə-sīn) a red azo dye, used as a cytoplasmic stain.

**Ce·ras·tes** (sĕ-ras′tēz) a genus of venomous snakes of the family Viperidae. *C. ceras′tes* is the horned viper.

**cer·a·sus** (ser′ə-səs) [L.] cherry.

**ce·rate** (se′rāt) [L. *ceratum,* from *cera* wax] a medicinal preparation for external application, made with a basis of fat or wax, or both, intermediate in consistency between an ointment and a plaster.
**simple c.,** a mixture of benzoinated lard and white wax, melted together.
**Turner's c.,** calamine ointment.

**cer·a·tec·to·my** (ser″ə-tek′tə-me) keratectomy.

**cer·a·tin** (ser′ə-tin) keratin.

**Ce·ra·ti·um** (sə-ra′she-əm) [Gr. *keration,* dim. of *keras* horn] a genus of plantlike, marine and freshwater protozoa (order Dinoflagellida, class Phytomastigophorea); like other dinoflagellates, when present in vast numbers they produce discoloration of the water (red tide).

**cerat(o)-** for words beginning thus, see also those beginning *kerato-.*

**cer·a·to·cri·coid** (ser″ə-to-kri′koid) pertaining to the inferior horn of the thyroid cartilage and the cricoid cartilage; see under *muscle.*

**cer·a·to·cri·coi·de·us** (ser″ə-to-kri-koi′de-əs) ceratocricoid.

**cer·a·to·hy·al** (ser″ə-to-hi′əl) pertaining to a cornu minus of the hyoid bone.

**Cer·a·to·nia** (ser″ə-to′ne-ə) a genus of trees of the family Leguminosae. *C. sili′qua* L. is the carob (carob bean or locust bean) tree, native to the Mediterranean region, whose dried ripe fruit is the source of carob used in pharmaceutical preparations.

**cer·a·to·pha·ryn·ge·us** (ser″ə-to-fə-rin′je-əs) pertaining to the inferior horn of the thyroid cartilage and the pharynx; see under *musculus.*

**Cer·a·to·phyl·lus** (ser″ə-to-fil′əs) [Gr. *keras* horn + *phyllon* leaf] a genus of fleas, now including only bird fleas, but formerly including those of birds and small mammals.
**C. acu′tus,** *Diamanus montanus.*
**C. fascia′tus,** *Nosopsyllus fasciatus.*
**C. galli′nae,** a species that attacks chickens and man.
**C. idahoen′sis,** *Oropsylla idahoensis.*
**C. monta′nus,** *Diamanus montanus.*
**C. punjaben′sis,** a rat flea of India.
**C. silantie′wi,** *Oropsylla silantiewi.*
**C. tesquo′rum,** a plague-transmitting flea of ground squirrels in the steppes of Central Asia.

**Cer·a·to·po·gon·i·dae** (ser″ə-to-po-gon′ĭ-de) [MeSH: Ceratopogonidae] Heleidae.

**ce·ra·tum** (sə-ra′təm) [L.] cerate.

**cer·ber·in, cer·ber·ine** (sər′bə-rin) a poisonous alkaloid from the Asian tree *Cerbera odallam;* it is cardiotonic.

**cer·ca·ria** (sər-kar′e-ə) pl. *cerca′riae* [Gr. *kerkos* tail] the final free-swimming larval stage of a trematode parasite, consisting of a body and tail. Some cercariae encyst on aquatic vegetation and penetrate the skin of a fish or the tissues of an aquatic arthropod to form encysted metacercariae. Cercariae of schistosomes penetrate directly into the skin of the definitive host without forming metacercariae.

**cer·car·i·ci·dal** (sər-kar″ĭ-si′dəl) destructive to cercariae.

**cer·car·i·en·hul·len·re·ak·tion** (sər-kar″e-ən-hul″ən-re-ak′shən) a test for *Schistosoma mansoni,* utilized in measuring the efficiency of chemotherapy against schistosomiasis. When cercariae of *S. mansoni* are placed *in vitro* in contact with sera of monkeys or men infected with *S. mansoni,* a transparent envelope is formed around each cercaria.

**cer·clage** (ser-klahzh′) [Fr. "an encircling"] encircling of a part with a ring or loop, such as encirclement of the incompetent cervix uteri with suture material, or the binding together of the ends of a fractured bone with a metal ring or wire loop (tiring).

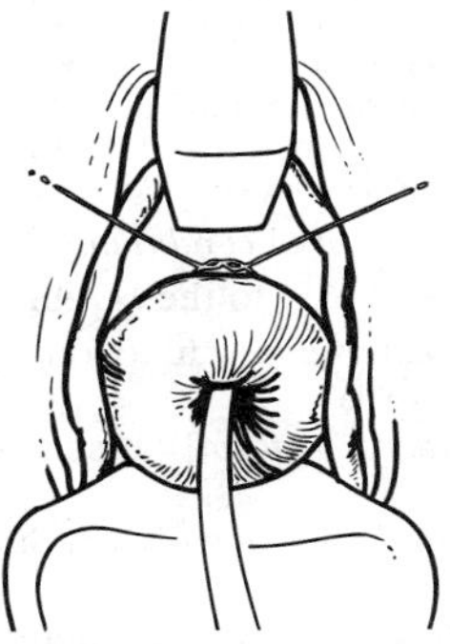

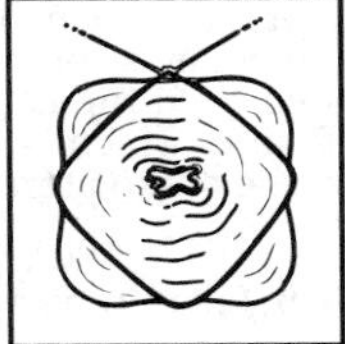

Cerclage of an incompetent cervix uteri, the inset showing the effect of the tightened suture.

**cerc(o)-** [Gr. *kerkos* tail] a combining form denoting a relationship to a tail or to a tail-like structure.

**cer·co·cys·tis** (sər″ko-sis′tis) cysticercoid.

**cer·coid** (sər′koid) the last stage in the development of a tapeworm.

**Cer·co·pith·e·ci·dae** (sər-ko-pĭ-thes′ĭ-de) [MeSH: Cercopithecidae] a family of Old World monkeys (superfamily Cercopithecoidea); some species of genus *Macaca* are used as laboratory animals.

**cer·co·pith·e·coid** (ser″ko-pith′ə-koid′″) any member of the family Cercopithecidae.

**Cer·co·pith·e·coi·dea** (ser″ko-pith″ə-koid′e-ə) a superfamily of the order Primates, including Old World monkeys (family Cercopithecidae) and human beings (family Hominidae); they have nostrils that are close together and pointed downward, and when a tail is present it is not prehensile. Formerly called *Catarrhina.*

**Cer·cos·po·ra** (sər-kos′pə-rə) a genus of Fungi Imperfecti of the form-class Hyphomycetes. *C. a′pii* is a species that causes celery blight and can cause hyphomycosis in humans.

**cer·cos·po·ra·my·co·sis** (sər-kos″spəro-mi-ko′sis) infection with *Cercospora apii.*

**cer·cus** (ser′kəs) pl. *cer′ci* [L., from Gr. *kerkos* tail] a rigid bristle-like appendage near the tail of most insects and some other arthropods, with varying functions including mechanoreception and copulation.

**ce·rea flex·i·bil·i·tas** (sēr′e-ə flex″sĭ-bil′ĭ-tas) [L. "waxy flexibility"] the rigidity of the body seen in some severe cases of catatonic schizophrenia, in which the patient maintains whatever body position he is placed in, the limbs having a heavy waxy malleability.

**ce·re·al** (sēr′e-əl) [L. *cerealis*] [MeSH: Cereals] 1. pertaining to edible grain. 2. any plant of the grass family (Gramineae) bearing an edible seed. 3. the seed or grain of such a plant.

**cer·e·bel·la** (ser″ə-bel′ə) [L.] plural of *cerebellum.*

**cer·e·bel·lar** (ser″ə-bel′ər) pertaining to the cerebellum.

**cer·e·bel·lif·u·gal** (ser″ə-bel-if′ə-gəl) [*cerebello-* + *-fugal*] tending or proceeding from the cerebellum.

**cer·e·bel·lip·e·tal** (ser″ə-be-lip′ə-təl) [*cerebello-* + *-petal*] tending or moving toward the cerebellum.

**cer·e·bel·li·tis** (ser″ə-bel-i′tis) inflammation of the cerebellum.

**cerebell(o)-** [L. *cerebellum,* q.v.] a combining form denoting relationship to the cerebellum.

**cer·e·bel·lof·u·gal** (ser″ə-bel-of′ə-gəl) cerebellifugal.

**cer·e·bel·lo·ol·i·vary** (ser″ə-bel″o-ol′i-var″e) conducting or proceeding from the cerebellum to the olivary body.

**cer·e·bel·lo·pon·tile** (ser″ə-bel″o-pon′tēl) cerebellopontine.

**cer·e·bel·lo·pon·tine** (ser″ə-bel″o-pon′tēn) conducting or proceeding from the cerebellum to the pons.

**cer·e·bel·lo·ru·bral** (ser″ə-bel″o-roo′brəl) conducting or proceeding from the cerebellum to the red nucleus.

**cer·e·bel·lo·ru·bro·spi·nal** (ser″ə-bel″o-roo″bro-spi′nəl) conducting or proceeding from the cerebellum, to the red nucleus, and then to the spinal cord.

**cer·e·bel·lo·spi·nal** (ser″ə-bel″o-spi′nəl) conducting or proceeding from the cerebellum to the spinal cord.

**cer·e·bel·lum** (ser″ə-bel′əm) [L. dim. of *cerebrum* brain] [TA] [MeSH: Cerebellum] the part of the metencephalon that occupies the posterior cranial fossa behind the brain stem and is concerned in the coordination of movements. It is a fissured mass consisting of a body, comprising a narrow middle strip (the vermis) and two lateral lobes (the hemispheres, connected with the brain stem by three pairs (caudal, middle, and rostral), of peduncles. Functionally, the cerebellum is subdivided into a cranial (anterior) lobe, which is separated from the caudal (posterior or median) lobe by the primary fissure, which is in turn separated from the flocculonodular lobe by the dorsolateral (posterolateral) fissure.

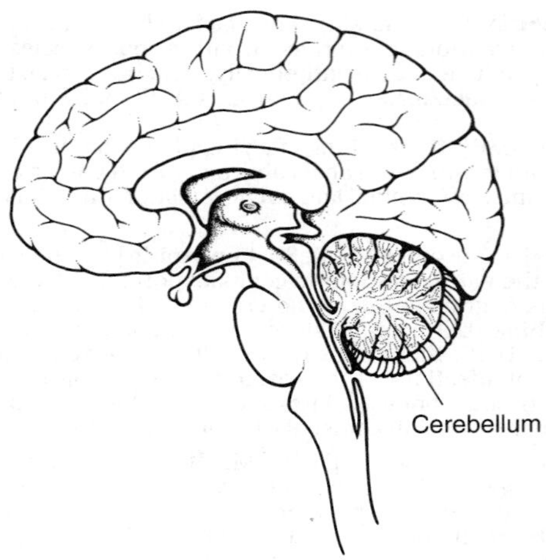


**cer·e·bra** (sə-re′brə, ser′e-brə) [L.] plural of *cerebrum.*

**cer·e·bral** (sə-re′brəl, ser′ə-brəl) pertaining to the cerebrum.

**cer·e·bra·tion** (ser″ə-bra′shən) [L. *cerebratio*] functional activity of the cerebrum; thinking; mental activity.

**cer·e·bri·form** (sə-re′brĭ-form) [*cerebro-* + *form*] resembling the surface of the cerebrum.

**cer·e·brif·u·gal** (ser″ə-brif′u-gəl) [*cerebro-* + *-fugal*] conducting or proceeding away from the brain, or cerebrum.

**cer·e·brip·e·tal** (ser″ə-brip′ə-təl) [*cerebro-* + *-petal*] conducting or proceeding toward the brain, or cerebrum.

**cerebr(o)-** [L. *cerebrum,* q.v.] a combining form denoting relationship to the cerebrum.

**cer·e·bro·car·di·ac** (ser″ə-bro-kahr′de-ak) [*cerebro-* + L. *cardia* heart] pertaining to the brain and heart.

**cer·e·bro·cer·e·bel·lar** (ser″ə-bro-ser″ə-bel′ər) pertaining to the cerebrum and the cerebellum.

**cer·e·bro·cu·pre·in** (ser″ə-bro-koo′prēn) a copper protein isolated from the human and bovine brain.

**cer·e·broid** (ser′ə-broid) resembling the cerebral substance.

**cer·e·brol·o·gy** (ser″ə-brol′ə-je) [*cerebro-* + *-logy*] the sum of knowledge regarding cerebral structure and function.

**cer·e·bro·mac·u·lar** (ser″ə-bro-mak′u-lər) maculocerebral.

**cer·e·bro·ma·la·cia** (ser″ə-bro-mə-la′shə) [*cerebro-* + *malacia*] abnormal softening of the substance of the cerebrum.

**cer·e·bro·me·nin·ge·al** (ser″ə-bro-mə-nin′je-əl) pertaining to the cerebrum and its membranes.

**cer·e·bro·men·in·gi·tis** (ser″ə-bro-men″in-ji′tis) meningoencephalitis.

**cer·e·bron·ic ac·id** (ser″ə-bron′ik) a fatty acid, the 2-hydroxy derivative of lignoceric acid, found in cerebrosides such as phrenosine.

**cer·e·bro-oc·u·lar** (ser″ə-bro-ok′u-lər) pertaining to the cerebrum and the eye.

**cer·e·bro·path·ia** (ser″ə-bro-path′e-ə) [L.] cerebropathy. **c. psy′chica toxe′mica,** Korsakoff's psychosis.

**cer·e·brop·a·thy** (ser″ə-brop′ə-the) [*cerebro-* + *-pathy*] any disorder of the cerebrum; cf. *encephalopathy.*

**cer·e·bro·phys·i·ol·o·gy** (ser″ə-bro-fiz″e-ol′ə-je) the physiology of the cerebrum.

**cer·e·bro·pon·tile** (ser″ə-bro-pon′tīl) pertaining to the cerebrum and pons.

**cer·e·bro·ra·chid·i·an** (ser″ə-bro″rə-kid′e-ən) cerebrospinal.

**cer·e·bro·scle·ro·sis** (ser″ə-bro″sklə-ro′sis) [*cerebro-* + *sclerosis*] morbid hardening of the substance of the cerebrum.

**cer·e·bro·side** (ser′ə-bro-sīd″) a sphingolipid in which the head group linked to ceramide is either of the monosaccharides glucose or galactose. Cerebrosides are abundant in cell membranes of brain and nervous tissue, especially the myelin sheath, but are also found in other tissues. See also *glucocerebroside* and *galactocerebroside.* **c. sulfate,** sulfatide.

**cer·e·bro·side sul·fa·tase** (ser′ə-bro″sīd sul′fə-tās) [EC 3.1.6.8] [MeSH: Cerebroside-Sulfatase] an enzyme of the hydrolase class that catalyzes the cleavage of sulfate residues from sulfatides to form cerebrosides. Deficiency of the enzyme, an autosomal recessive trait, is one of the causes of metachromatic leukodystrophy. Called also *arylsulfatase A.*

**cer·e·bro·si·do·sis** (ser″ə-bro″sĭ-do′sis) a lipoidosis in which the fatty accumulation in the body consists largely of kerasin, as in Gaucher's disease.

**cer·e·bro·sis** (ser″ə-bro′sis) cerebropathy.

**cer·e·bro·spi·nal** (ser″ə-bro-spi′nəl) pertaining to the brain and spinal cord; called also *encephalospinal* and *myeloencephalic.*

**cer·e·bro·spi·nant** (ser″ə-bro-spi′nənt) any medicine or agent that affects the brain and spinal cord.

**cer·e·bros·to·my** (ser″ə-bros′tə-me) [*cerebr-* + *ostomy*] the making of an artificial opening into the cerebrum.

**cer·e·bro·ten·di·nous** (ser″ə-bro-ten′dĭ-nəs) pertaining to the cerebrum and the tendons.

**cer·e·brot·o·my** (ser″ə-brot′ə-me) [*cerebr-* + *-otomy*] encephalotomy.

**cer·e·bro·to·nia** (ser″ə-bro-to′ne-ə) [*cerebro-* + *ton-* + *-ia*] a personality type associated with ectomorphy and characterized by love of privacy, introversion, emotional restraint, and intellectual intensity.

**cer·e·bro·vas·cu·lar** (ser″ə-bro-vas′ku-lər) pertaining to the blood vessels of the cerebrum, or brain.

**cer·e·brum** (ser′ə-brəm, sə-re′brəm) [L.] 1. the main portion of the brain, occupying the upper part of the cranial cavity; its two hemispheres (see *cerebral hemisphere,* under *hemisphere*), united by the corpus callosum, form the largest part of the central nervous system in man. It is derived (developed) from the telencephalon of the embryo. In official nomenclature, the term is considered an alternative to telencephalon [TA]. 2. a term sometimes applied to the postembryonic prosencephalon and mesencephalon together or to the entire brain.

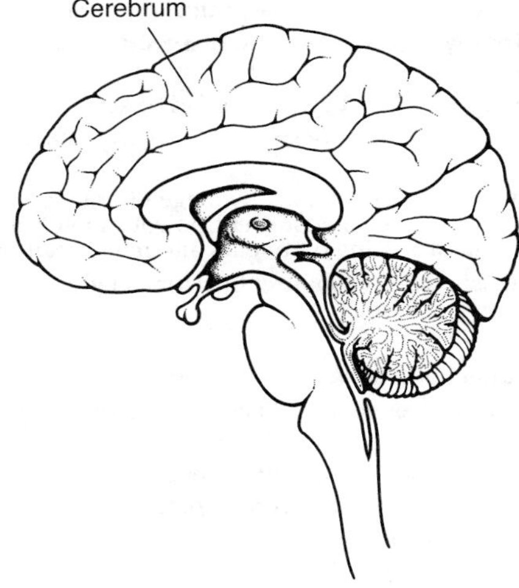


**cere·cloth** (sēr′kloth) cloth impregnated with wax and made antiseptic; used in dressings.

**Cer·e·dase** (ser′ədās) trademark for a preparation of alglucerase.

**Cer·en·kov radiation** (chĕ′reng-kof) [Pavel Aleksandrovich *Cherenkov* (or *Cerenkov*), Russian physicist, 1904–1990] see under *radiation.*

**cer·e·o·li** (se-re′o-li) plural of *cereolus.*

**cer·e·o·lus** (se-re′o-ləs) pl. *cere′oli* [L., dim. of *cereus* wax taper] a medicated bougie.

**Cer·e·tec** (ser′ə-tek″) trademark for a kit for the preparation of technetium Tc 99m exametazime.

**Cer·e·zyme** (ser′ə-zīm″) trademark for a preparation of imiglucerase.

**Cer·i·thid·ia** (ser″ĭ-thid′e-ə) a genus of spiral-shelled snails of the family Cerithiidae, subclass Streptoneura, found in brackish water in tropical and subtropical areas. *C. cingula′ta* is a Japanese species that is the chief intermediate host for the trematode *Heterophyes heterophyes.*

**ce·ri·um** (se′re-əm) [L.] [MeSH: Cerium] a metallic element: symbol, Ce; atomic number, 58; atomic weight, 140.12.

**cer·met** (sər′met) [*cer*amic *met*al] a type of metal ceramic that is a component of dental cements and heat-resistant solid materials.

**ce·ro·plas·ty** (se′ro-plas″te) [*cera* + *-plasty*] the making of anatomical models in wax.

**cer·ti·fi·a·ble** (sər″tĭ-fi′ə-bəl) capable of being certified; said of infectious diseases, cases of which must by law be reported to public health officers.

**Ce·ru·bi·dine** (sə-roo′bĭ-dēn) trademark for a preparation of daunorubicin hydrochloride.

**ce·ru·le·an** (sə-rōōl′yən) [L. *caeruleus*] blue; azure.

**ce·ru·le·in** (sə-roo′le-in) a decapeptide amide isolated from the skin of frogs; it is a peptide analogue of cholecystokinin and gastrin; in mammals it is a powerful stimulant of gallbladder contraction.

**ce·ru·le·us** (sə-roo′le-əs) variant spelling of *caeruleus* (q.v.).

**ce·ru·lo·plas·min** (sə-roo″lo-plaz′min) [MeSH: Ceruloplasmin] a deep blue $\alpha_2$-globulin with a single subunit, containing six atoms of copper and occurring in blood plasma. Although studied extensively, its functions *in vivo* remain unclear; it is believed to function in transport and maintenance of tissue levels of copper and to display ferroxidase activity, and it may oxidize additional unsaturated compounds. Ceruloplasmin levels are decreased in Wilson's disease. In EC nomenclature, called *ferroxidase.*

**ce·ru·men** (sə-roo′mən) [L. from *cera* wax] [MeSH: Cerumen] the waxlike secretion found within the external meatus of the ear; called also *earwax.*
**impacted c.,** accumulated cerumen forming a solid mass that adheres to the wall of the external auditory canal.
**inspissated c.,** dried earwax in the external canal of the ear.

**ce·ru·mi·nal** (sə-roo′mĭ-nəl) of or pertaining to the cerumen.

**ce·ru·min·ol·y·sis** (sə-roo″mĭ-nol′ə-sis) the solution or disintegration of cerumen in the external auditory meatus.

**ce·ru·mi·no·ly·tic** (sə-roo″mĭ-no-lit′ik) 1. pertaining to, characterized by, or promoting ceruminolysis. 2. an agent that dissolves cerumen in the external auditory canal.

**ce·ru·mi·no·ma** (sə-roo″mi-no′mə) tumor of the ceruminous glands.

**ce·ru·mi·no·sis** (sə-roo″mĭ-no′sis) excessive or disordered secretion of cerumen.

**ce·ru·mi·nous** (sə-roo′mĭ-nəs) ceruminal.

**ce·ruse** (se′rōōs) [L. *cerussa*] the basic carbonate of lead; white lead.

**cer·vi·cal** (sər′vĭ-kəl) [L. *cervicalis,* from *cervix* neck] 1. pertaining to the neck. 2. pertaining to the neck or cervix of any organ or structure.

**cer·vi·ca·lis** (sər″vĭ-ka′lis) [L.] cervical.

**cer·vi·cec·to·my** (sər″vĭ-sek′tə-me) excision of the cervix uteri; called also *trachelectomy.*

**cer·vi·ci·tis** (sər″vĭ-si′tis) [MeSH: Cervicitis] inflammation of the cervix uteri; called also *trachelitis.*
**granulomatous c.,** granulomatous infections of the cervix, including tuberculosis, syphilis, and granuloma inguinale.
**traumatic c.,** a nonspecific cervicitis resulting from such procedures as irradiation or cauterization.

**cervic(o)-** [L. *cervix* neck] a combining form denoting a neck or the cervix uteri.

**cer·vi·co·ax·il·lary** (sər″vĭ-ko-ak′sĭ-lar-e) pertaining to the neck and axilla.

**cer·vi·co·bra·chi·al** (sər″vĭ-ko-bra′ke-əl) pertaining to the neck and arm.

**cer·vi·co·bra·chi·al·gia** (sər″vĭ-ko-bra″ke-al′jə) pain in the neck radiating to the arm, due to compression of nerve roots of the cervical spinal cord.

**cer·vi·co·buc·cal** (sər″vĭ-ko-buk′əl) buccocervical.

**cer·vi·co·col·pi·tis** (sər″vĭ-ko-kol-pi′tis) inflammation of the cervix uteri and vagina.
**c. emphysemato′sa,** colpitis emphysematosa with similar lesions occurring beneath the squamous mucosa of the cervix uteri.

**cer·vi·co·dor·sal** (sər″vĭ-ko-dor′səl) pertaining to the neck and back.

**cer·vi·co·dyn·ia** (sər″vĭ-ko-din′e-ə) [*cervico-* + *-odynia*] pain in the neck; called also *trachelodynia.*

**cer·vi·co·fa·cial** (sər″vĭ-ko-fa′shəl) pertaining to the neck and face.

**cer·vi·co·la·bi·al** (sər″vĭ-ko-la′be-əl) labiocervical.

**cer·vi·co·lin·gual** (sər″vĭ-ko-ling′gwəl) linguocervical.

**cer·vi·co·oc·cip·i·tal** (sər″vĭ-ko-ok-sip′ĭ-təl) pertaining to the neck and occiput.

**cer·vi·co·plas·ty** (sər′vĭ-ko-plas″te) [*cervico-* + *-plasty*] plastic surgery on the neck.

**cer·vi·co·scap·u·lar** (sər″vĭ-ko-skap′u-lər) pertaining to the neck and scapula.

**cer·vi·co·tho·rac·ic** (sər″vĭ-ko-thə-ras′ik) pertaining to the neck and thorax.

**cer·vi·co·vag·i·ni·tis** (sər″vĭ-ko-vaj″ĭ-ni′tis) inflammation involving both the cervix uteri and vagina.

**cer·vi·co·ves·i·cal** (sər″vĭ-ko-ves′ĭ-kəl) vesicocervical.

**Cer·vi·dil** trademark for a preparation of dinoprostone.

**Cer·vi·lax·in** (sər″vĭ-lak′sin) trademark for a preparation of relaxin.

**cer·vix** (sər′viks) pl. *cer′vices* [L.] 1. TA alternative for *collum.* 2. [TA] a constricted portion of a body part or organ. 3. cervix uteri.
**c. of axon,** a constricted part of an axon, before the beginning of the myelin sheath.
**c. cor′nus dorsa′lis medul′lae spina′lis,** c. cornus posterioris medullae spinalis.
**c. cor′nus posterio′ris medul′lae spina′lis** [TA], neck of posterior horn of spinal cord: the constricted portion of the posterior horn of gray matter in the spinal cord between the base of the horn and the head. Called also *c. cornus dorsalis medullae spinalis* and *neck of dorsal horn of spinal cord.*
**c. den′tis** [TA], neck of tooth: the slightly constricted region of union of the crown and the root or roots of a tooth; called also *collum dentis* and *dental neck.*
**c. glan′dis,** collum glandis penis.
**incompetent c.,** one that is abnormally prone to dilate in the second trimester of pregnancy, resulting in premature expulsion of the fetus (middle trimester abortion).
**strawberry c.,** colpitis macularis.
**tapiroid c.,** a uterine cervix with a peculiarly elongated anterior lip.
**c. u′teri** [TA], **uterine c.,** neck or cervix of uterus: the lower and narrow end of the uterus, between the isthmus and the ostium uteri.
**c. vesi′cae** [TA], neck of urinary bladder: a constricted portion of the bladder, formed by the meeting of its inferolateral surfaces proximal to the opening of the urethra.

**ces** central excitatory state; see under *state.*

**ce·sar·e·an** (sə-zar′e-ən) [L. *caesus,* from *caedere* to cut] see under *section.*

**CESD** cholesteryl ester storage disease.

**ce·si·um** (se′ze-əm) [L. *caesium,* from *caesius* blue] [MeSH: Cesium] a rare univalent metallic element with an alkaline oxide; atomic number, 55; atomic weight, 132.905; symbol, Cs.

**Ces·tan's syndrome** (səs-tahnz′) [Raymond J. *Cestan,* French neurologist, 1872–1934] Cestan-Chenais syndrome.

**Ces·tan-Che·nais syndrome** (səs-tahn′shə-na′) [R. J. *Cestan;* Louis *Chenais,* French physician, 1872–1950] see under *syndrome.*

**Ces·tan-Ray·mond syndrome** (səs-tahn′ra-maw′) [R. J. *Cestan;* Fulgence *Raymond,* French neurologist, 1844–1910] Raymond-Cestan syndrome.

**ces·ti·ci·dal** (ses″tĭ si′dəl) destructive to cestodes.

**Ces·to·da** (səs-to′də) [MeSH: Cestoda] a subclass of Cestoidea comprising the true tapeworms, which have a head or scolex, and segments or proglottides. Adults are endoparasitic in the alimentary tract and associated ducts of various vertebrate hosts; their larval stages (cysticercus, coenurus, hydatid, sparganum) may be found in various organs or tissues. Of the eleven orders, two, Pseudophyllidea and Cyclophyllidea, contain species that parasitize humans and other animals. Called also *Eucestoda.*

**Ces·to·da·ria** (ses″to-dar′e-ə) a subclass of tapeworms, the unsegmented tapeworms of the class Cestoidea, which are endoparasitic in the intestines and coelom of various primitive fishes and rarely in reptiles.

**ces·tode** (ses′tōd) 1. tapeworm (q.v.); either any member of the subclass Cestoda or any member of the class Cestoidea. 2. cestoid.

**ces·to·di·a·sis** (ses″to-di′ə-sis) infection by cestodes.

**ces·to·dol·o·gy** (ses″to-dol′ə-je) the scientific study of cestodes.

**ces·toid** (ses′toid) [Gr. *kestos* girdle + *-oid*] resembling a tapeworm.

**Ces·toi·dea** (ses-toi′de-ə) a class of tapeworms (platyhelminths) characterized by the absence of a mouth and digestive tract and by the presence of a noncuticular layer covering their bodies. It comprises two subclasses: Cestodaria and Cestoda.

**Ces·trum** (ses′trum) a genus of tropical plants of the family Solanaceae. Several species cause hemorrhagic gastroenteritis and liver and kidney degeneration in cattle and other animals. *C. diur′num,* the day jasmine, is a West Indian plant that cause enzootic calcinosis in farm animals and gastroenteritis in humans who consume its fruit.

**ce·ta·ce·um** (sə-ta′se-əm) spermaceti.

**cet·al·ko·ni·um chlo·ride** (sət-əl-ko′ne-əm) a cationic quaternary ammonium surfactant, used as a topical anti-infective and disinfectant.

**ce·ta·nol** (se′tə-nol) a solid white alcohol, $C_{16}H_{33}OH$, from sperm oil; used as a constituent of ointments and creams.

**ce·ti·e·dil cit·rate** (sə-ti′ə-dil) a peripheral vasodilator, which has been used in the treatment of arteritis, Raynaud's disease, and acrocyanosis.

**ce·ti·ri·zine hy·dro·chlo·ride** (sə-tir′ĭ-zēn) an $H_1$-receptor antihistaminic that is a metabolite of hydroxyzine, used in the treatment of allergic rhinitis and chronic idiopathic urticaria, and as a treatment adjunct in asthma; administered orally.

**ce·to·cy·cline hy·dro·chlo·ride** (se″to-si′klēn) an antibacterial, $C_{22}H_{21}NO_7 \cdot HCl$.

**ce·tri·mide** (set′rĭ-mīd) cetrimonium bromide.

**cet·ri·mo·ni·um bro·mide** (set″rĭ-mo′ne-əm) a quaternary ammonium antiseptic and detergent composed of a mixture of tetradecyltrimethylammonium bromide with dodecyl- and hexadecyltrimethyl ammonium bromides, applied topically to the skin to cleanse wounds, as a preoperative disinfectant, and to treat seborrhea of the scalp; solutions are also used to cleanse utensils and store surgical instruments. Abbreviated CTBA. Called also *cetrimide* and *cetyltrimethylammonium bromide.*

**ce·tyl** (se′təl) a univalent alcohol radical, $CH_3(CH_2)_{14}CH_2$—.

**ce·tyl·pyr·i·din·i·um chlo·ride** (se″təl-pir″ĭ-din′e-əm) [USP] a cationic disinfectant, used as a local anti-infective administered sublingually or applied topically to intact skin and mucous membranes, and as a preservative in pharmaceutical preparations.

**ce·tyl·tri·meth·yl·am·mo·ni·um bro·mide** (se″təl-tri-meth″əl-ə-mo′ne-əm) cetrimonium bromide.

**ce·vi·tam·ic acid** (se-vi-tam′ik) ascorbic acid.

**Cey·lan·cy·clos·to·ma** (se″lan-si-klos′to-mə) *Ancylostoma braziliense.*

**ceys·sa·tite** (sa′sə-tīt) [*Ceyssat,* a village of France] a white earth from France, useful as an adsorbent powder in eczema and hyperhidrosis, and in preparing ointments and medicated pastes.

**CF** carbolfuchsin; cardiac failure; Christmas factor; citrovorum factor.

**Cf** symbol for *californium.*

**cf.** abbreviation for L. *confer* bring together, compare.

**cff** critical fusion frequency (flicker fusion threshold); see under *flicker.*

**CFT** complement fixation test; see under *fixation.*

**CFTR** cystic fibrosis transmembrane regulator.

**CFU** colony-forming unit, def. 2.

**CFU-C** colony-forming unit–culture.

**CFU-E** colony-forming unit–erythroid.

**CFU-GM** colony-forming unit–granulocyte-macrophage.

**CFU-S** colony-forming unit–spleen.

**CG** trademark for a preparation of indocyanine green.

**CGD** chronic granulomatous disease.

**cGMP** cyclic guanosine monophosphate.

**CGS, cgs** abbreviation for *centimeter-gram-second* system, a system of measurements in which the units are based on the centimeter as the unit of length, the gram as the unit of mass, and the second as the unit of time.

**cGy** centigray.

**CH** crown-heel (length of fetus).

**CH50, $CH_{50}$** see *CH50 assay,* under *assay,* and *CH50 unit,* under *unit.*

**Cha·ber·tia** (shah-ber′te-ə) a genus of nematodes of the family Strongylidae. *C. ovi′na* is a bowel worm parasitic in the colon of sheep, goats, and cattle.

**cha·ber·ti·a·sis** (shah-bər-ti′ə-sis) infection by *Chabertia ovina,* which is clinically apparent mainly in sheep; characteristics include edema and small hemorrhages of the colon with passage of feces containing large amounts of mucus.

**Chad·dock's reflex (sign)** (chad′əks) [Charles Gilbert *Chaddock,* American neurologist, 1861–1936] see under *reflex.*

**Chae·to·mi·um** (ke-to′me-əm) [MeSH: Chaetomium] a genus of fungi of the family Sordariaceae. *C. globo′sum* and other species have occasionally been found infecting human nails (onychomycosis) and skin (phaeohyphomycosis).

**Chad·wick's sign** (chad′wiks) [James Read *Chadwick,* American gynecologist, 1844–1905] see under *sign.*

**chafe** (chāf) to irritate the skin, as by the rubbing together of opposing folds.

**Cha·gas' disease** (shah'gəs) [Carlos Justiniano Ribeiro das *Chagas,* Brazilian physician, 1879–1934] see under *disease.*

**Cha·gas·ia** (chə-gās'e-ə) [C. J. R. das *Chagas*] a genus of mosquitoes of the tribe *Anophelini,* subfamily Anophelinae, native to Central and South America.

**cha·gas·ic** (chə-gās'ik) pertaining to or due to Chagas' disease.

**cha·go·ma** (chə-go'mə) an erythematous nodule appearing within a few days at the site of a bite by a reduviid bug carrying the parasite causing Chagas' disease; lymphatic vessels draining the site may become blocked with scar tissue and produce edema of the area.

**Cha·il·le·tia** (ka-il-e'she-ə) a genus of tropical trees and shrubs, some of which are poisonous to humans and other animals. *C. toxica'ria* is a West African species with poisonous seeds and fruit. *C. cymo'sa* has been reclassified as *Dichapetalum cymosum.*

**Chain** (chān) Ernst Boris. German-born British biochemist, 1906–1979; co-winner, with Sir Alexander Fleming and Sir Howard Walter Florey, of the Nobel prize for medicine or physiology in 1945 for his work on antibacterial substances produced by microorganisms.

**chain** (chān) a collection of objects linked together in linear fashion, or end to end, as the assemblage of atoms or radicals in a chemical compound, or an assemblage of individual bacterial cells.
**$\alpha$ c.,** a globin chain of 141 amino acids found in fetal hemoglobin and normal adult hemoglobin A.
**$\beta$ c.,** a globin chain of 146 amino acids found in normal adult hemoglobin A.
**branched c.,** an open chain of atoms, usually carbon, with one or more side chains attached to it.
**closed c.,** several atoms linked together so as to form a ring, which may be saturated, as in cyclopentane, or aromatic, as in benzene.
**$\delta$ c.,** a globin chain of 146 amino acids, found in normal adult hemoglobin $A_2$.
**$\epsilon$ c.,** a globin chain found in embryonic hemoglobin Gower and hemoglobin Portland.
**electron transport c.,** the series of electron carriers in the inner mitochondrial membrane that pass electrons from reduced coenzymes (NADH, $FADH_2$) to molecular oxygen via sequential redox reactions coupled to vectorial transduction of protons across the membrane. The chain is the final common pathway of biological oxidation, using $O_2$ for fuel combustion; the energy produced is utilized for ATP synthesis, ion translocation, and protein synthesis. See illustration. See also *oxidative phosphorylation.* Called also *respiratory c.*
**food c.,** a sequence of organisms through which energy is transferred from its ultimate source in a plant; each organism eats the preceding and is eaten by the following member in the sequence.
**$\gamma$ c.,** a globin chain of 146 amino acids, found in fetal hemoglobin and in small amounts in normal adult hemoglobin A.
**globin c.,** the polypeptide chain that makes up a globin; those found in adults are *$\alpha$, $\beta$, $\gamma$,* and *$\delta$ chains.*
**H c., heavy c.,** any of the larger polypeptide chains of antibody molecules, two identical heavy chains occurring (with two identical light chains) in each immunoglobulin monomer. The heavy chains determine the immunoglobulin class and subclass and are designated accordingly: $\gamma$, $\alpha$, $\mu$, $\epsilon$, and $\delta$, the heavy chains of IgG, IgA, IgM, IgE, and IgD. The subclass may be designated by a number, e.g., $\gamma 1$, the heavy chain of IgG1. Heavy chains have four homology regions of about 110 amino acid residues: one variable region ($V_H$) and three constant regions ($C_H1$, $C_H2$, $C_H3$) except for $\mu$ and $\epsilon$ chains which have an extra constant region ($C_H4$). See *immunoglobulin.*
**J c.,** [for "joining"] a 15-kilodalton polypeptide occurring in all immunoglobulin polymers, a single J chain occurring in each IgM pentamer and in each IgA dimer, trimer, or tetramer.
**kappa c.,** a type of light polypeptide chain of immunoglobulin molecules; see *light c.*
**L c.,** light c.
**lambda c.,** a type of light polypeptide chain found in immunoglobulin molecules; see *light c.*
**lateral c.,** side c.
**light c.,** any of the smaller polypeptide chains of antibody molecules, two identical light chains occurring (with two identical heavy chains) in each immunoglobulin monomer. There are two types,

Open chain

Closed chain

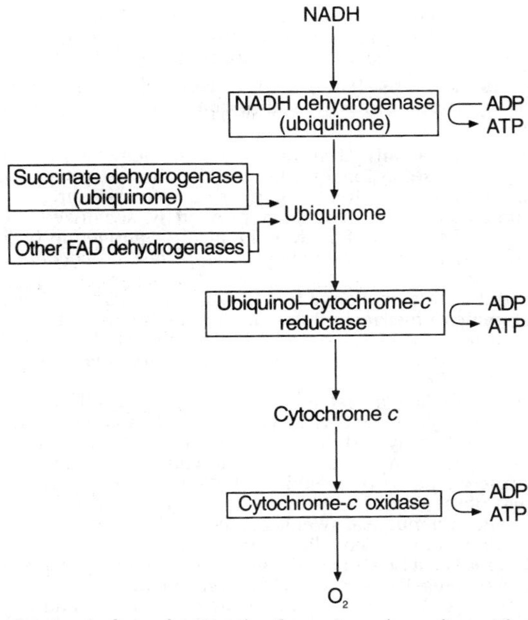

Electron transport chain showing the three sites of coupling with oxidative phosphorylation, generating adenosine triphosphate.

designated $\kappa$ and $\lambda$, both occurring in all immunoglobulin classes (in a ratio of about two $\kappa$ chains to one $\lambda$ chain in humans). Light chains have two homology regions of about 110 amino acid residues: one variable region ($V_L$) and one constant region ($C_L$). Called also *L c.* See *immunoglobulin.*
**nuclear c.,** a longitudinal array of nuclei occurring on an intrafusal fiber of muscle.
**open c.,** a series of atoms united in a straight line; compounds of this series are related to methane and are also called *fatty, aliphatic, acyclic,* or *paraffin* compounds.
**ossicular c.,** ossicula auditus.
**polypeptide c.,** the structural element of protein, consisting of a series of amino acid residues (peptides, q.v.) joined together by peptide bonds.
**respiratory c.,** electron transport c.
**side c.,** a group of atoms attached to a larger chain or to a ring; called also *lateral c.*
**sympathetic c.,** truncus sympathicus.
**$\zeta$ c.,** a globin chain of 141 amino acids, found in embryonic hemoglobin such as hemoglobin Gower and hemoglobin Portland.

**cha·la·sia** (kə-la'zhə) [Gr. *chalasis* relaxation] relaxation of a bodily opening, such as the cardiac sphincter of the esophagus, a cause of vomiting in infants.

**cha·la·za** (kə-la'zə) [Gr. "lump"] a spiral band of albumin extending from either end of the yolk of a bird's egg to the shell.

**cha·la·zia** (kə-la'zhə) [Gr.] plural of *chalazion.*

**cha·la·zi·on** (kə-la'ze-on) pl. *chala'zia* or *chalazions* [Gr. "small lump"] [MeSH: Chalazion] an eyelid mass that results from chronic inflammation of a meibomian gland and shows a granulomatous reaction to liberated fat when subjected to histopathological examination; sometimes called *meibomian* or *tarsal cyst.*

**cha·la·zo·der·mia** (kə-la"zo-dər'me-ə) cutis laxa.

**chal·ci·tis** (kal-si'tis) chalkitis.

**chal·co·sis** (kal-ko'sis) [Gr. *chalkos* copper] the presence of copper deposits in the tissues.
**c. cor'neae,** deposition of copper in the cornea resulting in a pigmented ring in the deeper layers.

**chal·i·co·sis** (kal-ĭ-ko'sis) [Gr. *chalix* gravel] pneumoconiosis in stonecutters due to the inhalation of stone dust. Called also *flint disease.*

**chalk** (chawk) [L. *calx*] 1. a natural calcium carbonate; the amorphous remains of minute marine organisms deposited on the sea bottom and decomposed by the action of acids and heat. Used as a polishing agent in dentistry and frequently as an ingredient in dentifrices. 2. any of various other substances physically resembling calcium carbonate.
**French c.,** talc (def. 1).
**precipitated c.,** precipitated calcium carbonate.

**prepared c.,** native calcium carbonate freed from most of its impurities by elutriation; used as an antacid, and has been used in the treatment of diarrhea and in the preparation of dentifrices.

**chal·ki·tis** (kal-ki'tis) [Gr. *chalkos* brass] inflammation of the eyes caused by rubbing the eyes after the hands have been used on brass.

**chal·lenge** (chal'ənj) 1. to administer a chemical substance to a patient for observation of whether the normal physiological response occurs. 2. in immunology, to administer antigen to evoke an immunologic response in a previously sensitized individual. 3. the administration of such a chemical or antigen in order to assess for a response. Called also *challenge test, provocative test,* and *provocation.*
**bronchial c.,** 1. a challenge test in which a nonspecific agent such as histamine or methacholine is applied to the bronchi and they are assessed for a bronchoconstriction reaction. Called also *bronchoprovocation, bronchial provocation,* and *bronchial challenge test.* 2. inhalational c.
**food c.,** a challenge test for determining food allergens; a small amount of a lyophilized preparation of the suspected allergen is administered orally and the patient is monitored for reactions such as rash, rhinorrhea, or diarrhea. Called also *food challenge test.*
**histamine c.,** a type of bronchial challenge done to assess responsiveness of the mucosa: histamine is applied to the nose or mucous membrane and mucosal swelling is monitored; allergic or otherwise susceptible subjects have lowered thresholds of reactivity.
**inhalational c.,** a type of challenge test done to determine reactivity to drugs or causative allergens in atopic or extrinsic asthma; a dilute concentrate of the suspected substance is inhaled and the patient is assessed for bronchial reactivity, which may be either early or late. Called also *inhalational provocation* or *challenge test.*
**methacholine c.,** a type of bronchial challenge or inhalational challenge used as a test for airway reactivity or atopic asthma; aerosolized methacholine is applied to the airways and the patient is assessed for responsiveness or hyperresponsiveness.

**chal·one** (kal'ōn) [Gr. *chalan* to relax] a group of tissue-specific (but not species-specific) water-soluble proteins that are produced within a tissue and that inhibit mitosis of cells of that tissue and whose action is reversible.

**cha·lon·ic** (kə-lon'ik) of or pertaining to a chalone.

**cha·lyb·e·ate** (kə-lib'e-āt) [L. *chalybs;* Gr. *chalyps* steel] ferruginous.

**cham·ae·ce·phal·ic** (kam″e-sə-fal'ik) pertaining to or characterized by chamaecephaly.

**cham·ae·ceph·a·ly** (kam″e-sef'ə-le) [Gr. *chamai* low + *-cephaly*] the condition of having a low flat head, that is, a cephalic index of 70 or less.

**cham·ae·pro·so·pic** (kam″ə-pro-sop'ik) pertaining to or characterized by chamaeprosopy.

**cham·ae·pros·o·py** (kam″ə-pros'ə-pe) [Gr. *chamai* low + *prosōpon* face] the condition of having a low, broad face, i.e., a facial index of 90 or less.

**cham·ber** (chām'bər) [L. *camera;* Gr. *kamara*] an enclosed space or antrum.
**Abbe-Zeiss counting c.,** Thoma-Zeiss counting c.
**acoustic c.,** a soundproof enclosure used in measuring hearing. See also *anechoic c.*
**air-equivalent ionization c.,** in radiology, a chamber in which the materials of the wall and electrodes are such that ionizing radiations produce ionization essentially similar to that in a free-air ionization chamber.
**altitude c.,** a vacuum chamber used to simulate the effects of high altitude and low atmospheric pressure.
**anechoic c.,** an acoustic chamber that is echo-free. Called also *anechoic room.*
**anterior c. of eye,** camera anterior bulbi.
**aqueous c.,** that part of the eyeball which is filled with aqueous humor; see *anterior c. of eye* and *posterior c. of eye.*
**Boyden c.,** a device consisting of two compartments separated by a micropore filter, used in tests for chemotaxis. Cells are placed in the upper compartment and the chemotactic agent in the lower; if cells are attracted to the agent, they migrate through the pores of the filter. The filter is then stained so that cell migration can be measured.
**counting c.,** hemacytometer.
**diffusion c.,** an apparatus for separating a substance by means of a semipermeable membrane.
**c's of eye,** the various spaces in the eyeball; see *anterior c. of eye, posterior c. of eye,* and *vitreous c.*
**Finn c.,** see under *test.*
**free-air ionization c.,** an ionization chamber in which the ionization in an accurately defined volume of free air is measured.
**Haldane c.,** an air-tight chamber in which animals may be confined for the performance of metabolic studies; called also *Haldane apparatus.*

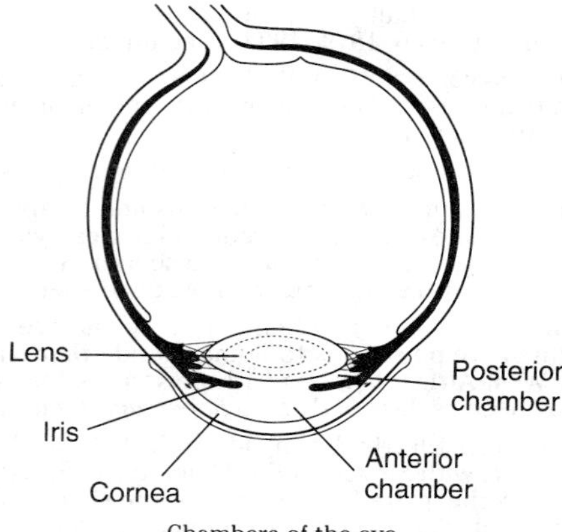

Chambers of the eye.

**c's of the heart,** the cavities of the atria and ventricles.
**hyperbaric c.,** a compartment in which the air pressure may be raised to more than normal atmospheric pressure; used in treatment of gas gangrene and other anaerobic infections, or other conditions in which a high concentration of oxygen is desirable, and for studying the effects of pressure and decompression in animals and man.
**ionization c.,** a device for measuring ionizing radiation by the measurement of the ionization of the gas contained in the chamber.
**lethal c.,** a chamber that may be filled with gas, for killing small animals.
**posterior c. of eye,** camera posterior bulbi.
**pulp c.,** cavitas coronalis.
**relief c.,** a recess in the impression surface of a denture to reduce or eliminate pressure or force from that area of the mouth. See also *relief,* defs. 3 and 4.
**Storm Van Leeuwen c.,** a room that can be kept free of airborne antigens for allergic patients.
**thimble c.,** a small, thin-walled ionization chamber, usually with walls of organic material; used as a dosimeter.
**Thoma-Zeiss counting c.,** a common kind of hemacytometer; called also *Abbe-Zeiss counting c.*
**tissue-equivalent ionization c.,** an ionization chamber in which the walls, electrodes, and gas are selected to produce ionization essentially equivalent to that which would occur in the tissue under consideration.
**vitreous c., vitreous c. of eye,** camera vitrea bulbi.
**Zappert's c.,** a type of hemacytometer.

**Cham·ber·len forceps** (chām'bər-lən) [Peter *Chamberlen,* English obstetrician, 1560–1631] see under *forceps.*

**cham·e·ce·phal·ic** (kam″ə-sə-fal'ik) chamaecephalic.

**cham·e·ceph·a·ly** (kam″ə-sef'ə-le) chamaecephaly.

**cham·e·pro·so·pic** (kam″ə-pro-sop'ik) chamaeprosopic.

**cham·e·pros·o·py** (kam″ə-pros'ə-pe) chamaeprosopy.

**cham·fer** (sham'fər) on an extracoronal cavity preparation, a marginal finish that makes a curve from an axial wall to the cavosurface.

**cham·o·mile** (kam'ə-mēl) 1. *Anthemis nobilis.* 2. *Matricaria chamomilla.* 3. the dried flower heads of either *Anthemis nobilis* or *Matricaria chamomilla,* used as a counterirritant externally and as a carminative internally in the form of a tea. The official preparation [NF] is from *M. chamomilla.*

**Chance fracture** (chans) [G.Q. *Chance,* British radiologist, 20th century] see under *fracture.*

**chan·cre** (shang'kər) [Fr. for "canker," a destructive sore, from L. *cancer* crab] [MeSH: Chancre] 1. the usually painless primary lesion of syphilis, occurring at the site of entry of the infection, typically presenting as a small red papule or crusted erosion that breaks down to become round or oval, indurated, and slightly elevated with an eroded surface that exudes a serous fluid, and gives rise to a nontender nonfluctuant, firm regional lymphadenopathy (bubo); it heals without scarring. Called also *hard c., hard sore, hunterian c.,* and *true c.* 2. any of various primary cutaneous lesions that are seen at the site of inoculation of infection in such diseases as herpes, sporotrichosis, tuberculosis, tularemia, and trypanosomiasis.
**hard c., hunterian c.,** chancre, def. 1.
**mixed c.,** a skin lesion due to simultaneous infection with *Treponema pallidum* (primary syphilis) and *Haemophilus ducreyi* (chancroid); called also *mixed sore.*
**monorecidive c.,** c. redux.

**c. re'dux,** the reappearance of a chancre after partial healing as a result of insufficient treatment, accompanied by lymphadenopathy and the presence of numerous spirochetes at the site of the lesion; called also *monorecidive c.*
**soft c.,** chancroid.
**true c.,** chancre, def. 1.
**tuberculous c.,** see *primary inoculation tuberculosis,* under *tuberculosis.*

**chan·cri·form** (shang'krĭ-form) resembling a chancre.

**chan·croid** (shang'kroid) [*chancre* + *-oid*] [MeSH: Chancroid] a sexually transmitted disease caused by *Haemophilus ducreyi,* characterized by a painful primary ulcer at the site of inoculation, usually on the external genitalia, associated with regional lymphadenitis. See also *mixed chancre.* Called also *soft chancre, soft sore,* and *soft ulcer.*
**phagedenic c.,** a variety attended by sloughing of the tissues.
**serpiginous c.,** a variety which tends to spread in curved lines.

**chan·croi·dal** (shang-kroi'dəl) pertaining to chancroid.

**chan·crous** (shang'krəs) of the nature of chancre.

**change** (chānj) an alteration.
**Armanni-Ebstein c.,** see under *lesion.*
**Crooke's c's, Crooke-Russell c's,** Crooke's hyalinization.
**fatty c.,** abnormal accumulation of fat within parenchymal cells; the term encompasses the older concepts defined as *fatty degeneration* and *fatty infiltration.*
**harlequin color c.,** transient reddening of one half of the body longitudinally with simultaneous blanching of the other half; a temporary vasomotor disorder of the newborn.
**hyaline c.,** a pale, eosinophilic, homogeneous glassy appearance seen in histologic specimens, especially of collagenous connective tissue and smooth muscle; it is a purely descriptive term and has a variety of causes.
**hydropic c.,** hydropic degeneration.
**personality c. due to a general medical condition,** [DSM-IV], persistent disturbance of personality due to the direct effects of a general medical condition and neither better accounted for by another mental disorder nor occurring exclusively during delirium.

**ch'ang shan** (chahng shahn) [Chinese] 1. *Dichroa febrifuga.* 2. the root of *D. febrifuga,* which contains the alkaloids dichroine, febrifugine, and isofebrifugine; used in Chinese medicine in the treatment of malaria because of its antiparasitic, emetic, and antipyretic properties.

**chan·nel** (chan'əl) [L. *canalis* a water pipe] 1. a passageway through which something flows; see also *canalis* and *groove.* 2. protein c.
**acetylcholine c.,** a ligand-gated protein channel in which the ligand acetylcholine opens the gate; it is important in the intercellular transmission of nerve cell signals.
**blood c's,** narrow passages with indistinct walls, containing blood; they are found in fresh granulation tissue.
**calcium c.,** a slow voltage-gated protein channel very permeable to calcium ions and slightly permeable to sodium ions, existing in three subtypes designated *L, M,* and *N* and located throughout the body; calcium channels are the main cause of action potentials in certain smooth muscles, and the N channels regulate neurotransmitter release.
**calcium-sodium c.,** calcium c.
**fast c.,** a protein channel, such as a sodium channel, that becomes activated relatively quickly; a fast voltage-gated channel has a much lower activation potential than does the slow type. Cf. *slow c.*
**gated c.,** see *voltage-gated c.* and *ligand-gated c.*
**ligand-gated c.,** a protein channel that opens in response to the binding of a molecule (the ligand) to the protein, which causes a conformational change in the protein molecule. Cf. *voltage-gated c.*
**lymph c's,** the smaller lymph sinuses; irregular in and about the lymphatic glands and around lymphatic vessels.
**perineural c.,** a lymph channel that surrounds a nerve trunk.
**potassium c.,** a voltage-gated slow protein channel selective for the passage of potassium ions, occurring on the surface of a wide variety of cells, including nerve, muscle, and secretory cells; its functions include regulation of cell membrane excitability, regulation of repetitive low frequency firing in some neurons, and recovery of the nerve fiber membrane at the end of the action potential.
**protein c.,** a watery pathway through the interstices of a protein molecule by which ions and small molecules can cross a membrane into or out of a cell by diffusion; protein channels play a vital role in depolarization and repolarization of nerve and muscle fibers, and may have physical characteristics such as shape or diameter that particularly attract certain ions.
**slow c.,** a protein channel, such as the calcium channel, that is slow to become activated; a slow voltage-gated channel has a much higher activation potential than does the fast type. Cf. *fast c.*
**sodium c.,** a protein channel selective for the passage of sodium ions. Voltage-gated sodium channels are the main causes of depolarization and repolarization of nerve membranes during the action potential.
**thoroughfare c.,** a channel between terminal arterioles and venules, larger than a capillary.
**voltage-gated c.,** a protein channel that can be opened or closed in response to changes in the electric potential across a cell membrane. Cf. *ligand-gated c.*
**water c.,** a channel in a cell membrane that permits passage of water molecules; chemical substances such as vasopressin cause the opening of new channels and increase permeability. See also *aggrephore.*

**Cha·o·bor·us** (ka″o-bor'əs) a genus of non–blood-sucking gnats of the family Culicidae; called also *Corethra. C. lacus'tris* is the Clear Lake gnat of California.

**Cha·os cha·os** (ka'os ka'os) *Pelomyxa carolinensis.*

**Cha·oul therapy, tube** (showl) [Henri *Chaoul,* Lebanese radiologist in Germany, 1887–1964] see under *therapy* and *tube.*

**chap·er·one** (shap'ər-ōn) someone or something that accompanies and oversees another.
**molecular c.,** any of a diverse group of proteins that oversee the correct intracellular folding and assembly of polypeptides without being components of the final structure. The group includes nucleoplasmins, chaperonins, other heat shock proteins, and various other unrelated proteins.

**chap·er·o·nin** (shap″ər-o'nin) any of various heat shock proteins that act as molecular chaperones in bacteria, plasmids, mitochondria, and eukaryotic cyotsol. They are large multi-subunit proteins with ring structures and act by enclosing unfolded proteins and preventing their nonspecific aggregation during assembly.

**chapped** (chapt) roughened and cracked, or split open by the cold or frequent wetting, as chapped hands or lips.

**char·ac·ter** (kar'ak-tər) [Gr. *charaktēr* an engraved or impressed mark or stamp] [MeSH: Character] 1. a quality or attribute indicative of the nature of an object or organism. 2. in genetics, the expression in the phenotype of a gene or group of genes; see also *gene* and *inheritance.* 3. in psychiatry, a term used, especially in the psychoanalytic literature, in much the same way as personality (q.v.), particularly for those personality traits that are shaped by life experiences and developmental processes. See also *temperament.*
**acquired c.,** a noninheritable modification produced in an animal as a result of its own activities or of environmental influences.
**imvic c's,** four important characters in the classification of the coliform organisms: they are indole, methyl-red, Voges-Proskauer, and citrate.
**primary sex c's,** those characters in the male or female that are directly involved in reproduction; the gonads and their accessory structures.
**secondary sex c's,** those characters specific to the male or female but not directly involved in reproduction. See also *masculinization* and *feminization.*

**char·ac·ter·is·tic** (kar″ak-tər-is'tik) 1. character. 2. typical of an individual or other entity.
**demand c's,** cues regarding the purpose of the study or the behavior expected that an experimental subject perceives and responds to.

**char·ac·ter·ol·o·gy** (kar″ak-tər-ol'ə-je) the study of character and personality.

**char·bon** (shahr-bo') [Fr. "coal"] old name for *anthrax.*

**char·coal** (chahr'kōl) [MeSH: Charcoal] carbon prepared by charring wood or other organic material.
**activated c.** [USP], the residue from the destructive distillation of various organic materials, treated to increase its adsorptive powers; used as a general purpose antidote. Called also *carbo activatus.*
**animal c.,** charcoal prepared from bone; called also *animal, ivory,* or *Paris black,* and *bone-black.*
**purified animal c.,** charcoal prepared from bone and purified by removal of materials dissolved by hot hydrochloric acid and water; adsorbent and decolorizer.

**Char·cot's arthropathy (disease, joint),** etc. (shahr-kōz') [Jean Martin *Charcot,* French neurologist, 1825–1893] see under *foot, gait, sign,* and *triad;* see *neuropathic arthropathy,* under *arthropathy;* see *primary biliary cirrhosis,* under *cirrhosis;* see *intermittent claudication,* under *claudication;* and see *intermittent hepatic fever,* under *fever.*

**Char·cot-Bou·chard aneurysm** (shahr-ko'boo-shahr') [J.M. *Charcot;* Charles Jacques *Bouchard,* French physician, 1837–1886] see under *aneurysm.*

**Char·cot-Ley·den crystals** (shahr-ko'li'dən) [J.M. *Charcot;* Ernst Victor von *Leyden,* German physician, 1832–1910] see under *crystal.*

**Char·cot-Ma·rie atrophy (syndrome)** (shahr-ko'mah-re') [J.M. *Charcot;* Pierre *Marie,* French physician, 1853–1940] Charcot-Marie-Tooth disease.

**Char·cot-Ma·rie-Tooth disease (atrophy)** (shahr-ko'mah-re'to͞oth) [J.M. *Charcot;* Pierre *Marie;* Howard Henry *Tooth,* English physician, 1856–1925] see under *disease.*

**Char·cot-Weiss-Bak·er syndrome** (shahr-ko'wīs-ba'kər) [J.M. *Charcot;* Soma *Weiss,* American physician, 1898–1942; James Porter *Baker,* American physician, born 1902] carotid sinus syndrome; see under *syndrome.*

**charge** (chahrj) a fundamental physical characteristic of elementary particles that determines the strength and nature of their interactions with the electromagnetic field. It is defined as positive or negative (or zero), existing only in integral numbers of charge quanta (e.g., proton, +1; electron, −1; neutron 0) each of which is $1.602 \times 10^{-19}$ coulomb. The charge of a body is the algebraic sum of the charges of its constituents. Symbol *Q* or *q.* Called also *electric charge.*

**char·la·tan** (shahr'lə-tən) [Fr.] a pretender to knowledge or skills that he does not possess; in medicine, a quack.

**char·la·tan·ism** (shahr'lə-tən-iz"əm) the pretension of knowledge and skills that one does not possess; in medicine, quackery.

**char·la·tan·ry** (shahr'lə-tən-re) charlatanism.

**Charles' law** (shahrlz) [Jacques Alexandre César *Charles,* French physicist, 1746–1823] see under *law.*

**char·ley horse** (chahr'le hors) soreness and stiffness in a muscle caused by overstrain or contusion; the term is usually restricted to injuries of the quadriceps muscle.

**Char·lin's syndrome** (chahr'lēnz) [Carlos *Charlin,* Chilean ophthalmologist, 1886–1945] see under *syndrome.*

**Charn·ley's hip arthroplasty, prosthesis** (charhn'lēz) [Sir John *Charnley,* British orthopedic surgeon, born 1911] see under *arthroplasty* and *prosthesis.*

**Char·rière scale** (shahr"e-ār') [Joseph Frédéric Benoit *Charrière,* Swiss-born instrument maker in France, 1803–1876] see under *scale.*

**Chart.** abbreviation for L. *char'ta,* paper.

**chart** (chahrt) 1. a simplified graphic representation of the fluctuation of some variable, as of pulse, temperature, and respiration, or a record of all the clinical data of a particular case. 2. to record graphically the fluctuation of some variable, or to record the clinical data of a particular case.
**alignment c.,** nomogram.
**Amsler c's,** a set of charts showing various geometric patterns in black and white, e.g., grids or parallel lines, used for detecting defects of the central visual field.
**Guibor's c.,** a chart containing outline pictures for orthoptic training.
**Liley c.,** a chart that uses the spectrographic measurement of amniotic fluid bilirubin levels plotted against gestational age to estimate the severity of fetal hemolysis resulting from Rh isoimmunization. The chart is divided into three zones; a measurement falling in zone 1 indicates no disease or mild disease, while one falling in zone 3 indicates severe disease with impending fetal death.
**reading c.,** a chart bearing material printed in type of gradually increasing sizes; used in testing acuity of near vision.
**Reuss' color c's,** charts with colored letters printed on colored backgrounds, used in testing color vision; called also *Reuss' tables.*
**Snellen's c.,** a chart imprinted with block letters (Snellen's test type) in gradually decreasing sizes, identified according to distances at which they are ordinarily visible; used in testing visual acuity. See also *Snellen's test type,* under *test type.*

**char·ta** (kahr'tə) pl. *char'tae* [L.; Gr. *chartēs*] 1. paper. 2. a piece of paper, medicated or otherwise.

**char·ta·ce·ous** (kahr-ta'shəs) papyraceous.

**char·tu·la** (kahr'tu-lə) pl. *char'tulae* [L. dim. of *charta* paper] a small piece of paper, as for containing a dose of a medicinal powder.

**chas·ma·to·plas·son** (kaz-mat'o-plas"on) [*chasma* + *plasson*] the protoplasm of a non-nucleated cell in an expanded condition. Cf. *pyknoplasson.*

**Chas·sai·gnac's tubercle** (shahs"ən-yahks') [Charles Marie Édouard *Chassaignac,* French surgeon, 1804–1879] *tuberculum caroticum.*

**chaude-pisse** (shōd-pēs) [Fr.] a burning sensation experienced during micturition.

**Chauf·fard's syndrome** (sho-fahrz') [Anatole Marie Emile *Chauffard,* French physician, 1855–1932] see under *syndrome.*

**Chauf·fard-Still syndrome** (sho-fahr'stil) [A. M. E. *Chauffard;* Sir George Frederick *Still,* English physician, 1868–1941] Chauffard's syndrome.

**Chau·liac** (sho"le-ahk') Guy de (1300–1368). French surgeon who practiced in Avignon; *Chirurgia magna,* his treatise on surgery, was regarded as a standard work until Paré's time.

**ChB** abbreviation for L. *Chirur'giae Baccalau'reus,* Bachelor of Surgery.

**CHD** 1. congenital heart disease. 2. coronary heart disease; see *ischemic heart disease,* under *disease.*

**ChD** abbreviation for L. *Chirur'giae Doc'tor,* Doctor of Surgery.

**ChE** cholinesterase.

**check-bite** (chek'bīt) check bite; see under *bite.*

**chec·ker·board** (chek'ər-bord) in genetics, a grid with margins which shows the gametes of each parent (in the margins) and their possible progeny (in the squares); called also *Punnett square.*

**Ché·di·ak-Hi·ga·shi syndrome (anomaly)** (cha'de-ahk he-gah'she) [Moisés *Chédiak,* Cuban physician, 20th century; Otakata *Higashi,* Japanese physician, 20th century] see under *syndrome.*

**Ché·di·ak-Stein·brinck-Hi·ga·shi anomaly** (cha'de-ahk shtīn'bringk he-gah'she) [M. *Chédiak;* W. *Steinbrinck,* German physician, 20th century; O. *Higashi*] Chédiak-Higashi syndrome.

**cheek** (chēk) [MeSH: Cheek] 1. bucca. 2. any fleshy protuberance resembling the cheek of the face.
**cleft c.,** facial cleft caused by developmental failure of union between the maxillary and frontonasal prominences.

**cheesy** (che'ze) caseous.

**Chei·lan·thes** (ki-lan'thēz) a genus of ferns. *C. sei'beri* is the rock fern, an Australian species that causes poisoning in cattle similar to bracken poisoning. *C. sinna'ta* is the jimmy fern, a North American species poisonous to cattle, sheep, and goats, causing convulsions.

**chei·lec·to·my** (ki-lek'tə-me) [*cheil-* + *-ectomy*] 1. excision of a lip. 2. the operation of chiseling off the irregular bony edges of a joint cavity that interfere with motion.

**chei·lec·tro·pi·on** (ki"lek-tro'pe-on) [*cheil-* + *ectropion*] eversion of the lip.

**chei·li·tis** (ki-li'tis) [*cheil-* + *-itis*] [MeSH: Cheilitis] inflammation affecting the lips. Spelled also *chilitis.* Cf. *cheilosis.*
**actinic c.,** painful swelling of the lip(s) and development of scaly crust and erosions on the vermilion border after overexposure to sun rays; it may be acute or chronic. Called also *solar c.*
**angular c.,** perlèche.
**apostematous c.,** see *c. glandularis.*
**commissural c.,** cheilitis affecting principally the angles (commissures) of the mouth. See also *perlèche.*
**c. exfoliati'va,** persistent exfoliation of the lip caused by inflammation of the mucous membrane, similar to but not identical with dermatitis seborrheica.
**c. glandula'ris,** a rare disease in which the lower lip becomes enlarged and later everted, exposing the openings of the accessory salivary glands, which are inflamed and dilated; the glands themselves are enlarged and sometimes nodular. It may be associated with carcinoma of the lip. There are three types: the *simple type* is characterized by multiple painless, pinhead-sized lesions, with central depressions and dilated canals, and may develop into one of the other types; the *superficial suppurative type* (called also *Baelz's disease*) is characterized by painless swelling, induration, crusting, and ulcerations of the lip; the *deep suppurative type* is a deep-seated infection with abscesses and fistulous tracts that eventually form scars. Called also *apostematous c., c. glandularis apostematosa,* and *myxadenitis labialis.*
**c. glandula'ris apostemato'sa,** see *c. glandularis.*
**c. granulomato'sa, granulomatous c.,** an inflammation of the lips characterized by granulomas and swelling; it is sometimes part of

| | | Affected parent A/a | |
|---|---|---|---|
| | Gametes | A | a |
| Normal parent a/a | a | A/a Affected | a/a normal |
| | a | A/a Affected | a/a normal |

Checkerboard diagramming the probabilities for inheritance of a hypothetical dominant trait upon crossing a heterozygote with a homozygote lacking the trait (normal).

Melkersson-Rosenthal syndrome. Called also *Miescher's granulomatous c.*
**impetiginous c.,** impetigo of the lips.
**Miescher's granulomatous c.,** granulomatous c.
**migrating c.,** perlèche.
**solar c.,** actinic c.
**c. venena'ta,** that due to a toxic substance.

**cheil(o)-** [Gr. *cheilos* lip] a combining form denoting relationship to the lip, or to an edge.

**chei·lo·an·gi·os·co·py** (ki″lo-an″je-os′kə-pe) [*cheilo-* + *angioscopy*] microscopical observation of the circulation in the blood vessels of the lip.

**chei·lo·car·ci·no·ma** (ki″lo-kahr-sĭ-no′mə) carcinoma of the lip.

**chei·lo·gnatho·pal·a·tos·chi·sis** (ki″lo-na″tho-pal″ə-tos′kĭ-sis) cheilognathouranoschisis.

**chei·lo·gnatho·pros·o·pos·chi·sis** (ki″lo-na″tho-pros″o-pos′kĭ-sis) [*cheilo-* + *gnatho-* + *prosoposchisis*] a developmental anomaly consisting of an oblique facial cleft continuing into the lip and upper jaw.

**chei·lo·gnath·os·chi·sis** (ki″lo-na-thos′kĭ-sis) [*cheilo-* + *gnathoschisis*] a developmental anomaly consisting of a cleft lip and jaw.

**chei·lo·gnatho·ura·nos·chi·sis** (ki-″lo-na″tho-u-rə-nos′kĭ-sis) [*cheilo-* + *gnatho-* + *uranoschisis*] a developmental anomaly consisting of a cleft lip, upper jaw, and palate.

**chei·lo·pha·gia** (ki″lo-fa′jə) [*cheilo-* + *-phagia*] biting of the lips.

**chei·lo·plas·ty** (ki′lo-plas″te) [*cheilo-* + *-plasty*] plastic surgery of the lip; called also *labioplasty.*

**chei·lor·rha·phy** (ki-lor′ə-fe) [*cheilo-* + *-rrhaphy*] the operation of suturing the lip, as in surgical repair of a congenitally cleft lip.

**chei·los·chi·sis** (ki-los′kĭ-sis) [*cheilo-* + Gr. *schisis* cleft] cleft lip.

**chei·lo·sis** (ki-lo′sis) [*cheil-* + *-osis*] a noninflammatory condition of the lips characterized by chapping and fissuring. Cf. *cheilitis.*
**angular c.,** perlèche.

**chei·lo·sto·ma·to·plas·ty** (ki″lo-sto-mat′o-plas″te) [*cheilo-* + *stomato-* + *-plasty*] plastic restoration of the mouth and lips.

**chei·lot·o·my** (ki-lot′ə-me) [*cheilo-* + *-tomy*] incision into the lip.

**Chei·ra·can·thi·um** (ki″rə-kan′the-əm) *Chiracanthium.*

**Chei·ra·can·thus** (ki″rə-kan′thəs) *Gnathostoma.*

**chei·ra·gra** (ki-rag′rə) [*cheir-* + *agra*] gout of the hand, especially tophaceous gout with torsion of the fingers.

**chei·ral·gia** (ki-ral′jə) pain in the hand.
**c. paresthe′tica,** isolated neuritis of the superficial ramus of the radial nerve.

**cheir·ar·thri·tis** (ki″rahr-thri′tis) [*cheir-* + *arthritis*] inflammation of the joints of the hand and fingers.

**cheir(o)-** [Gr. *cheir* hand] a combining form denoting relationship to the hand. For words beginning thus, see also those beginning *chir(o)-.*

**chei·ro·cin·es·the·sia** (ki″ro-sin″əs-the′zhə) cheirokinesthesia.

**chei·ro·kin·es·the·sia** (ki″ro-kin″əs-the′zhə) the subjective perception of the movements of the hand, especially in writing.

**chei·ro·kin·es·thet·ic** (ki″ro-kin″əs-thet′ik) pertaining to or characterized by cheirokinesthesia.

**chei·rol·o·gy** (ki-rol′ə-je) dactylology.

**chei·ro·meg·a·ly** (ki-ro-meg′ə-le) abnormal enlargement of the hands.

**chei·ro·plas·ty** (ki′ro-plas″te) [*cheiro-* + Gr. *-plasty*] plastic surgery on the hand.

**chei·ro·po·dal·gia** (ki″ro-po-dal′jə) [*cheiro-* + *podo-* + *-algia*] pain in the hands and feet.

**chei·ro·pom·pho·lyx** (ki″ro-pom′fo-liks) [*cheiro-* + *pompholyx*] pompholyx.

**chei·ro·scope** (ki′ro-skōp) [*cheiro-* + *-scope*] an instrument used in the training of binocular vision, by which the image of a test object seen reflected in a mirror by the sound eye is projected by the other eye to a drawing board, where it is traced with a pencil guided by the hand of the subject.

**chei·ro·spasm** (ki′ro-spaz″əm) [*cheiro-* + *spasm*] spasm of the muscles of the hand.

**che·late** (ke′lāt) [Gr. *chēlē* claw] 1. to combine with a metal in complexes in which the metal is part of a ring. 2. by extension, a chemical compound in which a metallic ion is sequestered and firmly bound into a ring within the chelating molecule. Chelates are used in chemotherapeutic treatments for metal poisoning.

**che·la·tion** (ke-la′shən) combination with a metal in complexes in which the metal is part of a ring.

**che·lic·era** (ke-lis′ər-ə) pl. chelic′erae [Gr. *chēlē* claw + *keras* horn] a pair of pincer-like head appendages of spiders, scorpions, and other arachnids. In certain arthropods, such as spiders, mites, and scorpions, anterior chelicerae serve as feeding appendages.

**Chel-Iron** (kēl′i-ərn) trademark for preparations of ferrocholinate.

**che·loid** (ke′loid) keloid.

**che·lo·ma** (ke-lo′mə) keloid.

**chel·on·i·an** (kel-o′ne-ən) [Gr. *chelōnē* tortoise] pertaining to turtles and tortoises (order Chelonia).

**chem·abra·sion** (kēm″ə-bra′zhən) superficial destruction and exfoliation of the epidermis and the upper layer of the dermis by application of a cauterant to the skin; done to remove scars, tattoos, pigmented nevi, etc. Called also *chemexfoliation* and *chemical peel.* See also *planing.*

**chem·ex·fo·li·a·tion** (kēm″eks-fo″le-a′shən) [MeSH: Chemexfoliation] chemabrasion.

**chemi-** see *chem(o)-.*

**chemi·at·ric** (kem″e-at′rik) iatrochemical.

**chemi·a·try** (kem′e-ə-tre) iatrochemistry.

**chem·i·cal** (kem′ĭ-kəl) 1. of, or pertaining to, chemistry. 2. a substance composed of chemical elements, or obtained by chemical processes.

**chemic(o)-** see *chem(o)-.*

**chem·i·co·bi·o·log·i·cal** (kem″ĭ-ko-bi″o-loj′ĭ-kəl) biochemical.

**chem·i·co·cau·tery** (kem″ĭ-ko-kaw′tər-e) chemocautery.

**chem·i·co·gen·e·sis** (kem″ĭ-ko-jen′ə-sis) [*chemico-* + *-genesis*] development of an oocyte (ovum) by chemical stimulation.

**chem·i·co·phys·i·cal** (kem″ĭ-ko-fiz′ə-kəl) pertaining to chemistry and physics; pertaining to physical chemistry.

**chem·i·co·phys·i·o·log·ic** (kem″ĭ-ko-fiz″e-o-loj′ik) pertaining to physiology and chemistry.

**chemi·lu·mi·nes·cence** (kem″ĭ-loo″mĭ-nes′əns) [MeSH: Chemiluminescence] luminescence produced by direct transformation of chemical energy into light energy.

**chemi·os·mo·sis** (kem″e-os-mo′sis) chemical action taking place through an intervening semipermeable membrane.

**chemi·os·mot·ic** (kem″e-os-mot′ik) pertaining to chemiosmosis.

**chem·io·tax·is** (kēm″e-o-tak′sis) chemotaxis.

**chem·io·ther·a·py** (kēm″e-o-ther′ə-pe) chemotherapy.

**chem·ism** (kem′izm) 1. chemical activity. 2. a chemical property or relationship.

**chemi·sorp·tion** (kem″ĭ-sorp′shən) the chemical adsorption of a gas or liquid onto the surface of a solid material, altering their molecular properties; in contrast to physical adsorption, which is characterized by weaker Van der Waals forces.

**chem·ist** (kem′ist) 1. an individual skilled in chemistry. 2. (British) a pharmacist.

**chem·is·try** (kem′is-tre) [Gr. *chēmeia*] [MeSH: Chemistry] the science that treats of the elements and atomic relations of matter, and of the various compounds of the elements.
**analytical c.,** chemistry that deals with analysis of different elements in a compound.
**applied c.,** the application of chemistry to industry and the arts; called also *industrial c.*
**biological c.,** biochemistry.
**colloid c.,** chemistry dealing with the nature and composition of colloids.
**ecological c.,** the study of those chemical compounds synthesized by plants that serve no metabolic purpose but which, by reason of their toxic effect on insects and higher animals, influence a community of interacting plants and animals.
**forensic c.,** use of chemical knowledge in the solution of legal problems.
**industrial c.,** applied c.
**inorganic c.,** that branch of the science of chemistry which deals with compounds that do not occur in the plant or animal worlds; called also *mineral c.*
**medical c.,** chemistry as it relates to medicine.
**metabolic c.,** biochemistry.
**mineral c.,** inorganic c.
**organic c.,** that branch of chemistry which deals with compounds that contain carbon.
**pharmaceutical c.,** chemistry that deals with the composition and preparation of substances used in treatment of patients or diagnostic studies.

**physical c.,** the branch of chemistry that uses a quantitative approach, applying the concepts and laws of physics, to describe and understand chemical properties.
**physiological c.,** biochemistry.
**surface c.,** the study of forces acting at the surfaces of gases, liquids, or solid, or the interfaces between two states.
**synthetic c.,** that branch of chemistry which deals with the building up of chemical compounds from simpler substances or from the elements.

**chem(o)-** [Gr. *chēmeia* alchemy] a combining form denoting relationship to chemistry, or to a chemical. Also, *chemi-, chemic(o)-*.

**che·mo·at·trac·tant** (ke″mo-ə-trak′tənt) a chemotactic factor that induces positive chemotaxis.

**che·mo·au·to·troph** (ke″mo-aw′to-trōf) a chemoautotrophic microorganism.

**che·mo·au·to·troph·ic** (ke″mo-aw″to-trōf′ik) [*chemo-* + *autotrophic*] requiring for growth only inorganic compounds with carbon dioxide as the sole source of carbon (autotrophic), and oxidizing inorganic chemical compounds as the source of energy; said of certain bacteria and protozoa. Cf. *photoautotrophic.*

**che·mo·bi·ot·ic** (ke″mo-bi-ot′ik) the combination of a chemotherapeutic agent and an antibiotic, as of one or more of the sulfonamide compounds with penicillin.

**che·mo·cau·tery** (ke″mo-kaw′tər-e) destruction of tissue by application of a caustic chemical substance. Called also *chemical cautery.*

**che·mo·ce·pha·lia** (ke″mo-sə-fa′le-ə) chamaecephaly.

**che·mo·ceph·a·ly** (ke″mo-sef′ə-le) chamaecephaly.

**che·mo·cep·tor** (ke′mo-sep-tor) chemoreceptor.

**che·mo·co·ag·u·la·tion** (ke″mo-ko-ag″u-la′shən) coagulation or destruction of tissue by the application of chemicals.

**che·mo·dec·to·ma** (ke″mo-dek-to′mə) [*chemo-* + *dektos* to be received or accepted + *-oma*] any benign, chromaffin-negative tumor of the chemoreceptor system; the most common types are the *carotid body tumor,* the *glomus jugulare tumor,* and the *glomus vagale tumor.* Called also *nonchromaffin paraganglioma.*

**che·mo·dif·fer·en·ti·a·tion** (ke″mo-dif″ər-ən-she-a′shən) the invisible point of decision which foreruns and controls the actual differentiation of cells into the rudimentary organs of the embryo.

**che·mo·dy·ne·sis** (ke″mo-di′nə-sis) the initiation of cytoplasmic streaming in plant cells by chemicals.

**che·mo·em·bo·li·za·tion** (ke″mo-em″bo-lĭ-za′shən) percutaneous introduction of a substance to occlude a vessel in combination with a chemotherapeutic agent, used in the treatment of cancer to deliver sustained therapeutic levels of the agent to a tumor.

**che·mo·en·do·crine** (ke″mo-en′do-krin) [*chemo-* + *endocrine*] chemohormonal.

**che·mo·het·ero·troph** (ke″mo-het′ər-o-trōf″) a chemoheterotrophic organism.

**che·mo·het·ero·troph·ic** (ke″mo-het″ər-o-trof′ik) heterotrophic; requiring preformed organic compounds as a source of carbon and oxidizing organic compounds as a source of energy.

**che·mo·hor·mo·nal** (ke″mo-hor-mo′nəl) pertaining to drugs having hormone activity.

**che·mo·im·mu·nol·o·gy** (ke″mo-im-u-nol′ə-je) immunochemistry.

**che·mo·kine** (ke′mo-kīn) any of a group of low molecular weight cytokines, such as interleukin-8, identified on the basis of their ability to induce chemotaxis or chemokinesis in leukocytes (or in particular populations of leukocytes) in inflammation, the group now divided into four subgroups on the basis of genetic, structural, and functional criteria. They function as regulators of the immune system and may also play roles in the circulatory and central nervous systems.

**che·mo·ki·ne·sis** (ke″mo-kĭ-ne′sis) [*chemo-* + *-kinesis*] increased nondirectional activity of cells due to presence of a chemical substance. Cf. *chemotaxis.*

**che·mo·ki·net·ic** (ke″mo-kĭ-net′ik) pertaining to or exhibiting chemokinesis.

**che·mo·litho·troph** (ke″mo-lith′o-trōf) a chemolithotrophic organism.

**che·mo·litho·troph·ic** (ke″mo-lith″o-trof′ik) chemoautotrophic; utilizing carbon dioxide as the sole source of carbon and deriving energy from the oxidation of inorganic compounds.

**che·mo·lu·mi·nes·cence** (ke″mo-loo″mĭ-nes′əns) chemiluminescence.

**che·mol·y·sis** (ke-mol′ĭ-sis) [*chemo-* + *-lysis*] chemical decomposition.

**che·mo·mor·pho·sis** (ke″mo-mor-fo′sis) [*chemo-* + *morphosis*] change of form or developmental stage due to chemical action.

**che·mo·nu·cle·ol·y·sis** (ke″mo-noo″kle-ol′ə-sis) [*chemo-* + *nucleo-* + *lysis*] dissolution of the nucleus pulposus of an intervertebral disk by injection of a proteolytic agent such as chymopapain; used especially in the treatment of herniation of an intervertebral disk (see under *herniation*).

**che·mo·or·gano·troph** (ke″mo-or′gə-no-trōf″) a chemo-organotrophic organism.

**che·mo·or·gano·troph·ic** (ke″mo-or″gə-no-trof′ik) heterotrophic; requiring preformed organic compounds as a source of carbon and oxidizing organic compounds as a source of energy; said of bacteria.

**che·mo·pal·li·dec·tomy** (ke″mo-pal″ĭ-dek′tə-me) [*chemo-* + *pallidectomy*] destruction of a portion of the globus pallidus by the introduction of a chemical agent.

**che·mo·pal·li·do·thal·a·mec·to·my** (ke″mo-pal″ĭ-do-thal″ə-mek′tə-me) destruction of a portion of the globus pallidus and thalamus by the introduction of a chemical agent.

**che·mo·phar·ma·co·dy·nam·ic** (ke″mo-fahr″mə-ko-di-nam′ik) denoting the relationship between chemical constitution and biologic or pharmacologic activity.

**che·mo·phys·i·ol·o·gy** (ke″mo-fiz″e-ol′ə-je) biochemistry.

**che·mo·pre·ven·tion** (ke″mo-pre-ven′shən) [MeSH: Chemoprevention] chemoprophylaxis.

**che·mo·pro·phy·lax·is** (ke″mo-pro″fə-lak′sis) [*chemo-* + *prophylaxis*] use of a chemotherapeutic agent as a means of preventing development of a specific disease. Called also *chemoprevention, chemical prophylaxis,* and *drug prophylaxis.*
**primary c.,** prophylactic use of a chemotherapeutic agent before infection has occurred in an individual.
**secondary c.,** prophylactic use of a chemotherapeutic agent in an individual after infection has occurred (with *Mycobacterium tuberculosis,* for example) but before disease has become manifest.

**che·mo·pro·tec·tant** (ke″mo-pro-tek′tənt) 1. providing protection against the toxic effects of chemotherapeutic agents. 2. an agent that provides protection against the toxic effects of chemotherapeutic agents.

**che·mo·psy·chi·a·try** (ke″mo-si-ki′ə-tre) the use of drugs in the treatment of mental and emotional disorders; psychopharmacology.

**che·mo·ra·dio·ther·a·py** (ke″mo-ra″de-o-ther′ə-pe) [*chemo-* + *radiotherapy*] combined modality therapy using chemotherapy and radiotherapy, designed to reduce the need for surgery by maximizing the interaction between the radiation and the therapeutic agent or agents.

**che·mo·re·cep·tion** (ke″mo-re-sep′shən) the process of being sensitive to or perceiving chemical stimuli in the surrounding medium.

**che·mo·re·cep·tor** (ke″mo-re-sep′tər) [*chemo-* + *receptor*] [MeSH: Chemoreceptors] 1. a receptor adapted for excitation by chemical substances, e.g., olfactory and gustatory receptors. 2. a sense organ such as the carotid body, the aortic bodies, or the glomus jugulare, which is sensitive to chemical changes in the blood stream, especially reduced oxygen content, and reflexly increases both respiration and blood pressure. See also *receptor,* def. 2 and *chemoreceptor system,* under *system.* 3. a supposed group of atoms in cell protoplasm having the power of fixing chemicals, in the same way as bacterial poisons are fixed. Called also *chemoceptor.*

**che·mo·re·sis·tance** (ke″mo-re-zis′təns) specific resistance acquired by cells to the action of chemicals.

**che·mo·sen·si·tive** (ke″mo-sen′sĭ-tiv) sensitive to changes in chemical composition of the environment.

**che·mo·sen·sory** (ke″mo-sen′sər-e) relating to the perception of chemical substances, as in odor detection.

**che·mo·se·ro·ther·a·py** (ke″mo-se″ro-ther′ə-pe) the treatment of disease with both drugs and serum.

**che·mo·sis** (ke-mo′sis) [Gr. *chēmōsis*] excessive edema of the ocular conjunctiva.

**chem·os·mo·sis** (ke″mos-mo′sis) chemiosmosis.

**chem·os·mot·ic** (ke″mos-mot′ik) chemiosmotic.

**che·mo·sorp·tion** (kem″o-sorp′shən) chemisorption.

**che·mo·sphere** (ke′mo-sfēr) the layer of the upper atmosphere where photochemical reactions become important (30–80 km).

**che·mo·stat** (ke′mo-stat) an apparatus in which the environment is so controlled that bacterial populations are maintained in a steady state of continuous cell division in a constant environment.

**che·mo·ster·il·ant** (ke″mo-ster′ĭ-lənt) a chemical compound the ingestion of which causes sterility of an organism; such compounds have been used as a means of controlling various insects and other pests by inducing sterility in the male.

**che·mo·sur·gery** (ke″mo-sər′jər-e) the destruction of tissue by chemical agents; originally applied to chemical fixation of malignant, gangrenous, or infected tissue, with the use of frozen sections to facilitate systematic microscopic control of the extent of ablation.
**Mohs' c.**, see *Mohs' technique,* under *technique.*

**che·mo·syn·the·sis** (ke″mo-sin′thə-sis) [*chemo-* + *synthesis*] the synthesis of carbohydrate from carbon dioxide and water as a result of the energy derived from chemical reactions, rather than from absorbed light. Such synthesis is carried out by certain bacteria and algae. Cf. *photosynthesis.*

**che·mo·syn·thet·ic** (ke″mo-sin-thet′ik) pertaining to or characterized by chemosynthesis.

**che·mo·tac·tic** (ke″mo-tak′tik) of or pertaining to chemotaxis.

**che·mo·tax·in** (ke″mo-tak′sin) chemotactic factor.

**che·mo·tax·is** (ke″mo-tak′sis) [*chemo-* + *-taxis*] [MeSH: Chemotaxis] orientation of a cell along a chemical concentration gradient or movement in the direction of the gradient, either toward (positive chemotaxis) or away from (negative chemotaxis) the greater concentration of the substance, referred to as a chemotactic factor, chemotactin, or chemoattractant. Macrophages, neutrophils, eosinophils, and lymphocytes exhibit chemotaxis in response to a wide variety of substances released at sites of inflammatory reactions, including lymphokines, mediators released by basophils and mast cells, bacterial products, and C5a and other activated complement components. Cf. *chemokinesis.*

**che·mo·thal·a·mec·to·my** (ke″mo-thal″ə-mek′tə-me) destruction of a portion of the thalamus by the introduction of a chemical agent.

**che·mo·ther·a·peu·tic** (ke″mo-ther″ə-pu′tik) pertaining to chemotherapy.

**che·mo·ther·a·peu·tics** (ke″mo-ther′ə-pu′tiks) chemotherapy.

**che·mo·ther·a·py** (ke″mo-ther′ə-pe) the treatment of disease by chemical agents; originally applied to use of chemicals that affect the causative organism unfavorably but do not harm the patient. Cf. *pharmacotherapy.*
**adjuvant c.**, cancer chemotherapy employed after the primary tumor has been removed by some other method.
**combination c.**, the use of several different agents at once in order to enhance effectiveness; seen particularly in cancer chemotherapy. Called also *polychemotherapy.*
**induction c.**, chemotherapy as the initial treatment for cancer, especially as part of combined modality therapy.
**neoadjuvant c.**, chemotherapy used as neoadjuvant therapy (q.v.) for cancer. Called also *preoperative c., presurgical c.,* and *primary c.*
**preoperative c., presurgical c.**, neoadjuvant c.
**primary c.**, neoadjuvant c.
**regional c.**, chemotherapy, especially for cancer, administered as a regional perfusion.

**che·mot·ic** (ke-mot′ik) 1. pertaining to or affected with chemosis. 2. an agent that increases the production of lymph in the ocular conjunctiva.

**che·mo·troph** (ke′mo-trōf) a chemotrophic organism.

**che·mo·troph·ic** (ke″mo-trof′ik) deriving energy from the oxidation of organic (chemo-organotrophic) or inorganic (chemolithotrophic) compounds; said of bacteria. Cf. *phototrophic.*

**che·mo·trop·ic** (ke″mo-trop′ik) of or pertaining to chemotropism.

**che·mot·rop·ism** (ke-mot′ro-piz-əm) [*chemo-* + *tropism*] tropism in response to a chemical stimulus.

**chem·ur·gy** (kem′ər-ge) [*chemo-* + Gr. *ergon* work] chemistry applied to the industrial use of raw organic products, especially agricultural products.

**Che·nix** (ke′niks) trademark for a preparation of chenodiol.

**che·no·de·oxy·cho·late** (ke″no-de-ok-se-ko′lāt) a salt or anionic form of chenodeoxycholic acid.

**che·no·de·oxy·cho·lic ac·id** (ke″no-de-ok″se-kol′ik) [MeSH: Chenodeoxycholic Acid] one of the primary bile acids in humans, usually occurring conjugated with glycine or taurine; it facilitates fat absorption and cholesterol excretion. The pharmaceutical preparation is called *chenodiol.*

**che·no·de·oxy·cho·lyl·gly·cine** (ke″no-de-ok″se-ko″ləl-gli′sēn) a bile salt, the glycine conjugate of chenodeoxycholic acid; called also *glycochenodeoxycholic acid.*

**che·no·de·oxy·cho·lyl·tau·rine** (ke″no-de-ok″se-ko″ləl-taw′rēn) a bile salt, the taurine conjugate of chenodeoxycholic acid; called also *taurochenodeoxycholic acid.*

**che·no·di·ol** (ke″no-di′ol) chenodeoxycholic acid used as an anticholelithic to dissolve radiolucent, noncalcified gallstones; administered orally.

**Che·no·po·di·um** (ke″no-po′de-əm) a genus of herbs of the family Chenopodiaceae, native to temperate regions, the source of chenopodium oil. *C. al′bum,* or white goosefoot, contains oxalates and nitrates and can cause oxalate poisoning and nitrite poisoning in ruminants.

**cher·ry** (cher′e) [L. *cerasus*] 1. any of various rosaceous trees and species of the genus *Prunus;* called also *cerasus.* 2. the fruit of one of these trees; used as a flavoring. See also under *juice* and *syrup.* 3. any of certain other trees resembling the cherry trees of genus *Prunus.*
**Barbados c.**, acerola.
**choke c.**, *Prunus virginiana,* a North American tree whose bark has sedative, pectoral, and astringent qualities and whose fruit is highly astringent. Its leaves and seeds contain cyanogenetic compounds and can cause cyanide poisoning in livestock.
**rum c.**, *Prunus serotina.*
**wild c.**, 1. *Prunus serotina,* a large American tree with dark bark and thick oval leaves that yields the flavoring wild cherry; both its leaves and its seeds contain cyanogenetic compounds and can cause cyanide poisoning in livestock. 2. the dried stem bark of *P. serotina,* used in a syrup as a flavored vehicle for drugs; see also *wild cherry syrup,* under *syrup.* Called also *wild black cherry bark.*

**cher·ub·ism** (cher′əb-iz-əm) [*cherub* + *-ism*] [MeSH: Cherubism] hereditary and progressive bilateral swelling at the angle of the mandible, sometimes involving the entire jaw. The swelling imparts a cherubic look to the face, in some cases enhanced by upturning of the eyes. Called also *fibrous dysplasia of jaw* and *familial bilateral giant cell tumor.*

**chest** (chest) thorax.
**alar c.**, flat c.
**barrel c.**, a rounded, bulging chest with abnormal increase in the anteroposterior diameter, showing little movement on respiration; seen in emphysema and in kyphosis.
**blast c.**, pulmonary concussion (q.v.) and hemorrhage occurring in blast injury (see under *injury*).
**cobbler's c.**, a chest showing a sinking in at the lower end of the sternum.
**flail c.**, one whose wall moves paradoxically with respiration, owing to multiple fractures of the ribs.
**flat c.**, deformity of the chest in which it is flattened from front to back; called also *alar c.* and *pterygoid c.*
**foveated c., funnel c.**, pectus excavatum.
**keeled c.**, pectus carinatum.
**paralytic c.**, a long and narrow chest with emaciation so that the ribs stand out sharply under the skin.
**pigeon c.**, pectus carinatum.
**pterygoid c.**, flat c.
**tetrahedron c.**, a chest that suggests a solid with four sides, each an equilateral triangle, the chest projecting in a peak between the nipples.

**chest·nut** (chest′nət) 1. *Castanea.* 2. the nut of any of various species of *Castanea.* 3. one of the masses of horn on the medial surface of the forearm of humans or on the distal part of the medial surface of the tarsus of horses.
**horse c.**, *Aesculus hippocastanum.*

**Chey·le·ti·el·la** (ki″lə-te-el′ə) a genus of nonburrowing mites of the family Cheyletiellidae. They mainly infest domestic animals, but some species cause a dermatosis in human beings. *C. bla′kei* infests cats; *C. parasito′vorax* infests rabbits; and *C. yas′guri* infests dogs.

**chey·le·ti·el·lo·sis** (ki″lə-te″el-o′sis) 1. infestation of dogs, cats, or rabbits with species of *Cheyletiella,* characterized by a pruritic dermatitis. Called also *walking dandruff.* 2. pruritic dermatitis in humans caused by a species of *Cheyletiella.*

**Chey·le·ti·el·li·dae** (ki″lə-te-el′ĭ-de) a family of mites that infest domestic mammals and occasionally humans. It includes the genus *Cheyletiella.*

**Cheyne's nystagmus** (chānz) [John *Cheyne,* Scottish physician, 1777–1836] see under *nystagmus.*

**Cheyne-Stokes nys·tag·mus, res·pi·ra·tion (sign)** (chān-stōks) [J. *Cheyne;* William *Stokes,* Irish physician, 1804–1878] see under *respiration.*

**CHF** congestive heart failure.

**chi** (ki) [X, χ] the twenty-second letter of the Greek alphabet.

**Chi·a·ri's network (reticulum), malformation (deformity), syndrome (disease)** (ke-ah′rēz) [Hans *Chiari,* Austrian pathologist, 1851–1916] see under *network* and *malformation,* and see *Budd-Chiari syndrome,* under *syndrome.*

**Chi·a·ri-Ar·nold syndrome** (ke-ah're-ahr'nold) [H. *Chiari;* Julius *Arnold,* German pathologist, 1835–1915] Arnold-Chiari malformation; see under *malformation.*

**Chi·a·ri-From·mel syndrome (disease)** (ke-ah're-from'əl) [Johann Baptist *Chiari,* German obstetrician, 1817–1854; Richard Julius Ernst *Frommel,* German gynecologist, 1854–1912] see under *syndrome.*

**chi·asm** (ki'az-əm) [L., Gr. *chiasma*] a decussation or X-shaped crossing; see *chiasma.*
**c. of digits of hand,** chiasma tendinum digitorum manus.
**optic c.,** chiasma opticum.
**tendinous c. of fingers,** chiasma tendinum digitorum manus.

**chi·as·ma** (ki-az'mə) pl. *chias'mata* [L.; Gr. a cross, crosspiece; from the shape of the letter *chi,* X] 1. [TA] a general term in anatomical nomenclature for a decussation or X-shaped crossing, such as of nerves. 2. in genetics, the places where pairs of homologous chromatids remain in contact during late prophase to anaphase of the first meiotic division, indicating where an exchange of homologous segments has taken place between non-sister chromatids by crossing over.
**optic c., c. op'ticum** [TA], optic chiasm: the part of the hypothalamus formed by the decussation, or crossing, of the fibers of the optic nerve from the medial half of each retina; called also *optic decussation.*

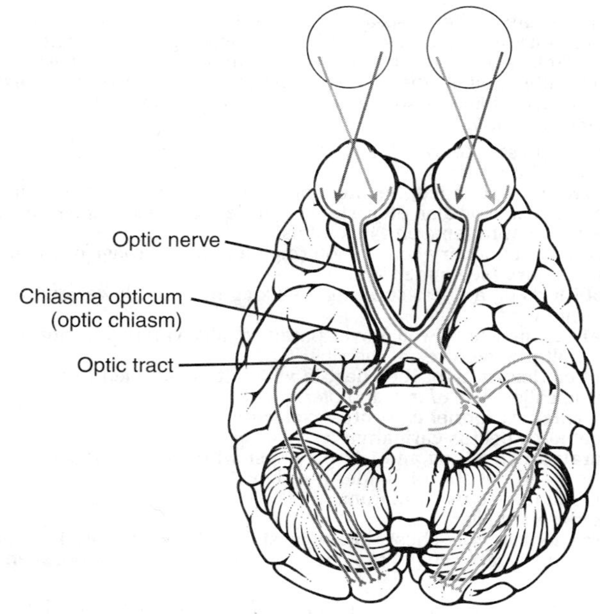


**c. ten'dinum digito'rum ma'nus** [TA], tendinous chiasm of fingers: the crossing of the tendons of the flexor digitorum profundus through the tendons of the flexor digitorum superficialis; called also *chiasm of digits of hand.*

**chi·as·mal** (ki-az'məl) chiasmatic.

**chi·as·ma·ta** (ki-az'mə-tə) [L.] plural of *chiasma.*

**chi·as·mat·ic** (ki-az-mat'ik) resembling a chiasm; crosswise.

**chi·as·ma·ty·py** (ki-az'mə-ti"pe) [*chiasma* + *type*] crossing over.

**chi·as·mic** (ki-az'mik) chiasmatic.

**chi·as·mom·e·ter** (ki"az-mom'ə-tər) chiastometer.

**chi·as·tom·e·ter** (ki"az-tom'ə-tər) [Gr. *chiastos* crossed + *-meter*] an apparatus for measuring any deviation of the optic axes from their normal parallelism; called also *chiasmometer.*

**Chi·ba needle** (che'bə) [*Chiba* University in Japan, where it was developed] see under *needle.*

**chick·en·pox** (chik'ən-poks) [MeSH: Chickenpox] varicella: a highly contagious infectious disease caused by human herpesvirus 3, usually affecting children, spread by direct contact or the respiratory route via droplet nuclei, and characterized by the appearance on the skin and mucous membranes of successive crops of typical pruritic vesicular lesions that are easily broken and become scabbed, and generally accompanied by mild constitutional symptoms. It is relatively benign in children except in those with severe underlying disease, but adult infection may be complicated by pneumonia and encephalitis. See also *herpes zoster.*

**chick·pea** (chik'pe) 1. the leguminous plant *Cicer arietinum* of Southern Europe. 2. the edible seed of *C. arietanum,* widely used as food but toxic to certain individuals. Called also *garbanzo.*

**Chi·do-Rod·gers blood group** (che'do roj'ərz) [from the names of propositi first observed in the 1960s] see under *blood group.*

**Chie·vitz's layer, organ** (che'vit-səz) [Johan Henrik *Chievitz,* Danish anatomist, 1850–1901] see under *layer* and *organ.*

**chig·ger** (chig'ər) [MeSH: Trombiculid Mites] the six-legged red larva of a mite of the family Trombiculidae; they infest many vertebrates, especially mammals, including humans. They attach to the skin of their hosts and their bites produce a wheal, usually with severe itching and dermatitis *(trombiculiasis).* Their habitat is tall grass and underbrush. *Eutrombicula alfreddugèsi* is the common chigger of the United States; *E. splendens* is found in the southeastern United States; and *Trombicula autumnalis* is a common European species. Some species in the East Asia–Pacific region are vectors of the rickettsiae of scrub typhus. Chiggers are to be distinguished from chigoes. Called also *bête rouge, harvest bug* or *mite, red bug* or *mite,* and *mower's mite.*

**chigo** (chig'o) chigoe.

**chig·oe** (chig'o) the flea *Tunga penetrans,* of tropical and subtropical America and Africa. The pregnant female flea burrows into the skin of the feet (often beneath the nail), legs, or other part of the body, causing intense irritation and ulceration, and sometimes leading to spontaneous amputation of a digit. Chigoes are to be distinguished from chiggers. Called also *burrowing flea, chigo, jigger,* and *sand flea.*

**chik·un·gun·ya** (chik"ən-gun'yə) [Swahili "that which bends up"] a self-limited disease resembling dengue, seen mainly in Africa and Southeast Asia, caused by an alphavirus transmitted chiefly by mosquitoes of the genus *Aedes;* its most prominent symptoms are musculoskeletal and it has occasionally been associated with hemorrhagic fever.

**Chi·lai·di·ti's sign, syndrome** (ke-lah-the'tēz) [Demetrios *Chilaiditi,* Austrian physician, born 1883] see under *sign* and *syndrome.*

**chil·blain, chil·blains** (chil'blān, chil'blānz) [L. *pernio*] a recurrent localized erythema and doughy subcutaneous swelling caused by exposure to cold associated with dampness, and accompanied by pruritus and a burning sensation, usually involving the hands, feet, ears, and face in children, the legs and toes in women, and the hands and fingers in men. Called also *erythema pernio* and *pernio.*

**child** (chīld) [MeSH: Child] the human young, from infancy to puberty.
**preschool c.,** a child between two and six years of age.
**school c.,** a child between six and ten to twelve years of age.

**child·birth** (chīld'bərth) the act or process of giving birth to a child, including both *labor* and *delivery.* Called also *parturition.*

**child·hood** (chīld'hood) the period of life of the human young generally considered to extend from infancy to puberty.

**chi·li·tis** (ki-li'tis) cheilitis.

**chill** (chil) [MeSH: Shivering] a shivering or shaking; an attack of involuntary contractions of the voluntary muscles, accompanied by a sense of cold and pallor of the skin; called also *ague.*
**brass c., brazier's c.,** brassfounder's fever.
**creeping c.,** a chilly sensation, without any definite tremor or chattering of the teeth.
**shaking c.,** a chill in which there is a definite tremor.
**spelter's c.,** see under *fever.*
**urethral c.,** a chilly sensation, with or without tremor, sometimes following the passage of a catheter.
**zinc c.,** spelter's fever.

**chil(o)-** for words beginning thus, see also words beginning *cheil(o)-.*

**Chi·lo·do·nel·la** (ki"lə-də-nel'ə) a genus of ciliophoran protozoa that infect goldfish, guppies, and other common aquarium fish, causing weakness, incoordination, and loss of skin near the gills, which can be fatal.

**Chi·log·na·tha** (ki-log'nə-thə) an order of millipedes, arthropods of the class Diplopoda.

**chi·lo·mas·ti·gi·a·sis** (ki"lo-mas"tĭ-gi'ə-sis) infection with *Chilomastix.*

**Chi·lo·mas·tix** (ki"lo-mas'tiks) [*chilo-* + Gr. *mastix* whip] a genus of pear- or lemon-shaped parasitic protozoa (order Retortamonadida, class Zoomastigophorea), having three flagella and a single nucleus, beside which the cytostome is located, and found in the intestines of various vertebrates, including humans. All species are considered nonpathogenic or only slightly so, but one species, *C. mesnili,* has been associated with rare cases of watery diarrhea.

**chi·lo·mas·tix·i·a·sis** (ki″lo-mas″tik-si′ə-sis) chilomastigiasis.

**Chi·lop·o·da** (ki-lop′ə-də) [Gr. *cheilos* lip + *pous* foot] the centipedes, a class of elongated arthropods of the superclass Myriapoda; they have one pair of legs to each body segment, with 15 to 173 pairs of legs. They paralyze and kill insects and small animals with their poison claws, which are modified legs of the first body segment. A few species of the genus *Scolopendra* are capable of penetrating human skin with a painful bite.

**chi·mae·ra** (ki-me′rə) chimera.

**chi·me·ra** (ki-me′rə) [Gr. *chimaira* a mythological fire-spouting monster with a lion's head, goat's body, and serpent's tail] [MeSH: Chimera] an individual organism whose body contains cell populations derived from different zygotes, of the same or of different species; it may occur spontaneously, as in twins (blood group chimeras), or be produced artificially, as an organism that develops from combined portions of different embryos, or one in which tissues or cells of another organism have been introduced. Cf. *mosaic.*
**heterologous c.,** a chimera in which the foreign cells or tissues are derived from an organism of a different species.
**homologous c.,** a chimera in which the foreign cells or tissues are derived from an organism of the same species but of a different genotype.
**isologous c.,** a chimera in which the foreign cells or tissues are derived from a different organism of the same genotype, such as an identical twin.
**radiation c.,** an organism that survives with immunologic characteristics of host and donor after a bone marrow graft from an antigenically different donor, the host having first been subjected to sublethal whole-body irradiation so that there is reduced or no immune response to foreign cells by the donor.

**chi·mer·ism** (ki-mēr′iz-əm) the quality of being a chimera; in genetics, the presence in an individual of cells of different origin, as of blood cells derived from a dizygotic co-twin. Cf. *mosaicism.*

**chim·pan·zee** (chim-pan-ze′, chim-pan′ze) [Kongo *chimpenzi* or *kimpenzi*] *Pan troglodytes,* an anthropoid ape that inhabits the tropical rain forests of Africa and is used for experimental purposes because of its susceptibility to some human diseases and in behavioral studies because of its high level of intelligence.

**chin** (chin) [MeSH: Chin] mentum.
**galoche c.** (gah-losh′) [Fr. "galosh"], a long pointed chin.

**chin·a·crine** (kin′ə-krēn) quinacrine.

**chin·cap** (chin′kap) an extraoral orthodontic appliance consisting of a caplike device fitted over the chin, which is connected to the headgear by elastics for the purpose of exerting upward and backward force on the mandible in the treatment of prognathism.

**chi·on·ablep·sia** (ki″o-nə-blep′se-ə) [Gr. *chiōn* snow + *ablepsia*] snow blindness.

**chip** (chip) a small piece, as of something broken off.
**bone c's,** small pieces of bone, usually cancellous, generally used to fill in bony defects to facilitate recalcification.

**Chi·ra·can·thi·um** (ki″rə-kan′the-əm) a genus of venomous spiders. Two species, *C. inclu′sum* in California and *C. diver′sium* in Hawaii, have produced local reactions in humans.

**chi·ral** (ki′rəl) exhibiting chirality.

**chi·ral·i·ty** (ki-ral′ĭ-te) [Gr. *cheir* hand] the property of handedness, of not being superimposable on a mirror image; the handedness of an asymmetric molecule, as specified by its optical rotation or absolute configuration. Cf. *stereoisomerism.*

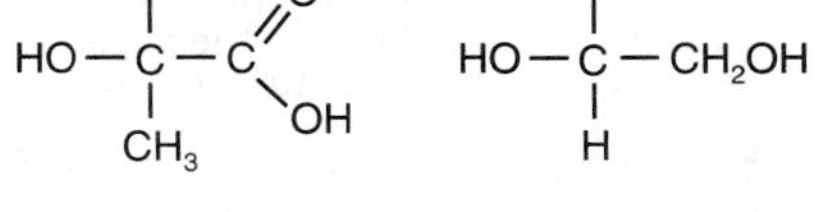

Lactic acid, its tetracoordinate carbon atom bearing four different substituents, is not superimposable on its mirror image. Ethylene glycol, with two identical substituents on its tetracoordinate carbon, can be superimposed on its mirror image.

**chir(o)-** [Gr. *cheir* hand] a combining form denoting relationship to the hand; for words beginning thus, see also those beginning *cheir(o)-.*

**chi·ro·bra·chi·al·gia** (ki″ro-bra″ke-al′jə) cheirobrachialgia.

**chi·rog·nos·tic** (ki″rog-nos′tik) cheirognostic.

**chi·ro·meg·a·ly** (ki″ro-meg′ə-le) cheiromegaly.

**Chi·ro·nex** (ki′rə-neks) a genus of cubomedusan jellyfish. *C. flec′keri* Southcott is a species of sea wasp found along the coast of Australia whose sting is highly lethal, killing humans and other animals within 15 minutes.

**Chi·ro·nom·i·dae** (ki″ro-nom′ĭ-de) [MeSH: Chironomidae] a family of the suborder Nematocera, order Diptera, that comprises the true midges.

**Chi·ron·o·mus** (ki-ron′ə-məs) a genus of gnatlike flies noted for their giant chromosomes.

**chi·ro·plas·ty** (ki′ro-plas″te) cheiroplasty.

**chi·ro·po·dal·gia** (ki″ro-po-dal′jə) cheiropodalgia.

**chi·ro·pod·i·cal** (ki″ro-pod′ĭ-kəl) pertaining to chiropody (now called *podiatry*).

**chi·rop·o·dist** (ki-rop′ə-dist) podiatrist.

**chi·rop·o·dy** (ki-rop′ə-de) podiatry.

**chi·ro·prac·tic** (ki″ro-prak′tik) [*chiro-* + Gr. *prassein* to do] [MeSH: Chiropractic] a science of applied neurophysiologic diagnosis based on the theory that health and disease are life processes related to the function of the nervous system: irritation of the nervous system by mechanical, chemical, or psychic factors is the cause of disease; restoration and maintenance of health depend on normal function of the nervous system. Diagnosis is the identification of these noxious irritants and treatment is their removal by the most conservative method.

**chi·ro·prac·tor** (ki″ro-prak′tər) a practitioner of chiropractic.

**chi·ro·prax·is** (ki″ro-prak′sis) chiropractic.

**Chi·ro·psal·mus** (ki″rə-sahl′məs) a genus of cubomedusan jellyfish. *C. quadra′tus* Haeckel is a species of sea wasp found in the Philippines whose sting can kill humans and other animals.

**chi·ro·scope** (ki′ro-skōp) cheiroscope.

**chi·ro·spasm** (ki′ro-spaz-əm) cheirospasm.

**chis·el** (chis′əl) 1. a wedgelike instrument with a cutting edge at the end of the blade. 2. a dental instrument whose cutting edge is in line with the center of the handle; used for planing or smoothing a surface, as during cavity preparation.
**periodontal c.,** a straight instrument that curves slightly as the blade extends from the shank, the straight cutting edge at the end of the instrument being beveled at a 45° angle. Used chiefly for scaling the proximal surfaces of teeth too closely spaced to permit the use of other scalers. Called also *chisel scaler.*
**Wedelstaedt c.,** any of various periodontal chisels whose blade is continuous with the shank and at a curve from it.

**chi-square** (ki′skwār) see under *distribution* and *test.*

**chi·tin** (ki′tin) [Gr. *chitōn* tunic] [MeSH: Chitin] a white, insoluble, linear homopolymer composed of *N*-acetylglucosamine residues in *β*-(1,4) linkage; it is widely distributed, forming the principal constituent of arthropod exoskeletons, and found in some plants, particularly fungi.

**chi·tin·ous** (ki′tin-əs) composed of or of the nature of chitin.

**chi·to·bi·ose** (ki″to-bi′ōs) a disaccharide, two *N*-acetylglucosamine moieties in *β*-(1,4) linkage, forming the basic repeating unit of chitin.

**chi·to·san** (ki′to-sən) a polysaccharide composed of repeating glucosamine units; obtained by de-acetylation of chitin and used to absorb heavy metals in water treatment.

**CHL** crown-heel length.

**chla·my·de·mia** (klam″ĭ-de′me-ə) the presence of chlamydiae in the blood.

**Chla·myd·ia** (klə-mid′e-ə) [Gr. *chlamys* cloak] [MeSH: Chlamydia] a genus of bacteria of the family Chlamydiaceae, order Chlamydiales, occurring as gram-negative, coccoid organisms that multiply only within a host cell and have a unique growth cycle (see *Chlamydiaceae*). They are common pathogens of animals and cause a variety of diseases in humans. Called also *PLT group* and, formerly, *Bedsonia, Chlamydozoon,* and *Miyagawanella.*
**C. pneumo′niae,** a species, formerly considered to be a strain of *C. psittaci,* that is an important cause of pneumonia, bronchitis, and sinusitis. See also Chlamydia pneumoniae *pneumonia,* under *pneumonia.*
**C. psit′taci,** a species, various strains of which cause psittacosis in humans and birds and a variety of diseases in farm animals and other mammals.
**C. tracho′matis,** a species occurring predominantly as a human pathogen, causing trachoma, inclusion conjunctivitis, nonspecific urethritis, proctitis, mouse pneumonitis, lymphogranuloma venereum, and *C. trachomatis* pneumonia.

**chla·myd·ia** (klə-mid′e-ə) pl. *chlamyd′iae* [MeSH: Chlamydia] Any member of the genus *Chlamydia.*

**Chla·myd·i·a·ceae** (klə-mid″e-a′se-e) [MeSH: Chlamydiaceae] a family of bacteria of the order Chlamydiales consisting of small coccoid microorganisms that have a unique, obligately intracellular developmental cycle and are incapable of synthesizing ATP. Infection occurs when the small, rigid-walled extracellular form (elementary body) enters the cell and changes into a larger, thin-walled form (initial body) that divides by fission. The daughter cells thus formed reorganize and condense to become elementary bodies that then infect other cells. The organisms are parasites of humans and other vertebrates, capable of producing a variety of diseases. They have also been found in arthropods. The family contains the genus *Chlamydia.*

**chla·myd·i·ae** (klə-mid′e-e) plural of *chlamydia.*

**chla·myd·i·al** (klə-mid′e-əl) pertaining to or caused by *Chlamydia.*

**Chla·myd·i·al·es** (klə-mid′e-a″lēz) [MeSH: Chlamydiales] an order of bacteria made up of coccoid, gram-negative, parasitic microorganisms that multiply only within the cytoplasm of vertebrate host cells by a unique developmental cycle. It includes the family Chlamydiaceae.

**chla·myd·i·o·sis** (klə-mid″e-o′sis) 1. any infection or disease caused by species of *Chlamydia.* 2. psittacosis, def. 1.

**chlam·y·do·co·nid·i·um** (klam″ĭ-do-kə-nid′e-əm) [Gr. *chlamys* cloak + *conidium*] a thick-walled intercalary or terminal asexual spore formed by the rounding up of a cell; it is not shed. See also *conidium.* Called also *chlamydospore.*

**chlam·y·do·spore** (klam′ĭdo-spor″) [Gr. *chlamys* cloak + *spore*] chlamydoconidium.

**Chlam·y·do·zo·a·ceae** (klam″ĭ-do″zo-a′se-e) Chlamydiaceae.

**Chlam·y·do·zo·on** (klam″ĭ-do-zo′on) *Chlamydia.*

**chlo·as·ma** (klo-az′mə) [Gr. *chloazein* to be green] melasma.

**chlor·a·ce·tic acid** (klor″ə-se′tik) chloroacetic acid.

**chlor·ac·ne** (klor-ak′ne) an acneiform eruption caused by exposure to chlorine compounds. Called also *chlorine acne.*

**chlo·ral** (klor′əl) [*chlor*ine + *-al*[3]] 1. a colorless, oily liquid, having a pungent, irritating odor; it is used in the manufacture of chloral hydrate and DDT. 2. c. hydrate.
**c. betaine,** an adduct formed by the reaction of chloral hydrate with betaine, having actions and uses similar to those of chloral hydrate but having the advantage of eliminating undesirable gastrointestinal symptoms sometimes associated with chloral hydrate; administered orally.
**c. hydrate** [USP], a hypnotic and sedative, administered orally.

**chlo·ral·ism** (klor′əl-iz-əm) a morbid condition caused by excessive use of chloral.

**chlo·ral·iza·tion** (klor″əl-ĭ-za′shən) 1. chloralism. 2. formerly, anesthesia by the use of chloral.

**chlo·ra·lose** (klor′ə-lōs) [MeSH: Chloralose] a compound of chloral and glucose, used as a rodenticide for mice and a bird repellent on grain. Called also *α-chloralose.*

**chlor·am·bu·cil** (klor-am′bu-sil) [USP] [MeSH: Chlorambucil] an alkylating agent of the nitrogen mustard group, which acts both by cross-linking of DNA and RNA and by inhibiting of protein synthesis, used as an antineoplastic in the treatment of chronic lymphocytic leukemia, Hodgkin's and non-Hodgkin's lymphomas, Waldenström's macroglobulinemia, and multiple myeloma; administered orally. It has also been used as an immunosuppressive in the treatment of steroid-resistant nephrotic syndrome.

**chlo·ra·mine-T** (klor′ə-mēn) a chlorine derivative, used in solution as a topical antiseptic to irrigate and dress wounds and as a mouthwash and used to sterilize drinking water.

**chlor·am·phen·i·col** (klor″əm-fen′ĭ-kol) [USP] [MeSH: Chloramphenicol] a broad-spectrum antibiotic, originally derived from *Streptomyces venezuelae* and later shown to be elaborated by other spirochetes, and produced synthetically. It is effective against rickettsiae, gram-positive and gram-negative bacteria, and certain spirochetes, being used especially in the treatment of typhus and other rickettsial infections and in typhoid, shigellosis, and related enteric diseases; used as an antibacterial, administered orally or applied topically to the conjunctiva, or as an antirickettsial, administered orally.
**c. palmitate** [USP], the monopalmitic ester of chloramphenicol, having the same actions and uses as the base; administered orally.
**c. sodium succinate** [USP], the sodium succinate derivative of chloramphenicol, having the same actions and uses as the base; administered intravenously. Sterile chloramphenicol sodium succinate [USP] conforms to FDA regulations concerning antibiotic drugs.

**chlo·rate** (klor′āt) any salt of chloric acid.

**chlor·bu·tol** (klor-bu′tol) chlorobutanol.

**chlor·cy·cli·zine hy·dro·chlo·ride** (klor-si′klĭ-zēn) an $H_1$ histamine receptor antagonist derived from piperazine, having anticholinergic, antiemetic, local anesthetic, and mild sedative properties; administered orally as a component of various cold and allergy preparations and topically as an antipruritic.

**chlor·dane** (klor′dān) [MeSH: Chlordan] a toxic chlorinated hydrocarbon insecticide; poisoning of humans or other animals may occur by percutaneous absorption, ingestion, or inhalation and consists of neurotoxic symptoms such as muscular spasms and seizures that can be fatal.

**chlor·dan·to·in** (klor-dan′to-in) an antifungal agent effective against various fungi, including *Candida albicans;* used topically in the treatment of fungal infections of the vulvovaginal region and of the skin.

**chlor·de·cone** (klor′də-kōn) [MeSH: Chlordecone] a polychlorinated ketone used as an insecticide; workers exposed to this nonbiodegradable compound have suffered neurologic symptoms, such as tremors and slurred speech.

**chlor·di·az·ep·ox·ide** (klor″di-az″ə-pok′sīd) [USP] [MeSH: Chlordiazepoxide] a benzodiazepine used as an anxiolytic in the treatment of anxiety disorders and for the short-term relief of anxiety symptoms, for the relief of acute alcohol withdrawal symptoms, and as an anti-tremor agent; administered orally.
**c. hydrochloride** [USP], the monohydrochloride salt of chlordiazepoxide, administered orally for the same indications as the base and intravenously or intramuscularly as an anxiolytic in the treatment of anxiety and panic disorders, the short-term relief of anxiety symptoms and of preoperative anxiety, and in the treatment of acute alcohol withdrawal symptoms.

**Chlo·rel·la** (klo-rel′ə) [MeSH: Chlorella] a genus of fresh-water green algae which are the source of chlorellin and are used in studies of photosynthesis.

**chlo·rel·lin** (klo-rel′in) a bacteriostatic substance derived from fresh water algae of the genus *Chlorella.*

**chlor·emia** (klor-e′me-ə) [*chlor-* + *-emia*] hyperchloremia.

**chlor·en·chy·ma** (klor-en′kĭ-mə) the chlorophyll-bearing tissue of plants.

**Chlo·re·si·um** (klo-re′ze-um) trademark for a preparation of chlorophyllin copper complex sodium.

**Chlo·re·tone** (klo′rə-tōn) trademark for a preparation of chlorobutanol.

**chlor·gua·nide** (klor-gwahn′īd) proguanil.

**chlor·hex·i·dine** (klor-heks′ĭ-dēn) [MeSH: Chlorhexidine] an antibacterial, effective against a wide variety of gram-negative and gram-positive organisms.
**c. acetate,** the diacetate salt of chlorhexidine, having the same actions as the base; used mainly as a preservative for eye drops.
**c. gluconate,** the digluconate salt of chlorhexidine, used as a topical anti-infective for the skin and mucous membranes.
**c. hydrochloride,** the dihydrochloride salt of chlorhexidine, having the same actions as the base; used as a topical anti-infective for the skin and mucous membranes.

**chlor·hy·dria** (klor-hi′dre-ə) hyperchlorhydria.

**chlo·ric** (klor′ik) [L. *chloricus*] derived from or containing pentavalent chlorine; a term used to distinguish those compounds which contain a smaller proportion of chlorine than the chlorous compounds, and forming salts known as chlorates.

**chlo·ric ac·id** (klor′ik) a strong oxidizing agent, $HClO_3 \cdot 7H_2O$, occurring only in aqueous solution; it is used as a catalyst and is strongly irritating to the skin and mucous membranes.

**chlo·ride** (klor′īd) a salt of hydrochloric acid; any binary compound of chlorine in which the latter is the negative element.
**acid c.,** a substance formed by substituting chlorine for hydroxyl in an acid molecule.
**chromic c.** [USP], the trichloride salt of chromium, $CrCl_3$, used as a supplement for the treatment of chromium deficiency; administered intravenously.
**cupric c.** [USP], a mineral supplement, $CuCl_2$, used in the treatment of copper deficiency; administered intravenously.
**mercuric c.,** mercury bichloride.
**mercurous c.,** calomel.
**thallous c. Tl 201** [USP], the form in which thallium 201 in solution is injected intravenously as a diagnostic aid in imaging of myocardial infarction, ischemic heart disease, parathyroid disorders, and neoplastic disease. Called also *thallium chloride* ($^{201}TlCl$).

**chlo·ri·dim·e·ter** (klor″ĭ-dim′ə-tər) [*chloride* + *-meter*] an instrument for measuring the chloride content of the urine or other fluid.

**chlo·ri·dim·e·try** (klor″ĭ-dim′ə-tre) the determination of the chloride content of fluids.

**chlo·rid·i·on** (klor″id-i′on) negatively ionic chlorine, the anion of hydrochloric acid and the chlorides.

**chlo•ri•dom•e•ter** (klor″ĭ-dom′ə-tər) chloridimeter.

**chlor•id•or•rhea** (klor″i-dor′e-ə) diarrhea with an excess of chlorides in the stool.
**familial c.**, familial chloride diarrhea.

**chlo•ri•du•ria** (klor″ĭ-du′re-ə) excess of chlorides in the urine.

**chlo•ri•nat•ed** (klor′ĭ-nat″əd) charged with chlorine.

**chlo•rine** (klor′ēn) [L. *chlorum* or *chlorinum,* from Gr. *chlōros* green] [MeSH: Chlorine] a yellowish green, gaseous element, of suffocating odor; symbol, Cl; atomic number, 17; atomic weight, 35.453; specific gravity, 1.56. It is a disinfectant, decolorant, and irritant poison. It is used for disinfecting, fumigating, and bleaching, either in an aqueous solution or in the form of chlorinated lime.
**c. dioxide,** an oxidizing and germicidal agent, $ClO_2$, used in the purification of water and for bleaching.

**chlor•io•dized** (klor-i′o-dīzd) containing chlorine and iodine.

**chlor•i•son•da•mine chlo•ride** (klor″i-son′də-mēn) an asymmetrical bisquaternary ammonium derivative with ganglionic blocking action, used as an antihypertensive.

**chlo•rite** (klor′īt) any salt of chlorous acid.

**chlor•mad•i•none ac•e•tate** (klor-mə′dĭ-nōn) [MeSH: Chlormadinone Acetate] a progestin, $C_{23}H_{29}ClO_4$, used in oral contraceptive products.

**chlor•mer•o•drin** (klor-mer′o-drin) [MeSH: Chlormerodrin] an orally effective mercurial diuretic. Labeled with radioisotopes of mercury, $^{197}Hg$ or $^{203}Hg$, it was used as a diagnostic agent in renal function determination, but has been superseded by other agents.

**chlor•meth•az•a•none** (klor″meth-az′ə-nōn) chlormezanone.

**chlor•mez•a•none** (klor-mez′ə-nōn) [MeSH: Chlormezanone] a muscle relaxant and tranquilizer, used in the treatment of anxiety disorders; administered orally.

**chlor(o)-** [Gr. *chlōros* green] a combining form meaning green, or denoting the presence of chlorine.

**chlo•ro•ac•et•al•de•hyde** (klor″o-as″et-al′də-hīd) a mutagenic metabolite produced by biotransformation of vinyl chloride in the liver.

**chlo•ro•ace•tic acid** (klor″o-ə-se′tik) a strong acid, $CH_2ClCOOH$, used as a laboratory reagent.

**chlo•ro•ac•e•to•phe•none** (klo″ro-as″ə-to-fe′nōn) a commonly used tear gas.

**chlo•ro•az•o•din** (klor″o-az′o-din) an antibacterial that has been used as an antiseptic.

***o*-chlo•ro•ben•zyl•i•dene•mal•o•ni•trile** (klo″ro-ben-zil″ĭ-dēn-mal″o-ni′trīl) a commonly used tear gas.

**Chlo•ro•bac•te•ri•um** (klor″o-bak-tēr′e-əm) [*chloro-* + *bacterium*] a complex of green phototrophic bacteria living symbiotically on the surface of protozoa such as amebae and flagellates.

**chlo•ro•bu•ta•nol** (klor″o-bu′tə-nol) [NF] [MeSH: Chlorobutanol] colorless to white crystals, with a camphoraceous odor and taste; used as an antimicrobial preservative in various pharmaceutical solutions, especially injectables. It has been used as a local dental analgesic, hypnotic, antipruritic, sedative, somnifacient, and antiseptic.

**Chlo•ro•chro•ma•ti•um** (klor″o-kro-ma′she-əm) [*chloro-* + Gr. *chroma* color] a complex of green phototrophic sulfur bacteria found in mud and stagnant waters containing hydrogen sulfide.

**2-chlorodeoxyadenosine** (klor″o-de-ok″se-ə-den′o-sēn) cladribine.

**chlo•ro•eth•ane** (klor″o-eth′ān) ethyl chloride.

**chlo•ro•eth•y•lene** (klor″o-eth′ə-lēn) vinyl chloride.
**c. oxide,** a toxic metabolite produced by biotransformation of vinyl chloride in the liver.

**chlo•ro•flu•o•ro•car•bon** (klo″ro-floo′o-ro-kahr″bən) any of a group of hydrocarbons in which some or all of the hydrogen atoms are replaced by chlorine or fluorine; some in this group were formerly widely used in aerosols, but their use is declining because of their destructive effect on stratospheric ozone.

**chlo•ro•form** (klor′ə-form) [MeSH: Chloroform] trichloromethane, $CHCl_3$, a colorless, volatile liquid with a strong ethereal odor and a sweetish, burning taste, a common laboratory solvent; it is hepatotoxic and nephrotoxic when ingested. It was once widely used as an inhalation anesthetic and analgesic, and as an antitussive, carminative, and counterirritant.
**acetone c.,** chlorobutanol.

**chlo•ro•form•ism** (klor′ə-form″iz-əm) 1. the habitual use of chloroform for its narcotic effect. 2. the anesthetic effect of the vapor of chloroform.

**chlo•ro•form•iza•tion** (klor″ə-form″ĭ-za′shən) the administration of chloroform.

**chlo•ro•gua•nide hy•dro•chlo•ride** (klor″o-gwahn′īd) proguanil hydrochloride.

**chlo•ro•labe** (klor′o-lāb) [*chloro-* + Gr. *lambanein* to take] name proposed for the pigment in retinal cones that is more sensitive to the green portion of the spectrum than are the other pigments (cyanolabe and erythrolabe).

**chlo•ro•leu•ke•mia** (klor″o-loo-ke′me-ə) chloroma.

**chlo•ro•ma** (klor-o′mə) [*chlor-* + *-oma*] a malignant green-colored tumor arising from myeloid tissue, associated with myelogenous leukemia and occurring anywhere in the body. Besides containing green pigment, which has no clear metabolic role and is principally myeloperoxidase, chloroma tissue demonstrates a bright red fluorescence under ultraviolet light. Cf. *myeloblastoma.* Called also *chloroleukemia, chloromatous sarcoma,* and *granulocytic sarcoma.*

***p*-chlo•ro•mer•cu•ri•ben•zo•ate** (klor″o-mər″ku-re-ben′zo-āt) a univalent organic mercury compound that reacts with sulfhydryl groups on proteins, or other molecules, thereby often inhibiting their activities.

**chlo•rom•e•try** (klor-om′ə-tre) the quantitative determination of chlorine.

**chlo•ro•mo•nad** (klor″o-mo′nad) [*chloro-* + *monad*] a protozoan of the order Chloromonadida.

**Chlo•ro•my•ce•tin** (klor″ə-mi-se′tin) trademark for preparations of chloramphenicol.

**chlo•ro•naph•tha•lene** (klor-o-naf′thə-lēn) chlorinated naphthalene.

**chlo•ro•phane** (klor′o-fān) [*chloro-* +Gr. *phainein* to show] a greenish yellow pigment obtainable from the retina.

***p*-chlo•ro•phe•nol** (klor″o-fe′nol) parachlorophenol.

**chlo•ro•phyll** (klor′o-fil) [*chloro-* + Gr. *phyllon* leaf] [MeSH: Chlorophyll] any of a group of green magnesium-containing porphyrin derivatives occurring in all photosynthetic organisms. Chlorophylls act as respiratory pigments, converting light energy to reducing potential; the reduction of $CO_2$ is the first step in the synthesis of hexoses in photosynthetic organisms. Chlorophyll *a* occurs in all organisms exhibiting aerobic photosynthesis (green plants, algae, and cyanobacteria), chlorophyll *b* in higher plants, chlorophylls $c_1$ and $c_2$ in diatoms and brown algae, and chlorophyll *d* in red algae. Bacteriochlorophylls occur in bacteria exhibiting anaerobic photosynthesis. Preparations of water soluble chlorophyll salts are used as deodorizers; see *chlorophyllin.*

**chlo•ro•phyl•lin** (klor′o-fəl-in) any of the water-soluble salts obtained by alkaline hydrolysis of chlorophyll with replacement of the methyl and phytyl ester groups by sodium or potassium; preparations of the salts are applied topically for the deodorization of skin lesions and administered orally to deodorize ulcerative skin lesions and the urine and feces in colostomy, ileostomy, or incontinence.
**c. copper complex,** a chlorophyllin in which copper has replaced the porphyrin magnesium; it is the most widely used form of chlorophyllin.

**Chlo•ro•phyl•lum** (klo-rof′ĭ-ləm) a genus of mushrooms of the family Agaricaceae. *C. molyb′dites* is similar in appearance to species of *Amanita* and contains small amounts of amatoxins, so that it occasionally causes mushroom poisoning (see under *poisoning*).

**chlo•ro•pia** (klor-ōp′e-ə) chloropsia.

**Chlo•rop•i•dae** (klor-op′ĭ-de) a family of small to minute flies (order Diptera); two medically important genera are *Hippelates* and *Siphunculina.*

**chlo•ro•plast** (klor′o-plast) [*chloro-* + *-plast*] [MeSH: Chloroplasts] any one of the chlorophyll-bearing bodies of plant cells; called also *chloroplastid.*

**chlo•ro•plas•tid** (klor″o-plas′tid) chloroplast.

**chlo•ro•prene** (klor′o-prēn) [MeSH: Chloroprene] an organic compound used in the synthesis of neoprene rubber; it is toxic by inhalation, ingestion, and skin absorption, causes lung and liver cancer, and has reproductive effects.

**chlo•ro•priv•ic** (klor″o-priv′ik) [*chlorine* + L. *privare* to deprive] deprived of chlorides; due to loss of chlorides.

**chlo•ro•pro•caine hy•dro•chlo•ride** (klor″o-pro′kān) [USP] a local anesthetic used in minor and general surgery for infiltration, field block, and regional nerve block, including caudal and epidural block.

**chlo•ro•pro•py•lene ox•ide** (klo″ro-pro′pə-lēn) epichlorohydrin.

**chlo•rop•sia** (klor-op′se-ə) [*chloro-* + *-opsia*] a chromatopsia in which all objects seen appear to have a greenish tinge, a symptom of digitalis poisoning.

**Chlor·op·tic** (klor-op'tik) trademark for preparations of chloramphenicol.

**chlo·ro·quine** (klor'o-kwin) [USP] [MeSH: Chloroquine] a 4-aminoquinoline compound with antiprotozoal and anti-inflammatory properties, used for the suppression and treatment of malaria, for the treatment of giardiasis and extraintestinal amebiasis, for suppression of lupus erythematosus, and as an anti-inflammatory in the treatment of rheumatoid arthritis.
**c. hydrochloride,** the dihydrochloride salt of chloroquine, used for suppression and treatment of malaria and for treatment of extraintestinal amebiasis; administered intramuscularly.
**c. phosphate** [USP], the phosphate salt of chloroquine, used for suppression and treatment of malaria, for treatment of extraintestinal amebiasis, and as a lupus erythematosus suppressant; administered orally.

**chlo·ro·sis** (klor-o'sis) a disorder that was common during the nineteenth century but has now disappeared, characterized by greenish yellow skin discoloration and hypochromic erythrocytes; it was usually seen in adolescent females and may have been associated with iron deficiency anemia.

**Chlo·ro·stig·ma** (klor"o-stig'mə) a genus of plants of the family Asclepiadaceae. *C. stuckertia'num* is the source of the alkaloid chlorostigmine.

**chlo·ro·stig·mine** (klor"o-stig'mēn) an alkaloid from plants of the genus *Chlorostigma,* especially *C. stuckertia'num,* which has been used to stimulate secretion of milk in nursing mothers.

**chlo·ro·thi·a·zide** (klor"o-thi'ə-zīd) [USP] [MeSH: Chlorothiazide] a thiazide diuretic, used for treatment of hypertension and edema; administered orally.
**c. sodium** [USP], the monosodium salt of chlorothiazide, having the same actions and uses as the base; administered intravenously.

**chlo·ro·thy·mol** (klor"o-thi'mol) a powerful germicide which has been used as a topical antibacterial and fungicide.

**chlo·ro·tri·an·i·sene** (klor"o-tri-an'ĭ-sēn) [MeSH: Chlorotrianisene] a synthetic estrogen used to suppress lactation in postpartum women, for palliative treatment in inoperable prostatic carcinoma, and for replacement therapy of estrogen deficiency; administered orally.

**chlo·rous** (klor'əs) derived from or containing trivalent chlorine, as in chlorous acid, $HClO_2$; a term used to distinguish those compounds which contain a larger proportion of chlorine than the chloric compounds, and forming salts known as chlorites.

**chlo·rous acid** (klor'əs) a weak inorganic acid, $HClO_2$.

**chlo·ro·vi·nyl·di·chlo·ro·ar·sine** (klor"o-vīn"əl-di-klor"o-ahr'sin) lewisite.

**chlo·rox·ine** (klor-ok'sēn) a synthetic antibacterial, used in the topical treatment of dandruff and seborrheic dermatitis of the scalp.

**chlo·ro·xy·le·nol** (klor"o-zi'lə-nol) an antibacterial active chiefly against streptococci; used mainly as a skin disinfectant.

**chlor·phen·e·sin** (klor-fen'ə-sin) [MeSH: Chlorphenesin] an antibacterial, antifungal, and antitrichomonal agent, used in the treatment of tinea pedis and other fungal infections of the skin and in fungal and trichomonal infections of the vagina, applied topically or intravaginally.
**c. carbamate,** a skeletal muscle relaxant used as an adjunct in the short-term treatment of skeletal muscle spasms, such as sprains, strains, and trauma to tendons and ligaments; administered orally.

**chlor·phen·ir·amine** (klor"fən-ir'ə-mēn) [MeSH: Chlorpheniramine] an antihistaminic derived from pheniramine.
**c. maleate** [USP], the maleate salt of chlorpheniramine, administered orally or by subcutaneous injection for therapy and prophylaxis of conditions in which antihistamines may be effective. Called also *chlorprophenpyridamine maleate.*

**chlor·phen·ox·amine hy·dro·chlo·ride** (klor"fen-ok'sə-mēn) an anticholinergic with weak antihistaminic action, used as a skeletal muscle relaxant in the treatment of Parkinson's disease; administered orally.

**chlor·phen·ter·mine hy·dro·chlo·ride** (klor-fen'tər-mēn) a sympathomimetic amine with properties similar to those of dextroamphetamine, formerly used as an anorexic agent.

**chlor·pro·ma·zine** (klor-pro'mə-zēn) [USP] [MeSH: Chlorpromazine] a phenothiazine derivative, used as an antiemetic and tranquilizer, administered by rectal suppository.
**c. hydrochloride** [USP], the hydrochloride salt of chlorpromazine, used as an antipsychotic and antiemetic, to control presurgical apprehension, to control the manic phase of bipolar disorder, to treat intractable hiccups, acute intermittent porphyria, and tetanus, and for the management of severe behavior disorders in children.

**chlor·pro·pa·mide** (klor-pro'pə-mīd) [USP] [MeSH: Chlorpropamide] a sulfonylurea compound used as a hypoglycemic in the treatment of type 2 diabetes mellitus; administered orally.

**chlor·pro·phen·py·rid·amine** (klor"pro-fən-pi-rid'ə-mēn) chlorpheniramine.

**chlor·pro·thix·ene** (klor"pro-thik'sēn) [MeSH: Chlorprothixene] a thioxanthene drug having sedative, antiemetic, antihistaminic, anticholinergic, and alpha-adrenergic blocking activity; used to control the symptoms of psychotic disorders, administered orally or by intramuscular injection.
**c. hydrochloride,** the hydrochloride salt of chlorprothixene, having the same actions as the base; administered intramuscularly.
**c. lactate and hydrochloride,** a combination of the lactate and hydrochloride salts of chlorprothixene, having the same actions as the base; administered orally.

**chlor·quin·al·dol** (klor-kwin'əl-dol) [MeSH: Chlorquinaldol] a bactericidal and fungicidal agent having properties similar to those of clioquinol, applied topically in the treatment of cutaneous and vaginal infections.

**chlor·tet·ra·cy·cline** (klor"tet-rə-si'klēn) [MeSH: Chlortetracycline] a broad-spectrum antibiotic, elaborated by *Streptomyces aureofaciens;* it was the first of the tetracycline group to be discovered.
**c. hydrochloride** [USP], the monohydrochloride salt of chlortetracycline, a broad-spectrum antibiotic used as an antibacterial and antiprotozoal, administered orally, by intravenous injection, or applied topically to the conjunctiva.

**chlor·thal·i·done** (klor-thal'ĭ-dōn) [USP] [MeSH: Chlorthalidone] a sulfonamide derivative that has a different chemical structure from but the same actions as the thiazide diuretics, used in the treatment of hypertension and edema; administered orally.

**Chlor-Tri·me·ton** (klor-tri'mə-ton) trademark for preparations of chlorpheniramine maleate.

**chlo·rum** (klor'əm) gen. *chlo'ri* [L.] chlorine.

**chlor·ure·sis** (klor"u-re'sis) [*chlor-* + *-uresis*] the excretion of chlorides in the urine.

**chlor·uret·ic** (klor"u-ret'ik) 1. promoting the excretion of chlorides in the urine. 2. an agent that promotes the excretion of chlorides in the urine.

**chlor·uria** (klor-u're-ə) [*chlor-* + *-uria*] presence of chlorides in the urine.

**chlor·zox·a·zone** (klor-zok'sə-sōn) [MeSH: Chlorzoxazone] a skeletal muscle relaxant, used to relieve discomfort of painful musculoskeletal disorders, administered orally.

**ChM** abbreviation for L. *Chirur'giae Magis'ter,* Master of Surgery.

**CHO** Chinese hamster ovary; see under *cell.*

**cho·a·na** (ko'ə-nə) pl. *cho'anae* [L.; Gr. *choanē* funnel] 1. any funnel-shaped cavity or infundibulum. 2. [TA] [pl.] the paired openings between the nasal cavity and the nasopharynx; called also *posterior nasal apertures* and *posterior nares.*
**primary c.,** the opening of the embryonic olfactory sac into the mouth.
**secondary c.,** the definitive choana after the formation of the palate.

**cho·a·nae** (ko'ə-ne) [L.] genitive and plural of *choana.*

**cho·a·nal** (ko'ə-nəl) pertaining to a choana.

**choan(o)-** [L., Gr. *choanē* funnel] a combining form denoting a relationship to a funnel or to a funnellike structure.

**cho·a·no·cyte** (ko'ə-no"sīt) [*choano-* + *-cyte*] a unique type of cell having a flagellum surrounded by a thin cytoplasmic collar; characteristic of sponges and certain protozoa.

**cho·a·noid** (ko'ə-noid) [*choan-* + *-oid*] funnel-shaped.

**cho·a·no·mas·ti·gote** (ko"ə-no-mas'tĭ-gōt) [choano- + Gr. *mastix* whip] any of the bodies representing the morphologic ("barleycorn") stage in the life cycle of trypanosomatid protozoa of the genus *Crithidia,* in which the kinetoplast and basal body are anterior to the nucleus and the flagellum emerges through a funnel-shaped depression at the anterior end of the cell. Cf. *amastigote, epimastigote, opisthomastigote, promastigote,* and *trypomastigote.*

**Cho·a·no·tae·nia** (ko-a"no-te'ne-ə) [Gr. *choanē* funnel + *taenia* (def. 2)] a genus of tapeworms. *C. infundi'bulum* is a common but nonpathogenic parasite of chickens and turkeys.

**choc·o·late** (chok'ə-lət) [Nahuatl *xocolatl*] cocoa.

**choke** (chōk) 1. to interrupt respiration by obstruction or compression. Called also *strangle.* 2. the condition resulting from interruption of respiration. Called also *strangulation.* 3. [pl.] a burning sensation experienced during decompression, beginning in the substernal region, with increasing uncontrollable urge to cough and a feeling of great apprehension, leading to vasovagal attack.
**water c.,** laryngeal spasm caused by fluid entering the larynx and especially by getting between the true and false vocal cords.

**chol·a·gog·ic** (ko″lə-goj′ik) stimulating the flow of bile to the duodenum.

**chol·a·gogue** (ko′lə-gog) [*chol-* + *-agogue*] an agent that stimulates the flow of bile into the duodenum.

**cho·la·ic ac·id** (ko-la′ik) cholyltaurine.

**Cho·lan-DH** (ko′lən) trademark for preparations of dehydrocholic acid.

**cho·la·ner·e·sis** (ko″lə-ner′ə-sis) increase in the output or elimination of bile acids, their conjugates, or their salts.

**cho·lan·ge·itis** (ko-lan″je-i′tis) cholangitis.

**cho·lan·gi·ec·ta·sis** (ko-lan″je-ek′tə-sis) dilatation of a bile duct.

**cholangi(o)-** [*chol-* + *angi(o)-*] a combining form denoting relationship to a bile duct.

**cho·lan·gio·ad·e·no·ma** (ko-lan″je-o-ad″ə-no′mə) bile duct adenoma.

**cho·lan·gi·o·car·ci·no·ma** (ko-lan″je-o-kahr″sĭ-no′mə) [MeSH: Cholangiocarcinoma] 1. an adenocarcinoma arising from the epithelium of the intrahepatic bile ducts, composed of eosinophilic cuboidal or columnar epithelial cells arranged in tubules or acini with abundant fibrous stroma; mucus may be secreted but not bile. 2. cholangiocellular carcinoma.
**hilar c.**, that arising from the major intrahepatic bile ducts; called also *Klatskin's tumor.*
**peripheral c.**, that arising from the small bile ducts in the periphery of the liver.

**cho·lan·gio·cho·le·cys·to·cho·le·do·chec·to·my** (ko-lan″je-o-ko″le-sis″to-ko″le-do-kek′tə-me) excision of hepatic duct, common bile duct, and gallbladder.

**cho·lan·gio·en·ter·os·to·my** (ko-lan″je-o-en″tər-os′tə-me) [*cholangio-* + *enterostomy*] surgical anastomosis of a bile duct to the intestine.

**cho·lan·gio·gas·tros·to·my** (ko-lan″je-o-gas-tros′tə-me) [*cholangio-* + *gastrostomy*] surgical anastomosis of a bile duct to the stomach.

**cho·lan·gio·gram** (ko-lan′je-o-gram″) a radiograph of the gallbladder and bile ducts.

**cho·lan·gi·og·ra·phy** (ko-lan″je-og′rə-fe) [*cholangio-* + *-graphy*] [MeSH: Cholangiography] radiography of the biliary ducts after administration or injection of a contrast medium, orally, intravenously, or percutaneously.
**fine needle transhepatic c. (FNTC)**, transhepatic cholangiography performed by means of a very fine, highly flexible steel needle (fine needle).
**operative c.**, cholangiography performed during a surgical procedure on the gallbladder.
**transhepatic c.**, cholangiography after introduction of radiopaque media into the biliary system by percutaneous puncture of a bile duct. See also *endoscopic retrograde cholangiopancreatography,* under *cholangiopancreatography.*
**transjugular c.**, cholangiography after catheterization of a hepatic vein via the internal jugular vein in the neck and entry into a bile duct by percutaneous puncture across the wall of the hepatic vein.

**cho·lan·gio·hep·a·ti·tis** (ko-lan″je-o-hep″ə-ti′tis) severe inflammation of the bile passages in humans, ruminants, or horses, often associated with liver fluke infestation that causes obstruction of the bile ducts.
**Oriental c.**, recurrent pyogenic cholangitis.

**cho·lan·gio·hep·a·to·ma** (ko-lan″je-o-hep″ə-to′mə) hepatocellular carcinoma of mixed liver cell and bile-duct cell origin; called also *hepatocholangiocarcinoma.*

**cho·lan·gio·je·ju·nos·to·my** (ko-lan″je-o-jə-joo-nos′to-me) surgical anastomosis of a bile duct to the jejunum.
**intrahepatic c.**, portoenterostomy.

**cho·lan·gi·o·lar** (ko″lan-je′o-lər) pertaining to a cholangiole.

**cho·lan·gi·ole** (ko-lan′je-ōl) [*cholangio-* + *-ole* diminutive suffix] one of the fine terminal elements of the bile duct system, leaving the portal canal, and pursuing a course at the periphery of a lobule of the liver; called also *bile* or *biliary ductule* and, rarely, *bile capillary.*

**cho·lan·gi·o·li·tis** (ko-lan″je-o-li′tis) inflammation of the cholangioles.

**cho·lan·gi·o·ma** (ko-lan″je-o′mə) [*cholangi-* + *-oma*] cholangiocellular carcinoma.

**cho·lan·gio·pan·cre·a·tog·ra·phy** (ko-lan″je-o-pan″kre-ə-tog′rə-fe) radiographic examination of the bile ducts and pancreas after administration of a contrast medium.
**endoscopic retrograde c. (ERCP)**, a procedure consisting of a combination of retrograde cholangiography and transhepatic cholangiography used to demonstrate all portions of the biliary tree, performed by cannulation of the common bile duct and pancreatic duct through the papilla of Vater by means of a flexible fiberoptic endoscope and retrograde injection of radiopaque contrast media.

**cho·lan·gi·os·to·my** (ko″lan-je-os′tə-me) [*cholangio-* + *-stomy*] creation of an opening into a bile duct; sometimes used to refer to a fistula into the bile duct.

**cho·lan·gi·ot·o·my** (ko″lan-je-ot′ə-me) [*cholangio-* + *-tomy*] incision into a bile duct.

**cho·lan·gi·tis** (ko″lan-ji′tis) [*cholangi-* + *-itis*] [MeSH: Cholangitis] inflammation of a bile duct.
**chronic nonsuppurative destructive c.**, primary biliary cirrhosis.
**c. len′ta**, chronic infectious cholangitis without gallstones or biliary tract obstruction.
**Oriental c.**, recurrent pyogenic c.
**primary sclerosing c.**, a progressive chronic fibrosing inflammation of the bile ducts of unknown cause, occurring most commonly in young men and frequently in association with chronic ulcerative colitis; it also occurs as a complication of HIV infection.
**progressive nonsuppurative c.**, primary biliary cirrhosis.
**recurrent pyogenic c.**, recurrent attacks of cholangitis with brown pigment gallstones in the common bile duct (choledocholithiasis), ductal stenosis, fever, and jaundice, a disorder often seen in eastern and southern Asia, sometimes associated with dietary deficiencies (high carbohydrate, low protein diet) or parasite infections such as with *Ascaris* or *Clonorchis.* Called also *Oriental c.* and *Oriental cholangiohepatitis.*
**sclerosing c.**, primary sclerosing c.

**cho·lan·ic ac·id** (ko-lan′ik) a steroidal acid, 5*β*-cholan-24-oic acid, which can be considered the parent compound of the bile acids.

**cho·lano·poi·e·sis** (ko″lə-no-poi-e′sis) the synthesis of bile acids or of their conjugates and salts by the liver.

**cho·lano·poi·et·ic** (ko″lə-no-poi-et′ik) 1. pertaining to or promoting cholanopoiesis. 2. an agent that promotes cholanopoiesis.

**cho·lan·threne** (ko-lan′thrēn) a carcinogenic pentacyclic hydrocarbon; see also *3-methylcholanthrene.*

**cho·late** (ko′lāt) a salt, anion, or ester of cholic acid.

**chole-** see *chol(o)-.*

**cho·le·bil·i·ru·bin** (ko″le-bil″e-roo′bin) a pigment, differing from bilirubin, occurring in gallbladder bile; it gives a direct reaction to the van den Bergh test.

**cho·le·cal·ci·fer·ol** (ko″lə-kal-sif′ər-ol) [MeSH: Cholecalciferol] 1. a hormone synthesized in the skin on irradiation of 7-dehydrocholesterol or obtained as a vitamin from dietary sources; it is activated when metabolized to 1,25-dihydroxycholecalciferol. See table. See also *ergocalciferol.* Called also *vitamin* $D_3$. 2. [USP] a preparation of this compound, derived from animal tissues and used in the prophylaxis and treatment of vitamin D deficiencies due to low intake, high requirement, or impaired absorption of the vitamin. It is also used in the treatment of hypocalcemic tetany and hypoparathyroidism. Called also *vitamin* $D_3$.

**Cholecalciferol and Related Metabolites of Vitamin D**

| Systematic Name | Vitamin | Abbreviation |
|---|---|---|
| 7-Dehydrocholesterol | Provitamin $D_3$ | — |
| Cholecalciferol | Vitamin $D_3$ | $D_3$ |
| 25-Hydroxycholecalciferol | 25-Hydroxyvitamin $D_3$ | $25(OH)D_3$ |
| 1,25-Dihydroxycholecalciferol | 1,25-Dihydroxyvitamin $D_3$ | $1,25(OH)_2D_3$ |
| 24,25-Dihydroxycholecalciferol | 24,25-Dihydroxyvitamin $D_3$ | $24,25(OH)_2D_3$ |

**cho·le·chro·mo·poi·e·sis** (ko″le-kro″mo-poi-e′sis) the synthesis of bile pigments.

**cho·le·cy·a·nin** (ko″le-si′ə-nin) bilicyanin.

**cho·le·cyst** (ko′le-sist) [*chole-* + *cyst*] vesica biliaris.

**cho·le·cyst·a·gog·ic** (ko″le-sis″tə-goj′ik) cholecystokinetic.

**cho·le·cyst·a·gogue** (ko″le-sis′tə-gog) a cholecystokinetic agent.

**cho·le·cys·tal·gia** (ko″le-sis-tal′jə) [*cholecyst* + *-algia*] 1. biliary colic. 2. pain due to inflammation of the gallbladder.

**cho·le·cys·tat·o·ny** (ko″le-sis-tat′ə-ne) atony of the gallbladder.

**cho·le·cys·tec·ta·sia** (ko″le-sis″tek-ta′zhə) [*cholecyst* + *ectasia*] distention of the gallbladder.

**cho·le·cys·tec·to·my** (ko″le-sis-tek′tə-me) [*cholecyst* + *-ectomy*] [MeSH: Cholecystectomy] surgical removal of the gallbladder.

**cho·le·cys·ten·ter·ic** (ko″le-sis″ten-ter′ik) pertaining to communication between the gallbladder and intestine; called also *cholecystointestinal.*

**cho·le·cyst·en·tero·anas·to·mo·sis** (ko″le-sis-ten″tər-o-ə-nas″tə-mo′sis) cholecystenterostomy.

**cho·le·cyst·en·ter·or·rha·phy** (ko″le-sis-ten″tər-or′ə-fe) suture of the gallbladder to the small intestine.

**cho·le·cyst·en·ter·os·to·my** (ko″le-sis″ten-tər-os′tə-me) [*cholecyst* + *enterostomy*] surgical anastomosis of the gallbladder to the intestine. Called also *cholecystenteroanastomosis* and *enterocholecystostomy.*

**cho·le·cyst·gas·tros·to·my** (ko″le-sist-gas-tros′tə-me) cholecystogastrostomy.

**cho·le·cys·tic** (ko″le-sis′tik) pertaining to the gallbladder.

**cho·le·cys·tis** (ko″le-sis′tis) [*chole-* + *cystis*] the gallbladder.

**cho·le·cys·ti·tis** (ko″le-sis-ti′tis) [*cholecyst* + *-itis*] [MeSH: Cholecystitis] inflammation of the gallbladder.
**acute c.,** a form usually due to obstruction of the gallbladder outlet, with signs ranging from mild edema and congestion to severe infection with gangrene and perforation.
**chronic c.,** inflammation of the gallbladder with relatively mild symptoms persisting over a long period.
**c. emphysemato′sa,** emphysematous c.
**emphysematous c.,** inflammation of the gallbladder caused by gas-producing organisms, characterized by gas in the gallbladder lumen and frequently infiltrating into the wall of the gallbladder and surrounding tissues; called also *gaseous c.*
**follicular c.,** inflammation of the gallbladder in which there is conspicuous formation of lymphoid follicles, which commonly contain germinal centers.
**gaseous c.,** emphysematous c.
**c. glandula′ris proli′ferans,** a thickening of the wall of the chronically inflamed gallbladder, with formation of crypts which may develop into cysts.

**cho·le·cyst·ne·phros·to·my** (ko′le-sist″nə-fros′tə-me) cholecystopyelostomy.

**cho·le·cys·to·cho·lan·gio·gram** (ko″le-sis″to-ko-lan′je-o-gram) radiograph of the gallbladder and bile ducts.

**cho·le·cys·to·co·lon·ic** (ko″le-sis″to-ko-lon′ik) pertaining to communication between the gallbladder and colon, as cholecystocolonic fistula.

**cho·le·cys·to·co·los·to·my** (ko″le-sis″to-ko-los′tə-me) surgical anastomosis of the gallbladder to the colon; called also *colocholecystostomy.*

**cho·le·cys·to·co·lot·o·my** (ko″le-sis″to-ko-lot′ə-me) surgical incision of the gallbladder and colon.

**cho·le·cys·to·du·o·de·nal** (ko″le-sis-to-doo″o-de′nəl) pertaining to communication between the gallbladder and duodenum.

**cho·le·cys·to·du·o·de·nos·to·my** (ko″le-sis″to-doo″o-də-nos′tə-me) surgical anastomosis of the gallbladder and the duodenum.

**cho·le·cys·to·en·ter·os·to·my** (ko″le-sis″to-en″tər-os′tə-me) cholecystenterostomy.

**cho·le·cys·to·gas·tric** (ko″le-sis″to-gas′trik) pertaining to communication between the gallbladder and stomach, as a cholecystogastric fistula.

**cho·le·cys·to·gas·tros·to·my** (ko″le-sis″to-gas-tros′tə-me) surgical anastomosis between the gallbladder and the stomach.

**cho·le·cys·to·gog·ic** (ko″le-sis″to-goj′ik) cholecystokinetic.

**cho·le·cys·to·gram** (ko″le-sis′to-gram) a radiograph of the gallbladder.

**cho·le·cys·tog·ra·phy** (ko″le-sis-tog′rə-fe) [*cholecyst* + *-graphy*] [MeSH: Cholecystography] radiography of the gallbladder.

**cho·le·cys·to·il·e·os·to·my** (ko″le-sis″to-il″e-os′tə-me) surgical anastomosis of the gallbladder and the ileum.

**cho·le·cys·to·in·tes·ti·nal** (ko″le-sis″to-in-tes′tĭ-nəl) cholecystenteric.

**cho·le·cys·to·je·ju·nos·to·my** (ko″le-sis″to-jə-joo-nos′tə-me) surgical anastomosis of the gallbladder and the jejunum.

**cho·le·cys·to·ki·net·ic** (ko″le-sis″to-kĭ-net′ik) causing or promoting contraction of the gallbladder.

**cho·le·cys·to·ki·nin (CCK)** (ko″le-sis″to-ki′nin) [*cholecyst* + *kinin*] [MeSH: Cholecystokinin] a polypeptide hormone secreted by the mucosa of the upper intestine and by the hypothalamus. It stimulates contraction of the gallbladder (with release of bile) and secretion of pancreatic enzymes; hypothalamic cholecystokinin is a neurotransmitter. Called also *pancreozymin.*

**cho·le·cys·to·li·thi·a·sis** (ko″le-sis″to-lĭ-thi′ə-sis) [*cholecyst* + *lithiasis*] the occurrence of gallstones (see *cholelithiasis*) within the gallbladder.

**cho·le·cys·to·litho·trip·sy** (ko″le-sis″to-lith′o-trip″se) [*cholecyst* + *lithotripsy*] the fragmentation of gallstones within the gallbladder.

**cho·le·cys·to·ne·phros·to·my** (ko″le-sis″to-nə-fros′tə-me) cholecystopyelostomy.

**cho·le·cys·top·a·thy** (ko″le-sis-top′ə-the) [*cholecyst* + *-pathy*] any gallbladder disease.

**cho·le·cys·to·pexy** (ko″le-sis′to-pek″se) [*cholecyst* + *-pexy*] suspension or fixation of the gallbladder by surgical means.

**cho·le·cys·top·to·sis** (ko″le-sis″top-to′sis) [*cholecyst* + *-ptosis*] downward or distal displacement of the gallbladder.

**cho·le·cys·to·py·elos·to·my** (ko″le-sis″to-pi″ə-los′tə-me) surgical anastomosis of the gallbladder to the pelvis of the kidney; called also *cholecystonephrostomy.*

**cho·le·cys·tor·rha·phy** (ko″le-sis-tor′ə-fe) [*cholecyst* + *-rrhaphy*] suture or repair of the gallbladder.

**cho·le·cys·to·sis** (ko″le-sis-to′sis) any noninflammatory disease of the gallbladder.
**hyperplastic c.,** abnormal increase in cellular structure of the gallbladder.
**percutaneous c.,** the insertion of a catheter into the gallbladder under radiologic guidance for drainage or the removal of gallstones.

**cho·le·cys·tot·o·my** (ko″le-sis-tot′ə-me) [*cholecyst* + *-tomy*] surgical incision of the gallbladder; done for exploration, drainage (cholecystostomy), or removal of calculi.

**cho·led·o·chal** (ko-led′ə-kəl) pertaining to the common bile duct.

**cho·le·do·chec·to·my** (kol″ə-do-kek′tə-me) [*choledoch-* + *-ectomy*] excision of a portion of the common bile duct.

**cho·le·do·chen·dy·sis** (kol″ə-do-ken′də-sis) [*choledoch-* + *endysis* entrance] choledochotomy.

**cho·le·do·chi·tis** (kol″ə-do-ki′tis) inflammation of the common bile duct (ductus choledochus).

**choledoch(o)-** [*choledochus*] a combining form denoting relation to the common bile duct.

**cho·led·o·cho·cele** (ko-led′ə-ko-sēl) a rare form of congenital cystic dilatation of the common bile duct in which the dilated portion is within the wall of the duct.

**cho·led·o·cho·chol·e·do·chos·to·my** (ko-led″o-ko-kol″ə-də-kos′tə-me) surgical formation of an anastomosis between two portions of the common bile duct.

**cho·led·o·cho·du·o·de·nos·to·my** (ko-led″o-ko-doo″o-də-nos′tə-me) surgical anastomosis of the common bile duct to the duodenum.

**cho·led·o·cho·en·ter·os·to·my** (ko-led′ə-ko-en′tər-os′tə-me) surgical anastomosis of the common bile duct to the intestine.

**cho·led·o·cho·gas·tros·to·my** (ko-led″ə-ko-gas-tros′tə-me) surgical anastomosis of the common bile duct and the stomach.

**cho·led·o·cho·gram** (ko-led′ə-ko-gram″) a radiograph of the common bile duct.

**cho·led·o·chog·ra·phy** (ko-led″ə-kog′rə-fe) [*choledocho-* + *-graphy*] radiography of the common bile duct after the administration of opaque material.

**cho·led·o·cho·hep·a·tos·to·my** (ko-led′ə-ko-hep″ə-tos′tə-me) surgical anastomosis of the common bile duct to the hepatic duct.

**cho·led·o·cho·il·e·os·to·my** (ko-led″ə-ko-il-e-os′tə-me) surgical anastomosis of the common bile duct and the ileum.

**cho·led·o·cho·je·ju·nos·to·my** (ko-led″ə-ko-jə-joo-nos′tə-me) surgical anastomosis of the common bile duct and the jejunum.

**cho·led·o·cho·lith** (ko-led′ə-ko-lith″) a gallstone or other calculus in the common bile duct. Called also *bile duct calculus.*

**cho·led·o·cho·li·thi·a·sis** (ko-led″ə-ko-lĭ-thi′-ə-sis) the occurrence of calculi (see *cholelithiasis*) in the common bile duct.

**cho·led·o·cho·li·thot·o·my** (ko-led″ə-ko-lĭ-thot′ə-me) incision of the common bile duct for the removal of stone.

**cho·led·o·cho·litho·trip·sy** (ko-led″o-ko-lith′o-trip″se) the crushing of a gallstone within the common bile duct.

**cho·led·o·cho·plas·ty** (ko-led″ə-ko-plas′te) the performance of a plastic operation on the common bile duct; plastic repair of the duct following injury.

**cho·led·o·chor·rha·phy** (ko-led″ə-kor′ə-fe) [*choledocho-* + *-rrhaphy*] suture or repair of the common bile duct.

**cho·led·o·cho·scope** (ko-led′ə-ko-skōp″) an instrument used during surgical exploration for direct inspection of the interior of the common bile duct.

**cho·led·o·chos·to·my** (ko-led″ə-kos′tə-me) [*choledocho-* + *-stomy*] [MeSH: Choledochostomy] surgical formation of an opening into the common bile duct and drainage by catheter or T-tube.

**cho·led·o·chot·o·my** (ko-led″ə-kot′ə-me) [*choledocho-* + *-tomy*] incision into the common bile duct for exploration or removal of a calculus; called also *choledochendysis.*

**cho·led·o·chus** (ko-led′ə-kəs) [*chole-* + Gr. *dochos* receptacle] ductus choledochus.

**Cho·le·dyl** (ko′lə-dil″) trademark for preparations of oxtriphylline.

**cho·le·glo·bin** (ko″le-glo′bin) a compound of globin and an open-ring iron porphyrin, being an intermediate in the formation of bile pigment from the catabolism of hemoglobin.

**cho·le·hem·a·tin** (ko″le-hem′ə-tin) phylloerythrin.

**cho·le·ic** (ko-le′ik) biliary.

**cho·le·ic ac·id** (ko-le′ik) any of the complexes formed between deoxycholic acid and a fatty acid or other lipid.

**cho·le·lith** (ko′lĕ-lith) [*chole-* + *-lith*] gallstone.

**cho·le·li·thi·a·sis** (ko″le-lĭ-thi′ə-sis) [*chole-* + *lithiasis*] [MeSH: Cholelithiasis] the presence or formation of gallstones; they may be either in the gallbladder *(cholecystolithiasis)* or in the common bile duct *(choledocholithiasis).*

**cho·le·lith·ic** (ko″le-lith′ik) pertaining to or caused by gallstones.

**cho·le·li·thot·o·my** (ko″le-lĭ-thot′ə-me) removal of gallstones through an incision in the gallbladder.

**cho·le·litho·trip·sy** (ko″le-lith′o-trip-se) [*chole-* + *litho-* + *-tripsy*] the crushing of gallstones.

**cho·le·li·thot·ri·ty** (ko″le-lĭ-thot′rĭ-te) cholelithotripsy.

**cho·lem·e·sis** (ko-lem′ə-sis) [*chole-* + *emesis*] vomiting of bile.

**cho·le·mia** (ko-le′me-ə) [*chole-* + *-emia*] the presence of bile or bile pigments in the blood.
**familial c., Gilbert c.,** Gilbert syndrome.

**cho·le·mic** (ko-le′mik) pertaining to, marked by, or due to cholemia.

**cho·le·mim·e·try** (ko″le-mim′ə-tre) determination of the amount of bile pigment in the blood.

**cho·le·peri·to·ne·um** (ko″le-per″ĭ-tə-ne′əm) [*chole-* + *peritoneum*] the presence of bile in the peritoneum resulting from rupture of the bile passages; called also *biliary* or *bile peritonitis,* and *choleperitonitis.*

**cho·le·peri·to·ni·tis** (ko″lĕ-per″ĭ-tə-ni′tis) choleperitoneum.

**cho·le·poi·e·sis** (ko″le-poi-e′sis) [*chole-* + *-poiesis*] 1. the manufacture and secretion by the liver of bile constituents other than water. 2. the manufacture and secretion of bile salts by the liver.

**cho·le·poi·et·ic** (ko″le-poi-et′ik) forming or secreting a constituent peculiar to bile; increasing the secretion of bile without a fall in its specific gravity.

**cho·le·pra·sin** (ko″le-pra′sin) one of the pigments of bile isolated from gallstones.

**chol·era** (kol′ər-ə) [Gr., from *cholē* bile] [MeSH: Cholera] 1. an acute infectious, sometimes fulminant, enteritis endemic in India and Southeast Asia and periodically spreading in epidemics or pandemics to other warm regions of the world; it is spread by feces-contaminated water and food. The cause is a potent enterotoxin (choleragen), elaborated by *Vibrio cholerae,* that acts on epithelial cells in the small intestine to cause copious secretion of isotonic fluid from the mucosal surface. Severe cases are marked by painless watery diarrhea (rice-water stools), which are diagnostic and result in massive fluid loss, saline depletion, acidosis, and shock; effortless vomiting; muscle cramps; and a peculiar faint high-pitched voice. 2. any of several infections that resemble this disease, particularly in veterinary medicine, but are not caused by *Vibrio cholerae.*
**Asiatic c.,** classic cholera; so called because the disease was originally confined to Asia.
**dry c.,** c. sicca.
**fowl c.,** an infection by *Pasteurella multocida,* seen in bird species around the world, including domestic fowl, canaries, waterfowl, seagulls, game birds, and birds of prey, occurring in acute, often fatal, forms and chronic forms; symptoms include abdominal hyperemia with petechiae and hemorrhage, fever, anorexia, ruffled feathers, diarrhea, increased respiratory rate, and sometimes pneumonia.
**c. gallina′rium,** fowl c.
**hog c.,** an epizootic infectious disease of swine caused by a togavirus; marked by fever, loss of appetite, emaciation, ulceration of the intestines, diarrhea, and ecchymoses in the kidney and on the skin of the ventral surface of the body. Called also *swine fever.*
**c. mor′bus,** former name for a type of acute gastroenteritis with diarrhea, cramps, and vomiting that occurred in summer or autumn; called also *summer c.*
**pancreatic c.,** Verner-Morrison syndrome.
**c. sic′ca,** a rare type of cholera in which ileus produces pooling of fluid in the gut, associated with profound shock with diarrhea; called also *dry c.*
**summer c.,** c. morbus.

**chol·er·a·gen** (kol′ər-ə-jen) the exotoxin produced by the cholera vibrio, which is thought to stimulate electrolyte and water secretion into the small intestine in Asiatic cholera.

**chol·e·ra·ic** (kol″ə-ra′ik) of, pertaining to, or of the nature of cholera.

**chol·er·a·phage** (kol′ər-ə-fāj) a bacteriophage that infects cholera bacilli.

**cho·ler·e·sis** (ko-ler′ə-sis) [*chole-* + Gr. *hairesis* a taking] the secretion of bile by the liver by either cholepoiesis or hydrocholeresis.

**cho·ler·et·ic** (ko″lər-et′ik) 1. stimulating the production of bile by the liver by either cholepoiesis or hydrocholeresis. 2. a choleretic agent.

**chol·er·ic** (kol′ər-ik) [Gr. *cholerikos,* from *chole* bile] hot-tempered, irascible, having the temperament that, according to the humoral theory of the ancient Greeks, is caused by an excess of yellow bile.

**cho·ler·i·form** (ko-ler′ĭ-form) choleroid.

**chol·er·i·gen·ic** (kol″ər-ĭ-jen′ik) causing cholera.

**chol·er·ig·e·nous** (kol″ər-ij′ə-nəs) cholerigenic.

**chol·er·oid** (kol′ər-oid) [Gr. *cholera* + *-oid*] resembling cholera.

**cho·le·scin·ti·gram** (ko″le-sin′tĭ-gram) the two-dimensional images of the biliary system obtained by cholescintigraphy.

**cho·le·scin·tig·ra·phy** (kol″e-sin-tig′rə-fe) scintigraphy of the biliary tract.

**cho·les·tane** (ko′ləs-tān) a saturated steroid hydrocarbon, with C-18 and C-19 methyl groups and an isooctyl side chain at C-17; obtained by reduction of cholesterol and other $C_{27}$ steroids.

**cho·les·tane·tri·ol** (ko-les″tān-tri′ol) a triply hydroxylated intermediate formed in the biosynthesis of bile acids from cholesterol.

**cho·les·tane·tri·ol 26-mono·oxy·ge·nase** (ko-les″tān-tri′ol mon″o-ok′sə-jən-ās) [EC 1.14.13.15] an enzyme of the oxidoreductase class that hydroxylates 5$\beta$-cholestane-3$\alpha$,7$\alpha$,12$\alpha$-triol (or any of several related intermediates) at the 26 position as a step in the major biosynthetic pathway of bile acids from cholesterol. Deficiency of the enzyme, an autosomal recessive trait, results in cerebrotendinous xanthomatosis. Called also *26-hydroxylase.*

**cho·les·ta·nol** (ko-les′tə-nol) [MeSH: Cholestanol] a compound, $C_{27}H_{47}OH$, formed by the reduction of cholesterol.
**beta-c.,** an isomer of coprosterol derived from cholesterol by bacterial action and found in the feces; called also *dihydrocholesterol.*

**cho·le·sta·sia** (ko″le-sta′zhə) cholestasis.

**cho·le·sta·sis** (ko″le-sta′sis) [*chole-* + *-stasis*] [MeSH: Cholestasis] stoppage or suppression of the flow of bile, having intrahepatic or extrahepatic causes.

**cho·le·stat·ic** (ko″le-stat′ik) pertaining to or characterized by cholestasis.

**cho·le·ste·a·to·ma** (ko″le-ste″ə-to′mə) [*chole-* + *steatoma*] [MeSH: Cholesteatoma] a cystlike mass or benign tumor lined with stratified squamous epithelium, usually keratinizing, and filled with desquamating debris often including cholesterol. Cholesteatomas are most common in the middle ear and mastoid region secondary to trauma or infection that heals improperly so that epithelium invaginates. A congenital variety (see *congenital c.*), resulting from embryonic inclusions, is less common.
**congenital c.,** a benign tumor resulting from inclusion of epidermal elements at the time of closure of the neural groove; it may be in or near the ear but more often is in the form of an intracranial cholesteatoma. See also *epidermoid cyst* (def. 2).

**intracranial c.,** a congenital cholesteatoma that is a type of epidermoid cyst of the skull, meninges, or brain; it grows slowly, often in the cisterns. Symptoms vary depending on what part of the brain is under pressure, but may become life-threatening.
**c. tym'pani,** a type of cholesteatoma usually associated with chronic infection of the middle ear, formed of the outer desquamating layers of stratified squamous epithelium which has extended inward and upward to line the tympanum, epitympanum, and antrum.

**cho•le•ste•a•to•ma•tous** (ko"le-ste"ə-to'mə-təs) relating to or of the nature of cholesteatoma.

**cho•le•ste•a•to•sis** (ko"le-ste"ə-to'sis) fatty deposits of cholesterol esters in a tissue.

**cho•les•ter•in** (ko-les'tər-in) cholesterol.

**cho•les•tero•gen•e•sis** (ko-les"tər-o-jen'ə-sis) [*cholesterol* + *-genesis*] synthesis of cholesterol.

**cho•les•tero•hy•dro•tho•rax** (ko-les"tər-o-hi"dro-thor'aks) a chyliform effusion (q.v.) that is high in cholesterol.

**cho•les•ter•ol** (kə-les'tər-ol") [*chole-* + *sterol*] [MeSH: Cholesterol] 1. a eukaryotic sterol that in higher animals is the precursor of bile acids and steroid hormones and a key constituent of cell membranes, mediating their fluidity and permeability. Most is synthesized by the liver and other tissues, but some is absorbed from dietary sources, with each kind transported in plasma by specific lipoproteins. Cholesterol can accumulate or deposit abnormally, as in some gallstones and in atheromas. 2. [NF] a preparation of cholesterol used as an emulsifying agent in pharmaceuticals.

**cho•les•ter•ol ac•yl•trans•fer•ase** (kə-les'tər-ol a"səl-trans'fər-ās) [MeSH: Cholesterol Acyltransferase] sterol *O*-acyltransferase.

**cho•les•ter•ol des•mol•ase** (kə-les'tər-ol dez'mol-ās) cholesterol monooxygenase (side-chain-cleaving).

**cho•les•ter•ol des•mo•lase de•fi•cien•cy** lipoid adrenal hyperplasia.

**cho•les•ter•ol•emia** (kə-les"tər-ol-e'me-ə) hypercholesterolemia.

**cho•les•ter•ol•er•e•sis** (kə-les"tər-ol-er'ə-sis) increased elimination of cholesterol in the bile.

**cho•les•ter•ol es•ter•ase** (kə-les'tər-ol es'tər-ās) [MeSH: Cholesterol Esterase] sterol esterase.

**cho•les•ter•ol•es•ter•sturz** (ko-les"tər-ol-es'tər-stoorts) [Ger.] decrease in the proportion of esters in the blood cholesterol.

**cho•les•ter•ol mono•oxy•gen•ase (side-chain-cleav•ing)** (kə-les'tə-rol mon"o-ok'sə-jən-ās sīd chān klēv'ing) [EC 1.14.15.6] [MeSH: Cholesterol Monooxygenase (Side-Chain-Cleaving)] an enzyme of the oxidoreductase class that catalyzes the NADPH-dependent conversion of cholesterol to pregnenolone in a series of three reactions, successive hydroxylations of the 20 and 22 positions followed by cleavage of the side chain. The enzyme is a mitochondrial cytochrome P-450 acting as a terminal oxidase in an electron transport chain that also contains adrenodoxin and a flavoprotein. The reaction is the first step in the conversion of cholesterol to steroid hormones. Deficiency of the enzyme, an autosomal recessive trait, causes lipoid adrenal hyperplasia, a type of congenital adrenal hyperplasia (type I). Called also *cholesterol desmolase* and *20,22-desmolase.*

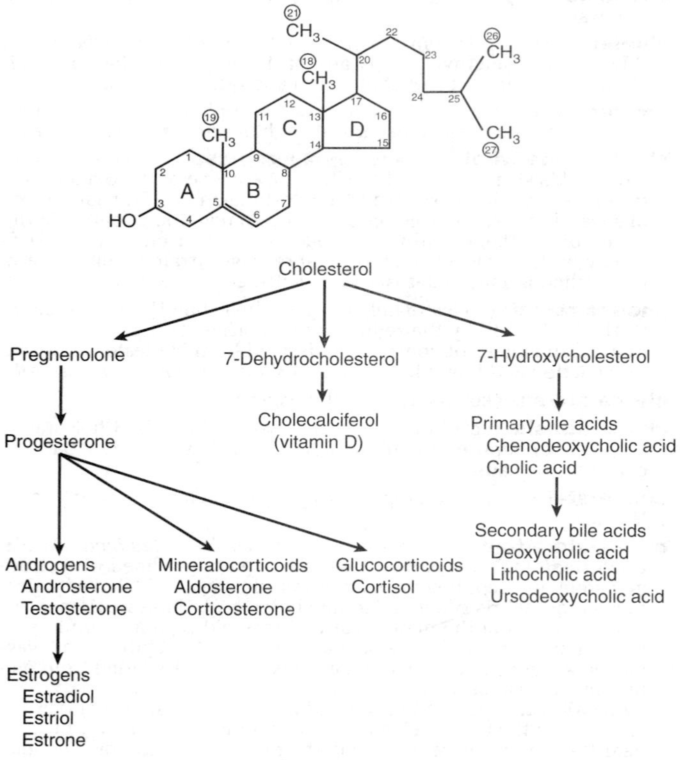

Cholesterol
Pregnenolone → Progesterone → Androgens (Androsterone, Testosterone) → Estrogens (Estradiol, Estriol, Estrone)
Progesterone → Mineralocorticoids (Aldosterone, Corticosterone)
Progesterone → Glucocorticoids (Cortisol)
7-Dehydrocholesterol → Cholecalciferol (vitamin D)
7-Hydroxycholesterol → Primary bile acids (Chenodeoxycholic acid, Cholic acid) → Secondary bile acids (Deoxycholic acid, Lithocholic acid, Ursodeoxycholic acid)

Structure and metabolism of cholesterol.

**cho•les•ter•olo•poi•e•sis** (kə-les"tər-ol"poi-e'sis) [*cholesterol* + *-poiesis*] the synthesis of cholesterol by the liver.

**cho•les•ter•ol•o•sis** (kə-les"tər-ol-o'sis) a condition in which cholesterol is deposited in tissues in abnormal quantities. Called also *cholesterosis.*

**cho•les•ter•ol sul•fa•tase** (kə-les'tər-ol sul'fə-tās) steryl sulfatase.

**cho•les•ter•ol•uria** (kə-les"tər-ol-u're-ə) the presence of cholesterol in the urine.

**cho•les•ter•o•sis** (kə-les"tər-o'sis) cholesterolosis.
**extracellular c.,** erythema elevatum dilutinum.

**cho•les•ter•yl** (kə-les'tə-rəl") the radical of cholesterol, formed by removal of the hydroxyl group.

**cho•le•sty•ra•mine** (ko"lə-sti'rə-mēn) [MeSH: Cholestyramine] see *cholestyramine resin,* under *resin.*

**Cho•le•tec** (ko'lə-tek") trademark for a kit for the preparation of technetium Tc 99m mebrofenin.

**cho•let•e•lin** (ko-let'ə-lin) [*chole-* + Gr. *telos* end] a yellow pigment, the oxidation product of bilirubin; bilixanthine.

**cho•le•ther•a•py** (ko-le-ther'ə-pe) [*chole-* + *therapy*] treatment by the administration of bile salts.

**cho•le•u•ria** (ko"le-u're-ə) [*chole-* + *-uria*] choluria.

**cho•le•ver•din** (ko"le-ver'din) biliverdin.

**cho•lic ac•id** (ko'lik) one of the primary bile acids in humans, usually occurring conjugated with glycine or taurine; it facilitates fat absorption and cholesterol excretion.

**cho•line** (ko'lēn) [MeSH: Choline] a water-soluble compound derivable from many animal and some vegetable tissues and produced synthetically. Considered to be a vitamin of the B complex, it is the basic constituent of lecithin and prevents the deposition of fat in the liver; the acetic acid ester of choline (acetylcholine) is essential in synaptic transmission of nerve impulses. Choline is also oxidized to form betaine in methionine biosynthesis.
**acetyl glyceryl ether phosphoryl c.,** platelet activating factor; see under *factor.*
**c. magnesium trisalicylate,** a combination of choline salicylate and magnesium salicylate, used as an antiarthritic.
**c. salicylate,** the choline salt of salicylic acid; used as an analgesic, antipyretic, and antirheumatic.
**c. theophyllinate,** oxtriphylline.

**cho•line acet•y•lase** (ko'lēn ə-set'ə-lās) choline *O*-acetyltransferase.

**cho•line *O*-ac•e•tyl•trans•fer•ase** (ko'lēn as"ə-tēl-trans'fər-ās) [EC 2.3.1.6] an enzyme of the transferase class that catalyzes the synthesis of acetylcholine, transferring the acetyl moiety from acetyl coenzyme A to choline. The enzyme occurs in synaptosomes of the autonomic nervous system and skeletal muscle, and in some regions of the central nervous system. Called also *choline acetylase.*

**cho•line es•ter•ase I** (ko'lēn es'tər-ās) acetylcholinesterase.

**cho•line es•ter•ase II (unspecific)** (ko'lēn es'tər-ās un"spə-sif'ik) cholinesterase.

**cho•lin•er•gic** (ko"lin-ər'jik) 1. stimulated, activated or transmitted by choline (acetylcholine): a term applied to the sympathetic and parasympathetic nerve fibers that liberate acetylcholine at a synapse when a nerve impulse passes. See also under *receptor.* 2. an agent that produces such effects. Called also *parasympathomimetic.* Cf. *adrenergic.*

**cho•lin•es•ter•ase** (ko"lin-es'tər-ās) [EC 3.1.1.8] an enzyme of the hydrolase class that catalyzes the cleavage of the acyl group from various esters of choline, including acetylcholine, and some related compounds (cf. *acetylcholinesterase*). The enzyme occurs primarily in the serum, liver, and pancreas; determination of enzyme activity is used to test liver function, succinylcholine sensitivity, and whether organophosphate insecticide poisoning has occurred. Called also *choline esterase II (unspecific), pseudocholinesterase (PCE),* and *serum c. (SChE).* Abbreviated CHS.
**serum c. (SChE),** cholinesterase.

**true c.**, acetylcholinesterase.

**cho·li·no·cep·tive** (ko″lin-o-sep′tiv) pertaining to the sites on effector organs that are acted upon by cholinergic transmitters.

**cho·li·no·cep·tor** (ko″lin-o-sep′tər) cholinergic receptor; see under *receptor.*

**cho·li·no·lyt·ic** (ko″lin-o-lit′ik) 1. blocking the action of acetylcholine, or of cholinergic agents. 2. an agent that blocks the action of acetylcholine in cholinergic areas, that is, organs supplied by parasympathetic nerves, and voluntary muscles.

**cho·li·no·mi·met·ic** (ko″lin-o-mi-met′ik) having an action similar to that of acetylcholine; parasympathomimetic.

**chol(o)-** [Gr. *cholē* bile] a combining form denoting relationship to the bile. Also, *chole-.*

**cholo·chrome** (kol′o-krōm) [*cholo-* + *-chrome*] any biliary pigment.

**cholo·cy·a·nin** (kol″o-si′ə-nin) [*cholo-* + Gr. *kyanos* blue] bilicyanin.

**cholo·ge·net·ic** (kol″o-jə-net′ik) [*cholo-* + Gr. *gennan* to produce] producing bile; cholepoietic.

**Cho·lo·gra·fin** (ko″lo-gra′fin) trademark for preparations of iodipamide.

**cholo·he·mo·tho·rax** (kol″o-he″mo-thor′aks) [*cholo-* + *hemothorax*] a pleural effusion containing bile and blood, usually due to a rupture in the intestinal wall.

**cholo·lith** (kol′o-lith) cholelith.

**cholo·li·thi·a·sis** (kol″o-lĭ-thi′ə-sis) cholelithiasis.

**cholo·lith·ic** (kol″o-lith′ik) cholelithic.

**cholo·poi·e·sis** (kol″o-poi-e′sis) cholepoiesis.

**cholo·tho·rax** (kol″o-thor′aks) [*cholo-* + *thorax*] a pleural effusion containing bile, usually due to a rupture in the intestinal wall. Cf. *cholohemothorax.*

**Cho·lox·in** (ko-lok′sin) trademark for a preparation of dextrothyroxine sodium.

**chol·uria** (kol-u′re-ə) [*chol-* + *-uria*] the presence of bile in the urine; discoloration of the urine with bile pigments.

**chol·uric** (kol-u′rik) pertaining to or marked by choluria.

**Cho·ly·bar** (ko′le-bahr) trademark for a preparation of cholestyramine resin.

**cho·lyl·gly·cine** (ko″ləl-gli′sēn) a bile salt, the glycine conjugate of cholic acid, called also *glycocholic acid.*

**cho·lyl·tau·rine** (ko″ləl-taw′rēn) a bile salt, the taurine conjugate of cholic acid, called also *taurocholic acid* and *cholaic acid.*

**Chon·do·den·dron** (kon″do-den′dron) a genus of climbing shrubs of the family Menispermaceae. *C. tomento′sum* Ruiz et Pavon is one of the sources of curare (q.v.).

**chon·dral** (kon′drəl) pertaining to cartilage.

**chon·dral·gia** (kon-dral′jə) chondrodynia.

**chon·dral·lo·pla·sia** (kon″dral-o-pla′zhə) [*chondr-* + *allo-* + *-plasia*] dyschondroplasia.

**chon·drec·to·my** (kon-drek′tə-me) [*chondr-* + *-ectomy*] surgical removal of cartilage.

**chon·dric** (kon′drik) cartilaginous; of or relating to cartilage.

**Chon·drich·thy·es** (kon-drik′the-ēz) [Gr. *chondros* cartilage + *ichthys* fish] a class of fishes with cartilaginous skeletons, including sharks, skates, and their allies. See also *elasmobranch.*

**chon·dri·fi·ca·tion** (kon″drĭ-fĭ-ka′shən) [*chondri-* + L. *facere* to make] the formation of cartilage; transformation into cartilage.

**chondri(o)-** [Gr. *chondrion* granule] a combining form denoting relationship to a granule.

**chon·dri·ome** (kon′dre-ōm) all of the mitochondria of a cell or organism considered as one structure.

**chon·drio·some** (kon′dre-o-sōm″) [*chondrio-* + *some*] mitochondrion.

**chon·dri·tis** (kon-dri′tis) [*chondr-* + *-itis*] inflammation of cartilage.
**costal c.**, Tietze's syndrome, def. 1.
**c. intervertebra′lis calca′nea**, calcinosis intervertebralis.

**chondr(o)-** [Gr. *chondros* cartilage] a combining form denoting relationship to cartilage.

**chon·dro·an·gi·o·ma** (kon″dro-an″je-o′mə) [*chondro-* + *angioma*] a benign mesenchymoma containing chondromatous and angiomatous elements.

**chon·dro·blast** (kon′dro-blast) [*chondro-* + *-blast*] a cell that arises from the mesenchyma and forms cartilage; called also *chondroplast.*

**chon·dro·blas·to·ma** (kon″dro-blas-to′mə) [*chondroblast* + *-oma*] [MeSH: Chondroblastoma] a usually benign tumor derived from immature cartilage cells, occurring primarily in the epiphyses of adolescents; it is characterized by fine, matrix-like calcifications arranged hexagonally, often resembling chicken wire, around closely packed cells.
**benign c.**, chondroblastoma.

**chon·dro·cal·ci·no·sis** (kon″dro-kal″sĭ-no′sis) [*chondro-* + *calcinosis*] [MeSH: Chondrocalcinosis] the presence of calcium salts, especially calcium pyrophosphate, in the cartilaginous structures of one or more joints.

**chon·dro·clast** (kon′dro-klast) [*chondro-* + *clast*] a giant cell of the class that is believed associated with the absorption of cartilage.

**Chon·dro·coc·cus** (kon″dro-kok′əs) [*chondro-* + Gr. *kokkos* berry] in former systems of classification, a genus of bacteria made up of organisms now assigned to the genera *Archangium, Flexibacter,* and *Myxococcus.*

**chon·dro·cos·tal** (kon″dro-kos′təl) [*chondro-* + *costal*] of or pertaining to the ribs and costal cartilages.

**chon·dro·cra·ni·um** (kon″dro-kra′ne-əm) [*chondro-* + *cranium*] [TA] that part of the neurocranium formed by endochondral ossification and comprising the bones of the base of the skull; called also *cartilaginous neurocranium.*

**chon·dro·cyte** (kon′dro-sīt) [*chondro-* + *-cyte*] a mature cartilage cell embedded in a lacuna within the cartilage matrix.
**isogenous c's**, cartilage cells that make up a single group.

**chon·dro·der·ma·ti·tis** (kon″dro-dər″mə-ti′tis) an inflammatory process involving cartilage and skin; used almost exclusively to mean chondrodermatitis nodularis chronica helicis.
**c. nodula′ris chro′nica he′licis**, a small, painful, scaly, nodular lesion on the helix of the ear, colored skin color, grayish, or translucent; multiple lesions may occur along the rim of the ear. Seen usually in middle-aged men and more often on the right ear. Called also *Winkler's disease.*

**chon·dro·dyn·ia** (kon″dro-din′e-ə) [*chondr-* + *-odynia*] pain in a cartilage.

**chon·dro·dys·pla·sia** (kon″dro-dis-pla′zhə) [*chondro-* + *dysplasia*] dyschondroplasia.
**hereditary deforming c.**, former name for multiple cartilaginous exostoses.
**metaphyseal c.**, see under *dysostosis.*
**c. puncta′ta**, a heterogeneous group of bone dysplasias, the common characteristic of which is stippling of the epiphyses in infancy. The group includes a severe autosomal recessive form (rhizomelic dwarfism), an autosomal dominant form (Conradi-Hünermann syndrome), and a milder X-linked form. Called also *chondrodystrophia calcificans congenita, chondrodystrophia congenita punctata, chondrodystrophia fetalis calcificans, Conradi's disease* or *syndrome, dysplasia epiphysealis punctata, hypoplastic fetal chondrodystrophy,* and *stippled epiphyses.*

**chon·dro·dys·tro·phia** (kon″dro-dis-tro′fe-ə) [*chondro-* + *dystrophy*] chondrodystrophy.
**c. calci′ficans conge′nita, c. conge′nita puncta′ta, c. feta′lis calci′ficans**, chondrodysplasia punctata.

**chon·dro·dys·tro·phy** (kon″dro-dis′trə-fe) a morbid condition characterized by abnormal development of cartilage.
**hyperplastic c.**, chondrodystrophy with excessive growth of the epiphyses.
**hypoplastic c.**, chondrodystrophy in which the bone is spongy and the epiphyses are irregularly developed.
**hypoplastic fetal c.**, chondrodysplasia punctata.
**c. mala′cia**, a form marked by softening of the epiphyseal cartilage.

**chon·dro·en·do·the·li·o·ma** (kon″dro-en″do-the″le-o′mə) [*chondro-* + *endothelioma*] a benign mesenchymoma containing chondromatous and endotheliomatous elements.

**chon·dro·epi·phys·e·al** (kon″dro-ep″ĭ-fiz′e-əl) pertaining to the epiphyseal cartilages.

**chon·dro·epi·phys·itis** (kon″dro-ep″ĭ-fiz-i′tis) inflammation involving the epiphyseal cartilages.

**chon·dro·fi·bro·ma** (kon″dro-fi-bro′mə) [*chondroma* + *fibroma*] a benign tumor with extensive fibrous and cartilaginous elements.

**chon·dro·gen·e·sis** (kon″dro-jen′ə-sis) [*chondro-* + *-genesis*] the formation of cartilage.

**chon·dro·gen·ic** (kon″dro-jen′ik) giving rise to or forming cartilage.

**chon·dro·glos·sus** (kon″dro-glos′əs) see under *musculus.*

**chon·drog·ra·phy** (kon-drog′rə-fe) [*chondro-* + *-graphy*] a description or account of the cartilages.

**chon·droid** (kon′droid) 1. resembling cartilage. 2. hyaline cartilage.

**chon·dro·it·ic** (kon″dro-it′ik) pertaining to, derived from, or resembling cartilage.

**chon·dro·i·tin sul·fate** (kon-dro′ĭ-tin) a glycosaminoglycan that predominates in the ground substance of cartilage, bone, and blood vessels but also occurs in other connective tissues. It consists of repeating disaccharide units in specific linkage, each composed of a glucuronic acid residue linked to a sulfated *N*-acetylgalactosamine residue. There are two forms: chondroitin 4-sulfate *(chondroitin sulfate A)* and chondroitin 6-sulfate *(chondroitin sulfate C)*, named for the position of the sulfate group on the sugar. One or both types accumulate abnormally in several mucopolysaccharidoses. *Chondroitin sulfate B* is now called *dermatan sulfate.*

**chon·dro·i·tin·uria** (kon-dro″ĭ-tin-u′re-ə) the presence of chondroitic acid in the urine.

**chon·dro·li·po·ma** (kon″dro-lĭ-po′mə) [*chondro-* + *lip-* + *-oma*] a benign mesenchymoma containing lipomatous and cartilaginous elements.

**chon·drol·o·gy** (kon-drol′ə-je) [*chondro-* + *-logy*] the sum of knowledge in regard to the cartilages.

**chon·drol·y·sis** (kon-drol′ĭ-sis) [*chondro-* + *-lysis*] the degeneration of cartilage cells that occurs in the process of intracartilaginous ossification.

**chon·dro·ma** (kon-dro′mə) pl. *chondromas, chondro′mata* [*chondr-* + *-oma*] [MeSH: Chondroma] a benign tumor or tumorlike growth of mature hyaline cartilage. It may remain centrally within the substance of a cartilage or bone *(enchondroma)* or may develop on the surface of a cartilage or bone *(juxtacortical chondroma)*, and usually occurs in adolescents or young adults in the small bones of the hands or feet, the femur, the humerus, or the ribs.
**joint c.**, a mass of cartilage in the synovial membrane of a joint; see *synovial chondromatosis.*
**juxtacortical c.**, an uncommon benign tumor of cartilage growing beneath the periosteum but external to the cortex of a bone, usually the small bones of the hands or feet. Called also *periosteal c.*
**periosteal c.**, juxtacortical c.
**synovial c.**, a cartilaginous body formed in a synovial membrane; see under *chondromatosis.*
**true c.**, enchondroma.

**chon·dro·ma·la·cia** (kon″dro-mə-la′shə) [*chondro-* + *-malacia*] softening of the articular cartilage, most frequently in the patella.
**c. feta′lis**, a condition in which the limbs of the stillborn fetus are soft and pliable due to softening of the epiphyseal cartilage.
**c. patel′lae**, pain and crepitus over the anterior aspect of the knee, particularly in flexion, with softening of the cartilage on the articular surface of the patella and, in later stages, effusion.

**chon·dro·ma·to·sis** (kon″dro-mə-to′sis) [MeSH: Chondromatosis] formation of multiple chondromas.
**synovial c.**, formation of multiple intrasynovial nodules resembling osteochondromas, resulting from proliferative changes in the synovial linings of joints; as the disorder progresses, nodules increasingly forsake the intrasynovial areas for the joint cavities.

**chon·dro·ma·tous** (kon-dro′mə-təs) pertaining to or of the nature of cartilage.

**chon·dro·mere** (kon′dro-mēr) [*chondro-* + *-mere*] a cartilaginous vertebra of the fetal vertebral column.

**chon·dro·meta·pla·sia** (kon″dro-met″ə-pla′zhə) a condition characterized by metaplastic activity of the chondroblasts.
**synovial c.**, synovial chondromatosis.
**tenosynovial c.**, synovial chondromatosis affecting the sheath of a tendon.

**chon·dro·mi·tome** (kon″dro-mi′tōm) [*chondro-* + *mitome*] the paranucleus.

**chon·dro·mu·cin** (kon″dro-mu′sin) chondromucoprotein.

**chon·dro·mu·coid** (kon″dro-mu′koid) chondromucoprotein.

**chon·dro·mu·co·pro·tein** (kon″dro-mu″ko-pro′tēn) the principal constituent of the ground substance of cartilage; it is a copolymer of a mucoprotein and chondroitin sulfates.

**chon·dro·my·o·ma** (kon″dro-mi-o′mə) [*chondro-* + *myoma*] a benign mesenchymoma containing myomatous and cartilaginous elements.

**chon·dro·myx·o·ma** (kon″dro-mik-so′mə) chondromyxoid fibroma.

**chon·dro·myxo·sar·co·ma** (kon″dro-mik″so-sahr-ko′mə) [*chondro-* + *myxo-* + *sarcoma*] a malignant mesenchymoma containing myxoid and cartilaginous elements.

**chon·dro·ne·cro·sis** (kon″dro-nə-kro′sis) necrosis of cartilage.

**chon·dro·os·se·ous** (kon″dro-os′e-əs) composed of cartilage and bone.

**chon·dro·path·ia** (kon″dro-path′e-ə) chondropathy.
**c. tubero′sa**, Tietze's syndrome.

**chon·dro·pa·thol·o·gy** (kon″dro-pə-thol′ə-je) the pathology of disease of cartilage.

**chon·drop·a·thy** (kon-drop′ə-the) [*chondro-* + *-pathy*] disease of a cartilage.

**chon·dro·phyte** (kon′dro-fīt) [*chondro-* + *-phyte*] a cartilaginous growth at the articular extremity of a bone.

**chon·dro·pla·sia** (kon″dro-pla′zhə) the formation of cartilage by specialized cells (chondrocytes).
**c. puncta′ta**, chondrodysplasia punctata.

**chon·dro·plast** (kon′dro-plast) [*chondro-* + *-plast*] chondroblast.

**chon·dro·plas·tic** (kon″dro-plas′tik) pertaining to plastic operations on cartilage.

**chon·dro·plas·ty** (kon′dro-plas″te) [*chondro-* + *-plasty*] plastic surgery on cartilage; repair of lacerated or displaced cartilage.

**chon·dro·po·ro·sis** (kon″dro-po-ro′sis) [*chondro-* + *porosis* (2)] the formation of spaces or sinuses in the cartilages; it occurs normally during ossification.

**chon·dro·sa·mine** (kon-dro′sə-mēn) older term for *galactosamine.*

**chon·dro·sar·co·ma** (kon″dro-sahr-ko′mə) [*chondro-* + *sarcoma*] [MeSH: Chondrosarcoma] a malignant tumor derived from cartilage cells or their precursors, but lacking direct osteoid formation; it occurs predominantly in the pelvis, femur, and shoulder girdle in middle-aged to older adults. It may be primary, arising from cartilage cells, or secondary to a pre-existing benign lesion.
**central c.**, one developing in the interior of a bone; it usually presents with dull pain but a mass is rare.
**clear cell c.**, a very rare form characterized by swollen, glycogen-rich clear cells, occurring usually in the femur, tibia, vertebrae, or pubis in adults; it is slow-growing and metastasizes only after multiple local recurrences.
**dedifferentiated c.**, a rare, fast-growing, very aggressive form of chondrosarcoma that contains additional malignant mesenchymal elements, such as areas of fibrosarcoma or spindle cells.
**juxtacortical c.**, that arising in relation to the cortex of the periosteum, occurring on the surface of the bone, particularly the femur or humerus, usually in adults.
**mesenchymal c.**, a rare, aggressive, malignant neoplasm composed of a small cell stroma containing islands of cartilaginous elements; it occurs primarily in flat bones, but also in soft tissue, and particularly in adolescents and young adults.
**myxoid c.**, chondromyxosarcoma.
**periosteal c.**, juxtacortical c.
**peripheral c.**, that arising on the surface of a bone; it may be either primary or secondary to underlying neoplasms, which are usually benign cartilage tumors, and generally presents as a large mass.

**chon·dro·sar·co·ma·to·sis** (kon″dro-sahr-ko″mə-to′sis) the formation of multiple chondrosarcomas.

**chon·dro·sar·co·ma·tous** (kon″dro-sahr-ko′mə-təs) pertaining to or of the nature of chondrosarcoma.

**chon·dro·sep·tum** (kon″dro-sep′təm) [*chondro-* + *septum*] pars cartilaginea septi nasi.

**chon·dro·sin** (kon′dro-sin) the basic disaccharide unit of chondroitin sulfate, comprising a molecule each of glucuronic acid and sulfated *N*-acetylgalactosamine in specific linkage.

**chon·dro·sis** (kon-dro′sis) [*chondro-* + *-sis*] the formation of cartilaginous tissue.

**chon·dro·skel·e·ton** (kon″dro-skel′ə-tən) 1. a cartilaginous skeleton, as in certain fish. 2. that part of the skeleton composed of cartilage.

**chon·dros·te·o·ma** (kon-dros″te-o′mə) osteochondroma.

**chon·dro·ster·nal** (kon″dro-stər′nəl) pertaining to the costal cartilages and the sternum.

**chon·dro·ster·no·plas·ty** (kon″dro-stər″no-plas′te) surgical correction of funnel chest.

**chon·dro·tome** (kon′dro-tōm) an instrument for cutting cartilage.

**chon·drot·o·my** (kon-drot′ə-me) [*chondro-* + *-tomy*] the dissection or surgical division of cartilage.

**chon·dro·troph·ic** (kon″dro-trof′ik) [*chondro-* + *-trophic*] having an influence on the formation or growth of cartilage.

**chon·dro·xi·phoid** (kon″dro-zi′foid) [*chondro-* + *xiphoid*] xiphisternal.

**Chon·drus** (kon′drəs) a genus of red algae. *C. cris′pus* (L.) Stackhouse is a source of carrageenan and chondrus.

**chon·drus** (kon′drəs) 1. any alga of the genus *Chondrus.* 2. dried and bleached algae, either *Chondrus crispus* or *Gigartina mammillosa,* which contain a polysaccharide widely used as a gel, thickening agent, emulsifier, and demulcent. Called also *carrageen, carragheen, killeen,* and *Irish, pearl,* or *salt rock moss.*

**cho·ne·chon·dro·ster·non** (ko″nə-kon″dro-stər′nən) pectus excavatum.

**CHOP** a regimen of cyclophosphamide, hydroxydaunomycin (doxorubicin), Oncovin (vincristine), and prednisone, used in cancer chemotherapy.

**CHOP-BLEO** a regimen of bleomycin, Adriamycin (doxorubicin), cyclophosphamide, Oncovin (vincristine), and prednisone, used in cancer chemotherapy.

**Cho·part's amputation (operation), articulation (joint)** (sho-pahrz′) [François *Chopart,* French surgeon, 1743–1795] see under *amputation,* and see *articulatio tarsi transversa.*

**cho·ran·gi·o·ma** (ko-ran″je-o′mə) chorioangioma.

**chord** (kord) cord.
**condyle c.,** condylar axis.

**chor·da** (kor′də) gen. and pl. *chor′dae* [L., from Gr. *chordē* cord] [TA] any cord or sinew.
**c. dorsa′lis,** notochord.
**c. guberna′culum,** gubernacular cord: a portion of the gubernaculum testis or of the round ligament of the uterus that develops in the inguinal crest and adjoining body wall.
**c. mag′na,** tendo calcaneus.
**c. obli′qua membra′nae interos′seae antebra′chii** [TA], a small ligamentous band extending from the lateral face of the tuberosity of the ulna to the radius a little distal to its tuberosity; called also *oblique cord of elbow joint,* and *Weitbrecht's cord* or *ligament.*
**c. sperma′tica,** funiculus spermaticus.
**chor′dae tendi′neae cor′dis** [TA], the tendinous cords that connect each cusp of the two atrioventricular valves to appropriate papillary muscles in the heart ventricles. The cords are of varying lengths and thicknesses and are frequently branched.
**c. tym′pani** [TA], a nerve originating from the facial nerve (nervus intermedius) and distributed to the submandibular, sublingual, and lingual glands and the anterior two-thirds of the tongue; modality: parasympathetic and special sensory. Called also *radix parasympathica ganglii submandibularis* [TA alternative] and *radix parasympathica ganglii sublingualis* [TA alternative].
**c. umbilica′lis,** umbilical cord.
**c. voca′lis,** plica vocalis.

**chor·dae** (kor′de) [L.] genitive and plural of *chorda.*

**chor·dal** (kor′dəl) pertaining to any chorda (chiefly used of the notochord).

**chor·da·meso·derm** (kor″də-mes′o-dərm) tissue of the dorsal lip of the blastopore, which gives rise to both notochord and mesoderm.

**Chor·da·ta** (kor-da′tə) [L. *chordatus* having a cord] [MeSH: Chordata] a phylum of the animal kingdom comprising all animals that have a notochord during some stage of their development. It includes the subphyla Cephalochordata, Urochordata, and Vertebrata.

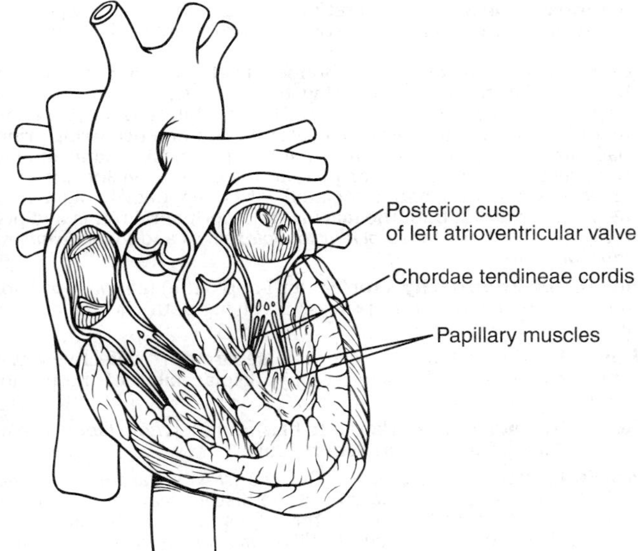


Chordae tendineae of the posterior cusps of atrioventricular valves in a cross-section of the heart.

**chor·date** (kor′dāt) 1. an animal belonging to the phylum Chordata. 2. having a notochord.

**chor·dec·to·my** (kor-dek′tə-me) [*chord-* + *-ectomy*] cordectomy.

**chor·dee** (kor′de, kor′da) [Fr. *cordée* corded] downward bowing of the penis as a result of a congenital anomaly (hypospadias) or a urethral infection (gonorrhea); called also *gryposis penis.*

**chor·di·tis** (kor-di′tis) inflammation of a vocal or spermatic cord.
**c. fibrino′sa,** acute laryngitis marked by the deposition of fibrin and the formation of erosions on the vocal cords.
**c. nodo′sa,** c. tuberosa.
**c. tubero′sa,** formation of small whitish nodules *(vocal cord nodules)* on one or both vocal cords, seen in persons who use their voices excessively; called also *c. nodosa.*
**c. voca′lis,** inflammation of the vocal cords.
**c. voca′lis infe′rior,** chronic subglottic laryngitis.

**chord(o)-** [L. *chorda,* q.v.] a combining form denoting relationship to a cord.

**chor·do·blas·to·ma** (kor″do-blas-to′mə) [*chordo-* + *blast-* + *-oma*] chordoma.

**chor·do·car·ci·no·ma** (kor″do-kahr″sĭ-no′mə) chordoma.

**chor·do·epi·the·li·o·ma** (kor″do-ep″ĭ-the″le-o′mə) chordoma.

**chor·doid** (kor′doid) resembling the notochord.

**chor·do·ma** (kor-do′mə) [*chord-* + *-oma*] [MeSH: Chordoma] a malignant tumor arising from the embryonic remains of the notochord, usually along the sella or in the sacrococcygeal region; called also *chordocarcinoma* and *chordoepithelioma.* Cf. *ecchondrosis physaliphora.*

**chor·do·pexy** (kor′do-pek″se) cordopexy.

**Chor·do·pox·vi·ri·nae** (kor″do-poks″vir-i′ne) [MeSH: Chordopoxvirinae] poxviruses of vertebrates: a subfamily of viruses of the family Poxviridae, containing the poxviruses that infect vertebrates. It includes the genera *Avipoxvirus, Capripoxvirus, Leporipoxvirus, Orthopoxvirus, Parapoxvirus, Suipoxvirus, Molluscipoxvirus,* and *Yatapoxvirus.*

**chor·do·sar·co·ma** (kor″do-sahr-ko′mə) chordoma.

**chor·do·skel·e·ton** (kor″do-skel′ə-ton) [*chordo-* + *skeleton*] that portion of the bony skeleton which is formed around the notochord.

**chor·dot·o·my** (kor-dot′ə-me) [*chordo-* + *-tomy*] cordotomy.

**cho·rea** (kə-re′-ə) [L.; Gr. *choreia* dance] [MeSH: Chorea] the ceaseless occurrence of a wide variety of rapid, highly complex, jerky, dyskinetic movements that appear to be well coordinated but are performed involuntarily.
**acute c.,** Sydenham's c.
**chronic c., chronic progressive hereditary c.,** Huntington's c.
**chronic progressive nonhereditary c.,** senile c.
**c. cor′dis,** chorea with great irregularity of the heart's action.
**dancing c.,** saltatory c.
**degenerative c.,** Huntington's c.
**c. dimidia′ta,** hemichorea.
**Dubini's c.,** an acute, fatal form due to acute infection of the central nervous system; called also *electric c.* and *Dubini's disease.*
**electric c.,** Dubini's c.
**fibrillary c.,** paramyoclonus.
**c. gravida′rum,** Sydenham's chorea occurring in the early months of pregnancy, with or without a previous history of rheumatic disease; it may recur in subsequent pregnancies.
**hemilateral c.,** hemichorea.
**hereditary c.,** Huntington's c.
**Huntington's c.,** an autosomal dominant disease characterized by chronic progressive chorea and mental deterioration terminating in dementia; the age of onset is variable but usually in the fourth decade of life, with death within 15 years. Called also *chronic progressive hereditary c., degenerative c., hereditary c.,* and *Huntington's disease.*
**hyoscine c.,** chorea-like movements occurring in acute hyoscine (scopolamine) intoxication.
**hysterical c.,** conversion disorder in which the symptoms are choreiform movements.
**juvenile c.,** Sydenham's c.
**methodic c.,** a variety in which the movements take place at regular intervals.
**mimetic c.,** that which is caused by imitation.
**c. mi′nor,** Sydenham's c.
**c. noctur′na,** chorea in which the movements continue during sleep.
**c. nu′tans,** nodding spasm, or chorea with nodding head movements.
**one-sided c.,** hemichorea.

**paralytic c.**, chorea in which immobility replaces movement; see *Huntington's c.*
**posthemiplegic c.**, a form that affects the partially paralyzed muscles after hemiplegia; see *athetosis.*
**saltatory c.**, any chorea, such as Sydenham's chorea, that involves involuntary jumping or dancing movements. See also *saltatory spasm.*
**senile c.**, a benign, usually mild disorder of the elderly, marked by choreiform movements unassociated with mental disturbance.
**simple c.**, Sydenham's c.
**Sydenham's c.**, an acute, usually self-limited disorder of early life, usually between the ages of 5 and 15, or during pregnancy, and closely linked with rheumatic fever. It is characterized by involuntary movements that gradually become severe, affecting all motor activities including gait, arm movements, and speech. A mild psychic component is usually present. The disorder may be limited to one side of the body (hemichorea) or may take the form of muscular rigidity (paralytic chorea). Called also *acute, juvenile,* or *simple c., c. minor,* and *St. Vitus' dance.*

**cho·re·al** (kor'e-əl) choreic.

**cho·re·ic** (ko-re'-ik) pertaining to, of the nature of, or characterized by chorea.

**cho·re·i·form** (ko-re'ĭ-form) [*chorea* + *form*] resembling chorea.

**cho·reo·acan·tho·cy·to·sis** (kor″e-o-ə-kan″tho-si-to'sis) [*chorea* + *acanthocytosis*] an autosomal recessive syndrome characterized by tics, chorea, and personality changes, with acanthocytes in the blood. Called also *neuroacanthocytosis.*

**cho·reo·ath·e·toid** (kor″e-o-ath'ə-toid) pertaining to or characterized by choreoathetosis.

**cho·reo·ath·e·to·sis** (kor″e-o-ath″ə-to'sis) a condition marked by choreic and athetoid movements.
**familial paroxysmal c.**, Mount-Reback syndrome.
**paroxysmal c.**, Mount-Reback syndrome.
**paroxysmal kinesigenic c.**, the most common form of Mount-Reback syndrome, with the choreoathetotic movements provoked by sudden movements or startling.

**cho·re·oid** (kor'e-oid) choreiform.

**cho·ri·al** (kor'e-əl) of or relating to the chorion.

**chori(o)-** [Gr. *chorion* membrane] a combining form denoting relationship to a membrane.

**cho·rio·ad·e·no·ma** (kor″e-o-ad″ə-no'mə) [*chorio-* + *adenoma*] an adenomatous tumor of the chorion.
**c. destru'ens**, a form of hydatidiform mole in which molar chorionic villi penetrate into the myometrium and/or parametrium or, rarely, are transported to distant sites, most often the lungs; called also *invasive* or *metastasizing mole.*

**cho·rio·al·lan·to·ic** (kor″e-o-al″an-to'ik) pertaining to the chorioallantois.

**cho·rio·al·lan·to·is** (kor″e-o-ə-lan'to-is) an extraembryonic structure derived from union of the chorion and allantois which by means of vessels in the associated mesoderm serves in gas exchange. In reptiles and birds, it is a membrane apposed to the egg shell; in many mammals, it forms the placenta.

**cho·rio·am·ni·o·ni·tis** (kor″e-o-am″ne-o-ni'tis) [MeSH: Chorioamnionitis] inflammation of the chorion and amnion.

**cho·rio·an·gio·fi·bro·ma** (kor″e-o-an″je-o-fi-bro'mə) angiofibroma of the chorion.

**cho·rio·an·gi·o·ma** (kor″e-o-an″je-o'mə) an angiomatous tumor of the chorion.

**cho·rio·blas·to·ma** (kor″e-o-blas-to'mə) choriocarcinoma.

**cho·rio·blas·to·sis** (kor″e-o-blas-to'sis) overgrowth of the chorion.

**cho·rio·cap·il·la·ris** (kor″e-o-kap″ĭ-lar'is) lamina choroidocapillaris.

**cho·rio·car·ci·no·ma** (kor″e-o-kahr″sĭ-no'mə) [*chorio-* + *carcinoma*] [MeSH: Choriocarcinoma] an epithelial malignancy of trophoblastic cells, formed by the abnormal proliferation of cuboidal and syncytial cells of the placental epithelium, without the production of chorionic villi. Almost all cases arise in the uterus, developing from hydatidiform mole, following abortion, or during normal pregnancy. The remainder occur in ectopic pregnancies and genital (ovarian and testicular) and extragenital teratomas. Called also *chorioblastoma, chorioepithelioma, chorionic carcinoma* or *epithelioma,* and *syncytioma malignum.*

**cho·rio·cele** (kor'e-o-sēl″) [*chorio-* + *-cele*[1]] protrusion of the eye through an aperture in the choroid.

**cho·rio·epi·the·li·o·ma** (kor″e-o-ep″ĭ-the″le-o'mə) choriocarcinoma.
**c. malig'num**, choriocarcinoma.

**cho·rio·gen·e·sis** (kor″e-o-jen'ə-sis) [*chorio-* + *-genesis*] the development of the chorion.

**cho·rio·gon·a·do·tro·pin** (ko″re-o-gon'ə-do-tro″pin) chorionic gonadotropin.

**cho·ri·oid** (kor'e-oid) choroid (def. 1).

**cho·ri·oi·dea** (kor″e-oi'de-ə) choroid (def. 1).

**chorioid(o)-** for words beginning thus, see those beginning *choroid(o)-.*

**cho·ri·o·ma** (kor″e-o'mə) [*chori-* + *-oma*] 1. any trophoblastic proliferation, benign or malignant. 2. choriocarcinoma.

**cho·rio·mam·mo·tro·pin** (ko″re-o-mam'o-tro″pin) human placental lactogen.

**cho·rio·men·in·gi·tis** (kor″e-o-men″in-ji'tis) cerebral meningitis with lymphocytic infiltration of the choroid plexuses.
**lymphocytic c.**, a form of meningitis caused by the lymphocytic choriomeningitis virus, usually occurring in adults 20 to 40 years of age during the late winter months. Infection results from contact with infected rodents and is usually asymptomatic or mild, although severe meningoencephalitis may occur.

**cho·ri·on** (kor'e-on) [Gr. "membrane"] [MeSH: Chorion] 1. in human embryology, the cellular, outermost extraembryonic membrane, composed of trophoblast lined with mesoderm; it develops villi about 2 weeks after fertilization, is vascularized by allantoic vessels a week later, gives rise to the placenta, and persists until birth. 2. in mammalian embryology, the cellular, outer extraembryonic membrane, not necessarily developing villi. 3. endometrial stroma. 4. in biology, the noncellular membrane covering eggs of various animals, including fish and insects. See illustration under *amnion.*
**c. frondo'sum**, the region of the chorion that bears villi; called also *shaggy c.* or *villous c.*
**c. lae've**, the smooth (nonvillous) and membranous part of the chorion. Called also *smooth c.*
**primitive c., primordial c.**, the chorion from its inception by addition of mesoderm to trophoblast through the stage in which it has many primordial villi.
**shaggy c.**, c. frondosum.
**smooth c.**, chorion laeve.
**villous c.**, c. frondosum.

**cho·ri·on·epi·the·li·o·ma** (kor″e-on-ep″ĭ-the″le-o'mə) choriocarcinoma.

**cho·ri·on·ic** (kor″e-on'ik) pertaining to the chorion.

**cho·rio·pla·cen·tal** (kor″e-o-plə-sen'təl) pertaining to the chorion and the placenta.

**Cho·ri·op·tes** (kor″e-op'tēz) a genus of parasitic mites of the family Psoroptidae, infesting the skin and hair of domestic animals and causing chorioptic mange.

**cho·ri·op·tic** (kor″e-op'tik) pertaining to or caused by *Chorioptes.*

**cho·rio·ret·i·nal** (kor″e-o-ret'ĭ-nəl) pertaining to the choroid and retina.

**cho·rio·ret·i·ni·tis** (kor″e-o-ret'ĭ-ni'tis) [*chorio-* + *retinitis*] [MeSH: Chorioretinitis] inflammation of the choroid and retina; retinochoroiditis.
**c. sclopeta'ria**, a concussive, nonpenetrating injury characterized by choroidal and retinal rupturing, hemorrhage, fibrosis and retinal destruction, and poor vision; caused by an orbital missile (gunshot).
**toxoplasmic c.**, a unilateral or bilateral condition occurring principally as a late sequel of congenital toxoplasmosis, manifested by recurrent episodes of ocular pain and decreased vision with progressive visual loss, and associated with deep, heavily pigmented, necrotic lesions in both the macular and peripheral retina and posterior uveitis. Called also *ocular toxoplasmosis* and *toxoplasmic retinochoroiditis.*

**cho·rio·ret·i·nop·a·thy** (kor″e-o-ret″ĭ-nop'ə-the) [*chorio-* + *retinopathy*] a noninflammatory process involving both choroid and retina.

**cho·ris·ta** (ko-ris'tah) [Gr. *chōristos* separated] defective development due to, or characterized by, displacement of the primordium.

**cho·ris·to·blas·to·ma** (kor-is″to-blas-to'mə) [*choristoma* + *blastoma*] [MeSH: Choristoma] choristoma.

**cho·ris·to·ma** (kor″is-to'mə) [Gr. *chōristos* separated + *-oma*] [MeSH: Choristoma] a mass of tissue histologically normal for an organ or part of the body other than the site at which it is located; called also *aberrant rest, choristoblastoma, heterotopia,* and *heterotopic tissue.*

**cho·roid** (kor'oid) [*chori-* + *-oid*] [MeSH: Choroid] 1. the thin, pigmented, vascular coat of the eye extending from the ora serrata to the optic nerve; it furnishes blood supply to the retina and conducts arteries and nerves to the anterior structures. Called also *chorioid, choroidea* [TA] and *chorioidea.* 2. resembling the chorion.

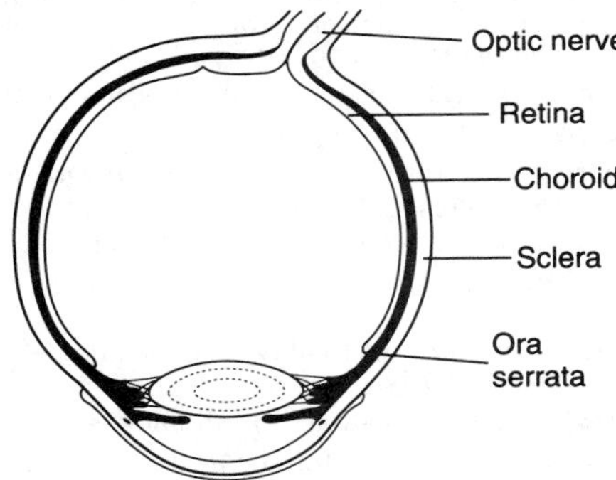


**cho·roid·al** (kor-oid′əl) pertaining to the choroid, def. 1.

**cho·roi·dea** (kor-oid′e-ə) [TA] choroid (def. 1).

**cho·roid·ec·to·my** (kor″oid-ek′tə-me) surgical removal or destruction of the choroid plexus of the lateral ventricles of the brain.

**cho·roid·er·e·mia** (kor″oid-ər-e′me-ə) [*choroid* + Gr. *erēmia* destitution] [MeSH: Choroideremia] hereditary primary choroidal degeneration, transmitted as an X-linked trait and beginning in the first decade of life. In males, the earliest symptom is usually night blindness, followed by constricted visual field and eventual blindness as the degeneration of the pigment epithelium of the retina progresses to complete atrophy. In females, it is nonprogressive; usually there is normal vision and often an atypical pigmentary retinopathy. Called also *progressive tapetochoroidal dystrophy.*

**cho·roid·itis** (kor″oid-i′tis) [*choroid* + *-itis*] [MeSH: Choroiditis] uveitis affecting the choroid, the posterior portion of the uveal tract.
**acute diffuse serous c.,** 1. a disease of sudden onset in adults, characterized by widespread, yellowish, fundal edema, by retinal detachment with loss of sight, and by later retinal reattachment with probable restoration of sight. 2. Harada's syndrome.
**anterior c.,** that in which there are points of inflammation in the peripheral choroid.
**areolar c., areolar central c.,** that which starts around or near the macula lutea and progresses toward the periphery. Unlike other forms of choroiditis, the lesions are pigmented at first and then lose their pigmentation. Called also *Förster's c.* or *disease.*
**central c.,** a variety in which the inflammation is in the region of the macula lutea.
**diffuse c.,** a widespread, exudative lesion of the choroid.
**disseminated c.,** exudative choroiditis with numerous isolated foci of inflammation on the fundus.
**Doyne's familial honeycombed c.,** a hereditary degenerative ocular abnormality marked by light-colored patches in the neighborhood of the optic disk and macula; called also *Doyne's familial colloid degeneration* and *Doyne's honeycomb degeneration.*
**exudative c.,** that which is characterized by scattered patches of an exudate.
**focal c.,** a localized choroiditis.
**Förster's c.,** areolar c.; called also *Förster disease.*
**c. gutta′ta seni′lis,** Tay's c.
**juxtapapillary c.,** choroiditis near the optic disk.
**macular c.,** choroiditis underlying the macula.
**metastatic c.,** a form due to metastasis in pyemia, meningitis, etc.
**senile macular exudative c.,** disciform macular degeneration.
**c. sero′sa,** glaucoma.
**suppurative c.,** that which leads to the formation of pus.
**Tay's c.,** degeneration of the choroid marked by irregular yellow spots around the macula lutea, and believed to be due to an atheromatous state of the arteries; seen in advanced life. Called also *c. guttata senilis* and *Tay's disease.*

**cho·roi·do·cyc·li·tis** (kor-oi″do-sik-li′tis) uveitis in the choroid and ciliary processes.

**cho·roi·do·iri·tis** (kor-oi″do-i-ri′tis) uveitis in the choroid coat and the iris.

**cho·roid·op·a·thy** (kor″oid-op′ə-the) [*choroid* + *-pathy*] choroiditis.

**cho·roi·do·ret·i·ni·tis** (kor-oi″do-ret″ĭ-ni′tis) chorioretinitis.

**Chot·zen's syndrome** (kot′zənz) [F. *Chotzen,* German psychiatrist, 20th century] see under *syndrome.*

**Christ-Sie·mens-Tou·raine syndrome** (krist-se′mənz-too-rān′) [Josef *Christ,* German dermatologist, 1871–1948; Hermann Werner *Siemens,* German dermatologist, 1891–1969; Henri *Touraine,* French dermatologist, 1883–1961] anhidrotic ectodermal dysplasia.

**Chris·ten·sen-Krab·be disease** (kris′tən-sən-krah′bə) [Erna *Christensen,* Danish pathologist, 1906–1967; Knud Haraldsen *Krabbe,* Danish neurologist, 1885–1961] Alpers' disease.

**Chris·tian's disease (syndrome)** (kris′chənz) [Henry Asbury *Christian,* American physician, 1876–1951] Hand-Schüller-Christian disease.

**Chris·tian-Web·er disease** (kris′chən-va′bər) [H. A. *Christian;* Frederick Parkes *Weber,* English physician, 1863–1962] relapsing febrile nodular nonsuppurative panniculitis.

**Christ·mas disease, factor** (kris′məs) [Stephen *Christmas,* 20th century Englishman, the first patient with the disease who was studied in detail] see *hemophilia B* and see *factor IX* at *coagulation factors,* under *factor.*

**chro·maf·fin** (kro-maf′in) [*chromium-* + L. *affinis* having affinity for] taking up and staining strongly with chromium salts; see *chromaffin cells,* under *cell.* Called also *chromaphil* and *pheochrome.*

**chro·maf·fin·i·ty** (kro″mə-fin′ĭ-te) the property of staining strongly with chrome salts.

**chro·maf·fi·no·ma** (kro-maf″ĭ-no′mə) any tumor containing chromaffin cells, such as a pheochromocytoma.
**medullary c.,** pheochromocytoma.

**chro·maf·fi·nop·a·thy** (kro-maf″ĭ-nop′ə-the) [*chromaffin* + *-pathy*] any disease of the chromaffin system.

**chro·ma·phil** (kro′mə-fil) [*chrom-* + *-phil*] chromaffin.

**chro·mar·gen·taf·fin** (kro″mahr-jen′tə-fin) [*chrom-* + *argentaffin*] staining with chromium salts and impregnable with silver; said of certain cells of the mucous membrane of the intestinal tract. Cf. *argentaffinoma.*

**chro·mate** (kro′māt) 1. any salt of chromic acid. 2. to subject to the action of a salt of chromic acid.

**chro·mat·ic** (kro-mat′ik) 1. pertaining to color; stainable with dyes. 2. pertaining to chromatin.

**chro·ma·tid** (kro′mə-tid) [MeSH: Chromatids] one of the paired chromosome strands, joined at the centromere, which make up a metaphase chromosome, resulting from chromosome reduplication during the S phase (DNA synthetic phase) of interphase.
**nonsister c's,** the two chromatids of one homologous chromosome with respect to those of the other homologue.
**sister c's,** the two chromatids of a chromosome held together by a centromere; dyads.

**chro·ma·tin** (kro′mə-tin) [Gr. *chrōma* color] [MeSH: Chromatin] the more readily stainable portion of the cell nucleus, forming a network of nuclear fibrils. It is a deoxyribonucleic acid attached to a protein (primarily histone) structure base and is the carrier of the genes in inheritance. It occurs in two states, euchromatin and heterochromatin, with different staining properties, and during cell division it coils and folds to form the metaphase chromosomes.
**nucleolar-associated c., nucleolus-associated c.,** heterochromatin containing DNA, situated around, and sometimes extending into, the nucleolus of a cell.
**sex c.,** a chromatin mass (Barr body) in the nucleus of female interphase cells of most mammalian species, including humans. It represents a single, inactive, condensed X chromosome. See *Lyon hypothesis,* under *hypothesis.*

**chro·ma·tin·ic** (kro″mə-tin′ik) of or pertaining to the chromatin.

**chro·ma·tin-neg·a·tive** (kro″mə-tin-neg′ə-tiv) lacking sex chromatin; characteristic of the nuclei of cells in a normal male or in other individuals with only one X chromosome.

**chro·ma·tin-pos·i·tive** (kro″mə-tin-poz′ĭ-tiv) having sex chromatin (Barr body) in the nuclei of somatic cells, a characteristic of the normal female or of other individuals with two (or more) X chromosomes.

**chro·ma·tism** (kro′mə-tiz″əm) abnormal pigment deposits.

**chro·ma·tize** (kro′mə-tīz) to charge with some chromium compound.

**chromat(o)-** [Gr. *chrōma,* gen. *chrōmatos* color] a combining form denoting relationship to (1) color, or (2) chromatin.

**chro·mato·blast** (kro-mat′o-blast) [*chromato-* + *-blast*] a cell that can become a chromatophore, or bearer of pigment.

**chro·ma·to·ci·ne·sis** (kro″mə-to-sĭ-ne′sis) chromatokinesis.

**chro·ma·tog·e·nous** (kro″mə-toj′ə-nəs) [*chromato-* + *-genous*] producing color or coloring matter.

**chro·mato·gram** (kro-mat′o-gram) [*chromato-* + *gram*] originally the pattern of bands of substances separated by column chromatography, so called because the technique was first used to separate plant pigments producing a pattern of colored bands; by extension, a permanent record produced by any form of chromatography, e.g., in paper or thin-layer chromatography, a dried and stained filter paper or plate and, in gas or high-performance liquid chromatography, the chart recorder output.

**chro·mato·graph** (kro-mat′o-graf) 1. the apparatus used in chromatography. 2. to analyze by chromatography.

**chro·ma·to·graph·ic** (kro″mə-to-graf′ik) pertaining to or produced by chromatography.

**chro·ma·tog·ra·phy** (kro″mə-tog′rə-fe) [MeSH: Chromatography] any of a diverse group of techniques used to separate mixtures of substances based on differences in the relative affinities of the substances for two different media, one (the mobile phase) a moving fluid and the other (the stationary phase or sorbent) a porous solid or gel or a liquid coated on a solid support; the speed at which each substance is carried along by the mobile phase depends on its solubility (in a liquid mobile phase) or vapor pressure (in a gas mobile phase) and on its affinity for the sorbent.
**adsorption c.,** that in which the stationary phase is a nonspecific adsorbent, such as silica gel, porous polymers, or charcoal.
**affinity c.,** that based on a highly specific biologic interaction such as that between antigen and antibody, enzyme and substrate, or receptor and ligand. Any of these substances, covalently linked to an insoluble support or immobilized in a gel, may serve as the sorbent allowing the interacting substance to be isolated from relatively impure samples; often a 1000-fold purification can be achieved in one step.
**column c.,** a type of chromatography using a sorbent packed in a column. The sample, dissolved in a solvent, is poured in the top. Some components are retained in the column bound to the sorbent. They are then washed out (eluted) in successive aliquots of the same solvent (more strongly bound components being eluted later) or of different solvents.
**gas c. (GC),** a type of automated chromatography in which the sample, dissolved in a solvent, is vaporized and carried by an inert gas through a column packed with a sorbent to any of several types of detector. Each component of the sample, separated from the others by passage through the column, produces a separate peak in the detector output, which is graphed by a chart recorder. The sorbent may be an inert porous solid *(gas-solid c.)* or a nonvolatile liquid coated on a solid support *(gas-liquid c.)*.
**gas-liquid c. (GLC),** see *gas c.*
**gas-solid c. (GSC),** see *gas c.*
**gel-filtration c., gel-permeation c.,** that in which the stationary phase consists of gel-forming hydrophilic beads containing pores of an accurately controlled size. As the sample is carried through the gel small molecules are frequently trapped in the pores and delayed while larger molecules pass unimpeded. Sample components are thus separated on the basis of size and shape. Called also *molecular exclusion c.* and *molecular sieve c.*
**high-performance liquid c., high-pressure liquid c. (HPLC),** a type of automated chromatography in which the mobile phase is a liquid, which is forced under high pressure through a column packed with a sorbent. As in gas chromatography, a detector at the end of the column coupled to a chart recorder graphs the sample efflux. Various separation methods, including adsorption, gel filtration, ion-exchange, and partition, are used.
**ion-exchange c.,** that in which the stationary phase is an ion-exchange resin. The mobile phase is an aqueous buffer solution that determines the degree of ionization of the sample components and thus their affinity for the stationary phase.
**liquid-liquid c.,** partition c.
**molecular exclusion c., molecular sieve c.,** gel-filtration c.
**paper c.,** a type of chromatography in which the stationary phase is a sheet of special-grade filter paper; it is in all other aspects similar to thin-layer chromatography (q.v.).
**partition c.,** that in which the stationary and mobile phases are immiscible liquids and the sample components are separated on the basis of their partition coefficients. Called also *liquid-liquid c.*
**thin-layer c. (TLC),** type of chromatography in which the stationary phase is a thin layer of an adsorbent, e.g., silica gel, coated on a rectangular plate and the mobile phase is a solvent mixture. The sample is applied to a small spot on the plate, and then the plate is stood on end with its lower edge in solvent. As the solvent rises by capillary action through the adsorbent, the components of the sample are carried along at different rates and can be visualized as a row of spots after the plate is dried and stained or viewed under ultraviolet light.

**chro·ma·toid** (kro′mə-toid) having the tinctorial properties of chromatin; see also under *body.*

**chro·ma·to·ki·ne·sis** (kro″mə-to-kĭ-ne′sis) [*chromato-* + *-kinesis*] movement of chromatin during the life and division of a cell.

**chro·ma·tol·o·gy** (kro″mə-tol′ə-je) [*chromato-* + *-logy*] the science of colors.

**chro·ma·tol·y·sis** (kro″mə-tol′ə-sis) [*chromato-* + *-lysis*] disintegration of the Nissl (chromophil) bodies of a nerve cell as the result of injury, or of fatigue or exhaustion; a part of the so-called axon reaction.

**chro·ma·tom·e·ter** (kro″mə-tom′ə-tər) [*chromato-* + *-meter*] an instrument for measuring color or color perception; called also *chromatoptometer, chromometer,* and *chromoptometer.*

**chro·ma·to·pec·tic** (kro″mə-to-pek′tik) chromopectic.

**chro·ma·to·pex·is** (kro″mə-to-pek′sis) chromopexy.

**chro·ma·toph·a·gus** (kro″mə-tof′ə-gəs) [*chromato-* + Gr. *phagein* to devour] destroying pigments.

**chro·ma·to·phil** (kro′mə-to-fil″) a cell or element that stains easily.

**chro·ma·to·phile** (kro′mə-to-fīl″) 1. chromatophil. 2. chromatophilic.

**chro·ma·to·phil·ia** (kro″mə-to-fil′e-ə) [*chromato-* + *-philia*] the condition of staining easily.

**chro·ma·to·phil·ic** (kro″mə-to-fil′ik) staining easily.

**chro·ma·toph·i·lous** (kro″mə-tof′ĭ-ləs) chromatophilic.

**chro·mato·phore** (kro-mat′o-for″) [*chromato-* + *-phore*] [MeSH: Chromatophores] any pigmentary cell or color-producing plastid, such as those of the cutis or deep layers of the epidermis.

**chro·ma·to·pho·ro·trop·ic** (kro″mə-to-for″o-trop′ik) having an influence or effect on chromatophores, as the pigmentary effect of melanocyte-stimulating hormone.

**chro·ma·to·plasm** (kro′mə-to-plaz″əm) the colored portions of the protoplasm of a pigmented cell.

**chro·ma·top·sia** (kro″mə-top′se-ə) [*chromato-* + *-opsia*] 1. a visual defect in which colored objects appear unnaturally colored and colorless objects appear tinged with color. The chromatopsias are named for the colors seen: cyanopsia, blue; chloropsia, green; erythropsia, red; xanthopsia, yellow. Chromatopsia may be caused by drugs, disturbance of the optic centers, cataract extraction, or dazzling light. 2. imperfect perception of color; anomalous color vision.

**chro·ma·top·tom·e·ter** (kro″mə-top-tom′ə-tər) chromatometer.

**chro·ma·top·tom·e·try** (kro″mə-top-tom′ə-tre) the testing of the power of discriminating colors.

**chro·mato·scope** (kro-mat′o-skōp) [*chromato-* + *-scope*] an instrument used in chromatoscopy (def. 1).

**chro·ma·tos·co·py** (kro″mə-tos′kə-pe) [*chromato-* + *-scopy*] 1. the testing of color vision. 2. diagnosis of renal function by the color of the urine following the administration of dyes.
**gastric c.,** diagnosis of gastric function by the color of the gastric contents; a test for achylia gastrica.

**chro·ma·to·ski·am·e·ter** (kro″mə-to-ski-am′ə-tər) [*chromato-* + *skia-* + *-meter*] chromatometer that uses colored shadows.

**chro·ma·to·tax·is** (kro″mə-to-tak′sis) [*chromato-* + *-taxis*] the attraction or influence of certain substances on the chromatin of a cell nucleus, causing destruction of the chromatin, while the cell body remains intact.

**chro·ma·to·trop·ism** (kro″mə-tot′rə-piz-əm) [*chromato-* + *tropism*] an orienting response to a color.

**chro·ma·tu·ria** (kro″mə-tu′re-ə) [*chromato-* + *-uria*] abnormal coloration of the urine.

**-chrome** [Gr. *chroma* color] a word termination denoting relationship to color.

**1,2-chro·mene** (kro′mēn) a plant pigment, a constituent of oxidized tocopherol; called also *1,2-benzopyran.*

**chro·mes·the·sia** (kro″mes-the′zhə) [*chrom-* + *esthesia*] the association of imaginary sensations of color with actual sensations of hearing, taste, or smell; see *photism.*

**chrom·hi·dro·sis** (kro″mĭ-dro′sis) [*chrom-* + *hidro-* + *-sis*] the secretion of colored sweat; called also *chromidrosis.*

**chro·mic ac·id** (kro′mik) the common name for chromium trioxide ($CrO_3$), although the term strictly refers to the species $H_2CrO_4$, which exists only in aqueous solution. It is a highly toxic, corrosive, strong oxidizing agent.

**chro·mi·cize** (kro′mĭ-sīz) to treat with a chromium compound.

**chro·mid·ro·sis** (kro″mid-ro′sis) chromhidrosis.

**chro·mi·um** (kro′me-əm) [L.; Gr. *chrōma* color] [MeSH: Chromium] a blue-white, brittle metal: atomic number, 24; atomic weight, 51.996; specific gravity, 7.1; symbol, Cr; several of its compounds are pigments, and the metal itself is used for weather-resistant plating; it is also an important component of most base metal alloys used in dentistry. Chromium plays a role in glucose metabolism and is considered essential in trace amounts in nutrition. Hexavalent chromium is carcinogenic.

**c. 51,** a radioactive isotope of chromium, atomic mass 51, having a half-life of 27.7 days; it decays by electron capture, emitting gamma rays (0.32 MeV), and is used to label red blood cells for measurement of red cell mass or volume, survival time, and sequestration studies, and for the diagnosis of gastrointestinal bleeding, and is used to label platelets to study their survival. It has also been used to label human serum albumin for measurements of gastrointestinal protein loss.
**c. picolinate** [NF], a biologically active form of chromium, used as a nutritional supplement.
**c. trioxide,** see *chromic acid.*

**chrom(o)-** [Gr. *chrōma* color] a combining form denoting relationship to color.

**Chro·mo·bac·te·ri·um** (kro″mo-bak-tēr′e-əm) [*chromo-* + *bacterium*] [MeSH: Chromobacterium] a genus of gram-negative, aerobic or facultatively anaerobic, usually nonpathogenic, rod-shaped bacteria, found in soil and water in tropical countries, characteristically producing violet pigment that is soluble in alcohol but not in water or chloroform.
**C. viola′ceum,** a species that may infect humans, causing abscesses, diarrhea, and urinary tract and systemic infections.

**chro·mo·blast** (kro′mo-blast) [*chromo-* + *-blast*] an embryonic cell that develops into a pigment cell.

**chro·mo·blas·to·my·co·sis** (kro″mo-blas″to-mi-ko′sis) [*chromo-* + *blasto-* + *mycosis*] [MeSH: Chromoblastomycosis] a chronic fungal infection of the skin, usually beginning at the site of a puncture wound or other trauma and affecting one leg or foot (mossy foot) but sometimes involving other areas of the body, producing wartlike nodules or papillomas that may or may not ulcerate; microscopically, the lesions are characterized by round, brown bodies (sclerotic bodies) that reproduce by equatorial splitting and not by budding. It is usually caused by *Phialophora verrucosa, Fonsecaea pedrosoi, F. compactum, Cladosporium carrionii,* or some other dematiaceous fungi. Called also *chromomycosis* and *verrucose* or *verrucous dermatitis.*

**chro·mo·cen·ter** (kro′mo-sen″tər) [*chromo-* + *center* (def. 1)] 1. karyosome. 2. a fused mass of heterochromatin with spokelike extensions of euchromatin, representing portions of the chromosomes in the salivary glands of some insects.

**chro·mo·cho·los·co·py** (kro″mo-ko-los′kə-pe) [*chromo-* + *cholo-* + *-scopy*] testing the biliary function by a pigment excretion test (methylthionine chloride).

**chro·mo·clas·to·gen·ic** (kro″mo-klas″to-jen′ik) giving rise to or inducing chromosomal disruption or damage.

**chro·mo·cys·tos·co·py** (kro″mo-sis-tos′kə-pe) [*chromo-* + *cystoscopy*] examination of the interior of the bladder after administration of indigo carmine or other dye which is excreted in the urine, for identification and study of the activity of the ureteral orifices; called also *chromoureteroscopy* and *cystochromoscopy.*

**chro·mo·cyte** (kro′mo-sīt) [*chromo-* + *-cyte*] any colored cell or pigmented corpuscle.

**chro·mo·dac·ry·or·rhea** (kro″mo-dak″re-o-re′ə) [*chromo-* + *dacryo-* + *-rrhea*] the shedding of bloody tears.

**chro·mo·di·ag·no·sis** (kro″mo-di″əg-no′sis) [*chromo-* + *diagnosis*] 1. diagnosis by change of color. 2. diagnosis of functional derangements by observing the rate at which coloring matters, such as methylthionine chloride, are excreted. 3. diagnostic examination made through colored glass or sheets of colored gelatin.

**chro·mo·fla·vine** (kro″mo-fla′vēn) acriflavine.

**chro·mo·gen** (kro′mo-jən) 1. a chemical compound, itself without color, that can be transformed into a colored compound, or can react with another material to form a colored compound. 2. a microorganism that produces pigment, e.g., certain strains of *Mycobacterium* that produce yellow to red colonies.
**Porter-Silber c.,** a 17-hydroxycorticosteroid with a dihydroxyacetone side chain; these react positively in the Porter-Silber reaction.

**chro·mo·gen·e·sis** (kro″mo-jen′ə-sis) [*chromo-* + *genesis*] the formation of pigments or colors, as by bacterial action.

**chro·mo·gen·ic** (kro″mo-jen′ik) producing a pigment or coloring matter.

**chro·mo·gran·in** (kro″mo-gran′in) any of a group of acidic polypeptides that are the major soluble protein constituents of the secretory granules of the chromaffin cells of the adrenal medulla; they are also widely distributed in endocrine tissues and tumor cells. Some are precursors of peptide hormones.

**chro·mo·isom·er·ism** (kro″mo-i-som′ər-iz-əm) [*chromo-* + *isomerism*] isomerism in which the isomers have different colors.

**chro·mo·lip·oid** (kro″mo-lip′oid) lipochrome.

**chro·mo·mere** (kro′mo-mēr) [*chromo-* + *-mere*] 1. any of the bead-like granules seen in prophase occurring in series along the chromonema of a chromosome; called also *idiomere.* 2. granulomere.

**chro·mom·e·ter** (kro-mom′ə-tər) 1. chromatometer. 2. colorimeter.

**chro·mo·my·co·sis** (kro″mo-mi-ko′sis) chromoblastomycosis.

**chro·mone** (kro′mōn) [Gr. *chrōma* color] coumarin.

**chro·mo·ne·ma** (kro″mo-ne′mə) pl. *chromone′mata* [*chromo-* + *nema*] the coiled central thread of a chromatid, as opposed to the more densely coiled chromomere regions.

**chro·mo·ne·mal** (kro″mo-ne′məl) of or pertaining to a chromonema.

**chro·mo·ne·ma·ta** (kro″mo-ne′mə-tə) plural of *chromonema.*

**chro·mo·neme** (kro′mo-nēm) chromonema.

**chro·mo·par·ic** (kro-mo-par′ik) [*chromo-* + L. *parere* to produce] producing or giving rise to color; chromogenic.

**chro·mo·pec·tic** (kro″mo-pek′tik) pertaining to, characterized by, or promoting chromopexy.

**chro·mo·pex·ic** (kro″mo-pek′sik) chromopectic.

**chro·mo·pexy** (kro′mo-pek″se) [*chromo-* + *-pexy*] the fixation of pigment, a term applied especially to the function of the liver in forming bilirubin.

**chro·mo·phage** (kro′mo-fāj) [*chromo-* + *-phage*] pigmentophage.

**chro·mo·phane** (kro′mo-fān) [*chromo-* + Gr. *phainein* to show] a retinal pigment found in some species of animals.

**chro·mo·phil** (kro′mo-fil) [*chromo-* + *-phil*] any easily stainable cell, structure, or tissue.

**chro·mo·phile** (kro′mo-fīl) 1. chromophil. 2. chromophilic.

**chro·mo·phil·ic** (kro-mo-fil′ik) readily or easily stained; said especially of certain leukocytes and other histologic elements.

**chro·moph·i·lous** (kro-mof′ĭ-ləs) chromophilic.

**chro·mo·phobe** (kro′mo-fōb) [*chromo-* + Gr. *phobein* to be affrighted by] any cell, structure, or tissue that does not stain readily; such as the nonstaining cells of the adenohypophysis.

**chro·mo·pho·bia** (kro″mo-fo′be-ə) the quality of staining poorly with dyes.

**chro·mo·phore** (kro′mo-for) any chemical group whose presence gives a decided color to a compound and which unites with certain other groups (auxochromes) to form dyes; called also *color radical.*

**chro·mo·phor·ic** (kro″mo-for′ik) [*chromo-* + Gr. *pherein* to bear] 1. bearing color; said of chromogenic bacteria when the pigment is a component of the bacterial cell itself. 2. pertaining to a chromophore.

**chro·moph·o·rous** (kro-mof′ər-əs) chromophoric.

**chro·mo·phose** (kro′mo-fōs) [*chromo-* +*phose*] a subjective sensation of a spot of color in the eye.

**chro·mo·pho·to·ther·a·py** (kro″mo-fo″to-ther′ə-pe) [*chromo-* + *photo-* + *therapy*] chromotherapy.

**chro·mo·plasm** (kro′mo-plaz-əm) [*chromo-* + *-plasm*] chromatin.

**chro·mo·plast** (kro′mo-plast) [MeSH: Plastids] chromoplastid.

**chro·mo·plas·tid** (kro″mo-plas′tid) [*chromo-* + *plastid*] any pigment-producing plastid other than a chloroplast.

**chro·mo·pro·tein** (kro″mo-pro′tēn) [*chromo-* + *protein*] a colored conjugated protein. Examples are the red hemoglobin of the higher animals, the blue hemocyanin of many lower animals, and the red and blue pigments of seaweeds. Chromoproteins have respiratory functions and are closely related to the green chlorophyll of the higher plants.

**chro·mop·sia** (kro-mop′se-ə) chromatopsia.

**chro·mop·tom·e·ter** (kro″mop-tom′ə-tər) chromatoptometer.

**chro·mo·ret·i·nog·ra·phy** (kro″mo-ret″ĭ-nog′rə-fe) [*chromo-* + *retina* + *-graphy*] color photography of the retina.

**chro·mo·rhi·nor·rhea** (kro″mo-ri″no-re′ə) [*chromo-* + *rhinorrhea*] the discharge of a pigmented secretion from the nose.

**chro·mo·san·to·nin** (kro″mo-san′to-nin) yellow santonin; an isomeric form produced when santonin is exposed to sunlight.

**chro·mo·scope** (kro′mo-skōp) chromatoscope.

**chro·mos·co·py** (kro-mos′kə-pe) chromatoscopy.

**chro·mo·so·mal** (kro″mo-sōm′əl) pertaining to chromosomes.

**chro·mo·some** (kro′mo-sōm) [*chromo-* + *-some*] [MeSH: Chromosomes] 1. in animal cells, a structure in the nucleus containing a linear thread of DNA, which transmits genetic information and is associated with RNA and histones; during cell division, the material

(chromatin) composing the chromosome is compactly coiled, making it visible with appropriate staining and permitting its movement in the cell with minimal entanglement. Each organism of a species normally has a characteristic number of chromosomes in its somatic cells, 46 being the number normally present in man, including the two (XX or XY) which determine the sex of the organism. See illustration. 2. in bacterial genetics, a closed circle of double-stranded DNA that contains the genetic material of the cell and is attached to the cell membrane; the bulk of the material forms a compact bacterial nucleus (called also *chromatinic body).*
**accessory c's,** supernumerary c's.
**acentric c.,** a chromosome with no centromere.
**acrocentric c.,** a chromosome with the centromere near one end. In humans such chromosomes have satellited short arms that carry genes for ribosomal RNA.
**B c.,** supernumerary c.
**bivalent c.,** see *bivalent,* def. 2.
**daughter c's,** the name for chromatids when they reach the poles of the cell in the anaphase stage of mitosis.
**dicentric c.,** a structurally abnormal chromosome with two centromeres.
**gametic c.,** chromosome of a haploid cell (gamete).
**giant c's,** 1. polytene c's. 2. lampbrush c's.
**heterotypical c's,** see *sex c's.*
**homologous c's,** a matching pair of chromosomes, one from each parent, with the same gene loci in the same order.
**lampbrush c's,** giant chromosomes of the oocytes of many lower animals arranged like a cylindrical brush.
**m-c.,** mitochondrial c.
**metacentric c.,** a chromosome with its centromere in the center and arms of equal length.
**mitochondrial c.,** a small single circular chromosome within each mitochondrion, capable of synthesizing protein since it contains ribosomal RNA, messenger RNA, and transfer RNA. The mitochondrial chromosome carries the genes for 13 proteins and is the basis for maternal inheritance (q.v.); some authorities consider it the 25th human chromosome in addition to the 22 autosomes and the X and Y chromosomes.
**nucleolar c's,** those in relation to which the nucleoli reorganize during the telophase of mitosis.
**odd c's,** see *sex c's.*
**Ph[1] c., Philadelphia c.,** an abnormality of chromosome 22, characterized by shortening of its long arms (the missing portion usually translocated to chromosome 9) and present in marrow cells of most patients with chronic granulocytic leukemia.
**polytene c's,** giant bundles of unseparated chromonemata occurring especially in the salivary glands of some insects; called also *giant c's.*
**ring c.,** a chromosome in which both ends have been lost (deletion) and the two broken ends have reunited to form a ring. Symbol r. See Plate 1.
**sex c's,** chromosomes that are associated with the determination of sex, in mammals constituting an unequal pair, the X and the Y chromosome.
**small c.,** m-c.
**somatic c.,** a chromosome of a diploid (tissue) cell of the body.
**submetacentric c.,** a chromosome with its centromere slightly off-center so that the arms are different in length.
**supernumerary c.,** one or more extra chromosomes found inconstantly in wild populations of certain species of animals; they are not homologous to members of the regular set of chromosomes and apparently exert little influence on the phenotypic effect. Called also *accessory* and *B c.*
**telocentric c.,** a chromosome with a terminal centromere; not normally found in humans.
**W c's,** the sex chromosomes of certain insects, birds, and fishes, in which the female is heterogametic (i.e., has a W and a Z chromosome) and the males are homogametic (having only Z chromosomes).
**X c.,** the female sex chromosome, being the differential sex chromosome carried by half the male gametes and all female gametes in man and other male-heterogametic species.
**Y c.,** the male sex chromosome, being the differential sex chromosome carried by half the male gametes and none of the female gametes in man and in some other male-heterogametic species in which the homologue of the X chromosome has been retained.
**yeast artificial c. (YAC),** a DNA segment, containing up to 1000 kilobase pairs and having a centromere and telomere, introduced into the yeast *Saccharomyces cerevisiae;* it allows the cloning and isolation of much larger DNA segments than is possible using bacterial cloning.
**Z c's,** see *W c's.*

**Symbols Used in Chromosome Nomenclature**

| Symbol | Meaning |
|---|---|
| A–G | Chromosome groups |
| 1–22 | Autosome numbers |
| X, Y | Sex chromosomes |
| / | Diagonal line separating cell lines in descriptions of mosaicism |
| ? | Identification of chromosome or chromosome structure questionable |
| + − | When placed before the chromosome number, these denote addition or loss of a whole chromosome; when placed after the chromosome number, they denote an increase or decrease in length of a chromosome part. |
| : | Break with no reunion |
| : : | Break with reunion |
| → | From . . . to . . . |
| ace | Acentric |
| cen | Centromere |
| del | Deletion |
| der | Derivative chromosome |
| dic | Dicentric |
| dup | Duplication |
| end | Endoreduplication |
| h | Secondary constriction or negatively staining region |
| i | Isochromosome |
| ins | Insertion |
| inv | Inversion |
| inv ins | Inverted insertion |
| mar | Marker chromosome |
| mat | Maternal origin |
| p | Short arm |
| pat | Paternal origin |
| q | Long arm |
| r | Ring chromosome |
| rep | Reciprocal translocation |
| rec | Recombinant chromosome |
| rob | Robertsonian translocation |
| s | Satellite |
| t | Translocation |
| ter | Terminal |

Repeated symbols denote duplication of chromosome structure.
Symbols for rearrangements are placed before the chromosome number and the rearranged chromosomes are placed in parenthesis, e.g., t(14q21q), r(18).

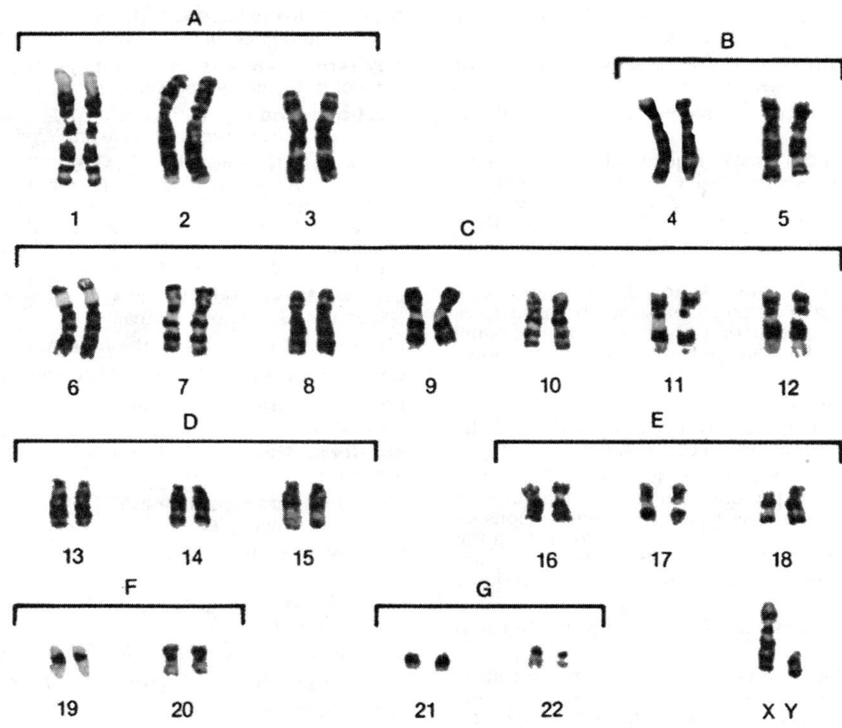


Human male chromosomes with Giemsa banding (Type G banding), arranged as a karyotype.

**chro·mo·sperm·ism** (kro″mo-spər′miz-əm) [*chromo-* + *sperm*] a colored condition of the sperm.

**chro·mo·ther·a·py** (kro″mo-ther′ə-pe) [*chromo-* + *therapy*] the therapeutic use of light of restricted areas of the spectrum; called also *beam therapy.*

**chro·mo·tox·ic** (kro″mo-tok′sik) [*chromo-* + *toxic*] destructive to hemoglobin or due to the destruction of hemoglobin.

**chro·mo·trich·ia** (kro″mo-trik′e-ə) [*chromo-* + *trich-* + *-ia*] coloration of the hair.

**chro·mo·trich·i·al** (kro″mo-trik′e-əl) pertaining to the coloration of the hair.

**chro·mo·trop·ic** (kro″mo-trop′ik) [*chromo-* + *-tropic*] turning to or attracting color or pigment.

**chro·mo·ure·ter·os·co·py** (kro″mo-u-re″tər-os′kə-pe) chromocystoscopy.

**chro·mo·uri·nog·ra·phy** (kro″mo-u″rĭ-nog′rə-fe) diagnosis by measuring the intensity of color and the time of appearance in the urine after injection of a dye.

**chro·nax·ie** (kro′nak-se) chronaxy.

**chro·naxy** (kro′nak-se) [*chron-* + Gr. *axios* fit] [MeSH: Chronaxy] the minimum time an electric current must flow at a voltage twice the rheobase to cause a muscle to contract.

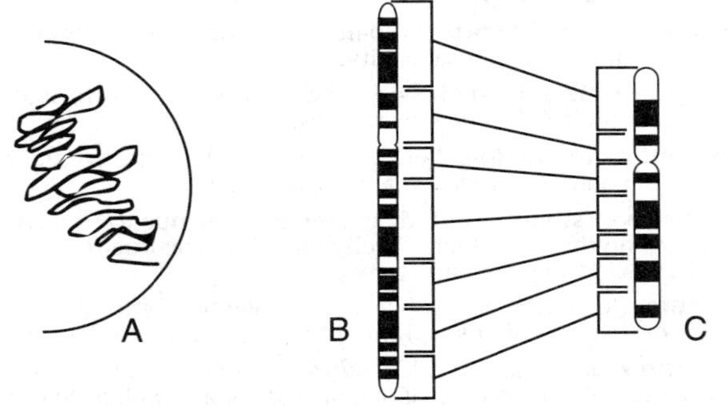


Chromosome. *(A)*, Long, threadlike interphase chromatin in nucleus. *(B)*, Giemsa-stained, partially condensed chromatid in late prophase. *(C)*, Giemsa-stained, fully condensed chromatid in metaphase; note that some of the of the sub-bands visible in late prophase have condensed into single bands. (In *B* and *C*, only one of a pair of sister chromatids is shown).

**chron·ic** (kron′ik) [L. *chronicus,* from Gr. *chronos* time] persisting over a long period of time.

**chro·nic·i·ty** (kro-nis′ĭ-te) the quality of being chronic.

**chron(o)-** [Gr. *chronos* time] a combining form denoting relationship to time.

**chron·o·bi·o·log·ic, chron·o·bi·o·log·i·cal** (kron″o-bi″o-loj′ik, kron″o-bi″o-loj′ĭ-kəl) pertaining to chronobiology; relating to the effects of time and biologic rhythms on living systems.

**chron·o·bi·ol·o·gist** (kron″o-bi-ol′ə-jist) a specialist in chronobiology.

**chron·o·bi·ol·o·gy** (kron″o-bi-ol′ə-je) [*chrono-* + *biology*] [MeSH: Chronobiology] the scientific study of the effect of time on living systems.

**chron·og·no·sis** (kron″og-no′sis) [*chrono-* + Gr. *gnōsis* knowledge] the subjective appreciation of the passage of time.

**chron·o·graph** (kron′o-graf) [*chrono-* + *-graph*] an instrument for recording small intervals of time.

**chro·nom·e·try** (kro-nom′ə-tre) [*chrono-* + *-metry*] the measurement of time or intervals of time.
**mental c.,** the measurement and study of the duration of mental processes.

**chron·o·pho·bia** (kron″o-fo′be-ə) [*chrono-* + *-phobia*] extreme, irrational fear of time; because it is so common in prisoners, it is sometimes called *prison neurosis* (q.v.).

**chron·o·pho·to·graph** (kron″o-fo′tə-graf) [*chrono-* + *photograph*] a photograph taken with a kinetoscope.

**chron·o·scope** (kron′o-skōp) [*chrono-* + *-scope*] an instrument for measuring minute intervals of time.

**chro·no·tar·ax·is** (kron″o-tər-ak′sis) [*chrono-* + Gr. *taraxis* confusion] disorientation for time; observed as a transient symptom following thalamic or frontal lobe lesions.

**chronotherapy** (kro′no-ther″ə-pe) [MeSH: Chronotherapy] treatment of certain sleep disorders by capitalizing on the natural phase delay in adults; the bedtime is successively advanced by one to several hours each day until the individual can retire, sleep, and arise at appropriate times.

**chron·o·trop·ic** (kron″o-trop′ik) [*chrono-* + *-tropic*] affecting the time or rate, as the rate of contraction of the heart.

**chro·not·ro·pism** (kro-not′ro-piz-əm) modulation of the regularity of a periodic movement, such as the heart beat.

**chro·to·plast** (kro′to-plast) [Gr. *chrōs* skin + *-plast*] a dermal or skin cell.

**chrys·a·lis** (kris′ə-lis) [L.] the pupa of some insects, especially of a moth or butterfly.

**Chry·san·the·mum** (krĭ-san′thə-məm) a genus of perennial flowering herbs of the family Compositae, native to the Balkans and the Middle East, some of which were formerly classified in genus *Pyrethrum.* They are a common cause of contact dermatitis, and their powdered flowers are insecticidal and scabicidal and a source of pyrethrins.

**chrys·a·ro·bin** (kris″ə-ro′bin) a brownish to yellow-orange microcrystalline powder consisting of a mixture of the neutral principles extracted from Goa powder; a reduction product of chrysophanic acid, it is used topically in the treatment of psoriasis and other chronic skin disease.

**chrys·a·zin** (kris′ə-zin) danthron.

**chry·sene** (kri′sēn) a carcinogenic tetracyclic hydrocarbon derived from coal tar by distillation and used in organic synthesis.

**chry·si·a·sis** (krĭ-si′ə-sis) [*chrys-* + *-iasis*] 1. deposition of gold particles in the tissues as a result of prolonged or excessive parenteral chrysotherapy, which commonly causes adverse reactions consisting primarily of dermatitis, stomatitis, or transient mild proteinuria; more serious toxicity involves the hematopoietic system, liver, kidney, eye (cornea, lens), or other vital organ. Called also *auriasis.* 2. chrysoderma.

**chrys(o)-** [Gr. *chrysos* gold] a combining form denoting relationship to gold.

**chryso·der·ma** (kris″o-dər′mə) [*chryso-* + *derma*] a manifestation of chrysiasis presenting as a permanent gray- to lilac-colored pigmentation on the face, eyelids, and other sun-exposed areas of the body. Called also *aurochromoderma* and *chrysiasis.*

**chryso·mo·nad** (kris″o-mo′nad) [*chryso-* + *monad*] a protozoan of the order Chrysomonadida.

**Chryso·mo·nad·i·da** (kris″o-mo-nad′ĭ-də) [*chryso-* + Gr. *monas* unit, from *monos* single] an order of free-swimming, flagellate, chiefly ameboid, plastic, plantlike, marine and freshwater protozoa (class Phytomastigophorea, subphylum Mastigophora) having two unequal flagella, golden-brown chloroplasts when present, and a cyst wall that is typically siliceous. *Synura* is a representative genus.

**Chryso·my·ia** (kris″o-mi′yə) [*chryso-* + Gr. *myia* fly] a genus of flies of the family Calliphoridae, found in Africa, Australia, and parts of Asia. Several species lay eggs on wounds or wool, causing cutaneous myiasis.
**C. al′biceps,** a South African species whose larvae (wool maggots) live in the soiled wool of sheep, causing cutaneous botfly myiasis.
**C. bezzia′na,** a species widely distributed in Asia and Africa; its maggots are frequently found in wounds of humans and other animals, such as in cutaneous blowfly myiasis of sheep; it may also cause a severe and disfiguring myiasis in man. Called also *Cochliomyia bezziana.*
**C. macella′ria,** *Cochliomyia hominivorax.*

**Chrys·ops** (kris′ops) [*chryso-* + Gr. *ōps* eye] a genus of small blood-sucking horse flies of warm regions, of the family Tabanidae.
**C. cecu′tiens,** a species that bites near the eyes of humans and other animals.
**C. dimidia′ta,** a species of southwestern Africa that is an intermediate host of *Loa loa;* called also *mango* or *mangrove fly.*
**C. disca′lis,** a common vector of tularemia in the western part of the United States; called also *deer fly.*
**C. sila′cea,** an intermediate host of *Loa loa.*

**Chryso·spor·i·um** (kris″o-spor′e-əm) [MeSH: Chrysosporium] a genus of Fungi Imperfecti of the form-class Hyphomycetes, keratinophilic soil fungi, related to the dermatophytes; some species have been isolated from dermatophytosis.

**chryso·ther·a·py** (kris″o-ther′ə-pe) [*chryso-* + *therapy*] treatment with gold salts; called also *aurotherapy.*

**chryso·tile** (kris′o-tīl) the most widely-used form of asbestos, a gray-green magnesium silicate in the serpentine class of asbestos; inhalation of its dust may cause asbestosis and, rarely, forms of mesothelioma and other lung cancers.

**Chryso·zo·na** (kris″o-zo′nə) [*chryso-* + Gr. *zōne* girdle] *Haematopota.*

**CHS** cholinesterase.

**Churg-Strauss syndrome (vasculitis)** (chərg-strous) [Jacob *Churg,* American pathologist, born 1910; Lotte *Strauss,* American pathologist, born 1913] see under *syndrome.*

**Chvos·tek's sign** (kvos′təks) [Franz *Chvostek,* Austrian surgeon, 1835–1884] see under *sign.*

**Chvos·tek-Weiss sign** (kvos′tək-vīs′) [F. *Chvostek;* Nathan *Weiss,* Austrian physician, 1851–1883] Chvostek's sign.

**chy·lan·gi·o·ma** (ki-lan″je-o′mə) [*chyle* + *angioma*] a tumor made up of intestinal lymph vessels.

**chyl·aque·ous** (ki-la′kwe-əs) [*chyle* + *aqueous*] both chylous and watery. See *chylous hydrocele* and *chylous hydrothorax.*

**chyle** (kīl) [L. *chylus* juice] [MeSH: Chyle] 1. the milky fluid taken up by the lacteals from the food in the intestine during digestion, consisting of lymph and droplets of triglyceride fat (chylomicrons) in a stable emulsion. It passes into the veins by the thoracic duct, becoming mixed with the blood. 2. turbid, milky fluid resembling that produced during digestion.

**chyl·ec·ta·sia** (ki″lek-ta′zhə) [*chyle* + *ectasia*] dilatation of a chylous vessel; e.g., of a lacteal.

**chy·le·mia** (ki-le′me-ə) the presence of chyle in the blood.

**chy·li·fa·cient** (ki″lĭ-fa′shənt) chylopoietic.

**chy·li·fac·tion** (ki″lĭ-fak′shən) [*chyle* +L. *facere* to make] chylopoiesis.

**chy·li·fac·tive** (ki″lĭ-fak′tiv) [*chyle* +L. *facere* to make] chylopoietic.

**chy·lif·er·ous** (ki-lif′ər-əs) [*chyle* + *-ferous*] 1. chylopoietic. 2. conveying chyle.

**chy·li·fi·ca·tion** (ki″lĭ-fĭ-ka′shən) [*chyle* + L. *facere* to make] chylopoiesis.

**chy·li·form** (ki′lĭ-form) resembling chyle; cf. *pseudochylous.* Called also *chyloid.*

**chy·lo·cele** (ki′lo-sēl) [*chyle* + *-cele*[1]] elephantiasis scroti.

**chy·lo·cyst** (ki′lo-sist) [*chyle* + *cyst*] cisterna chyli.

**chy·lo·der·ma** (ki″lo-dər′mə) [*chyle* + *derma*] elephantiasis.

**chy·loid** (ki′loid) chyliform.

**chy·lol·o·gy** (ki-lol′ə-je) the study of chyle.

**chy·lo·me·di·as·ti·num** (ki″lo-me″de-as-ti′nəm) the presence of chyle in the mediastinum.

**chy·lo·mi·cro·graph** (ki″lo-mi′kro-graf) a curve plotted from counts of chylomicrons.

**chy·lo·mi·cron** (ki″lo-mi′kron) [*chylo-* + Gr. *mikros* small] a class of lipoproteins that transport exogenous (dietary) cholesterol and triglycerides from the small intestine to tissues after meals. Synthesized in the intestinal mucosa and carried via the intestinal lacteals and lymphatic system to the blood stream, they are then degraded to chylomicron remnants (q.v.) in the capillaries of muscle and adipose tissue via cleavage of the majority of their triglycerides by endothelial lipoprotein lipase. These remnants are rapidly cleared by the liver via receptor-mediated endocytosis.

**chy·lo·mi·cro·ne·mia** (ki″lo-mi″krə-ne′me-ə) hyperchylomicronemia.

**chy·lo·peri·car·di·tis** (ki″lo-per″ĭ-kahr-di′tis) [*chyle* + *pericarditis*] pericarditis due to effusion of chyle into the pericardial sac.

**chy·lo·peri·car·di·um** (ki″lo-per″ĭ-kahr′de-əm) [*chyle* + *pericardium*] the presence of effused chyle in the pericardium, usually due to trauma to the thoracic duct.

**chy·lo·peri·to·ne·um** (ki″lo-per″ĭ-to-ne′əm) [MeSH: Chyloperitoneum] chyliform ascites.

**chy·lo·phor·ic** (ki″lo-for′ik) [*chyle* + Gr. *phoros* bearing] chyliferous (def. 2).

**chy·lo·pleu·ra** (ki″lo-ploor′ə) chylothorax.

**chy·lo·pneu·mo·tho·rax** (ki″lo-noo″mo-thor′aks) the presence of chyle and air in the pleural cavity.

**chy·lo·poi·e·sis** (ki″lo-poi-e′sis) [*chyle* + *-poiesis*] the formation of chyle; called also *chylifaction* and *chylification.*

**chy·lo·poi·et·ic** (ki″lo-poi-et′ik) concerned in the formation of chyle. Called also *chylifacient* and *chylifactive.*

**chy·lor·rhea** (ki″lo-re′ə) 1. discharge of chyle due to rupture of or injury to the thoracic duct. 2. chylous diarrhea, due to rupture of lymphatics in the small intestine.

**chy·lo·sis** (ki-lo′sis) the process of conversion of food into chyle *(chylopoiesis)* and of absorption of the latter into the tissues.

**chy·lo·tho·rax** (ki″lo-tho′raks) [*chyle* + *thorax*] [MeSH: Chylothorax] a pleural effusion consisting of chyle or a chylelike fluid. There are two types: *chylous effusion,* due to leakage of chyle from the thoracic duct, and *chyliform* or *pseudochylous effusion,* consisting of chylelike fluid, the result of a chronic disease such as tuberculosis. Called also *chylopleura, chylous hydrothorax,* and *chylous pleurisy.*
**congenital c.,** a chylous effusion due to some congenital defect of

the thoracic duct; affected infants can die from malnutrition or systemic infection.
**traumatic c.**, a chylous effusion resulting from traumatic damage to the thoracic duct; causes include surgery on thoracic organs or vessels and nonpenetrating trauma such as hyperextension of the spine.

**chy·lous** (ki'ləs) pertaining to, mingled with, or of the nature of chyle.

**chy·lu·ria** (kīl-u're-ə) [*chyle* + *-uria*] the presence of chyle in the urine, giving it a milky appearance, due to obstruction anywhere between the intestinal lymphatics and the thoracic duct, which causes rupture of renal lymphatics into the renal tubules. It may occur as a result of obstruction of the retroperitoneal lymphatics in bancroftian filariasis. Called also *chylous urine* and *galacturia.*

**chy·lus** (ki'ləs) [L. *juice*] chyle (def. 1).

**Chy·mar** (ki'mər) trademark for preparations of chymotrypsin.

**chy·mase** (ki'mās) [EC 3.4.21.39] an enzyme of the hydrolase class that catalyzes the hydrolysis of peptide bonds, with a specificity similar to that of chymotrypsin. It is a serine proteinase and is found in mast cell granules.

**chyme** (kīm) [Gr. *chymos* juice] the semifluid, homogeneous, creamy or gruel-like material produced by gastric digestion of food; called also *chymus.*

**Chy·mex** (ki'məks) trademark for a preparation of bentiromide.

**chy·mi·fi·ca·tion** (ki"mĭ-fĭ-ka'shən) [*chyme* + L. *facere* to make] the formation of chyme; gastric digestion.

**chy·mo·pa·pa·in** (ki"mo-pə-pān') [EC 3.4.22.6] [MeSH: Chymopapain] an enzyme of the hydrolase class, a cysteine endopeptidase, that catalyzes the hydrolysis of proteins and polypeptides. Its specificity is very close to that of papain and both occur in the latex of the tropical papaya tree, *Carica papaya.* The enzyme is used to break down the proteoglycan portion of the nucleus pulposus in the treatment of herniation of intervertebral disks by chemonucleolysis.

**chy·mor·rhea** (ki"mo-re'ə) [*chyme* + *-rrhea*] a discharge or flow of chyme.

**chy·mo·sin** (ki'mo-sin) [EC 3.4.23.4] [MeSH: Chymosin] an enzyme of the hydrolase class that catalyzes the cleavage of a single bond in casein to form soluble paracasein, which then reacts with calcium to form a curd, insoluble paracasein. It is found in the fourth stomach of the calf and other ruminants. A commercial preparation, rennet, is used for making cheese and rennet custards. Called also *rennin* (not to be confused with *renin*).

**chy·mo·sin·o·gen** (ki"mo-sin'o-jən) prochymosin.

**chy·mo·tryp·sin** (ki"mo-trip'sin) [MeSH: Chymotrypsin] 1. [EC 3.4.21.1] a serine endopeptidase that preferentially cleaves peptide bonds on the carboxyl side of amino acids with bulky hydrophobic residues, particularly tyrosine, tryptophan, phenylalanine and leucine. It is secreted by the pancreas as the inactive proenzyme chymotrypsinogen. 2. [USP] a proteolytic enzyme preparation crystallized from an extract of ox pancreas, used for enzymatic zonulolysis in intracapsular lens extraction. It has also been used to debride necrotic lesions and to reduce inflammation and edema; administered orally, buccally, or intramuscularly.

**chy·mo·tryp·sin·o·gen** (ki"mo-trip-sin'o-jən) [MeSH: Chymotrypsinogen] an inactive proenzyme secreted by the pancreas and cleaved by trypsin in the small intestine to yield the active enzyme chymotrypsin.

**chy·mous** (ki'məs) pertaining to chyme.

**chy·mus** (ki'məs) chyme.

**CI** cardiac index; Colour Index.

**Ci** curie.

**Ciac·cio's glands** (chah'chōz) [Giuseppe Vincenzo *Ciaccio,* Italian anatomist, 1824–1901] glandulae lacrimales accessoriae.

**Ciac·cio's method, stain** (chah'chōz) [Carmelo *Ciaccio,* Italian pathologist, 1877–1956] see under *stain.*

**cib.** abbreviation for L. *ci'bus,* food.

**ci·biso·tome** (sĭ-bis'o-tōm) cystitome.

**cic·a·trec·to·my** (sik"ə-trek'tə-me) excision of a cicatrix.

**ci·ca·tri·ces** (sĭ-ka'trĭ-sēz, sik"ə-tri'sēz) [MeSH: Cicatrix] plural of *cicatrix.*

**cic·a·tri·cial** (sik"ə-trish'əl) pertaining to or of the nature of a scar (cicatrix).

**cic·a·tri·cot·o·my** (sik"ə-tri-kot'o-me) [*cicatrix* + *-tomy*] incision of a cicatrix.

**cic·a·trix** (sik-a'triks, sik'ə-triks) pl. *cica'trices* [L.] [MeSH: Cicatrix] scar (def. 1).

**filtering c.**, a cicatrix following glaucoma operation through which the aqueous humor escapes.
**hypertrophic c.**, a hard, rigid tumor formed by hypertrophy of the tissue of a cicatrix.
**vicious c.**, a cicatrix that causes deformity or impairs the function of an extremity.

**cic·at·ri·zant** (sik-at'rĭ-zənt) an agent that promotes cicatrization.

**cic·a·tri·za·tion** (sik"ə-trĭ-za'shən) the formation of a cicatrix or scar.

**cic·a·trize** (sik'ə-trīz) to heal by the formation of a scar or cicatrix.

**Ci·cer** (si'sər) a genus of plants of the family Leguminosae, native to southern Europe and parts of Asia. *C. arieti'num* is the garbanzo or chickpea (q.v.).

**cic·lo·pir·ox ol·amine** (si"klo-pēr'oks) [USP] a broad-spectrum antifungal with activity similar to that of the imidazoles, used in the treatment of cutaneous infections caused by susceptible organisms; applied topically.

**Cic·u·ta** (sik'u-tə) the water hemlocks, a genus of plants of the family Umbelliferae that contain cicutoxin and are poisonous to humans and livestock. *C. macula'ta* L. is the American water hemlock, which has cicutoxin in its roots. *C. viro'sa* is the European water hemlock.

**cic·u·tox·in** (sik"u-toks'in) a highly toxic unsaturated higher alcohol found in species of *Cicuta;* it causes hyperactivity of the central nervous system with convulsions and respiratory failure in humans and other animals.

**-cide** [L. *-cida,* from *caedere* to kill] a word termination denoting a killer or a killing.

**Ci·dex** (si'dəks) trademark for a preparation of glutaraldehyde.

**ci·dof·o·vir** (sĭ-dof'o-vir) an antiviral nucleoside analogue used in the treatment of cytomegalovirus retinitis in patients with acquired immunodeficiency syndrome; administered by intravenous infusion.

**CIE** counterimmunoelectrophoresis.

**ci·gua·te·ra** (se"gwə-ta'rə) [Sp. (orig. Taino) *cigua* a poisonous snail + *-era* Sp. noun suffix] a form of ichthyosarcotoxism, marked by gastrointestinal and neurologic symptoms due to ingestion of tropical or subtropical marine fish such as the grouper and the snapper that have ciguatoxin in their tissues. The term was formerly applied to all types of fish poisoning in the West Indies.

**ci·gua·tox·in** (se"gwə-tok'sin) [MeSH: Ciguatoxin] a heat-stable ichthyosarcotoxin secreted by the dinoflagellate *Gambierdiscus toxicus* and concentrated in the tissues of certain marine fish; it affects sodium channels and is the cause of ciguatera.

**CIH** Certificate in Industrial Health.

**Ci-hr** curie-hour.

**cil·a·sta·tin so·di·um** (si"lə-stat'in) a renal dipeptidase inhibitor that blocks the metabolism of imipenem; used in combination with imipenem to increase urinary levels of imipenem. The official preparation is *sterile cilastatin sodium* [USP].

**cil·ia** (sil'e-ə) sing. *cil'ium* [L.] [MeSH: Cilia] 1. [TA] eyelashes: the hairs growing on the edges of the eyelids. 2. minute vibratile hairlike processes that project from the free surface of a cell and are composed of nine pairs of microtubules arrayed around a central pair. They are extensions of basal bodies and move in rhythmical beats *(ciliary beats)* that serve to move the cell around in its environment or to move fluid or mucous films over the cell surface. See also *flagellum* and *mucociliary clearance.*

**cil·i·a·ris** (sil"e-a'ris) [L., from *cilium*] see under *musculus.*

**cil·i·ar·i·scope** (sil"e-ar'ĭ-skōp) [*ciliary* + *-scope*] an instrument for examining the ciliary region of the eye.

**cil·i·ar·ot·o·my** (sil"e-ə-rot'ə-me) [*ciliary* + *-tomy*] surgical division of the ciliary zone for glaucoma.

**cil·i·ary** (sil'e-ar"e) [L. *ciliaris,* from *cilium*] 1. pertaining to or resembling any cilium. 2. pertaining to the eyelashes.

**Cil·i·a·ta** (sil"e-a'tə) in former systems of classification, a class of ciliophorans comprising those protozoa characterized by the presence of cilia throughout their life cycle.

**cil·i·ate** (sil'e-āt) 1. having cilia. 2. any protozoan of the phylum Ciliophora; a ciliophoran.

**cil·i·at·ed** (sil'e-āt"əd) provided with cilia or with a fringe of hairs.

**cil·i·ec·to·my** (sil"e-ek'tə-me) [*cili-* + *-ectomy*] 1. excision of a portion of the ciliary body. 2. excision of a portion of the ciliary margin of the eyelid with the roots of the lashes.

**cili(o)-** [L. *cilium* eyelid, eyelash] a combining form denoting cilia or a ciliary structure.

**cil·io·gen·e·sis** (sil″e-o-jen′ə-sis) [*cilio-* + *genesis*] the formation or development of cilia.

**Cil·i·oph·o·ra** (sil″e-of′ə-rə) [*cilio-* + Gr. *phoros* bearing] [MeSH: Ciliophora] a phylum of protozoa characterized by the presence of cilia or compound ciliary structures as locomotor or food-gathering organelles at some time during their life cycle, a subpellicular infraciliature composed of ciliary basal bodies and kinetodesmata (even when cilia are absent), and two types of nuclei, a macronucleus and a micronucleus (with rare exceptions); a contractile vacuole is typically present. Sexuality involves conjugation, autogamy, and cytogamy. Most ciliophorans are free living, many are commensals of vertebrates and invertebrates, and some are parasites. The phylum comprises three classes: Kinetofragminophorea, Oligohymenophorea, and Polyhymenophorea. Cf. *Opalinata.*

**cil·i·oph·o·ran** (sil″e-of′ə-rən) any protozoan of the phylum Ciliophora; a ciliate.

**cil·io·ret·i·nal** (sil″e-o-ret′ĭ-nəl) pertaining to the retina and the ciliary body.

**cil·io·scle·ral** (sil″e-o-skler′əl) pertaining to the ciliary apparatus and to the sclera.

**cil·io·spi·nal** (sil″e-o-spi′nəl) [*cilio-* + *spinal*] pertaining to the ciliary body and the spinal cord; see under *center* and *reflex.*

**cil·i·ot·o·my** (sil″e-ot′ə-me) [*cilio-* + *tomy*] surgical division of the ciliary nerves.

**cil·i·um** (sil′e-əm) [L.] 1. singular of *cilia.* 2. old term for the outer margin of an eyelid.
**olfactory cilia,** see under *hair.*

**cil·lo** (sil′o) cillosis.

**Cil·lo·bac·te·ri·um** (sil″o-bak-tēr′e-əm) in former systems of classification, a genus of bacteria of the family Lactobacillaceae, made up of nonsporulating, anaerobic, gram-positive, rod-shaped organisms. These organisms are now assigned to the genus *Eubacterium.*

**cil·lo·sis** (sil-o′sis) [L. from Fr. *ciller* to wink + *-osis*] a spasmodic quivering of the eyelid; called also *cillo.*

**cim·bia** (sim′be-ə) [L.] a white band running across the ventral surface of the crus cerebri.

**ci·met·i·dine** (si-met′ĭ-dēn) [MeSH: Cimetidine] an antagonist to histamine $H_2$ receptors, which inhibits gastric acid secretion in response to all stimuli, and is effective especially in the treatment of peptic ulcer; administered orally, intravenously, and by intravenous infusion.
**c. hydrochloride** [USP], the monohydrochloride salt of cimetidine, having the same actions and uses as the base; administered orally, intravenously, and intramuscularly.

**Ci·mex** (si′məks) [L. "bug"] a genus of insects, the bedbugs, of the family Cimicidae.
**C. boue′ti,** the tropical bedbug of West Africa and South America; called also *Leptocimex boueti.*
**C. hemip′terus,** *C. rotundatus.*
**C. lectula′rius,** the common bedbug that infests man in temperate areas; called also *Acanthia lectularia.*
**C. pilosel′lus,** an American species found in bats.
**C. pipistrel′la,** a species that transmits a trypanosome disease of bats.
**C. rotunda′tus,** a flattened, oval, reddish bedbug that infests man in the tropics; called also *C. hemipterus.*

**ci·mex** (si′məks) pl. *cim′ices* [L.] an individual of the genus *Cimex;* a bedbug.

**ci·mi·cid** (si′mĭ-sid) pertaining to insects of the family Cimicidae.

**Ci·mic·i·dae** (si-mis′ĭ-de) a family of wingless, blood-sucking, hemipterous insects of the suborder Heteroptera, including the bedbugs and related forms. *Cimex, Haematosiphon, Leptocimex,* and *Oeciacus* are medically important genera.

**Cim·i·cif·u·ga** (sim″ĭ-sif′u-gə) [L. *cimex* bug + *fugare* to put to flight] a genus of plants of the family Ranunculaceae. *C. racemo′sa* (L.) Nutt. is the black snakeroot or cohosh and has rootlets that are tonic and antispasmodic.

**cim·i·co·sis** (sim″ĭ-ko′sis) itching of the skin due to the bites of *Cimex lectularius* (bedbug).

**CIN** cervical intraepithelial neoplasia.

**cinch·ing** (sinch′ing) [Sp. *cincha* girdle] surgical shortening of an ocular muscle by plicating.

**Cin·cho·na** (sin-ko′nə) [named from a countess of *Chinchon*] [MeSH: Cinchona] a genus of South American trees of the family Rubiaceae, the source of the medicinal bark called *cinchona.* The major species used are *C. succiru′bra* Pavon et Klotzsch and its hybrids (red cinchona), *C. calisa′ya* Weddell, and *C. Ledgeria′na* (Howard) Moens et Trimen and its hybrids (yellow cinchona).

**cin·cho·na** (sin-ko′nə) [MeSH: Cinchona] 1. any tree of the genus *Cinchona.* 2. the dried bark of the stem or root of various species of *Cinchona,* the source of the medicinally important quinoline alkaloids quinine, quinidine, cinchonine, and cinchonidine; it was once widely used as an antimalarial but has been largely replaced by its alkaloids. Called also *calisaya bark, cinchona bark, Jesuit's bark, Peruvian bark,* and *quinquina.*

**cin·cho·ni·dine** (sin-ko′nĭ-dēn) an alkaloid of cinchona, used as an antimalarial, chiefly in the form of the sulfate salt; administered orally.

**cin·cho·nine** (sin′ko-nēn) [L. *cinchonina*] an alkaloid of cinchona used as an antimalarial, chiefly in the form of the sulfate salt; administered orally.

**cin·cho·nin·ic ac·id** (sin″ko-nin′ik) quinoline 4-carboxylic acid, an oxidation product of cinchona alkaloids.

**cin·cho·nism** (sin′ko-niz″əm) poisoning by the injudicious use of cinchona bark or its alkaloids, characterized by nausea, vomiting, headache, tinnitus, deafness, symptoms of cerebral congestion, vertigo, and visual disturbances.

**cin·cli·sis** (sin′klĭ-sis) [Gr. *kinklisis* a wagging] a rapidly repeated movement, such as rapid breathing, or rapid winking.

**cine-** [Gr. *kinēsis* movement] a combining form denoting relationship to movement.

**cine·an·gio·car·diog·ra·phy** (sin″ə-an″je-o-kahr″de-og′rə-fe) [*cine-* + *angiocardiography*] the photographic recording of fluoroscopic images of the heart and great vessels by motion picture techniques.

**cine·an·gio·graph** (sin″ə-an′je-o-graf) a motion picture camera for photographing fluoroscopic images.

**cine·an·gi·og·ra·phy** (sin″ə-an″je-og′rə-fe) [*cine-* + *angiography*] [MeSH: Cineangiography] the photographic recording of fluoroscopic images of the blood vessels by motion picture techniques.

**cine·den·sig·ra·phy** (sin″ə-dən-sig′rə-fe) the recording of movements of internal body structures by means of x-rays and radiosensitive cells.

**cine·flu·o·rog·ra·phy** (sin″ə-floo″or-og′rə-fe) cineradiography.

**cin·e·mat·ics** (sin″ə-mat′iks) kinematics.

**cine·mat·iza·tion** (sin″ə-mat′-ĭ-za′shən) kineplasty.

**cin·e·ma·tog·ra·phy** (sin″ə-mə-tog′rə-fe) cineradiography.

**cine·ma·to·ra·di·og·ra·phy** (sin″ə-mə-to-ra″de-og′rə-fe) cineradiography.

**cine·mi·crog·ra·phy** (sin″ə-mi-krog′rə-fe) the making of moving pictures of a small object through the lens system of a microscope.
**time-lapse c.,** the taking of motion pictures of a minute object through a microscope at a slower than normal speed, so that with projection at normal speed the movements of the object appear to occur more rapidly.

**cin·e·ol** (sin′e-ol) eucalyptol.

**cin·e·paz·et mal·e·ate** (sin″ə-paz′ət) a coronary vasodilator, which has been used in the treatment of angina of effort.

**cine·phle·bog·ra·phy** (sin″ə-flə-bog′rə-fe) cineradiography of the veins after administration of a contrast medium. In *ascending functional c.,* the contrast medium is introduced into a vein in the foot and its progress is observed as it courses through the tibial, popliteal, femoral, and iliac veins.

**cine·plas·tics** (sin″ə-plas′tiks) kineplasty.

**cin·e·plas·ty** (sin′ə-plas″te) kineplasty.

**cine·ra·dio·flu·o·rog·ra·phy** (sin″ə-ra″de-o-flo͞or-og′rə-fe) cineradiography.

**cine·ra·di·og·ra·phy** (sin″ə-ra″de-og′rə-fe) [MeSH: Cineradiography] the making of a motion picture record of the successive images appearing on a fluoroscopic screen; called also *cinefluorography, cinematography,* and *cinematoradiography.*

**ci·ne·rea** (sĭ-nēr′e-ə) [L. *cinereus* ashen hued] the gray matter of the nervous system.

**ci·ne·re·al** (sĭ-nēr′e-əl) pertaining to the gray matter of the brain or nervous system.

**cin·er·i·tious** (sin″ər-ish′əs) [L. *cineritius*] ashen gray; of the color of ashes.

**cin·es·al·gia** (sin″əs-al′jə) [*cinsi-* + *-algia*] pain in a muscle when it is brought into action.

**cinesi-** for words beginning thus, see those beginning *kinesi-.*

**cinet(o)-** for words beginning thus, see those beginning *kinet(o)-.*

**cine·urog·ra·phy** (sin″ə-u-rog′rə-fe) cineradiography of the urinary tract.

**cin·gu·la** (sing′gu-lə) [L.] plural of *cingulum.*

**cin·gu·late** (sing′gu-lāt) pertaining to a cingulum.

**cin·gule** (sing′gūl) cingulum.

**cin·gu·lec·to·my** (sing″gu-lek′tə-me) bilateral extirpation of the anterior half of the gyrus cinguli; cf. *cingulotomy.*

**cin·gu·lot·o·my** (sing″gu-lot′ə-me) the creation, by stereotaxic introduction of electrodes, of lesions in the gyrus cinguli for relief of intractable pain and in treatment of psychiatric disorders and addiction.

**cin·gu·lum** (sing′gu-ləm) pl. *cin′gula* [L. "girdle"] 1. an encircling structure or part; anything that encircles a body. Called also *cingule* and *girdle.* 2. [TA] a bundle of association fibers that partly encircles the corpus callosum not far from the median plane, the fibers of which interrelate the cingulate and hippocampal gyri. 3. the lingual lobe of an anterior tooth, making up the bulk of the cervical third of its lingual surface; called also *basal, linguocervical,* and *linguogingival ridge.*
**c. mem′bri inferio′ris,** TA alternative for *c. pelvicum.*
**c. mem′bri superio′ris,** TA alternative for *c. pectorale.*
**c. pectora′le** [TA], pectoral girdle: the encircling bony structure supporting the upper limbs, comprising the clavicles and scapulae, articulating with each other and with the sternum and vertebral column, respectively; called also *c. membri superioris* [TA alternative] and *shoulder girdle.*
**c. pel′vicum** [TA], pelvic girdle: the encircling bony structure supporting the lower limbs, comprising the two ossa coxae, articulating with each other and with the sacrum, to complete the essentially rigid bony ring; called also *c. membri inferioris* [TA alternative].

**cin·gu·lum·ot·o·my** (sing″gu-ləm-ot′ə-me) cingulotomy.

**C1 INH** C1 inhibitor.

**cin·na·mal·de·hyde** (sin″ə-mal′də-hīd) a yellowish oily liquid with a strong odor of cinnamon, used as a flavoring agent.

**cin·na·mene** (cin′ə-mēn) styrene.

**cin·nam·ic ac·id** (sĭ-nam′ik) a fragrant acid, phenylacrylic acid, occurring in cinnamon and balsams and other aromatic resins.

**cin·na·mol** (cin′ə-mol) styrene.

**Cin·na·mo·mum** (sin″ə-mo′məm) a genus of evergreen trees of the family Lauraceae, native to Asia. The wood of *C. cam′phora* is the source of camphor and the bark of *C. lourei′rii* is the source of cinnamon.

**cin·na·mon** (sin′ə-mən) [Gr. *kinnamon,* from Hebrew *quinnāmōn*] [MeSH: Cinnamon] the dried bark of *Cinnamomum loureirii,* containing, in each 100 gm, not less than 2.5 mL of volatile oil (see *cinnamon oil*); used as a flavor in pharmaceutical preparations.

**cin·nar·i·zine** (sĭ-nahr′ĭ-zēn) [MeSH: Cinnarizine] an antihistamine, used chiefly in the treatment of nausea and vertigo associated with labyrinthine disorders and in the prevention and treatment of motion sickness.

**ci·nol·o·gy** (sĭ-nol′ə-je) kinesiology.

**ci·nom·e·ter** (sĭ-nom′ə-tər) kinesimeter, def. 1.

**cino·plasm** (sin′o-plaz-əm) kinetoplasm.

**cin·ox·a·cin** (sin-ok′sə-sin) [MeSH: Cinoxacin] a broad-spectrum quinolone antibacterial agent, administered orally.

**cin·ox·ate** (sin-ok′sāt) a sunscreen effective against ultraviolet B, applied topically to the skin.

**Ci·o·nel·la** (si″o-nəl′ə) a genus of land snails of the family Cionellidae; they serve as hosts of the liver fluke *Dicrocoelium dendriticum* in North America.

**Ci·o·nel·li·dae** (si″o-nel′ĭ-de) a family of garden snails of the suborder Stylommatophora, subclass Euthyneura; they often serve as hosts of the liver fluke *Dicrocoelium dendriticum.*

**Cip·ro** (sip′ro) trademark for a preparation of ciprofloxacin hydrochloride.

**cip·ro·ci·no·nide** (sip″ro-si′no-nīd) an adrenocorticosteroid.

**ci·pro·fi·brate** (si″pro-fi′brāt) a fibric acid derivative having actions similar to those of clofibrate, used as a hypolipidemic in the treatment of certain hyperlipoproteinemias; administered orally.

**cip·ro·flox·a·cin** (sip″ro-flok′sə-sin) [USP] [MeSH: Ciprofloxacin] a fluorinated 4-quinolone antibacterial effective against many gram-positive and gram-negative bacteria, including some strains resistant to penicillins, cephalosporins, and aminoglycosides.
**c. hydrochloride** [USP], the monohydrated hydrochloride salt of ciprofloxacin, having the same actions as the parent compound and used to treat a wide variety of bacterial infections.

**cir·ca·di·an** (sər″kə-de′ən) [L. *circa* about + *dies* a day] pertaining to a period of about 24 hours; applied especially to the rhythmic repetition of certain phenomena in living organisms at about the same time each day (circadian rhythm).

**cir·can·nu·al** (sər-kan′u-əl) [L. *circa* about + *annus* year] occurring every year; applied especially to the rhythmic repetition of certain phenomena (e.g., the flowering of plants) in living organisms at about the same time each year.

**cir·cel·lus** (sər-səl′əs) [L., dim. of *circulus*] a small ring, or circle.

**cir·ci·nate** (sər′sĭ-nāt) 1. circular. 2. annular.

**cir·cle** (sər′kəl) [L. *circulus*] a round figure, structure, or part. See also *anulus* and *ring.*
**arterial c.,** circulus arteriosus.
**arterial c. of iris, greater,** circulus arteriosus iridis major.
**arterial c. of iris, lesser,** circulus arteriosus iridis minor.
**arterial c. of Willis,** circulus arteriosus cerebri.
**Berry's c's,** charts with circles on them for testing stereoscopic vision.
**c. of Carus,** see under *curve.*
**cerebral arterial c.,** circulus arteriosus cerebri.
**c. of confusion,** a disk representing the image of a theoretical point made by a lens.
**defensive c.,** the coexistence of two conditions that tend to have an antagonistic or inhibitory effect on each other.
**c. of dispersion, c. of dissipation,** the circular space on the retina within which the image of a luminous point is formed.
**c. of Haller,** circulus vasculosus nervi optici.
**c. of Hovius,** an intrascleral circular arrangement of anastomosing ciliary veins anterior to the vorticose veins, not far from the corneoscleral margin, occurring in mammals other than humans.
**Huguier's c.,** the circle formed about the junction of the cervix with the body of the uterus by the uterine arteries.
**c. of iris, greater,** anulus iridis major.
**c. of iris, lesser,** anulus iridis minor.
**Latham's c.,** a circle 5 cm in diameter covering the area of pericardial dullness and situated midway between the left nipple and the lower end of the sternum.
**Minsky's c's,** a series of circles used for the graphic recording of eye lesions.
**Robinson's c.,** an arterial circle formed by anastomoses between the abdominal aorta, common iliac, hypogastric, uterine, and ovarian arteries.
**vascular c.,** circulus vasculosus.
**vascular c. of optic nerve,** circulus vasculosus nervi optici.
**Vieth-Müller c.,** see under *horopter.*
**c. of Willis,** circulus arteriosus cerebri.
**c. of Zinn,** circulus vasculosus nervi optici.

**cir·clet** (sər′klət) circellus.

**cir·cling** (sər′kling) walking in a circle, as that done by animals with listeriosis and other central nervous system disorders.

**cir·cuit** (sər′kət) [L. *circuitus*] the round or course traversed by an electrical current. The circuit is said to be *closed* when it is continuous, so that the current may pass through it; it is *open, broken,* or *interrupted* when it is not continuous and the current cannot pass through it.
**gate c.,** gate.
**macroreentrant c.,** a reentry pathway involving the bundle branches of the conduction system of the heart.
**microreentrant c.,** a reentry pathway involving only a few myocardial cells.
**open c.,** a circuit having some break in it so that current is not passing or cannot pass.
**Papez c.,** a neuronal circuit in the limbic system, consisting of the hippocampus, fornix, mammillary body, anterior thalamic nuclei, and cingulate gyrus; postulated by Papez to be involved with the experiencing of emotions and responses to them.
**reentrant c.,** the circuit formed by the circulating impulse in reentry.
**reflex c.,** see under *arc.*
**reverberating c.,** a neuronal pathway arranged in a circle so that impulses are recycled to cause positive feedback or reverberation (q.v.).
**short c.,** 1. an unwanted low-resistance connection between two points in an electric circuit. 2. a communication between two portions of intestine, one above and the other below an obstruction.

**cir·cu·lar** (sər′ku-lər) [L. *circularis*] shaped like a circle or occurring in a circle. See also *annular.*

**cir·cu·la·tion** (sər″ku-la′shən) [L. *circulatio*] 1. movement of something through a circuitous course. 2. the movement of the blood through the heart and blood vessels.
**allantoic c.,** fetal circulation through the umbilical vessels; called also *umbilical c.*

**assisted c.**, pumping that aids the natural activity of the heart.
**collateral c.**, that which is carried on through secondary channels after obstruction of the principal vessel supplying the part; called also *compensatory c.*
**compensatory c.**, collateral c.
**coronary c.**, that within the coronary vessels of the heart.
**cross c.**, the circulation in a portion of the body of one animal of blood supplied from another animal.
**enterohepatic c.**, the recurrent cycle in which bile salts and other substances excreted by the liver pass through the intestinal mucosa and become reabsorbed by the hepatic cells and re-excreted.
**extracorporeal c.**, the circulation of blood outside the body, as through a heart-lung apparatus for carbon dioxide–oxygen exchange, or through an artificial kidney for removal of substances usually excreted in the urine.
**fetal c.**, that propelled by the fetal heart through the fetus, umbilical cord, and chorionic villi of the placenta.
**first c.**, primitive c.
**fourth c.**, the continuous movement of lymphocytes from their sources in all the hematopoietic and connective tissues to the blood passing through all the tissues and organs, then to the lymph nodes, then into the lymph of the thoracic duct, and into the blood again.
**greater c.**, systemic c.
**hypophysial portal c.**, **hypophysioportal c.**, hypothalamo-hypophysial portal system.
**intervillous c.**, the flow of maternal blood through the intervillous space.
**lesser c.**, pulmonary c.
**lymph c.**, the passage of the lymph through lymph vessels and glands.
**omphalomesenteric c.**, vitelline c.
**persistent fetal c.**, pulmonary hypertension in the postnatal period secondary to right-to-left shunting of the blood through the foramen ovale and ductus arteriosus.
**placental c.**, the fetal circulation; also, the maternal circulation through the intervillous space of the placenta.
**portal c.**, 1. the circulation of blood from the capillaries of one organ through larger vessels to the capillaries of another organ, before returning through larger veins back to the heart; see also *hypophysioportal c.* 2. the passage of the blood from capillaries of the gastrointestinal tract and spleen through capillaries of the liver before entering the hepatic vein. 3. hypothalamo-hypophysial portal system.
**portoumbilical c.**, Cruveilhier-Baumgarten syndrome.
**primitive c.**, **primordial c.**, the earliest circulation by which nutriment and oxygen are conveyed to the embryo; called also *first c.*

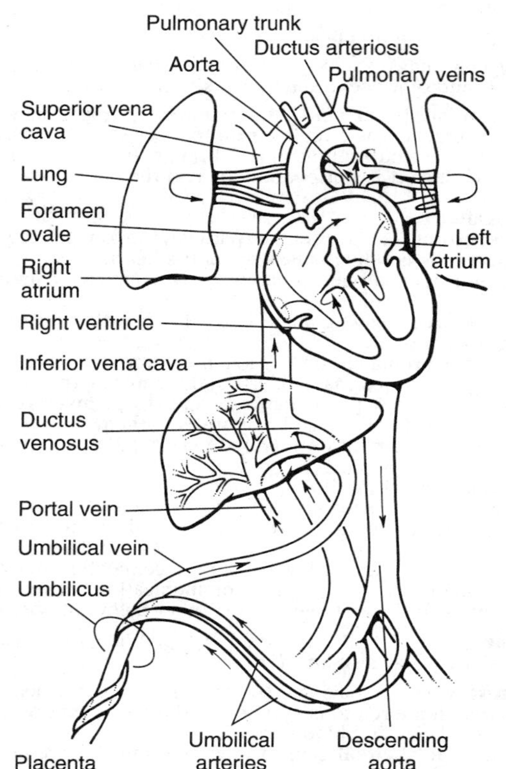

Schematic diagram of fetal circulation.

**pulmonary c.**, that carrying the venous blood from the right ventricle to the lungs, and returning oxygenated blood to the left atrium of the heart; called also *lesser c.*
**sinusoidal c.**, that occurring through the sinusoids.
**systemic c.**, the general circulation, carrying oxygenated blood from the left ventricle to various tissues of the body, and returning the venous blood to the right atrium of the heart; called also *greater c.*
**thebesian c.**, the circulation of blood through the venae cordis minimae (thebesian veins).
**umbilical c.**, allantoic c.
**vitelline c.**, the circulation through the blood vessels of the yolk sac; called also *omphalomesenteric c.*

**cir·cu·la·to·ry** (sər′ku-lə-tor″e) 1. pertaining to any circulation. 2. pertaining to the circulation of the blood. 3. containing blood; called also *sanguiferous.*

**cir·cu·lus** (sər′ku-ləs) pl. *cir′culi* [L. "a ring"] [TA] circle: general anatomical nomenclature for a ringlike arrangement, usually of arteries or veins.
**c. arterio′sus** [TA], arterial circle: a complete or incomplete circle of anastomosing arteries.
**c. arterio′sus ce′rebri** [TA], cerebral arterial circle: the important polygonal anastomosis formed by the internal carotid, the anterior and posterior cerebral arteries, the anterior communicating artery, and the posterior communicating arteries; called also *arterial circle of Willis, circle of Willis,* and *c. willisii.*
**c. arterio′sus i′ridis ma′jor** [TA], greater arterial circle of the iris: a circle of anastomosing arteries situated in the ciliary body along the ciliary margin of the iris.
**c. arterio′sus i′ridis mi′nor** [TA], lesser arterial circle of the iris: a circle of anastomosing arteries in the iris near the pupillary margin.
**c. arterio′sus [Willis′ii]**, c. arteriosus cerebri.
**c. articula′ris vasculo′sus**, an arrangement of anastomosing vessels encircling a joint.
**c. umbilica′lis**, an arterial plexus in the subperitoneal tissue surrounding the navel.
**c. vasculo′sus** [TA], vascular circle: a complete or incomplete circle of anastomosing blood vessels.
**c. vasculo′sus ner′vi op′tici** [TA], vascular circle of optic nerve: a circle of arteries in the sclera surrounding the site of entrance of the optic nerve; called also *circle of Haller* and *circle of Zinn.*
**c. veno′sus hal′leri**, plexus venosus areolaris.
**c. willis′ii**, c. arteriosus cerebri.

**circum-** [L.] a prefix signifying around or encircling.

**cir·cum·anal** (sər″kəm-a′nəl) surrounding the anus; cf. *perianal.*

**cir·cum·ar·tic·u·lar** (sər″kəm-ahr-tik′u-lər) around a joint.

**cir·cum·ax·il·lary** (sər″kəm-ak′sĭ-lar″e) around the axilla.

**cir·cum·bul·bar** (sər″kəm-bul′bər) surrounding the eyeball.

**cir·cum·cal·lo·sal** (sər″kəm-kə-lo′səl) surrounding the corpus callosum.

**cir·cum·cise** (sər′kəm-sīz) to perform circumcision.

**cir·cum·ci·sion** (sər″kəm-sizh′ən) [L. *circumcisio* a cutting around] [MeSH: Circumcision] the removal of all or part of the prepuce, or foreskin.
**female c.**, a general term encompassing both the excision of a portion of the external female genitalia (see *Sunna c.* and *pharaonic c.*) and infibulation (q.v.). Although it is associated with severe health risks and has been declared illegal in many places, it is widely practiced in a number of cultures, particularly in Africa.
**pharaonic c.**, a type of female circumcision comprising two procedures: a radical form in which the clitoris, labia minora, and labia majora are removed and the remaining tissues are approximated by clips or sutures, and a modified form in which the prepuce and glans of the clitoris and the adjacent labia minora are removed.
**Sunna c.**, a form of female circumcision in which the prepuce of the clitoris is removed.

**cir·cum·cor·ne·al** (sər″kəm-kor′ne-əl) around the cornea.

**cir·cum·cres·cent** (sər″kəm-kres′ənt) [*circum-* + L. *crescere* to grow] growing around and over.

**cir·cum·duc·tion** (sər″kəm-duk′shən) [L. *circumducere* to draw around] the active or passive circular movement of a limb or of the eye.

**cir·cum·fer·ence** (sər-kum′fər-əns) [*circum-* + L. *ferre* to bear] the outer limit or margin of a rounded body.
**articular c.**, circumferentia articularis.
**midarm c.**, **mid upper arm c.**, the circumference of the upper arm measured midway between the acromion and olecranon.

**cir·cum·fer·en·tia** (sər-kum″fər-en′shə) [L.] circumference.
**c. articula′ris**, articular circumference: the rounded surface of a bone which is received into a depression of another bone with which it articulates.
**c. articula′ris ca′pitis ra′dii** [TA], articular circumference of head

of radius: the rounded surface of the head or capitulum of the radius which articulates with the radial notch of the ulna.
**c. articula'ris ca'pitis ul'nae** [TA], articular circumference of head of ulna: the semilunar surface of the head of the ulna which articulates with the ulnar notch of the radius; called also *c. articularis capituli ulnae.*
**c. articula'ris capi'tuli ul'nae,** c. articularis capitis ulnae.

**cir·cum·fer·en·tial** (sər"kəm-fər-en'shəl) pertaining to forming a circumference.

**cir·cum·flex** (sər'kəm-fleks) [L. *circumflexus* bent about] curved like a bow.

**cir·cum·flex·us** (sər"kəm-flek'səs) [L.] bent about; circumflex.

**cir·cum·gem·mal** (sər"kəm-jem'əl) [*circum-* + *gemma* + *-al*[1]] surrounding a bud; a term applied to that form of nerve ending in which an end-bud is surrounded by fibrils.

**cir·cum·in·su·lar** (sər"kəm-in'su-lər) [*circum-* + *insular*] surrounding, situated, or occurring about the insula.

**cir·cum·in·tes·ti·nal** (sər"kəm-in-tes'tĭ-nəl) surrounding the intestine.

**cir·cum·len·tal** (sər"kəm-len'təl) situated or occurring around the lens.

**cir·cum·nu·cle·ar** (sər"kəm-noo'kle-ər) surrounding or occurring near a nucleus.

**cir·cum·oc·u·lar** (sər"kəm-ok'u-lər) surrounding or occurring around the eye.

**cir·cum·oral** (ser"kəm-or'əl) [*circum-* + *oral*] around or encircling the mouth; cf. *perioral.*

**cir·cum·or·bi·tal** (sər"kəm-or'bĭ-təl) situated around or occurring near an orbit.

**cir·cum·re·nal** (sər"kəm-re'nəl) perinephric.

**cir·cum·scribed** (sər'kəm-skrībd") [*circum-* + L. *scribere* to write] bounded or limited; confined to a limited space.

**cir·cum·scrip·tus** (sər"kəm-skrip'təs) [L.] circumscribed.

**cir·cum·stan·ti·al·i·ty** (sər"kəm-stan"she-al'ĭ-te) a disturbed pattern of speech or writing characterized by delay in getting to the point because of the interpolation of unnecessary details and irrelevant parenthetical remarks; seen in persons with schizophrenia and obsessive-compulsive disorders. Cf. *tangentiality.*

**Cir·cum·straint** (sər'kəm-strānt") trademark for a device used to hold a baby for circumcision.

**cir·cum·val·late** (sər"kəm-val'āt) [*circum-* + *vallate*] surrounded by a trench or by a ridge; see *vallate papilla,* under *papilla.*

**cir·cum·vas·cu·lar** (sər"kəm-vas'ku-lər) [*circum-* + *vascular*] around or encircling a vessel.

**cir·cum·ven·tric·u·lar** (sər"kəm-ven-trik'u-lər) located around a ventricle, particularly in the brain.

**cir·cum·vo·lute** (sər"kəm-vo'lūt) [*circum-* + *volute*] twisted about.

**cir·rhog·e·nous** (sĭ-roj'ə-nəs) producing cirrhosis or hardening.

**cir·rhon·o·sus** (sĭ-ron'ə-səs) [Gr. *kirrhos* orange yellow + *nosos* disease] a fetal disease characterized by a golden-yellow staining of the pleura and peritoneum.

**cir·rho·sis** (sĭ-ro'sis) [Gr. *kirrhos* orange-yellow] liver disease characterized by diffuse interlacing bands of fibrous tissue dividing the hepatic parenchyma into micronodular or macronodular areas. See also *c. of liver.*
**acholangic biliary c.,** a liver ailment affecting children up to 12 years old, due to complete or partial agenesis of the intrahepatic, intralobular bile ducts, with manifestations similar to those in obstructive biliary cirrhosis.
**acute juvenile c.,** chronic active hepatitis.
**alcoholic c.,** cirrhosis in the alcoholic, attributed by some to associated nutritional deficiency and by others to chronic excessive exposure to alcohol as a hepatotoxin.
**atrophic c.,** cirrhosis in which the liver is decreased in size; it may be seen in the alcoholic, but is more common in posthepatitic or postnecrotic cirrhosis.
**bacterial c.,** a variety said to be of microbic origin.
**biliary c.,** cirrhosis of the liver due to obstruction or infection of the major extra- or intrahepatic bile ducts (except in *primary biliary c.*). It is marked by jaundice, abdominal pain, steatorrhea, and enlargement of the liver and spleen. See *primary* and *secondary biliary c.*
**biliary c. of children,** secondary biliary cirrhosis due to congenital atresia of the bile ducts; called also *infantile liver.* See also *Indian childhood c.*
**calculus c.,** secondary biliary cirrhosis caused by the presence of gallstones.
**cardiac c.,** fibrosis of the liver, probably following central hemorrhagic necrosis, in association with congestive heart disease. It is characterized by scarring about the central veins of the hepatic lobules.
**Charcot's c.,** primary biliary c.
**congestive c.,** cirrhosis resulting from increased hepatic venous pressure or thrombosis; commonly due to congestive heart failure (cardiac c.) or to obstruction of the hepatic vein.
**Cruveilhier-Baumgarten c.,** see under *syndrome.*
**decompensated c.,** cirrhosis accompanied by ascites.
**fatty c.,** cirrhosis in which liver cells are infiltrated with fat (triglyceride), the infiltration usually being due to alcohol ingestion; Laënnec's c.
**Indian childhood c.,** cirrhosis of the liver of unknown etiology occurring in children in India, characterized typically by insidious onset, stunting of growth, hepatomegaly, and a low inconstant fever. In the late stages, portal hypertension with ascites, evidence of collateral circulation, hematemesis, splenomegaly, and edema may be seen. Cf. *veno-occlusive disease of the liver.*
**Laënnec's c.,** cirrhosis of the liver closely associated with chronic excessive alcohol ingestion. In the early stages, liver enlargement may reflect fatty infiltration of liver cells (fatty c.), with necrosis and inflammation due to acute alcohol injury; progressive fibrosis extending from portal areas separates uniform small regeneration nodules. See *c. of liver* for symptoms.
**c. of liver,** a group of chronic diseases of the liver characterized by loss of normal hepatic lobular architecture with fibrosis, and by destruction of parenchymal cells and their regeneration to form nodules. The disease has a lengthy latent period, usually followed by the sudden appearance of abdominal swelling and pain, hematemesis, dependent edema, or jaundice. In advanced stages, ascites, jaundice, portal hypertension, and central nervous system disorders, which may end in hepatic coma, become prominent. Called also *chronic interstitial hepatitis.*
**macronodular c.,** cirrhosis of the liver that follows subacute hepatic necrosis due to toxic or viral hepatitis. The reticulin framework of normal lobules collapses and may be replaced by broad bands of fibrous tissue separating regeneration nodules of various sizes. Called also *multilobular c., periportal c., postnecrotic c.,* and *toxic c.*
**malarial c.,** cirrhosis associated with malaria; the malaria is probably not an etiologic factor.
**metabolic c.,** cirrhosis of the liver associated with metabolic diseases, such as hemochromatosis, Wilson's disease, glycogen storage disease, galactosemia, and disorders of amino acid metabolism.
**multilobular c.,** macronodular c.
**periportal c.,** macronodular c.
**pigment c., pigmentary c.,** a condition marked by a slightly to moderately enlarged, chocolate-brown liver, the surface of which is diffusely nodular; it is the characteristic lesion of hemochromatosis.
**pipe stem c.,** cirrhosis of the liver characterized by fibrotic scars around the large portal vessels; seen in hepatic schistosomiasis, in which fibrosis surrounds parasites or ova trapped in branches of the portal vein.
**portal c.,** Laënnec's c.
**posthepatitic c.,** cirrhosis (usually macronodular) resulting as a sequela to acute hepatitis.
**postnecrotic c.,** macronodular c.
**primary biliary c.,** a rare form of biliary cirrhosis of unknown etiology in which small intrahepatic bile ducts are destroyed while the major intra- and extrahepatic ducts remain patent; 90 per cent of patients are female; most are middle-aged; it is characterized by chronic cholestasis with pruritus, jaundice, hypercholesterolemia and xanthomas, osteomalacia, and, in the later stages, by portal hypertension and liver failure. Almost all patients have circulating antimitochondrial antibodies.
**secondary biliary c.,** cirrhosis of the liver resulting from chronic bile obstruction due to congenital atresia or stricture.
**stasis c.,** a general term for cirrhosis due to obstruction of the outflow of the hepatic vein; see also *cardiac c., veno-occlusive disease,* and *Budd-Chiari syndrome.*
**syphilitic c.,** cirrhosis of the liver due to congenital or tertiary syphilis.
**Todd's c.,** primary biliary c.
**toxic c.,** macronodular c.
**unilobular c.,** primary biliary c.
**vascular c.,** cirrhosis of the liver following obstruction of the hepatic vein, portal vein, or general hepatic circulation.

**cir·rhot·ic** (sĭ-rot'ik) pertaining to or characterized by cirrhosis.

**cir·ri** (sər'i) plural of *cirrus.*

**cir·rus** (sər'əs) pl. *cir'ri* [L. "curl"] 1. any of various slender, usually flexible, appendages, such as one of the organelles used for locomotion by certain peritrichous ciliate protozoa; an eversible penis seen in flatworms; a fingerlike projection of a polychete parapodium; a branch of the thoracic leg of a barnacle; a lateral appendage on the stalk or aboral base of a crinoid; or one of the short projections around the mouth of a cephalochordate that together form a sieve to prevent large particles from entering the mouth. 2. a

coarse hair on an animal, longer than most body hair but less coarse than a tactile hair or a vibrissa.
**c. ca'pitis,** one of the long hairs in the forelock of a horse.
**c. cau'dae,** one of the long hairs in an animal's tail.

**cir·sen·chy·sis** (sər-sen'kĭ-sis) [*cirso-* + *enchysis* injection] sclerotherapy for treatment of varicose veins.

**cirs(o)-** [Gr. *kirsos* varix] a combining form denoting relationship to a varix. See also terms beginning with *varico-*.

**cir·so·cele** (sər'so-sēl) [*cirso-* + *-cele*[1]] varicocele.

**cir·soid** (sər'soid) [*cirso-* + *-oid*] varicoid.

**cir·som·pha·los** (sər-som'fə-los) [*cirso-* + Gr. *omphalos* navel] a varicose state of the navel; caput medusae.

**cir·soph·thal·mia** (sər″sof-thal'me-ə) [*cirso-* + Gr. *ophthalmos* eye] a varicose state of the conjunctival vessels.

***cis*** (sis) [L. "on this side"] 1. a prefix denoting on this side, on the same side, on the near side. 2. in organic chemistry, having certain atoms or radicals on the same side. 3. in genetics, denoting two or more loci, especially pseudoalleles, occurring on the same chromosome of a homologous pair. Cf. trans. See also cis-trans *test,* under *test.*

**cis-** a prefix denoting on this side, on the same side, on the near side.

**cisapride** (sis'ə-prīd) an agent that enhances the release of acetylcholine at the myenteric plexus, used to promote gastric emptying in the treatment of gastroesophageal reflux disease and gastroparesis; administered orally.

**cis·at·ra·cu·ri·um bes·y·late** (sis″at-rə-kūr'e-əm) a nondepolarizing neuromuscular blocking agent administered intravenously as an adjunct to general anesthesia to facilitate endotracheal intubation, induce skeletal muscle relaxation during surgery, and facilitate mechanical ventilation.

**cis·clo·mi·phene** (sis-klo'mĭ-fēn) enclomiphene.

**cis·plat·in** (sis'plat-in) [USP] [MeSH: Cisplatin] *cis*-dichlorodiammineplatinum, a platinum coordination complex capable of producing inter- and intrastrand DNA crosslinks and having a broad spectrum of antitumor activity, used in the treatment of a wide variety of neoplasms, particularly metastatic ovarian and testicular carcinoma and advanced carcinoma of the bladder; administered intravenously. Called also *cis-diamminedichloroplatinum, CDDP,* cis-*DDP,* and *DDP.*

**Cis·sam·pe·los** (sis-am'pə-los) [Gr. *kissos* ivy + *ampelos* vine] a genus of climbing vines of the family Menispermaceae. *C. capen'sis* of southern Africa is emetic and purgative. *C. parei'ra* L. is the false pareira or velvetleaf, used in tropical parts of the Americas to treat snakebites and as a diuretic, expectorant, emmenagogue, and febrifuge.

**cis·tern** (sis'tərn) a closed space serving as a reservoir for fluid; see also *cisterna.*
**ambient c.,** cisterna ambiens.
**basal c.,** cisterna interpeduncularis.
**c. of chiasma, chiasmatic c.,** cisterna chiasmatica.
**c. of fossa of Sylvius,** cisterna fossae lateralis cerebri.
**great c.,** cisterna cerebellomedullaris posterior.
**interpeduncular c.,** cisterna interpeduncularis.
**c. of lateral cerebral fossa,** cisterna fossae lateralis cerebri.
**c. of Pecquet,** cisterna chyli.
**pontine c.,** a large space ventral to the pons, continuous caudally with the spinal subarachnoid space and the cerebellomedullary cistern and rostrally with the interpeduncular space; the basilar artery runs through it.
**posterior c., posterior cerebellomedullary c.,** cisterna cerebellomedullaris posterior.
**subarachnoid c's,** cisternae subarachnoideae.
**terminal c's,** pairs of transversely oriented channels that are confluent with the sarcotubules, which together with an intermediate T tubule constitute a triad of skeletal muscle. See also *T system,* under *system; T tubule,* under *tubule;* and *triad of skeletal muscle.*

**cis·ter·na** (sis-tər'nə) gen. and pl. *cister'nae* [L.] [TA] cistern: a closed space serving as a reservoir for lymph or other body fluid, especially one of the enlarged subarachnoid spaces containing cerebrospinal fluid.
**c. am'biens** [TA], the subarachnoid space surrounding the midbrain; it connects the cisterna venae magnae cerebri with the cisterna interpeduncularis. Called also *c. mesencephalicum.*
**c. basa'lis,** c. interpeduncularis.
**c. cerebellomedulla'ris poste'rior** [TA], posterior cerebellomedullary cistern: the enlarged subarachnoid space between the inferior surface of the cerebellum and the posterior surface of the medulla oblongata, and continuous below with the spinal subarachnoid space. It can be tapped by means of a needle inserted through the posterior atlanto-occipital membrane (cisternal puncture). Called also *c. magna,* and *great* or *posterior cistern.*
**c. chiasma'tica** [TA], chiasmatic cistern: a subarachnoid space between the optic chiasma and the rostrum of the corpus callosum; called also *cistern of chiasma.*
**c. chy'li** [TA], a dilated portion of the thoracic duct at its origin in the lumbar region; it receives several lymph-collecting vessels, including the intestinal, lumbar, and descending intercostal trunks. Called also *ampulla chyli, chylocyst, cistern of Pecquet, receptaculum chyli,* and *receptaculum Pecqueti.*

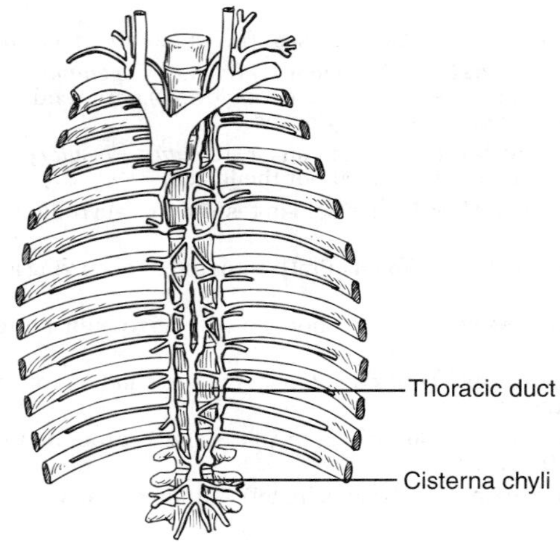


**cylindrical confronting cisternae,** cytoplasmic structures often associated with tuboreticular structures in cells in a variety of pathological conditions including immunologic and neoplastic disorders, neurodegenerative diseases, and viral infections.
**c. fos'sae latera'lis ce'rebri** [TA], cistern of lateral cerebral fossa: the space between the arachnoid and the lateral cerebral fossa; called also *c. fossae Sylvii,* and *cistern of fossa of Sylvius.*
**c. fos'sae Syl'vii,** c. fossae lateralis cerebri.
**c. interpeduncula'ris** [TA], interpeduncular cistern: a dilatation of the subarachnoid space between the cerebral peduncles; called also *basal cistern.*
**c. mag'na,** TA alternative for *c. cerebellomedullaris posterior.*
**c. mesencepha'licum,** c. ambiens.
**perinuclear c.,** the space separating the inner from the outer nuclear membrane; called also *perinuclear space.*
**c. pon'tis,** pontine cistern.
**c. retrothala'mica,** the subarachnoid space posterior to the thalamus.
**cister'nae subarachnoi'deae** [TA], subarachnoid cisterns: localized enlargements of the subarachnoid space, occurring in areas where the dura mater and arachnoid do not closely follow the contour of the brain with its covering pia mater, and serving as reservoirs of cerebrospinal fluid.
**subsarcolemmal cisternae,** hollow swellings of the tubules of the sarcoplasmic reticulum; they participate in the coupling of the sarcoplasmic reticulum with the sarcolemma in cardiac muscle.
**c. ve'nae mag'nae ce'rebri** [TA], the superior confluent of the subarachnoid space, lying in the angle between the splenium of the corpus callosum and the superior surfaces of the cerebellum and mesencephalon, and containing the great vein of the cerebrum.

**cis·ter·nae** (sis-tər'ne) [L.] genitive and plural of *cisterna.*

**cis·ter·nal** (sis-tər'nəl) pertaining to a cistern, especially the cisterna cerebellomedullaris.

**cis·ter·no·graph·ic** (sis″tər-no-graf'ik) pertaining to cisternography.

**cis·ter·nog·ra·phy** (sis″tər-nog'rə-fe) radiography of the basal cistern of the brain after subarachnoid injection of a contrast medium.
**air c.,** visualization of the cisterns of the brain following administration of approximately 5 mL of air by lumbar puncture; used in the evaluation of masses in the cerebellopontine angle and for detecting small acoustic tumors in the internal acoustic meatus.
**metrizamide c.,** visualization of the cisterns of the brain by computed tomography following intrathecal injection of metrizamide.
**radionuclide c.,** imaging of the cisterns of the brain following the intrathecal injection of a radiopharmaceutical.

**cis·tron** (sis'tron) [L. *cis* on this side + *trans* on the other side + Gr. *on* neuter ending] the smallest unit of genetic material that must be intact to function as a transmitter of genetic information, i.e., to determine the sequence of amino acids of one polypeptide chain. The cistron is identified by the *cis-trans* test. By one definition, the gene is identical to the cistron.

**ci·tal·o·pram hy·dro·bro·mide** (si-tal'o-pram) an antidepressant compound used in the treatment of major depressive disorder, administered orally.

**Ci·ta·nest** (si'tə-nest) trademark for preparations of prilocaine hydrochloride.

**Ci·tel·li's syndrome** (che-tel'ēz) [Salvatore *Citelli,* Italian laryngologist, 1875–1947] see under *syndrome.*

**Ci·tel·lus** (si-tel'əs) former name of *Spermophilus.*

**cit·rate** (sit'rāt) any anionic form, salt, or ester of citric acid.
**cupric c.,** a bluish green, crystalline powder; antiseptic and astringent.
**ferric c.,** garnet-red scales or brown granules, $FeC_6H_5O_7 \cdot xH_2O$, used as a reagent; called also *iron citrate.*
**c. phosphate dextrose (CPD),** anticoagulant citrate phosphate dextrose solution.
**c. phosphate dextrose adenine (CPDA-1),** anticoagulant citrate phosphate dextrose adenine solution.

**cit·rate con·dens·ing en·zyme** (sit'rāt kon-den'sing en'zīm) ATP citrate lyase.

**cit·rat·ed** (sit'rāt-əd) containing a citrate, especially potassium citrate.

**cit·rate *(si)*-syn·thase** (sit'rāt sin'thās) [EC 4.1.3.7] an enzyme of the lyase class that catalyzes the condensation of oxaloacetate and the acetyl group of acetyl coenzyme A to form citrate and coenzyme A. This is the initial reaction in the tricarboxylic acid cycle (see illustration at *tricarboxylic acid cycle*).

**ci·treo·vir·i·din** (sĭ"tre-o-vir'ĭ-din) a mycotoxin found in the fungus *Penicillium citreoviride,* which sometimes contaminates rice and can cause cardiac damage.

**cit·ric ac·id** (sit'rik) [MeSH: Citric Acid] a compound from citrus fruits that is an intermediate in the tricarboxylic acid (Krebs) cycle (q.v.). Citrate chelates calcium ions and prevents blood clotting and is used as an anticoagulant for stored whole blood and red cells and also for blood specimens.

**cit·ri·nin** (sit'rĭ-nin) [MeSH: Citrinin] a mycotoxin produced by *Aspergillus ochraceus, Penicillium citrinum,* and related species, which contaminate grain; it causes mycotoxic nephropathy in livestock and has been implicated as a cause of Balkan nephropathy in humans.

**Cit·ro·bac·ter** (sit"ro-bak'tər) [L. *citrus* lemon + Gr. *baktron* a rod] [MeSH: Citrobacter] a genus of gram-negative, facultatively anaerobic, rod-shaped bacteria of the family Enterobacteriaceae, made up of motile organisms that are able to use citrate as a sole carbon source. The organisms occur in water, food, feces, and urine. They have been associated with diarrhea and secondary infections in debilitated persons, occasionally causing severe primary septicemia.
**C. amalona'ticus,** a species that produces indole, does not ferment adonitol, and is not inhibited by potassium cyanide; found in humans as an opportunistic pathogen.
**C. diver'sus,** a species that produces indole, ferments adonitol, and is inhibited by potassium cyanide; it occasionally causes neonatal meningitis.
**C. freun'dii,** the most commonly isolated species. It does not produce indole or ferment adonitol and is not inhibited by potassium cyanide; found in soil, water, sewage and food, in clinical specimens from normal persons, and as an opportunistic pathogen.
**C. interme'dius,** a variant of *C. freundii.* Called also *Escherichia intermedia.*

**Ci·tro·my·ces** (sit"ro-mi'sēz) [*citric acid* + Gr. *mykes* fungus] former name for *Penicillium.*

**cit·ron** (sit'ron) [L. *citrus*] 1. *Citrus medica,* an orangelike tree. 2. the fruit of this tree.

**cit·ron·el·la** (sit"ron-el'ə) *Cymbopogon nardus,* the source of citronella oil.

**cit·ro·phos·phate** (sit"ro-fos'fāt) a compound of a citrate and a phosphate.

**cit·rul·line** (sit'rul-ēn) [MeSH: Citrulline] alpha-amino delta-carbamido normal valeric acid; it is formed from ornithine and is itself converted into arginine in the urea cycle.

**cit·rul·lin·emia** (sit-rul"in-e'me-ə) 1. argininosuccinate synthase deficiency. 2. excess of citrulline in the blood.

**Ci·trul·lus** (sĭ-trul'əs) a genus of plants of the family Cucurbitaceae, originally native to Africa. *C. colocyn'this* is the colocynth. *C. vulga'ris* is the watermelon.

**cit·rul·lin·uria** (sit-rul"in-u're-ə) 1. argininosuccinate synthase deficiency. 2. excretion of high levels of citrulline in the urine.

**Cit·rus** (sit'rəs) [L.] the citrus fruits, a genus of trees of the family Rutaceae, widely cultivated for their fruit; several of the fruits are rich in vitamin C and are sources of flavorings. *C. aurantifo'lia* is the lime; *C. auran'tium* L. is the orange; *C. berga'mia* is the bergamot; *C. li'mon* (Linné) Burmann filius is the lemon; *C. me'dica* is the citron; and *C. sinen'sis* is the sweet orange.

**Ci·vatte's poikiloderma** (se-vahts') [Achille *Civatte,* French dermatologist, 1877–1956] see under *body* and *poikiloderma.*

**Ci·vi·ni·ni's ligament, process (spine)** (che"ve-ne'nēz) [Filippo *Civinini,* Italian anatomist, 1805–1844] see *ligamentum pterygospinale* and *processus pterygospinosus.*

**CK** creatine kinase.

**Cl** symbol for *chlorine.*

**clad·i·o·sis** (klad"e-o'sis) name given to a single case of a fungal disease resembling sporotrichosis.

**Cla·do's anastomosis, band, ligament** (klah-dōz') [Spiro *Clado,* French gynecologist, 1862–1920] see under *anastomosis, band,* and *ligament.*

**Cla·dor·chis wat·so·ni** (klə-dor'kis wat-so'ni) *Watsonius watsoni.*

**clad·o·spo·ri·o·sis** (klad"o-spor"e-o'sis) a general term for infection with *Cladosporium,* including brain infections such as abscesses and meningitis, and skin infections such as chromoblastomycosis and tinea nigra.
**c. epider'mica,** tinea nigra.

**Clad·o·spo·ri·um** (klad"o-spor'e-əm) [Gr. *klados* branch + *spores* seed] [MeSH: Cladosporium] a genus of chiefly saprobic Fungi Imperfecti of the form-class Hyphomycetes, form-family Dematiaceae, having mainly aseptate, acropetal conidia.
**C. bantia'num,** a species that causes thick-walled abscesses of the brain and sometimes meningitis. Authorities differ on whether this and *C. trichoides* are the same species or different.
**C. carrio'nii,** a species that is an agent of chromoblastomycosis.
**C. manso'nii,** *Malassezia furfur.*
**C. trichoi'des,** a species that causes thick-walled abscesses of the brain and sometimes meningitis. Authorities differ on whether this and *C. bantianum* are the same species or different.
**C. wernec'kii,** *Exophiala werneckii.*

**Clad·o·thrix** (klad'o-thriks) [Gr. *klados* branch + *thrix* hair] a genus of bacteria made up of organisms now classified in the genera *Actinomyces, Bacterionema, Nocardia, Sphaerotilus,* and *Streptomyces.*

**clad·ri·bine** (kla'drĭ-bēn) [MeSH: Cladribine] a purine antimetabolite used as an antineoplastic in the treatment of hairy cell leukemia; administered intravenously. Called also *2-chlorodeoxyadenosine.*

**clair·voy·ance** (klār-voi'əns) [Fr.] a form of extrasensory perception in which knowledge of objective events is acquired without the use of the senses. Cf. *telepathy.*

**clamp** (klamp) 1. any device used to grip, join, compress, or fasten parts. 2. a surgical instrument for effecting compression. See also under *forceps.*
**Cope's c.,** a crushing clamp with several hinged segments for use in surgery of the colon and rectum.
**cotton roll rubber dam c.,** a rubber dam clamp with a buccal and lingual wing or flange to hold cotton rolls in position in the mouth; useful in the placement of direct gold or other restorative material in subgingival class V cavity preparations.
**Crile's c.,** a rubber-shod clamp to secure temporary hemostasis in suture of blood vessels.
**Doyen's c.,** a forceps with flexible blades for clamping tissues to

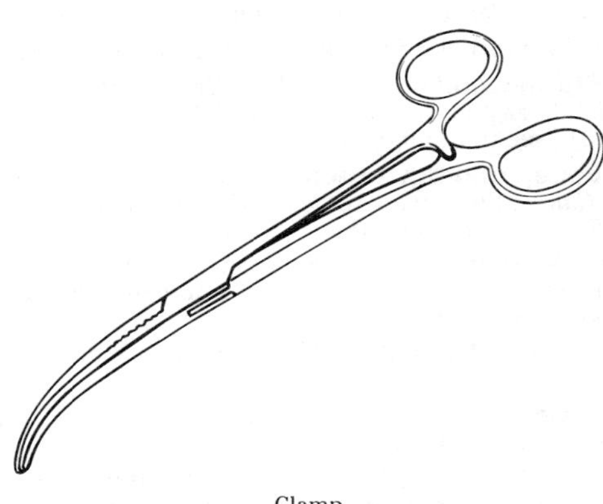
Clamp.

control bleeding temporarily during operations on the gastrointestinal tract.
**Gant's c.**, a right-angled clamp used in operating on hemorrhoids.
**gingival c.**, a clamp for retracting gingival tissues.
**Goldblatt's c.**, a clamp for the renal artery to produce experimental hypertension; see also *Goldblatt hypertension* and *Goldblatt kidney*, under *hypertension* and *kidney*.
**Joseph's c.**, a clamp used after a nasal operation to improve the alignment of the mobilized fragments of the bony framework of the nose.
**Martel's c.**, a crushing clamp used in resection of the colon.
**Mikulicz's c.**, a clamp used for crushing the septum between the proximal and distal segments of the colon after exteriorization.
**patch c.**, a type of voltage clamp in which a patch electrode is pressed against an area of the plasma membrane of a cell, forming an electrically tight seal so that the flow of current through individual ion channels can be measured.
**Payr c.**, a crushing clamp used in resections of the stomach, intestine, and colon.
**pedicle c.**, clamp forceps, def. 1; see under *forceps*.
**Potts' c.**, an atraumatic clamp used to grasp a blood vessel.
**Rankin c.**, a three-bladed clamp for crushing the colon during resection.
**rubber dam c.**, a device made of spring metal that is used to retain a rubber dam on a tooth; it has beveled jaws that contact the tooth and a bow that connects the jaws.
**Sehrt's c.**, a clamp for compressing the aorta or for compressing a limb to arrest hemorrhage; called also *Sehrt's compressor*.
**voltage c.**, an electronic technique employing the feedback principle to impose a fixed potential difference across a cell membrane. Voltage across the membrane is fixed at a set level and the current changes to counterbalance any induced flow of ions; the current change is a measure of the change in conductance of the membrane for one or more specific ions.
**Willett c.**, Willett forceps.
**Yellen c.**, a special clamp used for circumcision.

**clamping** (klamp'ing) in the measurement of insulin secretion and action, the infusion of a glucose solution at a rate adjusted periodically to maintain a predetermined blood glucose concentration.

**clang·ing** (klang'ing) a pattern of speech in which sound rather than sense governs word choice, and rhyming and punning *(clang association)* substitute for logic; commonly observed in schizophrenia and manic episodes.

**clap** (klap) popular name for gonorrhea.

**clap·o·tage** (klap″o-tahzh') clapotement.

**cla·pote·ment** (klah-pawt-maw') [Fr.] a splashing sound heard on succussion; called also *clapotage*.

**claque·ment** (klahk-maw') [Fr.] a clapping or snapping.
**c. d'ouverture**, opening snap.

**Cla·ra cells** (klah'rah) [Max *Clara*, Austrian anatomist, born 1899] see under *cell*.

**clar·if·i·cant** (klar-if'ĭ-kənt) an agent that clears liquids of turbidity.

**clar·i·fi·ca·tion** (klar″ĭ-fĭ-ka'shən) [L. *clarus* clear + *facere* to make] the clearing of a liquid from turbidity.

**clar·i·fy** (klar'ĭ-fi) [L. *clarificare* to render clear] to clear of turbidity or of suspended matter.

**cla·rith·ro·my·cin** (klə-rith″ro-mi'sin) [USP] [MeSH: Clarithromycin] a macrolide antibiotic effective against a wide spectrum of gram-positive and gram-negative bacteria, used in the treatment of respiratory tract infections and skin and soft tissue infections, and in conjunction with omeprazole in the treatment of duodenal ulcer associated with *Helicobacter pylori* infections; administered orally.

**Clar·i·tin** (klar'ĭ-tin) trademark for a preparation of loratadine.

**Clark-Col·lip method** (klahrk-kol'ip) [Earl Perry *Clark*, American biochemist, born 1892; James Bertram *Collip*, Canadian biochemist, 1892–1965] see under *method*.

**Clarke's cells, column (nucleus)** (klahrks) [Jacob Augustus Lockhart *Clarke*, English anatomist and physician, 1817–1880] see under *cell*, and see *nucleus thoracicus posterior*.

**Clarke-Had·field syndrome** (klahrk-had'fēld) [Cecil *Clarke*, British physician, 20th century; Geoffrey *Hadfield*, British physician, 1889–1968] see under *syndrome*.

**clas·mato·cyte** (klaz-mat'o-sit) [Gr. *klasma* a piece broken off + *-cyte*] old term for *macrophage*.

**clas·ma·to·sis** (klaz″mə-to'sis) [Gr. *klasma* a piece broken off] the breaking off of parts of a cell.

**clasp** (klasp) 1. a device by which something is held. 2. in dentistry, a part of an extracoronal direct retainer that retains and stabilizes the denture by attaching to abutment teeth.

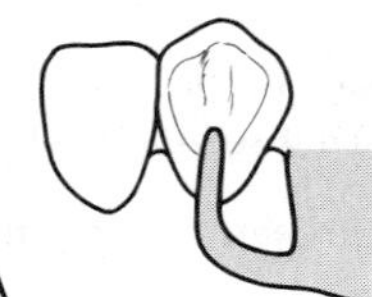

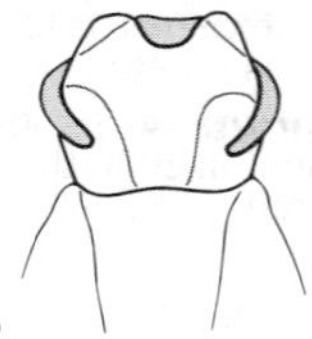

*(A)*, I-bar clasp; *(B)*, circumferential clasp.

**Adams c.**, a modified arrow clasp that utilizes buccal, mesial, and distal proximal undercuts of a tooth for retention.
**arrow c., arrowhead c.**, a clasp made by bending a piece of stainless steel wire in the shape of an arrowhead; used to stabilize an orthodontic appliance by holding the teeth in the interproximal areas.
**bar c.**, one whose arms are bar-type extensions from major connectors or from within the denture base; the arms approach the point of contact on the tooth in the cervico-occlusal direction.
**circumferential c.**, one that encircles more than 180° of a tooth, including opposite angles, and usually contacts the tooth throughout the extent of the clasp, at least one terminal being in the infrabulge area. See illustration.
**continuous c., continuous lingual c.**, one made of two or more stainless steel lingual clasps joined to each other and then joined to a major connector by two or more minor connectors; used to brace lingual upper teeth. Called also *continuous bar retainer, Kennedy bar*, and *lingual bar*.
**Crozat c.**, a metal attachment of a removable appliance adapted to the embrasure.
**I-bar c., infrabulge c.**, a bar clasp arm that approaches the crown of the tooth from an apical direction, without crossing the survey line, crossing the tooth-tissue junction at right angles and continuing in a straight line to the unattached mucosa before turning to a horizontal position. See illustration.

**class** (klas) 1. a taxonomic category subordinate to a phylum (or subphylum) and superior to an order. 2. in statistics, a subgroup of a population for which certain variables measured for individuals in the population fall within specific limits.

**clas·sic** (klas'ik) of first class or rank; standard.

**clas·si·fi·ca·tion** (klas″ĭ-fĭ-ka'shən) [MeSH: Classification] the systematic arrangement of similar entities on the basis of certain differing characteristics.
**adansonian c.**, numerical taxonomy.
**Angle's c.**, a classification of dental malocclusion based on the mesiodistal (anteroposterior) position of the mandibular dental arch and teeth relative to the maxillary dental arch and teeth; see under *malocclusion*.
**Arneth's c.**, classification of neutrophils according to the number of lobes in their nuclei for calculating the Arneth count.
**Bergey's c.**, a system of classification of bacteria in which the organisms are grouped according to Gram reaction, metabolism, and morphology, with each group being further subdivided into orders, families, genera, and species.
**Black's c.**, a classification of dental caries into five groups on the basis of similarity of treatment required. See table at *caries*.
**Borrmann's c.**, a classification of gastric carcinoma as either polypoid, ulcerating, ulcerating-infiltrating, or infiltrating.
**Broders' c.**, see under *index*.
**Caldwell-Moloy c.**, classification of female pelves as gynecoid, android, anthropoid, and platypelloid; see under *pelvis*.
**Chicago c.**, the classification of human chromosomes adopted by geneticists at Chicago in 1966 for the identification of chromosomal bands and regions and for the location of structural chromosomal abnormalities. See also *Denver c.* and *Paris c.*
**Denver c.**, a former classification of human chromosomes on the basis of size and centromere position, adopted by geneticists in Denver in 1960. The 23 pairs of chromosomes are arranged into seven groups, labeled A to G, in the order of decreasing length. See also *Chicago c.*
**Dukes' c.**, a three-class staging system that classifies colorectal carcinoma from A to C based on the extent of the tumor: A, penetration into but not through the bowel wall; B, penetration through the bowel wall; C, lymph node involvement regardless of extent of bowel wall penetration. Many modifications of this classification exist.
**FIGO c.**, any of the classification systems established by the International Federation of Gynecology and Obstetrics for the staging of gynecological cancers. Cancers at any particular site are staged from 0 to IV with 0 being precancerous or in situ and IV being highly malignant or invasive; subdivisions using letters may also be used, as IA, IB, IIA, IIB, and so on.
**Frankel C.**, a classification dividing spinal cord injuries into five groups according to severity of deficit below the level of injury: *Group A*, complete interruption of all sensation and motor function; *Group B*, incomplete interruption, with some sensation but no motor

function; *Group C,* incomplete interruption, with demonstrable voluntary motor function but at a minimal, nonuseful level; *Group D,* incomplete interruption, with some voluntary motor function that is useful to the patient; and *Group E,* recovery to normal functioning attained.

**Fredrickson and Lees c.,** a scheme for subdividing the familial hyperlipoproteinemias on the basis of phenotypes, which are classified as I–V. See table at *hyperlipoproteinemia.*

**French-American-British (FAB) c.,** a classification of acute leukemia produced by a three-nation joint collaboration; acute lymphocytic leukemia is subdivided into three types and acute myelogenous leukemia is subdivided into six types.

**Gell and Coombs c.,** a classification of immune mechanisms of tissue injury, called by Gell and Coombs "allergic reactions," comprising four types: *type I,* immediate hypersensitivity reactions, mediated by IgE antibody; *type II,* antibody-mediated hypersensitivity reactions, including complement-dependent lysis, antibody-dependent cell-mediated cytotoxicity (ADCC), and phagocytosis induced by opsonizing antibody; *type III,* immune complex–mediated hypersensitivity reactions, including serum sickness, Arthus reactions, and systemic lupus erythematosus; and *type IV,* cell-mediated hypersensitivity reactions, mediated by sensitized T lymphocytes either by release of lymphokines or by T-cell–mediated cytotoxicity, including contact dermatitis, allograft rejection, and graft-versus-host disease. Other authorities have added *type V,* antibody interference with the function of biologically active substances, including autoimmune diseases mediated by antireceptor antibodies and coagulation disorders mediated by antibodies to coagulation factors. The individual types I–IV are described under *hypersensitivity reaction,* under *reaction.*

**Kauffman-White c.,** a scheme for the serologic identification of species of *Salmonella* by classification of their reactions to O, H, and Vi antisera.

**Keith-Wagener-Barker c.,** a classification of hypertension and arteriolosclerosis based on retinal changes. *Group 1,* essential benign hypertension indicated by moderate arteriolar attenuation. *Group 2,* constant high blood pressure but no apparent effect on health, indicated by more definite arteriolar attenuation with localized constriction. *Group 3,* hypertension with retinal, renal, cerebral, and other symptoms, indicated by marked attenuation of the arterioles, cotton-wool exudates, and hemorrhages. *Group 4,* severe hypertension with severe nervous system, visual, and other organ disturbances, indicated by ophthalmoscopic signs of Group 3, with papilledema.

**Kennedy c.,** a classification of partially edentulous conditions and partial dentures, based on the location of the edentulous spaces in relation to the remaining teeth.

**Kiel c.,** a classification of non-Hodgkin's lymphomas, used primarily in Europe and based on morphologic and cytologic criteria. A later classification system is the Revised European American Lymphoma (REAL) Classification. Called also *Lennert's c.*

**Lancefield c.,** a serologic classification of the hemolytic streptococci, based on extraction and examination by a precipitin technique of group-specific carbohydrate antigens contained in the cell wall. Groups A through O have been established.

**Lennert's c.,** Kiel c.

**Lukes-Collins C.,** a classification of non-Hodgkin's lymphomas based on their presumed cells of origin. It stresses the distinction between B-cell, T-cell, and lymphocytic lymphomas, with the B-cell and T-cell types having several subtypes that can be arranged by grade of malignancy. A later classification is the Revised European American Lymphoma (REAL) Classification.

**Lund-Browder c.,** a classification of burn severity in children; it attaches percentages to different body surface areas similarly to the rule of nines used for adults and is modified according to the age of the child.

**McNeer c.,** Borrmann's c.

**Migula's c.,** a classification of bacteria drawn up by Migula in 1900.

**New York Heart Association (NYHA) c.,** a functional and therapeutic classification for prescription of physical activity for cardiac patients; see table.

**numerical c.,** see under *taxonomy.*

**Paris c.,** a modification made in Paris in 1971 of the Chicago classification of human chromosomes, providing more detailed cytogenetic information; see also *Denver c.*

**Rappaport C.,** a classification of non-Hodgkin's lymphomas based on histologic criteria; the categories it developed were *nodular lymphomas* and *diffuse lymphomas.* It was replaced by the Lukes-Collins Classification and the Kiel Classification.

**REAL C., Revised European American Lymphoma C.,** a classification of lymphomas based on histologic criteria, dividing them into three main categories: B-cell neoplasms, T- or NK-cell neoplasms, and Hodgkin's disease.

**Runyon c.,** a classification of mycobacteria based on the pigmentation and growth condition of the organisms. See *nontuberculous mycobacteria,* under *mycobacterium.*

**Rye C.,** a classification of Hodgkin's disease on the basis of histology and pathology into the categories of lymphocyte predominance type, mixed cellularity type, lymphocyte depletion type, and nodular sclerosis type.

**Skinner c.,** a method of classifying partially edentulous conditions and partial dentures, based on the location of the edentulous spaces in relation to the remaining teeth.

**New York Heart Association Classification of Cardiac Patients**

| Class | Limitation of activity | Symptoms |
|---|---|---|
| I(A) | None | None from ordinary activity |
| II(B) | Slight | On moderate or normal exertion |
| III(C) | Marked | On mild exertion |
| IV(D) | Complete | Even at rest, worsened by any exertion |

**-clast** [Gr. *-klastēs* breaker, from *klan* to break] a word termination denoting that which breaks or destroys.

**clas·tic** (klas′tik) [Gr. *klastos* broken + *-ic*] 1. causing or undergoing a division into parts. 2. separable into parts, as an anatomic model.

**clas·to·gen·ic** (klas″to-jen′ik) [Gr. *klastos* broken + *-genic*] giving rise to or inducing disruption or breakages, as of chromosomes.

**clas·to·thrix** (klas′to-thriks) [Gr. *klastos* broken + *-thrix*] trichorrhexis nodosa.

**clath·rate** (klath′rāt) [L. *clathare* to provide with a lattice] 1. having the shape or appearance of a lattice. 2. clathrate compound. 3. pertaining to a such a compound.

**clath·rin** (klath′rin) [MeSH: Clathrin] a 180,000-dalton protein that coats the cytoplasmic face of coated pits (q.v.) involved in receptor-mediated endocytosis of low-density lipoprotein (LDL), insulin, and other ligands.

**Claude** (klawd) Albert. Belgian-born American cytologist, born 1899; co-winner, with Christian René de Duve and George Emil Palade, of the Nobel prize for medicine or physiology in 1974 for their discoveries concerning the structural and functional organization of the cell.

**Claude's hyperkinesis sign, syndrome** (klōdz) [Henri *Claude,* French psychiatrist, 1869–1945] see under *sign* and *syndrome.*

**Claude Ber·nard** (klōd bār-nahr′) see *Bernard.*

**clau·di·cant** (klaw′dĭ-kənt) 1. pertaining to claudication; called also *claudicatory.* 2. affected by claudication. 3. affected by intermittent claudication.

**clau·di·ca·tion** (klaw′dĭ-ka′shən) [L. *claudicatio*] limping or lameness.

**intermittent c.,** a complex of symptoms characterized by pain, tension, and weakness in a limb when walking is begun, intensification of the condition until walking becomes impossible, and disappearance of the symptoms after a period of rest. It is seen in occlusive arterial diseases of the limbs, such as thromboangiitis obliterans, and in compression of the cauda equina. Called also *Charcot's syndrome* and *angina cruris.*

**jaw c.,** a complex of symptoms like those of intermittent claudication but seen in the muscles of mastication, occurring in giant cell arteritis.

**neurogenic c.,** claudication accompanied by pain and paresthesias in the back, buttocks, and legs that is relieved by stooping, caused by mechanical disturbances due to posture or by ischemia of the cauda equina.

**venous c.,** intermittent claudication caused by venous stasis.

**clau·di·ca·tory** (klaw′dĭ-kə-tor″e) claudicant (def. 1).

**Clau·di·us' cells** (klaw′de-əs) [Friedrich Matthias *Claudius,* German anatomist, 1822–1869] see under *cell.*

**claus·tra** (klaws′trə) [L.] plural of *claustrum.*

**claus·tral** (klaws′trəl) pertaining to the claustrum.

**claus·tro·pho·bia** (klaws″tro-fo′be-ə) [L. *claudere* to shut + *-phobia*] irrational fear of being shut in; fear of enclosed spaces, such as elevators and tunnels.

**claus·trum** (claws′trəm) pl. *claus′tra* [L. "a barrier"] [TA] the thin layer of gray matter lateral to the external capsule of the lentiform nucleus, separating the nucleus from the white substance of the insula; it is mainly composed of spindle cells. Called also *claustrum of insula.*

**clau·su·ra** (klaw-su′rə) [L. "closure"] atresia.

**cla·va** (kla′və) [L. "stick"] tuberculum gracile.

**cla·va·cin** (kla'və-sin) patulin.

**cla·val** (kla'vəl) pertaining to the clava (tuberculum gracile [TA]).

**cla·vate** (kla'vāt) [L. *clavatus* club] 1. claval. 2. club-shaped.

**Clav·i·ceps** (klav'ĭ-seps) [L. *clava* club + *caput* head] [MeSH: Claviceps] a genus of parasitic fungi of the family Clavicipitaceae that infest the seeds of various plants; several species are sources of ergot. *C. purpu'rea* infests rye and is the most common source of ergotism in humans. *C. pas'pali* infests paspalum grasses and causes paspalum staggers in ruminants.

**Clav·i·cip·i·ta·ceae** (klav"ĭ-sip"ĭ-ta'se-e) a family of fungi of the order Clavicipitales, having long cylindrical asci and long filiform ascospores; it includes the genera *Claviceps* and *Cordyceps.*

**Clav·i·cip·i·ta·les** (klav"ĭ-sip"ĭ-ta'lēz) an order of perfect fungi of the subphylum Ascomycotina, series Unitunicatae, characterized by perithecia formed in well-developed stroma and inoperculate asci. Most species are parasitic on insects or fungi; some are plant parasites. It includes the family Clavicipitaceae.

**clav·i·cle** (klav'ĭ-kəl) [MeSH: Clavicle] clavicula.

**clav·i·cot·o·my** (klav"ĭ-kot'ə-me) [*clavicle* + Gr. *-tomy*] the operation of cutting or dividing the clavicle.

**cla·vic·u·la** (klə-vik'u-lə) [L. dim. of *clavis* key] [TA] the clavicle: a bone, curved like the letter *f,* that articulates with the sternum and scapula, forming the anterior portion of the shoulder girdle on either side; called also *collar bone.*

**cla·vic·u·lar** (klə-vik'u-lər) pertaining to the clavicle.

**cla·vic·u·lus** (klə-vik'u-ləs) pl. *clavic'uli* [L. dim. of *clavus* nail] any one of Sharpey's fibers (a set of fibers that hold together the laminae of a bone).

**clav·i·for·min** (klav"ĭ-for'min) patulin.

**clav·i·pec·to·ral** (klav"ĭ-pek'tə-rəl) [L. *clavis* clavicle + *pectoral*] pertaining to the clavicle and thorax.

**Cla·vis·po·ra** (klə-vis'pə-rə) a genus of fungi of the order Endomycetales. *C. lusita'niae* is the perfect (sexual) stage of *Candida lusitaniae.*

**clav·u·la·nate po·tas·si·um** (klav'u-lə-nāt) a β-lactamase inhibitor used in combination with penicillins in treating infections caused by β-lactamase–producing organisms.

**cla·vus** (kla'vəs) pl. *cla'vi* [L. "nail"] corn (def. 1).
**c. du'rus,** hard corn.
**c. hyste'ricus,** a sharp, painful sensation as if a nail were being driven into the head; usually regarded as a manifestation of conversion.
**c. mol'lis,** soft corn.
**c. secali'nus,** ergot (def. 1).
**c. syphili'ticus,** a cornlike lesion seen on the palm or sole, a type of papular syphilid.

**claw** (klaw) a nail of an animal, particularly a carnivore, that is long and curved and has a sharp end. Called also *unguiculus.*

**claw·foot** (klaw'foot) gampsodactyly.

**claw·hand** (klaw-hand) flexion and atrophy of the hand and fingers; it occurs in lesions of the ulnar nerve, in leprosy, and in syringomyelia. Called also *main en griffe.*

**clay** (kla) a native hydrated aluminum silicate, resulting from the decomposition of rocks caused by weathering; various forms of clays have been used in medicine, both externally and internally, since earliest times.
**China c.,** kaolin.

**cla·zu·ril** (klaz'u-ril) a coccidiostat used in birds.

**clear** (klēr) 1. to remove cloudiness from microscopic specimens by the use of a clearing agent. 2. to remove a substance from the blood.

**clear·ance** (klēr'əns) 1. the process of removing a substance or an obstruction. 2. a quantitative measure of the rate at which a substance is removed from the blood by processes such as renal clearance, hepatic clearance, or hemodialysis; the volume of plasma that is completely cleared of the substance per unit time. Symbol *C.* 3. the space existing between opposed structures.

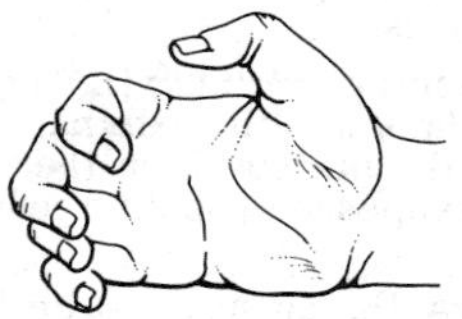
Clawhand.

***p*-aminohippurate c.,** the renal clearance of exogenously administered *p*-aminohippuric acid, accepted as the most accurate measurement of effective renal plasma flow (ERPF).
**blood-urea c.,** urea c.
**creatinine c.,** the renal clearance of endogenous creatinine, a commonly used clinical measurement that closely estimates the glomerular filtration rate (GFR).
**free water c.,** the net amount of solute-free water moved from the blood to the urine; the difference between the urine volume and the osmolal clearance.
**hepatic c.,** the removal of a substance from the blood via the liver.
**immune c.,** immune elimination.
**interocclusal c.,** see under *distance.*
**inulin c.,** the renal clearance of inulin maintained at a constant serum level by continuous infusion, accepted as the most accurate measurement and reference of the glomerular filtration rate (GFR).
**mucociliary c.,** the clearance of mucus and other material from the airways by the cilia of the epithelial cells, which move mucus cephalad with every beat. See also *ciliary beat,* under *beat.*
**occlusal c.,** a condition in which the opposing occlusal surfaces may glide over one another without any interfering projection.
**osmolal c.,** the amount of water cleared from the plasma, resulting in urine having the same osmolality as plasma, calculated as urine volume × urine osmolality ÷ plasma osmolality.
**plasma iron c.,** plasma iron clearance half-time.
**renal c.,** a measure of the rate at which a substance is removed from the blood via the kidneys; given by the formula $C = V \times U/P$, where $C$ is the clearance, $V$ the urine volume in mL/min, $U$ the urine concentration of the substance, and $P$ the plasma concentration. See also clearances of specific substances such as p-*aminohippurate c., creatinine c., inulin c.,* and *urea c.*
**total c.,** total body c.
**total body c.,** the total clearance of a substance via all the organs of the body. Cf. *hepatic c.* and *renal c.*
**urea c.,** clearance of urea from the blood, by either renal clearance or hemodialysis; the efficiency, or fractional urea clearance, of one hemodialysis session is expressed by the formula *KT/V* (q.v.). See also *urea kinetic modeling,* under *modeling.*
**whole body c.,** total body c.

**clear·er** (klēr'ər) a clearing agent; an agent used in microscopy to remove the cloudiness from a specimen.

**cleav·age** (klēv'əj) the mitotic segmentation of the zygote, the size of the structure remaining unchanged, as the cleavage cells, or blastomeres, become smaller and smaller with each division.
**accessory c.,** peripheral cleavage in telolecithal oocytes due to polyspermy.
**adequal c.,** a form in which the blastomeres are practically equal in size.
**complete c.,** holoblastic c.
**determinate c.,** cleavage following a precise pattern, each blastomere having a characteristic and unalterable fate, i.e., each blastomere becoming the precursor of a definite part of the embryo.
**discoidal c.,** cleavage limited to the animal pole of highly telolecithal oocytes.
**equal c.,** a form in which the blastomeres are equal in size.
**equatorial c.,** cleavage that occurs in a plane passing through the equator of the oocyte.
**holoblastic c.,** a form in which the entire oocyte participates in cell division; called also *complete* or *total c.*
**incomplete c.,** meroblastic c.
**indeterminate c.,** that following a less rigid cleavage pattern, the blastomeres having more developmental possibilities than they usually show, each of which, when isolated, being capable of developing into a normal embryo.
**latitudinal c.,** cleavage in planes passing at right angles to the oocyte axis.
**meridional c.,** cleavage in planes passing through the oocyte axis.
**meroblastic c., partial c.,** a form in which only the protoplasmic portions of the oocyte participate; called also *incomplete c.*
**progressive c.,** in the formation of spores within a sporangium, the production of a series of cleavage planes in succession, resulting first in formation of protospores and later in formation of sporangiospores.
**radial c.,** a cleavage pattern characteristic of vertebrates and echinoderms, in which the spindle axes are parallel or at right angles to the polar axis of the oocyte.
**spiral c.,** a cleavage pattern characteristic of such invertebrates as annelids and mollusks, in which the cleavage planes are oriented obliquely to the polar axis of the oocyte.
**superficial c.,** a form in which only the surface region of centrolecithal oocytes participate.
**total c.,** holoblastic c.
**unequal c.,** a form in which the blastomeres about the vegetal pole remain larger in size than those nearer the animal pole.

**cleft** (kleft) 1. a fissure or elongated opening, especially one occur-

ring in the embryo. 2. a pathologic fissure derived from a failure of parts to fuse during embryonic development.
**anal c.,** crena analis.
**branchial c.,** 1. any of the slitlike openings in the gills of fishes, formed between the branchial arches. 2. pharyngeal groove.
**cervical c's,** clefts in the endocervical mucosa.
**cholesterol c.,** a cleft in a section of tissue embedded in paraffin, due to the dissolving of cholesterol crystals.
**clunial c.,** crena analis.
**corneal c.,** see under *fissure.*
**facial c.,** 1. any of the clefts between the embryonic prominences that normally unite to form the face. 2. failure of union of a facial cleft, which, depending on its site, causes such developmental defects as cleft cheek, cleft lip, cleft mandible, oblique facial cleft, and lateral facial cleft. Called also *prosoposchisis.*
**facial c., lateral,** transverse facial cleft extending from the angle of the mouth toward the ear. See also *macrostomia.*
**facial c., oblique,** a rare form of facial cleft extending from the lip to the inner canthus of the eye. It may be superficial but usually separates the underlying bone and is associated with cleft lip, cleft palate, or lateral facial cleft. Called also *meloschisis* and *prosopoanoschisis.*
**facial c., transverse,** lateral facial c.
**genital c.,** a depression of the external genital region of the fetus, which develops into the male urethra or the female vestibule.
**gingival c.,** an area of isolated gingival recession occurring over a dehiscence of the bone covering the root.
**gluteal c.,** crena analis.
**hyobranchial c.,** the cleft between the hyoid and the next succeeding arch in the developing embryo; called also *posthyoidean c.*
**hyoid c.,** hyomandibular c.
**hyomandibular c.,** the cleft between the mandibular and hyoid arches in the developing embryo; called also *hyoid c.*
**interdental c.,** diastema.
**intergluteal c.,** crena analis.
**Lanterman's c's,** incisures of Lanterman.
**Larrey's c.,** trigonum sternocostale.
**Maurer's c's,** Maurer's dots.
**natal c.,** crena analis.
**posthyoidean c.,** hyobranchial c.
**primary synaptic c.,** synaptic trough.
**Schmidt-Lanterman c's,** incisures of Lanterman.
**secondary synaptic c's,** subneural c's.
**sternal c.,** cleft sternum.
**Stillman's c.,** a small apostrophe-shaped or slitlike fissure of the gingiva extending from the gingival margin to a depth of up to 5 to 6 cm.
**subneural c's,** evenly spaced lamella-like clefts within the primary synaptic cleft, formed by infoldings of the sarcolemma into the underlying sarcolemma of muscle; called also *subneural apparatus* and *secondary synaptic c's.*
**synaptic c.,** 1. a narrow extracellular cleft between the presynaptic and postsynaptic membranes. 2. synaptic trough.
**visceral c.,** pharyngeal groove.
**vulval c.,** rima pudendi.

**clei·dag·ra** (kli-dag'rə) [*cleid-* + *-agra*] gouty pain in the clavicle.

**clei·dal** (kli'dəl) pertaining to or affecting the clavicle.

**clei·dar·thri·tis** (kli"dahr-thri'tis) [*cleid-* + *arthritis*] gout in the clavicular region.

**cleid(o)-** [Gr. *kleis,* gen. *kleidos,* key, clavicle] a combining form denoting relationship to the clavicle.

**clei·do·cos·tal** (kli"do-kos'təl) pertaining to the clavicle and the ribs.

**clei·do·cra·ni·al** (kli"do-kra'ne-əl) [*cleido-* + *cranium*] pertaining to the clavicle and the head.

**clei·do·ic** (kli-do'ik) [Gr. *kleidouchos* holding the keys] isolated from the environment, self-contained, as the oocytes (ova) of reptiles, birds, and primitive mammals, which are self-sufficient, having become a closed system, and, except for oxygen intake, developing at the expense of the substances stored inside the oocyte itself, directly into miniature adults without passing through a larval stage.

**clei·do·mas·toid** (kli"do-mas'toid) pertaining to the clavicle and the mastoid process.

**clei·dot·o·my** (kli-dot'ə-me) [*cleido-* + *-tomy*] surgical division of the clavicle of the fetus in difficult labor, to facilitate passage of the shoulders through the birth canal.

**clei·sag·ra** (kli-sag'rə) cleidagra.

**cleis·to·the·ci·um** (klīs"to-the'se-əm) [Gr. *kleisis* closure + *theca*] the fruiting body (ascocarp) produced by certain ascomycetes, in which there is no pore for the escape of ascospores, the spores being released by rupture or decay of the body. Cf. *apothecium, gymnothecium,* and *perithecium.*

**clem·as·tine** (klem'əs-tēn) [MeSH: Clemastine] an ethanolamine derivative with antihistaminic effects.
**c. fumarate,** a salt of clemastine; an antihistaminic used in the treatment of allergic rhinitis and allergic skin disorders.

**Clem·a·tis** (klem'ə-tis) [Gr. *klēmatis*] a genus of flowering plants of the family Ranunculaceae. Most species contain ranunculin, which breaks down in the body to form the lethal toxin protoanemonin.

**clem·i·zole** (klem'ĭ-zōl) an antihistaminic compound; also used to produce a repository form of penicillin G.
**c. hydrochloride,** the hydrochloride salt of clemizole, used as an antihistaminic in the treatment of skin allergies, food and cosmetic hypersensitivities, and serum sickness; administered orally.
**c. penicillin,** see under *penicillin.*

**clen·bu·ter·ol** (klen-bu'tər-ol) [MeSH: Clenbuterol] a long-acting $\beta$-2 adrenergic agonist used to treat bronchospasms in the horse.

**clench·ing** (klench'ing) the clamping and pressing of the jaws and teeth together in centric occlusion, frequently associated with acute nervous tension or physical effort, such as pushing or lifting a heavy object or performing a difficult task. See also *bruxism.*

**Cle·o·cin** (kle'o-sin) trademark for preparations of clindamycin.

**cle·oid** (kle'oid) [Middle English *cle* claw + *-oid*] a claw-shaped nib used to carve amalgam restorations.

**Clé·ram·bault** see *de Clérambault.*

**Cleth·ri·on·o·mys** (kleth"re-on'ə-mis) a genus of rodents of the family Muridae, including voles.
**C. glare'olus,** the bank vole, a European species that is the natural host of Puumala virus.

**click** (klik) a brief sharp sound; see also *clicking.*
**ejection c's,** see under *sound.*
**midsystolic c.,** a high frequency sound in mid-systole, often associated with prolapse of a floppy mitral valve; it may be accompanied by a late systolic murmur.
**mitral c.,** mitral opening snap.
**nonejection systolic c.,** midsystolic c.
**Ortolani's c.,** see under *sign.*
**systolic c's,** short, dry, clicking heart sounds during systole; they are often indicative of various heart conditions associated with abnormal mitral or aortic valves but may have extracardiac causes. Their timing within systole may indicate the nature of the disorder; see *midsystolic c.* and *ejection sounds.*

**click·ing** (klik'ing) a series of clicks, such as the snapping, cracking, or crepitant noise evident on excursions of the mandibular condyle.

**cli·din·i·um bro·mide** (klĭ-din'e-əm) [USP] a quaternary ammonium anticholinergic with pronounced antispasmodic and antisecretory effects on the gastrointestinal tract, used as adjunctive therapy in the treatment of peptic ulcer and other gastrointestinal disorders, administered orally.

**clid(o)-** for words beginning thus, see those beginning *cleid(o)-.*

**cli·mac·ter·ic** (kli-mak'tər-ik) [Gr. *klimaktēr* rung of ladder, critical point in human life] [MeSH: Climacteric] 1. the syndrome of endocrine, somatic, and psychic changes occurring at the time of menopause in the female. 2. similar changes occurring in men owing to normal diminution of sexual drives with the aging process. Called also *climacterium.*

**Cli·ma·ra** (kli-mar'ə) trademark for a preparation of estradiol.

**cli·mac·te·ri·um** (kli"mak-tēr'e-əm) climacteric.
**c. prae'cox,** premature menopause.

**cli·ma·tol·o·gy** (kli"mə-tol'ə-je) [Gr. *klima* the supposed slope of the earth from the equator to the pole + *-logy*] the science devoted to the study of the conditions of the natural environment (rainfall, daylight, temperature, humidity, air movement) prevailing in specific regions of the earth.
**medical c.,** that concerned especially with the effect of climatic factors on man, on his functions and health, and on the treatment of his ills.

**cli·ma·to·ther·a·peu·tics** (kli"mə-to-ther"ə-pu'tiks) climatotherapy.

**cli·ma·to·ther·a·py** (kli"mə-to-ther'ə-pe) [*climate* + *therapy*] the treatment of disease by means of a favorable climate.

**cli·max** (kli'maks) [Gr. *klimax* a ladder, staircase] the acme, or period of greatest intensity, as in the course of a disease (crisis), or in sexual excitement (orgasm).

**cli·mo·graph** (kli'mo-graf) [*climate* + *-graph*] a diagram representing the effect of climate on man.

**clin·ar·thro·sis** (klin"ahr-thro'sis) [Gr. *klinein* to bend + *arthrosis*] abnormal deviation in the alignment of the bones at a joint.

**clin·da·my·cin** (klin"də-mi'sin) [USP] [MeSH: Clindamycin] a semi-

synthetic analogue of the natural antibiotic lincomycin from which it is produced by chlorination; it is effective primarily against gram-positive bacteria.
**c. hydrochloride** [USP], the hydrated hydrochloride salt of clindamycin; used primarily in the treatment of penicillin-resistant gram-positive infections and in patients allergic to penicillin; administered orally.
**c. palmitate hydrochloride** [USP], a water-soluble hydrochloride salt of the ester of clindamycin and palmitic acid, having the same actions and uses as the hydrochloride salt; it is suitable for the preparation of solutions for oral administration.
**c. phosphate** [USP], a water-soluble ester of clindamycin and phosphoric acid, having the same actions and uses as the hydrochloride salt; it is suitable for preparation of parenteral dosage forms, administered intramuscularly or intravenously.

**cline** (klīn) [Gr. *klinein* to cause to slope] a continuous series of differences in structure or function exhibited by the members of a species along a line extending from one part of their range to another.

**clin·ic** (klin'ik) [Gr. *klinikos* pertaining to a bed] 1. an establishment where patients are admitted for special study and treatment by a group of physicians practicing medicine together. 2. a clinical lecture; examination of patients before a class of students; instruction at the bedside.
**ambulant c.,** one for patients not confined to the bed.
**dry c.,** a clinical lecture with the presentation of case histories but without the presence of the patients described.

**clin·i·cal** (klin'ĭ-kəl) pertaining to a clinic or to the bedside; pertaining to or founded on actual observation and treatment of patients, as distinguished from theoretical or basic sciences.

**cli·ni·cian** (klĭ-nish'ən) an expert clinical physician and teacher.
**nurse c.,** see under *nurse.*

**clin·i·co·ge·net·ic** (klin″ĭ-ko-jə-net'ik) pertaining to the clinical manifestations of a chromosomal (genetic) abnormality.

**clin·i·co·patho·log·ic** (klin″ĭ-ko-path″-ə-loj'ik) pertaining both to the symptoms of disease and to its pathology.

**Clin·i·stix** (klin'ĭ-stiks) trademark for an enzyme-impregnated strip of plastic used to test for sugar in the urine. The strip is dipped into the urine and results of positive or negative are indicated by the color of the strip.

**Clin·i·test** (klin'ĭ-test) trademark for reagent tablets containing copper sulfate, used to test for the presence of sugar in the urine. Ten drops of water and 5 drops of urine are placed in a test tube. The tablet, which generates heat, is added and the solution is allowed to boil. After a few moments the color of the solution is compared to a color chart.

**cli·no·ceph·a·lism** (kli″no-sef'ə-liz-əm) clinocephaly.

**cli·no·ceph·a·ly** (kli″no-sef'ə-le) [Gr. *klinein* to bend + *-cephaly*] congenital flatness or concavity of the vertex of the head.

**cli·no·dac·tyl·ism** (kli″no-dak'təl-iz-əm) clinodactyly.

**cli·no·dac·ty·ly** (kli″no-dak'tə-le) [Gr. *klinein* to bend + *daktylos* finger] permanent lateral or medial deviation or deflection of one or more fingers.

**cli·nog·ra·phy** (klĭ-nog'rə-fe) [Gr. *klinē* bed + *-graphy*] a system of graphic representations of the temperature, symptoms, and pathologic manifestations exhibited by a patient.

**cli·noid** (klī'noid) [Gr. *klinē* bed + *-oid*] resembling a bed; bed-shaped, as the clinoid processes. See *processus clinoideus.*

**Clin·or·il** (klin'ə-ril) trademark for a preparation of sulindac.

**cli·no·stat·ic** (klĭ″no-stat'ik) occurring when the patient lies down.

**cli·no·stat·ism** (kli'no-stat″iz-əm) [Gr. *klinē* bed + *stasis* position] a lying-down position of the body.

**cli·no·ther·a·py** (klĭ-no-ther'ə-pe) treatment by keeping the patient in bed.

**cli·o·quin·ol** (kli″o-kwin'ol) [USP] [MeSH: Clioquinol] an antibacterial and antifungal agent with antieczematic and antipruritic properties, used as a local anti-infective in a wide range of dermatoses, including all types of eczema, and in vaginitis due to *Trichomonas vaginalis, Candida albicans, Trichophyton,* or mixed bacteria; administered topically or intravaginally. It was formerly administered orally in the treatment of amebic dysentery; this use has been discontinued because of associated neurotoxicity. Called also *iodochlorhydroxyquin.*

**CLIP** corticotropin-like intermediate lobe peptide.

**clip** (klip) [MeSH: Surgical Instruments] a metallic device for approximating the edges of a wound or for the prevention of bleeding from small individual blood vessels.

**clis·e·om·e·ter** (klis″e-om'ə-tər) [Gr. *klisis* inclination + *-meter*] an instrument for measuring the angle which the pelvic axis makes with the spinal column.

**Clis·tin** (klis'tin) trademark for preparations of carbinoxamine maleate.

**cli·tel·lum** (kli-tel'əm) [L. *clitellae* packsaddle] a saddle-like glandular segment in earthworms and leeches that secretes the cocoon in which the eggs are enclosed.

**clit·i·on** (klit'e-on) [Gr. *kleitys* slope, clivus] the midpoint of the anterior border of the clivus.

**Cli·to·cy·be** (kli-tos'ĭ-be) a genus of club fungi of the family Agaricaceae. Some species are poisonous and several contain muscarine. *C. nebula'ris* is the source of nebularine. Ingestion of *C. illu'dens,* the orange jack-o-lantern mushroom, causes mycetismus gastrointestinalis.

**clit·o·ral** (klit'ə-rəl, kli'tə-rəl, klĭ-tor'əl) pertaining to the clitoris.

**clit·o·rec·to·my** (klit″ə-rek'tə-me) clitoridectomy.

**clit·o·rid·auxe** (klit'ə-rid-awk″se) [*clitoris* + Gr. *auxe* increase] enlargement of the clitoris; clitorism.

**clit·o·rid·e·an** (klit″ə-rid'e-ən) clitoral.

**clit·o·ri·dec·to·my** (klit″ə-rĭ-dek'to-me) [*clitoris* + *-ectomy*] excision of the clitoris; called also *clitorectomy.*

**clit·o·ri·di·tis** (klit″ə-rĭ-di'tis) clitoritis.

**clit·o·ri·dot·o·my** (klit″ə-rĭ-dot'ə-me) [*clitoris* + *-tomy*] incision of the clitoris.

**clit·o·ri·meg·a·ly** (klit″ə-rĭ-meg'ə-le) [*clitoris* + *-megaly*] an enlarged clitoris.

**clit·o·ris** (klit'ə-ris, kli'tə-ris, klĭ-tor'is) [Gr. *kleitoris*] [TA] [MeSH: Clitoris] a small, elongated, erectile body, situated at the anterior angle of the rima pudendi; homologous with the penis in the male. Called also *coles femininus.*

**clit·o·rism** (klit'ə-riz″əm, kli'tə-riz″əm) 1. hypertrophy of the clitoris. 2. persistent and usually painful erection of the clitoris.

**clit·o·ri·tis** (klit″ə-ri'tis, kli″tə-ri'tis) inflammation of the clitoris.

**clit·o·ro·meg·a·ly** (klit″ə-ro-meg'ə-le) clitorimegaly.

**clit·o·ro·plas·ty** (klit'ə-ro-plas″te) plastic surgery of the clitoris.

**clit·o·rot·o·my** (klit″ə-rot'ə-me) [*clitoris* + *-tomy*] surgical incision of the clitoris.

**cli·val** (kli'vəl) pertaining to the clivus.

**cli·vog·ra·phy** (kli-vog'rə-fe) radiographic visualization of the clivus, or posterior cranial fossa.

**cli·vus** (kli'vəs) [L. "slope"] [TA] a bony surface in the posterior cranial fossa, sloping superiorly from the foramen magnum to the dorsum sellae, the inferior part being formed by a portion of the basilar part of the occipital bone (c. ossis occipitalis) and the superior part by a surface of the body of the sphenoid bone (c. ossis sphenoidalis). Called also *Blumenbach's c.* and *c. blumenbachii.*
**basilar c., c. basila'ris,** c. ossis occipitalis.
**Blumenbach's c., c. blumenba'chii,** clivus.
**c. monti'culi,** declive.
**c. os'sis occipita'lis** [TA], the lower part of the clivus, formed by the basilar portion of the occipital bone; called also *basilar c.* or *c. basilaris,* and *basilar groove of occipital bone.*
**c. os'sis sphenoida'lis,** the upper part of the clivus, formed by a surface of the body of the sphenoid bone; called also *basilar groove of sphenoid bone.*

**clo** (klo) a unit of measurement, being the insulation provided by man's normal everyday clothing and representing approximately the insulation provided by $\frac{1}{4}$ in. thickness of wool.

**clo·a·ca** (klo-a'kə) pl. *cloa'cae* [L. "drain"] [MeSH: Cloaca] 1. a common passage for fecal, urinary, and reproductive discharge in monotremes, birds, and lower vertebrates. See also *cloacal aperture,* under *aperture.* 2. in mammalian embryology, the terminal end of the hindgut before division into rectum, bladder, and genital primordia (see *sinus urogenitalis*). Failure to divide properly during development may result in persistent c. (q.v.). 3. in pathology, an opening in the involucrum of a necrosed bone.
**congenital c.,** persistent c.
**ectodermal c.,** that portion of the embryonic cloaca originally external to the cloacal membrane.
**entodermal c.,** that portion of the embryonic cloaca originally internal to the cloacal membrane.
**persistent c.,** the congenital persistence of a common cavity into which the intestinal, urinary, and reproductive ducts open; called also *congenital c.*

**clo·a·cal** (klo-a'kəl) pertaining to the cloaca.

**clo·a·ci·tis** (klo″ə-si'tis) inflammation of the cloaca of an animal.

**clo·a·co·gen·ic** (klo″ə-ko-jen′ik) originating from the cloaca or from persisting cloacal remnants.

**clo·ba·zam** (klo′bə-zəm) a benzodiazepine having actions and uses similar to those of diazepam.

**clo·be·ta·sol pro·pi·o·nate** (klo-ba′tə-sol) [USP] a synthetic corticosteroid, an analogue of prednisolone, used topically for the relief of inflammation and pruritus in corticosteroid-responsive dermatoses.

**clock** (klok) a device by which time may be measured.
**biological c.,** the physiologic mechanism that governs the rhythmic occurrence of certain biochemical, physiological, and behavioral phenomena in plants and animals.

**clo·cor·to·lone** (klo-kor′to-lōn) a glucocorticoid, available as the 21-acetate, and as the 21-pivalate, esters.

**clo·dro·nate disodium** (klo-dro′nāt) the disodium salt of clodronic acid; a diphosphonate calcium-regulating agent that inhibits bone resorption and is used to treat osteitis deformans and hypercalcemia related to malignancy. Administered orally or intravenously.

**clo·dron·ic ac·id** (klo-dron′ik) [MeSH: Clodronic Acid] a bone calcium regulator.

**clo·faz·i·mine** (klo-faz′ĭ-mēn) [USP] [MeSH: Clofazimine] an antibacterial, having leprostatic and tuberculostatic actions.

**clo·fen·am·ic acid** (klo″fən-am′ik) a fenamate analgesic, anti-inflammatory agent.

**clo·fi·brate** (klo-fi′brāt) [USP] [MeSH: Clofibrate] an antihyperlipidemic agent, used to reduce elevated serum lipids, administered orally.

**Clo·mid** (klo′mid) trademark for a preparation of clomiphene citrate.

**clo·mi·phene cit·rate** (klo′mĭ-fēn) [USP] a synthetic gonad-stimulating principle structurally related to the proestrogen chlorotrianisene, occurring as a white to pale yellow powder and consisting of a mixture of the *cis-* and *trans-* isomers; used to induce ovulation in certain forms of anovulatory infertility, administered orally.

**clo·mip·ra·mine hy·dro·chlo·ride** (klo-mip′rə-mēn) a tricyclic antidepressant of the dibenzazepine class, also having anxiolytic activity. It is also used investigationally to relieve the symptoms of obsessive-compulsive disorder.

**clon·al** (klōn′əl) of or pertaining to a clone.

**clo·nal·i·ty** (klo-nal′ĭ-te) the ability to form clones.

**clo·naz·e·pam** (klo-naz′ə-pam) [USP] [MeSH: Clonazepam] a benzodiazepine used as an anticonvulsant in the treatment of Lennox-Gastaut syndrome and of atonic and myoclonic seizures; administered orally.

**clone** (klōn) [Gr. *klōn* young shoot or twig] [MeSH: Clone Cells] 1. one or a group of genetically identical cells, organisms, or plants derived by vegetative reproduction from a single parent; also, a DNA population derived from a single hybrid DNA molecule (recombinant vector, q.v.) by replication in a eukaryotic or bacterial host cell. 2. used as a verb to denote the establishment of a clone.
**forbidden c.,** see *clonal deletion theory,* under *theory.*

**clon·ic** (klon′ik) [Gr. *klonos* turmoil] pertaining to or of the nature of clonus.

**clo·nic·i·ty** (klo-nis′ĭ-te) the condition of being clonic.

**clon·i·co·ton·ic** (klon″ĭ-ko-ton′ik) both clonic and tonic.

**clo·ni·dine hy·dro·chlo·ride** (klo′nĭ-dēn) [USP] an $\alpha_2$-adrenergic agonist-antagonist (its major actions are agonistic, but it acts as an antagonist if the concentration of norepinephrine is high) used as an oral antihypertensive; it is also used for the prophylaxis of migraine and in the treatment of dysmenorrhea, vasomotor symptoms of menopause, and opioid withdrawal.

**clon·ing** (klōn′ing) the formation of a clone.
**DNA c.,** in genetics, the production of many identical copies of a specific DNA fragment.

**clon·ism** (klon′iz-əm) [Gr. *klonos* turmoil] a succession of clonic spasms.

**clo·nis·mus** (klo-niz′məs) clonism.

**clo·no·gen·ic** (klo″no-jen′ik) [*clone* + *-genic*] giving rise to a clone of cells.

**Clon·o·pin** (klon′o-pin) former spelling for Klonopin.

**clo·nor·chi·a·sis** (klo″nor-ki′ə-sis) [MeSH: Clonorchiasis] opisthorchiasis in humans or other animals caused by infestation of biliary passages by the liver fluke *Opisthorchis sinensis (Clonorchis sinensis),* which may lead to inflammation of the biliary tree, proliferation of the biliary epithelium, progressive portal fibrosis, and sometimes biliary duct carcinoma; extension into the liver parenchyma may lead to fatty changes and cirrhosis. Called also *clonorchiosis.*

**clo·nor·chi·o·sis** (klo-nor″ki-o′sis) clonorchiasis.

**Clo·nor·chis** (klo-nor′kis) [Gr. *klōn* branch + *orchis* testicle] former name for a genus of trematodes, now considered identical to *Opisthorchis.*

**clono·spasm** (klon′o-spaz″əm) [*clonus* + *spasm*] clonic spasm.

**clo·no·type** (klo′no-tīp) [*clone* + *type*] a particular combination of immunoglobulin heavy and light chains, e.g., that produced by a single clone of plasma cells. A single organism produces a repertoire of about $10^7$ to $10^8$ clonotypes; a single antigenic determinant may react with $10^3$ to $10^4$ clonotypes.

**clo·nus** (klo′nəs) [Gr. *klonos* turmoil] 1. alternate muscular contraction and relaxation in rapid succession. 2. a continuous rhythmic reflex tremor initiated by the spinal cord below an area of spinal cord injury, set in motion by reflex testing.
**ankle c.,** a series of abnormal rhythmic reflex movements of the foot, induced by sudden dorsiflexion, which causes alternate contraction and relaxation of the triceps surae muscle (gastrocnemius and soleus muscles); called also *foot c.*
**foot c.,** ankle c.
**patellar c.,** rhythmic jerking movement of the patella produced by grasping it between the thumb and forefinger and pushing it suddenly and forcibly toward the foot; this is an abnormal reflex with alternate contraction and relaxation of the quadriceps muscle.
**wrist c.,** spasmodic movement of the hand, induced by suddenly and forcibly extending the hand at the wrist.

**clo·pa·mide** (klo-pă′mīd) [MeSH: Clopamide] a diuretic used in the treatment of edema associated with various disorders and in hypertension.

**clo·pen·thix·ol** (klo″pən-thik′səl) [MeSH: Clopenthixol] a compound, having sedative, tranquilizing, antiemetic, antihistaminic, anticholinergic, and alpha-adrenergic blocking properties; it has been used as a tranquilizer in the treatment of schizophrenia.

**clo·pid·o·grel bi·sul·fate** (klo-pid′o-grel) an inhibitor of platelet aggregation used as an antithrombotic for the prevention of myocardial infarction, stroke, and vascular death in patients with atherosclerosis; administered orally.

**clo·pi·dol** (klo′pĭ-dol) [MeSH: Clopidol] a coccidiostat for poultry.

**clo·pros·te·nol** (klo-pros′tə-nol) [MeSH: Cloprostenol] a prostaglandin, $C_{22}H_{28}ClO_6$. Also available as the sodium salt.

**Clo·quet's canal, fascia** etc. (klo-kāz′) [Jules Germain *Cloquet,* French surgeon, 1790–1883] see under *fascia* and *node,* and see *canalis hyaloideus, pectineal herniavestigium processus vaginalis,* and *septum femorale.*

**Clo·quet's ganglion (pseudoganglion)** (klo-kāz′) [Hippolyte *Cloquet,* French anatomist, 1787–1840] see under *ganglion.*

**clor·az·e·pate di·po·tas·sium** (klor-az′ə-pāt) [USP] [MeSH: Clorazepate Dipotassium] a benzodiazepine used as an anxiolytic for the short-term relief of anxiety symptoms, as an anticonvulsant in the treatment of complex partial seizures, and for the treatment of acute alcohol withdrawal symptoms; administered orally.

**clor·a·zep·ic ac·id** (klor′ə-zep′ik) the free acid of clorazepate.

**clor·ex·o·lone** (klor-ek′sə-lōn) a diuretic, used in the treatment of edema associated with various disorders and in hypertension.

**clor·o·phene** (klor′o-fēn) a disinfectant, effective against a wide variety of bacteria and fungi.

**Clor·pac·tin XCB** (klōr-pak′tin) trademark for a preparation of oxychlorosene.

**clor·pren·a·line hy·dro·chlo·ride** (klor-pren′ə-lēn) an adrenergic, $C_{11}H_{16}ClNO \cdot HCl \cdot H_2O$, used as a bronchodilator.

**clor·su·lon** (klor′su-lon) [USP] a sulfonamide used as a fasciolicide in humans and domestic animals.

**clor·ter·mine hy·dro·chlo·ride** (klor-tər′mēn) an adrenergic used as an oral anorexic in the short-term treatment of exogenous obesity.

**clo·san·tel** (klo′sən-təl) a salicylanilide anthelmintic used in cattle and sheep.

**clos·trid·ia** (klos-trid′e-ə) [L.] plural of *clostridium.*

**clos·trid·i·al** (klos-trid′e-əl) pertaining to or caused by clostridia.

**clos·trid·i·o·sis** (klos-trid″e-o′sis) any disease caused by infection with clostridia.
**equine intestinal c.,** acute, usually fatal, diarrhea in horses due to infection with large numbers of *Clostridium perfringens* type A.

**Clos·trid·i·um** (klos-trid′e-əm) [Gr. *klōstēr* spindle] [MeSH: Clostridium] a genus of bacteria of the family Bacillaceae, made up of obligate anaerobic or microaerophilic, gram-positive, spore-forming, rod-shaped bacilli, with spores of greater diameter than the vegetative cells. The spores may be central, terminal, or subterminal. Over one hundred species have been differentiated on the basis of physiology, morphology, and toxin formation; pathogenic species produce destructive exotoxins or enzymes. Different species are found in soil, in water, and in the intestinal tracts of humans and other animals.

**C. acetobuty'licum,** a species found widely distributed in agricultural soils but not found to be pathogenic.

**C. ag'ni,** former name for type B of *C. perfringens.*

**C. bifermen'tans,** a species found widely distributed in nature, occurring commonly in feces, sewage, and soil; it is sometimes associated with cases of gas gangrene.

**C. botuli'num,** the agent causing botulism in man, wild ducks, and other waterfowl, limberneck of fowl, certain forms of forage poisoning in cattle and horses in Australia, and lamziekte of cattle in South Africa. It produces a powerful exotoxin that is resistant to proteolytic digestion, and is divided into types A, B, C alpha and beta, D, E, F, and G on the basis of the immunologic specificity of the toxin. Formerly called *Bacillus botulinus.*

**C. buty'ricum,** a species isolated from the soil, fecal material, and dairy products.

**C. cada'veris,** a species found in feces and infections of animals and man.

**C. chauvoe'i,** the principal cause of blackleg in cattle and sheep; called also *C. feseri.*

**C. clostridiofor'me,** a weakly gram-positive species that is commonly isolated from clinical specimens; called also *Bacteroides clostridiiformis.*

**C. diffi'cile,** a species that is part of the normal colon flora in human infants and sometimes in adults. It produces a toxin that causes pseudomembranous enterocolitis in patients receiving antibiotic therapy.

**C. fe'seri,** *C. chauvoei.*

**C. haemoly'ticum,** a species isolated from the blood and other tissues of cattle dying with bacillary hemoglobinuria, thought by some to be a type of *C. novyi.*

**C. histoly'ticum,** a pathogenic species found in wounds and frequently associated with gas gangrene. It is commonly found in soil.

**C. inno'cuum,** a species of uncertain pathogenicity, commonly isolated from gas gangrene and other anaerobic infections.

**C. kluy'veri,** a species isolated from wetland soil of fresh and salt water, which has been used in studies of microbial synthesis and oxidation of fatty acids.

**C. limo'sum,** a toxicogenic species found in soil and in a variety of animal infections.

**C. no'vyi,** a species that is an important cause of gas gangrene in humans and a source of infection in other animals. Three immunologic types have been identified, designated A, B, and C. Formerly called *C. oedematiens* and *Bacillus oedematis maligni No. II.*

**C. oedema'tiens,** *C. novyi.*

**C. ovitox'icus,** former name for type D of *C. perfringens.*

**C. palu'dis,** former name for type C of *C. perfringens.*

**C. paraboṭuli'num e'qui,** *C. botulinum.*

**C. parabotuli'nus,** *C. botulinum* type C.

**C. paraputri'ficum,** a species found in soil and feces.

**C. pasteuria'num,** an anaerobic microorganism occurring in soil, which was the first nitrogen-fixing bacterium to be studied in pure culture.

**C. pastoria'num,** *C. pasteurianum.*

**C. perfrin'gens,** the most common etiologic agent of gas gangrene, differentiable, on the basis of the distribution of 12 different toxins, into several different types: *type A* causes gas gangrene, necrotizing colitis, and food poisoning in humans; *type B* causes lamb dysentery; *type C* causes enteritis necroticans in man and struck in sheep; *type D* causes enterotoxemia (pulpy kidney disease) in sheep; *type E* causes enterotoxemia in lambs and calves. *C. perfringens* is also a major cause of food poisoning; see *clostridial food poisoning,* under *poisoning.* Called also *C. welchii.*

**C. ramo'sum,** a species found in human and animal infections and in feces, one of the most commonly isolated clostridia in clinical specimens.

**C. sep'ticum,** a toxicogenic species commonly occurring in animal intestines and soil, strikingly pathogenic for various animals, causing diseases such as braxy and malignant edema; in humans it is reportedly associated with gas gangrene in only 20 per cent of cases. Six immunologic groups have been distinguished. Called also *Vibrio septicus* and *Ghon-Sachs bacillus.*

**C. sordel'lii,** a species of uncertain pathogenicity, found associated with infections of man and animals.

**C. sphenoi'des,** a species found in infected wounds in man.

**C. sporo'genes,** a species widely distributed in nature; a harmless saprophyte in pure culture, it is reportedly associated with pathogenic anaerobes in gangrenous infections.

**C. subtermina'le,** a species found in soil and wounds.

**C. ter'tium,** a species found widely distributed in feces, sewage, and soil, and associated with gas gangrene.

**C. te'tani,** a common inhabitant of soil and human and horse intestines, and the cause of tetanus in humans and domestic animals; its potent exotoxin is made up of two components, a neurotoxin, or tetanospasmin, and a hemolytic toxin, or tetanolysin. Formerly called *Bacillus tetani.*

**C. wel'chii,** British name for *C. perfringens.*

**clos·trid·i·um** (klos-trid'e-əm) pl. *clostrid'ia* [MeSH: Clostridium] A microorganism belonging to the genus *Clostridium.*

**clo·sure** (klo'zhər) 1. occlusion. 2. obstruction.

**flask c.,** the bringing together of the two halves or parts of a flask in which a denture base is formed.

**flask c., final,** the last closure of a flask before curing the denture-base material packed in the mold.

**flask c., trial,** preliminary closure of the flask, to eliminate excess material and to ensure that the mold is completely filled.

**velopharyngeal c.,** closure of nasal air escape by the elevation of the soft palate and contraction of the posterior pharyngeal wall. See also *velopharyngeal adequacy* and *velopharyngeal insufficiency.*

**clo·sy·late** (klo'sə-lāt) USAN contraction for *p*-chlorobenzenesulfonate.

**clot** (klot) 1. a semisolidified mass, as of blood or lymph; called also *coagulum.* 2. blood c. 3. coagulate.

**agonal c., agony c.,** a type of antemortem clot formed in the process of dying.

**antemortem c.,** a blood clot formed before death but found after death in the heart or in a large vessel.

**blood c.,** a coagulum in the blood stream formed of an aggregation of blood factors, primarily platelets, and fibrin with entrapment of cellular elements; see also *thrombus.* Some authorities differentiate thrombus formation from simple coagulation or clot formation. Called also *cruor.*

**chicken fat c.,** a blood clot that appears yellow because of the settling out of the erythrocytes before clotting occurred.

**sentinel c.,** a discrete protuberance within the crater of a peptic ulcer, usually representing a hemostatic clot in the vessel or a false aneurysm; pigmentation of the protuberance is often prognostic of rebleeding of the ulcer.

**currant jelly c.,** a blood clot of reddish color because of the presence of erythrocytes enmeshed in it.

**distal c.,** a clot formed in a blood vessel distal to a ligature.

**external c.,** a clot formed outside a blood vessel.

**heart c.,** postmortem coagulation within the heart.

**internal c.,** a blood clot formed within a blood vessel.

**laminated c.,** a blood clot formed by successive deposits of fibrin and whole blood, giving it a layered appearance; called also *stratified c.*

**marantic c.,** a blood clot formed because of enfeebled circulation, general wasting, or thromboplastic substances released by cancers.

**passive c.,** a clot formed in the sac of an aneurysm through which the blood has stopped circulating.

**plastic c.,** a clot formed on the intima of an artery at the point of ligation, permanently obstructing the artery.

**postmortem c.,** a blood clot formed in the heart or in a large blood vessel after death.

**proximal c.,** a clot formed in a blood vessel proximal to a ligature.

**spider-web c.,** the fine fibrin clot that forms when a sample of fluid from a subject with tuberculous meningitis is allowed to stand, especially when it is warmed to 37°C for a few hours.

**stratified c.,** laminated c.

**washed c., white c.,** a blood clot composed of fibrin and platelets; see also under *thrombus.*

**clo·trim·a·zole** (klo-trim'ə-zōl) [USP] [MeSH: Clotrimazole] an imidazole derivative used as a broad-spectrum antifungal agent, applied topically to the skin in the treatment of candidiasis and various forms of tinea, and administered intravaginally in the treatment of vulvovaginal candidiasis.

**clot·ting** (klot'ing) coagulation (def. 1).

**cloud·ing** (kloud'ing) loss of clarity.

**c. of consciousness,** a lowered level of consciousness (q.v.) with loss of ability to respond properly to external stimuli. See also *levels of consciousness,* under *level.* Called also *mental fog, obnubilation,* and *obtundation.*

**Cloud·man's melanoma S91** (kloud'mənz) [Arthur Mosher *Cloudman,* American zoologist, born 1901] see under *melanoma.*

**Clou·ston's syndrome** (klou'stonz) [H. R. *Clouston,* Canadian physician, 20th century] hidrotic ectodermal dysplasia.

**clove** (klōv) [L. *clavus* a nail or spike] 1. *Syzygium aromaticum.* 2. the dried flower bud of *Syzygium aromaticum,* used as an aromatic spice and flavoring and source of clove oil.

**clo·ver** (klo'vər) 1. any member of the genus *Trifolium;* called also *trefoil.* 2. any of various other members of the pea family, such as genus *Melilotus.*
**sweet c.,** any member of the genus *Melilotus;* see also *sweet clover disease,* under *disease.*

**clox·a·cil·lin so·di·um** (klok″sə-sil'in) [USP] a semisynthetic penicillinase-resistant penicillin, used primarily in the treatment of infections due to penicillinase-producing staphylococci, administered orally.

**clo·za·pine** (klo'zə-pēn) [MeSH: Clozapine] a sedative and antipsychotic agent, a dibenzodiazepine; used in the treatment of schizophrenia.

**club·bing** (klub'ing) a deformity produced by proliferation of the soft tissues about the terminal phalanges of the fingers or toes, with no constant osseous changes; seen in various types of chronic disease of the thoracic organs. Cf. *clubbed finger.*

**club·foot** (klub'foot) [MeSH: Clubfoot] talipes.

**club·hand** (klub'hand) a deformity of the hand due to congenital absence of the radius or ulna in which the hand is twisted out of shape or position; called also *talipomanus.*
**radial c.,** the most common type of clubhand in which the hand is deflected toward the radial side; when the hand is held in the anatomic position it is known as *manus valga* and when it is held in the opposite direction as *manus vara.* Called also *manus valga.* See also *Madelung deformity,* under *deformity.*
**ulnar c.,** clubhand in which the hand is deflected toward the ulnar side; when the hand is held in the anatomic position it is known as *manus vara* and when it is held in the opposite direction as *manus valga.* Called also *manus vara.*

**clump** (klump) an aggregation as of bacteria caused by the action of agglutinins (agglutination).

**clump·ing** (klump'ing) the aggregation of particles, such as bacteria, into irregular masses.

**clu·ne·al** (kloo'ne-əl) gluteal; spelled also *clunial.*

**clu·nes** (kloo'nēz) sing. *clu'nis* [L.] TA alternative for *nates.*

**clu·ni·al** (kloo'ne-əl) cluneal; used especially of the nervi clunium.

**clu·nis** (kloo'nis) pl. *clu'nes* [L.] a buttock; see *nates.*

**clu·pan·o·don·ic ac·id** (kloo-pan″o-don'ik) a 22-carbon fatty acid containing five double bonds that has been isolated from fish oil but may be an artifact of the isolation process.

**clu·pe·ine** (kloo'pe-in) [L. *clupea* herring] [MeSH: Clupeine] a protamine obtainable from the spermatozoa of the herring.

**clus·ter·in** (klus'tər-in) a multifunctional glycoprotein with roles in the metabolism and transport of lipids and membrane fragments, secretion of hormones, reproductive biology, inhibition of assembly of the membrane attack complex of complement activation, programmed cell death, and modulation of inter-cell interactions; its expression is enhanced in tissue injury and remodeling as well as in degenerative diseases such as Alzheimer's disease and scrapie. Called also *SP-40,40.*

**clut·ter·ing** (klut'ər-ing) hurried nervous speech marked by the dropping of syllables, usually seen in children. Cf. *logorrhea.*

**Clut·ton's joint** (klut'ənz) [Henry Hugh *Clutton,* English surgeon, 1850–1909] see under *joint.*

**cly·sis** (kli'sis) [Gr. *klysis*] 1. the administration other than by the oral route of any one of several solutions to replace lost body fluid, supply nutriment, or raise blood pressure. 2. the solution so administered.

**clys·ma** (kliz'mə) pl. *clys'mata* [Gr. *klysma*] enema.

**Cly·so·drast** (kli'so-drast) trademark for a preparation of bisacodyl tannex.

**clys·ter** (klis'tər) [Gr. *klystēr* a syringe] enema.

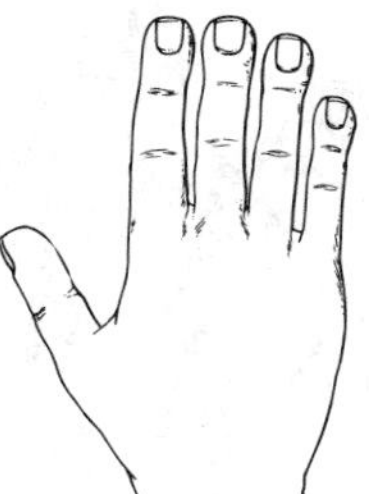
Clubbing of digits.

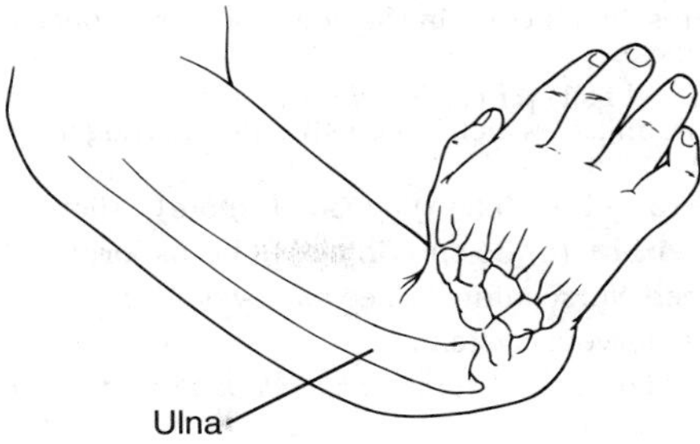

Radial clubhand; note absence of radius.

**clys·ter·ize** (klis'tər-īz) to treat with an enema.

**CM** abbreviation for L. *Chirur'giae Ma'gister,* Master in Surgery.

**Cm** symbol for *curium.*

**cM** symbol for *centimorgan.*

**cm** symbol for *centimeter.*

**cm²** symbol for *square centimeter.*

**cm³** symbol for *cubic centimeter.*

**CMA** Canadian Medical Association; Certified Medical Assistant.

**CMAP** compound muscle action potential.

**CMD** cerebromacular degeneration.

**CMF** a regimen of cyclophosphamide, methotrexate, and 5-fluorouracil, used in cancer chemotherapy.

**CMHC** community mental health center.

**cm $H_2O$** centimeter of water, a unit of pressure equal to that exerted by a column of water at 4°C one millimeter high at mean sea level; officially defined as the pressure exerted by a 1 cm column of fluid with a density of 1 g/cm³ in a gravitational field of 9.80665 m/s², which equals 9.80665 pascals.

**CMI** cell-mediated immunity.

**CML** cell-mediated lympholysis.

**c mm** symbol for *cubic millimeter.*

**C-MOPP** a regimen of cyclophosphamide, Oncovin (vincristine), procarbazine, and prednisone, used in cancer chemotherapy.

**CMP** cytidine monophosphate.

**CMR** cerebral metabolic rate.

**c.m.s.** abbreviation for L. *cras ma'ne sumen'dus,* to be taken tomorrow morning.

**CMT** Certified Medical Transcriptionist; California mastitis test.

**CMV** cytomegalovirus.

**c.n.** abbreviation for L. *cras noc'te,* tomorrow night.

**CNA** Canadian Nurses' Association.

**CN-Cbl** cyanocobalamin.

**C3 NeF** C3 nephritic factor.

**cne·mi·al** (ne'me-əl) tibial.

**Cne·mi·do·cop·tes** (ne″mĭ-do-kop'tēz) *Knemidokoptes.*

**cne·mis** (ne'mis) tibia.

**cne·mi·tis** (ne-mi'tis) inflammation of the tibia.

**cne·mo·sco·li·o·sis** (ne″mo-sko″le-o'sis) [Gr. *knēmē* leg + *scolio-* + *-sis*] a lateral bending of the leg.

**Cni·da·ria** (ni-dar'e-ə) [Gr. *knidē* a nettle] [MeSH: Cnidaria] a phylum of marine invertebrates that includes sea anemones, hydras, corals, and jellyfish (all of which were formerly assigned to the phylum Coelenterata), plus comb jellies or sea walnuts, characterized by a radially symmetrical body bearing tentacles around the mouth.

**cni·dar·i·an** (ni-dar'e-ən) [MeSH: Cnidaria] 1. pertaining or belonging to the phylum Cnidaria. 2. an individual of the phylum Cnidaria. See also *coelenterate* (def. 3).

**Cni·di·an** (ni'de-ən) pertaining to Cnidos, a Dorian Greek city on the southwest Asia Minor coast famous for its temple of healing, its medical school, and its libraries. The Cnidian school stressed thorough diagnosis and classification of diseases (especially pathology) to the extent of ignoring the patient. Cf. *Hippocrates of Cos.*

**cnid(o)-** [Gr. *knidē* a nettle] a combining form denoting a relationship to a nettle or nettle-like structure.

**cni·do·blast** (ni'do-blast) [*cnido-* + *-blast*] the epidermal cells of coelenterates which contain the nematocysts, especially numerous on the tentacles.

**cni·do·cil** (ni'do-sil) [*cnido-* + *cil*ium] a bristle-like process at one end of a cnidoblast, which, when stimulated, triggers the discharge of the nematocyst.

**Cni·dos·po·ra** (ni"dos'pə-rə) [*cnido-* + *spore*] Microspora.

**Cni·do·spo·rid·ia** (ni"do-spo-rid'e-ə) Microsporida.

**CNM** Certified Nurse-Midwife; see *nurse-midwife.*

**CNS** central nervous system.

**c.n.s.** abbreviation for L. *cras noc'te sumen'dus,* to be taken tomorrow night.

**CNV** contingent negative variation.

**CO** cardiac output.

**Co** symbol for *cobalt* and *coccygeal* (in vertebral formulas).

**co-** see *con-*.

**COA** Canadian Orthopaedic Association.

**CoA** coenzyme A.

**co·ac·er·vate** (ko-as'ər-vāt) [L. *coacervatus* heaped up] the viscous phase separating from a colloid-containing system in the phenomenon of coacervation.

**co·ac·er·va·tion** (ko-as"ər-va'shən) the separation of a mixture of two liquids, one or both of which are colloids, into two phases, one of which (the coacervate) contains the colloidal particles, the other being an aqueous solution, e.g., as when gum arabic is added to gelatin.

**Co·ac·tin** (ko-ak'tin) trademark for a preparation of amdinocillin.

**co·ad·ap·ta·tion** (ko-ad"ap-ta'shən) [*co-* + *adaptation*] the mutual, correlated, adaptive changes in two interdependent organs.

**co·ad·u·na·tion** (ko-ad"u-na'shən) [*co-* + *ad-* + L. *unus* one] union of dissimilar substances in one mass.

**co·ad·u·ni·tion** (ko-ad"u-nish'ən) coadunation.

**co·ag·glu·ti·na·tion** (ko"ə-gloo"tĭ-na'shən) the aggregation of particulate antigens combined with agglutinins of more than one specificity.

**co·ag·u·la·bil·i·ty** (ko-ag"u-lə-bil'ĭ-te) the state of being coagulable.

**co·ag·u·la·ble** (ko-ag'u-lə-bəl) capable of being formed into clots.

**co·ag·u·lant** (ko-ag'u-lənt) [L. *coagulans*] 1. promoting, accelerating, or making possible the coagulation of blood. 2. an agent that promotes or accelerates the coagulation of blood.

**co·ag·u·lase** (ko-ag'u-lās) [MeSH: Coagulase] a bacterial enzyme that reacts with a cofactor found in blood plasma to catalyze the formation of fibrin from fibrinogen. It is produced by *Staphylococcus aureus* and by *Yersinia pestis.*

**co·ag·u·late** (ko-ag'u-lāt) [L. *coagulare*] to undergo coagulation (q.v.); called also *clot.*

**co·ag·u·la·tion** (ko-ag"u-la'shən) [L. *coagulatio*] 1. in colloid chemistry, the solidification of a sol into a gelatinous mass; an alteration of a disperse phase or of a dissolved solid which causes the separation of the system into a liquid phase and an insoluble mass called the clot or curd; it is usually irreversible. Called also *clotting.* 2. blood c. 3. in surgery, the disruption of tissue by physical means to form an amorphous residuum, as in electrocoagulation and photocoagulation.
**blood c.,** the sequential process by which the multiple coagulation factors of the blood interact in the coagulation cascade, ultimately resulting in the formation of an insoluble fibrin clot. See also *extrinsic, intrinsic,* and *common pathways of coagulation.*
**diffuse intravascular c. (DIC), disseminated intravascular c.,** a bleeding disorder characterized by abnormal reduction in the elements involved in blood clotting due to their use in widespread intravascular clotting. It may be caused by any of numerous disorders; in the late stages, it is marked by profuse hemorrhaging. Called also *consumption coagulopathy, defibrination syndrome,* and *disseminated intravascular coagulation syndrome.*
**electric c.,** electrocoagulation.
**massive c.,** coagulation of the spinal fluid so as to form an almost solid clot; a condition seen in some cases of Froin's syndrome in meningomyelitis or tumor of the cord.

**co·ag·u·la·tive** (ko-ag'u-la"tiv) associated with coagulation or promoting a process of coagulation; of the nature of coagulation.

**co·ag·u·la·tor** (ko-ag"u-la'tər) a surgical device that utilizes electrical current or light to stop bleeding.

**co·ag·u·lo·gram** (ko-ag'u-lo-gram") a term used colloquially in clinical hematology to denote a series of laboratory tests measuring the various parameters of hemostasis.

**co·ag·u·lop·a·thy** (ko-ag"u-lop'ə-the) any disorder of blood coagulation.
**consumption c.,** diffuse intravascular coagulation.

**co·ag·u·lum** (ko-ag'u-ləm) pl. *coag'ula* [L.] clot (def. 1).
**closing c.,** Schlusskoagulum.

**co·a·les·cence** (ko"ə-les'əns) [L. *coalescere* to grow together] the fusion or blending of parts.

**co·a·li·tion** (ko"ə-lish'ən) [L. *coalescere* to grow together] the fusion of parts that are normally separate.
**calcaneocuboid c.,** an often asymptomatic tarsal coalition involving the calcaneus and the cuboid bone.
**calcaneonavicular c.,** one of the most common types of tarsal coalition, involving the calcaneus and the navicular bone.
**cubonavicular c.,** tarsal coalition involving the cuboid and navicular bones.
**naviculocuneiform c.,** tarsal coalition involving the navicular and cuneiform bones.
**talocalcaneal c.,** one of the most common types of tarsal coalition, involving the talus and calcaneus.
**talonavicular c.,** tarsal coalition involving the talus and the navicular bone.
**tarsal c.,** the fibrous, cartilaginous, or bony fusion of two or more of the tarsal bones, often resulting in talipes planovalgus, although other deformities occur and some patients are asymptomatic; it may be congenital or acquired as a response to trauma, infection, or joint disease. Called also *tarsal bar* or *bridge.*

**co·apt** (ko-apt') [L. *coaptare*] to approximate, as the edges of a wound or the ends of a fractured bone.

**co·arc·tate** (ko-ahrk'tāt) 1. to press close together or contract. 2. pressed together or restrained.

**co·arc·ta·tion** (ko"ahrk-ta'shən) [L. *coarctatio,* from *cum* together + *arctare* to make tight] stenosis.
**c. of aorta,** a localized malformation characterized by deformity of the aortic media, causing narrowing, usually severe, of the lumen of the vessel.
**c. of aorta, adult type,** a form characterized by a localized constriction at or below the insertion of the ductus arteriosus and distal to the aortic isthmus and left subclavian artery, with a closed ductus and absence of cyanosis.
**c. of aorta, infantile type,** a form usually seen in infants, characterized by cyanosis and diffuse involvement of the aortic isthmus, associated with other anomalies such as a patent ductus.
**reversed c.,** Takayasu's arteritis.

**coarse** (kōrs) not fine; not microscopic.

**co·ar·tic·u·la·tion** (ko"ahr-tik"u-la'shən) [*co-* + *articulation*] a synarthrosis.

**CoA-SH** coenzyme A.

**coat** (kōt) [L. *cotta* tunic] 1. tunica. 2. the layer or layers of protective protein surrounding the nucleic acid in a virus. Cf. *capsid.*
**adventitial c., adventitious c.,** tunica adventitia.
**adventitious c. of uterine tube,** tela subserosa tubae uterinae.
**albugineous c.,** tunica albuginea; see terms beginning thus under *tunica.*
**buffy c.,** the thin yellowish layer of leukocytes overlying the packed red cells in centrifuged blood; called also *leukocytic cream.*
**cremasteric c. of testis,** musculus cremaster.
**dartos c.,** tunica dartos.
**dry c.,** anhidrosis (def. 2).
**external c. of capsule of graafian follicle,** tunica externa thecae folliculi.
**external c. of esophagus,** tunica adventitia oesophagi.
**external c. of ureter,** tunica adventitia ureteris.
**external c. of vessels,** tunica externa vasorum.

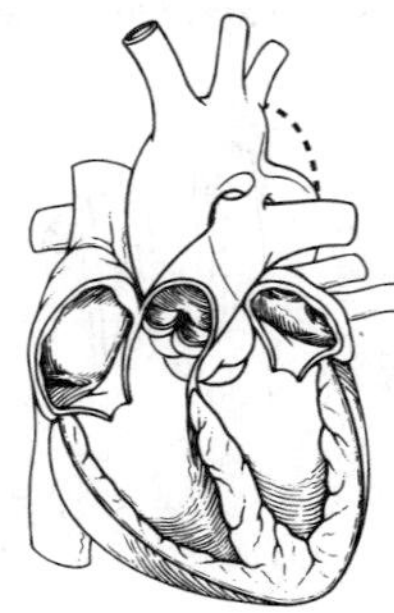

Coarctation of the aorta in the region of the ductus arteriosus. The dotted line indicates the normal aorta.

**external c. of viscera,** tunica adventitia.
**extraneous c.,** a cement-like structure, constituting a visible cell wall, in some animal cells; it generally plays no role in permeability, but has other important functions.
**fibrous c.,** tunica fibrosa; see terms beginning thus under *tunica.*
**fibrous c. of corpus cavernosum of penis,** tunica albuginea corporum cavernosorum.
**fibrous c. of eye,** tunica fibrosa bulbi.
**fibrous c. of ovary,** theca folliculi.
**fibrous c. of pharynx,** fascia pharyngobasilaris.
**fibrous c. of testis,** tunica albuginea testis.
**inner c. of vessels,** tunica intima vasorum.
**internal c. of capsule of graafian follicle,** tunica interna thecae folliculi.
**middle c. of vessels,** tunica media vasorum.
**mucous c.,** tunica mucosa.
**mucous c. of tympanic cavity,** tunica mucosa cavitatis tympanicae.
**muscular c.,** tunica muscularis; see terms beginning thus under *tunica.*
**outer c. of vessels,** tunica externa vasorum.
**pharyngobasilar c.,** fascia pharyngobasilaris.
**proper c.,** tunica propria.
**proper c. of corium, proper c. of dermis,** stratum reticulare dermidis.
**proper c. of testis,** tunica albuginea testis.
**sclerotic c.,** the sclera.
**serous c.,** tunica serosa; see terms beginning thus under *tunica.*
**submucous c.,** tela submucosa; see terms beginning thus under *tela.*
**subserous c.,** tela subserosa; see terms beginning thus under *tela.*
**uveal c.,** uvea; called also *vascular c. of eyeball.*
**vaginal c. of testis,** tunica vaginalis testis.
**vascular c. of eyeball,** uvea; called also *uveal c.*
**vascular c. of stomach,** tela submucosa ventriculi.
**vascular c. of viscera,** tela submucosa.
**villous c. of small intestine,** tunica mucosa intestini tenuis.
**white c.,** tunica albuginea.

**CoA-trans·fer·ase** (ko'a trans'fər-ās) [EC 2.8.3.] one of a sub-subclass of enzymes of the transferase class that catalyze the transfer of coenzyme A from one molecule to another.

**Coats' disease, retinitis** (kōts) [George *Coats,* English ophthalmologist, 1876–1915] exudative retinopathy.

**co·ax·i·al** (ko-ak'se-əl) having a common axis; said of two tubes mounted with one inside the other. Cf. *concentric.*

**co·bal·a·min** (ko-bal'ə-min) 1. in chemical nomenclature, a compound comprising the substituted corrin ring and 5,6-dimethylbenzimidazole–containing nucleotide that are characteristic of vitamin $B_{12}$, but lacking a ligand at the 6 position of the cobalt. 2. a term used generically to denote any substituted derivative of this compound, including cyanocobalamin, particularly one with vitamin $B_{12}$ activity.

**co·b(I)al·a·min ad·e·no·syl·trans·fer·ase** (ko-bal'ə-min ə-den″o-səl-trans'fər-ās) [EC 2.5.1.17] a mitochondrial enzyme of the transferase class that catalyzes the transfer of an adenosyl group to cobalamin from ATP, forming the coenzyme adenosylcobalamin. Deficiency of the enzyme, an autosomal recessive trait *(CblB),* leads to deficiency of methylmalonyl-CoA mutase activity and results in methylmalonicacidemia.

**co·bal·amin re·duc·tase** (ko-bal'ə-min re-duk'tās) either of two mitochondrial reductases that catalyze steps in the synthesis of adenosylcobalamin from hydroxocobalamin; deficiency of one or both is believed to be a cause of methylmalonicacidemia (q.v.).

**co·bal·oph·i·lin** (ko-bə-lof'ĭ-in) R protein.

**co·balt** (ko'bawlt) [L. *cobaltum*] [MeSH: Cobalt] a metal, atomic number, 27; atomic weight 58.9332; symbol Co; the metal is used in magnetic alloys, and the compounds afford pigments; inhalation of the dust can cause cobaltosis and exposure to the powder may cause dermatitis. See also *cobalt poisoning,* under *poisoning.* In animals, a deficiency of this element leads to anemia and an excess of normal dietary requirements leads to erythrocytosis. In humans, although cobalt has been used with limited transient effectiveness to treat the anemia of infection and renal disease, its sole physiologic function is probably as a constituent of vitamin $B_{12}$.
**c. 57,** a radioactive isotope of cobalt, atomic mass 57, having a half-life of 271.77 days and decaying in the form of electron capture and gamma rays (energy 0.122 MeV); used to label vitamin $B_{12}$ for the Schilling and other tests of intestinal absorption.
**c. 58,** a radioactive isotope of cobalt, atomic mass 58, having a half-life of 71.92 days and decaying in the form of electron capture, positrons (energy 0.48 MeV), and gamma rays (energy 0.811 MeV); used together with $^{57}Co$ in a test of intestinal vitamin $B_{12}$ absorption.
**c. 60,** a radioactive isotope of cobalt, atomic mass 60, having a half-life of 5.27 years and emitting beta particles (energy 0.318, 1.48 MeV) and gamma rays (energy 1.173, 1.332 MeV); used as a source of radiation in the treatment of malignancies. It has also been used to label vitamin $B_{12}$ for the Schilling and other tests of intestinal absorption.

**co·bal·to·sis** (ko″bawl-to'sis) pneumoconiosis due to inhalation of and tissue reaction to cobalt dust.

**co·bal·tous** (ko-bawl'təs) pertaining to or containing cobalt in its bivalent state.

**co·ba·mide** (ko'bə-mīd) 1. in chemical nomenclature, a derivative of cobalamin lacking the 5,6-dimethylbenzimidazole moiety. 2. a term sometimes used generically for any substituted compound containing this structure, particularly any *cobalamin* (def. 2).

**co·bra** (ko'brə) [Port. *cobra de capello* snake with a hood, from L. *coluber* snake] [MeSH: Cobra] any of several extremely poisonous elapid snakes of the large genus *Naja* and smaller genus *Ophiophagus,* commonly found in Africa, Asia, and India. They are capable of expanding the neck region to form a hood, and have two comparatively short, erect, deep grooved fangs. A serum obtained from animals inoculated with cobra venom is used in counteracting the effects of the venom. See table at *snake.*
**Asian c.,** any member of the species *Naja naja,* whose subspecies are widely distributed throughout Asia and nearby islands including Indonesia and the Philippines; among the Asian cobras are the Indian cobra, *N. naja naja,* and a spitting cobra found in Southeast Asia and the Philippines, *N. naja sputatrix.*
**black-necked c.,** *Naja nigricollis,* a type of spitting cobra found in southern Egypt, West Africa, and south through western Africa to South Africa.
**Cape c.,** *Naja nivea,* a species found in southern Africa.
**Egyptian c.,** *Naja haje,* a species found throughout Africa and the western part of the Arabian peninsula.
**Indian c.,** *Naja naja naja,* a yellowish to dark brown cobra with black and white markings resembling a pair of spectacles on its hood; it sometimes attains a length of 6 feet. Called also *N. naja.*
**king c.,** *Ophiophagus hannah,* a large cobra found from India to the Philippines, which may reach a length of 3.6 meters.
**Mozambique c.,** *Naja mossambica,* a type of spitting cobra found in southeastern Africa.
**spitting c.,** any of several cobras that have a venom canal opening forward in the fangs, so that the snake can eject a fine spray of venom over a distance of several meters ("spitting"). If the venom enters the eyes severe irritation results, and secondary infection may lead to blindness. The group includes the black-necked cobra, the Mozambique cobra, and *Naja naja sputatrix,* a subspecies of *N. naja.*

**co·bra·ism** (ko'brə-iz-əm) poisoning by cobra venom.

**co·bral·y·sin** (ko-bral'ĭ-sin) a hemolytic substance derived from the poison of the cobra.

**COBS** abbreviation for *cesarean-obtained barrier-sustained,* a term applied to animals delivered by cesarean section into a germ-free environment and maintained under the same conditions.

**COC** calcifying odontogenic cyst.

**co·ca** (ko'kə) [MeSH: Coca] 1. *Erythroxylon coca.* 2. the leaves of *E. coca,* widely used in parts of South America as a euphoriant masticatory. A central nervous system stimulant, it was once widely used medicinally and is a source of the crystalline extract cocaine.

**co·caine** (ko-kān') [USP] [MeSH: Cocaine] a crystalline alkaloid, obtained from leaves of *Erythroxylon coca* (coca leaves) and other *Erythroxylon species,* or by synthesis from ecgonine or its derivatives; used as a local anesthetic and vasoconstrictor applied topically to mucous membranes. Abuse of cocaine or its salts leads to dependence.
**crack c.,** a smokable form of cocaine prepared for illicit use, characterized by rapid absorption and onset of euphoric effects.
**c. hydrochloride** [USP], the hydrochloride salt of cocaine, used as a local anesthetic and vasoconstrictor, applied topically to mucous membranes.

**co·cain·iza·tion** (ko″kə-nĭ-za'shən) the act of putting under the influence of cocaine.

**co·cain·ize** (ko'kə-nīz) to put under the influence of cocaine.

**co·car·cin·o·gen** (ko-kahr-sin'ə-jən) promoter (def. 3).

**co·car·ci·no·gen·e·sis** (ko-kahr″sĭ-no-jen'ə-sis) [MeSH: Cocarcinogenesis] the development, according to one theory, of cancer only in preconditioned cells and as a result of conditions favorable to its growth.

**coc·cal** (kok'əl) resembling or pertaining to cocci.

**coc·ce·rin** (kok'sə-rin) a wax from *Coccus,* the cochineal insect, being an ester of cocceryl alcohol and two acids, 13-keto-n-dotriacontanoic acid and n-triacontanoic acid; used as a biological stain.

**coc·ci** (kok'si) [L.] plural of *coccus.*

**Coc·ci·dae** (kok'sĭ-de) a family of insects of the order Hemiptera; it includes the genera *Coccus* and *Laccifer*.

**Coc·cid·ia** (kok-sid'e-ə) [Gr. *kokkos* berry] [MeSH: Coccidia] a subclass of parasitic protozoa (class Sporozoea, phylum Apicomplexa) found in both vertebrates, including humans, and higher invertebrates; see *coccidiosis*. Their life cycle involves merogony, gametogony, and sporogony, and gamonts are usually present, with mature gamonts being small and typically intracellular, without an epimerite or mucron. Syzygy does not usually occur, but if it does, it involves anisogamous gametes. The subclass comprises three orders: Agamococcidiida, Protococcidiida, and Eucoccidiida.

**coc·cid·ia** (kok-sid'e-ə) [MeSH: Coccidia] plural of *coccidium*.

**coc·cid·i·al** (kok-sid'e-əl) coccidian, def. 1.

**coc·cid·i·an** (kok-sid'e-ən) 1. pertaining to Coccidia. 2. any protozoan of the order Coccidia.

**coc·cid·i·oi·dal** (kok-sid"e-oi'dəl) caused by fungi of the genus *Coccidioides*.

**Coc·cid·i·oi·des** (kok-sid"e-oi'dēz) [MeSH: Coccidioides] a pathogenic genus of Fungi Imperfecti of the form-class Hyphomycetes, form-family Moniliaceae. In soil it grows as a mycelium with arthrospores; in tissue as a spherule with endospores. *C. im'mitis* causes coccidioidomycosis.

**coc·cid·i·oi·din** (kok-sid"e-oi'din) [USP] [MeSH: Coccidioidin] a skin test antigen prepared from mycelial phase *Coccidioides immitis* organisms. Because most individuals in endemic areas are skin test positive it is not useful in diagnosis. A negative skin test (cutaneous anergy) occurs in many patients with disseminated disease and indicates a poor prognosis. Cf. *spherulin*.

**coc·cid·i·oi·do·ma** (kok-sid"e-oi-do'mə) a solid round focus of residual pulmonary granulomatous nodules, seen radiographically in coccidioidomycosis.

**coc·cid·i·oi·do·my·co·sis** (kok-sid"e-oi"do-mi-ko'sis) [MeSH: Coccidioidomycosis] a fungal disease caused by infection with *Coccidioides immitis*, occurring in both primary and secondary forms. Called also *California disease, coccidioidosis, coccidioidal granuloma, Posadas' disease* or *mycosis*, and *Posadas-Wernicke disease*.
**primary c.**, an acute, benign, self-limited respiratory infection due to inhalation of spores of *Coccidioides immitis*, seen primarily in the southwestern United States, northwestern Mexico, and parts of Central and South America. It varies in severity from a condition resembling a common cold to symptoms like those of influenza, sometimes with pneumonia, cavitation, high fever, and occasionally erythema nodosum *(bumps)*. Called also *desert* or *valley fever, San Joaquin* or *San Joaquin Valley fever*, and *desert rheumatism*.
**progressive c., secondary c.**, a virulent and severe chronic progressive granulomatous disease with involvement of the cutaneous and subcutaneous tissues, viscera, central nervous system, and lungs, with anemia, phlebitis, and a variety of allergic responses. It may be either a new infection or a reactivation of arrested primary disease, such as in immunocompromised patients.

**coc·cid·i·oi·do·sis** (kok-sid"e-oi-do'sis) coccidioidomycosis.

**coc·cid·i·o·sis** (kok"sid-e-o'sis) [MeSH: Coccidiosis] 1. in humans, infection by the coccidian protozoa *Isospora hominis* or *I. belli;* such infection is often asymptomatic and is found only upon testing of a stool sample, but occasionally it causes a severe watery mucous diarrhea, especially in immunocompromised patients. 2. in mammals such as cattle, sheep, rabbits, swine, cats, and dogs, infection by coccidia of the genera *Cystoisospora, Eimeria, Hepatozoon, Isospora*, or *Tyzzeria;* it especially affects young animals, causing destruction of the intestinal mucosa, accompanied by diarrhea, intestinal hemorrhage, emaciation, and sometimes fatal dysentery. Coccidial infections cause greatest damage to poultry; *Eimeria* species are particularly infective, producing high morbidity and mortality rates, especially in young birds.

**coc·cid·io·stat** (kok-sid'ĭ-o-stat") an agent that controls coccidiosis in animals; often administered as a feed additive or in drinking water. Called also *anticoccidial* and *coccidiostatic*.

**coc·cid·io·stat·ic** (kok-sid"ĭ-o-stat'ik) 1. inhibiting the growth of coccidia. 2. coccidiostat.

**Coc·cid·i·um** (kok-sid'e-əm) [L.; dim. of Gr. *kokkos* berry] in former systems of classification, a genus of coccidians, the organisms of which have been assigned to other genera.
**C. tenel'lum,** *Eimeria tenella*.

**coc·cid·i·um** (kok-sid'e-əm) pl. *coccid'ia*. Any protozoan of the subclass Coccidia.

**coc·ci·gen·ic** (kok"sĭ-jen'ik) caused by cocci.

**coc·ci·lla·na** (kok"sĭ-yah'nə) cocillana.

**coc·ci·nel·la** (kok"sĭ-nəl'ə) cochineal.

**coc·ci·nel·lin** (kok"sĭ-nəl'in) [L. *coccinellinum*] carmine; the coloring principle of cochineal.

**cocco-** [Gr. *kokkos* berry] a word element denoting a resemblance to a berry.

**coc·co·bac·il·lary** (kok"o-bas'ĭ-lar"e) pertaining to or resembling a coccobacillus.

**coc·co·ba·cil·li** (kok"o-bə-sil'i) plural of *coccobacillus*.

**Coc·co·ba·cil·lus** (kok"o-bə-sil'əs) [*cocco-* + *bacillus*] in former systems of classification, a genus of bacteria made up of organisms now classified in the genera *Bacteroides, Fusobacterium*, and *Haemophilus*.

**coc·co·ba·cil·lus** (kok"o-bə-sil'əs) pl. *coccobacil'li*. An oval bacterial cell intermediate between the coccus and bacillus forms.

**coc·co·bac·te·ria** (kok"o-bak-tēr'e-ə) [*cocco-* + *bacteria*] a common name for the spheroid bacteria, or for the various bacterial cocci.

**coc·code** (kok'ōd) a globular granule.

**coc·co·gen·ic** (kok"o-jen'ik) coccigenic.

**coc·co·gen·ous** (kok-oj'ə-nəs) [*cocco-* + *-genous*] coccigenic.

**coc·coid** (kok'oid) resembling a coccus; globose.

**coc·cu·lus in·di·cus** (kok'u-lus in'dĭkus) 1. *Anamirta cocculus*. 2. the seeds of *A. cocculus*, which contain picrotoxin.

**Coc·cus** (kok'əs) [L., from Gr. *kokkos* berry] a genus of hemipterous insects of the family Coccidae, order Hemiptera. *C. cac'ti* is a source of cochineal.

**coc·cus** (kok'əs) pl. *coc'ci* [L., from Gr. *kokkos* berry] a spherical bacterial cell, usually slightly less than 1 $\mu$m in diameter.

**coc·cy·al·gia** (kok"se-al'jə) coccygodynia.

**coc·cy·ceph·a·lus** (kok"se-sef'ə-ləs) [*coccyx* + *-cephalus*] a fetus whose head is beak shaped.

**coc·cy·dyn·ia** (kok"sə-din'e-ə) coccygodynia.

**coc·cy·gal·gia** (kok"sə-gal'jə) coccygodynia.

**coc·cyg·e·al** (kok-sij'e-əl) pertaining to or located in the region of the coccyx.

**coc·cy·gec·to·my** (kok"sĭ-jek'tə-me) [*coccyx* + *-ectomy*] excision of the coccyx.

**coc·cy·ge·rec·tor** (kok"sĭ-jə-rek'tər) the ventral sacrococcygeal muscle.

**coc·cyg·e·us** (kok-sij'e-əs) [L.] coccygeal.

**coc·cy·go·dyn·ia** (kok"sĭ-go-din'e-ə) [*coccyx* + *-odynia*] pain in the coccyx and neighboring region; called also *coccyalgia, coccydynia, coccygalgia*, and *coccyodynia*.

**coc·cy·got·o·my** (kok"sĭ-got'ə-me) [*coccyx* + *-tomy*] freeing the coccyx from its attachments.

**coc·cy·odyn·ia** (kok"se-o-din'e-ə) coccygodynia.

**coc·cyx** (kok'siks) [Gr. *kokkyx* cuckoo, whose bill it is said to resemble] [MeSH: Coccyx] TA alternative for *os coccygis*.

**coch·i·neal** (koch"ĭ-nēl') the dried female insects, *Coccus cacti*, enclosing the young larvae; formerly used as a coloring agent for pharmaceutical agents. It is the source of carmine and carminic acid.

**cochl.** abbreviation for L. *cochlea're*, a spoonful.
**c. amp.**, L. *cochlea're am'plum*, a heaping spoonful.
**c. mag.**, L. *cochlea're mag'num*, a tablespoonful.
**c. med.**, L. *cochlea're me'dium*, a dessertspoonful.
**c. parv.**, L. *cochlea're par'vum*, a teaspoonful.

**coch·lea** (kok'le-ə) [L. "snail shell"] [MeSH: Cochlea] 1. anything of a spiral form. 2. [TA] a spirally wound tube, resembling a snail shell, which forms part of the inner ear. Its base lies against the lateral end of the internal acoustic meatus and its apex is directed anterolaterally. It consists of the modiolus, a bony canal, and the osseous spiral lamina, which partially divides the cochlea into the essential organs of hearing, the scala vestibuli and scala tympani; the scalae communicate through the helicotrema.
**membranous c.**, ductus cochlearis.
**Mondini's c.**, the misshapen cochlea seen in Mondini's deformity.

**coch·le·ar** (kok'le-ər) of or pertaining to the cochlea.

**Coch·le·a·ria** (kok"le-ar'e-ə) [L.] a genus of plants of the family Cruciferae. *C. officina'lis* is scurvy grass, a species formerly used to treat scurvy. *C. armora'cia* is a former name for *Armoracia lapathifolia*, the horseradish plant.

**coch·le·ar·i·form** (kok"le-ar'ĭ-form) [L. *cochleare* spoon + *form*] shaped like a spoon.

**coch·le·itis** (kok"le-i'tis) inflammation of the cochlea.

**coch·leo·sac·cu·lot·o·my** (kok"le-o-sak"u-lot'ə-me) creation of a fistula between the saccule and cochlear duct by means of a pick introduced through the round window, in order to relieve endolymphatic hydrops.

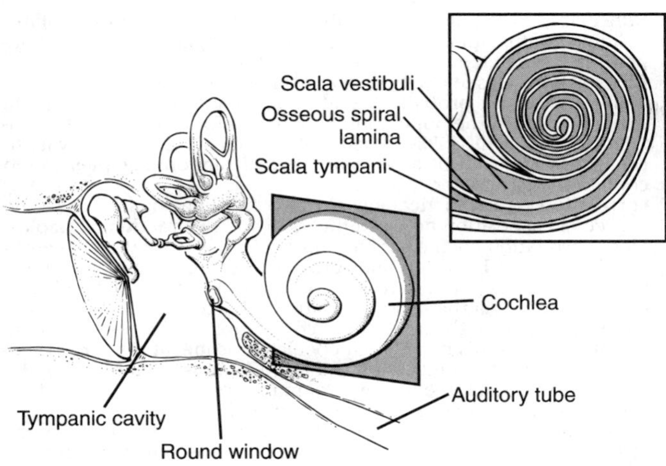


**coch·leo·top·ic** (kok″le-o-top′ik) relating to the organization of the auditory pathways and auditory area of the brain.

**coch·leo·ves·tib·u·lar** (kok″le-o-ves-tib′u-lər) pertaining to the cochlea and vestibule of the ear.

**Coch·li·ob·o·lus** (kok″le-ob′ə-ləs) a genus of fungi of the order Dothideales. It includes the perfect (sexual) stage of various species of *Bipolaris, Curvularia,* and *Drechslera.*

**Coch·lio·my·ia** (kok″le-o-mi′yə) [Gr. *kochlias* snail with a spiral shell + *myia* fly] a genus of flies of the family Calliphoridae.
**C. america′na,** *C. hominivorax.*
**C. bezzia′na,** *Chrysomyia bezziana.*
**C. hominivo′rax,** the screw-worm fly, a bluish green fly that deposits its eggs during the warmest hours of the day on wounds of animals; the larvae, known as screw-worms, after hatching, burrow into the wound and feed on living tissue. Called also *C. americana* and *Chrysomyia macellaria.*

**coch·li·tis** (kok-li′tis) cochleitis.

**co·ci·lla·na** (ko″se-yah′nə) the bark of *Guarea rusbyi,* used as an emetic, expectorant, and cathartic.

**Cock·ayne's syndrome** (kok-ānz′) [Edward Alfred *Cockayne,* English physician, 1880–1956] see under *syndrome.*

**cock·le·burr** (kok′əl-bər) any plant of the genus *Xanthium.*

**cock·roach** (kok′rōch) [Sp. *cucaracha*] any of various crawling winged insects with flat oval bodies of the order Blattaria. Many are household pests and reservoirs of disease. Common genera are *Blatta, Blattella,* and *Periplaneta.* Called also *roach.*
**American c.,** *Periplaneta americana,* a common household pest in the Northern hemisphere.
**Australian c.,** *Periplaneta australasiae,* a common household pest in warm regions of the world.
**German c.,** *Blattella germanica,* a small light brown species found as a household pest in North America and Europe. Called also *Croton bug.*
**Oriental c.,** *Blatta orientalis,* a black species originally seen in Asia but now found as a household pest in many parts of the world.

**cock·tail** (kok′tāl) a beverage concocted of various ingredients.
**lytic c.,** a concoction of various drugs used to block the function of the autonomic nervous system at every level, thus inhibiting the homeostatic defense reactions of the organism and producing the state known as artificial hibernation.
**McConckey c.,** an emulsion of cod liver oil and tomato juice.
**Philadelphia c.,** Rivers' c.
**Rivers' c.,** a solution of dextrose in isotonic saline solution, with thiamine chloride and insulin added, given by intravenous drip for detoxification in acute alcoholism.

**co·coa** (ko′ko) 1. a powder prepared from roasted, cured ripe seeds of *Theobroma cacao,* which contains caffeine and theobromine; used as a flavor in pharmaceutical preparations (see also *cocoa syrup,* under *syrup*). Dogs eating excessive amounts can become poisoned by the theobromine, with vomiting, diarrhea, muscle spasms, and coma. Called also *cacao, chocolate,* and *theobroma.* 2. cacao, def. 2.

**co·con·scious** (ko-kon′shəs) 1. not in the field of the conscious yet capable under favorable circumstances of being remembered; preconscious. 2. characterized by or pertaining to coconsciousness.

**co·co·nut** (ko′kə-nət) [MeSH: Coconut] the fruit of *Cocos nucifera,* a palm tree whose sap is used to make wine and whose nut is important as a food and a source of coconut oil (see under *oil*).

**Co·cos** (ko′kōs) a genus of palm trees (family Palmae). *C. nuci′fera* is the coconut palm, the source of coconuts and coconut oil.

**Coct.** abbreviation for L. *coc′tio,* boiling.

**coc·tion** (kok′shən) [L. *coctio,* a cooking] 1. the process of boiling. 2. digestion (def. 2).

**coc·to·an·ti·gen** (kok″to-an′tĭ-jən) an antigen modified by heat treatment.

**coc·to·im·mu·no·gen** (kok″to-ĭ-mu′no-jən) coctoantigen.

**coc·to·la·bile** (kok″to-la′bil) [L. *coctus* cooked + *labile*] destroyed or altered by heating to the boiling point of water.

**coc·to·pre·cip·i·tin** (kok″to-pre-sip′ĭ-tin) [L. *coctus* cooked + *precipitin*] a precipitin produced by immunization with a coctoantigen.

**coc·to·pro·tein** (kok″to-pro′tēn) a heated protein.

**coc·to·sta·bile** (kok″to-sta′bəl) [L. *coctus* cooked + *stabile*] not altered by heating to the temperature of boiling water.

**coc·to·sta·ble** (kok″to-sta′bəl) coctostabile.

**coc·u·line** (kok′u-lēn) sinomenine.

**co·cul·ti·va·tion** (ko″kəl-tĭ-va′shən) the culturing of cells (e.g., normal uninfected human cells) with infected or latently infected cells of the same kind.

**cod** (kod) *Gadus morrhua.*

**code** (kōd) [L. *codex* something written] 1. a set of rules governing one's conduct. 2. a system by which information can be communicated.
**degeneracy of c.,** see under *degeneracy.*
**genetic c.,** the manner in which information specifying the sequence of amino acid residues in the polypeptides synthesized by living organisms is encoded in the sequence of nucleotides in their genomes (see accompanying table). See also *codon, transcription,* and *translation.*
**triplet c.,** codon.

**co·deine** (ko′dēn) [L. *codeina*] [USP] [MeSH: Codeine] a narcotic alkaloid obtained from opium or prepared by methylating morphine, used as an analgesic and antitussive, administered orally. Called also *methylmorphine.*
**c. phosphate** [USP], the phosphate salt of codeine, used as a narcotic analgesic and antitussive; administered subcutaneously.
**c. sulfate** [USP], white crystals or white crystalline powder, used as a narcotic analgesic, administered orally.

**co·dex** (ko′deks) pl. *cod′ices* [L.] an authorized medicinal formulary; especially the French Pharmacopoeia, *Codex medicamentarium.*

**Cod·man's sign, triangle** (kod′mənz) [Ernest Amory *Codman,* American surgeon, 1869–1940] see under *sign* and *triangle.*

**co·do·cyte** (ko′do-sīt) target cell.

**co·dom·i·nance** (ko-dom′ĭ-nəns) codominant gene.

**co·dom·i·nant** (ko-dom′ĭ-nənt) see under *gene.*

**co·don** (ko′don) [MeSH: Codon] a set of three adjacent bases on a single strand of DNA or RNA. Of the 64 different codons, 61 direct the incorporation of a specific amino acid into a polypeptide chain and three signal chain termination (see table of the genetic code).
**chain-initiation c's,** the codons, AUG or GUG, occurring at the beginning of mRNA sequences coding for polypeptide chains. There they are recognized by the initiator tRNA, which carries the amino acid methionine (in the cytosol of eukaryotes) or *N*-formyl methionine (in prokaryotes, mitochondria, and chloroplasts). In the middle of a polypeptide chain these codons are recognized by other tRNAs so that AUG directs the incorporation of methionine and GUG of valine.
**chain-termination c's,** the three codons UAA, UAG, and UGA that cause termination of the synthesis of a growing polypeptide chain and its release from the ribosome. Called also *nonsense c's.*
**nonsense c's,** chain-termination c's.

**coe-** for words beginning thus, see also words beginning *ce-.*

**co·ef·fi·cient** (ko″ə-fish′ənt) 1. a numerical factor multiplying a term in an algebraic equation. 2. a number preceding a formula in a chemical equation, indicating the relative number of molecules of that species entering the reaction. 3. a unitless constant characterizing a chemical or physical process. 4. a unitless statistical parameter indicating the amount of change in an outcome under given conditions.
**absorption c.,** 1. absorptivity. 2. see *linear absorption c.* 3. see *mass absorption c.*
**activity c.,** the ratio of the activity (of an electrolyte) as measured by some property, such as the depression of the freezing point of a

**The Genetic Code**

| UUU | UCU | UAU | UGU |
|---|---|---|---|
| AAA | AGA | ATA | ACA |
| phe | ser | tyr | cys |
| UUC | UCC | UAC | UGC |
| GAA | GGA | GTA | GCA |
| phe | ser | tyr | cys |
| UUA | UCA | UAA | UGA |
| TAA | TGA | TTA | TCA |
| leu | ser | *term* | *term* |
| UUG | UCG | UAG | UGG |
| CAA | CGA | CTA | CCA |
| leu | ser | *term* | trp |
| CUU | CCU | CAU | CGU |
| AAG | AGG | ATG | ACG |
| leu | pro | his | arg |
| CUC | CCC | CAC | CGC |
| GAG | GGG | GTG | GCG |
| leu | pro | his | arg |
| CUA | CCA | CAA | CGA |
| TAG | TGG | TTG | TCG |
| leu | pro | gln | arg |
| CUG | CCG | CAG | CGG |
| CAG | CGG | CTG | CCG |
| leu | pro | gln | arg |
| AUU | ACU | AAU | AGU |
| AAT | AGT | ATT | ACT |
| ile | thr | asn | ser |
| AUC | ACC | AAC | AGC |
| GAT | GGT | GTT | GCT |
| ile | thr | asn | ser |
| AUA | ACA | AAA | AGA |
| TAT | TGT | TTT | TCT |
| ile | thr | lys | arg |
| AUG | ACG | AAG | AGG |
| CAT | CGT | CTT | CCT |
| met *(init)* | thr | lys | arg |
| GUU | GCU | GAU | GGU |
| AAC | AGC | ATC | ACC |
| val | ala | asp | gly |
| GUC | GCC | GAC | GGC |
| GAC | GGC | GTC | GCC |
| val | ala | asp | gly |
| GUA | GCA | GAA | GGA |
| TAC | TGC | TTC | TCC |
| val | ala | glu | gly |
| GUG | GCG | GAG | GGG |
| CAC | CGC | CTC | CCC |
| val *(init)* | ala | glu | gly |

Each grouping matches a messenger RNA codon *(top)*, its complementary DNA codon *(middle)*, and the amino acid they specify *(bottom)*. U = uracil; C = cytosine; A = adenine; G = guanine; T = thymine; see *amino acid* for amino acid symbols. The codons marked *term* are chain termination codons. Those marked *init* are chain initiation codons which code for methionine (in the cytosol of eukaryotic cells) or *N*-formylmethionine (in mitochondria and prokaryotes) at the beginning of polypeptide chains and for the indicated amino acid (methionine or valine) within polypeptide chains.

solution, to the true concentration (molality). It is usually less than 1 and increases as the solution becomes more dilute, approaching unity at infinite dilution, when the attractive forces between oppositely charged ions become negligible.
**binomial c.,** the number of different sets of size *k* that can be chosen from a set of *n* objects; denoted

$$\binom{n}{k}$$

or ${}_nC_k$, and equal to

$$\frac{n!}{k!(n-k)!}.$$

**biological c.,** the amount of potential energy consumed by the body when at rest.
**Bunsen c.,** the number of milliliters of gas dissolved in a milliliter of liquid at atmospheric pressure (760 mm Hg) and a specified temperature. Symbol, $\alpha$. Called also *solubility c.*
**Chick-Martin c.,** see *Chick-Martin m.,* under *method.*
**confidence c.,** the probability that a confidence interval will contain the true value of the population parameter. For example, if the confidence coefficient is .95, 95 per cent of the confidence intervals so calculated for each of a large number of random samples would contain the parameter.
**correlation c.,** a statistical measure which when squared gives the degree of association between the values of two random variables. Most correlation coefficients are normalized so that they have values between +1 (which indicates perfect correlation) and −1 (which indicates perfect inverse correlation); a value of 0 indicates no correlation. As the absolute value of the correlation coefficient increases, so does the strength of correlation. When not otherwise specified, Pearson's correlation coefficient is meant. The true theoretical correlation coefficient for a population is symbolized $\rho$; the sample correlation coefficient, computed from experimental data, estimates the theoretical and is symbolized *r.*
**creatinine c.,** the figure obtained by dividing the total of milligrams of creatinine in the day's urine by the body weight expressed in kilograms.
**cryoscopic c.,** the comparison of the freezing point depression of an electrolyte with that of an ideal nonelectrolyte of the same concentration (usually 1 molal of each).
**c. of demineralization,** the proportion of mineral matter to the total dry residue of the urine; it averages 30 per cent.
**dilution c.,** a number that expresses the effectiveness of a disinfectant for a given organism. It is calculated by the equation $tc^n = k$, where $t$ is the time required for killing all organisms, $c$ is the concentration of disinfectant, $n$ is the dilution coefficient, and $k$ is a constant. A low coefficient indicates the disinfectant is effective at a low concentration.
**distribution c.,** partition c.
**extinction c.,** absorptivity.
**Hill c.,** a coefficient occurring in the Hill equation, indicating the degree of cooperativity of the enzyme being examined; a Hill coefficient of 1.0 indicates independent binding while greater and lesser values indicate positive and negative cooperativity, respectively. The value for hemoglobin is 2.8.
**homogeneity c.,** in radiology, the ratio of the half-value layer to the second half-value layer; it is unity for radiation in which the photons all originate with the same energy.
**hygienic laboratory c.,** phenol c.
**c. of inbreeding,** an expression of the probability that an individual has received both alleles of a pair from a single ancestor common to both parents, or of the proportion of loci at which he is homozygous.
**Kendall's rank correlation c.,** a rank correlation coefficient used when both variables represent ordinal data in a limited number of grades, such as the categories none, mild, moderate, and severe, so that multiple samples can be assigned to each grade; called also *Kendall's tau.* See also *Spearman's rank correlation c.*
**Lancet c.,** phenol c.
**lethal c.,** that concentration of a disinfectant that will kill sporeless bacteria *(inferior lethal c.)* or bacterial spores *(superior lethal c.)* in water at a temperature of 20° to 25°C in the shortest period of time.
**linear absorption c.,** in radiation physics, the fraction of a beam of x-rays or gamma rays that is absorbed per unit thickness of the absorber.
**linear attenuation c.,** in radiation physics, the fraction of a beam of x-rays or gamma rays that is absorbed or scattered per unit thickness of the absorber. Symbol $\mu$.
**mass absorption c.,** in radiology, the linear absorption coefficient divided by the density of the absorber.
**mass attenuation c.,** the linear attenuation coefficient divided by the density of the absorbing material.
**molar absorption c., molar extinction c.,** molar absorptivity.
**olfactory c.,** Proetz test.
**osmotic c.,** a factor, $\phi$, which corrects for the deviation in the behavior of a solute in question from ideal behavior defined by the ideal gas equation as applied to osmotic pressure.
**partition c.,** the ratio in which a given substance distributes itself between two or more different phases; called also *distribution c.*
**Pearson's correlation c.,** the most common correlation coefficient; it is the covariance of two random variables divided by the product of their standard deviations. Called also *product-moment correlation c.* See also *correlation c.*
**phenol c.,** a measure of the bactericidal activity of a chemical compound in relation to phenol. The test is standardized (Rideal-Walker method, U. S. Department of Agriculture method). The coefficient is calculated by dividing the concentration of the test compound at which it kills the test organism in 10 minutes, but not in 5 minutes, by the concentration of phenol that kills the organism under the same conditions. It can be determined in the absence of organic

matter, or in the presence of a standard amount of added organic matter.
**product-moment correlation c.,** Pearson's correlation c.
**rank correlation c.,** the correlation coefficient of two variables calculated after ranks have been substituted for actual values. See also *Kendall's rank correlation c.* and *Spearman's rank correlation c.*
**c. of relationship,** an expression of the probability that two persons have inherited a certain gene from a common ancestor; or the proportion of all their genes that have been inherited from common ancestors.
**Rideal-Walker c.,** see *phenol c.*
**sample correlation c.,** see *correlation c.*
**sedimentation c.,** the velocity at which a particle sediments in a centrifuge divided by the applied centrifugal field, the result having units of time (velocity divided by acceleration), usually expressed in Svedberg units (S), which equal $10^{-13}$ second. Sedimentation coefficients are used to characterize the size of macromolecules, e.g., 5.8S rRNA, 22S rRNA; they increase with increasing mass and density and are higher for globular than for fibrous particles. Called also *sedimentation constant.*
**selection c.,** a measure of the disadvantage in survival value of a given genotype as compared with that of a standard genotype in a population.
**solubility c.,** Bunsen c.
**Spearman's rank correlation c.,** a rank correlation coefficient used when both variables represent ordinal data in an unlimited ranking, such as class standing, so that each sample is assigned a unique rank. Symbol $r_s$. Called also *Spearman's rho.* Cf. *Kendall's rank correlation c.*
**temperature c.,** a number indicating the effect of temperature upon the velocity constant of a chemical reaction. Symbol $Q_{10}$ because 10°C is the most commonly employed temperature change; see *van't Hoff's rule,* under *rule.*
**c. of thermal conductivity,** a number indicating the quantity of heat that passes in a unit of time through a unit thickness of a substance when the difference in temperature is 1°C.
**c. of thermal expansion,** the change in volume per unit volume of a substance produced by a 1°C temperature increase.
**c. of variation (CV),** the standard deviation divided by the mean, sometimes multiplied by 100; a unitless quantity indicating the variability around the mean in relation to the size of the mean.
**velocity c.,** a number expressing the rate of a reaction; the rate of transformation of a unit mass of a substance in a chemical reaction.
**c. of viscosity,** the force necessary to slide tangentially a unit of area of smooth surface at unit velocity on another parallel surface separated from the first surface by a unit layer of viscous substance.

**coe·la·ri·um** (se-lar'e-əm) [L., from Gr. *koilos* a hollow] the membrane that lines the body cavity of the embryo, or coelom; it consists of a parietal layer, the *exocoelarium,* and a visceral layer, the *endocoelarium.* Called also *mesothelium.*

**-coele** [Gr. *koilia* cavity] a word termination denoting a cavity or space; sometimes spelled *-cele* and *-coel.*

**Coe·len·ter·a·ta** (se-len"tər-a'tə) [Gr. *koilos* hollow + *enteron* intestine] former name for a phylum of marine invertebrates that included sea anemones, hydras, jellyfish, and corals, which are now assigned to the phylum Cnidaria. See also *coelenterate.*

**coe·len·ter·ate** (se-len'tər-āt) [MeSH: Cnidaria] 1. pertaining or belonging to the phylum Cnidaria. 2. an individual of the phylum Cnidaria; a cnidarian. 3. the cnidarians and ctenophores collectively.

**coe·len·ter·on** (se-len'tər-on) 1. archenteron. 2. gastrovascular cavity.

**coe·li·ac** (se'le-ak) abdominal.

**coel(o)-** [Gr. *koilos* hollow] a combining form denoting relationship to a cavity or space; sometimes spelled *cel(o)-.*

**coe·lo·blas·tu·la** (se"lo-blas'tu-lə) [*coelo-* + *blastula*] the common type of blastula, consisting of a hollow sphere composed of blastomeres.

**coe·lom** (se'lom) [Gr. *koilōma*] the body cavity. In the higher invertebrates, persists throughout life (cf. *Eucoelomata*). In the mammalian embryo, it is situated between the somatopleure and the splanchnopleure; it is both extraembryonic and intraembryonic. From the intraembryonic portion arise the principal cavities of the trunk. Also spelled *celom.* Called also *coeloma* and *somatic cavity.*
**extraembryonic c.,** the portion of the coelom external to the embryo, bordered by chorionic mesoderm and the mesoderm of the amnion and yolk sac; it communicates temporarily at the umbilicus with the intraembryonic coelom. Called also *exocoelom.*

**coe·lo·ma** (se-lo'mə) coelom.

**coe·lo·mate** (sēl'o-māt) 1. having a coelom. 2. eucoelomate.

**coe·lom·ic** (se-lom'ik) pertaining to the coelom.

**coe·lo·my·ar·i·an** (se"lo-mi-ar'e-ən) designating a type of nematode musculature in which the muscle fibers are next to the hypodermis and perpendicular to it; myofibrils extend varying distances up the side of the muscle cell, partially enclosing the sarcoplasm.

**Coe·lo·my·ce·tes** (se"lo-mi-se'tēz) a form-class of Fungi Imperfecti whose members produce conidia in pycnidia or acervuli; many of its members are saprobes or parasites on plants, animals, or other organisms. There are several different systems for dividing this group into orders and families. Medically important genera include *Colletotrichum, Diplodia, Hendersonula, Phoma, Pyrenochaeta,* and *Scytalidium.*

**coe·lo·so·my** (se"lo-so'me) celosomia.

**coe·lo·thel** (se'lo-thel) [*coelo-* + *thel*] mesothelium.

**coen(o)-** see *cen(o)-*[3].

**coe·no·cyte** (se'no-sīt") [*coen(o)-* + *-cyte*] 1. a multinucleate plant cell enclosed within a hollow wall, examples of which are found within the fungi and algae. 2. a multinucleate bit of cytoplasm in which the nuclei are not separated by walls. 3. a multinucleate plant protoplast. Spelled also *cenocyte.*

**coe·no·cyt·ic** (se"no-sit'ik) pertaining to or having the characteristics of a coenocyte.

**coe·nu·ri·a·sis** (se'nu-ri'ə-sis) 1. coenurosis, def. 1. 2. gid.

**coe·nu·ro·sis** (se"nu-ro'sis) 1. any infection by species of *Coenurus;* it is found only rarely in humans, nearly always in the form of central nervous system cysts that obstruct the outflow of cerebrospinal fluid and cause a rise in intracranial pressure that can be fatal. Called also *coenuriasis.* 2. gid.

**Coe·nu·rus** (se-nu'rəs) [Gr. *koinos* common + *oura* tail] a genus of tapeworm larvae consisting of semitransparent fluid-filled organisms that contain multiple scoleces attached to the inner surface of the cavity wall; they do not form brood capsules. *C. cerebra'lis,* the larva of *Taenia multiceps,* is found in the brains of sheep (causing gid), as well as in brains of goats, other ruminants, and occasionally humans.

**coe·nu·rus** (se-nu'rəs) a tapeworm larva of the genus *Coenurus;* cf. *cysticercus.* Called also *bladder worm.*

**co·en·zyme** (ko-en'zīm) an organic nonprotein molecule, frequently a phosphorylated derivative of a water-soluble vitamin, that binds with the protein molecule (apoenzyme) to form the active enzyme (holoenzyme).
**c. A,** a coenzyme in which phosphorylated pantothenic acid is covalently linked to β-mercaptoethylamine and adenosine 3',5'-bisphosphate. The terminal thiol group of the β-mercaptoethanolamine is enzymatically acylated to form high-energy thiol ester compounds such as the acetyl, acetoacetyl, and long chain fatty acid (acyl) compounds. These thiol esters play a central role in various metabolic reactions, e.g., the tricarboxylic acid cycle, the transfer of acetyl groups, and the oxidation of fatty acids. Abbreviated CoA and CoA-SH. See also *acetoacetyl coenzyme A, acetyl coenzyme A, acyl coenzyme A,* and *succinyl coenzyme A.*
**c. $B_{12}$,** adenosylcobalamin. See also *methylcobalamin.*
**c. Q,** former name for *ubiquinone.*

**coe·ru·le·us** (sə-roo'le-əs) [L.] variant spelling of *caeruleus* (q.v.).

**coeur** (kər) [Fr.] heart.
**c. en sabot,** (on să-bo'), a heart visible radiographically as having an increased transverse diameter, a convexity in the inferior line, and an elevation and rounded shape of the apex, so that its form suggests vaguely that of a wooden shoe; noted in tetralogy of Fallot.

**co·fac·tor** (ko'fak-tor) an element or principle, as a coenzyme, with which another must unite in order to function.
**heparin c. II,** a serine proteinase inhibitor of the serpin family; it is a single-chain glycoprotein, $M_r$ 65,000, that inhibits thrombin. It resembles antithrombin III in being markedly stimulated by heparin; it differs in that it binds and is activated by dermatan sulfate and in that it does not inhibit any other activated coagulation factors.
**platelet c. I,** factor VIII; see under *coagulation factors,* at *factor.*
**platelet c. II,** factor IX; see under *coagulation factors,* at *factor.*

**Cof·fea** (kaw'fe-ə) the coffee plants, a genus of small trees of the family Rubiaceae thought to have originated in Africa. *C. ara'bica* L. and *C. libe'rica* are cultivated in warm regions around the world as sources of coffee.

**cof·fee** (kof'e) [Ar. al-qahwah] [MeSH: Coffee] 1. the dried, roasted seeds of *Coffea arabica* or *C. liberica.* 2. a drink made by decoction or infusion of these seeds, which is invigorating, tonic, and conservant; useful in chronic asthma, headache, and opium poisoning. The active principles include caffeine (q.v.) in the seeds, coffee oil, sugars, protein, and numerous volatile flavoring oils.

**Cof·fin-Low·ry syndrome** (kof'in-lou're) [Grange S. *Coffin,* American pediatrician, born 1923; R. Brian *Lowry,* Irish-born Canadian physician, 20th century] see under *syndrome.*

**Cof·fin-Sir·is syndrome** (kof'in-sir'is) [G.S. *Coffin;* Evelyn *Siris,* American radiologist, 1914–1987] see under *syndrome.*

**Co·gan's oc·u·lo·mo·tor aprax·ia, syndrome** (ko'gənz) [David Glendenning *Cogan,* American ophthalmologist, 1908–1993] see under *apraxia* and *syndrome.*

**co·ge·ner** (ko'jə-nər) congener.

**Co·gen·tin** (ko-jen'tin) trademark for preparations of benztropine mesylate.

**Cog·nex** (kog'neks) trademark for a preparation of tacrine.

**cog·ni·tion** (kog-nish'ən) [L. *cognitio,* from *cognoscere* to know] [MeSH: Cognition] that operation of the mind by which one becomes aware of objects of thought or perception; it includes all aspects of perceiving, thinking, and remembering.

**cog·ni·tive** (kog'nĭ-tiv) of, pertaining to, or characterized by cognition.

**Co·hen** (ko'ən) Stanley, American biochemist, born 1922, co-winner with Rita Levi-Montalcini of the Nobel prize for medicine or physiology in 1986 for discoveries regarding the mechanisms by which growth factors regulate cell and organ growth.

**co·he·sion** (ko-he'zhən) [L. *cohaesio,* from *con* together + *haerere* to stick] the intermolecular attractive force that causes various particles of a single material to unite.

**co·he·sive** (ko-he'siv) uniting together, or characterized by cohesion.

**Cohn·heim's areas (fields), theory** (kōn'hīmz) [Julius Friedrich *Cohnheim,* German pathologist, 1839–1884] see under *area* and *theory.*

**co·ho·ba** (ko-ho'bə) [Sp.] parica.

**co·ho·ba·tion** (ko″ho-ba'shən) the repeated distilling of a liquid from the same material; redistillation.

**co·hort** (ko'hort) [L. *cohors* one of the ten units making up a Roman legion] 1. in epidemiology, a group of individuals who share a common characteristic, e.g., all of the individuals born in one year (a birth cohort) or a group of individuals entered in a prospective study or a clinical trial. The term always indicates observation of the individuals over time. 2. a taxonomic category approximately equivalent to a division, order, or suborder in various systems of classification.

**co·hosh** (ko-hosh') [Algonquian] any of various North American medicinal plants, such as *Actaea spicata,* or red cohosh; *Caulophyllum thalictroides,* or blue cohosh; and *Cimicifuga racemosa,* or black cohosh.

**co·con·scious·ness** (ko-kon'shus-nes) 1. a secondary consciousness coexisting with the main stream of consciousness, as in some dissociative disorders. 2. the edge of consciousness.

**coil** (koil) [Old Fr. *collier,* from L. *colligere* to gather together] a winding structure. See also *spiral* and *helix.*
**random c.,** a term used to refer to any protein secondary structure that does not have a regular repetitive pattern, e.g., $\alpha$-helix or $\beta$-sheet.

**co·in·fec·tion** (ko'in-fek″shən) simultaneous infection by separate pathogens, as by hepatitis B and hepatitis D viruses.

**coin(o)-** see *cen(o)-*[3].

**coi·no·site** (koi'no-sīt) [*coino-* + *sitos* food] a free or unfixed commensal organism; called also *cenosite.*

**co·iso·ge·ne·ic** (ko-i″so-jə-ne'ik) of or relating to strains of inbred animals that are constructed to be genetically identical except for a difference at a single genetic locus.

**co·i·so·gen·ic** (ko-i″so-jen'ik) congenic.

**co·i·tal** (ko'ĭ-təl) pertaining to coitus.

**co·i·tion** (ko-ish'ən) coitus.

**co·i·to·pho·bia** (ko″ĭ-to-fo'be-ə) [*coitus* + *-phobia*] irrational fear of coitus.

**co·i·tus** (ko'ĭ-tus) [L. *coitio* a coming together, meeting] [MeSH: Coitus] sexual connection per vaginam between male and female.
**c. incomple'tus, c. interrup'tus,** coitus in which the penis is withdrawn from the vagina before ejaculation; a widely used but unreliable method of contraception.
**c. reserva'tus,** coitus in which ejaculation is intentionally suppressed.

**Co·ke·ro·my·ces** (ko″kə-ro-mi'sēz) a genus of fungi of the family Thamnidiaceae. *C. recurva'tus* has been isolated occasionally from cases of mucormycosis and cystitis.

**Col.** abbreviation for L. *co'la,* strain.

**col** (kol) [Fr., from L. *collum* neck] a valley-like depression of the interdental gingiva, which connects the facial and lingual papillae and conforms to the shape of the interproximal contact area.

**col-** see *con-.*

**Co·lace** (ko'lās) trademark for a preparation of docusate sodium.

**co·la·mine** (ko'lə-min) monoethanolamine.

**co·las·pase** (kə-las'pās) BAN for asparaginase derived from *Escherichia coli.*

**Colat.** abbreviation for L. *cola'tus,* strained.

**co·la·tion** (ko-la'shən) [L. *colare* to strain] 1. the process of removing solids from liquids, by straining or filtration. 2. the product of such a process.

**col·a·to·ri·um** (kol″ə-tor'e-əm) [L. *colare* to strain] filter.

**co·la·ture** (ko'lə-chər) [L. *colatura,* from *colare* to strain] a liquid obtained by straining.

**Col·BEN·E·MID** (kol-ben'ə-mid) trademark for a preparation of probenecid with colchicine.

**col·chi·cine** (kol'chĭ-sēn) [USP] [MeSH: Colchicine] an alkaloid obtained from species of *Colchicum,* used in the treatment of gouty arthritis. It binds to microtubules and is used in the laboratory to arrest cell division by disrupting the mitotic spindle. Its action in gout may be due to inhibition of granulocyte migration into areas of inflammation.

**Col·chi·cum** (kol'chi-kəm) [MeSH: Colchicum] a genus of plants of the family Liliaceae, native to Europe and Asia; their corms or dried ripe seeds are sources of colchicine. *C. autumna'le* is the meadow saffron; cattle eating excessive amounts of it may suffer a fatal enteritis.

**COLD** chronic obstructive lung disease.

**cold** (kōld) [MeSH: Cold] 1. low in temperature, physiologic activity, or in radioactivity. 2. a catarrhal disorder of the upper respiratory tract, which may be viral, a mixed infection, or an allergic reaction. It is marked by acute rhinitis, a slight rise in temperature, and chilly sensations. Called also *common c.*
**common c.,** see *cold,* def. 2.

**cold·sore** (kōld'sor″) see *herpes simplex.*

**Cole's sign** (kōlz) [Lewis Gregory *Cole,* American roentgenologist, 1874–1954] see under *sign.*

**co·lec·to·my** (ko-lek'tə-me) [*colon* + *-ectomy*] [MeSH: Colectomy] excision of a portion of the colon *(partial c.)* or of the whole colon *(complete* or *total c.).*
**left c.,** see under *hemicolectomy.*
**right c.,** see under *hemicolectomy.*
**sigmoid c.,** sigmoidectomy.

**cole(o)-** [Gr. *koleos* sheath] a combining form denoting relationship to the vagina, or to a sheath.

**Col·e·op·tera** (kol″e-op'tər-ə) [*coleo-* + Gr. *pteron* wing] [MeSH: Coleoptera] the beetles, an order of insects having strong mouth parts for chewing and a pair of hard exterior wings that protect the body, are not used for flight, and cover the membranous flight wings.

**co·les** (ko'lēz) [Gr. *kōlē*] penis.
**c. femini'nus,** clitoris.

**Co·les·tid** (ko-les'tid) trademark for a preparation of colestipol hydrochloride.

**co·les·ti·pol hy·dro·chlo·ride** (ko-les'tĭ-pol) [USP] an insoluble, high-molecular-weight anion exchange resin that binds bile acids in the intestines to form a complex that is excreted in the feces; administered orally as an antihyperlipoproteinemic in the treatment of familial hyperlipoproteinemia, type IIa, pruritus associated with partial biliary obstruction, and diarrhea due to excess bile acids in the colon.

**Colet.** abbreviation for L. *cole'tur,* let it be strained.

**co·li·bac·il·le·mia** (ko″lĭ-bas-ĭ-le'me-ə) the presence of *Escherichia coli* in the blood.

**co·li·bac·il·lo·sis** (ko″lĭ-bas-ĭ-lo'sis) infection with *Escherichia coli.*
**enteric c., enterotoxigenic c.,** coliform gastroenteritis.
**c. gravida'rum,** severe infection with *Escherichia coli* during pregnancy.

**co·li·bac·il·lu·ria** (ko″lĭ-bas″ĭl-u're-ə) presence of *Escherichia coli* in the urine.

**co·li·bac·il·lus** (ko″lĭ-bə-sil'əs) *Escherichia coli.*

**col·ic** (kol'ik) [Gr. *kōlikos*] [MeSH: Colic] 1. acute abdominal pain; characteristically, intermittent visceral pain with fluctuations corresponding to smooth muscle peristalsis. 2. colonic.
**appendicular c.,** vermicular c.
**biliary c.,** paroxysms of pain and other severe symptoms due to the passage of gallstones along the bile duct; called also *gallstone* or *hepatic c.,* and *cholecystalgia.*
**bilious c.,** abdominal pain accompanied by the vomiting of bile.

**copper c.**, a severe colic due to copper poisoning.
**Devonshire c.**, lead c.
**endemic c.**, a dangerous form of colic peculiar to hot countries.
**equine c.**, intestinal pain in horses; causes may include excessive gas; blockage by an impaction, foreign body, or twisting or other malposition; or infection or enteritis.
**flatulent c.**, tympanites.
**gallstone c.**, biliary c.
**gastric c.**, gastrodynia.
**hepatic c.**, biliary c.
**infantile c.**, benign paroxysmal abdominal pain during the first three months of life.
**intestinal c.**, colic originating from the small bowel, characteristically periumbilical in location.
**lead c.**, colic due to lead poisoning; called also *Devonshire, painters', Poitou,* or *saturnine c.*
**menstrual c.**, dysmenorrhea.
**nephric c.**, renal c.
**ovarian c.**, oophoralgia.
**painters' c.**, lead c.
**pancreatic c.**, abdominal pain caused by obstruction of the excretory duct of the pancreas.
**Poitou c.**, lead c.
**renal c.**, pain produced by thrombosis or dissection of the renal artery, renal infarction, intrarenal mass lesions, the passage of a stone within the collecting system, or thrombosis of the renal vein; called also *nephric c.*
**sand c.**, chronic indigestion in horses and cattle due to the presence in the stomach or intestine of sand taken in with food or drink.
**saturnine c.**, lead c.
**stercoral c.**, intestinal colic due to accumulation of feces.
**tubal c.**, painful spasmodic contraction of the fallopian tube.
**ureteral c.**, colicky pains due to obstruction of the ureter.
**uterine c.**, hysteralgia.
**vermicular c.**, a condition of colic in the vermiform appendix occasioned by a catarrhal inflammation resulting from blocking of the outlet of the appendix; called also *appendicular c.*
**verminous c.**, colic due to the presence of intestinal worms; called also *worm c.*
**worm c.**, verminous c.
**zinc c.**, colic resulting from chronic zinc poisoning.

**col·i·cin** (kol'ĭ-sin) [*coli* (from *Escherichia coli*) + *-cin* (adapted from L. *caedere* to kill)] a bacteriocin secreted by colicinogenic strains of *Escherichia coli* and *Shigella sonnei* that is lethal to closely related bacterial strains. Specific colicins attach to specific receptors on cell membranes and impair systems of electron transport, membrane function, molecular synthesis, or energy production.

**col·i·cin·o·gen** (kol"ĭ-sin'o-jən) bacteriocinogen; a plasmid in some strains of *Escherichia coli* that induces secretion of the corresponding colicin. Some colicinogens also serve as sex factors.

**col·i·ci·nog·e·nic** (kol"ĭ-sĭ-noj'ə-nik) elaborating colicin; said of strains of *Escherichia coli.*

**col·i·ci·nog·e·ny** (kol"ĭ-sin-oj'ə-ne) the production of colicin; see *colicinogen.*

**col·icky** (kol'ik-e) pertaining to or affected by colic.

**col·i·co·ple·gia** (kol"ĭ-ko-ple'jə) [*colic* + *-plegia*] lead colic and lead paralysis together.

**co·li·cys·ti·tis** (ko"lĭ-sis-ti'tis) cystitis dependent upon the presence of *Escherichia coli.*

**co·li·cys·to·py·eli·tis** (ko"lĭ-sis-to-pi"ə-li'tis) [*colic* + *cystis* + *pyelo-* + *-itis*] inflammation of the bladder and kidney pelvis.

**col·i·form** (ko'lĭ-form) [L. *colum* a sieve] 1. a collective term denoting enteric, fermentative gram-negative rods, and sometimes restricted to the lactose-fermenting, gram-negative enteric bacilli, i.e., *Citrobacter, Edwardsiella, Enterobacter, Escherichia, Klebsiella,* and *Serratia.* 2. any organism of that group.

**co·lin·e·ar·i·ty** (ko"lin-e-ar'ĭ-te) the correspondence between the linear sequence of the nucleotide codons, the RNA, and the linear sequence of amino acids in the polypeptide coded for by that sequence; a concept implicit in the original Watson-Crick model of the DNA structure.

**co·lip·ase** (ko-li'pās) a cofactor of pancreatic lipase, secreted by pancreatic acinar cells as a proenzyme and activated via hydrolytic cleavage by trypsin.

**col·i·phage** (kol'ĭ-fāj) [MeSH: Coliphages] any bacteriophage that infects *Escherichia coli.*

**co·li·pli·ca·tion** (ko"lĭ-plĭ-ka'shən) coloplication.

**co·li·punc·ture** (ko'lĭ-pungk"chər) colocentesis.

**co·lis·ti·meth·ate so·di·um** (ko-lis"tĭ-meth'āt) [USP] chemical name: colistinmethanesulfonic acid pentasodium; the pentasodium salt of the methanesulfonate derivative of colistin, having actions and uses similar to those of the base (colistin); administered intramuscularly or intravenously.

**co·lis·tin** (ko-lis'tin) [MeSH: Colistin] a polypeptide antibiotic of the polymyxin (q.v.) group, produced by the growth of the soil bacterium *Bacillus polymyxa* var. *colistinus,* specifically effective against many gram-negative bacteria, especially *Pseudomonas aeruginosa,* but also useful against others, including *Escherichia coli* and species of *Aerobacter, Klebsiella, Shigella,* and *Brucella; Proteus* species are resistant.
**c. sulfate** [USP], the sulfate salt of colistin, occurring as a white to cream-colored, hygroscopic powder; used in the treatment of various systemic, urinary tract, gastrointestinal, ophthalmic, and otic infections due to susceptible gram-negative bacteria, administered orally, parenterally, and topically.

**co·lit·i·des** (ko-lit'ĭ-dēz) [MeSH: Colitis] plural of *colitis.* Inflammatory disorders of the colon considered collectively.

**co·li·tis** (ko-li'tis) [MeSH: Colitis] inflammation of the colon. See also *enterocolitis.*
**amebic c.**, see under *dysentery.*
**antibiotic-associated c.**, see under *enterocolitis.*
**balantidial c.**, colitis due to infestation with *Balantidium coli.*
**cathartic c.**, colitis due to chronic laxative abuse.
**chemical c.**, colitis that is a reaction to a chemical instilled per rectum.
**collagenous c.**, a type of colitis of unknown etiology characterized by deposits of collagenous material beneath the epithelium of the colon, with crampy abdominal pain and marked reduction in fluid and electrolyte absorption, leading to watery diarrhea; there is no mucosal ulceration.
**Crohn's c.**, see under *disease.*
**c. cys'tica profun'da**, a condition marked by mucous retention cysts in the colic submucosa that are characteristic of the healing of chronic lesions of bacillary dysentery.
**c. cys'tica superficia'lis**, a cystic condition of the colic mucous membrane sometimes seen in children with such chronic debilitating disease as leukemia, possibly the result of malnutrition and vitamin deficiency.
**diversion c.**, inflammation of a segment of distal colon that has been defunctionalized by diversion of the fecal stream by subtotal colectomy; it may be asymptomatic or may be marked by tenesmus, anorectal pain, and bloody rectal discharge. It resolves following reanastomosis of the intestine.
**equine ehrlichial c.**, equine monocytic ehrlichiosis.
**granulomatous c.**, transmural colitis with the formation of noncaseating granulomas.
**c. gra'vis**, ulcerative c.
**hemorrhagic c.**, a usually afebrile diarrheal disease caused by *Escherichia coli* serotype O157:H57, characterized by abdominal cramping and watery diarrhea that progresses to bloody diarrhea after one or two days; it is generally self-limited but may be complicated by hemolytic-uremic syndrome.
**infectious c.**, colitis caused by an infectious agent.
**irradiation c.**, radiation c.
**ischemic c.**, acute vascular insufficiency of the colon usually involving the portion supplied by the inferior mesenteric artery; symptoms include pain at the left iliac fossa, bloody diarrhea, low-grade fever, abdominal distention, and abdominal tenderness. The classic radiologic sign is thumbprinting due to localized elevation of the mucosa by submucosal hemorrhage or edema. Ulceration may follow.
**lymphocytic c., microscopic c.**, a form similar to collagenous colitis but without deposits in the subepithelial region; marked reduction in fluid absorption is present, with chronic diarrhea and without ulceration.
**mucous c.**, former term for *irritable bowel syndrome;* see under *syndrome.*
**necrotizing amebic c.**, see under *pancolitis.*
**c. polypo'sa**, ulcerative colitis associated with the formation of pseudopolyps (edematous, inflamed islands of mucosa between areas of ulceration).
**pseudomembranous c.**, see under *enterocolitis.*
**radiation c.**, colitis resulting from radiation therapy to the abdominal region, marked by tenesmus, pain, rectal bleeding, diarrhea, and telangiectasis which may progress to malabsorption, ulceration, and partial or complete obstruction. Called also *irradiation c.* and *radiation enteritis.*
**regional c., segmental c.**, transmural or granulomatous inflammatory disease of the colon; regional enteritis involving the colon. It may be associated with ulceration, strictures, or fistulas.
**soap c.**, inflammation of the colon as a reaction to a soapsuds enema.
**transmural c.**, inflammation of the full thickness of the bowel, rather than mucosal and submucosal disease, usually with the formation of noncaseating granulomas. It may be confined to the colon, segmentally or diffusely, or may be associated with small bowel disease (regional enteritis). Clinically, it may resemble ulcerative colitis, but

the ulceration is often longitudinal or deep, the disease is often segmental, stricture formation is common, and fistulas, particularly in the perineum, are a frequent complication.
**c. ulcerati'va, ulcerative c.,** chronic, recurrent ulceration in the colon, chiefly of the mucosa and submucosa, of unknown cause; it is manifested clinically by cramping abdominal pain, rectal bleeding, and loose discharges of blood, pus, and mucus with scanty fecal particles. Complications include hemorrhoids, abscesses, fistulas, perforation of the colon, pseudopolyps, and carcinoma.
**uremic c.,** colitis that results from the uremia of chronic renal failure.

**col·i·tose** (kol'ĭ-tōs) an unusual sugar found in the O-specific chains in the lipopolysaccharides of certain serotypes of *Salmonella* and *Escherichia coli.*

**co·li·tox·emia** (ko"lĭ-tok-se'me-ə) toxemia due to infection with *Escherichia coli.*

**co·li·tox·i·co·sis** (ko"lĭ-tok"sĭ-ko'sis) intoxication caused by *Escherichia coli.*

**co·li·tox·in** (ko"lĭ-tok'sin) a substance contained in *Escherichia coli* that is the cause of colitoxicosis.

**co·li·uria** (ko"lĭ-u're-ə) presence of *Escherichia coli* in the urine.

**col·la** (kol'ə) [L.] plural of *collum.*

**col·la·cin** (kol'ə-sin) degenerate collagenous tissue; collastin.

**col·la·gen** (kol'ə-jən) [Gr. *kolla* glue + *-gen*] [MeSH: Collagen] any of a family of extracellular, closely related proteins occurring as a major component of connective tissue, giving it strength and flexibility. At least 14 types exist, each composed of tropocollagen (q.v.) units that share a common triple-helical shape but that vary somewhat in composition between types, with the types being localized to different tissues, stages, or functions. In some types, including the most common, Type I, the tropocollagen rods associate to form fibrils or fibers; in other types the rods are not fibrillar but are associated with fibrillar collagens, while in others they form nonfibrillar, nonperiodic but structured networks. Collagen is converted to gelatin by boiling. See also under *disease, fiber,* and *fibril.*

**col·la·ge·nase** (kə-laj'ə-nās) an enzyme that catalyzes the hydrolysis of peptide bonds in triple helical regions of collagen.
***Clostridium histolyticum* c.,** any of several forms of microbial collagenase isolated from *Clostridium histolyticum* that catalyze the cleavage of collagen into small fragments, cleaving it in the triple helical region N-terminal to glycine residues. The extracellular $Zn^{2+}$ enzyme degrades the collagen framework of muscles, facilitating the spread of gas gangrene by *C. histolyticum.*
**interstitial c.** [EC 3.4.24.7], any of a group of enzymes of the hydrolase class that catalyze the cleavage of native collagen, usually at a glycine-leucine or glycine-isoleucine bond. The best studied are those that cleave the fibrillar collagens into a large N-terminal (75 per cent) and a small C-terminal fragment (25 per cent). The enzymes require zinc, occur widely in vertebrates, and are involved in the degradation of collagen during tissue repair or during embryonic and fetal development. Called also *vertebrate c.*
**microbial c.** [EC 3.4.24.3], any of various collagenases purified from a variety of microbes, particularly *Clostridium histolyticum* (see *C. histolyticum c.*); they preferentially cleave collagen on the N-terminal side of glycine residues and occur in several classes of differing specificity.
**vertebrate c.,** interstitial c.

**col·lag·e·na·tion** (kə-laj"ə-na'shən) the appearance of collagen in developing cartilage.

**col·la·gen·ic** (kol"ə-jen'ik) 1. collagenous. 2. collagenogenic.

**col·lag·e·no·blast** (ko-laj'ə-no-blast) a cell that arises from a fibroblast and that as it matures is associated with the production of collagen; it may form cartilage and bone by metaplasia. Collagenoblasts proliferate at the site of chronic inflammation. Sometimes called also *fibroblast.*

**col·lag·e·no·cyte** (ko-laj'ə-no-sīt") a mature collagen-producing cell; see *collagenoblast.*

**col·la·gen·o·gen·ic** (kol"ə-jən-o-jen'ik) pertaining to or characterized by the production of collagen; forming collagen or collagen fibers.

**col·la·gen·ol·y·sis** (kol"ə-jən-ol'ə-sis) dissolution or digestion of collagen.

**col·lag·e·no·lyt·ic** (ko-laj"ə-no-lit'ik) effecting the digestion of collagen.

**col·lag·e·nous** (ko-laj'ə-nəs) pertaining to collagen; forming or producing collagen.

**col·lapse** (kə-laps') [L. *collapsus*] 1. a state of extreme prostration and depression, with failure of circulation. 2. abnormal falling in of the walls of any part or organ.

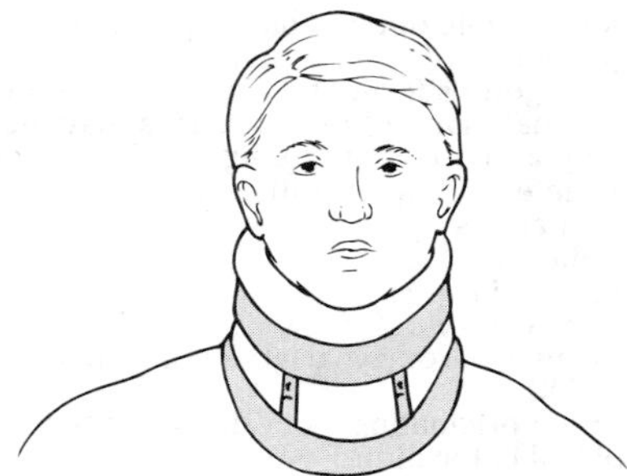

Philadelphia collar.

**circulatory c.,** shock; circulatory insufficiency without congestive heart failure.
**c. of the lung,** an airless or fetal state of all or a part of a lung, as seen in atelectasis from bronchial obstruction and in pneumothorax.
**massive c.,** a condition in which an entire lung becomes airless, often due to obstruction of a main bronchus.
**scapholunate advanced c. (SLAC),** a common form of arthritic degeneration of the wrist, with gradual loss of ligamentous support due to chronic malalignment of the scaphoid bone, resulting in a rotational deformity.

**col·lar** (kol'ər) an encircling band, generally around the neck.
**Casal's c.,** see under *necklace.*
**cervical c.,** cervical orthosis.
**circumaortic venous c.,** a rare vascular anomaly in which the left renal vein encircles the inferior vena cava and constricts it. Called also *circumaortic venous ring.*
**c. of pearls,** syphilitic leukoderma.
**periosteal bone c.,** a band of spongy bone that forms around the middle of the diaphysis of early bones.
**Philadelphia c.,** a type of cervical orthosis that restricts anterior-posterior cervical motion to a great degree but allows some normal rotation and lateral bending.
**Spanish c.,** paraphimosis.
**c. of Stokes,** edematous thickening of the neck and soft parts of the thorax in the superior vena cava syndrome.
**venereal c., c. of Venus,** syphilitic leukoderma.

**col·lar·ette** (kol"ər-et') 1. a narrow rim of loosened keratin overhanging the periphery of a circumscribed skin lesion, attached to the normal surrounding skin, especially in moniliasis and pityriasis rosea. 2. an irregular jagged line dividing the anterior surface of the iris into two regions. 3. in mycology, a ring around the apex of a phialide resulting from rupture during release of the first phialospore.

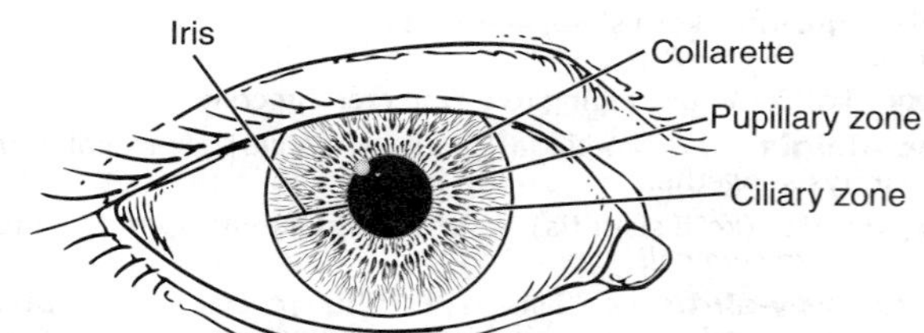


**Biett's c.,** a type of papular syphilid in which the central papule is surrounded by a ring of scales.

**col·las·tin** (kŏ-las'tin) degenerate collagenous tissue that stains like normal elastic tissue.

**col·lat·er·al** (ko-lat'ər-əl) [*co-* + *lateral*] 1. secondary or accessory; not direct or immediate. 2. a small side branch, as of a blood vessel or nerve.
**Schaffer c's,** branches of the axons of the stratum pyramidale of the hippocampus, some of which end on cells in the stratum oriens, but many of which pass into the stratum moleculare.

**Col·les' fascia, fragment, ligament, space** (kol'ēz) [Abraham *Colles,* Irish surgeon, 1773–1843] see *fascia diaphragmatis urogenitalis inferior* and *ligamentum inguinale reflexum,* and see under *fracture* and *space.*

**Col·let's syndrome** (ko-lāz') [Frédéric Justin *Collet,* French laryngologist, born 1870] see under *syndrome.*

**Col·let-Si·card syndrome** (ko-la'se-kahr') [F.J. *Collet;* Jean Athanase *Sicard,* French neurologist, 1872–1929] Collet's syndrome.

**Col·le·to·tri·chum** (kol"ə-to-trī'kəm) a genus of Fungi Imperfecti of the form-class Coelomycetes. Some species have been isolated from cases of phaeohyphomycosis.

**col·lic·u·lec·to·my** (ko-lik″u-lek′tə-me) [*colliculus* + *-ectomy*] excision of the colliculus seminalis.

**col·lic·u·li** (ko-lik′u-li) [L.] genitive and plural of *colliculus*.

**col·lic·u·li·tis** (ko-lik″u-li′tis) inflammation in or around the colliculus seminalis; called also *verumontanitis*.

**col·lic·u·lus** (ko-lik′u-ləs) pl. *collic′uli* [L.] a small elevation, or mound.
**c. of arytenoid cartilage,** c. cartilaginis arytenoideae.
**bulbar c.,** corpus spongiosum penis.
**c. cartila′ginis arytenoi′deae** [TA], colliculus of arytenoid cartilage: a small eminence on the anterior margin and anterolateral surface of the arytenoid cartilage; also written *colliculus cartilaginis arytaenoideae*.
**caudal c., c. cauda′lis,** c. inferior.
**c. cauda′tus,** nucleus caudatus.
**cervical c. of female urethra (of Barkow),** crista urethralis (def. 1).
**c. facia′lis** [TA], facial colliculus: an elevation of the medial eminence above the medullary striae in the rhomboid fossa, caused by the internal genu of the facial nerve as it loops backward around the abducent nucleus.
**c. infe′rior** [TA], inferior colliculus: either of the inferior (caudal) pair of rounded eminences symmetrically located in the tectum of the mesencephalon, containing reflex centers for auditory sensations; called also *caudal c.*
**rostral c., c. rostra′lis,** c. superior.
**c. semina′lis** [TA], seminal colliculus: a prominent portion of the urethral crest on which are the opening of the prostatic utricle and, on either side of it, the orifices of the ejaculatory ducts; called also *caput gallinaginis, seminal crest, seminal hillock,* and *verumontanum*.
**c. supe′rior** [TA], superior colliculus: either of the superior (rostral) pair of rounded eminences symmetrically located in the tectum of the mesencephalon, containing reflex centers for visual sensations; called also *rostral c.*

**col·li·ga·tive** (kol′ĭ-ga″tiv) in physical chemistry, depending on the number of molecules present in a given space, rather than on their size, molecular weight or chemical constitution. The colligative properties of solutions are osmotic pressure, boiling point elevation, freezing point depression, and vapor pressure lowering.

**col·li·ma·tion** (ko″lĭ-ma′shən) 1. in microscopy, the process of making light rays parallel; the process of aligning the optical axis of the optical system to the reference mechanical axes or surfaces of the instrument, or the adjustment of two or more optical axes with respect to each other. 2. in radiology, the elimination of the peripheral (more divergent) portion of an x-ray beam by means of metal tubes, cones, or diaphragms interposed in the path of the beam. 3. in nuclear medicine, the use of a perforated absorber to restrict the field of view of a detector and reduce scatter; the use of an absorber with converging or diverging perforations will also change the camera's angle of view.

**col·li·ma·tor** (kol′ĭ-ma″tər) a diaphragm or system of diaphragms made of an absorbing material, designed to define and restrict the dimensions and direction of a beam of radiation.

**Col·lin·so·nia** (kol″in-so′ne-ə) [Peter *Collinson,* 1694–1768] a genus of herbs of the family Labiatae. C. *canaden′sis,* the stoneroot or richweed, is tonic and diuretic.

**col·liq·ua·tive** (ko-lik′wə-tiv) [*co-* + L. *liquare* to melt] 1. characterized by an excessive fluid discharge. 2. marked by liquefaction of tissues.

**col·li·sion** (ko-lĭ′zhən) 1. in obstetrics, the contact *in utero* of any parts of one twin with those of the co-twin, so that engagement of either is prevented. 2. in nerve conduction studies, the meeting of two action potentials traveling toward each other along the same nerve; their refractory periods prevent propagation in either direction from the site of collision.

**col·lo·chem·is·try** (kol″o-kem′is-tre) the chemistry of colloids.

**col·lo·di·a·phys·e·al** (kol″o-di″ə-fiz′e-əl) [*collum* + *diaphyseal*] pertaining to the neck and shaft of a long bone, especially the femur.

**col·lo·di·on** (ko-lo′de-on) [L. *collodium,* from Gr. *kollōdēs* glutinous] [USP] [MeSH: Collodion] a clear or slightly opalescent, highly flammable, syrupy liquid compounded of pyroxylin, ether, and alcohol, which dries to a transparent, tenacious film; used as a topical protectant, applied to the skin to close small wounds, abrasions, and cuts, to hold surgical dressings in place, and to keep medications in contact with the skin.
**c. elastique,** flexible c.
**flexible c.** [USP], a preparation of camphor, castor oil, and collodion, used for the same purposes as collodion but providing a flexible, contracting film. Called also *c. elastique*.
**salicylic acid c.** [USP], a preparation containing 9.5–11.5 per cent salicylic acid in flexible collodion; used as a topical keratolytic for warts and corns.

**col·loid** (kol′oid) [Gr. *kollōdēs* glutinous] [MeSH: Colloids] 1. glutinous or resembling glue. 2. a substance comprising very small, insoluble particles, usually 1 to 1000 nm in diameter, that are uniformly dispersed or suspended in a finely divided state throughout a continuous dispersion medium, not settling readily; either phase can be solid, liquid, or gas. The particles are often called the *dispersed phase* and the dispersion medium the *continuous phase*. Colloid can refer specifically to the particles or to the system of particles plus dispersion medium. 3. thyroid c.
**antimony trisulfide c.,** antimony sulfide ($Sb_2S_3$), a pharmaceutic aid.
**association c.,** a colloid in which the dispersed particles are each made up of many molecules.
**bovine c.,** conglutinin.
**dispersion c.,** colloid, def. 2; sometimes specifically an unstable colloid system.
**emulsion c.,** 1. lyophilic c. 2. rarely, emulsion.
**hydrophilic c.,** a lyophilic colloid in which the solvent is water.
**hydrophobic c.,** a lyophobic colloid in which the solvent is water.
**irreversible c.,** a colloid that once precipitated cannot be dispersed. Cf. *reversible c.*
**lyophilic c.,** a stable colloid system in which the dispersed phase is relatively liquid, usually comprising highly complex organic substances, such as starch or glue, which readily absorb solvent, swell, and distribute uniformly through the medium.
**lyophobic c.,** an unstable colloid system in which the dispersed phase particles tend to repel liquids, are easily precipitated, and cannot be dispersed with additional solvent.
**lyotropic c.,** lyophilic c.
**protective c.,** a hydrophilic colloid polymer that is able to prevent the precipitation of another colloid by acting as a stabilizer, suspending or thickening agent, or emulsifier.
**reversible c.,** a colloid that can be dispersed after having been precipitated or a gel that can be converted into a sol.
**stable c.,** reversible c.
**stannous sulfur c.,** a sulfur colloid containing stannous ions, formed by reacting sodium thiosulfate with hydrochloric acid then adding stannous ions; complexed with technetium 99m it is used as a diagnostic aid (bone, liver, and spleen imaging).
**suspension c.,** lyophobic c.
**thyroid c.,** the colloid in the thyroid follicles; it contains several proteins, including thyroglobulin and $CA_2$. Called also *thyrocolloid*.

**col·loi·dal** (ko-loid′əl) of the nature of a colloid.

**col·loi·din** (ko-loid′in) a yellowish, translucent, jellylike product of colloid degeneration.

**col·loid·oph·a·gy** (kol″oi-dof′ə-je) [*colloid* + *-phagy*] resorption of colloid by macrophages under the influence of the thyroid-stimulating hormone.

**col·lum** (kol′əm) pl. *col′la* [L.] [TA] neck: the part of the body connecting the head and trunk; called also *cervix*.
**c. anato′micum hu′meri** [TA], anatomical neck of humerus: the somewhat constricted zone on the humerus just distal to the head, separating the articular surface from the tubercles.
**c. chirur′gicum hu′meri** [TA], surgical neck of humerus: the region on the humerus just below the tubercles, where the bone becomes constricted.
**c. cos′tae** [TA], neck of rib: the part of a rib extending from the head to the tubercle.
**c. den′tis,** cervix dentis.
**c. distor′tum,** torticollis.
**c. fe′moris** [TA], neck of femur: the heavy column of bone connecting the head of the femur and the shaft.
**c. folli′culi pi′li,** the narrow portion of a hair follicle between the hair bulb and the opening on the surface of the skin. Called also *neck of hair follicle*.
**c. glan′dis pe′nis** [TA], neck of the glans penis: the constricted por-

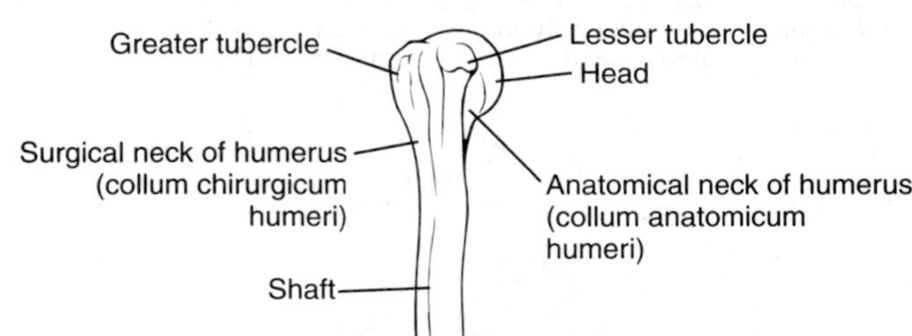

Anterior aspect of right humerus, showing the collum chirurgicum (surgical neck) and collum anatomicum (anatomical neck).

tion between the corona of the glans penis and the corpora cavernosa; called also *cervix glandis.*
**c. mal'lei** [TA], neck of malleus: the constricted portion of the malleus below its head.
**c. mandi'bulae** [TA], neck of mandible: the narrow portion supporting the condyle of the mandible; called also *c. processus condyloidei mandibulae.*
**c. os'sis fem'oris,** c. femoris.
**c. proces'sus condyloi'dei mandi'bulae,** c. mandibulae.
**c. ra'dii** [TA], neck of radius: the somewhat constricted portion of the radius just distal to the head.
**c. sca'pulae** [TA], neck of scapula: the somewhat constricted part of the scapula that surrounds the lateral angle.
**c. ta'li** [TA], neck of talus: the constriction between the head and body of the talus.
**c. val'gum,** coxa valga.
**c. vesi'cae bilia'ris** [TA], neck of gallbladder: the upper constricted portion of the gallbladder, between the body and the cystic duct; called also *c. vesicae felleae* [TA alternative].
**c. vesi'cae fel'leae,** TA alternative for *c. vesicae biliaris.*

**Collut.** abbreviation for L. *collutorium* (mouth wash).

**col·lu·to·ria** (kol″u-to're-ə) [L.] plural of *collutorium.*

**col·lu·to·ri·um** (kol″u-tor'e-əm) pl. *colluto'ria* [L.] collutory.

**col·lu·to·ry** (kol'u-tor″e) [L. *collutorium*] a mouthwash or gargle.

**Collyr.** abbreviation for L. *collyr'ium,* an eye wash.

**col·lyr·ia** (ko-lir'e-ə) [L.] plural of *collyrium.*

**Col·ly·ric·u·lum** (kol″ə-rik'u-ləm) a genus of trematode parasites. *C. fa'ba* forms subcutaneous cysts in chickens, turkeys, and sparrows.

**col·lyr·i·um** (kə-lir'e-əm) pl. *colly'ria* [L.; Gr. *kollyrion* eye salve] a lotion for the eyes; an eye wash.

**colo-** [Gr. *kolon* colon] a combining form denoting the colon.

**col·o·bo·ma** (kol″o-bo'mə) pl. *colobomas* or *colobo'mata* [L.; Gr. *kolobōma* defect, from *koloboun* to mutilate] [MeSH: Coloboma] 1. an absence or defect of tissue. 2. particularly, a defect of ocular tissue, usually due to malclosure of the fetal intraocular fissure, or sometimes from trauma or disease. Such anomalies range from a small pit in the optic disk to extensive defects in the iris, ciliary body, choroid, retina, or optic disk. A scotoma is usually present, corresponding to the area of the coloboma.
**atypical c's,** one not originating from the embryonic cleft nor located in the inferonasal quadrant of the eye; it is usually unilateral.
**bridge c.,** a narrow zone of normal fundus between a retinochoroidal coloboma and an optic nerve coloboma.
**c. of choroid,** fissure in the choroid, causing a scotoma on the retina, and often associated with defects of the ciliary body and iris.
**c. of ciliary body,** a white lesion surrounded by varying pigment and affecting the iris and lens. It is the most frequent congenital defect of the ciliary body and common in trisomy 13.
**complete c.,** a typical coloboma when it extends from the pupillary margin to the posterior pole, therefore involving the iris, ciliary body, choroid, retina, and optic disk.
**Fuchs' c.,** a small conus or crescent on the choroid, at the lower edge of the optic disk.
**c. of fundus,** retinochoroidal c.
**c. i'ridis, c. of iris,** a keyhole-shaped notch in the inferonasal quadrant of the eye; it may also result from an iridectomy.
**c. of lens, c. len'tis,** a cleft at the edge of the lens, extending down, with a defect in the zonule of Zinn in the same area.
**c. lo'buli,** fissure of the ear lobe, which may occur as a congenital defect, or be acquired.
**c. of optic disk, c. of optic nerve,** 1. a coloboma, mild or severe, within or at the optic nerve head. A mild coloboma may be a separate, isolated entity, unilateral, and limited to minor cupping in the optic disk. A severe coloboma may be part of a bridge coloboma or part of a complete coloboma, or it may enlarge the optic disk two to four times and thus affect the adjacent retina and choroid. Nystagmus, strabismus, severe impairment of vision, microphthalmia, cyclopia, and anencephaly may be present. 2. a defect attributed to the incomplete closure of the fetal fissure of the optic stalk.

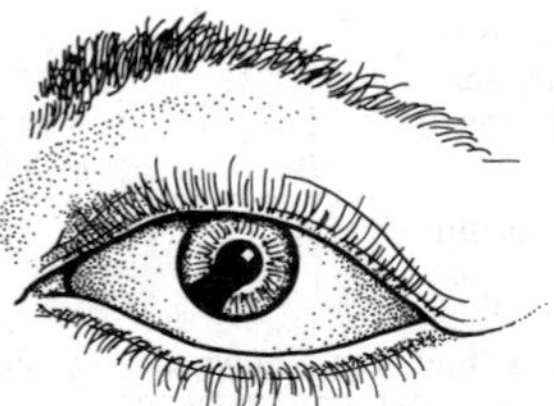

Coloboma of the iris.

**c. at optic nerve entrance,** a coloboma of the optic disk that affects only the optic nerve.
**c. palpebra'le,** a vertical fissure of an eyelid.
**peripapillary c.,** a chorioretinal defect surrounding or extending down from the optic disk.
**c. of retina, c. re'tinae,** a congenital fissure of the retina attributed to incomplete closure of the fetal fissure in the optic cup.
**retinochoroidal c.,** an absence of retinal and choroidal tissue, usually in the lower fundus, marked by a bright white ectatic zone of exposed sclera extending into and distorting the optic disk. Called also *c. of fundus.*
**typical c.,** a defect resulting from incomplete or irregular, or lack of fusion of the lips of the embryonic intraocular fissure by the end of the sixth or seventh week. A typical coloboma is found in the lower nasal quadrant of the eye and is often bilateral.
**c. of vitreous,** a notch in the lower border of the vitreous.

**co·lo·ce·cos·to·my** (ko″lo-se-kos'tə-me) [*colon* + *ceco-* + *-ostomy*] cecocolostomy.

**co·lo·cen·te·sis** (ko″lo-sen-te'sis) [*colon* + *-centesis*] surgical puncture of the colon for the withdrawal of fluid or gas; called also *colopuncture.*

**co·lo·cho·le·cys·tos·to·my** (ko″lo-ko″le-sis-tos'tə-me) cholecystocolostomy.

**co·lo·cly·sis** (ko″lo-kli'sis) [*colon* + *clysis*] irrigation of the colon.

**co·lo·clys·ter** (ko″lo-klis'tər) an enema injected into the colon through the rectum.

**co·lo·co·los·to·my** (ko″lo-ko-los'tə-me) [*colon* + *colostomy*] surgical formation of an anastomosis between two portions of the colon.

**co·lo·cu·ta·ne·ous** (ko″lo-ku-ta'ne-əs) pertaining to the colon and skin, or communicating with the colon and the cutaneous surface of the body, as colocutaneous fistula.

**colo·cynth** (kol'o-sinth) [L. *colocynthis;* Gr. *kolokynthē*] 1. *Citrullus colocynthus.* 2. the pulpy fruit of *C. colocynthus.* 3. the dried pulp of the full grown but unripe fruit of *C. colocynthus,* used as a drastic cathartic. Called also *bitter apple* and *bitter cucumber.*

**colo·cyn·thi·dism** (kol″o-sin'thĭ-diz-əm) poisoning by colocynth.

**colo·cyn·thin** (kol″o-sin'thin) a bitter, purgative glycoside, $C_{38}H_{54}O_{13}$, from colocynth.

**colo·cyn·this** (kol″o-sin'this) gen. *colocyn'thidis* [L.] colocynth.

**co·lo·dys·pep·sia** (ko″lo-dis-pep'se-ə) dyspepsia due to reflex disturbance set up by the constipated colon.

**co·lo·en·ter·itis** (ko″lo-en″tər-i'tis) [*colon* + *enteritis*] enterocolitis.

**co·lo·fix·a·tion** (ko″lo-fik-sa'shən) fixation or suspension of the colon.

**Col·o·gel** (kol'o-jəl) trademark for a preparation of methylcellulose.

**co·lo·hep·a·to·pexy** (ko″lo-hep'ə-to-pek″se) [*colon* + *hepato-* + *-pexy*] fixation of the colon to the liver to prevent the formation of adhesions between the liver and the stomach.

**co·lo·il·e·al** (ko″lo-il'e-əl) ileocolic.

**co·lol·y·sis** (ko-lol'ə-sis) [*colon* + *-lysis*] the division of pericolic adhesions.

**co·lo·me·trom·e·ter** (ko″lo-mə-trom'ə-tər) an apparatus for measuring the activity of the colon.

**co·lon** (ko'lon) [L., from Gr. *kolon*] [TA] [MeSH: Colon] that part of the large intestine which extends from the cecum to the rectum; sometimes used inaccurately as a synonym for the entire large intestine.
**c. ascen'dens** [TA], ascending colon: the portion of the colon between the cecum and the right colic flexure.
**c. descen'dens** [TA], descending colon: the portion of the colon between the left colic flexure and the sigmoid colon at the pelvic brim; the portion of the descending colon lying in the left iliac fossa is sometimes called the *iliac colon.*
**giant c.,** megacolon.
**iliac c.,** that part of the descending colon lying in the left iliac fossa and continuous with the sigmoid colon.
**irritable c.,** irritable bowel syndrome.
**lead-pipe c.,** a term applied to the radiologic appearance of a diseased colon which has become shortened, contracted, and rigid owing to inflammatory fibrosis. In such a colon the normal haustral pattern is lost and function may be impaired. This is usually a consequence of chronic ulcerative or granulomatous colitis.
**left c.,** the distal portion of the colon; it develops embryonically from the hindgut and functions in the storage and elimination of waste.
**pelvic c.,** sigmoid c.

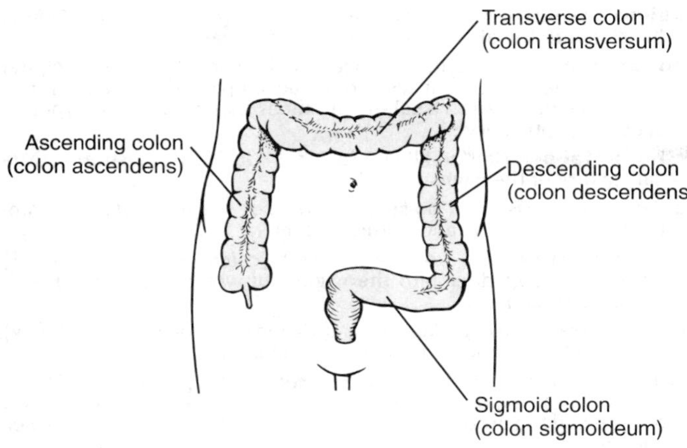


**right c.**, the proximal portion of the colon, extending from the ileocecal valve usually to a point proximal to the left colic flexure; it develops embryonically from the terminal portion of the midgut and functions in absorption.
**c. sigmoi'deum** [TA], sigmoid colon: the S-shaped part of the colon which lies in the pelvis, extending from the pelvic brim to the third segment of the sacrum, and continuous above with the descending (or iliac) colon and below with the rectum; called also *pelvic c.* and *sigmoid flexure.*
**spastic c.**, irritable bowel syndrome.
**c. transver'sum** [TA], transverse colon: the portion of the colon that runs transversely across the upper part of the abdomen, from the right to the left colic flexure.

**co•lon•al•gia** (ko″lon-al'jə) [*colon* + *-algia*] pain in the colon.

**co•lon•ic** (ko-lon'ik) pertaining to the colon. Called also *colic.*

**col•o•ni•za•tion** (kol″ə-nĭ-za'shən) 1. innidiation. 2. implantation and growth of a microorganism on a host.

**Co•lon•na's operation** (kŏ-lon'ah) [Paul *Colonna,* American orthopedic surgeon, 1892–1966] see under *operation.*

**co•lo•nop•a•thy** (ko″lo-nop'ə-the) [*colon* + *-pathy*] any disease or disorder of the colon.

**co•lon•or•rha•gia** (ko″lon-ə-ra'jə) hemorrhage from the colon.

**co•lono•scope** (ko-lon'o-skōp) [*colon* + *-scope*] an elongated flexible endoscope which permits visual examination of the entire colon; called also *coloscope.*

**co•lo•nos•co•py** (ko″lon-os'kə-pe) [MeSH: Colonoscopy] examination by means of the colonoscope. Called also *coloscopy.*

**col•o•ny** (kol'ə-ne) [L. *colonia*] a collection or group of bacteria in a culture derived from the increase of an isolated single organism or group of organisms.
**checker c.**, a round, steeply elevated colony with a flat top, resembling the disk used in a game of checkers. It is frequently seen in cultures of *Streptococcus pneumoniae* on blood agar.
**D c.**, dwarf c.
**daisy-head c.**, a round gray or black colony with a narrow translucent scalloped border, typically produced by *Corynebacterium diphtheriae* on tellurite blood agar.
**daughter c.**, a small bacterial colony formed as a papilla on the surface or in the margin of an older colony.
**dwarf c.**, a bacterial colony smaller than normal and containing poorly developed forms; called also *D c.*
**gregaloid c.**, a transient grouping of protozoa formed by union of previously independent organisms; seen in sarcodines and in the ameboid stages of certain other protozoa. Called also *gregaloid.*
**H c.**, (*Hauch,* q.v.), a type of bacterial colony that spreads in a thin film over the culture medium. Cf. *O c.*
**M c.**, mucoid c.
**motile c.**, one that moves across the surface of the culture plate leaving lines of bacterial cells on the paths of motion, typical of colonies of *Bacillus circulans.*
**mucoid c.**, one that is large, dome-shaped, and shiny, containing large quantities of capsular polysaccharide material that may be drawn out in viscous strings by a needle; called also *M c.*
**O c.**, (*ohne Hauch,* q.v.), a bacterial colony that is discrete and compact, as contrasted with an H colony.
**R c., rough c.**, a bacterial colony showing a rough, wrinkled, granular, flattened surface.
**S c.**, smooth c.
**satellite c.**, a bacterial colony that grows more vigorously in the immediate vicinity of a colony of some other organism, as *Hemophilus influenzae* near a colony of staphylococci; called also *bacterial satellite.*
**smooth c.**, a bacterial colony showing the smooth, glistening, rounded, regular surface, normally shown by colonies of organisms; called also *S c.*

**co•lop•a•thy** (ko-lop'ə-the) colonopathy.

**colo•pex•ia** (ko″lo-pek'se-ə) colopexy.

**co•lo•pex•ot•o•my** (ko″lo-pek-sot'ə-me) [*colon* + Gr. *pēxis* fixation + *-tomy*] incision and fixation of the colon.

**co•lo•pexy** (ko'lo-pek″se) [*colon* + *-pexy*] fixation or suspension of the colon by surgical means.

**co•loph•o•ny** (ko-lof'ə-ne) [L. *colophonia;* Gr. *Kolophōn* (Colophon) a city of Asia Minor] rosin.

**co•lo•pli•ca•tion** (ko″lo-plĭ-ka'shən) [*colon* + *plica*] the operation of infolding or taking tucks in the wall of the colon in cases of dilatation to shorten or decrease its lumen.

**co•lo•proc•tec•to•my** (ko″lo-prok-tek'tə-me) proctocolectomy.

**co•lo•proc•ti•tis** (ko″lo-prok-ti'tis) proctocolitis.

**co•lo•proc•tos•to•my** (ko″lo-prok-tos'tə-me) [*colon* + *proctostomy*] colorectostomy.

**co•lop•to•sis** (ko″lop-to'sis) [*colon* + *ptosis*] downward displacement of the colon, a term based on the outmoded concept that variations in the position of abdominal organs are pathologic.

**co•lo•punc•ture** (ko'lo-pungk″chər) colocentesis.

**Color.** abbreviation for L. *colore'tur,* let it be colored.

**col•or** (kul'ər) [L. *color, colos*] [MeSH: Color] 1. a property of a surface or substance resulting from absorption of certain of the incident light rays and reflection of others falling within the range of wavelengths (roughly 370–760 m$\mu$) adequate to excite the retinal receptors. 2. radiant energy within the range of adequate chromatic stimuli of the retina, that is, between the infrared and ultraviolet. 3. a sensory impression of one of the rainbow hues, excited by stimulation of the retinal receptors, notably the cones, by radiant energy of the appropriate wavelength.
**complementary c's**, two colors for which the sensory mechanisms are so linked that when they are mixed on the color wheel they cancel each other out, leaving neutral gray; they are also associated with each other in afterimage and contrast.
**confusion c's**, different colors that are likely to be mistakenly matched by individuals with defective color vision (e.g., violet and blue with defect of vision for red); for this reason they are combined in the design on charts used for detecting different types of color vision defects.
**contrast c.**, an illusory tinge of complementary hue or brightness induced by a vivid hue or luminance on the area surrounding it in the visual field.
**incidental c.**, that seen as an after-image.
**metameric c's**, colors that appear identical to the normal eye, but which are the resultants of different combinations of chromatic stimuli or wavelengths.
**Munsell's c's**, a set of standardized colors, representing 40 hues in varying degrees of brightness and saturation, identifiable by a simple letter-number formula.
**primary c's**, a small number of fundamental colors, usually referred to the retinal receptor cones, mixture of varying proportions of the approximate stimuli of which will yield the 150 discriminable hues of normal human vision. According to *(a)* the Newton theory, the seven rainbow hues: violet, indigo, blue, green, yellow, orange, red; *(b)* the painter and printer: blue (cyan), yellow, red (or magenta); *(c)* the Helmholtzian theory (old school): red, green, blue (or violet); *(d)* the Hering theory: four paired complementary hues, red-green and blue-yellow, plus a black-white pair. *(e)* Other theories list five to seven colors as primaries.
**pseudoisochromatic c's**, colors that appear the same to an individual with defective color vision; see *confusion c's.*
**pure c.**, a color whose stimulus consists of homogeneous wavelengths, with little or no admixture of other hues.
**saturation c.**, one that is high on the chroma or vividness scale, the farthest possible removed from gray.

**col•or•a•tion** (kul″or-a'shən) the state of being colored; an arrangement of colors distinguishing a species.
**protective c.**, coloration that blends with the background, making the organism less visible to predators.
**warning c.**, brilliant, conspicuous coloration of poisonous or unpalatable animals, as a warning to potential predators.

**co•lo•rec•tal** (ko″lo-rek'təl) pertaining to or affecting the colon and rectum.

**co•lo•rec•ti•tis** (ko″lo-rek-ti'tis) coloproctitis.

**co•lo•rec•tos•to•my** (ko″lo-rek-tos'tə-me) [*colon* + *recto-* + *-stomy*] formation of an artificial opening between the colon and rectum; called also *coloproctostomy.*

**co·lo·rec·tum** (ko″lo-rek′təm) the colon and rectum considered as a unit.

**col·or·im·e·ter** (kul″or-im′ə-tər) [*color* + *-meter*] an instrument for measuring the color or color intensity of a solution. Cf. *spectrophotometer.* Called also *chromometer.*
**Duboscq's c.**, an apparatus for measuring concentration by comparing the tint of the substance in question against that of a standard.
**titration c.**, a device using colorimetric technique to automatically stop titration at the endpoint.

**co·lor·rha·phy** (ko-lor′ə-fe) [*colon* + *-rrhaphy*] suture or repair of the colon.

**co·lor·rhea** (ko″lo-re′ə) a discharge of mucus from the colon.

**co·lo·scope** (kol′o-skōp) colonoscope.

**co·los·co·py** (ko-los′ko-pe) colonoscopy.

**co·lo·sig·moid·os·to·my** (ko″lo-sig″moi-dos′tə-me) surgical creation of an artificial opening between the sigmoid and the proximal portion of the colon.

**co·los·to·my** (kə-los′tə-me) [*colon* + *-stomy*] [MeSH: Colostomy] the surgical creation of an opening between the colon and the surface of the body; also used to refer to the opening, or stoma, so created.
**dry c.**, colostomy performed in the left half of the colon, the discharge from the stoma consisting of soft or formed fecal residue.
**Hartmann's c.**, see under *procedure.*
**ileotransverse c.**, surgical anastomosis between the ileum and the transverse colon.
**Mikulicz c.**, see under *operation* (def. 4).
**wet c.**, colostomy in *(a)* the right half of the colon, the drainage from which is liquid in character, or *(b)* the left half of the colon following anastomosis of the ureters to the sigmoid or descending colon so that urine is also expelled through the same stoma.

**co·los·tric** (kə-los′trik) pertaining to or occurring in colostrum.

**co·los·tror·rhea** (kə-los″tro-re′ə) [L. *colostrum* + *-rrhea*] spontaneous discharge of colostrum.

**co·los·trous** (kə-los′trəs) [L. *colostrosus*] containing or filled with colostrum.

**co·los·trum** (kə-los′trəm) [L.] [MeSH: Colostrum] the thin, yellow, milky fluid secreted by the mammary gland before or after parturition. It contains up to 20 per cent protein, predominant among which are immunoglobulins, representing the antibodies found in maternal blood. It contains more minerals and less fat and carbohydrate than does milk. It also contains many colostrum corpuscles and usually will coagulate on boiling due to a large amount of lactalbumin.
**c. gravida′rum,** the colostrum secreted before parturition, and especially that secreted during the first few days following delivery.
**c. puerpera′rum,** the colostrum secreted after labor.

**co·lot·o·my** (ko-lot′ə-me) [*colo-* + *-tomy*] incision into the colon for removal of a foreign body, polyp, or other benign tumor. Cf. *colostomy.*

**co·lo·vag·i·nal** (ko″lo-vaj′ĭ-nəl) pertaining to or communicating with the colon and vagina, as a colovaginal fistula.

**co·lo·ves·i·cal** (ko″lo-ves′ĭ-kəl) vesicocolonic.

**col·pal·gia** (kol-pal′jə) [*colp-* + *-algia*] vaginodynia.

**col·pa·tre·sia** (kol″pə-tre′zhə) [*colp-* + *atresia*] atresia or occlusion of the vagina.

**col·pec·ta·sia** (kol″pek-ta′zhə) [*colp-* + *ectasia*] distention or dilatation of the vagina.

**col·pec·ta·sis** (kol-pek′tə-sis) colpectasia.

**col·pec·to·my** (kol-pek′tə-me) [*colp-* + *-ectomy*] excision of the vagina.

**col·peu·ry·sis** (kol-pu′rĭ-sis) [*colp-* + *eury-* + *-sis*] dilation of the vagina, particularly with a bag or sac.

**col·pis·mus** (kol-piz′məs) [Gr. *kolpos* vagina] vaginismus.

**col·pi·tis** (kol-pi′tis) [*colpo-* + *-itis*] vaginitis.
**c. emphysemato′sa, emphysematous c.**, vaginitis emphysematosa.
**c. macularis,** punctate hemorrhage of the vaginal mucosa, often with small vesicles or papules, seen in trichomoniasis vaginalis; called also *strawberry cervix.*
**c. myco′tica,** vaginomycosis.

**colp(o)-** [Gr. *kolpos* vagina] a combining form denoting relationship to the vagina.

**col·po·cele** (kol′po-sēl) [*colpo-* + *-cele*[1]] vaginal hernia.

**col·po·ce·lio·cen·te·sis** (kol″po-se″le-o-sen-te′sis) puncture of the abdominal cavity through the vagina, usually the posterior vault.

**col·po·ce·li·ot·o·my** (kol″po-se″le-ot′ə-me) [*colpo-* + *celio-* + *-tomy*] incision into the abdomen through the vaginal wall.

**col·po·ceph·a·ly** (kol″po-sef′ə-le) enlargement of the occipital horns of the lateral ventricles, often accompanied by mental retardation, seizures, and visual disturbances that result from hypoplasia of the optic nerve.

**col·po·clei·sis** (kol″po-kli′sis) [*colpo-* + Gr. *kleisis* closure] surgical closure of the vaginal canal.

**col·po·cys·ti·tis** (kol″po-sis-ti′tis) [*colpo-* + *cyst* + *-itis*] inflammation of the vagina and of the bladder.

**col·po·cys·to·cele** (kol″po-sis′to-sēl) [*colpo-* + *cysto-* + *-cele*[1]] hernia of the bladder into the vagina, of which the anterior wall becomes prolapsed.

**col·po·cys·tot·o·my** (kol″po-sis-tot′ə-me) [*colpo-* + *cysto-* + *-tomy*] incision of the bladder through the vaginal wall.

**col·po·cys·to·ure·tero·cys·tot·o·my** (kol″po-sis″to-u-re″tər-o-sis-tot′ə-me) [*colpo-* + *cysto-* + *uretero-* + *cystotomy*] the operation of exposing the ureteral orifices by incising the walls of the bladder and vagina.

**col·po·cy·to·gram** (kol″po-si′to-gram) a tabulation of the various types of cells observed in smears taken from the mucous membrane of the vagina.

**col·po·cy·tol·o·gy** (kol″po-si-tol′ə-je) the quantitative and differential study of cells exfoliated from the epithelium of the vagina.

**Col·po·di·da** (kol-po′dĭ-də) [Gr. *kolpos* a bosom or fold] an order of mostly free-living, commonly in the soil, ciliate, often reniform protozoa (subclass Vestibuliferia, class Kinetofragminophorea).

**col·po·dyn·ia** (kol″po-din′e-ə) [*colpo-* + *-odynia*] vaginodynia.

**col·po·hy·per·pla·sia** (kol″po-hi″pər-pla′zhə) [*colpo-* + *hyperplasia*] excessive growth of the mucous membrane and wall of the vagina.
**c. cys′tica,** a variety characterized by the presence of cysts in the mucous membrane.
**c. emphysemato′sa,** a variety characterized by the presence of small gas-filled spaces in the mucous membrane.

**col·po·mi·cro·scope** (kol″po-mi′kro-skōp) an instrument especially designed for the microscopic examination of tissues of the cervix *in situ;* it has higher powers of magnification than the colposcope.

**col·po·mi·cro·scop·ic** (kol″po-mi″kro-skop′ik) pertaining to the colpomicroscope, or to colpomicroscopy.

**col·po·mi·cros·co·py** (kol″po-mi-kros′kə-pe) examination of tissues of the cervix in situ with the colpomicroscope.

**col·po·myo·mec·to·my** (kol″po-mi″o-mek′tə-me) [*colpo-* + *myomectomy*] vaginal myomectomy.

**col·po·per·i·neo·plas·ty** (kol″po-per″ĭ-ne′o-plas″te) [*colpo-* + *perineum* + *-plasty*] vaginoperineoplasty.

**col·po·per·i·ne·or·rha·phy** (kol″po-per″ĭ-ne-or′ə-fe) [*colpo-* + *perineum* + *-rrhaphy*] vaginoperineorrhaphy.

**col·po·pexy** (kol′po-pek″se) [*colpo-* + *-pexy*] suture of the prolapsed vagina to a surrounding structure such as the abdominal wall; called also *vaginofixation.*

**col·po·plas·ty** (kol′po-plas″te) [*colpo-* + *-plasty*] vaginoplasty.

**col·po·poi·e·sis** (kol″po-poi-e′sis) [*colpo-* + *-poiesis*] the creation of a vagina by plastic surgery.

**col·pop·to·sis** (kol″po-to′sis) [*colpo-* + *ptosis*] vaginocele, def. 2.

**col·po·rec·to·pexy** (kol″po-rek′to-pek″se) [*colpo-* + *recto-* + *-pexy*] suspension of a prolapsed rectum by suture to the vaginal wall.

**col·por·rha·gia** (kol″po-ra′jə) [*colpo-* + *-rrhagia*] vaginal hemorrhage.

**col·por·rha·phy** (kol-por′ə-fe) [*colpo-* + *-rrhaphy*] 1. the operation of suturing the vagina. 2. the operation of denuding and suturing the vaginal wall for the purpose of restructuring the vagina.

**col·por·rhex·is** (kol″po-rek′sis) [*colpo-* + *-rrhexis*] laceration of the vagina.

**col·po·scope** (kol′po-skōp) [*colpo-* + *-scope*] 1. an instrument for examination of the tissues of the vagina and cervix by means of a magnifying lens. Cf. *colpomicroscope.* 2. vaginoscope.

**col·po·scop·ic** (kol″po-skop′ik) relating to the colposcope or to colposcopy.

**col·pos·co·py** (kol-pos′kə-pe) [MeSH: Colposcopy] examination of the cervix and vagina by means of the colposcope.

**col·po·spasm** (kol′po-spaz-əm) [*colpo-* + *spasm*] vaginal spasm.

**col·po·stat** (kol′po-stat) [*colpo-* + *-stat*] an appliance for retaining something, such as radium, in the vagina.

**col·po·ste·no·sis** (kol″po-stə-no′sis) [*colpo-* + *-stenosis*] contraction or narrowing of the vagina.

**col·po·ste·not·o·my** (kol″po-stə-not′ə-me) [*colpo-* + *steno-* + *-tomy*] a cutting operation for stricture or atresia of the vagina.

**col·pot·o·my** (kol-pot′ə-me) [*colpo-* + *-tomy*] incision of the vagina with entry into the cul-de-sac; called also *vaginotomy.*
**posterior c.,** culdotomy.

**col·po·ure·tero·cys·tot·o·my** (kol″po-u-re″tər-o-sis-tot′ə-me) [*colpo-* + *uretero-* + *cystotomy*] the exposure of the orifices of the ureters by cutting through the walls of the vagina and bladder.

**col·po·ure·ter·ot·o·my** (kol″po-u-re″tər-ot′ə-me) incision of the ureter through the vagina, performed for the relief of ureteral stricture.

**col·po·xe·ro·sis** (kol″po-ze-ro′sis) [*colpo-* + *xerosis*] abnormal dryness of the vulva and vagina.

**col·te·rol** (kol′tə-rol) an adrenergic agent, specific for $\beta_2$-adrenergic receptors, to which the prodrug bitolterol is converted.

**Col·ti·vi·rus** (kol′tĭ-vi″rəs) [*Co*lorado *ti*ck fever + *virus*] a genus of viruses of the family Reoviridae, containing the Colorado tick fever virus and related viruses.

**Col·ton blood group** (kōl′tən) [from the name of the Norwegian propositus first reported on in 1965] see under *blood group.*

**Col·u·ber** (kol′u-bər) a genus of nonvenomous snakes of the family Colubridae, found in northeastern Asia and North America. *C. constric′tor* is the American blacksnake.

**col·u·brid** (kol′u-brid) 1. any snake of the family Colubridae. 2. of or pertaining to the family Colubridae.

**Col·u·bri·dae** (kol-u′brĭ-de) [L. *coluber* serpent] [MeSH: Colubridae] a family of snakes found in North America and Africa; most genera are harmless. It includes the nonvenomous genus *Coluber* and the venomous southern African genus *Dispholidus.* See table at *snake.*

**col·u·mel·la** (kol″u-mel′ə) pl. *columel′lae* [L. "small column," dim. of *columna* column] 1. any of various columnlike anatomical structures. 2. in certain fungi and protozoa, a sterile invagination of the sporangiophore into the fertile area of the sporangium. Called also *columnella.*
**c. coch′leae,** modiolus.
**c. na′si,** the fleshy distal margin of the nasal septum.

**col·u·mel·lae** (kol″u-mel′e) [L.] genitive and plural of *columella.*

**col·u·mel·late** (kol″u-mel′āt) of certain protozoa and fungi, having columellae.

**col·umn** (kol′əm) [L. *colum′na*] an anatomical part in the form of a pillarlike structure, sometimes used specifically for the gray column of the spinal cord; see also *columna.*
**c's of abdominal ring,** thickened fibers of the aponeurosis of the external oblique muscle around the superficial inguinal ring.
**anal c's,** columnae anales.
**anterior c. of fauces,** arcus palatoglossus.
**anterior c. of spinal cord,** columna anterior medullae spinalis.
**anterolateral c.,** funiculus lateralis medullae spinalis.
**autonomic c. of spinal cord,** columna intermediolateralis medullae spinalis.
**c's of Bertin,** columnae renales.
**c. of Burdach,** fasciculus cuneatus medullae spinalis.
**Clarke's c.,** nucleus thoracicus posterior.
**dorsal c.,** columna vertebralis.
**dorsal funicular c., dorsal gray c.,** nucleus proprius.
**dorsal c. of spinal cord,** columna posterior medullae spinalis.
**enamel c's,** prismata adamantina.
**c's of folds of tongue,** papillae foliatae.
**fornix c., c. of fornix,** columna fornicis.
**fractionating c.,** an apparatus for separating the volatile constituents of a solution by distillation.
**fundamental c.,** fasciculi proprii; see entries under *fasciculus.*
**c. of Goll,** fasciculus gracilis medullae spinalis.
**Gowers' c.,** tractus spinocerebellaris anterior.
**gray c's,** columnae griseae.
**gray c. of spinal cord, anterior,** columna anterior medullae spinalis.
**gray c. of spinal cord, lateral,** columna intermedia medullae spinalis.
**gray c. of spinal cord, posterior,** columna posterior medullae spinalis.
**intermediate c. of spinal cord,** columna intermedia medullae spinalis.
**interomediolateral c. of spinal cord,** columna intermediolateralis medullae spinalis.
**c. of Kölliker,** sarcostyle, def. 2.
**lateral c. of spinal cord,** columna intermedia medullae spinalis.
**c. of Lissauer,** tractus posterolateralis.
**c's of Morgagni,** columnae anales.
**muscle c.,** sarcostyle, def. 2.
**positive c.,** a pinkish stream of light seen when a current of high potential is passed through a tube from which the air has been partly exhausted.
**posterior c. of fauces,** arcus palatopharyngeus.
**posterior c. of spinal cord,** columna posterior medullae spinalis.
**posteromedian c. of medulla oblongata,** fasciculus gracilis medullae oblongatae.
**posteromedian c. of spinal cord,** fasciculus gracilis medullae spinalis.
**Rathke's c's,** two cartilages at the anterior end of the notochord.
**rectal c's,** columnae anales.
**renal c's of Bertin,** columnae renales.
**c. of Sertoli,** an elongated Sertoli cell in the parietal layer of the seminiferous tubules.
**spinal c.,** columna vertebralis.
**c. of Spitzka and Lissauer,** tractus posterolateralis.
**Stilling's c.,** nucleus thoracicus posterior.
**striomotor c.,** an efferent column of the anterior horn of the spinal cord supplying striated muscle.
**thoracic c.,** nucleus thoracicus posterior.
**Türck's c.,** tractus corticospinalis anterior.
**vaginal c's,** columnae rugarum vaginae.
**vaginal c., anterior,** columna rugarum anterior vaginae.
**vaginal c., posterior,** columna rugarum posterior vaginae.
**ventral c. of spinal cord,** columna anterior medullae spinalis.
**vertebral c.,** the columnar assemblage of the vertebrae from the cranium through the coccyx; called also *axon, columna vertebralis* [TA], *backbone, spine,* and *dorsal* or *spinal c.*
**white c's of spinal cord,** funiculi medullae spinalis.

**co·lum·na** (ko-lum′nə) gen. and pl. *colum′nae* [L.] [TA] column: in anatomical nomenclature, used to designate a pillarlike structure or part.
**colum′nae ana′les** [TA], **colum′ni a′ni,** anal columns: vertical ridges or folds of mucous membrane at the upper half of the anal canal; called also *columnae rectales [Morgagnii], rectal columns, columns of Morgagni,* and *mucous folds of rectum.*
**c. ante′rior medul′lae spina′lis** [TA], anterior column of spinal cord: the anterior portion of the gray substance of the spinal cord (see *columnae griseae medullae spinalis*); it contains neurons that innervate the skeletal muscles of the neck, trunk, and limbs. In transverse section it is seen as a horn *(cornu anterius medullae spinalis).* Called also *ventral column of spinal cord* and *c. ventralis medullae spinalis.*
**c. autono′mica medul′lae spina′lis,** c. intermediolateralis medullae spinalis.
**colum′nae berti′ni,** columnae renales.
**c. dorsa′lis medul′lae spina′lis,** c. posterior medullae spinalis.
**c. for′nicis** [TA], fornix column: either of the two columnar masses of fibers diverging from the anterior end of the body of the fornix to descend into the diencephalon; called also *anterior pillar of fornix,* and *column of fornix.*
**colum′nae gri′seae medul′lae spina′lis** [TA], gray columns of spinal cord: the three longitudinally oriented thickenings in the spinal cord *(columnae anterior, posterior,* and *intermedia medullae spinalis),* composed of the gray substance, and containing the nerve cell bodies. The columns are commonly referred to as *cornua anterius, posterius,* and *laterale,* respectively, because in transverse sections of the spinal cord they have the appearance of horns.
**c. interme′dia medul′lae spina′lis** [TA], intermediate column of spinal cord: the lateral portion of the gray matter of the spinal cord (see *columnae griseae medullae spinalis*), extending from the second thoracic to the first lumbar segment of the spinal cord; in transverse section it is seen as a horn *(cornu laterale medullae spinalis).* Called also *intermediate zone of spinal cord, c. lateralis medullae spinalis,* and *lateral column of spinal cord.*
**c. intermediolatera′lis medul′lae spina′lis,** intermediolateral column of spinal cord: the column of gray matter the cells of which (interomediolateral nucleus) form the intermediate column of the spinal cord; called also *autonomic column of spinal cord* and *c. autonomica medullae spinalis.*
**c. latera′lis medul′lae spina′lis,** c. intermedia medullae spinalis.
**c. na′si,** septum nasi.
**c. poste′rior medul′lae spina′lis** [TA], posterior column of spinal cord: the posterior portion of the gray substance of the spinal cord (see *columnae griseae medullae spinalis*); it contains groups of motoneurons that extend the length of the cord and two groups that are limited to the thoracic and upper lumbar segments. In transverse section it is seen as a horn *(cornu posterius medullae spinalis).* Called also *dorsal column of spinal cord* and *c. dorsalis medullae spinalis.*
**colum′nae recta′les [Morgagn′ii],** columnae anales.
**colum′nae rena′les** [TA], renal columns: inward extensions of the cortical structure of the kidney, between the renal pyramids; called also *columnae renales* [*Bertini*], *columnae bertini,* and *renal columns of Bertin.*

**colum′nae rena′les [Berti′ni],** columnae renales.
**c. ruga′rum ante′rior vagi′nae** [TA], anterior vaginal column: a well-marked longitudinal ridge on the anterior wall of the vagina.
**c. ruga′rum poste′rior vagi′nae** [TA], posterior vaginal column: a well-marked longitudinal ridge on the posterior wall of the vagina.
**colum′nae ruga′rum vagi′nae** [TA], vaginal columns: well-marked longitudinal ridges on either the anterior *(c. rugarum anterior vaginae)* or posterior *(c. rugarum posterior vaginae)* wall of the vagina.
**c. thora′cica,** nucleus thoracicus posterior.
**c. ventra′lis medul′lae spina′lis,** c. anterior medullae spinalis.
**c. vertebra′lis** [TA], the columnar assemblage of the vertebrae from the cranium through the coccyx; called also *axon, backbone, spine,* and *vertebral, dorsal,* or *spinal column.*

**co•lum•nae** (ko-lum′ne) [L.] genitive and plural of *columna.*

**co•lum•nel•la** (kol″ə-nel′ə) [L.] columella.

**col•um•ni•za•tion** (kol″əm-nĭ-za′shən) the supporting of the prolapsed uterus with tampons.

**Coly-My•cin M** (kol′e-mi″sin) trademark for preparations of colistimethate sodium.

**Coly-My•cin S** (kol′e-mi″sin) trademark for a preparation of colistin sulfate.

**co•ly•pep•tic** (ko″le-pep′tik) kolypeptic.

**com-** see *con-.*

**co•ma** (ko′mə) [L.; Gr. *kōma*] [MeSH: Coma] 1. a state of unconsciousness from which the patient cannot be aroused, even by powerful stimulation; called also *exanimation.* See also *consciousness.* 2. the optical aberration produced when an image is received upon a screen which is not exactly at right angles to the line of propagation of the incident light.
**agrypnodal c.,** old name for *locked-in syndrome.*
**alcoholic c.,** coma accompanying severe alcoholic intoxication.
**alpha c.,** coma in which there are electroencephalographic findings of dominant alpha-wave activity.
**diabetic c.,** the coma of severe diabetic acidosis, which is accompanied by Kussmaul's respiration.
**hepatic c., c. hepa′ticum,** coma accompanying hepatic encephalopathy.
**hyperosmolar nonketotic c.,** diabetic coma in which the level of ketone bodies is normal, due to hyperosmolarity of extracellular fluid resulting in dehydration of intracellular fluid; often a consequence of overtreatment with hyperosmolar solutions.
**irreversible c.,** brain death; see under *death.*
**Kussmaul's c.,** diabetic c.
**metabolic c.,** the coma accompanying metabolic encephalopathy.
**myxedema c.,** an often fatal complication of long-term hypothyroidism in which the patient is comatose with hypothermia, depression of respiration, bradycardia, and hypotension; usually seen in elderly patients during cold weather.
**nonketotic hyperosmolar c.,** hyperosmolar nonketotic c.
**uremic c.,** lethargic state due to uremia.
**c. vigil,** locked-in syndrome.

**com•a•tose** (ko′mə-tōs) pertaining to or affected with coma.

**Com•bi•pres** (kom′bĭ-pres) trademark for preparations of clonidine hydrochloride and chlorthalidone.

**Com•bi•vent** (kom′bĭ-vent) trademark for a preparation of ipratropium bromide plus albuterol sulfate.

**Com•bi•vir** (kom′bĭ-vir) trademark for a preparation of zidovudine plus lamivudine.

**com•bus•tion** (kəm-bus′chən) [L. *combustio*] rapid oxidation with emission of heat.

**com•e•do** (kom′ə-do) pl. *comedo′nes.* A noninflammatory lesion of acne, consisting of a plug of keratin and sebum within the dilated orifice of a hair follicle, frequently containing the bacteria *Propionibacterium acnes, Staphylococcus albus,* and *Malassezia furfur.* See also *acne vulgaris.*
**closed c.,** a comedo whose opening is not widely dilated, appearing as a small, flesh-colored papule; because the keratin and sebum produced cannot escape, it may rupture and cause an inflammatory lesion in the dermis. Called also *whitehead.*
**open c.,** a comedo with a widely dilated orifice in which the pigmented impaction is visible at the skin surface; called also *blackhead.*

**com•e•do•car•ci•no•ma** (kom″ə-do-kahr″sĭ-no′mə) [*comedo* + *carcinoma*] a type of ductal carcinoma in situ whose central cells are degenerated and easily expressed from the cut surface of the tumor.

**com•e•do•gen•ic** (kom″ə-do-jen′ik) producing comedones.

**com•e•do•mas•ti•tis** (kom″ə-do-mas-ti′tis) mammary duct ectasia.

**co•mes** (ko′mēz) pl. *com′ites* [L. "companion"] an artery or vein that accompanies another artery, a vein, or a nerve trunk; see also terms beginning *arteria comitans* and *vena comitans.*

**com•for•ti•za•tion** (kum″fər-tĭ-za′shən) the scientific application of physiological principles for the promotion of comfort in potentially stressful situations, as in aircraft design.

**com•frey** (kom′fre) *Symphytum officinale.*

**com•i•tes** (kom′ĭ-tēz) plural of *comes.*

**com•men•sal** (ko-men′səl) [*com-* + L. *mensa* table] 1. living on or within another organism, and deriving benefit without injuring or benefiting the other individual. 2. an organism living on or within another, but not causing injury to the host. See *symbiosis.*

**com•men•sal•ism** (ko-men′səl-iz″əm) symbiosis (q.v.) in which one population (or individual) gains from the association and the other is neither harmed nor benefited.

**com•mi•nut•ed** (kom′ĭ-nōōt′əd) [*com-* + L. *minuere* to diminish] broken or crushed into small pieces, as a comminuted fracture.

**com•mi•nu•tion** (kom″ĭ-nu′shən) [L. *comminutio*] the act of breaking, or condition of being broken, into small fragments, as of a fractured bone.

**Com•miph•o•ra** (kom-if′o-rə) a genus of trees of the family Burseraceae, native to Indonesia and Africa. *C. abyssi′nica* (Berg.) Engl. and other species yield myrrh. *C. opobal′samum* Engl. yields Mecca balsam.

**com•mis•su•ra** (kom″ĭ-su′rə) gen. and pl. *commissu′rae* [L. "a joining together"] [TA] commissure: a site of union of corresponding parts; a general term used to designate such a junction of corresponding anatomical structures, frequently, but not always, across the median plane of the body.
**c. al′ba ante′rior medul′lae spina′lis** [TA], anterior white commissure of spinal cord: the aggregate of fibers crossing from one side of the spinal cord to the other, anterior to the gray commissure. Called also *ventral white commissure of spinal cord.*
**c. al′ba poste′rior medul′lae spina′lis** [TA], posterior white commissure of spinal cord: the group of transverse myelinated nerve fibers crossing from one side of the spinal cord to the other posterior to the central canal, permeating the gray commissure; called also *dorsal white commissure of spinal cord.*
**c. ante′rior** [TA], anterior commissure: a bundle of myelinated nerve fibers passing transversely through the lamina terminalis and connecting symmetrical parts of the two cerebral hemispheres; it consists of a smaller anterior part *(pars anterior commissurae anterioris)* and a larger posterior part *(pars posterior commissurae anterioris).* Called also *c. rostralis* and *rostral commissure.*
**c. bulbo′rum vesti′buli** [TA], commissure of bulbs of vestibule: a narrow median band spanning the vaginal orifice to unite the bulbs of the vestibule. Called also *pars intermedia bulborum vestibuli.*
**c. colli′culi cauda′lis,** c. colliculi inferioris.
**c. colli′culi inferio′ris** [TA], commissure of inferior colliculus: a band of nerve fibers that connect the two inferior colliculi; called also *c. colliculi caudalis* and *commissure of caudal colliculus.*
**c. colli′culi rostra′lis,** c. colliculi superioris.
**c. colli′culi superio′ris** [TA], commissure of superior colliculus: a band of nerve fibers that connect the two superior colliculi; called also *c. colliculi rostralis* and *commissure of rostral colliculus.*
**c. epithala′mica,** TA alternative for *c. posterior.*
**c. for′nicis** [TA], commissure of fornix: a band of fibers connecting the hippocampi of the two sides through the body of the fornix; called also *hippocampal commissure.*
**c. gri′sea ante′rior/poste′rior medul′lae spina′lis,** anterior/posterior gray commissure of spinal cord: the transverse band of gray substance surrounding the central canal of the spinal cord external to the central gelatinous substance; it connects the intermediate, anterior, and posterior columns. Called also *gray commissure of spinal cord.*
**c. gri′sea ante′rior medul′lae spina′lis** [TA], anterior gray commissure of spinal cord: the portion of the gray commissure anterior to the central canal; see *c. grisea anterior/posterior medullae spinalis.* Called also *ventral gray commissure of spinal cord.*
**c. gri′sea poste′rior medul′lae spina′lis** [TA], posterior gray commissure of spinal cord: the portion of the gray commissure posterior to the central canal; see *c. grisea anterior/posterior medullae spinalis.* Called also *dorsal gray commissure of spinal cord.*
**c. habenula′rum** [TA], habenular commissure: a band of fibers of the stria medullaris that pass through the habenula of each side to decussate and terminate in the habenula of the other side.
**c. labio′rum ante′rior** [TA], anterior commissure of labia: the junction of the two labia majora anteriorly, at the lower border of the pubic symphysis.
**c. labio′rum o′ris** [TA], commissure of lips of mouth: the junction of the upper and lower lips at either side of the mouth.
**c. labio′rum poste′rior** [TA], posterior commissure of labia: the apparent junction of the labia majora posteriorly, formed by the forward projection of the tendinous center of the perineum into the pudendal cleft.

**c. labio'rum puden'di,** see *c. labiorum anterior* and *c. labiorum posterior.*
**c. latera'lis palpebra'rum** [TA], lateral commissure of eyelids: the junction of the upper and lower eyelids on the lateral side. Called also *lateral palpebral commissure.*
**c. mag'na ce'rebri,** corpus callosum.
**c. media'lis palpebra'rum** [TA], medial commissure of eyelids: the junction of the upper and lower eyelids on the medial side; called also *medial palpebral commissure.*
**c. oliva'rum,** see *fibrae arcuatae internae.*
**c. palpebra'rum latera'lis,** c. lateralis palpebrarum.
**c. palpebra'rum media'lis, c. palpebra'rum nasa'lis,** c. medialis palpebrarum.
**c. palpebra'rum tempora'lis,** c. lateralis palpebrarum.
**c. poste'rior** [TA], posterior commissure of cerebrum: a large fiber bundle that crosses the midline of the epithalamus just dorsal to the point where the cerebral aqueduct opens into the third ventricle; called also *c. epithalamica* [TA alternative] and *commissure of epithalamus.*
**c. rostra'lis,** c. anterior.
**c. supraop'tica dorsa'lis** [TA], dorsal supraoptic commissure: the more dorsal fiber bundle that crosses the midline of the brain dorsal to the caudal border of the optic chiasm; see also *supraoptic commissures,* under *commissure.*
**c. supraop'tica ventra'lis** [TA], ventral supraoptic commissure: the more ventral fiber bundle that crosses the midline of the brain dorsal to the caudal border of the optic chiasm; see also *supraoptic commissures,* under *commissure.*

**com·mis·su·rae** (kom″ĭ-su're) [L.] genitive and plural of *commissura.*

**com·mis·su·ral** (kə-mish'o͞o-rəl) pertaining to or acting as a commissure.

**com·mis·sure** (kom'ĭ-shoor) 1. a site of union of corresponding parts; see also *commissura.* 2. the site of junction between adjacent cusps of a heart valve.
**anterior c.,** commissura anterior.
**c. of bulbs of vestibule,** commissura bulborum vestibuli.
**c. of caudal colliculus,** commissura colliculi inferioris.
**cerebral c., posterior,** commissura posterior.
**c. of epithalamus,** commissura posterior.
**c. of fornix,** commissura fornicis.
**Ganser's c.,** the anterior supraoptic commissure; see *supraoptic c's.*
**gray c.,** substantia intermedia centralis medullae spinalis.
**gray c. of spinal cord,** the anterior and posterior gray commissures of spinal cord considered together; see *commissura grisea anterior/posterior medullae spinalis.*
**gray c. of spinal cord, anterior,** commissura grisea anterior medullae spinalis.
**gray c. of spinal cord, anterior/posterior,** commissura grisea anterior/posterior medullae spinalis.
**gray c. of spinal cord, dorsal,** commissura grisea posterior medullae spinalis.
**gray c. of spinal cord, posterior,** commissura grisea posterior medullae spinalis.
**gray c. of spinal cord, ventral,** commissura grisea anterior medullae spinalis.
**Gudden's c.,** the ventral, or inferior, supraoptic commissure; see *supraoptic c's.*
**c. of habenulae, habenular c.,** commissura habenularum.
**hippocampal c.,** commissura fornicis.
**c. of inferior colliculus,** commissura colliculi inferioris.
**c. of labia, anterior,** commissura labiorum anterior.
**c. of labia, posterior,** commissura labiorum posterior.
**laryngeal c.,** the region of junction (anterior or posterior) of the two sides of the larynx.
**lateral c. of eyelids, lateral palpebral c.,** commissura lateralis palpebrarum.
**c. of lips of mouth,** commissura labiorum oris.
**medial c. of eyelids, medial palpebral c.,** commissura medialis palpebrarum.
**Meynert's c.,** the dorsal, or superior, supraoptic commissure; see *supraoptic c's.*
**posterior c.,** commissura posterior.
**rostral c.,** commissura anterior.
**c. of rostral colliculus,** commissura colliculi superioris.
**c. of superior colliculus,** commissura colliculi superioris.
**supraoptic c's,** at least three fiber bundles situated dorsal to the optic chiasm, which have been associated with the names of Gudden (ventral or inferior), Meynert (dorsal or superior), and Ganser (anterior), and which have been referred to as commissures but are probably decussations; their connections in humans are uncertain. Only the dorsal and ventral bundles are recognized in official anatomical nomenclature: see *commissura supraoptica dorsalis* and *commissura supraoptica ventralis.*
**supraoptic c., dorsal,** commissura supraoptica dorsalis.
**supraoptic c., ventral,** commissura supraoptica dorsalis.
**white c. of spinal cord, anterior,** commissura alba anterior medullae spinalis.
**white c. of spinal cord, dorsal,** commissura alba posterior medullae spinalis.
**white c. of spinal cord, posterior,** commissura alba posterior medullae spinalis.
**white c. of spinal cord, ventral,** commissura alba anterior medullae spinalis.

**com·mis·su·ror·rha·phy** (kom″ĭ-shər-or'ə-fe) [*commissure* + *-rrhaphy*] suture of the component parts of a commissure, to decrease the size of the orifice.

**com·mis·sur·ot·o·my** (kom″ĭ-shər-ot'ə-me) [*commissure* + *-tomy*] surgical incision or digital disruption of the component parts of a commissure to increase the size of the orifice; commonly utilized to separate the adherent, thickened leaflets of a stenotic mitral valve.

**com·mit·ment** (kə-mit'mənt) civil commitment; the legal proceeding by which a person is involuntarily confined to a mental hospital or made to undergo outpatient treatment.

**com·mo·tio** (kə-mo'she-o) [L. "disturbance"] a concussion; a violent shaking, or the shock which results from it.
**c. ce'rebri,** concussion of the brain.
**c. re'tinae,** edema around the macular region of the retina, caused by a severe blow to the eyeball, and producing a permanent central scotoma as a result of destruction of the delicate cones in the fovea. Called also *Berlin's edema,* and *concussion of the retina.*
**c. spina'lis,** concussion of the spinal cord.

**com·mu·ni·ca·ble** (kə-mu'nĭ-kə-bəl) capable of being transmitted from one person or species to another, as a communicable disease; contagious. Cf. *infectious.*

**com·mu·ni·cans** (kə-mu'nə-kanz) [L.] communicating; used in anatomical nomenclature to denote a communicating structure, as a nerve.

**com·mu·nis** (kə-mu'nis) [L.] [TA] common: a general term denoting a structure serving several branches.

**com·mu·ni·ty** (kə-mu'nĭ-te) a body of individuals living in a defined area or having a common interest or organization.
**biotic c.,** an assemblage of populations living in a defined area.
**climax c.,** the final, stable, and mature community in a series that appears in succession, which is in equilibrium with the environmental conditions and is composed of a definite group of plant and animal species. The entire sequence of communities is called a *sere* and the individual transitional communities are *seral stages.*
**seral c.,** see under *stage.*
**therapeutic c.,** a specially structured mental treatment center employing group and milieu therapy and encouraging the patient to function within social norms.

**Com·ol·li's sign** (kom-ol'ēz) [Antonio *Comolli,* Italian pathologist, born 1879] see under *sign.*

**co·mor·bid** (ko-mor'bid) pertaining to a disease or other pathological process that occurs simultaneously with another.

**co·mor·bid·i·ty** (ko″mor-bid'ĭ-te) [MeSH: Comorbidity] 1. a comorbid disease or condition. 2. the state of being comorbid. 3. the extent to which two diseases or disorders occur together in a given population.

**Comp.** abbreviation for L. *compos'itus,* compound.

**com·pact** (kəm-pakt') dense; having a dense structure.

**com·pac·tion** (kəm-pak'shən) 1. a complication of labor in twin births in which there is simultaneous full engagement of the leading fetal poles of both twins, so that the true pelvic cavity is filled and further descent is prevented. Cf. *interlocking.* 2. in embryology, the process during which the blastomeres change their shape and align themselves tightly against each other to form a compact ball of cells (the morula).

**com·pa·ges** (kəm-pa'jēz) [L.] a joining together or that which is joined together.
**c. thora'cis,** skeleton thoracis.

**com·par·a·scope** (kəm-par'ə-skōp″) a device attached to a microscope for the purpose of comparing two slides.

**com·par·a·tor** (kəm-par'ə-tər) a simple colorimeter consisting of a block of wood with holes in which to place the test tubes to be compared, and transverse holes through which to view the colors; called also *comparator block.*

**com·par·ti·men·tum** (kəm-pahr″tĭ-men'təm) [L., from *compartiri* to share] [TA] compartment.
**c. superficiale perinei** [TA], superficial perineal compartment: the region between the perineal membrane and the superficial perineal fascia; called also *spatium superficiale perinei* [TA alternative] and *superficial perineal pouch* or *space.*

**com·part·ment** (kəm-pahrt'mənt) a small enclosure within a larger space.

**muscular c.,** lacuna musculorum.
**superficial perineal c.,** compartimentum superficiale perinei.
**vascular c.,** lacuna vasorum.

**com·part·men·ta·li·za·tion** (kəm-pahrt″men-tə-lĭ-za′shən) the natural partitioning within cells due to the selectively permeable membranes which enclose each of the separate parts (mitochondria, lysosomes, Golgi complex, etc.), enabling each part to regulate its own contents. Called also *compartmentation.*

**com·part·men·ta·tion** (kəm-pahrt″men-ta′shən) compartmentalization.

**com·pat·i·bil·i·ty** (kəm-pat″ĭ-bil′ĭ-te) the quality of being compatible.

**com·pat·i·ble** (kəm-pat′ĭ-bəl) [L. *compatibilis* accordant] 1. capable of harmonious coexistence; said of two or more medications that are suitable for simultaneous administration without nullification or aggravation of their effects. 2. denoting a donor and recipient of a blood transfusion in which there is no transfusion reaction. 3. histocompatible.

**Com·pa·zine** (kom′pə-zēn) trademark for preparations of prochlorperazine maleate.

**com·pen·sa·tion** (kom″pən-sa′shən) [L. *compensatio,* from *cum* together + *pensare* to weigh] 1. the counterbalancing of any defect of structure or function. 2. a conscious process or, more frequently, an unconscious defense mechanism by which a person attempts to make up for real or imagined physical or psychological deficiencies. 3. in the presence of disease, the maintenance of an adequate blood flow without distressing symptoms, accomplished by such cardiac and circulatory adjustments as tachycardia, cardiac hypertrophy or dilation, and increase of blood volume by sodium and water retention.
**dosage c.,** in genetics, the mechanism by which the effect of the two X chromosomes of the normal female is rendered identical to that of the one X chromosome of the normal male. See *Lyon hypothesis,* under *hypothesis.*

**com·pen·sa·to·ry** (kəm-pen′sə-tor″e) making good a defect or loss; restoring a lost balance.

**com·pe·tence** (kom′pə-təns) 1. the ability of an organ or part to perform adequately any function required of it. 2. in embryology, the ability of embryonic cells to differentiate into cell types determined by inductors.
**embryonic c.,** the ability of embryonic tissue to respond normally to the influence of an inductor.
**immunologic c.,** immunocompetence.

**com·pe·ti·tion** (kom″pə-tish′ən) the phenomenon in which two structurally similar molecules "compete" for a single binding site on a third molecule. See *competitive inhibition,* under *inhibition.*
**antigenic c.,** an altered response to an immunogen resulting from the simultaneous or close administration of two immunogens: the response to one is normal, while the response to the second is suppressed or diminished.

**com·plaint** (kəm-plānt′) symptom.
**chief c.,** presenting symptom.

**com·ple·ment** (kom′plə-mənt) [L. *complēre* to fill out or up] [MeSH: Complement] a term originally used to refer to the heat-labile factor in serum that causes immune cytolysis, the lysis of antibody-coated cells. It is now used to refer to the entire functionally related system comprising at least 20 distinct serum proteins, their cellular receptors, and related regulatory proteins that is the effector not only of immune cytolysis but also of other biologic functions including anaphylaxis, phagocytosis, opsonization, and hemolysis. Complement activation occurs by two different sequences, the classical and alternative pathways (qq.v.). All of the components of complement, designated C1 through C9, participate in the classical pathway; the alternative pathway lacks components C1, C2, and C4 but adds factors B and D and properdin. Regulatory proteins include factors H and I, clusterin, C3 nephritic factor, decay accelerating factor, homologous restriction factor, anaphylatoxin inactivator, C1 inhibitor, C4 binding protein, membrane cofactor protein, protectin, and vitronectin. Activation of the classical pathway triggers an enzymatic cascade involving C1, C4, C2, and C3; activation of the alternative pathway triggers a cascade involving C3 and factors B and D and properdin. Both result in the cleavage of C5 and the formation of the membrane attack complex, which in its final state creates a pore in the cell wall and causes cell lysis. See illustration. Complement activation also results in the formation of many biologically active complement fragments that act as anaphylatoxins, opsonins, or chemotactic factors. NOTE: Fragments resulting from proteolytic cleavage of complement proteins are designated with lower-case-letter suffixes, e.g., C3a. By convention, the smaller initial cleavage fragment is designated "a" and the larger "b," excepting the fragments C2a and C2b generated from C2, where the larger, active fragment has conventionally been designated C2a. Inactivated fragments are designated by the prefix "i," e.g., iC3b. Terminology of activated components or complexes with biologic activity is quite variable. A bar over the symbol is sometimes used, e.g., $C\overline{1}$ or $\overline{C4b,2a}$, and in designating multicomponent complexes, commas may or may not be present between components, and the "a" and "b" designations may or may not be used. Thus, C4b,2a may also be written $\overline{C4b,2a}$, C4b2a, $\overline{C4b2a}$, C42, or $C\overline{42}$. Some authors use the overbar for any activated component, while others reserve it specifically for those with enzymatic activity.
**C1,** the first component of the classical pathway of complement activation, a pentamolecular calcium-dependent complex comprising C1q and two molecules each of C1r and C1s.
**C1q,** a six-subunit molecule, comprising 18 polypeptide chains, having the shape of six parallel rods flaring apart from each other at one end to terminate in a flower bunch arrangement, the globular head of each rod resembling a tulip; binding of the heads to IgM or IgG initiates the classical complement pathway, which continues by binding of two molecules each of C1r and C1s by C1q.
**C1r,** a serine esterase component of C1 in the classical complement pathway, activated by cleavage of C1r bound to the stem of immunoglobulin-bound C1q; once activated, it can cleave and activate C1s. The activated state is sometimes specifically denoted by $C\overline{1r}$.
**C1s,** an enzyme that cleaves C4 into C4a and C4b and C2 into C2a and C2b, activated by cleavage of a peptide bond when C1 interacts with activators of the classical pathway; it is inhibited by C1 inhibitor. Called also *C1 esterase.* The activated state is sometimes specifically denoted by $C\overline{1s}$.
**C2,** a component of the classical complement pathway that binds surface-bound C4b; cleavage of C2 by C1s releases a small C2b fragment and leaves C2a bound to C4b to form the classical pathway C3 convertase (C4b,2a).
**C2a,** a constituent of the classical pathway C3 and C5 convertases (C4b,2a and C4b,2a,3b, respectively), generated by C1s-mediated cleavage of C2 bound to C4b. Because in most other cases the active fragment generated by cleavage of complement factors is designated the "b" fragment (e.g., C3b, C4b), some authors designate this active fragment as C2b, the small soluble fragment being thus C2a; in this case, the C3 and C5 convertases are designated C4b2b and C4b2b3b, respectively.
**C3,** a component of both the classical and alternative complement pathways; it can be cleaved spontaneously at low level (tickover) or by one of the C3 convertases (C4b,2a or C3b,Bb) to form C3a and C3b. Deficiency of C3 may be associated with repeated severe pyogenic bacterial infection.
**C3a,** an anaphylatoxin generated, along with C3b, when C3 is cleaved by one of the C3 convertases.
**C3b,** a constituent of the classical pathway C5 convertase and of the alternative pathway C3 and C5 convertases, generated by C3 convertases in both pathways and also continuously generated in the circulation in the small amounts required to initiate the alternative pathway (tickover); it is inactivated by variable combinations of factor H, factor I, membrane cofactor protein, decay accelerating factor, and complement receptor 1. C3b is also an opsonin having receptors on erythrocytes, B lymphocytes, granulocytes, monocytes, and macrophages.
**C3b,Bb,** the alternative pathway C3 convertase, which splits C3 into C3a and C3b; it is generated by the interaction of factor B and factor D with C3b deposited on activators of the alternative pathway and thus protected from inactivation by factor I and factor H. It is unstable until the addition of properdin. See also note at *complement.*
**C3b$_n$,Bb,** the alternative pathway C5 convertase, generated by addition of one or more C3b fragments to C3b,Bb; it is unstable until the addition of properdin. See also note at *complement.*
**C3b,P,Bb,** a more stable form of the alternative pathway C3 convertase, generated by addition of properdin to C3b,Bb. See also note at *complement.*
**C3b$_n$,P,Bb,** a more stable form of the alternative pathway C5 convertase, generated by addition of properdin to C3b$_n$,Bb. See also note at *complement.*
**C3d,** a B cell growth factor generated by inactivation of C3b by factor I and various cofactors, including complement receptor 1, membrane cofactor protein, and factor H; it interacts with complement receptor 2 on B lymphocytes.
**C4,** a component of the classical complement pathway; it binds C1 and is cleaved by C1s to generate the small anaphylatoxin C4a and the larger active fragment C4b.
**C4a,** a weak anaphylatoxin generated by cleavage of C4 by C1s in the classical pathway of complement activation.
**C4b,** a constituent of the classical pathway C3 convertase (C4b,2a), generated by cleavage of C4 by C1s; the active fragment C4b then binds C2 for cleavage of C2 by C1s. It is inactivated by factor I in the presence of C4 binding protein. C4b is also an opsonin that binds to the same receptors as C3b.
**C4b,2a,** the classical pathway C3 convertase, which cleaves C3 to C3a and C3b, a complex of C4b and C2a formed on cell membrane surfaces in the presence of $Mg^{2+}$. See also notes at *C2a* and *complement.*
**C4b,2a,3b,** the classical pathway C5 convertase, which cleaves C5

**Defects in Complement Components and Selected Regulatory Proteins**

| Defective Protein | Pathway Affected | Clinically Associated Disorders |
|---|---|---|
| C1 | Classical pathway | Autoimmune disorders; pyogenic infections |
| C2 | Classical pathway | Autoimmune disorders; pyogenic infections |
| C3 | Classical and alternative pathways | Autoimmune disorders; pyogenic infections |
| C4 | Classical pathway | Autoimmune disorders |
| C5–C9 | Membrane attack complex | Recurrent disseminated neisserial infection |
| Properdin | Alternative pathway | Neisserial and other pyogenic infections |
| Factor D | Alternative pathway | Neisserial and other pyogenic infections |
| C1 inhibitor | Deregulation of classical pathway | Hereditary angioneurotic edema; some autoimmune disorders |
| Factor I | Deregulation of alternative pathway | Autoimmune disorders; pyogenic infections |
| Factor H | Deregulation of classical pathway | Glomerulonephritis |

to C5a and C5b; the complex is formed by attachment of C3b to membrane-bound C4b,2a. See also notes at *C2a* and *complement.*
**C5,** a complement component that binds to the C3b component of both the classical and alternative pathway C5 convertases (C4b,2a,3b and $C3b_n$,P,Bb), being split by either convertase into the smaller anaphylatoxin C5a and the larger cell surface–bound C5b, the initial component of the membrane attack complex.
**C5a,** an anaphylatoxin and chemotactic factor for basophils, neutrophils, mast cells, macrophages, and endothelium generated in the cleavage of C5 by C5 convertases. It is a potent local mediator of inflammation and also induces smooth muscle contraction.
**C5b,** a constituent of the membrane attack complex generated by cleavage of C5 by the classical and alternative pathway C5 convertases; it can also be generated by the action of certain serum proteases, e.g., plasmin and trypsin.
**C5b,6,** the hydrophilic complex of C5b and C6 formed in the initial steps of formation of the membrane attack complex; it is loosely associated with the membrane until it is bound by C7.
**C5b,6,7,** a trimolecular complex of C5b, C6, and C7 that binds to cell membranes in the formation of the membrane attack complex; it can be inhibited by binding by vitronectin, which yields an inactivated complex unable to bind to membranes. C5b,6,7 is also a chemotactic factor for neutrophils. Sometimes abbreviated C5b–7.
**C5b,6,7,8,** a complex generated by binding of C8 to membrane-bound C5b,6,7; it causes a slow leakage of the cell membrane. Sometimes abbreviated C5b–8.
**C5b,6,7,8,9,** the complete membrane attack complex (cytolytic agent) of the complement system, generated by addition of multiple molecules of C9 to C5b,6,7,8; this complex has a hydrophilic center that allows the rapid passage of water and ions through the cell

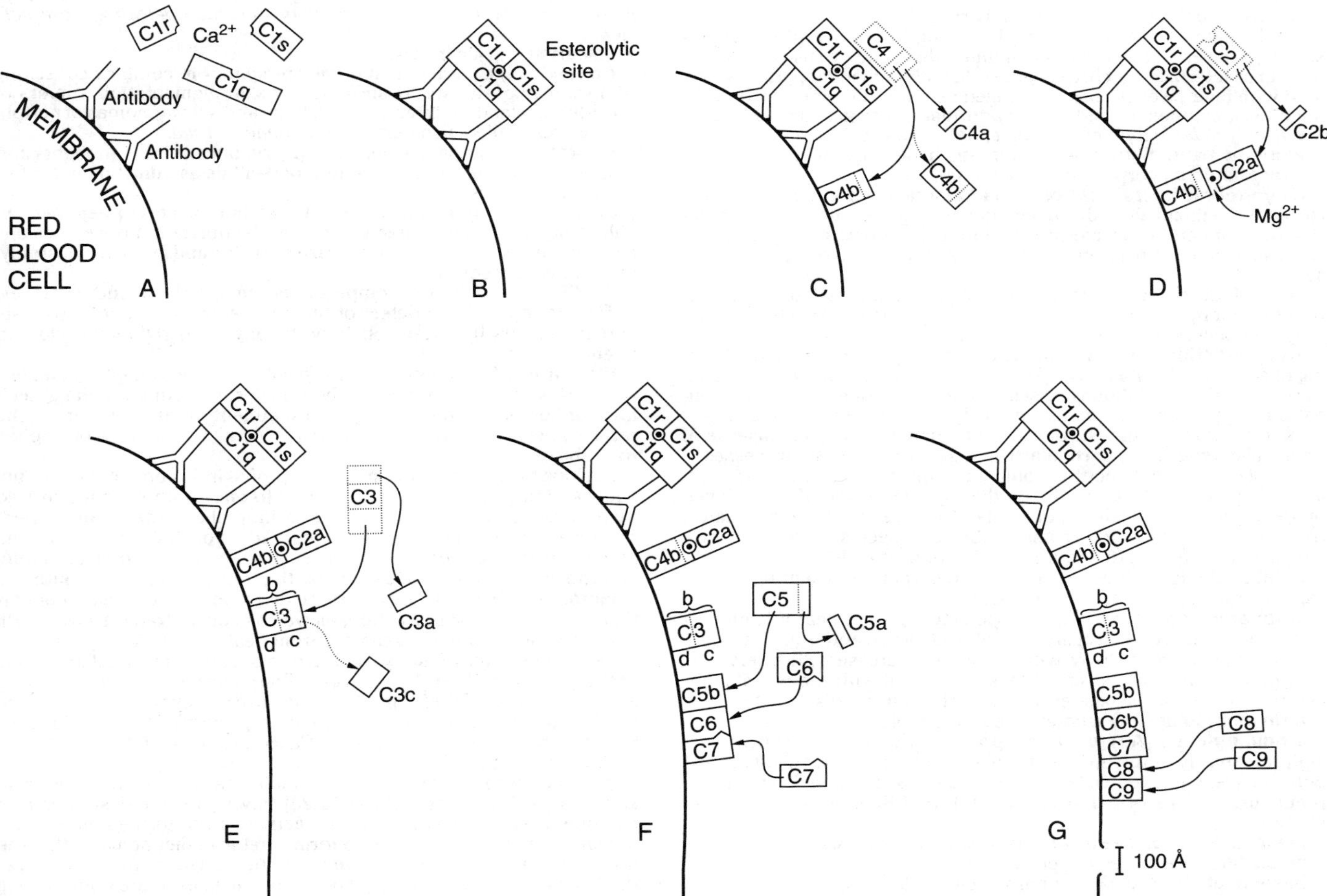


Schematic representation of the classical complement pathway. Two molecules of IgG, termed a "doublet," combine with homologous antigenic determinants on a red blood cell surface and activate the first complement component (C1) by interacting with C1q *(A)* followed by C1r and C1s *(B)*. The esterolytic site on C1s activates C4, splitting off C4b which binds the red cell surface *(C)*. The same site on C1s then activates C2, splitting off C2a which binds to C4b *(D)*. The C4b2a complex activates C3 by splitting off C3b, which binds to the red cell membrane *(E)*. The C4b2a3b complex (C5 convertase) cleaves C5 into C5a and C5b, and C5b, C6, and C7 attach to the red cell *(F)*. Activation and binding to the red cell membrane by C8 and C9 is followed by membrane rupture *(G)*.

membrane, causing osmotic lysis of the cell. Sometimes abbreviated C5b–9 or C5b–$9_n$.

**C6,** a component of the membrane attack complex, bound by C5b to form C5b,6.

**C7,** a component of the membrane attack complex, bound by C5b,6 to form the lipophilic intermediate C5b,6,7.

**C8,** a component of the membrane attack complex, bound by membrane-bound C5b,6,7 to form C5b,6,7,8, which is anchored in the cell membrane by C8. C8 can then induce the polymerization of C9.

**C9,** a component of the membrane attack complex; multiple molecules are bound by a single C5b,6,7,8 complex to form the final membrane attack complex. Although as few as 3 to 4 molecules of C9 are sufficient for full lytic activity on many substrates, 12 to 15 are necessary to form the usual doughnut-shaped pore in the membrane. $C9_n$ is often used to denote the multiple molecules of C9 in the membrane attack complex.

**total hemolytic c. (CH50, $CH_{50}$),** see *CH50 assay,* under *assay* and *CH50 unit,* under *unit.*

**com·ple·men·tal** (kom″plə-men′təl) complementary.

**com·ple·men·ta·ry** (kom″plə-men′tə-re) [L. *complēre* to fill out or up] supplying a defect, or helping to do so; making complete; accessory.

**com·ple·men·ta·tion** (kom″plə-men-ta′shən) [L. *complēre* to fill out or up] the interaction between two sets of cellular or viral genes introduced into the same cell, such that the cell can function even though each set of genes carries a mutated, nonfunctional gene; it indicates that the defects are not identical.

**interallelic c.,** intragenic c.

**intercistronic c., intergenic c.,** the essentially full restoration of wild-type function in a *cis-trans* test when two mutations are located in two different cistrons (genes).

**intracistronic c., intragenic c.,** the partial restoration of function sometimes seen in the *cis-trans* test when the two mutations are located at different sites within the same cistron.

**com·plex** (kom′pleks) [L. *complexus* woven together, encompassing] 1. the sum, combination, or collection of various things or related factors, like or unlike, e.g., a complex of symptoms. See also *syndrome.* 2. sequence (def. 2). 3. a group of interrelated ideas, mainly unconscious, that have a common emotional tone and strongly influence a person's attitudes and behavior. 4. that portion of an electrocardiographic tracing which represents the systole of an atrium or ventricle.

## Complex

**adrenochrome monosemicarbazone sodium salicylate c.,** carbazochrome salicylate.

**AIDS dementia c.,** HIV encephalopathy.

**AIDS-related c. (ARC),** a complex of signs and symptoms representing a severe stage of human immunodeficiency virus (HIV) infection, characterized by chronic generalized lymphadenopathy associated with fever, weight loss, prolonged diarrhea, minor opportunistic infections, cytopenias, and T-cell abnormalities associated with AIDS. See also *lymphadenopathy syndrome,* under *syndrome.*

**amniotic band disruption c.,** amniotic band sequence.

**amygdaloid c.,** corpus amygdaloideum.

**amyotrophic lateral sclerosis–parkinsonism–dementia c.,** an autosomal dominant disorder occurring among the Chamorro population of Guam and characterized by gradually progressing parkinsonism associated with progressive dementia and amyotrophic lateral sclerosis.

**anomalous c.,** in electrocardiography, an abnormal atrial or ventricular complex resulting from aberrant impulse conduction occurring over accessory conduction pathways.

**antigen-antibody c.,** the complex formed by the noncovalent binding of an antibody and an antigen. Complexes of antibodies belonging to certain immunoglobulin classes may activate complement. Antigen-antibody complexes are mediators of Type III immune responses (Arthus reactions, serum sickness, and immune complex diseases). Called also *immune c.,* particularly in discussing disease processes.

**apical c.,** an ultrastructural complex of apical organelles characteristic of apicocomplexan protozoa during some stage of their development, generally consisting of a polar ring(s), a conoid, micronemes, rhoptries, and subpellicular microtubules. It seems to function as a means of attachment to and penetration of host cells.

**atrial c.,** the P wave of the electrocardiogram, representing electrical activation of the atria. Cf. *ventricular c.*

**atrial premature c. (APC),** a single ectopic atrial beat arising prematurely, manifest electrocardiographically as an abnormally shaped premature P wave, usually with a slightly increased PR interval. It occurs in normal hearts, sometimes associated with the use of stimulants, but may be associated with structural heart disease.

**atrioventricular (AV) junctional escape c.,** see under *beat.*

**atrioventricular (AV) junctional premature c.,** an ectopic beat arising prematurely in the atrioventricular junction and traveling toward both the atria and ventricles if unimpeded, causing the P wave to be premature and abnormal or absent and the QRS complex to be premature.

**avian leukosis c.,** see *avian leukosis,* under *leukosis.*

**avian sarcoma c.,** see under *sarcoma.*

**basal c. of choroid,** lamina basalis choroideae.

**branched-chain α-keto acid dehydrogenase c.,** a multienzyme complex composed of 3-methyl-2-oxobutanoate dehydrogenase (lipoamide) [EC 1.2.4.4], dihydrolipoamide dehydrogenase [EC 1.8.1.4], and dihydrolipoamide acyltransferase, with thiamine pyrophosphate, lipoic acid, $NAD^+$, FAD, and coenzyme A as cofactors. The integrated complex catalyzes the oxidative decarboxylation of the keto acid analogues of the branched-chain amino acids leucine, isoleucine, and valine. Deficiency of any enzyme of the complex causes maple syrup urine disease. See also *lipoamide dehydrogenase deficiency.*

**calcarine c.,** calcar avis.

**Carney's c.,** an autosomal dominant symptom complex consisting of myxomas of the soft tissues, spotty skin pigmentation, tumors of the adrenal gland, pituitary, and testicle, and schwannomas of peripheral nerves. Called also *Carney's syndrome* or *triad.*

**castration c.,** in psychoanalytic theory, unconscious thoughts and motives stemming from fear of loss of genitals as punishment for forbidden sexual desires.

**chlorophyllin copper c. sodium,** the sodium salt of copper-chelated chlorophyllin, applied topically for the deodorization of skin lesions and administered orally to deodorize the urine and feces in colostomy, ileostomy, or incontinence.

**EAHF c.,** the symptom complex of eczema, asthma, and hay fever.

**Eisenmenger's c.,** a defect of the interventricular septum with severe pulmonary hypertension, hypertrophy of the right ventricle, and latent or overt cyanosis.

**Electra c.,** the counterpart in females of the Oedipus complex, which was originally applied only to males, involving the daughter's love for her father and jealousy or resentment toward her mother; the term is now rarely used since *Oedipus c.* (q.v.) has come to be applied to both sexes.

**eosinophilic granuloma c.,** a group of skin lesions in cats, of unknown etiology but apparently related to one another, characterized by lesions on the skin surface and eosinophilia of the dermis. There are three types: the mild *eosinophilic ulcer* on the lip; the circumscribed pruritic *eosinophilic plaque,* usually on the abdomen or groin; and the *linear granuloma,* usually on the thigh or near the mouth.

**factor IX c.** [USP], a sterile, freeze-dried powder consisting of partially purified factor IX fraction, as well as concentrated factor II, VII, and X fractions, of venous plasma from healthy human donors.

**feline respiratory disease c.,** a group of contagious viral infections of the upper respiratory tract in cats, characterized by fever, sneezing and coughing, and discharges from the nose and eyes. The usual cause is infection with a herpesvirus (feline herpesvirus 1) or a calicivirus. See also *feline viral rhinotracheitis.* Called also *feline influenza.*

**Ghon c.,** primary c.

**glucoamylase c.,** the two heat-stable maltases in humans, also known as α-glucosidases [EC 3.2.1.20] (q.v.); they are described as a complex because the two enzyme activities are formed as a single polypeptide which is cleaved to form a heterodimer active within the brush border of the intestinal mucosa; the enzyme activities catalyze the hydrolysis of α-1,4 linked glucose residues from the nonreducing ends of disaccharides and oligomers such as maltose, amylose, amylopectin, and glycogen.

**β-glycosidase c.,** the enzyme complex comprising lactase and glycosylceramidase (phlorhizin hydrolase) activities, occurring in the brush border membrane of the intestinal mucosa and hydrolyzing lactose as well as cellobiose and cellotriose; it is a single polypeptide, processed from a larger precursor, with two catalytic sites for the two enzyme activities. See also *lactase deficiency.*

**Golgi c.,** a complex cuplike structure within cells, made up of several elements, each consisting of a number of flattened sacs (cisternae) with associated vacuoles and vesicles. Golgi complexes are membrane sites of the formation of the carbohydrate side chains of glycoproteins and mucopolysaccharides, and of other substances. The secretion vacuoles migrate through the cell membrane and release the glycoproteins and mucopolysaccharides, and thus play a role in internal and external secretion. Cytochemical studies have shown that they are also sites of formation of primary lysosomes and give rise to the acrosome of spermatozoa and the nematocyst of *Hydra.* Called also *Golgi apparatus* and *Golgi body.*

**H-2 c.,** the murine major histocompatibility complex.

**hapten-carrier c.,** the antigen formed by the coupling of a hapten and a carrier protein.

**HLA c.,** the human major histocompatibility complex; see *HLA antigens,* under *antigen.*

**immune c.,** antigen-antibody c.

**inclusion c's,** compounds in which molecules of one type are enclosed within cavities in the crystalline lattice of another substance.

**inferiority c.,** unconscious feelings of inadequacy, producing timidity or, as a compensation, exaggerated aggressiveness and expression of superiority; based on Alfred Adler's concept that everyone is born with a feeling of inferiority stemming from real or imagined physical or psychological deficiency, with the manner in which the inferiority is handled determining behavior.

**interpolated ventricular premature c.,** a ventricular premature complex that does not block conduction of the next sinus beat and thus is not associated with a compensatory pause.

**jumped process c.,** dislocation of articular processes of spine.

**junctional c.,** the intercellular arrangement between adjacent columnar epithelial cells, consisting of the zonula occludens, the zonula adherens, and the desmosome.

**junctional premature c.,** atrioventricular junctional premature c.

**juvenile nephronophthisis–medullary cystic disease c.,** a term preferred by some authorities to denote familial juvenile nephronophthisis (def. 1, q.v.), on the grounds that although the diseases comprising the complex have identical clinical manifestations, the modes of inheritance and ages of onset are different. Four variants are recognized: a sporadic form; familial juvenile nephronophthisis (def. 2), inherited recessively; renal-retinal dysplasia, inherited recessively and associated with retinitis pigmentosa; and adult-onset medullary cystic disease, inherited dominantly.

**juxtaglomerular c.,** see under *apparatus.*

**K c.,** a burst of high-voltage slow waves seen on the electroencephalogram during sleep; it may occur spontaneously or in response to a sensory (usually auditory) stimulus.

**α-keto acid dehydrogenase c.,** any of the enzyme complexes catalyzing the oxidative decarboxylation of α-keto acids; see *branched-chain α-keto acid dehydrogenase c., α-ketoglutarate dehydrogenase c.,* and *pyruvate dehydrogenase c.*

**α-ketoglutarate dehydrogenase c.,** a multienzyme complex consisting of at least three distinct enzymes: oxoglutarate dehydrogenase (lipoamide) [EC 1.2.4.2], dihydrolipoamide *S*-succinyltransferase [EC 2.3.1.61], and dihydrolipoamide dehydrogenase [EC 1.8.1.4]. The integrated enzyme complex catalyzes the overall reaction α-ketoglutarate + coenzyme A + $NAD^+$ = succinyl coenzyme A + NADH + $CO_2$. Thiamine pyrophosphate, lipoic acid, and FAD are required as cofactors. The reaction is a part of the tricarboxylic acid cycle. (See illustration under *cycle.*) Deficiency of the last component causes lipoamide dehydrogenase deficiency.

**lactase–phlorhizin hydrolase c.,** β-glycosidase c.

**LCMV-LASV c.,** a group of antigenically related viruses comprising the Old World arenaviruses (Ippy, Lassa, lymphocytic choriomeningitis, Mobala, and Mopeia viruses). Lassa virus (Lassa fever) and lymphocytic choriomeningitis virus are pathogenic for humans.

**Lutembacher's c.,** see under *syndrome.*

**major histocompatibility c. (MHC),** the genes determining the major histocompatibility antigens, in all species a group of closely linked multiallelic genes located in a small region on one chromosome; designated the *HLA c.* in humans and the *H-2 c.* in mice.

**membrane attack c. (MAC),** the pentamolecular complex C5b,6,7,8,9 that is the cytolytic agent of the complement system; see under *complement.*

**Meyenburg's c's,** bile duct hamartomas.

**oculomotor nuclear c.,** nucleus nervi oculomotorius.

**Oedipus c.,** in psychoanalytic theory, the feelings and conflicts occurring in a child during the phallic phase of psychosexual development that result from sexual attraction to the opposite-sex parent, including envious, aggressive feelings toward the same-sex parent.

**olivary c., inferior,** complexus olivaris inferior.

**olivary c., superior,** nucleus olivaris superior.

**osteomeatal c.,** the area of the nasal cavity between the middle and inferior turbinates, where the drainages from the frontal, ethmoid, and maxillary sinuses have their confluence.

**perihypoglossal c., perihypoglossal nuclear c.,** nuclei perihypoglossales.

**pore c.,** a nuclear pore and its annulus considered together.

**posterior nuclear c. of thalamus,** nuclei posteriores thalami.

**primary c.,** 1. the combination of a parenchymal pulmonary lesion *(Ghon focus* or *tubercle)* and a corresponding lymph node focus, occurring in primary tuberculosis, usually in children; it may undergo cellular necrosis and eventually calcify. Similar lesions may also be associated with other mycobacterial infections and with fungal infections such as histoplasmosis and coccidioidomycosis. Called also *Ghon c.* and *Ranke c.* 2. the primary cutaneous lesion at the site of infection in the skin, e.g., chancre in syphilis and tuberculous chancre.

**primary inoculation c., primary tuberculous c.,** see under *tuberculosis.*

**pyruvate dehydrogenase c.,** a multienzyme complex consisting of at least three distinct enzymes: pyruvate dehydrogenase (lipoamide) [EC 1.2.4.1], dihydrolipoamide *S*-acetyltransferase [EC 2.3.1.12], and dihydrolipoamide dehydrogenase [EC 1.8.1.4]. The integrated enzyme complex requires the cofactors thiamine pyrophosphate, lipoic acid, coenzyme A, FAD, and $NAD^+$. It catalyzes the formation of acetyl coenzyme A from pyruvate and coenzyme A, using $NAD^+$ as an electron acceptor; the acetyl coenzyme A is used in fatty acid synthesis, for acetylations, and for oxidation via the tricarboxylic acid cycle. Deficiency of any component of the complex results in lacticacidemia, ataxia, and psychomotor retardation. See also *lipoamide dehydrogenase deficiency.*

**QRS c.,** the portion of the electrocardiogram comprising the Q, R, and S waves, together representing ventricular depolarization. See also *electrocardiogram.*

**QS c.,** in the electrocardiogram, a QRS complex in which the Q wave returns to baseline but does not produce a positive (R) wave; the entire ventricular complex is negative.

**Ranke c.,** primary c.

**sicca c.,** primary Sjögren's syndrome.

**sling ring c.,** tracheal stenosis caused by pulmonary sling syndrome combined with a fixed complete cartilaginous ring.

**stomatitis-pneumoenteritis c.,** peste des petits ruminants.

**sucrase-isomaltase c.,** the enzyme complex comprising sucrase and α-dextrinase (isomaltase) activities, occurring in the brush border of the intestinal mucosa and hydrolyzing maltose as well as maltotriose and some other glycosidic bonds; the enzymes are synthesized as a single polypeptide and cleaved to form a heterodimer, each possessing a separate catalytic site. See also *sucrase-isomaltase deficiency.*

**symptom c.,** a set of symptoms that occur together; the sum of signs of any morbid state; a syndrome.

**synaptonemal c.,** a thick, threadlike structure formed during the zygotene (synaptic) stage of meiosis by the intertwining of two leptotene chromosomes so that they are indistinguishable separately.

**Tacaribe c.,** a group of antigenically related viruses comprising the New World arenaviruses (Amapari, Flexal, Guanarito, Junin, Machupo, Parana, Pichinde, Tacaribe, and Tamiami viruses). Guanarito virus (Venezuelan hemorrhagic fever), Junin virus (Argentinian hemorrhagic fever), and Machupo virus (Bolivian hemorrhagic fever) are pathogenic for humans.

**ureterotrigonal c.,** ureterovesical junction.

**urobilin c.,** a hypothetical substance consisting of a number of urobilinogen molecules linked together, which is the form in which urobilinogen exists in the blood and tissues.

**VATER c.,** a nonrandom association of congenital anomalies consisting of *v*ertebral defects, imperforate *a*nus, *t*racheoesophageal fistula, and *r*adial and *r*enal dysplasia.

**ventral lateral c. of thalamus,** nuclei ventrales laterales thalami.

**ventral medial c. of thalamus,** nuclei ventrales mediales thalami.

**ventricular c.,** the combined QRS complex and T wave, together representing ventricular electrical activity. Cf. *atrial c.*

**ventricular premature c. (VPC),** an ectopic beat arising in the ventricles and stimulating the myocardium prematurely. It is characterized by an early, wide, oddly shaped QRS complex with an ST segment and T wave directed opposite to the QRS complex, usually without resetting of the sinus node, and with occasional fusion beats. It may occur in normal hearts but often is indicative of organic heart disease.

**ventrobasal c. of thalamus,** nuclei ventrobasales thalami.

**com·plex·ion** (kom-plek'shən) [L. *complexio* combination] the color and appearance of the skin of the face.

**com·plex·us** (kom-plek'səs) [L. "encompassing"] complex.
**c. basa'lis choroi'deae,** lamina basalis choroideae.
**c. oliva'ris infe'rior** [TA], inferior olivary complex: a folded band of gray matter that encloses a white core *(hilum nuclei olivaris inferioris)* and that produces the elevation called the *oliva* on the medulla oblongata. It is a nuclear complex that receives heavy projections from the spinal cord, mesencephalon, and cerebral cortex and projects fibers via the contralateral inferior cerebellar peduncle, mostly to the neocerebellum, with a few going to the vermis. Called also *nuclei olivares inferiores* [TA alternative], *inferior olivary nuclei, nuclei olivares caudales,* and *caudal olivary nuclei.*
**c. sti'mulans cor'dis** [TA], conducting system of heart: a system of specialized muscle fibers that generate and rapidly transmit cardiac impulses and serve to coordinate contractions, comprising the sinoatrial node, atrioventricular node, bundle of His and its right and left bundle branches, and the subendocardial branches (rami subendocardiales) of Purkinje fibers. Called also *systema conducens cordis* [TA alternative].

**com·pli·ance** (kom-pli'əns) [MeSH: Compliance] 1. the quality of yielding to pressure or force without disruption. 2. an expression of the ability to yield to pressure without disruption, such as the distensibility of an air- or fluid-filled organ, e.g., the lung or urinary bladder, measured in terms of unit of volume change per unit of pressure change. Symbol C. It is the reciprocal of *elastance.*
**dynamic c.,** compliance measured while an organ is expanding or contracting; in the lung it is a measure of the change in volume per change in inflation pressure during air flow into or out of the lung. Cf. *static c.*
**static c.,** compliance measured in the absence of any motion. Cf. *dynamic c.*

**com·pli·cat·ed** (kom'plĭ-kāt"əd) [L. *complicare* to infold] involved; associated with other injuries, lesions, or diseases.

**com·pli·ca·tion** (kom"plĭ-ka'shən) [L. *complicatio* from *cum* together + *plicare* to fold] 1. a disease or diseases concurrent with another disease. 2. the concurrence of two or more diseases in the same patient.

**Com·po·cil·lin-VK** (com"po-sil'in) trademark for a preparation of penicillin V potassium.

**com·po·mer** (kom'pə-mər) a hybrid resin matrix composite filling material that contains components of glass ionomer but whose hardening occurs by polymerization of the resin matrix.

**com·po·nent** (kom-po'nənt) 1. a constituent element or part. 2. in neurology, a series of neurons forming a functional system for conducting the afferent and efferent impulses in the somatic and splanchnic (visceral) mechanisms of the body.
**anterior c.,** Angle's term for "a forward propelling force which is the result of meshing and pounding of the occlusal inclined planes of the teeth and the mesial inclination of the teeth."
**complement c's, c's of complement,** see *complement.*
**group-specific c.,** vitamin D–binding protein, a serum protein of particular use in anthropological studies because of the great differences in gene frequency in different populations.
**M c.,** [*M*yeloma or *M*acroglobulinemia], an abnormal monoclonal immunoglobulin with a characteristic electrophoretic pattern, occurring in the serum of patients with plasma cell dyscrasias and formed by the proliferating concentrations of immunoglobulin-producing cells.
**plasma thromboplastin c. (PTC),** factor IX; see under *coagulation factors,* at *factor.*
**secretory c. (SC),** a 70,000 dalton glycopeptide occurring in secretory IgA; not synthesized by the plasma cell producing the IgA but added while the IgA is crossing the epithelium; it may protect secretory IgA from proteolytic attack after secretion, or it may play some role in the process of secretion. Secretory component deficiency has been seen in a few patients; there is complete lack of IgA in external secretions although serum IgA is normal. Called also *secretory piece.*
**somatic motor c.,** the system of neurons that conduct impulses to the somatic effectors (skeletal muscle) of the body.
**somatic sensory c.,** the system of neurons conducting impulses from the somatic receptors.
**splanchnic motor c.,** the system of neurons conducting impulses to the splanchnic (visceral) effectors (cardiac muscle, smooth muscle, and glands).
**splanchnic sensory c.,** the system of neurons conducting impulses from the splanchnic (visceral) receptors.
**visceral motor c.,** splanchnic motor c.
**visceral sensory c.,** splanchnic sensory c.

**Com·pos·i·tae** (kəm-poz'ĭ-te) a large family of flowering herbs, shrubs, and trees having composite flower heads in which a number of small florets are on each head; many well-known genera such as *Chrysanthemum,* the sunflowers, and the dandelions are in this family. Called also *Asteraceae.*

**composite** (kəm-poz'it) 1. made up of unlike parts. 2. resin matrix c.
**resin matrix c.,** a synthetic resin, usually acrylic based, to which a high percentage (about 75 to 80 per cent) of an inert filler has been added (such as glass beads or rods, borosilicate glass powder, or natural silica); filler particles are coated with a coupling agent that binds them to the resin matrix. Used chiefly in dental restorative procedures. Called also *composite* and *composite resin.*

**com·pos men·tis** (kom'pos men'tis) [L.] sound of mind; sane.

**com·pound** (kom'pound) [L. *componere* to place together] 1. in chemistry, a substance that consists of two or more chemical elements in union. 2. in genetics, a genotype in which there are two different mutant alleles at a locus, or a phenotype produced by such a genotype. Cf. *homozygote, homozygous.*
**acyclic c.,** an open-chain compound; see under *chain.*
**addition c.,** a compound formed by the union of two or more compounds or elements.
**aliphatic c.,** an open-chain compound that does not contain multiple bonds; a saturated compound. See *open chain,* under *chain.*
**APC c.,** a preparation of acetylsalicylic acid, phenacetin, and caffeine citrate.
**aromatic c.,** a closed-chain compound in which the ring contains several double bonds; see *closed chain,* under *chain.*
**benzene c's,** aromatic c's.
**benzoin tincture c.,** see under *tincture.*
**binary c.,** a compound whose molecule is composed of atoms of only two elements.
**clathrate c.,** a type of inclusion complex in which molecules of one type are trapped within cavities of another substance, such as within a crystalline lattice structure or large molecule; called also *occlusion c.*
**closed-chain c.,** see under *chain.*
**condensation c.,** a compound that is formed by union of substances with the loss of one or more molecules, usually of low molecular weight, as water or ammonia.
**cyclic c.,** a closed-chain compound; see *closed chain,* under *chain.*
**diazo c.,** a compound containing the group $—N_2—$.
**endothermic c.,** one whose formation is attended with absorption of heat from the environment.
**energy rich c's,** high energy c's.
**exothermic c.,** one whose formation is attended with loss of heat to the environment.
**Grignard c.,** see under *reagent.*
**heterocyclic c.,** a chemical substance that contains a ring-shaped nucleus composed of dissimilar elements.
**high energy c's,** compounds containing high energy bonds (q.v.); because they yield high levels of free energy on hydrolysis, the compounds are basic to the energy supply of living organisms. Important classes include acid anhydrides (e.g., adenosine triphosphate, aminoacyl adenylates), enol phosphates (e.g., phospho*enol*pyruvate), thioesters (e.g., acetyl coenzyme A), and phosphagens (e.g., phosphocreatine). Called also *energy rich c's.*
**Hurler-Scheie c.,** see under *syndrome.*
**inorganic c.,** a compound that contains no carbon.
**isocyclic c.,** a chemical substance that contains a ring-shaped nucleus composed of the same elements throughout.
**low energy c's,** compounds yielding relatively low levels of free energy on hydrolysis, such as adenosine monophosphate, glucose 1-phosphate, and glucose 6-phosphate. Cf. *high energy c's.*
**nonpolar c's,** compounds in which electrons are shared equally by the two atoms forming a bond and which therefore do not ionize in solution, e.g., the paraffins, olefins, and cyclic compounds.
**occlusion c.,** clathrate c.
**open-chain c.,** see under *chain.*
**organic c.,** a compound of chemical elements containing carbon atoms.
**organometallic c.,** one in which carbon is linked to a metal.
**polar c's,** compounds in which the electrons are unequally shared by the two atoms forming the bond and which therefore may act as dipoles or, in some instances, completely ionize. They include the alcohols, water, and ammonia.
**quaternary c.,** one composed of four elements.
**quaternary ammonium c.,** see *tetraethylammonium.*
**ring c.,** see *closed chain,* under *chain.*
**saturated c.,** a compound in which the combining capacities of all the elements are satisfied.
**substitution c.,** a compound formed by replacement of elements of a molecule by other elements.
**ternary c., tertiary c.,** a compound composed of three elements.
**unsaturated c.,** a compound in which the combining capacities of all the elements are not satisfied; see *unsaturated.*

**com·press** (kom'prəs) [L. *compressus*] a pad or bolster of folded gauze or other material, applied with pressure; it is sometimes medicated, and may be wet or dry, hot or cold.

**com·pres·si·bil·i·ty** (kom-pres″ĭ-bil′ĭ-te) 1. the capability of a substance to be condensed or reduced in volume. 2. the volume decrease per unit of a substance produced by a unit increase in pressure.

**com·pres·sion** (kom-presh′ən) [L. *compressio* from *comprimere* to squeeze together] 1. the act of pressing together; an action exerted upon a body by an external force which tends to diminish its volume and augment its density. 2. in embryology, the shortening or omission of certain stages during development.
**c. of the brain,** cerebral c.
**cardiac c.,** see under *massage.*
**cerebral c.,** any condition in which the brain is compressed, such as by a tumor or other mass, blood clot, or abscess. Called also *c. of the brain.*
**digital c.,** compression of a blood vessel by the fingers for the purpose of checking hemorrhage.
**instrumental c.,** compression of a blood vessel by instruments.
**nerve c.,** entrapment of a nerve; cf. *entrapment neuropathy.*
**spinal c., spinal cord c.,** a condition in which pressure is exerted on the spinal cord, as by a tumor, spinal fracture, etc.; its manifestations, which vary with location and degree of pressure, may include pain, paresthesias, and sensory and motor disturbances.

**com·pres·sor** (kom-pres′or) [L.] 1. an instrument that compresses a vessel. 2. a muscle that compresses or presses down on a part.
**Deschamps' c.,** an instrument for the direct compression of an artery.
**c. na′ris,** pars transversa musculi nasalis.
**Sehrt's c.,** see under *clamp.*
**shot c.,** a forceps for compressing split shot applied to sutures; see also *shotted suture,* under *suture.*
**c. ure′thrae,** musculus sphincter urethrae.
**c. vagi′nae,** the bulbospongiosus muscle in the female.

**com·pres·so·ri·um** (kom″pres-or′e-əm) pl. *compresso′ria* [L.] a device for applying graduated pressure upon objects under microscopic examination.

**Comp·ton effect, scattering** (komp′tən) [Arthur Holly *Compton,* American physicist, 1892–1962; winner of the Nobel prize in physics for 1927] see under *effect* and *scattering.*

**com·pul·sion** (kom-pul′shən) 1. a persistent and irresistible impulse to perform an irrational or apparently useless act. 2. a compulsive act or ritual; a repetitive and stereotyped action, such as hand-washing, touching, counting, and checking, that is engaged in for an unknown or unconscious purpose.
**repetition c.,** in psychoanalytic theory, the impulse to reenact earlier emotional experiences or traumatic behavior.

**com·pul·sive** (kom-pul′siv) 1. pertaining to or characterized by compulsion. 2. perfectionistic, rigid, stubborn, indecisive, preoccupied with work; the personality traits of obsessive-compulsive personality (disorder).

**con-** [L., from *cum* with] a prefix meaning with or together. It appears as *co-* before a vowel or *h; l* before another *l; m* before *b, m,* or *p;* and *r* before another *r.*

**ConA** concanavalin A.

**con·al·bu·min** (kon″al-bu′min) [MeSH: Conalbumin] a glucoprotein, formed by the acidification of egg white to pH 3.9, containing 2.1 per cent of mannose and 0.7 per cent of galactose; the noncrystalline part of egg albumin.

**co·na·tion** (ko-na′shən) in psychology, the power that impels to effort of any kind; the conscious tendency to act.

**con·a·tive** (kon′ə-tiv) pertaining to the basic strivings of a person, as expressed in his behavior and actions.

**con·a·van·ine** (kon″ə-van′in) a basic amino acid from soybean meal, $\alpha$-amino-$\gamma$-guanidinoxybutyric acid.

**c-*onc*** [cellular *onc*ogene] a proto-oncogene that has been activated within the host so that oncogenicity results. Cf. *v*-onc. See also table of oncogenes at *oncogene.*

**con·ca·nav·a·lin A** (kon″kə-nav′ə-lin) [*con-* + *canavalin*] [MeSH: Concanavalin A] a lectin isolated from the jack bean; it is a hemagglutinin that agglutinates mammalian erythrocytes and a mitogen that stimulates predominantly T lymphocytes. Abbreviated ConA.

**con·cas·sa·tion** (kon″kə-sa′shən) the act of breaking up roots or woods into small pieces in order that their active principles may be more easily extracted by solvents.

**con·cat·e·nate** (kən-kat′ə-nāt) [*con-* + L. *catena* chain] to fasten or link together, as in a chain.

**con·cat·e·na·tion** (kən-kat″ə-na′shən) a series of events or objects occurring together or in sequence.

**Con·ca·to's disease** (kon-kah′tōz) [Luigi Maria *Concato,* Italian physician, 1825–1882] see under *disease.*

**con·cave** (kon-kāv′) [L. *concavus*] having a rounded, somewhat depressed surface, resembling the hollowed inner surface of a segment of a sphere.

**con·cav·i·ty** (kon-kav′ĭ-te) [*con-* + *cavity*] a hollowed-out area on the surface of an organ or other structure.

**con·ca·vo·con·cave** (kən-ka″vo-kon′kāv) concave on each of two opposite surfaces.

**con·ca·vo·con·vex** (kən-ka″vo-kon′veks) concave on one surface and convex on the opposite one.

**con·ceive** (kən-sēv′) 1. to become pregnant. 2. to take in, grasp, or form in the mind.

**con·cen·trate** (kon′sən-trāt) [*con-* + *centrum*] 1. to bring to a common center; to gather together at one point. 2. to increase the strength by diminishing the bulk of, as of a liquid; to condense. 3. a drug or other preparation that has been strengthened by the evaporation of its nonactive parts.
**benzylpenicilloyl polylysine c.** [USP], a concentrated solution of benzylpenicilloyl polylysine with one or more suitable buffers; used as a diagnostic aid for penicillin sensitivity.
**lactulose c.** [USP], a solution of sugars prepared from lactose, consisting principally of lactulose, with small quantities of lactose and galactose and traces of other related sugars and water.
**liver c.,** a dried, unfractionated product produced from a water extract derived from mammalian liver; used as a hematopoietic.
**plant protease c.,** a concentrate of bromelains, proteolytic enzymes derived from pineapple plants; used to reduce inflammation and edema, and to accelerate tissue repair.
**vitamin c.,** a concentrated medicinal preparation of a vitamin or vitamins.

**con·cen·tra·tion** (kon″sən-tra′shən) [L. *concentratio*] 1. increase in strength by evaporation. 2. the ratio of the mass or volume of a solute to the mass or volume of the solution or solvent. Cf. *molarity, molality, normality,* and *mole fraction.*
**hydrogen ion c.,** the degree of concentration of hydrogen ions in a solution; it is inversely related to the pH of the solution by the equation $[H^+] = 10^{-pH}$.
**ionic c.,** the number of moles of an ion that are contained in the unit volume of a solution or in the unit mass of solvent.
**limiting isorrheic c. (LIC),** the upper limit of urinary concentration at which a steady state consistent with effective physiologic regulation of solute and water balance can be maintained.
**mass c.,** the mass of a constituent substance divided by the volume of the mixture, as milligrams per liter (mg/L), etc.
**maximum cell (MC) c.,** the maximum number of microorganisms that can be produced in a given volume of culture medium.
**maximum urinary c. (MUC),** the highest attainable concentration of a solute or of the collective solutes of the urine; in humans it is about 1200 mOsm/kg $H_2O$.
**mean corpuscular hemoglobin c. (MCHC),** the average hemoglobin concentration in erythrocytes, conventionally expressed in "per cent" meaning grams per deciliter of red cells, obtained by dividing the blood hemoglobin concentration (in g/dL) by the hematocrit (in L/L): MCHC = Hb/Hct.
**minimal alveolar c. (MAC),** the alveolar concentration of anesthetic that at a pressure of 1 atmosphere produces immobility in 50 per cent of subjects exposed to a noxious stimulus.
**minimal bactericidal c. (MBC),** the lowest concentration of a given antibiotic required to kill a specific organism. Called also *minimal lethal c.*
**minimal inhibitory c. (MIC),** the lowest concentration of a given antibiotic that inhibits the growth of a specific organism.
**minimal isorrheic c. (MIC),** the lower limit of urinary concentration at which a steady state consistent with effective physiologic regulation of solute and water balances can be maintained.
**minimal lethal c. (MLC),** minimal bactericidal c.
**molar c.,** the concentration of a substance expressed in terms of molarity; symbol *c.* See *molar*[1].

**con·cen·tric** (kən-sen′trik) [L. *concentricus,* from *con-* together + *centrum* center] having a common center; extending out equally in all directions from a common center.

**con·cept** (kon′sept) the image of a thing as held in the mind.

**con·cep·tion** (kən-sep′shən) [L. *conceptio*] 1. the onset of pregnancy, marked by fertilization of an oocyte by a sperm or spermatozoon; formation of a visible zygote. 2. concept.

**con·cep·tive** (kən-sep′tiv) 1. able to become pregnant. 2. pertaining to conception.

**con·cep·tus** (kən-sep′təs) [L.] the sum of derivatives of a fertilized oocyte (ovum) at any stage of development from fertilization until birth, including extraembryonic membranes as well as the embryo or fetus.

**con·cha** (kong'kə) pl. *con'chae* [L.; Gr. *konchē*] 1. a shell. 2. in anatomical nomenclature, a structure or part that resembles a sea shell in shape.
**c. auri'culae** [TA], **c. auricula'ris,** concha of auricle: the hollow of the auricle of the external ear, bounded anteriorly by the tragus and posteriorly by the anthelix.
**c. bullo'sa,** a cystic distention of the middle nasal concha, sometimes seen in chronic rhinitis.
**c. of cranium,** calvaria.
**ethmoidal c., inferior,** c. nasalis media.
**ethmoidal c., superior,** c. nasalis superior.
**ethmoidal c., supreme,** c. nasalis suprema.
**nasal c., inferior,** c. nasalis inferior.
**nasal c., middle,** c. nasalis media.
**nasal c., supreme,** c. nasalis suprema.
**nasal c., superior,** c. nasalis superior.
**c. nasa'lis infe'rior** [TA], c. nasi inferior.
**c. nasa'lis me'dia** [TA], c. nasi media.
**c. nasa'lis supe'rior** [TA], c. nasi superior.
**c. nasa'lis supre'ma** [TA], c. nasi suprema.
**c. na'si infe'rior** [TA], inferior nasal concha: a thin bony plate with curved margins, articulating with the ethmoid, maxilla, and lacrimal and palatine bones, and forming the lower part of the lateral wall of the nasal cavity, and the mucous membrane covering the plate; called also *inferior spongy bone, inferior turbinate bone,* and *inferior turbinate.*
**c. na'si me'dia** [TA], middle nasal concha: the lower of two bony plates projecting from the inner wall of the ethmoid labyrinth and separating the superior from the middle meatus of the nose, and the mucous membrane covering the plate; called also *inferior ethmoidal c., ethmoid cornu, middle turbinate bone,* and *middle turbinate.*
**c. na'si supe'rior** [TA], superior nasal concha: the upper of two bony plates projecting from the inner wall of the ethmoid labyrinth and forming the upper boundary of the superior meatus of the nose, and the mucous membrane covering the plate. Called also *superior ethmoidal c., superior turbinate bone, superior spongy bone,* and *superior turbinate.*
**c. na'si supre'ma** [TA], supreme nasal concha: a thin bony plate occasionally found projecting from the inner wall of the ethmoid labyrinth above the bony superior nasal concha, and the mucous membrane covering the plate; called also *highest* or *supreme turbinate bone, supreme ethmoidal c.,* and *supreme turbinate.*
**nasoturbinal c.,** agger nasi.
**c. sphenoida'lis** [TA], sphenoidal concha: a thin curved plate of bone at the anterior and lower part of the body of the sphenoid bone, on either side, forming part of the roof of the nasal cavity; called also *sphenoturbinal bone* or *ossicle* and *Bertin's bone* or *ossicle.*

**con·chae** (kong'ke) [L.] genitive and plural of *concha.*

**con·chi·form** (kong'kĭ-form) [*concha* + *form*] shaped like one half of a bivalve shell.

**con·chio·lin·os·teo·my·eli·tis** (kong-ki″ə-lin-os″te-o-mi″ə-li'tis) a form of osteomyelitis occurring in pearl workers.

**con·chi·tis** (kong-ki'tis) an inflammation of a concha.

**con·choi·dal** (kong-koi'dəl) like a shell.

**con·cho·scope** (kong'ko-skōp) [*concha* + *-scope*] a speculum for examining the walls of the nasal cavity.

**con·cho·tome** (kong'ko-tōm) [*concha* + *-tome*] turbinotome.

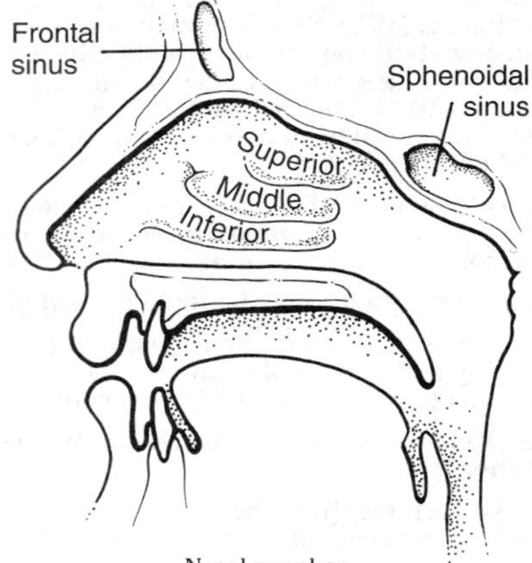


Nasal conchae.

**con·chot·o·my** (kong-kot'ə-me) turbinotomy.

**Concis.** abbreviation for L. *conci'sus,* cut.

**con·cli·na·tion** (kon″klĭ-na'shən) intorsion.

**con·coc·tion** (kən-kok'shən) [L. *concoctio*] 1. a mixture of medicinal substances usually prepared with the aid of heat. 2. the digestive process.

**con·com·i·tant** (kən-kom'ĭ-tənt) [L. *concomitans,* from *cum* together + *comes* companion] accompanying; accessory; joined with another. Cf. *concurrent.*

**con·cor·dance** (kən-kor'dəns) [L. *concordare* to agree] in genetics, the occurrence of a given trait in both members of a twin pair, as opposed to discordance.

**con·cor·dant** (kən-kor'dənt) 1. exhibiting concordance. 2. belonging to closely related species; said of transplanted tissue. See under *xenograft.*

**con·cre·ment** (kon'krə-mənt) [L. *concrementum,* from *concrescere* to grow together] a concretion, especially a calcified tubercle or similar mass.

**con·cres·cence** (kən-kres'əns) [*con-* + L. *crescere* to grow] 1. a growing together; a union of parts originally separate. 2. in embryology, the flowing together and piling up of cells. 3. in dentistry, the union of the roots of two approximating teeth by a deposit of cementum.

**con·cre·tio** (kən-kre'she-o) [L.] concretion.
**c. cor'dis, c. pericar'dii,** a form of adhesive pericarditis in which the pericardial cavity is obliterated.

**con·cre·tion** (kən-kre'shən) [L. *concretio,* from *concrescere* to grow together] 1. a calculus or inorganic mass in a natural cavity or in the tissues of an organism. 2. abnormal union of adjacent parts. 3. the process of becoming harder or more solid.
**calculous c.,** articular calculus.
**preputial c.,** a concretion formed beneath a tight foreskin through deposit of urinary salts on the accumulated smegma.
**prostatic c's,** rounded and often lamellated masses of amyloid-like material present in many prostatic alveoli.
**tophic c.,** tophus.

**con·cur·rent** (kon-kur'ənt) happening at the same time; simultaneous. Cf. *concomitant.*

**con·cus·sion** (kən-kush'ən) [L. *concussio*] a violent jar or shock, or the condition which results from such an injury.
**abdominal c., hydraulic,** abdominal injury produced in persons in the water by violent underwater explosions.
**air c.,** see under *blast*[2].
**c. of the brain,** loss of consciousness as the result of a blow to the head or sudden movement of the brain within the head as from violent shaking of the head. In *mild concussion* there is transient loss of consciousness with possible impairment of higher mental functions, such as retrograde amnesia and emotional lability. In *severe concussion* there is prolonged unconsciousness with impairment of the functions of the brain stem, such as transient loss of respiratory reflex, vasomotor activity, and dilatation of the pupils. Cf. *brain contusion,* under *contusion.*
**c. of the labyrinth,** trauma to the labyrinth, usually from a blow on or explosion near the ear, resulting in tinnitus and deafness.
**pulmonary c.,** mechanical damage to the lungs produced by an explosion. See *blast chest,* under *chest* and *blast injury,* under *injury.*
**c. of the retina,** commotio retinae.
**c. of the spinal cord,** transient spinal cord dysfunction due to mechanical injury.

**con·den·sa·tion** (kon″dən-sa'shən) [L. *condensare* to pack close together] 1. the act of rendering or the process of becoming more compact; compression. 2. the packing of dental filling material into a prepared tooth cavity. 3. a mental process in which one symbol stands for a number of components and contains all the emotion associated with them. 4. conversion from the gaseous state to the liquid or solid state; gas liquefaction.

**con·den·ser** (kən-den'sər) [L. *condensare* to make thick, press close together] 1. a vessel or apparatus for condensing gases or vapors. 2. the lens in a microscope located just above the light source that aligns all available light into one beam. 3. an apparatus by which charges of electricity can be accumulated, consisting of two conducting surfaces separated by a nonconductor. 4. in dentistry, an instrument used to pack a plastic filling material into the prepared cavity of a tooth.
**Abbe's c.,** as originally designed, a two-lens condenser combination placed below the stage of a microscope.
**automatic c.,** mechanical c.
**back-action c.,** one with a U-shaped shank so that the force applied is toward the operator. Called also *reverse c.*
**cardioid c.,** a special type of condenser for illuminating a specimen in darkfield microscopy.

**darkfield c.**, one with a central stop, permitting production of a hollow cone of light having its apex in the plane of the specimen.
**foot c.**, one with a long, angled, foot-shaped nib.
**gold c.**, one for compacting gold filling material into the prepared cavity in dental restorations.
**mechanical c.**, one equipped with a spring-activated, pneumatic, or electronic mechanism for compacting the restorative material in a prepared tooth cavity through repeated blows. Called also *automatic c.*
**paraboloid c.**, a special type of condenser for illuminating a specimen in darkfield microscopy.
**reverse c.**, back-action c.

**con·di·tion** (kən-dish'ən) to train; to subject to conditioning.

**con·di·tion·ing** (kon-dish'un-ing) 1. learning in which a stimulus initially incapable of evoking a certain response acquires the ability to do so by repeated pairing with another stimulus that does elicit the response. Called also *classical c., pavlovian c.,* and *respondent c.* 2. in physical medicine, improvement of physical condition with a program of exercises; called also *physical chemistry*
**aversive c.**, learning in which punishment or other unpleasant stimulation is used to associate negative feelings with an undesirable response and so reduce the frequency of that response.
**avoidance c.**, a form of operant conditioning in which an organism is trained to avoid certain responses or situations associated with negative consequences.
**classical c.**, conditioning (def. 1).
**instrumental c.**, learning in which the frequency of a particular voluntary response is altered by the application of positive or negative consequences; called also *operant c.*
**operant c.**, instrumental c.
**pavlovian c.**, conditioning (def. 1).
**respondent c.**, conditioning (def. 1).

**con·dom** (kon'dəm) [L. *condus* a receptacle; according to some authorities a corruption of *Condon,* the inventor] a sheath or cover for the penis, worn during coitus to prevent impregnation or infection.

**con·duc·tance** (kən-duk'təns) capacity for conducting or ability to convey; the unit of electrical conductance is the siemens. Symbol *G.*
**airway c.**, the reciprocal of airway resistance: the air flow divided by the mouth-to-alveoli pressure difference.

**con·duc·tion** (kən-duk'shən) [L. *conductio*] the transfer of sound waves, heat, nervous impulses, or electricity; see also under *system.*
**aberrant c.**, cardiac conduction through pathways not normally conducting cardiac impulses, particularly through ventricular tissue.
**aerial c.**, air c.
**aerotympanal c.**, the conduction of sound to the inner ear through the air and tympanum.
**air c.**, the conduction of sound to the inner ear through the external auditory canal and middle ear.
**anomalous c.**, conduction of the sinus impulse over accessory conducting pathways, thus avoiding the delay in passage through the normal atrioventricular node.
**anterograde c.**, transmission of a cardiac impulse in the normal direction, from the sinus node to the ventricles; used particularly to describe forward conduction through the atrioventricular node.
**antidromic c.**, the conduction of a nerve impulse in a direction contrary to the normal direction, as occurs in experimental conduction studies. It may occur naturally in some neurons of the dorsal roots of the spinal cord, although evidence suggests that the phenomenon may actually result from ephaptic transmission rather than backward transmission.
**avalanche c.**, the conduction of nerve impulses which takes place when the terminals of one neuron come in contact with the bodies of several neurons, resulting in widespread discharge following relatively little input.
**bone c.**, the conduction of sound to the inner ear through the bones of the skull; called also *cranial c., osteotympanic c.,* and *tissue c.*
**concealed c.**, incomplete penetration of a propagating impulse through the cardiac conducting system such that electrocardiograms reveal no evidence of transmission but the behavior of one or more subsequent impulses is somehow affected.
**concealed retrograde c.**, retrograde conduction blocked in the atrioventricular node; it does not produce an extra P wave but leaves the node refractory to the next normal sinus beat, manifest as lengthening of the PR interval of that beat.
**cranial c.**, bone c.
**decremental c.**, the delay or failure of propagation of an impulse in the atrioventricular node resulting from progressive decrease in the rate of the rise and amplitude of the action potential as it spreads through the node.
**delayed c.**, slowed cardiac impulse propagation resulting in an interval greater than 0.2 second between atrial and ventricular contractions, as occurs in first degree heart block.

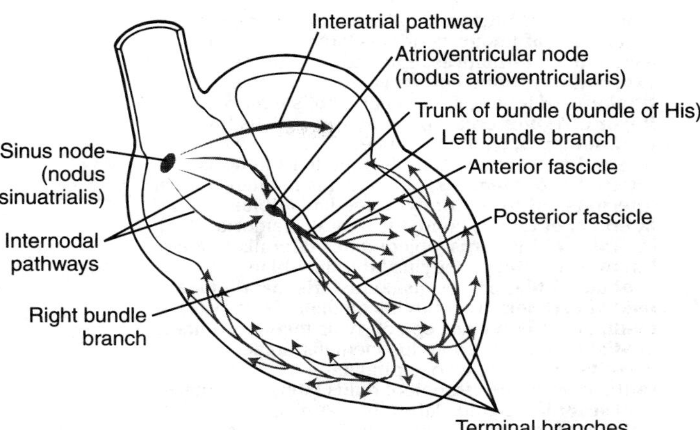

Diagrammatic view of the conducting system of the heart, showing anterograde conduction of the cardiac impulse.

**ephaptic c.**, the conduction of a nerve impulse across an ephapse, as opposed to synaptic conduction.
**osteotympanic c.**, bone c.
**retrograde c.**, transmission of a cardiac impulse backward in the ventricular to atrial direction; particularly, conduction from the atrioventricular node into the atria.
**saltatory c.**, the rapid passage of a potential from node (of Ranvier) to node of a myelinated nerve fiber, rather than along the full length of the membrane.
**synaptic c.**, the conduction of a nerve impulse across a synapse.
**tissue c.**, bone c.
**ventriculoatrial c.**, retrograde conduction, specifically that in which the impulse is conducted from ventricles to atria.
**volume c.**, in electromyography, the loss of measurable action potential because of spreading of current away from the source through conducting media such as extracellular fluid.

**con·duc·tiv·i·ty** (kon″dək-tiv'ĭ-te) the capacity of a body to transmit a flow of electricity or heat; it is the conductance per unit area of the body. When expressed in figures electrical conductivity is the reciprocal of resistivity.

**con·duc·tor** (kən-duk'tər) [L.] 1. a material that possesses conductivity; a substance that transmits electricity. 2. a grooved director for surgical use.

**con·du·it** (kon'doo-it) channel (def. 1).
**ileal c.**, the surgical anastomosis of the ureters to one end of a detached segment of ileum, the other end being used to form a stoma on the abdominal wall (see *ureteroileostomy*).

**con·du·pli·ca·to cor·po·re** (kən-doo″plĭ-kā'to kor'por-e) [L. "with the body doubled up"] spontaneous evolution.

**con·du·ran·gin** (kon″du-rang'gin) either of two glycosides from condurango; in large amounts they are poisonous but in small amounts they are used as a bitter in homeopathic medicine.

**con·du·ran·go** (kon″du-rang'go) [Spanish American] 1. *Marsdenia condurango.* 2. the bark of *Marsdenia condurango,* which contains condurangin and is normally poisonous but has been used as a bitter in homeopathic medicine.

**con·dy·lar** (kon'də-lər) pertaining to a condyle.

**con·dy·lar·thro·sis** (kon″dəl-ahr-thro'sis) [*condyle* + *arthrosis* (def. 1)] articulatio ellipsoidea.

**con·dyle** (kon'dīl) [L. *condylus;* Gr. *kondylos* knuckle] a rounded projection on a bone; see *condylus.*

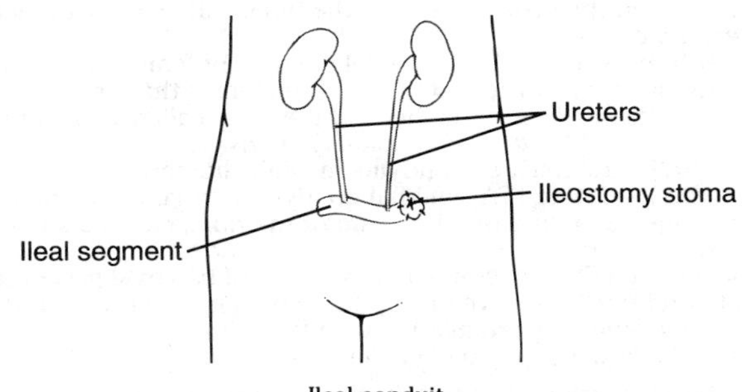

Ileal conduit.

**extensor c. of humerus,** epicondylus lateralis humeri.
**external c. of femur,** condylus lateralis femoris.
**external c. of humerus,** epicondylus lateralis humeri.
**external c. of tibia,** condylus lateralis tibiae.
**fibular c. of femur,** condylus lateralis femoris.
**flexor c. of humerus,** epicondylus medialis humeri.
**c. of humerus,** condylus humeri.
**internal c. of femur,** condylus medialis femoris.
**internal c. of humerus,** epicondylus medialis humeri.
**internal c. of tibia,** condylus medialis tibiae.
**lateral c. of femur,** condylus lateralis femoris.
**lateral c. of humerus,** epicondylus lateralis humeri.
**lateral c. of tibia,** condylus lateralis tibiae.
**c. of mandible,** processus condylaris mandibulae.
**medial c. of femur,** condylus medialis femoris.
**medial c. of humerus,** epicondylus medialis humeri.
**medial c. of tibia,** condylus medialis tibiae.
**occipital c.,** condylus occipitalis.
**radial c. of humerus,** epicondylus lateralis humeri.
**c. of scapula,** angulus lateralis scapulae.
**tibial c. of femur,** condylus medialis femoris.
**ulnar c. of humerus,** epicondylus medialis humeri.

**con·dy·lec·to·my** (kon′dəl-ek′tə-me) [*condyle* + *-ectomy*] excision of a condyle.

**con·dy·li** (kon′də-li) [L.] genitive and plural of *condylus.*

**con·dyl·i·cus** (kon-dil′ĭ-kəs) pertaining to a condyle; condylar.

**con·dyl·i·on** (kon-dil′e-ən) [Gr. *kondylion* knob] the most lateral point on the surface of the caput mandibulae.

**con·dy·loid** (kon′də-loid) [*condyle* + *-oid*] resembling a condyle or knuckle.

**con·dy·lo·ma** (kon″də-lo′mə) pl. *condylomas* or *condylo′mata* [Gr. *kondylōma,* knuckle or knob] 1. c. acuminatum. 2. rarely, c. latum.
**c. acumina′tum,** a papilloma with a central core of connective tissue in a treelike structure covered with epithelium, usually occurring on the mucous membrane or skin of the external genitals or in the perianal region; although the lesions are usually few in number, they may aggregate to form large cauliflower-like masses. Caused by the human papilloma virus, it is infectious, and autoinoculable. Called also *acuminate* or *venereal wart, moist* or *mucous papule,* and *verruca acuminata.*
**flat c.,** c. latum.
**giant c.,** Buschke-Löwenstein tumor.
**c. la′tum,** a broad and flat syphilitic condyloma located in warm, moist, intertriginous areas, especially about the anus and external genitals; it may become hypertrophic and erode to form a soft, red mass with a moist, weeping surface. Called also *flat c.*
**pointed c.,** c. acuminatum.

**con·dy·lo·ma·ta** (kon″də-lo′mə-tə) [L.] plural of *condyloma.*

**con·dy·lo·ma·toid** (kon″də-lo′mə-toid) resembling a condyloma.

**con·dy·lo·ma·to·sis** (kon″də-lo″mə-to′sis) the presence of numerous condylomas.

**con·dy·lom·a·tous** (kon″də-lom′ə-təs) of the nature of a condyloma.

**con·dy·lot·o·my** (kon″də-lot′ə-me) [*condyle* + *-tomy*] surgical incision or division of a condyle or of condyles.

**Con·dy·lox** (kon′dĭ-loks) trademark for preparations of podofilox.

**con·dy·lus** (kon′də-ləs) pl. *con′dyli* [L.; Gr. *kondylos* knuckle] [TA] condyle: a rounded projection on a bone, usually for articulation with another.
**c. hu′meri** [TA], condyle of humerus: the distal end of the humerus, including the various fossae as well as the trochlea and capitulum.
**c. latera′lis fe′moris** [TA], lateral condyle of femur: the lateral of the two surfaces at the distal end of the femur that articulate with the superior surfaces of the head of the tibia; called also *external* or *fibular condyle of femur.*
**c. latera′lis hu′meri,** epicondylus lateralis humeri.
**c. latera′lis ti′biae** [TA], lateral condyle of tibia: the lateral articular eminence on the proximal end of the tibia; called also *external condyle of tibia.*
**c. media′lis fe′moris** [TA], medial condyle of femur: the medial of the two surfaces at the distal end of the femur that articulate with the superior surfaces of the head of the tibia; called also *internal* or *tibial condyle of femur,* and *c. tibialis femoris.*
**c. media′lis hu′meri,** epicondylus medialis humeri.
**c. media′lis ti′biae** [TA], medial condyle of tibia: the medial articular eminence on the proximal end of the tibia; called also *internal condyle of tibia.*
**c. occipita′lis** [TA], occipital condyle: one of two oval processes on the lateral portions of the occipital bone, on either side of the foramen magnum, for articulation with the atlas.
**c. tibia′lis fe′moris,** c. medialis femoris.

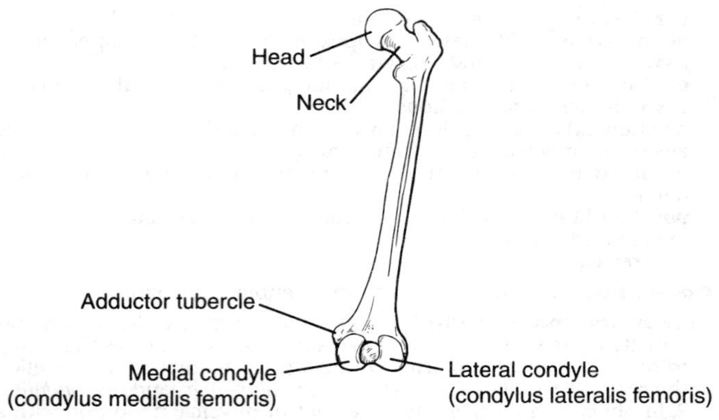


Posterior view of right femur, showing the medial (condylus medialis femoris) and lateral (condylus lateralis femoris) condyles.

**cone** (kōn) [L. *conus,* from Gr. *konos*] 1. a solid figure or body with a circular base tapering to a point; called also *conus* [TA]. 2. retinal c. 3. in radiology, a conical or open-ended cylindrical structure attached over the portal of the x-ray tube housing, used as an aid in centering the radiation beam on the target field and as a guide to source-to-film distance; also, often designed to collimate primary and/or scattered radiation, and/or to retain disks for added filtration. 4. in root canal therapy, a solid substance with a tapered form, usually made of gutta-percha or silver, fashioned to conform to the shape of a root canal. 5. a marine snail of the family Conidae.
**acrosomal c.,** an axial body of the spermatozoon between the acrosomal granule and the nucleus.
**antipodal c.,** the cone of rays opposite the spindle fibers of the amphiaster.
**arterial c.,** conus arteriosus.
**attraction c.,** fertilization c.
**bifurcation c.,** the cone-shaped structure at the bifurcation of a dendrite.
**cerebellar pressure c.,** a deformity of the brain caused by increased intracranial pressure, which forces the cerebellar tonsils downward into the spinal canal.
**ectoplacental c.,** the thickened trophoblast of the blastocyst in rodents that becomes the fetal portion of the placenta.
**elastic c.,** conus elasticus.
**ether c.,** an apparatus placed over the face for the administration of ether by inhalation.
**fertilization c.,** a bulging of the cytoplasm in the oocyte (ovum) at the site of contact of a spermatozoon, which gradually engulfs the spermatozoon and then retracts, carrying the spermatozoon inward; called also *attraction c.*
**growth c.,** a bulbous enlargement of the growing tip of an axon.
**gutta-percha c.,** in root canal therapy, a plastic radiopaque cone made from gutta-percha combined with other ingredients, available in standard sizes conforming to the dimensions of root canal reamers and files; used to fill and seal the canal in conjunction with sealer cements. Called also *gutta-percha point.*
**Haller's c's,** lobuli epididymidis.
**implantation c.,** axon hillock.
**c. of light,** the triangular reflection of light seen on the membrana tympani; called also *Politzer's c.* and *light reflex.*
**long c.,** in dental radiology, a tubular cone (see *cone,* def. 3) designed to establish an extended anode-to-skin distance, usually in a range of 10 to 25 cm or more.
**medullary c.,** conus medullaris.
**ocular c.,** a cone of light in the eye, the base being on the cornea, the apex on the retina; called also *visual c.*
**Politzer's c.,** c. of light.
**pressure c.,** the area of compression exerted by a mass in the brain, as in uncal or transtentorial herniation.
**primitive c.,** the conelike arrangement of the collecting tubules in the kidney.
**retinal c.,** a visual cell that serves light and color vision and visual acuity. The synaptic terminal is a broad, flattened pedicle. Outside the fovea the dendritic segments are relatively short and squat with blunt, rounded tips; within the fovea the segments are elongated and narrow and thus resemble rods. There are 6 million to 7 million cones, of which some 10 per cent are concentrated in the fovea, the remainder being fairly uniformly distributed over the rest of the retina. Called also *cone, cone cell,* and *visual c.* See also *visual cell,* under *cell,* and *retinal rod,* under *rod.*
**sarcoplasmic c.,** the conical mass of sarcoplasm at each end of the nucleus of a smooth or cardiac muscle fiber.
**short c.,** in dental radiology, a conical or tubular cone (see *cone,* def. 3) having as one of its functions the establishment of an anode-to-skin distance of up to 10 to 25 cm.

**silver c.**, see under *point.*
**terminal c. of spinal cord,** conus medullaris.
**twin c's,** cone cells of the retina in which two cells are blended.
**ureteral c.**, the upper conic part of the ureter; at ordinary rates of urine flow it is filled with urine during the resting phase of the renal pelvis and emptied during activity.
**visual c.**, 1. ocular c. 2. retinal c.
**Tyndall c.**, the murky cone of scattered light seen when a colloid is viewed at right angles to the incident beam, due to the Tyndall effect; it distinguishes colloids from crystalloids.

**cone-nose** (kōn'nōs″) cone-nose bug.

**Con·es·tron** (kon-es'tron) trademark for a preparation of conjugated estrogens.

**co·nex·us** (ko-nek'səs) pl. *conex'us* [L. "connection," from *conectere* to join together] *connexus.*

**co·ney** (ko'ne) hyrax.

**con·fab·u·la·tion** (kon″fab-u-la'shən) [l. *confabulari* to converse together] unconscious filling in of gaps in memory with fabricated facts and experiences, most commonly associated with organic pathology. It differs from lying in that the patient has no intention to deceive and believes the fabricated memories to be real. Called also *fabrication* and *fabulation.*

**con·fec·tion** (kən-fek'shən) [L. *confectio*] a medicated conserve, sweetmeat, or electuary.
**c. of senna,** a mild laxative containing powdered senna with other ingredients.

**con·fer·tus** (kən-fər'təs) [L.] close together; confluent.

**con·fi·den·ti·al·i·ty** (kon″fĭ-den″she-al'ĭ-te) [MeSH: Confidentiality] the principle in medical ethics that the information a patient reveals to a health care provider is private and has limits on how and when it can be disclosed to a third party; usually the provider must obtain permission from the patient to make such a disclosure.

**con·fig·u·ra·tion** (kən-fig″u-ra'shən) the arrangement of parts of a whole. In chemistry, the spatial arrangement of atoms in a molecule, the property that distinguishes a compound from its stereoisomers. Cf. *constitution.*
***cis* c.**, in genetics, arrangement of two or more loci, especially pseudoalleles, occurring on the same chromosome of a homologous pair. Cf. trans *c.*
***trans* c.**, in genetics, arrangement of two or more loci, especially pseudoalleles, on opposite chromosomes of a homologous pair. Cf. cis *c.*

**con·flict** (kon'flikt) in psychiatry, a psychic struggle, often unconscious, arising from the clash of incompatible or opposing impulses, wishes, drives, or external demands.
**approach-approach c.**, conflict resulting from two available goals which are desirable but incompatible.
**approach-avoidance c.**, conflict resulting from a single goal having both desirable and undesirable consequences or qualities.
**avoidance-avoidance c.**, conflict resulting from the desire to avoid two equally distasteful alternatives.
**extrapsychic c.**, conflict between a person's wishes or needs and the expectations or desires of others.
**intrapersonal c.**, intrapsychic c.
**intrapsychic c.**, conflict between incompatible and often unconscious wishes, impulses, needs, thoughts, or demands within one's own mind. Called also *intrapersonal c.*

**con·flu·ence** (kon'floo-əns) [L. *confluens* running together] 1. a place of running together; the meeting of streams. 2. in embryology, the flowing of cells, a component process of gastrulation.
**c. of sinuses,** confluens sinuum.

**con·flu·ens** (kon'floo-əns) [L., from *confluere* to run together] confluence.
**c. si'nuum** [TA], confluence of (venous) sinuses: the dilated point of confluence of the superior sagittal, straight, occipital, and two transverse sinuses of the dura mater, lodged in a depression at one side of the internal occipital protuberance; called also *torcular Herophili.*

**con·flu·ent** (kon'floo-ənt) [L. *confluens* running together] becoming merged; not discrete.

**con·fo·cal** (kon-fo'kəl) having the same focus.

**con·for·ma·tion** (kon″for-ma'shən) the particular shape of an entity. In chemistry, the spatial arrangement of atoms in a molecule produced by rotations about single bonds, the property that distinguishes different conformers (conformational isomers) from each other.

**con·form·er** (kon-for'mər) 1. any of the group of structures that are produced by rotations about single bonds in a molecule. 2. a device that covers the surface of a spherical eye implant, used following enucleation to preserve the shape of the conjunctival fornices prior to the fitting of a cosmetic prosthesis.

**con·found·er** (kən-foun'dər) a third variable that can indirectly distort the statistical relationship between two variables under manipulation or observation.

**con·found·ing** (kon-foun'ding) interference by a third variable so as to distort the association being studied between two other variables, because of a strong relationship with both of the other variables; a relationship between two causal factors such that their individual contributions can not be separated.

**con·fri·ca·tion** (kon″frĭ-ka'shən) [L. *confricatio*] the rubbing of a drug to the consistency of a powder.

**con·fron·ta·tion** (kon″frən-ta'shən) [*con-* + *frons* face] the act of facing or being made to face one's own attitudes and shortcomings, the way one is perceived, and the consequences of one's behavior, or of causing another to face these things; a therapeutic technique which demonstrates where change must begin, but which also has destructive potential.

**con·fu·sion** (kən-fu'zhən) [L. *confusus,* past participle of *confundere* to mix together] [MeSH: Confusion] disturbed orientation in regard to time, place, or person, sometimes accompanied by disordered consciousness.

**con·fu·sion·al** (kən-fu'zhən-əl) pertaining to, characterized by, or resulting in confusion.

**cong.** abbreviation for L. *con'gius,* gallon.

**con·ge·la·tion** (kon″jə-la'shən) [L. *congelatio*] frostbite or freezing.

**con·ge·ner** (kon'jə-nər) [*con-* + *genus* race] 1. something closely related to another thing, as a member of the same genus, a muscle having the same function as another, or a chemical compound closely related to another in composition and exerting similar or antagonistic effects, or something derived from the same source or stock. 2. a secondary product in alcohol fermentation that helps to determine the composition of the final product.

**con·ge·ner·ic** (kon″jə-ner'ik) pertaining to a congener.

**con·gen·er·ous** (kən-jen'ər-əs) [*con-* + *genus* race] having a common action or function; derived from the same source. See *congener.*

**con·gen·ic** (kən-jen'ik) [*con-* + L. *genus* race, kind] pertaining to two inbred strains of animals that are genetically identical except at a single locus or a few specified loci so that their known genetic differences are expressed in the same "genetic background." A congenic strain is produced by outbreeding a strain and then eliminating the background genes by many generations of backcrosses while maintaining the desired genetic differences by selection of progeny. Called also *coisogenic.*

**con·gen·i·tal** (kən-jen'ĭ-təl) [L. *congenitus* born together] existing at, and usually before, birth; referring to conditions that are present at birth, regardless of their causation. Cf. *hereditary.*

**con·gest·ed** (kən-jest'əd) overloaded, as with blood; in a state of congestion.

**con·ges·tin** (kən-jes'tin) a toxic substance derived from the tentacles of sea anemones which, when injected into dogs, causes intense congestion of the splanchnic vessels, and hemorrhage; originally called *actinocongestin.*

**con·ges·tion** (kən-jes'chən) [L. *congestio,* from *congerere* to heap together] excessive or abnormal accumulation of fluid, as of blood in a part. Cf. *hyperemia.*
**active c.**, accumulation of blood in a part on account of the dilatation of the lumen of its supplying blood vessels.
**functional c.**, increased vascularization and flow of blood to an organ during the performance of its function. Called also *physiologic c.*
**hypostatic c.**, congestion of the lowest part of an organ by reason of the action of gravity when the circulation is much enfeebled.
**neurotonic c.**, that which is due to irritation of the vasodilator nerves.
**passive c.**, the congestion of a part due to the obstruction to the escape of blood from the part; called also *venous c.*
**physiologic c.**, functional c.
**pulmonary c.**, engorgement of the pulmonary vessels, with transudation of fluid into the alveolar and interstitial spaces *(pulmonary edema)*; it occurs in cardiac disease, infections, and certain injuries.
**venous c.**, passive c.

**con·ges·tive** (kən-jes'tiv) pertaining to, characterized by, or resulting in congestion.

**con·gi·us** (kon'je-əs) [L.] a gallon; abbreviated C. or cong.

**con·glo·bate** (kon'glo-bāt) [L. *conglobatus*] forming a rounded mass or clump; said of certain glands and of a form of acne.

**con·glo·ba·tion** (kon″glo-ba'shən) the act of forming, or the state of being formed, into a rounded mass.

**con·glom·er·ate** (kən-glom'ər-āt) [L. *con-* together + *glomerare* to heap] heaped together.

**con·glu·tin** (kən-gloo′tin) a protein from almonds and from seeds of various leguminous plants.

**con·glu·ti·nant** (kən-gloo′tĭ-nənt) [L. *conglutinare* to glue together] promoting union, as of the edges of a wound.

**con·glu·ti·na·tio** (kən-gloo″tĭ-na′she-o) [L. *conglutinare* to glue together] conglutination (def. 2).
**c. orifi′cii exter′ni,** a condition in labor in which the circular fibers around the cervical os will not relax, and the cervix does not dilate.

**con·glu·ti·na·tion** (kən-gloo″tĭ-na′shən) 1. agglutination by conglutinin or immunoconglutinin of bacteria or erythrocytes in the presence of specific antibody or complement components. 2. abnormal adhesion; see *adhesion* (def. 2).

**con·glu·ti·nin** (kən-gloo′tĭ-nin) a nonimmunoglobulin bovine serum protein that aggregates immune complexes with conglutinogen activity (inactivated C3b) in the presence of divalent cations. It has been used as an indicator system, replacing complement fixation, in serologic tests, and in the detection of immune complexes. Not to be confused with *immunoconglutinin.* Called also *bovine colloid.*
**immune c.,** immunoconglutinin.

**con·glu·ti·no·gen** (kən-gloo′tĭ-no-jən) the capacity of certain immune complexes to react with conglutinin due to the fixation of the complement component C3 and the subsequent inactivation of C3b by factor I (formerly called *conglutinogen-activating factor [KAF]*).

**con·go·phil·ic** (kon″go-fil′ik) [*Congo red* + *-philic*] staining with Congo red.

**co·ni** (ko′ni) [L.] genitive and plural of *conus.*

**con·ic** (kon′ik) conical.

**con·i·cal** (kon′ĭ-kəl) cone-shaped.

**Co·ni·dae** (kon′ĭ-de) the cones, a family of gastropods of the order Neogastropoda that live in warm ocean water. Some members of the genus *Conus* have a poisonous bite.

**co·nid·ia** (ko-nid′e-ə) [L.] plural of *conidium.*

**co·nid·i·al** (ko-nid′e-əl) 1. pertaining to or of the nature of conidia. 2. bearing conidia.

**Co·ni·dio·bo·lus** (ko-nid″e-ob′o-ləs) [*conidium* + Gr. *bolos* a throw] a genus of fungi of the family Entomophthoraceae, having few septa in the mycelium and producing few zygospores but many chlamydospores and a large number of conidia that are ejected from the conidiophores. *C. corona′tus* is usually a saprobe but sometimes causes entomophthoromycosis in humans and horses. *C. incon′gruus* has been isolated from a few cases of human entomophthoromycosis.

**co·nid·io·gen·e·sis** (ko-nid″e-o-jen′ə-sis) the development of conidia; the two principal types are *blastic c.* and *thallic c.*
**blastic c.,** that in which a fertile hypha or conidiogenous cell enlarges or blows out to form a conidium before delimitation by a septa takes place; two types are distinguished, *holoblastic c.* and *enteroblastic c.*
**enteroarthric c.,** thallic-arthric c. in which conidia are formed from only the inner part of the wall of the conidiogenous cell.
**enteroblastic c.,** blastic c. in which only the inner part of the cell wall is used to form the conidium.
**holoarthric c.,** thallic-arthric c. in which conidia are formed from both walls of the conidiogenous cell.
**holoblastic c.,** blastic c. in which all of the cell wall is used to form the conidium.
**holothallic c.,** thallic c. in which just one portion of the conidiogenous cell disarticulates to form a conidium.
**thallic c.,** that in which an entire parent cell becomes a conidium with formation of a septum, without enlargement or new growth. Two types are distinguished: *holothallic c.* and *thallic-arthric c.*
**thallic-arthric c.,** thallic c. in which several conidia form by separation at the septa; two types are distinguished: *enteroarthric c.* and *holoarthric c.*

**co·nid·io·gen·ous** (kə-nid″e-oj′ə-nəs) producing conidia.

**co·ni·di·o·ma** (kə-nid″e-o′mə) pl. *conidio′mata.* A specialized, polyhyphal structure bearing conidia.

**co·nid·io·phore** (ko-nid′e-o-for) [*conidium* + *-phore*] the branch of the mycelium of a fungus that bears conidia.
**determinate c.,** one whose growth does not continue after a conidium has started to form.
**indeterminate c.,** one that continues to lengthen as sporulation continues.
**macronematous c.,** one noticeably different morphologically from its hypha.
**micronematous c.,** one similar morphologically to its hypha.

**co·nid·io·spore** (ko-nid′e-o-spor) [Gr. *konidion* a particle of dust + *spore*] conidium.

**co·nid·i·um** (kə-nid′e-əm) pl. *conid′ia* [L., from Gr. *konidion* a particle of dust] An asexual fungal spore that is deciduous (shed at maturity) and formed by budding or splitting off from the summit of a conidiophore. See also *aleurioconidium* and *chlamydoconidium.* Called also *conidiospore* and *exospore.*

**co·ni·ine** (co′ne-ēn) a poisonous alkaloid found in *Conium maculatum;* it causes gastrointestinal irritation and paralysis with respiratory failure in many animal species, including humans.

**coni(o)-** [Gr. *konis* dust] combining form denoting a relationship to dust.

**co·nio·fi·bro·sis** (ko″ne-o-fi-bro′sis) [*conio-* + *fibrosis*] a form of pneumoconiosis marked by an exuberant growth of connective tissue caused by a specific irritant, as in asbestosis, silicosis, and silicotuberculosis.

**co·ni·ol·o·gy** (ko-ne-ol′ə-je) [*conio-* + *-logy*] the scientific study of dust and its influence and its effects on plant and animal life.

**co·nio·lymph·sta·sis** (ko″ne-o-limf′stə-sis) a form of pneumoconiosis caused by dusts that act by blocking the lymphatics.

**co·ni·om·e·ter** (ko″ne-om′ə-tər) konimeter.

**co·nio·phage** (ko′ne-o-fāj″) [*conio-* + *-phage*] a macrophage that ingests dust particles.

**co·ni·o·sis** (ko″ne-o′sis) [Gr. *konis* dust] a disease state caused by the inhalation of dust, such as byssinosis or pneumoconiosis.

**Co·nio·spor·i·um** (ko″ne-o-spor′e-əm) *Cryptostroma.*

**co·nio·spo·ro·sis** (ko″ne-o-spo-ro′sis) maple bark disease.

**co·ni·ot·o·my** (ko″ne-ot′ə-me) cricothyrotomy.

**co·nio·tox·i·co·sis** (ko″ne-o-tok″sĭ-ko′sis) a form of pneumoconiosis in which the irritants affect the tissues directly.

**Co·ni·um** (ko-ni′əm) [L.; Gr. *kōneion*] a genus of plants of the family Umbelliferae. *C. macula′tum* L. is the poison hemlock; see under *hemlock.*

**con·iza·tion** (kon″ĭ-za′shən) [MeSH: Conization] the removal of a cone of tissue, as in partial excision of the cervix uteri.
**cold c.,** that done with a cold knife, as opposed to electrocautery.
**laser c.,** that done with a laser beam.

**con·joined** (kən-joind′) joined together; united; see *conjoined twins,* under *twins.*

**con·ju·gal** (kon′jo͞o-gəl) [*con-* + *jugal*] pertaining to marriage; pertaining to husband and wife.

**con·ju·gant** (kon′jo͞o-gənt) either individual of a pair of organisms or gametes during the process of conjugation; after separation, each is known as an *exconjugant.*

**con·ju·ga·ta** (kon″jo͞o-ga′tə) 1. conjugate (def. 1). 2. conjugata anatomica pelvis.
**c. anato′mica pel′vis** [TA], anatomical conjugate of pelvis: the anteroposterior diameter of the pelvic inlet (superior aperture of the pelvis), measured from the superior margin of the symphysis pubis to the sacrovertebral angle; called also *conjugata vera pelvis; anteroposterior* or *conjugate diameter of pelvis; anatomical, internal,* or *true conjugate diameter;* and *anatomical, internal,* or *true conjugate.*
**c. diagona′lis pel′vis** [TA], diagonal conjugate of pelvis: a diameter of the pelvic inlet; the distance from the posterior surface of the pubis to the tip of the sacral promontory. Called also *diagonal conjugate diameter.*
**c. exter′na pel′vis** [TA], external conjugate of pelvis: the distance from the depression under the last lumbar spine to the upper margin of the pubis; called also *external conjugate diameter* and *Baudelocque's diameter* or *line.*
**c. ve′ra pel′vis** [TA], c. anatomica pelvis.
**c. ve′ra obstet′rica,** obstetric conjugate diameter.

**con·ju·gate** (kon′jo͞o-gāt) [L. *conjugatus* yoked together] 1. the distance between two specified opposite points on the periphery of the pelvic inlet. Called also *conjugate diameter* and *pelvic c.* 2. conjugata anatomica pelvis. 3. the product of chemical conjugation.
**anatomical c., anatomical c. of pelvis,** conjugata anatomica pelvis.
**diagonal c.,** diagonal conjugate diameter.
**external c.,** conjugata externa pelvis.
**internal c.,** conjugata anatomica pelvis.
**obstetric c.,** obstetric conjugate diameter.
**pelvic c.,** conjugate (def. 1).
**true c.,** conjugata anatomica pelvis.

**con·ju·ga·tion** (kon″jo͞o-ga′shən) [L. *conjugatio* a blending] 1. the act of joining together or the state of being conjugated. 2. a sexual process seen in bacteria, ciliate protozoa, and certain fungi in which nuclear material is exchanged during the temporary fusion of two cells (conjugants). In *bacterial genetics,* a form of sexual reproduction in which a donor bacterium (male) contributes some, or all, of its DNA (in the form of a replicated set) to a recipient (female), which then incorporates differing genetic information into its own chromosome by recombination and passes the recombined set on to its progeny by replication. In *ciliate protozoa,* two conjugants of separate mating types exchange micronuclear material and then separate, each now being a fertilized cell. In certain fungi, the process involves fusion of two gametes, resulting in union of their nuclei and formation of a zygote. 3. in chemistry, the joining together of two compounds to produce another compound, such as the combination of a toxic product with some substance in the body to form a detoxified product that can then be eliminated, or the binding of tumor-specific monoclonal antibodies to cytotoxic drugs in immunotherapy.

**con·junc·ti·va** (kən-jənk′ti-və) pl. *conjunc′tivae* [L.] [MeSH: Conjunctiva] the delicate membrane that lines the eyelids *(palpebral conjunctiva)* and covers the exposed surface of the sclera *(bulbar* or *ocular conjunctiva);* called also *tunica conjunctiva* [TA].

**con·junc·ti·val** (kən-junk′tĭ-vəl) pertaining to the conjunctiva.

**con·junc·ti·vi·plas·ty** (kən-junk′tĭ-vĭ-plas″te) conjunctivoplasty.

**con·junc·ti·vi·tis** (kən-junk″tĭ-vi′tis) [MeSH: Conjunctivitis] inflammation of the conjunctiva, generally consisting of conjunctival hyperemia associated with a discharge.
**actinic c.,** conjunctivitis produced by ultraviolet (actinic) rays, as that of Klieg lights, therapeutic lamps, or acetylene torches.
**acute contagious c., acute epidemic c.,** a mucopurulent, epidemic conjunctivitis caused by *Haemophilus aegyptius,* occurring in the spring or fall, with the same symptoms as acute catarrhal conjunctivitis. Called also *pinkeye.*
**acute hemorrhagic c.,** a highly contagious disease, certain epidemics of which have been associated etiologically with enteroviruses, characterized by subconjunctival hemorrhage varying from minute petechiae to confluent hemorrhages, and by sudden swelling of the eyelids and congestion, redness, and pain in the eye.
**allergic c., anaphylactic c.,** hay fever.
**angular c.,** conjunctivitis with characteristic reddening at the canthi, usually due to Morax-Axenfeld bacillus or *Staphylococcus aureus;* called also *diplobacillary c.* and *Morax-Axenfeld c.*
**arc-flash c.,** actinic c.
**atopic c.,** allergic conjunctivitis of the immediate type, due to such airborne allergens as pollens, dusts, spores, and animal hair.
**atropine c.,** follicular conjunctivitis from continued use of atropine.
**blennorrheal c.,** gonorrheal c.
**calcareous c.,** c. petrificans.
**catarrhal c., acute,** an acute, infectious conjunctivitis associated with cold or catarrh and marked by vivid hyperemia, edema, loss of translucence, and mucous or mucopurulent discharge. Called also *mucopurulent c., simple c.,* and *simple acute c.*
**catarrhal c., chronic,** a mild, chronic conjunctivitis with only slight hyperemia and mucous discharge. It may be a sequel to acute catarrhal conjunctivitis, or the result of eyestrain, dust, glare, or ingrown lashes.
**chemical c.,** that due to exposure to chemical irritants.
**croupous c.,** pseudomembranous c.
**diphtheritic c.,** membranous conjunctivitis occurring as a primary infection caused by *Corynebacterium diphtheriae* or secondarily to diphtheria of the respiratory tract.
**diplobacillary c.,** angular c.
**eczematous c.,** phlyctenular c.
**Egyptian c.,** trachoma.
**epidemic c.,** acute contagious c.
**follicular c.,** a form characterized by dense localized infiltrations of lymphoid tissue that occur as a response to irritation.
**gonococcal c., gonorrheal c.,** a severe form caused by infection with gonococci, marked by greatly swollen conjunctivae and eyelids and by a profuse purulent discharge. The infection is bilateral in newborns, who acquire it from an infected vaginal passage; it is usually unilateral in adults, who acquire it by autoinoculation into the eye of other gonococcal infections, e.g., gonococcal urethritis, either in themselves or in others. Called also *blennorrheal c.* and *gonoblennorrhea.* Cf. *gonorrheal ophthalmia* and *ophthalmia neonatorum,* under *ophthalmia.*
**granular c.,** trachoma.
**inclusion c.,** conjunctivitis caused by an organism *(Chlamydia trachomatis)* of the psittacosis-lymphogranuloma venereum-trachoma group; it affects primarily newborn infants, beginning as an acute purulent conjunctivitis that leads to papillary hypertrophy of the palpebral conjunctiva. Called also *inclusion blennorrhea* and *swimming pool c.*
**infantile purulent c.,** ophthalmia neonatorum.
**Koch-Weeks c.,** acute contagious c.
**larval c.,** myiasis of the conjunctiva.
**lithiasis c.,** c. petrificans.
**c. medicamento′sa,** conjunctivitis due to medication.
**membranous c.,** severe conjunctivitis marked by the presence of a membrane on the inner surface of the lids formed by the profuse fibrinous exudation from the cul-de-sac, which on attempted removal leaves a raw, bleeding surface; it is caused by various bacteria, including *Corynebacterium diphtheriae,* streptococci, gonococci, and pneumococci. Cf. *pseudomembranous c.*
**meningococcus c.,** conjunctivitis occurring as a complication of epidemic cerebrospinal meningitis.
**molluscum c.,** conjunctivitis occurring as a complication of molluscum contagiosum.
**Morax-Axenfeld c.,** angular c.
**mucopurulent c.,** acute catarrhal c.
**necrotic infectious c.,** a unilateral, purulent, necrotic conjunctivitis marked by small, diffuse, elevated, white spots in the palpebral conjunctiva and fornices, with ipsilateral swelling of the preauricular, parotid, and submaxillary lymph glands. Called also *Pascheff's c.*
**neonatal c.,** ophthalmia neonatorum.
**c. nodo′sa, nodular c.,** ophthalmia nodosa.
**Parinaud's c.,** Parinaud's oculoglandular syndrome.
**Pascheff's c.,** necrotic infectious c.
**c. petri′ficans,** a variety of conjunctivitis marked by the formation of deposits of chalky concretions in the conjunctiva and attended with necrosis; called also *calcareous c., lithiasis c.,* and *uratic c.*
**phlyctenular c.,** a variety marked by small vesicles or ulcers, each surrounded by a reddened zone; called also *eczematous c.* and *scrofular c.* See also *phlyctenulosis.*
**pseudomembranous c.,** inflammation of the conjunctiva resembling membranous conjunctivitis except that the membrane can be removed without traumatizing the epithelium and in addition to being caused by bacterial infections can also be caused by toxic and allergic factors and various viral infections. Called also *croupous c.*
**purulent c.,** acute conjunctivitis caused by bacteria or viruses, particularly gonococci, meningococci, pneumococci, and streptococci, characterized by severe inflammation of the conjunctiva and copious discharge of pus.
**scrofular c.,** phlyctenular c.
**shipyard c.,** epidemic keratoconjunctivitis.
**simple c., simple acute c.,** acute catarrhal c.
**spring c.,** vernal c.
**swimming pool c.,** inclusion c.
**trachomatous c.,** trachoma.
**tularemic c.,** see *oculoglandular tularemia,* under *tularemia.*
**uratic c.,** c. petrificans.
**vaccinial c.,** autovaccinia affecting the eye.
**vernal c.,** bilateral conjunctivitis of seasonal occurrence, of unknown cause, affecting children, especially boys. Flattened papules and a thick, gelatinous exudate develop on the conjunctivae on the inside of the upper lid; itching and photophobia are present. The condition is usually self-limiting, but it may become severe if corneal vascularization and ulceration develop. Also called *vernal catarrh* and *spring ophthalmia.*
**welder's c.,** actinic c.
**Widmark's c.,** congestion of the inferior tarsal conjunctiva, with occasional slight stippling of the cornea.

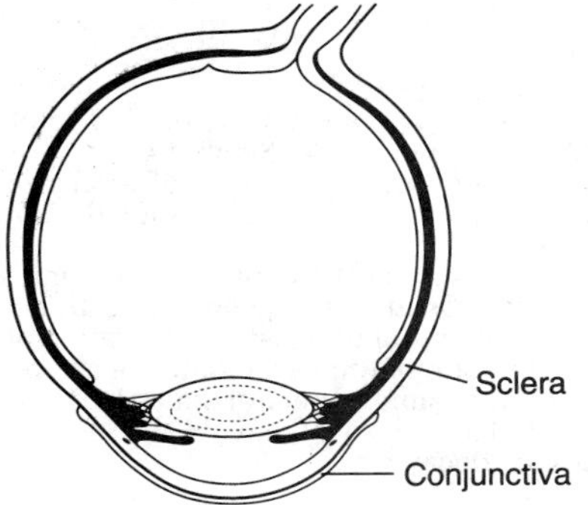


**con·junc·ti·vo·dac·ryo·cys·tos·to·my** (kən-junk″tĭ-vo-dak″re-o-sis-tos′tə-me) surgical connection of the lacrimal sac directly to the conjunctival sac.

**con·junc·ti·vo·ma** (kən-junk″tĭ-vo′mə) a tumor of the eyelid made up of conjunctival tissue.

**con·junc·ti·vo·plas·ty** (kən-junk′tĭ-vo-plas″te) [*conjunctiva* + *-plasty*] repair of a defect of the conjunctiva by plastic surgery.

**con·junc·ti·vo·rhi·nos·to·my** (kən-junk″tĭ-vo-ri-nos′tə-me) surgical correction of total lacrimal canalicular obstruction: a dacryocystorhinostomy is done by suturing the posterior flaps, and the lacrimal caruncle is dissected out, preserving the conjunctiva.

**Conn's syndrome** (konz) [Jerome W. *Conn,* American internist, born 1907] primary hyperaldosteronism.

**con·nec·tion** (kə-nek'shən) 1. the act of connecting or state of being connected. 2. anything that connects; a connector.
**clamp c.,** a short tubular branch connecting one cell of a hypha to another, formed by fusion during cell division in certain basidiomycetous fungi, and serving in the transfer of the two daughter nuclei of the parent cell to a newly formed cell.
**intertendinous c's,** connexus intertendinei.

**con·nec·tor** (kə-nek'tər) 1. anything serving as a link between two separate objects or units. 2. the part of a fixed partial denture that unites the retainer and the pontic; it may be rigid or nonrigid.
**major c.,** a rigid unit of a removable partial denture, serving as its chassis, which joins the parts of the prosthesis on one side of the dental arch to those on the other side, and to which all other components are attached. Called also *saddle c.* Cf. *connector bar.*
**minor c.,** a connecting link between the major connector or base of a partial denture and other units of the prosthesis, such as clasps, indirect retainers, and occlusal rests; called also *connector bar.*
**saddle c.,** major c.

**Con·nell's suture** (kon'əlz) [Frank Gregory *Connell,* American surgeon, 1875–1968] see under *suture.*

**con·nex·on** (kə-nek'son) the functional unit of a gap junction; it is the hexagonal array of membrane-spanning proteins around a central lumen that connects with its counterpart in an adjacent cell to form the intercellular pore of the gap junction.

**con·nex·us** (kə-nek'səs) gen. and pl. *connex'us* [L., variant of *conexus,* q.v.] [TA] a connecting structure; written also *conexus.*
**c. intertendi'nei** [TA], intertendinous connections: narrow bands extending obliquely between the tendons of insertion of the extensor digitorum muscles on the dorsum of the hand. Called also *juncturae tendinum* and *tendinous junctions.*
**c. interthala'micus,** adhesio interthalamica.

**cono-** [Gr. kōnos *cone*] a combining form denoting a relationship to a cone or to a conelike structure.

**co·noid** (ko'noid) [*cono-* + *-oid*] 1. resembling or shaped like a cone. 2. an electron-dense, protrusible, hollow region surrounded by polar rings and composed of spirally coiled microtubules that forms part of the apical complex of apicocomplexan protozoa.
**Sturm's c.,** the changing shapes of the diffusion images of a point in various forms of astigmatism; the image may be an ellipse, a circle, or a sharp line.

**co·no·my·oi·din** (ko"no-mi-oi'din) [*cono-* + *myoid*] a protoplasmic material within the cones of some retinas that expands and contracts under the influence of light, causing the cones to shift.

**con·oph·thal·mus** (kon"of-thal'məs) [*cono-* + *ophthalmus*] staphyloma corneae, def. 1.

**Co·no·po·di·na** (ko"no-po-di'nə) [Gr. *kōnos* cone] a suborder of ameboid protozoa (order Amoebida, subclass Gymnamoebia), characterized by the presence of digitiform or mammilliform, usually blunt, normally unbranched subpseudopodia, most commonly produced from a broad hyaline lobe. *Paramoeba* is a representative genus.

**Co·no·rhi·nus** (ko"no-ri'nəs) [*cono-* + Gr. *rhis* nose] a genus name formerly applied to insects of the family Reduviidae, now placed in the genera *Panstrongylus* and *Triatoma.*

**con·qui·nine** (kon-kwin'in) quinidine.

**Con·ra·di's disease (syndrome)** (kon-rah'dēz) [Erich *Conradi,* German physician, 20th century] see *chondrodysplasia punctata.*

**Con·ra·di's line** (kon-rah'dēz) [Andreas Christian *Conradi,* Norwegian physician, 1809–1869] see under *line.*

**Con·ra·di-Hün·er·mann syndrome** (kon-rah'de-hu'nər-mahn) [E. *Conradi;* Carl *Hünermann,* German physician, 20th century] see under *syndrome.*

**Con·ray** (kon'ra) trademark for a preparation of iothalamate meglumine.

**Cons.** abbreviation for L. *conser'va,* keep.

**con·san·guin·e·ous** (kon"san-gwin'e-əs) related by blood.

**con·san·guin·i·ty** (kon"san-gwin'ĭ-te) [L. *consanguinitas*] [MeSH: Consanguinity] kinship; relationship by blood.

**con·science** (kon'shəns) [MeSH: Conscience] the nontechnical term for the moral faculty of the mind, corresponding roughly to the psychoanalytic concept of the superego (q.v.), although, unlike the ordinary conception of conscience, the actions of the superego are often unconscious.

**con·scious** (kon'shəs) [L. *conscius* aware] 1. having awareness of one's self, acts, and surroundings. 2. a state of awareness or alertness characterized by response to external stimuli. 3. the part of the mind that is constantly within awareness, one of the systems of Freud's topographic model of the mind. Cf. *preconscious* and *unconscious.*

**con·scious·ness** (kon'shəs-nəs) [MeSH: Consciousness] 1. the state of being conscious, fully alert, aware, oriented, and responsive to the environment; having a clear or intact sensorium. 2. subjective awareness of the aspects of cognitive processing and the content of the mind. 3. the current totality of experience of which an individual or group is aware at any time. 4. in psychoanalysis, the conscious.
**colon c.,** a condition in which the patient is aware of the colon and its activities, because of disturbance of the normal defecation reflex, embracing chronic constipation.

**con·sen·su·al** (kən-sen'shoo-əl) excited by reflex stimulation; used especially to designate the similar reaction of both pupils to a stimulus applied to only one.

**con·sent** (kən-sent') [L. *consentire* to agree] 1. to assent or approve; to grant permission. 2. the granting of permission or agreement; assent; approval.
**informed c.,** voluntary permission given by a subject or guardian for participation in a study or investigation, or for medical care, after having been informed of the purpose, methods, procedures, benefits, and risks.

**con·ser·va·tive** (kən-sər'və-tiv) [L. *conservare* to preserve] designed to preserve health, restore function, and repair structures by nonradical methods, as conservative surgery. Cf. *radical.*

**con·serve** (kon'sərv) [L. *conserva*] a confection, electuary, or medicated sweetmeat.

**con·sis·ten·cy** (kən-sis'tən-se) coherence among parts; reliability of successive events or results.
**c. of an estimator,** the property of approaching the value of a population parameter as the sample size increases ad infinitum.

**con·sol·i·dant** (kən-sol'ĭ-dənt) [L. *consolidare* to make firm] 1. promoting the healing or union of parts. 2. an agent that promotes the healing or union of parts.

**con·sol·i·da·tion** (kən-sol"ĭ-da'shən) [L. *consolidatio*] solidification; the process of becoming or the condition of being solid, as when the lung becomes firm as air spaces are filled with exudate in pneumonia.

**con·so·lute** (kon'so-lo͞ot) perfectly miscible.

**con·spe·cif·ic** (kon"spə-sif'ik) 1. of or pertaining to the same species. 2. a member of the same species.

**con·stan·cy** (kon'stən-se) the state of being constant.
**cell c.,** an extreme example of mosaic development resulting in all individuals in a species having the same number of cells in comparable tissues performing similar functions.
**object c.,** 1. the ability to perceive an object as unchanging even under different conditions of observation. 2. see under *permanence.*

**con·stant** (kon'stənt) [L. *constans* standing together] 1. not failing; remaining unaltered. 2. a datum, fact, or principle that is not subject to change.
**absorption c.,** absorptivity.
**acid dissociation c.,** the dissociation constant describing the ionization of an acid. Symbol $K_a$. For an acid HA,

$$K_a = \frac{[H^+][A^-]}{[HA]}.$$

**association c.,** a measure of the extent of a reversible association between two molecular species; called also *binding c.*
**Avogadro's c.,** see under *number.*
**base dissociation c.,** the dissociation constant describing the ionization of a base. Symbol $K_b$. For a base BOH,

$$K_b = \frac{[B^+]\,[OH^-]}{[BOH]}.$$

**binding c.,** association c.
**Boltzmann's c.,** the gas constant divided by Avogadro's number; $1.38066 \times 10^{-23}$ joule per kelvin. Symbol *k.*
**decay c.,** the fraction of the number of atoms of a radionuclide which decay per unit time; symbol $\lambda$. Called also *disintegration c.* and *radioactive c.*
**dielectric c.,** a measure of the capability of a unit volume of a material to store electrostatic energy on application of a unit voltage; the ability of that material to resist the formation of an electric field within it. It is the ratio of the capacitance of a capacitor having the material versus the same capacitor having only a vacuum as the dielectric. Symbol $\kappa$.
**disintegration c.,** decay c.

**dissociation c.**, an equilibrium constant, expressed in concentrations, describing the dissociation of a molecule or ion into its components. Symbol $K_d$. See also *acid dissociation c.* and *base dissociation c.* Called also *ionization c.*
**equilibrium c.**, a constant, $K$ (or $K_{eq}$), describing the amounts of reactants and products of a chemical reaction at equilibrium at constant temperature; technically defined by thermodynamic activities, it is usually approximated using concentrations (and sometimes therefore denoted $K_c$) and is defined by the equation for the reaction quotient (q.v.). For gases, it can be approximated by partial pressures rather than concentrations (and denoted $K_p$). See also *dissociation c.*
**Faraday's c.**, faraday.
**gas c.**, the proportionality constant in the ideal gas law (q.v.); 8.3144 joules per mole kelvin or 1.987 calories per mole kelvin. Symbol *R*.
**gravitational c., c. of gravitation**, the constant of proportionality in the law of gravitation, equal to $6.67 \times 10^{-11}$ N·m²/kg²; symbol G.
**ionization c.**, dissociation c.
**Lapicque's c.**, the figure 0.37, used for converting noninductive resistance into direct current equivalents.
**Michaelis' c.**, a constant representing the substrate concentration at which the velocity of an enzyme-catalyzed reaction is half maximal; symbol $K_m$ or $K_M$. See also *Michaelis-Menten equation*, under *equation*.
**newtonian c. of gravitation**, gravitational c.
**Planck's c., quantum c.**, a constant, *h*, which represents the ratio of the energy of any quantum of radiation to its frequency; the value of *h* is $6.626 \times 10^{-34}$ joule second.
**radioactive c.**, decay c.
**rate c.**, a constant of proportionality, *k*, relating the rate of a single step of a reaction to the concentrations of the reactants, e.g., for a reaction $aA + bB \rightleftarrows yY + zZ$, the rate $(v) = k[A]^a[B]^b$. The rate constant for the forward reaction is $k_f$; for the reverse it is $k_r$.
**sedimentation c.**, see under *coefficient*.
**solubility product c.**, a derived equilibrium constant ($K_{sp}$) for the equilibrium existing between a slightly soluble compound and the solution it has saturated. Because so little compound dissolves, its concentration is considered constant and $K_{sp}$ is equivalent to the product of *K* (equilibrium constant) times the original concentration of the compound; it is thus equivalent to the ion product. Higher concentrations of ions cause precipitation.
**velocity c.**, rate c.

**con·sti·pat·ed** (kon'stĭ-pāt″əd) affected with constipation.

**con·sti·pa·tion** (kon″stĭ-pa'shən) [L. *constipatio* a crowding together] [MeSH: Constipation] infrequent or difficult evacuation of the feces.
**atonic c.**, constipation due to intestinal atony.
**gastrojejunal c.**, constipation due to reflex inhibition from some disease of the gastrointestinal tract.
**proctogenous c.**, constipation due to some abnormality of the defecation reflex resulting in failure of fecal masses in the rectum to excite impulses leading to their evacuation.
**spastic c.**, constipation marked by spasmodic constriction of a portion of the intestine; seen in neurasthenia and lead poisoning.

**con·sti·tu·tion** (kon″stĭ-too'shən) [L. *constituere* to set up] 1. the make-up or functional habit of the body, determined by the genetic, biochemical, and physiologic endowment of the individual, and modified in great measure by environmental factors. Cf. *diathesis, type*, and *genotype*. 2. in chemistry, the atoms making up a molecule and the way they are linked, the property that distinguishes a compound from its structural isomers. Cf. *configuration*.
**lymphatic c.**, a condition of hyperplasia of the lymphatic system.

**con·sti·tu·tion·al** (kon″stĭ-too'shən-əl) 1. affecting the whole constitution of the body; not local. 2. pertaining to the constitution.

**con·sti·tu·tive** (kon-stĭ-too'tiv, kon-stich'u-tiv) produced constantly or in fixed amounts, regardless of environmental conditions or demand; cf. *inducible*.

**con·stric·tion** (kən-strik'shən) [*con-* + *stringere* to draw] [MeSH: Constriction] a constricted part or place; a stricture.
**duodenopyloric c.**, the constriction marking the junction of the stomach and duodenum.
**primary c.**, centromere.
**secondary c.**, 1. in genetics, the narrowed heterochromatic area of the short arms of acrocentric autosomes by which a satellite is attached. 2. a nonfunctional centromere in a dicentric chromosome.

**con·stric·tive** (kən-strik'tiv) causing constriction or having a tendency to constriction.

**con·stric·tor** (kən-strik'tər) [L.] that which constricts, such as a muscle or an instrument by which a part may be constricted. See under *musculus*.
**c. na'ris**, pars transversa musculi nasalis.
**c. ure'thrae**, musculus sphincter urethrae.
**c. vagi'nae**, the musculus bulbospongiosus in the female.

**con·struc·tive** (kən-struk'tiv) pertaining to any process of construction; in physiology, anabolic.

**con·sult** (kən-sult') [L. *consultus*] to confer with another physician about a case.

**con·sul·tant** (kən-sul'tənt) [L. *consultare* to counsel] [MeSH: Consultants] a physician called in for advice and counsel.

**con·sul·ta·tion** (kon″səl-ta'shən) [L. *consultatio*] a deliberation by two or more physicians with respect to the diagnosis or treatment in any particular case.

**con·sump·tion** (kən-sump'shən) [L. *consumptio* a wasting] 1. the act of consuming, or the process of being consumed. 2. a wasting away of the body. 3. old name for *pulmonary tuberculosis*.

**con·sump·tive** (kən-sump'tiv) old term for a person with pulmonary tuberculosis; cf. *tubercular*.

**Cont.** abbreviation for L. *contu'sus*, bruised.

**con·tact** (kon'takt) [L. *contactus* a touching together] 1. a mutual touching of two bodies or persons. 2. an individual known to have been sufficiently near to an infected individual to have been exposed to the transfer of infectious material. 3. contactant.
**balancing c.**, the contact between the upper and lower occlusal surfaces of the teeth (of the natural or artificial dentition) on the side opposite the working contact.
**complete c.**, contact of the entire proximal surface of one tooth with the entire proximal surface of the adjacent tooth.
**deflective c.**, deflective occlusal c.
**direct c., immediate c.**, transmission of infection from an infected host or reservoir to a susceptible individual by physical contact.
**indirect c.**, transmission of infection to a susceptible host by means of formites or a vector or through the air in dust or droplet nuclei (see under *nucleus*); called also *mediate c.*
**initial c.**, initial occlusal c.
**mediate c.**, indirect c.
**occlusal c.**, the contact between the upper and lower teeth when the jaws are closed in habitual occlusion.
**occlusal c., deflective**, a form of occlusal interference in which the mandible is diverted from its normal path of closure to central jaw relation, or the denture slides or rotates on its basal seat. Called also *deflective c.* and *cuspal interference*.
**occlusal c., initial**, the initial normal, noninterfering occlusal contact and intercuspation occurring when the mandibular and maxillary teeth are brought together. In ideal occlusion, it takes place in centric occlusion. Called also *initial c.*
**occlusal c., interceptive**, an initial contact of the teeth that stops or deviates from the normal movement of the mandible.
**premature c.**, an occlusal contact or interference that occurs before a balanced and stable jaw-to-jaw relationship is reached in either centric relation or centric occlusion, or in the area between the two positions.
**proximal c., proximate c.**, touching of the proximal surfaces of two adjoining teeth.
**weak c.**, contact in which the proximal surface of one tooth barely touches that of the adjacent tooth, enhancing the packing of food between the teeth.
**working c.**, the contact between the upper and lower teeth (of the natural or artificial dentition) on the side toward which the mandible has been moved in mastication.

**con·tac·tant** (kən-tak'tənt) an allergen capable of inducing delayed contact-type hypersensitivity of the animal or human epidermis after one or more episodes of contact.

**con·tac·tol·o·gist** (kon″tak-tol'ə-jist) a craftsman in contactology.

**con·tac·tol·o·gy** (kon″tak-tol'ə-je) the craft of making and fitting contact lenses.

**con·ta·gion** (kən-ta'jən) [L. *contagio* contact, infection] 1. the communication of disease from one individual to another. 2. a contagious disease.
**psychic c.**, communication of psychological symptoms through mental influence.

**con·ta·gi·os·i·ty** (kən-ta″je-os'ĭ-te) the quality of being contagious.

**con·ta·gious** (kən-ta'jəs) [L. *contagiosus*] capable of being transmitted from one individual to another, as a contagious disease; communicable. Cf. *infectious*.

**con·tam·i·nant** (kən-tam'ĭ-nənt) something that causes contamination.

**con·tam·i·na·tion** (kən-tam″ĭ-na'shən) [L. *contaminatio*, from *con* together + *tangere* to touch] 1. the presence of any substance or organism that makes a preparation impure. 2. the soiling or pollution by inferior material, as by the introduction of organisms into a wound, or sewage into a stream. 3. the deposition of radioactive material where it is not desired, particularly where its presence may be harmful or constitute a radiation hazard.

**con·tent** (kon'tent) that which is contained within a thing.
**latent c.**, in freudian theory, the hidden and unconscious true meaning of a symbolic representation, such as a dream or fantasy, as opposed to the manifest content.
**manifest c.**, in freudian theory, the content of a dream or fantasy as it is experienced and remembered, and in which the latent content is disguised and distorted by displacement, condensation, symbolization, projection, and secondary elaboration.

**con·ti·gu·i·ty** (kon″tĭ-gu'ĭ-te) [L. *contiguus* in contact] contact or close proximity; the quality of being contiguous.

**con·tig·u·ous** (kən-tig'u-əs) [L. *contiguus*] in contact or nearly so.

**Contin.** abbreviation for L. *continue'tur,* let it be continued.

**con·ti·nence** (kon'tĭ-nəns) [L. *continentia*] the ability to refrain from yielding to desire, as self-restraint with respect to sexual indulgence.
**fecal c.**, the ability to retain the contents of the colon until conditions are proper for defecation.
**urinary c.**, the ability to retain the contents of the bladder until conditions are proper for urination.

**con·ti·nent** (kon'tĭ-nənt) able to refrain from yielding to normal impulses, as sexual desire, or from the urge to defecate or urinate.

**con·tin·ued** (kən-tin'ūd) having no remission, intermission, or interruption.

**con·ti·nu·i·ty** (kon″tĭ-nu'ĭ-te) [L. *continuitas,* uninterrupted succession] the quality of being without interruption or separation.

**con·tin·u·ous** (kən-tin'u-əs) [L. *continuus*] not interrupted; having no interruption. See under *variable.*

**con·tour** (kon'to͞or) [Fr.] 1. the normal outline or configuration of the body or of a part. 2. to shape a solid along certain desired lines.
**height of c.**, see under *height.*

**con·toured** (kon'to͞ord) having an irregularly undulating outline or surface; said of bacterial colonies.

**con·tour·ing** (kon-to͞or'ing) the process of forming a contour; shaping.
**occlusal c.**, correction by grinding of gross disharmonies of the occlusal tooth forms. See also under *adjustment.*

**contra-** [L. *contra* against] a prefix signifying against, opposed.

**con·tra·an·gle** (kon″trə-ang'gəl) an angulation by which the working point of a surgical instrument is brought close to the long axis of its shaft; it may involve two, three, or four bends, or angles, in its shank.

**con·tra·ap·er·ture** (kon″trə-ap'ər-chər) [*contra-* + *aperture*] a second opening made in an abscess to facilitate the discharge of its contents.

**con·tra·cep·tion** (kon″trə-sep'shən) [MeSH: Contraception] the prevention of conception or impregnation.
**intrauterine c.**, prevention of conception by use of a device inserted into the uterus; see under *device.*

**con·tra·cep·tive** (kon″trə-sep'tiv) 1. diminishing the likelihood of, or preventing, conception. 2. an agent that diminishes the likelihood of or prevents conception.
**barrier c.**, a contraceptive device, such as a condom or diaphragm, that physically prevents spermatozoa from entering the endometrial cavity and fallopian tubes.
**chemical c.**, a spermicidal agent inserted into the vagina before intercourse to prevent pregnancy.
**intrauterine c.**, see under *device.*
**oral c.**, a compound, usually hormonal, taken orally in order to block ovulation and prevent the occurrence of pregnancy.

**con·tract** (kən-trakt') [L. *contractus,* from *contrahere* to draw together] 1. to shorten, or reduce in size, as a muscle. 2. to acquire or incur.

**con·trac·tile** (kən-trak'tīl) [*con-* + L. *trahere* to draw] having the power or tendency to contract in response to a suitable stimulus.

**con·trac·til·i·ty** (kon″trak-til'ĭ-te) capacity for becoming shorter in response to a suitable stimulus.
**cardiac c.**, the intrinsic property, belonging to cardiac cells and tissues, of shortening in response to an appropriate stimulus. Cardiac contractility is variable and under the control of the autonomic nervous system and is also affected by other factors such as loading conditions; changes in contractility give rise to changes in the strength of contraction of the heart. It may be estimated by the end-systolic pressure-volume relationship, the change in either pressure or volume over time. Called also *inotropic state.*
**galvanic c.**, galvanocontractility.
**idiomuscular c.**, a contractility peculiar to wasted or degenerated muscles.
**neuromuscular c.**, normal, as distinguished from idiomuscular, contractility.

**con·trac·tion** (kən-trak'shən) [L. *contractus* drawn together] 1. a shortening or reduction in size; in connection with muscles contraction implies shortening and/or development of tension. 2. a morbid or pathologic shortening or shrinkage. 3. abnormal approximation of mandibular and maxillary structures to the median plane. See also *distraction,* def. 5.
**atrial premature c.**, see under *complex.*
**atrioventricular (AV) junctional premature c.**, see under *complex.*
**automatic ventricular c.**, ventricular escape beat.
**Braxton Hicks c's**, light, usually painless, irregular uterine contractions during pregnancy, gradually increasing in intensity and frequency and becoming more rhythmic during the late third trimester.
**carpopedal c.**, the condition resulting from chronic shortening of the muscles of the fingers, toes, arms, and legs in tetany.
**cicatricial c.**, wound c.
**clonic c.**, clonus.
**concentric c.**, shortening c.
**Dupuytren's c.**, Dupuytren's contracture.
**eccentric c.**, lengthening c.
**escaped ventricular c.**, ventricular escape beat.
**fibrillary c's**, abnormal spontaneous contractions occurring successively in different bundles of the fibers of a diseased muscle.
**hourglass c.**, contraction of an organ (as the stomach or uterus) at or near the middle.
**idiomuscular c.**, a contraction produced in a wasted or denervated muscle by direct electrical stimulation.
**isometric c.**, muscle contraction without appreciable shortening or change in distance between its origin and insertion.
**isotonic c.**, muscle contraction without appreciable change in the force of contraction; the distance between the muscle's origin and insertion becomes less.
**isovolumetric c., isovolumic c.**, see under *period.*
**junctional premature c.**, atrioventricular junctional premature complex.
**lengthening c.**, a muscle contraction in which the ends of the muscle move farther apart, as when a limb is forcibly flexed. Called also *eccentric c.*
**myotatic c.**, contraction or irritability of a muscle brought into play by sudden passive stretching or by tapping on its tendon. See also *stretch reflex* and *tendon reflex.*
**palmar c.**, Dupuytren's contracture.
**paradoxical c.**, the contraction of a muscle caused by the passive approximation of its extremities.
**postural c.**, that state of muscular tension and contraction which just suffices to maintain the posture of the body.
**premature c.**, extrasystole.
**segmentation c.**, see under *movement.*
**shortening c.**, a muscle contraction in which the ends of the muscle move closer together, as when a flexed limb is extended. Called also *concentric c.*
**supraventricular premature c.**, an ectopic beat arising prematurely from a focus within the atria or atrioventricular junction, e.g., an atrial premature complex or atrioventricular junctional premature complex.
**tetanic c.**, sustained contraction of a muscle without intervals of relaxation; see *tetanus* (def. 2). Called also *tonic c.*
**tonic c.**, tetanus, def. 2.
**twitch c.**, twitch.
**uterine c.**, contraction of the uterus.
**ventricular premature c.**, see under *complex.*
**wound c.**, the shrinkage and spontaneous closure of open skin wounds. Called also *cicatricial c.*

**con·trac·ture** (kən-trak'chər) [L. *contractura*] [MeSH: Contracture] a condition of fixed high resistance to passive stretch of a muscle, resulting from fibrosis of the tissues supporting the muscles or the joints, or from disorders of the muscle fibers.
**Dupuytren's c.**, shortening, thickening, and fibrosis of the palmar fascia, producing a flexion deformity of a finger; sometimes associated with long-standing epilepsy. Applied also to flexion deformity of a toe caused by involvement of the plantar fascia.
**ischemic c.**, contracture and degeneration of a muscle due to interference with the circulation from pressure, as by a tight bandage, or from injury or cold.
**organic c.**, one that is permanent and continuous.
**postpoliomyelitic c.**, any distortion of a joint following an attack of poliomyelitis, due to partial or complete paralysis of one muscle or group of muscles, allowing overuse of an opposing muscle or group of muscles, such as flexion contracture of the knee and paralysis of the quadriceps muscle group.
**Volkmann's c.**, contracture of the fingers and sometimes the wrist after severe injury in or near the elbow or improper use of a tourniquet interferes with the blood supply to the muscles. A similar phenomenon may develop in the lower leg and foot after similar vascular damage to leg muscles. Called also *ischemic muscular atrophy* and *Volkmann's syndrome.*

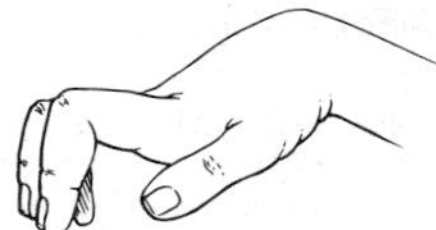
Volkmann's contracture.

**con·tra·fis·sure** (kon″trə-fish′ər) a fracture in a part opposite the site of a blow.

**con·tra·in·ci·sion** (kon″trə-in-sizh′ən) counterincision to promote drainage.

**con·tra·in·di·cant** (kon″trə-in′dĭ-kənt) rendering any particular line of treatment undesirable or improper.

**con·tra·in·di·ca·tion** (kon″trə-in″dĭ-ka′shən) any condition, especially any condition of disease, which renders some particular line of treatment improper or undesirable.

**con·tra·in·su·lar** (kon″trə-in′su-lər) having an inhibiting influence on the secretion of pancreatic insulin.

**con·tra·lat·er·al** (kon″trə-lat′ər-əl) [*contra-* + *lateral*] situated on, pertaining to, or affecting the opposite side, as opposed to ipsilateral.

**con·tra·sex·u·al** (kon″trə-sek′shoo-əl) 1. a term used to describe the repressed side of an individual, embodying those characteristics normally occurring in the opposite sex. 2. showing secondary sex characters of the opposite sex; called also *heterosexual.*

**con·trast** (kon′trast) [*contra-* + L. *stare* to stand] the degree to which light and dark areas of an image differ in brightness or in optical density. In radiology, the difference in optical density in a radiograph that results from a difference in radiolucency or penetrability of the subject.
**film c.,** contrast inherent in the film.
**high c.,** short-scale c.
**long-scale c., low c.,** an increased range of grays on a radiograph, which limits visual differentiation to those image densities produced by relatively disparate structural features.
**short-scale c.,** a reduced range of grays on a radiograph, which favors visual differentiation of image densities produced by objects or object components with relatively comparable structural features.
**subject c.,** contrast resulting from differences in absorption of radiation by various parts of the subject.

**con·tra·stim·u·lant** (kon″trə-stim′u-lənt) [*contra-* + *stimulant*] 1. counteracting or opposing stimulation. 2. a depressant medicine.

**con·tra·stim·u·lism** (kon″trə-stim′u-liz-əm) the systematic use of contrastimulant medicines or appliances.

**con·tra·stim·u·lus** (kon″trə-stim′u-ləs) [*contra-* + *stimulus*] a remedy, force, or agent that opposes stimulation.

**con·tre·coup** (kōn″trə-koo′) [Fr. "counterblow"] injury resulting from a blow on another site, especially of the brain, such as a fracture by contrecoup of the skull or a contrecoup contusion.

**con·trec·ta·tion** (kon″trek-ta′shən) [L. *contrectare* to handle] the act of touching and fondling, especially in the sense of foreplay.

**Cont. rem.** abbreviation for L. *continue′tur reme′dium,* let the medicine be continued.

**con·trol** (kən-trōl′) [Fr. *contrôle* a register] 1. the governing or limitation of certain objects or events. 2. a standard against which experimental observations may be evaluated; see *negative c.* and *positive c.* 3. a patient or group differing from that under study (the treated or case group) by lacking the disease or by having a different or absent treatment or regimen; the controls and case or treated subjects usually otherwise have certain similarities to allow or enhance comparison between them. 4. in psychiatry, the process of consciously restraining and regulating impulses and suppressing instincts and affects.
**aversive c.,** in behavior therapy, the use of unpleasant stimuli to change undesirable behavior.
**birth c.,** deliberate limitation of childbearing by measures designed to control fertility and to prevent conception; see also *contraception.*
**feedback c.,** a physiological control mechanism operating to regulate the metabolic processes of a cell and thus maintain a constant internal environment, in which the accumulation of the product of a reaction leads to a decrease in its rate of production, or a deficiency of the product leads to an increase in its rate of production.
**idiodynamic c.,** nerve impulses from the cells of the ventral gray column and the motor nuclei of the brain that maintain the muscles in their normal trophic condition.
**motor c.,** the systematic transmission of impulses from the motor cortex to motor units, resulting in coordinated muscular contractions.
**negative c.,** a laboratory procedure identical in all respects to an experimental procedure except for the absence of the one factor being studied.
**positive c.,** in an experimental study of a given substance, a sample of the substance with known values that can be used as a reference base.
**reflex c.,** control of muscular activity by nerve impulses transmitted to the muscles by one of the reflex arcs by which reflex action is maintained.
**Schick test c.** [USP], heat-inactivated diphtheria toxin used as a control in the Schick test. Formerly called *inactivated diagnostic diphtheria toxin.*
**sex c.,** regulation of the sex of future offspring by artificial means.
**stimulus c.,** any influence exerted by the environment on behavior.
**thought c.,** a delusion of control in which it is believed that one's thoughts are not one's own but come from another person or other outside source.
**tonic c.,** nerve impulses transmitted to the final common pathway through the reflex arc for the maintenance of muscle tone.
**vestibuloequilibratory c.,** nerve impulses from the semicircular canals, saccule, and utricle for the maintenance of body equilibrium.
**volitional c., voluntary c.,** impulses from the motor area of the cerebral cortex that direct muscular action under the influence of the will.

**Con·trolled Sub·stan·ces Act** a federal law enacted in 1970 that regulates the prescribing and dispensing of psychoactive drugs, including narcotics, according to five schedules based on their abuse potential, medical acceptance, and ability to produce dependence; it also establishes a regulatory system for the manufacture, storage, and transport of the drugs in each schedule. Drugs covered by this Act include opium and its derivatives, opiates, hallucinogens, depressants, and stimulants.

**con·tund** (kən-tund′) [L. *contundere*] to bruise.

**con·tuse** (kən-to͞oz′) to bruise.

**con·tu·sion** (kən-too′zhən) [L. *contusio,* from *contundere* to bruise] [MeSH: Contusions] an injury of a part without a break in the skin and with a subcutaneous hemorrhage. Called also *bruise.*
**brain c.,** contusion with loss of consciousness as a result of direct trauma to the head, usually associated with fracture of the skull. See also *concussion of the brain.*
**contrecoup c.,** a contusion resulting from a blow on one side of the head with damage to the cerebral hemisphere on the opposite side by transmitted force.
**myocardial c.,** contusion of the heart, most frequently due to impact against an automobile steering wheel or other blunt object; the trauma may cause arrhythmias, conduction disturbances, or clinical signs of infarction such as electrocardiographic abnormalities.
**c. of spinal cord,** organic injury to the cord due to a blow to the vertebral column, with resultant transient or prolonged dysfunction below the level of the lesion. See also *concussion of spinal cord.*

**con·tu·sive** (kən-too′siv) producing a bruise.

**con·u·lar** (kon′u-lər) conical.

**Co·nus** (ko′nəs) a genus of marine snails (cones) of the family Conidae. *C. geogra′phicus* (the geographic cone) and *C. texti′le* (the textile cone) are carnivorous species that live in tropical oceans and kill fish by punching a hole with a proboscis and injecting poison; occasionally humans have been killed in the same manner.

**co·nus** (ko′nəs) gen. and pl. *co′ni* [L.; Gr. *kōnos*] 1. [TA] cone: general anatomical nomenclature for a structure resembling a cone in shape. 2. posterior staphyloma of the myopic eye.
**c. arterio′sus** [TA], arterial cone: the anterosuperior portion of the right ventricle of the heart, which is delimited from the rest of the ventricle by the supraventricular crest and which joins the pulmonary trunk, thus forming the outflow tract for blood in the right ventricle. Called also *infundibulum.*
**distraction c.,** a crescentic white area at the temporal edge of the papilla of the optic nerve sometimes seen with the ophthalmoscope in myopic eyes.
**c. elas′ticus,** 1. [TA] elastic cone: the paired lateral portion of the fibroelastic laryngeal membrane, which extends upward in parallel thickenings from the cricoid cartilage to the vocal ligaments. Called also *lateral cricothyroid ligament, cricothyroid* or *cricovocal membrane,* and *membrana cricovocalis.* 2. cricothyroid ligament. 3. ligamentum cricothyroideum medianum.
**co′ni epididy′midis,** TA alternative for *lobuli epididymidis.*
**c. medulla′ris** [TA], medullary cone: the cone-shaped lower end of the spinal cord, at the level of the upper lumbar vertebrae; called also *c. terminalis* and *terminal cone of spinal cord.*
**myopic c.,** posterior staphyloma of the myopic eye.
**supertraction c.,** a gray or yellowish ring on the nasal side of the optic papilla sometimes seen with the ophthalmoscope, especially in myopic eyes.

**c. termina'lis,** c. medullaris.
**co'ni vasculo'si,** lobuli epididymidis.

**con·va·les·cence** (kon"və-les'əns) [L. *convalescere* to become strong] [MeSH: Convalescence] the stage of recovery following an attack of disease, a surgical operation, or an injury.

**con·va·les·cent** (kon"və-les'ənt) 1. pertaining to or characterized by convalescence. 2. a patient who is recovering from a disease, surgical operation, or injury.

**con·vec·tion** (kən-vek'shən) [L. *convectio,* from *convehere* to convey] [MeSH: Convection] transmission of heat in liquids or gases by a circulation carried on by bulk movement of the heated particles to a cooler area; See also *convection current,* under *current.*

**con·ver·gence** (kən-vər'jəns) [L. *convergere* to lean together] 1. in evolution, the development of similar structures or organisms in unrelated taxa. 2. in embryology, the movement of cells from the periphery toward the midline during gastrulation. 3. in ophthalmic physiology, the coordinated inclination of the two lines of sight toward their common point of fixation, or the point of fixation itself. 4. in neurology, the exciting of a single sensory neuron by incoming impulses from multiple other neurons, particularly in the central nervous system.
**accommodative c.,** that portion of convergence initiated by the stimulus to accommodation.
**amplitude of c.,** see under *amplitude.*
**far point of c.,** the point of intersection of the lines of sight at minimum convergence.
**fusional c.,** convergence resulting from the attempt to keep the visual stimulus on the fovea of both eyes.
**multimodal c.,** in neurology, convergence in which the incoming impulses are from neurons of different sensory modalities.
**multisensory c.,** multimodal c.
**near point of c.,** the point of intersection of the lines of sight at maximum convergence.
**negative c.,** outward vergence, or divergence, of the visual axes.
**positive c.,** inward deviation of the visual axes.
**proximal c.,** convergence induced by the sense of nearness of an object.
**tonic c.,** the continuous convergence maintained by the tone of the medial rectus muscle in the primary position.

**con·ver·gent** (kən-vər'jənt) [*con-* + *vergere* to incline] meeting at or tending toward a common point.

**con·ver·gi·om·e·ter** (kən-vər"je-om'ə-tər) [*convergence* (def. 3) + *-meter*] an instrument for measuring latent strabismus.

**Con·verse method** (kon'vərs) [John Marquis *Converse,* American plastic surgeon, 1909–1981] see under *method.*

**con·ver·sion** (kən-vər'zhən) [*con-* + *version*] 1. a shift from one form or state to another. 2. an unconscious defense mechanism by which the anxiety that stems from intrapsychic conflict is converted and expressed in a symbolic somatic manifestation; see also *conversion disorder* under *disorder.*
**internal c.,** in decay of an isomer, transition between two nuclear energy states not characterized by emission of a photon because the energy is instead transferred to an inner orbital electron, which is ejected from the atom.

**con·ver·tase** (kən-vər'tās) an enzyme of the complement system that activates specific components of the system.
**C3 c.,** an enzyme that splits the complement component C3 to C3a and C3b; the classical pathway C3 convertase is C4b,2a; the alternative pathway C3 convertases are C3b,Bb and C3b,P,Bb; see under *complement.*
**C3 proactivator c.,** former name for *factor D.*
**C5 c.,** an enzyme that splits the complement component C5 to C5a and C5b; the classical pathway C5 convertase is C4b,2a,3b; the alternative pathway C5 convertases are $C3b_n$,Bb and $C3b_n$,P,Bb; see under *complement.*

**con·ver·tin** (kən-vər'tin) the activated form of factor VII; see *coagulation factors,* at *factor.*

**con·vex** (kon-veks') [L. *convexus*] having a rounded, somewhat elevated surface, resembling a segment of the external surface of a sphere.

**con·vex·i·ty** (kon-vek'sĭ-te) [L. *convexitas*] 1. the condition of being convex. 2. a rounded, somewhat elevated area on the surface of an organ or other structure.

**con·vexo·ba·sia** (kon-vek"so-ba'zhə) [*convex* + *base* of the skull] a deformity of the occipital bone, which is bent forward by the spine; seen in osteitis deformans.

**con·vexo·con·cave** (kon-vek"so-kon'kāv) convex on one surface and concave on the other.

**con·vexo·con·vex** (kon-vek"so-kon'veks) convex on each of two opposite surfaces.

**con·vo·lut·ed** (kon"vo-lo͞ot'-əd) [L. *convolutus*] rolled together or coiled.

**con·vo·lu·tion** (kon"vo-loo'shən) [L. *convolutus* rolled together] a tortuous irregularity or elevation caused by a structure being infolded upon itself; see *gyri cerebri,* under *gyrus.*
**Broca's c.,** the inferior frontal gyrus of the left hemisphere of the cerebrum; called also *Broca's gyrus* or *region.*
**c's of cerebrum,** gyri cerebri.
**Heschl's c's,** gyri temporales transversi; see under *gyrus.*
**occipitotemporal c.,** either the gyrus occipitotemporalis lateralis or the gyrus occipitotemporalis medialis.
**Zuckerkandl's c.,** gyrus paraterminalis.

**con·vo·lu·tion·al** (kon"vo-loo'shən-əl) of or pertaining to a convolution or convolutions.

**con·vo·lu·tion·ary** (kon"vo-loo'shən-ar-e) convolutional.

**Con·vol·vu·la·ceae** (kon-vol"vu-la'se-e) the morning glory family, a large family of plants that includes vines, herbs, shrubs, and trees. Genera of medical interest include *Convolvulus* and *Ipomoea.*

**Con·vol·vu·lus** (kon-vol'vu-ləs) a genus of flowering plants of the family Convolvulaceae, native to Turkey and nearby areas of the Middle East. *C. scammo'nia* L. is scammony, a species whose root is medicinal.

**con·vul·sant** (kən-vul'sənt) 1. producing or causing convulsions. 2. an agent that causes convulsions.

**con·vul·si·bil·i·ty** (kən-vul"sĭ-bil'ĭ-te) capability of being convulsed.

**con·vul·sion** (kən-vul'shən) [L. *convulsio,* from *convellere* to pull together] [MeSH: Convulsions] 1. a violent involuntary contraction or series of contractions of the voluntary muscles. 2. seizure (def. 2).
**central c.,** a convulsion not excited by any external cause, but due to a lesion of the central nervous system; called also *essential c.*
**clonic c.,** a convulsion marked by alternating contracting and relaxing of the muscles.
**essential c.,** central c.
**febrile c's,** those associated with high fever, occurring in infants and children.
**hysterical c., hysteroid c.,** convulsions of psychogenic origin, as in conversion disorder.
**local c.,** any minor spasm affecting only one muscle or one part or member, as in jacksonian epilepsy.
**mimetic c., mimic c.,** facial spasm.
**puerperal c.,** involuntary spasms in women just before, during, or just after childbirth.
**salaam c's,** infantile spasms.
**tetanic c.,** a tonic spasm without loss of consciousness; see *tetanus* (def. 2) and *tetany* (def. 1).
**tonic c.,** prolonged contraction of the muscles, as a result of an epileptic discharge.
**uremic c.,** one due to uremia, or retention in the blood of material that should have been expelled by the kidneys.

**con·vul·si·vant** (kən-vul'sĭ-vənt) convulsant.

**con·vul·sive** (kən-vul'siv) pertaining to, characterized by, or of the nature of convulsion.

**Coo·ley's anemia, disease** (koo'lēz) [Thomas Benton *Cooley,* American pediatrician, 1871–1945] see *thalassemia.*

**Coo·lidge tube** (koo'lij) [William David *Coolidge,* American physicist, 1873–1977] see under *tube.*

**cool·ing** (ko͞ol'ing) the process of reducing the temperature, especially the body temperature of patients and experimental animals. See also *hypothermia.*

**Coombs' test** (ko͞omz) [Rorbert Royston Amos *Coombs,* British immunologist, born 1921] [MeSH: Coombs' Test] see *antiglobulin test,* under *test.*

**Coo·per's breast, fascia,** etc. (koo'pərz) [Sir Astley Paston *Cooper,* English surgeon, 1768–1841] see under *breast, fascia, hernia, ligament,* and *testis.*

**co·op·er·a·tiv·i·ty** (ko-op"ər-ə-tiv'ĭ-te) the phenomenon of alteration of binding of subsequent ligands upon binding of an initial ligand by an enzyme, receptor, or other molecule with multiple binding sites, such as frequently occurs in enzymes exhibiting allostery.
**negative c.,** cooperativity in which the dissociation constant for each successive ligand bound is higher than for the one preceding it, so that the binding affinity is successively decreased.
**positive c.,** cooperativity in which the dissociation constant for each successive ligand bound is lower than for the one preceding it, so that the binding affinity is successively increased.

**Coo·pe·ria** (koo-pe're-ə) a genus of nematodes of the family

Trichostrongylidae. *C. onco'phora, C. pectina'ta,* and *C. puncta'ta* are parasites found in the small intestines of cattle and other ruminants.

**coo·pe·ri·a·sis** (koo-pə-ri'ə-sis) infection of ruminants with nematodes of the genus *Cooperia.*

**coo·per·id** (koo'pər-id) a parasitic nematode of the genus *Cooperia.*

**Coo·per·nail's sign** (koo'pər-nālz) [George Peter *Coopernail,* American physician, 1876–1962] see under *sign.*

**co·or·di·nate** (ko-or'dĭ-nət) one of a set of numbers that locate a point in space.

**co·or·di·na·tion** (ko-or"dĭ-na'shən) the harmonious functioning of interrelated organs and parts; applied especially to the process of the motor apparatus of the brain which provides for the co-working of particular groups of muscles for the performance of definite adaptive useful responses.

**co·os·si·fi·ca·tion** (ko-os"ĭ-fĭ-ka'shən) the action or state of being joined together by ossification.

**co·os·si·fy** (ko-os'ĭ-fi) to grow together by ossification.

**COP** a regimen of cyclophosphamide, Oncovin (vincristine), and prednisone, used in cancer chemotherapy.

**co·pal** (ko-pal') [Mex.] the commercial name of many resinous substances of extremely varied origin and character; the original copals came from trees of tropical America, chiefly of the leguminous species *Hymeaea courbaril* L. and various species of *Trachylobium.* It is used in various varnishes and cements and in dentistry for modeling compounds and varnishes for cavities.

**co·par·af·fin·ate** (ko-par'ə-fin"āt) a mixture of water-insoluble isoparaffinic acids partially neutralized with isooctyl hydroxybenzyldialkyl amines; used as an anti-infective for the skin.

**COP-BLAM** a regimen of cyclophosphamide, Oncovin (vincristine), prednisone, bleomycin, Adriamycin (doxorubicin), and Matulane (procarbazine) used in cancer chemotherapy.

**COPD** chronic obstructive pulmonary disease.

**Cope's sign** (kōps) [Sir Vincent *Cope,* English surgeon, 1881–1974] see under *sign.*

**cope** (kōp) 1. the upper half of a flask used in the casting art; applied in prosthetic dentistry to the upper or cavity side of a denture flask. 2. coping.

**co·pe·pod** (ko'pə-pod) [Gr. *kōpē* oar + *pous* foot] any animal of the subclass Copepoda.

**Co·pep·o·da** (ko-pep'o-də) [Gr. *kōpē* oar + *pous* foot] a subclass of minute aquatic arthropods of the class Crustacea; some are intermediate hosts of the nematode *Diphyllobothrium* and others host the tapeworm *Dracunculus;* ingestion of copepods infected with the early larval stages of *Spirometra mansonoides* may cause human sparganosis.

**Co·per·ni·cia** (ko"pər-nish'e-ə) a genus of palms (family Palmae), native to the Americas. *C. ceri'fera* Mart. is the carnauba, a South American species that yields carnauba wax.

**cop·ing** (kōp'ing) a truncated cone-shaped metal cap that fits over the prepared natural tooth and serves as an abutment for dentures. Called also *cope* and *thimble.*

**transfer c.,** a covering or cap of metal, acrylic resin, or other material, used to position a die in an impression.

**copi·opia** (kop"e-o'pe-ə) [Gr. *kopos* fatigue + *-opia*] eyestrain from overwork or improper use of the eyes.

**Co·poly·mer 1** (ko-pol'ə-mər) trademark for a synthetic polypeptide consisting of alanine, glutamic acid, lysine, and tyrosine; it simulates myelin basic protein and is used experimentally in the treatment of relapsing and remitting multiple sclerosis, administered subcutaneously.

**co·poly·mer** (ko-pol'ə-mər) a polymer containing monomers of more than one kind.

**COPP** a regimen of cyclophosphamide, Oncovin (vincristine), procarbazine, and prednisone, used in cancer chemotherapy.

**cop·per** (kop'ər) [L. *cuprum;* Gr. *Kypros*] [MeSH: Copper] a reddish, malleable metal; atomic number, 29; atomic weight, 63.54; symbol Cu; with poisonous salts. Copper is essential in nutrition, being a component of various proteins, including ceruloplasmin, erythrocuprein, cytochrome *c* oxidase, and tyrosinase. Deficiency, which is rare, may result in hypochromic microcytic anemia, neutropenia, and bone changes. Excessive accumulation in the body may lead to copper poisoning (see under *poisoning*).

**c. 64,** a radioactive isotope of copper, atomic mass 64, with a half-life of 12.70 hours, emitting positrons (energy 0.657 MeV), beta particles (energy 0.571 MeV), and gamma rays (energy 1.34 MeV); used in brain scanning.

**c. 67,** a radioisotope of copper, atomic mass 67, with a half-life of 2.58 days, emitting beta particles (energy 0.395, 0.484, 0.577 MeV) and gamma rays (energy 0.185, 0.092 MeV); used in radiotherapy as well as for imaging, tracer kinetic studies, and dosimetry.

**c. acetoarsenite,** an emerald green powder derived by reaction of sodium arsenite, copper sulfate, and acetic acid; it is toxic by ingestion and is used as an insecticide and wood preservative. Called also *Paris green.*

**c. citrate,** see *cupric citrate,* under *citrate.*

**c. sulfate,** cupric sulfate; see under *sulfate.*

**cop·per·as** (kop'ər-əs) commercial ferrous sulfate, disinfectant and deodorizer. See also *ferrous sulfate,* under *ferrous.*

**cop·per·head** (kop'ər-hed) 1. *Agkistrodon contortrix,* a venomous snake of the United States that has a brown to copper-colored body with dark bands. Called also *highland moccasin.* 2. *Denisonia superba,* a highly venomous elapid snake found in Australia and the Solomon Islands. See table at *snake.*

**cop·ra·cra·sia** (kop"rə-kra'shə) [*copr-* + *a-*[1] + *-crasia*] fecal incontinence.

**cop·ra·gogue** (kop'rə-gog) [*copro-* + *agōgos* leading] cathartic.

**co·pre·cip·i·tin** (ko"pre-sip'ĭ-tin) a precipitin in the same serum with one or more other precipitins.

**cop·rem·e·sis** (kop-rem'ə-sis) [*copro-* + *emesis*] the vomiting of fecal material.

**Co·pri·na·ceae** (ko"prĭ-na'se-e) a family of mushrooms (order Agaricales); it includes the genus *Coprinus.*

**co·prine** (ko'prēn) a glutamic acid derivative found in the edible mushroom *Coprinus atramentarius;* its active metabolite is cyclopropanone hydrate.

**Co·pri·nus** (ko-pri'nəs) [MeSH: Coprinus] the ink caps or inky caps, a genus of mushrooms of the family Coprinaceae. *C. atramenta'rius* is an edible species that contains coprine and causes a disulfiram-like toxic response in the presence of alcohol.

**copr(o)-** [Gr. *kopros* dung] a combining form denoting relationship to feces.

**cop·ro·an·ti·body** (kop"ro-an'tĭ-bod'e) an antibody found in the feces, chiefly secretory IgA.

**Cop·ro·coc·cus** (kop"ro-kok'əs) [*copro-* + Gr. *kokkos* berry] a genus of bacteria, made up of gram-positive anaerobic cocci, occasionally isolated from human specimens.

**cop·ro·dae·um** (kop"ro-de'əm) [*copro-* + Gr. *hodiaos* on the way] the large dorsal passage in the proximal part of the cloaca in monotremes, into which the intestine opens.

**cop·ro·de·um** (kop"ro-de'əm) coprodaeum.

**cop·ro·lag·nia** (kop"ro-lag'ne-ə) [*copro-* + Gr. *lagneia* lust] sexual excitement occurring in association with feces or defecation.

**cop·ro·la·lia** (kop"ro-la'le-ə) [*copro-* + *lal-* + *-ia*] compulsive, stereotyped use of obscene, "filthy" language, particularly of words relating to feces; seen in some cases of schizophrenia and Gilles de la Tourette's syndrome. Called also *coprophrasia.*

**cop·ro·lith** (kop'ro-lith) [*copro-* + *-lith*] fecalith.

**cop·rol·o·gy** (kop-rol'ə-je) [*copro-* + *-logy*] scatology (def. 1).

**cop·ro·ma** (kop-ro'mə) [*copro-* + *-oma*] stercoroma.

**Cop·ro·mas·tix** (kop"ro-mas'tiks) a genus of coprozoic protozoa of the order Polymastigida, class Zoomastigophora, having four equally long anterior flagella and a trailing flagellum.

**C. prowaze'ki,** a species found in rat and human feces in Brazil.

**cop·ro·pha·gia** (kop"ro-fa'jə) [MeSH: Coprophagia] coprophagy.

**cop·roph·a·gous** (kop-rof'ə-gəs) feeding on dung, or feces.

**cop·roph·a·gy** (kop-rof'ə-je) [*copro-* + *-phagy*] the habitual ingestion of dung, or feces.

**cop·ro·phil** (kop'ro-fil) a coprophilous microorganism.

**cop·ro·phile** (kop'ro-fīl) 1. coprophil. 2. coprophilous.

**cop·ro·phil·ia** (kop"ro-fil'e-ə) [*copro-* + *-philia*] an absorbing interest in feces or filth, particularly a paraphilia in which sexual arousal or activity is linked to feces.

**cop·ro·phil·i·ac** (kop"ro-fil'e-ak) coprophilic, def. 1.

**cop·ro·phil·ic** (kop"ro-fil'ik) 1. pertaining to or characterized by coprophilia. 2. coprophilous.

**cop·roph·i·lous** (kop-rof'ĭ-ləs) living and growing on dung or feces or in feces-polluted water; said of certain microorganisms and fungi. Called also *coprophilic.*

**cop·ro·pho·bia** (kop"ro-fo'be-ə) [*copro-* + *-phobia*] abnormal repugnance to defecation and to feces.

**cop·ro·phra·sia** (kop″ro-fra′zhə) coprolalia.

**cop·ro·por·phy·ria** (kop″ro-por-fir′e-ə) the presence of coproporphyrin in the feces.
**erythropoietic c.**, an extremely rare erythropoietic porphyria characterized by mild skin photosensitivity and elevated erythrocyte coproporphyrin III levels.
**hereditary c. (HCP)**, a hepatic porphyria transmitted as an autosomal dominant trait, characterized by recurrent attacks of gastroenterologic and neurologic dysfunction similar to those of acute intermittent porphyria, and sometimes by cutaneous photosensitivity. Coproporphyrin III is excreted constantly in the feces and intermittently, with δ-aminolevulinic acid and porphobilinogen, in the urine. The disorder is caused by partial deficiency of coproporphyrinogen oxidase activity.

**cop·ro·por·phy·rin** (kop″ro-por′fə-rin) the porphyrin (q.v.) produced by oxidation of the methylene bridges in coproporphyrinogen. Coproporphyrin III is excreted in the feces and urine in hereditary coproporphyria and in variegate porphyria, particularly during acute attacks; coproporphyrin I is excreted in the feces and urine in congenital erythropoietic porphyria.

**cop·ro·por·phy·rin·o·gen** (kop″ro-por″fə-rin′o-jən) a porphyrinogen (q.v.) in which each pyrrole ring has one methyl side chain and one propionate side chain; it is formed by oxidative decarboxylation of uroporphyrinogen. Four isomers are possible but only two exist naturally, types I and III; the latter is a functional intermediate in heme biosynthesis while the former is produced in an abortive side reaction.

**cop·ro·por·phy·rin·o·gen ox·i·dase** (kop″ro-por″fə-rin′o-jən ok′sĭ-dās) [EC 1.3.3.3] [MeSH: Coproporphyrinogen Oxidase] an enzyme of the oxidoreductase class that catalyzes the conversion of coproporphyrinogen III to protoporphyrinogen IX. It occurs in mitochondria, and the reaction is a part of the pathway of heme biosynthesis. Deficiency of the enzyme, an autosomal dominant trait, results in hereditary coproporphyria.

**cop·ro·por·phy·rin·uria** (kop″ro-por″fər-in-u′re-ə) the presence of coproporphyrin in the urine.

**cop·ros·ta·nol** (kop-ros′tə-nol) a saturated sterol of the feces, formed by bacterial reduction of cholesterol in the intestines. Called also *coprosterol*.

**cop·ros·ta·sis** (kop-ros′tə-sis) [*copro-* + *-stasis*] impaction of the feces in the intestine.

**cop·ros·ter·ol** (kop-ros′tər-ol) coprostanol.

**cop·ro·zoa** (kop″ro-zo′ə) [*copro-* + Gr. *zōon* animal] protozoa which are found in fecal matter outside the body, but which do not inhabit the intestine.

**cop·ro·zo·ic** (kop″ro-zo′ik) living in fecal material; found in fecal material.

**cop·u·la** (kop′u-lə) [L.] 1. any connecting part or structure. 2. c. linguae.
**c. lin′guae**, a median ventral elevation on the embryonic tongue formed by union of the second pharyngeal arches; it represents the future root of the tongue.

**cop·u·la·tion** (kop″u-la′shən) [L. *copulatio*] [MeSH: Copulation] sexual union between male and female; the act transferring the sperm from male to female; used particularly for nonhuman animals.

**Coq.** abbreviation for L. *co′que,* boil.

**Coq. in s. a.** abbreviation for L. *co′que in sufficien′te a′qua,* boil in sufficient water.

**Coq. s. a.** abbreviation for L. *co′que secun′dum ar′tem,* boil properly.

**co·quille** (ko-kēl′) [Fr. "shell"] a glass or lens of uniform thickness shaped like a watch crystal.

**Co·quil·let·tid·ia** (ko-kwil′ə-tid′e-ə) a genus of large, mostly yellow fresh water mosquitoes of the tribe Mansoniini, subfamily Culicini that lay egg masses on stagnant water or weedy ponds and are vicious biters; some species have been implicated as vectors of disease.
**C. juxtamanso′nia**, a species that is a vector of *Wuchereria bancrofti* in Brazil.
**C. ochra′cea**, a species that is a vector of *Brugia malayi* in Southeast Asia.
**C. pertur′bans**, a species that is a vector of eastern equine encephalitis in North America.
**C. venezuelen′sis**, a South American species that is the vector of several arboviruses, including Oropouche virus.

**cor** (kor) gen. *cor′dis* [L.] [TA] the heart (q.v.): the muscular organ that maintains the circulation of the blood.
**c. adipo′sum**, fatty heart (def. 2).
**c. bilocula′re**, a congenital anomaly characterized by failure of formation of the interatrial and interventricular septa, the heart having only two chambers, a single atrium and a single ventricle, and a common atrioventricular valve.
**c. bovi′num**, [L. "ox heart"], a greatly enlarged heart resulting from a hypertrophied or dilated left ventricle; called also *c. taurinum, bovine heart,* and *ox heart.*
**c. dex′trum**, right heart.
**c. pulmonale, acute**, acute overload of the right ventricle due to pulmonary hypertension, usually resulting from acute pulmonary embolism.
**c. pulmonale, chronic**, heart disease characterized by hypertrophy and sometimes dilation of the right ventricle secondary to disease affecting the structure or function of the lungs, but excluding those pulmonary disorders resulting from congenital heart disease or from diseases primarily affecting the left side of the heart.
**c. sinis′trum**, left heart.
**c. tauri′num**, c. bovinum.
**c. triatria′tum**, a congenital anomaly caused by failure of resorption of the embryonic common pulmonary vein, resulting in division of the left atrium by a fibromuscular diaphragm, the posterosuperior chamber receiving the pulmonary venous return and the anteroinferior chamber communicating with the left atrial appendage and mitral orifice. The orifice between the two compartments may be reduced or absent, producing pulmonary venous obstruction.
**c. trilocula′re**, three-chambered heart.
**c. trilocula′re biatria′tum**, a congenital anomaly caused by failure of formation of the interventricular septum, the heart having two atria and a single ventricle.
**c. trilocula′re biventricula′re**, a developmental anomaly caused by failure of formation of the interatrial septum, the heart having one atrium and two ventricles.

**cor-** see *con-*.

**cor·a·cid·ia** (kor″ə-sid′e-ə) [L.] plural of *coracidium.*

**cor·a·cid·i·um** (kor″ə-sid′e-əm) pl. *coracid′ia* [L.] The individual free-swimming or free-crawling, spherical, ciliated embryo of tapeworms of the order Pseudophyllidea.

**cor·a·co·acro·mi·al** (kor″ə-ko-ə-kro′me-əl) pertaining to the coracoid and acromion processes.

**cor·a·co·cla·vic·u·lar** (kor″ə-ko-klə-vik′u-lər) pertaining to the coracoid process and the clavicle.

**cor·a·co·hu·mer·al** (kor″ə-ko-hu′mər-əl) pertaining to the coracoid process and the humerus.

**cor·a·coid** (kor′ə-koid) [Gr. *korakoeidēs* crowlike] 1. like a raven's beak. 2. the coracoid process (processus coracoideus scapulae [TA]).

**cor·a·coi·di·tis** (kor″ə-koi-di′tis) a painful condition in the region of the scapula and the coracoid process, with deltoid atrophy; attributed to injury of the coracoid process.

**cor·a·co·ra·di·a·lis** (kor″ə-ko-ra″de-a′lis) caput breve musculi bicipitis brachii.

**cor·a·co·ul·nar·is** (kor″ə-ko-əl-nar′is) the fibers of the biceps muscle attached to the fascia of the forearm.

**co·ral·li·form** (ko-ral′ĭ-form) [L. *corallum* coral + *form*] having the form of a coral; branching like a coral.

**cor·al·lin** (kor′ə-lin) aurin.
**yellow c.**, the sodium salt of aurin, occurring as yellow masses with a greenish metallic luster, which turns red in solution; called also *corallin yellow.*

**cor·al·loid** (kor′ə-loid) coralliform.

**Co·ra·mine** (ko′rə-mēn) trademark for preparations of nikethamide.

**Cor·bus′ disease** (kor′bəs) [Budd Clarke *Corbus,* American urologist, 1876–1954] balanitis gangrenosa.

**cord** (kord) [L. *chorda;* Gr. *chordē* string] any long, rounded, flexible structure; see also *chorda.*
**Bergmann's c's**, striae medullares ventriculi quarti; see under *stria.*
**Billroth's c's**, red pulp c's.
**dental c.**, a cordlike mass of cells from which the enamel organ develops.
**enamel c.**, a vertical extension of the enamel knot in a developing tooth, connecting the enamel knot with the outer dental epithelium, a temporary structure which disappears before enamel formation begins.
**farcy c's**, enlarged lymphatic vessels seen in farcy; called also *farcy pipes.*
**genital c.**, in the embryo, the midline fused caudal part of the two urogenital ridges, each containing a mesonephric and a paramesonephric duct.
**gubernacular c.**, chorda gubernaculum.
**hepatic c's**, anastomosing plates of hepatic cells radiating outward

from the central vein and composing the parenchyma of a hepatic lobule; called also *hepatic cell c's.*
**lateral c. of brachial plexus,** fasciculus lateralis plexus brachialis.
**lymph c's,** medullary c's (def. 1).
**medial c. of brachial plexus,** fasciculus medialis plexus brachialis.
**medullary c's,** 1. strands of dense lymphoid tissue surrounded by the sinuses of the medulla of a lymph node; called also *lymph c's.* 2. rete c's.
**nephrogenic c.,** a longitudinal cordlike part of the urogenital ridge, formed of fused or never separated nephrotome plates, that gives rise to the mesonephric tubule and part of the metanephric tubules.
**oblique c. of elbow joint,** chorda obliqua membranae interosseae antebrachii.
**ovigerous c's,** rete cords of the primordial ovary that resolve into eggs and their follicles.
**Pflüger's c's,** the ovarian tubes.
**posterior c. of brachial plexus,** fasciculus posterior plexus brachialis.
**red pulp c's,** the masses of red pulp of the spleen; called also *Billroth's c's* and *splenic c's.*
**rete c's,** strands of primordial cells in the medulla of the embryonic gonads that connect with some of the mesonephric tubules, and from which the rete ovarii or the rete testis develops; called also *medullary c's* and *sex c's.*
**retraction c.,** a cord impregnated with a chemical or medication, used in dental surgery for gingival retraction.
**scirrhous c.,** chronic fibrous enlargement of the stump of the spermatic cord of a castrated horse caused by bacterial infection, with discharge of pus and sometimes formation of a tumorlike mass with numerous weeping sinuses.
**sex c's,** rete c's.
**sexual c's,** the seminiferous tubules of the early fetus.
**spermatic c.,** funiculus spermaticus.
**spinal c.,** medulla spinalis.
**splenic c's,** red pulp c's.
**testis c's,** the rete cords of the embryonic testis.
**tethered c.,** see under *syndrome.*
**umbilical c.,** the flexible structure connecting the umbilicus of the embryo and fetus with the placenta and giving passage to the umbilical arteries and vein. In the newborn it measures about 50 cm in length. First formed during the fifth embryonic week from the connecting stalk, it contains the omphalomesenteric duct (yolk stalk) and the allantois. Called also *funiculus umbilicalis* [TA] and *chorda umbilicalis.*
**vocal c., false,** plica vestibularis.
**vocal c., true,** plica vocalis.
**Weitbrecht's c.,** chorda obliqua membranae interosseae antebrachii.
**Willis' c's,** numerous fibrous bands (dural trabeculae) that extend transversely across the inferior angle of the superior sagittal sinus.

**cord·al** (kor'dəl) pertaining to a cord; used specifically in referring to the vocal cord (*plica vocalis* [TA]).

**Cor·da·rone** (kor'də-rōn) trademark for a preparation of amiodarone.

**cor·date** (kor'dāt) [L. *cor* heart] heart-shaped.

**cor·dec·to·my** (kor-dek'tə-me) [*cord* + *-ectomy*] excision of all or part of a cord, as a vocal cord or the spinal cord.

**cor·dial** (kor'jəl) [L. *cordialis*] an aromatized alcoholic liqueur.

**cor·di·a·le** (kor-de-a'le) [L.] cordial.

**cor·di·form** (kor'dĭ-form) [*cor* + *form*] heart-shaped.

**cor·ding-up** (kōr″ding-up′) azoturia, def. 2.

**cor·di·tis** (kor-di'tis) inflammation of the spermatic cord.

**cor·do·cen·te·sis** (kor″do-sen-te'sis) [MeSH: Cordocentesis] percutaneous puncture of the umbilical vein under ultrasonographic guidance to obtain a fetal blood sample. Called also *percutaneous umbilical blood sampling.*

**cor·do·pexy** (kor'do-pek″se) [*cord* + *-pexy*] the operation of displacing outward the vocal cord for bilateral vocal cord paralysis.

**cor·dot·o·my** (kor-dot'ə-me) [MeSH: Cordotomy] 1. section of a vocal cord. 2. interruption of the lateral spinothalamic tract of the spinal cord, usually in the anterolateral quadrant, for relief of intractable pain. Also spelled *chordotomy.*
**open c.,** cordotomy (def. 2) done through an open incision; now largely replaced by percutaneous cordotomy.
**percutaneous c.,** cordotomy (def. 2) performed using percutaneous electrodes guided radiographically with stereotactic techniques; approaches used include lateral high cervical, posterior high cervical, and anterior low cervical.

**Cor·dran** (kor'dran) trademark for preparations of flurandrenolide.

**Cor·dy·ceps** (kor'dĭ-seps) a genus of fungi of the family Clavicipitaceae; certain species produce fatal disease of caterpillars.
**C. sinen'sis,** a parasite of insect larvae; in Chinese medicine it is used as a drug coagulant. Called also *Sphaeria sinensis.*

**Cor·dy·lo·bia** (kor″də-lo'be-ə) a genus of flies of the family Calliphoridae. *C. anthropo'phaga* (the tumbu fly) is a species found in Africa whose larvae (cayor worms) burrow under the skin of humans and other animals, causing myiasis.

**core** (kor) 1. the central part of anything, such as the central mass of necrotic matter in a boil. 2. a bar of iron around which a wire is wound to form an induction coil or electromagnet. 3. the central part of a virion, consisting of nucleic acid and sometimes protein. 4. cast c.
**cast c.,** a metal casting, usually with a post in the root canal, designed to support and retain an artificial crown.

**core-** [Gr. *korē* pupil] a combining form denoting relationship to the pupil of the eye; also, *cor(o)-.* See also words beginning *irid(o)-.*

**core·cli·sis** (kor″ə-kli'sis) [*core-* + Gr. *kleisis* closure] iridencleisis.

**cor·ec·ta·sis** (kor-ek'tə-sis) [*core-* + *ectasis*] dilatation of the pupil.

**cor·ec·tome** (kor-ek'tōm) [*core-* + *-tomy*] a cutting instrument used in performing iridectomy (corectomy).

**co·rec·to·me·di·al·y·sis** (ko-rek″to-me″de-al'ə-sis) [*core-* + *ectomy* + *dialysis*] the operation of forming an artificial pupil by detaching the iris from the ciliary ligament.

**co·rec·to·my** (ko-rek'tə-me) [*cor-* +*ectomy*] iridectomy.

**cor·ec·to·pia** (kor″ek-to'pe-ə) [*core-* + *ectopia*] abnormal situation of the pupil.

**core·di·al·y·sis** (kor″ə-di-al'ə-sis) [*core-* + *dialysis*] the surgical separation of the external margin of the iris from the ciliary body.

**core·di·as·ta·sis** (kor″ə-di-as'tə-sis) [*core-* + Gr. *diastasis* distention] the dilatation or a dilated state of the pupil.

**co·reg·o·nin** (ko-reg'o-nin) a protamine obtained from the sperm of the white fish.

**co·rel·y·sis** (ko-rəl'ə-sis) [*core-* + *lysis*] operative destruction of the pupil; especially the surgical detachment of adhesions of the pupillary margin of the iris from the lens.

**co·rem·i·um** (kə-re'me-əm) synnema.

**cor·e·mor·pho·sis** (kor″ə-mor-fo'sis) [*core-* + *morphosis*] the surgical formation of an artificial pupil.

**cor·en·cli·sis** (kor″en-kli'sis) [*core-* + Gr. *enkleiein* to inclose] iridencleisis.

**cor·e·om·e·ter** (kor″e-om'ə-tər) [*core-* + *-meter*] pupillometer.

**cor·e·om·e·try** (kor″e-om'ə-tre) pupillometry.

**cor·eo·plas·ty** (kor'e-o-plas″te) [*core-* + *-plasty*] any plastic operation on the iris.

**co·re·pres·sor** (ko″re-pres'or) a small molecule that combines with a protein aporepressor molecule to form an active substance, which then binds to an operator gene and inhibits the synthesis of an enzyme. The mechanism is a negative control in inducible enzyme systems.

**cor·e·ste·no·ma** (kor″e-stə-no'mə) [*core-* + Gr. *stenōma* contraction] an abnormally contracted state of the pupil.
**c. conge'nitum,** a congenital condition in which the pupil is partially occluded by excrescences which meet, leaving scattered small openings.

**Co·re·thra** (ko-re'thrə) *Chaoborus.*

**co·re·to·me·di·al·y·sis** (kor″ə-to″me-di-al'ə-sis) corectomedialysis.

**co·ret·o·my** (kor-et'ə-me) iridectomy.

**Cor·gard** (kor'gahrd) trademark for a preparation of nadolol.

**Co·ri** (ko're) Carl Ferdinand. Czechoslovakian-born American physician and biochemist, 1896–1984; co-winner, with his wife Gerty Theresa Radnitz Cori and Bernardo Alberto Houssay, of the Nobel prize for medicine or physiology in 1947 for their discovery of the catalytic conversion of glycogen to lactic acid.

**Co·ri** (ko're) Gerty Theresa Radnitz. Czechoslovakian-born American physician and biochemist, 1896–1957; co-winner, with her husband Carl Ferdinand Cori and Bernardo Alberto Houssay, of the Nobel prize for medicine or physiology in 1947 for their discovery of the catalytic conversion of glycogen to lactic acid.

**Co·ri cycle, disease, ester** (ko're) [Carl F. *Cori* and Gerty T.R. *Cori*] see under *cycle,* see *glycogen storage disease, type III,* under *disease,* and see *glucose 1-phosphate.*

**co·ri·a·ceous** (kor″e-a'shəs) [L. *corium* leather] resembling leather; leathery, tough; said of bacterial cultures.

**co·ri·a·myr·tin** (kor″e-ə-mər'tin) a toxic glycoside from *Coriaria* with neurostimulating activity, causing convulsions and death in humans and other animals.

**cor·i·an·der** (kor″e-an′dər) [Gr. *koriandron,* variant of *koriannon*] 1. *Coriandrum sativum.* 2. the dried ripe fruit of *C. sativum,* used as a flavoring and source of coriander oil.

**Co·ri·an·drum** (ko″re-an′drəm) a genus of plants of the family Umbelliferae. *C. sati′vum* is coriander, used as a flavoring and source of coriander oil.

**Co·ri·a·ria** (kor″e-ar′e-ə) a genus of trees and shrubs of the family Coriariaceae, native to Europe and Asia. Most species contain the toxin coriamyrtin, which causes vomiting, convulsions, and death in humans and other animals. They are also noted for their content of dyes and tannins.

**Cor·id** (kor′id) trademark for a preparation of amprolium.

**co·ri·in** (kor′e-in) a substance formed by treating fibrous connective tissue with alkalis.

**co·ri·um** (kor′e-əm) [L. "hide"] TA alternative for *dermis.*

**corm** (korm) [L. *cormus*] a solid bulblike expansion of a plant stem below the surface of the ground.

**Cor·mack** (kor′mak) Allan MacLeod. South African–born American physicist, born 1924; co-winner, with Godfrey Newbold Hounsfield, of the Nobel prize for medicine or physiology in 1979 for their development of computerized axial tomography.

**corn** (korn) [L. *cornu* horn] [MeSH: Corn] 1. a horny thickening of the stratum corneum of the skin of the toes, caused by friction and pressure from poorly fitting shoes or hose; it forms a conical mass pointing down into the corium, producing pain and inflammation. There are two kinds, the *hard c.* and the *soft c.* Called also *clavus.* 2. *Zea mays.* 3. the seeds of certain cereal grains, especially *Zea mays,* used as both animal and human food. See also *corn oil,* under *oil.* 4. a bruise on the bottom of a horse's foot between the wall of the heel and the bar. 5. a circumscribed hyperkeratosis of the footpad of dogs, sensitive to pressure.
**hard c.,** a firm type of corn, usually found on the outside of the little toe or the upper surface of a toe; called also *clavus durus* and *heloma durum.*
**soft c.,** a type of corn found between the toes and kept soft by moisture; called also *clavus mollis* and *heloma molle.*
**squirrel c., turkey c.,** *Dicentra canadensis.*

**corn cock·le** (kōrn kok′əl) *Agrostemma githago.*

**cornea** (kor′ne-ə) [L. *corneus* horny] [TA] [MeSH: Cornea] the transparent structure forming the anterior part of the sclera of the eye. It consists of five layers: (1) the anterior corneal epithelium, continuous with that of the conjunctiva; (2) the anterior limiting layer (Bowman's membrane); (3) the substantia propria, or stroma; (4) the posterior limiting layer (Descemet's membrane); and (5) the endothelium of the anterior chamber.
**conical c.,** keratoconus.
**c. farina′ta,** senile degeneration of the cornea marked by fine dustlike stippling.
**flat c.,** the configuration of the cornea when a shallow ocular chamber is present or when the eyeball is atrophic.
**c. globo′sa,** megalocornea.
**c. gutta′ta,** a degenerative condition of the cornea due to dystrophy of the endothelial cells; called also *dystrophia endothelialis corneae.*
**c. opa′ca,** the sclerotic coat of the eye.
**c. pla′na,** congenital flatness of the cornea.
**c. verticilla′ta,** Fleischer's vortex.

**cor·ne·al** (kor′ne-əl) pertaining to the cornea.

**cor·ne·itis** (kor″ne-i′tis) keratitis.

**Cor·ne·lia de Lange** (kor-na′le-ah da-lahng′ə) see *de Lange.*

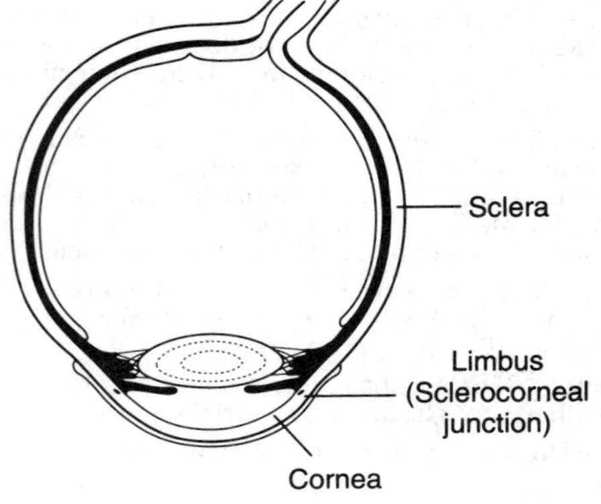


**cor·neo·bleph·a·ron** (kor″ne-o-blef′ə-ron) [*cornea* + Gr. *blepharon* eyelid] adhesion between the eyelid and cornea.

**cor·neo·cyte** (kor′ne-o-sīt″) the remains of a keratinocyte; it is shed by the stratum corneum.

**cor·neo·iri·tis** (kor″ne-o-i-ri′tis) inflammation of the cornea and iris.

**cor·neo·scle·ra** (kor″ne-o-skler′ə) the cornea and sclera regarded as forming one organ.

**cor·neo·scle·ral** (kor″ne-o-skler′əl) affecting or pertaining to both the cornea and the sclera.

**cor·ne·ous** (kor′ne-əs) [L. *corneus*] hornlike, or horny; consisting of keratin.

**cor·ner** (kor′nər) corner tooth.

**Cor·ner-Al·len test, unit** (kor′nər-al′ən) [George Washington *Corner,* American anatomist, 1889–1981; Willard Myron *Allen,* American gynecologist, born 1904] see under *test* and *unit.*

**Cor·net's forceps** (kor′nəts) [Georg *Cornet,* German bacteriologist, 1858–1915] a cover glass forceps.

**cor·ne·um** (kor′ne-əm) [L. "horny"] see *stratum corneum epidermidis* and *stratum corneum unguis.*

**cor·nic·u·late** (kor-nik′u-lāt) shaped like a small horn.

**cor·nic·u·lum** (kor-nik′u-ləm) [L. dim. of *cornu*] cartilago corniculata.

**cor·ni·fi·ca·tion** (kor″nĭ-fĭ-ka′shən) [*cornu* + L. *facere* to make] 1. conversion into keratin, or horn. 2. conversion of epithelium to the stratified squamous type.

**cor·ni·fied** (kor′nĭ-fīd) converted into horny tissue (keratin); keratinized.

**cor·noid** (kor′noid) [*cornu* + *-oid*] resembling horn; see under *lamella.*

**cor·nu** (kor′noo) pl. *cor′nua* [L. "horn"] 1. horn (def. 1). 2. a hornlike excrescence or projection. 3. [TA] in anatomical nomenclature, a structure resembling a horn in shape.
**c. ammo′nis** [L. "horn of Ammon"], hippocampus.
**c. ante′rius medul′lae spina′lis** [TA], anterior horn of spinal cord: the horn-shaped configuration presented by the anterior column of the spinal cord in transverse section; called also *c. ventrale medullae spinalis* and *ventral horn of spinal cord.*
**c. ante′rius ventri′culi latera′lis,** TA alternative for *c. frontale ventriculi lateralis.*
**cor′nua cartila′ginis thyroi′deae,** the horns of the thyroid cartilage; see *c. inferius cartilaginis thyroideae* and *c. superius cartilaginis thyroideae.*
**c. coccygea′le,** c. coccygeum.
**c. coccy′geum** [TA], **c. coccyx,** coccygeal horn: either of the cranial pair of rudimentary articular processes of the coccyx that articulate with the cornua of the sacrum. Called also *c. coccygeale.*
**c. cuta′neum,** cutaneous horn.
**c. dorsa′le medul′lae spina′lis,** c. posterius medullae spinalis.
**ethmoid c.,** concha nasalis media.
**c. fronta′le ventri′culi latera′lis** [TA], frontal horn of lateral ventricle: the part of the lateral ventricle that extends forward from the pars centralis into the frontal lobe; called also *anterior horn of lateral ventricle* and *c. anterius ventriculi lateralis* [TA alternative].
**c. infe′rius cartila′ginis thyroi′deae** [TA], inferior horn of thyroid cartilage: the inferior extension of the posterior border of the thyroid cartilage.
**c. infe′rius mar′ginis falcifor′mis** [TA], inferior horn of falciform margin: the distal edge of the falciform margin of the saphenous hiatus, deep to the great saphenous vein. Called also *crus inferius marginis falciformis* [TA alternative].
**c. infe′rius ventri′culi latera′lis,** TA alternative for *c. temporale ventriculi lateralis.*
**c. latera′le medul′lae spina′lis** [TA], lateral horn of spinal cord: the horn-shaped configuration presented by the intermediate column of the spinal cord in transverse section. See also *columnae griseae* and *columna intermedia medullae spinalis.*
**c. ma′jus os′sis hyoi′dei** [TA], greater horn of hyoid bone: a bony projection passing posteriorly and superiorly from either side of the body of the hyoid bone.
**c. mi′nus os′sis hyoi′dei** [TA], lesser horn of hyoid bone: a small conical eminence projecting superiorly on either side of the hyoid bone at the angle of junction between the body and the greater horn.
**c. occipita′le ventri′culi latera′lis** [TA], occipital horn of lateral ventricle: the part of the lateral ventricle that extends backward from the par centralis into the occipital lobe; called also *c. posterius ventriculi lateralis* [TA alternative] and *posterior horn of lateral ventricle.*
**cor′nua os′sis hyoi′dei,** the horns of the hyoid bone; see *c. majus ossis hyoidei* and *c. minus ossis hyoidei.*

**c. poste'rius medul'lae spina'lis** [TA], posterior horn of spinal cord: the horn-shaped configuration presented by the posterior column of the spinal cord in transverse section; called also *c. dorsale medullae spinalis* and *dorsal horn of spinal cord.*
**c. poste'rius ventri'culi latera'lis,** TA alternative for *c. occipitale ventriculi lateralis.*
**sacral c., c. sacra'le** [TA], sacral horn: either of the two hook-shaped processes extending downward from the arch of the last sacral vertebra; called also *coccygeal eminence.*
**cornua of spinal cord,** the horn-shaped structures seen in transverse section of the spinal cord; see *c. anterius medullae spinalis, c. laterale medullae spinalis,* and *c. posterius medullae spinalis.*
**c. supe'rius cartila'ginis thyroi'deae** [TA], superior horn of thyroid cartilage: the superior extension of the posterior border of the thyroid cartilage.
**c. supe'rius mar'ginis falcifor'mis** [TA], superior horn of falciform margin: the proximal end of the falciform margin of the saphenous hiatus; called also *crus superius marginis falciformis* [TA alternative] and *ligament of Scarpa.*
**c. tempora'le ventri'culi latera'lis** [TA], temporal horn of lateral ventricle: the part of the lateral ventricle that extends downward and forward from the pars centralis behind the thalamus and into the temporal lobe; called also *c. inferius ventriculi lateralis* [TA alternative] and *inferior horn of lateral ventricle.*
**c. u'teri** [TA], **c. uteri'num,** horn of uterus: either of the bluntly rounded superior lateral extremities of the body of the uterus that marks the entrance of the uterine tube.
**c. ventra'le medul'lae spina'lis,** c. anterius medullae spinalis.

**cor·nua** (kor'noo-ə) [L.] plural of *cornu.*

**cor·nu·al** (kor'noo-əl) pertaining to a cornu or to cornua.

**cor·nu·ate** (kor'nu-āt) cornual.

**cor·nu·com·mis·sur·al** (kor″noo-ko-mis'u-rəl) pertaining to a cornu and to a commissure.

**cor(o)-** see *core-.*

**co·ro·di·as·ta·sis** (kor″o-di-as'tə-sis) corediastasis.

**co·rol·la** (ko-rol'ə) [L. "little crown"] the inner set of leaves of a floral envelope, the individual portions of which are called *petals.*

**co·ro·na** (kə-ro'nə) pl. *coronas* or *coro'nae* [L.; Gr. *korōnē*] a crown; used in anatomical nomenclature to designate a crownlike eminence or encircling structure.
**c. cilia'ris** [TA], ciliary crown: the region on the anterior inner surface of the ciliary body of the eye from which radiate the ciliary processes; called also *pars plicata corporis ciliaris.*
**c. cli'nica** [TA], clinical crown: that portion of the tooth above the clinical root, i.e., the portion exposed beyond the gingiva, and thus visible in the oral cavity. Called also *extra-alveolar crown.*
**dental c., c. den'tis** [TA], crown of tooth: the upper part of the tooth, which joins the lower part, the root, at the cervix at the cementoenamel junction, and terminates as the grinding surface of molar or premolar teeth or the cutting edge of incisors. Called also *anatomical* or *dental crown.*
**c. glan'dis pe'nis** [TA], corona of glans penis: the rounded proximal border of the glans penis, separated from the corpora cavernosa penis by the neck of the glans.
**c. radia'ta,** 1. [TA] the radiating crown of projection fibers which pass from the internal capsule to every part of the cerebral cortex. 2. an investing layer of radially elongated follicular cells surrounding the zona pellucida of a secondary oocyte or ovum.
**c. ve'neris,** a ring of syphilitic sores around the forehead, sometimes deeply affecting the bones of the head.
**Zinn's c.,** circulus vasculosus nervi optici.

**co·ro·nad** (kor'ŏ-nad) toward the crown of the head or any corona.

**co·ro·nae** (kə-ro'ne) [L.] genitive and plural of *corona.*

**co·ro·nal** (kə-rōn'əl) [L. *coronalis*] 1. pertaining to the crown of the head, the crown of a tooth, or any other corona. 2. in the direction of the coronal suture; said of a longitudinal plane or section passing through the body at right angles to the median plane. See under *plane.* Called also *coronalis.*

**co·ro·na·le** (kor-o-na'le) 1. the point of the coronal suture at the end of the maximum frontal diameter. 2. os frontale.

**co·ro·na·lis** (kor″o-na'lis) [L.] [TA] coronal: general anatomical nomenclature denoting something situated in the direction of the coronal suture.

**cor·o·nary** (kor'ə-nar″e) [*corona*] encircling in the manner of a crown; a term applied to vessels, nerves, ligaments, etc. The term usually denotes the arteries that supply the heart muscle and, by extension, a pathologic involvement of them.

**Co·ro·na·vi·ri·dae** (kə-ro″nə-vir'ĭ-de) [MeSH: Coronaviridae] the coronaviruses and toroviruses: a family of RNA viruses having a pleomorphic virion 120–160 nm in diameter consisting of a lipid-containing membrane, with large peplomers, surrounding a helical (for coronaviruses) or tubular (for toroviruses) nucleocapsid. The genome consists of a single molecule of positive-sense single-stranded polyadenylated RNA (MW $5.5–6.1 \times 10^6$, size about 30 kb for coronaviruses and 20 kb for toroviruses). Viruses contain three major structural polypeptides and are resistant to trypsin but sensitive to lipid solvents, detergents, ultraviolet radiation, disinfectants, and heat. Replicating occurs in the cytoplasm and assembly is by budding, usually through intracytoplasmic membranes; virions are released by exocytosis or by cell destruction. Transmission is mechanical, including airborne particles, contaminated equipment, and contact with infected persons. Included here are the genera *Coronavirus* and *Torovirus.*

**Co·ro·na·vi·rus** (kə-ro'nə-vi″rus) [L. *corona* crown + *virus,* from the appearance of the virions on electron micrographs] [MeSH: Coronavirus] coronaviruses; a genus of viruses of the family Coronaviridae that cause respiratory disease and possibly gastroenteritis in humans, and hepatitis, gastroenteritis, encephalitis, and respiratory disease in other animals. In newborn calves and lambs it causes neonatal diarrhea.

**co·ro·na·vi·rus** (kə-ro'nə-vi″rəs) [MeSH: Coronavirus] any virus belonging to the family Coronaviridae.

**co·ro·ne** (kə-ro'ne) [L.; Gr. *korōnē* anything hooked or curved] the coronoid process of the mandible (processus coronoideus mandibulae [TA]).

**cor·o·ner** (kor'ə-nər) [MeSH: Coroners and Medical Examiners] an officer who holds inquests in regard to violent, sudden, or unexplained deaths.

**cor·o·net** (kor'ə-net) coronary band.

**co·ro·ni·on** (kə-ro'ne-on) the tip of the coronoid process of the mandible.

**cor·o·ni·tis** (kor-ə-ni'tis) inflammation of the coronary band or cushion, especially of the horse.

**cor·o·noid** (kor'ə-noid) [Gr. *korōnē* anything hooked or curved, a kind of crown + *-oid*] 1. shaped like a crow's beak. 2. crown-shaped.

**cor·o·noi·dec·to·my** (kor″ə-noi-dek'tə-me) surgical removal of the coronoid process of the mandible.

**cor·o·noi·dot·o·my** (kor″ə-noi-dot'ə-me) coronoidectomy.

**coro·par·el·cy·sis** (kor″o-pər-el'sə-sis) [*coro-* + Gr. *parelkein* to draw aside] the drawing aside of the pupil in partial corneal opacity in order to bring it under a transparent portion.

**coro·plas·ty** (kor'o-plas″te) coreoplasty.

**co·ros·co·py** (kə-ros'kə-pe) [*coro-* + *-scopy*] retinoscopy.

**co·rot·o·my** (kə-rot'ə-me) iridectomy.

**cor·po·ra** (kor'pə-rə) [L.] plural of *corpus.*

**cor·po·ral** (kor'po-rəl) corporeal.

**cor·po·re·al** (kor-por'e-əl) pertaining to the body.

**cor·por·ic** (kor-por'ik) [*corpus*] affecting the body, or corpus, of an organ.

**corps** (kor) [Fr., from L. *corpus*] 1. an organized body, or group of individuals. 2. corpus.
**medical c.,** the surgeon officers of the army or navy, comprising a surgeon general, medical directors, medical inspectors, surgeons, passed assistant surgeons, and assistant surgeons.
**c. ronds,** Darier's name for round, double-contoured bodies seen in keratosis follicularis.

**corpse** (korps) [*corpus*] a dead body; used to refer specifically to a human body in the early period after death. Cf. *cadaver.*

**cor·pu·len·cy** (kor'pu-len″se) [L. *corpulentia*] obesity.

**cor·pus** (kor'pəs) gen. *cor'poris,* pl. *cor'pora* [L. "body"] [TA] 1. body: a discrete mass of material, as of specialized tissue. 2. in anatomical nomenclature, the entire body of the organism, or the main portion of an anatomical part, structure, or organ.

## Corpus

Descriptions are given on TA terms, and include anglicized names of specific structures.

**c. adipo'sum buc'cae** [TA], buccal fat pad: an encapsulated mass of fat in the cheek, separated from the subcutaneous fascia by a facial cleft, and situated between the masseter and the external surface of the buccinator muscles; especially well developed in infants and said to aid in sucking. Called also *sucking cushion,* and *sucking* or *suctorial pad.*

**c. adipo'sum fos'sae ischioana'lis** [TA], **c. adipo'sum fos'sae ischiorecta'lis,** fat body of the ischioanal fossa: a pad of fat found in the ischioanal fossa.

**c. adipo'sum infrapatella're** [TA], infrapatellar fat pad: a mass of fibrous fatty tissue inferior to the patella, in the angle between the deep surface of the patellar ligament and the tibia. Called also *retropatellar fat pad.*

**c. adipo'sum or'bitae** [TA], orbital fat body: a mass of fatty tissue in the posterior part of the orbit, around the optic nerve, extraocular muscles, and vessels. Called also *retrobulbar fat.*

**c. adipo'sum pararena'le** [TA], pararenal fat body: a large mass of fat lying dorsal to the renal fascia; called also *paranephric body* and *paranephric* or *pararenal fat.*

**c. adipo'sum preepiglot'ticum** [TA], preepiglottic fat body: a mass of fatty tissue separating the lower anterior surface of the epiglottis from the thyroid cartilage and the thyrohyoid membrane.

**c. al'bicans** (pl. cor'pora albican'tia) [TA], white fibrous tissue that replaces the regressing corpus luteum in the human ovary in the latter half of pregnancy, or soon after ovulation when pregnancy does not supervene; called also *c. fibrosum.*

**c. alie'num,** a foreign body.

**cor'pora alla'ta,** a set of small endocrine glands in the head of insects just behind the brain, which inhibit metamorphosis by secretion of juvenile hormone.

**c. amygdaloi'deum** [TA], amygdaloid body: a small, ovoid complex of nuclei partly covered by the pyriform cortex, within the tip of the temporal lobe, anterior to the inferior horn of the lateral ventricle of the brain; it is part of the limbic system and is classified as a part of the basal nuclei. The amygdaloid body is divided into two main groups of nuclei, found in the basolateral and corticomedial parts (*pars basolateralis corporis amygdaloidei* and *pars corticomedialis corporis amygdaloidei*), and in a poorly differentiated transitional region, the anterior amygdaloid area. It has olfactory connections, is reciprocally connected to the limbic cortex, and projects fibers to the hippocampus, the septum, the thalamus, and especially the hypothalamus. Called also *amygdala, amygdaloid complex,* and *nucleus amygdalae.*

**cor'pora amyla'cea,** small basophilic, periodic acid–Schiff–positive, hyaline masses, 5–50 μm in diameter, derived from degenerate cells or inspissated secretions and consisting of a central nidus surrounded by concentric lamellae. They occur in the prostate, neuroglia, and pulmonary alveoli and become more numerous with advancing age; their significance is not known. Called also *amylaceous bodies* or *corpuscles, amyloid bodies* or *corpuscles, colloid corpuscles,* and *corpora versicolorata.*

**c. anococcy'geum** [TA], anococcygeal ligament: a fibrous band connecting the posterior fibers of the sphincter of the anus to the coccyx.

**cor'pora atre'tica,** ovarian follicles that never mature, but undergo degeneration.

**cor'pora bige'mina,** 1. two bodies in the brains of non-mammalian vertebrates that correspond to the superior colliculi of mammals; called also *optic lobes.* 2. two bodies in the brain of the human fetus that later split to become the corpora quadrigemina.

**c. calca'nei,** the body of the calcaneus.

**c. callo'sum** [TA], an arched mass of white matter, found in the depths of the longitudinal fissure, composed of three layers of fibers, the central layer consisting primarily of transverse fibers connecting the cerebral hemispheres; its subsections, from anterior to posterior, are called the rostrum, genu, trunk (truncus), and splenium. Called also *commissura magna cerebri.*

**c. caverno'sum clito'ridis** [TA], cavernous body of clitoris: a column of erectile tissue on either side (right and left), the two fusing to form the body of the clitoris (c. clitoridis).

**c. caverno'sum pe'nis** [TA], cavernous body of penis: one of the columns of erectile tissue forming the dorsum and sides of the penis; called also *spongy body of penis.*

**c. caverno'sum ure'thrae viri'lis,** c. spongiosum penis.

**c. cerebel'li** [TA], body of cerebellum: the main portion of the cerebellum, consisting of the two cerebellar hemispheres joined by a median strip, the vermis; see also *cerebellum.*

**c. cilia're** [TA], ciliary body: the thickened part of the vascular tunic of the eye anterior to the ora serrata, connecting the choroid with the iris; it is composed of the corona ciliaris, ciliary processes and folds, ciliary orbiculus, the ciliary muscle, and a basal lamina.

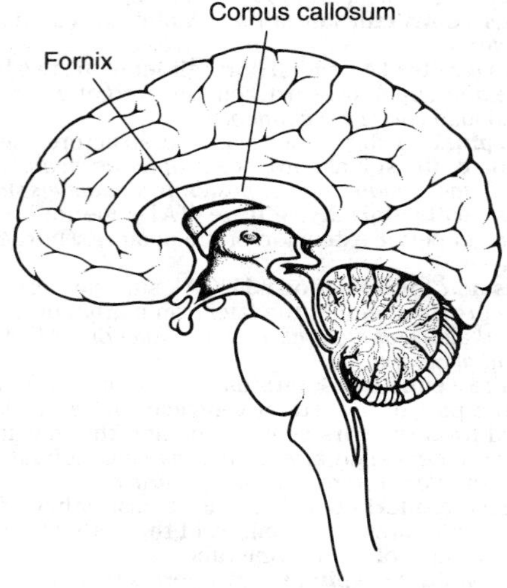


**c. clavi'culae** [TA], **c. clavicula're,** body of clavicle: the long curved central part of the clavicle, extending between the acromial and sternal extremities.

**c. clito'ridis** [TA], corpus of clitoris: the main part of the clitoris, formed by the two fused corpora cavernosa, which are embedded anteriorly in the floor of the vestibule of the vagina.

**c. coccy'geum,** glomus coccygeus.

**c. cos'tae** [TA], body of rib: the part of a rib extending between its dorsally placed tubercle and its ventral extremity; called also *shaft of rib.*

**c. epididy'midis** [TA], body of epididymis: the middle part of the epididymis, which is formed by the convolutions of the single ductus epididymidis.

**c. fibro'sum,** c. albicans.

**c. fi'bulae** [TA], body of fibula: the principal part or shaft of the fibula; called also *shaft of fibula.*

**c. fimbria'tum hippocam'pi,** fimbria hippocampi.

**c. for'nicis** [TA], body of fornix: the middle part of the fornix of the cerebrum, formed by fusion of the two lateral halves under the corpus callosum.

**c. gas'tricum** [TA], gastric body: that part of the stomach between the fundus and the pyloric part; called also *body of stomach, c. ventriculare,* and *c. ventriculi.*

**c. genicula'tum latera'le** [TA], lateral geniculate body: an eminence of the metathalamus produced by the underlying lateral geniculate nucleus, just lateral to the medial geniculate body. It relays visual impulses from the optic tract to the calcarine cortex and links visual inputs to the nearby midbrain. Called also *optic thalamus.*

**c. genicula'tum media'le** [TA], medial geniculate body: an eminence of the metathalamus produced by the underlying medial geniculate nucleus, just lateral to the superior colliculus. It relays auditory impulses from the lateral lemniscus to the auditory cortex.

**c. glan'dulae bulbourethra'lis,** the body of the bulbourethral gland.

**c. glan'dulae sudori'ferae,** body of sweat gland: the coiled secretory part of a sweat gland, found in the deep part of the corium; called also *coil* or *acinus of the sweat gland.*

**c. glandula're prosta'tae,** substantia glandularis prostatae.

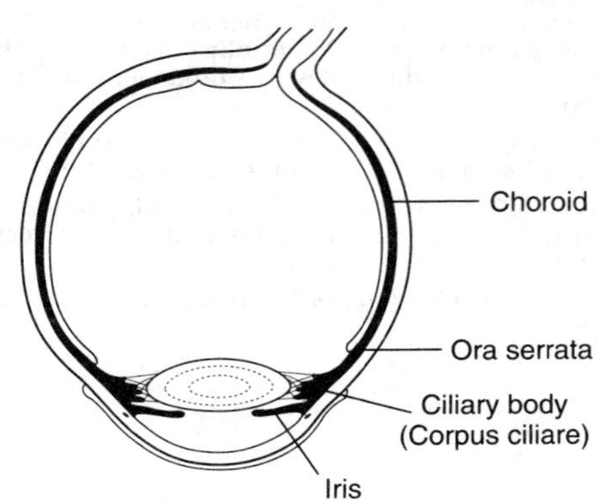

**c. hemorrha'gicum,** 1. an ovarian follicle containing blood. 2. a corpus luteum containing a blood clot.

**c. Highmo'ri, c. highmoria'num,** mediastinum testis.

**c. hu'meri** [TA], body of humerus: the long central part of the humerus; called also *shaft of humerus.*

**c. incu'dis** [TA], body of incus: the central part of the incus, which contains an excavation (facet for malleus) in which the head of the malleus articulates.

**c. lin'guae** [TA], the larger anterior part of the tongue, in the floor of the mouth.

**c. lu'teum** (pl. *cor'pora lu'tea*) [TA], yellow body of ovary: a yellow glandular mass in the ovary formed by an ovarian follicle that has matured and discharged its ovum; if the ovum has been impregnated, the corpus luteum increases in size and persists for several months *(true c. luteum, c. luteum of pregnancy, c. luteum graviditatis)*; if impregnation has not taken place, the corpus luteum degenerates and shrinks *(false c. luteum, c. luteum of menstruation, c. luteum menstruationis)*. The corpus luteum secretes progesterone. Cf. *c. albicans.*

**cor'pora lu'tea atre'tica,** corpora lutea in which regressive changes have occurred.

**c. mam'mae** [TA], the essential mass of the mammary gland, exclusive of the glandular elements, which is thickest beneath the nipple and thinner toward the periphery; see illustration accompanying *glandula mammaria.*

**c. mammilla're** [TA], mammillary body: either of the pair of small spherical masses situated close together in the interpeduncular space rostral to the posterior perforated substance in the posterior hypothalamic region, consisting of two main nuclei, lateral and medial, and smaller associated aggregations of gray matter. It forms a portion of the limbic system (see under *system*).

**c. mandi'bulae** [TA], body of mandible: the horizontal horseshoe-shaped portion of the mandible.

**c. maxil'lae** [TA], body of maxilla: the large central portion of the maxilla, roughly pyramidal in shape, to which four major processes are connected; it contains the maxillary sinus.

**c. medulla're cerebel'li** [TA], medullary body of cerebellum: the white substance of the cerebellum; called also *medullary center of cerebellum.*

**c. metacarpa'le,** corpus ossis metacarpi.

**c. metatarsa'le,** c. ossis metatarsi.

**c. nu'clei cauda'ti** [TA], the part of the caudate nucleus lying in the floor of the pars centralis of the lateral ventricle of the brain, extending posteriorly from the head and continuous with the tail.

**c. of Oken,** mesonephros.

**cor'pora oryzoi'dea** (sing. *cor'pus oryzoi'deum*), rice bodies.

**c. os'sis hyoi'dei** [TA], body of hyoid bone: the central portion of the hyoid bone to which the large and small horns are attached; called also *basihyal* and *basihyoid.*

**c. os'sis i'lii** [TA], **c. os'sis i'lium,** body of ilium: the inferior portion of the ilium, which forms roughly the superior two fifths of the acetabulum.

**c. os'sis is'chii** [TA], body of ischium: the thick, irregular, prismatic part of the ischium. Its superior end participates in the acetabulum, and from its inferior end the ramus of the ischium projects. It incorporates what was formerly called the superior ramus.

**c. os'sis metacarpa'lis, c. os'sis metacar'pi** [TA], body of metacarpal bone: the long central part of a metacarpal bone. Called also *c. metacarpale* and *shaft of metacarpal bone.*

**c. os'sis metatarsa'lis, c. os'sis metatar'si** [TA], body of metatarsal bone: the long central part of a metatarsal bone. Called also *c. metatarsale* and *shaft of metatarsal bone.*

**c. os'sis pu'bis** [TA], body of pubic bone: the irregular mass of the pubic bone that lies alongside the median plane, articulating with the similar portion of the opposite pubic bone. From it extend the superior and inferior rami of the pubic bone.

**c. os'sis sphenoida'lis** [TA], body of sphenoid bone: the central, cuboidal part of the sphenoid bone to which the greater wings, lesser wings, and pterygoid processes are attached; it contains the sphenoidal sinuses. Called also *c. sphenoidale.*

**c. pampinifor'me,** epoöphoron.

**c. pancre'atis** [TA], body of pancreas: the triangularly prismatic portion of the pancreas, extending from the neck on the right to the tail on the left.

**cor'pora paraaor'tica** [TA], para-aortic bodies: exclaves of glandular cells of sympathetic origin (chromaffin cells) found near the sympathetic ganglia along the aorta in the abdominal cavity; they serve as chemoreceptors responsive to oxygen, carbon dioxide, and hydrogen ion concentration, that help to control respiration. Called also *aortic, vagal,* or *Zuckerkandl's bodies* and *glomera aortica.*

**c. pe'nis** [TA], corpus of penis: the free part of the penis between the root and the glans, consisting chiefly of the paired corpora cavernosa and the unpaired corpus spongiosum penis; called also *shaft of penis.*

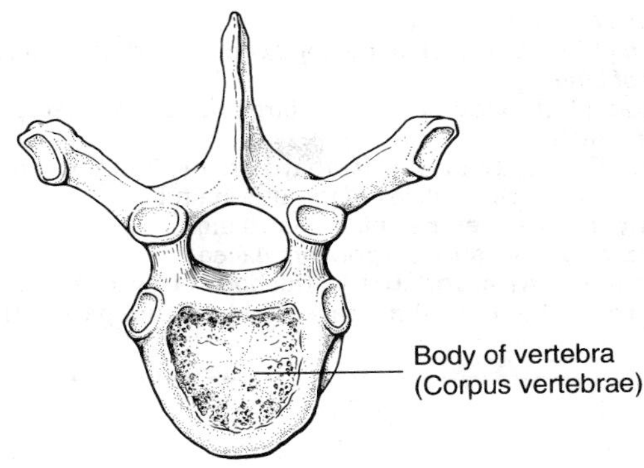


Corpus vertebrae.

**c. perinea'le** [TA], perineal body: the fibromuscular mass in the median plane of the perineum where converge and attach the bulbospongiosus and sphincter ani externus muscles, the two levatores ani, and the two deep and the two superficial transverse perineal muscles; called also *centrum perinei* [TA alternative] and *centrum tendineum perinei.*

**c. phalan'gis ma'nus** [TA], body of phalanx of hand: the long central part of a phalanx of the hand; called also *shaft of phalanx of hand.*

**c. phalan'gis pe'dis** [TA], body of phalanx of foot: the long central part of a phalanx of the foot; called also *shaft of phalanx of foot.*

**c. pinea'le,** TA alternative for *glandula pinealis.*

**cor'pora quadrige'mina,** the rostral and caudal colliculi of the tectum of the mesencephalon considered together.

**c. ra'dii** [TA], body of radius: the long central part of the radius; called also *shaft of radius.*

**c. restifor'me,** pedunculus cerebellaris caudalis.

**c. santoria'num,** cartilago corniculata.

**c. sphenoida'le,** c. ossis sphenoidalis.

**c. spongio'sum pe'nis** [TA], spongy body of penis: the column of erectile tissue that forms the urethral surface of the penis, and in which the urethra is found; its distal expansion forms the glans penis. Called also *c. cavernosum urethrae virilis* and *spongy body of male urethra.*

**c. ster'ni** [TA], body of sternum: the second or principal portion of the sternum, located between the manubrium above and the xiphoid process below; called also *gladiolus.*

**c. stria'tum** [TA], striate body: one of the components of the basal nuclei; specifically, a subcortical mass of gray and white substance in front of and lateral to the thalamus in each cerebral hemisphere. The gray substance of this structure is arranged in two principal masses, the caudate nucleus and the lentiform nucleus; its name denotes the striate appearance on section of the area, produced by connecting bands of gray substance passing from one of these nuclei to the other through the anterior limb of the internal capsule.

**c. subthala'micum,** nucleus subthalamicus.

**c. ta'li** [TA], body of talus: the roughly quadrilateral portion of the talus, which presents several surfaces for articulation with the calcaneus, tibia, and fibula.

**c. ti'biae** [TA], **c. tibia'le,** body of tibia: the long central part of the tibia; called also *shaft of tibia.*

**c. trapezoi'deum** [TA], trapezoid body: a mass of transverse fibers extending through the central part of the pons and forming a part of the path of the cochlear nerve.

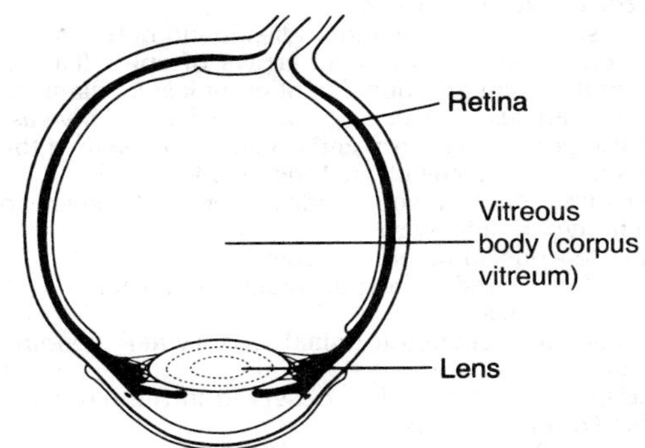


Corpus vitreum (vitreous body).

## Corpus *Continued*

**c. triti'ceum,** cartilago triticea.
**c. ul'nae** [TA], body of ulna: the long central part of the ulna; called also *shaft of ulna.*
**c. un'guis** [TA], body of nail: the large distal, exposed portion of the nail of a digit.
**c. u'teri** [TA], body of uterus: that part of the uterus above the isthmus and below the orifices of the uterine tubes.
**c. ventricula're, c. ventric'uli,** c. gastricum.
**cor'pora versicolora'ta,** corpora amylacea.
**c. ver'tebrae** [TA], **c. vertebra'le,** the body of a vertebra, consisting of the centrum, the ossified neurocentral joint and part of the vertebral arches, and the facets for the heads of the ribs. Called also *vertebral body.*
**c. vesi'cae bilia'ris** [TA], body of gallbladder: the portion of the gallbladder between the fundus and the neck; called also *c. vesicae felleae* [TA alternative].
**c. vesi'cae fel'leae,** TA alternative for *c. vesicae biliaris.*
**c. vesi'cae urina'riae** [TA], body of urinary bladder: that part of the bladder between the apex and the fundus.
**c. vi'treum** [TA], vitreous body: the transparent gel that fills the inner portion of the eyeball between the lens and the retina; called also *hyaloid body, humor cristallinus,* and *crystalline* or *vitreous humor.*
**c. Wolf'fi,** mesonephros.

**cor·pus·cal·lo·sot·o·my** (kor'pəs-kal-ə-sot'ə-me) [*corpus callos*um + *-otomy*] surgical transection of the fibers in the corpus callosum, done to gain access to third ventricular structures; formerly used to treat intractable epilepsy. Written also *corpus callosotomy.* Called also *callosotomy.* Cf. *split brain.*

**cor·pus·cle** (kor'pəs-əl) any small mass or body; see also *corpusculum.*
**amylaceous c's, amyloid c's,** corpora amylacea.
**articular c.,** a type of lamellated corpuscle found within joints.
**axile c., axis c.,** the central part of a tactile corpuscle.
**blood c.,** see under *cell.*
**blood c., red,** erythrocyte.
**blood c., white,** leukocyte.
**bone c.,** bone cell.
**bridge c.,** desmosome.
**bulboid c.,** corpusculum bulboideum.
**cartilage c.,** cartilage cell.
**chorea c's,** a name given peculiar round hyaline bodies, concentrically laminated and strongly refractile, found in the perivascular sheaths of the vessels of the corpora striata and internal capsule in chorea.
**chromophil c's,** Nissl bodies.
**chyle c.,** a lymphocyte found in chyle.
**colloid c's,** corpora amylacea.
**colostrum c's,** large rounded bodies in colostrum, containing droplets of fat and sometimes a nucleus; they apparently are phagocytic cells of the mammary gland, present for the first two weeks after parturition. Called also *Donné's bodies* or *corpuscles.*
**compound granular c.,** gitter cell.
**concentric c's,** Hassall's c's.
**corneal c's,** star-shaped connective tissue cells within the corneal spaces; called also *Toynbee's* and *Virchow's c's.*
**Dogiel's c.,** genital c.
**Donné's c's,** colostrum c's.
**dust c's,** hemoconia.
**genital c.,** a type of lamellated corpuscle found in the genital mucous membranes and in the skin around the nipples.
**Gierke's c's,** Hassall's c's.
**Gluge's c's,** granular corpuscles occurring in diseased nerve tissue.
**Golgi's c.,** Golgi tendon organ.
**Golgi-Mazzoni c's,** tactile corpuscles found in the subcutaneous tissue of the fingertips, resembling pacinian corpuscles, but possessing fewer lamellae and a relatively larger cone, and having the contained nerve fibers more extensively branched.
**Guarnieri's c's,** see under *body.*
**Hassall's c's,** spherical or ovoid bodies found in the medulla of the thymus, composed of concentric arrays of epithelial cells which contain keratohyalin and bundles of cytoplasmic filaments. Called also *Hassall's bodies, concentric c's, Leber's c's,* and *thymus c's.*
**Herbst's c's,** peculiar sensory end-organs in the skin of the bill and in the mucous membrane of the tongue of the duck.
**Jaworski's c's,** spiral mucous bodies seen in the secretion of the stomach in hyperchlorhydria.
**Krause's c.,** corpusculum bulboideum.
**lamellar c., lamellated c.,** corpusculum lamellosum.
**Leber's c's,** Hassall's c's.
**lingual c.,** an encapsulated terminal sensory nerve ending in a lingual papilla.
**Lostorfer's c's,** granular bodies observed in the blood in syphilis; called also *Lostorfer's bodies.*
**lymph c's,** lymphocytes observed in lymph.
**lymphoid c's,** lymphocytes observed in tissues.
**malpighian c's of kidney,** corpuscula renis.
**malpighian c's of spleen,** noduli lymphoidei splenici; see under *nodulus.*
**Mazzoni's c.,** corpusculum bulboideum.
**meconium c's,** epithelial cells containing many coarse yellow granules, observed in the distal part of the small intestine in a fetus.
**Meissner's c.,** corpusculum tactus.
**Merkel's c.,** see under *cell.*
**mucous c's,** bodies resembling leukocytes occurring in mucus.
**Norris' c's,** decolorized erythrocytes; see also *hypochromic erythrocyte.*
**pacchionian c's,** granulationes arachnoideae.
**Pacini's c., pacinian c.,** corpusculum lamellosum.
**paciniform c's,** rapidly adapting lamellar nerve endings (corpuscula lamellosa) that are more elongated and have fewer laminae than pacinian corpuscles; found in the vibrissae and epidermis of the nose, in joint capsules, in aponeuroses, and at myotendinous junctions associated with Golgi tendon organs. They respond to muscle stretch and light pressure. Called also *paciniform receptors.*
**Paschen's c's,** see under *body.*
**pessary c.,** see under *cell.*
**pus c's,** see under *cell.*
**Rainey's c.,** any of the uninucleate, crescentic or banana-shaped trophozoites found in sarcocysts in sarcocystosis.
**red c.,** erythrocyte.
**renal c's,** corpuscula renis.
**reticulated c.,** reticulocyte.
**Röhl's marginal c's,** small bodies seen in the margins of erythrocytes of animals after the administration of chemotherapeutic substances.
**Ruffini's c.,** a type of lamellated corpuscle in the dermis that is a slowly-adapting receptor for sensations of continuous pressure. Called also *Ruffini's cylinder* or *ending.*
**salivary c.,** a white blood cell that has migrated through the oral epithelium and is mixed in the saliva.
**Schwalbe's c.,** caliculus gustatorius.
**splenic c's,** noduli lymphoidei splenici; see under *nodulus.*
**tactile c.,** corpusculum tactus.
**taste c.,** caliculus gustatorius.
**tendon c's,** flattened cells of connective tissue occurring in rows between the primary bundles of the tendons.
**terminal nerve c.,** corpusculum nervosum terminale.
**thymus c's,** Hassall's c's.
**Timofeew's c.,** a specialized form of lamellated corpuscle found in the submucosa of the membranous and prostatic portions of the urethra.
**touch c.,** corpusculum tactus.
**Toynbee's c's,** corneal c's.
**Tröltsch's c's,** connective tissue spaces lined with flattened endothelial cells, and appearing like corpuscular bodies among the radial fibers of the membrana tympani.
**typhic c's,** cells of Peyer's patches that have undergone degeneration in typhoid fever.
**Valentin's c's,** small amyloid bodies sometimes found in nerve tissue.
**Vater's c., Vater-Pacini c.,** corpusculum lamellosum.
**Virchow's c's,** corneal c's.
**Weber's c.,** utriculus prostaticus.
**white c.,** leukocyte.

**cor·pus·cu·la** (kor-pus'ku-lə) [L.] plural of *corpusculum.*

**cor·pus·cu·lar** (kor-pus'ku-lər) pertaining to or of the nature of corpuscles.

**cor·pus·cu·lum** (kor-pus'ku-ləm) pl. *corpus'cula* [L. dim. of *corpus*] a small mass or body; used as a general term in anatomical nomenclature to designate certain small discrete masses of specialized tissue, especially of nerve tissue.
**c. articula're,** articular corpuscle.
**c. bulboi'deum,** bulboid corpuscle: a type of small encapsulated nerve ending found in the skin, mucous membranes, and conjunctiva, at varying levels; thought to function as either thermoreceptors for cold or as rapidly adapting receptors. Called also *bulb of Krause* and *Krause's corpuscle* or *end bulb.*
**c. genita'le,** genital corpuscle.
**c. lamello'sum,** lamellar or lamellated corpuscle: a type of large encapsulated nerve ending sensitive to pressure and vibration; the most complicated of the nerve endings, it is found throughout the body. Called also *Pacini's, pacinian, Vater's,* and *Vater-Pacini corpuscle.*
**c. nervo'sum termina'le,** terminal nerve corpuscle: a sensory nerve ending characterized by a fibrous capsule of varying thickness that is continuous with the endoneurium; for different named varieties, see under *corpuscle.* Called also *end bulb* and *encapsulated nerve ending.*
**corpus'cula re'nis,** renal corpuscles: bodies forming the beginnings of the nephrons, each consisting of a tuft of capillaries (the glomerulus), surrounded by an expanded portion of the renal tubule (the glomerular capsule); called also *malpighian corpuscles, acinus renalis [malpighii], acinus renis [malpighii],* and *malpighian bodies of kidneys.*
**c. tac'tus,** tactile corpuscle: a type of medium-sized encapsulated nerve ending found in the skin, most commonly in the palms and soles; called also *tactile cell, touch cell* or *corpuscle,* and *Meissner's corpuscle.*
**c. triti'ceum,** cartilago triticea.

**cor·rec·tion** (kə-rek'shən) [L. *correctio* straightening out; amendment] a setting right, as the provision of specific lenses for the improvement of vision, or an arbitrary adjustment made in values or devices in performance of experimental procedures.

**cor·rec·tor** (kə-rek'tər) something that corrects or sets right.
**function c.,** a removable orthodontic appliance utilizing oral and facial muscle forces to move teeth and possibly change the relationship of dental arches; called also *Fränkel appliance.*

**cor·re·la·tion** (kor"ə-la'shən) most generally, the degree to which one phenomenon or random variable is associated with or can be predicted from another. In statistics, correlation usually refers to the degree to which a linear predictive relationship exists between random variables, as measured by a correlation coefficient (q.v.). Correlation may be *positive* (but never larger than 1), i.e., both variables increase or decrease together; *negative* or *inverse* (but never smaller than −1), i.e., one variable increases when the other decreases; or zero, i.e., a change in one variable does not affect the other.

**cor·re·spon·dence** (kor"ə-spon'dəns) [L. *correspondēre* to answer, to correspond] [MeSH: Correspondence] the condition of being in agreement, or conformity.
**anomalous retinal c.,** a condition in which disparate points on the retinas of the two eyes come to be associated sensorially; abbreviated ARC.
**normal retinal c.,** the condition in which corresponding points on the retinas of the two eyes are associated sensorially; abbreviated NRC.
**retinal c.,** the relation between corresponding points on the retinas of the eyes such that simultaneous stimulation causes the sensation of a single object.

**Cor·ri·dor disease** (kor'ĭ-dor) [The *Corridor,* a region in South Africa where it was first reported] see under *disease.*

**Cor·ri·gan's disease,** etc. (kor'ĭ-gənz) [Sir Dominic John *Corrigan,* Irish physician, 1802–1880] see under *disease, line, pulse,*

**cor·ri·gent** (kor'ĭ-jənt) [L. *corrigens* correcting] 1. amending or rendering milder. 2. any agent that favorably modifies the action of a drug which is too powerful or harsh, or that improves its taste.

**cor·rin** (kor'in) a tetrapyrrole ring system resembling the porphyrin ring system of hemoglobin, but in which a pair of the rings is joined directly rather than through a methylene bridge, with cobalt being bound to the inner four nitrogen atoms. The cobalamins contain a corrin ring system.

**cor·rin·oid** (kor'in-oid) a compound, such as a cobalamin, containing a corrin ring system.

**cor·rode** (kə-rōd') [L. *corrodere* to gnaw] 1. to produce corrosion. 2. to undergo corrosion.

**cor·ro·sion** (kə-ro'zhən) [MeSH: Corrosion] 1. the gradual destruction of a metal or alloy by electrochemical reaction or of the body tissues by the action of a strong acid or alkali. 2. the product of a corrosive process.

**cor·ro·sive** (kə-ro'siv) 1. causing, or able to cause, corrosion. 2. a substance that causes corrosion. 3. a caustic or escharotic agent.

**cor·ru·ga·tor** (cor'ə-ga"tor) [*cor-* + *ruga*] that which wrinkles; a muscle that wrinkles.

**cor·sair** (kor'sar) any of various biting reduviid bugs of the genus *Melanolestes.*

**cor·set** (kor'sət) an orthopedic device that encircles and supports a part, as worn in certain spinal injuries or deformities. See also *spinal orthosis,* under *orthosis.*

**Cort.** abbreviation for L. *cor'tex,* bark.

**Cor·tate** (kor'tāt) trademark for preparations of desoxycorticosterone acetate.

**Cort-Dome** (kort'dōm) trademark for preparations of hydrocortisone.

**Cor·tef** (kor'təf) trademark for preparations of hydrocortisone.

**Cor·ten·e·ma** (kor-ten'ə-mə) trademark for a preparation of hydrocortisone.

**cor·tex** (kor'teks) gen. *cor'ticis,* pl. *cor'tices* [L. "bark, rind, shell"] 1. an external layer, as the bark of a tree, or the rind of a fruit. 2. [TA] the outer layer of an organ or other body structure, as distinguished from the internal substance.
**adrenal c., c. of adrenal gland,** c. glandulae suprarenalis.
**adrenal c., fetal,** fetal zone of adrenal cortex.
**agranular c.,** a type of cortex occurring in some parts of the neocortex, having very thin granular layers; seen in the motor area of the precentral gyrus and elsewhere.
**cerebellar c., c. cerebella'ris,** c. cerebelli.
**c. cerebel'li** [TA], **c. of cerebellum,** cerebellar cortex: the superficial gray matter of the cerebellum; it consists of three layers, the stratum moleculare, stratum granulosum, and stratum purkinjense. Called also *c. cerebellaris.*
**cerebral c., c. cerebra'lis,** c. cerebri.
**c. cere'bri** [TA], **c. of cerebrum,** cerebral cortex: the thin (about 3 mm) layer or mantle of gray substance covering the surface of each cerebral hemisphere, folded into gyri that are separated by sulci. It is responsible for the higher mental functions, for general movement, for visceral functions, perception, and behavioral reactions, and for the association and integration of these functions. Many classifications have been suggested: it has been divided into *archicortex, paleocortex,* and *neocortex* according to supposed phylogenetic and ontogenetic differences; into functional areas such as *motor areas, primary receptive* or *receiving areas,* and *association areas;* and into areas according to the presence of six cell layers (the *isocortex*) or of variable numbers and arrangements of cell and fiber layers (the *allocortex*). See also *layers of cerebral cortex.* Called also *c. cerebralis* and *pallium.* See illustration at *neocortex.*
**c. glan'dulae suprarena'lis** [TA], cortex of adrenal or suprarenal gland: the outer, firm yellowish layer that comprises the larger part of the adrenal gland, consisting of the zona glomerulosa, the zona fasciculata, and the zona reticularis; it secretes, in response to release of corticotropin by the pulmonary gland, many steroid hormones. Called also *adrenal* or *suprarenal cortex.*
**granular c.,** koniocortex.
**heterotypical c.,** allocortex.
**homotypical c.,** isocortex.
**c. of kidney,** renal c.
**c. len'tis** [TA], cortex of lens: the softer, external part of the lens of the eye; called also *substantia corticalis lentis* and *cortical substance of lens.*
**motor c.,** see under *area.*
**c. no'di lympha'tici,** TA alternative for *c. nodi lymphoidei.*
**c. no'di lymphoi'dei** [TA], cortex of lymph node: the outer portion of the node, consisting mainly of dense lymphatic tissue and follicles; called also *c. nodi lymphatici* [TA alternative] and *cortical substance of lymph node.*
**nonolfactory c.,** neocortex.
**olfactory c.,** archicortex.
**c. ova'rii** [TA], cortex of ovary: the dense layer of compact stroma forming the peripheral zone around the medulla of the ovary, in which the ovarian follicles are embedded.
**piriform c.,** the cortex of the piriform lobe or area.
**provisional c.,** fetal zone of adrenal cortex.
**renal c., c. rena'lis** [TA], **c. re'nis,** the outer part of the substance of the kidney, composed mainly of glomeruli and convoluted tubules; called also *cortical substance of kidney.*
**somesthetic c.,** somatosensory area.
**striate c.,** Brodmann's area 17: the part of the occipital lobe of the cerebral cortex that receives the fibers of the optic radiation from the lateral geniculate body and is the primary receptive area for vision; so called because of the prominent broad line or stria of Gennari. Called also *striate area* or *first visual area.*
**suprarenal c., c. of suprarenal gland,** c. glandulae suprarenalis.
**tertiary c.,** thymus-dependent area.

**c. thy'mi** [TA], **c. of thymus,** the outer part of each lobule of the thymus; it consists chiefly of closely packed lymphocytes (thymocytes) and surrounds the medulla.

**visual c.,** the area of the occipital lobe of the cerebral cortex concerned with vision; it consists of the *first visual area* or *striate c.* (Brodmann's area 17) and two other areas, the *second visual area* or *parastriate area* (Brodmann's area 18) and the *third visual area* or *peristriate area* (Brodmann's area 19).

**cor·tex·one** (kor-tek'sōn) 11-deoxycorticosterone.

**Cor·ti's arch, canal, cells,** etc. (kor'tēz) [Alfonso *Corti,* Italian anatomist, 1822–1888] see under *arch, canal, cell, fiber, ganglion, rod,* and *tunnel,* and see *membrana tectoria ductus cochlearis* and *organum spirale.*

**cor·ti·cal** (kor'tĭ-kəl) [L. *corticalis*] pertaining to or of the nature of a cortex or bark.

**cor·ti·cal·os·te·ot·o·my** (kor″tĭ-kəl-os″te-ot'ə-me) osteotomy through the bone cortex at the base of the dentoalveolar segment, which serves to weaken the resistance of the bone to the application of orthodontic forces.

**cor·ti·cate** (kor'tĭ-kāt) possessing a cortex or bark.

**cor·ti·cec·to·my** (kor″tĭ-sek'tə-me) topectomy.

**cor·ti·ces** (kor'tĭ-sēz) [L.] plural of *cortex.*

**cor·ti·cif·u·gal** (kor″tĭ-sif'ə-gəl) [*cortex* + L. *fugere* to flee] proceeding or conducting away from the cerebral cortex. Cf. *efferent.*

**cor·ti·cip·e·tal** (kor″tĭ-sip'ə-təl) [*cortic-* + L. *-petal*] proceeding or conducting toward the cortex. Cf. *afferent.*

**cortic(o)-** [L. *cortex,* q.v.] a combining form denoting relationship to a cortex.

**cor·ti·co·ad·re·nal** (kor″tĭ-ko-ə-dre'nəl) adrenocortical.

**cor·ti·co·af·fer·ent** (kor″tĭ-ko-af'ər-ent) corticipetal.

**cor·ti·co·au·to·nom·ic** (kor″tĭ-ko-aw″to-nom'ik) denoting the relationship of autonomic function to definite areas in the cerebral cortex.

**cor·ti·co·bul·bar** (kor″tĭ-ko-bul'bər) pertaining to or connecting the cerebral cortex and the medulla oblongata and/or brain stem.

**cor·ti·co·can·cel·lous** (kor″tĭ-ko-kan'sə-ləs) referring to bony tissue containing both cortical and cancellous elements.

**cor·ti·co·di·en·ce·phal·ic** (kor″tĭ-ko-di″en-sə-fal'ik) pertaining to or connecting the cerebral cortex and the diencephalon.

**cor·ti·co·ef·fer·ent** (kor″tĭ-ko-ef'ər-ent) corticifugal.

**cor·ti·cof·u·gal** (kor″tĭ-kof'u-gəl) corticifugal.

**cor·ti·coid** (kor'tĭ-koid) corticosteroid.

**cor·ti·co·lipo·trope** (kor″tĭ-ko-lip'o-trōp) corticotroph.

**cor·ti·co·mes·en·ce·phal·ic** (kor″tĭ-ko-mes″en-sə-fal'ik) pertaining to or connecting the cerebral cortex and the mesencephalon.

**cor·ti·co·pe·dun·cu·lar** (kor″tĭ-ko-pə-dung'ku-lər) pertaining to the cortex and the peduncles of the brain.

**cor·ti·cop·e·tal** (kor″tĭ-kop'ə-təl) corticipetal.

**cor·ti·co·pleu·ri·tis** (cor″tĭ-ko-plo͞o-ri'tis) pulmonary pleurisy.

**cor·ti·co·pon·tine** (kor″tĭ-ko-pon'tīn) pertaining to or connecting the cerebral cortex and the pons.

**cor·ti·co·spi·nal** (kor″tĭ-ko-spi'nəl) pertaining to or connecting the cortex of the brain and the spinal cord.

**cor·ti·co·ster·oid** (kor″tĭ-ko-ster'oid) any of the 21-carbon steroids elaborated by the adrenal cortex (excluding the sex hormones of adrenal origin) in response to adrenocorticotropic hormone (ACTH) released by the pituitary gland or to angiotensin II. They are divided, according to their predominant biologic activity, into two major groups: *glucocorticoids,* chiefly influencing carbohydrate, fat, and protein metabolism, and *mineralocorticoids,* affecting the regulation of electrolyte and water balance. Some corticosteroids exhibit both types of activity in varying degrees, and others exert only one type of effect. They are used clinically for hormonal replacement therapy, for suppression of ACTH secretion by the anterior pituitary, as antineoplastic, antiallergic, and anti-inflammatory agents, and to suppress immune responses. Called also *adrenocorticoid, corticoid, adrenal cortical* or *adrenocortical steroid,* and *adrenocortical* or *cortical hormone.*

**cor·ti·cos·ter·one** (kor″tĭ-kos'tər-ōn) [MeSH: Corticosterone] a glucocorticoid with moderate activity, having life-maintaining properties in adrenalectomized animals and several other activities peculiar to the adrenal cortex. Its actions closely resemble those of cortisol, except that it is not anti-inflammatory. It also shows some mineralocorticoid activity.

**cor·ti·cos·ter·one meth·yl ox·i·dase** (kor″tĭ-kos'tər-ōn meth'əl ok'sĭ-dās) corticosterone 18-monooxygenase.

**cor·ti·cos·ter·one meth·yl ox·i·dase de·fi·cien·cy** a disorder of steroidogenesis in which deficiency of a corticosterone 18-monooxygenase impairs the biosynthesis of aldosterone and causes salt wasting. It occurs as two types: *type I,* in which decreased hydroxylation of corticosterone results in corticosterone and deoxycorticosterone accumulation, and *type II,* in which decreased oxidation of the 18-hydroxy intermediate results in elevated levels of this compound and corticosterone. Called also *18-hydroxylase deficiency.*

**cor·ti·cos·ter·one 18-mono·oxy·ge·nase** (kor″tĭ-kos'tər-ōn mon″o-ok'sə-jən-ās) [EC 1.14.15.5] an enzyme of the oxidoreductase class that catalyzes hydroxylation of corticosteroids at the 18 position followed by oxidation of the 18-hydroxy intermediates, steps in the biosynthesis of aldosterone. The two reactions are sometimes considered separately as I (hydroxylation) and II (oxidation); defects in each reaction have been described and called corticosterone methyl oxidase deficiency, types I and II. The enzyme may be an activity of steroid 11$\beta$-monooxygenase (q.v.)

**cor·ti·co·ten·sin** (kor″tĭ-ko-ten'sin) a low-molecular-weight polypeptide purified from kidney extract that exhibits a vasopressor effect when given intravenously.

**cor·ti·co·tha·lam·ic** (kor″tĭ-ko-thə-lam'ik) pertaining to or connecting the cerebral cortex and the thalamus.

**cor·ti·co·trope** (kor'ti-ko-trōp) corticotroph.

**cor·ti·co·troph** (kor'tĭ-ko-trof″) a small, irregularly stellate, acidophilic cell of the adenohypophysis, having small, sparsely distributed secretory granules and secreting adrenocorticotropic hormone and $\beta$-endorphin, which are cleaved from a large prohormone called *pro-opiomelanocortin.* Called also *corticotrope, corticotroph-lipotroph, corticolipotrope, corticotrope cell,* and *corticotroph cell.*

**cor·ti·co·troph·ic** (kor″tĭ-ko-trof'ik) adrenocorticotropic.

**cor·ti·co·tro·phin** (kor'tĭ-ko-tro″fin) 1. corticotropin (def. 1). 2. adrenocorticotropic hormone.

**cor·ti·co·troph-li·po·troph** (kor'tĭ-ko-trof-lip'o-trof) corticotroph.

**cor·ti·co·trop·ic** (kor″tĭ-ko-trop'ik) adrenocorticotropic.

**cor·ti·co·tro·pin** (kor'tĭ-ko-tro″pin) [USP] [MeSH: Corticotropin] 1. a preparation of animal-derived adrenocorticotropic hormone, administered intravenously for diagnostic testing of adrenocortical function and subcutaneously or intramuscularly as an antiemetic in cancer chemotherapy and as an anticonvulsant. Called also *acortan, corticotrophin, adrenocorticotrophin,* and *adrenocorticotropin.* 2. adrenocorticotropic hormone.

**cor·ti·co·tro·pi·no·ma** (kor″tĭ-ko-tro″pĭ-no'mə) corticotroph adenoma.

**Cor·ti·fair** (kor'tĭ-far) trademark for preparations of hydrocortisone.

**cor·ti·lymph** (kor'tĭ-limf″) [organ of *Corti* + *lymph*] the fluid filling the intercellular spaces of the organ of Corti; it is similar in composition to perilymph.

**Cor·ti·na·ri·a·ceae** (kor″tĭ-nar″e-a'se-e) a family of mushrooms (order Agaricales). Some genera are edible, but genus *Galerina* contains amatoxins and can be deadly.

**Cor·ti·na·ri·us** (kor″tĭ-nar'e-əs) a large genus of mushrooms that includes many edible species; certain species found in Europe and Japan contain the toxins orelline and orellanine.

**cor·ti·sol** (kor'tĭ-sol) the major natural glucocorticoid synthesized in the zona fasciculata of the adrenal cortex; it affects the metabolism of glucose, protein, and fats and has appreciable mineralocorticoid activity. It also regulates the immune system and affects many other functions. When used as a pharmaceutical, it is usually referred to as hydrocortisone. For therapeutic uses, see *hydrocortisone.*

**cor·ti·sone** (kor'tĭ-sōn) [MeSH: Cortisone] a natural glucocorticoid that is metabolically convertible to cortisol. The human adrenal cortex secretes only minute amounts; most that is found in peripheral plasma is formed from cortisol by a reversible reaction. The synthetic hormone exerts its pharmaceutical effects through its metabolic conversion to cortisol.

**c. acetate** [USP], an ester of cortisone, having a slow onset but long duration of action, used in replacement therapy for adrenal insufficiency and as an anti-inflammatory and immunosuppressant in a wide variety of disorders; administered orally and intramuscularly.

**Cor·tone** (kor'tōn) trademark for preparations of cortisone acetate.

**Cor·tril** (kor'tril) trademark for preparations of hydrocortisone.

**Cor·tro·phin** (kor-tro'fin) trademark for preparations of corticotropin.

**Cor·tro·syn** (kor'tro-sin) trademark for a preparation of cosyntropin.

**co·run·dum** (ko-run′dəm) naturally occurring aluminum oxide; used in dentistry as an abrasive in grinding wheels and for points mounted on mandrels for the dental engine. See also *emery.*

**cor·us·ca·tion** (kor″əs-ka′shən) [L. *coruscatio* a flash] a glittering sensation, as of flashes of light before the eyes.

**Cor·vert** (kor′vərt) trademark for a preparation of ibutilide acetate.

**Cor·vi·sart's disease** (kor″ve-sahrz′) [Baron Jean Nicolas *Corvisart* des Marets, French physician, personal physician to Napoleon, 1755–1821] see under *disease.*

**co·ryd·a·line** (ko-rid′ə-lēn) an alkaloid from species of *Corydalis* and *Dicentra;* it is used as a diuretic and tonic in humans but can cause diarrhea and potentially fatal convulsions in other animals.

**Co·ry·da·lis** (ko-rid′ə-lis) [L. from Gr. *korys* helmet] a large genus of herbs found in temperate climates. *C. bulbo′sa* (DC.), *C. ca′va* (L.) Schweigg. & Korte (Fumariaceae), and other species contain bulbocapnine and cause neurotoxicity in animals. See also *bulbocapnine experiment,* under *experiment.*

**co·ryd·a·lis** (ko-rid′ə-lis) 1. any plant of the genus *Corydalis.* 2. the dried tuber of *Dicentra cucullaria* or *D. canadensis,* which contains bicuculline and several isoquinoline alkaloids, including corydaline, bulbocapnine, and corytuberine.

**co·rym·bi·form** (ko-rim′bĭ-form) [Gr. *korymbos* the cluster of ivy flower + *form*] clustered; said of lesions grouped around a single, usually larger, lesion, as in tinea versicolor or late secondary syphilis.

**co·rym·bose** (kor′im-bōs) corymbiform.

**co·ry·ne·bac·te·ria** (ko-ri″ne-bak-tēr′e-ə) plural of *corynebacterium.*

**Co·ry·ne·bac·te·ri·a·ceae** (ko-ri″ne-bak-te″re-a′se-e) in former systems of classification, a family of coryneform bacteria, related to the actinomycetes, consisting of the genera *Arthrobacter, Cellulomonas, Corynebacterium, Erysipelothrix, Listeria,* and *Microbacterium.* For current classification, see the specific genus.

**Co·ry·ne·bac·te·ri·um** (ko-ri″ne-bak-tēr′e-əm) [Gr. *korynē* club + *bacterium*] [MeSH: Corynebacterium] a genus of coryneform bacteria, made up of gram-positive, nonsporulating, nonmotile, straight to slightly curved rods. The catalase-positive organisms are irregularly staining, sometimes granular, and may be arranged in angular and palisade groups. They are widely distributed in nature and include human and animal parasites and pathogens, plant pathogens, and nonpathogens.
**C. ac′nes,** *Propionibacterium acnes.*
**C. diphthe′riae,** the specific etiologic agent of diphtheria, which also causes skin infections. The organisms are separated according to cultural characteristics into three biotypes: *mitis, intermedius,* and *gravis,* which apparently are not related to pathogenicity. Most strains produce a potent exotoxin. Called also *Klebs-Löffler bacillus.*
**C. diphtheroi′des,** *Eubacterium lentum.*
**C. e′qui,** *Rhodococcus equi.*
**C. genita′lium,** a species associated with genitourinary infections in humans.
**C. granulo′sum,** *Propionibacterium granulosum.*
**C. haemoly′ticum,** *Arcanobacterium haemolyticum.*
**C. hofman′nii,** *C. pseudodiphtheriticum.*
**C. infantisep′ticum,** *Listeria monocytogenes.*
**C. kut′scheri,** a species causing latent and overt infections in mice and rats.
**C. minutis′simum,** a species of uncertain affiliation that causes erythrasma in humans.
**C. murisep′ticum,** a diphtheria-like bacillus producing septicemic disease in mice, but apparently nonpathogenic for other animals.
**C. necro′phorum,** *Fusobacterium necrophorum.*
**C. o′vis,** *C. pseudotuberculosis.*
**C. par′vulum,** *Listeria monocytogenes.*
**C. par′vum,** 1. *Propionibacterium acnes.* 2. a heat-killed and formaldehyde-treated preparation of *C. parvum (P. acnes)* administered orally or parenterally as an experimental cancer immunotherapeutic agent, usually in conjunction with conventional chemotherapy. It appears to act by activating macrophages and also seems to depress T cell function.
**C. pseudodiphtheri′ticum,** a species normally present in the respiratory tract, which closely resembles *C. diphtheriae* but is nontoxigenic; it is sometimes an opportunistic pathogen. Called also *C. hofmannii* and *Hofmann's bacillus.*
**C. pseudotuberculo′sis,** a pathogenic toxin-producing species found in lower animals. It causes caseous lymphadenitis, abscesses, and chronic purulent infections, especially in sheep and goats, and contagious acne of horses. Occasional human disease may form from contact with infected animals or food. Called also *C. ovis* and *Preisz-Nocard bacillus.*
**C. pyo′genes,** a toxicogenic species closely related to group G streptococci. It causes acute pyogenic lesions in cattle, sheep, and pigs, interdigital dermatitis in sheep, and foot rot in pigs, and has been isolated from human pharyngitis and skin lesions.
**C. rena′le,** a species that causes contagious bovine pyelonephritis in cattle and enzootic balanoposthitis in sheep.
**C. te′nuis,** a nocardia-like species of uncertain affiliation that is the etiologic agent of trichomycosis axillaris.
**C. ul′cerans,** a toxigenic species of uncertain affiliation that causes nasopharyngeal infections in humans and acute mastitis in cattle.
**C. vesicula′re,** *Pseudomonas vesicularis.*
**C. xero′sis,** an opportunistic pathogenic species found in the conjunctival sac and on the skin and mucous membranes of humans.

**co·ry·ne·bac·te·ri·um** (ko-ri″ne-bak-tēr′e-əm) pl. *corynebacte′ria* [Gr. *korynē* club + *bacterium*] [MeSH: Corynebacterium] 1. any member of the family Corynebacteriaceae or of the genus *Corynebacterium.* 2. a bacterium that displays coryneform shape during some stage of its development on artificial media. See also *coryneform bacteria,* under *bacterium.*
**group 3 c.,** *Eubacterium lentum.*
**group JK c.,** a group of pathogenic diphtheroid bacteria cultured from blood, tissue, and wound infections of immunosuppressed patients.

**Co·ry·ne·form** (ko-ri′nə-form) a group of asporogenous, gram-positive, irregular rod-shaped bacteria containing the genera *Arthrobacter, Cellulomonas, Corynebacterium,* and *Kurthia.*

**co·ry·ne·form** (ko-ri′nə-form) [Gr. *korynē* club + L. *forma*] club-shaped; see under *bacteria.*

**Co·ry·nes·po·ra** (kor″ĭnes′pə-rə) a widespread genus of imperfect fungi of the form-order Moniliales.
**C. cassi′cola,** a species that is a cause of eumycotic mycetoma.

**cor·y·tu·ber·ine** (ko″re-too′bər-ēn) a crystalline alkaloid from commercial corydaline.

**co·ry·za** (ko-ri′zə) [L.; Gr. *koryza*] acute rhinitis.
**c. foe′tida,** ozena.
**infectious c., infectious avian c.,** an acute respiratory disease of chickens characterized by nasal discharge, sneezing, and edema of the face, and caused by *Haemophilus paragallinarum.* Infection of the lower respiratory tract sometimes occurs.

**COS** Canadian Ophthalmological Society.

**co·sen·si·tize** (ko-sen′sĭ-tīz) to sensitize to two or more sensitizing agents.

**Cos·me·gen** (kos′mə-jən) trademark for a preparation of dactinomycin.

**cos·me·sis** (koz-me′sis) [Gr. *kosmēsis* an arranging or adorning] 1. the preservation, restoration, or bestowing of bodily beauty. 2. the surgical correction of a disfiguring physical defect.

**cos·met·ic** (koz-met′ik) [Gr. *kosmētikos*] [MeSH: Cosmetics] 1. pertaining to cosmesis. 2. a beautifying substance or preparation.

**cos·mid** (koz′mid) [*co*hesive end *s*ito + plas*mid*] a vector constructed of plasmid DNA packaged in vitro into a phage, useful for cloning large (up to 50 kb) DNA fragments.

**cos·ta** (kos′tə) gen. and pl. *cos′tae* [L. "rib"] [TA] 1. rib: any one of the paired elastic arches of bone, twelve on either side *(costa I–costa XII),* extending from the thoracic vertebrae toward the median line on the anterior aspect of the trunk; they form the major part of the thoracic skeleton. The upper seven (I–VII) are called *costae verae* (true ribs) and are connected anteriorly with the sternum; the lower five (VIII–XII) are called *costae spuriae* (false ribs) and are not connected directly with the sternum. 2. the bony part of a rib. 3. a rodlike structure extending along the base of the undulating membrane in certain flagellate protozoa, such as trichomonads.
**c. cervica′lis** [TA], cervical rib: a supernumerary rib arising from a

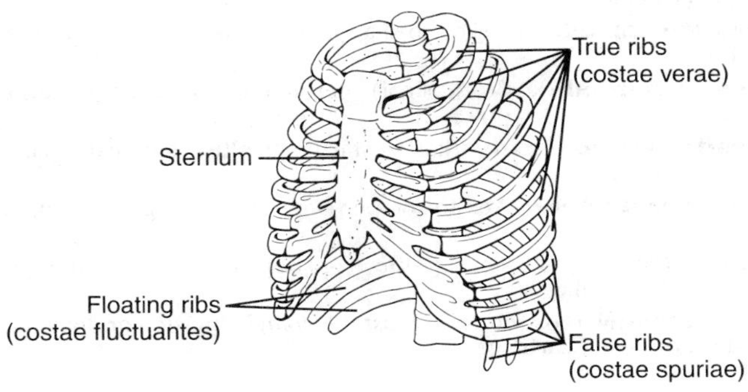

cervical vertebra, usually the seventh. See also *scalenus syndrome* and *cervical rib syndrome,* under *syndrome.*
**cos'tae fluctuan'tes, cos'tae fluitan'tes** floating ribs: the lower two ribs on either side *(costa XI* and *costa XII),* which ordinarily have no ventral attachment; called also *vertebral ribs.*
**c. pri'ma** [TA], first rib: costa I, the superior rib on either side.
**c. secun'da** [TA], second rib: costa II, the rib just inferior to the costa prima on either side.
**cos'tae spu'riae** [TA], false ribs: the lower five ribs on either side (costa VIII to costa XII); the ventral tips of the upper three connect with the costal cartilages of the superiorly adjacent ribs, and the ventral tips of the lower two (costae XI and XII) ordinarily have no attachment.
**cos'tae ve'rae** [TA], true ribs: the upper seven ribs on either side (costa I to costa VII), which are connected to the sides of the sternum by their costal cartilages. Called also *sternal ribs* and *vertebrosternal ribs.*

**cos·tae** (kos'te) [L.] genitive and plural of *costa.*

**cos·tal** (kos'təl) [L. *costalis*] pertaining to a rib or ribs.

**cos·tal·gia** (kos-tal'jə) [*cost-* + *-algia*] 1. pain in the ribs. 2. pain in the costal muscles; called also *pleurodynia.*

**cos·ta·lis** (kos-ta'lis) [L.] costal; used in anatomical nomenclature to denote relationship to a rib.

**cos·ta·tec·to·my** (kos"tə-tek'tə-me) costectomy.

**cos·tec·to·my** (kos-tek'tə-me) [*cost-* + *-ectomy*] the operation of excising or resecting a rib.

**Cos·ten's syndrome** (kos'tənz) [James Bray *Costen,* American otolaryngologist, 1895–1962] see under *syndrome.*

**cos·ti·car·ti·lage** (kos"tĭ-kahr'tĭ-ləj) [*cost-* + *cartilage*] the cartilage of a rib.

**cos·ti·cer·vi·cal** (kos"tĭ-sər'vĭ-kəl) pertaining to or connecting the ribs and the neck.

**cos·tif·er·ous** (kos-tif'ər-əs) [*cost-* + *-ferous*] bearing a rib, as the thoracic vertebrae of man.

**cos·ti·form** (kos'tĭ-form) shaped like a rib.

**cos·ti·spi·nal** (kos"tĭ-spi'nəl) pertaining to or connecting the ribs and spine.

**cos·tive** (kos'tiv) 1. pertaining to, characterized by, or producing constipation. 2. an agent that depresses intestinal motility.

**cos·tive·ness** (kos'tiv-nəs) constipation.

**cost(o)-** [L. *costa* rib] a combining form denoting relationship to the ribs.

**cos·to·cen·tral** (kos"to-sen'trəl) pertaining to a rib and the centrum (body) of a vertebra.

**cos·to·cer·vi·ca·lis** (kos"to-sər"vĭ-ka'lis) [*costo-* + *cervicalis*] musculus iliocostalis cervicis.

**cos·to·chon·dral** (kos"to-kon'drəl) pertaining to a rib and its cartilage.

**cos·to·cla·vic·u·lar** (kos"to-klə-vik'u-lər) pertaining to the ribs and clavicle.

**cos·to·cor·a·coid** (kos"to-kor'ə-koid) pertaining to the ribs and coracoid process.

**cos·to·gen·ic** (kos"to-jen'ik) [*costo-* + *-genic*] arising from a rib, especially from a defect of the marrow of the ribs.

**cos·to·in·fe·ri·or** (kos"to-in-fēr'e-ər) pertaining to the lower ribs.

**cos·to·phren·ic** (kos"to-fren'ik) pertaining to the ribs and diaphragm.

**cos·to·pleu·ral** (kos"to-ploor'əl) pertaining to the ribs and the pleura.

**cos·to·scap·u·lar** (kos"to-skap'u-lər) pertaining to the ribs and the scapula.

**cos·to·scap·u·lar·is** (kos"to-skap"u-lar'is) musculus serratus anterior.

**cos·to·ster·nal** (kos"to-stər'nəl) pertaining to a rib and to the sternum.

**cos·to·ster·no·plas·ty** (kos"to-stər'no-plas"te) surgical repair of funnel chest.

**cos·to·su·pe·ri·or** (kos"to-soo-pēr'e-ər) pertaining to the upper ribs.

**cos·to·tome** (kos'to-tōm) [*costo-* + *-tome*] a knife for dividing ribs or costal cartilages.

**cos·tot·o·my** (kos-tot'ə-me) [*costo-* + *-tomy*] incision or division of a rib or costal cartilage.

**cos·to·trans·verse** (kos"to-trans-vərs') lying between the ribs and transverse processes of the vertebrae.

**cos·to·trans·ver·sec·to·my** (kos"to-trans"vər-sek'tə-me) excision of a part of a rib with the transverse process of a vertebra.

**cos·to·ver·te·bral** (kos"to-vər'tə-brəl) pertaining to a rib and a vertebra.

**cos·to·xi·phoid** (kos"to-zi'foid) connecting the ribs and the xiphoid process.

**co·syn·tro·pin** (ko-sin-tro'pin) [MeSH: Cosyntropin] a synthetic polypeptide identical with the first 24 amino acids of corticotropin, having the corticotropic activity of corticotropin but lacking its allergenicity; used in the diagnosis of adrenal insufficiency by plasma cortisol response following subcutaneous, intramuscular, or intravenous injection.

**Co·tard's syndrome** (ko-tahrz') [Jules *Cotard,* French neurologist, 1840–1887] see under *syndrome.*

**Cot·a·zym** (kot'ə-zīm) trademark for a preparation of pancrelipase.

**co·throm·bo·plas·tin** (ko-throm"bo-plas'tin) [MeSH: Factor VII] factor VII; see under *coagulation factors,* at *factor.*

**co·ti·nine** (ko'tĭ-nēn) [MeSH: Cotinine] the major urinary metabolite of nicotine.
**c. fumarate,** an antidepressant, $(C_{10}H_{12}N_2O)_2 \cdot C_4H_4O_4$.

**co·trans·fec·tion** (ko"trans-fek'shən) simultaneous transfection with two separate, unrelated nucleic acid molecules, one of which may contain a gene that is easily assayed and acts as a marker.

**co·trans·port** (ko-trans'port) linking of the transport of one substance across a membrane with the simultaneous transport of a different substance in the same direction. Cf. *countertransport* and *symport.*

**Co·trel-Du·bous·set instrumentation, rod** (ko-trel'du-boo-sa') [Yves *Cotrel,* French orthopedic surgeon, 20th century; J. *Dubousset,* French orthopedic surgeon, 20th century] see under *instrumentation* and *rod.*

**co·tri·mox·a·zole** (ko"tri-moks'ə-zol) a mixture of trimethoprim and sulfamethoxazole.

**Cotte's operation** (kots) [Gaston *Cotte,* French surgeon, 1879–1951] see under *operation.*

**Cot·ting's operation** (kot'ingz) [Benjamin Eddy *Cotting,* American surgeon, 1812–1898] see under *operation.*

**cot·ton** (kot'ən) [Ar. *al-qoton* or *al-qutn*] [MeSH: Cotton] a textile material derived from the hair of the seeds of one or more of the cultivated varieties of *Gossypium.*
**absorbable c.,** oxidized cellulose.
**absorbent c.,** purified c.
**purified c.** [USP], cotton that has been purified, freed from fatty matter, bleached, and sterilized; used as a surgical dressing. Called also *absorbent c.,* and *gossypium asepticum, depuratum,* or *purificatum.*
**salicylated c.,** purified cotton charged with salicylic acid, an antiseptic dressing.
**styptic c.,** cotton impregnated with a styptic solution and dried.

**cot·ton·mouth** (kot'ən-mouth) water moccasin.

**cot·ton·pox** (kot'ən-poks) variola minor.

**cot·ton·seed** (kot'ən-sēd) the seeds of cultivated species of *Gossypium,* which are sources of cottonseed oil They are commonly made into cakes and fed to livestock, but must first be processed to remove the toxin gossypol, which could cause gossypol poisoning.

**cot·ton-wool** (kot'ən-wool) raw nonabsorbent cotton, especially the absorbent form prepared by removing the cottonseed oil.

**Co·tu·gno's disease** (ko-toon'yōz) [Domenico Felice Antonio *Cotugno,* Italian anatomist, 1736–1822] sciatica. See also *Cotunnius.*

**Co·tun·ni·us' aqueduct, canal, nerve, space** (ko-tun'e-əs) [Domenico *Cotugno (Cotunnius)*] see under *aqueduct, canal, nerve,* and *space.*

**co·tur·nism** (ko-too͝r'niz-əm) food poisoning caused by ingestion of meat of the European migratory quail, genus *Coturnix,* and marked by such symptoms as difficult breathing, impaired speech, nausea, weakness and loss of feeling in the legs, and partial paralysis, and sometimes resulting in death; the causative toxin, which occurs in only some of the quail, is unidentified.

**Co·tur·nix** (kə-too͝r'niks) [MeSH: Coturnix] a genus of birds of the family Phasianidae, including European migratory quails whose meat can be poisonous; see *coturnism.*

**co·twin** (ko-twin) a twin; usually applied in twin studies to identify pairs of twins.

**Cot•y•le•don** (kot″ə-le′dən) [MeSH: Cotyledon] a genus of herbaceous plants found in southern Africa; several species contain cotyledontoxin.

**cot•y•le•don** (kot″ə-le′don) [Gr. *kotylēdōn*] [MeSH: Cotyledon] 1. the seed leaf of the embryo of a plant. 2. any one of the subdivisions of the uterine surface of a discoidal placenta. 3. one of the tufted areas of a ruminant's placenta.

**cot•y•le•don•tox•in** (kot″ə-le″don-tok′sin) a neutral, nonalkaloidal, nonglucosidal, non-nitrogenous, amorphous substance toxic to humans and other animals, obtained from several species of the genus *Cotyledon;* see also *krimpsiekte.*

**Cot•y•lo•gon•i•mus** (kot″ə-lo-gon′ĭ-məs) [Gr. *kotylē* cup + *gonimos* productive] *Heterophyes.*

**cot•y•loid** (kot′ə-loid) [Gr. *kotyloeides* cup shaped] 1. cup-shaped. 2. pertaining to the cotyloid cavity (acetabulum).

**Co•ty•lo•pho•ron** (kot″ĭ-lof′ə-ron) a genus of trematodes of the family Paramphistomatidae that infest the rumen and intestines of ruminants, causing paramphistomiasis.

**cot•y•lo•pu•bic** (kot″ə-lo-pu′bik) relating to the cotyloid cavity (acetabulum) and the os pubis.

**cot•y•lo•sa•cral** (kot″ə-lo-sa′krəl) relating to cotyloid cavity (acetabulum) and the sacrum.

**co′type** (ko′tīp) any strain of microorganisms (of the same taxon), other than a holotype, from the collection of the bacteriologist who originally described the taxon.

**cough** (kawf) [L. *tussis*] [MeSH: Cough] 1. a sudden noisy expulsion of air from the lungs, usually produced to keep the airways of the lungs free of foreign matter; see also under *reflex.* Called also *tussis.* 2. to produce such an expulsion of air.
**aneurysmal c.,** cough associated with aortic aneurysm, sometimes with paralysis of one vocal cord.
**Balme's c.,** cough on lying down, seen in obstruction of the nasopharynx.
**barking c.,** a barklike cough of children, seen in croup and other conditions.
**brassy c.,** a cough with a metallic, barking quality due to inflammation of the trachea.
**dry c.,** one not accompanied by expectoration.
**ear c.,** a reflex cough caused by disease of the ear, when Arnold's nerve is stimulated.
**habit c.,** coughing, usually in children, that lacks a physical basis; it is a dry cough unaccompanied by other symptoms, seen only during waking hours, often lasting for weeks, and refractory to medication. Called also *psychogenic c.*
**hacking c.,** a short, frequent, shallow, and feeble cough. Called also *tussiculation.*
**kennel c.,** canine infectious tracheobronchitis.
**mechanical c.,** expulsion of air from the lungs produced by use of an exsufflator, with effects similar to those of a natural cough.
**privet c.,** an allergic cough noted in China and attributed to the pollen of privet.
**productive c.,** one that is effective in removing material from the respiratory tract. Called also *wet c.*
**psychogenic c.,** habit c.
**reflex c.,** a cough due to the irritation of some remote organ.
**trigeminal c.,** a cough due to irritation of the fibers of the trigeminal nerve distributed to the throat, nose, and external meatus of the ear.
**wet c.,** productive c.
**whooping c.,** pertussis.
**winter c.,** chronic bronchitis recurring in the winter.

**cou•lomb** (koo′lom) [after Charles Augustin de *Coulomb,* French physicist, 1736–1806] the SI unit of electric charge defined as the charge carried across a surface by a steady current of one ampere in one second; it is equivalent to $6.25 \times 10^{18}$ electrons. Symbol C.

**Coul•ter counter** (kōl′tər) [Wallace H. *Coulter,* American engineer, 20th century] see under *counter.*

**Cou•ma•din** (koo′mə-din) trademark for preparations of warfarin sodium.

**cou•ma•my•cin** (koo″mə-mi′sin) coumermycin.

**cou•ma•ric ac•id** (koo′mə-rik) an acid from coumarin, readily convertible into salicylic acid.

**cou•ma•rin** (koo′mə-rin) 1. a principle with a bitter taste and an odor like that of vanilla beans, derived from tonka bean, sweet clover, and other plants, and also prepared synthetically. It contains a factor, dicumarol, that inhibits the hepatic synthesis of the vitamin K–dependent coagulation factors (prothrombin, factors VII, IX, and X), and a number of its derivatives are used widely as anticoagulants in the treatment of disorders in which there is excessive or undesirable clotting, such as thrombophlebitis, pulmonary embolism, and certain cardiac conditions. 2. any derivative of coumarin or any synthetic compound with coumarin-like actions.

**cou•mer•my•cin** (koo″mər-mi′sin) an antibacterial agent isolated from *Streptomyces hazeliensis* var. *hazeliensis* and from *S. rishiriensis.*

**Coun•cil•man's bodies (lesions)** (koun′səl-mənz) [William Thomas *Councilman,* American pathologist, 1854–1933] see under *body.*

**count** (kount) [L. *computare* to reckon] a numerical computation or indication.
**Addis c.,** the determination of the number of red blood cells, white blood cells, epithelial cells, casts, and the protein content in an aliquot of a twelve-hour urine specimen, used in the diagnosis and management of kidney disease.
**Arneth c.,** a method of determining what percentages of neutrophils in a population have each number of nuclear lobes or segments between one and five; normally over 75 per cent should have two or three lobes. An increase in the percentages with fewer lobes, called a *shift to the left,* is seen in bacterial infections, whereas an increased number with hypersegmentation of the nuclei, called a *shift to the right,* is seen in cobalamin and folate deficiency. Called also *neutrophil lobe c.*
**blood c., blood cell c.,** determination of the number of formed elements in a cubic millimeter of blood; it may be a *complete blood count* or it may measure just one of the formed elements. Methods include manual counts with a hemacytometer and automated counts with a flow cytometer, a Coulter counter, or other means.
**blood c., complete,** a series of tests of the peripheral blood, including the erythrocyte count, erythrocyte indices, leukocyte counts, and sometimes platelet count.
**blood c., differential,** differential leukocyte count.
**erythrocyte c.,** determination of the number of erythrocytes in a unit volume of blood that has been diluted in an isotonic solution, done with an automatic counter such as a flow cytometer. Called also *red blood cell c.* and *red cell c.*
**filament-nonfilament c.,** in the differential leukocyte count, determination of the number of juvenile and mature leukocytes.
**leukocyte c.,** determination of the number of leukocytes in a unit volume of blood, usually after the erythrocytes have been lysed and the blood has been diluted; it may be done either manually with a hemacytometer or electronically. See *total leukocyte c.* and *differential leukocyte c.* Called also *white blood cell c.* and *white cell c.*
**leukocyte c., differential,** a leukocyte count that calculates the percentages of different types. Cf. *total leukocyte c.*
**leukocyte c., total,** a leukocyte count measuring the total number of all the types in a given volume of blood. Cf. *differential leukocyte c.*
**neutrophil lobe c.,** Arneth c.
**platelet c.,** determination of the number of platelets per cubic millimeter of blood; it may be either a *direct platelet count* with a hemacytometer and a microscope or an *indirect platelet count* in which the ratio of platelets to erythrocytes on a blood smear is determined and the number of platelets is computed from the erythrocyte count.
**red blood cell c., red cell c.,** erythrocyte c.
**reticulocyte c.,** a calculation of the number of reticulocytes in 1 cu mm of peripheral blood, recorded as an absolute number or as the percentage of the erythrocyte count. It provides a means of assessing the erythropoietic activity of the bone marrow.
**total lymphocyte c.,** a test that may be useful as an indicator of nutritional status and outcome.
**white blood cell c., white cell c.,** leukocyte c.

**coun•ter** (koun′tər) an instrument or apparatus by which numerical value is computed; in radiology, a device for enumerating ionizing events.
**Coulter c.,** an automated instrument for performing blood counts, based on the principle that cells are poor electrical conductors compared with saline solution.
**Geiger c., Geiger-Müller c.,** a radiation counter that uses a gas-filled tube to indicate the presence of ionizing particles; the type and energy of a particle cannot be determined because the degree of ionization produced is independent of them. It is highly sensitive to $\beta$ particles, but relatively insensitive to $\gamma$ and x-rays.
**proportional c.,** a gas-filled radiation detection tube in which the pulse produced is proportional to the number of ions formed in the gas by the primary ionizing particle; thus it is possible to discriminate among radiations of different energies or types.
**scintillation c.,** an instrument for indicating the emission of ionizing particles, making possible the determination of the concentration of radioactive isotopes in the body or other substance; the radiation is absorbed by a specific type of crystal or liquid that subsequently emits minute flashes of light, which are detected and amplified by a photomultiplier tube and counted if they fall within a preset window of energies characteristic of the radioisotope in question.

**coun•ter•bal•ance** (koun″tər-bal′əns) counterpoise; offset.

**renal c.**, compensatory hypertrophy of a normal kidney or part of a kidney accompanied by the tendency of its diseased mate or part to remain in a relatively atrophic state.

**coun·ter·ca·thex·is** (koun″tər-kə-thek′sis) anticathexis.

**coun·ter·cur·rent** (koun′tər-kər″ənt) flowing in an opposite direction; see also under *mechanism*.

**coun·ter·elec·tro·pho·re·sis** (koun″tər-e-lek″tro-fo-re′sis) counterimmunoelectrophoresis.

**coun·ter·ex·ten·sion** (koun″tər-eks-ten′shən) countertraction.

**coun·ter·im·mu·no·elec·tro·pho·re·sis** (koun″tər-im″u-no-e-lek″tro-fə-re′sis) [MeSH: Counterimmunoelectrophoresis] one-dimensional double electroimmunodiffusion; a technique in which antibody and antigen are placed in separate wells in an agar plate and driven toward each other by an applied electric field, because the gel is buffered at a pH between the isoelectric points of the antigen and antibody. It is more sensitive and faster than double immunodiffusion and is particularly useful for antigens that diffuse slowly in the gel. Abbreviated CIE. Called also *countercurrent immunoelectrophoresis* and *counterelectrophoresis*.

**coun·ter·in·ci·sion** (koun″tər-in-si′zhən) a second incision usually made to promote drainage, but occasionally to relieve tension on the edges of a clean wound during closure.

**coun·ter·in·vest·ment** (koun″tər-in-vest′mənt) anticathexis.

**coun·ter·ir·ri·tant** (koun″tər-ir′ĭ-tənt) 1. producing a counterirritation. 2. any agent which causes counterirritation.

**coun·ter·ir·ri·ta·tion** (koun″tər-ir″ĭ-ta′shən) a superficial irritation produced in one part of the body and intended to relieve an irritation in another part.

**coun·ter·open·ing** (koun″tər-o′pən-ing) a second incision made across an earlier one to promote drainage.

**coun·ter·pho·bia** (koun″tər-fo′be-ə) the state of seeking out of situations or objects which one fears or has feared, consciously or unconsciously.

**coun·ter·pho·bic** (koun″tər-fo′bik) pertaining to or characterized by counterphobia.

**coun·ter·poi·son** (koun′tər-poi″zon) a poison given to counteract another poison.

**coun·ter·pul·sa·tion** (koun″tər-pəl-sa′shən) [MeSH: Counterpulsation] a technique for assisting the circulation and decreasing the work of the heart, by synchronizing the force of an external pumping device with cardiac systole and diastole.
**intra-aortic balloon (IAB) c.**, circulatory support provided by a balloon inserted into the thoracic aorta, which is inflated during diastole (enhancing coronary perfusion pressure) and deflated during systole, resulting in a decrease in afterload and improvement in cardiac function.

**coun·ter·punc·ture** (koun″tər-punk′chər) counteropening.

**coun·ter·shock** (koun′tər-shok″) a high-intensity direct current shock delivered to the heart to interrupt ventricular fibrillation and restore synchronous electrical activity.

**coun·ter·stain** (koun′tər-stān) a stain applied to render the effects of another stain more discernible.

**coun·ter·trac·tion** (koun″tər-trak′shən) traction opposed to another traction; employed in the reduction of fractures.

**coun·ter·trans·fer·ence** (koun″tər-trans-fər′əns) a transference reaction of a psychoanalyst or other psychotherapist to a patient, i.e., an emotional reaction that is generally a reflection of the analyst's own inner needs and conflicts but also may be a reaction to the client's behavior. See *transference*.

**coun·ter·trans·port** (koun″tər-trans′port) the simultaneous transport of two substances across a membrane in opposite directions, either by the same carrier or by different carriers that are biochemically linked to each other. Cf. *antiport* and *cotransport*.
**sodium-lithium c.**, a transport pathway by which sodium ions enter erythrocytes and lithium ions leave in order to maintain sodium balance in the cells and in the plasma.

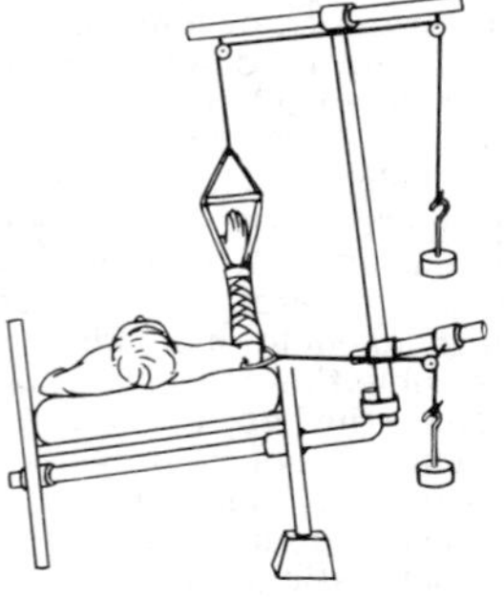

Countertraction.

**count·ing** (kownt′ing) the act of making a count.
**liquid scintillation c.**, determination of the concentration of radioisotopes in a body or sample by means of a scintillation counter (q.v.) that uses as a detector an organic liquid capable of emitting pulses of light when struck by radiation.

**coup** (koo) [Fr.] a blow or stroke.
**c. de fouet** (də-fwa′) [Fr. "stroke of the whip"], rupture of the plantaris muscle accompanied by a sharp disabling pain.
**c. de sabre, en c. de sabre** (də-sahb′, ahn-koo-də-sahb′) [Fr. "saber stroke"], a linear lesion of scleroderma involving the frontal or frontoparietal area of the forehead and scalp; it is often associated with facial hemiatrophy.
**c. de soleil** (də-so-la′), sunstroke.
**c. sur c.** (sur-koo′) [Fr. "blow on blow"], the administration of a drug in small doses at short intervals, to secure rapid, complete, or continuous action; abbreviated CSC.

**cou·ple** (kup′əl) [L. *copula* a bond] 1. two equal forces operating on an object in parallel but opposite directions. 2. an area of contact between two dissimilar metals, producing a difference in electrical potential.

**coup·let** (kup′lət) pair, def. 2.

**coup·ling** (kup′ling) 1. the joining together of two things. 2. in genetics, the occurrence on the same chromosome in a double heterozygote of the two mutant alleles of interest. Cf. *repulsion*. 3. in cardiology, the serial occurrence of a normal heart beat followed closely by a premature beat.
**excitation-contraction c.**, the coupling of the action potential to muscle constriction by means of calcium ions which diffuse rapidly into the myofibrils and catalyze the chemical reactions that promote the contractile sliding of actin and myosin filaments.
**fixed c.**, coupling in which the premature heart beats follow the preceding normal beats at identical intervals.
**variable c.**, coupling in which the interval between extrasystoles and the sinus beats preceding them is not constant.

**Cour·nand** (ko͞or-nahn′) André Frédéric. French-born American physiologist, born 1895; co-winner, with Werner Theodor Otto Forssmann and Dickinson Woodruff Richards, Jr., of the Nobel prize for medicine or physiology in 1956 for the development of cardiac catheterization.

**Cour·voi·si·er's law (sign)** (koor-vwah″ze-āz′) [Ludwig Georg *Courvoisier*, Swiss surgeon, 1843–1918] see under *law*.

**Cour·voi·si·er-Ter·rier syndrome** (koor-vwah″ze-a′-ter-ya′) [L. G. *Courvoisier;* Louis Félix *Terrier*, French surgeon, 1837–1908] see under *syndrome*.

**Cou·tard's method** (koo-tahrz′) [Henri *Coutard*, French radiologist in United States, 1876–1950] see under *method*.

**cou·vade** (koo-vahd′) a custom of certain societies in which the husband feigns illness during his wife's parturient and puerperal periods.

**Cou·ve·laire uterus** (koo″və-lār′) [Alexandre *Couvelaire*, French obstetrician, 1873–1948] see *uteroplacental apoplexy*, under *apoplexy*.

**cou·ver·cle** (koo′vər-kəl) [Fr.] hematoma.

**co·va·lence** (ko-va′ləns) 1. the number of electron pairs an atom can share with other atoms. 2. one or more chemical bonds formed by sharing of electron pairs between atoms.

**co·va·lent** (ko′va-lənt) see under *bond*.

**co·var·i·ance** (ko-vār′e-əns) [*co-* + *variance*] in statistics, a measure of the tendency of two random variables to vary together: the expected value of the product of the deviations of corresponding values of the variables from their respective means. It may be positive, with both variables increasing or decreasing together; negative, with one variable decreasing as the other increases; or zero, with one variable unaffected by changes in the other.

**co·va·ri·ate** (ko-var′e-ət) a variable that is related to a second variable.

**cov·er** (kov′ər) 1. to provide protection against, as by prophylaxis. 2. the prophylaxis so provided.

**cov·er·glass** (kov′ər-glas) a thin glass plate that covers a mounted microscopical object or a culture. Spelled also cover glass.

**cov·er·slip** (kov′ər-slip) coverglass.

**cow·age** (kou′əj) 1. *Mucuna pruriens*. 2. the hairs of the pods of

*M. pruriens,* which cause severe itching, and are used medicinally as a vermifuge, anthelmintic, and counterirritant mixed with such vehicles as honey. Also used as "itching powders" of joke-shop fame.

**Cow·den disease** (kou'dən) [*Cowden,* the family name of the first reported case] see under *disease.*

**Cow·dria** (kou'dre-ə) [Edmund Vincent *Cowdry,* American anatomist and zoologist, 1888–1975] [MeSH: Cowdria] a genus of bacteria of the tribe Ehrlichieae, family Rickettsiaceae, order Rickettsiales, occurring in the cytoplasm of vascular endothelial cells of ruminants.
**C. ruminan'tium,** the etiologic agent of heartwater (q.v.) of sheep, goats, and cattle; it is nonpathogenic for man.

**cow·dri·o·sis** (kow"dre-o'sis) heartwater.

**Cow·en's sign** (kou'ənz) [J.P. *Cowen,* American ophthalmologist, 20th century] see under *sign.*

**cowl** (koul) caul, def. 1.

**Cow·per's gland, ligament** (kou'pərz) [William *Cowper,* English surgeon, 1666–1709] see *glandula bulbourethralis* and *fascia pectinea.*

**cow·pe·ri·an** (kou-pēr'e-ən) described by or named in honor of William Cowper.

**cow·per·itis** (kou"pər-i'tis) inflammation of Cowper's glands (glandula bulbourethralis).

**cow·pox** (kou'poks) [MeSH: Cowpox] 1. a mild, self-limited, eruptive skin disease of milk cows, principally confined to the udder and teats, caused by a pox virus; milkers may spread the disease to uninfected animals. 2. human infection with the same virus, usually occurring accidentally, as while milking an infected animal; the primary lesions, vesicles, usually appear on the fingers, may rupture and spread to the hands or adjacent areas, and usually heal without scarring. Local edema, lymphangitis, and regional lymphadenitis with or without fever may be associated. Cowpox is not to be confused with *paravaccinia.* Cf. *vaccinia.* Edward Jenner first demonstrated vaccination in 1798 when he showed that inoculation with material from cowpox lesions conferred immunity against smallpox.

**Cox proportional hazards model** (koks) [David Roxbee *Cox,* British statistician, born 1924] see under *model.*

**coxa** (kok'sə) [L.] 1. [TA] hip (def. 1). 2. articulatio coxae.
**c. adduc'ta, c. flex'a,** c. vara.
**c. mag'na,** a condition marked by broadening of the head and neck of the femur.
**c. pla'na,** osteochondrosis of the capitular epiphysis of the femur; see *osteochondrosis.*
**c. val'ga,** deformity of the hip in which the angle formed by the axis of the head and the neck of the femur and the axis of its shaft is materially increased.
**c. va'ra,** deformity of the hip in which the angle formed by the axis of the head and neck of the femur and the axis of its shaft is materially decreased; called also *c. adducta* and *c. flexa.*
**c. va'ra lux'ans,** fissure of the neck of the femur with dislocation of the head developing from coxa vara.

**cox·al·gia** (kok-sal'jə) [*coxa* + *-algia*] 1. hip joint disease. 2. pain in the hip.

**cox·ar·thria** (kok-sahr'thre-ə) coxitis.

**cox·ar·thri·tis** (kok-sahr-thri'tis) coxitis.

**cox·ar·throc·a·ce** (kok"sahr-throk'ə-se) fungus disease of the hip joint.

**cox·ar·throp·a·thy** (kok"sahr-throp'ə-the) [*coxa* + *arthro-* + *-pathy*] hip joint disease.

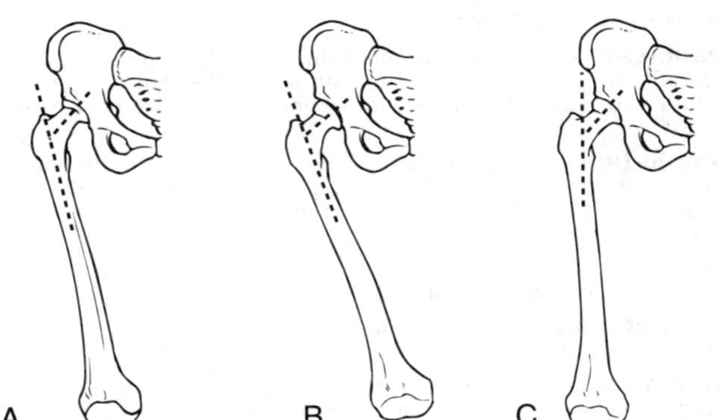

*(A)* Normal hip joint; *(B)* coxa vara; *(C)* coxa valga.

**cox·ar·thro·sis** (kok"sahr-thro'sis) degenerative joint disease or osteoarthritis of the hip joint.

**Cox·i·el·la** (kok"se-el'ə) [Herald Rae *Cox,* American bacteriologist, born 1907] [MeSH: Coxiella] a genus of bacteria of the tribe Rickettsieae, family Rickettsiaceae, order Rickettsiales, occurring as short rods in the vacuoles of host cells. The organisms have been found in various mammals and ticks worldwide, and have been isolated from milk and placentas of infected cattle, sheep, and goats and from the wool of infected sheep.
**C. burnet'ii,** the etiologic agent of Q fever, transmitted by *Haemaphysalis, Ixodes, Dermacentor,* and *Amblyomma* ticks. Human infection usually occurs from inhalation of infectious dust and aerosols derived from domestic livestock, and from contaminated wool in textile plants. Called also *Rickettsia burnetii* and *R. diaporica.*

**cox·itis** (kok-si'tis) inflammation of the hip joint; called also *coxarthritis.*
**c. fu'gax,** a transient benign coxitis.
**senile c.,** degenerative arthritis of the hip joint.

**cox·odyn·ia** (kok"so-din'e-ə) coxalgia, def. 2.

**coxo·fem·o·ral** (kok"so-fem'o-rəl) [*coxa* + *femoral*] pertaining to the hip and thigh.

**coxo·tu·ber·cu·lo·sis** (kok"so-too-bər"ku-lo'sis) [*coxa* + *tuberculosis*] tuberculous disease of the hip joint.

**cox·sack·ie·vi·rus** (kok-sak'e-vi"rəs) [*Coxsackie,* New York, where it was first identified] [MeSH: Coxsackieviruses] any of a heterogeneous group of viruses of the genus *Enterovirus* producing, in man, a disease resembling poliomyelitis but without paralysis, as well as a disease with fever and rash. It is separable into two groups: A (23 serotypes, 1–22 and 24, with 23 being identical to echovirus 9), producing degenerative lesions of striated muscle, and B (6 serotypes), producing leptomeningitis in infant mice. A number of different serotypes have also been identified. Also written *Coxsackie virus.*

**co·yo·ti·llo** (koi-o-te'yo) [Mexican Spanish "little coyote"] *Karwinskia humboldtiana.*

**Co·zaar** (ko'zahr) trademark for a preparation of losartan potassium.

**CP** chemically pure; candle power.

**cp** symbol for *centipoise.*

**C3PA** C3 proactivator, former name for *factor B.*

**CPAP** continuous positive airway pressure.

**CPC** clinicopathological conference.

**CPD** citrate phosphate dextrose; see *anticoagulant citrate phosphate dextrose solution,* under *solution.*

**CPDA-1** citrate phosphate dextrose adenine; see *anticoagulant citrate phosphate dextrose adenine solution,* under *solution.*

**CPDD** calcium pyrophosphate deposition disease.

**C Ped** Certified Pedorthist.

**CPH** Certificate in Public Health.

**CPI** congenital palatopharyngeal incompetence; California Personality Inventory.

**CPK** creatine phosphokinase; see *creatine kinase.*

**cpm** counts per minute, an expression of the rate of particle emission from a radioactive material.

**CPPD** calcium pyrophosphate dihydrate; see *calcium pyrophosphate deposition disease* under *disease.*

**CPR** cardiopulmonary resuscitation.

**CPS** carbamoyl phosphate synthetase.
**CPSI,** carbamoyl phosphate synthetase I; see *carbamoyl-phosphate synthase (ammonia).*
**CPSII,** carbamoyl phosphate synthetase II; see *carbamoyl-phosphate synthase (glutamine-hydrolyzing).*

**cps** cycles per second.

**CR** conditioned response; crown-rump (in embryology, the usual axis of measurement of an embryo or fetus); complement receptor.

**CR3** complement receptor type 3; see *glycoprotein Mac-1,* under *glycoprotein.*

**Cr** symbol for *chromium.*

**crab** (krab) [MeSH: Crabs] 1. any of various mollusks of the order Decapoda; see also *Potamon.* 2. a vernacular term for *Phthirus pubis.*

**crack** (krak) 1. an incomplete split, break, or fissure. 2. sand c.
**hoof wall c.,** sand c.
**quarter c.,** a sand crack on the quarter (medial aspect of the hoof).

**sand c.**, a crack originating at the ground level in a horse's hoof, sometimes causing lameness. Two types are the *quarter c.* and the *toe c.* Called also *hoof wall c.*
**toe c.**, a sand crack on the anterior part of the hoof.

**crack·le** (krak'əl) [MeSH: Respiratory Sounds] rale.

**cra·dle** (kra'dəl) a frame placed over the body of a bed patient for application of heat or cold or for protecting injured parts from contact with the bed clothes.
**electric c., heat c.**, a tunnel- or hood-shaped cradle equipped with electric light bulbs, for application of heat to the body of a patient.
**ice c.**, a device for lowering a patient's body temperature.

**Crafts' test** (krafts) [Leo Melville *Crafts*, American neurologist, 1863–1938] see under *test*.

**Crai·gia** (kra'ge-ə) [Charles Franklin *Craig*, U. S. Army surgeon, 1872–1950] *Paramoeba*.

**Cra·mer's splint** (krah'mərz) [Friedrich *Cramer*, German surgeon, 1847–1903] see under *splint*.

**cramp** (kramp) a painful spasmodic muscular contraction, especially a tonic spasm.
**accessory c.**, spastic torticollis due to a lesion of the accessory nerve.
**heat c.**, a form of heat exhaustion in which muscular spasm is attended by pains, dilated pupils, and weak pulse; seen in those who labor in intense heat (stokers, miners, cane-cutters) and lose much water and salt. Called also *Edsall's disease*.
**recumbency c's**, cramping of muscles in legs and feet occurring while resting or during light sleep.
**stoker's c.**, heat c.
**writers' c.**, a muscle cramp in the hand, a type of focal dystonia caused by excessive use in writing; called also *graphospasm, scriveners' palsy, paralysis notariorum, writers' paralysis*, and *writers' spasm*.

**Cramp·ton's muscle** (kramp'tənz) [Sir Philip *Crampton*, Irish surgeon, 1777–1858] see under *muscle*.

**Cramp·ton's test** (kramp'tənz) [Charles Ward *Crampton*, American physician, 1877–1964] see under *test*.

**cra·ni·ad** (kra'ne-ad) [*crani-* + *-ad*[1]] cephalad.

**cra·ni·al** (kra'ne-əl) [L. *cranialis*] 1. pertaining to the cranium. 2. toward the head end of the body; a synonym of *superior* in humans and other bipeds. In quadruped anatomy *anterior* is sometimes used as a synonym. Called also *cephalic*.

**cra·ni·a·lis** (kra″ne-a'lis) [L.] [TA] cranial.

**cra·ni·am·phit·o·my** (kra″ne-am-fit'ə-me) [*crani-* + *amphi-* + *-tomy*] division of the entire circumference of the skull to secure decompression.

**Cra·ni·a·ta** (kra″ne-a'tə) the subphylum of the Chordata containing the species with a true skull and spinal column; the vertebrates.

**cra·ni·ec·to·my** (kra″ne-ek'tə-me) [*crani-* + *-ectomy*] excision of a part of the skull.

**cra·nii** (kra'ne-i) genitive of *cranium*.

**crani(o)-** [L. *cranium*, q.v.] a combining form denoting relationship to the cranium or skull.

**cra·nio·acro·mi·al** (kra″ne-o-ə-kro'me-əl) pertaining to the cranium and acromion.

**cra·nio·au·ral** (kra″ne-o-aw'rəl) pertaining to the cranium and the ear.

**cra·nio·buc·cal** (kra″ne-o-buk'əl) pertaining to the cranium and the mouth.

**cra·nio·cele** (kra'ne-o-sēl″) [*cranio-* + *-cele*[1]] encephalocele.

**cra·nio·cer·e·bral** (kra″ne-o-sər-e'brəl) pertaining to the cranium and the cerebrum.

**cra·nio·cer·vi·cal** (kra″ne-o-sər'vĭ-kəl) pertaining to the cranium and the neck.

**cra·nio·did·y·mus** (kra″ne-o-did'ĭ-məs) [*cranio-* + *-didymus*] a fetus with two heads.

**cra·nio·fa·cial** (kra″ne-o-fa'shəl) pertaining to the cranium and the face.

**cra·nio·fe·nes·tria** (kra″ne-o-fə-nes'tre-ə) [*cranio-* + L. *fenestra* an opening] defective development of the calvaria of the fetal skull, with areas in which no bone is formed. Cf. *craniolacunia*.

**cra·ni·og·no·my** (kra-ne-og'nə-me) [*cranio-* + Gr. *gnōmōn* an interpreter or judge] the study of the shape of the head.

**cra·nio·graph** (kra'ne-o-graf″) [*cranio-* + *-graph*] an instrument for outlining the skull.

**cra·ni·og·ra·phy** (kra″ne-og'rə-fe) the study of the skull by means of photographs, charts, etc.

**cra·nio·la·cu·nia** (kra″ne-o-lə-koo'ne-ə) [*cranio-* + *lacuna* + *-ia*] defective development of the calvaria of the fetal skull with depressed areas on the inner surfaces. Cf. *craniofenestria*. Called also *lückenschädel*.

**cra·ni·ol·o·gy** (kra″ne-ol'ə-je) [*cranio-* + *-logy*] [MeSH: Craniology] the scientific study of skulls.

**cra·nio·ma·la·cia** (kra″ne-o-mə-la'shə) [*cranio-* + *-malacia*] abnormal softness of the skull.

**cra·nio·me·nin·go·cele** (kra″ne-o-mə-ning'go-sēl) cranial meningocele.

**cra·ni·om·e·ter** (kra″ne-om'ə-tər) [*cranio-* + *-meter*] an instrument for use in craniometry.

**cra·nio·met·ric** (kra″ne-o-met'rik) pertaining to craniometry.

**cra·ni·om·e·try** (kra″ne-om'ə-tre) [*cranio-* + *-metry*] [MeSH: Craniometry] the scientific measurement of the dimensions of the bones of the skull and face.

**cra·ni·op·a·gus** (kra″ne-op'ə-gəs) [*cranio-* + *-pagus*] conjoined twins united by the heads; called also *cephalopagus*.
**c. occipita'lis**, craniopagus in which fusion is in the occipital region.
**c. parasi'ticus**, craniopagus in which a parasitic head is attached to the head of the larger, more nearly normal twin.
**c. parieta'lis**, craniopagus in which fusion is in the parietal region.

**cra·ni·op·a·thy** (kra″ne-op'ə-the) [*cranio-* + *-pathy*] any disease of the skull.
**metabolic c.**, a condition characterized by lesions of the calvarium with multiple metabolic changes and marked by headache, obesity, and visual disturbances.

**cra·nio·pha·ryn·ge·al** (kra″ne-o-fə-rin'je-əl) pertaining to the cranium and the pharynx.

**cra·nio·pha·ryn·gi·o·ma** (kra″ne-o-fə-rin″je-o'mə) [MeSH: Craniopharyngioma] a tumor arising from cell rests derived from the hypophysial stalk or Rathke's pouch, frequently associated with increased intracranial pressure, and showing calcium deposits in the capsule or in the tumor proper. Deficits of pituitary hormones may also occur. Called also *craniopharyngeal duct tumor, Rathke's* or *Rathke's pouch tumor, suprasellar cyst*, and *pituitary adamantinoma* or *ameloblastoma*.

**cra·nio·phore** (kra'ne-o-for) [*cranio-* + *-phore*] a device for holding a skull during measurement of its diameters and angles.

**cra·nio·plas·ty** (kra'ne-o-plas″te) [*cranio-* + *-plasty*] any plastic operation on the skull; surgical correction of defects of the skull.

**cra·nio·punc·ture** (kra'ne-o-punk″chər) [*cranio-* + *puncture*] cephalocentesis.

**cra·nio·ra·chis·chi·sis** (kra″ne-o-rə-kis'kĭ-sis) [*cranio-* + *rhachis* + *schisis* fissure] congenital fissure of the skull and vertebral column; see *cranium bifidum* and *spina bifida*.

**cra·nio·sa·cral** (kra″ne-o-sa'krəl) 1. pertaining to the skull and the sacrum. 2. pertaining to the parasympathetic nerves.

**cra·ni·os·chi·sis** (kra″ne-os'kĭ-sis) [*cranio-* + Gr. *schisis* fissure] cranium bifidum.

**cra·nio·scle·ro·sis** (kra″ne-o-sklə-ro'sis) [*cranio-* + *sclerosis*] thickening of the bones of the skull.

**cra·nio·spi·nal** (kra″ne-o-spi'nəl) pertaining to the cranium and the vertebral column.

**cra·nio·ste·no·sis** (kra″ne-o-stə-no'sis) [*cranio-* + *stenosis*] deformity of the skull caused by craniosynostosis, with consequent cessation of skull growth; the nature of the deformity depends on the sutures involved in the process.

**cra·ni·os·to·sis** (kra″ne-os-to'sis) craniosynostosis.

**cra·nio·syn·os·to·sis** (kra″ne-o-sin″os-to'sis) [*cranio-* + *syn-* + *ostosis*] premature closure of the sutures of the skull, causing deformities such as oxycephaly and scaphocephaly. Called also *craniostosis*.

**cra·nio·ta·bes** (kra″ne-o-ta'bēz) [*cranio-* + *tabes*] reduction in the mineralization of the skull, with abnormal softness of the bone, usually located in the occipital and parietal bones along the lambdoidal sutures.

**cra·nio·tome** (kra'ne-o-tōm″) [*cranio-* + *-tome*] an instrument for use in performing craniotomy.

**cra·ni·ot·o·my** (kra″ne-ot'ə-me) [*cranio-* + *-tomy*] [MeSH: Craniotomy] any operation on the cranium; incision into the cranium.

**cra·nio·to·pog·ra·phy** (kra″ne-o-to-pog'rə-fe) [*cranio-* + *topography*] the study of the relations of the surface of the skull to the various parts of the brain beneath.

**cra·nio·try·pe·sis** (kra″ne-o-trĭ-pe'sis) [*cranio-* + *trypesis*] trephination of the skull.

**cra·nio·tym·pan·ic** (kra″ne-o-tim-pan′ik) pertaining to the skull and the tympanum.

**cra·ni·um** (kra′ne-əm) gen. *cra′nii,* pl. *cra′nia* [L., from Gr. *kranion* the upper part of the head] [TA] the large round superior part of the skull, enclosing the brain and made up of the cranial bones; see *ossa cranii,* under *os.*
**c. bi′fidum,** incomplete formation of the calvaria, with defective development of the brain and often an encephalocele or meningocele. Called also *cranioschisis.*
**c. bi′fidum occul′tum,** congenital cleft of the calvaria without associated abnormality of the brain or meninges, detectable only radiographically.
**cerebral c., c. cerebra′le,** those portions of the bones of the head that contribute to the calvaria.
**visceral c., c. viscera′le,** those portions of the bones of the head that form the skeleton of the face; see *facial bones,* under *bone*

**crap·u·lent, crap·u·lous** (krap′u-lənt, krap′u-ləs) [L. *crapulentus, crapulosis* drunken] due to excess in eating or drinking; see *hyperalimentation.*

**-crasia** [Gr. *krasis* mixture] combining form denoting a mixture of different elements.

**cras·sa·men·tum** (kras″ə-men′təm) [L.] clot (def. 1).

**Crast.** abbreviation for L. *cras′tinus,* for tomorrow.

**cra·ter** (kra′tər) a circular area of depression surrounded by an elevated margin.

**cra·ter·i·form** (kra-ter′ĭ-form) [*crater* + *form*] depressed or hollowed, like a bowl.

**cra·ter·iza·tion** (kra″tər-ĭ-za′shən) the operation of excising a craterlike piece from a bone.

**cra·vat** (krə-vaht′) [Fr. *cravate*] a bandage made by folding a triangular piece of cloth from its apex toward the base.

**craw** (kraw) crop.

**craw-craw** (kraw′kraw) a name for *onchocerciasis* in West Africa.

**craz·ing** (kra′zing) the appearance of minute cracks on the surface of artificial or natural teeth, porcelain, and resin denture bases.

**cream** (krēm) 1. the oily or fatty part of milk from which butter is prepared, or a fluid mixture of similar consistency. 2. in pharmaceutical preparations, a semisolid emulsion of the oil-in-water or water-in-oil type, ordinarily used topically.
**cold c.,** a preparation of spermaceti, white wax, mineral oil, sodium borate, and purified water; used as a topical emollient for minor skin irritations and as a water-in-oil emulsion ointment base.
**dienestrol c.** [USP], a mixture of dienestrol in a suitable water-miscible base; used topically for its estrogenic effect in the treatment of postmenopausal and senile vulvovaginitis, atrophic vaginitis, pruritus vulvae due to atrophic changes in the vulval epithelium, dyspareunia associated with atrophic vaginal epithelium, and prior to plastic pelvic surgery in menopausal cases.
**leukocytic c.,** buffy coat.
**Moynihan's c.,** a mixture consisting of as much bismuth carbonate in 1:1000 aqueous solution of mercuric iodide as will make a thick paste; used as a wound dressing.
**c. of tartar,** potassium bitartrate.

**Cream·a·lin** (krēm′ə-lin) trademark for preparations of aluminum hydroxide gel.

**crease** (krēs) a line or slight linear depression (in anatomical terminology).
**ear lobe c.,** a diagonal crease in the ear lobe associated with aging; when present in younger persons it may be a sign of coronary artery disease.
**flexion c., palmar c.,** any of the normal grooves across the palm which accommodate flexion of the hand by separating folds of tissue. In certain congenital anomalies, there is only a single transverse (simian) crease.
**simian c.,** a single transverse palmar crease formed by fusion of the proximal and distal palmar creases; frequently seen in congenital disorders such as Down syndrome and rarely in normal persons; called also *simian line.*

**cre·a·sote** (kre′ə-sōt) creosote.

**cre·at·i·nase** (kre-at′ĭ-nās) [EC 3.5.3.3] an amidohydrolase that catalyzes the conversion of creatine to sarcosine and urea.

**cre·a·tine** (kre′ə-tin) [Gr. *kreas* flesh] [MeSH: Creatine] an amino acid formed by methylation of guanidinoacetic acid and occurring in vertebrate tissues, particularly in muscle. Phosphorylated creatine (see *phosphocreatine*) is an important storage form of high energy phosphate, the energy source for muscle contraction.
**c. phosphate,** phosphocreatine.

**cre·a·tine ki·nase** (kre′ə-tin ki′nās) [EC 2.7.3.2] [MeSH: Creatine Kinase] an $Mg^{2+}$-activated enzyme of the transferase class that catalyzes the phosphorylation of creatine by ATP to form phosphocreatine. The reaction effectively stores the energy of ATP as phosphocreatine in muscle and brain tissue and holds the muscle concentration of ATP nearly constant during the initiation of exercise. It occurs as three isoenzymes, each having two components composed of M (muscle) and of B (brain) subunits. $CK_1$ (BB) is found primarily in brain, $CK_2$ (MB) primarily in cardiac muscle, and $CK_3$ (MM) primarily in skeletal muscle. Differential determination of isoenzymes is useful for clinical diagnoses. Abbreviated CK.

**cre·a·tin·emia** (kre″ə-tĭ-ne′me-ə) excess of creatine in the blood.

**cre·a·tine phos·pho·ki·nase** (kre′ə-tin-fos″fo-ki′nāse) former name for *creatine kinase.* Abbreviated CPK.

**cre·a·ti·ni·nase** (kre-at′ĭ-nin-ās) [EC 3.5.2.10] an amidohydrolase that catalyzes the conversion of creatinine to creatine.

**cre·at·i·nine** (kre-at′ĭ-nin) [MeSH: Creatinine] 1. the cyclic anhydride of creatine, produced as the final product of decomposition of phosphocreatine. It is excreted in the urine; measurements of excretion rates are used as diagnostic indicators of kidney function (see *creatinine clearance,* under *clearance*) and muscle mass and can be used to simplify other clinical assays. 2. [NF] a preparation of creatinine, used as a bulking agent in freeze-drying.

**cre·a·tin·uria** (kre″ah-tĭ-nu′reə) increased concentration of creatine in the urine.

**cre·a·tor·rhea** (kre″ə-to-re′ə) [Gr. *kreas* flesh + *-rrhea*] the presence of undigested muscle fibers in the feces.

**cre·a·to·tox·ism** (kre″ə-to-tok′siz-əm) meat poisoning.

**cre·a·tox·i·con** (kre″ə-tok′sĭ-kon) kreotoxicon.

**cre·a·tox·in** (kre″ə-tok′sin) kreotoxin.

**crèche** (kresh) [Fr.] a day nursery for infants.

**Cre·dé's method (maneuver)** (krĕ-dāz′) [Karl Sigmund Franz *Credé,* German gynecologist, 1819–1892] see under *method.*

**creep** (krēp) 1. a slow flow over time that occurs with materials under stress below their elastic limits, often due to warm temperature; it may occur with dental materials in the mouth. 2. the time-dependent strain in a tissue or body as a result of application and maintenance of a stress at a set level.

**CREG** cross-reactive group (of HLA antigens).

**cre·mas·ter** (kre-mas′tər) [L.; Gr. *kremasthai* to suspend] musculus cremaster.
**internal c. of Henle,** fibers of the gubernaculum testis, inserted in elements of the fetal spermatic cord.

**crem·as·ter·ic** (krem″as-ter′ik) pertaining to the cremaster.

**cre·ma·tion** (kre-ma′shən) [L. *crematio* a burning] the burning or incineration of dead bodies.

**cre·ma·to·ri·um** (kre″mə-tor′e-əm) an establishment for the burning of dead bodies.

**Crem·o·phor** (krem′o-for) trademark for a number of polyoxyl compounds used as lipid vehicles for solubilizing and emulsifying drugs.

**cre·mor** (kre′mor) [L.] cream.
**c. tar′tari,** ["cream of tartar"], potassium bitartrate.

**cre·na** (kre′nə) pl. *cre′nae* [L. "notch," from *crenare* to split] a notch or cleft.
**c. ana′lis** [TA], intergluteal cleft: the cleft between the buttocks on which the anus opens. Called also *anal, clunial, gluteal,* or *natal cleft, c. ani* or *c. interglutealis* [TA alternatives], *c. clunium, gluteal furrow, rima ani,* and *rima clunium.*
**c. a′ni,** TA alternative for *c. analis.*
**c. clu′nium,** c. analis.
**c. cor′dis,** sulcus interventricularis anterior.
**c. interglutea′lis,** TA alternative for *c. analis.*

**cre·nate** (kre′nāt) [L. *crenatus*] crenated.

**cre·nat·ed** (kre′nāt-əd) scalloped or notched; see *crenation.*

**cre·na·tion** (kre-na′shən) 1. the formation of abnormal notching in the edge of an erythrocyte; see *burr cell,* under *cell.* 2. the notched appearance of an erythrocyte caused by its shrinkage after suspension in a hypertonic solution. Cf. *echinosis.* Called also *crenulation.*

**cren·il·a·brin** (kren-il-a′brin) a protamine obtained from the sperm of the cunner (fish).

**cre·no·cyte** (kre′no-sīt) burr cell.

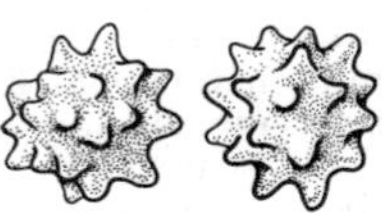

Crenated erythocytes.

**cre·no·cy·to·sis** (kre″no-si-to′sis) the presence of burr cells (crenocytes) in the blood; called also *echinosis.*

**Cre·no·so·ma** (kre″no-so′mə) a genus of nematodes of the family Crenosomatidae. *C. vul′pis* is a lungworm of dogs and other carnivores.

**Cre·no·so·mat·i·dae** (kre″no-so-mat′ĭ-de) a family of nematodes that includes the genera *Crenosoma* and *Troglostrongylus.* Several species infect the lungs or bronchioles of dogs or cats.

**cren·u·la·tion** (kren″u-la′shən) crenation.

**cre·oph·a·gism, cre·oph·a·gy** (kre-of′ə-jiz-əm, kre-of′ə-je) [Gr. *kreas* flesh + *phagein* to eat] the eating of flesh (meat); see also *carnivore.*

**cre·o·sol** (kre′o-sol) [*creosote* + L. *oleum* oil] a colorless oily liquid, the methyl ether of methyl catechol, one of the active constituents of creosote.

**cre·o·sote** (kre′o-sōt) [MeSH: Creosote] a colorless to yellowish, oily, refractive liquid, a mixture of phenols obtained by distilling wood tar, mainly beech *(Fagus sylvatica).* It was formerly used as an expectorant and external antiseptic and is now mainly used as a wood preservative. Animals may suffer skin irritation from wood recently treated with creosote, or ulceration of the esophagus if they chew on it.
**c. carbonate,** a clear, viscid liquid, a mixture of carbonates of various constituents of creosote, used as an expectorant and antiseptic.

**creo·tox·in** (kre″o-tok′sin) kreotoxin.

**creo·tox·ism** (kre″o-tok′siz-əm) kreotoxism.

**crep·i·tant** (krep′ĭ-tənt) [L. *crepitare* to rattle or crackle] rattling or crackling. See under *rale.*

**crep·i·ta·tion** (krep″ĭ-ta′shən) 1. a sound like that made by throwing salt into a fire. See *crepitant rale,* under *rale.* 2. the noise made by rubbing together the ends of a fractured bone.

**crep·i·tus** (krep′ĭ-təs) [L.] 1. the discharge of flatus from the bowels. 2. crepitation. 3. crepitant rale.
**articular c.,** joint c.
**bony c.,** the crackling sound produced by the rubbing together of fragments of fractured bone.
**false c.,** joint c.
**c. in′dux,** a crepitant rale, or crackling sound, heard in pneumonia at the beginning of the process of solidification of the lung.
**joint c.,** the grating sensation caused by the rubbing together of the dry synovial surfaces of joints; called also *articular c.*
**c. re′dux,** crepitus heard in the resolving stage of pneumonia.
**silken c.,** a sensation as of two pieces of silk rubbed between the fingers, felt on moving a joint affected with hydrarthrosis.

**cre·pus·cu·lar** (kre-pus′ku-lər) [L. *crepusculum* twilight] 1. referring to twilight, as a twilight state. 2. becoming active at twilight, as animals such as bats.

**cres·cent** (kres′ənt) [L. *crescens*] 1. shaped like a new moon. 2. a crescent-shaped structure.
**articular c.,** a crescent-shaped articular fibrocartilage.
**epithelial c.,** a more or less crescentic mass of cells between the glomerular tuft and the inside of Bowman's capsule in glomerulonephritis.
**c's of Giannuzzi,** crescent-shaped patches of serous cells surrounding the mucous tubules in seromucous glands, and formed by the outnumbered albuminous cells pushed to the blind ends of the terminal portions or into saccular outpocketings. Called also *demilunes of Heidenhain; Giannuzzi's bodies, cells,* or *demilunes; crescent, demilune,* or *marginal cells;* and *semilunar bodies.*
**glomerular c.,** epithelial c.
**gray c.,** an area on some amphibian eggs from which pigment retreats; it is dorsal and opposite to the point of sperm entry, giving the first visible sign of the dorsoventral axis.
**malarial c's,** the gametocytes of *Plasmodium falciparum;* they may be male (microgametocytes) or female (macrogametocytes). Called also *flagellated bodies.*
**myopic c.,** a crescentic posterior staphyloma in the fundus of the eye in myopia.
**sublingual c.,** the crescent-shaped area on the floor of the mouth, formed by the lingual wall of the mandible and the adjacent part of the floor of the mouth.

**cres·cen·tic** (krə-sen′tik) resembling a crescent.

**cre·sol** (kre′sol) a liquid obtained from coal tar and containing not more than 5 per cent phenol, ranging from colorless to yellow, brown, or pink, toxic to humans and many other animals; it is a corrosive mixture of three isomeric forms and is a more powerful disinfectant and antiseptic than phenol. Its primary use is for sterilizing instruments, dishes, utensils, and other inanimate objects. Called also *cresylic acid* and *tricresol.*

**cre·sol·phtha·lein** (kre″sol-thal′ēn) an acid-base indicator that is colorless at pH 7.2 and red at 8.8.

**cre·sor·cin** (kre-sor′sin) a crystalline derivative from cresol.

**cre·sor·cin·ol** (kre-sor′sin-ol) cresorcin.

**crest** (krest) [L. *crista*] a projection or projecting structure, or ridge, especially one surmounting a bone or its border; see also *crista* and *ridge.*
**acoustic c.,** crista ampullaris.
**acusticofacial c.,** the embryonic cell mass from which develop the ganglia of the seventh and eighth cranial nerves.
**alveolar c.,** the margin of compact bone on the coronal edge of a dental alveolus.
**ampullar c., ampullary c.,** crista ampullaris.
**anterior c. of fibula,** margo anterior fibulae.
**anterior c. of tibia,** margo anterior tibiae.
**arcuate c. of arytenoid cartilage,** crista arcuata cartilaginis arytenoideae.
**basilar c. of cochlear duct,** crista basilaris ductus cochlearis.
**basilar c. of occipital bone,** tuberculum pharyngeum.
**buccinator c.,** crista buccinatoria.
**cerebral c's of cranial bone,** juga cerebralia ossium cranii; see under *jugum.*
**c. of cochlear window,** crista fenestrae cochleae.
**conchal c. of body of maxilla,** crista conchalis corporis maxillae.
**conchal c. of palatine bone,** crista conchalis ossis palatini.
**deltoid c.,** tuberositas deltoidea humeri.
**dental c.,** the maxillary ridge passing along the alveolar processes of the fetal maxillary bones.
**ethmoid c. of maxilla,** crista ethmoidalis maxillae.
**ethmoid c. of palatine bone,** crista ethmoidalis ossis palatini.
**femoral c.,** linea aspera.
**fimbriated c.,** plica fimbriata.
**frontal c.,** crista frontalis.
**frontal c., external,** linea temporalis ossis frontalis.
**frontal c., internal,** crista frontalis.
**gingival c.,** the coronal border of the gingiva.
**gluteal c.,** tuberositas glutea femoris.
**c. of greater tubercle of humerus,** crista tuberculi majoris.
**c. of hypotrochanteric fossa,** tuberositas glutea femoris.
**iliac c.,** crista iliaca.
**iliopectineal c. of iliac bone,** linea arcuata ossis ilii.
**iliopectineal c. of pelvis,** linea terminalis pelvis.
**iliopectineal c. of pubis,** eminentia iliopubica.
**c. of ilium,** crista iliaca.
**infratemporal c.,** crista infratemporalis.
**infundibuloventricular c.,** crista supraventricularis.
**inguinal c.,** a prominence on the inguinal body wall in the embryo, participating in the formation of the gubernaculum testis.
**interosseous c. of fibula,** margo interosseus fibulae.
**interosseous c. of radius,** margo interosseus radii.
**interosseous c. of tibia,** margo interosseus tibiae.
**interosseous c. of ulna,** margo interosseus ulnae.
**intertrochanteric c.,** crista intertrochanterica.
**intertrochanteric c., anterior,** linea intertrochanterica.
**lacrimal c., anterior,** crista lacrimalis anterior.
**lacrimal c., posterior,** crista lacrimalis posterior.
**c. of larger tubercle,** crista tuberculi majoris.
**lateral c. of fibula,** margo posterior fibulae.
**c. of lesser tubercle,** crista tuberculi minoris.
**c. of little head of rib,** crista capitis costae.
**malar c. of greater wing of sphenoid bone,** margo zygomaticus alae majoris.
**c. of matrix of nail,** crista matricis unguis.
**medial c. of fibula,** crista medialis fibulae.
**mental c., external,** protuberantia mentalis.
**mitochondrial c's,** complex infoldings in the mitochondrial cavity which originate in a membrane outside the cavity.
**nasal c. of maxilla,** crista nasalis maxillae.
**nasal c. of palatine bone,** crista nasalis ossis palatini.
**c. of neck of rib,** crista colli costae.
**neural c.,** a cellular band dorsolateral to the neural tube that gives origin to the cranial and spinal ganglia and many other structures.
**obturator c. (anterior),** crista obturatoria.
**occipital c., external,** crista occipitalis externa.
**occipital c., internal,** crista occipitalis interna.
**orbital c.,** margo supraorbitalis ossis frontalis.
**palatine c., c. of palatine bone,** crista palatina.
**pectineal c. of femur,** linea pectinea.
**pharyngeal c. of occipital bone,** tuberculum pharyngeum.
**pubic c., c. of pubis,** crista pubica.
**radial c.,** margo interosseus radii.
**rough c. of femur,** linea aspera.
**sacral c.,** crista sacralis mediana.
**sacral c., articular,** crista sacralis medialis.
**sacral c., external,** crista sacralis lateralis.
**sacral c., intermediate,** crista sacralis medialis.
**sacral c., lateral,** crista sacralis lateralis.
**sacral c., medial,** crista sacralis medialis.

**sacral c., median,** crista sacralis mediana.
**seminal c.,** colliculus seminalis.
**c. of smaller tubercle,** crista tuberculi minoris.
**sphenoidal c.,** crista sphenoidalis.
**spinal c. of Rauber,** processus spinosus vertebrae.
**c. of spinous processes of sacrum,** crista sacralis mediana.
**spiral c.,** labium limbi vestibulare.
**spiral c. of cochlea, spiral c. of cochlear duct,** crista basilaris ductus cochlearis.
**supinator c., c. of supinator muscle,** crista musculi supinatoris.
**supracondylar c. of humerus, lateral,** crista supraepicondylaris lateralis humeri.
**supracondylar c. of humerus, medial,** crista supraepicondylaris medialis humeri.
**supraepicondylar c. of humerus, lateral,** crista supraepicondylaris lateralis humeri.
**supraepicondylar c. of humerus, medial,** crista supraepicondylaris medialis humeri.
**supramastoid c.,** crista supramastoidea.
**supraventricular c.,** crista supraventricularis.
**temporal c. of frontal bone,** linea temporalis ossis frontalis.
**terminal c. of right atrium,** crista terminalis atrii dextri.
**tibial c.,** margo anterior tibiae.
**transverse c. of internal acoustic meatus,** crista transversa meati acustici interni.
**trigeminal c.,** the embryonic cell mass from which the trigeminal ganglion develops.
**turbinal c. of maxilla, inferior,** crista conchalis corporis maxillae.
**turbinal c. of maxilla, superior,** crista ethmoidalis maxillae.
**turbinal c. of palatine bone, inferior,** crista conchalis ossis palatini.
**turbinal c. of palatine bone, superior,** crista ethmoidalis ossis palatini.
**ulnar c.,** margo interosseus ulnae.
**urethral c., female,** crista urethralis (def. 1).
**urethral c., male,** crista urethralis (def. 2).
**c. of vestibule,** crista vestibuli.
**zygomatic c. of greater wing of sphenoid bone,** margo zygomaticus alae majoris.

**cres·to·my·cin sul·fate** (kres-to-mi'sin) paromomycin sulfate.

**cre·syl·ic ac·id** (kre-sil'ik) cresol.

**cre·tin** (kre'tin, kret'in) [Fr.] a person affected with cretinism.

**cre·tin·ism** (kre'tin-iz-əm) [MeSH: Cretinism] a chronic condition due to congenital severe hypothyroidism; manifestations begin in late infancy and include arrested physical development (dwarfism), mental retardation, dystrophy of the bones and soft parts, and lowered basal metabolism.
**athyreotic c., athyrotic c.,** that due to thyroid aplasia or destruction of the thyroid of the fetus *in utero;* called also *sporadic nongoitrous c.*
**endemic c.,** a form seen in regions of severe endemic goiter; the two primary types are *neurologic cretinism* and *myxedematous cretinism.*
**myxedematous c.,** an uncommon type of endemic cretinism with delayed growth of long bones, myxedema, and sometimes goiter but with fewer neurologic problems than are seen in neurologic cretinism.
**neurologic c.,** the usual kind of endemic cretinism, characterized by delayed growth of long bones, neurologic complications such as deaf mutism, mental retardation, and spasticity, sometimes with goiter, but usually without myxedema. Cf. *myxedematous c.*
**spontaneous c., sporadic c.,** cretinism in a person not descended from cretins, and who has not lived in a region where goiter is endemic.
**sporadic goitrous c.,** a genetically determined condition in which enlargement of the thyroid gland is associated with deficient biosynthesis of and a consequently reduced supply of circulating thyroid hormone.
**sporadic nongoitrous c.,** athyrotic c.

**cre·tin·is·tic** (kre″tin-is'tik) cretinous.

**cre·tin·oid** (kre'tin-oid) 1. resembling a cretin. 2. resembling cretinism.

**cre·tin·ous** (kre'tin-əs) affected with cretinism.

**Creutz·feldt-Ja·kob disease** (kroits'fəlt-yah'kōp) [Hans Gerhard *Creutzfeldt,* German psychiatrist, 1885–1964; Alfons Maria *Jakob,* German psychiatrist, 1884–1931] see under *disease.*

**crev·ice** (krev'is) [Fr. *crever* to split] a longitudinal fissure.
**gingival c.,** a shallow trough or fissure surrounding the anatomic crown of a tooth; considered by some authorities to be the same as the *gingival sulcus* and by others to be two separate and distinct entities. Called also *subgingival space.*

**cre·vic·u·lar** (krə-vik'u-lər) pertaining to a crevice, especially the gingival crevice.

**CRH** corticotropin-releasing hormone.

**crib** (krib) [MeSH: Infant Equipment] 1. any racklike structure. 2. a removable anchorage from an orthodontic appliance. 3. a habit-breaking orthodontic appliance.
**clinical c.,** a crib in which an infant is placed for observation.
**Jackson c.,** see under *appliance.*

**crib·bing** (krib'ing) a nervous habit of some horses consisting of grasping the manger or another object with the incisor teeth, arching the neck and making other peculiar head movements, and swallowing quantities of air; called also *crib-biting* and *windsucking.*

**crib-bit·ing** (krib'bīt-ing) cribbing.

**crib·ra** (krib'rə) [L.] plural of *cribrum.*

**crib·ral** (krib'rəl) pertaining to the cribrum, or sievelike structure.

**crib·rate** (krib'rāt) [L. *cribratus*] perforated, as a sieve.

**crib·ra·tion** (krib-ra'shən) 1. the quality of being cribrate. 2. the process or act of sifting or passing through a sieve, as a drug.

**crib·ri·form** (krib'rĭ-form) [*cribrum* + *form*] perforated with small apertures like a sieve.

**crib·rum** (krib'rəm) pl. *crib'ra* [L. "sieve"] lamina cribrosa ossis ethmoidalis.

**Cri·ce·tu·lus** (kri-se'tu-ləs) [MeSH: Cricetulus] a genus of rodents of the family Muridae, one of several genera of hamsters. *C. gri'seus* is the Chinese hamster.

**Cri·ce·tus** (kri-se'təs) a genus of rodents of the family Muridae, one of several genera of hamsters; *C. crice'tus* is the European hamster.

**Crich·ton-Browne's sign** (kri'tən-brounz) [Sir James *Crichton-Browne,* Scottish physician, 1840–1938] see under *sign.*

**Crick** (krik) Francis Harry Compton. British biologist, born 1916; co-winner, with Maurice Wilkins and James Dewey Watson, of the Nobel prize in medicine and physiology for 1962, for discoveries concerning the molecular structure of nucleic acids and its significance for information transfer in living material.

**cri·co·ar·y·te·noid** (kri″ko-ahr″ĭ-te'noid) pertaining to or extending between the cricoid and arytenoid cartilages.

**cri·coid** (kri'koid) [Gr. *krikos* ring + *-oid*] 1. resembling a ring; ring-shaped. 2. the cricoid cartilage (cartilago cricoidea [TA]).

**cri·coi·dec·to·my** (kri″koi-dek'tə-me) excision of the cricoid cartilage.

**cri·coi·dyn·ia** (kri″koi-din'e-ə) [Gr. *krikos* ring + *-odynia*] pain in the cricoid cartilage.

**cri·co·pha·ryn·ge·al** (kri″ko-fə-rin'je-əl) pertaining to the cricoid cartilage and the pharynx.

**cri·co·thy·roid** (kri-ko-thi'roid) pertaining to or connecting the cricoid and thyroid cartilages.

**cri·co·thy·roi·dot·o·my** (kri″ko-thi″roi-dot'ə-me) cricothyrotomy.

**cri·co·thy·rot·o·my** (kri″ko-thi-rot'ə-me) tracheotomy involving incision through the skin and cricothyroid membrane to secure a patent airway for emergency relief of upper airway obstruction. Called also *inferior laryngotomy, intercricothyrotomy,* and *thyrocricotomy.*

**cri·cot·o·my** (kri-kot'ə-me) [Gr. *krikos* ring + *-tomy*] incision of the cricoid cartilage.

**cri·co·tra·che·ot·o·my** (kri″ko-tra″ke-ot'ə-me) tracheotomy with incision of the cricoid cartilage.

**cri du chat** (kre doo shah') [Fr. "cat's cry"] see under *syndrome.*

**Crig·ler-Naj·jar syndrome** (krig'lər-nah'jahr) [John Fielding *Crigler,* Jr., American pediatrician, born 1919; Victor Assad *Najjar,* Lebanese-born American microbiologist, born 1914] [MeSH: Crigler-Najjar Syndrome] see under *syndrome.*

**crim·i·nol·o·gy** (krim″ĭ-nol'ə-je) [L. *crimen* crime + *-logy*] [MeSH: Criminology] the scientific study of crime and criminals.

**cri·nes** (kri'nēz) [L.] plural of *crinis.*

**cri·nis** (kri'nis) pl. *cri'nes* [L.] hair.

**crin·oph·a·gy** (krin-of'ə-je) [Gr. *krinein* to separate + *-phagy*] the intracytoplasmic digestion of the contents (peptides, proteins) of secretory vacuoles, after the vacuoles fuse with lysosomes.

**Cri·num** (kri'nəm) a genus of plants of the family Amaryllidaceae. *C. asia'ticum* is an Indian species whose root has properties like those of squill.

**cris·an·tas·pase** (kris″ən-tas'pās) BAN for asparaginase derived from *Erwinia carotovora (E. chrysanthemi).*

**cri·sis** (kri'sis) pl. *cri'ses* [L.; Gr. *krisis*] 1. the turning point of a disease for better or worse; especially, a sudden change, usually for the better, in the course of an acute disease. A disease terminates

by crisis when recovery is indicated by a sudden and definite decrease in the intensity of the symptoms. Cf. *lysis* (def. 4). 2. a sudden paroxysmal intensification of symptoms in the course of a disease.
**addisonian c., adrenal c.,** acute onset of adrenocortical insufficiency or sudden worsening of Addison's disease; manifestations include anorexia, vomiting, abdominal pain, apathy, confusion, extreme weakness, renal loss of sodium and water, and hypotension progressing to shock and, if untreated, death. Called also *acute adrenocortical insufficiency* and *Bernard-Sergent syndrome.*
**anaphylactoid c.,** see under *reaction.*
**aplastic c.,** the most common type of sickle cell crisis, a transient condition marked by sudden disappearance of erythroblasts from the bone marrow; it develops under various circumstances, including certain hemolytic states and infections.
**blast c.,** a sudden, severe transformation of chronic myelogenous leukemia to a more aggressive course; the proportion of blast cells increases rapidly, and the clinical picture resembles that in acute myelogenous leukemia.
**bronchial c.,** a paroxysm of dyspnea in the course of a case of tabes dorsalis.
**carcinoid c.,** an episodic attack of the carcinoid syndrome.
**cardiac c.,** a severe paroxysm of palpitation of the heart occurring in tabes dorsalis.
**catathymic c.,** an isolated, nonrepetitive act of violence that develops as a result of intolerable tension.
**celiac c.,** an attack of severe watery diarrhea and vomiting producing dehydration and acidosis, which sometimes occurs in the infantile form of nontropical sprue.
**cholinergic c.,** muscular weakness resulting from depolarization block due to overdosage of anticholinesterase agents used for myasthenia gravis; similar to but different from myasthenic crisis.
**clitoris c.,** an attack of sexual excitement occurring in women with tabes dorsalis.
**deglobulinization c.,** a condition observed in congenital spherocytic anemia, characterized clinically by the acute onset of fever, abdominal pain, and vomiting, associated with reticulocytopenia, leukopenia, thrombocytopenia, and erythroblastopenia.
**Dietl's c.,** sudden severe attack of nephralgia or gastric pain, chills, fever, nausea and vomiting, and general collapse; said to be due to partial turning of the kidney upon its pedicle.
**false c.,** pseudocrisis.
**febrile c.,** an attack of chilliness, fever, and sweating.
**gastric c.,** a paroxysm of intense abdominal pain in tabes dorsalis.
**genital c. of newborn,** a condition characterized by hyperplasia of the breasts, estrinization of the vaginal mucosa, and sometimes vaginal bleeding, under the influence of transplacentally acquired estrogens.
**glaucomatocyclitic c.,** a relatively uncommon, recurrent, unilateral form of secondary open-angle glaucoma, lasting one to two weeks, and rarely producing permanent damage to the optic disk or to the outflow facility. It is characterized by high intraocular pressure and marked depression of outflow facility, with minimal inflammatory signs and symptoms.
**hemolytic c.,** a rare type of sickle cell crisis in which there is acute red cell destruction leading to jaundice.
**hepatic c.,** an attack of intense pain in the region of the liver.
**hypertensive c.,** dangerously high blood pressure of acute onset.
**identity c.,** a period in the psychosocial development of an individual, generally occurring during adolescence, usually manifested by a loss of the sense of the sameness and historical continuity of one's self, confusion over values, or an inability to accept the role the individual perceives as being expected of him by society.
**intestinal c.,** gastric c.
**laryngeal c.,** paroxysmal spasm of the larynx in the earlier course of tabes dorsalis.
**megaloblastic c.,** megaloblastic anemia due to deficiency of folic acid, seen in some patients with hereditary spherocytosis after an aplastic crisis or during pregnancy.
**myasthenic c.,** the sudden development of dyspnea requiring respiratory support in myasthenia gravis; the crisis is usually transient, lasting several days, and accompanied by fever.
**nefast c.,** the peculiar onset of severe and unaccountable symptoms in experimental icterogenous spirochetosis.
**nephralgic c.,** a paroxysm of pain in the ureter in a case of tabes dorsalis.
**ocular c.,** a sudden attack of intense pain in the eyes, with lacrimation, photophobia, etc.
**oculogyric c.,** a crisis occurring in epidemic encephalitis, postencephalitic parkinsonism, or secondary to use of antipsychotic agents; the eyeballs become fixed in one position, typically upwardly rotated, for minutes or hours.
**parkinsonian c.,** a condition sometimes observed in parkinsonism, superficially resembling akinetic mutism or coma vigil, the patient lying stiff and motionless, and making no spontaneous communication.
**pharyngeal c.,** a sudden attack occurring in tabes dorsalis, marked by peculiar sensations in the pharynx and involuntary swallowing movements.
**rectal c.,** a severe seizure of rectal pain in tabes dorsalis.
**renal c.,** an attack of pain resembling renal colic, occurring in tabes.
**salt-depletion c., salt-losing c.,** see under *syndrome.*
**sickle cell c.,** a broad term used to describe several different acute conditions occurring with sickle cell disease, including aplastic crisis, hemolytic crisis, and vaso-occlusive crisis.
**tabetic c.,** a painful paroxysm with functional disturbance occurring in the course of tabes dorsalis.
**thoracic c.,** an attack of pain resembling angina pectoris, but with spasmodic contracture of the muscles of the chest and arms in tabes dorsalis.
**thyroid c., thyrotoxic c.,** a sudden and dangerous increase of the symptoms of thyrotoxicosis. Called also *thyroid* or *thyrotoxic storm.*
**vaso-occlusive c.,** a type of sickle cell crisis in which there is severe pain due to infarctions, which may be in the bones, joints, lungs, liver, spleen, kidney, eye, or central nervous system.
**vesical c.,** a severe seizure of pain in the bladder in cases of tabes dorsalis.
**visceral c.,** a paroxysm of shooting pain in any viscus occurring in a case of tabes dorsalis.

**cris·pa·tion** (kris-pa'shən) [L. *crispare* to curl] slight convulsive or spasmodic muscular contractions producing a creeping sensation.

**cris·ta** (kris'tə) gen. and pl. *cris'tae* [L.] [TA] a projection or projecting structure, or ridge, especially one surmounting a bone or its border; called also *crest* and *ridge.*

## Crista

Descriptions are given on TA terms, and include anglicized names of specific structures.

**c. acus'tica,** c. ampullaris.
**c. ampulla'ris** [TA], ampullary crest: the most prominent part of a localized thickening of the membrane that lines the ampullae of the semicircular ducts, covered with neuroepithelium containing endings of the vestibular nerve; called also *c. acustica* and *acoustic crest.*
**c. ante'rior fi'bulae,** margo anterior fibulae.
**c. ante'rior ti'biae,** margo anterior tibiae.
**c. arcua'ta cartila'ginis arytenoi'deae** [TA], arcuate crest of arytenoid cartilage: a ridge on the external surface of the arytenoid cartilage between the triangular pit and the oblong pit.
**c. basila'ris duc'tus cochlea'ris** [TA], basilar crest of cochlear duct: the triangular eminence on the spiral ligament of the cochlea, providing a site of attachment for the basilar membrane. Called also *c. spiralis ductus cochlearis* [TA alternative] and *c. spiralis cochleae.*
**c. buccinato'ria,** buccinator crest: a ridge running from the base of the coronoid process of the mandible to a point near the last molar tooth, giving attachment to the buccinator muscle.
**c. ca'pitis cos'tae** [TA], **c. capi'tuli cos'tae,** crest of head of rib: a horizontal crest dividing the articular surface of the head of the rib into two facets, for articulation with the depression on the bodies of two adjacent vertebrae; called also *crest of little head of rib, cuneiform eminence of head of rib,* and *interarticular ridge of head of rib.*
**c. col'li cos'tae** [TA], crest of neck of rib: a crest on the superior border of the neck of a rib, giving attachment to the anterior costotransverse ligament; called also *ridge of neck of rib.*
**c. concha'lis cor'poris maxil'lae** [TA], conchal crest of body of maxilla: an oblique ridge on the nasal surface of the body of the maxilla, just anterior to the lacrimal sulcus, which articulates with the inferior nasal concha; called also *inferior turbinal crest of maxilla.*
**c. concha'lis os'sis palati'ni** [TA], conchal crest of palatine bone: a sharp transverse ridge, near the posterior edge of the palatine bone, which articulates with the inferior concha; called also *inferior turbinal crest of palatine bone.*
**cris'tae cu'tis** [TA], dermal ridges: ridges of the skin produced by the projecting papillae of the corium on the palm or sole, producing a fingerprint or footprint that is characteristic of the individual.

**c. divi'dens,** limbus foraminis ovalis.
**c. ethmoida'lis maxil'lae** [TA], ethmoidal crest of maxilla: a low, oblique ridge on the medial surface of the frontal process of the maxilla, which articulates with the middle nasal concha; called also *superior turbinal crest of maxilla.*
**c. ethmoida'lis os'sis palati'ni** [TA], ethmoidal crest of palatine bone: a ridge near the upper end of the medial surface of the palatine bone, which articulates with the middle concha; called also *superior turbinal crest of palatine bone.*
**c. falcifor'mis,** c. transversa meati acustici interni.
**c. fe'moris,** linea aspera.
**c. fenes'trae coch'leae** [TA], crest of cochlear window: the ledge of bone that overhangs the cochlear (round) window of the middle ear.
**c. fronta'lis** [TA], frontal crest: a median ridge on the internal surface of the frontal bone, extending superiorly from the foramen cecum to unite with the sulcus for the superior sagittal sinus; called also *internal frontal crest.*
**c. gal'li** [TA], a thick triangular process projecting superiorly from the cribriform plate of the ethmoid bone; the falx cerebri attaches to it.
**c. he'licis,** crus helicis.
**c. ili'aca** [TA], **c. i'lii,** iliac crest: the thickened, expanded upper border of the ilium; called also *crest of ilium.*
**c. infratempora'lis** [TA], infratemporal crest: a crest separating the temporal surface of the greater wing of the sphenoid bone into a superior temporal portion and an inferior infratemporal portion.
**c. interos'sea fi'bulae,** margo interosseus fibulae.
**c. interos'sea ra'dii,** margo interosseus radii.
**c. interos'sea ti'biae,** margo interosseus tibiae.
**c. interos'sea ul'nae,** margo interosseus ulnae.
**c. intertrochante'rica** [TA], intertrochanteric crest: a prominent ridge running obliquely downward and medialward from the summit of the greater trochanter on the posterior surface of the neck of the femur to the lesser trochanter; called also *intertrochanteric ridge, linea intertrochanterica posterior,* and *posterior intertrochanteric line.*
**c. lacrima'lis ante'rior** [TA], anterior lacrimal crest: the lateral margin of the groove on the posterior border of the frontal process of the maxilla.
**c. lacrima'lis poste'rior** [TA], posterior lacrimal crest: a vertical ridge dividing the lateral or orbital surface of the lacrimal bone into two parts, and forming one margin of the fossa for the lacrimal sac.
**c. latera'lis fi'bulae,** margo posterior fibulae.
**c. margina'lis** [TA], marginal ridge: one of the elevated convex crests that form the mesial and distal borders of the occlusal surfaces of posterior teeth and of the lingual surfaces of anterior teeth.
**c. ma'tricis un'guis,** crest of matrix of nail: a vascular longitudinal ridge in the nail matrix.
**c. media'lis fi'bulae** [TA], medial crest of fibula: the long crest on the posterior surface of the body of the fibula, which separates the origin of the tibialis posterior muscle from that of the flexor hallucis longus muscle; called also *oblique line of fibula* and *posterointernal border of fibula.*
**mitochondrial cristae, cris'tae mitochondria'les,** numerous narrow, transverse infoldings of the inner membrane of a mitochondrion.
**c. mus'culi supinato'ris** [TA], crest of supinator muscle: a strong ridge forming the posterior margin of the supinator fossa below the radial notch of the ulna, and with it giving attachment to the supinator muscle; called also *supinator crest* or *ridge.*
**c. nasa'lis maxil'lae** [TA], nasal crest of maxilla: a ridge, raised along the medial border of the palatine process of the maxilla, with which the vomer articulates.
**c. nasa'lis os'sis palati'ni** [TA], nasal crest of palatine bone: a thick ridge projecting superiorly from the medial part of the horizontal plate of the palatine bone and articulating with the posterior part of the vomer.
**c. obturato'ria** [TA], obturator crest: the inferior border of the superior ramus of the os pubis, a strong ridge of bone beginning near the pubic tubercle and extending to the anterior part of the gap in the rim of the acetabulum, forming part of the circumference of the obturator foramen, and giving attachment to the obturator membrane.
**c. occipita'lis exter'na** [TA], external occipital crest: a variable crest of bone that sometimes extends from the external occipital protuberance toward the foramen magnum; called also *median* or *middle nuchal line.*
**c. occipita'lis inter'na** [TA], internal occipital crest: a median ridge on the internal surface of the occipital bone extending from the midpoint of the cruciform eminence toward the foramen magnum.
**c. palati'na os'sis palati'ni** [TA], palatine crest of palatine bone: a transverse crest often seen on the inferior surface of the horizontal plate of the palatine bone a short distance anterior to the posterior border.
**c. pu'bica** [TA], pubic crest: the thick, rough, anterior border of the body of the pubic bone.
**c. sacra'lis articula'ris,** c. sacralis medialis.
**c. sacra'lis interme'dia,** c. sacralis medialis.
**c. sacra'lis latera'lis** [TA], lateral sacral crest: either of two series of tubercles lateral to the dorsal sacral foramina, representing the transverse processes of the sacral vertebrae; called also *external sacral crest.*
**c. sacra'lis me'dia,** c. sacralis mediana.
**c. sacra'lis media'lis** [TA], medial sacral crest: either of two indefinite crests just medial to the dorsal sacral foramina, formed by fusion of the articular processes of the sacral vertebrae; called also *articular sacral crest.*
**c. sacra'lis media'na** [TA], median sacral crest: a median ridge on the dorsal surface of the sacrum, formed by the remnants of the spinous processes of the upper four sacral vertebrae; called also *sacral crest, crest of spinous processes of sacrum,* and *tubercular ridge of sacrum.*
**c. sphenoida'lis** [TA], sphenoidal crest: a median ridge on the anterior surface of the body of the sphenoid bone, articulating with the perpendicular plate of the ethmoid.
**c. spira'lis,** labium limbi vestibulare.
**c. spira'lis coch'leae,** c. basilaris ductus cochlearis.
**c. spira'lis duc'tus cochlea'ris,** TA alternative for c. basilaris ductus cochlearis.
**c. supracondyla'ris latera'lis hu'meri,** TA alternative for *c. supraepicondylaris lateralis humeri.*
**c. supracondyla'ris media'lis hu'meri,** TA alternative for *c. supraepicondylaris medialis humeri.*
**c. supraepicondyla'ris latera'lis hu'meri** [TA], lateral supraepicondylar crest of humerus: a prominent curved ridge on the lateral surface of the humerus, giving attachment in front to the brachioradialis and extensor carpi radialis longus muscles; called also *c. supracondylaris lateralis humeri* [TA alternative] and *lateral supracondylar crest* or *ridge of humerus.*
**c. supraepicondyla'ris media'lis hu'meri** [TA], medial supraepicondylar crest of humerus: a prominent, curved ridge on the medial surface of the humerus, giving attachment to the brachialis muscle in front and to the medial head of the triceps behind; called also *c. supracondylaris medialis humeri* [TA alternative] and *medial supracondylar crest* or *ridge of humerus.*
**c. supramastoi'dea** [TA], supramastoid crest: a ridge on the temporal bone that is a continuation of the superior border of the posterior root of the zygomatic process of the temporal bone.
**c. supraventricula'ris** [TA], supraventricular crest: a ridge on the inner surface of the right ventricle of the heart, marking off the conus arteriosus or outflow tract from the remainder of the right ventricle, the inflow tract. Called also *infundibuloventricular crest.*
**c. tempora'lis,** linea temporalis ossis frontalis.
**c. tempora'lis mandi'bulae** [TA], a ridge on the medial aspect of the coronoid process, extending from near the apex of the coronoid process to the level of the last molar, that gives attachment to the temporalis muscle.
**c. termina'lis a'trii dex'tri** [TA], terminal crest of right atrium: a ridge on the internal surface of the right atrium of the heart, located to the right of the orifices of the superior and inferior venae cavae, and separating the sinus venarum cavarum from the atrium proper and auricle. The pectinate muscles of the right atrium are attached at this crest. It corresponds to a groove on the external surface, the sulcus terminalis. Called also *taenia terminalis.*
**c. transver'sa mea'ti acus'tici inter'ni** [TA], transverse crest of internal acoustic meatus: a ridge of bone that divides the fundus of the internal acoustic meatus into a superior and an inferior fossa; called also *c. falciformis.*
**c. transversa'lis** [TA], transverse ridge: an elevated crest coursing transversely across the occlusal surface of a mandibular premolar to link the apices of the buccal and lingual cusps. It comprises the buccal and lingual cusps and may be an uninterrupted prominence or may be sharply divided at its approximate midpoint by a groove.
**c. triangula'ris** [TA], triangular ridge: a ridge that descends from the tips of the cusps of molars and premolars toward the central part of the occlusal surface; so named because the slopes of each side of the ridge resemble two sides of a triangle. See also *oblique ridge* (def. 1), under *ridge,* and *c. transversalis.*
**c. tuber'culi majo'ris** [TA], crest of greater tubercle (of the humerus): a projection on the greater tubercle of the humerus, forming one lip of the intertubercular groove; called also *crest of larger tubercle, pectoral ridge,* and *external, outer,* or *posterior bicipital ridge.*
**c. tuber'culi mino'ris** [TA], crest of lesser tubercle (of the humerus): a projection on the lesser tubercle of the humerus, forming one lip of the intertubercular groove; called also *crest of smaller tubercle,* and *anterior* or *internal bicipital ridge.*
**c. tympa'nica,** a ridge on the tympanic ring.
**c. ul'nae,** margo interosseus ulnae.
**c. urethra'lis** [TA], urethral crest: 1. in the female, a prominent

longitudinal fold of the mucosa along the posterior wall of the urethra; called also *c. urethralis muliebris* and *cervical colliculus of female urethra (of Barkow).* 2. in the male, a median elevation along the posterior wall of the urethra, lying between the prostatic sinuses; called also *c. urethralis virilis.*

**c. urethra'lis mulie'bris,** c. urethralis (def. 1).
**c. urethra'lis vi'rilis,** c. urethralis (def. 2).
**c. vesti'buli** [TA], crest of vestibule: a ridge between the spherical and elliptical recesses of the vestibule, dividing posteriorly to bound the cochlear recess.

**cris·tae** (kris'te) [L.] genitive and plural of *crista.*

**cris·tal** (kris'təl) pertaining to a crest or ridge.

**cris·to·ba·lite** (kris-to'bə-līt) a translucent crystalline form of silica used in casting investments because it has a high capacity for thermal expansion and is resistant to being broken down by heat.

**cri·te·ri·on** (kri-tēr'e-on) [Gr. *kritērion* a means for judging] a standard by which something may be judged.
**Ranson's criteria,** a set of eleven signs, five of which are measured at admission to the hospital, and six in the first 48 hours after admission, for the assessment of severity of acute pancreatitis. Three or more positive signs indicate that systemic complications are likely; four or more are associated with significantly increased mortality. See accompanying table.

**crith** (krith) [Gr. *krithē* barleycorn, the smallest weight] the unit of weight for gases, being the weight of a liter of hydrogen gas at 0°C and pressure equivalent to that of a column of mercury 760 mm high.

**Cri·thid·ia** (krĭ-thid'e-ə) [Gr. *krithē* barleycorn] [MeSH: Crithidia] a genus of parasitic protozoa (suborder Trypanosomatina, order Kinetoplastida) found in the digestive tract of arthropods and other invertebrates. The adult form is similar to the leptomonads, but the flagellum arises from the kinetoplast just in front of the nucleus, and is attached to the body by an undulating membrane. During their life cycle the organisms pass through choanomastigote (promastigote) and amastigote stages.

**cri·thid·ia** (krĭ-thid'e-ə) [MeSH: Crithidia] 1. any protozoan of the genus *Crithidia.* 2. see *epimastigote.*

**cri·thid·i·al** (krĭ-thid'e-əl) 1. pertaining to the genus *Crithidia.* 2. denoting a morphologic stage in the life cycle of certain trypanosomid protozoa of the genus *Crithidia;* see *epimastigote.*

**crit·i·cal** (krit'ĭ-kəl) 1. pertaining to or of the nature of a crisis. 2. pertaining to a disease or other morbid condition in which there is danger of death. 3. in sufficient quantity as to constitute a turning point, as a critical mass or critical concentration.

**Crix·i·van** (krik'sĭ-van) trademark for a preparation of indinavir sulfate.

**CRL** crown-rump length.

**CRM** cross-reacting material.

**CRNA** Certified Registered Nurse Anesthetist.

**cRNA** complementary RNA.

**cro·cein** (kro'sēn) any one of a series of bright red stains.

**cro·ci·dis·mus** (kro″sĭ-diz'məs) [Gr. *krokē* a tuft of wool] flocculation.

**cro·cid·o·lite** (krə-sid'ə-līt) a sodium ferrosoferric silicate in the amphibole group of asbestos, bluish in color, used industrially but now restricted because it causes asbestosis and certain forms of cancer such as mesotheliomas. Called also *blue asbestos.*

**Ranson's Criteria for Severity of Acute Pancreatitis**

*At Admission*

- Age > 55 years
- White cell count > $16.0 \times 10^9$/L
- Blood glucose > 11 mmol/L
- Serum lactate dehydrogenase (LDH) > 350 IU/L
- Aspartate transaminase (SGOT) > 250 U/L

*During Initial 48 Hours*

- Hematocrit decrease > 10 percentage points
- Blood urea nitrogen (BUN) increase > 1.8 mmol/L as urea
- $PaO_2$ < 60 mm Hg
- Base deficit > 4 mEq/L
- Serum calcium < 2.0 mmol/L
- Fluid sequestration > 6 L

**cro·fil·con A** (kro-fil'kon) a contact lens material (hydrophobic).

**Crohn's disease** (krōnz) [Burrill Bernard *Crohn,* American physician, 1884–1983] see under *disease.*

**cro·mo·gly·cate** (kro″mo-gli'kāt) a salt of cromoglycic acid; the disodium salt, cromolyn sodium, is used in the treatment of bronchial asthma.

**cro·mo·gly·cic ac·id** (kro″mo-gli'sik) [BAN] cromolyn.

**cro·mo·lyn** (kro'mə-lin) an inhibitor of the release of histamine and other mediators of immediate hypersensitivity from mast cells; used as *c. sodium* [USP] by inhalation for prophylaxis of bronchial asthma. Called also *cromoglycic acid* [BAN].
**c. sodium** [USP], the disodium salt of cromoglycic acid, which interferes with allergic histamine release; administered by inhalation in the prophylactic treatment of bronchial asthmas and rhinitis associated with allergy, and as an ophthalmic solution for prevention and treatment of allergic conjunctivitis.

**Cro·nin method** (kro'nin) [Thomas Dillon *Cronin,* American plastic surgeon, born 1906] see under *method.*

**Cron·khite-Can·a·da syndrome** (krong'kĭt-kan'ə-də) [Leonard Wolsey *Cronkhite,* Jr., American internist, born 1919; Wilma Jeanne *Canada,* American radiologist, 20th century] see under *syndrome.*

**Crooke's changes** (krooks) [Arthur Carleton *Crooke,* British pathologist, born 1905] see *Crooke's hyaline degeneration,* under *degeneration.*

**Crookes' space** (krooks) [Sir William *Crookes,* English physicist, 1832–1919] see under *space.*

**crop** (krop) 1. in birds, a dilatation of the esophagus at the base of the neck where food is temporarily stored and softened by the uptake of water before digestion begins; it then is passed through the proventriculus and into the gizzard. Called also *craw* and *ingluvies.* 2. a similar organ of certain insects, earthworms, and other invertebrates.

**Cross syndrome** (kros) [Harold Eugene *Cross,* American physician, born 1937] see under *syndrome.*

**cross** (kros) 1. any figure or structure in the shape of a cross. 2. any organism produced by crossbreeding; a method of crossbreeding.
**phage c.,** 1. a phage (bacteriophage) having genes from two or more parental phages as a result of infection by the parent phages of a single bacterial cell; it is a result of recombination. 2. the process of formation of a phage cross.
**Ranvier's c's,** dark, cross-shaped markings at the nodes of Ranvier, seen on longitudinal section after staining with silver nitrate.
**silver c's,** Ranvier's c's.
**two-factor c.,** recombination involving two genetic markers.
**yellow c.,** 2,2′-dichlorodiethyl sulfide.

**cross·bite** (kros'bīt) malocclusion in which the mandibular teeth are in buccal version (or in complete lingual version in posterior segments) to the maxillary teeth, bilaterally, unilaterally, or involving only a pair of opposing teeth, so that opposing occlusal surfaces are not in contact in habitual occlusion. Also written *cross bite* and *X-bite.*
**anterior c.,** that in which one or more primary or permanent maxillary incisors are lingual to the mandibular incisors.
**buccal c.,** that in which the maxillary molar is buccal to its mandibular antagonist.
**lingual c.,** crossbite in which the maxillary or mandibular molar is lingual to its antagonist.
**posterior c.,** that in which one or more primary or permanent posterior teeth are locked in an abnormal relation with the opposing teeth of the opposite arch; it may be buccal or lingual crossbite and may be accompanied by a shift of the mandible.
**scissors-bite c., telescoping c.,** that in which the mandibular arch is entirely lingual to the maxillary arch.

**cross·breed·ing** (kros′brēd-ing) hybridization; the mating of animals or plants of different strains or species.

**cross-bridges** (kros-brij′əz) in A bands of myofibrils, the intertwining of the thick and the thin filaments to form the dark striations.

**cross-dress·ing** (kros′dres-ing) the wearing of clothing specific to or characteristic of the opposite sex.

**crossed** (krost) shaped or arranged like a cross; decussating.

**cross-eye** (kros′i) esotropia.

**cross·foot** (kros′foot) talipes varus.

**cross·ing over** (kros′ing o′vər) the exchanging of genetic material between nonsister chromatids of the paired homologous chromosomes during the pachytene stage of the first meiotic division, resulting in new combinations of genes; called also *chiasmatypy.*

**cross-link·ing** (kros′link″ing) establishment of chemical links between chains of molecules of a polymer, resulting in a single network that has greater strength and less solubility. See also *cross-linked polymer,* under *polymer.*

**cross·match** (kros′mach) 1. a test of the compatibility of donor and recipient blood performed before transfusion: red cells of the donor are placed in serum of the recipient *(major crossmatch)* and red cells of the recipient in serum of the donor *(minor crossmatch)* and antiglobulin is added to increase reactivity; the presence of hemolysis or agglutination indicates incompatibility. 2. a test for the presence in the serum of a prospective transplant recipient of cytotoxic antibodies against donor tissue antigens: donor lymphocytes are placed in serum of the recipient; the presence of cytolysis indicates incompatibility and the likelihood of hyperacute graft rejection. Called also *pretransplant crossmatch* and *HLA crossmatch.* Also written *cross match* and *cross-match.*

**cross·match·ing** (kros-mach′ing) the performance of a crossmatch.

**cross·over** (kros′o-vər) 1. the result of the reciprocal exchange of genetic material between chromosomes; see *crossing over.* 2. see under *trial.*

**cross-re·ac·ti·va·tion** (kros″re-ak″tĭ-va′shən) the activation of an inactive virus particle by another active or inactive virus particle in the same cell.

**cross-re·ac·tiv·i·ty** (kros″re-ak-tiv′ĭ-te) the degree to which an antibody or antigen participates in cross reactions (see under *reaction*).

**cross-re·sis·tance** (kros-re-zis′təns) multidrug resistance; see under *resistance.*

**cross-sen·si·ti·za·tion** (kros-sen″sĭ-tĭ-za′shən) sensitization to a substance induced by exposure to another substance having cross-reacting antigens.

**cross·talk** (kros′tawk) in cardiology, inappropriate detection of the atrial stimulus by the ventricular sensing mechanism, usually seen with dual-chamber pacemakers.

**cross-tol·er·ance** (kros′tol-ər-əns) extension of the tolerance for a substance to others of the same class, even those to which the body has not been exposed previously.

**cross·way** (kros′wa) the path by which something crosses; decussation.

**Cro·ta·la·ria** (kro″tə-lar′e-ə) [L. *crotalum* rattle or castanet] a large genus of leguminous herbs, most species of which grow in warm to tropical climates; many species contain pyrrolizidine alkaloids such as monocrotaline, which can cause crotalism in animals that consume them.

**crot·a·lid** (krot′ə-lid) [MeSH: Viperidae] 1. any snake of the family Crotalidae; a pit viper. 2. of or pertaining to the family Crotalidae.

**Cro·tal·i·dae** (kro-tal′ĭ-de) a family of venomous snakes, the pit vipers, characterized by front, movable, hollow fangs and a depression or pit between the nostril and the eye. Sometimes it is considered a subfamily of Viperidae and called Crotalinae. It includes the genera *Agkistrodon, Bothrops, Calloselasma, Crotalus, Lachesis, Sistrurus,* and *Trimeresurus.* See table at *snake.*

**Cro·tal·i·nae** (kro-tal′ĭ-ne) name given to the snake family Crotalidae when it is considered a subfamily under Viperidae.

**cro·ta·line** (kro′tə-lēn) crotalid.

**cro·tal·ism** (kro′təl-iz-əm) congestion and hemorrhage of the liver and spleen with emaciation, weakness, and stupor, seen in animals that consume plants of the genus *Crotalaria,* owing to poisonous pyrrolizidine alkaloids such as monocrotaline in the plants. Called also *bottom disease, Kimberley horse disease,* and *walkabout disease.*

**cro·ta·lo·tox·in** (kro″tə-lo-tok′sin) a poisonous substance from rattlesnake venom.

**Crot·a·lus** (krot′ə-ləs) [L. from Gr. *krotalon* rattle] [MeSH: Crotalus] a genus of venomous rattlesnakes of the family Crotalidae; numerous species are found in North America. *C. adaman′teus* is the eastern diamondback rattlesnake; *C. atrox′* is the western diamondback rattlesnake; *C. ceras′tes* is the sidewinder; *C. duris′sus terri′ficus* is the cascabel of Central and South America; *C. hor′ridus* is the timber rattlesnake; and *C. scutula′tus scutula′tus* is the Mojave rattlesnake. *C. vi′ridis* has many subspecies in the western and southwestern United States, such as *C. vi′ridis vi′ridis,* the prairie rattlesnake. See table at *snake.*

**cro·ta·mine** (kro′tə-mēn) a toxic protein occurring in the venom of some *Crotalus* species.

**cro·ta·mi·ton** (kro″tə-mi′ton) [USP] a scabicide, occurring as a light yellow, oily liquid; applied topically to the skin.

**cro·taph·i·on** (kro-taf′e-on) [Gr. *krotaphos* the temple] a craniometric point at the tip of the great wing of the sphenoid.

**cro·tin** (kro′tin) a phytotoxin derived from the seeds of *Croton tiglium,* which causes crotonism.

**Cro·ton** (kro′tən) [L.; Gr. *krotōn* tick] a genus of shrubs of the family Euphorbiaceae, some of which are popular as ornamentals. Certain species are used medically in Mexico and South America, and others, such as *C. texen′sis* and *C. capita′tus,* are poisonous to humans and livestock. *C. tig′lium* L., an Asian species, yields poisonous croton oil.

**cro·ton·ic ac·id** (kro-ton′ik) an unsaturated fatty acid, $CH_3CH{=}CHCOOH$, found in croton oil.

**cro·ton·ism** (kro′tən-iz-əm) poisoning of humans or other animals by croton oil, characterized by burning of the mouth and sometimes emesis with severe diarrhea and colic; it may be accompanied by headache, somnolence, vertigo, prostration, and collapse, with death from circulatory or respiratory failure.

**cro·tox·in** (kro-tok′sin) [MeSH: Crotoxin] a crystalline neurotoxic principle from the venom of the rattlesnake, *Crotalus terrificus.*

**croup** (kro͞op) [MeSH: Croup] a condition resulting from acute partial obstruction of the upper airway, seen mainly in infants and children; characteristics include resonant barking cough, hoarseness, and persistent stridor. It may be caused by a viral infection (usually a parainfluenzavirus), a bacterial infection (usually *Staphylococcus aureus, Streptococcus pneumoniae,* or *Streptococcus pyogenes*), an allergy, a foreign body, or new growth.
**bacterial c.,** see under *tracheitis.*
**false c.,** laryngismus stridulus.
**membranous c., pseudomembranous c.,** bacterial tracheitis.
**spasmodic c.,** laryngismus stridulus.

**croup·ous** (kroo′pəs) pertaining to or similar to croup.

**croupy** (kro͞op′e) affected with or resembling croup.

**Crou·zon's disease** (kroo-zonz′) [Octave *Crouzon,* French neurologist, 1874–1938] craniofacial dysostosis.

**Crow-Fu·ka·se syndrome** (kro-foo-kah′se) [R.S. *Crow,* British physician, 20th century; Masaichi *Fukase,* Japanese physician, 20th century] POEMS syndrome; see under *syndrome.*

**crowd·ing** (kroud′ing) [MeSH: Crowding] the condition in which the teeth are crowded and assume such altered positions as overlapping, displacement in various directions, torsiversion, etc.

**Crowe's sign** (krōz) [Frank W. *Crowe,* American physician, 20th century] see under *sign.*

**crown** (kroun) [L. *corona*] [MeSH: Crowns] 1. the topmost part of an organ or other structure, such as the top of the head, or the upper part of a tooth (corona dentis [TA]); see *anatomical c.* and *physiological c.* 2. artificial c.
**anatomical c.,** corona dentis.
**artificial c.,** a restoration made of metal alone, metal with a veneer of porcelain or resin, or porcelain or resin alone that reproduces the entire surface anatomy of the clinical crown of a tooth; it may be attached to a prepared tooth stump, to one partially rebuilt by a cast metal core alone, or to a cast core and a post, or it may be cemented to the remaining tooth structure. Colloquially called *cap.*

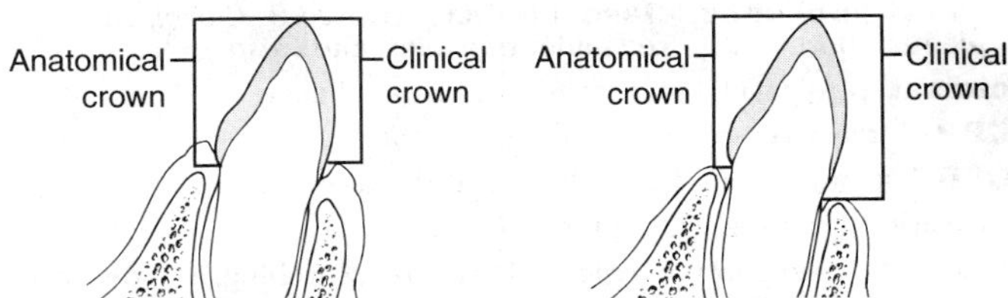

Anatomical and clinical crowns, demonstrating that the former are independent of the state of surrounding tissues while the latter depend on the height of the surrounding gingiva.

**basket c.,** an artificial gold crown fitted over a natural tooth with minimal removal of tissue, so called because added retention is provided by a thin band of labial metal similar in shape to a basket handle.
**bell c.,** a tooth crown whose circumference at the occlusal surface is larger than usual in relation to the size of the circumference at the crown cervix.
**Bonwill c.,** an artificial porcelain crown held to the tooth root by means of a threaded metal dowel extending through a hole in the porcelain, and upon which a nut is screwed.
**cap c.,** shell c.
**celluloid c.,** a temporary crown made of celluloid that facilitates the fabrication of a temporary crown during fixed prosthodontic procedures.
**ciliary c.,** corona ciliaris.
**clinical c.,** corona clinica.
**collar c.,** an artificial crown attached by a metal ferrule to a natural tooth root.
**complete c.,** full c.
**dental c.,** corona dentis.
**dowel c.,** an artificial crown that replaces the entire coronal portion of a tooth and is retained by a dowel extending into a filled root canal.
**extra-alveolar c.,** corona clinica.
**full c., full veneer c.,** a dental restoration that completely reproduces the clinical crown of a natural tooth. Called also *complete c.* and *full veneer c.*.
**half-cap c.,** open-face c.
**jacket c.,** a porcelain or acrylic resin restoration of the clinical crown of a tooth that usually terminates under the gingiva.
**open-face c.,** a gold crown that covers the labial or buccal cervical region in addition to the lingual, proximal, and occlusal surfaces, or the incisal edge of anterior teeth, the buccal or labial surface of the natural crown being left exposed through the opening. Called also *half-cap c.*
**overlay c.,** a cast metal artificial crown fitted over a prepared natural crown to support the walls around an inlay that are not strong or thick enough to withstand occlusal stresses, while leaving exposed the labial surface of the natural crown for esthetic purposes.
**physiological c.,** the portion of a tooth that is exposed beyond the gingival crevice or the margin of the gum. It may involve all of the part of a tooth covered by enamel (dental c.; see *corona dentis* [TA]) or a portion of it (clinical crown; see *corona clinica* [TA]), and it may also involve a portion of the part not covered by enamel (anatomical root).
**pinledge c.,** an artificial crown retained by means of pins that fit into prepared pinledges in a tooth.
**Richmond c.,** an artificial crown consisting of a metal base or cap, which fits the prepared face or a stump of a natural root and carries a post or pivot for insertion into the root canal, and a porcelain facing reinforced with metal backing.
**shell c.,** an artificial crown applied like a shell or cap over the remaining natural crown of a tooth; the space between the crown and the shell is filled with cement. Called also *cap c.*
**tapered c.,** an artificial crown seated over a tapered abutment so that it may be fitted in place and removed without obstruction.
**three-quarter c.,** an artificial crown covering mainly three surfaces of anterior teeth (mesial, distal, and lingual) and four surfaces of posterior teeth (mesial, distal, lingual, and occlusal); used as a retainer for a bridge or as a single-unit restoration on a carious fractured tooth. Called also *partial veneer c.*
**veneer c., complete,** a restoration of metal, porcelain, or acrylic resin that reproduces the entire surface anatomic form of the clinical crown and fits over a prepared tooth or root.
**veneer c., full,** full c.
**veneer c., partial,** three-quarter c.
**veneered c.,** an artificial crown that bears a thin layer of resin or porcelain on the buccal or labial surface, attached to or bonded to the metal casting; called also *window c.*
**window c.,** veneered c.

**crown·ing** (krown'ing) that phase in the second stage of labor when a large segment of the fetal scalp is visible at the vaginal orifice, the perineum being distended.

**Cro·zat appliance, clasp** (kro'zat) [George B. *Crozat,* American dentist, born 1876] see under *appliance* and *clasp.*

**cro·zat** (kro'zat) [G. B. *Crozat*] Crozat appliance.

**CRP** C-reactive protein; see under *protein.*

**CRRT** continuous renal replacement therapy.

**cru·ces** (kroo'sēz) [L.] plural of *crux.*

**cru·cial** (kroo'shəl) [L. *crucialis*] severe, searching, and decisive.

**cru·ci·ate** (kroo'she-āt) shaped like a cross.

**cru·ci·ble** (kroo'sĭ-bəl) [L. *crucibulum*] a vessel for melting refractory substances.

**cru·ci·form** (kroo'sĭ-form) [*crux* + *form*] shaped like a cross.

**crude** (kro͞od) [L. *crudus* raw] raw or unrefined.

**cru·fo·mate** (kroo'fo-māt) a veterinary anthelmintic.

**cru·or** (kroo'or) pl. *cruo'res* [L.] blood clot.

**cru·ra** (kroo'rə) [L.] plural of *crus.*

**cru·ral** (kro͞or'əl) pertaining to the leg or to a leglike structure (crus).

**cru·re·us** (kroo-re'əs) musculus vastus intermedius.

**cru·ris** (kroo'ris) genitive of *crus.*

**cru·rot·o·my** (kroo-rot'ə-me) surgical cutting of a crus of the stapes, usually the anterior crus.

**crus** (krus) gen. *cru'ris,* pl. *cru'ra* [L.] [TA] 1. the leg, from knee to foot. 2. a general term used to designate a leglike part.
**c. I,** lobulus semilunaris superior.
**c. II,** lobulus semilunaris inferior.
**ampullary membranous crura of semicircular duct,** crura membranacea ampullaria ductus semicircularis.
**ampullary osseous crura,** crura ossea ampullaria.
**anterior c. of anterior inguinal ring,** c. mediale annuli inguinalis superficialis.
**anterior c. of internal capsule,** c. anterius capsulae internae.
**anterior c. of stapes,** c. anterius stapedis.
**c. ante'rius cap'sulae inter'nae** [TA], anterior limb of internal capsule: the part of the internal capsule of the brain that separates the caudate and the lentiform nuclei; it contains the anterior thalamic radiations and the frontopalatine tract.
**c. ante'rius stape'dis** [TA], anterior crus of stapes: the anterior of the two bony limbs that connect the footplate and capitulum of the stapes; called also *anterior limb of stapes.*
**cru'ra anthe'licis** [TA], crura of anthelix: the two ridges on the external ear marking the superior termination of the anthelix and bounding the triangular fossa; called also *limbs of anthelix.*
**c. bre've incu'dis** [TA], short crus of incus: the backward-projecting process on the incus that is connected to the posterior wall of the tympanic cavity by the posterior incudal ligament; called also *short limb* or *process of incus.*
**c. ce'rebri,** 1. [TA] the part anterior to the substantia nigra, consisting of a large bundle of nerve fiber tracts called the *basis pedunculi cerebri.* Called also *pars anterior pedunculi cerebri* and *anterior part of cerebral peduncle.* 2. basis pedunculi cerebri.
**c. clito'ridis** [TA], crus of clitoris: the continuation of each corpus cavernosum clitoridis, diverging posteriorly to be attached to the ischiopubic rami.
**common membranous c. of semicircular duct,** c. membranaceum commune ductus semicircularis.
**common osseous c.,** c. osseum commune.
**c. commu'ne cana'lis semici'rcula'ris,** c. osseum commune.
**c. dex'trum diaphrag'matis** [TA], right crus of diaphragm; a fibromuscular band arising from the superior three or four lumbar vertebrae, and ascending along with the left crus, to insert into the central tendon of the diaphragm.
**c. dex'trum fascic'uli atrioventricula'ris** [TA], right crus of atrioventricular bundle: a discrete group of fascicles arising from the trunk of the bundle at the superior end of the muscular part of the interventricular septum; it descends to be distributed to the right ventricle of the heart as a terminal network of Purkinje fibers that become continuous with the ventricular cardiac muscle fibers. Called also *right bundle branch* and *right branch of atrioventricular bundle.*
**crura of diaphragm,** see *c. dextrum diaphragmatis* and *c. sinistrum diaphragmatis.*

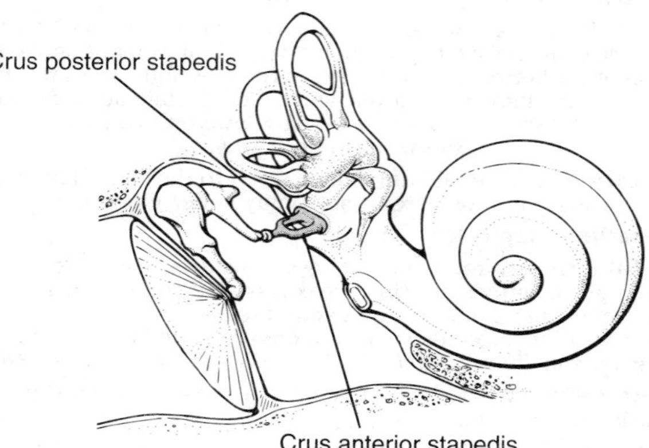

**c. of diaphragm, left,** c. sinistrum diaphragmatis.
**c. of diaphragm, right,** c. dextrum diaphragmatis.
**cru'ra diaphrag'matis,** see *c. dextrum diaphragmatis* and *c. sinistrum diaphragmatis.*
**external c. of anterior inguinal ring,** c. laterale anuli inguinalis superficialis.
**c. for'nicis** [TA], crus of fornix: either of the two flattened bands of white substance of the brain that are in close contact with the splenium and that unite under the posterior part of the body of the corpus callosum to form the body of the fornix.
**c. glan'dis clito'ridis,** frenulum clitoridis.
**c. he'licis** [TA], crus of helix: the anterior termination of the helix of the external ear located above the entrance to the external acoustic meatus; called also *crista helicis.*
**crura of incus,** see *c. breve incudis* and *c. longum incudis.*
**c. infe'rius an'nuli inguina'lis subcuta'nei,** c. laterale anuli inguinalis superficialis.
**c. infe'rius mar'ginis falcifor'mis,** TA alternative for *cornu inferius marginis falciformis.*
**internal c. of anterior inguinal ring,** c. mediale anuli inguinalis superficialis.
**internal c. of greater alar cartilage,** c. mediale cartilaginis alaris majoris.
**lateral c. of greater alar cartilage,** c. laterale cartilaginis alaris majoris.
**lateral c. of superficial inguinal ring,** c. laterale anuli inguinalis superficialis.
**c. latera'le a'nuli inguina'lis superficia'lis** [TA], lateral crus of superficial inguinal ring: the part of the superficial inguinal ring that blends with the inguinal ligament as it goes to the pubic tubercle; called also *c. inferius annuli inguinalis subcutanei,* and *external* or *posterior c. of anterior inguinal ring.*
**c. latera'le cartila'ginis ala'ris majo'ris** [TA], lateral crus of greater alar cartilage: the part of the greater alar cartilage that curves laterally around the naris and helps maintain its contour.
**left c. of atrioventricular bundle,** c. sinistrum fasciculi atrioventricularis.
**long c. of incus,** c. longum incudis.
**c. lon'gum incu'dis** [TA], long crus of incus: a process on the incus directed downward and inward, parallel with the manubrium of the malleus; called also *long limb* or *process of incus.*
**medial c. of external inguinal ring,** ligamentum inguinale reflexum.
**medial c. of greater alar cartilage,** c. mediale cartilaginis alaris majoris.
**medial c. of superficial inguinal ring,** c. mediale anuli inguinalis superficialis.
**c. media'le a'nuli inguina'lis superficia'lis** [TA], medial crus of superficial inguinal ring: the part of the superficial inguinal ring that is attached to the symphysis and that blends with the fundiform ligament of the penis; called also *superior colliculus of subcutaneous inguinal ring, c. superius annuli inguinalis subcutanei, anterior* or *internal callus of anterior inguinal ring,* and *anterior* or *internal inguinal ligament.*
**c. media'le cartila'ginis ala'ris majo'ris** [TA], medial crus of greater alar cartilage: the part of the greater alar cartilage, loosely attached to its fellow of the opposite side, and helping to form the mobile septum of the nose; called also *internal c. of greater alar cartilage.*
**cru'ra membrana'cea,** membranous crura: the two ends of each semicircular duct of the ear, both opening into the utricle. See *crura membranacea ampullaria ductus semicircularis, c. membranaceum commune ductus semicircularis,* and *c. membranaceum simplex ductus semicircularis.*
**cru'ra membrana'cea ampulla'ria duc'tus semicircula'ris** [TA], ampullary membranous crura of semicircular duct: the ends of the semicircular ducts of the ear, in which the membranous ampullae are situated.
**c. membrana'ceum commu'ne duc'tus semicircula'ris** [TA], common membranous crus of semicircular duct: an area consisting of the joined nonampullary ends of the anterior and posterior semicircular duct of the ear.
**c. membrana'ceum sim'plex duc'tus semicircula'ris** [TA], simple membranous crus of semicircular duct: the nonampullary end of the lateral semicircular duct of the ear, opening into the utricle.
**membranous crura,** crura membranacea.
**cru'ra os'sea,** osseous crura: those parts of the bony semicircular canals of the ear that lodge the correspondingly named parts of the membranous crura of the semicircular ducts; see *crura ossea ampullaria, c. osseum commune,* and *c. osseum simplex.*
**cru'ra os'sea ampulla'ria** [TA], ampullary osseous crura: the parts of the bony semicircular canals of the ear that lodge the crura membranacea ampullaria ductus semicircularis.
**c. os'seum commu'ne** [TA], common osseous crus: the part of a bony semicircular canal of the ear that lodges the crus membranaceum commune ductus semicircularis; called also *c. commune canalis semicircularis.*
**c. os'seum sim'plex** [TA], simple osseous crus: that part of a bony semicircular canal of the ear that lodges the crus membranaceum simplex ductus semicircularis; called also *c. simplex canalis semicircularis.*
**c. pe'nis** [TA], crus of penis: the continuation of each corpus cavernosum penis, diverging posteriorly to be attached to the pubic arch.
**posterior c. of anterior inguinal ring,** c. laterale anuli inguinalis superficialis.
**posterior c. of internal capsule,** c. posterius capsulae internae.
**posterior c. of stapes,** c. posterius stapedis.
**c. poste'rius cap'sulae inter'nae** [TA], posterior limb of internal capsule: the part of the internal capsule of the brain that separates the thalamus from the lentiform nucleus; its main known function is the conveyance of corticofugal efferent motor fibers from the cerebral cortex, but it also carries other fiber projections. It consists of thalamolenticular, sublentiform, and retrolentiform parts.
**c. poste'rius stape'dis** [TA], posterior crus of stapes: the posterior of the two bony limbs that connect the footplate and capitulum of the stapes; called also *posterior limb of stapes.*
**c. pri'mum lo'buli ansifor'mis,** TA alternative for *lobulus semilunaris superior.*
**right c. of atrioventricular bundle,** c. dextrum fasciculi atrioventricularis.
**c. secun'dum lo'buli ansifor'mis,** TA alternative for *lobulus semilunaris inferior.*
**short c. of incus,** c. breve incudis.
**simple membranous c. of semicircular duct,** c. membranaceum simplex ductus semicircularis.
**simple osseous c.,** c. osseum simplex.
**c. sim'plex cana'lis semicircula'ris,** c. osseum simplex.
**c. sinis'trum diaphrag'matis** [TA], left crus of diaphragm: a fibromuscular band arising from the superior two or three lumbar vertebrae, and ascending along with the right crus, to insert into the central tendon of the diaphragm.
**c. sinis'trum fasci'culi atrioventricula'ris** [TA], left crus of atrioventricular bundle: a dispersed array of fascicles arising from the trunk of the bundle at the superior end of the muscular part of the interventricular septum; they continue as a flattened sheet, generally diverging into anterior and posterior limbs, and descend to be distributed to the papillary muscles of the left ventricle of the heart as a terminal network of Purkinje fibers that become continuous with the ventricular cardiac muscle fibers. Called also *left bundle branch* and *left branch of atrioventricular bundle.*
**crura of stapes,** see *c. anterius stapedis* and *c. posterius stapedis.*
**superior c. of cerebellum,** pedunculus cerebellaris rostralis.
**superior c. of subcutaneous inguinal ring,** c. mediale annuli inguinalis superficialis.
**c. supe'rius an'nuli inguina'lis subcuta'nei,** c. mediale anuli inguinalis superficialis.
**c. supe'rius mar'ginis falcifor'mis,** TA alternative for *cornu superius marginis falciformis.*

**crust** (krust) [L. *crusta*] 1. a formed outer layer, especially an outer layer of solid matter formed by the drying of a bodily exudate or secretion. 2. scab (def. 1).
**milk c.,** crusta lactea.

**crus·ta** (krus'tah) gen. and pl. *crus'tae* [L.] a crust.
**c. lac'tea,** seborrhea of the scalp of nursing infants; called also *cradle cap* and *milk crust.*

**Crus·ta·cea** (krəs-ta'she-ə) [L. from *crusta* shell] [MeSH: Crustacea] a large class of arthropods including the lobsters, crabs, shrimps, wood lice, water fleas, and barnacles.

**crus·ta·ceo·ru·bin** (krəs-ta″she-o-roo'bin) a brown-black pigment (chromoprotein) found in lobster shells and eggs and in certain crabs; called also *zoonerythrin, tetraerythrin,* and *vitellorubin.*

**crus·tae** (krus'te) [L.] genitive and plural of *crusta.*

**crus·to·sus** (krəs-to'səs) [L.] crusted; said of certain lesions of the skin.

**crutch** (kruch) 1. a device of wood or metal, ordinarily long enough to reach from the armpit to the ground, with a concave surface fitting under the arm and a cross bar for the hand, used for supporting the weight of the body. 2. the perineal region, especially of a nonhuman animal.
**axillary c.,** any of several types of crutches that have a long, rigid vertical structure, a short padded horizontal bar that fits under the axilla, and another short bar at waist level that is used as a hand grip.
**Canadian c.,** triceps c.
**forearm c.,** a crutch whose top is at the level of the forearm, with a hand bar as well as a cuff that goes around the forearm to increase stability.
**Lofstrand c.,** the most common kind of forearm crutch, consisting of an aluminum tube that bends slightly posteriorly just above the hand grip.
**triceps c.,** a crutch consisting of two uprights extending halfway between the elbow and shoulder, with a cross piece for the hand

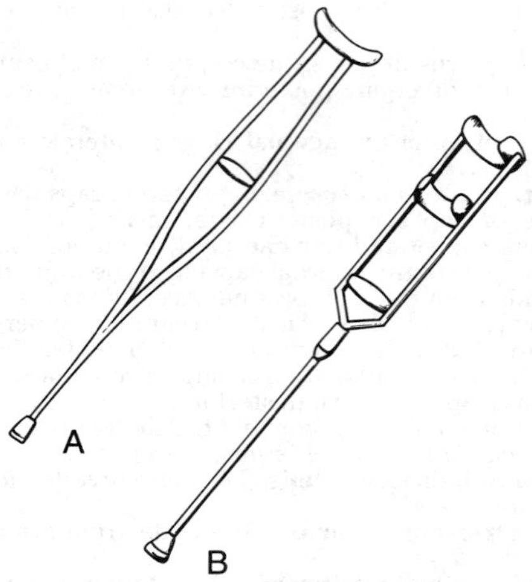

*(A)* Axillary crutch; *(B)* triceps crutch.

and a curved upper arm part against which the subject leans the upper arm.

**Cru·veil·hier's atrophy,** etc. (kroo-vāl-yāz') [Jean *Cruveilhier,* French pathologist, 1791–1874] see *spinal muscular atrophy* under *atrophy;* see *articulatio atlanto-occipitalis, fascia perinei superficialis, ligamenta palmaria articulationum interphalangealium manus,* and *ligamenta palmaria articulationum metacarpophalangealium;* and see under *disease.*

**Cru·veil·hier-Baum·gar·ten syndrome (cirrhosis)** (kroo-vāl-ya'boum'gahr-tən) [J. *Cruveilhier;* Paul Clemens von *Baumgarten,* German pathologist, 1848–1928] see under *syndrome.*

**crux** (kruks) pl. *cru'ces* [L.] cross.
**c. of heart,** the intersection of the walls separating the right and left sides and the atrial and ventricular chambers of the heart.
**cru'ces pilo'rum** [TA], crosslike figures formed by the pattern of hair growth, the hairs lying in opposite directions.

**cry** (kri) 1. a sudden loud, involuntary vocal sound. 2. to utter such a sound. 3. weep, def. 1.
**arthritic c., articular c.,** night c.
**cephalic c.,** a shrill, high-pitched penetrating cry of the newborn suggesting intracranial damage of some severity.
**epileptic c.,** a loud scream that often occurs at the onset of an epileptic attack.
**joint c.,** night c.
**night c.,** a shrill cry uttered by a child in sleep, often heard in beginning joint disease; called also *arthritic, articular,* or *joint c.*

**cry·al·ge·sia** (kri"əl-je'ze-ə) [*cryo-* + *algesia*] pain due to the application of cold; cf. *psychroalgia.*

**cry·an·es·the·sia** (kri-an"əs-the'zhə) [*cryo-* + *anesthesia*] loss of the power of perceiving cold; see *temperature sense,* under *sense.*

**Cry·er's elevator** (kri'ərz) [Matthew Henry *Cryer,* American surgeon, 1840–1921] see under *elevator.*

**cry·es·the·sia** (kri"əs-the'zhə) [*cryo-* + *esthesia*] abnormal sensitiveness to cold; cf. *crymodynia* and *psychroalgia.*

**crym(o)-** [Gr. *krymos* frost] a combining form denoting relationship to cold.

**cry·mo·dyn·ia** (kri"mo-din'e-ə) [*crymo-* + *-odynia*] rheumatic pain coming on in cold or damp weather. Cf. *cryesthesia* and *psychroalgia.*

**cry·mo·phil·ic** (kri"mo-fil'ik) psychrophilic.

**cry·mo·phy·lac·tic** (kri"mo-fə-lak'tik) cryophylactic.

**cry·mo·ther·a·py** (kri"mo-ther'ə-pe) cryotherapy.

**cry(o)-** [Gr. *kryos* cold] a combining form denoting relationship to cold.

**cryo·ab·la·tion** (kri"o-ab-la'shən) [*cryo-* + *ablation*] the removal of tissue by destroying it with extreme cold.

**cryo·an·al·ge·sia** (kri"o-an"əl-je'ze-ə) the relief of pain by application of cold by cryoprobe to peripheral nerves.

**cryo·an·es·the·sia** (kri"o-an"əs-the'zhə) [*cryo-* + *anesthesia*] local anesthesia produced by chilling the part to near freezing temperature; called also *frost* or *refrigeration anesthesia.*

**cryo·bank** (kri'o-bank") a facility for freezing and preserving substances at low temperatures, usually by immersion in liquid nitrogen at −196.5°C.

**cryo·bi·ol·o·gy** (kri"o-bi-ol'ə-je) [*cryo-* + *biology*] the science dealing with the effect of low temperatures on biological systems.

**cryo·car·dio·ple·gia** (kri"o-kahr"de-o-ple'jə) [*cryo-* + *cardioplegia*] cessation of contraction of the myocardium produced by cooling the heart during cardiac surgery.

**cryo·cau·tery** (kri"o-kaw'tər-e) [*cryo-* + *cautery*] cauterization by means of the application of a substance, such as liquid nitrogen or carbon dioxide snow, or an instrument that destroys tissue by freezing; called also *cold cautery.*

**cryo·crit** (kri'o-krit) the volume of sedimented cryoglobulin after cold centrifugation of serum at 4° to 5°C.

**cryo·ex·trac·tion** (kri"o-eks-trak'shən) the application of low temperature in the removal of a cataractous lens; it is accomplished with an instrument (cryoprobe) whose extremely cold tip forms an adhesion (iceball) with the lens, thus permitting removal of the lens.

**cryo·ex·trac·tor** (kri"o-eks-trak'tər) [*cryo-* + *extractor*] a cryoprobe used in cryoextraction.

**cry·o·fi·brin·o·gen** (kri"o-fi-brin'o-jən) [*cryo-* + *fibrinogen*] fibrinogen with the abnormal physical property of precipitating in the cold (4°C) and subsequently redissolving at 37°C.

**cryo·fi·brin·o·gen·emia** (kri"o-fi-brin"o-jə-ne'me-ə) the presence of cryofibrinogen in the blood.

**cryo·gam·ma·glob·u·lin** (kri"o-gam"ə-glob'u-lin) cryoglobulin.

**cry·o·gen** (kri'o-jən) [*cryo-* + *-gen*] a substance used for lowering temperatures.

**cry·o·gen·ic** (kri"o-jen'ik) pertaining to or causing the production of low temperatures.

**cryo·glob·u·lin** (kri"o-glob'u-lin) any of numerous serum globulins or globulin complexes, almost always an immunoglobulin, that precipitate at low temperature (around 4°C) and redissolve at 37°C; they are classified in three groups, called *type I, type II,* and *type III.* See also *cryoglobulinemia.*
**type I c's,** a group of monoclonal immunoglobulins sometimes found in plasma cell dyscrasias and lymphoproliferative disorders such as multiple myeloma and Waldenström's macroglobulinemia.
**type II c's,** a group of mixed immunoglobulin complexes with a monoclonal component that has antibody activity against polyclonal immunoglobulins, sometimes found in hepatitis, plasma cell dyscrasias, lymphoproliferative disorders, and autoimmune disorders such as rheumatoid arthritis, systemic lupus erythematosus, and Sjögren's syndrome.
**type III c's,** a group of immune complexes involving polyclonal immunoglobulins, usually globulin-antiglobulin complexes, found in infectious diseases and autoimmune disorders such as rheumatoid arthritis, systemic lupus erythematosus, and Sjögren's syndrome.

**cryo·glob·u·lin·emia** (kri"o-glob"u-lĭ-ne'me-ə) [MeSH: Cryoglobulinemia] the presence of cryoglobulin in the blood, associated with a variety of clinical manifestations including Raynaud's phenomenon, vascular purpura, cold urticaria, necrosis of extremities, bleeding disorders, vasculitis, arthralgia, neurologic manifestations, hepatosplenomegaly, and glomerulonephritis.
**essential mixed c.,** a rare condition characterized by deposition of type II cryoglobulins without a detectable cause, inducing cutaneous vasculitis, synovitis, and glomerulonephritis.

**cryo·hy·drate** (kri"o-hi'drāt) [*cryo-* + *hydrate*] 1. a salt containing water of crystallization at low temperatures. 2. a eutectic mixture, especially one having water as one of its constituents. 3. a crystal obtained by freezing a supersaturated solution and containing solute and solvent in the same ratio as occurred in solution.

**cryo·hy·po·phys·ec·to·my** (kri"o-hi"po-fiz-ek'tə-me) destruction of the hypophysis by the application of cold.

**cry·om·e·ter** (kri-om'ə-tər) [*cryo-* + *-meter*] a thermometer for measuring very low temperatures.

**cry·op·a·thy** (kri-op'ə-the) [*cryo-* + Gr. *-pathy*] any morbid condition caused by cold.

**cryo·phile** (kri'o-fīl") [*cryo-* + *-phile*] psychrophile.

**cryo·phil·ic** (kri"o-fil'ik) [*cryo-* + *-philic*] psychrophilic.

**cryo·phy·lac·tic** (kri"o-fə-lak'tik) [*cryo-* + *phylactic*] resistant to very low temperatures; said of bacteria.

**cryo·pre·cip·i·ta·bil·i·ty** (kri"o-pre-sip"ĭ-tə-bil'ĭ-te) ability to undergo cryoprecipitation.

**cryo·pre·cip·i·tate** (kri"o-pre-sip'ĭ-tāt) [*cryo-* + *precipitate*] any precipitate that results from cooling, such as cryoglobulin or antihemophilic factor.

**cryo·pre·cip·i·ta·tion** (kri"o-pre-sip"ĭ-ta'shən) precipitation of a substance in solution upon cooling, such as antihemophilic factor in blood plasma.

**cryo·pres·er·va·tion** (kri"o-pres"ər-va'shən) [*cryo-* + *preservation*]

[MeSH: Cryopreservation] the maintaining of the viability of excised tissue or organs by storing at very low temperatures.

**cryo·probe** (kri'o-prōb) an instrument for applying extreme cold to tissue.

**cryo·pro·tec·tive** (kri″o-pro-tek'tiv) capable of protecting against injury due to freezing, as glycerol protects frozen red blood cells.

**cryo·pro·tein** (kri″o-pro'tēn) [*cryo-* + *protein*] any blood protein that precipitates on cooling, such as cryoglobulin or cryofibrinogen.

**cryo·scope** (kri'o-skōp) an apparatus for performing cryoscopy.

**cryo·scop·i·cal** (kri″o-skop'ĭ-kəl) pertaining to cryoscopy.

**cry·os·co·py** (kri-os'kə-pe) [*cryo-* + *-scopy*] examination of liquids, based on the principle that the freezing point of solutions varies according to the amount and the nature of the solute.

**cryo·stat** (kri'o-stat) [*cryo-* + *-stat*] 1. a device by which temperature can be maintained at a very low level. 2. in pathology and histology, a chamber containing a microtome for sectioning frozen tissue.

**cryo·sur·gery** (kri″o-sər'jər-e) [MeSH: Cryosurgery] destruction of tissue by the application of extreme cold, used in some forms of intracranial and cutaneous surgery.

**cryo·thal·a·mec·to·my** (kri″o-thal″ə-mek'tə-me) cryothalamotomy.

**cryo·thal·a·mot·o·my** (kri″o-thal″ə-mot'ə-me) destruction of a portion of the thalamus by application of extreme cold.

**cryo·ther·a·py** (kri″o-ther'ə-pe) [*cryo-* + *therapy*] [MeSH: Cryotherapy] the therapeutic use of cold. Called also *crymotherapy* and *frigotherapy.*

**cryo·tol·er·ant** (kri″o-tol'ər-ənt) able to withstand unusually low temperatures.

**crypt** (kript) [L. *crypta,* from Gr. *kryptos* hidden] a blind pit or tube on a free surface; see also *crypta* [TA].
**anal c's,** sinus anales.
**bony c.,** the crypt in the developing alveolar bone that becomes the socket of the developing tooth.
**dental c.,** tooth c.
**enamel c.,** a space bounded by the dental ledges on either side and usually by the enamel organ; it is filled with mesenchyma.
**c's of Fuchs,** c's of iris.
**c's of Haller,** glandulae preputiales.
**c's of iris,** pitlike depressions found in the iris, in the region of the circulus arteriosus minor; called also *c's of Fuchs.*
**c's of Lieberkühn,** glandulae intestinales.
**c's of Littre,** glandulae preputiales.
**Luschka's c's,** deep indentations of the gallbladder mucosa which penetrate into the muscular layer of the organ.
**c. of Morgagni,** 1. fossa navicularis urethrae. 2. see *sinus anales.*
**mucous c's of duodenum,** glandulae duodenales.
**odoriferous c's of prepuce,** glandulae preputiales.
**c's of palatine tonsil,** 1. fossulae tonsillares tonsillae palatinae. 2. see *cryptae tonsillares tonsillae palatinae.*
**c's of pharyngeal tonsil,** 1. fossulae tonsillares tonsillae pharyngeae. 2. cryptae tonsillares tonsillae pharyngeae.
**synovial c.,** a pouch in the synovial membrane of a joint.
**c's of tongue,** cryptae tonsillares tonsillae lingualis.
**tonsillar c's of lingual tonsil,** cryptae tonsillares tonsillae lingualis.
**tonsillar c's of palatine tonsil,** cryptae tonsillares tonsillae palatinae.
**tonsillar c's of pharyngeal tonsil,** cryptae tonsillares tonsillae pharyngeae.
**tooth c.,** the depression in the alveolar bone occupied by the tooth germ and the tooth follicle. Called also *dental c.*
**c's of Tyson,** glandulae preputiales.

**cryp·ta** (krip'tə) gen. and pl. *cryp'tae* [L.] [TA] crypt: a blind pit or tube opening on a free surface.
**cryp'tae muco'sae,** see *mucous gland,* under *gland.*
**cryp'tae muco'sae duode'ni,** glandulae duodenales.
**cryp'tae odori'ferae, cryp'tae praeputia'les,** glandulae preputiales.
**cryp'tae tonsil'lae** [TA], **cryp'tae tonsilla'res,** tonsillar crypts: crypts associated with any of the four types of tonsils in the throat (lingual, palatine, pharyngeal, and tubal).
**cryp'tae tonsil'lae tonsil'lae palati'nae,** cryptae tonsillares tonsillae palatinae.
**cryp'tae tonsil'lae tonsil'lae pharyn'geae,** cryptae tonsillares tonsillae pharyngeae.
**cryp'tae tonsilla'res tonsil'lae lingua'lis** [TA], tonsillar crypts of lingual tonsil: deep, irregular invaginations from the surface of the lingual tonsils.
**cryp'tae tonsilla'res tonsil'lae palati'nae** [TA], tonsillar crypts of palatine tonsil: crypts within a palatine tonsil, representing the blind ends of the tonsillar fossulae.
**cryp'tae tonsilla'res tonsil'lae pharyn'geae** [TA], **cryp'tae tonsilla'res tonsil'lae pharyngea'lis,** tonsillar crypts of pharyngeal tonsil: crypts found within a pharyngeal tonsil, representing the blind ends of the tonsillar fossulae.
**cryp'tae tonsilla'res tonsil'lae tuba'riae** [TA], tonsillar crypts of tubal tonsil: small invaginations extending into a tubal tonsil.
**cryp'tae ure'thrae mulie'bris,** glandulae urethrales urethrae femininae.

**cryp·tae** (krip'te) [L.] genitive and plural of *crypta.*

**crypt·an·am·ne·sia** (kript″an-am-ne'zhə) cryptomnesia.

**cryp·tec·to·my** (krip-tek'tə-me) [*crypt-* + *-ectomy*] excision or obliteration of a crypt.

**cryp·ten·amine** (krip-ten'ə-mīn) a mixture of ester alkaloids derived from a nonaqueous extract of *Veratrum viride* Ait. (Liliaceae); it forms a white amorphous powder that has antihypertensive properties, and contains several alkaloids, including protoveratrines A and B, neogermitrine, germitrine, and germerine.
**c. acetates,** a mixture of the acetate salts of cryptenamine, administered intravenously or intramuscularly in the management of eclampsia and hypertensive encephalopathy.
**c. tannates,** a mixture of the tannate salts of cryptenamine, administered orally to control moderate to severe hypertension.

**cryp·tes·the·sia** (krip″təs-the'zhə) [*crypt-* + *esthesia*] clairvoyance.

**cryp·tic** (krip'tik) [Gr. *kryptikos* hidden] concealed, hidden, larval.

**cryp·ti·tis** (krip-ti'tis) inflammation of a crypt.
**anal c.,** inflammation of the anal crypts, with pain and tenderness (especially during bowel movements), pruritus, and spasm of the anal sphincter; it may progress to abscess of the crypt.

**crypt(o)-** [Gr. *kryptos* hidden] a combining form meaning hidden or concealed, or denoting relationship to a crypt.

**cryp·to·ceph·a·lus** (krip″to-sef'ə-ləs) [*crypto-* + *-cephalus*] microcephalus.

**Cryp·to·coc·ca·ceae** (krip″to-kŏ-ka'se-e) a form-family of Fungi Imperfecti, usually classified in the form-class Blastomycetes, although some authorities place it in Hyphomycetes; its members are yeastlike throughout most or all of their life cycle. It includes a number of pathogenic genera, such as *Candida, Cryptococcus, Geotrichum, Malassezia, Rhodotorula,* and *Trichosporon.*

**Cryp·to·coc·ca·les** (krip″to-kok-a'lēz) in some systems of classification, a form-order of Fungi Imperfecti, usually classified in form-class Blastomycetes although some authorities consider it part of Hyphomycetes. It includes the form-family Cryptococcaceae.

**cryp·to·coc·co·ma** (krip″to-kok-o'mə) a fungus ball consisting of *Cryptococcus neoformans.* Those in the brain often cause symptoms, while those in the lungs may be quiescent.

**cryp·to·coc·co·sis** (krip″to-kŏ-ko'sis) [MeSH: Cryptococcosis] infection by *Cryptococcus neoformans,* most commonly seen in immunocompromised patients and fatal if left untreated; the most common types are *cutaneous c., pulmonary c.,* and *cryptococcal meningitis.* There may also be invasion of the central nervous system, liver, spleen, and joints. Called also *torulosis* and *Buschke's* or *Busse-Buschke disease.*
**cutaneous c.,** a form manifested primarily by cutaneous lesions, usually acneiform in type. Called also *European blastomycosis.*
**pulmonary c.,** infection of the lungs with *Cryptococcus neoformans;* most cases are asymptomatic or characterized by cough, dull chest pain, and low grade fever, although a few cases are fulminant in the lungs or spread to become cryptococcal meningitis.

**Cryp·to·coc·cus** (krip″to-kok'əs) [*crypto-* + Gr. *kokkos* berry] [MeSH: Cryptococcus] a genus of yeastlike Fungi Imperfecti of the form-family Cryptococcaceae, which usually have a capsule and do not form pseudomycelia as do *Candida* species.
**C. al'bidus,** a species that has been found in a few cases of cryptococcosis; its perfect (sexual) stage is *Filobasidium floriforme.*
**C. capsula'tus,** former name for *Histoplasma capsulatum.*
**C. histoly'ticus, C. ho'minis, C. meningi'tidis,** 1. *C. neoformans.* 2. former names for *C. neoformans.*
**C. neofor'mans,** a species found around the world in nests and droppings of pigeons; it is the most common species causing cryptococcosis in humans, and it also infects cats. Its perfect (sexual) stage has been named *Filobasidiella neoformans.* Formerly called *C. histolyticus, C. hominis, C. meningitidis, Debaryomyces neoformans hominis,* and *Torula histolytica.*

**cryp·to·crys·tal·line** (krip″to-kris'tə-lēn) [*crypto-* + *crystalline*] composed of crystals of microscopic size.

**Cryp·to·cys·tis trich·o·dec·tis** (krip″to-sis'tis trik″o-dek'tis) former name for the larval form of *Dipylidium caninum.*

**cryp·to·de·ter·min·ant** (krip″to-de-tər'mĭ-nənt) hidden determinant.

**cryp·to·did·y·mus** (krip″to-did'ə-məs) [*crypto-* + *-didymus*] endadelphos.

**cryp·to·em·py·ema** (krip″to-em″pi-e′mə) [*crypto-* + *empyema*] empyema that is difficult to aspirate, being loculated or interlobar.

**cryp·to·gam** (krip′to-gam) [*crypto-* + Gr. *gamos* marriage] any one of the lower plants that have no true flowers, but propagate by spores, such as fungi, algae, mosses, and ferns.

**cryp·to·gam·ic** (krip″to-gam′ik) pertaining to cryptogams; reproducing by spores.

**cryp·to·ge·net·ic** (krip″to-jə-net′ik) cryptogenic.

**cryp·to·gen·ic** (krip″to-jen′ik) [*crypto-* + *-genic*] idiopathic.

**cryp·to·glan·du·lar** (krip″to-glan′du-lər) [*crypto-* + *glandular*] pertaining to or arising from an anal gland and an anal crypt.

**cryp·to·lith** (krip′to-lith) [*crypto-* + *-lith*] a calculus or concretion in a crypt.

**cryp·to·men·or·rhea** (krip″to-men″o-re′ə) [*crypto-* + *menorrhea*] a condition in which the symptoms of menstruation are experienced but no external bleeding occurs, as in cases of imperforate hymen.

**cryp·to·mere** (krip′to-mēr) [*crypto-* + *-mere*] a cystic or saclike condition.

**cryp·to·me·ro·ra·chis·chi·sis** (krip″to-me″ro-rə-kis′kĭ-sis) [*crypto-* + *mero-*[1] + *rhachischisis*] spina bifida occulta.

**cryp·tom·ne·sia** (krip″tom-ne′zhə) [*crypto-* + Gr. *mnasthai* to be mindful] the recall of memories not recognized as such but thought to be original creations.

**cryp·tom·ne·sic** (krip″tom-ne′sik) pertaining to or characterized by cryptomnesia.

**cryp·to·neu·rous** (krip″to-noo′rəs) [*crypto-* + *neuro-* + *-ous*] having no definite or distinct nervous system.

**cryp·toph·thal·mia** (krip″tof-thal′me-ə) cryptophthalmos.

**cryp·toph·thal·mos** (krip″tof-thal′mos) [*crypto-* + Gr. *ophthalmos* eye] a developmental anomaly in which the skin is continuous over the eyeball without any indication of the formation of eyelids.

**cryp·toph·thal·mus** (krip″tof-thal′məs) cryptophthalmos.

**cryp·to·pine** (krip′to-pin) [*crypto-* + Gr. *opion* opium] a minor alkaloidal constituent of opium, of *Corydalis sempervirens* (L.) Pers., and of *Dicentra* spp. (Fumariaceae).

**cryp·to·plas·mic** (krip″to-plaz′mik) having no apparent causative agent; said of an infection in which the infecting organism has concealed itself.

**cryp·to·po·dia** (krip″to-po′de-ə) [*crypto-* + Gr. *pous* foot] a condition characterized by swelling of the lower part of the leg and dorsum of the foot so as to cover all but the soles of the feet.

**cryp·to·py·ic** (krip″to-pi′ik) [*crypto-* + *py-* + *-ic*] characterized by concealed suppuration.

**cryp·tor·chid** (krip-tor′kid) [*crypto-* +Gr. *orchis* testis] 1. pertaining to or characterized by cryptorchidism. 2. an individual exhibiting cryptorchidism.

**cryp·tor·chi·dec·to·my** (krip″tor-kĭ-dek′tə-me) [*cryptorchid* + *-ectomy*] excision of an undescended testis.

**cryp·tor·chi·dism** (krip-tor′kĭ-diz″əm) [MeSH: Cryptorchidism] a developmental defect characterized by failure of one or both of the testes to descend into the scrotum. Called also *cryptorchism* and *undescended testis.*

**cryp·tor·chi·do·pexy** (krip-tor″kĭ-do-pek′se) orchiopexy.

**cryp·tor·chi·dy** (krip-tor′kĭ-de) cryptorchidism.

**cryp·tor·chism** (krip-tor′kiz-əm) cryptorchidism.

**cryp·to·scope** (krip′to-skōp) [*crypto-* + *-scope*] fluoroscope.
**Satvioni's c.,** one of the early forms of fluoroscope.

**cryp·tos·co·py** (krip-tos′kə-pe) fluoroscopy.

**cryp·to·spo·rid·i·o·sis** (krip″to-spo-rid″e-o′sis) [MeSH: Cryptosporidiosis] 1. infection of young farm animals (calves, lambs, foals, or piglets) with protozoa of the genus *Cryptosporidium,* which may be associated with or contribute to enteric disease. 2. human infection with *Cryptosporidium,* usually seen as a self-limited diarrhea in those who work with cattle; in immunocompromised patients it is much more serious, manifested as prolonged debilitating diarrhea, weight loss, fever, and abdominal pain, with occasional spread to the trachea and bronchial tree.

**Cryp·to·spo·ri·di·um** (krip″to-spo-rid′e-əm) [*crypto-* + *spore*] [MeSH: Cryptosporidium] a genus of minute homoxenous coccidian protozoa (suborder Eimeriina, order Eucoccidiida), characterized by the presence of oocysts with four sporozoites; they are parasitic in the intestinal tracts of many different vertebrates, including humans, causing cryptosporidiosis.

**Cryp·to·stro·ma** (krip″to-stro′mə) [*crypto-* + *stroma*] a genus of fungi of the form-class *Hyphomycetes;* called also *Coniosporium. C. cortica′le* grows under the bark of maple trees and inhalation of its spores causes maple bark disease in lumber workers.

**cryp·to·tia** (krip-to′she-ə) a rare anomaly in which the superior portion of the auricle is buried in the scalp.

**cryp·to·tox·ic** (krip″to-tok′sik) [*crypto-* + *toxic*] having hidden toxic properties; said of a solution normally nontoxic, but which may become toxic when the colloidal balance is disturbed.

**cryp·to·xan·thin** (krip″to-zan′thin) a yellow carotenoid widely distributed in nature (egg yolk, green grass, yellow corn, etc.), which can be converted into vitamin A in the body.

**cryp·to·zo·ite** (krip″to-zo′īt) [*crypto-* + Gr. *zōon* animal] a meront of certain sporozoan protozoa in the exoerythrocytic stage.

**cryp·toz·y·gous** (krip-toz′ə-gəs) [*crypto-* + Gr. *zygon* yoke] having the face no wider than the cranium, so that the zygomatic arches are concealed by the bulging of the cranium when the skull is viewed from above. Cf. *phenozygous.*

**Crys.** crystal.

**crys·tal** (kris′təl) [Gr. *krystallos* ice] a homogeneous angular solid formed from a chemical element, compound, or isomorphous mixture, having a definite form in which the ultimate units from which it is built up are systematically arranged.
**asthma c's,** Charcot-Leyden c's.
**blood c's,** hematoidin crystals in the blood.
**calcium pyrophosphate dihydrate (CPPD) c's,** microscopic crystals of calcium pyrophosphate dihydrate occurring in the synovial fluid in calcium pyrophosphate deposition disease.
**Charcot-Leyden c's,** elongated birefringent crystals in the form of two hexagonal pyramids joined base to base, derived from lysophospholipase released from the plasma membranes of disintegrating eosinophils; seen in serous fluids such as the bronchial secretions in asthma and in stools in some cases of intestinal parasitism. Called also *asthma c's.*
**coffin lid c's,** peculiar indented crystals of ammoniomagnesium phosphate from alkaline urine; called also *knife rest c's.*
**CPPD c's,** calcium pyrophosphate dihydrate c's.
**dumbbell c's,** crystals of calcium oxalate occurring in the urine.
**ear c.,** statoconium.
**hedgehog c's,** a spiny form of uric acid concretions.
**hydroxyapatite c.,** microscopic crystals of hydroxyapatite occurring in joints or bursae in a variety of connective tissue disorders. See also *apatite deposition disease,* under *disease.*
**knife rest c's,** coffin lid c's.
**liquid c's,** certain liquids which manifest some of the optical properties of crystals and the hydrodynamic properties of fluids, e.g., phosphatidylcholine.
**Lubarsch's c's,** crystals in the testis resembling sperm crystals.
**c's of Reinke,** see under *crystalloid.*
**rock c.,** quartz; a transparent form of silicon dioxide (silica), $SiO_2$; used for lenses.
**scintillation c.,** a substance that emits a flash of light (scintillation) when contacted by high-energy particles, such as alpha, beta, or gamma rays, such as a sodium iodide crystal with a trace impurity of thallium used in the Anger camera to detect gamma radiation.
**Teichmann's c's,** crystals of hemin, seen in microscopic tests for the presence of blood.
**thorn apple c's,** yellow or reddish brown spheres of ammonium urate which are covered with sharp spicules or prisms, as found in the urine.
**Virchow's c's,** yellow or orange crystals of hematoidin sometimes seen in extravasated blood.
**whetstone c's,** crystals of xanthine sometimes seen in urine.

**crys·tal·bu·min** (kris″təl-bu′min) 1. an albuminous substance found in an aqueous extract of the crystalline lens. 2. a general term for crystallizable albumins of the type of egg albumin and serum albumin.

**crys·tal·lin** (kris-tal′in) a globulin existing in the crystalline lens of the eye. *Alpha c.* is precipitated by dilute acetic acid; *beta carotene* is not.

**crys·tal·line** (kris′tə-lēn) resembling a crystal in nature or clearness.

**crys·tal·li·za·tion** (kris″təl-ĭ-za′shən) [MeSH: Crystallization] the formation of crystals; conversion to a crystalline form.
**fern-leaf c.,** crystallization of cervical mucus in a fernlike pattern, observable during the first half of the menstrual cycle and said to be most conspicuous at the time of ovulation.

**crys·tal·log·ra·phy** (kris″təl-og′rə-fe) [*crystal* + *-graphy*] [MeSH: Crystallography] the science dealing with the study of crystals.
**x-ray c.,** the determination of the three-dimensional structure of molecules by means of diffraction patterns produced by x-rays of crystals of the molecules.

**crys·tal·loid** (kris′tə-loid) [*crystal* + *-oid*] 1. resembling a crystal. 2. a substance smaller than a colloid, in solution passing readily

through semipermeable membranes, lowering the freezing point of the solvent containing it, and generally capable of being crystallized. Cf. *colloid,* def. 2.
**Charcot-Böttcher c's,** slender spindle-shaped crystals 10 to 25 μ long, commonly found in Sertoli cells of the human testis but not in other species.
**c's of Reinke,** conspicuous, variously shaped, crystal-like structures contained in Leydig cells.

**crys·tal·lu·ria** (kris″təl-u′re-ə) the excretion of crystals in the urine, producing renal irritation.

**Crys·ti·cil·lin** (kris″tĭ-sil′in) trademark for preparations of penicillin G procaine.

**Crys·to·dig·in** (kris″to-dij′in) trademark for preparations of digitoxin.

**CS** cesarean section; conditioned stimulus; coronary sinus.

**Cs** symbol for *cesium.*

**CSAA** Child Study Association of America.

**CSC** coup sur coup.

**CSF** cerebrospinal fluid; colony-stimulating factor.
**CSF-1,** macrophage colony-stimulating factor.

**CSGBI** Cardiac Society of Great Britain and Ireland.

**CSII** continuous subcutaneous insulin infusion; see *insulin pump,* under *pump.*

**CSM** cerebrospinal meningitis.

**CST** contraction stress test.

**CT** computed tomography.

**CTA** Canadian Tuberculosis Association.

**CTBA** cetrimonium bromide.

**ctei·no·phyte** (ti′no-fīt) [Gr. *kteinein* to kill + *-phyte*] a fungus that has a destructive influence upon its host; limited to chemical rather than parasitic activity.

**cteno-** [Gr. *kteis,* gen. *ktenos* comb] a combining form denoting relationship to a comb or comblike structure.

**Cte·no·ce·phal·i·des** (te″no-sə-fal′ĭ-dēz) [*cteno-* + *cephalo-* + *eidos* form, shape] a genus of fleas often found parasitic on domestic animals.
**C. ca′nis,** a species frequently found on dogs, which may transmit the dog tapeworm to humans.
**C. fe′lis,** a species commonly found on cats that transmits cat flea typhus and murine typhus.

**Cten·oph·o·ra** (ten-of′o-rə) [*cteno-* + Gr. *pherein* to bear] a phylum of marine invertebrates that includes the comb jellies or sea walnuts, whose bodies consist of two layers of cells enclosing a jellylike mass; eight rows of cilia, which resemble combs, cover the outer body surface and provide locomotor power.

**cten·o·phore** (ten′o-for) 1. pertaining or belonging to the phylum Ctenophora. 2. an individual of the phylum Ctenophora. See also *coelenterate* (def. 3).

**Cte·noph·thal·mus** (te″nof-thal′məs) [*cteno-* + Gr. *ophthalmos* eye] a genus of fleas. *C. agry′tes* is the European mouse flea.

**Cte·nus** (te′nəs) a genus of spiders. *C. fe′rus* is the wandering spider of South America.

**C-ter·mi·nal** (tər′mĭ-nəl) the end of the peptide chain carrying the free alpha carboxyl group of the last amino acid, conventionally written to the right.

**Cte·si·as of Cnidus** (te′se-əs) (5th century B.C.) a Greek physician and historian, a contemporary of Hippocrates of Cos. Ctesias was a long-time resident at, historian and apologist for, and physician to the royal Persian court.

**CTL** cytotoxic lymphocytes; cytotoxic T lymphocytes.

**CTP** cytidine triphosphate.

**CTP syn·thase** (sin′thās) [EC 6.3.4.2] an enzyme of the transferase class that catalyzes the transfer of an amino group to UTP to form CTP, using glutamine or ammonia as a donor. The reaction is part of pyrimidine nucleotide biosynthesis.

**Cu** symbol for *copper* (L. *cuprum*).

**cu·beb** (ku′bəb) [L. *cubeba;* Arabic *kabāba*] 1. the fruit of *Piper cubeba.* 2. the dried, unripe, almost fully grown fruit of *P. cubeba,* which contains 10 to 18 per cent volatile oil, cubebin, resins, fat, and wax. It was formerly used to stimulate healing of mucous membranes, and as a diuretic and urinary antiseptic. See also *cubebism.*

**cu·beb·ism** (ku′bəb-iz″əm) poisoning by cubeb *(Piper cubeba),* characterized by nausea, vomiting, diarrhea, fever with or without skin eruptions, prostration, arthralgia, irritation of the kidneys, soft pulse, loss of consciousness, miosis, delirium, and coma. In severe poisonings, death from respiratory failure may occur.

**cu·bi·cle** (ku′bĭ-kəl) a compartment in a larger area, such as a dormitory or a ward, separated from similar adjoining compartments and from the rest of the room by low partitions.

**cu·bi·tal** (ku′bĭ-təl) 1. pertaining to the elbow; called also *anconal* and *anconeal.* 2. pertaining to the ulna or to the forearm.

**cu·bi·ta·lis** (ku-bĭ-ta′lis) [L.] cubital.

**cu·bi·to·car·pal** (ku″bĭ-to-kahr′pəl) pertaining to the ulna and the carpus.

**cu·bi·to·ra·di·al** (ku″bĭ-to-ra′de-əl) pertaining to the ulna and the radius.

**cu·bi·tus** (ku′bĭ-təs) [L.] 1. [TA] elbow: the joint between the arm and forearm. 2. the upper limb distal to the humerus: the elbow, forearm, and hand. 3. ulna.
**c. val′gus,** deformity of the elbow (judged with the palm facing forward), in which it deviates away from the midline of the body when extended.
**c. va′rus,** deformity of the elbow, due to lateral angulation of the joint and accompanied by deviation of the forearm toward the midline of the body when the forearm is extended; called also *gun stock deformity.*

**cu·boid** (ku′boid) [Gr. *kyboeidēs*] 1. resembling a cube. 2. the cuboid bone (os cuboideum [TA]).

**cu·boi·dal** (ku-boi′dəl) resembling a cube.

**Cu·bo·me·du·sae** (ku″bo-mə-doo′sae) an order of jellyfish that have four-sided cup-shaped bodies; genera of medical importance include *Chironex* and *Chiropsalmus.*

**cu·bo·me·du·san** (ku″bo-mə-doo′sən) 1. pertaining to Cubomedusae. 2. a jellyfish of the order Cubomedusae.

**cu cm** cubic centimeter.

**cu·co·line** (ku′ko-lēn) sinomenine.

**cu·cul·la·ris** (ku″ku-lar′is) [L. *cucullus* hood] musculus trapezius.

**cu·cum·ber** (ku′kəm-bər) [L. *cucumis*] [MeSH: Cucumbers] 1. any of various species of the genus *Cucumis.* 2. the edible fruit of any of these species, chiefly *C. sativus;* their seeds are diuretic and their juice is used as an astringent in various cosmetic formulations.
**bitter c.,** colocynth.

**Cu·cum·is** (ku′kəm-is) a genus of plants of the family Curcurbitaceae. It includes several edible species and some that have medicinal properties, such as *C. sati′vus* L., the cucumber (q.v.).

**cu·cur·bi·tol** (ku-kər′bĭ-tol) a sterol, $C_{24}H_{40}O_4$, obtained from watermelon seeds.

**cud** (kud) the bolus of partially digested food that a ruminant casts back up from the rumen to be chewed a second time.

**cud·bear** (kud′bār) a red-brown powder, obtained from lichens, such as *Lecanora tartarea,* and used as a coloring matter in pharmacy.

**cud·ding** (kud′ing) rumination, def. 1.

**cuff** (kuf) a small bandlike structure encircling a part.
**musculotendinous c.,** one formed by intermingled muscle and tendon fibers; see *rotator c.*
**rotator c.,** a musculotendinous structure about the capsule of the shoulder joint, formed by the inserting fibers of the supraspinatus, infraspinatus, teres minor, and subscapularis muscles, blending with the capsule, and providing mobility and strength to the shoulder joint.

**cuff·ing** (kuf′ing) the formation of a cufflike surrounding border, such as collections of leukocytes surrounding blood vessels, noted in certain viral diseases.

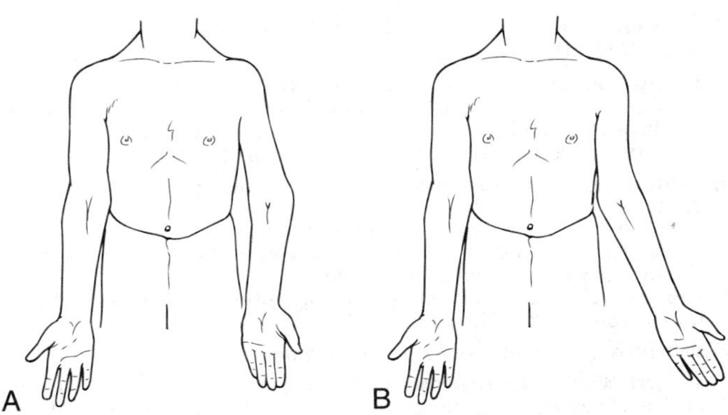

*(A)* Cubitus valgus; *(B)* cubitus varus.

**Cui·gnet's method** (kwēn-yāz') [Ferdinand Louis Joseph *Cuignet,* French ophthalmologist, 19th century] retinoscopy.

**cui·rass** (kwe-rahs') [Fr. *cuirasse* breastplate] a covering for the chest, such as the plastic shell or bubble used in a cuirass respirator (q.v.).
**tabetic c.,** an area of diminished sense of touch encircling the chest of a patient with tabes dorsalis.

**Cuj.** abbreviation for L. *cu'jus,* of which.

**cu·lard** (ku-lahrd') myofiber hyperplasia.

**cul-de-sac** (kul"də-sak') [Fr.] a blind pouch or cecum; a tubular cavity closed at one end, such as a diverticulum.
**conjunctival c.-d.-s.,** either of the conjunctival fornices; see *fornix conjunctivae inferior* and *fornix conjunctivae superior.*
**Douglas' c.-d.-s.,** excavatio rectouterina.

**cul·do·cen·te·sis** (kul"do-sən-te'sis) [*cul-de-*sac + *centesis*] aspiration of fluid from the rectouterine space by puncture of the apex of the vaginal wall.

**cul·do·scope** (kul'do-skōp) an endoscope for performing culdoscopy.

**cul·dos·co·py** (kəl-dos'kə-pe) [MeSH: Culdoscopy] visual examination of the female pelvic viscera by means of an endoscope introduced into the pelvic cavity through the posterior vaginal fornix.

**cul·dot·o·my** (kəl-dot'ə-me) [*cul-de-*sac + *-tomy*] incision into the cul-de-sac (pouch of Douglas); called also *posterior colpotomy.*

**Cu·lex** (ku'ləks) [L. "gnat"] [MeSH: Culex] a genus of mosquitoes of the tribe Culicini, subfamily Culicinae, having short palpi and holding their bodies parallel to the surface on which they rest. Many species around the world are vectors of disease-producing agents for humans and other animals. Species include *C. annuliros'tris, C. fa'tigans, C. moles'tus, C. pi'piens, C. quinquefascia'tus, C. tarsa'lis,* and *C. tritaeniorhyn'cus,* among many others.

**cu·lic·i·cide** (ku-lis'ĭ-sīd) culicide.

**Cu·lic·i·dae** (ku-lis'ĭ-de) [MeSH: Culicidae] the mosquitoes, a family of insects of the suborder Nematocerca, order Diptera. There are two subfamilies of particular medical interest: Anophelinae and Culicinae, containing tribes Anophelini, Aedini, Culicini, Mansoniini, and others

**cu·li·ci·dal** (ku"lĭ-si'dəl) destructive to gnats and mosquitoes.

**cu·li·cide** (ku'lĭ-sīd) [*culex* + *-cide*] an agent destructive to gnats and mosquitoes.

**cu·lic·i·fuge** (ku-lis'ĭ-fūj) [*culex* + *-fuge*] a preparation that repels gnats and mosquitoes.

**Cu·li·ci·nae** (ku"lĭ-si'ne) a subfamily of mosquitoes of the family Culicidae; genera of medical interest include *Aedes, Culex,* and *Mansonia.*

**cu·li·cine** (ku'lĭ-sin, ku'lĭ-sīn) 1. a member of the genus *Culex* or the tribe Culicini. 2. pertaining to, involving, or affecting mosquitoes of the genus *Culex* or the tribe Culicini.

**Cu·li·ci·ni** (ku-lĭ-si'ni) a tribe of mosquitoes of the subfamily Culicinae; genera of medical importance include *Culex* and *Culiseta.*

**Cu·li·coi·des** (ku-lĭ-koi'dēz) a genus of biting flies of the family Heleidae; some are vectors for viral diseases such as bluetongue and African horse sickness. *C. aus'teni* and *C. gra'hami* are intermediate hosts of the parasitic roundworm *Mansonella perstans. C. fu'rens* and possibly other species are intermediate hosts of *M. ozzardi.*

**Cu·li·se·ta** (ku"lĭ-se'tə) a genus of mosquitoes of the subfamily Culicinae, some of whom transmit disease viruses; formerly called *Theobaldia. C. inora'ta* is a vector of the Cache Valley virus and *C. melanu'ra* is a vector of the eastern and western equine encephalomyelitis viruses.

**Cul·len's sign** (kul'ənz) [Thomas Stephen *Cullen,* American surgeon, 1868–1953] see under *sign.*

**cull·ing** (kul'ing) the process of selective removal. The term is applied to the removal from the circulation, by the spleen, of abnormal erythrocytes, such as those occurring in congenital spherocytosis, or to the selective separation of other elements or organisms.

**cul·men** (kul'mən) pl. *cul'mina* [L.] 1. acme or summit. 2. c. cerebelli.
**c. cerebel'li** [TA], **c. of cerebellum,** the portion of the rostral lobe of the cerebellum that lies medially between the central lobule and the primary fissure; called also *culmen.*
**c. of left lung,** the nonlingular portion of the upper lobe of the left lung (see *lingula pulmonis sinistri*).

**cul·mi·na** (kul'mĭ-nə) [L.] plural of *culmen.*

**Culp-De Weerd ureteropelvioplasty** (kulp-de-wērd') [Ormond Skinner *Culp,* American surgeon, 1910–1977; James Henry *De Weerd,* American surgeon, born 1914] see under *ureteropelvioplasty.*

**cult** (kult) a system of treating disease based on some special and unscientific theory of disease causation.

**cul·ti·va·tion** (kul"tĭ-va'shən) [L. *cultivatio*] the propagation of living organisms, applied especially to the propagation of cells in artificial media.

**cul·tur·a·ble** (kul'chər-ə-bəl) capable of being cultured.

**cul·tur·al** (kul'chər-əl) pertaining to a culture.

**cul·ture** (kul'chər) [L. *cultura*] [MeSH: Culture] 1. the propagation of microorganisms or of living tissue cells in special media conducive to their growth. 2. a growth of microorganisms or other living cells. 3. to induce the propagation of microorganisms or living tissue cells in media conducive to their growth. See also *culture medium.*
**asynchronous c.,** one in which cells are randomly distributed with respect to the phase of cell division, as in an ordinary culture of bacteria or animal cells.
**attenuated c.,** a culture of pathogenic microorganisms whose virulence is weakened or abolished.
**blood c.,** microbiologic examination of a blood sample to check for presence of microorganisms.
**cell c.,** the maintenance or growth of animal cells *in vitro,* or a culture of such cells.
**chorioallantoic c.,** the cultivation of microorganisms, cells, or tissues on the chorioallantois of the developing chick.
**continuous flow c.,** the cultivation of bacteria in a continuous flow of fresh medium to maintain bacterial growth in logarithmic phase.
**direct c.,** a culture of microorganisms made by direct transfer from a natural source to an artificial medium.
**enrichment c.,** one grown on a medium, usually liquid, that has been supplemented to encourage the growth of a given type of organism.
**hanging-block c.,** one grown on a block of agar medium fastened to a coverglass, which is then inverted over a hollow slide.
**hanging-drop c.,** a culture in which the material to be cultivated is inoculated into a drop of fluid attached to a coverglass, which is inverted over a hollow slide.
**mixed c.,** one containing two or more kinds of microorganisms.
**mixed lymphocyte c. (MLC),** a type of lymphocyte proliferation test (q.v.) in which lymphocytes from two individuals are cultured together and the proliferative response (mixed lymphocyte reaction) is measured by $^{3}$H-labeled thymidine uptake. The test may be performed as a "two-way" MLC in which cells of both individuals can proliferate or as a "one-way" MLC in which the cells of one individual are prevented from responding by treatment with radiation or mitomycin. Three controls are used: cultures of syngeneic pairs, both untreated and radiation- or mitomycin-treated, and a culture of allogeneic irradiated or mitomycin-treated pairs. The primary clinical use of MLC is selection of compatible donors for bone marrow and living-related renal allotransplantation and for typing of HLA-D antigens; it is also used in diagnosis of immunodeficiency diseases.
**needle c.,** stab c.
**plate c.,** one grown on a medium, usually agar or gelatin, on a Petri dish.
**primary c.,** a cell or tissue culture made by direct transfer from a natural source to an artificial medium.
**pure c.,** one containing only one kind of microorganism, without any contaminants.
**radioisotopic c.,** a bacterial culture in a medium containing $^{14}$C-labeled carbohydrate. Metabolism is detected by the release of $^{14}CO_2$, offering earlier detection of growth than do conventional methods.
**roll-tube c.,** one made by inoculating a tube of molten agar medium and rotating it while it is solidifying, the medium being dispersed in a thin layer on the inner surface of the tube. The method is used for making colony counts, particularly of anaerobic bacteria.
**secondary c.,** one derived from a primary culture.
**selective c.,** one grown on a medium, usually solid, that has been supplemented to encourage the growth of a single species of microorganism. It may also include substances that inhibit the growth of other species.
**sensitized c.,** bacterial cells that have been incubated with specific antiserum.
**shake c.,** a culture made by inoculating warm liquid agar culture medium in a tube and shaking to distribute contents evenly. Incubation of the resolidified culture allows the development of separated colonies; especially applicable to obligate anaerobes.
**slant c.,** one made on a slanting surface of a solidified medium in a tube, the tube being tilted to provide a greater surface area for growth.
**slope c.,** slant c.
**stab c.,** one in which a tube of solid medium is inoculated by a needle thrust deep into the contents.
**stock c.,** a culture of microorganisms maintained in a viable state as a reference strain and subcultured into fresh medium as necessary.
**streak c.,** a culture in which the surface of a solid medium is inoc-

ulated by drawing across it, in a zigzag fashion, a wire inoculating loop carrying the inoculum.
**subculture c.**, one derived from an existing culture.
**suspension c.**, a culture in which cells multiply while suspended in a suitable medium.
**synchronized c.**, a culture of bacterial or animal cells in which all cells are in the same phase of cell division.
**tissue c.**, the maintaining or growing of tissue, organ primordia, or the whole or part of an organ *in vitro* so as to preserve its architecture and/or function.
**type c.**, a culture of any species of microorganism usually maintained in a central collection of type or standard cultures.

**cul·ture me·di·um** (kul'chər me'de-əm) any substance or preparation used for the cultivation of living cells.

## Culture Medium

Abbreviations used in this table are: a. = agar, b. = broth, ba. = base, c. = culture medium, m. = medium.

**agar c. m.**, one in which agar is used as the solidifying agent.
**Amies transport medium**, an agar medium containing sodium thioglycolate, sodium and potassium chloride, phosphate buffer, calcium chloride, magnesium chloride, and neutral charcoal, used for transport of specimens for anaerobic culture.
**antibiotic c. m. 3 FDA**, a broth medium containing peptone, yeast and beef extracts, sodium chloride, glucose, and potassium buffer, used for testing the activity of antibiotic agents against fungi.
**antibiotic c. m. 12 FDA**, an agar medium containing peptone, yeast and beef extracts, sodium chloride, and glucose, used for agar dilution susceptibility tests with antifungal antibiotics. Called also *nystatin assay a.*
**beef infusion c. m.**, see *infusion m.*
**Bennett agar**, an agar medium containing casein digest, yeast extract, beef extract, and glucose, used as an isolation medium for *Nocardia* and *Streptomyces.*
**bile-esculin agar**, an agar medium containing beef extract, peptone, oxgall, ferric citrate, and esculin, sometimes supplemented with horse serum, used for the identification of group D streptococci.
**birdseed agar**, Staib a.
**bismuth sulfite (BS) agar**, an agar culture medium containing beef extract, peptone, glucose, sodium sulfite, bismuth ammonium citrate, and brilliant green, used to isolate *Salmonella* species, especially *S. typhi*, from stool and other clinical specimens. Called also *Wilson-Blair c.*
**blood agar**, an agar medium containing heart infusion, peptone, and sodium chloride, autoclaved and enriched by the addition of sterile defibrinated blood, used for primary plating and subculturing, especially to determine bacterial hemolysis. The blood used may be sheep (for group A *Streptococcus*), rabbit (for *Haemophilus parahaemolyticus*), or horse.
**Bordet-Gengou (B-G) agar**, an agar base containing potato infusion, glycerol, and sodium chloride, enriched with blood, used for the isolation of *Bordetella pertussis* and *B. parapertussis.*
**brain-heart infusion (BHIA) medium**, an agar medium containing calf brain and beef heart infusion, peptone, glucose, and phosphate buffer; sheep blood may also be added. It is used for the cultivation of bacteria, actinomycetes, and fungi. A broth medium without the agar is used for cultivating the pneumococcus for the bile solubility test.
**brilliant green (BG) agar**, a highly selective primary isolation medium containing yeast extract, peptone, lactose, sucrose, sodium chloride, phenol red, and brilliant green in an agar base, used for the culture of salmonellae other than *Salmonella typhi.*
**Brucella agar**, an agar medium containing pancreatic digest of casein, peptic digest of animal tissue, yeast autolysate, and glucose, for the culture and isolation of *Brucella.* It may be supplemented by the addition of sheep blood and vitamin $K_1$ solution for the isolation of anaerobic bacteria.
**buffered glycerol-saline base (Sachs)**, a broth medium containing sodium chloride, phosphate buffer, phenol red, and glycerol, used to transport and preserve fecal specimen material.
**Campylobacter medium**, an agar medium containing pancreatic casein digest, peptic digest of animal tissues, yeast autolysate, glucose, sodium chloride, and sodium bisulfite, supplemented with sheep erythrocytes, vancomycin, trimethoprim, polymyxin, amphotericin, and cephalothin; used for isolating *Campylobacter* from specimens of fecal origin.
**carbohydrate broth**, a broth medium that contains heart infusion or peptone, sodium chloride, and an indicator supplemented with a single carbohydrate, used to test the ability to ferment various sugars.
**Cary-Blair transport medium**, an agar medium containing thioglycolate, phosphate, and sodium chloride, used for the collection and holding of clinical specimens containing gram-negative facultative organisms. The medium may be supplemented with calcium chloride, sodium bisulfite, and resazurin for culture of anaerobes.
**casein agar**, a medium containing dehydrated skim milk and agar, used for differentiation of *Nocardia* and *Streptomyces.*
**cetrimide agar**, an agar medium containing peptone, magnesium chloride, potassium sulfate, cetrimonium hydrochloride (cetrimide), and sometimes glycerol, used for the differentiation of strains of *Pseudomonas.*
**charcoal agar**, a beef heart infusion–peptone culture medium containing soluble starch, yeast extract, and charcoal. The base medium is supplemented with sheep blood and cephalexin for the selective culture of *Bordetella pertussis.*
**charcoal-yeast extract (CYE) agar**, an agar medium containing activated charcoal, L-cysteine, ferric pyrophosphate, and yeast extract, used for the culture of *Legionella.*
**charcoal-yeast extract diphasic blood c. m.**, a diphasic medium consisting of a lower solid slant containing charcoal and agar, partially covered with a liquid broth containing yeast extract, L-cysteine, and ferric nitrate. It is used for the culture of *Legionella.*
**chlamydospore agar**, an inorganic salt medium containing polysaccharide, biotin, and trypan blue, for the identification of *Candida albicans* by favoring the formation of chlamydospores which are stained blue by the dye.
**chocolate agar**, an agar medium containing casein digest, peptone, cornstarch, sodium chloride, and phosphate buffer; sterile hemoglobin or fresh blood is added and the medium heated until the color is chocolate brown. Other agar media may also be used as the base. It is used for the isolation of fastidious organisms, e.g., *Haemophilus influenzae* and *Neisseria* species.
**chopped meat (CM) broth**, a liquid medium containing chopped meat treated with sodium hydroxide, casein digest, yeast extract, phosphate buffer, and cysteine; it may also include hemin, vitamin $K_1$, glucose, and resazurin. It is used for the cultivation of anaerobic bacteria, especially *Clostridium* species.
**Christensen's urea agar**, an agar medium containing peptone or gelatin digest, sodium chloride, glucose, phenol red, urea, and phosphate buffer, used to detect urease production, especially in enteric bacteria such as species of *Proteus, Cryptococcus,* and aerobic actinomycetes. See also *urease test b.*
**citrate agar (Simmons)**, an agar medium containing sodium citrate, sodium chloride, magnesium sulfate, bromthymol blue, and phosphate buffer, used to determine the ability of gram-negative bacilli, particularly the Enterobacteriaceae, to utilize citrate as the sole carbon source.
**Columbia colistin–nalidixic acid (CNA) agar**, an agar medium containing peptone, cornstarch, sodium chloride, colistin, nalidixic acid, and sheep blood, used for the selective culture of gram-positive cocci, especially *Proteus* species.
**corn meal agar**, an agar medium containing corn meal infusion, used to stimulate sporulation in the identification of fungi. With the addition of Tween 80 it stimulates the production of chlamydospores by species of *Candida.* It may also be supplemented with glucose, sucrose, and yeast extract for the general culture of fungi.
**cycloserine cefoxitin fructose egg yolk agar**, an agar medium containing peptone, sodium chloride, magnesium sulfate, fructose, neutral red, and phosphate buffer, supplemented with cycloserine, cefoxitin, and egg yolk, used as a selective medium for *Clostridium difficile.*
**cystine-heart agar**, an agar medium containing beef heart infusion, peptone, glucose, sodium chloride, and L-cystine. The medium is supplemented with hemoglobin for the *in vitro* conversion of dimorphic hyaline molds.
**cystine-tellurite agar**, an agar medium containing meat infusion, po-

tassium tellurite, cystine, and agar enriched with blood, used for the isolation of *Corynebacterium diphtheriae.*

**cystine trypticase agar,** an agar medium containing cystine, pancreatic digest of casein, sodium chloride, sodium sulfite, and phenol red, an aerobic differential medium for the general culture of pathogenic bacteria, including fastidious organisms. It may be supplemented with specific sugars and used to test fermentation reactions in *Neisseria* species.

**Czapek-Dox agar, Czapek solution agar,** an agar medium containing sucrose, sodium nitrate, magnesium sulfate, potassium chloride, ferrous sulfate, and potassium buffer, used for the culture of *Nocardia, Streptomyces,* and fungi. Called also *Czapek-Dox solution.*

**decarboxylase broth,** a liquid culture medium containing beef extract, peptone, and glucose, to which is added an amino acid (commonly lysine, arginine, or ornithine), for the determination of the amino acid decarboxylase activity as a differential character of bacteria, especially Enterobacteriaceae.

**deoxycholate citrate (Leifson) (LDC) agar,** an agar medium containing meat infusion, peptone, lactose, sodium and ferric citrates, sodium deoxycholate, and neutral red, used for the primary culture and isolation of *Salmonella* and *Shigella.*

**deoxycholate (Leifson) (LD) agar,** an agar medium containing peptone, lactose, sodium citrate, ferric citrate, sodium chloride, sodium deoxycholate, neutral red, and potassium buffer, used for the isolation of Enterobacteriaceae and differentiation of lactose-fermenting and non–lactose-fermenting species.

**differential c. m.,** a culture medium, usually solid, that reveals the presence of two or more similar microorganisms by differences in the appearance of their colonies. Such a medium may or may not be selective also.

**DNase test agar,** an agar medium containing deoxyribonucleic acid, peptone, sodium chloride, and toluidine blue, used for differentiating strains of *Serratia, Enterobacter,* and *Staphylococcus.*

**egg-yolk agar,** an agar medium containing peptone, phosphate buffer, sodium chloride, magnesium sulfate, glucose, and egg-yolk emulsion, used for the culture of *Bacillus anthracis.* When supplemented with hemin or yeast extract it may be used for the culture of *Clostridium* and for the demonstration of lecithinase and lipase activity.

**enriched c. m.,** a basic medium to which specific nutrients, e.g., serum, blood, and vitamins, have been added to promote the growth of particular organisms.

**eosin–methylene blue (EMB) agar,** an agar medium containing peptone, lactose, eosin Y, methylene blue, and dipotassium phosphate; sucrose may be added. It is used for the primary isolation of species of Enterobacteriaceae.

**esculin c. m.,** an agar medium containing heart infusion, peptone, sodium chloride, ferric citrate, and esculin, used to differentiate *Escherichia* from *Shigella.*

**FDA medium,** 1. antibiotic c. 3 FDA. 2. antibiotic c. 12 FDA.

**Feeley-Gorman (F-G) agar,** an agar medium containing casein hydrolysate, beef extract, starch, L-cysteine, and ferric pyrophosphate, used for the culture of *Legionella.* A broth culture without the agar is also used for the same purpose.

**fermentation medium,** a basal medium containing no carbohydrate to which is added a single sugar to be tested for fermentability.

**Fildes enrichment agar,** a sterile enzymatic digest of sheep blood added to liquid or solid culture media for the cultivation and isolation of *Haemophilus influenzae* and fastidious streptococci.

**Fletcher medium,** a liquid culture medium containing peptone, and beef extract enriched with 20 per cent fresh pooled rabbit serum, for the isolation, cultivation, and maintenance of *Leptospira.*

**gelatin c. m.,** a medium containing extract or infusion broth solidified with 12 per cent gelatin, used to determine gelatinase activity in the identification of *Serratia* and *Clostridium.* The medium may be supplemented with thioglycolate for cultivation of *Clostridium* in an aerobic environment.

**gram-negative (GN) broth,** a liquid medium containing peptone, glucose, D-mannitol, sodium citrate, sodium desoxycholate, sodium chloride, and phosphate buffer, used as an enrichment medium for the primary culture of salmonellae and shigellae in fecal specimens.

**heart infusion agar,** an agar medium containing beef heart infusion, peptone, and sodium chloride, used as a base for blood agar and esculin agar.

**Hektoen enteric (HE) agar,** an agar medium containing peptone, bile salts, yeast extract, lactose, sucrose, salicin, sodium chloride, sodium thiosulfate, ferric ammonium citrate, acid fuchsin, and bromthymol blue. It is a selective medium used for the primary isolation and identification of enteric pathogens, especially coliform organisms, salmonellae, and shigellae.

**infusion medium,** a medium containing infusion of fresh meat (commonly veal or beef), peptone, and sodium chloride, used as a liquid medium (broth) or solidified with agar, used for the culture of fastidious bacteria and as a base for enriched media.

**kanamycin-vancomycin blood agar,** an agar medium containing casein digest, soybean meal digest, sodium chloride, yeast extract, sheep blood, L-cystine, vitamin $K_1$, kanamycin, and vancomycin, used for selective isolation of anaerobes, particularly *Bacteroides.*

**kanamycin-vancomycin laked blood (KVLB) agar,** an agar medium having the same ingredients as kanamycin-vancomycin blood agar except that the blood is laked (hemolyzed) by freezing and thawing. It is used to isolate the *Bacteroides melaninogenicus* group.

**Kligler iron agar,** triple sugar iron agar.

**laked blood (LB) agar,** a solid culture medium containing blood that has been hemolyzed to release hemin.

**litmus-milk c. m.,** milk culture medium containing sufficient litmus solution to give it a deep lavender color, used to determine lactose fermentation and production of gas in the identification of *Clostridium perfringens.*

**Littman agar,** an agar medium containing peptone, oxgall, glucose, and crystal violet. Streptomycin may be added to inhibit bacteria, and the medium may be supplemented with birdseed extract. It is used for the isolation and culture of fungi.

**Loeffler coagulated serum medium,** a culture medium containing veal infusion, beef serum, and glucose, solidified by coagulation of the serum, used for the isolation of *Corynebacterium diphtheriae.*

**Löwenstein-Jensen c. m.,** a solid medium containing asparagine, potato flour, glycerol, magnesium sulfate, malachite green, magnesium citrate, and whole eggs, used for the primary isolation of mycobacteria; the medium is solidified by heat coagulation of the egg.

**lysine-iron agar,** an agar medium containing peptone, yeast extract, glucose, L-lysine, ferric ammonium citrate, sodium thiosulfate, and bromcresol purple, used to determine lysine decarboxylase and lysine deaminase in the Enterobacteriaceae, especially for the genera *Proteus* and *Providencia.*

**McBride Listeria medium,** an agar medium containing peptone, beef extract, sodium chloride, glycine anhydride, lithium chloride, and phenylethanol, used for the cultivation of *Listeria.*

**MacConkey (MC) agar,** an agar medium containing peptone, lactose bile salts, sodium chloride, neutral red, and crystal violet, used to differentiate lactose fermenters (coliforms) from non–lactose fermenters among the enteric bacilli.

**malt extract agar,** an agar medium containing malt extract, peptone, and glucose, used for the cultivation of yeasts and molds.

**mannitol salt agar,** an agar medium containing beef extract, peptone, mannitol, phenol red, and 7.5 per cent sodium chloride, used for the selective isolation of pathogenic staphylococci.

**Martin-Lester agar, Martin-Lewis agar,** a modification of chocolate agar containing antibiotics, used for the transport and primary isolation of *Neisseria gonorrhoeae* and *N. meningitidis.*

**meat extract medium,** one prepared with an extract from meat.

**meat infusion medium,** see *infusion m.*

**methylene blue milk c. m.,** a liquid medium containing skim milk powder and methylene blue, used in the identification of *Streptococcus.*

**methyl red–Voges-Proskauer (MR-VP) broth,** a broth culture medium containing peptone, glucose, and phosphate, used for the culture of coliform bacteria and differentiation by the methyl red and Voges-Proskauer tests.

**Middlebrook 7H10 agar,** a complex agar medium containing ammonium sulfate, D-glutamic acid, sodium citrate, ferric ammonium phosphate, magnesium sulfate, pyridoxine, biotin, malachite green, and phosphate buffer. OADC enrichment, containing oleic acid, albumin, glucose, and beef catalase, is added. The medium is used for the primary isolation of mycobacteria and for antimicrobial susceptibility testing.

**milk c. m.,** fresh or dehydrated skim milk used as a culture medium. See also *litmus-milk c.* and *methylene blue milk c.*

**motility test medium,** a culture medium containing beef extract and peptone, partially solidified by the inclusion of 0.4 per cent agar, used for the detection of motility of Enterobacteriaceae. A medium containing pancreatic casein digest, yeast extract, sodium chloride, and 0.3 per cent agar is used to determine motility in nonfermenting gram-negative bacteria.

**MR-VP broth,** methyl red–Voges-Proskauer b.

**Mueller-Hinton medium,** an agar medium containing beef infusion, peptone, and starch, used for the primary isolation of *Neisseria gonorrhoeae* and *N. meningitidis,* and for antibiotic and sulfonamide susceptibility testing. A broth medium (MHB), prepared by omitting the agar, is used to determine antibiotic susceptibility by broth dilution testing.

**Mueller-Hinton-IH agar,** an agar medium containing beef infusion, casein hydrolysate, starch, hemoglobin, and a complex enrichment supplement, used for the culture of *Legionella.*

**Mycoplasma isolation c. m.,** an agar medium containing beef heart infusion, peptone, sodium chloride, horse extract, yeast extract, and penicillin; thallium acetate and amphotericin B may also be added to reduce bacterial and fungal contamination. A broth culture is made by omitting the agar. It is used for the culture and isolation of mycoplasmas.

**nitrate broth,** nutrient broth containing sodium nitrate, for testing for the bacterial reduction of nitrate to nitrite.

**nutrient c. m.,** a bacterial culture medium containing beef extract and peptone, used as a liquid medium (nutrient broth) or solidified with agar (nutrient agar, plain agar) for the culture of nonfastidious organisms.

**NYC medium,** [*N*ew *Y*ork *C*ity] an agar medium containing protease peptone, cornstarch, phosphate buffer, horse plasma, hemoglobin, glucose, yeast dialysate, vancomycin, colistin, nystatin or amphotericin, and trimethoprim lactate, used as a selective medium for *Neisseria.*

**nystatin assay agar,** antibiotic c. 12 FDA.

**oatmeal–tomato paste agar,** an agar medium containing strained oatmeal and tomato paste, used for the formation of ascospores in dermatophyte fungi.

**oxidation-fermentation (OF) medium,** an agar medium containing peptone, sodium chloride, bromthymol blue, potassium buffers, and glucose; lactose, mannitol, or sucrose may be used instead of glucose. The medium is used to distinguish oxidative from fermentative utilization of carbohydrates, a characteristic used to differentiate *Acinetobacter, Alcaligenes,* and *Pseudomonas* from the Enterobacteriaceae.

**peptone–yeast extract–glucose (PYG) medium,** a liquid medium containing peptone, yeast extract, glucose, resazurin, L-cysteine, and salts, used as a transport medium for anaerobes. It may be supplemented with hemin and vitamin $K_1$, and used to prepare broth cultures of anaerobes for gas-liquid chromatography.

**Petragnani c. m.,** a culture medium containing milk, potato flour, potato, whole egg and egg yolk, and malachite green, for the culture of tubercle bacilli; the medium is solidified by heat coagulation of the egg.

**phenol red medium,** a liquid medium containing peptone, sodium chloride, and phenol red, used as a base medium supplemented with various sugars for determining fermentation reactions.

**phenylalanine agar,** an agar medium containing yeast extract, DL-phenylalanine, disodium phosphate, and sodium chloride, used to test for phenylalanine deaminase activity by members of the Enterobacteriaceae, especially species of *Proteus* and *Providencia.*

**phenylethyl alcohol (PEA) blood agar,** an agar medium containing pancreatic digest of casein, papain digest of soybean meal, sodium chloride, and phenylethyl alcohol. Defibrinated blood may be added. It is used for the isolation of gram-positive cocci, especially in a mixed culture containing *Proteus* or other gram-negative bacilli.

**potato blood agar,** Bordet-Gengou a.

**potato dextrose agar,** a culture medium containing potato infusion and glucose (dextrose), for culturing and inducing sporulation in molds.

**PRAS medium,** prereduced and anaerobically sterilized media, used for the culture of anaerobes. See *Cary-Blair transport m.* and *peptone–yeast extract–glucose m.*

**purple broth base,** a broth medium containing peptone, beef extract, sodium chloride, and bromcresol purple, used as a base to which is added a sugar supplement for use in fermentation studies.

**rice grain medium,** a medium containing water and polished white rice that is autoclaved; used for the differentiation of species of *Microspora* and other dermatophytes.

**rice-Tween agar,** an agar medium containing cream of rice and Tween-80 (polysorbate 80), used for the development of chlamydospores in *Candida* and other fungi.

**Rogosa selective Lactobacillus (SL) agar,** a selective culture medium containing tryptone, yeast extract, glucose, arabinose, sucrose, acetate, citrate, sorbitan monooleate, phosphate buffer, and agar, used in the culture and presumptive identification of lactobacilli.

**Sabhi agar,** [*Sab*ouraud's dextrose and *b*rain *h*eart *i*nfusion] an agar medium containing brain infusion, heart infusion, gelatin digest, glucose, sodium chloride, peptone, and phosphate buffer; chloramphenicol may be added. It is used for isolating clinically important fungi.

**Sabouraud dextrose (SAB) agar,** an agar medium containing glucose, peptone, pancreatic digest of casein, and peptic digest of animal tissue; antibiotics may be added. Used for the cultivation and identification of fungi.

**Salmonella-Shigella (SS) agar,** a selective differential culture medium containing beef extract, peptone, lactose, bile salts, sodium and ferric citrates, thiosulfate neutral red, and brilliant green, used for the primary isolation of enteric bacilli, especially *Salmonella* and *Shigella.*

**selective c. m.,** a liquid or solid culture medium that contains inhibitory substances (antibiotics, dyes, tellurite, bile salts, etc.) that allow the growth of the desired microorganism while inhibiting the growth of contaminants.

**selenite broth,** a liquid medium containing peptone, lactose, phosphate, and sodium selenite, used as an enrichment medium for the isolation of *Salmonella* and *Shigella.*

**semisolid c. m.,** 1. a culture medium containing 0.3 to 0.5 per cent agar to give it a semisolid consistency; see *motility test medium.* 2. a culture medium containing agar or gelatin that is liquid in the warm state and solid when cooled.

**Simmons citrate agar,** citrate a. (Simmons).

**sodium chloride (6.5 per cent) c. m.,** a broth medium containing beef heart infusion, peptone, and 6.5 per cent sodium chloride, used for the selective culture of enterococci (especially group D streptococci) and other salt-tolerant organisms. Nutrient broth or soybean-casein digest agar supplemented with 6.5 per cent sodium chloride is also used for *Pseudomonas* and other nonfermenting gram-negative bacteria.

**soybean casein digest agar,** an agar medium containing pancreatic casein digest, papaic soybean meal digest, and sodium chloride; used as a general purpose primary isolation medium and as a base for blood agar.

**Staib agar,** an agar medium containing an extract of *Guizottia abyssinica* seeds, creatinine, glucose, chloramphenicol, and diphenyl, used for the identification of the yeast *Cryptococcus neoformans.* Called also *birdseed a.*

**starch agar,** an agar medium containing peptone, beef extract, sodium chloride, and soluble starch, used for determining hydrolysis of starch. Bromcresol purple may be included for identification of *Haemophilus vaginalis.*

**Stuart broth, modified,** a culture medium containing inorganic salts, asparagine, and glycerol, enriched with rabbit serum and used for the isolation and culture of *Leptospira.*

**tellurite taurocholate gelatin agar,** a selective agar medium containing sodium taurocholate, potassium tellurite, and sodium carbonate, used for the isolation of *Vibrio.*

**tetrathionate broth,** a liquid medium containing peptone, bile salts, calcium carbonate, and sodium thiosulfate, which is converted to tetrathionate by the addition of iodine immediately before use, used as a selective medium for the isolation of *Salmonella* other than *S. typhi.*

**Thayer-Martin (TM) agar,** chocolate agar enriched with vitamins and other supplements, to which is added antibiotic inhibitors (vancomycin, colistin, and nystatin), used for the transport and primary culture of *Neisseria gonorrhoeae* and *N. meningitidis.*

**thioglycolate (THIO) broth,** a liquid medium containing peptone, glucose, sodium chloride, sodium thioglycolate, L-cystine, sodium sulfite, and 0.7 per cent agar, enriched with rabbit serum. It is used as a general utility medium for the growth of both aerobic and anaerobic bacteria. Methylene blue may be added as a redox indicator, and the medium may be enriched with yeast extract, vitamin $K_1$, and hemin. Spelled also *thioglycollate b.*

**thiosulfate citrate bile salts sucrose (TCBS) agar,** a selective medium containing peptone, yeast extract, citrate, thiosulfate, oxgall, sodium cholate, sucrose, sodium chloride, ferric citrate bromthymol blue, and thymol blue, used for the isolation of *Vibrio cholerae* and *V. parahaemolyticus.*

**Tindale's agar,** a base composed of proteose-peptone, sodium chloride, and agar to which is added an enrichment of bovine serum, L-cystine, sodium thiosulfate, and potassium tellurite; used to detect *Corynebacterium diphtheriae,* which form grayish-black colonies surrounded by a black halo.

**Todd-Hewitt broth,** a liquid medium containing beef heart infusion, peptone, glucose, sodium chloride, sodium bicarbonate, and phosphate buffer, used for growing streptococci for serological grouping.

**transport medium,** a medium used for transport of clinical specimens for bacteriological examination. See *Amies transport m., buffered glycerol-saline ba. (Sachs), Cary-Blair transport m.,* and *peptone–yeast extract–glucose m.*

**triple sugar iron (TSI) agar,** an agar medium containing peptone, lactose, sucrose, glucose, ferrous ammonium sulfate, sodium thiosulfate, sodium chloride, and phenol red, used for the preliminary screening of Enterobacteriaceae. Production of hydrogen sulfide causes the formation of black ferrous sulfide along the stab line, gas production causes bubbles in the agar, and fermentation of the sugars is indicated by the amount of acid produced.

**trypticase soy broth with agar,** a medium containing a trypsin digest of soybean meal, peptone, sodium chloride, phosphate buffer, and glucose with 0.1 per cent agar, used for the primary culture of fastidious bacteria, including anaerobes.

**tyrosine xanthine agar,** an agar medium containing nutrient agar and tyrosine or xanthine, used for differentiation of species of aerobic actinomycetes.

**urea agar of Christensen,** Christensen's urea a.

**urease test broth,** the medium used in the urease test (q.v.); a liquid medium containing yeast extract, urea, phenol red, and phosphate buffer, used to determine urease activity in the differentiation of *Proteus* from *Salmonella* and *Shigella* in enteric infections. See also *Christensen's urea a.*

**veal infusion c. m.,** see *infusion m.*

**Wilson-Blair c. m.,** bismuth sulfite a.

**xylose-lysine-deoxycholate (XLD) agar,** an agar medium containing xylose, L-lysine, lactose, sucrose, sodium chloride, yeast extract, phenol red, sodium desoxycholate, sodium thiosulfate, and ferric ammonium citrate, used for isolating intestinal pathogens, especially *Shigella* and *Salmonella.*

**yeast extract agar,** an agar medium containing yeast extract and phosphate buffer, used for identification of *Histoplasma capsulatum, Blastomyces dermatitidis,* and *Coccidioides immitis.*

**cu mm** cubic millimeter.

**cu·mu·la·tive** (ku'mu-lə-tiv) [L. *cumulus* heap] increasing by successive additions, the total being greater than the expected sum of its parts.

**cu·mu·li** (ku'mu-li) [L.] genitive and plural of *cumulus.*

**cu·mu·lus** (ku'mu-ləs) pl. *cu'muli* [L.] a little mound, usually formed by a collection of cells.
**c. oo'phorus, ovarian c., c. ova'ricus,** a solid mass of follicular cells surrounding the ovum in the side of a developing vesicular ovarian follicle; called also *discus oophorus, ovigerus,* or *proligerus.*

**cu·ne·ate** (ku'ne-āt) [*cuneus* + *-ate*] wedge-shaped.

**cu·nei** (ku'ne-i) [L.] genitive and plural of *cuneus.*

**cu·ne·i·form** (ku-ne'ĭ-form) [*cuneus* + *form*] shaped like a wedge.

**cu·neo·cu·boid** (ku"ne-o-ku'boid) pertaining to the cuneiform and cuboid bones.

**cu·neo·na·vic·u·lar** (ku"ne-o-nə-vik'u-lər) pertaining to the cuneiform and navicular bones.

**cu·neo·scaph·oid** (ku"ne-o-skaf'oid) cuneonavicular.

**cu·ne·us** (ku'ne-əs) pl. *cu'nei* [L. "wedge"] [TA] a wedge-shaped lobule of the occipital lobe of the cerebrum on its medial aspect, between the parietooccipital and calcarine sulci.

**cu·nic·u·li** (ku-nik'u-li) [L.] genitive and plural of *cuniculus.*

**Cu·nic·u·lus** (ku-nik'u-ləs) a genus of burrowing rodents found in tropical parts of the Americas. *C. pa'ca* is the paca.

**cu·nic·u·lus** (ku-nik'u-ləs) pl. *cunic'uli* [L. "rabbit," "rabbit-burrow"] 1. a tunnel. 2. the burrow of an itch mite, *Sarcoptes scabiei,* in the skin.
**c. exter'nus,** outer tunnel.
**c. inter'nus,** inner tunnel.
**c. me'dius,** a fluid-filled canal in the organ of Corti between the pillar cells and the outer hair cells; called also *Nuel's space.*

**cun·ni·linc·tus** (kun"ĭ-link'təs) cunnilingus.

**cun·ni·lin·gus** (kun"ĭ-ling'əs) [*cunnus* + *lingere* to lick] oral stimulation of the female genitalia.

**Cun·ning·ha·mel·la** (kun"ing-ham-el'ə) a genus of fungi of the family Cunninghamellaceae, characterized by a lack of a sporangium and by conidia that arise from a vesicle. *C. berthole'tiae* is a species that causes opportunistic mucormycosis of the lung in debilitated or immunocompromised patients, with progressive vascular invasion, thrombosis, and infarction.

**Cun·ning·ha·mel·la·ceae** (kun"ing-ham-əl-a'ce-e) a family of fungi of the order Mucorales, that lacks sporangia; it includes one pathogenic genus, *Cunninghamella.*

**cun·nus** (kun'əs) [L.] pudendum femininum.

**cup** (kup) 1. a cupping glass. 2. a cup-shaped part or structure.
**Diogenes' c.,** poculum Diogenis.

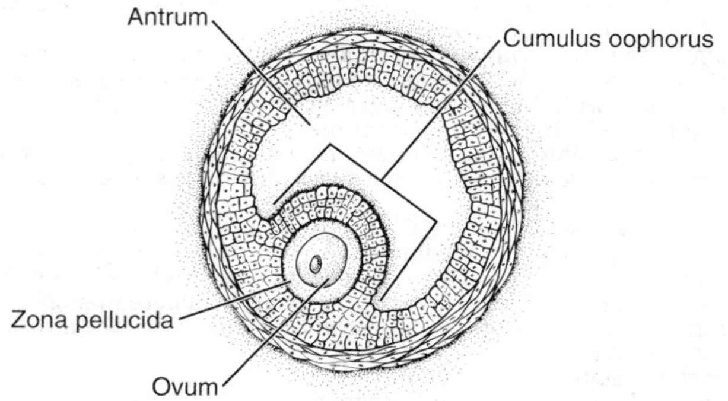


Cumulus oophorus surrounding an ovum in a developing ovarian follicle.

**dry c.,** a cupping glass applied to the intact skin in order to induce a flow of blood to the area; no longer used.
**glaucomatous c.,** a form of ocular disk depression peculiar to glaucoma; called also *glaucomatous excavation.*
**ocular c., ophthalmic c.,** caliculus ophthalmicus.
**optic c.,** 1. physiologic cup. 2. caliculus ophthalmicus.
**physiologic c.,** a depression in the center of the optic disk; called also *excavatio disci* [TA] and *optic c.*
**wet c.,** a cupping glass applied to the incised skin in order to abstract blood; no longer used.

**cu·po·la** (koo'pə-lə) cupula.

**cupped** (kupt) hollowed out like a cup.

**cup·ping** (kup'ing) 1. the application of a cupping glass. 2. the formation of a cup-shaped depression.
**pathologic c.,** depression of the optic disk due to disease.

**cu·pre·ine** (ku'pre-ēn) an alkaloid from cuprea bark that is related to cinchonidine and has antimalarial properties.

**cu·pre·mia** (koo-pre'me-ə) [L. *cuprum* copper + *-emia*] the presence of copper in the blood. See also *hypercupremia.*

**cu·pric** (koo'prik) containing copper in its divalent form (=Cu), and yielding divalent ions ($Cu^{2+}$) in aqueous solution. For cupric compounds, see under the salt, e.g., sulfate.

**Cup·ri·mine** (kup'rĭ-mēn) trademark for a preparation of penicillamine.

**cup·ri·myx·in** (kup"rĭ-mik'sin) a veterinary antibacterial and antifungal.

**cu·pri·uria** (koo"pre-u're-ə) the presence of copper in the urine.

**cu·pro·phane** (koo'pro-fān) a membrane made of regenerated cellulose, used in hemodialyzers.

**cu·prous** (koo'prəs) containing copper in its monovalent form ($Cu^{+}$).

**cu·pru·re·sis** (koo"proo-re'sis) [L. *cuprum* copper + *-uresis*] the urinary excretion of copper.

**cu·pru·ret·ic** (ku"proo-ret'ik) [L. *cuprum* copper + *uretic*] pertaining to or promoting the urinary excretion of copper.

**cu·pu·la** (koo'pu-lə) pl. *cu'pulae* [L.] a small inverted cup or dome-shaped cap over some structure.
**c. ampulla'ris** [TA], **c. of ampullary crest,** ampullary cupula: a cap of viscid, gelatinous fluid over the ampullary crest of the ear; in fixed material this cap stains slightly and is thus differentiated from the rest of the ampullar fluid. Called also *c. cristae ampullaris.*
**c. coch'leae** [TA], cupula of cochlea: the rounded or dome-shaped apex of the spiral cochlear duct.
**c. cris'tae ampulla'ris,** c. ampullaris.
**c. pleu'rae** [TA], **c. pleura'lis,** cupula of pleura: the domelike roof of the pleural cavity on either side, extending up through the superior aperture of the thorax.

**cu·pu·lae** (koo'pu-le) [L.] genitive and plural of *cupula.*

**cu·pu·lo·gram** (ku'pu-lo-gram") the record, in the form of a tracing, made during cupulometry.

**cu·pu·lo·li·thi·a·sis** (ku"pu-lo-lĭ-thi'ə-sis) the presence of calculi in the cupula of the posterior semicircular duct, a cause of benign paroxysmal positional vertigo.

**cu·pu·lom·e·try** (ku"pu-lom'ə-tre) a method of testing vestibular function in which subjects are accelerated and decelerated in a rotational chair and the duration of postrotational vertigo and nystagmus are plotted against angular deceleration.

**cu·ra·re** (koo-rah're) [South American Indian *Kurari*] [MeSH: Curare] a term applied to a wide variety of highly toxic extracts from numerous botanical sources, including various species of *Strychnos;* used originally as arrow poisons in South America. A form extracted from *Chondodendron tomentosum* has been used for the reduction of spasms in tetanus and in shock treatments, in plastic muscular rigidity, spastic paralysis, and similar conditions, and also as an adjunct to general anesthesia. Cf. *tubocurarine.*

**cu·ra·ri** (koo-rah're) curare.

**cu·ra·ri·form** (ku-rar′ĭ-form) resembling curare.

**cu·ra·ri·mi·met·ic** (koo-rah″re-mi-met′ik) having an action similar to that of curare, or producing similar effects.

**cu·rar·iza·tion** (ku″rər-ĭ-za′shən) administration of curare until the physiologic effect of the drug is produced.

**cur·a·tive** (kūr′ə-tiv) [L. *curare* to take care of] tending to overcome disease and promote recovery.

**curb** (kərb) a thickening of the metatarsocalcaneal ligament of the horse, causing a swelling at the back of the hock joint and resulting in lameness.

**Cur·cu·ma** (kər′ku-mə) a genus of plants of the family Zingiberaceae, native to India, China, and the East Indies. *C. lon′ga* L. is turmeric, which yields the coloring agent and condiment also called turmeric.

**cur·cu·min** (kər′ku-min) [MeSH: Curcumin] an orange-yellow crystalline substance, the coloring principle of turmeric.

**cure** (kūr) [L. *curatio,* from *cura* care] 1. the course of treatment of any disease, or of a special case. 2. the successful treatment of a disease or wound. 3. a system of treating diseases. 4. a medicine effective in treating a disease. 5. the preservation of a product, such as tobacco, meat, or fish. 6. the hardening of a material by the process of curing. 7. a procedure for polymerization of resins such as those used in denture base materials. See also *curing.*

**cu·ret** (ku-ret′) [Fr. *curette* scraper] 1. a spoon-shaped instrument for removing material from the wall of a cavity or other surface. 2. to remove growths or other material from the wall of a cavity or other surface with a spoon-shaped instrument.
**Hartmann's c.,** an instrument for removing adenoids.

**cu·ret·tage** (ku″rə-tahzh′) [Fr.] [MeSH: Curettage] the removal of growths or other material from the wall of a cavity or other surface, as with a curet; called also *curettement.*
**apical c.,** periapical c.
**gingival c.,** removal with a curet of the inflamed tissue wall of a periodontal pocket, including junctional and pocket epithelium and immediately underlying connective tissue. Called also *subgingival c.*
**medical c.,** the induction of bleeding from the endometrium by administration and withdrawal of any progestational agent.
**periapical c.,** removal with a curet of diseased pathological soft tissues in the bony crypt surrounding a tooth root apex and smoothing of the apical surface of a tooth without excision of the tooth tip. Called also *apical c.*
**subgingival c.,** 1. gingival curettage apical to the epithelial attachment to sever the connective tissue attachment down to the osseous crest without reflection of a flap. 2. gingival c.
**suction c.,** vacuum c.
**surgical c.,** a flap procedure to excise an inflamed periodontal pocket wall and the connective tissue attachment down to the osseous crest, followed by reattachment of the flap to the teeth. Called also *modified Widman flap.*
**ultrasonic c.,** removal of inflamed tissue from the tooth surface and wall of the gingival crevice with an ultrasonic scaler.
**vacuum c.,** removal of the uterine contents, after cervical dilation, by means of a hollow curet introduced into the uterus, through which suction is applied. Called also *suction c.* and *vacuum aspiration.*

**cu·rette** (ku-ret′) [Fr.] curet.

**cu·rette·ment** (ku-ret′ment) curettage.
**physiologic c.,** enzymatic débridement.

**Curie** (ku-re′) Marie Sklodowska. Polish-born chemist and physicist in France, 1867–1934. Discovered polonium and radium with her husband Pierre Curie and did pioneering work on radioactivity, including its medical use. Co-winner of Nobel prize in physics in 1903 with Pierre Curie and Henri Becquerel for studies on spontaneous radioactivity, and winner of Nobel prize in chemistry in 1911 for discovery and isolation of radium.

**Curie** (ku-re′) Pierre. French chemist and physicist, 1859–1906. Discovered polonium and radium with his wife Marie Curie and did pioneering work on radioactivity. Co-winner of Nobel prize in physics in 1903 with Marie Curie and Henri Becquerel for studies on spontaneous radioactivity.

**Cu·rie's law** (ku-rēz′) [P. *Curie*] see under *law.*

**cu·rie** (ku′re) [M. and P. *Curie*] a unit of radioactivity, defined as the quantity of any radioactive nuclide in which the number of disintegrations per second is $3.700 \times 10^{10}$. Abbreviated Ci (formerly c).

**cu·rie-hour** (ku′re-our″) a unit of cumulated radioactivity equal to the presence of 1 curie for 1 hour. Abbreviated Ci-hr.

**cu·rie·ther·a·py** (ku″re-ther′ə-pe) originally, radium or radon therapy; but now applied to therapy given by emanations from any radioactive source.

**cur·ing** (kūr′ing) a method for promoting and accelerating hardening processes through the use of dampness, heat, cold, chemical agents, electromagnetic radiation, or other agents.
**denture c.,** the process by which resinous denture base materials are polymerized; see also *resin.*

**cu·ri·os·co·py** (ku″re-os′kə-pe) the detection and mapping of objects by means of the nuclear radiations coming from them.

**cu·ri·um** (ku′re-əm) [Pierre and Marie *Curie*] [MeSH: Curium] the chemical element of atomic number 96, atomic weight 247, symbol Cm, obtained by cyclotron bombardment of uranium and plutonium.

**curl·ing** (kər′ling) shaped like a curl or coil, as the appearance of the esophagus in diffuse esophageal spasm.

**Cur·ra·ri·no's tri·ad** (koo″rə-re′nōz) [Guido *Currarino,* Italian-born American radiologist, born 1920] see under *triad.*

**Cur·ra·ri·no-Sil·ver·man syndrome** (kər″ə-re′no sil′vər-mən) [G. *Currarino;* Frederic Noah *Silverman,* American pediatrician, born 1914] see under *syndrome.*

**cur·rent** (kur′ənt) [L. *currens* running] 1. anything that flows. 2. electric c.
**action c.,** the current generated in a cell membrane of a nerve or muscle by the action potential; it serves to depolarize adjacent membrane areas beyond the threshold, thus initiating a repetition of the action potential process along the nerve fiber. Called also *nerve-action c.*
**alternating c.,** a current that periodically flows in opposite directions. Abbreviated AC.
**ascending c.,** centripetal c.
**axial c.,** the core of rapid flow *(laminar flow)* in the center of a channel, as in the lumen of a blood vessel, bordered or surrounded by a zone in which the elements move more slowly or do not move at all.
**centrifugal c.,** an electric current in the body with the positive pole near the nerve center and the negative at the periphery; called also *descending c.*
**centripetal c.,** an electric current passing through the body with the positive electrode on the nerve or at the periphery and the negative electrode near the nerve center: called also *ascending c.*
**coagulating c.,** an electric current applied by a needle, ball, or other type of electrode to coagulate tissue.
**convection c.,** a current caused by movement by convection of warmer fluid into an area of cooler fluid.
**d'Arsonval c.,** a high-frequency, low-voltage current of comparatively high amperage. See also *high-frequency c.*
**demarcation c.,** c. of injury.
**descending c.,** centrifugal c.
**direct c.,** a current that flows in one direction only. When used medically it is called the galvanic current; this current has distinct and important polarity and marked secondary chemical effects.
**electric c.,** the stream of electricity that moves along a conductor. Symbol *I.* An electric current is due to a difference of potential between two points, this difference being measured in volts. The volume of flow depends on the difference of potential and the resistance to be overcome and is measured in amperes. The quantity of current is measured in coulombs.
**electrotonic c.,** a current induced in the sheath of a nerve by a current passing through the conducting part of that nerve, or by an action potential in an adjacent nerve.
**fulguration c.,** high-frequency current used in destruction of superficial skin lesions.
**galvanic c.,** a steady direct current.
**high-frequency c.,** an alternating current having a frequency of interruption or change of direction sufficiently high so that tetanic contractions are not set up when it is passed through living contractile tissues; see *d'Arsonval c.*
**induced c.,** electricity in a circuit generated by proximity to another current, i.e., by induction.
**c. of injury,** a flow of electric current to or from the injured region of an ischemic heart, due to regional alteration in transmembrane potential. See also *diastolic c. of injury* and *systolic c. of injury.*
**c. of injury, diastolic,** net current flow from ischemic to normal cardiac tissue during diastole, due to more rapid repolarization of the injured region and thus a more positive transmembrane potential than in surrounding tissue. Cf. *systolic c. of injury.*
**c. of injury, systolic,** net current flow from normal to ischemic cardiac tissue during systole, due to a decrease in the amplitude and duration of the action potential so that the transmembrane potential of the ischemic tissue is less negative than that of surrounding tissue. Cf. *diastolic c. of injury.*
**nerve-action c.,** action c.
**pacemaker c.,** the small net positive current flowing into certain cardiac cells, such as those of the sinoatrial node, causing them to depolarize.
**saturation c.,** the amount of current in an x-ray tube when the voltage is sufficient to drive all the electrons produced from the cathode filament to the anode as fast as they are produced.

**sinusoidal c.,** an alternating current whose form is that of a sine wave.
**surgical c.,** an electric current used to achieve surgical dissection or fulguration.

**cur·ric·u·la** (kər-ik′u-lə) [L.] plural of *curriculum.*

**cur·ric·u·lum** (kər-ik′u-ləm) pl. *curric′ula* [L.] [MeSH: Curriculum] a regular and established course of study.

**Cursch·mann's spiral** (ko͞orsh′mahnz) [Heinrich *Curschmann,* German physician, 1846–1910] see under *spiral.*

**Cursch·mann-Bat·ten-Stei·nert syndrome** (koorsh′mahn bat′ən shti′nərt) [Hans *Curschmann,* German physician, 1875–1950; Frederick Eustace *Batten,* English ophthalmologist, 1865–1918; Hans *Steinert,* German physician, early 20th century] myotonic dystrophy; see under *dystrophy.*

**curse** (kərs) an infliction thought to be invoked by a malevolent spirit.
**Ondine's c.,** primary alveolar hypoventilation.

**Cur·ti·us' syndrome** (koor′te-us) [Friedrich *Curtius,* German internist, born 1896] see under *syndrome.*

**cur·va·tu·ra** (kər″və-tu′rə) gen. and pl. *curvatu′rae* [L.] [TA] curvature: a nonangular deviation from a straight course in a line or surface.
**c. gas′trica ma′jor,** c. major gastris.
**c. gas′trica mi′nor,** c. minor gastris.
**c. ma′jor gas′tris** [TA], greater curvature of stomach: the left or lateral and inferior border of the stomach, marking the inferior junction of the anterior and posterior surfaces. Called also *greater gastric curvature.*
**c. mi′nor gas′tris** [TA], lesser curvature of stomach: the right or medial border of the stomach, marking the superior junction of the anterior and posterior surfaces. Called also *lesser gastric curvature.*
**c. ventricula′ris ma′jor,** c. major gastris.
**c. ventricula′ris mi′nor,** c. minor gastris.

**cur·va·ture** (kər′və-chər″) [L. *curvatura*] deviation from a rectilinear direction.
**compensating c.,** see under *curve.*
**gastric c., greater,** curvatura major gastris.
**gastric c., lesser,** curvatura minor gastris.
**greater c. of stomach,** curvatura major gastris.
**lesser c. of stomach,** curvatura minor gastris.
**occlusal c.,** curve of occlusion (def. 1); see under *curve.*
**Pott's c.,** abnormal posterior curvature of the vertebral column caused by tuberculous caries.
**Spee's c., c. of Spee,** see under *curve.*
**spinal c.,** deviation of the spine from its normal direction or position; see *kyphosis, lordosis,* and *scoliosis.*

**curve** (kərv) [L. *curvum*] a nonangular deviation from a straight course in a line or surface.
**alignment c.,** the dental curve determined by a line passing through the center of the teeth and paralleling the dental arch.
**anti-Monson c.,** reverse c.
**audibility c.,** a plotting of the relationship between frequency and the intensity of sound waves necessary to elicit a sensation.
**Barnes' c.,** the segment of a circle whose center is the promontory of the sacrum, the concavity being directed dorsally.
**bell-shaped c.,** the curve of the probability density function of the normal distribution (q.v.).
**Bragg c.,** a curve showing the increase in intensity of ionization produced by an ionizing particle as it loses velocity and energy; see also *Bragg peak,* under *peak.*
**buccal c.,** the portion of the curve of occlusion from the mesial surface of the first premolar to the distal surface of the third molar.
**cardiac output c.,** a graphic representation of cardiac output as a function of atrial pressure; it is a measure of the pumping ability of the heart under specific conditions. See also *Starling c.* and *venous return c.*
**c. of Carus,** the normal axis of the pelvic outlet; called also *circle of Carus.*
**compensating c.,** the curve introduced in the construction of artificial dentures to compensate for the opening influence produced by the condylar and incisal guidances during lateral and protrusive mandibular excursive movements. Called also *compensating curvature.*
**dental c.,** 1. c. of occlusion (def. 1). 2. curvea occlusalis.
**dissociation c.,** see *oxygen dissociation c.*
**dose-effect c.,** a graphic representation of the effect (such as therapeutic response or the incidence of cancer) plotted against the dose of an agent (such as a drug or x-rays), showing the relationship of the effect to changes in the dose of the agent. See illustrations at *efficacy* and *potency.* Cf. *dose-frequency c.* and *dose-intensity c.*
**dose-frequency c.,** a graphic representation of the relationship of the number of responses (such as cases of cancer) in a population to changes in the dose of an agent.
**dose-intensity c.,** a graphic representation of the relationship of the intensity of effect (such as amount of vasodilation) in an individual to changes in the dose of an agent.
**dose-response c.,** dose-effect c.
**dromedary c.,** a temperature or other curve showing two phases of elevation separated by a phase of depression.
**dye dilution c.,** an indicator dilution curve in which the indicator is a dye, usually indocyanine green; it is used in studies of cardiac output and other aspects of cardiovascular function.
**Frank-Starling c.,** Starling c.
**gaussian c.,** bell-shaped c.
**growth c.,** the curve obtained by plotting increase in size or numbers against the elapsed time, as a measure of the growth of a child, or the multiplication of microorganisms.
**Harrison's c.,** see under *groove.*
**indicator dilution c.,** a graphic representation of the concentration of an indicator added in known quantity to the circulatory system and measured over time at a specific point in the system; the indicator is usually a dye (see *dye dilution c.*), radionuclide, or cold liquid (see *thermodilution*), and the curve is used in studies of cardiovascular function.
**isodose c's,** diagrams delimiting body areas receiving equal quantities of radiation in radiotherapy.
**isovolume pressure-flow c.,** a curve generated by plotting various values of pressures against the corresponding airflows at a single lung volume. At high lung volumes (approaching total lung capacity), the maximum flow or flow limitation is usually not reached. See illustration.
**Kaplan-Meier survival c.,** a consistent estimate of the survival curve that can be computed from randomly censored data. At each patient death (or other endpoint) the conditional probability of survival during the interval since the last death is calculated as the number of patients observed to survive beyond that point (i.e., those who have not yet died and have not left the trial for other reasons) divided by the number at risk. The value of the survival curve at that point is calculated as the product of the conditional probabilities of survival for all of the intervals up to that point. Called also *product-limit estimate.*
**labial c.,** that portion of the curve of occlusion between the distal surfaces of the two canine teeth in the dental arch.
**logistic c.,** an S-shaped curve that describes population growth under limiting conditions as a function of time; when the population is low, growth begins slowly, then becomes rapid and increases exponentially, finally slowing down and reaching equilibrium as the population reaches the maximum that the environment can support.
**maximal expiratory flow–volume c.,** a curve generated during forced expiration from total lung capacity to residual volume by plotting maximal expiratory flow against the corresponding lung volumes; it can also be constructed from a series of isovolume pressure-flow curves at different vital capacities. See illustration.
**Monson c.,** a curve of occlusion conforming to a segment of the surface of a sphere 8 inches in diameter, with its center in the region of the glabella. See also *compensating c.*
**normal c., normal c. of distribution,** bell-shaped c.
**occlusal c.,** curvea occlusalis.
**c. of occlusion,** 1. a curved surface that makes simultaneous contact with major portions of the incisal and occlusal prominences of the existing teeth. Called also *dental c.* and *occlusal curvature.* 2. curvea occlusalis.
**oxygen dissociation c.,** a graphic curve representing the normal variation in the amount of oxygen that combines with hemoglobin as a function of the partial pressure of oxygen. The curve is said to shift to the right *(the Bohr effect)* when less than a normal amount of oxygen is taken up by the blood at a given $Po_2$, and to shift to the left *(the Haldane effect)* when more than a normal amount is taken up. Factors influencing the shape of the curve include changes in

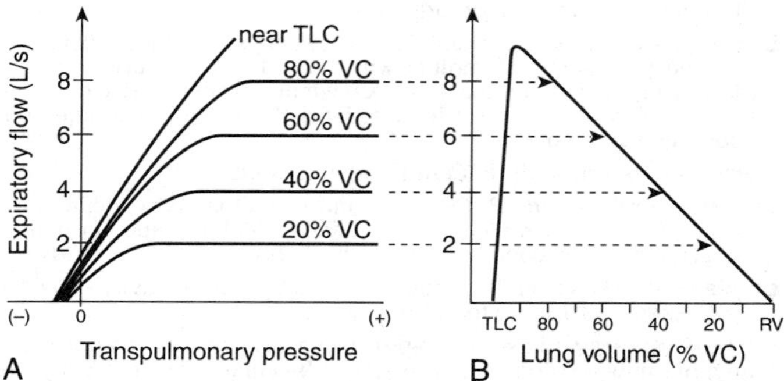


Series of isovolume pressure-flow curves *(A),* from which can be constructed a maximal expiratory flow-volume curve *(B).*

the blood pH, $P_{CO_2}$, and temperature, the presence of carbon monoxide, alterations in the constituents of the erythrocytes, and certain disease states. Called also *oxygen-hemoglobin dissociation c.*
**oxygen-hemoglobin dissociation c., oxyhemoglobin dissociation c.,** oxygen dissociation c.
**Price-Jones c.,** a frequency distribution curve of erythrocyte diameters, calculated electronically with a Coulter counter, a flow cytometer, or a similar instrument; it can detect conditions such as *macrocytic anemia* and *microcytic anemia.*
**pulse c.,** sphygmogram.
**receiver operating characteristic c.,** one plotting sensitivity versus [1 − specificity (or false-positive error rate)] to help determine the best cutoff point or points for demarcating dimensional data in diagnostic tests for disease, optimizing the balance between sensitivity and specificity.
**regression c.,** a curve describing the relation between the average value of one variable (the dependent variable) and the values of one or more independent variables; the regression curve of $Y$ on $X$ is the graph of the average value of $Y$ associated with each value of $X$.
**reverse c.,** in excessive wear of the teeth, obliteration of the cusps and formation of either flat or cupped-out occlusal surfaces, associated with reversal of the occlusal plane of the premolar and first and second molar teeth, so that the occlusal surfaces of the mandibular teeth slope facially instead of lingually, and those of the maxillary teeth incline lingually. Called also *anti-Monson c.*
**ROC c.,** receiver operating characteristic c.
**Spee c., c. of Spee,** anatomic curvature of the occlusal alignment of teeth, beginning at the tip of the lower canine, following the buccal cusps of the natural premolars and molars, and continuing to the anterior border of the ramus. Called also *Spee's curvature* and *curvature of Spee.*
**Starling c.,** a graphic representation of cardiac output, or other measure of ventricular performance, as a function of ventricular filling for a given level of contractility; as atrial pressure and venous return increase, cardiac output initially increases proportionately, then plateaus and decreases. Called also *ventricular function c.*
**strength-duration c.,** a graphic representation of the relationship between the intensity of an electric stimulus at the motor point of a muscle and the length of time it must flow to elicit a minimal contraction; see also *chronaxy* and *rheobase.*
**survival c.,** a graph of the probability of survival versus time, commonly used to present the results of clinical trials, e.g., a graph of the fraction of patients surviving (until death, relapse, or some other defined endpoint) at each time after a certain therapeutic procedure; see also *life table,* under *table.*
**temperature c.,** a graphic tracing showing variations in body temperature.
**tension c's,** lines observed in the arrangement of the cancellous tissue of bones, depending on the directions of tension exerted on the bones.
**thermal dilution c., thermodilution c.,** the graphic representation of results obtained with thermodilution.
**venous return c.,** a graphic representation of venous return as a function of atrial pressure; it measures the contributions of peripheral factors that affect the flow of blood from the veins to the heart. Multiple curves generated under varying conditions are combined with similarly obtained cardiac output curves (q.v.) to analyze cardiac regulation.
**ventricular function c.,** Starling c.
**visibility c.,** a plotting of the relationship between wavelength and the intensity of light necessary to elicit a sensation.
**c. of Wilson,** the curvature of the cusps of the teeth as projected on the frontal plane; that of the inferior dental arch is concave and that of the superior dental arch is convex.
**Wunderlich's c.,** the typical variation shown by the temperature in a patient with typhoid fever.

**cur·vea** (kər′ve-ə) curve.
**c. occlusa′lis** [TA], occlusal curve: the curve of a dentition on which the occlusal surfaces lie. Called also *curve of occlusion.*

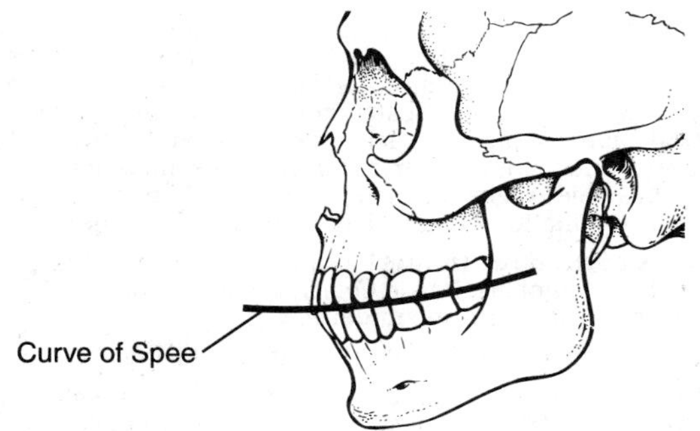


**Cur·vu·la·ria** (kər-vu-lar′e-ə) a genus of Fungi Imperfecti of the form-class Hyphomycetes, form-family Dematiaceae, commonly found in soil and elsewhere. *C. genicula′ta, C. luna′ta, C. palles′cens,* and *C. senegalen′sis* have been isolated from human eumycotic mycetoma and other infections. The perfect (sexual) stage of *Curvularia* species is in genus *Cochliobolus.*

**CUSA** [*C*avitron *U*ltrasonic *S*urgical *A*spirator] trademark for an ultrasonic dissector and aspirator used in hepatic resection.

**cus·cam·i·dine** (kəs-kam′ĭ-dēn) a cinchona alkaloid.

**cus·cam·ine** (kəs-kam′ēn) a cinchona alkaloid.

**Cush·ing's disease, phenomenon, syndrome, ulcer** (koosh′ingz) [Harvey Williams *Cushing,* American surgeon, 1869–1939] see under *disease, phenomenon, syndrome,* and *ulcer.*

**Cush·ing's suture** (koosh′ingz) [Hayward W. *Cushing,* American surgeon, 1854–1934] see under *suture.*

**Cush·ing-Ro·ki·tan·sky ul·cers** (koosh′ing ro″kĭ-tahn′ske) [Harvey W. *Cushing;* Karl Freiherr von *Rokitansky,* Austrian pathologist, 1804–1878] Rokitansky-Cushing ulcers.

**cush·ing·oid** (koosh′ing-oid) resembling the features, symptoms, and signs associated with Cushing's syndrome.

**cush·ion** (koosh′ən) a fleshy, padlike anatomical structure.
**coronary c.,** see under *band.*
**digital c.,** a wedge-shaped mass of white and elastic fibers, containing fat and cartilage, overlying the frog of a horse's foot. Called also *plantar c.*
**endocardial c's,** elevations of embryonic connective tissue covered by endothelium bulging into the atrioventricular canal of the embryonic heart, which later fuse with the free edge of the septum primum to separate the right and left atria.
**c. of epiglottis,** tuberculum epiglotticum.
**eustachian c.,** torus tubarius.
**intimal c's,** longitudinal thickenings of the intima of certain arteries, e.g., the penile arteries, formed by prominent local concentrations of smooth muscle fibers; they serve functionally as valves, controlling blood flow by occluding the lumen of the artery.
**Passavant's c.,** see under *bar.*
**plantar c.,** digital c.
**sucking c.,** corpus adiposum buccae.

**cusp** (kusp) [L. *cuspis* point] a tapering projection; especially one of the triangular segments of a cardiac valve or a dental cusp.
**anterior c. of mitral valve,** cuspis anterior valvae atrioventricularis sinistrae.
**anterior c. of pulmonary valve,** valvula semilunaris anterior valvae trunci pulmonalis.
**anterior c. of tricuspid valve.,** cuspis anterior valvae atrioventricularis dextrae.
**c's of aortic valve,** semilunar c's of aortic valve.
**Carabelli c.,** an accessory cusp on the lingual aspect of the mesiolingual cusp of an upper molar, which may be unilateral or bilateral and may vary considerably in size; it is common in Caucasians but quite rare in East Asians and certain other groups. Called also *Carabelli's tubercle.*
**commissural c's,** cuspides commissurales.
**dental c.,** cuspis dentis.
**infundibular c. of tricuspid valve,** cuspis anterior valvae atrioventricularis dextrae.
**left c. of aortic valve,** valvula semilunaris sinistra aortae.
**left c. of pulmonary valve,** valvula semilunaris sinistra valvae trunci pulmonalis.
**marginal c. of tricuspid valve,** cuspis posterior valvae atrioventricularis dextrae.
**medial c. of tricuspid valve,** cuspis septalis valvae atrioventricularis dextrae.
**posterior c. of aortic valve,** valvula semilunaris posterior aortae.
**posterior c. of mitral valve,** cuspis posterior valvae atrioventricularis sinistrae.
**posterior c. of tricuspid valve,** cuspis posterior valvae atrioventricularis dextrae.
**c's of pulmonary valve,** semilunar c's of pulmonary valve.
**right c. of aortic valve,** valvula semilunaris dextra valvae aortae.
**right c. of pulmonary valve,** valvula semilunaris dextra valvae trunci pulmonalis.
**semilunar c.,** any of the semilunar segments of the aortic or pulmonary valves; called also *valvula semilunaris.*
**semilunar c's of aortic valve,** the three semilunar cusps surrounding the orifice of the aortic valve. They are officially designated *right, left,* and *posterior* for their positions in the fetal heart (TA, *valvula semilunaris dextra aortae, sinistra aortae,* and *posterior aortae*), but they are sometimes termed *anterior, left posterior,* and *right posterior semilunar cusps,* respectively, for their positions in the adult heart, or *right coronary, left coronary,* and *non-coronary,* respectively, for their relations to orifices of the coronary sinuses.
**semilunar c's of pulmonary valve,** the three semilunar cusps sur-

rounding the orifice of the pulmonary trunk valve; officially designated *right, left,* and *anterior* for their positions in the fetal heart (TA, *valvula semilunaris dextra valvae trunci pulmonalis, sinistra valvae trunci pulmonalis,* and *anterior valvae trunci pulmonalis*), but they are sometimes termed *right anterior, posterior,* and *left anterior semilunar cusps,* respectively, for their positions in the adult heart.
**septal c. of tricuspid valve,** cuspis septalis valvae atrioventricularis dextrae.
**c. of tooth,** cuspis dentis.

**cus·pid** (kus′pid) [MeSH: Cuspid] 1. having one cusp or point. 2. canine tooth.

**cus·pi·date** (kus′pĭ-dāt) [L. *cuspidatus*] having a cusp or cusps.

**cus·pi·des** (kus′pĭ-dēz) [L.] plural of *cuspis.*

**cus·pis** (kus′pis) pl. *cus′pides* [L.] 1. [TA] a tapering projection or structure, applied especially to one of the triangular segments of a cardiac valve. 2. c. dentis.
**c. ante′rior val′vae atrioventricula′ris dex′trae** [TA], the anterior of the cusps of the right atrioventricular valve; called also *anterior cusp of tricuspid valve.*
**c. ante′rior val′vae atrioventricula′ris sinis′trae** [TA], the anterior of the cusps of the left atrioventricular valve; called also *anterior cusp of mitral valve.*
**cus′pides commisura′les** [TA], commissural cusps: two small cusps that form the two outer of the three scallops constituting the posterior cusp of the mitral valve. See also *c. posterior valvae atrioventricularis sinistrae.*
**c. coro′nae,** c. dentis.
**c. denta′lis, c. den′tis** [TA], cusp of tooth: an elevation or mound on the crown of a tooth making up part of the occlusal surface; called also *dental cusp* or *tubercle.* See also *tuberculum dentis.*
**c. poste′rior val′vae atrioventricula′ris dex′trae** [TA], the posterior of the cusps of the right atrioventricular valve; called also *posterior cusp of tricuspid valve.*
**c. poste′rior val′vae atrioventricula′ris sinis′trae** [TA], the posterior of the cusps of the left atrioventricular valve; the term is sometimes used to denote the entire three-scalloped region posterior to the anterior cusp of the mitral valve but at other times is restricted to the central scallop, with the two outer scallops called the cuspides commissurales. Called also *posterior cusp of mitral valve.*
**c. septa′lis val′vae atrioventricula′ris dex′trae** [TA], the cusp of the right atrioventricular valve which is attached to the membranous interventricular septum; called also *septal cusp of tricuspid valve.*

**cut** (kut) a narrow cleft or wound made by a sharp edge.

**cu·ta·ne·ous** (ku-ta′ne-əs) [*cutis*] pertaining to the skin; dermal; dermic.

**cut·down** (kut′doun) creation of a small incised opening over a vein to facilitate phlebotomy.

**Cu·ter·e·bra** (ku″tər-e′brə) a genus of botflies of the family Cuterebridae, whose larvae commonly infest rodents.

**Cu·te·reb·ri·dae** (ku″te-reb′rĭ-de) a family of New World botflies (order Diptera), the larvae of which parasitize various mammals, including humans. The one genus of medical interest is *Cuterebra.*

**cu·ti·cle** (ku′tə-kəl) [L. *cuticula,* from *cutis* skin] 1. a layer of more or less solid substance which covers the free surface of an epithelial cell. 2. eponychium (def. 1).
**dental c.,** cuticula dentis.
**enamel c.,** primary c.
**primary c.,** a film on the enamel of unerupted teeth, considered to be the final product of degenerating ameloblasts after completion of enamel formation; electron microscopy shows it to consist primarily of ameloblasts of the reduced enamel epithelium attached to the enamel by a basal lamina. Called also *enamel c.* Cf. *cuticula dentis.*
**c. of root sheath,** a layer of cells lining the hair follicles.

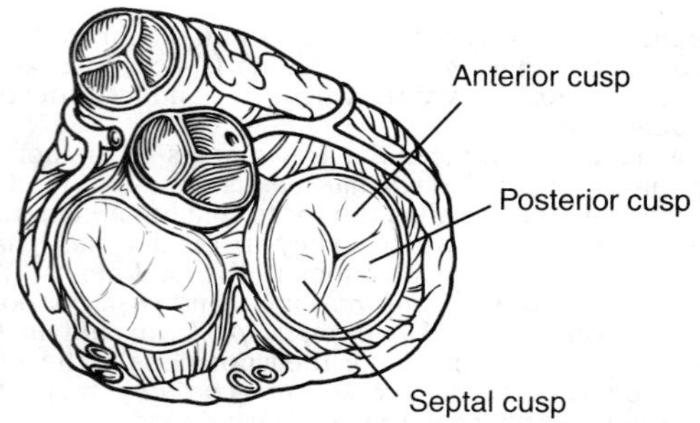

Cusps of the atrioventricular (tricuspid) valve.

**secondary c.,** cuticula dentis.

**cu·tic·u·la** (ku-tik′u-lə) pl. *cutic′ulae* [L. "little skin"] a horny secreted layer.
**c. den′tis,** dental cuticle: a film occurring on some teeth on both the enamel and the cementum, external to the primary cuticle, with which it combines, being deposited by the epithelial attachment as it migrates along the tooth and separates from the crown and root. It is not present on cementum to which the periodontal ligament is not attached. Some authorities consider it to be a nonkeratinized product of the epithelial attachment cells, probably contributed by the gingival fluid and saliva; others consider it as a pathologic product of inflamed gingiva, or a conglutinate of erythrocytes. Called also *secondary cuticle* and *Nasmyth's membrane.* Cf. *primary cuticle,* under *cuticle.*

**cu·tic·u·lae** (ku-tik′u-le) [L.] genitive and plural of *cuticula.*

**cu·ti·dure** (ku′tĭ-do͞or) coronary band.

**cu·ti·du·ris** (ku″tĭ-doo′ris) coronary band.

**cu·tin** (ku′tin) [*cutis*] a waxy substance which, combined with cellulose, forms the cuticle of plants.

**cu·ti·re·ac·tion** (ku″tĭ-re-ak′shən) [*cutis* + *reaction*] cutaneous reaction.

**cu·tis** (ku′tis) [L.] [TA] the skin: the outer protective covering of the body, consisting of the epidermis and dermis, or corium, and resting upon the subcutaneous tissues.
**c. anseri′na,** a transitory localized change in the skin surface caused by elevation of the hair follicles as a result of contraction of the arrectores pilorum muscles, a reflection of sympathetic nerve discharge. Called also *goose flesh.*
**c. hyperelas′tica,** Ehlers-Danlos syndrome.
**c. lax′a,** a group of connective tissue disorders in which the skin hangs in loose pendulous folds, believed to be associated with decreased elastic tissue formation as well as an abnormality in elastin formation, and usually occurring as a genetic disorder and occasionally in an acquired form. The *congenital form,* present at birth or developing soon afterwards, has several different varieties: an *autosomal recessive form* associated with severe complications, including pulmonary and cardiovascular manifestations, diverticula of the urinary and gastrointestinal tracts, and multiple hernias; an *autosomal dominant form,* essentially benign and of only cosmetic significance; and an *X-linked recessive form* (associated with decreased activity of lysyl oxidase, the enzyme responsible for the formation of aldehyde groups, which are essential for collagen cross linkages), characterized by bladder diverticula and dysfunction, growth of bony occipital horns, and relatively normal intelligence; the latter is also called *occipital horn syndrome* or *Ehlers-Danlos syndrome, type IX.* Affected individuals have a prematurely aged appearance, hooked nose with everted nostrils, long upper lip, everted lower eyelids, and sagging cheeks. The *acquired form,* which is often preceded by mild fever, usually presents after puberty and sometimes not until middle age or later. Called also *chalazodermia, dermatochalasis, dermatochalazia, dermatolysis, dermatomegaly, generalized elastolysis,* and *lax* or *loose skin.*
**c. marmora′ta,** a transient form of livedo reticularis occurring as a normal response to cold. Called also *marble skin.* Cf. *livedo reticularis.*
**c. rhomboida′lis nu′chae,** actinic elastosis occurring chiefly in men, in which the skin of the nape of the neck becomes thickened, tough, leathery, yellowish in color, and furrowed, acquiring a rhomboidal pattern.
**c. ver′ticis gyra′ta,** thickening of the skin of the scalp, most often involving the vertex, and forming folds and furrows resembling sulci and gyri of the brain. It may occur alone or it may be characteristic of another condition, such as pachydermoperiostosis. Called also *gyrate scalp.*

**Cu·ti·vate** (ku′tĭ-vāt″) trademark for a preparation of fluticasone propionate.

**cut·tle·bone** (kut′əl-bōn) sepium.

**cu·vette** (ku-vet′) [Fr. dim. of *cuve* vat or tub] a container with specific dimensions (particularly thickness) and optical properties, used to examine colored or colorless solutions that are free of turbidity, as well as the light scattering of turbid suspensions, such as bacterial suspensions. Its efficacy depends on its chemical composition; e.g., one made of quartz is used for examination of materials in the ultraviolet region of the spectrum and one made of Pyrex is used for examination of materials in the visible range.

**Cu·vier's canal, duct (sinus)** (ku-ve-āz′) [Georges Léopold Chrétien Frédéric Dagobert, Baron *Cuvier,* French naturalist, 1769–1832] see *ductus venosus,* and see under *duct.*

**CV** cardiovascular; coefficient of variation; closing volume.

**C.V.** abbreviation for L. *cras ves′pere,* tomorrow evening, and L. *conjuga′ta ve′ra,* true conjugate diameter of the pelvic inlet.

**CVA** costovertebral angle; cerebrovascular accident; cardiovascular accident.

**CVB** 1. a high-dose transplant regimen consisting of cyclophosphamide, VP = 16 (etoposide), and BCNU (carmustine). 2. a regimen of CCNU (lomustine), vinblastine, and bleomycin, used in cancer chemotherapy.

**CVID** common variable immunodeficiency.

**CVP** 1. central venous pressure. 2. a regimen of cyclophosphamide, vincristine, and prednisone, used in cancer chemotherapy.

**CVS** cardiovascular system; chorionic villus sampling.

**CX** circumflex artery; see *ramus circumflexus arteriae coronariae sinistrae.*

**Cx** cervix; convex.

**Cy** symbol for *cyanogen.*

**Cy·a·mop·sis** (si″ə-mop′sis) a genus of plants of the family Leguminosae. *C. tetragonolo′bus* (called also *C. psoraloi′des*) is the source of guar gum.

**cy·an·al·co·hol** (si″an-al′kə-hol) cyanohydrin.

**cy·an·amide** (si-an′ə-mīd) [MeSH: Cyanamide] 1. carbamic acid nitril, N≡C—$NH_2$. 2. HN=C=NH, the anhydride of urea. 3. calcium cyanamide.

**cy·an·he·mo·glo·bin** (si″an-he′mo-glo″bin) a complex of cyanide and hemoglobin; see also *cyanmethemoglobin.*

**cy·a·nide** (si′ə-nīd) the $CN^-$ anion or a salt containing this ion; all cyanides are extremely toxic; see *cyanide poisoning* under *poisoning.*

**cy·an·met·he·mo·glo·bin** (si″an-met″he′mo-glo″bin) a tightly bound complex of methemoglobin with the cyanide ion. The standard method of hemoglobinometry (measuring hemoglobin content) is determination of the amount of this compound via spectrophotometry; cyanmethemoglobin is produced quantitatively from oxyhemoglobin, deoxyhemoglobin, carboxyhemoglobin, and methemoglobin (but not sulfhemoglobin) by addition of Drabkin's solution.

**cy·an·met·myo·glo·bin** (si″an-met-mi′o-glo″bin) a compound formed from metmyoglobin by addition of the cyanide ion to yield reduction to the ferrous state.

**cyan(o)-** [Gr. *kyanos* blue] a combining form denoting blue.

**cy·a·no·ac·ry·late** (si″ə-no-ak′rĭ-lāt) an acrylate monomer or polymer that has substitution with one or more cyano group(s); see also under *adhesive* and *resin.*

**Cy·a·no·bac·te·ria** (si″ə-no-bak-tēr′e-ə) [*cyano-* + *bacteria*] [MeSH: Cyanobacteria] the blue-green bacteria (formerly called *blue-green algae*), a subgroup of the class Oxyphotobacteria, kingdom Procaryotae, unicellular or filamentous phototrophic organisms that use water as an electron donor and produce oxygen in the presence of light. Cells are enclosed by a rigid wall containing peptidoglycan, are generally motile, and reproduce by fission. Photopigments include chlorophyll *a* and phycobilin proteins. Cyanobacteria are the only organisms that fix both carbon dioxide (in the presence of light) and nitrogen. Most species are photosynthetic and many are strong nitrogen fixers. Several species are common causes of water pollution and are often used as indicators of eutrophication of lakes and streams; see *cyanobacteria poisoning,* under *poisoning.* Called also *Cyanophyceae* and *Schizophyceae.*

**cy·a·no·bac·te·ria** (si″ə-no-bak-te′re-ə) [MeSH: Cyanobacteria] plural of *cyanobacterium.*

**cy·a·no·bac·te·ri·um** (si″ə-no-bak-te′re-um) an individual bacterium of the group *Cyanobacteria.*

**cy·a·no·co·bal·a·min** (si″ə-no″-ko-bal′ə-min) 1. a cobalamin derivative in which the substituent is a cyanide ion; it is the form of vitamin $B_{12}$ first isolated and hence is the form chemically defined as and the form used as a synonym of that vitamin, although it is actually an artifact of isolation. 2. [USP] a preparation of cyanocobalamin used to treat disorders caused by deficiencies of vitamin $B_{12}$, particularly to prevent and treat pernicious anemia and other megaloblastic anemias and associated neuropathy; administered subcutaneously or intramuscularly or, occasionally, orally. Abbreviated CN-Cbl. Called also *vitamin* $B_{12}$.
**c. Co 57,** cyanocobalamin radioactively labeled with $^{57}Co$; official preparations are *c. Co 57 capsules* [USP] and *c. Co 57 oral solution* [USP], in which a portion of the molecules are radioactively labeled. The preparations are used in the diagnosis of pernicious anemia and other disorders of vitamin $B_{12}$ absorption. See also *Schilling test.*
**c. Co 58,** cyanocobalamin labeled with $^{58}Co$, used in the diagnosis of pernicious anemia and other disorders of vitamin $B_{12}$ absorption. See also *Schilling test.*
**c. Co 60,** cyanocobalamin in which a portion of the molecules are radioactively labeled with $^{60}Co$, used in the diagnosis of pernicious anemia and other disorders of vitamin $B_{12}$ absorption. See also *Schilling test,* under *test.*

**cy·a·no·crys·tal·lin** (si″ə-no-kris′tə-lin) a blue coloring matter from the integument of decapods.

**cy·an·o·gen** (si-an′o-jən) [*cyano-* + *-gen*] 1. the radical CN—; symbol Cy. 2. an extremely poisonous gas, NCCN; called also *ethanedinitrile.*.
**c. bromide,** a highly toxic lacrimatory war gas, BrCN.
**c. chloride,** a gas, ClCN, used for fumigating houses, ships, etc. It is as lethal for rats and other vermin as hydrocyanic acid, but less dangerous to man, as it also causes lacrimation, which makes it useful as a warning gas in fumigants.

**cy·a·no·gen·e·sis** (si″ə-no-jen′ə-sis) [*cyano-* + *-genesis*] the formation or production of cyanogen or hydrocyanic acid.

**cy·a·no·ge·net·ic** (si″ə-no-jə-net′ik) producing cyanogen or hydrocyanic acid.

**cy·a·no·hy·drin** (si″ə-no-hi′drin) a compound containing a cyano and a hydroxyl group; formed by the addition of hydrocyanic acid to an aldehyde group; called also *cyanalcohol.*

**cy·a·no·labe** (si′ə-no-lāb″) [*cyano-* + Gr. *lambanein* to take] name proposed for the pigment in retinal cones that is more sensitive to the blue range of the spectrum than are the other retinal pigments. Cf. *chlorolabe* and *erythrolabe.*

**cy·a·no·phil** (si-an′o-fil) 1. cyanophilous. 2. a cell or other histologic element readily stainable with blue.

**cy·a·noph·i·lous** (si″ə-nof′ĭ-ləs) [*cyano-* + Gr. *philein* to love] stainable with blue dyes.

**cy·a·no·phor·ic** (si″ə-no-for′ik) yielding hydrocyanic acid; e.g., the glycoside amygdalin yields HCN on hydrolysis.

**cy·a·no·phose** (si′ə-no-fōz) [*cyano-* + *phose*] a blue phose.

**Cy·a·no·phy·ceae** (si″ə-no-fi′se-e) [*cyano-* + Gr. *phykos* seaweed] Cyanobacteria.

**cy·a·nop·sia** (si″ə-nop′se-ə) [*cyano-* + *-opsia*] a chromatopsia in which all objects appear to have a blue tinge.

**cy·a·nop·sin** (si″ə-nop′sin) [*cyano-* + *opsin*] a visual pigment of bluish tint found in the retinal cones of some animals and important for vision.

**cy·a·nosed** (si′ə-nōsd) cyanotic.

**cy·a·no·sis** (si″ə-no′sis) [Gr. *kyanos* blue] [MeSH: Cyanosis] a bluish discoloration, especially of the skin and mucous membranes due to excessive concentration of deoxyhemoglobin in the blood.
**autotoxic c.,** enterogenous c.
**enterogenous c.,** a syndrome due to absorption of nitrites and sulfides from the intestine, principally marked by methemoglobinemia and/or sulfhemoglobinemia associated with cyanosis. It is accompanied by severe enteritis, abdominal pain, constipation or diarrhea, headache, dyspnea, dizziness, syncope, anemia, and, occasionally, digital clubbing and indicanuria. Called also *Stokvis-Talma syndrome, van den Bergh's disease,* and *autotoxic c.*
**false c.,** cyanosis due to the presence of a pigment such as methemoglobin and not to deficient oxygenation of the blood.
**hereditary methemoglobinemic c.,** cyanosis caused by a structural variant in the hemoglobin molecule, such as an M hemoglobin; see *methemoglobinemia.*
**c. lie′nis,** passive congestion of the spleen.
**pulmonary c.,** central cyanosis caused by poor oxygenation of the blood in the lungs.
**c. re′tinae,** distinct cyanosis of the retina, observable in some cases of cyanotic congenital heart disease, patent ductus arteriosus, and other congenital cardiac anomalies.
**shunt c.,** central cyanosis caused by mixing of unoxygenated blood with the arterial blood in the heart or great vessels.
**tardive c.,** cyanosis in congenital heart disease that appears only after cardiac failure has developed.

**cy·a·not·ic** (si″ə-not′ik) pertaining to or characterized by cyanosis.

**Cy·an·tin** (si-an′tin) trademark for a preparation of nitrofurantoin.

**cy·an·uria** (si″ən-u′re-ə) the passage of blue urine.

**cy·an·uric ac·id** (si″ən-u′rik) a cyclic compound formed by heating urea.

**cy·an·urin** (si″ən-u′rin) [*cyan-* + *urine*] indigo blue found in the urine on the addition of a mineral acid to it.

**Cyath.** abbreviation for L. *cy′athus,* a glassful.

**Cya·thos·to·ma** (si″ə-thos′tə-mə) a genus of nematodes of the family Syngamidae that parasitizes the upper respiratory tract of birds.

**cy·a·tho·sto·mi·a·sis** (si″ə-tho-sto-mi′ə-sis) infection of the large intestines of horses with nematodes of the genus *Cyathostomum;* characteristics include anemia with diarrhea that can be fatal.

**Cya·tho·sto·mum** (si″ə-tho-sto′mum) a genus of small nematodes of the family Strongylidae, which parasitize the large intestines of horses, causing cyathostomiasis.

**cy·ber·net·ics** (si″bər-net′iks) [Gr. *kybernētēs* helmsman] [MeSH: Cybernetics] the science of communication and control processes within systems. Control is based on communication both within the system and with the external environment and influences the actions of the system to bring it into some desired future state or to maintain homeostasis. Cybernetics includes the concepts of autoregulation and feedback (qq.v.), as well as the transmission and self-correction of information, and can be applied not only to machines like computers but also to living organisms, including humans, and to complex organizations and societies.

**CYC** cyclophosphamide.

**cy·cad** (si′kad) a palm tree of the genus *Cycas* or other closely related genera such as *Macrozamia* and *Zamia.* See also *zamia.*

**Cy·cas** (si′kəs) a genus of palms (family Palmae) found on Guam and other islands of the South Pacific. *C. circina′lis* L. and *C. revolu′tus* Thumb. have seeds that were formerly used as part of the diet on Guam and contain toxic glycosides such as cycasin and macrozamin. Cattle and sheep consuming the seeds may suffer fatal gastrointestinal and liver damage or the neurological condition known as *zamia staggers.*

**cy·ca·sin** (si′kə-sin) [MeSH: Cycasin] a toxic principle from the seeds of *Cycas revoluta* and *C. circinalis.* In humans it is neoplastic to the liver, kidneys, intestine, and lungs after hydrolysis by intestinal bacteria and yields the breakdown product methylazoxymethanol; in cattle it causes fatal gastrointestinal and liver damage.

**cy·cla·cil·lin** (si″klə-sil′in) [MeSH: Cyclacillin] an antibacterial agent effective against a wide range of gram-negative and gram-positive organisms.

**cy·cla·mate** (si′klə-māt) any salt of cyclamic acid. Cyclamate calcium and cyclamate sodium were once used widely as non-nutritive sweeteners, but because of an association with bladder tumors in animals they were banned as food additives in the United States in 1969.

**Cyc·la·men** (sik′lə-mən) [L.] a genus of plants of the family Primulaceae. *C. europae′um* L. is a common house plant in North America that has an acrid, cathartic root and contains the toxic alkaloid cyclamin.

**cy·clam·ic acid** (si-klam′ik) the free acid of cyclamate.

**cyc·la·min** (sik′lə-min) a toxic glycoside from *Cyclamen europaeum;* it is strongly purgative and emetic.

**Cy·cla·my·cin** (si′klə-mi″sin) trademark for a preparation of troleandomycin.

**cy·clan·de·late** (si-klan′də-lāt) [MeSH: Cyclandelate] an antispasmodic with a direct effect on vascular smooth muscle, occurring as a white to pale yellow, crystalline powder; used as a vasodilator mainly in peripheral vascular diseases, administered orally.

**cyc·lar·thro·di·al** (sik″lahr-thro′de-əl) pertaining to a cyclarthrosis.

**cyc·lar·thro·sis** (sik″lahr-thro′sis) [*cycl-* + *arthrosis*] a joint that permits rotation.

**cy·clase** (si′klās) an enzyme that catalyzes the formation of a cyclic compound.

**cy·cla·zo·cine** (si″klə-zo′sēn) [MeSH: Cyclazocine] a narcotic antagonist which has been used as an analgesic and in the treatment of narcotic dependence.

**cy·cle** (si′kəl) [Gr. *kyklos* circle] a round or succession of observable phenomena, recurring usually at regular intervals and in the same sequence.

**aberrant c.,** one that shows variation in the interval or the sequence of events.

**anovulatory c.,** a sexual cycle in which no ovum is discharged.

**asexual c.,** generation by budding or division of the parent organism.

**biliary c.,** Schiff's biliary c.

**Calvin c.,** a dark reaction occurring in photosynthesis in plants in which carbon dioxide is affixed to a five-carbon sugar molecule and subsequently reduced to form other sugars.

**carbon c.,** the steps by which carbon (in the form of carbon dioxide) is extracted from the atmosphere by living organisms and ultimately returned to the atmosphere. It comprises a series of interconversions of carbon compounds beginning with the production of carbohydrates by plants during photosynthesis, proceeding through animal consumption, and ending and beginning again in the decomposition of the animal or plant or in the exhalation of carbon dioxide by animals.

**cardiac c.,** a complete cardiac movement or heart beat. The period from the beginning of one heart beat to the beginning of the next; the systolic and diastolic movement, with the interval between them. See also accompanying illustration.

**cell c.,** the cycle of biochemical and morphological events occurring in a reproducing cell population; it consists of: the *S phase,* occurring toward the end of interphase, in which DNA is synthesized; the *$G_2$ phase,* a relatively quiescent period; the *M phase,* consisting of the four phases of mitosis; and the *$G_1$ phase* of interphase, which lasts until the *S phase* of the next cycle.

**chewing c.,** masticating c.

**citrate-pyruvate c.,** the mechanism by which acetyl groups and electrons are moved across the mitochondrial membrane during fatty acid synthesis.

**citric acid c.,** tricarboxylic acid c.

**Cori c.,** the mechanism by which lactate produced by muscles is carried to the liver, converted back to glucose via gluconeogenesis, and returned to the muscles.

**cytoplasmic c.,** that stage in the life of a parasite during which it lives in cytoplasm of the cells of the host.

**endogenous c.,** that portion of the life of a parasite which is spent within the body of its host.

**estrous c.,** the type of sexual cycle seen in most adult female mammals, with recurring periods that include estrus and the correlated changes in the reproductive tract from one period to the next. The stages are *proestrus, estrus, metestrus,* and *diestrus* (the latter sometimes including *anestrus* of varying lengths of time). Cf. *ovarian c.* and *menstrual c.*

**exogenous c.,** that part of the life of a parasite which is spent outside the body of its definitive host.

**forced c.,** a cardiac cycle that is interrupted by a forced beat.

**futile c.,** a combination of two or more biochemical reactions resulting only in the hydrolysis of ATP or other high-energy compounds; thermogenesis may result. Called also *substrate c.*

**gait c.,** the series of movements of the leg and foot between one touch of the heel on the ground and the next time the same heel touches. See also *stance phase* and *swing phase,* under *phase.*

**gastric c.,** rhythmic alterations in the shape of the stomach due to peristaltic waves.

**genesial c.,** the reproductive period of a woman's life.

**glucose-lactate c.,** Cori c.

**γ-glutamyl c.,** a metabolic cycle for transporting amino acids into cells. The reactions involve transfer of the γ-glutamyl group of glutathione to extracellular amino acids, enabling them to enter the cells; additional reactions recreate free amino acids and resynthesize glutathione.

**glyoxylate c.,** a metabolic pathway by which certain microorganisms and plants convert fat to carbohydrate, the enzymes of which are contained in microbodies known as *glyoxosomes;* it is a modification of the tricarboxylic acid cycle but differs in that two auxiliary enzymes (isocitratase and malate synthetase) are used and two molecules of acetyl coenzyme A instead of one are required.

**gonotrophic c.,** the interval in the life of an insect between the time of feeding to deposition of the ova.

**hair c.,** the successive phases in the production of hair, from initiation of its growth to its loss from the follicle, consisting of anagen, catagen, and telogen.

**heat c.,** estrous c.

**Hodgkin c.,** a regenerative, circular sequence of events between depolarization and permeability to sodium occurring in excitable cells: depolarization increases permeability to sodium, thus increasing the entry of sodium ($Na^+$) into the cell, and the increased concentration of $Na^+$ further depolarizes the membrane.

**isohydric c.,** the series of chemical reactions in the erythrocyte, in which the uptake of $CO_2$ and the release of $O_2$ are accomplished without the production of an excess of hydrogen ions ($H^+$). See also *buffer.*

**Krebs c.,** tricarboxylic acid c.

**Krebs-Henseleit c.,** urea c.

**life c.,** the successive events in the life history of an organism, for example, the entire life of a protozoan blood parasite, including the endogenous and exogenous cycles.

**mammary c.,** the rhythmic growth of mammary glands after menarche occurring in coordination with the ovarian cycle.

**masticating c., masticatory c.,** the complete pathway of the mandible performed in mastication of food. Called also *chewing c.*

**menstrual c.,** the type of sexual cycle seen in female humans and some other primates, with physiologic changes in the endometrium that recur at regular intervals during the reproductive years; it culminates in partial shedding of the endometrium and some bleeding per vagina (menstruation). Cf. *ovarian c.* and *estrous c.* See illustration.

**mosquito c.,** that period of the life of a malarial parasite that is spent in the body of the mosquito host.

**nitrogen c.,** the steps by which nitrogen is extracted from the nitrates of soil and water, incorporated as amino acids and proteins in living organisms, and ultimately reconverted to nitrates: (1) conversion of nitrogen to nitrates by bacteria; (2) the extraction of the nitrates by plants and the building of amino acids and proteins by addition of an amino group to the carbon compounds produced in photosynthesis; (3) the ingestion of plants by animals; and (4) the return of nitrogen to the soil in animal excretions or on the death and decomposition of plants and animals.

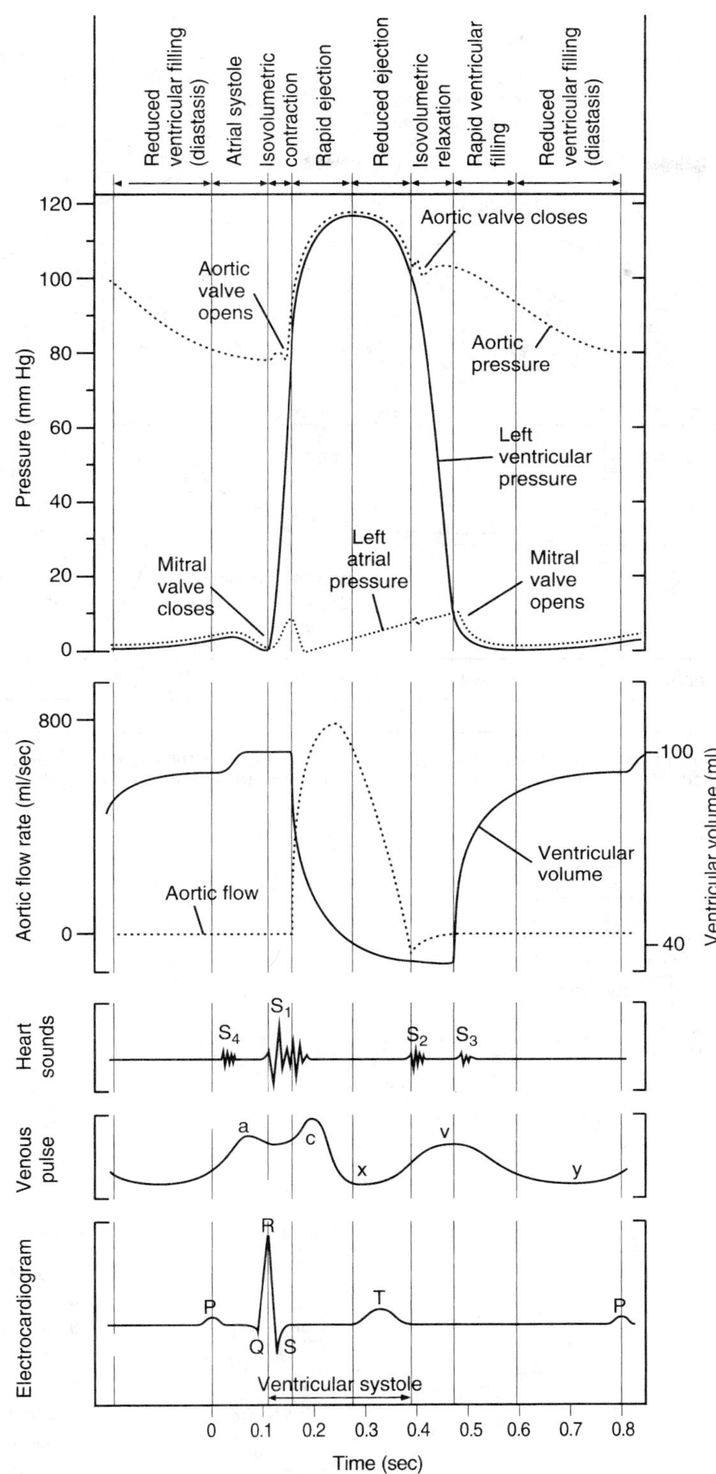


Events of the cardiac cycle. For the meaning of symbols, see individual entries and see illustrations at *electrocardiogram* and *venous pulse*.

**oogenetic c.,** ovarian c.
**ornithine c.,** urea c.
**ovarian c.,** the sequence of physiologic changes in the ovary, including development and rupture of the follicle, discharge of the ovum, and corpus luteum formation and regression; see also *menstrual c.* and *estrous c.* Called also *oogenetic c.*
**reproductive c.,** the cycle of physiologic changes occurring in the female reproductive organs, from the time of fertilization of the ovum through gestation and parturition.
**restored c.,** a cardiac cycle following a returning cycle and taking up the normal rhythm.
**returning c.,** a cardiac cycle that begins with an extrasystole.
**Schiff's biliary c.,** the cycle in which bile salts in the bile are absorbed by the intestinal villi and are then conveyed back to the liver, where they are used over again; see also *enterohepatic circulation,* under *circulation.*
**schizogenic c., schizogenous c.,** the asexual cycle in protozoa during which growth and segmentation occur.
**sex c., sexual c.,** 1. a series of recurring physiologic changes in the genital organs of female mammals; when pregnancy does not supervene, they typically come at regular intervals. The two types are the *menstrual c.* and the *estrous c.* See also *ovarian c.* 2. the period of sexual reproduction in an organism that also reproduces asexually.

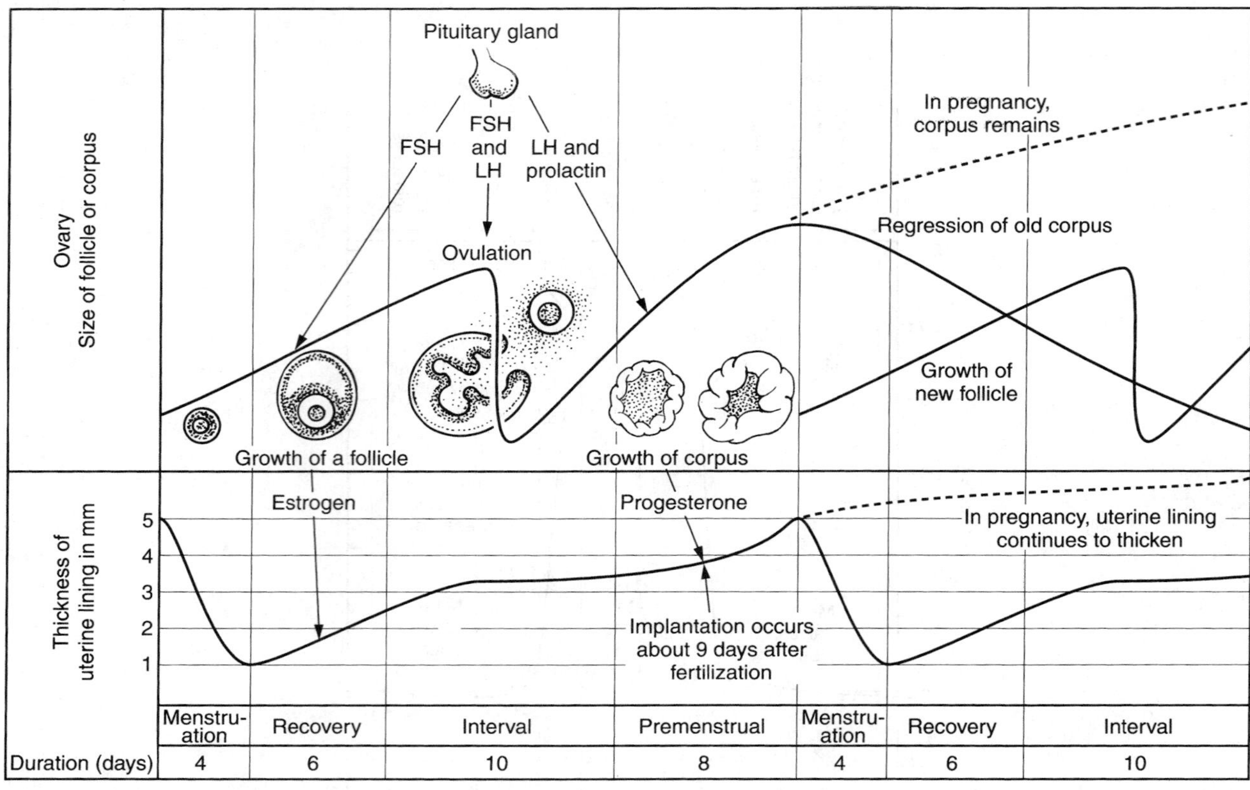


Changes in the menstrual cycle in the human female. Solid lines indicate the course of events when the ovum is not fertilized; dotted lines indicate the course of events when fertilization occurs. Arrows indicate the actions of hormones of the pituitary and the ovary in regulating the cycle.

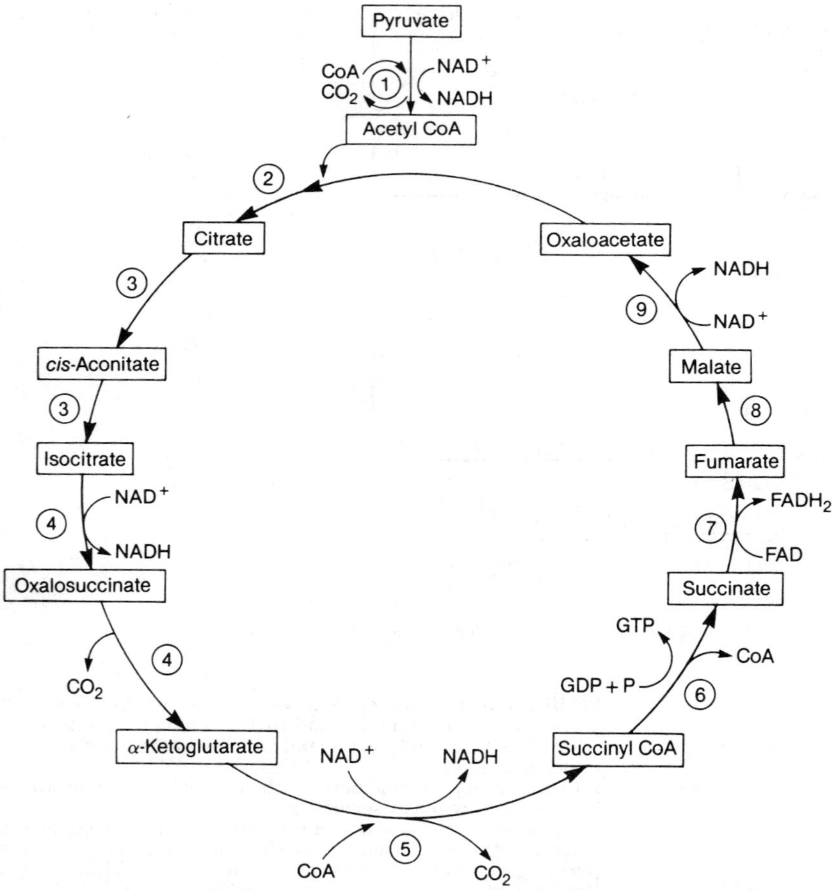

Pyruvate
CoA (1) $NAD^+$
$CO_2$ NADH
Acetyl CoA
(2)
Citrate
Oxaloacetate
(3)
NADH
(9) $NAD^+$
*cis*-Aconitate
Malate
(3)
(8)
Isocitrate
Fumarate
$NAD^+$
(4)
NADH
$FADH_2$
(7)
FAD
Oxalosuccinate
Succinate
GTP
$CO_2$ (4)
CoA
GDP + P (6)
α-Ketoglutarate
$NAD^+$ NADH
Succinyl CoA
(5)
CoA $CO_2$

KEY TO ENZYMES (Circled Numbers)

1. Pyruvate dehydrogenase complex
2. Citrate (*si*)-synthase
3. Aconitate hydratase
4. Isocitrate dehydrogenase ($NAD^+$)
5. α-Ketoglutarate dehydrogenase complex
6. Succinate-CoA ligase (GDP-forming)
7. Succinate dehydrogenase (ubiquinone)
8. Fumarate hydratase
9. Malate dehydrogenase

Tricarboxylic acid cycle. Diagrammatic representation of reactions by which carbon chains of sugars, fatty acids, and amino acids are metabolized to yield carbon dioxide. Water produced by the cycle and components of the high-energy phosphate pool generated by the associated electron chain are not shown.

**sporogenic c., sporogenous c.,** the sexual cycle in protozoa that is usually passed in another host, often an insect.
**substrate c.,** futile c.
**tricarboxylic acid c.,** the final common pathway for the oxidation to $CO_2$ of fuel molecules, most of which enter the cycle as acetyl coenzyme A; it also provides intermediates for biosynthetic reactions. The cycle occurs in mitochondria and generates ATP by providing electrons to the electron transport chain. See accompanying illustration. Called also *Krebs c.* and *citric acid c.*
**urea c.,** a series of metabolic reactions, occurring in the liver, by which ammonia is converted to urea using cyclically regenerated ornithine as a carrier. See illustration.
**uterine c.,** the phenomena occurring in the endometrium during the estrous or menstrual cycle, preparing it for implantation of the blastocyst.
**visual c.,** the cyclic association of 11-*cis* retinal with an opsin followed by photon-induced conformational changes in the compound protein (rhodopsin or an iodopsin) and dissociation of opsin and an all-*trans* isomeric form of retinal; the cycle is completed by direct or indirect reconversion of retinal to the 11-*cis* isomer. The conformational changes create an electric potential and initiate the cascade generating a sensory nerve impulse in vision. See illustration.

**cyc·lec·to·my** (sik-lek'tə-me) [*cycl-* + *-ectomy*] 1. excision of a piece of the ciliary body. 2. excision of a portion of the ciliary border of the eyelid.

**cyc·len·ceph·a·lus** (sik″len-sef'ə-ləs) [*cycl-* + *enkephalos* brain] a fetus with the cerebral hemispheres blended into one.

**cyc·lic** (sik'lik, si'klik) pertaining to or occurring in a cycle or cycles; the term is applied to chemical compounds that contain a ring of atoms in the nucleus. See *closed chain,* under *chain.*

**cyc·lic AMP** [MeSH: Cyclic AMP] cyclic adenosine monophosphate.

**cyc·lic-AMP-de·pen·dent pro·tein ki·nase** (si'klik de-pen'dent pro'tēn ki'nās) cAMP-dependent protein kinase.

**cyc·lic GMP** [MeSH: Cyclic GMP] cyclic guanosine monophosphate.

**3′,5′-cyc·lic GMP phos·pho·di·es·ter·ase** (si'klik fos″fo-di-es'tər-ās) [EC 3.1.4.35] an enzyme of the hydrolase class that catalyzes the cleavage of cyclic guanosine monophosphate to form guanosine monophosphate.

**cyc·li·cot·o·my** (sik″lĭ-kot'ə-me) cyclotomy.

**cyc·lin** (sik'lin) proliferating cell nuclear antigen.

**cyc·li·tis** (sik-li'tis) [*cycl-* + *-itis*] inflammation of the ciliary body.

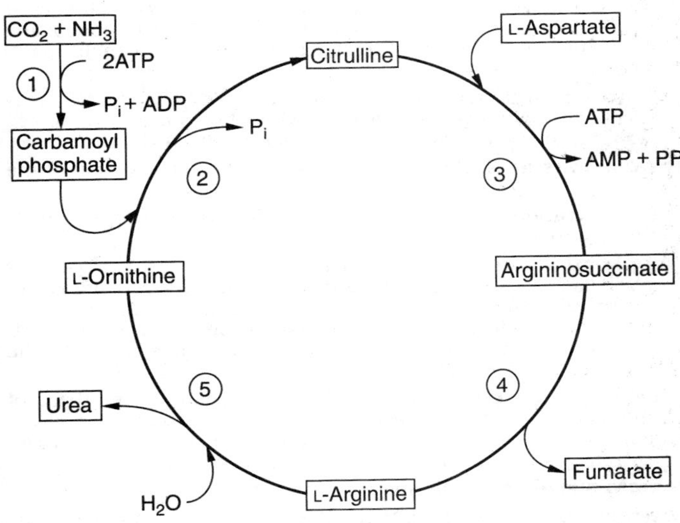


Urea cycle. Diagrammatic representation of reactions by which excess nitrogen in the form of ammonia is converted to soluble urea, using L-ornithine as a recyclable carrier.

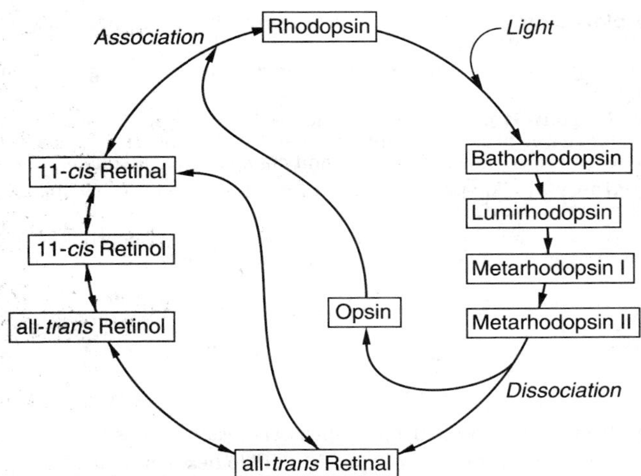


Visual cycle of retinal rod cells; an analogous cycle occurs with iodopsins in the cones.

**heterochromic c.,** chronic cyclitis producing difference in the color of the two irides, the inflamed eye having the lighter iris.
**plastic c.,** cyclitis with exudation of fibrinous matter into the anterior chamber.
**pure c.,** inflammation of the ciliary body without involvement of the iris.
**purulent c.,** suppuration in the ciliary body; it usually involves the entire uveal tract, constituting endophthalmitis.
**serous c.,** simple inflammation of the ciliary body.

**cy·cli·zine** (si'klĭ-zēn) [MeSH: Cyclizine] an antihistaminic, used in the form of the lactate salt as an antiemetic and antinauseant, especially for the prevention and relief of motion sickness, administered intramuscularly.
**c. hydrochloride** [USP], the monohydrochloride salt of cyclizine, having the same actions and uses as the base; administered orally.
**c. lactate,** see *cyclizine.*

**cycl(o)-** [Gr. *kyklos* circle] a combining form denoting round or recurring; see *cyclic.* Often used with particular reference to the eye, or to the ciliary body of the eye.

**cy·clo·bar·bi·tal** (si″klo-bahr'bĭ-təl) a short-acting barbiturate, mainly used as a hypnotic; administered orally.
**c. calcium,** the calcium salt of cyclobarbital, having actions and uses similar to those of the base; administered orally.

**cy·clo·ben·za·prine hy·dro·chlo·ride** (si″klo-ben'zə-prēn) [USP] a compound structurally related to the tricyclic antidepressants, used as a muscle relaxant; administered orally.

**cy·clo·ceph·a·lus** (si″klo-sef'ə-ləs) [*cyclo-* + *-cephalus*] cyclops.

**cy·clo·cer·a·ti·tis** (si″klo-sər″ə-ti'tis) cyclokeratitis.

**cy·clo·cho·roid·itis** (si″klo-ko″roid-i'tis) [*cyclo-* + *choroid*] inflammation of the choroid and ciliary body.

**Cy·clo·cort** (si'klo-kort″) trademark for preparations of amcinonide.

**cy·clo·cryo·ther·a·py** (si″klo-kri″o-ther'ə-pe) [*cyclo-* + *cryotherapy*] freezing of the ciliary body; done in the treatment of glaucoma.

**cy·clo·da·mia** (si″klo-da'me-ə) [*cyclo-* + Gr. *damazein* to subdue] subdued or suppressed accommodation of the eyes.

**cy·clo·dex·trin** (si″klo-deks'trin) any of a group of nonreducing cyclic compounds obtained by the enzymatic hydrolysis of starch, designated $\alpha$-, $\beta$-, and $\gamma$-cyclodextrins; used as complexing agents and in the study of enzyme action.
**beta c.,** betadex.

**cy·clo·di·al·y·sis** (si″klo-di-al'ə-sis) [*cyclo-* + *dialysis*] the operative formation of a communication between the anterior chamber of the eye and the suprachoroidal space; done in the treatment of glaucoma.

**cy·clo·di·a·ther·my** (si″klo-di'ə-thər″me) [*cyclo-* + *diathermy*] destruction of a portion of the ciliary body by diathermy; employed as therapy in cases of glaucoma.

**cy·clo·duc·tion** (si″klo-duk'shən) [*cyclo-* + *duction*] the duction of the eyeball produced by the oblique muscle.

**cy·clo·elec·trol·y·sis** (si″klo-e″lek-trol'ə-sis) [*cyclo-* + *electrolysis*] electrolysis of the ciliary body, used to lower intraocular pressure in glaucoma.

**cy·clog·e·ny** (si-kloj'ə-ne) [*cyclo-* + *-geny*] the developmental cycle of a microorganism.

**cy·clo·guan·ide em·bo·nate** (si-klo-gwahn'īd) cycloguanil pamoate.

**cy·clo·guan·il pam·o·ate** (si-klo-gwahn'əl) a metabolite of the antimalarial drug proguanil, and itself having potent antimalarial effects. Called also *c. embonate* and *cycloguanide embonate.*

**Cy·clo·gyl** (si'klo-jəl) trademark for a preparation of cyclopentolate hydrochloride.

**cy·clo·hex·ane** (si"klo-hek'sān) an alicyclic hydrocarbon, $C_6H_{12}$, existing in two forms, the "boat" and the "chair":

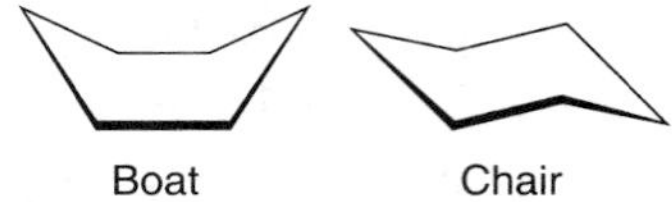


**cy·clo·hex·ane·hex·ol** (si"klo-heks"ān-heks'ol) inositol.

**cy·clo·hex·ane·sul·fam·ic ac·id** (si"klo-hek"sān-səl-fam'ik) cyclamic acid.

**cy·clo·hex·a·nol** (si"klo-hek'sə-nol) the monohydroxy derivative of cyclohexane; used as a solvent and blending agent.

**cy·clo·hex·i·mide** (si"klo-heks'ĭ-mīd) [MeSH: Cycloheximide] an antibiotic isolated from *Streptomyces griseus* and used as an agricultural fungicide and in selective media for fungi. It inhibits most saprobic fungi, while allowing dermatophytes and most systemic fungi to grow, and inhibits nuclear division of karyotic organisms but has no effect on prokaryotic cells (bacteria).

**cy·cloid** (si'kloid) characterized by alternating moods of elation and depression. The terms cycloid, cyclothymic, and manic-depressive overlap in meaning, although cycloid would generally be used for the least severe, and manic-depressive for the most severe conditions.

**cy·clo·isom·er·ase** (si"klo-i-som'ər-ās) a term used in the trivial names of intramolecular lipases of the isomerase class [EC 5.5.1] that catalyze certain rearrangements of a molecule to break or form a ring, e.g., the synthesis of *myo*-inositol phosphate from glucose 6-phosphate.

**cy·clo·ker·a·ti·tis** (si"klo-ker"ə-ti'tis) [*cyclo-* + *keratitis*] inflammation of the cornea and ciliary body; called also *Dalrymple's disease.*

**cy·clo·li·gase** (si"klo-li'gās) [EC 6.3.3] one of a sub-subclass of enzymes of the ligase class that catalyze the formation of carbon-nitrogen bonds to produce a heterocyclic ring, driven by the hydrolysis of adenosine triphosphate.

**cy·clo·mas·top·a·thy** (si"klo-mas-top'ə-the) [*cyclo-* + *masto-* + *-pathy*] an affection of the mammae, presenting excessive connective tissue overgrowth or epithelial proliferation or both in response to growth stimuli or as a manifestation of abnormal involution following normal response.

**cy·clo·oxy·gen·ase** (si"klo-ok'sə-jən-ās) an activity of prostaglandin endoperoxide synthase (q.v.).

**cy·clo·pen·tane** (si"klo-pen'tān) a hydrocarbon, $C_5H_{10}$, in which all five carbon atoms are in a single ring.

**cy·clo·pen·ta·no·per·hy·dro·phen·an·threne** (si"klo-pen"tə-no-pər-hi"dro-fə-nan'thrēn) the basic skeleton common to the steroids, consisting of a saturated phenanthrene ring (three fused six-member carbocyclic rings) joined to a cyclopentane.

**cy·clo·pen·thi·a·zide** (si"klo-pen-thi'ə-zīd) [MeSH: Cyclopenthiazide] an orally effective diuretic, used in the treatment of edema associated with various disorders and in hypertension.

**cy·clo·pen·to·late hy·dro·chlo·ride** (si"klo-pen'to-lāt) [USP] an anticholinergic, used to produce cycloplegia and mydriasis by instillation into the eye.

**cy·clo·pho·ria** (si"klo-for'e-ə) [*cyclo-* + *phoria*] heterophoria in which there is deviation of the eye from the anteroposterior axis in the absence of visual fusional stimuli. See *excyclophoria* and *incyclophoria.* Cf. *cyclotropia.*
**accommodative c.,** cyclophoria due to oblique astigmatism.
**minus c.,** incyclophoria.
**plus c.,** excyclophoria.

**cy·clo·pho·rom·e·ter** (si"klo-for-om'ə-tər) [*cyclophoria* + *-meter*] an instrument for measuring cyclophoria.

**cy·clo·phos·pha·mide** (si"klo-fos'fə-mīd) [USP] [MeSH: Cyclophosphamide] a cytotoxic alkylating agent of the nitrogen mustard group, used as an antineoplastic, often in combination with other agents, for a wide variety of conditions, including Hodgkin's disease, lymphosarcoma, acute lymphocytic leukemia, Burkitt's lymphoma, carcinoma of the breast, multiple myeloma, chronic lymphocytic leukemia, bronchogenic carcinoma, neuroblastoma, ovarian carcinoma, and carcinoma of the uterine cervix; also used as an immunosuppressive agent to prevent transplant rejection and in the treatment of certain diseases with abnormal immune function. Cyclophosphamide itself is pharmacologically inert; several active metabolites are produced by the microsomal enzyme systems in the liver.

**Cy·clo·phyl·lid·ea** (si"klo-fəl-id'e-ə) an order of tapeworms of the subclass Cestoda, class Cestoidea, comprising seven families that are habitually or accidentally parasitic in humans and domestic animals: Taeniidae, Hymenolepididae, Dipylidiidae, Davaineidae, Anoplocephalidae, Linstowiidae, and Mesocestoididae.

**cy·clo·pia** (si-klo'pe-ə) [*cycl-* + *-opia*] any developmental anomaly characterized by a single orbit; the globe may range from absent or rudimentary to apparently normal or duplicated, and the nose may be absent or present as a tubular appendage (proboscis) superior to the orbit.

**cy·clo·ple·gia** (si"klo-ple'je-ə) [*cyclo-* + *-plegia*] paralysis of the ciliary muscle; paralysis of accommodation.

**cy·clo·ple·gic** (si"klo-ple'jik) 1. pertaining to, characterized by, or causing cycloplegia. 2. an agent that causes cycloplegia.

**cy·clo·pro·pane** (si"klo-pro'pān) [USP] a colorless, flammable gas with a characteristic odor and pungent taste that is an inhalational anesthetic; now little used because of its flammability.

**cy·clo·pro·pa·none hy·drate** (si"klo-pro'pə-nōn hi'drāt) the active metabolite of the glutamic acid derivative coprine, which is found in the edible mushroom *Coprinus atramentarius;* for three to seven days after ingestion of the mushrooms, presence of coprine in the body results in a disulfiram-like toxic reaction if alcohol is ingested.

**Cy·clops** (si'klops) a genus of minute crustaceans, species of which are hosts to *Dracunculus* and *Diphyllobothrium.*

**cy·clops** (si'klops) [Gr. *kyklōps* one of a race of one-eyed giants] a fetus exhibiting cyclopia; called also *cyclocephalus.*
**c. hypogna'thus,** a modified cyclops, lacking the typical proboscis, with ears abnormally low, rudimentary mandible, and tiny mouth.

**cy·clo·ro·ta·ry** (si"klo-ro'tə-re) pertaining to cyclorotation (torsion).

**cy·clo·ro·ta·tion** (si"klo-ro-ta'shən) torsion (def. 3).

**cy·clo·ser·ine** (si"klo-ser'ēn) [USP] [MeSH: Cycloserine] a broad-spectrum antibiotic with tuberculostatic activity, produced by growth of *Streptomyces orchidaceus* or obtained by synthesis, occurring as a white to pale yellow, crystalline powder; effective against many gram-negative and gram-positive bacteria, it is used in the treatment of tuberculosis, pulmonary and extrapulmonary, and sometimes in urinary tract infections due to susceptible pathogens; administered orally.

**cy·clo·sis** (si-klo'sis) [Gr. *kyklōsis* a surrounding, enclosing] movement of the cytoplasm within a cell, without deformation of the cell wall; called also *cytoplasmic* or *protoplasmic streaming.*

**cy·clo·spasm** (si'klo-spaz-əm) spasm of accommodation of the eyes.

**Cy·clo·spas·mol** (si"klo-spaz'mol) trademark for preparations of cyclandelate.

**Cy·clo·spo·ra** (si-klos'pə-rə) [*cyclo-* + Gr. *spora* seed] a genus of coccidian protozoa (suborder Eimeriina, order Eucoccidiida) characterized by the presence of two sporocysts in each oocyst, which is covered by a bivalve shell, and two sporozoites in each sporocyst. *C. cayetanen'sis* is the most common species and is spread by the fecal-oral route. See also *cyclosporiasis.*

**cy·clo·spo·ri·a·sis** (si"klo-spə-ri'ə-sis) infection by protozoa of the genus *Cyclospora,* especially *C. cayetanen'sis,* seen especially in immunocompromised patients; the predominant symptoms are recurrent gastrointestinal disease and watery diarrhea.

**cy·clo·spor·in A** (si"klo-spor'in) cyclosporine.

**cy·clo·spor·ine** (si"klo-spor'ēn) [USP] [MeSH: Cyclosporine]a cyclic peptide produced as a metabolite by the soil fungus *Tolypocladium inflatum Gams* that selectively inhibits activation of helper T lymphocytes; used as an immunosuppressant to prevent rejection in organ transplant recipients.

**cy·clo·stat** (si'klo-stat") a cylinder of glass in which an experimental animal is rotated about its vertical axis.

**cy·clo·tate** (si'klo-tāt) USAN contraction for 4-methylbicyclo-[2.2.2]oct-2-ene-1-carboxylate.

**cy·clo·thi·a·zide** (si"klo-thi'ə-zīd) a thiazide diuretic, used in the treatment of hypertension; administered orally.

**cy·clo·thyme** (si'klo-thīm) an individual with a cyclothymic personality or exhibiting cyclothymic disorder.

**cy·clo·thy·mia** (si″klo-thi′me-ə) [*cyclo-* + *-thymia*] cyclothymic disorder.

**cy·clo·thym·i·ac** (si″klo-thim′e-ak) cyclothymic.

**cy·clo·thy·mic** (si″klo-thi′mik) pertaining to or characterized by cyclothymic disorder.

**cy·clo·tol** (si′klo-tol) a polyhydroxy cyclohexane, such as inositol.

**cy·clo·tome** (si′klo-tōm) [*cyclo-* + *-tome*] a cutting instrument for use in cyclotomy or other operations upon the eye.

**cy·clot·o·my** (si-klot′ə-me) [*cyclo-* + *-tomy*] division of or incision of the ciliary muscle.

**cy·clo·tron** (si′klo-tron) [MeSH: Cyclotrons] an apparatus for accelerating charged particles (e.g., protons, deuterons, or ions) to high energies by a combination of a constant magnet and an oscillating electric field.

**cy·clo·tro·pia** (si″klo-tro′pe-ə) [*cyclo-* + *tropia*] a form of strabismus in which there is permanent cyclophoria of an eye around the anteroposterior axis even in the presence of visual fusional stimuli, resulting in diplopia. Cf. *excyclotropia* and *incyclotropia.*

**cy·cri·mine hy·dro·chlo·ride** (si′krĭ-mēn) an anticholinergic, $C_{19}H_{29}NO·HCl$, used in the treatment of parkinsonism, administered orally.

**Cy·crin** (si′krin) trademark for a preparation of medroxyprogesterone acetate.

**cy·e·sis** (si-e′sis) [Gr. *kyēsis*] pregnancy.

**cy·es·tein** (si-es′tēn) a skinlike formation sometimes seen on the surface of urine of a pregnant woman.

**cy·es·thein** (si-es′thēn) cyestein.

**cyl** cylinder; cylindrical lens.

**Cy·lert** (si′lərt) trademark for a preparation of pemoline.

**cyl·i·cot·o·my** (sil″ĭ-kot′ə-me) cyclotomy.

**cyl·in·der** (sil′in-der) [Gr. *kylindros* a roller] 1. a solid body shaped like a column, 2. cylindrical lens.
**axis c.,** axon (def. 1).
**Bence Jones c's,** cylindrical gelatinous bodies forming the contents of the seminal vesicles; called also *Lallemand's, Lallemand-Trousseau,* or *Trousseau-Lallemand bodies.*
**crossed c's,** two cylindrical lenses at right angles to each other.
**Külz's c.,** coma cast.
**Leydig's c's,** bundles of muscular fibers separated by partitions of protoplasm.
**Ruffini's c.,** see under *corpuscle.*
**terminal c.,** Ruffini's corpuscle.
**urinary c.,** a urinary cast.

**cyl·in·drar·thro·sis** (sil″in-drahr-thro′sis) [*cylinder* + *arthrosis*] a joint in which the articular surfaces are cylindrical, as in the proximal radioulnar joint or the odontoid process and atlas.

**cy·lin·dri·cal** (sə-lin′drĭ-kəl) pertaining to or shaped like a cylinder.

**cy·lin·dri·form** (sə-lin′drĭ-form) cylindrical.

**Cy·lin·dro·car·pon** (sĭ-lin″dro-kahr′pon) a genus of Fungi Imperfecti of the form-class Hyphomycetes. Several species have been isolated from human infections such as hyalohyphomycosis and eumycotic mycetomas.

**cyl·in·dro·cel·lu·lar** (sil″in-dro-sel′u-lər) composed of or containing cylindrical cells.

**cyl·in·droid** (sil′in-droid) [Gr. *kylindroeidēs* cylindrical] 1. resembling, or shaped like, a cylinder. 2. a cast in the urine, of various origins and of various forms, generally resembling a hyaline cast, but differing from the latter in that it tapers to a slender tail which is often twisted or curled upon itself; called also *mucous* or *spurious (tube) cast.*

**cyl·in·dro·ma** (sil″in-dro′mə) [*cylinder* + *-oma*] 1. a usually benign tumor of either apocrine or eccrine origin generally arising in early life as single or multiple nodules located on the scalp and less often on the face and extremities, and consisting of cylindrical epithelial masses containing small basophilic and larger pale-staining cells surrounded by pink hyaline sheaths. Multiple lesions, which affect females more often and may completely cover the scalp (hence the descriptive term *turban tumor*), are usually dominantly inherited, and may also be associated with multiple trichoepitheliomas. 2. adenoid cystic carcinoma.

**cy·lin·drom·a·tous** (sil″in-drom′ə-təs) pertaining to or of the nature of cylindroma.

**Cy·lin·dro·tho·rax** (sə-lin″dro-tho′raks) a genus of beetles. *C. melanoce′phala* is an African blister beetle that secretes cantharidin.

**cyl·in·dru·ria** (sil″in-droo′re-ə) [*cylindroid* + *uria*] the presence of tube casts in the urine.

**cy·lite** (si′līt) benzyl bromide.

**cyl·lo·sis** (sə-lo′sis) [Gr. *kyllōsis*] clubfoot or similar deformity of the foot or leg.

**cyl·lo·so·ma** (sil″o-so′mə) [Gr. *kyllos* lame + *soma*] a fetus with lower lateral abdominal eventration and absence or imperfect development of the lower limb on the side having the eventration.

**cyl·lo·so·mus** (sil″o-so′məs) cyllosoma.

**cy·ma·rose** (si′mə-rōs) a rare sugar, 2,6-deoxy-3-methoxyaldohexose, from hydrolysis of various strophanthin glycosides.

**cym·ba** (sim′bə) pl. *cym′bae* [L., from Gr. *kymbē*] a boat-shaped structure.
**c. con′chae auri′culae** [TA], **c. concha′lis auri′culae,** the upper part of the concha of the auricle.

**cym·bi·form** (sim′bĭ-form) [*cymbo-* + *form*] boat-shaped; scaphoid.

**cymb(o)-** [Gr. *kymbē,* boat] a combining form meaning boat-shaped.

**cym·bo·ce·pha·lia** (sim″bo-sə-fā′le-ə) scaphocephaly.

**cym·bo·ce·phal·ic** (sim″bo-sə-fal′ik) [*cymbo-* + *cephalic*] scaphocephalic.

**cym·bo·ceph·a·lous** (sim″bo-sef′ə-ləs) scaphocephalic.

**cym·bo·ceph·a·ly** (sim″bo-sef′ə-le) scaphocephaly.

**Cym·bo·po·gon** (sim″bə-po′gon) a genus of grasses found in warm regions of Europe, Africa, and Asia. *C. nar′dus* (L.) Rendle is citronella, a fragrant species that is the source of citronella oil.

**cyme** (sīm) a type of inflorescence composed of a flat-topped cluster of blossoms.

**cy·mo·graph** (si′mo-graf) kymograph.

**cy·nan·thro·py** (sə-nan′thro-pe) [*cyn-* + Gr. *anthrōpos* man] a delusion in which the patient considers himself a dog or behaves like a dog.

**cyn·ic** (sin′ik) [Gr. *kynikos*] see *risus sardonicus.*

**cyn(o)-** [Gr. *kyōn,* gen. *kynos* dog] a combining form denoting relationship to a dog, or doglike.

**cy·no·ce·phal·ic** (si″no-sə-fal′ik) [*cyno-* + *cephalic*] having a head shaped like that of a dog.

**Cy·no·don** (si′nə-don) a genus of grasses (family Gramineae). *C. dac′tyon* is Bermuda grass, whose pollen causes hay fever.

**cy·no·dont** (si′no-dont) [*cyno-* + Gr. *odous* tooth] a canine tooth.

**cyn·o·mol·gus** (sin″o-mol′gəs) *Macaca cynomolgus.*

**Cy·no·my·ia** (si″no-mi′yə) a genus of blue-bottle flies that deposit their ova in decaying meat and in wounds.

**Cy·no·mys** (si′no-mis) the prairie dogs, a genus of the family Sciuridae; some species harbor plague-transmitting fleas.

**cy·no·pho·bia** (si″no-fo′be-ə) [*cyno-* + *-phobia*] irrational fear of dogs.

**cy·o·gen·ic** (si″o-jen′ik) [Gr. *kyos* fetus + *-genic*] producing pregnancy.

**Cy·on's experiment, nerve** (se′onz) [Elie de *Cyon* (Il′ia Faddeevich Tsion), Russian physiologist, 1842–1912] see under *experiment* and *nerve.*

**cy·o·pho·ria** (si″o-for′e-ə) [Gr. *kyos* fetus + *phoros* bearing] pregnancy.

**cy·o·phor·ic** (si″o-for′ik) pertaining to pregnancy.

**cy·ot·ro·phy** (si-ot′rə-fe) [Gr. *kyos* fetus + *-trophy*] nutrition of the embryo or fetus.

**Cy·pe·rus** (si-pe′rəs) [L.; Gr. *kypeiros* rush] a genus of plants of the family Cyperaceae, grasslike sedges or rushes. *C. articula′tus* is adrue, whose root has medicinal uses.

**cyph(o)-** for words beginning thus, see those beginning *kyph(o)-.*

**cyp·i·o·nate** (sip′e-o-nāt) USAN contraction for cyclopentanepropionate.

**cy·po·thrin** (si′po-thrin) a veterinary anthelmintic.

**cyp·ri·nin** (sip′rĭ-nin) a toxic substance derived from the milt of the carp, *Cyprinus carpio.*

**cy·pro·hep·ta·dine hy·dro·chlo·ride** (si″pro-hep′tə-dēn) [USP] a serotonin and histamine antagonist with anticholinergic and sedative properties, used as an antihistaminic for relief of symptoms of allergy and as an antipruritic for relief of itching associated with various skin disorders, administered orally.

**cy·pro·quin·ate** (si-pro-kwin′āt) a coccidiostat for poultry.

**cy·pro·ter·one ac·e·tate** (si-pro′tər-ōn) [MeSH: Cyproterone Acetate] a synthetic antiandrogenic steroid that has been used in the treatment of male sexual disorders.

**Cyr·i·ax's syndrome** (sĭ′re-ak-səz) [Edward F. *Cyriax,* British orthopedic surgeon, early 20th century] see under *syndrome.*

**cyrto-** [Gr. *kyrtos* bent] a combining form meaning bent or curved.

**cyr·to·sis** (sir-to′sis) [Gr. *kyrtōsis*] 1. kyphosis. 2. distortion of the bones.

**Cys** cysteine.

**Cys-Cys** cystine.

**cyst** (sist) [Gr. *kystis* sac, bladder] [MeSH: Cysts] 1. a bladder or sac in the body (see *vesica* [TA]). 2. an abnormal closed cavity in the body, lined by epithelium containing a liquid or semisolid material. 3. a stage in the life cycle of certain parasites, during which they are enclosed within a protective wall; see, for example, *hydatid c., multilocular c.,* and *pseudocyst* (def. 2).

## Cyst

**adventitious c.,** pseudocyst (def. 1).

**allantoic c.,** urachal c.

**alveolar c's,** dilatations of pulmonary alveoli, which may fuse by breakdown of their septa to form large air cysts (pneumatoceles).

**alveolar hydatid c.,** a hydatid cyst formed by the larvae of the tapeworm *Echinococcus multilocularis;* see *alveolar hydatid disease,* under *disease.*

**amnionic c.,** cystlike processes containing amniotic fluid resulting from adhesion of amnionic folds.

**aneurysmal bone c.,** a benign, rapidly growing, osteolytic lesion usually occurring in childhood or adolescence; it may be primary or secondary to an existing lesion and is characterized by blood-filled, often large, cystic spaces lined by bony or fibrous septa that contain osteoid and multinucleated giant cells.

**angioblastic c.,** an ingrowth of the mesenchymal tissue having blood-forming power in an embryo.

**apical c.,** an epithelium-lined cyst in the bone at the apex of a pulpless tooth.

**arachnoid c.,** a fluid-filled cyst between the layers of the leptomeninges, lined with arachnoid membrane, most commonly occurring in the sylvian fissure; called also *leptomeningeal c.*

**atheromatous c.,** epidermal c.

**Baker's c.,** a swelling behind the knee, caused by escape of synovial fluid which has become enclosed in a sac of membrane; popliteal bursitis; synovial cyst of the popliteal space.

**Bartholin's c.,** a mucin-filled cyst resulting from obstruction of the duct of the greater vestibular gland (Bartholin's gland).

**Blessig's c's,** cystic spaces that frequently appear at the periphery of the retina close to the ora serrata without significant effect on vision; called also *Blessig's lacunae, Blessig's spaces, cystoid degeneration,* and *Iwanoff's c's.*

**blue dome c.,** a benign retention cyst of the breast containing straw-colored fluid that shows a blue color when unopened; see *fibrocystic disease of breast,* under *disease.*

**Boyer's c.,** a painless and gradual enlargement of the subhyoid bursa.

**branchial c., branchial cleft c.,** a cyst arising in the lateral aspect of the neck, from epithelial remnants of a branchial cleft, usually between the second and third branchial arches. Called also *cervical lymphoepithelial c.* and *lymphoepithelial c.*

**branchiogenetic c., branchiogenous c.,** branchial cleft c.

**bronchial c.,** bronchogenic c.

**bronchogenic c.,** a spherical congenital cyst arising from anomalous budding during the formation of the tracheobronchial tree; it is usually found in the mediastinum or the lung and is lined with bronchial epithelium that may contain secretory elements. It may contain air, and if it communicates with the trachea or a bronchus it may periodically evacuate fluid contents into the air passages, resulting in attacks of voluminous expectoration. Infection leads to mediastinal or pulmonary abscess. Called also *bronchial c.*

**bronchopulmonary c.,** bronchogenic cyst of the lung.

**bursal c.,** a cyst derived from a serous bursa.

**calcifying odontogenic c.,** a slow-growing benign neoplasm either in the mandible or in the gingiva, varying from solid to soft and cystlike; the center contains a layer resembling stellate reticulum, with ghost cells, some of which have dystrophic calcification. Called also *Gorlin's c.*

**cervical c.,** a cyst in the neck; see *branchial c.* and *thyroglossal c.*

**cervical lymphoepithelial c.,** branchial c.

**chocolate c.,** one having dark, syrupy contents, resulting from collection of hemosiderin following local hemorrhage, such as sometimes occurs after mastectomy or in the ovary in ovarian endometriosis; called also *endometrial c.* and *Sampson's c.*

**choledochal c.,** a congenital cystic dilatation of the common bile duct, which may cause pain in the right upper quadrant, jaundice, fever, or vomiting, or be asymptomatic.

**choledochus c.,** a dilatation of the lower end of the common bile duct, usually recognized during childhood.

**chyle c.,** an abnormal sac of the mesentery containing chyle.

**colloid c.,** a cyst that contains jellylike material, particularly in the third ventricle.

**compound c.,** multilocular c.

**corpus luteum c.,** a cyst of the ovary formed by a serous accumulation developed from a corpus luteum.

**craniobuccal c's, craniopharyngeal c's,** Rathke's c's.

**daughter c.,** a small parasitic cyst developed from the wall of a larger one, as from the hydatid cyst of the tapeworm *Echinococcus granulosus;* called also *secondary c.*

**dental c.,** one derived from some portion of the odontogenic apparatus.

**dentigerous c.,** a fluid-containing odontogenic cyst surrounding the crown of an unerupted tooth, usually involving the crowns of normal permanent teeth.

**dermoid c.,** 1. an epidermal cyst, usually present at birth, representing a disorder of embryologic development, generally occurring along lines of embryonic fusion, with middorsal, midventral, and branchial cleft locations, most often involving the head, especially around the eyes, and the neck, and lined with stratified squamous epithelium containing cutaneous appendages, including hair. Called also *dermoid.* 2. a benign teratoma of the ovary, usually found in young women, presumably derived from the ectodermal differentiation of totipotential cells, lined by apparent skin and its associated adnexal structures, and typically filled with a sebaceous caseous material in which is found hair. Called also *benign cystic, cystic,* or *mature teratoma* and *dermoid.* Cf. *malignant teratoma.*

**dilatation c.,** a cyst formed by dilation of a previously existing cavity.

**distention c.,** a collection of watery fluid in a normal, but distended cavity.

**echinococcus c.,** hydatid c.

**endometrial c.,** 1. a chocolate cyst, particularly in the ovary, containing blood debris and endometrium. 2. endometrioma.

**endometriotic c.,** endometrial c. (def. 1).

**endothelial c.,** a cyst whose sac has an endothelial lining.

**enteric c., enterogenous c.,** a cyst of the intestine arising or developing from some fold or pouch along the intestinal tract. Called also *enterocyst* and *enterocystoma.*

**ependymal c.,** a circumscribed dilatation of some part of the ependyma.

**epidermal c.,** a benign cyst derived from the epidermis or the epithelium of the hair follicle, which is formed by cystic enclosures of epithelium within the dermis that become filled with keratin admixed with variable amounts of lipid-rich debris. The two main types are *epidermal inclusion c.* and *pilar c.,* with *dermoid c.* and *steatocystoma multiplex* being less common variants. Called also *epidermoid c., sebaceous c.,* and *wen.*

**epidermal inclusion c.,** a well-circumscribed mobile epidermal cyst occurring on the head, neck, and trunk, formed by keratinizing squamous epithelium with a granular layer, similar to the normal epithelium of the follicular infundibulum. Cf. *pilar c.*

**epidermoid c.,** 1. epidermal c. 2. a benign tumor formed by inclusion of epidermal elements, especially at the time of closure of the neural groove and located in the skull, meninges, or brain (see *intracranial cholesteatoma* ); it may grow gradually because of accumulations of desquamated debris and may become calcified. Called also *epidermoid, epidermoidoma,* and *epidermoid tumor.*

**epithelial c.,** 1. any cyst lined by keratinizing stratified squamous epithelium, found most often in the skin, and including epidermal, pilar, and dermoid cysts, milia, and steatomas. 2. epidermal c.

**eruption c.,** a dentigerous cyst presenting as a dilatation of the follicular space about the crown of the erupting deciduous or permanent teeth in children, caused by the accumulation of tissue fluid or blood.

**esophageal duplication c.,** a cystic formation, usually found in children, consisting of duplication of part or all of the thoracic esophagus.

**extravasation c.,** simple bone c.

**exudation c.,** a cyst formed by an exudate collected in a closed cavity.

**false c.,** pseudocyst (def.1).

**fissural c.,** inclusion c., def. 1.
**follicular c.,** 1. one due to the occlusion of the duct of a follicle or small gland. 2. a cyst formed by the enlargement of a graafian follicle as a result of accumulated transudate.
**ganglionic c.,** subchondral c.
**Gartner's c., Gartner's duct c., gartnerian c.,** a benign cystic vaginal tumor developed from remnants of either Gartner's duct, the embryonic mesonephros, or the wolffian duct system.
**gas c.,** a small cyst filled with gas, of bacterial origin.
**gingival c.,** an odontogenic cyst of the soft tissue of either the free or attached gingiva, presenting as a small, well-circumscribed, painless swelling, sometimes resembling a superficial mucocele.
**globulomaxillary c.,** an inclusion cyst of the maxillary bone, located in the globulomaxillary fissure, usually between the lateral incisor and cuspid teeth, which seldom presents any clinical manifestation.
**Gorlin's c.,** calcifying odontogenic c.
**granddaughter c.,** a cyst sometimes seen within a daughter cyst (q.v.).
**hemorrhagic c.,** simple bone c.
**heterotopic oral gastrointestinal c.,** a cyst lined by gastric or intestinal mucosa but occurring in the oral cavity, usually in the tongue, floor of the mouth, or neck, or adjacent to the submaxillary gland.
**hydatid c.,** the larval cyst stage of the tapeworms *Echinococcus granulosus* and *E. multilocularis,* which contains daughter cysts, each of which contains many scoleces; called also *echinococcus c.* and *hydatid.* See *unilocular hydatid disease,* under *disease.*
**hydatid c's, osseous,** hydatid cysts formed by the larvae of *Echinococcus granulosus* and occurring in bone, which may become weakened and eroded by the exuberant growth.
**implantation c.,** epidermal inclusion c.
**incisive canal c.,** median anterior maxillary c.
**inclusion c.,** 1. one formed by the inclusion of a small portion of epithelium or mesothelium within connective tissue along a line of fusion of embryonic processes; types found in the oral region are the median palatal cyst, median anterior maxillary cyst, globulomaxillary cyst, and nasoalveolar cyst. Called also *fissural c.* 2. epidermal inclusion c.
**intraepithelial c's,** round or oval cavities which develop in the epithelium of the ureter, bladder, and urethra and contain a peculiar colloid substance.
**intraluminal c's,** duplications of the bowel, or retention cysts, which are an infrequent cause of intrinsic obstruction in the newborn.
**intrapituitary c's,** Rathke's c's.
**involution c.,** mammary duct ectasia.
**Iwanoff's (Iwanow's) c's,** Blessig's c's.
**keratinizing c., keratinous c.,** any cyst containing keratinous material; see *epithelial c.*
**Klestadt's c.,** nasoalveolar c.
**lacteal c.,** a cyst of the breast due to obstruction of a lactiferous duct; called also *milk c.*
**lateral periodontal c.,** a cyst of the lateral periodontal membrane of an erupted tooth, usually occurring in the bicuspid region of the mandible.
**leptomeningeal c.,** arachnoid c.
**lutein c.,** a cyst of the ovary developed from a corpus luteum.
**lymphoepithelial c.,** branchial c.
**median anterior maxillary c.,** an inclusion cyst of the maxilla located in or near the incisive canal, which arises from proliferation of epithelial remnants of the nasopalatine duct. Called also *incisive canal c.* and *nasopalatine duct c.*
**median mandibular c.,** a rare inclusion cyst occurring in the midline of the mandible, believed to be caused by inclusion of the epithelium trapped in the central groove of the mandibular process, or by cystic degeneration of a supernumerary tooth germ.
**median palatal c.,** an inclusion cyst located in the midline of the hard palate between the lateral palatal processes.
**meibomian c.,** chalazion.
**mesenteric c.,** a congenital thin-walled cyst of the abdomen between the leaves of the mesentery, which may be of wolffian or lymphatic duct origin; as it enlarges, it may cause colicky pain and intestinal obstruction.
**milk c.,** lacteal c.
**morgagnian c.,** see *appendix testis* and *appendices vesiculosae epoophori.*
**mother c.,** a cyst enclosing other cysts, as in the cyst stage of *Echinococcus granulosus.*
**mucous c.,** a retention cyst that contains mucus.
**mucus retention c.,** a mucus-containing retention cyst caused by blockage of a salivary gland duct, visible as a small nodule on the oral mucosa; called also *mucocele.* Cf. *mucus extravasation phenomenon,* under *phenomenon.*
**multilocular c.,** 1. a cyst containing several loculi or spaces. 2. a hydatid cyst with many small irregular cavities that may contain scoleces but generally little fluid; it tends to enlarge by budding since it has a poorly developed hyaline cuticle, as in *Echinococcus multilocularis.* See also *alveolar carcinoma* 3. a thick-walled cyst in the kidney, found in clusters and usually unilaterally. In children it contains blastema and may develop into a Wilms tumor. A variety in adults has more fibrous tissue than the juvenile variety.
**myxoid c.,** a nodular lesion usually overlying a distal interphalangeal finger joint in the dorsolateral or dorsomesial position, consisting of focal mucinous degeneration of the collagen of the dermis; not a true cyst, lacking an epithelial wall, it does not communicate with the underlying synovial space. Called also *synovial c.* and *synovial ganglion.*
**Naboth's c's, nabothian c's,** Naboth's follicles.
**nasoalveolar c., nasolabial c.,** an inclusion cyst arising from epithelial remnants at the junction of the globular, lateral nasal, and maxillary processes, which clinically may cause a swelling in the mucolabial fold and in the floor of the nose and superficial erosion of the outer surface of the maxilla.
**nasopalatine duct c.,** median anterior maxillary c.
**necrotic c.,** a cyst containing necrotic matter.
**neural c.,** a cyst or cystlike structure occurring in the central nervous system, as a soapsuds cyst or a porencephalic cyst.
**neurenteric c.,** a cyst of the posterior mediastinum containing tissues from the nervous system and other organs, and connecting with the spinal dura mater.
**nevoid c.,** an abnormal cyst with vascular walls.
**odontogenic c.,** one derived from epithelium, usually containing fluid or semisolid material, which develops during various stages of odontogenesis. Nearly all odontogenic cysts are enclosed within bone. Primordial, dentigerous, periodontal, and gingival cysts are the specific types.
**oil c.,** a cyst containing oily matter, due to fatty degeneration of the epithelial lining.
**omental c's,** cysts similar in all respects to mesenteric ones except that they are confined to the omentum.
**oophoritic c.,** a cyst of the ovary proper.
**pancreatic c.,** a retention cyst of the pancreatic duct; called also *pancreatic ranula.* Cf. *pancreatic pseudocyst.*
**paranephric c.,** a cyst of the fatty tissue surrounding the kidney.
**parapyelitic c's,** apparently congenital cysts of uncertain etiology occurring in the kidney sinus, usually in a small cluster, and causing pelvic compression and local deformity, with pain, hematuria, infection, and pyuria.
**parasitic c.,** a cyst formed by the larva of a parasite, such as a hydatid cyst.
**parovarian c.,** a cyst of the epoöphoron.
**pearl c.,** a cyst or a solid mass of epithelial cells in the iris caused by implantation of an eyelash, cotton, or other foreign particle.
**periapical c.,** a periodontal cyst involving the apex of an erupted tooth, frequently a result of infection via the pulp chamber and root canal through carious involvement of the tooth. Called also *radicular c.*
**pericardial c.,** a benign collection of clear fluid, almost always located immediately adjacent to the pericardium; such cysts must be differentiated from the more serious mediastinal tumors.
**perineurial c.,** an outpouching of the perineurial space on the extradural portion of the posterior sacral or coccygeal nerve roots at the junction of the root and ganglion; it may cause low back pain and sciatica.
**periodontal c.,** one in the periodontal ligament and adjacent structures, usually at the apex *(periapical c.),* but sometimes along the lateral surfaces of the tooth *(lateral periodontal c.).*
**pilar c.,** an epidermal cyst usually occurring as a firm, well-circumscribed, subepidermal nodule, especially on the scalp, and formed by an outer wall of keratinizing epithelium without a granular layer, similar to the normal epithelium of the hair follicle at and distal to the sebaceous duct. Called also *sebaceous c., trichilemmal c.,* and *wen.* Cf. *epidermal inclusion c.*
**piliferous c., pilonidal c.,** pilonidal sinus.
**placental c.,** a grayish white, disklike cyst of the placenta, resulting from degeneration of trophoblastic cells.
**porencephalic c.,** a cyst occurring in the brain substance in porencephaly.
**preauricular c., congenital,** a cyst resulting from imperfect fusion of the branchial arches in formation of the auricle, communicating with an ear pit (q.v.) on the surface. See also *congenital preauricular fistula.*
**primordial c.,** a relatively uncommon type of odontogenic cyst that develops through cystic degeneration and liquefaction of the stellate reticulum in an enamel organ before any calcified enamel or dentin has been formed. Such cysts originate from supernumerary teeth, and are found in place of a tooth rather than being associated with one.
**pseudomucinous c.,** mucinous cystadenoma.
**pyelogenic renal c.,** calyceal diverticulum.
**radicular c.,** periapical c.

**Rathke's c's, Rathke's cleft c's,** groups of epithelial cells forming small colloid-filled cysts in the pars intermedia of the pituitary gland; they are vestiges of Rathke's pouch and are closely related to craniopharyngiomas. Called also *craniobuccal c's* and *craniopharyngeal c's.*
**residual c.,** a periodontal cyst that remains after or develops subsequent to tooth extraction.
**retention c.,** one caused by blockage of the excretory duct of a gland, so that glandular secretions are retained; called also *secretory c.*
**Sampson's c.,** chocolate c.
**sarcosporidian c.,** sarcocyst, def. 2.
**sebaceous c.,** 1. epidermal c. 2. pilar c.
**secondary c.,** a daughter cyst.
**secretory c.,** retention c.
**seminal c.,** a cyst containing semen.
**serous c.,** a cyst containing a thin liquid or serum.
**simple bone c.,** a unilocular, cystic, often asymptomatic bone lesion usually occurring in the long tubular bones of children and adolescents; it is hollow or fluid-filled, lacks an epithelial lining, and does not penetrate the cortex or extend into soft tissue. Its origin is debated, but it is postulated to occur secondary to traumatic hematoma formation. Called also *unicameral bone c.*
**soapsuds c's,** cysts that stud the cerebral cortex in cryptococcosis.
**solitary bone c.,** simple bone c.
**springwater c.,** pericardial c.
**sterile c.,** a true hydatid cyst that fails to produce brood capsules; called also *acephalocyst.*
**subchondral c.,** a bone cyst within the fused epiphysis beneath the articular plate; it is lined with a membrane (probably modified synovia) which contains a mucinous material. Called also *ganglionic c.*
**subepiglottic c.,** a congenital cyst in the subepiglottic mucosa of a horse, often associated with respiratory stridor.
**sublingual c.,** ranula.
**subsynovial c.,** one caused by the accumulation of synovial or inflammatory fluid beneath the synovium.
**suprasellar c.,** craniopharyngioma.
**synovial c.,** myxoid c.
**Tarlov c.,** perineurial c.
**tarry c.,** 1. a corpus luteum cyst resulting from hemorrhage into a corpus luteum. 2. a bloody cyst resulting from endometriosis.
**tarsal c.,** chalazion.
**thecal c.,** distention of a sheath of a tendon.
**theca-lutein c.,** a cyst of the ovary in which the cells lining the cystic cavity are theca-lutein cells.
**thymic c's,** rare unilocular or multilocular cysts of the upper anterior mediastinum containing tissue resembling that of the thymus; they are congenital in origin.
**thyroglossal c., thyrolingual c.,** a cyst in the neck caused by persistence of portions of, or by lack of closure of, the primitive thyroglossal duct.
**tissue c.,** see *cyst* (def. 2) and *pseudocyst* (def. 2).
**Tornwaldt's (Thornwaldt's) c.,** bursa pharyngealis.
**traumatic bone c.,** simple bone c.
**trichilemmal c.,** pilar c.
**trichilemmal c., proliferating,** see under *tumor.*
**true c.,** any cyst that is not a normal structure and is not formed by the dilatation of a passage or cavity.
**tubular c.,** tubulocyst.
**umbilical c.,** vitellointestinal c.
**unicameral c.,** unilocular c.
**unicameral bone c.,** simple bone c.
**unilocular c.,** a cyst containing but one cavity. Cf. *multilocular c.*
**urachal c.,** a form of cystic dilatation of the urachus; called also *allantoic c.*
**urinary c.,** a cyst containing urine.
**vitellointestinal c.,** a cystlike tumor at the umbilicus, caused by persistence of a portion of the umbilical duct; called also *umbilical c.*
**wolffian c.,** a cyst of the remnants of the wolffian duct (ductus mesonephricus).

**cys·tad·e·no·car·ci·no·ma** (sis-tad″ə-no-kahr″sĭ-no′mə) [*cyst-* + *adenocarcinoma*] [MeSH: Cystadenocarcinoma] adenocarcinoma characterized by tumor-lined cystic cavities; occurring usually in the ovaries but also in other sites such as the appendix, pancreas, or thyroid.
**mucinous c.,** pseudomucinous c.
**papillary c.,** a cystadenocarcinoma with papillary projections into the cystic lumina, usually occurring in the ovary.
**pseudomucinous c.,** cystadenocarcinoma in which the epithelium-lined cystic masses produce a sticky, gelatinous, glycoprotein-rich fluid; it usually occurs in the ovary and is often benign.
**serous c.,** cystadenocarcinoma in which the epithelium-lined cystic neoplasms are filled with serous fluid; it often occurs in the ovaries and may also be characterized by papillary projections from, or masses or thickenings of, the cavity walls.

**cys·tad·e·no·ma** (sis″tad-ə-no′mə) [*cyst-* + *adenoma*] [MeSH: Cystadenoma] adenoma characterized by epithelium-lined cystic masses that contain secreted material, usually serous or mucinous; it generally occurs in the ovary, salivary glands, or pancreas.
**apocrine c.,** see under *hidrocystoma.*
**bile duct c.,** a large multiloculated cystic tumor of the liver, usually in the right lobe and filled with clear or cloudy fluid.
**mucinous c.,** a multilocular tumor produced by the epithelial cells of the ovary and having mucin-filled cavities; the great majority of these tumors are benign.
**papillary c.,** 1. any tumor producing patterns which are both papillary and cystic. 2. a type of adenoma in which the acini are distended by fluid or by outgrowths of tissue. Called also *papillary cystic adenoma.*
**papillary c. lymphomato′sum,** adenolymphoma.
**papillary c. of thyroid,** a benign tumor of the thyroid gland with branching papillae and cystlike cavities; it may be an early stage of papillary carcinoma.
**pseudomucinous c.,** mucinous c.; so called because the cavity contents were thought to be pseudomucin.
**serous c.,** a cystic tumor of the ovary, containing thin, clear, yellow serous fluid and varying amounts of solid tissue, with a malignant potential several times greater than that of mucinous cystadenoma.

**Cys·ta·gon** (sis′tə-gon) trademark for a preparation of cysteamine hydrochloride.

**cys·tal·gia** (sis-tal′jə) [*cyst-* + *-algia*] pain in the urinary bladder; called also *cystodynia.*

**γ-cys·ta·thi·o·nase** (sis″tə-thi′o-nās) cystathionine γ-lyase.

**cys·ta·thi·o·nine** (sis″tə-thi′o-nēn) [MeSH: Cystathionine] an unsymmetrical thio-ether of homocysteine and serine that serves as an intermediate in the transfer of a sulfur atom from methionine to cysteine.

**cys·ta·thi·o·nine γ-ly·ase** (sis″tə-thi′o-nēn li′ās) [EC 4.4.1.1] an enzyme of the lyase class that catalyzes the cleavage of cystathionine to cysteine, α-ketoglutarate, and ammonia as a step in the metabolism of methionine. It is a pyridoxal-phosphate protein and the reaction occurs in the liver. Deficiency of the enzyme, an autosomal recessive trait, results in cystathioninuria. Called also *γ-cystathionase.*

**cys·ta·thi·o·nine β-syn·thase** (sis″tə-thi′o-nēn sin′thās) [EC 4.2.1.22] an enzyme of the lyase class that catalyzes the condensation of serine and homocysteine to form cystathionine as a step in the catabolism of methionine. It is a pyridoxal-phosphate protein, found in the mammalian liver.

**cys·ta·thi·o·nine β-syn·thase de·fi·cien·cy** an autosomal recessive aminoacidopathy characterized by homocystinuria accompanied by hypermethioninemia. Clinical abnormalities occur primarily in the eye and the skeletal, nervous, and vascular systems; ectopia lentis, osteoporosis, mental retardation, and thrombosis are the most common manifestations. In older literature, the disorder is sometimes called homocystinuria (q.v.).

**cys·ta·thi·o·nin·u·ria** (sis″tə-thi″o-ne-nu′re-ə) 1. an autosomal recessive aminoacidopathy characterized by excess of cystathionine in urine and body tissues but without other clinical manifestations; it is caused by deficiency of cystathionine γ-lyase. 2. excess of cystathionine in the urine.

**cys·ta·tro·phia** (sis″tə-tro′fe-ə) [*cyst-* + *atrophia*] atrophy of the bladder.

**cys·tau·che·ni·tis** (sis″taw-kə-ni′tis) [*cyst-* + Gr. *auchēn* neck + *-itis*] inflammation of the neck of the bladder.

**cys·tau·che·not·o·my** (sis″taw-kə-not′ə-me) [*cyst-* + Gr. *auchēn* neck + *-tomy*] surgical incision of the neck of the bladder.

**cys·te·amine** (sis'te-ə-mēn") [MeSH: Cysteamine] β-mercaptoethylamine.
**c. bitartrate,** the hydrochloride salt of cysteamine, used for the prevention of nephropathic cystinosis; administered orally.

**cys·tec·ta·sia, cys·tec·ta·sy** (sis"tek-ta'zhə, sis-tek'tə-se) [*cyst-* +Gr. *ektasis* dilatation] slitting of the membranous portion of the urethra and dilation of the neck of the bladder for the extraction of stone.

**cys·tec·to·my** (sis-tek'tə-me) [*cyst-* + *-ectomy*] [MeSH: Cystectomy] 1. excision of a cyst. 2. resection of the bladder.
**radical c.,** surgical treatment of invasive bladder cancer by removal of the bladder with its peritoneal covering, the lower ureters, pelvic lymph nodes, and surrounding organs and structures. In females it is a synonym of *anterior pelvic exenteration.* In males (called also *radical cystoprostatectomy*) the prostate, seminal vesicles, pelvic vas deferens and its ampulla, and sometimes part or all of the urethra are removed.

**cys·te·ic ac·id** (sis-te'ik) [MeSH: Cysteic Acid] an intermediate formed by oxidation of the thiol group of cysteine to a sulfo group, and precursor of taurine.

**cys·te·ine** (sis-te'ēn) [MeSH: Cysteine] chemical name: 2-amino-3-mercaptopropanoic acid. A sulfur-containing nonessential amino acid produced by the enzymatic or acid hydrolysis of proteins. It is easily oxidized to cystine, is sometimes found in the urine, and has limited detoxification properties. Symbols Cys and C. See also table at *amino acid.*
**c. hydrochloride** [USP], a compound suggested for the treatment of cutaneous ulcers.

**cys·te·ine en·do·pep·ti·dase** (sis-te'ēn en"do-pep'tĭ-dās) [EC 3.4.22] any of a group of endopeptidases containing at the active site a cysteine residue involved in catalysis; the group includes papain and several cathepsins. Called also *thiol endopeptidase.*

**cys·te·ine-type car·boxy·pep·ti·dase** (sis'te-ēn-tīp" kahr-bok"se-pep'tĭ-dās) [EC 3.4.18] 1. any exopeptidase that contains a cysteine residue at the active site and catalyzes the thiol-dependent hydrolytic cleavage of the terminal or penultimate peptide bond at the C-terminal end of a peptide or polypeptide. 2. [EC 3.4.18.1] a lysosomal carboxypeptidase with broad specificity but not acting on C-terminal proline residues. Called also *lysosomal carboxypeptidase B* and *cathepsin* $B_2$.

**cys·te·in·yl** (sis'tēn-il, sis-te'in-il) the acyl radical of cysteine.

**cys·tel·co·sis** (sis"təl-ko'sis) [*cyst-* + *elcosis*] ulceration of the bladder.

**cys·ten·ceph·a·lus** (sis"tən-sef'ə-ləs) [*cyst-* + Gr. *enkephalos* brain] a fetus with a membranous sac in place of a brain.

**cyst·er·e·thism** (sis-ter'ə-thiz-əm) [*cyst-* + Gr. *erethismos* irritation] irritability of the bladder.

**cyst·hy·per·sar·co·sis** (sist-hi"pər-sahr-ko'sis) [*cyst-* + *hyper-* + *sarco-* + *-sis*] a thickening of the muscular coat of the bladder.

**cysti-** see *cyst(o)-.*

**cys·tic** (sis'tik) 1. pertaining to a cyst. 2. pertaining to the urinary bladder or to the gallbladder. Cf. *vesical.*

**cys·ti·cer·ci** (sis"tĭ-sər'si) plural of *cysticercus.*

**cys·ti·cer·coid** (sis"tĭ-sər'koid) a form of larval tapeworm resembling *Cysticercus,* but having the cyst small, almost devoid of fluid, and provided with a caudal appendage, as in *Hymenolepis.*

**cys·ti·cer·co·sis** (sis"tĭ-sər-ko'sis) [MeSH: Cysticercosis] infection with cysticerci. In various animals it occurs as cysts found in striated muscles and causes no adverse symptoms (called also *beef measles, pork measles,* and *sheep measles*). Humans who eat incompletely cooked pork may become infected with larval forms of *Taenia solium* (formerly known as *Cysticercus cellulosae*), which penetrate the intestinal wall and invade such tissues as the subcutaneous tissue, brain, eye, muscle, heart, liver, lung, and peritoneum. Brain involvement results in neurocysticercosis (q.v.). Humans who eat incompletely cooked beef may become infected with *C. bovis (Taenia saginata),* which can grow to a tapeworm 12 to 25 feet long in the intestine.

**Cys·ti·cer·cus** (sis"tĭ-sər'kəs) [Gr. *kystis* bladder + *kerkos* tail] [MeSH: Cysticercus] a former genus of larval forms of tapeworms of the genus *Taenia.*
**C. bo'vis,** the larva of *Taenia saginata.*
**C. cellulo'sae,** the larva of *Taenia solium;* see also *cysticercosis.*
**C. o'vis,** the larva of *Taenia ovis.*
**C. tenuicol'lis,** the larva of *Taenia hydatigena.*

**cys·ti·cer·cus** (sis"tĭ-sər'kəs) pl. *cysticer'ci* [MeSH: Cysticercus] A larval form of tapeworm, consisting of a single scolex enclosed in a bladderlike cyst; cf. *hydatid cyst,* under *cyst.* Called also *bladder worm.*

**cys·ti·co·li·thec·to·my** (sis"tĭ-ko"lĭ-thek'tə-me) [*cysti-* + *lithectomy*] removal of a calculus from the cystic duct.

**cys·ti·co·li·tho·trip·sy** (sis"tĭ-ko-lith'o-trip-se) crushing of a calculus within the cystic duct.

**cys·ti·cor·rha·phy** (sis"tĭ-kor'ə-fe) [*cystic* duct + *-rrhaphy*] suture or repair of the cystic duct.

**cys·ti·cot·o·my** (sis"tĭ-kot'ə-me) [*cystic* duct + *-tomy*] incision into the cystic duct.

**cys·ti·des** (sis'tĭ-dēz) plural of *cystis.*

**cystid(o)-** see *cyst(o)-.*

**cys·ti·do·ce·li·ot·o·my** (sis"tĭ-do-se"le-ot'ə-me) cystidolaparotomy.

**cys·ti·do·lap·a·rot·o·my** (sis"tĭ-do-lap"ə-rot'ə-me) [*cystido-* + *laparotomy*] incision of the bladder through the abdominal wall.

**cys·ti·do·tra·chel·o·to·my** (sis"tĭ-do-tra"kəl-ot'ə-me) [*cystido-* + *trachlo-* + *-tomy*] incision of the neck of the bladder.

**cys·tif·er·ous** (sis-tif'ər-əs) cystigerous.

**cys·ti·form** (sis'tĭ-form) [*cysti-* + *form*] having the form or appearance of a cyst.

**cys·tig·er·ous** (sis-tij'ər-əs) [*cysti-* + L. *gerere* to bear] containing cysts.

**cys·tine** (sis'tēn, sis'tin) [MeSH: Cystine] chemical name: 3,3'-dithiobis(2-aminopropanoic acid). An amino acid produced by the digestion or acid hydrolysis of proteins. It is sometimes found in the urine and in the kidneys in the form of minute hexagonal crystals, frequently forming a cystine calculus in the bladder. Cystine is the chief sulfur-containing compound of the protein molecule and is readily reduced to two molecules of cysteine (hence, also called *dicysteine*).

**cys·tin·emia** (sis'tĭ-ne'me-ə) presence of cystine in the blood.

**cys·ti·no·sis** (sis"tĭ-no'sis) [MeSH: Cystinosis] lysosomal storage disorders of unknown molecular defect, characterized by widespread deposition of cystine crystals in reticuloendothelial cells. There are three clinical types: *early onset c., late onset juvenile c.,* and *benign c.* Called also *cystine storage disease* and *Lignac-Fanconi syndrome.*
**adolescent nephropathic c.,** late onset juvenile c.
**adult nephropathic c.,** benign c.
**benign c.,** a type of cystinosis that does not affect kidneys or shorten life span, is marked by deposition of cystine in the bone marrow, leukocytes, and corneas, and is diagnosed by ophthalmic examination. Called also *adult nephropathic c.*
**early onset c.,** the most common cause of the Fanconi syndrome (def. 2), a type marked by vitamin D–resistant rickets, chronic acidosis, polyuria, and dehydration, all resulting from proximal renal tubular dysfunction, and by corneal opacities, growth failure, uremia, and death before age ten. Called also *infantile nephropathic c.*
**infantile nephropathic c.,** early onset c.
**late onset juvenile c.,** a type that falls between the early onset type and the benign type; there are ocular and renal manifestations, but the kidney lesion does not always lead to renal insufficiency. Called also *adolescent nephropathic c.*

**cys·tin·uria** (sis"tĭ-nu're-ə) [MeSH: Cystinuria] a hereditary condition of persistent excessive urinary excretion of cystine and three other dibasic amino acids: lysine, ornithine, and arginine; it is due to impairment of renal transport in tubular reabsorption of these amino acids. The predominant clinical manifestation is the formation of urinary cystine calculi.

**cys·tin·uric** (sis"tin-u'rik) pertaining to or affected with cystinuria.

**cys·tir·rha·gia** (sis"tĭ-ra'je-ə) cystorrhagia.

**cys·tir·rhea** (sis"tĭ-re'ə) cystorrhea.

**cys·tis** (sis'tis) pl. *cys'tides* [Gr. *kystis*] 1. vesica. 2. cyst (def. 2).
**c. fel'lea,** vesica biliaris.

**cys·ti·stax·is** (sis"tĭ-stak'sis) [*cysti-* + *staxis*] oozing of blood from the mucous membrane into the bladder.

**cys·ti·tis** (sis-ti'tis) [MeSH: Cystitis] inflammation of the urinary bladder; called also *urocystitis.*
**allergic c.,** cystitis resulting from some unusual hypersensitivity, characterized by a large number of mononuclear leukocytes and eosinophils in the bladder mucosa and musculature, and in the urinary sediment.
**bacterial c.,** bacterial infection of the bladder.
**catarrhal c., acute,** cystitis resulting from injury, irritation by foreign bodies, gonorrhea, etc., and marked by burning in the bladder, pain in the urethra, and painful micturition.
**c. col'li,** inflammation involving the neck of the bladder.
**croupous c.,** diphtheritic c.
**cystic c., c. cys'tica,** cystitis with the formation of multiple submucosal cysts in the bladder wall.

**diphtheritic c.,** cystitis due to infection by *Corynebacterium diphtheriae,* and characterized by the formation of a false membrane; called also *croupous c.*
**c. emphysemato'sa,** an unusual inflammation of the bladder, characterized by the presence of gas-filled vesicles and cysts in the bladder mucosa and musculature.
**eosinophilic c.,** cystitis characterized by the presence of large numbers of eosinophils in the urinary sediment.
**exfoliative c.,** cystitis with sloughing of the bladder mucosa.
**c. follicula'ris,** cystitis in which the mucosa of the bladder is studded with nodules containing lymph follicles.
**c. glandula'ris,** cystitis in which the mucosa contains mucin-secreting glands, observed more frequently in cases of exstrophy of the bladder, and sometimes leading to malignant degeneration.
**hemorrhagic c.,** cystitis accompanied by severe hemorrhage, seen as a dose-limiting toxic condition with administration of ifosfamide and cyclophosphamide and as a complication of bone marrow transplantation.
**incrusted c.,** an intense cystitis characterized by deposition of phosphatic or other inorganic salts on the chronically inflamed bladder wall, generally at the site of ulcerations, granulations, or tumors.
**interstitial c., chronic,** a condition of the bladder occurring predominantly in women, with an inflammatory lesion, usually in the vertex, and involving the entire thickness of the wall, appearing as a small patch of brownish-red mucosa, surrounded by a network of radiating vessels. The lesions, known as Fenwick-Hunner or Hunner ulcers, may heal superficially, and are notoriously difficult to detect. Typically, there is urinary frequency and pain on bladder filling and at the end of micturition. Called also *panmural c., submucous c.,* and *panmural fibrosis of the bladder.*
**mechanical c.,** cystitis resulting from irritation by a vesical calculus, manipulation, or a foreign body in the bladder.
**panmural c.,** interstitial c., chronic.
**c. papillomato'sa,** cystitis characterized by the presence of papillomatous growths on the inflamed mucous membrane.
**c. seni'lis femina'rum,** a chronic cystitis occurring in elderly women, marked by abnormal frequency of micturition, with tenesmus and burning.
**submucous c.,** interstitial c., chronic.

**cys·ti·tome** (sis'tĭ-tōm) [*cysti-* + *-tome*] an instrument for opening the capsule of the lens of the eye; called also *cibisotome* and *kibisitome.*

**cys·tit·o·my** (sis-tit'ə-me) [*cysti-* + *-tomy*] the surgical division of the capsule of the lens; capsulotomy.

**cyst(o)-** a combining form denoting a relationship to a sac, cyst, or bladder, most frequently used in reference to the urinary bladder. Also, *cysti-* and *cystido-.*

**cys·to·ad·e·no·ma** (sis″to-ad″ə-no'mə) cystadenoma.

**cys·to·blast** (sis'to-blast) [*cysto-* + *-blast*] the layer of cells that lines the amniotic cavity of the early embryo on the side of the enveloping layer.

**Cys·to·cau·lus** (sis″to-kaw'lus) a genus of parasitic nematodes of the family Protostrongylidae, several species of which are lungworms of sheep and goats.

**cys·to·cele** (sis'to-sēl) [*cysto-* + *cele*[1]] hernial protrusion of the urinary bladder through the vaginal wall; called also *cystic hernia.*

**cys·to·chrome** (sis'to-krōm) [*cysto-* + *-chrome*] a mixture of indigo carmine and methenamine; used by intramuscular or intravenous injection for the indigo carmine test of renal function.

**cys·to·chro·mos·co·py** (sis″to-kro-mos'kə-pe) chromocystoscopy.

**cys·to·co·los·to·my** (sis″to-ko-los'tə-me) [*cysto-* + *colostomy*] the surgical creation of a permanent passage from the bladder to the colon.

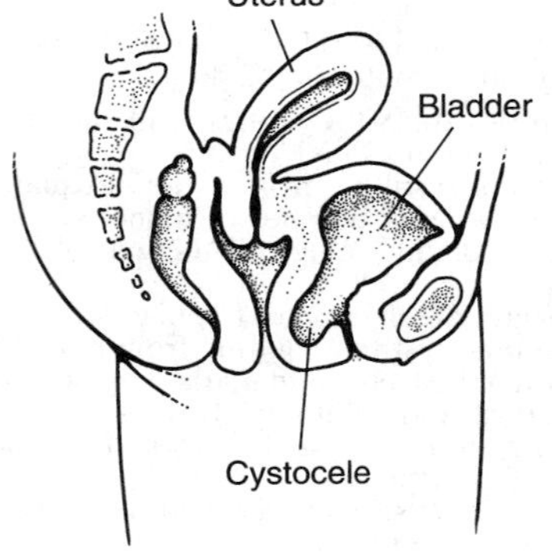


**cys·to·di·a·pha·nos·co·py** (sis″to-di″ə-fə-nos'kə-pe) [*cysto-* + *diaphanoscopy*] examination within, or transillumination of, the urinary bladder by means of a diaphanoscope.

**cys·to·du·od·e·nos·to·my** (sis″to-du″o-də-nos'tə-me) internal drainage of an adjacent cyst into the duodenum.

**cys·to·dyn·ia** (sis″to-din'e-ə) [*cysto-* + *-odynia*] cystalgia.

**cys·to·elyt·ro·plas·ty** (sis″to-e-lit'ro-plas″te) [*cysto-* + *elytro-* + *-plasty*] surgical repair of vesicovaginal injuries.

**cys·to·en·tero·cele** (sis″to-en'tər-o-sēl) hernia of a portion of the bladder and of the intestine.

**cys·to·epip·lo·cele** (sis″to-e-pip'lo-sēl) hernia of a portion of the bladder and of the omentum.

**cys·to·gas·tros·to·my** (sis″to-gas-tros'tə-me) internal drainage of an adjacent cyst into the stomach.

**cys·to·gen·e·sis** (sis″to-jen'ə-sis) formation of a cyst.

**cys·to·gram** (sis'to-gram) a radiograph of the bladder.

**cys·tog·ra·phy** (sis-tog'rə-fe) [*cysto-* + *-graphy*] radiography of the bladder after injection of the organ with opaque solution.
**delayed c.,** cystography in which film exposures are made at varying intervals up to 30 minutes or longer; useful in the study of urinary reflux.
**voiding c.,** radiography of the bladder while the patient is urinating.

**cys·toid** (sis'toid) [*cysto-* + *-oid*] 1. resembling a cyst. 2. a cystlike, circumscribed collection of softened material, differing from a true cyst in having no enclosing capsule.

**Cys·to·i·sos·po·ra** (sis″to-i-sos'pə-rə) a genus of coccidian protozoa that infect the intestines of dogs and cats; formerly classified as part of *Isospora.* Infections may be subclinical or may lead to mild coccidiosis. *C. fe'lis* and *C. rivol'ta* infect cats. *C. burrow'si, C. ca'nis, C. neorivol'ta,* and *C. ohioen'sis* infect dogs.

**cys·to·je·ju·nos·to·my** (sis″to-jə-joo-nos'tə-me) internal drainage of an adjacent cyst into the jejunum.

**cys·to·lith** (sis'to-lith) [*cysto-* + *-lith*] [MeSH: Bladder Calculi] vesical calculus.

**cys·to·li·thec·to·my** (sis″to-lĭ-thek'tə-me) [*cysto-* + *lithectomy*] the removal of a urinary calculus by cutting into the urinary bladder. The term has been used erroneously for excision of a gallstone from the gallbladder.

**cys·to·li·thi·a·sis** (sis″to-lĭ-thi'ə-sis) [*cysto-* + Gr. *lithos* stone] the development of calculi in the urinary bladder.

**cys·to·lith·ic** (sis″to-lith'ik) pertaining to vesical calculi.

**cys·to·li·thot·o·my** (sis″to-lĭ-thot'ə-me) cystolithectomy.

**cys·to·ma** (sis-to'mə) [*cysto-* + *-oma*] a cystic tumor.
**c. sero'sum sim'plex,** simple cyst of the ovary.

**cys·to·ma·tous** (sis-to'mə-təs) relating to or containing cystoma.

**cys·tom·e·ter** (sis-tom'ə-tər) [*cysto-* + *-meter*] an instrument for studying the neuromuscular mechanism of the bladder by means of measurements of pressure and capacity.

**cys·to·met·ro·gram** (sis″to-met'ro-gram) the tracing recorded by cystometrography.

**cys·to·me·trog·ra·phy** (sis″to-mə-trog'rə-fe) the graphic recording of the pressure exerted at varying degrees of filling of the urinary bladder.

**cys·tom·e·try** (sis-tom'ə-tre) the study of bladder efficiency by means of the cystometer.

**cys·to·mor·phous** (sis″to-mor'fəs) [*cysto-* + *morph-* + *-ous*] shaped like a cyst or bladder.

**cys·to·ne·phro·sis** (sis″to-nə-fro'sis) [*cysto-* + *nephro-* + *-sis*] cystiform dilatation or enlargement of the kidney.

**cys·to·neu·ral·gia** (sis″to-noor-al'jə) [*cysto-* + *neuralgia*] neuralgia of the bladder.

**cys·to·pa·ral·y·sis** (sis″to-pə-ral'ĭ-sis) cystoplegia.

**cys·to·pa·re·sis** (sis″to-pə-re'sis) cystoplegia.

**cys·to·pexy** (sis'to-pek″se) [*cysto-* + *-pexy*] fixation of the bladder to the abdominal wall in the treatment of cystocele; vesicofixation.

**cys·toph·o·rous** (sis-tof'ə-rəs) [*cysto-* + Gr. *phoros* bearing] containing cysts.

**cys·to·pho·tog·ra·phy** (sis″to-fo-tog'rə-fe) the photographing of the inside of the bladder.

**cys·toph·thi·sis** (sis-tof'thĭ-sis) [*cysto-* + *phthisis*] tuberculosis of the bladder.

**cys·to·plas·ty** (sis'to-plas″te) [*cysto-* + *-plasty*] any plastic or re-

constructive operation on the bladder. See also *gastrocystoplasty* and *ileocystoplasty*.
**augmentation c.**, enlargement of the bladder by grafting to it a detached segment of intestine (ileum, cecum, or sigmoid).
**sigmoid c.**, cystoplasty in which a portion of the sigmoid colon is used to reconstruct or augment the bladder.

**cys·to·ple·gia** (sis″to-ple′jə) [*cysto-* + *-plegia*] paralysis of the bladder; called also *cystoparalysis*.

**cys·to·proc·tos·to·my** (sis″to-prok-tos′tə-me) [*cysto-* + *proctostomy*] the surgical creation of a communication between the urinary bladder and rectum; called also *cystorectostomy*.

**cys·to·pros·ta·tec·to·my** (sis″to-pros-tə-tek′təme) [*cysto-* + prostatectomy] surgical removal of the urinary bladder and prostate gland.
**radical c.**, radical cystectomy in a male.

**cys·top·to·sis** (sis″top-to′sis) [*cysto-* + *-ptosis*] prolapse of a part of the inner coat of the bladder into the urethra.

**cys·to·py·eli·tis** (sis″to-pi″ə-li′tis) inflammation involving both the urinary bladder and the pelvis of the kidney.

**cys·to·py·elog·ra·phy** (sis″to-pi″ə-log′rə-fe) radiography of the urinary bladder and the pelvis of the kidney.

**cys·to·py·elo·ne·phri·tis** (sis″to-pi″ə-lo-nə-fri′tis) [*cysto-* + *pyelonephritis*] combined cystitis and pyelonephritis.

**cys·to·ra·di·og·ra·phy** (sis″to-ra″de-og′rə-fe) [*cysto-* + *radiography*] radiography of the bladder.

**cys·to·rec·tos·to·my** (sis″to-rek-tos′tə-me) cystoproctostomy.

**cys·tor·rha·gia** (sis″to-ra′jə) [*cysto-* + *-rrhagia*] hemorrhage from the bladder.

**cys·tor·rha·phy** (sis-tor′ə-fe) [*cysto-* + *-rrhaphy*] the operation of suturing the bladder.

**cys·tor·rhea** (sis″to-re′ə) [*cysto-* + *-rrhea*] catarrh of the bladder.

**cys·to·sar·co·ma** (sis″to-sahr-ko′mə) phyllodes tumor.
**c. phyllo′des**, phyllodes tumor.

**cys·tos·chi·sis** (sis-tos′kĭ-sis) [*cysto-* + *-schisis*] fissure of the bladder.

**cys·to·scle·ro·sis** (sis″to-skə-ro′sis) a cyst that has undergone sclerosis or fibrosis.

**cys·to·scope** (sis′to-skōp″) [*cysto-* + *-scope*] an endoscope for visual examination of the bladder.

**cys·to·scop·ic** (sis″to-skop′ik) pertaining to cystoscopy, or performed with the cystoscope.

**cys·tos·co·py** (sis-tos′kə-pe) [MeSH: Cystoscopy] direct visual examination of the urinary tract with a cystoscope.

**cys·tose** (sis′tōs) resembling or containing a cyst or cysts.

**cys·to·spasm** (sis′to-spaz-əm) [*cysto-* + *spasm*] spasm of the bladder.

**Cys·to·spaz** (sis′to-spaz) trademark for preparations of hyoscyamine.

**cys·to·sper·mi·tis** (sis″to-spər-mi′tis) [*cysto-* + *sperm-* + *-itis*] inflammation of a seminal vesicle.

**cys·to·stax·is** (sis″to-stak′sis) cystistaxis.

**cys·tos·to·my** (sis-tos′tə-me) [*cysto-* + *-stomy*] [MeSH: Cystostomy] the formation of an opening into the bladder. Called also *vesicostomy*.
**suprapubic c.**, surgical diversion of the urethra to an opening in the skin above the symphysis pubis for bladder drainage in cases of urethral stricture.
**tubeless c.**, cutaneous vesicostomy.

**cys·to·tome** (sis′to-tōm) [*cysto-* + *-tome*] 1. an instrument for incising the bladder. 2. cystitome.

**cys·tot·o·my** (sis-tot′ə-me) surgical incision of the urinary bladder; called also *vesicotomy*.
**suprapubic c.**, the operation of cutting into the bladder by an incision just above the pubic symphysis.

**cys·to·tra·chel·ot·o·my** (sis″to-tra″kəl-ot′ə-me) [*cysto-* + *trachelo-* + *-tomy*] surgical incision of the neck of the bladder.

**cys·to·ure·ter·itis** (sis″to-u-re″tər-i′tis) inflammation involving the urinary bladder and ureters.

**cys·to·ure·tero·gram** (sis″to-u-re′tər-o-gram) a radiograph of the urinary bladder and ureters.

**cys·to·ure·tero·py·eli·tis** (sis″to-u-re″tər-o-pi″ə-li′tis) inflammation involving the urinary bladder, ureter, and pelvis of the kidney.

**cys·to·ure·ter·o·py·elo·neph·ri·tis** (sis″to-u-re″tər-o-pi″ə-lo-nə-fri′tis) combined inflammation of the bladder, ureter, and pelvis and pyramids of the kidney.

**cys·to·ure·thri·tis** (sis″to-u″re-thri′tis) urethrocystitis.

**cys·to·ure·thro·cele** (sis″to-u-re′thro-sēl) prolapse of the female urethra and bladder.

**cys·to·ure·thro·gram** (sis″to-u-re′thro-gram) a radiograph of the urinary bladder and urethra.
**voiding c. (VCUG),** the radiograph made during voiding cystourethrography.

**cys·to·ure·throg·ra·phy** (sis″to-u″rə-thog′rə-fe) radiography of the urinary bladder and urethra.
**chain c.**, that in which a sterile beaded metal chain is introduced via a modified catheter into the bladder and urethra; used in evaluating anatomical relationships of the bladder and urethra.
**voiding c.**, cystourethrography in which radiographs are made before, during, and after voiding. Abbreviated VCU.

**cys·to·ure·thro·scope** (sis″to-u-re′thro-skōp″) an instrument for examining the bladder and posterior urethra.

**cys·tous** (sis′təs) cystose.

**cys·tyl** (sis′təl) the divalent acyl radical of cystine.

**Cy·ta·dren** (si′tə-drən) trademark for a preparation of aminoglutethimide.

**cyt·a·phe·re·sis** (sīt″ə-fə-re′sis) [*cyt-* + *apheresis*] [MeSH: Cytapheresis] apheresis of blood cells; see *erythrocytapheresis, leukocytapheresis,* and *thrombocytapheresis.*

**cy·tar·a·bine** (si-tar′ə-bēn) [USP] [MeSH: Cytarabine] a deoxycytidine analogue, cytosine arabinoside (ara-C), that is metabolically activated to the triphosphate nucleotide (ara-CTP), which acts as a competitive inhibitor of DNA polymerase and produces S phase–specific cytotoxicity; used as an antineoplastic, generally as part of a combination chemotherapy regimen, in the treatment of acute lymphocytic and acute myelogenous leukemia, the blast phase of chronic myelogenous leukemia, erythroleukemia, and non-Hodgkin's lymphoma, administered intravenously and subcutaneously, and for the prophylaxis and treatment of meningeal leukemia, administered intrathecally. Called also *ara-C* and *cytosine arabinoside.*

**cyt·ar·me** (sit-ahr′me) [*cyt-* + *armē* union] the flattening of rounded blastomeres at the conclusion of cleavage.

**cy·tas·ter** (si′tas-tər) [*cyt-* + *aster*] aster.

**Cy·taux·zo·on** (si″tawk-zo′on) [*cyt-* + *aux-* + Gr. *zōon* animal] a genus of parasitic protozoa (order Piroplasmida, subclass Piroplasmia) found in African ungulates and in the domestic cat in North America. *C. fe′lis* causes fatal cytauxzoonosis in cats.

**cy·taux·zoo·no·sis** (si″tawk-zo″o-no′sis) a rapidly fatal disease due to infection with protozoa of the genus *Cytauxzoon,* occurring in African ungulates and in domestic cats. The feline infection is caused by *Ctenocephalides felis* and is seen chiefly in cats roaming the wooded areas of the Gulf Coast states of North America. It is clinically characterized by fever, anemia, icterus, anorexia, lethargy, dehydration, and depression, and microscopically by huge reticuloendothelial cells packed with schizonts in the peripheral blood that nearly occlude the lumens of the small and medium-sized veins of the lungs, spleen, and lymph nodes.

**-cyte** [Gr. *kytos* hollow vessel] a word termination denoting a cell, the type of which is designated by the root to which it is affixed, as *elliptocyte, erythrocyte, leukocyte.*

**Cy·tel·lin** (si-tel′in) trademark for a preparation of sitosterols.

**cy·ti·dine** (si′tĭ-dēn) [MeSH: Cytidine] a purine nucleoside, cytosine linked by its N9 nitrogen to the C1 carbon of ribose. It is a component of ribonucleic acid and its nucleotides are important in the synthesis of a variety of lipid derivatives. Symbol C.
**c. diphosphate (CDP),** a nucleotide, the 5′-pyrophosphate of cytidine, that serves as a carrier for choline and ethanolamine in phospholipid synthesis.
**c. monophosphate (CMP),** a nucleotide, the 5′-phosphate of cytidine, that serves as a carrier for *N*-acetylneuraminic acid in glycoprotein synthesis. Called also *cytidylic acid.*
**c. triphosphate (CTP),** a nucleotide, the 5′-triphosphate of cytidine; it is an activated precursor in the synthesis of ribonucleic acid and of CDP- and CMP-linked compounds.

**cy·ti·dine de·am·i·nase** (si′tĭ-dēn de-am′ĭ-nās) [EC 3.5.4.5] [MeSH: Cytidine Deaminase] an enzyme of the hydrolase class that catalyzes the deamination of cytidine to form uridine. The reaction, occurring in animal tissues and bacteria, is part of the pyrimidine degradation pathway.

**cy·ti·dyl·ate** (si″tĭ-dil′āt) a dissociated form of cytidylic acid.

**cy·ti·dyl·ate ki·nase** (si″tĭ-dil′āt ki′nās) [EC 2.7.4.14] an enzyme of the transferase class that catalyzes the phosphorylation of CMP or dCMP to form the corresponding bisphosphate compound.

**cy·ti·dyl·ic ac·id** (si″tĭ-dil′ik) phosphorylated cytidine, usually cytidine monophosphate.

**cy·ti·dyl·yl** (si″tĭ-dil′əl) the radical formed by removal of OH from the phosphate group of cytidine monophosphate.

**cyt·i·sine** (sit′ĭ-sin) [Gr. *kytisos* laburnum] a highly toxic alkaloid from various members of the genus *Cytisus,* especially *C. laburnum;* it causes cytisism and was formerly used as an antiemetic and antitussive.

**cyt·i·sism** (sit′ĭ-siz-əm) poisoning by eating plants that contain cytisine, such as *Cytisus laburnum* or various members of the genus *Laburnum;* characteristics include burning in the mouth and pharynx, thirst, nausea, vomiting, diarrhea, prostration, an irregular pulse, and sometimes aphasia, visual disturbances, delirium, and unconsciousness with respiratory paralysis and death.

**Cyt·i·sus** (sit′ĭ-səs) a genus of trees of the family Leguminosae, native to Europe, northern Africa, and southern Asia. *C. scopa′rius* (L.) Link., or scotch broom, is the source of scoparin and scoparius and the cause of broom poisoning (q.v.). *C. labur′num* is a laburnum tree that contains cytisine and causes cyticism. Called also *Sarothamnus.*

**cyt(o)-** [Gr. *kytos* hollow vessel] a combining form denoting relationship to a cell.

**cy·to·an·a·ly·zer** (si″to-an′ə-li″zər) an electronic optical apparatus for the detection of malignant cells in smears.

**cy·to·ar·chi·tec·ton·ic** (si″to-ahr″kĭ-tek-ton′ik) pertaining to cytoarchitecture or to cytoarchitectonics.

**cy·to·ar·chi·tec·ton·ics** (si″to-ahr″kĭ-tek-ton′iks) 1. cytoarchitecture. 2. the study of cytoarchitecture.

**cy·to·ar·chi·tec·tu·ral** (si″to-ahr″kĭ-tek′chə-rəl) pertaining to cytoarchitecture.

**cy·to·ar·chi·tec·ture** (si″to-ahr′kĭ-tek′chər) the organization of cells in the structure of an organ or tissue such as the cerebral cortex.

**cy·to·bi·ol·o·gy** (si″to-bi-ol′ə-je) [*cyto-* + *biology*] the biology of cells.

**cy·to·bio·tax·is** (si″to-bi-o-tak′sis) [*cyto-* + *bio-* + *taxis*] cytoclesis.

**cy·to·cen·trum** (si″to-sen′trəm) [*cyto-* + Gr. *kentron* center] centrosphere, def. 1.

**cy·to·ce·ras·tic** (si″to-sə-ras′tik) cytokerastic.

**cy·to·chal·a·sin** (si″to-kal′ə-sin) any of a group of fungal metabolites that interfere with the formation of microfilaments and thus disrupt the cellular processes dependent on those filaments.
**c. B,** cytochalasin used to examine the role of microfilaments in the morphology and physiology of cells; it causes microfilaments to disappear by inhibiting the assembly of actin filaments, thus blocking numerous cell processes, e.g., cytokinesis, endocytosis, exocytosis, smooth muscle contraction, and cell migration.

**cy·to·chem·ism** (si″to-kem′iz-əm) [*cyto-* + *chemism*] chemical activity of cells.

**cy·to·chem·is·try** (si″to-kem″is-tre) [*cyto-* + *chemistry*] the study of the locations, structural relationships, and interactions of cellular constituents by means of methods such as electron microscopy, cell fractionation, and immunochemical techniques.

**cy·to·chrome** (si′to-krōm) [*cyto-* + *-chrome*] any electron transfer hemoprotein having a mode of action in which the transfer of a single electron is effected by a reversible valence change of the central iron atom of the heme prosthetic group between the +2 and +3 oxidation states; classified as cytochromes *a* when the heme contains a formyl side chain, cytochromes *b* when protoheme (or a closely similar heme) is not covalently bound to the protein, cytochromes *c* when protoheme or other heme is covalently bound to the protein, and cytochromes *d* when the iron-tetrapyrrole has fewer conjugated double bonds than the hemes have. Well-known cytochromes have been numbered consecutively within groups and are designated by subscripts (beginning with no subscript), e.g., cytochromes *c*, $c_1$, $c_2$, etc. New cytochromes are named according to the wavelength in nanometers of the absorption maximum of the α-band of the iron (II) form in pyridine, e.g., c-555.
**c. $aa_3$,** cytochrome-*c* oxidase.
**c. *b*,** a cytochrome in the inner mitochondrial membrane that, with cytochrome $c_1$ and an iron-sulfur protein, acts as the electron carrier of the enzyme ubiquinol–cytochrome-*c* reductase.
**c. $b_5$,** a cytochrome occurring in the endoplasmic reticulum that acts as an intermediate electron carrier in some reactions catalyzed by mixed function oxidases, e.g., fatty acid desaturation; it activates molecular oxygen for an attack on the substrate.
**c. *c*,** a cytochrome on the inner mitochondrial membrane that accepts electrons from ubiquinol–cytochrome-*c* reductase and transfers them to cytochrome-*c* oxidase, part of the electron transport chain (q.v.).
**c. $c_1$,** a cytochrome in the inner mitochondrial membrane that, with cytochrome *b* and an iron-sulfur protein, acts as the electron carrier of the enzyme ubiquinol–cytochrome-*c* reductase.
**c. P-450, c. $P_{450}$,** trivial name (P for pigment, 450 nm for the absorption maximum of the carbon monoxide derivative) for a cytochrome occurring in most tissues and containing a protoheme IX prosthetic group. It serves as the oxygenating catalyst in a wide variety of reactions catalyzed by monooxygenases, e.g., hydroxylation of steroid hormones and oxidations involved in the detoxification of many drugs; cytochrome P-450 activates molecular oxygen for an attack on the substrate.

**cy·to·chrome-$b_5$ re·duc·tase** (si′to-krōm re-duk′tas) [EC 1.6.2.2] an enzyme of the endoplasmic reticulum and erythrocytes that catalyzes several series of redox reactions transferring electrons from NADH to an acceptor via the intermediate electron carrier cytochrome $b_5$. It is a flavoprotein (FAD). In the endoplasmic reticulum, the enzyme is composed of polar and hydrophobic segments and is membrane-bound; the reduced cytochrome $b_5$ carries electrons in several reactions of fatty acid desaturation and fatty acid elongation. In the erythrocytes, the enzyme comprises the polar segment only and is soluble; the reduced cytochrome $b_5$ transfers electrons to methemoglobin, reducing it to hemoglobin. Deficiency of the enzyme, an autosomal recessive trait, results in hereditary methemoglobinemia; deficiency in erythrocytes only is characterized by cyanosis whereas deficiency also in leukocytes, and sometimes brain and muscle, has been linked to both cyanosis and mental retardation. Called also *NADH cytochrome* $b_5$ *reductase, NADH methemoglobin reductase,* and *methemoglobin reductase (NADH).*

**cy·to·chrome-*c* ox·i·dase** (si′to-krōm ok′sĭ-dās) [EC 1.9.3.1] an enzyme complex of the inner mitochondrial membrane that catalyzes the transfer of electrons from cytochrome *c* to oxygen, oxidizing the former and reducing the latter in the final step of the electron transport chain (q.v.) by which oxygen is used for fuel combustion. The enzyme contains cytochromes *a* and $a_3$ and two copper atoms and is associated with proton translocation and the resultant synthesis of ATP. The $Fe^{2+}$ in heme *a* has a strong affinity for CO; in the $Fe^{3+}$ state it binds $CN^-$, $S^{2-}$, and $N_3$. The binding of these compounds inactivates the enzyme, a cause of their extreme toxicity for all aerobic organisms. Called also *cytochrome* $aa_3$ and *cytochrome oxidase.*

**cy·to·chrome-*c* ox·i·dase de·fi·cien·cy** a hereditary defect in the cytochrome *c* oxidase complex that prevents the transfer of electrons from cytochrome *c* to molecular oxygen, ultimately halting the production of ATP. Manifestations are extremely variable and include myopathies, encephalopathies, ocular and cardiac defects, sensorineural deafness, Fanconi syndrome (def. 1), diabetes mellitus, and short stature. Inheritance may be autosomal recessive, X-linked, or, possibly, maternal (mitochondrial), depending on the part of the cytochrome *c* oxidase complex that is affected.

**cy·to·chrome ox·i·dase** (si′to-krōm ok′sĭ-dās) cytochrome-*c* oxidase.

**cy·to·chy·le·ma** (si″to-kə-le′mə) [*cyto-* + Gr. *chylos* juice] hyaloplasm, def. 1.

**cy·to·ci·dal** (si″to-si′dəl) destructive to cells; cf. *cytolytic* and *cytotoxic.*

**cy·to·cide** (si′to-sīd) [*cyto-* + *-cide*] an agent that destroys cells; see also *cytolytic* and *cytotoxic.*

**cy·to·ci·ne·sis** (si″to-sĭ-ne′sis) cytokinesis.

**cy·toc·la·sis** (si-tok′lə-sis) [*cyto-* + Gr. *klasis* a breaking] the destruction of cells.

**cy·to·clas·tic** (si″to-klas′tik) pertaining to, characterized by, or causing cytoclasis.

**cy·to·cle·sis** (si″to-kle′sis) [*cyto-* + Gr. *klēsis* a call] a form of energy, totally unrelated to electricity, light, heat, or sound, which is generated by living tissues; the vital principle in all living tissues (M. Kelly). The term was first introduced in 1923 by Frederic Wood Jones, who defined it as the influence of body cells on other body cells; the "call of cell to cell." Called also *cytobiotaxis.*

**cy·to·clet·ic** (si″to-klet′ik) pertaining to cytoclesis.

**cy·to·cu·prein** (si″to-koo′prēn) superoxide dismutase.

**cy·tode** (si′tōd) [*cyto-* + Gr. *eidos* form] a non-nucleated cell or cell element.

**cy·to·den·drite** (si″to-den′drīt) [*cyto-* + *dendrite*] dendrite.

**cy·to·des·ma** (si″to-dez′mə) [*cyto-* + Gr. *desma* band] the lamellar or bridgelike tissues binding animal cells together (Studnicka).

**cy·to·di·er·e·sis** (si″to-di-er′ə-sis) [*cyto-* + *dieresis*] cell division, i.e., meiosis or mitosis.

**cy·to·dif·fer·en·ti·a·tion** (si″to-dif″ə-ren″she-a′shən) the development of specialized structures and functions in embryonic cells.

**cy·to·dis·tal** (si″to-dis′təl) [*cyto-* + *distal*] denoting that part of an axon remote from the cell of origin.

**Cy·to·e·ce·tes** (si″to-ə-se′tez) suggested name for a genus of rickettsiae, which some consider members of *Ehrlichia*. *C. ondiri* (or *E. ondiri*), a species found in Kenya, causes bovine petechial fever.

**cy·to·gene** (si′to-jēn) plasmagene.

**cy·to·gen·e·sis** (si″to-jen′ə-sis) [*cyto-* + *-genesis*] the origin and development of cells.

**cytogenetic** (si″to-jə-net′ik) chromosome; cytogenetics. 1. chromosomal. 2. pertaining to cytogenetics.

**cy·to·ge·net·i·cal** (si″to-jə-net′ĭ-kəl) cytogenetic.

**cy·to·ge·net·i·cist** (si″to-jə-net′ĭ-sist) a specialist in cytogenetics.

**cy·to·ge·net·ics** (si″to-jə-net′iks) [MeSH: Cytogenetics] the branch of genetics devoted to study of the cellular constituents concerned in heredity, that is, the chromosomes.
**clinical c.**, the scientific study of the relationship between chromosomal aberrations and pathological conditions.

**cy·to·gen·ic** (si-to-jen′ik) 1. pertaining to cytogenesis. 2. forming or producing cells.

**cy·tog·e·nous** (si-toj′ə-nəs) [*cyto-* + *-genous*] producing cells.

**cy·tog·e·ny** (si-toj′ə-ne) 1. cytogenesis. 2. cell lineage.

**cy·to·glu·co·pe·nia** (si″to-gloo″ko-pe′ne-ə) cytoglycopenia.

**cy·to·gly·co·pe·nia** (si″to-gli″ko-pe′ne-ə) [*cyto-* + *glyco-* + *-penia*] deficient glucose content of body or blood cells.

**cy·tog·o·ny** (si-tog′ə-ne) [*cyto-* + Gr. *gonos* seed] cytogenic reproduction.

**cy·to·his·to·gen·e·sis** (si″to-his″to-jen′ə-sis) [*cyto-* + *histo-* + *-genesis*] the development of the structure of cells.

**cy·to·his·to·log·ic** (si″to-his″to-loj′ik) involving both cytologic and histologic methods.

**cy·to·his·tol·o·gy** (si″to-his-tol′ə-je) the combination of cytologic and histologic methods.

**cy·to·hor·mone** (si″to-hor′mōn) [*cyto-* + *hormone*] a cell hormone.

**cy·to·hy·a·lo·plasm** (si″to-hi′ə-lo-plaz″əm) [*cyto-* + *hyalo-* + *-plasm*] the clear substance of cytoplasm.

**cy·toid** (si′toid) [*cyto-* + *-oid*] resembling a cell.

**cy·to·kal·i·pe·nia** (si″to-kal″ĭ-pēn′e-ə) [*cyto-* + *kalium* + *-penia*] deficient potassium content of body or blood cells.

**cy·to·ke·ras·tic** (si″to-kə-ras′tik) [*cyto-* + Gr. *kerastos* mixed] pertaining to the development of cells from a lower to a higher order.

**cy·to·ker·a·tin** (si″to-ker′ə-tin) any of a group of proteins found in keratin filaments (q.v.).

**cy·to·kine** (si″to-kīn) [*cyto-* + *kinesis*] a generic term for nonantibody proteins released by one cell population (e.g., primed T lymphocytes) on contact with specific antigen, which act as intercellular mediators, as in the generation of an immune response. Examples include lymphokines and monokines.

**cy·to·ki·ne·sis** (si″to-kĭ-ne′sis) [*cyto-* + *-kinesis*] the changes that take place in the cytoplasm during cell division; division of the cytoplasm, a process synchronized in eukaryotic cells with nuclear division (mitosis).

**cy·to·ki·nin** (si″to-ki′nin) any of a class of phytohormones ($N^6$-substituted adenines) whose principal functions are the induction of cell division (cytokinesis) and the regulation of differentiation of tissue (organogenesis).

**cy·to·log·ic** (si″to-loj′ik) pertaining to cytology.

**cy·tol·o·gist** (si-tol′ə-jist) a specialist in cytology.

**cy·tol·o·gy** (si-tol′ə-je) [*cyto-* + *-logy*] [MeSH: Cytology] the study of cells, their origin, structure, function, and pathology.
**aspiration biopsy c. (ABC)**, the microscopic study of cells obtained from superficial or internal lesions by suction through a fine needle.
**exfoliative c.**, microscopic examination of cells desquamated from a body surface or lesion as a means of detecting malignancy to measure hormonal levels, etc. Such cells may be obtained by such procedures as aspiration, washing, smear, and scraping, and the technique may be applied to vaginal secretions, sputum, urine, abdominal fluid, prostatic secretion, etc.

**cy·to·lymph** (si′to-limf) [*cyto-* + *lymph*] hyaloplasm, def. 1.

**cy·tol·y·sate** (si-tol′ə-sāt) a preparation of lyzed cells.
**blood c.**, hemolysate.

**cy·tol·y·sin** (si-tol′ə-sin) a substance or antibody that produces cytolysis (dissolution of cells); those with a specific action for a certain type of cell are named accordingly, as *hemolysins*, etc.

**cy·tol·y·sis** (si-tol′ə-sis) [*cyto-* + Gr. *-lysis*] the dissolution or destruction of cells; see also *cytotoxicity*.
**immune c.**, cell lysis produced by antibody with the participation of complement.

**cy·to·ly·so·some** (si″to-li′so-sōm) autophagosome.

**cy·to·lyt·ic** (si″to-lit′ik) pertaining to, characterized by, or causing cytolysis; cf. *cytotoxic*.

**cy·to·me·gal·ic** (si″to-mə-gal′ik) pertaining to the greatly enlarged cells with intranuclear inclusions seen in cytomegalovirus infections.

**cy·to·meg·a·lo·vi·ru·ria** (si″to-meg″ə-lo-vi-roo′re-ə) presence in the urine of cytomegaloviruses.

**Cy·to·meg·a·lo·vi·rus** (si″to-meg′ə-lo-vi″rəs) [*cyto-* + *megalo-* + *virus*, from the appearance of infected cells] [MeSH: Cytomegalovirus] a genus of ubiquitous viruses of the subfamily Betaherpesvirinae (family Herpesviridae), containing the single species human herpesvirus 5, transmitted by multiple routes, that causes infection that is usually mild or subclinical but may be symptomatic (cytomegalic inclusion disease).

**cy·to·meg·a·lo·vi·rus (CMV)** (si″to-meg′ə-lo-vi″rəs) any virus of the subfamily Betaherpesvirinae, highly host-specific herpesviruses that infect man, monkeys, or rodents, with the production of unique large cells bearing intranuclear inclusions. Depending upon the age and the immune status of the host, cytomegaloviruses can cause a variety of clinical syndromes, collectively known as cytomegalic inclusion disease (see under *disease*), although the majority of infections are very mild or subclinical. Called also *salivary gland virus*.

**Cy·to·mel** (si′to-məl) trademark for a preparation of liothyronine sodium.

**cy·to·mere** (si′to-mēr) [*cyto-* + *-mere*] the multinucleate portion of the schizont of certain sporozoa that separates and gives rise to merozoites.

**cy·to·meta·pla·sia** (si″to-met″ə-pla′zhə) [*cyto-* + *metaplasia*] alteration in the form or function of a cell.

**cy·tom·e·ter** (si-tom′ə-tər) [*cyto-* + *-meter*] a device for counting cells, either visually, as a hemocytometer, or automatically, as a flow cytometer.
**flow c.**, an instrument used to perform flow cytometry.

**cy·tom·e·try** (si-tom′ə-tre) the characterization and measurement of cells and cellular constituents.
**flow c.**, a technique in which cells suspended in a fluid flow one at a time through a focus of exciting light, which is scattered in patterns characteristic to the cells and their components; they are often labeled with fluorescent markers so that light is first absorbed and then emitted at altered frequencies. A sensor detecting the scattered or emitted light measures the size and molecular characteristics of individual cells; tens of thousands of cells can be examined per minute and the data gathered are processed by computer.
**image c.**, a technique in which histologically prepared cells are imaged using a scanning technique that divides the whole image into many smaller elements and aspects, which can then be analyzed by a computer and compared between many different cells in a series.

**cy·to·mi·tome** (si″to-mi′tōm) [*cyto-* + *mitome*] a fibril or fibrillary structure in the cytoplasm.

**cy·to·mor·phol·o·gy** (si″to-mor-fol′ə-je) the morphology of cells.

**cy·to·mor·pho·sis** (si″to-mor-fo′sis) [*cyto-* + *morphosis*] the series of changes through which cells go in the process of formation, development, senescence, etc.

**cy·ton** (si′ton) perikaryon.

**cy·to·ne·cro·sis** (si″to-nə-kro′sis) death of individual cells.

**cy·to·path·ic** (si″to-path′ik) pertaining to or characterized by pathological changes in cells.

**cy·to·patho·gen·e·sis** (si″to-path″o-jen′ə-sis) the production of pathological changes in cells.

**cy·to·patho·ge·net·ic** (si″to-path″o-jə-net′ik) pertaining to or characterized by cytopathogenesis.

**cy·to·path·o·gen·ic** (si″to-path″o-jen′ik) capable of producing pathological changes in cells.

**cy·to·patho·ge·nic·i·ty** (si″to-path″o-jə-nis′ĭ-te) the quality of being capable of producing pathological changes in cells.

**cy·to·patho·log·ic, cy·to·patho·log·i·cal** (si″to-path″o-loj′ik, si″to-path″o-loj′ĭ-kəl) relating to cytopathology; denoting the changes in cells in disease.

**cy·to·pa·thol·o·gist** (si″to-pə-thol′ə-jist) an expert in the study of cells in disease; a cellular pathologist.

**cy·to·pa·thol·o·gy** (si″to-pə-thol′ə-je) [*cyto-* + *patho-* + *-logy*] the study of cells in disease; cellular pathology.

**cy·to·pe·nia** (si″to-pe′ne-ə) [*cyto-* + *-penia*] deficiency in number of any of the cellular elements of the blood; called also *hematocytopenia* and *hypocytosis*.

**Cy·toph·aga** (si-tof′ə-gə) [MeSH: Cytophaga] a genus of bacteria, gram-negative rods that are aerobic or facultatively anaerobic. *C. psychro′phila* is a species that prefers cold water and causes cold-water disease in fish. *C. columna′ris* is a species that prefers warm water and causes columnaris disease in fish.

**cy·to·phago·cy·to·sis** (si″to-fag″o-si-to′sis) cytophagy.

**cy·toph·a·gous** (si-tof′ə-gəs) [*cyto-* + *phag-* + *-ous*] devouring or consuming cells; said of phagocytes.

**cy·toph·a·gy** (si-tof′ə-je) the ingestion of cells by phagocytes.

**cy·to·phar·ynx** (si″to-far′inks) [*cyto-* + *pharynx*] a nonciliated gullet-like canal between the cytostome and the endoplasm of ciliate and certain other protozoa. See also *cytopharyngeal apparatus*, under *apparatus*.

**cy·to·phil** (si′to-fil) an element or substance that has an affinity for cells.

**cy·to·phil·ic** (si-to-fil′ik) [*cyto-* + *-philic*] having an affinity for cells, as cytophilic antibodies.

**cy·to·pho·tom·e·ter** (si″to-fo-tom′ə-tər) a photometer for measuring localization of organic compounds within cells by measuring the light intensity through selected stained areas of cytoplasm.

**cy·to·pho·to·met·ric** (si″to-fo″to-met′rik) pertaining to or accomplished by cytophotometry.

**cy·to·pho·tom·e·try** (si″to-fo-tom′ə-tre) [MeSH: Cytophotometry] the study of organic compounds within cells by means of the cytophotometer. Called also *microfluorometry*.

**cy·to·phy·lac·tic** (si″to-fə-lak′tik) pertaining to cytophylaxis.

**cy·to·phy·lax·is** (si″to-fə-lak′sis) [*cyto-* + *phylaxis*] 1. the protection of cells. 2. increase of cellular activity.

**cy·to·phy·let·ic** (si″to-fə-let′ik) [*cyto-* + *phyletic*] pertaining to the genealogy of cells.

**cy·to·phys·ics** (si″to-fiz′iks) the physics of cell activity.

**cy·to·phys·i·ol·o·gy** (si″to-fiz-e-ol′ə-je) [*cyto-* + *physiology*] the physiology of the cell.

**cy·to·pig·ment** (si″to-pig′mənt) any pigment found in cells.

**cy·to·pi·pette** (si″to-pi-pet′) a pipette for taking cytological smears.

**cy·to·plasm** (si′to-plaz″əm) [*cyto-* + *-plasm*] [MeSH: Cytoplasm] the protoplasm of a cell exclusive of that of the nucleus; it consists of a continuous aqueous solution (cytosol) and the organelles and inclusions suspended in it (phaneroplasm), and is the site of most of the chemical activities of the cell. Cf. *nucleoplasm*.

**cy·to·plas·mic** (si″to-plaz′mik) pertaining to or contained in the cytoplasm.

**cy·to·plast** (si′to-plast) a cell from which the nucleus has been removed and which remains viable for a time.

**cy·to·proct** (si′to-prokt) [*cyto-* + Gr. *prōktos* anus] a permanent posterior pore seen in certain ciliates, through which waste egesta can be eliminated. Called also *cytopyge*.

**cy·to·pro·tec·tant** (si″to-pro-tek′tənt) cytoprotective.

**cy·to·pro·tec·tion** (si″to-pro-tek′shən) enhancement of the ability of cells to resist injury.

**cy·to·pro·tec·tive** (si″to-pro-tec′tiv) 1. protecting cells from noxious chemicals or other stimuli. 2. an agent that so protects. Called also *cytoprotectant*.

**cy·to·prox·i·mal** (si″to-prok′sĭ-məl) [*cyto-* + *proximal*] denoting that part of an axon nearer to the cell of origin.

**cy·to·pyge** (si″to-pi′je) [*cyto-* + *pygē* rump] cytoproct.

**cytoreduction** (si″to-re-duk′shən) 1. decrease in the number of cells, such as in a tumor. 2. debulking.

**cy·to·re·duc·tive** (si″to-rə-duk′tiv) reducing the number of cells, as in surgery for a tumor; see *debulking*.

**cy·to·re·tic·u·lum** (si″to-rə-tik′u-ləm) [*cyto-* + *reticulum*] spongioplasm.

**cy·tor·rhyc·tes** (si″to-rik′tēz) [*cyto-* + Gr. *oryssein* to dig] cell inclusions, found in various diseases, which may be specific protozoan pathogens, or they may be manifestations of cell reactions to the parasite causing the disease, or they may be degenerations caused by the disease.

**Cy·to·sar-U** (si′to-sahr) trademark for preparations of cytarabine.

**cy·tos·co·py** (si-tos′kə-pe) [*cyto-* + *-scopy*] examination of cells.

**cy·to·sid·er·in** (si″to-sid′ər-in) intracellular pigment due probably to derangement of iron metabolism.

**cy·to·sine** (si′to-sēn) [MeSH: Cytosine] a pyrimidine base found in animal and plant cells, usually occurring condensed with ribose or deoxyribose to form the nucleosides cytidine and deoxycytidine, major constituents of nucleic acids. Symbol C. See also illustration at *pyrimidine bases*, under *base*.
**c. arabinoside,** cytarabine.

**cy·to·sine de·am·i·nase** (si′to-sēn de-am′ĭ-nās) [EC 3.5.4.1] an enzyme of the hydrolase class that catalyzes the deamination of cytosine to form uracil, a step in the degradation of pyrimidine nucleotides.

**cy·to·skel·e·tal** (si″to-skel′ə-təl) of or pertaining to the cytoskeleton.

**cy·to·skel·e·ton** (si″to-skel′ə-tən) [MeSH: Cytoskeleton] a conspicuous internal reinforcement in the cytoplasm of a cell, consisting of tonofibrils, terminal web, or other microfilaments.

**cy·to·sol** (si′to-sol) [MeSH: Cytosol] the liquid medium of the cytoplasm, i.e., cytoplasm minus organelles and nonmembranous insoluble components.

**cy·to·sol ami·no·pep·ti·dase** (si′to-sol ə-me″no-pep′ti-dās) leucyl aminopeptidase.

**cy·to·sol·ic** (si″to-sol′ik) pertaining to or contained in the cytosol.

**cy·to·some** (si′to-sōm) [*cyto-* + *-some*] 1. the body of a cell apart from its nucleus. 2. multilamellar body.

**cy·to·spon·gi·um** (si″to-spon′je-əm) [*cyto-* + Gr. *spongos* sponge] spongioplasm.

**cy·tost** (si′tost) [Gr. *kytos* hollow vessel] a specific toxin given off from a cell as a result of injury to it; a specific agent given off from broken-down tissue.

**cy·tos·ta·sis** (si-tos′tə-sis) [*cyto-* + *-stasis*] the closure of capillaries by white blood corpuscles in the early stages of inflammation.

**cy·to·stat·ic** (si″to-stat′ik) [*cyto-* + *-static*] 1. suppressing the growth and multiplication of cells. 2. an agent that suppresses cell growth and multiplication.

**cy·to·stome** (si′to-stōm) [*cyto-* + *stoma*] the mouth opening of ciliates and certain other protozoa, which opens into the cytopharynx, which in turn opens into the endoplasm.

**cy·to·stro·mat·ic** (si″to-stro-mat′ik) [*cyto-* + *stroma*] pertaining to the stroma of a cell.

**cy·to·tac·tic** (si″to-tak′tik) pertaining to cytotaxis.

**cy·to·tax·i·gen** (si″to-taks′ĭ-jən) a substance that mediates chemotaxis of cells indirectly by inducing cytotaxin formation; thus antigen-antibody complexes are cytotaxigenic because when added to serum they fix complement, resulting in the liberation of chemotactic factors derived from complement.

**cy·to·tax·in** (si″to-taks′in) chemotactic factor.

**cy·to·tax·is** (si-to-tak′sis) [*cyto-* + *taxis*] the movement and arrangement of cells with respect to a specific source of stimulation.

**Cy·to·tec** (si′to-tek) trademark for a preparation of misoprostol.

**cy·toth·e·sis** (si-toth′ə-sis) [*cyto-* + *thesis*] the restitution of injured cells to their normal condition.

**cy·to·tox·ic** (si″to-tok′sik) pertaining to or exhibiting cytotoxicity.

**cy·to·tox·ic·i·ty** (si″to-tok-sis′ĭ-te) the degree to which an agent possesses a specific destructive action on certain cells or the possession of such action; used particularly in referring to the lysis of cells by immune phenomena and to antineoplastic drugs that selectively kill dividing cells.
**antibody-dependent cell-mediated c. (ADCC), antibody-dependent cellular c.,** lysis of target cells coated with antibody by effector cells with cytolytic activity and Fc receptors, including K cells, macrophages, and granulocytes; a form of type II hypersensitivity reaction. ADCC involves binding of the effector cell by means of Fc receptors which bind to the Fc portion of the IgG molecule. Lysis of the target cell is extracellular, requires direct cell-to-cell contact, and does not involve complement.
**cell-mediated c.,** cytolysis of a target cell by effector lymphocytes, such as cytotoxic T lymphocytes or NK cells; it may be antibody-dependent (see *antibody-dependent cell-mediated c.*) or independent, as in certain type IV hypersensitivity reactions (q.v.).

**cy·to·tox·in** (si′to-tok″sin) [*cyto-* + *toxin*] a toxin or antibody that has a specific toxic action upon cells of special organs; cytotoxins are named according to the special variety of cell for which they are specific, as *nephrotoxin*.

**cy·to·tropho·blast** (si″to-trof′o-blast) [*cyto-* + *trophoblast*] 1. the cellular (inner) layer of the trophoblast; called also *Langhans′ layer*. 2. cytotrophoblastic cell.

**cy·to·tropho·blas·tic** (si″to-trof″o-blas′tik) pertaining to or of the nature of the cytotrophoblast.

**cy·to·trop·ic** (si″to-trop′ik) [*cyto-* + *-tropic*] attracting cells; possessing an affinity for cells; said especially of antibodies that attach to cell surfaces. See also under *antibody.*

**cy·to·tro·pism** (si-tot′ro-piz-əm) 1. cell movement in response to external stimulation. 2. the tendency of viruses, bacteria, drugs, etc., to exert their effect upon certain cells of the body.

**Cy·to·vene** (si′to-vēn″) trademark for preparations of ganciclovir.

**Cy·tox·an** (si-tok′sən) trademark for preparations of cyclophosphamide.

**cy·to·zo·ic** (si″to-zo′ik) living within or attached to cells; said of parasites.

**cy·tu·ria** (si-tu′re-ə) [*cyt-* + *-uria*] the presence of cells of any sort in the urine.

**Cza·pek-Dox agar (solution)** (chah′pek doks) [Friedrich Johann Franz *Czapek,* Czech botanist, 1868–1921; Arthur Wayland *Dox,* American chemist, 20th century] see under *culture medium.*

**Czer·mak's spaces (lines)** (cher′mahks) [Johann Nepomuk *Czermak,* Czech physician, 1828–1873] spatia interglobularia.

**Czer·ny's suture** (cher′nēz) [Vincenz *Czerny,* Czech surgeon in Germany, 1842–1916] see under *suture.*

**Czer·ny-Lem·bert suture** (cher′ne-lah-bār′) [V. *Czerny;* Antoine *Lembert,* French surgeon, 1802–1851] see under *suture.*

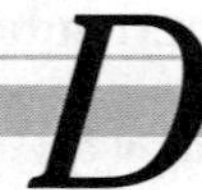

**D** symbol for *diffusing capacity, dalton, deciduous* (teeth; see under *tooth*), *density, deuterium, died, diopter, distal, dorsal vertebrae* (D1 through D12), *dose, duration, dwarf* (colony), and *decimal reduction time.*

**D.** abbreviation for L. *do'sis,* dose; *da,* give; *de'tur,* let it be given; and *dex'ter,* right.

**2,4-D** a toxic chlorphenoxy herbicide (2,4-dichlorophenoxyacetic acid) that acts as a growth-regulating hormone killing broadleaf plants by overstimulation.

**$D_{37}$** the dose necessary to reduce the surviving fraction, as of cells, to $e^{-1}$ or 0.37, where the biological activity declines exponentially as a function of dose.

**$D_L$** diffusing capacity of the lung; $D_{LO_2}$ denotes diffusing capacity for oxygen, $D_{LCO}$, diffusing capacity for carbon monoxide, etc.

**D-** a chemical prefix (small capital D) that specifies the relative configuration of an enantiomer, the mirror image configuration being specified as L-. Carbohydrates are designated as D or L depending on their configuration at the asymmetric carbon atom most distant from the carbonyl functional group; those with the same configuration as the D-glyceraldehyde (the arbitrarily chosen standard) are in the D (or $D_g$) configurational family. Amino acids are designated according to their configuration at the asymmetric carbon atom closest to the carbonyl group; D-serine is the standard and similarly configured amino acids are designated D or $D_s$. All of the $\alpha$-amino acids occurring in proteins have the L configuration; a few D-amino acids occur in short peptides produced by bacteria. The symbols *R* and *S,* indicating absolute configuration, are preferable.

**d** symbol for *day, deci-,* and *deoxyribose* (in specifying nucleosides and nucleotides, e.g., A is adenosine, dA is deoxyadenosine).

**d.** abbreviation for L. *da* (give), *de'tur* (let it be given), *dex'ter* (right), and *do'sis* (dose).

***d*** symbol for *density* and *diameter.*

***d*-** [abbreviation for *dextro* (right or clockwise)] a chemical prefix indicating an enantiomer that rotates the plane of polarization of a beam of light in the clockwise direction (dextrorotatory), the other enantiomer being specified as *l-* (for *levo*). NOTE: The prefixes *d-* and *l-* are now being replaced by (+)- and (−)-, respectively, especially when the prefixes D- and L- are also used, e.g., *l*-fructose is D-(−)-fructose.

**Δ** the Greek capital letter delta; symbol for an increment, e.g., $\Delta G$ (see *Gibbs free energy,* under *energy*); also used alone as an abbreviation for *change* (as in temperature).

**Δ-** a prefix designating the position of a double bond in a carbon chain, e.g., $\Delta^9$- indicates a double bond between carbons 9 and 10.

**δ** delta, the fourth letter of the Greek alphabet; symbol for the heavy chain of IgD (see *immunoglobulin*) and the δ chain of hemoglobin.

**δ-** a prefix designating (1) the fourth carbon along a chain starting with that adjacent to the principal functional group, e.g., δ-aminolevulinic acid (see *α-*); (2) one in a series of related entities or chemical compounds, e.g., δ-carotene or δ-ray. For terms prefixed with the symbol δ-, see the unprefixed form.

**DA** abbreviation for *developmental age* and *diphenylchlorarsine.*

**Da** symbol for *dalton.*

**da-** rarely used symbol for the metric prefix *deka-.*

**Daae's disease** (dah'əz) [Anders *Daae,* Norwegian physician, 1838–1910] epidemic pleurodynia; see under *pleurodynia.*

**Da·boia** (də-boi'ə) [Hindi "furtive mover"] Russell's viper.
**D. russel'li,** Russell's viper *(Vipera russelli).*

**DAC** decitabine.

**da·car·ba·zine** (də-kahr'bə-zēn") [USP] [MeSH: Dacarbazine] a cytotoxic alkylating agent used as an antineoplastic primarily for treatment of malignant melanoma and in combination chemotherapy for Hodgkin's disease and sarcomas; administered intravenously. Abbreviated DTIC.

**da·cliz·u·mab** (də-kliz'u-mab) an immunosuppressant used to prevent acute organ rejection in renal transplant patients; administered intravenously.

**d'Acos·ta** see *Acosta.*

**Da Cos·ta's syndrome** (də-kah'stəz) [Jacob Mendes *Da Costa,* American physician, 1833–1900] see *neurocirculatory asthenia,* under *asthenia.*

**Da·cron** (da'kron) trademark for a polyethylene terephthalate fiber. In fiber form, it is used as a suture material; in fabric form, it is used for vascular grafts and prostheses and for vascular catheters.

**dac·ry·ad·e·nal·gia** (dak"re-ad"ə-nal'jə) dacryoadenalgia.

**dac·ry·a·gog·atre·sia** (dak"re-ə-gog"ə-tre'zhə) [*dacry-* + *-agogue* + *atresia*] lacrimal duct atresia.

**dac·ry·cys·tal·gia** (dak"re-sis-tal'jə) dacryocystalgia.

**dac·ry·cys·ti·tis** (dak"re-sis-ti'tis) dacryocystitis.

**dac·ry·el·co·sis** (dak"re-əl-ko'sis) dacryohelcosis.

**dacry(o)-** [Gr. *dakryon* tear] a combining form denoting relationship to tears.

**dac·ryo·ad·e·nal·gia** (dak"re-o-ad"ə-nal'jə) [*dacryo-* + *aden-* + *-algia*] pain in a lacrimal gland.

**dac·ryo·ad·e·nec·to·my** (dak"re-o-ad"ə-nek'tə-me) [*dacryo-* + *aden-* + *ectomy*] excision of a lacrimal gland.

**dac·ryo·ad·e·ni·tis** (dak"re-o-ad"ə-ni'tis) inflammation of a lacrimal gland.

**dac·ryo·blen·nor·rhea** (dak"re-o-blen"o-re'ə) [*dacryo-* + *blennorrhea*] mucous discharge from the lacrimal ducts, as in chronic dacryocystitis.

**dac·ryo·cana·lic·u·li·tis** (dak"re-o-kan"ə-lik"u-li'tis) inflammation of the lacrimal ducts.

**dac·ryo·cele** (dak're-o-sēl") dacryocystocele.

**dac·ryo·cyst** (dak're-o-sist") [*dacryo-* + *cyst*] the lacrimal sac.

**dac·ryo·cys·tal·gia** (dak"re-o-sis-tal'jə) [*dacryocyst* + *-algia*] pain in a lacrimal sac.

**dac·ryo·cys·tec·ta·sia** (dak"re-o-sis"tek-ta'zhə) [*dacryocyst* + *ectasia*] dilatation of the lacrimal sac.

**dac·ryo·cys·tec·to·my** (dak"re-o-sis"tek'tə-me) [*dacryocyst* + *ectomy*] excision of the wall of the lacrimal sac.

**dac·ryo·cys·tis** (dak"re-o-sis'tis) [*dacryo-* + *cystis*] the lacrimal sac.

**dac·ryo·cys·ti·tis** (dak"re-o-sis-ti'tis) [MeSH: Dacryocystitis] inflammation of the lacrimal sac.

**dac·ryo·cys·ti·tome** (dak"re-o-sis'tĭ-tōm) [*dacryocyst* + *-tome*] an instrument for incising strictures of the lacrimal duct.

**dac·ryo·cys·to·blen·nor·rhea** (dak"re-o-sis"to-blen"o-re'ə) [*dacryocyst* + *blennorrhea*] a chronic catarrhal inflammation of the lacrimal sac, with constriction of the lacrimal duct.

**dac·ryo·cys·to·cele** (dak"re-o-sis'to-sēl) [*dacryocyst* + *-cele*¹] hernial protrusion of the lacrimal sac; called also *dacryocele.*

**dac·ryo·cys·top·to·sis** (dak"re-o-sis"top-to'sis) [*dacryocyst* + *ptosis*] prolapse or downward displacement of the lacrimal sac.

**dac·ryo·cys·to·rhi·no·ste·no·sis** (dak"re-o-sis"to-ri"no-stə-no'sis) narrowing of the duct leading from the lacrimal sac to the nasal cavity.

**dac·ryo·cys·to·rhi·nos·to·my** (dak"re-o-sis"to-ri-nos'tə-me) [*dacryocyst* + *rhino-* + *-stomy*] [MeSH: Dacryocystorhinostomy] surgical creation of a communication between the lacrimal sac and the nasal cavity; called also *dacryorhinocystotomy* and *Toti's operation.*

**dac·ryo·cys·to·rhi·not·o·my** (dak"re-o-sis"to-ri-not'ə-me) [*dacryocyst* + *rhino-* + *-tomy*] passage of a probe through the lacrimal sac into the nasal cavity.

**dac·ryo·cys·to·ste·no·sis** (dak"re-o-sis"to-stə-no'sis) narrowing of the lacrimal sac.

**dac·ryo·cys·tos·to·my** (dak"re-o-sis-tos'tə-me) [*dacryocyst* + *-stomy*] surgical creation of a new opening into the lacrimal sac.

**dac·ryo·cys·to·tome** (dak"re-o-sis'to-tōm) dacryocystitome.

**dac·ryo·cys·tot·o·my** (dak"re-o-sis-tot'ə-me) [*dacryocyst* + *-tomy*] incision of the lacrimal sac; called also *Ammon's operation,* def. 2.

**dac·ryo·cyte** (dak're-o-sīt) an abnormal erythrocyte shaped like a

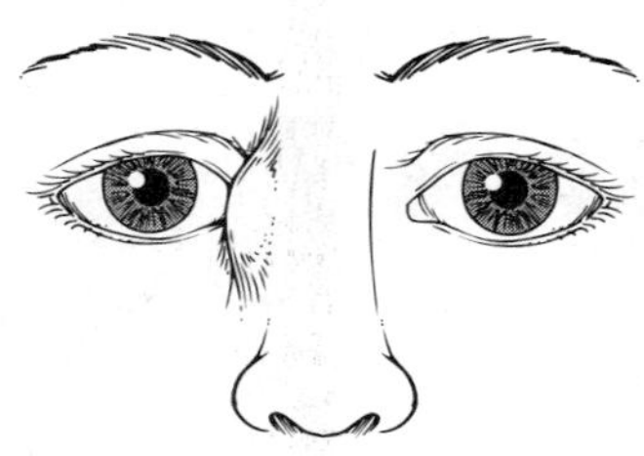

Dacryocystocele.

teardrop, seen in myelofibrosis and certain other myeloproliferative diseases. Called also *teardrop cell.*

**dac·ry·o·gen·ic** (dak″re-o-jen′ik) [*dacryo-* + *-genic*] promoting the secretion of tears.

**dac·ryo·hel·co·sis** (dak″re-o-həl-ko′sis) [*dacryo-* + *helcosis*] ulceration of the lacrimal sac or lacrimal duct.

**dac·ryo·hem·or·rhea** (dak″re-o-hem″o-re′ə) [*dacryo-* + *hemo-* + *-rrhea*] the discharge of tears mixed with blood.

**dac·ryo·lith** (dak′re-o-lith″) [*dacryo-* + *-lith*] a concretion in the lacrimal sac or duct.

**dac·ryo·li·thi·a·sis** (dak″re-o-lĭ-thi′ə-sis) [*dacryo-* + *lithiasis*] the presence of calculi in the lacrimal sac or duct.

**dac·ry·o·ma** (dak″re-o′mə) a tumor-like swelling caused by obstruction of the lacrimal duct.

**dac·ry·on** (dak′re-on) [Gr. *dakryon* tear] a cranial point at the juncture of the lacrimal and frontal bones, and the maxilla.

**dac·ry·ops** (dak′re-ops) [*dacry-* + Gr. *ōps* eye] 1. a watery state of the eye. 2. distention of a lacrimal duct by contained fluid.

**dac·ryo·py·or·rhea** (dak″re-o-pi″o-re′ə) [*dacryo-* + *pyorrhea*] the discharge of tears mixed with pus.

**dac·ryo·py·o·sis** (dak″re-o-pi-o′sis) [*dacryo-* + *pyosis*] suppuration of the lacrimal sac and duct.

**dac·ryo·rhi·no·cys·tot·o·my** (dak″re-o-ri″no-sis-tot′ə-me) dacryocystorhinostomy.

**dac·ry·or·rhea** (dak″re-o-re′ə) [*dacryo-* + *-rrhea*] an overabundant flow of tears.

**dac·ryo·scin·tig·ra·phy** (dak″re-o-sin-tig′rə-fe) scintigraphy of the lacrimal ducts.

**dac·ryo·si·nus·itis** (dak″re-o-si″nəs-i′tis) inflammation of the lacrimal duct and ethmoid sinus.

**dac·ryo·so·le·ni·tis** (dak″re-o″so-lə-ni′tis) [*dacryo-* + *solen-* + *-itis*] inflammation of a lacrimal duct.

**dac·ryo·ste·no·sis** (dak″re-o-stə-no′sis) [*dacryo-* + *stenosis*] stricture or narrowing of a lacrimal duct.

**dac·ryo·syr·inx** (dak″re-o-sir′inks) [*dacryo-* + *syrinx*] 1. a lacrimal duct (canaliculus lacrimalis [TA]). 2. a lacrimal fistula. 3. a syringe for irrigating the lacrimal ducts.

**DACT** dactinomycin.

**Dac·til** (dak′til) trademark for preparations of piperidolate hydrochloride.

**dac·ti·no·my·cin** (dak″tĭ-no-mi′sin) [USP] [MeSH: Dactinomycin] an antineoplastic antibiotic (actinomycin D) produced by *Streptomyces parvulus;* it consists of a phenoxazone ring and two cyclic pentapeptide side chains and acts by binding to DNA with the ring intercalated between adjacent guanine-cytosine base pairs, resulting in blocking of transcription by RNA polymerase. It is used as an antineoplastic agent for treatment of rhabdomyosarcoma and Wilms' tumor in children and is also effective against Ewing's sarcoma, Kaposi's sarcoma, osteogenic sarcoma and soft tissue sarcomas, testicular carcinoma, and choriocarcinoma; administered intravenously and by isolation-perfusion technique. Major side effects are nausea and vomiting, ulceration of the oral mucosa, and bone marrow depression. Abbreviated DACT.

**dac·tyl** (dak′təl) [Gr. *daktylos* a finger] digitus.

**Dac·ty·la·ria** (dak-tĭ-la′re-ə) a genus of Fungi Imperfecti of the form-family Dematiaceae. *D. gallopa′va* is a thermophilic species that causes encephalitis in chickens and turkeys, sometimes in epidemics, and has been found in opportunistic infections of humans.

**dac·ty·late** (dak′tə-lāt) digitate.

**dac·ty·le·de·ma** (dak″təl-ə-de′mə) edema or swelling of the fingers or toes.

**dac·tyl·i·on** (dak-til′e-on) syndactyly.

**dac·ty·li·tis** (dak″tə-li′tis) [*dactyl-* + *-itis*] inflammation of a finger or toe.

**dactyl(o)-** [Gr. *daktylos* finger] a combining form denoting relationship to a digit, usually referring to the fingers but sometimes to the toes.

**dac·ty·lo·camp·so·dyn·ia** (dak″tə-lo-kamp″so-din′e-ə) [*dactylo-* + Gr. *kampsis* bend + *-odynia*] painful flexure of the fingers.

**dac·tylo·gram** (dak-til′o-gram) [*dactylo-* + *-gram*] a fingerprint taken for purposes of identification.

**dac·ty·log·ra·phy** (dak″tə-log′rə-fe) [*dactylo-* + *-graphy*] the study of fingerprints.

**dac·ty·lo·gry·po·sis** (dak″tə-lo-grĭ-po′sis) [*dactylo-* + *gryposis*] a permanent curving of the fingers.

**Dac·ty·lo·gy·rus** (dak″tĭ-lo-ji′rus) a genus of trematodes that infect the skin and gills of aquarium fish, causing hyperactivity and breathing problems that can be fatal.

**dac·ty·lol·o·gy** (dak″tə-lol′ə-je) [*dactylo-* + *-logy*] use of movements of the hands and fingers as a means of communication between individuals; called also *cheirology, dactylophasia,* and *signing.*

**dac·ty·lol·y·sis** (dak″tə-lol′ĭ-sis) [*dactylo-* + *-lysis*] loss or amputation of a digit.
**d. sponta′nea,** ainhum.

**dac·ty·lo·meg·a·ly** (dak″tə-lo-meg′ə-le) [*dactylo-* + *-megaly*] abnormally large fingers or toes.

**dac·ty·lo·pha·sia** (dak″tə-lo-fa′zhə) [*dactylo-* + *-phasia*] dactylology.

**dac·ty·los·co·py** (dak″tə-los′kə-pe) [*dactylo-* + *-scopy*] examination of fingerprints for purposes of identification.

**Dac·ty·lo·so·ma** (dak″tə-lo-so′mə) [*dactylo-* + Gr. *soma* body] a genus of hematozoic protozoa (order Piroplasmida, subclass Piroplasmia) found in reptiles, amphibians, and fish.

**dac·ty·lo·spasm** (dak′tə-lo-spaz-əm) [*dactylo-* + *-spasm*] spasm or cramp of a finger or toe.

**dac·ty·lus** (dak′tə-ləs) [Gr. *daktylos* finger] a digit; a finger or toe.

**DAD** delayed afterdepolarization.

**DADDS** diacetyl diaminodiphenylsulfone; see *acedapsone.*

**dADP** deoxyadenosine diphosphate.

**DAF** decay accelerating factor.

**daf·fo·dil** (daf′ə-dil) *Narcissus pseudonarcissus.*

**Dag·e·nan** (dag′ə-nən) trademark for sulfapyridine.

**dahl·ia** (dahl′yə) the term for certain unspecified mixtures of methylated and ethylated pararosanilines and rosanilines; C.I.42530. Sometimes used as a basic dye for violet staining. Called also *Hofmann's* or *iodine violet.*
**d. B.,** see *gentian violet,* under *gentian.*

**dahl·in** (dahl′in) inulin.

**Da·kin's fluid (solution)** (da′kinz) [Henry Drysdale *Dakin,* English chemist in the United States, 1880–1952] diluted sodium hypochlorite solution.

**Da·kin-Car·rel method** (da′kin-kah-rel′) [H. D. *Dakin;* Alexis *Carrel,* French surgeon, 1873–1944] see *Carrel treatment*, under *treatment.*

**dak·ry·on** (dak′re-on) dacryon.

**Dal·a·lone** (dal′ə-lōn″) trademark for preparations of dexamethasone.

**Dale** (dāl) Sir Henry Hallett. British physiologist and pharmacologist, 1875–1968; co-winner, with Otto Loewi, of the Nobel prize for medicine or physiology in 1936 for their study of acetylcholine as an agent in the chemical transmission of nerve impulses.

**Dale's reaction (phenomenon)** (dāl) [Sir Henry Hallett *Dale*] see under *reaction.*

**Dal·gan** (dal′gan) trademark for a preparation of dezocine.

**Dal·mane** (dal′mān) trademark for a preparation of flurazepam hydrochloride.

**Dal·rym·ple's disease, sign** (dal′rim-pəlz) [John *Dalrymple,* English oculist, 1804–1852] see *cyclokeratitis,* and see under *sign.*

**dal·tep·a·rin so·di·um** (dal-tep′ə-rin) an antithrombotic prepared from heparin sodium derived from porcine intestinal mucosa; it enhances the inhibition of factor Xa and thrombin by antithrombin. It is administered subcutaneously for the prevention of pulmonary thromboembolism and deep venous thrombosis in patients who are at risk for thromboembolism undergoing abdominal surgery.

**Dal·ton's law** (dawl′tənz) [John *Dalton,* English chemist and physicist, 1766–1844, the founder of the atomic theory] see under *law.*

**Dal·ton-Hen·ry law** (dawl′tən-hen′re) [J. *Dalton;* Joseph *Henry,* American physicist, 1797–1878] see under *law.*

**dal·ton** (dawl′tən) [John *Dalton*] an arbitrary unit of mass, being $\frac{1}{12}$ the mass of the nuclide of carbon-12, equivalent to $1.657 \times 10^{-24}$ g. Symbol D or Da. Called also *atomic mass unit.*

**dal·ton·ism** (dawl′tən-iz-əm) [John *Dalton*] a name applied to defective perception of red and green; deuteranomaly or deuteranopia.

**Dam** (dahm) Carl Peter Henrik. Danish biochemist, 1895–1976; co-winner, with Edward Adelbert Doisy, of the Nobel prize for medicine or physiology in 1943, for the discovery of vitamin K.

**dam** (dam) 1. a barrier to obstruct the flow of water or other fluid. 2. a thin sheet of latex used in surgical procedures to separate certain tissues or structures. 3. rubber d.
**rubber d.,** a sheet of latex with punched-out holes that is placed

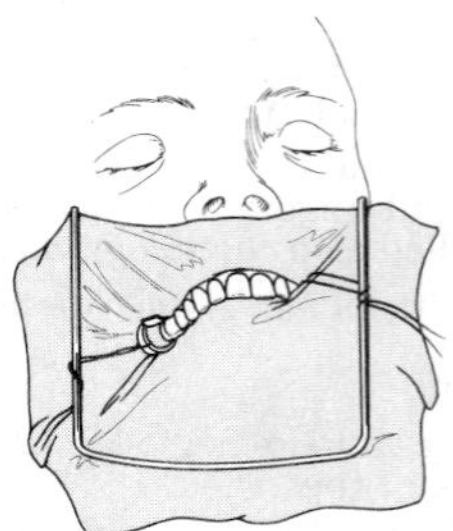

Rubber dam.

over the teeth during dental procedures to isolate the operative field from the rest of the oral cavity.

**Dam·a·lin·ia** (dam″ə-lin′e-ə) a genus of parasitic biting lice (order Mallophaga); several species were formerly classified in the genus *Trichodectes. D. bo′vis* infests cattle; *D. e′qui* and *D. pilo′sus* infest horses; *D. herm′si* and *D. o′vis* infest sheep; and *D. cap′rae, D. cras′sipes,* and *D. limba′ta* infest goats.

**D'Ama·to's sign** (dah-mah′tōz) [Luigi *D'Amato,* Italian physician, early 20th century] see under *sign.*

**da·mi·a·na** (dah″me-ah′nə) the leaves of the Mexican plants *Turnera aphrodisiaca (T. diffusa)* and *Haplopappus discoideus,* which are said to be tonic, analeptic, diuretic, and aphrodisiac. Called also *turnera.*

**dam·mar** (dam′ər) a transparent resin from tropical trees of the genera *Hopea, Shorea,* and others; used in varnishes, as a mounting medium in microscopy, and for the preservation of animal and vegetable specimens.

**dAMP** deoxyadenosine monophosphate.

**damp** (damp) foul air or noxious gas(es) in a mine.
**after-d.,** a gaseous mixture formed in a mine by the explosion of fire damp or dust; it contains nitrogen, carbon dioxide, and usually carbon monoxide.
**black d., choke d.,** a nonrespirable atmosphere sometimes formed in a mine by the gradual absorption of the oxygen and the giving off of carbon dioxide by the coal.
**cold d.,** foggy vapor charged with carbon dioxide.
**fire d.,** light explosive hydrocarbon gases, chiefly methane, $CH_4$, found in coal mines.
**white d.,** old name for *carbon monoxide.*

**damp·ing** (damp′ing) the steady diminution of the amplitude of vibration of a specific form of energy, as of electricity or sound waves.

**dan·a·zol** (dan′ə-zol) [USP] [MeSH: Danazol] an anterior pituitary suppressant that has been used in the treatment of endometriosis, gynecomastia, fibrocystic mastitis, precocious puberty, and pubertal breast hypertrophy.

**Dan·bolt-Closs syndrome** (dahn′bōlt-klos) [Niels Christian *Danbolt,* Norwegian dermatologist, born 1900; Karl *Closs,* Swedish physician, 20th century] acrodermatitis enteropathica; see under *acrodermatitis.*

**dance** (dans) movement of a rhythmic, or of an unusual or exaggerated type.
**brachial d.,** writhing of tortuous brachial arteries under the skin, sometimes observed in elderly arteriosclerotic patients.
**hilar d., hilus d.,** marked pulsations of the hilus shadows of both lungs on radiographic examination; seen in pulmonic regurgitation.
**St. Anthony's d., St. Guy's d., St. John's d., St. Vitus' d.,** Sydenham's chorea.

**D and C** dilatation and curettage (dilatation of the cervix and curettage of the uterus).

**dan·der** (dan′dər) small scales from the hair or feathers of animals, which may be the cause of allergy in sensitive persons.

**dan·druff** (dan′drəf) 1. dry scaly material desquamated from the scalp; the term is applied to that normally desquamated from the epidermis of the scalp as well as to the excessive scaly material associated with disease, as in seborrheic dermatitis. 2. seborrheic dermatitis of the scalp; called also *pityriasis sicca.*
**walking d.,** cheyletiellosis (def. 1).

**Dan·dy's operation** (dan′dēz) [Walter Edward *Dandy,* American surgeon, 1886–1946] see under *operation.*

**Dan·dy-Walk·er malformation (deformity, syndrome)** (dan′de-wawk′ər) [W. E. *Dandy;* Arthur Earl *Walker,* American surgeon, born 1907] see under *malformation.*

**Dane particle** (dān) [David M. S. *Dane,* British virologist, 20th century] see under *particle.*

**Dan·i·lone** (dan′ĭ-lōn) trademark for a preparation of phenindione.

**Dan·los' syndrome (disease)** (dahn-los′) [Henri Alexandre *Danlos,* French dermatologist, 1844–1912] Ehlers-Danlos syndrome.

**DANS** 5-dimethylamino-1-naphthalenesulfonic acid. See *dansyl chloride.*

**dan·syl chlo·ride** (dan′səl) [the acyl chloride of DANS] a fluorochrome that emits an apple green fluorescence when excited by ultraviolet light; used as a fluorescent label in immunofluorescence methods and in amino acid analysis.

**dan·thron** (dan′thron) a synthetic anthraquinone derivative used as a laxative; administered orally.

**Dan·tri·um** (dan′tre-əm) trademark for a preparation of dantrolene sodium.

**dan·tro·lene so·di·um** (dan′tro-lēn) a skeletal muscle relaxant used as an antispasmodic in conditions such as stroke, multiple sclerosis, and cerebral palsy.

**Dan·ysz's phenomenon (effect)** (dah′nish-əs) [Jan *Danysz,* Polish pathologist in France, 1860–1928] see under *phenomenon.*

**Daph·ne** (daf′ne) [Gr. *daphnē* bay tree] a genus of trees and shrubs of the family Thymelaeaceae. *D. gni′dium* and *D. meze′reum* L. are medicinal species that contain daphnin and mezerein and are vesicatory and purgative in small amounts but in larger amounts are poisonous, causing severe or even fatal irritation of the alimentary tract in humans and other animals.

**daph·ne·tin** (daf-ne′tin) 7,8-dihydroxycoumarin, the aglycon of daphnin.

**Daph·nia** (daf′ne-ə) [MeSH: Daphnia] a genus of fresh-water crustaceans, called water fleas, often used in biological research.

**daph·nin** (daf′nin) 7,8-dihydroxycoumarin-7-β-D-glucoside, a glycoside found in *Daphne mezereum.*

**daph·nism** (daf′niz-əm) poisoning of humans or other animals by species of *Daphne;* symptoms include severe enteritis with diarrhea.

**dap·sone** (dap′sōn) [USP] [MeSH: Dapsone] an antibacterial, the parent compound of a group of sulfonamide-like sulfones, including acedapsone, acetosulfone sodium, glucosulfone sodium, sulfoxone sodium, and solapsone. Dapsone and its derivatives are bacteriostatic for a broad spectrum of gram-negative and gram-positive organisms, including *Mycobacterium tuberculosis* and *M. leprae,* and have suppressive action on *Plasmodium falciparum.* Dapsone is used as a leprostatic, especially in tuberculoid and lepromatous leprosy, as a dermatitis herpetiformis suppressant, and in the prophylaxis of falciparum malaria; administered orally. Called also *diaminodiphenylsulfone* or *DDS.*

**Dar·a·nide** (dar′ə-nīd) trademark for a preparation of dichlorphenamide.

**Dar·a·prim** (dar′ə-prim) trademark for a preparation of pyrimethamine.

**Dar·bid** (dar′bid) trademark for a preparation of isopropamide iodide.

**Dar es Sa·laam bacterium** (dahr es sə-lahm′) [*Dar es Salaam,* now capital of Tanzania, where it was isolated in 1922] *Salmonella salamae.*

**Dar·i·con** (dar′ĭ-kon) trademark for a preparation of oxyphencyclimine hydrochloride.

**Da·rier's disease, sign** (dah-re-āz′) [Jean Ferdinand *Darier,* French dermatologist, 1856–1938] see *keratosis follicularis,* and see under *sign.*

**Da·rier-Rous·sy sarcoid** (dah-re-a′roo-se′) [J. F. *Darier;* Gustave *Roussy,* French pathologist and neurologist, 1874–1948] see under *sarcoid.*

**Da·rier-White disease** (dah-re-a′hwīt) [J. F. *Darier;* James Clarke *White,* American dermatologist, 1833–1916] keratosis follicularis.

**Dark·she·vich's nucleus** (dahrk-sha′vich-əz) [Liverij Osipovich *Darkshevich,* Russian neurologist, 1858–1925] see under *nucleus.*

**Dar·ling's disease** (dahr′lingz) [Samuel Taylor *Darling,* American physician, 1872–1925] histoplasmosis.

**dar·nel** (dahr′nəl) *Lolium temulentum.*

**d'Ar·son·val current** (dahr-saw-vahl′) [Jacques A. *d'Arsonval,* French physicist, 1851–1940] see under *current.*

**dar·to·ic** (dahr-to′ik) of the nature of a dartos; having a slow, involuntary contractility like that of the dartos.

**dar·toid** (dahr′toid) resembling the dartos.

**dar·tos** (dahr'tos) [Gr. "flayed"] 1. musculus dartos, def. 1. 2. tunica dartos, def. 1.

**Dar·vo·cet-N** (dahr'vo-set) trademark for preparations of propoxyphene napsylate and acetaminophen.

**Dar·von** (dahr'von) trademark for a preparation of propoxyphene hydrochloride.

**Dar·win's ear, tubercle** (dahr'winz) [Charles Robert *Darwin*, English biologist, 1809–1882] see under *ear* and see *tuberculum auriculare*.

**dar·win·ian** (dahr-win'e-ən) named for C. R. *Darwin*.

**dar·win·ism** (dahr'win-iz-əm) [C. R. *Darwin*] the theory of evolution according to which higher organisms have developed from lower ones through the influence of natural selection. Called also *darwinian theory*.

**das·sie** (das'e) rock hyrax.

**Das·y·proc·ta** (das"e-prok'tə) a genus of large rodents of tropical America, including various species of agouti (q.v.).

**da·ta** (da'tə) [L., plural of *datum*] the material or collection of facts on which a discussion or an inference is based.
**censored d.**, in statistics, observations whose final outcomes are not completely determined in a study, as, for example, data for patients who have not yet reached the study's endpoint (e.g., relapse or death) when the data are analyzed or who drop out of the study before reaching that endpoint.

**dATP** deoxyadenosine triphosphate.

**Da·tu·ra** (da-too'rə) a genus of plants of the family Solanaceae; several species contain the anticholinergic alkaloids hyoscyamine and scopolamine.
**D. me'tel**, a species that is a source of scopolamine; its seeds sometimes contaminate animal feed, causing daturism.
**D. stramo'nium**, the most common species of *Datura*; it is a source of hyoscyamine and scopolamine. Its seeds sometimes contaminate animal feed and cause daturism. Called also *Jimson weed, stramonium*, and *thorn apple*.

**da·tu·rine** (da-too'rin) hyoscyamine.

**da·tu·rism** (da-too'riz-əm) poisoning of humans or other animals by plants of the genus *Datura*, which contain solanaceous alkaloids such as atropine, hyoscyamine, and scopolamine.

**Dau·ben·ton's angle, plane (line)** (do-bon-tonz') [Louis Jean Marie *Daubenton*, French physician and naturalist, 1716–1800] see under *angle* and *plane*.

**Dau·cus** (daw'kəs) a genus of herbs of the family Umbelliferae, native to Europe and Asia. *D. caro'ta* is the carrot.

**daugh·ter** (daw'tər) [MeSH: Nuclear Family] 1. decay product. 2. arising from cell division, as a daughter cell.

**dau·no·my·cin** (daw-no-mi'sin) daunorubicin.

**dau·no·ru·bi·cin** (daw"no-roo'bĭ-sin) [MeSH: Daunorubicin] an anthracycline (q.v.) antibiotic produced by *Streptomyces coeruleorubidus* or *S. peucetius* and used as an antineoplastic.
**d. hydrochloride** [USP], the hydrochloride salt of daunorubicin, having the same actions as the base; used in the treatment of acute lymphocytic leukemia, acute myelogenous leukemia, acute monocytic leukemia, erythroleukemia, and neuroblastoma, administered intravenously.

**dau·no·sa·mine** (daw-nōs'ə-mēn) a six-carbon amino sugar found in anthracycline antibiotics.

**Dau·no·Xome** (daw'nok-sōm) trademark for a preparation of daunorubicin in a lipid complex for injection.

**Daus·set** (do-sa') Jean Baptiste Gabriel. French physician, born 1916; co-winner, with Baruj Benacerraf and George Davis Snell, of the Nobel prize for medicine or physiology in 1980 for their research on genetically determined structures of the cell surface that regulate immunological reactions. Dausset identified the first HLA (human leukocyte antigen) "MAC."

**Da·vai·nea** (da-va'ne-ə) [Casimir Joseph *Davaine*, French physician, 1812–1882] a genus of tapeworms of the family Davaineidae. *D. proglotti'na* causes severe enteritis in fowls.

**Da·vai·ne·i·dae** (da"va-ne'ĭ-de) a family of small tapeworms of the order Cyclophyllidea, subclass Cestoda, which parasitize mammals and birds. *Davainea* and *Raillietina* are medically important genera.

**Da·vid's disease** (dah-vēdz') [Jean Pierre *David*, French surgeon, 1737–1784] tuberculosis of the spine.

**Da·vid·off's (Da·vid·ov's) cells** (dah'vid-ofs) [M. von *Davidoff*, German histologist, died 1904] Paneth's cells.

**Da·vid·sohn differential absorption test** (da'vid-sən) [Israel Davidsohn, American pathologist, 1895–1979] Paul-Bunnell-Davidsohn test.

**Da·vi·el's operation, spoon** (dah-ve-elz') [Jacques *Daviel*, French oculist, 1696–1762, originator of treatment of cataract by extraction of the lens] see under *operation* and *spoon*.

**Da·vis graft** (da'vis) [John Staige *Davis*, American surgeon, 1872–1946] a pinch graft.

**Daw·barn's sign** (daw'barnz) [Robert Hugh Mackay *Dawbarn*, American surgeon, 1860–1915] see under *sign*.

**Day·pro** (da'pro) trademark for a preparation of oxaprozin.

**dB, db** decibel.

**DBA** dibenzanthracene.

**DBI** trademark for preparations of phenformin hydrochloride.

**DC** direct current; Doctor of Chiropractic.

**D & C** dilatation and curettage (dilatation of the cervix and curettage of the uterus).

**dC** deoxycytidine.

**DCA** desoxycorticosterone acetate.

**DCc** double concave.

**dCDP** deoxycytidine diphosphate.

**DCF** direct centrifugal flotation; see *Lane method*, under *method*.

**DCH** Diploma in Child Health.

**DCI** dichloroisoproterenol.

**DCIS** ductal carcinoma in situ.

**dCMP** deoxycytidine monophosphate.

**dCMP de·am·i·nase** (de-am'in-ās) [EC 3.5.4.12] [MeSH: DCMP Deaminase] an enzyme of the hydrolase class that catalyzes the deamination of dCMP to form dUMP, a step in the synthesis of dTTP from CDP.

**DCOG** Diploma of the College of Obstetricians and Gynaecologists (British).

**dCTP** deoxycytidine triphosphate.

**DCx** double convex.

**d.d.** abbreviation for L. *de'tur ad*, "let it be given to."

**DDAVP** trademark for preparation of desmopressin.

**ddC** zalcitabine (dideoxycytidine).

**DDD** [MeSH: DDD] TDE.

***o,p'*-DDD** mitotane.

**ddI** didanosine (dideoxyinosine).

**DDP, *cis*-DDP** cisplatin (*cis*-dichlorodiammineplatinum).

**DDS** diaminodiphenylsulfone (see *dapsone*); Doctor of Dental Surgery.

**DDSc** Doctor of Dental Science.

**DDT** [MeSH: DDT] dichlorodiphenyltrichloroethane, a chlorinated hydrocarbon pesticide moderately toxic to humans and other animals; it was formerly widely used but is now banned in the United States except for a few specialized purposes because of the ecological damage it causes.

**de-** [L. *de* away from, down from] a prefix often denoting negation or privation; it may signify down or away from, cessation, reversal, or removal. It sometimes has an intensive force.

**de·ac·e·tyl·la·nat·o·side C** (de-as"ə-tēl-lə-nat'o-sīd) deslanoside.

**de·acid·i·fi·ca·tion** (de"ə-sid"ĭ-fĭ-ka'shən) the act of correcting or destroying acidity or of neutralizing an acid.

**de·ac·ti·va·tion** (de-ak"tĭ-va'shən) the process of making or becoming inactive, as the removal or loss of radioactivity from a previously radioactive material.

**de·acyl·ase** (de-a'səl-ās) any enzyme of the hydrolase class that catalyzes the cleavage of an acyl group in ester or amide linkage.

**dead** (ded) 1. destitute of life; see also *death*. 2. numb.

**deaf** (def) lacking the sense of hearing or having profound hearing loss.

**de·af·fer·en·ta·tion** (de-af"ər-ən-ta'shən) the elimination or interruption of afferent nerve impulses, as by destruction of the afferent pathway.

**deaf-mute** (def-mūt) an individual who is unable to hear or speak.

**deaf-mut·ism** (def-mūt'iz-əm) the absence both of the sense of hearing and of the faculty of speech.

**deaf·ness** (def'nəs) [MeSH: Deafness] lack or significant deficiency of the sense of hearing. Called also *hearing loss*. See also *anakusis*.
**acoustic trauma d.**, noise-induced hearing loss caused by a single loud noise such as blast injury.

**Alexander's d.**, congenital deafness due to cochlear aplasia, involving chiefly the organ of Corti and adjacent ganglion cells of the basal coil of the cochlea; a high-frequency hearing loss results. Called also *Alexander's hearing loss.*
**bass d.**, deafness to certain low tones.
**boilermakers' d.**, noise-induced hearing loss in boilermakers.
**central d.**, deafness due to causes in the auditory pathways or in the auditory center.
**cochlear d.**, sensorineural deafness due to a defect in the receptor or transducing mechanisms of the cochlea.
**conduction d., conductive d.**, see under *hearing loss.*
**cortical d.**, deafness due to a lesion of the subcortical pathways immediately below an auditory area of the hemisphere dominant for speech and language, or of the auditory area itself.
**functional d.**, see under *hearing loss.*
**hysterical d.**, functional hearing loss.
**labyrinthine d.**, that due to disease of the labyrinth.
**Michel's d.**, congenital deafness due to total lack of development of the inner ear (Michel's aplasia).
**midbrain d.**, deafness dependent on injury of the fillet tract of the tegmentum.
**Mondini's d.**, congenital deafness due to dysgenesis of the organ of Corti, with partial aplasia of the bony and membranous labyrinth and a resultant flattened cochlea. See also *Mondini's deformity,* under *deformity.*
**music d.**, amusia.
**nerve d., neural d.**, that which is due to a lesion of the vestibulocochlear nerve or the central neural pathways.
**organic d.**, deafness due to defect in the ear or auditory apparatus.
**pagetoid d.**, that occurring in osteitis deformans (Paget's disease) of the bones of the skull.
**paradoxic d.**, see under *hearing loss.*
**perceptive d.**, sensorineural d.
**postlingual d.**, deafness acquired after the development of speech.
**prelingual d.**, deafness acquired before the development of speech.
**retrocochlear d.**, sensorineural deafness in which the lesion is proximal to the cochlea, i.e., in the vestibulocochlear nerve or one of the auditory areas of the brain.
**Scheibe's d.**, congenital deafness due to partial aplasia of the saccule and cochlear duct (Scheibe's aplasia).
**sensorineural d.**, deafness due to a lesion in either the cochlea (sensory mechanism of the ear), the vestibulocochlear nerve, the central neural pathways, or a combination of these structures. It is sometimes subdivided into *cochlear d.* and *retrocochlear d.* Called also *nerve d., perceptive d.,* and *transmission d.*
**tone d.**, sensory amusia.
**toxic d.**, ototoxic hearing loss.
**transmission d.**, sensorineural d.
**vascular d.**, that due to disease of blood vessels of the inner ear.
**word d.**, auditory aphasia.

**de·al·ba·tion** (de″al-ba′shən) bleaching.

**de·al·co·hol·iza·tion** (de-al″ko-hol″ĭ-za′shən) the removal of alcohol from an object or substance.

**de·al·ler·gi·za·tion** (de-al″ər-jĭ-za′shən) the desensitization of an allergic individual to any particular allergen.

**de·am·i·dase** (de-am′ĭ-dās) amidohydrolase.

**de·am·i·da·tion** (de-am″ĭ-da′shən) deamidization.

**de·am·i·di·za·tion** (de-am″ĭ-dĭ-za′shən) the removal of an amido group from a molecule.

**de·am·i·nase** (de-am′ĭ-nās) a term used in the trivial names of some aminohydrolases (q.v.), usually restricted to those deaminating cyclic amidines; the enzymes are generally named for their substrates (e.g., adenosine deaminase).

**de·am·i·na·tion** (de-am″ĭ-na′shən) [MeSH: Deamination] removal of the amino group, —$NH_2$, from a compound.

**de·am·i·ni·za·tion** (de-am″ĭ-nĭ-za′shən) deamination.

**Dea·ner** (de′nər) trademark for a preparation of deanol acetamidobenzoate.

**de·a·nol ac·et·am·i·do·ben·zo·ate** (de′ə-nol as″ət-am″ĭ-do-ben′zo-āt) a cerebral stimulant with parasympathomimetic activity, used as an antidepressant in the treatment of certain behavior and/or learning disorders in children.

**de·ar·te·ri·al·i·za·tion** (de″ahr-te″re-əl-ĭ-za′shən) the occluding or cutting off of the arterial supply to a part, causing ischemia; sometimes done in a transient fashion as a treatment for liver cancer.

**de·ar·tic·u·la·tion** (de″ahr-tik″u-la′shən) dislocation of a joint.

**death** (deth) [MeSH: Death] the cessation of life; permanent cessation of all vital bodily functions. For legal and medical purposes, the following definition of death has been proposed—the irreversible cessation of all of the following: (1) total cerebral function, (2) spontaneous function of the respiratory system, and (3) spontaneous function of the circulatory system.
**activation-induced cell d. (AICD),** recognition and deletion of T lymphocytes that have been induced to proliferate by receptor-mediated activation, preventing their overgrowth when responding to perception of a foreign agent. It is particularly important for regulation of lymphocytes that recognize self antigens.
**apparent d.**, a state of complete interruption of bodily processes from which the patient can be resuscitated.
**black d.**, bubonic plague (q.v.) thought to be associated with necrotic purpura and symmetrical gangrene.
**brain d.**, irreversible brain damage as manifested by absolute unresponsiveness to all stimuli, absence of all spontaneous muscle activity, including respiration, shivering, etc., and an isoelectric electroencephalogram for 30 minutes, all in the absence of hypothermia or intoxication by central nervous system depressants. Called also *irreversible coma* and *cerebral d.*
**cell d.**, complete disintegration or necrosis of cells.
**cerebral d.**, brain d.
**cognitive d.**, persistent vegetative state.
**cot d., crib d.**, sudden infant death syndrome.
**fetal d.**, death in utero; failure of the product of conception to show evidence of respiration, heart beat, or definite movement of a voluntary muscle after expulsion from the uterus, with no possibility of resuscitation. Called also *stillbirth.*
**fetal d., early,** fetal death occurring during the first 20 weeks of gestation.
**fetal d., intermediate,** fetal death occurring during the twenty-first to twenty-eighth weeks of gestation.
**fetal d., late,** fetal death occurring after 28 weeks of gestation.
**functional d.**, total, permanent destruction of cognition and related higher functions of the central nervous system, with vital functions being sustained by artificial means.
**genetic d.**, the failure of a mutation to be passed on to the next generation because of the mutation's damaging phenotypic effects.
**liver d.**, death due to failure of hepatic function.
**local d.**, death of a part of the body.
**molecular d.**, caries, or the last stage of a catabolic process.
**programmed cell d.**, the theory that particular cells are programmed to die at specific sites and during specific stages of development. Called also *apoptosis.*
**somatic d.**, cessation of all vital cellular activity.
**sudden cardiac d.**, unexpected natural death due to cardiac causes that occur rapidly after the onset of acute symptoms in a patient with or without known preexisting heart disease, in whom cardiac dysfunction produces abrupt loss of cerebral blood flow. The interval between the onset of symptoms and death is given variably as ranging from less than one hour to less than 24 hours.
**voodoo d.**, a phenomenon seen among certain cultural groups in which the affected individual dies after transgressing a taboo or becoming convinced that he is bewitched.

**Dea·ver's incision** (de′vərz) [John Blair *Deaver,* American surgeon, 1855–1931] see under *incision.*

**de·band·ing** (de-band′ing) the removal of the bands of a fixed orthodontic appliance.

**De·bary·o·my·ces** (de″bar-e-o-mi′sēz) a genus of fungi of the family Saccharomycetaceae. *D. hanse′nii* (formerly called *Saccharomyces hansenii*) changes sugars into oxalic acid and has occasionally been isolated from human infections. *D. ho′minis* and *D. neofor′mans* are former names for *Cryptococcus neoformans.*
**D. hanse′nii,** a species that changes sugars into oxalic acid; called also *Saccharomyces hansenii.*
**D. ho′minis, D. neofor′mans,** former name for *Cryptococcus neoformans.*

**de·bil·i·ty** (də-bil′ĭ-te) asthenia.

**dé·bouche·ment** (da-boosh-maw′) [Fr.] an opening out.

**de·branch·er en·zyme** (de-branch′ər en′zīm) see under *enzyme.*

**de·branch·er en·zyme de·fi·cien·cy** glycogen storage disease, type III.

**de·branch·ing en·zyme** (de-branch′ing en′zīm) see under *enzyme.*

**De·bré's phe·nom·e·non** (də-brāz′) [Robert *Debré,* French pediatrician and bacteriologist, 1882–1978] see under *phenomenon.*

**De·bré-Sé·mé·laigne syndrome** (də-bra′sa-ma-len′yə) [R. *Debré;* Georges *Sémélaigne,* French pediatrician, 20th century] see under *syndrome.*

**dé·bride** (da-brēd′) to remove foreign material and contaminated or devitalized tissue, usually by sharp dissection.

**dé·bride·ment** (da-brēd-maw′) [Fr.] the removal of foreign material and devitalized or contaminated tissue from or adjacent to a traumatic or infected lesion until surrounding healthy tissue is exposed. Cf. *épluchage.*
**enzymatic d.**, removal of fibrinous or purulent exudate by application of a nontoxic and nonirritating enzyme that is capable of lysing

fibrin, denatured collagen, and elastin but does not destroy normal tissue.
**surgical d.,** débridement by mechanical methods, usually sharp dissection.

**de•bris** (də-bre′) [Fr.] an accumulation of fragments of necrotic tissue or foreign material.

**De•bri•san** (də-bri′sən) trademark for dextranomer.

**deb•ris•o•quin sul•fate** (deb-ris′o-kwin) an antihypertensive agent having actions and uses similar to those of guanethidine; administered orally. Spelled also *debrisoquine* [BAN and INN].

**Deb. spis.** abbreviation for L. *deb′ita spissitu′dine,* of the proper consistency.

**debt** (det) something owed.
**oxygen d.,** the extra oxygen that must be used in the oxidative energy processes after a period of strenuous exercise to reconvert lactic acid to glucose, and decomposed ATP and creatine phosphate to their original states.

**de•bulk•ing** (de-bulk′ing) removal of a major portion of the material that composes a lesion, as the removal of most of a tumor so that there is less tumor load for subsequent treatment (e.g., by chemotherapy or radiation). Called also *cytoreduction* and *cytoreductive surgery.*

**Dec.** abbreviation for L. *decan′ta,* pour off.

**deca-** [Gr. *deka* ten] a combining form designating ten; used in naming units of measurement to indicate a quantity ten ($10^1$) times the unit designated by the root with which it is combined. Symbol, dk.

**Deca•derm** (dek′ə-dərm″) trademark for a preparation of dexamethasone.

**Deca•dron** (dek′ə-dron″) trademark for preparations of dexamethasone.

**Deca-Du•rab•o•lin** (dek″ə-dur″ə-bo′lin) trademark for a preparation of nandrolone decanoate.

**Deca•ject** (dek′ə-jekt″) trademark for preparations of dexamethasone.

**de•cal•ci•fi•ca•tion** (de-kal″sĭ-fĭ-ka′shən) 1. the loss of calcium salts from a bone or tooth. 2. the process of removing calcareous matter.

**de•cal•ci•fy** (de-kal′sĭ-fi) [*de-* + *calcify*] to deprive of calcium salts.

**dec•a•me•tho•ni•um** (dek″ə-mə-tho′ne-əm) a bisquaternary ammonium compound, structurally analogous to tubocurarine; used as a nondepolarizing muscle relaxant.
**d. bromide,** the bromide salt of decamethonium, used as a skeletal muscle relaxant during surgical anesthesia, to aid endotracheal intubation, in obstetrics, and in electroconvulsive therapy; administered intravenously.
**d. iodide,** the iodide salt of decamethonium, which has been used for the same purposes as the bromide salt.

**dec•ane** (dek′ān) a hydrocarbon, $C_{10}H_{22}$, from paraffin.

**de•can•nu•la•tion** (de-kan″u-la′shən) extubation, especially of a tracheostomy cannula.

**de•can•ta•tion** (de″kan-ta′shən) [*de-* + L. *canthus* tire of a wheel] the pouring of a clear supernatant liquid from a sediment.

**deca•pep•tide** (dek″ə-pep′tīd) a peptide containing ten amino acids.

**Deca•pep•tyl** (dek″ə-pep′təl) trademark for a preparation of triptorelin.

**de•cap•i•ta•tion** (de-kap″ĭ-ta′shən) [*de-* + L. *caput* head] the removal of the head, as of an animal, a fetus, or a bone; beheading.

**de•cap•i•ta•tor** (de-kap′ĭ-ta″tor) an instrument for removing the head of a fetus in embryotomy.

**De•ca•po•da** (de-kə-po′də) [Gr. *deka* ten + *pous* foot] an order of Crustacea, including the crabs, lobsters, and shrimps, whose members have five pairs of legs upon the thorax.

**Dec•a•pryn** (dek′ə-prin) trademark for preparations of doxylamine succinate.

**de•cap•su•la•tion** (de-kap″su-la′shən) capsulectomy.
**renal d.,** surgical removal of the capsule of the kidney; called also *renal capsulectomy, renal decortication,* and *nephrocapsectomy.*

**de•car•box•y•lase** (de″kahr-bok′sə-lās) a term used in the recommended names of enzymes of the sub-subclass carboxy-lyase [EC 4.1.1]; they catalyze the nonhydrolytic removal of carbon dioxide from carboxylic acids.

**de•car•box•y•la•tion** (de″kahr-bok″sə-la′shən) [MeSH: Decarboxylation] removal of the carboxyl group from a molecule.

**De•ca•spray** (dek′ə-spra″) trademark for a preparation of dexamethasone.

**deca•vi•ta•min** (dek″ə-vi′tə-min) a combination of vitamins in capsular or tablet form, each of which contains vitamins A and D, ascorbic acid, calcium pantothenate, cyanocobalamin, folic acid, niacinamide, pyridoxine hydrochloride, riboflavin, thiamine hydrochloride, and a suitable form of alpha tocopherol.

**de•cay** (de-ka′) [*de-* + L. *cadere* to fall] 1. the gradual decomposition of dead organic matter. 2. the process or stage of decline, as in aging.
**alpha d.,** a form of radioactive decay in which an alpha particle (two neutrons plus two protons) is emitted, decreasing both the size and the charge of the nucleus and yielding a daughter product that is a different element. It often occurs serially.
**beta d.,** disintegration of the nucleus of an unstable radionuclide in which the mass number is unchanged, but the atomic number is increased or decreased by 1, as result of emission of a negatively or positively charged (beta) particle and a neutrino.
**free induction d.,** the signal analyzed in magnetic resonance imaging or spectroscopy; it results from the emission of energy by nuclei after they are excited by a pulse of radio frequency waves.
**positron d.,** see under *emission.*
**radioactive d.,** disintegration of the nucleus of an unstable nuclide by the spontaneous emission of charged particles and/or photons; called also *radioactive disintegration.*
**tone d.,** the decrease in threshold sensitivity resulting from the presence of a barely audible continuous sound.
**tooth d.,** dental caries.

**de•ce•dent** (də-se′dənt) a person who has recently died.

**de•cel•er•a•tion** (de-sel′ər-a″shən) [MeSH: Deceleration] decrease in speed or rate.
**early d.,** in fetal heart rate monitoring, a transient decrease in heart rate that coincides with the onset of a uterine contraction.
**late d.,** in fetal heart rate monitoring, a transient decrease in heart rate occurring at or after the peak of a uterine contraction, which may result from fetal hypoxia.
**variable d's,** in fetal heart rate monitoring, a transient series of decelerations in heart rate that vary in duration, intensity, and relation to uterine contractions; they are abrupt in onset and cessation and result from vagus nerve firing in response to stimuli such as umbilical cord compression in the first stage of labor.

**de•cen•ter** (de-sen′tər) [*de-* + *center*] in optics, to design or make a lens such that the visual axis does not pass through the optical center of the lens.

**de•cen•tra•tion** (de″sen-tra′shən) the act or process of removing from a center.

**de•ce•ra•tion** (de′sə-ra′shən) [*de-* + L. *cera* wax] the removal of paraffin from a tissue section prepared for the microscope.

**de•cer•e•bel•la•tion** (de-ser″ə-bəl-a′shən) removal of the cerebellum or elimination of its functions.

**de•cer•e•brate** (de-ser′ə-brāt) 1. in an experimental animal, to eliminate cerebral function by transecting the brain stem between the superior colliculi and the vestibular nuclei or by ligating the common carotid arteries and the basilar artery at the center of the pons. 2. an animal so prepared. 3. a person with brain damage resulting in neurologic signs similar to those of a decerebrated animal; the human brain lesion may differ somewhat from that of an experimental animal. See also *decerebrate rigidity,* under *rigidity.*

**de•cer•e•bra•tion** (de-ser″ə-bra′shən) [*de-* + *cerebration*] the act of decerebrating.

**de•cer•e•brize** (de-ser′ə-brīz) to decerebrate (def. 1).

**de•chlo•ri•da•tion** (de-klor″ĭ-da′shən) the removal of chloride, or salt.

**de•cho•les•ter•ol•iza•tion** (de″kə-les″tər-ol-ĭ-za′shən) extraction of cholesterol from the blood.

**De•cho•lin** (de′ko-lin) trademark for preparations of dehydrocholic acid.

**deci-** [L. *decem* ten] a combining form designating one-tenth; used in naming units of measurement to indicate one-tenth ($10^{-1}$) of the unit designated by the root with which it is combined. Symbol, d.

**dec•i•bel** (des′ĭ-bəl) a unit of relative power intensity equal to one tenth of a bel, used for electric or acoustic power measurements. The decibel level is ten times the base ten logarithm of the ratio of the measured power to some reference power level. A one decibel change is an increase in the power level by a factor of 1.26, approximately the smallest change in sound level detectable by human ears; a ten decibel (one bel) change multiplies the power by a factor of ten and approximately doubles the perceived sound level. In audiometry the reference power level (0 db) corresponds to a root-mean-square sound pressure level of $2 \times 10^{-4}$ dyn/cm$^2$, which is approximately the threshold of hearing for healthy young persons. Symbol, dB.

**de•cid•ua** (də-sid′u-ə) [L., from *deciduus* falling off] [MeSH: Decidua]

the endometrium of the pregnant uterus, all of which, except the deepest layer, is shed at parturition. Called also *membranae deciduae, caduca, decidual* or *deciduous membrane,* and *tunica decidua.*
**d. basa'lis,** basal decidua: the portion of the decidua directly underlying the chorionic vesicle and attached to the myometrium; called also *d. serotina* and *membrana serotina.*
**d. capsula'ris,** capsular decidua: the portion of the decidua directly overlying the chorionic vesicle and facing the uterine cavity; called also *reflex d.* and *d. reflexa.*
**menstrual d., d. menstrua'lis,** the hyperemic mucosa of the uterus that is shed during the menstrual period.
**d. parieta'lis,** parietal decidua: the portion of the decidua lining the uterus elsewhere than at the site of attachment of the chorionic vesicle; called also *d. vera.*
**reflex d., d. reflex'a,** d. capsularis.
**d. seroti'na,** d. basalis.
**d. subchoria'lis,** the maternal component of the tissue comprising the closing ring of Winkler-Waldeyer.
**true d.,** d. parietalis.
**d. tubero'sa papulo'sa,** decidual cast.
**d. ve'ra,** d. parietalis.

**de·cid·u·al** (də-sid'u-əl) pertaining to the decidua.

**de·cid·u·ate** (də-sid'u-āt) characterized by shedding.

**de·cid·u·itis** (də-sid'u-i'tis) a bacterial disease leading to alterations in the decidua.

**de·cid·u·o·ma** (də-sid"u-o'mə) [*decidua* + *-oma*] an intrauterine mass containing decidual cells.
**Loeb's d.,** a tumor-like structure resembling the maternal placenta, produced in the uteri of guinea pigs by the action of progesterone.
**d. malig'num,** choriocarcinoma.

**de·cid·u·o·ma·to·sis** (də-sid"u-o-mə-to'sis) formation of decidual tissue in the nonpregnant state.

**de·cid·u·o·sis** (də-sid'u-o'sis) the presence of decidual tissue or of tissue resembling the endometrium of pregnancy in an ectopic site.

**de·cid·u·ous** (də-sid'u-əs) [L. *deciduus,* from *decidere* to fall off] falling off or shed at maturity; the term is used to designate the teeth of the first dentition in animals and humans.

**dec·ile** (des'īl) [*deca-* + *-ile* (by analogy with *quartile*)] any of the nine values that divide the range of a probability distribution into ten equal parts of equal probability, i.e., the 1st, 2nd, 3rd, etc.; deciles are the 10th, 20th, 30th, etc., percentiles.

**dec·i·li·ter** (des'ĭ-le"tər) one tenth of a liter; 100 milliliters.

**de·cip·a·ra** (də-sip'ə-rə) [*deca-* + *para*] a woman who has had ten pregnancies that resulted in viable offspring; also written para X.

**de·ci·ta·bine (DAC)** (de-si'tə-bēn") an S-phase specific cytotoxic compound used as an antineoplastic in the treatment of acute leukemia; administered by intravenous infusion.

**deck·platte** (dek'plah-tə) [Ger.] roof plate; see under *plate.*

**de·claw·ing** (de-klaw'ing) onychectomy.

**de Clé·ram·bault syndrome** (də kla"rahm-bo') [Gaetan Gatian *de Clérambault,* French psychiatrist, 1872–1934] see *erotomania.*

**dec·li·na·tion** (dek"lĭ-na'shən) [L. *declinare* to decline] deviation from a normally vertical position, as rotation of the eye about its anteroposterior axis so that its vertical meridian lies to the temporal *(positive d.)* or to the nasal side *(negative d.)* of its proper position. Cf. *extorsion* and *intorsion.*

**dec·li·na·tor** (dek'lĭ-na"tor) an instrument by which parts are retracted during an operation.

**de·cline** (de-klīn') 1. the period or stage of the abatement of a disease or paroxysm. 2. a gradual deterioration or wasting away of the physical and mental faculties.

**de·clive** (de-kli've) [L. neuter of *declivis* sloping downward] [TA] the part of the vermis of the cerebellum just caudal to the primary

**de·cli·vis** (de-kli'vis) [L.] declive.

**Dec·lo·my·cin** (dek'lo-mi"sin) trademark for preparations of demeclocycline.

**de·co·ag·u·lant** (de"ko-ag'u-lənt) 1. reducing the amount of existing coagulants or procoagulants in the blood. 2. a substance that has this quality and inhibits coagulation of blood.

**Decoct.** abbreviation for L. *decoc'tum,* a decoction.

**de·coc·tion** (de-kok'shən) [L. *decoctum,* from *de* down + *coquere* to boil] 1. the act or process of boiling. 2. a medicine or other substance prepared by boiling.

**de·col·la·tion** (de"ko-la'shən) [*de-* + *collum*] decapitation, chiefly of a dead fetus.

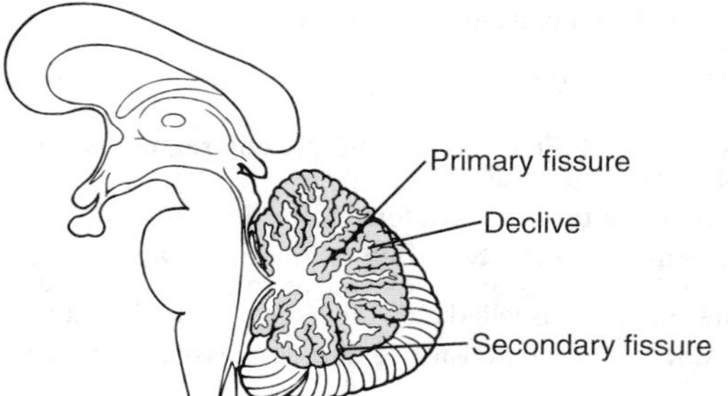

Median section of cerebellum, showing declive.

**de·col·or·a·tion** (de-kul-or-a'shən) 1. removal of color; bleaching. 2. lack or loss of color.

**de·col·or·ize** (de-kul'or-īz) to free from color; to bleach.

**de·com·pen·sa·tion** (de-kom"pən-sa'shən) 1. failure of compensation; cardiac decompensation is marked by dyspnea, venous engorgement, and edema. 2. in psychiatry, failure of defense mechanisms resulting in progressive personality disintegration.

**de·com·ple·men·tize** (de-kom'plə-men"tīz) to remove complement from.

**de·com·po·si·tion** (de"kom-pə-zish'ən) [*de-* + L. *componere* to put together] the separation of compound bodies into their constituent principles by whatever process.
**anaerobic d.,** the breakdown of organic compounds in the absence of oxygen. In animals, the process is known as *glycolysis;* in plants and microorganisms, *fermentation.*
**d. of movement,** a form of ataxia characterized by irregularity in the successive flexion and extension of joints in performing a movement with the limb.

**de·com·pres·sion** (de"kom-presh'ən) [MeSH: Decompression] 1. any removal of pressure. 2. the lessening of atmospheric pressure on deep-sea divers and caisson workers who return to normal pressure environments, or on persons ascending to great heights. If not controlled or artificially slowed, it can cause *decompression sickness.* 3. any technique for artificially controlling this process. 4. a surgical operation for the relief of pressure in a body compartment.
**abdominal d.,** the removal of pressure from the abdomen during the first stage of labor.
**cardiac d.,** d. of heart.
**cerebral d.,** removal of a flap of the skull and incision of the dura mater for relief of intracranial pressure.
**explosive d.,** decompression more rapid than that corresponding to a rate of ascent greater than 5000 feet per minute.
**d. of heart,** pericardiotomy with evacuation of blood or fluid; called also *d. of pericardium.*
**microvascular d.,** a microsurgical procedure for relief of trigeminal neuralgia; decompression of the sensory root of the trigeminal nerve is accomplished by insertion of a small nonabsorbable sponge to relieve pressure from small blood vessels where the root enters the pons. Called also *Jannetta procedure.*
**nerve d.,** relief of pressure on a nerve by surgical removal of the constricting fibrous or bony tissue.
**d. of pericardium,** d. of heart.
**d. of spinal cord,** relief of pressure on the spinal cord by means of surgery.
**suboccipital d.,** cerebral decompression by occipital craniectomy and opening of the dura.
**subtemporal d.,** cerebral decompression by removal of a portion of the temporal bone and opening of the dura.

**de·con·di·tion·ing** (de"kən-dish'ən-ing) a change in cardiovascular function after prolonged periods of weightlessness, probably related to a shift of a quantity of blood from the lower limbs to the thorax, resulting in reflex diuresis and a reduction of blood volume.

**de·con·ges·tant** (de"kən-jes'tənt) 1. tending to reduce congestion or swelling. 2. an agent that reduces congestion or swelling.

**de·con·ges·tive** (de"kən-jes'tiv) reducing congestion.

**de·con·tam·i·na·tion** (de"kən-tam"ĭ-na'shən) [MeSH: Decontamination] the freeing of a person or an object of some contaminating substance such as poisonous gas, radioactive material, etc.

**de·co·quin·ate** (de-ko-kwin'āt) [USP] [MeSH: Decoquinate] a coccidiostat for poultry, effective against *Eimeria.*

**de·cor·ti·ca·tion** (de-kor"tĭ-ka'shən) [*de-* + *cortex*] 1. the removal of bark, hull, husk, or shell from a plant, seed, or root, as in pharmacy. 2. removal of portions of the cortical substance of a structure or organ, as of the brain, kidney, or lung.

**chemical d., enzymatic d.,** removal of cortical substance by chemical agents or enzymes.
**d. of lung,** removal of constricting visceral pleura to permit the lung to expand.
**renal d.,** renal decapsulation.

**dec·re·ment** (dek'rə-mənt) [L. *decrementum*] 1. subtraction, or decrease; the amount by which a quantity or value is decreased. 2. the stage of decline of a disease; see *stadium decrementi.*

**de·crep·i·tate** (de-krep'ĭ-tāt) 1. to roast or calcine certain substances (salt, crystals, etc.) until crackling occurs, or until crackling ends. 2. to explode with a crackling noise upon heating, owing to the release of entrapped water as steam.

**de·crep·i·ta·tion** (de-krep"ĭ-ta'shən) the explosion or crackling of certain substances (salt, crystals, etc.) upon heating.

**de·cru·des·cence** (de"kroo-des'əns) diminution or abatement of the intensity of symptoms or physical signs.

**de·crus·ta·tion** (de"krəs-ta'shən) the detachment of a crust.

**Decub.** abbreviation for L. *decu'bitus,* lying down.

**de·cu·bi·tal** (de-ku'bĭ-təl) pertaining to decubitus (decubitus ulcer).

**de·cu·bi·tus** (de-ku'bĭ-təs) L. pl. *decu'bitus* [L. "a lying down"] 1. an act of lying down; also the position assumed in lying down. 2. decubitus ulcer; see under *ulcer.*
**Andral's d.,** decubitus on the sound side, a position assumed in the early stages of pleurisy.
**dorsal d.,** lying in the supine position.
**lateral d.,** lying on the side; used in radiologic examination, with the x-ray beam directed horizontally; designated *right lateral decubitus* when the subject lies on the right side and *left lateral decubitus* when on the left side.
**ventral d.,** lying on the stomach.

**de·cum·bin** (de-kum'bin) a toxic substance obtained from *Penicillium decumbens,* which causes respiratory distress and hemorrhage; the oral $LD_{50}$ for rats is about 275 mg/kg.

**de·cur·rent** (de-kur'ənt) [L. *decurrere* to run down] extending or moving from above downward.

**de·cus·sate** (de-kus'āt) [L. *decussare* to cross in the form of an X] 1. to cross or intersect in the form of the letter X. 2. crossing in the form of the letter X.

**de·cus·sa·tio** (de"kə-sa'she-o) pl. *decussatio'nes* [L.] [TA] decussation: a general term for the intercrossing of fellow parts or structures in the form of an X. See also *chiasma* and *commissura.*
**d. fibra'rum nervo'rum trochlea'rium** [TA], decussation of trochlear nerve fibers: the crossing of the fibers of the trochlear nerves in the superior medullary velum. Called also *d. trochlearis, d. nervorum trochlearis,* and *trochlear decussation.*
**d. lemnis'ci media'lis** [TA], decussation of medial lemniscus: the region at the caudal end of the medulla oblongata in which the fibers from the nucleus cuneatus and the nucleus gracilis on each side intersect as they cross the midline before ascending as the medial lemniscus.
**d. moto'ria,** d. pyramidum.
**d. nervo'rum trochlea'ris, d. nervo'rum trochlea'rium,** d. fibrarum nervorum trochlearium.
**d. pedunculo'rum cerebella'rium superio'rum** [TA], decussation of superior cerebellar peduncles: the crossing of the fibers of the peduncles within the tegmentum of the mesencephalon.
**d. pyra'midum** [TA], decussation of pyramids: the anterior part of the lower medulla oblongata in which most of the fibers of each pyramid intersect as they cross the midline and descend as the lateral corticospinal tracts. Called also *d. motoria, pyramidal decussation,* and *motor decussation.*
**d.'nes tegmenta'les** [TA], tegmental decussations: crossing fibers in the midbrain, including the decussatio tegmentalis anterior and the decussatio tegmentalis posterior.
**d. tegmenta'lis ante'rior** [TA], anterior tegmental decussation: the anterior portion of the decussation of the cerebellar peduncle, comprising fibers of the lateral third of the peduncle, which decussate immediately dorsal to the interpeduncular nucleus in the ventral tegmentum. The fibers merge with those of the decussatio tegmentalis posterior at the level of the caudal red nucleus.
**d. tegmenta'lis poste'rior** [TA], posterior tegmental decussation: the posterior portion of the decussation of the cerebellar peduncle, comprising fibers of the medial two thirds of the peduncle, which start to cross the midline at the level of the inferior colliculus, ventral to the medial longitudinal fasciculus. The fibers merge with those of the decussatio tegmentalis anterior at the level of the caudal red nucleus.
**d.'nes tegmen'ti, d.'nes tegmento'rum,** decussationes tegmentales.
**d. trochlea'ris,** d. fibrarum nervorum trochlearium

**de·cus·sa·tion** (de"kə-sa'shən) a crossing over; see *decussatio.*
**anterior tegmental d.,** decussatio tegmentalis anterior.
**dorsal tegmental d.,** decussatio tegmentalis posterior.
**Forel's d.,** decussatio tegmentalis anterior.
**fountain d. of Meynert,** decussatio tegmentalis posterior.
**d. of medial lemniscus,** decussatio lemnisci medialis.
**motor d.,** decussatio pyramidum.
**optic d.,** chiasma opticum.
**posterior tegmental d.,** decussatio tegmentalis posterior.
**pyramidal d., d. of pyramids,** decussatio pyramidum.
**rubrospinal d.,** decussatio tegmentalis anterior.
**sensory d.,** decussatio lemnisci medialis.
**d. of superior cerebellar peduncles,** decussatio pedunculorum cerebellarium superiorum.
**tectospinal d.,** decussatio tegmentalis posterior.
**tegmental d's, d's of tegmentum,** decussationes tegmentales.
**trochlear d., d. of trochlear nerves, d. of trochlear nerve fibers,** decussatio fibrarum nervorum trochlearium.
**ventral tegmental d.,** decussatio tegmentalis anterior.

**de·cus·sa·ti·o·nes** (de"kə-sa"she-o'nēz) [L.] plural of *decussatio.*

**de·den·ti·tion** (de"den-tish'ən) [*de-* + *dentition*] the shedding or loss of teeth.

**de·dif·fer·en·ti·a·tion** (de-dif'ər-en"she-a'shən) anaplasia.

**de d. in d.** abbreviation for L. *de di'e in di'em,* from day to day.

**ded·o·la·tion** (ded"o-la'shən) the removal of a thin piece of skin by an oblique cut.

**de Duve** see *Duve.*

**deep** (dēp) situated far beneath the surface; not superficial.

**de·epi·car·di·al·iza·tion** (de-ep"ĭ-kahr"de-əl"ĭ-za'shən) a surgical procedure formerly used for the relief of intractable angina pectoris, in which epicardial tissue is destroyed by phenolization or the application of other caustic agents to promote the development of collateral circulation.

**deet** (dēt) [MeSH: Deet] diethyltoluamide.

**Deet·jen's bodies** (dāt'yənz) [Hermann *Deetjen,* German physician, 1867–1915] blood platelets.

**DEF** see under *rate.*

**de·fat·i·ga·tion** (de-fat"ĭ-ga'shən) overstrain or fatigue of muscular or nervous tissue.

**de·fat·ted** (de-fat'əd) deprived of fat, as a food.

**de·faun·ate** (de-fawn'āt) [*de-* + *fauna*] to remove or destroy an animal population, especially parasites, such as by removing hookworms from the intestinal tract or delousing.

**de·faun·a·tion** (de-faw-na'shən) the process of defaunating; cf. *disinfestation.*

**def·e·ca·tion** (def"ə-ka'shən) [L. *defaecare* to deprive of dregs] [MeSH: Defecation] 1. the removal of impurities, as chemical defecation. 2. the evacuation of fecal material from the rectum.
**fragmentary d.,** the evacuation of small pieces of feces.

**def·e·cog·ra·phy** (def"ə-kog'rə-fe) [*defecation* + *-graphy*] the making of rapid-sequence radiographs or the recording of fluoroscopic images on videotape during defecation following the instillation of barium into the rectum; used in the evaluation of fecal incontinence.

**de·fect** (de'fekt) an imperfection, failure, or absence.
**acquired d.,** a non-genetic imperfection arising secondarily, after birth.
**aortic septal d.,** a congenital anomaly in which there is abnormal communication between the ascending aorta and pulmonary artery just above the semilunar valves; called also *aorticopulmonary fenestration, aorticopulmonary septal d.,* and *aorticopulmonary window.*
**aorticopulmonary septal d.,** aortic septal d.
**atrial septal d's, atrioseptal d's,** congenital cardiac anomalies in which there is persistent patency of the atrial septum due to failure of fusion between either the septum secundum or the septum primum and the endocardial cushions. In *ostium secundum d.* there is a rim of septum all around the defect. In *ostium primum d.,* which is an incomplete form of atrioventricularis communis, there is no septum at the base of the defect, between the mitral and tricuspid valves; it is usually associated with a cleft mitral cusp and occasionally with a cleft tricuspid valve or a ventricular septal defect.
**birth d.,** a defect present at birth; the term may refer to a morphological defect (dysmorphism) or to an inborn error of metabolism.
**congenital d.,** birth defect; a structural or chemical imperfection present at birth.
**cortical d.,** a benign, symptomless, circumscribed rarefaction of cortical bone, detected radiographically.
**ectodermal d., congenital,** anhidrotic ectodermal dysplasia.
**endocardial cushion d's,** a spectrum of septal defects resulting from imperfect fusion of the endocardial cushions and ranging from persistent ostium primum to persistent complete common atrioventricular canal; see *atrial septal d's* and *atrioventricularis communis.*
**fibrous cortical d.,** a small, asymptomatic, osteolytic, fibrous lesion

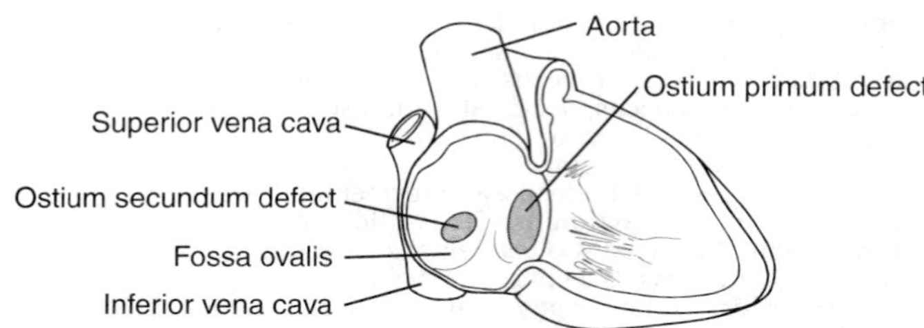


Atrial septal defects; cutaway composite view showing possible locations of ostium primum and secundum defects in the right atrium.

occurring within the bone cortex, particularly in the metaphyseal region of long bones in childhood. When large and actively growing, it is generally termed *nonossifying fibroma.* Called also *metaphyseal fibrous d.*
**filling d.,** any localized defect in the contour of the stomach, duodenum, or intestine, as seen in the radiograph after a barium enema, due to a lesion of the wall projecting into the lumen or to an object in the lumen.
**genetic d.,** see under *disease.*
**intercalary d. of pollical ray,** radial ray d.
**metaphyseal fibrous d.,** 1. fibrous cortical d. 2. nonossifying fibroma.
**neural tube d.,** a developmental anomaly consisting of failure of closure of the neural tube, resulting in conditions such as cranium bifidum, encephalocele, spina bifida, and myelomeningocele.
**ostium primum d.,** see *atrial septal d.*
**ostium secundum d.,** see *atrial septal d.*
**polytopic field d.,** a pattern of anomalies derived from the disturbance of a single developmental field.
**retention d.,** a defect in the power of recalling or remembering names, numbers, or events.
**salt-losing d.,** see under *syndrome.*
**septal d.,** a defect in one of the cardiac septa, resulting in an abnormal communication between the opposite chambers of the heart.
**ventricular septal d.,** a congenital cardiac anomaly in which there is persistent patency of the ventricular septum in either the muscular or fibrous (membranous) portions, most often due to failure of the bulbar septum to completely close the interventricular foramen.

**de·fec·tive** (de-fek′tiv) 1. imperfect. 2. a person lacking in some physical, mental, or moral quality.

**de·fem·i·ni·za·tion** (de-fem″ĭ-nĭ-za′shən) loss of female secondary sex characters; see also *masculinization.*

**de·fense** (de-fens′) the practice of, or measures taken to ensure, self-protection.
**character d.,** any character trait, e.g., a mannerism, attitude, or affectation, which serves as a defense mechanism.
**insanity d.,** a legal concept that a person cannot be convicted of a crime if he lacked criminal responsibility by reason of insanity at the time of commission. See *M'Naghten rule* and *Durham rule,* under *rule,* and *American Law Institute Formulation,* under *formulation.*
**muscular d.,** the muscular tension and rigidity that accompanies a localized inflammation (as in appendicitis) or passage of a kidney stone.

**de·fen·sin** (de-fen′sin) any of a group of small antimicrobial cationic peptides occurring in neutrophils and macrophages; they act by binding fungal and bacterial membranes and increasing membrane permeability.

**def·er·ens** (def′ər -enz) [L.] deferent; see *ductus deferens.*

**def·er·ent** (def′ər-ənt) [L. *deferens* carrying away] conveying anything away, as from a center.

**def·er·en·tec·to·my** (def″ər-ən-tek′tə-me) vasectomy.

**def·er·en·tial** (def″ər-en′shəl) pertaining to the ductus deferens.

**def·er·en·ti·tis** (def″ər-ən-ti′tis) inflammation of the ductus deferens.

**de·fer·ox·amine** (də-fər-oks′ə-mēn) [MeSH: Deferoxamine] a chelating agent, isolated from *Streptomyces pilosus,* which binds with iron to form a soluble complex. Called also *desferrioxamine.*
**d. hydrochloride,** the hydrochloride salt of deferoxamine, $C_{25}H_{48}N_6O_8{\cdot}HCl$.
**d. mesylate** [USP], the water-soluble mesylate salt of deferoxamine, having the same actions as the base; used as an antidote to iron poisoning, usually administered by intramuscular injection or by intravenous infusion.

**def·er·ves·cence** (def″ər-ves′əns) [L. *defervescere* to cease boiling] the abatement of fever.

**def·er·ves·cent** (def″ər-ves′ənt) 1. causing reduction of fever. 2. an agent that acts to reduce fever.

**de·fib·ril·la·tion** (de-fib″rĭ-la′shən) termination of atrial or ventricular fibrillation, usually by electroshock.

**de·fib·ril·la·tor** (de-fib″rĭ-la′tər) an electronic apparatus used to counteract atrial or ventricular fibrillation by the application of brief electroshock to the heart, either directly or through electrodes placed on the chest wall.
**automatic implantable cardioverter-d.,** see under *cardioverter.*

**de·fi·bri·nat·ed** (de-fi′brĭ-nāt″əd) characterized by defibrination.

**de·fi·bri·na·tion** (de-fi″brĭ-na′shən) removal of fibrin from a blood sample to prevent clotting; it also occurs pathologically in diffuse intravascular coagulation.

**de·fi·brino·gen·a·tion** (de″fi-brin″ə-jə-na′shən) induced defibrination, such as that caused by ancrod in thrombolytic therapy.

**de·fi·cien·cy** (de-fish′ən-se) a lack or defect. For deficiencies of specific enzymes, see under the enzyme name.
**brancher d.,** glycogen storage disease, type IV.
**debrancher d.,** glycogen storage disease, type III.
**disaccharidase d.,** less than normal activity of disaccharidases of the intestinal mucosa; it usually denotes a generalized deficiency of all such enzymes secondary to a disorder of the small intestine, which clinically may be manifest only as a deficiency of lactase activity, but is sometimes used to denote deficiency of a single enzyme or enzyme complex, e.g., lactase, sucrase-isomaltase, or trehalase. See also individual enzyme deficiencies and see *disaccharide intolerance,* under *intolerance.*
**familial apolipoprotein C-II (apo C-II) d.,** an autosomal recessive disorder due to lack of apo C-II, a necessary cofactor for lipoprotein lipase. It results in familial hyperchylomicronemia that is usually milder and of later onset than that caused by a defect in the enzyme itself. See also table at *hyperlipoproteinemia.*
**familial high-density lipoprotein (HDL) d.,** any of several inherited disorders of lipoprotein and lipid metabolism that result in decreased plasma levels of HDL, particularly Tangier disease.
**familial lipoprotein d.,** any inherited disorder of lipoprotein metabolism resulting in deficiency of one or more plasma lipoproteins; see *abetalipoproteinemia, Tangier disease* under *disease,* and *hypobetalipoproteinemia.*
**IgA d., isolated, IgA d., selective,** the most common immunodeficiency disorder: deficiency of IgA with normal levels of the other immunoglobulin classes and normal cellular immunity. It is marked by recurrent sinopulmonary infections and an increased incidence of allergy, gastrointestinal disease (celiac disease, ulcerative colitis, Crohn's disease), and autoimmune diseases (rheumatoid arthritis, systemic lupus erythematosus). Many patients have anti-IgA antibodies that can cause severe transfusion reactions.
**immune d.,** immunodeficiency.
**iron d.,** deficiency of iron in the system, usually caused by blood loss, low dietary levels of iron, or a disease condition that inhibits iron uptake. Three stages of severity are distinguished: *iron depletion, latent iron deficiency,* and *iron deficiency anemia.*
**iron d., latent,** a moderate form of iron deficiency in which the serum iron level drops but the hematocrit is unchanged and there is no anemia.
**iron d., prelatent,** iron depletion.
**leukocyte adhesion d.,** a rare autosomal recessive disorder in which the expression of the $\beta$ subunit of $\beta_2$ integrins is defective or absent, characterized by delayed umbilical cord separation, recurrent bacterial infections, impaired pus formation, poor wound healing, gingivitis, leukocytosis, and impairment of adhesion-dependent leukocyte functions. Two phenotypes, moderate and severe, occur and are related to the degree of the deficiency.
**mental d.,** see under *retardation.*
**molybdenum cofactor d.,** an autosomal recessive disorder in which

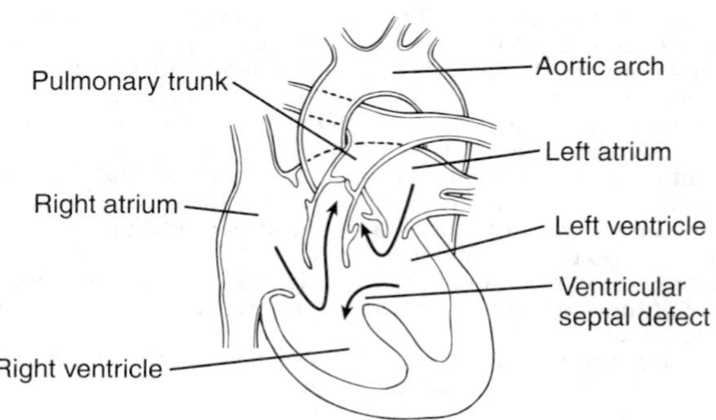


Abnormal communication between the ventricles in ventricular septal defect.

deficiency of the molybdenum cofactor causes deficiency of the molybdoenzymes sulfite oxidase, xanthine dehydrogenase, and aldehyde oxidase, resulting in severe neurologic abnormalities, dislocated ocular lenses, mental retardation, xanthinuria, and early death.
**multiple acyl CoA dehydrogenation d. (MADD),** glutaricaciduria, type II.
**oxygen d.,** see *anoxia, hypoxia,* and *hypoxemia.*
**plasma thromboplastin antecedent d., PTA d.,** hemophilia C.
**sucrase-α-dextrinase d., intestinal,** disaccharide intolerance I.
**sucrase-isomaltase d., congenital,** disaccharide intolerance I.
**vitamin d.,** see specific vitamins.
**vitamin E–selenium d.,** see under *syndrome.*

**def·i·cit** (def′ĭ-sit) a lack or deficiency.
**oxygen d.,** see *anoxia, hypoxemia,* and *hypoxia.*
**pulse d.,** the difference between the heart rate and the pulse rate in atrial fibrillation, resulting from failure of some of the ventricular contractions to produce peripheral pulse waves of sufficient magnitude to detect by palpation.
**reversible ischemic neurologic d. (RIND),** a type of cerebral infarction whose clinical course lasts longer than 24 hours but less than 72 hours; brain imaging usually reveals an infarct. Cf. *stroke in evolution.*
**saturation d.,** the difference between the amount of water vapor a given volume of air could contain at a specific temperature and the amount it actually contains.

**Def·i·nate** (def′ĭ-nāt) trademark for a preparation of docusate sodium.

**def·i·ni·tion** (def″ĭ-nish′ən) the clear determination of the limits of anything, as of a disease process or a microscopic image. See also *resolution,* def. 2.

**de·fin·i·tive** (de-fin′ĭ-tiv) established with certainty. In embryology, denoting acquisition of final differentiation or character. In parasitology, denoting the host in which a parasite reaches the sexual stage.

**de·flec·tion** (de-flek′shən) [L. *deflectere* to turn away] 1. deviation or movement from a straight line or given course. 2. in electrocardiography, any of the deviations from baseline, measured as the waves or complexes of the recording.
**H d., His bundle d.,** in the His bundle electrogram, the deflection due to advance of the depolarizing impulse through the bundle of His. See also illustration at *electrogram.*
**intrinsic d.,** the sharp reversal in polarity of surface electrical charge in a muscle, such as is registered in an electrode directly attached to muscle, as the dipole of an action potential passes the electrode during muscle activity.
**intrinsicoid d.,** the sharp deflection occurring between the onset of the Q wave and the peak of the R wave in electrocardiography using indirect surface leads, such as unipolar precordial leads.

**def·lo·ra·tion** (def″lo-ra′shən) [L. *deflora′tio*] the rupturing of the hymen in sexual intercourse, in vaginal examination, or by manipulation.

**de·flo·res·cence** (def″lo-res′əns) the disappearance of the eruption in any exanthematous disease.

**de·flu·vi·um** (de-floo′ve-əm) [L., from *defluere* to flow down] 1. a flowing down. 2. a disappearance.
**postpartum d.,** loss of hair by the mother after delivery.
**d. un′guium,** onychomadesis.

**de·flux·io** (de-fluk′se-o) [L., from *defluere* flow down] defluvium.

**de·flux·ion** (de-fluk′shən) [L. *defluxio*] 1. a sudden disappearance. 2. a copious discharge, as of catarrhal fluid. 3. a falling out, as of the hair.

**de·form·a·bil·i·ty** (de-form″ə-bil′ĭ-te) the ability of cells to change shape as they pass through narrow spaces, such as erythrocytes passing through the microvasculature.

**de·for·ma·tion** (de″for-ma′shən) [L. *deformatio* a disfiguring] 1. in dysmorphology, a type of structural defect characterized by the abnormal form or position of a body part, caused by a nondisruptive mechanical force. 2. the process of adapting in shape or form, as the change in shape of erythrocytes as they pass through capillaries.

**de·form·ing** (de-form′ing) causing or producing deformity.

**de·form·i·ty** (de-for′mĭ-te) [MeSH: Abnormalities] distortion of any part or general disfigurement of the body; malformation.
**Åkerlund d.,** a deformity of the duodenal cap in the radiograph in duodenal ulcer, consisting of an indentation (incisura) in addition to the niche.
**Arnold-Chiari d.,** see under *malformation.*
**boutonnière d.,** a deformity of the finger characterized by flexion of the proximal interphalangeal joint and hyperextension of the distal joint; called also *buttonhole d.*

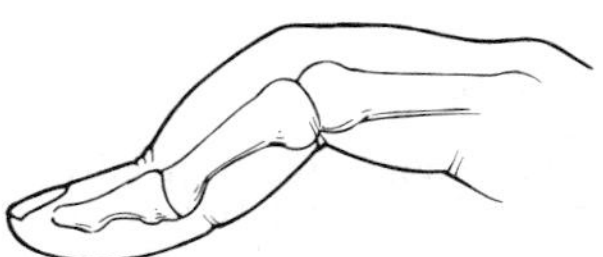

Boutonnière deformity.

**buttonhole d.,** boutonnière d.
**Chiari's d.,** see under *malformation.*
**crossbar d.,** the stiffening of a segment of the lesser curvature of the stomach, usually due to the healing of a deep penetrating ulcer.
**Dandy-Walker d.,** see under *malformation.*
**gun stock d.,** cubitus varus.
**Ilfeld-Holder d.,** prominent scapula with difficulty in raising the arm.
**lobster-claw d.,** cleft hand.
**Madelung's d.,** radial deviation of the hand secondary to overgrowth of the distal ulna or shortening of the radius; called also *carpus curvus.*
**Mondini's d.,** a misshapen cochlea with dysplasia or aplasia of the bony and membranous labyrinths, as seen in Mondini's deafness. Called also *Mondini's malformation.*
**pollybeak d.,** an iatrogenic bony deformity, occurring following rhinoplasty, in which the top of the nose is narrowed and the tip projects down over the lips, so that the nose resembles the beak of a parrot.
**recurvatum d.,** a deformity of the proximal interphalangeal joint in which the joint extends when pressure is exerted between the thumb and middle finger.
**reduction d.,** congenital absence of a portion or all of a body part, especially the limbs.
**rocker-bottom d.,** see under *foot.*
**rolled edge d.,** a highly characteristic deformity of the aortic valve cusps caused by syphilis.
**seal-fin d.,** ulnar deviation of the fingers in rheumatoid arthritis.
**silver fork d.,** the peculiar deformity seen in Colles' fracture; see illustration under *fracture.* Called also *Velpeau's d.*
**split-foot d.,** cleft foot.
**split-hand d.,** cleft hand.
**Sprengel's d.,** congenital elevation of the scapula, due to failure of descent of the scapula to its normal thoracic position during fetal life.
**swan-neck d.,** a finger deformity in which the proximal interphalangeal joint is hyperextended and the distal interphalangeal joint is flexed.
**thumb-in-palm d.,** adduction contracture of the thumb.
**ulnar drift d.,** ulnar deviation.
**uni-tip d.,** a deformity, resulting from nasal tip surgery, in which the domes of the lower lateral cartilages are pinched or overnarrowed and take on a uni-tip shape, while the tip of the nose has a normal bidomal appearance.
**Velpeau's d.,** silver fork d.
**Volkmann's d.,** see under *disease.*

**Deg** degeneration; degree.

**de·gas·sing** (de-gas′ing) 1. treatment of a person or an object subjected to the fumes of gas. 2. the volatilization of foreign matter from the surface of a metal, as in the heat treatment of gold foil in rendering it cohesive; called also *annealing* (see *anneal,* def. 3).

**de·gen·er·a·cy** (de-jen′ər-ə-se) 1. the state of being degenerate. 2. the process of degenerating. 3. d. of code.
**d. of code, code d.,** the presence in the genetic code of more than one codon that may specify for a single amino acid and lead to its insertion into a growing peptide chain.

**de·gen·er·ate** 1. (de-jen′er-āt) to change from a higher to a lower type or form. 2. (de-jen′er-it) characterized by degeneration.

**de·gen·er·a·tio** (de-jen″ər-a′she-o) [L.] degeneration.
**d. mi′cans,** glistening degeneration.

**de·gen·er·a·tion** (de-jen″ər-a′shən) [L. *degeneratio*] deterioration; change from a higher to a lower form; especially change of tissue to a lower or less functionally active form.

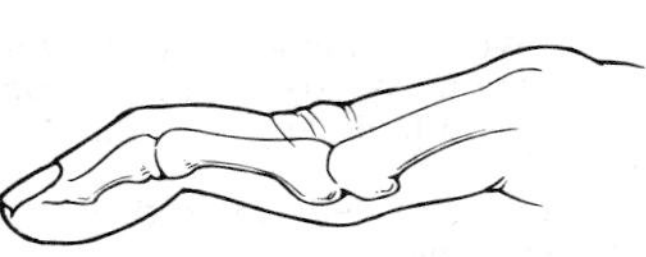

Swan-neck deformity.

**adipose d.,** fatty d.
**adiposogenital d.,** adiposogenital dystrophy.
**Alzheimer's neurofibrillary d.,** neurofibrillary tangles.
**angiolithic d.,** one characterized by mineral deposits and hyaline changes in the coats of the vessels.
**Armanni-Ebstein d.,** see under *lesion.*
**ascending d.,** wallerian degeneration affecting centripetal nerve fibers and progressing toward the brain or spinal cord.
**atheromatous d.,** atheroma.
**atrophic pulp d.,** pulp atrophy.
**axonal d.,** 1. axonal reaction. 2. wallerian d.
**ballooning d.,** hydropic d.
**blastophthoric d.,** blastophthoria.
**calcareous d.,** degeneration with infiltration of calcareous materials into the tissues; called also *earthy d.*
**caseous d.,** caseation, def. 2.
**cerebellar d., paraneoplastic, cerebellar d., paraneoplastic subacute,** the most common paraneoplastic syndrome affecting the brain, occurring most commonly with ovarian and breast carcinoma and Hodgkin's disease, characterized pathologically by severe loss of Purkinje cells and clinically by insidious and progressive truncal and appendicular ataxia, dysarthria, nystagmus, and occasionally dementia. In some women with gynecologic or breast carcinoma, it is associated with an autoantibody (anti-Yo).
**cerebellar d., primary progressive,** a familial disease marked by motor disorders and due to cerebellar degeneration, occurring in adults between the ages of thirty and forty and progressing slowly to a fatal termination; called also *Holmes' d.*
**cerebromacular d. (CMD), cerebroretinal d.,** 1. degeneration of brain cells and the macula luteae, as in Tay-Sachs disease. 2. any lipidosis with cerebral lesions and degeneration of the retinal macula. 3. any form of neuronal ceroid-lipofuscinosis.
**cheesy d.,** caseation, def. 2.
**colloid d.,** the assumption by the tissues of a gumlike or gelatinous character; called also *gelatiniform d.*
**colloid d. of choroid,** Tay's choroiditis.
**comma d.,** progressive degeneration of the nervous matter of the comma tract (interfascicular fasciculus).
**corticostriatal-spinal d.,** Creutzfeldt-Jakob disease.
**Crooke's hyaline d.,** Crooke's hyalinization.
**cystic d.,** degeneration with the formation of cysts.
**cystoid d.,** Blessig's cysts.
**descending d.,** wallerian degeneration extending peripherally along nerve fibers.
**Doyne's familial colloid d., Doyne's honeycomb d.,** see under *choroiditis.*
**dystrophic d.,** degeneration arising from defective or faulty nutrition.
**earthy d.,** calcareous d.
**elastoid d.,** amyloid degeneration of the elastic tissue of arteries.
**familial colloid d.,** Doyne's familial honeycombed choroiditis.
**fascicular d.,** degeneration of paralyzed muscles due to lesion in the motor ganglion cells of the central tube of gray matter of the cord.
**fatty d.,** deposit of fat globules in a tissue; an older term for a concept now included in *fatty change.*
**fibrinous d.,** necrosis with deposit of fibrin within the cells of the tissue.
**fibroid d.,** degeneration of a leiomyoma with subsequent fibrosis.
**fibrous d.,** fibrosis.
**gelatiniform d.,** colloid d.
**glassy d.,** a peculiar change occurring in the heart muscle and other muscles in fevers.
**glistening d.,** degeneration of glia tissue characterized by the formation of glistening masses; called also *degeneratio micans* and *Rosenthal's d.*
**glycogenic d.,** a form of degeneration in which abnormal amounts of glycogen accumulate in the cells, as in glycogenosis.
**Gombault's d.,** progressive hypertrophic neuropathy.
**granulovascular d.,** a condition in which the ganglion cells become filled with vacuoles containing condensed granules of protoplasm.
**gray d.,** degeneration of the white substance of the spinal cord, in which it loses myelin and assumes a gray color.
**hepatolenticular d.,** Wilson's disease.
**Holmes' d.,** primary progressive cerebellar d.
**Horn's d.,** degeneration with nuclear proliferation in striated muscles.
**hyaline d.,** a regressive cellular change in which the cytoplasm takes on a homogeneous glassy eosinophilic appearance. Also used loosely to describe the histologic appearance of tissues. Called also *vitreous d.* and *hyalinosis.*
**hydropic d.,** the swelling of cells caused by the accumulation of intracellular water in response to cell injury; called also *ballooning d.*
**lattice d. of retina,** a frequently bilateral, usually benign asymptomatic condition, characterized by patches of fine gray or white lines that intersect at irregular intervals in the peripheral retina, usually associated with numerous, round, punched-out areas of retinal thinning or retinal holes.
**lipoidal d.,** a condition somewhat resembling fatty change but in which the extraneous material is lipoid.
**macular d.,** degenerative changes in the macula retinae.
**macular d., congenital,** an autosomal dominant form of macular degeneration characterized by the presence of a cystlike lesion that in the early stages resembles egg yolk; called also *vitelliform* or *vitelline macular d., Best's disease, Best's macular dystrophy,* and *hereditary vitelliform dystrophy.*
**macular d., disciform,** a form of macular degeneration occurring in persons over 40 years of age, in which sclerosis involving the macula and retina is produced by hemorrhages between Bruch's membrane and the pigment epithelium; called also *macular disciform d., senile exudative macular d., senile macular exudative choroiditis, senile disciform d., Kuhnt-Junius disease, disciform retinitis,* and *central disk-shaped retinopathy.*
**macular d., senile exudative,** disciform macular d.
**macular d., Stargardt's,** Stargardt's disease.
**macular d., vitelliform, macular d., vitelline,** congenital macular d.
**macular disciform d.,** disciform macular d.
**Mönckeberg's d.,** see under *arteriosclerosis.*
**mucinoid d.,** a term used to include both mucoid and colloid degeneration; called also *mucinous d.* and *myelinic d.*
**mucinous d.,** mucous d.
**mucoid d.,** degeneration accompanied by deposition of myelin and lecithin in the cells.
**mucous d.,** a form in which mucus accumulates in epithelial tissues.
**myelinic d.,** mucoid d.
**myofibrillar d.,** contraction band necrosis.
**myxomatous d.,** degeneration in which mucus accumulates in connective tissues.
**Nissl d.,** axonal reaction.
**olivopontocerebellar d.,** see under *atrophy.*
**pallidal d.,** degeneration of the globus pallidus, as in juvenile paralysis agitans.
**pigmental d., pigmentary d.,** that in which cells of affected tissue become abnormally pigmented.
**red d.,** degeneration of a uterine leiomyoma during pregnancy, marked by the formation of soft red areas due to necrosis and edema.
**retrograde d.,** axonal reaction.
**rim d.,** degeneration of the spinal cord affecting the periphery only.
**Rosenthal's d.,** glistening d.
**sclerotic d.,** a variety of hyaline degeneration affecting connective tissue, especially the intima of arteries.
**secondary d.,** wallerian d.
**senile d.,** the widespread degenerative changes, principally fibrous and atheromatous, that occur in old age. Cf. *senile atrophy.*
**senile disciform d.,** disciform macular d.
**spongy d. of central nervous system, spongy d. of white matter,** a rare, autosomal recessive form of leukodystrophy, characterized by early onset, widespread demyelination and vacuolation of the cerebral white matter that gives rise to a spongy appearance, severe mental retardation, megalocephaly, atony of the neck muscles, spasticity of the arms and legs, and blindness, with death usually occurring at about 18 months of age. Called also *Canavan's disease* and *Canavan-van Bogaert-Bertrand disease.*
**striatonigral d.,** a form of multiple system atrophy in which nerve cell degeneration occurs mainly in the region of the substantia nigra and the neostriatum. Symptoms are similar to those of parkinsonism, with rigidity, slowing of movements, poor balance, and mumbling speech, but parkinsonian tremor is absent.
**subacute combined d. of spinal cord,** degeneration of both the posterior and lateral columns of the spinal cord caused by vitamin $B_{12}$ deficiency; a progressive disease, most often affecting persons over forty years of age, it is usually associated with pernicious anemia. The symptoms include paresthesias, ataxia, unsteadiness of gait, and sometimes emotional disorders. Called also *combined system disease, combined sclerosis, Lichtheim's disease* or *syndrome, Putnam-Dana syndrome,* and *posterolateral sclerosis.*
**tapetoretinal d.,** degeneration of the pigmented layer of the retina, as occurs in retinitis pigmentosa and other disorders.
**transneuronal d.,** atrophy of certain neurons after interruption of afferent axons or death of other neurons to which they send their efferent output.
**traumatic d.,** degeneration of a divided nerve up to the nearest node of Ranvier.
**Türck's d.,** secondary parenchymatous degeneration of nerve tracts of the cord.
**uratic d.,** degeneration marked by the deposit of urates or uric acid.
**vacuolar d.,** the formation of vacuoles in the cells of a tissue.
**vitelliform d. of Best,** congenital macular d.
**vitreous d.,** hyaline d.

**wallerian d.**, fatty degeneration of a nerve fiber that has been severed from its nutritive centers; cf. *dying-back*. Called also *secondary d.*
**Wilson's d.**, see under *disease*.
**Zenker's d.**, necrosis and hyaline degeneration of striated muscle; called also *Zenker's necrosis*.

**de·gen·er·a·tive** (de-jen′ər-ə-tiv) of or pertaining to degeneration.

**de·germ** (de-germ′) disinfect.

**de·glov·ing** (de-gluv′ing) intra-oral surgical exposure of the bony mandibular structures, as by rolling the lower lip and vestibular soft tissue over the chin to expose the symphysis. The operation can also be performed in the posterior region if necessary.

**Deglut.** abbreviation for L. *deglutia′tur,* let it be swallowed.

**de·glu·ti·ble** (de-gloo′tĭ-bəl) capable of being swallowed.

**de·glu·ti·tion** (deg″loo-tish′ən) [L. *deglutitio*] [MeSH: Deglutition] swallowing.

**de·glu·ti·tive** (de-gloo′tĭ-tiv) deglutitory.

**de·glu·ti·to·ry** (de-gloo′tĭ-to″re) pertaining to or promoting swallowing.

**de·glyc·er·ol·ize** (de-glis′ər-ol-īz) to remove the glycerol cryopreservative medium from frozen red blood cells and replace it with an isotonic solution for transfusion.

**De·gos' disease, syndrome** (də-gōz′) [Robert *Degos,* French dermatologist, born 1904] malignant atrophic papulosis.

**deg·ra·da·tion** (deg″rə-da′shən) the reduction of a chemical compound to one less complex, as by splitting off one or more groups. Cf. *lysis.*

**de·gran·u·la·tion** (de-gran″u-la′shən) the process of losing granules; said of certain granular cells.

**de·gree** (də-gre′) 1. a grade or rank within a series; especially, a rank awarded to scholars by a college or university. 2. a unit of measure of temperature. 3. a unit of measure of arcs and angles.
**d's of freedom,** the number of ways the members of a sample can vary independently; a numerical index of a family of probability distributions that corresponds to the number of independent variables in the definition of each member, e.g., the chi-squared distribution with $n$ degrees of freedom is the distribution of the sum of squares of $n$ standard normal deviations. Symbol $\nu$.
**prism d.,** centrad, def. 2.

**de·gus·ta·tion** (de″gəs-ta′shən) [L. *degustatio*] taste.

**de·hep·a·tized** (de-hep′ə-tīzd) having the liver removed.

**de·his·cence** (de-his′əns) [L. *dehiscere* to gape] a splitting open.
**Killian's d.,** a triangular area in the wall of the pharynx between the inferior constrictor muscle and the cricopharyngeus muscle; it represents a potentially weak spot where a pharyngoesophageal diverticulum is more likely. Called also *Killian's triangle.*
**root d.,** an isolated area in which the root of a tooth is denuded of bone from the margin to near the apex; it occurs most often on anterior teeth, usually on the vestibular surface rather than the oral surface.
**wound d.,** separation of the layers of a surgical wound; it may be partial and superficial only, or complete, with disruption of all layers.
**Zuckerkandl's d's,** small gaps occasionally seen in the layers of the ethmoid bone.

**de·hu·mid·i·fi·er** (de″hu-mid′ĭ-fi″ər) an apparatus by which the content of moisture in the air is reduced.

**de·hy·drant** (de-hi′drənt) 1. reducing hydration. 2. an agent that removes or reduces body water.

**de·hy·drase** (de-hi′drās) a term formerly applied to both the dehydrogenases and the dehydratases.

**de·hy·dra·tase** (de-hi′drə-tās) a term used in the usual recommended or trivial name for enzymes of the sub-subclass hydro-lyase (q.v.).

**de·hy·drate** (de-hi′drāt) to remove water from (a compound, the body, etc.).

**de·hy·dra·tion** (de″hi-dra′shən) [*de-* + *hydration*] [MeSH: Dehydration] 1. removal of water from a substance. 2. the condition that results from excessive loss of body water.
**absolute d.,** water content below the normal or below a standard amount.
**hypernatremic d.,** a condition in which electrolyte losses are disproportionately smaller than water losses.
**relative d.,** dehydration resulting from increased osmotic pressure of the body fluids.
**voluntary d.,** that resulting when thirst does not stimulate sufficient replacement of water loss.

**de·hy·dro·an·dros·ter·one** (de-hi″dro-an-dros′tər-ōn) former name for *dehydroepiandrosterone.*

**de·hy·dro·as·cor·bic ac·id** (de-hi″dro-ə-skor′bik) [MeSH: Dehydroascorbic Acid] the reversibly oxidized form of ascorbic acid, which has the same vitamin C activity as ascorbic acid when ingested.

**de·hy·dro·bil·i·ru·bin** (de-hi″dro-bil-ĭ-roo′bin) biliverdin.

**de·hy·dro·cho·lan·er·e·sis** (de-hi″dro-ko″lən-er′ə-sis) increase in the output of dehydrocholic acid in the bile.

**de·hy·dro·cho·late** (de-hi″dro-ko′lāt) a salt of dehydrocholic acid.

**7-de·hy·dro·cho·les·ter·ol** (de-hi″dro-kə-les′tər-ol) a sterol found in the skin; it is the provitamin of cholecalciferol, being converted to that compound upon irradiation by ultraviolet light.
**7-d., activated,** cholecalciferol.

**de·hy·dro·cho·lic ac·id** (de-hi″dro-ko′lik) [USP] [MeSH: Dehydrocholic Acid] a synthetic bile acid that acts as a hydrocholeretic, increasing bile output to clear the increased bile acid load; bile pigment secretion is not increased; used as a laxative and to produce choleresis after gallbladder surgery or in cholecystography.

**11-de·hy·dro·cor·ti·cos·ter·one** (de-hi″dro-kor″tĭ-kos′tər-ōn) an adrenocortical steroid made from, and convertible to, corticosterone; it is not directly active. Also produced synthetically, it is used like cortisone as a glucocorticoid and as an antiallergic agent.

**de·hy·dro·co·ryd·a·line** (de-hi″dro-ko-rid′ə-lēn) a yellowish crystalline alkaloid from the roots of species of *Corydalis.*

**de·hy·dro·em·e·tine** (de-hi″dro-em′ə-tēn) an antiprotozoal used like emetine hydrochloride, but causing fewer and milder adverse effects; available as *dehydroemetine hydrochloride.*

**de·hy·dro·epi·an·dros·ter·one (DHEA)** (de-hi″dro-ep″e-an-dros′tər-ōn) a steroid secreted by the adrenal cortex, the major androgen precursor in females; it is often present in excessive amounts in body fluids of patients with adrenal virilism. During pregnancy it diffuses into the syncytiotrophoblasts and is metabolized to form estrogen; by the third trimester it metabolizes at nine times the rate seen in a nonpregnant woman. Called also *dehydroisoandrosterone* and, formerly, *dehydroandrosterone.*

**de·hy·dro·gen·ase** (de-hi′dro-jən″ās) an enzyme of the oxidoreductase class [EC 1] that catalyzes the transfer of hydrogen or electrons from a donor, which becomes oxidized, to an acceptor compound, which becomes reduced. Dehydrogenases are usually designated according to the hydrogen donor.

**de·hy·dro·gen·ate** (de-hi′dro-jən-āt) to remove hydrogen from a molecule.

**de·hy·dro·gen·a·tion** (de-hi″dro-jə-na′shən) oxidation due to removal of hydrogen by the reaction of a hydrogen acceptor.

**de·hy·dro·iso·an·dros·ter·one** (de-hi″dro-i″so-an-dros′tər-ōn) dehydroepiandrosterone.

**de·hy·dro·mor·phine** (de-hi″dro-mor′fēn) pseudomorphine.

**de·hy·dro·ret·i·nol** (de-hi″dro-ret′ĭ-nol) a form of vitamin A, vitamin $A_2$, occurring with retinol in freshwater fish; it is similar in structure to retinol, but has an additional conjugated double bond and only approximately one third the biological activity.

**de·hyp·no·tize** (de-hip′no-tīz) to arouse from the hypnotic state.

**de·io·din·a·tion** (de-i″o-din-a′shən) the loss or removal of iodine from a compound.

**de·ion·iza·tion** (de-i″on-ĭ-za′shən) the production of a mineral-free state by the removal of ions, especially by use of ion-exchange resins.

**dei·ter·al** (di'tər-əl) pertaining to Deiters' nucleus.

**Dei·ters' cells,** etc. (di'terz) [Otto Friedrich Karl *Deiters,* German anatomist, 1834–1863] see under *cell, frame, nucleus, phalanx, process,* and see *tractus vestibulospinalis.*

**dé·jà en·ten·du** (da-zhah' on"ton-doo') [Fr. "already heard"] the feeling that one has heard or perceived something previously although it is in fact new to one's experience.

**dé·jà éprou·vé** (da-zhah' a"proo-va') [Fr. "already tested"] a feeling that one has previously engaged in or experienced something when one has not.

**dé·jà fait** (da-zhah' fa) [Fr. "already done"] a feeling that what is happening has happened before.

**dé·jà pen·sé** (da-zhah' pon-sa') [Fr. "already thought"] a feeling that one has thought the same thoughts before.

**dé·jà ra·con·té** (da-zhah' rah-kōn-ta') [Fr. "already told"] 1. a feeling when telling someone about an experience that one had previously related the same experience either to them or to someone else, when in fact one had not. 2. a feeling that a long-forgotten event that is being recalled was told to one before, when it was not.

**dé·jà vé·cu** (da-zhah' va-koo') [Fr. "already lived"] a feeling that a new experience has been encountered before, in a previous existence.

**dé·jà vou·lu** (da-zhah' voo-loo') [Fr. "already desired"] a feeling that one has entertained the same desires before.

**dé·jà vu** (da-zhah' voo') [Fr. "already seen"] an illusion in which a new situation is incorrectly viewed as a repetition of a previous situation.

**De·jean's syndrome** (də-zhahz') [M. C. *Dejean,* French physician, 20th century] orbital floor syndrome.

**de·jec·tion** (de-jek'shən) [L. *dejectio*] a mental state marked by sadness; the lowered mood characteristic of depression.

**De·je·rine's disease, sign, syndrome** (dĕ-zhĕ-rēnz') [Joseph Jules *Dejerine,* French neurologist, 1849–1917] see *progressive hypertrophic neuropathy,* under *neuropathy,* and see under *sign* and *syndrome.*

**De·je·rine-Klump·ke paralysis, syndrome** (dĕ-zhĕ-rēn' kloomp'kə) [Augusta *Dejerine-Klumpke,* French neurologist, 1859–1927] Klumpke's paralysis.

**De·je·rine-Lan·dou·zy dystrophy** (dĕ-zhĕ-rēn' lahn-doo-ze') [J. J. *Dejerine;* Louis Théophile Joseph *Landouzy,* French physician, 1845–1917] facioscapulohumeral muscular dystrophy.

**De·je·rine-Licht·heim phenomenon** (dĕ-zhĕ-rēn' likt'hīm) [J. J. *Dejerine;* Ludwig *Lichtheim,* German physician, 1845–1928] Lichtheim's sign.

**De·je·rine-Rous·sy syndrome** (dĕ-zhĕ-rēn' roo-se') [J. J. *Dejerine;* Gustav *Roussy,* French pathologist, 1874–1948] thalamic syndrome.

**De·je·rine-Sot·tas atrophy, disease** (dĕ-zhĕ-rēn' so-tahz') [J. J. *Dejerine;* Jules *Sottas,* French neurologist, 1866–1943] progressive hypertrophic neuropathy.

**De·je·rine-Thom·as syndrome** (dĕ-zhĕ-rēn' to-mahs') [J.J. *Dejerine;* André Antoine Henri *Thomas,* French neurologist, 1867–1943] olivopontocerebellar atrophy.

**deka-** [Gr. *deka* ten] a combining form meaning ten; for words beginning thus, see also those beginning *deca-.*

**de·la·cri·ma·tion** (de-lak"rĭ-ma'shən) [L. *delacrimatio* weeping] excessive and abnormal flow of tears.

**de·lac·ta·tion** (de"lak-ta'shən) 1. weaning. 2. the cessation of lactation.

**Del·a·field's fluid, hematoxylin** (del'ə-fēldz) [Francis *Delafield,* American pathologist, 1841–1915] see under *fluid,* and *stain.*

**Del·a·lu·tin** (del"ə-loo'tin) trademark for a preparation of hydroxyprogesterone caproate.

**de·lam·i·na·tion** (de-lam"ĭ-na'shən) [*de-* + *lamina*] separation into layers, as the separation of the inner cell mass or embryoblast into epiblast and hypoblast during early embryo development.

**de Lange's syndrome** (da lahng'əz) [Cornelia *de Lange,* Dutch pediatrician, 1871–1950] [MeSH: De Lange's Syndrome] see under *syndrome.*

**Del·a·tes·tryl** (del"ə-tes'trəl) trademark for a preparation of testosterone enanthate.

**de·layed-re·lease** (de-lād're-lēs') releasing a drug at a time later than immediately following the administration of the drug.

**Del·bet's sign** (del-bāz') [Pierre *Delbet,* French surgeon, 1861–1957] see under *sign.*

**Del·brück** (del'brik) Max. German-born American biologist, 1906–1981; co-winner, with Alfred Day Hershey and Salvador Edward Luria, of the Nobel prize for medicine or physiology in 1969 for research on the genetic structure of viruses.

**del Cas·ti·llo's syndrome** (dāl kahs-te'yōz) [E.B. *del Castillo,* Argentine physician, 20th century] Sertoli-cell–only syndrome; see under *syndrome.*

**de-lead** (de-led') to remove lead from a tissue, as from the bones in lead poisoning by the administration of edetate disodium calcium. See also *deleading therapy,* under *therapy.*

**DeLee catheter, forceps** (de-le') [Joseph Bolivar *DeLee,* American obstetrician and gynecologist, 1869–1942] see under *catheter* and *forceps.*

**DeLee-Hil·lis stethoscope** (de-le'-hil'is) [J.B. *DeLee;* David S. *Hillis,* American obstetrician and gynecologist, 1873–1942] see under *stethoscope.*

**Del·es·tro·gen** (del-es'tro-jən) trademark for a preparation of estradiol valerate.

**del·e·te·ri·ous** (del"ə-tēr'e-əs) [Gr. *dēlētērios*] hurtful; injurious.

**de·le·tion** (də-le'shən) [L. *deletio* destruction] in genetics, the loss of any portion of the genetic material on a chromosome, ranging from loss of a single nucleotide within, which can throw the reading frame out of register and cause a frameshift mutation if it is within a coding sequence, to loss of part or all of a gene, to loss of a microscopically visible portion of the chromosome, possibly involving multiple genes.
**antigenic d.,** loss or masking of antigenic determinants in daughter cells of cells whose parent tissue normally carries them; it may result from neoplastic or other mutational change in the parent tissue or may be due to loss or repression of genetic material from the cell.
**interstitial d.,** loss of a segment within a chromosome arm. See Plate 1.
**terminal d.,** loss of a segment from the end of a chromosome arm. See Plate 1.

**de·lim·i·ta·tion** (de-lim"ĭ-ta'shən) [*de-* + *limitation*] 1. the process of limiting or of becoming limited. 2. ascertainment of the limits and extent of some diseased tissue or process, or the spread of a disease in a host or a community.

**de·lin·quent** (də-ling'kwənt) [L. *delinquens,* present participle of *delinquere,* to offend] 1. failing to do that which is required by law or obligation. 2. a person who neglects a legal obligation.
**juvenile d.,** a juvenile offender; an individual who commits a violation of the law within the jurisdiction of the juvenile court system.

**del·i·ques·cence** (del"ĭ-kwes'əns) [L. *deliquescere* to grow moist] the condition of becoming moist or liquefied as a result of the absorption of water from the air.

**del·i·ques·cent** (del"ĭ-kwes'ənt) having a tendency to form an aqueous solution or become liquid by the absorption of moisture from the air.

**de·lir·ia** (də-lēr'e-ə) [L.] plural of *delirium.*

**de·lir·i·ant** (də-lēr'e-ənt) 1. capable of producing delirium. 2. a drug which may produce delirium. 3. a delirious person.

**de·lir·i·fa·cient** (də-lēr"ĭ-fa'shənt) [*delirium* + *-facient*] 1. capable of causing delirium. 2. a drug which may produce delirium.

**de·lir·i·ous** (de-lēr'e-əs) suffering from delirium.

**de·lir·i·um** (də-lēr'e-əm) pl. *delir'ia* [*de-* + L. *lira* furrow or track; i.e., "off the track"] [MeSH: Delirium] [DSM-IV] an acute, transient disturbance of consciousness accompanied by a change in cognition and having a fluctuating course. Characteristics include reduced ability to maintain attention to external stimuli and disorganized thinking as manifested by rambling, irrelevant, or incoherent speech; there may also be a reduced level of consciousness, sensory misperceptions, disturbance of the sleep-wake cycle and level of psychomotor activity, disorientation to time, place, or person, and

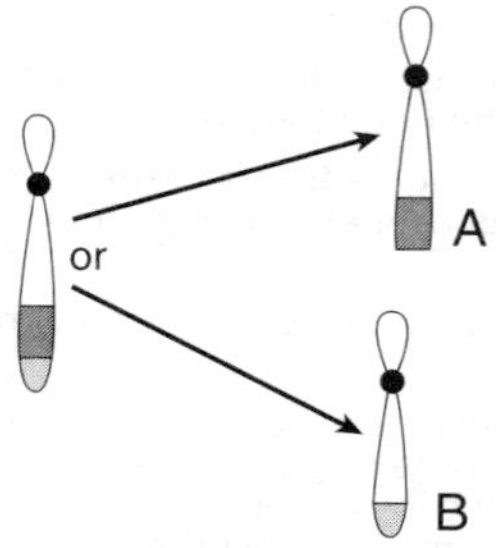


Examples of large-scale chromosomal deletions: *(A),* terminal; *(B),* interstitial.

memory impairment. Delirium may be caused by a number of conditions that result in derangement of cerebral metabolism, including systemic infection, cerebral tumor, poisoning, drug intoxication or withdrawal, seizures or head trauma, and metabolic disturbances such as fluid, electrolyte, or acid-base imbalance, hypoxia, hypoglycemia, or hepatic or renal failure; specific types are named according to etiology, e.g., delirium due to hypoglycemia.
**acute d.,** a suddenly appearing and severe delirium lasting only a short time.
**alcohol withdrawal d.** [DSM-IV], delirium caused by cessation or reduction in alcohol consumption, typically in alcoholics with 10 years or more of heavy drinking. Clinical manifestations include autonomic hyperactivity, such as tachycardia, sweating, and hypertension; a coarse, irregular tremor, and delusions; vivid hallucinations; and wild, agitated behavior. The onset is usually 2 or 3 days after cessation of drinking; the delirium and other withdrawal symptoms usually resolve in 3 or 4 days. Called also *d. tremens.*
**febrile d.,** the delirium of fever.
**low d.,** delirium marked by confusion of ideas and slowness of mental action rather than by excitement.
**postcardiotomy d.,** postcardiotomy psychosis syndrome.
**senile d.,** a form of senile dementia, usually of acute onset and characterized by disorientation, restlessness, insomnia, hallucinations, and aimless wandering.
**substance-induced d.** [DSM-IV], that associated with substance intoxication *(substance intoxication d.),* substance withdrawal *(substance withdrawal d.),* medication side effects, or exposure to toxins; individual cases are named for the specific substance involved, e.g., digitalis-induced delirium.
**substance intoxication d.,** that which can occur during intoxication with any of a variety of substances, including alcohol, amphetamines and related substances, cannabis, cocaine, hallucinogens, inhalants, opioids, phencyclidine and related substances, and sedatives, hypnotics, and anxiolytics; specific disorders are named for the substance involved.
**substance withdrawal d.,** that which can occur during withdrawal from any of a variety of substances, including alcohol and sedatives, hypnotics, and anxiolytics; specific disorders are named for the substance involved.
**toxic d.,** delirium caused by poisons.
**traumatic d.,** that which follows severe head injury; superficially the patient is alert, but there is marked disorientation, memory defect, and confabulation.
**d. tre'mens,** alcohol withdrawal d.

**del·i·tes·cence** (del″ĭ-tes′əns) [L. *delitescere* to lie hidden] 1. sudden disappearance of symptoms or of objective signs of a disease or of a lesion. 2. the period of latency or incubation of a poison or morbific agent.

**de·liv·er** (de-liv′ər) [Fr., from L. *deliberare* to set free] 1. to aid in the process of childbirth. 2. to remove, as the fetus or placenta, or the lens of the eye.

**de·liv·ery** (de-liv′ər-e) [MeSH: Delivery] 1. expulsion or extraction of the child and the afterbirth; see also *labor.* 2. removal of a part, as the lens of the eye.
**abdominal d.,** cesarean section.
**breech d.,** delivery of a fetus in breech presentation; see *breech extraction,* under *extraction.*
**forceps d.,** extraction of a fetus from the maternal passages by application of forceps to the child's head.
**forceps d., high,** forceps delivery in which the forceps is applied to the head before engagement has taken place.
**forceps d., low,** forceps delivery in which the forceps is applied when the leading point of the fetal skull is at station equal to or greater than +2 centimeters but not on the pelvic floor, and rotation is necessary.
**forceps d., outlet,** forceps delivery in which the forceps is applied when the scalp is or has been visible at the introitus without separating the labia and the skull has reached the pelvic floor, with the sagittal suture in the anteroposterior diameter of the pelvis; the fetus is in right or left occipitoanterior or occipitoposterior position.
**midforceps d.,** the application of forceps when the fetal head is engaged but station is above +2 centimeters.
**postmature d.,** delivery of a postmature infant; see under *infant.*
**postmortem d.,** birth of a fetus after the death of the mother.
**premature d.,** birth of a premature infant; see under *infant.*
**spontaneous d.,** birth of an infant without any mechanical, pharmacologic, or medical assistance.
**vaginal d.,** delivery of an infant through the normal openings of the uterus and vagina.

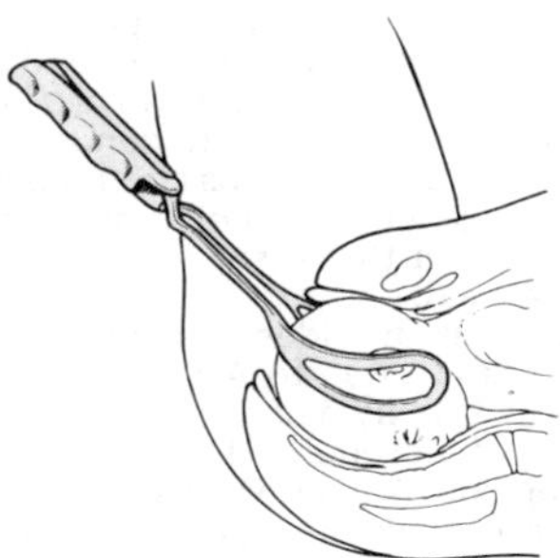
Forceps delivery.

**dell** (del′) a slight depression or dimple.

**del·le** (del′ə) the clear area in the center of a stained erythrocyte.

**del·len** (del′ən) [Ger. "dents"] saucer-shaped excavations at the periphery of the cornea, usually on the temporal side, probably caused by insufficiency of the limbal circulation; called also *Fuchs' dimples.*

**dell·ing** (del′ing) the formation of a slight depression; dimpling.

**del·mad·i·none ac·e·tate** (del-mad′ĭ-nōn) a veterinary progestin, antiandrogen, and antiestrogen; administered to male cats and dogs to control hypersexuality and other aggressive behavior and to treat prostatic hypertrophy and tumors, and to female cats as an estrus suppressant.

**de·lo·mor·phic** (del″o-mor′fik) delomorphous.

**de·lo·mor·phous** (del″o-mor′fəs) [Gr. *dēlos* evident + *morph-* + *-ous*] having definitely formed and well-defined limits, as a cell or tissue.

**de·lous·ing** (de-lous′ing) 1. the freeing of a human or animal from lice. 2. destruction of lice.

**Del·phi·an node** (del′fe-ən) [*Delphi,* a town in ancient Greece, site of a sanctuary and oracle of Apollo, because of the predictive nature of the node] see under *node.*

**del·phine** (del′fēn) delphinine.

**del·phi·nine** (del′fĭ-nēn) a poisonous alkaloid found in various species of *Delphinium,* causing larkspur poisoning in ruminants and other animals. Called also *delphine.*

**Del·phin·i·um** (del-fin′e-əm) [L.] a genus of plants of the family Ranunculaceae, including the larkspurs and delphinium, many of which contain delphinine and other toxic alkaloids and are common causes of poisoning in humans and other animals. See *larkspur poisoning,* under *poisoning. D. aja'cis* and *D. conso'lida* have seeds that are diuretic, emmenagogue, and poisonous. *D. staphisa'gria* is the lousewort or stavesacre, a poisonous species whose seeds, called staphisagria, were formerly used medicinally.

**del·phin·i·um** (del-fin′e-əm) any plant of the genus *Delphinium;* see also *larkspur.*

**del·phi·noid·ine** (del″fĭ-noid′in) a toxic alkaloid from the seeds of *Delphinium staphisagria.*

**del·phi·sine** (del′fĭ-sēn) a toxic alkaloid, isomeric with delphinine, from seeds of *Delphinium staphisagria.*

**del·ta** (del′tə) [Δ, δ] 1. the fourth letter of the Greek alphabet. See also Δ- and δ-. 2. a triangular space.
**d. mesosca'pulae,** the triangular area at the root of the spine of the scapula.

**Del·ta-Cor·tef** (del′tə-kor″təf) trademark for a preparation of prednisolone.

**del·ta·meth·rin** (del″tə-meth′rin) a pyrethroid insecticide applied topically to cattle and pigs.

**Del·ta·sone** (del′tə-sōn″) trademark for a preparation of prednisone.

**Del·ta·vi·rus** (del′tə-vi″rəs) [hepatitis *delta* + *virus*] a genus of satellite viruses that require a helper hepatitis B virus for their replication; an individual consists of spherical virion about 34 nm in diameter with an envelope derived from the helper virus surrounding a spherical core 18 nm in diameter; the genome consists of a single molecule of single-stranded, negative sense, circular RNA (size 1.7 kb). It contains a single species, hepatitis D virus.

**del·toid** (del′toid) [L. *deltoides* triangular] triangular in outline, as the deltoid muscle.

**Del·tra** (del′trə) trademark for prednisone.

**de·lu·sion** (də-loo′zhən) [L. *delusio,* from *de* from + *ludus* a game] [MeSH: Delusions] a false belief that is firmly maintained in spite of incontrovertible and obvious proof or evidence to the contrary and in spite of the fact that other members of the culture do not share the belief.
**d. of being controlled,** d. of control.

**bizarre d.**, a delusion that is patently absurd and has no possible basis in fact, such as delusions of being controlled or thought broadcasting.
**d. of control,** the delusion that one's thoughts, feelings, and actions are not one's own but are being imposed by someone else or by some external force.
**depressive d.**, a delusion that is congruent with a predominant depressed mood, such as a delusion that one is being persecuted because of one's sinfulness or inadequacy, somatic delusions of serious illness, nihilistic delusions, or delusions of poverty.
**encapsulated d.**, a delusion that has no significant effect on behavior.
**erotomanic d.**, a delusional conviction that some other person, usually of higher status and often famous, is in love with the individual; it is one of the subtypes of delusional disorder.
**expansive d.**, d. of grandeur.
**fragmentary d's,** unconnected delusions not organized around a coherent theme.
**d. of grandeur, grandiose d.**, a delusion involving an exaggerated concept of one's importance, power, or knowledge or that one is, or has a special relationship with, a deity or a famous person; it is one of the subtypes of delusional disorder.
**d. of jealousy,** a delusional belief that one's spouse or lover is unfaithful, based on erroneous inferences drawn from innocent events imagined to be evidence and often resulting in confrontation with the accused. It is one of the subtypes of delusional disorder.
**d. of misidentification,** delusional misidentification.
**mixed d.**, one in which no central theme predominates; one of the subtypes of delusional disorder.
**mood-congruent d.**, a delusion occurring as a manifestation of a mood disorder; see also *mood-congruent.*
**mood-incongruent d.**, a delusion occurring as a manifestation of a psychotic disorder; see also *mood-incongruent.*
**d. of negation, nihilistic d.**, a depressive delusion that the self or part of the self, part of the body, other persons, or the whole world has ceased to exist.
**paranoid d's,** an older term denoting delusion of grandeur and delusion of persecution; its use is discouraged.
**d. of persecution, persecutory d.**, a delusion that one is being attacked, harassed, cheated, persecuted, or conspired against; it is one of the subtypes of delusional disorder.
**d. of poverty,** a delusion that one is, or soon will be, bereft of material possessions.
**d. of reference,** a delusional conviction that ordinary events, objects, or behaviors of others have an unusual or peculiar meaning specifically for oneself. When less frequent or intense, or if not organized or systematized, such beliefs are called *ideas of reference.*
**somatic d.**, a delusion that there is some alteration in a bodily organ or its function; it is one of the subtypes of delusional disorder.
**systematized d's,** a group of delusions organized around a common theme.

**de·lu·sion·al** (də-loo'zhən-əl) pertaining to or characterized by delusions.

**Del·vi·nal** (del'vĭ-nəl) trademark for preparations of vinbarbital.

**De·ma·dex** (de'mə-deks) trademark for preparations of torsemide.

**De·man·sia** (de-man'se-ə) a genus of venomous snakes of the family Elapidae, including the brown snake of Australia and New Guinea. See table at *snake.*

**de·mar·ca·tion** (de″mahr-ka'shən) [L. *demarcare* to limit] the marking off or ascertainment of boundaries.
**surface d.**, any dividing line apparent on the surface of a solid body, such as the boundary between living and necrotic tissue.

**De·mar·quay's sign** (də-mahr-kāz') [Jean Nicholas *Demarquay,* French surgeon, 1814–1875] see under *sign.*

**de·mas·cu·lin·iza·tion** (de-mas″ku-lin″ĭ-za'shən) the loss of normal male secondary sex characters; when hormonal in nature it may be accompanied by testicular atrophy and involution of the prostate. See also *feminization.*

**De·mat·i·a·ceae** (de-mat″ĭ-a'se-e) in some systems of classification, a form-family of Fungi Imperfecti of the form-order Moniliales, producing simple conidiophores, and having dark brown or black conidia, spores, or hyphae. Genera of medical importance include *Acremoniella, Alternaria, Arthrographis, Aureobasidium, Bipolaris, Cladosporium, Curvularia, Dematium, Drechslera, Exophiala, Exserohilum, Fonsecaea, Madurella,* and *Phialophora.*

**de·mat·i·a·ceous** (de-mat″e-a'shəs) 1. dark brown to black in color; said of fungi. The color usually comes from pigment in the cell wall or other parts. 2. of or pertaining to a fungus of the family Dematiaceae.

**De·ma·ti·um** (de-ma'she-əm) a genus of soil and wood-rotting Fungi Imperfecti of the form-class Hyphomycetes, form-family Dematiaceae; some species have been reportedly isolated from human lesions.

**deme** (dēm) [Gk. *dēmos* common people] a population of very similar organisms interbreeding in nature and occupying a circumscribed area; called also *genetic population.*

**dem·e·ca·ri·um** (dem″ə-kar'e-əm) an anticholinesterase agent used topically to produce miosis, reduce intraocular pressure, and potentiate accommodation in the treatment of open-angle glaucoma and in the management of accommodative convergent strabismus.
**d. bromide** [USP], a potent, long-acting cholinesterase inhibitor, applied topically to the conjunctiva in the treatment of glaucoma and convergent strabismus.

**dem·e·clo·cy·cline** (dem″ə-klo-si'klēn) [USP] [MeSH: Demeclocycline] a broad-spectrum oral antibiotic of the tetracycline group, produced by a mutant strain of *Streptomyces aureofaciens* or semisynthetically. It also inhibits the effect of antidiuretic hormone on the renal tubules. Called also *demethylchlortetracycline.*
**d. hydrochloride** [USP], the monohydrochloride salt of demeclocycline, administered orally. It is also used as a diuretic.

**de·ment·ed** (də-men'təd) deprived of reason, mentally deteriorated; affected with dementia.

**de·men·tia** (də-men'shə) [*de-* + L. *mens* mind] [MeSH: Dementia] [DSM-IV] a general loss of cognitive abilities, including impairment of memory as well as one or more of the following: aphasia, apraxia, agnosia, or disturbed planning, organizing, and abstract thinking abilities. It does not include loss of intellectual functioning caused by clouding of consciousness (as in delirium), depression, or other functional mental disorder (pseudodementia). Causes include a large number of conditions, some reversible and some progressive, that result in widespread cerebral damage or dysfunction. The most common cause is Alzheimer's disease; others include cerebrovascular disease, central nervous system infection, brain trauma or tumors, vitamin deficiencies, anoxia, metabolic conditions, endocrine conditions, immune disorders, prion diseases, Wernicke-Korsakoff syndrome, normal-pressure hydrocephalus, Huntington's chorea, multiple sclerosis, and Parkinson's disease.
**alcoholic d.**, Korsakoff's syndrome.
**Alzheimer's d.**, see under *disease.*
**d. of the Alzheimer type** [DSM-IV], that occurring in Alzheimer's disease, being of insidious onset and gradually progressive course, with histopathological changes characteristic of Alzheimer's disease and not due to other central nervous system, systemic, or substance-induced conditions known to cause dementia. It is characterized as *early onset* or *late onset* depending on whether it begins by the age of 65, and is subcategorized on the basis of accompanying features, including delirium, delusions, depressed mood, behavioral disturbances, or none (uncomplicated).
**arteriosclerotic d.**, multi-infarct dementia as a result of cerebral arteriosclerosis.
**Binswanger's d.**, see under *disease.*
**boxer's d.**, a syndrome more serious than boxer's traumatic encephalopathy, the result of cumulative cerebral injuries in boxers; characterized by forgetfulness, slowness in thinking, dysarthric speech, and slow, uncertain movements, especially of the legs. Called also *d. pugilistica, punch-drunk encephalopathy,* and *punch-drunk.*
**dialysis d.**, see under *encephalopathy.*
**epileptic d.**, a progressive mental and intellectual deterioration that occurs in a small fraction of cases of epilepsy; it is thought by some to be caused by neuronal degeneration secondary to circulatory disturbances during seizures.
**multi-infarct d.**, vascular d.
**myoclonic d., d. myoclo'nica,** mental deterioration with myoclonus, as seen in disorders such as Alpers' disease, Creutzfeldt-Jakob disease, subacute sclerosing panencephalitis, and Alzheimer's disease.
**paralytic d., d. paraly'tica,** general paresis.
**posttraumatic d.**, dementia following head injury or other brain trauma; it may last from a few months to years. Cf. *boxer's d.* and *postconcussional syndrome.*
**d. prae'cox,** *(obs.)* schizophrenia.
**presenile d.**, that occurring in younger persons, usually in persons age 65 or younger; since most cases are due to Alzheimer's disease, the term is sometimes used as a synonym of *d. of the Alzheimer type, early onset,* and has also been used to denote *Alzheimer's disease.*
**primary degenerative d.**, severe loss of intellectual function of no discernible cause; it generally denotes dementia of the Alzheimer type but may be used for that associated with Pick's disease.
**d. pugilis'tica,** boxer's d.
**senile d.**, that occurring in older persons, usually over the age of 65; since most cases are due to Alzheimer's disease, the term is sometimes used as a synonym of *d. of the Alzheimer type, late onset.*
**subcortical d.**, any of a group of dementias thought to be caused by lesions affecting subcortical brain structures (e.g. the centrum ovale, basal ganglia, or thalamus) more than cortical ones, and characterized by memory loss with slowness in processing information or making intellectual responses. Included are vascular dementia

and dementias that accompany Huntington's chorea, Wilson's disease, paralysis agitans, and thalamic atrophies.
**substance-induced persisting d.** [DSM-IV], that resulting from exposure to or use or abuse of a substance, such as alcohol, sedatives, anxiolytics, anticonvulsants, lead, mercury, carbon monoxide, and organophosphate insecticides, but persisting long after exposure to the substance ends, usually with permanent and worsening deficits. Individual cases are named for the specific substance involved.
**toxic d.,** that due to excessive exposure to a toxic substance.
**vascular d.** [DSM-IV], dementia with a stepwise deteriorating course (a series of small strokes) and a patchy distribution of neurologic deficits (affecting some functions and not others) caused by cerebrovascular disease. It may be classified as uncomplicated or as occurring with delusions, delirium, or depressed mood. Called also *multi-infarct d.*

**Dem·er·ol** (dem′ər-ol) trademark for preparations of meperidine hydrochloride.

**de·meth·yl·a·tion** (de-meth″əl-a′shən) the removal of a methyl group, —$CH_3$, from a compound.

**de·meth·yl·chlor·tet·ra·cy·cline** (de-meth″əl-klor-tet″rə-si′klēn) demeclocycline.

**demi-** [Fr. *demi* half, from L. *dimidius*] a prefix meaning half.

**De·mi·a·noff's sign** (dem″e-ah-nofs′) [G.S. *Demianoff*, French physician, 20th century] see under *sign.*

**demi·bain** (dem′e-ban) [Fr.] sitz bath.

**demi·fac·et** (dem″e-fas′ət) a small plane surface on either of two bones which both articulate with a third bone.
**inferior d. for head of rib,** fovea costalis inferior.
**superior d. for head of rib,** fovea costalis superior.

**demi·gaunt·let** (dem″e-gawnt′lət) a form of bandage that covers the hand but leaves the fingers exposed.

**demi·lune** (dem′e-lo͞on) 1. a half moon, or crescent. 2. crescentic; crescent shaped.
**d's of Giannuzzi, d's of Heidenhain,** crescents of Giannuzzi.

**demi·mon·stros·i·ty** (dem″e-mon-stros′ĭ-te) malformation of a part which does not prevent the exercise of its function.

**de·min·er·al·iza·tion** (de-min″ər-əl-ĭ-za′shən) excessive elimination of mineral or inorganic salts, as in pulmonary tuberculosis, cancer, and osteomalacia.

**demi·pen·ni·form** (dem″e-pen′ĭ-form) feather-shaped as to one of the two margins; said of certain muscles.

**Demi-Reg·ro·ton** (dem′ĭ-reg′ro-ton) trademark for preparations of chlorthalidone and reserpine.

**De·moc·ri·tus** (de-mok′rĭ-təs) **of Abdera** [c. 460–c. 370 B.C.] a Greek philosopher who was the first to state that everything in nature, including the body and the soul, is made up of atoms of different sizes and shapes, the movements of which are the cause of life and mental activity. Democritus' only influential Greek follower was Epicurus (341–270 B.C.). Their mechanistic, atomistic theory was influential at Alexandria, and the Epicurean school of philosophy corresponds roughly to the Empiric school of medicine. See also *Asclepiades of Bithynia.*

**dem·o·dec·tic** (dem-o-dek′tik) pertaining to or caused by *Demodex.*

**Dem·o·dex** (dem′o-deks) [Gr. *dēmos* fat + *dēx* worm] a genus of acarid mites of the family Demodicidae, which cause demodectic mange.
**D. bo′vis,** a species causing mange in cattle.
**D. cap′ri,** a species causing mange in goats.
**D. ca′ti,** a species causing mange in cats.
**D. crice′ti,** a species causing mange in hamsters.
**D. folliculo′rum,** the hair follicle mite: a species found in hair follicles of humans, and in sebaceous secretions, especially of the face and nose; called also *Acarus folliculorum, face mite,* and *follicle mite.*
**D. o′vis,** a species causing mange in sheep.
**D. phylloi′des,** a species causing mange in swine.

**Dem·o·dic·i·dae** (dem″o-dis′ĭ-de) a family of minute follicular mites (order Acarina) that parasitize the skin of various mammals, including humans. It includes the genus *Demodex.*

**dem·o·dic·i·do·sis** (dem″o-dis″ĭ-do′sis) 1. demodicosis (def. 1). 2. demodectic mange.

**dem·o·di·co·sis** (dem″ə-dĭ-ko′sis) 1. any infestation by species of *Demodex;* called also *demodicidosis.* 2. demodectic mange.

**de·mo·gram** (de′mo-gram) a graphic representation, in grid form, of the population of a given area according to the time period and the age and sex of the individuals constituting it.

**de·mog·ra·phy** (de-mog′rə-fe) [Gr. *dēmos* people + *-graphy*] [MeSH: Demography] the statistical study of a population or of populations, including characteristics such as geographical distribution, physical environment, disease, sex and age composition, and birth and death rates.
**dynamic d.,** collective physiology of communities, with statistics of births, marriages, deaths, etc.
**static d.,** collective anatomy of communities and study of their environment.

**de·mo·ni·ac** (de-mo′ne-ak) 1. frenzied. 2. possessed by demons, the medieval conception of insanity.

**de·mono·pho·bia** (de″mən-o-fo′be-ə) [Gr. *daimōn* demon + *-phobia*] irrational fear of demons.

**dem·on·stra·tor** (dem′ən-stra″tər) [L.] an instructor who teaches individuals or small groups by using dissections or other aids.

**De Mor·gan's spots** (də-mor′gənz) [Campbell *De Morgan*, English physician, 1811–1876] cherry angiomas.

**de·mor·phin·iza·tion** (de-mor″fin-ĭ-za′shən) treatment of morphine addiction by gradual withdrawal of the drug.

**de Mor·si·er's syndrome** (də-mor-se-āz′) [Georges *de Morsier*, Swiss neurologist, 20th century] septo-optic dysplasia.

**de·mox·e·pam** (də-mok′sə-pam) a minor tranquilizer, which is an active metabolite of chlordiazepoxide.

**de·mu·co·sa·tion** (de-mu″ko-sa′shən) removal of the mucous membrane from a part.

**de·mul·cent** (de-mul′sənt) 1. soothing; bland; allaying the irritation of inflamed or abraded surfaces. 2. a soothing, mucilaginous, or oily medicine or application. Called also *lenitive.*

**de Mus·set** see *Musset.*

**de·mus·tard·iza·tion** (de-mus″tərd-ĭ-za′shən) 1. removal of mustard gas from a person. 2. treatment of a person subjected to the fumes of mustard gas.

**de·mu·ti·za·tion** (de-mu″tĭ-za′shən) [*de-* + L. *mutus* mute] the teaching of the deaf to communicate by lip reading or by dactylology.

**de·my·e·lin·ate** (de-mi′ə-lin′āt) to destroy or remove the myelin sheath of a nerve or nerves.

**de·my·e·lin·a·tion** (de-mi″ə-lĭn-a′shən) destruction, removal, or loss of the myelin sheath of a nerve or nerves. Called also *demyelinization, myelinolysis,* and *myelolysis.*
**segmental d.,** degeneration of the myelin sheath in segments between successive nodes of Ranvier, with preservation of the axon; seen in a variety of polyneuropathic conditions.

**de·my·e·lin·iza·tion** (de-mi″ə-lin-ĭ-za′shən) demyelination.

**de·nar·co·tize** (de-nahr′ko-tīz) 1. to deprive of a narcotic drug in the process of treating addiction. 2. to remove the narcotic element from an opiate.

**de·na·sal·i·ty** (de″na-zal′ĭ-te) hyponasality.

**de·na·tal·i·ty** (de″na-tal′ĭ-te) decrease in the number of births in proportion to the population.

**de·na·to·ni·um ben·zo·ate** (de″nə-to′ne-əm) [NF] an alcohol denaturant, used as a pharmaceutic aid.

**de·na·tur·ant** (de-na′chər-ənt) a denaturing agent.

**de·na·tur·a·tion** (de-na″chər-a′shən) the destruction of the usual nature of a substance, as the addition of methanol or acetone to alcohol to render it unfit for drinking, or the change in the physical properties of a substance, such as a protein or nucleic acid, caused by heat or certain chemicals that alter tertiary structure.
**protein d.,** disruption of the configuration (tertiary structure) of a protein, as by heat, change in pH, or other physical or chemical means, resulting in alteration of the physical properties and loss of biological activity of the protein.

**de·na·tured** (de-na′chərd) having undergone denaturation.

**Den·a·vir** (den′əvir) trademark for a preparation of penciclovir.

**den·dric** (den′drik) dendritic.

**Den·drid** (den′drid) trademark for a preparation of idoxuridine.

**den·dri·form** (den′drĭ-form) branched, or tree-shaped.

**den·drite** (den′drīt) [Gr. *dendron* tree] [MeSH: Dendrites] 1. one of the threadlike extensions of the cytoplasm of a neuron (q.v.), which typically branch into tree-like processes. In unipolar and bipolar neurons, there is a single dendrite, which proximally resembles an axon but branches distally; in multipolar neurons there are many short, branching dendrites. Dendrites compose most of the receptive surface of a neuron. Called also *dendron, neurodendrite,* and *neurodendron.* See illustration. 2. dendritic ulcer.
**apical d.,** a thick dendrite extending from the outer side of a pyramidal cell towards the surface of the cortex.

**den·drit·ic** (den-drit′ik) 1. branched like a tree. 2. pertaining to or possessing dendrites.

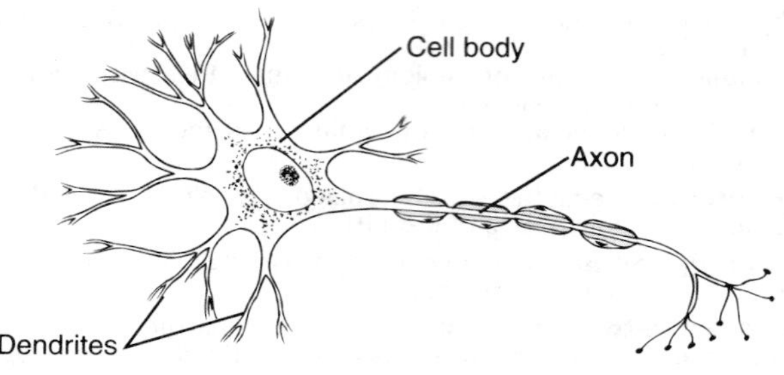

Dendrites in a multipolar neuron.

**dendr(o)-** [Gr. *dendron* tree] a combining form denoting relationship to a tree or treelike structure.

**Den·dro·as·pis** (den-dro-as'pis) a genus of extremely venomous African snakes of the family Elapidae, related to cobras but lacking a dilatable hood. *D. angus'ticeps* is the green mamba and *D. polyle'pis* is the black mamba. See table at *snake*.

**den·dro·den·drit·ic** (den″dro-den-drit'ik) referring to a synapse between dendrites of two neurons.

**den·dro·do·chio·tox·i·co·sis** (den-dro″do-ke-o-tok″sĭ-ko'sis) a form of mycotoxicosis caused by the fungus *Dendrodochium toxicum,* characterized by diarrhea, and hemorrhagic gastroenterocolitis; seen in Russia and adjacent areas in horses and occasionally in humans.

**Den·dro·do·chi·um** (den-dro-do'ke-əm) a genus of Fungi Imperfecti of the family Stilbellaceae. *D. tox'icum* is the etiologic agent of dendrodochiotoxicosis.

**Den·dro·hy·rax** (den″dro-hi'raks) a genus of tree hyraxes that live in forested areas of Ethiopia and Kenya; they are common reservoirs for *Leishmania aethiopica,* the cause of Ethiopian cutaneous leishmaniasis.

**den·droid** (den'droid) [*dendro-* + *-oid*] branching like a tree or shrub.

**den·dron** (den'dron) [Gr. "tree"] a dendrite.

**den·dro·phago·cy·to·sis** (den″dro-fag″o-si-to'sis) the absorption by microglia cells of broken portions of degenerating astrocytes.

**de·ner·vate** (de-ner'vāt) to deprive of a nerve supply.

**de·ner·va·tion** (de″nər-va'shən) [MeSH: Denervation] resection or removal of the nerves to an organ or part.

**den·gue** (deng'e; Spanish, dān'ga) [Sp.] [MeSH: Dengue] classically, an acute, self-limited disease (typically lasting 5 to 7 days), characterized by fever, prostration, headache, myalgia, rash, lymphadenopathy, and leukopenia, caused by four antigenically related but distinct types of the dengue virus. It occurs epidemically and sporadically in India, Japan, West Africa, the eastern Mediterranean area, Southeast Asia, Indonesia, northeastern Australia, Polynesia, the Caribbean, and northern South America. It is transmitted by the bite of infected mosquitoes of the genus *Aedes,* especially *A. aegypti, A. albopictus, and A. polynesiensis. Called also Aden, breakbone, dandy,* or *dengue fever.*
**hemorrhagic d.,** a syndrome affecting principally Southeast Asian children, distinguished from classic dengue by hemorrhagic manifestations such as thrombocytopenia and hemoconcentration, and caused by the same four serotypes of dengue virus. The World Health Organization distinguishes four types according to severity: *grade I,* fever, constitutional symptoms, and positive tourniquet test; *grade II,* grade I plus spontaneous bleeding into skin, gums, gastrointestinal tract, and other sites; *grade III,* grade II plus circulatory failure and agitation; and *grade IV,* profound shock with undetectable blood pressure and pulse. *Dengue shock syndrome* comprises grades III and IV. Called also *Philippine* or *Thai hemorrhagic fever.*

**de·ni·al** (də-ni'əl) in psychiatry, a defense mechanism in which the existence of unpleasant internal or external realities is kept out of conscious awareness; they by being so disavowed are prevented from causing anxiety.

**den·i·da·tion** (den″ĭ-da'shən) [*de-* + *nidation*] degeneration and expulsion of the uterine mucous membrane (endometrium) in the menstrual cycle.

**Den·is Browne splint** (den'is broun) [Sir *Denis* John *Browne,* Australian-born English pediatric surgeon, 1892–1967] see under *splint.*

**Den·i·so·nia** (den″ĭ-so'ne-ə) a genus of highly venomous snakes of the family Elapidae; *D. super'ba* is the copperhead of Australia and nearby Pacific islands. See table at *snake.*

**de·ni·tri·fi·ca·tion** (de-ni″trĭ-fĭ-ka'shən) the setting free of gaseous nitrogen from nitrites and nitrates, as by certain soil bacteria, which results in depletion of nitrogen for plant growth. Denitrification carried out by aquatic bacteria can be beneficial in ridding waste waters of excess nitrates.

**de·ni·tri·fi·er** (de-ni'trĭ-fi″ər) a bacterium that causes denitrification.

**de·ni·tri·fy** (de-ni'trĭ-fi) to remove nitrogen from any substance; see *denitrification.*

**de·ni·tro·ge·na·tion** (de-ni″tro-jən-a'shən) removal of the dissolved nitrogen from the body, as a preventive of caisson disease, aeroembolism, etc.

**Den·man's spontaneous evolution (version, method)** (den'mənz) [Thomas *Denman,* English obstetrician, 1733–1815] see under *evolution.*

**Den·nie's sign** (den'ēz) [Charles Clayton *Dennie,* American dermatologist, 1883–1971] see *Morgan's line,* under *line.*

**Den·nie-Mar·fan syndrome** (den'e-mahr-fă') [C.C. *Dennie;* Antoine Bernard Jean *Marfan,* French pediatrician, 1858–1947] see under *syndrome.*

**Den·ny-Brown's sensory neuropathy (sensory radicular neuropathy), syndrome** (den'e-broun) [Derek Ernest *Denny-Brown,* New Zealand-born neurologist in Great Britain and United States, 1901–1981] hereditary sensory radicular neuropathy; see under *neuropathy.*

**de·no·fun·gin** (de″no-fun'jin) an antibiotic substance produced by a variant of *Streptomyces hygroscopicus,* which has antifungal and antibacterial properties.

**De·non·vil·liers' aponeurosis, fascia, operation** (dĕ-naw-ve-yāz') [Charles Pierre *Denonvilliers,* French surgeon, 1808–1872] see *septum rectovesicale,* and see under *fascia* and *operation.*

**dens** (dens) pl. *den'tes* [L.] 1. [TA] tooth (q.v.): one of the small bonelike structures of the jaws of humans and other animals. 2. d. axis. 3. a toothlike structure.
**den'tes acus'tici** [TA], auditory teeth: elevations along the free surface and margin of the labium limbi vestibulare; called also *auditory teeth of Huschke.*
**d. acu'tus,** incisor tooth.
**d. ax'is** [TA], tooth of axis: the toothlike process that projects from the superior surface of the body of the axis, ascending to articulate with the atlas; called also *d. epistrophei, odontoid bone, odontoid apophysis, odontoid process of axis,* and *tooth of epistropheus.*
**d. cani'nus** [TA], canine tooth: the tooth immediately lateral to the lateral incisor; see under *tooth.*
**den'tes deci'dui** [TA], deciduous teeth: the teeth of the first dentition; see under *tooth.*
**d. epistro'phei,** d. axis.
**d. incisi'vus** [TA], incisor tooth: either of the two most frontal teeth of each jaw; see under *tooth.*
**d. in den'te,** a malformed tooth resulting from invagination of the crown before it is calcified; so named because severe invagination of enamel and dentin gives the appearance of a "tooth within a tooth." Called also *d. invaginatus* and *dilated odontoma.*
**d. invagina'tus,** d. in dente.
**d. mola'ris** [TA], molar tooth: one of the grinding, double teeth at the back of each jaw. See under *tooth.*
**d. mola'ris ter'tius** [TA], third molar tooth: the last tooth on each side of each jaw. See under *tooth.*
**den'tes permanen'tes** [TA], permanent teeth: the teeth of the second dentition; see under *tooth.*
**d. premola'ris** [TA], premolar tooth: either of the two permanent teeth between the canine teeth and the molars. See under *tooth.*
**d. sa'piens,** third molar tooth.
**d. seroti'nus,** TA alternative for *d. molaris tertius; see third molar tooth,* under *tooth.*

**den·sim·e·ter** (den-sim'ə-tər) densitometer, def. 1.

**den·si·tom·e·ter** (den″sĭ-tom'ə-tər) [L. *densus* dense + *-meter*] 1. an apparatus for determining the density of a liquid. Called also *densimeter.* 2. an instrument for determining the degree of darkening of developed photographic or x-ray film by means of a photocell which measures light transmission through a given area of the film. 3. an instrument for determining the density of deposits on electrophoresis strips and chromatographic plates by measuring light absorbancy.
**gas d.,** an apparatus for measuring specific gravity of a gas.

**den·si·tom·e·try** (den″sĭ-tom'ə-tre) [MeSH: Densitometry] determination of variations in density by comparison with that of another material, or with a certain standard.

**den·si·ty** (den'sĭ-te) [L. *densus* dense] 1. the quality of being compact or dense. 2. quantity per unit space, e.g., the mass of matter per unit volume. Symbol $\rho$ or *d.* 3. the degree of darkening of exposed and processed photographic or x-ray film, expressed as the logarithm of the opacity of a given area of the film.

**arciform d.,** a trough-shaped body separating the synaptic ribbon and the membrane of the cone pedicle or of the rod spherule in the retina.
**background d.,** in radiography, the density of a processed film due to factors other than the radiation exposure received through the recorded objects or structures, e.g., inherent (film) density, scatter radiation, or fogging.
**fiber d.,** 1. the number of muscle or nerve fibers in a unit area of tissue. 2. after a number of recordings of single fiber electromyography to the same muscle, the mean number of muscle fiber action potentials found to be single fiber action potentials and therefore to belong to the same motor unit; it is usually between 1.5 and 1.8.
**inherent d.,** the density of a processed film due to inherent factors such as the density of the film base, emulsion gelatin, etc.
**ionization d.,** the number of ion pairs per unit volume.
**magnetic flux d.,** a vector quantity that measures the magnitude of a magnetic field, given by the equation $F = qv\mathrm{B}$, where $F$ is the force exerted by the magnetic field on a moving charged particle, $q$ is the particle's charge, $v$ is the particle's velocity, and B is the magnetic flux density. Symbol B.
**optical d. (OD),** absorbance.

**den·tag·ra** (den-tag'rə, den'tə-grə) [*dent-* + *-agra*] 1. a forceps or key for extracting teeth. 2. toothache.

**den·tal** (den'təl) [L. *dentalis*] 1. pertaining to a tooth or teeth. 2. a speech sound such as *d, t,* or *th* that is made with the tongue against the front teeth; called also *linguodental.*

**den·tal·gia** (den-tal'jə) [*dent-* + *-algia*] toothache.

**den·ta·ta** (den-ta'tə) the second cervical vertebra or axis, so called from its toothlike process.

**den·tate** (den'tāt) [L. *dentatus*] having teeth or projections like saw teeth on the edges.

**den·ta·to·tha·lam·ic** (den-ta″to-thə-lam'ik) pertaining to or connecting the dentate nucleus and the thalamus.

**den·ta·tum** (den-ta'təm) [L. "toothed"] the nucleus dentatus.

**den·tes** (den'tēz) [L.] plural of *dens.*

**denti-** see *dent (o)-.*

**den·tia** (den'shə) [L.] a condition relating to development or eruption of the teeth. Used also as a combining form, denoting relationship to the teeth.
**d. prae'cox,** 1. premature teeth. 2. predeciduous teeth.
**d. tar'da,** delayed dentition.

**den·ti·buc·cal** (den″tĭ-buk'əl) pertaining to the teeth and cheek.

**den·ti·cle** (den'tĭ-kəl) [L. *denticulus* a little tooth] 1. a small toothlike process. 2. a calcified concretion that develops in the dental pulp as part of the aging process; called also *pulp stone.* 3. in mycology, a small process on which a conidium develops.
**adherent d., attached d.,** a calcified formation in a pulp chamber partially fused with the dentin.
**embedded d.,** interstitial d.
**false d.,** a calcified formation in the pulp chamber of a tooth that does not show the structure of true dentin.
**free d.,** a calcified formation in a tooth completely surrounded by the dental pulp.
**interstitial d.,** a calcified formation within a tooth, completely surrounded by dentin.
**true d.,** a calcified formation in the pulp chamber of a tooth that consists of dentin and shows traces of dentinal tubules and odontoblasts.

**den·tic·u·lat·ed** (den-tik'u-lāt″əd) [L. *denticulatus*] having minute teeth.

**den·ti·fi·ca·tion** (den″tĭ-fĭ-ka'shən) dentinogenesis.

**den·ti·form** (den'tĭ-form) shaped like a tooth.

**den·ti·frice** (den'tĭ-fris) [L. *dentifricium*] a preparation, usually a paste, gel, or powder, used with a toothbrush for cleaning the accessible surfaces of the teeth.

**den·tig·er·ous** (den-tij'ər-əs) [*denti-* + L. *gerere* to carry] bearing teeth.

**den·ti·la·bi·al** (den″tĭ-la'be-əl) [*denti-* + *labial*] pertaining to the teeth and lips.

**den·ti·lin·gual** (den″tĭ-ling'wəl) [*denti-* + *lingual*] pertaining to the teeth and tongue.

**den·tim·e·ter** (den-tim'ə-tər) [*denti-* + *-meter*] an instrument for measuring teeth.

**den·tin** (den'tin) [L. *dens* tooth] [MeSH: Dentin] the hard portion of the tooth surrounding the pulp, covered by enamel on the crown and cementum on the root, which is harder and denser than bone but softer than enamel. Called also *dentinum* [TA] and *substantia eburnea dentis.* Sometimes spelled *dentine.*
**adventitious d.,** secondary irregular d.
**calcified d.,** transparent d.
**circumpulpal d.,** the inner portion of the dentin, adjacent to the pulp chamber, consisting of thinner fibrils. See also *predentin.*
**cover d.,** mantle d.
**functional d.,** secondary regular d.
**hereditary opalescent d.,** the brown opalescent-appearing dentin observed in dentinogenesis imperfecta.
**interglobular d.,** imperfectly calcified dentinal matrix situated between the calcified globules near the periphery of the dentin.
**irregular d.,** secondary irregular d.
**mantle d.,** the peripheral portion of the dentin adjacent to the enamel or cementum, consisting mostly of coarse fibers (Korff's fibers). Called also *cover d.*
**opalescent d.,** dentin giving an unusual translucent or opalescent appearance to the teeth, as in dentinogenesis imperfecta.
**primary d.,** dentin formed subsequently to the time when the tooth takes its anatomic position in the oral cavity; it is separated from secondary dentin by a demarcation line, formed by a change in the directional path of the dentinal tubules.
**reparative d.,** secondary irregular d.
**sclerotic d.,** transparent d.
**secondary d.,** dentin formed and deposited in response to a normal or slightly abnormal stimulus, after the complete formation of the tooth. See *secondary irregular d.* and *secondary regular d.*
**secondary irregular d.,** dentin formed in response to stimuli associated with pathologic processes, such as caries or injury, or cavity preparation. Such dentin is usually irregular in nature, being composed of a few tubules that may be tortuous in appearance, and it often demonstrates cellular inclusions. Called also *adventitious d., irregular d., reparative d.,* and *tertiary d.*
**secondary regular d.,** dentin formed in response to stimuli associated with normal body processes. Called also *functional d.*
**tertiary d.,** secondary irregular d.
**transparent d.,** dentin in which some dentinal tubules have become sclerotic or calcified (dental sclerosis), producing the appearance of translucency, usually resulting from injury, abrasion, or normal aging processes. Called also *calcified d.* and *sclerotic d.*

**den·ti·nal** (den'tĭ-nəl) pertaining to dentin.

**den·tine** (den'tēn) dentin.

**den·ti·no·blast** (den'tĭ-no-blast) [*dentin* + *-blast*] a cell that forms dentin.

**den·ti·no·gen·e·sis** (den″tĭ-no-jen'ə-sis) [*dentin* + *-genesis*] [MeSH: Dentinogenesis] the formation of dentin; called also *dentification.*
**d. imperfec'ta,** an autosomal dominant disorder of tooth development characterized by opalescent dentin resulting in discoloration of the teeth, ranging from dusky blue to brownish. The dentin is poorly formed with an abnormally low mineral content; the pulp canal is obliterated, but the enamel is normal. The teeth usually wear down rapidly, leaving short, brown stumps. Called also *odontogenesis imperfecta.*

**den·ti·no·gen·ic** (den″tĭ-no-jen'ik) forming or producing dentin.

**den·ti·noid** (den'tĭ-noid) 1. resembling dentin. 2. predentin.

**den·ti·no·ma** (den″tĭ-no'mə) a tumor of odontogenic origin, composed of immature connective tissue, odontogenic epithelium, and dysplastic dentin.

**den·ti·nos·te·oid** (den″tĭ-nos'te-oid) osteodentinoma.

**den·ti·num** (den-ti'nəm) [L.] [TA] dentin: the chief substance or tissue of the teeth. See *dentin.*

**den·tip·a·rous** (den-tip'ə-rəs) bearing teeth.

**den·tist** (den'tist) [MeSH: Dentists] a person who has received a degree from an accredited school of dentistry and is licensed to practice dentistry by a state board of dental examiners. Called also *odontologist.*
**pediatric d.,** a specialist in pediatric dentistry (q.v.); called also *pedodontist.*

**den·tis·try** (den'tis-tre) [MeSH: Dentistry] 1. that department of the healing arts which is concerned with the teeth, oral cavity, and associated structures, including the diagnosis and treatment of their diseases and the restoration of defective and missing tissue. 2. the work done by dentists, such as the creation of restorations, crowns, and bridges, and surgical procedures performed in and about the oral cavity. Called also *odontoiatria, odontology,* and *oral medicine.*
**cosmetic d., esthetic d.,** that aspect of dental practice concerned with the repair and restoration of carious, broken, or defective teeth in such a manner as to improve their appearance.
**forensic d.,** that branch of dentistry that deals with the application of the art and science of dentistry to the purposes of law. *Dental jurisprudence* and *forensic d.* are sometimes used synonymously, but some authorities consider dental jurisprudence as a branch of law and forensic dentistry as a branch of dentistry.

**geriatric d.,** gerodontics.
**legal d.,** forensic d.
**operative d.,** that phase of dentistry concerned with restoration of parts of the teeth that are defective through disease, trauma, or abnormal development to a state of normal function, health, and esthetics, including preventive, diagnostic, biological, mechanical, and therapeutic techniques, as well as material and instrument science and application.
**pediatric d.,** the branch of dentistry concerned with the diagnosis and treatment of conditions of the teeth and mouth in children. Called also *pedodontia* and *pedodontics.*
**preventive d.,** that phase of dentistry concerned with the preservation of healthy teeth and the maintenance of oral structures in a state of optimal health for the longest period of time possible.
**prosthetic d.,** prosthodontics.
**psychosomatic d.,** that phase of dentistry which considers the mind-body relationship.
**restorative d.,** that phase of clinical dentistry concerned with the restoration of existing teeth that are defective through disease, trauma, or abnormal development to the state of normal function, health, and esthetics, including crown and bridgework. See also *restoration.*

**den·ti·tion** (den-tish'ən) [L. *dentitio*] [MeSH: Dentition] the teeth in the dental arch; ordinarily used to designate the natural teeth in position in their alveoli.
**artificial d.,** see *denture.*
**deciduous d.,** deciduous teeth; see under *tooth.*
**delayed d.,** eruption of the first deciduous teeth after the end of the thirteenth month of life or eruption of the first permanent teeth after the seventh year of life. Called also *retarded d., delayed eruption,* and *dentia tarda.*
**first d.,** deciduous teeth; see under *tooth.*
**mixed d.,** the complement of teeth in the jaws after eruption of some of the permanent teeth, before all of the deciduous teeth are shed; called also *transitional d.*
**natural d.,** the natural teeth in the dental arch, considered collectively; it may comprise deciduous or permanent teeth, or a mixture of the two, present at one time.
**permanent d.,** permanent teeth; see under *tooth.*
**precocious d.,** premature teeth; see under *tooth.*
**predeciduous d.,** see under *tooth.*
**premature d.,** see under *tooth.*
**primary d.,** deciduous teeth; see under *tooth.*
**retarded d.,** delayed d.
**secondary d.,** permanent teeth; see under *tooth.*
**temporary d.,** deciduous teeth; see under *tooth.*
**transitional d.,** mixed d.

**dent(o)-** [L. *dens* tooth] a combining form denoting relationship to a tooth or to the teeth. Also, *denti-.* Cf. *odont(o)-.*

**den·to·al·ve·o·lar** (den"to-al-ve'ə-lər) pertaining to a tooth and its alveolus.

**den·to·al·ve·o·li·tis** (den"to-al"ve-ə-li'tis) periodontal disease.

**den·to·fa·cial** (den"to-fa'shəl) of or pertaining to the teeth and alveolar process and the face.

**den·tog·ra·phy** (den-tog'rə-fe) odontography.

**den·toid** (den'toid) odontoid.

**den·to·le·gal** (den"to-le'gəl) pertaining to dental jurisprudence.

**den·to·ma** (den-to'mə) dentinoma.

**den·to·me·chan·i·cal** (den"to-mə-kan'ĭ-kəl) pertaining to the mechanics or to the biomechanics of dentistry.

**den·ton·o·my** (den-ton'ə-me) [*dent-* + Gr. *onoma* name] odontonomy.

**den·to·sur·gi·cal** (den"to-sər'jĭ-kəl) pertaining to or used in dentistry and oral surgery.

**den·to·trop·ic** (den"to-trop'ik) turning toward or having an affinity for tissues composing the teeth.

**den·tu·lous** (den'tu-ləs) possessing natural teeth.

**den·ture** (den'chər) [Fr., from L. *dens* tooth] [MeSH: Dentures] 1. an artificial or prosthetic replacement for missing natural teeth and adjacent tissues, such as a bridge, restoration, or dental prosthesis. 2. any set of teeth.
**clasp d.,** a removable partial denture retained with a clasp. See also *clasp* and *retainer.*
**complete d.,** a dental prosthesis replacing all natural teeth and associated mandibular and maxillary structures; it is completely supported by the tissues. Called also *full d.*
**conditioning d.,** a temporary denture used to condition the patient to wearing a denture. See also *interim d.*
**full d.,** complete d.
**immediate d., immediate-insertion d.,** a complete or removable partial denture made before all teeth are extracted, so constructed that it may be inserted immediately following the removal of the natural teeth.
**implant d.,** an artificial denture retained and stabilized through the use of a subperiosteal, intraperiosteal, or intraosseous implant, consisting of the framework (substructure) implanted in contact with the bone, and the overlying structure (superstructure).
**interim d.,** a denture to be used for a short interval of time for reasons of esthetics, mastication, occlusal support, convenience, or to condition the patient to the acceptance of an artificial substitute for missing natural teeth until more definite prosthetic dental treatment can be provided. Called also *provisional d.* See also *conditioning d.* and *transitional d.*
**overlay d.,** a removable tooth-supported partial or complete denture whose built-in secondary copings overlay or telescope over the primary copings that fit over the prepared natural crowns, posts, or studs. Called *overdenture* and *telescopic d.*
**partial d.,** a prosthetic appliance replacing one or more missing teeth in one jaw, and receiving its support and retention from the underlying tissues and/or some or all of the remaining teeth; it may be fixed or removable.
**partial d., cantilever fixed,** cantilever bridge.
**partial d., distal extension,** a removable partial denture that is retained by natural teeth only at the anterior end of the base segments, with part of the functional load carried by the residual ridge.
**partial d., fixed,** a prosthetic dental appliance that replaces lost teeth and is held in position by attachments to adjacent prepared natural teeth, roots, or implants. Called also *bridge* or *fixed bridge.*
**partial d., removable,** a denture replacing one or several of the natural teeth, made so that it can be readily removed from the mouth; it may be entirely supported by the residual teeth or supported by both the teeth and the tissue of the residual area. Called also *removable bridgework.*
**partial d., unilateral,** a partial denture for just one side of the dental arch.
**provisional d.,** interim d.
**telescopic d.,** overlay d.
**temporary d.,** an artificial denture that serves for a short time in a temporary or emergency situation. See *conditioning d., interim d., transitional d.,* and *trial d.*
**transitional d.,** a partial denture that serves temporarily, to which more teeth will be added later, and which will be replaced after postextraction tissue changes have occurred; it may become an interim denture when all the natural teeth have been removed from the dental arch.
**trial d.,** a denture for placement in the mouth to verify its esthetic qualities, make a record, or do other procedures before completion of the final denture.

**den·tur·ism** (den'chər-is-əm) the practice of fabrication and fitting of dentures by dental technologists without benefit of a dentist's expertise.

**den·tur·ist** (den'chər-ist) [MeSH: Denturists] a dental technologist who fabricates and fits dentures for patients without benefit of a dentist's expertise. Denturists practice in parts of Canada and the United States but in many states denturism is illegal.

**De·nu·cé's ligament** (də-nu-sāz') [Jean Henri Maurice *Denucé,* French surgeon, 1859–1924] see under *ligament.*

**de·nu·cle·at·ed** (de-noo'kle-āt"əd) deprived of the nucleus; called also *anucleated.*

**de·nu·da·tion** (den"u-da'shən) [L. *denudare* to make bare] the act of laying bare; removal of the epithelial covering from any surface, by surgery, trauma, or pathologic change.

**de·odor·ant** (de-o'dər-ənt) [*de-* + *odorant*] [MeSH: Deodorants] 1. removing undesirable or offensive odors. 2. a substance that masks offensive odors. Called also *antibromic.*

**de·odor·ize** (de-o'dər-īz) [*de-* + *odor* + *-ize*] to neutralize or absorb odor.

**de·odor·iz·er** (de-o'dər-īz"ər) a deodorizing agent.

**de·on·tol·o·gy** (de"on-tol'ə-je) [Gr. *deonta* things that ought to be done + *-logy*] the theory or study of professional duties and etiquette.

**de·op·pi·lant** (de-op'ĭ-lənt) removing obstructions.

**de·op·pi·la·tion** (de-op"ĭ-la'shən) [*de-* + L. *oppilatio* obstruction] the removal of obstructions.

**de·or·sum·duc·tion** (de-or"səm-duk'shən) infraduction.

**de·or·sum·ver·gence** (de-or"səm-vər'jəns) infravergence.

**de·or·sum·ver·sion** (de-or"səm-vər'zhən) infraversion (def. 3).

**de·os·si·fi·ca·tion** (de-os"ĭ-fĭ-ka'shən) [*de-* + *ossification*] loss of or removal of bone.

**de·ox·i·da·tion** (de-ok"sĭ-da'shən) [L. *de* from + *oxygen*] the removal of oxygen from a chemical compound.

**de·ox·i·dize** (de-ok′sĭ-dīz) to deprive of chemically combined oxygen.

**deoxy-** a prefix used in naming chemical compounds, to designate a compound containing one less atom of oxygen than the reference substance. For words beginning thus see also those beginning *desoxy-*.

**de·oxy·aden·o·sine** (de-ok″se-ə-den′o-sēn) a purine nucleoside, adenine linked by its N9 nitrogen to the C1 carbon of deoxyribose. Symbol dA.
**d. diphosphate (dADP),** a nucleotide, the 5′-pyrophosphate of deoxyadenosine.
**d. monophosphate (dAMP),** a nucleotide, the 5′-phosphate of deoxyadenosine, occurring in deoxyribonucleic acid.
**d. triphosphate (dATP),** a nucleotide, the 5′-triphosphate of deoxyadenosine; it is an activated precursor in DNA synthesis.

**de·oxy·ad·e·no·syl** (de-ok″se-ə-den′o-səl) the radical formed from deoxyadenosine on loss of an H or OH group.

**de·oxy·ad·e·no·syl·co·bal·a·min** (de-ok″se-ə-den″o-səl-ko-bal′ə-min) adenosylcobalamin.

**de·oxy·aden·yl·ate** (de-ok″se-ə-den′ə-lāt) a dissociated form of deoxyadenylic acid.

**de·oxy·ad·e·nyl·ic ac·id** (de-ok″se-ad″ə-nil′ik) deoxyadenosine monophosphate.

**de·oxy·ad·e·nyl·yl** (de-ok″se-ad″ə-nil′il) the radical formed by removal of OH from the phosphate group of deoxyadenosine monophosphate.

**de·ox·y·cho·lan·er·e·sis** (de-ok″se-ko″lən-er′ə-sis) increase in the output of deoxycholic acid in the bile.

**de·oxy·cho·late** (de-ok″se-ko′lāt) a salt, ester, or anionic form of deoxycholic acid.

**de·oxy·chol·ic ac·id** (de-ok″se-ko′lik) [MeSH: Deoxycholic Acid] a secondary bile acid formed by dehydroxylation of cholic acid in the intestine; it is a choleretic acid and is also used in biochemistry as a detergent.

**de·oxy·chol·yl·gly·cine** (de-ok″se-ko″ləl-gli′sēn) a bile salt, the glycine conjugate of deoxycholic acid.

**de·oxy·chol·yl·taur·ine** (de-ok″se-ko″ləl-taw′rēn) a bile salt, the taurine conjugate of deoxycholic acid.

**11-de·oxy·cor·ti·cos·ter·one (DOC)** (de-ok″se-kor″tĭ-kos′tər-ōn, -kor″tĭ-ko-ster′ōn) 21-hydroxypregn-4-ene-3,20-dione, a mineralocorticoid produced in small quantities by the human adrenal cortex, having about 3 per cent of the sodium-retaining activity of aldosterone. The acetate and pivalate salts are used for mineralocorticoid replacement therapy. Called also *cortexone, deoxycortone, desoxycorticosterone, desoxycortone,* and *21-hydroxyprogesterone.*
**11-d. acetate,** see under *desoxycorticosterone.*
**11-d. pivalate,** see under *desoxycorticosterone.*

**11-de·oxy·cor·ti·sol** (de-ok″se-kor′tĭ-sol) an intermediate formed in the conversion of cholesterol to cortisol in steroidogenesis.

**de·oxy·cor·tone** (de-ok″se-kor′tōn) 11-deoxycorticosterone.

**de·oxy·cy·ti·dine** (de-ok″se-si′tĭ-dēn) [MeSH: Deoxycytidine] a nucleoside, cytosine linked by its N1 nitrogen to the C1 carbon of deoxyribose. Symbol dC.
**d. diphosphate (dCDP),** a nucleotide, the 5′-pyrophosphate of deoxycytidine.
**d. monophosphate (dCMP),** a nucleotide, the 5′-phosphate of deoxycytidine, occurring in deoxyribonucleic acid.
**d. triphosphate (dCTP),** a nucleotide, the 5′-triphosphate of deoxycytidine; it is an activated precursor in the synthesis of DNA.

**de·oxy·cy·ti·dyl·ate** (de-ok″se-si-tĭ-dil′āt) a dissociated form of deoxycytidylic acid.

**de·oxy·cy·ti·dyl·ic ac·id** (de-ok″se-si″tĭ-dil′ik) deoxycytidine monophosphate.

**de·oxy·cy·ti·dyl·yl** (de-ok″se-si″tĭ-dil′əl) the radical formed by removal of OH from the phosphate group of deoxycytidine monophosphate.

**de·ox·y·gen·a·tion** (de-ok″sĭ-jən-a′shən) the act of depriving of oxygen.

**2-de·oxy-D-glu·cose** (de-ok″se-gloo′kōs) an antimetabolite of glucose that has antiviral properties by virtue of its inhibition of the glycosylation of glycoproteins and glycolipids; radioactive 2-deoxyglucose is also used to determine the rate of energy metabolism in cells, since cells (e.g., neurons) adjust their rate of glucose (or 2-deoxyglucose) uptake to fill their metabolic needs.

**de·oxy·guan·o·sine** (de-ok″se-gwahn′o-sēn) [MeSH: Deoxyguanosine] a purine nucleoside, guanine linked by its N9 nitrogen to the C1 carbon of deoxyribose.
**d. diphosphate (dGDP),** a nucleotide, the 5′-pyrophosphate of deoxyguanosine.
**d. monophosphate (dGMP),** a nucleotide, the 5′-phosphate of deoxyguanosine, occurring in deoxyribonucleic acid.
**d. triphosphate (dGTP),** a nucleotide, the 5′-triphosphate of deoxyguanosine; it is an activated precursor in the synthesis of DNA.

**de·oxy·guan·yl·ate** (de-ok″se-gwahn′əl-āt) a dissociated form of deoxyguanylic acid.

**de·oxy·guan·yl·ic ac·id** (de-ok″se-gwah-nil′ik) deoxyguanosine monophosphate.

**de·oxy·guan·yl·yl** (de-ok″se-gwah-nil′əl) the radical formed by removal of OH from the phosphate group of deoxyguanosine monophosphate.

**de·oxy·he·mo·glo·bin** (de-ok″se-he″mo-glo′bin) hemoglobin not combined with oxygen, formed when oxyhemoglobin releases its oxygen; called also *deoxygenated* or *reduced hemoglobin.*

**de·oxy·hex·ose** (de-ok″se-hek′sōs) any deoxy sugar formed from a hexose; one in which the 6 carbon is reduced (6-deoxyhexose) is also called a *methylpentose.*

**de·oxy·ni·val·e·nol** (de-ok″se-nĭ-val′ə-nol) a trichothecene mycotoxin produced by species of *Fusarium,* causing fusariotoxicosis with vomiting and hemorrhaging in domestic animals. Called also *vomitoxin.*

**de·oxy·pent·ose** (de-ok″se-pen′tōs) any deoxy sugar formed from a pentose, e.g., deoxyribose.

**de·oxy·ri·bo·nu·cle·ase** (de-ok″se-ri″bo-noo′kle-ās) any nuclease specifically catalyzing the cleavage of phosphate ester linkages in deoxyribonucleic acids; the deoxyribonucleases are grouped as those cleaving internal bonds (endodeoxyribonucleases) and those cleaving at termini (exodeoxyribonucleases). Called also *DNase.*
**d. I (DNase I)** [EC 3.1.21.1], an endonuclease that produces di- and oligonucleotides with 5′-phosphate groups. The enzyme occurs in tissues such as the pancreas and thymus.
**d. II (DNase II)** [EC 3.1.22.1], an endonuclease that produces di- and oligonucleotides with 3′-phosphate groups. The enzyme occurs in tissues such as the pancreas, liver, thymus, and gastric mucosa.

**de·oxy·ri·bo·nu·cle·ic ac·id** (de-ok″se-ri″bo-noo-kle′ik) DNA; the nucleic acid in which the sugar is deoxyribose, constituting the primary genetic material of all cellular organisms and the DNA viruses, and occurring predominantly in the nucleus. It is a linear or circular polymer with a backbone composed of deoxyribose moieties that are linked by phosphate groups attached to their 5′ and 3′ hydroxyls, with side chains composed of purine (adenine, guanine) and pyrimidine (cytosine, thymine) bases attached to the sugars. In double-stranded DNA (see illustration), adenine forms two hydrogen bonds with thymine, and cytosine forms three with guanine; these are complementary base pairs. The strands are twisted to form a double helix and are antiparallel. DNA is duplicated by replication, and it serves as a template for synthesis of ribonucleic acid (transcription). For specific types of DNA, see under *DNA.*

**de·oxy·ri·bo·nu·cleo·pro·tein** (de-ok″se-ri″bo-noo″kle-o-pro′tēn) a nucleoprotein in which the nucleic acid sugar is D-2-deoxyribose.

**de·oxy·ri·bo·nu·cleo·side** (de-ok″se-ri″bo-noo′kle-o-sīd) a nucleoside having a purine or pyrimidine base bonded to deoxyribose.

**de·oxy·ri·bo·nu·cleo·tide** (de-ok″se-ri″bo-noo′kle-o-tīd) a nucleotide consisting of a purine or a pyrimidine base bonded to deoxyribose, which in turn is bound to a phosphate group.

**de·oxy·ri·bose** (de-ok″se-ri′bōs) [MeSH: Deoxyribose] a deoxypentose found in deoxyribonucleic acids (DNA), deoxyribonucleotides, and deoxyribonucleosides.

**de·oxy·ri·bo·vi·rus** (de-ok″se-ri′bo-vi″rəs) DNA virus.

**de·oxy·thy·mi·dine** (de-ok″se-thi′mĭ-dēn) a pyrimidine nucleoside, thymine linked by its N1 nitrogen to the C1 carbon of deoxyribose. Symbol dT. Often called *thymidine* (q.v.).
**d. diphosphate (dTDP),** a nucleotide, the 5′-pyrophosphate of deoxythymidine.
**d. monophosphate (dTMP),** a nucleotide, the 5′-phosphate of deoxythymidine, occurring in deoxyribonucleic acid.
**d. triphosphate (dTTP),** a nucleotide, the 5′-triphosphate of deoxythymidine; it is an activated precursor in the synthesis of deoxyribonucleic acid.

**de·oxy·thy·mi·dyl·ate** (de-ok″se-thi″mĭ-dil′āt) a dissociated form of deoxythymidylic acid.

**de·oxy·thy·mi·dyl·ic ac·id** (de-ok″se-thi″mĭ-dil′ik) deoxythymidine monophosphate.

**de·oxy·thy·mi·dyl·yl** (de-ok″se-thi″mĭ-dil′əl) the radical formed by removal of OH from the phosphate group of deoxythymidine monophosphate.

**de·oxy·uri·dine** (de-ok″se-ūr′ĭ-dēn) [MeSH: Deoxyuridine] a pyrimidine nucleoside, uracil linked by its N1 nitrogen to the C1 carbon of deoxyribose. Symbol dU.
**d. monophosphate (dUMP),** a nucleotide, the 5′-phosphate of de-

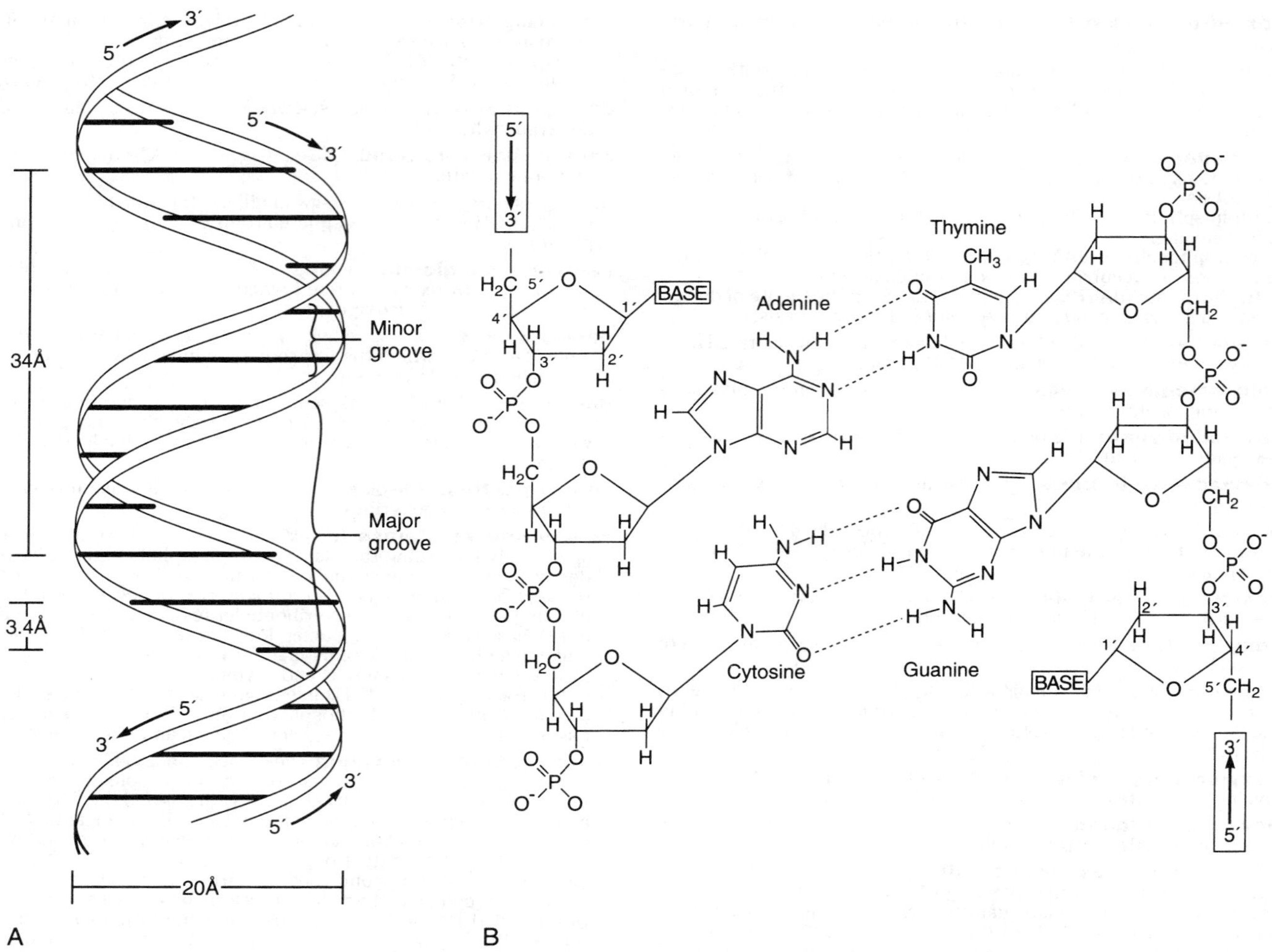


The DNA double helix. *A,* Diagrammatic model of the helical structure, showing its dimensions, the major and minor grooves, the periodicity of the bases, and the antiparallel orientation of the backbone chains (represented by ribbons). The base pairs (represented by rods) are perpendicular to the axis and lie stacked one on another. *B,* The chemical structure of the backbone and bases of DNA, showing the sugar phosphate linkages of the backbone and the hydrogen bonding between the base pairs. There are two hydrogen bonds between adenine and thymine, and three between cytosine and guanine.

oxyuridine; it is an intermediate in the synthesis of deoxythymidine triphosphate.

**d. triphosphate (dUTP),** a nucleotide, the 5′-triphosphate of deoxyuridine; it is an intermediate in the synthesis of deoxyribonucleotides.

**de·oxy·uri·dyl·ate** (de-ok″se-ūr″ĭ-dil′āt) a dissociated form of deoxyuridylic acid.

**de·oxy·uri·dyl·ic ac·id** (de-ok″se-ūr″ĭ-dil′ik) deoxyuridine monophosphate.

**Dep.** abbreviation for L. *depura′tus,* purified.

**Dep·a·kene** (dep′ə-kēn) trademark for preparations of valproic acid.

**De·pa·kote** (dep′ə-kōt) trademark for a preparation of divalproex sodium.

**De·pen** (dep′en) trademark for a preparation of penicillamine.

**de·pen·dence** (de-pen′dəns) 1. a state of relying on or requiring the aid of something, particularly for support or maintenance. 2. a state in which there is a compulsive or chronic need, as for a drug; see *substance d.*

**emotional d.,** psychological d.

**physical d., physiological d.,** substance dependence in which there is evidence of tolerance, withdrawal, or both.

**polysubstance d.** [DSM-IV], substance dependence in which three or more substances, excluding nicotine and caffeine, are used repeatedly, with none of them predominating.

**psychoactive substance d.,** substance abuse

**psychological d.,** substance dependence in which the drug is used to obtain relief from tension or emotional discomfort, rather than being associated with tolerance or withdrawal. Called also *emotional d.*

**substance d.** [DSM-IV], compulsive use of a substance despite significant problems resulting from such use. Although tolerance and withdrawal were previously defined as necessary and sufficient for dependence, they are currently only two of several possible criteria; others include taking the substance longer or in larger amounts than planned, repeatedly expressing a desire or attempting unsuccessfully to cut down or regulate use, and continuing use in the face of acknowledged substance-induced physical or mental problems. The term is sometimes used more narrowly to refer only to physiological dependence, and in this sense it may be considered to be a phenomenon distinct from tolerance. DSM-IV includes specific substance dependence disorders for alcohol, amphetamines or similarly acting sympathomimetics, cannabis, cocaine, hallucinogens, inhalants, nicotine, opioids, phencyclidines or similarly acting substances, and sedatives, hypnotics, or anxiolytics, as well as one for multiple substances (polysubstance).

**de·pen·den·cy** (de-pen′dən-se) a state of relying on another for love, affection, mothering, comfort, security, food, warmth, shelter, protection, and the like—the so-called dependency needs.

**de·pen·dent** (de-pen′dənt) 1. exhibiting dependence or dependency. 2. hanging down.

**De·pen·do·vi·rus** (də-pen′do-vi″rəs) [L. *dependere* to depend on + *virus*] [MeSH: Dependovirus] adeno-associated viruses; a genus of viruses of the subfamily Parvovirinae (family Parvoviridae) that require coinfection with an adenovirus or herpesvirus to provide helper functions for replication. If no helper virus is present, the genome can be integrated into the host cell DNA, resulting in latent infection. Asymptomatic infection is common in humans and in many animal species.

**de·pep·sin·ized** (de-pep′sin-īzd) deprived of pepsin; peptically inactivated: said of gastric juice.

**de·per·son·al·iza·tion** (de-pər″sən-əl-ĭ-za′shən) alteration in the perception of the self so that the usual sense of one's own reality is lost, manifested in a sense of unreality or self-estrangement, in changes of body image, or in a feeling that one does not control his own actions and speech; seen in disorders such as depersonalization disorder, depression, dissociative states, hypochondriasis, temporal lobe epilepsy, schizophrenic disorders, and schizotypal personality disorder. Some do not draw a distinction between depersonalization and derealization, using depersonalization to include both.

**de Pez·zer catheter** (də-pə-za′) [Oscar Michel Benvenuto *de Pezzer,* French surgeon, 1853–1917] see under *catheter.*

**de·phos·phor·y·la·tion** (de-fos″for-ə-la′shən) removal of a phosphate group from an organic molecule.

**de·pig·men·ta·tion** (de-pig″mən-ta′shən) removal or loss of pigment, especially melanin. Cf. *amelanosis, hypomelanosis,* and *hypopigmentation.*

**dep·i·late** (dep′ĭ-lāt) [*de-* + *pilus* (def. 2)] to remove hair from; called also *epilate.*

**dep·i·la·tion** (dep″ĭ-la′shən) the removal of hair by the roots; called also *epilation.*

**de·pil·a·to·ry** (de-pil′ə-tor″e) [*de-* + *pilus* (def. 2)] 1. having the power to remove the hair. 2. an agent for removing or destroying the hair.

**de·plas·mol·y·sis** (de″plaz-mol′ə-sis) return to the initial volume, after plasmolysis, of the protoplasm of a cell in hypertonic solution.

**de·plas·mo·lyze** (de-plaz′mo-līz) to undergo deplasmolysis.

**de·plete** (də-plēt′) [L. *deplere* to empty] to empty; to unload; to cause depletion.

**de·ple·tion** (də-ple′shən) [L. *deplere* to empty] 1. the act or process of emptying or removing, such as of fluid from a body compartment. 2. an exhausted state resulting from excessive loss of blood.
**iron d.,** the mildest form of iron deficiency, with depletion of bodily stores but no change in hematocrit or serum iron levels. Called also *prelatent iron deficiency.*

**de·po·lar·iza·tion** (de-pōl″ər-ĭ-za′shən) [*de-* + *polarization*] 1. the process or act of neutralizing polarity. 2. in electrophysiology, the reversal of the resting potential in excitable cell membranes when stimulated, i.e., the tendency of the cell membrane potential to become positive with respect to the potential outside the cell. See also *sodium channel,* under *channel.*
**atrial premature d. (APD),** see under *complex.*
**ventricular premature d. (VPD),** see under *complex.*

**de·po·lar·ize** (de-pōl′ər-īz) to reduce toward a nonpolarized condition; to deprive of polarity. See *depolarization.*

**de·po·lar·iz·er** (de-pōl′ə-r-īz″ər) 1. a chemical agent placed in a galvanic cell for reducing the polarization of an electrode. 2. a substance that reduces the voltage across a biological membrane. 3. a muscle relaxant that produces striated muscle paralysis by altering the electrical state of the muscle receptor, thus blocking muscle response to nerve impulse.

**de·poly·mer·iza·tion** (de″po-lim″ər-ĭ-za′shən) the conversion of a polymer into its component monomers.

**de·poly·mer·ize** (de″po-lim′ər-īz) to cause to undergo depolymerization.

**De·po-Med·rol** (de″po-med′rol) trademark for preparations of methylprednisolone acetate.

**De·po-Pro·vera** (de″po-pro-ver′ə) trademark for a preparation of medroxyprogesterone acetate for intramuscular injection.

**de·pos·it** (de-poz′it) [*de-* + L. *ponere* to place] 1. sediment or dregs. 2. extraneous inorganic matter collected in the tissues or in a viscus or cavity. 3. tooth d.
**tooth d.,** a hard or soft material deposited on a tooth surface, such as dental calculus or plaque and materia alba.

**de·pot** (de′po, dep′o) [Fr. *dépôt* from L. *depositum*] a body area in which a substance, e.g., a drug, can be accumulated, deposited, or stored and from which it can be distributed.
**fat d.,** a site in the body in which large quantities of fat are stored, as in adipose tissue.

**De·po-Tes·tos·ter·one** (de″po-tes-tos′tər-ōn) trademark for a sustained-action preparation of testosterone cypionate.

**dep·ra·va·tion** (dep″rə-va′shən) [L. *depravare* to vitiate; *de* down + *pravus* bad] deterioration; a change for the worse.

**L-de·pren·yl** (dep′rə-nəl) selegiline.

**de·pres·sant** (de-pres′ənt) 1. diminishing functional activity. 2. an agent that reduces functional activity and the vital energies in general by producing muscular relaxation and diaphoresis.
**cardiac d.,** an agent that depresses the rate or force of contraction of the heart.

**de·pressed** (de-prest′) carried below the normal level; associated with depression.

**de·pres·sion** (de-presh′ən) [L. *deprimere* to press down] [MeSH: Depression] 1. a hollow or depressed area; downward or inward displacement. 2. a lowering or decrease of functional activity. 3. a mental state of depressed mood characterized by feelings of sadness, despair, and discouragement. Depression ranges from normal feelings of "the blues" through dysthymic disorder to major depressive disorder. It in many ways resembles the grief and mourning that follow bereavement; there are often feelings of low self-esteem, guilt, and self-reproach, withdrawal from interpersonal contact, and somatic symptoms such as eating and sleep disturbances.
**agitated d.,** major depressive disorder with psychomotor agitation.
**anaclitic d.,** impairment of an infant's physical, social, and intellectual development resulting from absence of mothering.
**congenital chondrosternal d.,** a congenital, deep, funnel-shaped depression in the anterior chest wall.
**double d.,** a major depressive episode superimposed for a time on a chronic dysthymic disorder; after the episode ends the patient returns to the usual dysthymic state.
**endogenous d.,** a type of depression caused by somatic or biological factors rather than environmental influences, in contrast to a reactive depression (q.v.). It is usually identified with a specific symptom complex—psychomotor retardation, early morning awakening, weight loss, excessive guilt, and lack of reactivity to the environment—that is roughly equivalent to the symptoms of major depressive disorder.
**freezing point d.,** the depression of the freezing point of a solution below that of the pure solvent, proportional to the concentration of the solute in the solvent; see also *osmolality.*
**Leão's spreading d.,** depression of normal electrical rhythms recorded from the cerebral cortex, spreading outward from an area of stimulation or cortical damage; the rate of spread closely approximates the visual aura of a migraine. Called also *spreading d.*
**major d.,** major depressive disorder.
**neurotic d.,** any depression that is not a psychotic depression (q.v.); used sometimes broadly to indicate any depression without psychotic features and sometimes more narrowly to denote only milder forms of depression, which would be diagnosed as dysthymic disorder by DSM-IV criteria or as reactive (rather than endogenous) depression.
**otic d.,** auditory pit.
**pacchionian d's,** granular foveolae.
**postactivation d.,** a reduction in amplitude and area of the M wave upon additional stimulus a few minutes after a strong violent contraction or after tetanus produced by repetitive nerve stimulation (q.v.). See also *postactivation exhaustion,* under *exhaustion.*
**precordial d.,** epigastric fossa, def. 1.
**psychotic d.,** in the strict sense, major depressive disorder with psychotic features, such as hallucinations, delusions, mutism, or stupor. However, this term is commonly used in a broader sense to cover all severe depressions causing gross impairment of social or occupational functioning, i.e., as a rough equivalent of major depressive disorder or of endogenous depression. Cf. *neurotic d.*
**pterygoid d.,** pterygoid fovea.
**radial d.,** fossa radialis humeri.
**reactive d.,** a depression that is precipitated by a stressful life event or other environmental factor, in contrast to an endogenous depression, with an absence of significant vegetative disturbances; see also *neurotic d.* and *dysthymic disorder.*
**retarded d.,** major depressive disorder with psychomotor retardation.
**situational d.,** reactive d.
**spreading d.,** Leão's spreading d.
**supratrochlear d.,** a slight depression on the anterior surface of the femur, above the trochlea.
**tooth d.,** intrusion.
**unipolar d.,** that unaccompanied by episodes of mania or hypomania, as in major depressive disorder or dysthymic disorder; the term is sometimes used to denote the former specifically.
**ventricular d.,** that part of the venous pulse tracing which lies between the ventricular and atrial waves.

**de·pres·sive** (de-pres′iv) 1. tending to lower. 2. of or pertaining to depression.

**de·pres·so·mo·tor** (de-pres″o-mo′tər) 1. retarding or abating motion. 2. an agent which lessens or depresses motor activity.

**de·pres·sor** (de-pres′ər) [L., from *deprimere* to press down] 1. that which causes depression, as a muscle, agent, instrument, or apparatus. 2. tending to decrease blood pressure; said of nerves and chemical substances. 3. depressor nerve.
**d. an′guli o′ris,** see under *musculus.*
**d. epiglot′tidis,** musculus thyroepiglotticus.
**d. la′bii inferio′ris,** see under *musculus.*

**tongue d.**, an instrument for pressing the tongue against the floor of the mouth.

**dep·ri·mens oc·u·li** (dep'rĭ-mənz ok'u-le) [L.] musculus rectus inferior bulbi.

**dep·ri·va·tion** (dep"rĭ-va'shən) [*de-* + L. *privare* to remove] loss or absence of parts, organs, powers, or things that are needed.
**emotional d.**, deprivation of adequate and appropriate interpersonal or environmental experience in the early development years.
**maternal d.**, the result of premature loss or absence of the mother or of lack of proper mothering; see also *maternal deprivation syndrome,* under *syndrome.*
**sensory d.**, partial to total deprivation of visual, auditory, and tactile stimuli, such as may be produced experimentally or by solitary confinement, loss of sight or hearing, paralysis, or even hospital bed rest; it may result in some combination of anxiety, irritability, boredom, loss of ability to concentrate and organize thoughts, increased suggestibility, delusions, panic, and unpleasant vivid hallucinations.
**thought d.**, blocking (def. 2).
**water d.**, a method for testing the body's ability to concentrate urine when plasma osmolality is artificially increased; see *water deprivation test,* under *test.*

**de·pro·tein·iza·tion** (de-pro"tēn-ĭ-za'shən) removal of protein.

**dep·side** (dep'sīd) one of a class of compounds which are products of the condensation of two or more molecules of phenolic carboxylic acids, e.g., tannic acid.

**depth** (depth) an expression of the distance separating the upper and lower surfaces of an object.
**focal d., d. of focus,** the measure of the power of a lens to yield clear images of objects at different distances from it. Called also *penetration.*

**dep·u·la** (dep'u-lə) [L., from Gr. *depas* goblet] in zoology, the developing egg in the stage succeeding the blastula and preceding the gastrula.

**dep·u·rant** (dep'u-rənt) 1. cleansing or purifying. 2. an agent that cleanses or purifies.

**dep·u·rate** (dep'u-rāt) [L. *depurare* to purify] to cleanse, refine, or purify.

**dep·u·ra·tion** (dep"u-ra'shən) cleansing, purification; especially placement of shellfish in clean water to allow them to cleanse themselves of bacteria.

**dep·u·ra·tive** (dep'u-ra"tiv) tending to purify or cleanse; called also *pellant.*

**dep·u·ra·tor** (dep'u-ra"tor) an agent that cleanses or purifies.

**de Quer·vain's disease, fracture, thyroiditis** (də-kār-vaz') [Fritz *de Quervain,* Swiss physician, 1868–1940] see under *disease* and *fracture* and see *subacute granulomatous thyroiditis,* under *thyroiditis.*

**der·a·del·phus** (der"ə-del'fəs) [*der-* + *-adelphus*] conjoined twins fused at or near the umbilicus, and having only one head.

**de·rail·ment** (de-rāl'ment) disordered thought or speech characteristic of schizophrenia and marked by constant jumping around from one topic to another before the first is fully realized, the topics often being clearly but obliquely related or unrelated. The term is sometimes used synonymously with *loosening of associations.*

**der·an·en·ce·pha·lia** (der-an"ən-sə-fa'le-ə) [*der-* + *an-*[1] + *encephal-* + *-ia*] anencephaly marked by defect of the brain and upper part of the spinal cord.

**de·range·ment** (de-rānj'mənt) 1. older term for a mental disorder. 2. disarrangement of a part or organ.
**Hey's internal d.**, partial dislocation of the knee, marked by great pain and spasm of the muscles.

**Der·cum's disease** (der'kəmz) [Francis Xavier *Dercum,* American physician, 1856–1931] adiposis dolorosa.

**de·re·al·i·za·tion** (de-re"əl-ĭ-za'shən) a loss of the sensation of the reality of one's surroundings; the feeling that something has happened, that the world has been changed and altered, that one is detached from one's environment. It is seen most frequently in schizophrenic disorders. See also *depersonalization.*

**de·re·ism** (de're-iz-əm) [*de-* + *res* thing] dereistic thinking.

**de·re·is·tic** (de"re-is'tik) pertaining to or characterized by dereism.

**der·en·ceph·a·lo·cele** (der"en-sef'ə-lo-sēl) [*derencephalus* + *-cele*[1]] the brain substance that protrudes through the defect in the cervical vertebrae in a derencephalus.

**der·en·ceph·a·lus** (der"en-sef'ə-ləs) [*der-* + Gr. *enkephalos* brain] a fetus with rudimentary skull bones and bifid cervical vertebrae, the brain resting in the bifurcation.

**de·re·pres·sion** (de"re-presh'ən) removal of repression of an operon, so that gene transcription occurs or is enhanced. In prokaryotes, the mechanism involves inactivation of a repressor, either by inhibition of a corepressor or by the action of an inducer. In eukaryotes, the process appears to involve combinations of regulatory proteins and specific effectors, but has not been elucidated. The net result is frequently elevation of the level of a specific enzyme.

**De·ri·fil** (der'ĭ-fil) trademark for a preparation of chlorophyllin copper complex sodium.

**der·i·vant** (der'ĭ-vənt) derivative.

**de·riv·a·tive** (də-riv'ə-tiv) a chemical substance produced from another substance either directly or by modification or partial substitution.
**hematoporphyrin d.**, a material prepared by an acetic acid–sulfuric acid treatment of hematoporphyrin that concentrates selectively in metabolically active tumor tissue; used in photodynamic therapy.
**purified protein d. (PPD),** see under *tuberculin.*

**-derm** [Gr. *derma* skin] a word termination denoting skin, or a germ layer.

**der·ma** (dər'mə) [Gr.] the skin, usually with special reference to the dermis.

**derma-** see *dermat(o)-.*

**derm·abrad·er** (dər"mə-brād'ər) any device used for dermabrasion.

**derm·abra·sion** (dər"mə-bra'zhən) [MeSH: Dermabrasion] planing of the skin done by mechanical means, as by fine sandpaper or wire brushes. See *planing.*

**Der·ma·cen·tor** (dər"mə-sen'tər) [*derma-* + Gr. *kentein* to prick, stab] [MeSH: Dermacentor] a genus of ticks that are important as transmitters of disease.
**D. albipic'tus,** a species of brown ticks widely distributed in the United States, parasitic on cattle, horses, deer, elk, and moose. Called also *winter tick.*
**D. anderso'ni,** a reddish brown tick that is responsible for transmitting Rocky Mountain spotted fever, Colorado tick fever, and tularemia to humans and for causing tick paralysis. Its hosts include deer, elk, antelope, grizzly bear, porcupine, prairie dog, and various species of rabbits. Called also *D. venustus, Rocky Mountain wood tick,* and *wood tick.*
**D. hal'li,** a yellow-brown tick found on peccaries in Texas.
**D. hun'teri,** a brown tick found on Rocky Mountain sheep in the southwestern United States, particularly in southwestern Arizona.
**D. margina'tus,** a species that is the vector of a type of tick-borne hemorrhagic fever in Siberia.
**D. ni'tens,** *Anocentor nitens.*
**D. nuttal'lii,** a tick that transmits Siberian tick typhus.
**D. occidenta'lis,** a brown tick common along the West Coast of the United States, from southern Oregon to southern California, the principal hosts being the cow, horse, deer, dog, and human; called also *Pacific coast dog tick.*
**D. parumaper'tus,** a reddish brown tick which is found widely distributed in the southwestern United States, found on deer and coyotes, and abundant on various species of rabbits.
**D. reticula'tus,** a tick that attacks sheep and oxen, occurring in Europe, Asia, and America; a vector of canine babesiosis in southern Europe.
**D. sylva'rum,** a tick that transmits Siberian tick typhus.
**D. varia'bilis,** a dark brown tick found along the California coast and widely distributed east of the Rocky Mountains, the dog being the principal host of the adults, which are found also on cattle, horses, rabbits, and man; it is the principal vector of Rocky Mountain spotted fever in the central and eastern United States. Called also *American dog tick* and *dog tick.*
**D. venus'tus,** *D. andersoni.*

**Der·ma·cen·trox·e·nus** (dər"mə-sen"trok-se'nəs) [*Dermacentor* +

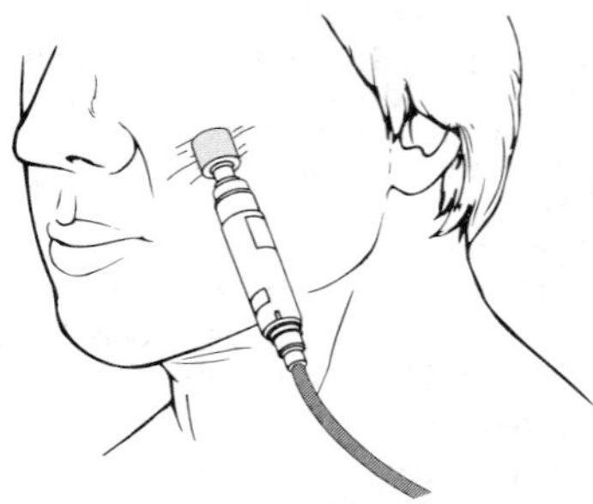

Dermabrader.

Gr. *xenos* a guest-friend] a genus name formerly given microorganisms parasitic in ticks, now included in the genus *Rickettsia*.
**D. rickett'si,** *Rickettsia rickettsii.*
**D. ty'phi,** *Rickettsia typhi (mooseri).*

**der·mad** (dər'mad) toward the skin or other integument.

**der·mal** (dər'məl) 1. pertaining to the dermis. 2. pertaining to the skin; cutaneous; dermic.

**der·ma·my·ia·sis** (der"mə-mi-i'ə-sis) [*derma-* + *myiasis*] myiasis linearis.

**Der·ma·nys·si·dae** (dər"mə-nis'ĭ-de) a family of mites (order Acarina) parasitizing mammals, reptiles, and birds, whose bite may cause a painful dermatitis in man; *Dermanyssus* is the type genus.

**Der·ma·nys·sus** (dər"mə-nis'əs) [*derma-* + Gr. *nyssein* to prick] a genus of mites of the family Dermanyssidae. *D. galli'nae,* the bird mite or chicken mite, infests poultry and sometimes humans.

**der·ma·skel·e·ton** (dər"mə-skel'ə-tən) exoskeleton.

**der·ma·tan sul·fate** (der"mə-tan) [MeSH: Dermatan Sulfate] a glycosaminoglycan found mostly in the skin but also in blood vessels, tendons, heart valves, and pulmonary connective tissues. It consists of repeating disaccharide units in specific linkage, each composed of a (C-4) sulfated *N*-acetylgalactosamine linked to a uronic acid, generally L-iduronic acid, which is sometimes sulfated. It is an accumulation product in several mucopolysaccharidoses.

**der·ma·tit·i·des** (dər"mə-tit'ĭ-dēz) [MeSH: Dermatitis] plural of *dermatitis.*

**der·ma·ti·tis** (der"mə-ti'tis) pl. *dermati'tides* [*dermato-* + *-itis*] [MeSH: Dermatitis] inflammation of the skin.

## Dermatitis

**acral lick d.,** a psychogenic skin condition in dogs in which they lick excessively on a distal part of a limb until a thickened plaque or ulcer forms; the usual cause is boredom from enforced inactivity, but sometimes the licked area may be overlying a fracture, arthritic lesion, or area of nerve damage. Called also *acral lick granuloma.*

**actinic d.,** dermatitis resulting from exposure to actinic radiation, such as that from the sun, ultraviolet waves, or x- or gamma radiation.

**allergic d.,** 1. atopic d. 2. allergic contact d.

**allergic contact d.,** contact dermatitis due to allergic sensitization to various substances that produce inflammatory reactions in the skin of those who have acquired hypersensitivity to the allergen as a result of previous exposure to it. Called also *allergic d., contact d.,* and *d. venenata.* Cf. *irritant d.*

**ammonia d.,** diaper d.

**d. artefac'ta,** factitial d.

**ashy d.,** erythema dyschromicum perstans.

**atopic d.,** a chronic type seen in those with a hereditary susceptibility to pruritus; it may be accompanied by allergic rhinitis, hay fever, and asthma. The extreme pruritus often leads to scratching and rubbing that in turn results in the typical lesions of eczema. In infants *(infantile eczema),* it usually occurs on the cheeks and then may extend to other areas; in older children and adults it is found chiefly on the flexural surfaces *(flexural eczema),* especially on the antecubital and popliteal areas, and on the neck, eyelids, and wrists and behind the ears. Called also *allergic d., allergic* or *atopic eczema,* and *Besnier's prurigo.*

**berlock d., berloque d.** [Fr. *berloque,* Ger. *Berlocke* pendant], phytophotodermatitis due to sequential exposure to cologne, perfume, or other toilet articles containing bergamot oil and then to sunlight. In women, the lesions usually present as brown pigmented patches on the sides of the neck, behind the ears, and sometimes on the face, breasts, shoulders, or elsewhere. Aftershave lotion containing bergamot oil or a related substance may cause a similar reaction in men. Called also *perfume d.*

**brown-tail moth d.,** a type of insect dermatitis produced by the hairs of the brown-tail moth, *Euproctis chrysorrhoea;* called also *brown-tail rash.*

**d. bullo'sa stria'ta praten'sis,** phytophotodermatitis manifested as a bizarrely arranged linear or streaky eruption of vesicles and bullae that heal with intense residual melanoderma, caused by contact with meadow grass, usually *Agrimonia eupatoria,* and then exposure to sunlight. Called also *grass disease, meadow d., meadow-grass d.,* and *d. striata pratensis bullosa.*

**d. calo'rica,** inflammation of the skin due to heat or cold. Cf. *erythema ab igne* and *cold erythema.*

**caterpillar d.,** insect dermatitis caused by caterpillar hairs.

**cercarial d.,** a severely pruritic papular eruption occurring in those who swim or wade in certain bodies of fresh or salt water, due to hypersensitivity to the cercariae of schistosomes in the water that penetrate the skin and die without gaining access to the circulation and deeper tissues, evoking an inflammatory reaction. Called also *clam diggers' itch, cutaneous schistosomiasis, schistosome d.,* and *swimmers' d.* or *itch.*

**chigger d.,** dermatitis due to infestation with chiggers; see also *trombiculiasis.*

**contact d.,** acute or chronic dermatitis caused by materials or substances coming in contact with the skin, which may involve either allergic or nonallergic mechanisms. See *allergic contact d.* and *irritant d.*

**contagious pustular d.,** 1. contagious acne of horses. 2. contagious ecthyma.

**cosmetic d.,** allergic contact dermatitis caused by some ingredient in a cosmetic preparation.

**dhobie mark d.,** dhobie mark itch.

**diaper d.,** irritant dermatitis in the area in contact with the diaper in infants, often sparing the genitocrural folds, occurring as a reaction to prolonged contact with urine and feces, retained soaps and topical preparations, and friction and maceration, and commonly associated with secondary bacterial and yeast infections, especially with *Candida albicans.* Some consider irritation by the ammoniac decomposition products of urine to be a contributing factor. Called also *diaper rash, ammonia* or *napkin d.,* and *Jacquet's d.* or *erythema.*

**eczematous d.,** eczema.

**d. exfoliati'va,** exfoliative d.

**d. exfoliati'va neonato'rum,** staphylococcal scalded skin syndrome.

**exfoliative d.,** widespread involvement of the skin by a scaly erythematous dermatitis occurring as a secondary or reactive process to an underlying cutaneous disorder (e.g., atopic dermatitis, psoriasis, scabies, lichen planus) or as a primary or idiopathic disorder, and often associated with loss of hair and nails, hyperkeratosis of the palms and soles, pruritus, and sometimes severe and debilitating secondary physiological effects. Called also *d. exfoliativa, erythroderma,* and *pityriasis rubra (Hebra).*

**exudative discoid and lichenoid d.,** a form of neurodermatitis occurring predominantly in middle-aged or older men of Jewish extraction, characterized by intense pruritus with exudative, weeping discoid and oval patches scattered irregularly over most of the body, many of which are of the eczematous type and undergo lichenification, or they may resemble lesions seen in various other cutaneous disorders such as mycosis fungoides or lichen planus. Called also *oid-oid disease* and *Sulzberger-Garbe syndrome.*

**factitial d.,** various types of self-inflicted lesions, usually produced by mechanical means, burning, or application of chemical irritants or caustics. Called also *d. artefacta.*

**filarial d.,** 1. stephanofilariasis. 2. elaeophoriasis.

**d. gangreno'sa infan'tum,** a gangrenous disease occurring as a primary condition or secondarily to varicella or another exanthematous disease, chiefly in children under the age of 3, in which multiple small erosive and pustular lesions coalesce to form extensive sloughs, usually over the lower back and buttocks.

**gangrenous d.,** necrotic d.

**d. herpetifor'mis,** a chronic, relapsing multisystem disease in which the primary clinical manifestations are cutaneous, presenting as an extremely pruritic eruption consisting of various combinations of grouped, erythematous, symmetrical, papular, papulovesicular, vesicular, eczematous, and bullous lesions, which frequently heal with hyperpigmentation or occasionally hypopigmentation and sometimes scarring. It usually occurs in association with an asymptomatic gluten-sensitive enteropathy. The cause is unknown, but immunogenetic factors are thought to play a role. Called also *Duhring's disease.*

**d. hiema'lis,** dermatitis coming on with cold weather; cf. *xerotic eczema.*

**industrial d.,** occupational d.

**infectious eczematous d.,** a condition arising from a primary lesion that is the source of an infectious exudate (e.g., a boil, surgical wound, draining ear or nose), spreads by autoinoculation, and has a tendency to the formation of circumscribed eczematous plaques that enlarge gradually, and in which vesicles and pustules may occur.

**insect d.,** a transient localized or widespread dermatitis caused by the toxin-containing irritant hairs of certain insects, especially moths and their caterpillars, which may be associated with severe conjunctivitis, pruritus, a burning sensation, and pain; clinical manifestations vary according to the species involved and the intensity of exposure.

**interdigital d.,** dermatitis of the interdigital skin of sheep, with exudate, varying amounts of necrotic skin, and lameness, due to infection with *Fusobacterium necrophorum, Corynebacterium pyogenes,* or *Bacteroides nodosus.* It is worse in cold or wet weather and may be a precursor of foot rot. Called also *scald* and *foot scald.*

**irritant d.,** a nonallergic type of contact dermatitis due to exposure to a substance that damages the skin. Called also *primary irritant d.* Cf. *allergic contact d.*

**Jacquet's d.,** diaper d.

**livedoid d.,** a condition due to temporary or prolonged local ischemia resulting from vasculitis or accidental arterial obliteration from intragluteal administration of medications, marked by severe local pain, swelling, livedoid changes, and local increase in temperature; fever, tachycardia, dyspnea, and albuminuria also occur, and gangrene may supervene.

**marine d.,** swimmer's itch occurring in persons wading or swimming in salt water; called also *seabather's eruption.*

**meadow d., meadow-grass d.,** d. bullosa striata pratensis.

**d. medicamento'sa,** drug eruption.

**moth d.,** insect dermatitis caused by moth hairs.

**napkin d.,** diaper d.

**nasal solar d.,** actinic dermatitis of the nonpigmented parts of the nose of a dog, especially the bridge or the nasal plane; it is worse in the summer and may become inflamed or ulcerated. A similar but not identical condition occurs as part of some types of lupus. Called also *nasal eczema* and *collie nose.*

**necrotic d.,** a contagious, usually fatal disease of young chickens in which there is gangrenous necrosis of the skin of the thighs and breast, caused by infection with *Clostridium septicum* or some other *Clostridium* species. Chickens suffering from infectious bursal disease are particularly susceptible. Called also *gangrenous cellulitis* and *gangrenous d.*

**nickel d.,** allergic contact dermatitis caused by contact with nickel or a nickel-containing alloy.

**nummular eczematous d.,** see under *eczema.*

**occupational d.,** contact dermatitis caused by primary or allergic contactants found in the work place. Called also *industrial d.* and *industrial dermatosis.*

**onion mite d.,** dermatitis affecting handlers of decaying onions, caused by the onion mite, *Acarus rhyzoglypticus hyacinthi.*

**d. papilla'ris capilli'tii,** a rare disease seen most commonly in black males, characterized by the development of persistent hard follicular plaques along the posterior hairline of the scalp that fuse to form a thick, sclerotic, hypertrophic, pseudokeloidal band extending across the occiput. Called also *acne keloid, folliculitis keloidalis, keloidal folliculitis,* and *sycosis nuchae.*

***Pelodera* d.,** rhabditic d.

**perfume d.,** berlock d.

**periocular d.,** see *perioral d.*

**perioral d.,** a papular eruption of unknown etiology that progresses to residual papular erythema and scaling usually confined to the area about the mouth, and almost exclusively occurring in young women; it may also be localized or extend to involve the eyelids and adjacent glabella area of the forehead *(periocular d.)*

**photoallergic contact d.,** the cutaneous manifestations of photoallergy, consisting of a papulovesicular, eczematous, or exudative dermatitis, and occurring chiefly on the light-exposed areas of the skin. Called also *photocontact d.*

**photocontact d.,** photoallergic contact d.

**phototoxic d.,** an exaggerated sunburn-like reaction, sometimes with vesiculation, resulting in hyperpigmentation and desquamation, which occurs on the light-exposed areas of the skin as the cutaneous manifestation of phototoxicity.

**phytophototoxic d.,** phytophotodermatitis.

**pigmented purpuric lichenoid d.,** a purpuric cutaneous eruption usually seen in men 40–60 years of age, occurring chiefly on the legs, thighs, and lower trunk, and characterized by the presence of minute, rust-colored, lichenoid papules that tend to fuse into plaques, which may contain variously pigmented papules. Called also *Gougerot-Blum syndrome.*

**poison ivy d., poison oak d., poison sumac d.,** see *rhus d.*

**precancerous d.,** Bowen's disease.

**primary irritant d.,** irritant d.

**proliferative d.,** dermatophilosis of sheep.

**radiation d.,** radiodermatitis.

**rat-mite d.,** dermatitis resulting from the bite of *Ornithonyssus bacoti.*

**d. re'pens,** acrodermatitis continua.

**rhabditic d.,** a type of dermatitis found in domestic animals and occasionally spread to humans, due to invasion of a break in the skin by larvae of the nematode *Rhabditis strongyloides,* often as a result of sleeping in a damp, filthy bed. Called also *Pelodera d.*

**rhus d.,** allergic contact dermatitis due to exposure to plants of the genus *Rhus (Toxicodendron)* (poison ivy, poison oak, poison sumac), which contain urushiol, a potent skin-sensitizing agent.

**roentgen-ray d.,** radiodermatitis.

**sabra d.,** a dermatitis somewhat resembling scabies, affecting those who handle the fruit of cacti (sabra or prickly pear) and Indian figs in Israel; thought to be due to the penetration of minute thorns or hairs into the skin.

**schistosome d.,** cercarial d.

**seborrheic d., d. seborrhe'ica,** a chronic inflammatory disease of the skin of unknown etiology, characterized by moderate erythema, dry, moist, or greasy scaling, and yellow crusted patches on various areas, including the mid-parts of the face, ears, supraorbital regions, umbilicus, genitalia, and especially the scalp, where it is manifested by small patches of scales that progress to involve the entire scalp, with exfoliation of an excessive amount of dry scales (dandruff). The condition is usually accompanied by itching. Called also *seborrheic eczema* and *seborrhea.*

**stasis d.,** an often chronic, usually eczematous dermatitis, which initially involves the inner aspect of the lower leg just above the internal malleolus and which later may involve the entire lower leg or portions thereof, characterized by edema, pigmentation, and commonly ulceration; it is due to venous insufficiency.

**d. stria'ta praten'sis bullo'sa,** d. bullosa striata pratensis.

**swimmers' d.,** cercarial d.

**trefoil d.,** a photosensitization condition, similar to trifoliosis but without liver damage, seen in livestock that have eaten *Medicago polymorpha* (burr trefoil).

**uncinarial d.,** ground itch.

**d. ve'getans,** a cutaneous reaction to secondary infection with an eczematous lesion, especially in moist areas of the body such as axillae, groin, genitalia, and lips, which is characterized by the development of exuberant hypertrophic granulation tissue that may erode to form ulcers. A variant involving the oral mucosa and associated with ulcerative colitis or other gastrointestinal disturbance is known as pyostomatitis vegetans. Called also *pemphigus vegetans, Hallopeau type.*

**d. venena'ta,** 1. allergic contact d. 2. former name for contact dermatitis due to exposure to sensitizing agents in plants.

**verminous d.,** stephanofilariasis.

**verrucose d., verrucous d.,** 1. chromoblastomycosis. 2. a proliferative lesion of the skin of the leg in cattle, extending downwards from the fetlock joint along the pastern, usually on the hind legs, with hyperkeratosis and papillomas forming cauliflowerlike lesions. It usually occurs in crowded unsanitary conditions as a result of a bacterial infection, such as with *Fusobacterium necrophorum.*

**vesicular d.,** 1. dermatitis with vesicle formation. 2. a sometimes fatal disease, believed to be a photosensitization following ingestion of certain plants and seeds, affecting young poultry that range over unbroken prairie sod, marked by the formation of blisters and scabs on the feet and legs.

**viral papular d.,** a type of dermatitis seen in horses in the United States, Great Britain, and Australia, characterized by formation of firm papules followed by a dry crust that detaches and leaves small areas of alopecia.

**x-ray d.,** radiodermatitis.

---

**dermat(o)-** [Gr. *derma,* gen. *dermatos* skin] a combining form denoting relationship to the skin. Also, *derma-, derm(o)-.*

**der·ma·to·ar·thri·tis** (dər″mə-to-ahr-thri′tis) [*dermato-* + *arthritis*] skin disease associated with arthritis.

**lipid d., lipoid d.,** multicentric reticulohistiocytosis.

**der·ma·to·au·to·plas·ty** (dər″mə-to-aw′to-plas″te) [*dermato-* + *autoplasty*] the grafting on denuded areas of skin taken from some other portion of the patient's own body.

**Der·ma·to·bia** (dər″mə-to′be-ə) [*dermato-* + Gr. *bios* life] a genus of botflies of the family Oestridae.
**D. ho′minis,** the human botfly of South America whose larvae are parasitic in the skin of humans, mammals, and birds; the eggs are deposited on the bodies of mosquitoes, flies, or ticks, which then transport them to the host.

**der·ma·to·bi·a·sis** (dər″mə-to-bi′ə-sis) the presence of *Dermatobia* in the body.

**der·ma·to·chal·a·sis, der·ma·to·chal·a·zia** (dər″mə-to-kal′ə-sis, dər″mə-to-kəl-a′zhə) [*dermato-* + Gr. *chalasthai* to become slack] cutis laxa.

**der·ma·to·con·junc·ti·vi·tis** (dər″mə-to-kən-junk″tĭ-vi′tis) inflammation of the conjunctiva and of the skin around the eyes.

**der·ma·to·dys·pla·sia** (dər″mə-to-dis-pla′zhə) [*dermato-* + *dysplasia*] abnormal development of the skin.

**der·ma·to·fi·bro·ma** (dər″mə-to-fi-bro′mə) [*dermato-* + *fibroma*] [MeSH: Dermatofibroma] a benign, circumscribed, erythematous to brown nodular neoplasm occurring in the dermis, particularly on the lower extremities of women, often after minor trauma; it is composed of histiocytes which may differentiate to resemble fibroblasts. It is a form of benign fibrous histiocytoma, and the two terms are sometimes used synonymously. NOTE: Related terms describe lesions variously said to be synonymous with, similar to, or variants of dermatofibroma and/or benign fibrous histiocytoma; e.g., *nodular subepidermal fibrosis* and *sclerosing hemangioma.*
**d. protu′berans,** see under *dermatofibrosarcoma.*

**der·ma·to·fi·bro·sar·co·ma** (dər″mə-to-fi″bro-sahr-ko′mə) [*dermato-* + *fibrosarcoma*] [MeSH: Dermatofibrosarcoma] a fibrosarcoma of the skin.
**d. protu′berans,** a bulky, protuberant, nodular, fibrotic neoplasm occurring in the dermis, usually on the trunk, often extending into the subcutaneous fat; it is locally aggressive and frequently recurs. It is sometimes classified as a type of malignant fibrous histiocytoma.

**der·ma·to·fi·bro·sis** (dər″mə-to-fi-bro′sis) a condition characterized by fibrotic changes in the skin.
**d. lenticula′ris dissemina′ta,** an autosomal dominant syndrome, present at birth or appearing before puberty, characterized by the development of connective tissue nevi of the elastic type in association with osteopoikilosis; the skin lesions are manifested as small, firm, yellowish or skin-colored papules or plaques distributed symmetrically, primarily on the lower trunk and extremities. Called also *Buschke-Ollendorff syndrome.*

**der·ma·to·glyph·ics** (dər″mə-to-glif′iks) [*dermato-* + Gr. *glyphein* to carve] [MeSH: Dermatoglyphics] the study of the patterns of ridges of the skin of the fingers, palms, toes, and soles; of interest in anthropology and law enforcement as a means of establishing identity and in medicine, both clinically and as a genetic indicator, particularly of chromosomal abnormalities.

**der·ma·to·graph·ic** (dər″mə-to-graf′ik) pertaining to or characterized by dermatographism.

**der·ma·tog·ra·phism** (dər″mə-tog′rə-fiz″əm) urticaria due to physical allergy, in which moderately firm stroking or scratching of the skin with a dull instrument produces a pale, raised welt or wheal, with a red flare on each side; see also *white d.* and *black d.*
**black d.,** black or greenish streaking of the skin caused by deposit of fine metallic particles abraded from jewelry by various dusting powders.
**white d.,** linear blanching of (usually erythematous) skin of persons with atopic dermatitis in response to firm stroking with a blunt instrument.

**der·ma·to·het·ero·plas·ty** (dər″mə-to-het′ər-o-plas″te) [*dermato-* + *heteroplasty*] the grafting of skin derived from a member of another species.

**der·ma·to·log·ic, der·ma·to·log·i·cal** (dər″mə-to-loj′ik, dər″mə-to-loj′ĭ-kəl) pertaining to dermatology; of or affecting the skin.

**der·ma·tol·o·gist** (dər″mə-tol′o-jist) a physician who limits his practice to the diagnosis and treatment of skin disorders.

**der·ma·tol·o·gy** (dər″mə-tol′o-je) [MeSH: Dermatology] the medical specialty concerned with the diagnosis and treatment of diseases of the skin.

**der·ma·tol·y·sis** (dər″mə-tol′ə-sis) [*dermato-* + *-lysis*] cutis laxa.
**d. palpebra′rum,** blepharochalasis.

**der·ma·tome** (dər′mə-tōm) [*derma-* + *-tome*] 1. an instrument for cutting thin skin slices for skin grafts. 2. the area of skin supplied with afferent nerve fibers by a single posterior spinal root; called also *dermatomic area.* 3. the lateral portion of a mesodermal somite; the cutis plate.
**Brown d.,** an electric dermatome, the first to be developed, for cutting split-thickness skin grafts; it enables the surgeon to rapidly remove long strips of skin.

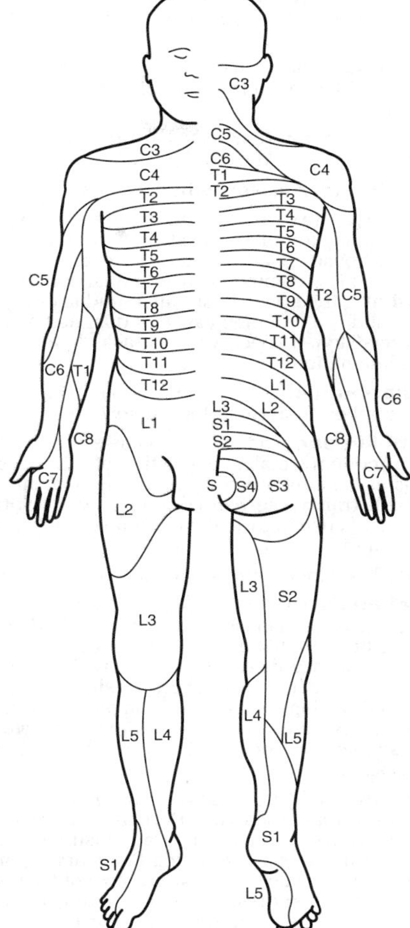

Anterior and posterior views of the dermatomes.

**Castroviejo d.,** an electric dermatome used for cutting mucous membrane grafts for the treatment of eyelid and socket deformities and as an adjunct in the removal of tattoos after the initial excision has been done using either the Brown or Padgett dermatomes. It has a tiny cutting head with special blades and skims to control the thickness of the cut.
**Padgett d.,** an instrument for rapid cutting of split-thickness skin grafts of any desired thickness.
**Reese d.,** an instrument for cutting split-thickness skin grafts that permits careful calibration of the thickness of the graft.

**der·ma·to·meg·a·ly** (dər″mə-to-meg′ə-le) cutis laxa.

**der·ma·to·mere** (dər′mə-to-mēr″) [*dermato-* + *-mere*] any segment or metamere of the embryonic integument.

**der·ma·tom·ic** (dər″mə-tom′ik) pertaining to a dermatome, def. 2.

**der·ma·to·my·co·sis** (dər″mə-to-mi-ko′sis) [*dermato-* + *mycosis*] a superficial infection of the skin or its appendages by fungi. The term includes dermatophytosis and the various clinical forms of tinea, as well as deep fungous infections. Called also *epidermomycosis.*
**d. furfura′cea,** tinea versicolor.

**der·ma·to·my·ia·sis** (dər″mə-to-mi-i′ə-sis) [*dermato-* + *myiasis*] myiasis linearis.

**der·ma·to·my·o·ma** (dər″mə-to-mi-o′mə) [*dermato-* + *myoma*] leiomyoma cutis.

**der·ma·to·myo·si·tis** (dər″mə-to-mi″ə-si′tis) [*dermato-* + *myositis*] [MeSH: Dermatomyositis] polymyositis occurring in association with characteristic inflammatory skin changes, including Gottron's sign (flat-topped violaceous papules over the dorsal aspects of the knuckles), which is pathognomonic; a violaceous or heliotrope rash on the upper eyelids accompanied by edema of the eyelids and periorbital tissue; and an erythematous rash on the forehead, neck, shoulders, trunk, and arms.

**der·ma·to·neu·rol·o·gy** (dər″mə-to-n͝oo-rol′ə-je) [*dermato-* + *neurology*] the study of the nerves of the skin in health and disease.

**der·ma·to·oph·thal·mi·tis** (dər″mə-to-of″thəl-mi′tis) inflammation of the skin and of the eye, including the conjunctiva, cornea, etc.

**der·ma·to·path·ic** (dər″mə-to-path′ik) pertaining or attributable to disease of the skin, as dermatopathic lymphadenopathy. Called also *dermopathic.*

**der·ma·to·pa·thol·o·gy** (dər″mə-to-pə-thol′ə-je) microscopic anatomic pathology of the skin.

**der·ma·top·a·thy** (dər″mə-top′ə-the) dermatosis.

**Der·ma·toph·a·goi·des** (dər″mə-tof″ə-goi′dēs) a genus of sarcoptiform mites, usually found on the skin of chickens.
**D. fari′nae,** the house dust mite found in North America, which acts as an antigen and is a common cause of dust asthma.
**D. pteronyssi′nus,** the house dust mite found in Europe, which acts as an antigen and is a common cause of dust asthma.
**D. scheremetew′skyi,** a species that attacks humans and causes a mangelike inflammation.

**der·ma·to·phar·ma·col·o·gy** (dər″mə-to-fahr″mə-kol′ə-je) pharmacology as applied to dermatologic disorders.

**Der·ma·to·phi·la·ceae** (dər″mə-to-fi-la′se-e) a family of bacteria of the order Actinomycetales, consisting of gram-positive aerobic microorganisms characterized by mycelial filaments or muriform thalli that divide transversely and in at least two longitudinal planes to form masses of coccoid or cuboid motile cells. It includes genera *Dermatophilus* and *Geodermatophilus.*

**der·ma·to·phi·li·a·sis** (dər″mə-to-fĭ-li′ə-sis) dermatophilosis.

**der·ma·to·phi·lo·sis** (dər″mə-to-fĭ-lo′sis) 1. infection with *Dermatophilus congolensis,* seen in cattle, sheep, horses, dogs, goats, deer, and sometimes humans. In humans it is characterized by nonpainful pustules on the hands and arms that later break down, forming shallow red ulcers that heal to leave scars. In sheep it is characterized by exudative red scaling lesions that form pyramidal masses. Called also *dermatophiliasis* and (in sheep) *lumpy wool, proliferative dermatitis,* and *strawberry foot rot.* 2. a term sometimes incorrectly used for *tungiasis.*

**Der·ma·toph·i·lus** (dər″mə-tof′ĭ-ləs) [*dermato-* + Gr. *philos* loving] 1. a genus of bacteria of the family Dermatophilaceae, consisting of aerobic or facultatively anaerobic, gram-positive, nonacid-fast organisms that form mycelia containing filaments segmenting transversely and longitudinally to produce coccoid cells in packets, which become motile spores. They are pathogenic for mammals, involving the uncornified epidermis. 2. *Tunga.*
**D. congolen′sis,** the etiologic agent of dermatophilosis; called also *Streptothrix bovis.*
**D. pe′netrans,** an incorrect name sometimes used for *Tunga penetrans.*

**der·ma·to·phyte** (dər′mə-to-fīt″) [*dermato-* + *-phyte*] any of a group of imperfect fungi parasitic on keratinized tissue (skin, nails, or hair) of humans (anthropophilic) or other animals (zoophilic); some usually found in soil (geophilic) will infect patients who are weak or immunocompromised. The three most common infecting genera are *Microsporum, Epidermophyton,* and *Trichophyton.*

**der·ma·to·phy·tid** (dər″mə-tof′ĭ-tid) [*dermatophyte* + *-id*] an id reaction associated with a dermatophytosis, which may be associated with various types of lesions but with the most common being vesicles occurring on the hands, wrists, and sides of the fingers in association with tinea pedis. Called also *epidermophytid* and *mycid.*

**der·ma·to·phy·to·sis** (dər″mə-to-fi-to′sis) [*dermatophyte* +*-osis*] 1. any superficial fungal infection caused by a dermatophyte and involving the stratum corneum of the skin, hair, and nails, including onychomycosis and the various forms of tinea. Called also *epidermomycosis* and *epidermophytosis.* 2. in veterinary medicine, infection of the skin of an animal by a fungus of either genus *Microsporum* or *Trichophyton;* called also *ringworm.* 3. tinea pedis.

**der·ma·to·plas·tic** (dər″mə-to-plas′tik) pertaining to dermatoplasty.

**der·ma·to·plas·ty** (dər′mə-to-plas″te) [*dermato-* + *-plasty*] a plastic operation on the skin; operative replacement of destroyed or lost skin.

**der·ma·to·poly·neu·ri·tis** (dər″mə-to-pol″e-noo͞-ri′tis) acrodynia.

**der·ma·tor·rha·gia** (dər″mə-to-ra′jə) discharge of blood into or from the skin.
**d. parasi′tica,** a disease of the skin of horses, other equids, and cattle in Europe and Asia, marked by hard elevations formed by accumulations of blood between skin layers; the cause is a parasitic worm, *Parafilaria multipapillosa* (in equids) or *P. bovicola* (in cattle). Called also *summer bleeding.*

**der·ma·tor·rhex·is** (der″mah-to-rek′sis) [*dermato-* + *-rrhexis*] rupture of the skin capillaries, as in Ehlers-Danlos syndrome.

**der·ma·to·scle·ro·sis** (der″mə-to-sklə-ro′sis) [*dermato-* + *sclerosis*] scleroderma.

**der·ma·to·sis** (der″mə-to′sis) pl. *dermato′ses* [*dermat-* + *-osis*] any skin disease, especially one not characterized by inflammation.
**acute febrile neutrophilic d.,** a condition usually seen on the upper body of middle-aged women, characterized by the presence of one or more large, rapidly extending, erythematous, tender or painful plaques, and occurring in association with fever and dense infiltration of neutrophilic leukocytes in the upper and middle dermis. Called also *Sweet's syndrome.*
**ashy d. of Ramirez,** erythema dyschromicum perstans.
**Bowen's precancerous d.,** Bowen's disease.
**d. cenicien′ta,** erythema dyschromicum perstans.
**chronic bullous d. of childhood,** an autoimmune skin disorder seen in infants and children up to age 5, characterized by deposition of immunoglobulin A in lines along the dermoepidermal junction, forming vesicular bulbous lesions. See also *linear IgA d. of adulthood.* Called also *linear IgA d. of childhood.*
**dermatolytic bullous d.,** epidermolysis bullosa dystrophica.
**industrial d.,** occupational dermatitis.
**lichenoid d.,** any skin disorder characterized by lichenification.
**linear IgA d. of adulthood,** an autoimmune skin disorder usually seen in adults over age 60, clinically resembling bullous pemphigoid. Characteristics include deposition of immunoglobulin A in lines along the dermoepidermal junction, forming vesicular bullous lesions. Cf. *chronic bullous d. of childhood.*
**linear IgA d. of childhood,** chronic bullous d. of childhood.
**d. papulo′sa ni′gra,** a variant of seborrheic keratosis seen almost exclusively in blacks, characterized by the development of small, pedunculated, pigmented papules on the malar regions, upper cheeks, or lateral orbital areas.
**precancerous d.,** any skin condition having a tendency to malignant change.
**progressive pigmentary d.,** Schamberg's disease.
**Schamberg's d., Schamberg's progressive pigmented purpuric d.,** see under *disease.*
**subcorneal pustular d.,** a chronic, superficial, pustular disorder with a chronic relapsing course, resembling dermatitis herpetiformis, and chiefly affecting women in middle life, with sterile pustular blebs beneath the horny layer of the epidermis on the trunk and in the major skin folds. Called also *Sneddon-Wilkinson disease.*
**transient acantholytic d.,** a self-limited papulovesicular disease occurring in middle-aged individuals and having a predilection for the trunk; the histologic changes are suggestive of keratosis follicularis or benign familial pemphigus. It may be an epidermal reaction to actinic injury.
**ulcerative d.,** an infectious viral skin disease of sheep characterized by skin ulcers around the mouth, nose, legs, and external genitalia; the genital ulcers are venereal in nature and may be so painful as to prevent copulation.
**d. ve′getans,** a hereditary disease of young pigs characterized by raised skin lesions, abnormalities of the hooves, and pneumonitis.

**der·ma·to·some** (dər′mə-to-sōm″) [*dermato-* + *-some*] a thickening on each spindle fiber in the equatorial region during mitosis.

**der·ma·to·spa·rax·is** (dər″mə-to-spə-rak′sis) [*dermato-* + Gr. *sparaxis, sparagmos* a tearing] cutaneous asthenia (def. 1).

**der·ma·to·ther·a·py** (dər″mə-to-ther′ə-pe) [*dermato-* + *therapy*] treatment of the skin and its diseases.

**der·ma·to·trop·ic** (dər″mə-to-trop′ik) [*dermato-* + *-tropic*] preferentially infecting, infesting, or affecting the skin; said of certain microorganisms. Called also *dermotropic.*

**der·ma·to·zo·ia·sis** (dər″mə-to-zo-i′ə-sis) dermatozoonosis.

**der·ma·to·zo·on** (dər″mə-to-zo′ən) [*dermato-* + Gr. *zōon* animal] any animal parasite of the skin; an ectoparasite.

**der·ma·to·zoo·no·sis** (dər″mə-to-zo″o-no′sis) [*dermato-* + *zoonosis*] a skin disease caused by a dermatozoon; called also *dermatozoiasis.*

**der·mic** (dər′mik) dermal; cutaneous.

**der·mis** (dər′mis) [Gr. *derma* skin, hide] [TA] the layer of the skin deep to the epidermis, consisting of a dense bed of vascular connective tissue; called also *corium* [TA alternative].

**derm(o)-** see *dermat(o)-.*

**der·mo·blast** (dər′mo-blast) [*dermo-* + *-blast*] that part of the mesoblast which develops into the true skin or corium.

**der·mo·cy·ma** (dər″mo-si′mə) [*dermo-* + Gr. *kyma* fetus] endadelphos.

**der·mo·cy·mus** (dər″mo-si′məs) endadelphos.

**der·mo·graph·ism** (dər″mo-graf′iz-əm) dermatographism.

**der·mo·hy·grom·e·ter** (dər″mo-hi-grom′ə-tər) an instrument for measuring skin resistance without inducing a constant current into the skin.

**der·moid** (dər'moid) [*derm-* + *-oid*] 1. resembling skin. 2. dermoid cyst.
**corneal d.,** a hairy tumorous growth on the cornea of certain mammals.

**der·moid·ec·to·my** (dər"moid-ek'tə-me) [*dermoid* + *-ectomy*] excision of a dermoid cyst.

**der·mo·li·pec·to·my** (dər"mo-lĭ-pek'tə-me) [*dermo* + *lipectomy*] resection of excess skin and fat, usually from the abdomen.

**der·mo·li·po·ma** (dər"mo-lĭ-po'mə) a congenital yellow fatty growth beneath the bulbar conjunctiva.

**der·mom·e·ter** (dər-mom'ə-tər) the instrument used in dermometry.

**der·mom·e·try** (dər-mom'ə-tre) [*dermo-* + *-metry*] the measurement of areas of skin resistance to a passage of direct electric current; these areas will correspond to the areas of sensory loss.

**der·mo·myo·tome** (dər"mo-mi'o-tōm) [*dermo-* + *myo-* + *-tome*] all but the sclerotome of a mesodermal somite; the primordium of skeletal muscle and, perhaps, of corium.

**der·mo·neu·ro·trop·ic** (dər"mo-noor"o-trop'ik) having an affinity for the skin and nervous tissue.

**der·mo·path·ic** (dər"mo-path'ik) dermatopathic; pertaining to dermopathy.

**der·mop·a·thy** (dər-mop'ə-the) dermatosis.
**diabetic d.,** any of several cutaneous lesions, usually manifestations of diabetes mellitus, consisting of papular, ulcerated, pigmented, macular, or cicatricial lesions of the shins *(shin spots);* similar lesions may occur after trauma in nondiabetic patients. The cause is apparently a type of angiitis of small cutaneous blood vessels. The term is sometimes broadened to include bullae on the feet or ankles of diabetic patients or necrobiosis lipoidica diabeticorum. Called also *diabetid.*
**infiltrative d.,** pretibial myxedema.

**der·mo·plas·ty** (dər'mo-plas"te) dermatoplasty.

**der·mo·re·ac·tion** (dər"mo-re-ak'shən) cutaneous reaction.

**der·mo·skel·e·ton** (dər"mo-skel'ə-tən) exoskeleton.

**der·mo·syn·o·vi·tis** (dər"mo-sin"o-vi'tis) [*dermo-* + *synovitis*] inflammation of skin overlying an inflamed bursa or tendon sheath.

**der·mo·tox·in** (dər"mo-tok'sin) a toxin produced by certain bacteria, especially staphylococci, which causes necrosis and other pathologic changes of the skin.

**der·mo·trop·ic** (dər"mo-trop'ik) dermatotropic.

**der·mo·vas·cu·lar** (dər"mo-vas'ku-lər) [*dermo-* + *vascular*] pertaining to the blood vessels of the skin.

**der(o)-** [Gr. *derē* neck] a combining form denoting relationship to the neck.

**der·o·did·y·mus** (der"o-did'ə-məs) dicephalus.

**der·ren·ga·de·ra** (da-rāng-gah-da'rah) [Sp. "crookedness" or "lameness"] murrina.

**der·ren·gue** (da-rāng'ga) [Sp. from *derrengar* to dislocate the hip] a fatal neuropathy of cattle seen in El Salvador following ingestion of the plant *Melochia pyramidata,* characterized by weakness and paralysis starting in the hindlimbs and progressing forward.

**der·ri·en·gue** (dar-yāng'ga) [Sp. from *derrengar* to dislocate the hip] rabies, usually of the paralytic form, transmitted by vampire bats in Mexico, South and Central America, and Trinidad. It is usually seen in cattle, but infected bats may attack other domestic animals and even humans.

**Der·ris** (der'is) a genus of woody vines of the family Leguminosae, native to Australia and other islands of the southern Pacific. *D. ellip'tica* yields the toxic insecticide rotenone.

**der·ris** (der'is) 1. any plant of the genus *Derris.* 2. the dried roots and rhizomes of *Derris elliptica,* a source of the toxic insecticide rotenone.

**DES** diethylstilbestrol.

**de·sal·i·na·tion** (de-sal"ĭ-na'shən) [*de-* + *sal*] the removal of salt from a substance.

**de·sal·i·va·tion** (de-sal"ĭ-va'shən) the depriving of saliva.

**des·am·i·do-NAD**$^+$ (des-ə-me'do) deaminated NAD$^+$, an intermediate in the biosynthesis of NAD$^+$. It is nicotinate ribonucleotide coupled in pyrophosphate linkage to adenosine monophosphate.

**De Sanc·tis-Cac·chi·o·ne syndrome** (da-sahngk'tis kah"keo'na) [Carlo *De Sanctis,* Italian psychiatrist, born 1888; Aldo *Cacchione,* Italian psychiatrist, 20th century] see under *syndrome.*

**de·sat·ur·ase** (de-sach'ə-rās) an enzyme that, complexed with cytochrome $b_5$ reductase and cytochrome $b_5$, catalyzes the desaturation of fatty acids, e.g., stearoyl-CoA desaturase.

**de·sat·u·ra·tion** (de-sach"ə-ra'shən) the process of converting a saturated compound to one that is unsaturated, such as the introduction of a double bond between carbon atoms of a fatty acid.

**De·sault's bandage (apparatus), sign** (də-sōz') [Pierre Joseph *Desault,* French surgeon, 1744–1795] see under *bandage* and *sign.*

**Des·cartes' law** (da-kahrts') [René *Descartes,* French mathematician and philosopher, 1596–1650] see under *law.*

**Des·ce·met's membrane** (des-ə-māz') [Jean *Descemet,* French anatomist, 1732–1810] [MeSH: Descemet's Membrane] lamina limitans posterior corneae.

**des·ce·me·ti·tis** (des"ə-mə-ti'tis) inflammation of Descemet's membrane.

**des·ce·me·to·cele** (des"ə-met'o-sēl) [*Descemet's membrane* + *-cele*[1]] herniation of Descemet's membrane.

**des·cen·dens** (de-sen'dənz) [L.] descending; a general term denoting a descending structure or part.
**d. cervica'lis, d. cer'vicis,** radix inferior ansae cervicalis.
**d. hypoglos'si,** radix superior ansae cervicalis.

**des·cend·ing** (de-send'ing) [L. *descendere* to go down] extending inferiorly.

**des·cen·sus** (de-sen'səs) pl. *descen'sus* [L.] the process of descending or falling.
**d. tes'tis,** the descent of the testis from its fetal position in the abdominal cavity to the scrotum; it normally occurs during the twenty-eighth week of fetal life and is essential to spermatogenesis.
**d. u'teri,** prolapse of the uterus.

**de·scent** (də-sent') [L. *descendere* to go down] the act or instance of descending.
**x d.,** see under *wave.*
**y d.,** see under *wave.*

**Des·champs' compressor, needle** (da-shahz') [Joseph François Louis *Deschamps,* French surgeon, 1740–1824] see under *compressor* and *needle.*

**de·sen·si·ti·za·tion** (de-sen"sĭ-tĭ-za'shən) 1. the prevention or reduction of immediate hypersensitivity reactions by administration of graded doses of allergen; called also *hyposensitization* and *immunotherapy.* 2. in behavior therapy, the treatment of phobias and related disorders by intentionally exposing the patient, in imagination or in real life, to a hierarchy of emotionally distressing stimuli. Common forms of desensitization include flooding, implosion, and systematic desensitization (qq.v.).
**systematic d.,** a form of desensitization therapy in which the patient is taught to relax and is then exposed, in imagination, to the mildest or least anxiety-provoking stimuli first; as treatment progresses he is exposed progressively to stronger anxiety-provoking stimuli until he can tolerate the most extreme stimuli.

**de·sen·si·tize** (de-sen'sĭ-tīz) 1. to deprive of sensation; paralysis of a sensory nerve by section or blocking. 2. to carry out desensitization.

**de·ser·pi·dine** (de-sər'pĭ-dēn) an alkaloid of *Rauwolfia canescens,* used as an antihypertensive and tranquilizer, administered orally.

**de·sex·u·al·ize** (de-sek'shoo-əl-īz") castrate.

**Des·fer·al** (des'fər-əl) trademark for a preparation of deferoxamine mesylate.

**des·fer·ri·ox·amine** (des-fer"e-oks'ə-mēn) deferoxamine.

**des·flu·rane** (des-floo'rān) [USP] an inhalational anesthetic used for induction and maintenance of general anesthesia.

**des·hy·dre·mia** (des"hi-dre'me-ə) [*de-* + *hydremia*] deficiency of the watery element of the blood, with resultant hemoconcentration.

**des·ic·cant** (des'ĭ-kənt) 1. promoting dryness; causing to dry up. 2. an agent that promotes dryness. Called also *exsiccant.*

**des·ic·cate** (des'ĭ-kāt) [L. *desiccare* to dry up] to render thoroughly dry.

**des·ic·ca·tion** (des"ĭ-ka'shən) [MeSH: Desiccation] the act of drying up.
**electric d.,** the treatment of a tumor or other disease by drying up the part by the application of a monopolar electric current (short spark) of high frequency and high tension.

**des·ic·ca·tive** (des'ĭ-ka"tiv) causing to dry up.

**des·ic·ca·tor** (des'ĭ-ka"tor) a closed vessel for containing apparatus or chemicals that are to be kept free from moisture.

**de·sip·ra·mine hy·dro·chlo·ride** (də-sip'rə-mēn) [USP] a metabolite of imipramine: a tricyclic antidepressant of the dibenzazepine class; used also in the treatment of anxiety, chronic pain, attention-deficit/hyperactivity disorder, cataplexy associated with narcolepsy, and bulimia. Administered orally.

**-desis** [Gr. *desis* "a binding together"] a word termination denoting a binding or fusion.

**Des·jar·dins' point** (da″zhahr-daz′) [Abel *Desjardins,* French surgeon, early 20th century] see under *point.*

**des·lan·o·side** (des-lan′o-sīd) [USP] [MeSH: Deslanoside] a digitalis glycoside derived from lanatoside C, having the same actions and uses as digitalis; administered intramuscularly or intravenously. Called also *deacetyllanatoside C.*

**des·mal·gia** (des-mal′jə) [*desmo-* + *-algia*] pain in a ligament; called also *desmodynia.*

**des·mec·ta·sis** (des-mek′tə-sis) [*desmo-* + *ektasis*] the stretching of a ligament.

**des·mep·i·the·li·um** (des-mep″ĭ-the′le-əm) [*desmo-* + *epithelium*] the endothelial lining of blood vessels, lymphatics, and synovial membranes.

**des·mid** (des′mid) unicellular, free-floating, aquatic algae characterized by symmetrical, curved, spiny or lacey bodies with a median constriction dividing the cell into two equal halves.

**des·min** (dez′min) [MeSH: Desmin] a protein that polymerizes to form the intermediate filaments of muscle cells; it is used as an immunohistochemical marker of these cells. See also *desmin filaments.*

**des·mi·og·nath·us** (des″me-o-nath′əs) [Gr. *desmios* binding + *gnathos* jaw] a fetus with a parasitic head attached to the jaw or neck; called also *dicephalus parasiticus.*

**des·mi·tis** (des-mi′tis) [*desmo-* + *-itis*] inflammation of a ligament.

**desm(o)-** [Gr. *desmos* band, ligament] a combining form denoting relationship to a band, bond, or ligament.

**des·mo·cra·ni·um** (des″mo-kra′ne-əm) [*desmo-* + *cranium*] [TA] the mass of mesoderm at the cranial end of the notochord in the early embryo, forming the earliest stage of the skull.

**des·mo·cyte** (des′mo-sīt) [*desmo-* + *-cyte*] fibroblast.

**des·mo·cy·to·ma** (des″mo-si-to′mə) fibroma.

**des·mo·don·ti·um** (des″mo-don′she-əm) [*desmo-* + Gr. *odous* tooth] [TA] periodontal ligament.

**Des·mo·dus** (dez-mo′dəs) a genus of vampire bats of South America, Central America, Mexico, and the West Indies.

**des·mo·dyn·ia** (des″mo-din′e-ə) [*desm-* + *-odynia*] desmalgia.

**des·mog·e·nous** (des-moj′ə-nəs) [*desmo-* + *-genous*] of ligamentous origin.

**des·mog·ra·phy** (des-mog′rə-fe) [*desmo-* + *-graphy*] a description of the ligaments.

**des·mo·he·mo·blast** (dez″mo-he′mo-blast) [*desmo-* + *hemoblast*] mesenchyma.

**des·moid** (dez′moid) [*desm-* + *-oid*] 1. fibrous or fibroid. 2. see under *tumor.*
**periosteal d.,** a benign tumorlike fibrous proliferation of the periosteum, occurring particularly in the medial femoral condyle in adolescents, and often disappearing spontaneously.

**des·mo·lase** (dez′mo-lās) a nonspecific term for an enzyme that catalyzes the cleavage of a carbon-carbon bond in a substrate with formation of two products by a process other than hydrolysis, i.e., an oxidoreductase, a lyase, or a transferase. Used especially for enzymes involved in synthesis of steroid hormones.
**17,20-d.,** 17$\alpha$-hydroxyprogesterone aldolase.
**20,22-d.,** cholesterol monooxygenase (side-chain-cleaving).

**des·mol·o·gy** (des-mol′ə-je) [*desmo-* + *-logy*] 1. the study of ligaments, their structure and function. 2. the art of bandaging.

**des·mo·ma** (dez-mo′mə) [*desm-* + *-oma*] desmoid tumor.

**des·mop·a·thy** (des-mop′ə-the) [*desmo-* + *-pathy*] any disease of the ligaments.

**des·mo·pla·sia** (des″mo-pla′zhə) the formation and development of fibrous tissue.

**des·mo·plas·tic** (des″mo-plas′tik) [*desmo-* + *-plastic*] characterized by or causing desmoplasia.

**des·mo·pres·sin ace·tate** (des″mo-pres′in) a potent synthetic analogue of vasopressin, used intranasally, intramuscularly, or intravenously as an antidiuretic in pituitary diabetes insipidus and intravenously to increase coagulation factor VIII activity before surgical procedures in patients with hemophilia and von Willebrand's disease.

**des·mor·rhex·is** (des″mo-rek′sis) [*desmo-* + *-rrhexis*] rupture of a ligament.

**des·mose** (des′mōs) [Gr. *desmos* band, ligament] a filament, fibril, or strand connecting intranuclear *(centrodesmose)* or extranuclear *(paradesmose)* basal bodies during mitosis; seen especially in certain protozoa (e.g., *Dientamoeba fragilis*). The terms *desmose, centrodesmose,* and *paradesmose* have been used synonymously by some authorities.

**des·mo·sine** (des′mo-sēn) [MeSH: Desmosine] one of two unusual amino acids found in elastin, the other being isodesmosine.

**des·mo·sis** (des-mo′sis) [*desm-* + *-osis*] a disease of the connective tissue.

**des·mo·some** (dez′mo-sōm) [*desmo-* + *-some*] [MeSH: Desmosomes] a type of adherent junction that links intermediate filaments and cell membranes within and between cells; it is a small, discrete, circular, dense body abundant in epithelial cells but occurring also in other cell types. It consists of local differentiations of the apposing cell membranes, with a dense cytoplasmic plaque underlying each membrane, toward which numerous tonofilaments converge; a dense lamina may occur within the intercellular gap. Called also *macula adherens.*
**belt d.,** zonula adherens; by extension sometimes also used for the fascia adherens.
**half d.,** hemidesmosome.
**spot d.,** desmosome.

**des·mos·ter·ol** (des-mos′tər-ol) [MeSH: Desmosterol] the immediate precursor of cholesterol in the biosynthetic pathway, 24-dehydrocholesterol; normally not present in the blood in amounts that can be detected by ordinary means.

**des·mot·o·my** (des-mot′o-me) [*desmo-* + *-tomy*] the cutting or division of ligaments.

**des·o·ges·trel** (dez″o-jes′trəl) [MeSH: Desogestrel] a progestational agent used in oral contraceptives.

**deso·leo·lec·i·thin** (des-o″le-o-les′ĭ-thin) one of the components, the other being oleic acid, into which lecithin is split by the action of cobra venom.

**des·o·nide** (des′ə-nīd) [MeSH: Desonide] a synthetic corticosteroid used topically for the relief of inflammation and pruritus in corticosteroid-responsive dermatoses.

**de·sorb** (de-sorb′) to remove a substance from the state of absorption or adsorption.

**de·sorp·tion** (de-sorp′shən) the process of being desorbed.

**Des·Owen** (des-o′wən) trademark for preparations of desonide.

**des·ox·i·met·a·sone** (des-ok″sĭ-met′ə-sōn) [USP] [MeSH: Desoximetasone] a synthetic corticosteroid used topically for the relief of inflammation and pruritus in corticosteroid-responsive dermatoses.

**desoxy-** older form for *deoxy-.*

**des·oxy·cor·ti·cos·ter·one** (des-ok″se-kor″tĭ-kos′tər-ōn) [MeSH: Desoxycorticosterone] 11-deoxycorticosterone.
**d. acetate** [USP], the acetate salt of 11-deoxycorticosterone; used as replacement therapy to treat adrenocortical insufficiency; administered by intramuscular injection.
**d. pivalate** [USP], the pivalate salt of 11-deoxycorticosterone, used as replacement therapy to treat adrenocortical insufficiency; administered by intramuscular injection.

**des·oxy·cor·tone** (des-ok″se-kor′tōn) 11-deoxycorticosterone.

**des·oxy·mor·phine** (des-ok″se-mor′fēn) a product of the reduction of morphine.

**Des·ox·yn** (des-ok′sən) trademark for preparations of methamphetamine hydrochloride.

**des·oxy·phe·no·bar·bi·tal** (des-ok″se-fe″no-bahr′bĭ-təl) primidone.

**de·spe·ci·ate** (de-spe′she-āt) to undergo despeciation; to subject to (as by chemical treatment), or to undergo, loss of species antigenic characteristics.

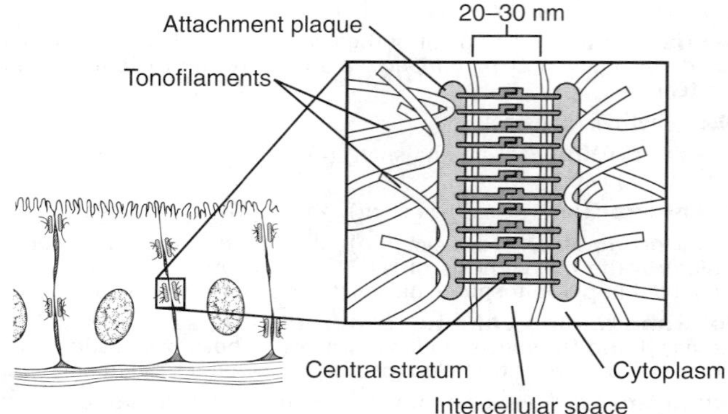


Desmosome.

**de·spe·ci·a·tion** (de-spe″she-a′shən) deviation from or loss of species characteristics.

**de·spe·ci·fi·ca·tion** (de-spes″ĭ-fĭ-ka′shən) the process of reducing the antigenicity of heterologous antisera used therapeutically, by treating them with enzymes such as pepsin to remove the antigenic Fc regions of the immunoglobulin molecules. This leaves $F(ab')_2$ fragments which contain both antigen binding regions of each immunoglobulin molecule.

**d'Es·pine's sign** (des-pēnz′) [Adolphe *d'Espine,* French physician, 1846–1930] see under *sign.*

**des·qua·ma·tion** (des″kwə-ma′shən) [*de-* + *squama*] the shedding of epithelial elements, chiefly of the skin, in scales or small sheets; exfoliation.
**furfuraceous d.,** desquamation in branlike scales.
**lamellar d. of the newborn,** see *collodion baby,* under *baby.*

**des·qua·ma·tive** (də-skwahm′ə-tiv) pertaining to or characterized by desquamation.

**des·qua·ma·to·ry** (də-skwahm′ə-to-re) desquamative.

**dest.** abbreviation for L. *destil'la* distil, and *destilla'tus,* distilled.

**destil.** abbreviation for L. *destil'la,* distil.

**de·sulf·hy·drase** (de″səlf-hi′drās) a term used in the recommended and trivial names of some carbon-sulfur lyases [EC 4.4], which catalyze the removal of hydrogen sulfide or substituted hydrogen sulfide from a compound.

**De·sul·fo·bul·bus** (de-sul″fo-bul′bəs) [*de-* + *sulfo-* + L. *bulbus* onion] a genus of anaerobic, ellipsoidal to onion-shaped nonspore-forming bacteria that reduce sulfate compounds to hydrogen sulfide, found in anaerobic sediments from fresh or brackish waters, in bovine rumen fluid, and in animal feces. The type species is *D. propio'nicus.*

**De·sul·fo·coc·cus** (de-sul″fo-kok′əs) [*de-* + *sulfo-* + *coccus*] a genus of anaerobic, gram-negative, nonspore-forming, spherical bacteria that reduce sulfate compounds to hydrogen sulfide, found in anaerobic sediments from fresh and marine waters and in sewage sludge. The type species is *D. multivo'rans.*

**De·sul·fo·mo·nas** (de-sul″fo-mo′nəs) [*de-* + *sulfo-* + Gr. *monas* unit, from *monos* single] a genus of bacteria made up of gram-negative, nonspore-forming, anaerobic bacilli that reduce sulfate to hydrogen sulfide. They are part of the normal flora of the oral cavity and the respiratory, intestinal, and urogenital tracts of humans and other animals. The type species is *D. pi'gra.*

**De·sul·fo·to·mac·u·lum** (de-sul″fo-tə-mak′u-ləm) [*de-* + *sulfo-* + L. *tomaculum* sausage] a genus of endospore-forming, rod-shaped bacteria of the family Bacillaceae, made up of anaerobic, gram-negative cells that reduce sulfates, sulfites, and other sulfur compounds. They are found in soil, water, and geothermal regions, and in the intestines of insects, and in the contents of animal rumens. The type species is *D. nigri'ficans.*

**De·sul·fo·vib·rio** (de-sul″fo-vib′re-o) [*de-* + *sulfo-* + *vibrio*] [MeSH: Desulfovibrio] a genus of gram-negative, nonspore-forming, anaerobic bacteria, consisting of actively motile curved rods that reduce sulfur compounds to hydrogen sulfide, found in animal intestines and feces, fresh and salt water, soil, and mud. The type species is *D. desulfu'ricans.*

**de·sul·fur·ase** (de-sul′fər-ās) desulfhydrase.

**Des·yr·el** (des′ir-əl) trademark for a preparation of trazodone hydrochloride.

**DET** diethyltryptamine.

**Det.** abbreviation for L. *de'tur,* let it be given.

**de·tach·ment** (de-tach′mənt) [Fr. *détacher* to unfasten; to separate] the condition of being unfastened, disconnected, or separated.
**d. of retina, retinal d.,** detached retina; see under *retina.*

**de·tec·tion** (de-tek′shən) discovery of the presence or existence of something.
**coincidence d.,** in positron emission tomography, collimation in detection of ionization events, limiting recognition to simultaneous events occurring in opposite directions, which occurs when the emitted positron collides with an electron, simultaneously emitting two photons in opposing directions.

**de·tec·tor** (de-tek′tər) a device by which the presence of something, or the existence of a certain condition, is discovered.
**lie d.,** polygraph.
**radiation d.,** any device for converting radiant energy to a form more readily observable.

**de·ter·gent** (de-tər′jənt) [L. *detergere* to cleanse] [MeSH: Detergents] 1. purifying, cleansing. 2. an agent which purifies or cleanses. 3. in biochemistry, any of a class of agents structurally consisting of a nonpolar hydrocarbon chain attached to a polar head group, which reduce the surface tension of water, emulsify, and aid in the solubilization of soil.

**de·ter·mi·nant** (de-tər′mĭ-nənt) [L. *determinare* to bound, limit, or fix] a factor that establishes the nature of an entity or event.
**allotypic d.,** allotope.
**antigenic d.,** a site on the surface of an antigen molecule to which a single antibody molecule binds; generally an antigen has several or many different antigenic determinants and reacts with antibodies of many different specificities. Called also *epitope.*
**hidden d.,** an antigenic determinant located in an unexposed region of a molecule so that it is prevented from interacting with receptors on lymphocytes, or with antibody molecules, and is unable to induce an immune response unless exposed by conformational change or stereochemical alteration of the molecule. Such hidden determinants may appear following stereochemical alterations of molecular structure.
**immunogenic d.,** the part of an immunogenic molecule that interacts with a helper T cell in triggering antibody production, as opposed to the antigenic determinant or hapten, which interacts with B cells.
**sequential d.,** a polymeric antigenic determinant with antigenic specificity determined by monomer sequence rather than monomer composition.

**de·ter·mi·na·tion** (de-tər′mĭ-na′shən) establishment of the exact nature of an entity or event.
**embryonic d.,** the loss of pluripotency in any part of an embryo and its start on the way toward an unalterable fate.
**sex d.,** the process by which the sex of an organism is fixed, associated, in man, with the presence or absence of the Y chromosome.

**de·ter·min·er** (de-tər′min-ər) determinant.

**de·ter·min·ism** (de-tər′min-iz-əm) the theory that all phenomena are the result of antecedent conditions, nothing occurs by chance, and there is no free will.
**psychic d.,** the concept, originated by Freud, that mental events do not occur by chance but have their antecedent mental causes, that even accidents, slips of the tongue, or whims commonly felt to be inexplicable result from unconscious mental processes.

**de·to·mi·dine** (de-to′mĭ-dēn) an analgesic and sedative used in horses.

**de To·ni-Fan·co·ni syndrome** (da to′ne-fahn-ko′ne) [Giovanni *de Toni,* Italian pediatrician, 1896–1973; Guido *Fanconi,* Swiss physician, 1892–1979] see *Fanconi's syndrome* (def. 2), under *syndrome.*

**Det. in 2 plo., Det. in dup.** abbreviations for L. *de'tur in du'plo,* let twice as much be given.

**de·tor·sion** (de-tor′shən) 1. the correction of a twisting or deformity, as the reduction of torsion of the testis. 2. a deficiency in a normal twisting as may occur in the early development of the heart.

**de·tox·i·cate** (de-tok′sĭ-kāt) detoxify.

**de·tox·i·ca·tion** (de-tok″sĭ-ka′shən) detoxification.

**de·tox·i·fi·ca·tion** (de-tok″sĭ-fĭ-ka′shən) 1. reduction of the toxic properties of poisons. 2. treatment designed to free an addict from his drug habit.
**metabolic d.,** reduction of the toxic properties of a substance by chemical changes induced in the body, producing a compound which is less poisonous or is more readily eliminated.

**de·tox·i·fy** (de-tok′sĭ-fi) to remove the toxic quality of a substance.

**de·tri·tion** (de-trish′ən) [*de-* + L. *terere* to wear] a wearing away, as of the teeth, by friction. See also *abrasion.*

**de·tri·tiv·o·rous** (de″trĭ-tiv′ə-rəs) subsisting on particulate matter (detritus), a mode of existence important in certain, such as aquatic, ecosystems.

**de·tri·tus** (de-tri′təs) [L., from *deterere* to rub away] particulate matter produced by or remaining after the wearing away or disintegration of a substance or tissue; designated as organic or nonorganic, depending on the nature of the original material. See also *biodetritus.*

**de·tru·sor** (de-troo′ser) [L., from *detrudere* to push down] [TA] a general term for any body part that pushes down; often used alone to denote the musculus detrusor vesicae.
**d. uri'nae,** musculus detrusor vesicae.

**D. et s.** abbreviation for L. *de'tur et signe'tur,* let it be given and labeled.

**de·tu·ba·tion** (de″too-ba′shən) extubation.

**de·tu·mes·cence** (de″too-mes′əns) [*de-* + *tumescence*] the subsidence of swelling, or turgor.

**Deur·sil** (de-ur′sil) trademark for a preparation of ursodiol.

**deu·tan** (doo′tən) 1. pertaining to deuteranomaly or deuteranopia. 2. a person with deuteranomaly or deuteranopia.

**deu·ter·anom·al** (doo″tər-ə-nom′əl) a person with deuteranomaly.

**deu·ter·anom·a·lous** (doo″tər-ə-nom′ə-ləs) pertaining to or characterized by deuteranomaly.

**deu·ter·anom·a·ly** (doo″tər-ə-nom′ə-le) [*deuter-* + *anomaly*] a type of anomalous trichromasy in which the second, green-sensitive, cones have decreased sensitivity; therefore a greater than normal proportion of thallium green light to lithium red light is required to match a fixed sodium yellow light. Deuteranomaly is an X-linked trait, affects about 5 per cent of white males and 0.25 per cent of females, and is the most common color vision deficiency.

**deu·ter·an·ope** (doo′tər-ə-nōp″) an individual exhibiting deuteranopia.

**deu·ter·an·o·pia** (doo″tər-ə-no′pe-ə) [*deuter-* + *an-*[1] + *-opia*] a dichromasy characterized by retention of the sensory mechanism for two hues only (blue and yellow) of the normal 4-primary quota, and lacking that for red and green and their derivatives, without loss of luminance or shift or shortening of the spectrum. It is an X-linked trait occurring in about 1 per cent of males, but only rarely in females.

**deu·ter·an·op·ic** (doo″tər-ə-nop′ik) pertaining to or characterized by deuteranopia.

**deu·ter·an·op·sia** (doo″tər-ə-nop′se-ə) deuteranopia.

**deu·te·ri·on** (doo-te′re-on) deuteron.

**deu·te·ri·um** (doo-te′re-əm) [Gr. *deuteros* second] [MeSH: Deuterium] the mass two isotope of hydrogen, symbol $^{2}$H, or D. It is available as a gas or as heavy water and has been used in metabolic studies; called also *heavy hydrogen* (see *hydrogen*). Cf. *protium* and *tritium*.
**d. oxide,** heavy water; see under *water*.

**deuter(o)-** [Gr. *deuteros* second] a combining form meaning second. Also, *deut(o)-*.

**deu·tero·co·ni·di·um** (doo″tər-o-ko-nid′e-əm) [*deutero-* + *conidium*] a reproductive element derived from a hemispore.

**deu·tero·my·cete** (doo″tər-o-mi′sēt) imperfect fungus.

**Deu·tero·my·ce·tes** (doo″tər-o-mi-se′tēz) [MeSH: Deuteromycetes] name given to Deuteromycota when it is considered a class.

**Deu·tero·my·co·ta** (doo″tər-o-mi-ko′tə) the imperfect fungi (Fungi Imperfecti), a large, heterogeneous group ordinarily treated as a phylum, distinguished by having no known sexual stage; in many cases the sexual stage is later discovered and can be shown to be an ascomycete or basidiomycete. This group includes many of the fungi pathogenic for humans and other animals. Deuteromycota are subclassified into form-classes, form-orders, and so on. For some fungi the name of the asexual stage is retained even though the sexual stage has been identified, so that the fungus has a different name for each stage of its life cycle; in such cases the name of the sexual stage is used to refer to the fungus in all its states. Some authorities consider this group a subphylum of the Eumycota and call it Deuteromycotina; others consider it a class and call it Deuteromycetes.

**Deu·tero·my·co·ti·na** (doo″tər-o-mi″ko-ti′nə) name given to Deuteromycota when it is considered a subphylum of Eumycota.

**deu·ter·on** (doo′tər-on) the nucleus of deuterium, or heavy hydrogen; deuterons are used as bombing particles for nuclear disintegration.

**deu·tero·path·ic** (doo″tər-o-path′ik) occurring secondarily to some other disease.

**deu·ter·op·a·thy** (doo″tər-op′ə-the) [*deutero-* + *-pathy*] a disease that is secondary to another disease.

**deu·tero·pine** (doo″tər-o′pēn) an alkaloid from opium.

**deu·tero·plasm** (doo′tər-o-plaz″əm) [*deutero-* + *-plasm*] the passive or inactive materials in protoplasm, especially reserve foodstuffs, such as yolk. Cf. *energid*.

**deu·tero·some** (doo′tər-o-sōm″) [*deutero-* + *-some*] a cytoplasmic organelle of ciliating epithelial cells that plays a role in the formation of ciliary basal bodies, being the precursor of the procentriole.

**deu·tero·stome** (doo′tər-o-stōm″) an animal belonging to the Deuterostomia.

**Deu·tero·sto·mia** (doo″tər-o-sto′me-ə) [*deutero-* + Gr. *stoma* mouth + *-ia*] a series of the Eucoelomata, including the echinoderms, hemichordates, and chordates, in all of which the site of the blastopore is posterior—far from the mouth, which forms a new structure unrelated to the blastopore. Cf. *Protostomia*.

**deu·tero·to·cia** (doo″tər-o-to′se-ə) [*deutero-* + Gr. *tokos* birth] asexual reproduction in which the female produces offspring of both sexes.

**deu·ter·ot·o·ky** (doo″tər-ot′ə-ke) deuterotocia.

**deu·thy·alo·some** (doo″thi-al′ə-sōm) [*deuto-* + *hyalo-* + *-some*] the matured nucleus of an ovum.

**deut(o)-** see *deuter(o)-*.

**deu·ton** (doo′ton) deuteron.

**deu·to·neph·ron** (doo″to-nef′ron) [*deuto-* + Gr. *nephron*] mesonephros.

**deu·to·plasm** (doo′to-plaz″əm) deuteroplasm.

**deu·to·plas·mol·y·sis** (doo″to-plaz-mol′ə-sis) destruction or disintegration of deutoplasm.

**Deutsch·län·der's disease** (doich′len-dərz) [Karl Ernst Wilhelm *Deutschländer*, German surgeon, 1872–1942] 1. see under *disease*. 2. march foot.

**DEV** duck embryo vaccine.

**de·val·u·a·tion** (de-val″u-a′shən) a defense mechanism in which emotional conflict or stressors are faced by attributing exaggerated negative qualities to the self or to others.

**de·vas·cu·lar·iza·tion** (de-vas″ku-lər-ĭ-za′shən) interruption of the circulation of blood to a part caused by obstruction or destruction of the blood vessels supplying it. See also *ischemia*.

**Dev·e·gan** (dev′e-gən) trademark for a preparation of acetarsone.

**de·vel·op·ment** (de-vel′əp-mənt) the process of growth and differentiation.
**arrested d.,** cessation of the development process at some stage prior to its normal completion.
**cognitive d.,** the development of intelligence, conscious thought, and problem solving ability that begins in infancy.
**mosaic d.,** the development of an embryo in a fixed, unalterable way, local regions being independent portions of a mosaic whole.
**postnatal d.,** that which occurs after birth.
**prenatal d.,** that which occurs before birth.
**psychosexual d.,** 1. a general term for the developing sexuality of the individual as affected by biological, cultural, and emotional influences from prenatal life onward through the life cycle. 2. in psychoanalysis, libidinal maturation from infancy through adulthood (in classic psychoanalysis including the oral, anal, and genital stages). One schema is Erikson's eight stages of development.
**psychosocial d.,** the development of the personality, including the acquisition of social attitudes and skills, from infancy through maturity.
**regulative d.,** the development of an embryo, the determination of the various organs and parts being gradually attained through the action of inductors.

**de·vel·op·men·tal** (de-vel″əp-men′təl) pertaining to development.

**de·vi·ant** (de′ve-ənt) [L. *deviare* to turn aside] 1. varying from a determinable standard. 2. an individual with characteristics varying from what is considered normal, or standard.
**sexual d.,** an individual exhibiting sexual deviation.

**de·vi·a·tion** (de″ve-a′shən) [L. *deviare* to turn aside] 1. a turning away from the regular standard or course. 2. in ophthalmology, strabismus. 3. in statistics, the difference between a sample value and the mean.
**animal d.,** the attracting of zoophilous mosquitos from human beings by the proximity of animals preferred by the insects.
**axis d.,** alteration in the direction of the mean QRS complex vector, determined from the electrocardiogram; it may be due to alteration in the anatomical position of the heart or to any of a variety of disorders such as ventricular hypertrophy or bundle branch block. Relative to the hexaxial reference system (q.v.), a normal axis is $-30°$ to $90°$; right axis deviation is $90°$ to $180°$; left axis deviation is $-30°$ to $-90°$; and $-90°$ to $180°$ is an indeterminate axis.
**complement d.,** inhibition of complement fixation or complement-mediated immune hemolysis in the presence of excess antibody. Called also *Neisser-Wechsberg phenomenon*.
**conjugate d.,** the deflection of two similar parts, as the eyes when turned in the same direction at the same time.
**Hering-Hellebrand d.,** the amount of deviation between any point on the Vieth-Müller horopter and the frontoparallel plane passing through the point of fixation.
**immune d.,** modification of the immune response to an antigen by previous inoculation of the same antigen.
**latent d.,** heterophoria.
**d. to the left,** shift to the left.
**left axis d. (LAD),** see *axis d.*
**manifest d.,** strabismus.
**minimum d.,** the smallest deflection of a ray of light that can be produced by a given prism.
**population standard d.,** standard d.

**primary d.**, deviation of the visual axis of the squinting eye in strabismus when the sound eye fixates.
**d. to the right**, shift to the right.
**radial d.**, a hand deformity sometimes seen in rheumatoid arthritis, in which the fingers are displaced to the radial side. Arthritic hands may be splinted into this position to counteract ulnar deviation. Called also *radial drift*.
**right axis d. (RAD)**, see *axis d.*
**sample standard d.**, an estimate of the population standard deviation, usually determined (from a sample of size *n*) by dividing the sum of the squared deviations from the sample mean by $n-1$ and taking the square root; $n-1$ is used (rather than *n*) in order to obtain an unbiased estimate of the population variance. Symbol *s*.
**secondary d.**, deviation of the visual axis of the sound eye in strabismus when the squinting eye fixates.
**sexual d.**, sexual behavior or fantasy outside that which is morally, biologically, or legally sanctioned, often specifically one of the paraphilias.
**skew d.**, downward and inward rotation of the eye on the side of the cerebellar lesion and upward and outward deviation on the opposite side. Called also *Hertwig-Magendie phenomenon, Magendie's sign*, and *Magendie-Hertwig sign*.
**spiral d. of the penis**, corkscrew penis.
**squint d.**, squint angle; see under *angle*.
**standard d. (SD)**, in statistics a measure of the amount by which each value deviates from the mean; equal to the square root of the variance, i.e., the square root of the average of the squared deviations from the mean. It is the most commonly used measure of dispersion of statistical data. Called also *population standard d.*. Symbol *σ*. See figure at *normal distribution*, and see also *sample standard d.*
**strabismic d.**, deviation of the visual axis of an eye in strabismus.
**ulnar d.**, a hand deformity, seen in chronic rheumatoid arthritis and lupus erythematosus, in which the swelling of the metacarpophalangeal joints causes the fingers to become displaced to the ulnar side. Called also *ulnar drift* and *ulnar drift deformity*. Cf. *radial d.*

**De·vic's disease** (də-vēks') [Eugène *Devic*, French physician, 1869–1930] neuromyelitis optica.

**de·vice** (də-vīs') [MeSH: Equipment and Supplies] something contrived for a specific purpose.
**assistive listening d's**, devices other than hearing aids that help the deaf to hear.
**biventricular assist d. (BVAD)**, a ventricular assist device with the combined functions of both left and right ventricular assist devices.
**central-bearing d.**, a device that provides a central point of bearing, or support, between upper and lower occlusion rims, consisting of a contacting point attached to one occlusion rim and a plate that provides the surface on which the bearing point rests or moves.
**central-bearing tracing d.**, one for determining the central bearing or support between maxillary and mandibular occlusion rims or dentures.
**contraceptive d.**, a device used to prevent conception, such as a barrier contraceptive, an intrauterine device, or a means of preventing ovulation (e.g., birth control pill).
**intrauterine d. (IUD)**, a plastic or metallic device inserted into the uterus to prevent pregnancy.
**left ventricular assist d. (LVAD)**, a ventricular assist device capable of augmenting left ventricular function; it consists of an external or implanted pump with afferent and efferent conduits attached to the left atrium or left ventricular apex and the ascending aorta, respectively. Implanted systems are sometimes called *left ventricular assist systems*. Cf. *biventricular assist d.* and *right ventricular assist d.*
**right ventricular assist d. (RVAD)**, a ventricular assist device capable of augmenting right ventricular function, consisting of a pump with afferent and efferent conduits attached to the right atrium and pulmonary artery, respectively. Cf. *biventricular assist d.* and *left ventricular assist d.*
**ventricular assist d. (VAD)**, a circulatory support device that augments function of the left ventricle, the right ventricle, or both; it consists of one or two implanted or extracorporeal pumps with afferent and efferent conduits attached so as to provide mechanically assisted pulsatile blood flow. See *left ventricular assist d., right ventricular assist d.*, and *biventricular assist d.*

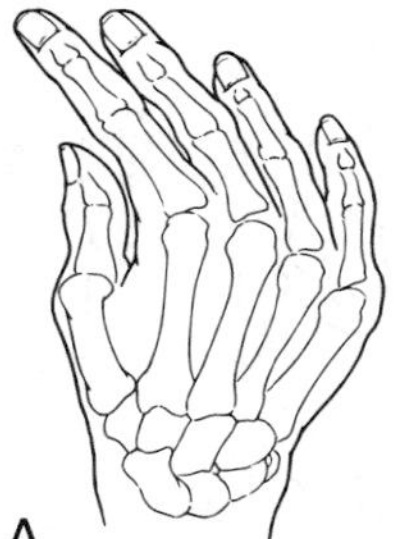


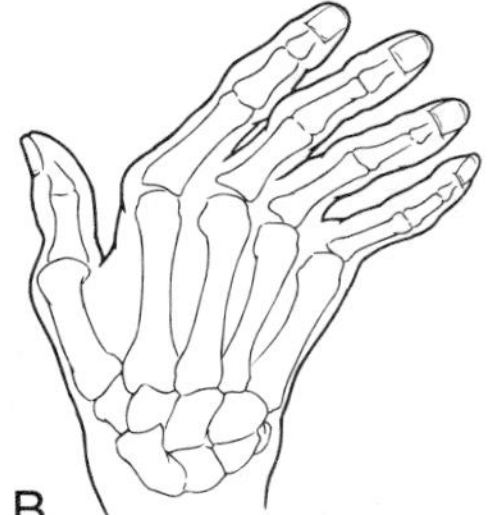


Radial *(A)* and ulnar *(B)* deviation of the digits.

**de·vi·om·e·ter** (de″ve-om'ə-tər) strabismometer.

**de·vis·cer·a·tion** (de-vis″ər-a'shən) evisceration.

**de·vi·tal·iza·tion** (de-vi″təl-ĭ-za'shən) the deprivation of vitality or life, as of a tissue.
**pulp d.**, the destruction of vitality of the pulp of a tooth.

**de·vi·tal·ize** (de-vi'təl-īz) [*de-* + *vital* + *-ize*] to deprive of vitality or of life.

**de·vit·ri·fi·ca·tion** (de-vit″rĭ-fĭ-ka'shən) [*de-* + *vitrification*] the changing of a supercooled liquid such as glass into a crystalline state.

**dev·o·lu·tion** (dev″o-loo'shən) [L. *de* down + *volvere* to roll] 1. the reverse of evolution. 2. catabolic change.

**Dew's sign** (dūz) [Sir Harold Robert *Dew*, Australian physician, 1891–1962] see under *sign*.

**de·wa·tered** (de-wah'tərd) having the water removed; a term applied to sludge from which the water has been removed by drying or pressing.

**dew·claw** (doo'klaw) a vestigial digit or claw, found in the feet of dogs, cats, and ruminants.

**dew·lap** (doo'lap) a heavy fold of skin on the ventral aspect of the neck in animals.

**de·worm·ing** (de-wərm'ing) the destruction and removal of worms from an infected person or animal; cf. *anthelmintic*.

**Dex·a·cen** (dek'sə-sen″) trademark for preparations of dexamethasone.

**dex·a·meth·a·sone** (dek″sə-meth'ə-sōn) [USP] [MeSH: Dexamethasone] a synthetic glucocorticoid, 25 times as potent as cortisol; used topically as an anti-inflammatory and administered orally in replacement therapy for adrenal insufficiency, as an anti-inflammatory and immunosuppressant in a wide variety of disorders, and as an antiemetic in cancer chemotherapy. It is also used as a diagnostic aid in the detection of Cushing's syndrome in the high-dose and low-dose dexamethasone suppression tests (see under *test*).
**d. acetate** [USP], an ester of dexamethasone, having actions similar to those of the base and used in replacement therapy in adrenal insufficiency and as an anti-inflammatory and immunosuppressant; administered by intra-arterial, intramuscular, intralesional, or soft-tissue injection.
**d. sodium phosphate** [USP], an ester of dexamethasone, having actions and uses similar to those of the base; administered by intra-articular, soft tissue, intravenous, or intramuscular injection, by inhalation, or applied topically to the skin and conjunctiva.

**Dex·a·sone** (dek'sə-sōn″) trademark for preparations of dexamethasone.

**dex·brom·phen·ir·a·mine** (deks″brom-fən-ēr'ə-mēn) the bromine analogue of dexchlorpheniramine, an antihistaminic drug.
**d. maleate** [USP], the maleate salt of dexbrompheniramine, administered orally for therapy and prophylaxis of conditions in which antihistamines may be effective.

**dex·chlor·phen·ir·a·mine** (deks″klor-fən-ēr'ə-mēn) the dextrorotatory isomer of chlorpheniramine, an antihistaminic drug.
**d. maleate** [USP], the maleate salt of dexchlorpheniramine, administered orally for therapy and prophylaxis of conditions in which antihistamines may be effective.

**dex·cla·mol hy·dro·chlo·ride** (deks'klə-mol) a sedative, $C_{24}H_{29}NO \cdot HCl$.

**Dex·e·drine** (dek'sə-drēn) trademark for preparations of dextroamphetamine sulfate.

**dex·et·i·mide** (dek-set'ĭ-mīd) [MeSH: Dexetimide] an anticholinergic which has been used as an antiparkinsonian agent.

**dex·fen·flur·a·mine hy·dro·chlor·ide** (deks″fen-floor'ə-mēn) an adrenergic used as an anorexic in the short-term treatment of exogenous obesity; administered orally.

**Dex·Fer·rum** (deks-fer'əm) trademark for a preparation of iron dextran injection.

**dex·io·car·dia** (dek″se-o-kahr'de-ə) dextrocardia.

**dex·io·trop·ic** (dek″se-o-trop'ik) [Gr. *dexios* on the right + *-tropic*] wound in a spiral from left to right, as a shell.

**Dex·on** (dek'son) trademark for a preparation of polyglycolic acid, a polymer used to make nonirritating absorbable sutures.

**Dex·one** (dek'sōn) trademark for a preparation of dexamethasone.

**dex·pan·the·nol** (deks-pan'thə-nol) the D(+) form of *panthenol* (pantothenyl alcohol), the alcoholic analogue of pantothenic acid. It is claimed to be a precursor of coenzyme A, and is administered intravenously or intramuscularly to increase peristalsis in atony and paralysis of the lower intestine and orally to help relieve gas retention and abdominal distention in certain conditions. It is also applied topically to the skin to stimulate healing of the lesions of various dermatologic lesions such as burns, infected wounds, eczema, diaper rash, etc.

**dex·pro·pran·o·lol hy·dro·chlo·ride** (deks″pro-pran′ə-lol) the dextrorotatory isomer of propranolol, having cardiac depressant properties similar to those of the parent compound; used as an antiarrhythmic.

**dex·ra·zox·ane** (deks″ra-zok′sān) a derivative of ethylenediaminetetraacetic acid (EDTA) used as a cardioprotectant in chemotherapy to counteract doxorubicin-induced cardiomyopathy; administered intravenously.

**dex·ter** (deks′tər) [L.] [TA] right: a term denoting the right-hand one of two similar structures, or the one situated on the right side of the body.

**dex·trad** (deks′trad) toward the right side.

**dex·tral** (deks′trəl) 1. right as opposed to left; right-handed. 2. a right-handed person.

**dex·tral·i·ty** (deks-tral′ĭ-te) [*dexter*] the preferential use, in voluntary motor acts, of the right member of the major paired organs of the body, as the right ear, eye, hand, or foot.

**dex·tran** (deks′trən) a high-molecular-weight polymer of D-glucose, produced by enzymes (glycosyltransferases) on the cell surface of certain lactic acid bacteria. Dextrans, formed from sucrose by bacteria in the mouth, adhere to the tooth surfaces and produce dental plaque, a major cause of dental caries. Uniform molecular weight dextrans from *Leuconostoc mesenteroides* preparations are used as plasma volume expanders. Specific preparations are designated, according to their average molecular weight in thousands, as *dextran 40 [USP], dextran 70 [USP],* and so on. Commercial preparations in bead form are also used in gel-filtration chromatography.

**dex·trano·mer** (deks-tran′o-mər) a preparation of highly hydrophilic dextran polymers occurring as small beads, used in débridement of secreting wounds, such as venous stasis ulcers; the sterilized beads are poured over secreting wounds to absorb wound exudates and prevent crust formation.

**dex·trates** (deks′trāts) a tablet binder and diluent, composed of a mixture of sugars (approximately 92 per cent dextrose monohydrate and 8 per cent high saccharides; dextrose equivalent is 95 to 97 per cent) resulting from the controlled enzymatic hydrolysis of starch.

**dex·trau·ral** (deks-traw′rəl) [*dextr-* + *aural*] hearing better with the right ear than with the left.

**dex·tri·fer·ron** (deks″trĭ-fer′on) a complex of ferric hydroxide and partially hydrolyzed dextrin used in the treatment of iron-deficiency anemia.

**dex·trin** (dek′strin) [L. *dexter* right] 1. any one, or the mixture, of the intermediate polysaccharides formed during the hydrolysis of starch, which are dextrorotatory, soluble in water, and precipitable in alcohol. They may be linear or branched, and include the amylodextrins, erythrodextrins, and achroodextrins. 2. [NF] an official preparation, from starch by heating; used as a suspending and viscosity-increasing agent, tablet binder, and tablet and capsule diluent.
**limit d.,** any of the small, nonreducing polymers remaining after exhaustive digestion of starch or glycogen with enzymes that catalyze the removal of terminal sugar residues but which cannot hydrolyze the linkages of branch points.

**dex·trin·ase** (dek′strin-ās) any enzyme that catalyzes the hydrolysis of dextrins.

**α-dex·trin·ase** (dek′strin-ās) an enzyme that catalyzes the hydrolysis of both α-1,6 and α-1,4 bonds in linear and branched oligoglucosides and maltose and isomaltose. It occurs on the brush border of the intestinal mucosa, completes the digestion of starch or glycogen to glucose, and is present as a complex with sucrase; absence of the enzyme complex activity, called sucrase-isomaltase deficiency, is a form of disaccharide intolerance. Called also *isomaltase* and *limit dextrinase.* In EC nomenclature called, *oligo-1,6-glucosidase.*

**dex·trin·ate, dex·trin·ize** (dek′strin-āt; dek′strin-īz) to convert into dextrin.

**dex·tri·no·sis** (dek″strĭ-no′sis) accumulation in the tissues of an abnormal polysaccharide.
**limit d.,** glycogen storage disease, type III.

**dex·trin·uria** (deks″trĭ-nu′re-ə) the presence of dextrin in the urine.

**dextr(o)-** [L. *dexter* right] 1. a combining form denoting relationship to the right. 2. chemical prefix used to designate the dextrorotatory enantiomorph of a substance; opposed to *levo-*. Symbol (+)- (formerly *d-;* sometimes Δ).

**dex·tro·am·phet·amine** (deks″tro-am-fet′ə-mēn) [MeSH: Dextroamphetamine] the dextrorotatory isomer of amphetamine, which has substantially more central nervous system–stimulating effect than the racemic form of amphetamine. Abuse of this drug may lead to dependence; see *amphetamine.*
**d. sulfate** [USP], the sulfate salt of dextroamphetamine, used orally in the treatment of narcolepsy and attention-deficit/hyperactivity disorder; it has been used as an anorexiant in the treatment of obesity but is no longer recommended for this purpose.

**dex·tro·car·dia** (deks″tro-kahr′de-ə) [*dextro-* + *cardia*] [MeSH: Dextrocardia] location of the heart in the right hemithorax, with the apex pointing to the right, occurring with transposition (situs inversus) of the abdominal viscera, or without such transposition.
**isolated d.,** mirror-image transposition of the heart without accompanying alteration of the abdominal viscera.
**mirror-image d.,** location of the heart in the right side of the chest, the atria being transposed and the right ventricle lying anteriorly and to the left of the left ventricle, usually associated with complete situs inversus.
**secondary d.,** displacement of the heart to the right as a result of disease of the pleura, diaphragm, or lungs.

**dex·tro·cer·e·bral** (deks″tro-sər′e-brəl) [*dextro-* + *cerebral*] pertaining to or situated in the right cerebral hemisphere.

**dex·tro·cli·na·tion** (deks″tro-klĭ-na′shən) [*dextro-* + L. *clinatus* leaning] rotation of the upper poles of the vertical meridians of the two eyes to the right; called also *dextrocycloduction* and *dextrotorsion.* Cf. *levoclination.*

**dex·tro·com·pound** (deks″tro-kom′pound) a dextrorotatory compound.

**dex·troc·u·lar** (deks-trok′u-lər) right eyed; affected with dextrocularity.

**dex·troc·u·lar·i·ty** (deks″trok-u-lar′ĭ-te) [*dextro-* + *oculus*] the condition of having greater visual power in the right eye and, therefore, using it more than the left.

**dex·tro·cy·clo·duc·tion** (deks″tro-si″klo-duk′shən) dextroclination.

**dex·tro·duc·tion** (deks″tro-duk′shən) [*dextro-* + *duction*] movement of either eye to the right.

**dex·tro·gas·tria** (deks″tro-gas′tre-ə) [*dextro-* + *gastr-* + *-ia*] displacement of the stomach to the right, being simple displacement or situs inversus.

**dex·tro·gy·ral** (deks″tro-ji′rəl) [*dextro-* + *gyrare* to turn] dextrorotatory.

**dex·tro·gy·ra·tion** (dek″stro-ji-ra′shən) [*dextro-* + *gyration*] a turning to the right or motion to the right; said of movements of the eye and of the plane of polarization.

**dex·tro·man·u·al** (deks″tro-man′u-əl) [*dextro-* + *manual*] right-handed.

**dex·tro·men·thol** (deks″tro-men′thol) an oxidation product of menthol.

**dex·tro·meth·or·phan** (deks″tro-məth-or′fan) [USP] [MeSH: Dextromethorphan] a nonopioid, synthetic derivative of morphine that acts on the cough center to suppress the cough reflex, used as an antitussive; administered orally.
**d. hydrobromide** [USP], the monohydrated hydrobromide salt of dextromethorphan, having the same action and use as the base; administered orally.

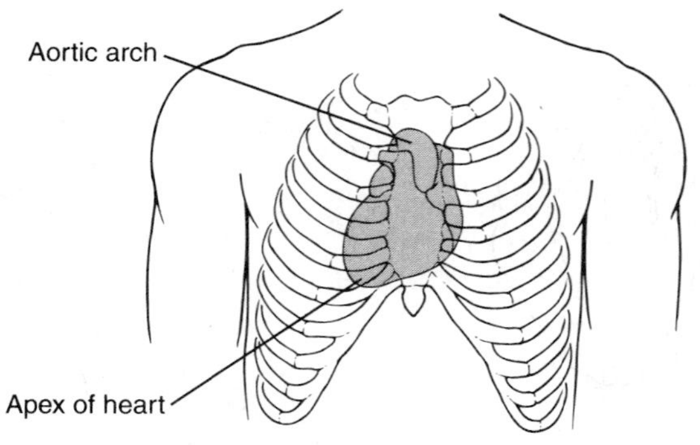


Dextrocardia.

**d. polistirex,** sulfonated styrene-divinylbenzene copolymer complex with dextromethorphan, administered orally as an extended-release antitussive.

**dex·trop·e·dal** (deks-trop'ə-dəl) [*dextro-* + *pedal*] using the right foot in preference to the left.

**dex·tro·po·si·tion** (dek″stro-pə-zish'ən) displacement to the right.

**dex·tro·pro·poxy·phene** (deks″tro-pro-pok'sə-fēn) propoxyphene.

**dex·tro·ro·ta·ry** (deks″tro-ro'tə-re) dextrorotatory.

**dex·tro·ro·ta·to·ry** (deks″tro-ro'tə-tor-e) [*dextro-* + *rotatory*] turning the plane of polarization, or rays of light, to the right; called also *dextrogyral.*

**dex·trose** (dek'strōs) chemical name: D-glucose monohydrate. A monosaccharide known as *glucose* (q.v.) in biochemistry and physiology. The official preparation [USP] is usually obtained by the hydrolysis of starch; it is used chiefly as a fluid and nutrient replenisher, usually administered by intravenous infusion. It is also used as a diuretic and alone or in combination with other agents for various other clinical purposes.

**dex·tro·sin·is·tral** (dek″stro-sin'is-trəl) [*dextro-* + *sinistral*] 1. extending from right to left. 2. a person naturally left-handed but trained to use the right hand in certain activities.

**Dex·tro·stix** (dek'stro-stiks) trademark for a reagent strip designed for determination of blood-glucose levels with the use of fingertip venous blood.

**dex·tros·uria** (deks″trōs-u're-ə) glycosuria.

**dex·tro·thy·rox·ine so·di·um** (deks″tro-thi-rok'sin) the sodium salt of the dextrorotatory isomer of thyroxine that acts as an antilipemic; used as an adjunct in the treatment of familial hyperlipoproteinemia type IIa in euthyroid patients; administered orally.

**dex·tro·tor·sion** (deks″tro-tor'shən) dextroclination.

**dex·tro·trop·ic** (deks″tro-trop'ik) [*dextro-* + *-tropic*] turning to the right; see also *dexiotropic.*

**dex·tro·ver·sion** (dek″stro-vər'zhən) [*dextro-* + *version*] 1. version to the right side; especially movement of the eyes to the right. 2. location of the heart in the right hemithorax, the left ventricle remaining on the left as in the normal position, but lying anterior to the right ventricle.

**dex·tro·vert·ed** (deks″tro-vərt'əd) turned to the right.

**dez·o·cine** (dez'o-sēn) an opioid analgesic, having both agonist and antagonist activity, used for the short-term relief of pain; administered intramuscularly or intravenously.

**DF-2** see *Capnocytophaga canimorsus.*

**DFDT** a powerful insecticide, difluoro-diphenyl-trichloroethane; called also *GIX.*

**DFP** diisopropyl fluorophosphate.

**dG** deoxyguanosine.

**dg** decigram.

**dGDP** deoxyguanosine diphosphate.

**dGMP** deoxyguanosine monophosphate.

**dGTP** deoxyguanosine triphosphate.

**DH** delayed hypersensitivity.

**DHA** docosahexaenoic acid.

**dha·va** (dah'və) [Hindi] *Anogeissus latifolia.*

**DHE 45** [MeSH: Dihydroergotamine] trademark for dihydroergotamine.

**DHEA** dehydroepiandrosterone.

**d'He·relle phenomenon** (də-rel') [Félix Hubert *d'Herelle,* Canadian bacteriologist in France, 1873–1949] Twort-d'Herelle phenomenon; see under *phenomenon.*

**DHF** dihydrofolate or dihydrofolic acid.

**DHFR** dihydrofolate reductase.

**DHg** Doctor of Hygiene.

**DHPG** 3,4-dihydroxyphenylglycol; see *ganciclovir.*

**DHT** dihydrotestosterone.

**dhur·rin** (doo'rin) a cyanogenetic glycoside from sorghum which hydrolyzes into parahydroxy benzaldehyde, glucose, and hydrocyanic acid.

**DHy** Doctor of Hygiene.

**di-** [Gr. *dis* twice] a prefix meaning twice. In chemical nomenclature, the use of *di-* is preferred to the use of *bi-* (q.v.).

**dia-** [Gr. *dia* through] a prefix meaning through, between, apart, across, or completely.

**DiaBeta** (di-ə-ba'tə) trademark for a preparation of glyburide.

**di·a·be·tes** (di″ə-be'tēz) [Gr. *diabētēs* a syphon, from *dia* through + *bainein* to go] 1. any of various disorders characterized by polyuria. 2. d. mellitus.
**alloxan d.,** an animal model for diabetes mellitus; administration of alloxan produces selective destruction of the beta cells of the pancreas, causing hyperglycemia and ketoacidosis.
**brittle d.,** type 1 diabetes mellitus that is characterized by wide, unpredictable fluctuations of blood glucose values and is difficult to control.
**bronze d., bronzed d.,** hemochromatosis.
**chemical d.,** former name for *impaired glucose tolerance.*
**gestational d.,** gestational d. mellitus.
**d. insi'pidus,** any of several types of polyuria in which the volume of urine exceeds 3 liters per day, causing dehydration and great thirst, as well as sometimes emaciation and great hunger. The underlying cause may be hormonal *(central d. insipidus)* or renal *(nephrogenic d. insipidus).*
**d. insipidus, central,** diabetes insipidus due to injury of the neurohypophyseal system, with a deficient quantity of antidiuretic hormone being released or produced, causing failure of renal tubular reabsorption of water. It may be inherited, acquired, or idiopathic. Called also *pituitary insipidus.*
**d. insipidus, nephrogenic,** diabetes insipidus caused by failure of the renal tubules to reabsorb water in response to antidiuretic hormone, without disturbance in the renal filtration and solute excretion rates; the condition does not respond to exogenous vasopressin. It may be inherited as an X-linked trait or be acquired as a result of drug therapy or systemic disease.
**d. insipidus, pituitary,** central d. insipidus.
**latent d.,** former name for *impaired glucose tolerance.*
**lipoatrophic d.,** total lipodystrophy.
**maturity-onset d. of youth (MODY),** an autosomal dominant variety of type 2 diabetes mellitus characterized by onset in late adolescence or early adulthood.
**d. mel'litus (DM),** a chronic syndrome of impaired carbohydrate, protein, and fat metabolism owing to insufficient secretion of insulin or to target tissue insulin resistance. It occurs in two major forms: *type 1 d. mellitus* and *type 2 d. mellitus,* which differ in etiology, pathology, genetics, age of onset, and treatment.
**d. mellitus, adult-onset,** type 2 d. mellitus.
**d. mellitus, gestational,** diabetes mellitus with onset or first recognition during pregnancy; this category does not include diabetics who become pregnant or women who become lactosuric.
**d. mellitus, growth-onset,** type 1 d. mellitus.
**d. mellitus, insulin-dependent (IDDM),** type 1 d. mellitus.
**d. mellitus, juvenile, d. mellitus, juvenile-onset,** type 1 d. mellitus.
**d. mellitus, ketosis-prone,** type 1 d. mellitus.
**d. mellitus, ketosis-resistant,** type 2 d. mellitus.
**d. mellitus, malnutrition-related (MRDM),** a rare type of diabetes mellitus associated with chronic malnutrition and characterized by beta-cell failure, insulinopenia, insulin resistance, and moderate to severe hyperglycemia, but without ketosis. Called also *tropical* or *tropical pancreatic d. mellitus.*
**d. mellitus, maturity-onset,** type 2 d. mellitus.
**d. mellitus, non–insulin-dependent (NIDDM),** type 2 d. mellitus.
**d. mellitus, tropical, d. mellitus, tropical pancreatic,** malnutrition-associated d. mellitus.
**d. mellitus, type 1,** one of the two major types of diabetes mellitus, characterized by abrupt onset of symptoms, insulinopenia, and dependence on exogenous insulin to sustain life; peak age of onset is 12 years, although onset can be at any age. It is due to lack of insulin production by the beta cells of the pancreas, which may result from viral infection, autoimmune reactions, and probably genetic factors; islet cell antibodies are usually detectable at diagnosis. When it is inadequately controlled, lack of insulin causes hyperglycemia, protein wasting, and production of ketone bodies owing to increased fat metabolism, and the hyperglycemia leads to overflow glycosuria, osmotic diuresis, hyperosmolarity, dehydration, and diabetic ketoacidosis. It is accompanied by angiopathy of blood vessels, particularly the small ones *(microangiopathy),* which affects the retinas, kidneys, and basement membrane of arterioles throughout the body. Other symptoms include polyuria, polydipsia, polyphagia, weight loss, paresthesias, blurred vision, and irritability; if untreated, diabetic ketoacidosis progresses to nausea and vomiting, stupor, and potentially fatal hyperosmolar coma. Called also *insulin-dependent d. mellitus, juvenile* or *juvenile-onset d. mellitus,* and *Type I d. mellitus.*
**d. mellitus, Type I,** type 1 d. mellitus.
**d. mellitus, type 2,** one of the two major types of diabetes mellitus, characterized by peak age of onset between 50 and 60 years, gradual onset with few symptoms of metabolic disturbance (glycosuria and its consequences), and no need for exogenous insulin; dietary control with or without oral hypoglycemics is usually effective. Obesity

and genetic factors may also be present. Diagnosis is based on laboratory tests indicating glucose intolerance. Basal insulin secretion is maintained at normal or reduced levels, but insulin release in response to a glucose load is delayed or reduced. Defective glucose receptors on the beta cells of the pancreas may be involved. It is often accompanied by disease of various sizes of blood vessels, particularly the large ones, which leads to premature atherosclerosis with myocardial infarction or stroke syndrome. Called also *adult-onset d. mellitus, maturity-onset d. mellitus, non–insulin-dependent d. mellitus,* and *Type II d. mellitus.*
**d. mellitus, Type II,** type 2 d. mellitus.
**preclinical d.,** former name for *impaired glucose tolerance.*
**puncture d.,** diabetes produced in an experimental animal by puncturing the floor of the fourth ventricle in the medulla oblongata; see *Bernard's puncture,* under *puncture.*
**renal d.,** renal glycosuria.
**steroid d., steroidogenic d.,** glucose intolerance or overt hyperglycemia induced by glucocorticoids or estrogens; it is due in part to target tissue insulin resistance and is characterized by a relatively low incidence of microvascular sequelae.
**subclinical d.,** former name for *impaired glucose tolerance.*
**thiazide d.,** glucose intolerance or overt hyperglycemia induced by thiazide diuretics, which inhibit insulin secretion, possibly through thiazide-induced hypokalemia.

**di•a•bet•ic** (di″ə-bet′ik) 1. pertaining to or affected with diabetes. 2. a person with diabetes.

**di•a•be•tid** (di″ə-be′tid) diabetic dermopathy.

**di•a•be•to•gen•ic** (di″ə-bet″o-jen′ik) [*diabetes* + *-genic*] producing diabetes.

**di•a•be•tog•e•nous** (di″ə-be-toj′ə-nəs) produced by diabetes.

**Di•ab•i•nese** (di-ab′ĭ-nēs) trademark for a preparation of chlorpropamide.

**di•a•bro•sis** (di″ə-bro′sis) [*dia-* + Gr. *brōsis* eating] perforation resulting from a corrosive process; perforating ulceration.

**di•a•brot•ic** (di″ə-brot′ik) [Gr. *diabrōtikos*] 1. ulcerative; caustic. 2. a corrosive or escharotic agent.

**di•ac•e•tate** (di-as′ə-tāt) acetoacetate.

**di•ac•e•te•mia** (di-as′ə-te′me-ə) the presence of acetoacetic acid (diacetic acid) in the blood.

**di•a•ce•tic ac•id** (di″ə-se′tik) acetoacetic acid.

**di•ac•e•ton•uria** (di-as″ə-to-nu′re-ə) diaceturia.

**di•a•ce•tox•y•scir•pe•nol** (di-as″ə-tok″se-sir′pə-nol) a trichothecene mycotoxin produced by species of *Fusarium* that contaminate grain and other foodstuffs, causing fusariotoxicosis and hemorrhaging in livestock.

**di•ac•et•uria** (di-as″ə-tu′re-ə) the excretion of acetoacetic acid (diacetic acid) in the urine.

**di•ac•e•tyl** (di-as′ə-təl) [MeSH: Diacetyl] a yellow liquid, 2,3-butanedione, having the odor of butter.
**d. peroxide,** acetyl peroxide.

**di•ac•e•tyl•mor•phine** (di″ə-se″təl-mor′fēn) [MeSH: Diacetylmorphine] heroin; a white, bitterish, crystalline powder, the diacetic acid ester of morphine, formerly used as an analgesic and narcotic. Because it is highly addictive, the importation of heroin and its salts into the United States, as well as its use in medicine, is illegal. Called also *acetomorphine* and *diamorphine.*

**Di•a•chlo•rus** (di-ə-klor′əs) a genus of South American biting flies of the family Tabanidae.

**di•a•cho•re•ma** (di″ə-ko-re′mə) [Gr. *diachōrēma*] excrement; feces.

**di•a•cho•re•sis** (di″ə-ko-re′sis) defecation.

**di•ac•id** (di-as′id) [*di-* + *acid*] having two replaceable hydrogen atoms; a dibasic acid, having the acid activity of two molecules of a monobasic acid.

**di•ac•la•sis** (di-ak′lə-sis) [*dia-* + Gr. *klasis* fracture] osteoclasis.

**di•ac•ri•nous** (di-ak′rĭ-nəs) [Gr. *diakrinein* to separate] giving off secretion directly, as from a filter; said of gland cells, as those of the kidney. Opposed to *ptyocrinous.*

**di•ac•ri•sis** (di-ak′rĭ-sis) [Gr. *diakrisis* separation] 1. diagnosis. 2. a disease marked by a morbid state of the secretions. 3. a critical discharge or excretion.

**di•a•crit•ic** (di″ə-krit′ik) [*dia-* + Gr. *krinein* to judge] distinguishing; diagnostic.

**di•ac•tin•ic** (di″ak-tin′ik) transmitting chemically active rays.

**di•ac•tin•ism** (di-ak′tin-izəm) [*dia-* + *actinism*] the property of transmitting chemically active rays.

**di•acyl•glyc•er•ol** (di-a″səl-glis′ər-ol) a diester of glycerol in which two fatty acids are linked to its hydroxyl groups, usually at positions 1 and 2. Diacylglycerols are triglyceride and phospholipid degradation products and are second messengers in calcium-mediated responses to hormones, activating protein kinase C isozymes.

**di•ac•yl•glyc•er•ol *O*-ac•yl•trans•fer•ase** (di-a″səl-glis′ər-ol a″səl-trans′fər-ās) [EC 2.3.1.20] an enzyme of the transferase class that catalyzes the transfer of an acyl group from acyl CoA to a diglyceride, forming a triglyceride. Called also *diglyceride acyltransferase.*

**di•ac•yl•glyc•er•ol ki•nase** (di-a″səl-glis′ər-ol ki′nās) [EC 2.7.1.107] an enzyme of the transferase class that catalyzes the phosphorylation of a diacylglycerol to form a phosphatidate, using ATP as a phosphate donor. Called also *diglyceride kinase.*

**Di•ad•e•ma** a genus of sea urchins. *D. seto′sum* is the black sea urchin, a venomous species.

**di•ad•o•cho•ci•ne•sia** (di-ad″ə-ko-sĭ-ne′zhə) diadochokinesia.

**di•ad•o•cho•ki•ne•sia** (di-ad″ə-ko-kĭ-ne′zhə) [Gr. *diadocha* in succession + *-kinesi-* + *-ia*] the function of arresting one motor impulse and substituting for it one that is diametrically opposite, to permit sequential alternating movements, as pronation and supination of the arm. Cf. *adiadochokinesia* and *dysdiadochokinesia.* Called also *diadochocinesia.*

**di•ad•o•cho•ki•ne•sis** (di-ad″ə-ko-kĭ-ne′sis) diadochokinesia.

**di•ad•o•cho•ki•net•ic** (di-ad″ə-ko-kĭ-net′ik) pertaining to diadochokinesia.

**Di•a•dol** (di′ə-dol) trademark for a preparation of allobarbital.

**di•ag•nose** (di′əg-nōs) to make a diagnosis of; to recognize the nature of an attack of disease.

**di•ag•no•sis** (di″əg-no′sis) [*dia-* + Gr. *gnōsis* knowledge] [MeSH: Diagnosis] 1. the determination of the nature of a case of disease. 2. the art of distinguishing one disease from another.
**biological d.,** diagnosis by tests performed on animals.
**clinical d.,** diagnosis based on signs, symptoms, and laboratory findings during life.
**cytohistologic d.,** cytologic d.
**cytologic d.,** the diagnosis of disease, both benign and malignant, by study of exfoliated cells; called also *cytohistologic d.*
**differential d.,** the determination of which one of two or more diseases or conditions a patient is suffering from, by systematically comparing and contrasting their clinical findings.
**direct d.,** pathologic diagnosis by observing structural lesions or pathognomonic symptoms.
**d. by exclusion,** recognition of a disease by excluding all other known diseases.
**d. ex juvan′tibus,** diagnosis based on the results of treatment.
**laboratory d.,** diagnosis based on the findings of various laboratory examinations or measurements.
**niveau d.,** [Fr. "level diagnosis"], localization of the exact level of a lesion; as, for instance, of an intervertebral tumor.
**pathologic d.,** diagnosis by observing the structural lesions present.
**physical d.,** determination of disease by inspection, palpation, percussion, and auscultation.
**provocative d.,** the induction of a condition for the purpose of diagnosis, as the induction of a seizure in a doubtful case of epilepsy.
**serum d.,** diagnosis by means of the analysis of serums; immunodiagnosis.

**di•ag•nos•tic** (di″əg-nos′tik) pertaining to or subserving diagnosis; distinctive of or serving as a criterion of a disease, as signs and symptoms.

**di•ag•nos•ti•cate** (di″əg-nos′tĭ-kāt) diagnose.

**di•ag•nos•ti•cian** (di″əg-nos-tish′ən) an expert in diagnosis.

**di•ag•nos•tics** (di″əg-nos′tiks) the science and practice of diagnosis of disease.

**di•a•gram** (di′ə-gram) a graphic representation, in simplest form, of an object or concept, made up of lines and lacking entirely any pictorial elements.
**scatter d.,** scatterplot.
**ladder d.,** a diagrammatic representation of the routes of cardiac conduction as determined by electrocardiographic recording, used in diagnosing arrhythmias. Vectors describing the origins and paths of individual normal or ectopic impulses as well as points of blocks to conduction are drawn across a series of horizontal lines representing the atria, atrioventricular node, ventricles, and sometimes additional regions of the conduction system. See illustration. Called also *laddergram.*
**vector d.,** a diagram representing the direction and magnitude of electromotive forces of the heart for one entire cycle, based on analysis of the scalar electrocardiogram.
**Wiggers d.,** a graphic representation of the events of the cardiac cycle, showing the changes in a variety of physical variables over the period of a heartbeat; it includes depictions of the electrocardiogram, the pressure in the cardiac chambers and aorta, the ven-

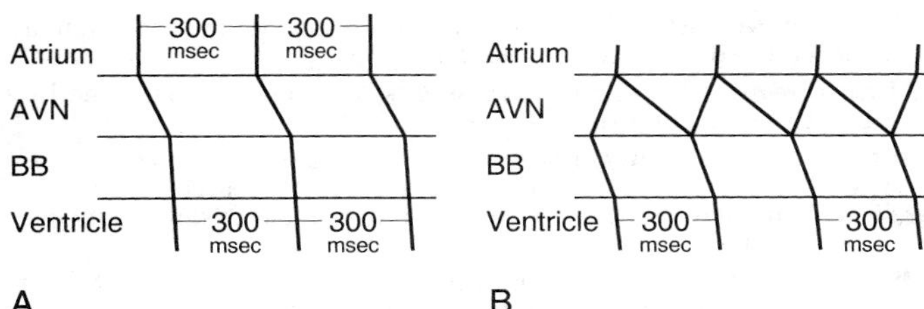


Ladder diagrams. *(A),* Sinus rhythm; *(B),* atrioventricular nodal reentrant tachycardia; AVN = atrioventricular node; BB = bundle branch.

tricular volume, and the heart sounds, and sometimes of the aortic flow rate and the venous pulse. See illustration at *cardiac cycle,* under *cycle.*

**di·a·gram·mat·ic** (di″ə-grə-mat′ik) pertaining to or of the nature of a diagram.

**di·a·graph** (di′ə-graf) [*dia-* + *-graph*] an instrument for recording outlines; used in craniometry, etc.

**di·a·ki·ne·sis** (di′ə-kĭ-ne′sis) [*dia-* + *-kinesis*] the stage of first meiotic prophase in which the nucleolus and nuclear envelope disappear and the spindle fibers form.

**di·al** (di′əl) [L. *dialis* daily, from *dies* day] a circular area with graduations around the circumference and a centrally fixed pointer for indicating values of time, pressure, etc.

**astigmatic d.,** a diagram arranged like the face of a watch used to determine the presence and axis of astigmatism.

**Di·a·lis·ter** (di″ə-lis′tər) a former genus of bacteria whose members have been reassigned to genus *Bacteroides.*

**di·al·lyl** (di-al′əl) any compound containing two allyl molecules.

**di·al·lyl·bis·nor·tox·i·fer·in di·chlo·ride** (di-al″əl-bis-nor-tok′sĭ-fər-in) alcuronium chloride.

**Di·a·log** (di′ə-log) trademark for a preparation of allobarbital and acetaminophen.

**Di·a·lume** (di′ə-lo͞om) trademark for a preparation of dried aluminum hydroxide gel.

**di·al·y·sance** (di-al′ə-səns) [*dialysis* + *-ance* suffix denoting action or process] the minute rate of net exchange of a substance between blood and bath fluid, per unit blood-bath concentration gradient; a parameter in artificial kidney kinetics (nonfiltration) functionally equivalent to the clearance of the natural kidney.

**di·al·y·sate** (di-al′ə-sāt) the material that passes through the membrane in dialysis.

**di·al·y·sis** (di-al′ə-sis) [Gr. "dissolution"] [MeSH: Dialysis] 1. the process of separating macromolecules from ions and low molecular weight compounds in solution by the difference in their rates of diffusion through a semipermeable membrane, through which crystalloids can pass readily but colloids pass very slowly or not at all. Two distinct physical processes are involved, diffusion and ultrafiltration (qq.v.). 2. hemodialysis.

**cross d.,** dialytic parabiosis.

**equilibrium d.,** a technique used to measure antibody-hapten affinities: solutions of pure antibody and hapten are placed in two cells separated by a semipermeable membrane and the hapten diffuses across until the free hapten concentration is the same on both sides. From the known total amounts of antibody and hapten and the measured free hapten concentration, the concentrations of free antibody and antibody-hapten complex and the dissociation constant are calculated.

**lymph d.,** removal of urea and other elements from lymph collected from the thoracic duct, treated outside the body, and later reinfused.

**peritoneal d.,** hemodialysis through the peritoneum, the dialyzing solution being introduced into and removed from the peritoneal cavity as either a continuous or an intermittent procedure. See also *intermittent peritoneal d.*

**peritoneal d., continuous ambulatory (CAPD),** a common method of peritoneal dialysis, involving the continuous presence of dialysis solution in the peritoneal cavity; drainage of the cavity and replacement with fresh solution is done 3 or 4 times daily and can be performed by patients themselves at home.

**peritoneal d., continuous cycling (CCPD),** a procedure similar to continuous ambulatory peritoneal dialysis but taking place at night using a machine to make several fluid exchanges automatically; two liters of dialysate fluid are left in the peritoneal cavity during the daytime to facilitate one additional fluid exchange.

**peritoneal d., intermittent (IPD),** an older form of peritoneal dialysis, in which dialysis solution is infused into the peritoneal cavity, allowed to equilibrate for 10 to 20 minutes, and then drained out; the process is repeated several times over a period of 24 hours at least twice a week.

**di·a·lyz·able** (di′ə-līz′ə-bəl) capable of dialysis or of passing through a membrane.

**di·a·lyzed** (di′ə-līzd) separated or prepared by dialysis.

**di·a·lyz·er** (di′ə-līz″ər) hemodialyzer.

**Di·a·ma·nus** (di″ə-ma′nəs) a genus of fleas. *D. monta′nus* infests rodents in the western United States and has been implicated in the transmission of sylvatic plague.

**di·am·e·ter** (di-am′ə-tər) the length of a straight line passing through the center of a circle and connecting opposite points on its circumference; hence the distance between two specified opposite points on the periphery of a structure such as the cranium or pelvis. Symbol *d.*

**anteroposterior d.,** the distance between a point on the anterior aspect and one on the posterior aspect of a structure, such as the true conjugate diameter of the pelvis, or the occipitofrontal diameter of the skull.

**anteroposterior d. of pelvis,** conjugata anatomica pelvis.

**anterotransverse d.,** (of the cranium), temporal d.

**Baudelocque's d.,** conjugata externa pelvis.

**bicristal d.,** the greatest distance between the external margins of the iliac crests.

**biischial d.,** transverse d. of pelvic outlet.

**biparietal d.,** the distance between the two parietal eminences.

**bisacromial d.,** the distance between the outermost points of the shoulder.

**bisiliac d.,** the distance between the two most remote points of the iliac crests.

**bispinous d.,** the distance between the opposite spines of the ischia.

**bitemporal d.,** the distance between the two extremities of the coronal suture.

**buccolingual d.,** the distance from the buccal to the lingual surface of a tooth crown at its widest point or greatest curvature.

**cervicobregmatic d.,** the distance between the center of the anterior fontanel and the junction of the neck with the floor of the mouth.

**coccygeopubic d.,** the distance from the tip of the coccyx to the under margin of the symphysis pubis.

**d. conjuga′ta pel′vis,** conjugata anatomica pelvis.

**conjugate d.,** 1. conjugate (def. 1). 2. conjugata anatomica pelvis.

**conjugate d., anatomical,** conjugata anatomica pelvis.

**conjugate d., diagonal,** conjugata diagonalis pelvis.

**conjugate d., external,** conjugata externa pelvis.

**conjugate d., internal,** conjugata anatomica pelvis.

**conjugate d., obstetric,** the shortest anteroposterior diameter of the pelvic inlet; the distance from a point 1 cm. below the top of the pubis to the tip of the sacral promontory, measuring 11 to 13 cm. in the normal pelvis. So called because it is intimately concerned in the process of labor. Called also *obstetric conjugate* and *conjugata vera obstetrica.*

**conjugate d., true,** conjugata anatomica pelvis.

**conjugate d. of pelvis,** 1. conjugata anatomica pelvis. 2. conjugate (def. 1).

**cranial d′s,** distances measured between certain landmarks of the skull, such as the *biparietal d., bitemporal d., cervicobregmatic d., frontomental d., occipitofrontal d., occipitomental d.,* and *suboccipitobregmatic d.*

**craniometric d.,** any line connecting two craniometric points of the same name.

**frontomental d.,** the distance from the forehead to the chin.

**fronto-occipital d.,** occipitofrontal d.

**intercristal d.,** distantia intercristalis.

**interspinous d.,** distantia interspinosa.

**intertuberal d.,** the distance between the sciatic notches.

**longitudinal d., inferior,** the distance from the foramen cecum to the internal occipital protuberance.

**mento-occipital d.,** occipitomental d.

**mentoparietal d.,** the distance from the chin to the vertex of the skull.

**d. obli′qua pel′vis** [TA], oblique diameter of pelvis: the oblique diameter across the pelvic inlet, measured from one sacroiliac articulation to the iliopubic eminence of the other side. Designated right or left depending on which sacroiliac joint is used for reference; the left is uniformly 0.5 cm. shorter than the right.

**occipitofrontal d.,** the distance from the external occipital protuberance to the most prominent midpoint of the frontal bone; called also *fronto-occipital d.*

**occipitomental d.,** the distance from the external occipital protuberance to the most prominent midpoint of the chin; called also *mento-occipital d.*

**parietal d.,** the distance between tuberosities of parietal bones; called also *posterotransverse d.*

**pelvic d.,** any diameter of the pelvis.

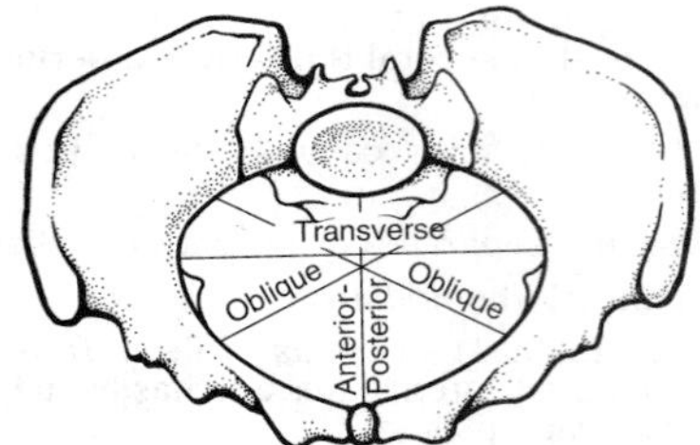

Diameters of pelvic inlet (see also pelvic planes).

**posterotransverse d.,** parietal d.
**pubosacral d.,** true conjugate d.
**pubotuberous d.,** the distance from the tuberosity of the ischium to a point on the superior ramus of the pubis which is located directly perpendicular to the tuberosity.
**sacropubic d.,** the distance from the tip of the sacrum or coccyx to the lower margin of the symphysis pubis.
**sagittal d.,** the distance from the glabella to the external occipital protuberance.
**suboccipitobregmatic d.,** the distance from the lowest posterior point of the occiput to the center of the anterior fontanel.
**temporal d.,** the distance between the tips of the alae magnae; called also *anterotransverse d.*
**d. transver'sa pel'vis** [TA], transverse diameter of pelvis: the greatest distance from side to side across the pelvic inlet.
**transverse d.,** the distance between two points located on the opposite sides of the body part being measured, such as the biparietal diameter of the head.
**transverse d. of pelvic outlet,** the distance between the medial surfaces of the ischial tuberosities (average length 11 cm.); called also *biischial d.*
**transverse d. of pelvis,** d. transversa pelvis.
**vertebromammary d.,** the anteroposterior diameter of the chest.
**vertical d.,** the distance between two points situated on the upper and lower aspects of the structure being measured, such as the distance between the occipital foramen and the vertex of the skull.

**di·amide** (di-am'īd) [*di-* + *amide*] [MeSH: Diamide] a compound that contains two amido groups.

**di·am·i·dine** (di-am'ĭ-dēn) a compound that contains two amidine groups.

**diamido-** a prefix indicating the possession of two amido groups.

**di·amine** (di'ə-mēn", -min') [*di-* + *amine*] a compound that contains two amino groups, sometimes specifically hydrazine.

**di·amine ox·i·dase** (di'ə-mēn" ok'sĭ-dās) amine oxidase (copper-containing).

**di·ami·no·ac·ri·dine** (di-ə-me"-no-ak'rĭ-din) proflavine.

***p*-di·ami·no·di·phen·yl** (di-ə-me"no-di-fen'əl) benzidine.

**di·ami·no·di·phen·yl·sul·fone** (di-am"ĭ-no-di-fen"əl-sul'fōn) dapsone.
**diacetyl d.,** acedapsone.

**di·am·in·uria** (di-am"ĭ-nu're-ə) the presence of diamines in the urine.

***cis*-di·am·mine·di·chlor·o·plat·i·num** (di"ə-mēn-di-klor"o-plat'ĭ-nəm) cisplatin.

**di·am·ni·on·ic** (di"am-ne-on'ik) having or developing within separate amniotic cavities.

**di·am·ni·ot·ic** (di-am"ne-ot'ik) diamnionic.

**Di·a·mond-Black·fan syndrome** (di'ə-mond-blak'fən) [Louis Klein *Diamond,* U.S. pediatrician, born 1902; Kenneth D. *Blackfan,* U.S. pediatrician, 1883–1941] see *congenital hypoplastic anemia,* under *anemia.*

**di·a·monds** (di'ə-məndz) the urticarial form of swine erysipelas.

**dia·mor·phine** (di"ə-mor'fēn) diacetylmorphine.

**Di·a·mox** (di'ə-moks) trademark for preparations of acetazolamide.

**di·am·tha·zole di·hy·dro·chlo·ride** (di-am'thə-zōl) an antifungal agent effective against species of *Trichophyton* and *Microsporum* and *Candida albicans;* it has been used in the treatment of various forms of tinea, applied topically.

**Di·an·a·bol** (di-an'ə-bol) trademark for methandrostenolone.

**di·an·hy·dro·an·ti·ar·i·gen·in** (di"an-hi"dro-an"te-ahr'ĭ-jen"in) an aglycone from antiarin.

**di·a·no·et·ic** (di"ə-no-et'ik) [*dia-* + *noetic*] pertaining to the intellectual functions, especially to reasoning.

**di·an·te·bra·chia** (di"ən-tə-bra'ke-ə) a developmental anomaly characterized by duplication of a forearm.

**Di·ap·a·rene** (di-ap'ə-rēn) trademark for preparations of methylbenzethonium chloride.

**di·a·pause** (di'ə-pawz) [*dia-* + *pause*] a state of inactivity and arrested development accompanied by greatly decreased metabolism, as in many eggs, insect pupae, and plant seeds; it is a mechanism for surviving adverse winter conditions.

**di·a·pe·de·sis** (di"ə-pə-de'sis) [*dia-* + Gr. *pēdan* to leap] the outward passage through intact vessel walls of cellular elements of the blood (erythrocytes or leukocytes). Called also *emigration, migration,* and *transmigration.*

**di·a·pe·det·ic** (di"ə-pə-det'ik) pertaining to or characterized by diapedesis.

**di·a·phane** (di'ə-fān) [Gr. *diaphanēs* transparent] a minute electric lamp for use in transillumination.

**di·a·pha·ne·i·ty** (di"ə-fə-ne'ĭ-te) transparency.

**di·aph·a·nog·ra·phy** (di-af"ə-nog'rə-fe) transillumination of the breast, with photography of the transilluminated light on infrared-sensitive film.

**di·aph·a·nom·e·ter** (di-af"ə-nom'ə-tər) [*diaphane* + *-meter*] an instrument for testing urine and other fluids by means of transmitted light.

**di·aph·a·nom·e·try** (di-af"ə-nom'ə-tre) the measurement of the transparency of a fluid.

**di·aph·a·no·scope** (de-af'ə-no-skōp") [*diaphane* + *-scope*] an instrument for transilluminating a body cavity; called also *electrodiaphane* and *electrodiaphanoscope.*

**di·aph·a·nos·co·py** (di-af'ə-nos'kə-pe) examination with the diaphanoscope; transillumination; called also *electrodiaphanoscopy.*

**di·aph·e·met·ric** (di-af'ə-met'rik) [*dia-* + Gr. *haphē* touch + *-metric*] pertaining to the measurement of tactile sensibility.

**di·aph·o·rase** (di-af'o-rās) any flavoprotein catalyzing the oxidation of reduced nicotinamide adenine dinucleotide (NAD) or reduced nicotinamide adenine dinucleotide phosphate (NADP) using a nonphysiological compound such as methylene blue as electron acceptor, but not oxygen or cytochromes. The reaction is an artifact arising from removal of the enzyme from the complexes in which it occurs naturally.

**di·a·pho·re·sis** (di"ə-fo-re'sis) [Gr. *diaphorēsis*] sweating, especially of a profuse type. Called also *sudoresis.*

**di·a·pho·ret·ic** (di"ə-fo-ret'ik) [Gr. *diaphorētikos*] 1. pertaining to, characterized by, or promoting sweating. 2. an agent that promotes sweating. Called also *sudorific.*

**di·a·phragm** (di'ə-fram) [MeSH: Diaphragm] 1. diaphragma (def. 1). 2. any separating membrane or structure. 3. a disk with one or more openings in it, or with an adjustable opening, mounted in relation to a lens or source of radiation by which part of the light or radiation may be excluded from the area. 4. a contraceptive device of molded rubber or other soft plastic material, fitted over the cervix uteri prior to intercourse to prevent the entrance of spermatozoa; for added efficacy, a spermicidal agent is usually placed within it. Called also *contraceptive d.* and *vaginal d.*
**accessory d.,** diaphragma urogenitale.
**antral d.,** see under *membrane.*
**contraceptive d.,** diaphragm (def. 4).
**epithelial d.,** an epithelial structure, evolving from the root sheath (sheath of Hertwig), that narrows the opening into the pulp chamber, diminishing its caliber. It is in close contact with the bone forming the fundus of the developing alveolus, from which it is separated by the dental sac.
**d. of mouth,** musculus mylohyoideus.
**oral d.,** musculus mylohyoideus.
**pelvic d., d. of pelvis,** diaphragma pelvis.
**polyarcuate d.,** one showing abnormal scalloping of margins on radiographic visualization.
**Potter-Bucky d.,** Bucky grid.
**pyloric d.,** see under *membrane.*

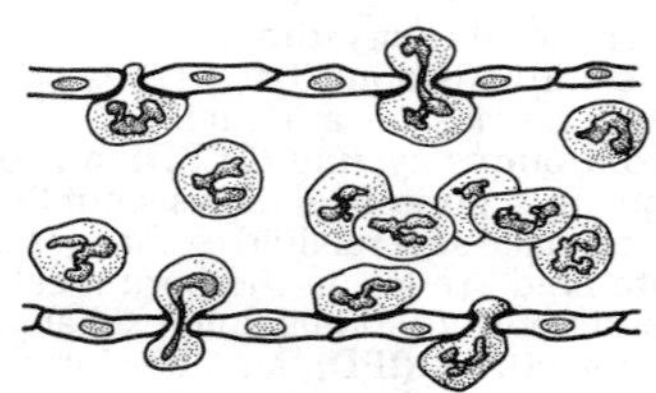
Diapedesis of leukocytes.

**respiratory d.**, diaphragma (def. 1).
**secondary d.**, diaphragma urogenitale.
**sellar d., d. of sella turcica,** diaphragma sellae.
**splinted d.**, inhibition of diaphragmatic movement, seen in a variety of disease processes. See also *paradoxical diaphragm phenomenon,* under *phenomenon.*
**thoracic d.**, diaphragma (def. 1).
**urogenital d.**, diaphragma urogenitale.
**vaginal d.**, diaphragm (def. 4).

**di·a·phrag·ma** (di″ə-frag′mə) pl. *diaphrag′mata* [Gr. "a partition-wall, barrier"] 1. [TA] diaphragm: the musculomembranous partition separating the abdominal and thoracic cavities, and serving as a major thoracic muscle. Called also *phren, midriff, diaphragmatic muscle,* and *thoracic* or *respiratory diaphragm.* 2. a term used in anatomical nomenclature to denote a separating structure.
**d. pel′vis** [TA], pelvic diaphragm: the portion of the floor of the pelvis formed by the coccygei and levatores ani muscles and their fasciae.
**d. sel′lae** [TA], sellar diaphragm: a ring-shaped fold of dura mater covering the sella turcica, and containing an aperture for passage of the infundibulum of the hypophysis.
**d. thoraco-abdomina′le,** diaphragma (def. 1).
**d. urogenita′le,** urogenital diaphragm: traditional but no longer valid concept that superior and inferior fascial layers enclose the sphincter urethrae and deep transverse perineal muscles and together form a musculomembranous sheet that extends between the ischiopubic rami. Called also *accessory* or *secondary diaphragm,* and *Camper's ligament. See also membrana perinei.*

**di·a·phrag·mal·gia** (di″ə-frag-mal′jə) phrenalgia.

**di·a·phrag·ma·ta** (di″ə-frag′mə-tə) [Gr.] plural of *diaphragma.*

**di·a·phrag·mat·ic** (di″ə-frag-mat′ik) 1. pertaining to or of the nature of a diaphragm. 2. phrenic.

**di·a·phrag·ma·ti·tis** (di″ə-frag″mə-ti′tis) phrenitis.

**di·a·phrag·mat·o·cele** (di″ə-frag-mat′o-sēl) [*diaphragm* + *-cele*[1]] diaphragmatic hernia.

**di·a·phrag·mi·tis** (de″ə-frag-mi′tis) phrenitis.

**di·aph·y·sary** (di-af′ə-zar-e) diaphyseal.

**di·a·phy·se·al** (di″ə-fiz′e-əl) pertaining to or affecting the shaft of a long bone (diaphysis).

**di·a·phys·ec·to·my** (di″ə-fiz-ek′tə-me) [*diaphysis* + *-ectomy*] excision of a portion of the shaft of a long bone.

**di·aph·y·ses** (di-af′ə-sēz) [Gr.] [MeSH: Diaphyses] plural of *diaphysis.*

**di·a·phy·si·al** (di″ə-fiz′e-əl) diaphyseal.

**di·aph·y·sis** (di-af′ə-sis) pl. *diaph′yses* [Gr. "the point of separation between stalk and branch"] 1. [TA] the elongated cylindrical portion (the shaft) of a long bone, between the ends or extremities (the epiphyses), which are usually articular and wider than the shaft; it consists of a tube of compact bone, enclosing the medullary (marrow) cavity. Called also *shaft.* 2. the portion of a long bone formed from a primary center of ossification.

**di·a·phys·itis** (di″ə-fiz-i′tis) inflammation of a diaphysis.
**tuberculous d.**, inflammation involving intermediate segments of the shafts of long bones, caused by the tubercle bacillus.

**di·a·pi·re·sis** (di″ə-pi-re′sis) [Gr. *diapeirein* to drive through] diapedesis.

**dia·pla·cen·tal** (di″ə-plə-sen′təl) through the placenta.

**di·a·poph·y·sis** (di″ə-pof′ə-sis) [*dia-* + *apophysis*] the superior or articular part of a transverse process of a vertebra.

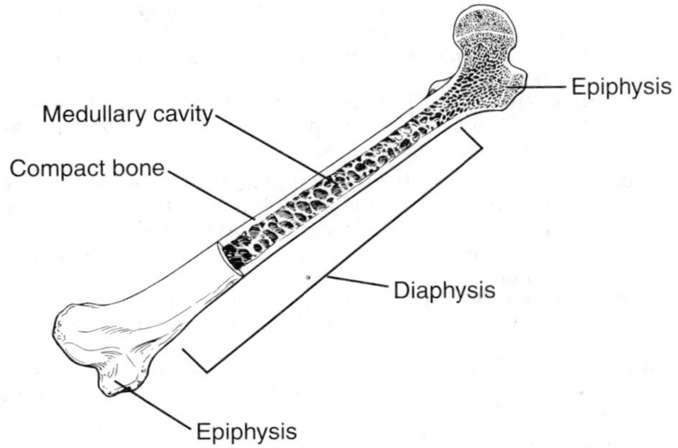


**Di·ap·to·mus** (di-ap′to-məs) a genus of copepod crustaceans, species of which act as hosts of the larvae of *Diphyllobothrium latum.*

**di·a·py·e·sis** (di″ə-pi-e′sis) suppuration.

**di·a·py·et·ic** (di″ə-pi-et′ik) promoting suppuration.

**di·ar·rhea** (di″ə-re′ə) [*dia-* + *-rrhea*] [MeSH: Diarrhea] abnormal frequency and liquidity of fecal discharges.
**bovine viral d., bovine virus d.,** an infectious disease of cattle, caused by a virus of the genus *Pestivirus;* marked by ulceration and hemorrhage of the alimentary tract with diarrhea and dehydration. Called also *mucosal disease.*
**cachectic d.,** diarrhea associated with cachexia; it may be due to malabsorption, or both the diarrhea and the cachexia may be manifestations of an underlying disease, e.g., neoplasm.
**calf d.,** diarrhea in calves; see *neonatal d.,* def. 2 and *white scours.* Called also *calf scours.*
**choleraic d.,** acute diarrhea with serous stools, accompanied by circulatory collapse, thus resembling cholera.
**chronic bacillary d.,** Johne's disease.
**d. chylo′sa,** diarrhea in which the discharge consists of a yellowish white, mucopurulent substance that resembles chyle in gross appearance.
**congenital chloride d.,** familial chloride d.
**dientameba d.,** a mild though chronic diarrhea caused by infection with *Dientamoeba fragilis.*
**dysenteric d.,** diarrhea with mucous and bloody stools.
**enteral d.,** diarrhea due to infection within the gastrointestinal tract.
**epidemic d. of newborn,** a contagious diarrhea occurring in epidemics among newborn infants in hospitals; called also *neonatal d.*
**familial chloride d.,** severe watery diarrhea with an excess of chloride in the stool, beginning in early infancy and marked by distended abdomen, lethargy, and retarded growth and mental development. It is accompanied by alkalosis and hypokalemia, and maternal hydramnios is often associated. The disorder is due to impairment of chloride-bicarbonate exchange in the lower bowel. Called also *congenital chloride d.* and *familial chloridorrhea.*
**fermental d., fermentative d.,** diarrhea caused by fermentation due to microorganisms.
**flagellate d.,** diarrhea marked by the presence of flagellate organisms *(Giardia)* in the stools.
**gastrogenic d.,** diarrhea due to gastric disorder.
**hill d.,** a chronic diarrhea peculiar to hot climates and occurring only at elevations of several thousand feet: named from the hill districts of India; it is considered by some to be identical with sprue.
**infantile d.,** summer d.
**inflammatory d.,** diarrhea in which there is an inflammation of the intestine due to bacterial action.
**irritative d.,** diarrhea due to irritation of the intestine by improper food, poisons, purgatives, etc.
**lienteric d.,** diarrhea with fluid stools containing undigested food.
**mechanical d.,** diarrhea due to mechanical obstruction to the portal circulation, producing gastrointestinal hyperemia.
**morning d.,** a condition marked by diarrhea in the morning only.
**mucous d.,** a kind characterized by the presence of mucus in stools.
**neonatal d.,** 1. epidemic diarrhea of the newborn. 2. any diarrhea seen in newborn animals, such as white scours; the most common cause is infection with *Escherichia coli, Coronavirus,* or *Rotavirus.*
**osmotic d.,** diarrhea resulting from the presence of osmotically active nonabsorbable solutes, e.g., magnesium sulfate, in the intestine.
**d. pancrea′tica,** the diarrhea that accompanies parenchymatous degeneration or cystic disease of the pancreas.
**pancreatogenous fatty d.,** a diarrhea in which the stools contain an excessive amount of fat owing to dysfunction of the pancreas.
**paradoxical d.,** stercoral d.
**parenteral d.,** diarrhea due to infections outside the gastrointestinal tract, such as tuberculosis, syphilis, etc.
**postweaning d.,** potentially fatal diarrhea in piglets just after they are weaned; causes may be allergies to ingredients of the new diet or intestinal infection, such as by a strain of *Escherichia coli* (see *coliform gastroenteritis*). Called also *weanling pig scours.*
**putrefactive d.,** diarrhea due to putrefaction of the intestinal contents.
**secretory d.,** watery, voluminous diarrhea resulting from increased stimulation of ion and water secretion, inhibition of their absorption, or both; stool osmolality approximates that of plasma, and diarrhea persists during fasting. Cf. *osmotic d.*
**serous d.,** diarrhea with copious serous fluid; called also *watery d.*
**stercoral d.,** diarrhea accompanied by colic and following two or three days of constipation; called also *paradoxical d.*
**summer d.,** acute diarrhea in children during great heat of summer; called also *infantile d.*
**toxigenic d.,** the watery, voluminous diarrhea caused by enterotoxins from enterotoxigenic bacteria such as *Vibrio cholerae* and ETEC strains of *Escherichia coli;* the enterotoxin is the primary pathogen and the bacteria do not invade the intestinal mucosa.
**traveler's d.,** diarrhea occurring among travelers, particularly in

those visiting tropical or subtropical areas where sanitation is suboptimal; it is caused by many different infectious agents, the most common being enterotoxigenic *Escherichia coli.* In Mexico, it is also called *turista.*
**tropical d.,** see *sprue,* def. 1.
**virus d.,** a specific infectious condition manifested by diarrhea in infants and by stomatitis and diarrhea in older children.
**watery d.,** serous d.
**weanling d.,** diarrhea in an infant when put on food other than its mother's milk, usually due to inadequate sanitation and infection with an enterotoxigenic strain of *Escherichia coli* or a rotavirus.
**white d.,** 1. a form in which the stools contain a thin, white mucus. 2. pullorum disease.

**di·ar·rhe·al** (di″ə-re′əl) pertaining to or marked by diarrhea.

**di·ar·rhe·ic** (di″ə-re′ik) diarrheal.

**di·ar·rhe·o·gen·ic** (di″ə-re″o-jen′ik) [*diarrhea* + *-genic*] giving rise to diarrhea.

**di·ar·thric** (di-ahr′thrk) [*di-* + *arthr-* + *-ic*] pertaining to or affecting two different joints.

**di·ar·thro·di·al** (di″ahr-thro′de-əl) of the nature of a diarthrosis (TA, *junctura synovialis*).

**di·ar·thro·ses** (di″ahr-thro′sēz) plural of *diarthrosis.*

**di·ar·thro·sis** (di″ahr-thro′sis) pl. *diarthro′ses* [Gr. *diarthrōsis* a movable articulation] TA alternative for *junctura synovialis.*
**d. rotato′ria,** a joint characterized by mobility in a rotary direction.

**di·ar·tic·u·lar** (di″ahr-tik′u-lər) diarthric.

**di·as·chi·sis** (di-as′kĭ-sis) [*dia-* + *-schisis*] the loss of function and electrical activity caused by cerebral lesions in areas remote from the lesion but neuronally connected to it; called also *Monakow's theory.*

**di·a·scope** (di′ə-skōp) [*dia-* + *-scope*] a glass or clear plastic plate, usually a flat blade or microscope slide, pressed against the skin to permit observation of changes produced in the underlying skin after the blood vessels are emptied and the skin is blanched.

**di·as·co·py** (di-as′kə-pe) 1. examination with the diascope. 2. transillumination.

**Di·a·sone** (di′ə-sōn) trademark for a preparation of sulfoxone sodium.

**di·as·pi·ro·nec·ro·bi·o·sis** (di-as″pĭ-ro-nek″ro-bi-o′sis) [*dia-* + Gr. *speirein* to sow + *necrobiosis*] disseminated necrobiosis.

**di·as·pi·ro·nec·ro·sis** (di-as″pĭ-ro-nə-kro′sis) disseminated necrosis.

**di·a·stase** (di′ə-stās) a mixture of amylolytic enzymes from malt, used to convert starch into simple sugars.

**di·as·ta·sic** (di″əs-ta′sik) diastatic.

**di·as·ta·sis** (di-as′tə-sis) [Gr. "separation"] 1. a form of dislocation in which there is separation of two bones normally attached to each other without the existence of a true joint; as in separation of the pubic symphysis. Also, separation beyond the normal between associated bones, as between the ribs, or the ulna and radius. 2. a relatively quiescent period of slow ventricular filling during the cardiac cycle; it occurs in mid-diastole, following the rapid filling phase and just prior to atrial systole. See illustration at *cardiac cycle,* under *cycle.*
**iris d.,** iridodiastasis.
**d. rec′ti abdo′minis,** separation of the rectus muscles of the abdominal wall, sometimes occurring during pregnancy.

**di·a·stas·uria** (di″ə-stās-u′re-ə) the presence of diastase in the urine.

**di·a·stat·ic** (di″ə-stat′ik) 1. pertaining to diastase. 2. pertaining to diastasis.

**di·a·stem** (di′ə-stem) diastema.

**di·a·ste·ma** (di″ə-ste′mə) pl. *diaste′mata* [Gr. *diastēma* an interval] [MeSH: Diastema] 1. a space or cleft. 2. [TA] a space between two adjacent teeth in the same dental arch. 3. a narrow zone in the equatorial plane through which the cytosome divides in mitosis.
**anterior d.,** a space between the incisor teeth, generally one between the maxillary central incisors.

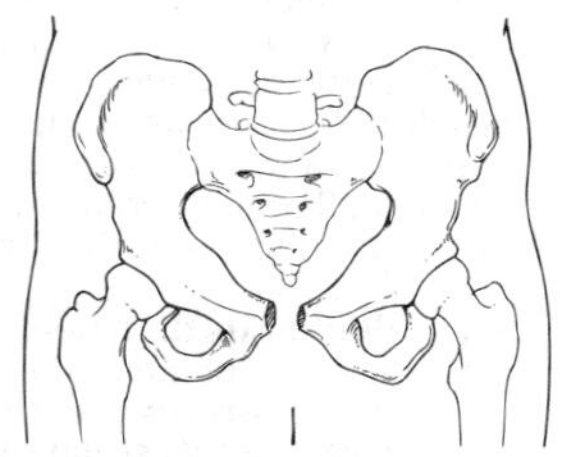

Diastasis of the pubic symphysis.

**di·a·stem·a·ta** (di″ə-stem′ə-tə) [Gr.] pl. of *diastema.*

**di·a·stem·a·to·cra·nia** (di″ə-stem″ə-to-kra′ne-ə) [*diastema* + *cranium*] congenital longitudinal fissure of the cranium.

**di·a·stem·a·to·my·e·lia** (di″-ə-stem″ə-to-mi-e′le-ə) [*diastema* + *myelo-* + *-ia*] a congenital anomaly, often associated with spina bifida, in which the spinal cord is split into halves by a bony spicule or fibrous band, each half being surrounded by a dural sac. Cf. *myeloschisis.*

**di·a·stem·a·to·py·e·lia** (di″ə-stem″ə-to-pi-e′le-ə) [*diastema* + *pyelos* pelvis + *-ia*] congenital median fissure of the pelvis.

**di·as·ter** (di′as-tər) [*di-* + *aster*] amphiaster.

**dia·ster·eo·iso·mer** (di″ə-ster″e-o-i′so-mər) diastereomer.

**dia·ster·eo·iso·mer·ic** (di″ə-ster″e-o-i″so-mer′ik) exhibiting diastereoisomerism.

**dia·ster·eo·isom·er·ism** (di″ə-ster″e-o″i-som′ər-iz-əm) the relationship between two or more stereoisomers whose molecules are not mirror images of each other, e.g., glucose and galactose or *cis* and *trans* isomers.

**dia·ster·eo·mer** (di″ə-ster′e-o″mər) one of a group of compounds having a diastereoisomeric relationship.

**Di·a·stix** (di′ə-stiks) trademark for a reagent strip designed for the quantitative determination of glucose in urine.

**di·as·to·le** (di-as′to-le) [Gr. *diastolē* a drawing asunder; expansion] [MeSH: Diastole] the dilatation, or period of dilatation, of the heart, especially of the ventricles; it coincides with the interval between the second and the first heart sound. Cf. *systole* and see illustration at *cardiac cycle,* under *cycle.*

**di·a·stol·ic** (di″ə-stol′ik) of or pertaining to diastole.

**di·as·to·my·e·lia** (di-as″to-mi-e′le-ə) diastematomyelia.

**di·a·stroph·ic** (di″ə-strof′ik) [Gr. *diastrephein* distortion] bent or curved; said of structures, such as bones, deformed in such manner.

**di·atax·ia** (di″ə-tak′se-ə) [*di-* + *ataxia*] ataxia affecting both sides of the body.
**cerebral d., d. cerebra′lis infanti′lis,** cerebral palsy with ataxia.

**di·a·ther·mal** (di″ə-thər′məl) pertaining to diathermy; heated by high-frequency electromagnetic radiation.

**di·a·ther·mic** (di″ə-thər′mik) pertaining to diathermy; permeable to high-frequency electromagnetic radiation.

**di·a·ther·my** (di′ə-thər″me) [*dia-* + Gr. *thermē* heat] [MeSH: Diathermy] heating of the body tissues due to their resistance to the passage of high-frequency electromagnetic radiation, electric currents, or ultrasonic waves. Tissues may be either simply warmed *(medical d.)* or coagulated and destroyed *(surgical d.).*
**medical d.,** application of currents of low tension and high amperage, which produce warmth in the deeper parts of the body; used particularly to promote muscle relaxation and to treat joint disorders including contractures. Called also *thermopenetration.*
**microwave d.,** medical diathermy using electromagnetic radiation by microwaves; it heats to a greater tissue depth than short-wave diathermy and is particularly effective in heating tissues with high water content such as muscles, subcutaneous fat, and fluid-filled cavities.
**short wave d.,** the therapeutic heating of the body tissues by means of an oscillating electromagnetic field of high frequency; the frequency varies from 10 million to 100 million cycles per second and the wavelength from 30 to 3 meters; it heats to a tissue depth of 2 to 3 cm and is used for heating large areas of body surface.
**surgical d.,** electrocoagulation.
**ultrashort wave d.,** diathermy in which the wavelength used is less than 10 meters.
**ultrasound d.,** medical diathermy using ultrasound; it heats to a tissue depth of 5 to 6 cm and is particularly used to warm areas around tissue interfaces such as joints.

**di·ath·e·sis** (di-ath′ə-sis) [Gr. "arrangement, disposition"] a constitution or condition of the body which makes the tissues react in special ways to certain extrinsic stimuli and thus tends to make the person more than usually susceptible to certain diseases. Cf. *constitution* (def. 1) and *type.*
**d. of connective tissue,** a congenital condition of bone and ligamentous tissue that leads to such disorders as recurrent dislocation of the elbow.
**exudative d.,** subcutaneous edema with surface exudation, seen in young pigs and chickens whose diet is deficient in selenium and vitamin E.
**gouty d.,** predisposition to gout.

**hemorrhagic d.**, a predisposition to abnormal hemostasis and hemorrhage.

**di·a·thet·ic** (di″ə-thet′ik) of or pertaining to a diathesis.

**di·a·tom** (di′ə-tom) any unicellular microscopical form of alga having a wall of silica and belonging to the family Diatomaceae. Several species are toxic, causing the "red blooms" or "red tides." The skeletal siliceous remains of many others are mined from deposits and used as filtering and abrasive agents; see *infusorial earth*, under *earth*.

**di·a·to·ma·ceous** (di″ə-to-ma′shəs) composed of diatoms; see *infusorial earth,* under *earth.*

**di·a·tom·ic** (di″ə-tom′ik) [*di-* + *atomic*] 1. made up of two atoms. 2. dibasic. 3. diatomaceous.

**di·at·o·mite** (di-at′ə-mīt) infusorial earth (diatomaceous earth) in a dry, compacted, stony form; workers inhaling its dust may suffer from diatomite fibrosis.

**dia·tri·zo·ate** (di″ə-tri-zo′āt) [MeSH: Diatrizoate] the most commonly used water-soluble, iodinated, radiopaque x-ray contrast medium; used as *d. meglumine* [USP] and *d. sodium* [USP] for all types of angiography; for splenoportography, hysterosalpingography, and arthrography; for cystography and intravenous and retrograde urography; for intravenous, operative, T-tube, and percutaneous transhepatic cholangiography; and for gastrointestinal tract studies.
**d. meglumine** [USP], a radiopaque medium, available in solution, consisting of diatrizoate meglumine in water for injection or of diatrizoic acid in water for injection, prepared with the aid of meglumine; used intra-arterially in angiocardiography,
**d. sodium** [USP], a radiopaque medium, available in solution, consisting of diatrizoate sodium in water for injection or of diatrizoic acid in water for injection, prepared with the aid of sodium hydroxide; used in cholangiography, intravenously in excretory urography, hysterosalpingography, and unilaterally in retrograde pyelography.

**dia·tri·zo·ic ac·id** (di″ə-tri-zo′ik) [USP] a white powder used in the preparation of certain radiopaque media; see *diatrizoate.*

**di·auch·e·nos** (di-awk′ə-nos) a dicephalic fetus with two necks.

**di·aux·ic** (di-awk′sik) pertaining to or characterized by diauxie; implying two periods of growth separated by a lag period.

**di·aux·ie** (di-awk′se) [*di-* + Gr. *auxein* to increase in size] a phenomenon of bacterial growth in which an organism given a mixture of organic compounds first grows exclusively on one until that compound is exhausted, and then, after a lag during which it forms induced enzymes for utilizing the second compound, resumes growth on the latter.

**dia·ver·i·dine** (di″ə-ver′ĭ-dēn) an antibacterial and coccidiostat used in poultry, especially against *Eimeria.*

**di·ax·on** (di-ak′son) [*di-* + *axon*] bipolar cell.

**di·az·e·pam** (di-az′ə-pam) [USP] [MeSH: Diazepam] a benzodiazepine used as an anxiolytic in the treatment of anxiety disorders and for short-term relief of anxiety symptoms, as a preoperative medication to relieve anxiety and tension, also as a skeletal muscle relaxant, anticonvulsant, antitremor agent, antipanic agent, and for treatment of symptoms of acute alcohol withdrawal; administered orally, intravenously, or intramuscularly.

**di·a·zine** (di-a′zēn) 1. any of a group of compounds derived from benzene by replacement of two carbon atoms by nitrogen atoms. 2. a suffix denoting a ring compound containing two nitrogen atoms.

**di·a·zi·quone (AZQ)** (di-a′zĭ-kwōn″) an alkylating agent that acts by cross-linking DNA, used as an antineoplastic in the treatment of primary brain malignancies, administered intravenously; it has also been used experimentally in the treatment of leukemia.

**diazo-** (di-az′o) a prefix indicating possession of the group —N═N—.

**di·azo·ben·zene·sul·fon·ic ac·id** (di-az″o-ben″zēn-səl-fon′ik) *p*-sulfobenzenediazonium hydroxide inner salt; white or slightly red crystals, prepared by the diazotization of sulfanilic acid and used in Ehrlich's diazo reaction.

**di·a·zo·ma** (di″ə-zo′mə) [Gr. *diazōma* that which is put round] the diaphragm.

**di·azo·meth·ane** (di-az″o-meth′ān) [MeSH: Diazomethane] an extremely poisonous yellow gas, $N_2CH_2$, used in organic synthesis.

**di·a·zo·nal** (di″ə-zo′nəl) 1. situated across or bridging two zones. 2. pertaining to a diazone.

**di·a·zone** (di′ə-zōn) one of the dark bands that alternate with light bands (parazones) to form the lines of Schreger, which are seen under reflected light in a ground section of a tooth; believed to be an area in which the enamel prisms have been cut in cross section.

**di·azo·sul·fo·ben·zol** (di-az″o-sul″fo-ben′zol) a substance which acts upon certain principles in the urine to form aniline colors.

**di·az·o·ti·za·tion** (di-az″o-tĭ-za′shən) conversion into a diazo compound.

**di·az·o·tize** (di-az′o-tīz) to introduce the diazo group into a compound.

**di·az·ox·ide** (di″əz-ok′sīd) [USP] [MeSH: Diazoxide] an antihypertensive, structurally related to chlorothiazide but having no diuretic properties, administered intravenously. Because it inhibits release of insulin, it is also administered orally in the treatment of hypoglycemia due to hyperinsulinism.

**di·ba·sic** (di-bā′sik) [*di-* + *basic*] containing two hydrogen atoms replaceable by bases, and thus yielding two series of salts, as $H_2SO_4$.

**Di·ben·amine** (di-ben′ə-mēn) [MeSH: Dibenamine] trademark for a preparation of dibenzylchlorethamine.

**di·ben·zan·thra·cene** (di″ben-zan′thrə-sēn) a polycyclic aromatic hydrocarbon consisting of anthracene with two benzene substitutions; when injected into the body it may produce epithelial tumors. Abbreviated DBA.

**di·ben·zaz·e·pine** (di-ben-zaz′ə-pēn) any of a group of structurally related drugs including the tricyclic antidepressants clomipramine, desipramine, imipramine, and trimipramine.

**di·ben·ze·pin hy·dro·chlo·ride** (di-ben′zə-pin) a tricyclic antidepressant having properties similar to those of amitriptyline; administered orally.

**di·ben·zo·cy·clo·hep·ta·di·ene** (di-ben″zo-si″klo-hep″tə-di′ēn) any of a group of structurally related drugs including the tricyclic antidepressants amitriptyline, nortriptyline, and protriptyline.

**di·ben·zo·di·az·e·pine** (di-ben″zo-di-az′ə-pēn) any of a group of structurally related drugs including the antipsychotic agent clozapine.

**di·ben·zo·thi·a·zine** (di-ben″zo-thi′ə-zēn) phenothiazine, def. 1.

**di·ben·zox·az·e·pine** (di-ben″zok-saz′ə-pēn) any of a class of structurally related, heterocyclic drugs, including the antipsychotic agent loxapine and the antidepressant amoxapine.

**di·ben·zox·e·pin** (di-ben-zok′sə-pin) dibenzoxepine.

**di·ben·zox·e·pine** (di-ben-zok′sə-pēn) any of a group of structurally related drugs including the tricyclic antidepressant doxepin.

**di·ben·zyl·chlo·reth·amine** (di-ben″zəl-klor-eth′ə-mēn) an alpha-adrenergic blocking agent which has been used in the treatment of peripheral vascular disorders and in the diagnosis of pheochromocytoma.

**Di·ben·zy·line** (di-ben′zə-lēn) trademark for a preparation of phenoxybenzamine hydrochloride.

**di·blas·tu·la** (di-blas′tu-lə) [*di-* + *blastula*] a blastula in which the ectoderm and endoderm are both present.

**di·both·rio·ceph·a·li·a·sis** (di-both″re-o-sef″ə-li′ə-sis) diphyllobothriasis.

**Di·both·rio·ceph·a·lus** (di-both″re-o-sef′ə-ləs) [*di-* + Gr. *bothrion* pit + *-cephalus*] *Diphyllobothrium.*

**di·bra·chia** (di-bra′ke-ə) [*di-* + *brachia*] a developmental anomaly characterized by duplication of an arm.

**di·bra·chi·us** (di-bra′ke-əs) conjoined twins having only two arms.

**di·bro·mide** (di-bro′mīd) any bromide which combines two atoms of bromine with one of another element or radical.

**di·bro·mo·chlo·ro·pro·pane** (di-bro″mo-klor″o-pro′pān) a colorless halogenated hydrocarbon formerly used as a pesticide, soil fumigant, and nematocide; its use is now restricted because of its carcinogenicity.

**di·bro·mo·dul·ci·tol** (di-bro″mo-dul′sĭ-tol) mitolactol.

**1,2-di·bro·mo·eth·ane** (di-bro″mo-eth′ān) ethylene dibromide.

**di·bro·mo·ke·tone** (di-bro″mo-ke′tōn) methyl dibromoethyl ketone, a war gas.

**di·brom·sa·lan** (di-brom′sə-lan) a bromsalan disinfectant with antibacterial and antifungal activities, used mainly in medicated soaps.

**di·bu·caine** (di′bu-kān) [USP] [MeSH: Dibucaine] a potent local anesthetic applied topically to the skin and mucous membranes. See also *dibucaine number,* under *number.*
**d. hydrochloride** [USP], the monohydrochloride salt of dibucaine, having the same actions as the base; administered in the form of an aerosol spray to produce anesthesia of the skin and mucous membranes or injected into the subarachnoid space to produce spinal anesthesia.

**Di·bu·line** (di′bu-lēn) trademark for a preparation of dibutoline sulfate.

**di·bu·to·line sul·fate** (di-bu′to-lēn) a quaternary ammonium anticholinergic, used as a cycloplegic and gastrointestinal antispasmodic, administered intramuscularly or subcutaneously.

**di·bu·tyl** (di-bu'təl) indicating the presence of two butyl groups.

**DIC** diffuse or disseminated intravascular coagulation.

**di·cac·o·dyl** (di-kak'o-dəl) cacodyl.

**di·cal·cic** (di-kal'sik) having in each molecule two atoms of calcium.

**di·cal·ci·um phos·phate** (di-kal'se-əm) dibasic calcium phosphate; see under *calcium.*

**di·car·bon·ate** (di-kahr'bon-āt) bicarbonate.

**di·car·box·yl·ic·ac·id·uria** (di″kahr-bok-sil″ik-as″id-u're-ə) urinary excretion of high levels of dicarboxylic acids, such as occurs in deficiencies of acyl-CoA dehydrogenase, when $\beta$-oxidation of fatty acids is blocked and $\omega$-oxidation is predominant.

**di·ce·lous** (di-se'ləs) [*di-* + *cel(o)-*[2] + *-ous*] 1. amphicelous. 2. having two cavities.

**Di·cen·tra** (di-sen'trə) a genus of perennial herbs of north central North America that have white or cream-colored flowers. *D. canaden'sis* (DC.) Walp. (squirrel or turkey corn) and *D. cuculla'ria* (L.) Bernh. (Fumariaceae) (Dutchman's breeches) are sources of the dried tuber called *corydalis* and contain bicuculline, bulbocapnine, corydaline, corytuberine, and other alkaloids that are toxic to livestock.

**di·cen·tric** (di-sen'trik) [*di-* + *center*] in genetics, a structurally abnormal chromosome with two centromeres.

**di·ceph·a·lous** (di-sef'ə-ləs) having two heads.

**di·ceph·a·lus** (di-sef'ə-ləs) [*di-* + *-cephalus*] a fetus with two heads.
**d. di'pus dibra'chius,** a fetus with two heads but only two feet and two arms.
**d. di'pus tetrabra'chius,** conjoined twins with only two legs, but with varying degrees of fusion of the upper trunk, each component having a head and pair of arms.
**d. di'pus tribra'chius,** a fetus with two heads, two feet, but with a median third arm or arm rudiment.
**d. dipy'gus,** anakatadidymus.
**d. parasi'ticus,** desmiognathus.
**d. tri'pus tribra'chius,** a fetus with a common trunk, but with two heads, three arms, and three legs, the third limbs being either rudimentary or complete.

**di·ceph·a·ly** (di-sef'ə-le) a developmental anomaly characterized by the presence of two heads.

**di·cha·pet·a·lum** (di″kə-pet'ə-lum) a genus of southern African trees. *D. cymo'sum* contains fluoroacetate and can cause fatal fluoroacetate poisoning in humans and livestock.

**di·chei·lia** (di-ki'le-ə) the appearance of a double lip, owing to folding of the oral mucosa.

**di·chei·ria** (di-ki're-ə) [*di-* + *cheir-* + *-ia*] a developmental anomaly characterized by duplication of a hand.

**di·chei·rus** (di-ki'rəs) an individual exhibiting dicheiria.

**Di·che·lo·bac·ter** (di-ke'lo-bak″tər) [Gr. *dichēlos* cloven-hoofed + *-bacter*] a genus of gram-negative, obligately anaerobic, nonmotile, non–spore-forming, rod-shaped bacteria. It includes organisms formerly included in the genus *Bacteroides.*
**D. nodo'sus,** a species that causes interdigital dermatitis and foot rot in sheep. Called also *Bacteroides nodosus.*

**di·chlo·ral·phen·a·zone** (di″klor-əl-fen'ə-zōn) [USP] a water-soluble complex of chloral hydrate and antipyrine (phenazone [INNrs]), into which it dissociates on administration; its properties are generally those of chloral hydrate, and it is used as a mild sedative and relaxant in combination with isometheptene mucate and acetaminophen in the treatment of migraine and tension headache.

**di·chlor·di·oxy·di·am·i·do·ar·seno·ben·zol** (di-klor″di-ok″se-di-am″ĭ-do-ahr″sə-no-ben'zol) arsphenamine.

**di·chlo·ride** (di-klor'id) a combination of a base or a metal with two atoms of chlorine.
**carbonic d.,** phosgene.

***o*-di·chlo·ro·ben·zene** (di-klor″o-ben'zēn) a solvent, fumigant, and insecticide, sometimes used as a spray; it is toxic if ingested or inhaled.

**3,3-di·chlo·ro·ben·zi·dine** (di-klor″o-ben'zĭ-dēn) a gray to purple crystalline solid used in the manufacture of dyes and plastics; it is carcinogenic.

**di·chlo·ro·di·eth·yl sul·fide** (di-klor″o-di-eth'əl) mustard gas, a vesicant gas once employed in war. It produces blistering and subsequent sloughing of the skin with involvement of the eyes and respiratory tract. Death results from bronchopneumonia. Called also *yellow cross* and *yperite.*

**di·chlo·ro·di·flu·o·ro·meth·ane** (di-klor″o-di-flo͞or″-o-meth'ān) [NF] a clear, colorless gas with a faint, ethereal odor, $CCl_2F_2$, used as an aerosol propellant, and also as a refrigerant.

**1,1-di·chlo·ro·eth·ane** (di-klor″o-eth'ān) ethylidene chloride.

**1,2-di·chlo·ro·eth·ane** (di-klor″o-eth'ān) ethylene dichloride.

**di·chlo·ro·iso·pro·ter·e·nol** (di-klor″o-i″so-pro-ter'ə-nol) a beta-adrenergic blocking agent used in the treatment of various cardiac disorders.

**di·chlo·ro·phen** (di-klor'o-fən) [MeSH: Dichlorophen] an anthelmintic used to treat infestations of large tapeworms in dogs and cats.

**2,4-di·chlo·ro·phen·oxy·ace·tic ac·id** (di-klor″o-fən-ok″se-ə-se'tic) [MeSH: 2,4-Dichlorophenoxyacetic Acid] 2,4-D.

**di·chlo·ro·tet·ra·flu·o·ro·eth·ane** (di-klor″o-tet″rə-flo͞or″-o-eth'ān) [NF] a clear, colorless gas with a faint ethereal odor, $CClF_2$-$CClF_2$, used as an aerosol propellant.

**di·chlor·phen·a·mide** (di″klor-fen'ə-mīd) [USP] [MeSH: Dichlorphenamide] a carbonic anhydrase inhibitor; used as an adjunct to reduce intraocular pressure in the treatment of glaucoma; administered orally.

**di·chlor·vos** (di-klor'vos) [MeSH: Dichlorvos] an organophosphorus insecticide, also used in veterinary medicine as an external parasiticide and anthelmintic.

**di·chog·e·ny** (di-koj'ə-ne) [Gr. *dicha* in two + *-geny*] development of tissues in different ways in accordance with changes in conditions affecting them.

**di·cho·ri·al** (di-kor'e-əl) dichorionic.

**di·cho·ri·on·ic** (di-kor″e-on'ik) having two distinct chorions; said of dizygotic twins.

**di·chot·o·mi·za·tion** (di-kot″ə-mĭ-za'shən) dichotomy.

**di·chot·o·my** (di-kot'ə-me) [Gr. *dicha* in two + *-tomy*] the process or result of division into two parts.

**Di·chroa** (di-kro'ə) a genus of plants of the family Saxifragaceae. *D. febrifu'ga* Lour. is a shrub found in China, India, Indonesia, and the Philippines, called *ch'ang shan* by the Chinese; its root, also called *ch'ang shan,* is used medicinally as a treatment for malaria.

**di·chro·ic** (di-kro'ik) exhibiting dichroism.

**di·chro·ine** (di-kro'ēn) an alkaloid from the plant *Dichroa febrifuga* (ch'ang shan); it has three isomeric forms: $\alpha$-, $\beta$-, and $\gamma$-dichroine.

**di·chro·ism** (di'kro-iz-əm) [*di-* + Gr. *chroa* color] the quality or condition of presenting one color in reflected and another in transmitted light.

**di·chro·ma·sy** (di-kro'mə-se) [*di-* + Gr. *chrōma* color] a defect in color vision in which one of the three cone pigments is missing altogether. The most common forms are protanopia and deuteranopia, each of which is transmitted by X-linked inheritance and affects about 1 per cent of white males. The third form, tritanopia, is very rare; and a fourth, tetartanopia, is of doubtful existence.

**di·chro·mat** (di'kro-mat) a person with dichromasy.

**di·chro·mate** (di-kro'māt) any salt containing the bivalent $Cr_2O_7$ radical.

**di·chro·mat·ic** (di″kro-mat'ik) pertaining to or characterized by dichromasy.

**di·chro·ma·tism** (di-kro'mə-tiz-əm) 1. the quality of existing in or exhibiting two different colors. 2. dichromasy.

**di·chro·ma·top·sia** (di″kro-mə-top'se-ə) dichromasy.

**di·chro·mic** (di-kro'mik) pertaining to two colors.

**di·chro·mo·phil** (di-kro'mo-fil) amphophilic; also, an amphophilic element.

**di·chro·moph·i·lism** (di″kro-mof'ĭ-liz-əm) capacity for double staining, that is, with both acid and basic dyes.

**Dick test (reaction), toxin** (dik) [George Frederick *Dick,* 1881–1967, and Gladys Rowena Henry *Dick,* 1881–1963, American physicians] see under *test,* and see *erythrogenic toxin,* under *toxin.*

**di·clo·fen·ac so·di·um** (di-klo'fən-ak) [USP] a nonsteroidal anti-inflammatory drug derived from phenylacetic acid, administered orally in the treatment of rheumatoid arthritis, osteoarthritis, and ankylosing spondylitis, and also for a variety of nonrheumatic inflammatory conditions.

**di·clox·a·cil·lin so·di·um** (di-klok″sə-sil'in) [USP] a semisynthetic penicillinase-resistant penicillin, used primarily in the treatment of infections due to penicillinase-producing staphylococci, administered orally.

**Di·co·did** (di-ko'did) trademark for preparations of hydrocodone bitartrate.

**di•coe•lous** (di-se'ləs) [*di-* + *coelo-* + *-ous*] 1. hollowed on each of two sides. 2. having two cavities.

**di•cot•y•le•don** (di-kot"əl-e'don) [*di-* + *cotyledon*] a flowering plant with embryos having two seed leaves, or cotyledons.

**di•cou•ma•rin** (di-koo'mə-rin) dicumarol (def. 1).

**dic•ro•ce•li•a•sis** (dik"ro-sə-li'ə-sis) hepatic fascioliasis due to infection with *Dicrocoelium dendriticum.*

**Dic•ro•coe•li•i•dae** (dik"ro-se-li'ĭ-de) a family of trematodes that includes the genera *Dicrocoelium, Eurytrema,* and *Platynosomum.* They infect the liver, pancreas, and bile ducts of various animals and occasionally humans.

**Dic•ro•coe•li•um** (dik"ro-se'le-əm) [Gr. *dikroos* forked + *koilia* bowel] [MeSH: Dicrocoelium] a genus of trematodes of the family Dicrocoeliidae.
**D. dendri'ticum,** the lancet fluke, a species that infests the liver of cattle and sheep in Europe, North and South America, and northern Africa, the cause of dicroceliasis; it has also been found in human biliary passages. Called also *D. lanceolatum.*
**D. hos'pes,** a species found in the gallbladder of cattle in the Sudan.
**D. lanceola'tum,** *D. dendriticum.*
**D. macrosto'mum,** a species found in the gallbladder of guinea fowl in Egypt.

**di•crot•ic** (di-krot'ik) [Gr. *dikrotos* double beating] pertaining to or characterized by dicrotism. See also anadicrotic and catadicrotic.

**di•cro•tism** (di'krŏ-tiz-əm) the presence of a dicrotic pulse.

**dicty(o)-** [Gr. *diktyon* net] a combining form denoting a relationship to a net or to a netlike structure.

**Dic•tyo•cau•lus** (dik"te-o-kaw'ləs) [*dictyo-* + Gr. *kaulos* stalk] [MeSH: Dictyocaulus] a genus of nematode lungworms of the family Trichostrongylidae, parasitic in the bronchial tree of horses, sheep, goats, deer, and cattle.
**D. arnfiel'di,** a species that invades the lungs of donkeys and horses and sometimes causes verminous bronchitis.
**D. fila'ria,** a species that infects the bronchial tree of sheep, goats, and cattle, and causes hoose; called also *Strongylus filaria.*
**D. vivipa'rus,** a species that infects the bronchial tree of cattle and deer, and causes hoose; called also *Strongylus micrurus.*

**dic•tyo•co•nid•i•um** (dik"te-o-kə-nid'e-əm) dictyospore.

**dic•tyo•ki•ne•sis** (dik"te-o-kĭ-ne'sis) [*dictyo-* + *kinesis*] the migration and distribution of the dictyosomes to the daughter cells in mitosis.

**dic•ty•o•ma** (dik"te-o'mə) [*dicty-* + *-oma*] diktyoma.

**dic•tyo•some** (dik'te-o-sōm) [*dictyo-* + *-some*] a stack of membranous lamellae or cisternae with attached tubules and vesicles in the cytoplasm of various cells; see also *Golgi complex,* under *complex.*

**dic•tyo•spore** (dik'te-o-spor) a spore that has both vertical and horizontal septa; called also *dictyoconidium.*

**dic•tyo•tene** (dik'te-o-tēn) [*dictyo-* + *-tene*] the protracted stage resembling suspended prophase in which the primary oocyte persists from late fetal life until discharged from the ovary at or after puberty.

**di•cu•ma•rol** (di-koo'mə-rol) [MeSH: Dicumarol] 1. a coumarin anticoagulant found in spoiled sweet clover; animals eating the clover may develop the hemorrhagic condition known as *sweet clover disease.* Called also *bishydroxycoumarin, dicoumarin,* and *melilotoxin.* 2. a synthetic preparation of the same substance, used as an oral anticoagulant; it acts by inhibiting the hepatic synthesis of vitamin K–dependent coagulation factors (prothrombin and factors VII, IX, and X).

**Di•cur•in** (di-kūr'in) trademark for a preparation of merethoxylline.

**di•cy•clic** (di-si'klik) 1. pertaining to or having two cycles. 2. in chemistry, having a molecular structure containing two rings.

**di•cy•clo•mine hy•dro•chlo•ride** (di-si'klo-mēn) [USP] an anticholinergic, used as an antispasmodic in the treatment of functional gastrointestinal disorders, administered orally or intramuscularly.

**di•cys•te•ine** (di"sis-te'in) cystine.

**di•dac•tic** (di-dak'tik) [Gr. *didaktikos*] conveying instruction by lectures and books rather than by practice.

**di•dac•tyl•ism** (di-dak'təl-iz-əm) [*di-* + *daktyl-* + *-ism*] the condition of having only two digits on a hand or foot.

**di•dac•ty•lous** (di-dak'tə-ləs) having only two digits on a hand or foot.

**di•dan•o•sine** (di-dan'o-sēn) [MeSH: Didanosine] 2'3'-dideoxyinosine, an analogue of dideoxyadenosine; an antiretroviral agent that is converted intracellularly into the active metabolite dideoxyadenosine triphosphate, which inhibits viral replication both by incorporation into the viral genome and by interference with the action of reverse transcriptase; used for the treatment of advanced HIV-I infection and acquired immunodeficiency syndrome, administered orally. Formerly called *dideoxyinosine (ddI).*

**di•del•phia** (di-del'fe-ə) [*di-* + Gr. *delphys* uterus] uterus didelphys.

**di•del•phic** (di-del'fik) pertaining to or possessing a double uterus.

**Di•del•phis** (di-del'fis) [*di-* + Gr. *delphys* uterus] the opossums, a genus of marsupials; some species in South America are reservoirs of *Trypanosoma cruzi.*

**2',3'-di•de•oxy•aden•o•sine** (di"de-ok"se-ə-den'o-sēn) a dideoxynucleoside in which the base is adenine, in plasma rapidly converted to 2',3'-dideoxyinosine by the enzyme adenosine deaminase; it is used as an antiretroviral agent in the treatment of acquired immunodeficiency syndrome.

**di•de•oxy•cy•ti•dine** (di"de-ok"se-si'tĭ-dēn) zalcitabine

**di•de•oxy•in•o•sine** (di"de-ok"se-in'o-sēn) didanosine.

**di•de•oxy•nu•cleo•side** (di"de-ok"se-noo'kle-o-sīd") any of a group of synthetic nucleoside analogs lacking two deoxy groups; several 2',3'-dideoxynucleosides inhibit the enzyme reverse transcriptase and thus have antiretroviral activity.

**di•der•mo•ma** (di"dər-mo'mə) [*di-* + *derm-* + *-oma*] a teratoma composed of cells and tissues derived from two cell layers.

**Di•di•ée's projection** (de-de-ā'z) [J. *Didiée,* French radiologist, 20th century] see under *projection.*

**Di•drex** (di'dreks) trademark for a preparation of benzphetamine hydrochloride.

**Di•dro•nel** (di-dro'nəl) trademark for preparations of etidronate disodium.

**did•y•mal•gia** (did"ə-mal'jə) orchialgia.

**did•y•mi•tis** (did"ə-mi'tis) orchitis.

**did•y•mo•dyn•ia** (did"ə-mo-din'e-ə) orchialgia.

**did•y•mo•spore** (did'ĭ-mo-spor) a spore with two cells and one septa, as in certain imperfect fungi.

**did•y•mous** (did'ə-məs) occurring in pairs.

**did•y•mus** (did'ə-məs) [Gr. *didymos* double, twofold, twain] testis.

**-didymus** [Gr. *didymos* twin] a word termination denoting conjoined twins or duplication of body parts. See also *-pagus.*

**die** (di) 1. a form to be used in the construction of something. 2. a positive reproduction of the form of a prepared tooth in a suitable hard substance, such as a metal, resin, or plaster of Paris.
**amalgam d.,** a model of a tooth made of amalgam; used in making dental prostheses.
**electroformed d.,** a die formed by electroplating an impression, forming a metallic positive reproduction of a prepared tooth. Often incorrectly called *electroplated d.* or *plated d.*
**electroplated d., plated d.,** incorrect terms for *electroformed d.*
**waxing d.,** a die or model to which wax is adapted for the fabrication of a wax pattern.

**Dieb. alt.** abbreviation for L. *die'bus alter'nis,* on alternate days.

**Dieb. tert.** abbreviation for L. *die'bus ter'tiis,* every third day.

**di•echo•scope** (di-ek'o-skōp) [*di-* + *echo* + *-scope*] an instrument for the simultaneous perception of two different sounds in auscultation.

**di•e•cious** (di-e'shəs) [*di-* + Gr. *oikos* house] sexually distinct; denoting species in which male and female genitals do not occur in the same individual. In botany, having staminate and pistillate flowers on separate plants.

**Dief•fen•bach's operation** (de'fən-bahks) [Johann Friedrich *Dieffenbach,* German surgeon, 1792–1847] see under *operation.*

**Di•e•go blood group** (de-a'go) [from the name of the Venezuelan propositus family first observed in 1955] see under *blood group.*

**di•el•drin** (di-el'drin) [MeSH: Dieldrin] a chlorinated hydrocarbon insecticide closely related to aldrin, used against the sheep tick *Melophagus ovinus* and to control vectors of insect-borne diseases, especially mosquitoes. Inhalation, ingestion, or absorption through the skin by humans or other animals may cause neurotoxic symptoms such as tremors and convulsions that can be fatal.

**di•elec•tric** (di"ə-lek'trik) 1. transmitting electric effects by induction, but not by conduction. The term is applied to an insulating substance through or across which electric force is acting or may act, by induction without conduction. 2. a dielectric substance.

**di•elec•trol•y•sis** (di"ə-lek-trol'ə-sis) [*dia-* + *electrolysis*] electrolysis of a drug, the current being passed through a diseased portion of the body, so that the drug passes through the part.

**di•em•bry•ony** (di-em'bre-on"e) [*di-* + *embryony*] the production of two embryos from a single zygote.

**di·en·ce·phal·ic** (di″ən-sə-fal′ik) pertaining to the diencephalon.

**di·en·ceph·a·lo·hy·po·phys·i·al** (di″ən-sef″ə-lo-hi″po-fiz′e-əl) pertaining to the diencephalon and the pituitary gland.

**di·en·ceph·a·lon** (di″ən-sef′ə-lon) [*dia-* + *encephalon*] [MeSH: Diencephalon] 1. [TA] the caudal part of the prosencephalon, which largely bounds the third ventricle and connects the mesencephalon to the cerebral hemispheres; each lateral half is divided by the hypothalamic sulcus into a dorsal part, comprising the epithalamus, dorsal thalamus, and metathalamus, and a ventral part, comprising the ventral thalamus (subthalamus) and hypothalamus. Called also *interbrain*. See Plate 11. See also *brainstem*. 2. the posterior of the two brain vesicles formed by specialization of the prosencephalon in the developing embryo.

**-diene** a suffix used in chemistry to denote an unsaturated hydrocarbon containing two double bonds.

**die·ner** (de′nər) [Ger. "man-servant"] a technician or man-of-all-work usually in a gross laboratory.

**di·en·es·trol** (di″ən-es′trol) [USP] [MeSH: Dienestrol] a synthetic estrogen, administered orally in the management of menopausal symptoms, in the treatment of functional uterine bleeding, as a postpartum antigalactagogue, for palliative therapy in certain female breast cancers, and in the management of prostatic carcinoma, and applied locally in the treatment of postmenopausal and senile vulvovaginitis, atrophic vaginitis, pruritus vulvae due to atrophic changes in the vulval epithelium, dyspareunia associated with atrophic vaginal epithelium, and prior to plastic pelvic surgery in menopausal patients.

**Di·ent·amoe·ba** (di″ent-ə-me′bə) [*di-* + *ent-* + *ameba*] [MeSH: Dientamoeba] a genus of small highly active, usually nonpathogenic or mildly pathogenic ameboid protozoa (superorder Parabasalidea, order Trichomonadida) parasitic in the large intestine of humans and certain monkeys, and typically characterized by the presence of two nuclei connected by a desmose and an endosome formed by four to eight chromatin granules. *D. fragilis* has been associated with human infection, which is manifested chiefly by diarrhea, abdominal pain, bloody, mucoid, or loose stools, and flatulence.

**di·er·e·sis** (di-er′ə-sis) [Gr. *diairesis* a taking] 1. the division or separation of parts normally united. 2. in surgery, the operative separation of parts by incision, electrosurgery, or cautery.

**di·esoph·a·gus** (di-ə-sof′ə-gəs) doubling of the esophagus.

**di·es·ter** (di-es′tər) a compound containing two ester groups.

**di·es·trum** (di-es′trəm) diestrus.

**di·es·trus** (di-es′trəs) [MeSH: Diestrus] 1. in female mammals that have estrous cycles, a period of sexual quiescence between metestrus and the next proestrus; it represents the phase of the mature corpus luteum. 2. anestrus, def. 2. Called also *diestrum*.
**gestational d.**, the period of sexual inactivity occurring during gestation in female mammals.
**lactational d.**, the period of sexual inactivity occurring during lactation in female mammals.

**di·et** (di′ət) [Gr. *diaita* way of living] [MeSH: Diet] the customary allowance of food and drink taken by any person from day to day, particularly one especially planned to meet specific requirements of the individual, and including or excluding certain items of food.
**absolute d.**, fasting.
**acid-ash d.**, a diet to produce acidification of the urine, consisting of meat, fish, eggs and cereals, with little fruit and vegetables and no cheese or milk.
**adequate d.**, one that enables an animal to grow, mature, and reproduce in a normal manner. Cf. *optimal d.*
**alkali-ash d.**, a diet of fruit, vegetables, and milk with as little as possible of meat, fish, eggs, and cereals.
**balanced d.**, one containing all the nutritive factors in proper proportion for adequate nutrition.
**basal d.**, one which is just sufficient to meet the caloric requirements of basal metabolism.
**basic d.**, a diet which contains a preponderant proportion of alkaline ash; used for some types of urinary calculus.
**bland d.**, one that is free from any irritating or stimulating foods.
**challenge d.**, a diet to which foods suspected of causing sensitivity in the patient are added, usually one at a time, and the results assessed. Cf. *provocative d.*
**diabetic d.**, one designed to prevent complications of diabetes mellitus by controlling the timing and amount of energy intake and minimizing the occurrence of ketosis or hypoglycemia; fat, carbohydrate, and protein ratios and amounts are controlled but specific diet plans vary.
**elemental d.**, one consisting of a well-balanced, residue-free mixture of all essential and nonessential amino acids combined with simple sugars, electrolytes, trace elements, and vitamins.
**elimination d.**, a procedure to identify food allergy in which foods are sequentially omitted in order to detect the one or ones responsible for symptoms.
**Feingold d.**, a controversial diet for hyperactive children which excludes artificial colors, artificial flavors, preservatives, and salicylates.
**formula d.**, one in which one or more meals consist of or are supplemented by a processed drink formulated to contain defined levels of specific vitamins, nutrients, and caloric level; it is usually used in weight reduction.
**Giordano-Giovannetti d.**, a low protein diet given to alleviate gastrointestinal symptoms of chronic renal failure.
**gluten-free d.**, a diet deficient in the cereal protein gluten; used as a specific treatment for celiac disease (gluten enteropathy).
**gouty d.**, one for mitigation of gout, restricting nitrogenous, especially high-purine foods, and substituting dairy products, with prohibition of wines and liquors.
**high calorie d.**, one that furnishes more calories than needed for the maintenance of weight, often more than 3500–4000 calories per day.
**high fat d.**, ketogenic d.
**high fiber d.**, one relatively high in dietary fibers, which decreases bowel transit time and relieves constipation.
**high protein d.**, one containing large amounts of protein, consisting largely of meats, fish, milk, legumes, and nuts.
**ketogenic d.**, one containing a large amount of fat with minimal amounts of protein and carbohydrate, the object of such a diet being to produce ketosis; called also *high fat d.*
**light d.**, a simple mixed diet suitable for convalescents.
**low calorie d.**, one containing fewer calories than needed for the maintenance of weight, e.g., less than 1200 calories per day for an adult.
**low fat d.**, one containing limited amounts of fat.
**low oxalate d.**, one with no potatoes, beans, or fiber vegetables,

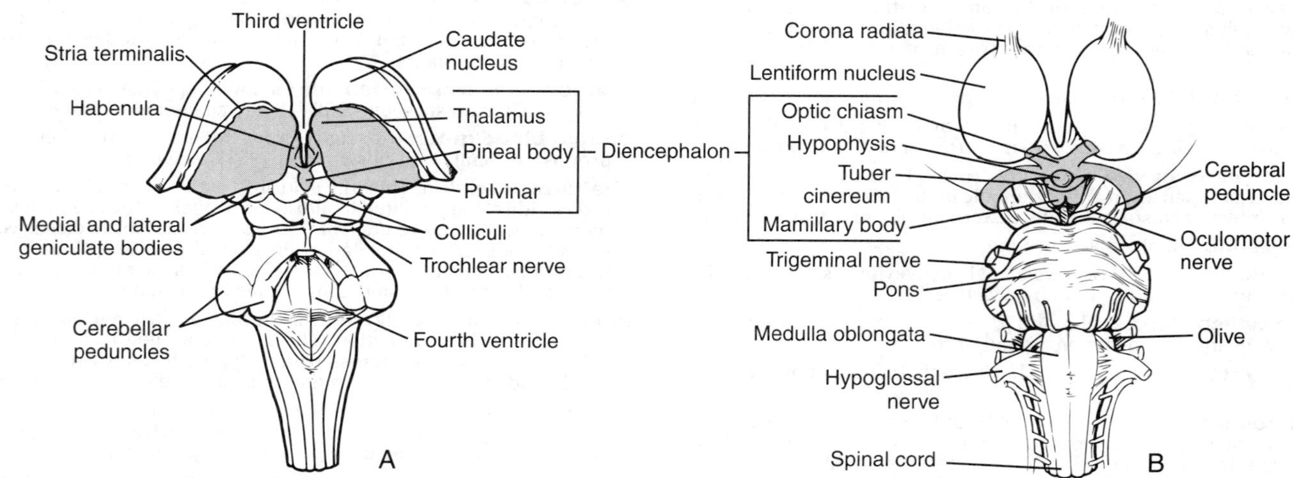


Diencephalon. Posterior (dorsal) *(A)* and anterior (inferior) *(B)* views of the base of the brain, showing the diencephalon in relation to the mesencephalon (midbrain) and rhombencephalon (hindbrain).

and no sweet fruit, tea, chocolate, or sweets; used for the prevention of oxalate stones in the urinary tract.
**low purine d.,** one for mitigation of gout, omitting meat, fowl, and fish and substituting milk, eggs, cheese, and vegetable protein.
**low residue d.,** a diet which gives the least possible fecal residue: such as gelatin, sucrose, glucose, broth, hard-boiled egg, meat, liver, rice, and cottage cheese.
**low salt d.,** a diet which contains very little sodium chloride; prescribed by some for hypertension and for edematous states.
**Moro-Heisler d.,** a diet of grated raw apple for diarrheal conditions in infants.
**nutraceutical d.,** a diet containing functional foods (nutraceuticals).
**optimal d.,** a diet that produces the most desirable growth, the most successful reproduction, and the maintenance of the best possible health; Cf. *adequate d.*
**protein-sparing d.,** one consisting only of liquid proteins or liquid mixtures of proteins, vitamins, and minerals, and containing no more than 600 calories; it is designed to maintain a favorable nitrogen balance.
**provocative d.,** a diet designed to include the most common allergenic foods, from which they are eliminated one by one, as a means of determining the offending substances in cases of food allergy. Cf. *challenge d.*
**purine-free d.,** see *low-purine d.*
**salt-free d.,** see *low-salt d.*
**Schemm d.,** a low-sodium, neutral and acid-ash diet for patients with congestive heart failure.
**Schmidt d.,** a daily diet consisting of 1.5 liters of milk, 100 gm. of zwieback, 2 eggs, 50 gm. of butter, 125 gm. of beef, 190 gm. of boiled potato, and gruel made from 80 gm. of oatmeal. It contains 102 gm. of protein, 111 gm. of fat, and 191 gm. of carbohydrate, giving 2234 calories. It is used to facilitate examination of the stools in various types of diarrhea.
**Schmidt-Strassburger d.,** Schmidt d.
**Sippy d.,** a diet formerly widely used to treat peptic ulcers, consisting of milk, cream, and other supposedly bland foods; it was later proved ineffective.
**smooth d.,** one which avoids the use of foods containing roughage.
**subsistence d.,** a diet on which one can just live.
**Taylor's d.,** a preparation of white of egg, olive oil, and sugar, given when the urine is to be tested for chlorides.
**test d.,** a diet designed to test allergy or sensitivity to certain foods by selectively omitting or including those foods, e.g., an elimination or a provocative diet.
**therapeutic d.,** one specifically formulated for use in the diagnosis or treatment of disease or deficiency.
**very low calorie d. (VLCD),** a diet providing 200 to 800 kilocalories per day, used for weight loss in markedly obese patients for whom other diet programs have been unsuccessful.

**di·e·tary** (di'ə-tar″e) a regular or systematic scheme of diet.

**di·e·tet·ic** (di″ə-tet'ik) [Gr. *diaitētikos*] pertaining to diet or proper food.

**di·e·tet·ics** (di″ə-tet'iks) [MeSH: Dietetics] the science or study and regulation of the diet.

**di·eth·a·nol·amine** (di″eth-ə-nol'ə-mēn) 1. 2,2′-iminobisethanol: an ethanolamine (see *monoethanolamine*) produced by the ammonolysis of ethylene oxide. 2. [NF] a mixture of ethanolamines consisting chiefly of diethanolamine, used as a pharmaceutic aid (alkalizing agent).

**di·eth·yl·car·bam·a·zine** (di-eth″əl-kahr-bam'ə-zēn) [MeSH: Diethylcarbamazine] an antifilarial agent effective against *Wuchereria* and *Loa loa* in humans, heartworms in dogs, and lungworms in cattle and sheep. It causes the disappearance of worms from the blood due to phagocytosis by macrophages of the reticuloendothelial system. Used as *diethylcarbamazine citrate.*

**di·eth·yl·ene·di·amine** (di-eth″əl-ēn-di'ə-mēn) piperazine.

**1,4-di·eth·yl·ene di·ox·ide** (di-eth'ə-lēn di-ok'sīd) dioxane.

**di·eth·yl·ene·tri·amine pen·ta·ace·tic ac·id** (di-eth'əl-ēn-tri'ə-mēn pen″tə-ə-se'tik as'id) DTPA; pentetic acid.

**di·eth·yl·pro·pi·on hy·dro·chlo·ride** (di-eth″əl-pro'pe-on) [USP] an adrenergic structurally related to amphetamine, methamphetamine, and ephedrine, occurring as a white to off-white, fine crystalline powder; used as an anorexic, administered orally.

**di·eth·yl·stil·bes·trol (DES)** (di-eth″əl-stil-bes'trol) [MeSH: Diethylstilbestrol] a synthetic nonsteroidal estrogen having activity similar to but greater than that of estrone. It is used for many purposes, including relief of menopausal symptoms; suppression of lactation; treatment of amenorrhea, dysmenorrhea, senile vaginitis, and pruritus vulvae; palliative treatment of female breast carcinoma; relief of symptoms of prostatic carcinoma; and formerly for prevention of threatened or habitual abortion and premature labor. Administered intramuscularly. It has been found to be an epigenetic carcinogen; women who have been exposed in utero to diethylstilbestrol show characteristic changes in the cervix and vagina and are subject to an increased risk of vaginal or cervical carcinoma. Called also *stilbestrol.*
**d. diphosphate** [USP], an ester of diethylstilbestrol, having the same actions as the base; used in the treatment of prostatic carcinoma, administered intravenously.
**d. dipropionate,** an ester of diethylstilbestrol, having actions and uses similar to those of the base; administered orally, intravaginally, or intramuscularly.

**di·eth·yl·tol·u·am·ide** (di-eth″əl-tol-u'ə-mīd) [USP] an arthropod repellent, occurring as a colorless liquid; applied topically to the skin and to the clothing.

**di·eth·yl·tryp·ta·mine** (di-eth″əl-trip'tə-mēn) a hallucinogenic substance closely related to dimethyltryptamine, but prepared synthetically. Abbreviated DET.

**di·e·ti·cian** (di″ə-tĭ'-shən) dietitian.

**di·e·ti·tian** (di″ə-tish'ən) a person trained in the scientific use of diet in health and disease.

**Die·tl's crisis** (de'təlz) [Józef *Dietl,* Polish physician, 1804–1878] see under *crisis.*

**di·e·to·ther·a·py** (di″ə-to-ther'ə-pe) diet therapy.

**di·e·to·tox·ic** (di″ə-to-tok'sik) having the quality of dietotoxicity.

**di·e·to·tox·i·ci·ty** (di″ə-to-tok-sis'ĭ-te) a quality in certain food substances which renders them toxic when used in an unbalanced diet.

**Dieu·la·foy's triad, vascular malformation (ulcer)** (dyo͞o-lah-fwahz') [Georges *Dieulafoy,* French physician, 1839–1911] see under *malformation.*

**di·fen·ox·in** (di″fən-ok'sin) an antiperistaltic that is the active metabolite of diphenoxylate.
**d. hydrochloride,** the hydrochloride salt of difenoxin, used as an antidiarrheal; administered orally.

**dif·fer·ence** (dif'ər-ens) the condition or magnitude of variation between two qualities or quantities.
**arteriovenous oxygen d.,** the difference in the oxygen content of blood between the arterial and venous systems, usually expressed in mL/L of blood.

**dif·fer·en·tial** (dif″ər-en'shəl) [L. *differre* to carry apart] pertaining to a difference or differences.

**dif·fer·en·ti·ate** (dif″ər-en'she-āt) 1. to distinguish, on the basis of differences. 2. to develop specialized form, character, or function differing from that of surrounding cytoplasm, cells, or tissue or from the original type.

**dif·fer·en·ti·a·tion** (dif″ər-en″she-a'shən) 1. the distinguishing of one thing or disease from another. 2. the act or process of acquiring completely individual characters, as occurs in the progressive diversification of cells and tissues of the embryo. 3. increase in morphological or chemical heterogeneity.
**correlative d.,** differentiation caused by factors outside the tissue itself, as by an inductor; called also *dependent d.*
**dependent d.,** correlative d.
**functional d.,** differentiation which results from the functioning of the tissue of a part.
**invisible d.,** the development toward a fixed fate, through chemodifferentiation, by cells that show no visible signs of this determination.
**regional d.,** the appearance of regional differences within a field of development.
**self d.,** differentiation produced by factors solely within the tissue or part.

**dif·flu·ence** (dif'loo-əns) the act of becoming fluid or of flowing readily.

**dif·flu·ent** (dif'loo-ənt) [L. *diffluere* to flow off] 1. easily flowing away or dissolving. 2. deliquescent.

**Diff-Quik** (dif'kwik) trademark for a Giemsa-type stain.

**dif·frac·tion** (dĭ-frak'shən) [*dis-*[1] + L. *frangere* to break] the bending of waves around small obstacles and the spreading out of waves past openings that are small compared to the wavelengths. See also under *grating.*
**x-ray d.,** a technique for studying the cell based on the diffraction of radiations when they encounter small obstacles; used especially in the study of inorganic and organic crystals, in which it is possible to determine the precise spatial relationships between the constituent atoms.

**dif·fu·sate** (dĭ-fu'zāt) 1. material that has passed through a membrane. 2. dialysate.

**dif·fuse** [*dis-*[1] + *fundere* to pour] 1. (dĭ-fūs') not definitely limited or localized; widely distributed. 2. (dĭ-fūz') to pass through or to spread widely through a tissue or structure.

**dif·fus·ible** (dĭ-fūz′ĭ-bəl) susceptible of becoming widely spread.

**dif·fu·si·om·e·ter** (dĭ-fu″ze-om′ə-tər) an apparatus for measuring the speed of diffusion.

**dif·fu·sion** (dĭ-fu′zhən) [MeSH: Diffusion] 1. the process of becoming diffused, or widely spread. 2. the spontaneous movement of molecules or other particles in solution, owing to their random thermal motion, to reach a uniform concentration throughout the solvent, a process requiring no addition of energy to the system. 3. in hemodialysis, the movement of solutes across semipermeable membranes down concentration gradients, the movement generally being of urea and low molecular weight toxins from the blood to the dialysate and of bicarbonate and acetate from the dialysate to the blood. 4. immunodiffusion.
**double d.**, immunodiffusion in which both the antigen and antibody diffuse through the medium toward each other.
**double d. in one dimension,** antiserum is placed in a test tube and overlaid with agar, which is allowed to solidify, and antigen is layered over the agar. Precipitin lines form where the concentrations of each antigen and antibody are equivalent. Called also *Oakley-Fulthorpe technique.*
**double d. in two dimensions,** double diffusion in which antigen and antiserum are placed in wells cut in an agar plate; antigen solutions to be compared are placed in wells equidistant from the antiserum well. Three principal types of reaction may occur, *reaction of identity, reaction of nonidentity,* and *reaction of partial identity* (see under *reaction*), each identified by a characteristic pattern of precipitin lines, indicating the extent to which the antigen samples a share antigenic determinants. Called also *Ouchterlony technique.*
**exchange d.**, the process in which diffusion of a molecule across a membrane in one direction is balanced by diffusion of another molecule in the opposite direction.
**facilitated d.**, diffusion across a plasma membrane or other biological membrane in which the molecules to be transported form complexes with specific transport proteins that shuttle them across the membrane and release them on the other side.
**free d.**, diffusion in which there is no obstacle such as a membrane.
**gel d.**, immunodiffusion.
**impeded d.**, diffusion in which the rate is slowed down by the difficulty of passing through a membrane.
**single d.**, immunodiffusion in which either the antibody or antigen remains fixed and the other reactant diffuses through it.
**single radial d.**, a quantitative immunodiffusion technique in which the antigen solutions are placed in wells cut in an agar plate containing antiserum; the area or diameter of the precipitin ring around an unknown solution is compared with the rings of a serial dilution of a standard antigen solution to determine the amount of antigen present in the unknown. Called also *radial immunodiffusion (RID).*
**thermal d.**, thermodiffusion.

**di·flor·a·sone di·ac·e·tate** (di-flor′ə-sōn) [USP] a synthetic corticosteroid used topically for the relief of inflammation and pruritus in corticosteroid-responsive dermatoses.

**Di·flu·can** (di′floo-kan) trademark for a preparation of fluconazole.

**di·flu·cor·to·lone va·ler·ate** (di″floo-kor′tə-lōn″) a synthetic corticosteroid used topically for the relief of inflammation and pruritus in corticosteroid-responsive dermatoses.

**di·flu·ni·sal** (di-floo′nĭ-səl) [USP] [MeSH: Diflunisal] a nonsteroidal antiinflammatory agent derived from salicyclic acid, having analgesic activity but lacking antipyretic activity; used for relief of mild to moderate pain.

**Dig.** abbreviation for L. *digera′tur,* let it be digested.

**di·gal·lic ac·id** (di-gal′ik) an incorrect term for tannic acid.

**di·ga·met·ic** (di″gə-met′ik) 1. pertaining to or producing gametes (germ or sex cells) of two different types, female (oocytes) and male (spermatozoa). 2. heterogametic.

**di·gas·tric** (di-gas′trik) [*di-* + *gastric*] 1. having two bellies. 2. musculus digastricus.

**di·gen·e·sis** (di-jen′ə-sis) alternation of generation.

**di·ge·net·ic** (di″jə-net′ik) [*di-* + *genetic*] having two stages of multiplication, one sexual in the mature forms, the other asexual in the larval stages; said of flukes and many other parasites.

**Di·George's syndrome** (dĭ-jor′jəz) [Angelo Mario *DiGeorge,* American pediatrician, born 1921] see under *syndrome.*

**di·ges·tant** (di-jes′tənt) 1. assisting or stimulating digestion. 2. an agent that assists or stimulates digestion.

**di·ges·tion** (di-jes′chən) [L. *digestio,* from *dis-* apart + *gerere* to carry] [MeSH: Digestion] 1. the process or act of converting food into chemical substances that can be absorbed and assimilated. 2. the subjection of a body to prolonged heat and moisture, so as to disintegrate and soften it.
**artificial d.**, that which is performed outside the body.
**biliary d.**, the digestive effect of the bile upon food.
**gastric d.**, that which is carried on in the stomach by aid of the gastric juice; called also *peptic d.* and *chymification.*
**gastrointestinal d.**, the gastric and intestinal digestions together; called also *primary d.*
**intercellular d.**, digestion carried on within an organ by secretions from the cells of the organ.
**intestinal d.**, that which is carried on in the intestine.
**intracellular d.**, digestion carried on within a single cell.
**lipolytic d.**, the splitting of fat into fatty acid and glycerol.
**pancreatic d.**, that which is performed by the pancreatic secretion.
**parenteral d.**, digestion taking place somewhere else in the body than in the alimentary canal, as in the blood or under the skin.
**peptic d.**, gastric d.
**primary d.**, gastrointestinal d.
**salivary d.**, the change of starch into maltose by the saliva.
**sludge d.**, the biochemical process by which organic matter in sludge is gasified, liquefied, mineralized, or converted into more stable organic matter.

**di·ges·tive** (di-jes′tiv) 1. pertaining to digestion. 2. digestant.

**Dig·i·bind** (dij′ĭ-bīnd″) trademark for a preparation of digoxin immune Fab (ovine).

**dig·it** (dij′it) [L. *digitus*] digitus.

**dig·i·tal** (dij′ĭ-təl) 1. of, pertaining to, or performed with, a finger. 2. resembling the imprint of a finger. 3. pertaining to numerical methods or discrete variables.

**dig·i·tal·in** (dij″ĭ-tal′in) 1. true digitalin; a cardiac glycoside, $C_{36}H_{56}O_{14}$, from the seeds of *Digitalis purpurea.* 2. any of several mixtures of digitalis glycosides extracted from the leaves or seeds.

**Dig·i·tal·ine Na·ti·velle** (dij″ĭ-tal′ēn na″tĭ-vel′) trademark for a preparation of digitoxin.

**Dig·i·tal·is** (dij″ĭ-tal′is) [L. from *digitus* finger, because of the finger-like leaves of the corolla of its flowers] [MeSH: Digitalis] a genus of herbs of the family Scrophulariaceae, native to Europe and Asia. *D. purpu′rea* is the purple foxglove whose leaves furnish digitalis. *D. lana′ta* is a Balkan species that yields digoxin and lanatoside.

**dig·i·tal·is** (dij″ĭ-tal′is) [MeSH: Digitalis] 1. [USP] the dried leaf of *Digitalis purpurea,* the purple foxglove, used to treat congestive heart failure, most supraventricular tachycardias, and cardiogenic shock. Digitalis and the digitalis glycosides act by increasing the force of myocardial contraction and by increasing the refractory period and decreasing the conduction rate of the atrioventricular node. When digitalis is prescribed, *powdered d.* (q.v.) is to be dispensed. 2. collectively, the digitalis glycosides or the cardiac glycosides. 3. [TA] a general term for any finger-like structure.
**d. leaf,** digitalis (def. 1).
**powdered d.** [USP], **prepared d.**, the standardized preparation to be dispensed when digitalis is prescribed; its actions and uses are as for digitalis; administered orally.

**dig·i·tal·iza·tion** (dij″ĭ-təl-ĭ-za′shən) the administration of digitalis or one of its glycosides in a dosage schedule designed to produce and then maintain optimal therapeutic concentrations of its cardiotonic glycosides.

**dig·i·tal·oid** (dij′ĭ-təl-oid) resembling or related to digitalis.

**dig·i·tate** (dij′ĭ-tāt) having finger-like processes. Called also *dactylate.*

**dig·i·ta·tio** (dij″ĭ-ta′she-o) pl. *digitatio′nes* [L.] a finger-like process.
**d.′nes hippocam′pi** [TA], pes hippocampi.

**dig·i·ta·tion** (dij″ĭ-ta′shən) 1. a finger-like process. 2. surgical creation of a functioning digit.

**dig·i·ta·ti·o·nes** (dij″ĭ-ta″she-o′nez) [L.] plural of *digitatio.*

**dig·i·ti** (dij′ĭ-ti) [L.] genitive and plural of *digitus.*

**dig·i·ti·form** (dij′ĭ-tĭ-form) resembling a finger; finger-like.

**dig·i·ti·grade** (dij′ĭ-tĭ-grād″) [*digitus* + L. *gradi* to walk] characterized by standing or walking on the toes, with the posterior part of the foot being raised; said of quadrupeds such as cats and dogs. Cf. *plantigrade* and *unguligrade.*

**dig·i·to·nin** (dij″ĭ-to′nin) [USP] [MeSH: Digitonin] a saponin obtained from *Digitalis purpurea;* it possesses no cardiotonic action and is used as a reagent to precipitate free cholesterol.

**dig·i·to·plan·tar** (dij″ĭ-to-plan′tər) [*digitus* + *plantar*] pertaining to the toes and the sole of the foot.

**di·gi·toxi·ge·nin** (dij″ĭ-tok″sĭ-je′nin) [MeSH: Digitoxigenin] the steroid nucleus that is the aglycone of digitoxin.

**dig·i·tox·in** (dij″ĭ-tok′sin) [USP] [MeSH: Digitoxin] a cardiac glycoside obtained from *Digitalis purpurea, D. lanata,* and other *Digitalis* species, containing 3 molecules of digitoxose linked to digitoxigenin; it has the same actions and uses as digitalis; administered orally, intramuscularly, or intravenously.

**dig·i·tox·ose** (dij″ĭ-tok′sōs) a hexose sugar that forms the carbohydrate moiety of the cardiac glycosides obtained from *Digitalis.*

**dig·i·tus** (dij′ĭ-təs) pl. *dig′iti* [L.] [TA] digit: a finger or a toe; see also *ossa digitorum manus* and *ossa digitorum pedis,* under *os*[2].
**d. anula′ris** [TA], ring finger: the fourth digit of the hand. Called also *d. quartus (IV) manus* [TA alternative].
**d. hippocra′ticus,** clubbed finger.
**d. mal′leus,** mallet finger.
**di′giti ma′nus** [TA], the digits of the hand; the fingers. See *pollex, index, d. medius, d. anularis,* and *d. minimus manus.*
**d. me′dius** [TA], middle finger: the third digit of the hand; called also *d. tertius (III) manus* [TA alternative].
**d. mi′nimus ma′nus** [TA], little finger: the fifth, and smallest, digit of the hand; called also *d. quintus (V) manus* [TA alternative].
**d. mi′nimus pe′dis** [TA], little toe: the fifth, and smallest, digit of the foot; called also *d. quintus (V) pedis* [TA alternative].
**d. mor′tuus,** [L.], dead finger.
**di′giti pe′dis** [TA], the digits of the foot; the toes. See *hallux, d. secundus pedis, d. tertius pedis, d. quartus pedis,* and *d. minimus pedis.*
**d. postmi′nimus,** an appendage ranging from a small round mass of fat and connective tissue to a longer mass containing bones and with a nail at its distal end, attached by a small pedicle to the soft tissue covering the lateral surface of the little finger or toe.
**d. pri′mus (I) ma′nus,** TA alternative for *pollex.*
**d. pri′mus (I) pe′dis,** TA alternative for *hallux.*
**d. quar′tus (IV) ma′nus,** TA alternative for *d. anularis.*
**d. quar′tus (IV) pe′dis** [TA], the fourth digit of the foot.
**d. quin′tus (V) ma′nus,** TA alternative for *d. minimus manus.*
**d. quin′tus (V) pe′dis,** TA alternative for *d. minimus pedis.*
**d. secun′dus (II) ma′nus,** TA alternative for *index.*
**d. secun′dus (II) pe′dis** [TA], the second digit of the foot.
**d. ter′tius (III) ma′nus,** TA alternative for *d. medius.*
**d. ter′tius (III) pe′dis** [TA], the third digit of the foot.
**d. val′gus,** deviation of a digit in the radial direction, or toward the digit of next lower number.
**d. va′rus,** deviation of a digit in the ulnar direction, or toward the digit of next higher number.

**di·glos·sia** (di-glos′e-ə) [*di-* + *gloss-* + *-ia*] bifid tongue.

**di·glyc·er·ide** (di′glis′ə-rīd) diacylglycerol.

**di·glyc·er·ide ac·yl·trans·fer·ase** (di-glis′ər-īd a″səl-trans′fər-ās) diacylglycerol *O*-acyltransferase.

**di·glyc·er·ide ki·nase** (di-glis′ər-īd ki′nās) diacylglycerol kinase.

**dig·na·thus** (dig-na′thəs) [*di-* + Gr. *gnathos* jaw] a fetus with two lower jaws; see also *myognathus.*

**di·goxi·ge·nin** (dĭ-jok″sĭ-je′nin) [MeSH: Digoxigenin] the steroid nucleus that is the aglycone of digoxin.

**di·gox·in** (dĭ-jok′sin) [USP] [MeSH: Digoxin] a cardiac glycoside obtained from the leaves of *Digitalis lanata,* containing 3 molecules of digitoxose linked to digoxigenin, and having the same actions and uses as digitalis; administered orally, intramuscularly, or intravenously.

**Di·gram·ma brau·ni** (di-gram′ə braw′ne) a larval tapeworm belonging to the family Diphyllobothriidae, reported from man in Romania; formerly called *Diplogonoporus brauni.*

**Di Gu·gli·el·mo's syndrome** (de goo-lyel′mōz) [Giovanni *Di Guglielmo,* Italian hematologist, 1886–1961] erythroleukemia.

**di·het·ero·zy·gote** (di-het″ər-o-zi′gōt) [*di-* + *heterozygote*] an individual heterozygous for two pairs of genes; called also *dihybrid.*

**di·hex·y·ver·ine hy·dro·chlo·ride** (di″heks-ĭ-ver′ēn) an anticholinergic which has been used as an antispasmodic in uterine hypermotility and intestinal muscle spasm.

**di·hy·brid** (di-hi′brid) diheterozygote.

**di·hy·drate** (di-hi′drāt) [*di-* + *hydrate*] 1. any compound containing two hydroxyl groups. 2. any compound containing two molecules of water.

**di·hy·drat·ed** (di-hi′drāt-əd) compounded with two molecules of water.

**di·hy·dric** (di-hi′drik) having two hydrogen atoms in each molecule.

**di·hy·dro·bi·op·ter·in** (di-hi″dro-bi-op′tər-in) a reduced pteridine derivative related to folic acid; its quinoid form is produced by oxidation of tetrahydrobiopterin in several biological hydroxylation reactions.

**di·hy·dro·bi·op·ter·in syn·the·tase de·fi·cien·cy** (di-hi″dro-bi-op′ter-in sin′thə-tās) older name for malignant hyperphenylalaninemia due to a defect in the biosynthesis of tetrahydrobiopterin.

**di·hy·dro·cho·les·ter·ol** (di-hi″dro-kə-les′tər-ol) cholestanol.

**di·hy·dro·co·deine** (di-hi″dro-ko′dēn) an opioid analgesic related to codeine; it has also been used as an antitussive; called also *drocode.*
**d. bitartrate** [USP], the acid tartrate of dihydrocodeine, used for the relief of moderate to moderately severe pain; administered orally.

**di·hy·dro·co·dei·none bi·tar·trate** (di-hi″dro-ko′de-nōn) hydrocodone bitartrate.

**di·hy·dro·di·eth·yl·stil·bes·trol** (di-hi″dro-di-eth″əl-stil-bes′trol) hexestrol.

**di·hy·dro·er·go·cor·nine** (di-hi″dro-er″go-kor′nin) an ergot derivative that has sympatholytic and adrenolytic properties.

**di·hy·dro·er·go·cris·tine** (di-hi″dro-er″go-kris′tin) an ergot derivative that has sympatholytic and adrenolytic properties.

**di·hy·dro·er·go·cryp·tine** (di-hi″dro-er″go-krip′tin) an ergot derivative that has sympatholytic and adrenolytic properties.

**di·hy·dro·er·got·amine mes·y·late** (di-hi″dro-ər-got′ə-mēn) [USP] an antiadrenergic produced by the catalytic hydrogenation of ergotamine; used as a vasoconstrictor in the treatment of migraine.

**di·hy·dro·fo·late** (di-hi″dro-fo′lāt) an ester or dissociated form of dihydrofolic acid. Abbreviated DHF.

**di·hy·dro·fo·late re·duc·tase** (di-hi″dro-fo′lāt re-duk′tās) [EC 1.5.1.3] an enzyme of the oxidoreductase class that catalyzes the reduction of dihydrofolate to tetrahydrofolate, using NADPH as an electron donor. The reaction produces reduced folate for amino acid metabolism, purine ring synthesis, and the formation of deoxythymidine monophosphate. Methotrexate and other folic acid antagonists used as chemotherapeutic drugs act by inhibiting this enzyme. Deficiency of the enzyme may be a cause of megaloblastic anemia responsive to therapy with reduced forms of folic acid. Abbreviated DHFR.

**di·hy·dro·fol·ic ac·id** (di-hi″dro-fo′lik) any of the folic acids in which the bicyclic pteridine structure is in the dihydro, partially reduced form; they are intermediates in folate metabolism and are reduced to their tetrahydro, reduced forms.

**di·hy·dro·in·do·lone** (di-hi″dro-in′do-lōn) any of a class of structurally related antipsychotic agents; the prototype is molindone.

**di·hy·drol** (di-hi′drol) the associated water molecule, $(H_2O)_2$.

**di·hy·dro·lipo·am·ide** (di-hi″dro-lip″o-am′īd) the reduced form of lipoamide, produced as an intermediate in the reactions in which lipoamide acts as a cofactor.

**di·hy·dro·lipo·am·ide *S*-ac·e·tyl·trans·fer·ase** (di-hi″dro-lip″o-am′īd as″ə-tēl-trans′fər-ās) [EC 2.3.1.12] an enzyme of the transferase class that is a component of the multienzyme pyruvate dehydrogenase complex (q.v.). The enzyme catalyzes the transfer of acetyl from acetyldihydrolipoamide to coenzyme A to form acetyl CoA; the enzyme is itself the physiological lipoamide in the reaction. Called also *dihydrolipoyltransacetylase.*

**di·hy·dro·lipo·am·ide ac·yl·trans·fer·ase** (di-hi″dro-lip″o-am′īd a″səl-trans′fər-ās) an enzyme of the transferase class that is the lipoamide component of the multienzyme branched-chain α-keto acid dehydrogenase complex (q.v.). The enzyme catalyzes the transfer of the decarboxylated branched-chain acyl moiety to coenzyme A via its own lipoic acid group.

**di·hy·dro·lipo·am·ide de·hy·dro·gen·ase** (di-hi″dro-lip″o-am′īd de-hi′dro-jən-ās) [EC 1.8.1.4] an enzyme of the oxidoreductase class that catalyzes the regeneration of lipoamide from dihydrolipoamide, reducing $NAD^+$. The enzyme contains FAD and is a component of several oxidative decarboxylation enzyme complexes: branched-chain α-keto acid dehydrogenase complex, α-ketoglutarate dehydrogenase complex, and pyruvate dehydrogenase complex; deficiency of the enzyme, an autosomal recessive trait, causes lipoamide dehydrogenase deficiency.

**di·hy·dro·lipo·am·ide *S*-suc·cin·yl·trans·fer·ase** (di-hi″dro-lip″o-am′īd suk″sin-əl-trans′fər-ās) [EC 2.3.1.61] an enzyme of the transferase class that is a component of the multienzyme α-ketoglutarate dehydrogenase complex (q.v.). The enzyme catalyzes the transfer of succinyl from succinyldihydrolipoamide to coenzyme A to form succinyl coenzyme A; the enzyme is itself the physiological lipoamide in the reaction. Called also *transsuccinylase.*

**di·hy·dro·lip·o·yl** (di-hi″dro-lip′o-əl) the acyl radical of dihydrolipoamide.

**di·hy·dro·lip·o·yl·trans·acet·y·lase** (di-hi″dro-lip″o-əl-trans″ə-set′ə-lās) dihydrolipoamide *S*-acetyltransferase.

**di·hy·dro·lu·ti·dine** (di-hi″dro-loo′tĭ-dēn) an oily, poisonous, caustic base from rancid cod liver oil.

**di·hy·dro·mor·phi·none hy·dro·chlo·ride** (di-hi″dro-mor′fĭ-nōn) hydromorphone hydrochloride.

**di·hy·dro·or·o·tase** (di-hi″dro-or′o-tās) [EC 3.5.2.3] [MeSH: Dihydroorotase] an enzyme activity of the trifunctional CAD protein (q.v.); it is a ligase that catalyzes the cyclization of carbamoylaspartate, creating the initial ring structure (dihydroorotate) in the biosynthesis of pyrimidine nucleotides.

**di·hy·dro·or·o·tate** (di-hi″dro-or′o-tāt) cyclized carbamoylaspartate, an intermediate in pyrimidine biosynthesis.

**di·hy·dro·pter·i·dine re·duc·tase** (di-hi″dro-ter′ĭ-dēn re-duk′tās) [EC 1.6.99.7] [MeSH: Dihydropteridine Reductase] an enzyme of the oxidoreductase class that catalyzes the NAD(P)H-dependent reduction of dihydrobiopterin to regenerate tetrahydrobiopterin, the coenzyme essential to the enzymes hydroxylating phenylalanine, tryptophan, and tyrosine and subsequently forming the corresponding neurotransmitters, such as dopamine. Deficiency of the enzyme, an autosomal recessive trait, causes malignant hyperphenylalaninemia.

**di·hy·dro·py·rim·i·dine de·hy·dro·gen·ase (NADP)** (di-hi″dro-pə-rim′ĭ-dēn de-hi′dro-jən-ās) [EC 1.3.1.2] an enzyme of the oxidoreductase class that catalyzes the dehydrogenation of uracil and of thymine, using NADPH as an electron donor; the reaction is a step in the catabolism of pyrimidines. Deficiency of the enzyme, an autosomal recessive disorder, results in elevated pyrimidine levels in plasma, urine, and cerebrospinal fluid; it is manifest clinically in children by cerebral dysfunction and in adults by hypersensitivity to the drug 5-fluorouracil.

**di·hy·dro·strep·to·my·cin sul·fate** (di-hi″dro-strep″to-mi′sin) [USP] [MeSH: Dihydrostreptomycin Sulfate] an aminoglycoside antibiotic produced by the hydrogenation of streptomycin; now used only in veterinary medicine because of its toxicity to humans.
**d. s. sulfate,** the sulfate salt of dihydrostreptomycin, used as a veterinary antibacterial.

**di·hy·dro·tach·ys·te·rol** (di-hi″dro-tak-is′tə-rol) [USP] [MeSH: Dihydrotachysterol] an analogue of ergocalciferol produced upon irradiation of ergosterol; it raises serum calcium levels via stimulation of intestinal absorption of calcium and mobilization of the mineral from bone in patients lacking renal function or parathyroid hormone. It is used in the treatment of hypocalcemic tetany, hypoparathyroidism, familial hypophosphatemia, and renal osteodystrophy.

**di·hy·dro·tes·tos·te·rone (DHT)** (di-hi″dro-tes-tos′tə-rōn) 7$\beta$-hydroxy-5$\alpha$-androstan-3-one, a powerful androgenic hormone, formed in peripheral tissue by the action of the enzyme 5$\alpha$-reductase on testosterone; it is thought to be the essential androgen responsible for formation of primary sex characters in males during embryogenesis, for development of most male secondary sex characters at puberty, and for adult male sexual function. A semisynthetic analog is called *stanolone.*

**di·hy·dro·ura·cil de·hy·dro·gen·ase (NADP$^+$)** (di-hi″dro-ūr′ə-sĭl de-hi′dro-jən-ās) dihydropyrimidine dehydrogenase (NADP).

**di·hy·droxy** (di″hi-drok′se) a term denoting a compound containing two molecules of the hydroxy (OH) radical; used also as a prefix (dihydroxy-) to denote such a compound.

**di·hy·droxy·ac·e·tone** (di″hi-drok″se-as″ĕ-tōn) [USP] [MeSH: Dihydroxyacetone] the simplest ketose, a triose; it is an isomer of glyceraldehyde. Formally called *glycerone.*
**d. phosphate,** an intermediate in glycolysis, the glycerol phosphate shuttle, and the biosynthesis of carbohydrates and of lipids.

**2,8-di·hy·droxy·ad·e·nine** (di″hi-drok″se-ad′ə-nēn) an insoluble purine produced in excess in deficiencies of the salvage pathway of adenine catalyzed by adenine phosphoribosyltransferase; accumulation can cause crystalluria and renal lithiasis.

**di·hy·droxy·alu·mi·num** (di″hi-drok″se-ə-loo′mĭ-nəm) an aluminum compound having two hydroxyl groups in the molecule.
**d. aminoacetate** [USP], a basic aluminum salt of aminoacetic acid used as a gastric antacid. Available in tablets and as a magma. Called also *aluminum aminoacetate.*
**d. sodium carbonate** [USP], an aluminum salt of sodium carbonate, used as a gastric antacid in tablet form.

**di·hy·droxy·cho·le·cal·cif·e·rol** (di″hi-drok″se-ko″le-kal-sif′ə-rol) a group of active metabolites of cholecalciferol, numbered according to the carbon atoms on which a hydroxyl group is substituted. See also table at *cholecalciferol.* Called also *dihydroxyvitamin $D_3$.*
**1,25-d.,** the most active metabolite of cholecalciferol, synthesized in the kidney from 25-hydroxycholecalciferol; it increases intestinal absorption of calcium and phosphate, enhances bone resorption, and prevents rickets. Because these activities occur at sites distant from its site of synthesis, it is considered a hormone. Called also *calcitriol* and *1,25-dihydroxyvitamin $D_3$.*
**24,25-d.,** a metabolite of cholecalciferol with an uncertain physiological role.

**di·hy·droxy·flu·o·rane** (di″hi-drok″se-floor′o-rān) fluorescein.

**3,4-di·hy·droxy·phen·yl·al·a·nine** (di″hi-drok″se-fen″əl-al′ə-nēn) dopa.

**3,4-di·hy·droxy·phen·yl·gly·col (DHPG)** (di″hi-drok″se-fen″il-gli′kol) ganciclovir.

**1,25-di·hy·droxy·vi·ta·min D** (di″hi-drok″se-vi′tə-min) either 1,25-dihydroxycholecalciferol, the corresponding dihydroxy-derivative of ergocalciferol, or both collectively. See also table at *cholecalciferol.*

**di·hy·droxy·vi·ta·min $D_3$** (di″hi-drok″se-vi′tə-min) dihydroxycholecalciferol.
**1,25-d. D.,** 1,25-dihydroxycholecalciferol.
**24,25-d. D.,** 24,25-dihydroxycholecalciferol.

**di·hys·te·ria** (di″his-te′re-ə) [*di-* + *hystero-* + *-ia*] the condition of having a double uterus.

**di·io·dide** (di-i′o-dīd) a combination of a base or a metal with two atoms of iodine.

**di·io·do·hy·droxy·quin** (di″i-o″do-hi-drok′sĭ-kwin) iodoquinol.

**3,5-di·io·do·thy·ro·nine** (di″i-o″do-thi′ro-nēn) an organic iodine-containing compound, used in the manufacture of thyroxine.

**di·io·do·ty·ro·sine** (di″i-o″do-ti′ro-sēn) [MeSH: Diiodotyrosine] an organic iodine-containing compound liberated from thyroglobulin in small amounts as a by-product of iodothyroglobulin hydrolysis. Called also *iodogorgoric acid.*

**di·iso·cy·anate** (di-i″so-si′ə-nāt) any of a group of compounds containing two isocyanate groups (—NCO), which are used in the manufacture of plastics and elastomers; diisocyanates can cause sensitization and are potent irritants of the eyes and respiratory system. See *isocyanate asthma,* under *asthma.*

**di·iso·pro·pyl flu·o·ro·phos·phate** (di-i″so-pro′pəl flo͞or″o-fos′fāt) DFP; a potent irreversible acetylcholinesterase inhibitor, widely used in biochemistry in the study of serine proteases; radiolabeled DF$^{32}$P has been used to label red and white blood cells in kinetics studies. DFP is also used (see *isoflurophate*) as an ophthalmic cholinergic agent.

**Di·karyo·my·co·ta** (di-kar″e-o-mi-ko′tə) in some systems of classification, a phylum of perfect fungi characterized by an extended dikaryon in the life cycle; it includes two subphyla, Ascomycotina and Basidiomycotina (which are variously considered phyla or classes, and renamed, in other systems).

**di·ka·ry·on** (di-kar′e-on) [*di-* + *karyon*] a growth stage in the mycelium of fungi, especially Basidiomycetes, in which each cell has two haploid nuclei.

**di·ka·ry·ote** (di-kar′e-ōt) a cell having two haploid nuclei.

**di·ka·ry·ot·ic** (di″kar-e-ot′ik) pertaining to the dikaryon or to a dikaryote.

**di·ke·tone** (di-ke′tōn) a ketone containing two carbonyl groups.

**di·ke·to·pi·per·a·zine** (di-ke″to-pi-per′ə-zēn) a closed-ring compound produced by the condensation of two amino acids, the carboxyl group of each combining with the amino group of the other.

**dik·ty·o·ma** (dik″te-o′mə) a medulloepithelioma of the pars ciliaris retinae; written also *dictyoma.*

**dik·wak·wadi** (dik″wak-wad′e) [Bantu] a South African term for *favus.*

**dil.** abbreviation for L. *dil′ue,* dilute or dissolve.

**di·lac·er·a·tion** (di-las″ər-a′shən) [L. *dilaceratio*] 1. a tearing apart, as of a cataract; see *discission.* 2. in dentistry, a condition due to injury to a tooth during its developmental period and characterized by a crease or band at the junction of the crown and root, or by tortuous roots with abnormal curvatures.

**Dil·a·cor** (dil′ə-kor″) trademark for a preparation of diltiazem hydrochloride.

**Di·lan·tin** (di-lan′tin) trademark for preparations of phenytoin.

**di·la·tan·cy** (di-la′tən-se) an unusual behavior observed in cytoplasm (and in some physical systems) during which its viscosity and applied force both increase.

**di·la·tant** (di-la′tənt) exhibiting dilatancy.

**dil·a·ta·tion** (dil″ə-ta′shən) [MeSH: Dilatation] 1. the condition, as of an orifice or tubular structure, of being dilated or stretched beyond the normal dimensions. 2. dilation (def. 1).
**digital d.,** digital dilation.
**gastric d.,** d. of the stomach.
**gastric d.-volvulus,** see under *volvulus.*
**d. of the heart,** enlargement of the cavities of the heart, with thinning of its walls.
**idiopathic d.,** dilatation of a vessel or other channel, especially of the pulmonary artery, without a known cause.
**poststenotic d.,** dilatation of a vessel distal to a stenosed segment or valve, often seen in the pulmonary artery distal to valvular pulmonary stenosis.

**prognathic d., prognathion d.,** dilatation of the pyloric end of the stomach greater than that of the fundus, giving a protruding appearance in the radiograph.
**d. of the stomach,** distention of the stomach with retained secretions, food, and/or gas due to obstruction, ileus, or denervation; called also *gastric d.*

**dil•a•ta•tor** (dil″ə-ta′tər) [L.] 1. something that dilates. 2. in anatomical terminology, referring to a structure (muscle) that dilates (musculus dilatator [TA]).

**di•late** (di′lāt) to stretch an opening or hollow structure beyond its normal dimensions; cf. *distend.*

**di•la•tion** (di-la′shən) 1. the act of dilating or stretching. 2. dilatation (def. 1).
**digital d.,** the expansion or stretching of a cavity or orifice by means of a finger.

**di•la•tor** (di-la′tər) 1. an instrument used in enlarging an orifice or canal by stretching. 2. dilatator, def. 2.
**anal d.,** an instrument for dilating or stretching the anal sphincter.
**Einhorn's d.,** a metal dilator used to stretch the cardioesophageal region in cardiospasm.
**Hegar d's,** a series of bougies of varying sizes for dilating the ostium uteri.
**Kollmann's d.,** a metallic, expandable urethral dilator.
**laryngeal d.,** a bougie-like instrument which is used for distending a stenosed larynx.
**d. naris,** pars alaris musculi nasalis.
**pneumatic d.,** a dilator for esophageal strictures, consisting of a bougie leading to an inflatable bag that straddles the stricture.
**d. pupillae,** musculus dilatator pupillae.
**Starck d.,** an expandable rubber-covered metal frame used to dilate the cardioesophageal region.

**Di•lau•did** (di-law′did) trademark for preparations of hydromorphone hydrochloride.

**di•le•ca•nus** (di″lə-ka′nəs) [*di-* + Gr. *lekanē* a dish] dipygus.

**Dil•e•pid•i•dae** (dil″ə-pid′ĭ-de) Dipylidiidae.

**dill** (dil) *Anethum graveolens.*

**dil•ti•a•zem hy•dro•chlo•ride** (dil-ti′ə-zəm) a calcium channel blocker that acts as a vasodilator; used in the treatment of angina pectoris and hypertension.

**Diluc.** abbreviation for L. *dilu′culo,* at daybreak.

**dil•u•ent** (dil′u-ənt) 1. diluting. 2. an agent that dilutes or renders less potent or irritant.

**dilut.** abbreviation for L. *dilu′tus,* diluted.

**di•lute** [L. *diluere* to wash] to make a mixture or solution less concentrated by adding a fluid.

**di•lu•tion** (di-loo′shən) 1. the art or process of diluting or the state of being diluted. 2. a diluted or attenuated medicine. 3. in homeopathy, the diffusion of a given quantity of a medicinal agent in ten or one hundred times the same quantity of water.
**doubling d.,** a serial dilution in which the dilution in each tube is double that of the preceding tube.
**nitrogen d.,** the addition of nitrogen to inspired air to lower its oxygen tension, producing an alveolar oxygen tension equal to a desired oxygen pressure.
**serial d.,** a set of dilutions in a mathematical sequence. In microbiological technique, serial dilutions are used to obtain a culture plate that yields a countable number of separate colonies. From this, a calculation of viable cells in the original suspension can be made, as a colony picked for pure culture.

**dim.** abbreviation for L. *dimid′ius,* one half.

**Di•mas•tig•amoe•ba** (di-mas″tig-ə-me′bə) *Naegleria.*

**di•me•fil•con A** (di″mə-fil′kon) a contact lens material (hydrophilic).

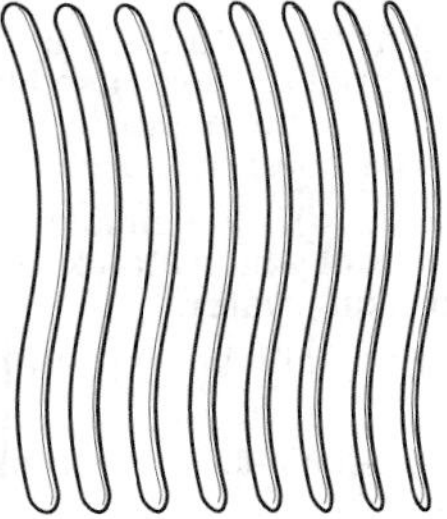
Hegar uterine dilators.

**di•meg•lu•mine** (di-meg′loo-mēn) any salt containing two meglumine molecules.

**di•me•lia** (di-me′le-ə) [*di-* + *-melia*] a developmental anomaly characterized by duplication of a limb.

**di•me•lus** (di-me′ləs) a fetus exhibiting dimelia.

**di•men•hy•dri•nate** (di″mən-hi′drĭ-nāt) [USP] [MeSH: Dimenhydrinate] an antiemetic, used in the treatment of motion sickness and in other conditions in which nausea may be a feature, administered orally.

**di•men•sion** (dĭ-men′shən) a numerical expression, in appropriate units, of a linear measurement of an object, such as an organ or body part.
**vertical d.,** the distance between two points, measured perpendicular to the horizontal. In prosthodontics, the length of the face determined by the distance of separation of the jaws. See *contact vertical d., postural vertical d.,* and *vertical d.*
**vertical d., contact, vertical d., occlusal,** the lower face height with the teeth in centric occlusion.
**vertical d., postural,** the vertical face height when the mandible is suspended in the postural resting position.
**vertical d., rest,** the lower face height measured from a chin point just below the nose, with the mandible in the rest position.

**di•men•sion•less** (dĭ-men′shən-ləs) denoting a numerical constant or variable that has no units of measurement.

**di•mer** (di′mər) 1. a compound formed by combination of two identical simpler molecules. 2. a capsomer having two structural subunits.
**D d.,** a fibrin degradation product containing a cross-link between two fibrin monomers; the cross-link does not occur in fibrinogen, so that tests for D-dimer are specific for fibrin. See *D-dimer assay,* under *assay.*
**thymine d.,** two adjacent thymine residues linked together by a covalent bond along a single polynucleotide of DNA, which may lead to inactivation of the DNA molecule. It results from exposure to ultraviolet radiation and may be reversed by photoreactivation.

**di•mer•cap•rol** (di″mər-kap′rol) [USP] [MeSH: Dimercaprol] a metal complexing agent, used as an antidote to poisoning by arsenic, gold, and mercury, and sometimes other metals, administered intramuscularly. It has also been used in the treatment of hepatolenticular degeneration.

**di•mer•ic** (di′mər-ik) exhibiting the characteristics of a dimer.

**dim•er•ous** (dim′ər-əs) [*di-* + *mero-*[1] + *-ous*] made up of two parts.

**di•me•tal•lic** (di″mə-tal′ik) containing two atoms or equivalents of a metallic element in the molecule.

**Di•me•tane** (di′mə-tān) trademark for preparations of brompheniramine maleate.

**di•me•thac•ry•late** (di″mə-thak′rĭ-lāt) a common resin matrix material; called also *BIS-GMA.*

**di•meth•i•cone** (di-meth′ĭ-kōn) 1. a silicone oil consisting of dimethylsiloxane polymers with viscosities from 0.65 to 3,000,000 centistokes at 25°C. The term is used with a numeric suffix which indicates the approximate viscosity of the various grades in centistokes, e.g., the viscosity of dimethicone 200 in centistokes is 190 to 210. Dimethicones are used as ingredients of ointments and other preparations for topical application to protect the skin against water-soluble irritants. 2. simethicone.
**d. 350,** a grade of dimethicone having a viscosity of approximately 350 centistokes at 25°C; a prosthetic aid for soft tissues.
**activated d.,** simethicone.

**di•me•thin•dene mal•e•ate** (di″mə-thin′dēn) an antihistaminic administered orally.

**di•me•thi•so•quin hy•dro•chlo•ride** (di″mə-thi′so-kwin) a local anesthetic applied topically to relieve pain, itching, and burning of the skin.

**di•me•this•ter•one** (di″mə-this′tər-ōn) [MeSH: Dimethisterone] an orally effective progestin, having actions and uses similar to those of progesterone; used alone or as the progestin component in combination with ethinyl estradiol as an oral contraceptive.

**2,5-di•me•thoxy-4-meth•yl•am•phet•amine** (di″mə-thok″se-meth″əl-am-fet′ə-mēn) a hallucinogenic compound derived from amphetamine; abbreviated DOM and popularly called STP.

**3,4-di•me•thoxy•phen•yl•eth•yl•amine** (di″mə-thok″se-fen″əl-eth″əl-am′ən) a substance found in the urine of schizophrenics but not controls in some studies; abbreviated DMPE.

**di•meth•yl•amine** (di-meth″əl-am′ən) a gaseous and liquid ptomaine, isolated from decaying nitrogenous plant and animal sources, particularly fish, and synthesized for use in industrial and pharmaceutical processes; it is a skin irritant.

***p*-di·meth·yl·a·mi·no·azo·ben·zene** (di-meth″əl-ə-me″no-a″zo-ben′zēn) a dicyclic carcinogenic compound used as an indicator in tests for and in Ehrlich's aldehyde reaction to detect urobilinogen. It has a pH range of 2.9 to 4, being red at 2.9 and yellow at 4. Called also *butter yellow* and *methyl yellow*.

**di·meth·yl·ami·no·pro·pio·ni·trile (DMAPN)** (di-meth″əl-ə-me″no-pro″pe-o-ni′tril) a colorless water-soluble liquid used in the manufacture of polyurethane foam; workers with excessive exposure to it are prone to urologic and neurologic disorders.

**di·meth·yl·ar·sine** (di-meth″əl-ahr′sēn) cacodyl hydride.

**di·meth·yl·ar·sin·ic ac·id** (di-meth″əl-ahr-sin′ik) cacodylic acid.

**7,12-di·meth·yl·benz[*a*]an·thra·cene** (di-meth″əl-benz-an′thrə-sēn) 9,10-dimethyl-1,2-benzanthracene; a highly carcinogenic polycyclic aromatic hydrocarbon produced during incomplete combustion of carbonaceous materials. It is a procarcinogen that requires metabolic activation to an epoxide intermediate to exert a mutagenic effect; it is widely used in research on chemical carcinogenesis. Abbreviated DMBA.

**di·meth·yl·ben·zene** (di-meth″əl-ben′zēn) xylene.

**5,6-di·meth·yl·ben·zi·mid·az·ole** (di″meth-əl-ben″zĭ-mid′ə-zōl) a derivative of benzimidazole doubly methylated on the benzene ring; it is an unusual base that together with a ribose 3′-phosphate moiety forms the nucleotide portion of the vitamin $B_{12}$ molecule.

**di·meth·yl·car·bam·yl chlo·ride** (di-meth″əl-kahr′bə-məl) a colorless liquid used as a chemical intermediate in the manufacture of pharmaceuticals, dyes, and pesticides; it is lacrimatory and possibly carcinogenic.

**di·meth·yl car·bate** (di-meth′əl kahr′bāt) a clear oily liquid used as an insect repellent; it has neurotoxic effects if ingested or inhaled.

**di·meth·yl·car·bi·nol** (di-meth″əl-kahr′bĭ-nol) isopropyl alcohol.

**di·meth·yl·eth·yl·pyr·role** (di-meth″əl-eth″əl-pir′ōl) a substituted pyrrole obtained from bilirubin.

**di·meth·yl·for·ma·mide (DMF)** (di-meth″əl-for′mə-mīd) [MeSH: Dimethylformamide] a solvent used in laboratories and in manufacturing acrylic resins; it is absorbed through the skin and by inhalation and is hepatotoxic.

***N,N*-di·meth·yl·gly·cine** (di-meth″əl-gli′sēn) an amino acid intermediate occurring as an immediate precursor of sarcosine in the metabolism of choline.

**di·meth·yl·gly·cine de·hy·dro·gen·ase** (di-meth″əl-gli′sēn de-hi′dro-jən-ās) [EC 1.5.99.2] a mitochondrial flavoprotein enzyme of the oxidoreductase class that catalyzes the oxidative demethylation of *N,N*-dimethylglycine to sarcosine in the metabolism of choline. It requires a folate cofactor and transfers electrons from its flavin moiety to electron transfer flavoprotein. The reaction occurs in the mitochondrial inner membrane in liver and kidney.

**di·meth·yl·ke·tone** (di-meth″əl-ke′tōn) acetone.

**di·meth·yl·ni·tro·sa·mine** (di-meth″əl-ni″trō′sə′mēn) [MeSH: Dimethylnitrosamine] *N*-nitrosodimethylamine.

**di·meth·yl·phe·nan·threne** (di-meth″əl-fə-nan′thrēn) a carcinogenic and weakly estrogenic hydrocarbon.

**di·meth·yl-*p*-phen·yl·ene·di·amine** (di-meth″əl-fen″əl-ēn-di′ə-mēn) a reddish-violet, crystalline, substituted aniline derivative, toxic by ingestion or inhalation; used in reagents for various biochemical and microbiological assays.

**di·meth·yl phthal·ate** (di-meth′əl thal′āt) a clear, colorless, oily liquid, the normal methyl ester of phthalic acid; used as an insect repellent.

**di·meth·yl sul·fate** (di-meth′əl sul′fāt) a colorless liquid used in adhesives and as a methylating agent for organic chemicals; it is severely irritant to the skin and mucous membranes and is carcinogenic.

**di·meth·yl sulf·ox·ide** (di-meth′əl sul-fok′sīd) [MeSH: Dimethyl Sulfoxide] 1. DMSO; a highly polar alkyl sulfoxide that is a powerful solvent and dissolves many organic and inorganic compounds; its biologic activities include the ability to penetrate plant and animal tissues and to preserve living cells during freezing. 2. [USP] a preparation used in veterinary medicine as a topical anti-inflammatory.

**di·meth·yl·tryp·ta·mine** (di-meth″əl-trip′tə-mēn) a hallucinogenic substance derived from the apocynaceous plant *Prestonia amazonica* (Benth.) Macbride *(Haemadictyon amazonicum* Spruce and Benth.) which is native to parts of South America and the West Indies. Abbreviated DMT.

**di·me·trid·a·zole** (di″mə-tri′də-zōl) [MeSH: Dimetridazole] an antiprotozoal drug used against histomoniasis of turkeys.

**di·min·a·zene ac·e·tu·rate** (dĭ-min′ə-zēn) a veterinary antibacterial and antiprotozoal used against *Babesia* and *Trypanosoma.*

**dim·i·nu·tion** (dim″ĭ-noo′shən) reduction or decrease in size or substance.

**Dim·mer's keratitis** (dim′ərz) [Friedrich *Dimmer,* Austrian ophthalmologist, 1855–1926] keratitis nummularis.

**Di·mo·cil·lin** (di-mo-sil′in) trademark for preparations of methicillin sodium.

**di·mor·phic** (di-mor′fik) dimorphous.

**di·mor·phism** (di-mor′fiz-əm) [*di-* + *morph-* + *-ism*] the property of having or existing in two forms, as fungi that can grow as molds or yeasts.

**physical d.,** the property of certain solids of existing in two crystalline or allotropic forms.

**sexual d.,** physical or behavioral differences associated with gender.

**di·mor·pho·bi·ot·ic** (di-mor″fo-bi-ot′ik) [*di-* + *morpho-* + *biotic*] showing alternation of generations and having a parasitic and a nonparasitic stage in the complete life history.

**di·mor·phous** (di-mor′fəs) [*di-* + *morpho-* + *-ous*] occurring in two distinct forms; having the property of dimorphism.

**di·mox·y·line phos·phate** (di-mok′sə-lēn) dioxyline phosphate.

**dim·ple** (dim′pəl) a slight depression, as in the flesh of the cheek, chin, or sacral region.

**Fuchs' d's,** dellen.

**postanal d.,** coccygeal foveola.

**dim·pling** (dim′pling) the formation of slight depressions or dimples.

**di·ner·ic** (di-ner′ik) [*di-* + Gr. *nēros* liquid] denoting a solution made up of two immiscible solvents with a single solute soluble in each.

**di·ni·trate** (di-ni′trāt) a compound of a base or a metal with two nitrate groups, as in lead dinitrate, $Pb(NO_3)_2$.

**di·ni·trat·ed** (di-ni′trāt-əd) compounded with or containing two nitrate ($NO_3$) or nitro ($NO_2$) groups.

**di·ni·tro·ami·no·phe·nol** (di-ni″tro-am″ĭ-no-fe′nol) a phenol found in the blood after poisoning with trinitrophenol, forming red granules, free or in the leukocytes. Called also *aminodinitrophenol.*

**di·ni·tro·ben·zene** (di-ni″tro-ben′zēn) a poisonous substance, $C_6H_4(NO_2)_2$, whose fumes may cause breathlessness and finally asphyxia.

**di·ni·tro·chlo·ro·ben·zene** (di-ni″tro-klor″o-ben′zēn) [MeSH: Dinitrochlorobenzene] a substance that produces a delayed-type hypersensitivity response (contact dermatitis) in sensitized individuals when applied to the skin; it is a commonly used sensitizing agent in laboratory immunology and has been used to test cellular immune function in evaluation of suspected immunodeficiency. Abbreviated DNCB.

**di·ni·tro-*o*-cre·sol** (di-ni″tro-kre′sol) a pesticide and herbicide used in agriculture; excessive exposure is highly toxic for humans and other animals, with central nervous system symptoms such as convulsions and coma, disruption of energy-producing metabolic processes, and sometimes fatal hyperpyrexia. Abbreviated DNOC.

**di·ni·tro·flu·o·ro·ben·zene** (di-ni″tro-flo͞or″o-ben′zēn) [MeSH: Dinitrofluorobenzene] a substance that induces a delayed-type hypersensitivity reaction (contact dermatitis) in sensitized individuals when applied to the skin; a commonly used sensitizing agent and hapten in laboratory immunology. Abbreviated DNFB.

**di·ni·tro·gen** (di-ni′tro-jən) containing two nitrogen atoms.

**d. monoxide,** nitrous oxide.

**di·ni·tro·phe·nol** (di-ni″tro-fe′nol) any one of six isomeric compounds used in making dyes. 2,4-Dinitrophenol is highly toxic and is used as a reagent and indicator and frequently as a hapten.

**di·ni·tro·re·sor·cin·ol** (di-ni″tro-re-sor′sin-ol) a green coal tar derivative, $C_6H_2(NO_2)_2(OH)_2$, used in preparing degenerated nerve tissue for study.

**di·ni·tro·tolu·ene** (di-ni″tro-tol′u-ēn) a highly toxic crystalline compound existing as three isomers, used in organic synthesis and the manufacture of dyes and explosives; it is readily absorbed through the skin and is a potential carcinogen.

**Di·nob·del·la** (di″nob-del′ə) a genus of leeches of the family Gnathobdellidae, species of which attack the larynx of cattle in India when swallowed in drinking water.

**Di·no·flag·el·la·ta** (di″no-flaj″ə-la′tə) [Gr. *dinos* whirl + L. *flagellum* whip] Dinoflagellida.

**di·no·flag·el·late** (di″no-flaj′ə-lāt) a protozoan of the order Dinoflagellida.

**Di·no·fla·gel·li·da** (di″no-flə-jel′ĭ-də) [Gr. *dinos* + L. *flagellum* whip]

[MeSH: Dinoflagellida] an order of minute, plantlike, chiefly marine protozoa of the class Phytomastigophorea, an important component of plankton. They have flagella in grooves, transverse and longitudinal, which cause them to rotate as they advance, as well as a cellulose covering and green, yellow, or brown chromatophores. They may be present in sea water in vast numbers, causing a discoloration known as red tide and resulting in the death of marine animals and fish by exhaustion of the oxygen supply. Some species secrete a powerful neurotoxin that can cause a severe reaction in humans who ingest shellfish that have fed on the toxin-producing organisms. Genera include *Ceratium, Gonyaulax, Gymnodinium,* and *Prorocentrum.* Called also *Dinoflagellata.*

**di·no·gun·el·lin** (di″no-gun′ə-lin) the toxic lipoprotein found in the roe of the Japanese blenny *Stichaeus (Dinogunellus) grigorjewi.*

**di·no·prost** (di′no-prost) [MeSH: Dinoprost] name given to prostaglandin $F_{2\alpha}$ when used as a pharmaceutical; used as an oxytocic for induction of abortion, for evacuation of the uterus in management of missed abortion, and in treatment of hydatidiform mole.
**d. trometanol,** d. tromethamine.
**d. tromethamine,** the tromethamine salt of dinoprost, having the same actions as the base; used as an oxytocic for induction of labor, termination of pregnancy, missed abortion, fetal death, and hydatidiform mole. It is administered intravenously, extra-amniotically, or intra-amniotically. Called also *d. trometanol* and *prostaglandin $F_{2\alpha}$ tromethamine.*

**di·no·prost·one** (di″no-pros′tōn) [MeSH: Dinoprostone] name given to prostaglandin $E_2$ when used pharmaceutically; used as an oxytocic for induction of abortion and for the induction of labor, to evacuate the uterus in the management of missed abortion, and in the treatment of hydatidiform mole.

**D. in p. aeq.** abbreviation for L. *divi′de in par′tes aequa′les,* divide into equal parts.

**din·sed** (din′səd) a coccidiostat for use in poultry.

**di·nu·cleo·tide** (di-noo′kle-o-tīd) one of the cleavage products into which a polynucleotide may be split; a dinucleotide itself may be split into two mononucleotides.

**Di·o·cles** (di′ŏ-klēz) **of Ca·rys·tus** [4th century B.C.] Greek physician and anatomist, a contemporary and student of Aristotle. Diocles was a founder of the Dogmatist school; he studied embryology, gynecology, and obstetrics, and he also performed animal dissections (e.g., on the womb of a mule). See also *Hippocrates* and *Praxagoras.*

**Di·oc·to·phyme** (di-ok′to-fīm) a genus of nematodes of the family Dioctophymidae.
**D. rena′le,** the kidney worm, a red species that is the largest nematode known; males are 35 cm long and females 103 cm (1.03m). It is found commonly in dogs, cattle, horses, and other animals, but rarely in humans. The usual location is in the pelvis of the kidney or free in the peritoneal cavity; it is highly destructive to kidney tissue and may cause death. Called also *Eustrongylus gigas.*

**Di·oc·to·phy·mi·dae** (di-ok″to-fi′mĭ-de) a family of nematodes found in the kidney and peritoneal cavity in mammals. It includes the single genus *Dioctophyma.*

**Di·oc·to·phy·moi·dea** (di-ok″to-fi″moi′de-ə) a superfamily of aphasmids, including the genus *Dioctophyma.*

**di·oc·tyl cal·ci·um sul·fo·suc·ci·nate** (di-ok′təl) docusate calcium.

**di·oc·tyl so·di·um sul·fo·suc·ci·nate** (di-ok′təl) docusate sodium.

**Di·o·don** (di′o-don) a genus of tetraodontiform fishes of the family Diodontidae; some species are poisonous when ingested.

**Di·o·do·quin** (di″o-do′kwin) trademark for a preparation of iodoquinol.

**di·oe·cious** (di″-o-e′shəs) diecious.

**di·ol·amine** (di-ol′ə-mēn) USAN contraction for diethanolamine.

**Di·on·o·sil** (di-on′o-sil) trademark for preparations of propyliodone.

**di·op·sim·e·ter** (di″op-sim′ə-tər) [*dia-* Gr. *opsis* sight + *-meter*] a device for measuring the field of vision.

**di·op·ter** (di-op′tər) [Gr. *dioptra* optical instrument for measuring angles] a unit of refractive power of lenses: the reciprocal of the focal length in meters is the refractive power in diopters. Symbol D.
**prism d.,** a unit of prismatic deviation; deflection of one centimeter at a distance of one meter.

**di·op·tom·e·ter** (di″op-tom′ə-tər) [*dioptric* + *-meter*] an instrument for use in testing ocular refraction.

**di·op·tom·e·try** (di″op-tom′ə-tre) the measurement of refraction and accommodation of the eye.

**di·op·tos·co·py** (di″op-tos′kə-pe) [*dioptric* + *-scopy*] measurement of ocular refraction by means of the ophthalmoscope.

**di·op·tre** (di-op′tər) diopter.

**di·op·tric** (di-op′trik) pertaining to refraction or to transmitted and refracted light; refracting.

**di·op·trics** (di-op′triks) the science of refracted light.

**di·op·trom·e·ter** (di″op-trom′ə-tər) dioptometer.

**di·op·trom·e·try** (di″op-trom′ə-tre) dioptometry.

**di·op·tros·co·py** (di″op-tros′kə-pe) dioptoscopy.

**di·op·try** (di′op-tre) diopter.

**di·os·cin** (di-os′kin) a saponin from *Dioscorea tokoro* Mal.; see *diosgenin.*

**Di·os·co·rea** (di″os-kor′e-ə) the Mexican yams, a genus of plants of the family Dioscoreaceae. *D. mexica′na* is a source of the steroid botogenin. Several species, such as *D. villo′sa, D. floribun′da,* and *D. toko′ro,* are sources of diosgenin. *D. villo′sa* L. contains saponin and acrid resins and was formerly used for its diaphoretic, expectorant, and diuretic properties.

**Di·os·cor·i·des** (di″ŏ-skor′ĭ-dēz) **of Ana·zar·bos** [1st century A.D.] a noted botanist and pharmacologist whose encyclopedia of materia medica was widely used for centuries after his death.

**di·ose** (di′ōs) any monosaccharide containing two carbon atoms; the only member of the class is glycoaldehyde (q.v.).

**di·os·gen·in** (di-os′jən-in) [MeSH: Diosgenin] an aglycone of the saponin dioscin. Obtained from several species of *Dioscorea,* it is a precursor in the synthesis of pregnenolone, progesterone, and other medically useful steroids.

**Di·o·van** (di′o-van) trademark for a preparation of valsartan.

**di·ov·u·la·to·ry** (di-ov′u-lə-tor″e) ordinarily discharging two ova in one ovarian cycle.

**di·ox·ane** (di-ok′sān) a colorless liquid prepared by treating ethylene glycol with sulfuric acid; used as a solvent for organic compounds and for dehydrating and clearing tissues prior to paraffin fixation. It is toxic if inhaled or absorbed through the skin and is carcinogenic. Called also *1,4-diethylene dioxide.*

**di·ox·ide** (di-ok′sīd) 1. a binary compound containing two oxide ions, such as silicon dioxide, $SiO_2$. 2. an oxide of a non-metal with a valence of four, such as sulfur dioxide, $SO_2$.

**di·ox·in** (di-ok′sin) any of the heterocyclic hydrocarbons present as a trace contaminant in herbicides, especially the chlorinated dioxin 2,3,7,8-tetrachlorodibenzo-*p*-dioxin; many are teratogenic and carcinogenic.

**di·oxy·ben·zone** (di-oks″ĭ-ben′zōn) [USP] an ultraviolet sunscreen applied topically to the skin.

**di·oxy·gen** (di-ok′sə-jən) molecular oxygen, $O_2$.

**di·oxy·gen·ase** (di-ok′sə-jən-ās) a term used in the recommended names of oxygenases specifically catalyzing incorporation of both atoms of oxygen from $O_2$ into a single substrate [EC 1.13.11]. A C=C bond is frequently cleaved; and most of these enzymes require either iron or copper for activity.

**di·oxy·line phos·phate** (di-ok′sə-lēn) a synthetic analogue of papaverine, used as a vasodilator, mainly in the treatment of vascular spasm associated with acute myocardial infarction, angina of effort, peripheral vascular disease in which there is a vasospastic element, and peripheral and pulmonary embolism, administered orally. Called also *dimoxyline phosphate.*

**Di·pax·in** (di-pak′sin) trademark for a preparation of diphenadione.

**di·pen·tene** (di-pen′tēn) a liquid terpene found in various volatile oils.

**Di·pen·tum** (di-pen′təm) trademark for a preparation of olsalazine sodium.

**di·pep·ti·dase** (di-pep′tĭ-dās) [EC 3.4.13] any member of a sub-subclass of enzymes of the hydrolase class that catalyzes the cleavage of the peptide linkage in a dipeptide.

**di·pep·tide** (di-pep′tīd) a peptide which on hydrolysis yields two amino acids.

**di·pep·ti·dyl car·boxy·pep·ti·dase I** (di-pep″tĭ-dəl kahr-bok″se-pep′tĭ-dās) peptidyl-dipeptidase A.

**di·pep·ti·dyl-pep·ti·dase** (di-pep″tĭ-dəl-pep′tĭ-dās) [EC 3.4.14] any member of a sub-subclass of enzymes of the hydrolase class that catalyze the cleavage of a dipeptide residue from a free N-terminal end of a peptide or polypeptide.

**di·pep·ti·dyl-pep·ti·dase I** (di-pep″tĭ-dəl-pep′tĭ-dās) [EC 3.4.14.1] an aminopeptidase that catalyzes the cleavage of a dipeptide from the N-terminus of a polypeptide. Called also *cathepsin C.*

**di·per·o·don** (di-per'o-don) a local anesthetic, applied topically to the skin for abrasions, irritations, and pruritus and intrarectally for relief of discomfort associated with hemorrhoids.
**d. hydrochloride,** the monohydrochloride salt of diperodon, having the same actions and uses as the base.

**Di·pet·a·lo·ne·ma** (di-pet"ə-lo-ne'mə) [MeSH: Dipetalonema] a genus of nematodes of the superfamily Filarioidea.
**D. per'stans,** *Mansonella perstans.*
**D. recondi'tum,** a species found in the perirenal fat pad of dogs; called also *Filaria recondita.*
**D. streptocer'ca,** *Mansonella streptocerca.*

**di·pet·a·lo·ne·mi·a·sis** (di-pet"ə-lo-ne-mi'ə-sis) mansonellosis.

**di·pha·ce·none** (di-fa'sə-nōn) diphenadione.

**di·phal·lia** (di-fal'e-ə) [*di-* + *phall-* + *-ia*] duplication of the penis.

**di·phal·lus** (di-fal'əs) a double penis.

**di·pha·sic** (di-fa'zik) [*di-* + Gr. *phasis* phase] occurring in two phases or stages. Cf. *monophasic* and *triphasic.*

**di·pheb·u·zol** (di-feb'u-zol) phenylbutazone.

**di·phe·ma·nil meth·yl·sul·fate** (di-fe'mə-nil) a quaternary ammonium anticholinergic, used in the treatment of peptic ulcer, gastric hyperacidity, and hypermotility in gastritis and pylorospasm, and in the treatment of hyperhidrosis, administered orally.

**di·phen·a·di·one** (di-fen"ə-di'ōn) an indanedione anticoagulant administered orally; it is also used as a rodenticide, causing fatal hemorrhaging in many mammals consuming sufficient doses. Called also *diphacenone.*

**di·phen·hy·dra·mine** (di"fen-hi'drə-mēn) [MeSH: Diphenhydramine] a potent antihistamine with anticholinergic, antitussive, antiemetic, and sedative actions.
**d. citrate** [USP], the citrate salt of diphenhydramine, used as a sedative and hypnotic; administered orally.
**d. hydrochloride** [USP], the hydrochloride salt of diphenhydramine, used for the symptomatic treatment of allergic symptoms, for the treatment of anaphylaxis, parkinsonism, and motion sickness, and as an antitussive and sedative; administered orally, intramuscularly, and intravenously.

**di·phen·i·dol** (di-fen'ĭ-dōl) an antiemetic used for the treatment of vertigo and to control nausea and vomiting; administered rectally.
**d. hydrochloride,** the hydrochloride salt of diphenidol, having the same actions and uses as the base; administered orally or intramuscularly.
**d. pamoate,** the pamoate salt of diphenidol, having the same actions as the base.

**di·phe·nol ox·i·dase** (di-fe'nol ok'sĭ-dās) see *catechol oxidase.*

**di·phen·ox·y·late hy·dro·chlo·ride** (di"fən-ok'sə-lāt) [USP] an antiperistaltic derived from meperidine, used as an antidiarrheal; administered orally.

**di·phe·nyl** (di-fe'nəl) a colorless toxic compound, comprising two linked benzene rings, used as a fungistat in containers for shipping citrus fruit. Called also *biphenyl.*

**di·phen·yl·amine** (di-fen"əl-am'ēn) [MeSH: Diphenylamine] a compound, used as a test for oxidizing agents, such as nitric acid and chlorine.

**di·phen·yl·amine chlor·ar·sine** (di-fen'əl-ə-mēn" klor"ahr'sēn) a toxic compound used as a gas in war and, as a compound with tear gas, in riot control; also used in some wood preserving solutions. It irritates the skin and respiratory tract and also causes nausea, vomiting, depression, and weakness. Called also *adamsite* and *phenarsazine chloride.* Symbol DM.

**di·phen·yl·a·mi·no·azo·ben·zene** (di-fen"əl-ə-me'no-a"zo-ben'zēn) an indicator with a pH range of 1.2 to 2.1.

**di·phen·yl·bu·tyl·pi·per·i·dine** (di-fen"əl-bu"təl-pi-per'ĭ-dēn) any of a class of structurally related antipsychotic agents that includes fluspirilene and pimozide.

**di·phen·yl·chlor·ar·sine** (di-fe"əl-klor-ahr'sin) sneezing gas, $(C_6H_5)_2AsCl$, a toxic war gas that causes sneezing, coughing, headache, salivation, and vomiting.

**di·phen·yl·di·i·mide** (di-fen"əl-di'ĭ-mīd) azobenzene.

**di·phen·yl·hy·dan·to·in** (di-fen"əl-hi-dan'to-in) phenytoin.

**di·phen·yl·ni·tros·amine** (di-fen"əl-ni-trōs'ə-mēn) *N*-nitrosodiphenylamine.

**di·phen·yl·pyr·a·line hy·dro·chlo·ride** (di-fen"əl-pēr'ə-lēn) an $H_1$ receptor antagonist with anticholinergic and sedative effects; used as an antihistaminic in the treatment of allergic symptoms, administered orally.

**di·pho·nia** (di fo'ne-ə) [*di-* + *phon-* + *-ia*] the production of two different tones in speaking; called also *double voice.*

**di·phos·gene** (di-fos'jēn) a gas which is intensely irritating to the lungs, producing pulmonary edema.

**di·phos·pha·ti·dyl·glyc·er·ol** (di"fos-fə-ti"dəl-glis'ər-ol) glycerol linked to two molecules of phosphatidic acid; 1,3-diphosphatidylglycerol is cardiolipin.

**2,3-di·phos·pho·glyc·er·ate** (di-fos'fo-glis'ər-āt) 2,3-bisphosphoglycerate.

**di·phos·pho·nate** (di-fos'fə-nāt) 1. a salt, ester, or anion of diphosphonic acid. While structurally similar to pyrophosphate, its P—C—P bonds give it enhanced stability to enzymatic and chemical hydrolysis. 2. any of a group of such compounds, having affinity for sites of osteoid mineralization and used as sodium salts to inhibit bone resorption as well as complexed with technetium Tc 99m for bone imaging; including alendronate, clodronate, etidronate, and pamidronate. Called also *bisphosphonate.*
**methylene d.,** medronate.

**di·phos·pho·nic ac·id** (di"fos-fon'ik) a dimer of phosphonic acid; structurally it is similar to pyrophosphoric acid, but with an organic substituent replacing the central oxygen atom of that molecule.

**di·phos·pho·pyr·i·dine nu·cleo·tide (DPN)** (di-fos'fo-pir'ĭ-dēn) former name of *nicotinamide adenine dinucleotide* (NAD).

**di·phos·pho·trans·fer·ase** (di-fos"fo-trans'fər-ās) [EC 2.7.6] any member of a sub-subclass of enzymes of the transferase class that catalyze the transfer of pyrophosphate (diphosphate) groups from one molecule to another. Called also *pyrophosphotransferase.*

**diph·the·ria** (dif-thēr'e-ə) [Gr. *diphthera* leather + *-ia*] [MeSH: Diphtheria] an acute infectious disease caused by toxigenic strains of *Corynebacterium diphtheriae,* acquired by contact with an infected person or a carrier; it is usually confined to the upper respiratory tract, and characterized by the formation of a tough *false membrane* attached firmly to the underlying tissue that will bleed if forcibly removed. In the most serious infections the membrane begins in the faucial area on one tonsil and may spread to the other tonsil, uvula, soft palate, and pharyngeal wall, followed by the larynx, trachea, and bronchial tree, where it may cause bronchial obstruction and death by hypoxia. Diphtheria also occurs in a cutaneous form and may rarely involve the eyes, middle ear, buccal mucosa, genitalia, and umbilical stump, usually secondarily. Systemic effects, chiefly myocarditis and peripheral neuritis, are caused by the exotoxin produced by *C. diphtheriae.*
**avian d.,** fowlpox.
**calf d.,** a contagious disease of young calves caused by infection with *Fusobacterium necrophorum;* symptoms include formation of grayish patches in the mouth or throat, foul-smelling breath, fever, cough, and dyspnea, often ending fatally. In the throat it is called also *necrotic laryngitis,* and in the mouth it is called also *necrotic stomatitis.*
**cutaneous d.,** a form of diphtheria involving the skin, occurring as a primary infection, usually seen in warm climates, characterized by a nonhealing, punched-out ulcer with a rolled border, surrounded by a zone of erythema, and sometimes covered by a hard, adherent membrane; or as a secondary infection of a preexisting lesion (burn, abrasion, cut, insect bite, etc.); or as a superinfection of various eczematous lesions.
**faucial d.,** diphtheria in the fauces, the most common type. Called also *pharyngeal d.*
**fowl d.,** fowlpox.
**laryngeal d., laryngotracheal d.,** diphtheria that has spread to the larynx.
**nasal d.,** diphtheria localized to the nasal mucosa, usually one or both of the anterior nasal septa of infants; characteristics include a serosanguineous discharge that becomes mucopurulent and causes skin erosion below the nostrils, and presence of a whitish membrane. Constitutional symptoms may be absent or slight.
**nasopharyngeal d.,** diphtheria that has spread to the nasopharynx.
**pharyngeal d.,** faucial d.
**umbilical d.,** diphtheria in the umbilical stump of an infant.

**diph·the·ri·al** (dif-thēr'e-əl) diphtheritic.

**diph·the·ric** (dif-thēr'ik) diphtheritic.

**diph·the·rin** (dif'the-rin) a polyvalent diphtheritic antigen for use in anaphylactic skin test.

**diph·the·rit·ic** (dif"the-rit'ik) pertaining to or resembling diphtheria or its characteristic false membrane. Called also *diphtherial* and *diphtheric.*

**diph·the·roid** (dif'thə-roid) 1. resembling diphtheria or the diphtheria bacillus. 2. any member of *Corynebacterium* other than *C. diphtheriae.* 3. pseudodiphtheria. 4. former name for organisms now in the genus *Propionibacterium.*

**diph·the·ro·tox·in** (dif"thə-ro-tok'sin) see *diphtheria toxin,* under *toxin.*

**diph·thon·gia** (dif-thon'je-ə) [*di-* + Gr. *phthongos* sound] the production of double vocal sounds; called also *diplophonia.*

**Di·phy·lets** (di'fĭ-ləts) trademark for a preparation of dextroamphetamine sulfate.

**Di·phyl·la** (di-fil'ə) a genus of vampire bats of South America, Central America, Mexico, and the West Indies.

**di·phyl·lo·both·ri·a·sis** (di-fil"o-both-ri'ə-sis) [MeSH: Diphyllobothriasis] infection with tapeworms of the genus *Diphyllobothrium;* formerly called *dibothriocephaliasis.*

**Di·phyl·lo·both·ri·i·dae** (di-fil"o-both-re'ĭ-de) a family of cestodes that are parasitic in man and other fish-eating vertebrates. The genera *Diphyllobothrium* and *Spirometra* are of medical importance.

**Di·phyl·lo·both·ri·um** (di-fil"o-both're-əm) [*di-* + Gr. *phyllon* leaf + *bothrion* pit] [MeSH: Diphyllobothrium] a genus of large tapeworms of the family Diphyllobothriidae; formerly called *Bothriocephalus* and *Dibothriocephalus.*
**D. corda'tum,** the heart-headed tapeworm; a small species found in dogs and in seals in Greenland and very rarely in humans.
**D. erina'cei,** a species found in the adult form in dogs and other carnivores; formerly called *D. mansoni.*
**D. la'tum,** the broad tapeworm or fish tapeworm, a large worm found in the intestines of humans, cats, dogs, mink, bears, and other fish-eating mammals, sometimes reaching a length of 9 meters. Its head has two grooves or suckers (bothria). It has two intermediate hosts: the first a crustacean, the second a fish. Human infection, acquired by eating inadequately cooked fish, may have a clinical picture like that of pernicious anemia. Called also *Dibothriocephalus latus,* and formerly *D. taenioides.* See accompanying illustration.
**D. manso'ni,** *D. erinacei.*
**D. mansonoi'des,** a species whose migrating larvae (spargana) are one of the causes of sparganosis.
**D. par'vum,** a species found in humans in Australia, Japan, Romania, Iran, and the northern United States; it may be identical with *D. latum.*
**D. taenioi'des,** *D. latum.*

**di·phy·odont** (di-fi'o-dont") [*di-* + Gr. *phyein* to produce + *odous* tooth] having two dentitions, a deciduous and a permanent, as in humans. Cf. monophyodont and polyphyodont.

**di·pip·a·none hy·dro·chlo·ride** (di-pip'ə-nōn) an analogue of methadone, used as an analgesic, administered subcutaneously, intramuscularly, and intravenously.

**di·piv·e·frin** (di-piv'ə-frin) an ester and prodrug of epinephrine; it is converted by enzyme hydrolysis in the eye to epinephrine, which lowers intraocular pressure by decreasing the production and increasing the outflow of aqueous humor.
**d. hydrochloride** [USP], the hydrochloride salt of dipivefrin, applied topically to the conjunctiva for the control of intraocular pressure in the treatment of open-angle glaucoma and secondary glaucoma.

**dip·la·cu·sia** (dip"lə-koo'ze-ə) diplacusis.

**dip·la·cu·sis** (dip"lə-koo'sis) [*diplo-* + *akousis* hearing] the perception of a single auditory stimulus as two sounds, as a result of cochlear pathology; called also *double disharmonic hearing.*
**binaural d.,** different perception of a single auditory stimulus by the two ears; the difference may be in tone (disharmonic d.) or in timing (echo d.).
**disharmonic d.,** a form of diplacusis in which a given pure tone is heard differently in the two ears.
**echo d.,** a form in which a sound of brief duration is heard in the one ear a fraction of a second later than in the other ear.
**monaural d., d. monaura'lis,** a form in which a pure tone is heard in the same ear as a split tone of two frequencies.

**di·plas·mat·ic** (di"plaz-mat'ik) [*di-* + *plasmatic*] containing substances besides protoplasm; said of cells.

**di·ple·gia** (di-ple'je-ə) [*di-* + *-plegia*] paralysis affecting like parts on both sides of the body; bilateral paralysis.
**atonic-astatic d.,** diplegic flaccid paralysis in infants; see *flaccid paralysis.* Called also *Förster's d.* or *syndrome.*
**facial d.,** paralysis affecting both sides of the face.
**facial d., congenital,** Möbius syndrome.
**Förster's d.,** atonic-astatic d.
**infantile d.,** birth palsy.

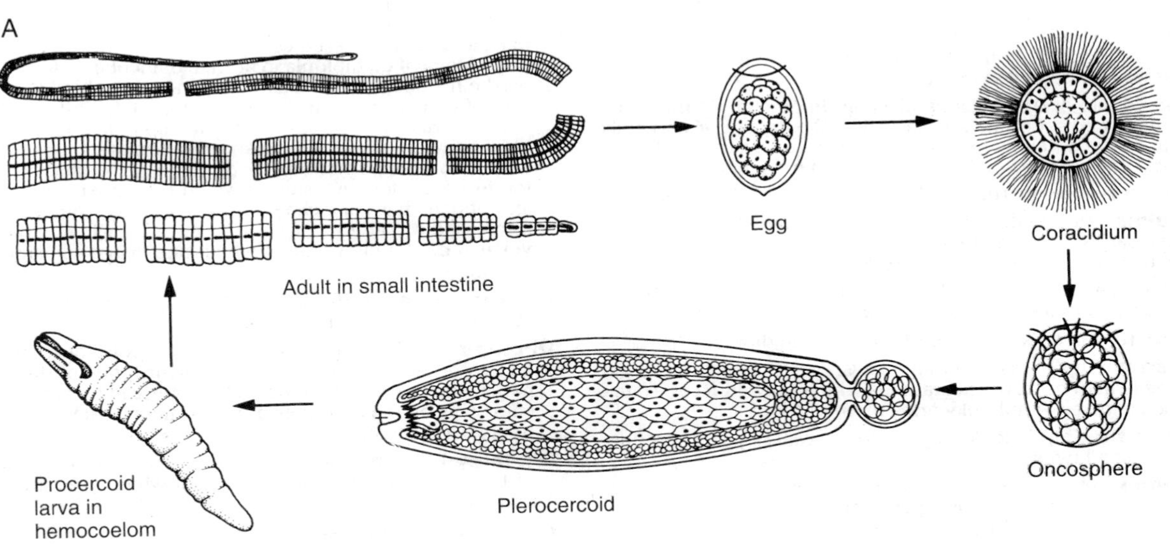


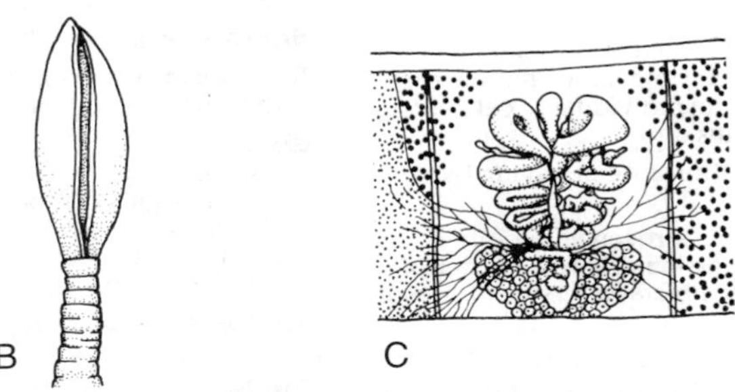


*(A),* Life cycle of *Diphyllobothrium latum.* *(B),* Scolex. *(C),* Gravid proglottid.

**masticatory d.**, paralysis of all the muscles which take part in mastication.
**spastic d.**, 1. Little's disease. 2. spastic paraplegia.

**di·ple·gic** (di-ple'jik) pertaining to or marked by diplegia.

**dipl(o)-** [Gr. *diploos* double] a combining form meaning double, twin, twofold, or twice.

**dip·lo·al·bu·min·uria** (dip"lo-al-bu"min-u're-ə) [*diplo-* + *albuminuria*] the presence of both physiologic and pathologic albuminuria.

**dip·lo·ba·cil·li** (dip"lo-bə-sil'i) [L.] plural of *diplobacillus.*

**dip·lo·ba·cil·lus** (dip"lo-bə-sil'əs) pl. *diplobacil'li* [*diplo-* + *bacillus*] a short, rod-shaped bacterium occurring in pairs, joined end to end; diplobacterium.
**Morax-Axenfeld d.**, *Moraxella lacunata.*

**dip·lo·bac·te·ria** (dip"lo-bak-tēr'e-ə) [L.] plural of *diplobacterium.*

**dip·lo·bac·te·ri·um** (dip"lo-bak-tēr'e-əm) pl. *diplobacte'ria* [*diplo-* + *bacterium*] a bacterial cell occurring as one of a pair of linked cells.

**dip·lo·blas·tic** (dip"lo-blas'tik) [*diplo-* + *blast-* + *-ic*] made up of two germ layers.

**dip·lo·ceph·a·lus** (dip"lo-sef'ə-ləs) dicephalus.

**dip·lo·ceph·a·ly** (dip"lo-sef'ə-le) dicephaly.

**dip·lo·coc·cal** (dip"lo-kok'əl) pertaining to or caused by diplococci.

**dip·lo·coc·ci** (dip"lo-kok'si) plural of *diplococcus.*

**dip·lo·coc·coid** (dip"lo-kok'oid) 1. resembling diplococci. 2. an organism that resembles a diplococcus.

**Dip·lo·coc·cus** (dip"lo-kok'əs) [*diplo-* + *coccus*] in former systems of classification, a genus of bacteria made up of organisms now assigned to various other genera.
**D. constella'tus,** *Peptococcus constellatus.*
**D. mag'nus,** *Peptococcus anaerobius.*
**D. muco'sus,** *Neisseria mucosa.*
**D. pneumo'niae,** *Streptococcus pneumoniae.*

**dip·lo·coc·cus** (dip"lo-kok'əs) pl. *diplococ'ci.* 1. a spherical bacterium occurring predominantly in pairs as a consequence of incomplete separation following cell division in a single plane. 2. an organism of the genus *Diplococcus.*
**d. of Morax-Axenfeld,** *Moraxella (Moraxella) lacunata.*
**d. of Neisser,** *Neisseria gonorrhoeae.*

**Dip·lo·dia** (dip-lo'de-ə) a genus of Fungi Imperfecti of the form-class Coelomycetes. Certain species cause the dry rot or cornstalk disease of corn; contaminated feed is thought to be a cause of cornstalk disease in horses and diplodiosis in other animals.

**dip·lo·di·a·tox·i·co·sis** (dip"lo-di"ə-tok"sĭ-ko'sis) diplodiosis.

**dip·lo·di·o·sis** (dip"lo-de-o'sis) a form of mycotoxicosis with temporary paralysis, seen in farm animals that eat corn containing *Diplodia* fungi. Called also *diplodiatoxicosis.*

**dip·loë** (dip'lo-e) [Gr. *diploē* fold] [TA] the loose osseous tissue between the two tables of the cranial bones.

**dip·lo·et·ic** (dip"lo-et'ik) of or pertaining to the diploë.

**Dip·lo·gas·ter** (dip'lo-gas"tər) [*diplo-* + Gr. *gastēr* stomach] a genus of free-living coprozoic nematodes which may, in fecal examination, be confused with hookworms or *Strongyloides.*

**dip·lo·gen·e·sis** (dip"lo-jen'ə-sis) [*diplo-* + *-genesis*] the production of conjoined twins.

**Dip·lo·go·nop·o·rus** (dip"lo-go-nop'ə-rəs) [*diplo-* + Gr. *gonos* seed + *poros* passage] a genus of tapeworms of the family Diphyllobothriidae, characterized by the possession of two sets of reproductive organs in each segment.
**D. brau'ni,** former name for *Digramma brauni.*
**D. gran'dis,** a common parasite of whales that has been found in man in Japan; it may be up to 10 meters long, and may cause diarrhea or constipation, and secondary anemia.

**dip·lo·ic** (dip-lo'ik) 1. double. 2. diploetic.

**dip·loid** (dip'loid) [Gr. *diploos* twofold] 1. having two sets of chromosomes, as normally found in the somatic cells of higher organisms. Cf. *haploid* (def. 1). Symbol 2n. 2. an individual or cell having two full sets of homologous chromosomes.

**dip·loi·dy** (dip'loi-de) [MeSH: Diploidy] the state of having two full sets of homologous chromosomes.

**dip·lo·mate** (dip'lo-māt) a person who has received a diploma or certificate. In medicine the term refers particularly to a holder of a certificate of the National Board of Medical Examiners or of one of the American Boards in the Specialties.

**dip·lo·mo·nad** (dip"lo-mo'nad) [*diplo-* + Gr. *monas* unit, from *monos,* single] 1. pertaining to or caused by protozoa of the order Diplomonadida. 2. a protozoan of the order Diplomonadida.

**Dip·lo·mo·nad·i·da** (dip"lo-mo-nad'ĭ-də) [*diplo-* + Gr. *monas* unit, from *monos* single] [MeSH: Diplomonadida] an order of mostly parasitic, bilaterally symmetrical protozoa (class Zoomastigophorea, subphylum Mastigophora) having one or two karyomastigonts, each with one to four flagella. It includes two suborders: Diplomonadina and Enteromonadina.

**Dip·lo·mo·na·di·na** (dip"lo-mo"nə-di'nə) a suborder of mostly parasitic protozoa (order Diplomonadida, class Zoomastigophorea) having two karyomastigonts, each containing four flagella. Representative genera include *Giardia, Hexamita,* and *Trepomonas.*

**dip·lo·my·e·lia** (dip"lo-mi-e'le-ə) [*diplo-* + *myel-* + *-ia*] lengthwise fissure and seeming doubleness of the spinal cord; cf. *diastematomyelia.*

**dip·lon** (dip'lon) [Gr. *diploos* double] deuteron.

**dip·lop·a·gus** (dip-lop'ə-gəs) [*diplo-* + *-pagus*] conjoined twins in which the component parts are equal to and the symmetrical equivalents of one another; called also *duplicitas symmetros.*

**dip·lo·phase** (dip'lo-fāz) that phase in the life history of certain organisms in which the nuclei are diploid.

**dip·lo·pho·nia** (dip"lo-fo'ne-ə) [*diplo-* + *phon-* + *-ia*] diphthongia.

**di·plo·pia** (dĭ-plo'pe-ə) [*diplo-* + *-opia*] [MeSH: Diplopia] the perception of two images of a single object; called also *ambiopia, double vision,* and *binocular polyopia.*
**binocular d.,** double vision in which the images of an object are formed on noncorresponding points of the retinas.
**crossed d.,** double vision in which the image belonging to the right eye is displaced to the left of the image belonging to the left eye, as occurs in exotropia (divergent squint). Called also *heteronymous d.*
**direct d.,** double vision in which the image belonging to the right eye appears to the right of the image belonging to the left eye, as occurs in esotropia (convergent squint). Called also *homonymous d.* and *uncrossed d.*
**heteronymous d.,** crossed d.
**homonymous d.,** direct d.
**horizontal d.,** diplopia in which the images lie in the same horizontal plane, being either crossed or direct.
**monocular d.,** the perception by the same eye of two images of a single object, due to double pupil, early cataract, irregular astigmatism, or displacement of the lens.
**paradoxical d.,** crossed d.
**physiological d.,** diplopia in normal binocular vision; all objects not on the horopter of the fixated object are doubled through stimulation of disparate points of the retinae outside the corresponding retinal areas. For nearer objects, the diplopia is crossed; for farther objects, uncrossed. Called also *stereoscopic d.*
**stereoscopic d.,** physiological d.
**torsional d.,** double vision in which the upper pole of the vertical axis of one image is inclined toward or away from that of the other.
**uncrossed d.,** direct d.
**vertical d.,** double vision in which one image appears to be above the other.

**di·plo·pi·om·e·ter** (dĭ-plo"pe-om'ə-tər) [*diplopia* + *-meter*] an instrument for measuring diplopia.

**Di·plop·o·da** (di-plop'o-də) [*diplo-* + Gr. *pous* foot] the millipedes, a class of more or less cylindrical arthropods of the order Chilognatha, superclass Myriapoda, characterized by having two pairs of short legs on most of their body segments; they may have from 13 to almost 200 pairs of legs.

**Dip·lo·py·lid·i·um** (dip"lo-pi-lid'e-əm) a genus of small tapeworms of the family Dipylidiidae, species of which are parasites of birds and mammals.

**dip·lo·scope** (dip'lo-skōp) [*diplo-* + *-scope*] an apparatus for the study of binocular vision.

**dip·lo·so·ma·tia** (dip"lo-so-ma'she-ə) [*diplo-* + *somat-* + *-ia*] symmetrical conjoined twins.

**dip·lo·some** (dip'lo-sōm) [*diplo-* + *-some*] the two centrioles of mammalian cells; called also *paired allosomes.*

**dip·lo·so·mia** (dip"lo-so'me-ə) symmetrical conjoined twins.

**Dip·lo·sto·ma·ti·dae** (dip"lo-sto-mat'ĭ-de) a family of trematodes that includes the genus *Alaria.*

**dip·lo·tene** (dip'lo-tēn) the stage of the first meiotic prophase, following the pachytene, in which the two chromosomes in each bivalent begin to repel one another and a split occurs between the chromosomes, which are then held together by regions where exchanges have taken place (chiasmata) during crossing over. See also *leptotene, pachytene,* and *zygotene.*

**dip·lo·ter·a·tol·o·gy** (dip"lo-ter"ə-tol'ə-je) [*diplo-* + *teratology*] the sum of what is known regarding conjoined twins.

**Dip·lur·i·dae** (dip-loo'rĭ-de) a family of spiders of the suborder Orthognatha; two genera, *Atrax* and *Trechona,* are harmful to humans.

**di·po·dia** (di-po'de-ə) [*di-* + *pod-* + *-ia*] 1. a developmental anomaly characterized by duplication of a foot. 2. dipodial symmelia.

**di·po·di·al** (di-po'de-əl) having symmelia with two feet present.

**di·pole** (di'pōl) 1. a molecule having charges of equal and opposite signs but in which the center of the positive charge does not coincide with that of the negative charge, a property which enables the molecule to be bound electrostatically by both positively and negatively charged groups. See *polar compounds,* under *compound.* 2. a pair of electric charges or magnetic poles separated by a short distance.

**di·po·tas·si·um phos·phate** (di"po-tas'e-əm) dibasic potassium phosphate; see under *potassium.*

**dip·ping** (dip'ing) 1. palpation of the liver by a quick depressing movement of the fingers with the hand flat across the abdomen. 2. the immersion of an animal in a large volume of dilute insecticide in order to kill external parasites.

**Di·pri·van** (di'prĭ-van) trademark for a preparation of propofol.

**Di·pro·lene** (di-pro'lene) trademark for preparations of betamethasone dipropionate.

**Di·pro·sone** (di-pro'sōn) trademark for preparations of betamethasone dipropionate.

**di·pros·o·pus** (di-pros'o-pəs) [*di-* + *prosopo-* + *-ous*] a fetus with a single trunk and normal limbs, but with varying degrees of duplication of the face.
**d. tetrophthal'mus,** a fetus having two fused faces, the median eye of each being fused into a common orbit.

**di·pro·tri·zo·ate** (di"pro-tri'zo-āt) chemical name: 3,5-dipropionamido-2,4,6-triiodobenzoate; used as a contrast medium in radiography of the urinary tract.

**dip·se·sis** (dip-se'sis) [Gr. *dipsēsis* a thirst, longing] thirst.

**dip·set·ic** (dip-set'ik) [Gr. *dipsētikos* thirsty; provoking thirst] pertaining to, characterized by, or producing dipsesis.

**dip·sia** (dip'se-ə) [Gr. *dipsa* thirst + *-ia*] thirst; often used as a word termination, denoting a condition relative to thirst, or the physiological state of the body leading to the ingestion of fluids.

**dip·so·gen** (dip'so-jən) [Gr. *dipsa* thirst + *-gen*] an agent or measure that induces thirst and promotes the ingestion of fluids.

**dip·so·gen·ic** (dip-so-jen'ik) engendering thirst.

**dip·so·sis** (dip-so'sis) [Gr. *dipsa* thirst + *-osis*] extreme thirst or a craving for unusual things to drink. Cf. *polydipsia.*

**dip·so·ther·a·py** (dip"so-ther'ə-pe) [Gr. *dipsa* thirst + *therapy*] treatment by strict limitation of the amount of water to be ingested.

**dip·stick** (dip'stik) a strip of cellulose chemically impregnated to render it sensitive to protein, glucose, or other substances in the urine.

**Dip·tera** (dip'tər-ə) [Gr. *dipteros* two winged] [MeSH: Diptera] an order of insects including the flies, gnats, and mosquitoes.

**dip·ter·ous** (dip'tər-əs) 1. having two wings. 2. pertaining to insects of the order Diptera.

**Dip·ter·yx** (dip'tər-iks) a genus of tropical and subtropical American trees. *D. odora'ta* Willd. (Leguminosae) is the tonka bean, a North American species.

**di·pus** (di'pəs) [*di-* + Gr. *pous* foot] sympus dipus.

**di·py·gus** (di-pi'gəs) [*di-* + Gr. *pygē* rump] a fetus with a double pelvis.
**d. parasi'ticus,** gastrothoracopagus dipygus.

**dip·y·li·di·a·sis** (dip"ə-lĭ-di'ə-sis) infection with *Dipylidium caninum.*

**Dip·y·li·di·i·dae** (dip"ə-lĭ-di'ĭ-de) a family of cestodes of the order Cyclophyllidea, which sometimes parasitize mammals, birds, and snakes. The genus *Dipylidium* is of medical interest. Formerly called Dilepididae.

**Dip·y·lid·i·um** (dip"ə-lid'e-əm) [Gr. *dipylos* having two entrances] a genus of tapeworms of the family Dipylidiidae, found in cats and other small carnivores.
**D. cani'num,** a common tapeworm of dogs and cats, the larval stage living in fleas *(Ctenocephalides canis)* and lice *(Trichodectes canis)* of dogs, as well as in *Pulex irritans,* which thus act as vectors; it has been found in man. Called also *Taenia elliptica.*

**di·py·rid·a·mole** (di"pĭ-rid'ə-mōl) [MeSH: Dipyridamole] a platelet inhibitor and coronary vasodilator used to prevent thromboembolism associated with mechanical heart valves, as prophylactic adjunct in the prevention of myocardial reinfarction, and as a diagnostic aid adjunct in myocardial perfusion imaging; administered orally and intravenously.

**di·py·rone** (di'pi-rōn) [MeSH: Dipyrone] a pyrazolone analgesic and antipyretic; now seldom used because it can cause agranulocytosis.

**di·rect** (dĭ-rekt') [L. *directus*] 1. straight; in a straight line. 2. performed immediately and without the intervention of subsidiary means.

**di·rec·tor** (dĭ-rek'tor) [L. *dirigere* to direct] any person, thing, or device that guides or directs.
**grooved d.,** a grooved instrument used to guide the direction and depth of a surgical incision.

**di·rhi·nic** (di-ri'nik) pertaining to both halves of the nasal cavity.

**dir·i·go·mo·tor** (dir"ĭ-go-mo'tor) [L. *dirigere* to direct + *motor*] controlling muscular activity.

**di·rith·ro·my·cin** (di-rith"ro-mi'sin) [USP] a macrolide antibiotic with activity similar to that of erythromycin, used in the treatment of bacterial infections of the respiratory tract, streptococcal pharyngitis, and skin and soft tissue infections; administered orally.

**Di·ro·fi·la·ria** (di"ro-fĭ-lar'e-ə) [MeSH: Dirofilaria] a genus of nematodes of the superfamily Filarioidea; they have very long filiform bodies and striated cuticles.
**D. immi'tis,** the heartworm, an important pathogen of dogs and other canids, which is of worldwide distribution in tropical and subtropical areas. Mosquitoes transmit the larvae, and adult worms are found in and may occlude the vessels of the heart, primarily the right ventricle and pulmonary artery, of affected animals.
**D. magalhae'si,** D. immitis.
**D. re'pens,** a species found in the subcutaneous connective tissues of dogs and occasionally of humans.

**di·ro·fil·a·ri·a·sis** (di"ro-fil"ə-ri'ə-sis) [MeSH: Dirofilariasis] infection with a parasite of the genus *Dirofilaria.* It is common in dogs, but in humans it is rare, manifesting with symptoms such as cough, chest pain, and sometimes hemoptysis.

**Dir. prop.** abbreviation for L. *directio'ne pro'pria,* with a proper direction.

**DIS** Diagnostic Interview Schedule.

**dis-**[1] [L.] a prefix denoting reversal or separation.

**dis-**[2] [Gr. *dis* twice] a prefix denoting duplication.

**dis·a·bil·i·ty** (dis"ə-bil'ĭ-te) 1. a lack of the ability to function normally, physically or mentally; incapacity. 2. anything that causes disability. 3. as defined by the federal government: "inability to engage in any substantial gainful activity by reason of any medically determinable physical or mental impairment which can be expected to last or has lasted for a continuous period of not less than 12 months."
**developmental d.,** a substantial handicap having its onset before the age of 18 years and of indefinite duration. Examples are mental retardation, autism, cerebral palsy, epilepsy, or other neuropathy.

**di·sac·cha·ri·dase** (di-sak'ə-ri-dās") an enzyme that hydrolyzes disaccharides. In humans, the disaccharidases, comprising the β-glycosidase (lactase–phlorhizin hydrolase) complex, sucrase-isomaltase complex; and trehalase, are located in the brush border membrane of the small intestine, hydrolyzing the oligo- and disaccharides produced after luminal digestion of starches and other dietary carbohydrates. See also under *deficiency* and see *disaccharide intolerance,* under *intolerance.*

**di·sac·cha·ride** (di-sak'ə-rīd) any of a class of sugars composed of two glycosidically linked monosaccharides; the term is most commonly used for those composed of hexoses, such as sucrose, lactose, and maltose.
**reducing d's,** disaccharides that can reduce Fehling's solution or other reagents, owing to the presence of a functional aldehyde group.

**di·sac·cha·rid·uria** (di-sak"ə-rīd-u're-ə) presence of a disaccharide (lactose or sucrose) in the urine.

**dis·ac·id·i·fy** (dis"ə-sid'ĭ-fi) to remove an acid from, or to neutralize an acid in, a mixture.

**Di·sal·cid** (di-sal'sid) trademark for preparations of salsalate.

**dis·ar·tic·u·la·tion** (dis"ahr-tik"u-la'shən) [*dis-* + *articulation*] [MeSH: Disarticulation] amputation or separation at a joint. Called also *exarticulation.*
**ankle d.,** amputation of the foot at the ankle joint; see also *Syme's amputation*
**elbow d.,** amputation of the upper limb through the elbow joint.
**hip d.,** amputation of the lower limb through the hip joint.
**knee d.,** amputation of the lower limb through the knee joint.
**shoulder d.,** amputation of the upper limb through the shoulder joint. Called also *Dupuytren's amputation* or *operation* and *Lisfranc's amputation* or *operation.*
**wrist d.,** amputation of the hand through the wrist joint.

**dis·as·sim·i·late** (dis"ə-sim'ĭ-lāt) dissimilate.

**dis·as·sim·i·la·tion** (dis″ə-sim″ĭ-la′shən) [*dis-* + *assimilation*] dissimilation.

**disc** (disk) [*discus*] disk.
**Bardeen's primitive d.,** the embryonic structure that develops into the intervertebral ligament.
**blastodermic d.,** the early embryonic disc during the period of cleavage.
**ectodermal d.,** an elongated plate of epithelial cells developed from the inner cell mass in the human blastocyst about a week after fertilization.
**embryonic d.,** a flattish area in a blastocyst in which the first traces of the embryo are seen, visible early in the second week in human development; called also *germ d., germinal d.,* and *gastrodisk.*
**germ d., germinal d.,** embryonic d.

**dis·cec·to·my** (dis-kek′tə-me) diskectomy.

**dis·charge** (dis-chahrj′) 1. a setting free, or liberation. 2. matter or force set free. 3. an excretion or substance evacuated. 4. release from a hospital or other course of care. 5. the passing of an action potential through a neuron, axon, or muscle fiber.
**bizarre high-frequency d., bizarre repetitive d.,** complex repetitive d.
**complex repetitive d.,** polyphasic or serrated formations seen on recordings of action potentials, having uniform amplitude and frequency and abrupt beginning and ending; seen in patients with muscular dystrophy and other motor unit diseases. Called also *bizarre high-frequency d., bizarre repetitive d.,* and *bizarre high-frequency potential.*
**disruptive d.,** the passing of a current through an insulating medium due to the breakdown of the medium under the electrostatic stress.
**double d.,** the repeated occurrence of two similar action potentials, separated by just a short interval, as part of a larger repeating pattern; called also *doublet.*
**epileptic d.,** the pathological discharge of multiple neurons in the central nervous system, signaling an attack of epilepsy.
**epileptiform d's,** see under *activity.*
**grouped d.,** 1. on an electroencephalogram, the occurrence of several motor unit action potentials together. 2. repetitive d.
**iterative d.,** repetitive d.
**multiple d.,** the repeated occurrence of four or more similar action potentials separated by short intervals, as part of a larger repeating pattern; called also *multiplet.*
**myokymic d.,** patterns of grouped or repetitive discharges of motor unit action potentials sometimes seen in myokymia. The most common type is groups of single units firing at a uniform rate interspersed with silent periods. A less common pattern is continuously recurring multiple discharges.
**myotonic d.,** high frequency repetitive discharges seen in myotonia and evoked by insertion of a needle electrode, percussion of a muscle, or stimulation of a muscle or its motor nerve; characterized by waxing and waning of frequency and amplitude. There are two types: one with biphasic spike potentials resembling fibrillation potentials and one with waves resembling positive sharp waves.
**nervous d., neural d.,** discharge, def. 4.
**periodic lateralized epileptiform d. (PLED),** a pattern of repetitive paroxysmal slow or sharp waves seen on an electroencephalogram from just one side of the brain.
**repetitive d.,** multiple recurrences of an action potential in similar forms; examples are *double d., triple d., multiple d., myokymic d.,* and *myotonic d.* Called also *iterative d.*
**triple d.,** the repeated occurrence of three similar action potentials separated by short intervals, near each other as part of a larger repeating pattern; called also *triplet.*

**dis·ci** (dis′i) [L.] genitive and plural of *discus.*

**dis·ci·form** (dis′ĭ-form) [*disc-* + *form*] in the form of a disk.

**dis·cis·sion** (dĭ-sizh′ən) [L. *discissio; dis-* apart + *scindere* to cut] incision, or cutting into, as of a soft cataract.
**d. of cataract,** the surgical rupturing of the capsule so that the aqueous humor may gain access to the lens of the eye.
**d. of cervix uteri,** incisions on each side of the cervix uteri, formerly done for the relief of stenosis of the cervix.
**posterior d.,** incision of the capsule of a cataract from behind.

**dis·ci·tis** (dis-ki′tis) [MeSH: Discitis] diskitis.

**dis·cli·na·tion** (dis″klĭ-na′shən) extorsion.

**disc(o)-** [L. *discus,* q.v.] a combining form denoting relationship to a disk, or disk-shaped. See also words beginning *disko-.*

**dis·co·blas·tic** (dis″ko-blas′tik) [*disco-* + *blast-* + *-ic*] pertaining to a discoblastula or to discoidal cleavage.

**dis·co·blas·tu·la** (dis″ko-blas′tu-lə) the specialized blastula formed by cleavage of a fertilized telolecithal ovum, consisting of a cellular cap (the *embryonic disc* or *blastoderm*) separated by the blastocoele from a floor of uncleaved yolk.

**dis·co·cyte** (dis′ko-sīt) an erythrocyte of the normal discoid shape, as opposed to a poikilocyte or other irregular form.

**dis·co·gas·tru·la** (dis″ko-gas′troo-lə) a modified, flattened gastrula formed by discoidal cleavage of a highly telolecithal ovum.

**dis·co·ge·net·ic** (dis″ko-jə-net′ik) discogenic.

**dis·co·gen·ic** (dis″ko-jen′ik) [*disco-* + *-genic*] caused by derangement of an intervertebral disk.

**dis·co·gram** (dis′ko-gram) diskogram.

**dis·cog·ra·phy** (dis-kog′rə-fe) diskography.

**dis·coid** (dis′koid) [*disc-* + *-oid*] 1. shaped like a disk. 2. a dental instrument with a circular blade around the entire periphery except where it meets the shank; used to carve dental restorations. 3. a disk-shaped dental excavator designed to remove the carious dentin of a decayed tooth.

**dis·coid·ec·to·my** (dis″koid-ek′tə-me) diskectomy.

**Dis·co·my·ces** (dis″ko-mi′sēz) [*disco-* + Gr. *mykēs* fungus] in former systems of classification, a genus of bacteria made up of organisms now assigned to the genera *Actinomyces, Nocardia,* and *Streptomyces.*

**dis·cop·a·thy** (dis-kop′ə-the) [*disco-* + *-pathy*] disease of an intervertebral cartilage (disk).
**traumatic d.,** herniation of an intervertebral disk due to trauma; see under *herniation.*

**dis·coph·o·rous** (dis-kof′ə-rəs) [*disco-* + Gr. *phoros* bearing] possessing a disklike organ or part.

**dis·co·pla·cen·ta** (dis″ko-plə-sen′tə) discoid placenta.

**dis·cord** (dis′kord) [L. *discordia*] a simultaneous assemblage of two or more inharmonious sounds.

**dis·cor·dance** (dis-kor′dəns) in genetics, the occurrence of a given trait in only one member of a twin pair, as opposed to *concordance.*

**dis·cor·dant** (dis-kor′dənt) 1. exhibiting discordance. 2. belonging to divergent species; said of transplanted tissue. See under *xenograft.*

**dis·co·ria** (dis-kor′e-ə) dyscoria.

**dis·co·spon·dy·li·tis** (dis″ko-spon″dĭ-li′tis) [*disco-* + *spondylitis*] inflammation of intervertebral disks in animals, often with osteomyelitis of adjacent vertebrae, caused by a bacterial infection or occasionally trauma. Resultant compression of the spinal cord can cause paralysis. It is most commonly seen in adult dogs but also affects pigs, horses, and cattle.

**dis·crep·an·cy** (dis-krep′ən-se) disagreement or inconsistency.
**tooth size d.,** lack of harmony of size of individual or groups of teeth when related to those within the same arch or the opposing arch.

**dis·crete** (dis-krēt′) [L. *discretus; discernere* to separate] made up of separated parts or characterized by lesions which do not become blended.

**dis·crim·i·na·tion** (dis-krim″ĭ-na′shən) the making of a fine distinction.
**speech d.,** ability to recognize spoken words, as measured by speech audiometry.

**dis·crim·i·na·tor** (dis-krim′ĭ-na″tər) a circuit in which output is a function of how the input signal compares with one or more standard or reference signals.

**dis·cus** (dis′kəs) pl. *dis′ci* [L.; Gr. *diskos*] a circular or rounded flat plate; used as a general term in anatomical nomenclature to designate such a structure. Called also *disc* or *disk.*
**d. articula′ris** [TA], articular disk: a pad composed of fibrocartilage or dense fibrous tissue found in some synovial joints; it extends into the joint from a marginal attachment at the articular capsule and in some cases completely divides the joint cavity into two separate compartments. Called also *interarticular disk.*
**d. articula′ris articulatio′nis acromioclavicula′ris** [TA], articular

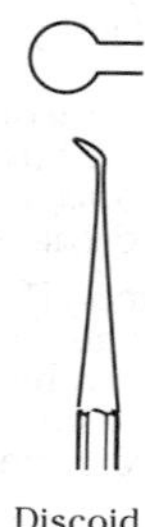

Discoid.

disk of acromioclavicular articulation: a pad of fibrocartilage, sometimes present, commonly imperfect, within the articular cavity of the acromioclavicular joint. Called also *Weitbrecht's cartilage* and *meniscus of acromioclavicular joint.*
**d. articula'ris articulatio'nis mandibula'ris,** d. articularis articulationis temporomandibularis.
**d. articula'ris articulatio'nis radioulna'ris dista'lis** [TA], articular disk of distal radioulnar articulation: a triangular pad of fibrocartilage, attached at its base to the radius and at its apex to the base of the styloid process of the ulna; it usually separates the articular cavity of the distal radioulnar joint from that of the radiocarpal joint. Called also *meniscus of inferior radioulnar joint* and *triquetrous* or *triquetral cartilage.*
**d. articula'ris articulatio'nis sternoclavicula'ris** [TA], articular disk of sternoclavicular articulation: a pad of fibrocartilage, the circumference of which is connected to the articular capsule of the sternoclavicular joint; it is attached superiorly to the clavicle and inferiorly to the first costal cartilage near its union with the sternum, and divides the joint cavity into two parts. Called also *meniscus of sternoclavicular joint.*
**d. articula'ris articulatio'nis temporomandibula'ris** [TA], articular disk of temporomandibular joint: a plate of fibrocartilage or fibrous tissue that divides the temporomandibular joint into two separate cavities; its circumference is connected to the articular capsule. Called also *d. articularis articulationis mandibularis* and *meniscus of temporomandibular joint.*
**d. interpu'bicus** [TA], interpubic disk: a midline plate of fibrocartilage interposed between the symphysial surfaces of the pubic bones, these surfaces being covered by a thin layer of hyaline cartilage; called also *lamina fibrocartilaginea interpubica.*
**dis'ci intervertebra'les** [TA], intervertebral disks: the 23 plates of fibrocartilage found, from the axis to the sacrum, between the bodies of adjacent vertebrae, each consisting of a fibrous ring (anulus fibrosus) enclosing a pulpy center (nucleus pulposus); called also *fibrocartilagines intervertebrales,* and *intervertebral cartilages, fibrocartilage,* or *ligaments.*
**d. ner'vi op'tici** [TA], the optic disk: the intraocular portion of the optic nerve formed by fibers converging from the retina and appearing as a pink to white disk; there are no sensory receptors in this region and hence no response to stimuli restricted to it. Called also *blind spot, optic papilla,* and *papilla nervi optici.*

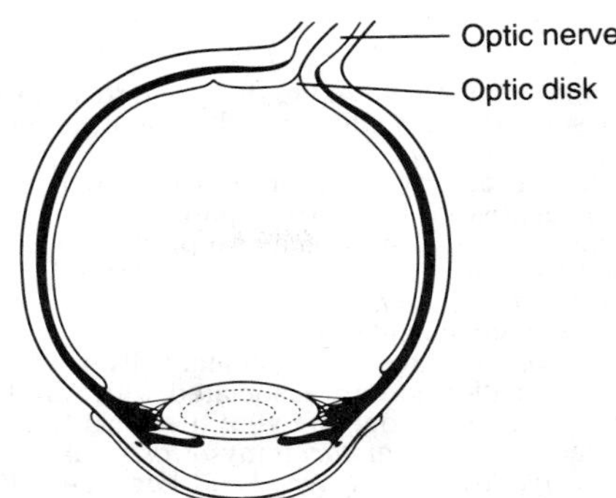


**d. oo'phorus,** cumulus oophorus.
**d. op'ticus,** d. nervi optici.
**d. ovi'gerus, d. proli'gerus,** cumulus oophorus.

**dis·cus·sive** (dis-kus'iv) discutient.

**dis·cu·ti·ent** (dis-ku'shənt) [L. *discutere* to dissipate] 1. scattering; causing a disappearance. 2. a remedy which so acts. Called also *discussive.*

**dis·di·a·clast** (dis-di'ə-klast) [*dis-*[2] + *dia-* + *-clast*] any of the doubly refracting elements of the contractile substance of muscle.

**dis·di·ad·o·cho·ki·ne·sia** (dis-di-ad"o-ko-kĭ-ne'zhə) dysdiadochokinesia.

**dis·ease** (dĭ-zēz') [Fr. *dès* from + *aise* ease] [MeSH: Disease] any deviation from or interruption of the normal structure or function of a part, organ, or system of the body as manifested by characteristic symptoms and signs; the etiology, pathology, and prognosis may be known or unknown.

## Disease

See also under *sickness* and *syndrome.*

**Acosta's d.,** acute mountain sickness.
**d's of adaptation,** a concept introduced by Hans Selye that certain diseases are by-products of physiologic adaptations to chronic stress *(general adaptation syndrome)*; he included in this category rheumatoid arthritis, peptic ulcer, and essential hypertension.
**Addison's d.,** a chronic type of adrenocortical insufficiency, characterized by hypotension, weight loss, anorexia, weakness, and a bronzelike hyperpigmentation of the skin. It is due to tuberculosis- or autoimmune-induced destruction of the adrenal cortex, which results in deficiency of aldosterone and cortisol and is fatal in the absence of replacement therapy. See also *addisonian crisis,* under *crisis.* Called also *chronic adrenocortical insufficiency* and *primary adrenal* or *primary adrenocortical insufficiency.*
**Adema d.,** inherited parakeratosis.
**adult celiac d.,** see *celiac d.*
**aftermath d.,** fog fever.
**airsac d.,** infectious sinusitis of turkeys.
**Akabane virus d.,** the symptom complex seen in fetal sheep or calves after their mothers have been bitten by insects and infected with the Akabane virus; fetuses have encephalomyelitis or defective brains (sometimes hydranencephaly) and arthrogryposis. See also *congenital articular rigidity,* under *rigidity.*
**akamushi d.,** scrub typhus.
**Akureyri d.,** epidemic neuromyasthenia.
**Åland eye d.,** Forsius-Eriksson syndrome.
**Albers-Schönberg d.,** osteopetrosis.
**Aleutian mink d.,** a chronic, progressive disease of mink, caused by a parvovirus, marked by inappetence, weight loss, lethargy, polydipsia, and hemorrhages; death may result from kidney failure.
**Alexander's d.,** an infantile form of leukodystrophy, characterized histologically by the presence of eosinophilic material at the surface of the brain and around its blood vessels, resulting in brain enlargement.
**alkali d.,** chronic selenium poisoning; see under *poisoning.*
**allogeneic d.,** graft-versus-host reaction occurring in immunosuppressed animals receiving injections of allogeneic lymphocytes.
**Almeida's d.,** paracoccidioidomycosis.
**Alpers' d.,** a rare disease of young children, characterized by neuronal degeneration of the cerebral cortex and elsewhere, accompanied by progressive mental deterioration, motor disturbances, seizures, and early death. Called also *Christensen-Krabbe disease, poliodystrophia cerebri,* and *progressive cerebral* or *progressive infantile poliodystrophy.*
**alpha chain d.,** the most common heavy chain disease, occurring predominantly in young adults in the Mediterranean area, and characterized by plasma cell infiltration of the lamina propria of the small intestine resulting in malabsorption with diarrhea, abdominal pain, and weight loss, or, exceedingly rarely, by pulmonary involvement. The gastrointestinal form is called also *immunoproliferative small intestine d.*
**altitude d.,** see under *sickness.*
**Alzheimer's d.,** a progressive degenerative disease of the brain of unknown etiology, characterized by diffuse atrophy throughout the cerebral cortex with distinctive lesions called *senile plaques* and clumps of fibrils called *neurofibrillary tangles.* There is a loss of choline acetyltransferase activity in the cortex, and many of the degenerating neurons seem to be cholinergic neurons projecting from the substantia innominata to the cortex. The first signs of the disease are slight memory disturbance or changes in personality; deterioration progresses to profound dementia over 5 to 10 years. Women are affected twice as often as men, and onset may occur at any age. It was originally called *presenile dementia* (i.e., in persons under 65) and opposed to *senile dementia* (i.e., that resulting from the aging process), but there is no clinical or pathophysiological distinction between the two classes of patients.
**Anders' d.,** adiposis tuberosa simplex.
**Andersen's d.,** glycogen storage d., type IV.
**Andes d.,** chronic mountain sickness.
**anti-GBM antibody d., anti–glomerular basement membrane antibody d.,** glomerulonephritis, usually of a generalized proliferative crescent-forming histologic type with a rapidly progressive course, marked by circulating anti-GBM antibodies and linear deposits of im-

munoglobulin and complement along the glomerular basement membrane. When associated with pulmonary hemorrhage the condition is called *Goodpasture's syndrome.*

**apatite deposition d.**, any acute or chronic connective tissue disorder marked by deposition of hydroxyapatite crystals in one or more joints or bursae; such deposition may be primary or it may be secondary to other disorders such as chronic renal failure. Called also *calcium hydroxyapatite deposition d.*

**Apert's d.**, acrocephalosyndactyly.

**Apert-Crouzon d.**, an autosomal dominant disorder, consisting of the hand and foot malformations associated with Apert's syndrome (see *acrocephalosyndactyly*) together with the facial characteristics of Crouzon's disease (see *craniofacial dysostosis,* under *dysostosis*). Called also *acrocephalosyndactyly type I* and *Vogt's cephalodactyly.*

**Aran-Duchenne d.**, spinal muscular atrophy.

**arc welder's d.**, welder's lung.

**Armstrong's d.**, lymphocytic choriomeningitis.

**arteriosclerotic cardiovascular d. (ASCVD),** atherosclerotic involvement of arteries to the heart and to additional organs, resulting in debility or death; the term is sometimes used more narrowly as a synonym of ischemic heart disease.

**arteriosclerotic heart d. (ASHD),** ischemic heart d.

**atopic d.**, atopy.

**Aujeszky's d.**, pseudorabies.

**Australian X d.**, Murray Valley encephalitis.

**autoimmune d.**, a disorder caused by an immune response directed against self antigens. Ideally there should be not only demonstrable circulating autoantibodies or cell-mediated immunity against autoantigens in conjunction with inflammatory lesions caused by immunologically competent cells or immune complexes in tissues containing the autoantigens but also clinical or experimental evidence that the autoimmune process is pathogenic not secondary to other tissue damage. In practice many diseases, such as systemic lupus erythematosus (SLE) and rheumatoid arthritis are often classified as autoimmune diseases although their pathogenesis is unclear.

**aviators' d.**, altitude sickness.

**Ayerza's d.**, a form of polycythemia vera associated with sclerosis of the pulmonary artery, marked by chronic cyanosis, dyspnea, bronchitis, bronchiectasis, enlargement of liver and spleen, and hyperplasia of bone marrow.

**Azorean d.**, a progressive degenerative disease of the central nervous system occurring in families of Portuguese-Azorean descent, having a variety of forms and inherited as an autosomal dominant trait. There are four major types: *Type I,* with pyramidal and extrapyramidal deficits; *Type II,* with cerebellar, pyramidal, and extrapyramidal deficits; *Type III,* with cerebellar deficits and distal sensorimotor neuropathy; *Type IV,* with parkinsonism and distal sensory neuropathy. Called also *Joseph d., Machado-Joseph d.,* and *Portuguese-Azorean d.*

**Baastrup's d.**, kissing spines.

**baby pig d.**, neonatal hypoglycemia.

**Baelz's d.**, see *cheilitis glandularis.*

**Baló's d.**, an atypical form of Schilder's disease in which the demyelination is arranged in concentric rings around a central circle; called also *encephalitis periaxialis concentrica, leukoencephalitis periaxialis concentrica,* and *concentric sclerosis.*

**Bamberger's d.**, 1. saltatory spasm. 2. Concato's d.

**Bamberger-Marie d.**, hypertrophic pulmonary osteoarthropathy.

**Bang's d.**, infectious abortion (def. 1).

**Bannister's d.**, angioedema.

**Banti's d.**, congestive splenomegaly.

**Barcoo d.**, desert sore.

**Barlow's d.**, infantile scurvy.

**barometer-maker's d.**, chronic mercurial poisoning in makers of barometers, due to the inhalation of the fumes of mercury.

**Barraquer's d.**, partial lipodystrophy.

**Basedow's d.**, Graves' d.

**Batten d., Batten-Mayou d.**, 1. Vogt-Spielmeyer d. 2. more generally, any or all of the group of disorders constituting neuronal ceroid-lipofuscinosis

**bauxite workers' d.**, bauxite pneumoconiosis.

**Bayle's d.**, general paresis.

**Bazin's d.**, see *erythema induratum.*

**Beck's d.**, Kashin-Bek d.

**Béguez César d.**, Chédiak-Higashi syndrome.

**Behr's d.**, degeneration of the macula retinae in adult life.

**Beigel's d.**, piedra.

**Bekhterev's (Bechterew's) d.**, ankylosing spondylitis.

**Benson's d.**, asteroid hyalosis.

**Berger's d.**, IgA nephropathy.

**Berlin's d.**, commotio retinae.

**Bernhardt's d., Bernhardt-Roth d.**, meralgia paresthetica.

**Besnier-Boeck d.**, sarcoidosis.

**Best's d.**, congenital macular degeneration.

**Bettlach May d.**, a fatal disease affecting adult honeybees, principally in Switzerland, marked by paralysis with inability to fly, caused by ingestion of the poisonous pollen of certain buttercups.

**Biedl's d.**, Bardet-Biedl syndrome.

**Bielschowsky-Janský d.**, Janský-Bielschowsky d.

**Bilderbeck's d.**, acrodynia.

**Billroth's d.**, traumatic meningocele.

**Binswanger's d.**, a degenerative dementia of presenile onset caused by thinning of the subcortical white matter of the brain; some have attributed it to sclerotic changes in the blood vessels. Called also *Binswanger's dementia* or *encephalitis, chronic subcortical encephalitis,* and *subcortical arteriosclerotic encephalopathy.*

**Birdsville d.**, poisoning of horses after eating either of the herbs *Indigofera dominii* or *I. linnaea*; characteristics include abdominal pain, stiffness and incoordination, and discharges from the nose and eyes.

**black d.**, infectious necrotic hepatitis.

**Blocq's d.**, astasia-abasia.

**Blount d.**, tibia vara.

**blue d.**, Rocky Mountain spotted fever.

**blue nose d.**, photosensitization of the face of a horse following ingestion of any of certain meadow plants; characteristics include blue discoloration of the muzzle, sloughing of nonpigmented skin, and frequently intense excitement.

**Boeck's d.**, sarcoidosis.

**border d. of sheep**, a highly fatal disease caused by a togavirus, affecting sheep on the English-Welsh border, as well as in Australia and New Zealand (where it is called *hairy shaker d.*); it is manifested by increased hair in the fleece, slow growth, diminished stature, abnormal head shape, and a swaying gait.

**Borna d.**, a fatal enzootic encephalitis of horses, cattle, and sheep, caused by the Borna disease virus; characteristics include tremor, lethargy, and flaccid paralysis. Called also *enzootic encephalitis of horses* and *equine encephalitis.*

**Bornholm d.**, epidemic pleurodynia.

**bottom d.**, crotalism.

**Bouchard's d.**, dilatation of the stomach from inefficiency of the gastric muscles.

**Bouchet-Gsell d.**, swineherd's d.

**Bourneville's d.**, tuberous sclerosis.

**Bowen's d.**, a squamous cell carcinoma in situ, often due to prolonged exposure to arsenic; it occurs as one or more sharply defined, slightly thickened, erythematous, scaly plaques, usually on sun-exposed areas of skin in older white males but sometimes found on mucous membranes. The corresponding lesion on the glans penis is termed erythroplasia of Queyrat. Called also *Bowen's precancerous dermatosis* and *precancerous dermatitis.*

**Bradley's d.**, epidemic nausea and vomiting.

**bran d.**, nutritional secondary hyperparathyroidism.

**Breisky's d.**, lichen sclerosus in women; see under *lichen.*

**Bright's d.**, a broad descriptive term once used for kidney disease with proteinuria, usually glomerulonephritis.

**Brill's d.**, Brill-Zinsser d.

**Brill-Symmers d.**, follicular lymphoma.

**Brill-Zinsser d.**, a recrudescence of epidemic typhus occurring years after the initial infection, in which the etiologic agent, *Rickettsia prowazekii,* persists in the body tissue in an inactive state (perhaps as long as 70 years), with humans as the reservoir. Compared with epidemic typhus, it is milder, the fever is not as high and is of shorter duration, the rash is less intense and is often absent, and the fatality rate is much lower. Called also *Brill's d.* and *latent* or *recrudescent typhus.*

**Brinton's d.**, linitis plastica.

**Brion-Kayser d.**, paratyphoid fever.

**brisket d.**, a disease seen in young cattle at altitudes above 7600 feet, resembling altitude sickness of humans and often progressing to fatal respiratory or cardiac failure; it is sometimes seen in sheep and has been produced experimentally in pigs.

**brittle bone d.**, osteogenesis imperfecta.

**broad beta d.**, familial dysbetalipoproteinemia; named for the electrophoretic mobility of the abnormal chylomicron and very-low-density lipoprotein remnants ($\beta$-VLDL) produced in this disorder.

**Brodie's d.**, 1. chronic synovitis, especially of the knee, with a pulpy degeneration of the parts affected. 2. hysterical pseudofracture of the spine.

**bronzed d.**, Addison's d.

**Brown-Symmers d.**, fatal acute serous encephalitis in children.

**Bruck's d.**, a condition marked by deformity of bones, multiple fractures, ankylosis of joints, and atrophy of muscles.

**Bruton's d.**, X-linked agammaglobulinemia.

**Buerger's d.**, thromboangiitis obliterans.

**Buhl's d.**, an acute sepsis affecting newborn infants, marked by hemorrhages into the skin, mucous membranes, and navel attended with cyanosis and jaundice; there are also hemorrhages in the intestinal organs.

**Buschke's d.,** cryptococcosis.
**bush d.,** see under *sickness.*
**Busquet's d.,** exostoses on the dorsum of the foot due to osteoperiostitis of the metatarsal bones.
**Buss d.,** encephalomyelitis with pleuritis affecting cattle in the United States, Japan, and parts of Europe, caused by infection with *Chlamydia psittaci;* characteristics include fever, labored breathing, cough, diarrhea, and neurological signs such as a staggering gait; sometimes there is drooling or a nasal discharge. Called also *sporadic bovine encephalomyelitis.*
**Busse-Buschke d.,** cryptococcosis.
**Cacchi-Ricci d.,** sponge kidney.
**Caffey's d.,** infantile cortical hyperostosis.
**caisson d.,** decompression sickness.
**calcium hydroxyapatite deposition d.,** apatite deposition d.
**calcium pyrophosphate deposition d. (CPDD),** an acute or chronic inflammatory arthropathy caused by deposition of calcium pyrophosphate dihydrate (CPPD) crystals in the joints and characterized by chondrocalcinosis and the presence of the crystals in synovial fluid. Clinically, it may resemble numerous connective tissue diseases, including osteoarthritis, rheumatoid arthritis, and gout, or it may be asymptomatic. While most commonly idiopathic, CPDD can also be hereditary or associated with a variety of metabolic diseases. Acute attacks are sometimes called *pseudogout.* Called also *CPPD d.*
**California d.,** coccidioidomycosis.
**caloric d.,** any disease due to exposure to high temperature.
**Calvé-Perthes d.,** osteochondrosis of the capitular epiphysis of the femur.
**Camurati-Engelmann d.,** diaphyseal dysplasia.
**Canavan's d., Canavan-van Bogaert-Bertrand d.,** spongy degeneration of the central nervous system; see under *degeneration.*
**canine parvovirus d.,** an acute, often fatal gastroenteritis of dogs caused by a parvovirus related to the virus of feline panleukopenia or of mink enteritis.
**Caroli's d.,** congenital dilatation of the intrahepatic bile ducts.
**Carrión's d.,** bartonellosis (def. 2).
**Castellani's d.,** hemorrhagic bronchitis.
**Castleman's d.,** a condition resembling lymphoma but without recognizable malignant cells; there are isolated masses of lymphoid tissue and lymph node hyperplasia, usually in the abdominal or mediastinal area. One variety has numerous small germinal centers near blood vessels with neovascularization; a second type consists of sheets of plasma cells and fewer but larger germinal centers. The disease may be either benign or premalignant. Called also *giant lymph node hyperplasia.*
**cat-scratch d.,** a usually benign, self-limited infectious disease of the regional lymph nodes, caused by *Bartonella henselae* and chiefly characterized by subacute painful regional lymphadenitis and mild fever of short duration. It is most often associated with close contact with a cat, the primary symptom being an isolated papule or pustule at the site of a cat scratch. Called also *benign lymphoreticulosis, cat-scratch fever,* and *regional lymphadenitis.*
**Cavare's d.,** familial periodic paralysis.
**celiac d.,** a malabsorption syndrome, thought to be hereditary, precipitated by the ingestion of gluten-containing foods. It is characterized by degeneration of intestinal villi with loss of their absorptive function; diarrhea and steatorrhea; abdominal distention; flatulence; weight loss; asthenia; deficiency of vitamins B, D, and K; and electrolyte depletion. The *infantile form* has an insidious onset, with irritability, loss of appetite, weakness, extreme wasting, growth retardation, and celiac crisis. The *adult form* is marked by fatigue, dyspnea, clubbing of fingers, bone pain, muscle cramps, tetany, megacolon and abdominal distention, tympanitis, and skin pigmentation. The two forms were formerly considered different entities but are now believed to be the same. Called also *gluten enteropathy* and *nontropical sprue.*
**central core d.,** an autosomal dominant form of myopathy characterized by dense, amorphous hyaline changes in the central portion of the myofibrils, which lack organelles. Onset is in infancy and causes delayed motor development, especially in the lower limbs. Called also *Shy-Magee syndrome.*
**Chagas' d.,** an acute, subacute, or chronic form of trypanosomiasis seen widely in Central and South America, caused by *Trypanosoma cruzi,* and transmitted by the bites of reduviid bugs of the genera *Triatoma, Panstrongylus,* and *Rhodnius;* the reservoir hosts are domestic and wild animals such as cats, dogs, rodents, armadillos, bats, and foxes. The *acute* form, prevalent in children, is marked initially by an erythematous nodule (chagoma) at the site of inoculation; high fever; unilateral swelling of the face with edema of the eyelid (Romaña's sign); regional lymphadenopathy; hepatosplenomegaly; and meningoencephalic irritation. If death does not occur, the disease may resolve completely, or the subacute or chronic form may follow. The *subacute* form may last for several months or years and is characterized by mild fever, severe asthenia, and generalized lymphadenopathy. The *chronic* form, which may or may not be preceded by an acute episode, is characterized principally by cardiac manifestations (myocarditis) and gastrointestinal manifestations (including megaesophagus and megacolon). Called also *American* or *South American trypanosomiasis.*
**Charcot's d.,** neuropathic arthropathy.
**Charcot-Marie-Tooth d.,** muscular atrophy of variable inheritance, beginning in the muscles supplied by the peroneal nerves and progressing slowly to involve the muscles of the hands and arms. Called also *Charcot-Marie atrophy* or *syndrome, peroneal* or *peroneal muscular atrophy, Marie-Tooth d.,* and *Tooth's d.*
**cheese handler's d., cheese washer's d.,** see under *lung.*
**Chester's d.,** xanthomatosis of the long bones with spontaneous fractures.
**Chiari-Frommel d.,** see under *syndrome.*
**Chicago d.,** blastomycosis (def.1).
**cholesteryl ester storage d. (CESD),** a relatively mild lysosomal storage disease caused by deficiency of the lysosomal sterol esterase; hepatomegaly may be the only clinical abnormality; hyperbetalipoproteinemia is common, and there is often severe premature atherosclerosis; patients may survive past 40.
**Christensen-Krabbe d.,** Alpers' d.
**Christian's d.,** Hand-Schüller-Christian d.
**Christian-Weber d.,** relapsing febrile nodular nonsuppurative panniculitis.
**Christmas d.,** hemophilia B.
**chronic granulomatous d. (CGD), chronic granulomatous d. of childhood,** any of a group of immunodeficiencies of X-linked or autosomal recessive inheritance, caused by failure of the respiratory or metabolic burst, resulting in deficient microbicidal ability. The clinical picture consists of frequent, severe, prolonged bacterial and fungal infections of the skin, oral and intestinal mucosa, reticuloendothelial system, bones, lungs, and genitourinary tract. The course of the disease varies: symptoms may appear in the neonate, with death during the first decade, or a patient may survive into middle age. There seem to be no physiologic differences between the X-linked and the autosomal recessive types.
**chronic obstructive lung d. (COLD), chronic obstructive pulmonary d. (COPD),** 1. any disorder characterized by persistent or recurring obstruction of bronchial air flow, such as chronic bronchitis, asthma, or pulmonary emphysema. 2. heaves.
**chronic respiratory d. of poultry,** a common respiratory disease of chickens caused by infection with *Mycoplasma gallisepticum,* and marked by distressed breathing, swelling of the face, and nasal discharge. Abbreviated CRD.
**circling d.,** listeriosis in domestic animals.
**climatic d.,** any disease thought to be produced by a change of climate.
**coast d.,** a type of enzootic marasmus seen in southeastern Australia, caused by cobalt and copper deficiencies.
**Coats' d.,** chronic progressive exudative retinopathy usually occurring in male children and young adults.
**coldwater d.,** infection of aquarium fish by *Cytophaga psycrophila;* symptoms include lumps or cottonlike lesions on the skin and gills with ulceration, necrosis, and hemorrhage. Called also *peduncle d.*
**collagen d.,** any of a group of diseases that, although clinically distinct and not necessarily related etiologically, have in common widespread pathologic changes in the connective tissue; they include lupus erythematosus, dermatomyositis, scleroderma, polyarteritis nodosa, rheumatic fever, and rheumatoid arthritis. Collagen disease is not to be confused with *collagen disorder* (q.v.).
**columnaris d.,** infection of warm-water fish by *Cytophaga columnaris,* with slimy or cottonlike skin lesions covering surface necrosis.
**comb d.,** favus of fowl.
**combined immunodeficiency d.,** 1. see under *immunodeficiency.* 2. an autosomal recessive disease of Arabian horses; foals lack their own cell-mediated immunity and seem normal only as long as they have passive immunity from the maternal blood acquired in utero. Soon after the age of two months, most die from uncontrollable infections, particularly respiratory.
**combined system d.,** subacute combined degeneration of spinal cord; see under *degeneration.*
**communicable d.,** an infectious disease transmitted from one individual to another, either by direct contact or indirectly by means of a vector or fomites; the terms *communicable d.* and *contagious d.* are used synonymously. Cf. *infectious d.*
**complicating d.,** one which occurs in the course of some other disease as a complication.
**compressed-air d.,** decompression sickness.
**Concato's d.,** progressive malignant polyserositis with large effusions into the pericardium, pleura, and peritoneum. Called also *Bamberger's d..*
**Conor and Bruch's d.,** boutonneuse fever.
**Conradi's d.,** chondrodysplasia punctata.

**constitutional d.,** one that involves a system of organs or one characterized by widespread symptoms.
**contagious d.,** communicable disease transmitted by contact; the terms *contagious d.* and *communicable d.* are used synonymously. Cf. *infectious d.*
**Cooley's d.,** thalassemia major.
**Corbus' d.,** gangrenous balanitis.
**Cori's d.,** glycogen storage d., type III.
**cork handler's d.,** suberosis.
**cornstalk d.,** moldy corn poisoning.
**coronary artery d. (CAD),** atherosclerosis of the coronary arteries, which may cause angina pectoris, myocardial infarction, and sudden death. Both genetically determined and avoidable risk factors contribute to the disease; they include hypercholesterolemia, hypertension, smoking, diabetes mellitus, and low levels of high density lipoproteins.
**coronary heart d. (CHD),** ischemic heart d.
**Corridor d.,** a tick-borne protozoal disease caused by infection with *Theileria lawrencei;* it resembles East Coast fever but is less severe, and is highly pathogenic for cattle, with buffalo serving as a reservoir of infection.
**Corrigan's d.,** aortic regurgitation.
**Corvisart's d.,** 1. tetralogy of Fallot associated with right aortic arch. 2. formerly, chronic hypertrophic myocarditis.
**Cotugno's d.,** sciatica.
**covering d.,** dourine.
**Cowden d.,** an autosomal dominant disorder comprising a combination of ectodermal, mesodermal, and endodermal anomalies, characterized by development of multiple hamartomatous lesions, especially in the skin, oral mucosa, breast, thyroid, colon, and intestines, and associated with a high incidence of malignancies in the organs involved. Called also *multiple hamartoma syndrome.*
**CPPD d.,** calcium pyrophosphate deposition d.
**crazy chick d.,** 1. avian encephalomalacia. 2. avian encephalomyelitis.
**creeping d.,** a condition marked by cutaneous lesions similar to those seen in larva migrans, but produced by nematodes of the genus *Gnathostoma.*
**Creutzfeldt-Jakob d.,** a rare prion disease, associated with a number of different mutations of the prion protein gene, existing in sporadic, familial (as an autosomal dominant), and infectious forms, with onset usually in middle life, and having a wide variety of clinical and pathological features. The most commonly seen are varying degrees of spongiform degeneration of neurons, neuronal loss, gliosis, and amyloid plaque formation, accompanied by rapidly progressive dementia, myoclonus, motor disturbances, and characteristic changes in the electroencephalogram. Death generally occurs within a year of onset, although longer courses up to 5 years are not uncommon. Sporadic cases account for 85–95 per cent of all occurrences. Infectious cases generally result from surgical procedures or injection of human growth hormone prepared from infected pituitary glands. Called also *Jakob's d.* and *Jakob-Creutzfeldt d.*
**Creutzfeldt-Jakob d., new variant (nvCJD),** a variant of Creutzfeldt-Jakob disease occurring almost exclusively in the United Kingdom, having a younger age of onset than is seen in Creutzfeldt-Jakob disease, and caused by the same agent that causes bovine spongiform encephalopathy.
**Crigler-Najjar d.,** see under *syndrome.*
**Crohn's d.,** a chronic granulomatous inflammatory disease of unknown etiology, involving any part of the gastrointestinal tract from mouth to anus, but commonly involving the terminal ileum with scarring and thickening of the bowel wall; it frequently leads to intestinal obstruction and fistula and abscess formation and has a high rate of recurrence after treatment. Called also *Crohn's colitis* and *regional* or *segmental enteritis.* When confined to the ileum it is also called *regional* or *terminal ileitis.*
**crooked calf d.,** a syndrome of congenital skeletal defects seen in calves in the western United States and Canada when their mothers have eaten certain species of *Lupinus* during pregnancy; characteristics include joint contractures, torticollis, and spinal deformities.
**Crouzon's d.,** craniofacial dysostosis.
**Cruveilhier's d.,** spinal muscular atrophy.
**Cushing's d.,** Cushing's syndrome in which the hyperadrenocorticism is secondary to excessive anterior pituitary secretion of adrenocorticotropic hormone, with or without a pituitary adenoma.
**cystic d. of breast,** fibrocystic d. of breast.
**cystic d. of kidney, acquired,** a disorder seen in patients with end stage renal disease; cysts develop in the formerly noncystic failing kidney, often containing oxalate and sometimes undergoing malignant transformation.
**cystic d. of lung,** a condition in which there are abnormally large air spaces in the lung parenchyma; the term is sometimes applied to cystic emphysema. Called also *pseudocysts of lung* and *pulmonary pseudocysts.*
**cysticercus d.,** cysticercosis.

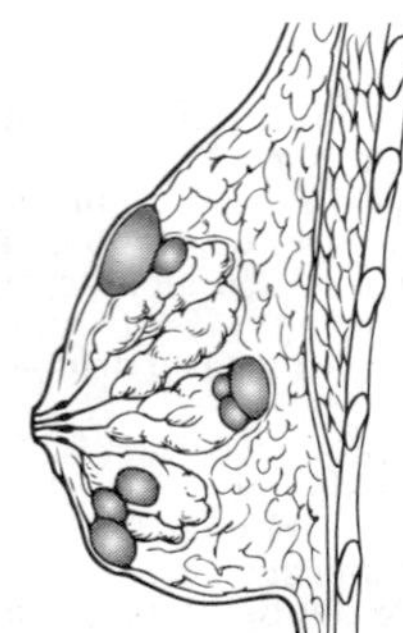

Cross-sectional view of cystic disease of the breast.

**cystine d., cystine storage d.,** cystinosis.
**cytomegalic inclusion d.,** any of a group of diseases caused by cytomegalovirus infection, marked by characteristic inclusion bodies in enlarged infected cells. The classic disease is congenital, being acquired in utero from the mother; infection can also be transmitted from mother to infant in passage through the birth canal or from ingestion of virus in the mother's milk. Most infected infants are asymptomatic, but in some there may be hepatosplenomegaly, jaundice, chorioretinitis, purpura, microcephaly, cerebral calcifications, and severe central nervous system sequelae with blindness, deafness, quadriplegia, and mental retardation. Acquired disease is transmitted via respiratory droplets, tissue or blood donation, or sexual transmission. The group also includes *cytomegalovirus mononucleosis;* in immunocompromised patients there may be a disseminated, sometimes fatal, infection as well as specific syndromes such as *cytomegalovirus encephalitis, cytomegalovirus pneumonia,* or *cytomegalovirus retinitis.*
**Czerny's d.,** periodic hydrarthrosis of the knee.
**Daae's d.,** epidemic pleurodynia.
**Dalrymple's d.,** cyclokeratitis.
**Darier's d., Darier-White d.,** keratosis follicularis.
**Darling's d.,** histoplasmosis.
**David's d.,** spinal tuberculosis.
**deficiency d.,** a condition produced by dietary or metabolic deficiency; the term includes all diseases—e.g., kwashiorkor, beriberi, scurvy, pellagra, calcium deficiency, etc.—caused by an insufficient supply of the essential nutrients, i.e., protein (or amino acids), vitamins, and minerals.
**degenerative joint d.,** osteoarthritis.
**Degos' d.,** malignant atrophic papulosis.
**Dejerine's d., Dejerine-Sottas d.,** progressive hypertrophic neuropathy.
**demyelinating d.,** any condition characterized by destruction of the myelin sheaths of nerves. Cf. *multiple sclerosis.*
**dense deposit d.,** type II membranoproliferative glomerulonephritis.
**Dent's d.,** tubulopathy of the proximal kidney tubules with low molecular weight proteinuria, hypercalciuria, hypokalemia, nephrocalcinosis, rickets, and progressive renal failure.
**deprivation d.,** deficiency d.
**de Quervain's d.,** painful tenosynovitis due to relative narrowness of the common tendon sheath of the abductor pollicis longus and the extensor pollicis brevis.
**Dercum's d.,** adiposis dolorosa.
**dermopathic herpesvirus d.,** a herpesvirus disease of cattle, characterized by ulcerative lesions in the skin; it resembles lumpy skin disease (q.v.).
**Deutschländer's d.,** 1. tumor of the metatarsal bones. 2. march foot.
**Devic's d.,** neuromyelitis optica.
**diamond skin d.,** the urticarial form of swine erysipelas.
**disappearing bone d.,** gradual, but often complete, resorption of a bone or group of bones, which may be associated with multiple hemangiomas; it usually occurs in children or young adults, sometimes following trauma, but its etiology is unknown.
**diverticular d.,** a general term embracing the prediverticular state, diverticulosis, and diverticulitis.
**Döhle d.,** syphilitic aortitis.
**drug d.,** 1. a morbid condition due to long-continued use of a drug. 2. in homeopathy, the group of symptoms seen after the administration of a drug for the purpose of proving.
**Dubini's d.,** see under *chorea.*
**Dubois' d.,** see under *abscess.*
**Duchenne's d.,** 1. spinal muscular atrophy. 2. bulbar paralysis. 3. tabes dorsalis. 4. Duchenne's muscular dystrophy.
**Duchenne-Aran d.,** spinal muscular atrophy.
**Duchenne-Griesinger d.,** Duchenne's muscular dystrophy.
**Duhring's d.,** dermatitis herpetiformis.

**Dukes' d.**, a mild febrile disease of childhood characterized by a bright rosy red, generalized exanthematous eruption, probably a viral exanthem of the Coxsackie-ECHO group; it was given the ordinal designation *fourth d.* to differentiate it from other exanthems (see *exanthem,* def. 2). Called also *Filatov-Dukes d.* and *scarlatinella.*

**Duncan's d.**, X-linked lymphoproliferative syndrome.

**Durand-Nicolas-Favre d.**, lymphogranuloma venereum.

**Durante's d.**, osteogenesis imperfecta.

**Duroziez's d.**, congenital mitral stenosis.

**Eales d.**, a condition marked by recurrent hemorrhages into the retina and vitreous, affecting mainly males in the second and third decades of life.

**Ebola d., Ebola virus d.**, a highly fatal, acute hemorrhagic fever, clinically very similar to Marburg virus disease, caused by the Ebola virus, and occurring in the Sudan and adjacent areas in northwestern Zaire; the natural reservoir and mode of transmission of the virus are unknown, but secondary infection is by direct contact with infected blood and other body secretions and by airborne particles.

**Ebstein's d.**, 1. hyaline degeneration and necrosis of the epithelial cells of the renal tubules; seen in diabetes. 2. see under *anomaly.*

**echinococcus d.**, hydatid d.

**Economo's d.**, lethargic encephalitis.

**edema d.**, enterotoxemia in recently weaned piglets caused by a strain of *Escherichia coli* that normally colonizes the small intestine; characteristics include edema in various parts of the body, with neurological signs such as circling and ataxia. See also *coliform gastroenteritis.* Called also *bowel edema, gut edema,* and E. coli enterotoxemia.

**Edsall's d.**, heat cramp.

**elevator d.**, a type of pneumoconiosis affecting persons who work in grain elevators.

**encephalomyocarditis virus d.**, a viral disease caused by a cardiovirus that usually occurs in rodents but is transmissible to other animals, especially pigs. It is often clinically inapparent but sometimes causes reproductive failure in young female pigs or encephalomyocarditis in various species, which can be fatal.

**endemic d.**, one present or usually prevalent in a population or geographical area at all times; such diseases usually have low mortality. Called also *endemia.* See also *holoendemic d.* and *hyperendemic d.* Cf. *epidemic d.*

**end-stage renal d. (ESRD)**, chronic, irreversible renal failure. See *renal failure,* under *failure.*

**Engelmann's d.**, diaphyseal dysplasia.

**Engel-Recklinghausen d.**, osteitis fibrosa cystica.

**English sweating d.**, anglicus sudor.

**eosinophilic endomyocardial d.**, Löffler's endocarditis.

**epidemic d.**, an infectious or other disease that suddenly affects individuals in a population or geographical area clearly in excess of the number of cases normally expected. Cf. *endemic d.*

**Epstein's d.**, pseudodiphtheria.

**Erb's d.**, Duchenne's muscular dystrophy.

**Erb-Charcot d.**, Erb's spastic paraplegia.

**Erb-Goldflam d.**, myasthenia gravis.

**Erdheim's d.**, cystic medial necrosis.

**Eulenburg's d.**, paramyotonia congenita.

**extensor process d.**, buttress foot.

**extrapyramidal d.**, any of a group of disorders marked by abnormal involuntary movements, alterations in muscle tone, and postural disturbances and involving lesions of the extrapyramidal tract; included are parkinsonism, chorea, athetosis, and others.

**Fabry's d.**, an X-linked lysosomal storage disease of glycosphingolipid catabolism, resulting from a deficiency of α-galactosidase A and leading to accumulation of ceramide trihexoside in the cardiovascular and renal systems. Clinical manifestations include telangiectases in the "bathing suit area," corneal opacities, burning pain in the palms, soles, and abdomen, chronic paresthesias of the hands and feet, cardiopulmonary involvement, edema of the legs, osteoporosis, retarded growth, and delayed puberty. Patients usually die of renal failure or cardiac or cerebrovascular disease. Called also *angiokeratoma corporis diffusum, diffuse angiokeratoma, α-galactosidase A deficiency,* and *ceramide trihexosidase deficiency.*

**Fahr-Volhard d.**, malignant nephrosclerosis.

**falling d.**, a condition seen in cattle with dietary copper deficiency, sometimes with molybdenum poisoning; affected animals suddenly throw up their heads, utter a loud cry, and usually quickly die. They may show earlier signs of dietary deficiency such as diarrhea and depigmentation of the hair.

**Farber's d.**, a lysosomal storage disease of ceramide metabolism due to defective ceramidase and marked by hoarseness, aphonia, and a brownish desquamating dermatitis beginning at about three months of age, followed by foam cell infiltration of bones and joints, resulting in deformations; granulomatous reaction in lymph nodes, heart, lungs, and kidneys, and psychomotor retardation. Called also *Farber's lipogranulomatosis,* and *ceramidase deficiency.*

**farmer's lung d. of cattle**, a disease in cattle similar to farmer's lung in humans, caused by hypersensitivity to moldy hay contaminated by *Micropolyspora faeni* or *Thermoactinomyces vulgaris.*

**fat-deficiency d.**, a condition characterized by cessation of growth and skin lesions that result when essential fatty acids (linolenic and linoleic acid) are absent from the diet.

**fatty liver d.**, 1. fatty liver in alcoholics; see under *liver.* 2. fat cow syndrome.

**Fauchard d.**, marginal periodontitis.

**Favre-Durand-Nicolas d.**, lymphogranuloma venereum.

**Fazio-Londe d.**, progressive bulbar palsy of childhood.

**Feer's d.**, acrodynia.

**Fenwick's d.**, idiopathic atrophic gastritis, first described by Fenwick in a patient with pernicious anemia.

**fibrocystic d., fibrocystic d. of breast**, a form of mammary dysplasia with formation of cysts of various size containing a semitransparent, turbid fluid that imparts a brown to blue color (blue dome cyst) to the unopened cysts; considered to be due to abnormal hyperplasia of the ductal epithelium and dilatation of the ducts of the mammary gland, occurring as a result of an exaggeration and distortion of the cyclic breast changes that normally occur in the menstrual cycle. Called also *chronic cystic mastitis, cystic d. of breast,* and *Schimmelbusch's d.*.

**fibrocystic d. of the pancreas**, cystic fibrosis.

**Fiedler's d.**, Weil's syndrome.

**fifth d.**, erythema infectiosum.

**Filatov's (Filatow's) d.**, infectious mononucleosis.

**Filatov-Dukes d.**, Dukes' d.

**file-cutters' d.**, lead poisoning from inhaling lead particles rising from the bed of lead used in file cutting.

**fish eye d.**, a less severe form of lecithin–cholesterol acyltransferase deficiency due to a partial defect in the enzyme activity; corneal opacities give the eye the appearance of the eye of a boiled fish, and lipoproteins show some abnormalities.

**fish-slime d.**, septicemia following a puncture wound made by the spine of a fish.

**Flajani's d.**, Graves' d.

**Flatau-Schilder d.**, Schilder's d.

**flax-dresser's d.**, byssinosis in flax-dressers.

**Flegel's d.**, hyperkeratosis lenticularis perstans.

**Fleischner's d.**, osteochondritis affecting the middle phalanges of the hand.

**flint d.**, chalicosis.

**floating beta d.**, familial dysbetalipoproteinemia.

**fluke d.**, trematodiasis.

**focal d.**, one which is localized at one or more foci.

**Følling d.**, phenylketonuria.

**foot-and-mouth d.**, an acute extremely contagious disease caused by a picornavirus, affecting wild and domestic animals, particularly ruminants and pigs, and occasionally humans. It is marked by an eruption of vesicles on the lips, buccal cavity, pharynx, legs, and feet; sometimes the skin of the udder or teats is involved. Called also *aftosa, aphthous fever, hoof-and-mouth d.,* and *contagious* or *epizootic aphthae.*

**foot process d.**, minimal change d.

**Forbes' d.**, glycogen storage d., type III.

**Fordyce's d.**, 1. see under *granule.* 2. Fox-Fordyce d.

**Forestier d.**, hyperostosis of the anterolateral vertebral column, especially in the thoracic region.

**Förster's d.**, see under *choroiditis.*

**Fournier's d.**, see under *gangrene.*

**fourth d.**, Dukes' d.

**fourth venereal d.**, 1. specific gangrenous and ulcerative balanoposthitis; see under *balanoposthitis.* 2. granuloma inguinale.

**Fox-Fordyce d.**, a chronic, usually pruritic disease chiefly seen in women, characterized by the development of small follicular papular eruptions of apocrine gland–bearing areas, especially the axillae and pubes, and caused by obstruction and rupture of the intraepidermal portion of the ducts of affected apocrine glands, resulting in alteration of the regional ductal epidermis, apocrine secretory tubule, and adjacent dermis. Called also *apocrine miliaria.*

**Francis' d.**, tularemia.

**Frei's d.**, lymphogranuloma venereum.

**Freiberg's d.**, osteochondrosis of the head of the second metatarsal.

**Friedländer's d.**, endarteritis obliterans.

**Friedreich's d.**, paramyoclonus multiplex.

**Frommel's d.**, Chiari-Frommel syndrome.

**functional d.**, see under *disorder.*

**functional cardiovascular d.**, neurocirculatory asthenia.

**Gaisböck's d.**, stress polycythemia.

**gamma chain d.**, a heavy chain disease occurring usually in elderly persons that clinically resembles a malignant lymphoma, with symptoms of lymphadenopathy, hepatosplenomegaly, and recurrent infections.

**Gamna's d.**, a form of splenomegaly, with thickening of the splenic capsule and the presence of small brownish areas (Gamna nodules) which are usually surrounded by a hematogenous zone; ferruginous pigment is deposited in the splenic pulp.

**Gamstorp's d.,** familial periodic paralysis II.

**Gandy-Nanta d.,** siderotic splenomegaly.

**Garré's d.,** sclerosing nonsuppurative osteomyelitis.

**gastroesophageal reflux d. (GERD),** any condition noted clinically or histopathologically that results from gastroesophageal reflux, ranging in seriousness from mild to life-threatening; principle characteristics are heartburn and regurgitation. When there is damage to the esophageal epithelium, it is known as *reflux esophagitis.*

**Gaucher's d.,** a lipidosis caused by deficient glucocerebrosidase (glucosylceramidase), with glucocerebroside (glucosylceramide) accumulation in Gaucher cells, storage cells in the liver, spleen, lymph nodes, alveolar capillaries, and bone marrow. There are three clinical types: *type 1,* called also chronic non-neuronopathic or "adult" type, may appear at any age and is associated with hypersplenism, thrombocytopenia, anemia, jaundice, and bone lesions; *type 2,* called also acute neuronopathic or "infantile" type, is associated with onset in infancy, hepatosplenomegaly, severe impairment of the central nervous system, and death usually within the first year; and *type 3,* called also subacute neuronopathic or "juvenile" type, is the most varied, having the same clinical features as types 1 and 2 but a longer course. Called also *glucosylceramide lipidosis.*

**Gee's d., Gee-Herter d., Gee-Herter-Heubner d.,** the infantile form of celiac disease.

**Gee-Thaysen d.,** the adult form of celiac disease.

**genetic d.,** a general term for any disorder caused by a genetic mechanism, comprising chromosome aberrations or anomalies, mendelian or monogenic or single-gene disorders, and multifactorial disorders.

**Gerhardt's d.,** erythromelalgia.

**Gerlier's d.,** an acute disease seen in farm workers and stablemen, characterized by vertigo, ptosis, and motor disorders; it is probably a form of vestibular neuronitis.

**gestational trophoblastic d.,** see under *neoplasia.*

**Gibney's d.,** see under *perispondylitis.*

**Gilbert's d.,** see under *syndrome.*

**Gilchrist's d.,** blastomycosis (def. 1).

**Gilles de la Tourette's d.,** see under *syndrome.*

**Glanzmann's d.,** see under *thrombasthenia.*

**Glasser's d.,** a disease of young pigs, caused by infection by *Haemophilus parasuis;* symptoms include swelling of the hocks or knee joints or both, accompanied by fever and lameness; severe cases may progress to neurological problems with disinclination to move, convulsions, and death. Called also *infectious porcine polyarthritis* and *porcine polyserositis.*

**glycogen storage d.,** any of a number of rare inborn errors of metabolism caused by defects in specific enzymes or transporters involved in the metabolism of glycogen.

**type I,** glucose-6-phosphatase deficiency: a severe hepatorenal form of the disease in which deficiency of glucose-6-phosphatase, an autosomal recessive trait, causes hepatomegaly, hypoglycemia, hyperuricemia, hyperlacticacidemia, hyperlipidemia, xanthomas, bleeding, and adiposity; patients frequently survive to adulthood.

**type IA,** glycogen storage disease, type I.

**type IB,** glucose-6-phosphatase translocase deficiency: an autosomal recessive disorder caused by a defect in the transport system for glucose 6-phosphate. Symptoms resemble those of the type I disorder, but patients are additionally predisposed to infection related to neutropenia and to chronic inflammatory bowel disease.

**type II,** lysosomal α-1,4-glucosidase deficiency: an autosomal recessive disorder caused by deficiency of the lysosomal enzyme glucan 1,4-α-glucosidase, with accumulation of glycogen in tissues. In infants, it is characterized by mild hepatomegaly, mental and motor retardation, hypotonia, and cardiomegaly and cardiorespiratory failure resulting in death; the adult form is usually characterized primarily by a gradual skeletal myopathy that sometimes causes respiratory problems.

**type III,** amylo-1,6-glucosidase deficiency: an autosomal recessive disorder caused by a defect in the debranching enzyme in muscle, liver, or both; defects in the liver enzyme are characterized by hepatomegaly and hypoglycemia while defects in the muscle enzyme are characterized by progressive muscle wasting and weakness. Heart and skeletal muscle are also frequently affected. Called also *debrancher deficiency.*

**type IV,** brancher enzyme deficiency: an autosomal recessive disorder caused by a defect in the glycogen branching enzyme 1,4-α-glucan branching enzyme; the most severe abnormalities are in the liver, with hepatosplenomegaly, early cirrhosis with portal hypertension, liver failure, and death in childhood. Neuromuscular abnormalities are also present.

**type V,** muscle phosphorylase deficiency: an autosomal recessive disorder caused by a defect in the skeletal muscle isozyme of glycogen phosphorylase; it is characterized by muscle cramps and fatigue during exercise.

**type VI,** hepatic phosphorylase deficiency: an autosomal recessive disorder caused by deficiency of the liver isozyme of glycogen phosphorylase; it is characterized by hepatomegaly, mild to moderate hypoglycemia, and mild ketosis. Phosphorylase b kinase deficiency was previously included in this type by some authors.

**type VII,** muscle phosphofructokinase deficiency: an autosomal recessive disorder caused by deficiency of the muscle isozyme of 6-phosphofructokinase; it is characterized by muscle weakness and cramping after exercise. Activity of the erythrocyte isozyme is also decreased, causing increased hemolysis.

**type VIII,** phosphorylase b kinase deficiency.

**Goldflam's d., Goldflam-Erb d.,** myasthenia gravis.

**Goldstein's d.,** hereditary hemorrhagic telangiectasia.

**Gorham's d.,** disappearing bone d.

**graft-versus-host d.,** disease caused by the immune response of histoincompatible, immunocompetent donor cells against the tissues of immunoincompetent host, which can occur as a complication of bone marrow transplantation or as a result of maternal-fetal blood transfusion or therapeutic blood transfusion in which the recipient has a cellular immunodeficiency disease. Clinical manifestations include skin disease ranging from a maculopapular eruption to epidermal necrosis, intestinal disease marked by diarrhea, malabsorption, and abdominal pain, and liver dysfunction caused by cholestatic hepatitis or veno-occlusive disease and marked by serum enzyme abnormalities. Called also *graft-versus-host reaction.*

**grass d.,** 1. see under *sickness.* 2. dermatitis bullosa striata pratensis.

**Graves' d.,** a syndrome of diffuse hyperplasia of the thyroid, with a female predominance; it usually has an autoimmune etiology and has been linked to autoimmune thyroiditis. Characteristics include hyperthyroidism (q.v.), usually with goiter and ophthalmic symptoms (*Graves' orbitopathy*). Most patients have circulating thyroid-stimulating immunoglobulins that cause excessive secretion of thyroid hormones by binding to TSH receptors on thyroid cells. Called also *Basedow's, Flajani's, Parry's d,* and *diffuse toxic goiter.*

**greasy pig d.,** seborrhea of piglets caused by infection of *Staphylococcus hyicus* through a cut or abrasion of the skin. Called also *exudative epidermitis.*

**Greenfield's d.,** former name for the late infantile form of metachromatic leukodystrophy.

**green muscle d.,** deep pectoral myopathy.

**grinder's d.,** pneumoconiosis of grinders.

**Gross d.,** encysted rectum; saccular dilatation of anal wall with retained inspissated feces.

**guinea worm d.,** dracunculiasis.

**Guinon's d.,** Gilles de la Tourette's syndrome.

**Gull's d.,** atrophy of the thyroid with myxedema.

**Gumboro d.,** infectious bursal d.

**Günther's d.,** congenital erythropoietic porphyria.

**GVH d.,** graft-versus-host d.

**H d.,** Hartnup d.

**Habermann's d.,** acute lichenoid pityriasis.

**Haff d.,** rhabdomyolysis following consumption of fish of certain types, caused by an as yet unidentified toxin, originally seen among fishermen of the Königsberg (or Frisches) Haff, a lagoon off the Baltic Sea during the 1920s.

**Haglund's d.,** bursitis in the region of the Achilles tendon.

**Hagner's d.,** hypertrophic pulmonary osteoarthropathy.

**Hailey-Hailey d.,** benign familial pemphigus.

**hairy shaker d.,** border d. of sheep.

**Hallervorden-Spatz d.,** a hereditary disorder characterized by marked reduction in the number of myelin sheaths of the globus pallidus and substantia nigra, with accumulations of iron pigment, progressive rigidity beginning in the legs, choreoathetoid movements, dysarthria, and progressive mental deterioration. Transmitted as an autosomal recessive trait, it usually begins in the first or second decade, with death usually occurring before the thirtieth year. Called also *status dysmyelinatus,* and *status dysmyelinisatus.*

**Haltia-Santavuori d.,** a rare infantile form of neuronal ceroid-lipofuscinosis, beginning about one year of age, with excessive storage of lipofuscin, failure to thrive, myoclonic seizures, muscular hypotonia, psychomotor developmental delay and deterioration, blindness with optic atrophy and cerebellar ataxia, and death within about 5 years.

**Hamman's d.,** pneumomediastinum.

**Hammond's d.,** athetosis.

**Hand's d.,** Hand-Schüller-Christian d.

**hand-foot-and-mouth d.,** a usually mild and self-limited exanthematous eruption most often caused by coxsackievirus A16, primarily seen in preschool children, and characterized by vesicles on the buccal mucosa, tongue, soft palate, gingivae, and hands and feet, including the palms and soles. Called also *hand-foot-and-mouth syndrome.*

**Hand-Schüller-Christian d.,** a chronic, progressive form of multifocal Langerhans cell histiocytosis, sometimes with accumulation of cholesterol, characterized by the triad of calvarial bone defects, exophthalmos, and diabetes insipidus. Called also *chronic idiopathic xanthomatosis.*

**Hansen's d.,** leprosy.

**d. of the Hapsburgs,** old term for *hemophilia.*

**Harada's d.,** Vogt-Koyanagi-Harada syndrome.

**hard metal d.,** a pneumoconiosis caused by inhalation of fine particles of cobalt, usually in conjunction with tungsten carbide. In early stages reversible hyperplasia and metaplasia of the bronchial epithelium are seen; later, subacute alveolitis and then chronic interstitial fibrosis develop. Called also *tungsten carbide d.* and *cobalt lung.*

**hard pad d.,** canine distemper.

**hardware d.,** 1. traumatic pericarditis (def. 2). 2. traumatic reticuloperitonitis.

**Hartnup d.,** an inborn error of metabolism characterized by cerebellar ataxia, a pellagra-like condition of the skin, and massive aminoaciduria involving a group of neutral monoaminomonocarboxylic amino acids sharing a common renal reabsorption mechanism; patients respond well to prolonged oral administration of nicotinamide.

**Hashimoto's d.,** a progressive type of autoimmune thyroiditis with lymphocytic infiltration of the gland and circulating antithyroid antibodies; patients have goiter and gradually develop hypothyroidism. It has a familial predisposition, usually affects women, and sometimes precedes the onset of Graves' disease or is manifested after the major symptoms subside. Called also *Hashimoto's, chronic lymphadenoid,* or *chronic lymphocytic thyroiditis,* and *lymphadenoid goiter.*

**heart d.,** any organic, mechanical, or functional abnormality of the heart, its structures, or the coronary arteries.

**heavy chain d's,** a group of rare malignant neoplasms of lymphoplasmacytic cells that secrete an M component consisting of monoclonal immunoglobulin heavy chains or heavy chain fragments; they are classified according to heavy chain type. See also *alpha chain d., gamma chain d.,* and *mu chain d.*

**Heberden's d.,** 1. rheumatism of the smaller joints, accompanied by nodules in or about the distal interphalangeal joints. 2. angina pectoris.

**Hebra's d.,** erythema multiforme minus.

**Heckathorn's d.,** a rare variant of hemophilia A in which the levels of coagulation factor VIII fluctuate; inherited as an X-linked recessive trait.

**Heerfordt's d.,** see under *syndrome.*

**Heine-Medin d.,** the major illness of poliomyelitis; see *poliomyelitis.*

**Heller-Döhle d.,** syphilitic aortitis.

**hemagglutinating encephalomyelitis virus d. of pigs,** vomiting and wasting d.

**hemoglobin d.,** any of the heredity conditions caused by the presence of abnormal hemoglobins in the blood, such as sickle cell anemia or various types of hemolytic anemia and thalassemia.

**hemoglobin C d.,** the state of being homozygous for hemoglobin C, characterized by splenomegaly, mild to moderate hemolytic anemia, recurrent jaundice, and increased numbers of target cells and reticulocytes in the peripheral blood.

**hemoglobin C–thalassemia d.,** a hereditary disorder involving simultaneous heterozygosity for hemoglobin C and thalassemia, manifested by mild hemolytic anemia and persistent splenomegaly; called also *hemoglobin C–thalassemia.*

**hemoglobin D d.,** the state of being homozygous for hemoglobin D, characterized by mild hemolytic anemia with numerous target cells in the peripheral blood.

**hemoglobin E d.,** the state of being homozygous for hemoglobin E; many patients are asymptomatic, but others have mild hemolytic anemia, usually without splenomegaly, and increased numbers of normochromic target cells in the peripheral blood.

**hemoglobin E–thalassemia d.,** a hereditary condition involving simultaneous heterozygosity for hemoglobin E and thalassemia, manifested by mild hemolytic anemia and persistent splenomegaly; called also *hemoglobin E–thalassemia.*

**hemoglobin H d.,** $\alpha$-thalassemia in individuals heterozygous for hemoglobin H, characterized by chronic hemolytic anemia associated with splenomegaly; red blood cell hypochromia, anisocytosis, and poililocytosis are accompanied by inclusion bodies detectable by supravital staining.

**hemoglobin SC d.,** sickle cell–hemoglobin C d.

**hemoglobin SD d.,** sickle cell–hemoglobin D d.

**hemolytic d. of the newborn,** erythroblastosis fetalis.

**hemorrhagic d. of the newborn,** a self-limited hemorrhagic disorder of the first days of life, caused by a deficiency of the vitamin K–dependent blood coagulation factors II, VII, IX, and X.

**Henderson-Jones d.,** osteochondromatosis characterized by the presence of numerous cartilaginous foreign bodies in the joint cavity or in the bursa of a tendon sheath.

**hepatic veno-occlusive d.,** veno-occlusive d. of the liver.

**hepatolenticular d.,** Wilson's d.

**hepatorenal glycogen storage d.,** glycogen storage d., type I.

**hereditary d.,** one that is transmitted genetically from parents to children.

**heredodegenerative d.,** any disease of the central nervous system characterized by specific loss of neural tissue due to hereditary influence.

**Herlitz's d.,** junctional epidermolysis bullosa.

**Hers' d.,** glycogen storage d., type VI.

**Herter's d., Herter-Heubner d.,** the infantile form of celiac disease.

**Heubner's d.,** syphilitic endarteritis of the cerebral vessels; called also *Heubner's endarteritis.*

**Heubner-Herter d.,** the infantile form of celiac disease.

**hip-joint d.,** tuberculosis of the hip joint.

**Hippel's d.,** see *von Hippel's d.*

**Hippel-Lindau d.,** see *von Hippel-Lindau d.*

**Hirschsprung's d.,** congenital megacolon.

**His' d., His-Werner d.,** trench fever.

**hock d.,** perosis.

**Hodgkin's d.,** a form of malignant lymphoma characterized by painless, progressive enlargement of the lymph nodes, spleen, and general lymphoid tissue; other symptoms may include anorexia, lassitude, weight loss, fever, pruritus, night sweats, and anemia. The characteristic histologic feature is presence of Reed-Sternberg cells. It affects twice as many males as females and is usually considered to be neoplastic in origin, although neither an infectious origin nor an immune response to Reed-Sternberg cells has been excluded. Four types have been distinguished according to histopathologic criteria, three with diffuse patterns *(lymphocyte predominance type, mixed cellularity type,* and *lymphocyte depletion type)* and one with a nodular pattern *(nodular sclerosis type).* Called also *Reed-Hodgkin d.* and *Hodgkin's lymphoma.* See also *non-Hodgkin's lymphoma,* under *lymphoma.*

**Hodgkin's d., lymphocyte depletion type,** a type of Hodgkin's disease characterized by a low number of lymphocytes and an abundance of Reed-Sternberg cells with fibrosis; it is the most aggressive of the three diffuse types of Hodgkin's disease. Called also *Hodgkin's sarcoma.*

**Hodgkin's d., lymphocyte predominance type,** a type of Hodgkin's disease characterized by a diffuse to slightly nodular infiltrate with abundant mature lymphocytes and varying numbers of benign histiocytes; there are few Reed-Sternberg cells and the degree of malignancy is low. Most patients are males under age 35. Called also *paragranuloma.*

**Hodgkin's d., mixed cellularity type,** a type of Hodgkin's disease intermediate between the lymphocyte predominance and lymphocyte depletion types; Reed-Sternberg cells are plentiful and there are more inflammatory cells, such as eosinophils and plasma cells, than in the lymphocyte predominance type.

**Hodgkin's d., nodular sclerosis type,** a type of Hodgkin's disease in which Reed-Sternberg cells are in the form of lacunar cells and bands of collagen divide the lymphoid tissue into nodules; there are varying numbers of lymphocytes and inflammatory cells such as eosinophils and plasma cells. This type is most common in young women and often has a low grade of malignancy.

**Hodgson's d.,** an aneurysmal dilatation of the proximal part of the aorta, often accompanied by dilatation or hypertrophy of the heart.

**Hoffa's d.,** traumatic proliferation of fatty tissue (solitary lipoma) in the knee joint.

**holoendemic d.,** an endemic disease occurring at a high level in a population so that most of the children are affected, the adults in the same population then being less so. Cf. *hyperendemic d.*

**hoof-and-mouth d.,** foot-and-mouth d.

**hookworm d.,** 1. in humans, infection with hookworms of the genera *Ancylostoma* and *Necator,* usually *A. duodenale* or *N. americanus.* It occurs in most tropical and subtropical countries, and in temperate regions it may occur in mines and tunnels where the temperature and moisture are similar to that in the tropics. The larvae live in soil and gain entrance to the digestive tract indirectly by way of the skin of the feet or legs or directly with contaminated food or water. The percutaneous infection is followed by a transitory eruption known as *ground itch.* From here the parasites are carried by the blood to the lungs, ascend the trachea, are swallowed, and settle in the small intestine, where they attach to the mucosa and ingest blood. Symptoms, which vary with diet and with severity of infection, may include abdominal pain, diarrhea, and colic or nausea. Anemia is seen only in moderate to severe infections or when other adverse nutritional factors operate in conjunction with the parasite-induced blood loss. See also *ancylostomiasis* and *necatoriasis.* 2. in mammals other than humans, infestation of the intestines with hookworms. Dogs and cats are usually infested by *Ancylostoma* or *Uncinaria,* and cattle and sheep by *Bunostomum.* See also *ancylostomiasis, bunostomiasis,* and *uncinariasis.*

**Horton's d.,** 1. cluster headache. 2. giant cell arteritis.

**Huchard's d.,** continued arterial hypertension, thought to be a cause of arteriosclerosis.

**hunger d., hungry d.,** excessive hunger accompanied by weakness and nervousness caused by the hypoglycemia of hyperinsulinism.

**Hunt's d.,** 1. dyssynergia cerebellaris myoclonica. 2. Ramsay Hunt syndrome (def. 1).

**Huntington's d.,** see under *chorea.*

**Hurler's d.,** see under *syndrome.*

**Hurst d.,** acute necrotizing hemorrhagic encephalomyelitis.

**Hutchinson's d.,** 1. prurigo estivalis. 2. angioma serpiginosum. 3. Tay's choroiditis.

**Hutinel's d.,** tuberculous pericarditis with cirrhosis of the liver in children.

**hyaline membrane d.,** respiratory distress syndrome of the newborn.

**hydatid d.,** an infection, usually of the liver or lungs, caused by larval forms (hydatid cysts) of tapeworms of the genus *Echinococcus,* and characterized by the development of expanding cysts; it occurs in humans, cattle, sheep, pigs, horses, and occasionally other mammals. The two types are *alveolar* and *unilocular.* Called also *hydatidosis, echinococcus d.,* and *echinococcosis.*

**hydatid d., alveolar,** infection with larval forms (hydatid cysts) of *Echinococcus multilocularis,* characterized by invasion and destruction of tissues as the cysts undergo endogenous budding to form an aggregate of small cysts that honeycomb the affected organ (usually the liver); they may metastasize later.

**hydatid d., unilocular,** infection with the larval forms (hydatid cysts) of *Echinococcus granulosus,* characterized by the formation of unilocular single or multiple expanding cysts; as the cysts expand they may give rise to symptoms of space-occupying lesions in the tissues or organs affected.

**hydrocephaloid d.,** a condition similar to hydrocephalus, but marked by depression of the fontanels, due to diarrhea or some other wasting disease with dehydration.

**hyperendemic d.,** an endemic disease equally prevalent in all age groups of a population. Cf. *holoendemic d.*

**hypophosphatemic bone d.,** an autosomal dominant disorder clinically resembling a mild form of X-linked hypophosphatemia and similarly due to a defect in renal tubular function, but usually showing osteomalacia without radiographic evidence of rickets and responding to calcitriol without supplemental phosphate in at least some cases.

**hypopigmentation-immunodeficiency d.,** Griscelli syndrome.

**Iceland d.,** chronic fatigue syndrome.

**I-cell d.,** mucolipidosis II.

**idiopathic d.,** one not consequent upon any other disease, and of which the cause is unknown.

**immune complex d.,** any of a variety of local or systemic diseases caused by the formation of circulating antibody-antigen immune complexes and their deposition in tissue, due to activation of complement and to recruitment and activation of leukocytes; see also *type III hypersensitivity reaction,* under *hypersensitivity reaction* at *reaction.*

**immunoproliferative small intestine d.,** the gastrointestinal form of alpha chain disease, characterized by diarrhea, malabsorption, abdominal pain, clubbing, plasma cell infiltration of the lamina propria of the small bowel, and presence of an abnormal alpha heavy chain fragment in the serum; it frequently evolves into primary malignant lymphoma. Called also *Mediterranean lymphoma.*

**inborn lysosomal d.,** lysosomal storage d.

**inclusion d.,** any disease in which cell inclusions are found.

**infantile celiac d.,** see *celiac d.*

**infectious d.,** a disease caused by a pathogenic microorganism; the etiologic agent may be a bacterium, virus, fungus, or animal parasite, and may be transmitted from another host or arise from the host's own indigenous microflora. See also *infection.* Cf. *communicable d.* and *contagious d.*

**infectious bursal d.,** a highly contagious acute disease of chickens, caused by the infectious bursal disease virus, characterized by edema and swelling of the cloacal bursa, soiled wet feathers, whitish watery diarrhea, listlessness, and trembling, progressing to extreme kidney damage and damage of the bursa of Fabricius, with resulting immunosuppression that can be fatal. Called also *Gumboro d.* and *infectious avian nephrosis.*

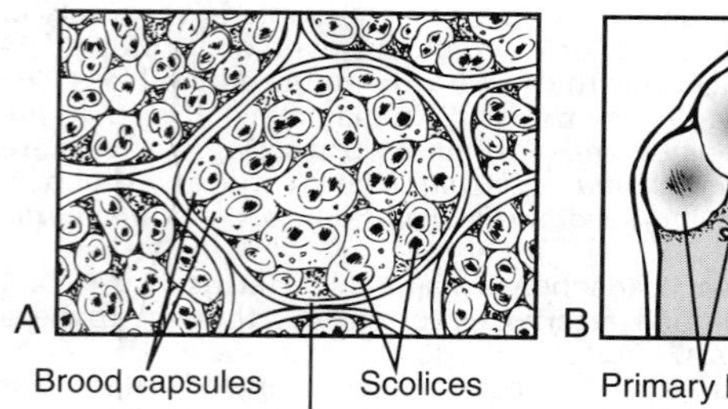
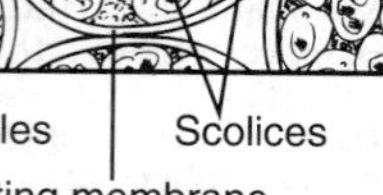
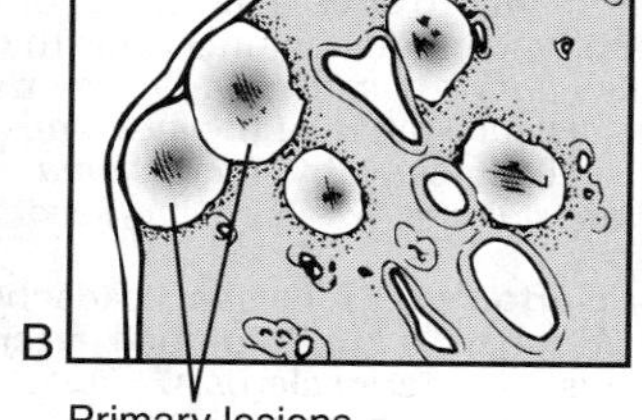


Alveolar hydatid disease. *(A),* Cross-section of cysts in the liver of a vole, a normal host. In humans, brood capsules and scolices are rarely present. *(B),* Sections of a human liver, showing primary lesions with central necrosis.

**inflammatory bowel d.,** a general term for those inflammatory diseases of the bowel of unknown etiology, including Crohn's disease and ulcerative colitis.

**inherited d.,** one transmitted genetically, from parents to offspring.

**intercurrent d.,** a disease occurring during the course of another disease with which it has no connection.

**interstitial d.,** one in which the stroma of an organ is mainly affected.

**interstitial lung d.,** a heterogeneous group of noninfectious, nonmalignant disorders of the lower respiratory tract, affecting primarily the alveolar wall structures but also often involving the small airways and blood vessels of the lung parenchyma; slowly progressive loss of alveolar-capillary units may lead to respiratory insufficiency and death.

**iron storage d.,** hemochromatosis.

**ischemic bowel d.,** ischemic colitis.

**ischemic heart d. (IHD),** any of a group of acute or chronic cardiac disabilities resulting from insufficient supply of oxygenated blood to the heart; it may be due to increased oxygen demand, to diminished blood oxygen transport, or most commonly to reduction in coronary blood flow because of arterial narrowing or obstruction such as that caused by atherosclerosis. It may manifest as angina pectoris, myocardial infarction, ventricular fibrillation, or sudden cardiac death.

**island d.,** scrub typhus.

**Isle of Wight d.,** paralysis of muscles of flight in honeybees due to tracheal infestation by the mite *Acarapis woodi.*

**Jaffe-Lichtenstein d.,** a form of polyostotic fibrous dysplasia characterized by an enlarged medullary cavity with a thin cortex, which is filled with fibrous tissue (fibroma). Called also *cystic osteofibromatosis.*

**Jakob's d., Jakob-Creutzfeldt d.,** Creutzfeldt-Jakob d.

**Jansen's d.,** metaphyseal dysostosis.

**Janský-Bielschowsky d.,** the late infantile form of neuronal ceroid-lipofuscinosis, occurring between two to four years of age and characterized by abnormal accumulation of lipofuscin; it begins as myoclonic seizures and progresses to neurologic and retinal degeneration and death, usually by the age of 8 to 12 years.

**Jensen's d.,** retinochoroiditis juxtapapillaris.

**Johne's d.,** a usually fatal form of chronic enteritis due to *Mycobacterium paratuberculosis,* affecting chiefly cattle but also sheep, goats, and deer. It remotely resembles a tuberculous infection, and is marked by intermittent or persistent diarrhea, progressive emaciation, anemia, and extreme weakness. Called also *chronic dysentery of cattle* and *paratuberculosis.*

**Johnson-Stevens d.,** see *Stevens-Johnson syndrome.*

**Joseph d.,** Azorean d.

**jumping d.,** any of several culture-specific disorders characterized by exaggerated responses to small stimuli, muscle tics including jumping, automatic obedience even to dangerous suggestions, and sometimes coprolalia or echolalia. It is unclear whether they are neurogenic or psychogenic in origin. See also *latah, myriachit, jumping Frenchmen of Maine syndrome,* and *Gilles de la Tourette's syndrome.*

**Kaiserstuhl d.,** a form of chronic arsenic poisoning that occurred prior to World War II among German workers in vineyards, due to arsenic-containing insecticides used on the grapes.

**Kashin-Bek (Kaschin-Beck) d.,** a slowly progressive, chronic, disabling, degenerative disease of the peripheral joints and spine, which principally occurs in children and is endemic in eastern Siberia, northern China, and Korea. It is believed to be caused by the ingestion of cereal grains infected with *Fusarium sporotrichiella.* Called also *osteoarthritis deformans endemica.*

**Katayama d.,** see under *fever.*

**Kawasaki d.,** mucocutaneous lymph node syndrome.

**Keshan d.,** a fatal, congestive cardiomyopathy caused by deficiency of essential trace elements in the diet; it primarily affects children and women of childbearing age, and occurs in areas with low soil trace elements, such as parts of China, New Zealand, and Finland.

**Kienböck's d.,** slowly progressive osteochondrosis of the semilunar (carpal lunate) bone; it may affect other bones of the wrist. Called also *lunatomalacia.*

**Kikuchi's d., Kikuchi-Fujimoto d.,** see under *lymphadenitis.*

**Kimberley horse d.,** crotalism.

**Kimura's d.,** a disease of the skin considered by some authorities to be synonymous with angiolymphoid hyperplasia with eosinophilia (q.v.) but differentiated by others on the basis of differences in the nature of the proliferating vascular cells.

**kinky hair d.,** Menkes' syndrome.

**Kinnier Wilson d.,** Wilson's d.

**kissing d.,** popular term for infectious mononucleosis.

**Klebs' d.,** glomerulonephritis.

**knight's d.,** infection of the perianal region following a minute abrasion of the skin, so called historically because of the frequency of its occurrence in horsemen.

**Köhler's bone d.,** 1. osteochondrosis of the tarsal navicular bone in children; called also *tarsal scaphoiditis, epiphysitis juvenilis, osteoarthrosis juvenilis,* and *os naviculare pedis retardatum.* 2. a disease of the second metatarsal bone, with thickening of its shaft and changes about its articular head, characterized by pain in the second metatarsophalangeal joint on walking or standing. Called also *Köhler's second d.,* and *juvenile deforming metatarsophalangeal osteochondritis.* See also *osteochondrosis.*

**Köhler's second d.,** Köhler's bone d. (def. 2).

**Köhler-Pellegrini-Stieda d.,** Pellegrini's d.

**Koshevnikoff's (Koschewnikow's, Kozhevnikov's) d.,** epilepsia partialis continua.

**Krabbe's d.,** a lysosomal storage disease due to a deficiency of galactosylceramidase. It begins in infancy with irritability, fretfulness, and rigidity, followed by tonic seizures, convulsions, quadriplegia, blindness, deafness, dysphagia, and progressive mental deterioration. Pathologically, there is rapidly progressive cerebral demyelination and large globoid bodies in the white substance. Called also *galactosylceramide lipidosis* and *globoid cell* or *Krabbe's leukodystrophy.*

**Krishaber's d.,** a syndrome characterized by tachycardia, insomnia, lightheadedness or vertigo, hyperesthesia, and a feeling of emptiness in the head; called also *cerebrocardiac syndrome.*

**Kufs' d.,** the adult form of neuronal ceroid-lipofuscinosis, beginning usually before the age of 40 and characterized by progressive neurologic degeneration, excessive storage of lipofuscin in the central nervous system, and shortened life expectancy. Unlike other forms of neuronal ceroid lipofuscinosis, it does not cause blindness.

**Kuhnt-Junius d.,** disciform macular degeneration.

**Kümmell's d., Kümmell-Verneuil d.,** compression fracture of vertebra; a complex of symptoms coming on in a few weeks after spinal injury, and consisting of pain in the spine, intercostal neuralgia, motor disturbances of the legs, and a gibbus of the spine which is painful on pressure and easily reduced by extension. Called also *post-traumatic spondylitis.*

**Kussmaul's d., Kussmaul-Maier d.,** polyarteritis nodosa.

**Kyasanur Forest d.,** a severe hemorrhagic fever marked by fever, hemorrhagic manifestations, and rash, occurring in the Mysore State of India, caused by a flavivirus and transmitted to humans from monkey and vole reservoirs by ticks of the genus *Haemaphysalis,* especially *H. spinigera.*

**Kyrle's d.,** a rare chronic disorder of keratinization characterized by a papular eruption with hyperkeratotic cone-shaped plugs in the hair follicles and eccrine ducts, which project through the epidermis into the dermis, producing a foreign body giant cell reaction and pain. The usually discrete lesions leave a depression on removal; they may coalesce to form patches, and coalescing plaques are often seen. Called also *hyperkeratosis penetrans.*

**Laënnec's d.,** see under *cirrhosis.*

**Lafora's d.,** Lafora's myoclonic epilepsy.

**Lancereaux-Mathieu d.,** Weil's syndrome.

**Landouzy's d.,** Weil's syndrome.

**Lane's d.,** chronic intestinal stasis; small bowel obstruction in chronic constipation.

**Larsen's d., Larsen-Johansson d.,** pain and tenderness over the lower pole of the patella, often accompanied by inflammation, with radiographic evidence of a secondary ossification center in the lower pole of the patella.

**Lauber's d.,** fundus albipunctatus.

**laughing d.,** kuru.

**Leber's d.,** 1. Leber's hereditary optic neuropathy. 2. Leber's congenital amaurosis.

**Legg's d., Legg-Calvé d.,** osteochondrosis of the capitular epiphysis of the femur.

**Legg-Calvé-Perthes d., Legg-Calvé-Waldenström d.,** Legg's d.

**legionnaires' d.,** a bacterial disease caused by infection with *Legionella pneumophila,* and not spread by person-to-person contact; it is characterized by pneumonia, high fever, gastrointestinal pain, headache, and sometimes involvement of the kidneys, liver, or nervous system.

**Leigh d.,** subacute necrotizing encephalomyelopathy.

**Leiner's d.,** a disorder of infancy characterized principally by generalized seborrheic-like dermatitis and erythroderma, intractable, severe diarrhea, recurrent infections, and failure to thrive. The cause is unclear, but familial cases associated with a dysfunction of the C5 component of complement, which results in decreased phagocytosis of the patient's serum (opsonic activity), have been reported. Called also *erythroderma desquamativum.*

**Lenègre's d.,** acquired complete heart block due to primary degeneration of the conduction system.

**Leriche's d.,** post-traumatic osteoporosis.

**Letterer-Siwe d.,** a Langerhans cell histiocytosis of early childhood, of autosomal recessive inheritance, characterized by cutaneous lesions resembling seborrheic dermatitis, hemorrhagic tendency, hepatosplenomegaly with lymph node enlargement, and progressive anemia. If untreated it is rapidly fatal. Called also *L-S d.* and *acute disseminated Langerhans cell histiocytosis.*

**Lev's d.,** acquired complete heart block due to sclerosis of the cardiac skeleton.

**Lewandowsky-Lutz d.,** epidermodysplasia verruciformis.

**Leyden's d.,** a form of periodic vomiting.

**Libman-Sacks d.,** see under *endocarditis.*

**Lichtheim's d.,** subacute combined degeneration of the spinal cord; see under *degeneration.*

**Lindau's d., Lindau-von Hippel d.,** von Hippel-Lindau d.

**lipid storage d.,** lipidosis.

**Lipschütz's d.,** ulcus vulvae acutum.

**Little's d.,** congenital spastic stiffness of the limbs, a form of cerebral palsy dating from birth and due to lack of development of the pyramidal tracts; it may be associated with various disorders, including birth trauma, fetal anoxia, or illness of the mother during pregnancy. Clinically, it is characterized by muscular weakness, walking difficulties, and, usually, by convulsions, bilateral athetosis, and mental deficiency. Called also *spastic diplegia.*

**Lobo's d.,** keloidal blastomycosis.

**Lobstein's d.,** osteogenesis imperfecta, type I.

**local d.,** a condition which originates in and remains confined to one part of the body.

**loco d., locoweed d.,** locoism.

**Lorain's d.,** hypophysial infantilism.

**Lou Gehrig d.,** amyotrophic lateral sclerosis.

**Lowe's d.,** oculocerebrorenal syndrome.

**L-S d.,** Letterer-Siwe d.

**Luft's d.,** a hypermetabolic disorder of striated muscle caused by an abnormal quantity and type of mitochondria producing excessive cellular respiration; it is characterized by profuse perspiration, asthenia, progressive weakness, and an abnormally increased basal metabolic rate.

**lumpy skin d.,** a highly infectious poxvirus disease indigenous to African cattle, which may result in permanent sterility or death, marked by the formation of nodules in the skin and sometimes in the mucous membranes. It resembles dermopathic herpesvirus disease (q.v.).

**lung fluke d.,** paragonimiasis.

**lunger d.,** 1. pulmonary adenomatosis (def. 2). 2. fog fever.

**Lutz-Splendore-Almeida d.,** paracoccidioidomycosis.

**Lyell's d.,** toxic epidermal necrolysis.

**Lyme d.,** a recurrent, multisystemic disorder caused by *Borrelia burgdorferi,* having the ticks *Ixodes scapularis* and *I. pacificus* as vectors. It begins in most cases with erythema chronicum migrans (at least 5 cm in diameter), followed by a variety of highly variable manifestations, including myalgia, arthritis of the large joints, and involvement of the nervous and cardiovascular systems.

**lymphocystic d. of fish, lymphocystis d.,** lymphocystis.

**lymphoproliferative d's,** see under *disorder.*

**lymphoreticular d's,** see under *disorder.*

**lysosomal storage d.,** any inborn error of metabolism having four characteristics: (1) a defect in a specific lysosomal hydrolase; (2) intracellular accumulation of the unmetabolized substrate; (3) clinical progression affecting multiple tissues and organs; (4) considerable phenotypic variation within a disease. All but two of the lysosomal storage disorders are of autosomal recessive inheritance. The term comprises the *mucolipidoses, mucopolysaccharidoses, disorders of glycoprotein degradation, lipase deficiencies, ceramidase deficiency (Farber's disease), α-galactosidase A deficiency (Fabry's disease), lipidoses,* and *gangliosidoses.* Called also *lysosomal enzymopathy* and *inborn lysosomal d.* See also *inborn errors of metabolism,* under *metabolism.*

**MAC d.,** Mycobacterium avium complex d.

**McArdle's d.,** glycogen storage d., type V.

**Machado-Joseph d.,** Azorean d.

**MacLean-Maxwell d.,** a chronic condition of the calcaneus marked by enlargement of its posterior third and attended by pain on pressure.

**Madelung's d.,** 1. see under *deformity.* 2. see under *neck.*

**Majocchi's d.,** purpura annularis telangiectodes.

**Malassez's d.,** cyst of the testis.

**Malibu d.,** surfers' nodules.

**Manchester wasting d.,** enzootic calcinosis.

**Manson's d.,** see under *schistosomiasis.*

**maple bark d., maple bark stripper's d.,** a type of hypersensitivity pneumonitis affecting logging and sawmill workers, caused by inhalation of the spores of the mold *Cryptostroma corticale,* which grows under the bark of maple logs.

**maple syrup urine d. (MSUD),** an autosomal recessive aminoacidopathy due to a defect in the second step in branched-chain amino acid (BCAA) catabolism; the decarboxylation of the corresponding α-keto acids by the branched-chain α-keto acid dehydrogenase complex. BCAAs and their keto acid analogues accumulate in blood and urine, causing severe ketoacidosis, seizures, coma, physical and mental retardation, and a characteristic smell of maple syrup in the urine and on the body. The disease can be divided into four clinical phenotypes: *classic,* the most severe, with neonatal onset and usually rapid death; *intermediate,* of lessened severity and usually later onset; *intermittent,* with normal periods punctuated by periods of ataxia and ketoacidosis; and *thiamine-responsive,* caused by decreased affinity of the dehydrogenase complex for the cofactor thiamine pyrophosphate. In at least some cases, MSUD is due to deficiency of one of the enzymes of the branched-chain α-keto acid dehydrogenase complex (see under *complex*). See also *lipoamide dehydrogenase deficiency.* Called also *branched-chain ketoaciduria.*

**marble bone d.,** osteopetrosis.

**Marburg d., Marburg virus d.,** an acute, often fatal hemorrhagic fever caused by the Marburg virus (family Filoviridae); characterized by fever, prostration, hemorrhagic manifestations, pancreatitis, and hepatitis. The first reported primary cases were in Marburg and Frankfurt, Germany, and Belgrade, Yugoslavia, in laboratory workers handling infected African green monkeys or their organs; secondary infection is acquired through direct physical contact with infected patients. It has been reported as occurring in Kenya, Zimbabwe, and South Africa.

**Marchiafava-Bignami d.,** progressive degeneration of the corpus callosum characterized by progressive intellectual deterioration, emotional disturbances, confusion, hallucinations, tremor, rigidity, and convulsions. It is a very rare disorder affecting chiefly middle-aged male alcoholics; also seen in patients with nutritional deficiency states.

**Marek's d.,** a lymphoproliferative disease of chickens, formerly included in the avian leukosis complex but now known to be caused by gallid herpesvirus 2. Lymphoid cell infiltrations are most common in the peripheral nerves and gonads, but widespread infiltrations may also be found in visceral organs, skin, muscle, and the iris; there is also frequently perivascular cuffing of blood vessels in the central nervous system. The location of the lesions dictates the clinical signs, such as paralysis, general depression, or blindness. When neurological symptoms predominate, it may be called *fowl* or *range paralysis, neural lymphomatosis,* or *neurolymphomatosis gallinarum.* When ocular or skin symptoms predominate, it may be called respectively *ocular lymphomatosis* and *skin leukosis.*

**margarine d.,** name given to an outbreak of erythema multiforme in Germany and Holland that was due to an emulsifier in margarine.

**Marie-Bamberger d.,** hypertrophic pulmonary osteoarthropathy.

**Marie-Strümpell d.,** ankylosing spondylitis.

**Marie-Tooth d.,** Charcot-Marie-Tooth d.

**Marion's d.,** congenital obstruction of the posterior urethra due to muscular hypertrophy of the bladder neck or absence of the plexiform dilator fibers in the urinary tract.

**Marsh's d.,** Graves' d.

**Medin's d.,** the major illness of poliomyelitis; see *poliomyelitis.*

**Mediterranean d.,** thalassemia major.

**medullary cystic d., medullary cystic kidney d.,** familial juvenile nephronophthisis.

**Meige's d.,** Milroy's d.

**Meleda d.,** mal de Meleda.

**Ménétrier's d.,** giant hypertrophic gastritis.

**Meniere's d.,** hearing loss, tinnitus, and vertigo resulting from nonsuppurative disease of the labyrinth with edema. Called also *endolymphatic hydrops, labyrinthine hydrops,* and *recurrent aural vertigo.*

**mental d.,** see under *disorder.*

**Merzbacher-Pelizaeus d.,** Pelizaeus-Merzbacher d.

**metabolic d.,** general term for diseases caused by disruption of a normal metabolic pathway because of a genetically determined enzyme defect.

**metazoan d.,** a disease caused by metazoan parasites, such as nematodes, cestodes, trematodes, and arthropods.

**Meyer's d.,** adenoid vegetations of the pharynx.

**Meyer-Betz d.,** a rare familial disease of unknown etiology, marked by attacks of myoglobinuria, which may be precipitated by strenuous exertion or possibly by an infection, and which results in tenderness, swelling, and weakness of muscles of varying intensity. It may occur with or without diffuse chronic myopathy or dystrophy. Called also *idiopathic,* or *familial myoglobinuria.*

**microdrepanocytic d.,** sickle cell–thalassemia d.

**Mikulicz's d.,** 1. a chronic, benign, usually painless inflammatory swelling of the lacrimal and salivary glands. See *benign lymphoepithelial lesion,* under *lesion.* 2. see under *syndrome.*

**Miller's d.,** osteomalacia.

**miller's d.,** nutritional secondary hyperparathyroidism.

**Milroy's d.,** congenital hereditary lymphedema of the legs caused by chronic lymphatic obstruction; other areas, including the arms, trunk, and face may be involved. Called also *Meige's d., Milroy's edema, Nonne-Milroy-Meige syndrome,* and *congenital lymphedema.*

**Milton's d.,** angioedema.

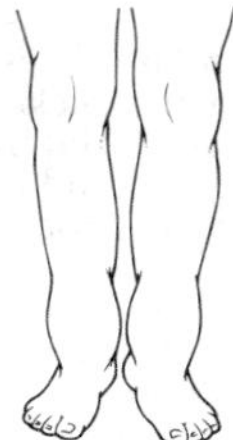

Lymphedema of the ankles in Milroy's disease.

**Minamata d.,** a severe neurologic disorder usually characterized by peripheral and circumoral paresthesia, ataxia, dysarthria, and loss of peripheral vision, and leading to severe permanent neurologic and mental disabilities or death; it is caused by alkyl mercury poisoning and was prevalent between 1953 and 1958 among those who ate seafood from a bay in Japan that was polluted with alkyl mercury compounds.

**minimal change d.,** subtle alterations in kidney function demonstrable by clinical albuminuria and the presence of lipid droplets in cells of the proximal tubules; abnormalities of foot processes of the glomerular epithelial cells are present but too subtle to be seen with light microscopy. It is seen primarily in children under 6 but sometimes in adults with the nephrotic syndrome, and may or may not progress to glomerulosclerosis or glomerulonephritis. Called also *foot process d., nil d., minimal change glomerulopathy* or *nephropathy,* and *lipid nephrosis.*

**Minor's d.,** hematomyelia involving the central parts of the spinal cord.

**Mitchell's d.,** erythromelalgia.

**mixed connective tissue d.,** a disorder combining features of scleroderma, myositis, systemic lupus erythematosus, and rheumatoid arthritis, and marked serologically by the presence of antibody against extractable nuclear antigen. Cf. *overlap syndrome.*

**Möbius' d.,** ophthalmoplegic migraine.

**Moeller-Barlow d.,** subperiosteal hematoma in rickets.

**molecular d.,** any disease in which the pathogenesis can be traced to a single molecule, usually a protein, which is either abnormal in structure or present in reduced amounts; the classical example is abnormal hemoglobin in sickle cell anemia.

**Monday morning d.,** azoturia (def. 2).

**Mondor's d.,** phlebitis affecting the large subcutaneous veins normally crossing the lateral chest region and breast from the epigastric or hypochondriac region to the axilla. Called also *sclerosing periphlebitis.*

**Monge's d.,** chronic mountain sickness.

**monoclonal immunoglobulin deposition d.,** light chain nephropathy.

**Morquio's d., Morquio-Ullrich d.,** see under *syndrome.*

**Morton's d.,** see under *neuralgia.*

**Moschcowitz's d.,** thrombotic thrombocytopenic purpura.

**motor neuron d.,** any disease of a motor neuron, including spinal muscular atrophy, progressive bulbar paralysis, amyotrophic lateral sclerosis, and lateral sclerosis.

**motor system d.,** motor neuron d.

**mountain d.,** see under *sickness.*

**moyamoya d.** [Jap. *moyamoya* foggy or smoky, from the angiographic appearance], cerebral ischemia due to occlusion of large arteries at the circle of Willis, with secondary proliferation of an abnormal network of vessels at the base of the brain, causing progressive neurologic disability; hemorrhage may occur from the dilated vessels.

**Mozer's d.,** myelosclerosis in adults.

**Mucha's d., Mucha-Habermann d.,** acute lichenoid pityriasis.

**mu chain d.,** the rarest heavy chain disease, found in patients with chronic lymphocytic leukemia, with symptoms of hepatomegaly and splenomegaly.

**mucosal d.,** bovine virus diarrhea.

**mulberry heart d.,** a form of vitamin E–selenium deficiency syndrome (q.v.) in pigs, characterized by subepicardial hemorrhaging, myocardial necrosis, and often death.

**mule-spinners' d.,** warts or ulcers of the skin, especially of the scrotum, which tend to become malignant (see *mule-spinners' cancer,* under *cancer*); so called because they were found chiefly among the operators of spinning mules in cotton mills.

**Münchmeyer's d.,** a diffuse progressive ossifying polymyositis.

**Murray Valley d.,** see under *encephalitis.*

**mushroom picker's d., mushroom worker's d.,** hypersensitivity pneumonitis in persons working with moldy compost prepared for growing mushrooms in closed areas, especially in those handling the dried material after harvesting, usually due to inhalation of spores of *Micropolyspora faeni.*

**mushy chick d.,** omphalitis of birds; see under *omphalitis.*

***Mycobacterium avium* complex d.,** systemic disease caused by infection with organisms of the *Mycobacterium avium-intracellulare* complex in patients with human immunodeficiency virus infection. Manifestations include bacteremia, fever, chills, fatigue, night sweats, weight loss, abdominal pain, anemia, and elevated alkaline phosphatase. Called also *MAC d.*

**myeloproliferative d's,** see under *disorder.*

**mystery pig d.,** porcine epidemic abortion and respiratory syndrome.

**Nairobi sheep d.,** an infectious disease of sheep and goats in East Africa, marked by acute hemorrhagic gastroenteritis, green, watery diarrhea, mucopurulent nasal discharge, and breathing difficulty; it is caused by a bunyavirus transmitted by the ticks *Rhipicephalus appendiculatus* and *Amblyomma variegatum.*

**nanukayami d.,** nanukayami.

**navicular d.,** necrotic inflammation of the navicular bone in horses, causing intermittent lameness. Called also *podotrochlitis* and *podotrochlosis.*

**Newcastle d.,** an influenzalike, often fatal, disease of birds, including domestic fowl, caused by a paramyxovirus; seen in several different forms, characterized variously by pneumonia and other respiratory symptoms, gastrointestinal symptoms, and encephalitic symptoms. It is transmissible to humans by contact with infected birds. Called also *avian influenza* and *avian pneumoencephalitis.*

**new duck d.,** infectious avian serositis in ducklings.

**Nicolas-Favre d.,** lymphogranuloma venereum.

**Niemann's d., Niemann-Pick d.,** a lysosomal storage disease due to a deficiency of sphingomyelin phosphodiesterase with sphingomyelin accumulation in the reticuloendothelial system. There are five types distinguished by age of onset and by the amount of CNS involvement and of sphingomyelin phosphodiesterase activity. *Type A* (acute neuronopathic) in the classic type, accounting for 85 per cent of the patients: onset is in early infancy; CNS damage is severe; death occurs by 4 years. *Type B* (chronic non-neuronopathic) has onset in early infancy but does not affect the CNS or intelligence; normal life-span is possible. *Type C* (chronic neuronopathic) has variable ages of onset (at 2 years or older) and of death (from age 5 to adulthood) and variable CNS involvement. *Type D* (the Nova Scotia variant) resembles type C; *type E* (the adult, non-neuronopathic form) may be a late-onset variant of type C. Called also *sphingolipidosis, sphingomyelin lipidosis,* and *sphingomyelinase deficiency.*

**nil d.,** minimal change d.

**nodular worm d., nodule d.,** a disease of sheep, cattle, and pigs caused by intestinal infestation with species of *Oesophagostomum,* the nodular worm, which infest the intestines and become embedded in the mucous membrane, causing the formation of nodules of varying size.

**Nonne-Milroy d.,** Milroy's d.

**Norrie's d.,** a congenital, X-linked disorder consisting of bilateral blindness from retinal detachment, hypoplasia, or dysplasia; and sometimes mental retardation and deafness developing later. Called also *atrophia bulborum hereditaria.*

**Norum-Gjone d.,** lecithin–cholesterol acyltransferase deficiency.

**nosema d.,** a protozoal infection of bees caused by *Nosema apis,* characterized by dysentery and paralysis. Cf. *pébrine.*

**notifiable d.,** one required to be reported to federal, state, or local health officials when diagnosed, because of infectiousness, severity, or frequency of occurrence; called also *reportable d.*

**Novy's rat d.,** a viral disease discovered by Novy in his stock of experimental rats.

**oasthouse urine d.,** methionine malabsorption syndrome.

**obstructive small airways d.,** chronic bronchitis with irreversible narrowing of the bronchioles and small bronchi with hypoxia and often hypercapnia.

**occupational d.,** one due to factors involved in one's employment, e.g., various forms of pneumoconiosis or dermatitis.

**Oguchi's d.,** a form of congenital night blindness and fundus discoloration following light adaptation.

**Ohara's d.,** in Japan, tularemia.

**oid-oid d.** [from disc*oid* and lichen*oid*], exudative discoid and lichenoid dermatitis.

**Ollier's d.,** enchondromatosis, particularly when involvement is unilateral.

**Ondiri d.,** bovine infectious petechial fever.

**Opitz's d.,** enlargement of the spleen due to thrombosis of the splenic vein; called also *thrombophlebitic splenomegaly.*

**organic d.,** one associated with demonstrable change in a bodily organ or tissue.

**Oriental lung fluke d.,** parasitic hemoptysis.

**Ormond's d.,** retroperitoneal fibrosis.

**Osgood-Schlatter d.,** osteochondrosis of the tuberosity of the tibia; called also *apophysitis tibialis adolescentium, Schlatter's d.,* and *Schlatter-Osgood d.* See also *osteochondrosis.*

**Osler's d.,** 1. polycythemia vera. 2. hereditary hemorrhagic telangiectasia.

**Osler-Vaquez d.,** polycythemia vera.

**Osler-Weber-Rendu d.,** hereditary hemorrhagic telangiectasia.

**Otto's d.,** arthrokatadysis.

**overeating d.,** pulpy kidney d.

**Owren's d.,** parahemophilia.

**ox-warble d.,** larva migrans.

**Paas's d.,** a familial disorder marked by skeletal deformities such as coxa valga, shortening of phalanges, scoliosis, spondylitis, etc.

**Pacheco's d.,** a highly fatal contagious disease of parrots caused by a herpesvirus; characteristics include hepatomegaly and diarrhea. Pigeons can get an almost identical disease, caused by a different herpesvirus.

**Paget's d.,** 1. intraductal carcinoma of the breast extending to involve the nipple and areola, characterized clinically by eczema-like inflammatory skin changes, and histologically by infiltration of the epidermis by malignant cells *(Paget's cells).* 2. a neoplasm of the vulva and sometimes the perianal region histologically and clinically quite similar to Paget's disease of the breast, but having less of a tendency to be associated with underlying invasive carcinoma. Called also *extramammary* or *vulvar Paget's d.* 3. osteitis deformans.

**Paget's d., extramammary,** Paget's d. (def. 2).

**Paget d., juvenile,** hyperostosis corticalis deformans juvenilis.

**Paget's d., vulvar,** Paget's d. (def. 2).

**Paget's d. of bone,** osteitis deformans.

**Panner's d.,** osteochondrosis of the capitellum of the humerus.

**parenchymatous d.,** one which attacks the parenchyma of an organ.

**Parkinson's d.,** paralysis agitans.

**Parrot's d.,** see under *pseudoparalysis.*

**parrot d.,** psittacosis.

**Parry's d.,** 1. Graves' d. 2. toxic multinodular goiter.

**Patella's d.,** pyloric stenosis in tuberculous patients following fibrous stenosis.

**Payr's d.,** constipation with left upper quadrant pain attributed to kinking of an adhesion between the transverse and descending colon with obstruction; probably a manifestation of the irritable colon syndrome rather than an organic lesion. Called also *splenic flexure syndrome.*

**pearl d.,** bovine tuberculosis of the peritoneum and mesentery in which the tubercles are calcified and pearllike.

**pearl-worker's d.,** recurrent inflammation of bone with hypertrophy, seen in persons who work in pearl dust.

**peduncle d.,** coldwater d.

**Pel-Ebstein d.,** see under *fever.*

**Pelizaeus-Merzbacher d.,** an X-linked leukoencephalopathy, occurring in early life and running a slowly progressive course into adolescence or adulthood. It is marked by nystagmus, ataxia, tremor, choreoathetoid movements, parkinsonian facies, dysarthria, and mental deterioration. Pathologically, there is diffuse demyelination in the white substance of the brain, which may involve the brain stem, cerebellum, and spinal cord. The cause is mutation of the gene on the long arm of the X chromosome that codes for proteolipid protein. Called also *Merzbacher-Pelizaeus d., familial centrolobar sclerosis,* and *Pelizaeus-Merzbacher sclerosis.*

**Pellegrini's d., Pellegrini-Stieda d.,** a condition characterized by a semilunar bony formation in the upper portion of the medial collateral ligament of the knee, due to traumatism; called also *Köhler-Pellegrini-Stieda d.* and *Stieda's d.*

**pelvic inflammatory d. (PID),** any pelvic infection involving the upper female genital tract beyond the cervix.

**periodic d.,** a condition characterized by regularly recurring and intermittent episodes of fever, edema, arthralgia, or gastric pain and vomiting, continuing for years without further development in otherwise healthy individuals.

**periodontal d.,** any of a group of pathological conditions that affect the surrounding and supporting tissues of the teeth, generally classified as inflammatory (gingivitis and periodontitis), dystrophic (periodontal trauma and periodontosis), and anomalies. Called also *dentoalveolitis.*

**Perrin-Ferraton d.,** snapping hip.

**Perthes' d.,** osteochondrosis of the capital femoral epiphysis; see *osteochondrosis.*

**Peyronie's d.,** induration of the corpora cavernosa of the penis, producing a fibrous chordee; called also *fibrous cavernitis, penis plastica,* and *penile induration.*

**Pfeiffer's d.,** infectious mononucleosis.

**Phocas' d.,** chronic glandular mastitis with the formation of numerous small nodules.

**phytanic acid storage d.,** 1. Refsum's d. 2. any of several disorders characterized by abnormal accumulation of phytanic acid in tissues.

**Pick's d.,** 1. [Arnold Pick] a rare progressive degenerative disease of the brain very similar in clinical manifestations and course to Alzheimer's disease but having a distinctive histopathology; cortical atrophy is confined to the frontal and temporal lobes; degenerating neurons contain globular intracytoplasmic filamentous inclusions (Pick bodies). Called also *circumscribed cerebral atrophy.* 2. [Ludwig Pick] Niemann-Pick d.

**Pictou d.,** a type of seneciosis in horses and cattle in Nova Scotia

**pink d.,** acrodynia.

**plaster-of-Paris d.,** atrophy of a limb which has been enclosed in a plaster-of-Paris splint.

**Plummer's d.,** toxic multinodular goiter.

**pneumatic hammer d.,** vibration d.

**policeman's d.,** tarsalgia.

**polycystic kidney d., polycystic d. of kidneys,** a heritable disorder marked by cysts scattered throughout both kidneys. It occurs in two unrelated forms: The *autosomal recessive* type (formerly called the *infantile* form) may be congenital or appear at any time during childhood. There is a high perinatal mortality rate, and almost all cases lead to hypertension. In older children cystic and fibrotic disease of the liver may be associated. The *autosomal dominant* type (formerly called the *adult* form) is marked by progressive deterioration of renal function. A similar acquired disease sometimes accompanies end-stage renal disease and is called *acquired cystic disease of kidney.* Called also *polycystic kidneys* and *polycystic renal d.*

**polycystic liver d.,** polycystic liver.

**polycystic ovary d.,** see under *syndrome.*

**polycystic renal d.,** polycystic kidney d.

**polyendocrine autoimmune d's, polyglandular autoimmune d's,** polyglandular autoimmune syndromes.

**polyhedral d's,** infectious diseases of insects, especially caterpillars, caused by viruses.

**Pompe's d.,** glycogen storage d., type II.

**Poncet's d.,** tuberculous arthritis.

**Portuguese-Azorean d.,** Azorean d.

**Posadas' d., Posadas-Wernicke d.,** coccidioidomycosis.

**Pott's d.,** tuberculosis of spine.

**Preiser's d.,** osteoporosis and atrophy of the carpal scaphoid due to trauma or a fracture which has not been kept immobilized.

**primary electrical d.,** a condition characterized by serious ventricular tachycardia, and sometimes ventricular fibrillation, in the absence of recognizable structural heart disease.

**Pringle's d.,** adenoma sebaceum (def. 1).

**prion d.,** any of a group of fatal, transmissible neurodegenerative diseases caused by abnormalities of prion protein metabolism, which may result from mutations in the prion protein gene or from infection with pathogenic isoforms of the protein (see *prion*). Characteristics include neuronal loss, gliosis, and extensive vacuolization of the cerebral cortex. Prion diseases may be sporadic, inherited as an autosomal dominant trait, or acquired. Human diseases include Creutzfeldt-Jakob disease, Gerstmann-Sträussler syndrome, fatal familial insomnia, and kuru; animal diseases include scrapie, bovine spongiform encephalopathy, and mink encephalopathy. Called also *transmissible neurodegenerative disease* and *subacute spongiform* or *transmissible spongiform encephalopathy.*

**puff d.,** anhidrosis (def. 2).

**pullorum d.,** an infectious disease of birds, including chickens, caused by *Salmonella enteritidis* serotype *pullorum* and marked by loss of appetite, dullness, diarrhea that leaves white lumps around the cloaca, reduced egg yield, and infertility of eggs. It is sometimes fatal, with moribund and dead birds found at hatching time. Called also *white diarrhea.*

**pulmonary veno-occlusive d.,** an idiopathic form of primary pulmonary hypertension, usually seen in children or young adults, characterized by dyspnea and syncope, sometimes with intimal fibrosis, hemoptysis, paroxysmal nocturnal dyspnea, and orthopnea.

**pulpy kidney d.,** a fatal enterotoxemia caused by *Clostridium perfringens* type B, usually seen in young animals, chiefly lambs, that are fed a high carbohydrate diet, although it may affect sheep, goats, and cattle of any age. Pathologically, the kidneys are mottled and soft in consistency and the cortex is jelly-like or almost semifluid; the liver is severely congested with small hemorrhages diffusely scattered over its surface. Called also *overeating d.*

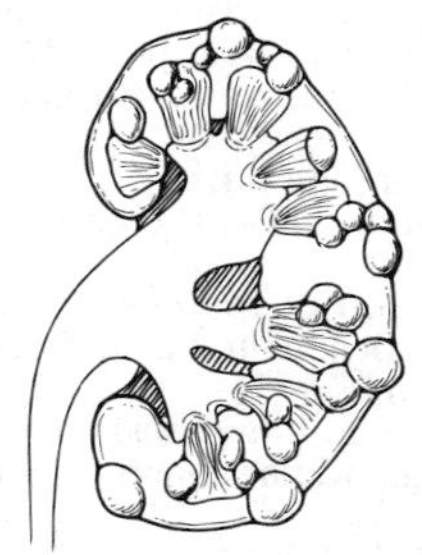

Polycystic kidney disease.

**pulseless d.,** Takayasu's arteritis.

**Purtscher's d.,** traumatic angiopathy of the retina with edema, hemorrhage, and exudation, usually following crush injuries of the chest; called also *Purtscher's angiopathic retinopathy.*

**Pyle's d.,** metaphyseal dysplasia.

**pyramidal d.,** buttress foot.

**Quervain's d.,** see *de Quervain's d.*

**Quincke's d.,** angioedema.

**rabbit hemorrhagic d.,** an acute infectious disease of wild and domestic rabbits and hares, caused by a calicivirus and characterized by necrotizing hepatitis and hemorrhagic lesions of many organs.

**ragpicker's d., ragsorter's d.,** inhalational anthrax.

**railroad d.,** transit tetany.

**rat-bite d.,** see under *fever.*

**Raynaud's d.,** a primary or idiopathic vascular disorder characterized by bilateral attacks of Raynaud's phenomenon; it affects females more often than males. Called also *Raynaud's gangrene.*

**Recklinghausen's d.,** 1. neurofibromatosis 1. 2. osteitis fibrosa cystica.

**Recklinghausen-Applebaum d.,** hemochromatosis.

**Recklinghausen's d. of bone,** osteitis fibrosa cystica.

**redwater d.,** bacillary hemoglobinuria.

**Reed-Hodgkin d.,** Hodgkin's d.

**Refsum's d.,** an autosomal recessive disorder of lipid metabolism in which deficiency of phytanic acid α-hydroxylase results in accumulation of phytanic acid; it is manifest chiefly by chronic polyneuritis, retinitis pigmentosa, cerebellar ataxia, and persistent elevation of protein in cerebrospinal fluid; there may also be ichthyosis, nerve deafness, and electrocardiographic abnormalities. Called also *phytanic acid storage d.,* and *heredopathia atactica polyneuritiformis.*

**remnant removal d.,** familial dysbetalipoproteinemia.

**reportable d.,** notifiable d.

**respiratory bronchiolitis–associated interstitial lung d.,** a mild interstitial lung condition seen in cigarette smokers, characterized by patchy inflammation of bronchioles with filling of their lumina as well as adjacent alveoli and alveolar ducts by pigmented macrophages, resulting in dyspnea and a productive cough; it is usually a benign condition that will clear up upon cessation of smoking.

**restrictive lung d.,** a general term comprising pulmonary diseases characterized by decreased total lung capacity, including those caused by disorders affecting the chest wall (e.g., poliomyelitis and scoliosis), and those caused by infiltrative interstitial and infiltrative diseases, such as adult respiratory distress syndrome.

**rheumatic heart d.,** the most important manifestation of and sequel to rheumatic fever (q.v.), consisting chiefly of valvular deformities.

**rheumatoid d.,** a systemic condition best known by its articular involvement (rheumatoid arthritis) but emphasizing nonarticular changes, e.g., pulmonary interstitial fibrosis, pleural effusion, and lung nodules.

**Rh hemolytic d.,** a hemolytic reaction in the blood of a fetus or newborn to anti-Rh antibodies in the mother's blood, such as occurs in erythroblastosis fetalis.

**Ribas-Torres d.,** variola minor.

**rice d.,** beriberi.

**Riedel's d.,** see under *thyroiditis.*

**Riga-Fede d.,** a small sublingual ulceration in infants with natal or neonatal teeth due to rubbing the lower central incisors; most often observed in whooping cough.

**Riggs' d.,** marginal periodontitis.

**Ritter's d.,** staphylococcal scalded skin syndrome.

**Roger's d.,** a ventricular septal defect; the term is usually restricted to small, asymptomatic defects.

**rolling d.,** a disease of laboratory mice characterized by lateral rolling movements, neurolysis, and a polymorphonuclear leukocytic reaction in the brain; it is caused by a potent neurolytic exotoxin produced by *Mycoplasma neurolyticum.*

**Romberg's d.,** facial hemiatrophy.

**Romney Marsh d.,** struck.

**Rosai-Dorfman d.,** a rare syndrome, seen usually in children or adolescents, in which cervical lymph nodes (and sometimes other lymph nodes) are massively swollen and contain large numbers of histiocytes; extranodal disease is common, sometimes with fever, anemia, neutrophilia, elevated erythrocyte sedimentation rate, and hypergammaglobulinemia. Called also *sinus histiocytosis with massive lymphadenopathy.*

**rose d.,** the urticarial form of swine erysipelas.

**Rossbach's d.,** hyperchlorhydria.

**Roth's (Rot's) d., Roth-Bernhardt (Rot-Bernhardt) d.,** meralgia paresthetica.

**Rougnon-Heberden d.,** angina pectoris.

**round heart d.,** a fatal type of cardiopathy seen in inbred strains of turkeys; the right heart becomes greatly enlarged.

**Rubarth's d.,** infectious canine hepatitis.

**runt d.,** graft-versus-host disease produced by injection of allogenic lymphocytes into immunologically immature experimental animals.

**Rust's d.,** tuberculous spondylitis of the cervical vertebrae.

**Ruysch's d.,** congenital megacolon.

**saccharine d.,** a term proposed for any disease resulting from the overconsumption of refined carbohydrate foods in combination with the removal of dietary fiber and protein, including diabetes, cardiovascular disease, constipation, obesity, peptic ulcer, etc.

**Sachs' d.,** Tay-Sachs d.

**sacroiliac d.,** chronic tuberculous inflammation of the sacroiliac joint.

**salivary gland d.,** cytomegalic inclusion d.

**Salla d.,** an autosomal recessive disorder of sialic acid metabolism characterized by mental retardation, delayed motor development, ataxia, and sialuria, with onset in childhood and slow progression in early adulthood. Sialic acid accumulates in lysosomes; the disorder is believed to be due to a defect in the carrier transporting sialic acid across the lysosomal membrane.

**Sanders' d.,** epidemic keratoconjunctivitis.

**Sandhoff's d.,** a type of $GM_2$ gangliosidosis (variant 0, or type II) with clinical features similar to Tay-Sachs disease and other forms of the B variant of $GM_2$ gangliosidosis but distinguished by the presence of stored or excreted *N*-acetylglucosamine-containing oligosaccharides, occasional organomegaly, and occurrence only in non-Jews. The underlying defect is deficiency of both hexosaminidase A and B isozymes due to a defect in the $\beta$ chain of the enzyme. It occurs as several forms (infantile, juvenile, and adult) decreasing in severity with increasing age of onset.

**sandworm d.,** cutaneous larva migrans.

**San Joaquin Valley d.,** primary coccidioidomycosis.

**Santavuori d., Santavuori-Haltia d.,** Haltia-Santavuori d.

**Saunders' d.,** a dangerous condition seen in infants having digestive disturbances to whom is given a large percentage of carbohydrates; it is marked by vomiting, cerebral symptoms, and depression of circulation.

**Schamberg's d.,** a chronic, asymptomatic dermatosis of the lower legs and feet of adolescent and young adult males, characterized by orange to tan macules with red puncta (cayenne pepper spots). Called also *progressive pigmentary dermatosis* and *Schamberg's dermatosis.*

**Schanz's d.,** traumatic inflammation of the tendo Achillis.

**Schaumann's d.,** sarcoidosis.

**Scheuermann's d.,** osteochondrosis of vertebral epiphyses in juveniles; see *osteochondrosis.*

**Schilder's d.,** a subacute or chronic form of leukoencephalopathy of children and adolescents. Clinical symptoms include blindness, deafness, bilateral spasticity, and progressive mental deterioration. There is massive destruction of the white substance of the cerebral hemispheres, cavity formation, and glial scarring. The disease as a separate diagnostic entity has been disputed. It usually occurs sporadically, but a familial form has been reported. Called also *encephalitis periaxialis diffusa, Flatau-Schilder d.,* and *Schilder's encephalitis.*

**Schimmelbusch's d.,** fibrocystic d. of breast.

**Schlatter's d., Schlatter-Osgood d.,** Osgood-Schlatter d.

**Schmorl's d.,** 1. herniation of the nucleus pulposus into an adjacent ventral body. 2. necrobacillosis in rabbits and rats, characterized by abscesses and areas of necrosis on the body, head, and interior of the mouth.

**Scholz's d.,** former name for the juvenile form of metachromatic leukodystrophy.

**Schönlein's d.,** see under *purpura.*

**Schottmüller's d.,** paratyphoid fever.

**Schroeder's d.,** a condition characterized by hypertrophic endometrium and excessive uterine bleeding.

**Schüller's d.,** 1. Hand-Schüller-Christian d.. 2. osteoporosis circumscripta cranii.

**Schüller-Christian d.,** Hand-Schüller-Christian d.

**Schwediauer's d.,** see *Swediaur's d.*

**secondary d.,** 1. a morbid condition occurring subsequent to or as a consequence of another disease. 2. one due to introduction of incompatible immunologically competent cells into a host rendered incapable of rejecting them by heavy exposure to ionizing radiation; see also *graft-versus-host d.*

**Seitelberger's d.,** infantile neuroaxonal dystrophy.

**self-limited d.,** one which by its very nature runs a limited and definite course.

**Selter's d.,** acrodynia.

**senecio d.,** cirrhosis of the liver occurring as the result of poisoning by the plant *Senecio.*

**septic d.,** one which arises from the development of pyogenic or putrefactive organisms.

**serum d.,** see under *sickness.*

**Sever's d.,** epiphysitis of the calcaneus.

**severe combined immunodeficiency d. (SCID),** see under *immunodeficiency.*

**sexually transmitted d.,** any of a diverse group of infections caused by biologically dissimilar pathogens and transmitted by sexual contact, which includes both heterosexual and homosexual behavior; sexual transmission is the only important mode of spread of some of the diseases in the group (e.g., the classic venereal diseases), while others (e.g., hepatitis viruses, shigellosis, amebiasis, giardiasis) can also be acquired by nonsexual means. See also *venereal d.*

**Shaver's d.,** bauxite pneumoconiosis.

**shimamushi d.,** scrub typhus.

**shuttlemaker's d.,** a condition in shuttlemakers, marked by faintness, shortness of breath, headache, nausea, etc., attributed to inhaling the dust of poisonous wood from which the shuttles (devices used in weaving) are made.

**sickle cell d.,** any of the diseases associated with the presence of hemoglobin S and sickle cells, including sickle cell anemia, sickle cell–hemoglobin C disease, sickle cell–hemoglobin D disease, and sickle cell–thalassemia disease.

**sickle cell–hemoglobin C d.,** a genetically determined anemia in which the erythrocytes contain both hemoglobin S and hemoglobin C; symptoms are similar to but less severe than those of sickle cell anemia and may include abdominal and skeletal pain, splenomegaly, splenic infarction, and infarctions or deformities of bone. Called also *hemoglobin SC d.*

**sickle cell–hemoglobin D d.,** a genetically determined anemia in which the erythrocytes contain both hemoglobin S and hemoglobin D, with symptoms like those of mild sickle cell anemia. Called also *hemoglobin SD d.*

**sickle cell–thalassemia d.,** any of several hereditary anemias involving simultaneous heterozygosity for hemoglobin S and a thalassemia gene; symptoms resemble those of sickle cell anemia. Called also *microdrepanocytosis, microdrepanocytic d., hemoglobin S–thalassemia, sickle cell–thalassemia,* and *thalassemia–sickle cell d.*.

**silo filler's d.,** see under *lung.*

**Simmonds' d.,** panhypopituitarism.

**Simons' d.,** partial lipodystrophy.

**Sinding-Larsen d., Sinding-Larsen-Johansson d.,** Larsen-Johansson d.

**sixth d.,** exanthema subitum.

**Sjögren's d.,** see under *syndrome.*

**Skevas-Zerfus d.,** sponge-diver's d.

**sleepy foal d.,** a usually fatal type of equulosis affecting foals within the first three days of life, characterized by sudden onset and extreme prostration.

**small airways d.,** chronic obstructive bronchitis with irreversible narrowing of the bronchioles and small bronchi. See also *obstructive small airways d.*

**Smith-Strang d.,** methionine malabsorption syndrome.

**Sneddon-Wilkinson d.,** subcorneal pustular dermatosis.

**specific d.,** any disease caused by a specific agent.

**specific heart muscle d.,** secondary cardiomyopathy.

**Spencer's d.,** a form (probably viral) of epidemic gastroenteritis.

**Spielmeyer-Vogt d.,** Vogt-Spielmeyer d.

**sponge-diver's d.,** a condition encountered by divers in the Mediterranean who come in contact with the stinging tentacles of sea anemones of the genera *Sagartia* and *Actinia,* which are frequently attached to the base of sponges; it is marked by burning, itching, erythema, necrosis, and ulceration. Called also *Skevas-Zerfus d.*

**Stargardt's d.,** hereditary degeneration of the macula lutea occurring between the ages of six and twenty, marked by rapid loss of visual acuity and by abnormal appearance and pigmentation of the macular area.

**startle d.,** hyperexplexia.

**Steinert's d.,** myotonic dystrophy.

**sterility d.,** a deficiency disease observed in experimental animals and due to a lack of vitamin E in the diet.

**Sternberg's d.,** Hodgkin's d.

**Sticker's d.,** erythema infectiosum.

**Stieda's d.,** Pellegrini's d.

**stiff lamb d.,** enzootic muscular dystrophy in lambs.

**Still's d.,** a variety of chronic polyarthritis affecting children and marked by enlargement of lymph nodes, generally of the spleen, with evanescent rash and irregular fever; see also *juvenile rheumatoid arthritis.*

**stone d.,** lithiasis.

**storage d.,** a metabolic disorder in which some substance accumulates or is stored in certain cells in unusually large amounts; the stored substances may be lipids, proteins, carbohydrates, or other substances. See, for example, *glycogen storage d., mucopolysaccharidosis,* and *proteinosis.*

**storage pool d.,** any of various blood coagulation disorders due to defects in the dense bodies of platelets, so that the platelets fail to release ADP in response to aggregating agents such as collagen, epinephrine, exogenous ADP, and thrombin. It is characterized by mild bleeding episodes, prolonged bleeding time, and reduced aggregation response to collagen or thrombin. One type is a component of the autosomal recessive condition Hermansky-Pudlak syndrome.

**structural d.,** any disease in which there are microscopic changes.

**Strümpell's d.,** 1. a hereditary form of lateral sclerosis in which the spasticity is principally limited to the legs. 2. cerebral poliomyelitis.

**Strümpell-Leichtenstern d.,** hemorrhagic encephalitis.

**Strümpell-Marie d.,** ankylosing spondylitis.

**Stuttgart d.,** a type of canine leptospirosis without jaundice, primarily caused by Leptospira interrogans serovar canicola; called also *canicola fever* and *canine typhus.*

**Sudeck's d.,** post-traumatic osteoporosis.

**Sutton's d.,** 1. halo nevus. 2. periadenitis mucosa necrotica recurrens. 3. granuloma fissuratum.

**Swediaur's (Schwediauer's) d.,** inflammation of the calcaneal bursa.

**sweet clover d.,** a hemorrhagic disease of animals, especially cattle, caused by ingestion of spoiled *Melilotus* (sweet clover), which contains the anticoagulant dicumarol.

**Swift's d., Swift-Feer d.,** acrodynia.

**swineherd's d.,** leptospirosis, manifested as a benign meningitis, caused by *Leptospira interrogans*, primarily serovars pomona and *tarassovi,* and affecting those who work with swine or pork or come in contact with the urine of carriers.

**Sylvest's d.,** epidemic pleurodynia.

**Symmers's d.,** follicular lymphoma.

**systemic d.,** one affecting a number of organs and tissues.

**Takahara's d.,** the symptomatic form of acatalasia (q.v.); it is characterized by oral ulcerations and gangrene.

**Takayasu's d.,** see under *arteritis.*

**Talfan d.,** infectious porcine encephalomyelitis.

**Talma's d.,** myotonia tarda.

**Tangier d.,** an autosomal recessive disorder of lipoprotein and lipid metabolism characterized by absence in plasma of normal high-density lipoproteins (HDL), deficiency of apolipoproteins A-I and A-II, low to normal low-density lipoproteins, and high triglycerides, and by accumulation in body tissues of cholesteryl esters. Clinical signs include enlargement and orange coloring of tonsils, pharyngeal mucosa, and rectal mucosa; recurrent peripheral neuropathy; splenomegaly; and corneal infiltration.

**Tarui's d.,** glycogen storage d., type VII.

**Tay's d.,** see under *choroiditis.*

**Tay-Sachs d. (TSD),** the most common ganglioside storage disease, occurring almost exclusively among northeast European Jews. TSD is a $GM_2$ gangliosidosis specifically characterized by infantile onset (3–6 months), doll-like facies, cherry-red macular spot (90+ per cent of the infants), early blindness, hyperacusis, macrocephaly, seizures, and hypotonia; the children die between 2 and 5 years of age. See also *Sandhoff's d. and see $GM_2$ gangliosidosis, variant B,* under *gangliosidosis.*

**teart d. of cattle,** molybdenum poisoning (q.v.) in cattle that graze on teart, a type of English pasture in which the grass contains high levels of molybdenum.

**Teschen d.,** infectious porcine encephalomyelitis.

**thalassemia–sickle cell d.,** sickle cell–thalassemia d.

**Thaysen's d.,** celiac d.

**Theiler's d.,** encephalomyelitis of mice caused by invasion of the nervous system by a picornavirus normally found in the intestinal tract; called also *mouse* or *murine encephalomyelitis, mouse* or *murine poliomyelitis,* and *Theiler's mouse encephalomyelitis.*

**Thiemann's d.,** familial avascular necrosis of the phalangeal epiphysis, beginning in childhood or adolescence and resulting in deformity of the interphalangeal joints; called also *familial osteoarthropathy of fingers.* Similar lesions may occur in the great toes and first tarsometatarsal joints, in which case the disorder is known as *osteochondritis ossis metacarpi et metatarsi.*

**Thomsen's d.,** myotonia congenita.

**Thomson's d.,** an autosomal recessive skin disorder similar to Rothmund-Thomson syndrome except that saddle nose and cataract are not manifestations.

**Thornwaldt's d.,** Tornwaldt's bursitis.

**thyrocardiac d., thyrotoxic heart d.,** heart disease associated with hyperthyroidism, marked by atrial fibrillation, cardiac enlargement, and congestive heart failure.

**Tietze's d.,** see under *syndrome.*

**Tillaux's d.,** fibrocystic d. of breast.

**Tommaselli's d.,** pyrexia and hematuria due to excessive use of quinine.

**Tooth's d.,** Charcot-Marie-Tooth d.

**Tornwaldt's (Thornwaldt's) d.,** see under *bursitis.*

**transmissible neurodegenerative d. (TND),** prion disease.

**Traum's d.,** brucellosis with abortion in swine.

**Trevor's d.,** dysplasia epiphysealis hemimelica.

**trophoblastic d.,** gestational trophoblastic neoplasia.

**tsutsugamushi d.,** scrub typhus.

**tubotympanic d.,** inflammatory disease of the middle ear resulting from eustachian tube dysfunction and decreased pressure in the tympanic cavity.

**tungsten carbide d.,** hard metal d.

**tunnel d.,** decompression sickness.

**twin-lamb d.,** pregnancy toxemia in ewes.

**twist d.,** whirling d.

**Tyzzer's d.,** a disease caused by *Bacillus piliformis* and characterized by necrotic lesions of the liver and intestine; originally described in Japanese waltzing mice, it also affects rats, rabbits, gerbils, dogs, and occasionally humans.

**Tzaneen d.,** a tick-borne protozoal disease, seen in South Africa, due to *Theileria mutans,* and occurring in cattle and water buffalo, which may manifest as a mild febrile disease or may be severe and fatal.

**Underwood's d.,** sclerema.

**Unna-Thost d.,** diffuse palmoplantar keratoderma.

**Unverricht's d., Univerricht-Lundborg d.,** Baltic myoclonic epilepsy.

**Urbach-Wiethe d.,** lipid proteinosis.

**uremic bone d.,** renal osteodystrophy.

**vagabonds' d., vagrants' d.,** discoloration of the skin in persons subjected to louse *(Pediculus humanus corporis)* bites over long periods; called also *parasitic melanoderma.*

**van Buren's d.,** Peyronie's d..

**van den Bergh's d.,** enterogenous cyanosis.

**Vaquez' d., Vaquez-Osler d.,** polycythemia vera.

**veld d., veldt d.,** heartwater.

**venereal d. (VD),** 1. sexually transmitted d. 2. a former classification of sexually transmitted diseases that included only gonorrhea, syphilis, chancroid, lymphogranuloma venereum, and granuloma inguinale.

**veno-occlusive d. of the liver,** symptomatic occlusion of the small hepatic venules, caused by ingestion of any of a variety of substances such as Senecio tea and certain chemotherapy agents (hepatotoxins) and by radiation. Many patients recover after withdrawal of the offending toxin; some progress to portal hypertension and liver failure, as in Budd-Chiari syndrome. Called also *hepatic veno-occlusive d.*

**vent d.,** rabbit syphilis.

**Verneuil's d.,** syphilitic disease of the bursae.

**Verse's d.,** calcinosis intervertebralis.

**vibration d.,** Raynaud's phenomenon with osteoarthritic changes and diminished flexion in joints of the arms and hands, seen in those who use vibrating tools for long periods. Called also *pneumatic hammer d.*

**vinyl chloride d.,** acro-osteolysis resulting from exposure to vinyl chloride, characterized by Raynaud's phenomenon, skin changes resembling scleroderma on the backs of the hands and on the forearms, and bony changes affecting the terminal phalanges of the fingers and toes, the styloid processes of the radius and ulna, the sacroiliac joints, and the patellae.

**Vogt-Spielmeyer d.,** the juvenile form of neuronal ceroid-lipofuscinosis with onset between 5 and 10 years of age, characterized by rapid cerebroretinal degeneration, massive loss of brain substance, excessive neuronal storage of lipofuscin, and death within 10 to 15 years.

**Volkmann's d.,** a congenital deformity of the foot due to a tibiotarsal dislocation; called also *Volkmann's deformity.*

**Voltolini's d.,** acute, painful inflammation of the inner ear followed by meningitis with deafness and unconsciousness.

**vomiting and wasting d.,** a disease of pigs caused by infection with the hemagglutinating encephalomyelitis virus; the virus is endemic in many parts of the world and only occasionally causes symptoms. The disease varies from acute encephalomyelitis that can be fatal in a few days to anorexia, vomiting, and wasting that can last for two or three weeks without being fatal. Called also *Ontario encephalitis* and *hemagglutinating encephalomyelitis virus d. of pigs.*

**von Economo's d.,** lethargic encephalitis.

**von Gierke's d.,** glycogen storage d., type I.

**von Hippel's d.,** hemangiomatosis confined principally to the retina; when associated with hemangioblastoma of the cerebellum, it is known as *von Hippel-Lindau d.* Called also *retinal hemangioblastoma* and *Hippel's d.*

**von Hippel-Lindau d.,** hereditary phakomatosis characterized by hemangiomas of the retina and hemangioblastomas of the cerebellum; there may also be similar lesions of the spinal cord and cysts of the pancreas, kidneys, and other viscera. Neurologic symptoms, including seizures and mental retardation, may be present. Called also *cerebroretinal* or *retinocerebral angiomatosis, angiophakomatosis,* and *Lindau's* or *Lindau-von Hippel d.*

**von Recklinghausen's d.,** 1. neurofibromatosis 1. 2. osteitis fibrosa cystica.

**von Willebrand's d.**, a congenital bleeding disorder, usually of autosomal dominant inheritance, characterized by deficiency of von Willebrand's factor, with prolonged bleeding time and often impairment of adhesion of platelets on glass beads, associated with epistaxis and increased bleeding after trauma or surgery, menorrhagia, and postpartum bleeding. Several different types have been distinguished, ranging from mild to severe. Called also *angiohemophilia, pseudohemophilia, vascular hemophilia, Minot-von Willebrand syndrome,* and *Willebrand's syndrome.*
**Vrolik's d.**, osteogenesis imperfecta (type II), recessive form; see *osteogenesis imperfecta.*.
**Waldenström's d.**, osteochondrosis of the capital femoral epiphysis.
**walkabout d.**, crotalism.
**Wartenberg's d.**, cheiralgia paresthetica.
**wasting d.**, any disease marked by wasting (progressive emaciation and weakness), such as the anorexia-cachexia syndrome.
**Weber's d.**, Sturge-Weber syndrome.
**Weber-Christian d.**, relapsing febrile nodular nonsuppurative panniculitis.
**Wegner's d.**, osteochondritic separation of the epiphyses in hereditary syphilis.
**Weil's d.**, see under *syndrome.*
**Weir Mitchell's d.**, erythromelalgia.
**Werdnig-Hoffmann d.**, Werdnig-Hoffmann spinal muscular atrophy.
**Werlhof's d.**, idiopathic thrombocytopenic purpura.
**Werner-His d.**, trench fever.
**Werner Schultz d.**, agranulocytosis.
**Wernicke's d.**, see under *encephalopathy.*
**Wesselsbron d.**, a viral disease of sheep and cattle in southern Africa, resembling Rift Valley fever but caused by a flavivirus. It causes death in newborn lambs and abortion in cows and ewes; human infection results in mild febrile illness.
**Weston Hurst d.**, acute necrotizing hemorrhagic encephalomyelitis.
**Westphal-Strümpell d.**, Wilson's d.
**wheat weevil d.**, miller's lung.
**Whipple's d.**, a malabsorption syndrome caused by *Tropheryma whippelii,* characterized by diarrhea, steatorrhea, skin pigmentation, arthralgia and arthritis, lymphadenopathy, and central nervous system lesions. The intestinal mucosa is infiltrated with macrophages containing PAS-positive material (the remnants of microorganisms which invade the lamina propria).
**whirling d.**, a highly fatal protozoal disease of young salmonid fish caused by *Myxosoma cerebralis,* characterized chiefly by cartilaginous damage in the axial skeleton and granuloma formation involving the auditory-equilibrium apparatus of the fish, causing it to swim rapidly in a circular pattern. Called also *twist d.*
**white heifer d.**, a congenital condition of heifers, most commonly white ones of the Shorthorn breed, in which there is a rubberlike sheet of fibrous tissue and membrane partially or completely covering the posterior part of the vagina. Called also *persistent hymen.*
**white muscle d.**, enzootic muscular dystrophy.
**white spot d.**, 1. lichen sclerosus. 2. guttate morphea. 3. a pustular eruption involving the skin, gills, and eyes of marine and freshwater fishes both in the wild and in aquaria, caused by the histophagous protozoan *Ichthyophthirius multifiliis,* and often leading to death, and sometimes to great economic loss. Called also *ich, ichthyophthiriasis,* and *ick.*
**Whitmore's d.**, former name for *melioidosis.*
**Whytt's d.**, tuberculous meningitis causing acute hydrocephalus.
**Wilson's d.**, a rare progressive disease, inherited as an autosomal recessive trait and due to a defect in the metabolism of copper, with accumulation of copper in the liver, brain, kidney, cornea, and other tissues. The resultant copper poisoning is characterized by cirrhosis of the liver and degenerative changes in the brain, particularly the basal ganglia. Liver disease is the most likely presenting manifestation in children; neurologic disease is most common in young adults. The characteristic ophthalmic feature is a pigmented ring (Kayser-Fleischer ring) at the outer margin of the cornea. Called also *hepatolenticular d.* or *degeneration, familial hepatitis,* and *Westphal-Strümpell d.* or *pseudosclerosis.*
**Winckel's d.**, a fatal disease of newborn infants characterized by jaundice, hemoglobinuria, hemorrhage, bloody urine, cyanosis, polyuria, collapse, and convulsions.
**Winiwarter-Buerger d.**, thromboangiitis obliterans.
**Winkler's d.**, chondrodermatitis nodularis chronica helicis.
**Witkop's d., Witkop-Von Sallmann d.**, hereditary benign intraepithelial dyskeratosis.
**Wolman's d.**, a lysosomal storage disease caused by deficiency of the lysosomal sterol esterase, with onset in early infancy and death before one year of age. Clinical features include hepatosplenomegaly, steatorrhea, abdominal distension, anemia, inanition, and adrenal calcification. Called also *primary familial* or *Wolman xanthomatosis.*
**woolsorter's d.**, inhalational anthrax.
**Woringer-Kolopp d.**, pagetoid reticulosis.
**x d.**, 1. aflatoxicosis. 2. former name for *hyperkeratosis* (def. 3).
**X-linked lymphoproliferative d.**, see under *syndrome.*
**yellow fat d.**, inflammation of adipose tissue in an animal whose diet is excessively high in unsaturated fats and low in vitamin E; it usually occurs in cats and mink fed certain kinds of fish. The body fat becomes hard, lumpy, and painful and the animal may be feverish or anorexic. Called also *steatitis* and *nutritional steatitis.*
**Zahorsky's d.**, exanthema subitum.
**Ziehen-Oppenheim d.**, dystonia musculorum deformans.

**dis·en·gage·ment** (dis″ən-gāj′mənt) liberation of the fetus, or parts thereof, from the vaginal canal.

**dis·equi·lib·ri·um** (dis-e″kwĭ-lib′re-əm) dysequilibrium.
**linkage d.**, the occurrence in a population of two linked alleles at a frequency higher (or lower) than the expected equilibrium frequency (which is the product of the frequencies of the two alleles).

**dis·es·the·sia** (dis″əs-the′zhə) dysesthesia.

**dis·ger·mi·no·ma** (dis-jər″mĭ-no′mə) dysgerminoma.

**dish** (dish) a shallow vessel of glass or other material for laboratory work.
**culture d.**, a shallow glass vessel for making bacterial cultures.
**dappen d.**, a small, heavy, solid glass, octagonal dish with a shallow depression to hold a few drops of medicaments or filling material.
**evaporating d.**, a laboratory vessel, usually wide and shallow, in which material is evaporated by exposure to heat.
**Petri d.**, a round, shallow, flat-bottomed transparent glass or plastic dish with vertical sides and a similar but slightly larger dish that forms a cover; used for the culture of microorganisms on solid media and for tissue cell cultures.
**Stender d's.**, vessels of various forms and sizes, used in preparing and staining histologic specimens.

**dis·har·mo·ny** (dis-hahr′mə-ne) lack of harmony; discord.
**occlusal d.**, a condition in which *(a)* contacts of opposing occlusal surfaces of teeth are not in harmony with other tooth contacts and with the anatomic and physiologic control of the mandible, or *(b)* occlusions do not coincide with their respective jaw relations.

**dis·im·pac·tion** (dis-im-pak′shən) removal of a fecal impaction, usually done digitally or with an enema.

**DISIDA** diisopropyl iminodiacetic acid; see *disofenin.*

**dis·in·fect** (dis″in-fekt′) [*dis-*[1] + L. *inficere* to corrupt] to free from pathogenic organisms, or to render them inert, especially as applied to the treatment of inanimate materials to reduce or eliminate infectious organisms.

**dis·in·fec·tant** (dis″in-fek′tənt) 1. freeing from infection. 2. an agent that disinfects; applied particularly to agents used on inanimate objects. Cf. *antiseptic.*
**coal-tar d.**, creosote.

**dis·in·fec·tion** (dis″in-fek′shən) [MeSH: Disinfection] the act of disinfecting.
**concomitant d., concurrent d.**, immediate disinfection and disposal of discharges and infective matter all through the course of a disease.
**terminal d.**, disinfection of a sick room and its contents at the termination of a disease.

**dis·in·fes·ta·tion** (dis″in-fəs-ta′shən) the extermination or destruction of insects, rodents, or other animal forms, especially those present on a person, an animal, or clothing; cf. *defaunation, delousing,* and *disparasitized.*

**dis·in·hi·bi·tion** (dis″in-hĭ-bish′ən) 1. removal of inhibitions, as reduction of the inhibitory function of the cerebral cortex by drugs such as ethyl alcohol or reduction in the severity of superego controls in psychotherapy. 2. in experimental psychology, the revival of an extinguished conditioned response by exposure to an unconditioned stimulus.

**dis·in·sect·ed** (dis″in-sek′təd) freed from unwanted insects.

**dis·in·sec·tion** (dis″in-sek′shən) disinsectization.

**dis·in·sec·ti·za·tion** (dis″in-sek″tĭ-za′shən) removal or extermination of unwanted insects.

**dis·in·sec·tor** (dis″in-sek′tər) an apparatus for the removal of insects or similar vermin from humans, animals, or clothing.

**dis·in·ser·tion** (dis″in-sər′shən) 1. rupture of a tendon from its insertion into a bone. 2. detachment of the retina at its periphery; retinodialysis.

**dis·in·te·grant** (dis-in′tə-grənt) disintegrator; an agent used in the pharmaceutical preparation of tablets, which causes them to disintegrate and release their medicinal substances on contact with moisture.

**dis·in·te·gra·tion** (dis′in″tə-gra′shən) [*dis-*[1] + L. *integer* entire] 1. the process of breaking up or decomposing. 2. disruption of integrative functions of personality in mental illness; disorganization of the psychic and behavioral processes.
**radioactive d.**, see under *decay*.

**Dis·i·pal** (dis′ĭ-pəl) trademark for a preparation of orphenadrine hydrochloride.

**dis·joint** (dis-joint′) to disarticulate.

**dis·junc·tion** (dis-junk′shən) 1. the act or state of being disjoined. 2. in genetics, the moving apart of bivalent chromosomes at first anaphase of meiosis, or the moving apart of daughter chromosomes at the second anaphase of meiosis or anaphase of mitosis.
**craniofacial d.**, Le Fort III fracture; see under *fracture*.

**disk** (disk) [L. *discus* quoit, from Gr. *diskos*] a circular or rounded flat plate; spelled also *disc* (q.v.).
**A d.**, A band; see under *band*.
**abrasive d.**, dental d.
**Amici's d.**, Z band; see under *band*.
**anangioid d.**, a retinal disk without blood vessels.
**anisotropic d., anisotropous d.**, A band; see under *band*.
**articular d.**, 1. a pad of fibrocartilage or dense fibrous tissue found in some synovial joints; see *discus articularis,* and for names of articular disks of particular joints, see entries beginning *discus articularis,* under *discus*. 2. meniscus articularis.
**Blake's d.**, a disk-shaped paper patch for a perforated tympanic membrane.
**blood d.**, platelet.
**Bowman's d's**, flat, disklike plates which make up striated muscle fibers.
**Carborundum d.**, a dental disk with Carborundum (silicon carbide) as the abrasive material.
**choked d.**, papilledema.
**ciliary d.**, orbiculus ciliaris.
**cloth d.**, rag wheel.
**contained d.**, herniation of intervertebral disk (see under *herniation*) in which the anulus fibrosus remains intact. Cf. *noncontained d.*
**cupped d.**, a pathologically depressed and enlarged optic disk, frequently seen in advanced glaucoma.
**cutting d.**, a dental disk with abrasive material attached to its surfaces or edge, used for grinding or reducing teeth.
**cuttlefish d.**, a dental disk with powdered cuttlefish bone bonded to its surface and edge.
**dental d.**, a thin, flat, oval, or concave circular plate with abrasive materials bonded to its surface or edge; used to polish and finish cavity preparations and for cutting or polishing dental restorations. Called also *abrasive d.*
**diamond d.**, a steel dental disk with diamond chips bonded to its surface or edge.
**emery d.**, a paper or resin dental disk with emery powder attached to its surface.
**Engelmann's d.**, H band; see under *band*.
**epiphyseal d.**, cartilago epiphysialis.
**extruded d.**, herniation of intervertebral disk (see under *herniation*) in which the nucleus pulposus protrudes through the anulus fibrosus and the nuclear material remains attached to the disk.
**gelatin d.**, a disk or lamella of gelatin, variously medicated; used chiefly in eye diseases.
**growth d.**, cartilago epiphysealis.
**Hensen's d.**, H band; see under *band*.
**herniated d.**, herniation of intervertebral disk see under *herniation*.
**I d.**, the light disk or band of a striated muscle fiber; called also *isotropic d.* or *J disk*.
**interarticular d.**, articular d., def. 1.
**intercalated d's**, dense bands running between myocardial cells both transversely and longitudinally, forming a stepped configuration. They contain intercellular junctions that link adjacent cells both electrically and mechanically; they are composed mainly of fascia adherens, but desmosomes and gap junctions are also present.
**intermediate d.**, Z band; see under *band*.
**interpubic d.**, discus interpubicus.
**intervertebral d's**, disci intervertebrales.

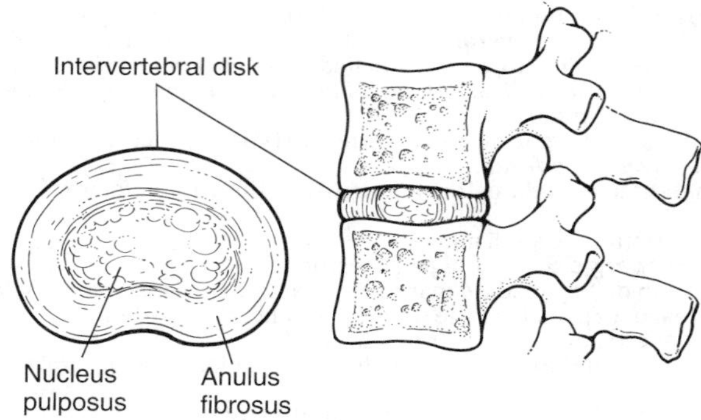


**intra-articular d's**, fibrous structures within the capsules of diarthrodial joints.
**isotropic d., J d.**, I band; see under *band*.
**M d.**, M band; see under *band*.
**Merkel's d.**, see under *cell*.
**micrometer d.**, a glass disk, engraved with a scale, used in an ocular in making microscopical measurements.
**Newton's d.**, a disk which is divided into seven sectors that are colored the seven primary colors of the spectrum and which, when rotated rapidly, appears to be white.
**noncontained d.**, herniation of intervertebral disk (see under *herniation*) in which there is rupture of the anulus fibrosus. Cf. *contained d.*
**optic d.**, discus nervi optici.
**Placido's d.**, a keratoscope.
**polishing d.**, a dental disk with a very fine abrasive material, used for finishing and polishing of surfaces.
**proligerous d.**, cumulus oophorus.
**protruded d.**, herniation of intervertebral disk; see under *herniation*.
**Q d.**, A band; see under *band*.
**Ranvier's tactile d's**, cup-shaped sensory nerve endings near the menisci tactus.
**Rekoss d.**, the rotating device for quickly changing the lenses in the ophthalmoscope.
**ruptured d.**, herniation of intervertebral disk; see under *herniation*.
**sandpaper d.**, a dental disk with pulverized silica as the abrasive material.
**sequestered d.**, a free fragment of the nucleus pulposus lying in the spinal canal outside of the annulus fibrosus and no longer attached to the intervertebral disk.
**slipped d.**, popular name for *herniation of intervertebral disk*.
**stenopeic d.**, an opaque disk having a narrow slit; used for testing for astigmatism.
**stroboscopic d.**, a revolving disk with alternate open and closed sections that gives successive views of a moving object.
**tactile d.**, see under *meniscus*.
**thin d.**, Z band; see under *band*.
**transverse d.**, A band; see under *band*.
**Z d.**, Z band; see under *band*.

**dis·kec·to·my** (dis-kek′tə-me) [MeSH: Diskectomy] excision of an intervertebral disk; called also *discectomy*.

**Disk·hal·er** (disk′hāl-ər) trademark for a type of dry powder inhaler that can deliver multiple doses of medication.

**dis·ki·form** (dis′kĭ-form) in the shape of a disk.

**dis·ki·tis** (dis-ki′tis) inflammation of a disk, particularly of an interarticular disk.

**disk(o)-** [Gr. *diskos* disk] a combining form denoting relationship to a disk, or disk-shaped. See also words beginning *disc(o)-*.

**dis·ko·gram** (dis′ko-gram) a radiograph of an intervertebral disk.

**dis·kog·ra·phy** (dis-kog′rə-fe) radiography of the spine for visualization of an intervertebral disk, after injection into the disk itself of an absorbable contrast medium.

**dis·lo·ca·tio** (dis″lo-ka′she-o) [L.] dislocation.
**d. erec′ta**, subglenoid dislocation of the shoulder with the arm in a vertical position and the hand on top of the head.

**dis·lo·ca·tion** (dis″lo-ka′shən) [*dis-*[1] + L. *locare* to place] [MeSH: Dislocations] the displacement of any part, more especially of a bone; see Plate 15. Called also *luxation*.

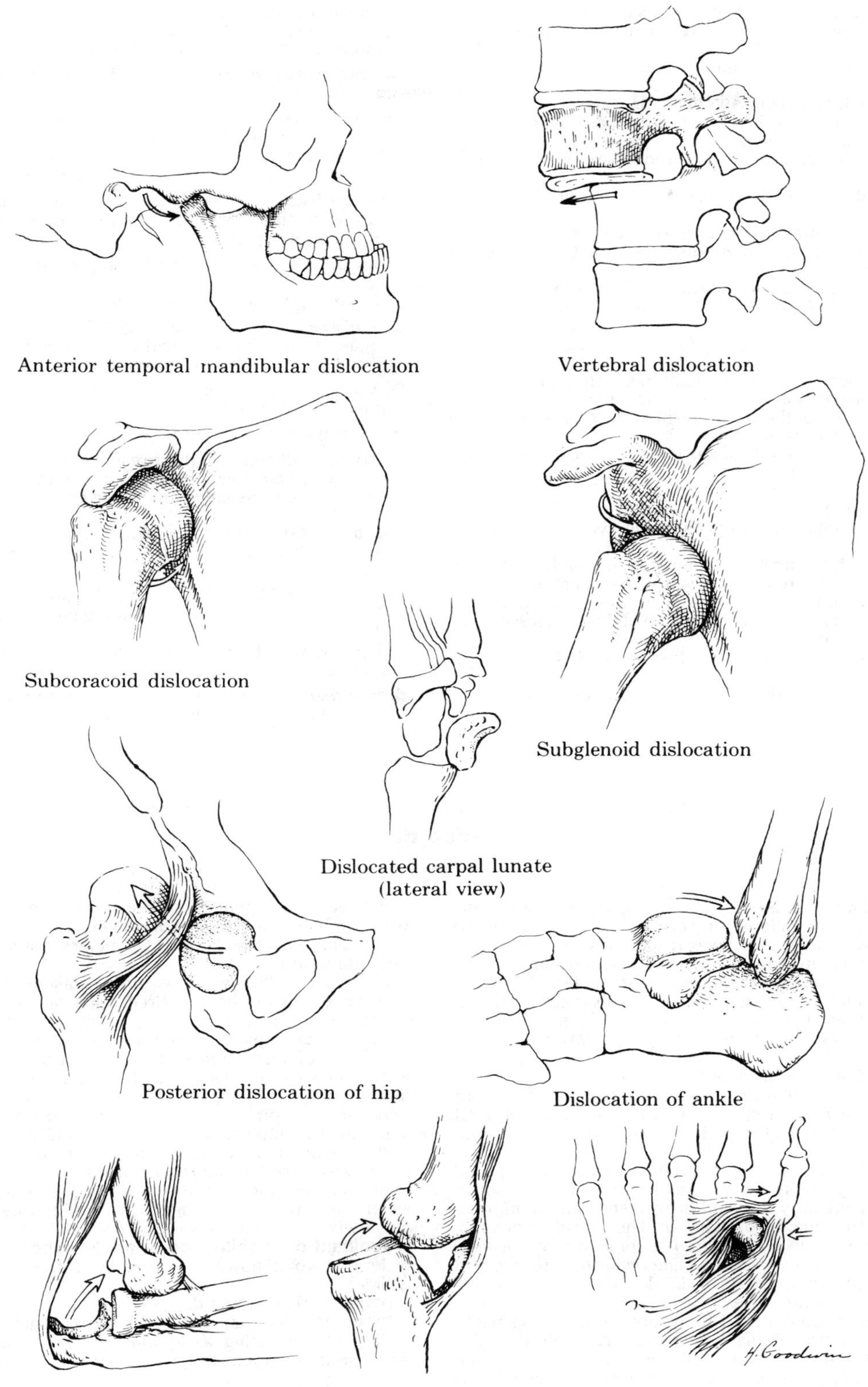


**PLATE 15**—VARIOUS TYPES OF DISLOCATION

**Bell-Dally d.,** nontraumatic dislocation of the atlas.
**closed d.,** simple d.
**complete d.,** one which completely separates the surfaces of a joint.
**complicated d.,** one which is associated with other important injuries.
**compound d.,** one in which the joint communicates with the external air.
**congenital d.,** one which exists from or before birth.
**consecutive d.,** one in which the luxated bone has changed its position since its first displacement.
**divergent d.,** one in which the ulna and radius are dislocated separately.
**fracture d.,** dislocation complicated by fracture of, or adjacent to, a joint.
**habitual d.,** one which often recurs after replacement.
**incomplete d.,** a subluxation; a slight displacement. Called also *partial d.*
**intrauterine d.,** one which occurs to the fetus in utero.
**Kienböck's d.,** isolated dislocation of the semilunar bone.
**d. of the lens,** displacement of the crystalline lens of the eye.
**Lisfranc's d.,** dislocation of the forefoot at the tarsometatarsal joints.
**Monteggia's d.,** dislocation of the hip joint in which the head of the femur is near the anterosuperior spine of the ilium.
**Nélaton's d.,** dislocation of the ankle in which the talus is forced up between the end of the tibia and the fibula.
**old d.,** a dislocation in which inflammatory or fibrotic changes have occurred.
**open d.,** compound d.
**partial d.,** incomplete d.
**pathologic d.,** one which results from paralysis, synovitis, infection, or other disease.
**primitive d.,** one in which the bones remain as originally displaced.
**recent d.,** one in which there is no complicating inflammation.
**simple d.,** one in which the joint is not penetrated by a wound.
**Smith's d.,** upward and backward dislocation of the metatarsals and the medial cuneiform bone.
**subastragalar d.,** separation of the calcaneus and the navicular bone from the talus.
**subcoracoid d.,** a type of dislocation of the head of the humerus. See Plate 15.
**subglenoid d.,** a type of dislocation of the head of the humerus. See Plate 15.
**subspinous d.,** dislocation of the head of the humerus into the space below the spine of the scapula.
**traumatic d.,** one due to an injury or to violence.

**dis·mem·ber·ment** (dis-mem′bər-mənt) amputation of a limb or a portion of it.

**dis·mu·ta·tion** (dis″mu-ta′shən) a reaction or reactions involving two identical molecules in which one gains what the other loses. For example, one may be oxidized and the other reduced, or one may be phosphorylated and the other dephosphorylated.

**dis·oc·clude** (dis″ŏ-klo͞od′) to cause loss of contact between opposing teeth as a result of tooth guidance, occlusal interferences, or occlusal adjustment.

**di·so·di·um** (di-so′de-əm) having two atoms of sodium in each molecule.
**d. cromoglycate,** cromolyn sodium.

**di·so·fen·in** (di″so-fen′in) DISIDA; a diisopropyl-substituted analogue of iminodiacetic acid (IDA); complexed with technetium Tc 99m it is used in hepatobiliary imaging. See also table at *technetium.*

**Di·so·mer** (di′so-mər) trademark for preparations of dexbrompheniramine maleate.

**di·so·mus** (di-so′məs) [*di-* + *soma*] synencephalus.

**di·so·my** (di′so-me) the presence of two chromosomes of a homologous pair in a karyotype or cell; in humans the normal state, with each pair usually comprising one chromosome from each parent.
**uniparental d.,** the abnormal state in which both chromosomes of the homologous pair are from the same parent, with none from the other parent.

**di·so·pyr·amide** (di″so-pir′ə-mīd) [MeSH: Disopyramide] a cardiac depressant with anticholinergic properties, used as an antiarrhythmic.
**d. phosphate** [USP], the phosphate salt of disopyramide, having the same actions and uses as the base, administered orally.

**dis·or·der** (dis-or′dər) a derangement or abnormality of function; a morbid physical or mental state.

## Disorder

**acute stress d.** [DSM-IV], an anxiety disorder characterized by development of anxiety and dissociative and other symptoms within one month following exposure to an extremely traumatic event, the symptoms including reexperiencing the event, avoidance of trauma-related stimuli, anxiety or increased arousal, and some or all of the following: a subjective sense of diminished emotional responsiveness, numbing, or detachment, derealization, depersonalization, and amnesia for aspects of the event. If persistent, it may become *posttraumatic stress disorder.*

**adjustment d.** [DSM-IV], a maladaptive reaction to identifiable stressful life events, such as divorce, loss of job, physical illness, or natural disaster; this diagnosis assumes that the condition will remit when the stress ceases or when the patient adapts to the situation.

**affective d's,** mood d's.

**amnestic d's** [DSM-IV], mental disorders characterized by acquired impairment in the ability to learn and recall new information, sometimes accompanied by inability to recall previously learned information, and not coupled to dementia or delirium. The disorders are subclassified on the basis of etiology as *amnestic disorder due to a general medical condition, substance-induced persisting amnestic disorder,* and *amnestic disorder not otherwise specified.* DSM-IV eliminates the distinction between this term and amnestic syndrome.

**anxiety d's** [DSM-IV], a group of mental disorders in which anxiety and avoidance behavior predominate. Included are panic disorder with and without agoraphobia, agoraphobia without history of panic disorder, specific phobia, social phobia, obsessive-compulsive disorder, posttraumatic stress disorder, acute stress disorder, generalized anxiety disorder, and substance-induced anxiety disorder.

**attention-deficit/hyperactivity d.** [DSM-IV], a childhood mental disorder characterized by inattention (such as distractibility, forgetfulness, not finishing tasks, and not appearing to listen), by hyperactivity and impulsivity (such as fidgeting and squirming, difficulty in remaining seated, excessive running or climbing, feelings of restlessness, difficulty awaiting one's turn, interrupting others, and excessive talking) or by both types of behavior. The disorder is subtyped as *predominantly hyperactive-impulsive type, predominantly inattentive type,* or *combined type,* depending on the criteria met. Behavior must interfere with academic, social, or work functioning, with impairment existing in at least two settings. Onset is before age seven but it can persist into adulthood.

**autistic d.** [DSM-IV], a severe pervasive developmental disorder with onset usually before three years of age and a biological basis related to neurologic or neurophysiologic factors; it is characterized by qualitative impairment in reciprocal social interaction (e.g., lack of awareness of the existence of feelings of others, failure to seek comfort at times of distress, lack of imitation), in verbal and nonverbal communication, and in capacity for symbolic play, and by restricted and unusual repertoire of activities and interests. Other characteristics sometimes include cognitive impairment, hyper- or hyporeactivity to certain stimuli, stereotypic behaviors, neurological abnormalities such as seizures or altered muscle tone, sleeping or eating pattern abnormalities, and severe behavioral problems. It is associated with several genetic conditions and pre- and perinatal risk factors. Called also *autism, infantile autism,* and *Kanner's syndrome.*

**avoidant d. of childhood or adolescence,** former name for a disorder that would now be included under the diagnosis of social phobia (DSM-IV).

**behavior d.,** conduct d.

**binge-eating d.,** an eating disorder characterized by repeated episodes of binge eating, as in bulimia nervosa, but not followed by inappropriate compensatory behavior such as purging, fasting, or excessive exercise.

**bipolar d's,** 1. [DSM-IV] mood disorders characterized by a history of manic, mixed, or hypomanic episodes, usually with concurrent or previous history of one or more major depressive episodes, including *bipolar I disorder, bipolar II disorder,* and *cyclothymic disorder.* Cf. *depressive d's.* 2. a term sometimes used in the singular to denote either *bipolar I d.* or *bipolar II d.,* or both.

**bipolar I d.** [DSM-IV], a type of bipolar disorder characterized by one or more manic or mixed episodes, often with a history of one or more major depressive episodes.

**bipolar II d.** [DSM-IV], a type of bipolar disorder characterized by one or more major depressive episodes accompanied by at least one hypomanic episode but without any manic or mixed episodes.

**body dysmorphic d.** [DSM-IV], a mental disorder in which a normal-appearing person is either preoccupied with some imagined defect in appearance or is overly concerned about some very slight physical anomaly.

**breathing-related sleep d.** [DSM-IV], any of several disorders characterized by sleep disruption due to some sleep-related breathing problem, resulting in excessive sleepiness or insomnia; included are central and obstructive sleep apnea syndromes (see *sleep apnea,* under *apnea*) and primary alveolar hypoventilation.

**brief psychotic d.** [DSM-IV], an episode of psychotic symptoms (incoherence, loosening of associations, delusions, hallucinations, disorganized or catatonic behavior) with sudden onset, lasting less than one month. If it occurs in response to a stressful life event, it may be called *brief reactive psychosis.*

**catatonic d.** [DSM-IV], catatonia due to the physiological effects of a general medical condition and neither better accounted for by another mental disorder nor occurring exclusively during delirium.

**character d's,** personality d's. See also *character.*

**childhood disintegrative d.** [DSM-IV], pervasive developmental disorder characterized by marked regression in a variety of skills, including language, social skills or adaptive behavior, play, bowel or bladder control, and motor skills, after at least two, but less than ten, years of apparently normal development.

**circadian rhythm sleep d.** [DSM-IV], a sleep disorder of the dyssomnia group, consisting of a lack of synchrony between the schedule of sleeping and waking required by the external environment and that of a person's own circadian rhythm. It usually has an environmental cause such as rotating shift work or long-distance air travel, although some individuals simply have natural circadian rhythms sharply different from the predominant one of their society.

**collagen d.,** any inborn error of metabolism involving abnormal structure or metabolism of collagen; the term includes Ehlers-Danlos syndrome, Marfan syndrome, cutis laxa, osteogenesis imperfecta, and epidermolysis bullosa. Collagen disorder is not to be confused with collagen disease (q.v.).

**communication d's** [DSM-IV], mental disorders characterized by difficulties in speech or language, severe enough to be a problem academically, occupationally, or socially; included are *expressive language disorder, mixed receptive-expressive language disorder, phonological disorder,* and *stuttering.*

**conduct d.** [DSM-IV], a type of disruptive behavior disorder of childhood and adolescence characterized by a persistent pattern of conduct in which rights of others or age-appropriate societal norms or rules are violated, with misconduct including aggression to people or animals, destruction of property, deceitfulness or theft, and serious violations of rules; it is classified as *childhood-onset* or *adolescent-onset* depending on whether the behavior begins before or after the age of ten.

**d. of consciousness,** a state of disordered attention and apperception, e.g., confusion or delirium.

**conversion d.** [DSM-IV], a mental disorder characterized by conversion symptoms (loss or alteration of voluntary motor or sensory functioning suggesting physical illness, such as seizures, paralysis, dyskinesia, anesthesia, blindness, or aphonia) having no demonstrable physiological basis and whose psychological basis is suggested by (1) exacerbation of symptoms at times of psychological stress, (2) relief from tension or inner conflicts (primary gain) provided by the symptoms, or (3) secondary gains (support, attention, avoidance of unpleasant responsibilities) provided by the symptoms. Many patients exhibit "la belle indifférence," a lack of concern about the impairment caused by the symptoms; histrionic personality traits are also common. Symptoms are neither intentionally produced nor feigned, and are not limited to pain or sexual dysfunction.

**cyclothymic d.** [DSM-IV], a mood disorder characterized by numerous alternating short cycles of hypomanic and depressive periods with symptoms like those of manic and major depressive episodes but of lesser severity. Called also *cyclothymia.*

**delusional d.** [DSM-IV], a mental disorder marked by well-organized, logically consistent delusions but lacking other psychotic symptoms. Most functioning is not markedly impaired, the criteria for schizophrenia have never been satisfied, and symptoms of a major mood disorder have been present only briefly if at all. DSM-IV distinguishes six types on the basis of the predominant delusional theme: persecutory, jealous, erotomanic, somatic, grandiose, and mixed.

**depersonalization d.** [DSM-IV], a dissociative disorder characterized by one or more severe episodes of depersonalization (feelings of unreality and strangeness in one's perception of the self or one's body image) not due to another mental disorder, such as schizophrenia. The perception of reality remains intact; patients are aware of their incapacitation. Episodes are usually accompanied by dizziness, anxiety, fears of going insane, and derealization.

**depressive d's** [DSM-IV], mood disorders in which depression is unaccompanied by manic or hypomanic episodes; e.g., major depressive disorder and dysthymic disorder. Cf. *bipolar d's.*

**developmental d's,** 1. developmental disabilities. 2. a former classification of chronic disorders of mental development with onset in childhood; such disorders are now classified as mental retardation, learning disorders, motor skills disorder, communication disorders, or pervasive developmental disorders.

**developmental coordination d.** [DSM-IV], problematic or delayed development of gross and fine motor coordination skills, not due to a neurological disorder or to general mental retardation; affected children appear to be clumsy rather than grossly impaired. It may persist into adulthood.

**disruptive behavior d's** [DSM-IV], a group of mental disorders of children and adolescents consisting of behavior that violates social norms, is disruptive, and may be illegal, often distressing others more than it does the person with the disorder. It includes *conduct disorder* and *oppositional defiant disorder* and is grouped with attention-deficit/hyperactivity disorder.

**dissociative d's** [DSM-IV], mental disorders characterized by sudden, temporary alterations in identity, memory, or consciousness, segregating normally integrated memories or parts of the personality from the dominant identity of the individual. This category includes *dissociative identity disorder, dissociative fugue, dissociative amnesia,* and *depersonalization disorder.*

**dissociative identity d.** [DSM-IV], a dissociative disorder characterized by the existence in an individual of two or more distinct personalities, each having unique memories, characteristic behavior, and social relationships. At least two of the personalities control the patient's behavior in turns, the transition often being abrupt. The host personality usually is totally unaware of the alternate personalities, experiencing only inexplicable gaps of time and inability to recall important personal information. Alternate personalities may or may not have awareness of the others. Called also *multiple personality d.*.

**dissociative trance d.,** a dissociative disorder characterized by an involuntary state of trance that is not a normal function of the person's cultural or religious practice and that causes impairment or distress.

**dream anxiety d.,** nightmare d.

**dysthymic d.** [DSM-IV], a mood disorder characterized by depressed feeling (sad, blue, low), loss of interest or pleasure in one's usual activities, and by at least some of the following: altered appetite, disturbed sleep patterns, lack of energy, low self esteem, poor concentration or decision-making skills, and feelings of hopelessness. Symptoms have persisted for more than two years but are not severe enough to meet the criteria for major depressive disorder.

**eating d.,** any of several disorders in which abnormal feeding habits are associated with psychological factors; in DSM-IV these include *anorexia nervosa, bulimia nervosa, pica,* and *rumination disorder.*

**emotional d.,** see under *illness.*

**expressive language d.** [DSM-IV], a communication disorder occurring in children and characterized by problems with the expression of language, either oral or signed. It includes difficulties such as limited speech or vocabulary, vocabulary errors, difficulty or hesitation in word selection, oversimplification of grammatical or sentence structure, omission of parts of sentences, unusual word order, and slowed acquisition of language skills. Two types are recognized, *acquired* and *developmental.*

**factitious d.** [DSM-IV], a mental disorder characterized by repeated, intentional simulation of physical or psychological signs and symptoms of illness for no apparent purpose other than obtaining treatment. It differs from malingering in that there is no recognizable motive for feigning illness. It is subtyped on the basis of whether the predominant signs and symptoms are physical (called also *Munchausen syndrome*), psychological, or both.

**factitious d. by proxy,** a form of factitious disorder in which one person intentionally fabricates or induces signs and symptoms of one or more physical *(Munchausen syndrome by proxy)* or psychological disorders in another person under their care and subjects that person to needless and sometimes dangerous or disfiguring diagnostic procedures or treatment, without any external incentives for the behavior. The dyad is usually that of mother and child.

**female orgasmic d.** [DSM-IV], a sexual dysfunction characterized by consistently delayed or absent orgasm in a female, even after a normal phase of sexual excitement and accounting for her age and sexual experience and the amount of stimulation, and causing significant distress or interpersonal difficulty.

**female sexual arousal d.** [DSM-IV], a sexual dysfunction involving failure by a female either to attain or maintain the lubrication and swelling response of sexual excitement during sexual activity, after adequate stimulation, causing significant distress or interpersonal difficulty. Both physiological and psychological factors may be involved. Formerly called *frigidity.* Cf. *male erectile d.*

**formal thought d.,** disturbance in the form, rather than the content, of thought; disruption in the flow of ideas or speech; inability to follow the normal semantic or syntactic rules in someone with adequate intelligence and education and the cultural background to do so.

**functional d.,** a disorder of physiological function having no known organic basis. Although not strictly correct, the term is often used in psychiatry as roughly equivalent to "psychogenic disorder"; in other branches of medicine, to "idiopathic disorder."

**gender identity d.** [DSM-IV], a disturbance of gender identification in which the affected person has an overwhelming desire to change their anatomic sex or insists that they are of the opposite sex, with persistent discomfort about their assigned sex or about filling its usual gender role; the disorder may become apparent in childhood or not appear until adolescence or adulthood. Individuals may attempt to live as members of the opposite sex and may seek hormonal and surgical treatment to bring their anatomy into conformity with their belief. Cf. *transvestism.*

**generalized anxiety d. (GAD)** [DSM-IV], an anxiety disorder characterized by the presence of excessive, uncontrollable anxiety and worry about two or more life circumstances, for six months or longer, accompanied by some combination of restlessness, fatigue, muscle tension, irritability, disturbed concentration or sleep, and somatic symptoms.

**genetic d.,** see under *disease.*

**hypoactive sexual desire d.** [DSM-IV], a sexual dysfunction consisting of persistently or recurrently low level or absence of sexual fantasies and desire for sexual activity, causing pronounced distress or interpersonal difficulties.

**identity d.,** former name for a disorder of adolescence that was defined as severe subjective distress about inability to reconcile aspects of the self into a relatively coherent whole and acceptable sense of self, with uncertainty about many social, academic, career, and moral choices. Lacking in substantiation, the disorder is no longer officially recognized, but similar uncertainty on multiple issues may be labeled as identity problem.

**impulse control d's** [DSM-IV], a group of mental disorders characterized by repeated failure to resist an impulse to perform some act harmful to oneself or to others. The person feels tension or an irresistible urge to perform the act which, even though ego-dystonic, gives pleasure or emotional release upon performance.

**induced psychotic d.,** shared psychotic d.

**intermittent explosive d.** [DSM-IV], an impulse control disorder characterized by multiple discrete episodes of loss of control of aggressive impulses resulting in serious assault or destruction of property that are out of proportion to any precipitating stressors; behavior in between such episodes lacks impulsiveness or aggressiveness.

**isolated explosive d.,** a former classification used to denote a single violent catastrophic act performed for no apparent reason and not attributable to any other disorder.

**late luteal phase dysphoric d.,** former name for *premenstrual dysphoric d.*

**LDL-receptor d.,** familial hypercholesterolemia.

**learning d's** [DSM-IV], a group of disorders characterized by academic functioning that is substantially below the level expected on the basis of the patient's age, intelligence, and education, interfering with academic achievement or other functioning. Included are *reading disorder, mathematics disorder,* and *disorder of written expression.*

**lymphoproliferative d's,** a group of malignant neoplasms arising from cells related to the common multipotential, primitive lymphoreticular cell that includes among others the lymphocytic, histiocytic, and monocytic leukemias, multiple myeloma, plasmacytoma, Hodgkin's disease, all lymphocytic lymphomas, and immunosecretory disorders associated with monoclonal gammopathy. An interrelationship with the myeloproliferative disorders (q.v.) is thought to exist. Called also *lymphoproliferative diseases* or *syndromes.*

**lymphoreticular d's,** a group of disorders of the lymphoreticular system, characterized by the proliferation of lymphocytes or lymphoid tissues; they may be either benign (e.g., lymphocytosis) or malignant (e.g., lymphocytic leukemias, multiple myeloma, or non-Hodgkin's lymphomas). See also *lymphoproliferative d's.* Called also *lymphoreticular diseases* or *syndromes.*

**major depressive d.** [DSM-IV], a mood disorder characterized by the occurrence of one or more major depressive episodes (q.v.) and the absence of any history of manic, mixed, or hypomanic episodes.

**major mood d's,** severe, full-blown mood disorders; e.g., major depressive disorder and bipolar I and II disorders.

**male erectile d.** [DSM-IV], a sexual dysfunction involving failure by a male to attain or maintain erection until completion of sexual relations, causing significant distress or interpersonal difficulty. Called also *psychogenic impotence.* Cf. *female sexual arousal d.*

**male orgasmic d.** [DSM-IV], a sexual dysfunction characterized by consistently delayed or absent orgasm in a male, even after a normal phase of sexual excitement and stimulation that is adequate for his age in focus, duration, and intensity, and which causes significant distress or interpersonal difficulty.

**manic-depressive d.,** former name for *bipolar d.*; see *bipolar d's* (def. 2).

**mathematics d.** [DSM-IV], a learning disorder (q.v.) in which the skill affected is mathematical calculation or reasoning.

**mendelian d.,** a genetic disease, showing a mendelian pattern of inheritance, and caused by a single mutation in the structure of DNA, which causes a single basic defect that has some pathological consequence or consequences. Called also *monogenic* or *single-gene d.* See also *inborn error of metabolism,* under *metabolism.*

**mental d.** [DSM-IV], any clinically significant behavioral or psychological syndrome characterized by the presence of distressing symptoms, impairment of functioning, or significantly increased risk of suffering death, pain, disability, or loss of freedom. Mental disorders are assumed to be the manifestation of a behavioral, psychological, or biological dysfunction in the individual. The concept does not include deviant behavior, disturbances that are essentially conflicts between the individual and society, or expected and culturally sanctioned responses to particular events.

**minor depressive d.** [DSM-IV], a mood disorder resembling closely major depressive disorder and dysthymic disorder but with symptoms intermediate in severity between the two and a course less protracted than that of dysthymic disorder.

**mixed anxiety-depressive d.,** a mental disorder characterized by symptoms of depression and of anxiety, but not meeting the full criteria for either a depressive disorder or an anxiety disorder.

**mixed receptive-expressive language d.** [DSM-IV], a communication disorder involving both the expression and the comprehension of language, either spoken or signed.Patients have difficulties with language production, such as in the selection of words and the creation of appropriate sentences, and also have trouble understanding words, sentences, or specific types of words.

**monogenic d.,** mendelian d.

**mood d's** [DSM-IV], mental disorders whose essential feature is a disturbance of mood manifested as one or more episodes of mania, hypomania, depression, or some combination. Functional mood disorders are subclassified as *bipolar disorders,* including bipolar I disorder, bipolar II disorder, and cyclothymic disorder; *depressive disorders,* including major depressive disorder and dysthymic disorder; *mood disorder due to a general medical condition*; and *substance-induced mood disorder.*

**motor skills d.** [DSM-IV], any disorder characterized by inadequate development of motor coordination severe enough to limit locomotion or restrict the ability to perform tasks, schoolwork, or other activities. Included is *developmental coordination d.*

**multifactorial d.,** a disorder caused by interaction of genetic factors and perhaps also nongenetic, environmental factors, e.g., some forms of birth defects and diabetes mellitus. See also *genetic disease,* under *disease.*

**multiple personality d.,** dissociative identity d.

**myeloproliferative d's,** a group of usually neoplastic diseases, which may be related histogenetically by a common multipotential stem cell, that includes among others acute and chronic granulocytic leukemias, acute and chronic myelomonocytic leukemias, polycythemia vera, and myelofibroerythroleukemia. An interrelationship with the lymphoproliferative disorders is thought to exist. Called also *myeloproliferative diseases* or *syndromes.*

**neurotic d.,** neurosis.

**nightmare d.** [DSM-IV], a sleep disorder of the parasomnia group, consisting of repeated episodes of nightmares that awaken the sleeper, who rapidly becomes fully oriented and alert and can vividly recall the dreams. Onset is usually in childhood or adolescence, and children often outgrow the disorder. Called also *dream anxiety d.*

**obsessive-compulsive d. (OCD)** [DSM-IV], an anxiety disorder characterized by recurrent obsessions or compulsions, which are severe enough to interfere significantly with personal or social functioning. Performing compulsive rituals may release tension temporarily, and resisting them causes increased tension. This disorder is not the same as *obsessive-compulsive personality d.,* which is a personality disorder.

**obsessive-compulsive personality d.** [DSM-IV], see under *personality.*

**oppositional defiant d.** [DSM-IV], a type of disruptive behavior disorder characterized by a recurrent pattern of defiant, hostile, disobedient, and negativistic behavior directed toward those in authority, including such actions as defying the requests or rules of adults, deliberately annoying others, arguing, spitefulness, and vindictiveness that occur much more frequently than would be expected on the basis of age and developmental stage.

**organic anxiety d.,** see under *syndrome.*

**organic mental d.,** a term formerly used to denote any mental disorder with a specifically known or presumed organic etiology; now discouraged because of the implication that other mental disorders do not have an organic basis. The term was also sometimes used to denote an organic mental syndrome (q.v.). Current classification divides these disorders into *delirium, dementia, and amnestic and other* *cognitive disorders; mental disorders due to a general medical condition;* and *substance-related disorders.*

**organic personality d.,** see under *syndrome.*

**orgasmic d's** [DSM-IV], sexual dysfunctions characterized by inhibited or premature orgasm; see *female orgasmic d., male orgasmic d.,* and *premature ejaculation.*

**overanxious d.,** former name for an anxiety disorder of childhood or adolescence, now subsumed by *generalized anxiety d.*.

**pain d.** [DSM-IV], a somatoform disorder characterized by a chief complaint of severe chronic pain that causes substantial distress or impairment in functioning; the pain is neither feigned nor intentionally produced, and psychological factors appear to play a major role in its onset, severity, exacerbation, or maintenance. It is subdivided into *pain d. associated with psychological factors* and *pain d. associated with both psychological factors and a general medical condition.* A third subtype, *pain d. associated with a general medical condition,* is not considered a mental disorder.

**panic d.** [DSM-IV], an anxiety disorder characterized by recurrent panic (anxiety) attacks, episodes of intense apprehension, fear, or terror associated with somatic symptoms such as dyspnea, palpitations, dizziness, vertigo, faintness, or shakiness and with psychological symptoms such as feelings of unreality (depersonalization or derealization) or fears of dying, going crazy, or losing control; there is usually chronic nervousness and tension between attacks. It is almost always associated with agoraphobia. (DSM-IV recognizes two types, *panic d. with agoraphobia* and *panic d. without agoraphobia.*) This disorder does not include panic attacks that may occur in phobias when the patient is exposed to the phobic stimulus.

**paranoid d.,** older term for *delusional d.*

**periodic limb movement d.,** nocturnal myoclonus.

**personality d's** [DSM-IV], a category of mental disorders characterized by enduring, inflexible, and maladaptive personality traits that deviate markedly from cultural expectations, are self-perpetuating, pervade a broad range of situations, and either generate subjective distress or result in significant impairments in social, occupational, or other functioning. Onset is by adolescence or early adulthood. For specific disorders, see under *personality.*

**pervasive developmental d's** [DSM-IV], a group of disorders characterized by impairment of development in multiple areas, including the acquisition of reciprocal social interaction, verbal and nonverbal communication skills, and imaginative activity and by stereotyped interests and behaviors; included are *autistic disorder, Rett syndrome, childhood disintegrative disorder,* and *Asperger's syndrome.*

**phagocytic dysfunction d's,** a group of immunodeficiency conditions characterized by disordered phagocytic activity; disorders may be *extrinsic* (e.g. suppression of the number of phagocytes by immunosuppressive agents, or dysfunction caused by corticosteroids) or *intrinsic* (related to enzyme deficiencies). They are marked by bacterial or fungal infections that range from mild recurrent skin infection to fatal systemic infection. For a list of disorders of this type, see table at *immunodeficiency.*

**phobic d's,** see *phobia.*

**phonological d.** [DSM-IV], a communication disorder of unknown etiology, characterized by failure to use age- and dialect-appropriate sounds in speaking, with errors occurring in the selection, production, or articulation of sounds. The most common errors are omissions, substitutions, and distortions of speech sounds.

**plasma cell d's,** see under *dyscrasia.*

**postconcussional d.,** see under *syndrome.*

**posttraumatic stress d. (PTSD)** [DSM-IV], an anxiety disorder caused by exposure to an intensely traumatic event; characterized by reexperiencing the traumatic event in recurrent intrusive recollections, nightmares, or flashbacks, by avoidance of trauma-associated stimuli, by generalized numbing of emotional responsiveness, and by hyperalertness and difficulty in sleeping, remembering, or concentrating. The onset of symptoms may be delayed for months to years after the event. Terms formerly used for disorders of this type include *gross stress reaction, shell shock,* and *combat* (or *battle* or *war*) *exhaustion, fatigue,* or *neurosis.*

**premenstrual dysphoric d.,** premenstrual syndrome viewed as a psychiatric disorder.

**primary mental d.** [DSM-IV], any of the mental disorders that are neither due to a general medical condition nor substance-induced.

**psychoactive substance–induced organic mental d's,** former name for *substance-induced d's.*

**psychoactive substance use d's,** substance use d's.

**psychogenic pain d.,** pain d.

**psychophysiologic d.,** psychosomatic d.

**psychosexual d's,** sexual d's (def. 2).

**psychosomatic d.,** a disorder in which the physical symptoms are caused or exacerbated by psychological factors, such as migraine headache, lower back pain, or irritable bowel syndrome. The synonym *psychophysiologic disorders,* used in previous official nomenclatures and defined as "physical disorders of presumably psychogenic origin," has been replaced in DSM-IV by the more neutral phrase *psychological factors affecting physical condition,* which may be applied to any physical condition judged to be adversely affected by one or more psychological or behavioral factors, and is subtyped on the basis of the specific factors involved.

**psychotic d.** [DSM-IV], psychosis (def. 1).

**rapid eye movement sleep behavior d.,** REM sleep behavior d.

**reactive attachment d.** [DSM-IV], a mental disorder of infancy or early childhood, characterized by notably unusual and developmentally inappropriate social relatedness, usually associated with grossly pathological care. It may be the *inhibited type,* with failure to initiate or respond to social interactions, or the *disinhibited type,* with indiscriminate sociability or attachment.

**reading d.** [DSM-IV], a learning disorder (q.v.) in which the skill affected is reading ability, including accuracy, speed, and comprehension.

**recurrent brief depressive d.,** short repeated episodes of depressive symptoms severe enough to qualify as major depressive episodes but of lesser duration, recurring at least once a month and not associated with the menstrual cycle.

**REM sleep behavior d. (RBD),** a sleep disorder of the parasomnia group characterized by abnormal electromyographic activity, altered dreams, and violent behaviors, often leading to self-injury, during REM sleep.

**rhythmic movement d.,** repetitive, rhythmic, stereotyped, large-muscle body or head movements occurring during the transition to sleep, such as in jactatio capitis nocturna; onset is usually in infancy and the disorder is usually outgrown by the age of five.

**rumination d.** [DSM-IV], an eating disorder seen in infants under one year of age; after a period of normal eating habits, the child begins excessive regurgitation and rechewing of food, which is then ejected from the mouth or reswallowed; if untreated, death from malnutrition may occur.

**schizoaffective d.** [DSM-IV], a mental disorder in which a major depressive episode, manic episode, or mixed episode occurs along with prominent psychotic symptoms characteristic of schizophrenia, the symptoms of the mood disorder being present for a substantial portion of the illness, but not for its entirety, and the disturbance not being due to the effects of a psychoactive substance.

**schizophreniform d.** [DSM-IV], a mental disorder with the signs and symptoms of schizophrenia but duration of less than 6 months.

**seasonal affective d. (SAD),** a cyclically recurring mood disorder characterized by depression, extreme lethargy, increased need for sleep, hyperphagia, and carbohydrate craving; it intensifies in one or more specific seasons, most commonly the winter months, and is hypothesized to be related to melatonin levels. In DSM-IV terminology called *mood disorder with seasonal pattern.*

**seasonal mood d.,** seasonal affective d.

**separation anxiety d.** [DSM-IV], excessive, prolonged, developmentally inappropriate anxiety and apprehension in a child concerning removal from parents, home, or familiar surroundings.

**sexual d's,** 1. any disorders involving sexual functioning, desire, or performance. 2. [DSM-IV] more specifically, any such disorders that are caused at least in part by psychological factors. Those characterized by decrease or other disturbance of sexual desire are called sexual dysfunctions, and those characterized by unusual or bizarre sexual fantasies, urges, or practices are called paraphilias. Called also *psychosexual d's.*

**sexual arousal d's** [DSM-IV], sexual dysfunctions characterized by alterations in sexual arousal; see *female sexual arousal d.* and *male erectile d.*

**sexual aversion d.** [DSM-IV], feelings of repugnance for and active avoidance of genital sexual contact with a partner, causing substantial distress or interpersonal difficulty.

**sexual desire d's** [DSM-IV], sexual dysfunctions characterized by alteration in sexual desire; see *hypoactive sexual desire d.* and *sexual aversion d.*

**sexual pain d's** [DSM-IV], sexual dysfunctions characterized by pain associated with intercourse; they include dyspareunia and vaginismus not due to a general medical condition.

**shared psychotic d.** [DSM-IV], a delusional system that develops in one or more persons as a result of a close relationship with someone who already has a psychotic disorder with prominent delusions. Most commonly it involves two people and is called *folie à deux.* Involvement of three people would be *folie à trois* and so on.

**simple deteriorative d.,** simple schizophrenia.

**single-gene d.,** mendelian d.

**sleep d's** [DSM-IV], chronic disorders involving sleep. Primary sleep disorders comprise dyssomnias and parasomnias; causes of secondary sleep disorders may include a general medical condition, mental disorder, or psychoactive substance.

**sleep terror d.** [DSM-IV], a sleep disorder of the parasomnia group, consisting of repeated episodes of pavor nocturnus (sleep terrors).

**sleep-wake schedule d.,** circadian rhythm sleep d.

**sleepwalking d.** [DSM-IV], a sleep disorder of the parasomnia group, consisting of repeated episodes of somnambulism.

**somatization d.** [DSM-IV], a mental disorder characterized by multiple somatic complaints that cannot be fully explained by any known general medical condition or the direct effect of a substance, but are not intentionally feigned or produced, beginning before the age of 30 and occurring over several years. Complaints comprise a combination of at least multiple pain symptoms, multiple gastrointestinal symptoms, a sexual symptom, and a neurological symptom. They are often presented in a dramatic, vague, or exaggerated way; many physicians become involved in the medical care; and numerous diagnostic evaluations and unnecessary medical treatment or surgery may be performed. Called also *Briquet's syndrome.*

**somatoform d's** [DSM-IV], mental disorders characterized by symptoms suggesting a general medical condition but neither fully explained by a general medical condition, the direct effects of a psychoactive substance, or another mental disorder nor under voluntary control; this category includes *body dysmorphic disorder, conversion disorder, hypochondriasis, pain disorder, somatization disorder,* and *undifferentiated somatoform disorder.*

**somatoform pain d.,** pain d.

**speech d.,** defective ability to speak; it may be either psychogenic (see *communication d.*) or neurogenic. See also *aphasia, aphonia, dysphasia,* and *dysphonia.* Called also *lalopathy* and *logopathy.*

**stereotypic movement d.** [DSM-IV], a mental disorder characterized by repetitive nonfunctional motor behavior, such as hand waving, rocking, head-banging, or self-biting, which often appears to be driven and can result in serious self-inflicted injuries.

**substance-induced d's** [DSM-IV], a subgroup of the substance-related disorders comprising a variety of behavioral or psychological anomalies resulting from ingestion of or exposure to a drug of abuse, medication, or toxin. Included are *substance intoxication, substance withdrawal, substance-induced delirium, substance-induced persisting dementia, substance-induced persisting amnestic disorder, substance-induced psychotic disorder, substance-induced mood disorder, substance-induced anxiety disorder, substance-induced sexual dysfunction,* and *substance-induced sleep disorder.* Specific disorders or groups are named on the basis of etiology, e.g., alcohol-induced disorders, alcohol intoxication. Cf. *substance use d's.*

**substance-induced anxiety d.** [DSM-IV], an anxiety disorder characterized by prominent anxiety, panic attacks, obsessions, or compulsions and directly due to the physiological effects of a psychogenic substance, including drugs of abuse, medications, and toxins. Individual cases are named for the specific substance involved.

**substance-induced mood d.** [DSM-IV], a prominent and lasting disturbance of mood, either manic, depressive, or both, due to direct physiological effects of a psychoactive substance, including medications, drugs of abuse, and toxins. Individual cases are named for the specific substance involved.

**substance-induced persisting amnestic d.** [DSM-IV], an amnestic disorder caused by the lasting effects of a drug of abuse, medication, or toxic substance, often remaining stable or even worsening long after exposure to the substance has ended. Individual cases are named for the specific substance involved.

**substance-induced psychotic d.** [DSM-IV], persistent delusions or hallucinations related to the use of a psychoactive substance, the patient being unaware of their etiology. Individual cases are named for the specific substance involved.

**substance-induced sleep d.** [DSM-IV], a disturbance of sleep due to the direct physiological effects of a psychoactive substance, including drugs of abuse, medications, and toxins; usually manifest as hypersomnia or insomnia but sometimes as a parasomnia or of mixed type. Individual disorders are named for the specific substance involved.

**substance-related d's** [DSM-IV], any of the mental disorders associated with excessive use of or exposure to psychoactive substances, including drugs of abuse, medications, and toxins. The group is divided into *substance use disorders* and *substance-induced disorders,* each of which is specified on the basis of etiology, e.g., alcohol use disorders. DSM-IV includes specific disorders for the classes alcohol, amphetamines or similarly acting sympathomimetics, caffeine, cannabis, cocaine, hallucinogens, inhalants, nicotine, opioids, PCP or similarly acting substances, and sedatives, hypnotics, or anxiolytics.

**substance use d's** [DSM-IV], a subgroup of the substance-related disorders (q.v.) in which psychoactive substance use or abuse repeatedly results in significantly adverse consequences. The group comprises *substance abuse* and *substance dependence*; specific disorders or groups of disorders are named on the basis of etiology, e.g., alcohol use disorders, alcohol abuse, and alcohol dependence.

**thought d.,** a disturbance in the thought process that is most narrowly defined as disorganized thinking with altered associations, as is characteristic of schizophrenia. The term is often used much more broadly to include any disturbance of thought, such as confusion, hallucinations, or delusions, which affects possession, quantity, or content of thought.

**undifferentiated somatoform d.** [DSM-IV], one or more physical complaints, not intentionally produced or feigned and persisting for at least six months, that cannot be fully explained by a general medical condition or the direct effects of a substance; the category comprises persisting disorders that do not completely satisfy the criteria for other somatoform disorders.

**unipolar d's,** depressive d's.

**d. of written expression** [DSM-IV], a learning disorder (q.v.) in which the affected skill is written communication, characterized by errors in spelling, grammar, or punctuation, by poor paragraph organization, or by poor story composition or thematic development.

---

**dis·or·gan·iza·tion** (dis-or″gən-ĭ-za′shən) the process of destruction of any organic tissue; any profound change in the tissues of an organ or structure which causes the loss of most or all of its proper characters.

**dis·or·i·en·ta·tion** (dis-or″e-ən-ta′shən) the loss of proper bearings, or a state of mental confusion as to time, place, or identity.

**spatial d.,** a condition in which a pilot or other air crew member is unable to determine accurately his spatial attitude in relation to the surface of the earth; it occurs only in conditions of poor visibility or when vision is otherwise restricted and results from vestibular illusions. Called also *pilot's vertigo.*

**dis·ox·i·da·tion** (dis″ok-sĭ-da′shən) deoxidation.

**dis·par** (dis′pahr) [L.] unequal.

**dis·par·a·si·tized** (dis-par′ə-sĭ-tīzd) freed from parasites. Cf. *disinfestation.*

**dis·pa·rate** (dis′pə-rāt) [L. *disparatus, dispar* unequal] not situated alike; not exactly paired; dissimilar in kind.

**dis·pen·sa·ry** (dis-pen′sə-re) [L. *dispensarium,* from *dispensare* to dispense] 1. a place where medical or dental skill, treatment, and remedies are provided for the indigent ambulant sick at little or no cost to them. 2. any place where drugs and medicines are actually dispensed.

**dis·pen·sa·to·ry** (dis-pen′sə-tor-e) [L. *dispensatorium*] [MeSH: Dispensatories] a treatise on the qualities and composition of medicines.

**D. of the United States of America,** a collection of monographs on unofficial drugs and drugs recognized by the United States Pharmacopoeia, the British Pharmacopoeia, and the National Formulary, and on general tests, processes, reagents, and solutions of the USP and NF, as well as drugs used in veterinary medicine.

**dis·pense** (dis-pens′) [L. *dispensare, dis-* out + *pensare* to weigh] to prepare and distribute medicines to those who are to use them.

**di·sper·my** (di′spər-me) the penetration of two sperms or spermatozoa into one oocyte.

**dis·per·sate** (dis′pər-sāt) a suspension of finely divided particles of a substance.

**dis·perse** (dis-pərs′) [*dis-*[1] + L. *spargere* to scatter] to scatter the component parts, as of a tumor or the fine particles in a colloid system; also the particles so dispersed.

**dis·per·si·ble** (dis-pər′sĭ-bəl) capable of being dispersed.

**dis·per·sion** (dis-pər′zhən) [L. *dispersio*] 1. the act of scattering or separating; the condition of being scattered. 2. the incorporation of the particles of one substance into the body of another, comprising solutions, suspensions, and colloid systems. 3. a colloid system, particularly an unstable one.

**colloid d.,** colloid system; see *colloid,* def. 2. Sometimes used specifically for an unstable colloid system.

**molecular d.,** solution, def. 1.

**temporal d.,** desynchronization of components of an evoked compound action potential as registered by the recording electrode, due to different rates of conduction of the fibers.

**dis·per·si·ty** (dis-pər'sĭ-te) the degree of dispersion of a colloid, i.e., the degree to which the dimensions of the disperse particles have been reduced.

**dis·per·soid** (dis-pər'soid) dispersion colloid.

**dis·pert** (dis'pərt) a medicinal preparation obtained from a vegetable drug or endocrine gland by extracting its therapeutic constituents in the cold and then reducing the product to a dry concentrated form.

**Dis·phol·i·dus** (dis-fol'ĭ-dəs) a genus of venomous snakes of the family Colubridae. *D. ty'pus* is the boomslang of South Africa. See table at *snake.*

**di·spi·ra** (di-spi'rə) [*di-* + Gr. *speira* coil] dispireme.

**di·spi·reme** (di-spi'rem, di-spi'rēm) [*di-* + *spireme*] the stage of cell division which follows the diaster; so called because the cytoplasm is divided into two parts, in each of which the chromatin appears to assume the form of a coil. See *mitosis.*

**dis·place·a·bil·i·ty** (dis-plās"ə-bil'ĭ-te) the quality of being susceptible to movement from an initial position, or the degree to which such movement is possible.

**dis·place·ment** (dis-plās'mənt) 1. malposition. 2. percolation. 3. a defense mechanism in which emotions, ideas, wishes, or impulses are unconsciously shifted from their original object to a more acceptable, usually less threatening, substitute. 4. in dentistry, the malposition of the crown and root of one or more teeth from the normal line of occlusion; also the deflection of the mandible from its normal path of closure, i.e., posterior displacement. 5. in a chemical reaction, the replacement of one atom or group in a molecule by another.

**character d.,** the adaptive characters that evolve and enable one species to exclude another from its ecological niche. See also *competitive exclusion,* under *exclusion.*

**condylar d.,** an abnormal position of the head of the mandibular condyle in the fossa due to a deviation or shift of the mandible, which is often the result of malocclusion.

**fetal d.,** a group of cells which, during fetal development, has become displaced from its normal relations.

**fish-hook d.,** a form of displacement of the stomach in which the orifice of the pylorus faces directly upward, and the duodenum runs upward and to the right to join the pylorus at an angle, producing a constricting hook; there is no evidence that such displacement causes symptoms.

**gallbladder d.,** wandering gallbladder.

**left d. of the abomasum,** LDA; displacement of the abomasum of a cow to the left, underneath the rumen, with abomasal atony, usually soon after birth of a calf. It may be due to previous pressure from the gravid uterus or to abomasal distention from a high-grain diet. Symptoms include anorexia, drop in milk production, and ketosis.

**right d. of the abomasum,** RDA; displacement of the abomasum of a cow to the right, with abomasal atony, usually soon after birth of a calf; it is sometimes due to obstruction of the pylorus. Symptoms include anorexia, drop in milk production, and a palpable fluid-filled organ on the right flank. It may progress to abomasal torsion, an emergency situation.

**tissue d.,** change in the position of tissues as the result of pressure or other force.

**di·spore** (di'spor) in fungi, either of the spores of a two-spored basidium; cf. *tetraspore.*

**di·spo·rous** (di'spor-əs) having two spores, as the basidia of the higher fungi.

**dis·po·si·tion** (dis"pə-zĭsh'ən) 1. a tendency, physical or mental, toward a disease. 2. the prevailing temperament or character, giving a degree of predictability to the response to a situation or other stimulus.

**dis·pro·por·tion** (dis"pro-por'shən) a lack of the proper relationship between two elements or factors.

**cephalopelvic d.,** a condition in which the head of the fetus is too large to permit passage through the pelvis of the mother.

**dis·rup·tion** (dis-rup'shən) [L. *diruptio* a bursting apart] a morphologic defect of an organ or larger region of the body, resulting from the extrinsic breakdown of, or interference with, an originally normal developmental process.

**dis·rup·tive** (dis-rup'tiv) bursting apart; rending.

**Dis·se's spaces** (dis'əz) [Joseph *Disse,* German anatomist, 1852–1912] see under *space.*

**dis·sect** (dĭ-sekt', di-sekt') [L. *dissecare* to cut up] 1. to cut apart or separate, as by surgery or trauma. 2. to expose structures of a cadaver for anatomical study.

**dis·sec·tion** (dĭ-sek'shən) [L. *dissectio*] [MeSH: Dissection] 1. the act of dissecting. 2. a part or whole of an organism prepared by dissecting.

**aortic d.,** dissecting aneurysm affecting the aorta, usually the thoracic aorta but sometimes the abdominal aorta.

**axillary d., axillary lymph node d.,** surgical removal of axillary lymph nodes, done as part of radical mastectomy.

**blunt d.,** dissection accomplished by separating tissues along natural cleavage lines, without cutting.

**lymph node d.,** lymphadenectomy.

**radical neck d.,** resection of a tumor in the neck along with an additional margin of at least 2 cm, as well as cervical lymphadenectomy.

**sharp d.,** dissection accomplished by incising tissues with a sharp edge.

**dis·sec·tor** (dĭ-sek'tor) 1. one who dissects. 2. a handbook used as a guide for the act of dissecting.

**ultrasonic d.,** an instrument with a metal tip that vibrates at ultrasonic frequency and fragments parenchymal cells while leaving vessels intact. Cf. *CUSA.*

**water-jet d.,** an instrument consisting of a nozzle that projects a fine stream of water under high pressure and a suction tube, used in hepatic resection to fragment liver parenchyma while sparing the hepatic vessels.

**dis·sem·i·nat·ed** (dĭ-sem'ĭ-nāt"əd) [*dis-* + *seminare* to sow] scattered; distributed over a considerable area.

**dis·sep·i·ment** (dĭ-sep'ĭ-mənt) partition; separation.

**dis·sim·i·late** (dĭ-sim'ĭ-lāt) [*dis-*[1] + *similare* to make alike] to decompose a substance into simpler compounds, for the production of energy or of materials that can be eliminated.

**dis·sim·i·la·tion** (dĭ-sim"ĭ-la'shən) the act or process of dissimilating (see *dissimilate*); the reverse of assimilation.

**dis·so·ci·able** (dĭ-so'shə-bəl) easily separable into component parts; separable from associations.

**dis·so·ci·a·tion** (dĭ-so"she-a'shən) [*dis-*[1] + *sociatio* union] 1. the act of separating or state of being separated. 2. the separation of a molecule into two or more fragments (atoms, molecules, ions, or free radicals) produced by the absorption of light or thermal energy or by solvation. 3. segregation of a group of mental processes from the rest of a person's usually integrated functions of consciousness, memory, perception, and sensory and motor behavior, as in the separation of the personality and aspects of memory or subpersonalities in the dissociative disorders (q.v.) or in the segregation of an idea or object from its emotional significance, as is sometimes seen in schizophrenia.

**albuminocytologic d.,** increase of protein with normal cell count in the spinal fluid.

**atrial d.,** independent beating of the left and right atria, each with normal rhythm or with various combinations of normal rhythm, atrial flutter, or atrial fibrillation.

**atrioventricular (AV) d.,** control of the atria by one pacemaker and of the ventricles by another, independent pacemaker; it may be due to heart block, to severe slowing of the sinus rhythm with activation of an ectopic pacemaker, to acceleration of an ectopic pacemaker that usurps control of the ventricles, or to a combination of factors. See also *interference atrioventricular d.* and *isorhythmic atrioventricular d.*

**bacterial d.,** the change, due to mutation and selection, in colonial morphology (usually from mucoid or smooth to rough) of bacteria in culture on laboratory media; called also *microbic d.* See also *smooth-rough variation,* under *variation.*

**electromechanical d.,** continued electrical rhythmicity of the heart in the absence of effective mechanical function; it may be due to uncoupling of ventricular muscle contraction from electrical activity or may be secondary to a disorder that causes cessation of cardiac venous return.

**interference d., interference atrioventricular d.,** a form of atrioventricular dissociation in which an accelerated junctional or ventricular pacemaker usurps control of the ventricles and rapidly bombards the atrioventricular node from below, rendering the node refractory to supraventricular impulses.

**isorhythmic atrioventricular d.,** a form of atrioventricular dissociation in which the atria and ventricles beat at similar rates, although independently; it usually results from severe sinus bradycardia in which the sinus node discharge rate drops just below that of the atrioventricular junctional tissue.

**microbic d.,** bacterial d.

**syringomyelic d.,** loss of pain and temperature sense due to a lesion in the region of the central canal of the spinal cord implicating the spinothalamic fibers with preservation of other sensory modalities.

**tabetic d.,** disturbance of the vibratory and muscle-tendon sensibility due to lesion of the dorsal columns.

**dis·sog·e·ny** (dĭ-soj'ə-ne) [Gr. *dissos* twofold + *-geny*] the state of having sexual maturity in both a larval and an adult stage.

**dis·so·lu·tion** (dĭ″so-loo′shən) [L. *dissolvere* to dissolve] 1. the process in which one substance is dissolved in another. 2. separation of a compound into its components by chemical action. 3. liquefaction. 4. the process of loosening, or of relaxing. 5. death.

**dis·solve** (dĭ-zolv′) 1. to cause a substance to pass into solution. 2. to pass into solution.

**dis·sol·vent** (dĭ-zol′vənt) 1. a solvent medium. 2. a medicine capable of dissolving concretions within the body. 3. solvent; capable of dissolving substances.

**dis·so·nance** (dis′o-nəns) discord or disagreement.
**cognitive d.**, anxiety or other unpleasant feelings resulting from a lack of agreement between a person's established ideas, beliefs, and attitudes and some more recently acquired information or experience.

**Dist.** abbreviation for L. *distil′la,* distil.

**dis·tad** (dis′tad) in a distal direction.

**dis·tal** (dis′təl) [L. *distans* distant] remote; farther from any point of reference; opposed to proximal. In dentistry, used to designate a position on the dental arch farther from the median line of the jaw. Symbol D.

**dis·ta·lis** (dis-ta′lis) [TA] distal; a term denoting remoteness from the point of origin or attachment of an organ or part.

**dis·tal·ly** (dis′tə-le) in a distal direction.

**dis·tance** (dis′təns) the measure of space intervening between two objects or two points of reference.
**angular d.**, the aperture of the angle made at the eye by lines drawn from the eye to two objects.
**focal d.**, the distance from the focal point to the optical center of a lens or the surface of a concave mirror.
**infinite d.**, in ophthalmology, a distance of 20 feet or more: so called because rays entering the eye from an object at that distance are practically as parallel as if they came from a point at an infinite distance.
**interarch d.**, 1. the vertical distance between the maxillary and mandibular arches (alveolar or residual) under certain conditions of vertical dimension that must be specified. 2. the vertical distance between the maxillary and mandibular ridges; called also *interridge d.*
**interocclusal d.**, the distance between the occluding surfaces of the maxillary and mandibular teeth when the mandible is in physiologic rest position; called also *freeway space* and *interocclusal clearance, gap,* and *space.*
**interocular d.**, the distance between the two eyes, usually used in reference to the interpupillary distance.
**interpediculate d.**, the distance between the vertebral pedicles as measured on the radiograph.
**interpupillary d.**, the distance between the centers of the pupils of the two eyes when the visual axes are parallel; in practice usually measured from the lateral margin of one pupil to the medial margin of the other.
**interridge d.**, interarch d.
**map d.**, the distance between two genetic loci on a linkage map, measured in centimorgans.
**source-skin d. (SSD)**, the distance from the focal spot on the target of the x-ray tube to the skin of the subject, as measured along the central ray.
**target-skin d.**, source-skin d.
**working d.**, the distance between the front lens of a microscope and the object when the instrument is correctly focused.

**dis·tan·tia** (dis-tan′shə) distance.
**d. intercrista′lis** [TA], intercristal distance: the distance between the middle points of the iliac crests; called also *intercristal diameter.*
**d. interspino′sa** [TA], interspinous distance: the greatest width between the anterior superior iliac spines; called also *interspinous diameter.*

**dis·tem·per** (dis-tem′pər) [MeSH: Distemper] a name for several infectious diseases of animals, especially canine distemper.
**canine d.**, an infectious respiratory and sometimes gastrointestinal disease of dogs, caused by a paramyxovirus and characterized by fever, dullness, loss of appetite, and a discharge from the eyes and nose. It is caused by a virus and it is also infectious for foxes and ferrets. Called also *hard pad disease.*
**cat d.**, panleukopenia.
**colt d., equine d.**, strangles (def. 1).
**feline d.**, panleukopenia.
**horse d.**, strangles (def. 1).

**dis·tem·per·oid** (dis-tem′pər-oid) an attenuated canine distemper virus that has been subjected to several passages in ferrets; called also *Green's distemperoid.*

**dis·tend** (dis-tend′) to expand outward owing to pressure from within; cf. *dilate.*

**dis·ten·si·bil·i·ty** (dis-ten″sĭ-bil′ĭ-te) 1. capability of being distended. 2. elastance.

**dis·ten·tion** (dis-ten′shən) the state of being distended or enlarged; the act of distending.

**dis·tich·ia** (dis-tik′e-ə) distichiasis.

**dis·ti·chi·a·sis** (dis″tĭ-ki′ə-sis) [Gr. *distichia* a double line] the presence of a double row of eyelashes on an eyelid, one or both of which are turned in against the eyeball.

**dis·ti·chous** (dis′tĭ-kəs) arranged in two vertical rows; said of the arrangement of leaves where the leaf at one node is opposite to those just above and below it.

**dis·til, dis·till** (dis-til′) [L. *destillare; de* from + *stillare* to drop] to volatilize by heat and then cool and condense the evaporated matter, as to purify a substance or to separate a volatile substance from other less volatile substances.

**dis·til·late** (dis′til-āt) material that has been obtained by distillation.

**dis·til·la·tion** (dis″tĭ-la′shən) the process of vaporizing and condensing a substance to purify the substance or to separate a volatile substance from less volatile substances. Called also *vaporization.*
**destructive d., dry d.**, decomposition of a solid by heating in the absence of air, which results in volatile liquid products.
**fractional d.**, that which is attended by the successive separation of volatilizable substances in the order of their respective volatility.
**molecular d.**, a process of purification applied to drugs and pharmaceuticals during which the crude material is evaporated under high vacuum of about one millionth of an atmosphere, and the condensate is caught on a cooled surface held close in front of the evaporating layer. The process is applied currently to vitamins A, D, and E, to animal and vegetable sterols and hormones, and to drugs and intermediates.
**vacuum d.**, distillation under reduced pressure to avoid the decomposition which might occur at atmospheric pressure.

**dis·to·ax·io·gin·gi·val** (dis″to-ak″se-o-jin′jĭ-vəl) 1. pertaining to the line angle formed by the axial and gingival walls of a cavity preparation on the distal aspect of a tooth. 2. axiodistogingival.

**dis·to·ax·io·in·ci·sal** (dis″to-ak″se-o-in-si′zəl) pertaining to or formed by the distal, axial, and incisal walls of a tooth cavity preparation.

**dis·to·ax·io·oc·clu·sal** (dis″to-ak″se-o-ə-kloo′zəl) pertaining to or formed by the distal, axial, and occlusal walls of a tooth cavity preparation.

**dis·to·buc·cal** (dis″to-buk′əl) pertaining to or formed by the distal and buccal surfaces of a tooth, or by the distal and buccal walls of a tooth cavity preparation. Called also *buccodistal.*

**dis·to·buc·co·oc·clu·sal** (dis″to-buk″o-ə-kloo′zəl) pertaining to or formed by the distal, buccal, and occlusal surfaces of a tooth.

**dis·to·buc·co·pul·pal** (dis″to-buk″o-pul′pəl) pertaining to or formed by the distal, buccal, and pulpal walls of a tooth cavity preparation.

**dis·to·cer·vi·cal** (dis″to-sər′vĭ-kəl) 1. pertaining to the distal surface of the neck of a tooth. 2. distogingival.

**dis·to·cli·na·tion** (dis″to-klĭ-na′shən) deviation of a tooth from the vertical, in the direction of the tooth next distal (posterior) to it in the dental arch.

**dis·to·clu·sal** (dis″to-kloo′zəl) disto-occlusal.

**dis·to·clu·sion** (dis″to-kloo′zhən) malocclusion in which the mandibular arch is in a posterior (distal) position in relation to the maxillary arch. Generally considered as identical with Class II in Angle's classification of malocclusion (see *malocclusion*). Called also *disto-occlusion, posterior occlusion, posteroclusion,* and *retrusive occlusion.*

**dis·to·gin·gi·val** (dis″to-jin′jĭ-vəl) pertaining to or formed by the distal and gingival walls of a tooth cavity preparation; called also *distocervical.*

**dis·to·la·bi·al** (dis″to-la′be-əl) pertaining to or formed by the distal and labial surfaces of a tooth, or the distal and labial walls of a tooth cavity preparation.

**dis·to·la·bio·in·ci·sal** (dis″to-la″be-o-in-si′zəl) pertaining to or formed by the distal, labial, and incisal surfaces of a tooth.

**dis·to·lin·gual** (dis″to-ling′gwəl) pertaining to or formed by the distal and lingual surfaces of a tooth, or the distal and lingual walls of a tooth cavity preparation.

**dis·to·lin·guo·in·ci·sal** (dis″to-ling″gwo-in-si′zəl) pertaining to or formed by the distal, lingual, and incisal surfaces of a tooth.

**dis·to·lin·guo·oc·clu·sal** (dis″to-ling″gwo-o-kloo′zəl) pertaining to or formed by the distal, lingual, and occlusal surfaces of a tooth.

**dis·to·lin·guo·pul·pal** (dis″to-ling″gwo-pul′pəl) pertaining to or formed by the distal, lingual, and pulpal walls of a tooth cavity preparation.

**Dis·to·ma** (dis′to-mə) [*di-* + Gr. *stoma* mouth] former name of a genus of trematode worms; members of this genus have been assigned to other genera.

**di·sto·mia** (di-sto′me-ə) the presence of two mouths.

**dis·to·mi·a·sis** (dis″to-mi′ə-sis) trematodiasis.
**pulmonary d.**, paragonimiasis.

**dis·to·mo·lar** (dis″to-mo′lər) a supernumerary molar; any tooth found distal to a third molar.

**di·sto·mus** (di-sto′məs) [*di-* + *stoma*] a fetus having a double mouth.

**dis·to·oc·clu·sal** (dis″to-ə-kloo′zəl) pertaining to or formed by the distal and occlusal surfaces of a tooth, or the distal and occlusal walls of a tooth cavity preparation; called also *distoclusal.*

**dis·to·oc·clu·sion** (dis″to-ə-kloo′zhən) distoclusion.

**dis·to·place·ment** (dis″to-plās′mənt) displacement of a tooth distally.

**dis·to·pul·pal** (dis″to-pul′pəl) pertaining to or formed by the distal and pulpal walls of a tooth cavity preparation.

**dis·to·pul·po·la·bi·al** (dis″to-pul″po-la′be-əl) pertaining to or formed by the distal, pulpal, and labial walls of a tooth cavity preparation.

**dis·to·pul·po·lin·gual** (dis″to-pul″po-ling′gwəl) pertaining to or formed by the distal, pulpal, and lingual walls of a tooth cavity preparation.

**dis·tor·tion** (dis-tor′shən) [*dis-*[1] + *torsio* a twisting] 1. the state of being twisted out of a natural or normal shape or position. 2. in psychiatry, the process of altering or disguising unconscious ideas or impulses so that they become acceptable to the conscious mind. 3. in optics or radiology, deviation of an image from the true outline or shape of an object or structure.
**barrel d.**, outward bowing of gridded straight lines in an image, resulting from lens distortion such that the lateral magnification at the center of the image is greater than that at the edges. Cf. *pincushion d.*
**parataxic d.**, Harry Stack Sullivan's term for distortions in judgment and perception, particularly in interpersonal relations, based upon the perception of objects and relationships in accord with patterns from earlier experience.
**pincushion d.**, inward bowing of gridded straight lines in an image as a result of lens distortion, the image of a square object thus resembling a pincushion or pillow. Cf. *barrel d.*

**dis·tor·tor** (dis-tor′tər) [L.] that which distorts.
**d. o′ris**, musculus zygomaticus minor.

**dis·to·ver·sion** (dis″to-vər′zhən) the position of a tooth which is farther than normal from the median line of the face along the dental arch.

**dis·trac·ti·bil·i·ty** (dis-trak″tĭ-bil′ĭ-te) inability to focus one's attention on the task at hand; the attention is too frequently drawn to irrelevant and unimportant environmental stimuli.

**dis·trac·tion** (dis-trak′shən) [L. *distrahere* to draw apart] 1. a state in which the attention is diverted from the main portion of an experience or is divided among various portions of it. 2. a form of dislocation in which the joint surfaces have been separated without rupture of their binding ligaments and without displacement. 3. excessive space between fracture fragments due to interposed tissue or too forceful traction. 4. surgical separation of the two parts of a bone after the bone is transected. 5. unusual width of the dental arch; placement of the teeth or other maxillary or mandibular structures farther than normal from the median plane. See also *contraction,* def. 3.

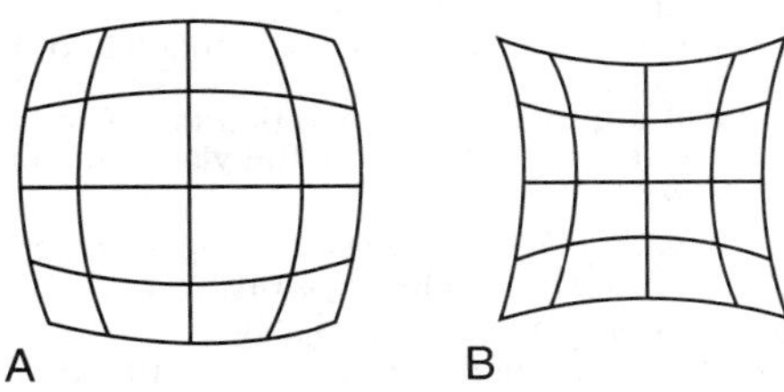

*(A),* Barrel distortion; *(B),* pincushion distortion.

**dis·tress** (dis-tres′) [L. *distringere* to draw apart] physical or mental anguish or suffering.
**idiopathic respiratory d. of newborn**, respiratory distress syndrome of newborn.

**dis·tri·bu·tion** (dis″trĭ-bu′shən) [L. *distributio*] 1. the specific location or arrangement of continuing or successive objects or events in space or time. 2. the extent of a ramifying structure such as an artery or nerve and its branches. 3. the geographical range of an organism or disease. 4. probability d. 5. in statistics, a synonym for *law;* for entries not found here, see under *law.*
**Bernoulli d.**, binomial d.
**binomial d.**, the probability distribution that describes the frequencies of the different possible combinations of two alternative outcomes in a series of $n$ independent trials; it is given by expansion of the binomial $(p + q)^n$, where one of the two alternative outcomes has probability of $p$ and the other of $q = 1 - p$.
**$\chi^2$ d., chi-square d.**, a theoretical probability distribution of the sum of the squares of a number *(k)* of normally distributed variables whose mean is 0 and standard deviation is 1; the parameter $k$ is the number of degrees of freedom. Cf. *chi-square test.*
**density d.**, frequency d.
**dose d.**, in radiology, a representation of the variation of dose with position in any region of an irradiated object.
**exponential d.**, a skewed probability distribution with right tail extending to infinity and having the density function

$$f(x) = \lambda e^{-\lambda x}$$

for $x \geq 0$ and $\lambda > 0$. The mean is $1/\lambda$ and the variance is $(1/\lambda)^2$. The mode is at zero and the larger the parameter $\lambda$, the more clustered the distribution toward zero. The exponential distribution arises in medicine and reliability as the time to mortality/morbidity or failure; $\lambda$ is often interpreted as the force of mortality or failure.
**F-d.**, the ratio of two independent chi-square distributions; the exact sampling distribution of the ratio of variances from two independent samples from identical normal distributions.
**frequency d.**, a presentation, such as a table or graph, describing the relative frequency or theoretical probability of a random variable assuming any value in the range of possible values.
**gaussian d.**, normal d.
**log-normal d.**, a distribution of a random variable $x$ such that $y = \ln x$ has a normal distribution; it is often used to model incubation times for diseases.
**normal d.**, a symmetric, bell-shaped probability distribution having the density function

$$f(x) = \frac{1}{\sqrt{2\pi}\sigma} e^{-(x-\mu)^2/2\sigma^2}$$

where $x$ is the abscissa, $f(x)$ is the ordinate, $e$ is the base of natural logarithms (2.718), $\mu$ is the mean, and $\sigma$ is the standard deviation. The normal distribution is entirely dependent on $\mu$ and $\sigma$; it is symmetric about the mean, with both tails extending to infinity; and the mean, the median, and the mode are identical. Roughly speaking, the normal distribution characterizes a random variable that is the sum of a large number of independent random effects. More precisely, it is typically the limiting distribution of a standardized sum of an infinite series of random variables with finite variance, each making a negligible contribution to the total variance (a fact known as the central limit theorem, q.v.). For this reason it is common statistical practice to assume that random sampling distributions of statistical measures are "approximately normal" and apply tests (e.g., *t*-test, analysis of variance) based on the normal distribution. See illustration. Called also *gaussian d.*

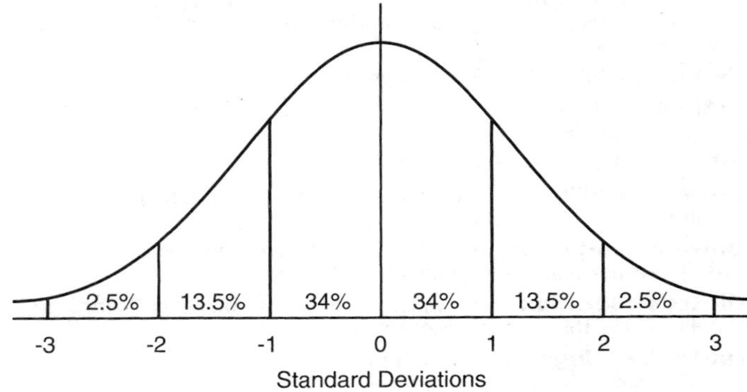

Normal distribution. The approximate percentage of the area (or frequency) lying under the curve between standard deviations is indicated.

**Poisson d.**, the probability distribution that describes counts of events randomly distributed in time or space, such as radioactive decay or blood cell counts. The probability of observing exactly *k* events in a fixed time period or region is

$$f(k) = \frac{\lambda^k e^{-\lambda}}{k!}$$

where $\lambda$ is the average density of events in a period or region of that size and *e* is the base of natural logarithms (2.718). The mean and variance of the distribution are both equal to $\lambda$, thus the coefficient of variation for a Poisson distribution is

$$1/\sqrt{\lambda}$$

(the variability of the count is inversely proportional to the square root of the average count).
**probability d.**, a mathematical function that assigns to each measurable event in a sample space the probability that the event will occur.
**skew d.**, a frequency distribution that is asymmetric.
**standard normal d.**, the normal distribution with mean 0 and standard deviation 1.
***t*-d.**, the probability distribution of the statistic

$$t = \frac{\bar{X} - \mu}{s/\sqrt{n}},$$

where $\bar{X}$ and *s* are the mean and standard deviations of a sample of size *n* taken from a population with a normal distribution having mean $\mu$; used in the *t*-test (q.v.). It is symmetric about zero and approaches the normal distribution as the sample size increases.
**Weibull d.**, a skewed unimodal probability distribution for nonnegative variables, characterized by the parameters of shape and scale. It can be used for negatively skewed data; common uses include modeling lifespans of materials and modeling incubation times for diseases such as AIDS.

**dis·tri·chi·a·sis** (dis″trĭ-ki′ə-sis) [*dis*[2] + *trich-* + *-iasis*] a condition in which two hairs grow from a single follicle.

**dis·trix** (dis′triks) [*dis*[2] + *thrix*] the splitting of hairs at their distal ends.

**dis·tur·bance** (dis-tər′bəns) a departure or divergence from that which is considered normal.
**emotional d.**, see under *illness.*
**transient situational d.**, acute stress reaction.

**di·sub·sti·tut·ed** (di-sub′stĭ-to͞ot″əd) having two atoms in each molecule replaced by other atoms or radicals.

**di·sul·fate** (di-sul′fāt) a compound containing two sulfate ions or radicals, as in titanium disulfate, $Ti(SO_4)_2$ (not to be confused with bisulfate).

**di·sul·fide** (di-sul′fīd) a compound of a base with two atoms of sulfur; see also under *bond.*

**di·sul·fide isom·er·ase** (di-sul′fīd i-som′ər-ās) protein disulfide-isomerase.

**di·sul·fi·ram** (di-sul′fĭ-rəm) [USP] [MeSH: Disulfiram] an antioxidant that inhibits the oxidation of the acetaldehyde metabolized from alcohol, resulting in high concentrations of acetaldehyde in the body. Extremely uncomfortable symptoms occur when alcohol is ingested subsequent to the oral administration of disulfiram (see *mal rouge*); used to produce an aversion to alcohol in the treatment of chronic alcoholism. Called also *triethylthiuram disulfide.*

**di·thi·az·a·nine io·dide** (di″thi-az′ə-nēn) a dark green crystalline powder, $C_{23}H_{23}IN_2S_2$, used as an anthelmintic against strongylids and whipworms.

**di·thio** (di-thi′o) the chemical group $—S_2—$.

**di·thi·ol** (di-thi′ol) a chemical compound containing two sulfhydryl (thiol) radicals.

**dith·ra·nol** (dith′rə-nol) anthralin.

**Di·tro·pan** (di′tro-pən) trademark for a preparation of oxybutynin chloride.

**Di·tro·pe·no·tus au·reo·vir·i·dis** (di″tro-pə-no′təs aw″re-o-vir′ĭ-dis) former name for *Pyemotes ventricosus.*

**Dit·tel's operation** (dit′əlz) [Leopold Ritter von *Dittel,* Vienna urologist, 1815–1898] see under *operation.*

**Dit·trich's plugs** (dit′riks) [Franz *Dittrich,* German pathologist, 1815–1859] see under *plug.*

**Dit·y·len·chus** (dit″ə-len′kəs) a genus of small nematodes.
**D. dip′saci,** the stem and bulb eelworm, a parasite of various grains, grasses, and bulbs, such as lilies, hyacinths, gladioli, narcissi, and onions; when ingested with the latter, it may be found as a pseudoparasite in the feces. Called also *Anguillulina putrefaciens.*

**Di·u·car·din** (di″u-kahr′din) trademark for preparations of hydroflumethiazide.

**Di·u·lo** (di′u-lo) trademark for preparations of metolazone.

**Di·u·pres** (di′u-prəs) trademark for preparations of chlorothiazide and reserpine.

**di·ure·ide** (di-u′re-īd) see *ureide.*

**di·urese** (di″u-rēs′) the act of effecting diuresis.

**di·ure·ses** (di″u-re′sēz) [MeSH: Diuresis] plural of *diuresis.*

**di·ure·sis** (di″u-re′sis) pl. *diure′ses* [Gr. *diourein* to urinate, to pass in urine] [MeSH: Diuresis] increased excretion of urine. Cf. *polyuria.*
**osmotic d.**, diuresis resulting from the presence of nonabsorbable or poorly absorbable, osmotically active substances (mannitol, urea, glucose, etc.) in the renal tubules.

**di·uret·ic** (di″u-ret′ik) [Gr. *diourētikos* promoting urine] 1. increasing the excretion of urine. 2. an agent that promotes the excretion of urine.
**high-ceiling d's,** loop d's.
**loop d's,** agents that inhibit the reabsorption of sodium and water in the thick ascending limb of the loop of Henle. They promote a high level of diuresis and their effect is not altered by acid-base imbalances or hypoalbuminemia. Used in the treatment of edema associated with congestive heart failure or hepatic or renal disease and, alone or in combination with other drugs, in the treatment of hypertension. Called also *high-ceiling d's.*
**mercurial d's,** a group of organometallic compounds, now rarely used, that inhibit tubular reabsorption of sodium and chloride.
**osmotic d.**, a substance, e.g., mannitol, that is filtered at the glomerulus and reabsorbed in the renal tubule only to a limited extent; it thus increases the amount of osmotically active solute in the urine with a corresponding increase in urine volume. Such compounds also increase the osmolality of plasma, thus increasing the diffusion of water from the intraocular and cerebrospinal fluids and are used for reducing the pressure and volume of these fluids.
**potassium sparing d's,** a class of drugs that block the exchange of sodium for potassium and hydrogen ions in the distal tubule, causing an increase in the excretion of sodium and chloride with a negligible increase in potassium excretion; used primarily as adjuncts to enhance the action and counteract the kaliuretic effects of thiazide and loop diuretics in the treatment of renal disease and in the treatment of hypertension.
**thiazide d.**, any of a group of synthetic compounds that effect diuresis by enhancing the excretion of sodium and chloride.

**di·uria** (di-u′re-ə) [L. *dies* day + *urine*] frequency of urination during the day.

**Di·uril** (di′u-ril) trademark for preparations of chlorothiazide.

**di·ur·nal** (di-ər′nəl) [L. *dies* day] occurring during the day.

**di·ur·nule** (di-ər′nūl) [L. *diurnus* daily] a pill or other preparation containing the complete allowance of a medicine for one day.

**Di·u·ten·sen** (di″u-ten′sən) trademark for preparations of cryptenamine with methyclothiazide (Diutensen-R also contains reserpine).

**Div.** abbreviation for L. *div′ide,* divide.

**di·va·ga·tion** (di″və-ga′shən) rambling, incoherent speech and thought.

**di·va·lent** (di-va′lent) [*di-* + *valence*] having a valence of two. Called also *bivalent.*

**di·val·pro·ex so·di·um** (di-val′pro-eks) a coordination compound of valproate sodium and valproic acid in a 1:1 molar relationship, used in the treatment of migraine, manic episodes associated with bipolar disorder, and epileptic seizures, particularly absence seizures; administered orally.

**di·var·i·ca·tion** (di-var″ĭ-ka′shən) 1. divergence. 2. diastasis.

**di·ver·gence** (di-vər′jəns) a spreading or tending apart; in ophthalmology, the simultaneous abduction of both eyes.
**negative vertical d. (−V.D.),** the condition in which the visual line of the left eye deviates upward or the visual line of the right eye deviates downward.
**positive vertical d. (+V.D.),** the condition in which the visual line of the right eye deviates upward, or the visual line of the left eye deviates downward.

**di·ver·gent** (di-vər′jənt) [L. *divergens; dis-* apart + *vergere* to tend] tending apart; deviating or radiating away from a common point.

**di·ver·sion** (dĭ-ver′zhən) a turning aside.
**antigenic d.**, the change in the antigenic structure of tumor cells or tissue to that normally found in different cells or tissue.

**di·ver·tic·u·la** (di″vər-tik′u-lə) [L.] plural of *diverticulum.*

**di·ver·tic·u·lar** (di″vər-tik′u-lər) pertaining to or resembling a diverticulum.

**di·ver·tic·u·lar·iza·tion** (di″vər-tik″u-lər-ĭ-za′shən) the act of forming diverticula or pockets.

**di·ver·tic·u·lec·to·my** (di″vər-tik″u-lek′tə-me) [*diverticulum* + *-ectomy*] excision of a diverticulum.

**di·ver·tic·u·li·tis** (di″vər-tik″u-li′tis) [MeSH: Diverticulitis] inflammation of a diverticulum, especially inflammation related to colonic diverticula, which may undergo perforation with abscess formation. Sometimes called *left-sided* or *L-sided appendicitis.*

**di·ver·tic·u·lo·gram** (di″vər-tik′u-lo-gram) [*diverticulum* + *-gram*] a radiograph of a diverticulum.

**di·ver·tic·u·lo·pexy** (di″vər-tik″u-lo-pek′se) surgical fixation of a diverticulum in a new position following its separation from the initial adjacent or adherent structures.

**di·ver·tic·u·lo·sis** (di″vər-tik″u-lo′sis) the presence of diverticula, particularly of colonic diverticula, in the absence of inflammation. Cf. *diverticulitis.*

**di·ver·tic·u·lum** (di″vər-tik′u-ləm) pl. *diverti′cula* [L. *divertere* to turn aside] [MeSH: Diverticulum] a circumscribed pouch or sac of variable size occurring normally or created by herniation of the lining mucous membrane through a defect in the muscular coat of a tubular organ.
**acquired d.,** any diverticulum produced secondarily, mechanically, or by disease.
**allantoic d.,** the endodermal sacculation that becomes the allantois; in humans it is an outpouching of the caudal wall of the yolk sac that becomes the urachus and remains throughout life as the median umbilical ligament. Called also *allantoic vesicle.*
**diverti′cula ampul′lae duc′tus deferen′tis** [TA], sacculations in the wall of the ampulla of the ductus deferens.
**caliceal d., calyceal d.,** an epithelial-lined cavity in the kidney, situated peripherally to a calix and connected to it by a narrow isthmus, the lining of the cavity being continuous with that of the calix.
**cervical d.,** a diverticulum in the neck, such as in the pharynx or esophagus.
**diverticula of colon, colonic diverticula,** acquired herniations of the mucosa of the colon through the muscular layers of the bowel wall, which may become inflamed (see *diverticulitis*).
**false d.,** pseudodiverticulum.
**functional d.,** a benign radiological entity, in which a diverticulum-like shadow is demonstrated by contrast medium, although subsequent laparotomy shows no sign of any corresponding anomaly.
**ganglion d.,** a hernial protrusion of the synovial membrane through a tendon sheath.
**Ganser's d.,** multiple pulsion diverticula of the sigmoid flexure.
**giant d.,** a large (6–29 cm) air-filled cyst formed following the perforation of a diverticulum as a complication of diverticulitis.
**Graser's d.,** false diverticulum of the sigmoid flexure.
**Heister's d.,** bulbus superior venae jugularis.
**hepatic d.,** one arising from the embryonic duodenum and forming the liver, gallbladder, and bile ducts.
**d. ilei verum,** Meckel's d.
**intestinal d.,** a pouch or sac formed by hernial protrusion of the mucous membrane through a defect in the muscular coat of the intestine.
**Kirchner's d.,** a diverticulum of the eustachian tube.
**laryngeal d.,** a diverticulum of the laryngeal mucous membrane.
**Meckel's d.,** an occasional sacculation or appendage of the ileum, derived from an unobliterated yolk stalk; called also *d. ilei verum.*
**metanephric d.,** ureteric bud.
**Nuck's d.,** processus vaginalis peritonei.
**pancreatic diverticula,** two outgrowths or buds from the embryonic duodenum, later forming the pancreas and its ducts.
**Pertik's d.,** an unusually deep recessus pharyngeus.
**pharyngoesophageal d.,** a diverticulum at the junction of the pharynx and esophagus, at the point of Killian's dehiscence; called also *Zenker's d.*
**pituitary d.,** Rathke's pouch.
**pressure d., pulsion d.,** a sac or pouch formed by hernial protrusion of the mucous membrane through the muscular coat (as of the colon or esophagus) as a result of pressure from within.
**Rokitansky's d.,** a traction diverticulum of the esophagus.
**supradiaphragmatic d.,** a diverticulum of the esophagus situated just above the diaphragm.
**synovial d.,** a hernial protrusion of the synovial membrane of a joint or a tendon sheath.
**thyroid d.,** an outpouching of the ventral floor of the embryonic pharynx that becomes the thyroid gland.
**diverticula of trachea, tracheal diverticula,** pouches projecting from the trachea.
**traction d.,** a localized distortion, angulation, or funnel-shaped bulging of the full thickness of the wall of the esophagus, caused by adhesions resulting from some external lesion.
**vesical d.,** diverticulum of the bladder.
**Zenker's d.,** pharyngoesophageal d.

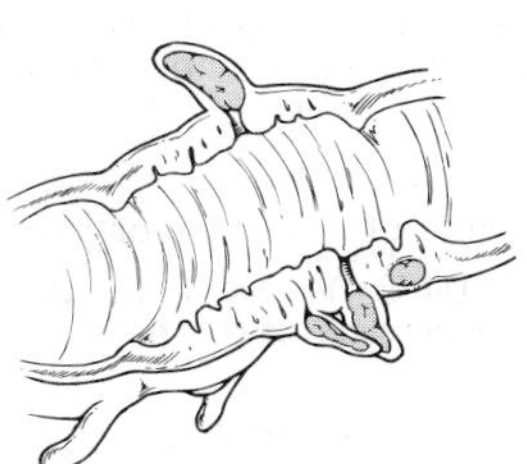
Colonic diverticula.

**di·vi·cine** (di-vi′sin) a toxic pyrimidine aglycone produced by endogenous degradation of vicine by $\beta$-glucosidase in fava beans; it is believed to be important in the pathogenesis of favism.

**divi-divi** (div″e-div′e) the leguminous pods of *Caesalpinia coriaria* (Jacq.) Willd., plants of South America; the seeds contain tannin and gallic acid and have been used as an astringent and in tanning.

**di·vi·nyl·ben·zene** (di″vi″nəl-ben′zēn) a toxic liquid hydrocarbon, $C_6H_4(CH{=}CH_2)_2$, a monomer used in polymerization reactions.

**di·vi·sio** (dĭ-viz′e-o) pl. *divisio′nes* [L.] 1. the act or process of separating or sectioning into two or more parts. 2. a section or part of a larger structure.
**divisio′nes anterio′res plex′us brachia′lis** [TA], anterior divisions of brachial plexus: the three anterior divisions into which each of the three trunks (superior, medial, and inferior) of the brachial plexus splits (see also *divisio′nes posteriores plexus brachialis*). The anterior divisions of the superior and medial trunks unite to form the lateral fasciculus; and the anterior division of the inferior trunk forms the medial fasciculus of the plexus.
**d. autono′mica systema′tis nervo′si periphe′rici** [TA], autonomic division of peripheral nervous system: the autonomic portion of the nervous system, concerned with regulation of activity of cardiac muscle, smooth muscle, and glands; called also *autonomic nervous system* (q.v.), *systema nervosum autonomicum, pars autonomica systematis nervosi peripherici* [TA alternative], and *autonomic part of peripheral nervous system.* See Plate 48.
**divisio′nes posterio′res plex′us brachia′lis** [TA], posterior divisions of brachial plexus: the three posterior divisions into which each of the three trunks (superior, medial, and inferior) of the brachial plexus splits (see also *divisio′nes anteriores plexus brachialis*). All three posterior divisions unite to form the posterior fasciculus of the plexus.

**di·vi·sion** (dĭ-vizh′ən) [L. *dividere* to separate] 1. the act or process of separation or sectioning into two or more parts. 2. a section or part of a larger structure. 3. in the taxonomy of plants, a primary grouping composed of classes; the equivalent of *phylum* in the animal kingdom. 4. in the taxonomy of fungi, former term for *phylum.*
**anterior d's of brachial plexus,** divisiones anteriores plexus brachialis.
**autonomic d. of peripheral nervous system,** divisio autonomica systematis nervosi peripherici.
**cell d.,** the fission of a cell.
**cell d., direct,** see *amitosis.*
**cell d., indirect,** see *meiosis* and *mitosis.*
**craniosacral d.,** parasympathetic nervous system.
**dorsal d's of trunks of brachial plexus,** divisiones posteriores plexus brachialis.
**equational d.,** the second meiotic division, essentially mitotic in type, characterized by the separation of sister chromatids. The latter are genetically identical except where recombination with the homologous chromosome has occurred in the first meiotic division.
**mandibular d.,** nervus mandibularis.
**maturation d.,** meiosis.
**maxillary d.,** nervus maxillaris.
**posterior d's of brachial plexus,** divisiones posteriores plexus brachialis.
**reduction d.,** the first meiotic division, so called because at this stage the chromosome number per cell is reduced from diploid to haploid.
**thoracicolumbar d., thoracolumbar d.,** sympathetic nervous system.
**ventral d's of trunks of brachial plexus,** divisiones anteriores plexus brachialis.

**di·vi·si·o·nes** (dĭ-viz″e-o′nēz) [L.] plural of *divisio.*

**di·vulse** (dĭ-vuls′) to pull apart forcibly.

**di·vul·sion** (dĭ-vul′shən) [*dis-*[1] + *vellere* to pluck] the act of forcibly separating or pulling apart.

**di·vul·sor** (dĭ-vul′sər) an instrument for dilating the urethra.

**Dix·on Mann** see *Mann.*

**di·zy·got·ic** (di″zi-got′ik) pertaining to or derived from two separate zygotes, as dizygotic (fraternal) twins.

**di·zy·gous** (di-zi′gəs) dizygotic.

**diz·zi·ness** (diz′e-nəs) [MeSH: Dizziness] a disturbed sense of relationship to space; a sensation of unsteadiness with a feeling of movement within the head. See also *dysequilibrium* and *vertigo.* Called also *giddiness.*

**djen·kol·ic acid** (jeng-kol′ik) a sulfur-containing amino acid found in djenkol beans, the cause of djenkol bean poisoning.

**djen·kol·ism** (jeng′kol-iz-əm) djenkol bean poisoning.

**DL-** chemical prefix (small capital D and L) used with the D and L convention to indicate a racemic mixture of enantiomers.

***dl*-** chemical prefix used with the *d* and *l* convention to indicate a racemic mixture of enantiomers; the prefix (+)- is used with the same meaning.

**DLE** discoid lupus erythematosus.

**DM** diabetes mellitus; diphenylamine chlorarsine.

**DMAPN** dimethylaminopropionitrile.

**DMBA** 7,12-dimethylbenz[a]anthracene.

**DMD** Doctor of Dental Medicine.

**DMF** dimethylformamide; decayed, missing, filled (see under *rate).*

**DMFO** eflornithine.

**DMPE** 3,4-dimethoxyphenylethylamine.

**DMRD** Diploma in Medical Radio-Diagnosis (British).

**DMRT** Diploma in Medical Radio-Therapy (British).

**DMSA** succimer.

**DMSO** dimethyl sulfoxide.

**DMT** dimethyltryptamine.

**DN** dibucaine number.

**DNA** [MeSH: DNA] deoxyribonucleic acid.
**B-DNA,** the usual double helical structure assumed by double-stranded DNA; see illustration at *deoxyribonucleic acid.*
**complementary DNA, copy DNA (cDNA),** synthetic DNA transcribed from a specific RNA through the reaction of the enzyme reverse transcriptase.
**DNA library,** see *library.*
**mitochondrial DNA (mtDNA),** the DNA of the mitochondrial chromosome, existing in several thousand copies per cell and inherited exclusively from the mother. Its code differs both from that of nuclear DNA and from that of any present day prokaryote, and it evolves 5 to 10 times more rapidly than nuclear DNA.
**nuclear DNA (nDNA),** the DNA of the chromosomes found in the nucleus of a eukaryotic cell.
**recombinant DNA,** a DNA molecule composed of linked sequences not normally occurring within the same molecule, such as a bacterial plasmid into which has been inserted a segment of viral DNA.
**repetitive DNA,** nucleotide sequences occurring multiply within a genome; they are characteristic of eukaryotes and generally do not encode polypeptides. Sequences may be clustered or dispersed, and repeated moderately (10 to $10^4$ copies per genome) to highly ($\geq 10^6$ copies per genome). Moderately repetitive DNA sequences encode some structural genes for ribosomal RNA and histones; highly repetitive sequences are mostly satellite DNA. Cf. *single copy DNA.*
**satellite DNA,** short, highly repeated DNA sequences found in eukaryotes, usually in clusters in constitutive heterochromatin and generally not transcribed.
**single copy DNA (scDNA),** nucleotide sequences present once in the haploid genome, as are the majority of the gene sequences encoding polypeptides in eukaryotes.
**spacer DNA,** the nucleotide sequences occurring between genes, in eukaryotes often long and including many repetitive sequences; particularly, the DNA occurring between the genes encoding ribosomal RNA.
**Z-DNA,** a form of DNA in which the phosphate groups form a dinucleotide repeating unit zigzagging up a left-handed helix with a single, deep groove; it is particularly likely to occur in stretches of alternating purines and pyrimidines. Cf. *B-DNA.*

**DNA-di·rect·ed DNA pol·y·mer·ase** (dĭ-rek′təd pə-lim′ər-ās) [EC 2.7.7.7] any of the enzymes of the transferase class that catalyze the template-directed, step-by-step addition of deoxyribonucleotides to the 3′ end of an RNA primer or growing DNA chain, using a single-stranded DNA template. The reaction is important in the replication and repair of deoxyribonucleic acids. Called also *DNA polymerase.*

**DNA-di·rect·ed RNA pol·y·mer·ase** (dĭ-rek′təd pə-lim′ər-ās) [EC 2.7.7.6] any of the enzymes of the transferase class that catalyze the template-directed step-by-step addition of ribonucleotides to the 3′ end of a growing RNA chain, using a single-stranded DNA template. The reaction is important in the flow of information from DNA to proteins. Prokaryotes have a single such polymerase while eukaryotes have three: *type I* transcribes most ribosomal RNA genes; *type II* synthesizes messenger and heterogeneous nuclear RNA molecules; and *type III* transcribes the genes for one species of ribosomal RNA and for transfer RNA molecules. Called also *RNA polymerase.*

**DNA gyrase** (ji′rās) [MeSH: DNA Topoisomerase (ATP-Hydrolysing)] DNA topoisomerase (ATP-hydrolyzing).

**DNA li·gase (ATP)** (li′gās) [EC 6.5.1.1] an enzyme of the ligase class that catalyzes the ATP-driven linkage of a double-stranded DNA chain with a free 3′ hydroxyl group to one with a 5′ phosphate group, forming a phosphodiester bond between them. The reaction is important in the repair of damaged DNA and in the joining of Okazaki fragments during DNA replication. The enzyme is used extensively in vitro in the formation of recombinant molecules. Called also *polydeoxyribonucleotide synthase (ATP).*

**DNA nu·cleo·tid·yl·exo·trans·fer·ase** (noo″kle-o-tīd′əl-ek″so-trans′fər-ās) [EC 2.7.7.31] [MeSH: DNA Nucleotidylexotransferase] an enzyme of the transferase class that acts as a DNA polymerase, specifically catalyzing the sequential addition of single deoxynucleotide residues, as nucleoside triphosphates, to the ends of nucleotide chains. The enzyme is often found in the blast cells of patients with acute lymphocytic leukemia; its presence is used in the differential diagnosis of this disease as well as to monitor response to treatment. Called also *terminal deoxynucleotidyl transferase.*

**DNA nu·cleo·tid·yl·trans·fer·ase** (noo″kle-o-tīd″əl-trans′fər-ās) older name for *DNA polymerase.*

**DNA po·ly·mer·ase** (pə-lim′ər-ās) 1. a general term denoting any enzyme catalyzing the template-directed incorporation of deoxyribonucleotides into a DNA chain; see *DNA-directed DNA polymerase* and *RNA-directed DNA polymerase.* 2. DNA-directed DNA polymerase.

**DNase** deoxyribonuclease.

**DNA topo·isom·er·ase** (to″po-i-som′ər-ās) [EC 5.99.1.2] [MeSH: DNA Topoisomerase] an enzyme of the isomerase class that catalyzes the ATP-independent breakage, passage, and rejoining of a single strand of DNA, altering the topology of the molecule by single-step changes in linking number. The enzyme removes superhelical turns and interconverts other topoisomers, such as simple and knotted single-stranded rings. Called also *type I topoisomerase.*

**DNA topo·isom·er·ase (ATP-hy·dro·lyz·ing)** (to″po-i-som′ər-ās hi′dro-li-zing) [EC 5.99.1.3] an enzyme of the isomerase class that catalyzes the ATP-dependent breakage, passage, and rejoining of both strands of a DNA helix simultaneously, altering the topology of the molecule by changing the linking number in steps of two. The enzyme removes and introduces superhelical turns and in prokaryotes is believed to be important in replication, transcription, recombination, and other processes. Called also *type II topoisomerase* and *DNA gyrase.*

**DNB** dinitrobenzene; Diplomate of the National Board (of Medical Examiners).

**DNCB** dinitrochlorobenzene.

**DNFB** dinitrofluorobenzene.

**DNOC** dinitro-*o*-cresol.

**DNR** do not resuscitate.

**DO** Doctor of Osteopathy.

**DOA** dead on arrival.

**Do·bie's globule, layer (line)** (do′bēz) [William Murray *Dobie,* English physician, 1828–1915] see under *globule,* and see *Z band,* under *band.*

**do·bu·ta·mine** (do-bu′tə-mēn) [MeSH: Dobutamine] a synthetic catecholamine used as an adrenergic with cardiotonic actions.
**d. hydrochloride** [USP], the hydrochloride salt of dobutamine, having the same actions as the base.

**DOC** 11-deoxycorticosterone.

**Do·ca** (do′kə) trademark for desoxycorticosterone acetate.

**do·ce·tax·el** (do″sə-tak′səl) an antineoplastic agent used in chemotherapy for carcinoma of the breast; administered by intravenous infusion.

**Doch·mi·us du·o·de·na·lis** (dok′me-əs du″o-də-na′lis) former name for *Ancylostoma duodenale.*

**Do·ci·bin** (do'si-bin) trademark for a crystalline preparation of vitamin $B_{12}$; see *cyanocobalamin.*

**dock** (dok) to perform a caudectomy on an animal.

**do·co·na·zole** (do-ko'nə-zōl) an antifungal, $C_{26}H_{22}Cl_2N_2O_3$.

**do·co·sa·hexa·eno·ic ac·id** (do-ko"sə-hek"sə-e-no'ik) [MeSH: Docosahexaenoic Acids] all *cis*-4,7,10,13,16,19-docosahexaenoic acid, an omega-3, polyunsaturated, 22-carbon fatty acid found almost exclusively in fish and marine animal oils; it is a substrate for cyclooxygenase. Abbreviated DHA. See also table accompanying *fatty acid.*

**doc·tor** (dok'tər) [L. "teacher"] 1. a practitioner of the healing arts, one who has received a degree from a college of medicine, osteopathy, chiropractic, optometry, podiatry, pharmacy, dentistry, or veterinary medicine, licensed to practice by a state. 2. a holder of a diploma of the highest degree from a university, qualified as a specialist in a particular field of learning.

**doc·trine** (dok'trin) a theory supported by authorities and having general acceptance.
**Arrhenius' d.,** see under *theory.*
**Monro-Kellie d.,** the central nervous system and its accompanying fluids are enclosed in a rigid container whose total volume tends to remain constant; an increase in volume of one component, e.g., brain, blood, or cerebrospinal fluid, will elevate pressure and decrease the volume of one of the other elements.
**neuron d.,** the doctrine that the nervous system is entirely cellular, that its cells are distinctive as to morphological type and functional characteristics, and that its cells are not in protoplasmic continuity but are juxtaposed without a significant amount of intervening extracellular substance.

**doc·u·sate** (dok'u-sāt) any of a group of anionic surfactants widely used as emulsifying, wetting, and dispersing agents.
**d. calcium** [USP], an anionic surfactant used as a stool softener; administered orally.
**d. potassium** [USP], an anionic surfactant used as a stool softener; administered orally.
**d. sodium** [USP], an anionic surfactant used as a stool softener, administered orally or rectally; as a tablet disintegrant because of its solubilizing action; and as an emulsifier and dispersant in topical preparations.

**do·de·ce·no·yl-CoA Δ-isom·er·ase** (do"də-sə-no'əl-ko-a' i-som'ər-ās) [EC 5.3.3.8] an enzyme of the isomerase class that catalyzes the shift of a *cis* double bond at C-2 of an unsaturated fatty acyl CoA to one *trans* at C-3; the reaction is necessary for oxidation of unsaturated fatty acids. Called also *enoyl CoA isomerase.*

**Dö·der·lein's bacillus** (dər'der-līnz) [Albert Siegmund Gustav *Döderlein,* German obstetrician and gynecologist, 1860–1941] see under *bacillus.*

**dog·bane** (dog'bān) any plant of the genus *Apocynum.*

**Do·gi·el's corpuscles** (do'ge-elz) [Alexander Stanislavovich *Dogiel,* Russian histologist, 1852–1922] see under *corpuscle.*

**dog·ma** (dog'mə) a belief or an opinion, or a system of beliefs or opinions, formally stated, defined, and held to be true.

**Dog·ma·tist** (dog'mə-tist) a school of medicine formed by Diocles of Carystus. The school put Aristotelian language, system, and speculation into Hippocratic medicine to discover the hidden causes of the constitution of man and of disease: such knowledge, they thought, was necessary for the practice of medicine. See also *Empiric* and *Praxagoras.*

**Do·her·ty** (do'ər-te) Peter C. Australian immunologist in the United States, born 1941. Co-winner, with Rolf M. Zinkernagel, of the Nobel prize for medicine or physiology in 1996 for their discovery about how the immune system detects virus-infected cells.

**Döh·le's disease, bodies (inclusion bodies)** (dər'ləz) [Karl Gottfried Paul *Döhle,* German pathologist, 1855–1928] see *syphilitic aortitis,* under *aortitis,* and see under *body.*

**Döh·le-Hel·ler aortitis** (dər'lə-hel'er) [K.G.P. *Döhle;* Arnold Ludwig Gotthilf *Heller,* German pathologist, 1840–1913] syphilitic aortitis.

**doigt** (dwah) [Fr.] finger or toe.
**d. mort** [Fr.], dead finger.

**Doi·sy** (doi'se) Edward Adelbert. An American biochemist, 1893–1986; co-winner, with Carl Peter Henrik Dam, of the Nobel prize for medicine and physiology in 1943, for the isolation and synthesis of vitamin K.

**dol** (dōl) [L. *do'lor* pain] a unit of pain intensity.

**do·lab·rate** (do-lab'rāt) [L. *dolabra* ax] ax-shaped.

**do·lab·ri·form** (do-lab'rĭ-form) dolabrate.

**do·las·e·tron mes·y·late** (do-las'ə-tron) a selective serotonin receptor antagonist, used for the prevention of nausea and vomiting associated with chemotherapy and for the prevention and treatment of postoperative nausea and vomiting; administered orally and intravenously.

**dolich(o)-** [Gr. *dolichos* long] a combining form meaning long.

**dol·i·cho·ce·pha·lia** (dol"ĭ-ko-sə-fa'le-ə) dolichocephaly.

**dol·i·cho·ce·phal·ic, dol·i·cho·ceph·a·lous** (dol"i-ko-sə-fal'ik, dol"ĭ-ko-sef'ə-ləs) [*dolicho-* + *cephalic*] long headed; having a cephalic index of 75.9 or less. Called also *mecocephalic.*

**dol·i·cho·ceph·a·lism** (dol"ĭ-ko-sef'ə-liz-əm) dolichocephaly.

**dol·i·cho·ceph·a·ly** (dol"ĭ-ko-sef'ə-le) the quality of being dolichocephalic.

**dol·i·cho·co·lon** (dol"ĭ-ko-ko'lon) [*dolicho-* + *colon*] an abnormally long colon.

**dol·i·cho·cra·ni·al** (dol"ĭ-ko-kra'ne-əl) having a cranial index of 74.9 or less.

**dol·i·cho·der·us** (dol"ĭ-ko-dēr'əs) [*dolicho-* + Gr. *dere* neck] an individual with a long neck.

**dol·i·cho·fa·cial** (dol"ĭ-ko-fa'shəl) having a long face.

**dol·i·cho·hi·er·ic** (dol"ĭ-ko-hi-er'ik) having a sacral index below 100.

**dol·i·cho·ker·kic** (dol"ĭ-ko-ker'kik) having a radiohumeral index above 80.

**dol·i·cho·kne·mic** (dol"ĭ-ko-ne'mik) having a tibiofemoral index of 83 or above.

**dol·i·cho·mor·phic** (dol"ĭ-ko-mor'fik) [*dolicho-* + Gr. *morphē* form] built along lines that tend toward the slender or longer type.

**dol·i·cho·pel·lic, dol·i·cho·pel·vic** (dol"ĭ-ko-pel'ik; dol"ĭ-ko-pel'vik) [*dolicho-* + *pelvic*] having a pelvic index of 95 or above.

**dol·i·cho·pro·sop·ic** (dol"ĭ-ko-pro-sop'ik) dolichofacial.

**dol·i·cho·steno·me·lia** (dol"ĭ-ko-sten"o-me'le-ə) [*dolicho-* + *steno-* + *-melia*] 1. the condition of having unusually long, thin extremities. 2. arachnodactyly.

**Döl·ling·er's tendinous ring** (dər'ling-erz) [Johann Ignaz Josef *Döllinger,* German physiologist, 1770–1841] see under *ring.*

**Do·lo·bid** (do'lo-bid) trademark for a preparation of diflunisal.

**Do·lo·phine** (do'lo-fēn) trademark for preparations of methadone hydrochloride.

**do·lor** (do'lor) pl. *dolo'res* [L.] pain; one of the cardinal signs of inflammation.
**d. ca'pitis,** headache.
**d. coxae,** coxalgia, def. 2.

**Do·lo·rac** (do'lə-rak) trademark for a preparation of capsaicin cream.

**do·lo·res** (do-lor'ēz) [L.] plural of *dolor.*

**do·lor·if·ic** (do"lor-if'ik) producing or causing pain.

**do·lor·im·e·ter** (do"lor-im'ə-tər) an instrument for measuring pain in dols.

**do·lor·im·e·try** (do"lor-im'ə-tre) [*dolor* + *-metry*] the measurement of pain.

**do·lor·o·gen·ic** (do-lor"o-jen'ik) dolorific.

**DOM** [MeSH: DOM] 2,5-dimethoxy-4-methylamphetamine.

**Do·magk** (do'mahk) Gerhard Johannes Paul. German physician and biochemist, 1895–1964; winner of the Nobel prize for medicine or physiology in 1939 for his discovery of the effectiveness of Prontosil, the predecessor of sulfa drugs, in treating streptococcal infections.

**do·main** (do-mān') a compact globular structure composed of one section of a polypeptide chain that constitutes a recognizable unit of the tertiary structure of a protein. Domains may fold up independently and maintain their native conformation when the connecting sections of the chain are broken.
**immunoglobulin d's.,** see *homology regions* under *region.*
**kringle d.,** a cysteine-rich, triply disulfide-bonded sequence of amino acids folded into a characteristic shape resembling the looped Scandinavian pastry; such domains occur in plasminogen and contain the binding sites for fibrin. Similar domains are found in other proteins.

**Dom·brock blood group** (dom'brok) [from the name of the propositus patient first observed in 1965] see under *blood group.*

**Dome·boro** (dōm'bor-o) trademark for preparations of aluminum subacetate.

**dom·i·cil·i·ary** (dom"ĭ-sil'e-ar"e) [L. *domus* house] pertaining to or carried on in the house or place of permanent residence, as domiciliary treatment.

**dom·i·nance** (dom'ĭ-nəns) [L. *dominari* to govern] 1. the state of being dominant. 2. in genetics, the full phenotypic expression of a gene in both heterozygotes and homozygotes; see also *Mendel's law,* under *law.* See also *codominant gene,* under *gene,* and also *quasidominance.* 3. in coronary artery anatomy, the state of supplying the posterior diaphragmatic part of the interventricular septum and the diaphragmatic surface of the left ventricle. In 85 percent of the population, the right coronary artery is dominant; in the remainder, the left coronary artery is dominant.
**cerebral d.,** the dominance of one cerebral hemisphere over the other in cerebral functions, demonstrated by laterality in voluntary motor acts.
**incomplete d.,** failure of one gene to be completely dominant, the heterozygotes showing a phenotype intermediate between the two parents; called also *partial d.* and *semidominance.*
**lateral d.,** the preferential use, in voluntary motor acts, of ipsilateral members of the major paired organs of the body (arm, ear, eye, and leg).
**ocular d.,** the preferential use of one eye over the other in vision.
**one-sided d.,** lateral d.
**partial d.,** incomplete d.

**dom·i·nant** (dom'ĭ-nənt) 1. exerting a ruling or controlling influence. 2. in genetics, capable of expression when carried by only one of a pair of homologous chromosomes. 3. a dominant allele or trait. 4. in coronary artery anatomy, supplying the posterior diaphragmatic part of the interventricular septum and the diaphragmatic surface of the left ventricle; used of the right and left coronary arteries.

**do·mi·phen bro·mide** (do'mĭ-fən) a quaternary ammonium compound effective against a wide range of gram-negative and gram-positive bacteria and against certain fungi; used as a topical anti-infective and to disinfect instruments and utensils.

**dom·o·ic ac·id** (dom'o-ik as'id) a neuroexcitatory, neurotoxic amino acid structurally similar to L-glutamic acid, occurring in *Nitzschia pungens* and other varieties of marine vegetation; ingestion of mussels contaminated by it has resulted in a type of shellfish poisoning characterized by gastrointestinal symptoms and neurologic abnormalities, including confusion, disorientation, and short-term memory loss.

**dom·per·i·done** (dom-per'ĭ-dōn) [MeSH: Domperidone] an antiemetic.

**Do·nath-Land·stein·er antibody, test** (do'naht-land'sti-nər) [Julius *Donath,* Austrian immunologist, 1870–1950; Karl *Landsteiner,* Austrian physician in United States, 1868–1943] see under *antibody* and *test.*

**do·nax·ine** (do-nak'sēn) gramine.

**Don·ders' glaucoma, law** (don'dərz) [Franciscus Cornelius *Donders,* Dutch physician and ophthalmologist, 1818–1889] see *advanced open-angle g.* and see under *law.*

**Donec alv. sol. fuerit** abbreviation for L. *do'nec al'vus solu'ta fu'erit,* until the bowels are opened (i.e., until a bowel movement occurs).

**do·nee** (do-ne') recipient; host (def. 2).

**do·nep·e·zil hy·dro·chlo·ride** (do-nep'ə-zil) a reversible acetylcholinesterase inhibitor used for the treatment of mild to symptoms of dementia of the Alzheimer type; administered orally.

**Don Juan·ism** (don hwahn'iz-əm) hypersexuality in a man.

**Don·nan's equilibrium** (don'ənz) [Frederick George *Donnan,* English chemist, 1870–1956] see under *equilibrium.*

**Don·a·tal** (don'ə-tal) trademark for preparations of atropine sulfate, hyoscyamine sulfate, phenobarbital, and scopolamine hydrobromide.

**Donné's corpuscles (bodies)** (do-nāz') [Alfred *Donné,* French bacteriologist, 1801–1878] see *colostrum corpuscles,* under *corpuscles.*

**Don·o·hue's syndrome** (don'ə-hūz) [William Leslie *Donohue,* Canadian physician, born 1906] leprechaunism.

**do·nor** (do'nər) [MeSH: Tissue Donors] 1. an individual organism that supplies living tissue to be used in another body, as a person who furnishes blood for transfusion, or an organ for transplantation in a histocompatible recipient. Organs for donation usually come from cadavers (see *cadaveric donor transplantation,* although kidneys and certain other organs may be from living donors (see *living related donor transplantation* and *living unrelated donor transplantation*). 2. in chemistry, a substance or compound which contributes part of itself, as an atom or radical, to another substance (acceptor).
**F d.,** in bacterial genetics, a cell that donates the F plasmid by means of bacterial conjugation.
**hydrogen d.,** a substance or compound that gives up hydrogen to another substance (the hydrogen acceptor).
**universal d.,** a person whose blood is type O in the ABO blood group system; such blood is sometimes used in emergency transfusion.

**Don·o·van bodies** (don'ə-vən) [Charles *Donovan,* Irish physician, 1863–1951] 1. *Calymmatobacterium granulomatis.* 2. Leishman-Donovan bodies.

**Don·o·va·nia gran·u·lo·ma·tis** (don"ə-va'ne-ə gran"u-lo'mə-tis) [C. *Donovan*] *Calymmatobacterium granulomatis.*

**don·o·va·no·sis** (don"ə-və-no'sis) granuloma inguinale.

**do·pa** (do'pə) [MeSH: Dopa] 3,4-dihydroxyphenylalanine, an amino acid produced by oxidation of tyrosine by monophenol monooxygenase; it is the precursor of dopamine and an intermediate product in the biosynthesis of norepinephrine, epinephrine, and melanin. The naturally occurring form is L-dopa (see *levodopa* [USP]).

**do·pa·mine** (do'pə-mēn) [MeSH: Dopamine] 3,4-dihydroxyphenylethylamine, a catecholamine formed in the body by the decarboxylation of dopa; it is an intermediate product in the synthesis of norepinephrine, and acts as a neurotransmitter in the central nervous system. It is also produced peripherally and acts on peripheral receptors, e.g., in blood vessels. Called also *3-hydroxytyramine.*
**d. hydrochloride,** the hydrochloride salt of dopamine, used to correct hemodynamic balance in the treatment of shock syndrome; administered intravenously.

**do·pa·mine β-hy·drox·y·lase** (do"pə-mēn hi-drok'sə-lās) dopamine β-monooxygenase.

**do·pa·mine β-mono·oxy·gen·ase** (do"pə-mēn mon"o-oks'ə-jən-ās) [EC 1.14.17.1] an enzyme of the oxidoreductase class that catalyzes the hydroxylation of dopamine to norepinephrine, simultaneously oxidizing ascorbate. It is a copper protein occurring in nervous tissue and the adrenal medulla. Called also *dopamine β-hydroxylase.*

**do·pa·min·er·gic** (do"pə-mēn-er'jik) 1. activated or transmitted by dopamine. 2. pertaining to tissues or organs affected by dopamine. 3. pertaining to neurons that release dopamine and to the effects exerted thereby.

**do·pa·quin·one** (do"pə-kwin'ōn) an oxidation product of dopa; it is an intermediate in the synthesis of melanin pigments from tyrosine.

**Do·par** (do'pər) trademark for a preparation of levodopa.

**dop·pel·len·der** (dop'əl-en"dər) myofiber hyperplasia.

**Dop·pler** (dop'lər) Doppler ultrasonography.
**color D.,** color flow Doppler imaging.

**Dop·pler effect (phenomenon, principle)** (dop'lər) [Christian *Doppler,* Austrian physicist and mathematician, 1803–1853] see under *effect.*

**Do·pram** (do'prəm) trademark for a preparation of doxapram hydrochloride.

**Dor·al** (dor'al) trademark for a preparation of quazepam.

**Do·rel·lo's ca·nal** (do-rel'ōz) [Primo *Dorello,* Italian anatomist, born 1872] see under *canal.*

**Dor·en·dorf's sign** (dor'ən-dorfs) [Hans *Dorendorf,* German physician, 1866–1953] see under *sign.*

**Dor·i·den** (dor'ĭ-dən) trademark for preparations of glutethimide.

**dor·man·cy** (dor'mən-se) [L. *dormire* to sleep] 1. the state of being dormant. 2. in bacteriology, the property exhibited by some bacteria, and especially by bacterial spores, of remaining viable for an extended time with minimal physical or chemical change, often in response to unfavorable growth conditions.

**dor·mant** (dor'mənt) [L. *dormire* to sleep] sleeping, inactive, quiescent.

**dor·mi·fa·cient** (dor"mĭ-fa'shənt) [L. *dormire* to sleep + *-facient*] hypnotic (defs. 1 and 3).

**dor·sa** (dor'sə) [L.] plural of *dorsum.*

**dor·sad** (dor'sad) toward the back or dorsal aspect.

**dor·sal** (dor'səl) [L. *dorsalis,* from *dorsum* back] 1. pertaining to the back or to any dorsum. 2. denoting a position more toward the back surface than some other object of reference; a synonym of *posterior* in human anatomy and of *superior* in the anatomy of quadrupeds.

**dor·sal·gia** (dor-sal'jə) [*dors-* + *-algia*] pain in the back.

**dor·sa·lis** (dor-sa'lis) [L.] [TA] dorsal.

**dor·si** (dor'si) genitive of *dorsum.*

**dorsi-** see *dors(o)-.*

**dor·si·duct** (dor'sĭ-dəkt) [*dorsi-* + *duct*] to draw toward the back or dorsum.

**dor·si·flex·ion** (dor"sĭ-flek'shən) [*dorsi-* + *flexion*] flexion or bending toward the extensor aspect of a limb, as of the hand or foot.

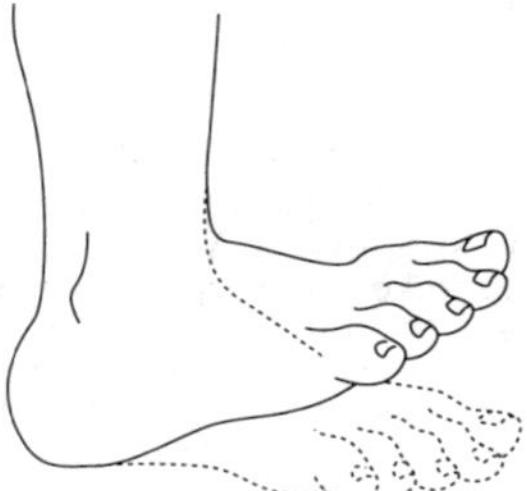
Dorsiflexion of foot.

**dor·si·mes·al** (dor″sĭ-mes′əl) dorsomesial.

**dor·si·spi·nal** (dor″sĭ-spi′nəl) pertaining to the back and vertebral column.

**dors(o)-** [L. *dorsum* back] combining form denoting relationship to a dorsum or to the back (posterior) aspect of the body. Also, *dorsi-*.

**dor·so·an·te·ri·or** (dor″so-an-tēr′e-ər) having the back of the fetus toward the front of the mother.

**dor·so·ceph·a·lad** (dor″so-sef′ə-lad) [*dorso-* + *cephalad*] directed toward the back of the head.

**dor·so·dyn·ia** (dor″so-din′e-ə) dorsalgia.

**dor·so·in·ter·cos·tal** (dor″so-in″tər-kos′təl) situated in the back and between the ribs.

**dor·so·lat·er·al** (dor″so-lat′ər-əl) pertaining to the back and the side.

**dor·so·lum·bar** (dor″so-lum′bahr) pertaining to the back and the loins, especially the region of the lower thoracic and upper lumbar vertebrae.

**dor·so·me·di·an** (dor″so-me′de-ən) the median line of the back.

**dor·so·me·si·al** (dor″so-me′se-əl) pertaining to the median line of the back.

**dor·so·na·sal** (dor″so-na′səl) pertaining to the dorsum of the nose or to the bridge of the nose.

**dor·so·nu·chal** (dor″so-noo′kəl) pertaining to the back of the neck.

**dor·so·pos·te·ri·or** (dor″so-pos-tēr′e-ər) having the back of the fetus directed toward the mother's back.

**dor·so·ra·di·al** (dor″so-ra′de-əl) pertaining to the radial or lateral side of the back of the forearm or hand.

**dor·so·scap·u·lar** (dor″so-skap′u-lər) pertaining to the posterior surface of the scapula.

**dor·so·ven·trad** (dor″so-ven′trəd) [*dorso-* + *ventrad*] directed from the dorsal toward the ventral aspect.

**dor·so·ven·tral** (dor″so-ven′trəl) 1. pertaining to the back and belly surfaces of the body. 2. passing from the back to the belly surface.

**dor·sum** (dor′səm )gen. *dor′si,* pl. *dor′sa* [L.] [TA] 1. the back. 2. the aspect of an anatomical part or structure corresponding in position to the back; posterior, in the human.
**d. of foot,** d. pedis.
**d. of hand,** d. manus.
**d. lin′guae** [TA], dorsum of the tongue: the upper or posterosuperior surface of the tongue.
**d. ma′nus** [TA], back of hand: the hand surface opposite the palm.
**d. na′si** [TA], dorsum of nose: that part of the external surface of the nose formed by junction of the lateral surfaces.
**d. pe′dis** [TA], the upper surface of the foot; the surface opposite the sole. Called also *regio dorsalis pedis* [TA alternative].
**d. pe′nis** [TA], **d. of penis,** the anterior, more extensive surface of the dependent penis, opposite the urethral surface.
**d. of scapula, d. sca′pulae,** facies posterior scapulae.
**d. sel′lae** [TA], the quadrilateral plate on the sphenoid bone that forms the posterior boundary of the sella turcica; the posterior clinoid processes project from its superior extremity, and it is continuous inferiorly with the clivus.
**d. of testis,** margo posterior testis.
**d. of tongue,** d. linguae.

**dor·zo·la·mide hy·dro·chlo·ride** (dor-zo′lə-mīd) a carbonic acid anhydrase inhibitor, used as an antiglaucoma agent in the treatment of open-angle glaucoma and ocular hypertension; administered topically to the conjunctiva.

**dos·age** (do′səj) the determination and regulation of the size, frequency, and number of doses.

**dose** (dōs) [*dosis*] 1. a quantity to be administered at one time, such as a specified amount of medication. 2. in radiology, the amount of energy absorbed per unit mass of tissue at a given site.
**absorbed d.,** the amount of energy from ionizing radiations absorbed per unit mass of matter, expressed in rads.
**air d.,** air exposure.
**average d.,** the quantity of an agent which will usually produce the therapeutic effect for which it is administered.
**booster d.,** a dose of an active immunizing agent, usually smaller than the initial dose, given to maintain immunity.
**cumulative d., cumulative radiation d.,** the total dose resulting from repeated exposures to radiation.
**curative d.,** a dose that is sufficient to restore normal health.
**curative d., median,** a dose that abolishes symptoms in 50 per cent of the test subjects. Abbreviated $CD_{50}$.
**daily d.,** the total amount of a drug administered in a 24-hour period.
**depth d.,** the intensity of radiation at a given depth in an irradiated body, expressed as a percentage of that at the surface of the body nearest the portal of entry.
**divided d.,** fractional d.
**doubling d.,** in radiation biology, the dose of ionizing radiation which will result in a doubling of the current rate of spontaneous biological changes, such as mutations or cancers of various kinds, in a population.
**effective d.,** that quantity of a drug which will produce the effects for which it is administered; abbreviated ED.
**effective d., median,** a dose that produces the desired effect in 50 per cent of a population. Abbreviated $ED_{50}$.
**epilating d.,** the amount of radiation necessary to cause temporary or permanent loss of hair.
**erythema d.,** the amount of radiation which, when applied to the skin, causes temporary reddening of the skin.
**exit d.,** the intensity of radiation emerging from the body at the surface opposite the portal of entry.
**exposure d.,** see *exposure,* def. 3.
**fatal d.,** lethal d.
**fractional d., fractionated d.,** a fraction of the total dose prescribed of a drug or therapeutic radiation; called also *divided d.*
**immunizing d., median,** the dose of vaccine or antigen sufficient to provide immunity in 50 per cent of test subjects.
**infective d.,** that amount of pathogenic microorganisms that will cause infection in susceptible subjects. Abbreviated ID.
**infective d., median,** the amount of pathogenic microorganisms that will produce demonstrable infection in 50 per cent of the test subjects. Abbreviated $ID_{50}$.
**integral d., integral absorbed d.,** in radiation biology, the total energy absorbed by an individual or other biological object during exposure to radiation, expressed in gram-rads (100 ergs).
**L+ d.,** $L_+$ **d.,** the limes tod (death) dose, the smallest amount of diphtheria toxin that will kill a 250-gm. guinea pig within four days when mixed with one unit of diphtheria antitoxin before being injected subcutaneously. Cf. *lethal d.*
**L0 d.,** $L_0$**d.,** the limes nul or zero dose; the largest amount of diphtheria toxin that when mixed with one standard unit of antitoxin produces no perceptible reaction when injected subcutaneously into a guinea pig.
**lethal d.,** the amount of an agent, such as a toxin or radiation, that will or may be sufficient to cause death. Called also *fatal d.* Cf. *L+ d.*
**lethal d., median,** the amount of pathogenic bacteria, bacterial toxin, or other poisonous substance required to kill 50 per cent of uniformly susceptible animals inoculated with it. In radiology, the amount of ionizing radiation that will kill, within a specified period, 50 per cent of individuals in a large group or population. Abbreviated $LD_{50}$.
**lethal d., minimum (MLD),** 1. the smallest amount of a toxic substance that can cause the death of a laboratory animal. 2. the smallest quantity of diphtheria toxin that will kill a guinea pig of 250 g weight in four to five days when injected subcutaneously.
**Lf d.,** the limes flocculating dose; the amount of diphtheria toxin that in the shortest time produces precipitation when mixed with one standard unit of antitoxin.
**limes nul d., limes zero d.,** L0 d.
**Lr d.,** the limes reacting dose; the amount of diphtheria toxin that, when mixed with one standard unit of antitoxin, will produce a minimal skin reaction in a guinea pig.
**maintenance d.,** a dose (often a daily dose or dosage regimen) sufficient to maintain at the desired level the influence of a drug achieved by earlier administration of larger amounts.
**maximum d.,** the largest quantity of an agent that may be safely administered to the average patient. Cf. *tolerance d.*
**maximum permissible d.,** MPD; the largest amount of ionizing radiation that may be received by a person in a specified period without expectation of appreciable bodily injury, according to recommended limits in current radiation protection guides; specific amounts vary with age and circumstance.
**maximum tolerated d.,** MTD; tolerance dose.
**median tissue culture infective d.,** that quantity of a cytopatho-

genic agent (virus) that will produce a cytopathic effect in 50 per cent of the cultures inoculated. Abbreviated $TCID_{50}$.
**minimal d., minimum d.,** the smallest quantity of an agent that is likely to produce an appreciable effect.
**optimal d., optimum d.,** the quantity of an agent which will produce the effect desired without unfavorable effects.
**organ tolerance d.,** in radiology, that amount of radiation which can be administered without appreciable damage to a normal organ; abbreviated OTD.
**permissible d.,** maximum permissible d.
**priming d.,** a quantity several times larger than the maintenance dose, used at the initiation of therapy to rapidly establish the desired blood and tissue levels of the drug.
**radiation absorbed d.,** see *absorbed d.* and *rad,* def. 1.
**reacting d.,** the second dose of sensitizing antigen administered to an animal; it is followed by an immediate hypersensitive (e.g., anaphylactic or allergic) response. Cf. *sensitizing d.*
**reference d.,** an estimate of the daily exposure to a substance for humans that is assumed to be without appreciable risk; it is calculated using the no observed adverse effect level and is more conservative than the older margin of safety.
**sensitizing d.,** the first dose of sensitizing antigen (e.g., protein) administered to an animal in the induction of a hypersensitivity (e.g., anaphylactic or allergic) response; cf. *reacting d.*
**skin d. (SD),** 1. the air dose of radiation at the skin surface, comprising primary radiation plus backscatter. 2. the absorbed dose in the skin.
**therapeutic d.,** a quantity several times larger than the maintenance dose, used in vitamin therapy when a marked deficiency exists.
**threshold d.,** the minimum dose of ionizing radiation, a chemical, or a drug that will produce a detectable degree of any given effect.
**threshold erythema d.,** the single skin dose that will produce in 80 per cent of those tested, a faint but definite erythema within 30 days, and in the other 20 per cent, no visible reaction. Abbreviated TED.
**tissue d.,** the absorbed dose of radiation in a tissue or organ, expressed in rads.
**tolerance d.,** the largest quantity of an agent, such as a drug or radiotherapy, that may be administered without harm. Called also *maximum tolerated d.*
**toxic d.,** the amount of an agent which will cause toxic symptoms.
**volume d.,** integral d.

**do·sim·e·ter** (do-sim′ə-tər) in radiology, an instrument used to detect and measure exposure to radiation of either personnel or radiotherapy patients. See also *film badge.* Called also *dosage meter.*

**do·si·met·ric** (do″sĭ-met′rik) of or pertaining to dosimetry.

**do·sim·e·trist** (do-sim′ə-trist) one who plans an optimum radiotherapy dosage pattern or establishes a summation isodose pattern for the radiotherapy by means of isodose curves or other data supplied by a radiation physicist.

**do·sim·e·try** (do-sim′ə-tre) [*dose* + *-metry*] the determination by scientific methods of the amount, rate, and distribution of radiation emitted from a source of ionizing radiation.
**biological d.,** the determination of the level of exposure to ionizing radiation by measurement of radiation-induced changes such as cytogenetic abnormalities, lymphopenia, and agranulocytosis; the dose is estimated by comparison of the measurements under consideration to those observed in prior radiation accidents.
**physical d.,** the determination of the level of exposure to ionizing radiation by means of radiation measuring instruments such as environmental monitoring devices or individual dosimeters.

**do·sis** (do′sis) [L., Gr. "a giving"] dose.
**d. curati′va,** the minimum amount of a therapeutic agent that will effect a cure.
**d. ef′ficax,** d. curativa.
**d. refrac′ta,** fractional dose.
**d. tolera′ta,** the largest amount of a therapeutic agent that can be given with safety.

**dos·sier** (dos′e-a) [Fr.] the accumulated records of a patient's case history.

**dot** (dot) a small spot or speck.
**Gunn's d's,** white dots seen about the macula lutea on oblique illumination.
**Marcus Gunn's d's,** Gunn's d's.
**Maurer's d's,** irregular dots, staining red with Leishman's stain, seen in erythrocytes from malarial patients infected with *Plasmodium falciparum;* called also *Maurer's clefts.*
**Mittendorf's d.,** a congenital anomaly manifested as a small gray or white opacity just inferior and nasal to the posterior pole of the lens, representing the remains of the lenticular attachment of the hyaloid artery; it does not affect vision.
**Schüffner's d's,** minute granules observed in erythrocytes infected with *Plasmodium vivax* when stained by certain methods, such as Romanowsky's or Wright's stain; called also *Schüffner's granules* or *punctuation.*
**Trantas' d's,** small, white calcareous looking dots in the limbus of the conjunctiva in vernal conjunctivitis.

**dot·age** (do′təj) deterioration of mental faculties, usually with age. It may be used to denote senile dementia.

**Do·thi·de·a·les** (do-thid″e-a′lēz) [Gr. *dothiēn* a boil] an order of perfect fungi of the subphylum Ascomycotina, series Bitunicatae, characterized by flasklike ascocarps in which the hymenium is exposed at maturity and by double-walled asci that develop in cavities in a preformed stroma. It is a large and varied order, and a number of different classifications have been proposed for it. It includes the family Piedraiaceae. Called also *Myriangiales.*

**do·thi·e·pin hy·dro·chlo·ride** (do-thi′ə-pin) a tricyclic antidepressant having actions and uses similar to those of amitriptyline; administered orally.

**dou·ble blind** (dub′əl blīnd) pertaining to a clinical trial or other experiment in which neither the subject nor the person administering treatment knows which treatment the subject is receiving. The term *double mask* is sometimes preferred to avoid confusion associated with the use of the term "blind."

**dou·ble mask** (dub′əl mask) double blind.

**doub·let** (dub′lət) [Middle English, from Old Fr. *double*] 1. a fixed combination of two lenses, as in a telescope or microscope, for reducing aberration and increasing power. 2. double discharge.
**Wollaston's d.,** a microscopical lens consisting of a combination of two planoconvex lenses for correcting chromatic aberration.

**douche** (dōōsh) [Fr.] a stream of water or gas directed against a part of the body or into a cavity.
**air d.,** a current of air blown into a cavity, particularly into the tympanum for opening the eustachian tube.

**Doug·las bag** (dug′ləs) [Claude Gordon *Douglas,* English physiologist, 1882–1963] see under *bag.*

**Doug·las' septum,** etc. (dug′ləs) [James *Douglas,* Scottish anatomist in London, 1675–1742] see under *septum,* and see *excavatio rectouterina, plica rectouterina,* and *linea arcuata vaginae musculi recti abdominis.*

**doug·las·cele** (dug′lə-sēl) posterior vaginal hernia.

**doug·la·si·tis** (dug″lə-si′tis) inflammation of Douglas' pouch (excavatio rectouterina).

**dou·rine** (doo-rēn′) [Fr.] [MeSH: Dourine] venereal trypanosomiasis affecting horses and asses in Africa, Asia, and certain regions of North and South America, caused by *Trypanosoma equiperdum;* characteristics include edematous swelling of the external genitalia, a mucopurulent discharge from the urethra or vagina, cutaneous plaques, and progressive emaciation and weakness. Called also *covering disease* and *equine* or *horse syphilis.*

**Do·vo·nex** (do′və-neks) trademark for a preparation of calcipotriene.

**dow·el** (dou′əl) a post or a pin, usually metal, fitted into a prepared posthole within the root canal and cemented in place, serving to retain a dental restoration, such as a crown. Called also *post.*

**Down syndrome (disease)** (doun) [John Langdon Haydon *Down,* English physician, 1828–1896] see under *syndrome.*

**down** (doun) lanugo.

**down-reg·u·la·tion** (doun reg-u-la′shən) a decrease in the number of receptors for a chemical or drug on cell surfaces in a given area, usually due to long-term exposure to the agent. See also *up-regulation.*

**Downs' analysis, Y axis** (dounz) [W.B. *Downs,* American orthodontist, 1899–1966] see under *analysis* and see *Y axis,* under *axis.*

**down·stream** (doun′strēm″) in molecular biology, a term used to denote a region of DNA or RNA that is located to the 3′ side of a gene or region of interest.

**dox·a·cu·ri·um chlo·ride** (dok″sə-ku′re-əm) a long-acting nondepolarizing neuromuscular blocking agent used to provide skeletal muscle relaxation during surgery and endotracheal intubation; administered by intravenous injection.

**dox·a·pram hy·dro·chlo·ride** (dok′sə-pram) [USP] a respiratory stimulant used in the treatment of postanesthetic respiratory depression, administered intravenously.

**dox·azo·sin mes·y·late** (dok″sa′-zo-sin) a quinazoline derivative that blocks certain of the α-adrenergic receptors and has a longer half life than that of prazosin; used as an antihypertensive agent.

**dox·e·pin hy·dro·chlo·ride** (dok′sə-pin) [USP] a tricyclic antidepressant of the dibenzoxepine class, also having significant anxiolytic activity; administered orally. It is also used orally to treat chronic pain, peptic ulcer, pruritus, and idiopathic cold urticaria and topically to treat pruritus. In veterinary medicine it is used as an antipruritic.

**Dox·il** (dok'sil) trademark for a preparation of doxorubicin hydrochloride in a liposome preparation for injection.

**Dox·i·nate** (dok'sĭ-nāt) trademark for a preparation of dioctyl sodium sulfosuccinate.

**doxo·ru·bi·cin** (dok″so-roo'bĭ-sin) [MeSH: Doxorubicin] an anthracycline (q.v.) antibiotic produced by *Streptomyces peucetius* var. *caesius* having one of the widest spectrums of antitumor activity of any antineoplastic agent.
**d. hydrochloride** [USP], the hydrochloride salt of doxorubicin, having the same actions as the base, used for the treatment of acute lymphocytic and acute myelogenous leukemia; Hodgkin's disease and non-Hodgkin's lymphomas; rhabdomyosarcoma and osteogenic, Ewing's, and soft tissue sarcomas; neuroblastoma; Wilms' tumor; carcinoma of the breast, bladder, prostate, testes, ovary, cervix, endometrium, thyroid, lung, liver, pancreas, and stomach; squamous cell carcinoma of the head and neck; hepatoma; and multiple myeloma. Administered intravenously.

**doxy·cy·cline** (dok″se-si'klēn) [USP] [MeSH: Doxycycline] a semisynthetic broad-spectrum antibacterial of the tetracycline group, derived from methacycline; administered orally.
**d. calcium,** a complex prepared from doxycycline hyclate and calcium chloride, having the same actions and uses as the hyclate salt; administered orally.
**d. hyclate** [USP], **d. hydrochloride,** a salt having the antibacterial effects of other tetracyclines; administered orally.

**Doxy·II** (dok'se) trademark for a preparation of doxycycline.

**dox·yl·amine suc·ci·nate** (dok-sil'ə-mēn) [USP] an orally administered antihistaminic.

**Doy·en's clamp** (dwah-yahz') [Eugène Louis *Doyen,* French surgeon, 1859–1916] see under *clamp.*

**Doyne's familial honeycombed choroiditis** (doinz) [Robert Walter *Doyne,* English ophthalmologist, 1857–1916] see under *choroiditis.*

**DP** abbreviation for L. *directio'ne prop'ria,* "with proper direction"; Doctor of Pharmacy; Doctor of Podiatry.

**DPH** Diploma in Public Health.

**DPM** Diploma in Psychological Medicine; Doctor of Podiatric Medicine.

**DPN** diphosphopyridine nucleotide; former name for *nicotinamide adenine dinucleotide* (NAD).

**DPT** diphtheria-pertussis-tetanus (vaccine).

**DR** reaction of degeneration; see under *reaction.*

**dr** dram.

**drachm** (dram) [Gr. *drachmē*] dram.

**drac·on·ti·a·sis** (drak″ən-ti'ə-sis) [Gr. *drakontion* (little dragon) tapeworm] dracunculiasis.

**dra·cun·cu·lar** (drə-kung'ku-lər) pertaining to or caused by nematodes of the genus *Dracunculus.*

**dra·cun·cu·li·a·sis** (drə-kung″ku-li'ə-sis) [MeSH: Dracunculiasis] infection with nematodes of the genus *Dracunculus;* called also *dracontiasis, dracunculosis,* and *guinea worm disease.*

**Dra·cun·cu·li·dae** (drə-kəng-ku'lĭ-de) a family of nematodes often parasitic to humans and domestic animals. It contains one genus of medical interest, *Dracunculus.*

**Dra·cun·cu·loi·dea** (drə-kung″ku-loi'de-ə) [MeSH: Dracunculoidea] a superfamily of phasmid nematodes including the genus *Dracunculus.*

**dra·cun·cu·lo·sis** (drə-kung″ku-lo'sis) dracunculiasis.

**Dra·cun·cu·lus** (drə-kung'ku-ləs) [L. "little dragon"] [MeSH: Dracunculus] a genus of nematode parasites of the family Dracunculidae.
**D. insig'nis,** a species that parasitizes dogs, cats, raccoons, and other carnivores.
**D. medinen'sis,** a threadlike worm 30 to 120 cm long that inhabits the subcutaneous and intermuscular tissues of humans and domestic animals in India, Africa, and the Arabian peninsula, causing dracunculiasis. Its embryos are discharged through an opening in the skin upon contact with water; from the water they enter the body of a small crustacean, *Cyclops,* where they undergo larval development. Called also *dragon worm, guinea worm, Medina worm,* and *serpent worm.*

**draft** (draft) a potion; dose.
**black d.,** the compound infusion of senna.

**drag** (drag) the lower or cast side of a denture flask to which the cope is fitted.

**dra·gée** (drah-zha') [Fr. "sugar-plum"] a sugar-coated pill, or medicated confection.

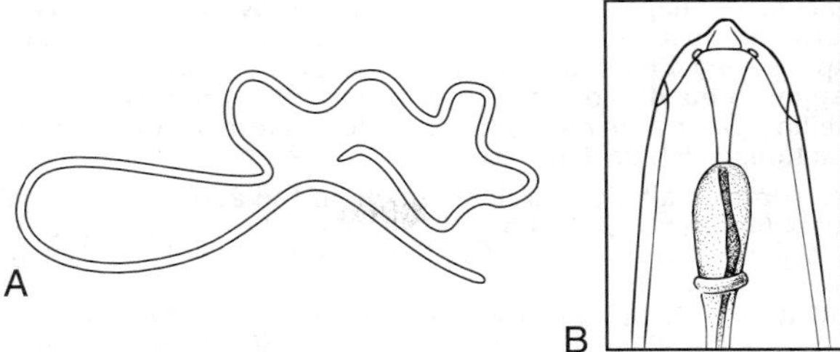


*Dracunculus medinensis.* Body *(A)* and head *(B)* of adult female.

**drain** (drān) any device by which a channel or open area may be established for the exit of fluids or purulent material from any cavity, wound, or infected area.
**cigarette d.,** a drain made by drawing a strip of gauze or surgical sponge into the lumen of a rubber tube.
**controlled d.,** a drain made by pressing a square of gauze into the wound and then packing with gauze strips, the ends of which, together with the corners of the square, are left projecting from the wound.
**Mikulicz d.,** a drain formed by pushing a single layer of gauze into a wound or cavity, then packing with several thick wicks of gauze as the original layer is forced farther and farther into the defect.
**Penrose d.,** a thin rubber tube, usually 0.5 to 1 inch in diameter.
**stab wound d.,** drainage accomplished by bringing out the drain through a small separate wound adjacent to the major operative incision.
**sump d.,** a double-lumen drain that allows air to enter the drained area through the smaller lumen and displace fluid into the larger lumen.
**sump-Penrose d.,** a triple-lumen drain formed by placing a double-lumen tube within a Penrose drain.

**drain·age** (drān'əj) [MeSH: Drainage] the systematic withdrawal of fluids and discharges from a wound, sore, or cavity.
**basal d.,** withdrawal of the cerebrospinal fluid from the basal subarachnoid space for the relief of intracranial pressure.
**button d.,** drainage of a peritoneal transudate by means of a special button affixed to all layers of the abdominal wall.
**capillary d.,** drainage effected by strands of hair, surgical gut, spun glass, or other material of tiny diameter which induces capillary attraction.
**closed d.,** airtight drainage of a cavity carried out so that the entrance of air or contaminants is prevented.
**continuous suction d.,** see *Wangensteen d.*
**open d.,** drainage of a cavity through an opening into which one or more rubber drainage tubes are inserted, the opening not being sealed against the entrance of outside air.
**percutaneous d.,** drainage of an abscess or collection of fluid by means of a catheter inserted through the skin and positioned under the guidance of computed tomography or ultrasonography.
**postural d.,** removal of secretions in bronchiectasis and lung abscess by changes in the patient's position with accompanying repetitive striking of the chest.
**suction d.,** closed drainage of a cavity, with a suction apparatus attached to the drainage tube.
**through d.,** drainage achieved by passing a perforated tube or other type of drain through a cavity, so that irrigation may be effected by injecting fluid into one aperture and letting it escape through another.

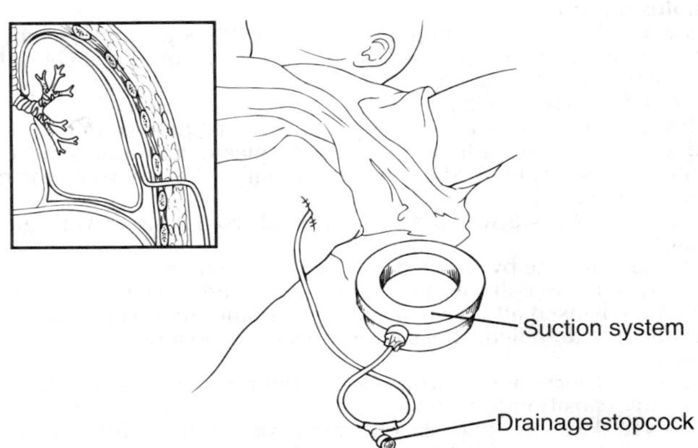


Closed drainage using a portable suction system.

**tidal d.,** drainage of the urinary bladder by an apparatus which alternately fills the bladder to a predetermined extent and then empties it by a combination of siphonage and gravity flow.
**Wangensteen d.,** continuous drainage by suction through an indwelling gastric or duodenal tube; for treatment of intestinal obstruction, paralytic ileus, etc.

**dram** (dram) a unit of weight which, in the apothecaries' system, equals 60 grains, or $\frac{1}{8}$ ounce; in the avoirdupois system it equals 27.34 grains, or $\frac{1}{16}$ ounce. Symbol ʒ; abbreviated dr. Called also *drachm.*
**fluid d.,** a unit of capacity (liquid measure) of the apothecaries' system, being 60 minims, or the equivalent of 3.697 mL. Abbreviated fl dr.

**Dram·a·mine** (dram'ə-mēn) trademark for preparations of dimenhydrinate.

**Dra·schia** (dră'she-ə) a genus of nematodes of the family Habronematidae. *D. megasto'ma* (formerly called *Habronema megastoma*) infects the stomach of horses, and its larvae form nodules in the stomach walls (see *gastric habronemiasis*).

**Drash syndrome** (drash) [Allan Lee *Drash,* American pediatrician, born 1931] see under *syndrome.*

**dras·tic** (dras'tik) [Gr. *drastikos* effective] 1. acting powerfully or thoroughly. 2. a violent purgative.

**draught** (draft) draft.

**dream** (drēm) [MeSH: Dreams] 1. a mental phenomenon occurring during sleep in which images, emotions, and thoughts are experienced with a sense of reality. Dreaming occurs during REM sleep; typically there are four or five such periods a night having a total duration of about 90 minutes. Freud originated psychological interpretation of dreams, theorizing that dreams enable the conscious expression of repressed unconscious impulses and wishes. 2. to experience such a phenomenon.
**day d.,** wishful, purposeless reveries, without regard to reality.
**wet d.,** a slang term for *nocturnal emission.*

**Drechs·le·ra** (dreks'lə-rə) a genus of Fungi Imperfecti of the form-class Hyphomycetes, form-family Dematiaceae, closely related to *Bipolaris* and *Exserohilum. D. bisepta'ta* has been isolated from a human brain abscess. The perfect (sexual) stage of *Drechslera* species is in genus *Cochliobolus.*

**drench** (drench) a draft of medicine given to an animal by pouring it into its mouth.

**Drep·a·nido·tae·nia** (drep"ə-nid-o-te'ne-ə) former name for a genus of cestodes; now classified as part of *Hymenolepis.*

**drep·a·no·cyte** (drep'ə-no-sīt) [Gr. *drepanē* sickle + *-cyte*] sickle cell.

**drep·a·no·cyt·ic** (drep"ə-no-sit'ik) having or pertaining to sickle cells.

**drep·a·no·cy·to·sis** (drep"ə-no-si-to'sis) old name for *sickle cell anemia.*

**Dres·bach's syndrome** (dres'bahks) [Melvin *Dresbach,* American physician, 1874–1946] elliptocytosis.

**dress·er** (dres'ər) a surgical assistant who dresses wounds, etc.

**dress·ing** (dres'ing) [MeSH: Bandages] 1. any of various materials utilized for covering and protecting a wound. See also *bandage.* 2. the putting on of clothing.
**adhesive absorbent d.,** a sterile individual dressing consisting of a plain absorbent compress affixed to a film or fabric coated with a pressure-sensitive adhesive substance.
**antiseptic d.,** a dressing of gauze impregnated with an antiseptic material.
**bolus d.,** tie-over d.
**cocoon d.,** a dressing of gauze affixed to the surrounding skin by collodion or other liquid adhesive in such fashion that its elevated appearance resembles a cocoon.
**cross d.,** cross-dressing.
**dry d.,** dry gauze or absorbent cotton applied to a wound.
**fixed d.,** a dressing impregnated with plaster of Paris, starch, or silicate of soda, utilized to secure fixation of the part when the material dries.
**occlusive d.,** one which seals a wound from contact with air or bacteria.
**pressure d.,** one by which pressure is exerted on the area covered to prevent the collection of fluids in the underlying tissues; most commonly used after skin grafting and in the treatment of burns.
**protective d.,** a light dressing to prevent exposure to injury or infection.
**stent d.,** a dressing in which is incorporated a mold or stent, to maintain position of a graft.
**tie-over d.,** a dressing placed over a skin graft or other sutured wound, and tied on by the sutures which have been made of sufficient length for that purpose; called also *bolus d.*

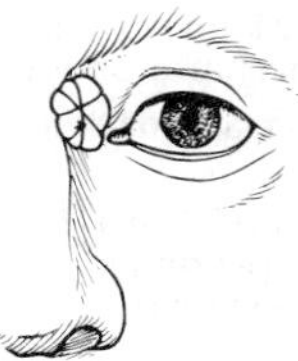
Tie-over dressing.

**Dress·ler's syndrome** (dres'lərz) [William *Dressler,* Polish-born American physician, 1890–1969] postmyocardial infarction syndrome.

**Drey·er and Ben·nett hypothesis** (dri'ər; ben'ət) [William J. *Dreyer,* American immunologist, born 1928; Joe Claude *Bennett,* American rheumatologist, born 1933] see *recombinational germline theory,* under *theory.*

**DRG** Diagnosis-Related Group.

**drift** (drift) [A.S. *drifan* to drive] 1. slow movement away from the normal or original position. 2. a chance variation, as in gene frequency between populations; the smaller the population, the greater the chance of random variations. Called also *genetic d.* or *random genetic d.*
**antigenic d.,** relatively minor changes in the antigenic structure of a virus strain, probably resulting from natural selection of virus variants circulating among an immune or partially immune population. Cf. *antigenic shift,* under *shift.*
**genetic d.,** see *drift,* def. 2.
**physiologic d.,** physiologic tooth migration.
**radial d.,** see under *deviation.*
**random genetic d.,** see *drift,* def. 2.
**ulnar d.,** see under *deviation.*

**drill** (dril) 1. a rotating cutting instrument for making holes in hard substances, such as bones or teeth. 2. bur, def. 1.
**cannulated d.,** a drill with a hole through the center of its long axis, to be used over a guide wire.

**drill·ing** (dril'ing) the act or process of boring holes with a rotary instrument; the term is sometimes used in connection with cavity preparation.

**drink** (drink) 1. a quantity of liquid taken in orally and swallowed. 2. to take in and swallow a liquid.
**sham d.,** a drink, as by an esophagostomized dog, in which swallowed water fails to be ingested or retained in the stomach.

**Drink·er respirator** (dring'kər) [Philip *Drinker,* American public health engineer, 1894–1972] see under *respirator.*

**drip** (drip) the slow, drop by drop, infusion of a liquid.
**intravenous d.,** continuous intravenous instillation, drop by drop, of saline or other solution.
**nasal d.,** a method of giving fluid slowly to dehydrated infants through a catheter inserted into the nose and pushed down into the esophagus.
**postnasal d.,** the dripping of discharges from the postnasal region into the pharynx due to hypersecretion of mucus in the nasal or nasopharyngeal mucosa or to chronic sinusitis.

**Dris·dol** (driz'dol) trademark for preparations of ergocalciferol.

**Dritho·creme** (drith'o-krēm") trademark for a preparation of anthralin.

**Dritho-Scalp** (drith'o-skalp") trademark for a preparation of anthralin.

**drive** (drīv) [MeSH: Drive] 1. the force which activates human impulses. 2. to activate or cause to move.
**aggressive d.,** death instinct.
**sexual d.,** life instinct.

**driv·en·ness** (driv'ən-nəs) hyperactivity (def. 2).
**organic d.,** hyperactivity seen in brain-damaged individuals as a result of injury to and disorganization of cerebellar structures.

**driv·ing** (drīv'ing) an effect seen on an electroencephalogram, by which certain repetitive sensory stimuli cause changes in amplitude of brain waves. Cf. *following.*
**photic d.,** driving in which alpha rhythms from the occipital cortex are altered when the eye is exposed to a rhythmically flashing light.

**dro·car·bil** (dro-kahr'bil) a mixture of acetarsone and arecoline, used as a veterinary anthelmintic.

**dro·code** (dro'kod) dihydrocodeine.

**drom(o)-** [Gr. *dromos* a course, race] a combining form denoting relationship to conduction, to running, or to speed.

**dromo·graph** (drom'o-graf) [*dromo-* + *-graph*] an instrument for recording conduction or flow.

**dro·mo·stan·o·lone pro·pio·nate** (dro″mo-stan′o-lōn) an androgenic, anabolic steroid, used as an antineoplastic agent in the palliative treatment of advanced metastatic, inoperable breast cancer in certain postmenopausal women; administered intramuscularly.

**drom·o·trop·ic** (drom″o-trop′ik) affecting the conductivity of a nerve fiber.

**dro·mot·ro·pism** (dro-mot′ro-piz-əm) [*dromo-* + *tropism*] the quality or property of affecting the conductivity of a nerve fiber.
**negative d.,** the property of diminishing the conductivity of a nerve.
**positive d.,** the property of increasing the conductivity of a nerve.

**dro·nab·i·nol** (dro-nab′in-ol) [USP] $\Delta^9$-tetrahydrocannabinol, one of the major active substances in cannabis; used to treat the nausea and vomiting associated with cancer chemotherapy. Because of its psychotomimetic activity, it is subject to abuse and its use as an antiemetic is limited to patients resistant to more conventional agents.

**Dron·cit** (dron′cit) trademark for preparations of praziquantel.

**drop** (drop) [L. *gutta*] 1. a minute sphere of liquid as it hangs or falls. 2. to descend or cause to descend. 3. a descent or falling.
**ear d's,** medicated oil or water to be dropped into the external auditory meatus.
**enamel d.,** enameloma.
**eye d's,** a medicated solution to be dropped into the conjunctival sac.
**foot d.,** footdrop.
**nose d's,** a medicated solution to be dropped into the nose.
**d. phalangette,** a condition in which the terminal phalanx of a finger or toe is permanently flexed, as in baseball finger or mallet finger.
**wrist d.,** wristdrop.

**drop·a·cism** (drop′ə-siz-əm) [Gr. *drōpax* plaster] the removal of hairs by means of a plaster or wax.

**dro·per·i·dol** (dro-per′ĭ-dol) [USP] [MeSH: Droperidol] a drug of the butyrophenone series, used for its antianxiety, sedative, and antiemetic effects as a premedication prior to surgery and during induction and maintenance of anesthesia, administered intravenously or intramuscularly. A combination of droperidol and fentanyl citrate is administered intramuscularly to produce neuroleptanalgesia.

**drop·let** (drop′lət) a diminutive drop, such as one of the particles of moisture expelled from the mouth in coughing, sneezing, or speaking, which may carry infection to others through the air. See also under *nucleus.*

**drop·per** (drop′ər) a pipet or tube for dispensing liquid in drops.

**drop·si·cal** (drop′sĭ-kəl) edematous.

**drop·sy** (drop′se) [L. *hydrops,* from Gr. *hydōr* water] edema.
**abdominal d.,** ascites.
**d. of amnion,** hydramnios.
**articular d.,** hydrarthrosis.
**d. of belly,** ascites.
**d. of chest,** hydrothorax.
**cutaneous d.,** edema.
**epidemic d.,** a sometimes fatal condition seen in India, Fiji, South Africa, and elsewhere, characterized by edema of the extremities; dilatation of vessels of the skin, subcutaneous tissues, and uveal tract, resulting in glaucoma; cardiac insufficiency; and liver abnormalities. It is caused by contamination of cooking oil by argemone oil (q.v.), which contains the toxic glycoside sanguinarine.
**peritoneal d.,** ascites.
**salpingian d.,** hydrosalpinx.
**wet d.,** beriberi.

**drop·wort** (drop′wōrt) any plant of the genus *Oenanthe.*

**Dro·soph·i·la** (dro-sof′ĭ-lə) [Gr. *drosos* dew + *philein* to love] [MeSH: Drosophila] a genus of flies; the pomace flies (often erroneously called fruit flies).
**D. melanogas′ter,** a small fly often seen about decaying fruit; used extensively in experimental genetics.

**dro·sop·ter·in** (dro-sop′tər-in) any of a group of bright red pteridine pigments of the eye of *Drosophila* which are readily decomposed by light.

**dro·stan·o·lone pro·pi·o·nate** (dro-stan′ə-lōn″) INN and BAN for *dromostanolone propionate.*

**drown·ing** (droun′ing) [MeSH: Drowning] suffocation and death resulting from filling of the lungs with water or other substance or fluid, so that gas exchange becomes impossible.
**near d.,** survival for any length of time after submersion in water and temporary suffocation; it sometimes ends with secondary drowning.
**secondary d.,** delayed death from drowning, due to such complications as pulmonary alveolar inflammation.

**drox·i·fil·con A** (drok″sĭ-fil′kon) a hydrophilic contact lens material.

**DrPH** Doctor of Public Health.

**drug** (drug) 1. a chemical substance that affects the processes of the mind or body. 2. any chemical compound used on or administered to humans or animals as an aid in the diagnosis, treatment, or prevention of disease or other abnormal condition, for the relief of pain or suffering, or to control or improve any physiologic or pathologic condition. 3. a substance used recreationally for its effects on the central nervous system, such as a narcotic; abuse may lead to dependence or addiction. 4. to administer a drug to.
**antagonistic d.,** one that tends to counteract or neutralize the effect of another.
**crude d.,** the whole drug with all its ingredients.
**designer d.,** a new drug of abuse similar in action to an older abused drug, usually created by making a slight alteration in the chemical structure of the older one so that it is no longer a controlled substance.
**mind-altering d.,** one that produces an altered state of consciousness, e.g., mescaline and lysergic acid diethylamide (LSD).
**nonsteroidal antiinflammatory d.,** NSAID; any of a large, chemically heterogeneous group of drugs that inhibit cyclooxygenase activity, resulting in decreased synthesis of prostaglandin and thromboxane precursors from arachidonic acid. All NSAIDs have analgesic, antipyretic, and antiinflammatory actions. Called also *nonsteroidal antiinflammatory analgesic.*
**orphan d.,** a drug that has limited commercial appeal because of the rarity of the condition it is used to treat.
**psychoactive d., psychotropic d.,** see under *substance.*

**drug-fast** (drug′fast″) drug-resistant.

**drug·gist** (drug′ist) pharmacist.

**drug-re·sis·tant** (drug′re-zis″tənt) resistant to the action of drugs; said of microorganisms. Called also *drug-fast.*

**drum** (drum) membrana tympanica.

**drum·head** (drum′hed) membrana tympanica.

**Drum·mond's marginal artery, sign** (drum′əndz) [Sir David *Drummond,* English physician, 1852–1932] see *arteria marginalis coli* and see under *sign.*

**drum·stick** (drum′stik) a nuclear lobule attached by a slender strand to the nucleus of a small proportion of polymorphonuclear leukocytes of normal females but not of normal males.

**drunk·en·ness** (drung′kən-nəs) inebriation.
**sleep d.,** a condition of prolonged transition from sleep to waking, with partial alertness, disorientation, drowsiness, and poor coordination; sometimes also characterized by excited or violent behavior.

**drupe** (dro͞op) [L. *drupa* an overripe olive] any of several stone fruits in which the outer part of the ovary wall forms a skin, the middle part becomes fleshy and juicy, and the inner part forms a hard pit or stone around the seed; e.g., peaches, plums, apricots.

**dru·sen** (droo′zən) sing. *druse* [Ger. "bumps"] 1. hyaline excrescences in Bruch's membrane (lamina basalis choroideae); they usually result from aging, but sometimes occur with pathologic conditions. 2. rosettes of granules occurring in the lesions of actinomycosis.

**Dry·op·te·ris** (dri-op′tə-ris) a large genus of ferns of the family Polypodiaceae; called also *Aspidium. D. filix-mas* is the male or male shield fern (called also *filix mas*), a species that is violently poisonous if ingested but also yields oil of male fern, an oleoresin used as an anthelmintic.

**DSC** Doctor of Surgical Chiropody.

**dsDNA** double-stranded DNA.

**dsRNA** double-stranded RNA.

**DT** diphtheria and tetanus toxoids for pediatric use.

**Dt** duration tetany.

**dT** deoxythymidine.

**DTaP** diphtheria and tetanus toxoids and acellular pertussis vaccine.

**D.T.D.** abbreviation for L. *da′tur ta′lis do′sis,* give of such a dose.

**dTDP** deoxythymidine diphosphate.

**DTH** delayed-type hypersensitivity.

**DTIC, Dtic** dacarbazine.

**DTIC-Dome** (dōm) trademark for a preparation of dacarbazine.

**dTMP** deoxythymidine monophosphate.

**dTMP ki·nase** (ki′nās) [EC 2.7.4.9] an enzyme of the transferase class that catalyzes the phosphorylation of dTMP to form dTDP, a step in the synthesis of dTTP from dUMP.

**DTP** diphtheria and tetanus toxoids and pertussis vaccine.

**DTPA** [MeSH: DTPA] diethylenetriamine pentaacetic acid; see *pentetic acid.*

**dTTP** deoxythymidine triphosphate.

**dU** deoxyuridine.

**du·al·ism** (doo'əl-iz-əm) [L. *duo* two] 1. dualistic theory; see under *theory.* 2. the theory that human beings are made up of two independent systems, mind and body, and that psychic and physical phenomena are fundamentally independent and different in nature.

**Duane's syndrome, test** (dwānz) [Alexander *Duane,* American ophthalmologist, 1858–1926] see under *syndrome* and *test.*

**du·azo·my·cin** (doo-az"o-mi'sin) an antibiotic substance with antineoplastic properties, produced by *Streptomyces ambofaciens.* **d. B,** former name for *azotomycin.*

**Du·bin-John·son syndrome** (doo'bən jon'sən) [Isidore Nathan *Dubin,* American pathologist, 1913–1981; Frank B. *Johnson,* American pathologist, born 1919] see under *syndrome.*

**Du·bin-Sprinz syndrome** (doo'bən shprintz) [I.N. *Dubin;* Helmuth *Sprinz,* German-born American pathologist, born 1911] Dubin-Johnson syndrome.

**Du·bi·ni's chorea (disease)** (doo-be'nēz) [Angelo *Dubini,* Italian physician, 1813–1902] see under *chorea.*

**Du·bois' abscess (disease), sign** (du-bwahz') [Paul *Dubois,* French obstetrician, 1795–1871] see under *abscess* and *sign.*

**Du·boi·sia** (doo-boi'se-ə) a genus of plants of the family Solanaceae. *D. myoporoi'des* is the corkwood tree, which contains hyoscyamine and scopolamine and can cause neurotoxicity in livestock.

**Du·boscq colorimeter** (du-bosk') [Louis Jules *Duboscq,* French optician, 1817–1886] see under *colorimeter.*

**Du·breu·il-Cham·bar·del's syndrome** (du-broo-e' shahm-bahr-delz') [Louis *Dubreuil-Chambardel,* French dentist, 1879–1927] see under *syndrome.*

**Du·chenne's disease,** etc. (du-shenz') [Guillaume Benjamin Amand *Duchenne,* French neurologist, 1806–1875] see under *disease, paralysis,* and *sign,* see *pseudohypertrophic muscular dystrophy,* under *dystrophy,* and see *progressive bulbar palsy,* under *palsy.*

**Du·chenne-Aran muscular atrophy (disease)** (du-shen'ah-rah') [G.B.A. *Duchenne;* François Amilcar *Aran,* French physician, 1817–1861] spinal muscular atrophy; see under *atrophy.*

**Du·chenne-Erb paralysis, syndrome** (du-shen' ārb) [G.B.A. *Duchenne;* Wilhelm Heinrich *Erb,* German internist, 1840–1921] Erb-Duchenne paralysis.

**Du·chenne-Grie·sing·er disease** (du-shen' gre'sing-er) [G.B.A. *Duchenne;* Wilhelm *Griesinger,* German neurologist, 1817–1868] Duchenne's muscular dystrophy.

**Du·chenne-Lan·dou·zy dystrophy** (du-shen' lahn-doo-ze') [G.B.A. *Duchenne;* Louis Théophile Joseph *Landouzy,* French physician, 1845–1917] facioscapulohumeral muscular dystrophy.

**Duck·worth's phenomenon (sign)** (duk'wərths) [Sir Dyce *Duckworth,* British physician, 1840–1928] see under *phenomenon.*

**Du·co·bee** (doo'ko-be) trademark for preparations of vitamin $B_{12}$; see *cyanocobalamin.*

**Du·crey's bacillus** (doo-krāz') [Augusto *Ducrey,* Italian dermatologist, 1860–1940] *Haemophilus ducreyi.*

**duct** (dukt) [L. *ductus,* from *ducere* to draw or lead] a passage with well-defined walls; called *ductus* [TA]. Cf. *ductule.*

## Duct

For descriptions of anatomic structures not found here, see under *ductus.*

**aberrant d.,** any duct that is not usually present or that takes an unusual course or direction, such as the ductulus aberrans superior.
**accessory d. of Santorini,** ductus pancreaticus accessorius.
**acoustic d.,** meatus acusticus externus.
**adipose d.,** an elongated sac in the cellular tissue filled with fat.
**alimentary d.,** thoracic d.
**allantoic d.,** allantoic stalk.
**alveolar d's,** ductuli alveolares.
**d. of Arantius,** ductus venosus.
**archinephric d.,** pronephric d.
**arterial d.,** ductus arteriosus.
**Bartholin's d.,** ductus sublingualis major.
**Bellini's d.,** ductus papillaris.
**Bernard's d.,** ductus pancreaticus accessorius.
**bile d.,** any of the ducts that convey bile in and from the liver; called also *biliary d.* and *gall d.* See *ductus choledochus, ductus cysticus, ductus hepaticus dexter,* and *ductus hepaticus sinister.*
**bile d., common,** ductus choledochus.
**bile d's, interlobular,** ductuli interlobulares.
**biliary d.,** 1. bile d. 2. ductus choledochus.
**Blasius' d.,** ductus parotideus.
**Bochdalek's d.,** ductus thyroglossalis.
**d. of Botallo,** ductus arteriosus.
**branchial d's,** drawn-out branchial grooves 2, 3, and 4, which open into the temporary cervical sinus of the embryo.
**canalicular d's,** ductus lactiferi.
**cervical d.,** the opening from the exterior into the temporary cervical sinus of the embryo.
**choledochous d.,** ductus choledochus.
**chyliferous d.,** thoracic d.
**cloacal d.,** Reichel's cloacal d.
**cochlear d.,** ductus cochlearis.
**collecting d.,** tubulus renalis colligens; see under *tubulus.*
**common bile d.,** the duct formed by union of the cystic duct and the hepatic duct; called also *ductus choledochus* [TA].
**cortical collecting d.,** see under *tubule.*
**cowperian d.,** ductus glandulae bulbourethralis.
**craniopharyngeal d.,** hypophysial d.
**d's of Cuvier,** common cardinal veins.
**cystic d.,** ductus cysticus.
**deferent d.,** ductus deferens.
**efferent d.,** a duct that gives outlet to a glandular secretion.
**ejaculatory d.,** ductus ejaculatorius.
**endolymphatic d.,** ductus endolymphaticus.
**d. of epididymis,** ductus epididymidis.
**d. of epoöphoron,** ductus longitudinalis epoöphori.
**excretory d.,** one that is merely conductive and not secretory.
**excretory d. of seminal gland, excretory d. of seminal vesicle,** ductus excretorius glandulae vesiculosae.
**excretory d. of testis,** ductus deferens.
**frontonasal d.,** a duct in the lateral wall of the nasal cavity extending from the frontal sinus to the infundibulum of the ethmoid bone; called also *nasofrontal d.*
**galactophorous d's,** ductus lactiferi.
**gall d.,** bile d.
**d. of gallbladder,** ductus cysticus.
**Gartner's d.,** ductus longitudinalis epoöphori.
**gasserian d.,** ductus paramesonephricus.
**genital d.,** genital canal.
**Guérin's d's,** ductus paraurethrales urethrae femininae.
**guttural d.,** tuba auditiva.
**Haller's aberrant d.,** a small coiled tube extending from the lower part of the canal of the epididymis; called also *ductus aberrans halleri.*
**Hensen's d.,** ductus reuniens.
**hepatic d., common,** ductus hepaticus communis.
**hepatic d., left,** ductus hepaticus sinister.
**hepatic d., right,** ductus hepaticus dexter.
**hepaticopancreatic d.,** ductus pancreaticus.
**hepatocystic d.,** ductus choledochus.
**d. of His,** ductus thyroglossalis.
**hypophysial d.,** an embryonic structure composed of the elongated Rathke's pouch joining the infundibulum of the embryonic hypophysis; called also *craniopharyngeal d.*
**incisive d., incisor d.,** ductus incisivus.
**intercalated d.,** a slender initial portion of the duct system interposed between an acinus of a gland and a secretory duct.
**interlobular d's,** channels located between different lobules of a gland; see *ductuli interlobulares.*
**lacrimal d.,** canaliculus lacrimalis.
**lacrimonasal d.,** ductus nasolacrimalis.
**lactiferous d's,** ductus lactiferi.
**Leydig's d.,** ductus mesonephricus.
**lingual d.,** a depression on the dorsum of the tongue at the apex of the terminal sulcus.
**longitudinal d. of epoöphoron,** ductus longitudinalis epoöphori.
**Luschka's d's,** tubular structures in the wall of the gallbladder, some connected with bile ducts but none connected with the lumen of the gallbladder; they may be aberrant bile ducts.
**lymphatic d's,** channels for conducting lymph.
**lymphatic d., left,** thoracic d.
**lymphatic d., right,** ductus lymphaticus dexter.
**mammary d's, mammillary d's,** ductus lactiferi.
**medullary collecting d.,** see under *tubule.*
**mesonephric d.,** ductus mesonephricus.

**metanephric d.**, ureter.
**milk d's**, ductus lactiferi.
**d. of Müller, müllerian d.**, ductus paramesonephricus.
**müllerian d., persistent**, the persistence in otherwise normal males of müllerian structures that normally should regress in utero. See *persistent müllerian duct syndrome,* under *syndrome.*
**nasal d.**, ductus nasolacrimalis.
**nasofrontal d.**, frontonasal d.
**nasolacrimal d.**, ductus nasolacrimalis.
**nephric d.**, ureter.
**omphalomesenteric d.**, the narrow tube connecting the umbilical vesicle of the yolk sac with the midgut of the embryo; called also *omphalomesenteric canal, umbilical duct, vitelline duct, vitellointestinal duct,* and *yolk stalk.*
**ovarian d.**, tuba uterina.
**pancreatic d.**, ductus pancreaticus.
**pancreatic d., accessory, pancreatic d., minor**, ductus pancreaticus accessorius.
**papillary d.**, ductus papillaris.
**paramesonephric d.**, ductus paramesonephricus.
**paraurethral d's of female urethra**, ductus paraurethrales urethrae femininae.
**paraurethral d's of male urethra**, ductus paraurethrales urethrae masculinae.
**parotid d.**, ductus parotideus.
**d. of Pecquet**, thoracic d.
**perilymphatic d.**, aqueductus cochleae.
**primordial d.**, ductus paramesonephricus.
**pronephric d.**, the duct of the pronephros, which later serves as the mesonephric duct (ductus mesonephricus); called also *archinephric d.* or *canal.*
**d's of prostate gland, prostatic d's**, ductuli prostatici.
**Rathke's d.**, that part of the ductus paramesonephricus lying between its main part and the sinus pocularis.
**Reichel's cloacal d.**, the cleft between Douglas' septum and the cloaca in the embryo.
**renal d.**, ureter.
**d's of Rivinus**, ductus sublinguales minores.
**Rokitansky-Aschoff d's**, see under *sinus.*
**sacculoutricular d.**, ductus utriculosaccularis.
**salivary d's**, the ducts that convey the saliva: they are the ductus parotideus, ductus submandibularis, ductus sublingualis major, and ductus sublinguales minores.
**d. of Santorini**, ductus pancreaticus accessorius.
**Schüller's d's**, ductus paraurethrales urethrae femininae.
**secretory d.**, a smaller duct that is tributary to an excretory duct of a gland and that also has a secretory function.
**semicircular d's**, ductus semicirculares.
**semicircular d., anterior**, ductus semicircularis anterior.
**semicircular d., lateral**, ductus semicircularis lateralis.
**semicircular d., posterior**, ductus semicircularis posterior.
**semicircular d., superior**, ductus semicircularis anterior.
**seminal d's**, passages for the conveyance of spermatozoa and semen, including the ductus deferens, ductus excretorius glandulae vesiculosae, and ductus ejaculatorius.
**d. of seminal gland, d. of seminal vesicle**, ductus excretorius glandulae vesiculosae.
**Skene's d's**, ductus paraurethrales urethrae femininae.
**spermatic d.**, ductus deferens.
**d. of Steno, Stensen's d.**, ductus parotideus.
**sublingual d's**, the ducts of the sublingual salivary glands, including the ductus sublingualis major and ductus sublinguales minores.
**sublingual d., major**, ductus sublingualis major.
**sublingual d's, minor**, ductus sublinguales minores.
**submandibular d., submaxillary d. of Wharton**, ductus submandibularis.
**sudoriferous d., sweat d.**, ductus sudoriferus.
**tear d's**, the ducts conveying the secretion of the lacrimal glands.
**testicular d.**, ductus deferens.
**thoracic d.**, the canal that ascends from the cisterna chyli to the junction of the left subclavian and left internal jugular veins; called also *ductus thoracicus* [TA], *alimentary d., chyliferous d., d. of Pecquet, left lymphatic d.,* and *Van Hoorne's canal.*
**thoracic d., right**, see *ductus lymphaticus dexter.*
**thyroglossal d., thyrolingual d.**, ductus thyroglossalis.
**umbilical d.**, yolk stalk.
**urogenital d's**, the ductus paramesonephricus and ductus mesonephricus.
**utriculosaccular d.**, ductus utriculosaccularis.
**d. of Vater**, ductus thyroglossalis.
**vitelline d., vitellointestinal d.**, yolk stalk.
**Walther's d's**, ductus sublinguales minores.
**Wharton's d.**, ductus submandibularis.
**d. of Wirsung**, ductus pancreaticus.
**d. of Wolff, wolffian d.**, ductus mesonephricus.

---

**duc·tal** (duk'təl) pertaining to a duct.

**duc·tile** (duk'til) [L. *ductilis,* from *ducere* to draw, to lead] susceptible of being drawn out, as into a wire.

**duc·tion** (duk'shən) [L. *ductio,* from *ducere* to lead] in ophthalmology, the rotation of an eye by the extraocular muscles around its horizontal, vertical, or anteroposterior axis, the direction of the movement of the eye being indicated by prefixes. See *infraduction, supraduction, abduction, adduction,* and *cycloduction,* and see also *vergence* (def. 2) and *version* (def. 5).

**duct·less** (dukt'ləs) having no excretory duct.

**duc·to·pe·nia** (duk″to-pe-nia) deficiency in the number of ducts, particularly bile ducts; it may be focal or generalized.

**duct·ule** (duk'tūl) a minute duct; called also *ductulus* [TA].
**aberrant d's**, 1. ductules that are not usually present, or that follow an unusual course or direction. 2. ductuli aberrantes.
**aberrant d., inferior**, ductulus aberrans inferior.
**aberrant d., superior**, ductulus aberrans superior.
**alveolar d's**, ductuli alveolares.
**bile d's, biliary d's**, 1. ductuli biliferi. 2. cholangioles.
**efferent d's of testis**, ductuli efferentes testis.
**excretory d's of lacrimal gland**, ductuli excretorii glandulae lacrimalis.
**interlobular d's**, ductuli interlobulares.
**d's of prostate**, ductuli prostatici.
**transverse d's of epoöphoron**, ductuli transversi epoöphori.

**duc·tu·lus** (duk'tu-ləs) gen. and pl. *duc'tuli* [L.] [TA] ductule: a general term for a minute duct; applied especially to branches of ducts nearest to the alveoli of a gland, or the smallest beginnings of the duct system of an organ.
**duc'tuli aberran'tes** [TA], aberrant ductules: blind vestiges of mesonephric tubules near the epididymis; see *d. aberrans inferior* and *d. aberrans superior.*
**d. aber'rans infe'rior** [TA], inferior aberrant ductule: a narrow, coiled tube often connected with the first part of the ductus deferens, or with the lower part of the duct of the epididymis.
**d. aber'rans supe'rior** [TA], superior aberrant ductule: a narrow tube of variable length that lies in the epididymis and is connected with the rete testis; called also *ductus aberrans.*
**duc'tuli alveola'res**, alveolar ductules: small passages connecting the respiratory bronchioles and the alveolar sacs; see Plate 49. Called also *alveolar ducts.*
**duc'tuli bili'feri**, biliary ductules: the small channels that connect the interlobular ductules with the right and left hepatic ducts; called also *bile ductules* or *vessels* and *ductus biliferi.*
**duc'tuli efferen'tes tes'tis** [TA], efferent ductules of testis: ductules entering the head of the epididymis from the rete testis.
**duc'tuli excreto'rii glan'dulae lacrima'lis** [TA], excretory ductules of lacrimal gland: numerous ductules that traverse the palpebral part of the lacrimal gland and open into the superior fornix of the conjunctiva.
**duc'tuli interlobula'res**, interlobular ductules: small channels between the hepatic lobules, draining into the bile ductules; called also *ductus interlobulares,* and *interlobular biliary canals* or *bile ducts.*
**duc'tuli prosta'tici** [TA], ductules of prostate gland: minute ducts from the prostate gland that open on either side into or near the prostatic sinuses on the posterior wall of the urethra: called also *ductus prostatici, ducts of prostate gland,* and *prostatic ducts.*
**duc'tuli transver'si epoö'phori** [TA], **duc'tuli transver'si epoöphoron'tis**, transverse ductules of epoöphoron: the vestigial remains of the mesonephric ducts, which open into the longitudinal duct of the epoophoron.

**duc·tus** (duk'təs) gen. and pl. *duc'tus* [L.] [TA] a duct: a general term for a passage with well-defined walls, especially such a channel for the passage of excretions or secretions.

## Ductus

Descriptions of structures are given on TA terms, and include the anglicized names of specific ducts.

**d. aber'rans,** ductulus aberrans superior.
**d. aber'rans hal'leri,** Haller's aberrant duct.
**d. Aran'tii,** d. venosus.
**d. arterio'sus** [TA], arterial duct: a fetal blood vessel connecting the left pulmonary artery directly to the descending aorta; called also *arterial canal, duct of Botallo,* and *pulmoaortic canal.*
**d. bilia'ris,** TA alternative for *d. choledochus.*
**d. bili'feri,** ductuli biliferi.
**d. chole'dochus** [TA], choledochous duct: the duct formed by union of the common hepatic and the cystic ducts which empties into the duodenum at the major duodenal papilla, along with the pancreatic duct; called also *biliary duct, common bile duct, d. biliaris* [TA alternative], *hepatic funiculus,* and *hepatocystic duct.*
**d. cochlea'ris** [TA], cochlear duct: a spirally arranged membranous tube in the bony canal of the cochlea along its outer wall, lying between the scala tympani below and the scala vestibuli above; called also *cochlear canal, membranous cochlea, scala media,* and *scala of Löwenberg.*
**d. cuvi'eri,** common cardinal veins.
**d. cys'ticus** [TA], cystic duct: the passage connecting the neck of the gallbladder and the common bile duct; called also *duct of gallbladder.*
**d. de'ferens** [TA], deferent duct: the excretory duct of the testis, which unites with the excretory duct of the seminal vesicle to form the ejaculatory duct; called also *vas deferens, excretory duct of testis, spermatic duct,* and *testicular duct.*
**d. de'ferens vestigia'lis** [TA], the vestigial remnants of the mesonephric duct in the female.
**d. ejaculato'rius** [TA], ejaculatory duct: the canal formed by union of the ductus deferens and the excretory duct of the seminal vesicle. It enters the prostatic part of the urethra on the colliculus seminalis.
**d. endolympha'ticus** [TA], endolymphatic duct: the membranous tube connecting the utriculosaccular duct with the endolymphatic sac, located within the bony vestibular aqueduct.
**d. epididy'midis** [TA], duct of epididymis: the single tube into which the coiled ends of the efferent ductules of the testis open; the convolutions of which make up the greater part of the epididymis; called also *canal of epididymis.*
**d. epoöph'ori longitudina'lis, d. epoöphoron'tis longitudina'lis,** d. longitudinalis epoöphori.
**d. excreto'rius glan'dulae semina'lis,** TA alternative for *d. excretorius glandulae vesiculosae.*
**d. excreto'rius glan'dulae vesiculo'sae** [TA], excretory duct of seminal gland: the duct that drains the seminal vesicle and unites with the ductus deferens to form the ejaculatory duct. Called also *d. excretorius glandulae seminalis* and *d. excretorius vesiculae seminalis* [TA alternatives].
**d. excreto'rius vesi'culae semina'lis,** TA alternative for *d. excretorius glandulae vesiculosae.*
**d. glan'dulae bulbourethra'lis** [TA], duct of bulbourethral gland: a duct passing from the bulbourethral gland through the urogenital diaphragm into the bulb of the penis and entering the spongy part of the urethra; called also *cowperian duct.*
**d. hepa'ticus commu'nis** [TA], common hepatic duct: the duct which is formed by union of the right and left hepatic ducts, and in turn joins the cystic duct to form the common bile duct.
**d. hepa'ticus dex'ter** [TA], right hepatic duct: the duct that drains the right lobe and part of the caudate lobe of the liver.

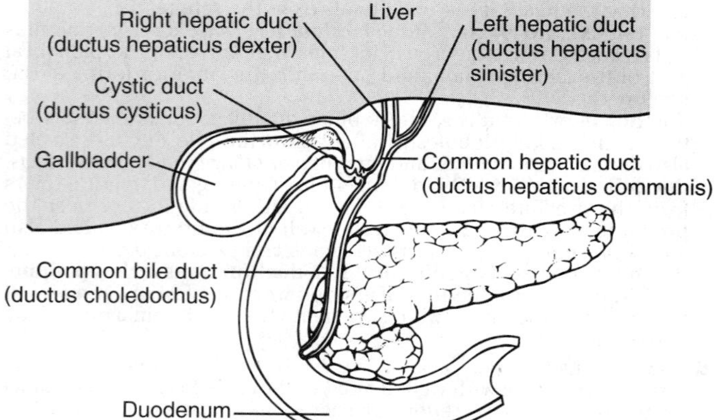


**d. hepa'ticus sinis'ter** [TA], left hepatic duct: the duct that drains the left and quadrate lobes and part of the caudate lobe of the liver.
**d. inci'sivus** [TA], incisive duct: a passage sometimes found in the incisive canal that interconnects the nasal and oral cavities during embryonic development; it occasionally fails to close. Called also *incisor canaliculus* and *incisor duct.*
**d. interlobula'res,** ductuli interlobulares.
**d. lacrima'lis,** canaliculus lacrimalis.
**d. lacti'feri** [TA], lactiferous ducts: channels conveying the milk secreted by the lobes of the breast to and through the nipples; called also *galactophorous tubules, lactiferous tubules,* and *mammary ducts.*
**d. lo'bi cauda'ti dex'ter** [TA], the right duct of the caudate lobe of the liver.
**d. lo'bi cauda'ti sinis'ter** [TA], the left duct of the caudate lobe of the liver.
**d. longitudina'lis epoö'phori** [TA], longitudinal duct of epoöphoron: a closed rudimentary duct lying parallel to the uterine tube into which the transverse ducts of the epoöphoron open; it is a remnant of the part of the mesonephros that participates in formation of the reproductive organs. Called also *duct of epoöphoron, d. epoöphorontis longitudinalis,* and *Gartner's canal* or *duct.*
**d. lympha'tici,** lymphatic ducts: the main lymph channels, the right lymphatic duct, thoracic duct, and cisterna chyli (when present), into which the converging lymph vessels drain, which in turn empty into the blood stream.
**d. lympha'ticus dex'ter** [TA], right lymphatic duct: a vessel draining the lymph from the upper right side of the body, typically formed by the right jugular, subclavian, and bronchomediastinal lymphatic trunks, any one of which may, however, end separately in the right brachiocephalic vein; when all three lymphatic vessels unite, a right lymphatic duct (called also *d. thoracicus dexter* [TA alternative] and *right thoracic duct*) is formed, which empties directly into the junction of the internal jugular and subclavian veins.
**d. mesoneph'ricus,** mesonephric duct: an embryonic duct which, initiated in association with rudiments of the pronephric kidney, is taken over as an excretory duct by the mesonephros, and develops into the epididymis, the ductus deferens and its ampulla, the seminal vesicles, and the ejaculatory duct in the male and into vestigial structures in the female. Called also *d. Wolffi, wolffian duct, duct of Wolff, Leydig's duct,* and *canal of Oken.*
**d. muel'leri,** d. paramesonephricus.
**d. nasolacrima'lis** [TA], nasolacrimal duct: the passage that conveys the tears from the lacrimal sac into the inferior nasal meatus; called also *lacrimonasal* or *nasal duct.*
**d. pancrea'ticus** [TA], pancreatic duct: the main excretory duct of the pancreas, which usually unites with the common bile duct before entering the duodenum at the major duodenal papilla; called also *duct* or *canal of Wirsung,* and *hepaticopancreatic duct.*
**d. pancrea'ticus accesso'rius** [TA], accessory pancreatic duct: a small inconstant duct draining a part of the head of the pancreas into the minor duodenal papilla; called also *minor pancreatic duct,* and *duct of Santorini* or *Bernard.*
**d. papilla'ris,** papillary duct: a wide terminal tubule in the renal pyramid, formed by the union of several straight collecting tubules and emptying into the renal pelvis in the area cribrosa. Called also *Bellini's duct* or *tubule.*
**d. paramesoneph'ricus,** paramesonephric duct: either of the paired embryonic ducts arising as a peritoneal pocket, extending caudally to join the urogenital sinus, and developing into uterine tubes and the uterus in the female and into a vestigial structure (appendix testis) in the male. Called also *d. muelleri, duct of Müller, müllerian duct,* and *gasserian* or *primordial duct.*
**d. paraurethra'les ure'thrae femini'nae** [TA], paraurethral ducts of female urethra: inconstantly present ducts in the female, which drain a group of the urethral glands into the vestibule; called also *Guérin's glands, Schüller's ducts* or *glands, Skene's ducts, glands,* or *tubules,* and *paraurethral glands of female urethra.*
**d. paraurethra'les ure'thrae masculi'nae** [TA], paraurethral ducts of male urethra: the ducts of the urethral glands situated in the spongy portion of the male urethra; called also *canales paraurethrales urethrae masculinae* and *paraurethral canals of male urethra.*
**d. paroti'deus** [TA], parotid duct: the duct that drains the parotid gland and empties into the oral cavity opposite the second superior molar; called also *Blasius' duct, Stensen's canal* or *duct,* and *duct* or *canal of Steno.*
**patent d. arteriosus (PDA),** abnormal persistence of an open lumen in the ductus arteriosus after birth, the direction of flow being from the aorta to the pulmonary artery, resulting in recirculation of arterial blood through the lungs.
**d. perilympha'tici, d. perilymphaticus,** aqueductus cochleae.
**d. prosta'tici,** ductuli prostatici.
**d. reu'niens** [TA], a small canal leading from the saccule to the

cochlear duct; called also *canalis reuniens, Hensen's canal* or *duct,* and *Reichert's canal.*

**d. semicircula'res** [TA], semicircular ducts: the long ducts of the membranous labyrinth of the ear, corresponding to the semicircular canals of the bony labyrinth and designated anterior, posterior, and lateral, according to the canal they occupy. Their diameter is only one-fourth that of the bony canals containing them, and each is affixed by one wall to the endosteal lining of the canal. They give information about angular acceleration and deceleration. Called also *membranous semicircular canals.*

**d. semicircula'ris ante'rior** [TA], anterior semicircular duct: the semicircular duct occupying the anterior semicircular canal; called also *d. semicircularis superior,* or *superior semicircular duct.* See *d. semicirculares.*

**d. semicircula'ris latera'lis** [TA], lateral semicircular duct: the semicircular duct occupying the lateral semicircular canal; see *d. semicirculares.*

**d. semicircula'ris poste'rior** [TA], posterior semicircular duct: the semicircular duct occupying the posterior semicircular canal; see *d. semicirculares.*

**d. semicircula'ris supe'rior,** d. semicircularis anterior.

**d. sperma'ticus,** d. deferens.

**d. sublingua'lis ma'jor** [TA], major sublingual duct: the duct that drains the sublingual gland and opens alongside the submandibular duct on the sublingual caruncle; called also *Bartholin's duct.*

**d. sublingua'les mino'res** [TA], minor sublingual ducts: the ducts that drain the sublingual gland and open along the crest of the sublingual fold; called also *canals* or *ducts of Rivinus,* and *Walther's ducts.*

**d. submandibula'ris** [TA], **d. submaxilla'ris [Wharto'ni],** submandibular duct: the duct that drains the submandibular gland and opens at the sublingual caruncle; called also *submaxillary duct of Wharton* and *Wharton's duct.*

**d. sudori'ferus,** sudoriferous duct: the duct that leads from the body of a sweat gland to the surface of the skin; called also *sweat duct.*

**d. thora'cicus** [TA], thoracic duct: the largest lymph channel in the body, which collects lymph from the portions of the body below the diaphragm and from the left side of the body above the diaphragm; it begins in the abdomen *(pars abdominalis)* at the junction of the intestinal, lumbar, and descending intercostal trunks (which consists of a plexus or the *cisterna chyli)* at about the level of the second lumbar vertebra, enters the thorax through the aortic hiatus of the diaphragm *(pars thoracica),* ascends to cross the posterior mediastinum, and enters the neck *(pars cervicalis),* where it forms a downward arch *(arcus ductus thoracici)* across the subclavian artery, and ends at the junction of the subclavian and internal jugular veins.

**d. thora'cicus dex'ter,** TA alternative for *d. lymphaticus dexter.*

**d. thyroglossa'lis** [TA], thyroglossal duct: a duct in the embryo extending between the thyroid primordium and the posterior part of the tongue, which opens as the foramen caecum; the distal part usually differentiates to form the pyramidal lobe the thyroid and the remainder becomes obliterated, but occasionally persists into adult life, giving rise to cysts, fistulas, or sinuses. Called also *duct of His* or *Vater, Bochdalek's duct, His canal,* and *thyrolingual duct.*

**d. utriculosaccula'ris** [TA], utriculosaccular duct: a tiny Y-shaped duct in the membranous labyrinth with one branch to the utricle, one branch to the saccule, and one branch to the ductus endolymphaticus. Called also *sacculoutricular duct* or *canal* and *utriculosaccular canal.*

**d. veno'sus,** a major blood channel that develops through the embryonic liver from the umbilical vein to the inferior vena cava; called also *canal* or *duct of Arantius, canal of Cuvier,* and *d. Arantii.*

**d. Wolf'fi,** d. mesonephricus.

---

**Duf·fy blood group** (duf'e) [from the name of the propositus first observed in 1950] see under *blood group.*

**Du·gas' test (sign)** (doo-gahz') [Louis Alexander *Dugas,* American physician, 1806–1884] see under *test.*

**Du·ha·mel operation** (du-ah-mel') [Bernard Georges *Duhamel,* French surgeon, born 1917] see under *operation.*

**Du·hot's line** (du-ōz') [Robert *Duhot,* Belgian urologist and dermatologist, late 19th century] see under *line.*

**Duh·ring's disease** (doo'ringz) [Louis Adolphus *Duhring,* American dermatologist, 1845–1913] dermatitis herpetiformis.

**Dührs·sen's incisions, operation** (dēr'sən z) [Alfred *Dührssen,* German gynecologist, 1862–1933] see under *incision* and *operation.*

**Duke's test (method)** (do͞oks) [William Waddell *Duke,* American pathologist, 1882–1946] see under *test.*

**Dukes' disease** (do͞oks) [Clement *Dukes,* English physician, 1845–1925] see under *disease.*

**Dukes' classification** (do͞oks) [Cuthbert Esquire *Dukes,* English pathologist, 1890–1977] see under *classification.*

**Dul·bec·co** (dool-bek'o) Renato. Italian-born American biologist, born 1914; co-winner, with David Baltimore and Howard Temin, of the Nobel prize for medicine or physiology for 1975, for discoveries concerning the interaction between tumor viruses and the genetic material of host cells and the role of reverse transcriptase.

**dul·ci·tol** (dul'sĭ-tol) [L. *dulcis* sweet] [MeSH: Dulcitol] galactitol.

**dull** (dul) not resonant on percussion.

**dull·ness** (dul'nəs) diminished resonance on percussion; also a peculiar percussion sound which lacks the normal resonance.

**Gerhardt's d.,** see under *triangle.*

**shifting d.,** dullness on abdominal percussion, the level of which shifts as the patient is rolled from side to side; indicative of free fluid in the abdominal cavity.

**tympanitic d.,** resonance of a dull and diminished quality.

**dumb·bell** (dum'bel") a mass consisting of two spherical portions connected by a narrow isthmus.

**d's of Schäfer,** microscopic bodies found in striated muscular tissue.

**Dum·dum fever** (dum'dum) [*Dum Dum,* India, area of Calcutta where some of the first cases were observed in the early 20th century.] visceral leishmaniasis.

**dum·my** (dum'e) 1. pontic. 2. placebo. 3. a foal with neonatal maladjustment syndrome.

**dUMP** deoxyuridine monophosphate.

**dump·ing** (dump'ing) see under *syndrome.*

**Dun·can disease, syndrome** (dung'kən) [*Duncan,* the original kindred in which the disease was described] X-linked lymphoproliferative syndrome; see under *syndrome.*

**Dun·can's folds, position, ventricle** (dung'kənz) [James Matthews *Duncan,* British gynecologist, 1826–1890] see under *fold* and *position,* and see *cavum septi pellucidi.*

**Dun·ferm·line scale** (dun'fərm-līn) [*Dunfermline,* Scotland, where the scheme was devised] see under *scale.*

**dun·siek·te** (dun-sēk'tə) [Afrikaans] crotalism in horses in South Africa.

**du·o·de·nal** (doo"o-dē'nəl) of, pertaining to, or situated in the duodenum.

**du·o·de·nec·to·my** (doo"o-də-nek'tə-me) [*duoden-* + *-ectomy*] excision of the duodenum, total or partial.

**du·od·e·ni·tis** (doo"o-də-ni'tis) [MeSH: Duodenitis] inflammation of the duodenal mucosa.

**duoden(o)-** [L. *duodenum,* q.v.] a combining form denoting relationship to the duodenum.

**du·o·de·no·cho·lan·ge·itis** (doo"o-de'no-ko-lan"je-i'tis) inflammation of the duodenum and common bile duct.

**du·o·de·no·cho·le·cys·tos·to·my** (doo"o-de"no-ko"le-sis-tos'tə-me) cholecystoduodenostomy.

**du·o·de·no·cho·led·o·chot·o·my** (doo"o-de"no-ko"led-o-kot'ə-me) surgical incision of the duodenum and common bile duct.

**du·o·de·no·col·ic** (doo"o-de"no-kol'ik) pertaining to the duodenum and colon.

**du·o·de·no·cys·tos·to·my** (doo"o-de"no-sis-tos'tə-me) cholecystoduodenostomy.

**du·o·de·no·du·o·de·nos·to·my** (doo"o-de"no-doo"o-də-nos'tə-me) anastomosis of the two portions of a divided duodenum.

**du·o·de·no·en·ter·os·to·my** (doo"o-de"no-en"tər-os'tə-me) surgical formation of a communication from the duodenum to another part of the small intestine.

**du·o·de·no·gram** (doo-o-de′no-gram) a radiograph of the duodenum.

**du·o·de·no·he·pat·ic** (doo-o-de′no-hə-pat′ik) pertaining to the duodenum and the liver.

**du·o·de·no·il·e·os·to·my** (doo″o-de″no-il″e-os′tə-me) surgical formation of a communication between the duodenum and the ileum.

**du·o·de·no·je·ju·nos·to·my** (doo″o-de″no-jə-joo-nos′tə-me) surgical formation of a communication between the duodenum and the jejunum.

**du·o·de·nol·y·sis** (doo″o-də-nol′ə-sis) the operation of loosening the duodenum from adhesions.

**du·o·de·no·pan·cre·a·tec·to·my** (doo″o-de″no-pan″kre-ə-tek′tə-me) pancreatoduodenectomy.

**du·o·de·nor·rha·phy** (doo″o-də-nor′ə-fe) [*duodeno-* + *-rrhaphy*] the operation of suturing the duodenum.

**du·o·de·no·scope** (doo″o-de′no-skōp) a fiberoptic endoscope inserted via the mouth for examining the duodenum.

**du·o·de·nos·co·py** (doo″o-də-nos′kə-pe) [*duodeno-* + *-scopy*] [MeSH: Duodenoscopy] endoscopic examination of the duodenum.

**du·o·de·nos·to·my** (doo″o-də-nos′tə-me) [*duodeno-* + *-stomy*] [MeSH: Duodenostomy] surgical formation of a permanent orifice into the duodenum.

**du·o·de·not·o·my** (doo″o-də-not′ə-me) [*duodeno-* + *-tomy*] incision of the duodenum.

**du·o·de·num** (doo″o-de′nəm, doo-od′ə-nəm) [L. *duode′ni* twelve at a time] [TA] [MeSH: Duodenum] the first or proximal portion of the small intestine, extending from the pylorus to the jejunum; so called because it is about 12 fingerbreadths in length.

**du·o·par·en·tal** (doo″o-pə-ren′təl) biparental.

**Du·pha·lac** (doo′fə-lak) trademark for a preparation of lactulose.

**Du·phas·ton** (doo-fas′ton) trademark for a preparation of dydrogesterone.

**Du·play's operation** (du-plāz′) [Simon Emanuel *Duplay,* French surgeon, 1836–1924] see under *operation.*

**du·pli·ca·tion** (doo″plĭ-ka′shən) [L. *duplicatio* doubling] 1. in genetics, the presence in the genome of additional genetic material (a chromosome or segment thereof, a gene or part thereof). 2. abnormal doubling of a body part; see *duplicitas.*
**incomplete d. of spinal cord,** diastematomyelia.

**du·pli·ci·tas** (doo-plis′ĭ-təs) [L.] a doubling, or duplication.
**d. ante′rior,** katadidymus.
**d. asym′metros,** heteropagus.
**d. comple′ta,** conjoined twins in which each component is completely or almost completely developed.
**d. crucia′ta,** conjoined twins with fused heads, each face being a joint product whose midplane forms a right angle with that of the body.
**d. incomple′ta,** conjoined twins in which the two components are not completely developed.
**d. infe′rior,** anadidymus.
**d. me′dia,** conjoined twins in which the duplication is restricted to the middle region of the body.
**d. paralle′la,** conjoined twins consisting of two components united in the sagittal plane.
**d. poste′rior,** anadidymus.
**d. supe′rior,** katadidymus.
**d. sym′metros,** diplopagus.

**dupp** (dup) a syllable used to represent the second sound of the heart in auscultation; it is shorter and higher pitched than the first sound. See *lubb* and *lubb-dupp.*

**Du·puy-Du·temps' operation** (du-pwe′du-tah′) [Louis *Dupuy-Dutemps,* Paris ophthalmologist, 1871–1946] see under *operation.*

**Du·puy·tren's contracture,** etc. (du-pwe-trahz′) [Baron Guillaume *Dupuytren,* French surgeon, 1777–1835] see under *contracture, fracture, hydrocele,* and *sign,* see *shoulder disarticulation* under *disarticulation,* and see *aponeurosis palmaris.*

**du·ra** (doo′rə) [L. "hard"] dura mater.

**Du·rab·o·lin** (doo-rab′o-lin) trademark for a preparation of nandrolone phenpropionate.

**Du·ra·cil·lin** (doo″rə-sil′in) trademark for preparations of penicillin G procaine.

**Du·ra·ge·sic** (doo″rə-je′zik) trademark for a preparation of fentanyl citrate.

**du·ral** (doo′rəl) pertaining to the dura mater.

**du·ra ma·ter** (doo′rə ma′tər) [L. "hard mother"] [TA] [MeSH: Dura Mater] the outermost, toughest, and most fibrous of the three membranes (meninges) covering the brain and spinal cord; called also *pachymeninx.*
**d. m. of brain, d. m. crania′lis** [TA], cranial dura mater: the dura mater covering the brain, composed of two mostly fused layers: an endosteal outer layer (endocranium) adherent to the inner aspect of the cranial bones, analogous to the periosteum of the bony skeleton, and an inner meningeal layer. Venous sinuses and the trigeminal ganglion are located between the layers. Called also *d. m. encephali* [TA alternative].
**d. m. ence′phali,** TA alternative for *d. m. cranialis.*
**d. m. of spinal cord, d. m. spina′lis** [TA], spinal dura mater: the dura mater covering the spinal cord; it is separated from the periosteum of the enclosing vertebrae by an epidural space containing blood vessels and fibrous and areolar tissue.

**Du·rand-Ni·co·las-Fa·vre disease** (du-rah′ ne-ko-lah′ fahv′rə) [J. *Durand,* French physician, born 1876; Joseph *Nicolas,* French physician, 1868–1960; Maurice Jules *Favre,* French physician, 1876–1954] lymphogranuloma venereum.

**Du·ra·nest** (doo′rə-nəst) trademark for a preparation of etidocaine hydrochloride.

**Du·ran-Rey·nals' permeability factor** (doo-rahn′ ra-nahlz′) [Francisco *Duran-Reynals,* American bacteriologist, 1899–1958] hyaluronidase.

**Du·ran·te's disease** (du-rahnts′) [Gustave *Durante,* French physician, 1865–1934] osteogenesis imperfecta; see under *osteogenesis.*

**dur·ap·a·tite** (door-ap′ə-tīt) [MeSH: Durapatite] a crystalline form of the compound $(Ca_3(PO_4)_2)_3 \cdot Ca(OH)_2$ (see *hydroxyapatite*), used as a prosthetic aid.

**du·ra·plas·ty** (doo′rə-plas″te) [*dura* mater + *-plasty*] a plastic operation on the dura mater; graft of the dura.

**du·ra·tion** (do͞o-ra′shən) [L. *durare* to last or remain] 1. a period of time, such as the length of time an electrical stimulus is being applied. 2. the length of time covered by one waveform, usually measured from a point at which it leaves the baseline to the next point at which it returns to a corresponding position on the baseline.

**Dürck's nodes** (dērks) [Hermann Ludwig Friedrich Franz *Dürck,* German pathologist, 1869–1941] see under *node.*

**Dur. dolor.** abbreviation for L. *duran′te dolo′re,* while the pain lasts.

**Du·ret's hemorrhages** (du-rāz′) [Henri *Duret,* French neurological surgeon, 1849–1921] see under *hemorrhage.*

**Dur·ham rule** (do͞or′əm) [*Durham,* surname of an American felon judged to be criminally insane in 1954] see under *rule.*

**Dur·ham's tube** (do͞or′əmz) [1. Arthur Edward *Durham,* English surgeon, 1834–1895. 2. Herbert Edward *Durham,* English bacteriologist, 1866–1945] see under *tube.*

**Du·ri·cef** (door′ĭ-sef) trademark for preparations of cefadroxil.

**du·ro·ar·ach·ni·tis** (doo″ro-ar″ak-ni′tis) inflammation of the dura mater and arachnoid.

**Du·ro·zi·ez's disease, murmur (sign)** (du-ro″ze-āz′) [Paul Louis *Duroziez,* French physician, 1826–1897] see under *disease* and *murmur.*

**dust** (dust) [MeSH: Dust] fine, dry particles of earth or any other substance small enough to be blown by the wind. See also *coniosis* and *pneumoconiosis.*
**blood d.,** hemoconia.
**chromatin d.,** small red granules, smaller than Howell's bodies, sometimes seen at the periphery of stained erythrocytes.

**dust-borne** (dust′born″) spread through the air in dust particles, as an infectious disease; see under *infection.*

**Dutch·er body** (duch′er) [Thomas F. *Dutcher,* American pathologist, born 1923] see under *body.*

**dUTP** deoxyuridine triphosphate.

**dUTP py·ro·phos·pha·tase** (pi-ro-fos′fə-tās) [EC 3.6.1.23] an enzyme of the hydrolase class that catalyzes the cleavage of dUTP to form dUMP and pyrophosphate. The dUMP so formed is a substrate for the reaction producing dTMP.

**Dut·ton's relapsing fever, spirochete** (dut′ənz) [Joseph Everett *Dutton,* English physician, 1877–1905] see under *fever,* and see *Borrelia duttonii.*

**Dut·to·nel·la** (dut″o-nel′ə) [J. Everett *Dutton*] in some systems of classification a subgenus of salivarian trypanosomes including *Trypanosoma uniforme* and *T. vivax.*

**Duve** (do͞ov) Christian René de. British-born Belgian cytologist, born 1917; co-winner, with Albert Claude and George E. Palade, of the Nobel prize for medicine or physiology for 1974, for their discoveries concerning the structural and functional organization of the cell.

**Du·ver·ney's foramen, gland** (du-vər-nāz') [Joseph Guichard *Duverney,* French anatomist, 1648–1730] see *foramen epiploicum* and *glandula bulbourethralis.*

**Du·void** (doo'void) trademark for preparations of bethanechol chloride.

**dv** double vibrations (a unit for the measurement of the frequency of sound waves).

**DVA** Department of Veterans Affairs (formerly the Veterans Administration).

**DVM** Doctor of Veterinary Medicine. Also abbreviated VMD.

**DVT** deep venous thrombosis.

**dwale** (dwāl) belladonna (def. 1).

**dwarf** (dworf) [A.S. *dweorh*] 1. a person who is unusually short. Called also *nanus.* 2. an animal or plant that is small in size.
**achondroplastic d.,** 1. a type of dwarf having a relatively large head with saddle nose and brachycephaly, short extremities, and usually lordosis; see also *achondroplasia.* 2. a calf with short legs, a wide head, a protruding mandible, and a malformed maxilla that partially obstructs the respiratory passages so that breathing is stertorous. Called also *snorter d.*
**Amsterdam d.,** a dwarf affected with de Lange's syndrome.
**asexual d.,** an adult dwarf with deficient sexual development.
**ateliotic d.,** a dwarf whose skeleton is infantile with persistent nonunion between epiphyses and diaphyses.
**bird-headed d.,** a dwarf with Seckel's syndrome; called also *nanocephalic d.* and *Seckel's bird-headed d.*
**Brissaud's d., cretin d.,** hypothyroid d.
**diastrophic d.,** a dwarf with progressive structural deformities of the bones and joints, including scoliosis, bilateral clubfoot, deformity of the thumb, micromelia, joint contractures and subluxations, malformation of the pinna with calcification of the cartilage, premature calcification of the costal cartilages, and cleft palate.
**geleophysic d.,** a dwarf with a peculiar facial appearance and bone dysplasia, especially of the hands and feet.
**hypophysial d.,** pituitary d.
**hypothyroid d.,** a dwarf with hypothyroidism, usually accompanied by cretinism. Called also *Brissaud's d.* and *cretin d.*
**infantile d.,** a dwarf with infantilism, such as hypophysial infantilism.
**Laron d.,** a dwarf whose skeletal growth retardation results from impaired ability to synthesize insulin-like growth factor I; see *Laron syndrome,* under *syndrome.*
**Lévi-Lorain d., Lorain-Lévi d.,** pituitary d.
**micromelic d.,** a dwarf with very small limbs.
**nanocephalic d.,** bird-headed d.
**normal d.,** a person who is unusually short (more than 3 standard deviations below mean height for age in a child) but is not deformed. Called also *midget* and *physiologic, primordial, pure,* or *true d.*
**phocomelic d.,** a dwarf in whom the diaphyses of the long bones are abnormally short.
**physiologic d.,** normal d.
**pituitary d.,** a dwarf with hypophysial infantilism. Called also *hypophysial d.* and *Lévi-Lorain* or *Lorain-Lévi d.*
**primordial d., pure d.,** normal d.
**rachitic d.,** a person dwarfed by rickets, having a high forehead with prominent bosses, bent long bones, and Harrison's sulcus or groove.
**renal d.,** a dwarf with renal dwarfism.
**rhizomelic d.,** one with an autosomal recessive form of chondrodysplasia punctata, characterized by symmetric shortening of the extremities, cataracts, optic atrophy, mental retardation, fibrous joint contractures, and ichthyosis; it is lethal in early childhood.
**Russell d.,** a dwarf with Silver-Russell syndrome.
**Seckel's bird-headed d.,** bird-headed d.
**sexual d.,** a dwarf with normal sexual development.
**Silver d.,** Russell d.
**snorter d.,** achondroplastic d. (def. 2).
**thanatophoric d.,** a micromelic dwarf having very short ribs and bones of the limbs, and vertebral bodies that are greatly reduced in height with wide intervertebral spaces; death usually occurs during the first few hours after birth. See also under *dysplasia.*
**true d.,** normal d.

**dwarf·ish** (dwor'fish) pertaining to or like a dwarf; called also *nanoid* and *nanous.*

**dwarf·ism** (dworf'iz-əm) [MeSH: Dwarfism] the state of being a dwarf; underdevelopment of the body. See various forms under *dwarf* and *infantilism.* Called also *microplasia, nanism,* and *nanosomia.*
**bird-headed d.,** Seckel's syndrome.
**camptomelic d.,** dwarfism due to camptomelia of the lower limbs, often accompanied by cleft palate, retrognathia, and other abnormalities.
**deprivation d.,** severe growth retardation in infants as a result of emotional deprivation, as in maternal deprivation syndrome.
**hypophysial d.,** see under *infantilism.*
**Laron d.,** see under *syndrome.*
**Lévi-Lorain d., Lorain-Lévi d., pituitary d.,** hypophysial infantilism.
**psychosocial d.,** deprivation d.
**renal d.,** dwarfism resulting from renal failure such as that of renal osteodystrophy.
**Robinow d.,** see under *syndrome.*
**Russell d., Russell-Silver d., Silver-Russell d.,** Silver-Russell syndrome.
**Seckel d.,** see under *syndrome.*
**symptomatic d.,** dwarfism with defective ossification, dentition, and sexual development.
**Walt Disney d.,** geroderma osteodysplastica.

**Dwy·er instrumentation** (dwi'ər) [Allen Frederick *Dwyer,* American orthopedic surgeon, 1920–1975] see under *instrumentation.*

**Dy** symbol for *dysprosium.*

**dy·ad** (di'ad) [Gr. *dyas* the number two, from *dyo* two] a double chromosome resulting from the halving of a tetrad in the first meiotic division.

**dy·as·ter** (di'əs-tər) amphiaster.

**Dy·a·zide** (di'ə-zīd) trademark for preparations of triamterene with hydrochlorothiazide.

**Dy·clone** (di'klōn) trademark for preparations of dyclonine hydrochloride.

**dy·clo·nine hy·dro·chlo·ride** (di'klo-nēn) [USP] a local anesthetic having significant bactericidal and fungicidal activity, applied topically to the skin and mucous membranes.

**dy·dro·ges·ter·one** (di″dro-jes'tər-ōn) [MeSH: Dydrogesterone] an orally effective, synthetic progestin occurring as a white to pale yellow, crystalline powder; used mainly in the diagnosis and treatment of primary amenorrhea and severe dysmenorrhea, and in combination with estrogen in dysfunctional menorrhagia.

**dye** (di) any of various colored substances that contain auxochromes and thus are capable of coloring substances to which they are applied; used for staining and coloring, as test reagents, and as therapeutic agents in medicine.
**acid d., acidic d.,** one which is acidic in reaction and usually unites with positively charged ions of the material acted upon; called also *anionic d.*
**amphoteric d.,** one containing both reactive basic and reactive acidic groups, and staining both acidic and basic elements.
**anionic d.,** acid d.
**azo d.,** any of a large group of synthetic dyes whose chromophore group is the structure —N═N—.
**basic d.,** one which is basic in reaction and unites with negatively charged ions of material acted upon; called also *cationic d.*
**cationic d.,** basic d.
**metachromatic d.,** a dye that stains tissues two or more colors.
**orthochromatic d.,** a dye that stains tissues a single color.
**vital d.,** one that penetrates living cells and colors certain structures, without serious injury to the cells.

**dy·ing** [di'ing] a stage in life; the process of approaching death. It is sometimes divided into the stages of denial and disbelief, anger, bargaining, depression, and acceptance.

**dy·ing-back** (di'ing bak) degeneration of an axon beginning distally and progressing to more proximal areas. Cf. *wallerian degeneration.*

**Dy·me·lor** (di'mə-lor) trademark for a preparation of acetohexamide.

**dyn** dyne.

**Dy·na·bac** (di'nə-bak) trademark for a preparation of dirithromycin.

**Dy·na·Circ** (di'nə-sərk) trademark for a preparation of isradipine.

**dy·nam·ic** (di-nam'ik) [*dynam-* + *-ic*] pertaining to or manifesting force.

**dy·nam·ics** (di-nam'iks) that phase of mechanics which deals with the motions of material bodies taking place under different specific conditions.

**dynam(o)-** [Gr. *dynamis* power] a combining form denoting relationship to power or strength.

**dy·na·mo·gen·e·sis** (di″nə-mo-jen'ə-sis) [*dynamo-* + *genesis*] the development of energy or force, as in muscle or nerves.

**dy·na·mo·gen·ic** (di″nə-mo-jen′ik) [*dynamo-* + *-genic*] producing or favoring the development of power; pertaining to the development of power, as in muscle or nerves.

**dy·na·mog·e·ny** (di″nə-moj′ə-ne) dynamogenesis.

**dy·namo·graph** (di-nam′o-graf) [*dynamo-* + *-graph*] a self-registering dynamometer.

**dy·na·mom·e·ter** (di″nə-mom′ə-tər) [*dynamo-* + *-meter*] an instrument for measuring the force of muscular contraction.
**grip d.**, squeeze d.
**squeeze d.**, one by which the grip of the hand is measured.

**dy·namo·path·ic** (di-nam″o-path′ik) [*dynamo-* + *path-* + *-ic*] functional.

**dy·namo·phore** (di-nam′o-for) [*dynamo-* + *-phore*] food or any substance that supplies energy to the body.

**dy·namo·scope** (di-nam′o-skōp) [*dynamo-* + *-scope*] a device for performing dynamoscopy.

**dy·na·mos·co·py** (di″nə-mos′kə-pe) the observation of the performance of function by an organ or structure, as of muscle action or of kidney function by ureteral catheterization.

**Dy·na·pen** (di′nə-pen) trademark for a preparation of dicloxacillin sodium.

**dyne** (dīn) the CGS unit of force, being that amount of force which, when acting continuously upon a mass of 1 gm, will impart to it an acceleration of 1 $cm \cdot s^{-2}$. Abbreviated dyn.

**dy·ne·in** (di′nēn) [Gr. *dynamis* power] a large protein playing several key roles in movement associated with microtubules. Attached to the microtubules of cilia and flagella, its ATPase activity drives a cyclic interaction that moves along the tubulin subunits and produces the bending movement of cilia and flagella by alternately forming and releasing cross-bridges between adjacent tubulin subunits. In the presence of specific cytoplasmic proteins, it also moves vesicles proximally along microtubules. Cf. *kinesin*. In EC nomenclature, called *dynein ATPase*.

**dy·ne·in ATP·ase** (di′nēn) [EC 3.6.1.33] [MeSH: Dynein ATPase] EC nomenclature for the ATP-hydrolyzing activity of dynein.

**dy·nor·phin** (di-nor′fin) [*dynamo-* + *morphine*] any of a family of opioid peptides found throughout the central and peripheral nervous systems; most are agonists at opioid receptor sites. Some are probably involved in pain regulation at the levels of the spinal cord and medulla and others may aid hypothalamic regulation of eating and drinking. See also *endorphin* and *enkephalin*.

**dy·phyl·line** (di′fəl-in) [USP] [MeSH: Dyphylline] a derivative of theophylline, used as a bronchodilator in the prevention and treatment of symptoms of asthma and of reversible bronchospasm associated with chronic bronchitis or emphysema; administered orally or intramuscularly.

**Dy·ren·i·um** (di-ren′e-əm) trademark for a preparation of triamterene.

**dys-** [Gr. "bad"] a combining form signifying difficult, painful, bad, disordered, abnormal; the opposite of *eu-*.

**dys·acou·sia** (dis″ə-koo′ze-ə) [*dys-* + Gr. *akousis* hearing + *-ia*] dysacusis.

**dys·acou·sis** (dis″ə-koo′sis) dysacusis.

**dys·acous·ma** (dis″ə-ko͞oz′mə) dysacusis.

**dys·acu·sis** (dis″ə-koo′sis) [*dys-* + Gr. *akousis* hearing] 1. a hearing impairment in which there is distortion of frequency or intensity. 2. a condition in which certain sounds produce discomfort; called also *auditory dysesthesia*. Defs. 1 and 2 called also *dysacousia* and *dysacousis*.

**dys·ad·ap·ta·tion** (dis″ad-ap-ta′shən) dysaptation.

**dys·ad·re·nal·ism** (dis″ad-re′nəl-iz-əm) adrenalism.

**dys·al·li·log·na·thia** (dis-al″ĭ-log-na′the-ə) disproportion of the maxilla and mandible.

**dys·an·ag·no·sia** (dis″an-ag-no′zhə) a form of dyslexia in which certain words cannot be recognized.

**dys·an·ti·graph·ia** (dis″an-tĭ-graf′e-ə) dysgraphia in which the ability to copy writing is lost.

**dys·aphia** (dis-a′fe-ə) [*dys-* + Gr. *haphē* touch] paraphia.

**dys·ap·ta·tion** (dis″ap-ta′shən) defective power of accommodation of the iris and retina to light variations.

**dys·ar·te·ri·ot·o·ny** (dis″ahr-tēr″eot′ə-ne) [*dys-* + *arteriotony*] abnormality of blood pressure.

**dys·ar·thria** (dis-ahr′thre-ə) [*dys-* + *arthr-*[2] + *-ia*] [MeSH: Dysarthria] a speech disorder consisting of imperfect articulation due to loss of muscular control after damage to the central or peripheral nervous system. Cf. *anarthria* and *aphasia*.
**ataxic d.**, dysarthria seen in patients with cerebellar lesions, characterized by slowness of speech, slurring, a monotonous tone, and scanning.
**flaccid d.**, lower motor neuron d.
**hyperkinetic d.**, loud, harsh speech with peculiar stresses, seen in extrapyramidal diseases such as myoclonus and chorea that involve hyperkinesia.
**hypokinetic d.**, low-pitched, monotonous speech with slurred words and incomplete sentences, seen in parkinsonism and other extrapyramidal diseases that involve hypokinesia.
**lower motor neuron d.**, a disorder of articulation caused by weakness or paralysis of the articulatory muscles and marked by a rasping, monotonous voice and, in advanced forms, shriveling and flaccidity of the tongue and laxness and tremulousness of the lips, seen in advanced cases of lesions of motor nuclei of the lower pons or medulla oblongata. Called also *flaccid d.*
**spastic d.**, dysarthria accompanying paresis of the tongue and facial muscles, usually with increased facial reflexes such as the jaw reflex; it occurs with bilateral lesions of the corticobulbar tracts.

**dys·ar·thric** (dis-ahr′thrik) characterized by or pertaining to dysarthria.

**dys·ar·thro·sis** (dis″ahr-thro′sis) [*dys-* + *arthrosis*] deformity or malformation of a joint.

**dys·au·to·no·mia** (dis″aw-to-no′me-ə) [*dys-* + Gr. *autonomia* autonomy] malfunction of the autonomic nervous system.
**familial d.**, an autosomal recessive disease of childhood characterized by defective lacrimation, skin blotching, emotional instability, motor incoordination, total absence of pain sensation, and hyporeflexia; seen almost exclusively in Ashkenazi Jews. Called also *familial autonomic dysfunction, Riley-Day syndrome, hereditary sensory and autonomic neuropathy (type III)*, and *HSAN-III.*
**feline d.**, a neurological disorder of cats, characterized by decreased numbers of neurons in autonomic and cranial nerve ganglia, resulting in mydriasis, dry mucous membranes, megaesophagus, bradycardia, and constipation. Called also *Key-Gaskell syndrome.*

**dys·bar·ism** (dis′bər-iz-əm) a general term applied to any clinical syndrome caused by difference between the surrounding atmospheric pressure and the total gas pressure in the various tissues, fluids, and cavities of the body, including such conditions as barotitis media, barosinusitis, or expansion of gases in the hollow viscera.

**dys·ba·sia** (dis-ba′zhə) [*dys-* + Gr. *basis* step] difficulty in walking, especially that due to a nervous lesion. Cf. *abasia.*
**d. lordo′tica progressi′va**, dystonia musculorum deformans.

**dys·be·ta·lipo·pro·tein·emia** (dis-ba″tə-lip″o-pro″te-ne′me-ə) 1. the presence in the blood of abnormal $\beta$-lipoproteins. 2. familial d.
**familial d.**, an inherited disorder of lipoprotein metabolism caused by interaction of homozygous inheritance of a specific mutant apolipoprotein E (apo E) with genetic and environmental factors tending to cause hypertriglyceridemia. It is characterized biochemically by accumulation of $\beta$-VLDL (chylomicron and very-low-density lipoprotein remnants) enriched in mutant apo E, with equally elevated cholesterol and triglycerides; the phenotype is thus that of a type III hyperlipoproteinemia. Clinical manifestations include tuberous or planar xanthomas, particularly of the palmar crease (xanthoma striatum palmare), and premature coronary and peripheral atherosclerosis. The term is sometimes used for all patients with this mutant apo E, although the majority are normolipidemic and clinically normal. Called also *broad beta* or *floating beta disease.*

**dys·bo·lism** (dis′bo-liz-əm) [*dys-* + *metabolism*] a condition arising from an error in metabolism not necessarily of a disease nature, as in incomplete oxidation of tyrosine, giving a reddish color to the urine.

**dys·cal·cu·lia** (dis″kal-ku′le-ə) impairment of the ability to do mathematical problems because of brain injury or disease. Cf. *acalculia.*

**dys·ceph·a·ly** (dĭ-sef′ə-le) malformation of the cranial and facial bones.
**mandibulo-oculofacial d.**, oculomandibulofacial syndrome.

**dys·che·sia** (dis-ke′shə) dyschezia.

**dys·che·zia** (dis-ke′zhə) [*dys-* + Gr. *chezein* to defecate + *-ia*] difficult or painful evacuation of feces from the rectum.

**dys·chi·a·sia** (dis-ki-a′zhə) any disorder of sense localization.

**dys·chi·ria** (dis-ki′re-ə) [*dys-* + *chir-* + *-ia*] derangement of the power to tell which side of the body has been touched; see *allochiria* and *synchiria.*

**dys·cho·lia** (dis-ko′le-ə) [*dys-* + *chol-* + *-ia*] a disordered condition of the bile.

**dys·chon·dro·pla·sia** (dis″kon-dro-pla′zhə) [*dys-* + *chondroplasia*] 1. enchondromatosis. 2. formerly, a general term encompassing both enchondromatosis and exostosis, which has caused some synonyms of one disorder to become incorrectly associated with the other disorder.

**dys·chon·dro·ste·o·sis** (dis″kon-dros″te-o′sis) a form of dyschondroplasia that may produce micromelia.

**dys·chro·ma·sia** (dis″kro-ma′zhə) dyschromatopsia.

**dys·chro·ma·top·sia** (dis-kro″mə-top′se-ə) [*dys-* + *chromat-* color + *-opsia*] disorder of color vision.

**dys·chro·mia** (dis-kro′me-ə) [*dys-* + *chrom-* + *-ia*] any disorder of pigmentation of the skin or hair.

**dys·chro·nism** (dis-kro′niz-əm) [*dys-* + *chron-* + *-ism*] separation in time; disturbance of any time relation.

**dys·chy·lia** (dis-ki′le-ə) disorder of the chyle.

**dys·ci·ne·sia** (dĭ-sĭ-ne′zhə) dyskinesia.

**dys·con·trol** (dis″kən-trōl′) inability to control one's behavior.
**episodic d.**, dyscontrol syndrome.

**dys·co·ria** (dis-kor′e-ə) [*dys-* + *cor-* + *-ia*] abnormality of the form or shape of the pupil or in the reaction of the two pupils.

**dys·cor·ti·cism** (dis-kor′tĭ-siz-əm) disordered functioning of the adrenal cortex; see *hyperadrenocorticism* and *adrenocortical insufficiency.*

**dys·cra·sia** (dis-kra′zhə) [*dys-* + *-crasia*] a term formerly used to indicate an abnormal mixture of the four humors; in surviving usages it now is roughly synonymous with "disease" or "pathologic condition."
**blood d.**, a pathologic condition of the blood, usually referring to disorders of the cellular elements of the blood.
**plasma cell d's**, a diverse group of neoplastic diseases involving proliferation of a single clone of cells producing a serum M component (a monoclonal immunoglobulin or immunoglobulin fragment); the cells usually have plasma cell morphology, but may have lymphocytic or lymphoplasmacytic morphology; this group includes multiple myeloma, Waldenström's macroglobulinemia, the heavy chain diseases, benign monoclonal gammopathy, and immunocytic amyloidosis. Called also *dysproteinemias, monoclonal gammopathies* or *immunoglobulinopathies,* and *paraproteinemias.*

**dys·cra·sic** (dis-kra′sik) dyscratic.

**dys·crat·ic** (dis-krat′ik) [Gr. *dyskratos*] pertaining to or characterized by dyscrasia.

**dys·di·ad·o·cho·ci·ne·sia** (dis″di-ad″o-ko″sĭ-ne′zhə) dysdiadochokinesia.

**dys·di·ad·o·cho·ki·ne·sia** (dis″di-ad″ŏ-ko-kĭ-ne′zhə) [*dys-* + *diadochokinesia*] a dyskinesia consisting of impaired ability to perform the rapid alternating movements of diadochokinesia. Called also *dysdiadochocinesia.*

**dys·di·ad·o·cho·ki·net·ic** (dis″di-ad″o-ko-kĭ-net′ik) pertaining to or characterized by dysdiadochokinesia.

**dys·dip·sia** (dis-dip′se-ə) [*dys-* + Gr. *dipsa* thirst] difficulty in drinking.

**dys·ec·dy·sis** (dis-ek′dĭ-sis) [*dys-* + *ecdysis*] incomplete or otherwise disordered shedding of the skin (ecdysis) by a reptile, such as due to malnutrition or an excessively dry or cold environment.

**dys·eco·ia** (dis″ə-koi′ə) dysacusis.

**dys·em·bry·o·ma** (dis-em″bre-o′mə) teratoma.

**dys·em·bryo·pla·sia** (dis-em″bre-o-pla′zhə) [*dys-* + *embryo* + *-plasia*] an anomaly occurring during embryonic life.

**dys·en·ce·pha·lia splanch·no·cys·ti·ca** (dis-en″sə-fa′le-ə splank″no-sis′tĭ-kə) Meckel's syndrome.

**dys·en·ter·ic** (dis″ən-ter′ik) pertaining to or of the nature of dysentery.

**dys·en·ter·i·form** (dis″ən-ter′ĭ-form) resembling dysentery.

**dys·en·tery** (dis′ən-ter″e) [L. *dysenteria,* from Gr. *dys-* + *enteron*] [MeSH: Dysentery] any of various disorders marked by inflammation of the intestines, especially of the colon, and attended by pain in the abdomen, tenesmus, and frequent stools containing blood and mucus. Causes include chemical irritants, bacteria, protozoa, or parasitic worms.
**amebic d.**, dysentery due to ulceration of the bowel caused by severe amebiasis; it may be associated with spread of the infection to the liver and other distant sites. Called also *amebic colitis* and *intestinal amebiasis.*
**bacillary d.**, an infectious disease caused by bacteria of the genus *Shigella,* and marked by intestinal pain, tenesmus, diarrhea with mucus and blood in the stools, and more or less toxemia; it is especially prevalent in tropical countries, but it frequently occurs elsewhere. Called also *Flexner's d.* and *Japanese d.*
**balantidial d.**, dysentery caused by *Balantidium coli.*
**bilharzial d.**, dysentery caused by the parasitic worm *Schistosoma haematobium (Bilharzia haematobia).*
**catarrhal d.**, sprue, def. 1.
**chronic d. of cattle**, Johne's disease.
**ciliary d., ciliate d.**, dysentery due to ciliate organisms, such as *Balantidium coli.*
**epidemic d.**, a variety that becomes epidemic and is often fatal.
**flagellate d.**, dysentery due to a flagellate organism, such as *Giardia lamblia* or *Trichomonas.*
**Flexner's d.**, bacillary d.
**fulminant d.**, bacillary dysentery marked by collapse and toxemia and followed by death.
**institutional d.**, bacillary dysentery affecting patients in an institution, especially in mental hospitals.
**Japanese d.**, bacillary d.
**lamb d.**, a highly fatal form of enterotoxemia affecting young lambs, caused by *Clostridium perfringens* type B, and marked by ulcerative inflammation of the intestine and fetid diarrhea, sometimes tinged with blood. A similar condition is frequently seen in young foals and calves.
**malarial d.**, that which is complicated with intermittent febrile attacks.
**malignant d.**, a form in which the symptoms are all very intense and progress rapidly to a fatal ending.
**protozoal d.**, amebic and balantidial dysentery.
**schistosomal d.**, dysentery accompanying intestinal schistosomiasis.
**scorbutic d.**, that which is an accompaniment of scurvy.
**Sonne d.**, bacillary dysentery occurring in temperate regions, caused by group D dysentery bacillus, *Shigella sonnei.*
**spirillar d.**, dysentery caused by spirilla in the intestines.
**sporadic d.**, dysentery occurring in scattered cases that have apparently no connection.
**swine d.**, a contagious form of enteritis in young swine, caused by *Treponema hyodysenteriae* and marked by grayish feces. Called also *bloody scours.*
**viral d.**, a virus-caused dysentery occurring in epidemics and marked by acute watery diarrhea.
**winter d.**, the black scours (q.v.) type of dysentery occurring in cattle when stabled for the winter. Called also *winter scours.*

**dys·equi·lib·ri·um** (dis″e-kwĭ-lib′re-əm) 1. any derangement of the sense of equilibrium; see *sense of equilibrium,* under *sense.* Cf. *dizziness* and *vertigo.* 2. disturbance of a state of equilibrium; see *equilibrium.*
**dialysis d.**, dialysis dysequilibrium syndrome.

**dys·er·gia** (dis-er′jə) [*dys-* + *erg-* + *-ia*] motor incoordination due to defect of efferent nerve impulse.

**dys·e·ryth·ro·poi·e·sis** (dis-ə-rith″ro-poi-e′sis) [*dys-* + *erythropoiesis*] defective development of erythrocytes, such as *anisocytosis* and *poikilocytosis.* See also *congenital dyserythropoietic anemia,* under *anemia.*

**dys·es·the·sia** (dis″es-the′zhə) [*dys-* + *esthesia*] 1. distortion of any sense, especially of that of touch. See also *paraphia.* 2. an unpleasant abnormal sensation produced by normal stimuli. Cf. *paresthesia.*
**auditory d.**, dysacusis (def. 2).

**dys·es·thet·ic** (dis″es-thet′ik) pertaining to or characterized by dysesthesia.

**dys·fi·brin·o·ge·ne·mia** (dis-fi-brin″o-jə-ne′me-ə) the presence in the blood of abnormal fibrinogen; both autosomal dominant and recessive forms are known.

**dys·flu·en·cy** (dis-floo′ən-se) the quality of being dysfluent; see also *stuttering.*

**dys·flu·ent** (dis-floo′ənt) proceeding with difficulty; said of speech disorders such as stuttering.

**dys·func·tion** (dis-funk′shən) disturbance, impairment, or abnormality of the functioning of an organ.
**constitutional hepatic d.**, Gilbert syndrome.
**erectile d.**, impotence, def. 2.
**familial autonomic d.**, familial dysautonomia.
**minimal brain d.**, former name for *attention-deficit/hyperactivity disorder.*
**myofascial pain d.**, Costen's syndrome.
**sexual d.** [DSM-IV], any of a group of sexual disorders characterized by disturbance either of sexual desire or of the psychophysiological changes that usually characterize sexual response. Included are sexual desire disorders, sexual arousal disorders, orgasmic disorders, sexual pain disorders, substance-induced sexual dysfunction, and sexual dysfunction due to a general medical condition.

**substance-induced sexual d.** [DSM-IV], any of various sexual dysfunctions, such as impaired desire, arousal, or orgasm, due to direct physiological effects of a psychoactive substance, including medications, drugs of abuse, and toxins. Individual cases are named for the specific substance and specific dysfunction involved.
**d. of uterus,** inertia uteri.

**dys·ga·lac·tia** (dis″gə-lak′te-ə) [*dys-* + *galact-* + *-ia*] disordered milk secretion.

**dys·gam·ma·glob·u·lin·emia** (dis-gam″ə-glob″u-lin-e′me-ə) [MeSH: Dysgammaglobulinemia] an immunological deficiency state characterized by selective deficiencies of one or more, but not all, classes of immunoglobulins. See also *hypogammaglobulinemia.*
**hyper-IgM d.,** hyperimmunoglobulin-M syndrome.

**dys·gen·e·sis** (dis-jen′ə-sis) defective development; see also *dysplasia* and *dyspoiesis.*
**epiphyseal d.,** a condition in which epiphyseal centers may be irregularly formed or appear to be fragmented or stippled.
**gonadal d.,** 1. defective development of the gonads. 2. Turner's syndrome.
**gonadal d., mixed,** a condition in which there is a testis on one side and a streak gonad on the other; those affected typically show some degree of virilization and ambiguous genitalia, and a uterus, vagina, and at least one fallopian tube are usually present. The most common karyotype is a mosaic, 45,XO/46,XY.
**gonadal d., pure,** the gonadal lesions of Turner's syndrome occurring without the somatic features.
**gonadal d., 46,XY,** an extreme form of male pseudohermaphroditism in which phenotypic females have a 46, XY karyotype with streak gonads, sexual infantilism, and primary amenorrhea; there are both sporadic types and hereditary X-linked types. Called also *Swyer syndrome.*
**reticular d.,** the most severe form of severe combined immunodeficiency (q.v.), of autosomal recessive inheritance and caused by a hematopoietic stem cell defect that results in absence of granulocytes, macrophages, and lymphocytes.
**seminiferous tubule d.,** Klinefelter's syndrome.

**dys·gen·ic** (dis-jen′ik) detrimental to the race or tending to counteract race improvement.

**dys·gen·ics** (dis-jen′iks) [*dys-* + Gr. *gennan* to produce] the study of racial deterioration. Cf. *eugenics.*

**dys·gen·i·tal·ism** (dis-jen′ĭ-təl-iz-əm) any abnormality of genital development.

**dys·ger·mi·no·ma** (dis″jər-mĭ-no′mə) [*dys-* + *germ* + *-oma*] [MeSH: Dysgerminoma] the most common malignant ovarian germ cell tumor, composed of large round or polygonal cells with much glycogen, which are frequently radiosensitive and located bilaterally. It is the counterpart of the classical seminoma of the testis. The term *germinoma* is now used to encompass both the female and male neoplasms.

**dys·geu·sia** (dis-goo′zhə) [*dys-* + Gr. *geusis* taste + *-ia*] [MeSH: Dysgeusia] parageusia.

**dys·glob·u·lin·emia** (dis-glob″u-lin-e′me-ə) [*dys-* + *globulin* + *emia*] any disorder of the blood globulins; see also *hyperglobulinemia* and *dysgammaglobulinemia.*

**dys·gly·ce·mia** (dis″gli-se′me-ə) [*dys-* + *glyc-* + *-emia*] any derangement of the content of glucose in the blood; see *hyperglycemia* and *hypoglycemia.*

**dys·gna·thia** (dis-na′the-ə) [*dys-* + *gnath-* + *-ia*] an abnormality of the oral cavity and teeth that also involves the jaws. Cf. *eugnathia.*

**dys·gnath·ic** (dis-nath′ik) [*dys-* + *gnathic*] pertaining to or characterized by dysgnathia.

**dys·go·ne·sis** (dis″go-ne′sis) [*dys-* + *gon-* + *-esis*] a functional disorder of the genital organs.

**dys·gon·ic** (dis-gon′ik) [*dys-* + *gon-* + *-ic*] seeding poorly; said of bacterial cultures, especially of species of *Mycobacterium,* that grow sparsely on culture media. Cf. *eugonic.*

**dys·gram·ma·tism** (dis-gram′ə-tiz-əm) agrammatism.

**dys·graph·ia** (dis-graf′e-ə) [*dys-* + *graph-* + *-ia*] difficulty in writing; cf. *agraphia.*

**dys·he·ma·to·poi·e·sis** (dis-he″mə-to″poi-e′sis) defective blood formation; called also *dyshemopoiesis.*

**dys·he·ma·to·poi·e·tic** (dis-he″mə-to-poi-et′ik) pertaining to or characterized by dyshematopoiesis.

**dys·he·mo·poi·e·sis** (dis-he″mo-poi-e′sis) dyshematopoiesis.

**dys·he·mo·poi·et·ic** (dis-he″mo-poi-et′ik) dyshematopoietic.

**dys·he·pa·tia** (dis-hə-pa′shə) [*dys-* + *hepat-* + *-ia*] disordered liver function.
**lipogenic d.,** a liver disorder of children due to excessive fats in the diet.

**dys·he·sion** (dis-he′zhən) [*dys* - + L. *haesio,* from *haerere* to stick] 1. disordered cell adherence. 2. loss of intercellular cohesion, a characteristic of malignancy, as determined by aspiration biopsy cytology.

**dys·hi·dro·sis** (dis-hi-dro′sis) [*dys-* + *hidro-* + *-sis*] 1. pompholyx; so called because it was formerly thought that the condition was a sweat retention disorder. 2. any disorder of the eccrine sweat glands. Spelled also *dyshydrosis.*

**dys·hy·dro·sis** (dis-hi-dro′sis) dyshidrosis.

**dys·idro·sis** (dis-id-ro′sis) dyshidrosis.

**dys·junc·tion** (dis-junk′shən) disjunction.

**dys·kary·o·sis** (dis-kar″e-o′sis) abnormal changes in cell nuclei, such as those observed in epithelial cells of the cervix during pregnancy.

**dys·kary·ot·ic** (dis″kar-e-ot′ik) [*dys-* + *karyo-* + *-ic*] pertaining to, characterized by, or promoting dyskaryosis.

**dys·ker·a·to·ma** (dis-ker″ə-to′mə) [*dys-* + *keratoma*] a dyskeratotic tumor.
**warty d.,** a benign, usually solitary, typically flesh-colored to brown elevated papule with a depressed and crusted center containing a keratotic plug, occurring in association with the pilosebaceous unit, especially on the scalp, face, neck, and axilla, and principally seen in older men. Histologically, it resembles the individual lesion of keratosis follicularis. Called also *isolated dyskeratosis follicularis.*

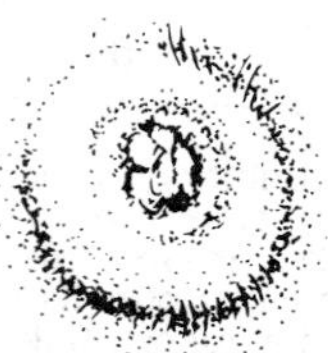

Warty dyskeratoma.

**dys·ker·a·to·sis** (dis-ker″ə-to′sis) abnormal, premature, or imperfect keratinization of the keratinocytes.
**d. conge′nita, congenital d.,** an X-linked syndrome with onset in childhood, characterized by nail dystrophy, reticular cutaneous hyperpigmentation, mucosal leukokeratosis, and pancytopenia resembling that of Fanconi's syndrome. Called also *Zinsser-Cole-Engman syndrome.*
**hereditary benign intraepithelial d.,** a congenital hereditary disease, transmitted as an autosomal dominant trait, characterized by foamy gelatinous plaques on the conjunctiva and white thickenings resembling leukoplakia on the oral mucosa; photophobia is common in children, and blindness may occur. Called also *Witkop's* or *Witkop-Von Sallmann disease.*
**isolated d. follicularis,** warty dyskeratoma.

**dys·ker·a·tot·ic** (dis-ker″ə-tot′ik) of, relating to, or affected by dyskeratosis.

**dys·ki·ne·sia** (dis″kĭ-ne′zhə) [Gr. *dyskinēsia* difficulty of moving] distortion or impairment of voluntary movement, as in tic, spasm, or myoclonus.
**biliary d.,** derangement of the filling and emptying mechanism of the gallbladder.
**d. intermit′tens,** disability of the limbs, coming on intermittently, and due to impairment of the circulation.
**orofacial d.,** facial movements resembling those of tardive dyskinesia, seen in elderly patients who are edentulous and demented; cf. *Meige's syndrome* (def. 2).
**primary ciliary d.,** any of a group of hereditary syndromes characterized by delayed or absent mucociliary clearance from the airways; often there is also lack of motion of sperm. One variety is Kartagener's syndrome. Called also *dyskinetic* or *immotile cilia syndrome.*
**tardive d.,** an iatrogenic extrapyramidal disorder caused by long-term use of antipsychotic drugs; it is characterized by oral-lingual-buccal dyskinesias that usually resemble continual chewing motions with intermittent darting movements of the tongue; there may also be choreoathetoid movements of the extremities. It is more common in women than in men and in the elderly than in the young, and incidence is related to drug dosage and duration of treatment. In some patients symptoms disappear within a few months after the drugs are withdrawn; in others symptoms may persist indefinitely. Two minor variants are *withdrawal-emergent d.* and *tardive dystonia.*
**withdrawal-emergent d.,** a variant of tardive dyskinesia in which symptoms appear after the drug has been withdrawn abruptly.

**dys·ki·net·ic** (dis″kĭ-net′ik) pertaining to or characterized by dyskinesia.

**dys·la·lia** (dis-la′le-ə) [*dys-* + *lal-* + *-ia*] paralalia.

**dys·lex·ia** (dis-lek′se-ə) [*dys-* + *lexis* word + *-ia*] [MeSH: Dyslexia] inability to read, spell, and write words, despite the ability to see and recognize letters; a familial disorder with autosomal dominant inheritance that occurs more frequently in males. Cf. *alexia.*

**dys·lip·id·e·mia** (dis-lip″id-e′me-ə) [*dys-* + *lipid* + *-emia*] abnormality in, or abnormal amounts of, lipids and lipoproteins in the blood; see also *hyperlipidemia* and *hypolipemia.*

**dys·lip·i·do·sis** (dis″lip-ĭ-do′sis) a disturbance of fat metabolism; it may be either localized or systemic.

**dys·lip·oi·do·sis** (dis-lip″oi-do′sis) dyslipidosis.

**dys·lipo·pro·tein·emia** (dis-lip″o-pro″te-ne′me-ə) the presence of abnormal concentrations of lipoproteins, or of abnormal lipoproteins, in the blood. See also *hyperlipoproteinemia* and *hypolipoproteinemia.*

**dys·lo·chia** (dis-lo′ke-ə) [*dys-* + *lochia*] disordered lochial discharge.

**dys·lo·gia** (dis-lo′jə) [*dys-* + *log-* + *-ia*] impairment of speech due to a mental disorder.

**dys·ma·ture** (dis″mə-cho͞or′) showing disordered development; said of infants with the dysmaturity syndrome.

**dys·ma·tur·i·ty** (dis-mə-cho͞or′ĭ-te) 1. disordered development. 2. dysmaturity syndrome; see under *syndrome.*
**pulmonary d.,** Wilson-Mikity syndrome.

**dys·meg·a·lop·sia** (dis-meg″ə-lop′se-ə) [*dys-* + *megal-* + *-opsia*] a disturbance of the visual appreciation of the size of objects, in which they appear larger than they are.

**dys·me·lia** (dis-me′le-ə) [*dys-* + *-melia*] anomaly of a limb or limbs as a result of a disturbance in embryonic development; the term includes defects of excessive development as well as reduction deformities. See also *amelia, meromelia,* and *phocomelia.*

**dys·men·or·rhea** (dis-men″ə-re′ə) [*dys-* + *menorrhea*] [MeSH: Dysmenorrhea] painful menstruation.
**acquired d.,** secondary d.
**congestive d.,** that which is accompanied by congestion of the uterus.
**essential d.,** primary d.
**inflammatory d.,** that which comes from or is due to inflammation.
**d. intermenstrua′lis,** intermenstrual pain.
**mechanical d.,** that which is believed to be due to mechanical interference with the flow, as from clots or flexion of the uterus.
**membranous d.,** that which is characterized by membranous exfoliations derived from the uterus.
**obstructive d.,** that which is due to mechanical obstruction to the discharge of the menstrual fluid.
**ovarian d.,** neuralgic pain which is due to ovarian disease.
**primary d.,** painful menstruation usually not associated with pelvic pathology and beginning near the time of menarche; called also *essential d.*
**secondary d.,** dysmenorrhea usually associated with pelvic pathology and arising some time after menarche.
**spasmodic d.,** that which is due to spasmodic uterine contractions.
**tubal d.,** that which is due to disease of the oviduct, such as chronic salpingitis.
**uterine d.,** that which arises from a uterine lesion.

**dys·me·tab·o·lism** (dis″mə-tab′o-liz-əm) defective metabolism.

**dys·me·tria** (dis-me′tre-ə) [*dys-* + Gr. *metron* measure] a condition in which there is improper estimation of distance in muscular acts, with disturbance of the power to control the range of muscular movement, often resulting in overreaching. See also *hypermetria* and *hypometria.*
**ocular d.,** an error in ocular fixation consisting of overshooting the desired focus followed by oscillations of focus until fixation is achieved; the cause is a cerebellar lesion, usually of the vermis.

**dys·met·rop·sia** (dis″mə-trop′se-ə) [*dys-* + Gr. *metron* measure + *-opsia*] defect in the visual appreciation of the measure or size of objects.

**dys·mne·sia** (dis-ne′zhə) [*dys-* + Gr. *mnēmē* memory] impaired memory, as in the amnestic syndrome; cf. *paramnesia.*

**dys·mne·sic** (dis-ne′zik) characterized by impairment or disorder of memory.

**dys·mor·phic** (dis-mor′fik) 1. pertaining to dysmorphology. 2. characterized by dysmorphism (def. 1); malformed.

**dys·mor·phism** (dis-mor′fiz-əm) [*dys-* + *morph-* + *-ism*] 1. an abnormality in morphological development, such as a congenital anomaly. 2. allomorphism. 3. ability to appear in different morphological forms.

**dys·mor·phol·o·gist** (dis″mor-fol′ə-jist) a specialist in dysmorphology.

**dys·mor·phol·o·gy** (dis″mor-fol′ə-je) [*dys-* + *morpho-* + *-logy*] a branch of clinical genetics concerned with the diagnosis and interpretation of patterns of the three types of structural defects—malformation, disruption, and deformation (qq.v.)

**dys·mor·pho·pho·bia** (dis-mor″fo-fo′be-ə) [*dys-* + *morpho-* + *-phobia*] body dysmorphic disorder.

**dys·mor·phop·sia** (dis″mor-fop′se-ə) [*dys-* + *morpho-* + *-opsia*] defective vision, with distortion of the shape of objects perceived.

**dys·mor·pho·sis** (dis″mor-fo′sis) [*dys-* + *morphosis*] malformation.

**dys·my·eli·na·tion** (dis″mi-ə-lin-a′shən) breakdown or defective formation of a myelin sheath, usually involving biochemical abnormalities.

**dys·my·e·lo·poi·e·sis** (dis-mi″ə-lo-poi-e′sis) [*dys-* + *myelopoiesis*] myelodysplasia.

**dys·myo·to·nia** (dis″mi-o-to′ne-ə) [*dys-* + *myotonia*] dystonia.

**dys·no·mia** (dis-no′me-ə) anomic aphasia.

**dys·odon·ti·a·sis** (dis″o-don-ti′ə-sis) [*dys-* + *odonto-* + *-iasis*] imperfect or defective dentition; defective, delayed, or difficult eruption of the teeth.

**dys·on·to·gen·e·sis** (dis″on-to-jen′ə-sis) [*dys-* + *ontogenesis*] defective embryonic development.

**dys·on·to·ge·net·ic** (dis″on-to-jə-net′ik) pertaining to or characterized by dysontogenesis.

**dys·opia** (dis-o′pe-ə) [*dys-* + *-opia*] defective vision.
**d. al′gera,** disturbances of vision due to pains in the eyes and head on looking at objects.

**dys·op·sia** (dis-op′se-ə) dysopia.

**dys·orex·ia** (dis″o-rek′se-ə) [*dys-* + Gr. *orexis* appetite] impaired or deranged appetite.

**dys·or·gano·pla·sia** (dis-or″gən-o-pla′shə) [*dys-* + *organo-* + *-plasia*] disordered development of an organ.

**dys·os·mia** (dis-oz′me-ə) [*dys-* + *osm-*[1] + *-ia*] parosmia.

**dys·os·teo·gen·e·sis** (dis-os″te-o-jen′ə-sis) defective bone formation; dysostosis.

**dys·os·to·sis** (dis″os-to′sis) [*dys-* + *ostosis*] defective ossification; defect in the normal ossification of fetal cartilages.
**cleidocranial d.,** a rare autosomal dominant condition in which there is defective ossification of the cranial bones, with large fontanels and delayed closing of the sutures; complete or partial absence of the clavicles, so that the shoulders may be brought together, or nearly together, in front; wide pubic symphysis; short middle phalanges of the fifth fingers; and dental and vertebral anomalies. Called also *cleidocranial dysplasia.*
**craniofacial d.,** an autosomal dominant disorder characterized by acrocephaly, exophthalmos, hypertelorism, strabismus, parrot-beaked nose, and hypoplastic maxilla with relative mandibular prognathism. Called also *Crouzon's disease.*
**d. enchondra′lis epiphysa′ria,** dysplasia epiphysealis multiplex.
**mandibulofacial d.,** a hereditary disorder occurring in two forms:

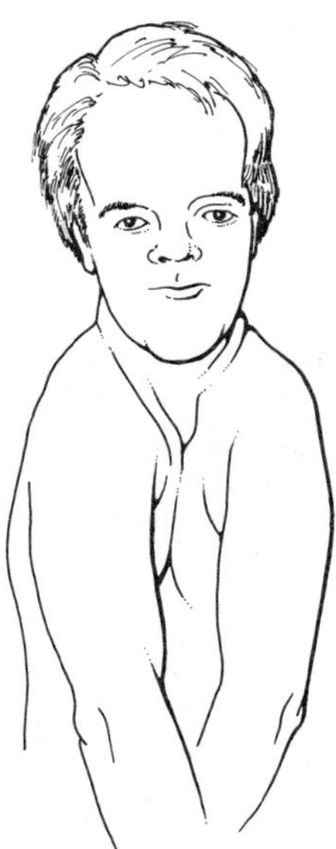

Cleidocranial dysostosis.

the complete form (Franceschetti's syndrome) is autosomal dominant and consists of antimongoloid slant of the palpebral fissures, coloboma of the lower lid, micrognathia, hypoplasia of the zygomatic arches, and microtia. The incomplete form (Treacher Collins syndrome) consists of the same anomalies in less pronounced degree; it occurs sporadically and autosomal dominance is suspected.
**mandibulofacial d. with epibulbar dermoids,** oculoauriculovertebral dysplasia.
**metaphyseal d.,** a skeletal abnormality in which the epiphyses are normal, or nearly so, and the metaphyseal tissues are replaced by masses of cartilage, producing interference with enchondral bone formation, and expansion and thinning of the metaphyseal cortices. Called also *Jansen's disease* and *metaphyseal chondrodysplasia.*
**d. mul'tiplex,** a term for the widespread skeletal manifestations typical of the mucopolysaccharidoses.
**Nager's acrofacial d.,** a congenital condition in which mandibulofacial dysostosis is associated with limb deformities consisting of absence of the radius, radioulnar synostosis, and hypoplasia or absence of the thumbs.
**orodigitofacial d.,** oral-facial-digital syndrome.
**postaxial acrofacial d.,** Miller syndrome.

**dys·pa·reu·nia** (dis″pə-roo′ne-ə) [Gr. *dyspareunos* badly mated] [MeSH: Dyspareunia] difficult or painful coitus.

**dys·pep·sia** (dis-pep′se-ə) [*dys-* + Gr. *peptein* to digest] [MeSH: Dyspepsia] impairment of the power or function of digestion; usually applied to epigastric discomfort following meals.
**acid d.,** a variety associated with excessive acidity of the stomach.
**appendicular d., appendix d.,** dyspeptic symptoms occurring in chronic appendicitis.
**catarrhal d.,** a variety accompanied by gastric inflammation.
**chichiko d.,** a condition of farinaceous malnutrition found in badly nourished infants who are fed mostly on solutions of polished rice powder.
**cholelithic d.,** the sudden dyspeptic attacks characteristic of gallbladder disturbance.
**colon d.,** functional disturbance of the large intestine, giving rise to the symptoms of dyspepsia.
**fermentative d.,** that characterized by the fermentation of ingested food.
**flatulent d.,** that which is associated with the formation of gas in the stomach, especially upper abdominal discomfort accompanied by frequent belching.
**gastric d.,** that which originates within the stomach.
**intestinal d.,** that which arises in the intestines.
**nonulcer d.,** dyspepsia in which the symptoms resemble those of peptic ulcer, although no ulcer is detectable.

**dys·pep·tic** (dis-pep′tik) pertaining to or affected with dyspepsia.

**dys·per·i·stal·sis** (dis-per″ĭ-stal′sis) [*dys-* + *peristalsis*] painful or abnormal peristalsis.

**dys·pha·gia** (dis-fa′je-ə) [*dys-* + *phag-* + *-ia*] difficulty in swallowing; see also *aphagia.* Called also *aphagopraxia.*
**contractile ring d.,** dysphagia due to an overactive interior esophageal sphincteric mechanism which gives rise to painful sticking sensations under the lower sternum.
**esophageal d.,** dysphagia caused by an abnormality in the esophagus, such as a smooth muscle disorder that interferes with peristalsis or an obstruction from external compression or a stricture.
**d. inflammato′ria,** dysphagia due to inflammation of the pharynx or esophagus.
**d. luso′ria,** dysphagia resulting from compression of the esophagus caused by an anomalous right subclavian artery that arises from the descending aorta and passes behind the esophagus.
**d. nervo′sa,** diffuse esophageal spasm.
**oropharyngeal d.,** dysphagia caused by difficulty in initiating the swallowing process, so that solids and liquids cannot move out of the mouth properly.
**d. paraly′tica,** dysphagia due to paralysis of the pharyngeal or esophageal muscles.
**sideropenic d.,** Plummer-Vinson syndrome.
**d. spas′tica,** diffuse esophageal spasm.
**vallecular d.,** dysphagia caused by the lodgment of food in the valleculae.

**dys·pha·gy** (dis′fə-je) dysphagia.

**dys·pha·sia** (dis-fa′zhə) [*dys-* + *-phasia*] impairment of speech, consisting in lack of coordination and failure to arrange words in their proper order, due to a central lesion; called also *dysphrasia* and *dysgrammatism.* See also *aphasia* and *paraphasia.*

**dys·phe·mia** (dis-fe′me-ə) [*dys-* + *-phemia*] stuttering or other speech disorder of psychogenic origin.

**dys·pho·nia** (dis-fo′ne-ə) [*dys-* + *phon-* + *-ia*] any impairment of voice; a difficulty in speaking. See also *aphonia, hyperphonia,* and *hypophonia.*
**d. clerico′rum,** clergyman's sore throat.
**dysplastic d.,** chronic hoarseness due to malformation of the larynx.
**d. pli′cae ventricula′ris,** a condition in which phonation is performed with the false vocal cords (ventricular folds).
**d. pu′berum,** the harsh, irregular utterance of puberty, and of the change of voice in youth.
**spasmodic d., spastic d., d. spas′tica,** difficulty in speaking due to excessively vigorous adduction, or rarely abduction, of the vocal cords against each other, so that the voice is hoarse, soft, and strained.

**dys·phon·ic** (dis-fon′ik) pertaining to or characterized by dysphonia.

**dys·pho·ret·ic** (dis″for-et′ik) 1. dysphoric. 2. dysphoriant.

**dys·pho·ria** (dis-for′e-ə) [Gr. "excessive pain, anguish, agitation"] disquiet; restlessness; malaise.
**gender d.,** unhappiness with one's biological sex or its usual gender role, with the desire for the body and role of the opposite sex.

**dys·pho·ri·ant** (dis-for′e-ənt) 1. producing a condition of dysphoria. 2. an agent that produces dysphoria.

**dys·phor·ic** (dis-for′ik) pertaining to or characterized by dysphoria.

**dys·phra·sia** (dis-fra′zhə) dysphasia.

**dys·pig·men·ta·tion** (dis-pig″mən-ta′shən) a disorder of pigmentation of the skin or hair.

**dys·pla·sia** (dis-pla′zhə) [*dys-* + *-plasia*] abnormality of development; in pathology, alteration in size, shape, and organization of adult cells. See also *dysgenesis* and *dyspoiesis.*

## Dysplasia

**anteroposterior facial d.,** defective development resulting in abnormal anteroposterior relationship of the maxilla and mandible to each other or to the cranial base with secondary malocclusion.
**arrhythmogenic right ventricular d.,** a congenital cardiomyopathy in which transmural infiltration of adipose tissue results in weakness and aneurysmal bulging of the infundibulum, apex, and posterior basilar region of the right ventricle and leads to ventricular tachycardia arising in the right ventricle.
**arteriohepatic d.,** Alagille syndrome.
**bronchopulmonary d.,** a chronic lung disease of infants, possibly related to oxygen toxicity or barotrauma, characterized by bronchiolar metaplasia and interstitial fibrosis.
**canine hip d.,** a bone disorder seen in dogs, particularly in large breeds, in which it may be hereditary; the acetabulum is shallow, the femoral head may be deformed or small, and there is excessive movement at the hip joint, which eventually becomes inflamed and weakened.
**cervical d., d. of cervix,** cellular deviations from the normal in the epithelium of the uterine cervix, which may begin as basal cell hyperplasia and progress through more disorderly epithelial changes toward anaplasia; it is considered a precursor to carcinoma.
**chondroectodermal d.,** achondroplasia occurring in association with defective development of skin, hair, and teeth, polydactyly, and defect of the cardiac septum; called also *Ellis-van Creveld syndrome.*
**cleidocranial d.,** see under *dysostosis.*
**cortical d.,** dysplasia of the cerebral cortex, such as is seen in polymicrogyria and ulegyria.
**craniocarpotarsal d.,** see under *dystrophy.*
**craniodiaphyseal d.,** an autosomal recessive condition in which progressive cranial and facial hyperostosis results in significant distortion of the shape of the head.
**craniometaphyseal d.,** metaphyseal dysplasia associated with overgrowth of the head bones, leontiasis ossea, and hypertelorism.
**cretinoid d.,** the abnormal development characteristic of cretinism, consisting of dwarfism, retarded ossification, and immaturity of the internal and sex organs.

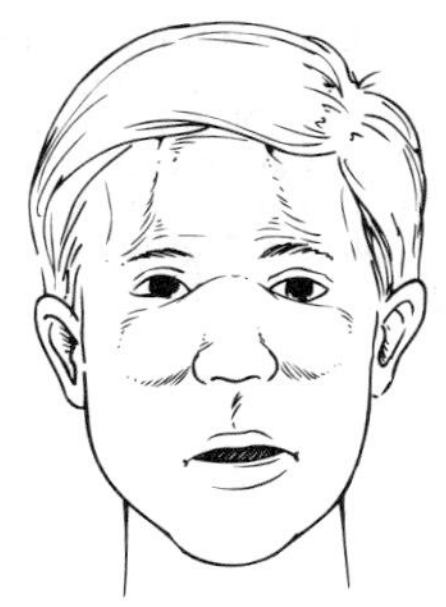

Craniometaphyseal dysplasia.

**cystic renal d.,** see *renal d.*

**dental d.,** dentoalveolar d..

**dentinal d.,** an apparently hereditary disorder of dentin formation, marked by a normal appearance of coronal dentin associated with pulpal obliteration, faulty root formation, and a tendency for periapheral lesions without obvious cause. The teeth become loose and are exfoliated prematurely, probably because of the short pointed roots and periapical granulomas and cysts that are a common complication. Called also *rootless teeth.*

**dentoalveolar d.,** abnormal development of two or more teeth within one or both jaws, producing disharmonious relationships between the teeth and their immediate supporting bone and periodontal structures, and resulting in malocclusion. Called also *dental d.*

**diaphyseal d.,** a condition characterized by thickening of the cortex of the mid-shaft area of the long bones, progressing toward the epiphyses, the thickening sometimes occurring also in the flat bones; excessive growth in length of bones of the extremities usually results in abnormal stature. Called also *diaphyseal sclerosis* and *Engelmann's disease.*

**ectodermal d's,** a group of hereditary disorders involving tissues and structures derived from the embryonic ectoderm; ectodermal dysplasia is a component of various syndromes, including anhidrotic and hidrotic ectodermal dysplasia and the EEC syndrome.

**ectodermal d., anhidrotic,** a congenital X-linked disorder fully expressed in males, or rarely as an autosomal recessive trait with full expression in both sexes, characterized by ectodermal dysplasia associated with aplasia or hypoplasia of the sweat glands, hypothermia, alopecia, anodontia, conical teeth, and typical facies with frontal bossing, midfacial hypoplasia, saddle nose, large chin, and thick lips. Called also *Christ-Siemens-Touraine syndrome, congenital ectodermal defect,* and *hypohidrotic ectodermal d.*

**ectodermal d., hidrotic,** an autosomal dominant disorder, characterized by ectodermal dysplasia associated with dystrophic, hypoplastic, or absent teeth, hypotrichosis, hyperpigmentation of the skin over joints, hyperkeratosis of the palms and soles, and occasionally small teeth with extensive decay. Called also *Clouston's syndrome.*

**ectodermal d., hypohidrotic,** anhidrotic ectodermal d.

**encephalo-ophthalmic d.,** Krause syndrome.

**epiphyseal d.,** faulty growth and ossification of the epiphyses, with radiographically apparent stippling and decreased stature, not associated with thyroid disease. See *d. epiphysealis hemimelica, d. epiphysealis multiplex,* and *chondrodysplasia punctata.*

**d. epiphysea'lis hemime'lica,** a rare condition characterized by swellings in the extremities, usually on the inner and outer aspects of the ankles and knees, made up of bone covered with epiphyseal cartilage, and leading to limitation of motion of the joints. Called also *tarsoepiphyseal aclasis* and *Trevor's disease.*

**d. epiphysea'lis mul'tiplex,** a developmental abnormality of various epiphyses, which appear late and are mottled, flattened, fragmented, and usually hypoplastic; the digits are short and thick, with blunt ends, and stature may be diminished owing to flattening deformities at the hips, knees, and ankles. Called also *dysostosis enchondralis epiphysaria.*

**d. epiphysea'lis puncta'ta,** chondrodysplasia punctata.

**faciogenital d.,** Aarskog syndrome.

**familial white folded mucosal d.,** white sponge nevus.

**fibromuscular d.,** dysplasia with fibrosis of the muscular layer of an artery wall, causing stenosis and hypertension; it occurs most often in the renal arteries, causing renovascular hypertension (q.v.).

**fibrous d., monostotic,** fibrous dysplasia of bone involving only one bone. Called also *osteitis fibrosa localisata.*

**fibrous d., polyostotic,** a later stage of fibrous dysplasia of bone in which several or many bones are involved; when associated with skin and endocrine disorders, it is known as *Albright's syndrome.* Called also *osteitis fibrosa disseminata.*

**fibrous d. of bone,** a disease of bone marked by thinning of the cortex and replacement of bone marrow by gritty fibrous tissue containing bony spicules, producing pain, disability, and gradually increasing deformity. Two types or stages are distinguished: *monostotic fibrous d.* and *polyostotic fibrous d.*

**fibrous d. of jaw,** cherubism.

**florid osseous d.,** an exuberant form of periapical cemental dysplasia that resembles diffuse sclerosing osteomyelitis but differs in being a dysplastic rather than inflammatory process: cysts are present and there is no inflammatory cell infiltrate. Patients are generally asymptomatic.

**frontonasal d.,** median cleft facial syndrome.

**hereditary bone d.,** a heterogeneous group of more than 80 distinct skeletal disorders associated with abnormalities in the size, shape, and proportions of the limbs, trunk, and skull, often resulting in short, disproportionate stature.

**d. linguofacia'lis,** oral-facial-digital syndrome.

**metaphyseal d.,** a disturbance in enchondral bone growth, failure of modeling causing the ends of the shafts to remain larger than normal in circumference; called also *Pyle's disease.* See also *craniometaphyseal d.*

**multiple epiphyseal d.,** d. epiphysealis multiplex.

**neuronal colonic d., neuronal intestinal d.,** a malformation of enteric plexuses resulting in neurons in abnormal locations such as in intestinal smooth muscles or lamina propria. One complex of symptoms includes enterocolitis, diarrhea, and bloody stools and another includes megacolon, decreased motility, constipation, and development of fecalomas. See also *congenital megacolon,* under *megacolon.*

**oculoauricular d., oculoauriculovertebral (OAV) d.,** a congenital condition in which colobomas of the upper eyelid, epibulbar dermoids, bilateral accessory auricular appendages anterior to the ears, and vertebral anomalies are frequently associated with characteristic facies, consisting of asymmetry of the skull, prominent frontal bossing, low hairline, mandibular hypoplasia, low-set ears, and sometimes hemifacial microstomia. Called also *Goldenhar's syndrome, mandibulofacial dysostosis with epibulbar dermoids,* and *OAV syndrome.*

**oculodentodigital (ODD) d., oculodento-osseous d. (ODOD),** a rare hereditary condition transmitted as an autosomal dominant trait, characterized by bilateral microphthalmos, abnormally small nose with anteverted nostrils, hypotrichosis, dental anomalies, camptodactyly, syndactyly, and missing phalanges of the toes. Called also *dysplasia oculodentodigitalis syndrome, Meyer-Schwickerath and Weyers syndrome, oculodentodigital* or *oculodento-osseous syndrome,* and *ODD syndrome.*

**ophthalmomandibulomelic d.,** an autosomal dominant syndrome consisting of blindness caused by corneal opacities, temporomandibular fusion, absent coronoid process, obtuse mandibular angle, radiohumeral and radioulnar dislocations, and aplasia of the lateral condyle of the humerus, radial head, and distal ulna. Called also *OMM syndrome.*

**periapical cemental d.,** a non-neoplastic condition characterized by the formation of areas of fibrous connective tissue, bone, and cementum around the apex of a tooth, particularly of a mandibular incisor. Patients are generally asymptomatic and affected teeth remain vital.

**primary adrenocortical nodular d.,** nodular adrenal hyperplasia

**progressive diaphyseal d.,** diaphyseal d.

**renal d.,** a congenital disorder of the kidney, characterized by the persistence of cartilage, undifferentiated mensenchyme, and immature collecting tublules and by abnormal lobar organization; it may be unilateral or bilateral, total or subtotal, and is nearly always cystic. Total bilateral dysplasia is rapidly fatal in the neonatal period, while milder disease may be asymptomatic.

**renal-retinal d.,** a recessively inherited syndrome of familial juvenile nephronophthisis (def. 1, q.v.) and retinal dysplasia; considered by some authorities to be a part of the juvenile nephronophthisis–medullary cystic disease complex.

**retinal d.,** 1. a general term for a congenital defect resulting from the abnormal growth and differentiation of a retina that fails to develop into functioning tissue and forms tubular, acinic rosettes. Further ocular defects, e.g. microphthalmos, may be present; syndromic abnormalities may accompany retinal changes. 2. amaurosis congenita. 3. a synonym for, or a conspicuous feature of, Krause syndrome and Patau syndrome.

**septo-optic d.,** a syndrome of hypoplasia of the optic disk with other ocular abnormalities, absence of the septum pellucidum, and hypopituitarism leading to growth deficiency. Called also *de Morsier's syndrome.*

**spondyloepiphyseal d.,** a hereditary dysplasia of the vertebrae and extremities resulting in dwarfism of the short-trunk type, often with shortened limbs due to epiphyseal abnormalities. In the delayed onset form, the principal feature is precocious osteoarthritis. There are several forms, including autosomal dominant, autosomal recessive, and X-linked forms, the dominant form often being associated with such ocular anomalies as myopia and detached retina.

**spondylothoracic d.,** Jarcho-Levin syndrome.

## Dysplasia *Continued*

**Streeter's d.,** congenital ringlike concentric bands on the limbs or trunk.

**thanatophoric d.,** a uniformly fatal type of skeletal dysplasia presenting as extreme shortening of limbs, thoracic cage deformity, and relative cephalomegaly. See also under *dwarf.*

**thymic d.,** any of a group of hereditary disorders, some transmitted as an autosomal recessive trait and others as an X-linked recessive trait, characterized by faulty development of the thymus, which may be associated with *(a)* normal serum immunoglobulin levels and impaired cell-mediated immunity (Nezelof's syndrome), *(b)* Swiss type agammaglobulinemia and impairment of both cell-mediated and humoral immunity, or *(c)* variable deficiencies of immunoglobulins, the severity being dependent on the degree of the deficiency.

**ureteral neuromuscular d.,** megaloureter.

---

**dys·plas·tic** (dis-plas'tik) marked by dysplasia.

**dysp·nea** (disp'ne-ə) [*dys-* + *-pnea*] [MeSH: Dyspnea] breathlessness or shortness of breath; difficult or labored breathing.
**cardiac d.,** distressful breathing caused by heart disease.
**exertional d.,** dyspnea provoked by physical effort or exertion.
**expiratory d.,** difficulty in breathing caused by hindrance to the free expiration of air from the lungs.
**functional d.,** respiratory distress not attributable to organic disease, often associated with anxiety states.
**inspiratory d.,** difficulty in breathing caused by hindrance to the free inspiration of air into the lungs.
**nocturnal d.,** respiratory distress that is minimal in the morning, and may gradually progress until it becomes quite disturbing at night.
**nonexpansional d.,** difficulty in breathing caused by inadequate expansion of the chest.
**orthostatic d.,** difficulty in breathing experienced when in the erect position.
**paroxysmal nocturnal d.,** episodes of respiratory distress that awaken patients from sleep and are related to posture (especially reclining at night), usually attributed to congestive heart failure with pulmonary edema but sometimes occurring in patients with chronic pulmonary diseases.
**renal d.,** difficulty in breathing attributable to anemia or volume overload associated with kidney disease.

**dysp·ne·ic** (disp-ne'ik) pertaining to or characterized by dyspnea.

**dys·poi·e·sis** (dis″poi-e'sis) 1. dysgenesis. 2. dyshematopoiesis.

**dys·pon·der·al** (dis-pon'dər-əl) [*dys-* + *ponderal*] pertaining to disorder of weight, either obesity or underweight.

**dys·po·ne·sis** (dis″po-ne'sis) [*dys-* + Gr. *ponēsis* toil, exertion] a reversible physiopathologic state consisting of unnoticed, misdirected neurophysiologic reactions to various agents (environmental events, bodily sensations, emotions, and thoughts) and the repercussions of these reactions throughout the organism. These errors in energy expenditure, which are capable of producing functional disorders, consist mainly of covert errors in action-potential output from the motor and premotor areas of the cortex and the consequences of that output. See also *hyperponesis* and *hypoponesis.*

**dys·pra·gia** (dis-pra'je-ə) [Gr. *dyspragia* ill luck] painful performance of any function.
**d. intermit'tens angiosclero'tica intestina'lis,** intestinal (abdominal) angina.

**dys·prax·ia** (dis-prak'se-ə) [Gr. *dyspraxia* ill luck] partial loss of ability to perform coordinated acts. Cf. *apraxia.*

**dys·pro·si·um** (dis-pro'se-əm) [MeSH: Dysprosium] one of the rare earth elements, atomic number 66, atomic weight 162.50, symbol Dy.

**dys·pros·o·dy** (dis-pros'o-de) [*dys-* + *prosody*] disturbance of stress, pitch, and rhythm of speech; lack of normal prosody. See also *aprosody, hyperprosody,* and *hypoprosody.*

**dys·pro·tein·emia** (dis-pro″tēn-e'me-ə) [*dys-* + *protein* + *-emia*] 1. derangement of the protein content of the blood. 2. (in plural) plasma cell dyscrasias.

**dys·ra·phia** (dis-ra'fe-ə) [*dys-* + *raphe* + *-ia*] incomplete closure of a raphe; defective fusion, particularly of the neural tube. See also *status dysraphicus* and *neural tube defect.* Called also *dysraphism.*

**dys·ra·phism** (dis-rāf'iz-əm) dysraphia.

**dys·re·flex·ia** (dis″re-flek'se-ə) disordered response to stimuli, as in *hyperreflexia* and *hyporeflexia.* Called also *parareflexia.*
**autonomic d.,** a syndrome affecting persons with lesions of the spinal cord above the mid-thoracic level, characterized by paroxysmal hypertension, bradycardia, excessive sweating, facial flushing, nasal congestion, pilomotor responses, and headache. It is due to an exaggerated autonomic response to such stimuli as distention of the bladder or rectum.

**dys·rha·phia, dys·rha·phism** (dis-ra'fe-ə, dis'rə-fiz-əm) dysraphia.

**dys·rhyth·mia** (dis-rith'me-ə) [*dys-* + *rhythm* + *-ia*] 1. disturbance of rhythm. 2. an abnormal cardiac rhythm; the term *arrhythmia* is usually used, even for abnormal but regular heart rhythms. For subentries, see under *arrhythmia.*
**cerebral d.,** disturbance or irregularity in the rhythm of the brain waves as recorded by electroencephalography; called also *electroencephalographic d.*
**electroencephalographic d.,** cerebral d.
**esophageal d.,** diffuse esophageal spasm.
**d. pneumophra'sia,** abnormality of speech rhythm due to defective breath grouping.
**d. proso'dia,** abnormality of speech rhythm due to defective placement of stress.
**d. to'nia,** abnormality of speech rhythm due to defective inflection.

**dys·se·ba·cea** (dis″se-ba'shə) dyssebacia.

**dys·se·ba·cia** (dis″ə-ba'shə) [*dys-* + *sebum*] a condition clinically indistinguishable from seborrheic dermatitis, due to alteration of the pattern of sebaceous gland retention, usually occurring as a manifestation of ariboflavinosis, and characterized by greasy scaling lesions involving the alae nasi, malar areas, canthi of the eyes, and earlobes and sometimes the scrotum or vulva.

**dys·som·nia** (dis-som'ne-ə) [*dys-* + *somn-* + *-ia*] [DSM-IV] a category of disorders consisting of disturbances in the quality, amount, or timing of sleep, due to abnormalities in the mechanisms generating the sleep/wake state or of the timing of sleep and wakefulness; included are primary insomnia, primary hypersomnia, narcolepsy, breathing-related sleep disorder, and circadian rhythm sleep disorder. Cf. *parasomnia.*

**dys·sper·mia** (dis-sper'me-ə) [*dys-* + *sperm-* + *-ia*] impairment of the spermatozoa, or of the semen.

**dys·sta·sia** (dis-sta'shə) [*dys-* + *-stasis*] difficulty in standing; called also *dystasia.*

**dys·stat·ic** (dis-stat'ik) pertaining to or characterized by dysstasia.

**dys·sym·bo·lia** (dis″-sim-bo'le-ə) failure of conceptual thinking so that thoughts cannot be intelligently formulated in language; it may be a form of asymbolia or a sign of schizophrenia.

**dys·sym·bo·ly** (dis-sim'bo-le) dyssymbolia.

**dys·sym·me·try** (dis-sim'ə-tre) a condition characterized by absence of symmetry.

**dys·syn·er·gia** (dis″sin-ər'je-ə) [*dys-* + *synergia*] disturbance of muscular coordination. See also *asynergy.*
**biliary d.,** failure of coordinated action of the different parts of the biliary system. Cf. *biliary dyskinesia.*
**d. cerebella'ris myoclo'nica,** dyssynergia cerebellaris progressiva associated with myoclonus epilepsy; called also *Hunt's disease.*
**d. cerebella'ris progressi'va,** a condition marked by generalized intention tremors associated with disturbance of muscle tone and of muscular coordination; due to disorder of cerebellar function. Called also *Ramsay Hunt syndrome.*
**detrusor–external sphincter d.,** detrusor-sphincter d.
**detrusor-sphincter d.,** contraction of the sphincter muscle of the urethra at the same time the detrusor muscle of the bladder is contracting, resulting in obstruction of normal urinary outflow; it may accompany detrusor hyperreflexia or detrusor instability.
**detrusor–striated sphincter d.,** detrusor-sphincter d.
**vesico-sphincter d.,** detrusor-sphincter d.

**dys·ta·sia** (dis-ta'zhə) [*dys-* + *(s)tasis*] dysstasia.

**hereditary areflexic d., Roussy-Lévy hereditary areflexic d.,** Roussy-Lévy syndrome.

**dys•tax•ia** (dis-tak′se-ə) [*dys-* + Gr. *taxis* arrangement] difficulty in controlling voluntary movements; partial ataxia.

**dys•tec•tia** (dis-tek′she-ə) [*dys-* + L. *tectum* roof] neural tube defect.

**dys•te•le•ol•o•gy** (dis-te″-le-ol′ə-je) 1. the study of apparently useless organs or parts. 2. lack of purposefulness, or of contribution to the final result.

**dys•thy•mia** (dis-thi′me-ə) [*dys-* + Gr. *thymos* mind] dysthymic disorder.

**dys•thy•mic** (dis-thi′mik) 1. depressed. 2. pertaining to dysthymia.

**dys•thy•re•o•sis** (dis-thi″re-o′sis) dysthyroidism.

**dys•thy•roid** (dis-thi′roid) denoting defective functioning of the thyroid gland.

**dys•thy•roid•al** (dis″thi-roi′dəl) dysthyroid.

**dys•thy•roid•ism** (dis-thi′roid-iz-əm) imperfect development or function of the thyroid gland; see also *hyperthyroidism* and *hypothyroidism.*

**dys•tith•ia** (dis-tith′e-ə) [*dys-* + Gr. *tithēnē* a nurse + *-ia*] difficulty in breast feeding.

**dys•to•cia** (dis-to′shə) [*dys-* + *toc-* + *-ia*] [MeSH: Dystocia] abnormal or difficult labor.
**cervical d.,** dystocia caused by mechanical obstruction at the ostium uteri.
**constriction ring d., contraction ring d.,** dystocia caused by contraction of an area of circular muscle fibers, which may occur at various levels of the parturient uterus.
**fetal d.,** dystocia due to the shape, size, or position of the fetus.
**maternal d.,** dystocia due to some condition inherent in the mother.
**placental d.,** difficulty in delivering the placenta.

**dys•to•nia** (dis-to′ne-ə) [*dys-* + *ton-* + *-ia*] [MeSH: Dystonia] dyskinetic movements due to disordered tonicity of muscle. Cf. *myotonia* and *paratonia.*
**d. defor′mans progressi′va,** d. musculorum deformans.
**d. lenticula′ris,** dystonia due to a lesion of the lenticular nucleus.
**d. musculo′rum defor′mans,** a rare, chronic, genetic disease marked by involuntary, irregular, clonic contortions of the muscles of the trunk and extremities. The symptoms appear chiefly on walking, at which time the contortions twist the body forward and sideways in a grotesque fashion. An autosomal recessive form occurs before puberty, principally among Jews; the autosomal dominant form has a later onset and is not as consistent in severity. Called also *Ziehen-Oppenheim disease, d. deformans progressiva, dysbasia lordotica progressiva, progressive torsion spasm, torsion d.,* and *torticpelvis.*
**oromandibular d.,** spasmodic contraction of the muscles of the mouth and jaw, causing involuntary movements of the mouth and lips; cf. *Meige's syndrome* (def. 2).
**tardive d.,** a variant of tardive dyskinesia in which there are dystonic rather than choreic movements.
**torsion d.,** d. musculorum deformans.

**dys•ton•ic** (dis-ton′ik) pertaining to or characterized by dystonia.

**dys•to•pia** (dis-to′pe-ə) [*dys-* + *top-* + *-ia*] malposition.

**dys•top•ic** (dis-top′ik) misplaced; out of its normal place.

**dys•to•py** (dis′to-pe) dystopia.

**dys•tro•phia** (dis-tro′fe-ə) [L.] dystrophy.
**d. adipo′sa cor′neae,** primary fatty degeneration of the cornea; called also *xanthomatosis corneae.*
**d. adiposogenita′lis,** adiposogenital dystrophy.
**d. brevicol′lis,** a condition of dwarfism characterized especially by shortness of the neck.
**d. endothelia′lis cor′neae,** cornea guttata.
**d. epithelia′lis cor′neae,** dystrophy of the epithelium of the cornea marked by erosions; called also *Fuchs' dystrophy.*
**d. media′na canalifor′mis,** d. unguis mediana canaliformis.
**d. mesoderma′lis conge′nita hyperplas′tica,** Weill-Marchesani syndrome.
**d. myoto′nica,** myotonic dystrophy; see under *dystrophy.*
**d. un′guis media′na canalifor′mis,** a deep longitudinal split or canal in the nail plate, sometimes showing lateral branches. Called also *d. mediana canaliformis* and *solenonychia.*
**d. un′guium,** dystrophy of the nails; changes in the color, texture, and structure of the nails. Called also *onychodystrophy.*
**d. un′gulae,** seedy toe.

**dys•troph•ic** (dis-trof′ik) pertaining to or characterized by dystrophy.

**dys•troph•in** (dis′trə-fin) [MeSH: Dystrophin] a protein found in skeletal and cardiac muscle, normally in a tightly bound complex with sarcolemmal glycoproteins; it is lacking in Duchenne's muscular dystrophy.

**dys•tropho•neu•ro•sis** (dis-trof″o-nōō-ro′sis) [*dys-* + *tropho-* + *neurosis*] 1. any nervous disorder due to poor nutrition. 2. impairment of nutrition which is caused by nervous disorder.

**dys•tro•phy** (dis′trə-fe) [L. *dystrophia,* from *dys-* + *-trophy*] 1. any disorder arising from defective or faulty nutrition. 2. muscular d.
**adiposogenital d.,** a condition seen in adolescent boys characterized by fat distribution of the feminine type and genital hypoplasia associated with lesions of the hypothalamus or pituitary gland. Called also *adiposogenital degeneration* or *syndrome, Fröhlich's syndrome,* and *Babinski-Fröhlich syndrome.*
**Albright's d.,** see under *syndrome.*
**asphyxiating thoracic d. (ATD),** a congenital hereditary syndrome transmitted as an autosomal recessive trait, characterized by chondrodystrophy of the rib cage that usually causes asphyxia early in the newborn period, in association with defects of the phalanges and pelvis; called also *Jeune's syndrome* and *thoracic-pelvic-phalangeal dystrophy.*
**Becker's muscular d., Becker type muscular d.,** a form closely resembling Duchenne's muscular dystrophy but having late onset and a slowly progressive course; it is transmitted as an X-linked trait.
**Best's macular d.,** a form of early macular degeneration.
**Biber-Haab-Dimmer d.,** lattice d.
**corneal d.,** see *granular corneal d., lattice d., macular corneal d., Salzmann's nodular corneal d., cornea guttata, dystrophia epithelialis corneae,* and *dystrophia adiposa corneae.*
**craniocarpotarsal d.,** a congenital anomaly transmitted as an autosomal dominant trait, consisting of characteristic flattened, masklike facies; microstomia, the lips protruding as in whistling; deep-set eyes with hypertelorism; camptodactyly with ulnar deviation of the fingers; and talipes equinovarus. Called also *Freeman-Sheldon syndrome, whistling face syndrome,* and *whistling face–windmill vane hand syndrome.*
**Dejerine-Landouzy d.,** facioscapulohumeral muscular d.
**distal muscular d.,** late distal hereditary myopathy.
**Duchenne's d.,** Duchenne's muscular d.
**Duchenne's muscular d., Duchenne type muscular d.,** the most common and severe type of pseudohypertrophic muscular dystrophy; chronic and progressive, it begins in early childhood. It is characterized by increasing weakness in the pelvic and shoulder girdles, with pseudohypertrophy of the muscles followed by atrophy, lordosis, and a peculiar swaying gait with the legs kept wide apart. It is transmitted as an X-linked trait, and affected individuals, predominantly males, rarely survive to maturity; death is usually due to respiratory weakness or heart failure. Called also *Duchenne's d., Duchenne's* or *Duchenne-Griesinger disease, Erb's atrophy* or *Erb's d.,* and *Zimmerlin's atrophy.* Cf. *Becker's muscular d.*
**Duchenne-Landouzy d.,** facioscapulohumeral muscular d.
**Emery-Dreifuss muscular d.,** a rare X-linked form of muscular dystrophy that begins early in life and involves slowly progressive weakness of the upper arm and pelvic girdle muscles, with cardiomyopathy and flexion contractures of the elbows; muscles are not hypertrophied. Called also *scapuloperoneal muscular d.*
**enzootic muscular d.,** myodegeneration in calves, lambs, and colts caused by deficiency of selenium or vitamin E in the diet. Symptoms include dyspnea, cardiac arrhythmias, and difficulty walking. Called also *white muscle disease* and (in lambs) *stiff lamb disease.*
**Erb's d., Erb's muscular d.,** 1. Duchenne's muscular d. 2. limb-girdle muscular d.
**facioscapulohumeral muscular d.,** a relatively benign autosomal dominant form of muscular dystrophy in which there is marked atrophy of the muscles of the face, shoulder girdle, and arm, producing a facial expression called myopathic face. Most patients enjoy a normal life-span. Called also *facioscapulohumeral muscular atrophy, Dejerine-Landouzy d., Duchenne-Landouzy d., Landouzy d., Landouzy-Dejerine d.,* and *Landouzy-Dejerine atrophy.*
**familial osseous d.,** Morquio's syndrome.
**Fuchs' d.,** dystrophia epithelialis corneae.
**Fukuyama type congenital muscular d.,** an autosomal recessive type of muscular dystrophy evident in infancy; muscle abnormalities resemble those of Duchenne's muscular dystrophy, and patients are mentally retarded with polymicrogyria and other cerebral abnormalities. Called also *Fukuyama's syndrome.*
**Gowers' muscular d.,** late distal hereditary myopathy.
**granular corneal d.,** a dominantly transmitted form of corneal dystrophy occurring during the first decade and characterized by the presence of small opacities in the superficial layers of the cornea, which form a granular disk. Called also *Groenouw's type I corneal d.*
**Groenouw's type I corneal d.,** granular corneal d.
**Groenouw's type II corneal d.,** macular corneal d.
**hereditary vitelliform d.,** congenital macular degeneration.
**infantile neuroaxonal d.,** progressive hereditary degenerative encephalopathy transmitted as an autosomal recessive trait, begin-

ning in infancy with muscular hypotonia and arrest of development in late infancy, followed by dementia, blindness, spasticity, and ataxia. Pathologically it is characterized by widespread focal swellings and degeneration of the axons with scattered spheroids in the brain. In some, but not all, cases it is caused by a deficiency of $\alpha$-*N*-acetylgalactosaminidase. Called also *Seitelberger's disease.*
**Landouzy d., Landouzy-Dejerine d., Landouzy-Dejerine muscular d.,** facioscapulohumeral muscular d.
**lattice d. (of cornea),** hereditary dystrophy of the cornea marked clinically by linear lesions having a filamentous interwoven appearance and histologically by fusiform areas of hyaline degeneration and dense deposits of hyalin between the epithelium and Bowman's membrane; called also *Biber-Haab-Dimmer d.*
**Leyden-Möbius muscular d.,** limb-girdle muscular d.
**limb-girdle muscular d.,** a slowly progressive form of muscular dystrophy affecting either sex and beginning usually in childhood, but sometimes in maturity or later; it is characterized by weakness and wasting in the pelvic girdle *(pelvifemoral muscular dystrophy)* or shoulder girdle *(scapulohumeral muscular dystrophy).* Called also *Leyden-Möbius muscular d.*
**macular corneal d.,** a recessively transmitted form of corneal dystrophy occurring during the first or second decade and characterized by the presence of macular opacities with indistinct irregular borders, between which the stroma is cloudy. Called also *Groenouw's type II corneal d.*
**muscular d.,** a group of genetic degenerative myopathies characterized by weakness and atrophy of muscle without involvement of the nervous system. There are three main types: pseudohypertrophic muscular dystrophy, facioscapulohumeral dystrophy, and limb-girdle muscular dystrophy. Other forms include distal muscular dystrophy, ocular myopathy, and myotonic dystrophy.
**myotonic d.,** a rare, slowly progressive, hereditary disease transmitted as an autosomal dominant trait, characterized by myotonia followed by atrophy of the muscles (especially those of the face and neck), cataracts, hypogonadism, frontal balding, and cardiac abnormalities; called also *dystrophia myotonica, myotonia atrophica,* and *Steinert's disease.*
**neuraxonal d., neuroaxonal d.,** 1. see *infantile neuroaxonal d.* 2. an inherited neurological disorder in sheep, dogs, and horses, characterized by ataxia and proprioceptive difficulties, usually with death at an early age.
**oculocerebrorenal d.,** see under *syndrome.*
**oculopharyngeal d., oculopharyngeal muscular d.,** an autosomal dominant disorder with onset in adult life, characterized by weakness of the external ocular and pharyngeal muscles that causes ptosis, ophthalmoplegia, and dysphagia; weakness of trunk and limb muscles may follow. Called also *oculopharyngeal syndrome.*
**pelvifemoral muscular d.,** limb-girdle muscular dystrophy affecting primarily the pelvic girdle.
**progressive muscular d.,** muscular d.
**progressive tapetochoroidal d.,** choroideremia.
**pseudohypertrophic muscular d.,** a group of muscular dystrophies characterized by enlargement (pseudohypertrophy) of muscles. All are X-linked and affect mainly males. The most common types are *Duchenne's muscular d.* and *Becker's muscular d.*
**reflex sympathetic d.,** a series of changes caused by the sympathetic nervous system, marked by pallor or rubor, pain, sweating, edema, or osteoporosis, following muscle sprain, bone fracture, or injury to nerves or blood vessels. When limited to the upper extremity it is called *shoulder-hand syndrome.* Called also *algodystrophy.* See also *post-traumatic osteoporosis.*
**Salzmann's nodular corneal d.,** a progressive hypertrophic degeneration of the epithelial layer of the cornea, Bowman's membrane, and the outer portion of the corneal stroma.
**scapulohumeral muscular d.,** limb-girdle muscular dystrophy affecting primarily the shoulder girdle.
**scapuloperoneal muscular d.,** Emery-Dreifuss muscular d.
**Simmerlin's d.,** limb-girdle muscular d.
**tapetochoroidal d.,** choroideremia.
**thoracic-pelvic-phalangeal d.,** asphyxiating thoracic d.
**wound d.,** a syndrome of defective protein metabolism (hypoproteinemia) that sometimes develops after severe injury.

**dys·tryp·sia** (dis-trip'se-ə) [*dys-* + *trypsin* + *-ia*] derangement of intestinal or pancreatic digestion due to lack of trypsin.

**dys·ure·sia** (dis″u-re'zhə) dysuria.

**dys·uria** (dis-u're-ə) [*dys-* + *uria*] painful or difficult urination.
**spastic d.,** difficult urination due to spasm of the bladder.

**dys·uriac** (dis-u're-ək) an individual exhibiting dysuria.

**dys·uric** (dis-u'rik) pertaining to dysuria.

**dys·vas·cu·lar** (dis-vas'ku-lər) having a defective blood supply; cf. *ischemic.*

**dys·vi·ta·min·o·sis** (dis-vi″tə-min-o'sis) a disorder due to an excess or deficiency of a vitamin.

**dys·zoo·sper·mia** (dis-zo-o-sper'me-ə) [*dys-* + *zoospermia*] a disorder of spermatozoon formation.

# E

**E** symbol for *emmetropia, enzyme,* and *exa-.*

***E*** symbol for *elastance, energy, expectancy, electromotive force, illumination, electric intensity,* and *redox potential.*

***E-*** [Ger. *entgegen* opposite] a stereodescriptor used to specify the absolute configuration of rigid compounds, such as those having double bonds. The substituents attached to the double-bonded carbons are ranked according to the Cahn-Ingold-Prelog sequence rules; then if the higher priority substituents are on the same side of the double bond the configuration is *Z*, otherwise *E*. In the simple case when both carbons have the same pair of substitutents, *Z-* is equivalent to *cis-*, *E-* to *trans-*.

**$E_1$** estrone.

**$E_2$** estradiol.

**$E_3$** estriol.

**$E_4$** estetrol.

**$E_h$** symbol for *redox potential.*

**$E°$** standard reduction potential.

**e** symbol for *electron.*

**e-** [L. *e* out of, away from] a prefix meaning away from, without, or outside.

***e*** symbol for an elementary unit of electric charge (see *charge*) and for the base of natural logarithms (approximately 2.7182818285).

**$e^+$** symbol for *positron.*

**$e^-$** symbol for *electron.*

**$\epsilon$** epsilon, the fifth letter of the Greek alphabet; symbol for *molar absorptivity,* the heavy chain of IgE (see *immunoglobulin*), and the $\epsilon$ chain of hemoglobin.

**$\epsilon$-** a prefix designating (1) the fifth carbon along a chain starting with that adjacent to the principal functional group, e.g., $\epsilon$-aminocaproic acid (see $\alpha$-); (2) one in a series of related entities or chemical compounds.

**$\eta$** eta, the seventh letter of the Greek alphabet; symbol for *absolute viscosity.*

**EAC** symbol for *erythrocyte, antibody, and complement,* sometimes used to denote complement complexes, e.g., EAC1 4b2a.

**EACA** epsilon-aminocaproic acid; see *$\epsilon$-aminocaproic acid.*

**EAD** early afterdepolarization.

**ead.** abbreviation for L. *ea'dem,* the same.

**EAE** experimental allergic encephalomyelitis.

**Ea·gle-Bar·rett syndrome** (e'gəl bar'ət) [J.F. *Eagle,* Jr., American physician, 20th century; Norman Rupert *Barrett,* British physician, born 1903] see under *syndrome.*

**EAHF** *e*czema, *a*sthma, *h*ay *f*ever; see *EAHF complex,* under *complex.*

**Eales' disease** (ēlz) [Henry *Eales,* British physician, 1852–1913] see under *disease.*

**EAP** epiallopregnanolone.

**Ea. R.** abbreviation for Ger. *Entartungs-Reaktion,* reaction of degeneration.

**ear** (ēr) [L. *auris;* Gr. *ous*] [MeSH: Ear] the organ of hearing and of equilibrium, consisting of the external ear, the middle ear, and the internal ear; called also *auris* [TA]. See Plate 16.
**aviator's e.,** barotitis media.
**Aztec e.,** an ear in which the lobule is wanting, the whole ear looking as if it were pushed forward and downward.
**bat e.,** lop e.
**beach e.,** otitis externa caused by irritation from ocean water and other beach conditions.
**Blainville e's,** asymmetry of the two ears.
**Cagot e.,** an ear in which the lobule is wanting.
**cat's e.,** an ear that is folded over on itself.
**cauliflower e.,** a partially deformed auricle caused by injury and subsequent perichondritis.
**cup e.,** a protruding, cup-shaped ear. Milder forms present with a poorly developed anthelical crus with deficient development of the superior helix and overdevelopment of its deep concave concha. In the severe forms, the ear is smaller than normal and the helical rim is shortened to such an extent that the helix margin cups forward over the scapha as a hood.
**Darwin's e.,** an ear having an eminence on the edge of the helix.
**diabetic e.,** mastoiditis complicating diabetes.
**external e.,** auris externa.
**glue e.,** a chronic condition marked by a collection of fluid of high viscosity in the middle ear, due to obstruction of the eustachian tube with or without tympanic membrane atelectasis (q.v.).
**hairy e's,** hypertrichosis pinnae auris.
**Hong Kong e., hot weather e.,** otomycosis.
**inner e.,** auris interna.
**internal e.,** auris interna.
**lop e.,** deformity of the external ear in which the conchal portion grows at a right angle to the head; called also *bat e.*
**middle e.,** auris media.
**Morel e.,** a deformed ear marked by abnormal development of the helix, anthelix, and scaphoid fossa, so that the folds of the ear seem obliterated, and the ear is smooth, large, and often prominent, with a thin edge.
**Mozart e.,** congenital fusion of the crura of the anthelix and the helix.
**outer e.,** auris externa.
**prizefighter e.,** cauliflower e.
**satyr e.,** one with a pointed pinna.
**scroll e.,** one in which the pinna is rolled up.
**Singapore e.,** otomycosis.
**swimmer's e., tank e.,** acute otitis externa.
**tropical e.,** otomycosis.
**Wildermuth's e.,** a deformed ear with prominent anthelix and poorly developed helix.

**ear·ache** (ēr'āk) [MeSH: Earache] otalgia.

**ear·drum** (ēr'drəm) membrana tympanica.

**ear-mind·ed** (ēr'mīnd-əd) audile.

**earth** (ərth) 1. the soil and other pulverulent substances forming the ground. 2. any amorphous, easily pulverizable mineral.
**alkaline e.,** any oxide of the alkaline earth metals.
**diatomaceous e.,** infusorial e.
**fuller's e.,** an impure aluminum silicate, consisting mainly of attapulgite, having decolorizing and purifying properties. See also *fuller's e. pneumoconiosis,* under *pneumoconiosis.*
**infusorial e.,** a silicon-rich earth composed mostly of fragments of diatoms; by boiling with dilute hydrochloric acid, washing, and calcining, it can be so purified as to be a very pure form of silica *(terra silicea purificata).* It is often mixed with clay and used in various industries. See also *diatomite.* Called also *diatomaceous e.*
**siliceous e., purified** [NF], a form of silica *(infusorial e.),* $SiO_2$, purified by boiling with acid, washing, and calcining; used as a pharmaceutical filtering agent.

**ear·wax** (ēr'waks) cerumen.

**eat·ing** (ēt'ing) [MeSH: Eating] the act of ingestion.
**binge e.,** uncontrolled ingestion of large quantities of food in a discrete interval, often with a sense of lack of control over the activity. It is sometimes followed by purging.

**Ea·ton-Lam·bert syndrome** (e'ton-lam'bərt) [Lealdes McKendree *Eaton,* American neurologist, 1905–1958; Edward H. *Lambert,* American physiologist, born 1915] see under *syndrome.*

**EB** elementary body.

**EBCT** electron beam computed tomography.

**Eberth's lines** (a'bərts) [Karl Joseph *Eberth,* German pathologist, 1835–1926] see under *line.*

**Eber·thel·la** (e"bər-thel'ə) [K. J. *Eberth*] a genus of bacteria of the family Enterobacteriaceae, made up of organisms now classified in various other genera.

**EBL** enzootic bovine leukosis.

**Eb·ner's gland, line, reticulum** (eb'nərz) [Victor *Ebner* von Rofenstein, Austrian histologist, 1842–1925] see under *gland, line,* and *reticulum.*

**Eb·o·la virus, virus disease (hemorrhagic fever)** (eb'o-lə) [*Ebola* River in northern Zaïre, where the disease was first observed in 1976] see under *virus* and *disease.*

**ebo·na·tion** (e"bo-na'shən) [L. *e* out + *bone*] the removal of bone fragments from a wound.

**ébranle·ment** (a-brahn-lə-maw') [Fr.] removal of a polyp by twisting the pedicle of the tumor.

**ebri·e·ty** (e-bri'ə-te) drunkenness; inebriety.

**Eb·stein's angle, anomaly, disease** (eb'shtīnz) [Wilhelm *Ebstein,* German physician, 1836–1912] see *cardiohepatic angle,* under *angle,* and see under *anomaly* and *disease.*

**eb·ul·li·tion** (eb"u-lish'ən) [L. *ebullire* to boil] 1. the process or condition of boiling. 2. the motion of a boiling liquid.

**ebur** (e'bər) [L.] ivory.
**e. den'tis,** dentin.

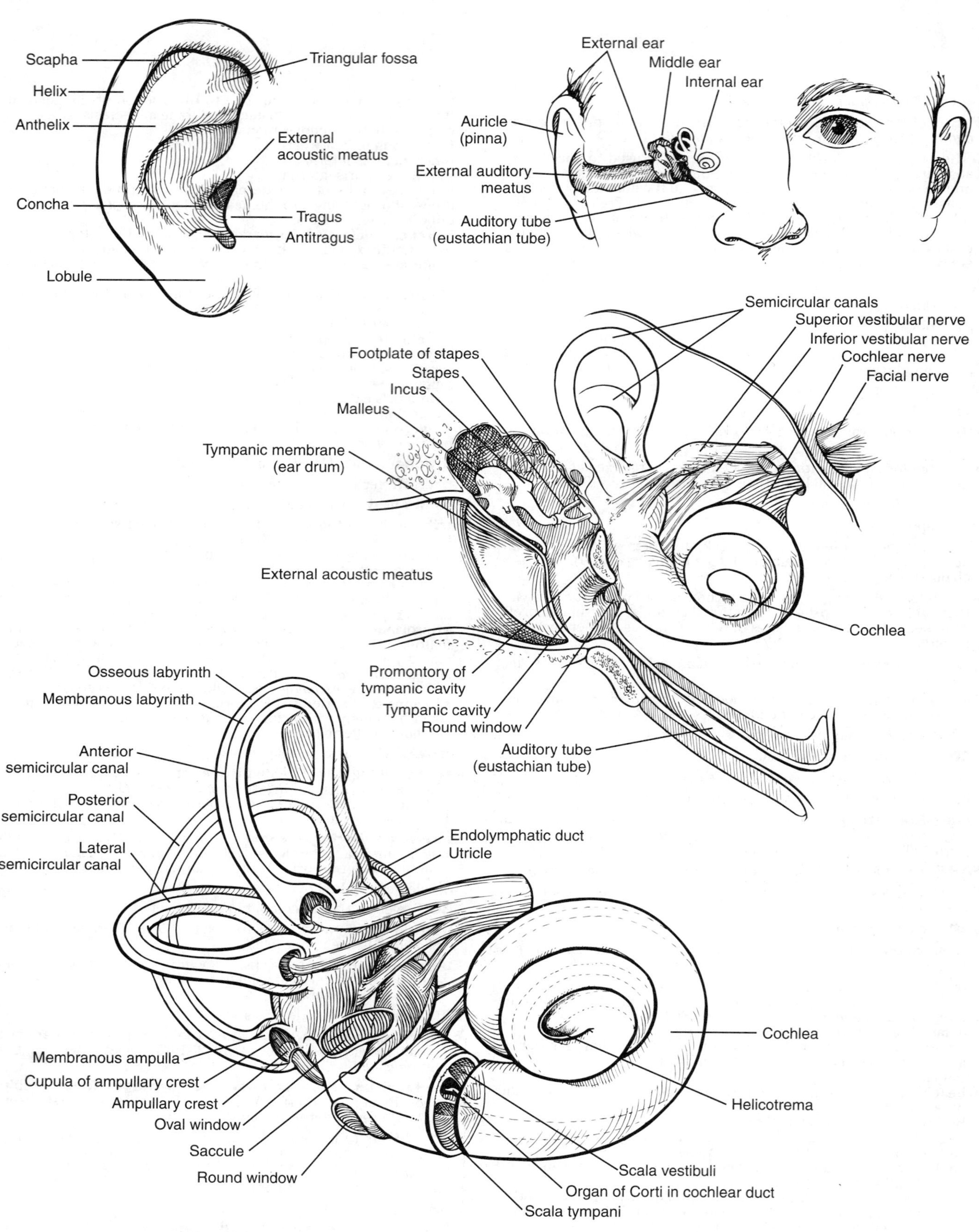


**PLATE 16**—EXTERNAL AND INTERNAL STRUCTURES OF THE EAR

**ebur·na·tion** (e″bər-na′shən) [L. *ebur* ivory] 1. the conversion of a bone into an ivory-like mass. In osteoarthritis, the thinning and loss of the articular cartilage resulting in exposure of the subchondral bone, which becomes denser and the surface of which becomes worn and polished. 2. e. of dentin.
**e. of dentin,** a condition observed in arrested dental caries, characterized by a large open cavity, usually on the occlusal surface of the deciduous and permanent teeth, in which decalcified dentin is burnished and takes a brown-stained, polished appearance.

**ebur·ne·ous** (e-bur′ne-əs) resembling ivory.

**ebur·ni·tis** (e″bər-ni′tis) [L. *eburnus* of ivory + *-itis*] increased hardness and density of dentin, generally occurring in exposed dentin, which may also undergo gradual discoloration, to yellow, to brown, and eventually to black.

**EBV** Epstein-Barr virus.

**EC** abbreviation for *Enzyme Commission.*

**écar·teur** (a-kahr-tər′) [Fr.] a retractor.

**ecau·date** (e-kaw′dāt) [*e-* + *caudate*] acaudate.

**ec·bol·ic** (ek-bol′ik) [Gr. *ekbolikos* throwing out] oxytocic.

**ec·bo·vi·rus** (ek′bo-vi″rəs) [from enteric cytopathic bovine orphan + *virus*] former name of *bovine enterovirus.*

**ec·cen·tric** (ek-sen′trik) 1. situated or occurring away from a center. 2. proceeding from a center.

**ec·cen·tro·chon·dro·pla·sia** (ek-sen″tro-kon″dro-pla′zhə) Morquio's syndrome.

**ec·cen·tro·os·teo·chon·dro·dys·pla·sia** (ek-sen″tro-os″te-o-kon″dro-dis-pla′zhə) [Gr. *ekkentros* from the center + *osteo-* + *chondro-* + *dys-* + *-plasia*] Morquio's syndrome.

**ec·chon·dro·ma** (ek″on-dro′mə) pl. *ecchondromas, ecchondro′mata* [Gr. *ek* out + *chondroma*] a hyperplastic growth of cartilage tissue developing on the surface of a cartilage or projecting under the periosteum of a bone; called also *ecchondrosis.*

**ec·chon·dro·sis** (ek″on-dro′sis) ecchondroma.
**e. physali′phora,** gelatinous nodules of heterotopic notochordal tissue projecting from the clivus or dorsum sellae. True tumors (chordomas) may arise from these or from intraosseous remnants of the notochord.

**ec·chon·dro·tome** (ə-kon′dro-tōm) [Gr. *ek* out + *chondro-* + *-tome*] a knife for excising cartilaginous tissue.

**ec·chy·mo·ma** (ek-ĭ-mo′mə) a swelling due to a bruise and formed by subcutaneous extravasation of blood.

**ec·chy·mosed** (ek′ĭ-mōsd) characterized by ecchymosis.

**ec·chy·mo·ses** (ek″ĭ-mo′sēz) [Gr.] [MeSH: Ecchymosis] plural of *ecchymosis.*

**ec·chy·mo·sis** (ek″ĭ-mo′sis) pl. *ecchymo′ses* [Gr. *ekchymōsis*] [MeSH: Ecchymosis] a small hemorrhagic spot, larger than a petechia, in the skin or mucous membrane forming a nonelevated, rounded or irregular, blue or purplish patch.
**cadaveric e's,** stains seen on the more dependent portions of the body after death, giving the appearance of bruises.

**ec·chy·mot·ic** (ek-ĭ-mot′ik) pertaining to or of the nature of an ecchymosis.

**Ec·cles** (ek′əlz) Sir John Carew. Australian physiologist, 1903–1997; co-winner, with Alan Lloyd Hodgkin and Andrew Fielding Huxley, of the Nobel prize in medicine or physiology for 1963, for discoveries concerning the ionic mechanisms involved in excitation and inhibition in the peripheral and central portions of the nerve cell membrane.

**ec·crine** (ek′rin) exocrine, with special reference to ordinary sweat glands.

**ec·cri·sis** (ek′rĭ-sis) [Gr. *ek* out + *krisis* separation] the excretion or expulsion of waste products.

**ec·crit·ic** (ek-rit′ik) [Gr. *ekkritikos*] 1. promoting excretion. 2. an agent that promotes excretion.

**ec·cy·e·sis** (ek″si-e′sis) [Gr. *ek* out + *cyesis* pregnancy] ectopic pregnancy.

**ECD** ethyl cysteinate dimer; see *bicisate.*

**ec·dem·ic** (ek-dem′ik) [Gr. *ekdēmos* gone on a journey] of or pertaining to an infectious disease introduced into a population or geographic area from without.

**ec·dy·si·asm** (ek-di′se-az-əm) [Gr. *ekdyein* to strip off one's clothes] an abnormal tendency to take off one's clothes in order to cause unsatisfied arousal in an observer.

**ec·dy·sis** (ek′dĭ-sis) [Gr. *ekdysis* a getting out] desquamation or sloughing; especially the shedding of an outer covering and the development of a new one such as occurs in certain arthropods, crustaceans, lizards, and snakes. Called also *molting.*

**ec·dy·sone** (ek-di′son) [Gr. *edkysis* a getting out] [MeSH: Ecdysone] the hormone produced in the prothoracic glands of arthropods that induces molting (ecdysis) and metamorphosis.

**ECF** extracellular fluid; eosinophil chemotactic factor, extended care facility.

**ECF-A** eosinophil chemotactic factor of anaphylaxis; see under *factor.*

**ECG** electrocardiogram.

**ec·go·nine** (ek′go-nin) the final basic product obtained by hydrolysis of cocaine and several related alkaloids. See also *e. methyl ester* and *benzoylecgonine.*
**e. methyl ester,** the major hydrolytic metabolite of cocaine detectable in blood by laboratory testing, accounting for approximately 49 per cent of cocaine metabolism.

**echid·nase** (e-kid′nās) [Gr. *echidna* viper + *-ase*] an enzyme found in the venom of vipers.

**echid·nin** (e-kid′nin) [Gr. *echidna* viper] serpent venom, or a nitrogenous poisonous principle from it.

**Ech·id·noph·a·ga** (ek″id-nof′ə-gə) a genus of fleas. *E. gallina′cea,* the sticktight flea, collects in dense masses on the heads of chickens, in the ears of other animals, and sometimes on the skin of humans.

**echid·no·tox·in** (e-kid″no-tok′sin) a poisonous principle in the venom of vipers.

**echid·no·vac·cine** (e-kid″no-vak′sēn) [Gr. *echidna* viper + *vaccine*] viper venom that has been deprived of its poisonous power by heating; it is used as a vaccine against venom.

**ech·i·nate** (ek′ĭ-nāt) echinulate.

**echin(o)-** [Gr. *echinos* hedgehog] a combining form denoting relationship to spines or to something spiny.

**Ech·i·no·chas·mus** (e-ki″no-kaz′məs) [*echino-* + Gr. *chasma* open mouth] a genus of parasitic intestinal flukes of the family Echinostomatidae. *E. perfolia′tus* is a cause of echinostomiasis in Japan.

**echi·no·chrome** (e-ki′no-krōm) a brown respiratory pigment found in sea urchins.

**echi·no·coc·ci·a·sis** (e-ki″no-kok-si′ə-sis) hydatid disease.

**echi·no·coc·co·sis** (e-ki″no-kok-o′sis) [MeSH: Echinococcosis] hydatid disease.

**echi·no·coc·cot·o·my** (e-ki″no-kok-ot′o-me) [*echinococcus* + *-tomy*] evacuation of an echinococcus (hydatid) cyst.

**Echi·no·coc·cus** (e-ki″no-kok′əs) [*echino-* + Gr. *kokkos* berry] [MeSH: Echinococcus] a genus of small tapeworms of the family Taeniidae.
**E. alveola′ris,** *E. multilocularis.*
**E. granulo′sus,** a small tapeworm parasitic in dogs and wolves and occasionally in cats. Its larva may develop in nearly any mammal, forming hydatid cysts in the liver, lungs, kidneys, and other organs. See *unilocular hydatid disease,* under *disease.*
**E. multilocula′ris,** a species whose adults usually parasitize the fox and wild rodents, although man is sporadically infected. It resembles *E. granulosis,* but the larvae form alveolar or multilocular cysts rather than unilocular cysts. See *alveolar hydatid disease,* under *disease.*
**E. voge′lii,** a species found in Central America and northern South America; its adult form parasitizes canids and its larvae have as intermediate hosts the paca, agouti, and other rodents.

**echi·no·coc·cus** (e-ki″no-kok′əs) pl. *echinococ′ci* [MeSH: Echinococcus] an individual organism of the genus *Echinococcus.*

**echi·no·cyte** (e-ki′no-sīt) [*echino-* + *-cyte*] burr cell.

**echi·no·derm** (e-ki′no-dərm) any animal of the phylum Echinodermata.

**Echi·no·der·ma·ta** (e-ki″no-dər′mə-tə) [*echino-* + Gr. *derma* skin] [MeSH: Echinodermata] a phylum of the animal kingdom, including starfishes, sea urchins, and related groups.

**Echi·noi·dea** (e-kĭnoi′de-ə) a class of the phylum Echinodermata, including the sea urchins. Genera include *Diadema* and *Echinothrix.*

**Echi·no·lae·laps** (e-ki″no-le′ləps) a genus of mites found on rats and in stable litter; its bite causes intense itching. Called also *Laelaps* or *Lelaps. E. echidni′nus* acts as an intermediate host of *Hepatozoon muris* and *H. perniciosum.*

**echin·oph·thal·mia** (e-kin″of-thal′me-ə) [*echino-* + *ophthalmia*] inflammation of the eyelids marked by projection of the lashes.

**Echi·no·rhyn·chus** (e-ki″no-ring′kəs) [*echino-* + Gr. *rhynchos* beak] a former genus of parasitic acanthocephalans.

**E. gi′gas, E. ho′minis,** *Macracanthorhynchus hirudinaceus.*
**E. monilifor′mis,** *Moniliformis moniliformis.*

**ech·i·no·sis** (ek″ĭ-no′sis) [*echin-* + *-osis*] 1. crenation. 2. crenocytosis.

**Ech·i·nos·to·ma** (ek″ĭ-nos′to-mə) [*echino-* + Gr. *stoma* mouth] [MeSH: Echinostoma] a genus of parasitic flukes of the family Echinostomatidae. *E. revolu′tum* is found in the intestines of ducks and geese and has been reported in humans in Taiwan and Indonesia. *E. iloca′num* has been found in human feces in Indonesia and the Philippines. *E. lindoen′sis* occurs in Indonesia; *E. perfolia′tum* is found in Japan.

**Echi·no·sto·mat·i·dae** (ek″ĭ-no-sto-mat′ĭ-de) a family of trematodes, including the genera *Echinochasmus* and *Echinostoma.*

**echi·no·sto·mi·a·sis** (e-kin″o-sto-mi′ə-sis) [MeSH: Echinostomiasis] infection by flukes of the genus *Echinostoma* or of related genera.

**Echi·no·thrix** (e-ki′no-thriks) a venomous genus of sea urchins.

**echin·u·late** (e-kin′u-lāt) [L. *echinus* hedgehog] having small prickles or spines; applied in bacteriology to cultures showing toothed or pointed outgrowths.

**Echis** (e′kis) a genus of snakes of the family Viperidae, small venomous vipers found from India to northern Africa as far south as Ghana and Nigeria; *E. carina′tus* and *E. colora′tus* are both called *carpet viper* or *saw-scaled viper* and their bites are often fatal to humans and other animals.

**echo** (ek′o) [Gr. *ēchō* a returned sound] repetition of a sound as a result of reverberation of sound waves; also the reflection of ultrasonic, radio, and radar waves. Sometimes used to refer to repetition of movement.
**amphoric e.,** a resonant repetition of a sound heard on auscultation of the chest, occurring at an appreciable interval after the vocal sound.
**metallic e.,** a peculiar ringing repetition of the heart sounds sometimes heard in patients with pneumopericardium and pneumothorax.
**spin e.,** a signal generated by a previously magnetized substance a short time after the components of magnetization have been refocused or rephased by application of a pulse of radio frequency energy or by a rapid change in gradient; when received by a radio antenna it can be used to generate a magnetic resonance image.

**echo·acou·sia** (ek″o-ə-koo′ze-ə) [*echo* + Gr. *akousis* hearing + *-ia*] the subjective experience of hearing echoes after normally heard sounds.

**echo·car·dio·gram** (ek″o-kahr′de-o-gram″) the record produced by echocardiography.

**echo·car·di·og·ra·phy** (ek″o-kahr″de-og′rə-fe) [MeSH: Echocardiography] a method of graphically recording the position and motion of the heart walls or the internal structures of the heart and neighboring tissue by the echo obtained from beams of ultrasonic waves directed through the chest wall. Called also *ultrasonic cardiography.*
**contrast e.,** that in which the ultrasonic beam detects tiny intravascular bubbles produced by intravascular injection of a liquid, such as the patient's blood, saline, or dextrose in water, or of small amounts of carbon dioxide gas; bubble movement can demonstrate abnormalities of blood flow.
**Doppler e.,** an echocardiographic technique that records the flow of red blood cells through the cardiovascular system by means of Doppler ultrasonography (q.v.).
**Doppler e., color,** color flow Doppler imaging.
**Doppler e., continuous wave,** that employing continuous wave Doppler ultrasonography to record the flow of blood through the cardiovascular system.
**Doppler e., pulsed wave,** that employing pulsed wave Doppler ultrasonography to record the flow of blood through the cardiovascular system.
**M-mode e.,** that recording the amplitude and rate of motion (M) of a moving structure in real time by repeatedly measuring the distance of the structure from the single transducer at a given moment. It yields a monodimensional image often called an "icepick" view of the heart.
**transesophageal e. (TEE),** the introduction of a transducer attached to a fiberoptic endoscope into the esophagus to provide two-dimensional cardiographic images or Doppler information.
**two-dimensional e.,** that performed by moving the ultrasonic beam in a sector, using multiple transducers or a rotating transducer; computer reconstruction yields a two-dimensional image of a specific plane of the heart.

**echo·gen·ic** (ek″o-jen′ik) in ultrasonography, giving rise to reflections (echoes) of ultrasound waves.

**echo·ge·ni·ci·ty** (ek″o-jen-is′ĭ-te) in ultrasonography, the extent to which a structure gives rise to reflections of ultrasound waves.

**echo·gram** (ek′o-gram) ultrasonogram.

**echo·graph·ia** (ek″o-graf′e-ə) [*echo* + *graph-* + *-ia*] a type of dysgraphia in which the patient can copy writing, but cannot write to express ideas. Called also *pseudoagraphia.*

**echog·ra·phy** (ə-kog′rə-fe) ultrasonography.

**echo·ki·ne·sis** (ek″o-kĭ-ne′sis) [*echo* + *-kinesis*] echopraxia.

**echo·la·lia** (ek″o-la′le-ə) [*echo* + *lal-* + *-ia*] [MeSH: Echolalia] stereotyped repetition of another person's words or phrases, seen in catatonic schizophrenia, Gilles de la Tourette's syndrome, and neurological disorders such as transcortical aphasia; called also *echophrasia.*

**echo·lu·cent** (ek″o-loo′sənt) permitting the passage of ultrasonic waves without giving rise to echoes, the representative areas appearing black on the sonogram.

**echo·ma·tism** (ĕ-ko′mə-tiz-əm) [*echo* + Gr. *matizein* to strive to do] echopraxia.

**echo·mim·ia** (ek″o-mim′e-ə) [*echo* + Gr. *mimia* imitation] echopraxia.

**echo·mo·tism** (ek′o-mo′tiz-əm) [*echo* + L. *motio* movement] echopraxia.

**echop·a·thy** (ĕ-kop′ə-the) [*echo* + *-pathy*] stereotyped repetition of the words or actions of others; echolalia or echopraxia.

**echo·pho·no·car·di·og·ra·phy** (ek″o-fo″no-kahr″de-og′rə-fe) the combined use of echocardiography and phonocardiography.

**echoph·o·ny** (ek-of′ə-ne) [*echo* + Gr. *phōne* voice] an echolike sound heard immediately after a voice sound on auscultation of the chest.

**echo·phot·o·ny** (ek″o-fot′o-ne) [*echo* + *photo-* + *-tony*] the association of certain colors with certain sounds.

**echo·phra·sia** (ek″o-fra′zhə) echolalia.

**echo·prax·ia** (ek″o-prak′se-ə) [*echo* + Gr. *praxia* action, from *prassein* to perform] stereotyped imitation of the movements of another person; seen sometimes in catatonic schizophrenia and Gilles de la Tourette's syndrome.

**echo·prax·is** (ek″o-prak′sis) echopraxia.

**echo·rang·ing** (ek″o-rānj′ing) in ultrasonography, the determining of the position or depth of a body structure on the basis of the time interval between the moment an ultrasonic pulse is transmitted and the moment its echo is received.

**echo·thi·o·phate io·dide** (ek″o-thi″o-fāt) [USP] [MeSH: Echothiophate Iodide] an anticholinesterase agent applied topically to produce miosis, decrease intraocular pressure, and potentiate accommodation in treatment of open-angle glaucoma and accommodative convergent strabismus.

**echo·vi·rus** (ek′o-vi″rəs) [*e*nteric *c*ytopathic *h*uman *o*rphan + *virus*] [MeSH: Echoviruses] species of the genus *Enterovirus,* separable into 29 serotypes (1–7, 9, 11–18, 20–27, 29–34; 8 is identical to 1 and 10, 19, and 28 have been reclassified), that is pathogenic for humans, causing primarily aseptic meningitis or a febrile rash.

**ECI** electrocerebral inactivity.

**Eck's fistula** (eks) [Nicolai Vladimirovich *Eck,* Russian physiologist, 1847–1908] see under *fistula.*

**Eck·er's fissure** (ek′ərz) [Alexander *Ecker,* German anatomist, 1816–1887] see under *convolution* and *fissure.*

**eclamp·sia** (ə-klamp′se-ə) [Gr. *eklampein* to shine forth] [MeSH: Eclampsia] 1. convulsions occurring in a pregnant or puerperal woman, associated with preeclampsia, i.e., with hypertension, proteinuria, or edema. 2. puerperal tetany.
**puerperal e.,** that occurring after childbirth.
**uremic e.,** eclampsia with uremia.

**eclamp·tic** (ə-klamp′tik) pertaining to or of the nature of eclampsia.

**eclamp·to·gen·ic** (ə-klamp″to-jen′ik) causing convulsions.

**eclec·tic** (ə-klek′tik) [Gr. *eklektikos* selecting] designating a sect or school which professes to select what is best from all other systems of medicine. See *eclecticism.*

**eclec·ti·cism** (ə-klek′tĭ-siz-əm) [MeSH: Eclecticism] a nineteenth-century medicinal cult popular in North America that treated diseases by the application of single remedies to known pathological conditions, without reference to nosology, special attention being given to developing indigenous plant remedies.

**eclipse** (e-klips′) in virology, that period of the infective cycle during which infected bacterial cells contain no detectable infective bacteriophage.

**ECM** extracellular matrix.

**ECMO** extracorporeal membrane oxygenation.

**ec•mo•vi•rus** (ek″mo-vi′rəs) [from *e*nteric *c*ytopathic *m*onkey *o*rphan + *virus*] former name for *simian enterovirus.*

**eco•ge•net•ics** (ek″o-jə-net′iks) the study of the relationship between genetic factors and the nature of response to an environmental agent.

**ecol•o•gist** (e-kol′o-jist) an individual skilled in ecology.

**ecol•o•gy** (e-kol′o-je) [Gr. *oikos* house + *-logy*] [MeSH: Ecology] the science of organisms as affected by the factors of their environments; study of the environment and life history of organisms.
**human e.,** application of the ecologic approach to the study of human societies.

**econ•a•zole ni•trate** (ə-kon′ə-zōl) [USP] an imidazole derivative used as a broad-spectrum antifungal agent, applied topically to the skin in the treatment of cutaneous candidiasis and various forms of tinea.

**Econ•o•mo's disease (encephalitis)** (a-kon′o-mōz) [Constantin von *Economo,* Austrian neurologist, 1876–1931] encephalitis lethargica.

**econ•o•my** (e-kon′ə-me) [Gr. *oikos* house + *nomos* law] the management of domestic affairs.
**token e.,** a program of treatment in behavior therapy, usually conducted in a hospital setting, in which the patient may earn tokens by engaging in appropriate personal and social behavior, or lose tokens by inappropriate or antisocial behavior; tokens may be exchanged for tangible rewards (food snacks, clothing, etc.) or for special privileges (watching television, passes to leave the hospital, etc.).

**écor•ché** (a″kor-sha′) [Fr.] a painting or sculpture of a man or other animal exhibited as deprived of its skin, so that the muscles are exposed for study.

**ecos•tate** (e-kos′tāt) [*e-* without + *costa*] ribless; without ribs.

**eco•sys•tem** (ek″o-sis′təm) [MeSH: Ecosystem] the fundamental unit in ecology, comprising the living organisms and the nonliving elements interacting in a certain defined area.

**eco•tax•is** (ek′o-tak″sis) [Gr. *oikos* house + *taxis* arrangement] the "homing" of recirculating lymphocytes to specific compartments of peripheral lymphoid tissues, with B cells going to B-dependent areas and T cells to T-dependent areas.

**eco•tone** (ek′o-tōn) a transition region where adjacent biomes blend, containing some organisms from each of the adjacent biomes plus some that are characteristic of, and perhaps restricted to, the ecotone; this region tends to have more species and to be more densely populated than either adjacent biome.

**Ec•o•trin** (ek′o-trin) trademark for a preparation of aspirin.

**eco•trop•ic** (e″ko-trop′ik) [Gr. *oikos* house + *-tropic*] pertaining to a virus that infects and replicates in cells from only the original host species. Cf. *xenotropic.*

**écou•vil•lon** (a-koo″ve-yaw′) [Fr.] a stiff brush or swab used for swabbing cavities and inflammatory lesions.

**écou•vil•lo•nage** (a-koo″ve-yo-nahzh′) [Fr.] the scrubbing of a cavity or an infected area.

**écrase•ment** (a-krahz-maw′) [Fr.] removal by means of the écraseur.

**écra•seur** (a-krah-zər′) [Fr. "crusher"] an instrument containing a chain or cord to be looped about a part and then tightened in order to transect the portion enclosed within the loop.

**ECS** electrocerebral silence.

**ec•so•mat•ics** (ek″so-mat′iks) [Gr. *ek* out + *somatic*] the study by laboratory methods of the materials removed from the body.

**ec•so•vi•rus** (ek″so-vi′rəs) [from *e*nteric *c*ytopathic *s*wine *o*rphan + *virus*] former name for *porcine enterovirus.*

**Ec•sta•sy** (ek′-stə-se) popular name for *3,4-methylenedioxymethamphetamine.*

**ec•sta•sy** (ek′stə-se) [Gr. *ekstasis*] a state of rapture and trancelike elation.

**ec•stat•ic** (ek-stat′ik) pertaining to or characterized by ecstasy.

**ec•stro•phy** (ek′stro-fe) [Gr. *ekstrephein* to turn inside out] exstrophy.

**ECT** electroconvulsive therapy.

**ec•ta•co•lia** (ek″tə-ko′le-ə) ectasia of a portion of the colon.

**ec•tad** (ek′təd) [*ect-* + *-ad*[1]] outward; the reverse of inward.

**ec•tal** (ek′təl) [*ect-* + *-al*[1]] superficial or external.

**ec•ta•sia** (ek-ta′zhə) [Gr. *ektasis* dilatation + *-ia*] dilatation, expansion, or distention.
**alveolar e.,** overdistention of the pulmonary alveoli.
**annuloaortic e.,** dilatation of the proximal aorta and the fibrous ring of the heart at the aortic orifice, marked by aortic regurgitation and, when severe, by dissecting aneurysm; it is often associated with Marfan's syndrome.
**corneal e.,** keratectasia.
**diffuse arterial e.,** racemose aneurysm.
**hypostatic e.,** dilatation of a blood vessel from the effect of gravity on the blood.
**mammary duct e.,** a condition characterized chiefly by dilatation of the collecting ducts of the mammary gland, inspissation of breast secretion, intraductal inflammation, and marked periductal and interstitial chronic inflammatory reaction in which plasma cells are prominent; a benign process associated with atrophy of the duct epithelium, it generally occurs during or after the menopause.
**papillary e.,** a circumscribed dilatation of the capillaries, forming a red spot on the skin.
**scleral e.,** see under *staphyloma.*
**tubular e.,** congenital, usually bilateral and diffuse dilation of collecting tubules and medullary cysts in the renal medulla.

**ec•ta•sis** (ek′tə-sis) ectasia.

**ec•ta•sy** (ek′tə-se) ectasia.

**ec•tat•ic** (ek-tat′ik) characterized by ectasia.

**ec•ten•tal** (ek-ten′təl) [*ect-* + *ental*] pertaining to the ectoderm and endoderm, and to their line of junction.

**ec•teth•moid** (ek-teth′moid) [*ect-* + *ethmoid*] labyrinthus ethmoidalis.

**ec•thy•ma** (ek-thi′mə) [Gr. *ekthyma*] [MeSH: Ecthyma] an ulcerative pyoderma usually caused by group A beta-hemolytic streptococcal infection at the site of minor trauma, predominantly involving the shins and dorsal feet, and generally healing with variable scar formation.
**contagious e.,** 1. an endemic infectious disease of sheep and goats caused by a poxvirus, characterized by the development on non-wool-bearing areas, especially the lips and oral mucosa, of an erythematous vesiculopustular eruption, the lesions of which may coalesce and crust over, forming large scabs that fall off, followed by healing of the tissues without scarring. Called also *contagious pustular dermatitis, orf, sore mouth,* and *ulcerative stomatitis of sheep.* 2. in humans, presence of a small number of painless pustules on a finger; if lesions become disseminated, systematic symptoms such as lymphadenitis and fever may occur. Human infection usually occurs only by contact with infected animals.
**e. gangreno′sum,** a condition most often seen in debilitated patients in association with septicemia caused by gram negative organisms (e.g., gonococcus, meningococcus, *Escherichia coli, Klebsiella, Pseudomonas*), characterized by lesions that begin as vesicles that rapidly progress to pustulation and gangrenous ulcers with undermined purpuric edges.

**ec•thy•mi•form** (ek-thi′mĭ-form) resembling ecthyma.

**ect(o)-** [Gr. *ektos* outside] a prefix meaning outside, or situated on the outside.

**ec•to•an•ti•gen** (ek″to-an′tə-jən) an antigen which seems to be loosely attached to the outside of bacteria so that it can be readily removed by shaking them in physiologic sodium chloride solution; also an antigen formed in the ectoplasm of a bacterium.

**ec•to•bi•ol•o•gy** (ek″to-bi-ol′ə-je) the study of the properties and biochemical constitution of the cell surface and the specific enzymes at the surface.

**ec•to•blast** (ek′to-blast) [*ecto-* + *-blast*] 1. the ectoderm. 2. an external membrane; a cell wall.

**ec•to•car•dia** (ek″to-kahr′de-ə) [*ecto-* + Gr. *kardia* heart] congenital displacement of the heart, either inside or outside the thorax.

**ec•to•cer•vi•cal** (ek″to-sər′vĭ-kəl) of or pertaining to the ectocervix.

**ec•to•cer•vix** (ek″to-sər′viks) portio vaginalis cervicis.

**ec•to•co•lon** (ek″to-ko′lon) [*ectasia* + *colon*] dilatation of the colon.

**ec•to•com•men•sal** (ek″to-kə-men′səl) a commensal organism that lives outside the body of its symbiotic companion, but cannot be separated from it.

**ec•to•con•dyle** (ek″to-kon′dīl) the external condyle of a bone.

**ec•to•cu•ne•i•form** (ek″to-ku-ne′ĭ-form) the lateral cuneiform bone.

**ec•to•cy•tic** (ek″to-si′tik) [*ecto-* + *cyt-* + *-ic*] outside the cell.

**ec•to•derm** (ek′to-dərm) [*ecto-* + *derm*] [MeSH: Ectoderm] the outermost layer of cells of the three primary germ layers of the embryo. From it are developed the epidermis and the epidermal tissues, such as the nails, hair, enamel of teeth, and glands of the skin, the nervous system, the external sense organs such as the ear and eye, and the mucous membrane of the mouth and anus. Cf. *endoderm* and *mesoderm.*

**amniotic e.**, the inner layer of the amnion (and covering of the umbilical cord) that is continuous with body ectoderm.
**basal e.**, trophoblast covering the eroded uterine tissue that faces the placental sinuses.
**blastodermic e.**, the external layer of a blastula or blastodisk; called also *primitive* or *primordial e.*
**chorionic e.**, the trophoblast.
**extraembryonic e.**, a derivative of epiblast or ectoderm located outside the body of the embryo.
**neural e.**, neuroderm.
**primitive e., primordial e.**, blastodermic e.

**ec·to·der·mal** (ek″to-dər′məl) [*ecto-* + *derma*] pertaining to or derived from the ectoderm.

**ec·to·der·ma·to·sis** (ek″to-dər″mə-to′sis) ectodermosis.

**ec·to·der·mic** (ek″to-dər′mik) ectodermal.

**ec·to·der·moid·al** (ek″to-dər-moid′əl) of the nature of or resembling the ectoderm.

**ec·to·der·mo·sis** (ek″to-dər-mo′sis) a disorder based on congenital maldevelopment of the organs of ectodermal derivation, i.e., nervous system, retina, eyeball, and skin. Called also *ectodermatosis.* See also *phakomatosis.*
**e. erosi′va pluriorificia′lis**, Stevens-Johnson syndrome.

**ec·to·en·tad** (ek″to-en′tad) from without inward.

**ec·to·en·zyme** (ek″to-en′zīm) an enzyme secreted from a cell into the surrounding medium; an extracellular enzyme. Cf. *endoenzyme.*

**ec·to·gen·ic** (ek″to-jen′ik) ectogenous.

**ec·tog·e·nous** (ek-toj′ə-nəs) [*ecto-* + *-genous*] introduced from without; arising from causes outside the organism, as an infectious disease.

**ec·tog·lia** (ek-tog′le-ə) [*ecto-* + *-glia*] the thin, external marginal layer of the early neural (medullary) tube of the embryo.

**ec·tog·o·ny** (ek-tog′o-ne) the influence exerted on the mother by the developing embryo. Improperly called *metaxenia.*

**ec·to·hor·mone** (ek″to-hor′mōn) a hormone secreted to the outside of the body, such as a pheromone.

**ec·to·lec·i·thal** (ek″to-les′ĭ-thəl) [*ecto-* + *lecithal*] having the yolk situated peripherally; see under *ovum.*

**ec·tol·y·sis** (ek-tol′ə-sis) [*ecto*plasm + *lysis*] lysis of the ectoplasm.

**ec·to·mere** (ek′to-mēr) [*ecto-* + *-mere*] any of the blastomeres which share in the formation of the ectoderm.

**ec·to·mes·en·chyme** (ec″to-mes′eng-kīm) mesenchyme originating from the ectoderm, particularly from the neural crest.

**ec·to·meso·blast** (ek″to-mes′o-blast) the layer of cells which has not yet become differentiated into ectoblast and mesoblast.

**-ectomize** [*-ectomy,* q.v.] word termination meaning to surgically remove, used following a root designating the structure removed. By extension, used in terms to designate destruction or deprivation by other methods as well.

**ec·to·morph** (ek′to-morf) an individual having a type of body build in which tissues derived from the ectoderm predominate: there is a preponderance of linearity and fragility, with large surface area, thin muscles and subcutaneous tissue, and slightly developed digestive viscera, as contrasted with endomorph and mesomorph.

**ec·to·mor·phic** (ek″to-mor′fik) pertaining to or characteristic of an ectomorph.

**ec·to·mor·phy** (ek′to-mor″fe) [*ectoderm* + Gr. *morphē* form] the condition of being an ectomorph.

**ec·to·my** (ek′tə-me) [Gr. *ektomē*] excision or resection.

**-ectomy** [Gr. *ektomē* excision, from *ektemnein* to cut out] word termination meaning surgical excision, used following a root designating the structure or organ removed. By extension, used in terms to designate destruction or deprivation by other methods as well.

**ec·to·nu·cle·ar** (ek′to-noo′kle-ər) outside the nucleus of a cell.

**ec·top·a·gus** (ek-top′ə-gəs) [*ecto-* + *-pagus*] conjoined twins connected along the side of the body, so that the components are definitely right and left, the inner arms and/or legs being represented by a bilateral median limb.

**ec·to·par·a·site** (ek″to-par′ə-sīt) [*ecto-* + *parasite*] a parasite that lives on the outside of the body of the host.

**ec·to·par·a·sit·i·cide** (ek″to-par″ə-sit′ĭ-sīd) [*ectoparasite* + *-cide*] an agent destructive to ectoparasites.

**ec·to·pec·to·ra·lis** (ek″to-pek″to-ra′lis) musculus pectoralis major.

**ec·to·peri·to·ne·al** (ek″to-per″ĭ-to-ne′əl) relating to the external or abdominal surface of the peritoneum.

**ec·to·peri·to·ni·tis** (ek″to-per″ĭ-to-ni′tis) [*ecto-* + *peritonitis*] inflammation of the external or abdominal side of the peritoneum.

**ec·to·phyte** (ek′to-fīt) [*ecto-* + *-phyte*] a vegetable parasite or species living on the outside of the body of its host.

**ec·to·pia** (ek-to′pe-ə) [Gr. *ektopos* displaced + *-ia*] malposition, especially if congenital.
**e. cloa′cae**, exstrophy of cloaca.
**e. cor′dis**, congenital displacement of the heart outside the thoracic cavity because of maldevelopment of the pericardium and sternum.
**e. cor′dis, pectoral**, location of the heart outside the thoracic wall, through a cleft in the lower sternum.
**e. cor′dis abdomina′lis**, a rare anomaly in which the heart is located in the abdominal cavity.
**crossed renal e.**, a condition in which the two kidneys are on the same side of the body, one ureter crossing the midline.
**e. len′tis**, displacement of the crystalline lens of the eye.
**e. pupil′lae conge′nita**, congenital displacement of the pupil.
**renal e., e. re′nis**, displacement of the kidney.
**e. tes′tis**, dislocation of the testicle.
**e. vesi′cae**, exstrophy of the bladder.

**ec·top·ic** (ek-top′ik) 1. pertaining to or characterized by ectopia. 2. located away from normal position, as in ectopic pregnancy. 3. arising in an abnormal site or tissue.

**ec·to·pla·cen·ta** (ek″to-plə-sen′tə) [*ecto-* + *placenta*] the actively growing trophoblast that becomes the placenta in rodents.

**ec·to·plasm** (ek′to-plaz-əm) [*ecto-* + *plasm*] plasma membrane.

**ec·to·plas·mat·ic** (ek″to-plaz-mat′ik) pertaining to ectoplasm.

**ec·to·plast** (ek′to-plast) cell membrane.

**ec·to·py** (ek′to-pe) ectopia.

**ec·tos·co·py** (ek-tos′ko-pe) [*ecto-* + *-scopy*] a diagnostic method based on observation of chest and abdominal movements, and said to be capable of determining the outlines of the lungs and of localized internal conditions.

**ec·to·skel·e·ton** (ek″to-skel′ə-ton) exoskeleton.

**ec·to·sphere** (ek′to-sfēr) the outer zone of the centrosome.

**ec·tos·te·al** (ek-tos′te-əl) pertaining to or situated on the outside of a bone.

**ec·to·sto·sis** (ek″to-sto′sis) [*ecto-* + *ostosis*] ossification beneath the perichondrium of a cartilage or the periosteum of a bone.

**ec·to·sym·bi·ont** (ek″to-sim′be-ont) a symbiont that lives outside the body of the organism with which it is biologically related.

**ec·to·therm** (ek′to-thərm) [*ecto-* + *therm*] 1. an animal that exhibits ectothermy. 2. poikilotherm.

**ec·to·therm·ic** (ek″to-thərm′ik) 1. pertaining to or characterized by ectothermy. 2. poikilothermic.

**ec·to·ther·my** (ek″to-thər′me) 1. the regulation of body temperature by the external environment rather than by internal metabolism, with thermoregulation being accomplished by behavioral means; i.e., the animal seeks an appropriate environmental temperature. Cf. *endothermy* (def. 2). 2. poikilothermy.

**ec·to·thrix** (ek′to-thriks) [*ecto-* + *-thrix*] a fungus that grows inside the hair shaft and also produces a sheath of arthrospores on the outside of the hair.
**large-spored e.**, one that forms chains or sheaths of large spores; this type includes *Microsporum fulvum, M. gypseum, M. nanum, M. vanbreuseghemii,* and *Trichophyton gallinae.*
**small-spored e.**, one that forms small spores in sheaths, mosaic masses, or occasionally chains; this type includes *Microsporum audouinii, M. canis, M. ferrugineum,* and *Trichophyton mentagrophytes.*

**Ec·to·tri·choph·y·ton** (ek″to-tri-kof′ĭ-ton) a former genus of fungi now included in the genus *Trichophyton.*

**ec·to·zoa** (ek″to-zo′ə) [Gr.] plural of *ectozoon.*

**ec·to·zo·al** (ek″to-zo′əl) pertaining to or caused by ectozoa.

**ec·to·zo·on** (ek″to-zo′on) pl. *ectozo′a* [*ecto-* + Gr. *zōon* animal] ectoparasite.

**ectr(o)-** [Gr. *ektrōsis* miscarriage] a combining form denoting congenital absence of a part.

**ec·tro·dac·tyl·ia** (ek′tro-dak-til′e-ə) ectrodactyly.

**ec·tro·dac·ty·lism** (ek′tro-dak′tə-liz-əm) ectrodactyly.

**ec·tro·dac·ty·ly** (ek″tro-dak′tə-le) [*ectro-* + *daktylos* finger] congenital absence of a digit or part of a digit; see also *EEC syndrome,* under *syndrome.*

**ec·tro·gen·ic** (ek″tro-jen′ik) pertaining to or characterized by ectrogeny.

**ec·trog·e·ny** (ek-troj′ə-ne) [*ectro-* + *-geny*] congenital absence or defect of a part.

**ec·tro·me·lia** (ek″tro-me′le-ə) [*ectro-* + *-melia*] [MeSH: Ectromelia] gross hypoplasia or aplasia of one or more long bones of one or more limbs; the term includes amelia, hemimelia, and meromelia.
**infectious e.,** a disease of mice caused by a poxvirus and characterized by gangrene and often loss of one or more of the feet and sometimes of other external parts, and by necrotic areas in the liver, spleen, and other organs; called also *mousepox.*

**ec·tro·mel·ic** (ek″tro-mel′ik) pertaining to or characterized by ectromelia.

**ec·trom·e·lus** (ek-trom′ə-ləs) [*ectros-* + *melos* limb] an individual exhibiting ectromelia.

**ec·tro·meta·car·pia** (ek″tro-met″ə-kahr′pe-ə) [*ectro-* + *metacarpus* + *-ia*] congenital absence of a metacarpal bone.

**ec·tro·meta·tar·sia** (ek″tro-met″ə-tahr′se-ə) [*ectro-* + *metatarsus* + *-ia*] congenital absence of a metatarsal bone.

**ec·tro·pha·lan·gia** (ek″tro-fə-lan′je-ə) congenital absence of one or more phalanges of a digit.

**ec·tro·pi·on** (ek-tro′pe-on) [Gr. "an everted eyelid"; *ektropē* a turning aside] [MeSH: Ectropion] 1. eversion (def. 1). 2. specifically, eversion of the eyelid, resulting in exposure of the palpebral conjunctiva.
**atonic e.,** eversion due to loss of skin tone or of muscle tone, especially of the orbicularis oculi muscle.
**cervical e.,** eversion of the uterine cervical canal, with columnar epithelium being farther outside the external os of the cervix.
**cicatricial e.,** eversion of the margin of an eyelid caused by contraction of scar tissue in the lid or by contraction of the skin.
**flaccid e.,** ectropion of the lower lid resulting from reduced tone of the orbicularis oculi muscle.
**e. luxu′rians,** e. sarcomatosum.
**paralytic e.,** eversion of the margin of the lower eyelid as a result of paralysis of the facial nerve, and loss of contractile power of the orbicularis oculi muscle.
**e. of pigment layer,** proliferation of the cells in the posteriorly situated pigment layer of the iris, leading to their migration around the pupillary margin to encroach upon the anterior surface of the iris.
**e. sarcomato′sum,** eversion of an eyelid resulting from chronic thickening of the palpebral conjunctiva; called also *e. luxurians.*
**senile e.,** eversion of the lower eyelid associated with relaxation of the fibers of the palpebral portion of the orbicularis oculi muscle as a concomitant of age, or occurring as a result of atrophic changes in the skin.
**spastic e.,** ectropion caused by tonic spasm of the orbicularis oculi muscle.
**e. u′veae,** eversion of the margin of the pupil, often congenital *(e. u′veae conge′nitum),* and frequently due to the presence of a newly formed membrane on the anterior layer of the iris, or to the formation of connective tissue in the stroma, particularly in diabetes. Called also *iridectropium.*

**ec·tro·pi·o·nize** (ek-tro′pe-ŏ-nīz″) to put into a state of eversion.

**ec·tro·pi·um** (ek-tro′pe-əm) ectropion.

**ec·tro·sis** (ek-tro′sis) [Gr. *ektrōsis*] 1. abortion. 2. treatment that arrests the development of disease.

**ec·tro·syn·dac·tyl·ia** (ek″tro-sin″dak-til′e-ə) ectrosyndactyly.

**ec·tro·syn·dac·ty·ly** (ek″tro-sin-dak′tə-le) [*ectro-* + *syndactyly*] a condition in which some of the digits are missing and those that remain are webbed, so that they are more or less attached.

**ec·trot·ic** (ek-trot′ik) 1. pertaining to or producing abortion. 2. arresting the development of a disease.

**ec·ze·ma** (ek′zə-mə) [Gr. *ekzein* to boil out] [MeSH: Eczema] a pruritic papulovesicular dermatitis occurring as a reaction to many endogenous and exogenous agents, characterized in the acute stage by erythema, edema associated with a serous exudate between the cells of the epidermis (spongiosis) and an inflammatory infiltrate in the dermis, oozing and vesiculation, and crusting and scaling; and in the more chronic stages by lichenification or thickening or both, signs of excoriations, and hyperpigmentation or hypopigmentation or both. Atopic dermatitis is the most common type of dermatitis. Called also *eczematous dermatitis.*
**allergic e.,** atopic dermatitis.

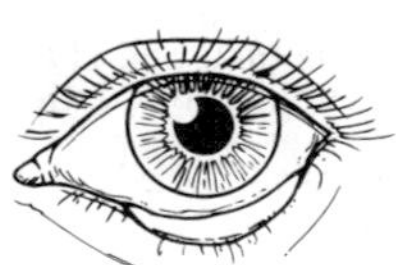

Ectropion.

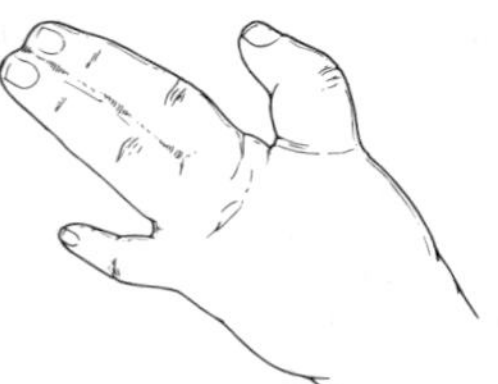

Ectrosyndactyly.

**asteatotic e.,** xerotic e.
**atopic e.,** see under *dermatitis.*
**e. craquelé** (krah-kĕ-la′) [Fr. "marred with cracks"], xerotic e.
**dyshidrotic e.,** pompholyx.
**facial e. of ruminants,** a type of hepatogenous photosensitization in ruminants, particularly in New Zealand, due to ingestion of grass or grain contaminated with the mold *Pithomyces chartarum,* which contains sporidesmin; it is often accompanied by hepatitis or biliary obstruction, which can be fatal. See also *pithomycotoxicosis.*
**flexural e.,** see *atopic dermatitis,* under *dermatitis.*
**e. herpe′ticum,** Kaposi's varicelliform eruption due to infection with the herpes simplex virus superimposed on a preexisting skin condition, usually atopic dermatitis. Cf. *e. vaccinatum.*
**infantile e.,** see *atopic dermatitis,* under *dermatitis.*
**e. intertri′go,** intertrigo.
**e. margina′tum,** tinea cruris.
**nasal e.,** nasal solar dermatitis.
**nummular e.,** eczema presenting in discrete coin-shaped or annular lesions that may coalesce to form large patches that may ooze and crust over, typically on the extensor surfaces of the extremities, lower legs, chest, back, and buttocks. It tends to occur in older men and young women. Called also *exudative* or *nummular neurodermatitis* and *nummular eczematous dermatitis.*
**seborrheic e.,** see under *dermatitis.*
**e. vaccina′tum,** Kaposi's varicelliform eruption due to infection with the vaccinia virus superimposed upon a preexisting skin condition, usually atopic dermatitis. Cf. *e. herpeticum.*
**xerotic e.,** a dehydrated condition of the skin characterized by erythema, dry scaling, fine cracking, and pruritus, which occurs chiefly during the winter when low humidity in heated rooms causes excessive water loss from the stratum corneum. Called also *asteatosis, asteatotic eczema, eczema craquelé, pruritus hiemalis, winter itch,* and *xerosis cutis.*

**ec·zem·a·ti·za·tion** (ek-zem″ə-tĭ-za′shən) persistent eczema-like lesions of the skin, usually due to the continued trauma of scratching.

**ec·zem·a·to·gen·ic** (ek-zem″ə-to-jen′ik) causing eczema.

**ec·zem·a·toid** (ek-zem′ə-toid) resembling eczema.

**ec·zem·a·tous** (ek-zem′ə-təs) affected with or of the nature of eczema.

**ED** erythema dose; effective dose.

**$ED_{50}$** median effective dose; a dose that produces the desired effect in 50 per cent of a population.

**edath·a·mil** (ə-dath′ə-mil) edetate.
**calcium disodium e.,** edetate calcium disodium.
**e. disodium,** edetate disodium.

**Ed·dowes' syndrome** (ed′ōz) [Alfred *Eddowes,* British physician, 1850–1946] osteogenesis imperfecta (type I); see under *osteogenesis.*

**Ed·e·bohls' position** (ed′ə-bōlz) [George Michael *Edebohls,* New York surgeon, 1853–1908] see under *position.*

**Edec·rin** (ə-dek′rin) trademark for preparations of ethacrynic acid.

**Edel·man** (ed′əl-mən) Gerald Maurice. American biochemist, born 1929; co-winner, with Rodney Porter, of the Nobel prize for medicine or physiology in 1972 for his work in separating and identifying the heavy and light chains in the antibody molecule.

**ede·ma** (ə-de′mə) [Gr. *oidēma* swelling] [MeSH: Edema] the presence of abnormally large amounts of fluid in the intercellular tissue spaces of the body, usually referring to demonstrable amounts in the subcutaneous tissues. It may be localized, due to venous or lymphatic obstruction or increased vascular permeability, or systemic, due to heart failure or renal disease. Edema is sometimes designated according to the site, e.g., *ascites* (peritoneal cavity), *hydrothorax* (pleural cavity), or *hydropericardium* (pericardial sac); massive generalized edema is called *anasarca.* Called also *dropsy* and *hydrops.*
**alimentary e.,** nutritional e.

**alveolar e.,** pulmonary edema in the alveoli, usually with hypoxemia and dyspnea.
**angioneurotic e.,** angioedema.
**Berlin's e.,** commotio retinae.
**bowel e.,** edema disease.
**brain e.,** cerebral e.
**brown e.,** pulmonary edema in which the fluid is a brown color, owing to chronic congestion.
**e. bullo'sum vesi'cae,** a condition of the mucous lining of the bladder marked by the formation of clear vesicles with small white particles floating between them.
**Calabar e.,** Calabar swellings.
**e. ca'lidum,** inflammatory e.
**cardiac e.,** a manifestation of congestive heart failure, caused by increased venous and capillary pressures and often associated with the retention of sodium by the kidneys.
**cerebral e.,** excessive accumulation of fluid in the brain substance; causes include trauma, tumor, and increased permeability of capillaries as a result of anoxia or exposure to toxic substances. Called also *brain e.* and *wet brain.*
**circumscribed e.,** angioedema.
**cytotoxic e.,** cerebral edema caused by hypoxic injury to brain tissue and decreased functioning of the sodium pump, so that the cellular elements take in fluid and swell.
**dependent e.,** edema affecting most seriously the lowermost or dependent parts of the body.
**famine e.,** nutritional e.
**e. fri'gidum,** noninflammatory e.
**e. fu'gax,** transient accumulation of fluid in a specific region.
**gaseous e.,** edema accompanied with gas formation, as in gas bacillus infection and subcutaneous emphysema.
**giant e.,** angioedema.
**gut e.,** edema disease.
**hepatic e.,** edema due to faulty functioning of the liver.
**hereditary angioneurotic e. (HANE),** hereditary angioedema.
**hunger e.,** nutritional e.
**hydremic e.,** edema in conditions marked by hydremia.
**idiopathic e.,** edema of unknown cause, usually affecting women, occurring intermittently over a period of years, and usually worse during the premenstrual phase; it is associated with increased aldosterone secretion.
**inflammatory e.,** a form due to inflammation, and accompanied by redness and pain.
**insulin e.,** edema which sometimes follows the injection of insulin.
**interstitial e.,** 1. an increase in interstitial fluid in the brain associated with hydrocephalus. 2. pulmonary edema in the interstitial tissues; there is dyspnea and sometimes hypoxemia.
**invisible e.,** the accumulation of a considerable amount of fluid in the subcutaneous tissues before it becomes demonstrable.
**e. of lung,** pulmonary e.
**lymphatic e.,** edema associated with obstruction of the lymph vessels.
**malignant e.,** 1. a form of cutaneous anthrax in which massive spreading edema develops around a necrotic eschar. 2. inflammatory edema in gas gangrene. 3. a usually fatal form of toxemia with fever, skin discoloration, and swelling, seen in farm animals with a wound contaminated by *Clostridium* species, especially *C. septicum.* Cf. *gas gangrene* and *blackleg.* 4. braxy.
**Milroy's e.,** see under *disease.*
**Milton's e.,** angioedema.
**mucous e.,** myxedema.
**e. neonato'rum,** a disease of premature and feeble infants that resembles sclerema and is marked by spreading edema with cold, livid skin.
**nephrotic e.,** edema occurring as a consequence of volume overload associated with nephrosis and in the intermediate stage of diffuse nephritis.
**neuraxial e.,** a hereditary disease of calves in which they are unable to stand up and their legs and neck become vigorously extended upon certain types of stimulation.
**noninflammatory e.,** edema without redness and pain, occurring from passive congestion or from lowered serum osmolarity.
**nonpitting e.,** edema in which the tissues cannot be pitted by pressure.
**nutritional e.,** a disorder of nutrition due to long-continued diet deficiency of protein and/or calories, and marked by anasarca and edema; called also *alimentary e., famine e., hunger e.,* and *war e.*
**passive e.,** edema occurring because of obstruction to vascular or lymphatic drainage from the area.
**periodic e.,** angioedema.
**periretinal e.,** central serous retinopathy.
**pitting e.,** edema in which the tissues show prolonged existence of the pits produced by pressure.
**placental e.,** the presence of fluid in the villi of the placenta, the villi being club-shaped and irregularly swollen.
**prehepatic e.,** edema occurring in prehepatic hypoproteinemia.
**pulmonary e.,** abnormal, diffuse, extravascular accumulation of fluid in the pulmonary tissues and air spaces due to changes in hydrostatic forces in the capillaries or to increased capillary permeability; it is characterized clinically by intense dyspnea and, in the intra-alveolar form, by voluminous expectoration of frothy pink serous fluid and, if severe, by cyanosis. Called also *wet lung.*
**pulmonary e., high-altitude,** pulmonary edema caused by hypoxia from excessive physical exertion after ascending quickly to a high altitude without acclimatization. See also *high-altitude sickness,* under *sickness.*
**pulmonary e., paroxysmal,** pulmonary edema marked by attacks of difficult respiration, audible rales, wheezes, and cough, caused by acute left ventricular failure, usually associated with hypertensive or ischemic heart disease.
**pulmonary e., re-expansion,** that occurring in a lung that has been rapidly reinflated after a period of collapse due to a pneumothorax or pleural effusion.
**pulmonary e., solid,** a rubbery consistency and gelatinous appearance of the lungs sometimes associated with hypertensive left ventricular failure and uremia.
**purulent e.,** a swelling due to the effusion of a purulent fluid.
**Quincke's e.,** angioedema.
**Reinke's e.,** inflammation and edema of the neck area called Reinke's space after prolonged irritation, usually the result of chronic misuse of the voice, smoking, or excessive exposure to dry air or dust.
**renal e.,** edema due to nephritis and the consequent hypoproteinemia.
**rheumatismal e.,** painful red edematous swellings on the limbs in rheumatism, due to subcutaneous exudation.
**salt e.,** edema produced by an increase of sodium chloride in the diet.
**solid e.,** myxedema.
**terminal e.,** pulmonary edema that develops just prior to death, from circulatory failure.
**toxic e.,** edema caused by a poison.
**vasogenic e.,** a type of cerebral edema seen in the area around tumors, largely confined to the white matter; it often results from increased permeability of capillary endothelial cells and less often is due to toxic injury to the vessels.
**venous e.,** edema in which the effused liquid comes from the blood.
**villous e.,** accumulation of fluid in the chorionic villi, resulting in compression of the blood vessels; reduced blood flow and gas exchange lead to fetal hypoxia.
**war e.,** nutritional e.

**ede·ma·gen** (ə-de'mə-jen) an irritant that elicits edema by causing capillary damage but not the cellular response of true inflammation. Cf. *inflammagen.*

**edem·a·tig·e·nous** (ə-dem″ə-tij'ə-nəs) edematogenic.

**edem·a·ti·za·tion** (ə-dem″ə-tī-za'shən) the process of becoming or of making edematous.

**edem·a·to·gen·ic** (ə-dem″ə-to-jen'ik) producing or causing edema.

**edem·a·tous** (ə-dem'ə-təs) pertaining to or affected by edema.

**Eden·ta·ta** (e″dən-ta'tə) [MeSH: Edentata] an order of mammals including armadillos, tree sloths, and anteaters.

**eden·tate** (e-den'tāt) edentulous.

**eden·tia** (e-den'shə) [*e-* + *dentia*] anodontia.

**eden·tu·late** (e-den'tu-lāt) edentulous.

**eden·tu·lism** (e-den'tu-liz-əm) anodontia.

**eden·tu·lous** (e-den'tu-ləs) without teeth; having lost some or all natural teeth. Called also *edentate* and *edentulate.*

**ed·e·tate** (ed'ə-tāt) nonproprietary drug name for salts of EDTA (ethylenediaminetetraacetic acid), a chelating agent used as *e. calcium disodium* [USP], *e. disodium* [USP], *e. sodium,* and *e. trisodium* in the diagnosis and treatment of lead poisoning and for emergency treatment of hypercalcemia. Formerly called *edathamil.*
**e. calcium disodium** [USP], **calcium disodium e.,** a metal complexing agent, consisting of a mixture of the dihydrate and tetrahydrate calcium disodium salt of edetic acid, used intramuscularly or intravenously in the diagnosis and treatment of lead poisoning. Called also *calcium disodium edathamil.*
**e. disodium** [USP], **disodium e.,** a metal complexing agent, used as a chelating pharmaceutic aid. It is also used in poisoning with lead and other heavy metals and, because of its affinity for calcium, in the treatment of hypercalcemia. Called also *edathamil disodium.*
**e. sodium,** the tetrasodium salt of edetic acid, used as a chelating agent.
**e. trisodium,** the trisodium salt of edetic acid, sometimes used similarly to edetate disodium.

**edet·ic ac·id** (ə-det'ik) [MeSH: Edetic Acid] EDTA; the free acid of edetate.

**edge** (ej) a thin side or border.

**cutting e.,** the angle formed by the merging of two flat surfaces, by which something may be cut, such as the blade of a knife, or the incisal surface of an anterior tooth.
**denture e.,** see under *border.*
**incisal e.,** the junction of the labial surface of an anterior tooth with a flattened linguoincisal surface created by occlusal wear.

**edge-strength** (ej strength) the ability of fine edges to resist fracture or abrasion; applied especially to such resistance in dental restorations.

**Ed·ing·er's nucleus** (ed'ing-gərz) [Ludwig *Edinger,* German neurologist, 1855–1918] nuclei accessorii nervi oculomotorii.

**Ed·ing·er-West·phal nucleus** (ed'ing-gər-vest'fahl) [L. *Edinger;* Carl Friedrich Otto *Westphal,* German neurologist, 1833–1890] nuclei accessorii nervi oculomotorii.

**ed·i·pism** (ed'i-piz-əm) oedipism.

**edis·y·late** (ə-dis'ə-lāt) USAN contraction for 1,2-ethanedisulfonate.

**EDR** effective direct radiation; electrodermal response.

**EDRF** endothelium-derived relaxing factor.

**ed·ro·pho·ni·um chlo·ride** (ed″ro-fo'ne-əm) [USP] an anticholinesterase agent with a duration of action of approximately 10 minutes; used for differential diagnosis and evaluation of treatment requirements in myasthenia gravis and as an antagonist to nondepolarizing neuromuscular blocking agents (e.g., tubocurarine).

**Ed·sall's disease** (ed'səlz) [David Linn *Edsall,* American physician, 1869–1945] heat cramp.

**EDTA** ethylenediaminetetraacetic acid; European Dialysis and Transplant Association.

**ed·u·ca·ble** (ej'u-kə-bəl) capable of being educated; formerly used to describe persons with mild mental retardation (IQ 50–70). See *mental retardation,* under *retardation.*

**edul·co·rant** (e-dul'ko-rənt) sweetening.

**edul·co·rate** (e-dul'ko-rāt) to sweeten.

**EDV** end-diastolic volume.

**Ed·wards' syndrome** (ed'wərdz) [J.H. *Edwards,* British physician, 20th century] trisomy 18 syndrome.

**Ed·ward·si·el·la** (ed-wahrd″se-el'ə) [Philip R. *Edwards,* American bacteriologist, 1901–1966] a genus of gram-negative, facultatively anaerobic bacteria of the family Enterobacteriaceae, made up of small rods that are mostly motile with peritrichous flagella. The organisms are pathogenic for aquatic animals and an occasional opportunistic pathogen for humans.
**E. hoshi'nae,** a motile species that, isolated from animals and humans, does not produce indole.
**E. ic'taluri,** a nonmotile species that does not produce indole, occurring as a pathogen of catfish.
**E. tar'da,** an indole-producing species found in the intestinal tract of snakes, and occasionally isolated from the urine, blood, and feces of humans. It can cause acute gastroenteritis and serious septic infections.

**Ed·ward·si·el·leae** (ed-ward″se-el'e-e) in some systems of classification, a tribe of gram-negative, facultatively anaerobic, rod-shaped bacteria of the family Enterobacteriaceae, made up of the genus *Edwardsiella.*

**EEE** eastern equine encephalomyelitis.

**EEG** electroencephalogram.

**eel·worm** (ēl'wərm) nematode.

**EENT** eye-ear-nose-throat.

**EERP** extended endocardial resection procedure.

**E.E.S.** trademark for a preparation of erythromycin ethylsuccinate.

**EFA** essential fatty acids.

**E-Fer·ol** (e-fer'ol) trademark for a preparation of an intravenous vitamin E supplement.

**ef·face·ment** (ə-fās'mənt) the taking up or obliteration of the cervix in labor when it is so changed that only the thin external os remains.

**ef·fect** (ə-fekt') the result produced by an action.
**additive e.,** the combined effect produced by the action of two or more agents, being equal to the sum of their separate effects.
**Anrep e.,** abrupt elevation of aortic pressure results in a positive inotropic effect, augmented resistance to outflow in the heart; also called *homeometric autoregulation* because it is independent of muscle length.
**Bayliss e.,** increased perfusion pressure and subsequent stretch of vascular smooth muscle causes muscle contraction and increased resistance, which returns blood flow to normal in spite of the elevated perfusion pressure.
**Blinks e's,** brief enhancement in photosynthesis which follows shifts from a long wavelength to a shorter wavelength.
**Bohr e.,** high concentrations of carbon dioxide and hydrogen ions, such as occur in the capillaries in metabolically active tissue, decrease the affinity of hemoglobin for oxygen, so that the oxygen dissociation curve shifts to the right. Cf. *Haldane e.*
**Bruce e.,** the blocking of pregnancy in a newly impregnated female mouse by a pheromone (the odor of a strange male).
**calorigenic e.,** obligatory thermogenesis.
**clasp-knife e.,** see under *rigidity.*
**Compton e.,** the change in the wavelength of gamma or x-rays due to interaction of an incident photon with an orbital electron of an atom, which produces a recoil electron and a scattered photon of reduced energy.
**contrary e.,** Hata's phenomenon.
**Crabtree e.,** the inhibition of oxygen consumption on the addition of glucose to tissues or microorganisms having a high rate of aerobic glycolysis; the converse of the Pasteur effect.
**cumulative e.,** see under *action.*
**cyclosporine e.,** perimyocytic fibrosis (with interstitial cellular infiltrates) occurring in transplanted hearts, due to the use of cyclosporine.
**cytoprotective e.,** an effect produced by an agent, such as prostaglandin $E_2$, that enhances the ability of cells to resist injury.
**Danysz e.,** see under *phenomenon.*
**Deelman e.,** scarification of the skin in artificial carcinogenesis tends to localize the subsequent carcinomata at the scarified area.
**Doppler e.,** the relationship of the apparent frequency of waves, as of sound, light, and radio waves, to the relative motion of the source of the waves and the observer, the frequency increasing as the two approach each other and decreasing as they move apart.
**Emerson e.,** the photosynthetic efficiency of a long wavelength of light is enhanced by simultaneous exposure of plant cells to shorter wavelengths of light.
**experimenter e's,** see *demand characteristics,* under *characteristic.*
**Fahraeus-Lindqvist e.,** blood viscosity is lower in small vessels (diameter less than 1.5 mm) than in large vessels, the viscosity in capillaries being less than half that in large vessels; the effect is due to red cells moving together in single file through the small vessels.
**Haldane e.,** high concentration of oxygen, such as occurs in the alveolar capillaries of the lungs, promotes the dissociation of carbon dioxide and hydrogen ions from hemoglobin, so that the oxygen dissociation curve shifts to the left. Cf. *Bohr e.*
**Hallberg e.,** the crests and troughs of ultrashort standing-wave field have opposite electrical signs.
**Hallwachs e.,** photoelectrical e.
**heel e.,** in radiology, variation in intensity through the cross section of the useful beam due to differential attenuation of x-rays emerging at varying angles from beneath the focal spot; the intensity is greater on the cathode side.
**isomorphic e.,** Koebner's phenomenon.
**McCollough e.,** an aftersensation of color; following exposure to vertical and horizontal lines of differing colors, a grid of vertical and horizontal black lines may be seen as edged with the previously seen colors.
**Mierzejewski e.,** the disharmonious development of gray and white matter of the brain, the gray being in excess.
**Nagler e.,** gas-filled tubes, placed in high frequency fields, will act as rectifiers, causing a unidirectional current.
**Orbeli e.,** see under *phenomenon.*
**Pasteur e.,** the decrease in the rate of glucose utilization (glycolysis) and the suppression of lactate accumulation by tissues or microorganisms in the presence of oxygen. Cf. *Crabtree e.*
**photechic e.,** Russell e.
**photoelectric e.,** the ejection of electrons from matter when light of short wavelengths falls upon it; called also *Hallwachs e.*
**placebo e.,** the sum total of all nonspecific effects, both good and adverse, of medical treatment, primarily psychological and psychophysiological effects associated with the physician-patient relationship and the patient's expectations and apprehensions concerning the treatment.
**position e.,** in genetics, the changed effect produced by alteration of the relative positions of various genes on the chromosomes.
**pressure e.,** the sum of the changes that are due to obstruction of tissue drainage by pressure.
**Purkinje e.,** see under *phenomenon.*
**Raman e.,** when a substance is irradiated with monochromatic light, the spectrum which the substance scatters contains, in addition to a line of the same wavelength as the incident radiation, lines which are satellites of the primary line moving with it when the wavelength of the primary radiation is altered.
**Russell e.,** the rendering of a photographic plate developable by agents other than light; called also *photechic e.*
**side e.,** see under *S.*
**Somogyi e.,** see under *phenomenon.*

**Soret e.**, when a solution is maintained for some time in a temperature gradient, a difference in concentration of one component develops along the temperature gradient.
**specific dynamic e.**, former name for *obligatory thermogenesis.*
**Staub-Traugott e.**, a second dose of glucose by mouth to a normal person one hour after a first dose does not elevate the blood glucose level. See also *Staub-Traugott phenomenon,* under *phenomenon.* Called also *Staub-Traugott test.*
**thermic e.**, obligatory thermogenesis.
**Tyndall e.**, a strong beam of light passes through a true solution invisibly but is clearly outlined passing through a colloidal solution because the light is reflected by the surfaces of the moving colloid particles. Called also *Tyndall phenomenon.*
**Whitten e.**, initiation and synchronization of the estrous cycles and reduction of the frequency of reproductive abnormalities in female mice by the odor (pheromone) of a male mouse placed among them; when more than four female mice are placed together in a cage their estrous cycles become very erratic.
**Wolff-Chaikoff e.**, inhibition of the synthesis of thyroid hormone by high concentrations of iodide.
**Zeeman e.**, separation of a single line in the spectrum by suitable magnetic fields.

**ef·fec·tive·ness** (ə-fek'tiv-nəs) 1. the ability to produce a specific result or to exert a specific measurable influence. 2. the ability of an intervention to produce the desired beneficial effect in actual use; cf. *efficacy.*
**relative biological e.**, an expression of the effectiveness of other types of radiation in comparison with that of gamma or x-rays. Abbreviated RBE.

**ef·fec·tor** (ə-fek'tor) 1. an agent that mediates a specific effect, e.g., an allosteric effector or an effector cell. 2. an organ that produces an effect, e.g., contraction or secretion, in response to nerve stimulation. Called also *effector organ.*
**allosteric e.**, an enzyme inhibitor or activator that has its effect at a site other than the catalytic site of the enzyme; see also under *site,* and see *allostery.*

**ef·fem·i·na·tion** (ə-fem"ĭ-na'shən) feminization (def. 2).

**ef·fer·ent** (ef'ər-ənt) [L. *ex* out + *ferre* to bear] 1. conveying away from a center; called also *centrifugal.* 2. something that so conducts; see under *fiber* and *nerve.* Cf. *corticifugal.*

**ef·fer·en·tial** (ef"ər-en'shəl) efferent.

**ef·fer·ves·cent** (ef"ər-ves'ənt) [L. *effervescens*] bubbling; sparkling; giving off gas bubbles.

**Ef·fex·or** (əfek'sor) trademark for a preparation of venlafaxine hydrochloride.

**ef·fi·ca·cy** (ef'ĭ-kə-se) [L. *efficax* effectual] 1. the ability of an intervention to produce the desired beneficial effect in expert hands and under ideal circumstances. Cf. *effectiveness.* 2. in pharmacology, the ability of a drug to produce the desired therapeutic effect; it is independent of *potency,* which expresses the amount of the drug necessary to achieve the desired effect.
**maximal e., maximum e.**, the greatest therapeutic effect that can be achieved with a given drug.

**ef·fic·ien·cy** (ə-fish'ən-se) [MeSH: Efficiency] 1. the ratio of the useful output of a system to the total input. 2. in statistics, the tendency of a procedure to make optimal use of the data.

**ef·fleu·rage** (ef-loo-rahzh') [Fr.] stroking movement in massage; frottage.

**ef·flo·res·cence** (ef"lo-res'əns) [L. *efflorescentia*] a rash or eruption; any skin lesions, especially numerous and conspicuous lesions.

**ef·flo·res·cent** (ef"lo-res'ənt) [L. *efflorescere* to bloom] becoming powdery in consequence of losing water of crystallization.

**ef·fluve** (ə-flo͞ov') a conductive discharge of a high voltage current through a dielectric.

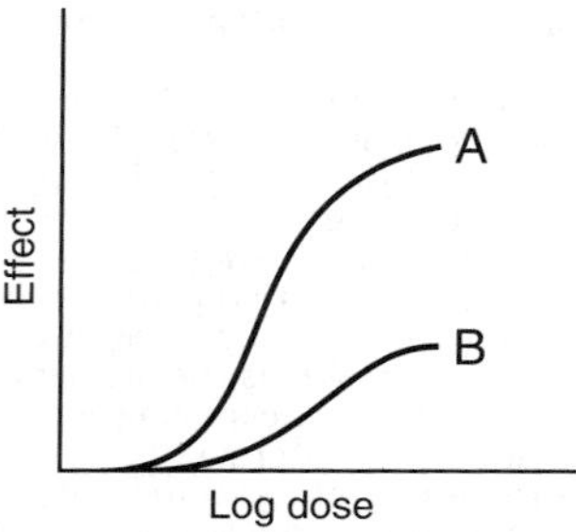


Dose-effect curve for two drugs of different efficacy: The efficacy of drug *A* is greater than that of drug *B.*

**ef·flu·vi·um** (ə-floo've-əm) pl. *efflu'via* [L. "a flowing out"] 1. an outflowing, or shedding, especially of the hair. 2. an exhalation or emanation, applied especially to one of the noxious emanations formerly believed to cause disease.
**anagen e.**, abnormal loss of hair during the anagen phase, which may occur following administration of certain cancer chemotherapeutic agents or exposure to certain chemicals, or in association with various other factors and diseases.
**telluric e.**, an emanation arising from the earth; see *miasma* and *tellurism.*
**telogen e.**, the early, excessive, temporary loss of normal club hairs from normal resting follicles in the scalp as a result of traumatization by some stimulus (e.g., surgery, starvation diet, parturition, drugs, traction, high fever, certain diseases, or psychogenic stress) that prematurely precipitates the anagen phase into catagen and telogen phases, altering the normal hair cycle.

**ef·frac·tion** (ə-frak'shən) a breaking open; a weakening.

**ef·fuse** [L. *effusus,* from *ex* out + *fundere* to pour] 1. (ə-fūs') spread out, profuse; said of bacterial growth that is thin, veillike, and unusually wide spread. 2. (ə-fūz') to pour out and spread widely.

**ef·fu·sion** (ə-fu'zhən) [L. *effusio* a pouring out] 1. the escape of fluid into a part or tissue, as an exudation or a transudation. 2. an effused material, which may be classified according to protein content as an exudate or transudate.
**chyliform e.**, chylothorax consisting of milky chylelike fluid that is low in fat but usually high in cholesterol; it often results from a chronic disease process such as tuberculosis or pleurisy. Called also *pseudochylous e.* and *pseudochylothorax.*
**chylous e.**, chylothorax consisting of chyle that has leaked from the thoracic duct.
**hemorrhagic e.**, an effusion of bloody liquid.
**parapneumonic e.**, a pleural effusion seen as a complication of pneumonia.
**pericardial e.**, the accumulation of an abnormally large amount of pericardial fluid in the pericardium.
**pleural e.**, the presence of fluid in the pleural space; types include *chylothorax, hemothorax, hydrothorax,* and *pyothorax (empyema).* See also *pleurisy with effusion.*
**pseudochylous e.**, chyliform e.
**tuberculous e., tuberculous pleural e.**, an exudative pleural effusion resulting from pulmonary tuberculosis.

**ef·lor·ni·thine hy·dro·chlo·ride** (ef-lor'nĭ-thēn") an irreversible inhibitor of the enzyme ornithine decarboxylase used in the treatment of African trypanosomiasis, administered intravenously. It has also been used experimentally as an antineoplastic agent. Called also *DMFO.*

**Ef·u·dex** (ef'u-deks) trademark for preparations of fluorouracil.

**ega·grop·i·lus** (e"gə-grop'ĭ-ləs) [Gr. *aigagros* wild goat + *pilos* felt] trichobezoar.

**EGD** esophagogastroduodenoscopy.

**eges·ta** (e-jes'tə) [*e-* out + *gerere* to bear] undigested material thrown out from the body.

**eges·tion** (e-jes'chən) the casting out of material which is indigestible.

**EGF** epidermal growth factor.

**egg** (eg) [L. *ovum*] 1. ovum (def. 1). 2. oocyte. 3. a female reproductive cell at any stage before fertilization; after fertilization and fusion of the pronuclei it is called a *zygote.*

**egg-bound** (eg'bownd) 1. unable to discharge eggs in the normal manner; said of a hen or other egg-laying animal. 2. inability of an egg-laying animal to discharge eggs in the normal manner.

**Eg·gers' plate** (eg'ərz) [George William Nordholtz *Eggers,* American orthopedic surgeon, 1896–1963] see under *plate.*

**egi·lops** (e'jĭ-lops) [Gr. *aix* goat + *ōps* eye] perforating abscess at the inner canthus of the eye.

**egland·u·lous** (e-glan'du-ləs) [*e-* + *glandulous*] having no glands.

**ego** (e'go) [L. "I"] [MeSH: Ego] in modern psychoanalytic theory, the psychologic segment of the personality, dominated by the reality principle, comprising integrative and executive aspects that function to adapt the forces and pressures exerted by the impulses of the id, the demands of the superego, and the requirements of external reality through conscious perception, thought, reasoning, learning, and all other activities necessary to interact effectively with the world. Cf. *id*[1] and *superego.*

**ego-ali·en** (e"go-āl'yən) ego-dystonic.

**ego·bron·choph·o·ny** (e"go-brong-kof'o-ne) [Gr. *aix* goat + *bronchophony*] egophony.

**ego·cen·tric** (e"go-sen'trik) [*ego* + *centric*] self-centered, conceited, egotistical; preoccupied with one's own interests and needs; lacking concern for others.

**ego·dys·ton·ic** (e″go-dis-ton′ik) denoting aspects of a person's thoughts, impulses, attitudes, and behavior that are felt to be repugnant, distressing, unacceptable, or inconsistent with the rest of their personality. Cf. *ego-syntonic.*

**ego·ide·al** (e′go-i′del) see under *ideal.*

**ego·ism** (e′go-iz-əm) 1. any of several ethical doctrines that morality is founded in self-interest or that self-interest is the appropriate motive for all conduct. 2. excessive preoccupation with oneself, self-interest with disregard for the needs of others. 3. egotism.

**ego·ma·nia** (e″go-ma′ne-ə) [*ego* + *mania*] extreme self-centeredness; extreme egotism.

**egoph·o·ny** (e-gof′o-ne) [Gr. *aix* goat + *phōnē* voice] increased resonance of voice sounds, with a high-pitched nasal or bleating quality, heard especially over lung tissue that is compressed or consolidated by pleural effusion. Called also *bronchoegophony, egobronchophony, tragophonia, tragophony,* and *voix de polichinelle.*

**ego·syn·ton·ic** (e″go-sin-ton′ik) denoting aspects of a person's thoughts, impulses, attitudes, and behavior that are felt to be acceptable and consistent with the rest of their personality. Cf. *ego-dystonic.*

**ego·tism** (e′go-tiz-əm) 1. conceit, selfishness, self-centeredness, with an inflated sense of one's importance. 2. egoism (def. 2).

**EGTA** egtazic acid; a tetracarboxylic acid chelator similar in structure and action to EDTA (ethylenediaminetetraacetic acid), but with a higher affinity for calcium than for magnesium. It is used in biochemical assays and as a pharmaceutic aid.

**eg·ta·zic ac·id** (əg-tāz′ik) [MeSH: Egtazic Acid] ethylene glycol-bis(β-aminoethyl ether)-*N,N*-tetraacetic acid; see *EGTA.*

**EHBF** estimated hepatic blood flow.

**EHDP** ethane-1-hydroxy-1,1-diphosphonate; see *etidronate.*

**Eh·lers-Dan·los syndrome (disease)** (a′lərz-dahn-los′) [Edvard *Ehlers,* Danish dermatologist, 1863–1937; Henri Alexandre *Danlos* French dermatologist, 1844–1912] [MeSH: Ehlers-Danlos Syndrome] see under *syndrome.*

**Ehr·en·rit·ter's ganglion** (ār′ən-rit″ərz) [Johann *Ehrenritter,* Austrian anatomist, 18th century] ganglion superius nervi glossopharyngei.

**Ehr·lich** (ār′lik) Paul. German physician and bacteriologist, 1854–1915; co-winner, with Elie Metchnikoff, of the Nobel prize for medicine or physiology in 1908 for developing the side chain theory.

**Ehr·lich's reaction,** etc. (ār′liks) [Paul *Ehrlich*] see under *reaction* and *theory.*

**Ehr·lich-Heinz granules** (ār′lik hīnts) [Paul *Ehrlich;* Robert *Heinz,* German pathologist, 1865–1924] Ehrlich's granules.

**Ehr·lich·ia** (ār-lik′e-ə) [Paul *Ehrlich*] [MeSH: Ehrlichia] a genus of bacteria of the tribe Ehrlichieae, family Rickettsiaceae, order Rickettsiales that produce disease in dogs, cattle, sheep, and humans.
**E. ca′nis,** a species causing canine ehrlichiosis, transmitted by the tick *Rhipicephalus sanguineus;* human infection is marked by symptoms similar to those of Rocky Mountain spotted fever.
**E. chaffeen′sis,** a species, transmitted by the ticks *Amblyomma americanum* and *Dermacentor variablis,* that causes human monocytic ehrlichiosis.
**E. e′qui,** a species that causes equine ehrlichiosis.
**E. ondi′ri,** see *Cytoecetes.*
**E. phagocyto′phila,** a species that causes ehrlichiosis in sheep and cattle.
**E. pla′tys,** a species that causes infectious cyclic thrombocytopenia in dogs.
**E. risti′cii,** a species that causes equine monocytic ehrlichiosis.
**E. sennet′su,** a species that is the etiologic agent of Sennetsu fever.

**ehr·lich·ia** (ār-lik′e-ə) [MeSH: Ehrlichia] an individual organism of the genus *Ehrlichia.*

**ehr·lich·i·al** (ār-lik′e-əl) pertaining to or caused by *Ehrlichia.*

**Ehr·lich·i·eae** (ār″lĭ-ki′e-e) [MeSH: Ehrlichieae] a tribe of bacteria of the family Rickettsiaceae, order Rickettsiales, made up of rickettsia-like organisms adapted to existence in invertebrates, chiefly arthropods, and pathogenic for certain mammals, including humans. It includes the genera *Cowdria, Ehrlichia,* and *Neorickettsia.*

**ehr·lich·i·osis** (ar-lik″e-o′sis) [MeSH: Ehrlichiosis] a tick-borne febrile illness caused by infection with bacteria of the genus *Ehrlichia.* In humans it is characterized by fever, headache, and malaise, with leukopenia and thrombocytopenia, and ranges in severity from asymptomatic to severe, with death occasionally occurring.
**canine e.,** an often fatal febrile disease of dogs caused by *Ehrlichia canis,* which is spread by the tick *Rhipicephalus sanguineus* and infects the circulating lymphocytes; it occurs chiefly in warm regions of the world. There are three phases: the *acute phase,* characterized by fever, serous or mucopurulent discharge from the eyes and nose, anorexia, dyspnea, lymphadenopathy, and central nervous system signs resulting from inflammation of the meninges; the *subclinical phase,* in which clinical signs disappear but antigenemia, thrombocytopenia, and anemia persist; and the *chronic phase,* characterized by depression, weight loss, abdominal tenderness, hemorrhage, ocular lesions, ataxia, paralysis, and cranial nerve deficits.
**equine e.,** a usually nonfatal infection of horses with *Ehrlichia equi,* seen in California and eastward into the midwestern United States; characteristics include fever, limb edema, and anemia.
**equine monocytic e.,** an often fatal infection of horses with *Ehrlichia risticii,* seen in Virginia, Maryland, and Pennsylvania; characteristics include fever, diarrhea, and anorexia. Called also *Potomac horse fever.*
**human granulocytic e. (HGE),** a sometimes fatal human ehrlichiosis, occurring in the United States and Europe, caused by a species of *Ehrlichia* antigenically related to *E. equi* and *E. phagocytophila* and transmitted by ticks of the genus *Ixodes;* it is characterized by nonspecific flulike symptoms and involves predominantly neutrophils.
**human monocytic e. (HME),** a sometimes fatal human ehrlichiosis, occurring in the United States, Europe, and Africa, caused by *Ehrlichia chaffeensis* and transmitted by the ticks *Amblyomma americanum* and *Dermacentor variabilis;* it is characterized by nonspecific flulike symptoms and involves predominantly fixed tissue mononuclear phagocytes.

**EI** erythema infectiosum.

**EIA** enzyme immunoassay.

**Eich·horst's atrophy** (īk′horsts) [Hermann Ludwig *Eichhorst,* German physician in Switzerland, 1849–1921] see under *atrophy.*

**Eic·ken's method** (i′kənz) [Carl Otto von *Eicken,* German laryngologist and otologist, 1873–1960] see under *method.*

**ei·co·nom·e·ter** (i″kŏ-nom′ə-tər) eikonometer.

**ei·co·sa·no·ate** (i-ko″sə-no′āt) arachidate.

**ei·co·sa·no·ic ac·id** (i″ko-sə-no′ik) systematic name for *arachidic acid;* see table at *fatty acid.*

**ei·co·sa·noid** (i-ko′sə-noid) any of the biologically active substances derived from arachidonic acid, including the prostaglandins and leukotrienes.

**ei·co·sa·pen·ta·eno·ic ac·id** (i-ko″sə-pen″tə-e-no′ik) all *cis*-5,8,11,14,17-eicosapentaenoic acid, an omega-3, polyunsaturated, 20-carbon fatty acid found almost exclusively in fish and marine animal oils; it is a substrate for cyclooxygenase. Abbreviated EPA. See also table accompanying *fatty acid.*

**ei·det·ic** (i-det′ik) [Gr. *eidos* that which is seen; form or shape] pertaining to or characterized by exact visualization of events or of objects previously seen. By extension, sometimes used to designate an individual possessing such an ability.

**ei·do·gen** (i′do-jen) [Gr. *eidos* form + *-gen*] a substance elaborated by a second grade inductor, which is capable of modifying the form of an embryonic organ already in the process of formation.

**ei·dop·tom·e·try** (i″dop-tom′ə-tre) [Gr. *eidos* form + *opto-* + *-metry*] measurement of the acuteness of vision for the perception of form.

**Eijk·man** (īk′mən) Christiaan. Dutch physiologist, 1858–1930; co-winner, with Sir Frederick Gowland Hopkins, of the Nobel prize for medicine or physiology in 1929 for his discovery of the antineuritic vitamin, thiamine.

**Ei·ken·el·la** (i″kən-el′ə) [M. *Eiken,* Scandinavian biologist, 20th century] [MeSH: Eikenella] a genus of gram-negative, facultatively anaerobic, rod-shaped bacteria. The organisms are part of the normal flora of the human oral cavity and upper respiratory tract but may cause infections of the head, neck, and abdominal area and general systemic disease. The single species is *E. corrodens.*

**ei·ko·nom·e·ter** (i″ko-nom′ə-tər) [Gr. *eikōn* image + *-meter*] an instrument used in making an examination for aniseikonia.

**ei·loid** (i′loid) [Gr. *eilein* to roll up + *-oid*] having a coiled appearance.

**Ei·me·ria** (i-me′re-ə) [Gustav Heinrich Theodor *Eimer,* German zoologist, 1843–1898] [MeSH: Eimeria] a genus of homoxenous coccidian protozoa (suborder Eimeriina, order Eucoccidiida) found principally as parasites of the gastrointestinal tract of birds and herbivorous mammals, characterized by the presence of four spores in each oocyst and two sporozoites in each spore, the oocysts being passed in the feces. It comprises numerous species, many of which are of economic importance. Some of the common pathogenic species found in domestic animals are *E. bovis, E. ellipsoidalis,* and *E. zuernii* in cattle; *E. arloingi* A *(ovina), E. weybridgensis (E. arloingi* B), *E. crandallis, E. ahsata, E. ovinoidalis,* and *E. gilruthi* in sheep; *E. debliecki, E. scabra,* and *E. perminuta* in swine; *E. leukarti* in horses and donkeys; *E. arloingi, E. faurei, E. caprina,* and *E. ninakohlyakimovae* in goats; *E. magna, E. stieda, E. sciurorum,* and *E. perforans* in rabbits; and *E.* acervulina, E. maxima, E. meleagridis, E. necatrix, and *E. tenella* in poultry. See also *coccidiosis.*

**Ei·me·ri·i·na** (i″me-ri′ī-nə) [MeSH: Eimeriina] a suborder of homoxenous or heteroxenous protozoa (order Eucoccidiida, subclass Coccidia), usually parasitizing the gut epithelium of the host, in which the macrogamete and microgametocyte develop independently, syzygy does not occur, the microgametocyte gives rise to numerous biflagellated microgametes, the zygont is not mobile, and the sporozoites are typically enclosed in an oocyst. Representative genera include *Aggregata, Besnoitia, Cryptosporidium, Eimeria, Isospora, Sarcocystis, Toxoplasma,* and *Tyzzeria.*

**Ein·horn string test** (īn′hornz) [Max *Einhorn,* Russian-born American physician, 1862–1953] see under *test.*

**ein·stei·ni·um** (īn-sti′ne-əm) [Albert *Einstein,* theoretical physicist, born in Germany, became a naturalized citizen of Switzerland, then of the United States, 1879–1955; winner of the Nobel prize for physics in 1921] [MeSH: Einsteinium] the chemical element of atomic number 99, atomic weight 254, symbol Es, originally discovered in debris from a thermonuclear explosion in 1952.

**Ein·tho·ven** (īn′to-vən) Willem. Dutch physiologist, 1860–1927; winner of the Nobel prize for medicine or physiology in 1924 for his invention of a string galvanometer to produce the electrocardiogram.

**Ein·tho·ven's galvanometer, law (formula), triangle** (īn′to-vənz) [W. *Einthoven*] see under *galvanometer, law,* and *triangle.*

**eis·an·the·ma** (īs-an′thə-mə) [Gr. *eis* into + *anthein* to bloom] an eruption on a mucous membrane.

**Ei·se·nia** (i-se′ne-ə) a genus of lumbricoid worms. *E. foe′tida* is a species reportedly found in the urine of man.

**Ei·sen·men·ger's complex, syndrome** (i′sən-meng″ərz) [Victor *Eisenmenger,* German physician, 1864–1932] see under *complex* and *syndrome.*

**ei·sod·ic** (i-sod′ik) [Gr. *eis* into + *hodos* way] afferent or centripetal.

**EIT** erythrocyte iron turnover.

**ejac·u·late** (e-jak′u-lāt) 1. to expel suddenly, especially semen. 2. the semen expelled in a single ejaculation; ejaculum.

**ejac·u·la·tio** (e-jak″u-la′she-o) [L.] ejaculation.
**e. defi′ciens,** defective ejaculation.
**e. prae′cox,** premature ejaculation.
**e. retarda′ta,** male orgasmic disorder.

**ejac·u·la·tion** (e-jak″u-la′shən) [L. *ejaculatio*] [MeSH: Ejaculation] a sudden act of expulsion, as of the semen.
**premature e.,** ejaculation consistently occurring either prior to, upon, or immediately after penetration and before it is desired, taking into account factors such as age, novelty of the specific situation, and recent frequency of the sexual act. Used officially [DSM-IV], it denotes also significant resulting distress or interpersonal difficulty.
**retarded e.,** male orgasmic disorder.
**retrograde e.,** ejaculation in which semen travels up the urethra toward the bladder instead of to the outside of the body; seen with spinal cord injury, after prostatectomy or bladder neck surgery, and in other conditions.

**ejac·u·la·tor** (e-jak′u-la″tor) [L.] that which or one who ejaculates.
**e. se′minis,** musculus bulbospongiosus.

**ejac·u·la·to·ry** (e-jak′u-lə-to″re) [L. *ejaculatorius*] pertaining to ejaculation.

**ejac·u·lum** (e-jak′u-ləm) the semen discharged in a single ejaculation in the male, consisting of the secretions of Cowper's gland, epididymis, ductus deferens, seminal vesicles, and prostate, and containing the spermatozoa. Called also *ejaculate.*

**ejec·ta** (e-jek′tə) [L. "things cast out," from *eicere* to cast out] 1. feces. 2. discharge (def. 3).

**ejec·tion** (e-jek′shən) [L. *ejectus,* past participle of *ejicere* to cast out] 1. the act of casting out or the state of being cast out, as of excretions, secretions, or other bodily fluids. 2. something cast out; see *discharge* (def. 3). 3. the discharge of blood from the heart; see under *period.*
**milk e.,** let-down reflex.

**Ejusd.** abbreviation for L. *ejus′dem,* of the same.

**eka-** [Sanskrit, "one" or "first"] a prefix added to the name of a known chemical element as a provisional designation of the unknown element which should occur next in the same group in the periodic system.

**Ek·bom syndrome** (ek′bom) [Karl Axel *Ekbom,* Swedish neurologist, born 1907] [MeSH: Restless Legs] restless legs syndrome.

**EKG** electrocardiogram.

**eki·ri** (ə-ke′re) an acute cerebral and cardiovascular disorder occurring in children with shigellosis in Japan.

**Ek·man's syndrome** (ek′mahnz) [Olof Jacob *Ekman,* Swedish physician, 1764–1839] osteogenesis imperfecta (type I); see under *osteogenesis.*

**Ek·man-Lob·stein syndrome** (ek′mahn-lōb′shtīn) [O.J. *Ekman;* Johann Friedrich Georg Christian *Lobstein,* German physician, 1777–1835] osteogenesis imperfecta (type I); see under *osteogenesis.*

**EKY** electrokymogram.

**elab·o·rate** (e-lab′o-rāt) [L. *elabora′re* to work out] to produce complex substances out of simpler materials.

**elab·o·ra·tion** (e-lab″ə-ra′shən) 1. the process of producing complex substances out of simpler materials. 2. in psychiatry, an unconscious mental process of expansion and embellishment of detail, especially of a symbol or representation in a dream; called also *secondary eye.*

**el·a·cin** (el′ə-sin) degenerated elastic tissue.

**elae(o)-** see *ele(o)-.*

**El·ae·oph·ora** (el″e-of′ə-rə) a genus of filariae of the family Onchocercidae. *E. schnei′deri* is found in the arteries of deer and sheep in the western United States, sometimes causing fatal brain disease (see *elaeophoriasis*).

**elae·o·pho·ria·sis** (el″e-of″ə-ri′ə-sis) infection of the arteries and facial and ocular capillaries of deer or sheep by microfilariae of *Elaeophora schneideri*; larvae are spread from animal to animal by the bites of *Tabanus* and *Hybomitra* horseflies. If the parasites spread to the leptomeningeal arteries they may cause necrosis of brain tissue, blindness, and death. Called also *elaeophorosis, filarial dermatitis,* and *sorehead.*

**elae·o·pho·ro·sis** (el″e-of″ə-ro′sis) elaeophoriasis.

**elai(o)-** see *ele(o)-.*

**el·a·id·ate** (el″ə-id′āt) a salt, ester, or anionic form of elaidic acid.

**el·a·id·ic ac·id** (el″ə-id′ik) the *trans* isomer of oleic acid; it does not occur naturally but can be synthesized from oleic acid.

**elai·o·ma** (e-la-o′mə) eleoma.

**elai·om·e·ter** (e″la-om′ə-tər) eleometer.

**el·aio·plast** (e-la′o-plast) [Gr. *elaion* oil + *-plast*] a fat-producing plastid.

**Elant's triangle** (a-loz′) [Léon Josef Stephaan *Elant,* Belgian anatomist, 20th century.] see under *triangle.*

**el·an·trine** (el′an-trēn) an anticholinergic which has been used in the treatment of drug-induced extrapyramidal syndrome.

**el·a·pid** (el′ə-pid) 1. any snake of the family Elapidae. 2. of or pertaining to the family Elapidae.

**Elap·i·dae** (e-lap′ĭ-de) [MeSH: Elapidae] a family of usually terrestrial, venomous snakes, which have cylindrical tails and front fangs that are short, stout, immovable, and grooved. It includes the genera *Acanthophis, Bungarus, Dendroaspis, Micruroides, Micrurus, Naja, Notechis,* and *Oxyuranus.* See table at *snake.*

**Elaps** (e′laps) *Micrurus.*

**elas·mo·branch** (e-las′mo-brank) [Gr. *elasmos* plate + *branchia*] [MeSH: Elasmobranchii] 1. any cartilaginous fish having platelike gills, each gill slit opening independently on the body surface, such as sharks, skates, rays, and sawfish. See also *Chondrichthyes.* 2. of or pertaining to such fish.

**elas·tance** (e-las′təns) 1. the quality of recoiling without disruption upon removal of pressure. 2. an expression of the ability to recoil without disruption when pressure is removed, such as that of an air- or fluid-filled organ, e.g., the lung or urinary bladder, measured in terms of unit of pressure change per unit of volume change. Symbol *E.* It is the reciprocal of *compliance.*

**elas·tase** (e-las′tās) any of a group of serine endopeptidases, secreted by neutrophils, macrophages, mast cells, the pancreas, and certain bacteria, that catalyze the cleavage of elastin and other proteins, preferentially cutting polypeptide chains at bonds involving the carbonyl groups of amino acids. Elastase activity is specifically inhibited by alpha$_1$-antitrypsin. See also *leukocyte elastase* and *pancreatic elastase II.*

**elas·tic** (e-las′tik) [L. *elasticus*] 1. susceptible of resisting and recovering from stretching, compression, or distortion applied by a force. Cf. *resiliency.* 2. an elastic band, usually of rubber, used in orthodontic therapy.
**intermaxillary e.,** an elastic band used to produce traction between the upper and lower teeth in orthodontic therapy.
**intramaxillary e.,** an elastic band applied within the same dental arch to achieve space closure.
**vertical e.,** an elastic band applied in a direction perpendicular to

the occlusal plane, connecting one arch wire to the other, usually for approximating teeth to improve intercuspation.

**elas·ti·ca** (e-las'tĭ-kə) [L.] 1. a general term for elastic tissue of the body. 2. either the internal or the external elastic membrane.

**elas·ti·cin** (e-las'tĭ-sin) elastin.

**elas·tic·i·ty** (e″las-tis'ĭ-te) [MeSH: Elasticity] the quality or condition of being elastic.
**physical e. of muscle,** the physical quality of muscle of being elastic, of yielding to passive physical stretch.
**physiologic e. of muscle,** the biologic quality, unique to muscle, of being able to change and resume size under neuromuscular control.
**total e. of muscle,** the combined effect of physical and physiologic elasticity of muscle.

**elas·tin** (e-las'tin) [MeSH: Elastin] a yellow scleroprotein, the essential constituent of yellow elastic connective tissue: it is brittle when dry, but when moist is flexible and elastic.

**elast(o)-** [L. *elasticus,* from late Gr. *elastos,* beaten, ductile, from Gr. *elaunein* to beat out] a combining form denoting relationship to flexibility, to elastin, or to elastic tissue.

**elas·to·fi·bro·ma** (e-las″to-fi-bro'mə) [*elasto-* + *fibroma*] a rare, benign, firm, unencapsulated tumor consisting of abundant sclerotic collagen mixed with thick irregular elastic fibers, usually occurring in the subscapular region in older adults and believed to be a fibrous reaction to injury. Called also *e. dorsi.*

**elas·toid** (e-las'toid) a substance formed by the hyaline degeneration of the internal elastic lamina of blood vessels; seen in the vessels of the uterus after delivery.

**elas·toi·do·sis** (e-las″toi-do'sis) changes in the skin resembling elastosis.
**nodular e.,** nodular elastosis of Favre and Racouchot.

**elas·tol·y·sis** (e″las-tol'ə-sis) [*elasto-* + *-lysis*] a defect in the elastic tissue, resulting in atrophy and laxity of the skin. See *anetoderma, atrophoderma,* and *cutis laxa.*
**generalized e.,** cutis laxa.
**perifollicular e.,** see under *anetoderma.*
**postinflammatory e.,** see under *anetoderma.*

**elas·to·lyt·ic** (e-las″to-lit'ik) [*elasto-* + *-lytic*] capable of catalyzing the digestion of elastic tissue.

**elas·to·ma** (e″las-to'mə) [*elast-* + *-oma*] a tumor or focal excess of elastic tissue fibers or abnormal collagen fibers of the skin.
**juvenile e.,** connective tissue nevus.

**elas·to·mer** (e-las'to-mər) [MeSH: Rubber] a synthetic rubber; any of various soft, elastic, rubber-like polymers; used in dentistry as an impression material and for maxillofacial extraoral prostheses.

**elas·tom·e·ter** (e″las-tom'ə-tər) [*elasto-* + *-meter*] an instrument for determining the elasticity of tissues, and thus measuring the degree of edema.

**elas·tom·e·try** (e″las-tom'ə-tre) [*elasto-* + *-metry*] the measurement of elasticity.

**elas·top·a·thy** (e″las-top'ə-the) [*elasto-* + *-pathy*] deficiency of elastic tissue.

**Elas·to·plast** (e-las'to-plast) trademark for an elastic bandage.

**elas·tor·rhex·is** (e-las″to-rek'sis) [*elasto-* + *-rrhexis*] rupture of elastic fibers.

**elas·to·sis** (e″las-to'sis) 1. degeneration of elastic tissue. 2. degenerative changes in the dermal connective tissue with increased amounts of elastotic material having the staining properties of elastin. 3. any disturbance of the dermal connective tissue.
**actinic e.,** premature aging of the skin due to prolonged exposure to sunlight, occurring especially in light-skinned individuals, and chiefly characterized by inelasticity, thinning or sometimes thickening, wrinkling, dryness with fine scaling, and variable hyperpigmentation, often with development of cherry angiomas, telangiectasis, senile lentigines, ecchymosis, milia, and senile keratosis. See also *nodular e. of Favre and Racouchot.* Called also *farmers'* or *sailors' skin* and *senile* or *solar e.*
**nodular e. of Favre and Racouchot,** a type of actinic e. usually seen in elderly men, in which giant comedones, pilosebaceous cysts, and large folds of furrowed and yellowish skin are seen in the periorbital region. Called also *Favre-Racouchot syndrome* and *nodular elastoidosis.*
**e. per'forans serpigino'sa, perforating e.,** a chronic disorder of the dermal connective tissue, usually occurring in males below 30 years of age, alone or in association with more widespread disease, typically characterized by the development of a skin-colored keratopapular eruption consisting of clustered arciform serpiginous lesions that gradually form a circular or horseshoe-shaped pattern, especially on the sides and nape of the neck but sometimes also on the upper arms, face, trunk, and other areas of the body. Elongated tortuous channels in the epidermis into which abnormal elastic tissue perforates and is extruded into the dermis are the most significant histopathologic features.
**senile e.,** 1. senile atrophy of skin. 2. actinic e.
**solar e.,** actinic e.

**elas·tot·ic** (e″las-tot'ik) 1. pertaining to or characterized by elastosis. 2. resembling elastic tissue; having the staining properties of elastin.

**el·a·ter** (el'ə-tər) a specialized structure of certain plants, such as liverworts and slime molds, which aids in the distribution of spores.

**ela·tion** (e-la'shən) emotional excitement marked by speeding up of mental and bodily activity, with extreme joy and an overly optimistic attitude even in the face of negative circumstances.

**El·a·vil** (el'ə-vil) trademark for preparation of amitriptyline hydrochloride.

**el·bow** (el'bo) [L. *cubitus*] [MeSH: Elbow] 1. the joint between the distal end of the humerus and the proximal ends of the radius and ulna; called also *cubitus* [TA]. 2. any angular bend.
**baseball pitchers' e.,** a disorder of the elbow in baseball pitchers due to a piece of cartilage or bone torn from the head of the radius.
**capped e.,** a hygroma of the elbow or a hard, fibrous mass on the point of the elbow in horses or cattle; cf. *capped hock.* Called also *shoe boil.*
**dropped e.,** radial paralysis (def. 2).
**golfer's e.,** pain due to medial epicondylitis, the lesion being in the origin of the flexor muscles.
**little leaguer's e.,** medial epicondylitis of the elbow due to repeated stress on the flexor muscles of the forearm, a frequent problem of adolescent ballplayers.
**miners' e.,** enlargement of the bursa over the point of the elbow (olecranon bursitis) caused by resting the weight of the body on the elbow as in mining.
**nursemaids' e.,** pulled e.
**pulled e.,** subluxation of the head of the radius distally under the annular ligament, produced by sudden traction on the hand with the elbow extended and the forearm pronated; called also *nursemaids' e., Goyrand's injury,* and *Malgaigne's luxation.*
**tennis e.,** a painful condition localized to the outer aspect of the elbow, due to inflammation or irritation of the extensor tendon attachment to the lateral humeral condyle; called also *external humeral epicondylitis, lateral epicondylitis* and *radiohumeral bursitis* or *epicondylitis.*

**el·co·sis** (el-ko'sis) ulceration.

**El·da·dryl** (el'də-drəl) trademark for a preparation of diphenhydramine hydrochloride.

**El·de·pryl** (el'də-prəl) trademark for a preparation of selegiline hydrochloride.

**el·der** (el'dər) any tree of the genus *Sambucus.*

**El·do·dram** (el'do-dram) trademark for a preparation of dimenhydrinate.

**El·do·paque** (el'do-pāk) trademark for preparations of hydroquinone.

**El·do·quin** (el'do-kwin) trademark for a preparation of hydroquinone.

**elec·tive** (e-lek'tiv) 1. tending to combine with or act on one substance rather than another. 2. subject to the choice or decision of the patient or physician; applied to procedures that are advantageous to the patient but not urgent.

**Elec·tra com·plex** (e-lek'trə) [*Electra,* character in Greek legend who incited her brother to kill their mother and stepfather for having murdered their father] see under *complex.*

**electro-** [Gr. *ēlektron* amber, because an electric charge can be produced in amber by rubbing] a combining form denoting relationship to electricity.

**elec·tro·acu·punc·ture** (e-lek″tro-ak″u-punk'chər) [MeSH: Electroacupuncture] acupuncture in which the needles are stimulated electrically.

**elec·tro·af·fin·i·ty** (e-lek″tro-ə-fin'ĭ-te) electronegativity.

**elec·tro·an·al·ge·sia** (e-lek″tro-an″əl-je'ze-ə) the reduction of pain by electrical stimulation of a peripheral nerve or the dorsal column of the spinal cord.

**elec·tro·anal·y·sis** (e-lek″tro-ə-nal'ə-sis) chemical analysis performed by the aid of the electric current.

**elec·tro·an·es·the·sia** (e-lek″tro-an″əs-the'zhə) anesthesia, either local or general, induced by electricity.

**elec·tro·bi·ol·o·gy** (e-lek″tro-bi-ol'o-je) [*electro-* + *biology*] the study of electric phenomena in living tissue.

**elec·tro·bi·os·co·py** (e-lek″tro-bi-os'ko-pe) [*electro-* + *bio-* + *-scopy*] the determination of the presence or absence of life by means of an electric current.

**elec·tro·blot** (e-lek'tro-blot") a blot, usually a Western blot, in which transfer of solutes from gel to membrane or other substrate is effected by electrophoresis rather than capillary action.

**elec·tro·car·dio·gram** (e-lek"tro-kahr'de-o-gram") [*electro-* + *cardiogram*] a graphic tracing of the variations in electrical potential caused by the excitation of the heart muscle and detected at the body surface. The normal electrocardiogram is a scalar representation that shows deflections resulting from atrial and ventricular activity as changes in the magnitude of voltage and polarity (positive and negative) with time. The first deflection, the P wave, is due to excitation of the atria; the QRS complex of deflections, to excitation (depolarization) of the ventricles; and the T wave, to recovery of the ventricles (repolarization). Abbreviated ECG or EKG. See also *lead*[2] and see under *wave, complex,* and *interval.*
**esophageal e.,** see under *electrogram.*
**intracardiac e.,** see under *electrogram.*
**scalar e.,** see *electrocardiogram.*

**elec·tro·car·di·o·graph** (e-lek"tro-kahr'de-o-graf") an instrument for performing electrocardiography, i.e., for making electrocardiograms.

**elec·tro·car·di·og·ra·phy** (e-lek"tro-kahr"de-og'rə-fe) [*electro-* + *cardio-* + *-graphy*] [MeSH: Electrocardiography] the making of graphic records of the variations in electrical potential caused by electrical activity of the heart muscle and detected at the body surface, as a method for studying the action of the heart muscle; see also *electrocardiogram* and *electrogram.*
**intracavitary e.,** that in which electrodes are placed within the cardiac cavities.
**12-lead e.,** that performed using the twelve standard leads: the three standard bipolar limb leads, the three augmented unipolar limb leads ($aV_F$, $aV_L$, and $aV_R$), and the six standard precordial leads ($V_1$ to $V_6$).
**precordial e.,** that in which potentials over the chest wall near the surface of the heart are recorded; see *precordial leads,* under *lead*[2].

**elec·tro·ca·tal·y·sis** (e-lek"tro-kə-tal'ə-sis) the catalytic effect produced by electricity on the bodily processes.

**elec·tro·cau·ter·i·za·tion** electrocautery (def. 2).

**elec·tro·cau·tery** (e-lek"tro-kaw'tər-e) 1. an apparatus for cauterization of tissue, consisting of a holder with a metal wire that is heated to a red or white heat when the instrument is activated by an electric current. See also *electrocoagulation* 2. the cauterization of tissue using such an instrument; see also *electrocoagulation.* Called also *electrocauterization.*

**elec·tro·chem·is·try** (e-lek"tro-kem'is-tre) [MeSH: Electrochemistry] the study of relationships and transformations between chemical and electrical energy.

**elec·tro·chro·ma·tog·ra·phy** (e-lek"tro-kro"mə-tog'rə-fe) electrophoresis.

**elec·tro·co·ag·u·la·tion** (e-lek"tro-ko-ag"u-la'shən) [MeSH: Electrocoagulation] coagulation of tissue usually by means of an electrocautery with a biterminal high frequency electric current. Called also *electric coagulation.*

**elec·tro·coch·leo·gram** (e-lek"tro-kok'le-o-gram) the record obtained by electrocochleography.

**elec·tro·coch·leo·graph·ic** (e-lek"tro-kok"le-o-graf'ik) pertaining to or accomplished by electrocochleography.

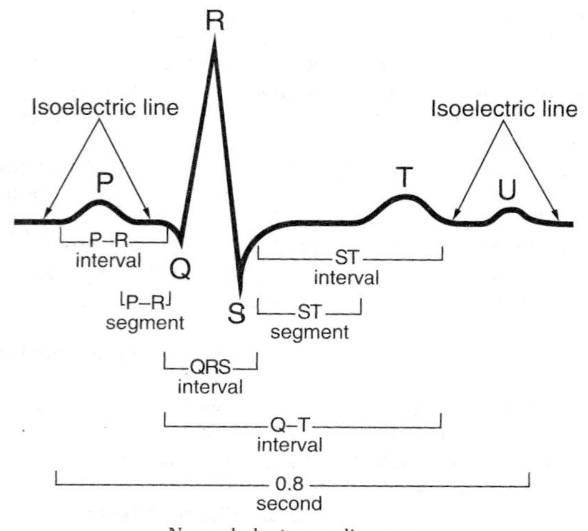

Normal electrocardiogram.

**elec·tro·coch·le·og·ra·phy** (e-lek"tro-kok"le-og'rə-fe) measurement of electrical potentials (cochlear microphonics, summating potentials, and action potentials of the eighth cranial nerve) in response to acoustic stimuli measured by an electrode in the external acoustic canal, on the tympanic membrane, or through the tympanic membrane applied to the promontory or the round window.

**elec·tro·con·trac·til·i·ty** (e-lek"tro-kon"trak-til'ĭ-te) contractility in response to electric stimulation.

**elec·tro·con·vul·sive** (e-lek"tro-kən-vul'siv) inducing convulsions by means of electric shock; see under *therapy.*

**elec·tro·cor·ti·co·gram** (e-lek"tro-kor'tĭ-ko-gram") the record obtained by electrocorticography.

**elec·tro·cor·ti·cog·ra·phy** (e-lek"tro-kor"tĭ-kog'rə-fe) electroencephalography with the electrodes applied directly to the cortex of the brain.

**elec·tro·cu·tion** (e-lek"tro-ku'shən) the taking of life by passage of electric current through the body.

**elec·tro·cys·tog·ra·phy** (e-lek"tro-sis-tog'rə-fe) the recording of changes of electric potential in the human urinary bladder.

**elec·trode** (e-lek'trōd) [*electro-* + *hodos* way] [MeSH: Electrodes] 1. a medium used between an electric conductor and the object to which the current is to be applied. 2. in electrotherapy, an instrument with a point or surface from which to transmit an electric current to the body of a patient or to another instrument. 3. in electrodiagnosis, a needle or metal plate used to stimulate or record the electrical activity of tissue; see also *lead*[2].
**active e.,** the term used in electromyography for an exploring electrode.
**bifilar needle e.,** bipolar needle e.
**bipolar needle e.,** a needle electrode consisting of two insulated wires inside a single cylinder, with neither one acting as the reference electrode; variations in voltage can be noted between the areas the wires touch.
**bipolar stimulating e.,** a stimulating electrode that has the two terminals attached together and near each other.
**calomel e.,** an electrode capable of both collecting and giving up chloride ions in neutral or acidic aqueous media, consisting of mercury in contact with mercurous chloride; used as a reference electrode in pH measurements.
**coaxial needle e.,** concentric needle e.
**concentric needle e.,** a recording electrode consisting of an insulated metal wire inside a hollow stainless steel cannula; differences in potential are measured using the needle shaft as reference and the wire tip as the exploring electrode.
**earth e.,** ground e.
**esophageal e., esophageal pill e.,** a pill electrode designed to lodge in the esophagus at the level of the atrium; it is used for obtaining esophageal electrograms and for delivering pacing stimuli.
**exploring e.,** in electrodiagnosis, the electrode, usually small, placed nearest to the site of the bioelectric activity being recorded; it determines the potential in only that localized area.
**ground e.,** an electrode that is connected to a ground; called also *earth e.*
**indifferent e.,** reference e.
**monopolar needle e.,** a needle electrode consisting of a single piece of stainless steel wire coated with insulating material except at the tip; it must be accompanied by another electrode as a reference.
**monopolar stimulating e.,** a stimulating electrode that has the two terminals attached separately and relatively far apart.
**multilead e.,** an electrode composed of a number of insulated wires inside a metal cannula, with their bare tips at apertures flush with the outer circumference of the cannula; used to determine the territory of a motor unit. Called also *multielectrode.*
**needle e.,** a thin, cylindrical electrode with an outer shaft beveled to a sharp point, enclosing a wire or series of wires that can explore the activity of single motor or nerve units or stimulate them.
**patch e.,** a tiny electrode with a blunt tip, used in studies of membrane potentials. See also *patch clamp* and *microelectrode.*
**pill e.,** an electrode usually enclosed within a gelatin capsule and attached to a flexible slender wire so that it may be swallowed, such as an esophageal electrode.
**recording e.,** an electrode used to measure electric potential change in body tissue; for recording, two electrodes must be used, the *exploring e.* and the *reference e.* (qq.v.).
**reference e.,** an electrode whose placement is remote from the source of recorded activity, so that it is presumed to be at either a negligible or constant potential.
**scalp e.,** an electrode placed on or just below the surface of the scalp; the most common type used in electroencephalography.
**single fiber needle e.,** a needle electrode with a small recording surface for the recording of individual muscle fiber action potentials. See also *single fiber electromyography.*
**stimulating e.,** an electrode used to apply electric current to tissue;

it must include both a negative terminal and a positive terminal. See also *bipolar stimulating e.* and *monopolar stimulating e.*
**surface e.,** one placed on the skin surface and used to stimulate or record electrical activity in the underlying tissue.

**elec·tro·der·mal** (e-lek″tro-dər′məl) pertaining to the electrical properties of the skin, especially to changes in its resistance.

**elec·tro·der·ma·tome** (e-lek″tro-dər′mə-tōm) an electrical dermatome for cutting off even layers of large areas of skin in a short time; used in skin grafting, shaving scars, etc.

**elec·tro·des·ic·ca·tion** (e-lek″tro-des″ĭ-ka′shən) dehydration of tissue by the use of a high frequency electric current; see *fulguration.*

**elec·tro·di·ag·no·sis** (e-lek″tro-di″əg-no′sis) [MeSH: Electrodiagnosis] the use of electrical devices in the diagnosis of pathologic conditions.

**elec·tro·di·ag·nos·tics** (e-lek″tro-di″əg-nos′tiks) the science and practice of electrodiagnosis.

**elec·tro·di·al·y·sis** (e-lek″tro-di-al′ə-sis) dialysis occurring under the influence of an electric field.

**elec·tro·di·a·ly·zer** (e-lek″tro-di″ə-li′zər) a hemodialyzer that uses an applied electric field and semipermeable membranes for separating the colloids from the solution.

**elec·tro·di·aph·a·ke** (e-lek″tro-di-af′ə-ke) [*electro-* + *dia-* + Gr. *phakos* lentil] an instrument for removing the lens by diathermy.

**elec·tro·di·a·phane** (e-lek″tro-di′ə-fān) [*electro-* + *diaphane*] diaphanoscope.

**elec·tro·di·aph·a·no·scope** (e-lek″tro-di-af′ə-no-skōp″) diaphanoscope.

**elec·tro·di·aph·a·nos·co·py** (e-lek″tro-di-af″ə-nos′kə-pe) diaphanoscopy.

**elec·tro·ejac·u·la·tion** (e-lek″tro-e-jak″u-la′shən) induction of ejaculation by application of a gradually increasing electrical current delivered through a probe inserted into the rectum; used in animal husbandry and for collection of sperm for insemination from men with spinal cord injuries and other conditions that prevent ejaculation.

**elec·tro·en·ceph·a·lo·gram (EEG)** (e-lek″tro-en-sef′ə-lo-gram″) a recording of the potentials on the skull generated by currents emanating spontaneously from nerve cells in the brain. The dominant frequency of these potentials is about 8 to 10 cycles per second and the amplitude about 10 to 100 microvolts. Fluctuations in potential are seen in the form of waves, which correlate well with different neurologic conditions and so are used as diagnostic criteria. See also *brain waves,* under *wave.*
**flat e., isoelectric e.,** one in which no brain waves are recorded, indicating a complete lack of brain activity.

**elec·tro·en·ceph·a·lo·graph** (e-lek″tro-ən-sef′ə-lo-graf″) an instrument for performing electroencephalography.

**elec·tro·en·ceph·a·log·ra·phy** (e-lek″tro-ən-sef′ə-log′rə-fe) [MeSH: Electroencephalography] the recording of the electric currents developed in the brain, by means of electrodes applied to the scalp, to the surface of the brain *(intracranial e.),* or placed within the substance of the brain *(depth e.).* See *electroencephalogram.*

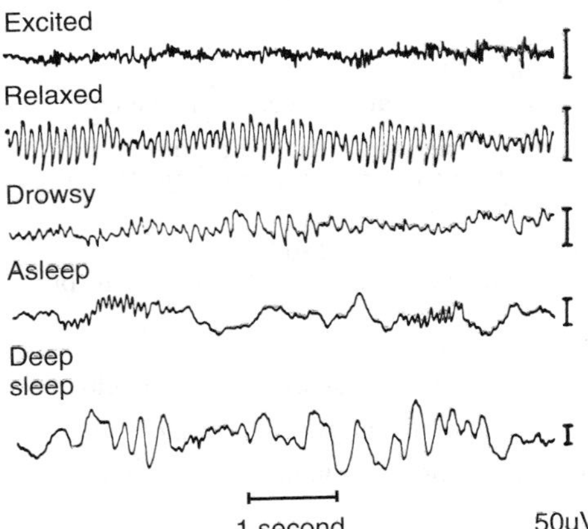


Electroencephalogram. Recordings made while the subject was excited, relaxed, and in various stages of sleep. During excitement the brain waves are rapid and of small amplitude, whereas in sleep they are much slower and of greater amplitude.

**elec·tro·en·ceph·a·lo·scope** (e-lek″tro-ən-sef′ə-lo-skōp) an instrument for detecting brain potentials at many different sections of the brain and displaying them on a cathode-ray tube.

**elec·tro·en·dos·mo·sis** (e-lek″tro-en″dos-mo′sis) 1. endosmosis under the influence of an electric field. 2. electro-osmosis.

**elec·tro·ex·ci·sion** (e-lek″tro-ek-sĭ′zhən) excision performed by electrosurgical means.

**elec·tro·fo·cus·ing** (e-lek″tro-fo′kəs-ing) isoelectric focusing.

**elec·tro·gas·tro·gram** (e-lek″tro-gas′tro-gram) the graphic record obtained by electrogastrography.

**elec·tro·gas·tro·graph** (e-lek″tro-gas′tro-graf) an instrument for recording the electrical activity of the stomach by means of swallowed gastric electrodes.

**elec·tro·gas·trog·ra·phy** (e-lek″tro-gas-trog′rə-fe) the recording of the electrical activity of the stomach as measured between its lumen and the surface of the body.

**elec·tro·gen·ic** (e-lek″tro-jen′ik) [*electro-* + *-genic*] pertaining to a process by which net charge is transferred to a different location so that hyperpolarization is set up, as in the pumping of ions across a membrane. See also under *pump.*

**elec·tro·go·ni·om·e·ter** (e-lek″tro-go″ne-om′ə-tər) an electrical goniometer.

**elec·tro·gram** (e-lek′tro-gram) [*electro-* + *-gram*] any record produced by changes in electric potential, such as an electrocardiogram or electroencephalogram.
**atrial e.,** see *intra-atrial e.* and *high right atrial e.*
**coronary sinus (CS) e.,** an intracardiac electrogram that records electrical potentials within the coronary sinus; it is used for indirect monitoring of left atrial and left ventricular sites.
**esophageal e.,** one recorded by an esophageal electrode; it is used for enhanced detection of P waves and elucidation of complex arrhythmias.
**high right atrial (HRA) e.,** an intracardiac electrogram that records electrical potentials within the upper region of the right atrium, obtained by introduction of electrodes high in the atrium near the sinus node; used in localizing conduction blocks and diagnosing arrhythmias. See also illustration.
**His bundle e. (HBE),** an intracardiac electrogram of potentials in the lower right atrium, atrioventricular node, and His-Purkinje system, obtained by positioning intracardiac electrodes near the tricuspid valve; it is used to pinpoint the site, extent, and mechanisms of arrhythmias and conduction defects. See also illustration.
**intra-atrial e.,** an intracardiac electrogram of potentials within the atrium; used particularly for monitoring P waves.
**intracardiac e.,** a record of changes in the electric potentials of specific cardiac loci as measured by electrodes placed within the heart via cardiac catheters; it is used for loci that cannot be assessed by body surface electrodes, such as the bundle of His or other regions within the cardiac conducting system. See also illustration.
**right ventricular e.,** an intracardiac electrogram obtained by placing electrodes in the right ventricle; used to assess ventricular activity and response to stimuli.
**right ventricular apical e.,** an intracardiac electrogram obtained by placing electrodes in the apex of the right ventricle; it is used in mapping ventricular arrhythmias.
**sinus node e.,** an intracardiac electrogram obtained by placing electrodes near the sinus node; it is used in examining the time for impulse conduction from the node to the atrium.

**elec·tro·graph** (e-lek′tro-graf) electrogram.

**elec·trog·ra·phy** (e″lek-trog′rə-fe) [*electro-* + *-graphy*] the graphic recording of changes in electric potential, as in electrocardiography, electroencephalography, etc.

**elec·tro·gus·tom·e·try** (e-lek″tro-gəs-tom′ə-tre) the testing of the sense of taste by application of galvanic stimuli to the tongue.

**elec·tro·he·mos·ta·sis** (e-lek″tro-he-mos′tə-sis) [*electro-* + *hemostasis*] the arrest of hemorrhage by the application of a high frequency current to coagulate the bleeding point or surface.

**elec·tro·hys·tero·gram** (e-lek″tro-his′tər-o-gram) the graphic record obtained by electrohysterography.

**elec·tro·hys·ter·og·ra·phy** (e-lek″tro-his″tər-og′rə-fe) the recording of the changes in electric potential associated with contractions of the uterine muscle.

**elec·tro·im·mu·no·dif·fu·sion** (e-lek″tro-im″u-no-dif-u′zhən) the combination of immunodiffusion with electrophoresis, using an applied electric field to speed up the migration of antigen and antibody. Two such techniques have achieved widespread use: *counterimmunoelectrophoresis* (one-dimensional double electroimmunodiffusion) and *Laurell's rocket immunoelectrophoresis* (one-dimensional single electroimmunodiffusion).

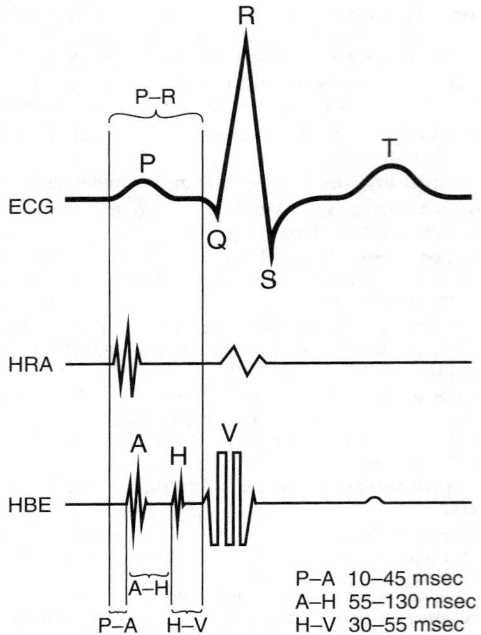


Intracardiac electrograms. Schematic illustrations of several intracardiac electrograms contrasted with a conventional body-surface electrocardiogram (ECG). HRA = high right atrial electrogram; HBE = His bundle electrogram, in which A = low right atrial activity, H = His bundle activity, and V = ventricular septal activity; also shown are the P–R, P–A, A–H, and H–V intervals.

**elec·tro·ky·mo·gram** (e-lek″tro-ki′mo-gram) the graphic record produced by electrokymography; abbreviated EKY.

**elec·tro·ky·mo·graph** (e-lek″tro-ki′mo-graf) an instrument for graphically recording motion of or changes in density of organs by recording variations in intensity of a small beam of x-rays; it consists of three essential parts—a fluoroscope, a pick-up unit, and a recording instrument; used especially for showing motion of the cardiac silhouette.

**elec·tro·ky·mog·ra·phy** (e-lek″tro-ki-mog′rə-fe) [MeSH: Electrokymography] the photography on x-ray film of the motion of the heart or of other moving structures which can be visualized radiologically. See *electrokymograph.*

**elec·tro·lar·ynx** (e-lek″tro-lar′inks) artificial larynx.

**elec·tro·li·thot·ri·ty** (e-lek″tro-lĭ-thot′rĭ-te) the disintegration of calculi by the application of electric current.

**elec·trol·y·sis** (e″lek-trol′ə-sis) [*electro-* + *-lysis*] [MeSH: Electrolysis] destruction by passage of a galvanic electric current, as in disintegration of a chemical compound in solution or removal of excessive hair from the body.

**elec·tro·lyte** (e-lek′tro-līt) [*electro-* + Gr. *lytos* that may be dissolved] a substance that dissociates into ions when fused or in solution, and thus becomes capable of conducting electricity; an ionic solute.
**amphoteric e.,** a compound containing at least one group that can act as a base and at least one that can act as an acid; called also *ampholyte.*
**colloidal e.,** an electrolyte in which one or more of the ionic components is of macromolecular dimensions.

**elec·tro·lyt·ic** (e-lek″tro-lit′ik) pertaining to or characterized by electrolysis.

**elec·tro·lyz·a·ble** (e-lek″tro-līz′ə-bəl) susceptible of being decomposed by electric current.

**elec·tro·mag·net** (e-lek″tro-mag′nət) a temporary magnet made by passing an electric current through a coil of wire surrounding a core of soft iron.

**elec·tro·mag·net·ic** (e-lek″tro-mag-net′ik) [MeSH: Electromagnetics] involving both electricity and magnetism.

**elec·tro·mag·net·ism** (e-lek″tro-mag′nə-tiz-əm) 1. magnetism produced by an electric current. 2. the branch of physics relating electricity and magnetism.

**elec·tro·ma·nom·e·ter** (e-lek″tro-man-om′ə-tər) an electronic instrument for measuring the pressure of gases or liquids.

**elec·trom·e·ter** (e″lek-trom′ə-tər) [*electro-* + *-meter*] an electrostatic instrument for measuring the difference in potential between two points. In radiology, it is used to measure changes in the potential of charged electrodes due to ionization occasioned by radiation.

**elec·tro·met·ro·gram** (e-lek″tro-met′ro-gram) [*electro-* + *metro-* + *-gram*] an apparatus for recording changes in electric potential associated with contraction of the uterine muscle.

**elec·tro·mi·gra·to·ry** (e-lek″tro-mi′grə-tor″e) moving under the influence of electric current.

**elec·tro·mo·tive** (e-lek″tro-mo′tiv) causing electric activity to be propagated along a conductor.

**elec·tro·myo·gram** (e-lek″tro-mi′o-gram) the record obtained by electromyography.

**elec·tro·myo·graph** (e-lek″tro-mi′o-graf) the instrument used in electromyography.

**elec·tro·my·og·ra·phy (EMG)** (e-lek″tro-mi-og′rə-fe) [*electro-* + *myography*] [MeSH: Electromyography] an electrodiagnostic tech-

**Types of Multiple Electrolytes Injection**

| Preparation | Ingredients |
|---|---|
| Multiple Electrolytes Injection Type 1 | Sodium, potassium, magnesium, chloride<br>May also contain acetate, acetate and gluconate, or acetate, gluconate, and phosphate |
| Multiple Electrolytes Injection Type 2 | Sodium, potassium, magnesium, chloride<br>May also contain either acetate and citrate or acetate and lactate |
| Multiple Electrolytes and Dextrose Injection Type 1 | Dextrose, sodium, potassium, magnesium, calcium, chloride<br>May also contain acetate, acetate and gluconate, acetate and phosphate, phosphate and lactate, or phosphate and sulfate |
| Multiple Electrolytes and Dextrose Injection Type 2 | Dextrose, sodium, potassium, magnesium, chloride<br>May also contain acetate, acetate and citrate, acetate and lactate, or gluconate and sulfate |
| Multiple Electrolytes and Dextrose Injection Type 3 | Dextrose, sodium, potassium, chloride<br>May also contain ammonium, acetate and phosphate, or phosphate and lactate |
| Multiple Electrolytes and Dextrose Injection Type 4 | Dextrose, sodium, magnesium, calcium, chloride, gluconate, sulfate |
| Multiple Electrolytes and Invert Sugar Injection Type 1 | Equal amounts of dextrose and sucrose*, sodium, potassium, magnesium, chloride, phosphate, lactate |
| Multiple Electrolytes and Invert Sugar Injection Type 2 | Equal amounts of dextrose and sucrose*, sodium, potassium, magnesium, calcium, chloride, lactate |
| Multiple Electrolytes and Invert Sugar Injection Type 3 | Equal amonts of dextrose and sucrose*, sodium, potassium, chloride, ammonium |

* Or an equivalent solution produced by hydrolysis of sucrose.

nique for recording the extracellular activity (action potentials and evoked potentials) of skeletal muscles at rest, during voluntary contractions, and during electrical stimulation; performed using any of a variety of surface electrodes, needle electrodes, and devices for amplifying, transmitting, and recording the signals.
**single fiber e. (SFEMG),** electromyography using a needle electrode to record the action potential of one muscle fiber at a time.
**ureteral e.,** recording of the action potentials produced by peristalsis of the ureter.

**elec·tron** (e-lek'tron) [Gr. *ēlektron* amber, because an electric charge can be produced in amber by rubbing] [MeSH: Electrons] an elementary particle possessing the unit quantum of (negative) electric charge, $1.6 \times 10^{-19}$ coulomb, with mass 1/1836 that of a proton, or $9.11 \times 10^{-31}$ kilogram. Electrons can exist as atomic constituents or in the free state; flowing in a conductor they constitute an electric current; when ejected from a radioactive substance, they constitute beta rays; and when revolving about the nucleus of an atom they determine all of its physical and chemical properties except mass and radioactivity. Symbol e or $e^-$. See also *atom.*
**Auger e.,** a low-energy electron emitted when an inner electron shell vacancy is created, such as by electron capture or internal conversion.
**emission e.,** one of the electrons released from the atom during radioactive decay.
**free e.,** an electron which is not bound to the nucleus of an atom but may move from one atom nucleus to another.
**valence e.,** one of the electrons in the outermost shell of an atom and thus able to participate in chemical reactions and the formation of chemical bonds.

**elec·tro·nar·co·sis** (e-lek"tro-nahr-ko'sis) [MeSH: Electronarcosis] a treatment for psychiatric disorders using passage of an electric current through the brain via scalp electrodes, conditions being such as to produce a tonic phase similar to that of electroconvulsive therapy but limited or absent convulsions; it is both less effective and more likely to cause side effects than is electroconvulsive therapy.

**elec·tron-dense** (e-lek'tron-dens") in electron microscopy, having a density that prevents electrons from penetrating.

**elec·tro·neg·a·tive** (e-lek"tro-neg'ə-tiv) bearing a negative electric charge.

**elec·tro·neg·a·tiv·i·ty** (e-lek"tro-neg"ə-tiv'ĭ-te) the relative power of an atom or molecule to attract electrons.

**elec·tro·neu·rog·ra·phy** (e-lek"tro-noo-rog'rə-fe) the measurement of the conduction velocity and latency of peripheral nerves.

**elec·tro·neu·rol·y·sis** (ə-lek"tro-noo-rol'ə-sis) [*electro-* + *neuro-* + *-lysis*] destruction of nerve tissue with an electric needle or electric current.

**elec·tro·neu·ro·my·og·ra·phy** (e-lek"tro-noo"ro-mi-og'rə-fe) electromyography in which the nerve of the muscle under study is stimulated by application of an electric current.

**elec·tron·ic** (e"lek-tron'ik) [MeSH: Electronics] pertaining to or carrying electrons.

**elec·tron·ics** (e"lek-tron'iks) [MeSH: Electronics] the science which treats of the conduction of electricity through gases, solids, or a vacuum.

**elec·tron-mi·cro·scop·ic** (e-lek'tron-mi-kro-skop'ik) visible under the electron microscope.

**elec·tron-mi·cro·scop·i·cal** (e-lek'tron-mi"kro-skop'ĭ-kəl) observable with the aid of an electron microscope; of such size as to be so observed.

**elec·trono·graph** (e"lek-tron'o-graf) electron micrograph.

**elec·tron trans·fer fla·vo·pro·tein:ubiq·ui·none ox·i·do·re·duc·tase** (e-lek'tron trans'fər fla"vo-pro'tēn u-bik'wə-nōn ok"sĭ-do-re-duk'tās) a component of a side chain of redox reactions by which certain electrons are funneled to ubiquinone and hence to the electron transport chain; the oxidoreductase catalyzes the transfer of electrons from electron transfer flavoprotein (q.v.) to ubiquinone via its FAD prosthetic group and iron-sulfur center. Deficiency of the oxidoreductase, an autosomal recessive trait, causes glutaricaciduria, type II.

**elec·tro·nys·tag·mo·gram** (e-lek"tro-nis-tag'mo-gram) the record obtained by electronystagmography.

**elec·tro·nys·tag·mo·graph** (e-lek"tro-nis-tag'mo-graf) an instrument for recording eye movements induced by electrical stimulation; abbreviated ENG.

**elec·tro·nys·tag·mog·ra·phy** (e-lek"tro-nis"tag-mog'rə-fe) [MeSH: Electronystagmography] the recording of changes in the corneoretinal potential due to eye movements, providing objective documentation of induced and spontaneous nystagmus.

**elec·tro·oc·u·lo·gram** (e-lek"tro-ok'u-lo-gram") the electroencephalographic tracings made by moving the eyes a constant distance between two fixation points, inducing a deflection of fairly constant amplitude; abbreviated EOG.

**elec·tro·oc·u·log·ra·phy** (e-lek"tro-ok"u-log'rə-fe) the production and interpretation of electro-oculograms.

**elec·tro·ol·fac·to·gram** (e-lek"tro-ol-fak'to-gram) a recording of electrical potential changes detected by an electrode placed on the surface of the olfactory mucosa as the mucosa is subjected to an odorous stimulus. Abbreviated EOG.

**elec·tro·os·mo·sis** (e-lek"tro-os-mo'sis) the movement through a membrane of the solvent phase of a colloidal solution when an electric potential is applied by electrodes positioned on either side of the membrane; see also *iontophoresis.*

**elec·tro·para·cen·te·sis** (e-lek"tro-par"ə-sən-te'sis) puncture of the eyeball with a needle, using galvanic current and holding the needle in position until bubbles of hydrogen appear in the aqueous humor.

**elec·tro·pa·thol·o·gy** (e-lek"tro-pə-thol'o-je) [*electro-* + *pathology*] the study of pathologic conditions of the body as revealed by electricity.

**elec·tro·phero·gram** (e-lek"tro-fer'o-gram) electrophoretogram.

**elec·tro·phile** (e-lek'tro-fīl) an electron acceptor that is covalently bonded to a nucleophile.

**elec·tro·phil·ic** (e-lek"tro-fil'ik) having an affinity for electrons; serving as an electrophile.

**elec·tro·pho·re·gram** (e-lek"tro-fo'rə-gram) electrophoretogram.

**elec·tro·pho·re·sis** (e-lek"tro-fə-re'sis) [*electro-* + *phoresis*] [MeSH: Electrophoresis] the separation of ionic solutes based on differences in their rates of migration in an applied electric field.
**agarose gel e.,** a type of gel electrophoresis with agarose as the support medium; used extensively to separate proteins, lipoproteins, nucleic acids, and other substances.
**cellulose acetate e.,** a method of zone electrophoresis in which the support medium is a sheet of cellulose acetate; used mainly in clinical chemistry to analyze or purify serum proteins.
**counter e.,** counterimmunoelectrophoresis.
**disc e.,** a method of polyacrylamide gel electrophoresis involving discontinuous (hence the name) gel layers. A discontinuity in pore size and pH between the layers is used to prevent diffusion and maximize separation of the components.
**gel e.,** a type of zone electrophoresis in which the support medium is a gel, in the form of tubes or a thin slab; it is usually composed of agarose, polyacrylamide, or starch and is so named. Specific types are used to separate certain classes of molecules on the basis of change, size, or both.
**moving boundary e.,** the original method of electrophoresis, in which the movement of the solvent is unrestricted and all of the particles of a species move at the same rate, maintaining a sharp boundary which can be optically monitored.
**paper e.,** an older method of zone electrophoresis in which the support medium is paper, mainly used to separate serum proteins.
**polyacrylamide gel e. (PAGE),** gel electrophoresis using a polymerized polyacrylamide matrix to separate molecules on the basis of size, charge, or both; usually used to separate proteins or sequence nucleic acids. Gels are usually discontinuous (see *disc e.*) but may be a single layer, and are either nondenaturing to examine native molecules or denaturing as in SDS-PAGE.
**pulsed-field e.,** a method of gel electrophoresis used to separate fragments of DNA as long as several million bases by subjecting the gel to an electrical current alternately delivered from two angles in timed intervals, which minimizes diffusion of large molecules.
**SDS–polyacrylamide gel e. (SDS-PAGE),** a type of polyacrylamide gel electrophoresis in which the anionic detergent sodium dodecyl sulfate (SDS) is used to denature the sample proteins into linear monomers, rendering their charge proportional to their length so that migration is a function of size.
**starch gel e.,** an older form of gel electrophoresis using a hydrolyzed starch support matrix to separate macromolecules, particularly proteins.
**two-dimensional gel e.,** a method for improved separation of complex mixtures of molecules by subjecting the support medium to electrophoresis in two directions, usually at right angles to each other; e.g., isoelectric focusing followed by SDS–polyacrylamide gel electrophoresis.
**zone e.,** any of several methods of electrophoresis in which an inert support medium holds the molecules as they migrate in the conducting medium, thus preventing convection and diffusion.

**elec·tro·pho·ret·ic** (e-lek"tro-fə-ret'ik) pertaining to electrophoresis.

**elec·tro·pho·reto·gram** (e-lek"tro-fə-ret'o-gram) the record produced on or in a supporting medium by bands of material which have been separated by the process of electrophoresis. Called also *electropherogram* and *electrophoregram.*

**elec·troph·o·rus** (e″lek-trof′o-rəs) [*electro-* + Gr. *phoros* bearing] [MeSH: Electrophorus] an instrument for obtaining static electricity by means of induction.

**elec·tro·pho·tom·e·ter** (e-lek″tro-fo-tom′ə-tər) an instrument equipped with a photoelectric sensor for colorimetric determinations.

**elec·tro·phren·ic** (e-lek″tro-fren′ik) pertaining to electrical stimulation of the phrenic nerve or diaphragm; see under *respiration.*

**elec·tro·phys·i·o·log·ic** (e-lek″tro-fis″ĭ-o-loj′ik) pertaining to electrophysiology.

**elec·tro·phys·i·ol·o·gy** (e-lek″tro-fiz″e-ol′ə-je) [MeSH: Electrophysiology] 1. the study of the mechanisms of production of electrical phenomena, particularly in the nervous system and their consequences in the living organism. 2. the study of the effects electricity has on physiologic phenomena.
**cardiac e., clinical cardiac e.,** the mechanisms, functions, and performance of the electrical activities of specific regions of the heart; the term is usually used in describing studies of such phenomena by invasive (intracardiac) recording of spontaneous activity as well as of cardiac responses to programmed stimuli. The studies are performed to assess complex arrhythmias, elucidate symptoms, evaluate abnormal electrocardiograms, assess risk, and design treatment; they increasingly include therapeutic methods in addition to diagnostic and prognostic procedures.

**elec·tro·plat·ing** (e-lek″tro-plāt′ing) [MeSH: Electroplating] plating or coating of an object with a layer of metal through the use of electrolytic processes. See also *electroplated die,* under *die.*

**elec·tro·plexy** (e-lek′tro-plek″se) [*electro-* + *-plexy*] electric shock.

**elec·tro·po·ra·tion** (e-lek″tro-pə-ra′shən) [MeSH: Electroporation] the application of an electric field to cause a reversible creation of pore-like openings in the plasma membrane of a cell, through which nucleic acids may be introduced.

**elec·tro·pos·i·tive** (e-lek″tro-poz′ĭ-tiv) [*electro-* + *positive*] bearing a positive electric charge.

**elec·tro·ra·di·om·e·ter** (e-lek″tro-ra″de-om′ə-tər) an electroscope for measuring radiant energy.

**elec·tro·re·sec·tion** (e-lek″tro-re-sek′shən) excision by electrosurgical means.

**elec·tro·ret·i·no·gram** (e-lek″tro-ret′ĭ-no-gram) the record obtained by electroretinography; abbreviated ERG.

**elec·tro·ret·in·o·graph** (e-lek″tro-ret′ĭ-no-graf) an instrument for measuring the electrical response of the retina to light stimulation; abbreviated ERG.

**elec·tro·ret·i·nog·ra·phy** (e-lek″tro-ret″ĭ-nog′rə-fe) [MeSH: Electroretinography] the recording of the changes in electric potential in the retina after stimulation by light.

**elec·tro·sa·li·vo·gram** (e-lek″tro-sə-li′vo-gram) [*electro-* + *saliva* + *-gram*] a graphic record or curve showing the action potential of the salivary glands, obtained with an electrically operated instrument.

**elec·tro·scis·sion** (e-lek″tro-sizh′ən) cutting tissue by use of the electrocautery.

**elec·tro·scope** (e-lek′tro-skōp) [*electro-* + *-scope*] an instrument for measuring the intensity of radiation by detecting the motion imparted to charged strips suspended from a conductor.

**elec·tro·sec·tion** (e-lek″tro-sek′shən) an incision made by electrosurgical means.

**elec·tro·se·le·ni·um** (e-lek″tro-sə-le′ne-əm) a form of colloidal selenium.

**elec·tro·shock** (e-lek′tro-shok) [MeSH: Electroshock] shock produced by application of electric current to the brain; see *electroconvulsive therapy,* under *therapy.*

**elec·tro·sleep** (e-lek′tro-slēp) the use of low-intensity electricity, below the threshold for inducing convulsions, in the treatment of insomnia, anxiety, or depression.

**elec·tro·sol** (e-lek′tro-sol) a colloidal solution of a metal obtained by passing electric sparks through distilled water between poles formed of the metal.

**elec·tro·spec·tro·gram** (e-lek″tro-spek′trə-gram) a record produced in electrospectrography.

**elec·tro·spec·trog·ra·phy** (e-lek″tro-spek-trog′rə-fe) the isolation and recording of the constituent wave systems that are merged in an electroencephalogram.

**elec·tro·spi·no·gram** (e-lek″tro-spi′no-gram) a tracing of the action potential of the spinal cord.

**elec·tro·stat·ic** (e-lek″tro-stat′ik) pertaining to static electricity.

**elec·tro·ste·nol·y·sis** (e-lek″tro-stə-nol′ə-sis) the oxidation and reduction which occur on opposite surfaces of a high resistance membrane in a solution when there is a steep electric potential gradient across the membrane, reduction occurring on the surface facing the anode.

**elec·tro·stim·u·la·tion** (e-lek″tro-stim″u-la′shən) electrical stimulation of tissues, as for therapeutic or experimental purposes.

**elec·tro·stri·a·to·gram** (e-lek″tro-stri-āt′o-gram) a record of waves derived by the bipolar technique from the several structures of the corpus striatum.

**elec·tro·sur·gery** (e-lek″tro-sər′jər-e) [MeSH: Electrosurgery] surgery performed by electrical methods.

**elec·tro·syn·the·sis** (e-lek″tro-sin′thə-sis) chemical reactions effected by means of electricity.

**elec·tro·tax·is** (e-lek″tro-tak′sis) [*electro-* + *-taxis*] the movement of organisms or cells under the influence of electric currents.

**elec·tro·tha·na·sia** (e-lek″tro-thə-na′zhə) [*electro-* + Gr. *thanatos* death] death by electricity; electrocution.

**elec·tro·ther·a·pist** (e-lek″tro-ther′ə-pist) a person trained in using electricity for therapeutic purposes.

**elec·tro·ther·a·py** (e-lek″tro-ther′ə-pe) treatment of disease by means of electricity.
**cerebral e.,** electrosleep.

**elec·tro·therm** (e-lek′tro-thərm) [*electro-* + *therm*] an electrosurgical appliance used for cutting.

**elec·tro·tome** (e-lek′tro-tōm) [*electro-* + *-tome*] an electric surgical cutting instrument.

**elec·trot·o·my** (e-lek-trot′ə-me) electroexcision with low current, high voltage, and high frequency; a procedure in which the tissues are not coagulated.

**elec·tro·ton·ic** (e-lek″tro-ton′ik) 1. pertaining to electrotonus. 2. denoting the direct spread of current in tissues by electrical conduction, without the generation of new current by action potentials.

**elec·trot·o·nus** (e-lek-trot′ə-nəs) the altered electrical state of a nerve or muscle cell when a constant electric current is passed through it.

**elec·trot·ro·pism** (e″lek-trot′ro-piz-əm) [*electro-* + *tropism*] the tendency of a cell or organism to react in a definite manner in response to an electric stimulus.
**negative e.,** the tendency of a cell to be repelled by an electric stimulus.
**positive e.,** the tendency of a cell to be attracted by an electric stimulus.

**elec·tro·ul·tra·fil·tra·tion** (e-lek″tro-ul″trə-fil-tra′shən) ultrafiltration in an electric field.

**elec·tro·ure·tero·gram** (e-lek″tro-u-re′tər-o-gram) the record obtained by electroureterography.

**elec·tro·u·re·ter·og·ra·phy** (e-lek″tro-u-re″tər-og′rə-fe) electromyography in which the action potentials produced by peristalsis of the ureter are recorded.

**elec·tro·va·go·gram** (e-lek″tro-va′go-gram) vagogram.

**elec·tro·va·lence** (e-lek″tro-va′ləns) 1. the number of charges an atom acquires by the gain or loss of electrons in forming an ionic bond. 2. the ionic bonding resulting from such a transfer of electrons.

**elec·tro·va·lent** (e-lek″tro-va′lənt) pertaining to electrovalence or to an electrovalent (ionic) bond.

**elec·tro·ver·sion** (e-lek″tro-vər′zhən) the act of electrically terminating a cardiac dysrhythmia.

**elec·tro·vert** (e-lek′tro-vərt) to apply electricity to the heart or precordium to depolarize the heart and terminate a cardiac dysrhythmia.

**elec·tu·a·ry** (e-lek′tu-ar-e) [L. *electuarium,* from *e* out + *legere* to select] a medicinal preparation consisting of a powdered drug made into a paste with honey or syrup; a confection. Called also *lincture* and *linctus.*
**e. of senna,** a mixture of senna, syrup, and tamarind pulp.

**el·e·doi·sin** (el-ə-doi′sin) [MeSH: Eledoisin] an endecapeptide from the posterior salivary gland of a species of small octopus *(Eledone),* which is a precursor of a large group of biologically active peptides. It has vasodilator, hypotensive, and extravascular smooth muscle stimulant properties.

**el·e·i·din** (el-e′ĭ-din) a protein chemically related to keratin, found in the cells of the stratum lucidum of the skin.

**el·e·ment** (el′ə-mənt) [L. *elementum*] 1. any of the primary parts

or constituents of a thing. 2. in chemistry, a simple substance which cannot be decomposed by chemical means and which is made up of atoms which are alike in their peripheral electronic configurations and so in their chemical properties, and also in the number of protons in their nuclei, but which may differ in the number of neutrons in their nuclei and so in their atomic weight and in their radioactive properties. See accompanying table.
**anatomic e.,** morphologic e.
**appendicular e's,** a set of cartilaginous rods attached to the chondral skull of the embryo; from them are developed the auditory ossicles, the hyoid, and the styloid process.
**electronegative e.,** any chemical element that adds electrons (or tends to add electrons) during chemical combination.
**electropositive e.,** a chemical element that loses electrons (or tends to lose electrons) during chemical combination.
**F e.,** see under *plasmid.*
**formed e's of the blood,** the blood cells; see under *cell.*
**labile e.,** tissue cells which continue to multiply during the life of the individual.
**morphologic e.,** any cell, fiber, or other of the ultimate structures which go to make up tissues and organs.
**radioactive e.,** a chemical element which spontaneously transmutes

**Table of Elements**

| Name* | Symbol | At. No. | At. Wt.† | Name* | Symbol | At. No. | At. Wt.† |
|---|---|---|---|---|---|---|---|
| Actinium | Ac | 89 | (227.028) | Magnesium | Mg | 12 | 24.305 |
| Aluminum | Al | 13 | 26.982 | Manganese | Mn | 25 | 54.938 |
| Americium | Am | 95 | (243.061) | Mendelevium | Md | 101 | (258.10) |
| Antimony | Sb | 51 | 121.760 | Mercury | Hg | 80 | 200.59 |
| Argon | Ar | 18 | 39.948 | Molybdenum | Mo | 42 | 95.94 |
| Arsenic | As | 33 | 74.922 | Neodymium | Nd | 60 | 144.24 |
| Astatine | At | 85 | (209.987) | Neon | Ne | 10 | 20.180 |
| Barium | Ba | 56 | 137.327 | Neptunium | Np | 93 | (237.048) |
| Berkelium | Bk | 97 | (247.070) | Nickel | Ni | 28 | 58.693 |
| Beryllium | Be | 4 | 9.012 | Niobium | Nb | 41 | 92.906 |
| Bismuth | Bi | 83 | 208.980 | Nitrogen | N | 7 | 14.007 |
| Boron | B | 5 | 10.811 | Nobelium | No | 102 | (259.101) |
| Bromine | Br | 35 | 79.904 | Osmium | Os | 76 | 190.2 |
| Cadmium | Cd | 48 | 112.411 | Oxygen | O | 8 | 15.999 |
| Calcium | Ca | 20 | 40.078 | Palladium | Pd | 46 | 106.42 |
| Californium | Cf | 98 | (251.080) | Phosphorus | P | 15 | 30.974 |
| Carbon | C | 6 | 12.011 | Platinum | Pt | 78 | 195.08 |
| Cerium | Ce | 58 | 140.115 | Plutonium | Pu | 94 | (244.064) |
| Cesium | Cs | 55 | 132.905 | Polonium | Po | 84 | (209.982) |
| Chlorine | Cl | 17 | 35.453 | Potassium | K | 19 | 39.098 |
| Chromium | Cr | 24 | 51.996 | Praseodymium | Pr | 59 | 140.908 |
| Cobalt | Co | 27 | 58.933 | Promethium | Pm | 61 | (144.913) |
| Copper | Cu | 29 | 63.546 | Protactinium | Pa | 91 | (231.039) |
| Curium | Cm | 96 | (247.070) | Radium | Ra | 88 | (226.025) |
| Dysprosium | Dy | 66 | 162.503 | Radon | Rn | 86 | (222.018) |
| Einsteinium | Es | 99 | (252.087) | Rhenium | Re | 75 | 186.207 |
| Element 104 | Unq | 104 | (261.11) | Rhodium | Rh | 45 | 102.906 |
| Element 105 | Unp | 105 | (262.114) | Rubidium | Rb | 37 | 85.468 |
| Element 106 | Unh | 106 | (263.118) | Ruthenium | Ru | 44 | 101.07 |
| Element 107 | Uns | 107 | (262.12) | Samarium | Sm | 62 | 150.36 |
| Element 108 | Uno | 108 | | Scandium | Sc | 21 | 44.956 |
| Element 109 | Une | 109 | | Selenium | Se | 34 | 78.96 |
| Erbium | Er | 68 | 167.26 | Silicon | Si | 14 | 28.086 |
| Europium | Eu | 63 | 151.965 | Silver | Ag | 47 | 107.868 |
| Fermium | Fm | 100 | (257.095) | Sodium | Na | 11 | 22.990 |
| Fluorine | F | 9 | 18.998 | Strontium | Sr | 38 | 87.62 |
| Francium | Fr | 87 | (223.020) | Sulfur | S | 16 | 32.066 |
| Gadolinium | Gd | 64 | 157.25 | Tantalum | Ta | 73 | 180.948 |
| Gallium | Ga | 31 | 69.723 | Technetium | Tc | 43 | (97.907) |
| Germanium | Ge | 32 | 72.61 | Tellurium | Te | 52 | 127.60 |
| Gold | Au | 79 | 196.967 | Terbium | Tb | 65 | 158.925 |
| Hafnium | Hf | 72 | 178.49 | Thallium | Tl | 81 | 204.383 |
| Helium | He | 2 | 4.003 | Thorium | Th | 90 | 232.038 |
| Holmium | Ho | 67 | 164.930 | Thulium | Tm | 69 | 168.934 |
| Hydrogen | H | 1 | 1.008 | Tin | Sn | 50 | 118.710 |
| Indium | In | 49 | 114.818 | Titanium | Ti | 22 | 47.867 |
| Iodine | I | 53 | 126.904 | Tungsten | W | 74 | 183.84 |
| Iridium | Ir | 77 | 192.217 | Uranium | U | 92 | 238.029 |
| Iron | Fe | 26 | 55.845 | Vanadium | V | 23 | 50.942 |
| Krypton | Kr | 36 | 83.80 | Xenon | Xe | 54 | 131.29 |
| Lanthanum | La | 57 | 138.906 | Ytterbium | Yb | 70 | 173.04 |
| Lawrencium | Lw | 103 | (262.11) | Yttrium | Y | 39 | 88.906 |
| Lead | Pb | 82 | 207.2 | Zinc | Zn | 30 | 65.39 |
| Lithium | Li | 3 | 6.941 | Zirconium | Zr | 40 | 91.224 |
| Lutetium | Lu | 71 | 174.967 | | | | |

* Multiple, and sometimes conflicting, names have been proposed for elements 104–108. The symbols given for elements 104–109 are based on the IUPAC systematic names.

† Atomic weights are corrected to conform with the 1993 values of the International Union of Pure and Applied Chemistry, expressed to the fourth decimal point, rounded off to the nearest thousandth. The numbers in parentheses are the mass numbers of the most stable or most common isotope for certain radioactive elements.

into another element with emission of corpuscular or electromagnetic radiations. The natural radioactive elements are all those with atomic number above 83, and some other elements, such as potassium (at. no. 19) and rubidium (at. no. 37), which are very weakly radioactive.
**rare earth e's,** elements of the lanthanum series, comprising elements with atomic numbers 57 to 71.
**sarcous e.,** any of the elementary granules into which the primordial fibril of an elementary muscle fiber is divisible.
**stable e.,** 1. a chemical element which does not spontaneously transmute into another element with emission of corpuscular or electromagnetic radiations; the stable elements are those with atomic number below 84, except for a few, such as potassium and rubidium, which are weakly radioactive. 2. a tissue cell of mature tissues which does not alter by mitosis.
**tissue e.,** morphological e.
**trace e's,** chemical elements that are distributed throughout the tissues in very small amounts and are essential in nutrition, such as cobalt, copper, magnesium, manganese, selenium, and zinc; for optimal bioavailability they must be in a balanced mixture, and they may be harmful or toxic in excess.
**transcalifornium e's,** the elements with atomic numbers higher than that of californium, and discovered subsequent to its discovery in 1950. They are einsteinium 99, fermium 100, mendelevium 101, nobelium 102, and lawrencium 103.
**transposable e.,** see *transposon.*
**transuranic e's, transuranium e's,** the elements with atomic numbers higher than that of uranium. Applied originally to neptunium 93, plutonium 94, americium 95, curium 96, berkelium 97, and californium 98, the term now, by definition, includes the transcalifornium elements as well.

**el·e·men·ta·ry** (el″ə-men′tə-re) not resolvable or divisible into simpler parts or components; see also under *particle.*

**ele(o)-** [Gr. *elaion* oil] combining form denoting relationship to oil.

**el·e·o·ma** (el″e-o′mə) [*eleo-* + *-oma*] a tumor or swelling caused by the injection of oil into the tissues.

**el·e·om·e·ter** (el″e-om′ə-tər) [*eleo-* + *-meter*] an instrument for determining the percentage of oil in a mixture, also the specific gravity of oils.

**el·e·op·a·thy** (el″e-op′ə-the) elaiopathy.

**el·eo·plast** (el-e′o-plast) [*eleo-* + *-plast*] a globular body made up of granular protoplasm.

**el·e·op·tene** (el″e-op′tēn) [*eleo-* + Gr. *ptēnos* volatile] the more volatile constituent of a volatile oil, as distinguished from its stearoptene.

**el·eo·sac·cha·rum** (el″e-o-sak′ə-rəm) pl. *eleosacch′ara* [*eleo-* + *sakcharon* sugar] a mixture of sugar with a volatile oil; an oil sugar. Called also *oleosaccharum.*

**el·eo·ther·a·py** (el″e-o-ther′ə-pe) [*eleo-* + *therapy*] oleotherapy.

**el·e·phan·ti·as·ic** (el″ə-fan″te-as′ik) pertaining to elephantiasis.

**el·e·phan·ti·a·sis** (el″ə-fən-ti′ə-sis) [Gr. *elephas* elephant + *-iasis*] [MeSH: Elephantiasis] 1. chronic obstruction of the lymphatics with hypertrophy of the skin and subcutaneous tissues (pachyderma), usually affecting dependent areas such as the legs, arms, or external genitalia; it is a filarial disease generally seen in the tropics due to infection of the lymphatics with any of the nematodes *Wuchereria bancrofti, Brugia malayi,* or *B. timori.* It begins with lymphangitis and enlargement of the part, along with chills and fever (elephantoid fever), followed by formation of ulcers and tubercles, with thickening, discoloration, and fissuring of the skin. See also *bancroftian filariasis* and *Malayan filariasis,* under *filariasis.* 2. hypertrophy and thickening of the tissues from any cause.

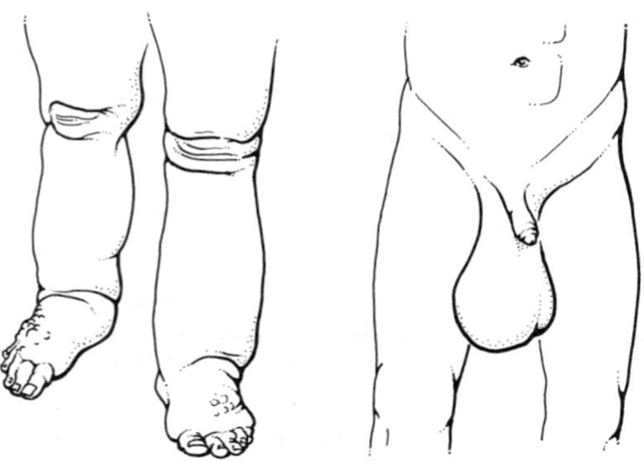
Elephantiasis of the legs and of the scrotum.

**e. chirur′gica,** massive edema of the arm after mastectomy.
**congenital e.,** Milroy's disease.
**e. gingi′vae,** fibromatosis gingivae.
**lymphangiectatic e.,** elephantiasis of a part due to lymphangiectasis.
**e. neuromato′sa,** neurofibroma.
**e. nos′tras,** that due to either chronic recurrent streptococcal erysipelas or chronic recurrent cellulitis.
**e. o′culi,** thickening and protrusion of the eyelids.
**e. scro′ti,** that in which the scrotum is the principal seat of the disease; called also *chylocele* and *lymph scrotum.*

**el·e·phan·toid** (el″ĕ-fan′toid) relating to or resembling elephantiasis.

**El·et·ta·ria** (el″ə-ta′re-ə) a genus of herbs of the family Zingiberaceae, native to Indonesia. *E. cardamo′mum* is cardamom, the usual source of the spice called cardamom. See also *cardamom oil,* under *oil.*

**el·e·va·tion** (el″ə-va′shən) a raised area, or point of greater height.
**tactile e's,** toruli tactiles.

**el·e·va·tor** (el′ə-va″tor) [L. *elevare* to lift] [MeSH: Elevators and Escalators] an instrument for lifting tissues, removing bony fragments, or removing roots of teeth.
**angular e.,** one in which the blade angles from the shank to the right or to the left.
**apical e.,** an instrument for removing fractured root tips retained in the apex of the tooth socket following tooth extraction; its shank has an angle to provide access within the socket and its tip has a barb for reaching a fractured root tip. Called also *apical pick* and *root pick.*
**cross bar e.,** one in which the handle is at a right angle to the shank. Called also *T-bar e.*
**Cryer e.,** a dental instrument for removing the roots of molar teeth; furnished in pairs, one for mesial and one for distal roots, which are reversed for use on opposite sides of the jaw.
**dental e.,** an instrument having a blade that engages the teeth or their roots and extracts teeth by elevating them from their alveoli through leverage applied to the handle.
**malar e.,** an instrument used to elevate or reposition the zygomatic bone and/or arch.
**periosteum e.,** a flat steel bar for separating the attachments of the periosteum to bone.
**root e.,** a dental elevator for extracting a fractured root of a tooth; they may be designed in pairs, a right and a left, and as single, straight, mitered, or double ended.
**screw e.,** a dental instrument designed to be screwed into a root canal for subsequent removal of the root, usually of the apical third.
**straight e.,** one in which the shank continues in a straight line with the handle.
**T-bar e.,** cross bar e.
**wedge e.,** one used as a lever in tooth extraction, being placed in a hole drilled into the root of the tooth below the investing bony tissue to rework a tooth.

**el·faz·e·pam** (el-faz′ə-pəm) a benzodiazepine used as a veterinary appetite stimulant.

**elim·i·nant** (e-lim′ĭ-nənt) 1. causing an evacuation. 2. an agent that promotes evacuation.

**elim·i·na·tion** (e-lim″ĭ-na′shən) [L. *eliminatio,* from *e* out + *limen* threshold] 1. the act of expulsion or of extrusion, especially of expulsion from the body. See *excretion, defecation, urination,* and *clearance.* 2. omission or exclusion, as in an elimination diet.
**immune e.,** the period of accelerated degradation of antigen (e.g., foreign gamma globulin) as a result of its removal and destruction by antibodies. Also, a technique for determining antibody response by measuring the rate of removal of labeled antigen from the circulation of an immunized animal. Called also *immune clearance.*

**el·i·nin** (el′ĭ-nin) a lipoprotein fraction of red cells containing the Rh and A and B factors.

**El·i·on** (el′e-ən) Gertrude Belle. American pharmacologist, born 1918. Co-winner with Sir James W. Black and George H. Hitchings of the Nobel prize for medicine or physiology in 1988 for discoveries made with Hitchings about the structure and activity of normal and abnormal cells, facilitating the development of drugs active against specific disease states.

**Elip·ten** (e-lip′-tən) trademark for a preparation of aminoglutethimide.

**ELISA** (e-li′sə) [*E*nzyme-*L*inked *I*mmuno*S*orbent *A*ssay] any enzyme immunoassay utilizing an enzyme-labeled immunoreactant (antigen or antibody) and an immunosorbent (antigen or antibody bound to a solid support). A variety of methods (e.g., competitive binding between the labeled reactant and unlabeled unknown or a sandwich technique in which the unknown binds both the immunosorbent and labeled antibody) may be used to measure the unknown concentration.

**elix·ir** (e-lik'sər) [L., from Arabic] a clear, sweetened, usually hydroalcoholic liquid containing flavoring substances and sometimes active medicinal agents, used orally as a vehicle or for the effect of the medicinal agent contained.

**aromatic e.** [NF], a preparation containing orange, lemon, coriander, and anise oils, syrup, talc, and alcohol in purified water; used as a flavored vehicle for pharmaceutical preparations.

**aromatic e., red,** aromatic elixir colored by addition of amaranth solution.

**benzaldehyde e., compound** [USP], a preparation of benzaldehyde, vanillin, orange flower water, alcohol, syrup, and purified water; used as a vehicle for pharmaceutical preparations.

**gentian e., glycerinated,** a preparation of gentian and taraxacum fluidextracts, compound cardamom tincture, raspberry syrup, sweet orange peel tincture, phosphoric acid, ethyl acetate, glycerin, sucrose, and alcohol, in purified water; used as a flavored vehicle for drugs.

**high-alcoholic e.,** see *iso-alcoholic e.*

**iso-alcoholic e.,** a mixture of low-alcoholic elixir and high-alcoholic elixir to produce a solution whose strength is suitable for the medicament for which it serves as a vehicle. *Low-alcoholic e.:* compound orange spirit 10 mL, alcohol 100 mL, glycerin 200 mL, sucrose 320 gm, and sufficient purified water to make a total of 1000 mL. *High-alcoholic e.:* compound orange spirit 4 mL, saccharin 3 gm, glycerin 200 mL, and sufficient alcohol to make a total of 1000 mL.

**low-alcoholic e.,** see *iso-alcoholic e.*

**pepsin e., lactated,** a water preparation containing a proteolytic enzyme from the glandular layer of the fresh stomach of the hog, with lactic acid, glycerin, alcohol, orange oil, and amaranth solution.

**terpin hydrate and codeine e.** [USP], 2 gm of codeine dissolved in a sufficient quantity of terpin hydrate elixir to make 1000 mL; used as an expectorant and antitussive.

**terpin hydrate and dextromethorphan hydrobromide e.,** 2 gm of dextromethorphan hydrobromide dissolved in a sufficient quantity of terpin hydrate elixir to make 1000 mL; used as an expectorant and antitussive.

**Elix·o·phyl·lin** (e-lik"sə-fil'in) trademark for preparations of theophylline.

**El·ko·sin** (el'kə-sin) trademark for preparations of sulfisomidine.

**el·ko·sis** (el-ko'sis) ulceration.

**El·li·ot's operation** (el'e-əts) [Col. Robert Henry *Elliot,* English ophthalmologist in India, 1864–1936] see under *operation.*

**El·li·ot's position** (el'e-əts) [John Wheelock *Elliot,* American surgeon, 1852–1925] see under *position.*

**El·li·ot's sign** (el'e-əts) [George T. *Elliot,* American dermatologist, 1851–1935] see under *sign.*

**el·lip·sin** (e-lip'sin) the insoluble constituents of cells which remain after the removal of the soluble proteins.

**el·lip·soid** (e-lip'soid) [Gr. *ellipēs (kyklos),* defective (circle) + *-oid*] 1. any structure shaped like a spindle or an ellipse. 2. Schweigger-Seidel sheath. 3. in ophthalmology, the acidophilic outer region of the inner segment of the dendritic process of a retinal rod or cone, lying between the cilium and the myoid, and containing some glycogen and many mitochondria; called also *visual cell e.*

**el·lip·to·cy·ta·ry** (e-lip"to-si'tə-re) pertaining to elliptocytes.

**el·lip·to·cyte** (e-lip'to-sīt) an abnormal oval or elliptical erythrocyte, as seen in elliptocytosis. Called also *cameloid cell* and *ovalocyte.*

**el·lip·to·cy·to·sis** (e-lip"to-si-to'sis) presence of large numbers of elliptocytes in the blood; called also *ovalocytosis.*

**hereditary e.,** any of a number of hereditary disorders in which 30 to 100 per cent of the erythrocytes are elliptocytes. In many patients there are no symptoms, but others show varying degrees of erythrocyte destruction and hemolytic anemia. Both autosomal dominant and recessive varieties are known. Called also *Dresbach's syndrome* and *elliptocytary, elliptocytic,* or *elliptocytotic anemia.*

**spherocytic e.,** a hereditary condition characterized by both elliptocytes and spherocytes that are osmotically and mechanically fragile; most patients have moderate hemolytic anemia and are at risk for aplastic crises.

**el·lip·to·cy·tot·ic** (e-lip"to-si-tot'ik) pertaining to or characterized by elliptocytosis.

**El·lis-van Crev·eld syndrome** (el'is-vahn kre'veld) [Richard White Bernhard *Ellis,* Scottish pediatrician, 1902–1966; Simon *van Creveld,* Dutch pediatrician, 1894–1971] [MeSH: Ellis-Van Creveld Syndrome] see *chondroectodermal dysplasia,* under *dysplasia.*

**elm** (elm) 1. any tree of the genus *Ulmus.* 2. [USP] slippery elm bark; the dried inner bark of the slippery elm *Ulmus rubra,* used as a demulcent.

**slippery e.,** a deciduous tree of eastern North America, *Ulmus rubra* Muhlenberg (*U. fulva* Michaux), the source of elm [USP]; see also under *bark.*

**El·o·con** (el'o-kon) trademark for preparations of mometasone furoate.

**Eloes·ser flap** (el-es'ər) [Leo *Eloesser,* American surgeon, 1881–1976] see under *flap.*

**elon·ga·tion** (e"long-a'shən) 1. the act, process or condition of increasing in length. 2. pathologic migration of a tooth in the occlusal or incisal direction. 3. radiographic distortion in which the image is proportionately longer than that which is being x-rayed.

**El·o·rine** (el'o-rēn) trademark for a preparation of tricyclamol chloride.

**Els·berg's test** (els'bərgz) [Charles Albert *Elsberg,* New York surgeon, 1871–1948] see under *test.*

**Elsch·nig's bodies (pearls)** (elsh'nigz) [Anton Philipp *Elschnig,* Austrian ophthalmologist, 1863–1939] see under *body.*

**El·spar** (el'spahr) trademark for a preparation of L-asparaginase derived from *Escherichia coli.*

**El Tor vibrio** (el tor) [*El Tor* Quarantine Station on the Egyptian Sinai Peninsula, where it was first isolated in 1960] *Vibrio cholerae* biotype *eltor.*

**el·u·ate** (el'u-āt) the substance separated out by, or the product of, elution or elutriation.

**elu·ent** (e-loo'ənt) a solution used in elution.

**elu·tion** (e-loo'shən) [L. *e* out + *luere* to wash] in chemistry, the separation of material by washing, as in the freeing of an enzyme from its absorbent.

**membrane e.,** a method of selecting cells in which a culture of cells is collected on a membrane filter, over which a fresh warm culture fluid is then slowly passed, washing off excess cells and leaving only adsorbed cells at a particular developmental stage.

**elu·tri·a·tion** (e-loo"tre-a'shən) [L. *elutriare* to wash out] the operation of pulverizing substances and mixing them with water in order to separate the heavier constituents, which settle out in solution, from the lighter constituents.

**Ely's test (sign)** (e'līz) [Leonard Wheeler *Ely,* American orthopedic surgeon, 1868–1944] see under *test.*

**elytr(o)-** [Gr. *elytron* a covering, sheath] a combining form denoting relationship to the vagina or to a sheath; for words beginning thus, see those beginning *colp(o)-.*

**Em** emmetropia.

**ema·ci·a·tion** (e-ma"she-a'shən) [L. *emaciare* to make lean] [MeSH: Emaciation] excessive leanness; a wasted condition of the body.

**em·an** (em'ən) a unit for expressing the concentration of radium emanation in solution: it is the concentration present when one tenth of a millimicrocurie of radium emanation is dissolved in 1 liter of air or water, or $10^{-10}$ curie.

**em·a·na·tion** (em"ə-na'shən) [L. *e* out + *manare* to flow] that which is given off, such as a gaseous disintegration product given off from radioactive substances or an effluvium.

**actinium e.,** one member of the radioactive series derived from actinium. It is produced from actinium X, has an atomic weight of 218, its atomic number is 86, and by the loss of alpha particles it becomes actinium A. Called also *actinon.*

**thorium e.,** one member of the radioactive series derived from thorium. It is produced from thorium X, has an atomic weight of 220, its atomic number is 86, and by the loss of alpha particles it changes into thorium A. Called also *thoron.*

**eman·ci·pa·tion** (e-man"sĭ-pa'shən) [L. *emancipare* to release, give up] the establishment of local autonomy within restricted fields of a developing embryo.

**emas·cu·late** (e-mas'ku-lāt) to castrate a male.

**emas·cu·la·tion** (e-mas"ku-la'shən) [L. *emasculare* to castrate] male castration.

**em·balm·ing** (em-bahm'ing) [MeSH: Embalming] the treatment of the dead body with antiseptics and preservatives, to prevent putrefaction.

**em·bar·rass** (əm-bar'əs) to impede the function of; to obstruct.

**Emb·den es·ter** (em'dən) [Gustav Georg *Embden,* German biochemist, 1874–1933] see under *ester.*

**Emb·den-Mey·er·hof pathway** (em'dən-mi'ər-hof) [G.G. *Embden;* Otto Fritz *Meyerhof,* German physiologist, 1884–1951] see under *pathway.*

**Emb·den-Mey·er·hof-Par·nas pathway** (em'den-mi'ər-hof-pahr'nahs) [G.G. Embden; O.F. *Meyerhof;* Jakub Karol *Parnas,* Polish biochemist, 1884–1949] see *Embden-Meyerhof pathway,* under *pathway.*

**em·bed·ding** (əm-bed'ing) the fixation of a tissue specimen in a firm medium, in order to keep it intact during the cutting of thin sections.

**Em·be·lia** (em-be'le-ə) a genus of East Indian climbing plants of the family Myrsinaceae. *E. ri'bes* (called also *E. robus'ta*) is a species whose fruit has been used for its anthelminthic and cathartic principles.

**em·boite·ment** (ahm-bwaht-maw') [Fr. "encasement"] the supposed encasement of miniature individuals within the germ cells of predecessors, advanced as one theory of preformation.

**em·bo·la·lia** (em"bo-la'le-ə) embololalia.

**em·bole** (em'bə-le) [Gr. *embolē* a throwing in] 1. the reducing of a dislocated limb. 2. emboly.

**em·bo·lec·to·my** (em"bə-lek'tə-me) [*embolus* + *-ectomy*] [MeSH: Embolectomy] surgical removal of an embolus.

**em·bo·li** (em'bə-li) [L.] plural of *embolus.*

**em·bo·lia** (em-bo'le-ə) embole.

**em·bol·ic** (em-bol'ik) pertaining to an embolus or to embolism.

**em·bol·i·form** (em-bol'ĭ-form) resembling an embolus.

**em·bo·lism** (em'bə-liz-əm) [L. *embolismus,* from *embolus* + *-ism*] [MeSH: Embolism] the sudden blocking of an artery by a clot or foreign material which has been brought to its site of lodgment by the blood current.
**air e.,** that due to air bubbles entering the veins from trauma, surgical procedures, or severe decompression sickness. Called also *aeroembolism.*
**amniotic fluid e.,** embolism due to amniotic fluid in the maternal circulation.
**bacillary e.,** obstruction of a vessel by an aggregation of bacilli.
**bland e.,** that in which the thrombotic plug is composed of nonseptic material.
**bone marrow e.,** embolism caused by material from a fractured long bone.
**capillary e.,** blocking of the capillaries with bacteria.
**cerebral e.,** embolism of a cerebral artery.
**coronary e.,** embolism of one of the coronary arteries.
**crossed e.,** paradoxical e.
**direct e.,** embolism occurring in the direction of the bloodstream.
**fat e.,** an embolism caused by fat that has entered the circulation, especially after fractures of large bones, or after corticosteroid administration. Called also *oil e.*
**infective e.,** embolism in which the embolus is infective.
**lymph e., lymphogenous e.,** embolism of a lymph vessel.
**miliary e.,** one affecting many small vessels at the same time.
**multiple e.,** embolism by a number of small emboli.
**oil e.,** fat e.
**pantaloon e.,** saddle e.
**paradoxical e.,** blockage of a systemic artery by a thrombus originating in a systemic vein, which has passed through a defect that permits direct communication between the right and the left side of the heart, usually an open foramen ovale. Called also *crossed e.*
**pulmonary e.,** the closure of the pulmonary artery or one of its branches by an embolus, sometimes associated with pulmonary infarction (q.v.).
**retinal e.,** embolism of the central artery of the retina.
**saddle e.,** an embolism at the bifurcation of the aorta, causing sudden severe pain of the legs, abdomen, and back, with numbing and coldness. Called also *pantaloon e.*
**spinal e.,** embolism of an artery in the spinal cord.
**trichinous e.,** embolism due to trichinae.
**tumor e.,** embolism due to tumor fragments.
**venous e.,** one in which the material originates in the veins.

**em·bo·li·za·tion** (em"bə-lĭ-za'shən) 1. the process or condition of becoming an embolus. 2. therapeutic introduction of a substance into a vessel in order to occlude it; called also *embolotherapy.*

**em·bo·lo·la·lia** (em"bə-lo-la'le-ə) [*embolus* + *-lalia*] the interpolation of meaningless or unintelligible words into the speech; called also *embolalia* and *embolophrasia.*

**em·bo·lo·my·cot·ic** (em"bə-lo-mi-kot'ik) pertaining to or marked by an infective embolism.

**em·bo·lo·phra·sia** (em"bə-lo-fra'zhə) embololalia.

**em·bo·lo·ther·a·py** (em"bo-lo-ther'ə-pe) embolization, def. 2.

**em·bo·lus** (em'bo-ləs) pl. *em'boli* [Gr. *embolos* plug, from *en* in + *ballein* to throw] 1. a mass, which may be a blood clot or some other material, that is brought by the bloodstream through the vasculature, lodging in a vessel or bifurcation too small to allow it to pass, obstructing the circulation; see illustration. See also *embolism.* 2. nucleus emboliformis.
**air e.,** one composed of an air bubble; see also under *embolism.*
**bullet e.,** migration of a bullet within a blood vessel; arterial emboli cause ischemia and possibly limb amputation and venous emboli may travel to the pulmonary artery or heart, causing bacterial endocarditis, pericardial effusion, myocardiac irritability, or valve mechanism interference.

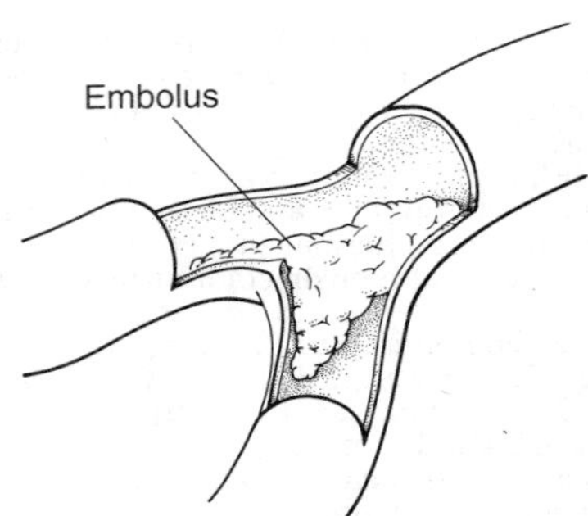

Embolus impacted at the site of branching of an artery.

**cancer e.,** tumor e.
**fat e.,** one composed of oil or fat. See also under *embolism.*
**foam e.,** one formed by a mixture of a gas and blood.
**obturating e.,** one completely blocking a vessel.
**riding e., saddle e., straddling e.,** one at the bifurcation of an artery, blocking both branches. See also *saddle embolism,* under *embolism.*
**tumor e.,** one composed of tumor cells; see also under *embolism.* Called also *cancer e.*

**em·bo·ly** (em'bə-le) [Gr. *embolē* a throwing in] the invagination of the blastula by which the gastrula is formed.

**em·bouche·ment** (ahm-bo͞osh-maw') [Fr.] the opening of one vessel into another.

**em·bra·sure** (em-bra'zhər) a space continuous with an interproximal space, produced by curvatures of teeth in contact in the same arch, that provides a channel or passage through which food escapes from the occlusal surfaces of the teeth during mastication. Called also *spillway.*
**buccal e.,** the embrasure opening out toward the cheek between molar and premolar teeth.
**incisal e.,** occlusal e.
**interdental e.,** the space formed by the interproximal contours of adjoining teeth, beginning at the contact area and extending lingually, facially, occlusally, and apically.
**labial e.,** the embrasure that widens out from the area of contact toward the lips between the canine and incisor teeth.
**lingual e.,** the embrasure that widens out from the area of contact toward the lingual sides of the teeth.
**occlusal e.,** the space bounded by the marginal ridges as they join the cusps and incisal ridges. Called also *incisal e.*

**em·bro·ca·tion** (em"bro-ka'shən) [L. *embrocatio*] 1. the application of a liquid medicament to the surface of the body. 2. a liquid medicine for external use.

**em·bry·ec·to·my** (em"bre-ek'tə-me) [*embryo* + *-ectomy*] excision of the embryo in extrauterine pregnancy.

**em·bryo** (em'bre-o) [Gr. *embryon*] [MeSH: Embryo] 1. in plants, the element of the seed that develops into a new individual. 2. in animals, those derivatives of the zygote that will eventually become the offspring, during their period of most rapid development, i.e., from the time the long axis appears until all major structures are represented. 3. in humans, the developing organism from the fourth day after fertilization to the end of the eighth week. Cf. *fetus.*
**hexacanth e.,** the six-hooked embryo, or onchosphere, characteristic of most tapeworms of humans and domestic animals.
**Janošík's e.,** a human embryo having three aortic arches and two pharyngeal pouches.
**presomite e.,** the embryo at any stage prior to the appearance of the first pair of somites.
**previllous e.,** the conceptus before the chorionic villi of the placenta develop.
**somite e.,** the embryo at any stage between the appearances of the first and the last pairs of somites.
**Spee's e.,** a 1.5 mm human embryo, horizon IX, about 20 days old as described by Spee.

**em·bryo·blast** (em'bre-o-blast") [*embryo* + *-blast*] inner cell mass.

**em·bry·oc·to·ny** (em"bre-ok'tə-ne) [*embryo* + Gr. *kteinein* to kill] the artificial destruction of the living embryo, or fetus.

**em·bryo·gen·e·sis** (em"bre-o-jen'ə-sis) [*embryo* + *genesis*] 1. the production of an embryo. 2. the development of a new individual by means of sexual reproduction, that is, from a zygote; called also *embryogeny* and *embryony.*

**em·bryo·ge·net·ic** (em"bre-o-jə-net'ik) embryogenic.

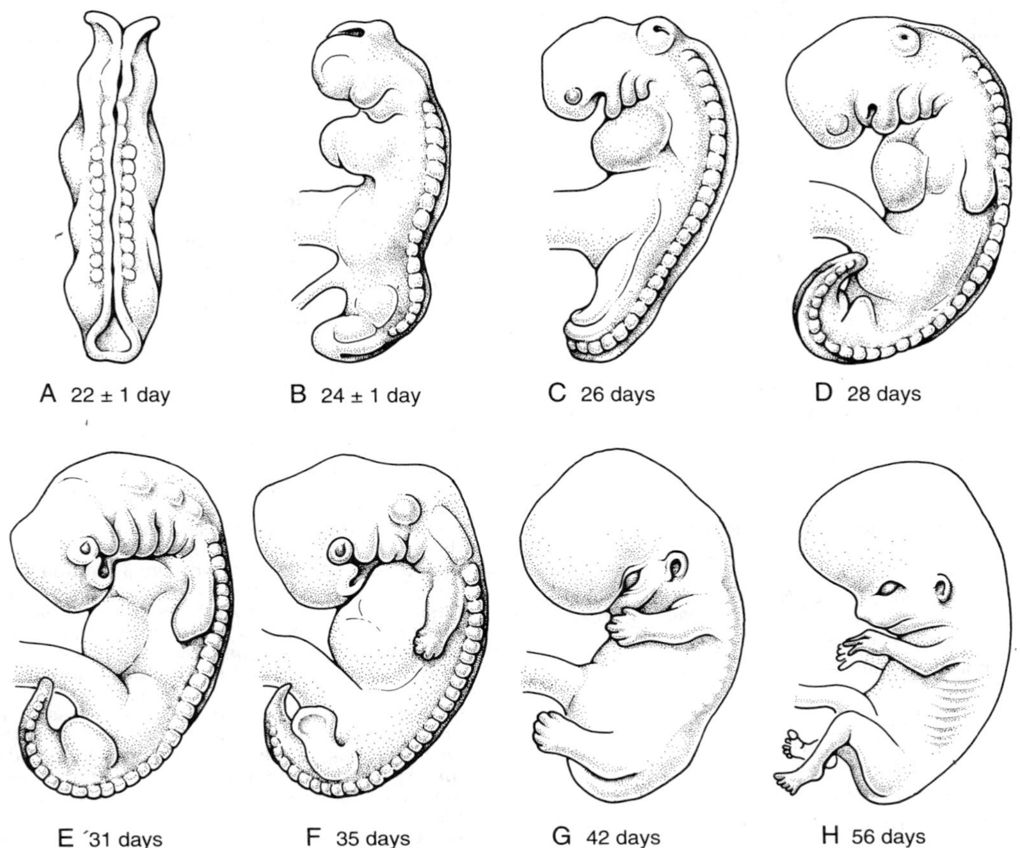


Human embryo at various stages of development. The relative size has been distorted to emphasize correspondence of parts.

**em·bry·o·gen·ic** (em″bre-o-jen′ik) 1. pertaining to the development of the embryo. 2. producing an embryo.

**em·bry·og·e·ny** (em″bre-oj′ə-ne) [*embryo* + *-geny*] embryogenesis.

**em·bryo·graph** (em′bre-o-graf) [*embryo* + *-graph*] a combination of a microscope and a camera lucida, used to draw sketches of the embryo.

**em·bry·og·ra·phy** (em″bre-og′rə-fe) [*embryo* + *-graphy*] 1. a treatise or description of the embryo. 2. the sketching of an embryo by means of the embryograph.

**em·bry·oid** (em′bre-oid) [*embryo* + *-oid*] resembling an embryo.

**em·bryo·ism** (em′bre-o-iz-əm) the condition of being an embryo.

**em·bryo·le·thal·i·ty** embryotoxicity that causes death of the embryo.

**em·bry·ol·o·gist** (em″bre-ol′ə-jist) an expert in embryology.

**em·bry·ol·o·gy** (em″bre-ol′ə-je) [*embryo* + *-logy*] [MeSH: Embryology] the science of the development of the individual during the embryonic stage and, by extension, in several or even all preceding and subsequent stages of the life cycle.
**causal e.,** experimental e.
**comparative e.,** embryology applied with a comparative view to various species studied with reference to their taxonomy and the principle that ontogeny recapitulates phylogeny.
**descriptive e.,** the study of embryos and fetuses and their components with reference to anatomical and chronological sequence so as to define stages and report the course of development.
**experimental e.,** analysis of the factors and relations in development, obtained by subjecting embryos to experimental procedures; called also *causal e.*

**em·bry·o·ma** (em″bre-o′mə) any neoplasm thought to be derived from embryonic cells or tissues, such as a dermoid cyst, teratoma, primitive neuroectodermal tumor, embryonal carcinoma or sarcoma, nephroblastoma, or hepatoblastoma. Called also *embryonal tumor.*
**e. of kidney,** Wilms' tumor.

**em·bryo·mor·phous** (em″bre-o-mor′fəs) [*embryo* + *morph-* + *-ous*] having a form suggestive of an embryo; said of certain abnormal tissue elements supposed to be remnants of an embryo.

**em·bry·o·nal** (em′bre-o″nəl) embryonic.

**em·bry·o·nate** (em′bre-o-nāt) 1. pertaining to or resembling an embryo. 2. containing an embryo. 3. impregnated; fecundated.

**em·bry·on·ic** (em″bre-on′ik) of or pertaining to the embryo.

**em·bry·on·i·form** (em″bre-on′ĭ-form) embryoid.

**em·bry·o·nism** (em′bre-o-niz-əm) embryoism.

**em·bry·o·ni·za·tion** (em″bre-o′nĭ-za′shən) reversion to the embryonic form on the part of a tissue or cell.

**em·bry·o·noid** (em′bre-o-noid″) embryoid.

**em·bry·o·ny** (em′bre-o-ne) embryogenesis.

**em·bryo·pa·thol·o·gy** (em″bre-o-pə-thol′o-je) the study of abnormal embryos or of defective development.

**em·bry·op·a·thy** (em″bre-op′ə-the) [*embryo* + *-pathy*] [MeSH: Fetal Diseases] a morbid condition of the embryo or a disorder resulting from abnormal embryonic development. Cf. *fetopathy.*
**rubella e.,** congenital anomalies in an infant due to rubella in the mother during early pregnancy. See also *congenital rubella syndrome,* under *syndrome.*

**em·bryo·phore** (em′bre-o-for) the inner egg shell surrounding the embryo, as seen in the eggs of *Taenia* found in the feces.

**em·bryo·plas·tic** (em″bre-o-plas′tik) [*embryo* + *plastic*] embryogenic.

**em·bryo·scope** (em″bre-o-skōp) [*embryo* + *-scope*] an instrument for observing the embryo.

**em·bryo·tome** (em′bre-o-tōm) a cutting instrument used in embryotomy.

**em·bry·ot·o·my** (em″bre-ot′o-me) [*embryo* + *-tomy*] 1. the dismemberment of a fetus in the uterus or vagina to facilitate delivery that is impossible by natural means. 2. the dissection of embryos and fetuses.

**em·bryo·tox·ic·i·ty** toxic effects on the embryo of a substance that crosses the placental membrane. See also *embryolethality.*

**em·bryo·tox·on** (em″bre-o-tok′son) arcus corneae; see under *arcus.*
**anterior e.,** arcus corneae.
**posterior e.,** Axenfeld's anomaly.

**em·bryo·troph** (em'bre-o-trōf") [*embryo* + Gr. *trophē* nourishment] the total nutriment (histotroph and hemotroph) available to the embryo.

**em·bry·ot·ro·phy** (em"bre-ot'rə-fe) [*embryo* + *-trophy*] the nutrition of the embryo.

**EMC** encephalomyocarditis (virus).

**Em·cyt** (em'sīt) trademark for a preparation of estramustine.

**emed·ul·late** (e-med'u-lāt) [*e-* + *medulla*] to extract bone marrow.

**emeio·cy·to·sis** (e"me-o-si-to'sis) emiocytosis.

**emer·gence** (e-mər'jəns) the process of coming out of a former state, as the restoration to a normal physiological state of an anesthetized patient.

**emer·gen·cy** (e-mər'jən-se) [L. *emergere* to raise up] [MeSH: Emergencies] an unlooked for or sudden occasion; an accident; an urgent or pressing need.

**emer·gent** (e-mər'jənt) 1. pertaining to an emergency. 2. coming into being through consecutive stages of development, as in emergent evolution.

**Em·er·i·cel·la** (em"ər-ĭ-sel'ə) a genus of fungi of the family Trichocomaceae. *E. ni'dulans* is the perfect (sexual) stage of *Aspergillus nidulans.*

**Eme·ri·cel·lop·sis** (em"ər-ĭ-sə-lop'sis) a teleomorph of *Acremonium*; *E. minimum* (formerly *Cephalosporium acremonium*) is the source of cephalosporin C.

**Em·ery-Drei·fuss muscular dystrophy** (em'ə-re-dri'fəs) [Alan Eglin Heathcote *Emery,* British geneticist, born 1928; F.E. *Dreifuss,* British physician, 20th century] see under *dystrophy.*

**em·ery** (em'ər-e) impure crystalline corundum mixed with iron oxide; used as an abrasive.

**eme·sia** (ə-me'zhə) vomiting.

**em·e·sis** (em'ə-sis) [Gr. *emein* to vomit] vomiting.
**e. gravida'rum,** vomiting of pregnancy.

**-emesis** a word termination denoting vomiting.

**em·e·ta·tro·phia** (em"ə-tə-tro'fe-ə) [Gr. *emetos* vomiting + *atrophia*] atrophy or wasting due to persistent vomiting.

**Emete·con** (ə-met'ə-kon") trademark for a preparation of benzquinamide hydrochloride.

**emet·ic** (ə-met'ik) [Gr. *emetikos;* L. *emeticus*] 1. bringing on or causing the act of vomiting. 2. an agent that causes vomiting.
**central e.,** one carried by the bloodstream to the vomiting center, upon which it acts; called also *indirect e.* and *systemic e.*
**direct e.,** one that acts directly on the stomach; called also *mechanical e.*
**indirect e.,** central e.
**mechanical e.,** direct e.
**systemic e.,** central e.

**emet·i·col·o·gy** (e-met"ĭ-kol'ə-je) the sum of knowledge regarding emetics.

**em·e·tine** (em'ə-tēn) [MeSH: Emetine] an alkaloid, obtained from ipecac or prepared by methylation of cephaeline.
**e. and bismuth iodide,** a complex iodide of emetine and bismuth, occurring as a reddish-orange powder; used as an antiamebic in amebic dysentery, administered orally.
**e. hydrochloride** [USP], the dihydrochloride salt of emetine, used as an antiamebic, administered subcutaneously or intramuscularly.

**em·e·to·ca·thar·tic** (em"ə-to-kə-thahr'tik) 1. both emetic and cathartic. 2. an agent that is both emetic and cathartic.

**em·e·to·gen·ic** (em"ə-to-jen'ik) [Gr. *emetos* vomiting + *-genic*] emetic (def. 1).

**em·e·tol·o·gy** (em"ə-tol'ə-je) emeticology.

**EMF** electromotive force.

**EMG** *electromyogram.*

**-emia** [Gr. *haima* blood + *-ia*] a word termination denoting the presence of a substance in the blood.

**em·i·gra·tion** (em"ĭ-gra'shən) diapedesis.

**Em·in·ase** (em'in-ās) trademark for a preparation of anistreplase.

**em·i·nec·to·my** (em"ĭ-nek'tə-me) resection of the articular eminence of the temporal bone.

**em·i·nence** (em'ĭ-nəns) a prominence or projection, especially one upon the surface of a bone; called also *eminentia* [TA].
**antithenar e.,** hypothenar (def. 1).
**arcuate e.,** eminentia arcuata.
**articular e. of temporal bone,** tuberculum articulare ossis temporalis.
**bicipital e.,** tuberositas radii.
**canine e.,** a prominent bony ridge overlying the root of either canine tooth on the labial surface of both the maxilla and the mandible.
**capitate e.,** capitulum humeri.
**caudate e. of liver,** processus caudatus hepatis.
**coccygeal e.,** cornu sacrale.
**cochlear e. of sacral bone,** promontorium ossis sacri.
**collateral e. of lateral ventricle,** eminentia collateralis ventriculi lateralis.
**e. of concha,** eminentia conchae.
**cruciate e., cruciform e. of occipital bone,** eminentia cruciformis.
**cuneiform e. of head of rib,** crista capitis costae.
**deltoid e.,** tuberositas deltoidea humeri.
**facial e. of eminentia teres,** colliculus facialis.
**frontal e.,** tuber frontale.
**genital e.,** see under *tubercle.*
**gluteal e. of femur,** tuberositas glutea femoris.
**e. of humerus,** capitulum humeri.
**hypobranchial e.,** copula linguae.
**hypoglossal e.,** trigonum nervi hypoglossi.
**hypothenar e.,** hypothenar (def. 1).
**iliopectineal e., iliopubic e.,** eminentia iliopubica.
**intercondylar e., intercondyloid e., intermediate e.,** eminentia intercondylaris.
**jugular e.,** tuberculum jugulare ossis occipitalis.
**maxillary e.,** tuber maxillae.
**medial e. of rhomboid fossa,** eminentia medialis fossae rhomboideae.
**median e.,** the raised area on the infundibulum hypothalami at the floor of the third ventricle of the brain. Continuous below with the infundibular stem or stalk of the pituitary gland, it contains the primary capillary network of the hypophysial portal system. In some anatomical classification systems it is included as part of the neurohypophysis and in others as part of the tuber cinereum. See also *circumventricular organs,* under *organ.*
**oblique e. of cuboid bone,** tuberositas ossis cuboidei.
**occipital e.,** a ridge on the lateral ventricle of the embryonic brain, corresponding to the occipital fissure in the adult.
**olivary e. of sphenoid bone,** tuberculum sellae turcicae.
**omental e. of body of pancreas,** tuber omentale corporis pancreatis.
**orbital e. of zygomatic bone,** eminentia orbitalis ossis zygomatici.
**parietal e.,** tuber parietale.
**postchiasmatic e.,** an inconstant protuberance on the floor of the third ventricle posterior to the optic chiasm; called also *postfundibular e.*
**postfundibular e.,** postchiasmatic e.
**pyramidal e.,** eminentia pyramidalis.
**radial e. of wrist,** eminentia carpi radialis.
**e. of scapha,** eminentia scaphae.
**e. of superior semicircular canal,** eminentia arcuata.
**terete e.,** eminentia medialis fossae rhomboideae.
**thenar e.,** thenar (def. 1).
**thyroid e.,** prominentia laryngea.
**triangular e., e. of triangular fossa of auricle,** eminentia fossae triangularis auriculae.
**trigeminal e.,** tuberculum trigeminale.
**e. of triquetral fossa,** eminentia fossae triangularis auriculae.
**trochlear e.,** trochlea humeri.
**ulnar e. of wrist,** eminentia carpi ulnaris.

**em·i·nen·tia** (em"ĭ-nen'shə) gen. and pl. *eminen'tiae* [L.] [TA] eminence: a general term for a prominence or projection, especially one on the surface of a bone.
**e. arcua'ta** [TA], arcuate eminence: an arched prominence on the internal surface of the petrous part of the temporal bone in the floor of the middle cranial fossa, marking the position of the superior semicircular canal. It is particularly prominent in young skulls. Called also *eminence of superior semicircular canal.*
**e. articula'ris os'sis tempora'lis,** tuberculum articulare ossis temporalis.
**e. capita'ta,** capitulum humeri.
**e. car'pi radia'lis,** an eminence on the palmar surface of the radial side of the wrist, formed by the tubercles on the scaphoid and trapezium bones; called also *radial eminence of wrist.*
**e. car'pi ulna'ris,** an eminence on the palmar surface of the ulnar side of the wrist, formed by the pisiform bone and the hook of the hamate bone; called also *ulnar eminence of wrist.*
**e. collatera'lis ventri'culi latera'lis** [TA], collateral eminence of lateral ventricle: an elevation in the floor of the temporal horn of the lateral ventricle, produced by the collateral sulcus.
**e. con'chae** [TA], eminence of concha: the projection on the medial surface of the auricle that corresponds to the concha on the lateral surface.
**e. crucia'ta,** e. cruciformis.
**e. crucifor'mis** [TA], cruciform eminence of occipital bone: the cross-shaped bony prominence on the internal surface of the squama of the occipital bone, at the intersection of the ridges as-

sociated with the sulci of the superior sagittal sinus and the transverse sinuses. Called also *e. cruciata* and *cruciate line*.
**e. fos'sae triangula'ris auri'culae** [TA], eminence of triangular fossa of auricle: the protuberance on the medial surface of the auricle of the ear that corresponds to the triangular fossa on the lateral surface. Called also *triangular eminence*.
**e. fronta'lis,** TA alternative for *tuber frontale*.
**e. hypothena'ris,** TA alternative for *hypothenar* (def. 1).
**e. iliopecti'nea,** e. iliopubica.
**e. iliopu'bica** [TA], iliopubic eminence: a diffuse enlargement just anterior to the acetabulum, marking the junction of the ilium with the superior ramus of the pubis; called also *e. iliopectinea, iliopectineal eminence* or *tubercle,* and *iliopubic tuber* or *tubercle*.
**e. intercondyla'ris** [TA], **e. intercondyloi'dea, e. interme'dia,** intercondylar eminence: an eminence on the proximal extremity of the tibia, surmounted on either side by a prominent tubercle, on to the sides of which the articular facets are prolonged; called also *intermediate eminence* and *tuberculum intercondyloideum*.
**e. jugula'ris,** tuberculum jugulare ossis occipitalis.
**e. maxil'lae,** TA alternative for *tuber maxillae*.
**e. maxilla're, e. maxilla'ris,** tuber maxillae.
**e. media'lis fos'sae rhomboi'deae** [TA], medial eminence of rhomboid fossa: an eminence in the medial part of the floor of the fourth ventricle, bounded laterally by the sulcus limitans and produced by the facial colliculus and the trigone of the hypoglossal nerve. Called also *e. teres* and *terete eminence*.
**e. orbita'lis os'sis zygoma'tici,** orbital eminence of zygomatic bone: a small tubercle that is usually present on the orbital surface of the frontal process of the zygomatic bone, within the orbital opening inferior to the frontozygomatic suture.
**e. parieta'lis,** TA alternative for tuber parietale.
**e. pyramida'lis** [TA], pyramidal eminence: an elevation in the posterior wall of the middle ear, which contains the stapedius muscle.
**e. sca'phae** [TA], eminence of scapha: the prominence on the medial side of the auricle of the external ear that corresponds to the scapha on the lateral side.
**e. sym'physis,** the prominent lower border of the middle of the chin.
**e. te'res,** e. medialis fossae rhomboideae.
**e. thena'ris,** TA alternative for *thenar* (def. 1).

**emio·cy·to·sis** (e″me-o-si-to'sis) the ejection of material from a cell. Cf. *exocytosis* (def. 1).

**emis·sa·ri·um** (em″ĭ-sar'e-əm) pl. *emissa'ria* [L.] vena emissaria.
**e. condyloi'deum,** vena emissaria condyloidea.
**e. mastoi'deum,** vena emissaria mastoidea.
**e. occipita'le,** vena emissaria occipitalis.
**e. parieta'le,** vena emissaria parietalis.

**em·is·sa·ry** (em'ĭ-sar″e) [L. *emissarium* drain] 1. affording an outlet, as an emissary vein. 2. vena emissaria.

**emis·sion** (e-mish'ən) [L. *emissio,* a sending out] 1. a discharge. 2. an involuntary discharge of semen.
**nocturnal e.,** reflex emission of the semen during sleep.
**otoacoustic e's (OAE),** subtle sounds produced by amplifying processes in the cochlea during normal hearing and transmitted through the middle ear to the external auditory canal.
**positron e.,** a form of radioactive decay in which a positron ($\beta^+$) and neutrino are ejected from the nucleus as a proton is transformed into a neutron. Collision of the positron with an electron causes annihilation of both particles and conversion of their masses into energy in the form of two 0.511 MeV gamma rays.
**thermionic e.,** the emission of electrons and ions by incandescent bodies.
**transient evoked otoacoustic e's (TEOAE),** sounds produced by the cochlea in response to sound stimuli, measured by a microphone placed in the external auditory canal; used to test the integrity of the cochlea in screening neonates for sensorineural hearing loss.

**emis·siv·i·ty** (e″mĭ-siv'ĭ-te) the ratio of emissive power (of radiant energy) of a surface to that of a black surface having the same temperature.

**EMIT** (e-mit') [*E*nzyme-*M*ultiplied *I*mmunoassay *T*echnique] trademark for a homogeneous (single phase) enzyme immunoassay which utilizes the change in enzyme activity of an enzyme-labeled hapten that occurs on binding with antibody to determine the amount of unlabeled hapten (the unknown) present in a biologic specimen.

**em·men·a·gog·ic** (ə-men″ə-goj'ik) inducing menstruation.

**em·men·a·gogue** (ə-men'ə-gog) [Gr. *emmēna* menses + *-agogue*] an agent or measure that induces menstruation.
**direct e.,** an agent that induces menstruation by acting directly upon the reproductive organs.
**indirect e.,** an agent or measure that acts to induce menstruation by relieving another condition of which amenorrhea is a secondary result.

**em·me·nia** (ə-men'e-ə) [Gr. *emmēna*] menses.

**em·men·ic** (ə-men'ik) menstrual.

**em·me·ni·op·a·thy** (ə-me″ne-op'ə-the) [Gr. *emmēnios* menses + *-pathy*] any disorder of menstruation.

**em·me·nol·o·gy** (em″ə-nol'ə-je) [Gr. *emmēna* menses + *-logy*] the sum of knowledge regarding menstruation and its disorders.

**Em·met's operation, retractor** (em'əts) [Thomas Addis *Emmet,* American gynecologist, 1828–1919] see under *operation* and *retractor*.

**em·me·trope** (em'ə-trōp) an individual who has no refractive error of vision.

**em·me·tro·pia** (em″ə-tro'pe-ə) [Gr. *emmetros* in proper measure + *-opia*] a state of proper correlation between the refractive system of the eye and the axial length of the eyeball, rays of light entering the eye parallel to the optic axis being brought to a focus exactly on the retina. Symbol E.

**em·me·trop·ic** (em″ə-trop'ik) pertaining to or characterized by emmetropia.

**Em·mon·sia** (ĕ-mon'se-ə) a genus of saprobic Fungi Imperfecti of the form-family Moniliaceae. Two species, *E. cres'cens* and *E. par'va,* cause adiaspiromycosis in rodents and humans. Called also *Haplosporangium*.

**em·o·din** (em'o-din) [from *Rheum emodi,* a Himalayan rhubarb] [MeSH: Emodin] a purgative compound, trihydroxymethyl anthraquinone, from rhubarb, aloes, senna, and cascara sagrada.

**emol·li·ent** (e-mol'e-ənt) [L. *emolliens* softening, from *e* out + *mollis* soft] 1. softening or soothing; called also *malactic*. 2. an agent which softens or soothes the skin, or soothes an irritated internal surface; called also *malagma*.

**emo·tion** (e-mo'shən) [L. *emovere* to disturb] [MeSH: Emotions] a strong feeling state, such as excitement, distress, happiness, sadness, love, hate, fear, or anger, arising subjectively and directed toward a specific object, with physiological, somatic, and behavioral components. In psychoanalytic theory, it is a state of tension associated with an instinctual drive. The external manifestation of emotion is called *affect;* a pervasive and sustained emotional state, *mood*.

**emo·tion·al** (e-mo'shən-əl) pertaining to the emotions.

**Emp.** abbreviation for L. *emplas'trum,* a plaster.

**em·pa·cho** (em-pah'cho) a Mexican term for chronic indigestion in children with diarrhea.

**em·pas·ma** (em-paz'mə) [Gr. *en* in + *passein* to sprinkle] a powder for external use.

**em·path·ic** (em-path'ik) pertaining to or characterized by empathy.

**em·pa·thize** (em'pə-thīz) to experience or feel empathy.

**em·pa·thy** (em'pə-the) [Gr. *en* into + *-pathy*] [MeSH: Empathy] intellectual and emotional awareness and understanding of another person's thoughts, feelings, and behavior, even those that are distressing and disturbing. *Empathy* emphasizes understanding, *sympathy* emphasizes sharing, of another person's feelings and experiences.

**Em·ped·o·cles** (em-ped'o-klēz) (c. 493 to c. 433 B.C.) a Greek philosopher born in Acragas, Sicily. He accepted and combined pneumatism with his own theories of the four "roots" (earth, air, fire, and water) and of the two opposite, complementary forces (love and strife), which unite and reunite or separate and disintegrate the four roots in diverse proportions to form or destroy matter; thus health is a balance, disease an imbalance, of the roots by the forces. See also *Alcmaeon* and *humoralism*.

**em·phrax·is** (em-frak'sis) [Gr.] a stoppage or obstruction.

**em·phy·se·ma** (em″fə-se'mə) [Gr. "an inflation"] [MeSH: Emphysema] 1. a pathological accumulation of air in tissues or organs. 2. pulmonary e.
**acute bovine pulmonary e.,** fog fever.
**alveolar duct e.,** distention of the alveolar ducts as seen in elderly individuals, often producing little or no functional disturbance.
**atrophic e.,** senile e.
**bullous e.,** single or multiple large cystic alveolar dilatations of lung tissue; see also *paraseptal e.* Called also *cystic e.*

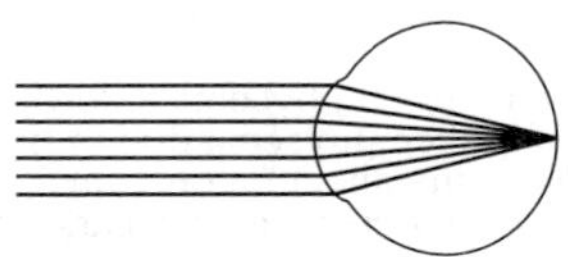

Emmetropia.

**centriacinar e., centrilobular e.,** one of the types of pulmonary emphysema, characterized by enlargement of air spaces in the proximal part of the acinus, primarily at the level of the respiratory bronchioles. See also *bronchiolectasis* and *coal workers' pneumoconiosis.*
**chronic hypertrophic e.,** panacinar e.
**compensating e., compensatory e.,** overdistention of lung tissue, which fills a void produced by contraction, atelectasis, surgical resection, fibrosis, or otherwise reduced volume of another part of the lung.
**cutaneous e.,** subcutaneous e.
**cystic e.,** bullous e.
**diffuse e.,** panacinar e.
**distal acinar e.,** one of the types of pulmonary emphysema, limited to the distal ends of the alveoli along the interlobular septa and beneath the pleura, forming bullae; see also *bullous e.* Called also *interlobular* or *paraseptal e.*
**ectatic e.,** panacinar e.
**false e.,** deformity of the thoracic cage simulating that associated with pulmonary emphysema (increased anterior-posterior diameter, elevated rib angle, etc.); the lungs may or may not be normal. Called also *skeletal e.*
**focal e., focal dust e.,** centriacinar emphysema associated with inhalation of environmental dusts, producing dilatation of the terminal and respiratory bronchioles.
**generalized e.,** pulmonary emphysema affecting all portions of both lungs in a similar manner.
**glass blower's e.,** emphysema of the lungs attributed to overstrain in glass blowers.
**hypoplastic e.,** pulmonary emphysema due to a developmental abnormality resulting in reduced number of alveoli, which are abnormally large; it may affect a pulmonary segment, lobe, or an entire lung.
**idiopathic unilobar e.,** a syndrome characterized by emphysematous expansion of one lobe of the lung, with the production of dyspnea and cyanosis.
**interlobular e.,** distal acinar e.
**interstitial e.,** escape of air into the connective tissue of the lung, mediastinum (see *pneumomediastinum*), or subcutaneous tissue (see *subcutaneous e.*); it results from a tear or rupture of the respiratory passages or alveoli, which may occur in association with bronchiolar obstruction, positive pressure ventilation, or a penetrating wound of the chest wall or lung.
**intestinal e.,** pneumatosis cystoides intestinalis.
**lobar e.,** emphysema involving fewer than all the lobes of the affected lung. Cf. *unilateral e.*
**lobar e., congenital, lobar e., infantile,** a condition characterized by overinflation, commonly affecting one of the upper lobes and causing respiratory distress in early life; called also *congenital lobar overinflation.*
**e. of lungs,** pulmonary e.
**mediastinal e.,** pneumomediastinum.
**obstructive e.,** overinflation of the lungs associated with partial bronchial obstruction which interferes with exhalation.
**obstructive e., localized,** overinflation of a lobe or segment of lung, often due to partial bronchial obstruction; called also *obstructive pulmonary overinflation.*
**panacinar e., panlobular e.,** one of the types of pulmonary emphysema, characterized by relatively uniform enlargement of air spaces throughout the acini. Called also *chronic hypertrophic e., diffuse e., ectatic e., generalized e.,* and *vesicular e.*
**paracicatricial e.,** alveolar distention occurring in the vicinity of pulmonary scars.
**paraseptal e.,** distal acinar e.
**pulmonary e.,** a condition of the lung characterized by increase beyond normal in the size of air spaces distal to the terminal bronchioles. Types named according to location of the damage include *centriacinar e., distal acinar e.,* and *panacinar e.*
**pulmonary e. of cattle, acute,** fog fever.
**pulmonary interstitial e. (PIE),** a condition occurring mainly in premature infants, in which air leaks from the alveoli of the lungs into the interstitial spaces; it is often associated with underlying lung disease or with the use of mechanical ventilation.
**senile e.,** pulmonary emphysema due to atrophic changes and dilatation of the alveoli occurring with age. Called also *atrophic e.*
**skeletal e.,** false e.
**small-lunged e.,** atrophic e.
**subcutaneous e.,** interstitial emphysema characterized by the presence of air in the subcutaneous tissue, usually caused by intrathoracic injury, and in most instances associated with pneumothorax and pneumomediastinum. Called also *cutaneous e.* and *pneumoderma.*
**surgical e.,** subcutaneous emphysema following surgical operation.
**traumatic e.,** interstitial emphysema due to trauma.
**unilateral e.,** emphysema affecting only one lung; it may be either congenital (such as from defects in circulation) or acquired *(Swyer-James syndrome).* Cf. *lobar e.* Called also *hyperlucent lung.*
**vesicular e.,** panacinar e.

**em·phy·sem·a·tous** (em″fə-sem′ə-təs) of the nature of or affected with emphysema.

**Em·pir·ic** (em-pir′ik) [Gr. *empeirikos* experienced] the second of the post-hippocratic schools of medicine, which arose in the second century B.C., under the leadership of Philinos of Cos and Serapion of Alexandria. As opposed to the Dogmatists, the Empirics declared that the search for the ultimate causes of phenomena was vain, but they were active in endeavoring to discover the immediate causes. They paid particular attention to the totality of symptoms. In their search for a line of treatment to benefit a particular set of symptoms they employed the "tripod of the Empirics": (1) their own chance observations—their own experience; (2) learning obtained from contemporaries and predecessors—the experience of others; and (3) in cases of new diseases, the formation of conclusions from other diseases which they resembled—analogy. The Empirics paid great attention to clinical observation, and were guided in their methods of treatment almost entirely by experience.

**em·pir·ic** (em-pir′ik) 1. empirical. 2. a practitioner whose skill is based on experience.

**em·pir·i·cal** (em-pir′ĭ-kəl) based on experience.

**em·pir·i·cism** (em-pir′ĭ-siz-əm) [MeSH: Empiricism] 1. the method of the Empiric school of medicine; opposed to rational medicine. 2. reliance on mere experience; empirical practice. 3. quackery.

**em·plas·tic** (em-plas′tik) [Gr. *emplastikos* stopping up] 1. adhesive or glutinous. 2. a constipating medicine.

**em·plas·trum** (em-plas′trəm) [L.; Gr. *emplastron*] plaster (def. 2).

**em·po·ri·at·rics** (em-por″e-at′riks) [Gr. *emporos* one who goes on shipboard as a passenger + *-iatrics*] that branch of medicine which treats of the health problems of international travelers.

**em·pros·thot·o·nos** (em″pros-thot′ə-nəs) [Gr. *emprosthen* forward + *tonos* tension] a form of tetanic spasm in which the head and feet are brought forward and the body is rendered tense; called also *episthotonos.*

**em·pros·thot·o·nus** (em″pros-thot′ə-nəs) emprosthotonos.

**em·py·e·ma** (em″pi-e′mə) [Gr. *empyema*] [MeSH: Empyema] 1. abscess. 2. a pleural effusion (q.v.) containing pus; called also *thoracic e., purulent* or *suppurative pleurisy,* and *pyothorax.*
**e. arti′culi,** acute suppurative synovitis.
**e. benig′num,** latent e.
**e. of the chest,** empyema (def. 2).
**e. of gallbladder,** cholecystitis in which the contents of the acutely inflamed gallbladder are turbid or appear to be frankly purulent.
**interlobar e.,** thoracic empyema situated between two lobes of the lung.
**latent e.,** thoracic empyema unaccompanied by any symptoms. Called also *e. benignum.*
**loculated e.,** thoracic empyema in which the pus is trapped in an enclosed space.
**mastoid e.,** suppurative inflammation of the mucous lining of the cavities of the mastoid process.
**metapneumonic e.,** thoracic empyema developing some time after the subsidence of the pneumonia; cf. *synpneumonic e.*
**e. necessita′tis,** thoracic empyema in which the pus can make a spontaneous escape toward the chest wall.
**e. of pericardium,** purulent pericarditis.
**pneumococcal e.,** thoracic empyema due to infection with *Streptococcus pneumoniae.*
**pulsating e.,** thoracic empyema in which the movements of the heart produce a visible vibration of the chest wall.
**putrid e.,** thoracic empyema in which the pus has become more or less decomposed.
**streptococcal e.,** thoracic empyema due to infection with *Streptococcus pyogenes.*
**synpneumonic e.,** thoracic empyema arising during the course of pulmonary inflammation. Cf. *metapneumonic e.*
**thoracic e.,** empyema (def. 2).
**tuberculous e.,** thoracic empyema due to infection with *Mycobacterium tuberculosis.*

**em·py·emic** (em″pi-e′mik) pertaining to or of the nature of empyema.

**em·py·e·sis** (em″pi-e′sis) [Gr. *empyēsis* suppuration] 1. a pustular eruption. 2. any disease characterized by phlegmonous vesicles becoming filled with purulent fluid.

**em·pyo·cele** (em′pi-o-sēl) [Gr. *empyein* to suppurate + *-cele*[1]] a collection of pus at the umbilicus.

**em·py·reu·ma** (em″pi-roo′mə) [Gr. *empyreuma* a live coal] the distinctive odor of animal or vegetable matter when charred in a closed vessel.

**em·py·reu·mat·ic** (em-pi′roo-mat′ik) pertaining to empyreuma;

pertaining to or produced by destructive distillation of organic matter.

**EMS** Emergency Medical Service.

**emul.** abbreviation for L. *emul'sum* emulsion.

**emul·gent** (e-mul'jənt) [L. *emulgere* to milk or drain out] 1. causing a straining or purifying process. 2. a medicine that stimulates the flow of bile or urine.

**emul·si·fi·er** (e-mul'sĭ-fi″ər) an agent used to produce an emulsion.

**emul·si·fy** (e-mul'sĭ-fi) to convert or to be converted into an emulsion.

**emul·sion** (e-mul'shən) [L. *emulsio, emulsum*] a preparation of one liquid distributed in small globules throughout the body of a second liquid. The dispersed liquid is the discontinuous phase, and the dispersion medium is the continuous phase. When oil is the dispersed liquid and an aqueous solution is the continuous phase, it is known as an oil-in-water emulsion, whereas when water or aqueous solution is the dispersed phase and oil or oleaginous substance is the continuous phase, it is known as a water-in-oil emulsion. Pharmaceutical emulsions for which official standards have been promulgated include cod liver oil emulsion, cod liver oil emulsion with malt, liquid petrolatum emulsion, and phenolphthalein in liquid petrolatum emulsion.
**hexachlorophene cleansing e.** [USP], an emulsion containing hexachlorophene in a suitable aqueous vehicle; used as a topical anti-infective and detergent.
**kerosene e.,** an emulsion of kerosene in soap solution, used as an insecticide.
**liquid petrolatum e.,** mineral oil e.
**mineral oil e.** [USP], an emulsion of mineral oil, acacia, syrup, vanillin, and alcohol in purified water, used as a cathartic; called also *liquid petrolatum e.*
**photographic e.,** a light- and radiation-sensitive gelatinous coating incorporating silver halide which is applied to film.

**emul·sive** (e-mul'siv) 1. capable of emulsifying a substance. 2. susceptible of being emulsified. 3. affording an oil on pressure.

**emul·soid** (e-mul'soid) 1. lyophilic colloid 2. rarely, emulsion.

**emul·sum** (e-mul'səm) pl. *emul'sa* [L.] an emulsion.

**emunc·to·ry** (e-munk'tə-re) [L. *emungere* to cleanse] 1. excretory or depurant. 2. any excretory organ or duct.

**E-My·cin** (e-mi'sin) trademark for a preparation of erythromycin.

**ENA** extractable nuclear antigens.

**enal·a·pril** (ə-nal'ə-pril) [MeSH: Enalapril] an angiotensin-converting enzyme inhibitor used as an antihypertensive; available as *enalapril maleate.*

**enal·a·pril·at** (ə-nal'ə-pril″ət) [USP] [MeSH: Enalaprilat] an angiotensin-converting enzyme inhibitor, the active metabolite of enalapril, administered intravenously in the treatment of hypertensive crisis or when oral administration of enalapril maleate is impractical.

**enam·el** (ə-nam'əl) [O.F. *esmail*] 1. the glazed surface of baked porcelain, metal, or pottery. 2. any hard, smooth, glossy coating. 3. dental e.
**curled e.,** dental enamel in which the columns are bent and are wavy and intertwined with one another. Called also *gnarled e.* Cf. *straight e.*
**dental e.,** a hard, thin, translucent layer of calcified substance that envelops and protects the dentin of the crown of the tooth; it is the hardest substance in the body and is almost entirely composed of calcium salts. Called also *adamantine layer, enamel, enamelum* [TA], and *substantia adamantina dentis.*
**dwarfed e.,** nanoid e.
**gnarled e.,** curled e.
**hereditary brown e.,** amelogenesis imperfecta.
**hypoplastic e.,** enamel hypoplasia.
**mottled e.,** a chronic endemic form of hypoplasia of the dental enamel caused by drinking water with a high fluorine content during the time of tooth formation, and characterized by defective calcification that gives a white chalky appearance to the enamel, which gradually undergoes brown discoloration. Called also *dental fluorosis* and *mottled teeth.*
**nanoid e.,** imperfectly formed dental enamel that is thinner than normal. Called also *dwarfed e.*
**straight e.,** dental enamel in which the rods are straight. Cf. *curled e.*

**enam·elo·blast** (ə-nam'əl-o-blast) ameloblast.

**enam·elo·blas·to·ma** (ə-nam″əl-o-blas-to'mə) ameloblastoma.

**enam·el·o·ma** (ə-nam″əl-o'mə) [*enamel* + *-oma*] a non-neoplastic excrescence sometimes found at the bifurcation of a multirooted tooth, at the end of an enamel spur, or on the root surface, which may be composed only of enamel, contain a small dentin nucleus, or contain a minute strand of dentin and pulp. Called also *enamel drop* and *enamel pearl.*

**enam·e·lo·plas·ty** (ə-nam'ə-lo-plas″te) contouring of the enamel surface of a tooth to remove superficial grooves and other defects.

**enam·e·lum** (ə-nam'əl-əm) [L.] [TA] dental enamel.

**en·an·thate** (ə-nan'thāt) the anionic form of enanthic acid; the term is used as a USAN contraction for heptanoate.

**en·an·them** (ə-nan'thəm) enanthema.

**en·an·the·ma** (en″ən-the'mə) pl. *enanthe'mas, enanthem'ata* [Gr. *en* in + *anthema* a blossoming] an eruption upon a mucous surface.

**en·an·them·a·tous** (en″ən-them'ə-təs) pertaining to or of the nature of an enanthema.

**enan·thic ac·id** (ə-nan'thik) a saturated seven-carbon fatty acid, heptanoic acid, not definitely occurring in nature but producible by oxidation of fats.

**en·an·tio·bio·sis** (en-an″te-o-bi-o'sis) [Gr. *enantios* opposite + *biosis*] the condition in which organisms living together antagonize one another's development. Cf. *symbiosis,* def. 1.

**en·an·tio·mer** (en-an'te-o″mər) one of a pair of compounds having a mirror image relationship. Called also *enantiomorph.*

**en·an·ti·om·er·ism** (en-an″te-om'ər-iz-əm) [Gr. *enantios* opposite + *mero-* + *-ism*] the relationship between two stereoisomers having molecules that are mirror images of each other. Enantiomers have identical chemical and physical properties in an achiral environment. However, they form different products when reacted with other chiral molecules, and they exhibit optical activity. The enantiomer that rotates the plane of polarization of a beam of polarized light in the clockwise direction is indicated by the prefix (+)-, formerly *d-* or dextro-. The other enantiomer rotates the plane of polarization an equal amount in the counterclockwise direction and is indicated by the prefix (−)-, formerly *l-* or levo-. Two conventions are used to designate the actual configurations of enantiomers. The D, L system (see D-) is used to denote the configuration of carbohydrates relative to D-(+)-glyceraldehyde and of amino acids relative to L-(−)-serine. The *R,S* system (see *R-*) is a more general system used to specify the absolute configuration at every asymmetric carbon atom. An equimolar mixture of enantiomers (a racemic form or racemic modification) is optically inactive and is designated by the prefixes (±)-, DL-, or *dl-.*

**en·an·tio·morph** (en-an'te-o-morf″) enantiomer.

**en·an·tio·mor·phic** (en-an″te-o-mor'fik) pertaining to or exhibiting the characteristics of an enantiomorph.

**en·an·tio·mor·phism** (en-an″te-o-mor'fiz-əm) enantiomerism.

**en·ar·thri·tis** (en″ahr-thri'tis) inflammation of an enarthrosis.

**en·ar·thro·di·al** (en″ahr-thro'de-əl) of or pertaining to an enarthrosis; see *articulatio spheroidea.*

**en·ar·thro·sis** (en″ahr-thro'sis) [Gr. *en* in + *arthrosis*] articulatio spheroidea.

**en bloc** (ahn blok') [Fr.] in a lump; as a whole.

**en·cain·ide hy·dro·chlo·ride** (en-ka'nīd) a sodium channel blocker that acts on the Purkinje fibers and myocardium, used in the treatment of life-threatening arrhythmias; administered orally.

**en·can·this** (en-kan'this) [Gr., from *en* in + *kanthos* the angle of the eye] a small red excrescence on the semilunar fold of the conjunctiva and inner lacrimal caruncle.

**en·cap·su·lat·ed** (en-kap'su-lāt-əd) [Gr. *en* in + *capsula* + *-ate*] enclosed within a capsule.

**en·cap·su·la·tion** (ən-kap″su-la'shən) 1. any act of inclosing in a capsule. 2. a physiologic process of inclosure in a sheath made up of a substance not normal to the part.

**en·cap·suled** (en-kap'səld) encapsulated.

**en·car·di·tis** (en″kahr-di'tis) endocarditis.

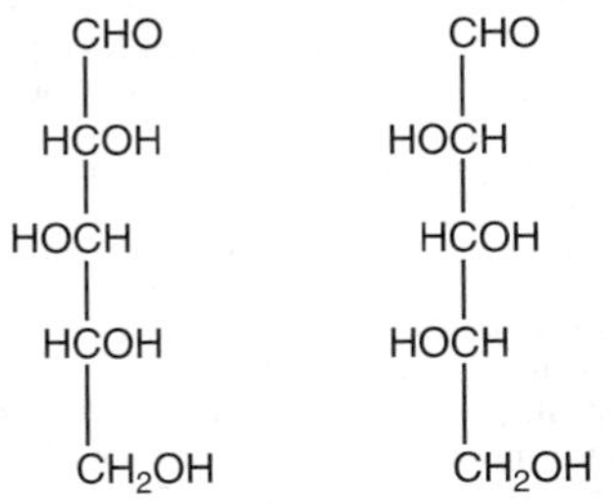

| | |
|---|---|
| CHO | CHO |
| HCOH | HOCH |
| HOCH | HCOH |
| HCOH | HOCH |
| $CH_2OH$ | $CH_2OH$ |

Enantiomerism.

**en·ca·tar·rha·phy** (en″kə-tahr′ə-fe) [Gr. *enkatarrhaptein* to sew in] the operation of burying a structure by suturing together the sides of the tissues adjacent to it.

**en·ce·li·al·gia** (en″se-le-al′jə) [Gr. *en* in + *celi-* + *-algia*] pain in an abdominal viscus.

**en·ce·li·itis** (en-se″le-i′tis) [Gr. *en* in + *celi-* + *-itis*] inflammation of an intra-abdominal organ.

**en·ce·li·tis** (en″se-li′tis) enceliitis.

**en·ceph·a·lal·gia** (en-sef″ə-lal′jə) [*encephal-* + *-algia*] headache.

**en·ceph·a·lat·ro·phy** (en-sef″ə-lat′ro-fe) [*encephalo-* + *atrophy*] atrophy of the brain.

**en·ceph·a·lauxe** (en″sef-ə-lawk′se) [*encephal-* + Gr. *auxē* increase] macrencephaly.

**en·ce·phal·ic** (en″sə-fal′ik) 1. pertaining to the encephalon. 2. within the skull.

**en·ceph·a·lit·ic** (en-sef″ə-lit′ik) pertaining to or affected with encephalitis.

**en·ceph·a·lit·i·des** (en-sef″ə-lit′ĭ-dēz) [Gr.] [MeSH: Encephalitis] plural of *encephalitis.*

**en·ceph·a·li·tis** (en-sef″ə-li′tis) pl. *encephalit′ides* [*encephalo-* + *-itis*] [MeSH: Encephalitis] inflammation of the brain.
**e. A,** lethargic e.
**acute disseminated e.,** see under *encephalomyelitis.*
**acute necrotizing e.,** encephalitis characterized by a particularly destructive reaction in the brain; cf. *herpes simplex e.* and *acute necrotizing hemorrhagic encephalomyelitis.*
**Australian X e.,** Murray Valley e.
**e. B,** Japanese B e.
**benign myalgic e.,** epidemic neuromyasthenia.
**Binswanger's e.,** see under *disease.*
**bovine e.,** Buss disease.
**e. C,** St. Louis e.
**California e.,** a usually mild form of encephalitis caused by a bunyavirus and transmitted chiefly by the mosquito *Aedes melanimon;* it primarily affects children.
**caprine arthritis-e.,** a disease of goats caused by a lentivirus. In kids it is characterized by encephalitis with paresis that is often fatal. In adults it takes the form of chronic arthritis with swollen carpal joints, giving it its nickname of *big knee.*
**Central European e.,** the milder form of tick-borne encephalitis, first noted in Central Europe.
**chronic subcortical e.,** Binswanger's disease.
**cytomegalovirus e.,** opportunistic infection of the brain by cytomegalovirus, seen in patients with immunodeficiency. Variable symptoms include seizures, clouding of consciousness, and other symptoms similar to those of the AIDS dementia complex.
**Dawson's e.,** subacute sclerosing panencephalitis.
**eastern equine e.,** see under *encephalomyelitis.*
**Economo's e.,** lethargic e.
**enzootic e. of horses,** Borna disease.
**epidemic e., e. epide′mica,** any viral encephalitis that occurs in epidemics; common types are *Japanese B e., St. Louis e.,* and *tick-borne e.* See also *equine encephalomyelitis.*
**equine e.,** 1. equine encephalomyelitis. 2. Borna disease.
**forest-spring e.,** tick-borne e.
**fox e.,** a disease of foxes, raccoons, and coyotes, considered to be a form of infectious canine hepatitis.
**granulomatous amebic e.,** a chronic type of encephalitis, usually seen in debilitated or immunocompromised persons, caused by infection with species of *Acanthamoeba;* characteristics include focal granulomas, often with headaches, seizures, nausea, and vomiting.
**hemorrhagic e.,** encephalitis in which there is inflammation of the brain with hemorrhagic foci and perivascular exudate; common types are herpes simplex encephalitis and acute necrotizing hemorrhagic encephalomyelitis. Called also *Strümpell-Leichtenstern e.*
**herpes e., herpes simplex e., herpetic e.,** the most common form of acute encephalitis, caused by herpesvirus and characterized by hemorrhagic necrosis of parts of the temporal and frontal lobes. Onset is over several days and involves fever, headache, seizures, stupor, and often coma, frequently with a fatal outcome.
**HIV e.,** see under *encephalopathy.*
**Ilheus e.,** a viral encephalitis transmitted by mosquitoes in Brazil. See also under *virus.*
**influenzal e.,** encephalitis occurring as a complication of influenza.
**Japanese e., Japanese B e.,** a form of epidemic encephalitis caused by a flavivirus and transmitted by the bites of infected mosquitoes, especially *Culex tritaeniorhyncus,* in eastern and southern Asia and nearby islands. It may occur as a symptomless subclinical infection or as an acute meningoencephalomyelitis with cortical damage and cord lesions resembling those of poliomyelitis. Called also *e. B* and *Russian autumnal e.* See also under *virus.*
**La Crosse e.,** encephalitis caused by the La Crosse virus, transmitted by *Aedes triseriatus,* and occurring primarily in children, chiefly in the midwestern United States.
**lead e.,** see under *encephalopathy.*
**Leichtenstern's e.,** hemorrhagic e.
**lethargic e., e. lethar′gica,** a form of epidemic encephalitis, the original type described by von Economo, characterized by increasing languor, apathy, and drowsiness, passing into lethargy; observed in various parts of the world between 1915 and 1926. Called also *e. A, Economo's e.* or *disease, Vienna e.,* and *von Economo's e.* or *disease.*
**limbic e.,** encephalitis of the limbic system of the rhinencephalon, a type similar to herpes encephalitis, characterized by degenerative changes of the hippocampus and amygdaloid nuclei with memory loss, confusion, seizures, and progressive dementia. There is sometimes an association with tumors elsewhere in the body, although some authorities speculate a link to chemotherapy or other tumor treatments.
**microglial nodular e.,** a manifestation of cytomegalovirus encephalitis that appears earlier than cytomegalovirus ventriculoencephalitis and is characterized by acute onset with confusion and delirium.
**Murray Valley e.,** a viral encephalitis that occurred epidemically in 1950 and 1951 in the Murray Valley, Victoria, Australia, and was later proved to be a recurrence of the Australian X encephalitis of the 1920's. It is caused by a flavivirus that infects birds and mosquitoes, most often in northern Australia and New Guinea. Epidemics are infrequent and children are the most seriously affected. See also under *virus.*
**Ontario e.,** vomiting and wasting disease.
**e. periaxia′lis concen′trica,** Baló's disease.
**e. periaxia′lis diffu′sa,** Schilder's disease.
**postinfectious e., postvaccinal e.,** acute disseminated encephalomyelitis.
**Powassan e.,** a form of viral encephalitis reported in Ontario in 1958, caused by the Powassan virus and closely resembling Russian spring-summer encephalitis.
**purulent e., pyogenic e.,** suppurative e.
**Russian autumnal e.,** Japanese B e.
**Russian endemic e., Russian forest-spring e.,** tick-borne e.
**Russian spring-summer e.,** the severe form of tick-borne encephalitis, occurring mainly in the far eastern part of Russia.
**Russian tick-borne e., Russian vernal e.,** tick-borne e.
**St. Louis e.,** a form of epidemic encephalitis caused by a flavivirus, first observed in Illinois in 1932; it is similar to western equine encephalomyelitis clinically, occurring in late summer and early fall and transmitted usually by mosquitoes of the genus *Culex.* It ranges from an abortive type of infection to severe disease and affects the elderly most often. Called also *e. C.*
**Schilder's e.,** see under *disease.*
**Semliki Forest e.,** a form due to a virus transmitted by mosquitoes in western Uganda. See also under *virus.*
**Strümpell-Leichtenstern e.,** hemorrhagic e.
**subacute inclusion body e.,** subacute sclerosing panencephalitis.
**e. subcortica′lis chron′ica,** Binswanger's disease.
**summer e.,** Japanese B e.
**suppurative e.,** encephalitis accompanied by suppuration and abscess formation; called also *purulent e.* and *pyogenic e.*
**tick-borne e.,** a form of epidemic encephalitis usually spread by the bites of ticks *(Ixodes persulcatus)* infected with flaviviruses; occasionally it may be spread via raw milk from goats, sheep, or cows infected with the virus. It ranges in severity from mild to fatal and there may be degenerative changes in organs other than those of the nervous system. The more common, severe form is *Russian spring-summer e.;* a milder form is called *Central European e.* Called also *Russian endemic, Russian forest-spring, Russian tick-borne,* or *Russian vernal e.*
**toxoplasmic e.,** see under *meningoencephalitis.*
**van Bogaert's e.,** subacute sclerosing panencephalitis.
**Venezuelan equine e.,** see under *encephalomyelitis.*
**vernal e., vernoestival e.,** tick-borne e.
**Vienna e.,** lethargic e.
**von Economo's e.,** lethargic e.
**western equine e.,** see under *encephalomyelitis.*
**West Nile e.,** a mild, febrile, sporadic disease caused by the flavivirus West Nile virus, transmitted by *Culex* mosquitoes, occurring chiefly in the summer; frequently, infection does not lead to encephalitis. It may be of sudden onset, and symptoms may include drowsiness, severe frontal headache, maculopapular rash, abdominal pain, loss of appetite, nausea, and generalized lymphadenopathy. It was first reported in Uganda, but is widespread elsewhere in Africa and also occurs in southern Europe, the Middle East, and southern Asia.
**woodcutter's e.,** tick-borne e.

**en·ceph·a·lit·o·gen** (en-sef″ə-lit′o-jen) any agent that causes encephalitis and related conditions; cf. *experimental allergic encephalomyelitis.*

**en·ceph·a·lit·o·gen·ic** (en-sef″ə-lit-o-jen′ik) [*encephalitis* + *-genic*] causing encephalitis.

**En·ce·phal·i·to·zo·on** (en″sə-fal″ĭ-to-zo′on) [*encephal-* + Gr. *zōon* animal] [MeSH: Encephalitozoon] a genus of parasitic protozoa (suborder Apansporoblastina, order Microsporida), formerly thought to be identical with *Nosema,* first reported in the brains of rabbits.
**E. cuni′culi,** a species causing encephalitozoonosis in various mammals, including rabbits, mice, rats, guinea pigs, dogs, and cats; in humans it attacks mainly immunocompromised patients. It involves chiefly the brain and kidney but also such other organs as the liver and spleen. Called also *Nosema cuniculi.*
**E. hel′lem,** a species causing encephalitozoonosis in immunocompromised patients, mainly causing eye infections.
**E. intestina′lis,** a species causing encephalitozoonosis in immunocompromised patients, mainly causing gastrointestinal infections with severe diarrhea and wasting.

**en·ce·phal·i·to·zoo·no·sis** (en″sə-fal″ĭ-to-zo″o-no′sis) [*encephal-* + *zoonosis*] [MeSH: Encephalitozoonosis] infection with protozoa of the genus *Encephalitozoon.* It was formerly seen more in other animals than in humans, and the most common infection was with *E. cuniculi,* but now other species are seen as opportunistic pathogens of immunocompromised human patients. Different species cause different types of infections. Formerly called *nosematosis.*

**en·ceph·a·li·za·tion** (en-sef″ə-lĭ-za′shən) the developmental process by which the cerebral cortex has taken over the functions of the lower (spinal) centers.

**encephal(o)-** [L. *encephalon,* q.v.] a combining form denoting relationship to the brain.

**en·ceph·a·lo·cele** (en-sef′ə-lo-sēl″) [*encephalo-* + *cele*[1]] [MeSH: Encephalocele] hernia of part of the brain and meninges through a skull defect (cranium bifidum); it may be congenital, traumatic, or postoperative in origin. Called also *cephalocele, craniocele, encephalomeningocele,* and *meningoencephalocele.* Cf. *cranial meningocele* and *encephalocystocele.*
**basal e.,** an encephalocele in the region of the base of the skull.
**frontal e.,** encephalocele in the region of the frontal bone; seen more commonly in Asia and Africa than in the Western Hemisphere.
**occipital e.,** an encephalocele in the occipital region, the most common kind seen in the Western Hemisphere.

**en·ceph·a·lo·clas·tic** (en-sef″ə-lo-klas′tik) [*encephalo-* + *clastic*] exhibiting the residues of a destructive lesion in the brain; see *porencephaly.*

**en·ceph·a·lo·cys·to·cele** (en-sef″ə-lo-sis′to-sēl) [*encephalo-* + *cysto-* + *-cele*[1]] hydroencephalocele.

**en·ceph·a·lo·di·al·y·sis** (en-sef″ə-lo-di-al′ə-sis) [*encephalo-* + *dialysis*] encephalomalacia.

**en·ceph·a·lo·du·ro·ar·te·ri·o·syn·an·gi·o·sis** (en-sef″ə-lo-du″ro-ahr-te″re-o-sin-an-je-o′sis) a surgical treatment for moyamoya disease, consisting of transfer of a pedicle graft containing the superficial temporal artery onto the pia mater. In time, arterial linkages form between donor scalp artery branches and recipient brain surface artery branches to revascularize the cerebrum.

**en·ceph·a·lo·dys·pla·sia** (en-sef″ə-lo-dis-pla′zhə) any congenital anomaly of the brain.

**en·ceph·a·log·ra·phy** (en-sef″ə-log′rə-fe) [*encephalo-* + *-graphy*] radiography demonstrating the intracranial fluid-containing spaces after the withdrawal of cerebrospinal fluid and introduction of air or other gas; it includes pneumoencephalography and ventriculography.

**en·ceph·a·loid** (en-sef′ə-loid) [*encephalo-* + *-oid*] 1. resembling the brain or brain substance. 2. medullary carcinoma.

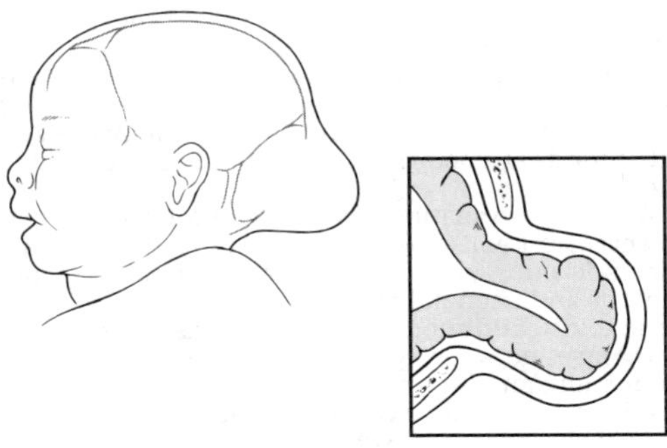

Encephalocele.

**en·ceph·a·lo·lith** (en-sef′ə-lo-lith″) [*encephalo-* + *-lith*] a brain calculus.

**en·ceph·a·lo·ma** (en-sef″ə-lo′mə) 1. any swelling or tumor of the brain. 2. medullary carcinoma.

**en·ceph·a·lo·ma·la·cia** (en-sef″ə-lo-mə-la′shə) [*encephalo-* + *-malacia*] [MeSH: Encephalomalacia] softening of the brain, especially that caused by an infarct.
**avian e.,** a disease of young chickens due to vitamin E deficiency, in which there is ataxia, incoordination, paralysis, and severe encephalomalacia in several areas of the brain, especially the cerebellum. It must be differentiated from avian encephalomyelitis. Called also *crazy chick disease.*
**nigropallidal e.,** neurotoxicity in horses that have spent an extended period grazing on *Centaurea repens* or *C. solstitialis,* which cause necrosis of the substantia nigra and globus pallidus; characteristics include wandering around in a confused manner and rigidity of facial muscles so that the animals cannot chew and may starve to death.

**en·ceph·a·lo·men·in·gi·tis** (en-sef″ə-lo-men″in-ji′tis) [*encephalo-* + *meningitis*] meningoencephalitis.

**en·ceph·a·lo·me·nin·go·cele** (en-sef″ə-lo-mə-ning′go-sēl) encephalocele.

**en·ceph·a·lo·men·in·gop·a·thy** (en-sef″ə-lo-men″in-gop′ə-the) meningoencephalopathy.

**en·ceph·a·lo·mere** (en-sef′ə-lo-mēr) [*encephalo-* + *-mere*] any one of the succession of segments which make up the embryonic brain.

**en·ceph·a·lom·e·ter** (en-sef″ə-lom′ə-tər) [*encephalo-* + *-meter*] an instrument used in locating certain of the regions of the brain.

**en·ceph·a·lo·my·eli·tis** (en-sef″ə-lo-mi″ə-li′tis) [MeSH: Encephalomyelitis] inflammation involving both the brain and the spinal cord. Called also *myeloencephalitis.*
**acute disseminated e.,** an acute or subacute encephalomyelitis or myelitis characterized by perivascular lymphocyte and mononuclear cell infiltration and demyelination; it occurs most commonly following an acute viral infection, especially measles, but may occur without a recognizable antecedent, and formerly occurred as a complication of rabies vaccination before the introduction of duck embryo and human diploid vaccines and of smallpox vaccination. It is believed to be a manifestation of an autoimmune attack on the myelin of the central nervous system. Clinical manifestations include fever, headache, vomiting, and drowsiness progressing to lethargy and coma; tremor, seizures, and paralysis may also occur; mortality ranges from 5 to 20 per cent; many survivors have residual neurologic deficits. Called also *acute perivascular myelinoclasis, postinfectious e., postvaccinal e.,* and *acute disseminated, postinfectious,* or *postvaccinal encephalitis.*
**acute necrotizing hemorrhagic e.,** a rare, fatal postinfection or allergic demyelinating disease of the central nervous system, having a fulminating course and occurring mainly in young adults. It is characterized by destruction of the white matter to the point of liquefaction; widespread necrosis of blood vessel walls leading to the formation of multiple small hemorrhages in the involved areas and the exudation of fibrin into the surrounding tissue; and cellular infiltration of the necrotic areas. Onset is abrupt and marked by headache, stiff neck, and confusion; these are followed by focal seizures, paralysis, progressively deepening coma, and death.
**autoimmune e.,** acute disseminated e.
**avian e.,** a viral disease of chickens under six weeks old, caused by an enterovirus and marked by weakness of the legs followed by partial or complete paralysis of the legs, trembling of the head and neck, and degeneration of the neurons in the pons, medulla, and anterior horns of the spinal cord. Clinically, it resembles avian encephalomalacia and must be differentiated from that condition. Called also *crazy chick disease* and *epidemic tremor.*
**benign myalgic e.,** chronic fatigue syndrome.
**bovine e.,** Buss disease.
**eastern equine e. (EEE),** a form of equine encephalomyelitis that occurs in the United States from New Hampshire west to Wisconsin and south to Texas, as well as in Canada, Mexico, the Caribbean, and parts of Central and South America. In humans it affects mainly children and the elderly; symptoms are fever, headache, and nausea followed by drowsiness, convulsions, and coma. Mortality is high in both humans and horses. Called also *eastern equine encephalitis.*
**equine e.,** a type of encephalomyelitis in horses and mules, caused by an alphavirus and spread to humans by mosquitoes; it occurs in summer epizootics in the Western Hemisphere. Three forms are recognized: *eastern equine e., western equine e.,* and *Venezuelan equine e.* Called also *equine encephalitis.* See also under *virus.*
**experimental allergic e. (EAE),** an animal model for acute disseminated encephalomyelitis in which the characteristic pathophysiology and clinical signs of this disease are produced by immunization of an animal with extracts of brain tissue or with myelin basic protein together with Freund's complete adjuvant; it is transferable by adoptive transfer of lymphocytes but not by serum.

**infectious porcine e.,** a type of encephalomyelitis of swine, seen primarily in Europe and caused by a picornavirus. It varies widely in severity; the severe form consists of a flaccid ascending paralysis similar to the paralysis of human poliomyelitis. Called also *porcine e., porcine poliomyelitis, Talfan disease,* and *Teschen disease.*
**Mengo e.,** a type of encephalomyelitis seen in monkeys and mongooses in East Africa, caused by an encephalomyocarditis virus.
**mouse e., murine e.,** Theiler's disease.
**porcine e., porcine viral e.,** infectious porcine e.
**postinfectious e., postvaccinal e.,** acute disseminated e.
**sporadic bovine e.,** Buss disease.
**Theiler's mouse e.,** Theiler's disease.
**toxoplasmic e.,** see under *meningoencephalitis.*
**Venezuelan equine e. (VEE),** a form of equine encephalomyelitis seen first in Colombia and Venezuela in the 1930's and later in Central America and the southwestern United States. The infection in humans resembles influenza, with only occasional central nervous system involvement; mortality is low. Called also *Venezuelan equine encephalitis.*
**viral e., virus e.,** encephalomyelitis caused by a virus.
**western equine e. (WEE),** a form of equine encephalomyelitis seen in the western United States, Canada, and from Mexico to South America; it is less severe and has a lower mortality rate than the eastern type. In humans it usually affects young children; symptoms are fever, drowsiness, and convulsions. Called also *western equine encephalitis.*

**en·ceph·a·lo·my·elo·cele** (en-sef″ə-lo-mi-′ə-lo-sēl) [*encephalo-* + *myelo-* + *-cele*[1]] abnormality of the foramen magnum and absence of the laminae and spinous processes of the cervical vertebrae, with herniation of meninges, brain substance, and spinal cord.

**en·ceph·a·lo·my·elo·neu·rop·a·thy** (en-sef″ə-lo-mi″ə-lo-noo-rop′ə-the) disease involving the brain, spinal cord, and peripheral nerves.

**en·ceph·a·lo·my·elop·a·thy** (en-sef″ə-lo-mi″əl-op′ə-the) [*encephalo-* + *myelopathy*] any disease or diseased condition of the brain and spinal cord.
**postinfection e.,** acute disseminated encephalomyelitis.
**postvaccinial e.,** acute disseminated encephalomyelitis.
**subacute necrotizing e.,** an encephalopathy of unclear clinical and pathological criteria, causing neuropathologic damage like that of the Wernicke-Korsakoff syndrome. It occurs in two forms: The *infantile form,* which may be the same as pyruvate carboxylase deficiency, is characterized by degeneration of gray matter with necrosis and capillary proliferation in the brain stem; hypotonia, seizures, and dementia; anorexia and vomiting; slow or arrested development; and ocular and respiratory disorders. Death usually occurs before age 3. The *adult* form usually first manifests as bilateral optic atrophy with central scotoma and colorblindness; then there is a quiescent period of up to 30 years; and then late symptoms appear such as ataxia, spastic paresis, clonic jerks, grand mal seizures, psychic lability, and mild dementia. Called also *subacute necrotizing encephalopathy* and *Leigh disease.*

**en·ceph·a·lo·my·elo·ra·dic·u·li·tis** (en-sef″ə-lo-mi″ə-lo-rə-dik″u-li′tis) inflammation of the brain, spinal cord, and spinal nerve roots.

**en·ceph·a·lo·my·elo·ra·dic·u·lop·a·thy** (en-sef″ə-lo-mi″ə-lo-rə-dik″u-lop′ə-the) disease involving the brain, spinal cord, and spinal nerve roots.

**en·ceph·a·lo·myo·car·di·tis** (en-sef-ə-lo-mi″o-kahr-di′tis) a viral disease of pigs and certain nonhuman primates, caused by a cardiovirus and characterized by degenerative and inflammatory changes in skeletal and cardiac muscle, and lesions of the central nervous system resembling those of poliomyelitis.

**en·ceph·a·lo·my·op·a·thy** (en-sef″ə-lo-mi-op′ə-the) any disease involving the brain and muscles.
**mitochondrial e.,** any of a group of diseases characterized by abnormal mitochondrial function with involvement of the central nervous system and skeletal muscle and, in most cases, lactic acidosis. Diseases in this group, which includes subacute necrotizing encephalomyelitis, Leber's hereditary optic neuropathy, MELAS syndrome, and MERRF syndrome, may also be classified as mitochondrial myopathies or mitochondrial encephalopathies.

**en·ceph·a·lon** (en-sef′ə-lon) [L., from Gr. *enkephalos,* from *en-* in + *kephalē* head] [TA] the brain: that part of the central nervous system contained within the cranium, comprising the prosencephalon, mesencephalon, and rhombencephalon; it is derived (developed) from the anterior part of the embryonic neural tube. See illustration accompanying *brain.* See also *cerebrum.*

**en·ceph·a·lo·nar·co·sis** (en-sef″ə-lo-nahr-ko′sis) [*encephalo-* + *narcosis*] stupor due to brain disease.

**en·ceph·a·lo·path·ic** (en-sef″ə-lo-path′ik) pertaining to encephalopathy.

**en·ceph·a·lop·a·thy** (en-sef″ə-lop′ə-the) [*encephalo-* + *-pathy*] any degenerative disease of the brain.
**AIDS e.,** HIV e.
**anoxic e.,** hypoxic e.
**biliary e.,** kernicterus.
**bilirubin e.,** kernicterus.
**bovine spongiform e.,** a prion disease of adult cattle that is epizootic in Great Britain and Northern Ireland, characterized by apprehensive behavior, hyperesthesia, and ataxia. It is transmitted by feed containing protein in the form of meat and bone meal derived from infected animals. The etiologic agent is also the cause of new variant Creutzfeldt-Jakob disease.
**boxer's e., boxer's traumatic e.,** a syndrome due to cumulative head blows absorbed in the boxing ring, characterized by general slowing of mental function, occasional bouts of confusion, and scattered memory loss. It may progress to the more serious *boxer's dementia.* Called also *traumatic e.* Cf. *postconcussional syndrome.*
**cytomegalovirus e.,** see under *encephalitis.*
**demyelinating e.,** any encephalopathy accompanied by demyelination; see *Schilder's disease,* under *disease.*
**dialysis e.,** a degenerative disease of the brain associated with long-term use of hemodialysis, marked by speech disorders and constant myoclonic jerks, progressing to global dementia, with associated psychological changes; it is often accompanied by osteomalacia and is due to high levels of aluminum in the water used in the dialysis fluid or to aluminum-containing compounds given to control phosphorus levels. Called also *progressive dialysis e.* and *dialysis dementia.*
**hepatic e.,** a condition usually occurring secondarily to advanced disease of the liver but also seen in the course of any severe disease or in patients with portacaval shunts. It is marked by disturbances of consciousness which may progress to deep coma (hepatic coma), psychiatric changes of varying degree, flapping tremor, and fetor hepaticus. Called also *portal-systemic e.*
**HIV e., HIV-related e.,** a progressive primary encephalopathy caused by human immunodeficiency virus type I infection; it involves principally the subcortical white matter and deep gray nuclei and is manifested by a variety of cognitive, motor, and behavioral abnormalities. Called also *AIDS dementia complex, AIDS e.,* and *HIV encephalitis.*
**hypernatremic e.,** a severe hemorrhagic encephalopathy induced by the hyperosmolarity accompanying hypernatremia and dehydration.
**hypertensive e.,** a complex of cerebral phenomena (headache, convulsions, coma, etc.) occurring in the course of malignant hypertension.
**hypoglycemic e.,** metabolic encephalopathy induced by severe hypoglycemia, as in glycogen storage disease, oversecretion or overdose of insulin, etc.
**hypoxic e.,** encephalopathy caused by hypoxia from either decreased rate of blood flow or decreased oxygen content of arterial blood; symptoms in mild cases include intellectual, visual, and motor disturbances. Severe cases, such as with cardiac arrest or blocking of the airways, can cause permanent damage within five minutes. Called also *anoxic e.*
**hypoxic-ischemic e.,** encephalopathy resulting from asphyxia. In infants presumed to have suffered prenatal or perinatal asphyxia, common symptoms are lethargy, feeding difficulties, and convulsions; serious cases may involve necrosis of neurons in the brain with psychomotor retardation and spastic motor deficits such as cerebral palsy. In adults, syndromes range from cortical blindness to irreversible coma.
**lead e.,** a condition caused by excessive ingestion of lead compounds, seen especially in young children. Pathological characteristics are edema and central demyelination; symptoms include vomiting and apathy followed by stupor, seizures, coma, and death. See also *lead poisoning,* under *poisoning.* Called also *lead encephalitis* and *saturnine e.*
**metabolic e.,** neuropsychiatric disturbances due to metabolic brain disease. It may occur primarily as a result of hypoxia, ischemia, or hypoglycemia, or secondarily to disease of other organs, such as the kidney, lung, or liver.
**mink e.,** a type of prion disease seen in minks, characterized by locomotor incoordination that progresses to semicoma and death.
**mitochondrial e.,** any of numerous encephalopathies associated with mitochondrial abnormalities, such as cytochrome-*c* oxidase deficiency.
**multicystic e.,** the formation of large, multilocular cavities throughout the cerebral hemispheres, occurring in the perinatal period; causes include anoxia, necrotizing viral encephalitis (especially herpes simplex), and neonatal meningitis.
**myoclonic e. of childhood,** a neurologic disorder of unknown etiology with onset between ages one and three, characterized by myoclonus of trunk and limbs and by opsoclonus, with ataxia of gait and intention tremor; some cases have been associated with occult neuroblastoma. Called also *Kinsbourne syndrome.*

**portal-systemic e., portasystemic e.,** hepatic e.
**progressive dialysis e.,** dialysis e.
**progressive subcortical e.,** Schilder's disease; see under *disease.*
**punch-drunk e.,** boxer's dementia.
**saturnine e.,** lead e.
**subacute necrotizing e.,** see under *encephalomyelopathy.*
**subacute spongiform e.,** prion disease.
**subcortical arteriosclerotic e.,** Binswanger's disease.
**transmissible spongiform e. (TSE),** prion disease.
**traumatic e.,** 1. postconcussional syndrome. 2. boxer's traumatic e.
**uremic e.,** cerebral symptoms seen in patients with uremia, including lethargy, fatigue, inattentiveness, irritability, confusion, sensory disturbances, and sometimes seizures.
**Wernicke's e.,** a neurological disorder characterized by confusion, apathy, drowsiness, ataxia of gait, nystagmus, and ophthalmoplegia. It was first described by Wernicke in 1881 and is now known to be due to thiamine deficiency, usually from chronic alcohol abuse. It is almost invariably accompanied by or followed by Korsakoff's syndrome (organic amnesia) and frequently accompanied by other nutritional polyneuropathies. Called also *Wernicke's disease* or *syndrome.* See also *Wernicke-Korsakoff syndrome,* under *syndrome.*

**en·ceph·a·lo·punc·ture** (en-sef″ə-lo-pungk′chər) surgical puncture of the brain.

**en·ceph·a·lo·py·o·sis** (en-sef″ə-lo-pi-o′sis) [*encephalo-* + *pyo-* + *-sis*] suppuration or abscess of the brain.

**en·ceph·a·lo·ra·chid·i·an** (en-sef″ə-lo-rə-kid′e-ən) [*encephalo-* + *rhachidian*] cerebrospinal.

**en·ceph·a·lo·ra·dic·u·li·tis** (en-sef″ə-lo-rə-dik′u-li″tis) inflammation of the roots of spinal nerves and of the brain.

**en·ceph·a·lor·rha·gia** (en-sef″ə-lo-ra′jə) [*encephalo-* + *-rrhagia*] hemorrhage within the brain or from the brain, especially cerebral pericapillary hemorrhage.
**pericapillary e.,** brain purpura.

**en·ceph·a·lo·scle·ro·sis** (en-sef″ə-lo-sklə-ro′sis) [*encephalo-* + *sclerosis*] hardening of the brain.

**en·ceph·a·lo·scope** (en-sef′ə-lə-skōp) an instrument for examining a cavity (such as an abscess cavity) in the brain.

**en·ceph·a·los·co·py** (en-sef″ə-los′kə-pe) [*encephalo-* + *-scopy*] inspection or examination of the brain.

**en·ceph·a·lo·sep·sis** (en-sef″ə-lo-sep′sis) [*encephalo-* + *sepsis*] gangrene of brain tissue.

**en·ceph·a·lo·sis** (en-sef″ə-lo′sis) encephalopathy.

**en·ceph·a·lo·spi·nal** (en-sef″ə-lo-spi′nəl) cerebrospinal.

**en·ceph·a·lo·thlip·sis** (en-sef″ə-lo-thlip′sis) [*encephalo-* + Gr. *thlipsis* pressure] compression of the brain.

**en·ceph·a·lo·tome** (en-sef′ə-lə-tōm) an instrument for performing encephalotomy.

**en·ceph·a·lot·o·my** (en-sef″ə-lot′ə-me) [*encephal-* + *-otomy*] incision of the brain; called also *cerebrotomy.*

**en·chon·dral** (en-kon′drəl) endochondral.

**en·chon·dro·ma** (en″kon-dro′mə) pl. *enchondromas, enchondromata* [Gr. *en* in + *chondroma*] a benign growth of cartilage arising in the metaphysis of a bone; called also *true chondroma.*
**multiple congenital e's,** enchondromatosis.

**en·chon·dro·ma·to·sis** (en-kon″dro-mə-to′sis) [MeSH: Enchondromatosis] a condition characterized by hamartomatous proliferation of cartilage cells within the metaphysis of several bones, causing thinning of the overlying cortex and distortion of the growth in length; it may undergo malignant transformation, particularly to chondrosarcoma. Called also *multiple* or *skeletal e.,* and *Ollier's disease.* See also *Maffucci's syndrome.*
**multiple e., skeletal e.,** enchondromatosis.

**en·chon·dro·ma·tous** (en″kon-drōm′ə-təs) of the nature of or pertaining to enchondroma.

**en·chon·dro·sar·co·ma** (en-kon″dro-sahr-ko′mə) central chondrosarcoma.

**en·chon·dro·sis** (en″kon-dro′sis) 1. an outgrowth from cartilage. 2. enchondroma.

**en·chy·le·ma** (en″ki-le′mə) [Gr. *en* in + *chylos* juice] hyaloplasm, def. 1.

**en·chy·ma** (en′kə-mə) [Gr. *en* in + *chymos* juice] the substance elaborated from absorbed nutritive materials; the formative juice of the tissues.

**en·clave** (en′klāv, ahn-klahv′) [Fr.] a tissue detached from its normal connection and enclosed within another organ or tissue.

**en·clo·mi·phene** (en-klo′mĭ-fēn) the *cis*-isomer of the gonad-stimulating principle clomiphene citrate; called also *cisclomiphene.* Cf *zuclomiphene.*

**en·col·pism** (en-kol′piz-əm) [Gr. *en* in + *colpo-* + *-ism*] medication administered via the vagina.

**en·co·pre·sis** (en-ko-pre′sis) [MeSH: Encopresis] fecal incontinence that does not have an organic cause.

**en·cra·ni·us** (en-kra′ne-əs) [Gr. *en* in + *kranion* skull] in asymmetrical conjoined twins, a parasitic twin located within the cranium of the larger twin.

**en·cy·e·sis** (en″si-e′sis) [Gr. *en* in + *cyesis*] normal uterine pregnancy.

**en·cyo·py·eli·tis** (en-si″o-pi″ə-li′tis) [*encyesis* + *pyelitis*] dilatation of the ureters and/or renal pelvis during normal pregnancy with associated edema, but seldom with all the classical signs of inflammation.

**en·cyst·ed** (en-sist′əd) [Gr. *en* in + *kystis* sac, bladder] enclosed in a sac, bladder, or cyst.

**en·cyst·ment** (en-sist′mənt) the process or condition of being or becoming encysted.

**end·a·del·phos** (end″ə-del′fos) [*end-* + *-adelphus*] asymmetrical conjoined twins in which a parasitic fetus is enclosed within the body of or within a tumor upon the larger twin. Cf. *fetus in fetu.*

**end·an·gi·itis** (en-an″je-i′tis) inflammation of the tunica intima; called also *endoangiitis, endovasculitis,* and *intimitis.*

**end·aor·tic** (en″da-or′tik) pertaining to the interior of the aorta.

**end·aor·ti·tis** (end″a-or-ti′tis) inflammation of the tunica intima of the aorta; called also *endoaortitis.*
**bacterial e.,** the formation of bacterial vegetations on the endothelial surface of the aorta.

**end·ar·ter·ec·to·my** (end-ahr″tər-ek′tə-me) [MeSH: Endarterectomy] excision of the thickened, atheromatous tunica intima of an artery. See also *atherectomy.*
**aortoiliac e.,** one performed on the abdominal aorta and common iliac arteries, done for disease localized around their junctions.
**carotid e.,** endarterectomy of the carotid artery, done for the prevention of stroke.
**common femoral e.,** one performed on the common femoral artery, done to relieve ischemia of the lower limb.
**gas e.,** endarterectomy done with high-pressure carbon dioxide to remove plaque deposits from the coronary blood vessels in treatment of atherosclerosis.
**transluminal e.,** that done using a cutting device inside a catheter that is inserted through the lumen of a vessel; see *transluminal endarterectomy catheter,* under *catheter.* Called also *transluminal atherectomy.*
**vertebral e.,** endarterectomy of the vertebral artery, done to treat some types of vertebrobasilar insufficiency.

**end·ar·te·ri·al** (end″ahr-tēr′e-əl) intra-arterial.

**end·ar·ter·itis** (end-ahr″tər-i′tis) [*end-* + *arteritis*] [MeSH: Endarteritis] inflammation of the tunica intima of an artery; intimitis. Cf. *arteritis* and *periarteritis.*
**Heubner's e.,** see under *disease.*
**e. obli′terans,** endarteritis in which the lumina of the smaller vessels become narrowed or obliterated as a result of proliferation of the tissue of the intimal layer; called also *arteritis obliterans* and *Friedländer's disease.* See also *arteriosclerosis obliterans.*
**e. proli′ferans,** overgrowth of fibrous tissue in the internal layers of the aorta or some other artery.

**end·ar·te·ri·um** (end″ahr-tēr′e-əm) [*end-* + *arteria*] the tunica intima of an artery.

**end·ar·ter·op·a·thy** (end-ahr″tər-op′ə-the) a disorder of the tunica intima of an artery.
**digital e.,** disorder of the tunica intima of the arteries of the digits, associated with Raynaud's phenomenon and nutritional lesions of the pulp of the fingers.

**end·au·ral** (end-aw′rəl) within the ear.

**end·brain** (end′brān) telencephalon.

**end-brush** (end′brush) telodendron.

**end-bud** (end′bud) see under *bud.*

**end-bulb** (end′bulb) corpusculum nervosum terminale.

**end·chon·dral** (end-kon′drəl) endochondral.

**en·deic·tic** (en-dīk′tik) [Gr. *endeixis* a pointing out] symptomatic.

**en·de·mia** (en-de′me-ə) any endemic disease.

**en·de·mi·al** (en-de′me-əl) endemic.

**en·dem·ic** (en-dem′ik) [Gr. *endēmos* dwelling in a place] present or usually prevalent in a population or geographical area at all times; said of a disease or agent. Called also *endemial*. See also *holoendemic* and *hyperendemic*. Cf. *epidemic*.

**en·de·mo·ep·i·dem·ic** (en″də-mo-ep″ĭ-dem′ik) endemic, but occasionally becoming epidemic.

**end·epi·der·mis** (end″ep-ĭ-dər′mis) epithelium.

**end·er·gon·ic** (end″ər-gon′ik) [*end-* + Gr. *ergon* work] characterized by or accompanied by the absorption of energy; said of reactions, particularly biochemical reactions, that require energy in order to proceed, so that the products have a higher free energy than the reactants. Opposed to *exergonic*.

**en·der·on** (en′dər-on) [Gr. *en* in + *deros* skin] the deeper part of the skin or mucous membrane, as distinguished from the epithelium or epidermis.

**en·der·on·ic** (en″dər-on′ik) pertaining to the enderon or derived from it.

**En·ders** (en′dərz) John Franklin. American microbiologist, 1897–1985; co-winner with Thomas Huckle Weller and Frederick Chapman Robbins, of the Nobel prize in medicine or physiology for 1954, for the discovery that many viruses (specifically, poliomyelitis viruses) can be grown in tissue culture and thereby studied and isolated, making possible the production of vaccines.

**end-foot** (end′foot) bouton terminal; see under *bouton*.

**end·ing** (end′ing) 1. a termination or finish 2. nerve ending.
**annulospiral e's,** wide, ribbon-like sensory nerve endings wrapped around the center of intrafusal fibers of a muscle spindle; called also *primary e's*. See also *flower-spray e's*.
**club e. of Bartelmez,** a type of nerve fiber ending in the vertebrate central nervous system, terminating abruptly on the dendrite of another neuron.
**encapsulated nerve e.,** corpusculum nervosum terminale.
**epilemmal e's,** sensory nerve endings in striated muscle in which the nerve endings are in close contact with the muscle fibers.
**flower-spray e's,** branched sensory nerve endings on intrafusal fibers of muscle spindles; their axons are more slender than those of annulospiral endings and they are at more peripheral locations or are confined to nuclear fibers. Called also *secondary e's*.
**free nerve e.,** terminatio nervorum libera.
**grape e's,** nerve endings in muscle which have the form of terminal swellings.
**nerve e's,** the fine branchlike terminations of neurons. Sensory nerve endings are the beginnings of afferent pathways of myelinated fibers of pseudounipolar neurons. They are classified as either free (see *terminatio nervorum libera* under *terminatio*) or encapsulated (see *corpusculum nervosum terminale* under *corpusculum*). Motor nerve endings are the endings of axons and are called *motor end plates;* see under *end plate*.
**nonencapsulated nerve e.,** free nerve e.
**primary e's,** annulospiral e's.
**Ruffini's e.,** see under *corpuscle*.
**secondary e's,** flower-spray e's.

**end-nu·clei** (end-noo′kle-i) terminal nuclei; see under *nucleus*.

**end(o)-** [Gr. *endon* within] prefix denoting an inward situation, within.

**en·do·ab·dom·i·nal** (en″do-ab-dom′ĭ-nəl) pertaining to the interior of the abdomen.

**en·do·am·y·lase** (en″do-am′ə-lās) an amylase that catalyzes the cleavage of $\alpha$-1,4-glucosidic bonds not necessarily at the nonreducing end of the polysaccharide. Cf. *exoamylase*.

**en·do·an·eu·rys·mor·rha·phy** (en″do-an″u-riz-mor′ə-fe) [*endo-* + *aneurysmorrhaphy*] a formerly common type of aneurysmoplasty done by opening the aneurysmal sac and narrowing the internal lumen by suture; called also *Matas' operation*.

**en·do·an·gi·itis** (en″do-an-je-i′tis) endangiitis.

**en·do·aor·ti·tis** (en″do-a″or-ti′tis) endaortitis.

**en·do·ap·pen·di·ci·tis** (en″do-ə-pen″dĭ-si′tis) inflammation of the mucous membrane lining the vermiform appendix.

**en·do·ar·ter·itis** (en″do-ahr″tər-i′tis) endarteritis.

**en·do·aus·cul·ta·tion** (en″do-aws″kəl-ta′shən) auscultation of the stomach and thoracic organs by means of a tube passed into the stomach.

**en·do·bac·il·lary** (en″do-bas′ĭ-lar-e) contained within a bacillus.

**en·do·bi·ot·ic** (en″do-bi-ot′ik) [*endo-* + *biotic*] living parasitically within the tissues of the host.

**en·do·blast** (en′do-blast) [*endo-* + *-blast*] endoderm.

**en·do·blas·tic** (en″do-blas′tik) endodermic.

**en·do·bron·chi·tis** (en″do-brong-ki′tis) inflammation of the epithelial lining of the bronchi.

**en·do·car·di·al** (en″do-kahr′de-əl) [*endo-* + *cardi-*(1) + *-al*[1]] pertaining to the endocardium.

**en·do·car·di·op·a·thy** (en″do-kahr″de-op′ə-the) [*endocardium* + *-pathy*] a disorder or disease of the endocardium.

**en·do·car·di·o·sis** (en″do-kahr″de-o′sis) chronic fibrosis of atrioventricular valves in dogs, usually the mitral valve; it may lead to congestive heart failure.

**en·do·car·dit·ic** (en″do-kahr-dit′ik) pertaining to endocarditis.

**en·do·car·di·tis** (en″do-kahr-di′tis) [*endocardium* + *-itis*] [MeSH: Endocarditis] exudative and proliferative inflammatory alterations of the endocardium, usually characterized by the presence of vegetations on the surface of the endocardium or in the endocardium itself, and most commonly involving a heart valve, but sometimes affecting the inner lining of the cardiac chambers or the endocardium elsewhere. It may occur as a primary disorder or as a complication of or in association with another disease.
**acute bacterial e. (ABE),** see *infective e.*
**atypical verrucous e.,** Libman-Sacks e.
**bacterial e.,** infectious endocarditis (q.v.) caused by any of various bacteria, including streptococci, staphylococci, enterococci, gonococci, or gram-negative bacilli.
***Candida* e.,** mycotic e. caused by a species of *Candida;* called also *endocardial candidiasis*.
**e. benig′na,** Libman-Sacks e.
**e. chorda′lis,** endocarditis affecting particularly the chordae tendineae.
**constrictive e.,** Löffler's e.
**fungal e.,** mycotic e.
**infectious e., infective e.,** endocarditis caused by infection with microorganisms, especially bacteria and fungi. It has been classified according to course as acute and subacute: the *acute* form is usually due to staphylococci, pneumococci, gonococci, or streptococci, involves a normal heart valve, and has a short history and rapid course; the *subacute* form usually is due to viridans or fecal streptococci or to fungi, affects damaged heart valves, and has a prolonged course. Because underlying causes and available therapies have changed, this division has little current clinical validity and has been largely replaced by classification on the basis of etiology or underlying anatomy.
**e. len′ta,** the subacute form of infective endocarditis.
**Libman-Sacks e.,** nonbacterial thrombotic endocarditis associated with systemic lupus erythematosus; the vegetations consist of necrotic debris, fibrinoid material, and trapped, disintegrating, fibroblastic and inflammatory cells, usually on the atrioventricular valves. Called also *Libman-Sacks disease* and *atypical verrucous* or *nonbacterial verrucous e.*
**Löffler's e., Löffler's parietal fibroplastic e.,** endocarditis associated with eosinophilia, marked by fibroplastic thickening of the endocardium, and resulting in congestive heart failure, persistent tachycardia, hepatomegaly, splenomegaly, serous effusions into the pleural cavity, edema of the legs, and edema and ascites of the arms; called also *constrictive e.* and *eosinophilic endomyocardial disease*.
**malignant e.,** older term for *infective endocarditis*.
**marantic e.,** nonbacterial thrombotic e.
**mural e.,** a form affecting the lining of the walls of the heart chambers, rather than the valvular, chordal, trabecular, or papillary tissue. Called also *parietal e.*
**mycotic e.,** infectious endocarditis, usually subacute, due to various fungi, most commonly *Candida* (especially *C. albicans*), *Aspergillus*, and *Histoplasma*. Called also *fungal e.*
**native valve e.,** infective endocarditis involving one or more of the natural heart valves, in contrast to *prosthetic valve e.*
**nonbacterial thrombotic e. (NBTE),** endocarditis usually occurring in chronic debilitating disease, particularly malignancy; it is characterized by noninfected vegetations composed of fibrin and other blood elements, generally located on the line of closure of the mitral and aortic valves and susceptible to embolization.
**nonbacterial verrucous e.,** Libman-Sacks e.
**parietal e.,** mural e.
**prosthetic valve e.,** infective endocarditis as a complication of implantation of a prosthetic valve in the heart; the vegetations usually occur along the line of suture.
**rheumatic e.,** endocarditis associated with rheumatic fever. Involvement may be mural but is usually valvular and involves the entire valve; it is then more accurately termed rheumatic valvulitis (q.v.).
**rickettsial e.,** endocarditis caused by invasion of the heart valves with *Coxiella burnetii;* it is a sequela of Q fever, usually occurring in persons who have had rheumatic fever.
**right-side e.,** primary acute endocarditis of the right side of the heart.
**septic e.,** infective e.
**staphylococcal e.,** infective endocarditis caused by staphylococcal invasion of the heart valves.

**streptococcal e.,** infective endocarditis caused by streptococcal invasion of the heart valves.
**subacute bacterial e. (SBE),** see *infective e.*
**syphilitic e.,** endocarditis resulting from extension of syphilitic infection from the aorta.
**tuberculous e.,** a rare form of endocarditis in which the endocardium is involved by extension of a tuberculous perimyocarditis or of miliary tuberculosis.
**ulcerative e.,** infective endocarditis characterized by rapid ulceration of the valvular lesions.
**valvular e.,** endocarditis affecting the membrane over the valves of the heart, rather than the mural, chordal, trabecular, or papillary tissue.
**vegetative e., verrucous e.,** endocarditis, infectious or noninfectious, the characteristic lesions of which are vegetations or verrucae on the endocardium.
**viridans e.,** a subacute form of infective endocarditis due to infection with viridans streptococci.

**en·do·car·di·um** (en″do-kahr′de-um) [*endo* + Gr. *kardia* heart] [TA] [MeSH: Endocardium] the endothelial lining membrane of the cavities of the heart and the connective tissue bed on which it lies. This subendothelial connective tissue contains varying amounts of elastic and collagen fibers and smooth muscle cells.

**en·do·ce·li·ac** (en″do-se′le-ak) [*endo-* + Gr. *koilia* cavity] inside one of the body cavities.

**en·do·cel·lu·lar** (en″do-sel′u-lər) intracellular.

**en·do·cer·vi·cal** (en″do-sər′vĭ-kəl) pertaining to the interior of the cervix uteri.

**en·do·cer·vi·ci·tis** (en″do-sər″vĭ-si′tis) [*endo-* + *cervicitis*] inflammation of the mucous membrane of the cervix uteri; called also *endotrachelitis.*

**en·do·cer·vix** (en″do-sər′viks) 1. the mucous membrane lining the canal of the cervix uteri. 2. the region of the opening of the uterine cervix into the uterine cavity.

**en·do·chon·dral** (en″do-kon′drəl) situated, formed, or occurring within cartilage.

**en·do·cho·ri·on** (en″do-kor′e-on) [*endo-* + *chorion*] the inner chorionic layer.

**en·do·chrome** (en′do-krōm) [*endo-* + *-chrome*] the coloring matter within a cell.

**en·do·co·li·tis** (en″do-ko-li′tis) inflammation of the mucous membrane of the colon.

**en·do·com·men·sal** (en″do-kə-men′səl) a commensal organism which lives inside the body of its symbiotic companion.

**en·do·co·nid·io·tox·i·co·sis** (en″do-ko-nĭd″e-o-tok″sĭ-ko′sis) mycotoxicosis from ingestion of fungi of the genus *Endoconidium;* see *darnel poisoning,* under *poisoning.*

**En·do·co·ni·di·um** (en″do-kə-nid′e-um) a genus of Fungi Imperfecti of the form-class Hyphomycetes. *E. temulen′tum* sometimes contaminates the grass *Lolium temulentum* and causes darnel poisoning.

**en·do·cor·pus·cu·lar** (en″do-kor-pus′ku-lər) intracorpuscular.

**en·do·cra·ni·al** (en″do-kra′ne-əl) intracranial.

**en·do·cra·ni·o·sis** (en″do-kra″ne-o′sis) Morgagni's term for hyperostosis frontalis interna.

**en·do·cra·ni·tis** (en″do-kra-ni′tis) inflammation of the endocranium.

**en·do·cra·ni·um** (en″do-kra′ne-əm) [*endo-* + Gr. *kranion* skull] the endosteal outer layer of the dura mater of the brain.

**en·do·crine** (en′do-krīn, en′do-krin) [*endo-* + Gr. *krinein* to separate] 1. secreting internally (as opposed to *exocrine*), applied to organs and structures that release their products into the blood or lymph, and to substances *(hormones)* that exert specific effects on other organs. See also under *system.* Called also *endosecretory.* 2. hormonal.

**en·do·cri·nol·o·gist** (en″do-krĭ-nol′ə-jist) a specialist in endocrinology.

**en·do·cri·nol·o·gy** (en″do-krĭ-nol′ə-je) [*endocrine* + *-logy*] [MeSH: Endocrinology] 1. the study of hormones, the endocrine system, and their role in the physiology of the body. 2. a medical specialty concerned with the diagnosis and treatment of disorders of the endocrine system.

**en·do·crino·path·ic** (en″do-krin″o-path′ik) pertaining to or characterized by endocrinopathy.

**en·do·cri·nop·a·thy** (en″do-krĭ-nop′ə-the) [*endocrine* + *-pathy*] any disease due to a disorder of the endocrine system (hormonal imbalance). Called also *endocrinosis.*

**en·do·cri·no·sis** (en″do-krĭ-no′sis) endocrinopathy.

**en·do·cri·no·ther·a·py** (en″do-krĭ″no-ther′ə-pe) endocrine therapy.

**en·do·cu·ti·cle** (en″do-ku′tĭ-kəl) [*endo-* + L. *cuticula*] the inner layer of the procuticle in certain crustaceans and arthropods, which is almost entirely composed of protein and chitin.

**en·do·cyc·lic** (en″do-sik′lik) a term applied to cyclic compounds in which the bond occurs in the ring.

**en·do·cyst** (en′do-sist) the inner, germinative, or embryonic membrane of the hydatid cyst.

**en·do·cys·ti·tis** (en″do-sis-ti′tis) inflammation of the lining membrane of the bladder.

**en·do·cyte** (en′do-sīt) [*endo-* + *-cyte*] any cell inclusion.

**en·do·cy·to·sis** (en″do-si-to′sis) [*endo-* + *cyt-* + *-osis*] [MeSH: Endocytosis] the uptake by a cell of material from the environment by invagination of its plasma membrane; it includes both phagocytosis and pinocytosis.

**en·do·de·oxy·ri·bo·nu·cle·ase** (en″do-de-ok″se-ri″bo-noo′kle-ās) [EC 3.1.21–25] any member of several sub-subclasses of enzymes of the hydrolase class that catalyze the hydrolysis of interior bonds of deoxyribonucleic acids, producing oligonucleotides or polynucleotides.

**en·do·derm** (en′do-dərm) [*endo-* + *-derm*] [MeSH: Endoderm] the innermost of the three primary germ layers of the embryo; from it are derived the epithelium of the pharynx, respiratory tract (except the nose), digestive tract, bladder, and urethra. Called also *entoderm, endoblast,* and *entoblast.* Cf. *ectoderm* and *mesoderm.*

**en·do·der·mal** (en″do-dər′məl) pertaining to or derived from the endoderm.

**En·do·der·moph·y·ton** (en″do-dər-mof′ĭ-ton) former name for *Trichophyton.*

**en·do·don·tics** (en″do-don′tiks) [*end-* + *odont-* + *-ics*] [MeSH: Endodontics] that branch of dentistry concerned with the etiology, prevention, diagnosis, and treatment of diseases and injuries affecting the dental pulp, tooth root, and periapical tissue. In current usage, this term has a more restrictive meaning than *endodontology,* which refers to study of the pulp in both health and disease, although sometimes the terms are used interchangeably.
**surgical e.,** the treatment of diseases and injuries of the dental pulp through surgical means.

**en·do·don·tist** (en″do-don′tist) a dentist who specializes in endodontics; called also *endodontologist.*

**en·do·don·ti·um** (en″do-don′she-əm) pulpa dentis.

**en·do·don·tol·o·gist** (en″do-don-tol′ə-jist) endodontist.

**en·do·don·tol·o·gy** (en″do-don-tol′ə-je) [*end-* + *odont-* + *-logy*] the scientific study of the dental pulp and associated processes in health and disease. In current usage, this term has a broader sense than *endodontics,* which is restricted to the pulp in situations of injury or disease. Sometimes the terms are used interchangeably.

**en·do·dy·og·e·ny** (en″do-di-oj′ə-ne) reproduction by the formation of two daughter cells within the wall of the mother cell (internal budding), the progeny being released by rupture of the mother cell, as in the protozoan *Toxoplasma.*

**en·do·ec·to·thrix** (en″do-ek′to-thriks) a fungus that produces spores both on the interior and exterior of the hairs.

**en·do·en·ter·itis** (en″do-en″tər-i′tis) inflammation of the mucous membrane of the intestine.

**en·do·en·zyme** (en″do-en′zīm) an intracellular enzyme; an enzyme that is retained in a cell and does not normally diffuse out of the cell into the surrounding medium. Cf. *ectoenzyme.*

**en·do·epi·der·mal** (en″do-ep″ĭ-dər′məl) within the epidermis.

**en·do·epi·the·li·al** (en″do-ep″ĭ-the′le-əl) within the epithelium.

**en·do·er·gic** (en″do-er′jik) 1. endergonic. 2. endothermic.

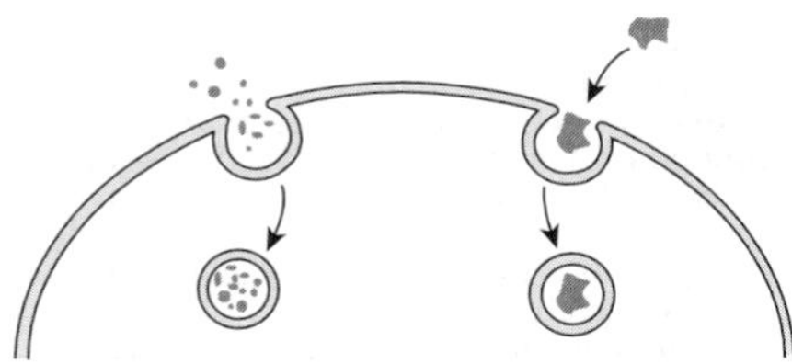

Endocytosis. Shown are pinocytosis of small fluid droplets *(left)* and phagocytosis of a large particle *(right).*

**en·do·esoph·a·gi·tis** (en″do-e-sof″ə-gi′tis) inflammation of the lining membrane of the esophagus.

**en·do·exo·ter·ic** (en″do-ek″so-ter′ik) [*endo-* + *exoteric*] resulting from certain causes internal to the body, and from others of external origin.

**en·do·far·a·dism** (en″do-far′ə-diz-əm) the application of alternating current to an internal organ, as to the stomach.

**en·do·gal·va·nism** (en″do-gal′və-niz-əm) the application of direct current to an internal organ, as to the stomach.

**en·dog·a·mous** (ən-dog′ə-məs) characterized by endogamy.

**en·dog·a·my** (en-dog′ə-me) [*endo-* + Gr. *gamos* marriage] 1. fertilization by the union of separate cells having the same genetic ancestry; called also *pedogamy.* Cf. *autogamy* (def. 1) and *exogamy.* 2. restricting marriage to persons within the community; inbreeding.

**en·do·gas·tric** (en″do-gas′trik) pertaining to the interior of the stomach.

**en·do·gas·tri·tis** (en″do-gas-tri′tis) inflammation of the mucous membrane of the stomach.

**en·do·ge·net·ic** (en″do-jə-net′ik) endogenous.

**en·do·gen·ic** (en″do-jen′ik) endogenous.

**en·do·ge·note** (en″do-je′nōt) in bacterial genetics, the recipient cell's own complement of genetic information, as opposed to the exogenote introduced by transduction.

**en·dog·e·nous** (en-doj′ə-nəs) [*endo-* + *-genous*] 1. growing from within. 2. developing or originating within the organism, or arising from causes within the organism.

**en·do·glo·bar** (en″do-glo′bər) intracorpuscular.

**en·do·glob·u·lar** (en″do-glob′u-lər) intracorpuscular.

**en·do·gna·thi·on** (en″do-na′the-on) [*endo-* + *gnathion*] the inner segment of the incisive bone.

**en·do·go·nid·i·um** (en″do-go-nid′e-əm) a gonidium developed within a cell, especially in the algal component of a lichen.

**en·do·her·ni·or·rha·phy** (en″do-hər″ne-or′ə-fe) surgical repair of a hernia by suture of the interior of its sac.

**en·do·in·tox·i·ca·tion** (en″do-in-tok″sĭ-ka′shən) poisoning caused by an endogenous toxin.

**en·do·la·ryn·ge·al** (en″do-lə-rin′je-əl) [*endo-* + Gr. *larynx*] located or occurring within the larynx; called also *intralaryngeal.*

**en·do·lymph** (en′do-limf) [MeSH: Endolymph] endolympha.

**en·do·lym·pha** (en″do-lim′fə) [*endo-* + *lympha*] [TA] endolymph: the fluid contained in the membranous labyrinth of the ear; it is entirely separate from the perilymph. Called also *Scarpa's fluid* and *liquor of Scarpa.*

**en·do·lym·phat·ic** (en″do-lim-fat′ik) pertaining to the endolymph.

**en·dol·y·sin** (en-dol′ĭ-sin) [*endo-* + *lysin*] a bactericidal substance existing in cells, acting directly on bacteria, e.g., leukin.

**en·dol·y·sis** (en-dol′ĭ-sis) [*endo-* + *-lysis*] dissolution or breaking up of the cytoplasm of a cell.

**en·do·mas·toid·itis** (en″do-mas″toi-di′tis) mastoiditis.

**en·do·meso·derm** (en″do-mes′o-dərm) [*endo-* + *mesoderm*] mesoderm originating from the endoderm of the two-layered blastodisc.

**en·do·me·tria** (en″do-me′tre-ə) [Gr.] plural of *endometrium.*

**en·do·me·tri·al** (en″do-me′tre-əl) pertaining to the endometrium.

**en·do·me·tri·oid** (en″do-me′tre-oid) resembling endometrium.

**en·do·me·tri·o·ma** (en″do-me″tre-o′mə) a solitary, non-neoplastic mass containing endometrial tissue and blood.

**en·do·me·tri·o·sis** (en″do-me″tre-o′sis) [*endometrium* + *-osis*] [MeSH: Endometriosis] a condition in which tissue containing typical endometrial granular and stromal elements occurs aberrantly in various locations in the pelvic cavity or some other area of the body; called also *adenomyosis externa* and *e. externa.*
**e. exter′na,** endometriosis.
**e. inter′na,** adenomyosis.
**ovarian e., e. ova′rii,** occurrence in the ovary of tissue resembling the uterine mucous membrane, either in the form of small superficial islands or in the form of endometrial ("chocolate") cysts of various sizes.
**stromal e.,** adenomyosis in which nearly all of the tissue infiltrating the myometrium consists of stroma.
**e. ve′sicae,** endometriosis involving the bladder.

**en·do·me·tri·ot·ic** (en″do-me″tre-ot′ik) pertaining to or characterized by endometriosis.

**en·do·me·tri·tis** (en″do-me-tri′tis) [*endometrium* + *-itis*] [MeSH: Endometritis] inflammation of the endometrium.
**bacteriotoxic e.,** endometritis caused by the toxins of bacteria, as distinguished from that caused by the presence of the organisms themselves.
**decidual e.,** inflammation of the decidua of pregnancy.
**exfoliative e.,** endometritis with the casting off of portions of the membrane.
**glandular e.,** endometritis of the uterine glands.
**membranous e.,** endometritis with an exudate which forms a false membrane.
**puerperal e.,** endometritis following childbirth.
**syncytial e.,** a post-pregnancy condition consisting of a benign tumor-like lesion with infiltration of the uterine wall by large syncytial trophoblastic cells; called also *syncytioma.*
**tuberculous e.,** inflammation of the endometrium due to infection by *Mycobacterium tuberculosis,* with the presence of tubercles; usually the uterine tubes are also involved.

**en·do·me·tri·um** (en″do-me′tre-əm) pl. *endome′tria* [L. from *endo-* + *metra*] [MeSH: Endometrium] TA alternative for *tunica mucosa uteri.*
**Swiss-cheese e.,** hyperplasia of the endometrium, under the influence of progesterone, in which the glands vary in size and shape, producing an appearance like that of Swiss cheese, with its large and small holes.

**en·dom·e·try** (en-dom′ə-tre) [*endo-* + *-metry*] the measurement of the capacity of a cavity.

**en·do·mi·to·sis** (en″do-mi-to′sis) reproduction of nuclear elements not followed by chromosome movements and cytoplasmic division; called also *endopolyploidy.*

**en·do·mi·tot·ic** (en″do-mi-tot′ik) pertaining to or characterized by endomitosis.

**en·do·morph** (en′do-morf) an individual having a body build in which tissues derived from the endoderm predominate: there is relative preponderance of soft roundness throughout the body, with large digestive viscera and accumulations of fat, and with large trunk and thighs and tapering extremities, as contrasted with ectomorph and mesomorph (def. 1).

**en·do·morph·ic** (en″do-mor′fik) pertaining to or characteristic of an endomorph.

**en·do·mor·phy** (en′do-mor″fe) [*endo*derm + Gr. *morphē* form] the condition of being an endomorph.

**En·do·my·ces** (en″do-mi′sēz) [*endo-* + Gr. *mykēs* fungus] a genus of fungi of the order Endomycetales that includes a number of yeasts from soil, nectar, and decaying fruit. *E. al′bicans* is a former name for *Candida albicans.*

**En·do·my·ce·ta·les** (en″do-mi″sə-ta′lēz) [MeSH: Endomycetales] in some systems of classification, an order of perfect fungi (yeasts) of the subphylum Ascomycotina, mostly saprobes, in which the zygote results from fusion of two cells and immediately forms an ascus; it includes the family Saccharomycetaceae.

**en·do·myo·car·di·al** (en″do-mi″o-kahr′de-əl) pertaining to the endocardium and the myocardium.

**en·do·myo·car·di·tis** (en″do-mi″o-kahr-di′tis) [*endo-* + *myocarditis*] inflammation of the endocardium and myocardium.

**en·do·my·si·al** (en″do-mis′e-əl) pertaining to the endomysium.

**en·do·mys·i·um** (en″do-mis′e-əm) [*endo-* + Gr. *mys* muscle] [TA] the sheath of delicate reticular fibrils which surrounds each muscle fiber.

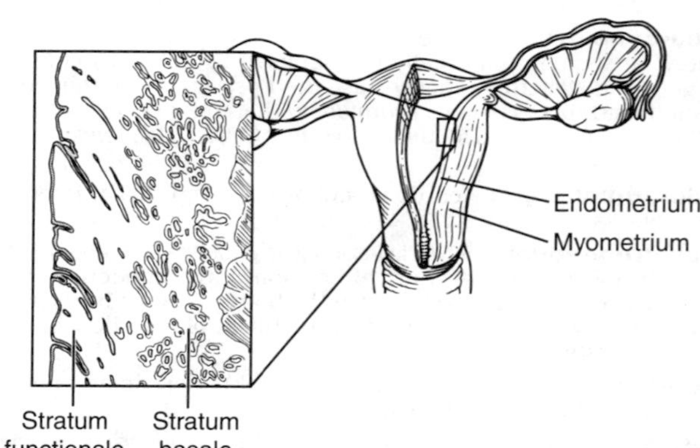

Endometrium, comprising the stratum functionale and stratum basale.

**en·do·na·sal** (en″do-na′zəl) intranasal.

**en·do·neu·ral** (en″do-noor′əl) within a nerve. Called also *intraneural.*

**en·do·neu·ri·al** (en″do-noor′e-əl) pertaining to the endoneurium.

**en·do·neu·ri·tis** (en″do-noo͞-ri′tis) inflammation of the endoneurium.

**en·do·neu·ri·um** (en″do-noor′e-um) [*endo-* + Gr. *neuron* nerve] [TA] the innermost layer of connective tissue in a peripheral nerve, forming an interstitial layer around each individual fiber outside the neurilemma; called also *epilemma, sheath of Henle,* and *sheath of Key and Retzius.* See also *epineurium* and *perineurium.*

**en·do·neu·rol·y·sis** (en″do-noo͞-rol′ə-sis) [*endo-* + *neurolysis*] hersage.

**en·do·nu·cle·ar** (en″do-noo′kle-ər) within a cell nucleus.

**en·do·nu·cle·ase** (en″do-noo′kle-ās) any nuclease specifically catalyzing the hydrolysis of interior bonds of ribonucleotide or deoxyribonucleotide chains, producing poly- or oligonucleotides. Cf. *exonuclease.*
**restriction e.,** an endonuclease that hydrolyzes deoxyribonucleic acid, cleaving it at an individual site of a specific base pattern. Thus, the enzyme degrades DNA foreign to a cell but spares the cell's own DNA, which is protected by methylation at the recognition site. Restriction endonucleases isolated from bacterial sources are used extensively for sequencing of DNA and recombinant technology.

**en·do·nu·cle·o·lus** (en″do-noo-kle′o-ləs) a nonstaining spot near the center of the nucleolus of a cell.

**en·do·par·a·site** (en″do-par′ə-sīt) [*endo-* + *parasite*] a parasite that lives within the body of its host.

**en·do·pel·vic** (en″do-pel′vik) intrapelvic.

**en·do·pep·ti·dase** (en″do-pep′tĭ-dās) [EC 3.4.21–24; 3.4.99] any peptidase that catalyzes the cleavage of internal peptide bonds in a polypeptide or protein; they are divided into subclasses on the basis of catalytic mechanism and comprise the serine endopeptidases, cysteine endopeptidases, aspartic endopeptidases, metalloendopeptidases, and other endopeptidases.

**en·do·peri·car·di·al** (en″do-per″ĭ-kahr′de-əl) pertaining to the endocardium and pericardium.

**en·do·peri·car·di·tis** (en″do-per″ĭ-kahr-di′tis) [*endo-* + *pericarditis*] inflammation involving both the endocardium and pericardium.

**en·do·peri·myo·car·di·tis** (en″do-per″ĭ-mi″o-kahr-di′tis) [*endo-* + *peri-* + *myocarditis*] inflammation of the endocardium, pericardium, and myocardium.

**en·do·peri·neu·ri·tis** (en″do-per″ĭ-noo-ri′tis) inflammation of the endoneurium and perineurium.

**en·do·peri·to·ne·al** (en″do-per″ĭ-to-ne′əl) within the peritoneum.

**en·do·peri·to·ni·tis** (en″do-per″ĭ-to-ni′tis) inflammation of the serous lining of the peritoneal cavity.

**en·do·per·ox·ide** (en″do-pə-rok′sīd) a peroxide in which the —O—O— group is attached as a bridge, joining two atoms within the molecule.

**en·do·per·ox·ide-D-isom·er·ase** (en″do-pə-rok′sīd i-som′ə-rās) prostaglandin-D synthase.

**en·do·per·ox·ide-E-isom·er·ase** (en″do-pə-rok′sīd i-som′ə-rās) prostaglandin-E synthase.

**en·do·per·ox·ide re·duc·tase** (en″do-pə-rok′sīd re-duk′tās) an enzyme of the oxidoreductase class that catalyzes the conversion of the intermediate prostaglandin $H_2$ ($PGH_2$) to prostaglandin $F_{2\alpha}$($PGF_{2\alpha}$). See also illustration at *prostaglandin.*

**en·do·phle·bi·tis** (en″do-flə-bi′tis) [*endo-* + *phlebitis*] inflammation of the intima of a vein; called also *endovenitis.*
**e. hepa′tica obli′terans,** Budd-Chiari syndrome.
**proliferative e.,** phlebosclerosis.

**en·do·pho·to·co·ag·u·la·tion** (en″do-fo″to-ko-ag′u-la-shən) photocoagulation performed within the vitreous, after vitrectomy, in the treatment of vitreous hemorrhage.

**en·doph·thal·mi·tis** (en″dof-thəl-mi′tis) [*end-* + *ophthalmitis*] [MeSH: Endophthalmitis] inflammation involving the ocular cavities and their adjacent structures; called also *entophthalmia.*
**phacoanaphylactic e.,** phacoantigenic uveitis.

**en·do·phyte** (en′do-fīt) [*endo-* + *-phyte*] a parasitic plant organism living within the body of its host.

**en·do·phyt·ic** (en″do-fit′ik) [*endo-* + Gr. *phyein* to grow] 1. pertaining to an endophyte. 2. growing inward; proliferating on the interior or inside of an organ or other structure, as a tumor.

**en·do·plasm** (en′do-plaz″əm) [*endo-* + *plasm*] the central portion of the cytoplasm of a cell. Cf. *ectoplasm.*

**en·do·plas·mic** (en″do-plas′mik) composed of or pertaining to endoplasm; see under *reticulum.*

**en·do·poly·ploid** (en″do-pol′e-ploid) having reduplicated chromatin within an intact nucleus, with or without an increase in the number of chromosomes (applied only to cells and tissues); see also *endomitosis.*

**en·do·poly·ploi·dy** (en″do-pol″e-ploi′de) [*endo-* + *polyploidy*] 1. endomitosis. 2. polysomaty. 3. autopolyploidy resulting from a previous endomitotic cycle. See also *polysomaty.*

**en·do·pred·a·tor** (en″do-pred′ə-tor) an individual or species that lives within the body of an organism of another species which it feeds upon and destroys.

**en·do·pros·the·sis** (en″do-pros-the′sis) [*endo-* + *prosthesis*] 1. a hollow stent. 2. a hollow stent in a bile duct, allowing biliary drainage across an obstruction.

**en·do·ra·di·og·ra·phy** (en″do-ra″de-og′rə-fe) the radiographic demonstration of the condition of internal organs and cavities by means of radiopaque materials.

**en·do·ra·dio·sonde** (en″do-ra″de-o-sond′) a small radio transmitter inserted within a body cavity or tube, as within the intestinal lumen to measure the pressure.

**en·do·re·du·pli·ca·tion** (en″do-re-doo″plĭ-ka′shən) replication of the chromosomes without subsequent cell division.

**end-or·gan** (end-or′gən) one of the larger, encapsulated endings of the sensory nerves, such as a lamellated, tactile, or terminal nerve corpuscle.

**en·do·ri·bo·nu·cle·ase** (en″do-ri″bo-noo′kle-ās) [EC 3.1.26–27] any member of two sub-subclasses of enzymes of the hydrolase class that catalyze the hydrolysis of interior bonds of ribonucleotides, producing oligonucleotides or polynucleotides.

**en·dor·phin** (en-dor′fin, en′dor-fin) [*endo*genous + mor*phine*] any of three neuropeptides, amino acid residues of β-lipotropin; they bind to opioid receptors in the brain and have potent analgesic activity. *β-Endorphin* is the C-terminal 30–amino acid residue and is found in the adenohypophysis, hypothalamus, and other sites in the brain; one function appears to be mediation of pain perception. *α-Endorphin* and *γ-endorphin* are the N-terminal 16 and 17 amino acid residues, respectively. See also *enkephalin* and *dynorphin.*

**en·do·sal·pin·gi·tis** (en″do-sal″pin-ji′tis) [*endosalpinx* + *-itis*] inflammation of the endosalpinx.

**en·do·sal·pin·go·ma** (en″do-sal″pin-go′mə) adenomyoma of the uterine tube.

**en·do·sal·pinx** (en″do-sal′pinks) [*endo-* + *salpinx*] tunica mucosa tubae uterinae.

**en·do·sarc** (en′do-sahrk″) endoplasm.

**en·do·scope** (en′do-skōp) [*endo-* + *-scope*] an instrument for examination of the interior of a cavity or hollow viscus; there are both rigid and flexible types. See also *fiberscope.*

**en·do·scop·ic** (en″do-skop′ik) performed by means of an endoscope; pertaining to endoscopy.

**en·dos·co·py** (en-dos′ko-pe) [MeSH: Endoscopy] visual inspection of any cavity of the body by means of an endoscope.
**peroral e.,** examination of organs accessible to observation through an endoscope passed through the mouth.
**transcolonic e.,** examination of the lumen of the colon by means of an endoscope inserted through an incision in its wall.

**en·do·se·cre·to·ry** (en″do-se′krə-tor-e) endocrine.

**en·do·sep·sis** (en″do-sep′sis) septicemia originating within the organism.

**en·do·skel·e·ton** (en″do-skel′ə-ton) [*endo-* + Gr. *skeleton*] the bony and cartilaginous skeleton of the body, exclusive of that part of the skeleton which is of dermal origin; called also *neuroskeleton.*

**en·dos·mom·e·ter** (en″dos-mom′ə-tər) [*endosmosis* + *-meter*] an instrument for determining the rate and extent of endosmosis.

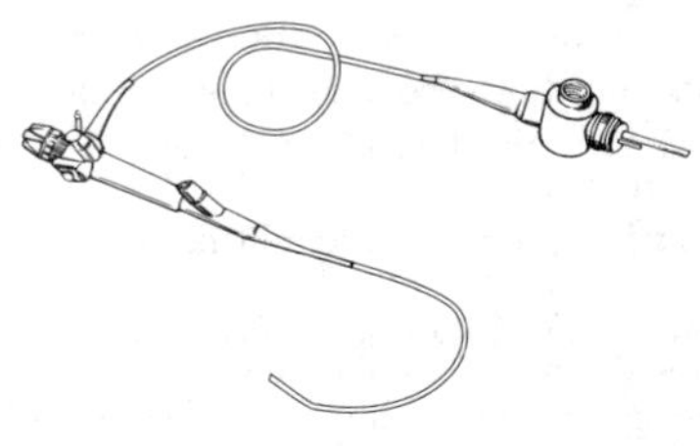

Endoscope.

**en·dos·mo·sis** (en″dos-mo′sis) [*end-* + *osmosis*] a movement in liquids separated by a membranous or porous septum, by which one fluid passes through the septum into the cavity which contains another fluid of a different density. Cf. *exosmosis.*

**en·dos·mot·ic** (en″dos-mot′ik) of the nature of endosmosis.

**en·do·some** (en′do-sōm) [*endo-* + *-some*] [MeSH: Endosomes] 1. in endocytosis, a vesicle that has lost its coat of clathrin. 2. a nucleolus-like, intranuclear, RNA-containing organelle of certain flagellate protozoa that persists during mitosis.

**en·do·so·nog·ra·phy** (en″do-sə-nog′rə-fe) [MeSH: Endosonography] ultrasonography in which the ultrasound transducer is incorporated into the tip of a fiberoptic endoscope that is inserted into the lumen of a cavity or organ. See also *endoscopic ultrasonography* and *endorectal ultrasonography.*

**en·do·sperm** (en′do-spərm) a substance containing reserve food materials, formed within the embryo sac of plants.

**en·do·spore** (en′do-spor) [*endo-* + *spore*] 1. a thick-walled body formed within the vegetative cells of certain bacteria (e.g., *Bacillus, Clostridium, Sarcina*) that is able to withstand adverse environmental conditions for prolonged periods; under favorable conditions it will germinate to form a vegetative bacterium. See also *spore.* 2. an asexual fungal spore produced within the hyphae or cell, as in a spherule of *Coccidioides immitis* or in a sporangium.

**en·do·spor·i·um** (en″do-spor′e-əm) the inner layer of the envelope of a spore.

**en·dos·te·al** (en-dos′te-əl) pertaining to the endosteum; occurring or located within a bone.

**en·dos·te·itis** (en-dos″te-i′tis) inflammation of the endosteum.

**en·dos·te·o·ma** (en-dos″te-o′mə) [*endo-* + *oste-* + *-oma*] a tumor in the medullary cavity of a bone.

**en·do·stetho·scope** (en″do-steth′o-skōp) a stethoscope passed into the esophagus for auscultating the heart.

**en·dos·te·um** (en-dos′te-əm) [*endo-* + *osteon*] [TA] the tissue lining the medullary cavity of a bone.

**en·dos·ti·tis** (en″dos-ti′tis) endosteitis.

**en·dos·to·ma** (en″dos-to′mə) endosteoma.

**en·do·sym·bi·ont** (en″do-sim′be-ont) [*endo-* + *symbiont*] a symbiont which lives within the cells of its partner.

**en·do·sym·bi·o·sis** (en″do-sim″be-o′sis) the state achieved between a virus and its host cell in which cellular division is inhibited but the cell is not immediately destroyed.

**en·do·ten·din·e·um** (en″do-tən-din′e-əm) [*endo-* + L. *tendo, tendines,* after Gr. *tenōn*] the delicate connective tissue separating the secondary bundles (fascicles) of a tendon.

**en·do·ten·on** (en″do-ten′on) [*endo-* + Gr. *tenōn* tendon] endotendineum.

**en·do·the·lia** (en″do-the′le-ə) [Gr.] plural of *endothelium.*

**en·do·the·li·al** (en″do-the′le-əl) pertaining to or made up of endothelium.

**en·do·the·li·al·iza·tion** (en″do-the″le-əl-ĭ-za′shən) the healing of the inner surfaces of vessels or grafts by endothelial cells.

**en·do·the·li·itis** (en″do-the-le-i′tis) inflammation of the endothelium.

**en·do·thel·in** (en″do-the′lin) a potent vasoconstrictor 21–amino acid polypeptide produced by endothelial cells; it is a contractile factor that may play a role in controlling blood pressure and may also function as a neurotransmitter.

**en·do·the·lio·blas·to·ma** (en″do-the″le-o-blas-to′mə) [*endothelium* + *blastoma*] a tumor derived from primitive vasoformative tissue with formation of usually small and slitlike vascular spaces lined by prominent endothelial cells; the term, which now includes hemangioendothelioma, angiosarcoma, lymphangioendothelioma, and lymphangiosarcoma, was applied formerly to such tumors arising from mesothelial tissue as well.

**en·do·the·lio·cho·ri·al** (en″do-the″le-o-kor′e-əl) [*endothelium* + *chorial*] denoting a type of placenta in which syncytial trophoblast embeds maternal vessels bared to their endothelial lining.

**en·do·the·li·oid** (en″do-the′le-oid) resembling endothelium.

**en·do·the·li·ol·y·sin** (en″do-the″le-ol′ə-sin) a cytolysin capable of lysing endothelial cells.

**en·do·the·lio·lyt·ic** (en″do-the″le-o-lit′ik) capable of destroying endothelial tissue.

**en·do·the·li·o·ma** (en″do-the″le-o′mə) [*endothelium* + *-oma*] a general term for any tumor, particularly a benign tumor, that originates from the endothelial linings of blood vessels *(hemangioendothelioma)* or lymphatics *(lymphangioendothelioma).*
**e. angiomato′sum,** angioma.
**dural e.,** a former name for meningioma; of historic interest.
**perithelial e.,** hemangiopericytoma.

**en·do·the·li·o·ma·to·sis** (en″do-the″le-o-mə-to′sis) the formation of multiple and diffuse endotheliomas in a tissue.

**en·do·the·lio·sar·co·ma** (en″do-the″le-o-sahr-ko′mə) Kaposi's sarcoma.

**en·do·the·li·o·sis** (en″do-the″le-o′sis) proliferation of endothelium.
**glomerular capillary e.,** a renal lesion typical of eclampsia; it is characterized by deposition of fibrous material in and beneath the cells of the grossly swollen glomerular capillary endothelium, resulting in near or total occlusion of the capillaries.

**en·do·the·lio·tox·in** (en″do-the″le-o-tok′sin) a specific toxin which acts on the endothelium of capillaries and small veins, producing hemorrhage. Cf. *hemorrhagin.*

**en·do·the·li·um** (en″do-the′le-əm) pl. *endothe′lia* [*endo-* + Gr. *thēlē* nipple] [MeSH: Endothelium] the layer of epithelial cells that lines the cavities of the heart, the lumina of blood and lymph vessels, and the serous cavities of the body; it originates from the mesoderm.
**anterior e. of cornea, e. ante′rius cor′neae,** epithelium posterius corneae.
**e. ca′merae anterio′ris bul′bi,** epithelium posterius corneae.
**corneal e., e. cornea′le,** epithelium posterius corneae.
**extraembryonic e.,** endothelium which arises outside of the body of the embryo, such as that lining the vitelline vessels.

**en·do·therm** (en′do-thərm″) [*endo-* + *therm*] 1. an animal that exhibits endothermy (def. 2). 2. homeotherm.

**en·do·ther·mal** (en″do-thər′məl) endothermic.

**en·do·ther·mic** (en″do-thər′mik) 1. characterized by or accompanied by the absorption of heat, as a chemical reaction accompanied by absorption of heat and to which heat must be supplied if it is to proceed; storing up heat or energy in a potential form. Cf. *exothermic.* 2. pertaining to or characterized by endothermy (def. 2). 3. homeothermic.

**en·do·ther·my** (en″do-thər′me) [*endo-* + Gr. *thermē* heat] 1. diathermy. 2. thermoregulation accomplished by internal heat production. Cf. *ectothermy* (def. 1). 3. homeothermy.

**en·do·tho·rac·ic** (en″do-tho-ras′ik) within the thorax; situated internal to the ribs.

**en·do·thrix** (en′do-thriks) [*endo-* + *-thrix*] a dermatophyte whose growth and spore production are confined chiefly within the shaft of the hair, without formation of conspicuous external spores; such fungi include *Trichophyton tonsurans* and *T. violaceum.*

**en·do·tox·e·mia** (en″do-tok-se′me-ə) [MeSH: Endotoxemia] the presence of endotoxins in the blood, which may result in shock.

**en·do·tox·in** (en″do-tok′sin) [*endo-* + *toxin*] a heat-stable toxin associated with the outer membranes of certain gram-negative bacteria, including the brucellae, the enterobacteria, neisseriae, and vibrios. Endotoxins are not secreted but are released only when the cells are disrupted; they are less potent and less specific than the exotoxins; and they do not form toxoids. They are composed of complex lipopolysaccharide molecules, of which the polysaccharide unit (somatic O antigen) is responsible for antigenicity, occurring in hundreds of variations, and the phospholipid moiety (lipid A) is the source of toxicity. When injected in large quantities the endotoxins produce hemorrhagic shock and severe diarrhea; smaller amounts cause fever, altered resistance to bacterial infection, leukopenia followed by leukocytosis, and numerous other biologic effects. Called also *bacterial pyrogen.* See also *toxin.*

**en·do·tra·che·al** (en″do-tra′ke-əl) [*endo-* + *tracheal*] 1. within or through the trachea. 2. performed by passage through the lumen of the trachea.

**en·do·tra·chel·itis** (en″do-tra″kəl-i′tis) [*endo-* + *trachelitis*] endocervicitis.

**en·do·ure·thral** (en″do-u-re′thrəl) within the urethra.

**en·do·urol·o·gy** (en″do-ūr-ol′ə-je) [*endo-* + *urology*] the branch of urologic surgery concerned with closed procedures for visualizing or manipulating the urinary tract; it may refer to procedures involving any part of the urinary tract or may be limited to procedures involving only the kidney or ureter.

**en·do·uter·ine** (en″do-u′tər-in) within the uterus.

**en·do·vac·ci·na·tion** (en″do-vak″sĭ-na′shən) [*endo-* + *vaccination*] the administration of vaccines by mouth.

**en·do·vas·cu·lar** (en″do-vas′ku-lər) intravascular.

**en·do·vas·cu·li·tis** (en″do-vas″ku-li′tis) endangiitis.

**en·do·ve·ni·tis** (en″do-ve-ni′tis) endophlebitis.

**en·do·ve·nous** (en″do-ve′nəs) intravenous.

**En·dox·an** (en-dok′sən) trademark for a preparation of cyclophosphamide.

**en·do·zo·ite** (en″do-zo′īt) tachyzoite.

**end plate** (end plāt) a flat termination. Spelled also *end-plate.*
**motor e. p.,** the discoid expansion of a terminal branch of the axon of a motor nerve fiber, which apposes the subneural apparatus of a skeletal muscle fiber, forming the neuromuscular junction (q.v.).

**end-plea·sure** (end′plezh-ər) the pleasure produced by the sexual orgasm, as contrasted with the fore-pleasure which precedes it.

**end point** (end point) in titration, the highest dilution of a substance that produces a reaction with a given volume of another substance.

**end prod·uct** (end prod′əkt) the chemical compound resulting from the completion of a sequence of metabolic reactions.

**En·drate** (en′drāt) trademark for preparations of edetate disodium.

**en·drin** (en′drin) [MeSH: Endrin] a highly toxic chlorinated hydrocarbon insecticide; if ingested or absorbed through the skin by a human or other animal, it can cause potentially fatal neurotoxicity such as tremors and convulsions.

**en·dry·sone** (en′drĭ-sōn) a topical anti-inflammatory for use in ophthalmology.

**end-tidal** (end-ti′dəl) pertaining to or occurring at the end of expiration of a normal tidal volume.

**En·du·ron** (en′du-ron) trademark for a preparation of methyclothiazide.

**En·dur·o·nyl** (en-dūr′o-nəl) trademark for preparations of methyclothiazide with reserpine.

**-ene** a suffix used in chemistry to indicate an unsaturated hydrocarbon containing one double bond.

**en·e·ma** (en′ə-mə) pl. *enemas* or *enema′ta* [Gr.] [MeSH: Enema] a liquid injected or to be injected into the rectum; called also *clysma* and *clyster.*
**barium e.,** a suspension of barium injected into the intestine as a contrast agent for radiological examination; see also *double-contrast examination,* under *examination.* Called also *contrast e.*
**blind e.,** the insertion of a soft-rubber tube into the rectum to aid in the expulsion of flatus.
**contrast e.,** barium e.
**double-contrast e.,** see under *examination.*
**Fleet e.,** trademark for an enema containing, in each 100 mL, 16 g sodium biphosphate and 6 g sodium phosphate, packaged in a plastic squeeze bottle fitted with a prelubricated rectal tube 5 cm long.
**hydrocortisone e.** [USP], an aqueous solution of hydrocortisone administered rectally as an anti-inflammatory in the treatment of ulcerative colitis.
**small bowel e.,** enteroclysis, def. 2.
**soapsuds e.,** an enema made by dissolving 2 oz of soap in a pint of warm water.
**sodium phosphate and biphosphate e., sodium phosphates e.** [USP], a solution of sodium phosphate and sodium biphosphate, or sodium phosphate and phosphoric acid, in purified water; used as a cathartic.
**theophylline olamine e.,** an enema containing an amount of anhydrous theophylline equivalent to 72 to 78 per cent of the labeled amount of theophylline olamine and an amount of monoethanolamine equivalent to 22 to 28 per cent of the labeled amount of theophylline olamine.

**en·e·ma·tor** (en′ə-ma″tor) an apparatus for giving enemas.

**en·er·get·ics** (en″ər-jet′iks) the study of energy; the science of energy.

**en·er·gid** (en′ər-jid) living, active protoplasm, as distinguished from deuteroplasm.

**en·er·gom·e·ter** (en″ər-gom′ə-tər) an apparatus for studying the pulse.

**en·er·gy** (en′ər-je) [Gr. *energeia*] the capacity to operate or work; the capacity to produce motion, to overcome resistance, and to effect physical changes. Symbol *E.*
**activation e.,** in a chemical reaction, the energy that must be supplied to the reactants in order to form an activated complex or transition state, which then breaks down to form the products.
**atomic e.,** energy that can be liberated by changes in the nucleus of an atom (as by fission of a heavy nucleus or fusion of light nuclei into heavier ones with accompanying loss of mass).
**binding e.,** the amount of energy that would be necessary to separate an atomic nucleus into its component protons and neutrons.
**chemical e.,** energy evolved or absorbed by chemical reactions.
**free e., Gibbs free e. (*G*),** the thermodynamic function $G = H - TS$, where $H$ is enthalpy, $T$ absolute temperature, and $S$ entropy. For chemical reactions occurring at a constant temperature and pressure, the free energy change $\Delta G = \Delta H - T\Delta S$ determines the direction in which a reaction proceeds; $\Delta G$ is negative for a spontaneous (exergonic) reaction; $\Delta G$ is positive for a nonspontaneous (endergonic) reaction. The free energy change can be determined from the equation $\Delta G = \Delta G° + RT \ln Q$, where $R$ is the gas constant, $Q$ is the reaction quotient (q.v.), and $\Delta G°$ is the standard free energy change (the difference between the sum of the free energies of the products and the sum of the free energies of the reactants when all products and reactants are in their standard states; solids and liquids are pure substances; gases are at 1 atm pressure; the temperature is 25°C; and all solutions have a concentration of 1M). For a reaction at equilibrium, $\Delta G = 0$; thus $\Delta G° = -RT \ln K$, where $K$ is the equilibrium constant.
**kinetic e.,** energy of motion; equal to one-half the mass of a body times the square of its velocity.
**nuclear e.,** atomic e.
**potential e.,** the energy that a body has due to its position, equal to the work required to move the body to that position from some reference position; e.g., a body has a gravitational potential energy equal to its mass times the acceleration due to gravity times its height above the reference position.
**radiant e.,** the energy of electromagnetic waves, such as radio waves, visible light, x-rays, and gamma rays.

**en·er·va·tion** (en″ər-va′shən) [L. *enervatio,* from *ex* out + *nervus* nerve] 1. lack of nervous energy; languor. 2. neurectomy.

**en·flag·el·la·tion** (en-flaj″ə-la′shən) flagellation (def. 2).

**en·flu·rane** (en′floo-rān) [USP] [MeSH: Enflurane] a potent inhalational anesthetic agent, widely used for induction and maintenance of general anesthesia; it is nonflammable, induction and recovery are smooth and rapid, and the depth of anesthesia is rapidly altered; the incidence of arrhythmias and postoperative nausea and vomiting are somewhat less than with halothane or methoxyflurane.

**ENG** electronystagmography.

**en·gage·ment** (en-gāj′mənt) in obstetrics, the entrance of the fetal head, or presenting part, into the superior pelvic strait and beginning descent through the pelvic canal so that its biparietal plane is below the plane of the pelvic inlet.

**en·gas·tri·us** (en-gas′tre-əs) [Gr. *en* in + *gastēr* belly] asymmetrical conjoined twins with the parasitic twin contained within the abdomen of the larger twin.

**En·gel-Reck·ling·hau·sen disease** (eng′gəl-rek′ling-hou′zən) [Gerhard *Engel,* German physician, 19th century; Friedrich Daniel von *Recklinghausen,* German pathologist, 1833–1910] osteitis fibrosa cystica; see under *osteitis.*

**Eng·el·mann's disease** (eng′gəl-mahnz) [Guido *Engelmann,* Austrian surgeon, born 1876] diaphyseal dysplasia.

**Eng·el·mann's disk** (eng′gəl-mahnz) [Theodor Wilhelm *Engelmann,* German physiologist, 1843–1909] H band; see under *band.*

**Eng·en orthosis** (eng′en) [Thorkild Jensen *Engen,* American prosthetist, born 1924] see under *orthosis.*

**en·gine** (en′jin) a machine by which energy is converted into mechanical motion.
**dental e.,** a machine operated by electricity, water, or compressed air that provides power for rotary dental instruments.

**en·gi·neer·ing** (en″jĭ-nēr′ing) [MeSH: Engineering] the application of physical, mathematical, and mechanical principles to practical purposes.
**biomedical e.,** the use of engineering in biomedical technology such as the analysis of movement of body parts or prosthetics. Called also *bioengineering.*
**tissue e.,** application of the methods and principles of engineering to gain an understanding of the relationship between structure and function in both normal and pathological tissue and to develop possible substitutes for pathological tissue.

**en·globe** (en-glōb′) phagocytose.

**en·gorged** (en-gorjd′) distended or swollen with fluids.

**en·gorge·ment** (en-gorj′mənt) 1. local congestion; excessive fullness of any organ, vessel, or tissue due to accumulation of fluids. 2. hyperemia.

**en·graft·ment** (ən-graft′mənt) incorporation of grafted tissue into the body of the host.

**en·gram** (en′gram) [Gr. *en* in + *-gram*] 1. a lasting mark or trace. 2. the permanent trace left by a stimulus in nerve tissue; see also *pattern generator.* 3. in psychology, the lasting trace left in the psyche by any experience; a latent memory picture.

**en·graph·ia** (en-graf′e-ə) the process hypothesized in the theory that stimuli leave definite traces (engrams) on the protoplasm which, when regularly repeated, induce a habit that persists after the stimuli cease.

**en·hance·ment** (en-hans'mənt) prolonged survival of tumor cells in animals previously immunized with antigens of the tumor owing to the presence of "enhancing" or "facilitating" antibodies that prevent an immune response against these antigens; called also *immunologic enhancement.*
**edge e.,** a sharp increase in contrast on a xeroradiograph where there is an abrupt difference in the tissue densities of adjacent structures.

**en·hanc·er** (en-hans'ər) 1. something that promotes or augments. 2. in eukaryotes, a specific DNA sequence that increases the expression of a gene; it can be positioned to either side of the gene or within the coding region and can occur on template or coding strand. It is activated upon binding by regulatory proteins. Specific enhancers are effective only in particular types of cells.
**penetration e.,** a physical change performed on skin or a chemical applied to the skin that results in increased absorption of a topically applied drug.

**En·hy·dri·na** (en"hi-dri'nə) a genus of sea snakes (family Hydrophiidae). *E. schisto'sa* is a venomous species found in the Indian and southern Pacific Oceans.

**En·kaid** (en'kād) trademark for a preparation of encainide hydrochloride.

**en·ka·tar·rha·phy** (en"kə-tahr'ə-fe) encatarrhaphy.

**en·keph·a·lin** (en-kef'ə-lin) either of two simple pentapeptides having the formula $H_2N$-Tyr-Gly-Gly-Phe-X, where X is leucine or methionine, referred to as *leu-enkephalin* and *met-enkephalin.* Although met-enkephalin is the N-terminal 5 residues of the endorphins and both enkephalins and endorphins bind to opioid receptors, the two groups derive from functionally and anatomically distinct groups of neurons. The enkephalins function as neurotransmitters or neuromodulators at many locations in the brain and spinal cord and play a part in pain perception, movement, mood, behavior, and neuroendocrine regulation; they are also found in nerve plexuses and exocrine glands of the gastrointestinal tract.

**en·keph·a·lin·er·gic** (en-kef"ə-lin-ər'jik) denoting synaptic transmission by enkephalin neurotransmitters.

**en·large·ment** (en-lahrj'mənt) 1. an increase in the size of an organ or part; see *hypertrophy* and *hyperplasia.* 2. in anatomy, a prominence or swelling; an intumescence.
**atrial e.,** a term used in electrocardiography to denote increased size of one or both atria, due to hypertrophy, dilatation, or both; it is manifest in the morphology of the P waves. See also *P mitrale* and *P pulmonale.*
**cardiac e.,** dilatation or hypertrophy of the heart, due to compensatory mechanisms or secondary to disease.
**cervical e.,** intumescentia cervicalis.
**choroidal e.,** glomus choroideum.
**gingival e.,** hyperplastic enlargement of the gingival tissue. It may occur as a result of inflammatory or fibrous lesions resulting from irritation or injury brought about by mechanical or chemical factors or systemic or localized pathologic processes. See also *fibromatosis gingivae* and *gingival hyperplasia.*
**e. of heart,** cardiac e.
**lumbar e., lumbosacral e.,** intumescentia lumbosacralis.
**tympanic e.,** intumescentia tympanica.

**en·ni·a·tin** (en-e-a'tin) a cyclic polypeptide antibiotic with a ring of 18 atoms, produced by a fungus of the genus *Fusarium.* It is active against certain gram-positive bacteria, functioning as an ionophore and altering membrane permeability.

**enol** (e'nol) [contraction from ethyl*ene* + alcoh*ol*] an organic compound in which one carbon of a double-bonded pair is also attached to a hydroxyl group; it is thus a tautomer of a ketone (see *keto-enol tautomerism* at *tautomerism*). The term is also used as a prefix or infix, often italicized.

**eno·lase** (e'no-lās) phosphopyruvate hydratase.
**neuron-specific e.,** an isozyme of enolase that is found in normal neurons and in all the cells of the diffuse neuroendocrine system; it serves as a marker for neuroendocrine differentiation in tumors.

**en·oph·thal·mos** (en"of-thal'mos) [Gr. *en* in + *ophthalmos* eye] [MeSH: Enophthalmos] a backward displacement of the eyeball into the orbit.

**en·oph·thal·mus** (en"of-thal'məs) enophthalmos.

**en·or·gan·ic** (en"or-gan'ik) existing as a permanent quality of the organism.

**en·os·to·sis** (en"os-to'sis) [Gr. *en* in + *ostosis*] a morbid bony growth developed within the cavity of a bone or on the internal surface of the bone cortex.

**En·o·vid** (en-o'vid) trademark for preparations of mestranol and norethynodrel.

**enox·a·par·in** (e-nok"sə-par'in) [MeSH: Enoxaparin] a low molecular weight heparin, prepared from porcine intestinal mucosa, that binds to and potentiates the action of antithrombin III, used to prevent pulmonary embolism and deep venous thrombosis following hip or knee replacement or high-risk abdominal surgery; administered subcutaneously.

**enox·i·mone** (en-ok'sĭ-mōn) [MeSH: Enoximone] a phosphodiesterase inhibitor similar to amrinone, having positive inotropic and vasodilator effects; used as a cardiotonic in the short-term management of congestive heart failure, administered intravenously.

**enoyl CoA** (e'no-əl ko-a') enoyl coenzyme A.

**enoyl-CoA hy·dra·tase** (e'no-əl ko-a' hi'drə-tās) [EC 4.2.1.17] [MeSH: Enoyl-CoA Hydratase] an enzyme of the lyase class that catalyzes the stereospecific hydration of the double bond in enoyl coenzyme A, forming the L-hydroxy derivative of acyl coenzyme A from the *trans* isomer of enoyl coenzyme A. The reaction is a step in the beta oxidation of fatty acids.

**enoyl CoA isom·er·ase** (e'no-əl ko-a' i-som'ə-rās) dodecenoyl-CoA Δ-isomerase.

**enoyl co·en·zyme A** (e'no-əl ko-en'zīm) dehydrogenated acyl coenzyme A; in the beta oxidation of fatty acids, the *trans* isomer of enoyl coenzyme A, with the double bond between carbons C-2 and C-3, is an intermediate.

**en plaque** (ahn-plak') [Fr.] in the form of a plaque or plate.

**en·rich·ment** (ən-rich'mənt) the addition of nutrients, as to culture media; the medium resulting from such addition.

**en·ro·flox·a·cin** (en"ro-flok'sə-sin) a veterinary quinolone antibiotic with actions and uses similar to those of ciprofloxacin in humans.

**En·roth's sign** (en'rots) [Emil Emanuel *Enroth,* Finnish physician, 1879–1953] see under *sign.*

**en·si·form** (en'sĭ-form) [L. *ensis* sword + *form*] sword-shaped; xiphoid.

**en·sis·ter·num** (en"sis-tər'nəm) [L. *ensis* sword + *sternum*] xiphoid process (processus xiphoideus [TA]).

**en·som·pha·lus** (ən-som'fə-ləs) [Gr. *en* in + *soma* + *omphalos* navel] conjoined twins with blended bodies, two separate navels, and two umbilical cords.

**en·stro·phe** (en'stro-fe) entropion.

**ENT** ears, nose, and throat; see *otorhinolaryngology.*

**en·tad** (en'tad) toward the center; inwardly.

**en·tal** (en'təl) [Gr. *entos* within] internal; inner; central.

**ent·ame·bi·a·sis** (en"tə-me-bi'ə-sis) infection with *Entamoeba.*

**Ent·amoe·ba** (en"tə-me'bə) [*ent-* + *ameba*] [MeSH: Entamoeba] a genus of naked ameboid protozoa (suborder Tubulina, order Amoebida) parasitic in invertebrates and vertebrates, including humans, and characterized by the presence of a vesicular nucleus with a comparatively small central karyosome with a number of peripheral chromatin granules attached to the nuclear membrane.
**E. bucca'lis,** *E. gingivalis.*
**E. co'li,** a very common nonpathogenic species found in the human intestinal tract.
**E. dis'par,** a species virtually identical to *E. histolytica* but nonpathogenic.
**E. gingiva'lis,** a species often found in the mouth of humans with periodontal disease; it has not been shown to be pathogenic. Called also *E. buccalis.*
**E. hartman'ni,** a nonpathogenic species found in the human intestinal tract that is almost indistinguishable from but smaller than *E. histolytica;* it was formerly designated "small race" *E. histolytica.*
**E. histoly'tica,** the only species of *Entamoeba* with the potential for producing human amebiasis; it is transmitted through ingestion of cysts in contaminated food and water. Trophozoites may invade the tissue of the large intestine and may be spread to extraintestinal sites such as the liver, spleen, brain, lungs, and pericardium.
**E. inva'dens,** the only pathogenic species of the genus *Entamoeba* other than *E. histolytica,* producing lesions of the stomach, colon, duodenum, ileum, colon, and liver in reptiles.
**E. polec'ki,** an intestinal parasite of hogs, sheep, monkeys, cattle, and occasionally humans.

**ent·epi·con·dyle** (en-tep"ĭ-kon'dīl) the internal epicondyle of the humerus.

**en·te·que** (en-ta'ka) enzootic calcinosis.

**en·ter·ad·en** (en-ter'ad-ən) [*enter-* + Gr. *adēn* gland] any intestinal gland.

**en·ter·ad·e·ni·tis** (en″tər-ad″ə-ni'tis) [*enteraden* + *-itis*] inflammation of the intestinal glands.

**en·ter·al** (en'tər-əl) [Gr. *enteron* intestine] enteric.

**en·ter·al·gia** (en″tər-al'jə) [*enter-* + *-algia*] pain or neuralgia of the intestine. Called also *enterodynia.*

**en·ter·ec·ta·sis** (en″tər-ek'tə-sis) [*enter-* + *ectasis*] distention of the intestines.

**en·ter·ec·to·my** (en″tər-ek'tə-me) [*enter-* + *-ectomy*] excision of a part of the intestine; resection of the intestine.

**en·ter·epip·lo·cele** (en″tər-ə-pip'lo-sēl) enteroepiplocele.

**en·ter·ic** (en-ter'ik) [Gr. *enterikos* intestinal] within or pertaining to the small intestine. Called also *enteral.*

**en·ter·ic-coat·ed** (en-ter'ik-kōt'əd) a term designating a special coating applied to tablets or capsules which prevents release and absorption of their contents until they reach the intestines.

**en·ter·i·tis** (en″tər-i'tis) [*enter-* + *-itis*] [MeSH: Enteritis] inflammation of the intestine, usually referring only to the small intestine; see also *enterocolitis.*
**cat e.,** panleukopenia.
**choleriform e.,** an acute, cholera-like diarrheal disease with a high case fatality rate, prevalent in epidemic and endemic form in the Western Pacific area since 1938, caused by the El Tor or Celebes vibrio, immunologically identical with the cholera vibrio.
**chronic cicatrizing e.,** Crohn's disease.
**e. cys'tica chro'nica,** a form marked by cystic dilatation of the intestinal glands, due to closure of the openings of their ducts.
**diphtheritic e.,** enteritis characterized by the presence of a false membrane and severe ulceration of the mucosa beneath the membrane.
**duck virus e.,** duck plague.
**feline e.,** panleukopenia.
**granulomatous e.,** a type of enteritis seen in horses and dogs, with granuloma formation under the muscularis mucosa, especially in the jejunum and ileum; symptoms include hypoproteinemia, weight loss, edema, and diarrhea.
**e. gra'vis,** an often fatal disease characterized by acute onset of severe abdominal pain, nausea, vomiting, and bloody diarrhea, with mucosal necrosis and hemorrhage and edema of the submucosa, most prominent in the jejunum and proximal ileum.
**infectious feline e.,** panleukopenia.
**lymphocytic-plasmacytic e.,** infiltration of the walls of the stomach and intestines of dogs by lymphocytes and plasma cells, with malabsorption, protein-losing enteropathy, and diarrhea.
**mink viral e.,** a highly contagious viral disease of mink resembling feline panleukopenia and caused by a closely related parvovirus.
**mucous e.,** former term for irritable bowel syndrome.
**necrotic e.,** 1. a type of porcine proliferative enteritis in which the intestinal walls become necrotic. 2. enterotoxemia in chickens, often with fatal hemorrhaging, due to infection by *Clostridium perfringens* type A or C.
**e. necro'ticans,** an inflammation of the intestines in humans, caused by *Clostridium perfringens* type C, and characterized by necrosis.
**e. nodula'ris,** enteritis with enlargement of the lymph nodes.
**phlegmonous e.,** a condition with symptoms resembling those of peritonitis; it may be secondary to other intestinal diseases, as chronic obstruction, strangulated hernia, carcinoma, etc.
**e. polypo'sa,** enteritis marked by polypoid growths in the intestine, due to proliferation of the connective tissue.
**porcine proliferative e.,** a disease of young pigs in which the walls of the intestines lose villi, immature epithelial cells proliferate, and the lamina propria becomes inflamed, resulting in diarrhea and anorexia. The cause is thought to be infection by *Campylobacter sputorum* or *C. hyointestinalis.* It is usually self-limiting, but it may develop into necrotic enteritis or proliferative hemorrhagic enteropathy that can be fatal.
**protozoan e.,** enteritis in which the intestine is infested with protozoan organisms of various species.
**pseudomembranous e.,** pseudomembranous enterocolitis.
**radiation e.,** see *colitis.*
**regional e., segmental e.,** Crohn's disease.
**streptococcus e.,** primary phlegmonous enteritis, due to *Streptococcus pyogenes.*
**terminal e.,** Crohn's disease.
**tuberculous e.,** enteritis secondary to advanced pulmonary tuberculosis, believed to be caused by the swallowing of large amounts of positive sputum; now rare due to antibiotic tuberculosis therapy.

**enter(o)-** [Gr. *enteron* intestine] a combining form denoting relationship to the intestines.

**en·tero·anas·to·mo·sis** (en″tər-o-ə-nas″to-mo'sis) enteroenterostomy.

**en·tero·ar·thric** (en″tər-o-ahr'thrik) said of thallic-arthric conidiogenesis in which only the inner part of the cell wall forms the conidia.

**En·tero·bac·ter** (en″tər-o-bak'tər) [*entero-* + Gr. *baktron* a rod] [MeSH: Enterobacter] a genus of gram-negative, facultatively anaerobic rod-shaped bacteria of the family Enterobacteriaceae, made up of motile, peritrichously flagellated cells, some being encapsulated. The organisms, widely distributed in nature, occur in the intestinal tract of humans and animals. They are frequently a cause of nosocomial infections, arising from contaminated medical devices and personnel.
**E. aero'genes,** a species isolated from feces, sewage, soil, and dairy products; it can cause nosocomial pneumonia (see Enterobacter *pneumonia,* under *pneumonia*) in debilitated patients. Called also *Aerobacter aerogenes* and *Bacterium aerogenes.*
**E. agglo'merans,** a species found on plants, in water, and in the human intestinal tract. It is a potential pathogen, causing a variety of infections, including those of nosocomial origin. Called also *Erwinia herbicola.*
**E. amni'genus,** a species found in natural waters but not identified as a pathogen of humans.
**E. cloa'cae,** the most commonly occurring species, found in feces, soil, and water and, less commonly, in urine, pus, and pathological material; it can cause nosocomial pneumonia in debilitated patients (see Enterobacter *pneumonia,* under *pneumonia*). Called also *Aerobacter cloacae* and *Bacterium cloacae.*
**E. gergo'viae,** a species that is lysine decarboxylase positive, a cause of human urinary, pulmonary, and bloodstream infections.
**E. haf'nia,** *Hafnia alvei.*
**E. sakaza'kii,** a species that produces a yellow pigment at 25°C, found in environment and foods, but rarely in human clinical specimens.

**En·tero·bac·te·ri·a·ceae** (en″tər-o-bak-te″re-a'se-e) [MeSH: Enterobacteriaceae] a family of gram-negative, facultatively anaerobic, rod-shaped bacteria, usually motile with peritrichous flagella, made up of saprophytes and plant and animal parasites of worldwide distribution, found in soil, water, and plants and in animals from insects to humans. Many species are important economically, causing disease in agricultural, fish, cattle, and poultry industries. In humans, disease is produced by both invasive action and production of toxin, and species not normally associated with disease may be opportunistic pathogens. Members of this family are responsible for as many as half of the nosocomial infections reported annually in the United States, especially species of *Enterobacter, Escherichia, Klebsiella, Proteus, Providencia,* and *Serratia.* Other genera in the family are *Buttiauxella, Cedecea, Citrobacter, Edwardsiella, Erwinia, Hafnia, Kluyvera, Morganella, Obesumbacterium, Rahnella, Salmonella, Shigella, Tatumella, Xenorhabdus,* and *Yersinia;* two additional genera are proposed: *Ewingella* and *Levinea.*

**en·tero·bi·a·sis** (en″ter-o-bi'ə-sis) [MeSH: Enterobiasis] infection with nematodes of the genus *Enterobius,* especially *E. vermicularis.*

**en·tero·bil·i·ary** (en″tər-o-bil'e-ar-e) pertaining to the small intestine and the bile passages.

**En·tero·bi·us** (en″tər-o'be-əs) [*entero-* + Gr. *bios* life] [MeSH: Enterobius] a genus of intestinal nematodes of the family Oxyuridae.
**E. vermicula'ris,** the seatworm, threadworm, or pinworm, a small white worm parasitic in the upper part of the human large intestine, and occasionally in the female genitals and bladder. Infection is frequent in children, sometimes causing itching. Formerly called *Ascaris vermicularis* and *Oxyuris vermicularis.*

**en·tero·blas·tic** (en″tər-o-blas'tik) said of blastic conidiogenesis in which only the inner part of the cell wall is used to form the conidium.

**en·tero·cele** (en'tər-o-sēl″) [*entero-* + *-cele*[1]] 1. a hernia containing intestine; see entries under *hernia.* 2. posterior vaginal hernia.

**en·tero·cen·te·sis** (en″tər-o-sən-te'sis) [*entero-* + *-centesis*] surgical puncture of the intestine.

**en·tero·cho·le·cys·tost·o·my** (en″tər-o-ko″le-sis-tos'tə-me) [*entero-* + *chole-* + *cysto-* + *-stomy*] cholecystenterostomy.

**en·tero·cho·le·cys·tot·o·my** (en″tər-o-ko″le-sis-tot'ə-me) [*entero-* + *cholecystotomy*] incision into the gallbladder and the intestine.

**en·ter·o·chro·maf·fin** (en″tər-o-kro'mə-fin) pertaining to cells in the gastrointestinal tract having granules that stain readily with silver and chromium salts; see *enterochromaffin cells,* under *cell.*

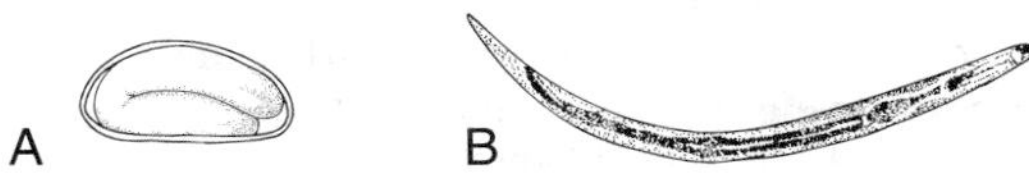

Enterobius vermicularis. *(A),*egg; *(B),* adult female.

**en·tero·ci·ne·sia** (en″tər-o-sĭ-ne′zhə) [*entero-* + *cinesi-* + *-ia*] peristalsis.

**en·tero·ci·net·ic** (en″tər-o-sĭ-net′ik) pertaining to or stimulating peristalsis.

**en·tero·clei·sis** (en″tər-o-kli′sis) [*entero-* + Gr. *kleisis* closure] 1. closure of a wound in the intestine. 2. occlusion of the lumen of the intestine.
**omental e.**, closure of an intestinal perforation by suturing the omentum over the defect.

**en·ter·oc·ly·sis** (en″tər-ok′lə-sis) [*entero-* + *clysis*] 1. the injection of a nutrient or medicinal liquid into the bowel. 2. the introduction of barium directly into the small bowel through a nasogastric tube whose end is positioned beyond the duodenojejunal junction; used in radiographic examination of the small bowel. Called also *small bowel enema.*

**en·tero·coc·ce·mia** (en″tər-o-kok-se′me-ə) [*enterococcus* + *-emia*] the presence of enterococci in the blood.

**En·tero·coc·cus** (en″tər-o-kok′əs) [*entero-* + *coccus*] [MeSH: Enterococcus] a genus of gram-positive, facultatively anaerobic bacteria of the family Streptococcaceae, formerly classified in the genus *Streptococcus.* Organisms are round to ovoid, found in pairs or short chains, catalase-negative, non–spore forming, and generally nonmotile. Members of this genus are common flora of the intestinal tract of humans and animals.
**E. a′vium,** a species found primarily in the feces of chickens; it is occasionally associated with appendicitis, otitis, and brain abscesses in humans.
**E. faeca′lis,** a widespread species that is a normal inhabitant of the human intestinal tract; it causes urinary tract infections, infective endocarditis, and bacteremia that is often fatal. Formerly called *Streptococcus faecalis.*
**E. fae′cium,** a widespread species that is a normal inhabitant of the human intestinal tract; it occasionally causes urinary tract infections, infective endocarditis, and bacteremia. Formerly called *Streptococcus faecium.*

**en·tero·coc·cus** (en″tər-o-kok′əs) pl. *enterococ′ci* [MeSH: Enterococcus] An organism belonging to the genus *Enterococcus;* formerly, an organism belonging to a group of streptococci that are normal inhabitants of the intestinal tract in humans and animals and are now assigned to the genus *Enterococcus.*

**en·tero·coel** (en′tər-o-sēl″) enterocoele.

**en·tero·coele** (en″tər-o-se′le) [*entero-* + Gr. *koilia* belly] the body cavity formed by the outpouchings from the archenteron, typically found in echinoderms and chordates.

**en·tero·coe·lom** (en″tər-o-se′lom) enterocoele.

**en·tero·coel·om·ate** (en″tər-o-sēl′o-māt) 1. having an enterocoele. 2. any of a group of animals, such as echinoderms and chordates, having a body cavity (enterocoele) derived from the archenteron.

**en·tero·co·lec·to·my** (en″tər-o-ko-lek′tə-me) resection of the intestines, including the ileum, cecum, and ascending colon.

**en·tero·co·li·tis** (en″tər-o-ko-li′tis) [*entero-* + *colitis*] [MeSH: Enterocolitis] inflammation involving both the small intestine and the colon; see also *enteritis* and *colitis.*
**antibiotic-associated e.,** that in which treatment with antibiotics alters the bowel flora and results in diarrhea or pseudomembranous enterocolitis. Called also *antibiotic-associated colitis.*
**hemorrhagic e.,** an inflammation of the small intestine and colon, characterized by hemorrhagic breakdown of the intestinal mucosa with inflammatory-cell infiltration. At least some cases have been linked to verotoxins produced by *Escherichia coli* 0157:H7.
**necrotizing e.,** pseudomembranous e.
**pseudomembranous e.,** an acute inflammation of the bowel mucosa with the formation of pseudomembranous plaques overlying an area of superficial ulceration, and the passage of the pseudomembranous material in the feces; it may result from shock and ischemia or be associated with antibiotic therapy. Called also *necrotizing e.* and *pseudomembranous colitis* or *enteritis.*
**regional e.,** Crohn's disease.

**en·tero·co·los·to·my** (en″tər-o-ko-los′tə-me) [*entero-* + *colostomy*] the surgical formation of a communication between the small intestine and the colon; also, the opening so constructed.

**en·tero·cu·ta·ne·ous** (en″tər-o-ku-ta′ne-əs) pertaining to or communicating with the intestine and the cutaneous surface of the body, as an enterocutaneous fistula.

**en·tero·cyst** (en′tər-o-sist″) [*entero-* + *cyst*] enteric cyst.

**en·tero·cys·to·cele** (en″tər-o-sis′to-sēl) [*entero-* + *cysto-* + *-cele*[1]] hernia of the bladder and intestine.

**en·tero·cys·to·ma** (en″tər-o-sis-to′mə) [*entero-* + *cyst* + *-oma*] enteric cyst.

**en·tero·cyte** (en′tər-o-sīt″) an intestinal epithelial cell.

**En·tero·cy·to·zo·on** (en″tər-o-si″to-zo′ən) a genus of protozoa of the order Microsporida. *E. bieneu′si* has been found in enterocytes of immunocompromised patients, causing diarrhea.

**en·ter·odyn·ia** (en″tər-o-din′e-ə) [*enter-* + *-odynia*] enteralgia.

**en·tero·en·ter·os·to·my** (en″tər-o-en″tər-os′tə-me) surgical anastomosis between two segments of the intestine. Called also *enteroanastomosis.*

**en·tero·epip·lo·cele** (en″tər-o-ə-pip′lo-sēl) [*entero-* + *epiplocele*] hernia of the small intestine and omentum.

**en·tero·gas·tric** (en″tər-o-gas′trik) gastrointestinal.

**en·tero·gas·tri·tis** (en″tər-o-gas-tri′tis) [*entero-* + *gastritis*] gastroenteritis.

**en·tero·gas·trone** (en″tər-o-gas′trōn) any of various hormones that mediate the humoral inhibition of gastric secretion and motility.

**en·ter·og·e·nous** (en″tər-oj′ə-nəs) [*entero-* + *-genous*] 1. arising from the primitive foregut. 2. originating within the small intestine.

**en·tero·glu·ca·gon** (en″tər-o-gloo′kə-gon) [*entero-* + *glucagon*] [MeSH: Enteroglucagon] any of several glucagon-like hyperglycemic peptides released by special cells of the mucosa of the upper intestine in response to the ingestion of food; the major ones are glicentin and oxyntomodulin. They are immunologically distinct from pancreatic glucagon but display some similar properties. Called also *gut glucagon* and *glucagon-like immunoreactivity.*

**en·tero·gram** (en′tər-o-gram″) a tracing made by an instrument of the movements of the intestine.

**en·tero·graph** (en′tər-o-graf″) [*entero-* + *-graph*] an instrument for recording the intestinal movements.

**en·ter·og·ra·phy** (en″tər-og′rə-fe) 1. recording of the intestinal movements by means of an enterograph. 2. a description of the intestines.

**en·tero·hep·a·ti·tis** (en″tər-o-hep″ə-ti′tis) [*entero-* + *hepatitis*] 1. inflammation of the bowel and liver. 2. histomoniasis.

**en·tero·hep·a·to·cele** (en″tər-o-hep′ə-to-sēl″) an infantile umbilical hernia which contains intestines and liver.

**en·tero·hy·dro·cele** (en″tər-o-hi′dro-sēl) [*entero-* + *hydrocele*] hernia with hydrocele.

**en·ter·oi·dea** (en″tər-oi′de-ə) enteric fevers; see under *fever.*

**en·tero·in·tes·ti·nal** (en″tər-o-in-tes′tĭ-nəl) [*entero-* + *intestine*] intestino-intestinal.

**en·tero·ki·nase** (en″tər-o-ki′nās) former name for *enteropeptidase.*

**en·tero·ki·ne·sia** (en″tər-o-kĭ-ne′zhə) peristalsis.

**en·tero·ki·net·ic** (en″tər-o-kĭ-net′ik) pertaining to or stimulating peristalsis.

**en·tero·lith** (en′tər-o-lith″) [*entero-* + *-lith*] any concretion found in the intestine; called also *intestinal calculus.*

**en·tero·li·thi·a·sis** (en″ter-o-lĭ-thi′ah-sis) [*entero-* + *lithiasis*] the presence of calculi (enteroliths) in the intestine.

**en·ter·ol·o·gy** (en″tər-ol′o-je) [*entero-* + *-logy*] the sum of what is known regarding the intestines.

**en·ter·ol·y·sis** (en″tər-ol′ə-sis) [*entero-* + *-lysis*] the operative division of adhesions between loops of intestine or between the intestine and abdominal wall.

**en·tero·me·ga·lia** (en″tər-o-mə-ga′le-ə) enteromegaly.

**en·tero·meg·a·ly** (en″tər-o-meg′ə-le) [*entero-* + *-megaly*] enlargement of the intestine.

**en·tero·mere** (en′tər-o-mēr″) [*entero-* + *-mere*] any segment of the embryonic alimentary tract.

**en·tero·me·ro·cele** (en″tər-o-me′ro-sēl) [*entero-* + *mero-*[2] + *-cele*[1]] femoral hernia.

**En·tero·mo·na·di·na** (en″tər-o-mo″nə-di′nə) a suborder of parasitic protozoa (order Diplomonadida, class Zoomastigophorea) having one karyomastigont containing one to four flagella. *Enteromonas* is a representative genus.

**En·tero·mo·nas** (en″tər-o-mo′nəs) [*entero-* + Gr. *monas* unit, from *monos* single] a genus of nonpathogenic parasitic intestinal protozoa (suborder Enteromonadina, order Diplomonadida) having four anterior flagella, one of which passes along the body and emerges and extends posteriorly.

**en·tero·my·co·der·mi·tis** (en″tər-o-mi″ko-dər-mi′tis) [*entero-* + *myco-* + *derm-* + *-itis*] endoenteritis.

**en·tero·my·co·sis** (en″tər-o-mi-ko′sis) [*entero-* + *myco-* + *-osis*] disease of the intestine due to bacteria or fungi.

**e. bacteria'cea,** a general name for certain infections of the intestine due to nonspecific bacteria.

**en·tero·my·ia·sis** (en″tər-o-mi-i'ə-sis) [*entero-* + *myiasis*] presence of fly larvae in the intestine.

**en·ter·on** (en'tər-on) [Gr.] 1. digestive tract. 2. intestinum tenue.

**en·tero·neu·ri·tis** (en″tər-o-noo-ri'tis) inflammation of the nerves of the intestine.

**en·tero·ni·tis** (en″tər-o-ni'tis) enteritis.

**en·tero·pa·re·sis** (en″tər-o-pə-re'sis) [*entero-* + Gr. *paresis* relaxation] relaxation of the intestine resulting in dilatation.

**en·ter·o·path·o·gen** (en″tər-o-path'o-jən) a microorganism which causes a disease of the intestines.

**en·tero·patho·gen·e·sis** (en″tər-o-path″o-jen'ə-sis) the production of disease or disorder of the intestines.

**en·ter·o·path·o·gen·ic** (en″tər-o-path″o-jen'ik) pertaining to or effective in production of disease of the intestines.

**en·ter·op·a·thy** (en″tər-op'ə-the) [*entero-* + *-pathy*] any disease of the intestine.
**gluten e.,** celiac disease.
**proliferative hemorrhagic e.,** a frequently fatal type of porcine proliferative enteritis characterized by anemia, diarrhea, and hemorrhagic intestinal lesions.
**protein-losing e.,** a nonspecific term referring to conditions associated with excessive enteric loss of plasma protein. It occurs in extensive ulceration (e.g., inflammatory bowel disease), diffuse mucosal disease (e.g., adult celiac disease) in which there is more rapid desquamation of mucosal epithelial cells, and in intestinal lymphatic obstruction (intestinal lymphangiectasia).

**en·tero·pep·ti·dase** (en″tər-o-pep'tĭ-dās) [EC 3.4.21.9] [MeSH: Enteropeptidase] a serine endopeptidase that catalyzes the cleavage of a specific peptide bond near the N-terminus of trypsinogen, converting it to the active form trypsin. The enzyme is secreted by the small intestine.

**en·tero·pexy** (en'tər-o-pek″se) [*entero-* + *-pexy*] surgical fixation of the intestine to the anterior or posterior abdominal wall, or occasionally of one segment to another.

**en·tero·plas·ty** (en'tər-o-plas″te) [*entero-* + *-plasty*] plastic surgery of the intestine, especially to enlarge the caliber of a constricted segment or area of bowel. Cf. *strictureplasty.*

**en·tero·ple·gia** (en″tər-o-ple'jə) [*entero-* + *-plegia*] adynamic ileus.

**en·tero·pty·chia, en·tero·pty·chy** (en″tər-o-ti'ke-ə, en″tər-o-ti'ke) [*entero-* + Gr. *ptychē* a fold] plication of the intestine, an operation for the prevention of intestinal adhesions.

**en·tero·re·nal** (en″tər-o-re'nəl) pertaining to the intestine and the kidney.

**en·ter·or·rha·gia** (en″tər-o-ra'jə) [*entero-* + *-rrhagia*] hemorrhage from the intestine.

**en·ter·or·rha·phy** (en″tər-or'ə-fe) [*entero-* + *-rrhaphy*] repair or suture of the intestine.
**circular e.,** the suturing of two completely divided portions of intestine after invaginating one segment over the other so that they are joined end to end.

**en·ter·or·rhea** (en″tər-o-re'ə) diarrhea.

**en·ter·or·rhex·is** (en″tər-o-rek'sis) [*entero-* + *-rrhexis*] rupture of the intestine.

**en·tero·scope** (en'tər-o-skōp) [*entero-* + *-scope*] an endoscope for examining the lumen of the intestine.

**en·tero·sep·sis** (en″tər-o-sep'sis) [*entero-* + *sepsis*] intestinal sepsis due to putrefaction of the contents of the intestines.

**en·tero·spasm** (en'tər-o-spaz″əm) [*entero-* + *spasm*] a spasm of the intestine.

**en·tero·sta·sis** (en″tər-o-sta'sis) [*entero-* + *stasis*] intestinal stasis.

**en·tero·stax·is** (en″tər-o-stak'sis) [*entero-* + *staxis*] slow hemorrhage through the intestinal mucous membrane.

**en·tero·ste·no·sis** (en″tər-o-stə-no'sis) [*entero-* + *stenosis*] narrowing or stricture of the intestine.

**en·tero·sto·mal** (en″tər-o-sto'məl) relating to or having undergone enterostomy.

**en·ter·os·to·my** (en″tər-os'tə-me) [*entero-* + *-stomy*] [MeSH: Enterostomy] the formation of a permanent opening into the intestine through the abdominal wall, usually by surgical means; also, the opening so created.
**gun-barrel e.,** enterostomy in which the two segments of the divided intestine are parallel to one another as they emerge through the abdominal wall, like the tubes of a double-barreled shotgun.

**en·tero·tome** (en'tər-ə-tōm″) [*entero-* + *-tome*] an instrument for cutting the intestine.

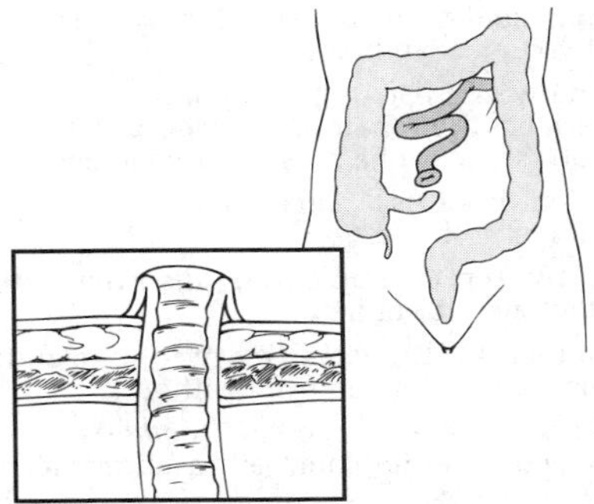

Ileostomy, with inset showing in cross-section the protrusion of the everted ileal terminus through the abdominal wall, forming the stoma.

**en·ter·ot·o·my** (en″tər-ot'ə-me) [*entero-* + *-tomy*] incision into the intestine.

**en·ter·o·tox·e·mia** (en″tər-o-tok-se'me-ə) [MeSH: Enterotoxemia] any of several usually fatal conditions in domestic animals characterized by presence in the blood of toxins or bacteria that are normally found in the intestines.
***Escherichia coli* e.,** edema disease.
**hemorrhagic e.,** struck.
**infectious e. of sheep,** pulpy kidney disease in sheep.

**en·ter·o·tox·i·gen·ic** (en″tər-o-tok″sĭ-jen'ik) producing or containing a toxin specific for the cells of the intestinal mucosa.

**en·tero·tox·in** (en″tər-o-tok'sin) [*entero-* + *toxin*] a toxin specifically affecting cells of the intestinal mucosa, causing vomiting and diarrhea, e.g., those elaborated by species of *Bacillus, Clostridium, Escherichia, Staphylococcus,* and *Vibrio.* See also *toxin.*
**cholera e.,** choleragen.

**en·tero·trop·ic** (en″tər-o-trop'ik) [*entero-* + *-tropic*] having a special affinity for or exerting its principal effect upon the intestines.

**en·tero·vag·i·nal** (en″tər-o-vaj'ĭ-nəl) pertaining to or communicating with the intestine and the vagina, as an enterovaginal fistula.

**en·tero·ve·nous** (en″tər-o-ve'nəs) communicating between the intestinal lumen and the lumen of a vein.

**en·tero·ves·i·cal** (en″tər-o-ves'ĭ-kəl) vesicointestinal.

**En·tero·Vi·o·form** (en″tər-o-vi'o-form) trademark for a preparation of iodochlorhydroxyquin.

**en·tero·vi·ral** (en″tər-o-vi'rəl) pertaining to or caused by enteroviruses.

**En·tero·vi·rus** (en'tər-o-vi″rəs) [*entero-* + *virus*] [MeSH: Enterovirus] enteroviruses; a genus of viruses of the family Picornaviridae that preferentially inhabit the intestinal tract. Infection is usually asymptomatic or mild but may result in a variety of disease syndromes. Human enteroviruses were originally classified as polioviruses, coxsackieviruses, or echoviruses and numbered sequentially within each group; because the boundaries between these groups have become indistinct, new enteroviruses are designated by a continuous numbering system, beginning with human enterovirus 68. The original groups continue to be used for previously discovered viruses. Enteroviruses also infect a wide range of animals and are grouped by host.

**en·tero·vi·rus** (en'tər-o-vi″rəs) [MeSH: Enterovirus] any virus of the genus *Enterovirus.*
**bovine e.,** a species of viruses of the genus *Enterovirus,* separable into two serotypes, that have been associated with infertility and abortion in cattle. Formerly called *ecbovirus.*
**porcine e.,** a species of viruses of the genus *Enterovirus,* separable into eleven serotypes, that are normal inhabitants of the intestinal tract of swine but may cause infectious porcine encephalomyelitis. Formerly called *ecsovirus.*
**simian e.,** a species of viruses of the genus *Enterovirus,* separable into 18 serotypes, that causes usually asymptomatic infection in monkeys. Formerly called *ecmovirus.*

**en·tero·zo·ic** (en″tər-o-zo'ik) relating to or caused by an enterozoon.

**en·tero·zo·on** (en″tər-o-zo'on) pl. *enterozo'a* [*entero-* + Gr. *zōon* animal] an animal parasite or species inhabiting or infecting the intestinal canal.

**en·ter·uria** (en″tər-u're-ə) [*entero-* + *-uria*] the presence of fecal constituents in the urine.

**en·thal·py** (en'thəl-pe) [Gr. *en* within + *thalpein* to warm] the heat content or chemical energy of a physical system; it is a thermody namic function equal to the internal energy plus the product of the pressure and volume. Symbol *H*.

**en·the·sis** (en-the′sis) [Gr. "a putting in; insertion"] 1. the use of artificial material in the repair of a defect or deformity of the body. 2. the site of attachment of a muscle or ligament to bone.

**en·the·si·tis** (en″thə-si′tis) inflammation of the muscular or tendinous attachment to bone.

**en·the·sop·a·thy** (en″thə-sop′ə-the) disorder of the muscular or tendinous attachment to bone.

**en·thet·ic** (en-thet′ik) [Gr. *enthetikos* fit for implanting] 1. pertaining to enthesis. 2. introduced from without.

**en·theto·bio·sis** (en-thet″o-bi-o′sis) [*enthesis* + *biosis*] dependency on a mechanical implant, as on an artificial cardiac pacemaker.

**en·thla·sis** (en′thlə-sis) [Gr. "a dent caused by pressure"] comminuted fracture of the skull, with depression of the bony fragments.

**en·tire** (en-tīr′) smooth and continuous with no projections or indentations; used to describe the border of a bacterial colony.

**en·ti·ris** (en-ti′ris) [*ent-* + *iris*] the posterior pigment layer of the iris.

**en·ti·ty** (en′tĭ-te) [L. *ens* being] an independently existing thing; a reality.

**ent(o)-** [Gr. *entos* inside] a prefix signifying within, or inner.

**en·to·blast** (en′to-blast) [*ento-* + *-blast*] endoderm.

**en·to·chon·dros·to·sis** (en″to-kon″dros-to′sis) [*ento-* + *chondro-* + *ostosis*] the development of bone taking place within cartilage.

**en·to·cho·roid·ea** (en″to-ko-roid′e-ə) lamina choroidocapillaris.

**en·toc·ne·mi·al** (en″tok-ne′me-əl) on the inner side of the tibia.

**en·to·cor·nea** (en″to-kor′ne-ə) [*ento-* + *cornea*] lamina limitans posterior cornea.

**en·to·cu·ne·i·form** (en″to-ku-ne′ĭ-form) os cuneiforme mediale.

**en·to·cyte** (en′to-sīt) [*ento-* + *-cyte*] the cell contents.

**en·to·derm** (en′to-dərm) [*ento-* + *-derm*] endoderm.
**primitive e., primordial e.,** the primary internal layer of the gastrula that becomes both gut and yolk sac.
**yolk-sac e.,** the epithelial lining of the yolk sac.

**en·to·der·mal** (en″to-dər′məl) endodermal.

**en·to·der·mic** (en″to-dər′mik) endodermal.

**En·to·di·nio·mor·phi·da** (en″to-di″ne-o-mor′fĭ-də) [*ento-* + Gr. *dinos* a whirling + *morphē* form] an order of ciliate protozoa (subclass Vestibuliferia, class Kinetofragminophorea) found as commensals in mammalian herbivores, including anthropoid apes. The somatic ciliature is reduced to unique tufts or bands and the oral ciliature is conspicuous, with the adoral zone being composed of membranelles that spiral toward the cytostome; the oral area is sometimes retractable, the pellicle is generally firm and may be drawn out into processes, and skeletal plates are present in many species.

**en·to·ec·tad** (en″to-ek′tad) [*ento-* + *ektad*] directed or proceeding from within outward.

**en·to·mere** (en′to-mēr) [*ento-* + *-mere*] a blastomere destined to become endoderm.

**en·to·meso·derm** (en″to-mes′o-dərm) endomesoderm.

**en·to·mi·on** (en-to′me-on) [Gr. *entomē* notch] the point at the tip of the mastoid angle of the parietal bone in the parietal notch of the temporal bone.

**entom(o)-** [Gr. *entomon* insect] a combining form denoting relationship to an insect, or to insects.

**En·to·mo·brya** (en″to-mo-bri′ə) a genus of insects, the spring tails, of the order Collembola, Australian species of which cause irritation by their bite.

**en·to·mog·e·nous** (en″to-moj′ə-nəs) [*entomo-* + *-genous*] 1. derived from insects, their bites, emanations, etc. 2. growing in the body of an insect.

**en·to·mol·o·gist** (en″to-mol′o-jist) an expert in entomology.

**en·to·mol·o·gy** (en″to-mol′o-je) [*entomo-* + *-logy*] [MeSH: Entomology] that branch of zoology which deals with the study of insects.
**medical e.,** that concerned with insects that cause disease or serve as vectors of microorganisms that cause disease in humans.

**En·to·moph·tho·ra** (en″to-mof′thə-rə) [*entomo-* + Gr. *phthora* destruction, death] [MeSH: Entomophthora] a former genus of fungi of the family Entomophthoraceae, now divided into several separate genera. *E. corona′ta* is now called *Conidiobolus coronata*.
**E. corona′ta,** *Conidiobolus coronatus*.

**En·to·moph·tho·ra·ceae** (en″to-mof″thə-ra′se-e) a family of fungi of the order Entomophthorales, found as saprobes and as parasites on higher fungi and insects; one genus, *Conidiobolus*, contains organisms pathogenic for humans and horses.

**En·to·moph·tho·ra·les** (en″to-mof″thə-ra′lēz) an order of perfect fungi of the phylum Zygomycota, class Zygomycetes, which are typically parasites of insects, although they can also infect humans (see *entomophthoromycosis*). Pathogenic organisms are found in the families Entomophthoraceae and Basidiobolaceae.

**en·to·moph·tho·ra·my·co·sis** (en″tə-mof″thə-rə-mi-ko′sis) entomophthoromycosis.

**en·to·moph·tho·ro·my·co·sis** (en″tə-mof″thə-ro-mi-ko′sis) 1. any disease in humans or other animals caused by fungi of the order Entomophthorales; human infections usually occur in apparently physiologically and immunologically normal individuals, although opportunistic infections also occur. 2. infection of the skin, oral mucosa, or nasal mucosa of horses by fungi of the order Entomophthorales, causing nodules or ulcerative granulomatous lesions. It is sometimes confused with cutaneous habronemiasis or pythiosis. See also *swamp cancer*.
**e. basidio′bolae,** a chronic infection caused by *Basidiobolus ranarum,* in which gradually enlarging granulomas form in the subcutaneous tissues of the arms, chest, and trunk. Multiple purulent ulcers may develop. It occurs in Indonesia, central Africa, and India, affecting chiefly children and adolescents. Unlike the other zygomycoses, it is unassociated with any apparent predisposing factors. Called also *basidiobolomycosis, subcutaneous phycomycosis* and *subcutaneous zygomycosis*.
**e. conidio′bolae,** infection by *Conidiobolus coronatus,* a form of zygomycosis usually involving the nose and paranasal sinuses *(rhinoenotmophthoromycosis)*. Sometimes, especially in weak or immunocompromised patients, it can spread to the central nervous system and cause fatal rhinocerebral zygomycosis.

**en·toph·thal·mia** (en″tof-thal′me-ə) endophthalmitis.

**en·to·phyte** (en′to-fīt) [*ento-* + *-phyte*] endophyte.

**en·top·ic** (en-top′ik) [Gr. *en* in + *topos* place] occurring in the proper place, as opposed to ectopic.

**en·to·plasm** (en′to-plaz-əm) [*ento-* + *-plasm*] endoplasm.

**en·top·tic** (en-top′tik) [*ent-* + *optic*] denoting visual phenomena which have their seat within the eye.

**en·top·to·scope** (en-top′to-skōp) an instrument for examining the media of the eyes, to ascertain their transparency.

**en·top·tos·co·py** (en″top-tos′ko-pe) [*ent-* + *opto-* + *-scopy*] the observation of the interior of the eye and its light and shadows.

**en·to·ret·i·na** (en″to-ret′ĭ-nə) [*ento-* + *retina*] the internal or nervous portion of the retina, disposed in five layers, which are named respectively outer molecular, inner nuclear, inner molecular, ganglion, and nerve fiber layers. See illustration at *retina*.

**ent·or·gan·ism** (ent-or′gə-niz-əm) [*ento-* + *organism*] endoparasite.

**en·to·rhi·nal** (en″to-ri′nəl) interior to the rhinal sulcus.

**en·to·sarc** (en′to-sahrk) [*ento-* + Gr. *sarx* flesh] endoplasm.

**ent·os·to·sis** (ent″os-to′sis) [*ent-* + *ostosis*] enostosis.

**en·to·tym·pan·ic** (en″to-tim-pan′ik) within the tympanum of the ear.

**en·to·zoa** (en″to-zo′ə) [Gr.] plural of *entozoon*.

**en·to·zo·al** (en″to-zo′əl) pertaining to or caused by entozoa.

**en·to·zo·on** (en″to-zo′on) pl. *entozo′a* [*ento-* + Gr. *zōon* animal] a parasitic animal organism living within the body of its host.

**en·train** (en-trān′) to modulate the cardiac rhythm by gaining control of the rate of the pacemaker, cardiac or ectopic, with an external stimulus.

**en·train·ment** (en-trān′mənt) 1. a technique for identifying the slowest pacing necessary to terminate an arrhythmia, particularly atrial flutter; as the pacing rate is slowly increased incrementally, the electrocardiographic appearance of the flutter waves shifts incrementally away from a flutter morphology until the arrhythmia is terminated. 2. the synchronization and control of cardiac rhythm by an external stimulus.

**en·trap·ment** (en-trap′ment) compression of a nerve or vessel by adjacent tissue, such as the walls of a fibrous or osseofibrous tunnel, muscle, tendon, or other tissue; see also *entrapment neuropathy*.

**en·tro·pi·on** (en-tro′pe-on) [Gr. *en* in + *tropein* to turn] [MeSH: Entropion] the turning inward (inversion) of an edge or margin, as of the margin of the eyelid, with the tarsal cartilage turned inward toward the eyeball; called also *blepharelosis, enstrophe,* and *trichoma*.
**cicatricial e.,** inversion of the margin of an eyelid caused by con-

traction of scar tissue in the palpebral conjunctiva or underlying tarsus.
**spastic e.,** inversion of the eyelid caused by tonic spasm of the orbicularis oculi muscle.
**e. u'veae,** inversion of the margin of the pupil, usually the result of an iritis attended with exudate, and occurring rarely as a congenital condition.

**en·tro·pi·on·ize** (en-tro'pe-o-nīz) to put into a state of entropion or inversion; to turn inward.

**en·tro·pi·um** (en-tro'pe-əm) entropion.

**en·tro·py** (en'tro-pe) [Gr. *entropē* a turning inward] [MeSH: Entropy] 1. the measure of that part of the heat or energy of a system which is not available to perform work; entropy increases in all natural (spontaneous and irreversible) processes. Symbol *S*. 2. the tendency of any system to move toward randomness or disorder. 3. diminished capacity for spontaneous change, as occurs in the psyche in aging.

**ent·wick·lungs·me·cha·nik** (ent"vik-loongs"mə-kahn'ik) [Ger. "developmental mechanics"] mechanisms of embryological development, as revealed by experimental study.

**en·ty·py** (en'ti-pe) [Gr. *entypē* pattern] a method of gastrulation in which the endoderm lies external to the amniotic ectoderm.

**enu·cle·ate** (e-noo'kle-āt) [L. *enucleare*] to remove whole and clean, as a tumor from its envelope or the eyeball; see *enucleation*.

**enu·cle·at·ed** (e-noo'kle-āt"əd) removed; said of an organ, tumor, or cell nucleus.

**enu·cle·a·tion** (e-noo"kle-a'shən) [L. *e* out + *nucleus* kernel] the removal of an organ, of a tumor, or of another body in such a way that it comes out clean and whole, like a nut from its shell. Used in connection with the eye, it denotes removal of the eyeball after the eye muscles and optic nerve have been severed.

**en·ure·sis** (en"u-re'sis) [Gr. *enourein* to void urine] [MeSH: Enuresis] urinary incontinence after the age at which urinary control should have been achieved; often used alone with specific reference to that occurring during sleep at night *(bed-wetting; nocturnal enuresis)*.

**en·uret·ic** (en"u-ret'ik) 1. pertaining to enuresis. 2. an agent which causes enuresis. 3. a person who exhibits enuresis.

**en·ve·lope** (en'və-lōp) [Old Fr. *enveloper* to wrap up] 1. an encompassing structure or membrane. 2. in virology, a lipoprotein bilayer surrounding the capsid of some viruses, acquired by budding through the cell membrane of the host cell; the lipids are derived from the host cell and the proteins are encoded by the virus. Called also *peplos*. 3. in bacteriology, the cell wall and the plasma membrane considered together.
**cell e.,** the plasma membrane and the cell wall considered together.
**egg e.,** see under *membrane*.
**nuclear e.,** the condensed double layer of lipids and proteins enclosing the cell nucleus and separating it from the cytoplasm; its two concentric membranes, inner and outer, are separated by a perinuclear space. Called also *nuclear membrane*.

**en·ven·om·a·tion** (en-ven"o-ma'shən) poisoning by venom.

**en·vi·ron·ment** (en-vi'ron-mənt) [Fr. *environner* to surround, to encircle] [MeSH: Environment] the sum total of all the conditions and elements which make up the surroundings and influence the development and actions of an individual.

**en·vy** (en've) a desire to have another's possessions or qualities for oneself.
**penis e.,** in psychoanalysis, the concept that the female envies the male his possession of a penis, first described by Freud as occurring during the phallic stage in little girls as they become aware of anatomical differences between the sexes; sometimes used to denote a woman's generalized envy of men or their characteristics.

**En·zac·tin** (en-zak'tin) trademark for preparations of triacetin.

**en·zo·ot·ic** (en"zo-ot'ik) [Gr. *en* in + *zootic*] 1. present in an animal community at all times, but occurring in only small numbers of cases. 2. a disease of low morbidity which is constantly present in an animal community. Cf. *epizootic*.

**En·zo·pride** (en'zo-prīd) trademark for a preparation of nadide.

**en·zy·got·ic** (en"zi-got'ik) developed from the same zygote.

**en·zy·mat·ic** (en"zi-mat'ik) relating to, caused by, or of the nature of an enzyme.

**en·zyme** (en'zīm) [Gr. *en* in + *zymē* leaven] a protein molecule that catalyzes chemical reactions of other substances without itself being destroyed or altered upon completion of the reactions. Symbol E. Enzymes are classified according to the recommendations of the Nomenclature Committee of the International Union of Biochemistry. Each enzyme is assigned a recommended name and an Enzyme Commission (EC) number. They are divided into six main groups: oxidoreductases, transferases, hydrolases, lyases, isomerases, and ligases. For individual enzymes, see under the specific name, e.g., *glucose-6-phosphate dehydrogenase*.
**adaptive e.,** induced e.
**allosteric e.,** an enzyme whose catalytic activity is altered by binding of specific ligands at sites other than the substrate binding site.
**brancher e., branching e.,** 1,4-α-glucan branching enzyme.
**constitutive e.,** one produced constantly, irrespective of environmental conditions or demand.
**cryptic e.,** in bacteriology, an enzyme that can attack added substrate in a cell lysate but not in intact cells, owing to selective action of a permeability barrier.
**debrancher e., debranching e.,** 1. amylo-1,6-glucosidase. 2. a term used to describe any enzyme removing branches from macromolecules, usually polysaccharides, by cleaving at branch points.
**extracellular e.,** exoenzyme.
**fat-splitting e.,** lipase.
**hydrolytic e.,** hydrolase.
**induced e., inducible e.,** one whose production can be stimulated by another compound, often a substrate or a structurally related compound (inducer). The inducers studied first were substrates whose utilization thus became possible; hence these enzymes were known earlier as *adaptive enzymes*. Cf. *constitutive e.*
**intracellular e.,** endoenzyme.
**proteolytic e.,** peptidase.
**receptor-destroying e. (RDE),** one that renders red cells insusceptible to viral hemolysis by destroying its receptors.
**redox e.,** oxidoreductase.
**repressible e.,** one whose rate of formation is decreased by an increased concentration of one or more end products. The process serves as a control mechanism in certain bacterial and mammalian metabolic systems.
**respiratory e.,** one that is part of an electron transport (respiratory) chain.
**restriction e.,** restriction endonuclease.
**yellow e's,** any of a number of enzymes having a flavin as a prosthetic group. Historically, NADPH dehydrogenase (occurring in plants and yeast) was called the *old yellow enzyme* to distinguish it from D-amino acid oxidase, known as the *new yellow enzyme*. See also *flavoprotein*.

**En·zyme Com·mis·sion (EC)** the International Commission on Enzymes, a committee established in 1956 by the International Union of Biochemistry to standardize enzyme classification and nomenclature.

**en·zym·ic** (en-zim'ik) enzymatic.

**en·zy·mol·o·gy** (en"zi-mol'o-je) the study of enzymes and enzymatic action.

**en·zy·mop·a·thy** (en"zi-mop'ə-the) an inborn error of metabolism consisting of defective or absent enzymes, as in the glycogen storage diseases or the mucopolysaccharidoses.
**lysosomal e.,** lysosomal storage disease.

**EOG** electro-olfactogram.

**eo·sin** (e'o-sin) [Gr. *ēōs* dawn] a rose-colored stain or dye: typically the sodium salt of tetrabromofluorescein, $C_{20}H_6Br_4Na_2O_5$, C.I. 45380. Commercially, several other red coal tar dyes are called eosin. All the eosins are bromine derivatives of fluorescin. Eosin is an important plasma stain, used especially with hematoxylin, methylene blue, and methyl green.
**e. B, e. I bluish,** dibromodinitrofluorescein, a dye having staining properties similar to eosin, but of a distinctly bluer shade.
**ethyl e.,** the ethyl ester of eosin.
**water-soluble e., e. W or W S, yellowish e., e. Y,** eosin.

**eo·sin·o·cyte** (e"o-sin'o-sīt) eosinophil.

**eo·sin·o·pe·nia** (e"o-sin-o-pe'ne-ə) [*eosinophil* + *-penia*] abnormal deficiency of eosinophils in the blood; called also *hypoeosinophilia*.

**eo·sin·o·phil** (e"o-sin'o-fil) [*eosin* + *-phil*] [MeSH: Eosinophils] 1. a granular leukocyte with a nucleus that usually has two lobes connected by a slender thread of chromatin, and cytoplasm containing coarse, round granules that are uniform in size. Called also *eosinocyte* and *eosinophilic leukocyte*. 2. any structure, cell, or histologic element readily stained by eosin.

**eo·sin·o·phile** (e"o-sin'o-fīl) 1. eosinophil. 2. eosinophilic.

**eo·sin·o·phil·ia** (e"o-sin"o-fil'e-ə) [*eosin* + *-philia*] [MeSH: Eosinophilia] 1. the formation and accumulation of an abnormally large number of eosinophils in the blood; see also *hypereosinophilia*. Called also *eosinophilic leukocytosis*. 2. the condition of being readily stained with eosin.
**Löffler's e.,** see under *syndrome*.
**pulmonary infiltration e.,** pulmonary infiltration with eosinophilia; see under *infiltration*.
**simple pulmonary e.,** Löffler's syndrome.
**tropical e., tropical pulmonary e.,** a subacute or chronic form of occult filariasis, usually involving *Brugia malayi, Wuchereria ban-*

*crofti,* or filariae that infect animals; it occurs in the tropics, especially in India, where some groups may have a genetic predisposition for the disease. It is characterized by episodic nocturnal wheezing and coughing, strikingly elevated eosinophilia, and diffuse reticulonodular infiltrations of the lung. Microfilariae are seldom detected in peripheral blood films since the parasites are confined primarily to the lungs. However, there is evidence of both humoral and cellular immunity to the filariae, and the illness often improves following antifilarial chemotherapy. Called also *filarial hypereosinophilia* and *Weingarten's syndrome.*

**eo·sin·o·phil·ic** (e″o-sin″o-fil′ik) 1. readily stainable with eosin. 2. pertaining to eosinophils. 3. pertaining to or characterized by eosinophilia.

**eo·sin·o·philo·poi·e·tin** (e″o-sin″o-fil″o-poi′ə-tin) a peptide of low molecular weight that induces production of eosinophils.

**eo·sin·o·phi·lo·sis** (e″o-sin″o-fĭ-lo′sis) eosinophilia (def. 1).

**eo·sin·oph·i·lous** (e″o-sin-of′ĭ-ləs) eosinophilic.

**eo·sin·o·phil·uria** (e″o-sin″o-fil-u′re-ə) the presence of eosinophils in the urine.

**eo·sin·o·tac·tic** (e″o-sin″o-tak′tik) [*eosinophil* + *tactic*] exhibiting an influence on eosinophils, either repelling them *(negatively e.)* or attracting them *(positively e.).*

**eo·so·late** (e-ŏ′sə-lāt) acetyl guaiacol trisulfonate; the silver salt is used as an antiseptic.

**EP** evoked potential.

**ep-** see *epi-*.

**EPA** Environmental Protection Agency.

**ep·ac·mas·tic** (ep″ak-mas′tik) pertaining to the epacme.

**ep·ac·me** (əp-ak′me) [Gr. *epakmazein* to come to its height] in evolution, the stage or period of development.

**epac·tal** (e-pak′təl) [Gr. *epaktos* brought in] 1. supernumerary. 2. (in the plural) ossa suturalia.

**ep·al·lo·bi·o·sis** (əp-al″o-bi-o′sis) [*epi-* + *allo-* + *biosis*] dependency on an external life-support system, as on a heart-lung machine or hemodialyzer.

**ep·ar·sal·gia** (ep″ahr-sal′jə) [Gr. *epairein* to lift + *-algia*] any painful disorder due to overstrain of a part, including dilatation of the heart, hernia, enteroptosis, coughing, etc.

**ep·ar·te·ri·al** (ep″ahr-te′re-əl) [*epi-* + *arterial*] over an artery; applied especially to the first branch of the right primary bronchus which is so situated.

**ep·ax·i·al** (əp-ak′se-əl) [*epi-* + *axial*] situated upon or above an axis, such as the axis of a limb.

**ep·en·dop·a·thy** (ep″ən-dop′ə-the) ependymopathy.

**epen·dy·ma** (ə-pen′də-mə) [Gr. *ependyma* upper garment] [TA] [MeSH: Ependyma] the lining membrane of the ventricles of the brain and of the central canal of the spinal cord.

**epen·dy·mal** (ə-pen′də-məl) pertaining to or composed of ependyma.

**epen·dy·mi·tis** (ə-pen″də-mi′təs) inflammation of the ependyma.

**epen·dy·mo·blast** (ə-pen′də-mo-blast) an embryonic ependymal cell; an ependymal spongioblast.

**epen·dy·mo·blas·to·ma** (ə-pen′də-mo-blas-to′mə) a rare malignant tumor composed of primitive ependymal cells. Some neuropathologists classify such tumors as malignant forms of ependymoma but some consider them a type of primitive neuroectodermal tumor.

**epen·dy·mo·cyte** (ə-pen′də-mo-sīt″) [*ependyma* + *-cyte*] an ependymal cell.

**epen·dy·mo·cy·to·ma** (ə-pen″də-mo-si-to′mə) ependymoma.

**epen·dy·mo·ma** (ə-pen″də-mo′mə) [MeSH: Ependymoma] a neoplasm composed of differentiated ependymal cells; most ependymomas are slow growing and benign, but malignant varieties occur.

**epen·dy·mop·a·thy** (ə-pen″də-mop′ə-the) disease of the ependyma.

**Ep·eryth·ro·zo·on** (ep″ə-rith″ro-zo′on) [*epi-* + *erythros-* + Gr. *zoon* animal] [MeSH: Eperythrozoon] a genus of rickettsiae of the family Anaplasmataceae that sometimes cause disease in rodents, cattle, sheep, and swine. The type species is *E. coccoi′des.*

**ep·eryth·ro·zoo·no·sis** (ep″ə-rith″ro-zo″o-no′sis) [MeSH: Eperythrozoonosis] infection with rickettsiae of the genus *Eperythrozoon.*

**ephapse** (ə-faps′) [Gr. *ephapsis* a touching] electrical synapse.

**ephap·tic** (ə-fap′tik) pertaining to an electrical synapse (ephapse) or to conduction across it.

**ep·har·mo·ny** (ep-hahr′mo-ne) development in complete harmony with environment; harmonic relation between structure and environment.

**ephe·bi·at·rics** (ə-fe″be-at′riks) [Gr. *ephēbos* one arrived at puberty + *-iatrics*] a branch of medicine consisting of the diagnosis and treatment of diseases of youth (18–25 years).

**Ephed·ra** (e-fed′rə) [Gr. *epi* upon + *hedra* seat] a genus of low, branching shrubs of the family Gnetaceae, indigenous to China and India. *E. equiseti′na* Bunge., *E. sini′ca* Stapf., *E. vulga′ris,* and other species (all called *ma huang* in China) are sources of ephedrine.

**ephed·rine** (ə-fed′rin, ef′ə-drin) [USP] [MeSH: Ephedrine] an adrenergic obtained from *Ephedra* species or prepared synthetically. Its principal uses, in the form of the hydrochloride or sulfate salt, are: to decongest the nasal mucosa in allergic states and to relax bronchiolar muscles in bronchial asthma; to stimulate the central nervous system in narcolepsy and in poisoning by central nervous system depressants; to prevent hypotension during spinal and infiltration anesthesia; and as a mydriatic.
**e. hydrochloride** [USP], the hydrochloride salt of ephedrine, having the same actions, uses, and routes of administration as the sulfate salt.
**e. sulfate** [USP], the sulfate salt of ephedrine, having the same actions as the base; administered orally, parenterally, or intranasally.
**e. tannate,** the tannate salt of ephedrine, used as a bronchodilator; administered orally.

**ephel·i·des** (ə-fel′ĭ-dēz) [Gr.] plural of *ephelis.*

**ephe·lis** (ə-fe′lis) pl. *ephel′ides* [Gr. *ephēlis*] a freckle.

**ephem·era** (ə-fem′ər-ə) [Gr. *ephēmeros* short-lived] a transitory condition or thing.

**ephem·er·al** (ə-fem′ər-əl) short-lived; transient.

**Ephe·mer·i·da** (e″fə-mer′i-də) a family of flies whose exuviae may cause sensitization and severe asthmatic paroxysms when inhaled.

**Ephem·er·op·tera** (e-fem″ər-op′tər-ə) [Gr. *ephemeros* short-lived + *pteron* wing] the mayflies, an order of elongated insects with net-veined paired wings, and two or three caudal filiform appendages; the adults have only vestigial mouth parts and starve to death soon after laying their eggs. See also *Hexagenia bilineata.*

**Ephem·ero·vi·rus** (e-fem′ər-o-vi″rəs) [Gr. *ephemeros* short-lived + *virus*] a genus of viruses of the family Rhabdoviridae that includes bovine ephemeral fever virus and related viruses.

**Eph·y·nal** (ef′ə-nəl) trademark for a preparation of vitamin E; see *tocopherol.*

**epi-** [Gr. *epi* on] a prefix meaning upon, above, or beside. In chemistry, it denotes a chemical compound or group that is related to another chemical compound or group. Also, *ep-*.

**epi·al·lo·preg·nan·o·lone** (ep″e-al″o-preg-nan′ə-lōn) a 21-carbon corticoid hormone present in pregnancy urine, thought to originate in the fetal adrenal cortex; probably a precursor of C19 androgens.

**epi·an·dros·ter·one** (ep″e-an-dros′tər-ōn) chemical name: 3β-hydroxy-17-androstan-17-one; an androgenic steroid, one of the urinary 17-ketosteroids, less active than androsterone and excreted in small amounts in normal human urine. Called also *isoandrosterone.*

**epi·blast** (ep′ĭ-blast) [*epi-* + *-blast*] 1. the upper layer of the bilaminar embryonic disc present during the second week; it gives rise to ectoderm. 2. ectoderm. 3. the ectoderm except for the neural plate.

**epi·blas·tic** (ep″ĭ-blas′tik) pertaining to or arising from the epiblast; ectodermal.

**epi·bleph·a·ron** (ep″ĭ-blef′ə-ron) [*epi-* + Gr. *blepharon* eyelid] a developmental anomaly in which a horizontal fold of skin stretches across the border of the eyelid, pressing the eyelashes inward against the eyelid.

**epib·o·le** (e-pib′o-le) epiboly.

**epib·o·ly** (e-pib′o-le) [Gr. *epibolē* cover] a method of gastrulation by which the smaller blastomeres at the animal pole of the fertilized ovum grow over and enclose the cells of the vegetal hemisphere.

**epi·bul·bar** (ep″ĭ-bul′bər) upon the eyeball.

**epi·can·thal, epi·can·thic** (ep″ĭ-kan′thəl, ep″ĭ-kan′thik) 1. pertaining to the epicanthus. 2. overlying the canthus.

**epi·can·thine** (ep″ĭ-kan′thīn) epicanthal.

**epi·can·thus** (ep″ĭ-kan′thəs) [*epi-* + *canthus*] a vertical fold of skin on either side of the nose, sometimes covering the inner canthus. It is present as a normal characteristic in persons of certain races and sometimes occurs as a congenital anomaly in others. Called also *epicanthal* or *palpebronasal fold,* and *plica palpebronasalis* [TA].

**ep·i·car·cin·o·gen** (ep″ĭ-kahr-sin′o-jən) epigenetic carcinogen.

**epi·car·dia** (ep″ĭ-kahr′de-ə) the lower portion of the esophagus, extending from the hiatus esophagi to the cardia.

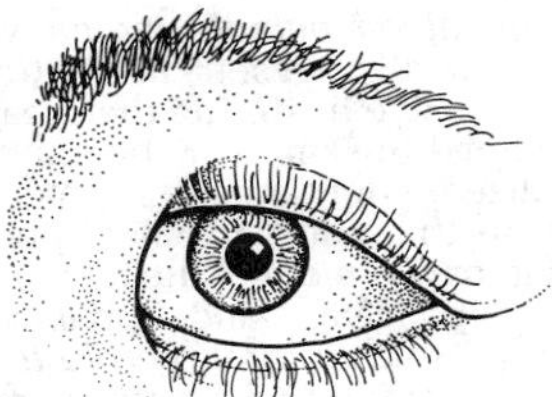
Epicanthus.

**epi·car·di·al** (ep″ĭ-kahr′de-əl) pertaining to the epicardium or to the epicardia.

**epi·car·di·ec·to·my** (ep″ĭ-kahr″de-ek′tə-me) [*epicardium* + *-ectomy*] surgical removal of the epicardium, usually performed in constrictive pericarditis to permit greater diastolic filling of the heart.

**epi·car·di·um** (ep″ĭ-kahr′de-um) [*epi-* + Gr. *kardia* heart] lamina visceralis pericardii serosi.

**epi·cau·ma** (ep″ĭ-kaw′mə) [*epi-* + Gr. *kauma* a burn] a superficial burn or ulcer on the eye.

**Ep·i·cau·ta** (ep″ĭ-kaw′tə) a genus of blister beetles (family Meloidae) that secrete cantharidin and can cause cantharidin poisoning in ruminants. *E. pennsylva′nica* and *E. vitta′ta* are found in the eastern United States, *E. cine′rea* in the southwestern United States, and *E. tormento′sa* and *E. sapphiri′na* in Africa.

**epi·cen·tral** (ep″ĭ-sen′trəl) attached to the centrum of a vertebra.

**epi·chlo·ro·hy·drin** (ep″-ə-klor″o-hi′drin) [MeSH: Epichlorohydrin] a solvent for resins, paints, varnishes, and other organic compounds; it is strongly irritant to the skin and is carcinogenic. Called also *chloropropylene oxide.*

**epi·chor·dal** (ep″ĭ-kor′dəl) situated dorsad of the notochord.

**epi·cho·ri·on** (ep″ĭ-kor′e-on) [*epi-* + *chorion*] that part of the uterine mucosa which encloses the implanted conceptus.

**epi·cil·lin** (ep-ĭ-sil′in) an antibacterial effective against various gram-negative and gram-positive organisms.

**epi·coe·lo·ma** (ep″ĭ-se-lo′mə) the portion of the coeloma nearest the notochord.

**epic·o·mus** (e-pik′o-məs) [*epi-* + Gr. *komē* hair] asymmetrical conjoined twins with the parasitic twin joined at the summit of the head of the larger twin.

**epi·con·dy·lal·gia** (ep″ĭ-kon″də-lal′jə) [*epicondyle* + *-algia*] pain in the muscles or tendons attached to the epicondyle of the humerus; see also *tennis elbow,* under *elbow.*

**epi·con·dyle** (ep″ĭ-kon′dīl) [*epi-* + *condyle*] an eminence upon a bone, above its condyle; called also *epicondylus [*NA].
**external e. of femur,** epicondylus lateralis femoris.
**external e. of humerus,** epicondylus lateralis humeri.
**internal e. of femur,** epicondylus medialis femoris.
**internal e. of humerus,** epicondylus medialis humeri.
**lateral e. of femur,** epicondylus lateralis femoris.
**lateral e. of humerus,** epicondylus lateralis humeri.
**medial e. of femur,** epicondylus medialis femoris.
**medial e. of humerus,** epicondylus medialis humeri.

**epi·con·dy·li** (ep″ĭ-kon′də-li) [L.] plural of *epicondylus.*

**epi·con·dyl·i·an, epi·con·dyl·ic** (ep″ĭ-kon-dil′e-ən, ep″ĭ-kon-dil′ik) pertaining to an epicondyle.

**epi·con·dy·li·tis** (ep″ĭ-kon″də-li′tis) inflammation of the epicondyle or of the tissues adjoining the epicondyle of the humerus.
**external humeral e., lateral e., radiohumeral e.,** tennis elbow.

**epi·con·dy·lus** (ep″ĭ-kon′də-ləs) pl. *epicon′dyli* [L.] [TA] epicondyle: a general term for an eminence upon a bone, above its condyle.
**e. latera′lis fe′moris** [TA], lateral epicondyle of femur: a projection from the distal end of the femur, above the lateral condyle, for the attachment of collateral ligaments of the knee. Called also *external epicondyle of femur.*
**e. latera′lis hu′meri** [TA], lateral epicondyle of humerus: a projection from the distal end of the humerus, giving attachment to a common tendon of origin of the extensor carpi radialis brevis, extensor digitorum communis, extensor digiti quinti proprius, extensor carpi ulnaris, and supinator muscles. Called also *external epicondyle of humerus, external, extensor, lateral,* or *radial condyle of humerus,* and *condylus lateralis humeri.*
**e. media′lis fe′moris** [TA], medial epicondyle of femur: a projection from the distal end of the femur, above the medial condyle, for the attachment of collateral ligaments of the knee; called also *internal epicondyle of femur.*
**e. media′lis hu′meri** [TA], medial epicondyle of humerus: a projection from the distal end of the humerus, giving attachment to the pronator teres above; a common tendon of origin of the flexor carpi radialis, palmaris longus, flexor digitorum sublimis, and flexor carpi ulnaris muscles in the middle, and the ulnar collateral ligament below. Called also *condylus medialis humeri, internal epicondyle of humerus,* and *flexor, internal, medial,* or *ulnar condyle of humerus.*

**epi·cor·a·coid** (ep″ĭ-kor′ə-koid) situated above the coracoid process.

**epi·cor·nea·scle·ri·tis** (ep″ĭ-kor″ne-ə-sklə-ri′tis) a chronic inflammatory condition affecting the cornea and sclera.

**epi·cos·tal** (ep″ĭ-kos′təl) [*epi-* + *costal*] situated upon a rib.

**epi·cot·yl** (ep″ĭ-kot′əl) the part of the stem of a plant embryo or seedling above the cotyledons and below the leaves.

**epi·cra·ni·um** (ep″ĭ-kra′ne-əm) [*epi-* + *cranium*] the integument, aponeurosis, and muscular expansions of the scalp.

**epi·cra·ni·us** (ep″ĭ-kra′ne-əs) [L.] pertaining to the epicranium; see under *musculus.*

**epi·cri·sis** (ep′ĭ-kri″sis) [*epi-* + *crisis*] 1. a second or supplementary crisis. 2. a critical analysis or discussion of a case of disease after its termination.

**epi·crit·ic** (ep″ĭ-krit′ik) [Gr. *epikrisis* determination] relating to or serving the purpose of accurate determination; applied to cutaneous nerve fibers that serve the purpose of perceiving fine variations of touch or temperature. See under *sensibility.*

**epi·cu·ti·cle** (ep″ĭ-ku′tĭ-kəl) [*epi-* + L. *cuticula*] the thin, flexible, colorless, outermost layer of the exoskeleton of certain crustaceans and arthropods, composed of wax and cuticulin.

**epi·cys·ti·tis** (ep″ĭ-sis-ti′tis) [*epi-* + *cystitis*] inflammation of the structures above the bladder.

**epi·cys·tot·o·my** (ep″ĭ-sis-tot′o-me) [*epi-* + *cysto-* + *-tomy*] suprapubic cystotomy.

**epi·cyte** (ep′ĭ-sīt) [*epi-* + *cyte*] the cell membrane covering gregarine trophozoites.

**ep·i·dem·ic** (ep″ĭ-dem′ik) [Gr. *epidēmios* prevalent] [MeSH: Disease Outbreaks] occurring suddenly in numbers clearly in excess of normal expectancy; said especially of infectious diseases but applied also to any disease, injury, or other health-related event occurring in such outbreaks. Cf. *endemic* and *sporadic.*

**ep·i·de·mic·i·ty** (ep″ĭ-də-mis′ĭ-te) the state or quality of being epidemic.

**ep·i·de·mi·og·ra·phy** (ep″ĭ-de″me-og′rə-fe) [*epidemic* + *-graphy*] a treatise upon or an account of epidemics.

**ep·i·de·mi·ol·o·gist** (ep″ĭ-de″me-ol′o-jist) one who specializes in epidemiology.

**ep·i·de·mi·ol·o·gy** (ep′ĭ-de″me-ol′o-je) [*epidemic* + *-logy*] [MeSH: Epidemiology] the science concerned with the study of the factors determining and influencing the frequency and distribution of disease, injury, and other health-related events and their causes in a defined human population for the purpose of establishing programs to prevent and control their development and spread. Also, the sum of knowledge gained in such a study.

**epi·derm** (ep′ĭ-dərm) epidermis.

**epi·der·mal** (ep″ĭ-dər′məl) 1. pertaining to or resembling epidermis. Called also *epidermic.* 2. epidermoid, def. 1.

**epi·der·ma·ti·tis** (ep″ĭ-dər″mə-ti′tis) a term sometimes used to denote an inflammation restricted to the epidermis; in actuality the inflammation also invariably affects the dermis. Called also *epidermitis.*

**epi·der·ma·to·plas·ty** (ep″ĭ-dər-mat′o-plas″te) [*epidermis* + *-plasty*] skin grafting done by transplanting pieces of epidermis to denuded areas.

**epi·der·mic** (ep″ĭ-dər′mik) epidermal, def. 1.

**epi·der·mic·u·la** (ep″ĭ-dər-mik′u-lə) a very thin membrane or cuticula, such as that covering a hair.

**epi·der·mi·dal·iza·tion** (ep″ĭ-dər″mid-ə-lĭ-za′shən) development of epidermic cells (stratified epithelium) from mucous cells (columnar epithelium).

**epi·der·mi·des** (ep″ĭ-dər′mĭ-dēz) [Gr.] plural of *epidermis.*

**epi·der·mis** (ep″ĭ-dər′mis) pl. *epider′mides* [*epi-* + *dermis*] [TA] [MeSH: Epidermis] the outermost and nonvascular layer of the skin, derived from the embryonic ectoderm, varying in thickness from 0.07 to 0.12 mm, except on the palms and soles where it may be 0.8 and 1.4 mm, respectively. On the palmar and plantar surfaces, it exhibits maximal cellular differentiation and layering, and comprises, from within outward, five layers: the *basal layer (stratum basale epidermidis),* the *prickle cell* or *spinous layer (stratum spinosum epidermidis),* the *granular layer (stratum granulosum epidermidis),* the *clear layer (stratum lucidum epidermidis),* and the *horny layer (stratum corneum epidermidis).* In the thinner epidermis of the general body surface, the basal, prickle cell, and horny layers are constantly present and the granular layer is usually identifiable, but the clear layer is usually absent. Called also *cuticle.*

**epi·der·mi·tis** (ep″ĭ-dər-mi′tis) epidermatitis.
**exudative e.,** greasy pig disease.

**epi·der·mi·za·tion** (ep″ĭ-dər″mĭ-za′shən) 1. the process of covering or of becoming covered with epidermis. 2. skin grafting.

**epi·der·mo·dys·pla·sia** (ep″ĭ-dər″mo-dis-pla′shə) faulty development of the epidermis.
**e. verrucifor′mis,** the widespread and persistent, sometimes for decades, dissemination of verruca plana associated with a tendency to malignant degeneration. It typically begins in early childhood with the development of flat-topped papules, varying in color from pink and flesh to gray or brown, which increase in number and coalesce to form large plaques, especially on the knees, elbows, and trunk. Familial occurrence, parental consanguinity, and mental retardation are often associated with the disorder. Called also *Lewandowsky-Lutz disease.*

**epi·der·moid** (ep″ĭ-dər′moid) 1. resembling the epidermis. Called also *epidermal.* 2. epidermal, def. 1. 3. epidermoid cyst.

**epi·der·moi·do·ma** (ep″ĭ-dər″moi-do′mə) epidermoid cyst (def. 2).

**epi·der·mol·y·sin** (ep″ĭ-dər-mol′ə-sin) exfoliatin.

**epi·der·mol·y·sis** (ep″ĭ-dər-mol′ə-sis) [*epidermis* + *-lysis*] a loosened state of the epidermis, with formation of blebs and bullae either spontaneously or after trauma.
**e. bullo′sa,** a group of heterogeneous, chronic, mostly hereditary, mechanobullous dermatoses. The group has been classified in four major types: *acquired epilepsy bullosa, e. bullosa dystrophica, e. bullosa simplex,* and *junctional e. bullosa.* Called also *e. bullosa hereditaria.*
**e. bullosa, acquired, e. bullo′sa acquisi′ta,** a form of epidermolysis bullosa presenting in adulthood with evidence of genetic transmission, and occurring in association with such diseases as diabetes mellitus, tuberculosis, amyloidosis, colitis, and multiple myeloma and with penicillamine therapy. The blisters, which occur most often on the pressure areas of the hands and feet but can occur anywhere on the body, heal leaving atrophic scars and milia; nail dystrophy and lesions of the oral mucosa are often seen. There is evidence of deposition of immunoglobulin on the dermal side of the dermal-epidermal basement membrane.
**e. bullosa, junctional,** an autosomal recessive disorder having onset at birth or during the neonatal period, characterized clinically by severe generalized blistering, particularly on the perioral area, scalp, legs, diaper area, and trunk, and extensive denudation that may be associated with secondary infection and death from septicemia, nail dystrophy, and dental dysplasia; growth retardation and refractory anemia are frequent findings in those who survive. On electron microscopy, a cleavage plane between the plasma membranes of the basal cells and the basement membrane is seen. Called also *e. bullosa letalis* and *Herlitz disease.*
**e. bullo′sa dystro′phica,** a generalized form of epidermolysis bullosa often present at birth or in early infancy, and marked by atrophy of previously blistered areas, severe scarring after healing, and dystrophy or absence of the nails. It occurs in autosomal dominant and recessive forms. Called also *dermatolytic bullous dermatosis.*
**e. bullosa dystrophica, albopapuloid,** the Pasini variant of dominant epidermolysis bullosa dystrophica.
**e. bullosa dystrophica, dominant,** the relatively mild autosomal dominant form of epidermolysis dystrophica, occurring in two main variants: The *Pasini (albopapuloid) variant,* which is the more severe of the two, is usually present at birth or in infancy, and is characterized by extensive blistering that heals with atrophic scarring, primarily confined to skin over the joints and extremities but sometimes generalized; spontaneous flesh-colored, scarlike (albopapuloid) lesions on the trunk, usually appearing during adolescence; and frequent involvement of the mucous membranes, including the oral, esophageal, and pharyngeal mucosa. The *Cockayne-Touraine (dysplastic* or *hyperplastic) variant* usually occurs in infancy or early childhood, and is characterized by keratotic lesions that may show ichthyotic changes, generally confined to the extremities, which may heal with hypertrophic rather than atrophic scars. See also *Bart's syndrome,* under *syndrome.*
**e. bullosa dystrophica, dysplastic,** the Cockayne-Touraine variant of dominant epidermolysis bullosa dystrophica.
**e. bullosa dystrophica, hyperplastic,** the Cockayne-Touraine variant of dominant epidermolysis bullosa dystrophica.
**e. bullosa dystrophica, polydysplastic,** recessive e. bullosa dystrophica.
**e. bullosa dystrophica, recessive,** the autosomal recessive form of epidermolysis bullosa dystrophica, tending to be more severe than the dominant disorder, characterized by the presence of extensive denuded hemorrhagic erosions and blisters on all body surfaces at birth or in early infancy, including mucous membranes, the subsequent healing of which produces esophageal strictures that may impair feeding and atrophic scars that may restrict mobility owing to fusion of the digits, mitten-like deformity of the hands and feet, and flexion contractures of joints. Called also *polydysplastic e. bullosa dystrophica.*
**e. bullo′sa heredita′ria,** e. bullosa.
**e. bullo′sa leta′lis,** junctional e. bullosa.
**e. bullo′sa sim′plex,** a dominantly inherited, relatively benign, nonscarring form of epidermolysis bullosa, most often involving the extremities, and usually presenting during the first few years of life; blistering may cease in adulthood. It occurs in two forms: generalized and localized.
**e. bullosa simplex, generalized,** a form of epidermolysis bullosa simplex present at birth or occurring in early infancy, in which the lesions, consisting of vesicles, bullae, and milia, are usually located on areas subjected to repeated minor trauma, such as the elbows, knees, hands, and feet.
**e. bullosa simplex, localized,** a form of epidermolysis bullosa primarily confined to the hands and feet, especially the palms and soles, appearing in infancy or later life, and often associated with hyperhidrosis. It may be exacerbated by unusual trauma such as prolonged walking. Called also *Weber-Cockayne syndrome.*
**toxic bullous e.,** toxic epidermal necrolysis.

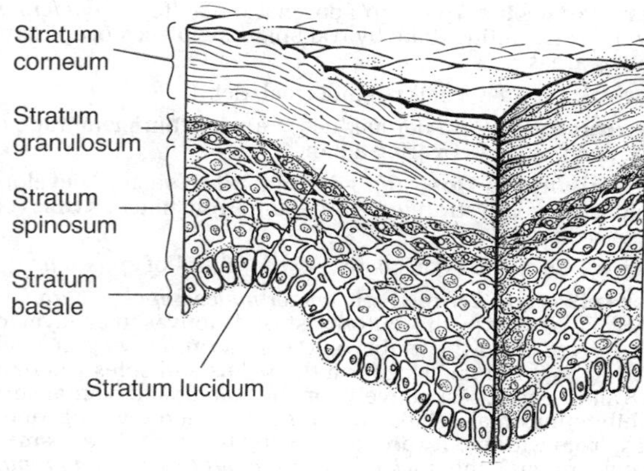

Section of epidermis.

**epi·der·mo·lyt·ic** (ep″ĭ-dər″mo-lit′ik) pertaining to or characterized by epidermolysis.

**epi·der·mo·my·co·sis** (ep″ĭ-dər″mo-mi-ko′sis) dermatophytosis.

**epi·der·moph·y·tid** (ep″ĭ-dər-mof′ə-tid) dermatophytid.

**Epi·der·moph·y·ton** (ep″ĭ-dər-mof′ĭ-ton) [*epidermis* + Gr. *phyton* plant] [MeSH: Epidermophyton] a genus of Fungi Imperfecti of the form-class Hyphomycetes, form-family Moniliaceae. *E. flocco′sum* is a species of dermatophytes that attacks skin and nails but not hair; it causes tinea cruris, tinea pedis, and onychomycosis.

**epi·der·mo·phy·to·sis** (ep″ĭ-dər″mo-fi-to′sis) 1. dermatophytosis. 2. infection by fungi of the genus *Epidermophyton.*

**epi·did·y·mal** (ep″ĭ-did′ə-məl) pertaining to the epididymis.

**epi·did·y·mec·to·my** (ep″ĭ-did″ə-mek′tə-me) [*epididymis* + *-ectomy*] surgical removal of the epididymis.

**ep·i·did·y·mis** (ep″ĭ-did′ə-mis) pl. *epididym′ides* [Gr., from *epi-* + *didymos* testis] [TA] [MeSH: Epididymis] the elongated cordlike structure along the posterior border of the testis, whose elongated coiled duct provides for storage, transit, and maturation of spermatozoa and is continuous with the ductus deferens. It consists of a head (caput epididymis), body (corpus epididymis), and tail (cauda epididymis). Called also *parorchis.*

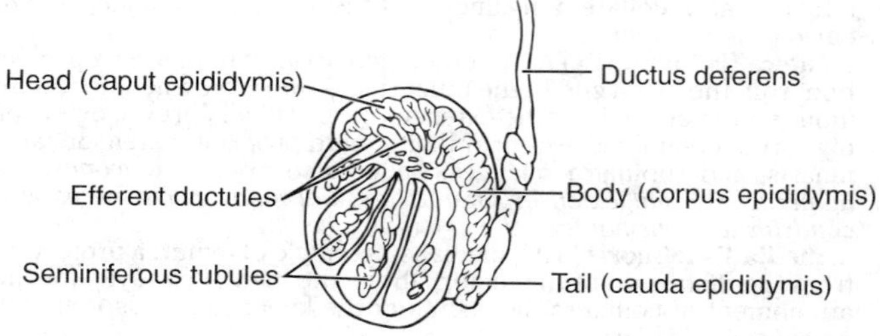

Vertical section of testis showing the head, body, and tail of the epididymis.

**epi•did•y•mi•tis** (ep″ĭ-did″ə-mi′tis) [MeSH: Epididymitis] inflammation of the epididymis.
**spermatogenic e.,** an inflammatory reaction to spermatozoa that have escaped from the lumen of the epididymal tubules into the tissues of the epididymis.

**epi•did•y•mo•def•er•en•tec•to•my** (ep″ĭ-did″ə-mo-def″ər-ən-tek′tə-me) epididymovasectomy.

**epi•did•y•mo•def•er•en•tial** (ep″ĭ-did″ə-mo-def″ər-en′shəl) pertaining to the epididymis and ductus deferens.

**epi•did•y•mo•or•chi•tis** (ep″ĭ-did″ə-mo-or-ki′tis) inflammation of the epididymis and testis.

**epi•did•y•mot•o•my** (ep″ĭ-did″ə-mot′ə-me) [*epididymis* + *-tomy*] incision of the epididymis.

**epi•did•y•mo•vas•ec•to•my** (ep″ĭ-did″ə-mo-və-sek′tə-me) excision of the epididymis and a large portion of the ductus deferens.

**epi•did•y•mo•vas•os•to•my** (ep″ĭ″-did″ə-mo-və-sos′tə-me) [*epididymo-* + *vaso-* + *-stomy*] surgical creation of a new communication between the epididymis and a formerly distal portion of the vas (ductus) deferens.

**epi•du•ral** (ep″ĭ-doo′rəl) situated upon or outside the dura mater.

**epi•du•rog•ra•phy** (ep″ĭ-doo-rog′rə-fe) radiography of the spine after a radiopaque medium has been injected into the epidural space.

**epi•es•tri•ol** (ep″e-es′tre-ol) any epimer of estriol found in the urine of pregnant women and originating in the fetoplacental unit.

**epi•fas•cial** (ep″ĭ-fash′əl) upon a fascia.

**epi•gas•ter** (ep″ĭ-gas′tər) [*epi-* + *gaster*] the hindgut: the embryonic structure from which the large intestine is formed.

**epi•gas•tral•gia** (ep″ĭ-gəs-tral′jə) [*epigastrium* + *-algia*] pain in the epigastrium.

**epi•gas•tric** (ep″ĭ-gas′trik) [*epi-* + *gastric*] pertaining to the epigastrium.

**epi•gas•tri•um** (ep″ĭ-gas′tre-əm) [Gr. *epigastrion*] [TA] the upper middle region of the abdomen, located within the infrasternal angle; called also *antecardium, anticardium, regio epigastrica* [TA alternative] and *epigastric region* or *zone.*

**epi•gas•tri•us** (ep″ĭ-gas′tre-əs) [*epi-* + *gaster*] asymmetrical conjoined twins in which the parasitic twin forms a tumor upon the epigastrium of the larger twin.

**epi•gas•tro•cele** (ep″ĭ-gas′tro-sēl) [*epigastrium* + *-cele*[1]] hernia in the epigastric region.

**epi•gen•e•sis** (ep″ĭ-jen′ə-sis) [*epi-* + *genesis*] the development of an organism from an undifferentiated cell, consisting in the successive formation and development of organs and parts that do not preexist in the zygote; opposed to the erroneous theory of preformation.

**epi•ge•net•ic** (ep″ĭ-jə-net′ik) 1. pertaining to epigenesis. 2. altering the activity of genes without changing their structure; cf. *genotoxic.*

**epi•ge•net•ics** (ep″ĭ-jə-net′iks) the science concerned with the analysis of development.

**epi•glot•tec•to•my** (ep″ĭ-glot-ek′tə-me) epiglottidectomy.

**epi•glot•tic** (ep″ĭ-glot′ik) pertaining to the epiglottis.

**epi•glot•tid•e•an** (ep″ĭ-glot-id′e-ən) epiglottic.

**epi•glot•ti•dec•to•my** (ep″ĭ-glot″ĭ-dek′tə-me) [*epiglottis* + *-ectomy*] excision of the epiglottis.

**epi•glot•ti•di•tis** (ep″ĭ-glot″ĭ-di′tis) epiglottitis.

**epi•glot•tis** (ep″ĭ-glot′is) [*epi-* + *glottis*] [TA] [MeSH: Epiglottis] the lidlike cartilaginous structure overhanging the entrance to the larynx and serving to prevent food from entering the larynx and trachea while swallowing.

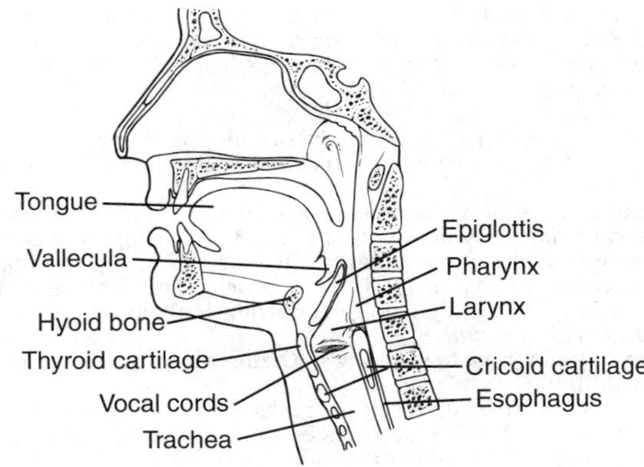


Epiglottis in a sagittal section of the head and neck.

**epi•glot•ti•tis** (ep″ĭ-glŏ-ti′tis) [MeSH: Epiglottitis] inflammation of the epiglottis, usually in children as a component of croup; it may lead to life-threatening upper airway obstruction. See also *supraglottitis.* Called also *epiglottiditis.*

**epi•glot•to•plas•ty** (ep″ĭ-glot′o-plas″te) plastic surgery of the epiglottis, such as trimming back its folds to correct laryngeal stridor in infants.

**epig•na•thous** (ə-pig′nə-thəs) of the nature of an epignathus.

**epig•na•thus** (ə-pig′nə-thəs) [*epi-* + Gr. *gnathos* jaw] a fetal tumor arising from the soft or hard palate in the region of the hypophyseal pouch (Rathke's pouch), filling the buccal cavity and protruding from the mouth. Because the tumor sometimes shows a certain degree of organization, it has been considered a parasitic fetus.

**epig•o•nal** (ə-pig′o-nəl) [*epi-* + *gon-* + *-al*[1]] situated on an embryonic gonad.

**epi•hy•drin•al•de•hyde** (ep″ĭ-hi″drin-al′də-hīd) a chemical compound, one of the substances that give rancid fats their disagreeable odor.

**epi•hy•oid** (ep″ĭ-hī′oid) situated upon the hyoid bone.

**epi•ker•a•to•pha•kia** (ep″ĭ-ker″ə-to-fa′ke-ə) [*epi-* + *kerato-* + *phak-* + *-ia*] [MeSH: Epikeratophakia] overlaying of a piece of donor cornea on the patient's cornea to change its curvature in order to correct refractive error.

**epi•la•mel•lar** (ep″ĭ-lə-mel′ər) situated upon the basement membrane.

**ep•i•late** (ep′ĭ-lāt) depilate.

**ep•i•la•tion** (ep″ĭ-la′shən) [L. *e* out + *pilus* hair] depilation.

**ep•i•lem•ma** (ep″ĭ-lem′ə) [*epi-* + *-lemma*] the endoneurium.

**ep•i•lem•mal** (ep″ĭ-lem′əl) pertaining to the epilemma (endoneurium).

**ep•i•lep•sia** (ep″ĭ-lep′se-ə) [L.; Gr. *epilēpsia*] epilepsy.
**e. partia′lis conti′nua,** a form of status epilepticus with focal motor seizures, marked by continuous clonic movements of a limited part of the body. Called also *simple partial status.*

**ep•i•lep•sy** (ep′ĭ-lep″se) [Gr. *epilēpsia* seizure] [MeSH: Epilepsy] any of a group of syndromes characterized by paroxysmal transient disturbances of the brain function that may be manifested as episodic impairment or loss of consciousness, abnormal motor phenomena, psychic or sensory disturbances, or perturbation of the autonomic nervous system. A single episode is called a *seizure* (q.v.). Many types of epilepsy are combinations of different kinds of seizures. Epilepsy is classified as either *symptomatic* or *idiopathic* according to whether the cause is known or unknown. Both of these types may be further subdivided into *partial* and *generalized* types depending on whether the seizures are due to a localized, limited brain lesion or to widespread brain lesions, respectively.
**abdominal e.,** paroxysmal abdominal pain, the expression of an abnormal neuronal discharge from the brain; called also *Moore's syndrome.*
**absence e.,** epilepsy characterized by absence seizures, usually having its onset in childhood or adolescence; called also *petit mal, petit mal e., absence,* and *minor e.*
**acquired e.,** symptomatic e.
**activated e.,** epileptic seizures induced by electrical or drug stimulation for the purpose of observing the pattern of clinical and electroencephalographic response.
**audiogenic e.,** reflex epilepsy caused by auditory stimuli.
**benign e. with centrotemporal spikes, benign rolandic e., benign e. with rolandic spikes,** a self-limited, autosomal dominant disorder of childhood consisting of partial seizures manifested by facial movements and grimaces, often followed by tonic-clonic seizures. The electroencephalogram from the primary somatomotor area (rolandic area) shows characteristic repetitive high-voltage spikes. Called also *rolandic e.*
**Bravais-jacksonian e.,** jacksonian e.
**chronic focal e.,** epilepsia partialis continua.
**cortical e.,** seizure phenomena originating in the cerebral cortex.
**cryptogenic e.,** idiopathic e.
**diurnal e.,** epileptic attacks occurring in the daytime or when the patient is awake.
**essential e.,** idiopathic e.
**focal e.,** epilepsy consisting of focal seizures.
**gelastic e.,** temporal lobe epilepsy in which the automatisms consist of fits of uncontrollable mirthless laughter.
**generalized e.,** epilepsy in which the seizures are generalized; they may have a focal onset or be generalized from the beginning.

**generalized flexion e.,** hypsarrhythmia.
**grand mal e.,** a symptomatic form of epilepsy often preceded by an aura; characterized by loss of consciousness with generalized tonic-clonic seizures (q.v.). Called also *grand mal, major e.,* and *haut mal e.*
**haut mal e.,** grand mal e.
**idiopathic e.,** epilepsy of unknown origin, possibly associated with some inherited predisposition for seizures; called also *cryptogenic e.* or *essential e.*
**jacksonian e.,** epilepsy characterized by focal motor seizures with unilateral clonic movements that start in one group of muscles and spread systematically to adjacent groups, reflecting the march of the epileptic activity through the motor cortex. The seizures are due to a discharging focus in the contralateral motor cortex; called also *Bravais-jacksonian e.*
**Koshevnikoff's (Koschewnikow's, Kozhevnikov's) e.,** epilepsia partialis continua.
**larval e.,** unerupted epileptic seizures, represented only by characteristic waves in the electroencephalogram; called also *latent e.*
**late e.,** epilepsy beginning in middle age or later.
**latent e.,** larval e.
**localized e.,** focal e.
**major e.,** grand mal e.
**matutinal e.,** epileptic seizures occurring in the morning on awakening.
**menstrual e.,** epileptic seizures associated with menstruation.
**minor e.,** absence e.
**minor focal e.,** simple partial seizures; see under *seizure.*
**musicogenic e.,** reflex epilepsy occurring in response to a musical stimulus.
**myoclonic e., myoclonus e.,** any form of epilepsy accompanied by myoclonus, such as *juvenile myoclonic e., Baltic myoclonic e.,* and *Lafora's myoclonic e.* See also *progressive familial myoclonic e.*
**myoclonic e., Baltic,** a progressive, autosomal recessive form of myoclonic epilepsy seen in Finland. Onset is between the ages of 6 and 13 and there are degenerative changes in the brain without presence of Lafora bodies. Mental deterioration is milder and survival is longer than in Lafora's myoclonic epilepsy. Called also *Unverricht's* or *Unverricht-Lundborg disease.*
**myoclonic e., juvenile,** a syndrome of sudden myoclonic jerks, occurring particularly in the morning or under conditions of stress or fatigue; seen primarily in children and adolescents. Occasionally the jerks may progress to generalized tonic-clonic seizures, but there is no mental deterioration. Called also *Janz syndrome.*
**myoclonic e., Lafora's,** a slowly progressive autosomal recessive form of epilepsy beginning in childhood and characterized by attacks of intermittent or continuous clonus of muscle groups, resulting in difficulties in voluntary movement; there is mental deterioration, sometimes progressing to complete dementia, and the presence of Lafora bodies in various cells, including those of the nervous system, retina, heart, muscle, and liver. Called also *Lafora's disease.* See also *myoclonic e.*
**myoclonic e., progressive familial,** myoclonic epilepsy that is hereditary; see *Baltic myoclonic e.* and *Lafora's myoclonic e.*
**nocturnal e.,** epileptic attacks occurring at night or while the patient is asleep.
**organic e.,** symptomatic e.
**partial e.,** focal e.
**petit mal e.,** absence e.
**photic e., photogenic e.,** reflex epilepsy in which seizures are induced by a flickering light.
**physiologic e.,** biologic or electrobiologic seizures based on physiologic and not on organic or structural abnormalities of the brain.
**post-traumatic e.,** epileptic seizures that occur after head injury; called also *traumatic e.*
**procursive e.,** temporal lobe epilepsy in which the automatisms consist of aimless running.
**psychic e., psychomotor e.,** temporal lobe e.
**reading e.,** reflex epilepsy that is triggered when the patient tries to read.
**reflex e.,** epileptic seizures occurring in response to sensory (tactile, visual, auditory, or musical) stimuli; called also *sensory e.* See also *audiogenic e., musicogenic e., photogenic e.,* and *reading e.*
**rolandic e.,** benign rolandic e.
**rotatory e.,** temporal lobe epilepsy in which the automatisms consist of rotating body movements.
**sensory e.,** 1. seizures manifested by paresthesias or hallucinations of sight, smell, or taste; see also *somatosensory e., uncinate e.,* and *visual e.* 2. reflex e.
**somatosensory e.,** sensory epilepsy with paresthesias such as tingling, numbness, or burning.
**symptomatic e.,** acquired epileptic seizures caused by disease of the central nervous system itself; a generalized systemic disorder, such as hypoglycemia or uremia; or poisoning, as with lead or pentylenetetrazol; called also *organic e.*
**tardy e.,** late e.
**temporal lobe e.,** a form of epilepsy characterized by complex partial seizures; called also *psychomotor e.*
**traumatic e.,** post-traumatic e.
**uncinate e.,** temporal lobe epilepsy caused by a lesion in the uncinate region and therefore associated with hallucinations of smell and taste.
**vertiginous e.,** focal seizures giving rise to a sensation of vertigo; occasionally these are auras of more general seizures. See also *vertiginous aura.*
**visual e.,** sensory epilepsy in which there are visual hallucinations such as flashes of light or colors.

**ep·i·lep·tic** (ep″ĭ-lep′tik) [Gr. *epilēptikos*] 1. pertaining to or affected with epilepsy. 2. a person affected with epilepsy.

**ep·i·lep·ti·form** (ep″ĭ-lep′tĭ-form) [*epileptic* + *form*] 1. resembling epilepsy or its manifestations. 2. occurring in severe or sudden paroxysms.

**epi·lep·to·gen·e·sis** (ep″ĭ-lep″to-jen′ə-sis) the production or development of epilepsy.

**ep·i·lep·to·gen·ic** (ep″ĭ-lep-to-jen′ik) [*epilepsy* + *-genic*] producing epileptic attacks.

**ep·i·lep·tog·e·nous** (ep″ĭ-lep-toj′ə-nəs) epileptogenic.

**ep·i·lep·toid** (ep″ĭ-lep′toid) epileptiform.

**ep·i·lep·tol·o·gist** (ep″ĭ-lep-tol′ə-jist) one who specializes in epileptology.

**ep·i·lep·tol·o·gy** (ep″ĭ-lep-tol′ə-je) the study, diagnosis, and treatment of epilepsy.

**ep·i·loia** (ep″ĭ-loi′ə) tuberous sclerosis.

**epi·man·dib·u·lar** (ep″ĭ-man-dib′u-lər) [*epi-* + *mandibular*] situated upon the lower jaw.

**epi·mas·ti·gote** (ep″ĭ-mas′tĭ-gōt) [*epi-* + Gr. *mastix* whip] any of the bodies representing the morphologic (crithidial) stage in the life cycle of certain trypanosomatid protozoa resembling the typical adult form of members of the genus *Crithidia,* in which the kinetoplast and basal body are located anterior to the central vesicular nucleus of the slender elongate cell and the flagellum is attached to the body up to the anterior end by a short undulating membrane before becoming free-flowing. Cf. *amastigote, choanomastigote, opisthomastigote, promastigote,* and *trypomastigote.*

**epi·men·or·rha·gia** (ep″ĭ-men″o-ra′je-ə) too frequent and too excessive menstruation.

**epi·men·or·rhea** (ep″ĭ-men″o-re′ə) abnormally frequent menstruation; menstrual irregularity in which the patient has a menstrual cycle less than the normal 28 days.

**ep·i·mer** (ep′ĭ-mər) either of two diastereomers that differ in the configuration around one asymmetric carbon atom.

**epim·er·ase** (ə-pim′ə-rās) a term used in the names of some enzymes of the subclass racemases and epimerases [EC 5.1] to denote those that catalyze inversion of the configuration about an asymmetric carbon atom in a substrate having more than one center of asymmetry; thus epimers are interconverted.

**ep·i·mere** (ep′ĭ-mēr) [*epi-* + *-mere*] the dorsal portion of a somite, from which is formed muscles innervated by the dorsal ramus of a spinal nerve.

**epim·er·iza·tion** (ə-pim″ər-ĭ-za′shən) the changing of one epimeric form of a compound into another, as by enzymatic action.

**epi·mes·trol** (ep″ĭ-mes′trol) [MeSH: Epimestrol] the 3-methyl ether of 17-epiestriol, an anterior pituitary activator used to stimulate ovulation.

**epi·mor·phic** (ep″ĭ-mor′fik) pertaining to or characterized by epimorphosis.

**epi·mor·pho·sis** (ep″ĭ-mor-fo′sis) [*epi-* + *morphosis*] the regeneration of a part of an organism by proliferation at the cut surface.

**Ep·i·mys** (ep′ĭ-mis) [*epi-* + Gr. *mys* mouse] *Rattus.*

**epi·mys·i·ot·omy** (ep″ĭ-mis″e-ot′ə-me) [*epimysium* + *-tomy*] incision of the epimysium.

**epi·mys·i·um** (ep″ĭ-mis′e-əm) [*epi-* + Gr. *mys* muscle] [TA] the fibrous sheath about an entire muscle; called also *perimysium externum* or *external perimysium.*

**Ep·i·nal** (ep′ĭ-nəl) trademark for a preparation of epinephryl borate.

**epi·neph·rine** (ep″ĭ-nef′rin) [MeSH: Epinephrine] 1. a catecholamine hormone secreted by the adrenal medulla and a neurotransmitter, released by certain neurons and active in the central nervous system. It is stored in the chromaffin granules and is released in response to hypoglycemia, stress, and other stimuli. It is a potent stimulator of the adrenergic receptors of the sympathetic nervous system and a powerful cardiac stimulant that accelerates the heart rate and increases cardiac output. It also promotes glycogenolysis and exerts other metabolic effects. 2. [USP] a synthetic prep-

aration of the levorotatory form of epinephrine, used chiefly as a topical vasoconstrictor, cardiac stimulant, and bronchodilator; administered intranasally, orally, parenterally, or by inhalation. Called also *adrenaline*.
**e. bitartrate** [USP], the bitartrate salt of epinephrine, having the same actions as the base; applied topically to the conjunctiva to reduce intraocular pressure in the management of chronic simple (open-angle) glaucoma and administered by inhalation as a bronchodilator.

**epi·neph·rin·emia** (ep″ĭ-nef″rĭ-ne′me-ə) the presence of epinephrine in the blood.

**epi·neph·ros** (ep″ĭ-nef′ros) [*epi-* + Gr. *nephros* kidney] an adrenal gland (glandula suprarenalis [TA]).

**epi·neph·ryl bo·rate** (ep″ĭ-nef′rəl) a compound containing epinephrine as a borate complex; used as an adrenergic in ophthalmology.

**epi·neu·ral** (ep″ĭ-noo′rəl) situated upon a neural arch.

**epi·neu·ri·al** (ep″ĭ-noo′re-əl) pertaining to the epineurium.

**epi·neu·ri·um** (ep″ĭ-noor′e-um) [epi- + Gr. *neuron* nerve] [TA] the outermost layer of connective tissue of a peripheral nerve, surrounding the entire nerve and containing its supplying blood vessels and lymphatics. See also *perineurium* and *endoneurium*.

**epi·or·chi·um** (ep″e-or′ke-əm) lamina visceralis tunicae vaginalis testis.

**epi·ot·ic** (ep″e-ot′ik) [*epi-* + *otic*] situated on or above the ear.

**ep·i·pas·tic** (ep″ĭ-pas′tik) [*epi-* + Gr. *passein* to sprinkle] 1. suitable for use as a dusting powder. 2. a powder to be sprinkled upon the surface of the body.

**epi·pha·ryn·ge·al** (ep″ĭ-fə-rin′je-əl) nasopharyngeal.

**epi·phar·yn·gi·tis** (ep″ĭ-far″in-ji′tis) nasopharyngitis.

**epi·phar·ynx** (ep″ĭ-far′inks) pars nasalis pharyngis.

**epi·phe·nom·e·non** (ep″ĭ-fə-nom′ə-non) [*epi-* + *phenomenon*] an accessory, exceptional, or accidental occurrence in the course of an attack of any disease.

**epiph·o·ra** (ə-pif′ə-rə) [Gr. *epiphora* sudden burst] an abnormal overflow of tears down the cheek, mainly due to stricture of the lacrimal passages; called also *illacrimation*.

**epi·phys·e·al** (ep″ĭ-fiz′e-əl) pertaining to or of the nature of an epiphysis.

**epi·phys·e·od·e·sis** (ep″ĭ-fiz″e-od′ə-sis) epiphysiodesis.

**epiph·y·ses** (ə-pif′ə-sēz) [Gr.] [MeSH: Epiphyses] plural of *epiphysis*.

**epi·phys·i·al** (ep″ĭ-fiz′e-əl) epiphyseal.

**epi·phys·i·od·e·sis** (ep″ĭ-fiz″e-od′ə-sis) [*epiphysis* + *-desis*] the operation of premature fusion of an epiphysis to arrest growth.

**epi·phys·i·oid** (ep″ĭ-fiz′e-oid) resembling epiphyses; a term applied to carpal and tarsal bones which develop like epiphyses from centers of ossification.

**epi·phys·i·ol·y·sis** (ep″ĭ-fiz″e-ol′ə-sis) [*epiphysis* + *-lysis*] separation of an epiphysis from its bone; especially slipping of the upper femoral epiphysis.

**epi·phys·i·om·e·ter** (ep″ĭ-fiz″e-om′ə-tər) an instrument for measuring the epiphyses, used in the diagnosis of rickets.

**epi·phys·i·op·a·thy** (ep″ĭ-fiz″e-op′ə-the) [*epiphysis* + *-pathy*] 1. any disease of the pineal body. 2. any disease of an epiphysis of a bone.

**epiph·y·sis** (ə-pif′ə-sis) pl. *epi′physes* [Gr. "an ongrowth; excrescence"] [TA] the expanded articular end of a long bone, developed from a secondary ossification center, which during the period of growth is either entirely cartilaginous or is separated from the shaft by the epiphyseal cartilage. Called also *apophysis ossium*.
**annular e's**, secondary growth centers occurring as rings at the periphery of the superior and inferior surfaces of the vertebral body.
**capital e.**, the epiphysis at the head of a long bone.
**e. ce′rebri**, glandula pinealis.
**slipped e.**, dislocation of the epiphysis of a bone, as of the epiphysis of the head of the femur.
**stippled e's**, chondrodysplasia punctata.

**epiph·y·si·tis** (ə-pif″ə-si′tis) inflammation of an epiphysis or of the cartilage that separates it from the main bone.
**e. juveni′lis**, Köhler's bone disease (def.1).
**vertebral e.**, osteochondrosis (q.v.) of the vertebra.

**ep·i·phyte** (ep′ĭ-fīt) [*epi-* + *-phyte*] 1. a plant organism growing upon another plant. 2. a plant organism parasitic upon the exterior of the human or an animal body.

**ep·i·phyt·ic** (ep″ĭ-fit′ik) pertaining to or caused by epiphytes.

**epi·pia** (ep″ĭ-pi′ə) [*epi-* + *pia*] the part of the pia mater adjacent to the arachnoid mater, as distinguished from the pia-glia.

**epi·pi·al** (ep″ĭ-pi′əl) 1. situated on the pia mater. 2. pertaining to the epipia.

**epi·pleu·ral** (ep″ĭ-ploor′əl) situated on a pleural element, or pleurapophysis.

**epipl(o)-** [Gr. *epiploon* omentum] a combining form denoting relationship to the omentum.

**epip·lo·cele** (ə-pip′lo-sēl) [*epiplo-* + *-cele*[1]] a hernia that contains omentum.

**epip·lo·ec·to·my** (ə-pip″lo-ek′tə-me) [*epiplo-* + *-ectomy*] omentectomy; excision of the omentum.

**epip·lo·en·tero·cele** (ə-pip″lo-en′tər-o-sēl) [*epiplo-* + *entero-* + *-cele*[1]] hernia containing intestine and omentum.

**epi·plo·ic** (ep″ĭ-plo′ik) omental.

**epip·lo·itis** (ə-pip″lo-i′tis) omentitis.

**epip·lo·me·ro·cele** (ə-pip″lo-me′ro-sēl) [*epiplo-* + *mero-*[2] + *-cele*[1]] femoral hernia containing omentum.

**epi·plom·phalo·cele** (ep″ĭ-plom-fal′o-sēl″) [*epiplo-* + *omphalo-* + *-cele*[1]] umbilical hernia containing omentum.

**epip·lo·on** (ə-pip′lo-on) [Gr.] the omentum.
**great e.**, omentum majus.
**lesser e.**, omentum minus.

**epip·lo·pexy** (ə-pip′lo-pek″se) [*epiplo-* + *-pexy*] omentopexy.

**epip·lo·plas·ty** (ə-pip′lo-plas″te) [*epiplo-* + *-plasty*] omentoplasty.

**epip·lor·rha·phy** (ep″ip-lor′ə-fe) [*epiplo-* + *-rrhaphy*] omentorrhaphy.

**epip·los·cheo·cele** (ep″ip-los′ke-o-sēl″) [*epiplo-* + *oscheo-* + *-cele*[1]] scrotal hernia containing omentum.

**epi·podo·phyl·lo·tox·in** (ep″ĭ-pod″o-fil″o-tok′sin) [*epi-* + *podophyllotoxin*] a chemical derivative of podophyllotoxin from which the antineoplastic drugs etoposide and teniposide are derived.

**epi·py·gus** (ep″ĭ-pi′gəs) pygomelus.

**epi·pyr·a·mis** (ep″ĭ-pir′ə-mis) a small supernumerary carpal bone sometimes found between the triquetrum, lunate, hamate, and capitate bones; called also *epitriquetrum*.

**epi·ro·tu·li·an** (ep″ĭ-ro-too′le-ən) [*epi-* + L. *rotula* patella] upon the patella.

**epi·ru·bi·cin** (ep″ĭ-roo′bĭ-sin) [MeSH: Epirubicin] an anthracycline antibiotic that is a stereoisomer of doxorubicin, having the same antineoplastic actions as but lower toxicity than doxorubicin; used in the treatment of carcinoma of the breast, ovary, stomach, colon, and rectum, leukemia, lymphoma, and multiple myeloma, administered intravenously. Available as *epirubicin hydrochloride*.

**epi·scle·ra** (ep″ĭ-skler′ə) the loose connective tissue forming the external surface of the sclera.

**epi·scle·ral** (ep″ĭ-skler′əl) 1. overlying the sclera. 2. of or pertaining to the episclera.

**epi·scle·ri·tis** (ep″ĭ-sklə-ri′tis) inflammation of tissues overlying the sclera; also inflammation of the outermost layers of the sclera.
**e. partia′lis fu′gax**, sudden hyperemia of the sclera and overlying conjunctiva, lasting a short time.

**epi·scle·ro·ti·tis** (ep″i-skler″o-ti′tis) episcleritis.

**episi(o)-** [Gr. *epision* pubic region] a combining form denoting relationship to the vulva.

**epis·io·per·i·neo·plas·ty** (ə-piz″e-o-per″ĭ-ne′o-plas″te) [*episio-* + *perineoplasty*] plastic repair of the vulva and perineum.

**epis·io·per·i·ne·or·rha·phy** (ə-piz″e-o-per″ĭ-ne-or′ə-fe) [*episio-* + *perineum* + *-rrhapy*] the suturing of the vulva and perineum.

**epis·io·plas·ty** (ə-piz′e-o-plas″te) [*episio-* + *-plasty*] plastic repair of the vulva.

**epis·i·or·rha·phy** (ə-piz″e-or′ə-fe) [*episio-* + *-rrhaphy*] the suturing of the labia majora for repair of the vulva and perineum.

**epis·io·ste·no·sis** (ə-piz″e-o-stə-no′sis) [*episio-* + *stenosis*] the narrowing of the vulvar orifice.

**epis·i·ot·o·my** (ə-piz″e-ot′o-me) [*episio-* + *-tomy*] [MeSH: Episiotomy] surgical incision into the perineum and vagina to prevent traumatic tearing during delivery.

**ep·i·sode** (ep′ĭ-sōd) a noteworthy happening or series of happenings occurring in the course of continuous events, as an episode of illness; a separate but not unrelated incident.
**acute schizophrenic e.**, acute schizophrenia.
**hypomanic e.** [DSM-IV], a period during which there is elevated, expansive, or irritable mood, with symptoms resembling those of a

manic episode but less severe and not including any psychotic features.

**major depressive e.** [DSM-IV], a period of daily and day-long depressed mood or loss of interest or pleasure in virtually all activities; in children or adolescents the mood may be irritable. Also present is some combination of the following symptoms: altered appetite, weight, or sleep patterns, psychomotor agitation or retardation, diminished capacity for thinking, concentration, or decisiveness, lack of energy and fatigue, feelings of worthlessness, self-reproach, or inappropriate guilt, recurrent thoughts of death or suicide, and plans or attempts to commit suicide.

**manic e.** [DSM-IV], a period of predominantly elevated, expansive, or irritable mood accompanied by some of the following symptoms: inflated self-esteem or grandiosity, decreased need for sleep, talkativeness, flight of ideas, distractibility, hyperactivity or psychomotor agitation, hypersexuality, and reckless behavior.

**mixed e.** [DSM-IV], a period during which the criteria are met both for a major depressive episode and for a manic episode nearly every day, with rapidly alternating moods and with symptoms characteristic of each type of episode.

**ep·i·some** (ep'ĭ-sōm) in bacterial genetics, any accessory extrachromosomal replicating genetic element that can exist either autonomously or integrated with the chromosome, e.g., the F factor, colicinogens, and (drug) resistance transfer factor. See also *plasmid.*

**epi·spa·dia** (ep″ĭ-spa'de-ə) [MeSH: Epispadias] epispadias.

**epi·spa·di·ac** (ep″ĭ-spa'de-ak) pertaining to or exhibiting epispadias; by extension, sometimes used to designate an individual exhibiting epispadias.

**epi·spa·di·al** (ep″ĭ-spa'de-əl) pertaining to epispadias.

**epi·spa·di·as** (ep″ĭ-spa'de-əs) [*epi-* + Gr. *spadōn* a rent] [MeSH: Epispadias] congenital absence of the upper wall of the urethra, occurring in various degrees of severity in both sexes, but affecting males more commonly, the urethral opening being anywhere on the dorsum of the penis, and manifested as a groove or cleft without a covering.

**balanic e., balanitic e.,** incomplete epispadias in which the urethral opening is above and behind the glans, the dorsum of the penis usually being indented to its tip, but the opening may end at the corona or proximal to it. Called also *glandular e.*

**clitoric e.,** incomplete epispadias in which the urethra opens cephalad to the clitoris or into it.

**complete e.,** epispadias in which the urethra is entirely open to the bladder neck in males, and there may be complete failure of fusion of the anterior urethral wall in the female; it is frequently associated with exstrophy of the bladder.

**glandular e.,** balanic e.

**incomplete e.,** epispadias in which the bladder does not entirely open to the outside; designated according to the location of urethral opening in the male as *balanic* and *penile,* and in the female as *clitoric* and *subsymphyseal.*

**penile e.,** incomplete epispadias in which the urethral orifice is somewhere between the postglandular sulcus and the suspensory ligament, but is usually at the base of the penis.

**penopubic e.,** complete epispadias in which the urethral opening is at the junction of the penis and pubis; unless associated with exstrophy of the bladder, the urethral passage emerges between the corpora cavernosa under the pubic symphysis.

**subsymphyseal e.,** incomplete epispadias in which the urethral opening is beneath the symphysis.

**epi·spi·nal** (ep″ĭ-spi'nəl) situated upon the spinal cord or the vertebral (spinal) column.

**epi·sple·ni·tis** (ep″ĭ-splə-ni'tis) [*epi-* + *splen-* + *-itis*] inflammation of the capsule of the spleen.

**epis·ta·sis** (ə-pis'tə-sis) [*epi-* + *stasis*] 1. suppression of a secretion or excretion, as of blood, menses, or lochia. 2. a scum or pellicle on the surface of urine. 3. the interaction between genes at different loci, as a result of which one hereditary character is unexpressed, or is masked by the superimposition of another upon it. Cf. *dominance.*

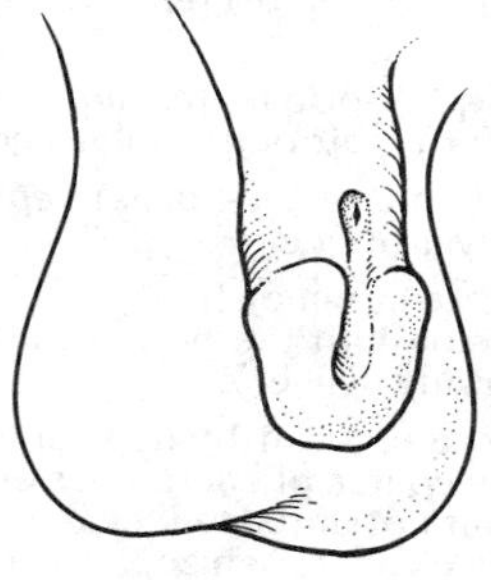

Epispadias.

**epis·ta·sy** (ə-pis'tə-se) epistasis.

**epi·stat·ic** (ep″ĭ-stat'ik) 1. pertaining to or characterized by epistasis. 2. superimposed.

**ep·i·stax·is** (ep″ĭ-stak'sis) [Gr.] [MeSH: Epistaxis] hemorrhage from the nose; called also *nosebleed* and *nasal hemorrhage.*

**anterior e.,** bleeding from the anterior part of the nasal cavity, more common in children than in older patients.

**Gull's renal e.,** essential hematuria.

**posterior e.,** bleeding from the posterior part of the nasal cavity, more common in older patients than in children; mild cases may go undetected because the blood does not exit through the nares.

**epis·te·mol·o·gy** (ep″ĭ-stə-mol'ə-je) [Gr. *epistēmē* knowledge + *-logy*] the science of the methods and validity of knowledge.

**epi·ster·nal** (ep″ĭ-stər'nəl) 1. situated on or over the sternum. 2. pertaining to the episternum.

**epi·ster·num** (ep″ĭ-stər'nəm) [*epi-* + *sternum*] a bone present in reptiles and monotremes that may be represented as part of the manubrium, or first piece of the sternum.

**epis·thot·o·nos** (e″pis-thot'ə-nos) emprosthotonos.

**epi·stro·phe·us** (ep″ĭ-stro'fe-əs) [Gr. "the pivot"] the second cervical vertebra (*axis* [TA]).

**epi·tar·sus** (ep″ĭ-tahr'səs) [*epi-* + *tarsus*] a congenital anomaly of the eye consisting of a fold of conjunctiva passing from the fornix to near the lid border; called also *congenital pterygium.*

**epi·taxy** (ep″ĭ-tak'se) the oriented growth and binding of a crystalline substance on a substrate of another crystalline compound, as in the embryonic formation of bone.

**epi·te·la** (ep″ĭ-te'lə) [*epi-* + *tela*] the delicate tissue of the rostral medullary velum.

**epi·ten·din·e·um** (ep″ĭ-tən-din'e-əm) vagina tendinis.

**epi·te·non** (ep″ĭ-te'non) [*epi-* + Gr. *tenōn* tendon] the connective tissue covering a tendon within its sheath.

**epi·tha·lam·ic** (ep″ĭ-thə-lam'ik) 1. overlying the thalamus. 2. pertaining to the epithalamus.

**epi·thal·a·mus** (ep″ĭ-thal'ə-məs) [TA] [MeSH: Epithalamus] the caudal part of the roof and the adjoining lateral walls of the third ventricle of the diencephalon, comprising the habenular nuclei and their commissure, pineal body, and commissure of the epithalamus.

**epi·tha·lax·ia** (ep″ĭ-thə-lak'se-ə) [*epithelium* + Gr. *allaxis* exchange] desquamation of the epithelium, especially of the intestinal mucosa.

**ep·i·the·lia** (ep″ĭ-the'le-ə) plural of *epithelium.*

**ep·i·the·li·al** (ep″ĭ-the'le-əl) pertaining to or composed of epithelium.

**ep·i·the·li·al·iza·tion** (ep″ĭ-the″le-əl-ĭ-za'shən) healing by the growth of epithelium over a denuded surface.

**ep·i·the·li·a·lize** (ep″ĭ-the'le-əl-īz″) to cover with epithelium.

**ep·i·the·li·itis** (ep″ĭ-the″le-i'tis) inflammation of epithelium.

**epitheli(o)-** [L. *epithelium,* q.v.] a combining form denoting relationship to the epithelium.

**ep·i·the·lio·chor·i·al** (ep″ĭ-the″le-o-ko're-əl) [*epithelio-* + *chorial*] denoting a type of placenta in which the chorion is apposed to the uterine epithelium but does not erode it.

**ep·i·the·lio·fi·bril** (ep″ĭ-the'le-o-fi″bril) one of the fibrils which run through the cytoplasm of epithelial cells.

**epi·the·lio·gen·e·sis** (ep″ĭ-the″le-o-jen'ə-sis) the forming of new epithelium.

**e. imperfec'ta lin'guae bo'vis,** smooth tongue.

**e. imperfec'ta,** aplasia cutis congenita.

**ep·i·the·lio·ge·net·ic** (ep″ĭ-the″le-o-jə-net'ik) [*epithelio-* + *genetic*] due to epithelial proliferation.

**ep·i·the·li·o·gen·ic** (ep″ĭ-the″le-o-jen'ik) tending to produce epithelium.

**ep·i·the·lio·glan·du·lar** (ep″ĭ-the″le-o-glan'du-lər) pertaining to the epithelial cells of a gland.

**ep·i·the·li·oid** (ep″ĭ-the'le-oid) resembling epithelium.

**ep·i·the·li·ol·y·sin** (ep″ĭ-the″le-ol'ə-sin) a cytolysin formed in the serum of an animal when epithelial cells from an animal of a different species are injected. The epitheliolysin has the power of destroying epithelial cells of an animal of the same species as that from which the epithelial cells were originally taken.

**ep·i·the·li·ol·y·sis** (ep″ĭ-the″le-ol′ə-sis) [*epithelio-* + *-lysis*] destruction of epithelial cells.

**ep·i·the·lio·lyt·ic** (ep″ĭ-the″le-o-lit′ik) pertaining to, characterized by, or causing epitheliolysis.

**ep·i·the·li·o·ma** (ep″ĭ-the″le-o′mə) [*epithelio-* + *-oma*] 1. a neoplasm of epithelial origin, ranging from benign (adenoma and papilloma) to malignant (carcinoma). 2. loosely and incorrectly, a carcinoma.
**e. adenoi′des cys′ticum,** multiple trichoepithelioma; see *trichoepithelioma.*
**basal cell e.,** see under *carcinoma.*
**benign calcifying e.,** pilomatricoma.
**calcified e., calcifying e., calcifying e. of Malherbe,** pilomatricoma.
**chorionic e.,** choriocarcinoma.
**diffuse e.,** infiltrating carcinoma.
**Ferguson Smith e.,** self-healing squamous e.
**Malherbe's calcifying e.,** pilomatricoma.
**malignant e.,** carcinoma.
**multiple self-healing squamous e.,** self-healing squamous e.
**sebaceous e.,** yellowish, papular or nodular, sometimes ulcerated lesions occurring on the scalp, face, and neck of older adults and closely resembling basal cell carcinoma clinically; lesions are characterized histologically by oval nests of irregular basaloid cells and sebaceous cells.
**self-healing squamous e.,** an autosomal dominant form of multiple keratoacanthoma, characterized by a succession of lesions resembling those of squamous cell carcinoma; they heal spontaneously with scarring and are most common on the face and extremities of male adolescents and young adults. Called also *Ferguson Smith e.*

**ep·i·the·li·o·ma·to·sis** (ep″ĭ-the″le-o-mə-to′sis) the state of being subject to or afflicted with epitheliomas.

**ep·i·the·li·o·ma·tous** (ep″ĭ-the″le-o′mə-təs) pertaining to or of the nature of epithelioma.

**ep·i·the·lio·mus·cu·lar** (ep″ĭ-the″le-o-mus′ku-lər) composed of epithelium and muscle.

**ep·i·the·lio·tox·in** (ep″ĭ-the″le-o-tok′sin) a cytotoxin which destroys epithelial cells.

**ep·i·the·lite** (ep″ĭ-the′līt) a lesion produced as a reaction to irradiation, in which the epithelium is replaced by a fibrous exudate.

**ep·i·the·li·um** (ep″ĭ-the′le-əm) pl. *epithe′lia* [*epi-* + Gr. *thēlē* nipple] [TA] [MeSH: Epithelium] the covering of internal and external surfaces of the body, including the lining of vessels and other small cavities. It consists of cells joined by small amounts of cementing substances. Epithelium is classified into types on the basis of the number of layers deep and the shape of the superficial cells.
**e. ante′rius cor′neae** [TA], anterior epithelium of cornea: the outer epithelial layer of the cornea, consisting of stratified squamous epithelium continuous with that of the conjunctiva; called also *e. corneae* or *corneal e.*
**Barrett's e.,** the metaplastic columnar epithelium of the esophagus seen in Barrett's syndrome.
**capsular e.,** the outer, or parietal, layer of the renal glomerular capsule, composed of simple squamous epithelium, and separated from the inner, or visceral, layer by the capsular space. Cf. *glomerular e.*
**ciliated e.,** any type bearing vibratile cilia on the free surface.
**columnar e.,** a type composed of tall prismatic cells.
**e. cor′neae, corneal e.,** e. anterius corneae.
**cubical e., cuboidal e.,** a type composed of cells which have a cubical shape.
**e. duc′tus semicircula′ris,** the inner, simple, low epithelium lining the semicircular ducts.
**enamel e.,** in the developing tooth, the inner or internal layer of cells (ameloblasts) of the enamel organ that deposit the organic matrix of enamel, plus the outer or external layer of cuboidal cells. The reduced enamel epithelium is the remains of both layers after enamel formation is complete.
**false e.,** the lining of joint cavities.
**germinal e.,** thickened peritoneal epithelium covering the gonad from earliest development; formerly thought to give rise to the germ cells, hence the name.
**gingival e.,** the stratified squamous epithelial covering of the gingival tissues, varying in architecture according to location, functional demands, and adaptation.
**glandular e.,** epithelium made up of glandular or secreting cells.
**glomerular e.,** the inner, or visceral, layer of the renal glomerular capsule, overlying the capillaries, composed of podocytes, and separated from the outer, or parietal, layer by the capsular (Bowman's) space. Cf. *capsular e.*
**junctional e.,** a collarlike band of stratified squamous epithelium adhering on one side to the free gingiva and on the other to the crown of a tooth.
**laminated e.,** stratified e.

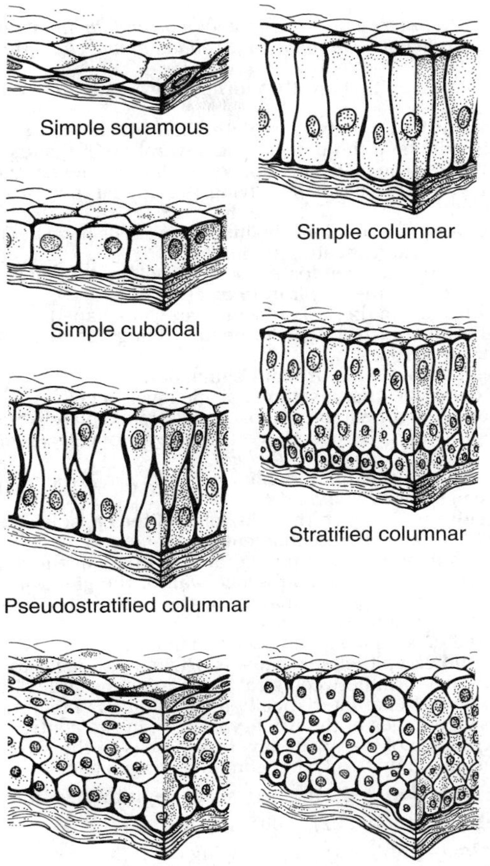

Epithelium of different types.

**e. len′tis** [TA], epithelium of lens: the cuboidal epithelium on the front of the lens; called also *subcapsular e.*
**mesenchymal e.,** the epithelium which lines the subdural and subarachnoid spaces, the perilymphatic spaces in the inner ear, and the chamber of the eye.
**e. muco′sae,** the epithelium that lines the tunica mucosa.
**olfactory e.,** pseudostratified epithelium lining the olfactory region of the nasal cavity, and containing the receptors for the sense of smell.
**pavement e.,** simple squamous epithelium.
**pigmentary e., pigmented e.,** epithelium containing granules of pigment.
**e. pigmento′sum i′ridis** [TA], pigmented epithelium of iris: the anterior epithelium of the iris, situated just posterior to the stroma, that contains pigment cells.
**e. poste′rius cor′neae** [TA], posterior epithelium of cornea: the mesothelial layer covering the posterior surface of the posterior limiting lamina of the cornea; it was once believed to extend to the anterior surface of the stroma of the iris. Called also *anterior endo-*

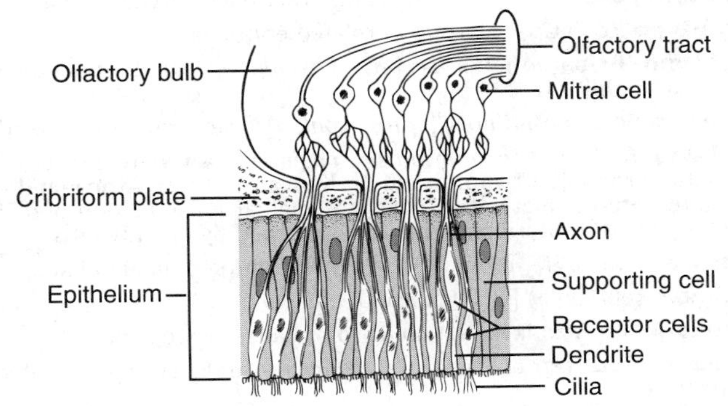

Schematic diagram of the receptors in the olfactory epithelium.

*thelium of cornea, corneal endothelium, endothelium anterius corneae, endothelium corneale,* and *endothelium camerae anterioris bulbi.*

**protective e.,** epithelium that forms a protective covering, as the epidermis.

**pseudostratified e.,** a type of epithelium which occurs in the large excretory ducts of the parotid and several other glands and in the male urethra. The nuclei are spaced at different levels and the cells are quite variable in shape, giving the appearance of a stratified epithelium.

**pyramidal e.,** columnar epithelium whose cells have been modified by pressure into truncated pyramids.

**respiratory e.,** the pseudostratified epithelium that lines all but the finer divisions of the respiratory tract.

**rod e.,** epithelium the cells of which are rod-shaped.

**seminiferous e.,** stratified epithelium lining the seminiferous tubules of the testis.

**sense e., sensory e.,** neuroepithelium, def. 1.

**simple e.,** a type composed of a single layer of cells.

**squamous e.,** epithelium composed of flattened platelike cells. Squamous epithelium composed of a single layer of cells *(simple epithelium)* is called *pavement epithelium.*

**stratified e.,** epithelium in which the cells are arranged in several layers; called also *laminated e.*

**subcapsular e.,** 1. the epithelioid lining of the capsule of a ganglion; cf. *satellite cell.* 2. epithelium lentis.

**sulcal e., sulcular e.,** the parakeratinized part of the gingival epithelium that covers the soft tissue wall of the gingival sulcus, extending from the gingival margin to the line of attachment of the epithelium to the tooth surface.

**tessellated e.,** simple squamous epithelium.

**transitional e.,** epithelium that was originally thought to represent a transitional form between stratified squamous and columnar epithelium, found characteristically in the mucous membrane of the excretory passages of the urinary system; in the contracted condition it consists of many cell layers, whereas in the stretched condition usually only two layers can be distinguished.

**ep·i·the·li·za·tion** (ep″ĭ-the″lĭ-za′shən) epithelialization.

**ep·i·the·lize** (ep″ĭ-the′līz) epithelialize.

**epith·e·sis** (ə-pith′ə-sis) [Gr. "a laying on"] 1. the surgical correction of deformity or of crooked limbs. 2. a splint or other appliance to be worn.

**ep·i·ton·ic** (ep″ĭ-ton′ik) [Gr. *epitonos* strained] abnormally tense or tonic; exhibiting an abnormal degree of tension or of tone.

**ep·i·tope** (ep′ĭ-tōp) antigenic determinant.

**Ep·i·trate** (ep′ĭ-trāt) trademark for a preparation of epinephrine bitartrate.

**ep·i·trich·i·um** (ep″ĭ-trik′e-əm) [*epi-* + Gr. *trichion* hair] periderm, def. 1.

**epi·tri·que·trum** (ep″ĭ-trĭ-kwe′trəm) epipyramis.

**epi·troch·lea** (ep″ĭ-trok′le-ə) [*epi-* + *trochlea*] the inner condyle of the humerus.

**epi·troch·le·ar** (ep″ĭ-trok′le-ər) 1. pertaining to the epitrochlea. 2. above a trochlea, such as the trochlea of the humerus.

**epi·tu·ber·cu·lo·sis** (ep″ĭ-too-bər″ku-lo′sis) a form of primary tuberculosis in children, producing mild symptoms despite large, usually lobar, consolidations as seen radiographically; probably due to bronchial compression by enlarged hilar lymph nodes, with atelectasis.

**epi·tym·pan·ic** (ep″ĭ-tim-pan′ik) 1. situated upon or over the tympanum. 2. pertaining to the epitympanum (recessus epitympanicus [TA]).

**epi·tym·pa·num** (ep″ĭ-tim′pə-nəm) recessus epitympanicus.

**ep·i·type** (ep′i-tīp) a group of related epitopes.

**epi·typh·li·tis** (ep″ĭ-tif-li′tis) [*epi-* + *typhlo-* + *-itis*] 1. appendicitis. 2. paratyphlitis.

**epi·ty·phlon** (ep″ĭ-ti′flon) [*epi-* + *typhlon*] the vermiform appendix.

**epi·vag** (ep′ĭ-vag) [*epididymitis* + *vaginitis*] a venereal disease of cattle, probably of viral origin, in Kenya, southern Africa, and the United States, marked in cows by vaginal inflammation and discharge and by sterility. In bulls it is marked by epididymitis.

**Epi·vir** (ep′ĭ-vir″) trademark for a preparation of lamivudine.

**epi·zoa** (ep″ĭ-zo′ə) [Gr.] plural of *epizoon.*

**epi·zo·ic** (ep″ĭ-zo′ik) pertaining to or caused by epizoa.

**epi·zo·i·cide** (ep″ĭ-zo′ĭ-sīd) [*epizoon* + *-cide*] an agent that destroys epizoa.

**epi·zo·on** (ep″ĭ-zo′on) pl. *epizo′a* [*epi-* + Gr. *zōon* animal] an animal parasite living upon the exterior of the body of the host.

**epi·zo·ot·ic** (ep″ĭ-zo-ot′ik) 1. attacking many animals in any region at the same time; widely diffused and rapidly spreading. 2. a disease of high morbidity which is only occasionally present in an animal community. Cf. *enzootic.*

**epi·zo·ot·i·ol·o·gy** (ep″ĭ-zo-ot″e-ol′ə-je) the study of the factors determining frequencies and distributions of infectious diseases among animals other than humans; animal epidemiology. See also *epizootic.*

**éplu·chage** (a″ploo-shahzh′) [Fr. "cleaning," "picking"] removal of the contused and contaminated tissues of a wound. Cf. *débridement.*

**epo·e·tin** (e-po′ə-tin) a 165–amino acid glycoprotein produced by recombinant DNA technology. It has the same amino acid sequence and mechanism of action as endogenous erythropoietin and is used in treatment of anemia; administered intravenously or subcutaneously. Available in two forms, designated *epoetin alfa* and *epoetin beta.* Called also *recombinant human erythropoietin (rHuEPO).*

**Ep·o·gen** (e′po-jən) trademark for a preparation of epoetin alfa.

**epon·tic** (ə-pon′tik) growing on any surface, plant, animal, or mineral.

**ep·o·nych·i·um** (ep″o-nik′e-əm) [*epi-* + *onyx*] 1. [TA] the narrow band of epidermis that extends from the nail wall onto the nail surface; called also *cuticle* and *perionychium.* 2. the horny fetal epidermis at the site of the future nail.

**ep·o·oph·o·rec·to·my** (ep″o-of″ə-rek′tə-me) [*epi-* + *oophoro-* + *-ectomy*] surgical removal of the epoophoron.

**ep·oöph·o·ron** (ep″o-of′ə-rən) [*epi-* + *oophoron*] [TA] a vestigial structure associated with the ovary, consisting of a more cranial group of mesonephric tubules and a corresponding portion of the mesonephric duct; called also *corpus pampiniforme, pampiniform body, parovarium,* and *Rosenmüller's organ.* Spelled also *epoophoron.*

**ep·o·pro·sten·ol** (ep″o-pro′stən-ol) [MeSH: Epoprostenol] name given to prostacyclin when used pharmaceutically.

**ep·or·ni·thol·o·gy** (ep-or″nĭ-thol′ə-je) the scientific study of diseases of high morbidity that are only occasionally present in bird communities.

**ep·or·nit·ic** (ep″or-nit′ik) [*epi-* + Gr. *ornis* bird] 1. attacking many birds in a region at the same time. 2. a disease of high morbidity that is only occasionally present in a bird population.

**epox·ide** (ə-pok′sīd) an organic compound containing a reactive group resulting from the union of an oxygen atom with two other atoms, usually carbon, that are themselves joined together. Commonly referred to as *epoxy.* See also *epoxy resin,* under *resin.*

**epoxy** (ə-pok′se) 1. epoxide. 2. see under *resin.*

**ep·oxy·tro·pine tro·pate** (e-pok″se-tro′pēn tro′pāt) methscopolamine.

**EPP** erythrohepatic or erythropoietic protoporphyria; see *protoporphyria.*

**Ep·py** (ep′e) trademark for a preparation of epinephryl borate.

**EPR** electron paramagnetic resonance; electrophrenic respiration.

**Ep·ro·lin** (ep′ro-lin) trademark for a preparation of vitamin E, consisting of a concentrate of distilled natural tocopherols.

**ep·si·lon** (ep′si-lon) [E,ϵ] the fifth letter of the Greek alphabet. See also ϵ-.

**EPSP** excitatory postsynaptic potential.

**Ep·stein's disease, pearls** (ep′stīnz) [Alois *Epstein,* Czech pediatrician, 1849–1918] see *pseudodiphtheria,* and see under *pearl.*

**Ep·stein's nephrosis, syndrome** (ep′stīnz) [Albert Arthur *Epstein,* New York physician, 1880–1965] see under *nephrosis,* and see *nephrotic syndrome,* under *syndrome.*

**Ep·stein-Barr virus** (ep′stīn-bahr′) [Michael Anthony *Epstein,* English physician, born 1921; Yvonne M. *Barr,* English virologist, 20th century] see under *virus.*

**ep·ta·tre·tin** (ep″tə-tre′tin) a potent cardiostimulant obtained from the branchial heart of the Pacific hagfish *Eptatretus stouti* and reported to be a highly unstable aromatic amine. Its chemical structure has not been fully defined, but it is not a catecholamine or other commonly occurring biochemical.

**epu·li·des** (ə-pu′lĭ-dēz) [Gr.] plural of *epulis.*

**epu·lis** (ə-pu′lis) pl. *epu′lides* [Gr. *epoulis* gumboil] 1. a nonspecific term applied to tumors and tumor-like masses of the gingiva. 2. peripheral ossifying fibroma.

**congenital e.,** a benign, nonencapsulated soft, pedunculated tumor of the mucosa of the jaws, usually the maxilla, of newborn infants. It is often found in the incisor region, arising on the crest of the alveolar ridge or process. Microscopically, it resembles granular cell tumor. Called also *e. of newborn.*

**e. fibromato′sa, fibromatous e.,** 1. a fibroma arising from the alve-

olar periosteum and the periodontal ligament. 2. a benign fibromatous tumor arising in periodontal stroma on the gum of a dog, usually an older animal. Some breeds are more susceptible than others, suggesting a genetic component. Called also *fibromatosis gingivae.*
**e. fissura'ta,** fibrous inflammatory hyperplasia.
**giant cell e., e. gigantocellula'ris,** a sessile or pedunculated lesion of the gingiva, or less often the mucous membrane covering edentulous ridges, which represents inflammatory reactions to injury or hemorrhage, and is not considered a true neoplasm. Histologically, it is composed of a spindle cell stroma punctuated by multinucleate giant cells. Called also *peripheral giant cell granuloma.*
**e. granulomato'sa,** a pyogenic granuloma on the gingiva resulting from mechanical or other irritation.
**e. of newborn,** congenital e.

**ep·u·lo·fi·bro·ma** (ep"u-lo"fi-bro'mə) a fibroma of the gingiva.

**ep·u·loid** (ep'u-loid) resembling an epulis.

**ep·u·lo·sis** (ep"u-lo'sis) [Gr. *epoulōsis*] cicatrization.

**ep·u·lot·ic** (ep"u-lot'ik) [Gr. *epoulōtikos*] pertaining to, characterized by, or promoting cicatrization.

**Equa·nil** (ek'wə-nil) trademark for preparations of meprobamate.

**equate** (e-kwāt') to make equal or equivalent. In color vision, the physiologic faculty of combining two colors to match a third, as to combine red and green to make a homogeneous yellow.

**equa·tion** (e-kwa'zhən) [L. *aequatio,* from *aequare* to make equal] an expression made up of two members connected by the sign of equality, =.
**Arrhenius e.,** an equation describing the temperature dependence of a reaction rate constant,

$$k = Ae^{-\Delta E_a/RT},$$

where $k$ is the rate constant, $e$ is the base of natural logarithms, $\Delta E_a$ the activation energy, $R$ the gas constant, $T$ the absolute temperature, and $A$ is a constant called the frequency factor, representing the frequency of encounters between reactant molecules.
**chemical e.,** an equation that expresses a chemical reaction, the symbols on the left of the equation denoting the substances before, and those on the right those after, the reaction.
**Harden and Young e.,** an equation showing the chemical reaction in the fermentation of glucose to carbon dioxide, alcohol, and hexose diphosphate.
**Henderson-Hasselbalch e.,** an equation giving the pH of a buffer system:

$$\mathrm{pH} = \mathrm{pK_a} + \log \frac{[\mathrm{A^-}]}{[\mathrm{HA}]}$$

where [HA] is the concentration of the free acid, $[A^-]$ is the concentration of the ionized form, and $pK_a$ is the negative logarithm of the acid dissociation constant ($K_a$).
**Hill e.,** an equation used in enzyme characterization, describing the fraction of the enzyme saturated by ligand as a function of the ligand concentration; it is used in determining the degree of cooperativity of the enzyme.
**Lineweaver-Burk e.,** a rearrangement of the Michaelis-Menten equation of enzyme kinetics to give

$$\frac{1}{v} = \frac{K_M}{V_{max}[S]} + \frac{1}{V_{max}}$$

where $v$ is the reaction velocity, [S] is the substrate concentration, $V_{max}$ is the maximum velocity, and $K_M$ is the Michaelis constant. If an enzyme reaction follows Michaelis-Menten kinetics, then a plot of $1/v$ against 1/[S] results in a straight line with defined slope and intercepts; see *Lineweaver-Burk plot,* under *plot.*
**Michaelis-Menten e.,** a fundamental equation of enzyme kinetics:

$$v = \frac{V_{max}[S]}{K_M + [S]}$$

where $v$ is the "initial velocity" of an enzyme-catalyzed reaction (the velocity when the product concentration is near zero); [S] is the substrate concentration; and $V_{max}$ and $K_M$ are two constants that characterize a specific enzyme: $V_{max}$, the maximum velocity, is the initial velocity seen when the enzyme is completely saturated with substrate, and $K_M$ is the Michaelis constant, defined operationally as the substrate concentration at which $v = V_{max}/2$. The Michaelis-Menten equation does not apply to allosteric enzymes for which the binding of the substrate at the active site is altered by binding of the substrate at a second (allosteric) site. See also *Lineweaver-Burk e.*
**Nernst e.,** an equation for the voltage produced by an electrochemical reaction:

$$E = E° - \frac{RT}{zF} \ln Q$$

where $E$ is the voltage produced, $E°$ is the standard reduction potential for the reaction, $R$ is the gas constant, $T$ the absolute temperature, $z$ the number of electrons transferred in the reaction, $F$ Faraday's constant, $Q$ the reaction quotient (q.v.), and ln the natural logarithm. The same formula gives the membrane potential produced by a concentration of a diffusible ion across a membrane; in this case $E°$ is zero, $z$ is the ionic charge, and $Q$ is the ratio of the concentrations on the two sides of the membrane.
**Poiseuille's e.,** see under *law.*
**Ussing e.,** a method for determining active transport across a biologic membrane, by considering the unidirectional fluxes.

**equa·tor** (e-kwa'tər) [L. *aequator* equalizer] an imaginary line encircling a globe, equidistant from the poles. Used in anatomical nomenclature to designate such a line on a spherical organ, dividing the surface into two approximately equal parts. Called also *aequator.*
**e. bul'bi o'culi** [TA], equator of eyeball: an imaginary line encircling the eyeball equidistant from the anterior and the posterior poles, dividing the eye into anterior and posterior halves.
**e. of cell,** the boundary of the plane of separation of a dividing cell.
**e. of crystalline lens,** e. lentis.
**e. of eyeball,** e. bulbi oculi.
**e. len'tis** [TA], equator of lens: the rounded peripheral margin of the lens at which the anterior and posterior surfaces meet.

**equa·to·ri·al** (e"kwə-tor'e-əl) pertaining to an equator; occurring at the same distance from each extremity of an axis.

**equi·an·al·ge·sic** (e"kwĭ-an"əl-je'sik) having the same analgesic effect as a given dose of another analgesic agent.

**equi·ax·i·al** (e"kwĭ-ak'se-əl) having axes of the same length.

**equi·ca·lor·ic** (e"kwĭ-kə-lor'ik) isocaloric.

**Equi·dae** (ek'wĭ-de) [L. *equus* horse] [MeSH: Equidae] a family of perissodactylous mammals containing a single living genus, *Equus,* which includes horses, asses, zebras, and onagers.

**equi·lat·er·al** (e"kwĭ-lat'ər-əl) having sides that are equal or identical; called also *isolateral.*

**equi·li·bra·tion** (e-kwil"ĭ-bra'shən) the achievement of a balance between opposing elements or forces.
**mandibular e.,** 1. the act or acts performed to place the mandible in equilibrium. 2. a condition in which all of the forces acting upon the mandible are neutralized. 3. a term applied to adjustive grinding of an interfering tooth structure during the functional stroke.
**occlusal e.,** see under *adjustment.*

**equi·li·bra·tor** (e-kwil"ĭ-bra'tor) an apparatus used to produce or maintain a state of balance between opposing forces.

**equi·li·bri·um** (e"kwĭ-lib're-əm) [L. *aequus* equal + *libra* balance] [MeSH: Equilibrium] 1. a condition in which opposing forces exactly counteract each other. 2. postural balance of the body; see *sense of equilibrium,* under *sense.*
**acid-base e.,** see under *balance.*
**body e.,** the condition in which the materials taken into the body are balanced by corresponding excretions.
**carbon e.,** the condition in which the total carbon of the excreta is balanced by the carbon of the food.
**Donnan's e.,** the conditions which exist at equilibrium when two solutions are separated by a membrane permeable to some but not all of the ions of the solutions. There is a complex distribution of the ions between the two solutions, an electrical potential develops between the two sides of the membrane, and the two solutions vary in osmotic pressure. Called also *Gibbs-Donnan e.*
**dynamic e.,** the condition of balance between varying, shifting, and opposing forces which is characteristic of living processes.
**fluid e.,** see under *balance.*
**genetic e.,** the condition that exists when the gene pool in a population is constant in successive generations (unless altered by selection or mutation); i.e., the frequency of each allele in the population remains unchanged in successive generations.
**Gibbs-Donnan e.,** Donnan e.
**Hardy-Weinberg e.,** genetic e.
**linkage e.,** in genetics, the situation in which the coupling and repulsion phases for two linked loci are equally frequent, so that the frequency of each combination of alleles is equal to the product of their individual frequencies.
**nitrogen e., nitrogenous e.,** the condition in which the body is metabolizing and excreting as much nitrogen as it is receiving in the food; cf. *nitrogen balance,* under *balance.* Called also *protein e.*
**nutritive e.,** physiologic e.
**physiologic e.,** the condition in which the amount of material taken into the body exactly equals the amount discharged.
**protein e.,** nitrogen e.
**radioactive e.,** the fixed ratio between a radioactive element and

one of its disintegration products that results after the lapse of a suitable time, owing to their half value periods. That of uranium and radium is 2,380,000:1.
**water e.,** fluid balance.

**equil·in** (ek'wil-in) [MeSH: Equilin] an estrogen, $C_{18}H_{20}O_2$, with both rings A and B aromatized, isolated from urine of pregnant horses.

**equi·mo·lar** (e"kwĭ-mo'lər) containing the same number of moles, or having the same molarity.

**equi·mo·lec·u·lar** (e"kwĭ-mo-lek'u-lər) containing the same number of molecules; said of solutions.

**equine** (e'kwīn) [L. *equus* a horse] pertaining to, characteristic of, or derived from the horse.

**equi·no·pho·bia** (e-kwi"no-fo'be-ə) [L. *equinus* relating to horses + *phobia*] irrational fear of horses.

**equi·no·val·gus** (e-kwi"no-val'gəs) talipes equinovalgus.

**equi·no·va·rus** (e-kwi"no-va'rəs) talipes equinovarus.

**equi·nus** (e-kwi'nəs) talipes equinus.

**equi·po·ten·tial** (e"kwĭ-po-ten'shəl) [L. *aequus* equal + *potential*] possessed of similar and equal power; capable of developing in the same way and to the same extent.

**equi·po·ten·ti·al·i·ty** (e"kwĭ-po-ten"she-al'ĭ-te) the quality or state of having similar and equal power; the capacity for developing in the same way and to the same extent.

**equi·se·to·sis** (ek"wĭ-sə-to'sis) incoordination and cardiac irregularities due to thiamine deficiency in horses or other animals that consume hay contaminated with *Equisetum.*

**equi·se·tum** (ek"wĭ-se'təm) the horsetails, a genus of plants of the family Equisetaceae. *E. arven'se* and *E. palus'tre* contain a thiamine antagonist that causes equisetosis in horses that eat them along with hay.

**equiv·a·lence** (e-kwiv'ə-ləns) 1. the condition of being equivalent; having equal valence. 2. in immunology, the ratio of antigen to antibody concentration at which maximal antigen-antibody combination takes place, yielding a precipitate or aggregate; see also *precipitin reaction,* under *reaction.*

**equiv·a·lent** (e-kwiv'ə-lent) [L. *aequivalens,* from *aequus* equal + *valere* to be worth] 1. having the same value; neutralizing or counterbalancing each other. 2. see under *weight.* 3. in medicine, a symptom that replaces one that is usual in a given disease.
**alpha-tocopherol e.,** the specific biological activity of 1.0 milligram of *d*-alpha-tocopherol. See also *international unit of vitamin E.*
**aluminum e.,** the thickness of pure aluminum affording the same radiation attenuation, under specified conditions, as the material or materials being considered.
**combustion e.,** the heat value of a gram of fat or carbohydrate burned outside the body. It measures the amount of potential energy of the substance available, in the form of food, for the production of heat or the supply of energy.
**concrete e.,** the thickness of concrete having a density of 2.35 g/cm$^3$ which would afford the same radiation attenuation, under specified conditions, as the material or materials being considered.
**dose e.,** in radiation biology, the product of absorbed dose in rads and the modifying factors, namely the quality factor (QF), distribution factor (DF), and any other necessary factors. The unit of dose equivalent is the rem.
**gold e.,** the amount of protective colloid, expressed in milligrams, which is just enough to prevent the precipitation of 10 mL of a 0.0055 per cent gold solution by 1 mL of a 10 per cent sodium chloride solution.
**gram e.,** equivalent weight.
**isodynamic e.,** the ratio, from a food-energy standpoint, between carbohydrate and fat. It is 9.3 to 4.1, or 2.3 to 1; that is, one part of fat is equivalent to 2.3 parts of sugar or starch.
**Joule's e.,** an expression of the relationship between mechanical energy and heat; numerically 4.186 joules = 1 calorie.
**lead e.,** the thickness of pure lead which would afford the same radiation attenuation, under specified conditions, as the material or materials under consideration.
**lethal e.,** a gene carried in the heterozygous state which, if homozygous, would be lethal, or any combination of genes which would be lethal to 100 percent of homozygotes; for example, a combination of two genes in the heterozygous state either of which in the homozygous state would have 50 per cent lethality.
**migraine e.,** migraine aura without headache; see under *aura.*
**neutralization e.,** the equivalent weight of an acid as determined by neutralization with a base regarded as a primary standard.
**protein e.,** the protein content of a food plus the nonprotein content that can be converted into protein in the animal body.
**psychic e.,** temporal lobe epilepsy.
**retinol e. (RE),** the specific biological activity of 1.0 microgram of all-*trans* retinol, 6.0 micrograms of *β*-carotene, or 12.0 micrograms of other provitamin A carotenoids; it is equivalent to 3.3 international units of vitamin A activity from retinol (10 from *β*-carotene).
**starch e.,** a number (nearly 2.4) expressing the amount of oxygen which a given weight of fat will require for its complete combustion as compared with the amount required by the same weight of starch.
**toxic e.,** the amount of poison per kilogram of body weight necessary to kill an animal.
**ventilation e., ventilatory e.,** the ratio of the total volume of ventilation to the volume of oxygen absorbed by the lungs per unit of time.
**water e.,** the product of the weight of an animal by its specific heat, it being also the number which represents the specific thermal capacity of an equal weight of water.

**equu·lo·sis** (ek"wə-lo'sis) [L. *equulus* a foal + *-osis*] actinobacillosis in horses and sometimes pigs, usually seen in the first few weeks of life, involving infection with *Actinobacillus equuli.* Symptoms in foals are purulent arthritis, synovitis, and enteritis, often with kidney abscesses and death; in piglets the symptoms are septicemia, fever, listlessness, and often death. When foals show extreme prostration, the condition is called *sleepy foal disease.*

**Eq·uus** (ek'wəs) the single living genus of the family Equidae, including horses, asses, and zebras.

**Eq·va·lan** (ek'və-lan) trademark for a preparation of ivermectin.

**ER** endoplasmic reticulum; estrogen receptor.

**Er** symbol for *erbium.*

**erab·u·tox·in** (ə-rab"u-tok'sin) the active toxic principle of the venom of the sea snake *Laticauda semifasciata.*

**Er·a·sis·tra·tus** (er"ə-sis'trə-təs) [c. 300 to c. 250 B.C.] a Greek physician born on Ceos, who studied at Alexandria and was a contemporary of Herophilus. Though believing bodily functions to be mechanical, Erasistratus adopted pneumatism to explain physiology, and rejected humoralism; he also invoked an external force, Nature, as shaper of the ends to which the body works. Erasistratus reputedly performed human vivisection and post mortems; he inferred that the greater number and complexity of convolutions in the human brain than in the animal implied greater intelligence (opposing Aristotle); and he distinguished the cerebrum from the cerebellum and the sensory from the motor nerves. Erasistratus ascribed disease to plethora, hyperemia from indigested food, yet he opposed phlebotomy and purgation (and other violent remedies) and advocated Hippocratic-like diet, exercise, and steam baths. See also *Alcmaeon of Crotona* and *Democritus.*

**Er·a·ty·rus** (er"ə-ti'rəs) a genus of reduviid bugs that transmit Chagas' disease.

**Erb's spastic paraplegia,** etc. (erbz) [Wilhelm Heinrich *Erb,* German neurologist, 1840–1921] see under *paraplegia* and *point,* see *primary lateral sclerosis* under *sclerosis,* and see *Duchenne muscular dystrophy,* under *dystrophy.*

**Erb-Char·cot disease** (erb-shahr-ko') [W. H. *Erb;* Jean Martin *Charcot,* French neurologist, 1825–1893] Erb's spastic paraplegia.

**Erb-Du·chenne paralysis** (erb-du-shen') [W.H. *Erb;* Guillaume Benjamin Amand *Duchenne,* French neurologist, 1806–1875] see under *paralysis.*

**Erb-Gold·flam disease** (erb-golt'flahm) [W. H. *Erb;* Samuel V. *Goldflam,* Polish neurologist, 1852–1932] myasthenia gravis.

**Er·ben's reflex (phenomenon, sign)** (er'bənz) [Siegmund *Erben,* Austrian neurologist, born 1863] see under *reflex.*

**ERBF** effective renal blood flow.

**er·bi·um** (ər'be-əm) [MeSH: Erbium] a rare metallic element: symbol, Er; atomic number, 68; atomic weight, 167.26.

**ERCP** endoscopic retrograde cholangiopancreatography.

**Erd·heim's disease (cystic medial necrosis)** (ərd'hīmz) [Jakob *Erdheim,* Austrian physician, 1874–1937] cystic medial necrosis.

**erec·tile** (ə-rek'tīl) capable of erection; see under *tissue.*

**erec·tion** (ə-rek'shən) [L. *erectio*] the condition of being made rigid and elevated, such as in erectile tissue when filled with blood.

**erec·tor** (ə-rek'tər) [L., from *erigere* to set up] something that erects, such as a muscle that raises or holds up a part.

**er·e·ma·cau·sis** (er"ə-mə-kaw'sis) [Gr. *ērema* gently + *kausis* burning] the slow oxidation, combustion, or decay of organic matter.

**er·e·mo·pho·bia** (er"ə-mo-fo'be-ə) [Gr. *erēmos* solitary + *-phobia*] irrational fear of being alone.

**Ereth·ma·pod·i·tes** (ə-reth"mə-pod'ĭ-tēs) a genus of mosquitoes, species of which transmit Rift Valley fever.

**ereuth(o)-** [Gr. *ereuthos* redness] for words beginning thus, see those beginning *erythr(o)-.*

**ERG** electroretinogram.

**erg** (erg) [Gr. *ergon* work] the CGS unit of work or energy, being the work performed when a force of 1 dyne moves its point of operation through a distance of 1 centimeter; equivalent to $2.4 \times 10^{-8}$ gram calorie, or to $0.624 \times 10^{12}$ electron volts.

**Er·ga·mi·sol** (ər-gam′ĭ-sol) trademark for a preparation of levamisole hydrochloride and 5-fluorouracil.

**er·ga·sia** (ər-ga′zhə) [Gr. "work"] Adolf Meyer's term for the total activity or functioning of a person, encompassing both behavior and mental activity.

**er·gas·to·plasm** (ər-gas′to-plaz-əm) [*ergasia* + *plasm*] granular endoplasmic reticulum.

**erg(o)-** [Gr. *ergon* work] a combining form denoting relationship to work.

**er·go·ba·sine** (er″go-ba′sin) ergonovine.

**er·go·cal·cif·er·ol** (er″go-kal-sif′ər-ol) [USP] a sterol occurring naturally in fungi and some fish oils and synthesized by irradiation or electronic bombardment of ergosterol; it is administered orally or added to food (e.g., milk) as a dietary source of vitamin D. It is also used in the treatment of rickets, hypoparathyroidism, hypocalcemia, and familial hypophosphatemia, administered orally or parenterally. The activity and metabolism of ergocalciferol are similar to those of cholecalciferol (q.v.). Called also *vitamin* $D_2$.

**er·go·cor·nine** (ər″go-kor′nēn) a toxic ergot alkaloid of the ergotoxine group.

**er·go·cris·tine** (ər″go-kris′tēn) a toxic ergot alkaloid of the ergotoxine group.

**er·go·cryp·tine** (ər″go-krip′tēn) a toxic ergot alkaloid of the ergotoxine group.

**er·go·dy·namo·graph** (er″go-di-nam′o-graf) [*ergo-* + *dynamo-* + *-graph*] an apparatus for recording the force exhibited and the work done in muscular contraction.

**er·go·es·the·sio·graph** (er″go-es-the′ze-o-graf) [*ergo-* + *esthesio-* + *-graph*] an apparatus for recording graphically muscular reactions to various stimuli.

**er·go·gen·ic** (er″go-jen′ik) [*ergo-* + *-genic*] tending to increase work output.

**er·go·gram** (er′go-gram) [*ergo-* + *-gram*] a tracing made by an ergograph.

**er·go·graph** (er′go-graf) [*ergo-* + *-graph*] an instrument for recording work done in muscular exertion.
**Mosso's e.**, an apparatus for recording the force and frequency of flexion of the fingers.

**er·go·graph·ic** (er″go-graf′ik) pertaining to the ergograph.

**er·go·loid mes·y·lates** (er′go-loid) [USP] [MeSH: Ergoloid Mesylates] a mixture consisting of equal proportions by weight of the methanesulfonate salts of the hydrogenated ergot alkaloids dihydroergocristine, dihydroergocornine, and dihydroergocryptine; administered orally in the treatment of idiopathic decline in mental function in the elderly.

**Er·go·mar** (er′go-mar) trademark for a preparation of ergotamine tartrate.

**er·gom·e·ter** (er-gom′ə-tər) [*ergo-* + *-meter*] dynamometer.
**bicycle e.**, a bicyclelike apparatus for measuring the muscular, metabolic, and respiratory effects of exercise; used to determine cardiac status. See also *bicycle ergometer exercise test,* under *test.*

**er·go·met·rine** (er″go-met′rin) ergonovine.

**er·go·nom·ics** (ər″go-nom′iks) [*ergo-* + Gr. *nomos* law] the science relating to humans and their work, embodying the anatomic, physiologic, psychologic, and mechanical principles affecting the efficient use of human energy.

**er·go·no·vine** (er″go-no′vin) [MeSH: Ergonovine] a water-soluble alkaloid, from ergot or produced synthetically; used as an oxytocic and to relieve migraine headache. Called also *ergobasine, ergometrine, ergostetrine,* and *ergotocine.*
**e. maleate** [USP], the bimaleate salt of ergonovine, occurring as a grayish white to faintly yellow odorless powder; used as an oxytocic, administered orally, intramuscularly, or intravenously. It is also used in the treatment of migraine and as a provocative test in detection of variant angina due to coronary artery spasm.

**er·go·plasm** (er′go-plaz″əm) ergastoplasm.

**er·go·some** (er′go-sōm) polyribosome.

**er·go·stat** (er′go-stat) a machine to be worked for muscular exercise.

**er·gos·te·rol** (er-gos′tə-rol″) [MeSH: Ergosterol] a sterol occurring mainly in yeast and forming ergocalciferol (vitamin $D_2$) upon irradiation by ultraviolet light or electronic bombardment. Called also *provitamin* $D_2$.
**activated e., irradiated e.**, ergocalciferol.

**er·go·stet·rine** (er″go-stet′rin) ergonovine.

**er·got** (er′got) [Fr.; L. *ergota*] 1. the dried sclerotium of *Claviceps purpurea,* which is developed on rye plants *(Secale cereale);* it is the source of the ergot alkaloids (q.v.). 2. a small mass of horn in the tuft of hair at the flexion surface of the fetlock in horses.

**er·got·amine** (er-got′ə-min) [MeSH: Ergotamine] an alkaloid derived from ergot, consisting of lysergic acid, ammonia, proline, phenylalanine, and pyruvic acid combined in amide linkages; used in the treatment of migraine.
**e. tartrate** [USP], the tartrate salt of ergotamine, used as an analgesic in the treatment of migraine.

**er·go·tam·i·nine** (er″go-tam′ĭ-nēn) an isomer of ergotamine.

**er·go·ther·a·py** (er″go-ther′ə-pe) [*ergo-* + *therapy*] treatment of disease by physical effort.

**er·go·thi·o·ne·ine** (er″go-thi″o-ne′in) [MeSH: Ergothioneine] the trimethylbetaine of thiolhistidine, originally found in ergot and later isolated from human blood; it occurs in abnormal amounts in the urine of cancer patients; called also *erythrothioneine, thiazine, thioneine,* and *thiozine.*

**er·got·ism** (er′got-iz-əm) [MeSH: Ergotism] poisoning of humans or other animals from excessive or misdirected medicinal use of ergot, or from eating ergotized grain; it is marked by cerebrospinal symptoms, spasms, cramps, and sometimes a kind of dry gangrene. Called also *ergot poisoning* and *ergotoxicosis.*

**er·got·ized** (er′got-īzd) diseased or otherwise affected by ergot.

**er·go·to·cine** (er″go-to′sēn) ergonovine.

**er·go·tox·i·co·sis** (er″go-tok″sĭ-ko′sis) ergotism.

**er·go·tox·ine** (er″go-tok′sēn) a mixture of three toxic ergot alkaloids, ergocornine, ergocristine, and ergocryptine, formerly used medicinally for its oxytocic and adrenergic blocking effects but no longer used because of the variability of these effects.

**Er·go·trate** (er′go-trāt) trademark for preparations of ergonovine maleate.

**Er·ich·sen's sign (test)** (er′ik-sənz) [Sir John Eric *Erichsen,* English surgeon, 1818–1896] see under *sign.*

**Er·i·o·dic·ty·on** (er″e-o-dik′te-on) [Gr. *erion* wool + *diktyon* net] a genus of resinous shrubs of the family Hydrophyllaceae that grow in the southwestern United States and Mexico. The most important species is *E. califor′nicum,* the source of the flavoring called eriodictyon. Called also *mountain balm* and *yerba santa.*

**er·i·o·dic·ty·on** (er″e-o-dik′te-on) 1. any plant of the genus *Eriodictyon.* 2. the dried leaf of *E. californicum;* its fluidextract is used as a flavoring and its aromatic syrup as a vehicle for dispensing drugs. See under *fluidextract* and *syrup.*

**er·i·o·nite** (er′e-o-nīt) a common form of zeolite used as an absorbent and filtering material; excessive inhalation of its dust can cause pulmonary fibrosis or silicatosis.

**er·is·i·phake** (er-is′ĭ-fāk) erysiphake.

**Er·is·ta·lis** (er-is′tə-lis) a genus of flies, the hover flies, of the family Syrphidae. *E. te′nax* is the drone fly; it breeds in drains and its maggots (rat-tail maggots) occasionally cause intestinal or nasal myiasis.

**Er·lan·ger** (er′lang-gər) E. Joseph. American physiologist, 1874–1965, noted for his work on the nervous system; co-winner, with Herbert S. Gasser, of the Nobel prize for medicine or physiology in 1944.

**Er·len·mey·er flask** (er′lən-mi″ər) [Emil Richard August Carl *Erlenmeyer,* German chemist, 1825–1909] see under *flask.*

**erode** (e-rōd′) to wear away.

**erog·e·nous** (ə-roj′ə-nəs) erotogenic; arousing erotic feelings.

**erose** (e-rōs′) [L. *erodere* to eat away] having an irregularly toothed edge.

**ero·sio** (e-ro′se-o) [L., from *erodere* to eat away] erosion.
**e. interdigita′lis blastomyce′tica,** candidal intertrigo manifested by an area of macerated white skin in the interdigital webs between and extending onto the sides of the fingers, and particularly involving the webs between the third and fourth fingers of those whose hands are frequently or continually immersed in water such as domestic, laundry, and cannery workers, bartenders, and dishwashers.

**ero·sion** (e-ro′zhən) [L. *erosio,* from *erodere* to eat out] 1. an eating away; destruction of the surface of a tissue, material, or structure. 2. progressive loss of the hard substance of a tooth by chemical processes that do not involve bacterial action. See also *abrasion* and *attrition.* 3. a gradual breakdown or very shallow ulceration of the skin which involves only the epidermis and heals without scarring.

**ero·sive** (e-ro'siv) 1. causing, characterized by, or producing erosion. 2. an agent that produces erosion.

**erot·ic** (ə-rot'ik) [Gr. *erōtikos*] 1. charged with sexual feeling. 2. pertaining to sexual desire.

**erot·i·cism** (ə-rot'ĭ-siz-əm) erotism.

**erot·i·cize** (ə-rot'ĭ-sīz) erotize.

**er·o·tism** (er'o-tizm) a sexual instinct or desire; the expression of one's instinctual energy or drive, especially the sex drive.
**anal e.,** fixation of libido at (or regression to) the anal phase of infantile development, said in psychoanalytic theory to produce egotistic, dogmatic, stubborn, miserly character.
**genital e.,** achievement and maintenance of libido at the genital phase of psychosexual development, said in psychoanalytic theory to permit acceptance of normal adult relationships and responsibilities.
**oral e.,** 1. fixation of libido at (or regression to) the oral phase of infantile development, said in psychoanalytic theory to produce passive, insecure, sensitive character. 2. the pleasure derived from the use of the mouth for other than nutritional satisfactions.

**er·o·tize** (er'o-tīz) to endow with erotic or libidinous meaning or significance.

**erot(o)-** [Gr. *erōs,* gen. *erōtos* sexual desire] a combining form denoting relationship to sexual desire.

**ero·to·gen·e·sis** (ə-rot"o-jen'ə-sis) the formation or production of erotic feeling.

**ero·to·gen·ic** (ə-rot"o-jen'ik) erogenous.

**ero·to·ma·nia** (ə-rot"o-ma'ne-ə) [*eroto-* + *-mania*] 1. a disorder in which the subject believes that a person, usually older and of higher social status, is deeply in love with them; failure of the object of the delusion to respond to the subject's advances are rationalized, and pursuit and harassment of the object of the delusion may occur. 2. occasionally, hypersexuality.

**ero·to·pho·bia** (ə-rot"o-fo'be-ə) [*eroto-* + *-phobia*] fear of love, especially of sexual feelings and activity.

**ERP** endocardial resection procedure.

**ERPF** effective renal plasma flow; see under *flow.*

**er·rat·ic** (ə-rat'ik) [L. *errare* to wander] 1. roving or wandering. 2. eccentric; deviating from an accepted course of thought or conduct.

**er·rhine** (er'īn) [Gr. *en* in + *rhis* nose] 1. promoting a nasal discharge. 2. a medicine that promotes nasal discharge or secretion.

**er·ror** (er'ər) a defect in structure or function; a deviation.
**alpha e.,** Type I e.
**beta e., false-negative e.,** Type II e.
**false-positive e.,** Type I e.
**inborn e. of metabolism,** see under *metabolism.*
**nondifferential e.,** random e.
**random e.,** indefiniteness or error in a measurement process that varies unsystematically or unpredictably from measurement to measurement; its magnitude may be quantifiable by statistical methods.
**standard e.,** in statistics, a measure of the variability that the calculated parameter estimate shows as repeated random samples are taken from the same population.
**standard e. of the mean,** an indication of how well a sample mean estimates the population mean by measurement of the standard deviation of a sampling distribution of the means. It is approximately equal to

$$s/\sqrt{n},$$

where $s$ is the sample estimate of the standard deviation and $n$ is the sample size.
**systematic e.,** reproducible inaccuracy; error in a measurement process that is predictable or in the same direction in all measurements; it may not be detectable by statistical methods. Called also *bias.*
**Type I e.,** in a hypothesis test, the rejection of the null hypothesis when it is true; the probability of a Type I error (the significance level) is denoted by $\alpha$.
**Type II e.,** in a hypothesis test, failing to reject the null hypothesis when it is false; the probability of a Type II error is denoted by $\beta$.

**Er·tron** (er'tron) trademark for preparations of ergocalciferol (vitamin $D_2$).

**eru·cic ac·id** (ə-roo'sik) a monounsaturated 22-carbon fatty acid occurring as a major constituent of most rapeseed and mustard oils. Because erucic acid has been linked to cardiac muscle damage, edible canola oil products are prepared from low erucic acid varieties of rapeseed plants. See also table accompanying *fatty acid.*

**eruc·ta·tion** (ə-rək-ta'shən) [L. *eructatio*] [MeSH: Eructation] the casting up of wind from the stomach through the mouth. Called also *belching.*

**erup·tion** (e-rup'shən) [L. *eruptio* a breaking out] 1. the act of breaking out, appearing, or becoming visible, as eruption of the teeth (see *tooth e.*). 2. visible efflorescent lesions of the skin due to disease, especially an exanthematous disease, and marked by redness and prominence; a rash. See also *exanthem.*
**active e.,** the continued eruption of the teeth after complete formation of their dentinal roots, consisting of movement of the teeth in the direction of the occlusal plane, and being coordinated with attrition.
**continuous e.,** a concept that tooth eruption continues throughout life and does not cease when teeth meet their functional antagonists. See also *active e.* and *passive e.*
**creeping e.,** 1. the development of migratory lesions corresponding to the movements of various parasites beneath the skin of a human or other animal, such as occurs in cutaneous larva migrans and cutaneous myiasis. 2. cutaneous larva migrans.
**delayed e.,** see under *dentition.*
**drug e.,** an adverse cutaneous reaction produced by ingestion, parenteral use, or local application of a drug, which may produce various morphologic patterns and types of lesions. Called also *dermatitis medicamentosa* and *drug rash.*
**fixed e.,** a circumscribed inflammatory skin lesion(s) that recurs at the same site(s) over a period of months or years; each attack lasts only a few days but leaves residual pigmentation which is cumulative.
**fixed drug e.,** a drug eruption that recurs at the same site; see *fixed e.*
**Kaposi's varicelliform e.,** a generalized and serious vesiculopustular, umbilicated eruption of viral origin, superimposed upon a preexisting atopic dermatitis; it may be caused by the virus of herpes simplex (eczema herpeticum) or vaccinia (eczema vaccinatum). Called also *pustulosis vacciniformis* (or *varioliformis*) *acuta.*
**passive e.,** the apparent eruption of a tooth that is actually the exposure of the crown of the tooth by separation of the epithelial attachment from the enamel and migration to the cementoenamel junction.
**polymorphous light e.,** a cutaneous eruption occurring after exposure to sunlight without evidence of any other precipitating factor, which may consist of papular, papulovesicular, nodular, eczematoid, or plaquelike lesions.
**seabather's e.,** marine dermatitis.
**serum e.,** an eruption or exanthem accompanying serum sickness.
**surgical e.,** surgical removal of tissue blocking an unerupted tooth to permit eruption.
**tooth e.,** the final stage of odontogenesis, in which a tooth breaks out from its crypt through surrounding tissue.

**erup·tive** (e-rup'tiv) pertaining to or characterized by eruption.

**ERV** expiratory reserve volume; see under *volume.*

**Er·win·ia** (ər-win'e-ə) [*Erwin* F. Smith, American bacteriologist, 1854–1927] [MeSH: Erwinia] a genus of gram-negative, facultatively anaerobic, rod-shaped bacteria of the family Enterobacteriaceae, made up of plant pathogens, epiphytes, and saprophytes. The genus includes organisms formerly classified as *Pectobacterium.*
**E. amylo'vora,** a species that causes fire blight of apples and pears, rarely isolated from humans.
**E. caroto'vora,** a species that causes soft spots in carrots, potatoes, and other plants; not found in clinical specimens; asparaginase derived from cultures of *E. carotovora* is used as an antineoplastic.
**E. herbi'cola,** a species found on plant surfaces, and occasionally isolated from human clinical specimens. It has been associated with nosocomial septicemia. Called also *Enterobacter agglomerans.*

**Er·win·i·eae** (er"wĭ-ni'e-e) in some systems of classification, a tribe of gram-negative, facultatively anaerobic, rod-shaped bacteria of the family Enterobacteriaceae, made up of the genera *Erwinia* and *Pectobacterium.*

**er·y·sip·e·las** (er"ə-sip'ə-ləs) [Gr. *erythros* red + *pella* skin] [MeSH: Erysipelas] an acute superficial form of cellulitis involving the dermal lymphatics, usually caused by infection with group A streptococci, and chiefly characterized by a peripherally spreading hot, bright red, edematous, brawny, infiltrated, and sharply circumscribed plaque with a raised indurated border. Formerly called *St. Anthony's fire.* Cf. *cellulitis* and *phlegmon,* def. 1.
**coast e.,** (Sp. *erisipela de la costa*), a cutaneous manifestation of onchocerciasis seen in Central America, so called because of its resemblance to streptococcal erysipelas, characterized by an erythematous macular rash and edema of the face; in chronic cases the skin loses its elasticity, atrophies, becomes wrinkled, and causes leonine facies.
**gangrenous e.,** necrotizing fasciitis.
**e. gra've inter'num,** erysipelas in the vagina, uterus, and peritoneum; a form of puerperal fever.
**malignant e.,** one of the forms of puerperal fever.

**necrotizing e.**, see under *fasciitis.*
**swine e.**, a contagious disease of swine caused by *Erysipelothrix rhusiopathiae.* It is of great economic importance around the world and occurs in four clinical forms: an *acute septicemic form,* marked by high fever, lesions of the internal organs and viscera, and a high mortality rate; an *urticarial form* (called also *diamonds* or *diamond skin disease*), the mildest form, rarely fatal, marked by sudden onset, high fever, general debility, red to purple blotches on the neck and body, and sometimes involvement of the viscera; a *chronic form,* sometimes fatal, marked by difficulty in breathing and vegetative endocarditis; and an *arthritic form,* not usually fatal, marked by stunting of growth; this form may occur alone or as a complication of other forms.

**er·y·si·pel·a·tous** (er″ə-sĭ-pel′ə-təs) pertaining to or of the nature of erysipelas.

**er·y·sip·e·loid** (er″ə-sip′ə-loid) [*erysipelas* + *-oid*] [MeSH: Erysipeloid] 1. bacterial cellulitis due to infection with *Erysipelothrix rhusiopathiae,* usually occurring as an occupational disease associated with the handling of infected fish, shellfish, meat, or poultry. It presents in three forms: in a usually self-limited, mild localized form manifested by an erythematous and painful swelling at the site of inoculation, which spreads peripherally with central clearing; in a generalized or diffuse form, which may be accompanied by fever and arthritis symptoms, and resolves spontaneously; and in a rare and sometimes fatal systemic form associated with endocarditis. 2. loosely, erysipelas-like.

**Er·y·sip·e·lo·thrix** (er″ə-sip′ə-lo-thriks″) [*erysipelas* + Gr. *thrix* hair] [MeSH: Erysipelothrix] a genus of bacteria of uncertain affiliation, consisting of gram-positive, asporogenous, rod-shaped organisms that form long filaments. They occur as parasites in mammals, birds, and fish.
**E. insidio′sa**, *E. rhusiopathiae.*
**E. rhusiopa′thiae**, a commonly seen species that causes swine erysipelas in swine and erysipeloid in humans. Called also *E. insidiosa* and *swine rotlauf bacillus.*

**er·y·sip·e·lo·tox·in** (er″ə-sip′ə-lo-tok′sin) the toxin produced by certain strains of *Streptococcus pyogenes* in bacterial erysipelas.

**Er·ys·i·pha·ceae** (er-is″ĭ-fa′se-e) a family of fungi of the order Erysiphales, consisting of plant pathogens; it includes the genus *Erysiphe.*

**er·ys·i·phake** (er-is′ĭ-fāk) [Gr. *erysis* a drawing + *phakos* lentil] an instrument for removing the lens in cataract by suction. Cf. *phacoerysis.*

**Er·ys·i·pha·les** (er-is″ĭ-fa′lēz) the powdery mildews, an order of perfect fungi of the subphylum Ascomycotina, series Bitunicatae, which are parasitic on higher plants such as grapes and usually have closed ascocarps and large spherical stalked asci; it includes the family Erysiphaceae.

**Er·ys·i·phe** (er-is′ĭ-fe) a genus of powdery mildews, fungi of the family Erysiphaceae. *E. polygo′ni* attacks many species of fruits and vegetables. The imperfect (sexual) stage is *Oidium.*

**er·y·the·ma** (er″ə-the′mə) [Gr. *erythēma* flush upon the skin] [MeSH: Erythema] redness of the skin produced by congestion of the capillaries.
**e. annula′re**, 1. gyrate erythema in which the lesions are ring shaped. 2. e. marginatum rheumaticum.
**e. annula′re centri′fugum**, an often mild but chronic and recurrent form of gyrate erythema characterized by the occurrence of crops of annular wheal-like lesions with edematous, sometimes vesicular, borders and commonly a yellowish central region that exhibits a fine branny scaling, which may coalesce. Called also *e. figuratum perstans* and *e. gyratum perstans.*
**e. annula′re rheuma′ticum**, e. marginatum rheumaticum.
**e. arthri′ticum epide′micum**, Haverhill fever.
**e. calo′ricum**, that caused by exposure to heat or cold. See *e. ab igne* and *cold e.*
**e. chro′micum figura′tum melanoder′micum**, e. dyschromicum perstans.
**e. chro′nicum mi′grans**, a deep form of gyrate erythema caused by the spirochete *Borrelia burgdorferi,* with the tick *Ixodes ricinus* as the vector, characterized by the development at the site of a tick bite of a red papule that expands slowly, producing an annular lesion with central clearing, and often associated with systemic symptoms, including chills, fever, headache, malaise, vomiting, backache, and stiff neck. See also *Lyme disease,* under *disease.*
**e. circina′tum, e. circina′tum rheuma′ticum**, e. marginatum rheumaticum.
**cold e.**, a congenital hypersensitivity to cold seen in children, characterized by localized pain, widespread erythema, occasional muscle spasms, and vascular collapse on exposure to cold, and vomiting after drinking cold liquids.
**diaper e.**, see under *dermatitis.*
**e. dyschro′micum per′stans**, an idiopathic dermatosis occurring predominantly in dark-skinned individuals, particularly in Latin Americans, characterized by the presence of single or multiple sharply demarcated ashen macules of variable size and shape, which in their acute phase have a fine erythematous border. Called also *ashy dermatitis, ashy dermatosis of Ramirez, dermatosis cenicienta,* and *e. chromicum figuratum melanodermicum.*
**e. eleva′tum diu′tinum**, a benign cutaneous, small vessel vasculitis of unknown etiology characterized by the development of red, brown, purple, and orange-yellow nodules and plaques, usually on the acral extremities and buttocks, which are sometimes associated with erosions, ulcers, and vesiculopustules. The lesions exhibit polymorphonuclear neutrophils and nuclear fragments infiltrating vessel walls in association with fibrinoid material, and lymphocytes, plasma cells, and eosinophils can be seen in perivascular and stromal locations. Intracellular and extracellular lipid deposits, chiefly cholesterol esters, occur in chronic lesions. See also *extracellular cholesterosis,* under *cholesterosis.*
**epidemic e.**, acrodynia.
**epidemic arthritic e.**, Haverhill fever.
**figurate e., e. figura′tum**, gyrate e.
**e. figura′tum per′stans**, e. annulare centrifugum.
**e. fu′gax**, redness of the skin that comes and goes quickly.
**gyrate e., e. gyra′tum**, erythema multiforme characterized by the development of gyrate, figurate, circinate, annular, arcuate, polycyclic, serpiginous, or reticulate lesions that tend to migrate and spread peripherally with central clearing. There are three basic types: *e. annulare centrifugum, erythema chronicum migrans,* and *e. gyratum repens.* Called also *figurate e.* and *e. figuratum.*
**e. gyra′tum per′stans**, e. annulare centrifugum.
**e. gyra′tum re′pens**, a superficial form of gyrate erythema almost always associated with internal malignancy, which is characterized by the presence of migratory wavy bands of slightly elevated erythema with a scaly collarette over the entire body, and sometimes accompanied by pruritus.
**e. ab ig′ne**, permanent erythema or a brown to red reticulated residual pigmentation produced by prolonged exposure to excessive nonburning heat. It is seen most often on the legs of women, but under appropriate environmental circumstances, it can occur anywhere on the body in either sex.
**e. indura′tum**, a type of panniculitis seen in young and middle-aged women, characterized by granulomas, vasculitis, and caseation necrosis; it was formerly considered the tuberculous counterpart of nodular vasculitis, but has been found to occur without tuberculous causation, although of uncertain etiology. It is initiated or exacerbated by cold weather, usually presenting as recurrent erythrocyanotic nodules or plaques on the calves, which may progress to form deep-seated indurations, ulcerations, and scars. Cases of tuberculous origin are called also *Bazin's disease, tuberculosis cutis indurativa,* and *tuberculosis indurativa.*
**e. infectio′sum**, a moderately contagious, often benign epidemic disease seen mainly in children and caused by B19 virus, characterized by a rash of abrupt onset with three stages: livid erythema of the cheeks, which appear to have been slapped; then an erythematous maculopapular rash on the trunk and extremities; and then fading of the rash with central clearing, leaving a lacelike pattern. More severe cases may be seen in immunocompromised patients. Called also *fifth disease* and *Sticker's disease.*
**e. i′ris**, the characteristic bull's eye or targetlike lesion of erythema multiforme.
**Jacquet's e.**, diaper dermatitis.
**e. margina′tum**, e. marginatum rheumaticum.
**e. margina′tum rheuma′ticum**, a superficial, often asymptomatic, form of gyrate erythema associated with some cases of rheumatic fever, which is characterized by the presence on the trunk and extensor surfaces of the extremities of a transient eruption of flat to slightly indurated, nonscaling, and usually multiple lesions. Called also *e. annulare, e. annulare rheumaticum, e. circinatum, e. circinatum rheumaticum,* and *e. marginatum.*
**e. mi′grans**, 1. geographic tongue. 2. e. chronicum migrans.
**e. multifor′me**, a symptom complex representing a reaction pattern of the skin and mucous membranes secondary to various known, suspected, and unknown factors, including infections, ingestants, physical agents, malignancy, and pregnancy. The conditions in the complex are characterized by the sudden onset of an erythematous macular, bullous, papular, nodose, or vesicular eruption, the characteristic lesion being the iris, bull's eye, or target lesion, which consists of a central papule with two or more concentric rings. The complex comprises a mild self-limited mucocutaneous form *(e. multiforme minus)* and a severe, sometimes fatal, multisystem form *(Stevens-Johnson syndrome).*
**e. multifor′me ma′jus**, Stevens-Johnson syndrome.
**e. multifor′me mi′nus**, a mild self-limited mucocutaneous form of erythema multiforme that may have a prodrome of fever, cough, and pharyngitis. In addition to the characteristic iris lesions, erythematous macules and papules, purpura, and occasional vesicu-

lobullous lesions may be present, which are usually asymptomatic, but may burn or itch slightly. Called also *Hebra's disease.*

**necrolytic migratory e.,** a generalized symmetrical scaling eczematous dermatitis, followed by migratory necrolysis of the upper epidermis, liquefaction of the granular layer, and subcorneal clefting, flaccid bulla formation, erosions, crusts, and postinflammatory hyperpigmentation It is usually seen on the central third of the face, lower abdomen, perineum, groin, buttocks, thighs, and distal extremities in association with a glucagon-secreting tumor of the alpha cells of the pancreas. See also *glucagonoma syndrome,* under *syndrome.*

**e. necro'ticans,** Lucio's phenomenon.

**e. nodo'sum,** a type of panniculitis occurring usually as a hypersensitivity reaction to multiple provoking agents, including various infections, especially beta-hemolytic streptococcal infections and tuberculosis; drugs, especially oral contraceptives and sulfonamides; sarcoidosis; and certain enteropathies. It may also be of idiopathic origin. It most often affects young women and is characterized by the development of crops of transient, inflammatory, nonulcerating nodules that are usually tender, multiple, and bilateral, and most commonly located on the shins; the lesions involute slowly, leaving bruiselike patches without scarring. The acute disease is often associated with mild constitutional symptoms, including fever, malaise, and arthralgias. A chronic variant sometimes occurs without any serious associated systemic disease. See also *e. nodosum migrans.*

**e. nodo'sum lepro'sum,** a recurrent lepra reaction resembling an Arthus reaction, occurring during chemotherapy for lepromatous leprosy, sometimes in the borderline form, and occasionally spontaneously, usually characterized histologically by vasculitis and clinically by the appearance of crops of small erythematous, tender cutaneous nodules or plaques, which are widely distributed, especially on the extremities and face; it may be associated with severe systemic symptoms and visceral manifestations. Cf. *Lucio's phenomenon.*

**e. nodo'sum mi'grans,** a variant of erythema nodosum in which the lesions are asymmetrical, often unilateral, usually less acute and less numerous than those in the classic disorder, and characterized by the coalescence and clearing of older central nodules and formation of new lesions nearby, which gives the appearance of migration. *Subacute nodular migratory panniculitis* may be the same variant.

**palmar e., e palma're,** persistent redness of the palms, which may be seen in pregnancy, liver disease, rheumatoid arthritis, regional ileitis, and certain skin diseases, e.g., psoriasis, pityriasis rubra pilaris, and genodermatoses, and rarely as an autosomal dominant condition.

**e. per'nio,** chilblain.

**e. strepto'genes,** pityriasis alba.

**toxic e., e. tox'icum,** a generalized, diffuse erythematous eruption or a widespread erythematomacular eruption occurring as a result of hypersensitivity to certain foods or drugs, or caused by bacterial or other toxins, or associated with various systemic diseases.

**e. tox'icum neonato'rum,** a benign, idiopathic, very common, generalized, transient eruption occurring in infants during the first week of life, usually consisting of small papules or pustules that become sterile, yellow-white, firm vesicles surrounded by an erythematous halo and some edema.

**er·y·them·a·to·edem·a·tous** (er″ĭ-thēm″ə-to″ĕ-dem'ətəs) pertaining to or affected by both erythema and edema.

**er·y·them·a·tous** (er″ə-them'ə-təs) characterized by erythema.

**er·y·the·mo·gen·ic** (er″ĭ-the″mo-jen'ik) causing erythema.

**er·y·thral·gia** (er″ə-thral'jə) [*erythro-* + *-algia*] erythromelalgia.

**er·y·thras·ma** (er″ə-thraz'mə) [MeSH: Erythrasma] a chronic, superficial bacterial infection of the skin involving the body folds and toe webs, sometimes becoming generalized, caused by *Corynebacterium minutissimum,* and characterized by the presence of sharply demarcated, dry, brown, slightly scaly, and slowly spreading patches.

**er·y·thre·mia** (er″ə-thre'me-ə) [*erythro-* + *-emia*] polycythemia vera.

**eryth·re·mo·mel·al·gia** (er-ith″rə-mo-məl-al'jə) [*erythrema* + *melalgia*] erythromelalgia.

**Er·y·thri·na** (er″ə-thri'nə) [MeSH: Erythrina] a genus of tropical shrubs and trees of the family Leguminosae, long used in folk medicine; several species yield the alkaloids $\alpha$-erythroidine and $\beta$-erythroidine.

**eryth·rism** (ə-rith'riz-əm) redness of the hair and beard with a ruddy complexion.

**er·y·thris·tic** (er″ə-thris'tik) characterized by erythrism. Called also *rufous.*

**eryth·ri·tol** (ə-rith'rĭ-tol) [MeSH: Erythritol] a four-carbon sugar formed from erythrose by reduction of the carbonyl group and occurring in algae, lichens, grasses, and several fungi; it is about twice as sweet as sucrose. Called also *erythrol.* See also *erythrityl.*

**eryth·ri·tyl** (ə-rith'rĭ-təl) the univalent radical $C_4H_9$ from erythritol.

**e. tetranitrate,** a synthetic compound, with actions similar to those of nitroglycerin, used in diluted form as a coronary vasodilator in the prophylaxis of angina pectoris and in long-term treatment of coronary insufficiency, administered orally or sublingually. Percussion or excessive heat can cause undiluted erythrityl tetranitrate to explode.

**erythr(o)-** [Gr. *erythros* red] a combining form denoting a relationship to red or to erythrocytes.

**eryth·ro·blas·te·mia** (ə-rith″ro-blas-te'me-ə) erythroblastosis (def. 1).

**eryth·ro·blas·tic** (ə-rith″ro-blas'tik) of, or relating to, erythroblasts.

**eryth·ro·blas·to·ma** (ə-rith″ro-blas-to'mə) a tumorlike mass composed of erythroblasts.

**eryth·ro·blas·to·pe·nia** (ə-rith″ro-blas″to-pe'ne-ə) abnormal deficiency of the erythroblasts, such as in an aplastic crisis.

**transient e. of childhood,** temporary aplasia of erythropoietic tissue in young children, usually with anemia; the etiology is unknown, although there has often been a viral illness within the previous two months. The condition almost always resolves spontaneously without recurring.

**eryth·ro·blas·to·sis** (ə-rith″ro-blas-to'sis) 1. the presence in the peripheral blood of abnormally large numbers of erythroblasts (nucleated red cells); called also *erythroblastemia.* 2. one of the avian leukosis complex of diseases, a condition of fowl marked by increased erythroblasts in the circulating blood, with weakness, pallor, diarrhea, and spontaneous hemorrhages. Called also *erythroid leukosis* and *erythroleukosis.*

**e. feta'lis, e. neonato'rum,** a type of hemolytic anemia of the fetus or newborn infant, caused by the transplacental transmission of maternally formed antibody, usually secondary to an incompatibility between the blood group of the mother and that of her offspring. The most common and frequently fatal type occurs when the baby or fetus is Rh positive and the mother is Rh negative. Another type is found in babies or fetuses of blood groups A and B whose mothers have type O blood; it is much milder than the Rh type because anti-A and anti-B antibodies only occasionally cross the placenta. Characteristics include accelerated destruction of erythrocytes, causing jaundice, increased red cell regeneration (nucleated red cells in the blood), and hepatosplenomegaly. In infants with severe jaundice, kernicterus may result. The most severe form is *hydrops fetalis.* Called also *congenital* or *hemolytic anemia of newborn* and *hemolytic disease of the newborn.*

**eryth·ro·blas·tot·ic** (ə-rith″ro-blas-tot'ik) pertaining to or characterized by erythroblastosis.

**eryth·ro·ca·tal·y·sis** (ə-rith″ro-kə-tal'ə-sis) hemolysis.

**eryth·ro·chro·mia** (ə-rith″ro-kro'me-ə) [*erythro-* + *chrom-* + *-ia*] hemorrhagic pigmentation of the spinal fluid, giving it a red color.

**Eryth·ro·cin** (ə-rith'ro-sin) trademark for a preparation of erythromycin.

**er·y·throc·la·sis** (er″ə-throk'lə-sis) [*erythro-* + Gr. *klasis* a breaking] fragmentation or splitting up of erythrocytes. Cf. *hemolysis.*

**eryth·ro·clast** (ə-rith'ro-klast) [*erythro-* + *-klast*] ghost cell.

**eryth·ro·clas·tic** (ə-rith″ro-klas'tik) pertaining to, characterized by, or producing erythroclasis.

**eryth·ro·cru·o·rin** (ə-rith″ro-kroo'ə-rin) a respiratory protein from the blood of the marine worm, *Spirographis spallanzanii,* and certain other worms.

**eryth·ro·cu·prein** (ə-rith″ro-koo'prēn) superoxide dismutase.

**eryth·ro·cy·a·no·sis** (ə-rith″ro-si″ə-no'sis) [*erythro-* + *cyanosis*] a condition seen in young girls and women following prolonged exposure to cold, characterized by the presence of a slight swelling and a bluish pink tint of the skin of the legs and thighs.

**eryth·ro·cy·ta·phe·re·sis** (ə-rith″ro-si″tə-fə-re'sis) [*erythrocyte* + *apheresis*] the withdrawal of blood, separation and retention of red blood cells, and retransfusion of the remainder into the donor.

**eryth·ro·cyte** (ə-rith'ro-sīt) [*erythro-* + *-cyte*] [MeSH: Erythrocytes] one of the elements found in peripheral blood. In humans the normal mature form is a non-nucleated, yellowish, biconcave disk, adapted by virtue of its configuration and its hemoglobin content to the transport of oxygen. For immature forms, see *erythrocytic series,* under *series.* Called also *red blood cell* or *corpuscle* and *red cell* or *corpuscle.*

**achromic e.,** achromocyte.

**basophilic e.,** an abnormal erythrocyte that takes on basic stains; see *basophilia* (def. 1).

**burr e., crenated e.,** burr cell.

**hypochromic e.,** one with less than the normal concentration of hemoglobin, thus appearing paler than normal; it is usually also microcytic. Cf. *normochromic e.*
**immature e.,** 1. normoblast. 2. erythroblast.
**Mexican hat e.,** target cell.
**normochromic e.,** one of normal color with a normal concentration of hemoglobin, as opposed to a hypochromic erythrocyte. See also *orthochromatic erythroblast.*
**nucleated e.,** 1. normoblast. 2. erythroblast.
**polychromatic e., polychromatophilic e.,** an erythrocyte that, on staining, shows various shades of blue, combined with tinges of pink.
**target e.,** see under *cell.*

**eryth·ro·cy·the·mia** (ə-rith″ro-si-the′me-ə) polycythemia.

**eryth·ro·cyt·ic** (ə-rith″ro-sit′ik) 1. pertaining to, characterized by, or of the nature of erythrocytes. 2. pertaining to the erythrocytic series; see under *series.*

**eryth·ro·cy·to·blast** (ə-rith″ro-si′to-blast) erythroblast.

**eryth·ro·cy·tol·y·sin** (ə-rith″ro-si-tol′ə-sin) hemolysin.

**eryth·ro·cy·tol·y·sis** (ə-rith″ro-si-tol′ə-sis) [*erythrocyte* + *-lysis*] hemolysis.

**eryth·ro·cy·tom·e·ter** (ə-rith″ro-si-tom′ə-tər) [*erythrocyte* + *-meter*] a device for measuring or counting erythrocytes.

**eryth·ro·cy·tom·e·try** (ə-rith″ro-si-tom′ə-try) the measurement or counting of erythrocytes.

**eryth·ro·cy·to·op·so·nin** (ə-rith″ro-si″to-op-so′nin) [*erythrocyte* + *opsonin*] hemopsonin.

**eryth·ro·cy·to·pe·nia** (ə-rith″ro-si″to-pe′ne-ə) erythropenia.

**eryth·ro·cy·toph·a·gous** (ə-rith″ro-si-tof′ə-gəs) erythrophagocytic.

**eryth·ro·cy·toph·a·gy** (ə-rith″ro-si-tof′ə-je) [*erythrocyte* + *-phagy*] erythrophagocytosis.

**eryth·ro·cy·to·poi·e·sis** (ə-rith″ro-si″to-poi-e′sis) erythropoiesis.

**eryth·ro·cy·tor·rhex·is** (ə-rith″ro-si″to-rek′sis) [*erythrocyte* + *-rrhexis*] partial erythrocytoschisis with splitting off of particles and escape from the cells of round, shiny granules. Called also *erythrorrhexis.*

**eryth·ro·cy·tos·chi·sis** (ə-rith″ro-si-tos′kĭ-sis) [*erythrocyte* + *-schisis*] a morphological change in erythrocytes consisting of their degeneration into disklike bodies similar to platelets. See also *schistocytosis.*

**eryth·ro·cy·to·sis** (ə-rith″ro-si-to′sis) secondary polycythemia.
**benign e., stress e.,** stress polycythemia.

**eryth·ro·cy·tu·ria** (ə-rith″ro-si-tu′re-ə) hematuria.

**eryth·ro·de·gen·er·a·tive** (ə-rith″ro-de-jen′ər-a″tiv) characterized by degeneration of erythrocytes; see also *hemolysis.*

**eryth·ro·der·ma** (ə-rith″ro-dər′mə) [*erythro-* + *derma*] 1. abnormal redness of the skin, usually applied to a condition of abnormal redness over widespread areas of the body. 2. exfoliative dermatitis. Called also *erythrodermia.*
**congenital ichthyosiform e., bullous,** epidermolytic hyperkeratosis.
**congenital ichthyosiform e., nonbullous,** former name for *lamellar ichthyosis.*
**e. desquamati′vum,** Leiner's disease.
**e. psoria′ticum,** erythrodermic psoriasis.
**Sézary e.,** see under *syndrome.*

**eryth·ro·der·mia** (ə-rith″ro-dər′me-ə) erythroderma.

**eryth·ro·dex·trin** (ə-rith″ro-deks′trin) any of the class of water-soluble dextrins staining red with iodine and formed by partial hydrolysis of starch.

**eryth·ro·don·tia** (ə-rith″ro-don′shə) [*erythro-* + *odont-* + *-ia*] reddish brown pigmentation of the teeth.

**eryth·ro·gen** (ə-rith′ro-jən) a fatty, crystalline compound from diseased bile.

**eryth·ro·gen·e·sis** (ə-rith″ro-jen′ə-sis) erythropoiesis.
**e. imperfec′ta,** congenital hypoplastic anemia (def. 1).

**eryth·ro·gen·ic** (ə-rith″ro-jen′ik) [*erythro-* + *-genic*] 1. erythropoietic. 2. producing a sensation of red. 3. erythemogenic.

**er·y·throid** (er″ĭ-throid) 1. of a red color; reddish. 2. pertaining to any of the cells in the developmental series ending in erythrocytes; see *erythrocytic series, under series.*

**β-eryth·roi·dine** (ə-rith′roi-din) an alkaloid, from *Erythrina americana;* it has a curare-like action.

**eryth·ro·ka·tal·y·sis** (ə-rith″ro-kə-tal′ə-sis) hemolysis.

**eryth·ro·ker·a·to·der·mia** (ə-rith″ro-ker″ə-to-dər′me-ə) a reddening and hyperkeratosis of the skin.
**e. varia′bilis,** a very rare autosomal dominant form of ichthyosis characterized by the presence at birth of two types of lesions: transient, migratory areas of discrete macular erythroderma with angular, arcuate, gyrate, and circinate configurations as well as fixed hyperkeratotic plaques.

**eryth·ro·ki·net·ics** (ə-rith″ro-kĭ-net′iks) [*erythro-* + *kinetics*] the kinetics of erythrocytes, described by laboratory measurements of total red cell volume, rate of red cell production, and red cell life-span (rate of destruction).

**er·yth·rol** (er′ith-rol) erythritol.
**e. tetranitrate,** erythrityl tetranitrate.

**eryth·ro·labe** (ə-rith′ro-lāb) [*erythro-* + Gr. *lambanein* to take] name proposed for the pigment in retinal cones that is more sensitive to the red range of the spectrum than are the other pigments (chlorolabe and cyanolabe).

**er·y·thro·lein** (er″ə-thro′lēn) the ether-soluble fraction of the acid-precipitable part of the water-soluble pigments of litmus, occurring as a red oily substance.

**eryth·ro·leu·ke·mia** (ə-rith″ro-loo-ke′me-ə) a malignant blood dyscrasia, one of the myeloproliferative disorders, characterized by neoplastic proliferation of erythroblastic and myeloblastic elements, with atypical erythroblasts and myeloblasts in the peripheral blood. Symptoms are progressive anemia, myeloblastic erythroid hyperplasia, myeloid dysplasia, hepatosplenomegaly, and hemorrhagic phenomena. It may follow an acute or chronic course. Called also *Di Guglielmo's syndrome* and *erythremic myelosis.*
**acute e.,** a form of acute myelogenous leukemia representing erythroleukemia in which malignant leukoblasts have proliferated and become predominant; called also *di Guglielmo's syndrome.*

**eryth·ro·leu·ko·blas·to·sis** (ə-rith″ro-loo″ko-blas-to′sis) icterus gravis neonatorum.

**eryth·ro·leu·ko·sis** (ə-rith″ro-loo-ko′sis) erythroblastosis (def. 2).

**eryth·ro·lit·min** (e-rith″ro-lit′min) the alcohol-soluble fraction of the acid-precipitable part of the water-soluble pigments of litmus, occurring as a bright red powder.

**er·y·throl·y·sin** (er″ə-throl′ə-sin) hemolysin.

**er·y·throl·y·sis** (er″ə-throl′ə-sis) hemolysis.

**eryth·ro·mel·al·gia** (ə-rith″ro-məl-al′jə) [*erythro-* + *melalgia*] [MeSH: Erythromelalgia] a disease affecting the feet and sometimes the hands, marked by paroxysmal, bilateral vasodilation with burning pain, increased skin temperature, and redness. Called also *acromelalgia, red neuralgia,* and *Gerhardt's, Mitchell's,* or *Weir Mitchell's disease.*
**e. of the head,** cluster headache.

**er·y·throm·e·ter** (er″ə-throm′ə-tər) [*erythro-* + *-meter*] 1. an instrument or color scale for measuring degrees of redness. 2. erythrocytometer.

**er·y·throm·e·try** (er″ə-throm′ə-tre) 1. the measurement of the degree of redness. 2. erythrocytometry.

**eryth·ro·my·cin** (ə-rith″ro-mi′sin) [USP] [MeSH: Erythromycin] an intermediate spectrum macrolide antibiotic, produced by *Streptomyces erythreus,* effective against most gram-positive and certain gram-negative bacteria, such as *Neisseria* species and *Haemophilus influenzae,* and against spirochetes, some rickettsias, and *Entamoeba;* it is also highly effective against *Mycoplasma pneumoniae.* It is used especially in patients allergic to penicillin and in those with penicillin-resistant infections and legionnaires' disease; administered orally or topically.
**e. B,** berythromycin.
**e. estolate** [USP], the lauryl sulfate ester of propionyl erythromycin, having the same actions and uses as the base; administered orally.
**e. ethylcarbonate,** a salt of erythromycin, used for oral administration.
**e. ethylsuccinate** [USP], a salt of erythromycin, occurring as a white or slightly yellow crystalline powder, having the same actions and uses as the base; administered orally or intramuscularly.
**e. gluceptate,** a salt of erythromycin, having the same actions and uses as the base; administered by intravenous infusion.
**e. lactobionate** [USP], a salt of erythromycin, having the same actions and uses as the base; administered by intravenous infusion.
**e. propionate,** a salt of erythromycin, suitable for oral use.
**e. propionate lauryl sulfate,** former name for *e. estolate.*
**e. stearate** [USP], a salt of erythromycin, suitable for oral use.

**eryth·ro·my·e·lo·blas·to·sis** (ə-rith″ro-mi″ə-lo-blas-to′sis) myeloblastosis (def. 2).

**er·y·thron** (er′ə-thron) [Gr. *erythros* red] the circulating erythrocytes in the blood, their precursors, and all the elements of the body concerned in their production. Cf. *leukon* and *thrombon.*

**eryth·ro·neo·cy·to·sis** (ə-rith″ro-ne″o-si-to′sis) [*erythro-* + *neo-* + *-cyte* + *-osis*] the presence of immature erythrocytes in the blood. Cf. *erythroblastosis.*

Cf. *erythroblastosis.*

**eryth·ro·par·a·site** (ə-rith″ro-par′ə-sīt) a parasite of erythrocytes.

**eryth·ro·pe·nia** (ə-rith″ro-pe′ne-ə) [*erythro-* + *-penia*] deficiency in the number of erythrocytes; see also *anemia* and *pancytopenia.* Called also *erythrocytopenia.*

**eryth·ro·phage** (ə-rith′ro-fāj) [*erythro-* + *-phage*] a phagocyte that takes up erythrocytes and blood pigments.

**eryth·ro·pha·gia** (ə-rith″ro-fa′jə) erythrophagocytosis.

**eryth·ro·phago·cyt·ic** (ə-rith″ro-fag″o-sit′ik) characterized by erythrophagocytosis; called also *erythrocytophagous.*

**eryth·ro·phago·cy·to·sis** (ə-rith″ro-fag″o-si-to′sis) [*erythro*cyte + *phagocytosis*] the engulfment or consumption of erythrocytes by macrophages. Called also *erythrocytophagy* and *erythrophagia.*

**er·y·throph·a·gous** (er″ĭ-throf′ə-gəs) erythrophagocytic.

**eryth·ro·phil** (ə-rith′ro-fil) [*erythro-* + *-phil*] 1. a cell or other element that is easily stained red. 2. erythrophilous.

**er·y·throph·i·lous** (er″ĭ-throf′ĭ-ləs) easily stained with red.

**Eryth·ro·phloe·um** (ə-rith″ro-fle′əm) [*erythro-* + Gr. *phloios* bark] a genus of trees of the family Leguminosae. *E. guineen′se* affords casca or Mancona bark, an African ordeal poison.

**eryth·ro·pho·bia** (ə-rith″ro-fo′be-ə) [*erythro-* + *-phobia*] 1. irrational fear of the color red, often accompanied by fear of blood (hematophobia). 2. fear of blushing; a distressing tendency to blush frequently.

**eryth·ro·pho·bic** (ə-rith″ro-fo′bik) having no affinity for red dye (acid fuchsin).

**eryth·ro·phore** (ə-rith′ro-for) [*erythro-* + *-phore*] a chromatophore containing granules of a red or brown alcohol-resistant pigment; called also *allophore.*

**eryth·ro·phose** (ə-rith′ro-fōz) [*erythro-* + *phose*] any red phose.

**eryth·ro·phyll** (ə-rith′ro-fəl) [*erythro-* + Gr. *phyllon* leaf] a red coloring matter occurring in plants.

**er·y·thro·pia** (er″ə-thro′pe-ə) erythropsia.

**eryth·ro·pla·kia** (ə-rith″ro-pla′ke-ə) [*erythro-* + Gr. *plax* plate + *-ia*] a slow growing, erythematous, velvety red lesion with well-defined margins, occurring on a mucous membrane, most often in the oral cavity. It is usually associated with severe dysplasia or carcinoma, and occurs in middle-aged to older adults. See also *erythroplasia of Queyrat.*
**speckled e.,** a lesion in the oral cavity with characteristics of both erythroplakia and leukoplakia, yielding a speckled appearance. Called also *speckled leukoplakia.*

**eryth·ro·pla·sia** (ə-rith″ro-pla′zhə) [MeSH: Erythroplasia] a condition of the mucous membrane characterized by erythematous papular lesions.
**e. of Queyrat,** a form of epithelial dysplasia, which may range in severity from mild disorientation of epithelial cells with variable cellular pleomorphism to changes of carcinoma in situ and even invasive carcinoma, usually found on the uncircumcised glans penis and prepuce, and occasionally on the vulva. It is typically characterized by the development of a slowly growing, circumscribed, erythematous, usually moist, velvety, and shiny patch. The term is sometimes used to denote the corresponding lesion of the oral mucosa, erythroplakia (q.v.).
**Zoon's e.,** balanitis circumscripta plasmacellularis.

**eryth·ro·plas·tid** (ə-rith″ro-plas′tid) an erythrocyte that has no nucleus, such as the type normal in mammals.

**eryth·ro·poi·e·sis** (ə-rith″ro-poi-e′sis) [*erythro-* + *-poiesis*] [MeSH: Erythropoiesis] the production of erythrocytes; in the fetus and neonate it takes place in the spleen and bone marrow, but in older individuals it is confined to the bone marrow. Called also *erythrocytopoiesis* and *erythrogenesis.*

**eryth·ro·poi·et·ic** (ə-rith″ro-poi-et′ik) pertaining to, characterized by, or promoting erythropoiesis. Called also *erythrogenic.*

**eryth·ro·poi·e·tin** (ə-rith″ro-poi′ə-tin) [MeSH: Erythropoietin] a glycoprotein hormone secreted chiefly by the kidney in the adult and by the liver in the fetus, which acts on the bone marrow cells to stimulate erythropoiesis. Called also *hematopoietin* and *hemopoietin.*
**recombinant human e. (r-HuEPO),** epoetin.

**eryth·ro·pros·o·pal·gia** (ə-rith″ro-pros″o-pal′jə) [*erythro-* + *prosopalgia*] a disorder similar to erythromelalgia, but with the redness and pain in the face.

**er·y·throp·sia** (er″ə-throp′se-ə) [*erythro-* + *-opsia* ] a chromatopsia in which all objects appear to have a red tinge, a symptom of aphakia.

**er·y·throp·sin** (er″ə-throp′sin) [*erythro-* + *opsin*] rhodopsin.

**eryth·ro·pyk·no·sis** (ə-rith″ro-pik-no′sis) [*erythro-* + *pyknosis*] pyknosis of red cells.

**eryth·ror·rhex·is** (ə-rith″ro-rek′sis) [*erythro-* + *-rrhexis*] erythrocytorrhexis.

**er·y·throse** (ĕ-rith′rōs) an aldotetrose occurring in phosphorylated form (erythrose 4-phosphate) as an intermediate in the pentose phosphate pathway.

**éry·throse** (a-rī-thrōz′) [Fr.] erythrosis.
**é. péribuccale pigmentaire of Brocq** (pa-re-bu-kahl′ pēg-man-tār′), a patchy facial melanoderma seen chiefly in women that may involve an inflammatory photosensitivity, perhaps phototoxic, reaction, and characterized by the presence of a combination of erythema and a diffuse brownish red pigmentation of the perioral region.

**eryth·ro·sin** (ə-rith′ro-sin) a red compound, used as a histologic stain.

**eryth·ro·sine so·di·um** (ə-rith′ro-sēn) a coloring agent used to disclose plaque on teeth; applied topically in solution, or tablets containing erythrosine sodium are chewed, after which the mouth is rinsed with water.

**er·y·thro·sis** (er″ə-thro′sis) a reddish or purplish discoloration of the skin and mucous membranes seen in polycythemia vera.

**eryth·ro·sta·sis** (ə-rith″ro-sta′sis) the stoppage of erythrocytes in the capillaries, as in sickle cell anemia.

**eryth·ro·thi·o·neine** (ə-rith″ro-thi′ə-nēn) ergothioneine.

**Eryth·ro·vi·rus** (ərith′ro-vi″rəs) [*erythro-* + *virus*] a genus of viruses of the subfamily Parvovirinae (family Parvoviridae) containing viruses that infect erythrocyte progenitor cells; there is a single species, B19 virus.

**Ery·throx·y·lon** (er-ĭ-throk′sə-lon) a genus of South American trees and shrubs. *E. co′ca* is a shrub native to Andean regions whose leaves are a source of coca.

**eryth·ru·lose** (ə-rith′roo-lōs) the sole ketotetrose, an isomer of erythrose.

**er·y·thru·ria** (er″ith-u′re-ə) [*erythr-* + *-uria*] the passing of red urine.

**Es** symbol for *einsteinium.*

**es·cape** (əs-kāp′) the act of becoming free.
**aldosterone e.,** a secondary response to the continuous presence of mineralocorticoids, in which the usual renal sodium-retaining effects of mineralocorticoids are time-limited, so that excessive retention of salt and water is limited.
**atrioventricular junctional e.,** the occurrence of one or more escape beats in which the atrioventricular node acts as the cardiac pacemaker; see also under *beat* and *rhythm.*
**nodal e.,** atrioventricular junctional e.
**vagal e.,** the exhaustion of or adaptation to neural chemical mediators in the regulation of systemic arterial pressure.
**ventricular e.,** the occurrence of one or more ectopic beats in which a ventricular pacemaker becomes effective before the sinoatrial pacemaker; it usually occurs with slow sinus rates and often, but not necessarily, with increased vagal tone. See also under *beat* and *rhythm.*

**es·char** (es′kahr) [Gr. *eschara* scab] 1. a slough produced by a thermal burn, by a corrosive application, or by gangrene. 2. the lesion seen in certain rickettsioses; see *tache noire.*

**es·cha·rot·ic** (es″kə-rot′ik′) [Gr. *escharōtikos*] 1. corrosive; capable of producing an eschar. 2. a corrosive or caustic agent.

**es·cha·rot·o·my** (es″kə-rot′ə-me) surgical incision of the constricting eschar of a circumferentially burned limb in order to permit the cut edges to separate and restore blood flow to unburned tissue distal to the eschar.

**Esch·er·ich's bacillus, sign (reflex)** (esh′ər-iks) [Theodor *Escherich,* German physician, 1857–1911] see *Escherichia coli,* and see under *sign.*

**Esch·e·rich·i·eae** (esh″ə-rik′e-e) in some systems of classification, a tribe of gram-negative, facultatively anaerobic, rod-shaped bacteria of the family Enterobacteriaceae, made up of the genera *Escherichia* and *Shigella.*

**Esch·e·rich·ia** (esh″ər-ik′e-ə) [T. *Escherich*] [MeSH: Escherichia] a genus of gram-negative, facultatively anaerobic, rod-shaped bacteria of the tribe Escherichieae, family Enterobacteriaceae, found in the large intestine of warm-blooded animals. The organisms are nonpathogenic or opportunistic pathogens. They are members of the "coliform" group of bacteria, their presence in water supplies being used as an indicator of fecal contamination.
**E. aures′cens,** a variant of *E. coli,* characterized by the production of yellow-orange carotenoid pigments.
**E. blat′tae,** a species isolated from cockroaches.
**E. co′li,** the principal species of the genus and the predominant facultative organism of the intestine of humans and other animals. The organisms are characteristically positive to indole and methyl

red and negative to the Voges-Proskauer and citrate tests; serotypes are based on the distribution of heat-stable O antigens, envelope K antigens of varying heat stability, and flagellar H antigens that are heat labile. They are usually nonpathogenic, but pathogenic strains producing pyogenic infections and diarrhea are common (see *colibacillosis*. The pyogenic strains are found in infections in the urinary tract, abscesses, conjunctivitis, and occasionally septicemia, such as the hemorrhagic septicemia in newborn infants known as *Winckel's disease*. The enteropathogenic strains (EPEC) produce intestinal disease and diarrhea, especially in hospitalized infants and other baby animals. The enterotoxicogenic species (ETEC) cause diarrhea in piglets and calves and a cholera-like disease in human infants and adults. Enteroinvasive serogroups (EIEC) related to *Shigella* invade the epithelial cells of the human colon, causing dysentery, sometimes associated with food poisoning. They often become the predominant bacteria in the flora of the mouth and throat during antibiotic therapy. Enterohemorrhagic groups (EHEC) cause acute bloody diarrhea. A preparation of asparaginase derived from type EC-2 is used as an antineoplastic. See Plate 8. Called also *Bacterium coli, B. coli commune, colibacillus, colon bacillus, and Escherich's bacillus.*
**E. ferguso'nii,** a species (enteric group 10) found in human clinical specimens.
**E. freun'dii,** *Citrobacter freundii.*
**E. herma'nii,** a species that produces a yellow pigment, found in human clinical specimens.
**E. interme'dia,** *Citrobacter intermedius.*
**E. vul'neris,** a species found in human clinical specimens.

**Esch•scholt•zia** (ə-shōlt'se-ə) a genus of plants of the family Papaveraceae. *E. califor'nica* Cham. is the California poppy, which is hypnotic and anodyne.

**es•cin** (es'kin) [MeSH: Escin] a strongly hemolytic saponin derived from the horse chestnut.

**Es•co•bar syndrome** (es-ko-bahr') [Victor *Escobar,* American dentist, 20th century] see under *syndrome.*

**es•cor•cin** (es-kor'sin) a brown powder, prepared from a substance extracted from the horse chestnut; used in detecting corneal and conjunctival lesions.

**es•cu•la•pi•an** (es″ku-la'pe-ən) aesculapian.

**es•cu•lent** (es'ku-lənt) edible.

**es•cu•lin** (es'ku-lin) [L. *aesculus* horse-chestnut] [MeSH: Esculin] a coumarin glycoside found in species of *Aesculus;* it has febrifuge properties but causes toxicity in livestock.

**es•cutch•eon** (es-kuch'ən) [L. *scutum* a shield] 1. a shield or something shaped like a shield. 2. the shieldlike pattern of distribution of the pubic hair.

**esep•tate** (e-sep'tāt) having no septa.

**es•er•ine** (es'ər-in) [*esere,* an African name of the Calabar bean] physostigmine.

**ESF** erythropoietic stimulating factor.

**Es•i•drix** (es'ĭ-driks) trademark for a preparation of hydrochlorothiazide.

**Es•i•mil** (es'ĭ-mil) trademark for preparations of guanethidine monosulfate with hydrochlorothiazide.

**-esis** [Gr.] a word termination denoting action, process, or condition; see also *-sis.*

**Es•ka•barb** (es'kə-bahrb) trademark for a preparation of phenobarbital.

**Es•ka•di•a•zine** (es″kə-di'ə-zēn) trademark for a preparation of sulfadiazine.

**Es•ka•lith** (es'kə-lith) trademark for a preparation of lithium carbonate.

**Es•march's bandage (tourniquet), tube** (es'mahrks) [Johann Friedrich August von *Esmarch,* German surgeon, 1823–1908] see under *bandage,* and *tourniquet.*

**es•march** (es'mahrk) an Esmarch bandage.

**ESMO** European Society for Medical Oncology.

**es•mo•lol hyd•ro•chlo•ride** (es'mo-lol) a short-acting, cardioselective $beta_1$-blocker used as an antiarrhythmic in the short-term control of atrial fibrillation, atrial flutter, and noncompensatory sinus tachycardia; administered by intravenous infusion.

**eso-** [Gr. *esō* inward] a combining form meaning within.

**eso•cata•pho•ria** (es″o-kat″ə-for'e-ə) [*eso-* + *cataphoria*] a phoria in which the visual axes turn downward and inward.

**eso•cine** (es'o-sēn) a protamine from the sperm of the pike, *Esox lucius.*

**eso•de•vi•a•tion** (es″o-de″ve-a'shən) 1. esophoria. 2. esotropia.

**eso•eth•moi•di•tis** (es″o-eth″moi-di'tis) [*eso-* + *ethmoiditis*] ethmoid sinusitis; see *sinusitis.*

**eso•gas•tri•tis** (es″o-gas-tri'tis) [*eso-* + *gastritis*] inflammation of the mucous membrane of the stomach.

**esoph•a•gal•gia** (ə-sof″ə-gal'ge-ə) [*esophagus* + *-algia*] pain in the esophagus.

**esoph•a•ge•al** (ə-sof″ə-je'əl) pertaining to or belonging to the esophagus.

**esoph•a•gec•ta•sia** (ə-sof-ə-jek-ta'shə) [*esophagus* + *ectasia*] dilatation of the esophagus.

**esoph•a•gec•ta•sis** (ə-sof″ə-jek'tə-sis) esophagectasia.

**esoph•a•gec•to•my** (ə-sof″ə-jek'tə-me) [*esophagus* + *-ectomy*] [MeSH: Esophagectomy] excision of part *(partial)* or all *(total)* of the esophagus.
**transhiatal e.,** removal of the thoracic part of the esophagus by blunt dissection superiorly through a cervical incision and inferiorly with a transhiatal approach through an abdominal incision.

**esoph•a•gism** (ə-sof'ə-jiz-əm) diffuse esophageal spasm.

**esoph•a•gis•mus** (ə-sof″ə-jiz'məs) diffuse esophageal spasm.

**esoph•a•gi•tis** (ə-sof″ə-ji'tis) [*esophagus* + *-itis*] [MeSH: Esophagitis] inflammation of the esophagus.
***Candida* e.,** fungal esophagitis caused by *Candida* species.
**chronic peptic e.,** reflux e.
**e. dis'secans superficia'lis,** infection of the esophagus, with sloughing of the squamous epithelial lining in the form of a tubular cast.
**fungal e.,** esophagitis caused by invasion of the epithelium by a fungus, usually a species of *Candida;* the incidence is increased among those with diabetes mellitus, hypoparathyroidism, adrenal insufficiency, and immunosuppression.
**pill e.,** esophagitis resulting from irritation by pills that pass more slowly than expected through the esophagus.
**reflux e.,** a serious and sometimes life-threatening type of gastroesophageal reflux disease that involves damage to the esophageal mucosa, often with erosion, ulceration, and infiltration by neutrophils or eosinophils. Stricture, scarring, and occasional perforation may occur in serious cases. Called also *chronic peptic e.*
**viral e.,** esophagitis in which the infecting agent is a virus, usually herpes simplex virus, cytomegalovirus, or varicella zoster virus; the incidence is sharply increased among immunocompromised patients.

**esoph•a•go•bron•chi•al** (ə-sof″ə-go-brong'ke-əl) bronchoesophageal.

**esoph•a•go•car•dio•my•ot•o•my** (ə-sof″ə-go-kahr″de-o-mi-ot'ə-me) incision of the muscular coats of the esophagus and cardiac part of the stomach performed for relief of achalasia of the esophagus. The original procedure involved a myotomy on both anterior and posterior walls of the esophagus; in the currently used modification, only an extramucosal anterior myotomy is done. Called also *cardiomyotomy* and *Heller's cardiomyotomy, esophagomyotomy, myotomy,* or *operation.*

**esoph•a•go•cele** (ə-sof'ə-go-sēl″) [*esophagus* + *-cele*[1]] abnormal distention of the esophagus; hernia of the esophagus: protrusion of the mucous and submucous coats of the esophagus through a rupture in the muscular coat, producing a pouch or diverticulum.

**esoph•a•go•co•lo•gas•tros•to•my** (ə-sof″ə-go-ko″lo-gas-tros'tə-me) surgical creation of a new connection between the esophagus and stomach, by interposition of a segment of colon.

**esoph•a•go•co•lo•plas•ty** (ə-sof″ə-go-ko'lo-plas″te) excision of a portion of the esophagus and its replacement by a segment of the colon.

**esoph•a•go•du•o•de•nos•to•my** (ə-sof″ə-go-doo″o-de-nos'tə-me) surgical anastomosis between the esophagus and the duodenum.

**esoph•a•go•dyn•ia** (ə-sof″ə-go-din'e-ə) [*esophagus* + *-odynia*] pain in the esophagus.

**esoph•a•go•en•ter•os•to•my** (ə-sof″ə-go-en″tər-os'tə-me) [*esophagus* + *enterostomy*] surgical formation of an anastomosis between the esophagus and small intestine after total gastrectomy.

**esoph•a•go•esoph•a•gos•to•my** (ə-sof″ə-go-ə-sof″ə-gos'tə-me) anastomosis between two parts of the esophagus.

**esoph•a•go•fun•do•pexy** (ə-sof″ə-go-fun″do-pek'se) surgical fixation of the fundus of the stomach to the esophagus.

**esoph•a•go•gas•trec•to•my** (ə-sof″ə-go-gas-trek'tə-me) excision of the esophagus and stomach, usually the distal portion of the esophagus and the proximal stomach.

**esoph•a•go•gas•tric** (ə-sof″ə-go-gas'trik) pertaining to the esophagus and the stomach.

**esoph•a•go•gas•tro•anas•to•mo•sis** (ə-sof-ə-go-gas″tro-ə-nas″to-mo'sis) surgical formation of an anastomosis between the esophagus and the stomach.

**esoph·a·go·gas·tro·du·o·de·nal** (ə-sof″ə-go-gas″tro-doo″o-de′nəl) pertaining to the esophagus, stomach, and duodenum.

**esoph·a·go·gas·tro·du·od·enos·co·py** (ə-sof″ə-go-gas″tro-doo″od-ə-nos′kə-pe) EGD; endoscopic examination of the esophagus, stomach, and duodenum.

**esoph·a·go·gas·tro·my·ot·o·my** (ə-sof-ə-go-gas″tro-mi-ot′ə-me) esophagocardiomyotomy.

**esoph·a·go·gas·tro·plas·ty** (ə-sof″ə-go-gas′tro-plas″te) plastic repair of the esophagus and stomach; cardioplasty.

**esoph·a·go·gas·tros·co·py** (ə-sof″ə-go-gas-tros′kə-pe) [*esophagus* + *gastro-* + *-scopy*] endoscopic examination of the esophagus and the stomach.

**esoph·a·go·gas·tros·to·my** (ə-sof″ə-go-gas-tros′tə-me) [*esophagus* + *gastro-* + *-stomy*] surgical creation of a communication between the stomach and esophagus.

**esoph·a·go·gram** (ə-sof′ə-go-gram) a radiograph of the esophagus.

**esoph·a·gog·ra·phy** (ə-sof″ə-gog′rə-fe) radiography of the esophagus.

**esoph·a·go·je·ju·no·gas·tros·to·mo·sis** (ə-sof″ə-go-jə-joo″no-gas″tros-tə-mo′səs) esophagojejunogastrostomy.

**esoph·a·go·je·ju·no·gas·tros·to·my** (ə-sof″ə-go-jə-joo″no-gas-tros′tə-me) the operation of mobilizing an isolated segment of jejunum and anastomosing its proximal end to the esophagus and its distal end to the stomach.

**esoph·a·go·je·ju·no·plas·ty** (ə-sof″ə-go-jə-joo′no-plas′te) replacement of the esophagus with a segment of jejunum.

**esoph·a·go·je·ju·nos·to·my** (ə-sof-ə-go-je″joo-nos′tə-me) surgical anastomosis between the esophagus and the jejunum.

**esoph·a·go·lar·yn·gec·to·my** (ə-sof″ə-go-lar″in-jek′tə-me) en bloc excision of the upper cervical esophagus and larynx.

**esoph·a·gol·o·gy** (ə-sof″ə-gol′ə-je) the study and treatment of diseases of the esophagus.

**esoph·a·go·ma·la·cia** (ə-sof″ə-go-mə-la′shə) [*esophagus* + *-malacia*] softening of the walls of the esophagus.

**esoph·a·go·my·co·sis** (ə-sof″ə-go-mi-ko′sis) [*esophagus* + *mycosis*] any disease of the esophagus caused by fungi. See *fungal esophagitis, under esophagitis.*

**esoph·a·go·my·ot·o·my** (ə-sof″ə-go-mi-ot′ə-me) incision through the muscular coat of the esophagus, the term usually referring to incision through the muscular coat of the distal part of the esophagus.
**Heller's e.,** esophagocardiomyotomy.

**esoph·a·go·plas·ty** (ə-sof′ə-go-plas″te) [*esophagus* + *-plasty*] [MeSH: Esophagoplasty] a plastic operation on the esophagus.

**esoph·a·go·pli·ca·tion** (ə-sof″ə-go-plī-ka′shən) the operation of narrowing the esophagus by folding in its wall.

**esoph·a·gop·to·sis** (ə-sof″ə-gop-to′sis) [*esophagus* + *-ptosis*] prolapse of the esophagus.

**esoph·a·go·res·pi·ra·to·ry** (ə-sof″ə-go-rə-spir′ə-to″re) pertaining to or communicating with the esophagus and respiratory tract (the trachea or a bronchus).

**esoph·a·go·scope** (ə-sof′ə-go-skōp) [*esophagus* + *-scope*] a flexible or rigid instrument for inspecting the lumen of the esophagus and carrying out diagnostic and therapeutic maneuvers such as taking biopsy specimens and removing foreign bodies.

**esoph·a·gos·co·py** (ə-sof″ə-gos′ko-pe) [MeSH: Esophagoscopy] endoscopic examination of the esophagus.

**esoph·a·go·spasm** (ə-sof′ə-go-spaz″əm) [*esophagus* + *spasm*] diffuse esophageal spasm.

**esoph·a·go·ste·no·sis** (ə-sof″ə-go-stə-no′sis) [*esophagus* + *stenosis*] stricture or constriction of the esophagus.

**esoph·a·gos·to·ma** (e″sof-ə-gos′tə-mə) [*esophagus* + *stoma*] the external opening of an artificial opening leading into the esophagus.

**esoph·a·go·sto·mi·a·sis** (ə-sof″ə-go-sto-mi′ə-sis) oesophagostomiasis.

**esoph·a·gos·to·my** (ə-sof″ə-gos′tə-me) [*esophagus* + *-stomy*] [MeSH: Esophagostomy] the creation of an opening into the esophagus.

**esoph·a·go·tome** (ə-sof′ə-go-tōm) a cutting instrument for use in esophagotomy.

**esoph·a·got·o·my** (ə-sof″ə-got′ə-me) [*esophagus* + *-tomy*] incision of the esophagus.

**esoph·a·go·tra·che·al** (ə-sof″ə-go-tra′ke-əl) tracheoesophageal.

**esoph·a·gram** (ə-sof′ə-gram) esophagogram.

**esoph·a·gus** (ə-sof′ə-gəs) [Gr. *oisophagos,* from *oisein* to carry + *phagēma* food] [MeSH: Esophagus] the musculomembranous passage extending from the pharynx to the stomach; spelled also *oesophagus* [TA]. See also *pars cervicalis oesophagi, pars thoracica oesophagi,* and *pars abdominalis oesophagi.* Called also *gullet.*
**abdominal e.,** pars abdominalis oesophagi.
**Barrett's e.,** see under *syndrome.*
**cervical e.,** pars cervicalis oesophagi.
**nutcracker e.,** a motility disorder characterized by high-amplitude peristaltic contractions, often of prolonged duration, arising from the distal esophagus.
**thoracic e.,** pars thoracica oesophagi.

**eso·pho·ria** (es″o-fo′re-ə) [*eso-* + *phoria*] a form of heterophoria in which there is a deviation of the visual axis of an eye toward that of the other eye after the visual fusional stimuli have been eliminated; called also *esodeviation.*

**eso·phor·ic** (es″o-for′ik) pertaining to or characterized by esophoria.

**eso·sphe·noid·itis** (es″o-sfe″noi-di′tis) [*eso-* + *sphenoid* + *-itis*] osteomyelitis of the sphenoid bone.

**eso·tro·pia** (es″o-tro′pe-ə) [*eso-* + *tropia*] [MeSH: Esotropia] strabismus in which there is manifest deviation of the visual axis of an eye toward that of the other eye, resulting in diplopia. Called also *cross-eye* and *convergent* or *internal strabismus.*

**eso·trop·ic** (es″o-trop′ik) pertaining to or characterized by esotropia.

**ESP** extrasensory perception.

**es·pun·dia** (es-pōōn′-jah) [Port. "sponge"] mucocutaneous leishmaniasis.

**es·quil·lec·to·my** (es″kwī-lek′tə-me) [Fr. *esquille* fragment + *-ectomy*] excision of fragments of bone following fractures caused by projectiles.

**ESR** erythrocyte sedimentation rate; electron spin resonance.

**ESRD** end-stage renal disease.

**es·sence** (es′əns) [L. *essentia* quality or being] 1. that which is or necessarily exists as the cause of the properties of a body. 2. a solution of a volatile oil in alcohol.
**e. of peppermint,** peppermint spirit; see under *spirit.*

**es·sen·tial** (ə-sen′shəl) [L. *essentialis*] 1. constituting the necessary or inherent part of a thing; giving a substance its peculiar and necessary qualities. 2. idiopathic; said of a disease. 3. indispensable; required in the diet, as essential fatty acids.

**Es·ser's graft, operation** (es′ərz) [Johannes Fredericus Samuel *Esser,* Dutch surgeon, 1877–1946] see under *graft,* and see *epithelial inlay,* under *inlay.*

**EST** electric shock therapy; electroshock therapy.

**es·ter** (es′tər) a compound formed by removal of water from an acid and an alcohol, e.g., carboxylic acid esters, R—O—CO—R′, and phosphoric acid esters (organic phosphates), $R—PO_4^{2-}$; esters are named as if they were salts of the parent acid, e.g., methyl acetate, glucose 6-phosphate.
**cholesteryl e.,** an ester formed from cholesterol and an acid; those in which the acid is a long chain fatty acid are major constituents of lipoproteins.
**Cori e.,** glucose 1-phosphate.
**Embden e.,** an equilibrium mixture of 75–80 per cent glucose 6-phosphate and 20–25 per cent fructose 6-phosphate.
**Harden-Young e.,** fructose 1,6-bisphosphate.

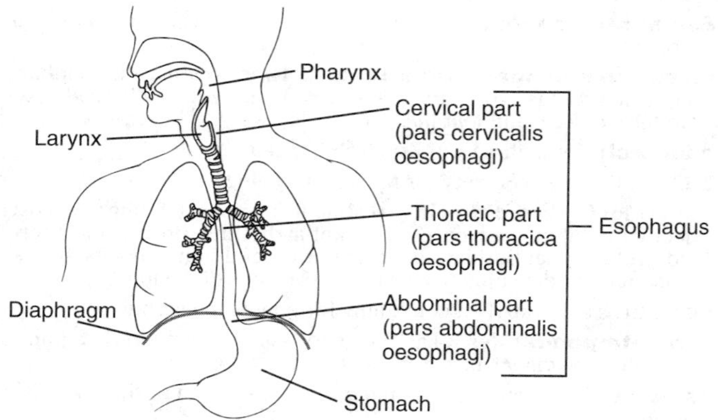

Esophagus, comprising cervical, thoracic, and abdominal parts.

**Neuberg e.,** fructose 6-phosphate.
**Robison e.,** glucose 6-phosphate.

**es·ter·a·pe·nia** (es"tər-ə-pe'ne-ə) [*esterase* + *-penia*] deficiency in the cholinesterase content of the blood.

**es·ter·ase** (es'tər-ās) 1. a term used in the recommended and trivial names of the hydrolases that act on ester bonds [EC 3.1] to produce an alcohol and an acid. 2. a general term used for any enzyme catalyzing this reaction.
**C1 e.,** C1s; see under *complement.*

**es·ter·i·fi·ca·tion** (es-ter"ĭ-fĭ-ka'shən) [MeSH: Esterification] the process of converting an acid into an ester.

**es·ter·i·fy** (es-ter'ĭ-fi) to combine with an alcohol with elimination of a molecule of water, forming an ester.

**es·ter·ize** (es'ter-īz) to convert, or be converted, into an ester.

**es·ter·ol·y·sis** (es"tər-ol'ə-sis) [*ester* + *-lysis*] the hydrolysis of an ester into its alcohol and acid.

**es·tero·lyt·ic** (es"tər-o-lit'ik) effecting or pertaining to esterolysis.

**Es·tes' operation** (es'tēz) [William Lawrence *Estes,* Jr., American surgeon, 1885–1940] see under *operation.*

**es·te·trol** (es'tə-trol) [MeSH: Estetrol] 15$\alpha$, 16$\alpha$, 17$\beta$-estetrol, an estrogen produced in the fetoplacental unit by 15$\alpha$-hydroxylation of estriol or estrogen precursors and found in the maternal serum, amniotic fluid, and urine.

**es·them·a·tol·o·gy** (es"them-ə-tol'ə-je) [Gr. *aisthēma* sensation + *-logy*] the science of the senses and sense organs.

**es·the·sia** (es-the'zhə) [*esthesi-* + *-ia*] perception, feeling, or sensation.

**es·the·sic** (es-the'sik) pertaining to the mental perception of sensations.

**esthesi(o)-** [Gr. *aisthēsis* perception, sensation] a combining form denoting relationship to feeling or to perception. Spelled also *aesthesi(o)-.*

**es·the·sio·blast** (es-the'ze-o-blast") [*esthesio-* + *-blast*] ganglioblast.

**es·the·si·od·ic** (es-the"ze-od'ik) esthesodic.

**es·the·si·o·gen·ic** (es-the"ze-o-jen'ik) producing sensation.

**es·the·si·ol·o·gy** (es-the"ze-ol'ə-je) [*esthesio-* + *-logy*] the science of sensation and the senses.

**es·the·si·om·e·ter** (es-the"ze-om'ə-tər) [*esthesio-* + *-meter*] an instrument for measuring tactile sensibility; tactometer.

**es·the·sio·neure** (es-the'ze-o-no͞or) [*esthesio-* + *neure*] a sensory neuron.

**es·the·sio·neu·ro·blas·to·ma** (es-the"ze-o-noo"ro-blas-to'mə) [MeSH: Esthesioneuroblastoma] olfactory neuroblastoma.

**es·the·sio·phys·i·ol·o·gy** (es-the"ze-o-fiz"e-ol'ə-je) the physiology of sensation and the sense organs.

**es·the·sod·ic** (es"thə-zod'ik) [*esthesio-* + Gr. *hodos* path] conducting or pertaining to the conduction of sensory impulses.

**es·thet·ic** (es-thet'ik) [Gr. *aisthēsis* sensation] [MeSH: Esthetics] 1. pertaining to esthesia; called also *esthesic.* 2. pertaining to beauty, or the improvement of appearance. Also spelled *aesthetic.*

**es·the·tics** (es-thet'iks) [MeSH: Esthetics] in dentistry, a philosophy concerned especially with the appearance of a dental restoration, as achieved through its color and/or form. Also spelled *aesthetics.*

**es·ti·mate**[1] (es'tĭ-mət) [L. *aestimare* to value, to estimate] 1. a rough calculation or one based on incomplete data. 2. a statistic used to characterize the value of a population parameter. Called also *estimator.*
**biased e.,** a point estimate that is not unbiased, i.e., a point estimate that for some reason should tend to be wrong in a given direction.
**consistent e.,** a statistic that converges to the true value of the parameter being estimated (population parameter) as the sample size increases; i.e., the estimate value can be made as statistically close to the true value as desired by taking a large enough sample.
**interval e.,** a statistical estimate that states with a specified degree of confidence that the parameter lies within a specified interval. Cf. *point e.*
**maximum likelihood e.,** the estimate of a parameter describing a population distribution that makes the likelihood function take its maximum value; an estimate of the parameter that maximizes the probability of obtaining the sample values actually observed.
**point e.,** a statistical estimate that specifies a value for the parameter. Cf. *interval e.*
**product-limit e.,** Kaplan-Meier survival curve.
**unbiased e.,** a point estimate having a sampling distribution with a mean equal to the parameter being estimated; i.e., the estimate will be greater than the true value as often as it is less than the true value.

**es·ti·mate**[2] (es'tĭ-māt) 1. to produce or use a rough calculation. 2. to measure or calculate a statistic for characterization of a population parameter.

**es·ti·ma·tor** (es'tĭ-ma"tər) estimate[1] (def. 2).

**Es·ti·nyl** (es'tĭ-nəl) trademark for a preparation of ethinyl estradiol.

**es·ti·val** (es'tĭ-vəl, ə-sti'vəl) [L. *aestivus,* from *aestas* summer] pertaining to or occurring in summer.

**es·ti·va·tion** (es"tĭ-va'shən) [L. *aestivus,* from *aestas* summer] [MeSH: Estivation] the dormant state of decreased metabolism in which certain animal species, as some tropical amphibians, survive a hot, dry summer; summer dormancy. Cf. *hibernation.*

**es·ti·vo·au·tum·nal** (es"tĭ-vo-aw-tum'nəl) pertaining to the summer and autumn; formerly applied, in the United States, to a form of malaria; see *falciparum malaria,* under *malaria.*

**Est·lan·der's operation** (est'lahnd-ərz) [Jakob August *Estlander,* Finnish surgeon, 1831–1881] see under *operation.*

**es·to·late** (es'to-lāt) USAN contraction for propionate lauryl sulfate.

**Es·trace** (es'trās) trademark for preparations of estradiol.

**Es·tra·derm** (es'trə-derm) trademark for a preparation of estradiol.

**es·tra·di·ol** (es"trə-di'ol, es-tra'de-ol) [MeSH: Estradiol] 1. the most potent naturally occurring ovarian and placental estrogen in mammals; it prepares the uterus for implantation of the fertilized ovum and promotes the maturation of and maintenance of the female accessory reproductive organs and secondary sex characters. It has also been produced semisynthetically. It exists in two isomeric forms: the active isomer is *estradiol-17$\beta$* and the inactive is *estradiol-17$\alpha$* (formerly called *$\beta$-estradiol* and *$\alpha$-estradiol* respectively). 2. [USP] a preparation of estradiol used in estrogen replacement therapy for conditions such as female hypogonadism, ovariectomy, or primary ovarian failure, and in treatment of abnormal uterine bleeding, vasomotor menopausal symptoms, postmenopausal osteoporosis, atrophic vaginitis or urethritis, vulvar squamous metaplasia, and certain advanced breast or prostatic carcinomas; administered orally, transdermally, intravaginally, or by intramuscular injection.
**e. benzoate,** an ester of estradiol, injected intramuscularly in oil solution.
**e. cypionate** [USP], an ester of estradiol, injected intramuscularly in oil solution.
**e. dipropionate,** an ester of estradiol, injected intramuscularly in oil solution.
**e. enanthate,** an ester of estradiol, injected intramuscularly in oil solution.
**ethinyl e.** [USP], an orally effective semisynthetic derivative of estradiol, one of the most potent estrogens. It is a component of many oral contraceptives and is also used in estrogen replacement therapy.
**e. undecylate,** an ester of estradiol, injected intramuscularly in oil solution.
**e. valerate** [USP], an ester of estradiol, injected intramuscularly in oil solution.

**es·tra·mus·tine phos·phate** (es"trə-mus'tēn) an antineoplastic agent consisting of estradiol joined to nitrogen mustard by a carbamate link, phosphorylated to make it water soluble; used for palliative treatment of metastatic or progressive carcinoma of the prostate. Available as *estramustine phosphate sodium.*

**es·trane** (es'trān) the 18-carbon tetracyclic hydrocarbon nucleus that is the parent structure of the estrogenic steroids; used for steroid hormone nomenclature.

**Es·tra·val** (es'trə-vəl) trademark for preparations of estradiol valerate.

**es·traz·i·nol hy·dro·bro·mide** (es-traz'ĭ-nol) an estrogen, $C_{20}H_{25}NO_2 \cdot HBr$.

**es·tri·a·sis** (es-tri'ə-sis) oestriasis.

**Es·tri·dae** (es'trĭ-de) Oestridae.

**es·trin** (es'trin) estrogen.

**es·trin·iza·tion** (es"trin-ĭ-za'shən) production of the cellular changes in the vaginal epithelium characteristic of estrus.

**es·tri·ol** (es'tre-ol) [MeSH: Estriol] 1. an oxidation product of estradiol and estrone, having relatively weak estrogenic activity and detectable in high concentrations in the urine, especially human pregnancy urine. 2. [USP] the official preparation of the hormone, now rarely used; administered orally. Called also *trihydroxyestrin.*

**es·tro·fur·ate** (es-tro-fūr'āt) an estrogen, $C_{24}H_{26}O_4$.

**es·tro·gen** (es'tro-jən) a generic term for any estrus-producing

steroid. In humans estrogens are formed in the ovary, possibly the adrenal cortex, the testis, and the fetoplacental unit and have various functions in both sexes. They are responsible for the development of the female secondary sex characters, and during the menstrual cycle they act on the female genitalia to produce an environment suitable for the fertilization, implantation, and nutrition of the early embryo. Exogenous estrogens are used in oral contraceptives; in treatment of some kinds of advanced breast and prostate carcinoma; in replacement therapy for female hypogonadism, ovariectomy, primary ovarian failure, atrophic vaginitis, vasomotor menopausal symptoms, and vulvar squamous hyperplasia, treatment of atrophic urethritis and abnormal uterine bleeding, and prophylaxis of osteoporosis. Common naturally occurring ones are *estradiol* and *estrone.* Called also *estrin* and *female sex hormone.*
**conjugated e's** [USP], a mixture of the sodium salts of the sulfate esters of estrone and equilin, derived from pregnant mares' urine or prepared synthetically from estrone and equilin; the actions and uses are those of estrogens, administered orally.
**esterified e's** [USP], a mixture of the sodium salts of esters of estrogenic substances, principally estrone, having the the actions and uses of estrogens; administered orally.

**es·tro·gen·ic** (es-tro-jen'ik) 1. producing estrus. 2. pertaining to, having the effects of, or similar to an estrogen. Called also *estrogenous.*

**es·tro·ge·nic·i·ty** (es″tro-jə-nis'ĭ-te) the quality of exerting or the ability to exert an estrus-producing or an estrogenic effect.

**es·trog·e·nous** (es-troj'ə-nəs) estrogenic.

**es·trone** (es'trōn) [MeSH: Estrone] 1. an oxidation product of estradiol, the first of the estrogens isolated in pure form, found in human pregnancy urine, male human urine, human plasma, mare pregnancy urine, stallion urine, human ovarian follicular fluid and placenta, and palm kernel oil; also produced synthetically. It is less potent than estradiol but more so than estriol and is metabolically convertible to estradiol; it is secreted by the ovary but circulating estrone is for the most part derived from peripheral metabolism of estradiol and especially androstenedione. 2. [USP] an official preparation of estrone, occurring as a sterile suspension or a vaginal cream; used as replacement therapy in cases of hypogonadism, ovariectomy, primary ovarian failure, atrophic vaginitis, vasomotor menopausal symptoms, and vulvar squamous hyperplasia and in the treatment of abnormal uterine bleeding and advanced prostatic carcinoma. Called also *ketohydroxyestrin.*

**es·tro·phil·in** (es″tro-fil'in) a cell protein that acts as a receptor for estrogen, found in estrogenic target tissue and in estrogen-dependent tumors and metastases.

**es·tro·pi·pate** (es'tro-pĭ-pāt) [USP] a compound of estrone sulfate and piperazine.

**es·trous** (es'trəs) pertaining to estrus.

**es·tru·al** (es'troo-əl) estrous.

**es·tru·a·tion** (es″troo-a'shən) estrus.

**Es·tru·gen·one** (es″troo-jen'on) trademark for a preparation of estrone.

**es·trum** (es'trəm) estrus.

**es·trus** (es'trəs) [L. *oestrus* gadfly; Gr. *oistros* anything that drives mad, any vehement desire] [MeSH: Estrus] the recurrent, restricted period of sexual receptivity in female mammals other than human females, marked by intense sexual urge. See also *estrous cycle,* under *cycle.* Called also *estruation, estrum, heat,* and *rut.* Also spelled *oestrus.*
**silent e.,** follicular development and ovulation occurring without the usual behavior of estrus.

**esu** electrostatic unit.

**ESV** end-systolic volume.

**es·y·late** (es'ə-lāt) USAN contraction for ethanesulfonate.

**Et** ethyl group.

**eta** (a'tə) [H, η] the seventh letter of the Greek alphabet.

**eta·fed·rine hy·dro·chlo·ride** (a″tə-fed'rēn) an adrenergic, administered orally in the treatment of bronchial asthma.

**eta·fil·con A** (ā″tə-fil'kon) a hydrophilic contact lens material.

**Et·a·mon** (at'ə-mon) trademark for a preparation of tetraethylammonium chloride.

**état** (a-tah') [Fr.] state; used in reference to morbid conditions. See also *status.*
**é. criblé** (krēb-la'), status cribralis.
**é. lacunaire** (lah-ku-nār'), status lacunaris.
**é. mammelonné** (mah-mel-un-a'), hyperplasia of the mucous membrane of the stomach in chronic gastritis, resulting in the formation of small elevations.
**é. marbré** (mar-bra'), status marmoratus.

**etch·ing** (ech'ing) [Old High Ger. *ezzen* to eat] the cutting of a hard surface such as metal or glass by a corrosive chemical, usually an acid, in order to create a design.
**acid e.,** etching of dental enamel with an acid in order to roughen the surface, increase retention of resin sealant, and promote mechanical retention.

**Eter·nod's sinus** (a-tər-nōz') [Auguste François Charles *Eternod,* Swiss histologist, 1854–1932] see under *sinus.*

**ETF** electron transfer flavoprotein.

**eth·a·cryn·ate so·di·um** (eth″ə-krin'āt) [USP] the sodium salt of ethacrynic acid (q.v.), having the same actions and uses as the base; administered intravenously.

**eth·a·cryn·ic ac·id** (eth-ə-krin'ik) [USP] [MeSH: Ethacrynic Acid] a loop diuretic used in the treatment of edema associated with congestive heart failure or hepatic or renal disease and in the treatment of hypertension, usually in combination with other drugs; administered orally.

**etham·bu·tol hy·dro·chlo·ride** (ə-tham'bu-tol) [USP] an antibacterial, specifically effective against *Mycobacterium,* including *M. tuberculosis;* used in conjunction with one or more other antituberculous drugs in the treatment of pulmonary tuberculosis, administered orally.

**eth·am·i·van** (eth-am'ĭ-van″) a central nervous system stimulant and analeptic, used as a respiratory stimulant, administered intravenously.

**etham·sy·late** (ə-tham'sə-lāt) [MeSH: Ethamsylate] a hemostatic agent that acts by maintaining capillary wall stability, used for the prophylaxis and treatment of hemorrhage from small blood vessels; administered orally, intramuscularly, and intravenously.

**eth·a·nal** (eth'ə-nal) acetaldehyde.

**eth·ane** (eth'ān) [MeSH: Ethane] a hydrocarbon of the methane series, $C_2H_6$, forming a constituent of natural gas, which occurs as a colorless, odorless, flammable gas.

**eth·ane·di·al** (eth″ān-di'al) glyoxal.

**eth·ane·di·ni·trile** (eth″ān-di-ni'tril) cyanogen, def. 2.

**eth·a·no·ic acid** (eth″ə-no'ik) systematic name for acetic acid.

**eth·a·nol** (eth'ə-nol) a primary alcohol existing as a transparent, colorless, volatile, flammable liquid, miscible with water, methanol, ether, chloroform and acetone; it is formed by microbial fermentation of carbohydrates or by synthesis from ethylene. Excessive ingestion results in acute intoxication, with psychological, gastrointestinal, neurological, and motor abnormalities; ingestion during pregnancy can harm the fetus. Called also *alcohol* (q.v.) and *ethyl* or *grain alcohol.*

**eth·a·nol·amine** (eth″ə-nol'ə-mēn) monoethanolamine.
**e. oleate,** a combination of monoethanolamine and oleic acid, used as a sclerosing agent in treatment of varicose veins.

**eth·a·nol·ism** (eth'ə-nol″iz-əm) alcoholism.

**eth·a·ver·ine hy·dro·chlo·ride** (et″ə-ver'ēn) the tetrahydroxy analogue of papaverine, used as an antispasmodic in peripheral and vascular insufficiency associated with arterial spasm and as a smooth muscle relaxant in spasticity of the gastrointestinal and genitourinary tracts; administered orally.

**eth·chlor·vy·nol** (eth-klor'və-nol) [USP] [MeSH: Ethchlorvynol] a nonbarbiturate sedative and hypnotic, used for the short-term treatment of insomnia; administered orally.

**eth·e·noid** (eth'ə-noid) containing an ethylene linkage.

**ether** (e'thər) [L. *aether,* Gr. *aithēr* "the upper and purer air"] 1. an organic compound having an oxygen atom bonded to two carbon atoms; general formula, R—O—R'. 2. [USP] diethyl e.
**anesthetic e.,** diethyl ether; also any other ether inhalational anesthetic.
**diethyl e.,** ethyl ether, ether [USP], a colorless, volatile, flammable liquid, $C_2H_5OC_2H_5$, with a characteristic odor; the first inhalational anesthetic used for surgical anesthesia (1846), now little used because of its flammability.
**diethylene glycol monoethyl e.** [NF], a condensation product of ethylene oxide and alcohol, used as a solvent in pharmaceutical preparations.
**petroleum e.,** see under *petroleum.*
**thio e.,** thioether.

**ethe·re·al** (ə-the're-əl) 1. pertaining to, prepared with, containing, or resembling ether. 2. evanescent; delicate.

**ether·i·fi·ca·tion** (e″thər-ĭ-fĭ-ka'shən) the formation of an ether from alcohol.

**ether·iza·tion** (e″thər-ĭ-za'shən) the administration of ether by inhalation, and the consequent production of anesthesia.

**ether·ize** (e'thər-īz) to put under the anesthetic influence of ether.

**eth·i·cal** (eth'ĭ-kəl) 1. in accordance with the principles which govern right conduct. 2. pertaining to ethics in general or to the discipline of ethics.

**eth·ics** (eth'iks) [Gr. *ēthos* the manner and habits of man or of animals] [MeSH: Ethics] 1. the rules or principles which govern right conduct. 2. the branch of philosophy that studies such principles.
**clinical e.,** the application of ethical analysis to decision making in the care of individual patients.
**medical e.,** the values and guidelines that should govern decisions in medicine.

**ethid·i·um** (ə-thid'e-əm) [MeSH: Ethidium] a fluorochrome that intercalates across double-stranded nucleic acids, particularly DNA. Its bromide salt is used to detect DNA after electrophoresis or in cytochemical preparations. In veterinary pharmacology, it is used as a trypanosomicide and is usually called *homidium.*

**ethin·a·mate** (ə-thin'ə-māt) [USP] a short-acting nonbarbiturate sedative, used as a hypnotic, administered orally.

**eth·i·nyl** (eth'ĭ-nəl) the radical HC≡C—, derived from acetylene.
**e. estradiol,** see under *estradiol.*

**ethi·on·am·ide** (ə-thi″ən-am'īd) [USP] [MeSH: Ethionamide] an antibacterial, effective against *Mycobacterium tuberculosis;* used in conjunction with one or more other antituberculous drugs in the treatment of pulmonary tuberculosis, administered orally.

**ethi·o·nine** (ə-thi'ə-nēn) [MeSH: Ethionine] the ethyl homologue of methionine.

**ethis·ter·one** (ə-this'tər-ōn) [MeSH: Ethisterone] a semisynthetic progestin, which may be considered a derivative of both progesterone and of testosterone. Called also *anhydrohydroxyprogesterone, pregneninolone,* and *ethinyl testosterone.*

**eth·mo·ceph·a·lus** (eth″mo-sef'ə-ləs) [Gr. *ēthmos* sieve + *-cephalus*] a fetus with an imperfect head, more or less union of the eyes, and a rudimentary nose, which may often be displaced upward.

**eth·mo·fron·tal** (eth″mo-fron'təl) pertaining to the ethmoid and frontal bones.

**eth·moid** (eth'moid) [Gr. *ēthmos* sieve + *-oid*] 1. cribriform; sieve-like, as the ethmoid bone. 2. ethmoidal.

**eth·moi·dal** (eth-moi'dəl) of or pertaining to the ethmoid bone. Called also *ethmoid.*

**eth·moid·ec·to·my** (eth″moid-ek'tə-me) [*ethmoid* + *-ectomy*] excision of the ethmoid cells or of a portion of the ethmoid bone.

**eth·moid·itis** (eth″moi-di'tis) ethmoid sinusitis.

**eth·moid·ot·o·my** (eth″moi-dot'ə-me) surgical incision into the ethmoid sinus.

**eth·mo·lac·ri·mal** (eth″mo-lak'rĭ-məl) pertaining to the ethmoid and the lacrimal bones.

**eth·mo·max·il·lary** (eth″mo-mak'sĭ-lar-e) pertaining to the ethmoid and maxillary bones.

**eth·mo·na·sal** (eth″mo-na'zəl) pertaining to the ethmoid and nasal bones.

**eth·mo·pal·a·tal** (eth″mo-pal'ə-təl) pertaining to the ethmoid and palatine bones.

**eth·mo·sphe·noid** (eth″mo-sfe'noid) sphenoethmoid.

**eth·mo·tur·bi·nal** (eth″mo-tər'bĭ-nəl) pertaining to the superior and middle nasal conchae.

**eth·mo·vo·mer·ine** (eth″mo-vo'mər-ēn) pertaining to the ethmoid bone and the vomer.

**eth·nic** (eth'nik) [Gr. *ethnikos* of a nation; national] pertaining to a social group who share cultural bonds (religious, national, etc.) or physical (racial) characteristics.

**eth·nics** (eth'niks) [Gr. *ethnikos* of a nation; national] ethnology.

**eth·no·bi·ol·o·gy** (eth″no-bi-ol'ə-je) the scientific study of physical characteristics of different races of mankind.

**eth·nog·ra·phy** (eth-nog'rə-fe) [Gr. *ethnos* race + *-graphy*] a description of the races of man. Cf. *anthropography.*

**eth·nol·o·gy** (eth-nol'ə-je) [Gr. *ethnos* race + *-logy*] [MeSH: Ethnology] the science which deals with the races of humankind, their descent, relationship, etc.

**etho·hep·ta·zine cit·rate** (eth″o-hep'tə-zēn) an analgesic, used to control mild or moderate pain; administered orally.

**etho·hex·a·di·ol** (eth″o-hek″sə-di'ol) an arthropod repellent, applied topically to the skin and clothing.

**eth·o·log·i·cal** (eth″o-loj'ĭ-kəl) pertaining to ethology.

**eth·ol·o·gist** (e-thol'ə-jist) an individual skilled in ethology.

**eth·ol·o·gy** (e-thol'ə-je) [Gr. *ēthos* the manners and habits of man, or of animals + *-logy*] [MeSH: Ethology] The scientific study of animal behavior, particularly in the natural state, the evolution of behavior, and its biologic significance.

**etho·pab·ate** (eth″o-pab'āt) [USP] an antiprotozoal agent used in veterinary practice for the control of coccidiosis.

**etho·pro·pa·zine hy·dro·chlo·ride** (eth″o-pro'pə-zēn) a phenothiazine derivative, having anticholinergic, antihistaminic, adrenergic-blocking, ganglion-blocking, local anesthetic, and central nervous system depressant effects; used as an antiparkinsonian agent, administered orally. Called also *isothiazine hydrochloride* and *phenopropazine hydrochloride.*

**etho·sux·i·mide** (eth″o-suk'sĭ-mīd) [USP] [MeSH: Ethosuximide] an anticonvulsant used in the treatment of petit mal epilepsy, administered orally.

**etho·to·in** (ə-tho'to-in) an anticonvulsant used in the treatment of grand mal epilepsy and psychomotor seizures, administered orally. Called also *ethylphenylhydantoin.*

**ethox·a·zene hy·dro·chlo·ride** (ə-thok'sə-zēn) a local analgesic used to relieve pain associated with urinary tract infections, administered orally.

**eth·ox·zol·amide** (eth″oks-zol'ə-mīd) [MeSH: Ethoxzolamide] a carbonic anhydrase inhibitor, used in the treatment of glaucoma and edema.

**Eth·rane** (eth'rān) trademark for a preparation of enflurane.

**Eth·ril** (eth'ril) trademark for preparations of erythromycin stearate.

**eth·y·benz·tro·pine** (eth″ə-benz-tro'pēn) an anticholinergic with high antihistaminic action which has been used as an antiparkinsonian agent and in the treatment of drug-induced extrapyramidal syndrome.

**eth·yl** (eth'əl) [*ether* + *-yl*] the univalent alcohol radical, $CH_3$—$CH_2$—. Symbol Et.
**e. acetate** [NF], a transparent, colorless liquid used as a flavoring agent in pharmaceutical preparations.
**e. aminobenzoate,** benzocaine.
**e. biscoumacetate,** one of the synthetic, orally effective coumarin anticoagulants.
**e. butyrate,** the butyric acid ester of ethyl alcohol, with the odor of pineapple, used in flavoring extracts and as a solvent.
**e. chloride** [USP], a colorless, extremely volatile, flammable liquid, $C_2H_5Cl$, sprayed on skin to produce local anesthesia by superficial freezing caused by its rapid evaporation; formerly used as an inhalational anesthetic.
**e. dibunate,** an antitussive.
**e. ether,** see *diethyl ether.*
**e. mercaptan,** a thioalcohol which has a revolting odor and contributes to the odor of feces.
**e. oleate** [NF], a mobile, practically colorless liquid consisting of esters of ethyl alcohol and high-molecular-weight fatty acids; used as a vehicle for pharmaceutical preparations.
**e. orange,** a dye, the sodium salt of diethylaniline-azo-benzene-sulfonic acid; used as an indicator, being turned red by acids and yellow by alkalis.

**eth·yl·al·de·hyde** (eth″əl-al'də-hīd) acetaldehyde.

**eth·yl·ate** (eth'əl-āt) any compound of ethyl alcohol in which the hydrogen of the hydroxyl is replaced by a base.

**eth·yl·a·tion** (eth″əl-a'shən) the act of combining or causing to combine with the ethyl radical.

**eth·yl·cel·lu·lose** (eth″əl-sel'u-lōs) [NF] chemical name: cellulose ethyl ester. A free-flowing, white to light tan powder, used as a tablet binder in pharmaceutical preparations.

**eth·y·lene** (eth'ə-lēn) $CH_2$=$CH_2$, a colorless, flammable gas with a sweet taste and odor, formerly used as an inhalational anesthetic.
**e. dibromide,** a derivative of bromine and ethylene used as a fumigant and gasoline additive; it is irritating to the skin and mucous membranes and carcinogenic. Called also *1,2-dibromoethane.*
**e. dichloride,** a colorless heavy liquid with a pungent odor, used as a solvent, gasoline additive, and intermediate; it is irritating to the eyes and respiratory tract and can cause central nervous system disturbances and renal and hepatic damage. Excessive exposure can be carcinogenic. Called also *1,2-dichloroethane.*
**e. glycol,** a solvent with a sweetish, acrid taste, used as an antifreeze. Acute poisoning by ingestion can result in central nervous system depression, vomiting, hypotension, coma, convulsions, renal damage, and death.
**e. oxide,** a gas used in the manufacture of ethylene glycol, acrylonitrile, and other compounds and as a fumigant, fungicide, and sterilizing agent. It is highly irritating to the eyes and mucous membranes and is carcinogenic. Called also *oxirane.*

**eth·y·lene·di·a·mine** (eth″ə-lēn-di'ə-mēn) [USP] a clear, colorless or slightly yellow liquid having an ammonia-like odor and a strong alkaline reaction; used as a component of aminophylline injection.

**eth·y·lene·di·a·mine·tet·ra·ac·e·tate** (eth″ə-lēn-di″ə-mēn-tet-rə-as′ə-tāt) a salt of ethylenediaminetetraacetic acid (EDTA). Called also *edetate.*

**eth·y·lene·di·a·mine·tet·ra·a·ce·tic ac·id** (eth″ə-lēn-di′ə-mēn-tet″rə-ə-se′tik) EDTA; a chelating agent that binds calcium and heavy metal ions; used as an anticoagulant for blood specimens and also (see *edetate*) for treatment of lead poisoning and hypercalcemia.

**eth·yl·ene·i·mine** (eth″əl-ēn′ĭ-mēn) ethylenimine.

**eth·yl·en·i·mine** (eth″əl-en′ĭ-mēn) a toxic and carcinogenic compound, $C_2H_5N$, occurring as a colorless oily liquid with a strong odor of ammonia, used as an intermediate in a variety of industrial processes. Derivatives include alkylating agents used as antineoplastics. Spelled also *ethyleneimine.*

**eth·yl·es·tre·nol** (eth″əl-es′trə-nol) [MeSH: Ethylestrenol] $C_{20}H_{32}O$, an androgen and anabolic steroid; administered orally.

**ethyl·ic** (ə-thil′ik) pertaining to or derived from ethyl.

**eth·yl·i·dene** (eth′əl-ĭ-dēn) the bivalent radical, $CH_3CH=$; called also *ethidene.*

**e. chloride,** 1,1-dichloroethane; an oily liquid with a chloroformlike odor, used as a solvent and fumigant; it is irritating to the eyes and respiratory system and can cause central nervous system disturbances and renal and hepatic damage.

**eth·yl·ism** (eth′əl-iz-əm) poisoning or intoxication by ethyl alcohol.

**eth·yl·ma·lon·ic-adip·ic·ac·id·uria** (eth′əl-mə-lon′ik ə-dip″ik-as-ĭ-du′re-ə) glutaricaciduria, type II.

**eth·yl·mor·phine hy·dro·chlo·ride** (eth″əl-mor′fēn) the chloride salt of the ethyl ester of morphine, having some of the actions of morphine and codeine; used as a chemotic in the treatment of glaucoma, iritis, and corneal ulcers, applied topically to the conjunctiva. It has also been used as an antitussive.

**eth·yl·nor·a·dren·a·line** (eth″əl-nor-ə-dren′ə-lin) ethylnorepinephrine.

**eth·yl·nor·epi·neph·rine hy·dro·chlo·ride** (eth″əl-nor-ep″ĭ-nef′rin) a synthetic adrenergic, used for the relief of bronchospasm in bronchial asthma; administered intramuscularly or subcutaneously.

**eth·yl·nor·su·pra·ren·in** (eth″əl-nor-soo″prə-ren′in) ethylnorepinephrine.

**eth·yl·par·a·ben** (eth″əl-par′ə-ben) [NF] an antifungal compound, closely related to butylparaben and methylparaben, used as a preservative in pharmaceutic preparations.

**eth·yl·phen·yl·hy·dan·to·in** (eth″əl-fen″əl-hi-dan′to-in) ethotoin.

**eth·yl·stib·amine** (eth″əl-stib′ə-mēn) neostibosan.

**ethy·no·di·ol di·ac·e·tate** (ə-thi″no-di′ol) [USP] [MeSH: Ethynodiol Diacetate] a progestin used in combination with an estrogen as an oral contraceptive.

**eth·y·nyl** (eth′ə-nəl) ethinyl.

**Eth·y·ol** (eth′e-ol) trademark for a preparation of amifostine.

**eti·do·caine hy·dro·chlo·ride** (ə-te′do-kān) a local anesthetic of the amide type used for percutaneous infiltration anesthesia, peripheral nerve blocks, and caudal and epidural blocks.

**eti·dro·nate** (e-tĭ-drō′nāt) EHDP; a hydroxyethylidene-substituted diphosphonate compound that inhibits the resorption and deposition of hydroxyapatite crystals in bone and is used for treatment of osteitis deformans; usually prescribed as the disodium salt. Because of its affinity for sites of osteoid mineralization, it is also used as a complex with technetium 99m in bone scanning; see table at *technetium.*

**e. disodium** [USP], the disodium salt of etidronate, a diphosphonate used to treat osteitis deformans and hypercalcemia of malignancy; administered orally or intravenously.

**eti·dro·nic acid** (e-ti-dro′nik) an acid used as a bone calcium regulator.

**etio·cho·lan·o·lone** (e″te-o-ko-lan′o-lōn) [MeSH: Etiocholanolone] a degradation product of testosterone, androstenedione, and dehydroepiandrosterone excreted in the urine.

**eti·o·gen·ic** (e″te-o-jen′ik) [Gr. *aitia* cause + *-genic*] causative.

**eti·o·la·tion** (e″te-o-la′shən) [Fr. *étioler* to blanch] 1. a blanching or paleness of color in a plant due to lack of chlorophyll when grown in the dark. 2. the process by which the skin becomes pale when deprived of sunlight.

**eti·o·log·ic, eti·o·log·i·cal** (e″te-o-loj′ik, e″te-o-loj′ĭ-kəl) pertaining to etiology, or to the causes of disease.

**eti·ol·o·gy** (e″te-ol′ə-je) [Gr. *aitia* cause + *-logy*] the study or theory of the factors that cause disease and the method of their introduction to the host; the causes or origin of a disease or disorder. Cf. *pathogenesis.*

**etio·pa·thol·o·gy** (e″te-o-pə-thol′ə-je) pathogenesis.

**etio·por·phyr·in** (e″te-o-por′fə-rin) a porphyrin (q.v.) in which each pyrrole ring has one methyl and one ethyl side chain.

**eti·o·trop·ic** (e″te-o-trop′ik) [Gr. *aitia* cause + *-tropic*] directed against the cause of a disease.

**ET-NANB** enterically transmitted non-A, non-B hepatitis; see *hepatitis E,* under *hepatitis.*

**eto·do·lac** (e-to-do′lak) [USP] [MeSH: Etodolac] a nonsteroidal anti-inflammatory drug prescribed as an analgesic and anti-inflammatory, especially to treat arthritis; administered orally. Called also *etodolic acid.*

**eto·do·lic acid** (e-to-do′lik) etodolac.

**eto·fen·a·mate** (e-to-fen′ə-māt) a nonsteroidal anti-inflammatory agent of the fenamate class.

**etom·i·date** (ə-tom′ĭ-dāt) [MeSH: Etomidate] a sedative-hypnotic, administered intravenously for the induction and maintenance of anesthesia and as a sedative for critically ill patients.

**eto·po·side** (e″tə-po′sīd) [USP] [MeSH: Etoposide] a semisynthetic derivative of podophyllotoxin used as an antineoplastic in the treatment of carcinoma of the testes, lung, and bladder, lymphoma, acute myelocytic leukemia, Ewing's sarcoma, and AIDS-associated Kaposi's sarcoma; administered orally or intravenously.

**eto·zo·lin** (et″ə-zo′lin) a loop diuretic with properties similar to those of furosemide but with a longer duration of effect; administered orally.

**etret·i·nate** (e-tret′ĭ-nāt) [MeSH: Etretinate] a tretinoin derivative used in the treatment of severe, recalcitrant psoriasis and various other skin disorders; administered orally.

**Eu** symbol for *europium.*

**eu-** [Gr. *eu* well] a combining form meaning well, easily, or good; the opposite of *dys-.*

**eu·adre·no·cor·ti·cism** (u″ə-dre″no-kor′tĭ-siz-əm) the normal state of secretion by the adrenal cortex, as distinguished from hypoadrenocorticism and hyperadrenocorticism.

**eu·bac·te·ria** (u″bak-te′re-ə) plural of *eubacterium.*

**Eu·bac·te·ri·a·les** (u″bak-te″re-a′lēz) in former systems of classification, an order of the class Schizomycetes, made up of the so-called true bacteria, i.e., bacteria that possess peritrichous flagella; cf. *Pseudomonadales.*

**Eu·bac·te·ri·um** (u″bak-te′re-əm) [*eu-* + Gr. *baktērion* small rod] [MeSH: Eubacterium] a genus of bacteria of the family Propionibacteriaceae, consisting of nonsporulating, gram-positive, anaerobic rod-shaped organisms found as saprophytes in soil and water. They are normal inhabitants of the skin and cavities of humans and other mammals, occasionally causing infections of soft tissues.

**E. alactoly′ticum,** a species isolated from dental tartar, various infections, and abscesses.

**E. len′tum,** a species isolated from various infections, including infected postoperative wounds and abscesses, and from human blood and feces. Called also *Bifidobacterium cornutum, Corynebacterium diphtheroides,* and *group 3 corynebacterium.*

**E. limo′sum,** a species that synthesizes vitamin $B_{12}$. It has been isolated from the feces of humans and other animals, from human infections, and from mud.

**eu·bac·te·ri·um** (u″bak-te′re-əm) pl. *eubacte′ria.* [MeSH: Eubacterium] 1. an organism of the genus *Eubacterium.* 2. formerly, an organism of the order Eubacteriales.

**eu·bi·ot·ics** (u″bi-ot′iks) [*eu-* + *biotics*] the science of healthy living.

**eu·caine** (u′kān) a substance closely resembling cocaine in action and composition, but less depressant to the heart; formerly used as a local anesthetic. Called also *benzamine.*

**eu·ca·lyp·tol** (u″kə-lip′tol) [USP] a colorless liquid with a camphoraceous odor and a cooling, pungent taste, obtained from eucalyptus oil and other sources, used as a flavoring agent, expectorant, and local antiseptic. Used in veterinary medicine as an inhalant and expectorant. Called also *cajeputol* and *cineol.*

**Eu·ca·lyp·tus** (u″kə-lip′təs) [*eu-* + Gr. *kalyptos* covered] [MeSH: Eucalyptus] a genus of trees and shrubs of the family Myrtaceae, chiefly native to Australia. *E. glo′bulus* is the blue gum, source of eucalyptus oil. *E. calophyl′la, E. camaldulen′sis,* and *E. rostra′ta* are all known as red gum and yield the medicinal substance red gum.

**eu·cap·nia** (u-kap′ne-ə) [*eu-* + *capn-* + *-ia*] the condition in which the carbon dioxide tension of the blood is normal. Called also *normocapnia.*

**eu·cap·nic** (u-kap'nik) pertaining to or characterized by eucapnia.

**eu·cary·on** (u-kar'e-on) eukaryon.

**eu·cary·o·sis** (u"kər-e-o'sis) eukaryosis.

**Eu·cary·o·tae** (u-kar"e-o'te) [*eu-* + Gr. *karyon* nucleus] in some systems of classification, a proposed kingdom of organisms that would include everything except the Procaryotae (q.v.), i.e. all plants, animals, fungi, and protozoa, and most algae (except blue-green algae), grouping together all the organisms that are made up of eukaryotic cells, i.e., that have a true nucleus. Also written *Eukaryotae.*

**eu·cary·ote** (u-kar'e-ōt) eukaryote.

**eu·cary·ot·ic** (u"kər-e-ot'ik) eukaryotic.

**eu·cat·ro·pine hy·dro·chlo·ride** (u-kat'ro-pēn) [USP] an anticholinergic used as a mydriatic, applied topically to the eye.

**Eu·ces·to·da** (u-səs-to'də) Cestoda.

**Eu·cheu·ma** (u-ku'mə) a genus of red algae that is a source of carrageenan.

**eu·chlor·hy·dria** (u"klor-hi'dre-ə) [*eu-* + *chlorhydric acid*] the presence of the normal proportion of free hydrochloric acid in the gastric juice.

**eu·cho·lia** (u-ko'le-ə) [*eu-* + *chol-* + *-ia*] normal condition of the bile.

**eu·chro·mat·ic** (u-kro-mat'ic) of or relating to euchromatin.

**eu·chro·ma·tin** (u-kro'mə-tin) [*eu-* + *chromatin*] the condensed state of chromatin in which it stains lightly, is genetically active, and is partially or fully uncoiled, being the interphase form of the chromosome or the material of most chromosome arms during metaphase. Cf. *heterochromatin.*

**eu·chro·ma·top·sy** (u-kro'mə-top"se) [*eu-* + *chromat-* + *-opsia*] normal color vision.

**eu·chyl·ia** (u-kil'e-ə) [*eu-* + Gr. *chylos* chyle] a normal condition of the chyle.

**Eu·coc·ci·di·ida** (u-kok"sĭ-di'ĭ-də) [*eu-* + Gr. *kokkos* berry] [MeSH: Eucoccidiida] an order of parasitic protozoa (subclass Coccidia, class Sporozoea) found in the blood and epithelial cells of invertebrates and vertebrates, and having a life cycle involving merogony. Human pathogens are included in the suborders Eimeriina and Haemosporina.

**eu·coe·lom** (u-se'lom) [*eu-* + *coelom*] coelom.

**Eu·coe·lo·ma·ta** (u"se-lo-ma'tə) the major division of the higher invertebrates, including mollusks, annelids, arthropods, echinoderms, and chordates, which all have a separate mouth and anus, a true coelom, and a well-developed circulatory system. It is divided into two series, the Deuterostomia and the Protostomia.

**eu·coe·lo·mate** (u-se'lə-māt") any member of the Eucoelomata; called also *coelomate.*

**eu·col·loid** (u-kol'oid) a colloid in which each dispersed particle consists of a single large molecule.

**eu·cra·sia** (u-kra'zhə) [*eu-* + *-crasia*] 1. a state of health; proper balance of different factors constituting a healthy state. 2. a state in which there is a decreased bodily reaction to ingested or injected drugs, proteins, etc.

**eu·di·om·e·ter** (u"de-om'ə-tər) [Gr. *eudia* fine weather + *-meter*] an instrument used in testing the purity of the air.

**eu·dip·sia** (u-dip'se-ə) [*eu-* + *-dipsia*] ordinary, mild thirst.

**Eu·flag·el·la·ta** (u-flaj"ə-la'tə) [*eu-* + L. *flagellum whip*] former name for Mastigophora.

**eu·fla·vine** (u-fla'vin) acriflavine.

**eu·ga·my** (u'gə-me) [*eu-* + *gamos* marriage] the union of gametes, each of which contains the proper (haploid) complement of chromosomes.

**Eu·ge·nia** (u-je'ne-ə) [Prince *Eugene* of Savoy, French-born Austrian general, 1663–1736] a genus of tropical trees and shrubs of the family Myrtaceae. *E. caryophyl'lus* is now called *Syzygium aromaticum.*

**eu·gen·ic acid** (u-jen'ik) eugenol.

**eu·gen·i·cist** (u-jen'ĭ-sist) a person who is versed in eugenics.

**eu·gen·ics** (u-jen'iks) [*eu-* + *-genic*] [MeSH: Eugenics] the improvement of a population by selection of its best specimens for breeding; called also *orthogenics.* Cf. *dysgenics.*
**negative e.,** that concerned with prevention of reproduction (procreation) by individuals possessing inferior or undesirable traits.
**positive e.,** that concerned with promotion of optimal reproduction of individuals possessing superior or desirable traits.

**eu·gen·ist** (u-jen'ist) eugenicist.

**eu·gen·ol** (u'jən-ol) [USP] [MeSH: Eugenol] a dental analgesic, obtained from clove oil or other natural sources; applied topically to dental cavities and also used as a component of dental protectives. Called also *allylguaiacol* and *eugenic acid.* See also *zinc oxide–eugenol cement.*

**eu·gle·nid** (u-gle'nid) a protozoan of the order Euglenida; euglenoid.

**Eu·gle·ni·da** (u-gle'nĭ-də) [MeSH: Euglenida] an order of plantlike, flagellate protozoa (class Phytomastigophorea, subphylum Mastigophora) having green chromatophores when present; one or two, rarely more, flagella protruding from an anterior invagination; and a small stigma located anteriorly in colored forms. The organisms are usually found in fresh water, although some inhabit salt or brackish water, and a few are parasitic. See also *euglenoid movement,* under *movement.*

**eu·gle·noid** (u-gle'noid) pertaining to the order Euglenida; see also under *movement.*

**eu·glob·u·lin** (u-glob'u-lin) one of a class of globulins characterized by being insoluble in water but soluble in saline solutions; see *globulin.*

**eu·gly·ce·mia** (u"gli-se'me-ə) a blood glucose level that is within the normal range. Called also *normoglycemia.*

**eu·gly·ce·mic** (u"gli-se'mik) pertaining to, characterized by, or conducive to euglycemia; called also *normoglycemic.*

**eu·gna·thia** (u-na'the-ə) [*eu-* + *gnath-* + *-ia*] an abnormality of the oral cavity which is limited to the teeth and their immediate alveolar supports and does not include the jaws. Cf. *dysgnathia.*

**eu·gnath·ic** (u-nath'ik) [*eu-* + *gnathic*] pertaining to or characterized by eugnathia.

**eu·gno·sia** (u-no'se-ə) [*eu-* + *gnosia*] ability to recognize and synthesize sensory stimuli into a normal perception.

**eu·gnos·tic** (u-nos'tik) pertaining to eugnosia.

**eu·gon·ic** (u-gon'ik) [*eu-* + Gr. *gonē* seed] growing luxuriantly; said of bacterial cultures, especially of species of *Mycobacterium,* that produce heavy growth on culture media. Cf. *dysgonic.*

**eu·hy·dra·tion** (u-hi-dra'shən) a normal state of body water content; absence of absolute or relative hydration or of dehydration.

**eu·kary·on** (u-kar'e-on) [*eu-* + *karyon*] 1. a highly organized nucleus bounded by a nuclear membrane, a characteristic of cells of higher organisms. Cf. *prokaryon.* 2. eukaryote.

**eu·kary·o·sis** (u"kər-e-o'sis) [*eu-* + *karyo-* + *-osis*] the state of having a true nucleus, the nuclear material being surrounded by a membrane and the cytoplasm containing organelles; generally a characteristic of all cell types except bacteria. Cf. *prokaryosis.*

**Eu·kary·o·tae** (u-kar"e-o'te) Eucaryotae.

**eu·kary·ote** (u-kar'e-ōt) [*eu-* + *karyon*] an organism whose cells have a true nucleus, i.e., one bounded by a nuclear membrane, within which lie the chromosomes, combined with proteins and exhibiting mitosis; eukaryotic cells also contain many membrane-bound compartments (organelles) in which cellular functions are performed. The cells of higher plants and animals, fungi, protozoa, and most algae are eukaryotic. See also *Eucaryotae.* Cf. *prokaryote.*

**eu·kary·ot·ic** (u"kər-e-ot'ik) pertaining to a eukaryon or a eukaryote or to eukaryosis.

**eu·ker·a·tin** (u-ker'ə-tin) a true keratin found in hair, nails, feathers, and horns.

**eu·ki·ne·sia** (u"kĭ-ne'zhə) [*eu-* + *kinesi-* + *-ia*] the state of possessing normal or proper motor function or activity; normal or proper mobility.

**eu·ki·ne·sis** (u"kĭ-ne'sis) eukinesia.

**eu·ki·net·ic** (u"kĭ-net'ik) pertaining to or characterized by eukinesia.

**eu·lam·i·nate** (u-lam'ĭ-nāt) having the normal number of lamina, as certain areas of the cerebral cortex.

**Eu·len·burg's disease** (oi'lən-bərgz) [Albert *Eulenburg,* German neurologist, 1840–1917] paramyotonia congenita.

**Eu·ler** (oi'lər) Ulf Svante von. Swedish physiologist, 1905–1983; co-winner, with Julius Axelrod and Sir Bernard Katz, of the Nobel prize for medicine or physiology in 1970 for his discovery of noradrenaline, showing that it is a chemical intermediary for neurotransmission in the sympathetic nervous system.

**Eu·lex·in** (u-lek'sin) trademark for a preparation of flutamide.

**eu·men·or·rhea** (u"mən-o-re'ə) [*eu-* + *menorrhea*] normal menstruation.

**eu·me·tria** (u-me'tre-ə) [Gr. "good measure," "good proportion"] a normal condition of nerve impulse, so that a voluntary movement just reaches the intended goal; the proper range of movement.

**eu·mor·phism** (u-mor′fiz-əm) [*eu-* + *morph-* + *-ism*] retention of the normal form of a cell.

**Eu·my·ce·tes** (u″mi-se′tēz) Eumycota.

**eu·my·ce·to·ma** (u″mi-se-to′mə) [*eu-* + *mycetoma*] eumycotic mycetoma.

**Eu·my·co·ta** (u″mi-ko′tə) [*eu-* + Gr. *mykēs* fungus] the true fungi, a phylum in some systems of classification, consisting of fungi whose trophic phase is not motile but whose reproductive cells may be motile. Subphyla grouped under Eumycota are Ascomycotina, Basidiomycotina, Deuteromycotina, Mastigomycotina, and Zygomycotina.

**eu·nuch** (u′nək) [Gr. *eunouchos*] a man or boy deprived of the testes or the external genital organs, especially one castrated before puberty so that male secondary sex characters characteristics fail to develop.

**eu·nuch·ism** (u′nək-iz-əm) [Gr. *eunouchismos* castration] [MeSH: Eunuchism] 1. the condition of being a eunuch. 2. eunuchoidism.

**eu·nuch·oid** (u′nə-koid) [Gr. *eunouchoeidēs*] 1. resembling or having the characteristics of a eunuch. 2. a male with hypogonadism and deficient secondary sex characters.

**eu·nuch·oid·ism** (u′nə-koi″diz-əm) hypogonadism in a male, with deficiency of the testes or testicular secretions and secondary sex characters.

**female e.,** a type of hypogonadism in females in which the ovaries fail to function at puberty, resulting in absence of secondary sex characters with infantile sexual organs and excessive growth of the long bones.

**hypergonadotropic e.,** conditions caused by androgen deficiency that are associated with high levels of gonadotropins. See *hypergonadotropic hypogonadism,* under *hypogonadism.*

**hypogonadotropic e.,** see under *hypogonadism.*

**eu·os·mia** (u-os′me-ə) [*eu-* + *osm-*[1] + *-ia*] 1. normal state of the sense of smell. 2. a pleasant odor.

**eu·pan·cre·a·tism** (u-pan′kre-ə-tiz″əm) a normal condition of the pancreatic function.

**Eu·pa·to·ri·um** (u″pə-tor′e-əm) a genus of composite-flowered plants (family Compositae). *E. ayapa′na* (called also *Eupato′rium tripliner′ve*) is a Brazilian shrub whose leaves are used medicinally and called *ayapana* (q.v.). *E. rugo′sum* (called also *E. urticaefo′lium*) is the white snakeroot, which contains the toxic principle tremetol and causes trembles in cattle and sheep.

**eu·pep·sia** (u-pep′se-ə) [*eu-* + Gr. *pepsis* digestion + *-ia*] good digestion; particularly the presence of a normal amount of pepsin in the gastric juice. Cf. *dyspepsia.*

**eu·pep·sy** (u′pep-se) eupepsia.

**eu·pep·tic** (u-pep′tik) pertaining to, characterized by, or promoting eupepsia. Cf. *dyspeptic.*

**eu·peri·stal·sis** (u-per″ĭ-stal′sis) normal or painless peristalsis.

**Eu·phor·bia** (u-for′be-ə) the spurges, a large genus of trees, shrubs, and herbs of the family Euphorbiaceae, whose sap is emetic and cathartic and in some species poisonous. *E. antisyphili′tica* Zucca. is candelilla, a shrub that yields candelilla wax.

**eu·pho·ret·ic** (u″fə-ret′ik) 1. producing euphoria. 2. euphoric. 3. an agent that produces euphoria.

**eu·pho·ria** (u-for′e-ə) [Gr. "the power of bearing easily"] [MeSH: Euphoria] an exaggerated feeling of physical and mental well-being, especially when not justified by external reality. Euphoria may be induced by drugs such as opioids, amphetamines, and alcohol and is also a feature of mania.

**eu·pho·ri·ant** (u-for′e-ənt) euphoretic.

**eu·phor·ic** (u-for′ik) characterized by euphoria. Called also *euphoretic.*

**eu·phor·i·gen·ic** (u-for″ĭ-jen′ik) euphoretic (def. 1).

**eu·pho·ris·tic** (u″fə-ris′tik) euphoretic (def. 1).

**eu·plas·tic** (u-plas′tik) [*eu-* + *plastic*] readily becoming organized; adapted to the formation of tissue, as in embryonic development or wound healing.

**eu·ploid** (u′ploid) [*eu-* + *-ploid*] 1. having a balanced set or sets of chromosomes, in any number. 2. an individual or cell having a balanced set or sets of chromosomes, in any number, that is an exact multiple of the haploid number.

**eu·ploi·dy** (u-ploi′de) the state of being euploid.

**eup·nea** (ūp-ne′ə) [*eu-* + *-pnea*] easy or normal respiration.

**eup·ne·ic** (ūp-ne′ik) pertaining to or characterized by eupnea.

**eu·prac·tic** (u-prak′tic) pertaining to, characterized by, or promoting eupraxia.

**eu·prax·ia** (u-prak′se-ə) [Gr. *eupraxin* success, from *en* well + *prassein* to do] intactness of reproduction of acquired, skilled movements.

**eu·prax·ic** (u-prak′sik) 1. concerned in the proper performance of a function. 2. eupractic.

**Eu·proc·tis** (u-prok′tis) a genus of moths. *E. chrysorrhoe′a* (called also *E. phaeorrhoe′a*) is the brown-tail moth, which causes brown-tail moth dermatitis.

**eu·py·rene** (u-pi′rēn) having a normal nucleus or chromatic material; said of certain spermatozoa.

**eu·py·rex·ia** (u″pĭ-rek′se-ə) a slight fever in the early stage of an infection, regarded as an attempt on the part of the individual to combat the infection.

**eu·py·rous** (u′pĭ-rəs) eupyrene.

**Eu·rax** (u′rəks) trademark for preparations of crotamiton.

**Eu·re·sol** (u′rə-sol) trademark for a preparation of resorcinol monoacetate.

**eu·rhyth·mia** (u-rith′me-ə) [Gr. "harmony"] harmonious relationships in body or organ development.

**eu·ro·pi·um** (u-ro′pe-əm) [MeSH: Europium] a rare element, atomic number 63, atomic weight 151.965, symbol Eu.

**Eu·ro·ti·a·ceae** (u-ro″she-a′se-e) Trichocomaceae.

**Eu·ro·ti·a·les** (u-ro″she-a′lēz) in some systems of classification, an order of mainly saprobic perfect fungi of the subphylum Ascomycotina, in which unitunicate asci are irregularly arranged within the primitive cleistothecium; it includes the family Trichocomaceae, which has human pathogens.

**Eu·ro·ti·um** (u-ro′she-əm) [Gr. *eurōs* mold] a genus of fungi or molds of the family Trichocomaceae; several species are perfect (sexual) stages of species of *Aspergillus. E. re′pens,* the sexual stage of *Aspergillus repens,* is sometimes found as a bread mold and occasionally infects human lungs.

**eury-** [Gr. *eurys* wide] a combining form meaning wide or broad.

**eu·ry·ce·phal·ic** (u″re-sə-fal′ik) [*eury-* + *cephalic*] brachycephalic.

**eu·ry·cra·ni·al** (u″re-kra′ne-əl) [*eury-* + *cranial*] brachycranic.

**eu·ryg·nath·ic** (u″rig-nath′ik) pertaining to or characterized by eurygnathism.

**eu·ryg·na·thism** (u-rig′nə-thiz-əm) [*eury-* + *gnatho-* + *-ism*] the state of having a wide jaw.

**eu·ry·on** (u′re-on) [Gr. *eurys* wide] the point on the right and left parietal bones marking the greatest transverse diameter of the skull or head.

**Eu·ry·pel·ma** (u″re-pel′mə) a genus of large spiders. *E. hent′zii* is the American tarantula.

**eu·ry·ther·mal** (u″re-thər′məl) [*eury-* + *thermal*] able to grow in a wide range of temperature, said of bacteria capable of good growth from 28°C to 50°C and above.

**eu·ry·ther·mic** (u″re-thər′mik) [*eury-* + *thermic*] eurythermal.

**Eu·ry·tre·ma** (u-re-tre′mə) a genus of trematodes of the family Dicrocoeliidae. *E. coeloma′ticum* and *E. pancrea′ticum* are found in the pancreatic ducts of sheep and cattle; humans occasionally become infected by eating inadequately cooked livers of other animals.

**Eu·scor·pi·us** (u-skor′pe-əs) a genus of scorpions. *E. ita′licus* is the black scorpion.

**Eu·si·mu·li·um** (u″sĭ-mu′le-əm) a genus of flies of the family Simuliidae, various species of which are common hosts of *Onchocerca volvulus,* a filarial worm parasitic in humans.

**eu·sit·ia** (u-sit′e-ə) [*eu-* + *sit-* + *-ia*] normal appetite.

**eu·splanch·nia** (u-splank′ne-ə) [*eu-* + *splanchno-* + *-ia*] a normal condition of the internal organs.

**eu·sple·nia** (u-sple′ne-ə) normal splenic function.

**eu·sta·chi·an** (u-sta′ke-ən) named for Bartolommeo *Eustachio* (L. *Eustachius*), Italian anatomist, 1524–1574, such as the eustachian muscle, tube, or valve.

**eu·sta·chi·tis** (u″stə-ki′tis) salpingitis, def. 2.

**eu·sthen·ia** (u-sthen′e-ə) [*eu-* + *stheno-* + *-ia*] a condition of normal strength and activity.

**eu·sthen·uria** (u″sthə-nu′re-ə) [*eu-* + *stheno-* + *-uria*] a normal state of the urine as regards osmolality.

**Eu·stron·gy·lus** (u-stron′jə-ləs) *Dioctophyma.*

**eu·sys·to·le** (u-sis′to-le) [*eu-* + *systole*] a normal state of the systole of the heart.

**eu·sys·tol·ic** (u″sis-tol′ik) pertaining to or characterized by eusystole.

**Eu·tam·i·as** (u-tam′e-əs) a genus of North American rodents, the western chipmunks, which can harbor the plague-infected flea *Monopsyllus eumolpi* and have sometimes been found infected with plague.

**eu·tec·tic** (u-tek′tik) [Gr. *eutēktos* easily melted or dissolved] 1. easily melted; used specifically of a mixture that melts at a lower temperature than any of its ingredients. 2. a solution or alloy of two or more components having the lowest possible melting temperature that could be obtained by manipulating the ratios of the components. 3. pertaining to such a solution, or to the lowest melting temperature so obtained.

**eu·telo·lec·i·thal** (u-tel″o-les′ĭ-thəl) [*eu-* + *telolecithal*] having deutoplasm greatly in excess of the cell protoplasm; said of the ova of birds and many reptiles. Cf. *oligolecithal* and *telolecithal.*

**eu·tha·na·sia** (u″thə-na′zhə) [*eu-* + Gr. *thanatos* death] [MeSH: Euthanasia] 1. an easy or painless death. 2. mercy killing; the deliberate ending of the life of a person suffering from an incurable and painful disease.

**eu·ther·a·peu·tic** (u-ther″ə-pu′tik) [*eu-* + *therapeutic*] having good therapeutic properties.

**Eu·the·ria** (u-the′re-ə) [*eu-* + Gr. *thērion* beast, animal] in some systems of classification, a subclass of the Mammalia and in others an infraclass of the subclass Theria, including all the true placental mammals, and excluding the monotremes and marsupials.

**eu·the·ri·an** (u-the′re-ən) any member of the Eutheria.

**eu·ther·mic** (u-thər′mik) [Gr. *euthermos* very warm] characterized by the proper temperature; promoting warmth.

**eu·thy·mia** (u-thi′me-ə) [*eu-* + Gr. *thymos* mind] a state of mental tranquility and well-being; neither depressed nor manic.

**Eu·throid** (u′throid) trademark for a preparation of liotrix.

**eu·thy·mism** (u-thi′miz-əm) a normal condition of thymus activity.

**Eu·thy·neu·ra** (u″thə-nu′rə) a subclass of gastropods, including snails and slugs found chiefly in fresh water or terrestrial habitats; many species are primary or intermediate hosts of trematodes and other pathogens. It includes the order Pulmonata.

**eu·thy·roid** (u-thi′roid) characterized by euthyroidism.

**eu·thy·roid·ism** (u-thi′roid-iz-əm) the condition of having normal thyroid function, as opposed to hyperthyroidism and hypothyroidism.

**eu·to·cia** (u-to′shə) [Gr. *eutokia*] normal labor, or childbirth.

**Eu·to·nyl** (u′tə-nəl) trademark for a preparation of pargyline hydrochloride.

**eu·top·ic** (u-top′ik) [*eu-* + *top-* + *-ic*] situated normally; arising from the normal site or tissue. Cf. *ectopic.*

**Eu·tri·at·o·ma** (u″tre-at′ə-mə) a genus of reduviid bugs, species of which transmit Chagas′ disease.

**Eu·trom·bic·u·la** (u″trom-bik′u-lə) a subgenus of the mite genus *Trombicula.*
**E. alfreddugè′si,** a species whose larval form is the common chigger of the United States, a cause of dermatitis *(trombiculiasis)* in many species of birds and mammals, including humans. Called also *Trombicula alfreddugèsi* and *T. irritans.*
**E. splen′dens,** a species whose chigger causes trombiculiasis in humans and other animals in the southeastern United States; called also *Trombicula splendens.*

**Eu·tron** (u′tron) trademark for preparations of pargyline hydrochloride and methyclothiazide.

**eu·tro·phia** (u-tro′fe-ə) [*eu-* + *tropho-* + *-ia*] a state of normal (good) nutrition.

**eu·troph·ic** (u-trof′ik) pertaining to, characterized by, or conducive to good nutrition.

**eu·tro·phi·ca·tion** (u″tro-fĭ-ka′shən) [MeSH: Eutrophication] the promotion of excessive growth of an organism to the disadvantage of other organisms in the same ecosystem by oversupplying the former with nutrients; e.g., the stimulation of excessive growth of plants and algae in natural waters by an oversupply of inorganic nitrogen and phosphate compounds found in fertilizers.

**eu·vo·lia** (u-vo′le-ə) normal water content or volume of a given body compartment, e.g., extracellular euvolia. Cf. *normovolemia.*

**eV, ev** electron volt.

**evac·u·ant** (e-vak′u-ənt) [L. *evacuans*] 1. emptying. 2. cathartic (def. 1). 3. a remedy that empties any organ, such as a cathartic, emetic, or diuretic.

**evac·u·a·tion** (e-vak″u-a′shən) [L. *evacuatio*] 1. an emptying. 2. purgation. 3. feces.

**evac·u·a·tor** (e-vak′u-a-tər) an instrument for removing fluid or small particles from a body cavity or container; formerly applied to one for compelling evacuation of the bowels or bladder.

**evag·i·na·tion** (e-vaj″ĭ-na′shən) an outpouching of a layer or part.
**optic e.,** vesicula ophthalmica.

**ev·a·nes·cent** (ev″ə-nes′ənt) [L. *evanescere* to vanish away] vanishing; passing away quickly; unstable; unfixed.

**Ev·ans′ syndrome** (ev′ənz) [Robert Sherman *Evans,* American physician, born 1912] see under *syndrome.*

**evap·o·ra·tion** (e-vap″o-ra′shən) [L. *e* out + *vaporare* to steam] conversion of a liquid or solid into vapor.

**eva·sion** (e-va′zhən) in psychiatry, suppression of an idea that would come next in a thought sequence and substitution of a closely related idea; a form of paralogia.

**even·tra·tion** (e″ven-tra′shən) [L. *eventratio* disembowelment, from *e* out + *venter* belly] 1. an intestinal hernia; see *hernia.* 2. evisceration, def. 2.
**diaphragmatic e.,** elevation of the dome of the diaphragm, usually the result of paralysis of a phrenic nerve.
**umbilical e.,** omphalocele.

**Evers·busch′s operation** (a′vərz-boosh″əz) [Oskar *Eversbusch,* German ophthalmologist, 1853–1912] see under *operation.*

**ever·sion** (e-ver′zhən) [L. *eversio*] 1. a turning inside out. Called also *ectropion.* 2. a turning outward, as of the sole of the foot or the eyelid.

**evert** (e-vərt′) [L. *e* out + *vertere* to turn] 1. to turn inside out. 2. to turn outward, as the sole of the foot or the eyelid.

**ever·tor** (ə-vər′tər) a muscle that turns a part outward.

**Evex** (e′vəks) trademark for a preparation of esterified estrogens.

**évide·ment** (a-vēd-maw′) [Fr.] the operation of scooping out a cavity or diseased portion of an organ.

**évi·deur** (a-ve-dər′) [Fr.] an instrument for performing évidement.

**evil** (e′vil) disease.
**poll e.,** an abscess behind the ears of a horse, caused by a dual infection of the supra-atlantal bursa by *Brucella* and *Actinomyces;* this condition is virtually identical to fistulous withers.
**quarter e.,** blackleg.

**evi·ra·tion** (e″vĭ-ra′shən) [L. *e* out + *vir* man] 1. castration. 2. feminization. 3. a delusional belief of a man that he has become a woman.

**evis·cer·a·tion** (e-vis″ər-a′shən) [*e-* + *viscus*] 1. extrusion of viscera outside the body, especially through a surgical incision. See also *hernia.* 2. removal of viscera. Called also *devisceration* and *eventration.* 3. in ophthalmology the removal of the contents of the eyeball, with the sclera being left intact.

**Evis·ta** (e-vis′tə) trademark for a preparation of raloxifene hydrochloride.

**evo·ca·tion** (ev″o-ka′shən) [L. *e* out + *vocare* to call] the calling forth of morphogenetic potentialities through contact with organizer material.

**evo·ca·tor** (ev′o-ka″tər) a chemical substance emitted by an organizer region of an embryo that evokes a specific morphogenetic response from competent embryonic tissue in contact with it.

**evo·lu·tion** (ev″ə-loo′shən) [L. *evolutio,* from *e* out + *volvere* to roll] [MeSH: Evolution] 1. an unrolling. 2. a process of development in which an organ or organism becomes more and more complex by the differentiation of its parts; a continuous and progressive change according to certain laws and by means of resident forces. 3. preformation. Cf. *devolution.*
**bathmic e.,** evolution due to something in the organism itself independent of environment; called also *orthogenic e.*
**convergent e.,** the appearance of similar forms and/or functions in two or more lines not sufficiently related phylogenetically to account for the similarity.
**Denman′s spontaneous e.,** a mechanism of spontaneous version in shoulder presentations in which the head rotates behind, and as the breech descends the shoulder ascends in the pelvis, the breech

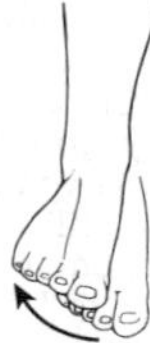

Eversion.

finally coming down and emerging. Called also *Denman's spontaneous version.*
**determinate e.,** orthogenesis, def. 2.
**emergent e.,** the assumption that each step in evolution produces something new and something that could not be predicted from its antecedents.
**organic e.,** the origin and development of species; the theory that existing organisms are the result of descent with modification from those of past times.
**orthogenic e.,** bathmic e.
**parallel e.,** the independent evolution of similar structures in two or more rather closely related organisms.
**saltatory e.,** evolution showing sudden changes; mutation or saltation.

**evul·sio** (e-vul'se-o) [L., from *evellere* to pull out] evulsion.

**evul·sion** (e-vul'shən) [L. *evulsio*] forcible extraction; see *avulsion.*

**Ew·art's sign** (u'ərts) [William *Ewart,* English physician, 1848–1929] see under *sign.*

**Ew·ing's tumor (sarcoma)** (u'ingz) [James *Ewing,* American pathologist, 1866–1943] see under *tumor.*

**Ew·ing·el·la** (u"ing-el'ə) [W. H. *Ewing,* American bacteriologist] a proposed genus of gram-negative, facultatively anaerobic, rod-shaped bacteria of the family Enterobacteriaceae. The organisms belong to enteric group 40. The type species is *E. america'na.*

**ex-** [L. *ex* out of, away from] a prefix meaning away from, without, or outside; it is sometimes used to denote completely, as in *exacerbation.*

**exa-** [Gr. *hexa* because it is sixth in the series of prefixes for multiples] a combining form used in naming units of measurement to indicate a quantity one quintillion ($10^{18}$) times the unit designated by the root with which it is combined. Symbol E.

**ex·ac·er·ba·tion** (eg-zas"ər-ba'shən) [*ex-* + L. *acerbus* harsh] increase in the severity of a disease or any of its symptoms.

**ex·air·e·sis** (ek-sār'ə-sis) [Gr. "a taking out"] exeresis.

**ex·al·ta·tion** (eg"zawl-ta'shən) a feeling of extreme elation, often associated with delusions of grandeur.

**ex·a·meta·zime** (eks"ə-met'ə-zēm) HMPAO; hexamethylpropyleneamine oxime, a neutral lipophilic compound that traverses the blood-brain barrier and localizes in the brain; complexed with technetium 99m it is used for imaging of cerebral regional blood flow in the detection of altered regional perfusion in stroke, identification of Alzheimer's disease, evaluation of epilepsy, and diagnosis of brain death. The same complex can also be used to label autologous leukocytes for diagnostic studies of intra-abdominal inflammatory lesions and bowel disease. See table at *technetium.*

**ex·am·i·na·tion** (eg-zam"ĭ-na'shən) [L. *examinare*] inspection, palpation, auscultation, percussion, or other means of investigation, especially for diagnosing disease, qualified according to the methods employed, as physical examination, radiologic examination, diagnostic imaging examination, or cystoscopic examination.
**double-contrast e.,** radiologic examination of the stomach or intestine using first a high concentration of contrast medium and, after most of that has been evacuated, injection of air or an effervescent substance to inflate the organ; the light coating of contrast medium on the mucosal surface reveals clearly any abnormalities. In the intestine this is called a *double-contrast enema.* See also *mucosal relief radiography* under *radiography.*
**Mental Status E.,** MSE; a component of the medical examination comprising the systematic evaluation of the mental status of the patient, including appearance, psychomotor behavior, speech, thinking and perception, emotional state including affect and mood, insight and judgment, intelligence, sensorium, attention and concentration, and memory.
**Present State E.,** a nondiagnostic semi-structured interview administered by a professional and measuring psychiatric symptoms in a variety of areas, concentrating on the one month interval preceding the interview.

**ex·a·nia** (ek-sa'ne-ə) [*ex-* + *anus*] prolapse of the rectum.

**ex·an·i·ma·tion** (eg-zan"ĭ-ma'shən) unconsciousness; coma.

**ex·an·them** (eg-zan'thəm) [Gr. *exanthēma*] 1. a skin eruption or rash. 2. a disease in which skin eruptions or rashes are a prominent manifestation. Classically, six exanthems (or exanthematous diseases) were described that had similar rashes; they were numbered in the order in which they were reported: first *(measles),* second *(scarlet fever),* third *(rubella),* fourth *(Dukes' disease),* fifth *(erythema infectiosum),* and sixth *(exanthema subitum);* only the latter three ordinal designations are still used.
**Boston e.,** a mild febrile exanthematous illness caused by echovirus 16, an epidemic of which occurred in Boston, Massachusetts.
**e. su'bitum,** exanthema subitum.

**ex·an·the·ma** (eg"zan-the'mə) pl. *exanthemas, exanthem'ata* [Gr. *exanthēma*] [MeSH: Exanthema] exanthem.
**equine coital e.,** a benign venereal disease of horses, caused by a herpesvirus, characterized by vesicles and ulcers on the external genitalia, and occasionally on the lips, nares, and conjunctiva, that heal within a few weeks.
**e. su'bitum,** an acute, short-lived disease of infants and young children, caused by human herpesvirus 6; after a high fever of 3 to 4 days' duration the temperature suddenly drops to normal; either shortly before, simultaneously with, or shortly after this happens, a macular or maculopapular rash appears on the trunk and spreads to other areas. The disease was given the ordinal designation *sixth disease* to differentiate it from other exanthems (see *exanthem,* def. 2.). Called also *exanthem subitum, roseola,* and *roseola infantum.*
**vesicular e.,** a disease of swine that was seen in 1959; it was caused by a calicivirus and was marked by vesicles on the snout, lips, tongue, feet, and teats.

**ex·an·them·a·ta** (eg"zan-them'ə-tə) [Gr.] plural of *exanthema.*

**ex·an·them·a·tous** (eg"zan-them'ə-təs) pertaining to, characterized by, or of the nature of an exanthem.

**ex·an·thrope** (ek'san-thrōp) [*ex-* + Gr. *anthrōpos* man] any source of disease not situated within the human body.

**ex·an·throp·ic** (ek"san-throp'ik) of the nature of an exanthrope; not situated within the human body.

**ex·ar·tic·u·la·tion** (eks"ahr-tik"u-la'shən) [*ex-* + *articulation*] disarticulation.

**ex·ca·la·tion** (eks"kə-la'shən) absence or exclusion of one member of a normal series, such as a vertebra.

**ex·car·na·tion** (eks"kahr-na'shən) [*ex-* + L. *caro, carnis* flesh] removal of superfluous fleshy tissue from a preparation.

**ex·ca·va·tio** (eks"kə-va'she-o) pl. *excavatio'nes* [L., from *ex* out + *cavus* hollow] [TA] excavation: a general term for a hollowed-out space, or pouchlike cavity.
**e. dis'ci** [TA], excavation of optic disk: a depression in the center of the optic disk; called also *optic* or *physiological cup* and *e. papillae nervi optici.*
**e. papil'lae ner'vi op'tici,** e. disci.
**e. rectouteri'na** [TA], rectouterine excavation: a sac or recess formed by a fold of the peritoneum dipping down between the rectum and the uterus; called also *Douglas' cul-de-sac, pouch of Douglas, Douglas' space,* and *rectouterine, rectovaginal, uterovesical,* or *vesicouterine pouch.*
**e. rectovesica'lis** [TA], rectovesical excavation: the space between the rectum and the bladder in the peritoneal cavity of the male; called also *rectovesical pouch.*
**e. vesicouteri'na** [TA], vesicouterine excavation: the space between the bladder and the uterus in the peritoneal cavity; called also *uterovesical* or *vesicouterine pouch.*

**ex·ca·va·tion** (eks"kə-va'shən) [L. *excavatio*] 1. the act of hollowing out. 2. a hollowed-out space, or pouchlike cavity.
**atrophic e.,** the cupping of the optic disk, caused by atrophy of the optic nerve fibers.
**dental e.,** removal of carious material from a tooth in preparation for restoration. See also *cavity preparation,* under *preparation,* and *prepared cavity,* under *cavity.*
**glaucomatous e.,** see under *cup.*
**ischiorectal e.,** fossa ischioanalis.
**e. of optic disk, physiologic e.,** excavatio disci.
**rectoischiadic e.,** fossa ischioanalis.
**rectouterine e.,** excavatio recto-uterina.
**rectovesical e.,** excavatio rectovesicalis.
**vesicouterine e.,** excavatio vesico-uterina.

**ex·ca·va·ti·o·nes** (eks"kə-va"she-o'nēz) [L.] plural of *excavatio.*

**ex·ca·va·tor** (eks'kə-va"tor) 1. an instrument for hollowing out something by removing the center or inner part, or for making a hole or cavity. 2. a scoop or gouge for surgical use.
**dental e.,** a handcutting instrument designed for removing the carious dentin of a decayed tooth. See also *discoid,* def. 4.
**hatchet e.,** hatchet.
**spoon e.,** a dental excavator having a spoonlike blade with the entire margin tapered and sharpened to cut carious dentin out of tooth cavities. Called also *spoon.*

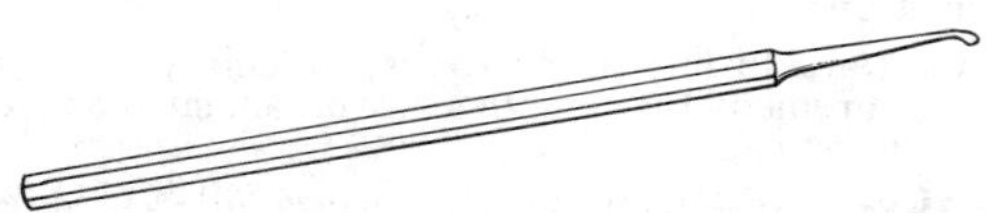

Excavator.

**ex·cer·e·bra·tion** (ek″ser-ə-bra′shən) [*ex-* + L. *cerebrum* brain] the removal of the brain, chiefly that of the fetus in embryotomy.

**ex·cer·nent** (ek-ser′nənt) [L. *excernere* to sift, to separate] causing an evacuation or discharge.

**ex·cess** (ek-ses′, ek′ses) the state of exceeding that which is normal, sufficient, or needed; superfluous.
**antibody e.,** see *prozone.*
**antigen e.,** see *precipitin reaction,* under *reaction.*
**base e.,** the deviation from normal of the concentration of titratable base when blood or plasma is titrated to a plasma pH of 7.40 at a $pCO_2$ of 40 mm Hg at 37°C; it is 1.2 times the deviation of the standard bicarbonate from normal. Positive values indicate metabolic alkalosis; negative values, metabolic acidosis.

**ex·change** (eks-chānj) 1. the substitution of one thing for another. 2. to substitute one thing for another.
**plasma e.,** the removal of plasma from withdrawn blood, usually to a greater extent than in plasmapheresis, with retransfusion of the formed elements into the donor; done for removal of circulating antibodies or abnormal plasma constituents. The plasma removed is replaced by type-specific frozen plasma or albumin.
**sister chromatid e.,** the exchange of segments of DNA between sister chromatids, which occurs very often in patients with Bloom syndrome.

**ex·chang·er** (eks-chānj′ər) an apparatus by which something may be exchanged.
**heat e.,** a device which is placed in the circuit of extracorporeal circulation to induce rapid cooling and rewarming of blood.

**ex·cip·i·ent** (ek-sip′e-ənt) [L. *excipiens,* from *ex* out + *capere* to take] any more or less inert substance added to a prescription in order to confer a suitable consistency or form to the drug; called also *vehicle.*

**ex·cise** (ek-sīz′) to cut out or off.

**ex·ci·sion** (ek-sizh′ən) [L. *excisio,* from *ex* out + *caedere* to cut] removal, as of an organ, by cutting. Called also *resection* and *ectomy.*
**intracapsular e.,** in surgery for soft tissue sarcoma, removal of the tumor alone by direct incision of the tumor capsule; of diagnostic value only since it leaves some gross tumor intact.
**marginal e.,** surgical removal of an entire lesion, including only a very small margin of surrounding tissue.
**radical e.,** in surgery for soft tissue sarcoma, removal of the entire anatomic compartment containing the tumor, as well as the origins and insertions of all muscles, bones, and joints contained in the compartment; frequently it involves the amputation of a limb.
**wide e.,** in surgery for neoplasms, removal of both the tumor and a margin of apparently normal surrounding tissue; the limb, breast, or other body structure that is the site of the tumor is not amputated.

**ex·ci·ta·bil·i·ty** (ek-sīt″ə-bil′ĭ-te) 1. readiness to respond to a stimulus; irritability. 2. the capacity of a cell to depolarize and form an action potential when in the presence of a stimulus stronger than a threshold value.

**ex·ci·ta·ble** (ek-sīt′ə-bəl) [L. *excitabilis*] susceptible of stimulation; responding to a stimulus.

**ex·cit·ant** (ek-sīt′ənt) any agent that produces excitation of the vital functions, or of those of the brain.

**ex·ci·ta·tion** (ek″si-ta′shən) [L. *excitatio,* from *ex* out + *citare* to call] an act of irritation or stimulation or of responding to a stimulus; the addition of energy, as the excitation of a molecule by absorption of photons.
**direct e.,** electrostimulation of a muscle by placing the electrode on the muscle itself.
**indirect e.,** electrostimulation of a muscle by placing the electrode on its nerve.
**reentrant e.,** reexcitation of cardiac tissue due to reentry; sometimes used synonymously with reentry.

**ex·ci·ta·to·ry** (ek-si′tə-tor″e) tending to excitation or stimulation.

**ex·cite·ment** (ek-sīt′ment) response to stimuli, often used specifically to denote excessive responsiveness to stimuli, particularly of an emotional nature, and often leading to impulsive activity.
**catatonic e.,** periods of uncontrollable, unorganized, and apparently purposeless motor activity, without euphoria or other symptoms of mania; characteristic of catatonic schizophrenia.
**psychomotor e.,** see under *acceleration.*

**ex·ci·to·an·a·bol·ic** (ek-si″to-an″ə-bol′ik) stimulating anabolism.

**ex·ci·to·cat·a·bol·ic** (ek-si″to-kat″ə-bol′ik) stimulating catabolism.

**ex·ci·to·glan·du·lar** (ek-si″to-glan′du-lər) causing glands to secrete.

**ex·ci·to·met·a·bol·ic** (ek-si″to-met″ə-bol′ik) producing metabolic changes.

**ex·ci·to·mo·tor** (ek-si″to-mo′tər) 1. tending to produce motion or motor function. 2. an agent that induces motion or functional activity.

**ex·ci·to·mus·cu·lar** (ek-si″to-mus′ku-lər) stimulating muscular activity.

**ex·ci·tor** (ek-si′tər) a nerve that when stimulated excites greater action in the part it supplies.

**ex·ci·to·se·cre·to·ry** (ek-si″to-se-kre′to-re) producing increased secretion.

**ex·ci·to·tox·ic** (ek-si″to-tok′sik) having a toxic excitatory effect on the nervous system; see *excitotoxin.*

**ex·ci·to·tox·in** (ek-si″to-tok′sin) any of a group of neurotoxic substances found in certain plants or made synthetically; they are analogous to glutamic acid and mimic its excitatory effects on neurons of the central nervous system as well as producing lesions on the perikarya; several of them are used experimentally to study the excitatory mechanisms of glutamate transmitters. They include ibotenic acid, kainic acid, quisqualic acid, and *N*-methyl-D-aspartate (NMDA).

**ex·ci·to·vas·cu·lar** (ek-si″to-vas′ku-lər) causing vascular changes.

**ex·clave** (eks′klāv) [*ex-* + L. *clavis* key, by analogy with *enclave*] a detached part of an organ, as of the pancreas, thyroid, or other gland.

**ex·clu·sion** (eks-kloo′zhən) [L. *exclusio,* from *ex* out + *claudere* to shut] 1. elimination, rejection, or extrusion. 2. an operation in which a portion of an organ is separated from the remainder but is not removed from the body.
**allelic e.,** a mechanism that allows the expression of only one of a set of alleles; seen in the expression of a single immunoglobulin by any one B lymphocyte or plasma cell and in the expression of a single T cell receptor by any one T lymphocyte.
**competitive e.,** the tendency for the better adapted species to exclude another related species from its particular ecological niche. See also *character displacement,* under *displacement.*

**ex·coch·le·a·tion** (eks-kok″le-a′shən) [*ex-* + L. *cochlea* spoon] the operation of curetting or scooping out a cavity.

**ex·con·ju·gant** (eks-kon′jo͞o-gənt) [*ex-* + L. *conjugare* to join] either member of a pair of ciliate protozoa or bacteria (conjugants) after separation following conjugation.

**ex·co·ri·a·tion** (eks-kor″e-a′shən) [L. *excoriare* to flay, from *ex* out + *corium* skin] a scratch or abrasion of the skin.
**neurotic e.,** a self-induced skin lesion, inflicted by the fingernails or other physical means.

**ex·cre·ment** (eks′krə-mənt) [L. *excrementum,* from *ex* out + *cernere* to sift, to separate] 1. matter cast out as waste from the body; see also *discharge* (def. 3). 2. feces.

**ex·cre·men·ti·tious** (eks″krə-mən-tish′əs) 1. pertaining to excrement. 2. fecal.

**ex·cres·cence** (eks-kres′əns) [*ex-* + L. *crescere* to grow] any abnormal outgrowth; a projection of morbid origin.
**fungating e., fungous e.,** a fungous growth in the umbilicus after separation of the umbilical cord; granuloma of the umbilicus.
**Lambl's e's,** small papillary projections on the cardiac valves seen post mortem on many adult hearts.

**ex·cres·cent** (eks-kres′ənt) resembling or of the nature of an excrescence.

**ex·cre·ta** (eks-kre′tə) [L., pl.] excretion (def. 2).

**ex·crete** (eks-krēt′) [L. *excernere*] to throw off or eliminate by a normal discharge, such as waste matter. Called also *void.*

**ex·cre·tin** (eks-kre′tin) a crystalline compound, $C_{20}H_{36}O$, derivable from human feces.

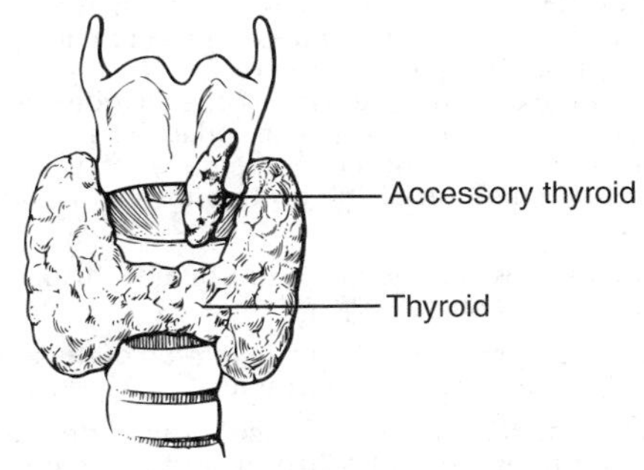

The accessory thyroid is an exclave of the thyroid.

**ex·cre·tion** (eks-kre'shən) [L. *excretio*] 1. the act, process, or function of excreting. 2. material that is excreted. Cf. *elimination.*
**pseudouridine e.**, increased excretion of pseudouridine in the urine of gouty patients, the significance of which remains to be established; a greater turnover of some forms of RNA has been suggested, possibly adding to the hyperuricemia of gout.

**ex·cre·to·ry** (eks'krə-tor-e) of, pertaining to, or subserving excretion.

**ex·cur·rent** (eks-kər'ənt) excretory; efferent.

**ex·cur·sion** (eks-kər'zhən) [L. *excurrere* to run out from] movements occurring from a normal, or rest, position of a movable part in performance of a function, as those of the mandible to attain functional contact between the cusps of the mandibular and maxillary teeth in mastication, or of the chest wall in respiration. Called also *excursive movements.*
**lateral e.**, sideward movement of the mandible between the position of closure and that in which the tips of the cusps of opposing teeth are in vertical proximity.
**protrusive e.**, movement of the mandible between the position of closure and that in which the incisal edges of the anterior teeth are in vertical approximation.
**retrusive e.**, the slight backward and return movement of the mandible between the position of closure and one slightly posterior, more often present with mandibular overclosure.

**ex·cur·sive** (eks-kər'siv) pertaining to or characterized by excursion.

**ex·cy·clo·pho·ria** (ek-si"klo-for'e-ə) [*ex-* + *cyclophoria*] cyclophoria in which the upper pole of the vertical axis of the eye deviates away from the midline of the face and toward the temple; called also *positive* (or *plus*) *cyclophoria.* Cf. *incyclophoria.*

**ex·cy·clo·tro·pia** (ek-si"klo-tro'pe-ə) [*ex-* + *cyclotropia*] cyclotropia in which the upper pole of the vertical axis of the eye deviates away from the midline of the face, and toward the temple; called also *positive* (or *plus*) *cyclotropia.*

**ex·cys·ta·tion** (ek"sis-ta'shən) escape from a cyst or envelope; especially a stage in the life cycle of parasites occurring after the cystic form has been swallowed by the host.

**Ex·el·derm** (ek'sel-dərm") trademark for a preparation of sulconazole nitrate.

**ex·e·mia** (eg-se'me-ə) [*ex-* + *-emia*] loss of fluid from the blood vessels, with resultant hemoconcentration.

**ex·en·ce·pha·lia** (ek"sən-sə-fa'le-ə) exencephaly.

**ex·en·ceph·a·lon** (ek"sən-sef'ə-lon) exencephalus.

**ex·en·ceph·a·lous** (ek"sən-sef'ə-ləs) characterized by exencephaly.

**ex·en·ceph·a·lus** (ek"sən-sef'ə-ləs) [*ex-* + Gr. *enkephalos* brain] a fetus exhibiting exencephaly.

**ex·en·ceph·a·ly** (ek"sən-sef'ə-le) [*ex-* + Gr. *enkephalos* brain] a developmental anomaly characterized by acrania with the brain exposed.

**ex·en·ter·a·tion** (ek-sen"tər-a'shən) [*ex-* + Gr. *enteron* bowel] 1. surgical removal of the inner organs; commonly used to indicate radical excision of the contents of a body cavity, as of the pelvis. 2. in ophthalmology, removal of the entire contents of the orbit.
**pelvic e.**, excision of the organs and adjacent structures of the pelvis.
**pelvic e., anterior**, excision en masse of the bladder, lower ureters, vagina, adnexa, pelvic lymph nodes, and pelvic peritoneum, with implantation of the ureters into the intact pelvic colon or an ileal conduit. See also *radical cystectomy,* under *cystectomy.*
**pelvic e., posterior**, excision en masse of the pelvic colon, uterus, vagina, and adnexa, with or without pelvic lymph node excision, the lower urinary tract being undisturbed.
**pelvic e., total**, excision en masse of the bladder, lower ureters, vagina, uterus, adnexa, and the pelvic and lower sigmoid colon, with excision of the pelvic lymph nodes, removal of all the pelvic peritoneum, and replantation of the ureters into an isolated ileal segment.

**ex·en·ter·a·tive** (ek-sen'tər-ə-tiv) pertaining to or requiring exenteration, as exenterative surgery.

**ex·en·ter·itis** (ek-sen"tər-i'tis) inflammation of the peritoneal covering of the intestine; visceral peritonitis.

**ex·er·cise** (ek'sər-sīz) [MeSH: Exercise] the performance of physical exertion for improvement of health or the correction of physical deformity.
**active e.**, motion imparted to a part by voluntary contraction and relaxation of the muscles controlling the part. Called also *free e.*
**active assisted e.**, motion imparted to a part of the body by voluntary contraction of muscles controlling the part, assisted by a therapist or by some other means.
**aerobic e.**, systematic exercise designed to increase oxygen consumption and improve the functioning of the respiratory and cardiovascular systems.
**breathing e's**, exercises to improve respiration, used both in primary respiratory disorders and in those due to musculoskeletal malformations, including relaxation techniques for slower, more efficient breathing patterns and techniques for better diaphragmatic, abdominal, and intercostal muscle coordination.
**corrective e.**, therapeutic e.
**endurance e.**, any exercise that involves the use of several large groups of muscles and is thus dependent on the delivery of oxygen to the muscles by the cardiovascular system; used in both physical fitness programs and testing of cardiovascular and pulmonary function.
**flexion back e's**, an exercise regimen designed to decrease low back pain by flexing the lumbosacral spine and strengthening the muscles in the region.
**free e.**, active e.
**Frenkel's e's**, a series of movements of increasing difficulty and precision to be performed by ataxic patients for restoration of coordination.
**isokinetic e.**, dynamic muscle activity performed at a constant angular velocity; torque and tension remain constant while muscles shorten or lengthen.
**isometric e.**, active exercise performed against stable resistance, without change in the length of the muscle. Called also *muscle-setting e.* and *static e.*
**isotonic e.**, active exercise without appreciable change in the force of muscular contraction, with shortening of the muscle.
**Kegel e's**, exercises performed to strengthen the pubococcygeal muscle, for controlling or preventing stress incontinence, improving sexual response, and diminishing a variety of problems and discomfort in pregnancy.
**muscle-setting e.**, isometric e.
**passive e.**, motion imparted to a segment of the body by another individual, machine, or other outside force, or produced by voluntary effort of another segment of the patient's own body.
**progressive resistance e., progressive resistive e.**, a physical therapy method of strengthening debilitated muscles by increasing the amount of the resisting force at regular time intervals.
**range of motion e.**, the putting of a joint through its full range of normal movements; it may be either active or passive.
**relaxation e.**, any exercise designed to decrease muscle tension, whether due to psychogenic causes, excess of physical exertion, or an organic neurologic condition; it may involve breathing exercise or the rhythmic shaking of the affected part.
**resistance e., resistive e.**, that performed by the patient against resistance supplied either by a weight or by the muscle power of the therapist.
**static e.**, isometric e.
**therapeutic e.**, the scientific use of bodily movement to restore normal function in diseased or injured tissues or to maintain a state of well being. Called also *corrective e.*
**underwater e.**, exercise performed in a pool or a large tub of water. The buoyancy of the water allows much freer movement of weakened body parts than is possible under normal atmospheric conditions; water temperature and water currents can be varied for different therapeutic effects. Cf. *Hubbard tank.*
**Williams' e's, Williams' flexion e's**, widely used flexion back exercises involving flexion of the neck, trunk, pelvis, and legs; designed to alleviate lower back pain by stretching the extensor muscles in the lower back and strengthening flexors such as the rectus abdominis and gluteus maximus.

**ex·er·e·sis** (ek-ser'ə-sis) [Gr. *exairesis* a taking out] surgical removal or excision.

**ex·er·gon·ic** (ek"sər-gon'ik) [*ex-* + Gr. *ergon* work] characterized or accompanied by the release of energy; said of reactions, particularly biochemical reactions, that release free energy, yielding products having a lower free energy than did the reactants. Opposed to *endergonic.*

**ex·e·sion** (eg-ze'zhən) [L. *exedere* to eat out] the gradual destruction of superficial parts of a tissue.

**ex·fe·ta·tion** (eks"fe-ta'shən) [*ex-* + L. *fetus*] ectopic or extrauterine pregnancy.

**ex·flag·el·la·tion** (eks-flaj"ə-la'shən) [*ex-* + L. *flagellum*] the rapid formation in the gut of the insect vector of microgametes from the microgamont in *Plasmodium* and certain other sporozoan protozoa.

**ex·fo·li·a·tin** (eks-fo″le-a′tin) [*ex-* + L. *folium* leaf] an erythrogenic, epidermolytic, heat-stabile, acid-labile exotoxin produced by certain strains of *Staphylococcus aureus* (phage group II), which causes intraepidermal separation by disturbing the adhesive forces between cells in the stratum granulosum to give rise to the clinical manifestations of the scalded skin syndrome. Called also *epidermolysin.*

**ex·fo·li·a·tio** (eks″fo-le-a′she-o) [L., from *ex* away from + *folium* leaf] exfoliation.
**e. area′ta lin′guae,** benign migratory glossitis.

**ex·fo·li·a·tion** (eks-fo″le-a′shən) [L. *exfoliatio*] 1. a falling off in scales or layers. 2. the normal loss of deciduous teeth following loss of their root structure.
**lamellar e. of newborn,** see *collodion baby,* under *baby.*

**ex·fo·li·a·tive** (eks-fo′le-ə-tiv″) characterized by exfoliation.

**ex·ha·la·tion** (eks″hə-la′shən) [L. *exhalatio,* from *ex* out + *halare* to breathe] 1. the act of breathing out. 2. the giving off of watery or other vapor; see also *effluvium.* 3. a vapor or effluvium that is exhaled or given off. Defs. 1, 2, and 3 called also *expiration.*

**ex·hale** (eks′hāl) [*ex-* + L. *halare* to breathe] 1. to expel from the lungs by breathing. 2. to give off a watery or other vapor. Defs. 1 and 2 called also *expire.*

**ex·haus·tion** (eg-zaws′chən) [*ex-* + L. *haurire* to drain] 1. a state of extreme mental or physical fatigue. 2. the state of being drained, emptied, consumed, or used up.
**combat e.,** older term for a form of posttraumatic stress disorder in which the traumatic event is combat-related.
**heat e.,** an effect of excessive exposure to heat, occurring among workers in hot places such as furnace rooms and foundries and sometimes in those under prolonged exposure to the sun's heat. It is marked by subnormal temperature, with dizziness, headache, nausea, and sometimes delirium or collapse. Distinguished from *heat stroke* and *sunstroke,* in which the body temperature may be dangerously elevated. Called also *heat prostration.*
**postactivation e., posttetanic e.,** changes at the cellular level, such as decreased neuromuscular transmission, seen when repetitive nerve stimulation is performed a few minutes after intense neuromuscular activity; see also *postactivation depression* and *postactivation facilitation.*

**Exhib.** abbreviation for L. *exhibea′tur,* let it be given.

**ex·hi·bi·tion·ism** (eg″zĭ-bish′ə-niz-əm) [DSM-IV] [MeSH: Exhibitionism] a paraphilia characterized by recurrent intense sexual urges and sexually arousing fantasies of exposing the genitals to an unsuspecting stranger. Exhibitionism occurs almost exclusively in males.

**ex·hi·bi·tion·ist** (eg″zĭ-bish′ə-nist) a person affected with exhibitionism.

**ex·hu·ma·tion** (eg″zu-ma′shən) [*ex-* + L. *humus* earth] disinterment; removal of the dead body from the earth after burial.

**ex·i·tus** (eg′sĭ-təs) pl. *exitus* [L. "a going out"] 1. death. 2. an exit or outlet.
**e. pel′vis,** apertura pelvis inferior.

**Ex·na** (eks′nə) trademark for a preparation of benzthiazide.

**Ex·ner's plex·us** (eks′nərz) [Siegmund *Exner,* Austrian physiologist, 1846–1926] see under *plexus.*

**exo-** [Gr. *exō* outside] a prefix meaning outside, or outward.

**exo·am·y·lase** (ek″so-am′ə-lās) an amylase that catalyzes the cleavage of α-1,4-glucosidic bonds only at the nonreducing termini of polysaccharide chains. Cf. endoamylase.

**exo·an·ti·gen** (ek″so-an′tə-jən) ectoantigen.

**exo·car·dia** (ek″so-kahr′de-ə) ectocardia.

**exo·carp** (ek′so-kahrp) the outer layer of the pericarp of a flower.

**exo·cata·pho·ria** (ek″so-kat″ə-for′e-ə) [*exo-* + *cataphoria*] a phoria in which the visual axes turn downward and outward.

**exo·cele** (ek′so-sēl) extraembryonic coelom.

**exo·cel·lu·lar** (ek″so-sel′u-lər) external to the cell membrane, yet still attached, e.g., flagella, capsule.

**exo·cer·vix** (ek″so-sər′viks) portio vaginalis cervicis.

**exo·cho·ri·on** (ek″so-kor′e-on) that part of the chorion which is derived from the ectoderm, as in those species in which extraembryonic membranes form by folding.

**exo·coe·lom** (ek″so-se′ləm) [*exo-* + *coelom*] extraembryonic coelom.

**exo·coe·lo·ma** (ek″so-se-lo′mə) extraembryonic coelom.

**exo·co·li·tis** (ek″so-ko-li′tis) [*exo-* + *colitis*] inflammation of the outer coat of the colon.

**exo·crine** (ek′so-krin) [*exo-* + Gr. *krinein* to separate] 1. secreting outwardly, via a duct; Cf. *endocrine.* 2. denoting such a gland or its secretion. See also under *gland.*

**exo·cri·nol·o·gy** (ek″so-krĭ-nol′ə-je) the study of substances secreted externally by individual organisms which effect integration of a group of organisms.

**exo·cri·nos·i·ty** (ek″so-krĭ-nos′ĭ-te) the quality or state of secreting externally.

**exo·cu·ti·cle** (ek″so-ku′tĭ-kəl) [*exo-* + L. *cuticula*] the outer layer of the procuticle of certain crustaceans and arthropods, which contains cuticulin, chitin, and phenolic substances that are oxidized to produce the dark pigment of the cuticle.

**exo·cyc·lic** (ek″so-sik′lik) denoting one or more atoms attached to a ring structure but outside it.

**exo·cy·to·sis** (ek″so-si-to′sis) [MeSH: Exocytosis] 1. the discharge from a cell of particles that are too large to diffuse through the wall; the opposite of endocytosis. 2. the aggregation of migrating leukocytes in the epidermis as part of the inflammatory response.

**exo·de·oxy·ri·bo·nu·cle·ase** (ek″so-de-ok″se-ri″bo-noo′kle-ās) [EC 3.1.11] any of a sub-subclass of enzymes of the hydrolase class that catalyze the hydrolysis of terminal bonds of deoxyribonucleic acids, releasing mononucleotides.

**exo·de·vi·a·tion** (ek″so-de″ve-a′shən) 1. exophoria. 2. exotropia.

**ex·odon·tia** (ek″so-don′shə) exodontics.

**ex·odon·tics** (ek″so-don′tiks) that branch of dentistry dealing with extraction of the teeth. Called also *exodontia.*

**ex·odon·tist** (ek″so-don′tist) a dentist who practices exodontics.

**exo·en·zyme** (ek″so-en′zīm) an extracellular enzyme; an enzyme that acts outside of the cells in which it originates.

**exo·er·gic** (ek″so-ər′jik) 1. exergonic. 2. exothermic.

**exo·eryth·ro·cyt·ic** (ek″so-ə-rith″ro-sit′ik) outside the erythrocyte, a term applied to stages in the development of malarial parasites which takes place in tissue cells instead of in erythrocytes.

**ex·og·a·my** (ek-sog′ə-me) [*exo-* + Gr. *gamos* marriage] fertilization by the union of elements that are not derived from the same cell. Cf. *autogamy* (def. 1) and *endogamy* (def. 1).

**exo·gas·tric** (ek″so-gas′trik) pertaining to the external surface of the stomach.

**exo·gas·tri·tis** (ek″so-gas-tri′tis) inflammation of the external coat of the stomach.

**exo·gas·tru·la** (ek″so-gas′troo-lə) [*exo-* + *gastrula*] a gastrula in which invagination is hindered and the mesentoderm bulges outward.

**exo·gas·tru·la·tion** (ek″so-gas″troo-la′shən) the evagination to the exterior (or turning inside out) of the gut due to an interference with the normal processes of gastrulation, which can occur if the morula is cut transversely below the equator. It is usually followed by a migration of mesenchyme cells into the interior.

**exo·ge·net·ic** (ek″so-jə-net′ik) [*exo-* + *genetic*] exogenous.

**ex·o·gen·ic** (ek″so-jen′ik) exogenous.

**ex·og·e·note** (eks″oj′ə-nōt) in bacterial genetics, the extra piece of genetic information introduced by transduction into the recipient cell by the donor cell. Cf. *endogenote.*

**ex·og·e·nous** (ek-soj′ə-nəs) [*exo-* + *-genous*] 1. developed or originating outside the organism, as exogenous disease. 2. growing by additions to the outside.

**ex·og·na·thia** (ek″sog-na′the-ə) prognathism.

**ex·og·na·thi·on** (ek″sog-na′the-on) [*exo-* + Gr. *gnathos* jaw] the maxilla exclusive of the premaxilla.

**ex·om·pha·los** (ek-som′fə-los) [*ex-* + Gr. *omphalos* navel] umbilical hernia.

**exo·mys·i·um** (ek″so-mis′e-əm) perimysium.

**ex·on** (ek′son) [MeSH: Exons] a coding sequence in a gene; see *intron.*

**exo·nu·cle·ase** (ek″so-noo′kle-ās) [EC 3.1.11.16] any nuclease specifically catalyzing the hydrolysis of terminal bonds of deoxyribonucleotide or ribonucleotide chains, releasing mononucleotides. Cf. *endonuclease.*

**exo·path·ic** (ek″so-path′ik) of the nature of an exopathy; originating outside the body.

**ex·op·a·thy** (ek-sop′ə-the) [*exo-* + *-pathy*] a disease originating in some cause lying outside the organism; exogenous disease.

**exo·pep·ti·dase** (ek″so-pep′tĭ-dās) [EC 3.4.11–19] any peptidase that catalyzes the cleavage of the terminal or penultimate peptide bond, releasing a single amino acid or dipeptide from the peptide chain. Exopeptidases are classified as aminopeptidases, carboxypeptidases, dipeptidases, and omega peptidases.

**Exo·phi·a·la** (ek″so-fi′ə-lə) [MeSH: Exophiala] a widespread genus of saprobic Fungi Imperfecti of the form-class Hyphomycetes, form-family Dematiaceae. *E. jeansel′mei* (called also *Phialophora jeanselmei* and *Torula jeanselmei*) is commonly found in soil and sewage and causes eumycotic mycetoma and opportunistic infections in humans. *E. spini′fera* (called also *P. spinifera*) occasionally causes phaeohyphomycosis of the skin. *E. wernec′kii* is the cause of tinea nigra; because it is so variable, some authorities have proposed dividing it into more than one species.

**exo·pho·ria** (ek-so-for′e-ə) [*exo-* + *phoria*] a form of heterophoria in which there is deviation of the visual axis of one eye away from that of the other eye in the absence of visual fusional stimuli. Called also *exodeviation.*

**exo·phor·ic** (ek″so-for′ik) pertaining to or characterized by exophoria.

**ex·oph·thal·mic** (ek″sof-thal′mik) of or pertaining to or characterized by exophthalmos.

**ex·oph·thal·mo·gen·ic** (ek″sof-thal″mo-jen′ik) causing or producing exophthalmos.

**ex·oph·thal·mom·e·ter** (ek″sof-thəl-mom′ə-tər) an instrument for measuring the amount of exophthalmos; called also *ophthalmostatometer, orthometer, proptometer, protometer,* and *statometer.*

**ex·oph·thal·mo·met·ric** (ek″sof-thal″mo-met′rik) pertaining to exophthalmometry.

**ex·oph·thal·mom·e·try** (ek″sof-thəl-mom′ə-tre) [*exophthalmos* + *-metry*] measurement of the extent of protrusion of the eyeball in exophthalmos.

**ex·oph·thal·mos** (ek″sof-thal′mos) [*ex-* + Gr. *ophthalmos* eye] [MeSH: Exophthalmos] abnormal protrusion of the eyeball. Spelled also *exophthalmus;* called also *exorbitism* and *proptosis.*
**endocrine e.,** exophthalmos associated with disorder of an endocrine gland; the most common type is thyrotoxic exophthalmos.
**malignant e.,** the severe exophthalmos of Graves' orbitopathy, in which there is marked edema and infiltration of the orbital tissues and extraocular muscles, protrusion, and stare. It was formerly attributed to overactivity of thyrotropin and was called *thyrotropic e.*
**pulsating e.,** exophthalmos with pulsation and bruit, often due to aneurysm pushing the eye forward.
**thyrotoxic e.,** exophthalmos due to thyrotoxicosis; see also *dysthyroid orbitopathy,* under *orbitopathy.*
**thyrotropic e.,** former name for *malignant e.*

**ex·oph·thal·mus** (ek″sof-thal′məs) exophthalmos.

**exo·phyt·ic** (ek″so-fit′ik) [*exo-* + *phyt-* + *-ic*] growing outward; in oncology, proliferating on the exterior or surface epithelium of an organ or other structure, in which the growth originated.

**exo·plasm** (ek′so-plaz-əm) plasma membrane.

**ex·or·bi·tism** (eg-sor′bĭ-tiz-əm) exophthalmos.

**exo·ri·bo·nu·cle·ase** (ek″so-ri-bo-noo′kle-ās) [EC 3.1.13–14] any member of two sub-subclasses of enzymes of the hydrolase class that catalyze the hydrolysis of terminal bonds of ribonucleotides, producing mononucleotides.

**exo·sep·sis** (ek″so-sep′sis) [*ex-* + *sepsis*] septic poisoning which does not originate within the organism.

**exo·se·ro·sis** (ek″so-se-ro′sis) an oozing of serum or exudate, as in moist skin diseases and edema.

**exo-α-si·al·i·dase** (ek″so-si-al′ĭ-dās) [EC 3.2.1.18] EC nomenclature for *sialidase* (def. 1).

**exo·skel·e·ton** (ek″so-skel′ə-ton) [*exo-* + *skeleton*] a hard structure developed on the outside of the body, as the shell of a crustacean. In vertebrates the term is applied to structures produced by the epidermis, as hair, nails, hoofs, teeth, etc.

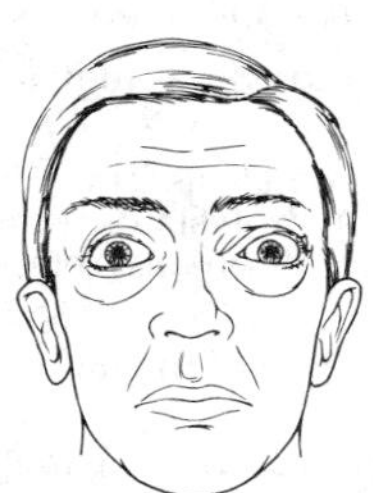
Exophthalmos.

**ex·os·mose** (ek′sos-mōs) to diffuse from within outward.

**ex·os·mo·sis** (ek″sos-mo′sis) [*ex-* + *osmosis*] diffusion or osmosis from within outward; movement outward through a diaphragm or through vessel walls. Cf. *endosmosis.*

**exo·spore** (ek′so-spor) conidium.

**exo·spo·ri·um** (ek″so-spor′e-əm) the external layer of the envelope of a spore.

**ex·os·to·sec·to·my** (ek-sos″to-sek′tə-me) excision of an exostosis.

**ex·os·to·sis** (ek″sos-to′sis) [*ex-* + *ostosis*] 1. a benign bony growth projecting outward from the surface of a bone. 2. osteochondroma.
**e. bursa′ta,** an exostosis from the epiphyseal portion of a bone, consisting of bone and cartilaginous tissue covered by a connective-tissue capsule.
**e. cartilagi′nea,** a variety of osteoma consisting of a layer of cartilage developing beneath the periosteum of a bone.
**hereditary multiple e's,** multiple cartilaginous exostoses.
**ivory e.,** compact osteoma.
**multiple e's, multiple cartilaginous e's, multiple osteocartilaginous e's,** 1. an autosomal dominant disorder characterized by exostoses near the extremities of diaphyses of long bones, which may be cartilaginous or osteocartilaginous growths; it is generally benign, although sarcomatous changes have occurred. Called also *diaphyseal aclasis* and *hereditary multiple e's.* 2. a bone disease in dogs (in whom it may be hereditary) and occasionally cats, characterized by exostoses on bones such as the ribs, long bones, or vertebrae. They may impinge on nerves, blood vessels, or the spinal cord; in the latter case the result may be paresis or paralysis.
**osteocartilaginous e.,** osteochondroma.
**subungual e.,** a cartilage-capped reactive bone spur occurring on the distal phalanx, usually of the great toe, particularly in women.

**ex·os·tot·ic** (ek″sos-tot′ik) pertaining to or of the nature of exostosis.

**exo·ter·ic** (ek″so-ter′ik) [Gr. *exōterikos* outer] generated or developed outside the organism; exogenous.

**exo·ther·mal** (ek″so-thər′məl) exothermic.

**exo·ther·mic** (ek″so-thər′mik) [*exo-* + *thermic*] characterized or accompanied by the evolution of heat, as in a chemical reaction during and by which heat is released; liberating heat or energy from its potential forms. Cf. *endothermic.*

**ex·ot·ic** (eg-zot′ik) of foreign origin; not native.

**exo·tox·ic** (ek″so-tok′sik) [*exo-* + *toxic*] pertaining to or produced by an exotoxin.

**exo·tox·in** (ek″so-tok′sin) [*exo-* + *toxin*] a toxic substance formed by species of certain bacteria (e.g., *Bacillus, Bordetella, Clostridium, Corynebacterium, Escherichia, Pseudomonas, Staphylococcus, Streptococcus, Vibrio, Salmonella, Shigella, Yersinia*) that is found outside the bacterial cell, or free in the culture medium. Exotoxins are heat-labile and protein in nature. They are detoxified with retention of antigenicity by treatment with formaldehyde (formol toxoid), and are the most poisonous substances known to humans; the $LD_{50}$ of crystalline botulinum type A toxin for the mouse is $4.5 \times 10^{-9}$ mg.
**streptococcal pyrogenic e.,** an exotoxin, existing in several antigenically distinct types, produced by *Streptococcus pyogenes*; it causes fever, the rash of scarlet fever, organ damage, increased permeability of the blood-brain barrier, and alterations in immune response, including increased susceptibility to endotoxic shock and changes in T cell function. Formerly called *erythrogenic toxin.*

**exo·tro·pia** (ek″so-tro′pe-ə) [*exo-* + *tropia*] [MeSH: Exotropia] strabismus in which there is permanent deviation of the visual axis of one eye away from that of the other, resulting in diplopia; called also *divergent* or *external strabismus,* and *walleye.*

**ex·o·trop·ic** (ek″so-tro′pik) pertaining to or characterized by exotropia.

**ex·pan·der** (ek-span′dər) [L. *expandere* to spread out] extender.
**plasma volume e.,** artificial plasma extender.

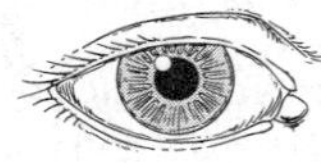
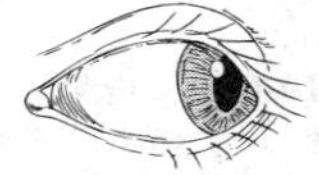
Exotropia.

**subperiosteal tissue e. (STE),** a fillable tube inserted temporarily into the subperiosteal tissue prior to reconstruction of the alveolar ridge with hydroxylapatite granules; by progressively inflating the tube the periosteal mucosa can be expanded to create space for the granules.

**ex·pan·sion** (ek-span′shən) [L. *expandere* to spread out] 1. the process or state of being increased in extent, surface, or bulk. 2. a region or area of increased bulk or surface.
**e. of the arch,** maxillary e.
**clonal e.,** an immunological response in which lymphocytes stimulated by antigen proliferate and amplify the population of relevant cells.
**cubical e.,** increase in volume by an increase in all dimensions.
**hygroscopic e.,** an increase in dimensions of a body or substance as a result of absorption of moisture.
**maxillary e.,** an orthodontic method of correcting narrow or collapsed maxillary arches and functional posterior crossbite, whereby increased maxillary arch width is obtained with the use of various appliances that provide laterally expansive force resulting in orthopedic and orthodontic movements. Called also *e. of the arch.*
**setting e.,** the increase in dimensions of a material, such as plaster of Paris, which occurs concurrently with its hardening.
**thermal e.,** an increase in dimensions of a body or substance as a result of an increase in its temperature; used in dentistry to enlarge an investment mold to compensate for shrinkage of the metal casting.
**wax e.,** a type of thermal expansion consisting of an increase in the dimensions of a wax pattern for a dental restoration to compensate for shrinkage of the gold during the casting process.

**ex·pan·sive·ness** (ek-span′siv-nəs) behavior marked by euphoria, loquacity, and grandiosity.

**ex·pec·tan·cy** (ek-spek′tən-se) the expected value or probability of occurrence for a specific event. Symbol *E.*
**life e.,** 1. the number of years, based on statistical averages, that a given person of a specific age, class, or other demographic variable may be expected to continue living. 2. the average length of survival expected for an organism from a given point in its life cycle.

**ex·pec·to·rant** (ek-spek′tə-rənt) [*ex-* + L. *pectus* breast] 1. promoting the ejection, by spitting, of mucus or other fluids from the lungs and trachea. 2. an agent that promotes the ejection of mucus or exudate from the lungs, bronchi, and trachea; sometimes extended to all remedies that quiet cough (antitussives).
**liquefying e.,** an expectorant that promotes the ejection of mucus from the respiratory tract by decreasing its viscosity.
**stimulant e.,** an expectorant that stimulates secretion of mucus by the respiratory tract mucosa.

**ex·pec·to·ra·tion** (ek-spek″tə-ra′shən) 1. the act of coughing up and spitting out materials from the lungs, bronchi, and trachea. 2. sputum.

**ex·per·i·ment** (ek-sper′ĭ-mənt) [L. *experimentum* "proof from experience"] a procedure done in order to discover or to demonstrate some fact or general truth.
**bulbocapnine e.,** the experimental injection of the alkaloid bulbocapnine into animals, which produces in them the motor phenomena typical of catatonia.
**check e.,** crucial e.
**control e.,** an experiment that is made under standard conditions, to test the correctness of other observations; see also *control.*
**crucial e.,** an experiment so designed and so prepared for by previous work that it will definitely settle some point.
**Cyon's e.,** the application of a stimulus to an intact anterior spinal nerve root, which induces a stronger contraction of muscle than the same stimulus to the peripheral end of a divided nerve root.
**defect e.,** observation of an embryo, after destruction of a region or part, to ascertain the effect on development.
**Goltz's e.,** the striking of a frog on the abdomen, which produces stoppage of the heart's action.
**Küss's e.,** injection of a solution of opium or belladonna into the bladder, which produces no symptoms of poisoning and thus proves the impermeability of the bladder epithelium to these substances.
**Mariotte's e.** (an experiment to demonstrate the blind spot of the eye): the eye is fixed on the center of a cross marked on a card on which is also marked a large spot; the card is moved to or from the face, and at a certain distance the image of the spot will disappear.
**Müller's e.,** see under *maneuver.*
**Nussbaum's e.,** ligation of the renal arteries of an animal in order to isolate the glomeruli of the kidneys from the circulation.
**Scheiner's e.,** an experiment in accommodation: one looks at an object through two pinholes closer together than pupil diameter in a card. If the object is in focus, only one image is observed; if it is not, two or more images are seen.
**Stensen's e.,** the experiment of cutting off the blood supply from the lumbar region of the spinal cord of an animal by compressing the abdominal aorta; it produces paralysis of the posterior parts of the body.
**Toynbee's e.,** see under *maneuver.*
**Valsalva's e.,** Valsalva's maneuver (def. 1).

**ex·pi·rate** (eks′pĭ-rāt) expired gas (or air); the gas expired in one expiration is called *single expirate.*

**ex·pi·ra·tion** (ek″spĭ-ra′shən) [*ex-* +L. *spirare* to breathe] 1. exhalation (def. 1). 2. termination, or death.

**ex·pi·ra·to·ry** (ek-spi′rə-tor″e) subserving or pertaining to expiration.

**ex·pire** (ek-spīr′) 1. exhale. 2. to die, or terminate.

**ex·plant** 1. (eks-plant′) to take from the body and place in an artificial medium for growth. 2. (eks′plant) tissue taken from its original site and transferred to an artificial medium for growth.

**ex·plan·ta·tion** (eks″plan-ta′shən) the removal of an implant.

**ex·plode** (ek-splōd′) [L. *explodere,* from *ex* out +*plaudere* to clap the hands] 1. to undergo sudden and violent decomposition or combustion; see also *blast.* 2. to burst; to spread rapidly, as an epidemic.

**ex·plo·ra·tion** (ek″splə-ra′shən) [L. *exploratio,* from *ex* out + *plorare* to cry out] investigation or examination, sometimes including surgery, for diagnostic purposes.

**ex·plor·a·to·ry** (ek-splor′ə-tor″e) [L. *exploratorius*] pertaining to exploration or investigation.

**ex·plor·er** (ek-splor′ər) 1. an instrument for use in exploration, particularly for foreign bodies. 2. an instrument with a flexible, sharp point, used to examine the crown of a tooth for defects or caries.

**ex·plo·sion** (ek-splo′zhən) [L. *explosio*] [MeSH: Explosions] 1. the act of exploding. 2. a sudden and violent outbreak, as of emotion.

**ex·plo·sive** (ek-splo′siv) characterized by explosions.

**ex·po·nent** (ek-spo′nənt) a number or symbol placed above and to the right of another number or symbol indicating the number of times that that value is to be multiplied by itself; a negative exponent indicates the reciprocal of the quantity arrived at by multiplication. For example, $3^3 = 3 \times 3 \times 3 = 27$, and $x^{-2} = 1/(x \times x)$.

**ex·po·nen·tial** (ek″spə-nen′shəl) denoting a mathematical function in which the variable or variables appear in exponents, e.g., $y = a^x$, where $a$ is a constant and $x$ is a variable.

**ex·po·sure** (ek-spo′zhər) [L. *exponere* to put out] 1. the act of laying open, as surgical exposure. 2. the condition of being subjected to something, as to infectious agents, extremes of weather or radiation, which may have a harmful effect. 3. in radiology, a measure of the x-ray or gamma radiation at a certain place based on its ability to cause ionization. The unit of exposure is the roentgen. Symbol X. Called also *exposure dose.* 4. in radiology, the product of the intensity of x-rays and the time the film is exposed.
**acute e.,** radiation exposure of short duration, usually referring to a heavy dose. See also *acute radiation syndrome,* under *syndrome.*
**air e.,** radiation exposure measured in a small mass of air, excluding backscatter from irradiated objects; called also *air dose.*
**chronic e.,** a long-term radiation exposure, either continuous *(protraction exposure)* or intermittent *(fractionation exposure),* usually referring to exposure to low-intensity radiation; effects may include accelerated aging, neoplastic disease, and genetic damage.

**ex·pres·sate** (ek-spres′āt) the material forced out by expression.

**ex·pres·sion** (ek-spresh′ən) [L. *expressio*] 1. the aspect or appearance of the face as determined by the physical or emotional state. 2. the act of squeezing or evacuating by pressure. 3. gene e.
**gene e.,** 1. the flow of genetic information from gene to protein. 2. the process, or the regulation of the process, by which the effects of a gene are manifested. 3. the manifestation of a heritable trait in an individual carrying the gene or genes that determine it.

**ex·pres·siv·i·ty** (ek″sprĕ-siv′ĭ-te) in genetics, the extent to which an inherited trait appears in an individual.
**variable e.,** expressivity that ranges in its manifestation from mild to severe but is never completely lacking in those who have the corresponding genotype.

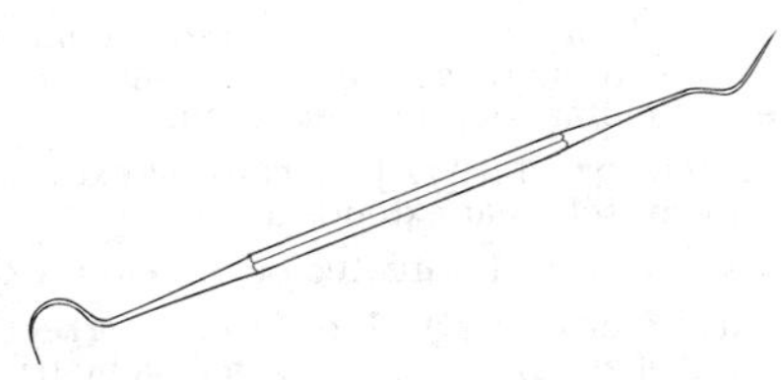

Explorer.

**ex·pul·sive** (ek-spul'siv) [*ex-* + L. *pellere* to drive] driving or forcing out; tending to expel.

**ex·san·gui·nate** (ek-sang'wĭ-nāt) [*ex-* + L. *sanguis* blood] 1. to deprive of blood. 2. bloodless (def. 1).

**ex·san·gui·na·tion** (ek-sang"wĭ-na'shən) extensive loss of blood due to hemorrhage.

**ex·san·guine** (ek-sang'win) bloodless (def. 1).

**ex·san·gui·no·trans·fu·sion** (ek-sang"wĭ-no-trans-fu'zhən) exchange transfusion.

**ex·sect** (ek-sekt') to excise; to cut out.

**ex·sec·tion** (ek-sek'shən) excision.

**ex·sec·tor** (ek-sek'tor) a cutting instrument for use in performing exsections (excisions).

**Ex·se·ro·hi·lum** (ek"sər-o-hi'ləm) a genus of Fungi Imperfecti of the form-class Hyphomycetes, form-family Dematiaceae, closely related to *Bipolaris* and *Drechslera*. *E. longirostra'tum*, *E. macgin'nisii*, and *E. rostra'tum* have been isolated from humans with sinusitis and meningitis.

**ex·sic·cant** (ek-sik'ənt) desiccant.

**ex·sic·cate** (ek'sĭ-kāt) [L. *exsiccare*, from *ex* out + *siccus* dry] desiccate.

**ex·sic·ca·tion** (ek"sĭ-ka'shən) the act of drying; in chemistry, the deprival of a crystalline substance of its water of crystallization.

**ex·sorp·tion** (ek-sorp'shən) the movement of substances out of cells, especially the movement of substances out of the blood, through the intestinal epithelial cells, and into the intestinal lumen.

**ex·stro·phy** (ek'stro-fe) [*ex-* + Gr. *strephein* to turn oneself] the congenital eversion or turning inside out of an organ, as the bladder.
**e. of the bladder,** a developmental anomaly marked by absence of a portion of the lower abdominal wall and the anterior vesical (urinary bladder) wall, with eversion of the posterior vesical wall through the deficit and with an open pubic arch and widely separated ischia connected by a fibrous band. Called also *ectopia vesicae*.
**e. of cloaca, cloacal e.,** a developmental anomaly in which two segments of bladder (hemibladders) are separated by an area of intestine with a mucosal surface, which appears as a large red tumor in the midline of the lower abdomen. Called also *ectopia cloacae*.

**ex·suf·fla·tion** (ek"sə-fla'shən) [*ex-* + L. *sufflatio* a blowing up] the act of removing the air from a cavity by artificial or mechanical means, especially such action upon the lungs by means of an exsufflator.

**ex·suf·fla·tor** (ek"sə-fla'tor) an apparatus that produces sudden negative pressure in order to reproduce in the bronchial tree the effects of a natural, vigorous cough.

**ext.** extract.

**ex·tend·ed-re·lease** (ek-stend'əd-re-lēs') allowing a twofold or greater reduction in frequency of administration of a drug in comparison with the frequency required by a conventional dosage form.

**ex·ten·der** (ek-sten'dər) [*ex-* + L. *tendere* to stretch] something that enlarges or prolongs; called also *expander*.
**artificial plasma e.,** a substance that can be transfused to maintain fluid volume of the blood in an emergency, supplemental to the use of whole blood and plasma.

**ex·ten·sion** (ek-sten'shən) [L. *extensio*] 1. the movement that straightens or increases the angle between the bones or parts of the body. 2. the bringing of the members of a limb into or toward a straight relation. 3. enlargement or prolongation.
**Buck's e.,** the extension of a fractured leg by weights, the foot of the bed being raised so that the body makes counterextension.
**nail e.,** extension exerted on the distal fragment of a fractured bone by means of a nail or pin driven into the fragment.
**e. per contiguita'tem,** the spreading of a morbid process through one tissue or part into one adjacent to it.
**e. per continuita'tem,** the spreading of a morbid process throughout a single tissue or part.
**e. per sal'tam,** the spreading of a morbid condition from one part to a part or tissue distant from it, with normal tissues intervening; metastasis.
**ridge e.,** an intraoral surgical operation for deepening the vestibular and oral sulci so as to increase the relative intraoral height of the alveolar ridge to facilitate denture retention.

**ex·ten·sor** (ek-sten'sər) [L.] [TA] 1. causing extension. 2. a general term for any muscle that extends a joint.

**ex·te·ri·or** (ek-stēr'e-ər) [L.] situated on or near the outside; outer.

**ex·te·ri·or·ize** (ek-stēr'e-ə-rīz") 1. to form a correct mental reference of the image of an object seen. 2. in psychiatry, to turn one's interest outward. 3. to transpose an internal organ to the exterior of the body.

**ex·tern** (ek'stərn) a medical student or graduate in medicine who assists in the care of patients in a hospital but does not reside in the hospital.

**ex·ter·nal** (ek-stər'nəl) [L. *externus* outside] situated or occurring on the outside; many anatomical structures formerly called external are now more correctly termed lateral.

**ex·ter·nal·iza·tion** (ek-stər"nəl-ĭ-za'shən) 1. the tendency to perceive in the external world and external objects components of one's own personality, including instinctual impulses, conflicts, moods, attitudes, and ways of thinking. 2. the process of learning the difference between self and non-self in childhood. 3. the process by which external rather than internal stimuli become capable of arousing a drive.

**ex·terne** (ek'stərn) extern.

**ex·ter·nus** (ek-stər'nəs) [TA] external: a term denoting a structure or an aspect farther from the center of a part or cavity.

**ex·tero·cep·tive** (ek"stər-o-sep'tiv) pertaining to exteroceptors and the stimuli they receive.

**ex·tero·cep·tor** (ek"stər-o-sep'tor) a sensory nerve terminal which is stimulated by the immediate external environment, such as those in the skin and mucous membranes; cf. *interoceptor*, *proprioceptor*, and *receptor* (def. 2).

**ex·tero·ges·tate** (ek"stər-o-jes'tāt) 1. developing outside the uterus, but still requiring complete care to meet all physical needs. 2. an infant during the period of exterior gestation.

**ex·ti·ma** (ek'stĭ-mə) [L.] outermost.

**ex·tinc·tion** (ek-stink'shən) in psychology, the disappearance or reduction in frequency of a conditioned response as a result of nonreinforcement; also, the process by which the disappearance is accomplished.

**ex·tin·guish** (ek-sting'wish) [L. *extinguere*] to render extinct.

**ex·tir·pa·tion** (ek"stər-pa'shən) [L. *extirpare* to root out, from *ex* out + *stirps* root] complete removal or eradication of an organ or tissue; see also *excision* and *resection*.
**dental pulp e.,** pulpectomy.

**ex·tor·sion** (ek-stor'shən) [*ex-* + *torsion*] outward rotation of the upper pole of the vertical meridian of each eye; called also *obtorsion* and *disclination*. Cf. *intorsion*.

**ex·tor·tor** (eks-tor'tər) [L. *extorquēre* to twist outward] 1. an outward rotator. 2. an extraocular muscle that produces extorsion, i.e. the inferior oblique or the inferior rectus muscle. Cf. *intorter*.

**extra-** [L. *extra* outside] a prefix meaning outside of, beyond, or in addition.

**ex·tra·adre·nal** (eks"trə-ə-dre'nəl) situated or occurring outside the adrenal gland.

**ex·tra·an·a·tom·ic** (eks"trə-an"ə-tom'ik) not following the normal anatomic path; said of certain arterial bypass procedures.

**ex·tra·an·throp·ic** (eks"trə-an-throp'ik) exanthropic.

**ex·tra·ar·tic·u·lar** (eks"trə-ahr-tik'u-lər) [*extra-* + L. *articulus* joint] situated or occurring outside a joint.

**ex·tra·bron·chi·al** (eks"trə-brong'ke-əl) outside or independent of the bronchial tubes; usually used in contrast to intrabronchial.

**ex·tra·buc·cal** (eks"trə-buk'əl) outside the mouth or cheek.

**ex·tra·bul·bar** (eks"trə-bul'bər) outside or away from a bulb, as the medulla oblongata or the urethral bulb.

**ex·tra·cap·su·lar** (eks"trə-kap'su-lər) situated or occurring outside a capsule.

**ex·tra·car·di·al** (eks"trə-kahr'de-əl) outside the heart.

**ex·tra·car·pal** (eks"trə-kahr'pəl) just outside the region of the wrist.

**ex·tra·cel·lu·lar** (eks"trə-sel'u-lər) outside a cell or cells.

**ex·tra·cer·e·bral** (eks"trə-ser'ə-brəl) situated or having its origin outside the cerebrum.

**ex·tra·cor·po·ral** (eks"trə-kor'pər-əl) extracorporeal.

**ex·tra·cor·po·re·al** (eks"trə-kor-por'e-əl) [*extra-* + *corporeal*] situated or occurring outside the body.

**ex·tra·cor·pus·cu·lar** (eks"trə-kor-pus'ku-lər) outside or on the exterior of the blood corpuscles.

**ex·tra·cor·ti·co·spi·nal** (eks"trə-kor"tĭ-ko-spi'nəl) outside the corticospinal tract; see under *tract*.

**ex·tra·cra·ni·al** (eks"trə-kra'ne-əl) outside the cranium.

**ex·tract** (ek'strakt) [L. *extractum*] a concentrated preparation of a vegetable or animal drug obtained by removing the active constituents therefrom with a suitable menstruum, evaporating all or nearly all the solvent, and adjusting the residual mass or powder to a prescribed standard. Extracts are prepared in three forms: semiliquid or of syrupy consistency, pilular or solid, and as dry powder.
**allergenic e.,** an extract of allergenic components from a crude preparation of an allergen, e.g., weed, grass, or tree pollen, molds, house dust, or animal dander, used for diagnostic skin testing or for immunotherapy (hyposensitization) of allergy.
**belladonna e.** [USP], a preparation, available in pilular and powdered form, containing alkaloids of belladonna leaf; used as an anticholinergic for the same purposes as atropine and hyoscyamine.
**cascara sagrada e.** [USP], a powdered preparation of cascara sagrada, used as a cathartic. Called also *Rhamnus purshiana e.*
**cell-free e.,** the solution obtained by rupturing cells and removing all particulate matter.
***Chondodendron tomentosum* e.,** an alcoholic extract of curare obtained from *Chondodendron tomentosum;* used in producing relaxation of skeletal muscle. See also *tubocurarine hydrochloride.*
**chondrus e.,** a tan powder prepared from chondrus, used as a protective; called also *Irish moss e.*
**compound e.,** one prepared from more than one drug.
**dry e.,** powdered e.
**glycyrrhiza e.,** a brown powder prepared from the rhizome and roots of species of *Glycyrrhiza,* used as a flavoring agent; called also *licorice root e.*
**glycyrrhiza e., pure,** preparation of the dried rhizome and roots of varieties of *Glycyrrhiza glabra,* used in the compounding of aromatic cascara sagrada fluidextract; called also *pure licorice root e.*
**henbane e.,** hyoscyamus e.
**hyoscyamus e.,** a preparation of hyoscyamus, formerly used as an anticholinergic for the same purposes as atropine.
**Irish moss e.,** chondrus e.
**licorice root e.,** glycyrrhiza e.
**licorice root e., pure,** glycyrrhiza e., pure.
**liver e.,** a brownish, somewhat hygroscopic powder prepared from mammalian livers; used as a hematopoietic.
**liver e., liquid,** liver solution.
**e. of male fern,** see under *oil.*
**malt e.,** an extract of malt, used as an emulsifying and flavoring agent.
**ox bile e.,** a brownish to greenish yellow powder or granules, with a characteristic odor and bitter taste, prepared from the fresh bile of the ox and containing not less than 45 per cent of cholic acid; used as a choleretic.
**oxgall e., powdered,** ox bile e.
**pilular e.,** an extract prepared as a plastic mass, with liquid glucose, malt extract, or glycerin being used as a diluent.
**poison ivy e.,** an extract of the fresh leaves of poison ivy, *Rhus radicans,* used in desensitization for prevention of rhus dermatitis due to poison ivy.
**poison ivy e., alum precipitated,** a repository form of a pyridine extract of poison ivy, *Rhus radicans,* used to counteract rhus dermatitis due to poison ivy.
**poison oak e.,** an extract of the fresh leaves of poison oak, *Rhus diversiloba,* used for desensitization in prevention of rhus dermatitis due to poison oak.
**pollen e.,** a preparation of the pollen of certain plants, such as ragweed, used in the diagnosis and treatment of inhalant allergy.
**powdered e.,** an extract prepared in a dry powdered form, with starch, sucrose, lactose, powdered glycyrrhiza, magnesium carbonate, magnesium oxide, or calcium phosphate being used as a diluent. Called also *dry e.*
**pyrethrum e.** [USP], a mixture of pyrethrin I and pyrethrin II, used as a pediculicide.
***Rhamnus purshiana* e.,** cascara sagrada e.
**semiliquid e.,** one evaporated to a syrupy consistency.
**solid e.,** pilular e.
**trichinella e.,** an aqueous extract of specially treated larvae of *Trichinella spiralis,* usually obtained from inoculated rodents; used as a skin test for trichinella infection.
**yeast e.,** a powder prepared from a water-soluble, peptonelike derivative of yeast cells; see under *culture medium.*

**ex·trac·tion** (ek-strak'shən) [*ex-* + *traction*] 1. the process or act of pulling or drawing out. 2. the preparation of an extract. 3. tooth e.
**breech e.,** extraction of the infant from the uterus in breech presentation, i.e., when the buttocks of the fetus are presented in labor.
**breech e., partial,** extraction of the remainder of the infant's body after it has been extruded from the uterus by natural forces as far as the umbilicus.
**breech e., total,** extraction of the entire body of the infant from the uterus in cases of breech presentation.
**cataract e.,** the surgical removal of a cataractous lens.
**cataract e., extracapsular,** the surgical removal of the anterior capsule of a cataractous lens and of the lens contents (cortex and nucleus).
**cataract e., intracapsular,** the surgical removal of a cataractous lens and its capsule.
**flap e.,** extraction of cataract by an incision which makes a flap of cornea.
**progressive e.,** serial e.
**selected e.,** serial e.
**serial e.,** the selective extraction of deciduous teeth during the stage of mixed dentition in accordance with the shedding and eruption of the teeth; it is done over an extended period to allow autonomous adjustment to relieve crowding of the dental arches during the eruption of the lateral incisors, canines, and premolars, eventually involving the extraction of the first premolar teeth. Called also *selected e.* and *progressive e.*
**tooth e.,** the surgical removal of a tooth; odontectomy.

**ex·trac·tive** (ek-strak'tiv) any substance present in an organized tissue, or in a mixture in a small quantity, and requiring to be extracted by a special method.

**ex·trac·tor** (ek-strak'tor) an instrument used for removing a calculus or foreign body.
**basket e.,** a device for removal of calculi from the upper urinary tract, consisting of a network of filaments on a catheter that is passed into the ureter through a ureteroscope; the filaments surround the calculus and snare it so that it is withdrawn when the catheter is withdrawn.
**vacuum e.,** a device to assist delivery consisting of a metal or plastic traction cup that is attached to the fetus' head; negative pressure is applied and traction is made.

**ex·trac·tum** (eks-trak'təm) gen. *extrac'ti,* pl. *extrac'ta* [L., from *ex* out + *trahere* to draw] an extract.
**e. fel'lis bo'vis,** ox bile extract.
**e. hep'atis,** liver extract.

**ex·tra·cys·tic** (eks"trə-sis'tik) outside a cyst or the bladder.

**ex·tra·du·ral** (eks"trə-doo'rəl) situated or occurring outside the dura mater.

**ex·tra·em·bry·on·ic** (eks"trə-em"bre-on'ik) external to the embryo proper, as the extraembryonic coelom or extraembryonic membranes.

**ex·tra·epi·phys·e·al** (eks"trə-ep"ĭ-fiz'ə-əl) away from, or unconnected with, an epiphysis.

**ex·tra·gen·i·tal** (eks"trə-jen'ĭ-təl) unrelated to, not originating in, or remote from the genital organs.

**ex·tra·glo·mer·u·lar** (eks"trə-glo-mer'u-lər) outside of or remote from a glomerulus.

**ex·tra·he·pat·ic** (eks"trə-hə-pat'ik) situated or occurring outside the liver.

**ex·tra·lig·a·men·tous** (eks"trə-lig"ə-men'təs) occurring outside a ligament.

**ex·tra·lym·phat·ic** (ek"strə-lim-fat'ik) situated or occurring outside the lymphatic system.

**ex·tra·mal·le·o·lus** (eks"trə-mə-le'o-ləs) the outer malleolus of the ankle joint.

**ex·tra·mas·toi·di·tis** (eks"trə-mas"toi-di'tis) inflammation of the outer surface of the mastoid process and of the superincumbent tissues.

**ex·tra·med·ul·la·ry** (eks"trə-med'u-lar"e) situated or occurring outside any medulla, especially the medulla oblongata.

**ex·tra·me·nin·ge·al** (eks"trə-mə-nin'jəl) occurring outside the meninges.

**ex·tra·mu·ral** (eks"trə-mu'rəl) [*extra-* + *mural*] situated or occurring outside the wall of an organ or structure.

**ex·tra·ne·ous** (ek-stra'ne-əs) [L. *extraneus* external] existing or belonging outside the organism.

**ex·tra·nu·cle·ar** (eks"trə-noo'kle-ər) situated or occurring outside a cell nucleus.

**ex·tra·oc·u·lar** (eks"trə-ok'u-lər) situated outside the eye.

**ex·tra·os·se·ous** (eks"trə-os'e-əs) occurring outside a bone or bones.

**ex·tra·pan·cre·at·ic** (ek"strə-pan"kre-at'ik) outside the pancreas.

**ex·tra·pa·ren·chy·mal** (eks"trə-pə-ren'kə-məl) occurring or formed outside the parenchyma.

**ex·tra·pel·vic** (eks"trə-pel'vik) unconnected with the pelvis.

**ex·tra·peri·car·di·al** (eks"trə-per"ĭ-kahr'de-əl) outside the pericardium.

**ex·tra·per·i·ne·al** (eks″trə-per″ĭ-ne′əl) away from, or not connected with, the perineum.

**ex·tra·peri·os·te·al** (eks″trə-per″e-os′te-əl) outside or independent of the periosteum.

**ex·tra·peri·to·ne·al** (eks″trə-per″ĭ-to-ne′əl) situated or occurring outside the peritoneal cavity.

**ex·tra·pla·cen·tal** (eks″trə-plə-sen′təl) outside of or independent of the placenta.

**ex·tra·plan·tar** (eks″trə-plan′tər) on the outside of the sole of the foot.

**ex·tra·pleu·ral** (eks″trə-ploor′əl) outside the pleural cavity.

**ex·trap·o·la·tion** (ek-strap″o-la′shən) inference of one or more unknown values on the basis of that which is known or has been observed; usually applied to estimation beyond the upper and lower ranges of observed data. Cf. *interpolation.*

**ex·tra·pros·tat·ic** (eks″trə-pros-tat′ik) not connected with the prostate gland.

**ex·tra·pros·ta·ti·tis** (eks″trə-pros″tə-ti′tis) paraprostatitis.

**ex·tra·psy·chic** (eks″trə-si′kik) occurring outside the mind; taking place between the mind and the external environment.

**ex·tra·pul·mo·na·ry** (eks″trə-pul′mo-nar″e) not connected with the lungs.

**ex·tra·py·ram·i·dal** (eks″trə-pĭ-ram′ĭ-dəl) outside of the pyramidal tracts; see under *system.*

**ex·tra·rec·tus** (eks″trə-rek′təs) musculus rectus lateralis bulbi.

**ex·tra·se·rous** (eks″trə-se′rəs) outside a serous cavity.

**ex·tra·so·mat·ic** (eks″trə-so-mat′ik) unconnected with the body.

**ex·tra·stim·u·lus** (ek″strə-stim′u-ləs) a premature stimulus delivered, singly or in a group of several stimuli, at precise intervals during a tachyarrhythmia in order to terminate it. Delivery of stimuli may be synchronous or asynchronous with the arrhythmia; if synchronous, delivery may be preprogrammed or adaptive to the tachycardia cycle length. Premature stimuli may also be delivered during cardiac electrophysiologic testing to initiate supraventricular or ventricular tachycardia.

**ex·tra·su·pra·re·nal** (eks″trə-soo″prə-re′nəl) extra-adrenal.

**ex·tra·sys·to·le** (eks″trə-sis′to-le) a premature contraction of the heart that is independent of the normal rhythm and arises in response to an impulse in some part of the heart other than the sinoatrial node; called also *premature beat* or *systole.*
**atrial e.,** atrial premature complex.
**atrioventricular (AV) e.,** atrioventricular junctional premature complex.
**infranodal e.,** ventricular e.
**interpolated e.,** see under *beat.*
**junctional e.,** atrioventricular junctional premature complex.
**nodal e.,** atrioventricular e.
**retrograde e.,** a premature ventricular contraction followed by a premature atrial contraction, due to transmission of the stimulus backward, usually over the bundle of His.
**ventricular e.,** ventricular premature complex.

**ex·tra·tho·rac·ic** (eks″trə-thor-as′ik) outside the thorax.

**ex·tra·tra·che·al** (eks″trə-tra′ke-əl) situated or occurring outside the trachea.

**ex·tra·tu·bal** (eks″trə-too′bəl) outside a tube.

**ex·tra·tym·pan·ic** (eks″trə-tim-pan′ik) outside the tympanum of the ear.

**ex·tra·uter·ine** (eks″trə-u′tər-in) situated or occurring outside the uterus.

**ex·tra·vag·i·nal** (eks″trə-vaj′ĭ-nəl) outside the vagina.

**ex·trav·a·sa·tion** (ek-strav″ə-sa′shən) [*extra-* + L. *vas* vessel] 1. a discharge or escape of blood or some other fluid normally found in a vessel or tube, into the surrounding tissues. 2. the process of being so discharged. 3. fluid that has been so discharged.
**punctiform e.,** extravasation which causes a tissue to be covered with minute bloody points.

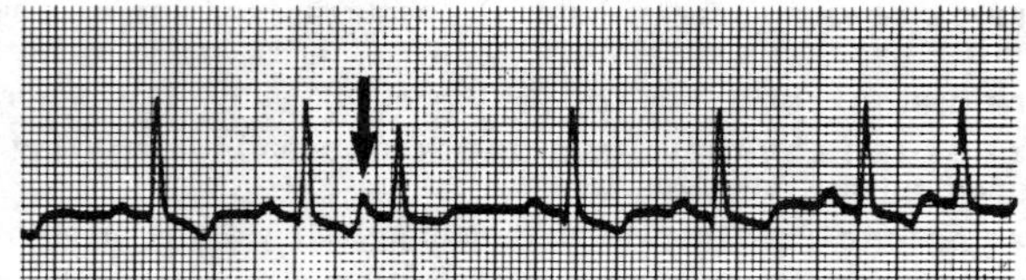
Atrial extrasystole measured in lead II. The arrow marks the position of the atrial premature complex, which is followed by a noncompensatory pause.

**ex·tra·vas·cu·lar** (eks″trə-vas′ku-lər) situated or occurring outside a vessel or the vessels.

**ex·tra·ven·tric·u·lar** (eks″trə-vən-trik′u-lər) situated or occurring outside a ventricle.

**ex·tra·ver·sion** (eks″trə-vər′zhən) extroversion.

**ex·tra·vert** (eks′trə-vərt) extrovert.

**ex·trem·i·tal** (ek-strem′ĭ-təl) pertaining to or situated at an extremity.

**ex·trem·i·tas** (ek-strem′ĭ-təs) pl. *extremita′tes* [L.] 1. [TA] extremity: a general term denoting the distal or terminal portion of elongated or pointed structures. 2. membrum (def. 2).
**e. acromia′lis clavi′culae** [TA], acromial extremity of clavicle: the lateral end of the clavicle, which articulates with the acromion of the scapula; called also *external* or *scapular extremity of clavicle.*
**e. ante′rior lie′nis,** TA alternative for *e. anterior splenis.*
**e. ante′rior sple′nis** [TA], anterior extremity of spleen: the lower pole of the spleen, which is situated anterior to the upper pole; called also *e. anterior lienis* [TA alternative] and *e. inferior lienis.*
**e. infe′rior,** membrum inferius.
**e. infe′rior lie′nis,** e. anterior splenis.
**e. infe′rior re′nis** [TA], inferior extremity of kidney: the lower, smaller pole of the kidney.
**e. infe′rior tes′tis** [TA], inferior extremity of testis: the lower end of the testis, which is attached to the tail of the epididymis.
**e. posterior lienis,** TA alternative for *e. posterior splenis.*
**e. poste′rior sple′nis** [TA], posterior extremity of spleen: the uppermost pole of the spleen, situated somewhat posterior to the lower pole; called also *caput lienis, e. posterior lienis* [TA alternative] and *e. superior lienis,* and *head of spleen.*
**e. sterna′lis clavi′culae** [TA], sternal extremity of clavicle: the medial end of the clavicle, which articulates with the sternum; called also *internal extremity of clavicle.*
**e. supe′rior,** membrum superius.
**e. supe′rior lie′nis,** e. posterior splenis.
**e. supe′rior re′nis** [TA], superior extremity of kidney: the upper, larger pole of the kidney.
**e. supe′rior tes′tis** [TA], **e. tuba′ria ova′rii** [TA], superior extremity of testis: the upper end of the testis, which is attached to the head of the epididymis.
**e. tuba′lis ova′rii,** tubal extremity of ovary: the upper end of the ovary, related to the free end of the uterine tube.
**e. uteri′na ova′rii** [TA], uterine extremity of ovary: the lower end of the ovary, directed toward the uterus; called also *pelvic extremity.*

**ex·trem·i·ta·tes** (ek-strem″ĭ-ta′-tēz) [L.] plural of *extremitas.*

**ex·trem·i·ty** (ek-strem′ĭ-te) [MeSH: Extremities] 1. extremitas. 2. an upper or lower limb; see *membrum.* 3. a hand or foot.
**cartilaginous e. of rib,** cartilago costalis.
**external e. of clavicle,** extremitas acromialis claviculae.
**fimbriated e. of fallopian tube,** fimbria ovarica.
**internal e. of clavicle,** extremitas sternalis claviculae.
**lower e.,** lower limb (*membrum inferius* [TA]).
**pelvic e. of ovary,** extremitas uterina ovarii.
**proximal e. of phalanx of finger,** basis phalangis digitorum manus.
**proximal e. of phalanx of toe,** basis phalangis digitorum pedis.
**scapular e. of clavicle,** extremitas acromialis claviculae.
**upper e.,** lower limb (*membrum superius* [TA]).
**uterine e. of ovary,** extremitas uterina ovarii.

**ex·trin·sic** (ek-strin′zik) [L. *extrinsecus* situated on the outside] coming from or originating outside; having relation to parts outside the organ or limb in which found.

**extro-** [L. *extra* outside] a prefix meaning outward, outside.

**ex·tro·gas·tru·la·tion** (eks″tro-gas″troo-la′shən) malformation resulting from exogastrulation.

**ex·tro·phia** (ek-stro′fe-ə) exstrophy.

**ex·tro·ver·sion** (eks″tro-vər′shən) [L. *extroversio,* from *extra* outside + *vertere* to turn] extraversion; 1. a turning inside out, as of an organ. 2. the turning outward to the external world of one's interest; cf. *introversion.* 3. in orthodontics, malocclusion in which the teeth or other maxillary structures are further from the median plane than normal, resulting in a wide dental arch. Cf. *intraversion.*

**ex·tro·vert** (eks′tro-vərt) 1. a person whose interest is turned outward to the external world. 2. to turn one's interest outward to the external world.

**ex·trude** (eks-trood′) 1. to force, thrust, or press out. 2. to force out, or to occupy a position mesial, distal, labial or buccal, or lingual or palatal to that normally occupied. 3. to occupy a position occlusal to that normally occupied, said of an overerupted tooth.

**ex·tru·sion** (ek-stroo′zhən) 1. thrusting or pushing out; expulsion by force. 2. the overeruption or movement of a tooth beyond its

normal occlusal plane in the absence of opposing occlusal force. 3. an orthodontic technique for the elongation or elevation of a tooth. Cf. *intrusion.*
**disk e.,** see *extruded disk,* under *disk.*

**ex·tu·bate** (eks-too'bāt) [*ex-* + L. *tuba* tube] to remove a tube from.

**ex·tu·ba·tion** (eks"too-ba'shən) the removal of a previously inserted tube; called also *detubation.* Cf. *decannulation.*

**ex·u·ber·ant** (eg-zoo'bər-ənt) [L. *exuberare* to be very fruitful] copious or excessive in production; showing excessive proliferation.

**ex·u·date** (eks'u-dāt) [L. *exsudare* to sweat out] [MeSH: Exudates and Transudates] material, such as fluid, cells, or cellular debris, which has escaped from blood vessels and has been deposited in tissues or on tissue surfaces, usually as a result of inflammation. An exudate, in contrast to a transudate, is characterized by a high content of protein, cells, or solid materials derived from cells.
**cotton-wool e's,** see under *spot.*

**ex·u·da·tion** (eks"u-da'shən) 1. the escape of fluid, cells, and cellular debris from blood vessels and their deposition in or on the tissues, usually as the result of inflammation. 2. an exudate.

**ex·u·da·tive** (ek-soo'də-tiv) of or pertaining to a process of exudation.

**ex·ul·cer·ans** (ek-sul'sər-ənz) [L.] ulcerating.

**ex·ul·cer·a·tio** (eks-ul"sər-a'she-o) [L.] ulceration.
**e. sim'plex,** superficial ulceration.

**ex·um·bil·i·ca·tion** (ek"səm-bil"ĭ-ka'shən) [*ex-* + *umbilicus*] 1. marked protrusion of the navel. 2. umbilical hernia.

**ex·u·vi·a·tion** (eks-u"ve-a'shən) [L. *exuere* to divest oneself of] the shedding of any epithelial structure, as of the deciduous teeth.

**ex vi·vo** (eks ve'vo) [L.] outside the living body, such as removal of an organ for reparative surgery, after which it is returned to its original site.

**eye** (i) [L. *oculus;* Gr. *ophthalmos*] [MeSH: Eye] the organ of vision; called also *oculus* [TA]. In shape the eyeball (bulbus oculi [TA]) is a large sphere, with the segment of a smaller sphere, the cornea, in front. It is composed of three coats: the external tough *fibrous tunic* or *layer,* consisting of the white sclera over most of the eyeball and the cornea on the anterior surface; the middle *vascular tunic* or *uvea,* consisting of the choroid, the ciliary body, and the iris; and the *internal tunic,* which is neural and sensory and consists primarily of the retina. Within the three coats are the refracting media: the *aqueous humor,* the *crystalline lens,* and the *vitreous humor.* The lens is a double convex transparent body between the vitreous and aqueous humors; its convexity is altered by the ciliary muscle during accommodation. Posteriorly, fibers of the optic nerve enter the ganglionic layer and receive sensations from the visual cells of the retina (the *retinal rods* and *retinal cones*). The arteries of the eye are the short ciliary, the long ciliary, the anterior ciliary, and the central artery of the retina. The nerves are the optic and the long and short ciliary nerves. See Plate 17.
**aphakic e.,** an eye lacking the crystalline lens; see also *aphakia.*
**artificial e.,** a ready-made (stock) or custom-made prosthesis of glass or plastic shaped and colored to resemble the anterior portion of a normal eye and inserted for cosmetic reasons in the socket of an enucleated or eviscerated eye.
**black e.,** ecchymosis of the eyelids and surrounding area.
**blear e.,** blepharitis ciliaris.
**cherry e.,** hypertrophy and prolapse of the gland of the nictitating membrane of a dog, with conjunctivitis and swelling in the form of a red mass.
**cinema e.,** Klieg e.
**compound e.,** the multifaceted eye of arthropods composed of units (ommatidia), each of which contains all of the structural and functional elements of the eye (including lens, retina, and photoreceptor cells).
**crab's e.,** 1. *Abrus precatorius.* 2. jequirity bean.
**crossed e's,** esotropia.
**cystic e.,** a malformed eye consisting of a cystic structure.
**dark-adapted e.,** an eye that has undergone the changes produced by adequate exposure to darkness; it is more sensitive to very weak light.
**deviating e.,** in strabismus, the nonfixating eye; called also *following e.*
**dry e.,** keratoconjunctivitis sicca.
**epiphyseal e.,** a modification of the parapineal organ of certain lower vertebrates to form an eyelike structure lying subepidermally on the median dorsal aspect of the head; it is a photoreceptor rather than an image forming eye, enabling the organism to respond to darkness or to light. Called also *parietal e., parietal body,* and *pineal e.*
**exciting e.,** the eye that is primarily injured and from which the influences start which involve the other eye in sympathetic ophthalmia; called also *primary e.*
**fixating e.,** in strabismus, the eye directed toward the object of vision.
**following e.,** deviating e.
**hop e.,** conjunctivitis in hop pickers caused by irritation from the spinelike hairs of the hop plant.
**Klieg e.,** a condition marked by conjunctivitis, edema of the eyelids, lacrimation, and photophobia due to exposure to intense lights (Klieg lights); called also *cinema e.*
**light-adapted e.,** an eye that has undergone the changes produced by adequate exposure to rather strong light; it is less sensitive to weak light.
**median e.,** an organ on the top of the head of many reptiles; it plays an important role in the response to light.
**monochromatic e.,** an eye that can perceive only one color.
**parietal e.,** epiphyseal e.
**pineal e.,** epiphyseal e.
**pink e.,** 1. acute contagious conjunctivitis. 2. infectious keratoconjunctivitis.
**primary e.,** exciting e.
**pseudophakic e.,** an eye with an intraocular lens implant.
**reduced e.,** a mathematical model of the eye in which the optical systems are diagrammatically reduced to one refracting unit.
**schematic e.,** 1. a diagrammatic illustration of the ideal normal eye, with constants for curvature, indices of refraction, and distances between the optical elements. 2. a model of the eye, usually simplified and enlarged, showing its anatomical and mechanical features.
**secondary e.,** sympathizing e.
**shipyard e.,** epidemic keratoconjunctivitis.
**Snellen's reform e.,** an artificial eye composed of two concavoconvex plates with an empty space between.
**squinting e.,** in strabismus, the eye the visual axis of which deviates from the object of vision while the sound eye fixates.
**sympathizing e.,** the uninjured eye which becomes secondarily involved in sympathetic ophthalmia; called also *secondary e.*
**wall e.,** 1. leukoma of the cornea. 2. exotropia.

**eye·ball** (i'bawl) bulbus oculi.

**eye·brow** (i'brow) [MeSH: Eyebrows] 1. the transverse elevation at the junction of the forehead and the upper eyelid, consisting of five layers: skin, subcutaneous tissue, a layer of interwoven fibers of the orbicularis oculi and occipitofrontalis muscles, a submuscular areolar layer, and pericranium; called also *supercilium* [TA]. 2. the hairs growing on the transverse elevation at the junction of the forehead and the upper eyelid; called also *supercilia* [TA].

**eye·cup** (i'kəp) 1. a small vessel for the application of cleansing or medicated solution to the exposed area of the eyeball. 2. physiologic cup. 3. caliculus ophthalmicus.

**eye·glass** (i'glas) a lens for aiding the sight.

**eye·ground** (i'ground) the fundus of the eye as revealed by ophthalmoscopic examination.

**eye·lash** (i'lash) one of the hairs growing at the edge of an eyelid; collectively called *cilia.*

**eye·let** (i'lət) an orthodontic attachment, usually used with an edgewise appliance, welded or soldered for better rotational control.

**eye·lid** (i'lid) [MeSH: Eyelids] either of the two movable folds (upper and lower) that protect the anterior surface of the eyeball; called also *palpebra.*
**third e.,** nictitating membrane.

**eye-mind·ed** (i'mīnd-əd) visile.

**eye·piece** (i'pēs) the lens or system of lenses in a microscope (or telescope) that is nearest to the eye of the user and that serves to further magnify the image produced by the objective.
**comparison e.,** an eyepiece which presents, as though in juxtaposition, the images of separate objects being transmitted through two different objectives.
**compensating e.,** an eyepiece especially designed to correct chromatic and spherical aberrations of the light rays produced by the objective.
**demonstration e.,** a device consisting of two eyepieces which may be affixed to the eyepiece tube of a microscope, permitting two observers to see the same field simultaneously.
**high-eyepoint e.,** one with an eyepoint higher than usual, which may be used by viewers wearing eyeglasses.
**huygenian e.,** a negative eyepiece consisting of two planoconvex lenses, the convexities being directed toward the objective.
**negative e.,** a combination of two lenses, one of which is below the

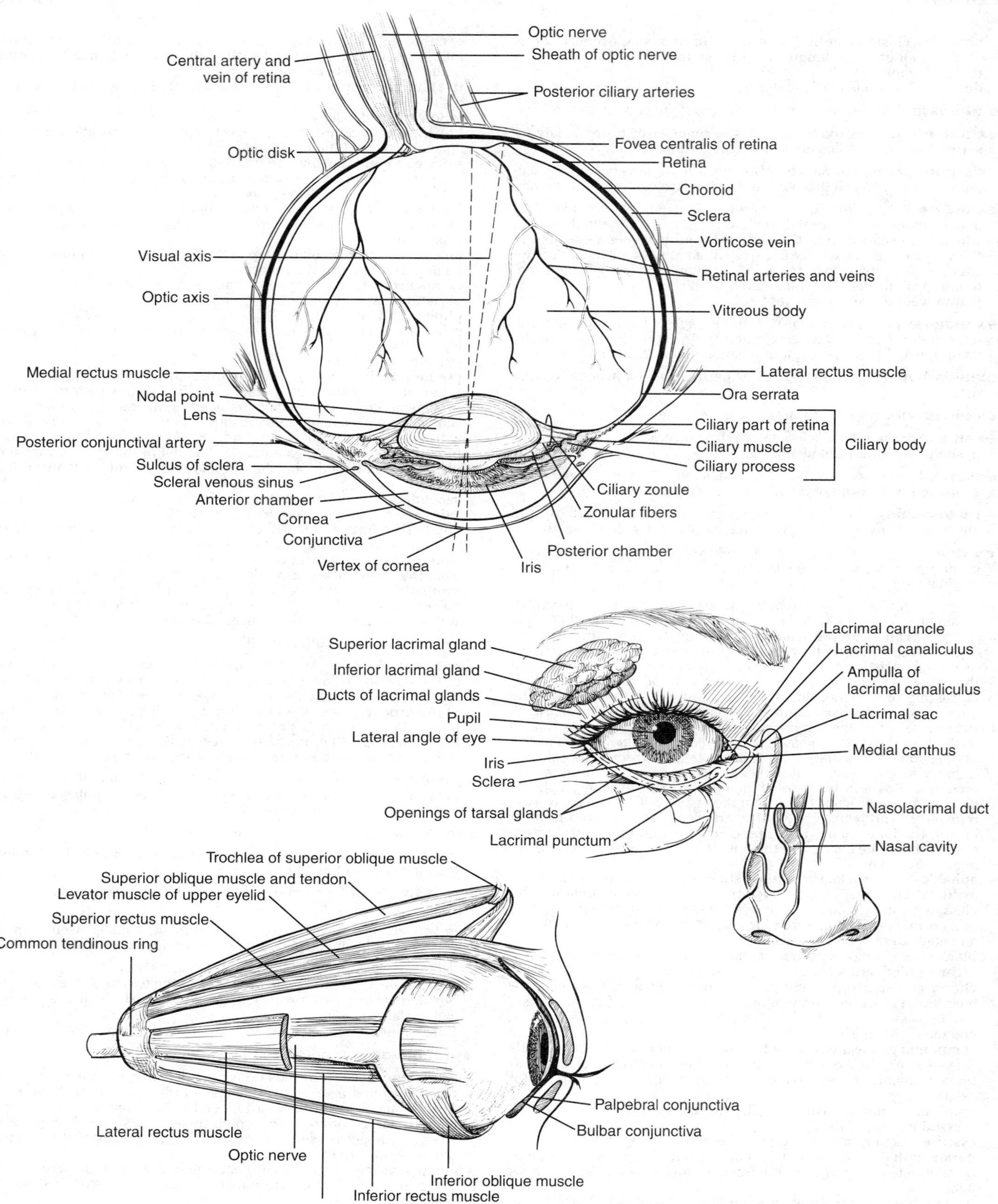


**PLATE 17**—THE EYE AND RELATED STRUCTURES

plane in which the real image from the objective is formed.
**positive e.,** a single lens combination, consisting of two planoconvex lenses or of an achromatic doublet or triplet, the combination being above the plane in which the real image from the objective is formed.
**Ramsden's e.,** a positive eyepiece consisting of two planoconvex lenses with the convexities turned toward each other.
**widefield e.,** a positive eyepiece consisting of a doublet and a single element, giving a wider field of view than that afforded by other eyepieces.

**eye·point** (i′point) the point above a microscope eyepiece where the image is focused and where the eye should be positioned for viewing.

**eye·spot** (i′spot) 1. a light-sensitive pigmented spot with a visual function occurring in various invertebrates. See also *stigma* (def. 5) and *ocellus* (def. 1). 2. eye spot; see under *spot*.

**eye·strain** (i′strān) fatigue of the eye from overuse or from uncorrected defect in focus of the eye.

**eye·worm** (i′wərm) see under *worm*.

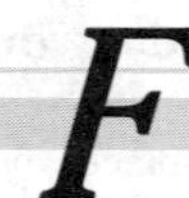

**F** symbol for *fluorine, farad, fertility* (see under *plasmid*), *visual field, formula,* and *French* (see under *scale*).

**F.** symbol for L. *fiat,* let there be made.

***F*** symbol for *faraday* and *force.*

**$F_1$** symbol for *first filial generation.*

**$F_2$** symbol for *second filial generation.*

**°F** symbol for degree Fahrenheit.

**f** symbol for *femto-* and *focal length.*

***f*** symbol for *frequency,* def. 2.

**FA** fatty acid; fluorescent antibody.

**FAB** French-American-British; see under *classification.*

**Fab** [*f*ragment, *a*ntigen-*b*inding] originally, either of two identical fragments, each containing an antigen combining site, obtained by papain cleavage of the IgG molecule; now generally used as an adjective, e.g., Fab region, segment, to refer to an "arm" of any immunoglobulin monomer, i.e., one light chain and the adjoining heavy chain $V_H$ and $C_H1$ domains. Cf. *Fc.*
**digoxin immune F. (ovine),** a preparation of antigen-binding fragments derived from specific antidigoxin antibodies produced in sheep that have been immunized with digoxin coupled as a hapten to human serum albumin, used as an antidote to life-threatening digoxin and digitoxin overdose; administered intravenously.

**F(ab′)$_2$** the fragment, containing both Fab regions and the hinge region connecting them by interchain disulfide bonds, obtained by pepsin cleavage of the IgG molecule; called also *F(ab′)$_2$ fragment.*

**fa·bel·la** (fə-bel′ə) pl. *fabel′lae* [L. "little bean"] a sesamoid fibrocartilage occasionally found on the gastrocnemius muscle; it is visible radiographically as a small bony shadow behind the knee joint.

**Fa·ber's syndrome** (fah′bərz) [Knud Helge *Faber,* Danish physician, 1862–1956] hypochromic anemia.

**fa·bism** (fa′biz-əm) [L. *faba* bean] favism.

**fab·ri·ca·tion** (fab″rĭ-ka′shən) confabulation.

**Fa·bri·ci·us** (fə-bris′e-əs) **ab Aqua·pen·den·te** Hieronymus. Italian anatomist and surgeon, 1537–1619; *(See format at Fibiger entry, p. 669)* the pupil and successor (at Padua) of Gabriele Falloppio. He was the teacher of William Harvey, and the first demonstrator of the valves of the veins.

**Fa·bri·ci·us' bursa** (fə-bris′e-əs) [H. *Fabricius*] see under *bursa.*

**Fa·bry's disease** (fah′brēz) [Johannes *Fabry,* German dermatologist, 1860–1930] [MeSH: Fabry's Disease] see under *disease.*

**fab·u·la·tion** (fab″u-la′shən) confabulation.

**Facb** [*f*ragment, *a*ntigen-and-*c*omplement-*b*inding] the fragment, containing both light chains and the $V_H$ $C_H2$ domains of both heavy chains, obtained by plasmin cleavage of an IgG molecule.

**FACD** Fellow of the American College of Dentists.

**face** (fās) [L. *facies*] [MeSH: Face] 1. the anterior, or ventral, aspect of the head from the forehead to the chin, including the eyes, nose, mouth, cheeks, and chin but excluding the auricles. Called also *facies* [TA]. 2. facies (def. 2).
**adenoid f.,** adenoid facies.
**bovine f.,** facies bovina.
**cleft f.,** see *lateral facial cleft* and *oblique facial cleft,* under *cleft.*
**cow f.,** facies bovina.
**dish f., dished f.,** a facial deformity characterized by a prominence of the forehead, a recession of the midface and lower half of the nose, a lengthening of the upper lip, and a prognathic chin; called also *facies scaphoidea.*
**frog f.,** flatness of the face due to intranasal disease.
**hippocratic f.,** facies hippocratica.
**moon f., moon-shaped f.,** the peculiar rounded face observed in various conditions, such as Cushing's disease, or following administration of corticosteroids; called also *moon facies.*

**face-bow** (fās′bo) a caliper-like device used in dentistry to record the positional relationship of the maxillary arch to the temporomandibular joints (or opening axis of the jaw) and to orient dental casts in this same relationship to the opening axis of the articulator.
**adjustable axis f.-b.,** a face-bow with caliper ends that can be adjusted in such a way as to permit location of the hinge axis of rotation of the mandible. Called also *hinge-bow* and *kinematic f.-b.*
**kinematic f.-b.,** adjustable axis f.-b.

**face-lift** (fās′lift) popular term for *rhytidectomy.*

**face·om·e·ter** (fās-om′ə-tər) an instrument for measuring the dimensions of the face.

**fac·et** (fas′ət) [Fr. *facette*] a small plane surface on a hard body, as on a bone; see also *fovea.*
**articular f.,** a small plane surface on a bone at the site where it articulates with another structure; see terms beginning *facies articularis,* under *facies.*
**articular f. of atlas, circular,** fovea dentis atlantis.
**articular f. of atlas, inferior,** facies articularis inferior atlantis.
**articular f. of atlas, superior,** facies articularis superior atlantis.
**articular f. of dens of axis, anterior,** facies articularis anterior dentis.
**articular f's for rib cartilages,** incisurae costales sterni.
**f. of calcaneus, medial posterior,** facies articularis talaris media calcanei.
**clavicular f.,** incisura clavicularis sterni.
**costal f., anterior, costal f., inferior,** facies articularis tuberculi costae.
**costal f., posterior, costal f., superior,** 1. facies articularis capitis costae. 2. fovea articularis capitis costae.
**costal f's of sternum,** incisurae costales sterni.
**costal f. of vertebra, superior,** fovea costalis superior.
**f. for incus,** the cartilage-covered surface on the head of the malleus that articulates with the body of the incus.
**lateral f's of sternum,** incisurae costales sterni.
**locked f's of spine,** dislocation of articular processes of the spine.
**malleolar f. of tibia, internal,** facies articularis malleoli medialis.
**f. for malleus,** the cartilage-covered surface on the body of the incus that articulates with the malleus.
**squatting f.,** a smooth area observed on the anterior surface of the lower end of the tibia in races whose members habitually sit in the squatting position.
**f. for tubercle of rib,** fovea costalis processus transversalis.

**fac·e·tec·to·my** (fas″ə-tek′tə-me) [*facet* + *-ectomy*] excision of the articular facet of a vertebra.

**fa·cette** (fah-set′) [Fr.] facet.

**fa·cial** (fa′shəl) [L. *facialis,* from *facies* face] pertaining to or directed toward the face.

**-facient** [L. *faciens,* present participle of *facere* to do, to make] a word termination meaning making or causing to become.

**fa·ci·es** (fa′she-ēz) pl. *fa′cies* [L.] [MeSH: Facies] 1. [TA] the face. 2. [TA] [TA] a specific surface of a body structure, part, or organ. 3. the expression or appearance of the face.

## Facies

Descriptions of anatomic structures are given on TA terms, and include anglicized names of specific structures.

**f. abdomina′lis,** the expression of the face characteristic of abdominal disease: it is pinched, anxious, and furrowed, with the nose and upper lip drawn up.
**adenoid f.,** the dull expression, with open mouth, sometimes seen in children with hypertrophy of the pharyngeal tonsils ("adenoids").
**antebrachial f., anterior,** regio antebrachii anterior.
**antebrachial f., posterior,** regio antebrachii posterior.
**f. antebrachia′lis ante′rior,** regio antebrachii anterior.
**f. antebrachia′lis poste′rior,** regio antebrachii posterior.
**f. ante′rior cor′dis,** f. sternocostalis cordis.
**f. ante′rior cor′neae** [TA], the anterior surface of the cornea.
**f. ante′rior cor′poris maxil′lae** [TA], anterior surface of body of maxilla: the surface of the body of the maxilla that is directed forward and somewhat laterally; it is bounded roughly by the infraorbital margin, root of the frontal process, nasal notch, alveolar process, and zygomatic process.

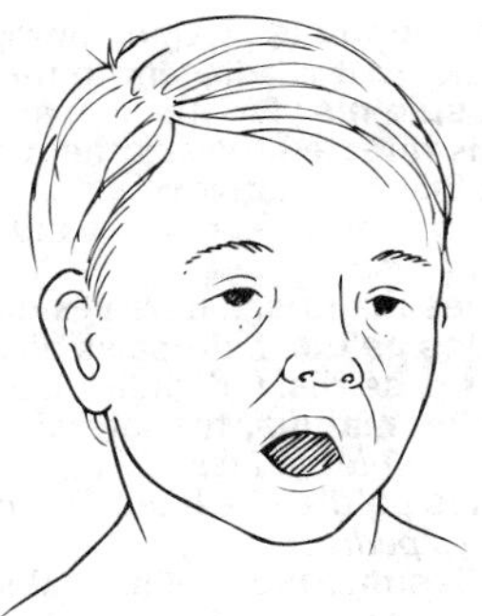

Adenoid facies.

**f. ante′rior cor′poris pancre′atis,** anterior surface of body of pancreas; see *f. anterosuperior* and *f. anteroinferior corporis pancreatis.*

**f. ante′rior den′tium premola′rium et mola′rium,** the mesial surfaces of the premolar and molar teeth.

**f. ante′rior glan′dulae suprarena′lis** [TA], the anterior surface of the adrenal (suprarenal) gland, where the hilum is located.

**f. ante′rior i′ridis** [TA], the anterior surface of the iris, directed toward the anterior chamber of the eye.

**f. ante′rior latera′lis hu′meri,** f. anterolateralis humeri.

**f. ante′rior len′tis** [TA], the surface of the lens directed toward the anterior surface of the eye.

**f. ante′rior media′lis hu′meri** [TA], anteromedial surface of humerus; it begins above at the intertubercular groove and spreads out inferiorly to form the wide smooth area for origin of the brachialis muscle. Called also *f. anteromedialis humeri* [TA alternative].

**f. ante′rior pal′pebrae** [TA], anterior surface of eyelid: the exterior surface of the eyelid.

**f. ante′rior palpebra′lis, f. ante′rior palpebra′rum,** f. anterior palpebrae.

**f. ante′rior par′tis petro′sae os′sis tempora′lis** [TA], anterior surface of petrous part of temporal bone: the surface of the petrous part of the temporal bone that forms the posterior portion of the floor of the middle cranial fossa; called also *f. anterior pyramidis ossis temporalis.*

**f. ante′rior patel′lae** [TA], anterior surface of patella: the slightly convex, longitudinally striated front surface of the patella, which is perforated by small openings for the nutrient vessels.

**f. ante′rior prosta′tae** [TA], the anterior surface of the prostate, separated from the pubic symphysis by the pudendal venous plexus.

**f. ante′rior pyra′midis os′sis tempora′lis,** f. anterior partis petrosae ossis temporalis.

**f. ante′rior ra′dii** [TA], anterior surface of radius; it gives attachment to the flexor pollicis longus and pronator quadratus muscles; called also *f. volaris radii.*

**f. ante′rior re′nis** [TA], anterior surface of kidney: the peritoneum-covered surface of the kidney which is directed toward the viscera.

**f. ante′rior sca′pulae,** TA alternative for *f. costalis scapulae.*

**f. ante′rior ul′nae** [TA], the anterior surface of the ulna; called also *f. volaris ulnae.*

**f. anteroinfe′rior cor′poris pancre′atis** [TA], the anteroinferior surface of the body of the pancreas.

**f. anterolatera′lis cartilag′inis arytenoi′deae** [TA], anterolateral surface of arytenoid cartilage: the external surface of the cartilage, which bears the triangular pit, the oblong pit, and the arcuate crest.

**f. anterolatera′lis hu′meri** [TA], anterolateral surface of humerus: the surface that provides attachment to the deltoid muscle and lateral part of the brachialis muscle. Called also *f. anterior lateralis humeri.*

**f. anteromedia′lis hu′meri** [TA], anteromedial surface of humerus: a surface beginning at the intertubercular groove and spreading out inferiorly to form the wide smooth area for origin of the brachialis muscle. Called also *f. anterior medialis humeri.*

**f. anterosupe′rior cor′poris pancre′atis** [TA], the anterosuperior surface of the body of the pancreas.

**f. approxima′lis den′tis** [TA], approximal surface: the area where the mesial and distal surfaces of the teeth touch each other; called also *centric stop, contact area* or *surface,* and *f. contactus dentis.*

**f. articula′ris acromia′lis clavi′culae** [TA], acromial articular surface of clavicle: the smooth area on the lateral end of the clavicle for articulation with the acromion of the scapula.

**f. articula′ris acromia′lis sca′pulae,** f. articularis acromii scapulae.

**f. articula′ris acro′mii sca′pulae,** articular surface of acromion: a small variable area on the acromion, for articulation with the acromial end of the clavicle; called also *f. articularis acromialis scapulae.*

**f. articula′ris ante′rior calca′nei,** f. articularis talaris anterior calcanei.

**f. articula′ris ante′rior den′tis** [TA], **f. articula′ris ante′rior epistro′phei,** anterior articular surface of dens: an oval facet on the anterior surface of the dens of the axis, articulating with the fovea dentis of the atlas; called also *anterior articular facet of dens of axis.*

**f. articula′ris arytenoi′dea cartila′ginis cricoi′deae** [TA], arytenoid articular surface of cricoid cartilage: the surface that articulates with the arytenoid cartilage.

**f. articula′ris calca′nea ante′rior ta′li** [TA], anterior calcaneal articular surface of talus: the small surface on the head of the talus that rests upon the anterior articular surface of the calcaneus.

**f. articula′ris calca′nea me′dia ta′li** [TA], middle calcaneal articular surface of talus: the convex part of the head of the talus that articulates with the sustentaculum tali of the calcaneus.

**f. articula′ris calca′nea poste′rior ta′li** [TA], posterior calcaneal articular surface of talus: a transverse concavity on the inferior surface of the talus, articulating with the calcaneus.

**f. articula′ris ca′pitis cos′tae** [TA], articular surface of head of rib: the surface on the head of a rib where it articulates with the body of a vertebra. Typically it is divided into two facets by a transverse crest, the lower facet articulating with the corresponding vertebra, and the upper facet with the suprajacent vertebra. The articular surfaces of the heads of the first, tenth, eleventh, and twelfth ribs generally consist of only one facet. Called also *f. articularis capituli costae,* and *posterior* or *superior costal facet.*

**f. articula′ris ca′pitis fi′bulae** [TA], articular surface of head of fibula: the medial surface of the head of the fibula, which articulates with the lateral condyle of the tibia; called also *f. articularis capituli fibulae.*

**f. articula′ris capi′tuli cos′tae,** f. articularis capitis costae.

**f. articula′ris capi′tuli fi′bulae,** f. articularis capitis fibulae.

**f. articula′ris carpa′lis ra′dii** [TA], carpal articular surface of radius: the convex surface of the distal end of the radius, which articulates with the lunate and scaphoid bones. Called also *f. articularis carpi radii.*

**f. articula′ris car′pi ra′dii,** f. articularis carpalis radii.

**f. articula′ris cartila′ginis arytenoi′dea** [TA], articular surface of arytenoid cartilage: the surface that articulates with the cricoid cartilage.

**f. articula′ris cuboi′dea calca′nei** [TA], cuboid articular surface of calcaneus: the saddle-shaped area on the anterior surface of the calcaneus where it articulates with the cuboid bone.

**f. articula′ris fibula′ris ti′biae** [TA], fibular articular surface of tibia: surface on the posteroinferior aspect of the lateral condyle of the tibia that articulates with the head of the fibula.

**f. articula′ris fos′sae mandibula′ris** [TA], articular surface of mandibular fossa: the articular surface found in the deep part of the mandibular fossa. Called also *f. articularis ossis temporalis.*

**f. articula′ris infe′rior atlan′tis** [TA], inferior articular surface of atlas: either of the two inferior articular surfaces found on the lateral masses of the atlas. Called also *inferior articular facet, fossa,* or *fovea of atlas.*

**f. articula′ris infe′rior ti′biae** [TA], inferior articular surface of tibia: the surface on the distal end of the tibia where it articulates with the talus.

**f. articula′ris infe′rior ver′tebrae** [TA], inferior articular surface of vertebra: the articulating surface on the inferior articular process of a vertebra.

**f. articula′ris malle′oli latera′lis** [TA], articular surface of lateral malleolus: the anterosuperior surface of the lateral malleolus, which articulates with the lateral side of the talus; called also *lateral malleolar fovea of fibula.*

**f. articula′ris malle′oli media′lis** [TA], articular surface of medial malleolus: the lateral aspect of the medial malleolus, which articulates with the talus; called also *fovea of lateral malleolus* and *internal malleolar facet of tibia.*

**f. articula′ris me′dia calca′nei,** f. articularis talaris media calcanei.

**f. articula′ris navicula′ris ta′li** [TA], navicular articular surface of talus: the surface of the head of the talus that articulates with the navicular bone.

**f. articula′ris os′sium,** articular surface of bone: the surface by which a bone articulates with another.

**f. articula′ris os′sis tempora′lis,** f. articularis fossae mandibularis.

**f. articula′ris patel′lae** [TA], articular surface of patella: the posterior surface of the patella, which is largely covered by a thick cartilaginous layer.

**f. articula′ris poste′rior den′tis** [TA], posterior articular surface of dens: a smooth groove on the posterior surface of the dens of the axis, which lodges the transverse ligament of the atlas.

**f. articula′ris sterna′lis clavi′culae** [TA], sternal articular surface of clavicle: a triangular surface on the medial end of the clavicle for articulation with the sternum.

**f. articula′ris supe′rior atlan′tis** [TA], superior articular surface of atlas: the large oval facet on the superior aspect of either lateral mass of the atlas; called also *superior articular facet, fossa,* or *fovea of atlas.*

**f. articula′ris supe′rior ti′biae** [TA], superior articular surface of tibia: the surface on the proximal end of the tibia that articulates with the condyles of the femur; called also *condyloid surface of tibia.*

**f. articula'ris supe'rior ver'tebrae** [TA], superior articular surface of vertebra: the articulating surface on the superior articular process of a vertebra.

**f. articula'ris tala'ris ante'rior calca'nei** [TA], anterior talar articular surface of calcaneus: the small area on the superior surface of the calcaneus just anterior to the middle articular surface, which articulates with the talus; called also *f. articularis anterior calcanei.*

**f. articula'ris tala'ris me'dia calca'nei** [TA], middle talar articular surface of calcaneus: the area on the superior surface of the calcaneus just in front of the calcaneal sulcus, which articulates with the talus; called also *f. articularis media calcanei* and *medial posterior facet of calcaneus.*

**f. articula'ris tala'ris poste'rior calca'nei** [TA], posterior talar articular surface of calcaneus: the area on the superior surface of the calcaneus just posterolateral to the calcaneal sulcus, which articulates with the talus.

**f. articula'ris thyroi'dea cartila'ginis cricoi'deae** [TA], thyroid articular surface of cricoid cartilage: the surface that articulates with the thyroid cartilage.

**f. articula'ris tuber'culi cos'tae** [TA], articular surface of tubercle of rib: the convex facet on the costal tubercle that articulates with the transverse process of a vertebra; called also *anterior* or *inferior costal facet.*

**f. auricula'ris os'sis i'lii** [TA], **f. auricula'ris os'sis i'lium,** auricular surface of ilium: a somewhat ear-shaped area on the sacropelvic surface of the ilium, which articulates with the auricular surface of the sacrum to form the sacroiliac joint.

**f. auricula'ris os'sis sa'cri** [TA], auricular surface of sacrum: the broad irregular surface on the superior half of the lateral aspect of the sacrum, which articulates with the ilium.

**f. bovi'na,** [L. "cow face"], a term sometimes applied to the appearance of the face in craniofacial dysostosis; called also *bovine* or *cow face.*

**brachial f., anterior,** regio brachii anterior.

**brachial f., posterior,** regio brachii posterior.

**f. brachia'lis ante'rior,** regio brachii anterior.

**f. brachia'lis poste'rior,** regio brachii posterior.

**f. bucca'lis den'tis** [TA], buccal surface: the vestibular surface of the molars and premolars that faces the cheek. See also *f. vestibularis dentis.*

**f. cerebra'lis a'lae mag'nae, f. cerebra'lis a'lae majo'ris** [TA], cerebral surface of greater wing: the smooth, concave part of the greater wing of the sphenoid bone that forms the anterior part of the floor of the middle cranial fossa, lying anterior to the petrous and squamous parts of the temporal bone.

**f. cerebra'lis os'sis fronta'lis,** f. interna ossis frontalis.

**f. cerebra'lis os'sis parieta'lis,** f. interna ossis parietalis.

**f. cerebra'lis par'tis squamo'sae os'sis tempora'lis** [TA], cerebral surface of squamous part of temporal bone: the inner surface of the squamous part forming the lateral wall of the middle cranial fossa.

**f. co'lica lie'nis,** TA alternative for *f. colica splenis.*

**f. co'lica sple'nis** [TA], the surface of the spleen in contact with the colon; called also *f. colica lienis* [TA alternative].

**f. contac'tus den'tis,** f. approximalis dentis.

**f. costa'lis pulmo'nis** [TA], costal surface of lung: the convex surface of each lung in close adaptation to the curvatures of the ribs and the costal cartilages, which joins the mediastinal surface at the anterior and posterior borders and the diaphragmatic surface at the inferior border. It is related behind to the sides of the vertebral bodies (pars vertebralis faciei costalis pulmonis).

**f. costa'lis sca'pulae** [TA], costal surface of scapula: the anteromedially facing, concave surface of the scapula; called also *anterior* or *ventral surface of scapula, f. anterior scapulae* [TA alternative], and *f. ventralis scapulae.*

**f. crura'lis ante'rior,** regio cruris anterior.

**f. crura'lis poste'rior,** regio cruris posterior.

**cubital f., anterior,** regio cubitalis anterior.

**cubital f., posterior,** regio cubitalis posterior.

**f. cubita'lis ante'rior,** regio cubitalis anterior.

**f. cubita'lis poste'rior,** regio cubitalis posterior.

**f. diaphragma'tica cor'dis** [TA], diaphragmatic surface of heart: the surface of the heart (within the pericardium) that rests on the diaphragm and is directed inferiorly and somewhat posteriorly; it is formed by the two ventricles, the left ventricle contributing a little more than the right; called also *f. inferior cordis.*

**f. diaphragma'tica he'patis** [TA], diaphragmatic surface of liver: the surface of the liver that is in contact with the diaphragm, being composed of the superior, anterior, right, and posterior parts (pars superior, pars anterior, pars dexter, and pars posterior).

**f. diaphragma'tica lie'nis,** TA alternative for *f. diaphragmatica splenis.*

**f. diaphragma'tica pulmo'nis** [TA], diaphragmatic surface of lung: the surface of each lung that is adjacent to the diaphragm.

**f. diaphragma'tica sple'nis** [TA], the convex posterolateral surface of the spleen which is directed toward the diaphragm; called also *f. diaphragmatica lienis* [TA alternative].

**f. digita'les,** the digital surfaces of the hand *(f. digitales manus),* or of the foot *(f. digitales pedis).*

**f. digita'les dorsa'les ma'nus,** f. dorsales digitorum manus.

**f. digita'les dorsa'les pe'dis,** f. dorsales digitorum pedis.

**f. digita'les fibula'res pe'dis,** f. digitales laterales pedis.

**f. digita'les latera'les ma'nus,** the lateral surfaces of the fingers; called also *f. digitales radiales manus.*

**f. digita'les latera'les pe'dis,** the lateral surfaces of the toes; called also *f. digitales fibulares pedis.*

**f. digita'les media'les ma'nus,** the medial surfaces of the fingers; called also *f. digitales ulnares manus.*

**f. digita'les media'les pe'dis,** the medial surfaces of the toes; called also *f. digitales tibiales pedis.*

**f. digita'les palma'res ma'nus,** f. palmares digitorum manus.

**f. digita'les planta'res pe'dis,** f. plantares digitorum pedis.

**f. digita'les radia'les ma'nus,** f. digitales laterales manus.

**f. digita'les tibia'les pe'dis,** f. digitales mediales pedis.

**f. digita'les ulna'res ma'nus,** f. digitales mediales manus.

**f. digita'les ventra'les ma'nus,** f. palmares digitorum manus.

**f. digita'les ventra'les pe'dis,** f. plantares digitorum pedis.

**f. dista'lis den'tis** [TA], distal surface: the proximal or contact surface of a tooth that is farthest from the midline of the dental arch.

**f. doloro'sa,** the facial expression of a patient experiencing pain or severe sickness.

**f. dorsa'les digito'rum ma'nus** [TA], the posterior or dorsal surfaces of the fingers; called also *f. digitales dorsales manus.*

**f. dorsa'les digito'rum pe'dis** [TA], the dorsal or superior surfaces of the toes; called also *f. digitales dorsales pedis.*

**f. dorsa'lis os'sis sac'ri** [TA], dorsal surface of sacral bone: the markedly convex and rough posterior, or dorsal, surface of the sacrum, which gives origin to the sacrospinalis and multifidus muscles; called also *posterior surface of sacral bone.*

**f. dorsa'lis ra'dii,** f. posterior radii.

**f. dorsa'lis sca'pulae,** f. posterior scapulae.

**f. dorsa'lis ul'nae,** f. posterior ulnae.

**f. exter'na os'sis fronta'lis** [TA], the external surface of the squama of the frontal bone; called also *f. frontalis ossis frontalis* and *outer table of frontal bone.*

**f. exter'na os'sis parieta'lis** [TA], the externally directed surface of the parietal bone; called also *f. parietalis ossis parietalis.*

**f. facia'lis den'tis,** f. vestibularis dentis.

**f. femora'lis ante'rior,** regio femoris anterior.

**f. femora'lis poste'rior,** regio femoris posterior.

**f. fronta'lis os'sis fronta'lis,** f. externa ossis frontalis.

**f. gas'trica lie'nis,** TA alternative for *f. gastrica splenis.*

**f. gas'trica sple'nis** [TA], the surface of the spleen in contact with the stomach; called also *f. gastrica lienis* [TA alternative].

**f. glu'tea os'sis i'lii** [TA], **f. glutea'lis os'sis i'lii,** gluteal surface of ilium: the large external, or posterior, surface of the ala of the ilium, on which are located the three gluteal lines.

**f. hepa'tica,** a thin face with sunken eyeballs, sallow complexion, and yellow conjunctivae, characteristic of certain chronic disorders of the liver.

**f. hippocra'tica,** a drawn, pinched, and pale appearance of the face, indicative of approaching death.

**Hutchinson's f.,** a peculiar appearance in ophthalmoplegia externa, the eyeballs being fixed, the eyebrows raised, and the lids drooping.

**f. infe'rior ce'rebri,** inferior surface of cerebrum: the inferior surfaces of the two hemispheres, considered as a unit; see *f. inferior hemispherii cerebri.* Called also *base of brain* and *basis cerebri.*

**f. infe'rior cor'dis,** f. diaphragmatica cordis.

**f. infe'rior hemisphe'rii cerebel'li,** inferior surface of hemisphere of cerebellum: a surface formed by the inferior semilunar lobule, the biventral lobule, the tonsilla, and the flocculus.

**f. infe'rior hemisphe'rii ce'rebri,** inferior surface of hemisphere of cerebrum: the part of the cerebral hemisphere that rests on the tentorium and in the anterior and middle cranial fossae. See *f. medialis et inferior hemispherii cerebri.*

**f. infe'rior he'patis,** f. visceralis hepatis.

**f. infe'rior lin'guae** [TA], inferior surface of tongue: the under surface of the body of the tongue.

**f. infe'rior pancre'atis,** f. anteroinferior corporis pancreatis.

**f. infe'rior par'tis petro'sae os'sis tempora'lis** [TA], **f. infe'rior pyram'idis os'sis tempora'lis,** inferior surface of petrous part of temporal bone: that surface of the petrous part of the temporal bone which appears on the external surface of the base of the cranium.

**f. inferolatera'lis prosta'tae** [TA], the inferolateral surface of the prostate, which is convex and separated from the superior fascia of the pelvic diaphragm by a venous plexus.

**f. infratempora'lis cor'poris maxil'lae** [TA], infratemporal surface of body of maxilla: the posterior convex surface of the body of the maxilla, bounded roughly by the inferior orbital fissure, the zygomatic process and associated ridge, maxillary tuberosity, and posterior margin of the nasal surface.

**f. interloba'ris pulmo'nis** [TA], interlobar surface of lung: the surface of each lung lying within the oblique and horizontal fissures.

**f. inter'na os'sis fronta'lis** [TA], internal surface of frontal bone: the vertically situated, concave cerebral surface of the frontal bone; in its midline the sagittal sulcus is seen superiorly and the frontal crest inferiorly. Called also *f. cerebralis ossis frontalis* and *inner table of frontal bone.*

**f. inter'na os'sis parieta'lis** [TA], the internal, or cerebral, surface of the parietal bone; called also *f. cerebralis ossis parietalis* and *cerebral surface of parietal bone.*

**f. intervertebra'lis** [TA], the surface of the vertebral body adjacent to the intervertebral disk, having an elevated rim (the annular apophysis) surrounding a rough center.

**f. intestina'lis u'teri** [TA], intestinal surface of uterus: the convex posterior surface of the uterus, adjacent to the intestine.

**f. labia'lis den'tis** [TA], labial surface: the vestibular surface of the incisors and canines that faces the lips. See also *f. vestibularis dentis.*

**f. latera'lis den'tium incisivo'rum et canino'rum,** the distal surfaces of incisors and canines.

**f. latera'lis fi'bulae** [TA], lateral surface of fibula: the area between the anterior and posterior borders of the body of the fibula.

**f. latera'lis os'sis zygoma'tici** [TA], lateral surface of zygomatic bone: the more anterior surface, which is convex; called also *f. malaris ossis zygomatici.*

**f. latera'lis ova'rii** [TA], lateral surface of ovary: the surface of the ovary in contact with the lateral pelvic wall.

**f. latera'lis ra'dii** [TA], lateral surface of radius: the surface of the radius that gives attachment to the supinator and pronator teres muscles proximally, and underlies the tendons of the extensor carpi radialis longus and brevis muscles distally.

**f. latera'lis tes'tis** [TA], lateral surface of testis: the surface of the testis that is directed away from its fellow of the opposite side.

**f. latera'lis ti'biae** [TA], lateral surface of tibia: the surface of the body of the tibia between the interosseous and anterior borders; called also *external border of tibia.*

**leonine f., f. leonti'na** ["lion's face"], a peculiar, deeply furrowed, lionlike appearance of the face, seen in certain cases of advanced lepromatous leprosy (see *leontiasis*) and in other diseases associated with facial edema such as coast erysipelas, a cutaneous manifestation of onchocerciasis seen in Central America.

**f. lingua'lis den'tis** [TA], lingual surface: the surface of a tooth that faces inward toward the tongue (oral cavity), and opposite the vestibular (or facial) surface. Called also *oral surface.*

**f. luna'ta aceta'buli** [TA], lunate surface of acetabulum: the articular portion of the acetabulum.

**f. mala'ris os'sis zygoma'tici,** f. lateralis ossis zygomatici.

**f. malleola'ris latera'lis ta'li** [TA], lateral malleolar surface of talus: the large triangular facet on the talus that articulates with the lateral malleolus.

**f. malleola'ris media'lis ta'li** [TA], medial malleolar surface of talus: the narrow facet on the talus continuous with the superior surface; it articulates with the medial malleolus.

**Marshall Hall's f.,** the facies of hydrocephalus: a triangular face with a broad forehead and prominent frontal bones.

**f. masticato'ria den'tis,** 1. f. occlusalis dentis. 2. working occlusal surface.

**f. maxilla'ris a'lae mag'nae, f. maxilla'ris a'lae majo'ris** [TA], maxillary surface of greater wing of sphenoid bone: a small surface on the inferior part of the greater wing superior to the pterygoid processes; it is perforated by the foramen rotundum. Called also *f. sphenomaxillaris alae magnae.*

**f. maxilla'ris la'minae perpendicula'ris os'sis palati'ni** [TA], maxillary surface of perpendicular plate of palatine bone: the lateral surface of the perpendicular plate of the palatine bone, which is in relation to the maxilla. Posteriorly and inferiorly it contains the greater palatine sulcus, which forms the greater palatine canal with a corresponding groove on the maxilla.

**f. media'lis cartila'ginis arytenoi'deae** [TA], medial surface of arytenoid cartilage: the surface that faces medially toward the opposite arytenoid cartilage.

**f. media'lis den'tium incisivo'rum et canino'rum,** the contact surface of the incisor and canine teeth that is directed toward the midline of the dental arch.

**f. media'lis fi'bulae** [TA], medial surface of fibula: the narrow area on the body of the fibula between the interosseous and anterior borders.

**f. media'lis hemisphe'rii ce'rebri,** medial surface of hemisphere of cerebrum: the surface of the cerebral hemisphere parallel to and facing both the median plane and the corresponding surface of the opposite hemisphere. See *f. medialis et inferior hemispherii cerebri.*

**f. media'lis et infe'rior hemisphe'rii ce'rebri** [TA], the medial and inferior surfaces of the cerebral hemisphere considered as a unit.

**f. media'lis ova'rii** [TA], medial surface of ovary: the side of the ovary in contact with the fimbriated end of the uterine tube and the intestine.

**f. media'lis pulmo'nis,** f. mediastinalis pulmonis.

**f. media'lis tes'tis** [TA], medial surface of testis: the surface of the testis that is directed toward its fellow of the opposite side.

**f. media'lis ti'biae** [TA], medial surface of tibia: the slightly convex surface of the body of the tibia between the anterior and medial borders.

**f. media'lis ul'nae** [TA], medial surface of ulna: the smooth, rounded, internal surface of the ulna.

**f. mediastina'lis pulmo'nis** [TA], mediastinal surface of lung: the surface of each lung lying medially to the vertebral column and mediastinum; it contains the cardiac impression. Called also *f. medialis pulmonis.*

**f. mesia'lis den'tis** [TA], mesial surface: the contact or proximal surface of a tooth that is closest to the midline of the dental arch.

**mitral f., mitrotricuspid f.,** the appearance of the face of some patients with mitral stenosis of long duration, marked by rosy, flushed cheeks and dilated capillaries.

**moon f.,** see under *face.*

**myasthenic f.,** the characteristic facial expression in myasthenia gravis, caused by ptosis and weakness of the facial muscles.

**myopathic f.,** the peculiar facial expression produced by relaxation of the facial muscles, as in Landouzy-Dejerine dystrophy.

**f. nasa'lis cor'poris maxil'lae** [TA], nasal surface of body of maxilla: the surface of the body of the maxilla that helps form the lateral wall of the nasal cavity; it is bounded roughly by the following: medial margin of the orbital surface, medial margin of the infratemporal surface, the palatine process, and the nasal notch.

**f. nasa'lis la'minae horizonta'lis os'sis palati'ni** [TA], nasal surface of horizontal plate of palatine bone: the superior surface of the horizontal plate, which forms the posterior part of the floor of the nasal cavity.

**f. nasa'lis la'minae perpendicula'ris os'sis palati'ni** [TA], nasal surface of perpendicular plate of palatine bone: the medial surface of the perpendicular plate; it articulates with the middle and inferior nasal conchae.

**f. occlusa'lis den'tis** [TA], occlusal surface of teeth: the surface of the posterior or artificial teeth coming in contact with those of the opposite jaw during the act of occlusion. In natural teeth, restricted to the anatomic tooth surfaces of the posterior teeth limited mesially and distally by the marginal ridges and buccally and lingually by the buccal and lingual boundaries of the cusp eminences. By extension, the term *occlusal surface* is used to designate the incisal surface (q.v.) of the anterior teeth. Called also *f. masticatoria dentis* and *masticatory surface.*

**f. orbita'lis a'lae mag'nae, f. orbita'lis a'lae majo'ris** [TA], orbital surface of greater wing: the quadrilateral surface on the greater wing of the sphenoid bone that forms the major part of the lateral wall of the orbit; called also *orbital border of sphenoid bone.*

**f. orbita'lis cor'poris maxil'lae** [TA], orbital surface of body of maxilla: a triangular surface on the body of the maxilla that forms the greater part of the floor of the orbit.

**f. orbita'lis os'sis fronta'lis** [TA], orbital surface of frontal bone: the triangular plates of the frontal bone that form most of the roof of each orbit and the floor of the anterior cranial fossa; they are separated by the ethmoidal notch.

**f. orbita'lis os'sis zygoma'tici** [TA], orbital surface of zygomatic bone: the part of the zygomatic bone that helps form the lateral wall of the orbit.

**f. palata'lis den'tis** [TA], palatal surface: the lingual surface of a maxillary tooth.

**f. palati'na la'minae horizonta'lis os'sis palati'ni** [TA], palatine surface of horizontal plate of palatine bone: the inferior surface of the horizontal plate, forming the posterior part of the hard palate.

**f. palma'res digito'rum ma'nus** [TA], the anterior or palmar surfaces of the fingers; called also *f. digitales palmares manus* and *f. digitales ventrales manus.*

**f. parieta'lis os'sis parieta'lis,** f. externa ossis parietalis.

**Parkinson's f., parkinsonian f.,** a stolid masklike expression of the face, with infrequent blinking, pathognomonic of parkinsonism; see also *parkinsonian syndrome,* under *syndrome,* and see *paralysis agitans.*

**f. patella'ris fe'moris** [TA], the smooth anterior continuation of the condyles that forms the surface of the femur articulating with the patella; called also *anterior intercondylar fossa of femur* and *patellar fossa of femur.*

**f. pel'vica os'sis sa'cri** [TA], **f. pelvi'na os'sis sac'ri,** pelvic surface of sacrum: the smooth, concave, ventrocaudally directed surface of the sacrum that helps form the posterior wall of the pelvis; called also *anterior surface of sacral bone.*

**f. planta′res digito′rum pe′dis** [TA], the plantar or inferior surfaces of the toes; called also *f. digitales plantares pedis* and *f. digitales ventrales pedis.*

**f. popli′tea fe′moris** [TA], popliteal surface of femur: the triangular lower third of the posterior surface of the femur, between the medial and lateral supracondylar lines, which forms the superior part of the floor of the popliteal fossa; called also *planum popliteum femoris.*

**f. poste′rior cartila′ginis arytenoi′deae** [TA], posterior surface of arytenoid cartilage: the concave dorsal surface, to which various laryngeal muscles are attached.

**f. poste′rior cor′neae** [TA], the posterior surface of the cornea, which forms the anterior boundary of the anterior chamber.

**f. poste′rior cor′poris pancre′atis** [TA], posterior surface of body of pancreas: the pancreatic surface directed toward the posterior part of the body.

**f. poste′rior den′tium premola′rium et mola′rium,** the distal surfaces of premolar and molar teeth.

**f. poste′rior fi′bulae** [TA], posterior surface of fibula: the large area between the posterior and interosseous borders of the body of the fibula, presenting the medial crest.

**f. poste′rior glan′dulae suprarena′lis** [TA], the posterior surface of the adrenal (suprarenal) gland, which borders the peritoneum.

**f. poste′rior he′patis,** pars posterior faciei diaphragmaticae hepatis.

**f. poste′rior hu′meri** [TA], posterior surface of humerus: the surface of the humerus that is subdivided obliquely by the radial groove to give attachment to the lateral and medial heads of the triceps muscle.

**f. poste′rior i′ridis** [TA], the posterior surface of the iris, directed toward the posterior chamber of the eye.

**f. poste′rior len′tis** [TA], the posterior surface of the lens, directed toward the vitreous body of the eye.

**f. poste′rior pal′pebrae** [TA], posterior surface of eyelid: the inner surface of the eyelid, which is covered with conjunctiva and in contact with the eyeball.

**f. poste′rior palpebra′lis, f. poste′rior palpebra′rum,** f. posterior palpebrae.

**f. poste′rior par′tis petro′sae os′sis tempora′lis** [TA], the surface of the petrous part of the temporal bone that forms part of the anterior portion of the floor of the posterior cranial fossa; called also *f. posterior pyramidis ossis temporalis.*

**f. poste′rior prosta′tae** [TA], the posterior surface of the prostate, separated by fascia from the anterior wall of the rectum.

**f. poste′rior pyra′midis os′sis tempora′lis,** f. posterior partis petrosae ossis temporalis.

**f. poste′rior ra′dii** [TA], posterior surface of radius: a surface giving attachment to the supinator, abductor pollicis longus, and extensor pollicis brevis muscles; called also *f. dorsalis radii.*

**f. poste′rior re′nis** [TA], posterior surface of kidney: the surface directed toward the posterior body wall, and not covered by peritoneum.

**f. poste′rior sca′pulae** [TA], posterior surface of scapula: the convex posterior surface of the scapula, which is divided into two unequal parts by the spine of the scapula. Called also *dorsal surface of scapula, dorsum of scapula, dorsum scapulae,* and *f. dorsalis scapulae.*

**f. poste′rior ti′biae** [TA], posterior surface of tibia: the surface of the body of the tibia between the medial and interosseous borders; in the proximal third it presents the soleal line.

**f. poste′rior ul′nae** [TA], posterior surface of ulna: the posterolaterally directed surface of the ulna; called also *f. dorsalis ulnae.*

**Potter f.,** the characteristic facial appearance seen with oligohydramnios sequence (q.v.), consisting of a flattened nose, receding chin, wide interpupillary space, large, low-set ears, and less commonly other anomalies.

**f. pulmona′lis cor′dis, f. pulmona′lis dex′tra/sinis′tra cor′dis** [TA], right/left pulmonary surface of heart: the surface of the heart that faces either of the lungs.

**f. rena′lis glan′dulae suprarena′lis** [TA], renal surface of adrenal gland: the surface directed toward the kidney, being separated from it by a layer of fat; called also *basis glandulae suprarenalis* and *inferior margin of suprarenal gland.*

**f. rena′lis lie′nis,** TA alternative for *f. renalis splenis.*

**f. rena′lis sple′nis** [TA], the surface of the spleen in contact with the left kidney; called also *f. renalis lienis* [TA alternative].

**f. sacropel′vica os′sis i′lii** [TA], **f. sacropelvi′na os′sis i′lii,** sacropelvic surface of ilium: an irregular area on the inner surface of the ala of the ilium, posterior to the iliac fossa; it contains the iliac tuberosity and the auricular surface.

**f. scaphoi′dea,** dish face.

**f. sphenomaxilla′ris a′lae mag′nae, f. sphenomaxilla′ris a′lae majo′ris,** f. maxillaris alae majoris.

**f. sternocosta′lis cor′dis** [TA], sternocostal surface of heart: the convex surface of the heart, which in general is directed anteriorly and somewhat superiorly, being formed mainly by the right ventricle, and to a lesser degree by the left ventricle and the atria; called also *f. anterior cordis.*

**f. supe′rior hemisphe′rii cerebel′li,** the superior surface of the cerebellar hemisphere, consisting of the ala of the lobulus centralis, the lobulus quadrangularis, the lobulus simplex, and the superior semilunar lobule.

**f. supe′rior he′patis,** pars superior faciei diaphragmaticae hepatis.

**f. supe′rior troch′leae ta′li** [TA], superior surface of trochlea of talus: the broad, smooth surface of the talus that articulates with the tibia.

**f. superolatera′lis ce′rebri, f. superolatera′lis hemisphe′rii ce′rebri** [TA], superolateral surface of hemisphere of cerebrum: the convex outer surface of the cerebrum, which faces the calvaria.

**f. symphy′seos os′sis pu′bis, f. symphysia′lis os′sis pu′bis** [TA], symphysial surface of pubic bone: the rough, ovoid, medial surface of the body of the pubic bone, by which it articulates at the pubic symphysis with its fellow of the opposite side.

**f. tempora′lis a′lae mag′nae, f. tempora′lis a′lae majo′ris** [TA], temporal surface of greater wing: the lateral and inferior surface of the greater wing of the sphenoid bone, divided by the infratemporal crest into a superior part that forms a portion of the wall of the temporal fossa, and an inferior part that forms part of the wall of the infratemporal fossa.

**f. tempora′lis os′sis fronta′lis** [TA], temporal surface of frontal bone: the slightly concave surface of the frontal bone that forms the superior part of the wall of the temporal fossa and gives attachment to the anterosuperior part of the temporalis muscle.

**f. tempora′lis os′sis zygomat′ici** [TA], temporal surface of zygomatic bone: the internal, concave surface of the bone, facing the temporal and infratemporal fossae.

**f. tempora′lis par′tis squamo′sae os′sis tempora′lis** [TA], temporal surface of squamous part of temporal bone: the external surface of the squamous part, the anterior part of which forms a portion of the temporal fossa.

**f. urethra′lis pe′nis** [TA], urethral surface of penis: the surface of the penis overlying the urethra, and opposite the dorsum penis.

**f. ventra′lis sca′pulae,** f. costalis scapulae.

**f. vesica′lis u′teri** [TA], vesical surface of uterus: the flat anterior surface of the uterus, adjacent to the urinary bladder.

**f. vestibula′ris den′tis** [TA], vestibular surface: the surface of a tooth that is directed outward toward the vestibule of the mouth, including the buccal and labial surfaces, and opposite the lingual (or oral) surface. Called also *f. facialis dentis* and *facial surface.*

**f. viscera′lis he′patis** [TA], the posteroinferior surface of the liver, which is in contact with various abdominal viscera; called also *f. inferior hepatis.*

**f. viscera′lis lie′nis,** TA alternative for *f. visceralis splenis.*

**f. viscera′lis sple′nis** [TA], the surface of the spleen which comes in contact with various other viscera, including the colon (facies colica), kidney (facies renalis), and stomach (facies gastrica); called also *f. visceralis lienis* [TA alternative].

**f. vola′ris ra′dii,** f. anterior radii.

**f. vola′ris ul′nae,** f. anterior ulnae.

**fa·cil·i·ta·tion** (fə-sil″ĭ-ta′shən) [L. *facilis* easy] 1. the promotion or hastening of any natural process; the reverse of inhibition. 2. in neurophysiology, the effect of a nerve impulse acting across a synapse, resulting in increased postsynaptic action potential of subsequent impulses in that nerve fiber or in other convergent nerve fibers. See *law of facilitation.*

**postactivation f., posttetanic f.,** facilitation at the neuromuscular junction, consisting of a decreased decrementing response or in-creased amplitude of the M wave, when nerve stimulation is repeated a few seconds after a strong voluntary contraction or after tetanus has occurred. See also *postactivation depression* and *postactivation exhaustion.*

**proprioceptive neuromuscular f.,** a system of therapeutic exercise for the inhibition of spasticity, with emphasis on the training of specific diagonal or spiral body movements against resistance in synergistic patterns; long repetition of involuntary reflex movements is aimed at the eventual development of greater voluntary motor control.

**Wedensky f.**, facilitation across a block; when there is a complete block to nerve conduction the threshold of the nerve below the block to electric stimulation is lowered.

**fa·cil·i·ta·tive** (fə-sil′ĭ-ta″tiv) in pharmacology, denoting a reaction arising as an indirect result of drug action, as development of an infection after the normal microflora has been altered by an antibiotic.

**fac·ing** (fās′ing) a porcelain reproduction of the labial or buccal surface of a tooth; it may be constructed with or without pins and is soldered or cemented to a metal backing.

**faci(o)-** [L. *facies* face] a combining form denoting relationship to the face.

**fa·cio·bra·chi·al** (fa″she-o-bra′ke-əl) [*facio-* + *brachial*] pertaining to the face and arm.

**fa·cio·ceph·a·lal·gia** (fa″she-o-sef″ə-lal′jə) [*facio-* + *cephalalgia*] neuralgic pain in the face and neck attributed to disorders of the autonomic nervous system.

**fa·cio·cer·vi·cal** (fa″she-o-sər′vĭ-kəl) [*facio-* + *cervical*] pertaining to or affecting the face and neck.

**fa·cio·lin·gual** (fa″she-o-ling′wəl) [*facio-* + *lingual*] pertaining to the face and tongue.

**fa·cio·plas·ty** (fa″she-o-plas′te) [*facio-* + *-plasty*] plastic surgery of the face.

**fa·cio·ple·gia** (fa″she-o-ple′jə) [*facio-* + *-plegia*] facial paralysis.

**fa·cio·scap·u·lo·hu·mer·al** (fa″she-o-skap″u-lo-hu′mər-əl) pertaining to the face, scapula, and arm.

**fa·cio·ste·no·sis** (fa″she-o-stə-no′sis) failure of the midface to grow.

**FACOG** Fellow of the American College of Obstetricians and Gynecologists.

**FACP** Fellow of the American College of Physicians.

**FACR** Fellow of the American College of Radiology.

**FACS** fluorescence-activated cell sorter; Fellow of the American College of Surgeons.

**FACSM** Fellow of the American College of Sports Medicine.

**F-act·in** see *actin.*

**fac·ti·tial** (fak-tish′əl) produced by artificial means; unintentionally produced.

**fac·ti·tious** (fak-tish′əs) [L. *factitiosus*] artificial; not natural.

**fac·tor** (fak′tor) [L. "maker"] 1. any of several substances or activities that are necessary to produce a result, e.g., a coagulation factor. Often, use of the term "factor" indicates that the chemical nature of the substance or its mechanism of action is unknown, as in endocrinology, where "factors" are renamed as "hormones" when their chemical nature is determined. 2. one of two or more quantities that multiplied together form a product. 3. a coefficient or conversion factor, a number by which a quantity is multiplied to produce a change of units of measurement. 4. a gene (hereditary factor).

## Factor

**f. I**, see under *coagulation f's.*
**f. II**, see under *coagulation f's.*
**f. III**, see under *coagulation f's.*
**f. IV**, see under *coagulation f's.*
**f. V**, see under *coagulation f's.*
**f. VI**, see under *coagulation f's.*
**f. VII**, see under *coagulation f's.*
**f. VIII**, see under *coagulation f's.*
**f. IX**, see under *coagulation f's.*
**f. X**, see under *coagulation f's.*
**f. XI**, see under *coagulation f's.*
**f. XII**, see under *coagulation f's.*
**f. XIII**, see under *coagulation f's.*

**f. A**, former name for the alternative pathway complement factor *C3;* see under *complement.*

**accelerator f.**, f. V; see under *coagulation f's.*

**activation f.**, f. XII; see under *coagulation f's.*

**angiogenesis f.**, a substance that causes the growth of new blood vessels, found in tissues with high metabolic requirements such as cancers and the retina; it is also released by hypoxic macrophages at the edges or outer surface of a wound and initiates revascularization in wound healing.

**antigen-specific T-cell helper f.**, a soluble factor produced by helper T cells that activates other lymphocytes that are specific for the stimulating antigen; it may itself bind antigen.

**antigen-specific T-cell suppressor f.**, a soluble factor produced by suppressor T cells following immunization; it produces antigen-specific suppression of the immune response and may itself bind antigen.

**antihemophilic f.**, 1. f. VIII, see under *coagulation f's.* Abbreviated AHF. 2. [USP] a sterile freeze-dried powder containing the Factor VIII fraction prepared from human venous plasma; used to arrest hemorrhage or to prevent hemorrhage during surgery or other procedures in patients with hemophilia A; administered intravenously.

**antihemophilic f. A**, f. VIII; see under *coagulation f's.*

**antihemophilic f. B**, f. IX; see under *coagulation f's.*

**antihemophilic f. C**, f. XI; see under *coagulation f's.*

**antihemophilic f. (human)**, antihemophilic f. (def. 2).

**antihemophilic f. (porcine)**, a highly purified sterile freeze-dried concentrate of porcine factor VIII:C; it is less antigenic than human factor VIII:C and is used in the treatment of hemophilia in patients with circulatory antibodies to factor VIII:C and in patients with spontaneously acquired inhibitors to human factor VIII:C; administered by intravenous infusion.

**antinuclear f. (ANF)**, see under *antibody.*

**atrial natriuretic f. (ANF)**, 1. atrial natriuretic peptide. 2. sometimes more specifically, the prohormone form of atrial natriuretic peptide.

**autocrine growth f.**, a polypeptide, produced endogenously by a cell free from usual external growth controls, that may act on its producer cell to cause malignant transformation.

**f. B**, a complement component that participates in the alternative pathway of complement activation (see *complement*), binding to C3b to form C3bB, which is a substrate for factor D.

**basophil chemotactic f. (BCF)**, a lymphokine produced by activated lymphocytes that is chemotactic for basophils, possibly responsible for the influx of basophils into sites of inflammation (Jones-Mote reaction).

**B-cell differentiation f's (BCDF)**, factors derived from T cells that stimulate B cells to differentiate into antibody-secreting cells. Cf. *B-lymphocyte stimulatory f's.*

**B-cell growth f's (BCGF)**, factors derived from T cells that stimulate B cells to proliferate in vitro but (unlike B-cell differentiation factors) do not stimulate antibody secretion. Cf. *B-lymphocyte stimulatory f's.*

**blastogenic f. (BF)**, lymphocyte mitogenic f.

**B-lymphocyte stimulatory f's (BSF)**, a system of nomenclature for factors that stimulate B cells, replacing individual factor names (e.g., B-cell differentiation factor). Each factor is designated by BSF and a number, BSF1, BSF2, etc., with the letter p prefixed to the number for factors that have not been purified or whose structure has not been identified. BSF1 is interleukin-4 and BSF2 is interleukin-6.

**bone f.**, in periodontal disease, the systemic influence on alveolar bone loss in response to local inflammatory processes.

**C f.**, a factor found in the soluble part of cytoplasm which promotes the contraction of mitochondria.

**CAMP f.**, see under *test.*

**Castle's intrinsic f.**, intrinsic f.

**chemotactic f.**, a substance that induces chemotaxis. Called also *chemoattractant* and *chemotaxin.*

**Christmas f.**, f. IX; see under *coagulation f's.*

**citrovorum f.**, folinic acid.

**C3 nephritic f. (C3 NeF)**, an autoantibody that binds the alternative complement pathway C3 convertase C3b,Bb and prevents its inactivation by factor H, resulting in chronic fluid phase alternative pathway activation and complete consumption of plasma C3; found in the serum of many patients with type II membranoproliferative glomerulonephritis.

**coagulation f's**, substances in the blood that are essential to the clotting process and hence, to the maintenance of normal hemostasis. They are designated by Roman numerals, to which the notation "a" is added to indicate the activated state. Platelet factors (q.v.) also play a role in coagulation.

**f. I**, fibrinogen: a high-molecular-weight plasma protein which is converted to fibrin through the action of thrombin. Deficiency of this factor results in afibrinogenemia or hypofibrinogenemia.

**f. II,** prothrombin: a plasma protein that is converted to the active form thrombin (factor IIa) by cleavage by activated factor X (Xa) in the common pathway of blood coagulation; thrombin then cleaves fibrinogen to its active form fibrin. Deficiency of the factor leads to hypoprothrombinemia.
**f. III,** tissue thromboplastin: a lipoprotein functioning in the extrinsic pathway of blood coagulation, activating factor X. Called also *tissue f.*
**f. IV,** calcium: a factor required in many phases of blood coagulation.
**f. V,** proaccelerin: a heat- and storage-labile material, present in plasma but not in serum, functioning in both the intrinsic and extrinsic pathways of blood coagulation, catalyzing the cleavage of prothrombin to the active thrombin. Deficiency of this factor, an autosomal recessive trait, leads to a rare hemorrhagic tendency, parahemophilia, of variable severity. Called also *accelerator globulin (AcG)* and *labile f.*
**f. VI,** a factor (accelerin) previously thought to be an activated form of factor V. It no longer is considered in the scheme of hemostasis, and hence it is currently assigned neither a name nor a function.
**f. VII,** proconvertin: a heat- and storage-stable factor participating in the extrinsic pathway of blood coagulation. It is activated by contact with calcium and in concert with factor III (tissue thromboplastin) activates factor X. Deficiency of this factor, which may be hereditary (autosomal recessive) or acquired (associated with vitamin K deficiency), results in a hemorrhagic tendency. Called also *serum prothrombin conversion accelerator (SPCA)* and *stable f.* The activated form is called also *convertin.*
**f. VIII,** antihemophilic factor (AHF): a relatively storage-labile factor participating in the intrinsic pathway of blood coagulation, acting (in concert with von Willebrand factor) as a cofactor in the activation of factor X. Deficiency, an X-linked recessive trait, causes hemophilia A (classical hemophilia). Called also *antihemophilic globulin (AHG)* and *antihemophilic f. A.*
**f. IX,** plasma thromboplastin component (PTC): a relatively storage-stable substance involved in the intrinsic pathway of blood coagulation; upon activation, it activates factor X. Deficiency results in a hemorrhagic syndrome called hemophilia B, resembling hemophilia A. Called also *autoprothrombin II, Christmas f.,* and *antihemophilic f. B.*
**f. X,** Stuart factor: a storage-stable factor that participates in both the intrinsic and extrinsic pathways of blood coagulation, uniting them to begin the common pathway of coagulation. Once activated, it forms a complex with calcium, phospholipid, and factor V; the complex (prothrombinase) can cleave and activate prothrombin to thrombin. Deficiency of this factor may cause a systemic coagulation disorder. Called also *autoprothrombin C, Prower factor, and Stuart-Prower factor.* The activated form is called also *thrombokinase.*
**f. XI,** plasma thromboplastin antecedent (PTA): a stable factor involved in the intrinsic pathway of blood coagulation; once activated, it activates factor IX. Deficiency of this factor results in a systemic blood-clotting defect called hemophilia C, which may resemble hemophilia A. Called also *antihemophilic f. C.*
**f. XII,** Hageman factor: a stable factor activated by contact with glass or other foreign surfaces, which initiates the intrinsic process of blood coagulation by activating factor XI and participates in activation of the kinin and fibrinolytic pathways. Deficiency of this factor results in a tendency toward thrombotic disorders, due to lack of activation of the fibrinolytic pathway. Called also *glass, contact,* or *activation f.*
**f. XIII,** fibrin-stabilizing factor (FSF): a factor that polymerizes fibrin monomers so that they become stable and insoluble in urea, thus enabling fibrin to form a firm blood clot. Deficiency of this factor produces a clinical hemorrhagic diathesis. Called also *fibrinase, protransglutaminase,* and *Laki-Lorand f.* The activated form is also called *transglutaminase.*

**colony-stimulating f's,** a group of glycoprotein lymphokine growth factors produced by blood monocytes, tissue macrophages, and stimulated lymphocytes; they are required for differentiation of stem cells into granulocyte and monocyte cell colonies, and were originally named according to their ability to stimulate the production of morphologically distinguishable myeloid cell colonies *in vitro. In vivo,* they stimulate the production of granulocytes and macrophages and enhance the actions of mature cells. Colony-stimulating factors can be produced by recombinant DNA techniques and have been used experimentally as anticancer agents and for the restoration of hematopoietic function after myelosuppression in transplantation and cancer chemotherapy.

**contact f.,** f. XII; see under *coagulation f's.*

**cord f.,** a mycoside produced by those strains of *Mycobacterium tuberculosis* that characteristically grow in long serpentine cords.

**cryoprecipitated antihemophilic f.** [USP], a sterile, frozen concentrate of human antihemophilic factor prepared from the coagulation factor VIII–rich cryoprotein fraction of human venous plasma; used for autologous replacement of factor VIII in patients with hemophilia A, administered intravenously.

**crystal-induced chemotactic f. (CCF),** a glycoprotein produced by neutrophils upon ingestion of monosodium urate or calcium pyrophosphate crystals, which is directly chemotactic for neutrophils and is thought to be involved in the inflammatory process in gouty arthritis.

**f. D,** a serine protease of the alternative complement pathway that cleaves factor B bound to C3b. The reaction releases Ba while leaving Bb bound to C3b to form the C3bBb that is the C3 convertase of the alternative pathway.

**decay accelerating f. (DAF),** a protein of most blood cells as well as endothelial and epithelial cells, CD55; it protects the cell membranes from attack by autologous complement, either by preventing assembly of convertase on the cell surface or by accelerating its decay once bound.

**diabetogenic f.,** see under *hormone.*

**diffusion f., Duran-Reynals f.,** hyaluronidase.

**elongation f.,** one of two soluble proteins (EF-1 and EF-2) involved in the addition of each amino acid to the growing polypeptide chain in protein synthesis (see *translation).*

**endothelial-derived relaxant f., endothelium-derived relaxing f. (EDRF),** nitric oxide.

**eosinophil chemotactic f. (ECF),** 1. eosinophil chemotactic f. of anaphylaxis. 2. a lymphokine produced by activated lymphocytes that is chemotactic for eosinophils.

**eosinophil chemotactic f. of anaphylaxis (ECF-A),** eosinophil chemoattractants released by basophils and mast cells in immediate hypersensitivity reactions. ECF-A activity is associated with two acidic tetrapeptides (Ala-Gly-Ser-Glu and Val-Gly-Ser-Glu) and with less well characterized larger peptides, which are chemotactic for eosinophils and, to a lesser degree, for neutrophils. Some ECF-A activity is due to arachidonic acid metabolites (leukotriene B, 12-HETE, and 12-HHT). Called also *eosinophil chemotactic f. (ECF).*

**epidermal growth f. (EGF),** a mitogenic polypeptide originally extracted from the submandibular glands of male mice; it is produced by many cell types and is made in large amounts by some tumors. It promotes growth and differentiation, is essential in embryogenesis, and is also important in wound healing. It has been found to be part of a family of compounds that includes human epidermal growth factor, transforming growth factors, and amphiregulin.

**epidermal growth f., human,** a mitogenic polypeptide found in humans that is 70 per cent homologous with the epidermal growth factor of mice; it promotes growth and differentiation, is essential in embryogenesis, and is important in wound healing. It is produced by many normal cell types and is made in large amounts by some tumors; the kidneys are the major source of the circulating factor. Called also *urogastrone.*

**epithelial growth f.,** human epidermal growth f.

**erythropoietic stimulating f. (ESF),** erythropoietin.

**extrinsic f.,** vitamin $B_{12}$ (cyanocobalamin).

**F f., fertility f.,** F plasmid.

**fibrin-stabilizing f. (FSF),** f. XIII; see under *coagulation f's.*

**fibroblast growth f.,** see under *hormone..*

**Fitzgerald f.,** high-molecular-weight kininogen.

**Fletcher f.,** prekallikrein.

**glass f.,** f. XII; see under *coagulation f's.*

**glucose tolerance f.,** a biologically active complex of chromium and nicotinic acid that facilitates the reaction of insulin with receptor sites on tissues.

**granulocyte colony-stimulating f. (G-CSF),** a colony-stimulating factor, secreted by stimulated endothelial cells, fibroblasts, and macrophages, that stimulates the production of neutrophils from precursor cells.

**granulocyte-macrophage colony-stimulating f. (GM-CSF),** a colony-stimulating factor, secreted by activated T lymphocytes and macrophages and by stimulated endothelial cells, that binds to a specific receptor found on stem cells and most myelocytes and stimulates their differentiation into granulocytes and macrophages. GM-CSF also enhances the function of mature granulocytes and macrophages *in vitro.* A recombinant form, sargramostim, is used as an adjuvant in myelosuppressive cancer therapy to accelerate recovery of the hematopoietic system.

**growth f.,** an imprecise term denoting any of numerous substances that promote normal or pathological growth of cells or tissue, including the epidermal growth factors, insulin-like growth factors, nerve growth factors, platelet-derived growth factors, and transforming growth factors.

**f. H,** a glycoprotein that binds to C3b (see under *complement*) and acts as an alternative pathway complement inhibitor by interfering with the binding of factor B to C3b; it also acts as a cofactor in the conversion of C3b to the inactive form iC3b by factor I.

**Hageman f. (HF),** f. XII; see under *coagulation f's.*

**hematopoietic growth f's,** a group of substances with the ability to support hematopoietic colony formation in vitro, including erythropoietin, interleukin-3, and colony-stimulating factors. All except erythropoietin stimulate mature cells, have overlapping capabilities to affect progenitor cells of several blood cell lines, and also affect cells outside the hematopoietic system.

**hepatocyte growth f. (HGF),** a potent mitogen and inducer of hepatocyte proliferation, produced by nonparenchymal cells in the liver and by mesenchymal cells in many other organs.

**high-molecular-weight neutrophil chemotactic f. (HMW-NCF),** neutrophil chemotactic f.

**histamine-releasing f. (HRF),** a lymphokine, believed to be produced by macrophages and B lymphocytes, that induces the release of histamine by IgE-bound basophils occurring in late phase allergic reaction in sensitive individuals.

**homologous restriction f. (HRF),** a regulatory protein that binds to the membrane attack complex factor C8 of autologous cells and by preventing C9 insertion into the membrane and subsequent polymerization so inhibits the final stages of complement activation.

**hydrazine-sensitive f. (HSF),** former name for alternative pathway complement factor *C3;* see under *complement.*

**hyperglycemic-glycogenolytic f. (HGF),** 1. glucagon. 2. the hyperglycemic component of growth hormone extracts.

**f. I,** a plasma enzyme that regulates both classical and alternative pathways of complement activation (see *complement*). In the classical pathway, it blocks the formation of C3 convertase by catabolizing C4b; in the alternative pathway, it inactivates C3b by cleaving it to form iC3b, requiring also a cofactor such as factor H, MCP (membrane cofactor protein), or CR1 (complement receptor 1).

**immunoglobulin-binding f. (IBF),** a lymphokine having the ability to bind IgG complexed with antigen and prevent complement activation, possibly Fc receptors shed from T cells.

**inhibiting f's,** factors elaborated by one structure (such as the hypothalamus) that inhibit the release of hormones by other structures (such as the anterior pituitary gland). The term is applied to substances of unknown chemical structure, while substances of established chemical identity are called *inhibiting hormones.*

**initiation f.,** one of three soluble proteins (IF-1, IF-2, and IF-3) involved in the binding of mRNA and the first aminoacyl-tRNA to the small ribosomal subunit and the attachment of the small subunit to the large subunit at the beginning of protein synthesis (see *translation*).

**insulin-like growth f's (IGF),** serum peptides with insulin-like actions, formerly called *somatomedins* (q.v.). IGF-I (formerly *somatomedin C*) is an important growth hormone–dependent mediator of cell growth and replication. IGF-II (formerly *somatomedin A*) appears to be essential for normal embryonic development and may play special roles in the central nervous system. Both are similar in sequence and structure to proinsulin.

**intrinsic f.,** a glycoprotein secreted by the parietal cells of the gastric glands, necessary for the absorption of vitamin $B_{12}$ (cyanocobalamin, extrinsic factor). Lack of intrinsic factor, with consequent deficiency of vitamin $B_{12}$, results in pernicious anemia.

**labile f.,** f. V; see under *coagulation f's.*

**Laki-Lorand f.,** f. XIII; see under *coagulation f's.*

**LE f.,** an antinuclear antibody present in the blood serum in systemic lupus erythematosus, having a sedimentation rate of 7S and reacting with leukocyte nuclei in the LE cell test.

**leukocyte inhibitory f. (LIF),** a lymphokine that inhibits the migration of polymorphonuclear leukocytes but not macrophages.

**lymph node permeability f. (LNPF),** a vasoactive factor, distinct from histamine, serotonin, bradykinin, and kallikrein, that is released without immunologic stimulus from many tissues, including lymph nodes, spleen, kidney, liver, and muscle.

**lymphocyte-activating f.,** interleukin-1.

**lymphocyte blastogenic f. (BF),** lymphocyte mitogenic f.

**lymphocyte mitogenic f. (LMF), lymphocyte-transforming f. (LTF),** a nondialyzable heat-stable macromolecule, mol. wt. approximately 20,000–30,000, released by lymphocytes stimulated by specific antigen, that causes nonstimulated lymphocytes to undergo blast transformation and cell division.

**macrophage-activating f. (MAF),** interferon-$\gamma$.

**macrophage chemotactic f. (MCF),** a lymphokine produced by activated lymphocytes that is chemotactic for macrophages.

**macrophage colony-stimulating f. (M-CSF),** a colony-stimulating factor, secreted by macrophages, stimulated endothelial cells, and most tissues, that stimulates the production of macrophages from precursor cells and maintains the viability of mature macrophages *in vitro.*

**macrophage-derived growth f.,** a substance released by macrophages below the surface of a wound that induces the proliferation of fibroblasts, with consequent deposition of collagen, fibronectin, and glycosaminoglycan.

**macrophage growth f. (MGF),** any of various glycoproteins that permit macrophages harvested from peritoneal exudates to proliferate in liquid-suspension cultures and form colonies consisting solely of mononuclear phagocytes.

**macrophage inhibitory f., migration inhibition f.,** a lymphokine that inhibits macrophage migration.

**mitogenic f.,** lymphocyte mitogenic f.

**müllerian duct inhibitory f., müllerian inhibiting f., müllerian regression f.,** antimüllerian hormone.

**multiple f's,** in heredity, two or more genes or environmental variants that act in combination to produce a certain trait.

**myocardial depressant f. (MDF),** a peptide putatively formed in response to a fall in systemic blood pressure related to sepsis; it has a negatively inotropic effect on myocardial muscle fibers.

**necrotizing f.,** necrotoxin.

**nerve growth f. (NGF),** a protein consisting of two identical polypeptide chains associated with two gamma subunits (enzymes) and two alpha subunits; first isolated from mouse sarcoma and later from snake venom and mouse salivary glands, it stimulates the growth of sensory and sympathetic nerve cells and of the adrenal medulla and has been found to be secreted by a variety of normal and neoplastic cells, including those in humans.

**neutrophil chemotactic f. (NCF),** 1. a poorly characterized chemotactic factor, mol. wt. approximately 750,000, that attracts neutrophils but not eosinophils or monocytes and is released by basophils or mast cells in immediate hypersensitivity reactions. Called also *high-molecular-weight neutrophil chemotactic f. (HMW-NCF).* 2. a lymphokine produced by activated lymphocytes that is chemotactic for neutrophils.

**osteoclast-activating f. (OAF),** a lymphokine that stimulates bone resorption; it is a small protein unrelated to parathyroid hormone and may be involved in the bone resorption associated with multiple myeloma and other hematologic neoplasms or inflammatory disorders such as rheumatoid arthritis and periodontal disease.

**f. P,** properdin.

**pellagra-preventive f.,** niacin.

**platelet f's,** factors important in hemostasis which are contained in or attached to the platelets; they act together with coagulation factors.

**platelet f. 1,** adsorbed factor V from the plasma.

**platelet f. 2,** an accelerator of the thrombin-fibrinogen reaction, attached to platelets.

**platelet f. 3,** a lipoprotein, extracted from platelets, which contributes to the interaction of activated plasma coagulation factors IX and VIII to produce activated factor X as well as of activated factors X and V to cleave and activate prothrombin.

**platelet f. 4,** an intracellular protein component of blood platelets, capable of neutralizing the antithrombic activity of heparin in the fibrinogen-fibrin reaction and the inhibitory effect of heparin in the thromboplastin generation test.

**platelet-activating f. (PAF),** a substance released by basophils and mast cells in immediate hypersensitivity reactions and macrophages and neutrophils in other inflammatory reactions that is an extremely potent mediator of bronchoconstriction and of the platelet aggregation and release reactions. It differs from other known biochemical mediators in being a phospholipid. Called also *PAF-acether* or *AGEPC* (acetyl glyceryl ether phosphoryl choline).

**platelet-derived growth f.,** a substance found in the alpha granules of platelets, capable of inducing proliferation of vascular endothelial cells, vascular smooth muscle cells, fibroblasts, and glia cells; its action contributes to the repair of damaged vascular walls.

**P.-P. f.,** niacin.

**prolactin-inhibiting f. (PIF),** see under *hormone.*

**prolactin-releasing f. (PRF),** see under *hormone.*

**Prower f.,** f. X; see under *coagulation f's.*

**R f.,** R plasmid.

**recruitment f.,** lymphocyte mitogenic f.

**releasing f's,** 1. factors elaborated in one structure (such as the hypothalamus) that effect the release of hormones from another structure (such as anterior pituitary gland). The term is applied to substances of unknown chemical structure, while substances of established chemical identity are called *releasing hormones* (see under *hormone*). 2. two soluble proteins (RF-1 and RF-2) involved in the release of the completed polypeptide chain from the ribosome when a chain-termination codon is encountered during protein synthesis (see *translation*). RF-1 recognizes the termination codon UAA or UAG and RF-2 recognizes UAA or UGA.

**resistance-inducing f.,** see *Rubin's test* (def. 2), under *test.*

**resistance transfer f. (RTF),** the portion of an R plasmid in a bacterial cell that contains the genes for conjugation and replication.

**Rh f., Rhesus f.,** any of numerous antigens (agglutinogens) that may be present on the membrane of erythrocytes and that determine the Rh blood group system; the most common ones are called (in one system) Rh 1, Rh 3, Rh 4, Rh 5, and Rh 21. See *Rh blood group,* under *blood group.* Called also *Rh antigen.*

**rheumatoid f. (RF),** antibodies directed against antigenic determinants, i.e., Gm, in the Fc region of IgG, found in the serum of about 80 per cent of patients with classical or definite rheumatoid arthritis but in only about 20 per cent of patients with juvenile rheumatoid arthritis; rheumatoid factors may be IgM, IgG, or IgA antibodies, although serologic tests measure only IgM. Rheumatoid factors also occur in other connective tissue diseases and infectious diseases (Sjögren's syndrome, systemic lupus erythematosus, sarcoidosis, subacute bacterial endocarditis, infectious hepatitis, leprosy).

**risk f.,** a clearly defined occurrence or characteristic that has been associated with the increased rate of a subsequently occurring disease; causality may or may not be implied.

**sex f.,** F plasmid.

**Simon's septic f.,** decrease of eosinophils and increase of neutrophils in the blood in pyogenic infections.

**skeletal growth f.,** a protein that stimulates growth of osteocytes.

**Factor** *Continued*

**skin reactive f. (SRF),** a lymphokine derived from antigen-stimulated lymphocytes that augments the delayed hypersensitivity skin reaction, increasing capillary permeability and infiltration of monocytes; perhaps a mixture of other lymphokines.
**somatotropin release–inhibiting f. (SRIF),** old name for somatostatin.
**spreading f.,** hyaluronidase.
**stable f.,** f. VII; see under *coagulation f's.*
**Stuart f., Stuart-Prower f.,** f. X; see under *coagulation f's.*
**sulfation f's,** former name for *insulin-like growth f's.*
**T-cell growth f.,** former name for *interleukin-2.*
**tissue f.,** f. III; see under *coagulation f's.*
**transfer f. (TF),** 1. a dialyzable extract obtained from lysates of peripheral blood lymphocytes that is capable of transferring antigen-specific cell-mediated immunity (delayed-type hypersensitivity) from donor to recipient and also has nonspecific immunostimulatory activity; it appears to contain both protein and RNA but not DNA and consist of small molecules (mol. wt. less than 10,000). TF is nonantigenic and does not transfer humoral immunity. It has been used in the treatment of a variety of immunodeficiency diseases. 2. elongation f.
**transforming growth f. (TGF),** any of several proteins secreted by transformed cells and stimulating growth of normal cells, although not causing transformation. *TGF-α* binds the epidermal growth factor receptor and also stimulates growth of microvascular endothelial cells. *TGF-β* exists as several subtypes, all of which are found in hematopoietic tissue, stimulate wound healing, and *in vitro* are antagonists of lymphopoiesis and myelopoiesis.
**tumor-angiogenesis f.,** a factor produced by cancer cells of solid tumors that stimulates the growth of blood vessels into the tumor.
**tumor necrosis f. (TNF),** a lymphokine produced by macrophages capable of causing *in vivo* hemorrhagic necrosis of certain tumor cells, but not affecting normal cells; it has been used as an experimental anticancer agent. It can also induce shock when bacterial endotoxins cause its release. Called also *cachectin.*
**V f.,** an accessory substance required for the growth of certain species of *Haemophilus,* replaceable by nicotinamide-adenine dinucleotide (NAD) or nicotinamide-adenine dinucleotide phosphate (NADP) and present in red blood cells. Cf. *X f.*
**von Willebrand's f. (vWF),** a glycoprotein synthesized in endothelial cells and megakaryocytes that circulates complexed to factor VIII (see under *coagulation f's*); it mediates adhesion of platelets to damaged epithelial surfaces and may participate in platelet aggregation. Deficiency results in the prolonged bleeding time seen in von Willebrand's disease. NOTE: this factor was originally considered to be part of factor VIII, so that in older terminology the term factor VIII generally refers to the complex of the two factors.
**X f.,** an accessory substance required for the aerobic growth of certain species of *Haemophilus* replaceable by hemin or other iron porphyrin compounds, and present in red blood cells. It is heat stable and is not destroyed by autoclaving. Cf. *V f.*

**Fac·trel** (fak'trəl) trademark for a preparation of gonadorelin hydrochloride.

**fac·ul·ta·tive** (fak'əl-ta"tiv) 1. not obligatory; capable of adaptation to different conditions. 2. in bacteriology, a bacterium that can grow either aerobically or anaerobically.

**fac·ul·ty** (fak'əl-te) [L. *facultas*] [MeSH: Faculty] 1. any normal power or function, especially a mental one. 2. the corps of professors and instructors of a college or university.
**fusion f.,** the power of blending into one the two images viewed by the two eyes.

**FAD** [MeSH: FAD] flavin adenine dinucleotide, sometimes used specifically for the oxidized form.

**FADH$_2$** the reduced form of flavin adenine dinucleotide.

**fad·ing** (fād'ing) progressive weakness in puppies, so that suckling is impossible; it is usually accompanied by a falling body temperature, paddling movements, and death within a few days of birth. The cause may be a viral infection, a bacterial infection, or adverse environmental conditions.

**fae-** for words beginning thus, see those beginning *fe-.*

**fag·op·y·rism** (fəg-op'ĭ-riz-əm) [L. *fagopyrum* buckwheat] photosensitization in humans or animals that eat excessive amounts of buckwheat *(Fagopyrum esculentum).*

**Fag·o·py·rum** (fag"o-pi'rəm) a genus of herbs of the family Polygonaceae, native to temperate regions of Europe and Asia. *F. esculen'tum* is buckwheat, a food and fodder crop that can cause fagopyrism in humans or animals if eaten in large quantities.

**Fahr·en·heit scale, thermometer** (far'ən-hīt) [Gabriel Daniel *Fahrenheit,* German physicist, 1686–1736] see under *scale* and *thermometer.*

**fail·ure** (fāl'yər) inability to perform or to achieve a desired outcome.
**acute congestive heart f.,** rapidly occurring deficiency in cardiac output marked by venocapillary congestion, hypertension, and edema, usually pulmonary edema.
**backward heart f.,** a concept of heart failure stating that imbalance of performance of the ventricles due to dysfunction of one results in a rise in pressure behind that ventricle, with backward transmission of the increased pressure and consequent rise in venous pressure and distention. Cf. *forward heart f.*
**bone marrow f.,** failure of the hematopoietic function of the bone marrow; see also bone marrow suppression, under *suppression.*
**cardiac f.,** heart f.
**congestive heart f. (CHF),** a clinical syndrome due to heart disease, characterized by breathlessness and abnormal sodium and water retention, often resulting in edema. The congestion may occur in the lungs or peripheral circulation or both, depending on whether the heart failure is right-sided or general.
**diastolic heart f.,** heart failure due to a defect in ventricular filling caused by an abnormality in diastolic function.
**forward heart f.,** a concept of heart failure that emphasizes the inadequacy of cardiac output relative to body needs; edema is attributed primarily to renal retention of sodium and water, and venous distention is considered a secondary feature.
**heart f.,** inability of the heart to pump blood at an adequate rate to fill tissue metabolic requirements or the ability to do so only at an elevated filling pressure. It can be defined clinically as a syndrome of ventricular dysfunction accompanied by reduced exercise capacity and other characteristic hemodynamic, renal, neural, and hormonal responses.
**high-output heart f.,** heart failure in which the cardiac output remains high enough to maintain a brisk circulation with warm extremities but is inadequate to meet demand; it is most often associated with hyperthyroidism, anemia, arteriovenous fistulas, beriberi, osteitis deformans, or sepsis.
**kidney f.,** renal f.
**lactation f. in swine,** a variable syndrome in sows with agalactia occurring during the first two days after they have given birth; it may be accompanied by mastitis with fever, anorexia, and increased respiratory and heart rates, and occasionally by metritis with a vaginal discharge. Called also *farrowing fever* and *mastitis-metritis-agalactia.*
**left-sided heart f., left ventricular f.,** failure of adequate output by the left ventricle despite an increase in distending pressure and in end-diastolic volume, with dyspnea, orthopnea, and other signs and symptoms of pulmonary congestion and edema.
**low-output heart f.,** heart failure in which cardiac output is decreased, as in most forms of heart disease, leading to clinical manifestations of impaired peripheral circulation and peripheral vasoconstriction (cold, pale extremities, cyanosis, narrowed pulse pressure).
**renal f.,** the inability of a kidney to excrete metabolites at normal plasma levels under conditions of normal loading or the inability to retain electrolytes under conditions of normal intake. In the acute form, it is marked by uremia and usually by oliguria or anuria, with hyperkalemia and pulmonary edema. Chronic forms result from a wide variety of conditions and may require hemodialysis or transplantation.
**respiratory f.,** a condition resulting from respiratory insufficiency, in which there is persistent abnormally low arterial oxygen tension ($Pa_{O_2}$) or abnormally high carbon dioxide tension ($Pa_{CO_2}$). Called also *ventilatory f.*
**right-sided heart f., right ventricular f.,** failure of proper functioning of the right ventricle, with venous engorgement, hepatic enlargement, and subcutaneous edema; it is often combined with left-sided heart failure.
**systolic heart f.,** heart failure due to a defect in expulsion of blood caused by an abnormality in systolic function.
**ventilatory f.,** respiratory f.

**faint** (fānt) syncope.

**Fa•jer•sztajn's crossed sciatic sign** (fah-zher-stīnz') [Jean *Fajersztajn,* French neurologist, early 20th century] see under *sign.*

**fal•cate** (fal'kāt) falciform.

**fal•ces** (fal'sēz) [L.] plural of *falx.*

**fal•cial** (fal'shəl) pertaining to a falx.

**fal•ci•form** (fal'sĭ-form) [*falx* + *form*] shaped like a sickle.

**fal•cu•lar** (fal'ku-lər) [*falx*] sickle-shaped.

**fall•ing-out** (fawl'ing out) a culture-specific syndrome occurring primarily in southern United States and Caribbean groups, characterized by an episode of sudden collapse, sometimes without forewarning, with temporary inability to speak, see, or move.

**fal•lo•pi•an aqueduct, artery, ligament, tube** (fə-lo'pe-ən) [Gabriele *Fallopio* (L. *Fallopius*), Italian anatomist, pupil of Vesalius, 1523–1562] see *canalis facialis, arteria uterina, ligamentum inguinale,* and *tuba uterina.*

**Fal•lot's pentalogy, tetralogy (tetrad), trilogy** (fə-lōz') [Étienne-Louis Arthur *Fallot,* French physician, 1850–1911] see under *pentalogy, tetralogy,* and *trilogy.*

**false-neg•a•tive** (fawls'neg'ə-tiv) 1. denoting a test result that wrongly excludes an individual from a diagnostic or other category, e.g., one that labels a diseased person as healthy in screening for detection of that disease. 2. an individual so excluded. 3. an instance of a false-negative result.

**false-pos•i•tive** (fawls'pos'ĭ-tiv) 1. denoting a test result that wrongly assigns an individual to a diagnostic or other category, e.g., one that labels a healthy person as diseased in screening for detection of that disease.. 2. an individual so categorized. 3. an instance of a false-positive result.
**biologic f.-p. (BFP),** a positive result on a serologic test when the disease itself is not present. Acute BFP is usually associated with infectious disease, e.g., bacterial and mycoplasma pneumonias, subacute bacterial endocarditis, varicella, infectious mononucleosis, and scarlet fever. Chronic BFP is usually associated with immune complex diseases, systemic lupus erythematosus, and leprosy.

**fal•si•fi•ca•tion** (fawl"sĭ-fĭ-ka'shən) an often deliberate misstatement or misrepresentation.
**retrospective f.,** unconscious distortion of memories of past experiences to conform to present emotional needs.

**falx** (falks) pl. *fal'ces* [L. "sickle"] a general term in anatomical nomenclature for a sickle-shaped organ or structure.
**aponeurotic f., f. aponeuro'tica,** f. inguinalis.
**f. cerebel'li** [TA], **f. of cerebellum,** cerebellar falx: the small fold of dura mater in the midline of the posterior cranial fossa, projecting forward toward the vermis of the cerebellum.
**f. ce'rebri** [TA], **f. of cerebrum,** cerebral falx: the fold of dura mater, sickle-shaped when viewed in sagittal section, that extends downward in the longitudinal cerebral fissure and separates the two cerebral hemispheres.
**f. inguina'lis** [TA], inguinal falx: the united tendons of the transverse and internal oblique muscles going to the linea alba and pectineal line of the pubic bone; called also *Henle's ligament* and *tendo conjunctivus* [TA alternative].
**ligamentous f., f. ligamento'sa,** processus falciformis ligamenti sacrotuberosi.
**f. sep'ti,** valvula foraminis ovalis.

**fam•ci•clo•vir** (fam-si'klo-vir) a prodrug of penciclovir that is converted to the active drug by cellular kinases following administration, used in the treatment of herpes zoster and herpes genitalis and of mucocutaneous herpes simplex in immunocompromised patients; administered orally.

**fa•mes** (fa'mēz) [L.] hunger.

**fa•mil•i•al** (fə-mil'e-əl) [L. *familia* family] occurring in or affecting more members of a family than would be expected by chance.

**fam•i•ly** (fam'ĭ-le) [MeSH: Family] 1. a group of individuals descended from a common ancestor. 2. a taxonomic subdivision subordinate to an order (or suborder) and superior to a tribe (or subfamily). 3. a group of related objects of any kind.
**secretin f.,** a group of peptides related to secretin, several of which are active in the alimentary tract; it includes secretin, glucagon, growth hormone–releasing hormone, glucose-dependent insulinotropic polypeptide, and vasoactive intestinal polypeptide.
**systematic f.,** see *family* (def. 2).
**tachykinin f.,** a family of hormones that are potent, rapidly acting secretagogues and cause smooth muscle contraction and vasodilation; it includes substance P and several less common peptides.

**fam•o•ti•dine** (fam-o'tĭ-dīn) [MeSH: Famotidine] a histamine $H_2$ antagonist used in the treatment of duodenal ulcers.

**Fam•vir** (fam'vir) trademark for a preparation of famciclovir.

**fan** (fan) an area, figure, or structure in the shape of a sector of a circle containing less than a semicircle.

**Fan•co•ni syndrome (anemia, pancytopenia)** (fahn-ko'ne) [Guido *Fanconi,* Swiss pediatrician, 1892–1979] [MeSH: Fanconi Syndrome] see under *syndrome.*

**F and R** force and rhythm (of pulse).

**fang** (fang) 1. a large canine tooth of a carnivore. 2. the envenomed tooth of a snake.

**Fan•nia** (fan'e-ə) a genus of flies (family Muscidae), the larvae of which have caused both intestinal and urinary myiasis in man. In some systems of classification, it is included in the family Anthomyiidae.
**F. canicula'ris,** the lesser housefly: a species of small grayish flies, visibly different from the housefly; they lay their eggs on decaying vegetable matter or animal manure, from which the eggs or larvae may gain access to human hosts.
**F. scala'ris,** a species of flies, the latrine flies, similar to but larger than *F. canicularis,* and commonly depositing their eggs on excrement, rather than on vegetable matter.

**fan•ta•sy** (fan'tə-se) [Gr. *phantasia* imagination; the power by which an object is made apparent to the mind] [MeSH: Fantasy] a consciously or unconsciously imagined situation or sequence of events, such as a daydream. Fantasy can serve as a realistic rehearsal of future events; it may also serve as an unconscious defense mechanism providing wish-fulfillment, gratification of repressed impulses, and resolution of unconscious conflicts.
**autistic f.,** a defense mechanism characterized by excessive daydreaming as a solution for emotional conflict or stressors, substituting for human relationships or for more effective actions.

**FAPHA** Fellow of the American Public Health Association.

**Far•a•beuf's amputation, triangle** (fahr"ə-boofs') [Louis Hubert *Farabeuf,* French surgeon, 1841–1910] see under *amputation* and *triangle.*

**far•ad** (far'əd) [M. *Faraday*] the International System (SI) unit of electrical capacitance. The capacitance of a condenser which, charged with 1 coulomb, gives a difference of potential of 1 volt. Symbol F. This unit is so large that one-millionth part of it has been adopted as a practical unit called a microfarad.

**Far•a•day's constant, law** (far'ə-dāz) [Michael *Faraday,* English physicist, 1791–1867] see under *constant* and *law.*

**far•a•day** (far'ə-da) [M. *Faraday*] the electric charge carried by one mole of electrons or one equivalent of ions, equal to $9.649 \times 10^4$ coulombs. Symbol *F.* Called also *Faraday's constant.*

**fa•rad•ic** (fə-rad'ik) pertaining to faradism.

**far•a•dim•e•ter** (far"ə-dim'ə-tər) [*farad* + *-meter*] an instrument for measuring faradic electricity.

**far•a•dism** (far'ə-diz-əm) 1. induced current. 2. induced current in a rapidly alternating current. 3. faradization.
**surging f.,** a faradic current of gradually increasing and decreasing amplitude; obtained by introducing a rhythmically varying series resistance into the circuit.

**far•a•di•za•tion** (far"ə-dĭ-za'shən) the therapeutic use of an interrupted current, derived from an induction coil; principally for the stimulation of muscles and nerves.

**Far•ber's disease (lipogranulomatosis, syndrome)** (fahr'bərz) [Sidney *Farber,* American pediatrician, 1903–1973] see under *disease.*

**Far•ber-Uz•man syndrome** (fahr'bər o͞oz'mən) [S. *Farber;* Lahut *Uzman,* American physician, 20th century] Farber's disease.

**far•cy** (fahr'se) 1. the more chronic and constitutional lymphatic form of glanders, marked by thickening of the superficial lymph vessels. 2. any of several other animal diseases that resemble this condition.
**bovine f.,** a benign type of nocardiosis in cattle, caused by infection with *Nocardia farcinica* and characterized by formation of nodules in subcutaneous tissues and organs. Called also *cattle f.*
**button f.,** farcy in which there are small tubercular nodules *(farcy buds)* on the skin.
**cattle f.,** bovine f.
**Japanese f., Neapolitan f.,** lymphangitis epizootica.

**far•cy pipes** (fahr'se pīps) farcy cords; see under *cord.*

**Farr's law** (fahrz) [William *Farr,* English medical statistician, 1807–1883] see under *law.*

**Farre's tubercles** (fahrz) [John Richard *Farre,* English physician, 1775–1862] see under *tubercle.*

**Farre's white line** (fahrz) [Arthur *Farre,* British obstetrician, 1811–1887] see under *line.*

**far•sight•ed** (fahr'sīt-əd) hyperopic.

**far·sight·ed·ness** (fahr-sīt′əd-nəs) hyperopia.

**fasc.** abbreviation for L. *fascic′ulus,* bundle.

**fas·cia** (fash′e-ə) gen. and pl. *fas′ciae* [L. "band"] [TA] [MeSH: Fascia] a sheet or band of fibrous tissue such as lies deep to the skin or forms an investment for muscles and various other organs of the body.

## Fascia

Descriptions of anatomic structures are given on TA terms, and include anglicized names of specific fasciae.

**abdominal f., internal,** f. transversalis.
**Abernethy's f.,** f. iliaca.
**f. adhe′rens,** an extensive adherent junction analogous to the zonula adherens but occurring in cardiac myocytes, primarily in the transverse portions of intercalated disks; it has multiple dense attachment plaques acting as sites of insertion of actin filaments into the sarcolemma and thus linking the cellular membrane and contractile apparatus with those of adjacent cells.
**alar f.,** an ancillary layer of the deep cervical fascia, anterior to the prevertebral fascia and extending from the base of the skull to the level of the second thoracic vertebra, where it merges with the pretracheal fascia.
**anal f.,** f. inferior diaphragmatis pelvis.
**anoscrotal f.,** f. perinei superficialis.
**antebrachial f., f. antebra′chii** [TA], the investing fascia of the forearm; called also *f. of forearm* and *deep f. of forearm.*
**aponeurotic f.,** f. profunda.
**f. of arm,** f. brachii.
**f. axilla′ris** [TA], **axillary f.,** the investing fascia of the armpit which passes between the lateral borders of the pectoralis major and latissimus dorsi muscles.
**bicipital f.,** aponeurosis musculi bicipitis brachii.
**brachial f., f. brachia′lis,** f. brachii.
**f. bra′chii** [TA], the investing fascia of the arm.
**buccinator f., f. buccopharyn′gea** [TA], **buccopharyngeal f., f. buccopharyngea′lis** [TA], buccopharyngeal fascia: a fibrous membrane forming the external covering of the constrictor muscles of the pharynx, and passing forward superiorly to the surface of the buccinator muscle.
**Buck's f.,** the deep fascia of the penis, being continuous with Colles' fascia of the perineum and with Scarpa's fascia of the abdominal wall.
**bulbar f., f. bul′bi [Teno′ni],** vagina bulbi.
**f. of Camper,** the superficial layer of the superficial fascia of the abdomen.
**cervical f.,** f. cervicalis.
**cervical f., deep,** deep layers of cervical fascia.
**cervical f., superficial,** 1. a thin layer of cervical fascia just beneath the skin, investing the platysma. 2. lamina superficialis fasciae cervicalis.
**f. cervica′lis** [TA], cervical fascia: the fascia of the neck, consisting of a thin superficial layer, three deep layers *(lamina superficialis, lamina pretrachealis,* and *lamina prevertebralis fasciae cervicalis),* and the carotid sheath *(vagina carotica fasciae cervicalis).*
**clavipectoral f., f. clavipectora′lis** [TA], a fascial sheet investing the subclavius muscle, attached to the clavicle above and continuing to the pectoralis minor muscle below; called also *f. coracoclavicularis* and *coracoclavicular f.*

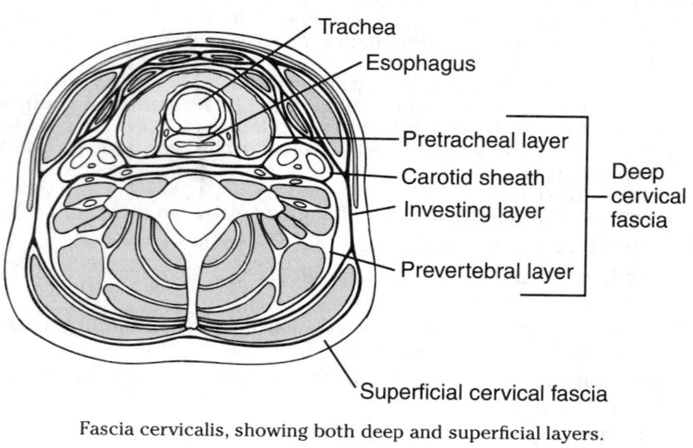

Fascia cervicalis, showing both deep and superficial layers.

**f. clito′ridis** [TA], **f. of clitoris,** the dense fibrous tissue that encloses the two corpora cavernosa of the clitoris.
**Cloquet's f.,** the condensation of extraperitoneal tissue closing the femoral ring (septum femorale).
**Colles' f.,** membrana perinei.
**f. col′li,** f. cervicalis.
**fasciae of colon,** teniae coli.
**Cooper's f.,** 1. f. cremasterica. 2. see *fibrae intercrurales.*
**coracoclavicular f., f. coracoclavicula′ris, coracocostal f.,** f. clavipectoralis.
**cremasteric f., f. cremaste′rica** [TA], the thin covering of the spermatic cord formed by the investing fascia of the cremasteric muscle; it is adjacent to the external surface of the internal spermatic fascia. Called also *Cooper's f.* and *intercolumnar f.*
**cribriform f.,** 1. f. cribrosa. 2. septum femorale.
**f. cribro′sa** [TA], cribriform fascia: the part of the superficial fascia of the thigh that covers the saphenous opening; called also *Hesselbach's f.*
**crural f., f. cru′ris** [TA], the investing fascia of the leg; called also *crural aponeurosis.*
**Cruveilhier's f.** [TA], f. perinei superficialis.
**dartos f. of scrotum,** tunica dartos.
**deep f.,** f. profunda.
**deep f. of arm,** f. brachii.
**deep f. of back,** f. thoracolumbalis.
**deep f. of forearm,** f. antebrachii.
**deep f. of perineum,** diaphragma urogenitale.
**deep f. of thigh,** f. lata.
**deltoid f., f. deltoi′dea** [TA], the deep fascia covering the deltoid muscle of the shoulder.
**Denonvilliers' f.,** septum rectovesicale.
**f. diaphrag′matis pel′vis infe′rior,** f. inferior diaphragmatis pelvis.
**f. diaphrag′matis pel′vis supe′rior,** f. superior diaphragmatis pelvis.
**f. diaphrag′matis urogenita′lis infe′rior,** membrana perinei.
**f. diaphrag′matis urogenita′lis supe′rior,** see *diaphragma urogenitale.*
**dorsal f., deep,** f. thoracolumbalis.
**dorsal f. of foot,** f. dorsalis pedis.
**dorsal f. of hand, f. dorsa′lis ma′nus** [TA], the investing fascia of the back of the hand.
**f. dorsa′lis pe′dis** [TA], the investing fascia on the dorsum of the foot.
**Dupuytren's f.,** aponeurosis palmaris.
**endoabdominal f.,** f. transversalis.
**endopelvic f.,** f. pelvis parietalis.
**f. endopelvi′na,** TA alternative for *f. pelvis parietalis.*
**endothoracic f., f. endothora′cica** [TA], the extrapleural fascial sheet beneath the serous lining of the thoracic cavity; called also *parietal fascia of thorax* and *fascia parietalis thoracis* [TA alternative].
**external intercostal f.,** f. thoracica.
**extraperitoneal f., f. extraperitonea′lis,** the thin layer of areolar connective tissue separating the parietal peritoneum from the abdominal walls; called also *extraperitoneal tissue, subperitoneal f.,* and *f. subperitonealis.*
**femoral f.,** f. lata.
**fibroareolar f.,** f. superficialis.
**f. of forearm,** f. antebrachii.
**fusion f.,** a double connective tissue band derived from the fusion of closely apposed surfaces of peritoneum as a result of degeneration of the lubricating serous layer between them; such fasciae are seen in the pelvic and abdominal cavities where crowding of organs occurs.
**f. of Gerota, Gerota's f.,** f. renalis.
**Hesselbach's f.,** f. cribrosa.
**hypogastric f.,** f. pelvis.
**iliac f.,** 1. f. iliaca. 2. arcus iliopectineus.
**f. ili′aca** [TA], a strong fascia covering the inner surface of the iliac and psoas muscles.
**f. iliopecti′nea, iliopectineal f.,** arcus iliopectineus.
**f. infe′rior diaphrag′matis pel′vis** [TA], inferior fascia of diaphragm

of pelvis: the fascia that covers the lower surface of the coccygeus and levator ani muscles, forming the medial wall of the ischiorectal fossa; called also *ischiorectal f.* or *aponeurosis, f. diaphragmatis pelvis inferior,* and *inferior layer of pelvic diaphragm.*

**infundibuliform f.,** f. spermatica interna.

**intercolumnar f.,** 1. f. cremasterica. 2. see *fibrae intercrurales.*

**ischiorectal f.,** f. inferior diaphragmatis pelvis.

**f. la'ta** [TA], the external investing fascia of the thigh.

**f. of leg,** f. cruris.

**longitudinal f., anterior,** ligamentum longitudinale anterius.

**longitudinal f., posterior,** ligamentum longitudinale posterius.

**lumbodorsal f., f. lumbodorsa'lis,** f. thoracolumbalis.

**masseteric f., f. massete'rica** [TA], a layer of fascia covering the masseter muscle.

**muscular fasciae of eye, fas'ciae muscula'res bul'bi** [TA], **fas'ciae muscula'res oc'uli,** the sheets of fascia investing the extraocular muscles, continuous with the vagina bulbi.

**f. of nape,** f. nuchae.

**f. of neck,** f. cervicalis.

**f. nu'chae** [TA], **nuchal f., f. nucha'lis,** the fascia on the muscles in the dorsal region of the neck.

**obturator f., f. obturato'ria** [TA], the part of the parietal fascia of the pelvis covering the internal obturator muscle.

**orbital fasciae, fas'ciae orbita'les,** fibrous tissue surrounding the posterior part of the eyeball, supporting and binding together the structures within the orbit.

**palmar f.,** aponeurosis palmaris.

**palpebral f., f. palpebra'lis,** septum orbitale.

**parietal f. of pelvis,** f. pelvis parietalis.

**parietal f. of thorax,** f. endothoracica.

**f. parieta'lis thora'cis,** TA alternative for *f. endothoracica.*

**parotid f., f. parotide'a** [TA], an extension of the deep cervical fascia that splits to enclose the parotid gland and sends extensions into the gland that become continuous with its stroma.

**f. parotideomasseter'ica,** the fascia enclosing the parotid gland and masseter muscle; separately called *f. parotidea* [TA] and *f. masseterica* [TA].

**f. pecti'nea, pectineal f.,** the pubic portion of the fascia lata; called also *Cowper's ligament.*

**pectoral f., f. pectora'lis** [TA], the sheet of fascia investing the pectoralis major muscle.

**pelvic f.,** f. pelvis.

**pelvic f., parietal,** f. pelvis parietalis.

**pelvic f., visceral,** f. pelvis visceralis.

**f. pel'vica,** TA alternative for *f. pelvis.*

**f. pel'vica parieta'lis,** f. pelvis parietalis.

**pelviprostatic f.,** f. prostatae.

**f. pel'vis** [TA], pelvic fascia: an inclusive term for the fascia that forms part of the general layer lining the walls of the pelvis and invests the pelvic organs; called also *f. pelvica* [TA alternative] and *hypogastric f.*

**f. pel'vis parieta'lis** [TA], parietal fascia of pelvis: the fascia on the wall of the pelvis that covers the muscles which pass from the interior of the pelvis to the thigh. Called also *f. pelvica parietalis.*

**f. pel'vis viscera'lis** [TA], visceral fascia of pelvis: the fascia that covers the organs and vessels of the pelvis.

**penile f., deep,** f. penis profunda.

**penile f., superficial,** f. penis superficialis.

**f. pe'nis profun'da** [TA], deep penile fascia: the firm inner fascial layer that surrounds the corpora cavernosa and the corpus spongiosum collectively.

**f. pe'nis superficia'lis** [TA], superficial penile fascia: the loose external layer of fascial tissue of the penis, continuous with the tunica dartos and with the superficial perineal fascia.

**perineal f., deep,** diaphragma urogenitale.

**perineal f., middle,** f. diaphragmatis urogenitalis superior.

**perineal f., superficial,** f. perinei superficialis.

**f. perine'i superficia'lis** [TA], superficial fascia of perineum: the subcutaneous tissue of the urogenital region, comprising a superficial fatty and a deep membranous layer; called also *Cruveilhier's f.*

**peritoneoperineal f., f. peritoneoperinea'lis,** the fusion fascia that passes from the front of the rectum to form the floor of the rectovesical or rectovaginal pouch, contributing to the rectovesical or rectovaginal septum.

**f. pharyngobasila'ris** [TA], pharyngobasilar fascia: a strong fibrous membrane in the wall of the pharynx, lined internally with mucous membrane and incompletely covered on its outer surface by the overlapping constrictor muscles of the pharynx. It blends with the periosteum at the base of the skull. Called also *pharyngeal* or *pharyngobasilar aponeurosis, aponeurosis pharyngis* or *pharyngobasilaris,* and *fibrous coat* or *layer of pharynx.*

**phrenicopleural f., f. phrenicopleura'lis** [TA], the fascial layer on the upper surface of the diaphragm, beneath the pleura.

**plantar f.,** aponeurosis plantaris.

**pretracheal f.,** lamina pretrachealis fasciae cervicalis.

**prevertebral f., f. prevertebra'lis,** lamina prevertebralis fasciae cervicalis.

**f. profun'da,** deep fascia: a dense, firm, fibrous membrane investing the trunk and limbs, and giving off sheaths to the various muscles; called also *aponeurotic f.*

**f. pro'pria coo'peri,** f. spermatica interna.

**f. prosta'tae** [TA], **f. of prostate,** the reflection of the superior fascia of the pelvic diaphragm onto the prostate.

**rectal f.,** f. superior diaphragmatis pelvis.

**rectoabdominal f.,** vagina musculi recti abdominis.

**rectovesical f.,** f. superior diaphragmatis pelvis.

**renal f., f. rena'lis** [TA], a thin membranous sheath that encloses the kidney, formed by condensation of the fibroareolar tissue surrounding the kidney and the perirenal fat; called also *f. of Gerota, Gerota's f.,* and *Gerota's capsule.*

**Richet's f.,** a fold of extraperitoneal fascia enveloping the obliterated umbilical vein.

**scalene f.,** membrana suprapleuralis.

**Scarpa's f.,** 1. the deep, membranous layer of subcutaneous abdominal fascia. 2. see *fibrae intercrurales.*

**semilunar f.,** aponeurosis musculi bicipitis brachii.

**Sibson's f.,** membrana suprapleuralis.

**spermatic f., external,** f. spermatica externa.

**spermatic f., internal,** f. spermatica interna.

**f. sperma'tica exter'na** [TA], external spermatic fascia: the thin outer covering of the spermatic cord, which is continuous with the investing fascia of the external oblique muscle.

**f. sperma'tica inter'na** [TA], internal spermatic fascia: the thin innermost covering of the spermatic cord, derived from the transversalis fascia of the abdominal wall.

**subperitoneal f., f. subperitonea'lis,** f. extraperitonealis.

**superficial f.,** 1. f. superficialis. 2. subcutaneous tissue.

**superficial f. of perineum,** f. perinei superficialis.

**f. superficia'lis,** a fascial sheet lying directly beneath the skin.

**f. superficia'lis perine'i,** f. perinei superficialis.

**f. supe'rior diaphrag'matis pel'vis** [TA], superior fascia of diaphragm of pelvis: the fascia on the upper surface of the levator ani and coccygeus muscles. Called also *f. diaphragmatis pelvis superior* and *superior layer of pelvic diaphragm.*

**f. of Tarin,** gyrus dentatus, def. 1.

**temporal f., f. tempora'lis** [TA], a strong fibrous sheet covering the temporal muscle, consisting of deep and superficial layers *(lamina profunda* and *lamina superficialis),* which attach inferiorly to the zygomatic arch. Called also *temporal aponeurosis.*

**f. of Tenon,** vagina bulbi.

**f. of thigh,** f. lata.

**thoracic f., f. thora'cica** [TA], the deep fascia that covers the outside of the thoracic cavity; called also *external intercostal f.*

**f. thoracolumba'lis** [TA], **thoracolumbar f.,** the fascia of the back that attaches medially to the spinous processes of the vertebral column for its entire length and blends laterally with the aponeurosis of the transversus abdominis muscle; inferiorly it attaches to the iliac crest and the sacrum. Called also *f. lumbodorsalis* and *lumbodorsal f.*

**f. transversa'lis** [TA], **transverse f.,** part of the inner investing layer of the abdominal wall, continuous with the fascia of the other side behind the rectus abdominis and the rectus sheath, and continuous also with the diaphragmatic fascia, the iliac fascia, and the parietal pelvic fascia.

**triangular f. of abdomen,** ligamentum inguinale reflexum.

**triangular f. of Macalister,** musculus pyramidalis.

**triangular f. of Quain,** ligamentum inguinale reflexum.

**Treitz's f.,** fascia posterior to the head of the pancreas.

**Tyrrell's f.,** septum rectovesicale.

**f. of urogenital diaphragm, inferior,** membrana perinei.

**f. of urogenital diaphragm, superior,** see *diaphragma urogenitale.*

**f. of urogenital trigone,** diaphragma urogenitale.

**visceral f. of pelvis,** f. pelvis visceralis.

**volar f.,** aponeurosis palmaris.

**fas·ciae** (fash'e-e) [L.] genitive and plural of *fascia.*

**fas·cial** (fash'e-əl) pertaining to or of the nature of a fascia.

**fas·cia·plas·ty** (fash'e-ə-plas"te) [*fascia* + *-plasty*] a plastic operation on fascia.

**fas·ci·cle** (fas'ĭ-kəl) fasciculus.

**fas·cic·u·lar** (fə-sik'u-lər) 1. pertaining to a fasciculus. 2. fasciculated.

**fas·cic·u·lat·ed** (fə-sik'u-lāt-əd) clustered together or occurring in bundles.

**fas·cic·u·la·tion** (fə-sik"u-la'shən) [MeSH: Fasciculation] 1. the formation of fasciculi. 2. a small local contraction of muscles, visible through the skin, representing a spontaneous discharge of a number of fibers innervated by a single motor nerve filament. **contraction f's,** brief, rhythmic twitching of a muscle during weak voluntary or postural contractions; seen in some elderly patients and those with neurogenic muscle atrophy.

**fas·cic·u·li** (fə-sik'u-li) [L.] genitive and plural of *fasciculus.*

**fas·cic·u·lo·ven·tric·u·lar** (fə-sic"u-lo-ven-trik'u-lər) [*fasciculus* + *ventricular*] connecting the bundle of His to the ventricle.

**fas·cic·u·lus** (fə-sik'u-ləs) gen. and pl. *fasci'culi* [L. dim. of *fascis* bundle] 1. a fascicle; a small bundle or cluster. 2. [TA] a small bundle of nerve, muscle, or tendon fibers. 3. a tract, bundle, or group of nerve fibers that are more or less associated functionally; see also under *bundle, lemniscus, tract,* and *tractus.*

## Fasciculus

Descriptions of anatomic structures are given on TA terms, and include anglicized names of specific fasciculi.

**f. aberrans of Monakow,** tractus rubrospinalis.
**alvear f.,** a bundle of fibers that originates in the medial part of the entorhinal area and extends to the alveus of the hippocampus, where it has synapses with fibers that go to the dentate gyrus; called also *alvear path.*
**anterior f. proprius of spinal cord,** f. proprius anterior medullae spinalis.
**arcuate f.,** f. longitudinalis superior cerebri.
**f. arcua'tus,** TA alternative for *f. longitudinalis superior cerebri.*
**f. atrioventricula'ris** [TA], atrioventricular bundle; a small band of atypical cardiac muscle fibers originating in the atrioventricular node and comprising the trunk of the bundle of His and the left and right bundle branches; see *bundle of His.*
**f. of Burdach,** 1. f. longitudinalis superior cerebri. 2. pars temporalis radiationis corporis callosi. 3. f. cuneatus medullae spinalis.
**cuneate f. of Burdach,** f. cuneatus medullae spinalis.
**cuneate f. of medulla oblongata,** f. cuneatus medullae oblongatae.
**cuneate f. of spinal cord,** f. cuneatus medullae spinalis.
**f. cunea'tus medul'lae oblonga'tae** [TA], cuneate fasciculus of medulla oblongata: the continuation into the medulla oblongata of the fasciculus cuneatus of the spinal cord.
**f. cunea'tus medul'lae spina'lis** [TA], cuneate fasciculus of spinal cord: the lateral portion of the posterior funiculus of the spinal cord, composed of ascending fibers that terminate in the nucleus cuneatus of the medulla oblongata; called also *cuneate f. of Burdach.*
**dorsal f. proprius of spinal cord,** f. proprius posterior medullae spinalis.
**dorsolateral f., f. dorsolatera'lis,** tractus posterolateralis.
**f. exi'lis,** a cluster of muscle fibers connecting the flexor pollicis longus with the medial condyle of the humerus, or with the coronoid process of the ulna.
**fibrous f. of biceps muscle,** aponeurosis musculi bicipitis brachii.
**f. of Foville,** stria terminalis.
**fronto-occipital f.,** f. subcallosus.
**f. of Goll,** f. gracilis medullae spinalis.
**Gowers' f.,** tractus spinocerebellaris anterior.
**gracile f. of medulla oblongata,** f. gracilis medullae oblongatae.
**gracile f. of spinal cord,** f. gracilis medullae spinalis.
**f. gra'cilis medul'lae oblonga'tae** [TA], the continuation into the medulla oblongata of the fasciculus gracilis of the spinal cord; called also *posteromedian column of medulla oblongata.*
**f. gra'cilis medul'lae spina'lis** [TA], the median portion of the posterior funiculus of the spinal cord, composed of ascending fibers that terminate in the nucleus gracilis of the medulla oblongata; called also *column of Goll.*
**f. interfascicula'ris** [TA], interfascicular fasciculus: a collection of fibers situated between the fasciculus gracilis and the fasciculus cuneatus, containing some of the descending branches of the fibers of the medial division of the posterior roots of the spinal nerves; called also *comma tract of Schultze, f. semilunaris* [TA alternative], *Schultze's tract,* and *semilunar f.* or *tract.*
**intersegmental f. of spinal cord, anterior,** f. proprius anterior medullae spinalis.
**intersegmental f. of spinal cord, dorsal,** f. proprius posterior medullae spinalis.
**intersegmental f. of spinal cord, lateral,** f. proprius lateralis medullae spinalis.
**intersegmental f. of spinal cord, posterior,** f. proprius posterior medullae spinalis.
**intersegmental f. of spinal cord, ventral,** f. proprius anterior medullae spinalis.
**lateral f. of brachial plexus, f. latera'lis plex'us brachia'lis** [TA], lateral cord of brachial plexus: the lateral bundle of fibers of the brachial plexus, formed by the union of the anterior divisions of the superior and middle trunks, C5 through C7, and from which arise the lateral pectoral and musculocutaneous nerves and the lateral root of the median and the ulnar nerves.
**lateral f. proprius of spinal cord,** f. proprius lateralis medullae spinalis.
**f. lenticula'ris** [TA], lenticular fasciculus: a bundle of pallidofugal nerve fibers that arise from the dorsal surface of the globus pallidus, pass through the internal capsule, traverse field $H_2$ of Forel, join and mingle with the fibers of the ansa lenticularis, and continue to the nuclei of the ventral thalamus.
**longitudinal f., dorsal,** f. longitudinalis posterior.
**longitudinal f., medial,** f. longitudinalis medialis.
**longitudinal f., posterior,** f. longitudinalis posterior.
**longitudinal f. of cerebrum, inferior,** f. longitudinalis inferior cerebri.
**longitudinal f. of cerebrum, superior,** f. longitudinalis superior cerebri.
**longitudinal fasciculi of colon,** see *teniae coli.*
**longitudinal fasciculi of cruciform ligament,** fasciculi longitudinales ligamenti cruciformis atlantis.
**longitudinal f. of medulla oblongata, medial,** f. longitudinalis medialis medullae oblongatae.
**f. longitudina'lis dorsa'lis,** TA alternative for *f. longitudinalis posterior.*
**f. longitudina'lis infe'rior ce'rebri** [TA], inferior longitudinal fasciculus of cerebrum: a bundle of assumed association fibers interconnecting the cortex of the occipital and temporal lobes, extending through the occipital and temporal lobes of the cerebrum, and consisting chiefly of geniculocalcarine projection fibers.
**fasci'culi longitudina'les ligamen'ti crucifor'mis atlan'tis** [TA], longitudinal fasciculi of cruciform ligament: vertical midline longitudinal fibers that, together with the transverse ligament of the atlas, form the cruciform ligament of the atlas. The fibers arise in two groups from the root of the dens—one group extending cranially to the anterior margin of the foramen magnum, the other caudally to the body of the axis.
**f. longitudina'lis media'lis** [TA], medial longitudinal fasciculus: a fiber tract extending between the mesencephalon and the upper part of the spinal cord; it lies close to the median plane, just ventral to the central gray matter, and interconnects the vestibular nuclei with motor nuclei, chiefly those of the third, fourth, sixth, and eleventh cranial nerves.
**f. longitudina'lis media'lis medul'lae oblonga'tae,** the portion of the fasciculus longitudinalis medialis within the medulla oblongata.
**f. longitudina'lis media'lis pon'tis,** the portion of the fasciculus longitudinalis medialis within the pons.
**f. longitudina'lis poste'rior** [TA], posterior longitudinal fasciculus: a lightly myelinated fiber bundle that runs in the periventricular gray substance throughout the extent of the mesencephalon, near the medial longitudinal fasciculus; called also *Schütz's bundle* or *tract, f. longitudinalis dorsalis* [TA alternative], and *dorsal longitudinal f.*
**f. longitudina'lis supe'rior ce'rebri** [TA], superior longitudinal fasciculus of cerebrum: a bundle of association fibers in the cerebrum, extending from the frontal lobe to the posterior end of the lateral sulcus, and interrelating the cortex of the frontal, temporal, parietal, and occipital lobes; called also *f. arcuatus* [TA alternative] and *arcuate f.*
**maculary f.,** a system of nerve fibers originating in the macula lutea;

some are uncrossed (on the temporal side) and others are crossed fibers (on the nasal side of the retina).

**f. mammillotegmenta'lis** [TA], mammillotegmental fasciculus: a bundle of fibers from the mammillary body to the tegmental nuclei of the reticular formation of the mesencephalon; called also *mammillotegmental tract.*

**f. mammillothala'micus** [TA], mammillothalamic fasciculus: a stout bundle of fibers from the mammillary body to the anterior nucleus of the thalamus; called also *mammillothalamic tract, thalamomammillary bundle,* and *thalamomammillary f.*

**medial f. of brachial plexus,** f. medialis plexus brachialis.

**medial prosencephalic f., medial telencephalic f.,** f. medialis telencephali.

**f. media'lis plex'us brachia'lis** [TA], medial cord of brachial plexus: the medial bundle of fibers of the brachial plexus, formed by the anterior division of the inferior trunk, C8 through T1, and from which arise the medial pectoral, medial brachial cutaneous, and medial antebrachial cutaneous nerves, and the medial root of the ulnar and the median nerves.

**f. media'lis telencepha'li** [TA], medial forebrain bundle: a fiber system that is the main pathway for longitudinal connection in the hypothalamus; it runs through the lateral hypothalamic region, connecting the tegmentum of the mesencephalon and elements of the limbic system. Called also *f. prosencephalicus medialis, medial prosencephalic f.,* and *medial telencephalic f.*

**Meynert's f.,** tractus habenulointerpeduncularis.

**f. of middle cerebellar peduncle, deep,** the most dorsal part of the transverse fibers of the pons, connecting pontine nuclei with the folia on the anterior superior surface of the cerebellum.

**f. of middle cerebellar peduncle, inferior,** the most caudal portion of the transverse fibers of the pons, connecting pontine nuclei with the cerebellar folia near the vermis.

**f. of middle cerebellar peduncle, superior,** the most rostral portion of the transverse fibers of the pons, connecting pontine nuclei with inferior lobules and posterior and lateral margins of the cerebellum.

**Monakow's f.,** tractus rubrospinalis.

**occipitofrontal f., inferior,** f. occipitofrontalis inferior.

**occipitofrontal f., superior,** f. occipitofrontalis superior.

**f. occipitofronta'lis infe'rior** [TA], inferior occipitofrontal fasciculus: a collection of association fibers in the inferior part of the extreme capsule near the uncinate fasciculus, connecting various inferior gyri of the temporal and frontal lobes.

**f. occipitofronta'lis supe'rior** [TA], superior occipitofrontal fasciculus: a collection of association fibers lying just internal to the intersection of the internal capsule and corpus callosum, interconnecting the cortex of the occipital and temporal lobes with that of the insula and frontal lobe, and probably comprising a significant part of the tapetum. Called also *f. subcallosus* [TA alternative] and *subcallosal f.*

**olivocochlear f.,** tractus olivocochlearis.

**f. parieto-occipitoponti'nus,** a bundle of nerve fibers that arise in the parietal and occipital lobes and pass through the retrolenticular part of the posterior limb of the internal capsule to end in the pontine nuclei.

**perforating f.,** perforant pathway.

**posterior f. of brachial plexus, f. poste'rior plex'us brachia'lis** [TA], posterior cord of brachial plexus: the posterior bundle of fibers of the brachial plexus, formed by the union of the posterior divisions of the superior, middle, and inferior trunks, C5 through C8 and sometimes T1, and from which arise the subscapular, thoracodorsal, radial, and axillary nerves.

**posterior f. proprius of spinal cord,** f. proprius posterior medullae spinalis.

**f. pro'prius ante'rior medul'lae spina'lis** [TA], anterior fasciculus proprius of spinal cord: any of the bundles of white substance in the anterior funiculus of the spinal cord, consisting of intersegmental fibers, some of which pass from the contralateral side, and probably also reticulospinal and descending autonomic fibers. Called also *anterior* or *ventral intersegmental f. of spinal cord, ventral f. proprius of spinal cord,* and *anterior* or *ventral intersegmental tract of spinal cord.*

**f. pro'prius dorsa'lis medul'lae spina'lis,** f. proprius posterior medullae spinalis.

**f. pro'prius latera'lis medul'lae spin'alis** [TA], lateral fasciculus proprius of spinal cord: any of the bundles of white substance in the lateral funiculus of the spinal cord, consisting of intersegmental fibers, some of which have passed from the contralateral side, and probably reticulospinal and autonomic fibers; called also *lateral intersegmental f. of spinal cord* and *lateral intersegmental tract of spinal cord.*

**f. pro'prius poste'rior medul'lae spina'lis** [TA], posterior fasciculus proprius of spinal cord: any of the bundles of white substance in the deepest part of the posterior funiculus of the spinal cord, consisting chiefly of intersegmental fibers derived from the cells of the posterior gray column, which divide into ascending and descending association fibers that reenter the gray substance and ramify in it. Called also *dorsal* or *posterior intersegmental f. of spinal cord, dorsal f. proprius of spinal cord,* and *dorsal* or *posterior intersegmental tract of spinal cord.*

**f. pro'prius ventra'lis medul'lae spina'lis,** f. proprius anterior medullae spinalis.

**f. prosencepha'licus media'lis,** f. medialis telencephali.

**pyramidal f. of medulla oblongata, f. pyramida'lis medul'lae oblonga'tae,** tractus pyramidalis (def. 1).

**f. retroflex'us,** TA alternative for *tractus habenulo-interpeduncularis.*

**Schütz's f.,** f. longitudinalis posterior.

**semilunar f.,** f. interfascicularis.

**f. semiluna'ris,** TA alternative for *f. interfascicularis.*

**septomarginal f., f. septomargina'lis** [TA], a bundle of nerve fibers situated along the dorsal periphery of the dorsal funiculus of the spinal cord in the thoracic region and bordering the dorsal median septum in the lumbar region; called also *septomarginal tract.*

**solitary f.,** tractus solitarius medullae oblongatae.

**subcallosal f.,** f. occipitofrontalis superior.

**f. subcallo'sus,** TA alternative for *f. occipitofrontalis superior.*

**f. subthala'micus** [TA], subthalamic fasciculus: a bundle of fibers passing through the internal capsule and connecting the subthalamic nucleus with the globus pallidus and putamen.

**f. sulcomargina'lis** [TA], sulcomarginal fasciculus: a layer of descending branches from the midbrain tectum situated in the ventral funiculus of the spinal cord, along the border of the ventral median fissure.

**thalamic f., f. thala'micus** [TA], a bundle of nerve fibers ascending through field H of Forel to pass dorsal to and partly through the zona incerta, crossing the lower portion of the posterior limb of the internal capsule to reach some of the ventral nuclei of the thalamus; it contains continuations of the ansa lenticularis and the fasciculus lenticularis and dentatothalamic, rubrothalamic, and thalamostriate fibers. See also *fields of Forel,* under *field.*

**thalamomammillary f.,** f. mammillothalamicus.

**fasci'culi transver'si aponeuro'sis palma'ris,** transverse fasciculi of palmar aponeurosis: the transverse fascial bands that support the webs between the fingers.

**fasci'culi transver'si aponeuro'sis planta'ris** [TA], transverse fasciculi of plantar aponeurosis: transverse bundles in the plantar aponeurosis near the toes.

**f. of Türck,** tractus corticospinalis anterior.

**unciform f., uncinate f., f. uncina'tus** [TA], a collection of association fibers which interconnect the cortex of the orbital surface of the frontal lobe with the parahippocampal gyrus and perhaps with the amygdala; other temporofrontal connections probably also exist.

**ventral f. proprius of spinal cord,** f. proprius anterior medullae spinalis.

**f. of Vicq d'Azyr,** f. mamillothalamicus.

**fas·ci·ec·to·my** (fas″e-ek'tə-me) [*fascia* + *-ectomy*] excision of fascia.

**fas·ci·od·e·sis** (fas″e-od'ə-sis) [*fascia* + *-desis*] the operation of suturing a fascia to skeletal attachment.

**Fas·ci·o·la** (fə-si'o-lə) [L. *fasciola* a band] [MeSH: Fasciola] a genus of flukes of the family Fasciolidae.

**F. cer'vi,** former name for *Paramphistomum cervi.*

**F. gigan'tica,** a giant liver fluke that infects cattle, sheep, wild animals, and occasionally humans in Africa, Asia, and Hawaii.

**F. hepa'tica,** the common liver fluke of sheep, oxen, goats, horses, and other herbivorous animals. It is occasionally found in the human liver, where it may cause dangerous symptoms by obstructing the biliary passages and by invasion of the liver parenchyma. Several snails of the genus *Lymnaea* act as invertebrate hosts. Called also *Distoma hepaticum.*

**F. hetero'phyes,** *Heterophyes heterophyes.*

**F. mag'na,** *Fascioloides magna.*

**fas·ci·o·la** (fə-si'o-lə) pl. *fasci'olae* [L., dim. of *fascia*] [MeSH: Fasciola] 1. a small band or striplike structure. 2. a small bandage.

**f. cine'rea, f. cine'rea cin'guli,** gyrus fasciolaris.

**fas·ci·o·lae** (fah-si'o-le) [L.] genitive and plural of *fasciola.*

**fas·ci·o·lar** (fə-si'o-lər) pertaining to a fasciola.

**fas·cio·li·a·sis** (fas″e-o-li'ə-sis) [MeSH: Fascioliasis] infection with *Fasciola hepatica* or *F. gigantica.*

**fas·ci·o·li·cide** (fas″e-o'lĭ-sīd) a substance lethal to flukes of the genus *Fasciola.*

**Fas·ci·o·li·dae** (fas″e-o'lĭ-de) [MeSH: Fasciolidae] a family of trematodes parasitic to mammals and birds; genera include *Fasciola, Fascioloides,* and *Fasciolopsis.*

**Fas·ci·o·loi·des** (fas″e-o-loi'dēz) a genus of flukes of the family Fasciolidae. *F. mag'na* is a large fluke found in the liver and lungs of herbivorous animals in North America.

**fas·ci·o·lop·si·a·sis** (fas″e-o-lop-si'ə-sis) the state of being infected with flukes of the genus *Fasciolopsis.*

**Fas·ci·o·lop·sis** (fas″e-o-lop'sis) [*fasciola* + Gr. *opsis* appearance] a genus of trematodes of the family Fasciolidae.
**F. bus'ki,** a trematode found in the small intestine of humans and pigs in many parts of Asia. It is the largest of the intestinal flukes, and may cause nausea, diarrhea, and a malabsorption syndrome if present in large numbers. The intermediate hosts are the snails *Planorbis coenosus* and various species of *Segmentina.*

**fas·cio·plas·ty** (fash'e-o-plas″te) plastic operation on fascia.

**fas·ci·or·rha·phy** (fash″e-or'ə-fe) [*fascia* + *-rrhaphy*] suture of lacerated fascia.

**fas·ci·ot·o·my** (fash″e-ot'ə-me) [*fascia* + *-tomy*] surgical incision or transection of fascia.

**fas·ci·tis** (fə-si'tis) fasciitis.

**fast** (fast) [A.S. *faest* firm; *faestan* to abstain from food] 1. immovable, or unchangeable; resistant to the action of a specific drug, stain, or destaining agent, as in acid-fast. 2. abstention from food.

**fas·tid·i·ous** (fas-tid'e-əs) in bacteriology, a microorganism having complex nutritional or cultural requirements for growth.

**fas·ti·ga·tum** (fas″tĭ-ga'təm) [L.] pointed; sharpened to a point.

**fas·tig·i·al** (fas-tij'e-əl) of or pertaining to the fastigium.

**fas·tig·i·um** (fas-tij'e-əm) [L. "gable end"] 1. [TA] the highest point in the roof of the fourth ventricle of the brain, at the junction between the superior medullary velum and the nodulus. 2. the acme, or highest point, as of a fever.

**fast·ness** (fast'nəs) the quality, in bacteria, of being resistant to the action of specific stains or inhibitors.

**fat** (fat) 1. adipose tissue; a white or yellowish tissue which forms soft pads between various organs of the body, serves to smooth and round out bodily contours, and furnishes a reserve supply of energy. 2. an ester of glycerol with fatty acids, usually oleic acid, palmitic acid, or stearic acid; triglyceride; neutral fat.
**bound f.,** masked f.
**brown f.,** brown adipose tissue.
**chyle f.,** fat in the form of an extremely fine emulsion taken into the chyle by the lymphatics of the intestine.
**corpse f.,** adipocere.
**fetal f.,** a term sometimes used in pathology to refer to brown adipose tissue.
**grave f.,** adipocere.
**masked f.,** fat that can be detected in a cell or tissue by chemical methods but is not revealed by staining methods; called also *bound f.*
**milk f.,** the suspension in milk which tends to separate out as cream.
**molecular f.,** fat occurring in fine specks within the cells.
**moruloid f., mulberry f.,** brown adipose tissue.
**neutral f.,** see *fat* (def. 2).
**paranephric f., pararenal f.,** corpus adiposum pararenale.
**perinephric f., perirenal f.,** capsula adiposa renis.
**polyunsaturated f.,** a fat containing polyunsaturated fatty acids.
**retrobulbar f.,** corpus adiposum orbitae.
**saturated f.,** a fat containing saturated fatty acids.
**unsaturated f.,** a fat containing unsaturated fatty acids.
**wool f.,** anhydrous lanolin.
**wool f., hydrous,** lanolin.
**wool f., refined,** anhydrous lanolin.

**fa·tal** (fa'təl) causing death; called also *mortal* and *lethal.*

**fate** (fāt) [L. *fatum* what is ordained by the gods] 1. the ultimate disposition or decreed outcome; see also *fate map,* under *map.* 2. in pharmacology, the intermediate and ultimate disposition of a drug in the body.
**prospective f.,** the development normally achieved by any region of the zygote or early embryo when there is no interference.

**fat·i·ga·bil·i·ty** (fat″ĭ-gə-bil'ĭ-te) easy susceptibility to fatigue.

**fa·tigue** (fə-tēg') [Fr.; L. *fatigatio*] [MeSH: Fatigue] 1. a state of increased discomfort and decreased efficiency resulting from prolonged or excessive exertion; loss of power or capacity to respond to stimulation. 2. the gradual fracturing of a material due to repetitive or cyclic stress.
**battle f., combat f.,** older terms for posttraumatic stress disorder in which the traumatic event is combat-related.
**pseudocombat f.,** a term applied to psychiatric combat casualties whose functional impairment is attributed to preexisting personality disorder rather than to reaction to combat stress.
**stimulation f.,** an increase in the threshold of a neural element due to repeated stimulation.
**vocal f.,** phonasthenia.

**fat·ty** (fat'e) pertaining to or characterized by fat.

**fat·ty ac·id** (fat'e) any straight chain monocarboxylic acid, especially those naturally occurring in fats. Fatty acids are classified as saturated or unsaturated; the latter are further classified as polyunsaturated or monounsaturated. The absolute and relative amounts of the various fatty acids consumed have been linked to plasma lipid levels, atherosclerosis, and coronary artery disease. See also accompanying table and illustration.
**essential f. a.,** any fatty acid that cannot be synthesized by the human body and must be obtained from dietary sources, e.g., linoleic acid and linolenic acid.
**free f. a's (FFA),** nonesterified f. a's.
**monounsaturated f. a's,** unsaturated fatty acids containing a single double bond; they occur predominantly as oleic acid, in peanut, olive, and canola oils. Monounsaturated fatty acids have been shown to reduce low-density lipoprotein levels and thus the blood cholesterol level.
**n-3 f. a's,** ω-3 f. a's.
**nonesterified f. a's (NEFA),** the fraction of plasma fatty acids that are not in the form of glycerol esters. Called also *free fatty a's* (a misnomer because they are transported complexed with albumin).
**ω-3 f. a's, omega-3 f. a's,** unsaturated fatty acids in which the double bond closest to the methyl (omega) terminus of the molecule occurs at the third carbon from that end; they are present in marine animal fats and some vegetable oils. These fatty acids can modulate leukotriene composition, alter prostaglandin synthesis, inhibit platelet aggregation, and increase the ratio of high-density to low-density lipoproteins while lowering overall plasma lipid levels (particularly of triglycerides). There is evidence that they may inhibit some cancers. See also accompanying table and illustration.
**ω-6 f. a's, omega-6 f. a's,** unsaturated fatty acids in which the double bond closest to the methyl (omega) terminus of the molecule occurs at the sixth carbon from that end; they are present predominantly in vegetable and seed oils. Diets in which the ratio of omega-6 to omega-3 fatty acids is high have been linked to promotion of some cancers. See also accompanying table and illustration.
**ω-9 f. a's,** polyunsaturated fatty acids from animal and vegetable fats.
**polyunsaturated f. a's (PUFA),** unsaturated fatty acids (q.v.) containing two or more double bonds; they occur predominantly as linoleic, linolenic, and arachidonic acids, in vegetable and seed oils. Dietary polyunsaturated fatty acids can lower plasma lipid levels and thus lower serum cholesterol; however, they have been shown to lower both low-density and high-density lipoprotein levels, and excessive consumption of these fatty acids has also been linked to cancer.
**saturated f. a's,** fatty acids without double bonds in their chains; they occur predominantly in animal fats and tropical oils and can be produced by hydrogenation of unsaturated fatty acids. Fats composed of saturated fatty acids increase serum low-density lipoproteins and blood cholesterol levels. See also accompanying table and illustration.
***trans*–f. a's,** stereoisomers of the naturally occurring *cis*–fatty acids, found in margarines and shortenings as artifacts after hydrogenation; pregnant women and certain other individuals should restrict intake of these.
**unsaturated f. a's,** fatty acids containing one (monounsaturated) or multiple (polyunsaturated) double bonds; they predominate in most plant-derived fats. The number and position of each double bond can be specified, as in the systematic names, or the position of the double bond closest to the methyl (omega) terminus can be specified to denote functional subdivisions of the overall group, e.g., omega-3 fatty acids (see illustration). The numbers and positions of the double bonds have been linked to effects on plasma lipid, triglyceride, and cholesterol levels; see also *polyunsaturated f. a's, monounsaturated f.a's,* and accompanying table.

**fat·ty-ac·id syn·thase** (fat'e as'id sin'thās) [EC 2.3.1.85] an enzyme complex that catalyzes the synthesis of long-chain fatty acids. Two-carbon units are successively added to the growing chain in a process similar to fatty acid oxidation in reverse, with each unit added via a series of condensation and decarboxylation, reduction, and dehydration reactions. The overall reaction is: acetyl CoA + $n$ malonyl CoA + $2n$ NADPH = long-chain fatty acid anion + $n$ $CO_2$ + $2n$ $NADP^+$ + $(n + 1)$ CoA. Palmitate is the preferred product of the

**Some Naturally Occurring Fatty Acids**

| Symbol* | Common Name | Systematic Name | Structural Formula |
|---|---|---|---|
| *Saturated* | | | |
| $C_{4:0}$ | Butyric acid | Butanoic acid | $CH_3(CH_2)_2COOH$ |
| $C_{6:0}$ | Caproic acid | Hexanoic acid | $CH_3(CH_2)_4COOH$ |
| $C_{8:0}$ | Caprylic acid | Octanoic acid | $CH_3(CH_2)_6COOH$ |
| $C_{10:0}$ | Capric acid | Decanoic acid | $CH_3(CH_2)_8COOH$ |
| $C_{12:0}$ | Lauric acid | Dodecanoic acid | $CH_3(CH_2)_{10}COOH$ |
| $C_{14:0}$ | Myristic acid | Tetradecanoic acid | $CH_3(CH_2)_{12}COOH$ |
| $C_{16:0}$ | Palmitic acid | Hexadecanoic acid | $CH_3(CH_2)_{14}COOH$ |
| $C_{18:0}$ | Stearic acid | Octadecanoic acid | $CH_3(CH_2)_{16}COOH$ |
| $C_{20:0}$ | Arachidic acid | Eicosanoic acid | $CH_3(CH_2)_{18}COOH$ |
| $C_{22:0}$ | Behenic acid | Docosanoic acid | $CH_3(CH_2)_{20}COOH$ |
| $C_{24:0}$ | Lignoceric acid | Tetracosanoic acid | $CH_3(CH_2)_{22}COOH$ |
| *Unsaturated* | | | |
| $C_{16:1\ \omega\text{-}7}$ | Palmitoleic acid | *cis*-9-Hexadecenoic acid | $CH_3(CH_2)_5CH{=}CH(CH_2)_7COOH$ |
| $C_{18:1\ \omega\text{-}9}$ | Oleic acid | *cis*-9-Octadecenoic acid | $CH_3(CH_2)_7CH{=}CH(CH_2)_7COOH$ |
| $C_{18:1\ \omega\text{-}7}$ | Vaccenic acid | 11-Octadecenoic acid | $CH_3(CH_2)_5CH{=}CH(CH_2)_9COOH$ |
| $C_{18:2\ \omega\text{-}6}$ | Linoleic acid | *cis,cis*-9,12-Octadecadienoic acid | $CH_3(CH_2)_4(CH{=}CHCH_2)_2(CH_2)_6COOH$ |
| $C_{18:3\ \omega\text{-}3}$ | Linolenic acid | all *cis*-9,12,15-Octadecatrienoic acid | $CH_3CH_2(CH{=}CHCH_2)_3(CH_2)_6COOH$ |
| $C_{20:4\ \omega\text{-}6}$ | Arachidonic acid | all *cis*-5,8,11,14-Eicosatetraenoic acid | $CH_3(CH_2)_4(CH{=}CHCH_2)_4(CH_2)_2COOH$ |
| $C_{20:5\ \omega\text{-}3}$ | — | all *cis*-5,8,11,14,17-Eicosapentaenoic acid | $CH_3(CH_2CH{=}CH)_5(CH_2)_3COOH$ |
| $C_{22:1\ \omega\text{-}9}$ | Erucic acid | *cis*-13-Docosenoic acid | $CH_3(CH_2)_7CH{=}CH(CH_2)_{11}COOH$ |
| $C_{22:6\ \omega\text{-}3}$ | — | all *cis*-4,7,10,13,16,19-Docosahexaenoic acid | $CH_3(CH_2CH{=}CH)_6(CH_2)_2COOH$ |
| $C_{24:1\ \omega\text{-}9}$ | Nervonic acid | *cis*-15-Tetracosenoic acid | $CH_3(CH_2)_7CH{=}CH(CH_2)_{13}COOH$ |

* Symbol subscripts denote *carbon chain length: number of double bonds;* in unsaturated fatty acids *position of the initial double bond relative to the ω-carbon* is also indicated.

mammalian liver enzyme complex, which includes catalytic sites for the seven sequential reactions.

**fat·ty ac·id thio·ki·nase** (fat'e as'id thi"o-ki'nās) acyl CoA synthetase, def. 1.

**fau·ces** (faw'sēz) [L., pl. of *faux* "a gorge, narrow pass"] [TA] the passage from the mouth to the pharynx, including both the lumen and its boundaries; called also *throat.*

**Fau·chard's disease** (fo-shahrz') [Pierre *Fauchard,* French dentist, 1678–1761] marginal periodontitis.

**fau·cial** (faw'shəl) pertaining to the fauces; called also *guttural.*

**fau·ci·tis** (faw-si'tis) inflammation of the fauces; called also *sore throat.*

**fau·na** (faw'nə) [L. *Faunus* mythical deity of herdsmen] the animal life present in or characteristic of a given region or locality. It may be discernible with the unaided eye (macrofauna), or only with the aid of a microscope (microfauna).

**fa·va** (fa'və) *Vicia faba* L. (Leguminosae).

**fa·ve·o·lar** (fa-ve'o-lər) foveolar.

**fa·ve·o·late** (fa-ve'o-lāt) alveolate.

**fa·ve·o·lus** (fa-ve'o-ləs) pl. *fave'oli* [L.] foveola.

**fa·vid** (fa'vid) a secondary skin eruption due to allergy in favus.

**fa·vism** (fa'vis-əm) [Italian *fava* bean] [MeSH: Favism] an acute hemolytic anemia caused by ingestion of fava beans or inhalation of the pollen of the plant *Vicia faba (fava),* occurring in susceptible individuals usually as a result of a hereditary deficiency of glucose-6-phosphate dehydrogenase in erythrocytes; see *glucose-6-phosphate dehydrogenase deficiency.*

**Fav·re-Du·rand-Nic·o·las disease** (fahv'rə-doo-rah'ne-ko-lah') [Maurice Jules *Favre,* French physician, 1876–1954; J. *Durand,* French physician, 20th century; Joseph *Nicolas,* French physician, 1868–1960] lymphogranuloma venereum.

Saturated: (Palmitic acid, $C_{16:0}$)

16 . . . . . . . 3 2 1
$CH_3(CH_2)_{12}CH_2CH_2COOH$
ω . . . . . . . . β α

Unsaturated: (Palmitoleic acid, $C_{16:1\ \omega\text{-}7}$)

16 . . . . . . 10 9 . . . . . . . 2 1
$CH_3(CH_2)_5CH{=}CH(CH_2)_6CH_2COOH$
ω . . . . . . . . . . . . . . . . . . . . α
ω-1 . . . . . . . ω-7 ω-8 . . . . ω-16

Palmitoleic acid is designated an ω-7 fatty acid, specifically *cis*-9-hexadecenoic acid.

Fatty acid numbering and nomenclature.

**Fav·re-Ra·cou·chot nodular elastosis (syndrome)** (fahv'rə rah-koo-sho') [M. J. *Favre;* Jean *Racouchot,* French physician, born 1908] see under *elastosis.*

**fa·vus** (fa'vəs) [L. "honeycomb"] a type of ringworm seen in humans and other animals, caused by species of *Trichophyton.* In humans the fungus is usually *T. schoenleinii* and is in the scalp, although it may also affect glabrous skin; the infection is characterized by formation of yellow cup-shaped crusts called *scutula,* which may enlarge and coalesce to form honeycomb-like masses, sometimes associated with hair loss, cutaneous atrophy, and scarring. Called also *honeycomb ringworm* and *tinea favosa.* Local names include *witkop* and *white head.*
**f. of fowl,** a chronic dermatomycosis affecting the comb of fowl, usually in male birds, caused by *Trichophyton gallinae;* called also *comb disease* and *honeycomb ringworm.*
**f. herpetifor'mis, mouse f., f. mu'rium,** a skin disease in mice caused by infection with a strain of the fungus *Trichophyton mentagrophytes;* it can be transmitted to humans, causing ringworm.

**Fay method** (fa) [T. *Fay,* American physical therapist, 20th century] see under *method.*

**Fa·zio-Londe atrophy, disease** (fahz'e-o lōnd) [E. *Fazio,* Italian physician, 1849–1902; P.F.L. *Londe,* French neurologist, 1864–1944] progressive bulbar palsy of childhood.

**5-FC** flucytosine.

**Fc** [*f*ragment, *c*rystallizable] originally, the fragment, not containing antigen combining sites, obtained by papain cleavage of the IgG molecule; now generally used as an adjective, e.g., Fc region, segment, to refer to the part of any immunoglobulin monomer comprising the hinge region and $C_H2$, $C_H3$, and $C_H4$ domains of both heavy chains. The Fc region contains the allotypic markers and mediates all biologic activities including complement activation, binding to cell-surface receptors (Fc receptors, IgE receptors), and transplacental transport of IgG. Cf. *Fab.*

**Fc'** a fragment produced in minute quantities by papain digestion of IgG molecules, a noncovalently bonded dimer containing most of the $C_H3$ domains of both heavy chains.

**fCi** femtocurie.

**Fd** the heavy chain portion of an Fab fragment.

**FDA** fronto-dextra anterior (right frontoanterior, a position of the fetus); Food and Drug Administration.

**FDI** abbreviation for *Fédération Dentaire Internationale* [Fr. International Dental Association].

**FDP** fibrin degradation products or fibrinogen degradation products; fronto-dextra posterior (right frontoposterior, a position of the fetus).

**FDT** fronto-dextra transversa (right frontotransverse, a position of the fetus).

**F-duc·tion** (ef-duk'shən) in bacterial genetics, the process whereby part of the bacterial chromosome is attached to the autonomous F factor (fertility factor) and thus is transferred with high frequency from the donor (male) bacterium to the recipient (female) bacterium. Called also *sexduction.*

**F-dUMP** 5-fluorodeoxyuridine monophosphate; see under *floxuridine.*

**$FE_{Na}$** excreted fraction of filtered sodium; see under *test.*

**Fe** symbol for *iron* (L. *ferrum*).

**fear** (fēr) [MeSH: Fear] the unpleasant emotional state consisting of psychological and psychophysiological responses to a real external threat or danger, including agitation, alertness, tension, and physiological mobilization of the alarm reaction. Cf. *anxiety.*

**feb·an·tel** (feb'ən-təl) a benzimidazole prodrug that is a precursor of fenbendazole; used as an anthelmintic in sheep, cattle, and horses.

**Feb. dur.** abbreviation for L. *feb're duran'te,* while the fever lasts.

**feb·ri·cant** (feb'rĭ-kənt) pyrogenic.

**feb·ri·cide** (feb'rĭ-sīd) [*febris* + *-cide*] antipyretic (def. 2).

**fe·bric·i·ty** (fə-bris'ĭ-te) feverishness.

**fe·bric·u·la** (fə-brik'u-lə) [L.] a slight or temporary attack of fever of indefinite origin or pathology.

**feb·ri·fa·cient** (feb"rĭ-fa'shənt) pyrogenic.

**fe·brif·ic** (fə-brif'ik) pyrogenic.

**fe·brif·u·gal** (fəb-rif'ə-gəl) [*febri-* + *-fugal*] antipyretic (def. 1).

**feb·ri·fuge** (feb'rĭ-fūj) antipyretic (def. 2).

**feb·rif·u·gine** (fə-brif'u-jin) an antimalarial alkaloid from the plant *Dichroa febrifuga* (ch'ang shan).

**feb·rile** (feb'ril) [L. *febrilis*] 1. pertaining to fever. 2. characterized by fever. Called also *feverish, pyrectic, pyretic,* and *pyrexial.*

**fe·bris** (fe'bris) [L.] fever.
**f. meliten'sis,** brucellosis.

**fe·cal** (fe'kəl) pertaining to or of the nature of feces. Called also *stercoral* and *stercorous.*

**fe·ca·lith** (fe'kə-lith) [*fecal* + *-lith*] an intestinal concretion of fecal matter. Called also *coprolith* and *stercolith.*

**fe·cal·oid** (fe'kəl-oid) resembling fecal matter.

**fe·ca·lo·ma** (fe'kə-lo'mə) [*feces* + *-oma*] stercoroma.

**fe·cal·u·ria** (fe"kəl-u're-ə) [*feces* + *-uria*] the presence of fecal matter in the urine.

**fe·ces** (fe'sēz) [L. *faeces,* pl. of *faex* refuse] [MeSH: Feces] the excrement discharged from the intestines, consisting of bacteria, cells exfoliated from the intestines, secretions, chiefly of the liver, and a small amount of food residue.

**fec·u·la** (fek'u-lə) [L. *faecula* lees, dregs] 1. lees or sediment. 2. starch; also the starchy part of a seed.

**fec·u·lent** (fek'u-lənt) [L. *faeculentus*] 1. having dregs or a sediment. 2. fecal.

**fe·cun·date** (fe'kən-dāt) [L. *fecundare* to fertilize] fertilize.

**fe·cun·da·tio** (fe"kən-da'she-o) [L., from *fecundare* to fertilize] fertilization.
**f. ab ex'tra,** impregnation occurring without entrance of the penis into the vagina.

**fe·cun·da·tion** (fe"kən-da'shən) [L. *fecundatio*] fertilization.
**artificial f.,** artificial insemination.

**fe·cun·di·ty** (fə-kun'dĭ-te) [L. *fecunditas*] ability to produce offspring rapidly and in large numbers. In demography, the physiological ability to reproduce, as opposed to fertility.

**Fe·de·ri·ci's sign** (fĕ-də-re'chēz) [Cesare *Federici,* Italian physician, 1838–1892] see under *sign.*

**fee·ble·mind·ed·ness** (fe"bəl-mīnd'əd-nəs) former name for *mental retardation.* The feebleminded were divided into three grades: idiots, with a mental age below two years; imbeciles, with a mental age between two and seven years; and morons, with a mental age between seven and twelve years.

**feed·back** (fēd'bak) [MeSH: Feedback] the return of some of the output of a system as input so as to exert some control in the process; see also *endproduct inhibition,* under *inhibition.*
**alpha f.,** see under *biofeedback.*
**negative f.,** the condition of maintaining a constant output of a system by exertion of an inhibitory control on a key step in the system by a product of that system.
**positive f.,** a condition causing the output of a system to increase continually by exertion of a stimulatory effect on a key step in the system by a product of that system.

**feed·for·ward** (fēd-for'wərd) the anticipatory effect that one intermediate in a metabolic or endocrine control system exerts on another intermediate further along in the pathway; such effect may be stimulatory (positive f.) or inhibitory (negative f.).

**feed·ing** (fēd'ing) the taking or giving of food.
**artificial f.,** feeding of a baby with food other than mother's milk.
**breast f.,** breast-feeding.
**extrabuccal f.,** the administration of nutriment other than by mouth.
**Finkelstein's f.,** feeding of infants based upon decrease in the milk sugar of the food.
**forced f., forcible f.,** the administration of food by force to those who cannot or will not receive it.
**sham f.,** 1. an experimental procedure that has been performed on dogs, in which food is chewed and swallowed but does not enter the stomach, because of diversion to the exterior by an esophageal fistula or other device. 2. see under *test.*

**Feer's disease** (fārz) [Emil *Feer,* Swiss pediatrician, 1864–1955] acrodynia.

**fee-split·ting** (fe'-split"ing) the division of moneys received by a specialist, such as a surgeon, between himself and the physician who referred the patient to him.

**feet** (fēt) see *foot.*

**FEF** forced expiratory flow.

**Feh·ling's solution** (fa'lingz) [Hermann Christian von *Fehling,* German chemist, 1812–1885] see under *solution.*

**fel** (fel) [L. "bile"] bile.
**f. bo'vis,** ox bile.
**f. bo'vis purifica'tum, f. tau'ri purifica'tum,** ox bile extract.

**Fel·dene** (fel'dēn) trademark for preparations of piroxicam.

**Fel·der·struk·tur** (fel"dər-shtrook'tər) [Ger.] the term used to describe the pattern of organization of the myofilaments in cardiac and red skeletal muscles, in which the myofilaments are not associated in discrete myofibrils, but instead form a continuous field interrupted by mitochondria. Cf. *Fibrillenstruktur.*

**Fel·i·co·la** (fel-ĭ-ko'lə) a genus of parasitic biting lice (order Mallophaga); *F. subros'trata* infests cats.

**fe·line** (fe'līn) [L. *feles* cat] pertaining to, characteristic of, or derived from a cat.

**Fe·lix-Weil reaction** (fa'liks-vīl) [Arthur *Felix,* Polish-born bacteriologist, 1887–1956; Edmund *Weil,* Austrian physician in Czechoslovakia, 1880–1922] Weil-Felix reaction.

**fel·la·tio** (fə-la'she-o) [L. *fellare* to suck] oral stimulation or manipulation of the penis.

**fe·lo·di·pine** (fə-lo'dĭ-pēn) [MeSH: Felodipine] a calcium channel blocker used as a vasodilator in the treatment of hypertension; administered orally.

**fel·on** (fel'ən) an extremely painful abscess on the palmar aspect of the fingertips, occurring as the result of infection in the closed space of the terminal phalanx, usually following inoculation into the skin of a pathogenic microorganism. Called also *whitlow.*

**Fel·sules** (fel'səlz) trademark for a preparation of chloral hydrate.

**Fel·ton's phenomenon** (fel'tənz) [Lloyd D. *Felton,* American physician, 1885–1953] see under *phenomenon.*

**felt·work** (felt'wərk) a complex of closely interwoven fibers, as of nerve fibrils.
**Kaes' f.,** Kaes-Bekhterev layer.

**Fel·ty's syndrome** (fel'tēz) [Augustus Roi *Felty,* American physician, 1895–1963] [MeSH: Felty's Syndrome] see under *syndrome.*

**fe·male** (fe'māl) [L. *femella* young woman] [MeSH: Female] 1. an individual organism of the sex that bears young or that produces ova or eggs. 2. feminine.

**fem·i·nine** (fem'ĭ-nin) 1. pertaining to the female sex. 2. having qualities normally asociated with females.

**fem·i·nin·i·ty** (fem"ĭ-nin'ĭ-te) possession of normal female qualities by a girl or woman.

**fem·i·nism** (fem'ĭ-niz-əm) old term for *feminization* (def. 2).

**fem·i·ni·za·tion** (fem"ĭ-nĭ-za'shən) [MeSH: Feminization] 1. the normal development of primary and secondary sex characters in females. 2. the induction or development of female secondary sex characters in the male. Called also *effemination.*
**testicular f.,** complete androgen resistance; see under *resistance.*

**testicular f., incomplete,** incomplete androgen resistance.

**fem•i•niz•ing** (fem'ĭ-nīz″ing) causing feminization.

**Fem•i•none** (fem'ĭ-nōn) trademark for a preparation of ethinyl estradiol.

**fem•i•no•nu•cle•us** (fem″ĭ-no-noo'kle-əs) female pronucleus.

**Fem. intern.** abbreviation for L. *femo'ribus inter'nus,* at the inner side of the thighs.

**Fem•o•gen** (fem'o-gən) trademark for preparations of esterified estrogens.

**fem•o•ra** (fem'o-rə) [L.] plural of *femur.*

**fem•o•ral** (fem'or-əl) [L. *femoralis*] pertaining to the femur, or to the thigh.

**femor(o)-** combining form denoting relationship to the femur.

**fem•o•ro•cele** (fem'o-ro-sēl″) [*femoro-* + *-cele*] femoral hernia.

**fem•o•ro•fem•o•ral** (fem″ə-ro-fem'ə-rəl) pertaining to both the right and left femoral arteries.

**fem•o•ro•fem•o•ro•pop•lit•e•al** (fem″ə-ro-fem″ə-ro-pop-lit'e-əl) pertaining to the left femoral, right femoral, and popliteal arteries.

**fem•o•ro•il•i•ac** (fem″o-ro-il'e-ak) pertaining to the femur and the ilium.

**fem•o•ro•pop•lit•e•al** (fem″ə-ro-pop-lit'e-əl) pertaining to the femoral and popliteal arteries.

**fem•o•ro•tib•i•al** (fem″o-ro-tib'e-əl) pertaining to the femur and the tibia.

**Fem•stat** (fem'stat) trademark for a preparation of butoconazole nitrate.

**femto-** [Danish *femten* fifteen] a combining form used in naming units of measurement to indicate one-quadrillionth ($10^{-15}$) of the unit designated by the root with which it is combined. Symbol f.

**fem•to•cu•rie** (fem″to-ku're) a unit of radioactivity, being one-quadrillionth ($10^{-15}$) curie, or the quantity of radioactive material in which the number of nuclear disintegrations is $3.7 \times 10^{-5}$ per second. Abbreviated fCi.

**fe•mur** (fe'mər) pl. *fem'ora, femurs* [L.] [MeSH: Femur] 1. [TA] the bone that extends from the pelvis to the knee, being the longest and largest bone in the body; its head articulates with the acetabulum of the hip bone, and distally, the femur, along with the patella and tibia, forms the knee joint. Called also *femoral bone, os femoris* [TA alternative], *os femorale,* and *thigh bone.* See also Plate 45. 2. the thigh; see also *regio femoris.*

**fen•a•mate** (fen'ə-māt) any of a class of analgesic and antiinflammatory agents derived from *N*-phenylanthranilic acid.

**fen•ben•da•zole** (fən-ben'də-zōl) [MeSH: Fenbendazole] a benzimidazole used as an anthelmintic in humans, sheep, cattle, and horses.

**fen•bu•fen** (fən-bu'fən) a nonsteroidal antiinflammatory drug derived from propionic acid, used for the relief of pain in musculoskeletal and joint disorders; administered orally.

**fe•nes•tra** (fə-nes'trə) gen. and pl. *fenes'trae* [L. "window"] 1. [TA] window (def. 1). 2. an opening in a bandage or cast. 3. an opening in the blade of a forceps.

**f. coch'leae** [TA], fenestra or window of cochlea: a round opening in the inner wall of the middle ear inferior to and a little posterior to the fenestra vestibuli; it is covered by the secondary tympanic membrane. Called also *f. rotunda, cochlear window,* and *round window.*

**f. nov-ova'lis,** a surgically created oval window in the lateral semicircular canal in Lempert's fenestration operation.

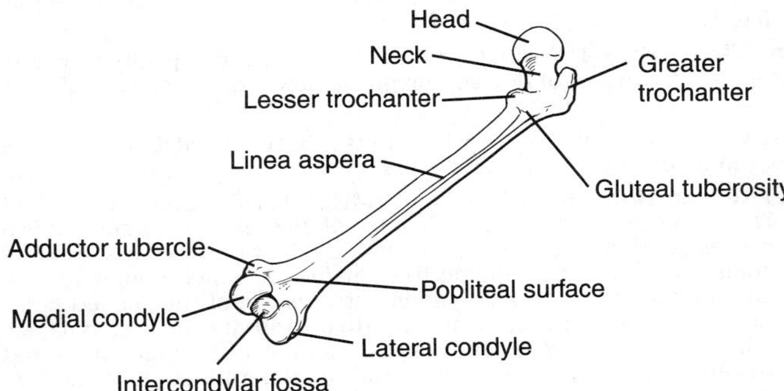

Posterior view of right femur.

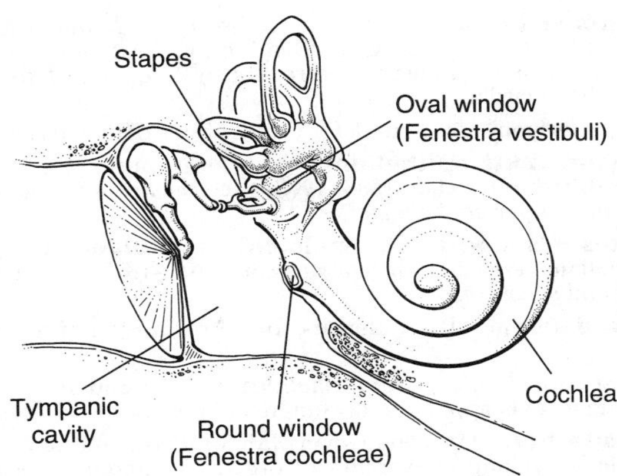


**f. ova'lis,** f. vestibuli.

**f. rotun'da,** f. cochleae.

**f. vesti'buli** [TA], fenestra or window of vestibule: an oval opening in the inner ear, which is closed by the base of the stapes; called also *f. ovalis, oval window,* and *vestibular window.*

**fe•nes•trae** (fə-nes'tre) [L.] genitive and plural of *fenestra.*

**fen•es•trate** (fen'əs-trāt) to pierce with one or more openings.

**fen•es•trat•ed** (fen'əs-trāt″əd) [L. *fenestratus*] pierced with one or more openings.

**fen•es•tra•tion** (fen″əs-tra'shən) [L. *fenestratus* furnished with windows] 1. the act of being perforated. 2. the presence of perforations or windows; see *fenestra.* 3. the surgical creation of a new opening in the labyrinth of the ear for the restoration of hearing in cases of otosclerosis; see *Lempert's fenestration operation,* under *operation.*

**alveolar plate f.,** apical f.

**aorticopulmonary f.,** aortic septal defect.

**apical f.,** a condition seen in children, consisting of round or oval openings perforating the cortical plate of bone that overlies part of a pulpless primary tooth; it may involve all the primary teeth but usually affects only the upper primary incisors. Called also *alveolar plate f.*

**fen•flur•amine hy•dro•chlo•ride** (fən-flo͞or'ə-mēn) an adrenergic used as an anorexic in the short-term treatment of exogenous obesity; administered orally.

**fen•met•o•zole hy•dro•chlo•ride** (fən-met'ə-zōl) an antidepressant and narcotic antagonist, $C_{10}H_{10}Cl_2N_2O{\cdot}HCl$.

**fen•nel** (fen'əl) 1. *Foeniculum vulgare.* 2. the edible seeds of *F. vulgare,* used as a flavoring agent and source of fennel oil.

**fen•o•pro•fen cal•ci•um** (fen″o-pro'fən) [USP] a nonsteroidal antiinflammatory agent that is a propionic acid derivative; used in the treatment of rheumatoid arthritis and osteoarthritis.

**fen•o•ter•ol hy•dro•bro•mide** (fen″o-ter'ol) [MeSH: Fenoterol] a *β*-adrenergic agent used as a bronchodilator for the treatment and prophylaxis of reversible bronchospasm in obstructive airway disease; administered by inhalation.

**fen•spir•ide hy•dro•chlo•ride** (fən-spēr'īd) 8-(2-phenethyl)-1-oxa-3,8-diazaspiro[4.5]decan-2-one monohydrochloride. An antiadrenergic compound, $C_{15}H_{20}N_2O_2{\cdot}HCl$, used as a bronchodilator.

**fen•ta•nyl cit•rate** (fen'tə-nəl) [USP] a narcotic analgesic derivative of piperidine, used mainly preoperatively, postoperatively, and during surgery, administered intravenously or intramuscularly. A combination of fentanyl citrate and droperidol (known as *Innovar*) is administered to produce neuroleptoanalgesia.

**fen•ti•clor** (fen'tī-klor) a topical anti-infective which has been used in candidal and dermatophytic infections of the skin and mucous membranes.

**fen•u•greek** (fen'u-grēk) [L. *faenum graecum* Greek hay] 1. *Trigonella foenumgraecum.* 2. the seeds of *T. foenumgraecum,* widely used as a flavoring agent, including in veterinary medicine to flavor powdered feed additives. See also *trigonelline.*

**Fen•wick's disease** (fen'wiks) [Samuel *Fenwick,* English physician, 1821–1902] see under *disease.*

**Fe•o•sol** (fe'o-sol) trademark for preparations of ferrous sulfate.

**FEP** free erythrocyte protoporphyrin.

**fe•ral** (fe'rəl) [L. *feralis*] savage; wild; living in the wild state, especially after having been domesticated.

**fer-de-lance** (fār-də-lahs') [Fr. "lance head"] 1. *Bothrops lanceolatus,* a large venomous pit viper found in the West Indies. See table at *snake.* 2. name sometimes erroneously given to *Bothrops atrox,* the barba amarilla.

**Fer·gon** (fer'gon) trademark for preparations of ferrous gluconate.

**Fer·gu·son Smith epithelioma** (fer'gə-sən"smith) [John *Ferguson Smith,* British physician, 1888–1978] see *self-healing squamous epithelioma,* under *epithelioma.*

**Fer·gus·son's operation (incision), speculum** (fər'gə-sənz) [Sir William *Fergusson,* British surgeon, 1808–1877] see under *incision* and *speculum.*

**Fer-In-Sol** (fer'in-sol) trademark for a preparation of ferrous sulfate.

**fer·ment** (fər-ment') [L. *fermentum* leaven] to undergo fermentation; the term is applied to decomposition of carbohydrates.

**fer·men·ta·tion** (fər"mən-ta'shən) [MeSH: Fermentation] the anaerobic enzymatic conversion of organic compounds, especially carbohydrates, to simpler compounds, especially to ethyl alcohol, resulting in energy in the form of adenosine triphosphate (ATP); the process is used in the production of alcohol, bread, vinegar, and other food or industrial products. It differs from respiration in that organic substances rather than molecular oxygen are used as electron acceptors. Fermentation occurs widely in bacteria and yeasts, the process usually being identified by the product formed; e.g., acetic, alcoholic, butyric, and lactic fermentation are those that result in the formation of acetic acid, alcohol, butyric acid, and lactic acid, respectively.
**heterolactic f.,** one that produces lactic acid and one or more additional products, such as ethanol, acetic acid, and carbon dioxide.
**homolactic f.,** one that produces only lactic acid as a product.
**mixed acid f.,** a type carried out by most Enterobacteriaceae, in which acetic, lactic, succinic, and formic acids are formed in proportions varying by species and growth conditions.
**stormy f.,** the rapid fermentation of milk produced by *Clostridium perfringens,* marked by rupture of the clotted milk by the pressure of the gas which develops.

**fer·mi·um** (fər'me-əm) [Enrico *Fermi,* Italian physicist, 1901–1954; winner of the Nobel prize for physics in 1938] [MeSH: Fermium] the chemical element number 100, atomic weight 253, symbol Fm, originally discovered in debris from a thermonuclear explosion in 1952.

**fern** (fərn) any of a large number of flowerless, seedless plants that reproduce by spores; some are toxic.
**bracken f.,** *Pteridium aquilinum;* see *bracken.*
**jimmy f.,** *Cheilanthes sinnata.*
**maidenhair f.,** any of several ferns of the genus *Adiantum,* including *A. pedatum,* which is used as an expectorant and demulcent.
**male f.,** *Dryopteris filix-mas.*
**male shield f.,** *Dryopteris filix-mas.*
**rock f.,** *Cheilanthes seiberi.*

**fern·ing** (fərn'ing) the appearance of a fernlike pattern in a dried specimen, due to the presence of sodium chloride and other electrolytes. In a specimen of cervical mucus this indicates presence of estrogen that is not being counteracted by progesterone. In a specimen of vaginal fluid not contaminated by cervical mucus, it indicates presence of amniotic fluid.

**-ferous** [L. *ferre* to bear] a word termination meaning bearing or producing.

**fer·pen·te·tate** (fər-pen'tə-tāt) a chelate of iron and ascorbate with pentetic acid; complexed with technetium 99m it is used in renal scanning.

**Fer·ra·ta's cell** (fə-rah'təz) [Adolfo *Ferrata,* Italian physician, 1880–1946] blast cell (def. 2).

**fer·rat·ed** (fer'āt-əd) charged with iron.

**fer·re·dox·in** (fer"ə-dok'sin) a nonheme iron-containing protein, also having a high sulfide content and a very low redox potential; the ferredoxins participate in electron transport in photosynthesis, nitrogen fixation, and various other biological processes.

**Fer·rein's canal,** etc. (fer-az') [Antoine *Ferrein,* French physician, 1693–1769] see under *canal, foramen, ligament, pyramid, tube,* and *tubule.*

**fer·ri** (fer'e) [L., gen. of *ferrum*] see *iron.*

**fer·ri·al·bu·min·ic** (fer"e-al-bu-min'ik) containing iron and albumin.

**fer·ric** (fer'ik) [L. *ferrum*] containing iron in its plus-three oxidation state, Fe(III) (sometimes designated $Fe^{3+}$).
**f. chloride,** orange-yellow or brownish yellow crystalline pieces, $FeCl_3 \cdot 6H_2O$, very soluble in water; used as a reagent and as a diagnostic aid in phenylketonuria; it was formerly used as a hematinic in the treatment of iron deficiency anemias, and has been used as a topical astringent and styptic. Called also *iron chloride.*
**f. fructose,** an oral iron preparation used in the treatment of iron deficiency.

**fer·ri·heme** (fer'e-hēm) hematin.

**fer·ri·tin** (fer'ĭ-tin) [MeSH: Ferritin] the iron-apoferritin complex, one of the chief forms in which iron is stored in the body; it occurs at least in the gastrointestinal mucosa, liver, spleen, bone marrow, and reticuloendothelial cells generally. See also *immunoferritin.*

**fer·ro·che·la·tase** (fer"o-ke'lə-tās) [EC 4.99.1.1] [MeSH: Ferrochelatase] a mitochondrial enzyme of the lyase class that catalyzes the insertion of ferrous iron into protoporphyrin IX to form protoheme IX, the heme of hemoglobin. Inhibition of the enzyme in lead poisoning results in accumulation of protoporphyrin IX. Deficiency of the enzyme, an autosomal dominant trait, results in protoporphyria.

**fer·ro·cho·lin·ate** (fer"o-ko'lin-āt) a chelate prepared by reacting equimolar quantities of freshly precipitated ferric chloride with choline dihydrogen citrate, the metallic ion being sequestered and firmly bound into a ring within the molecule; used in the treatment of iron deficiency anemias. Called also *iron choline citrate.*

**fer·ro·floc·cu·la·tion** (fer"o-flok"u-la'shən) a flocculation test for malaria, performed with a fine-grained iron antigen; see *Henry's test,* under *tests.*

**fer·ro·heme** (fer'o-hēm) the Fe(II) chelate of heme; sometimes called simply *heme.*

**fer·ro·ki·net·ic** (fer"o-kĭ-net'ik) pertaining to ferrokinetics.

**fer·ro·ki·net·ics** (fer"o-kĭ-net'iks) the movement of iron in the body from plasma transferrin to red cell precursors in bone marrow to circulating red cells to macrophages in the reticuloendothelial system and back to plasma transferrin. Ferrokinetic studies, using the radioisotope iron-59 as a tracer, measure kinetic parameters helpful in evaluating certain anemias and in detecting abnormal iron storage or extramedullary hematopoiesis by external counting over the liver, spleen, and bone marrow. Studies include *plasma iron clearance half-time, plasma iron turnover, red cell utilization,* and *erythrocyte iron turnover.*

**Fer·ro·lip** (fer'o-lip) trademark for preparations of ferrocholinate.

**fer·ro·pro·tein** (fer"o-pro'tēn) a protein combined with an iron-containing radical; the ferroproteins are respiratory carriers. Cf. *cytochrome* (def. 1).

**fer·ro·so·fer·ric** (fər-o"so-fer'ik) combining a ferrous with a ferric compound; containing iron in two different oxidation states, as in the oxide $Fe_3O_4$.

**fer·ro·ther·a·py** (fer"o-ther'ə-pe) [*ferrum* + *therapy*] therapeutic use of iron and iron compounds.

**fer·rous** (fer'əs) containing iron in its plus-two oxidation state, Fe(II) (sometimes designated $Fe^{2+}$).
**f. fumarate** [USP], an oral iron preparation used in the treatment of iron deficiency.
**f. gluconate** [USP], an oral iron preparation used in the treatment of iron deficiency.
**f. sulfate** [USP], an oral iron preparation used in the treatment of iron deficiency.

**fer·rox·i·dase** (fer-ok'sĭ-dās) [EC 1.16.3.1] 1. an enzyme or enzyme activity that catalyzes the oxidation of ferrous to ferric ions prior to their transport in the blood by transferrins. 2. EC nomenclature for *ceruloplasmin.*

**fer·ru·gi·nous** (fə-roo'jĭ-nəs) [L. *ferruginosus; ferrugo* iron rust] 1. containing iron or iron rust; called also *chalybeate* or *martial.* 2. of the color of iron rust.

**fer·rum** (fer'əm) [L.] iron.

**Fer·ry-Por·ter law** (fer'e-por'tər) [Ervin Sidney *Ferry,* American physicist, 1868–1956; Thomas Cunningham *Porter,* English scientist, late 19th century] see under *law.*

**fer·tile** (fər'til) [L. *fertilis*] 1. fruitful; having the capacity to produce. 2. capable of developing into a new individual; said of a zygote.

**fer·til·i·ty** (fər-til'ĭ-te) [MeSH: Fertility] 1. the capacity to conceive or induce conception. 2. see under *rate.*

**fer·ti·li·za·tion** (fər'tĭ-lĭ-za'shən) [MeSH: Fertilization] the act of rendering gametes fertile or capable of further development; it is a sequence of events that begins with contact between a spermatozoon and an oocyte, leading to their fusion, which stimulates the completion of oocyte maturation with release of the second polar body. Male and female pronuclei then form and merge; synapsis follows, which restores the diploid number of chromosomes and results in biparental inheritance and the determination of sex. The process of fertilization leads to the formation of a zygote and ends with the initiation of its cleavage. Called also *fecundation* and *impregnation.*

**cross f.**, the fertilization of one flower by the pollen of another; allogamy.
**external f.**, union of the gametes outside the bodies of the originating organisms, as in most fish.
**internal f.**, union of the gametes inside the body of the female, the sperm having been transferred from the body of the male by an accessory sex organ or other means.
**in vitro f.**, removal of a secondary oocyte, fertilization of it in a culture medium in the laboratory, and placement of the dividing zygote into the uterus.

**fer·ti·lize** (fər'tĭ-līz) to render a gamete fertile; see *fertilization.* Called also *fecundate* and *impregnate.*

**fer·ti·li·zin** (fər"tĭ-li'zin) a substance of the plasma membrane and gelatinous coat of the ovum of some species. It is considered to possess the specific receptor groups that bind the spermatozoon to the ovum. In sea-urchins, it has been characterized chemically as a glycoprotein of about 300,000 molecular weight.

**Fe·ru·la** (fə-roo'lə) [MeSH: Ferula] a genus of umbelliferous plants. *F. asafoe'tida* is a source of asafetida. *F. commu'nis* is a species found in Mediterranean regions that contains an anticoagulant and can cause fatal hemorrhaging in ruminants.

**Ferv.** abbreviation for L. *fer'vens,* boiling.

**fer·ves·cence** (fər-ves'əns) [L. *fervescere* to become hot] development of an increased body temperature, or fever.

**FES** functional electrical stimulation; functional endoscopic sinus surgery.

**fes·cue** (fes'ku) 1. any grass of the genus *Festuca.* 2. fescue foot.

**Fe·so·tyme** (fe'so-tīm) trademark for a preparation of ferrous sulfate.

**fes·ter** (fes'tər) to suppurate superficially.

**fes·ti·nant** (fes'tĭ-nənt) accelerating; characterized by festination.

**fes·ti·na·tion** (fes"tĭ-na'shən) [L. *festinatio*] an involuntary tendency to take short accelerating steps in walking; see *festinating gait,* under *gait.*

**fes·toon** (fes-to͞on') a carving in the base material of a denture that simulates the contours of the natural tissues being replaced by the denture.
**gingival f.**, the contour of the gingiva and oral mucosa over the roots of teeth with a thin alveolar process.
**McCall's f.**, a lifesaver-like enlargement of the marginal gingiva occurring on the vestibular surface, most commonly in the canine and premolar areas.

**Fes·tu·ca** (fes-too'kə) a genus of grasses (family Gramineae). *F. arundina'cea* is tall fescue, a species found in New Zealand, Australia, and the United States, sometimes host to the endophytic fungus *Acremonium coenophialum,* which causes fescue foot in cattle.

**fe·tal** (fe'təl) of or pertaining to a fetus; pertaining to *in utero* development after the embryonic period.

**fe·tal·ism** (fe'təl-iz-əm) fetalization.

**fe·tal·iza·tion** (fe"təl-ĭ-za'shən) the retention, into adult life, of bodily characters which at some earlier stage of evolutionary history were actually only infantile and were rapidly lost as the organism attained maturity.

**fe·ta·tion** (fe-ta'shən) 1. the development of a fetus within the uterus. 2. pregnancy.

**fe·ti·cide** (fe'tĭ-sīd) [*fetus* + *-cide*] the destruction of the fetus.

**fet·id** (fe'tid) [L. *foetidus*] having a rank or disagreeable smell.

**fet·ish** (fet'ish, fe'tish) [Fr. *fétiche,* from Port. *feitico* charm, sorcery] 1. a material object, such as an idol, charm, or talisman, believed to have supernatural powers. 2. an inanimate object used to obtain sexual gratification.

**fet·ish·ism** (fet'ish-iz-əm) 1. the worship of fetishes. 2. [DSM-III-R] a paraphilia characterized by recurrent, intense sexual urges and sexually arousing fantasies of the use of inanimate objects (fetishes), most commonly articles of feminine clothing such as shoes, earrings, or undergarments, as a preferred or necessary adjunct to sexual arousal or orgasm.
**transvestic f.**, [DSM-IV] a paraphilia of heterosexual males, characterized by recurrent, intense sexual urges, arousal, or orgasm associated with fantasized or actual cross-dressing. Called also *transvestism.*

**fet·ish·ist** (fet'ish-ist, fe'tish-ist) a person who obtains sexual gratification from a fetish.

**fet·lock** (fet'lok) the metacarpophalangeal and metatarsophalangeal regions in the horse.

**fet(o)-** [L. *fetus,* q.v.] a combining form denoting relationship to the fetus.

**fe·tog·ra·phy** (fe-tog'rə-fe) [*fetus* + *-graphy*] radiography of the fetus *in utero.*

**fe·tol·o·gy** (fe-tol'ə-je) that branch of medicine dealing with the fetus *in utero.*

**fe·tom·e·try** (fe-tom'ə-tre) [*fetus* + *-metry*] the measurement of the fetus, especially of the diameters of its head.
**roentgen f.**, measurement of the fetal head in the uterus by means of the x-ray.

**fe·top·a·thy** (fe-top'ə-the) a disease or disorder seen in a fetus; cf. *embryopathy.*

**fe·to·pla·cen·tal** (fe"to-plə-sen'təl) pertaining to the fetus and placenta.

**α-fe·to·pro·tein** (fe"to-pro'tēn) see *alpha-fetoprotein.*

**fe·tor** (fe'tor) [L.] stench, or offensive odor.
**f. ex o're**, halitosis.
**f. hepa'ticus**, the peculiar odor of the breath characteristic of hepatic disease; liver breath.
**f. o'ris**, halitosis.

**fe·to·scope** (fe'to-skōp) 1. a specially designed stethoscope for listening to the fetal heartbeat. 2. an endoscope for viewing the fetus *in utero.*

**fe·to·scop·ic** (fe"to-skop'ik) pertaining to or accomplished by fetoscopy.

**fe·tos·co·py** (fe-tos'kə-pe) [MeSH: Fetoscopy] viewing of the fetus *in utero* by means of the fetoscope.

**fe·tu·in** (fe'tu-in) a low-molecular-weight globulin that constitutes nearly the total globulin in the blood of the fetus and newborn of ungulates.

**fe·tus** (fe'təs) [L.] [MeSH: Fetus] the unborn offspring of any viviparous animal; specifically, the unborn offspring in the postembryonic period, after major structures have been outlined, in humans from nine weeks after fertilization until birth. Cf. *embryo.*
**f. acardi'acus**, acardius.
**f. amor'phus**, holoacardius amorphus.
**calcified f.**, lithopedion.
**f. compres'sus**, f. papyraceus.
**harlequin f.**, a fetus covered with thick, horny armorlike plates as a result of an autosomal recessive keratinizing disorder; it may also be a severe form of collodion baby or it may represent the extreme form of lamellar ichthyosis. Those affected are usually stillborn or die within days after birth.
**f. in fe'tu**, a well-differentiated fetal teratoma having axial formation of limbs and organs. Cf. *endadelphos.*
**mummified f.**, a shriveled and dried-up fetus.
**paper-doll f., papyraceous f.**, f. papyraceus.
**f. papyra'ceus**, a dead fetus pressed flat by the growth of a living twin.
**parasitic f.**, in asymmetrical conjoined twins, an incomplete minor fetus attached to the larger, more completely developed twin.
**f. sanguinolen'tis**, a dead fetus which has undergone maceration.
**sireniform f.**, sirenomelus.

**Feu·er·stein-Mims syndrome** (foi'ər-stīn mimz) [Richard C. *Feuerstein,* American physician, 20th century; Leroy C. *Mims,* American physician, 20th century] sebaceous nevus.

**Feul·gen reaction** (foil'gən) [Robert *Feulgen,* German physiologic chemist, 1884–1955] see under *reaction.*

**FEV** forced expiratory volume.

**fe·ver** (fe'vər) [L. *febris*] [MeSH: Fever] 1. elevation of body temperature above the normal; it may be due to physiological stresses such as ovulation, excess thyroid hormone secretions, or vigorous exercise; to central nervous system lesions or infection by microorganisms; or to any of a host of noninfectious processes, such as inflammation or the release of certain materials, as in leukemia. Called also *pyrexia.* 2. any disease characterized by elevated body temperature.

**Aden f.,** dengue.
**adynamic f.,** asthenic f.
**African Coast f.,** East Coast f.
**African swine f.,** a highly contagious, usually fatal disease of pigs in Africa, Southern Europe, and Brazil, transmitted by the African swine fever virus; symptoms closely resemble those of hog cholera. Transmission of the virus is by ticks of the genus *Ornithodoros,* by direct contact, by fomites, or by ingestion of infected meat. In Africa warthogs serve as a reservoir.
**African tick f.,** relapsing fever caused by *Borrelia duttonii.*
**aphthous f.,** foot-and-mouth disease.
**Argentine hemorrhagic f., Argentinian hemorrhagic f.,** a hemorrhagic fever primarily affecting agricultural field hands in northern Argentina, and caused by the Junin virus, transmitted by contact with the excreta of infected rodents, especially of the genus *Calomys.* It is characterized chiefly by high fever, leukopenia, thrombocytopenia, generalized myalgia, hemorrhagic manifestations, exanthema, renal involvement, neurologic disturbances, and shock. Called also *Junin f.*
**artificial f.,** elevation of bodily temperature produced by artificial means, as by external heat or the injection of typhoid vaccine or malarial parasites.
**aseptic f.,** fever associated with aseptic wounds, presumably due to the disintegration of leukocytes or to the absorption of avascular or traumatized but uninfected tissue.
**asthenic f.,** a fever with nervous depression, feeble pulse, and a cool, moist skin.
**Australian Q f.,** Q f.
**autumn f.,** 1. nanukayami. 2. mud f. (def. 1).
**biliary f. of dogs,** canine babesiosis.
**biliary f. of horses,** equine babesiosis.
**black f.,** 1. Rocky Mountain spotted f. 2. visceral leishmaniasis.
**blackwater f.,** a severe complication of malaria characterized by intravascular hemolysis, hemoglobinuria, renal failure, and passage of dark brown or red urine, seen in association with intermittent quinine therapy, with *Plasmodium falciparum* infection in the nonimmune, or with interrupted exposure in the partially immune. The hemolysis is believed to be caused primarily by an autoimmune response to the infection. Called also *malarial hemoglobinuria.*
**blue f.,** Rocky Mountain spotted f.
**Bolivian hemorrhagic f.,** a hemorrhagic fever occurring in rural areas of northeastern Bolivia, caused by the Machupo virus, the clinical manifestations and epidemiology of which are almost identical with those of Argentine hemorrhagic fever (q.v.).
**boutonneuse f.,** an acute febrile disease caused by *Rickettsia conorii,* transmitted by the bites of various ixodid ticks, with dogs and rodents being the chief hosts; characterized by a primary lesion (tache noire) at the site of the tick bite, maculopapular or petechial rash, headache, arthralgia, myalgia, chills, fever, and photophobia, usually without sequelae. It occurs around the Mediterranean, Black, and Caspian Seas, with variant forms in Africa and on the Indian subcontinent. Called also *boutonneuse* and *Conor and Bruch's disease.* There are other names based on geographical area, such as *South African tickbite f.* and *Indian tick typhus.*
**bovine ephemeral f., bovine epizootic f.,** an acute viral disease of cattle in Africa, parts of Asia, and Australia, caused by a rhabdovirus transmitted by insect vectors; its symptoms resemble those of mild African horse sickness and include high fever lasting about three days, stiffness, and lameness. Called also *stiff sickness* and *three-day sickness.*
**bovine infectious petechial f., bovine petechial f.,** a disease of cattle in Kenya, characterized by hemorrhages of the visible mucous membranes, fever, and diarrhea; there may be severe conjunctivitis, protrusion of the eyeball, and death within three days. The cause is believed to be a Rickettsia, *Cytoecetes ondiri* (or *Ehrlichia ondiri*), spread by a biting insect. Called also *Ondiri disease.*
**brassfounder's f.,** metal fume fever caused by fumes of any of several metals, most commonly zinc, copper, or magnesium; called also *brassfounder's ague* and *brass* or *brazier's chill.*
**Brazilian purpuric f.,** an acute illness in children characterized by fever, abdominal pain, vomiting, petechiae, purpura, and a recent history of conjunctivitis.
**Brazilian spotted f.,** Rocky Mountain spotted f.
**breakbone f.,** dengue.
**Bullis f.,** a febrile, probably rickettsial, disease transmitted by the tick *Amblyomma americanum,* observed in soldiers who had been at Camp Bullis, Texas, in 1942, marked by very low leukocyte count with neutropenia, headache, and constant lymphadenitis. Called also *Lone Star f.* and *Texas tick f.*
**Bwamba f.,** a mild, mosquito-borne, febrile infection, caused by a bunyavirus, occurring in eastern, central, western, and parts of southern Africa.
**cachectic f., cachexial f.,** visceral leishmaniasis.
**camp f.,** epidemic typhus.
**cane-field f.,** mild leptospirosis transmitted by rodents and caused by *Leptospira interrogans* (formerly believed to be caused specifically by the serovar *L. australis*).
**canicola f.,** Stuttgart disease.
**cat-scratch f.,** see under *disease.*
**central f.,** sustained fever resulting from damage to the thermoregulatory centers of the hypothalamus.
**cerebrospinal f.,** meningococcal meningitis.
**Charcot's f.,** intermittent hepatic f.
**childbed f.,** puerperal f.
**Choix f.,** Rocky Mountain spotted f.
**Colombian tick f.,** Rocky Mountain spotted f.
**Colorado tick f.,** an acute, benign febrile infection caused by an arenavirus, transmitted by the bite of the wood tick, *Dermacentor andersoni,* occurring in areas in which the tick is distributed, i.e., the Rocky Mountain area and Pacific slope of the United States and Canada, and characterized chiefly by a biphasic course and leukopenia. Called also *mountain tick f.*
**Congo red f.,** murine typhus.
**continued f.,** one which does not vary more than 1.0° to 1.5°F in twenty-four hours.
**continuous f.,** persistently elevated body temperature, showing no or little variation and never falling to normal during any 24-hour period.
**cotton-mill f.,** 1. mill f. (def. 1). 2. byssinosis.
**Crimean-Congo hemorrhagic f.,** a hemorrhagic fever caused by the Crimean-Congo hemorrhagic fever virus, transmitted by ticks, especially those of the genus *Hyalomma,* and by contact with blood, secretions, or fluids from infected humans or domestic animals; it occurs in the Crimea, Central Asia, Bulgaria, and West, Central, and East Africa.
**dandy f.,** dengue.
**deer fly f.,** tularemia.
**dehydration f.,** 1. inanition f. 2. fever due to loss of body water or inadequate fluid intake, sometimes occurring as a postoperative complication.
**dengue f.,** dengue.
**dengue hemorrhagic f.,** hemorrhagic dengue.
**desert f.,** primary coccidioidomycosis.
**digestive f.,** a slight rise of temperature during the process of digestion.
**drug f.,** a febrile reaction marked by prolonged temperature elevation during the course of administration of a drug, such as an antibiotic, antineoplastic, vaccine, etc.; it may be associated with vasculitis affecting small vessels, and usually disappears rapidly on discontinuance of the drug.
**duck f.,** a type of hypersensitivity pneumonitis caused by sensitivity to duck proteins contained in duck feathers.
**Dumdum f.,** visceral leishmaniasis.
**Dutton's relapsing f.,** the central African form of relapsing fever caused by *Borrelia duttonii.*
**East Coast f.,** a highly fatal form of theileriasis, seen in cattle from South Africa north to Kenya, caused by *Theileria parva* and transmitted by ticks of *Rhipicephalus* and *Hyalomma* spp.; characteristics include high fever, dyspnea, emaciation, lymphadenopathy, and tarry feces. Called also *African Coast f., bovine theileriasis, Rhodesian f., Rhodesian redwater f.,* and *Rhodesian tick f.*
**Ebola hemorrhagic f.,** Ebola virus disease.
**elephantoid f.,** a recurrent acute febrile condition occurring with filariasis; it may be associated with elephantiasis or lymphangitis.
**Elokomin fluke f.,** a mild form of salmon poisoning (q.v.) in dogs, usually not fatal; the infective agent is an unidentified rickettsia. Characteristics include fever, anorexia, and diarrhea.
**enteric f.,** any of a group of febrile illnesses associated with enteric symptoms caused by salmonellae, especially *typhoid f.* (the prototype of the severe enteric salmonellal infections) and *paratyphoid f.* Cf. *salmonellosis.*
**entericoid f.,** any fever which resembles typhoid fever in its clinical manifestations.
**ephemeral f.,** a slight fever persisting or lasting only a day or two.
**ephemeral f. of cattle,** bovine ephemeral f.
**epidemic hemorrhagic f.,** an acute, febrile viral disease occurring in epidemics in northeastern Asia, and in a milder form in the former Soviet Union, Eastern Europe, Scandinavia, and the southwestern United States. Symptoms include fever, prostration, vomiting, hemorrhagic phenomena, shock, and renal failure. It is caused by viruses of the genus *Hantavirus,* which are believed to be transmitted to humans by direct or indirect contact with the excreta of infected rodents. Called also *Far East* or *Korean hemorrhagic f., hemorrhagic* or *Korean hemorrhagic nephrosonephritis, hemorrhagic f. with renal syndrome, Korin f.,* and *nephrosonephritis.*
**equine biliary f.,** equine babesiosis.
**eruptive f.,** any fever accompanied by an eruption on the skin.
**essential f.,** fever for which no cause has been found.
**exanthematous f.,** eruptive f.

**familial Mediterranean f.**, a hereditary, autosomal recessive disease usually occurring in Armenians and Sephardic Jews, characterized by short recurrent attacks of fever with pain in the abdomen, chest, or joints and erythema resembling that seen in erysipelas; it is sometimes complicated by reactive systemic amyloidosis (q.v.). Called also *benign paroxysmal peritonitis, periodic peritonitis, familial recurrent polyserositis,* and *periodic* or *recurrent polyserositis.*

**Far East hemorrhagic f.**, epidemic hemorrhagic f.

**farrowing f.**, lactation failure in swine (see under *failure*).

**fatigue f.**, a febrile attack due to overexercise and the absorption of waste products.

**field f.**, 1. harvest f. 2. mud f. See also *cane-field f.* and *rice-field f.*

**five-day f.**, trench f.

**Flinders Island spotted f.**, an acute infection occurring during the summer months in Australia, caused by *Rickettsia honei* and characterized by fever, myalgia, and headache and by the appearance of an eschar and rash.

**fog f.**, an often fatal acute adenomatoid reaction in the lungs of cattle, believed to be a response to chemicals generated in the rumen after being fed cut second-growth grass *(aftermath* or *fog).* Called also *acute bovine pulmonary emphysema, acute pulmonary emphysema of cattle, aftermath disease, atypical interstitial pneumonia,* and *lunger disease.*

**Fort Bragg f.**, pretibial f.

**foundryman's f.**, metal fume f.

**glandular f.**, infectious mononucleosis.

**grain f.**, a syndrome of malaise, fever, chills, and myalgia, occurring in grain elevator workers and others who have heavy exposure to grain dust; the cause is usually inhalation of endotoxins or contaminants such as mites. In some workers there is chronic asthma. See also *grain handler's lung,* under *lung.*

**Hankow f.**, schistosomiasis japonica.

**harvest f.**, a form of leptospirosis affecting harvest workers; it is marked by fever, conjunctivitis, stupor, diarrhea, vomiting, and abdominal pains, and is caused by Leptospira interrogans (formerly believed to be caused specifically by the serovar *L. grippotyphosa*); called also *field f.*

**Hasami f.**, mild leptospirosis caused by *Leptospira interrogans* (formerly believed to be caused specifically by the serovar *L. autumnalis*) in Japan.

**Haverhill f.**, the bacillary form of rat-bite fever (q.v.), caused by *Streptobacillus moniliformis,* and transmitted through contaminated raw milk and its products. Called also *epidemic arthritic erythema* and *erythema arthriticum epidemicum.*

**hay f.**, a type of allergic rhinitis that occurs at the same time every year, marked by acute conjunctivitis with lacrimation and itching, swelling of the nasal mucosa, sneezing, and often asthmatic symptoms. It is regarded as an anaphylactic or allergic condition excited by an allergen such as a pollen to which the individual is sensitized. Called also *pollen allergy, seasonal allergic rhinitis,* and *pollinosis.*

**hay f., nonseasonal, hay f., perennial,** nonseasonal allergic rhinitis.

**hectic f.**, a fever that recurs each day, with profound sweating, chills, and facial flushing.

**hemoglobinuric f.**, malaria attended with hemoglobinuria; see *blackwater f.*

**hemorrhagic f's**, a group of diverse, severe epidemic viral infections, found in many parts of the world, mainly in tropical climates; causative viruses are often geographically restricted. They are usually transmitted to humans by arthropod bites or contact with virus-infected rodents; all the infections share certain clinicopathological features, including fever, hemorrhagic manifestations, thrombocytopenia, shock, and neurologic disturbances. The group comprises Argentine hemorrhagic fever, Bolivian hemorrhagic fever, chikungunya, Crimean-Congo hemorrhagic fever, dengue hemorrhagic fever, Ebola virus disease, epidemic hemorrhagic fever, Kyasanur Forest disease, Lassa fever, Marburg virus disease, Omsk hemorrhagic fever, Rift Valley fever, and yellow fever. Called also *viral hemorrhagic f's.*

**hemorrhagic f. with renal syndrome,** epidemic hemorrhagic f.

**herpetic f.**, primary infection with herpes simplex virus, with diffuse involvement of mucous membranes of the mouth and lips and the surrounding skin; fever and sometimes chills occur.

**horse sickness f.**, a mild nonfatal form of African horse sickness, characterized by a slow onset of fever with only slight respiratory distress.

**humidifier f.**, a syndrome of malaise, fever, cough, and myalgia, caused by inhalation of air that has been passed through humidifiers, dehumidifiers, or air conditioners contaminated by fungi, amebas, or thermophilic actinomycetes. See also *humidifier lung,* under *lung.*

**inanition f.**, a transitory fever that frequently occurs in infants during the first few days of life; it is believed to be due to dehydration and is also called *dehydration f.*

**intermittent f.**, an attack of malaria or other fever characterized by recurring paroxysms of elevated temperature separated by intervals during which the temperature is normal.

**intermittent hepatic f.**, a fever occurring intermittently as the result of intermittent impaction of stone in the common duct and inflammation of the bile ducts; called also *Charcot's f.* or *syndrome.*

**inundation f., island f.**, scrub typhus.

**jail f.**, epidemic typhus.

**Japanese flood f., Japanese river f.**, scrub typhus.

**jungle f.**, old name for *malaria.*

**jungle yellow f.**, a form of yellow fever endemic in parts of Africa and South America; it occurs in or near uncut forest or jungle.

**Junin f.**, Argentine hemorrhagic f.

**Katayama f.**, acute systemic schistosomiasis causing a distinct serum sickness–like syndrome, usually associated with heavy infection by *Schistosoma japonicum,* characterized by fever, chills, nausea and vomiting, cough, headache, urticaria, hepatosplenomegaly, lymphadenopathy, marked eosinophilia, and usually increased levels of IgE and IgG.

**Kedani f.**, scrub typhus.

**Kew Gardens spotted f.**, rickettsialpox.

**Kinkiang f.**, schistosomiasis japonica.

**Korean hemorrhagic f., Korin f.**, epidemic hemorrhagic f.

**land f.**, a set of symptoms resembling seasickness sometimes experienced when, after an ocean voyage, the ship enters a relatively landlocked body of water.

**Lassa f.**, an acute febrile disease caused by an arenavirus (Lassa virus), endemic throughout West Africa and spread by contact with the multimammate mouse, which sheds the virus in its urine, or by interpersonal contact; most infections are subclinical or mild, although severe cases resulting in death occur. Symptoms include fever of insidious onset, headache, dry cough, back pain, vomiting, diarrhea, pharyngitis, facial edema, and occasionally a maculopapular rash; in severe cases there is a sudden drop in blood pressure on the seventh day, with death resulting from shock, hypotension, peripheral vasoconstriction, hypovolemia, and anuria. Sensorineural deafness, which may be permanent, sometimes results.

**lechuguilla f.**, a disease of sheep and goats in western Texas, marked by toxic encephalitis, nephritis, photosensitization, listlessness, icterus, and a yellow discharge from the eyes and nostrils; it is caused by eating the plant *Agave lechuguilla.* Commonly called *swellhead.*

**Lone Star f.**, Bullis f.

**malarial f.**, old name for *malaria.*

**malignant catarrhal f.**, a highly fatal viral disease of cattle and other ungulates, characterized by exudative inflammation of mucous membranes, especially in the mouth, digestive tract, and respiratory tract, with corneal opacities, encephalitis, and enlargement of lymph nodes. The cause is thought to be a herpesvirus. Called also *bovine malignant catarrh* and *malignant catarrh of cattle.*

**Malta f.**, brucellosis, def. 1.

**Marburg hemorrhagic f.**, Marburg disease.

**Marseilles f.**, boutonneuse f.

**marsh f.**, 1. mud f. (def. 1). 2. old name for *malaria.*

**Mediterranean f.**, 1. brucellosis, def. 1. 2. boutonneuse f.

**Mediterranean Coast f.**, tropical theileriasis.

**metal fume f.**, an occupational disorder occurring in those engaged in welding and other metallic operations and due to inhalation of volatilized metals; it is characterized by sudden onset of thirst and a metallic taste in the mouth, followed by high fever, muscular aches and pains, shaking chills, headache, weakness, diaphoresis, and leukocytosis. The symptoms usually subside within 24 to 48 hours, but repeated attacks are common. The disorder includes *brassfounder's f.* and *spelter's f.* A related condition is *polymer fume f.* Called also *foundryman's f.*

**Meuse f.**, trench f.

**milk f.**, 1. a fever said to attend the establishment of lactation after delivery. 2. parturient paresis. 3. an endemic fever said to be caused by the use of unwholesome cow's milk.

**mill f.**, 1. fever and nausea in cotton mill workers, a rare manifestation of byssinosis. Called also *cotton-mill f.* 2. byssinosis.

**Mossman f.**, scrub typhus.

**mountain tick f.**, Colorado tick f.

**mud f.**, 1. leptospirosis occurring in the summer and late autumn in Germany and Russia, caused by *Leptospira interrogans* (formerly believed to be caused specifically by serovar *L. grippotyphosa*), transmitted by a field mouse, *Microtus arvalis,* and affecting workers in flooded fields or in swamps. Called also *autumn f., marsh f., slime f.,* and *swamp f.* 2. a disease of horses consisting of dermatophilosis, leptospirosis, and greasy heel.

**Murchison-Pel-Ebstein f.**, Pel-Ebstein f.

**nanukayami f.**, nanukayami.

**nine-mile f.**, Q f.

**Omsk hemorrhagic f.**, a hemorrhagic fever similar in its clinical manifestations to Kyasanur Forest disease, endemic in a forested region of western Siberia, and caused by a flavivirus, transmitted to humans by the bites of infected ticks of the genus *Dermacentor* or by direct contact with infected muskrats, as by fur trappers.

**o'nyong-nyong f.,** o'nyong-nyong.

**Oriental spotted f.,** an acute infection occurring in Japan and caused by *Rickettsia japonica,* characterized by fever and headache and the appearance of an eschar and rash.

**Oroya f.,** the first or acute stage of bartonellosis, marked by muscle pains, chills, fever, and severe hemolytic anemia that can be fatal. Called also Bartonella anemia.

**Pahvant Valley f.,** tularemia.

**pappataci f.,** phlebotomus f.

**paratyphoid f.,** a prolonged febrile illness clinically indistinguishable from but usually less severe than typhoid fever, caused by *Salmonella* serotypes other than *S. typhi,* especially *S. enteritidis* serotypes *paratyphi A* and *B* and *S. choleraesuis;* occasionally, the symptoms of paratyphoid fever may occur following an attack of salmonella food poisoning. Called also *Brion-Kayser disease, paratyphoid,* and *Schottmüller's disease.*

**parenteric f.,** a disease clinically resembling typhoid fever and paratyphoid fever, but not caused by *Salmonella.*

**parrot f.,** psittacosis.

**parturient f.,** see under *paresis.*

**Pel-Ebstein f.,** a cyclic fever occasionally seen in Hodgkin's disease and also associated with other diseases, characterized by irregular episodes of pyrexia of several days' duration, with intervening afebrile periods lasting for days or weeks. Called also *Murchison-Pel-Ebstein f.* and *Pel-Ebstein pyrexia.*

**periodic f.,** a hereditary condition characterized by repetitive febrile episodes and autonomic disturbances, occurring in precise or irregular cycles of days, weeks, or months. Transmitted as an autosomal dominant trait, it may begin at any time of life and may last for decades with temporary remissions, or may cease. See also *familial Mediterranean f.*

**Pfeiffer's glandular f.,** infectious mononucleosis.

**pharyngoconjunctival f.,** a febrile disease caused by an adenovirus, occurring in epidemic form, largely in school children, and characterized by fever, pharyngitis, rhinitis, conjunctivitis, and enlarged cervical lymph nodes.

**Philippine hemorrhagic f.,** hemorrhagic dengue.

**phlebotomus f.,** an acute, self-limited, febrile viral disease occurring chiefly during the warm months in parts of the Mediterranean littoral, central Asia, the Middle East, and Central and South America. It is caused by any of several types of *Phlebovirus* and transmitted by the urban sandfly *Phlebotomus papatasii,* except in the Americas, where the vectors are sylvan sandflies (genus *Lutzomyia*). Called also *pappataci f., sandfly f.,* and *three-day f.*

**pinta f.,** Rocky Mountain spotted f.

**polymer fume f.,** an occupational disorder due to exposure to the products of combustion of polymers, chiefly polytef (also known as Teflon); manifestations are similar to those of metal fume fever. Called also *Teflon shakes.*

**Pomona f.,** leptospirosis, which is caused by *Leptospira interrogans*; the term is used to denote disease formerly believed to be caused specifically by the serovar *L. pomona.*

**Pontiac f.,** an influenzalike disease caused by infection with a strain of *Legionella pneumophila;* characteristics include fever, chills, cough, muscle pain, headache, chest pain, and pleurisy.

**Potomac horse f.,** equine monocytic ehrlichiosis.

**pretibial f.,** leptospirosis marked by a rash on the pretibial region accompanied by lumbar and postorbital pain, malaise, coryza, and fever; it is caused by *Leptospira interrogans* (formerly believed to be caused specifically by the serovar *L. autumnalis*). Called also *Fort Bragg f.*

**prison f.,** epidemic typhus.

**protein f.,** heightened temperature produced by the injection of protein material into the body.

**puerperal f.,** septicemia accompanied by fever, in which the focus of infection is the uterus; the etiologic agent is frequently a streptococcus. Called also *childbed f.,* and *puerperal sepsis* or *septicemia.*

**Q f.,** an acute, generally self-limited rickettsial infection caused by *Coxiella burnetii,* characterized by fever, chills, headache, myalgia, malaise, and very rarely rash, and sometimes complicated by mild pneumonia (*Q fever pneumonia,* q.v.), hepatitis, and endocarditis. In humans, it is usually acquired by inhalation of airborne organisms in infected dust or aerosols derived from infected domestic animals, with no vector being involved in transmission as in other rickettsial diseases. Called also *Australian Q f.* and *nine-mile f.*

**quartan f.,** a fever that occurs every fourth day, associated with *Plasmodium malariae* infections; see under *malaria.*

**quintan f.,** trench f.

**quotidian f.,** a fever that recurs every day, associated with *Plasmodium falciparum* infections; see under *malaria.*

**rabbit f.,** tularemia.

**rat-bite f.,** either of two clinically similar but etiologically distinct acute infectious diseases, usually transmitted through the bite of a rat: (1) The *bacillary form* is caused by *Streptobacillus moniliformis* and has a latent period of about a week, during which the initial wound heals without inflammation; however, later the bite site becomes inflamed and indurated, and this is followed by adenitis, chills, vomiting, headache, high fever, morbilliform eruption, especially on the hands and feet, and polyarthritis that is often severe. This form may also be caused by ingestion of contaminated raw milk or its products *(Haverhill fever),* in which case there is no initial wound and the first symptoms are systemic. (2) The *spirillary form* (called also *sodoku*) is caused by *Spirillum minus* and has a latent period of usually more than ten days. Inflammation recurs at the primary wound site; the rash is less evident than in the bacillary form; arthritis is rare; and the fever is commonly of the relapsing type.

**recurrent f.,** 1. relapsing f. 2. recurrent paroxysmal fever occurring in various diseases, including tularemia, meningococcemia, malaria, and rat-bite fever.

**redwater f.,** bovine babesiosis.

**relapsing f.,** an acute infectious, systemic, usually self-limited disease of worldwide distribution, caused by various species of the genus *Borrelia;* it may be either endemic or epidemic and is transmitted by the bites of either the body louse *(Pediculus humanus corporis),* for which humans are the reservoir, or *Ornithodoros* ticks, for which rodents and other animals are reservoirs. Characteristics include alternating periods with and without fever and spirochetemia, each lasting for several days. During the febrile period, symptoms include chills, headache, fatigue, myalgia, arthralgia, anorexia, cough, abdominal pain, and sometimes coagulation disturbance, hepatosplenomegaly, psychic disturbances, petechial rash, and vomiting; treatment may be complicated by severe Jarisch-Herxheimer reaction. Both epidemiological forms of the disease are known by various descriptive and local names, including *recurrent,* or *spirillum f.*

**remittent f.,** a fever in which the diurnal variation is 2° F. or more, but in which the temperature never falls to a normal level; see *malaria.*

**rheumatic f.,** a febrile disease occurring as a delayed sequela of infections with group A beta-hemolytic streptococci and characterized by multiple focal inflammatory lesions of connective tissue, especially of the heart (rheumatic heart disease), blood vessels, and joints (polyarthritis), and by Aschoff bodies in the myocardium and skin. Onset is usually signaled by sudden fever and joint pain, followed by manifestations of heart and pericardial disease, abdominal pain, skin changes, and chorea. Atypical manifestations may also be seen, particularly in adults. Called also *acute articular rheumatism, acute rheumatic fever* or *arthritis,* and *polyarthritis rheumatica acuta.*

**Rhodesian f., Rhodesian redwater f., Rhodesian tick f.,** East Coast f.

**rice-field f.,** leptospirosis, which is caused by *Leptospira interrogans*; the term denotes disease formerly believed to be caused specifically by the serovar *L. bataviae.*

**Rift Valley f.,** an acute febrile infection of sheep and cattle, zoonotic in humans, caused by a bunyavirus and transmitted mainly by mosquitoes of the genera *Aedes, Culex,* and *Anopheles;* it is also spread by contact with infected tissues and secretions, particularly blood or amniotic fluid from aborting animals. In humans, it may be in a mild form, with nonspecific influenzalike symptoms, or in a severe form associated with encephalitis, retinitis, or hemorrhagic fever. In animals, it is characterized by fever, listlessness, hepatitis, melena, bloodstained nasal discharge, and abortion in pregnant animals. First observed in the Rift Valley of Kenya, it is now seen throughout southern and eastern Africa to Egypt.

**Rocky Mountain spotted f.,** an acute, infectious, sometimes fatal disease caused by *Rickettsia rickettsii,* usually transmitted by the bite of an infected ixodid tick, usually *Dermacentor andersoni* (wood tick) or *D. variabilis* (dog tick); it occurs only in North and South America. It is characterized by sudden onset; chills; fever lasting 2 to 3 weeks; a cutaneous rash that generally appears between the second and sixth days and spreads from the distal extremities to the proximal extremities, trunk, and face; myalgias; severe headache; and prostration. Called also *black, blue,* or *pinta f., blue disease,* and *tick-borne typhus.* It is also known by many local names including *Brazilian spotted, Choix, Colombian tick,* or *Tobia f.,* and *São Paulo typhus.*

**rose f.,** hay fever caused by grass pollens or rose pollen.

**salt f.,** fever associated with excess of salt in the body, due to the retention by the salt of the water normally eliminated in perspiration.

**sandfly f.,** phlebotomus f.

**San Joaquin f., San Joaquin Valley f.,** primary coccidioidomycosis.

**scarlet f.,** infection with group A $\beta$-hemolytic streptococci, now usually milder than in the past when septic complications were common, such as otitis media, mastoiditis, and suppurative lymphadenitis. It is characterized by pharyngitis and tonsillitis, with an erythematous rash produced by an erythrogenic toxin elaborated by the streptococci, progressing from the trunk and neck to the arms, legs, forehead, and face, with flushed face and circumoral pallor, red or white strawberry tongue, and lines of hyperpigmentation (Pastia's sign) in the body creases; the rash disappears and is followed by desquamation of the skin. Similar clinical manifestations, but usually with involvement of the pharynx and tonsils, may follow infection of wounds, burns, or the skin with group A β-hemolytic streptococci, or with any strain of streptococci that elaborates an erythrogenic toxin. Called also *scarlatina.*

**Schottmüller's f.,** paratyphoid f.

**Sennetsu f.,** a febrile disease occurring in Japan and Malaysia and caused by *Ehrlichia sennetsu;* symptoms include headache, nausea or vomiting, lymphocytosis, and postauricular and posterior lymphadenopathy.

**septic f.,** fever due to septicemia.

**seven-day f.,** 1. a fever affecting Europeans in India, and marked by symptoms similar to those of dengue. 2. benign leptospirosis. 3. nanukayami.

**shin bone f.,** trench f.

**ship f.,** epidemic typhus.

**shipping f.,** a disease of the respiratory tract of cattle caused by *Pasteurella haemolytica* in association with a virus; infection occurs when the resistance of the animal is lowered by stress. Characteristics include fever, pneumonialike symptoms, and sometimes death. Called also *stockyards f.* and *pneumonic pasteurellosis.*

**shoddy f.,** a febrile disease, with cough, dyspnea, and headache, caused by inhalation of dust in shoddy factories.

**Sindbis f.,** an epidemic-endemic febrile disease caused by an alphavirus, transmitted by mosquitoes of the genus *Culex,* and occurring in southern and eastern Africa, Egypt, Israel, India, the Philippines, and eastern Australia; symptoms include macular rash and arthritis.

**slime f.,** mud f. (def. 1).

**Songo f.,** epidemic hemorrhagic f.

**South African tickbite f.,** see *boutonneuse f.*

**spelter's f.,** metal fume fever caused by fumes in zinc smelters; called also *spelter's chill, zinc chill,* and *zinc fume f.*

**spirillum f.,** the spirillary form of rat-bite fever.

**splenic f.,** old name for *anthrax.*

**spotted f.,** a febrile disease typically characterized by a skin eruption, such as typhus, epidemic cerebral meningitis, and the infections caused by tick-borne rickettsiae (Rocky Mountain spotted fever, boutonneuse fever, and others).

**sthenic f.,** fever characterized by a full, strong pulse, hot and dry skin, high temperature, thirst, and active delirium.

**stockyards f.,** shipping f.

**swamp f.,** 1. mud f. (def. 1). 2. equine infectious anemia. 3. old name for *malaria.*

**swine f.,** hog cholera.

**tertian f.,** a fever that occurs every third day, associated with *Plasmodium vivax* or *P. ovale* infections; see under *malaria.*

**Texas f., Texas cattle f.,** bovine babesiosis.

**Texas tick f.,** Bullis f.

**Thai hemorrhagic f.,** hemorrhagic dengue.

**therapeutic f.,** pyretotherapy, def. 1.

**thermic f.,** sunstroke.

**three-day f.,** phlebotomus f.

**threshing f.,** grain f.

**tick f.,** any infectious disease of humans or other animals transmitted by the bite of a tick. The causative parasite may be a rickettsia, as in Rocky Mountain spotted fever; a bacterium such as *Anaplasma, Babesia,* or *Borrelia;* or a virus, as in Colorado tick fever.

**tick-borne f.,** bovine infectious petechial f.

**Tobia f.,** Rocky Mountain spotted f.

**trench f.,** a self-limited louse-borne rickettsial disease due to *Bartonella quintana,* transmitted by the body louse, *Pediculus humanus corporis,* and characterized by intermittent fever, generalized aches and pains, particularly severe in the shins, chills, sweating, vertigo, malaise, typhuslike rash, and multiple relapses. It was first recognized during the trench warfare of World War I and also was a major problem among military personnel in Europe in World War II, and is endemic in Mexico, North Africa, eastern Europe, and parts of Asia. Called also *five-day f., Meuse f., quintan f., shin bone f., Wolhynia f., His' disease, His-Werner disease,* and *Werner-His disease.*

**tsutsugamushi f.,** scrub typhus.

**typhoid f.,** an acute generalized, systemic febrile illness caused by *Salmonella typhi,* usually spread by ingestion of contaminated food and water, and characterized by sustained bacteremia and invasion by the pathogen and multiplication within the mononuclear phagocytic cells of the liver, spleen, lymph nodes, and Peyer's patches of the ileum, associated with prolonged hectic fever, malaise, transient characteristic skin rash (rose spots), abdominal pain, splenomegaly, bradycardia, delirium, and leukopenia; significant intestinal hemorrhages and frank perforation may be late complications. See also *paratyphoid f.* Called also *typhoid.*

**typhus f.,** typhus.

**undulant f.,** brucellosis, def. 1.

**urethral f., urinary f.,** fever following the use of the urethral bougie, catheter, or sound.

**uveoparotid f.,** Heerfordt's syndrome.

**valley f.,** primary coccidioidomycosis.

**Venezuelan hemorrhagic f.,** a hemorrhagic fever occurring in west central Venezuela, primarily in settlers moving into areas of cleared forest, caused by the Guanarito virus; the major reservoir is the cotton rat *Sigmodon alstoni.*

**viral hemorrhagic f's,** hemorrhagic f's.

**war f.,** epidemic typhus.

**West Nile f.,** see under *encephalitis.*

**Whitmore's f.,** melioidosis.

**Wolhynia f.,** trench f.

**Yangtze Valley f.,** schistosomiasis japonica.

**yellow f.,** an acute infectious disease caused by a flavivirus, transmitted to man by mosquitoes which acquire the infection either from man (urban type) or from animals (jungle type). In its severe form it is marked by fever, jaundice, hemorrhage, and renal damage, the jaundice resulting from necrosis of the liver; it may also occur as a mild febrile illness, with inapparent infections being frequent. Yellow fever occurs endemically and epidemically in tropical regions of the Americas and Africa. *Urban yellow fever* affects chiefly persons living in close contact with one another, and is transmitted by *Aedes aegypti,* which usually breeds near human habitations. *Jungle yellow f.* most often affects those working in or living near forests; it has a variety of mosquito vectors, including several species of *Haemagogus* in South America, and *A. africanus* and *A. simpsoni* in Central Africa.

**zinc fume f.,** spelter's f.

---

**fe·ver·few** (fe′və-fu″) [A.S. *feferfuge,* febrifuge, from L. *febrifugia*] [NF] the dried leaves of *Tanacetum parthenium,* used for migraine, arthritis, rheumatic diseases, and allergy; it has a wide variety of uses in folk medicine.

**fe·ver·ish** (fe′vər-ish) febrile.

**Fèv·re-Langue·pin syndrome** (fev′rə lahn-gə-pă′) [Marcel Paul Louis Edmond *Fèvre,* French physician, born 1897; Anne *Languepin,* French pediatrician, 20th century] see under *syndrome.*

**fex·o·fen·a·dine hy·dro·chlo·ride** (fek″so-fen′ə-dēn) an $H_1$-receptor antagonist used as an antihistaminic in the treatment of seasonal allergic rhinitis; administered orally.

**FFA** free fatty acids.

**FFT** flicker fusion threshold.

**F.h.** abbreviation for L. *fi′at haus′tus,* let a draught be made.

**FIA** fluoroimmunoassay; fluorescence immunoassay; fluorescent immunoassay.

**FIAC** Fellow of the International Academy of Cytology.

**fi·at** (fi′ət) pl. *fi′ant* [L.] let there be made. Symbol F.

**fi·ber** (fi′bər) 1. an elongated, threadlike structure; see also *fibra* [TA]. 2. nerve fiber; for bundles or tracts of nerve fibers, see under *bundle, fasciculus, lemniscus, tract,* and *tractus.* 3. in nutrition, the sum of the constituents of the diet that are not digested by gastrointestinal enzymes; see *dietary f.*

For anatomic structures not listed here, see under *fibra* and see under the terms listed in def. 2 above.

**A f's,** myelinated afferent or efferent fibers of the somatic nervous system having a diameter of 1$\mu$ to 22$\mu$ and a conduction velocity of 5 to 120 meters per second; they include the alpha, beta, delta, and gamma fibers.

**accelerating f's, accelerator f's,** adrenergic fibers that transmit the impulses that accelerate the heartbeat; called also *augmentor f's* and *cardiac accelerator f's.*

**accessory f's,** those fibers of the zonule of Zinn running perpendicularly to the chief fibers and not reaching the lens of the eye; supporting the fibers running from the ciliary body to the chief fibers and bracing them, including the interciliary fibers and the orbiculociliary fibers. Called also *auxiliary f's.*

**A delta f's,** a type of small myelinated afferent A fibers that respond to pressure, temperature, or chemical stimuli, conducting from the cutaneous tissues the initial stimulus perceived as the primary painful event. Their conducting velocity is slow, about the same as that of B fibers.

**adrenergic f's,** nerve fibers, usually sympathetic, that release epinephrine or related substances as neurotransmitters.

**afferent f's, afferent nerve f's,** neurofibrae afferentes.

**alpha f's,** motor and proprioceptive fibers of the A type having conduction velocities of 70 to 120 meters per second and ranging from 13$\mu$ to 22$\mu$ in diameter. See also under *motoneuron.*

**alveolar f's,** fibers of the periodontal ligament extending from the cementum of the tooth root to the walls of the alveolus, distinguished as alveolar crest, horizontal, oblique, and apical fibers. Called also *cementoalveolar f's.*

**alveolar crest f's,** fibers of the periodontal ligament extending from the cementum of the tooth root to the alveolar crest.

**aminergic f's,** nerve fibers that liberate one of the biogenic amines at a synapse as a nerve impulse passes; nearly all nerve fibers are this type. Cf. *peptidergic f's.*

**amygdalofugal f's,** the fibers of the ventral amygdalofugal tract and the stria terminalis.

**anastomosing f's, anastomotic f's,** fibers extending from one muscle bundle or nerve trunk to another.

**apical f's,** fibers of the periodontal ligament extending from the cementum to the fundus of the alveolus.

**archiform f's,** fibrae intercrurales.

**arcuate f's,** association fibers that follow arc-shaped paths; see *fibrae arcuatae cerebri, fibrae arcuatae internae,* and *fibrae arcuatae externae posteriores* and *anteriores,* under *fibra.*

**arcuate f's, anterior external,** fibrae arcuatae externae ventrales.

**arcuate f's, dorsal external,** fibrae arcuatae externae posteriores.

**arcuate f's, internal,** fibrae arcuatae internae.

**arcuate f's, long,** long association f's.

**arcuate f's, posterior external,** fibrae arcuatae externae posteriores.

**arcuate f's, short,** short association f's.

**arcuate f's, ventral external,** fibrae arcuatae externae anteriores.

**arcuate f's of cerebrum,** fibrae arcuatae cerebri.

**argentaffin f's, argentophil f's, argentophilic f's,** reticular f's.

**association f.,** fibra associationis.

**association f's of telencephalon,** fibrae associationis telencephali.

**association f's, long,** fibrae associationis longae.

**association f's, short,** fibrae associationis breves.

**association nerve f.,** fibra associationis.

**astral f.,** see under *ray.*

**augmentor f's,** accelerating f's.

**autonomic f's,** neurofibrae autonomicae.

**autonomic afferent f's,** see *neurofibrae autonomicae.*

**autonomic efferent f's,** see *neurofibrae autonomicae.*

**autonomic nerve f's,** neurofibrae autonomicae.

**auxiliary f's,** accessory f's.

**axial f.,** axon (def. 1).

**B f's,** myelinated preganglionic autonomic axons having a fiber diameter $\leq 3\mu m$ and a conduction velocity of 3 to 15 meters per second; these include only efferent fibers.

**bag f.,** nuclear bag f.

**basilar f's,** fibers that form the middle layer of the zona arcuata and the zona pectinata of the basilar membrane in the inner ear.

**Bergmann's f's,** processes which radiate from the molecular layer of the cerebellum and enter the pia.

**beta f's,** motor and proprioceptive fibers of the A type having conduction velocities of 30 to 70 meters per second and ranging from 8$\mu$ to 13$\mu$ in diameter. See also *beta motoneuron.*

**bone f's,** Sharpey's f's (def. 1).

**Brücke's f's,** fibrae meridionales musculi ciliaris.

**bulbospiral f's,** spiral muscle fibers that begin near the root of the aorta and spiral upward in bundles within the ventricles.

**Burdach's f's,** fasciculus cuneatus medullae spinalis.

**C f's,** unmyelinated nerve fibers, having a smaller diameter (0.3 $\mu$ to 1.3 $\mu$) and a slower conduction velocity (0.6 to 2.3 meters per second) than alpha fibers. They are found as postganglionic (efferent) fibers of the autonomic nervous system, and as afferent fibers at posterior roots, receiving impulses from free nerve endings that act as thermoreceptors, nociceptors, and interoceptors.

**cardiac accelerator f's,** accelerating f's.

**cardiac depressor f's,** vagal fibers to the heart which when activated cause a decrease in cardiac output.

**cardiac pressor f's,** sympathetic nerve fibers to the heart which when activated cause an increase in cardiac output.

**cemental f's,** the fibers of the periodontal ligament extending from the cementum to the zone of the intermediate plexus, where their terminations are interspersed with the terminations of the alveolar group of periodontal fibers.

**cementoalveolar f's,** alveolar f's.

**cerebellovestibular f's,** fibers in the fastigiobulbar tract that run from the cerebellar cortex to the vestibular nuclei.

**cerebrospinal f's,** fibrae corticospinales.

**chain f.,** nuclear chain f.

**chief f's,** those fibers of the zonule of Zinn which run from the ciliary body to the lens, including the orbiculoposterocapsular, the orbiculoanterocapsular, the cilioposterocapsular, and cilioequatorial fibers; called also *main* or *principal f's.*

**cholinergic f's,** nerve fibers that liberate acetylcholine as a neurotransmitter.

**chromatic f.,** the long fiber of chromatin into which the nucleus is resolved during the early stages of karyokinesis and which afterward separates into the chromosomes.

**chromosomal f.,** traction f.

**cilioequatorial f's,** those chief fibers which pass from the summits of the ciliary processes to the equator of the lens.

**cilioposterocapsular f's,** the most numerous of the chief zonular fibers, arising from the tips and sides of the ciliary processes, passing posteriorly and crossing the anteriorly directed fibers, to insert into the posterior capsule anterior to the insertion of the orbiculoposterocapsular fibers.

**circular f's,** 1. gingival fibers that pass through the connective tissue of the marginal and interdental gingivae and encircle the tooth in ringlike fashion. 2. fibrae circulares musculi ciliaris. 3. circular f's of eardrum.

**circular f's of ciliary muscle,** fibrae circulares musculi ciliaris.

**circular f's of eardrum,** the fibers in the stratum circulare membranae tympanicae.

**climbing f's, clinging f's,** afferent fibers arising in part from the middle cerebellar peduncle and passing through the granular layer of the cerebellar cortex to terminate on Purkinje cell dendrites. Called also *tendril f's.* Cf. *mossy f's.*

**collagen f's, collagenous f's,** the soft, flexible, white fibers which are the most characteristic constituent of all types of connective tissue, consisting of the protein collagen, and composed of bundles of fibrils that are in turn made up of smaller units (unit fibrils or microfibrils) which show a characteristic crossbanding with a major periodicity of approximately 65 nm. In describing the hierarchy of arrangement of collagen structure, the terms fiber and fibril are sometimes loosely interchanged; see also under *fibril.*

**collateral f's of Winslow,** fibrae intercrurales.

**commissural f.,** fibra commissuralis.

**commissural f's of telencephalon,** fibrae commissurales telencephali.

**cone f.,** a fiberlike extension of a retinal cone, running from the inner segment of the dendrite to the nucleus to the pedicle.

**continuous f's,** the spindle fibers in mitosis which extend from pole to pole.

**Corti's f's,** pillar cells.

**corticobulbar f's, corticonuclear f's,** fibrae corticonucleares.

**corticopontine f's,** fibrae corticopontinae.

**corticoreticular f's,** fibrae corticoreticulares.

**corticorubral f's,** fibrae corticorubrales.

**corticospinal f's,** fibrae corticospinales.

**corticostriate f's,** afferent fibers originating in many parts of the cerebral cortex and descending to the caudate nucleus and putamen in the corpus striatum.

**corticothalamic f's,** fibrae corticothalamicae.

**crude f.,** the fiber that remains after food is digested with alkali and acid, which destroys all soluble and some insoluble fiber; it comprises mainly lignin and cellulose.

**dark f's,** muscle fibers rich in sarcoplasm and having a dark appearance.

**decussating f's,** any set of interconnecting fibers.
**dentatorubral f's,** fibrae dentatorubrales.
**dentatothalamic f's,** nerve fibers in the cranial cerebellar peduncle that make up the dentatothalamic tract.
**dentinal f.,** process of odontoblast.
**dentinogenic f's,** Korff's f's.
**depressor f's,** 1. nerve fibers which, when stimulated reflexly, cause a diminished vasomotor tone and thereby a decrease in arterial pressure. 2. cardiac depressor f's.
**dietary f.,** that part of whole grains, vegetables, fruits, and nuts that resists digestion in the gastrointestinal tract; it includes soluble fibers such as pectins, gums, mucilages, and some hemicelluloses and insoluble fibers such as cellulose, some hemicelluloses, and lignin.
**Edinger's f's,** fibers in the cerebrum of amphibia, forming part of the visual paths.
**efferent f's, efferent nerve f's,** neurofibrae efferentes.
**elastic f's,** yellowish fibers of elastic quality traversing the intercellular substance of connective tissue; called also *yellow f's.*
**endogenous f's,** nerve fibers of the spinal cord which arise from cells the bodies of which are situated inside the cord.
**exogenous f's,** fibers of the spinal cord which arise from cells the bodies of which are situated outside the cord.
**extraciliary f's,** see *fleece.*
**extrafusal f's,** ordinary muscle fibers, as opposed to the intrafusal fibers of the muscle spindle.
**fasciculoventricular f's,** Mahaim fibers that connect the bundle of His directly to the ventricular myocardium.
**frontopontine f's,** fibrae frontopontinae.
**fusimotor f's,** efferent A fibers that innervate the intrafusal fibers of the muscle spindle; see also *gamma f's.* Called also *fusimotor axons.*
**gamma f's,** any A fibers that conduct at velocities of 15 to 40 meters per second and range from 3$\mu$ to 7$\mu$ in diameter; the only such fibers are the fusimotor fibers. See also under *loop* and *motoneuron.*
**geniculostriate f's,** the fibers of the optic radiation; see *radiatio optica* under *radiatio.*
**Gerdy's f's,** the fibers of the superficial ligament connecting the clefts of the palmar surfaces of the fingers.
**gingival f's,** the collagen fibers which make up the gingival corium and support the gingiva. They are attached and adapted to the tooth surface and act as a barrier to the apical migration of the epithelial attachment.
**gingivodental f's,** gingival fibers of the vestibular, oral, and interproximal surfaces, embedded in the cementum just beneath the epithelium at the base of the gingival crevice.
**Goll's f's,** fasciculus gracilis medullae spinalis.
**Gratiolet's radiating f's,** radiatio optica.
**gray f's,** unmyelinated nerve fibers, found largely, but not exclusively, in the sympathetic nerves.
**hair f.,** any one of the horny fibers, each containing relics of a nucleus, which make up the main substance of a hair.
**half-spindle f's,** spindle fibers in mitosis which extend from one pole to the chromosomes.
**Henle's f's,** the fibers of either of the elastic membranes of an artery.
**Herxheimer's f's,** minute spiral fibers in the stratum mucosum of the skin; called also *Herxheimer's spirals.*
**heterodesmotic f's,** nerve fibers connecting dissimilar structures of the central nervous system. Cf. *homodesmotic f's.*
**homodesmotic f's,** nerve fibers connecting similar structures of the central nervous system. Cf. *heterodesmotic f's.*
**horizontal f's,** fibers of the periodontal ligament extending horizontally from the cementum of the tooth root to the walls of the alveolus.
**impulse-conducting f's,** Purkinje f's.
**insoluble f.,** that not soluble in water, composed mainly of lignin, cellulose, and hemicelluloses and primarily found in the bran layers of cereal grains; its actions include increasing fecal bulk and decreasing free radicals in the gastrointestinal tract.
**interciliary f's,** those accessory fibers running between the ciliary processes.
**intercolumnar f's,** fibrae intercrurales.
**intercrural f's,** fibrae intercrurales.
**internuncial f's,** nerve fibers connecting two or more neurons.
**intersegmental f's,** see *fasciculus proprius posterior medullae spinalis, fasciculus proprius lateralis medullae spinalis,* and *fasciculus proprius anterior medullae spinalis.*
**interzonal f's,** the delicate fibers of achromatin forming the central spindle during karyokinesis.
**intrafusal f's,** modified muscle fibers which, surrounded by fluid and enclosed in a connective tissue envelope, compose the muscle spindle.
**intrasegmental f's,** fibers in the white commissures of the spinal cord that link neurons to contralateral neurons at the same level.
**intrathalamic f's,** fibrae intrathalamicae.
**James f's,** junctional tissue or a tract which bypasses the atrioventricular node, thus permitting ventricular preexcitation.
**Korff f's,** collagen fibrils extending from fibroblasts (preodontoblasts), which project their processes toward the inner enamel epithelium (preameloblasts), whence they reach the area of aperiodic fibrils and basal lamina, where they form bundles and make up the matrix for dentin, particularly the mantle dentin.
**lattice f's,** reticular f's.
**f's of lens,** fibrae lentis.
**light f's,** muscle fibers poor in sarcoplasm and therefore more transparent than dark fibers.
**longitudinal f's of ciliary muscle,** fibrae meridionales musculi ciliaris.
**longitudinal pontine f's,** fibrae pontis longitudinales.
**Luschka's f's,** fibers of the levator ani muscle that meet between the anus and the vagina in the perineal body.
**macular f's,** the fibers of the maculary fasciculus.
**Mahaim f's,** specialized tissue connecting components of the conduction system directly to the ventricular septum, usually important functionally only when abundant; they are often classified as *fasciculoventricular f's* and *nodoventricular f's.*
**main f's,** chief f's.
**mantle f.,** any one of the cytoplasmic filaments which assist in drawing the daughter chromosomes toward the poles of the central spindles.
**Mauthner's f.,** an axon that extends from the metencephalon to the caudal end of the spinal cord of fishes and amphibians, and provides the final common path for impulses to the tail.
**medullated f's, medullated nerve f's,** myelinated f's.
**meridional f's of ciliary muscle,** fibrae meridionales musculi ciliaris.
**Monakow's f's,** tractus rubrospinalis.
**moss f's, mossy f's,** thick afferent nerve fibers arising from the inferior cerebellar peduncle and passing into the cerebellar cortex to terminate in numerous branches or mosslike appendages around the cells of the granular layer. Cf. *climbing f's.*
**motor f.,** an efferent fiber from a motoneuron to a muscle.
**Müller's f's,** elongated neuroglial cells traversing all the layers of the retina and forming its most important supporting element; called also *sustentacular f's, cells of Müller, radial cells of Müller,* and *retinal gliocytes.*
**muscle f.,** any of the cells of skeletal or cardiac muscle tissue. Skeletal muscle fibers are cylindrical multinucleate cells containing contracting myofibrils, across which run transverse striations, enclosed in a sarcolemma. Cardiac muscle fibers contain one or sometimes two nuclei and myofibrils and are separated from one another by an intercalated disk; although striated, cardiac muscle fibers branch to form an interlacing network. See also *muscle cell,* under *cell.*
**muscle f's, fast twitch,** paler-colored muscle fibers of larger diameter than slow twitch fibers, and having less sarcoplasm and more prominent cross-striping; used for forceful and rapid contractions over short periods of time.
**muscle f's, intermediate,** muscle fibers having characteristics intermediate between red and white muscle fibers.
**muscle f's, red,** slow twitch muscle f's.
**muscle f's, slow twitch,** small dark muscle fibers rich in mitochondria, myoglobin, and sarcoplasm and with only faint cross-striping; designed for slow but repetitive contractions over long periods of time.
**muscle f's, type I,** slow twitch muscle f's.
**muscle f's, type II,** fast twitch muscle f's.
**muscle f's, white,** fast twitch muscle f's.
**myelinated f's, myelinated nerve f's,** grayish white nerve fibers whose axons are encased in a myelin sheath, which may in turn be enclosed by a neurilemma; called also *medullated f's* and *medullated nerve f's.* Cf. *unmyelinated f's.*
**nerve f.,** neurofibra.
**neuroglial f.,** one of the fibrillar structures embedded in the cytoplasm and expansions of neuroglial cells, particularly fibrous astrocytes.
**nigrostriate f's,** the fibers of the nigrostriate tract.
**nodoventricular f's,** Mahaim fibers that connect the atrioventricular node directly to the ventricle.
**nonmedullated f's, nonmedullated nerve f's,** unmyelinated f's.
**nuclear bag f.,** an intrafusal fiber that contains a nuclear bag; it is longer and thicker and contracts more slowly than a nuclear chain fiber.
**nuclear chain f.,** an intrafusal fiber that contains a nuclear chain; it is shorter and thinner and contracts more rapidly than a nuclear bag fiber.
**oblique f's,** the largest fibers of the periodontal ligament, extending from the cementum in a coronal direction obliquely to the apical two

thirds of the alveolus; they suspend and anchor the tooth in its socket and resist surface tooth pressures.

**oblique f's of ciliary muscle,** fibrae radiales musculi ciliaris.

**oblique gastric f's, oblique f's of stomach,** fibrae obliquae gastricae.

**occipitopontine f's,** see *fibrae corticopontinae,* under *fibra.*

**odontogenic f's,** fibers of connective tissue (periodontium and pulp) contributing to the matrix of dentin and cementum.

**olivocerebellar f's,** tractus olivocerebellaris.

**orbiculoanterocapsular f's,** those chief fibers which have the most posterior and internal position, lying in close relation to the anterior boundary of the vitreous.

**orbiculociliary f's,** those accessory fibers which pass from the pars orbicularis to the ciliary processes.

**orbiculoposterocapsular f's,** those chief fibers which spring from the prolongation of the hyaloid membrane investing the ciliary ring.

**osteocollagenous f's,** fibers gathered together into bundles and united by a special binding substance in the interstitial substance of bone.

**osteogenetic f's, osteogenic f's,** precollagenous fibers formed by osteoclasts and becoming the fibrous component of bone matrix.

**oxytalan f.,** 1. a connective tissue fiber, resistant to acid hydrolysis, found in structures subjected to mechanical stress, such as tendons, ligaments, adventitia, and connective tissue sheaths that surround the skin appendages. 2. oxytalan.

**pallidofugal f's,** fibers conducting impulses from the globus pallidus across the internal capsule and fields of Forel to the thalamus and nearby areas; see also *ansa lenticularis* and *fasciculus lenticularis.*

**parallel f's,** axons of granule cells in the cerebellum that cross the molecular layer at a right angle and synapse with gemmules of Purkinje cell dendrite; many thousands of parallel fibers may innervate a single Purkinje cell.

**paraventricular f's,** fibrae paraventriculohypophysiales.

**parietopontine f's,** fibrae parietopontinae.

**parietotemporopontine f's,** fibrae parietotemporopontinae.

**peptidergic f's,** nerve fibers that secrete neuropeptides as neurotransmitters. Cf. *aminergic f's.*

**perforating f's,** Sharpey's f's (def. 2).

**periventricular f's,** fibrae periventriculares.

**pilomotor f's,** unmyelinated nerve fibers going to the small muscles of the hair follicles.

**pontocerebellar f's,** fibrae pontocerebellares.

**postcommissural f's,** the fibers of the commissure of the epithalamus that lie behind the pineal body.

**postganglionic f's, postganglionic nerve f's,** neurofibrae postganglionicae.

**precollagenous f's,** a name given reticular fibers on the supposition that they are immature collagenous fibers.

**preganglionic f's, preganglionic nerve f's,** neurofibrae preganglionicae.

**pressor f's,** 1. nerve fibers which, when stimulated reflexly, cause or increase vasomotor tone. 2. cardiac pressor f's.

**principal f's,** 1. chief f's. 2. fibers of the periodontal ligament, which are collagen fibers arranged in bundles along the length of the root of a tooth that suspend and anchor the tooth to the alveolus. They include the transseptal, alveolar crest, horizontal, oblique, and apical fibers.

**projection f., projection nerve f's,** fibra projectionis.

**Prussak's f's,** two short fibers from the end of the short process of the malleus to the notch of Rivinus.

**Purkinje f's,** modified cardiac fibers composed of Purkinje cells, occurring as an interlaced network in the subendocardial tissue and constituting the terminal ramifications of the conducting system of the heart. The term is sometimes used loosely to denote the entire system of conducting fibers. See also *rami subendocardiales* and *systema conducens cordis.*

**radial f's of ciliary muscle,** fibrae radiales musculi ciliaris.

**radiating f's of anterior chondrosternal ligaments,** ligamenta sternocostalia radiata.

**radiating f's of eardrum,** the fibers in the stratum radiatum membranae tympanicae.

**radicular f's,** fibers in the roots of the spinal nerves.

**ragged red f's,** muscle fibers characterized by large collections of structurally abnormal mitochondria below the sarcolemmal surface and within the fiber itself that stain red with Gomori trichrome stain; seen in mitochondrial myopathy and occasionally in other myopathic disorders.

**Rasmussen's nerve f's,** tractus olivocochlearis.

**Reissner's f.,** a highly refractive longitudinal fiber in the central canal of the spinal cord.

**reticular f's,** immature connective tissue fibers, staining with silver, forming the reticular framework of lymphoid and myeloid tissue and occurring also in the interstitial tissue of glandular organs, the papillary layer of the skin, and elsewhere; called also *argentaffin f's, argentophilic f's, lattice f's,* and *Gitterfasern.*

**retinothalamic projection f's,** fibers that connect the visual receptors of the retina with the thalamus, forming part of the optic nerve and optic tract.

**Retzius' f's,** the stiff filaments of Deiters' cells in the organ of Corti.

**ring f.,** a band of circumferentially oriented myofibrils located beneath the sarcolemma of a muscle fiber and encircling the longitudinally oriented myofibrils within the fiber; seen in myotonic dystrophy.

**Ritter's f.,** a fiber in the axis of a retinal rod, probably a nerve fiber.

**rod f.,** a fiberlike extension of a retinal rod, running from the inner segment of the dendrite to the nucleus to the spherule.

**Rosenthal f's,** eosinophilic masses seen throughout the central nervous system, particularly just under the pia mater and near blood vessels, in Alexander's disease; they may be the remains of degenerated neuroglial cells.

**Sappey's f's,** smooth muscle fibers in the check ligaments of the eye near their orbital attachments.

**Sharpey's f's,** 1. collagenous fibers that pass from the periosteum and are embedded in the outer circumferential and interstitial lamellae of bone; called also *bone f's.* 2. terminal portions of principal fibers that insert into the cementum of a tooth. Called also *perforating f's.*

**sinospiral f's, sinuspiral f's,** spiral muscle fibers that begin near the posterior aspect of one or both atrioventricular fibrous rings and spiral upward in bundles within one or both ventricles.

**soluble f.,** that with an affinity for water, either dissolving or swelling to form a gel; it includes gums, pectins, mucilages, and some hemicelluloses, and is primarily found in fruits, vegetables, oats, barley, legumes, and seaweed. It acts to decrease the rate of stomach emptying and increase transit time, and also binds bile acids, increasing their excretion.

**somatic f's,** neurofibrae somaticae.

**somatic afferent f's,** see *neurofibrae somaticae.*

**somatic efferent f's,** see *neurofibrae somaticae.*

**somatic nerve f's,** neurofibrae somaticae.

**sphincter f's of ciliary muscle,** fibrae circulares musculi ciliaris.

**spindle f's,** the microtubules radiating from the centrioles during mitosis and forming a spindle-shaped configuration. See *spindle.*

**Stilling's f's,** nerve fibers in the reticular formation of the medulla oblongata.

**f's of stria terminalis,** fibrae striae terminalis.

**striatonigral f's,** the fibers of the strionigral tract.

**sudomotor f's,** unmyelinated nerve fibers going to the sweat glands.

**supraoptic f's,** fibrae supraopticohypophysiales.

**sustentacular f's,** Müller's f's.

**T f.,** a nerve fiber that branches at right angles from the axon, as seen in pseudounipolar neurons.

**tangential f's, tangential nerve f's,** neurofibrae tangentiales.

**temporopontine f's,** fibrae temporopontinae.

**tendril f's,** climbing f's.

**terminal conducting f's of Purkinje,** Purkinje f's.

**thalamocortical f's,** sensory nerve fibers that connect the dorsal thalamus to the cerebral cortex, which together form the peduncles of the thalamus; called also *thalamic radiations, radiations of thalamus,* and *thalamocortical projections.*

**thalamoparietal f's,** fibrae thalamoparietales.

**Tomes' f.,** process of odontoblast.

**traction f's,** the fibers of the spindle in mitosis along which the daughter chromosomes move apart; called also *chromosomal f's.*

**transseptal f's,** fibers of the periodontal ligament extending interproximally over the alveolar crest and embedding in the cementum of adjacent teeth; they support the interproximal gingiva and secure the adjacent tooth.

**transverse pontine f's,** fibrae pontis transversae.

**trigeminothalamic f's,** nerve fibers that convey sensory information from the spinal tract and the nuclei of the trigeminal nerve to the sensory nuclei of the thalamus.

**ultraterminal f.,** the thin unmyelinated twig that is the last ramification of the axon at the motor end plate.

**unmyelinated f's, unmyelinated nerve f's,** nerve fibers (axons) that lack the myelin sheath but may be enclosed by a neurilemma. Called also *nonmedullated f's* and *nonmedullated nerve f's.* Cf. *myelinated f's.*

**varicose f's,** certain myelinated fibers which have no neurilemma; after death a fluid accumulates between the myelin and the axon, giving the fibers a varicose appearance.

**vasomotor f's,** unmyelinated nerve fibers going chiefly to arteriolar muscles.

**visceral f's,** neurofibrae autonomicae.

**visceral afferent f's,** autonomic affererent f's; see *neurofibrae autonomicae.*

**visceral efferent f's,** autonomic effererent f's; see *neurofibrae autonomicae.*

**visceral nerve f's,** neurofibrae autonomicae.
**von Monakow's f's,** tractus rubrospinalis.
**Weissmann's f's,** fibers within the muscle spindle.
**white f's,** collagenous f's.
**yellow f's,** elastic f's.
**zonular f's,** fibrae zonulares.

**fi·ber·co·lono·scope** (fi″bər-ko-lon′o-skōp) a fiberoptic instrument for viewing the colon.

**Fi·ber·Con** (fi′bər-kon) trademark for a preparation of calcium polycarbophil.

**fi·ber·gas·tro·scope** (fi″bər-gas′tro-skōp) a fiberoptic instrument for viewing the stomach.

**fi·ber·il·lu·mi·nat·ed** (fi′bər-ĭ-loo′mĭ-nāt″əd) transmitting light by means of bundles of glass or plastic fibers, utilizing a lens system to transmit the image; said of endoscopes of such design.

**fi·ber·op·tic** (fi″bər-op′tik) 1. pertaining to fiberoptics. 2. coated with glass or plastic fibers having special optical properties.

**fi·ber·op·tics** (fi″bər-op′tiks) 1. the transmission of an image along flexible bundles of coated parallel glass or plastic fibers that propagate light by internal reflections. 2. the branch of optics dealing with such transmission.

**fi·ber·scope** (fi′bər-skōp) a flexible fiberoptic endoscope. See also *fiberoptics.*

**Fi·bi·ger** (fe′bĭ-gər) Johannes Andreas Grib. Danish pathologist, 1867–1928; winner of the Nobel prize in medicine or physiology for 1926 for his discovery of the Spiroptera carcinoma and thus of a method for the experimental induction of cancer.

**fi·bra** (fi′brə) gen. and pl. *fi′brae* [L.] [TA] fiber: a general term designating an elongated, threadlike structure. See also *neurofibra.*

**fi′brae annula′res,** see *pars anularis vaginae fibrosae digitorum manus* and *pars anularis vaginae fibrosae digitorum pedis.*

**fi′brae arcua′tae cer′ebri** [TA], arcuate fibers of cerebrum: short association fibers within the cerebral cortex, connecting adjacent gyri; called also *fibrae propriae.*

**fi′brae arcua′tae exter′nae anterio′res** [TA], anterior external arcuate fibers: fibers that arise from the arcuate nuclei, emerging from the anterior median fissure; they run laterally, backward, and upward over the medulla oblongata to reach the cerebellum by way of the inferior cerebellar peduncle. Called also *ventral external arcuate fibers* and *fibrae arcuatae externae ventrales.*

**fi′brae arcua′tae exter′nae dorsa′les,** fibrae arcuatae externae posteriores.

**fi′brae arcua′tae exter′nae posterio′res** [TA], posterior external arcuate fibers: fibers that arise from the accessory cuneate nucleus and enter the cerebellum by way of the ipsilateral inferior cerebellar peduncle; called also *dorsal external arcuate fibers* and *fibrae arcuatae externae dorsales.*

**fi′brae arcua′tae exter′nae ventra′les,** fibrae arcuatae externae anteriores.

**fi′brae arcua′tae inter′nae** [TA], internal arcuate fibers: fibers that arise from the nucleus cuneatus and nucleus gracilis and pass ventromedially around the central gray substance of the medulla oblongata to form the decussation of the medial lemnisci.

**f. associatio′nis** [TA], association fiber: one of the nerve fibers connecting different cortical areas within one hemisphere. Called also *association neurofiber* and *neurofibra associationis.* See also *fibrae associationis telencephali.*

**fi′brae associatio′nis bre′ves** [TA], short association fibers: association fibers that connect adjacent areas of the cortex; called also *short arcuate fibers.*

**fi′brae associatio′nis lon′gae** [TA], long association fibers: association fibers connecting areas of the cortex that are not adjacent; called also *long arcuate fibers.*

**fi′brae associatio′nis telence′phali** [TA], association fibers of telencephalon: nerve fibers that interconnect portions of the cerebral cortex within a hemisphere. See *fibrae associationis breves, fibrae associationis longae,* and *fibrae arcuatae cerebri.*

**fi′brae circula′res mus′culi cilia′ris** [TA], circular fibers of ciliary muscle: the most internal fibers of the ciliary muscle that form a discrete portion of the ciliary muscle and extend around the apex of the ciliary body close to the root of the iris. Called also *Müller fibers* or *muscle* and *sphincteric fibers of ciliary muscle.*

**f. commissura′lis** [TA], commissural fiber: one of the nerve fibers which pass between the cortex of opposite hemispheres of the brain, or between two sides of the brain stem or spinal cord. Called also *commissural neurofiber* and *neurofibra commissuralis.* See also *fibrae commissuralis telencephali.*

**fi′brae commissura′les telence′phali** [TA], commissural fibers of telencephalon: the nerve fibers that interconnect regions of the two hemispheres, crossing the median plane.

**fi′brae corticonuclea′res,** corticonuclear fibers: longitudinal fibers of the pyramidal tract (q.v.) that arise in the cerebral cortex, descend in the internal capsule, and synapse in the various motor nuclei of the mesencephalon, pons, and medulla oblongata. Together they form the corticonuclear tract. Called also *corticobulbar fibers.*

**fi′brae corticoponti′nae** [TA], corticopontine fibers: nerve fibers that arise in the cerebral cortex of the frontal, temporal, parietal, and occipital lobes, descend in the internal capsule and cerebral peduncle, and terminate at different levels in the pontine nuclei where they are relayed chiefly to the opposite cerebellar hemisphere. Collectively called *corticopontine tract* or *tractus corticopontinus.*

**fi′brae corticoreticula′res** [TA], corticoreticular fibers: nerve fibers that arise chiefly in the sensorimotor areas of the cerebral cortex, descend with corticospinal fibers, and synapse with cells of the reticular formation, especially in the pons and medulla oblongata.

**fi′brae corticorubra′les** [TA], corticorubral fibers: nerve fibers that descend from the cortex of the frontal lobe through the posterior limb of the internal capsule to terminate in the red nucleus.

**fi′brae corticospina′les** [TA], corticospinal fibers: longitudinal fibers that arise in the cerebral cortex, descend in the internal capsule, mesencephalon, pons, and pyramids of the medulla oblongata, and which form, upon reaching the spinal cord, the lateral and ventral corticospinal tracts; see also *tractus pyramidalis.*

**fi′brae corticothala′micae** [TA], corticothalamic fibers: nerve fibers that project from the cerebral cortex through the centrum semiovale to terminate in the thalamus.

**fi′brae dentatorubra′les,** dentatorubral fibers: afferent nerve fibers received by the red nucleus from the contralateral dentate nucleus.

**fi′brae frontoponti′nae** [TA], frontopontine fibers: nerve fibers that arise in the frontal lobe of the cerebral hemisphere and traverse the internal capsule and peduncle, ending in the pontine nuclei. Together they form the frontopontine tract (tractus frontopontinus).

**fi′brae intercrura′les** [TA], intercrural fibers: fibers joining the medial and lateral crura of the superficial inguinal ring; called also *Cooper's* or *Scarpa's fascia, Todd's process,* and *collateral fibers of Winslow.*

**fi′brae len′tis** [TA], fibers of lens: long bands, derived from the epithelium, that make up the substance of the lens; called also *cellulae lentis.*

**fi′brae longitudina′les mus′culi cilia′ris,** fibrae meridionales musculi ciliaris.

**fi′brae meridiona′les mus′culi cilia′ris** [TA], meridional fibers of ciliary muscle: the most external fibers of the ciliary muscle that run meridionally or longitudinally from the reticulum trabeculae toward the ciliary processes. Called also *Brücke's fibers* and *longitudinal fibers of ciliary muscle.*

**fi′brae obli′quae gas′tricae** [TA], **fi′brae obli′quae ventri′culi,** oblique gastric fibers: the inner obliquely coursing fibers of the muscular coat of the stomach; called also *oblique fibers of stomach.*

**fi′brae paraventricula′res, fi′brae paraventriculohypophysia′les** [TA], paraventricular fibers: the efferent fiber components of the hypothalamicohypophysial tract that arise in the paraventricular nucleus and form the paraventriculohypophysial tract.

**fi′brae parietoponti′nae** [TA], parietopontine fibers: nerve fibers that arise in the cerebral cortex of the parietal lobe, descend in the sublentiform part of the posterior limb of the internal capsule to become constituent fibers of the basis pedunculi cerebri of the ventral part of the cerebral peduncle, and end in the pontine nuclei.

**fi′brae parietotemporoponti′nae,** parietotemporopontine fibers: the fibrae parietopontinae and fibrae temporopontinae considered together.

**fi′brae periventricula′res** [TA], periventricular fibers: fibers that arise from the hypothalamus, then descend in the central gray matter through the tegmentum of the mesencephalon and the reticular formation of the pons and medulla oblongata; some are found in the dorsal longitudinal fasciculus.

**fi′brae pon′tis longitudina′les** [TA], longitudinal pontine fibers: a group of longitudinal nerve fibers that arise in the crus cerebri and run to the ventral part of the pons, where they become dispersed into smaller bundles, separated by the nuclei of the pons and the transverse fibers of the pons. The group includes the corticospinal, corticonuclear, corticoreticular, and corticopontine fibers.
**fi′brae pon′tis profun′dae,** the more deeply situated of the fibrae pontis transversae.
**fi′brae pon′tis superficia′les,** the more superficial of the fibrae pontis transversae.
**fi′brae pon′tis transver′sae** [TA], transverse pontine fibers: fibers within the ventral part of the pons which arise from the pontine nuclei and run laterally to form the middle cerebellar peduncles. Most of these fibers cross the midline. They are part of the frontopontocerebellar pathway.
**fi′brae pontocerebella′res** [TA], pontocerebellar fibers: longitudinal fibers in the ventral part of the pons that terminate in the vermis of the cerebellum.
**f. projectio′nis** [TA], projection fiber: one of the nerve fibers that connect the cerebral cortex with the subcortical centers, the brain stem, and the spinal cord; called also *projection neurofiber* and *neurofibra projectionis.*
**fi′brae radia′les mus′culi cilia′ris** [TA], radial fibers of ciliary muscle: the fibers of the ciliary muscle lying between the meridional (external) fibers and the circular (internal) fibers; they run in a radial or oblique direction from one to another and may form a fibrous network. Called also *oblique fibers of ciliary muscle.*
**fi′brae stri′ae termina′lis** [TA], fibers of stria terminalis: the myelinated nerve fibers that make up the stria terminalis.
**fi′brae supraop′ticae, fi′brae supraopticohypophysia′les** [TA], supraoptic fibers: the efferent fiber components of the hypothalamicohypophysial tract that arise in the supraoptic nucleus and form the supraopticohypophysial tract.
**fi′brae temporoponti′nae** [TA], temporopontine fibers: nerve fibers that arise in the cerebral cortex of the temporal lobe, descend in the sublentiform part of the posterior limb of the internal capsule to become constituent fibers of the basis pedunculi cerebri of the ventral part of the cerebral peduncle, and end in the pontine nuclei.
**fi′brae thalamoparieta′les** [TA], thalamoparietal fibers: nerve fibers that project from the parietal lobe through the posterior limb of the internal capsule to end in the thalamus.
**fi′brae zonula′res** [TA], zonular fibers: the fibers that anchor the lens capsule to the ciliary body and the retina; called also *aponeurosis of Zinn.*

**fi·brae** (fi′bre) [L.] genitive and plural of *fibra.*

**fi·bre** (fi′bər) fiber.

**fi·bric ac·id** (fi′brik) any of a group of compounds structurally related to clofibrate that can reduce plasma levels of triglycerides and cholesterol; used to treat hypertriglyceridemia and hypercholesterolemia.

**fi·bril** (fi′bril) [L. *fibrilla*] a minute fiber or filament; often a component of a compound fiber.
**anchoring f.,** a Type VII collagen fibril having a central cross-banded region and a fanlike group of filaments at each end that attach the dermis to the basement membrane by interweaving with collagen fibers in the dermis and lamina densa; such fibers also occur in the gingiva, where they attach the epithelium to the lamina propria.
**border f′s,** myoglia.
**collagen f′s,** delicate fibrils of collagen in connective tissue, composed of molecules of tropocollagen in linear arrays. In Type I collagen, the most common type, the tropocollagen molecules are associated in periodic, staggered arrays that give the appearance of cross-banding, with a period of approximately 65 nm in the unit fibril (or microfibril); these unit fibrils are aggregated in bundles to form larger fibrils, with longitudinal striations, which may themselves be aggregated into fibers. Some other types of collagen also associate into fibrils (e.g., Types II, III, VI) but may not aggregate to show cross-banding or to form fibers. The terms fiber and fibril are sometimes interchanged loosely in descriptions of the hierarchy of collagen aggregation. See also illustration.
**dentinal f′s,** component fibrils of the dentinal matrix.
**fibroglia f′s,** see *fibroglia.*
**muscle f., muscular f.,** myofibril.
**nerve f.,** neurofibril.
**side f. of Golgi,** a twig that branches off at a right angle near the beginning of an axon of a ganglion cell.
**Tomes′ f.,** process of odontoblast.

**fi·bril·la** (fi-bril′ə) gen. and pl. *fibril′lae* [L., dim. of *fibra*] a fibril.

**fi·bril·lae** (fi-bril′e) [L.] genitive and plural of *fibrilla.*

**fi·bril·lar, fi·bril·lary** (fi′brĭ-lər, fi′bri-lar″e) pertaining to a fibril or to fibrils.

**fi·bril·lat·ed** (fī′brĭ-lāt″əd) made up of fibrils.

**fi·bril·la·tion** (fī-brĭ-la′shən) 1. the quality of being fibrillar. 2. a small, local, involuntary contraction of muscle, invisible under the skin, resulting from spontaneous activation of single muscle cells or muscle fibers whose nerve supply has been damaged or cut off. 3. the initial degenerative changes in osteoarthritis, characterized by softening of the articular cartilage and development of vertical clefts between groups of cartilage cells.
**atrial f.,** an arrhythmia in which minute areas of the atrial myocardium are in various uncoordinated stages of depolarization and repolarization due to multiple reentry circuits within the atrial myocardium; instead of intermittently contracting, the atria quiver continuously in a chaotic pattern, causing a totally irregular, often rapid ventricular rate. Abbreviated AF or AFib.
**ventricular f.,** arrhythmia characterized by fibrillary contractions of the ventricular muscle due to rapid repetitive excitation of myocardial fibers without coordinated contraction of the ventricle; it is an expression of randomized circus movement or of an ectopic focus with a very rapid cycle. Abbreviated VF or VFib.

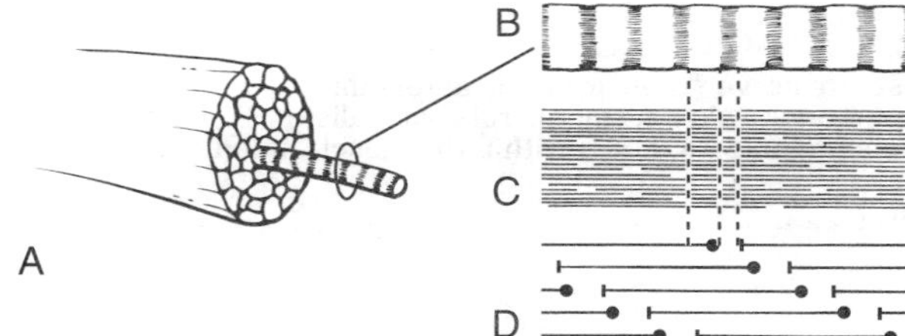

Type I collagen fibril *(A);* it is composed of unit fibrils, here shown negatively stained *(B).* The unit fibrils themselves comprise tropocollagen molecules in regular staggered arrays *(C, D).*

**Fi·bril·len·struk·tur** (fe-bril″en-shtrook′tər) [Ger.] the term used to describe the pattern of separate myofibrils that is typical of white skeletal muscles. Cf. *Felderstruktur.*

**fi·bril·lin** (fi-bril′in) a 350-kilodalton glycoprotein that is the main component of extracellular microfibrils; abnormal fibrillin metabolism results in a variety of connective tissue disorders, including Marfan syndrome.

**fi·bril·lo·blast** (fi-bril′o-blast) [*fibril* + *-blast*] odontoblast.

**fi·bril·lo·gen·e·sis** (fi-bril″o-jen′ə-sis) the formation of fibrils.

**fi·bril·lol·y·sis** (fi″brĭl-ol′ə-sis) the destruction or dissolution of fibrils or fibrillae.

**fi·bril·lo·lyt·ic** (fi″bril-o-lit′ik) destroying or dissolving fibrillae.

**fi·brin** (fi′brin) [MeSH: Fibrin] the insoluble protein formed from fibrinogen by the proteolytic action of thrombin during normal clotting of blood. Fibrin forms the essential portion of the blood clot.
**stroma f.,** fibrin obtained from the stroma of blood corpuscles.

**fi·brin·ase** (fi′brin-ās) [MeSH: Factor XIII] factor XIII; see under *coagulation factors,* at *factor.*

**fi·bri·no·cel·lu·lar** (fi″brĭ-no-sel′u-lər) made up of fibrin and cells.

**fi·brin·o·gen** (fi-brin′o-jən) [*fibrin* + *-gen*] [MeSH: Fibrinogen] factor I; see under *coagulation factors,* at *factor.*
**f., human,** a sterile fraction of normal human plasma, dried from the frozen state; administered by intravenous infusion to increase the coagulability of the blood.

**fi·brin·og·en·ase** (fi″brin-oj′ə-nās) [*fibrinogen* + *-ase*] thrombin.

**fi·brin·o·gen·emia** (fi-brin″o-jə-ne′me-ə) hyperfibrinogenemia.

**fi·bri·no·gen·e·sis** (fi″brĭ-no-jen′ə-sis) the production or formation of fibrin.

**fi·bri·no·gen·ic** (fi″brĭ-no-jen′ik) producing or causing the formation of fibrin; called also *fibrinogenous.*

**fi·bri·no·ge·nol·y·sis** (fi″brĭ-no-jə-nol′ə-sis) [*fibrinogen* + *-lysis*] the dissolution or inactivation of fibrinogen in the blood.

**fi·bri·no·geno·lyt·ic** (fi″brĭ-no-jen″o-lit′ik) pertaining to or inducing fibrinogenolysis.

**fi·brino·geno·pe·nia** (fi-brin″o-jen″o-pe′ne-ə) hypofibrinogenemia.

**fi·bri·nog·e·nous** (fi″brĭ-noj′ə-nəs) 1. fibrinogenic. 2. caused by fibrin, or resulting from the formation of fibrin.

**fi·brin·oid** (fi′brin-oid) [*fibrin* + *-oid*] 1. resembling fibrin. 2. a homogeneous, eosinophilic, refractile, relatively acellular material with some of the tinctorial properties of fibrin.

**fi·bri·nol·y·sin** (fi″brĭ-nol′ə-sin) plasmin.

**fi·bri·nol·y·sis** (fi″brĭ-nol′ə-sis) [*fibrin* + *-lysis*] [MeSH: Fibrinolysis] the dissolution of fibrin by enzymatic action.

**fi·bri·no·lyt·ic** (fi″brĭ-no-lit′ik) pertaining to, characterized by, or causing fibrinolysis.

**fi·bri·no·pep·tide** (fi″brĭ-no-pep′tid) either of two substances *(fibrinopeptide A* and *fibrinopeptide B)* split off from fibrinogen during coagulation, by the action of thrombin.

**fi·bri·no·plate·let** (fi″brĭ-no-plāt′lət) composed of fibrin and platelets, as a blood clot.

**fi·bri·no·pu·ru·lent** (fi″brĭ-no-pu′roo-lənt) characterized by the presence of both fibrin and pus.

**fi·bri·nor·rhea** (fi″brĭ-no-re′ə) a profuse discharge containing fibrin.

**fi·bri·nos·co·py** (fi-brĭ-nos′kə-pe) [*fibrin* + *-scopy*] inoscopy.

**fi·brin·ous** (fi′brin-əs) pertaining to or of the nature of fibrin.

**fi·brin·uria** (fi″brĭ-nu′re-ə) the presence of fibrin in the urine.

**fibr(o)-** [L. *fibra* fiber] a combining form denoting relationship to fibers.

**fi·bro·ad·e·no·ma** (fi″bro-ad″ə-no′mə) [MeSH: Fibroadenoma] adenoma containing fibrous tissue.
**giant f. of the breast,** phyllodes tumor.
**intracanalicular f.,** a fibroadenoma of the breast with irregularly shaped clefts within a fibrous stroma that contains strands or cords of epithelial tissue; polypoid masses grow inward and compress the ducts.
**pericanalicular f.,** a fibroadenoma of the breast with glandlike or cystlike spaces lined by epithelial cells in single or multiple layers.

**fi·bro·ad·e·no·sis** (fi″bro-ad″ə-no′sis) a nodular condition of the breast not due to neoplasm.

**fi·bro·ad·i·pose** (fi″bro-ad′ĭ-pōs) both fibrous and fatty.

**fi·bro·an·gi·o·ma** (fi″bro-an″je-o′mə) [*fibro-* + *angioma*] an angioma containing much fibrous tissue.
**nasopharyngeal f.,** juvenile nasopharyngeal angiofibroma.

**fi·bro·are·o·lar** (fi″bro-ə-re′o-lər) [*fibro-* + *areolar*] both fibrous and areolar.

**fi·bro·at·ro·phy** (fi″bro-at′ro-fe) a combination of fibrosis and atrophy.

**fi·bro·blast** (fi′bro-blast) [*fibro-* + *-blast*] [MeSH: Fibroblasts] 1. a connective tissue cell; a flat elongated cell with cytoplasmic processes at each end, having a flat, oval, vesicular nucleus. Fibroblasts, which differentiate into chondroblasts, collagenoblasts, and osteoblasts, form the fibrous tissues in the body including tendons, aponeuroses, supporting and binding tissues of all sorts. Called also *fibrocyte* and *desmocyte.* 2. collagenoblast.
**pericryptal f's,** flattened fibroblasts forming a sheath around the intestinal glands of the colon.

**fi·bro·blas·tic** (fi″bro-blas′tik) 1. pertaining to fibroblasts. 2. fibroplastic.

**fi·bro·blas·to·ma** (fi″bro-blas-to′mə) [*fibroblast* + *-oma*] a tumor arising from fibroblasts, divided into fibromas and fibrosarcomas.
**perineural f.,** neurilemoma.

**fi·bro·bron·chi·tis** (fi″bro-brong-ki′tis) fibrinous bronchitis.

**fi·bro·cal·cif·ic** (fi″bro-kal-sif′ik) pertaining to or characterized by partially calcified fibrous tissue.

**fi·bro·car·ci·no·ma** (fi″bro-kahr″sĭ-no′mə) scirrhous carcinoma.

**fi·bro·car·ti·lage** (fi″bro-kahr′tĭ-ləj) a type of cartilage made up of typical cartilage cells (chondrocytes), with parallel thick, compact collagenous bundles forming the interstitial substances, separated by narrow clefts enclosing the encapsulated cells; called also *stratified cartilage.* For names of specific structures composed of such tissue, see under *fibrocartilago.*
**basal f.,** fibrocartilago basalis.
**basilar f.,** synchondrosis spheno-occipitalis.
**circumferential f.,** fibrocartilage that forms a rim about a joint cavity.

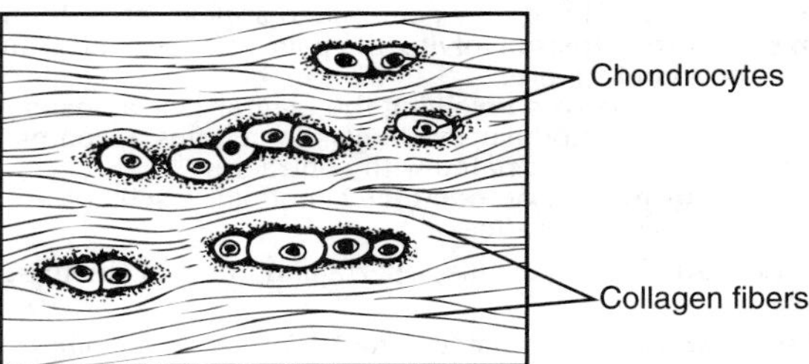

Fibrocartilage.

**connecting f.,** a disk of fibrocartilage that attaches opposing bones to each other by synchondrosis; called also *spongy f.*
**cotyloid f.,** labrum acetabulare.
**elastic f.,** fibrocartilage containing elastic fibers.
**interarticular f.,** an articular disk (def. 1); see terms beginning *discus articularis,* under *discus.*
**intervertebral f's,** disci intervertebrales.
**semilunar f's,** crescent-shaped structures resting on the articulating surfaces of the upper end of the tibia, increasing the concavity of the tibial condyles and acting as cushions or shock absorbers; the lateral and medial menisci.
**spongy f.,** connecting f.
**stratiform f.,** cartilage such as that lining the bony grooves lodging certain tendons.
**white f.,** fibrocartilage in which strong bundles of white fibrous tissue predominate.
**yellow f.,** fibrocartilage containing bundles of yellow elastic fibers but with little or no white fibrous tissue.

**fi·bro·car·ti·lag·i·nes** (fi″bro-kahr″tĭ-laj′ĭ-nēz) [L.] plural of *fibrocartilago.*

**fi·bro·car·ti·lag·i·nous** (fi″bro-kahr″tĭ-laj′ĭ-nəs) pertaining to or composed of fibrocartilage.

**fi·bro·car·ti·la·go** (fi″bro-kahr″tĭ-lah′go) pl. *fibrocartilag′ines* [L.] fibrocartilage: a general term for an anatomical structure composed of cartilage, the matrix of which contains a considerable amount of fibrous tissue; called also *stratified cartilage.*
**f. basa′lis,** basal fibrocartilage: the cartilage that fills the foramen lacerum of the skull.
**f. basila′ris,** synchondrosis spheno-occipitalis.
**fibrocartila′gines intervertebra′les,** disci intervertebrales.
**f. navicula′ris,** a fibrocartilaginous facet on the dorsal surface of the plantar calcaneonavicular ligament that helps form the articular cavity for the head of the talus.

**fi·bro·ca·seous** (fi″bro-ka′shəs) both fibrous and caseous.

**fi·bro·cel·lu·lar** (fi″bro-sel′u-lər) partly fibrous and partly cellular.

**fi·bro·chon·dri·tis** (fi″bro-kon-dri′tis) [*fibro-* + *chondritis*] inflammation of a fibrocartilage.

**fi·bro·chon·dro·ma** (fi″bro-kon-dro′mə) chondrofibroma.

**fi·bro·col·lag·e·nous** (fi″bro-ko-laj′ə-nəs) both fibrous and collagenous; pertaining to or composed of fibrous tissue mainly composed of collagen.

**fi·bro·cys·tic** (fi″bro-sis′tik) characterized by the development of cystic spaces, especially in relation to some duct or gland, accompanied by an overgrowth of fibrous tissue.

**fi·bro·cyte** (fi′bro-sīt) [*fibro-* + *-cyte*] fibroblast.

**fi·bro·cy·to·gen·e·sis** (fi′bro-si″to-jen′ə-sis) [*fibrocyte* + *-genesis*] the development of connective tissue fibrils.

**fi·bro·dys·pla·sia** (fi″bro-dis-pla′zhə) fibrous dysplasia.
**f. ossi′ficans progressi′va,** myositis ossificans progressiva.

**fi·bro·elas·tic** (fi″bro-e-las′tik) composed of fibrous and elastic tissue.

**fi·bro·elas·to·ma** (fi″bro-e-las-to′mə) a neoplasm consisting of fibroelastic elements.
**papillary f.,** the most common heart valve tumor, commonly seen post mortem, composed of a characteristic cluster of hairlike projections consisting of collagen surrounded by elastic fibers and connective tissue and covered by endothelium, attached to a valve or to the papillary muscles, chordae tendineae, or endocardium.

**fi·bro·elas·to·sis** (fi″bro-e″las-to′sis) overgrowth of fibroelastic elements.
**endocardial f.,** diffuse patchy thickening of the mural endocardium, particularly in the left ventricle, due to proliferation of collagenous and elastic tissue. It usually occurs in infants without other cardiac defects, but may occur in adolescents and adults, usually in association with congenital cardiac malformations. Thickening and incompetence of mitral and aortic valves is often associated. It is usually classified as *dilated* if the left ventricle is enlarged and hypertrophied or *contracted* if the left ventricle is of normal or reduced size.
**primary endocardial f.,** a congenital form of endocardial fibroelastosis, manifest in infancy and occurring unassociated with other cardiac defects.

**fi·bro·en·chon·dro·ma** (fi″bro-en″kon-dro′mə) [*fibro-* + *enchondroma*] enchondroma containing fibrous elements.

**fi·bro·ep·i·the·li·o·ma** (fi″bro-ep″ĭ-the″le-o′ma) a tumor composed of fibrous and epithelial elements.
**premalignant f.,** an uncommon, usually indolent, variant of basal cell carcinoma presenting as a firm sessile to pedunculated papule, usually located on the lower trunk or lumbosacral area in middle-aged or older adults. Histologically it is characterized by prominent

stromal fibrosis with long anastomosing cords of basal cells. Called also *premalignant fibroepithelial tumor.*

**fi·bro·fas·ci·tis** (fi″bro-fə-si′tis) fibrositis.

**fi·bro·fat·ty** (fi″bro-fat′e) both fibrous and fatty.

**fi·bro·fi·brous** (fi″bro-fi′brəs) joining or connecting fibers.

**fi·bro·fol·lic·u·lo·ma** (fi″bro-fə-lik″u-lo′mə) [*fibro-* + *folliculus* + *-oma*] a benign tumor of the perifollicular connective tissue, occurring as one or more yellowish-white, smooth, dome-shaped papules, usually on the face, and characterized histologically by proliferation of strands of follicular epithelium extending into the stroma. Multiple lesions usually occur as part of an autosomal dominant syndrome; see *Birt-Hogg-Dubé syndrome,* under *syndrome.*

**fi·bro·gen·e·sis** (fi″bro-jen′ə-sis) [*fibro-* + *genesis*] the development of fibers.
**f. imperfec′ta os′sium,** a rare collagen disorder causing osteomalacia, with progressive skeletal pain and tenderness.

**fi·bro·gen·ic** (fi″bro-jen′ik) conducive to the development of fibers.

**fi·brog·lia** (fi-brog′le-ə) [*fibro-* + *-glia*] border fibrils in close relation to the surface of fibroblasts, and thought by some to be transformations of the ectoplasm.

**fi·bro·hem·or·rhag·ic** (fi″bro-hem″o-raj′ik) attended with hemorrhage and fibrin formation.

**fi·bro·his·tio·cyt·ic** (fi″bro-his″te-o-sit′ik) having fibrous and histiocytic elements.

**fi·broid** (fi′broid) [*fibr-* + *-oid*] 1. having a fibrous structure; resembling a fibroma. 2. fibroma. 3. leiomyoma. 4. in the plural, a colloquial clinical term for uterine leiomyoma.

**fi·broid·ec·to·my** (fi″broid-ek′tə-me) [*fibroid* + *-ectomy*] uterine myomectomy.

**fi·bro·in** (fi-bro′in) [MeSH: Fibroin] a white albuminoid, $C_{15}H_{23}N_3O_6$, from spiders' webs and the cocoons of insects.

**fi·bro·la·mel·lar** (fi″bro-lə-mel′ər) characterized by the formation of fibers of collagen arranged in layers.

**fi·bro·li·po·ma** (fi″bro-lĭ-po′mə) [*fibro-* + *-lipoma*] lipoma containing an excess of fibrous tissue.

**fi·bro·li·po·ma·tous** (fi″bro-lĭ-po′mə-təs) pertaining to fibrolipoma.

**fi·bro·ma** (fi-bro′mə) pl. *fibromas, fibro′mata* [*fibr-* + *-oma*] [MeSH: Fibroma] a tumor composed mainly of fibrous or fully developed connective tissue; called also *fibroid* and *fibroid tumor.*
**ameloblastic f.,** an odontogenic tumor characterized by the simultaneous proliferation of both epithelial and mesenchymal tissue, without the formation of enamel or dentin.
**f. caverno′sum,** a cavernous hemangioma containing an excess of fibrous tissue.
**cementifying f.,** a tumor usually occurring in the mandible of older persons and consisting of fibroblastic tissue containing masses of cementum-like tissue.
**cemento-ossifying f.,** ossifying fibroma, particularly when characterized by globular cementoid calcifications.
**chondromyxoid f.,** a rare, benign, slowly growing tumor of bone of chondroblastic origin, usually affecting the large long bones of the lower extremity; it is characterized by chondroid, myxoid, and fibrous areas in a lobular pattern and often has a deceptively malignant histologic appearance resembling chondrosarcoma.
**cutaneous f.,** fibroma of the skin.
**cystic f.,** a fibroma that has undergone cystic degeneration.
**desmoplastic f.,** a rare, benign, fibrous, osteolytic neoplasm usually occurring in the mandible, in long tubular bones, or in the hip bone; it is characterized by abundant collagen formation and an absence of significant cellularity or pleomorphism.
**f. du′rum,** hard f.
**hard f.,** one composed of fibrous tissue with few cells; called also *f. durum.*
**intracanalicular f.,** see under *fibroadenoma.*
**juvenile nasopharyngeal f.,** see under *angiofibroma.*
**f. mol′le,** soft f.
**f. mollus′cum,** small subcutaneous nodules scattered over the body surface, seen in some forms of neurofibromatosis.
**f. myxomato′des,** myxofibroma.
**nonossifying f., nonosteogenic f.,** an osteolytic, proliferative, sometimes painful lesion comprising a focus of fibrous tissue in the metaphyseal region of long bones, particularly of the lower extremities, usually occurring in late childhood or adolescence; it is similar to fibrous cortical defect (q.v.) but is generally larger and actively growing. Called also *metaphyseal fibrous defect.*
**odontogenic f.,** a rare, benign, unencapsulated, odontogenic central tumor of the jaw, usually the mandible, occurring predominantly in women and characterized by islands of odontogenic epithelium within fibrous connective tissue and occasionally by calcifications.
**odontogenic f., peripheral,** an extraosseous counterpart to a central odontogenic fibroma; it is a gingival mass composed of vascularized fibrous connective tissue that contains strands of odontogenic epithelium. See also *odontogenic f.*
**ossifying f., ossifying f. of bone,** a benign, relatively slow-growing, central bone tumor, usually of the jaws, especially the mandible, which is composed of fibrous connective tissue within which bone is formed.
**ossifying f., peripheral,** a fibroma, usually of the gingiva, showing areas of calcification or ossification. Called also *epulis.*
**parasitic f.,** see under *leiomyoma.*
**f. pen′dulum,** soft f.
**perifollicular f.,** one or more small, flesh-colored, papular follicular lesions on the head and neck, characterized by hyperplastic, well-differentiated connective tissue surrounding the hair follicles.
**periungual f.,** one of multiple smooth, firm, protruding nodules, histologically angiofibromas, occurring at the nail folds and considered to be pathognomonic of tuberous sclerosis. Called also *Koenen's tumor.*
**rabbit f.,** a benign viral disease of the wild cottontail rabbit, caused by a poxvirus, transmissible to laboratory rabbits, and marked by the development of fibromas that regress; called also *Shope f.*
**recurrent digital f. of childhood,** infantile digital fibromatosis.
**Shope f.,** rabbit f.
**soft f.,** a large pedunculated acrochordon. Called also *f. pendulum.*
**telangiectatic f.,** angiofibroma.
**f. thecocellula′re xanthomato′des,** theca cell tumor.
**f. xantho′ma,** fibroxanthoma.

**fi·bro·ma·to·gen·ic** (fi-bro″mə-to-jen′ik) producing or causing the formation of fibroma.

**fi·bro·ma·toid** (fi-bro′mə-toid) resembling fibroma; fibroma-like.

**fi·bro·ma·to·sis** (fi-bro″mə-to′sis) pl. *fibromatoses* 1. the formation of a fibrous, tumorlike nodule arising from the deep fascia with a tendency to local recurrence, as in desmoid tumor. 2. a condition characterized by the formation of multiple fibromas.
**aggressive f.,** desmoid, particularly an extra-abdominal desmoid.
**f. col′li,** a firm, fusiform, fibrous mass in the midportion of the sternocleidomastoid muscle, usually occurring between two weeks and two months of age, and commonly disappearing in four to eight months; in some instances, torticollis may develop. It is believed by some to be a small hematoma due to injury to the muscle at birth.
**congenital generalized f.,** a condition in which multiple small, firm, spherical or ovoid fibromas of the subcutaneous and muscle tissues, the viscera, and the osseous systems are characteristically present at birth. Visceral involvement may be responsible for various symptoms, such as intestinal obstruction, diarrhea due to diffuse involvement of the intestines, and respiratory disturbances. Death frequently occurs during the neonatal period or early infancy. Called also *infantile myofibroma* and *juvenile myofibromatosis.*
**f. gingi′vae, gingival f.,** 1. generalized or localized diffuse fibrous overgrowth of the gingival tissue, usually transmitted as an autosomal dominant trait, but some cases are idiopathic and others produced by drugs (see *Dilantin gingivitis,* under *gingivitis*). The enlarged gingiva is pink, firm, and leatherlike with a minutely pebbled surface and in severe cases the teeth are almost completely covered and the enlargement projects into the oral vestibule. Called also *elephantiasis gingivae, keloid of gums,* and *macrogingivae.* 2. fibromatous epulis, def. 2.
**infantile digital f.,** a rare, often recurrent, condition, usually occurring in infants less than a year old, in which one or more small, smooth, dome-shaped, skin-colored to slightly red nodules occur on the lateral or dorsal aspects of the fingers and toes; histologically, the lesions are composed of fibrous connective tissue and abundant collagen, and contain characteristic viruslike, black intracellular inclusions. Called also *recurring digital fibrous tumors of childhood.*
**juvenile hyaline f.,** a rare disorder, of autosomal recessive inheritance, characterized by multiple painless cutaneous papules containing spindle-shaped cells in an amorphous, acidophilic ground substance, occurring on the head, back, and extremities; lesions recur after removal and may continue to appear into adulthood.
**palmar f.,** fibromatosis involving the palmar fascia, and resulting in Dupuytren's contracture.
**plantar f.,** fibromatosis involving the plantar fascia, manifested as single or multiple nodular swellings, sometimes accompanied by pain but usually unassociated with contractures.
**subcutaneous pseudosarcomatous f.,** nodular fasciitis.
**f. ventri′culi,** linitis plastica.

**fi·bro·ma·tous** (fi-bro′mə-təs) pertaining to or of the nature of fibroma.

**fi·bro·mec·to·my** (fi″bro-mek′tə-me) [*fibroma* + *-ectomy*] 1. excision of a fibroma. 2. uterine myomectomy.

**fi·bro·mem·bra·nous** (fi″bro-mem′brə-nəs) composed of membrane containing much fibrous tissue.

**fi·bro·mus·cu·lar** (fi″bro-mus′ku-lər) composed of fibrous and muscular tissue.

**fi·bro·my·al·gia** (fi″bro-mi-al′jə) pain and stiffness in the muscles and joints that is either diffuse or has multiple trigger points.

**fi·bro·my·itis** (fi″bro-mi-i′tis) [*fibro-* + *myitis*] inflammation and fibrous degeneration of a muscle.

**fi·bro·my·o·ma** (fi″bro-mi-o′mə) [*fibro-* + *myoma*] leiomyoma.
**f. u′teri,** leiomyoma uteri.

**fi·bro·myo·mec·to·my** (fi″bro-mi″o-mek′tə-me) uterine myomectomy.

**fi·bro·myo·si·tis** (fi″bro-mi″o-si′tis) [*fibro-* + *myositis*] inflammation of fibromuscular tissue.
**nodular f.,** a disease marked by inflammation and the formation of nodules in the muscles.

**fi·bro·myx·o·ma** (fi″bro-mik-so′mə) myxofibroma.

**fi·bro·myx·o·sar·co·ma** (fi″bro-mik″so-sahr-ko′mə) [*fibro-* + *myxo-* + *sarcoma*] sarcoma containing fibromatous and myxomatous elements.

**fi·bro·nec·tin** (fi″bro-nek′tin) [*fibro-* + *nexus*] any of several related adhesive glycoproteins. One form circulates in plasma, acting as an opsonin; another is a cell-surface protein that mediates cellular adhesive interactions. Fibronectins are important in connective tissue, where they cross-link to collagen, and are also involved in aggregation of platelets.

**fi·bro·neu·ro·ma** (fi″bro-noo͝-ro′mə) neurofibroma.

**fi·bro·nu·cle·ar** (fi″bro-noo′kle-ər) made up of nucleated fibers.

**fi·bro-odon·to·ma** (fi″bro-o″don-to′mə) [*fibro-* + *odont-* + *oma*] a tumor containing both fibrous and odontogenic elements.
**ameloblastic f.-o.,** a variant form of ameloblastic fibroma in which enamel and dentin are formed.

**fi·bro·os·se·ous** (fi″bro-os′e-əs) composed of both fibrous and bony tissue.

**fi·bro·os·te·o·ma** (fi″bro-os″te-o′mə) [*fibroma* + *osteoma*] ossifying fibroma.

**fi·bro·pap·il·lo·ma** (fi″bro-pap″ĭ-lo′mə) fibroepithelial papilloma.

**fi·bro·pi·tu·i·cyte** (fi″bro-pĭ-too′ĭ-sīt) see *pituicyte.*

**fi·bro·pla·sia** (fi″bro-pla′zhə) the formation of fibrous tissue, as occurs normally in the healing of wounds and abnormally in some tissues.
**retrolental f. (RLF),** retinopathy of prematurity.

**fi·bro·plas·tic** (fi″bro-plas′tik) [*fibro-* + *plastic*] giving origin to fibrous tissue.

**fi·bro·plate** (fi′bro-plāt) an interarticular fibrocartilage.

**fi·bro·poly·pus** (fi″bro-pol′ə-pəs) a polyp containing fibrous elements.

**fi·bro·pu·ru·lent** (fi″bro-pu′roo-lənt) characterized by the presence of both fibers and pus.

**fi·bro·re·tic·u·late** (fi″bro-rə-tik′u-lāt) composed of a network of fibers.

**fi·bro·sar·co·ma** (fi″bro-sahr-ko′mə) [*fibro-* + *sarcoma*] [MeSH: Fibrosarcoma] a malignant tumor composed of cells and fibers derived from fibroblasts, which produce collagen but otherwise lack cellular differentiation; it is grossly grayish white and firm, invades locally, and metastasizes hematogenously. Several varieties occur: an aggressive *adult* form, a rarely metastasizing *infantile* or *congenital* form, an *inflammatory* form, and a *postirradiation* form.
**ameloblastic f.,** an odontogenic tumor that is the malignant counterpart to an ameloblastic fibroma, within which it usually arises. Called also *ameloblastic sarcoma.*
**odontogenic f.,** a malignant tumor of the jaws, originating from one of the mesenchymal components of the tooth or tooth germ, and histologically identical with other fibrosarcomas; the malignant counterpart of odontogenic fibroma.

**fi·bro·scle·ro·sis** (fi″bro-sklə-ro′sis) fibrosis associated with sclerosis.
**multifocal f.,** any of a group of disorders of unknown etiology characterized by fibrosis, including mediastinal, hilar, and retroperitoneal fibrosis, Riedel's struma, and sclerosing cholangitis.

**fi·brose** (fi′brōs) 1. to form fibrous tissue. 2. fibrous.

**fi·bro·se·rous** (fi″bro-se′rəs) composed of both fibrous and serous elements.

**fi·bro·sis** (fi-bro′sis) [MeSH: Fibrosis] the formation of fibrous tissue, as in repair or replacement of parenchymatous elements.
**African endomyocardial f.,** endomyocardial f.
**congenital hepatic f.,** a developmental disorder of the liver marked by formation of irregular broad bands of fibrous tissue containing multiple cysts formed by disordered terminal bile ducts, chiefly in the portal areas, resulting in vascular constriction, which leads to portal hypertension. It may be associated with polycystic renal disease.
**cystic f., cystic f. of the pancreas,** an autosomal recessive disorder of infants, children, and young adults in which there is widespread dysfunction of the exocrine glands, with signs of chronic pulmonary disease (due to excess mucus production in the respiratory tract), pancreatic deficiency, abnormally high levels of electrolytes in the sweat, and occasionally biliary cirrhosis. Pathologically, the pancreas shows obstruction of its ducts by amorphous eosinophilic concretions, with consequent deficiency of pancreatic enzymes, resulting in steatorrhea and azotorrhea. The degree of involvement of organs and glandular systems may vary greatly, with consequent variations in the clinical picture. Called also *fibrocystic disease of the pancreas* and *mucoviscidosis.*
**diatomite f.,** a form of silicosis caused by inhalation of the dust of diatomite (hard, dry infusorial earth).
**diffuse interstitial pulmonary f.,** idiopathic pulmonary f.
**endomyocardial f.,** idiopathic myocardiopathy occurring endemically in various regions of Africa and rarely in other areas, characterized by cardiomegaly, marked thickening of the endocardium with dense, white fibrous tissue that frequently extends to involve the inner third or half of the myocardium, and congestive heart failure. Called also *African endomyocardial f.*
**graphite f.,** see under *pneumoconiosis.*
**idiopathic pulmonary f.,** chronic inflammation and progressive fibrosis of the pulmonary alveolar walls, with steadily progressive dyspnea, resulting finally in death from oxygen lack or right heart failure. Sometimes it is a component of bronchiolitis obliterans with organizing pneumonia (see under *bronchiolitis*).The acute, rapidly fatal form is called *acute interstitial pneumonia* or *Hamman-Rich syndrome.* Called also *chronic fibrous pneumonia, interstitial* or *usual interstitial pneumonia, diffuse interstitial pulmonary f., fibrosing alveolitis,* and *interstitial* or *interstitial pulmonary f.*
**idiopathic retroperitoneal f.,** retroperitoneal f.
**interstitial f., interstitial pulmonary f.,** idiopathic pulmonary f.
**mediastinal f.,** development of whitish, hard fibrous tissue in the upper mediastinum, causing compression, distortion, or obliteration of the superior vena cava, and sometimes constriction of the bronchi and large pulmonary vessels.
**neoplastic f.,** proliferative f.
**nodular subepidermal f.,** the formation beneath the epidermis of multiple fibrous nodules as a result of productive inflammation. It is a form of benign fibrous histiocytoma, and the two terms are sometimes used synonymously; alternatively, it is sometimes used synonymously with dermatofibroma.
**panmural f. of the bladder,** chronic interstitial cystitis.
**periureteric f.,** progressive development of fibrous tissue, spreading laterally from the great midline vessels, gradually engulfing, distorting, and finally causing strangulation of one or both ureters.
**pipestem f.,** fibrosis around hepatic portal veins, seen as a complication of hepatic schistosomiasis. Called also *Symmers's f.*
**pleural f.,** fibrosis of the visceral pleura so that part or all of a lung becomes covered with a plaque or a thick layer of nonexpansible fibrous tissue. The more extensive form is called *fibrothorax.*
**postfibrinous f.,** fibrosis occurring in tissues in which fibrin has been deposited.
**progressive massive f.,** a complication of silicosis or coal workers' pneumoconiosis in which there is at least one dense lung lesion more than 1 cm in diameter; there are usually multiple lesions in the upper parts of the lungs, and they grow larger and more dense over time. The condition may be accompanied by emphysema or ischemia adjacent to the lesions.
**proliferative f.,** fibrosis in which the fibrous elements continue to proliferate after the original causative factor has ceased to operate; called also *neoplastic f.*
**pulmonary f.,** see *idiopathic pulmonary f.*
**replacement f.,** the development of fibrous tissues to replace tissue that has been damaged.
**retroperitoneal f.,** deposition of fibrous tissue in the retroperitoneal space, producing vague abdominal discomfort, and often causing blockage of the ureters, with resultant hydronephrosis and impaired renal function, which may result in renal failure.
**root sleeve f.,** fibrosis and thickening of the dura mater resulting from prolonged nerve root pressure.
**Symmers' f.,** pipestem f.

**fi·bro·si·tis** (fi″bro-si′tis) [*fibro-* + *-itis* ] inflammation especially of the muscle sheaths and fascial layers of the locomotor system; it is marked by pain and stiffness. Called also *fibrofascitis* and *muscular rheumatism.*

**fi·bro·tho·rax** (fi″bro-thor′aks) adhesion of the two layers of pleura, so that the lung is covered by a thick layer of nonexpansible fibrous tissue (see *dry pleurisy*). It is often a consequence of traumatic hemothorax or of pleural effusion.

**fi•brot•ic** (fi-brot′ik) pertaining to or characterized by fibrosis.

**fi•brous** (fi′brəs) composed of or containing fibers.

**fi•bro•vas•cu•lar** (fi″bro-vas′ku-lər) both fibrous and vascular.

**fi•bro•xan•tho•ma** (fi″bro-zan-tho′mə) [*fibro-* + *xanthoma*] a type of xanthoma containing fibromatous elements; it is sometimes described as synonymous with or a subtype of either benign or malignant fibrous histiocytoma.
**atypical f. (AFX),** a small nodular cutaneous neoplasm usually occurring on sun-exposed areas of the face and neck in older white adults; it contains cells resembling histiocytes and fibroblasts and is sometimes considered to be related to or a subtype of either benign or malignant fibrous histiocytoma.

**fi•bro•xan•tho•sar•co•ma** (fi″bro-zan″tho-sahr-ko′mə) [*fibro-* + *xanthosarcoma*] malignant fibrous histiocytoma.

**fib•u•la** (fib′u-lə) [L. "buckle"] [TA] [MeSH: Fibula] the outer and smaller of the two bones of the leg, which articulates proximally with the tibia and distally is joined to the tibia in a syndesmosis. See Plate 45.

**fib•u•lar** (fib′u-lər) pertaining to the fibula; peroneal.

**fib•u•la•ris** (fib′u-lar′is) [TA] fibular, peroneal; a term designating relationship to the fibula. Called also *peronealis* [TA alternative].

**fib•u•lo•cal•ca•ne•al** (fib″u-lo-kal-ka′ne-əl) pertaining to the fibula and calcaneus.

**fi•cain** (fi′kān) [EC 3.4.22.3] an enzyme of the hydrolase class that catalyzes the cleavage of proteins on the carboxyl side of lysine, alanine, tyrosine, glycine, asparagine, leucine, and valine bonds. It is a cysteine endopeptidase derived from the sap of fig trees. Because it enhances the agglutination of red blood cells with IgG antibodies, it is used in the determination of the Rh factor; it is also used as a protein digestant in a variety of industrial applications.

**FICD** Fellow of the International College of Dentists.

**fi•cin** (fi′sin) [MeSH: Ficin] ficain.

**Fick's first law of diffusion, formula,** etc. (fiks) [Adolph Eugen *Fick*, German physiologist, 1829–1901] see under *formula, law, method,* and *principle.*

**FICS** Fellow of the International College of Surgeons.

**Fi•cus** (fi′kəs) the figs, a genus of tropical shrubs and trees of the family Moraceae. *F. cari′ca* is the common fig tree. *F. anthelmin′tica* Mart. is a wild species native to Central and South America whose sap, *leche de higuerón,* is medicinal. *F. bengalen′sis* is the banyan or banian, a species native to India and the East Indies whose branches send down auxiliary trunks that take root in the soil; its seeds and bark are tonic, antipyretic, and diuretic. *F. elas′ticus* is the source of one kind of rubber.

**fi•dic•i•na•les** (fi-dis″ĭ-na′lēz) [pl., from L. *fidicen, fidicinis,* a player on the harp] musculi lumbricales manus.

**Fied•ler's disease, myocarditis** (fēd′lərz) [Carl Ludwig Alfred *Fiedler,* German physician, 1835–1921] see *Weil's syndrome,* under *syndrome,* and see *acute isolated myocarditis,* under *myocarditis.*

**field** (fēld) 1. an area or open space, as an operative field or visual field. 2. a range of specialization in knowledge, study, or occupation. 3. in embryology, the developing region within a range of modifying factors.
**auditory f.,** the space or range within which stimuli may be perceived as sound.
**Cohnheim's f's,** see under *area.*
**dark-f.,** see under *microscope,* and see *ultramicroscope.*
**electric f.,** a region of space in which an electric intensity exists at every point, causing charged bodies to be attracted to or repelled from each other; it is associated with an electromagnetic wave or a changing magnetic field.
**electromagnetic f.,** a field of force resulting from electric charge in motion and having associated electric and magnetic components.
**extended f.,** in radiotherapy, as for malignant lymphoma, an area of irradiation beyond the involved field.
**eye f.,** see *frontal eye f.* and *occipital eye f.*
**f. of fixation,** the region bounded by the utmost limits of central or clear vision, the eye being allowed to move, but the head being fixed.
**Flechsig's f.,** myelinogenetic f.
**f's of Forel, Forel's f's,** three areas in the ventral thalamus that are rich in nerve fibers and associated with cell groups. They are designated *fields H, $H_1$,* and *$H_2$*. Called also *areas of Forel.*
**frontal eye f.,** an area in the precentral and frontal gyri (Brodmann areas 8, part of 6, and part of 9) concerned with the control of conjugate eye movements. Cf. *occipital eye f.*
**gamma f.,** any area subjected to radiation from an unshielded or slightly shielded gamma radiation source.
**f. H, f. H of Forel,** one of the fields of Forel, lying medial to the subthalamic nucleus, immediately rostral to the red nucleus; it is a large area in which pallidofugal, dentatothalamic, and rubrothalamic fibers and associated nuclei merge, uniting fields $H_1$ and $H_2$. Called also *prerubral f.* and *tegmental f.*
**f. $H_1$, f. $H_1$ of Forel,** one of the fields of Forel; it is the area occupied by the thalamic fasciculus, although the term is sometimes used synonymously with thalamic fasciculus.
**f. $H_2$, f. $H_2$ of Forel,** one of the fields of Forel; it is the area along the course of the lenticular fasciculus where the fibers of the fasciculus merge with the dorsal aspect of the subthalamic nucleus and the ventral aspect of the zona incerta.
**high-power f.,** the area of a slide visible under the high magnification system of a microscope.
**individuation f.,** a region in which an organizer influences adjacent tissue to become a part of a total embryo.
**inverted Y f.,** in radiotherapy, as for malignant lymphoma, a circumscribed area of irradiation below the diaphragm, covering the spleen, extending down the midline, and branching inferiorly to form tails across the inguinal areas.
**involved f.,** in radiotherapy, as for malignant lymphoma, the irradiated area when irradiation has been limited to sites of detectable macroscopic disease.
**low-power f.,** the area of a slide visible under the low magnification system of a microscope.
**magnetic f.,** that portion of space about a magnet in which its action is perceptible.
**mantle f.,** in radiotherapy, as for malignant lymphoma, a circumscribed area of irradiation around the shoulders and chest, including the neck, clavicular regions, axillae, and mediastinum.
**f. of a microscope,** the area that can be seen through a microscope at one time. The *high-power f.* is that area which is visible under the high-power objective; the *low-power f.* is that which is visible under low power.
**morphogenetic f.,** an embryonic region, larger than its main derivatives, out of which definite structures normally develop.
**myelinogenetic f.,** a collection of fibers in the neuraxis which at a definite stage of development receive myelin sheaths; called also *Flechsig's f.*
**occipital eye f.,** any of several motor areas of the visual cortex that control voluntary or involuntary movements of the eye muscles. Cf. *frontal eye f.*
**operative f.,** an isolated area where surgery is performed; it must be kept sterile by aseptic techniques (q.v.). Called also *surgical f.*
**para-aortic f.,** in radiotherapy, as for malignant lymphoma, an area of irradiation below the diaphragm, covering the spleen and extending down the midline but ending before the pelvic area.
**penumbra f.,** the region of free space which is irradiated by primary photons coming from only part of the radiation source.
**prerubral f.,** f. H.
**primary nail f.,** a flat area on the terminal phalanx in the embryo where the nail is to develop.
**sterile f.,** an operative field that is properly sterile according to aseptic techniques (q.v.).
**surgical f.,** operative f.

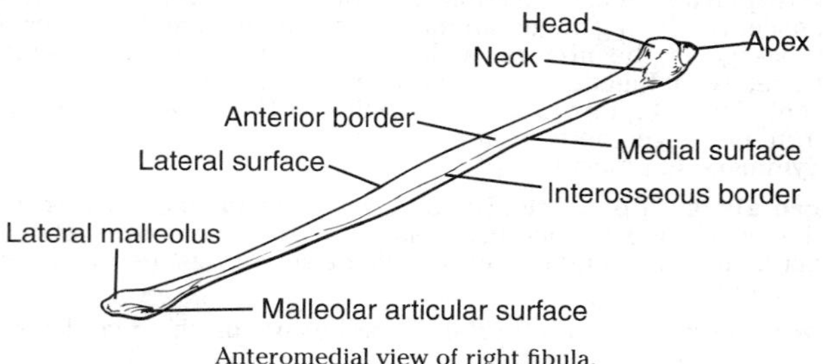

Anteromedial view of right fibula.

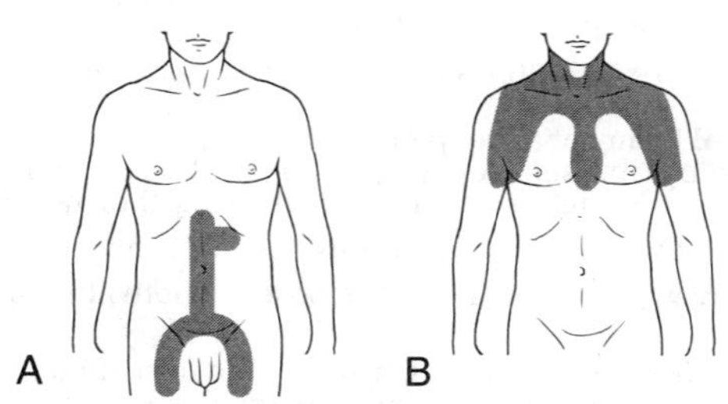

*(A),* Inverted Y field; *(B),* mantle field.

**surplus f.**, the portion of the field of vision in partial hemianopia which passes beyond the point of fixation.
**tegmental f.**, f. H.
**f. of vision**, visual f.
**f. of vision, cribriform**, a field of vision over which a number of isolated scotomas lie dispersed.
**visual f.**, the area within which stimuli produce the sensation of sight with the eye in a straight-ahead position; also called *f. of vision.* Symbol F or vf.
**Wernicke's f.**, see under *area.*

**Fies·sing·er-Le·roy-Rei·ter syndrome** (fe′sing-er-lə-rwah′ rī′tər) [Noël Armand *Fiessinger,* French physician, 1881–1946; Emile *Leroy,* French physician, born 1873; Hans Conrad *Reiter,* German physician, 1881–1969] Reiter's syndrome.

**fièv·re** (fe-ev′rə) [Fr.] fever.
**f. boutonneuse** (boo-tən-ooz′), boutonneuse fever.

**FIGLU** formiminoglutamic acid.

**FIGO** Fédération Internationale de Gynécologie et d'Obstétrique (International Federation of Gynecology and Obstetrics); see under *classification.*

**fig·u·ra·tum** (fig″u-ra′təm) [L.] figured; said of skin lesions that have geometric patterns.

**fig·ure** (fig′yər) [L. *figura,* from *fingere* to shape or form] 1. an object of a particular form. 2. a number, or numeral.
**flame f.**, a skin lesion seen with Wells' syndrome, in which eosinophils and histiocytes surround collagenous masses and form small areas of necrosis.
**fortification f's**, fortification spectra; see under *spectrum.*
**Minkowski's f.**, a numerical expression of the relation between glucose and nitrogen in the urine on a pure meat diet, and when fasting. It is 2.8:1.
**mitotic f's**, stages of chromosome aggregation exhibiting a pattern characteristic of mitosis.
**Purkinje f's**, patterns of shadows of retinal blood vessels cast onto the retina by obliquely projected light; called also *Purkinje's shadows.*
**Stifel's f.**, a black disk having a white spot in the center, used for locating and measuring the blind spot in the eye.
**Zöllner's f's**, see under *line.*

**fi·la** (fi′lə) [L.] plural of *filum.*

**fi·la·ceous** (fi-la′shəs) made up of filaments.

**fil·a·ment** (fil′ə-mənt) [L. *filamentum,* from *filum* thread] a delicate fiber or thread.
**acrosomal f.**, a long, thin, rigid filament projecting from the head of a spermatozoon; it is formed by elongation of the central part of the acrosome in preparation for the fertilization process, and is used to make contact with and to penetrate the cell membrane of the oocyte.
**actin f.**, one of the thin contractile myofilaments in a myofibril, composed mainly of actin; each actin filament is surrounded by three myosin filaments.
**axial f.**, axoneme.
**desmin f's**, intermediate filaments composed of desmin and occurring in muscle cells; they provide a cytoskeletal framework to hold myofibrils in place and thus coordinate contraction of the cells.
**glial f's**, intermediate filaments composed of glial fibrillary acidic protein and occurring in nonneuronal cells of the central nervous system, particularly astrocytes; they provide a framework for the cells and their cytoplasmic processes.
**intermediate f's**, a class of cytoplasmic filaments 8–11 nm in diameter that predominantly act as structural components of the cytoskeleton and also effect various movements in cellular processes. The proteins forming the different filaments are diverse and tissue specific. See also *desmin f's, glial filaments, keratin filaments, vimentin filaments, neurofilament,* and *lamin.*
**keratin f's**, intermediate filaments composed of cytokeratins; they are usually heteropolymers formed from one acidic and one basic cytokeratin and are present in most epithelial cells. The cytokeratin composition varies in different types, states, and degrees of differentiation of the epithelia and has been used as an immunohistochemical marker. Keratin filaments form a cytoskeletal framework, anchoring other elements and inserting into sites of cell-to-cell contact and are thus tonofilaments (q.v.).
**linin f.**, a network of linin spread throughout the cell nucleus.
**lymphatic anchoring f's**, filaments that attach the endothelial cells of lymphatic capillaries to the connective tissue between surrounding tissue cells.
**meningeal f., f. of meninges**, filum terminale.
**muscle f.**, myofilament.
**myosin f.**, one of the thick contractile myofilaments in a myofibril, composed mainly of myosin; each myosin filament is surrounded by six actin filaments.
**pial f. of filum terminale**, pars pialis fili terminalis.
**polar injecting f.**, polar tube.
**root f's of spinal nerve**, fila radicularia nervi spinalis.
**spermatic f.**, end piece.
**spinal f.**, filum terminale.
**terminal f.**, 1. filum terminale. 2. end piece.
**terminal f., dural, terminal f., external**, pars duralis fili terminalis.
**terminal f., internal, terminal f., pial**, pars pialis fili terminalis.
**terminal f. of spinal dura mater**, pars duralis fili terminalis.
**thick f's**, bipolar myosin filaments, 12–14 nm in diameter and 1.6 μm in length, occurring in striated muscle; the term may also be used to denote filaments, often much shorter, occurring elsewhere. See also *myofilament.*
**thin f's**, actin filaments, 7–9 nm in diameter and 1 μm in length, attached to the Z-disks in striated muscle; they are composed of F-actin associated with troponin and tropomyosin. See also *myofilament.*
**vimentin f's**, intermediate filaments composed of vimentin and occurring in a variety of cells derived from embryonic mesenchyme; they act as cytoskeletal support structures, play a role in mitosis, and are clustered particularly around the nucleus, probably helping to control its location. In cells containing more than one type of intermediate filament, vimentin filaments are always present.

**fil·a·men·ta** (fil″ə-men′tə) [L.] plural of *filamentum.*

**fil·a·men·tous** (fil″ə-men′təs) composed of long, threadlike structures; said of bacterial colonies.

**fil·a·men·tum** (fil″ə-men′təm) pl. *filamen′ta* [L.] a filament.

**fil·a·min** (fil′ə-min) an actin-binding protein found in smooth muscle and other cells; it helps bind actin filaments into loose bundles that are not disrupted in the presence of calcium.

**fi·lar** (fi′lər) [L. *filum* thread] threadlike; filamentous.

**Fi·la·ria** (fī-lar′e-ə) [L. *filum* thread] a name formerly used as a genus to include some members of the superfamily Filarioidea, now classified in a variety of genera.
**F. bancrof′ti**, *Wuchereria bancrofti.*
**F. demarquay′i**, *Mansonella ozzardi.*
**F. diur′na**, *Loa loa.* The name was actually applied to the microfilaria *(microfilaria diurna).*
**F. equi′na**, *Setaria equina.*
**F. immit′is**, *Dirofilaria immitis.*
**F. jun′cea**, *Mansonella ozzardi.*
**F. lo′a**, *Loa loa.*
**F. medinen′sis**, former name for *Dracunculus medinensis.*
**F. noctur′na**, *Wuchereria bancrofti.*
**F. ozzar′di**, *Mansonella ozzardi.*
**F. per′stans**, *Mansonella perstans.*
**F. recon′dita**, *Dipetalonema reconditum.*
**F. san′guinis-ho′minis**, *Wuchereria bancrofti.*
**F. vol′vulus**, *Onchocerca volvulus.*

**fi·la·ria** (fī-lar′e-ə) pl. *fila′riae* [L. *filum* thread] a nematode worm of the superfamily Filarioidea.
**Bancroft's f.**, *Wuchereria bancrofti.*
**Brug's f.**, *Brugia malayi.*

**fi·la·riae** (fī-lar′e-e) [L.] plural of *filaria.*

**fi·la·ri·al** (fī-lar′e-əl) pertaining to, caused by, or denoting filariae.

**fil·a·ri·a·sis** (fil″ə-ri′ə-sis) [MeSH: Filariasis] infestation by filariae.
**bancroftian f.**, infection with the filarial worm *Wuchereria bancrofti,* the adults of which reside in the lymphatic system, producing recurrent lymphangitis with fibrosis and obstruction. In extensive obstruction, chronic edema may result, progressing to elephantiasis. Microfilariae circulate in the blood, where they are transmitted to feeding mosquitoes, the vector and intermittent host.
**brugian f.**, infection with filarial worms of the species *Brugia malayi* and *B. timori,* the adult forms of which reside in the lymphatics, lymph nodes, and connective tissue; symptoms range from asymptomatic adenitis, to periodic attacks of fever and lymphangitis, to elephantiasis, especially of the legs and feet. Microfilariae circulate in the blood, where they are transmitted to feeding mosquitoes, the vector and intermediate host.
**lymphatic f.**, a general term comprising bancroftian and brugian filariasis.
**Malayan f.**, brugian filariasis caused by *Brugia malayi.*
**occult f.**, a condition in which microfilariae are present in the tissues but not in the blood; see *tropical pulmonary eosinophilia,* under *eosinophilia.*
**Ozzard's f.**, infection with *Mansonella ozzardi.*
**Timorian f.**, brugian filariasis caused by *Brugia timori.*

**fi·lar·i·cid·al** (fī-lar″ĭ-sīd′əl) [*filaria* + L. *caedere* to kill] destructive to filariae.

**fi·lar·i·cide** (fī-lar′ĭ-sīd) an agent that is destructive to filariae.

**fi·lar·i·form** (fī-lar′ĭ-form) threadlike; resembling filariae; denoting that developmental stage in the life cycle of certain nematodes which is characterized by the possession of an esophagus of uniform diameter and which is often, as in hookworms, the infective stage.

**Fi·lar·i·oi·dea** (fī-lar″e-oi′de-ə) [MeSH: Filarioidea] a superfamily or order of nematode parasites, the adults being threadlike worms which invade the tissues and body cavities where the female deposits embryonated eggs (prelarvae) known as microfilariae. These microfilariae are ingested by blood-sucking insects in whom they pass their developmental stage and are returned to man by the bites of such insects. Genera infecting humans include *Brugia, Dipetalonema, Loa, Mansonella, Onchocerca,* and *Wuchereria.* Those infecting domestic animals include *Dirofilaria, Parafilaria, Setaria,* and *Stephanofilaria.*

**Fi·la·roi·des** (fil″ə-roi′dēz) a genus of nematodes of the family Filaroididae. *F. hir′thi* and *F. os′leri* are lungworms that cause verminous bronchitis and occasionally verminous pneumonia in dogs.

**Fil·a·roi·di·dae** (fil″ə-roi′dĭ-de) a family of nematodes that infest the respiratory tract of mammals. It includes one genus of veterinary interest, *Filaroides.*

**Fi·lat·ov's (Fi·lat·ow's) disease** (fe-lah′tofs) [Nils Fedorovich *Filatov,* Russian pediatrician, 1847–1902] infectious mononucleosis.

**Fi·lat·ov-Dukes disease** (fī-lah′tof-dōōks) [N. F. *Filatov;* Clement *Dukes,* English physician, 1845–1925] Dukes' disease.

**Fil·des enrichment agar** (fil′dəz) [Sir Paul Gordon *Fildes,* English bacteriologist, 1882–1971] see under *culture medium.*

**file** (fīl) a surgical or a dental instrument with a finely serrated surface, for reducing surplus hard substance such as bone or materials used in dental restorations, or for smoothing roughened surfaces.
**endodontic f.,** root canal f.
**root canal f.,** one used in root canal therapy for cleaning and shaping the canal. Called also *endodontic f.*

**fil·gras·tim** (fil-gras′tim) [MeSH: Filgrastim] a human granulocyte colony-stimulating factor (G-CSF) produced by recombinant DNA technology, used to stimulate neutrophil production, reduce the duration of neutropenia, and reduce the incidence of infection in patients receiving myelosuppressive chemotherapy for non-myeloid malignancies; administered subcutaneously or intravenously.

**fil·i·cin** (fil′ĭ-cin) a compound found in oil of male fern.

**fil·i·form** (fil′ĭ-form, fi′lĭ-form) [*filum* + *form*] 1. thread shaped. 2. an extremely slender bougie.

**fil·io·pa·ren·tal** (fil″e-o-pə-ren′təl) pertaining to the relationships between children and their parents.

**Fi·li·po·vitch's (Fi·li·po·wicz's) sign** (fe-le-po′vich-əz) [Casimir *Filipovitch,* Polish physician, 19th century] see under *sign.*

**fi·lix mas** (fi′liks mas) [L. "male fern"] *Dryopteris filix-mas,* the male fern.

**fil·let** (fil′et) 1. a loop, as of cord or tape, for making traction on the fetus. 2. lemniscus.

**fill·ing** (fil′ing) 1. the material inserted into a prepared tooth cavity, usually gold, amalgam, cement, or a synthetic resin. 2. the process of inserting, condensing, shaping, and finishing a filling in a prepared tooth cavity or root canal. Called also *restoration.*
**complex f.,** a filling for a complex cavity.
**composite f.,** a filling that consists of a composite resin.
**compound f.,** a filling for a cavity that involves two surfaces of a tooth.
**direct f.,** one that is formed and completed directly in the prepared tooth cavity.
**direct resin f.,** a direct filling made from a synthetic resin.
**ditched f.,** the marginal failure of an amalgam restoration due to fracture of either the material or the tooth structure itself in the affected area.
**indirect f.,** one that is constructed on a die that has been made from an accurate impression of the tooth and that is then inserted into the tooth cavity.
**permanent f.,** a filling intended to provide complete function while the tooth remains in the oral cavity.
**retrograde f.,** in root canal therapy, an amalgam or other restoration placed in the apical portion of the canal to seal it after surgical removal of a periapical lesion; this is done through the apex, approached through the alveolar bone. Called also *retrograde amalgam.*
**reverse f.,** retrofilling.
**root canal f.,** 1. in root canal therapy, material(s) placed inside the canal to obturate or seal it. 2. canal obturation.
**root-end f.,** retrofilling.
**temporary f.,** a filling placed in a tooth cavity with the intention of removing it within a short period of time.
**treatment f.,** a filling used to allay sensitive dentin prior to final preparation of the cavity.

**film** (film) 1. a thin layer or coating. 2. a thin transparent sheet of cellulose acetate or similar material coated on one or both sides with an emulsion that is sensitive to light or radiation.
**bite-wing f.,** one with a central protruding tab or wing to be held between the upper and lower teeth; used in dental radiography.
**fixed blood f.,** a thin film of blood spread on a slide, dried quickly, and fixed.
**gelatin f., absorbable** [USP], a sterile, nonantigenic, absorbable, water-insoluble gelatin film, used as a local hemostatic.
**lateral jaw f.,** a radiograph showing either the ramus or the body of the mandible.
**occlusal f.,** a radiograph showing topographic and cross-sectional views of the maxillary or mandibular dental structure and adjacent tissue.
**periapical f.,** one used in radiography of the root apex of a tooth and the surrounding structures.
**plain f.,** a radiograph made without the use of a contrast medium.
**spot f.,** a radiograph of a small anatomic area obtained either by rapid exposure during fluoroscopy to provide a permanent record of a transiently observed abnormality, or by limitation of radiation passing through the area to improve definition and detail of the image produced.
**sulfa f.,** a film made from an emulsion of sulfadiazine, sulfanilamide, and methyl cellulose; used as a dressing for burns, cuts, and skin grafts.
**x-ray f.,** a film specially prepared for use in radiography; also, a radiograph.

**film badge** (film baj) a pack of radiographic film or films, usually worn on the body during potential exposure to radiation in order to detect and quantitate the dosage of exposure.

**Fi·lo·ba·sid·i·el·la** (fi″lo-bə-sid″e-el′ə) a genus of fungi classified in either order Ustilaginales or order Sporidiales. *F. neofor′mans* is the perfect (sexual) stage of *Cryptococcus neoformans,* the cause of cryptococcosis.

**Fi·lo·ba·sid·i·um** (fi″lo-bə-sid′e-əm) a genus of fungi classified in either order Ustilaginales or order Sporidiales. *F. florifor′me* is the perfect (sexual) stage of *Cryptococcus albidus.*

**fi·lo·po·di·um** (fi″lo-po′de-əm) pl. *filopo′dia* [*filum* + Gr. *pous* foot] a slender filamentous pseudopodium with a pointed end, branched or unbranched, consisting mostly of ectoplasm. Cf. *axopodium, lobopodium,* and *reticulopodium.*

**fi·lo·pres·sure** (fi′lo-presh″ər) [*filum* + *pressure*] the compression of a blood vessel by a thread.

**fi·lo·var·i·co·sis** (fi′lo-var″ĭ-ko′sis) the development of varicosities on the axon of a nerve fiber.

**Fi·lo·vi·ri·dae** (fi″lo-vir′ĭ-de) [MeSH: Filoviridae] Marburg and Ebola viruses: a family of RNA viruses having enveloped filamentous virions, sometimes branching or U- or 6-shaped, 80 nm in diameter and varying greatly in length, with large peplomers, surrounding a helical nucleocapsid. The genome consists of a single molecule of negative-sense single-stranded RNA (MW $4.2\times10^6$, size 19.1 kb). Viruses contain seven major polypeptides and are sensitive to heat, ultraviolet and gamma radiation, beta-propiolactone, and formalin. Replication occurs in the cytoplasm and assembly is by budding through the plasma membrane. There is a single genus, *Filovirus.*

**Fi·lo·vi·rus** (fi′lo-vi″rəs) [L. *filum* thread + *virus*] [MeSH: Filovirus] Marburg and Ebola viruses; a genus of viruses of the family Filoviridae that cause hemorrhagic fevers (Marburg virus disease, Ebola virus disease).

**fil·ter** (fil′tər) [L. *filtrum*] 1. a membrane or other porous substance or device for the separation of impurities or particulate matter from liquid or gas. 2. to pass liquid or gas through such a device or material. 3. a device used to absorb electromagnetic radiation, particularly light, of specific wavelengths. 4. in radiology, a solid screen usually of varying thickness of metal (aluminum, copper, tin, lead, etc.) which when placed in the pathway of the radiation beam prevents transmission of beta particles and photons of longer wavelengths.
**bird's nest f.,** an inferior vena cava filter consisting of four long, thin stainless steel wires with many bends, attached to struts that are fixed into place.
**collodion f.,** a synthetic cellulose nitrate membrane with uniform pore sizes, used as a microbiological filter and for estimating the size of viral particles.
**Greenfield f.,** an umbrella filter consisting of six stainless steel struts; small hooks on the ends of the struts anchor the filter in the vena cava when it is opened. Called also *Kimray-Greenfield f.*
**Hemming f.,** a bacterial filter that uses centrifugal force to move liquid through a filter pad into a receiving vessel.
**inferior vena cava f.,** a filter used in transvenous vena caval interruption for the prevention of pulmonary embolism; the most common type is the umbrella filter. Called also *vena cava* or *vena caval f.*
**intermittent sand f.,** a sand filter to which sewage is applied for

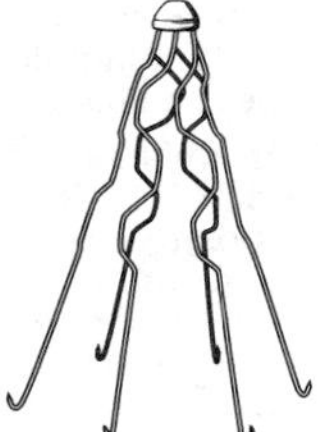
Greenfield filter.

only a short time and then is allowed to drain away so that aeration and oxidation may take place.
**Kimray-Greenfield f.,** Greenfield f.
**mechanical f.,** a filter of sand or other porous material through which water is forced rapidly to remove gross particles; these particles may be the precipitate caused by the addition of some coagulant.
**membrane f.,** a filter made up of a thin film of collodion, cellulose acetate, or other material, available in a wide range of defined pore sizes, the smaller ones being capable of retaining all the known viruses.
**Millipore f.,** trademark for any of a variety of membrane filters.
**Mobin-Uddin f.,** an umbrella filter consisting of six stainless steel spokes connected to a hub and covered by a perforated, heparin-impregnated Silastic membrane.
**percolating f.,** trickling f.
**roughing f., scrubbing f.,** a coarse-grained filter through which turbid water is passed to remove the larger particles and thus protect the sand filter from clogging.
**sintered glass f.,** a filter of sintered glass, available in various porosities, sometimes designated C (coarse), M (medium), F (fine), and UF (ultrafine); only the ultrafine is bacteria-proof.
**slow sand f.,** a filter made of sand and gravel through which water passes slowly and is purified largely by the action of the microorganisms growing on the surface of the grains of sand near the top of the filter.
**sprinkling f.,** a trickling filter in which sewage is applied by spray.
**trickling f.,** beds of porous material on which sewage is distributed and allowed to percolate through to drains laid on a tight floor; the purpose is to so oxidize the organic material as to make it nonputrescible. Called also *percolating f.*
**umbrella f.,** the most common kind of vena cava filter for prevention of pulmonary embolism; it is inserted in a folded position and springs open like an umbrella to engage the caval wall. Common types are the Greenfield and Mobin-Uddin filters.
**vena cava f., vena caval f.,** a filter used in transvenous vena caval interruption for the prevention of pulmonary embolism; the most common type is the umbrella filter. Called also *inferior vena cava f.*
**Wood's f.,** see under *light.*

**fil·ter·a·ble** (fil′tər-ə-bəl) capable of passing through the pores of a filter; usually referring to living infectious agents (i.e., viruses) able to pass through a filter that retains the usual pathogenic bacteria.

**fil·tra·ble** (fil′trə-bəl) filterable.

**fil·trate** (fil′trāt) a liquid or gas that has passed through a filter.
**glomerular f.,** the ultrafiltrate of plasma that passes across the membranes of the malpighian corpuscles of the kidney to the lumen of Bowman's capsule.

**fil·tra·tion** (fil-tra′shən) [MeSH: Filtration] 1. the passage of a liquid or gas through a filter. 2. in radiology, the use of a solid screen usually made of metal (aluminum, copper, tin, lead, etc.) to absorb beta particles and photons of longer wavelengths.
**gel f.,** column chromatography in which high molecular weight substances are separated according to molecular size.

**fil·trum ven·tric·u·li** (fil′trəm ven-trik′u-li) [L.] a depression between the two projections formed in the lateral wall of the vestibule of the larynx by the arytenoid and cuneiform cartilages.

**fi·lum** (fi′ləm) pl. *fi′la* [L.] [TA] a threadlike structure or part.
**fi′la anastomo′tica ner′vi acus′tici,** an anastomotic filament between the vestibulocochlear and facial nerves in the internal acoustic meatus.
**f. corona′rium,** a tapering collagenous bundle that forms part of the fibrous annulus at each atrioventricular orifice; in the mitral valve one extends anteriorly and one posteriorly from the right fibrous trigone, partially encircling the orifice, and in the tricuspid valve they extend similarly from the left fibrous trigone.
**f. du′rae ma′tris spina′le,** pars duralis fili terminalis.
**fi′la olfacto′ria** [TA], olfactory nerves (1st cranial): the nerves of smell, consisting of about 20 bundles which arise in the olfactory epithelium and pass through the cribriform plate of the ethmoid bone to the olfactory bulb.
**fi′la radicula′ria ner′vi spina′lis** [TA], rootlets of spinal nerve: the threadlike filaments by which the anterior and posterior roots of each spinal nerve are attached to the spinal cord. Called also *root filaments of spinal nerve.*
**f. spina′le,** f. terminale.
**f. termina′le** [TA], terminal filum: a slender threadlike filament of connective tissue that descends from the conus medullaris to the base of the coccyx; divided into a pial part *(pars pialis fili terminalis)* and a dural part *(pars duralis fili terminalis)*, the dividing line being the lower border of the second sacral vertebra. Called also *f. spinale, meningeal filament, filament of meninges, spinal filament,* and *terminal filament.*
**f. termina′le dura′le, f. termina′le exter′num,** pars duralis fili terminalis.
**f. termina′le inter′num, f. termina′le pia′le,** pars pialis fili terminalis.

**fim·bria** (fim′bre-ə) [L. *fimbriae* (pl.) a fringe] 1. [TA] a general term for a fringe, border, or edge. 2. pilus (def. 2).
**f. hippocam′pi** [TA], the band of white matter along the medial edge of the ventricular surface of the hippocampus; called also *corpus fimbriatum hippocampi.*
**f. ova′rica** [TA], ovarian fimbria: the longest of the processes that make up the fimbriae tubae uterinae, extending along the free border of the mesosalpinx; it is fused to the ovary, so that the ostium of the tube relates to the ovary. Called also *fimbriated extremity.*

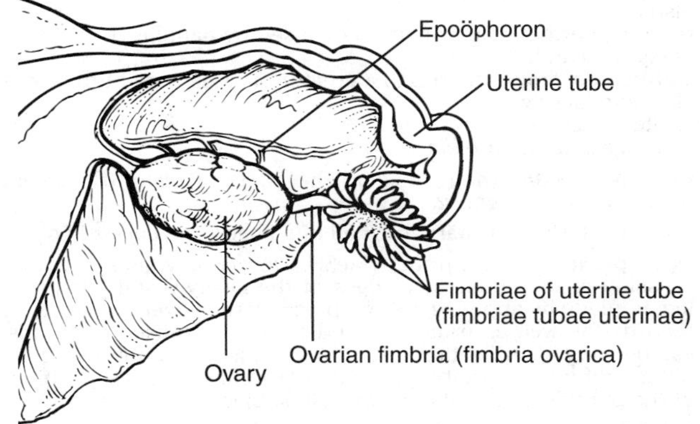


**fimbriae of tongue,** plica fimbriata.
**fim′briae tu′bae uteri′nae** [TA], fimbriae of uterine tube: the numerous divergent fringelike processes on the distal part of the infundibulum of the uterine tube.

**Fim·bri·a·ria** (fim″bre-ar′e-ə) a genus of tapeworms of the family Hymenolepididae, which are parasites of anseriform birds. *F. fasciola′ris* infects wild and domestic fowl.

**fim·bri·at·ed** (fim′bre-āt″əd) [L. *fimbriatus*] fringed.

**fim·bri·a·tion** (fim″bre-a′shən) the formation of or the possession of fimbriae.

**fim·bri·a·tum** (fim″bre-a′təm) [L.] fringed.

**fim·brin** (fim′brin) an actin-binding protein found in the epithelial brush border microvilli; it helps bind actin filaments into tight bundles that are not disrupted in the presence of calcium.

**fim·brio·cele** (fim′bre-o-sēl″) [*fimbria* + *-cele*] hernia containing fimbriae of the uterine tube.

**fi·nas·te·ride** (fĭ-nas′tər-īd) [MeSH: Finasteride] an inhibitor of 5α-reductase, used in the treatment of benign prostatic hyperplasia; administered orally.

**find·er** (fīnd′ər) a device on a microscope to facilitate the finding of some object in the field.

**find·ing** (fīnd′ing) an observation; a condition discovered.

**fin·ger** (fing′gər) [MeSH: Fingers] any of the five digits of the hand. See *pollex, index, digitus medius, digitus anularis,* and *digitus minimus.*
**baseball f.,** mallet f.
**blubber f.,** seal f.
**bolster f's,** the swollen fingers that result from a *Candida* infection in workers who handle sugar.
**clubbed f.,** clubbing (q.v.) in a finger. Called also *drumstick f.*
**dead f.,** a numb, mottled finger, as one seen in acrocyanosis.
**drop f.,** mallet f.
**drumstick f.,** clubbed f.
**fifth f.,** digitus minimus manus.
**first f.,** pollex.
**fourth f.,** digitus anularis.
**giant f.,** megalodactyly of the fingers.

**hammer f.,** mallet f.
**hippocratic f's,** enlargement of the terminal phalanges, with coarse nails curving over the ends of the fingers (hippocratic nails); see *hypertrophic pulmonary osteoarthropathy,* under *osteoarthropathy.*
**index f.,** index (def. 1).
**little f.,** digitus minimus manus.
**lock f.,** one that is fixed in a flexed position, owing to the presence of a small fibrous growth in the sheath of the flexor tendon.
**Madonna f's,** the thin, delicate fingers seen in acromicria.
**mallet f.,** partial permanent flexion of the terminal phalanx of a finger caused by a ball or other object striking the end or back of the finger, resulting in rupture of the attachment of the extensor tendon. Called also *baseball f., drop f.,* and *hammer f.*
**middle f.,** digitus medius manus.
**ring f.,** digitus anularis.
**seal f.,** a cellulitis of the hand, of unknown etiology and clinically resembling erysipeloid, occurring in handlers of seals and seal skins; called also *blubber f.*
**second f.,** index (def. 1).
**snapping f.,** trigger f.
**spider f.,** arachnodactyly.
**spring f.,** a condition in which flexion and extension of the finger beyond certain points are difficult.
**third f.,** digitus medius.
**trigger f.,** a finger liable to have a momentary spasmodic arrest of flexion or extension followed by a snapping into place, due either to stenosing tendovaginitis or to a nodule in the flexor tendon. See also *lock f.*
**tulip f's,** dermatitis of the fingers caused by handling tulip bulbs.
**waxy f.,** dead f.
**webbed f's,** fingers united to a greater or lesser extent by a fold of skin; syndactyly.
**white f.,** dead f.
**zinc f.,** see under *protein.*

**fin·ger·ag·no·sia** (fing"gər-ag-no'zhə) [*finger* + *agnosia*] finger agnosia; see under *agnosia.*

**fin·ger·nail** (fing'gər-nāl) the nail of a finger; see *unguis* [TA].

**fin·ger·print** (fing'gər-print) [MeSH: Dermatoglyphics] 1. an impression of the cutaneous ridges of the fleshy distal portion of a finger, made by applying ink and pressing the finger on paper; such records (as well as prints of hand or foot) are used as means of establishing identification. 2. in biochemistry, a photomicrograph obtained by fingerprinting (q.v.). 3. the characteristic positioning of the peptide fragments of a protein subjected to fingerprinting.

**fin·ger·print·ing** (fing'gər-print"ing) a technique for determining the structure of a protein in which the protein is split into peptides by digestion with a protease and the fragments are separated in one direction by electrophoresis and at right angles by chromatography. After staining, the peptide fragments are seen to be in characteristic locations.

**fin·ish** (fin'ish) a desired surface texture given to something, such as a denture or an artificial crown.

**Fin·kel·stein's feeding** (fing'kəl-shtīnz) [Heinrich *Finkelstein,* German pediatrician, 1865–1942] see under *feeding.*

**Fink·ler-Pri·or spirillum** (fing'klər-pri'or) [Dittmar *Finkler,* German bacteriologist, 1852–1912; J. *Prior,* German bacteriologist, 19th century] *Vibrio metschnikovii.*

**Fin·ney's pyloroplasty (operation)** (fin'ēz) [John Miller Turpin *Finney,* American surgeon, 1863–1942] see under *pyloroplasty.*

**Fi·no·chi·et·to's stirrup** (fe-no"ke-et'ōz) [Enrique *Finochietto,* Argentine surgeon, 1881–1948] see under *stirrup.*

**Fin·sen** (fin'sən) Niels Ryberg. Danish physician, 1860–1904; winner of the Nobel prize for medicine or physiology in 1903 for his discovery of the curative effects of ultraviolet rays, especially for lupus vulgaris.

**fire** (fīr) fever; inflammation.
**St. Anthony's f.,** 1. former name for *ergotism* (in humans). 2. former name for *erysipelas.*

**fir·ing** (fīr'ing) 1. the sintering of powder to produce porcelain, such as for a dental restoration. 2. the initiation of a nerve impulse.

**Fir·mac·u·tes** (fir-mak'u-tēz, fir"mə-ku'tēz) Firmicutes.

**Fir·mi·bac·te·ria** (fir"mĭ-bak-tēr'e-ə) [L. *firmus* strong + *bacteria*] a class of bacteria of the division Firmicutes, consisting of simple, gram-positive, asporogenous and sporogenous rods and cocci, including the medically important families: Micrococcaceae, Streptococcaceae, Peptococcaceae, Bacillaceae, and Lactobacillaceae.

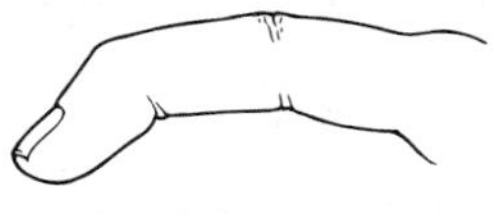

Mallet finger.

**Fir·mic·u·tes** (fir-mik'u-tēz, fir"mĭ-ku'tēz) [L. *firmus* strong + *cutis* skin] a division of bacteria of the kingdom Procaryotae made up of organisms with a gram-positive type of cell wall that consists of a thick layer of peptidoglycan containing muramic acid. The division includes simple asporogenous and sporogenous rods and cocci (Firmibacteria) as well as the actinomycetes and related organisms (Thallobacteria). Called also *Firmacutes.*

**first aid** (fərst ād) [MeSH: First Aid] emergency care and treatment of an injured or ill person before definitive medical and surgical management can be secured.

**Fisch·er** (fish'ər) Edmond Henri. American biochemist, born 1920. Co-winner with Erwin Gerhard Krebs of the Nobel prize for medicine or physiology in 1992 for their work on protein kinases in cell metabolism.

**Fish·berg concentration test** (fish'bərg) [Arthur Maurice *Fishberg,* American physician, 1898–1992] see under *test.*

**Fish·er exact test** (fish'ər) [Sir Ronald Aylmer *Fisher,* British statistician, 1890–1962] see under *test.*

**Fish·er syndrome** (fish'er) [C. Miller *Fisher,* American neurologist, 20th century] see under *syndrome.*

**fish·pox** (fish'poks) a hyperplastic epidermal disease of viral origin occurring in fresh-water and marine fish.

**fis·sile** (fis'il) capable of being split; fissionable.

**fis·sion** (fish'ən) [L. *fissio*] 1. the act of splitting. 2. a form of asexual reproduction in which the cell divides into two or more daughter parts of equal size, each of which becomes a new, independent organism; it is seen chiefly in unicellular organisms, such as bacteria. See also *binary f.* and *multiple f.*
**binary f.,** fission of a cell in which the cell divides into two approximately equal daughter parts.
**cellular f.,** see *fission,* def 2.
**multiple f.,** fission of a cell in which the cell divides into a number of daughter cells.
**nuclear f.,** the splitting of the nucleus of an atom, releasing a great quantity of kinetic energy.

**fis·sion·a·ble** (fish'ən-ə-bəl) capable of undergoing fission.

**fis·sip·a·rous** (fĭ-sip'ə-rəs) [L. *fissus* cleft + *parere* to produce] propagated by fission.

**fis·su·la** (fis'u-lə) [L., dim. of *fissura*] a little cleft.
**f. an'te fenes'tram,** an irregular ribbon of connective tissue that extends through the bony otic capsule from the vestibule just anterior to the oval window, to the tympanic cavity near the processus cochleariformis.

**fis·su·ra** (fis-u'rə) gen. and pl. *fissu'rae* [L., from *findere* to split] [TA] fissure: a general term for a cleft or groove, especially a deep fold in the cerebral cortex that involves its entire thickness. Cf. *sulcus.*
**f. in a'no,** anal fissure.
**f. antitragohelici'na** [TA], antitragohelicine fissure: a fissure in the auricular cartilage between the cauda helicis and the antitragus; called also *posterior fissure of auricle.*
**f. au'ris conge'nita,** congenital preauricular fistula.
**fissu'rae cerebel'li** [TA], cerebellar fissures: the numerous shallow grooves in the cortex of the cerebellum, on the surface and within the deep fissures, which divide the cortex into folia.
**f. choroi'dea ventri'culi latera'lis** [TA], choroid fissure of lateral ventricle: the medially located line in the lateral ventricle along which the choroid plexus invaginates.
**f. dorsolatera'lis cerebel'li,** f. posterolateralis cerebelli.
**f. horizonta'lis cerebel'li** [TA], horizontal fissure of cerebellum: the fissure that separates the cranial from the caudal semilunar lobule of the cerebellum. Called also *f. intercruralis cerebelli* [TA alternative], *horizontal sulcus of cerebellum,* and *great horizontal fissure.*
**f. horizonta'lis pulmo'nis dex'tri** [TA], horizontal fissure of right lung: the cleft that extends forward from the oblique fissure in the right lung, separating the upper and middle lobes.
**f. intercrura'lis cerebel'li,** TA alternative for *f. horizontalis cerebelli.*
**f. ligamen'ti te'retis** [TA], fissure for ligamentum teres: the fossa on the visceral surface of the liver lodging the ligamentum teres in the adult, and helping separate the right and left lobes of the liver; called also *fossa venae umbilicalis, fissure of round ligament,* and *umbilical fissure.*
**f. ligamen'ti veno'si** [TA], fissure for ligamentum venosum: a fossa on the posterior part of the diaphragmatic surface of the liver lodging the ligamentum venosum in the adult.
**f. longitudina'lis cerebra'lis, f. longitudina'lis ce'rebri** [TA], longitudinal cerebral fissure: the deep fissure between the cerebral hemispheres extending inferiorly to the corpus callosum.
**f. media'na ante'rior medul'lae oblonga'tae** [TA], anterior median fissure of medulla oblongata: the longitudinal fissure in the median

plane of the anterior aspect of the medulla oblongata, continuous with the anterior median fissure of the spinal cord; it separates the pyramids and is partially obliterated below by their decussation. Called also *anteromedian groove of medulla oblongata* and *f. mediana ventralis medullae oblongatae.*

**f. media'na ante'rior medul'lae spina'lis** [TA], anterior median fissure of spinal cord: the deep longitudinal fissure in the median plane of the anterior aspect of the spinal cord; it contains the anterior spinal artery ensheathed in the linea splendens. Called also *anteromedian groove of spinal cord, f. mediana ventralis medullae spinalis, Haller's line,* and *sulcus ventralis medullae spinalis.*

**f. media'na ventra'lis medul'lae oblonga'tae,** f. mediana anterior medullae oblongatae.

**f. media'na ventra'lis medul'lae spina'lis,** f. mediana anterior medullae spinalis.

**f. obli'qua pulmo'nis** [TA], oblique fissure of lung: 1. the cleft that separates the lower from the middle and upper lobes in the right lung. 2. the cleft that separates the upper from the lower lobe in the left lung.

**f. orbita'lis infe'rior** [TA], inferior orbital fissure: a cleft in the inferolateral wall of the orbit bounded by the great wing of the sphenoid and the orbital process of the maxilla; it transmits the infraorbital and zygomatic nerves and the infraorbital vessels.

**f. orbita'lis supe'rior** [TA], superior orbital fissure: an elongated cleft between the small and great wings of the sphenoid bone, which transmits various nerves and vessels.

**f. petrooccipita'lis** [TA], petrooccipital fissure: a fissure extending posteriorly from the foramen lacerum to the jugular foramen, between the basioccipital area and the posterior and inner border of the petrous portion of the temporal bone; called also *petrobasilar fissure.*

**f. petrosquamo'sa** [TA], petrosquamous fissure: a slight fissure of varying distinctness in the floor of the middle cranial fossa, marking the line of fusion between the squamous and petrous portions of the temporal bone.

**f. petrotympa'nica** [TA], petrotympanic fissure: a narrow transversely running slit just posterior to the articular surface of the mandibular fossa of the temporal bone; an arteriole and the chorda tympani nerve pass through it, and it lodges a portion of the malleus. Called also *glaserian fissure.*

**f. posterolatera'lis cerebel'li** [TA], posterolateral fissure of cerebellum: the fissure separating the nodulus from the uvula of the vermis and the flocculus from the tonsilla of the cerebellar hemisphere; called also *f. dorsolateralis cerebelli* and *dorsolateral fissure of cerebellum.*

**f. postpyramida'lis,** TA alterntive for *f. secunda cerebelli.*

**f. precliva'lis,** TA alternative for *f. prima cerebelli.*

**f. pri'ma cerebel'li** [TA], primary fissure of cerebellum: the fissure that separates the cranial from the caudal lobe in the cerebellum; it lies between the culmen and declive of the vermis, and between the quadrangular lobule and the lobulus simplex in the hemisphere of the cerebellum. Called also *f. preclivalis* [TA alternative] and *preclival fissure.*

**f. pterygoi'dea,** incisura pterygoidea.

**f. pterygomaxilla'ris** [TA], pterygomaxillary fissure: a cleft just posterior to the inferior orbital fissure between the lateral pterygoid plate and the maxilla; called also *pterygopalatine fissure.*

**f. secun'da cerebel'li** [TA], secondary fissure of cerebellum: a fissure that lies between the uvula of the cerebellum and the pyramid; called also *f. postpyramidalis* [TA alternative] and *postpyramidal fissure.*

**f. sphenooccipita'lis,** sphenooccipital fissure: the fissure between the basilar part of the occipital bone and the body of the sphenoid bone; called also *basilar* or *occipitosphenoidal fissure.*

**f. sphenopetro'sa** [TA], sphenopetrosal fissure: a fissure in the floor of the middle cranial fossa between the posterior edge of the greater wing of the sphenoid bone and the petrous part of the temporal bone; called also *angular* or *petrosphenoidal fissure.*

**f. transver'sa cerebra'lis, f. transver'sa ce'rebri** [TA], transverse cerebral fissure: the fissure between the dorsal surface of the diencephalon and the ventral surface of the cerebral hemispheres, produced by the folding back of the hemispheres during their development; called also *great* or *great transverse fissure of cerebrum* and *fissure of Bichat.*

**f. tympanomastoi'dea** [TA], tympanomastoid fissure: an external fissure on the inferior and lateral aspect of the skull between the tympanic portion and the mastoid process of the temporal bone; the auricular branch of the vagus nerve often passes through it. Called also *petromastoid fissure.*

**f. tympanosquamo'sa** [TA], tympanosquamous fissure: a line seen on the posterior wall of the external acoustic meatus at the junction between the tympanic and squamous parts of the temporal bone. Called also *squamotympanic fissure.*

**fis·su·rae** (fi-su're) [L.] genitive and plural of *fissura.*

**fis·su·ral** (fish'u-rəl) pertaining to a fissure.

**fis·sure** (fish'ər) [L. *fissura*] 1. fissura. 2. any cleft, groove, or sulcus, normal or otherwise. 3. a deep cleft in the tooth surface, usually due to imperfect fusion of the enamel of the adjoining dental lobes. Cf. *pit.* Considered as belonging to Class I in Black's classification (see table at *caries*). Called also *enamel f.*

## Fissure

For descriptions of specific anatomic structures not listed here, see under *fissura.*

**abdominal f.,** a congenital cleft in the abdominal wall. See also *gastroschisis* and *thoracoceloschisis.* Called also *celoschisis.*

**accessory f.,** any of various inconstant fissures on the lung surface; the most common one is the azygos fissure.

**adoccipital f.,** an inconstant sulcus which crosses the caudal part of the precuneus and joins the occipital fissure.

**Ammon's f.,** a pear-shaped aperture in the sclera at an early fetal period.

**amygdaline f.,** a slight groove inconstantly present near the extremity of the temporal lobe.

**anal f., f. in ano,** a painful linear ulcer at the margin of the anus.

**angular f.,** fissura sphenopetrosa.

**antitragohelicine f.,** fissura antitragohelicina.

**f. of aqueduct of vestibule,** apertura externa aqueductus vestibuli.

**f. of auricle, posterior,** fissura antitragohelicina.

**auricular f. of temporal bone,** fissura tympanomastoidea.

**azygos f.,** an inconstant fissure at the apex of the right lung, produced when the azygos vein arches over the superior part of the lung instead of near the hilum; it sets off the azygos lobe.

**basilar f.,** fissura spheno-occipitalis.

**basisylvian f.,** the part of the lateral sulcus between the temporal lobe and the orbital surface of the frontal bone.

**f. of Bichat,** fissura transversa cerebri.

**branchial f.,** 1. branchial cleft (def. 1). 2. pharyngeal groove.

**Broca's f.,** a term loosely applied to the anterior and ascending rami of the cerebral lateral sulcus which invade the left inferior frontal gyrus.

**Burdach's f.,** the groove between the lateral surface of the insula and the inner surface of the operculum.

**calcarine f.,** sulcus calcarinus.

**callosal f.,** sulcus corporis callosi.

**callosomarginal f.,** sulcus cinguli.

**central f.,** sulcus centralis cerebri.

**cerebellar f's,** fissurae cerebelli.

**cerebral f's,** 1. sulci cerebri. 2. see *fissura longitudinalis cerebri* and *fissura transversa cerebri.*

**cerebral f., great, cerebral f., great transverse,** fissura transversa cerebri.

**cerebral f., lateral,** sulcus lateralis cerebri.

**cerebral f., longitudinal,** fissura longitudinalis cerebri.

**cerebral f., transverse,** fissura transversa cerebri.

**f's of cerebrum,** 1. sulci cerebri. 2. see *fissura longitudinalis cerebri* and *fissura transversa cerebri.*

**choroid f.,** 1. fissura choroidea ventriculi lateralis. 2. optic f.

**choroid f. of lateral ventricle,** fissura choroidea ventriculi lateralis.

**collateral f.,** sulcus collateralis.

**corneal f.,** the cleft or groove in the scleral margin into which the limbus corneae fits; called also *corneal cleft.*

**craniofacial f.,** a vertical fissure separating the mesethmoid bone into two parts.

**cutaneous f.,** a fistula opening on the surface of the body.

**dentate f.,** sulcus hippocampalis.

**dorsolateral f. of cerebellum,** fissura posterolateralis cerebelli.

**f. of ductus venosus,** fossa ductus venosi.

**Ecker's f.,** sulcus occipitalis transversus.

**enamel f.,** fissure, def. 2.

**entorbital f.,** a sulcus occasionally seen between the orbital and olfactory sulci.

**glaserian f.,** fissura petrotympanica.
**f. of glottis,** rima glottidis.
**great f. of cerebrum, great transverse f. of cerebrum,** fissura transversa cerebri.
**great horizontal f.,** fissura horizontalis cerebelli.
**hippocampal f., f. of hippocampus,** sulcus hippocampalis.
**horizontal f. of cerebellum,** fissura horizontalis cerebelli.
**horizontal f. of right lung,** fissura horizontalis pulmonis dextri.
**intercrural f. of cerebellum,** fissura horizontalis cerebelli.
**inferofrontal f.,** sulcus frontalis inferior.
**interparietal f.,** sulcus intraparietalis.
**intratonsillar f.,** fossa supratonsillaris.
**lacrimal f.,** sulcus lacrimalis ossis lacrimalis.
**lateral f. of cerebrum,** sulcus lateralis cerebri.
**f. for ligamentum teres,** fissura ligamenti teretis.
**f. for ligamentum venosum,** fissura ligamenti venosi.
**longitudinal f.,** 1. fissura longitudinalis cerebri. 2. taenia omentalis.
**longitudinal f. of cerebellum,** vallecula cerebelli.
**longitudinal f. of cerebrum,** fissura longitudinalis cerebri.
**mandibular f's,** the two lowest facial fissures of the embryo.
**median f., anterior,** see *fissura mediana anterior medullae oblongatae* and *fissura mediana anterior medullae spinalis.*
**median f., posterior,** see *sulcus medianus posterior medullae oblongatae* and *sulcus medianus posterior medullae spinalis.*
**median f. of medulla oblongata, anterior,** fissura mediana anterior medullae oblongatae.
**median f. of medulla oblongata, dorsal, median f. of medulla oblongata, posterior,** sulcus medianus posterior medullae oblongatae.
**median f. of medulla oblongata, ventral,** fissura mediana anterior medullae oblongatae.
**median f. of spinal cord, anterior,** fissura mediana anterior medullae spinalis.
**median f. of spinal cord, dorsal, median f. of spinal cord, posterior,** sulcus medianus posterior medullae spinalis.
**median f. of spinal cord, ventral,** fissura mediana anterior medullae spinalis.
**f. of Monro,** sulcus hypothalamicus.
**oblique f. of lung,** fissura obliqua pulmonis.
**occipitosphenoidal f.,** fissura spheno-occipitalis.
**optic f.,** in the embryo, a ventral fissure formed by invagination of the optic vesicle and its stalk, permitting the ingrowth of the mesoblast. Called also *choroid f.*
**oral f.,** rima oris.
**orbital f., inferior,** fissura orbitalis inferior.
**orbital f., superior,** fissura orbitalis superior.
**f. of palpebrae, palpebral f.,** rima palpebrarum.
**Pansch's f.,** sulcus intraparietalis.
**parietooccipital f.,** sulcus parietooccipitalis.
**parietosphenoid f.,** incisura parietalis ossis temporalis.
**petrobasilar f.,** fissura petrooccipitalis.
**petromastoid f.,** fissura tympanomastoidea.
**petrooccipital f.,** fissura petrooccipitalis.
**petrosphenoidal f.,** fissura sphenopetrosa.
**petrosquamosal f., petrosquamous f.,** fissura petrosquamosa.
**petrotympanic f.,** fissura petrotympanica.
**portal f.,** porta hepatis.
**postcentral f.,** 1. sulcus postcentralis. 2. a fissure separating the central lobule of the cerebellum with its alae from the more dorsal culmen and quadrangular lobules.
**postclival f., posterior superior f.,** a fissure of the cerebellum between the declive and the folium vermis. Called also *postlunate f.*.
**posterolateral f. of cerebellum,** fissura posterolateralis cerebelli.
**postlingual f.,** a fissure in the anterior part of the superior vermis of the cerebellum, separating the lingula from the central lobule.
**postlunate f.,** postclival f.
**postpyramidal f.,** fissura secunda cerebelli.
**precentral f.,** sulcus precentralis.
**preclival f.,** fissura prima cerebelli.
**precuneal f.,** a sulcus in the precuneus.
**prepyramidal f.,** a fissure between the pyramis vermis and the tuber vermis.
**presylvian f.,** the anterior branch of the lateral cerebral sulcus.
**primary f. of cerebellum,** fissura prima cerebelli.
**pterygoid f.,** incisura pterygoidea.
**pterygomaxillary f.,** fissura pterygomaxillaris.
**pterygopalatine f.,** fissura pterygomaxillaris.
**pterygopalatine f. of palatine bone,** sulcus palatinus major ossis palatini.
**pudendal f., f. of pudendum,** rima pudendi.
**retrocuticular f.,** a fissure in the oral epithelium made by a tooth at the time of eruption.
**retrotonsillar f.,** either of a pair of curving fissures in the inferior cerebellum, lateral continuations of the sulcus valleculae, between the tonsils and the biventral lobes.
**f. of Rolando,** sulcus centralis cerebri.
**f. of round ligament,** fissura ligamenti teretis.
**sagittal f. of liver,** fossa sagittalis sinistra hepatis.
**Santorini's f's,** the two notches in cartilage of acoustic meatus; see *incisura cartilaginis meatus acustici.*
**Schwalbe's f.,** fissura choroidea ventriculi lateralis.
**secondary f. of cerebellum,** fissura secunda cerebelli.
**spheno-occipital f.,** fissura spheno-occipitalis.
**sphenopetrosal f.,** fissura sphenopetrosa.
**squamotympanic f.,** fissura tympanosquamosa.
**subfrontal f.,** sulcus frontalis inferior.
**subtemporal f.,** an occasional fissure in the inferior and middle temporal convolutions.
**superfrontal f.,** sulcus frontalis superior.
**supertemporal f.,** sulcus temporalis superior.
**sylvian f., f. of Sylvius,** sulcus lateralis cerebri.
**transtemporal f.,** an occasional short fissure on the lateral surface of the temporal lobe.
**transverse f.,** porta hepatis.
**transverse f. of cerebrum,** fissura transversa cerebri.
**transverse occipital f.,** sulcus occipitalis transversus.
**tympanic f.,** fissura petrotympanica.
**tympanomastoid f.,** fissura tympanomastoidea.
**tympanosquamous f.,** fissura tympanosquamosa.
**umbilical f.,** fissura ligamenti teretis.
**f. of the venous ligament,** fossa ductus venosi.
**f. of the vestibule,** rima vestibuli.
**zygal f.,** a cerebral fissure that consists of two portions united by a short perpendicular third portion.

---

**fis·su·rel·la** (fis″ə-rel′ə) the keyhole limpets, a genus of snaillike marine gastropods of the subclass Streptoneura, order Aspidobranchiae. See *keyhole-limpet hemocyanin,* under *hemocyanin.*

**fis·tu·la** (fis′tu-lə) pl. *fistulas* or *fis′tulae* [L. "pipe"] [MeSH: Fistula] an abnormal passage or communication, usually between two internal organs, or leading from an organ to the surface of the body; see illustration. Such passages may also be created experimentally to obtain body secretions for physiologic study.

**abdominal f.,** an abnormal passage leading from one of the hollow abdominal viscera to the surface of the abdomen.

**amphibolic f.,** an opening made into the gallbladder of an animal in order to obtain bile for study, with the common bile duct left intact so that the bile may flow through it when the fistula is closed.

**anal f., f. in a′no,** one opening on the cutaneous surface near the anus, which may or may not communicate with the rectum. See illustration.

**aortocaval f.,** communication between the abdominal aorta and inferior vena cava caused by erosion of an aortic aneurysm into the vena cava.

**aortoenteric f.,** communication between the aorta and intestine caused by erosion of an abdominal aortic aneurysm into the duodenum; it may be primary or it may be a late complication of prosthetic reconstruction of the aorta and the iliac arteries.

**arteriovenous f.,** 1. a communication, sometimes congenital but often traumatic, between an artery and a vein in which the blood flows directly into a neighboring vein *(aneurysmal varix)* or else is carried into such a vein by a connecting sac *(varicose aneurysm).* 2. a surgically created arteriovenous connection that provides a site for arteriovenous access (q.v.).

**f. au′ris conge′nita,** congenital preauricular f.

**biliary f.,** an abnormal passage communicating with the biliary tract.

**f. bimuco′sa,** a complete fistula of the anus, both ends of which open on the mucous surface of the anal canal.

**blind f.,** a fistula that is open at one end only; it may open only upon the cutaneous surface of the body *(external blind f.)* or on an internal mucous surface *(internal blind f.).* Called also *incomplete f.*

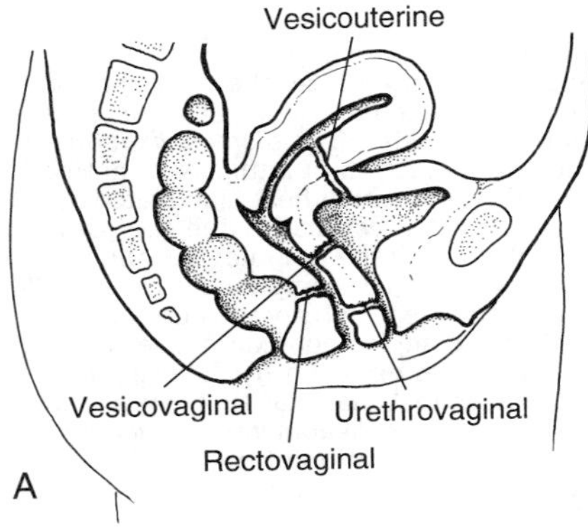


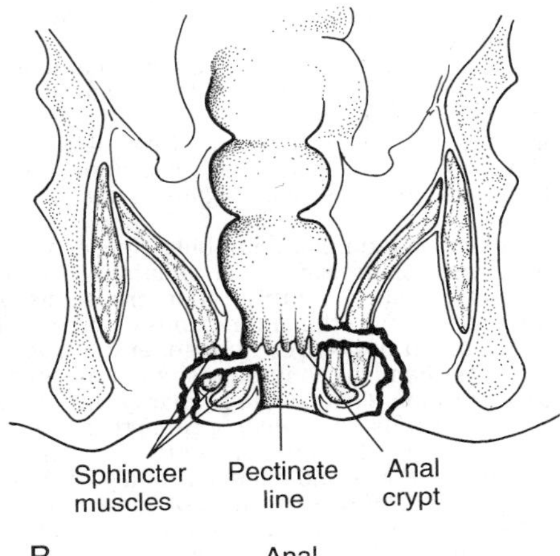


Various types of fistulae, designated according to site or to the organs with which they communicate. *(A)*, Genitourinary fistulae; *(B)*, anal fistulae.

**brachiocephalic f.,** an arteriovenous fistula for hemodialysis, connecting the brachial artery and the cephalic vein.
**branchial f.,** an abnormal passage opening on the side of the neck and leading into the pharynx, resulting from failure of closure of the second pharyngeal (branchial) groove and second pharyngeal pouch; called also *cervical f.*
**Brescia-Cimino f.,** an arteriovenous fistula for hemodialysis, consisting of a side-to-side anastomosis of the cephalic vein and radial artery. Called also *radiocephalic f.*
**bronchocavitary f.,** a fistula connecting a bronchus and a cavity within the lung.
**bronchopleural f.,** a fistula between a bronchus and the pleural cavity, sometimes seen after lung surgery or as a complication of empyema, fibrosis, or pneumonia.
**carotid cavernous f.,** communication between an injured internal carotid artery and the cavernous sinus or the orbital veins; the veins may swell and press against various ocular nerves, causing visual symptoms.
**cerebrospinal fluid f.,** a fistula between the subarachnoid space and a body cavity, with leakage of cerebrospinal fluid, usually in the form of rhinorrhea or otorrhea; causes include head trauma and bone erosion caused by a mass or other pathologic process.
**cervical f.,** 1. branchial f. 2. an abnormal passage communicating with the canal of the cervix uteri.
**f. col'li conge'nita,** branchial f.
**colonic f.,** an abnormal passage communicating with the colon and the cutaneous surface of the body *(external colonic f.)*, or with the colon and another hollow organ *(internal colonic f.)*.
**complete f.,** an abnormal passage in the body, each end of which opens on a mucous surface or on the cutaneous surface of the body.
**f. cor'neae,** an orifice remaining after failure of a corneal ulcer to heal.
**coronary arteriovenous f.,** a congenital condition in which there is an abnormal communication between a coronary artery and a cardiac chamber, pulmonary trunk or vein, coronary sinus, or vena cava, particularly between the right artery and the right heart.
**coronary artery f.,** coronary arteriovenous f.
**craniosinus f.,** a fistula between the intracranial space and one of the paranasal sinuses, permitting the escape of cerebrospinal fluid into the nose.
**Eck's f.,** an artificial communication made between the end of the portal vein and the side of the inferior vena cava; used in animal experiments, and in humans for the treatment of esophageal varices in portal hypertension.
**Eck's f. in reverse,** an artificial communication created to route all the blood from the posterior (lower) part of the body through the portal vein and liver; used in animal experiments.
**external f.,** an abnormal communication between a hollow organ and the external surface of the body.
**fecal f.,** a colonic fistula opening on the external surface of the body and discharging feces.
**gastric f.,** an abnormal passage communicating with the stomach; often applied to an artificially created opening through the abdominal wall into the stomach (gastrostoma).
**gastrocolic f.,** a fistula connecting the stomach and the colon.
**genitourinary f.,** an abnormal communication between organs of the urogenital system or between organs of the urogenital system and some other system. See illustration.
**hepatic f.,** an abnormal communication between the liver and another body part or organ.
**horseshoe f.,** a semicircular fistulous tract near the anus, both openings being on the cutaneous surface.
**incomplete f.,** blind f.
**internal f.,** an abnormal communication between two internal organs.
**intestinal f.,** 1. an abnormal passage communicating with the intestine. 2. an artificially created opening through the abdominal wall into the intestine.
**labyrinthine f.,** circumscribed labyrinthitis.
**lacrimal f.,** an abnormal passage communicating with the lacrimal sac or duct.
**lymphatic f., f. lympha'tica,** an abnormal passage communicating with a lymphatic vessel.
**Mann-Bollman f.,** an artificial opening into an isolated segment of intestine, the proximal end of which is sutured to the abdominal wall and the distal end attached by end-to-side anastomosis to the duodenum or other part of the small intestine; used in animal experiments.
**oroantral f.,** a fistula connecting the oral cavity and the maxillary antrum, usually as a result of extraction of a molar during which a small piece of bone is accidentally also extracted.
**parietal f.,** an abnormal passage in the body wall, ending blindly or communicating with an internal organ or body cavity.
**perianal f.,** anal f.
**perilymph f., perilymphatic f.,** rupture of the round window with leakage of perilymph into the middle ear, causing sensorineural deafness; it usually results from trauma such as barotrauma or from an erosive disease process.
**perineal f.,** a congenital malformation of the anus and rectum in which the anus is imperforate and there is a fistula exiting via a tiny hole in the perineum.
**pharyngeal f.,** an abnormal passage communicating with the pharynx. Cf. *branchial f.*
**pilonidal f.,** see under *sinus.*
**preauricular f., congenital,** an epidermis-lined tract communicating with an ear pit (q.v.) on the skin; it results from imperfect fusion of the first and second branchial arches in formation of the auricle; see also *congenital preauricular cyst.* Called also *f. auris congenita.*
**pulmonary f.,** an abnormal passage communicating with the lung.
**pulmonary arteriovenous f.,** a congenital anomaly consisting of a direct communication between the pulmonary arterial and venous systems, allowing unoxygenated blood to enter the systemic circulation.
**radiocephalic f.,** Brescia-Cimino f.
**rectovaginal f.,** one between the rectum and vagina. See illustration.
**rectovesical f.,** one between the rectum and urinary bladder.
**rectovestibular f.,** a congenital malformation of the anus and rectum of females in which the anus is imperforate and there is a fistula exiting via a hole in the vestibule of the vagina. Called also *vestibular f.*
**salivary f.,** one between a salivary duct or gland and the cutaneous surface, or into the oral cavity through other than a normal pathway.
**saphenous loop f.,** an arteriovenous fistula for hemodialysis, connecting the saphenous vein and the side of the femoral artery.
**spermatic f.,** an abnormal passage communicating with the seminal ducts.
**stercoral f.,** fecal f.
**submental f.,** a salivary fistula opening below the chin.
**Thiry's f.,** an artificial opening into an isolated segment of intestine, the proximal end of which is sutured to the abdominal wall and the distal end is closed; used in animal experiments.
**Thiry-Vella f.,** an artificial opening into an internal closed loop of intestine, which communicates with the abdominal wall through an

intestinal segment interposed between the surface and the loop; used in animal experiments.
**thoracic f.**, an abnormal passage communicating with the thoracic cavity.
**tracheal f.**, an abnormal passage communicating with the trachea.
**tracheocutaneous f.**, an abnormal connection between the trachea and the surface of the neck, due to epithelialization of a tracheotomy opening.
**tracheoesophageal f.**, a fistula between the trachea and the esophagus; it may be either pathological (the result of trauma or a congenital anomaly) or surgically created (see *tracheoesophageal puncture*).
**umbilical f.**, an abnormal passage communicating with the gut or with the urachus at the umbilicus.
**urachal f.**, an abnormal passage resulting from a patent urachus communicating with the umbilicus and urinary bladder.
**urethrovaginal f.**, one between the urethra and vagina. See illustration.
**urinary f.**, an abnormal passage communicating with the urinary tract.
**Vella's f.**, an artificial opening into an isolated segment of intestine, both open ends of which are sutured to the abdominal wall; used in animal experiments.
**vesical f.**, an abnormal passage communicating with the urinary bladder.
**vesicouterine f.**, one between the urinary bladder and uterus. See illustration.
**vesicovaginal f.**, one from the bladder to the vagina. See illustration.
**vestibular f.**, rectovestibular f.

**fis·tu·lae** (fis'tu-le) [L.] genitive and plural of *fistula*.

**fis·tu·la·tome** (fis'tu-lə-tōm) [*fistula* + *-tome*] an instrument for incising a fistula; syringotome.

**fis·tu·lec·to·my** (fis″tu-lek'tə-me) [*fistula* + *-ectomy*] excision of a fistulous tract.

**fis·tu·li·za·tion** (fis″tu-lĭ-za'shən) 1. the process of becoming fistulous. 2. the surgical creation of an opening into a hollow organ, cavity, or abscess; the creation of a communication between two structures which were not previously connected.

**fis·tu·lo·en·ter·os·to·my** (fis″tu-lo-en″tər-os'tə-me) the operation of making a fistula empty permanently into the intestine.

**fis·tu·lot·o·my** (fis″tu-lot'ə-me) incision of a fistula.

**fis·tu·lous** (fis'tu-ləs) [L. *fistulosus*] pertaining to or of the nature of a fistula.

**fit** (fit) 1. seizure, def. 2. 2. the adaptation of one structure into another, as the adaptation of any dental restoration to its site in the mouth.

**FITC** fluorescein isothiocyanate.

**fit·ness** (fit'nəs) in genetics, the probability of transmitting one's genes to the next generation and having them survive in that generation and be passed on to the next, relative to the average probability for the population.

**Fitz-Hugh–Cur·tis syndrome** (fitz'hu-kər'tis) [Thomas *Fitz-Hugh* Jr., American physician, 1894–1963; Arthur H. *Curtis*, American gynecologist, 1881–1955] see under *syndrome*.

**fix** (fiks) to fasten or hold firm; see *fixation*.

**fix·a·tion** (fik-sa'shən) [L. *fixatio*] 1. the act or operation of holding, suturing, or fastening in a fixed position. 2. the condition of being held in a fixed position. 3. in psychiatry, a term with two related meanings: *(a)* arrest of development at a particular stage, which if temporary is a normal reaction to difficulties but if continued is a cause of emotional problems; and *(b)* a close and suffocating attachment to another person, especially a childhood figure, such as a parent. Both meanings are derived from psychoanalytic theory and refer to "fixation" of libidinal energy either in a specific erogenous zone, hence fixation at the oral, anal, or phallic stage, or in a specific object, hence mother or father fixation. 4. the use of a fixative (q.v.) to preserve histological or cytological specimens. 5. in chemistry, the process whereby a substance is removed from the gaseous or solution phase and localized, as in carbon dioxide fixation or nitrogen fixation. 6. in ophthalmology, direction of the gaze so that the visual image of the object falls on the fovea centralis. 7. in film processing, the chemical removal of all undeveloped salts of the film emulsion, leaving only the developed silver to form a permanent image.
**autotrophic f.**, the cyclic mechanism whereby carbon dioxide is fixed into organic linkage by autotrophic organisms, e.g., plants and autotrophic bacteria.
**bifoveal f., binocular f.**, training both eyes on the same object as in ordinary vision.
**Bovin f.**, an acetic fixation which destroys the mitochondria of the cell.
**carbon dioxide f.**, conversion of atmospheric carbon dioxide to organic carbon compounds, as in photosynthesis.
**complement f., f. of complement**, the consumption of complement upon reaction with immune complexes containing complement-fixing antibodies, the basis of *complement fixation tests*, widely used procedures for the detection of antigens or antibodies. These are two-stage procedures in which heat-inactivated antiserum (or antigen) is reacted with the test material in the presence of a known amount of complement. If the homologous antigen (or antibody) is present in the test material, complement is fixed. Then sheep red blood cells and antisheep erythrocyte antibody are added; lack of hemolysis indicates complement fixation, i.e., a positive test result. Quantitative results are obtained by determining the highest dilution of antiserum or test material that gives a positive reaction. Called also *Bordet-Gengou phenomenon* or *reaction*.
**elastic band f.**, the stabilization of fractured segments of the jaws by means of intermaxillary elastic bands applied to splints or appliances.
**external pin f.**, in oral surgery, a method for stabilizing fractures by means of pins drilled into the bony parts through the overlying skin and connected by metal bars.
**external pin f., biphase**, external pin fixation in which the rigid metal bar connector is replaced with an acrylic bar adapted at the time of the reduction.
**internal f., intraosseous f.**, the open reduction and stabilization of fractured bony parts by direct fixation to one another with surgical wires, screws, pins, and plates.
**maxillomandibular f.**, the fixation of fractures of the maxilla or mandible in a functional relationship with the opposing dental arch, through the use of elastics, wire ligatures, arch bars, or other splints.
**nasomandibular f.**, mandibular immobilization, especially for edentulous jaws, using maxillomandibular splints; a circummandibular wire is connected with an intraoral interosseous wire passed through a hole drilled into the anterior nasal spine of the maxilla.
**nitrogen f.**, the union of the free atmospheric nitrogen with other elements to form chemical compounds, such as ammonia and nitrates or amino groups. This occurs primarily through the action of soil bacteria of the genus *Rhizobium* or *Bradyrhizobium* in symbiosis with leguminous plants. Nonbiological nitrogen fixation processes include electrical methods and chemical catalysis (Haber process).
**ossicular f.**, the fixing of one or more of the auditory ossicles by fibrous adhesion, tympanosclerosis, or bony fixation; it may be congenital or secondary to infection or trauma.
**skeletal f.**, immobilization of the ends of a fractured bone by metal wires or plates applied directly to the bone *(internal skeletal fixation)* or on the body surface *(external skeletal fixation)*.

**fix·a·tive** (fik'sə-tiv) a fluid, often a mixture of several reactive chemicals, into which histological or cytological specimens are placed so that, by processes such as denaturation and cross-linking of proteins, autolysis is prevented, the specimen is hardened to withstand further processing, and the specimen is preserved in a close facsimile of the living state in regard to both cellular morphology and the location of subcellular constituents. A standard fixative for routine use is buffered neutral formalin. A wide variety of fixatives, containing ingredients such as formalin, glutaraldehyde, and other aldehydes, ethanol, methanol, and other alcohols, acetone, acetic acid, chromates, mercuric salts, and picric acid, are used for special purposes. Osmium tetroxide and glutaraldehyde are standard fixatives for processing specimens for electron microscopy.
**glutaraldehyde f.**, a fixative used in specimen preparation for electron microscopy that does not simultaneously stain the tissue.
**Kaiserling's f.**, see under *solution*.
**Maximow's f.**, a solution composed of Zenker's fixative, formol, and osmic acid, used in preserving vertebrate cells for study with the visible light microscope.
**Zenker's f.**, a fixative solution containing corrosive mercuric chloride, potassium bichromate, sodium sulfate, glacial acetic acid, and water; the sodium sulfate is frequently omitted. The most widely

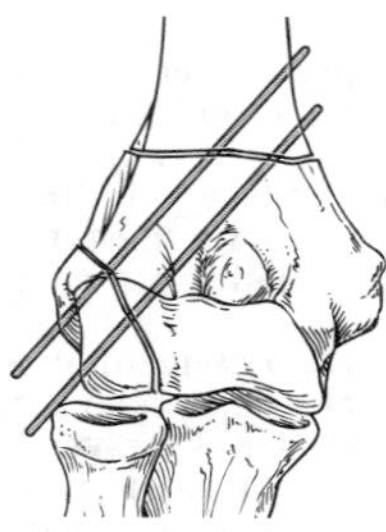

Internal fixation.

used variations of this fixative are the modifications by Maximow, by Helly, and by Custer, in which formalin replaces the acetic acid.
**Zenker-formol f.,** a solution composed of Zenker's fixative with added formalin; see *Helly's fluid,* under *fluid.*

**fix·a·tor** (fik'sa-tər) see under *muscle.*

**Fl.** fluid.

**FLA** fronto-laeva anterior (left frontoanterior—a position of the fetus).

**F.l.a.** abbreviation for L. *fi'at le'ge ar'tis,* let it be done according to rule.

**Flab·el·li·na** (flab″ə-li'nə) [L. *flabellum* fan] a suborder of ameboid protozoa (order Amoebida, class Lobosea) having a flattened, broad, sometimes discoid body with an extensive hyaline zone but no obvious pellicle-like layer.

**flac·cid** (flak'sid) [L. *flaccidus*] 1. weak or soft. 2. atonic.

**fla·che·rie** (flă-shre') [Fr.] a fatal disease of silkworms occurring in two forms: an infectious form due to a small nonoccluded virus and a noninfectious form due to environmental changes, such as a sudden increase in temperature and humidity. It is marked by diarrhea, weakness, flaccidity, and death, after which the body quickly turns dark and the tissues liquefy. See also *gattine.*

**Flack's node, test** (flaks) [Martin William *Flack,* British physiologist, 1882–1931] see *nodus sinuatrialis* and see under *test.*

**fla·gel·la** (flə-jel'ə) [L.] [MeSH: Flagella] plural of *flagellum.*

**flag·el·lan·tism** (flaj'ə-lən-tiz″əm) a type of sadomasochism characterized by the practice of whipping or being whipped for sexual arousal or gratification.

**fla·gel·lar** (flə-jel'ər) of or relating to a flagellum.

**Flag·el·la·ta** (flaj″ə-la'tə) former name for Mastigophora.

**flag·el·late** (flaj'ə-lāt) 1. any microorganism having flagella as organs of locomotion. 2. any protozoan of the subphylum Mastigophora. 3. having flagella. 4. to practice flagellation.
**animal-like f.,** any protozoan of the class Zoomastigophorea.
**plantlike f.,** any protozoan of the class Phytomastigophorea.

**flag·el·la·tion** (flaj″ə-la'shən) 1. the act or instance of whipping or beating, particularly as a sexual excitant. 2. the formation of flagella. 3. the arrangement of flagella on an organism or surface.

**fla·gel·li·form** (flə-jel'ĭ-form) [*flagellum* + *form*] shaped like a flagellum, or lash.

**fla·gel·lin** (flə-jel'in) [MeSH: Flagellin] a protein (mol. wt. approximately 40,000) occurring in the flagella of bacteria, which is composed of subunits arranged in several-stranded helix formation somewhat resembling myosin in structure, and sometimes containing ε-N-methyl lysine. Its composition varies with the species; thus flagellin antibodies are species-specific.

**flag·el·lo·sis** (flaj″ə-lo'sis) infection with flagellate protozoa.

**fla·gel·lo·spore** (flə-jel'o-spor) zoospore.

**fla·gel·lum** (flə-jel'əm) pl. *flagel'la* [L. "whip"] a long, mobile, whiplike projection from the free surface of a cell, serving as a locomotor organelle. In eukaryotes, it is composed of nine pairs of microtubules arrayed around a central pair. Arising from basal bodies, flagella are common to all mastigophoran protozoa and occur in such specialized cells as spermatozoa. Bacterial flagella are thinner and simpler, being composed of strands of flagellin tightly woven in a helical filament, attached to a basal body in the cell wall. Based on the configuration of their flagella, bacteria are characterized as either *monotrichous, lophotrichous, amphitrichous,* or *peritrichous.* See also *cilia* (def. 3).

**Flag·yl** (flag'əl) trademark for a preparation of metronidazole.

**flail** (flāl) exhibiting abnormal or paradoxical mobility, as flail joint, flail chest, or flail valve.

**Fla·jani's disease** (flə-jah'nēz) [Giuseppe *Flajani,* Italian surgeon, 1741–1808] Graves' disease.

**flame** (flām) 1. the luminous, irregular appearance usually accompanying combustion caused by the light emitted from energetically excited chemical species, or an appearance resembling it. 2. to render an object sterile by exposure to a flame.

**flange** (flanj) that part of the denture base which extends from the cervical ends of the teeth to the border of the denture. Called also *denture f.*
**buccal f.,** the portion of the flange of a denture that occupies the buccal vestibule of the mouth and extends distally from the buccal notch.
**denture f.,** flange.
**labial f.,** the portion of the flange of a denture that occupies the labial vestibule of the mouth.
**lingual f.,** the portion of the flange of a mandibular denture which occupies the space adjacent to the residual ridge and next to the tongue.

**flank** (flank) the side of the body inferior to the ribs and superior to the ilium; called also *latus* [TA].

**flap** (flap) [MeSH: Surgical Flaps] 1. a mass of tissue for grafting, usually including skin, only partially removed from one part of the body so that it retains its own blood supply during its transfer to a new location; used to repair defects in an adjacent or distant part of the body. 2. an uncontrolled movement.
**Abbe f.,** a triangular, full-thickness flap from the median portion of the lower lip used to fill a defect in the upper lip.
**advancement f.,** a local flap carried to its new position by a sliding technique of surgical advancement; called also *sliding f.*
**axial pattern f.,** a myocutaneous flap containing an artery in its long axis. Cf. *random pattern f.*
**bilobed f.,** a surgical flap consisting of a large lobe, which is transposed into the primary defect, and a smaller second lobe, which is transposed to fill the secondary defect produced by mobilization of the large lobe.
**bipedicle f.,** a pedicle flap with two vascular attachments.
**Boari f.,** in a ureteroneocystostomy, a flap of bladder wall that is fashioned into a tube and attached to a remnant ureter to replace a missing ureteral segment.
**bone f.,** craniotomy involving elevation of a section of skull; used to correct skull abnormalities or to allow surgical access to a relatively large area of the brain.
**cross-arm f.,** a surgical flap cut from one arm and attached to the other to repair a defect.
**cross-leg f.,** a surgical flap cut from one leg and attached to the other to repair a defect.
**delayed transfer f.,** a surgical flap that is partially raised from its donor bed and then replaced; done to permit development of collateral circulation through the pedicle.
**deltopectoral f.,** an axial pattern flap whose blood supply is the internal mammary artery and its branches; tissue is transferred from the deltoid and pectoral regions to the neck.
**direct transfer f.,** immediate transfer f.
**distant f.,** a pedicle flap brought from a distant area and transplanted by bringing the donor area and the recipient site into close approximation; called also *Italian f.*
**double pedicle f.,** bipedicle f.
**Eloesser f.,** a flap of skin created over the ribs for open drainage of chronic empyema.
**envelope f.,** a mucoperiosteal flap retracted from a horizontal linear incision (as along the free gingival margin) with no vertical component of that incision.
**Estlander f.,** a triangular flap from the side of the lower lip used to fill a defect in the lateral upper lip.
**free f.,** an island flap detached from the body and reattached at the distant recipient site by microvascular anastomosis.
**French f.,** advancement f.
**gauntlet f.,** pedicle f.
**Gillies' f.,** tube f.
**immediate transfer f.,** a surgical flap that is applied to the recipient site immediately after it is elevated from its bed; called also *direct transfer f.*
**Indian f.,** interpolated f.
**interpolated f.,** a local pedicle flap that is twisted or rotated on its base and placed into a contiguous area; called also *Indian f.*
**island f.,** a skin flap consisting of the skin and subcutaneous tissue with a pedicle made up of only the nutrient vessels.
**Italian f.,** distant f.
**jump f.,** a flap cut from the abdomen and attached to the forearm; the flap is transferred later to some other part of the body to fill a defect there.
**Langenbeck's pedicle mucoperiosteal f.,** von Langenbeck's bipedicle mucoperiosteal f.
**lingual tongue f.,** a combination flap used to repair fistulae of the hard palate: a palatal flap forms the floor of the nose, and a flap taken from the back or edge of the tongue forms the palatal surface.
**liver f.,** asterixis.
**local f.,** a surgical flap cut from tissue neighboring the defect, such as an advancement flap or some kinds of pedicle flaps.
**mucoperiosteal f.,** a flap of mucosal tissue, including the periosteum, reflected from bone.
**musculocutaneous f., myocutaneous f.,** a compound flap of skin and muscle with adequate vascularity to permit sufficient tissue to be transferred to the recipient site.
**pedicle f.,** a flap consisting of the full thickness of the skin and the subcutaneous tissue, attached by tissue through which it receives its blood supply. See also *local f.* and *distant f.*
**random pattern f.,** a myocutaneous flap with a random pattern of arteries, as opposed to an axial pattern flap.
**rope f.,** tube f.
**rotation f.,** a local pedicle flap whose width is increased by having the edge distal to the defect form a curved line; the flap is then

rotated and a counterincision is made at the base of the curved line, which increases the mobility of the flap. See illustration.
**skin f.,** a full-thickness mass or flap of tissue containing epidermis, dermis, and subcutaneous tissue.
**sliding f.,** advancement f.
**TRAM f.,** an autogenous myocutaneous flap that uses transverse rectus abdominal muscle (TRAM) to carry lower abdominal skin and fat to the breast for reconstruction.
**tube f., tubed pedicle f.,** a bipedicle flap made by elevating a long strip of tissue from its bed except at the two ends, the cut edges then being sutured together to form a tube; called also *rope* or *tunnel f.* and *Gillies' f.*
**tunnel f.,** tube f.
**tympanomeatal f.,** a flap made by an incision of the inferior part of the external auditory meatus, including the tympanum and part of the meatus, created surgically for access to the middle ear.
**von Langenbeck's bipedicle mucoperiosteal f.,** a bipedicle flap of the conjoined mucoperiosteal tissues, used for closure of a cleft palate.
**V-Y f.,** a flap in which the incision is made in the shape of a V and is sutured in the shape of a Y so as to lengthen an area of tissue; or conversely the incision is Y-shaped and the closure V-shaped to shorten an area of tissue.
**Widman f., modified,** see *surgical curettage,* under *curettage.*
**Z-f.,** a flap in which the incision is made in the shape of a Z so as to distribute contraction in more than one direction; often used to correct scars.
**Zimany's bilobed f.,** bilobed f.

**flare** (flār) 1. the red outermost zone of the "triple response" (Sir Thomas Lewis) urticarial wheal reaction, a manifestation of immediate, as opposed to delayed, allergy or hypersensitivity. 2. a spreading flush or area of redness on the skin, spreading out around an infective lesion or extending beyond the main point of reaction to an irritant. 3. sudden exacerbation of a disease.

**flash** (flash) excess material extruded from a mold, as in the packing of a denture by the compression technique.

**flash·lamp** (flash'lamp) a lamp that produces an intense light in pulses with alternate on and off phases of a few microseconds each; used with pulsed dye lasers.

**flask** (flask) 1. a container, such as a narrow-necked vessel of glass for containing liquid. 2. a metal case in which the materials used in the creation of artificial dentures are placed for processing. 3. to place a denture in a flask for processing.
**casting f.,** refractory f.
**crown f.,** denture f.
**denture f.,** a sectional, boxlike metal, ceramic, or polymer case that can be tightly closed, and with which sectional molds of plaster of Paris or dental stone are used to compress and form a resinous denture base or crown material during curing. Called also *crown f.*
**Erlenmeyer f.,** a glass flask with a conical body, broad base, and narrow neck.
**refractory f.,** a metal tube in which a refractory mold is made for casting metal dental restorations or appliances; called also *casting f.*
**volumetric f.,** a narrow-necked vessel of glass calibrated to contain or deliver an exact volume at a given temperature.

**flask·ing** (flask'ing) 1. the act of investing in a flask. 2. the process of investing the cast and a wax denture in a flask preparatory to molding the denture base material into the form of the denture.

**flat** (flat) 1. lying in one plane; having an even surface. 2. having little or no resonance. 3. slightly below the normal pitch of a musical tone.
**optical f.,** a glass plate so perfectly flat that only an interferometer can measure its unevenness.

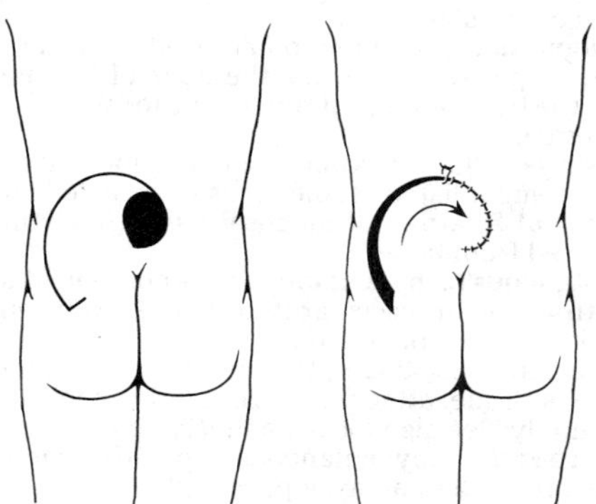

Rotation flap.

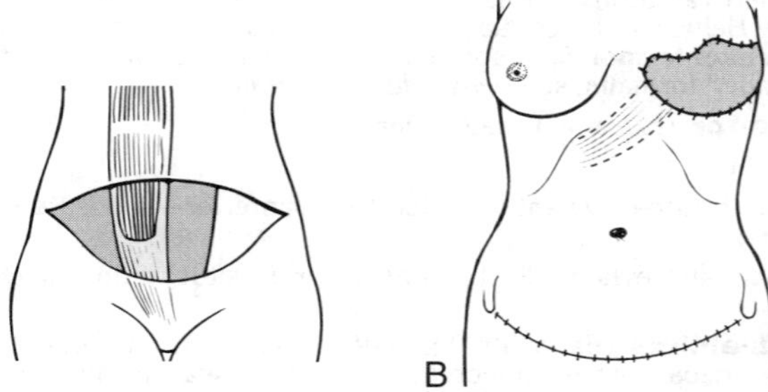


TRAM flap. *(A),* Rectus abdominis muscle and the attached skin and subcutaneous tissue *(shaded),* which will be used to form the flap. *(B),* The skin and tissue on the muscle pedicle have been transferred to the contralateral chest wall via a subcutaneous tunnel in the abdomen and chest, then sculpted and sutured to reconstruct the breast.

**Fla·tau's law** (flah'touz) [Edward *Flatau,* Polish neurologist, 1869–1932] see under *law.*

**Fla·tau-Schil·der disease** (flah'tou-shil'dər) [E. *Flatau;* Paul Ferdinand *Schilder,* German-born American psychiatrist, 1886–1940] see *Schilder's disease,* under *disease.*

**flat·foot** (flat'foot) [MeSH: Flatfoot] a condition in which one or more of the arches of the foot have been lowered and flattened out; called also *pes planovalgus, pes planus,* and *pes valgus.*
**rocker-bottom f.,** see under *foot.*
**spastic f.,** a painful form of flatfoot due to spasm of the peroneal muscles.

**flat·ness** (flat'nəs) a peculiar sound lacking resonance, heard on percussing a part that is abnormally solid.

**flat·ten·ing** (flat'ə-ning) making flat; diminishing.
**f. of affect,** see under *affect.*

**flat·u·lence** (flat'u-ləns) [L. *flatulentia*] [MeSH: Flatulence] the presence of excessive amounts of air or gas in the stomach or intestine, leading to distention of the organs.

**flat·u·lent** (flat'u-lənt) [L. *flatulentus*] pertaining to or characterized by flatulence; distended with gas.

**Flat·u·lex** (flat'u-leks) trademark for a preparation of simethicone and activated charcoal.

**fla·tus** (fla'təs) [L. "a blowing"] 1. gas or air in the gastrointestinal tract. 2. gas or air expelled through the anus.
**f. vagina'lis,** noisy expulsion of gas from the vagina.

**flat·worm** (flat'wərm) platyhelminth.

**fla·vec·to·my** (fla-vek'tə-me) [*flavo-* + *-ectomy*] excision of the ligamentum flavum.

**fla·ves·cent** (flə-ves'ənt) [L. *flavescere* to become gold colored] yellowish.

**fla·vin** (fla'vin) [L. *flavus* yellow] any one of a group of compounds containing the isoalloxazine nucleus, especially riboflavin. Flavin compounds are characterized by a yellow color and intense green fluorescence in the oxidized form; the reduced form is colorless.
**f. adenine dinucleotide (FAD),** a coenzyme composed of riboflavin 5′-phosphate (FMN) and adenosine 5′-phosphate linked by a pyrophosphate bond; it forms the prosthetic group of many flavoprotein enzymes, including D-amino acid oxidase and xanthine oxidase, serving as an electron carrier by being alternately oxidized (FAD) and reduced ($FADH_2$). It is important in electron transport in mitochondria and the endoplasmic reticulum.
**f. mononucleotide (FMN),** riboflavin 5′-phosphate; it acts as a coenzyme for a number of oxidative enzymes, including NADH dehydrogenase, serving as an electron carrier by being alternately oxidized (FMN) and reduced ($FMNH_2$).

**fla·vin mono·oxy·ge·nase** (fla'vin mon″o-ok'sə-jən-ās) unspecific monooxygenase.

**Fla·vi·vi·ri·dae** (fla″vĭ-vir'ĭ-de) [MeSH: Flaviviridae] the flaviviruses: a family of RNA viruses having a virion 40–60 nm in diameter consisting of a lipid envelope, with fine peplomers, surrounding a spherical nucleocapsid. The genome consists of a single molecule of positive-sense single-stranded RNA (MW $4 \times 10^6$, size 9.5–12.5 kb). Viruses contain two or three major structural polypeptides and are sensitive to lipid solvents, detergents, ultraviolet radiation, and heat. Replication occurs in the cytoplasm and assembly is by budding through the plasma membrane. It includes the genera *Flavivirus, Pestivirus,* and Hepacivirus.

**Fla·vi·vi·rus** (fla'vĭ-vi″rəs) [*flavo-* + *virus*] [MeSH: Flavivirus] a genus of viruses of the family Flaviviridae of worldwide distribution, containing about 75 species in 9 serogroups, many members of which cause disease in humans and animals. Important human pathogens include the yellow fever, dengue, West Nile, St. Louis encephalitis, Japanese encephalitis, Murray Valley encephalitis, tick-borne encephalitis, Kyasanur Forest disease, and Omsk hemorrhagic fever viruses. Mosquitoes are the most common vector, with some species being tick-borne and some species having no known vector. Formerly called group B arboviruses.

**fla·vi·vi·rus** (fla′və-vi″rəs) [MeSH: Flavivirus] any virus belonging to the family *Flaviviridae.*

**flav(o)-** [L. *flavus* yellow] a combining form meaning yellow.

**Fla·vo·bac·te·ri·um** (fla″vo-bak-tēr′e-əm) [*flavo-* + *bacterium*] [MeSH: Flavobacterium] a genus of gram-negative, aerobic or facultatively anaerobic, rod-shaped bacteria of uncertain affiliation, characterized by production of a yellow pigment. The organisms occur widely in soil and water, and are opportunistic pathogens in humans.
**F. bre′ve,** a species of uncertain pathogenicity, occasionally recovered from clinical specimens.
**F. meningosep′ticum,** a pathogenic species that is a major cause of nosocomial infections, producing meningitis and septicemia with a high fatality rate in premature and newborn infants. In adults, it causes a milder bacteremia.
**F. odora′tum,** a pathogenic species usually producing yellow pigment and a fruity odor, recovered from infections of wounds and the urinary tract.

**fla·vo·en·zyme** (fla″vo-en′zīm) any enzyme that is a flavoprotein.

**fla·vo·noid** (fla′və-noid) any of a group of compounds containing a characteristic aromatic trimeric heterocyclic nucleus, usually occurring in glycosidic form and widely distributed in plants, often as a pigment. A subgroup with biological activity in mammals is termed the bioflavonoids (q.v.).

**fla·vo·pro·tein** (fla″vo-pro′tēn) a protein containing a flavin nucleotide (FAD or FMN) as a prosthetic group. Most flavoproteins are enzymes; many are found in complexes containing metal ions and an iron-sulfur complex or a heme. They catalyze a wide variety of oxidation-reduction reactions.

**fla·vor** (fla′vor) 1. that quality of any substance which affects the taste. 2. a pharmaceutical or other preparation for improving the taste of a food or medicine.

**fla·vo·xan·thin** (fla″vo-zan′thin) a minor, yellow, carotenoid pigment from the petals of ranunculaceous plants, structurally related to vitamin A but having no vitamin A activity.

**fla·vox·ate hy·dro·chlo·ride** (fla-voks′āt) a smooth muscle relaxant used as an antispasmodic for the urinary system, administered orally.

**flax** (flaks) any of various plants of the genus *Linum,* especially *L. usitatis′simum.*

**Flax·e·dil** (flak′sə-dil) trademark for a preparation of gallamine triethiodide.

**flax·seed** (flak′sēd) linseed.

**fld** fluid.

**fl dr** fluid dram.

**flea** (fle) [MeSH: Fleas] any insect of the order *Siphonaptera;* many are parasitic and may act as carriers of disease. Genera of medical importance include *Cediopsylla, Ceratophyllus, Ctenocephalides, Ctenophthalmus, Diamanus, Echidnophaga, Hoplopsyllus, Leptopsylla, Monopsyllus, Neopsylla, Nosopsyllus, Oropsylla, Pulex, Rhopalopsyllus, Tunga,* and *Xenopsylla.*
**Asiatic rat f.,** *Xenopsylla cheopis.*
**burrowing f.,** chigoe.
**cat f.,** *Ctenocephalides felis.*
**cavy f.,** *Rhopalopsyllus cavicola.*
**chigoe f.,** chigoe.
**common human f.,** *Pulex irritans.*
**common rat f.,** *Nosopsyllus fasciatus.*
**dog f.,** *Ctenocephalides canis.*
**European mouse f.,** *Ctenophthalmus agrytes.*
**European rat f.,** *Nosopsyllus fasciatus.*
**human f.,** *Pulex irritans.*
**Indian rat f.,** *Xenopsylla astia.*
**jigger f.,** chigoe.
**mouse f.,** *Leptopsylla segnis.*
**rat f.,** any of various species of *Nosopsyllus* and *Xenopsylla.*
**sand f.,** chigoe.
**squirrel f.,** *Hoplopsyllus anomalus.*
**sticktight f.,** *Echidnophaga gallinacea.*
**suslik f.,** any of several species of fleas that infest the suslik (Russian ground squirrel) and are vectors of plague.
**tropical rat f.,** *Xenopsylla cheopis.*

**fle·cai·nide ace·tate** (fle-ka′nīd) [USP] a sodium channel blocker that decreases the rate of cardiac conduction and increases the ventricular refractory period; used in the treatment of life-threatening arrhythmias.

**Flech·sig's cuticulum, field,** etc. (flek′sigz) [Paul Emil *Flechsig,* German neurologist, 1847–1929] see under *cuticulum* and *zone* and see *myelinogenetic field* under *field* and *tractus spinocerebellaris posterior.*

**fleck** (flek) a flake, particle, speckle, or spot.
**tobacco f's,** Gamna nodules.

**fleck·fie·ber** (flek-fe′bər) [Ger.] epidemic typhus; see under *typhus.*

**fleck·milz** (flek′milts) [Ger.] a condition of the spleen in myeloid leukemia and other leukemic or lymphomatous diseases characterized by multiple pale ischemic infarcts.

**fleece** (flēs) 1. the thick, woolly or hairy coat of a sheep or other animal. 2. a network of interlacing fibers; see *neuropil.*
**f. of Stilling,** the lacework of myelinated fibers surrounding the dentate nucleus.

**Fle·gel's disease** (fla′gəlz) [Heinz *Flegel,* German physician, born 1923] hyperkeratosis lenticularis perstans; see under *hyperkeratosis.*

**Fleisch·ner's disease** (flīsh′nərz) [Felix *Fleischner,* Austrian-born American radiologist, 1893–1969] see under *disease.*

**Flem·ing** (flem′ing) Sir Alexander. Scottish bacteriologist, 1881–1955; co-winner, with Ernst Boris Chain and Sir Howard Walter Florey, of the Nobel prize for medicine or physiology for 1945 for the discovery of penicillin.

**Flem·ming's center, solution (fixing fluid)** (flem′ingz) [Walther *Flemming,* German anatomist, 1843–1905] see *germinal center,* under *center,* and see under *solution.*

**fler·ox·a·cin** a fluoroquinolone antibiotic having actions and uses similar to those of ciprofloxacin; administered orally or by intravenous infusion.

**flesh** (flesh) [A.S. *flaesc*] 1. muscular tissue. 2. skin.
**goose f.,** cutis anserina.
**proud f.,** exuberant amounts of soft, edematous, granulation tissue that may develop during the healing of large surface wounds.

**flet·cher·ism** (flech′ər-iz-əm) [Horace *Fletcher,* American dietitian, 1849–1919] the thorough mastication of solid food and the taking of liquids by sips.

**fleur·ette** (floor-et′) [Fr. "small flower"] a type of cell found in clusters in retinoblastomas and retinocytomas, representing differentiation of tumor cells into photoreceptors; eosinophilic processes project through the cell membrane so that the cell resembles a flower with petals.

**flex** (fleks) [L. *flexus* bent] to bend or put in a state of flexion.

**Flex·er·il** (flek′sə-ril) trademark for a preparation of cyclobenzaprine hydrochloride.

**Flex·i·bac·ter** (flek′se-bak″tər) a genus of gram-negative bacteria closely related to *Cytophaga.*
**F. columna′ris,** *Cytophaga columnaris.*

**flex·i·bil·i·tas** (flek″sĭ-bil′ĭ-təs) [L.] flexibility.
**ce′rea f.,** see under *C.*

**flex·i·bil·i·ty** (flek″sĭ-bil′ĭ-te) [L. *flexibilitas*] the quality of being flexible.
**waxy f.,** cerea flexibilitas.

**flex·i·ble** (flek′sĭ-bəl) [L. *flexibilis, flexilis*] readily bent without tendency to break.

**flex·ile** (fleks′īl) flexible.

**flex·ion** (flek′shən) [L. *flexio*] 1. the act of bending or condition of being bent. 2. in gynecology, a displacement of the uterus in which the organ is bent so far anteriorly or posteriorly that an acute angle forms between the fundus and the cervix. See *version* (def. 3). 3. in obstetrics, the normal bending forward of the head of the fetus in the uterus or the birth canal.
**plantar f.,** bending of the toes or foot downward toward the sole.

**Flex·ner's bacillus, dysentery** (fleks′nərz) [Simon *Flexner,* American pathologist, 1863–1946] see *Shigella flexneri,* and see *bacillary dysentery,* under *dysentery.*

**Flex·ner-Win·ter·stei·ner rosette** (fleks′nər vin′tər-shti″nər) [S. *Flexner;* Hugo *Wintersteiner,* Austrian ophthalmologist, 1865–1918] see under *rosette.*

**flex·or** (flek′sor) [L.] [TA] 1. causing flexion. 2. any muscle that flexes a joint; see under *musculus.*

**f. retina'culum,** see *retinaculum musculorum flexorum manus* and *retinaculum musculorum flexorum pedis.*

**flex·or·plas·ty** (flek'sor-plas"te) plastic surgery of flexor muscles.

**flex·u·ose** (flek'su-ōs) winding or wavy.

**flex·u·ra** (flek-shoo'rə) gen. and pl. *flexu'rae* [L.] [TA] flexure: a bending; a general term for a bent portion of a structure or organ.
**f. anorecta'lis rec'ti** [TA], anorectal flexure of rectum: the dorsal and caudal bend at the caudal end of the rectum; called also *f. perinealis recti* [TA alternative] and *perineal flexure of rectum.*
**f. co'li dex'tra** [TA], right flexure of colon: the bend in the large intestine at which the ascending colon becomes the transverse colon; called also *f. coli hepatica* [TA alternative], *f. hepatica coli,* and *hepatic flexure of colon.*
**f. co'li hepa'tica,** TA alternative for *f. coli dextra.*
**f. co'li sinis'tra** [TA], left flexure of colon: the bend in the large intestine at which the transverse colon becomes the descending colon; called also *f. lienalis coli* and *splenic flexure of colon.*
**f. co'li sple'nica,** TA alternative for *f. coli sinistra.*
**f. duode'ni infe'rior** [TA], inferior flexure of duodenum: the bend in the duodenum at which the descending duodenum becomes horizontal or transverse. Called also *inferior angle of duodenum.*
**f. duode'ni supe'rior** [TA], superior flexure of duodenum: the bend in the first or superior part of the duodenum; called also *superior angle of duodenum.*
**f. duodenojejuna'lis** [TA], duodenojejunal flexure: the bend in the small intestine at the junction between the duodenum and jejunum; the suspensory muscle of the duodenum attaches to this point.
**f. hepa'tica co'li,** f. coli dextra.
**f. liena'lis co'li,** f. coli sinistra.
**f. perinea'lis rec'ti,** TA alternative for *f. anorectalis recti.*
**f. sacra'lis rec'ti** [TA], sacral flexure of rectum: the dorsal first bend in the rectum.

**flex·u·rae** (flek-shoo're) [L.] genitive and plural of *flexura.*

**flex·ur·al** (flek'shər-əl) pertaining to or affecting a flexure.

**flex·ure** (flek'shər) a bending; a bent portion of a structure or organ; see *flexura.*
**anorectal f. of rectum,** flexura anorectalis recti.
**basicranial f.,** pontine f.
**caudal f.,** the bend at the aboral (caudal) end of the embryo; called also *sacral f.*
**cephalic f.,** the curve in the midbrain (mesencephalon) of the neural tube; called also *cranial f.* and *mesencephalic f.*
**cerebral f., cervical f.,** a bend in the neural tube of the embryo at the junction of the brain and spinal cord; called also *head bend, neck bend,* and *nuchal f.*
**cranial f.,** cephalic f.
**dorsal f.,** one of the flexures of the embryo in the mid-dorsal region.
**duodenojejunal f.,** flexura duodenojejunalis.
**hepatic f. of colon,** flexura coli dextra.
**inferior f. of duodenum,** flexura duodeni inferior.
**left f. of colon,** flexura coli sinistra.
**lumbar f.,** the ventral curvature of the back in the lumbar region.
**mesencephalic f.,** cranial f.
**nuchal f.,** cervical f.
**perineal f. of rectum,** flexura anorectalis recti.
**pontine f.,** a flexure in the hindbrain of the embryo; called also *basicranial f.*
**right f. of colon,** flexura coli dextra.
**sacral f.,** caudal f.
**sacral f. of rectum,** flexura sacralis recti.
**sigmoid f.,** sigmoid colon.
**splenic f. of colon,** flexura coli sinistra.
**superior f. of duodenum,** flexura duodeni superior.

**flick·er** (flik'ər) [A.S. *flicorian* to flutter] the visual sensation produced by regular flashes of light; the flashes may appear to flutter or to be steady according to the rate of interruption; called also *flicker phenomenon.* See also *critical fusion frequency,* under *frequency.*

**flight of ideas** (flīt of i-de'əz) a nearly continuous flow of rapid speech that jumps from topic to topic, usually based on discernible associations, distractions, or plays on words, but in severe cases so rapid as to be disorganized and incoherent. It is most commonly seen in manic episodes but may also occur in other mental disorders such as in manic phases of schizophrenia.

**Flin·ders Is·land spotted fever** (flin'dərz i'lənd) [*Flinders Island,* northeast of Tasmania, Australia] see under *fever.*

**Flint's arcade, law** (flints) [Austin *Flint,* Jr., American physiologist, 1836–1915] see under *arcade* and *law.*

**Flint's murmur** (flints) [Austin *Flint,* American physician, 1812–1886] see under *murmur.*

**float·ers** (flo'tərz) "spots before the eyes"; deposits in the vitreous of the eye, usually moving about and probably representing fine aggregates of vitreous protein occurring as a benign degenerative change. Called also *vitreous f's* and *muscae volitantes.*

**floc·cil·la·tion** (flok"sĭ-la'shən) [L. *floccilatio*] the aimless picking at bedclothes by a patient with delirium, dementia, fever, or exhaustion; called also *carphology, crocidismus,* and *tilmus.*

**floc·cose** (flok'ōs) [L. *floccosus* full of flocks of wool] woolly; said of a bacterial growth which is composed of short, curved chains variously oriented.

**floc·cu·lar** (flok'u-lər) pertaining to the flocculus.

**floc·cu·la·tion** (flok"u-la'shən) [MeSH: Flocculation] 1. a colloid phenomenon in which the disperse phase separates in discrete, usually visible, fleecy particles rather than in a continuous mass, as in coagulation. 2. in immunology, the formation of downy masses of precipitate in a precipitin test or of agglutinated bacteria in an agglutination test for the H antigens of *Salmonella* species.

**floc·cule** (flok'ūl) flocculus.
**toxoid-antitoxin f.,** a suspension of the precipitate formed when toxoid and antitoxin are mixed.

**floc·cu·lent** (flok'u-lənt) containing downy or flaky masses.

**floc·cu·lus** (flok'u-ləs) pl. *floc'culi* [L. "tuft"] 1. a small tuft, as of wool or similar material, or a small mass of other fibrous material such as one of the flakes of a flocculent solution. 2. [TA] one of the small paired, partially detached lateral lobules continuous with the nodulus of the cerebellum, separated from each cerebellar hemisphere by the dorsolateral fissure, and forming part of the flocculonodular lobe.
**accessory f.,** paraflocculus.

**floc·ta·fen·ine** (flok"tə-fen'ēn) a nonsteroidal antiinflammatory drug derived from anthranilic acid, used for the short-term relief of pain; administered orally.

**Flo·nase** (flo'nās) trademark for a preparation of fluticasone propionate.

**Flood's ligament** (fludz) [Valentine *Flood,* Irish surgeon, 1800–1847] see under *ligament.*

**flood·ing** (flud'ing) in behavior therapy, a form of desensitization for the treatment of phobias and related disorders in which the patient is repeatedly exposed to highly distressing stimuli without being able to escape but without danger, until the lack of reinforcement of the anxiety response causes its extinction. In general, the term is used for actual exposure to the stimuli, with *implosion* used for imagined exposure, but the two terms are sometimes used synonymously to describe either or both types of exposure. Cf. *systematic densensitization.*

**floor** (flor) [A.S. *flōr*] the inferior inner surface of a hollow organ or other space.
**cavity f.,** f. of prepared cavity.
**f. of fourth ventricle,** fossa rhomboidea.
**f. of lateral ventricle,** the inferior interior surface of the lateral ventricle, formed by the caudate nucleus, the stria terminalis, the thalamostriate veins, the collateral eminence, and the superior surfaces of the thalamus, the rostrum of the corpus callosum, and the hippocampus.
**f. of nasal cavity,** the inferior surface of the cavity, formed by the palatine process of the maxilla and the horizontal plate of the palatine bone.
**f. of orbit,** paries inferior orbitae.
**f. of pelvis,** the layer of tissue just below the outlet of the pelvis, formed by the coccygeal and levator ani muscles and the perineal fascia. See also *diaphragma pelvis.*
**f. of prepared cavity,** the bottom or enclosing base wall of a prepared cavity, which the restoration material rests on.
**f. of third ventricle,** the inferior interior surface of the third ventricle, formed by the optic chiasm, the tuber cinereum, the infundibulum, the mammillary bodies, and the posterior perforated substance.
**f. of tympanic cavity,** paries jugularis cavitatis tympani.

**Flor.** abbreviation for L. *flo'res,* flowers.

**flo·ra** (flor'ə) [L. *Flora,* the goddess of flowers] 1. the plant life present in or characteristic of a special location; it may be discernible with the unaided eye (macroflora), or only with the aid of a microscope (microflora). 2. the bacteria and fungi, both normally occurring and pathological, found in or on an organ.
**intestinal f.,** the bacteria normally residing within the lumen of the intestine.
**resident f.,** flora occurring in or on an organ over a protracted period.

**flor·an·ty·rone** (flor-an'tĭ-rōn) a hydrocholeretic agent administered orally in the treatment of chronic cholecystitis, cholangitis, and biliary dyskinesia, and in the prevention of cholelithiasis.

**Flor·a·quin** (flor'ə-kwin) trademark for a preparation of iodoquinol.

**flo·res** (flo′rēz) [L., pl. of *flos* flower] 1. the blossoms or flowers of a plant. 2. a drug after sublimation.
**f. benzoi′ni,** benzoic acid.
**f. sul′furis,** sublimed sulfur.

**Flo·rey** (flor′e) Sir Howard Walter. Australian-born British pathologist, 1898–1968; co-winner, with Ernst Boris Chain and Sir Alexander Fleming, of the Nobel prize for medicine or physiology in 1945 for the discovery of penicillin.

**flor·id** (flor′id) [L. *floridus* blossoming] 1. in full bloom; occurring in fully developed form. 2. having a bright red color.

**Flor·i·din** (flor′ĭ-din) trademark for a preparation of fuller's earth.

**Flor·i·nef** (flor′ĭ-nef) trademark for preparations of fludrocortisone acetate.

**Flor·one** (flor′ōn) trademark for preparations of diflorasone diacetate.

**Flor·o·pryl** (flor′o-pril) trademark for preparations of isoflurophate.

**Flo·vent** (flo′vent) trademark for a preparation of fluticasone propionate.

**flow** (flo) 1. the movement of a liquid or gas. 2. the rate at which a fluid passes through an organ or part, expressed as volume per unit of time. Called also *flow rate.*
**blood f.,** 1. circulation (def. 2). 2. circulation rate.
**forced expiratory f. (FEF),** the rate of airflow recorded in measurements of forced vital capacity, usually calculated as an average flow over a given portion of the expiratory curve; the portion between 25 and 75 per cent of forced vital capacity is called the *maximal* or *maximum midexpiratory f.*
**gene f.,** the movement of genes between populations due to migration and interbreeding.
**laminar f.,** the movement of corresponding parts of a fluid along parallel and relatively smooth paths; it has a lower Reynolds number than turbulent flow. See also *axial current,* under *current.*
**maximal expiratory f.,** maximum expiratory f.
**maximal midexpiratory f.,** maximum midexpiratory f.
**maximum expiratory f.,** the rate of airflow during a forced vital capacity maneuver, often specified at a given volume; see also *forced expiratory f.* Called also *maximal expiratory f.*
**maximum midexpiratory f.,** the average rate of airflow measured between expired volumes of 25 and 75 per cent of the vital capacity during a forced expiration. See also *forced expiratory f.* Called also *maximal midexpiratory f.* and *maximal* or *maximum midexpiratory flow rate.*
**peak expiratory f. (PEF),** the greatest rate of airflow that can be achieved during forced expiration beginning with the lungs fully inflated. Called also *peak expiratory f. rate.*
**renal blood f., effective (ERBF),** that portion of the total renal blood flow that perfuses functional renal tissue such as the glomeruli.
**renal plasma f. (RPF),** the amount of plasma that perfuses the kidneys per unit time, approximately 10 per cent greater than the effective renal plasma flow.
**renal plasma f., effective (ERPF),** the amount of plasma that perfuses the renal tubules per unit time, generally measured by the *p*-aminohippurate clearance.
**turbulent f.,** the movement of corresponding parts of a fluid through chaotic, nonparallel paths; it has a higher Reynolds number than laminar flow.

**Flow·er's index** (flou′ərz) [Sir William Henry *Flower,* British zoologist, 1831–1899] dental index; see under *index.*

**flow·ers** (flou′ərz) 1. the blossoms of a plant. 2. a sublimed drug.
**f. of arsenic,** arsenic trioxide.
**f. of benzoin,** benzoic acid.
**f. of camphor,** powdered camphor prepared by sublimation.
**pyrethrum f's,** the dried powdered flowers of certain species of *Chrysanthemum,* formerly used as an insecticide and scabicide because they contain pyrethrins. Called also *Dalmatian,* or *Persian, insect powder.*
**f. of sulfur,** sublimed sulfur.

**flow·me·ter** (flo′me-tər) [MeSH: Rheology] an apparatus for measuring the rate of flow of liquids or gases. See also *velocimetry.*
**blood f.,** an instrument for determining the rate of blood flow in the arteries or veins.
**Doppler ultrasonic f., Doppler ultrasound f.,** a device for measuring blood flow by noting the Doppler effect in ultrasonic waves reflected off moving red blood cells. Called also *ultrasonic* or *ultrasound Doppler f.*
**electromagnetic f.,** a flowmeter in which blood flow is examined by application of a magnetic field to a blood vessel and analysis of the voltage resulting in the vessel; the voltage is perpendicular to the direction of movement and to the magnetic field and is proportional to the velocity of movement.
**laser Doppler f.,** a flowmeter in which blood flow is examined by a laser beam; the light is shifted by moving objects, mostly red blood cells, in accordance with the Doppler effect and the scattered light detected with a photodetector.
**ultrasonic f.,** ultrasound f.
**ultrasonic Doppler f.,** Doppler ultrasonic f.
**ultrasound f.,** any of various types of flowmeters that use ultrasound techniques to measure blood flow, such as the *Doppler ultrasonic f.*
**ultrasound Doppler f.,** Doppler ultrasonic f.

**flox·a·cil·lin** (flok″sə-sil′in) [MeSH: Floxacillin] a penicillinase-resistant, semisynthetic penicillin which has been used primarily in the treatment of infections due to benzylpenicillin-resistant staphylococci. Called also *flucloxacillin.*

**Flox·in** (flok′sin) trademark for preparations of ofloxacin.

**flox·uri·dine** (floks-ūr′ĭ-dēn) [USP] [MeSH: Floxuridine] a fluoropyrimidine that is metabolically activated to the monophosphate nucleotide (F-dUMP), the metabolite of 5-fluorouracil (q.v.) that blocks DNA synthesis; FUDR is also metabolized to 5-fluorouracil; it is used as an antineoplastic by intra-arterial administration for treatment of liver metastases from gastrointestinal malignancies.

**fl oz** fluid ounce.

**FLP** fronto-laeva posterior (left frontoposterior—a position of the fetus).

**FLT** fronto-laeva transversa (left frontotransverse—a position of the fetus).

**flu** (floo) popular name for *influenza.*
**trimellitic anhydride (TMA) f.,** influenzalike symptoms in workers inhaling excessive amounts of trimellitic anhydride fumes. See also *trimellitic anhydride pneumonitis.*

**flu·ben·da·zole** (floo-ben′də-zōl) a benzimidazole anthelmintic used to treat roundworm infestations of humans and pigs.

**flu·clor·o·nide** (floo-klor′o-nīd) a synthetic glucocorticoid used in the treatment of steroid-responsive dermatoses.

**flu·clox·a·cil·lin** (floo-klok″sə-sil′in) floxacillin.

**flu·con·a·zole** (floo-kon′ə-zōl) [MeSH: Fluconazole] an antifungal agent used in the systemic treatment of candidiasis and cryptococcal meningitis; administered orally or intravenously.

**Flu·cort** (floo′kort) trademark for preparations of flumethasone.

**fluc·tu·ant** (fluk′choo-ənt) 1. showing varying levels. 2. conveying the sensation of or exhibiting wavelike motion on palpation, owing to a liquid content.

**fluc·tu·a·tion** (fluk″choo-a′shən) [L. *fluctuatio*] 1. a variation, as about a fixed value or mass. 2. a wavelike motion, as of a fluid in a cavity of the body after succussion.

**flu·cy·to·sine** (floo-si′to-sēn″) [USP] [MeSH: Flucytosine] an antifungal used in the treatment of serious infections, such as septicemia, endocarditis, and urinary tract infections, due to *Candida* and *Cryptococcus* species; administered orally.

**Flu·da·ra** (floo-dar′ə) trademark for a preparation of fludarabine phosphate.

**flu·dar·a·bine phos·phate** (floo-dar′ə-bēn) an adenine analogue and purine antimetabolite that inhibits DNA synthesis, used as an antineoplastic in the treatment of chronic lymphocytic leukemia; administered intravenously.

**flu·da·zo·ni·um chlo·ride** (floo″də-zo′ne-əm) a topical anti-infective, $C_{26}H_{20}Cl_5FN_2O_2$.

**flu·de·oxy·glu·cose F 18** (floo″de-ok″se-gloo′kōs) [USP] 2-deoxy-D-glucose labeled with $^{18}F$; used in positron emission tomography in the diagnosis of brain disorders, cardiac disease, and tumors of various organs. Called also *fluorodeoxyglucose.*

**flu·dro·cor·ti·sone ac·e·tate** (floo″dro-kor′tĭ-sōn) [USP] the acetate salt of a synthetic steroid with potent mineralocorticoid and high glucocorticoid activity, used in replacement therapy for primary or secondary adrenocortical insufficiency in Addison's disease and for the treatment of salt-losing adrenogenital syndrome.

**flu·ent** (floo′ənt) [L. *fluens* flowing] flowing effortlessly; said of speech.

**flu·fen·am·ic ac·id** (floo-fən-am′ik) [MeSH: Flufenamic Acid] an anthranilic acid derivative with analgesic, anti-inflammatory, and antipyretic properties.

**flügel·platte** (fle″gəl-plah′tə) [Ger.] lamina alaris.

**flu·id** (floo′id) [L. *fluidus*] 1. a liquid or a gas. 2. composed of elements or particles which freely change their relative positions without separating. See also *humor, liquid, liquor,* and *solution.*
**allantoic f.,** the fluid contained in the allantois.
**Altmann's f.,** a histologic fixing fluid composed of equal parts of 2 per cent osmic acid solution and a 5 per cent potassium dichromate solution.
**amniotic f.,** fluid within the amniotic cavity produced by the amnion

during the early embryonic period, and later by the lungs and kidneys; at first crystal clear, it later becomes cloudy. It protects the embryo and fetus from injury. The amount at term normally varies from 500 to 1500 mL. Called also *aqua amnii, liquor amnii,* and, popularly, *waters.*
**ascitic f.,** the serous fluid which accumulates in the peritoneal cavity in ascites.
**bleaching f.,** a fluid prepared by passing chlorine gas into an emulsion of calcium hydrate.
**Bouin's f.,** a histologic fixing fluid consisting of formaldehyde solution, glacial acetic acid, and saturated solution of trinitrophenol (picric acid).
**Callison's f.,** a solution of distilled water, Löffler's methylene blue, formaldehyde solution, glycerin, ammonium oxalate, and sodium chloride; used as a diluent in counting erythrocytes.
**Carrel-Dakin f.,** diluted sodium hypochlorite solution.
**cerebrospinal f. (CSF),** liquor cerebrospinalis.
**chlorpalladium f.,** a decalcifying fluid for anatomical and other specimens, containing palladium chloride and hydrochloric acid; called also *Waldeyer's f.*
**Condy's f.,** a disinfecting solution of sodium and potassium permanganates.
**Dakin's f.,** sodium hypochlorite solution, diluted.
**decalcifying f.,** a solution of formic acid and formalin.
**Delafield's f.,** a fixing fluid for delicate histologic tissues, containing osmic acid, chromic acid, acetic acid, and alcohol.
**extracellular f.,** a general term for all the body fluids outside the cells, including the interstitial fluid, plasma, lymph, cerebrospinal fluid, etc. Extracellular fluid consists of ultrafiltrates of the blood plasma and transcellular fluid, i.e., fluid produced by active cellular secretion. It provides a constant external environment for the cells.
**Flemming's fixing f.,** Flemming's solution.
**follicular f.,** liquor folliculi.
**formol-Müller f.,** Müller's fluid to which formaldehyde has been added.
**Helly's f.,** a histologic fixative consisting of Zenker's fluid in which the glacial acetic acid is replaced by formalin; the most widely used formula consists of 9 parts Zenker stock solution and 1 part neutral formalin (Zenker-Helly-Maximow) and is usually called *Zenker-formol fixative.*
**interstitial f.,** the extracellular fluid that bathes the cells of most tissues but which is not within the confines of the blood or lymph vessels and is not a transcellular fluid; it is formed by filtration through the blood capillaries and is drained away as lymph. It is the extracellular fluid volume minus the lymph volume, the plasma volume, and the transcellular fluid volume.
**intracellular f.,** the portion of the total body water with its dissolved solutes which is within the cell membranes.
**Kaiserling's f.,** see under *solution.*
**labyrinthine f.,** perilympha.
**Lang's f.,** a hardening fluid containing corrosive mercuric chloride, sodium chloride, and acetic acid, in water.
**Locke's f.,** see under *solution.*
**Müller's f.,** a hardening solution consisting of potassium dichromate, sodium sulfate, and water.
**Parker's f.,** a hardening fluid composed of formaldehyde and alcohol.
**pericardial f.,** a fluid found in small amounts in the potential space between the parietal and visceral laminae of the serous pericardium.
**Piazza's f.,** a blood-coagulating fluid composed of sodium chloride and ferric chloride in water.
**Scarpa's f.,** endolympha.
**Schaudinn's f.,** a hardening fluid consisting of mercury bichloride, alcohol, and distilled water.
**seminal f.,** semen, def. 2.
**serous f.,** normal lymph of a serous cavity.
**synovial f.,** synovia.
**Tellyesniczky's f.,** a fixing solution consisting of potassium dichromate, water, and glacial acetic acid.
**Thoma's f.,** a decalcifying fluid for histologic work, consisting of alcohol and pure nitric acid.
**tissue f.,** interstitial f.
**Toison's f.,** see under *solution.*
**transcellular f.,** that portion of the extracellular fluid produced by active cellular secretion.
**ventricular f.,** that portion of the cerebrospinal fluid contained in the cerebral ventricles.
**Waldeyer's f.,** chlorpalladium f.
**Wickersheimer's f.,** a fluid composed of arsenic trioxide, sodium chloride, and the sulfate, carbonate, and nitrate of potassium in a mixture of water, alcohol, and glycerin; used for preserving anatomical specimens.
**Zenker's f.,** see under *fixative.*

**flu·id·ex·tract** (floo″id-ek′strakt) a liquid preparation of a vegetable drug, prepared by percolation, containing alcohol as a solvent or as a preservative, or both, of such strength that each milliliter contains the extraction of 1 g of the standard drug which it represents.
**aromatic cascara f.** [USP], one prepared from cascara sagrada with the addition of pure glycyrrhiza extract; used as a cathartic.
**cascara sagrada f.** [USP], one prepared from cascara sagrada; used as a cathartic.
**eriodictyon f.,** one prepared from eriodictyon; used as a flavoring for drugs and in the preparation of aromatic eriodictyon syrup.
**glycyrrhiza f.,** one prepared from glycyrrhiza; used as a flavoring for drugs.
**senna f.** [USP], one prepared from senna; used as a laxative and in the preparation of senna syrup.

**flu·id·ounce** (floo-id-ouns′) fluid ounce; see under *ounce.*

**flu·i·drachm**[1] (floo″ĭ-dram′) fluid dram; see under *dram.*

**flu·i·dram**[2] (floo″ĭ-dram′) fluid dram; see under *dram.*

**fluke** (flo͞ok) trematode.
**blood f.,** *Schistosoma.*
**conical f.,** paramphistome.
**intestinal f's,** flukes that inhabit the intestines of humans or other animals, such as those of the families Fasciolidae, Heterophyidae, and Paramphistomatidae.
**lancet f.,** *Dicrocoelium dendriticum.*
**liver f.,** one found in the liver, such as species of *Clonorchis, Dicrocoelium, Fasciola, Fascioloides,* or *Opisthorchis.*
**lung f.,** see *Paragonimus.*
**rumen f., ruminal f.,** the usual type of paramphistome, found in the rumen of a ruminant.

**flu·like** (floo′līk) 1. resembling influenza. 2. characterized by symptoms resembling those of influenza.

**flu·ma·ze·nil** (floo′ma-zə-nil″) [MeSH: Flumazenil] a specific agonist to benzodiazepines that binds competitively to central nervous system benzodiazepine receptors, used to reverse the effects of benzodiazepines following sedation, general anesthesia, or overdose; administered intravenously.

**flu·men** (floo′mən) pl. *flu′mina* [L.] a stream.
**flu′mina pilo′rum** [TA], hair streams: continuous lines formed by the pattern of hair growth on various parts of the body, the hairs lying in the same direction.

**flu·me·quine** (floo′mə-kwin) a quinolone antibacterial with actions and uses similar to those of nalidixic acid; administered orally.

**flu·meth·a·sone** (floo-meth′ə-sōn″) [MeSH: Flumethasone] a synthetic corticosteroid used in veterinary medicine as an anti-inflammatory for a variety of corticosteroid-responsive conditions; administered intramuscularly, intravenously, intra-arterially, and orally.
**f. pivalate** [USP], the pivalate salt of flumethasone, used topically for the relief of inflammation and pruritus in corticosteroid-responsive dermatoses.

**flu·mi·na** (floo′mĭ-nə) [L.] plural of *flumen.*

**flu·nar·i·zine hy·dro·chlo·ride** (floo-nar′ĭ-zēn) a calcium channel blocker with antihistaminic activity, derived from cinnarizine, used for the prophylaxis of migraine and the treatment of subarachnoid hemorrhage; administered orally.

**flu·nis·o·lide** (floo-nis′o-līd″) [USP] a synthetic glucocorticoid administered by inhalator for the treatment of bronchial asthma and intranasally for the treatment of perennial and seasonal rhinitis.
**f. acetate,** the 21-acetate ester of flunisolide; an anti-inflammatory.

**flu·ni·traz·e·pam** (floo″nĭ-traz′ə-pam) [MeSH: Flunitrazepam] a short-acting benzodiazepine with properties similar to those of diazepam, administered orally as a hypnotic and intramuscularly as an induction agent in anesthesia.

**flu·nix·in** (floo-nik′sin) an anti-inflammatory and analgesic.
**f. meglumine** [USP], the meglumine salt of flunixin, used as a veterinary anti-inflammatory and analgesic.

**flu·o·cin·o·lone acet·o·nide** (floo″ə-sin′ə-lōn) [USP] [MeSH: Fluocinolone Acetonide] a synthetic corticosteroid used topically for the relief of inflammation and pruritus in corticosteroid-responsive dermatoses.

**flu·o·cin·o·nide** (floo″ə-sin′ə-nīd) [USP] [MeSH: Fluocinonide] a synthetic corticosteroid used topically for the relief of inflammation and pruritus in corticosteroid-responsive dermatoses.

**Flu·o·gen** (floo′o-jən) trademark for a preparation of influenza virus vaccine.

**Flu·o·nid** (floo′ə-nid) trademark for preparations of fluocinolone acetonide.

**flu·or** (floo′or) [L. "a flow"] a discharge.
**f. al′bus,** leukorrhea.

**flu·or·ane** (floor′ān) the parent compound of fluorescein and related dyes; 9-hydroxy-9-xanthene-*o*-benzoic acid lactone.

**flu·o·res·ce·in** (flo͞o-res′ēn) [USP23] the simplest of the fluorane dyes and the parent compound of eosin; used as a diagnostic indicator in assessing corneal trauma and fitting contact lenses.
**f. isothiocyanate (FITC),** a form capable of being conjugated to proteins, particularly antibodies, and hence used as a fluorescent label for these molecules in various assays.
**f. sodium** [USP], an odorless, water-soluble, orange-red powder used in dilute solution to reveal corneal trauma, in contact lens fitting, and in retinal angiography. Called also *uranin.*
**soluble f.,** f. sodium.

**flu·o·res·ce·in·uria** (flo͞o-res″e-nu′re-ə) the presence of fluorescein in the urine.

**flu·o·res·cence** (flo͞o-res′əns) [first observed in *fluorspar*] [MeSH: Fluorescence] the property of emitting light while exposed to light, the wavelength of the emitted light being only slightly longer than that of the light absorbed. Cf. *phosphorescence.*
**secondary f.,** fluorescence in tissues which is induced by staining with fluorescent dyes *(fluorochromes).* Cf. *autofluorescence.*

**flu·o·res·cent** (flo͞o-res′ənt) exhibiting fluorescence.

**flu·o·res·cin** (floo″o-res′in) a reduced form of fluorescein used to detect oxidative activity. As the sodium salt, it may be used for the same purposes as sodium fluorescein.

**flu·o·ri·da·tion** (floor″ĭ-da′shən) [MeSH: Fluoridation] treatment with fluorides; specifically, the addition of fluoride to the public water supply as part of the public health program to prevent or reduce the incidence of dental caries.

**flu·o·ride** (floor′īd) a binary compound of fluorine. See also *stannous fluoride,* under *stannous.*

**flu·o·rim·e·ter** (flo͞o-rim′ə-tər) fluorometer.

**flu·o·rim·e·try** (flo͞o-rim′ə-tre) fluorometry.

**flu·o·rine** (floor′ēn) [from *fluorspar,* from which it is derived] [MeSH: Fluorine] a nonmetallic, gaseous element, belonging to the halogen group; symbol, F; atomic number, 9; atomic weight, 18.998. Fluorine, in the form of fluoride, is incorporated into the structure of bone and teeth and provides protection against dental caries; an excess of fluorine may result in fluorosis.
**f. 18,** a radioactive isotope of fluorine, atomic mass 18, having a half-life of 1.8925 hours; it decays primarily by positron emission, with energy 0.635 MeV and is used as a tracer in positron emission tomography.

**flu·o·ro·ac·e·tate** (floor″o-as′ə-tāt) a salt of fluoroacetic acid; the sodium salt and others are used in rodenticides and are toxic to many mammalian species. See *fluoroacetate poisoning,* under *poisoning.*

**flu·o·ro·ace·tic ac·id** (floor″o-ə-se′tik) a toxin from a South African tree, used as a rodenticide; see *sodium fluoroacetate.*

**flu·o·ro·car·bon** (floor′-o-kahr″bən) an organic compound consisting of carbon and fluorine only; fluorocarbons are analogous to hydrocarbons but with the hydrogen atoms replaced by fluorine. Fluorocarbon emulsions dissolve oxygen and carbon dioxide and can be used in place of red blood cell preparations in the prevention and treatment of ischemia.

**flu·o·ro·chrome** (floor′o-krōm) any fluorescent dye used as a stain or label, e.g., fluorescein isothiocyanate attached to an antibody.

**flu·o·ro·cyte** (floor′o-sīt) a reticulocyte showing red fluorescence.

**flu·o·ro·de·oxy·glu·cose** (floor″o-de-ok″se-gloo′kōs) fludeoxyglucose F 18.

**flu·o·ro·do·pa F 18** (floor″o-do′pə) [USP] a compound containing fluorine and levodopa, in which some of the molecules are labeled with $^{18}$F; used for positron emission tomography of the cerebrum.

**flu·o·rog·ra·phy** (flo͞o-rog′rə-fe) photofluorography.

**flu·o·ro·im·mu·no·as·say (FIA)** (floor″o-im″u-no-as′a) [MeSH: Fluoroimmunoassay] fluorescence immunoassay.

**flu·o·rom·e·ter** (flo͞o-rom′ə-tər) the instrument used in fluorometry, consisting of an energy source (e.g., a mercury arc lamp or xenon lamp) to induce fluorescence, filters or monochromators for selection of the wavelength, and a detector; called also *fluorimeter.*

**flu·o·ro·meth·o·lone** (floor″o-meth′ə-lōn) [USP] [MeSH: Fluorometholone] a synthetic glucocorticoid used topically in the treatment of corticosteroid-responsive allergic and inflammatory conditions of the eye.

**flu·o·rom·e·try** (flo͞o-rom′ə-tre) [MeSH: Fluorometry] an analytical technique for identifying and characterizing minute amounts of a substance by excitation of the substance with a beam of ultraviolet light and detection and measurement of the characteristic wavelength of fluorescent light emitted. Called also *fluorimetry.*

**flu·o·ro·neph·e·lom·e·ter** (floor″o-nef″ə-lom′ə-tər) an instrument for analysis of a solution by measuring the light scattered or emitted by it. Called also *nefluorophotometer.*

**Fluor-Op** (floor′op) trademark for a preparation of fluorometholone.

***p*-flu·o·ro·phen·yl·al·a·nine** (floor″o-fen″əl-al′ə-nēn) a modified molecule of phenylalanine that binds to enzymes but is incapable of performing the functions of the natural molecule and thus acts as an antagonist.

**flu·o·ro·phos·phate** (floor″o-fos′fāt) a salt or ester containing fluorine and phosphorus.
**diisopropyl f.,** isoflurophate.

**flu·o·ro·pho·tom·e·try** (floor″o-fo-tom′ə-tre) [MeSH: Fluorophotometry] fluorometry.
**vitreous f.,** the measurement of light given off by intravenously injected fluorescein that has leaked through the retinal vessels into the vitreous; done to detect the breakdown of the blood-retinal barrier, an early ocular change in diabetes mellitus.

**Flu·or·o·plex** (floor′o-pleks″) trademark for preparations of fluorouracil.

**flu·o·ro·py·rim·i·dine** (flo͞or″o-pə-rim′ĭ-dēn) any of a group of uracil analogues having fluorine substitutions at the 5 position and demonstrating antineoplastic activity, including fluorouracil and floxuridine.

**flu·o·ro·quin·o·lone** (floor″o-kwin′o-lōn) any of a subgroup of quinolones that have a piperazinyl group and a fluorine atom at position 6 and a broader spectrum of activity than nalidixic acid, including ciprofloxacin, norfloxacin, and ofloxacin. Called also fluorinated 4-quinolone.

**flu·o·ro·ra·di·og·ra·phy** (floor″o-ra″de-og′rə-fe) photofluorography.

**flu·o·ro·scope** (floor′o-skōp) a device used for examining deep structures by means of x-rays; it consists of a screen *(fluorescent screen)* covered with crystals of calcium tungstate on which are projected the shadows of x-rays passing through the body placed between the screen and the source of irradiation.
**biplane f.,** a fluoroscope by which examinations can be made in two planes, horizontal and vertical.

**flu·o·ro·scop·i·cal** (floor″o-skop′ĭ-kəl) pertaining to fluoroscopy.

**flu·o·ros·co·py** (flo͞o-ros′kə-pe) [MeSH: Fluoroscopy] examination by means of the fluoroscope.

**flu·o·ro·sil·i·cate** (floor″o-sil′ĭ-kāt) a compound of silicon and some other base with fluorine, such as sodium silicofluoride; fluorosilicates are sometimes used as insecticides, and are very toxic when ingested. Called also *silicofluoride.*

**flu·o·ro·sis** (flo͞o-ro′sis) 1. a condition in humans due to exposure to excessive amounts of fluorine or its compounds, resulting from accidental ingestion of certain insecticides and rodenticides, chronic inhalation of industrial dusts or gases, or prolonged ingestion of water containing large amounts of fluorides. It is characterized by skeletal changes such as *osteofluorosis* and by *mottled enamel* when exposure occurs during enamel formation. 2. a condition in cattle, sheep, and other livestock, similar to fluorosis in humans and due to the same factors, in addition to ingestion of feed containing toxic levels of fluorides, or grazing on pastures contaminated from industrial dusts or gases. Called also *chronic endemic f.* and *chronic fluoride* or *fluorine poisoning.*
**dental f.,** mottled enamel.
**endemic f., chronic,** fluorosis.

**flu·o·ro·ura·cil** (floor″o-ūr′ə-sil″) [USP] [MeSH: Fluorouracil] 5-fluorouracil (5-FU); a fluoropyrimidine metabolically activated like uracil; used intravenously as an antineoplastic for the treatment of solid tumors, especially palliative treatment of carcinomas of the breast and gastrointestinal tract, for the treatment of malignant effusions, and also as a component of combination chemotherapy regimens. It is also used topically for treatment of actinic keratoses and other precancerous skin conditions and for superficial basal cell and squamous cell skin carcinoma.

**Flu·o·sol** (floo′o-sol) trademark name for a frozen perfluorochemical used as a temporary carrier of oxygen in the blood.

**Flu·o·thane** (floo′o-thān) trademark for a preparation of halothane.

**flu·ox·e·tine** (floo-ok′sə-tēn) [USP] [MeSH: Fluoxetine] a selective serotonin uptake inhibitor used in the treatment of depression, obsessive-compulsive disorder, and bulimia nervosa; administered orally.
**f. hydrochloride** [USP], the hydrochloride salt of fluoxetine, having the same actions and uses as the base.

**flu·oxy·mes·ter·one** (floo-ok″se-mes′tər-ōn) [USP] [MeSH: Fluoxymesterone] an androgen used in the treatment of male hypogonadism and in the palliative therapy of inoperable female breast cancer in selected patients, administered orally.

**flu·pen·thix·ol** (floo″pen-thik′sol) [MeSH: Flupenthixol] a thioxanthene derivative used in the treatment of the symptoms of psychotic disorders.

**flu·pen·tix·ol** (floo″pen-tik′sol) INN for flupenthixol.

**flu·phen·a·zine** (floo-fen′ə-zēn) [MeSH: Fluphenazine] the 2-trifluromethyl derivative of perphenazine, $C_{22}H_{26}F_3N_3OS$, the most potent of the phenothiazine tranquilizers.
**f. decanoate** [USP], the decanoate ester of fluphenazine, having the same actions as the hydrochloride salt, but of longer duration; administered subcutaneously or intramuscularly in maintenance therapy for psychotic disorders.
**f. enanthate** [USP], the enanthate ester of fluphenazine, having the same uses as the hydrochloride salt, but of longer duration; administered intramuscularly and subcutaneously.
**f. hydrochloride** [USP], the dihydrochloride salt of fluphenazine, used as a tranquilizer in the treatment of manifestations of psychotic disorders, and as an antiemetic; administered orally and intramuscularly.

**flu·pred·nis·o·lone** (floo″pred-nis′o-lōn) [MeSH: Fluprednisolone] a synthetic glucocorticoid used in the treatment of various conditions responsive to the anti-inflammatory actions of glucocorticoids, administered orally.
**f. valerate,** an ester of fluprednisolone with actions similar to those of the base.

**flu·pros·te·nol so·di·um** (floo-pros′tə-nol) a prostaglandin of the F series used in the treatment of infertility.

**flur·an·dren·o·lide** (floor″ən-dren′ə-līd) a synthetic corticosteroid used topically for the relief of inflammation and pruritus in corticosteroid-responsive dermatoses.

**flu·raz·e·pam hy·dro·chlo·ride** (flo͞o-raz′ə-pam) [USP] a benzodiazepine used as a sedative and hypnotic in the treatment of insomnia; administered orally.

**flur·bip·ro·fen** (floor-bip′ro-fen) [MeSH: Flurbiprofen] a nonsteroidal anti-inflammatory agent derived from propionic acid and structurally related to ibuprofen; administered orally in the treatment of rheumatoid arthritis and osteoarthritis and applied topically to the conjunctiva to inhibit miosis during ophthalmic surgery.

**Flur·ess** (flo͞o-res′) trademark for a preparation of benoxinate hydrochloride and fluorescein sodium.

**Flur·o·bate** (floor′o-bāt) trademark for preparations of betamethasone benzoate.

**Flur·o-Eth·yl** (floor″o-eth′əl) trademark for a preparation of ethyl chloride.

**flu·ro·thyl** (floor′o-thəl) [MeSH: Flurothyl] an inhalant convulsive agent, hexafluorodiethyl ether.

**flush** (flush) 1. transient, episodic redness of the face and neck caused by certain diseases, ingestion of certain drugs or other substances, heat, emotional factors, or physical exertion. See also *erythema.* 2. to wash out with fluid.
**atropine f.,** flushing and dryness of the skin of the face and neck from overdosage with atropine.
**breast f.,** a condition sometimes occurring in the early puerperium consisting of a tense and flushed state of the breasts with prominent veins.
**carcinoid f.,** extensive blotchy red or bluish flushing on the face or trunk, often associated with diarrhea and abdominal pain and sometimes bronchospasm; it is possibly due to vasoactive kinins or other peptides associated with carcinoid tumor.
**hectic f.,** a persistent or chronic flush associated with a hectic fever (q.v.).
**histamine f.,** sudden symmetric erythema of the face and upper trunk, usually associated with throbbing headache and bounding pulse, and histaminuria; seen in urticaria pigmentosa, it may also occur a few minutes after eating fish of the scombroid family (red snapper or mahimahi) contaminated by *Proteus* during cold storage prior to cooking.
**malar f.,** flushing, such as a hectic flush, at the malar eminence.

**flu·spir·i·lene** (floo-spēr′ĭ-lēn) [MeSH: Fluspirilene] a diphenylbutylpiperidine antipsychotic, used for the treatment of schizophrenia; administered intramuscularly.

**flu·ta·mide** (floo′tə-mīd) [USP] [MeSH: Flutamide] a nonsteroidal antiandrogen, administered orally in the treatment of metastatic prostatic carcinoma and to increase the flow of urine in benign prostatic hypertrophy.

**flu·ti·a·zin** (floo-ti′ə-zin) a veterinary anti-inflammatory agent.

**flu·tic·a·sone pro·pi·o·nate** (floo-tik′ə-sōn″) a synthetic corticosteroid used topically as an anti-inflammatory and antipruritic in the treatment of corticosteroid-responsive dermatoses, intranasally in the treatment of allergic rhinitis, and by inhalation in the treatment of asthma.

**flut·ter** (flut′ər) a rapid vibration or pulsation.
**atrial f.,** a condition of cardiac arrhythmia in which the atrial contractions are rapid (250 to 350 per minute), but regular. In many instances, a circus movement caused by reentry is probably present. The ventricles are unable to respond to each atrial impulse, so that at least a partial atrioventricular block must develop and the ventricular rate is usually approximately 150 beats per minute.
**diaphragmatic f.,** peculiar, wavelike fibrillations of the diaphragm of unknown cause; the condition may be paroxysmal or persist indefinitely.
**impure f.,** an arrhythmia in which the electrocardiogram shows alternating periods of atrial flutter and fibrillation or periods not clearly distinguishable as one versus the other.
**mediastinal f.,** a condition of abnormal motility of the mediastinum during respiratory movements.
**pure f.,** atrial f.
**ventricular f. (VFl),** a ventricular tachyarrhythmia characterized electrocardiographically by smooth undulating waves with QRS complexes merged with T waves, and a rate of approximately 250 per minute. If untreated it usually progresses to ventricular fibrillation.

**flut·ter-fib·ril·la·tion** (flut′ər-fib″rĭ-la′shən) impure flutters that vary from moment to moment in their resemblance to flutter or fibrillation, respectively.

**flu·vox·amine** (floo-vok′sə-mēn) [MeSH: Fluvoxamine] an inhibitor of serotonin reuptake used to relieve the symptoms of obsessive-compulsive disorder; administered orally.

**flux** (fluks) [L. *fluxus*] 1. an excessive flow or discharge. 2. a substance that maintains the cleanliness of metals to be united and facilitates the easy flow and attachment of solder.
**celiac f.,** diarrhea accompanied by the discharge of undigested food.
**ceramic f.,** a type of flux used in manufacturing of powdered silicate and porcelain for dental materials.
**ionic f.,** the number of mols per second passing through an area of 1 cm oriented perpendicularly to the direction of flow of the substance.
**luminous f.,** the rate of flow of radiant energy, specifically that of the visible spectrum; its SI unit is the lumen.
**magnetic f.,** a quantitative measure of a magnetic field, equal to the integral over a specified surface of the magnetic flux density perpendicular to the surface. Symbol $\Phi$.
**menstrual f.,** the menses.
**neutral f.,** a fusible material, usually an inorganic salt, which does not unite with the combined oxygen in the metal but merely dissolves the metal oxide (barium chloride, sodium chloride).
**oxidizing f.,** a material which, when heated, gives up oxygen that may unite with base metals and form oxides (as potassium nitrate, potassium chlorate).
**reducing f.,** a material that unites with the oxygen of metallic oxides and frees the metal from such combinations.

**flux·ion** (fluk′shən) a flowing; especially an abnormal or excessive flow of fluid to a part.

**fly** (fli) [MeSH: Diptera] general term for any of numerous two-winged insects of the order Diptera. Called also *musca.*
**black f.,** any of various insects of the family Simuliidae.
**blackbottle f.,** see *Phormia.*
**bloodsucking f's,** see *Chrysops* and *Tabanus.*
**blow f.,** 1. any member of the genus *Calliphora.* 2. any member of the family Calliphoridae that lays its eggs on injured or decayed animal flesh and causes cutaneous myiasis; this includes most species of *Calliphora* and *Phaenicia* and some of *Cochliomyia* and *Phormia.*
**bluebottle f.,** *Calliphora vomitoria.*
**bot f.,** botfly.
**caddis f.,** a fly of the order Trichoptera; hairs and scales from these flies are a cause of allergic symptoms in susceptible persons.
**cheese f.,** see *Piophila.*
**deer f.,** *Chrysops discalis.*
**drone f.,** *Eristalis tenax.*
**dung f.,** *Sepsis violacea.*
**eye f.,** any fly which attacks the eye; see *Hippelates* and *Siphunculina funicola.*
**face f.,** *Musca autumnalis.*
**filth f.,** *Musca domestica.*
**flesh f.,** any member of the family Sarcophagidae.
**fruit f.,** see *Drosophila.*
**gad f.,** tabanid.
**greenbottle f.,** see *Phaenicia.*
**head f.,** *Hydrotaea irritans.*
**heel f.,** see *Hypoderma.*
**horn f.,** *Haematobia irritans.*

**horse f.**, tabanid.
**house f.**, *Musca domestica.*
**hover f's**, flies of the family Syrphidae.
**lake f.**, *Hexagenia bilineata.*
**latrine f.**, *Fannia scalaris.*
**mango f.**, **mangrove f.**, *Chrysops dimidiata.*
**moth f.**, a fly of the family Psychodidae.
**nose f.**, **nostril f.**, *Oestrus ovis.*
**owl f.**, any member of the family Psychodidae.
**ox-warble f.**, *Hypoderma bovis* or *H. lineatum.*
**phlebotomus f.**, see *Phlebotomus.*
**pomace f.**, see *Drosophila.*
**Russian f.**, *Lytta.*
**sand f.**, see *sandfly.*
**screw-worm f.**, *Cochliomyia hominivorax.*
**Seroot f.**, *Tabanus gratus.*
**sheep maggot f.**, a fly whose larvae are sheep maggots.
**snipe f.**, a fly of the family *Rhagionidae.*
**soldier f.**, *Hermetia illucens.*
**Spanish f.**, 1. *Lytta vesicatoria.* 2. cantharides.
**stable f.**, *Stomoxys calcitrans.*
**tick f.**, see *Hippobosca.*
**tsetse f.**, see *Glossina.*
**tumbu f.**, *Cordylobia anthropophaga.*
**warble f.**, *Hypoderma.*

**Flynn-Aird syndrome** (flin-ard) [P. *Flynn,* American physician, 20th century; R.B. *Aird,* American physician, 20th century] see under *syndrome.*

**F.M.** abbreviation for L. *fi'at mistu'ra,* make a mixture.

**Fm** symbol for *fermium.*

**FML** trademark for preparations of fluorometholone.

**FMN** [MeSH: FMN] flavin mononucleotide, sometimes used specifically for the oxidized form.

**FMN ad·e·nyl·yl·trans·fer·ase** (ad″ə-nəl″əl-trans′fər-ās) [EC 2.7.7.2] an enzyme of the transferase class that catalyzes the formation of flavin adenine dinucleotide (FAD) by transferring AMP from ATP to flavin mononucleotide (FMN).

**$FMNH_2$** the reduced form of flavin mononucleotide.

**FNH** focal nodular hyperplasia.

**FNTC** fine needle transhepatic cholangiography.

**foam** (fōm) [A.S. *fām*] 1. a dispersion of gas in a liquid or solid, e.g., whipped cream or pumice. 2. frothy saliva, produced particularly on exertion or pathologically. 3. the frothy sweat of an equine. 4. to produce, or cause to produce, foam.

**fo·cal** (fo'kəl) pertaining to or occupying a focus.

**fo·ci** (fo'si) [L.] genitive and plural of *focus.*

**fo·cil, fo·cile** (fo'sil, fo'sĭ-le) [L. *fusillus,* a little spindle] one of the bones of the forearm or leg.

**fo·cim·e·ter** (fo-sim'ə-tər) [*focus* + *-meter*] an apparatus for finding the focus of a lens.

**fo·cus** (fo'kəs) pl. *fo'ci* [L. "fire-place"] 1. the point of convergence of light rays or of the waves of sound. 2. the chief center of a morbid process.
**aplanatic f.**, that focus or point from which diverging rays pass the lens without spherical aberration.
**Assmann f.**, the early exudative lesion of pulmonary tuberculosis, occurring most frequently in the subapical region; called also *Assmann's tuberculous infiltrate.*
**conjugate f.**, the point at which rays that come from some definite point are brought together.
**dysplastic f.**, a collection, less than 1 mm in diameter, of dysplastic hepatocytes, occurring as a precancerous condition in the liver. Cf. *dysplastic nodule,* under *nodule.*
**epileptogenic f.**, the area of the cerebral cortex responsible for causing epileptic seizures.
**epileptogenic f., secondary**, a second focus that develops in a different part of the brain because of a spread of the pathologic process outward from the original epileptogenic focus; it may develop into a new, independent focus that continues to operate after the original one has been treated.
**Ghon f.**, the primary parenchymal lesion of primary pulmonary tuberculosis in children; when associated with a corresponding lymph node focus, it is known as the *primary* or *Ghon complex.* Called also *Ghon's primary lesion* and *Ghon tubercle.*
**mirror f.**, a type of secondary epileptogenic focus that develops in the opposite hemisphere as an approximate mirror image of the original focus.
**principal foci**, points of convergence of rays parallel with the principal axis of a lens, or system: in the eye (approx.) 18 mm from the anterior nodal point, and 24 mm from the posterior nodal point, and holding the ratio of the indices of air and vitreum.
**real f.**, the point at which convergent rays intersect.
**Simon's foci**, hematogenous areas in the apices of the lungs of children regarded as precursors of apical tuberculosis in later life.
**virtual f.**, the point at which divergent rays would intersect if prolonged backward.

**fo·cus·ing** (fo'kəs-ing) the act of converging at a point.
**isoelectric f.**, electrophoresis in which the protein mixture is subjected to an electric field in a gel medium in which a pH gradient has been established; each protein then migrates until it reaches the site (or focus) at which the pH is equal to its isoelectric point. Called also *electrofocusing.*

**fo·drin** (fo'drin) a protein similar to spectrin in structure and function but found in cells of the brain and intestinal microvilli; it helps form and dismantle microfilaments, thus aiding or inhibiting cell movements.

**foe-** for words beginning thus, see those beginning *fe-.*

**Foe·nic·u·lum** (fe-nik'u-ləm) a genus of flowering herbs of the family Umbelliferae, native to Europe and Asia. *F. vulga're* is fennel, the source of fennel oil.

**Foer·ster** see *Förster.*

**fog** (fog) 1. a colloid system in which the dispersion medium is a gas and the disperse particles are liquid, e.g., a cloudlike mass of water droplets dispersed in air. 2. aftermath.
**mental f.**, clouding of consciousness.

**Fo·gar·ty catheter** (fo'gər-te) [Thomas J. *Fogarty,* American thoracic surgeon, born 1934] see under *catheter.*

**fog·ging** (fog'ing) in ophthalmology, a method employed in determining the refractive error, the patient being first made artificially myopic by means of plus spheres, in order to relax all accommodation before using cylinders.

**fo·go** (faw'goo) [Port. "fire"] a skin condition in Brazil.
**f. selva'gem** (sāl-vah'zha) [Port. "wild fire"], a progressive, sometimes fatal variant of pemphigus foliaceus endemic in certain areas of Brazil; it usually affects children and is characterized by a burning sensation with blisters that rupture to form erosions with peripheral rolls of epidermis. Called also *Brazilian, South American,* or *wildfire pemphigus.*

**foil** (foil) metal in the form of an extremely thin, pliable sheet.
**gold f.**, pure gold beaten and/or rolled into thin sheets, used as a direct filling material in dental restorations; gold foil used in direct restorations has a thickness of 0.5 μm or less. Occasionally used loosely to refer to mat gold and powdered gold.
**gold f., cohesive**, gold foil that has been rendered cohesive by the process of annealing or degassing; pieces of cold gold foil are welded together into a desired shape or thinness. Called also *cohesive gold.*
**mat f.**, foil produced by sandwiching mat gold (see under *gold*) between two sheets of cohesive gold foil; used as a direct filling dental material.
**platinum f.**, a very thin foil of pure platinum, suitable for use as a matrix to provide internal forms for porcelain restorations during their fabrication.
**tin f.**, a thin sheet rolled from tin, used as a protective wrapping; also used as a separating material between the cast and denture base material during flasking and curing. Written also *tinfoil.*

**Foix syndrome** (fwah) [Charles *Foix,* French neurologist, 1882–1927] cavernous sinus syndrome.

**Foix-Ala·jou·a·nine syndrome** (fwah ah-lah-zhoo-ah-nēn') [C. *Foix;* Théophile *Alajouanine,* French neurologist, 1890–1980] see under *syndrome.*

**Fol.** abbreviation for L. *fo'lia,* leaves.

**fo·la·cin** (fo'lə-sin) older name for folic acid or derivatives with similar vitamin activity.

**fo·late** (fo'lāt) 1. the anionic form of folic acid. 2. more generally, any of the pteroylglutamate derivatives having various levels of reduction of the bicyclic pteridine portion, substitutions of this structure, and numbers of glutamate residues.
**f. polyglutamate**, pteroylpolyglutamate.

**fold** (fōld) a thin, recurved margin, or doubling; called also *plica.*

## Fold

For descriptions of specific anatomic structures not found here, see under *plica*.

**alar f's,** plicae alares.
**amniotic f.,** the folded edge of the amniotic membrane where it rises over and finally encloses the embryo.
**aryepiglottic f.,** plica aryepiglottica.
**axillary f., anterior,** the fold of skin and muscle produced by the lower border of the pectoralis major muscle, forming the anterior boundary of the fossa axillaris. Called also *plica axillaris anterior.*
**axillary f., posterior,** the fold of skin and muscle produced by the latissimus dorsi and teres major muscles, forming the posterior boundary of the fossa axillaris. Called also *plica axillaris posterior.*
**Brachet's mesolateral f.,** mesolateral f.
**bulboventricular f.,** a fold between the bulbus cordis and the ventricle that disappears as the bulbus cordis is absorbed into the right ventricle.
**caval f.,** a ridge that contains the superior segment of the embryonic inferior vena cava.
**cecal f's,** plicae caecales.
**cholecystoduodenocolic f.,** an occasionally present fold of peritoneum sometimes uniting the colon, duodenum, and gallbladder.
**ciliary f's,** plicae ciliares.
**circular f's, circular f's of Kerckring,** plicae circulares.
**conjunctival f.,** the cul-de-sac formed where the conjunctiva is reflected from the eyeball to the upper or lower eyelid; called also *palpebral f.* and *retrotarsal f.*
**costocolic f.,** ligamentum phrenicocolicum.
**Douglas' f.,** 1. plica recto-uterina. 2. linea arcuata vaginae musculi recti abdominis.
**Duncan's f's,** the loose folds of peritoneum which cover the uterus immediately following delivery.
**duodenojejunal f.,** plica duodenalis superior.
**duodenomesocolic f.,** plica duodenalis inferior.
**epicanthal f., epicanthine f.,** epicanthus.
**epigastric f.,** plica umbilicalis lateralis.
**falciform f. of fascia lata,** margo falciformis hiatus saphenus.
**fimbriated f.,** plica fimbriata.
**gastric f's,** plicae gastricae.
**gastropancreatic f., left,** plica gastropancreatica.
**gastropancreatic f., right,** plica hepatopancreatica.
**genital f.,** genital ridge.
**glossoepiglottic f., lateral,** plica glosso-epiglottica lateralis.
**glossoepiglottic f., median,** plica glosso-epiglottica mediana.
**gluteal f.,** sulcus glutealis.
**Guérin's f.,** a fold of mucous membrane occasionally seen in the fossa navicularis of the urethra.
**Hasner's f.,** plica lacrimalis.
**head f.,** a crescentic, ventral fold of the embryonic disk at the future head end of the embryo.
**Heister's f.,** plica spiralis.
**Hensing's f.,** see under *ligament.*
**hepatopancreatic f.,** plica hepatopancreatica.
**horizontal f's of rectum,** plicae transversae recti.
**ileocecal f.,** plica ileocaecalis.
**ileocolic f.,** a crescentic fold of peritoneum forming a part of the mesentery, mesocecum, and mesocolon.
**incudal f.,** plica incudialis.
**inferior duodenal f.,** plica duodenalis inferior.
**interarticular f. of hip,** ligamentum capitis femoris.
**interarytenoid f.,** plica interarytenoidea.
**interdigital f.,** the free border of the web connecting the bases of adjoining digits.
**interureteric f.,** plica interureterica.
**iridial f's,** plicae iridis.
**Jonnesco's f., Juvara's f.,** parietoperitoneal f.
**Kerckring's (Kerkring's) f's (of small intestine),** plicae circulares.
**Kohlrausch's f's,** plicae transversae recti.
**lacrimal f.,** plica lacrimalis.
**f's of large intestine,** plicae semilunares coli.
**longitudinal f. of duodenum,** plica longitudinalis duodeni.
**malleolar f. of mucous coat of tympanic cavity, anterior,** plica mallearis anterior tunicae mucosae cavitatis tympanicae.
**malleolar f. of mucous coat of tympanic cavity, posterior,** plica mallearis posterior tunicae mucosae cavitatis tympanicae.
**malleolar f. of tympanic membrane, anterior,** plica mallearis anterior membranae tympanicae.
**malleolar f. of tympanic membrane, posterior,** plica mallearis posterior membranae tympanicae.
**mammary f.,** the bandlike thickening of ectoderm that is the primordium of the mammary gland in the early embryo; it extends from just below the axilla to the inguinal region.
**Marshall's f.,** plica venae cavae sinistrae.
**medullary f.,** neural f.
**mesolateral f.,** the right lamella of the primordial mesentery running to the right lobe of the liver; called also *Brachet's mesolateral f.*
**mesonephric f.,** mesonephric ridge.
**mesouterine f.,** a fold of peritoneum supporting the uterus.
**mucobuccal f.,** the cul-de-sac formed where the mucous membrane is reflected from the upper or lower jaw to the cheek.
**mucolabial f.,** the line of flexure of the oral mucous membrane as it passes from the mandible or maxilla to the lip.
**mucosal f.,** a fold of mucous membrane; called also *mucous f.*
**mucosobuccal f.,** mucobuccal f.
**mucous f.,** mucosal f.
**mucous f's of rectum,** columnae anales.
**nail f.,** the fold of palmar skin around the base and sides of the nail.
**nasopharyngeal f.,** plica salpingopalatina.
**Nélaton's f.,** a transverse fold of mucous membrane in the rectum, marking the junction of its lower and middle thirds.
**neural f.,** one of the paired folds of the neural plate, lying one on either side of the neural groove, that fuse to form the neural tube; called also *medullary f.*
**opercular f.,** a fold of tissue constituting an adhesion between the tonsil and the anterior pillar of the fauces.
**palatine f's, palatine f's, transverse,** plicae palatinae transversae.
**palmate f's,** plicae palmatae.
**palpebral f.,** conjunctival f.
**palpebronasal f.,** epicanthus.
**pancreaticogastric f., left,** plica gastropancreatica.
**paraduodenal f.,** plica paraduodenalis.
**parietocolic f.,** Hensing's ligament.
**parietoperitoneal f.,** a fold of peritoneum in the fetus, arising at the left side of the ascending colon and attached to the parietal peritoneum at the right of the ascending colon; called also *Jonnesco's f.* and *Juvara's f.*
**pharyngoepiglottic f.,** plica glosso-epiglottica lateralis.
**primitive f.,** one of the two ridges flanking the primitive groove in the primitive streak, one on either side.
**Rathke's f's,** two fetal folds of mesoderm which unite at the median line to form Douglas' septum and to render the rectum a complete canal.
**rectal f's,** plicae transversae recti.
**rectouterine f.,** plica recto-uterina.
**rectovaginal f.,** a fold of peritoneum interposed between the rectum and vagina.
**rectovesical f.,** plica recto-uterina.
**retrotarsal f.,** conjunctival f.
**Rindfleisch's f's,** folds in the serous surface of the pericardium around the beginning of the aorta.
**sacrogenital f.,** plica recto-uterina.
**salpingopalatine f.,** plica salpingopalatina.
**salpingopharyngeal f.,** plica salpingopharyngea.
**Schultze's f.,** a sickle-shaped fold of the amnion extending from the point of insertion of the cord into the placenta to the remains of the umbilical vesicle.
**semilunar f's of colon,** plicae semilunares coli.
**semilunar f. of conjunctiva,** plica semilunaris conjunctivae.
**semilunar f. of fauces,** plica semilunaris faucium.
**semilunar f. of transversalis fascia,** ligamentum interfoveolare.
**serosal f., serous f.,** a fold of serous membrane.
**sigmoid f's of colon,** plicae semilunares coli.
**skin f.,** skinfold.
**spiral f., spiral f. of cystic duct,** plica spiralis.
**stapedial f.,** plica stapedialis.
**sublingual f.,** plica sublingualis.
**superior duodenal f.,** plica duodenalis superior.
**synovial f.,** plica synovialis.
**synovial f., infrapatellar,** plica synovialis infrapatellaris.
**synovial f., mediopatellar,** plica synovialis mediopatellaris.
**synovial f., patellar,** plica synovialis infrapatellaris.
**synovial f., suprapatellar,** plica synovialis suprapatellaris.
**synovial f. of hip,** ligamentum capitis femoris.
**tail f.,** a crescentic, ventral fold of the embryonic disk at the future caudal end of the embryo.
**transverse f's of rectum,** plicae transversae recti.
**Treves' f.,** plica ileocaecalis.
**triangular f.,** plica triangularis.
**tubal f's of uterine tube,** plicae tubariae tubae uterinae.
**umbilical f., lateral,** plica umbilicalis lateralis.
**umbilical f., medial,** plica umbilicalis medialis.
**umbilical f., median, umbilical f., middle,** plica umbilicalis mediana.
**urogenital f.,** urogenital ridge.
**vaginal f's,** rugae vaginales.
**vascular cecal f.,** plica caecalis vascularis.
**Vater's f.,** a fold in the mucous membrane of the duodenum superior to the hepatopancreatic ampulla.
**ventricular f.,** plica vestibularis.

**vesical f., transverse,** plica vesicalis transversa.
**vestibular f.,** plica vestibularis.
**vestigial f. of Marshall,** plica venae cavae sinistrae.
**villous f's of stomach,** plicae villosae gastris.
**vocal f.,** plica vocalis.
**vocal f., false,** plica vestibularis.

**Fo·lex** (fo'leks) trademark for preparations of methotrexate.

**Fo·ley catheter** (fo'le) [Frederic Eugene Basil *Foley,* American urologist, 1891–1966] see under *catheter.*

**fo·lia** (fo'le-ə) plural of *folium.*

**fo·li·a·ceous** (fo″le-a'shəs) [L. *folia* leaves] having, pertaining to, or resembling leaves.

**fo·li·an** (fo'le-ən) named for Caecelius Folius, Italian anatomist, 1615–1660; see under *process.*

**fo·lic ac·id** (fo'lik) [MeSH: Folic Acid] 1. a water-soluble vitamin of the B complex composed of pteroic acid linked to L-glutamic acid (pteroylglutamic acid); more generally, any derivatives having various levels of reduction of the bicyclic pteridine portion, substitutions at this structure, and number of glutamate residues. Folic acid is necessary for hematopoiesis and is found in liver, green vegetables, and yeast. After absorption, it is successively reduced to dihydrofolic acid and then tetrahydrofolic acid (q.v.), the parent compound of the derivatives that act as coenzyme carriers of one-carbon groups in various metabolic reactions. Deficiency of folic acid results in anemia (see *folic acid deficiency anemia,* under *anemia*). 2. [USP] a preparation of folic acid administered orally or parenterally in the treatment of folic acid deficiency and megaloblastic anemia.

**fo·lie** (fo-le') [Fr.] psychosis; insanity.
**f. à deux** (ah-do͞o'), mental disorder affecting two persons who share the same delusions; classified as *shared psychotic disorder* (q.v.) by DSM-IV.
**f. du doute** (doo do͞ot'), older term for pathologic inability to make even the most trifling decisions, an extreme obsessive-compulsive reaction.
**f. du pourquoi** (doo-poor-kwah'), psychopathologic constant questioning.
**f. gémellaire** (zha″mĕ-lār'), psychosis occurring simultaneously in twins.
**f. raisonnante** (rez-un-ahnt'), f. du doute.

**Fol·in's method** (fol'inz) [Otto Knut Olof *Folin,* American physiologic chemist, 1867–1934] see under *method.*

**fo·lin·ic ac·id** (fo-lin'ik) the 5-formyl derivative of tetrahydrofolic acid; it can act as a coenzyme carrier in certain folate-mediated reactions but does not require dihydrofolate reductase activity and thus it is used, as the calcium salt leucovorin calcium, in treating some disorders of folic acid deficiency. Called also *leucovorin* and *citrovorum factor.*

**fo·li·um** (fo'le-əm) pl. *fo'lia* [L. "leaf"] [TA] a general term for a leaflike structure, especially one of the leaflike subdivisions of the cerebellar cortex.
**fo'lia cerebel'li** [TA], folia of cerebellum: the numerous long narrow folds of the cerebellar cortex, separated by sulci and supported by white laminae; they are aggregated into the various subdivisions of the cerebellum. Called also *gyri cerebelli.*
**lingual folia,** papillae foliatae.
**f. ver'mis** [TA], the part of the vermis of the cerebellum between the declive and the tuber vermis.

**Fo·li·us' muscle, process** (fo'le-əs) [Caecilius *Folius,* Italian anatomist, 1615–1660] see *ligamentum mallei laterale* and *processus anterior mallei.*

**fol·li·cle** (fol'ĭ-kəl) 1. a sac or pouchlike depression or cavity; see also *folliculus.* 2. nodulus lymphoideus.
**aggregated f's, aggregated lymphatic f's,** aggregated lymphoid nodules; see terms beginning *noduli lymphoidei aggregati,* under *nodulus.*
**antral f's,** folliculi ovarici vesiculosi.
**atretic f.,** an ovarian follicle which has involuted.
**dental f.,** tooth f.
**Fleischmann's f.,** an occasional follicle in the mucosa of the floor of the mouth, near the anterior border of the genioglossus muscle.
**gastric f's,** 1. fundic glands. 2. folliculi lymphatici gastrici.
**graafian f's,** folliculi ovarici vesiculosi.
**hair f.,** folliculus pili.
**intestinal f's,** glandulae intestinales.
**lenticular f's,** folliculi lymphatici gastrici.
**Lieberkühn's f's,** glandulae intestinales.
**lingual f's,** noduli lymphoidei tonsillae lingualis.
**lymph f.,** 1. nodulus lymphoideus. 2. lymphatic nodule (def. 2).
**lymph f's of stomach,** folliculi lymphatici gastrici.
**lymphatic f.,** 1. nodulus lymphoideus. 2. lymphatic nodule (def. 2).
**lymphatic f's, laryngeal,** folliculi lymphatici laryngei.
**lymphatic f's, solitary,** noduli lymphoidei solitarii; see under *nodulus.*
**lymphatic f's of large intestine, solitary,** see *noduli lymphoidei solitarii,* under *nodulus.*
**lymphatic f's of Peyer, aggregated,** noduli lymphoidei aggregati intestini tenuis.
**lymphatic f's of small intestine, aggregated,** noduli lymphoidei aggregati intestini tenuis.
**lymphatic f's of small intestine, solitary,** see *noduli lymphoidei solitarii,* under *nodulus.*
**lymphatic f's of tongue,** noduli lymphoidei tonsillae lingualis.
**lymphatic f's of vermiform appendix, aggregated,** noduli lymphoidei aggregati appendicis vermiformis.
**lymphoid f.,** nodulus lymphoideus.
**lymphoid f's, solitary,** noduli lymphoidei solitarii; see under *nodulus.*
**lymphoid f's of large intestine, solitary,** see *noduli lymphoidei solitarii,* under *nodulus.*
**lymphoid f's of small intestine, aggregated,** noduli lymphoidei aggregati intestini tenuis.
**lymphoid f's of small intestine, solitary,** see *noduli lymphoidei solitarii,* under *nodulus.*
**lymphoid f's of vermiform appendix, aggregated,** noduli lymphoidei aggregati appendicis vermiformis.
**Montgomery's f's,** Naboth's f's.
**Naboth's f's, nabothian f's,** cystlike formations caused by occlusion of the lumina of glands in the mucosa of the uterine cervix, causing them to be distended with retained secretion; called also *Montgomery's f's* and *Naboth's cysts* or *glands.*
**ovarian f.,** the egg and its encasing cells, at any stage of its development.
**ovarian f's, primary,** folliculi ovarici primarii.
**ovarian f's, vesicular,** folliculi ovarici vesiculosi.
**primordial f.,** an ovarian follicle consisting of an egg enclosed by a single layer of cells.
**sebaceous f.,** a hair follicle supplied with a relatively large sebaceous gland, and producing a relatively insignificant hair.
**secondary f's,** folliculi ovarici vesiculosi.
**solitary f's,** see *folliculi lymphatici solitarii intestini crassi* and *folliculi lymphatici solitarii intestini tenuis.*
**f. of Stannius,** a lymphoid unit in chicks, resembling the thymus and developing from nodules formed by proliferation of points of the epithelium of the bursa of Fabricius.
**thyroid f's, f's of thyroid gland,** folliculi glandulae thyroideae.
**f's of tongue,** noduli lymphoidei tonsillae lingualis.
**tooth f.,** the structure within the developing alveolar bone of the jaws enclosing the tooth germ. Called also *dental f.*
**unilaminar f.,** primordial f.

**fol·li·clis** (fol'ĭ-klis) a term applied to a superficial form of papulonecrotic tuberculid with a predilection for the dorsa of the hands, feet, forearms, and legs.

**fol·lic·u·lar** (fo-lik'u-lər) [L. *follicularis*] of or pertaining to a follicle or follicles.

**fol·lic·u·li** (fo-lik'u-li) [L.] genitive and plural of *folliculus.*

**fol·lic·u·li·tis** (fo-lik″u-li'tis) [MeSH: Folliculitis] inflammation of a follicle or follicles; used ordinarily in reference to hair follicles, but sometimes in relation to follicles of other kinds.
**f. absce'dens et suffo'diens,** perifolliculitis capitis abscedens et suffodiens.
**agminate f.,** inflammation of a number of follicles in one area.
**f. bar'bae,** sycosis barbae.
**f. decal'vans,** a rare, localized, spreading, suppurative folliculitis of unknown cause, leading to scarring, with permanent hair loss.
**eosinophilic pustular f.,** a rare pruritic dermatosis marked by the

appearance of pruritic sterile pustules on the face, trunk, and extremities, which coalesce to form plaques that tend toward central clearing and residual hyperpigmentation; the lesions undergo spontaneous exacerbation and remission. Histological features include spongiosis of the follicular epithelium and leukocytic infiltration of the hair follicle sheath and perifollicular dermis, resulting in destruction of the follicle and sometimes the formation of eosinophilic abscesses.
**f. gonorrhoe'ica,** littritis caused by gonococci.
**gram-negative f.,** a superinfection complicating long-term systemic antibiotic treatment of acne vulgaris, particularly tetracyclines, usually caused by species of *Enterobacter, Klebsiella,* or *Proteus.* Infection with the first two species is manifested by a superficial pustular eruption, often occurring around the nares; deep nodular cysts, usually on the back, are associated with *Proteus* infections.
**keloidal f., f. keloida'lis,** dermatitis papillaris capillitii.
**f. na'res per'forans,** inflammation of a hair follicle in the nose, with pustulation and destruction of the follicle, leading to extension of the process through the tissues to the external surface.
**f. ulerythemato'sa reticula'ta,** atrophodermia vermiculata usually confined to the cheek but sometimes spreading to involve the ears, forehead, and scalp. Called also *atrophoderma reticulatum symmetricum faciei.* See also *ulerythema ophryogenes.*
**f. variolifor'mis,** see under *acne.*

**fol·lic·u·lo·ma** (fo-lik″u-lo'mə) [*folliculus* + *-oma*] granulosa–theca cell tumor; see under *tumor.*
**f. lipidique,** a granulosa–theca cell tumor in which streamers or trabeculae of tall, columnar, lipid-laden cells are interspersed among the more characteristic collections of granulosa cells.

**fol·lic·u·lo·sis** (fə-lik″u-lo'sis) a disease characterized by excessive development of lymph follicles.

**fol·lic·u·lo·stat·in** (fo-lik″u-lo-stat'in) [*follicle*-stimulating hormone + *-statin*] follistatin.

**fol·lic·u·lus** (fo-lik'u-ləs) gen. and pl. *folli'culi* [L., dim. of *follis* a leather bag] [TA] follicle: a general term for a very small excretory or secretory sac or gland.
**folli'culi glan'dulae thyroi'deae,** follicles of thyroid gland: discrete, cystlike units of the thyroid gland that are lined with cuboidal epithelium and are filled with a colloid substance; there are about 30 to each lobule. Called also *thyroid acini* and *thyroid follicles.*
**folli'culi lingua'les,** noduli lymphoidei tonsillae lingualis.
**f. lympha'ticus,** nodulus lymphoideus.
**folli'culi lympha'tici aggrega'ti,** noduli lymphoidei aggregati intestini tenuis.
**folli'culi lympha'tici aggrega'ti appen'dicis vermifor'mis,** noduli lymphoidei aggregati appendicis vermiformis.
**folli'culi lympha'tici gas'trici,** lymph follicles of stomach: small lymphocytic aggregates in the interstitial tissue of the lamina propria of the stomach, especially in the pyloric region; called also *lenticular glands of stomach, lymphatic nodules of stomach,* and *noduli lymphatici gastrici.*
**folli'culi lympha'tici laryn'gei,** laryngeal lymphatic follicles: lymphatic aggregations in the mucosa of the ventricle of the larynx and on the posterior surface of the epiglottis; called also *noduli lymphatici laryngei.*
**folli'culi lympha'tici liena'les,** noduli lymphoidei splenici; see under *nodulus.*
**folli'culi lympha'tici rec'ti,** concentrations of lymphoid tissue in the tunica mucosa of the rectum; called also *noduli lymphatici recti.*
**folli'culi lympha'tici solita'rii,** noduli lymphoidei solitarii; see under *nodulus.*
**folli'culi lympha'tici solita'rii intesti'ni cras'si,** the solitary lymphatic nodules of the large intestine; see *noduli lymphoidei solitarii.*
**folli'culi lympha'tici solita'rii intesti'ni ten'uis,** the solitary lymphatic nodules of the small intestine; see *noduli lymphoidei solitarii.*
**folli'culi lympha'tici sple'nici,** noduli lymphoidei splenici; see under *nodulus.*
**folli'culi oo'phori prima'rii,** folliculi ovarici primarii.
**folli'culi oo'phori vesiculo'si [Graa'fi],** folliculi ovarici vesiculosi.
**folli'culi ova'rici prima'rii,** primary ovarian follicles: immature ovarian follicles, each comprising an immature ovum and the specialized epithelial cells (follicle cells) that surround it; called also *folliculi oophori primarii.*
**folli'culi ova'rici vesiculo'si** [TA], vesicular ovarian follicles: maturing ovarian follicles among whose cells fluid has begun to accumulate, leading to the formation of a single cavity or antrum and leaving the ovum eccentrically located in a hillock of follicle cells, the cumulus oophorus; called also *folliculi oophori vesiculosi* [*Graafi*], and *graafian follicles* or *vesicles.*
**f. pi'li** [TA], hair follicle: one of the tubular invaginations of the epidermis that enclose the hairs, and from which the hairs grow. It is divided into upper and lower segments: the upper comprises the infundibulum, extending from the free surface to the sebaceous gland, and the isthmus, extending from the sebaceous gland to the arrector pili; the lower comprises the stem and the bulb. At the level of the stem, the hair cuticle is surrounded successively by the inner and outer root sheaths, which are enclosed by a dermal sheath.

**fol·li·stat·in** (fol'ĭ-stat″in) [*follicle*-stimulating hormone + *-statin*] a peptide that suppresses the secretion of follicle-stimulating hormone; called also *folliculostatin.*

**Fol·lis·tim** (fol'is-tim) trademark for a preparation of follitropin beta.

**fol·li·tro·pin** (fol'ĭ-tro″pin) follicle-stimulating hormone.
**f. beta,** a synthetic isoform of follicle-stimulating hormone derived from genetically modified Chinese hamster ovary cells, used to stimulate the development of ovarian follicles in the treatment of female infertility and to induce ovulation in women undergoing an assisted reproductive technology procedure; administered subcutaneously or intramuscularly.

**fol·low·ing** (fol'o-ing) an effect seen on an electroencephalogram, in which brain waves change their frequencies in response to certain repetitive sensory stimuli. Cf. *driving.*

**Fol·lu·te·in** (fol'u-tēn) trademark for a preparation of chorionic gonadotropin.

**Foltz's valve** (fōltz'əz) [Jean Charles Eugène *Foltz,* French ophthalmologist, 1822–1876] see under *valve.*

**Fol·vite** (fol'vīt) trademark for preparations of folic acid.

**fo·men·ta·tion** (fo″mən-ta'shən) [L. *fomentatio; fomentum,* a poultice] treatment by warm and moist applications; also the substance thus applied.

**fo·mep·i·zole** (fo-mep'ĭ-zōl) an alcohol dehydrogenase inhibitor, used as an antidote to poisoning by methanol or ethylene glycol. Called also *4-methyl-1H-pyrazole.*

**fo·mes** (fo'mēz) pl. *fo'mites* [L. "tinder"] fomite.

**fo·mite** (fo'mīt) an object, such as a book, wooden object, or an article of clothing, that is not in itself harmful, but is able to harbor pathogenic microorganisms and thus may serve as an agent of transmission of an infection. Called also *fomes.*

**fom·i·tes** (fo'mĭ-tēz) plural of *fomes.*

**Fon·se·caea** (fon-se-se'ə) [O. da *Fonseca,* Brazilian physician, 20th century] a genus of Fungi Imperfecti of the form-class Hyphomycetes, form-family Dematiaceae; some species were formerly included in the genera *Hormodendrum* and *Cladosporium. F. compac'tum* and *F. pedro'soi* are etiologic agents of chromoblastomycosis.

**Fon·tan procedure** (fawn-tă') [François Maurice *Fontan,* French heart surgeon, born 1929] [MeSH: Fontan Procedure] see under *procedure.*

**Fon·tana's markings, spaces** (fon-tah'nəz) [Felice *Fontana,* Italian naturalist and physiologist, 1730–1805] see under *marking* and see *spatia anguli iridocornealis,* under *spatium.*

**fon·ta·nel** (fon″tə-nel') fontanelle.

**fon·ta·nelle** (fon'tə-nel') [Fr., dim. of *fontaine* spring, filter] a soft spot, such as one of the membrane-covered spaces (*fonticuli cranii* [TA]) remaining in the incompletely ossified skull of a fetus or infant. See also *fonticulus.*
**anterior f.,** fonticulus anterior.
**anterolateral f.,** fonticulus sphenoidalis.
**bregmatic f.,** fonticulus anterior.

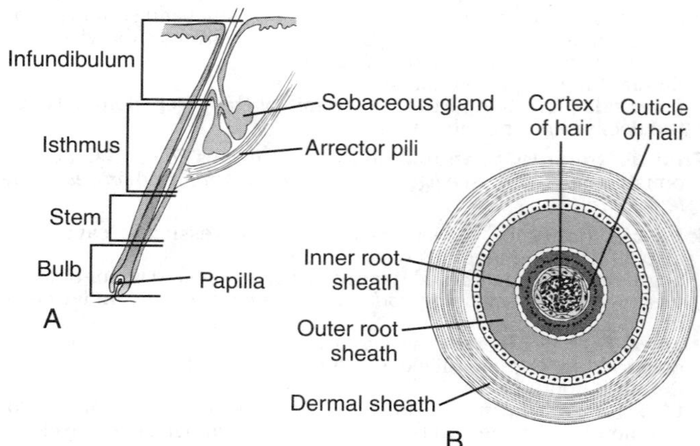


Folliculus pili (hair follicle). *(A),* longitudinal section, comprising the infundibulum, isthmus, stem, and bulb; *(B),* transverse section of follicle, showing the hair shaft and surrounding follicular sheaths.

**Casser's f., casserian f., Casserio's f.,** fonticulus mastoideus.
**cranial f's,** fonticuli cranii.
**frontal f.,** fonticulus anterior.
**Gerdy's f.,** a fontanelle occasionally occurring in the sagittal suture; called also *sagittal f.*
**mastoid f.,** fonticulus mastoideus.
**occipital f., posterior f.,** fonticulus posterior.
**posterolateral f., posterotemporal f.,** fonticulus mastoideus.
**quadrangular f.,** fonticulus anterior.
**sagittal f.,** Gerdy's f.
**sphenoidal f.,** fonticulus sphenoidalis.
**triangular f.,** fonticulus posterior.

**fon·tic·u·li** (fon-tik'u-li) [L.] genitive and plural of *fonticulus.*

**fon·tic·u·lus** (fon-tik'u-ləs) pl. *fontic'uli* [L., dim. of *fons* fountain] [TA] fontanelle; a soft spot; one of the membrane-covered spaces remaining in the incompletely ossified skull of the fetus or infant.
**f. ante'rior** [TA], anterior fontanelle: the unossified area of the skull situated at the junction of the frontal, coronal, and sagittal sutures; called also *forceps frontalis* [*major*], and *frontal fontanelle.*
**f. anterolatera'lis,** TA alternative for *f. sphenoidalis.*
**fontic'uli cra'nii** [TA], the membrane-covered spaces, or soft spots, remaining at the incomplete angles of the parietal and adjacent bones, until ossification of the skull is completed; called also *fontanelles.*
**f. fronta'lis [major],** f. anterior.
**f. guttu'ris,** fossa jugularis.
**f. ma'jor,** f. anterior.
**f. mastoi'deus** [TA], mastoid fontanelle: the unossified area of the skull at the junction of the lambdoidal, parietomastoid, and occipitomastoid sutures. Called also *posterolateral fontanelle, f. posterolateralis* [TA alternative], and *posterotemporal fontanelle.*
**f. mi'nor,** f. posterior.
**f. occipita'lis, f. poste'rior** [TA], posterior fontanelle: the unossified area of the skull at the junction of the sagittal and lambdoidal sutures; called also *f. minor,* and *occipital* or *triangular fontanelle.*
**f. posterolatera'lis,** TA alternative for *f. mastoideus.*
**f. sphenoida'lis** [TA], sphenoidal fontanelle: the unossified area at the junction of the parietal and frontal bones, the greater wing of the sphenoidal, and the squamous part of the temporal bones. Called also *anterolateral fontanelle* and *f. anterolateralis* [TA alternative].

**food** (fo͞od) [MeSH: Food] anything which, when taken into the body, serves to nourish or build up the tissues or to supply body heat; aliment; nutriment.
**functional f's,** foods and food supplements marketed for presumed health benefits, such as vitamin supplements and certain herbs; called also *nutraceuticals.*
**isodynamic f's,** foods which generate equal amounts of energy in heat units.

**foot** (foot) [L. *pes;* from A.S. *fōt*] [MeSH: Foot] 1. the distal portion of the leg, upon which an individual stands and walks. It consists, in man, of the tarsus, metatarsus, and phalanges and the tissues encompassing them. 2. something resembling this structure. 3. a unit of linear measure, 12 inches, being the equivalent of 30.48 cm.
**athlete's f.,** tinea pedis.
**broad f.,** metatarsus latus.
**burning feet,** 1. burning sensations in the soles of the feet; there are many causes such as the hyperalgesia of diabetes, alcoholism, or toxicity. 2. Gopalan's syndrome.
**buttress f.,** periostitis or ostitis in the region of the pyramidal process of the coffin bone of the horse, with fracture of the process,

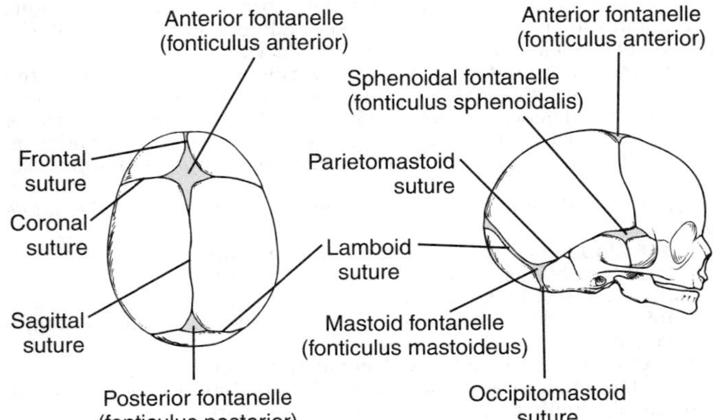

Neonatal skull showing the four fonticuli cranii (cranial fontanelles): the anterior, mastoid, posterior, and sphenoidal.

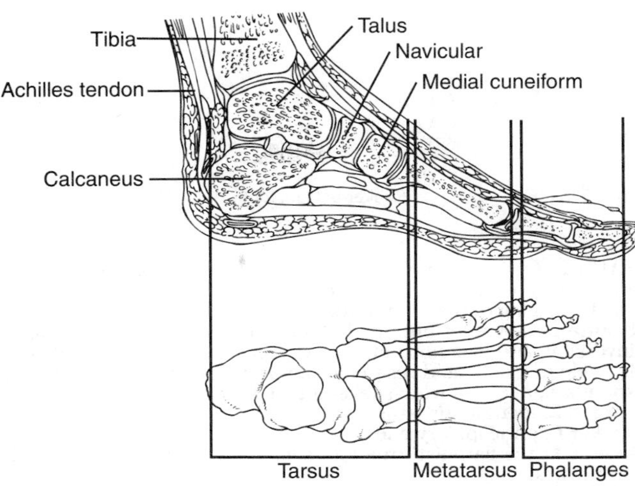

Foot. *(Top),* Longitudinal section; *(bottom),* dorsal aspect.

deformity of the hoof, and alteration of the normal angle of the joint. Called also *extensor process disease, pyramidal disease,* and *low ringbone.*
**Charcot's f.,** the deformed foot seen in tabetic arthropathy.
**cleft f.,** a congenitally deformed foot in which the division between the third and fourth toes extends into the metatarsal region, often with ectrodactyly. Called also *split-foot deformity.* See also *EEC syndrome,* under *syndrome.*
**club f.,** see *talipes.*
**contracted f.,** see under *hoof.*
**dangle f., drop f.,** footdrop.
**end f., end-f.,** bouton terminal; see under *bouton.*
**fescue f.,** a condition seen in cattle and sheep in Australia, New Zealand, and North America after they graze on tall fescue *(Festuca arundinacea)* contaminated by the fungus *Acremonium coenophialum,* which contains a toxic principle similar to that of ergot; characteristics include lameness of the hind feet that may progress to necrosis and dry gangrene and may spread to the ears and tail. Called also *fescue lameness* or *toxicosis, tall fescue lameness,* and *fescue.*
**flat f.,** flatfoot.
**Flex-F.,** trademark for a type of ankle-foot prosthesis that includes a flexible rod replacing the lower leg and foot as well as a heel replacement component allowing push-off.
**forced f.,** a painful swelling of the feet of soldiers after forced marches, due to fracture of a metatarsal bone.
**Friedreich's f.,** pes cavus, with hyperextension of the toes; seen in hereditary ataxia.
**Hong Kong f.,** an infectious mycotic disease (dermatophytosis) of the foot occurring in China.
**immersion f.,** a condition resembling trench foot occurring in persons who have spent long periods in water.
**immersion f., tropical,** maceration, blanching, and wrinkling of the skin of the feet and swelling of the soles with ridging of the surface, caused by prolonged immersion of the feet in warm water.
**Madura f.,** mycetoma of the foot.
**march f.,** painful swelling of the forefoot, often associated with fracture of one of the metatarsal bones, following excessive foot strain.
**Morand's f.,** a foot having eight toes.
**Morton's f.,** see under *neuralgia.*
**mossy f.,** chromoblastomycosis involving the foot.
**pericapillary end f.,** a pyramidal expansion of a process of an astrocyte against the wall of a capillary in the central nervous system; called also *perivascular f., sucker f., sucker process,* and *vascular foot plate.*
**perivascular f.,** pericapillary end f.
**pricked f.,** a condition in the horse in which the soft tissue of the foot has been punctured either by a horseshoe nail or by a nail or other object the animal has stepped on, causing pain and lameness. A nail that is near, but not into, the soft tissue may cause *nail bind.* Called also *nail prick.*
**red f.,** redfoot.
**reel f.,** talipes.
**rocker-bottom f.,** 1. congenital convex pes valgus, due to primary dislocation of the talonavicular joint; it may occur as an isolated primary deformity or be associated with autosomal trisomy, including trisomy 13–15 and trisomy 18; called also *rocker-bottom flatfoot.* 2. talipes equinovarus in which the foot is shaped like a rocker of a rocking chair, occurring as a result of a transverse break in the midtarsal area; called also *rocker-bottom deformity.* See illustration.

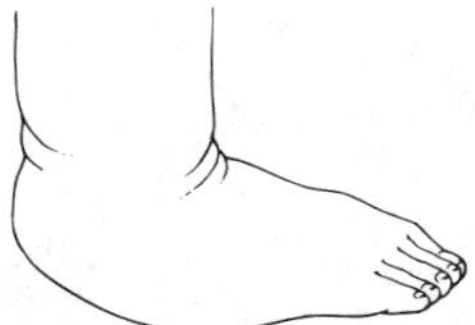

Rocker-bottom foot.

**SACH f.,** (*s*olid *a*nkle *c*ushion *h*eel) a type of prosthetic foot that allows flexion, extension, inversion, and eversion.
**sag f.,** sagging of the arch of the foot.
**Seattle f.,** a type of prosthetic foot that allows flexion, extension, inversion, and eversion, and allows some push-off when walking; it is made of plastic and resembles a normal human foot.
**spatula f.,** a foot in which several toes are fused together.
**spread f.,** metatarsus latus.
**sucker f.,** pericapillary end f.
**tabetic f.,** the flat, distorted foot seen in tabes, and due to disease of the tarsus.
**taut f.,** a shortening and contraction of the calf muscles and plantar flexors of the foot, due to high-heeled shoes.
**trench f.,** a condition of the feet resembling frostbite. It is due to the prolonged action of water on the skin combined with circulatory disturbance due to cold and inaction.
**weak f.,** an early stage of flatfoot.

**foot-can·dle** (foot'kan"dəl) a unit of illumination being 1 lumen per square foot or equivalent to 1.0764 milliphots. Cf. *lux.*

**foot·drop** (foot'drop) dropping of the foot from a peroneal or tibial nerve lesion that causes paralysis of the anterior muscles of the leg; see also *steppage gait.* Called also *dangle foot* and *drop foot.*

**foot lam·bert** (foot lam'bərt) see *lambert.*

**foot·plate** (foot'plāt) basis stapedis.
**floating f.,** abnormal mobilization of the stapedial footplate.
**stapedial f.,** basis stapedis.

**foot-pound** (foot-pound') the work done in raising a mass of one pound the distance of one foot against gravity. Abbreviated p.

**foot·print·ing** (foot'print-ing) a technique for determining the location of binding between a protein and a DNA molecule; the two are bound, enzymes or chemicals are used to hydrolyze unbound, unprotected DNA, and the resulting protected DNA fragments can be identified electrophoretically.

**fo·ra·men** (fo-ra'mən) pl. *fora'mina* [L.] 1. a natural opening or passage. 2. [TA] a general term for such a passage, especially one into or through a bone.

## Foramen

Descriptions of anatomic structures are given on TA terms, and include anglicized names of specific foramina.

**accessory f.,** a lateral or accessory orifice, other than the main apical foramen, opening into the root canal of a tooth; called also *lateral f.*
**alveolar foramina of maxilla, fora'mina alveola'ria maxil'lae** [TA], the openings of the alveolar canals at the deepest portion of the tooth sockets in the maxilla.
**aortic f.,** hiatus aorticus.
**apical f. of root of tooth, apical f. of tooth, f. a'picis den'tis** [TA], apical foramen of root of tooth: a minute aperture usually at or near the apex of a root of a tooth but on occasion located on a side of a root, which gives passage to the vascular, lymphatic, and neural structures supplying the pulp; the main foramen sometimes branches near the apex to form two or more apical ramifications. Called also *f. radicis dentis, pulpal f.,* and *root f.*
**auditory f., external,** meatus acusticus externus.
**auditory f., internal,** porus acusticus internus.
**f. of Bochdalek,** hiatus pleuroperitonealis.
**f. cae'cum lin'guae** [TA], foramen cecum of tongue: a depression on the dorsum of the tongue at the end of the median sulcus, representing the remains of the superior end of the thyroglossal duct of the embryo.
**f. cae'cum medul'lae oblonga'tae** [TA], a small triangular expansion at the lower border of the pons, formed by the termination of the anterior median fissure of the medulla oblongata; called also *f. caecum posterius, Schwalbe's f.,* and *f. of Vicq d'Azyr.*
**f. cae'cum os'sis fronta'lis** [TA], foramen cecum of frontal bone: a blind opening formed between the frontal crest and the crista galli, which sometimes transmits a vein from the nasal cavity to the superior sagittal sinus; called also *cecal f.*
**f. cae'cum poste'rius, f. caecum of Vicq d'Azyr,** f. caecum medullae oblongatae.
**caroticoclinoid f.,** the foramen between the anterior and middle clinoid processes in the minority of sphenoid bones where those processes meet at their outer ends.
**caroticotympanic foramina,** canaliculi caroticotympanici.
**carotid f.,** the inferior aperture of the carotid canal, giving passage to the carotid vessels.
**caval f.,** foramen venae cavae.
**cecal f.,** see *f. caecum linguae, f. caecum medullae oblongatae,* and *f. caecum ossis frontalis.*
**f. cecum of frontal bone,** f. caecum ossis frontalis.
**f. cecum of medulla oblongata,** f. caecum medullae oblongatae.
**f. cecum of tongue,** f. caecum linguae.
**f. centra'le,** one of the foramina of the tractus spiralis foraminosus, transmitting nerve filaments and continuing as a canal through the middle of the modiolus to the apex.
**condyloid f., anterior,** canalis nervi hypoglossi.
**condyloid f., posterior,** canalis condylaris.
**conjugate f.,** a foramen formed by a notch in each of two opposed bones.
**f. costotransversa'rium** [TA], **costotransverse f.,** the narrow space between the dorsal surface of the neck of a rib and the ventral surface of the transverse process of the corresponding vertebra.
**cotyloid f.,** a passage between the margin of the acetabulum and the transverse ligament.
**cribroethmoid f.,** f. ethmoidale anterius.
**fora'mina cribro'sa os'sis ethmoida'lis** [TA], the openings in the cribriform plate of the ethmoid bone for passage of the olfactory nerves. Called also *olfactory foramina.*
**dental foramina,** see *foramina alveolaria maxillae* and *foramina mandibulae.*
**f. diaphrag'matis [sel'lae],** the opening in the center of the diaphragm of the sella through which the infundibulum passes.
**Duverney's f.,** f. omentale.
**emissary f.,** any foramen in a cranial bone that gives passage to an emissary vein.
**emissary f., sphenoidal,** foramen venosum.
**epiploic f.,** *f. omentale.*
**f. epiplo'icum,** TA alternative for *f. omentale.*
**esophageal f.,** hiatus oesophageus.
**ethmoidal f., anterior,** f. ethmoidale anterius.
**ethmoidal f., posterior,** f. ethmoidale posterius.
**f. ethmoida'le ante'rius** [TA], anterior ethmoidal foramen: the anterior of two small grooves found as a pair crossing the superior surface on both sides of the ethmoid labyrinth, at its junction with the roof of each orbit; it transmits the nasal branch of the ophthalmic nerve and the anterior ethmoid artery and vein. Called also *anterior ethmoidal canal* and *anterior internal orbital canal.*
**f. ethmoida'le poste'rius** [TA], posterior ethmoidal foramen: the posterior of two small grooves found as a pair crossing the superior surface on both sides of the ethmoid labyrinth, at its junction with the roof of each orbit; it transmits the posterior ethmoid artery and vein. Called also *posterior ethmoidal canal* and *posterior internal orbital canal.*
**fora'mina ethmoida'lia,** see *f. ethmoidale anterius* and *f. ethmoidale posterius.*
**f. of Fallopio,** hiatus canalis nervi petrosi majoris.
**Ferrein's f.,** hiatus canalis nervi petrosi majoris.
**frontal f., f. fronta'le** [TA], see incisura frontalis.
**frontoethmoidal f.,** a foramen lying on the line of the frontoethmoidal suture.
**glandular foramina of Littre,** lacunae urethrales.
**Hartigan's f.,** a foramen said to exist in the base of the transverse process of a lumbar vertebra but seldom persisting to adult life.
**Huschke's f.,** a passage formed by union of the tubercles of the tympanic ring; it normally becomes ossified and disappears during childhood. Called also *Huschke's canal.*

**fora'mina incisi'va** [TA], incisive foramen: one of the openings in the incisive fossa of the hard palate that transmit the nasopalatine nerves. Called also *foramina of Stensen.* See also *canales incisivi.*
**incisor f., median,** Scarpa's f.
**infraorbital f., f. infraorbita'le** [TA], the opening of the infraorbital canal on the anterior surface of the maxilla giving passage to the infraorbital nerve and vessels; called also *suborbital f.*
**infrapiriform f.,** an opening below the piriformis muscle through which the inferior gluteal vessels and nerve pass out of the pelvis.
**interatrial f. primum,** ostium primum.
**interatrial f. secundum,** ostium secundum.
**intersacral foramina,** foramina intervertebralia ossis sacri.
**interventricular f., f. interventricula're** [TA], a passage through which the lateral and third ventricles communicate.
**f. intervertebra'le** [TA], intervertebral foramen: the passage formed by the inferior and superior notches on the pedicles of adjacent vertebrae; it transmits a spinal nerve and vessels.
**fora'mina intervertebra'lia os'sis sa'cri** [TA], intervertebral foramina of sacrum: the four short, forked tunnels in each lateral wall of the sacral canal, connecting it with the pelvic and dorsal sacral foramina; called also *intersacral canals* or *foramina.*
**ischiadic f., greater,** f. ischiadicum majus.
**ischiadic f., lesser,** f. ischiadicum minus.
**f. ischia'dicum ma'jus** [TA], greater sciatic foramen: a hole converted from the major sciatic notch by the sacrotuberal and sacrospinal ligaments; called also *f. sciaticum minus, greater ischiadic f.,* and *large sacrosciatic f.*
**f. ischia'dicum mi'nus** [TA], lesser sciatic foramen: a hole converted from the minor sciatic notch by the sacrotuberal and sacrospinal ligaments; called also *f. sciaticum minus, lesser ischiadic f.,* and *small sacrosciatic f.*
**ischiopubic f.,** f. obturatum.
**jugular f., f. jugula're** [TA], the opening formed by the jugular notches on the temporal and occipital bones, for the transmission of various veins, arteries, and nerves.
**f. of Key and Retzius,** apertura lateralis ventriculi quarti.
**lacerate f., anterior,** fissura orbitalis superior.
**lacerate f., middle,** f. lacerum.
**lacerate f., posterior,** f. jugulare.
**f. la'cerum** [TA], an irregular gap formed at the junction of the base of the greater wing of the sphenoid bone, the tip of the petrous part of the temporal bone, and the basilar part of the occipital bone; in life, it does not exist, being occupied by an unossified part of the petrous part of the temporal bone.
**Lannelongue's foramina,** foramina venarum minimarum atrii dextri.
**lateral f.,** accessory f.
**left f., inferior,** hiatus aorticus.
**left f., superior,** hiatus oesophageus.
**f. of Luschka,** apertura lateralis ventriculi quarti.
**f. of Magendie,** apertura mediana ventriculi quarti.
**f. mag'num** [TA], the large opening in the anterior and inferior part of the occipital bone, interconnecting the vertebral canal and the cranial cavity; called also *f. occipitale magnum* and *great occipital f.*
**malar f.,** f. zygomaticofaciale.
**f. mandi'bulae** [TA], **f. mandibula're,** mandibular foramen: the opening on the medial surface of the ramus of the mandible, leading into the mandibular canal.
**mastoid f., f. mastoi'deum** [TA], a prominent opening in the temporal bone posterior to the mastoid process and near its occipital articulation; an artery and vein usually pass through it.
**maxillary f.,** hiatus maxillaris.
**maxillary f., internal, maxillary f., posterior,** f. mandibulae.
**maxillary f., superior,** f. rotundum ossis sphenoidalis.
**medullary f.,** f. vertebrale.
**mental f., f. menta'le** [TA], an opening on the lateral part of the body of the mandible, opposite the second bicuspid tooth, for passage of the mental nerve and vessels.
**f. of Monro,** f. interventriculare.

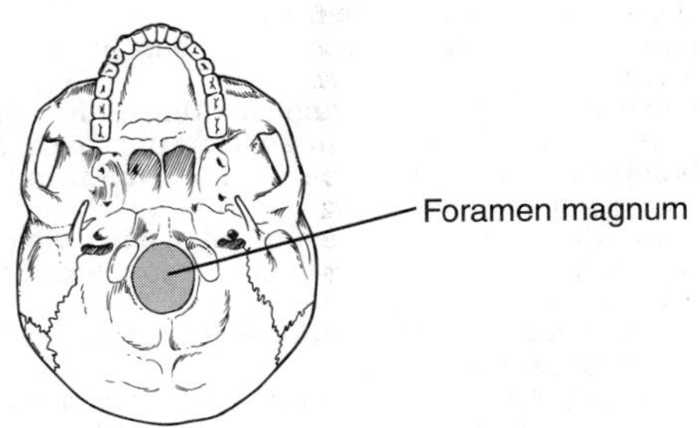

Inferior view of the base of the skull, showing the foramen magnum.

**Morgagni's f., morgagnian f.,** 1. a small defect on either side, between the sternal and costal portions of the diaphragm, allowing passage of the superior epigastric blood vessels and a few lymphatic vessels; called also *pleuroperitoneal f.* 2. f. caecum linguae. 3. f. singulare.
**nasal foramina, fora'mina nasa'lia** [TA], openings on the outer surface of each nasal bone for the transmission of blood vessels.
**fora'mina nervo'sa** [TA], **fora'mina nervo'sa la'minae spira'lis,** numerous small openings in the labium limbi tympanicum for the passage of the cochlear nerves; called also *habenulae perforatae.*
**neural f.,** f. intervertebrale.
**f. nutri'cium** [TA], **f. nu'triens, nutrient f.,** any one of the passages that admit the nutrient vessels to the medullary cavity of a bone.
**obturator f., f. obturato'rium, f. obtura'tum** [TA], the large opening between the os pubis and the ischium.
**occipital f., great, occipital f., inferior, f. occipita'le mag'num,** f. magnum.
**olfactory foramina,** foramina cribrosa ossis ethmoidalis.
**omental f., f. omenta'le** [TA], the opening connecting the greater and the lesser peritoneal sacs, situated below and behind the porta hepatis; called also *epiploic f.* and *f. epiploicum* [TA alternative].
**optic f. of sclera,** lamina cribrosa sclerae.
**optic f. of sphenoid bone, f. op'ticum os'sis sphenoida'lis,** canalis opticus.
**orbitomalar f.,** f. zygomatico-orbitale.
**oval f. of fetal heart, oval f. of fetus,** f. ovale cordis.
**oval f. of hip bone,** f. obturatum.
**f. ova'le cor'dis** [TA], the aperture in the septum secundum of the fetal heart that provides a communication between the atria; called also *oval f. of fetal heart* and *oval f. of fetus.*
**f. ova'le os'sis sphenoida'lis** [TA], foramen ovale of sphenoid: an opening in the posterior part of the medial portion of the greater wing of the sphenoid bone; it transmits the mandibular branch of the trigeminal nerve and some vessels.
**f. of Pacchioni, pacchionian f.,** f. diaphragmatis [sellae].
**palatine f., greater,** f. palatinum majus.
**palatine foramina, lesser,** foramina palatina minora.
**palatine f., posterior,** f. palatinum majus.
**foramina of palatine tonsil,** fossulae tonsillares tonsillae palatinae.
**f. palati'num ma'jus** [TA], greater palatine foramen: the inferior opening of the great palatine canal, found laterally on the horizontal plate of each palatine bone opposite the root of each third molar tooth; it transmits a palatine nerve and artery. Called also *posterior palatine f., pterygopalatine f.,* and *sphenopalatine f.*
**fora'mina palati'na mino'ra** [TA], lesser palatine foramina: the openings of the lesser palatine canals behind the palatine crest and the greater palatine foramina.
**fora'mina papilla'ria re'nis** [TA], **papillary foramina of kidney,** minute openings in the summit of each renal papilla, the orifices of the collecting tubules; called also *foveolae papillae.*
**parietal f., f. parieta'le** [TA], an opening on the posterior part of the superior portion of the parietal bone near the sagittal suture, for the passage of a vein and arteriole.
**f. petro'sum** [TA], petrosal foramen: a small opening sometimes present posterior to the oval foramen for transmission of the lesser petrosal nerve; called also *canaliculus innominatus* and *innominate canaliculus.*
**pleuroperitoneal f.,** 1. hiatus pleuroperitonealis. 2. Morgagni's f. (def. 1).
**f. proces'sus transver'si,** f. transversarium.
**pterygopalatine f., f. pterygopalati'num,** 1. f. palatinum majus. 2. f. sphenopalatinum.
**pulpal f.,** f. apicis dentis.
**quadrate f.,** f. venae cavae.
**f. ra'dicis den'tis,** f. apicis dentis.
**Retzius' f.,** apertura lateralis ventriculi quarti.
**right f.,** f. venae cavae.
**root f.,** f. apicis dentis.
**f. rotun'dum os'sis sphenoida'lis** [TA], round foramen of sphenoid bone: a round opening in the medial part of the greater wing of the sphenoid bone that transmits the maxillary branch of the trigeminal nerve; called also *superior maxillary f.* or *canal.*
**sacral foramina, anterior,** foramina sacralia anteriora.
**sacral foramina, dorsal,** foramina sacralia posteriora.
**sacral foramina, internal,** foramina sacralia anteriora.
**sacral foramina, posterior,** foramina sacralia posteriora.
**sacral foramina, ventral,** foramina sacralia anteriora.
**f. of sacral canal,** hiatus sacralis.
**fora'mina sacra'lia anterio'ra** [TA], anterior sacral foramina: the eight openings (four on each side) on the pelvic surface of the sacral bone for the ventral rami of the sacral nerves. Called also *internal* or *ventral sacral foramina, foramina sacralia pelvica, foramina sacralia pelvina,* and *foramina sacralia ventralia.*
**fora'mina sacra'lia dorsa'lia,** foramina sacralia posteriora.

**fora'mina sacra'lia pel'vica, fora'mina sacra'lia pelvi'na,** foramina sacralia anteriora.
**fora'mina sacra'lia posterio'ra** [TA], posterior sacral foramina: the eight openings (four on each side) on the dorsal surface of the sacral bone for the dorsal rami of the sacral nerves. Called also *dorsal sacral foramina* and *foramina sacralia dorsalia.*
**fora'mina sacra'lia ventra'lia,** foramina sacralia anteriora.
**sacrosciatic f., large,** f. ischiadicum majus.
**sacrosciatic f., small,** f. ischiadicum minus.
**f. of saphenous vein,** hiatus saphenus.
**Scarpa's f.,** one of the two foramina, one behind either upper medial incisor, for transmission of the nasopalatine nerves; called also *median incisor f.*
**Schwalbe's f.,** f. caecum medullae oblongatae.
**sciatic f., greater,** f. ischiadicum majus.
**sciatic f., lesser,** f. ischiadicum minus.
**f. scia'ticum ma'jus,** f. ischiadicum majus.
**f. scia'ticum mi'nus,** f. ischiadicum minus.
**f. singula're** [TA], singular foramen: the opening in the inferior vestibular area of the fundus of the internal acoustic meatus that gives passage to the nerves of the ampulla of the posterior semicircular duct; called also *Morgagni's* or *morgagnian f.* and *singular canal.*
**foramina of smallest veins of heart,** foramina venarum minimarum atrii dextri.
**sphenopalatine f.,** 1. f. sphenopalatinum. 2. f. palatinum majus.
**f. sphenopalati'num** [TA], sphenopalatine foramen: an opening on the medial wall of the pterygopalatine fossa, interconnecting this fossa with the nasal cavity, and transmitting the sphenopalatine artery and nasal nerves. Called also *pterygopalatine f.*
**sphenotic f.,** f. lacerum.
**spinal f., f. of spinal cord,** f. vertebrale.
**f. spino'sum** [TA], spinous foramen: an opening in the greater wing of the sphenoid bone, near its posterior angle, for the middle meningeal artery.
**Spöndel's f.,** a small transient foramen in the cartilaginous base of the developing skull between the ethmoid bone and the lesser wings of the sphenoid.
**foramina of Stensen,** 1. foramina incisiva. 2. canales incisivi.
**stylomastoid f., f. stylomastoi'deum** [TA], a foramen on the inferior part of the temporal bone between the styloid and mastoid processes, for the facial nerve and the stylomastoid artery.
**suborbital f.,** f. infraorbitale.
**supraorbital f., f. supraorbita'le** [TA], an opening in the frontal bone in the supraorbital margin, giving passage to the supraorbital artery and nerve; it is often present as a notch *(incisura supraorbitalis)* bridged only by fibrous tissue.
**suprapiriform f.,** an opening above the piriformis muscle through which the gluteal vessels and superior gluteal nerve pass out of the pelvis.
**temporomalar f.,** f. zygomaticotemporale.
**thebesian foramina,** foramina venarum minimarum atrii dextri.
**thyroid f.,** f. thyroideum.
**f. thyroi'deum** [TA], thyroid foramen: an inconstantly present opening in the upper part of the lamina of the thyroid cartilage, resulting from incomplete union of the fourth and fifth branchial cartilages.
**tonsillar foramina,** see *fossulae tonsillares tonsillae palatinae* and *pharyngeae.*
**f. transversa'rium** [TA], transverse foramen: the passage in either process of a cervical vertebra that, in the upper six vertebrae, transmits the vertebral vessels; it is small or may be absent in the seventh. Called also *f. processus transversi, f. of transverse process, f. vertebroarteriale,* and *vertebroarterial f.*
**f. of transverse process,** f. transversarium.
**f. ve'nae ca'vae** [TA], caval opening: the opening in the diaphragm that transmits the inferior vena cava and some branches of the right vagus nerve. Called also *caval foramen.*
**fora'mina vena'rum minima'rum a'trii dex'tri** [TA], foramina of smallest veins of heart: minute openings in the walls of the heart, through which small veins, the venae cardiacae minimae, empty their blood directly into the heart; they are most numerous in the right atrium and ventricle, occasional in the left atrium, and rare in the left ventricle. Called also *Lannelongue's foramina, Vieussens' foramina,* and *thebesian foramina.*
**f. veno'sum** [TA], sphenoidal emissary foramen: an opening occasionally found medial to the foramen ovale of the sphenoid for the passage of a vein from the cavernous sinus; called also *f. of Vesalius* and *f. Vesalii.*
**venous f.,** 1. f. venae cavae. 2. f. venosum.
**f. vertebra'le** [TA], vertebral foramen: the large opening in a vertebra formed by its body and arch; called also *medullary f.,* and *spinal f.* or *aperture.*
**vertebroarterial f., f. vertebroarteria'le,** f. transversarium.
**f. Vesa'lii, f. of Vesalius,** f. venosum.
**f. of Vicq d'Azyr,** f. caecum medullae oblongatae.
**Vieussens' foramina,** foramina venarum minimarum atrii dextri.
**Weitbrecht's f.,** an opening in the capsule of the shoulder joint through which passes the synovial membrane to the bursa that lines the under surface of the subscapularis muscle.
**f. of Winslow,** f. epiploicum.
**zygomatic f., anterior, zygomatic f., facial,** f. zygomaticofaciale.
**zygomatic f., orbital,** f. zygomatico-orbitale.
**zygomatic f., posterior,** f. zygomaticotemporale.
**zygomatic f., temporal,** f. zygomaticotemporale.
**zygomatic f. of Arnold, internal,** f. zygomatico-orbitale.
**zygomatic f. of Meckel, internal,** f. zygomaticotemporale.
**zygomaticofacial f., f. zygomaticofacia'le** [TA], the opening on the anterior surface of the zygomatic bone for the zygomaticofacial nerves and vessels.
**zygomatico-orbital f., f. zygomaticoorbita'le** [TA], either of the two openings on the orbital surface of each zygomatic bone, which transmit branches of the zygomatic branch of the trigeminal nerve and branches of the lacrimal artery.
**zygomaticotemporal f., f. zygomaticotempora'le** [TA], the opening on the temporal surface of the zygomatic bone for passage of the zygomaticotemporal nerve.

**fo·ram·i·na** (fo-ram'ĭ-nə) [L.] plural of *foramen.*

**fo·ram·i·nif·er·ous** (fo-ram″ĭ-nif'ər-əs) [*foramen* + *-ferous*] having foramina.

**fo·ram·i·not·o·my** (fo-ram″ĭ-not'ə-me) [*foramina* + *-tomy*] the operation of removing the roof of intervertebral foramina, done for the relief of nerve root compression.

**fo·ra·min·u·lum** (for″ə-min'u-ləm) pl. *foramin'ula* [L.] a minute foramen.

**For·ane** (for'ān) trademark for preparations of isoflurane.

**Forbes' disease** (forbz) [Gilbert Burnett *Forbes,* American pediatrician, born 1915] glycogen storage disease, type III; see under *disease.*

**For·bes-Al·bright syndrome** (forbz-awl'brīt) [Anne Poppenheimer *Forbes,* American physician, 1911–1992; Fuller *Albright,* American physician, 1900–1969] see under *syndrome.*

**force** (fors) [L. *fortis* strong] any influence that acts to change the motion of an object, either accelerating or decelerating it, including changes in direction of motion. Symbol *F.*
**bite f.,** masticatory f.
**catabolic f.,** energy derived from the metabolism of food.
**chewing f.,** masticatory f.
**electromotive f.,** the force which, by reason of differences in potential, causes a flow of electricity from one place to another, giving rise to an electric current; it is measured in volts. Abbreviated EMF. Symbol *E.*
**extraoral f.,** force applied by orthodontic anchorage units (calvarial, occipital, or cervical) outside the oral cavity.
**field f's,** hypothetical forces which have a part in the individuation processes of the early embryo.
**G f., g f.,** the unit of force exerted on a resting body that is equal to the force on it due to gravity. An accelerating body experiences multiple units of this force, symbolized *G* or *g* following the number of units.
**masticatory f.,** the degree of force applied against the occlusal surfaces of the teeth by the muscles of mastication during the chewing of food. Called also *chewing f.*
**occlusal f.,** the force exerted on opposing teeth when the jaws are brought into approximation.
**reciprocal f.,** a force applied by an orthodontic anchorage in which the resistance of one or more dental units is utilized to move one or more opposing dental units. Cf. *reciprocal anchorage.*

**reserve f.**, energy above that required for normal functioning; in the heart it is the power which will take care of the additional circulatory burden imposed by bodily exertion.
**rest f.**, the power of the heart necessary to maintain the circulation when the patient is at rest.
**van der Waals f's**, the relatively weak, short-range forces of attraction existing between atoms and molecules and arising from brief shifts of orbital electrons on one side of the atom or molecule and the corresponding electron shifts in adjacent molecules; it results in the attraction of nonpolar organic compounds to each other.
**vital f.**, the energy which characterizes a living organism.

**force·plate** (fors'plāt) force platform.

**for·ceps** (for'seps) [L.] 1. an instrument with two blades and a handle for compressing or grasping tissues in surgical operations, and for handling sterile dressings and other surgical supplies. 2. [TA] an organ or part shaped like the surgical instrument, particularly the terminal fibers of the corpus callosum.
**alligator f.**, a long, sharply angled forceps with a jawlike mechanism at the tip.
**Allis f.**, one with opposing serrated edges with short teeth, used for grasping fascia.
**f. ante'rior**, f. minor.
**artery f.**, forceps for grasping and compressing an artery.
**Asch f.**, forceps used for reduction and fixation of nasal fractures.
**axis-traction f.**, specially jointed obstetrical forceps so constructed that traction may be applied in the line of the pelvic axis.
**Bailey-Williamson f.**, a form of obstetrical forceps.
**Barton f.**, an obstetrical forceps with a hinge in one blade, which can be applied correctly to the fetal head without disturbing its relationship to the pelvic axis; used mainly for deep transverse arrests in a flat pelvis.
**bayonet f.**, a forceps whose blades are offset from the axis of the handle.
**bulldog f.**, spring forceps for seizing an artery to arrest or prevent hemorrhage; the jaws are usually covered with rubber tubing to prevent injury to the vascular wall.
**bullet f.**, a forceps for extracting bullets.
**capsule f.**, forceps for removing the lens capsule in membranous cataract.
**chalazion f.**, a thumb forceps with a flattened plate at the end of one arm and a matching ring on the other; it is an ophthalmologic instrument, also used for isolation of lip and cheek lesions to facilitate removal.
**Chamberlen f.**, the original form of obstetrical forceps, invented by Peter Chamberlen (1560–1631), and disclosed by Hugh Chamberlen (1664–1728).
**clamp f.**, 1. a forceps with an automatic lock, used for compressing arteries, the pedicle of a tumor, etc.; called also *pedicle clamp.* 2. rubber dam f.
**clip f.**, a double-action forceps for applying wound clips; also used to designate a McKenzie forceps for applying brain clips.
**Cornet's f.**, a forceps for holding a coverglass.
**DeLee f.**, a modified Simpson forceps.
**dental f.**, forceps for the extraction of teeth. Called also *extracting f.*
**disk f.**, a forceps for grasping the scleral disk in trephining the eyeball.
**dressing f.**, forceps with scissorlike handles for grasping lint, drainage tubes, etc., in dressing wounds.
**ear f.**, delicate forceps for ear surgery or extraction of foreign bodies from the ear.
**Elliot f.**, a form of obstetrical forceps used in vaginal delivery and breech presentations with aftercoming head.
**epilating f.**, forceps for use in plucking out hairs.
**extracting f.**, dental f.
**fixation f.**, forceps for holding a part during an operation.
**frontal f.**, f. minor.
**f. fronta'lis**, TA alternative for *f. minor.*
**galea f.**, Willett f.
**Garrison's f.**, an obstetrical forceps with unfenestrated blades; called also *Luikart f.*
**Haig Ferguson f.**, a form of obstetrical forceps.
**Hawks-Dennen f.**, a form of obstetrical forceps.
**hemostatic f.**, forceps for controlling hemorrhage.
**high f.**, see *forceps delivery, high,* under *delivery.*
**Kazanjian f.**, cutting forceps used for resection of the nasal dorsal hump.
**Kielland's (Kjelland's) f.**, obstetrical forceps having no pelvic curve, a marked cephalic curve, and an articulation permitting a gliding movement of one blade over the other, thus allowing the blades to adapt to the sides of the fetal head when the head lies with its long diameter in the transverse diameter of the pelvis.
**Kocher f.**, a strong forceps with sharp points at the tips and transverse serrations along the full length for holding tissues during operation or for compressing bleeding tissue.
**Koeberlé's f.**, hemostatic f.
**Laufe's f.**, a form of obstetrical forceps.
**Levret's f.**, modified Chamberlen forceps, curved to correspond with the curve of the parturient canal.
**lithotomy f.**, forceps for removing stone from the bladder in lithotomy.
**low f.**, see *forceps delivery, low,* under *delivery.*
**Löwenberg's f.**, forceps for removing adenoid growths.
**Luikart f.**, Garrison's f.
**f. ma'jor** [TA], major forceps: the terminal fibers of the corpus callosum that pass from the splenium into the occipital lobes; called also *f. occipitalis* [TA alternative], and *occipital f.*
**McKenzie f.**, a forceps for applying silver clips.
**mid f.**, see *midforceps delivery,* under *delivery.*
**f. mi'nor** [TA], minor forceps: the terminal fibers of the corpus callosum that pass from the genu into the frontal lobes; called also *frontal f.*, and *f. frontalis* [TA alternative].
**mosquito f.**, a small hemostatic forceps.
**mouse-tooth f.**, forceps with one or more fine teeth at the tip of each blade.
**obstetrical f.**, an instrument designed to extract the fetus by the head from the maternal passages without injury to it or to the mother.
**occipital f.**, f. major.

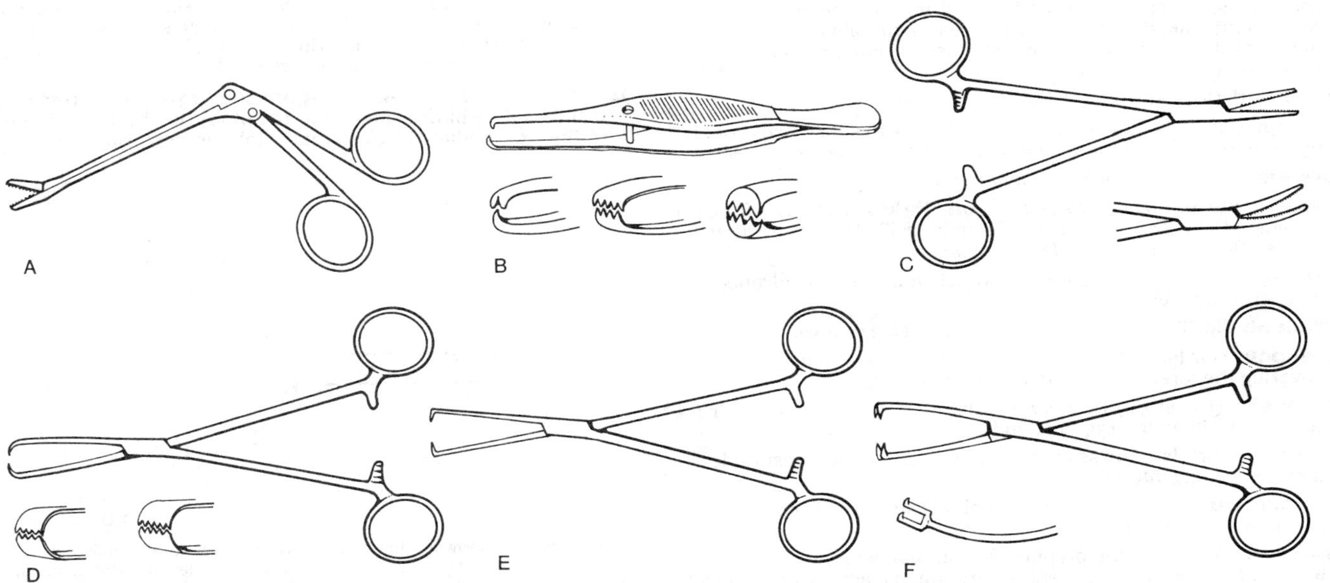

Some types of forceps. *(A)*, Alligator forceps; *(B)*, tissue forceps; *(C)*, Halsted mosquito forceps (straight and curved); *(D)*, Allis forceps; *(E)*, Schroeder tenaculum forceps; *(F)*, Schroeder vulsellum forceps (with side view of blade).

**f. occipita'lis,** TA alternative for *f. major.*
**Péan's f.,** a curved or straight clamp for hemostasis.
**Piper f.,** a special obstetrical forceps for an aftercoming head.
**point f.,** forceps used in root canal therapy to securely hold the cones or points during placement.
**f. poste'rior,** f. major.
**rongeur f.,** a forceps designed for use in cutting bone.
**rubber dam f., rubber dam clamp f.,** one for placing rubber dam clamps in position. Called also *clamp f.*
**sequestrum f.,** forceps with small but strong serrated jaws for removing the portions of bone forming a sequestrum.
**Simpson's f.,** a form of obstetrical forceps.
**speculum f.,** long slender forceps for use through a speculum.
**suture f.,** forceps used to hold the needle in passing a suture; a needle holder.
**Tarnier's f.,** a form of axis-traction forceps.
**tenaculum f.,** forceps having a sharp hook at the end of each jaw.
**thumb f.,** tissue f.
**tissue f.,** forceps with one or more fine teeth at the tip of each blade, designed for handling tissues with minimal trauma during surgery; called also *thumb f.*
**torsion f.,** forceps for making torsion on an artery to arrest hemorrhage.
**Tucker-McLean f.,** a long obstetrical forceps with a solid blade.
**volsella f., vulsellum f.,** a forceps with teeth for grasping tissues and applying traction.
**Walsham f's,** forceps used for reduction and fixation of nasal fractures.
**Willett f.,** a vulsellum for applying scalp traction in the control of hemorrhage from placenta previa; called also *galea f.* and *Willett clamp.*

**for·ci·pate** (for'sĭ-pāt) shaped like forceps.

**For·ci·po·my·ia** (for"sĭ-po-mi'yə) a genus of midges, family Chironomidae. *F. townsen'di* and *F. u'tae* were once thought to transmit mucocutaneous leishmaniasis.

**for·ci·pres·sure** (for'sĭ-presh"ər) pressure with forceps, chiefly for the arrest of hemorrhage.

**For·dyce's disease, granule (spot)** (for'dīs-əz) [John Addison *Fordyce,* New York dermatologist, 1858–1925] see *Fox-Fordyce disease,* under *disease,* and see under *granule.*

**fore·arm** (for'ahrm) [MeSH: Forearm] the part of the upper limb of the body between the elbow and the wrist; called also *antebrachium* [TA].

**fore·brain** (for'brān) prosencephalon.

**fore·con·scious** (for-kon'shəs) preconscious.

**fore·fin·ger** (for'fin-gər) index (def. 1).

**fore·foot** (for'foot) 1. the foot on the foreleg of a quadruped. 2. the fore part of the foot.

**fore·gild·ing** (for'gild-ing) the treatment of fresh nerve tissue with gold salts.

**fore·gut** (for'gət) 1. the endodermal canal of the embryo cephalic to the junction of the yolk stalk; it gives rise to the pharynx, lung, esophagus, stomach, liver, and part of the duodenum. 2. the anterior, chitin-lined, ectodermal portion of the alimentary tract of invertebrates, such as arthropods; it usually comprises a pharynx, crop, and proventriculus.

**fore·head** (for'hed) [MeSH: Forehead] frons.

**for·eign** (fahr'ən) in immunology, pertaining to substances not recognized as "self" and capable of inducing an immune response.

**fore·kid·ney** (for-kid'ne) pronephros.

**Fo·rel's commissure, decussation, fields (areas)** (fo-relz') [Auguste Henri *Forel,* Swiss psychiatrist, 1848–1931] see *decussationes tegmentorum,* under *decussationes.*

**fore·leg** (for'leg) the front leg (thoracic limb) of a quadruped. Cf. *hind leg,* under *leg.*

**fore·limb** (for'lim) [MeSH: Forelimb] a foreleg or a wing.

**fore·lock** (for'lok) the anterior portion of the mane of a horse, covering the forehead. Called also *foretop.*

**fo·ren·sic** (fo-ren'zik) [L. *forēnsis* relating to a market place or forum] pertaining to or applied in legal proceedings.

**fore·play** (for'pla) the sexually stimulating, usually pleasurable activity preceding intercourse.

**fore·pleas·ure** (for'plezh-ər) sexual pleasure which precedes orgasm. Cf. *end-pleasure.*

**fore·skin** (for'skin) the prepuce (preputium penis).
**hooded f.,** absence of the ventral foreskin, usually associated with hypospadias.

**Fo·res·tier's disease** (fo"res-te-āz') [Jacques *Forestier,* French neurologist, born 1890] see under *disease.*

**fore·stom·ach** (for'stum-ək) any of the first three stomachs of a ruminant, i.e., the rumen, reticulum, or omasum.

**fore·top** (for'top) forelock.

**fore·wa·ters** (for'wawt-ərz) the amniotic fluid that presents at the cervix uteri.

**For·his·tal** (for-his'təl) trademark for preparations of dimethindene maleate.

**fork** (fork) a pronged instrument.
**replication f.,** a site on a DNA molecule at which unwinding of the helices and synthesis of daughter molecules are both occurring.
**tuning f.,** a fork-shaped metal instrument with two tines, which produces harmonic vibration when the tines are struck; used to test hearing by air and bone conduction. See also *tuning fork tests,* under *test.*

**form** (form) [L. *forma*] 1. the characteristic of a structure or entity generally determined by its shape and size, or other external or visible feature. 2. in taxonomy, a prefix indicating that the taxon to which it is affixed is composed of organisms whose sexual phase is nonexistent or unknown; used in the classification of the *Deuteromycota* (Fungi Imperfecti).
**accolé f.** (ak"o-la'), appliqué f.
**appliqué f.** (ap"le-ka'), a term used to describe the early trophozoite of *Plasmodium falciparum* that does not assume a ring form but lies spread out along the periphery of the infected cell where it appears to have been "applied." Called also *accolé f.*
**arch f.,** the shape and contour of a dental arch.
**band f.,** see under *cell.*
**involution f.,** an abnormally shaped bacterial cell that occurs in an old culture or one that has been exposed to unfavorable conditions.
**juvenile f.,** metamyelocyte.
**L-f.,** L-phase variant; see under *variant.*
**racemic f.,** racemate.
**retention f.,** adaptation of the form of a tooth cavity in such a way as to help maintain the filling material in the cavity.
**ring f.,** the early trophozoite in the erythrocytic stage of the life cycle of hemosporian protozoa, which after Romanovsky staining has blue cytoplasm surrounding a clear zone with a red nucleus at one side, giving the cell the appearance of a signet ring. Called also *ring stage* and *signet ring.*
**spherical f. of occlusion,** an arrangement of teeth which places their occlusal surfaces on the surface of an imaginary sphere (usually 8 inches in diameter) with its center above the level of the teeth.
**tooth f.,** the characteristic contour of a tooth, with its curves, lines, and angles, which permits the tooth to be differentiated from other teeth and its identity to be established.
**young f.,** metamyelocyte.

**For·mad's kidney** (for'madz) [Henry F. *Formad,* American physician, 1847–1892] see under *kidney.*

**for·mal·de·hyde** (for-mal'də-hīd) [MeSH: Formaldehyde] a gas formerly used as a strong disinfectant; an aqueous solution called *formaldehyde solution* (see under *solution*) is used as a disinfectant and as a preservative and fixative for pathologic specimens. The gas is toxic if inhaled or absorbed through the skin and is carcinogenic. Called also *methanal* and *formic aldehyde.*

**for·mal·de·hyde de·hy·dro·gen·ase (glu·ta·thi·one)** (for-mal'də-hīd de-hi'dro-jən-ās gloo"tə-thi'ōn) [EC 1.2.1.1] an enzyme of the oxidoreductase class that catalyzes the formation of a com-

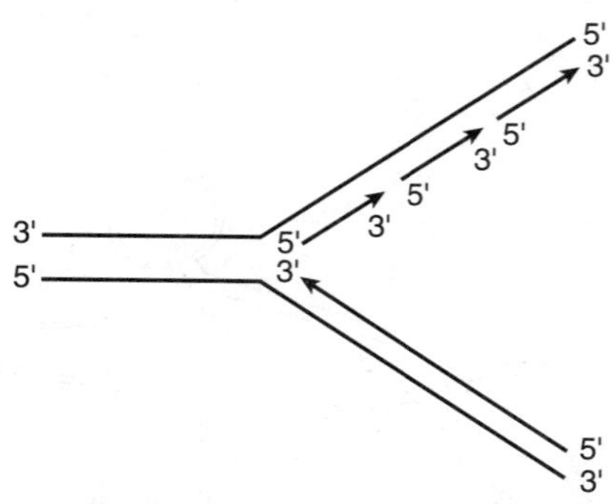


Replication fork, showing simultaneous synthesis of both strands; since synthesis occurs in the 5′ to 3′ direction, one strand, the leading strand, can be synthesized continuously while the other, the lagging strand, must be synthesized discontinuously in short fragments which are later joined.

plex between formaldehyde and glutathione, using $NAD^+$ as an electron acceptor. The reaction occurs in mitochondria and is the first step in the production of formate, important in folate metabolism.

**for·mal·de·hyd·o·gen·ic** (for-mal″də-hīd″o-jen′ik) producing formaldehyde; pertaining to the production of formaldehyde by certain compounds when subjected to chemical reactions (i.e., steroids with $\alpha$-ketol grouping in the C-17 position which on treatment with periodic acid liberate formaldehyde).

**for·ma·lin** (for′mə-lin) formaldehyde solution.

**for·ma·lin·ize** (for′mə-lin-īz) to treat with formaldehyde.

**for·mam·i·dase** (for-mam′ĭ-dās) 1. [EC 3.5.1.49] an enzyme of the hydrolase class that catalyzes the deamination of formamide to produce formate. The enzyme also acts on similar amides. 2. arylformamidase.

**for·ma·mide** (for′mə-mīd) the simplest amide, $HCONH_2$, derived from formic acid.

**for·mam·i·dox·im** (for-mam′ĭ-dok″sim) isouretin.

**form·ant** (for′mənt) a combination of tones produced in the articulation of a vowel sound.

**for·mate** (for′māt) any salt of formic acid.

**for·mate de·hy·dro·gen·ase** (for′māt de-hi′dro-jən-ās) [EC 1.2.1.2] an enzyme of the oxidoreductase class that catalyzes the oxidation of formate to $CO_2$, using $NAD^+$ as an electron acceptor. The reaction occurs in bacteria but not in mammals. The fact that bacteria containing the enzyme (e.g., *Escherichia coli* ) produce gas in mixed acid fermentations, and those that do not form the enzyme (e.g., *Shigella*) produce acid but no gas, is the basis for a test for the identification of Enterobacteriaceae.

**for·mate–tet·ra·hy·dro·fo·late li·gase** (for′māt tet″rə-hi″dro-fo′lāt li′gās) [EC 6.3.4.3] an enzyme activity of the ligase class that catalyzes the ATP-dependent synthesis of 10-formyltetrahydrofolate from formate and tetrahydrofolate, a step in the system of folate-mediated one-carbon transfer reactions. The enzyme activity is part of a trifunctional enzyme that also includes methenyltetrahydrofolate cyclohydrolase (q.v.) and methylenetetrahydrofolate dehydrogenase ($NADP^+$) activities.

**for·ma·tio** (for-ma′she-o) pl. *formatio′nes* [L.] [TA] formation: a general term designating a structure of definite shape.
**f. reticula′ris** [TA], reticular formation: any of several diffuse networks of cells and fibers in the spinal cord and brainstem; subdivided into the reticular formations of the spinal cord, medulla oblongata, mesencephalon, and pons.
**f. reticula′ris medul′lae oblonga′tae,** reticular formation of medulla oblongata: the phylogenetically old part of the medulla oblongata which has a reticular structure, i.e., which is structurally composed of diffuse aggregations of nerve cells in the midst of a wealth of nerve fibers and, with certain exceptions, lacks circumscribed cell groups; it fills the spaces between the major nuclei and fiber tracts.
**f. reticula′ris medul′lae spina′lis,** formatio reticularis spinalis.
**f. reticula′ris mesence′phali, f. reticula′ris pedun′culi ce′rebri,** f. reticularis tegmenti mesencephali.
**f. reticula′ris pon′tis,** f. reticularis tegmenti pontis
**f. reticula′ris spina′lis** [TA], spinal reticular formation: numerous small islets of gray matter and intersecting white fibers which together constitute part of the intermediate gray substance of the spinal cord; in the thoracic cord, the formation occurs immediately dorsal to the lateral horn. Called also *reticular formation of spinal cord* and *f. reticularis medullae spinalis.*
**f. reticula′ris tegmen′ti mesence′phali** [TA], reticular formation of mesencephalon: the part of the mesencephalon that has a reticular structure like that of the medulla oblongata; it lies between the substantia nigra and the central gray matter. Called also *f. reticularis mesencephali.*
**f. reticula′ris tegmen′ti pon′tis** [TA], reticular formation of pons: the part of the pars dorsalis pontis, anterior to the central gray matter, that has a structure similar to that of the reticular formation of the medulla oblongata. Called also *f. reticularis pontis.*

**for·ma·tion** (for-ma′shən) 1. the process of giving shape or form; the creation of an entity, or of a structure of definite shape. 2. a structure of definite shape; see *formatio.*
**coffin f.,** the surrounding of dead nerve cells by satellite cells in neuronophagia.
**compromise f.,** in psychoanalysis, a disguised idea or act representing and permitting partial expression of a repressed conflict.
**Gothic arch f.,** Henning's sign.
**hippocampal f.,** the gyrus dentatus, hippocampus, and gyrus parahippocampalis considered as a unit.
**palisade f.,** arrangement of cells in a palisade; see *palisade.*
**reaction f.,** a defense mechanism in which a person adopts conscious attitudes, interests, or feelings that are the opposites of his unconscious feelings, impulses, or wishes.
**reticular f.,** formatio reticularis.
**reticular f. of brainstem,** see *formatio reticularis medullae oblongatae, formatio reticularis tegmenti pontis,* and *formatio reticularis tegmenti mesencephali.*
**reticular f. of medulla oblongata,** formatio reticularis medullae oblongatae.
**reticular f. of mesencephalon,** formatio reticularis tegmenti mesencephali.
**reticular f. of pons,** formatio reticularis tegmenti pontis
**reticular f. of spinal cord,** formatio reticularis spinalis.
**rouleau f., f. of rouleaux,** the aggregation of erythrocytes in structures resembling piles of coins, caused by adhesion of their flat surfaces. Called also *impilation, pseudoagglutination,* and *pseudohemagglutination.*
**spinal reticular f.,** formatio reticularis spinalis.

**for·ma·ti·o·nes** (for-ma-she-o′nēz) [L.] plural of *formatio.*

**for·ma·tive** (for′mə-tiv) concerned in the origination and development of an organism, part, or tissue.

**for·ma·zan** (for′mə-zan) reduced nitroblue tetrazolium that is dark blue and water-insoluble; the reduction process is the basis of the nitroblue tetrazolium test (q.v.).

**form·board** (form′bord) a board containing variously shaped cutouts into which blocks corresponding to the cutouts are to be fitted; used as a test in mental retardation.

**form-class** (form-klas) an artificial taxonomic category comparable to a class, to which organisms are provisionally assigned, as are imperfect fungi until their perfect (sexual) stages are identified. Form-classes are subdivided into form-orders, form-families, and so on.

**forme** (form) pl. *formes* [Fr.] form.
**f. fruste** (froost) pl. *formes frustes* [Fr. "defaced"], an atypical, especially a mild or incomplete, form, as of a disease or anomaly.
**f. tardive** (tahr-dēv′) [Fr. "late"], a late-occurring form of a disease that usually makes its appearance at an earlier age.

**form-fam·i·ly** (form-fam′ĭ-le) see *form-class.*

**For·mi·ca** (for-mi′kə) a genus of ants (family Formicidae), including most of those that are household pests of humans.

**for·mic ac·id** (for′mik) $HCO_2H$, an acid from the distillation of ants and derivable from oxalic acid, glycerin, and the oxidation of formaldehyde. Formic acid resembles acetic acid in its actions but is far more irritating and pungent and is dangerously caustic to skin. The acid and its sodium and calcium salts are used as food preservatives.

**for·mi·ca·tion** (for″mĭ-ka′shən) [L. *formica* ant] a tactile hallucination in which there is a sensation of tiny insects crawling over the skin; most commonly seen in cocaine or amphetamine intoxication. Called also *Magnan's sign.*

**for·mi·ci·a·sis** (for″mĭ-si′ə-sis) [L. *formica* ant] poisoning resulting from ant bites.

**For·mic·i·dae** (for-mis′ĭ-de) the ants, a family of usually crawling insects of the order Hymenoptera, having a complex social organization with castes; some females become temporarily winged. Some varieties are human pests or reservoirs for disease, and others have venomous bites. Genera include *Formica* and *Solenopsis.*

**For·mi·coi·dea** (for″mĭ-koi-de′ə) a superfamily of the order Hymenoptera, containing a single family, Formicidae; the ants.

**for·mim·i·no** (for-mim′ĭ-no) the group —CH=NH.

**for·mim·i·no·glu·ta·mate** (for-mim″ĭ-no-gloo′tə-māt) the anionic form of formiminoglutamic acid.

**for·mim·i·no·glu·tam·ic ac·id** (for-mim″ĭ-no-gloo-tam′ik) [MeSH: Formiminoglutamic Acid] an intermediate in the catabolic pathway from histidine to glutamate. It may be excreted in the urine in liver disease, in vitamin $B_{12}$ or folic acid deficiency, or in glutamate formiminotransferase deficiency. Abbreviated FIGLU.

**5-for·mim·i·no·tet·ra·hy·dro·fo·late** (for-mim″ĭ-no-tet″rə-hi″dro-fo′lāt) a substituted derivative of tetrahydrofolate, carrying a formimino group; it is an intermediate in the degradation of histidine.

**for·mim·i·no·tet·ra·hy·dro·fo·late cy·clo·de·am·i·nase** (for-mim″ĭ-no-tet″rə-hi″dro-fo′lāt si″klo-de-am′ĭ-nās) [EC 4.3.1.4] an enzyme of the lyase class that catalyzes the deamination of 5-formiminotetrahydrofolate to form 5,10-methenyltetrahydrofolate, a step in the degradation of histidine. The enzyme activity occurs in a bifunctional enzyme, along with glutamate formiminotransferase (q.v.) activity.

**for·mim·i·no·trans·fer·ase** (for-mim″ĭ-no-trans′fər-ās) any enzyme that transfers a formimino group; usually used to refer to glutamate formiminotransferase.

**for·mim·i·no·trans·fer·ase de·fi·cien·cy** deficiency of glutamate formiminotransferase.

**For·min** (for′min) trademark for preparations of methenamine.

**for·mo·cor·tal** (for″mo-kor′tәl) a glucocorticoid, $C_{29}H_{38}ClFO_8$.

**for·mol** (for′mol) formaldehyde solution.

**form-ord·er** (form-or′dәr) see *form-class.*

**for·mot·er·ol fu·ma·rate** (for-mot′ә-rol) a long-acting sympathomimetic $\beta$-receptor agonist prescribed for treatment of asthma, administered intranasally as a mist.

**for·mu·la** (for′mu-lә) pl. *formulas* or *for′mulae* [L., dim. of *forma* form] a specific statement, using numerals and other symbols, of the composition of, or of the directions for preparing, a compound, such as a medicine, or of a procedure to follow for obtaining a desired value or result; a simplified statement, using numerals and symbols, of a single concept. See also *chemical f.*
**Arneth's f.**, see under *count.*
**Arrhenius' f.**, $\log x = \theta c$, in which $x$ is the viscosity of the solution relative to that of the medium of suspension, $c$ the percentage of volume occupied by the suspended particles, and $\theta$ a constant.
**Bazett's f.**, a formula correcting the Q–T interval for heart rate by dividing the duration of the Q–T interval by the square root of the duration from the R wave to the one preceding; i.e., $Q\text{–}Tc = (Q\text{–}T)/\sqrt{R\text{–}R}$.
**Beckmann's f.**, a formula used in cryoscopy, $\Delta T = K \times m$, in which $\Delta T$ is the difference in freezing points of the pure solvent and the solution containing a solute at molality $m$, and $K$ is a constant characteristic of the particular solvent.
**Berkow f.**, an adaptation of the rule of nines to burned children, taking into account the difference in proportional size of body parts between children and adults.
**chemical f.**, a combination of symbols used to express the chemical constitution of a substance; in practice, different types of formulas, of varying complexity, are employed. See *empirical f., molecular f., spatial f., structural f.*
**configurational f.**, spatial f.
**constitutional f.**, structural f.
**dental f.**, an expression in symbols of the number and arrangement of teeth in the jaws. Letters represent the various types of teeth: I, *incisor;* C, *canine;* P, *premolar;* M, *molar.* Each letter is followed by a horizontal line. Numbers above the line represent maxillary teeth; those below, mandibular teeth. The human dental formula is $I\frac{2}{2}C\frac{1}{1}M\frac{2}{2} = 10$ (one side only) for deciduous teeth, and $I\frac{2}{2}C\frac{1}{1}P\frac{2}{2}M\frac{3}{3} = 16$ (one side only) for permanent teeth.
**digital f.**, a formula expressing the relative lengths of the digits, usually $3 > 4 > 2 > 5 > 1$, or $3 > 2 > 4 > 5 > 1$, for the fingers, and $1 > 2 > 3 > 4 > 5$, or $2 > 1 > 3 > 4 > 5$, for the toes.
**Einthoven's f.**, see under *law.*
**empirical f.**, a chemical formula which expresses the proportions of the elements present in a substance. For substances composed of discrete molecules, it expresses the relative numbers of atoms present in a molecule of the substance in the smallest whole numbers. For example, the *empirical f.* for ethane is written $CH_3$, whereas its actual *molecular f.* is $C_2H_6$.
**Fick f.**, the equation used to determine cardiac output in the Fick method.
**Fischer projection f.**, a type of projection formula used to depict chirality, particularly for monosaccharides; in reference to the plane of symmetry defined by the central carbon chain, horizontal lines are drawn to depict substituents falling in front of the plane, or toward the viewer, while vertical lines depict substituents falling behind the plane, or away from the viewer.

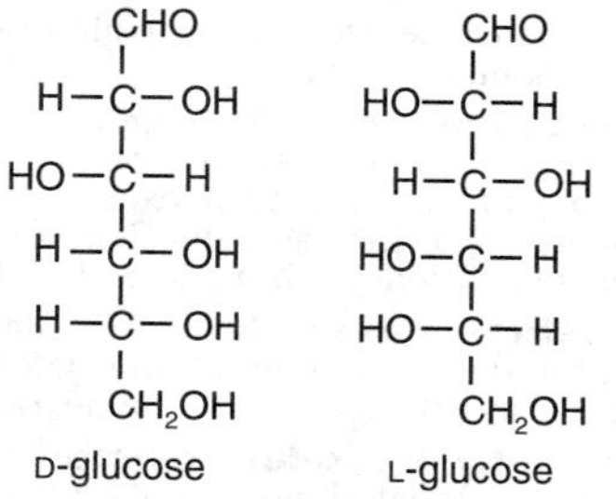

```
      CHO              CHO
       |                |
   H—C—OH         HO—C—H
       |                |
  HO—C—H           H—C—OH
       |                |
   H—C—OH         HO—C—H
       |                |
   H—C—OH         HO—C—H
       |                |
     CH2OH            CH2OH

   D-glucose        L-glucose
```

Fischer projection formula depicting the enantiomers D- and L-glucose.

**Gompertz's f.**, see under *law.*
**Gorlin f.**, a formula yielding an estimated area of the opening of a cardiac valve by calculating flow through the opening and pressure gradient across the valve.
**graphic f.**, a term occasionally used to describe a "complete" structural formula, i.e., one in which every individual atom and bond is represented in the formula. The distinction is made because structural formulas are frequently written in a simplified or shortened form. See *structural f.*
**Hamilton-Stewart f.**, a formula for measuring cardiac output following the rapid intravenous injection of an indicator dye: $F = i/ct$, in which $F$ represents the blood flow in liters per minute; $i$, the injected substance in milligrams; $c$, the average dye concentration of the primary curve; and $t$, the duration of the primary curve in seconds, i.e., the time from appearance to disappearance of the dye at a fixed site if there were no recirculation of the dye.
**molecular f.**, a chemical formula giving the number of atoms of each element present in a molecule of a substance, without indicating how they are linked.
**official f.**, one officially established by a pharmacopeia or other recognized authority.
**projection f.**, a planar, and therefore simplified, representation of a spatial formula.
**rational f.**, structural f.
**spatial f.**, a chemical formula giving the numbers of atoms of each element present in a molecule of a substance, which atom is linked to which, the types of linkages involved, and the relative positions of the atoms in space.
**stereochemical f.**, spatial f.
**structural f.**, a chemical formula telling how many atoms of each element are present in a molecule of a substance, which atom is linked to which, and the type of linkages involved; for convenience, abbreviated structural formulas are sometimes used. Called also *constitutional f., graphic f.,* and *rational f.*

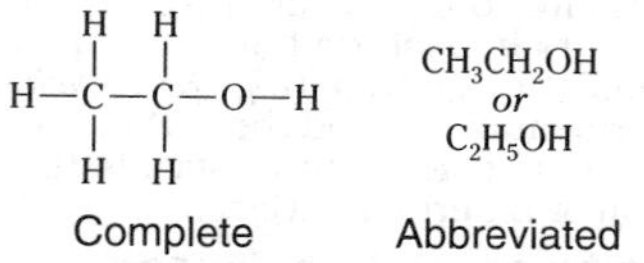

```
     H  H
     |  |              CH3CH2OH
  H—C—C—O—H              or
     |  |               C2H5OH
     H  H

   Complete          Abbreviated
```

Structural formulas for ethanol.

**Van Slyke's f.**, the urinary coefficient of various substances is equal to $D/(Bl \times \sqrt{Wt} \times V)$, in which $D$ is the daily output in grams of the substance in the urine; $Bl$, the grams of the same substance per liter of blood; $Wt$, the weight of the patient in kilograms; and $V$, the total volume of urine in 24 hours.
**vertebral f.**, an expression in symbols of the number of vertebrae in each region of the spinal column; for man it is C7 T12 L5 S5 Cd4 = 33.

**for·mu·lary** (for′mu-lar″e) [MeSH: Formularies] a collection of recipes, formulas, and prescriptions.
**National F.**, see under *N.*

**for·mu·late** (for′mu-lāt) 1. to state in the form of a formula. 2. to prepare in accordance with a prescribed or specified method.

**for·mu·la·tion** (for″mu-la′shәn) the act or product of formulating.
**American Law Institute f.**, a section of the American Law Institute Model Penal Code: "A person is not responsible for criminal conduct if at the time of such conduct as a result of mental disease or defect he lacks substantial capacity either to appreciate the criminality [wrongfulness] of his conduct or to conform his conduct to the requirements of the law . . . the terms 'mental disease or defect' do not include an abnormality manifested only by repeated criminal or otherwise antisocial conduct [antisocial personality]." This test of criminal responsibility or closely related rules have been adopted by many state and federal jurisdictions.
**Working F., Working F. of National Cancer Institute,** Working F. of Non-Hodgkin's Lymphomas for Clinical Usage.
**Working F. of Non-Hodkgin's Lymphomas for Clinical Usage,** a classification of non-Hodgkin's lymphomas that updated the Lukes-Collins Classification and others; it grouped lymphomas by pathologic classification, then assigned them to one of three clinical prognostic groups (low, intermediate, and high grade). It has been superseded by the Revised European American Lymphoma (REAL) Classification.

**for·myl** (for′mәl) [L. *formic* +Gr. *hylē* matter] the radical, HCO—, of formic acid.

**for·myl·ase** (form′әl-ās) arylformamidase.

**for·myl·ky·nu·re·nine** (for″mәl-kīn′u-rә-nēn″) the intermediate formed in tryptophan catabolism by oxidative cleavage of the indole ring of tryptophan.

**for·myl·tet·ra·hy·dro·fo·late** (for″mәl-tet″rә-hi″dro-fo′lāt) any derivative of tetrahydrofolate that carries a formyl group substitution. The 5-formyl derivative is folinic acid (q.v.); the 10-formyl derivative is important in purine synthesis and in the liver-mediated release of excess one-carbon units.

**5-for·myl·tet·ra·hy·dro·fo·late cy·clo·li·gase** (form″әl-tet″rә-hi″dro-fo′lāt si″klo-li′gās) [EC 6.3.3.2] an enzyme of the ligase class that catalyzes the ATP-dependent formation of 5,10-methenyltetrahydrofolate from 5-formyltetrahydrofolate (folinic acid). The reaction provides a means of utilization of folinic acid in the absence of dihydrofolate reductase activity. Called also *5,10-methenyltetrahydrofolate synthetase.*

**for·myl·tet·ra·hy·dro·fo·late de·hy·dro·gen·ase** (form″əl-tet″rə-hi″dro-fo′lāt de-hi′dro-jən-ās) [EC 1.5.1.6] an enzyme of the oxidoreductase class that catalyzes the oxidative decarboxylation of 10-formyltetrahydrofolate to produce tetrahydrofolate, using $NADP^+$ as an electron acceptor. The reaction occurs in liver to release excess active one-carbon fragments and maintain sufficient tetrahydrofolate for metabolism.

**for·myl·trans·fer·ase** (for″məl-trans′fər-ās) a term used in the names of some of the enzymes of the sub-subclass hydroxymethyl-, formyl-, and related transferases [EC 2.1.2] to denote those that catalyze the transfer of a formyl group from a donor to an acceptor compound. Cf. *hydroxymethyltransferase.*

**for·ni·cate** (for′nĭ-kāt) [L. *fornicatus* arched] shaped like an arch.

**for·nix** (for′niks) pl. *for′nices* [L. "arch"] 1. a general term for an archlike structure or the vaultlike space created by such a structure. 2. [TA] fornix of brain: the efferent pathway of the hippocampus, projecting chiefly to the mammillary bodies and habenular nuclei; each fornix of the pathway is an arched tract that is united under the corpus callosum with the other fornix, so that together they comprise two columns, a body, and two crura.

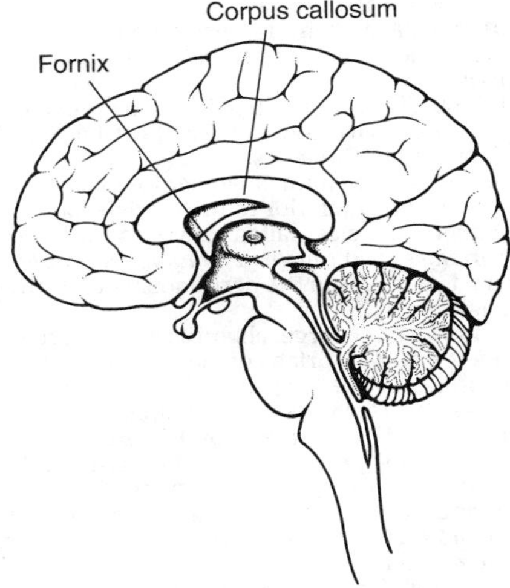


**anterior f.**, pars anterior fornicis vaginae.
**f. of brain,** fornix (def. 2).
**f. conjuncti′vae infe′rior** [TA], inferior conjunctival fornix: the inferior line of reflection of the conjunctiva from the eyelid to the eyeball.
**f. conjuncti′vae supe′rior** [TA], superior conjunctival fornix: the superior line of reflection of the conjunctiva from the eyelid to the eyeball; it receives the openings of the lacrimal duct.
**f. gas′tricus** [TA], gastric fornix: a term used in radiographic anatomy to refer to the arch of the fundus of the stomach. Called also *f. of stomach, f. ventricularis,* and *f. ventriculi.*
**lateral f.**, pars lateralis fornicis vaginae.
**f. pharyn′gis** [TA], pharyngeal fornix: the archlike roof of the nasopharynx; called also *vault of pharynx* and *roof of nasopharynx.*
**posterior f.**, pars posterior fornicis vaginae.
**f. sac′ci lacrima′lis** [TA], fornix of lacrimal sac: the upper, blind extremity of the lacrimal sac.
**f. of stomach,** f. gastricus.
**f. vagi′nae** [TA], the recess formed between the vaginal wall and the vaginal part of the cervix; sometimes subdivided into anterior *(pars anterior fornicis vaginae),* posterior *(pars posterior fornicis vaginae),* and lateral *(pars lateralis fornicis vaginae)* fornices, depending on the relation of the recess to the wall of the vagina; called also *fundus vaginae* and *fundus of vagina.*
**f. ventricula′ris, f. ventri′culi,** f. gastricus.

**For·o·blique** (for″o-blek′) trademark for an obliquely forward visual telescopic system used in panendoscopes.

**For·si·us-Eriks·son syndrome** (for′se-əs-er′ik-sən) [Henrik *Forsius,* Finnish physician, born 1921; Aldur W. *Eriksson,* Finnish geneticist, 20th century] see under *syndrome.*

**Fors·sell's sinus** (for′səlz) [Gösta *Forssell,* Swedish radiologist, 1876–1950] see under *sinus.*

**Forss·man's antigen** (fors′mənz) [John *Forssman,* Swedish pathologist, 1868–1947] see under *antigen.*

**Forss·mann** (fors′mən) Werner Theodor Otto. German surgeon, 1904–1979; co-winner, with André Frédéric Cournand and Dickinson Woodruff Richards, Jr., of the Nobel prize for medicine or physiology in 1956 for developing cardiac catheterization.

**För·ster's choroiditis (disease), photometer** (fer′stərz) [Carl Friedrich Richard *Förster,* German ophthalmologist, 1825–1902] see under *choroiditis,* and see *photoptometer.*

**För·ster's diplegia (syndrome, atonic-astatic syndrome)** (fer′stərz) [Otfrid *Förster,* German neurosurgeon, 1873–1941] atonic-astatic diplegia.

**For·taz** (for′taz) trademark for a preparation of ceftazidime.

**For·to·vase** (for′to-vās) trademark for a preparation of saquinavir mesylate.

**fos·car·net so·di·um** (fos-kahr′net) a virostatic agent used in the treatment of cytomegalovirus retinitis in immunocompromised patients.

**fos·fo·my·cin tro·meth·amine** (fos-fo-mi′sin) [MeSH: Fosfomycin] an antibacterial agent derived from phosphonic acid, active against a wide range of gram-positive and gram-negative bacteria, used in the treatment of urinary tract infection; administered orally.

**Fo·shay's test** (fo-shāz′) [Lee *Foshay,* American bacteriologist, 1896–1961] see under *test.*

**fo·sin·o·pril sodium** (fo-sin′o-pril) an angiotensin-converting enzyme inhibitor administered orally in tablet form to treat hypertension; it may be used alone or in combination with a thiazide diuretic.

**fos·pi·rate** (fos′pĭ-rāt) a veterinary anthelmintic.

**fos·sa** (fos′ə) gen. and pl. *fos′sae* [L.] [TA] a trench, channel, or hollow place.

## Fossa

Descriptions are given on TA terms, and include anglicized names of specific fossae.

**acetabular f., f. acetabula′ris,** f. acetabuli.
**f. aceta′buli** [TA], fossa of acetabulum: a rough nonarticular area in the floor of the acetabulum above the acetabular notch. Called also *acetabular f.* and *f. acetabularis.*
**adipose fossae,** spaces in the female breast, just beneath the skin, which contain fat.
**anconal f., anconeal f.,** f. olecrani.
**antecubital f.,** f. cubitalis.
**f. anthe′licis, f. of antihelix,** f. antihelica.
**f. antihe′lica** [TA], antihelical fossa: the depression on the medial surface of the auricle of the ear that corresponds to the antihelix on the lateral surface. Called also *f. anthelicis* and *f. of antihelix.*
**articular f. of atlas, inferior,** facies articularis inferior atlantis.
**articular f. of atlas, superior,** facies articularis superior atlantis.
**articular f. of mandible,** f. mandibularis.
**articular f. for odontoid process of axis,** fovea dentis atlantis.
**articular f. of temporal bone,** f. mandibularis.
**f. axilla′ris** [TA], axillary fossa: the small hollow underneath the arm where it joins the body at the shoulder.
**Biesiadecki's f.,** f. iliacosubfascialis.
**Broesike's f.,** parajejunal f.
**f. caeca′lis,** a peritoneal recess at the beginning medial to and behind the cecum; it is formed by the cecal folds.
**f. cani′na** [TA], canine fossa: a wide depression on the external surface of the maxilla superolateral to the canine tooth socket; the levator anguli oris muscle arises from it. Called also *maxillary f.*
**f. capitel′li,** facet for malleus.
**f. ca′pitis fe′moris,** fovea capitis femoris.
**f. caro′tica,** trigonum caroticum.
**f. cerebella′ris** [TA], cerebellar fossa: either of a pair of depressions in the internal surface of the occipital bone posterior to the foramen

magnum, separated from one another by the internal occipital crest, that lodge the hemispheres of the cerebellum.

**f. cerebra'lis** [TA], cerebral fossa: either of a pair of depressions in the internal surface of the occipital bone, posterior to the cerebellar fossae, that house the occipital lobes of the cerebrum.

**f. chor'dae duc'tus veno'si,** f. ductus venosi.

**f. condyla'ris** [TA], condylar fossa: either of two pits situated on the lateral portions of the occipital bone, one on either side of the foramen magnum, posterior to the occipital condyle. Called also *f. condyloidea, postcondyloid f.,* and *posterior condyloid f.*

**condyloid f., posterior,** fossa condylaris.

**condyloid f. of atlas,** fovea articularis superior atlantis.

**condyloid f. of mandible, condyloid f. of temporal bone,** f. mandibularis.

**f. condyloi'dea,** f. condylaris.

**f. coronoi'dea hu'meri** [TA], coronoid fossa of humerus: the cavity in the humerus that receives the coronoid process of the ulnar when the elbow is flexed. Called also *ulnar f.*

**f. of coronoid process,** f. coronoidea humeri.

**costal f., inferior,** fovea costalis inferior.

**costal f., superior,** fovea costalis superior.

**costal f. of transverse process,** fovea costalis processus transversus.

**cranial f., anterior,** f. cranii anterior.

**cranial f., middle,** f. cranii media.

**cranial f., posterior,** f. cranii posterior.

**f. crania'lis ante'rior,** f. cranii anterior.

**f. crania'lis me'dia,** f. cranii media.

**f. crania'lis posterior,** f. cranii posterior.

**f. cra'nii ante'rior** [TA], anterior cranial fossa: the anterior subdivision of the floor of the cranial cavity, supporting the frontal lobes of the brain, and composed of portions of three bones: the ethmoid, frontal, and sphenoid. Called also *f. cranialis anterior.*

**f. cra'nii me'dia** [TA], middle cranial fossa: the middle subdivision of the floor of the cranial cavity, supporting the temporal lobes of the brain and the pituitary gland; it is composed of the body and greater wings of the sphenoid bone and the squamous and petrous portions of the temporal bone. Called also *f. cranialis media.*

**f. cra'nii poste'rior** [TA], posterior cranial fossa: the posterior subdivision of the floor of the cranial cavity, lodging the cerebellum, pons, and medulla oblongata; it is formed by portions of the sphenoid, temporal, parietal, and occipital bones. Called also *f. cranialis posterior.*

**crural f.,** anulus femoralis.

**cubital f.,** 1. f. cubitalis. 2. f. coronoidea humeri.

**f. cubita'lis** [TA], cubital fossa: the depression in the anterior region of the elbow.

**f. cys'tidis fel'leae,** f. vesicae biliaris.

**digastric f.,** 1. f. digastrica. 2. incisura mastoidea ossis temporalis.

**f. digas'trica** [TA], digastric fossa: a depression on the internal surface of the body of the mandible on each side of the symphysis to which is attached the anterior belly of the digastric muscle; called also *f. musculi biventeris,* and *digastric fovea* or *impression.*

**digital f., inferior,** anulus femoralis.

**digital f., superior,** f. inguinalis lateralis.

**digital f. of femur,** f. trochanterica.

**f. duc'tus veno'si,** fossa of ductus venosus: an impression on the posterior part of the diaphragmatic surface of the liver in the fetus, lodging the ductus venosus.

**duodenal f., inferior,** recessus duodenalis inferior.

**duodenal f., superior,** recessus duodenalis superior.

**duodenojejunal f.,** recessus duodenalis superior.

**epigastric f.,** 1. fossa epigastrica. 2. urachal f.

**f. epigas'trica,** 1. epigastric fossa: a fossa in the epigastric region; called also *scrobiculus cordis* and *fovea cardiaca.* 2. [TA] epigastrium. See illustration at *abdomen.*

**ethmoid f.,** a groove situated in the cribriform plate of the ethmoid bone; it lodges the olfactory bulb of the brain. Called also *olfactory f.* or *groove.*

**femoral f.,** anulus femoralis.

**floccular f.,** f. subarcuata ossis temporalis.

**f. of gallbladder,** f. vesicae biliaris.

**Gerdy's hyoid f.,** trigonum caroticum.

**f. glan'dulae lacrima'lis** [TA], fossa of lacrimal gland: a shallow depression in the lateral part of the roof of the orbit, lodging the lacrimal gland; called also *lacrimal f.*

**glandular f. of frontal bone,** f. glandulae lacrimalis.

**glenoid f.,** 1. cavitas glenoidalis. 2. f. mandibularis.

**glenoid f. of scapula,** cavitas glenoidalis.

**glenoid f. of temporal bone,** f. mandibularis.

**greater f. of Scarpa,** trigonum femorale.

**Gruber's f.,** a diverticulum of the suprasternal space alongside of the inner end of the clavicle.

**Gruber-Landzert f.,** a recess in the peritoneum in the same situation as the superior duodenal recess, but extending downward behind the duodenojejunal angle.

**harderian f.,** the orbital depression in which the harderian glands are lodged.

**f. of head of femur,** fovea capitis femoris.

**f. he'licis,** scapha.

**f. hyaloi'dea** [TA], hyaloid fossa: a depression on the anterior surface of the vitreous body, in which the lens is lodged; called also *lenticular f. of vitreous body* and *patellar f.*

**hypogastric f.,** f. inguinalis medialis.

**f. hypophy'seos, f. hypophysia'lis** [TA], hypophysial fossa: a deep depression in the middle of the sella turcica of the sphenoid bone, lodging the hypophysis cerebri; called also *pituitary f.* and *sellar f.*

**ileocecal f., inferior,** recessus ileocaecalis inferior.

**ileocecal f., superior,** recessus ileocaecalis superior.

**ileocolic f.,** recessus ileocaecalis superior.

**f. ili'aca** [TA], iliac fossa: a large, smooth concave area occupying much of the inner surface of the ala of the ilium, especially anteriorly; from it arises the iliacus muscle.

**f. iliacosubfascia'lis,** iliacosubfascial fossa: an inconstant depression on the inner surface of the abdomen between the psoas muscle and the crest of the ilium; called also *Biesiadecki's f.*

**f. iliopecti'nea,** iliopectineal fossa: a depression between the iliopsoas and pectineus muscles in the center of the femoral triangle; called also *lesser f. of Scarpa.*

**implantation f.,** a shallow depression at the site where the tail of a spermatozoon attaches to the head.

**incisive f. of maxilla,** a slight depression on the anterior surface of the maxilla above the incisor teeth; called also *myrtiform f., f. praenasalis,* and *prenasal f.*

**incudal f., f. incu'dis** [TA], fossa of incus: a groove in the posterior wall of the tympanic cavity, lodging the short limb of the incus and the posterior ligament of the incus.

**f. infraclavicula'ris** [TA], infraclavicular fossa: the triangular region of the thorax or chest just inferior to the clavicle, between the deltoid and pectoralis major muscles; called also *infraclavicular triangle, Mohrenheim's f.* or *triangle,* and *trigonum deltoideopectorale.*

**infraduodenal f.,** a recess in the peritoneum below the third portion of the duodenum.

**f. infraspina'ta** [TA], the large, slightly concave area below the spinous process on the dorsal surface of the scapula; it is the site of origin of the infraspinatus muscle.

**f. infraspino'sa, infraspinous f.,** f. infraspinata.

**f. infratempora'lis** [TA], infratemporal fossa: the area on the side of the cranium limited superiorly by the infratemporal crest, posteriorly by the mandibular fossa, anteriorly by the infratemporal surface of the maxilla, and laterally by the zygomatic arch and part of the ramus of the mandible; called also *zygomatic f., infratemporal region,* and *regio infratemporalis.*

**inguinal f., external,** f. inguinalis lateralis.

**inguinal f., internal,** f. inguinalis medialis.

**inguinal f., lateral,** f. inguinalis lateralis.

**inguinal f., medial, inguinal f., middle,** f. inguinalis medialis.

**f. inguina'lis latera'lis** [TA], lateral inguinal fossa: the depression on the inside of the anterior abdominal wall lateral to the lateral umbilical fold; called also *external inguinal f.* or *fovea, fovea inguinalis lateralis,* and *lateral inguinal fovea.*

**f. inguina'lis media'lis** [TA], medial inguinal fossa: the depression on the inside of the anterior abdominal wall between the medial and lateral umbilical folds; called also *internal inguinal f.* or *fovea, fovea inguinalis medialis,* and *medial* or *middle inguinal fovea.*

**intercondylar f. of femur,** f. intercondylaris femoris.

**intercondylar f. of femur, anterior,** facies patellaris femoris.

**intercondylar f. of tibia, anterior,** area intercondylaris anterior tibiae.

**intercondylar f. of tibia, posterior,** area intercondylaris posterior tibiae.

**f. intercondyla'ris fe'moris** [TA], intercondylar fossa of femur: the posterior depression between the condyles of the femur; called also *f. intercondyloidea femoris, intercondylar notch of femur,* and *popliteal notch* or *incisure.*

**f. intercondy'lica,** f. intercondylaris femoris.

**intercondyloid f.,** see *f. intercondylaris femoris, area intercondylaris anterior tibiae,* and *area intercondylaris posterior tibiae.*

**f. intercondyloi'dea ante'rior ti'biae,** area intercondylaris anterior tibiae.

**f. intercondyloi'dea fe'moris,** f. intercondylaris femoris.

**f. intercondyloi'dea poste'rior ti'biae,** area intercondylaris posterior tibiae.

**f. intermesoco'lica transver'sa,** a recess of the peritoneum in the same situation as the recessus duodenalis superior, but extending transversely.

**f. interpeduncula'ris** [TA], interpeduncular fossa: a depression between the two cerebral peduncles, the floor of which is the posterior perforated substance; called also *Tarin's f.*

**intersigmoid f.,** recessus intersigmoideus.

**f. ischioana'lis** [TA], ischioanal fossa: the potential space between the pelvic diaphragm and the skin inferior to it; an anterior recess extends a variable distance between the pelvic and urogenital diaphragms, sometimes reaching the retropubic space. Called also *ischiorectal f., f. ischiorectalis,* and *perineal f.*

**ischiorectal f., f. ischiorecta'lis,** f. ischioanalis.

**Jobert's f.,** the fossa in the popliteal region bounded above by the adductor magnus and below by the gracilis and sartorius, best seen when the knee is bent and the thigh strongly rotated outward.

**f. of Jonnesco,** the duodenojejunal fossa between the superior and inferior duodenal folds.

**jugular f., f. jugula'ris,** 1. f. supraclavicularis minor. 2. f. jugularis ossis temporalis.

**f. jugula'ris os'sis tempora'lis** [TA], jugular fossa of temporal bone: a prominent depression on the inferior surface of the petrous part of the temporal bone, forming the major part of the jugular notch; it forms the anterior and lateral wall of the jugular foramen and lodges the superior bulb of the internal jugular vein.

**lacrimal f.,** 1. f. glandulae lacrimalis. 2. sulcus lacrimalis ossis lacrimalis.

**f. of lacrimal gland,** f. glandulae lacrimalis.

**f. of lacrimal sac,** f. sacci lacrimalis.

**Landzert's f.,** recessus paraduodenalis.

**lateral f. of cerebrum,** f. lateralis cerebralis.

**f. of lateral malleolus,** f. malleoli lateralis.

**f. latera'lis cerebra'lis** [TA], **f. latera'lis ce'rebri,** lateral cerebral fossa: a depression, in fetal life, on the lateral surface of each cerebral hemisphere at the bottom of which lies the insula; later it is closed over by the operculum, the edges of which form the lateral sulcus. Called also *sylvian f., f. of Sylvius,* and *vallecula sylvii.*

**lenticular f., lenticular f. of vitreous body,** f. hyaloidea.

**lesser f. of Scarpa,** f. iliopectinea.

**f. for ligamentum teres,** fissura ligamenti teretis.

**f. of little head of radius,** fovea capituli radii.

**longitudinal fossae of liver, right,** fossae sagittales dextrae hepatis.

**f. longitudina'lis he'patis,** f. sagittalis sinistra hepatis.

**Luschka's f.,** recessus ileocaecalis superior.

**Malgaigne's f.,** trigonum caroticum.

**f. malle'oli latera'lis** [TA], fossa of lateral malleolus: a depression on the medial aspect of the lateral malleolus behind its articular surface.

**f. mandibula'ris** [TA], mandibular fossa: a prominent depression in the inferior surface of the squamous part of the temporal bone at the base of the zygomatic process, in which the condyloid process of the mandible rests. Called also *articular f. of mandible* or *of temporal bone, condyloid f. of mandible* or *of temporal bone,* and *glenoid f. of temporal bone.*

**mastoid f., mastoid f. of temporal bone,** foveola suprameatica.

**maxillary f.,** f. canina.

**mesentericoparietal f.,** parajejunal f.

**mesogastric f.,** recessus duodenalis superior.

**Mohrenheim's f.,** f. infraclavicularis.

**f. of Morgagni,** f. navicularis urethrae.

**f. mus'culi biven'teris,** f. digastrica.

**mylohyoid f. of mandible,** fovea sublingualis.

**myrtiform f.,** incisive f. of maxilla.

**nasal f.,** the portion of the nasal cavity anterior to the middle meatus.

**navicular f. of Cruveilhier,** f. scaphoidea ossis sphenoidalis.

**navicular f. of male urethra,** f. navicularis urethrae.

**navicular f. of sphenoid bone,** f. scaphoidea ossis sphenoidalis.

**f. navicula'ris ure'thrae** [TA], **f. navicula'ris ure'thrae [Morgagnii],** navicular fossa of male urethra: the lateral expansion of the urethra in the glans penis. Called also *crypt, fossa,* or *fovea of Morgagni.*

**f. navicula'ris [vesti'buli vagi'nae],** f. vestibuli vaginae.

**f. olec'rani** [TA], **olecranon f.,** fossa of olecranon: a depression on the posterior surface of the humerus, above the trochlea, for lodging the olecranon of the ulna when the elbow is extended.

**olfactory f.,** ethmoid f.

**f. of omental sac, inferior,** recessus inferior bursae omentalis.

**f. of omental sac, superior,** recessus superior bursae omentalis.

**oral f.,** stomodeum.

**oval f. of heart,** f. ovalis cordis.

**oval f. of thigh,** hiatus saphenus.

**f. ova'lis cor'dis** [TA], oval fossa of heart: an oval depression in the right atrium on the lower part of the interatrial septum, within a triangular area bounded by the openings of the two venae cavae and the coronary sinus. It represents the remains of the fetal foramen ovale, its floor composed of the fetal septum primum.

**f. ova'lis fe'moris,** hiatus saphenus.

**f. ova'rica** [TA], ovarian fossa: a shallow pouch on the posterior surface of the broad ligament, in which the ovary is located.

**paraduodenal f.,** recessus duodenalis superior.

**parajejunal f.,** a pouch of peritoneum below the lower end of the first part of the jejunum.

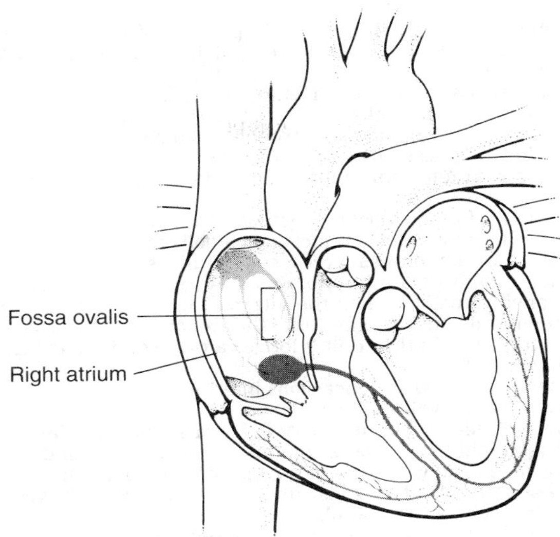


**f. paravesica'lis** [TA], paravesical fossa: the fossa formed by the peritoneum on each side of the urinary bladder.

**parietal f.,** the deepest portion of the inner surface of the parietal bone.

**patellar f.,** f. hyaloidea.

**patellar f. of femur,** facies patellaris femoris.

**patellar f. of tibia,** area intercondylaris anterior tibiae.

**perineal f.,** f. ischioanalis.

**petrosal f., f. for petrosal ganglion,** fossula petrosa.

**piriform f.,** recessus piriformis.

**pituitary f.,** f. hypophysialis.

**f. popli'tea** [TA], **popliteal f.,** the depression in the posterior region of the knee; called also *popliteal cavity.*

**popliteal f. of femur,** f. intercondylaris femoris.

**popliteal f. of tibia,** area intercondylaris posterior tibiae.

**postcondyloid f.,** f. condylaris.

**posterior f. of humerus,** f. olecrani.

**f. praenasa'lis, prenasal f.,** incisive f. of maxilla.

**prescapular f., prespinous f.,** a depression in the anterior surface of the spine of the scapula.

**pterygoid f. of inferior maxillary bone,** fovea pterygoidea mandibulae.

**f. pterygoi'dea os'sis sphenoida'lis** [TA], pterygoid fossa of sphenoid bone: the posteriorly facing fossa which is formed by the divergence of the medial and lateral pterygoid plates of the sphenoid bone, and lodges the origins of the internal pterygoid muscle and tensor veli palatini muscle.

**pterygomaxillary f.,** f. pterygopalatina.

**f. pterygopalati'na** [TA], pterygopalatine fossa: a small space between the anterior aspect of the root of the pterygoid process of the sphenoid bone and the posterior aspect of the maxilla. Called also *pterygomaxillary f.*

**f. radia'lis hu'meri** [TA], radial fossa of humerus: a depression on the anterior surface of the humerus just above the capitulum.

**retrocecal f.,** recessus retrocaecalis.

**retroduodenal f.,** a pouch of peritoneum below and behind the third portion of the duodenum.

**f. retromandibula'ris,** retromandibular fossa: the depression posterior to the angle of the mandible, on either side, inferior to the auricle.

**f. rhomboi'dea** [TA], rhomboid fossa: the floor of the fourth ventricle of the brain, made up of the dorsal surfaces of the medulla oblongata and pons. It is divided into superior, intermediate, and inferior parts.

**Rosenmüller's f.,** recessus pharyngeus.

**f. sac'ci lacrima'lis** [TA], the fossa that lodges the lacrimal sac, formed by the lacrimal sulcus of the lacrimal bone and the frontal process of the maxilla; called also *lacrimal groove.*

**fos'sae sagitta'les dex'trae he'patis,** a longitudinal fissure in the right lobe of the liver.

**fos'sae sagitta'les he'patis,** see *fossae sagittales dextrae hepatis* and *f. sagittalis sinistra hepatis.*

**f. sagitta'lis sinis'tra he'patis,** a longitudinal fissure in the left lobe of the liver, composed of the fossa venae umbilicalis in front and the fossa ductus venosi dorsally.

**scaphoid f.,** 1. f. scaphoidea ossis sphenoidalis. 2. scapha.

**f. scaphoi'dea os'sis sphenoida'lis** [TA], scaphoid fossa of sphenoid bone: a depression on the superior part of the posterior portion

of the medial plate of the pterygoid process of the sphenoid bone, giving attachment to the tensor veli palatini muscle. Called also *navicular f. of Cruveilhier* or *of sphenoid bone.*
**f. scar'pae ma'jor,** trigonum femorale.
**sellar f.,** f. hypophysialis.
**semilunar f. of ulna,** incisura trochlearis ulnae.
**sigmoid f.,** sulcus sinus transversi.
**sigmoid f. of temporal bone,** sulcus sinus sigmoidei ossis temporalis.
**sigmoid f. of ulna,** incisura trochlearis ulnae.
**sigmoid f. of ulna, lesser,** incisura radialis ulnae.
**splenic f. of omental sac,** recessus splenicus.
**f. subarcua'ta os'sis tempora'lis** [TA], subarcuate fossa of temporal bone: a small fossa on the internal surface of the petrous part of the temporal bone just inferior to the arcuate eminence, most prominent in the fetus. In the adult it lodges a piece of dura and transmits a small vein.
**subcecal f.,** recessus ileocaecalis inferior.
**sublingual f.,** fovea sublingualis.
**submandibular f., submaxillary f.,** fovea submandibularis.
**subpyramidal f.,** a fossa on the inferior wall of the middle ear, inferior to the round window and posterior to the pyramid.
**f. subscapula'ris** [TA], subscapular fossa: the concave ventral surface of the body of the scapula.
**subsigmoid f.,** a fossa between the mesentery of the sigmoid flexure and that of the descending colon.
**supraclavicular f., greater,** fossa supraclavicularis major.
**supraclavicular f., lesser,** fossa supraclavicularis minor.
**f. supraclavicula'ris ma'jor** [TA], greater supraclavicular fossa: a depression on the surface of the body, located superior and posterior to the clavicle, lateral to the tendon of the sternocleidomastoid muscle. See also *trigonum omoclaviculare.*
**f. supraclavicula'ris mi'nor** [TA], lesser supraclavicular fossa: the region of the neck in the depression posterior to the clavicle, about the interval between the two tendons of the sternocleidomastoid muscle; called also *Zang's space.*
**supracondyloid f.,** a depression on the femur between the internal tuberosity and the internal supracondyloid tubercle.
**supramastoid f.,** foveola suprameatica.
**suprasphenoidal f.,** f. hypophysialis.
**f. supraspina'ta** [TA], the deeply concave area above the spinous process on the dorsal surface of the scapula from which the supraspinous muscle takes origin.
**f. supraspino'sa, supraspinous f.,** f. supraspinata.
**f. supratonsilla'ris** [TA], supratonsillar fossa: the triangular space between the palatoglossal and palatopharyngeal arches superior to the tonsil.
**supratrochlear f., posterior,** f. olecrani.
**f. supravesica'lis** [TA], supravesical fossa: the depression on the inside of the anterior abdominal wall between the median and the medial umbilical fold; called also *fovea supravesicalis peritonaei.*
**sylvian f., f. of Sylvius,** 1. f. lateralis cerebralis. 2. sulcus lateralis cerebri.
**Tarin's f.,** f. interpeduncularis.
**f. tempora'lis** [TA], temporal fossa: the area on the side of the cranium outlined posteriorly and superiorly by the temporal lines, anteriorly by the frontal and zygomatic bones, laterally by the zygomatic arch, and inferiorly by the infratemporal crest.
**terminal f.,** f. navicularis urethrae.
**tibiofemoral f.,** a palpable space between the articular surfaces of the tibia and femur; it may be either medial *(internal tibiofemoral f.)* or lateral *(external tibiofemoral f.)* to the inferior pole of the patella.
**f. tonsilla'ris** [TA], tonsillar fossa: the depression between the palatoglossal and palatopharyngeal arches in which the palatine tonsil is located; called also *tonsillar sinus.*
**f. transversa'lis he'patis,** porta hepatis.
**f. of Treitz,** recessus duodenalis superior.
**f. triangula'ris auri'culae** [TA], triangular fossa of auricle: the cavity just above the concha of the ear between the crura of the anthelix.
**f. trochante'rica** [TA], trochanteric fossa: a deep depression on the medial surface of the greater trochanter that receives the insertion of the tendon of the obturator externus muscle.
**trochlear f., f. trochlea'ris,** fovea trochlearis.
**ulnar f.,** f. coronoidea humeri.
**umbilical f., medial,** f. inguinalis medialis.
**f. umbilica'lis he'patis,** fissura ligamenti teretis.
**urachal f.,** a depression on the inner surface of the anterior abdominal wall, between the urachus and the hypogastric artery; called also *epigastric f.*
**f. ve'nae ca'vae,** sulcus venae cavae.
**f. ve'nae umbilica'lis,** fissura ligamenti teretis.
**vermian f.,** a small fossa sometimes present on the interior surface of the occipital bone at the inferior end of the internal occipital crest; it houses part or all of the inferior cerebellar vermis.
**f. vesi'cae bilia'ris** [TA], fossa of gallbladder: the fossa on the posteroinferior surface of the liver that lodges the gallbladder and helps to separate the right and left lobes. Called also *f. vesicae felleae* [TA alternative].
**f. vesi'cae fel'leae,** TA alternative for *f. vesicae biliaris.*
**vestibular f., f. vesti'buli vagi'nae** [TA], fossa of vestibule of vagina: the part of the vestibule between the orifice of the vagina and the frenulum of the pudendal labia; called also *fossa navicularis [vestibuli vaginae].*
**Waldeyer's f.,** the recessus duodenalis inferior and recessus duodenalis superior considered as one space.
**zygomatic f.,** f. infratemporalis.

**fos·sae** (fos'e) [L.] genitive and plural of *fossa.*

**Fos·sa·max** (fos'ə-maks) trademark for a preparation of alendronate sodium.

**fos·sette** (fos-et') [Fr.] 1. a small depression. 2. a small and deep corneal ulcer.

**fos·su·la** (fos'u-lə) gen. and pl. *fos'sulae* [L., dim. of *fossa*] [TA] a small fossa; a general term for a slight depression in the surface of a structure or organ.
**f. of cochlear window,** f. fenestrae cochleae.
**costal f., inferior,** fovea costalis inferior.
**costal f., superior,** fovea costalis superior.
**f. fenes'trae coch'leae** [TA], fossula of cochlear window: a depression on the medial wall of the tympanic cavity, at the bottom of which is the fenestra cochleae; called also *f. of round window* and *niche of round window.*
**f. fenes'trae vesti'buli** [TA], fossula of vestibular window: a depression on the medial wall of the tympanic cavity, at the bottom of which is the fenestra vestibuli; called also *f. of oval window.*
**f. of oval window,** f. fenestrae vestibuli.
**f. petro'sa** [TA], **f. of petrous ganglion,** petrosal fossula: a small depression on the inferior surface of the petrous portion of the temporal bone, on a small ridge separating the jugular fossa from the external carotid foramen.
**f. post fenes'tram,** a connective tissue tract just behind the oval window, resembling the fissula ante fenestram, but smaller and less constant.
**f. of round window,** f. fenestrae cochleae.
**fos'sulae tonsil'lae tonsil'lae palati'nae,** fossulae tonsillares tonsillae palatinae.
**fos'sulae tonsil'lae tonsil'lae pharyn'geae, fos'sulae tonsil'lae tonsil'lae pharyngea'lis,** fossulae tonsillares tonsillae pharyngealis.
**tonsillar fossulae of palatine tonsil,** fossulae tonsillares tonsillae palatinae.
**tonsillar fossulae of pharyngeal tonsil,** fossulae tonsillares tonsillae pharyngeae.
**fos'sulae tonsilla'res tonsil'lae palati'nae** [TA], tonsillar fossulae of palatine tonsil: the mouths of the tonsillar crypts of the palatine tonsils. Called also *fossulae tonsillae tonsillae palatinae.*
**fos'sulae tonsilla'res tonsil'lae pharyn'geae** [TA], **fos'sulae tonsilla'res tonsil'lae pharyngea'lis,** tonsillar fossulae of pharyngeal tonsil: the mouths of the tonsillar crypts of the pharyngeal tonsil.
**f. of vestibular window,** f. fenestrae vestibuli.
**f. of window of cochlea,** f. fenestrae cochleae.
**f. of window of vestibule,** f. fenestrae vestibuli.

**fos·su·lae** (fos'u-le) [L.] genitive and plural of *fossula.*

**fos·su·late** (fos'u-lāt) marked by a small fossa; hollowed or grooved.

**Fos·ter Ken·ne·dy** see *Kennedy.*

**Foth·er·gill's operation** (foth'ər-gilz) [William Edward *Fothergill,* Manchester gynecologist, 1865–1926] see *Manchester operation,* under *operation.*

**Fou·chet's test** (foo-shāz') [André *Fouchet,* French chemist, born 1894] see under *test.*

**foul·brood** (foul'brood) a contagious disease of honeybees in which larvae are abnormal; the two kinds are *American foulbrood,* caused by *Bacillus larvae,* and *European foulbrood,* caused by *B. alvei.*

**foul in the foot** foot rot of cattle.

**foun·da·tion** (foun-da'shən) [MeSH: Foundations] the structure or basis on which something is built.
**denture f.,** denture-bearing area.

**found·er** (foun'dər) laminitis, def. 2.
**grain f.,** laminitis in the horse with indigestion or an overloaded stomach, probably due to overeating that results in metabolic disturbance.

**four·chette** (foor-shet') [Fr. "a fork-shaped object"] frenulum labiorum pudendi.

**Four·neau 309** (foor'no) trademark for a preparation of suramin sodium.

**Four·nier's gangrene (disease)** (foor-ne-āz') [Jean Alfred *Fournier,* French dermatologist, 1832–1914] see under *gangrene, sign,* and *tests.*

**fo·vea** (fo've-ə) gen. and pl. *fo'veae* [L. "a pit"] [TA] 1. pit or depression: a general term for a small pit in the surface of a structure or organ. 2. fovea centralis retinae.
**anterior f. of humerus, greater,** fossa coronoidea humeri.
**anterior f. of humerus, lesser,** fossa radialis humeri.
**articular f. of atlas, inferior,** facies articularis inferior atlantis.
**articular f. of atlas, superior,** facies articularis superior atlantis.
**articular foveae for rib cartilages,** incisurae costales sterni.
**f. articula'ris ca'pitis ra'dii** [TA], articular fovea of head of radius: a depression on the proximal surface of the head of the radius for articulation with the capitulum of the humerus.
**f. articula'ris infe'rior atlan'tis,** facies articularis inferior atlantis.
**f. articula'ris supe'rior atlan'tis,** facies articularis superior atlantis.
**calcaneal f.,** sulcus calcanei.
**f. ca'pitis fe'moris** [TA], fovea of head of femur: a depression in the head of the femur where the ligamentum teres is attached; called also *fossa capitis femoris* and *fossa of head of femur.*
**f. capi'tuli ra'dii,** a shallow cup on the upper surface of the head of the radius for articulation with the capitulum of the humerus.
**f. cardi'aca,** fossa epigastrica.
**caudal f., f. cauda'lis,** f. inferior.
**f. centra'lis re'tinae** [TA], central fovea of retina: a tiny pit, about 1 degree wide, in the center of the macula lutea, which in turn presents an extremely small depression (foveola) containing rodlike elongated cones; it is the area of most acute vision, because here the layers of the retina are spread aside, permitting light to fall directly on the cones. Called also *Soemmering's foramen.*

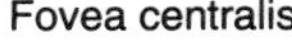


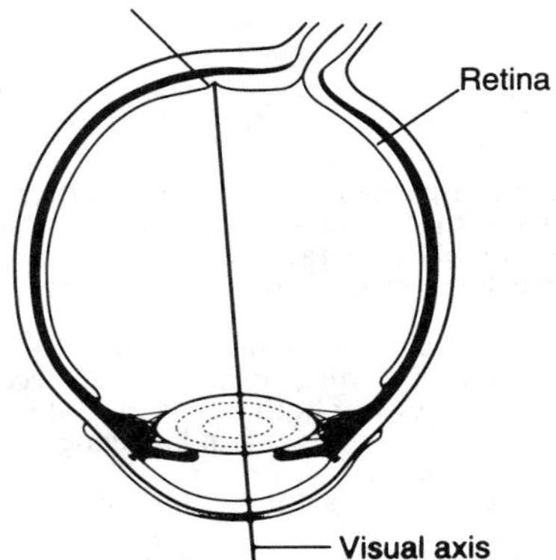


**f. of condyloid process,** f. pterygoidea mandibulae.
**f. of coronoid process,** fossa coronoidea humeri.
**costal f., inferior,** f. costalis inferior.
**costal f., superior,** f. costalis superior.
**costal f., transverse,** f. costalis transversi.
**costal foveae of sternum,** incisurae costales sterni.
**f. costa'lis infe'rior** [TA], inferior costal fovea: a small facet on the lower edge of the body of a vertebra articulating with the head of a rib; called also *inferior costal fossa* or *fossula.*
**f. costa'lis proces'sus transver'si** [TA], transverse costal fovea: a facet on the transverse process of a vertebra for articulation with the tubercle of a rib; called also *costal fossa of transverse process.*
**f. costa'lis supe'rior** [TA], superior costal fovea: a small facet on the upper edge of the body of a vertebra articulating with the head of a rib; called also *superior costal facet, fossa,* or *fossula.*
**cranial f., f. crania'lis,** f. superior.
**crural f.,** anulus femoralis.
**dental f. of atlas, f. den'tis atlan'tis** [TA], fovea for dens: the facet on the inner surface of the anterior arch of the atlas for the articulation of the dens of the axis.
**digastric f.,** fossa digastrica.
**femoral f.,** anulus femoralis.
**f. of fourth ventricle,** see *f. cranialis* and *f. caudalis.*
**glandular foveae of Luschka,** foveolae granulares.
**f. of head of femur,** f. capitis femoris.
**f. for head of radius,** fossa radialis humeri.
**f. hemiellip'tica,** recessus ellipticus vestibuli.
**f. hemisphe'rica,** recessus sphericus vestibuli.
**f. infe'rior** [TA], inferior fovea: a slight depression in the inferior part of the floor of the fourth ventricle, at the upper end of the vagal triangle, marking the end of the sulcus limitans. Called also *caudal f.* and *f. caudalis.*
**inguinal f., external,** fossa inguinalis lateralis.
**inguinal f., internal,** fossa inguinalis medialis.
**inguinal f., lateral,** fossa inguinalis lateralis.
**inguinal f., medial,** fossa inguinalis medialis.
**inguinal f., middle,** fossa inguinalis medialis.
**f. inguina'lis latera'lis,** fossa inguinalis lateralis.
**f. inguina'lis media'lis,** fossa inguinalis medialis.
**interligamentous f. of peritoneum,** fossa supravesicalis.
**f. of lateral malleolus,** facies articularis malleoli lateralis.
**f. lim'bica,** a sulcus marking the lateral border of the lateral area olfactoria and gyrus hippocampi in lower mammals.
**f. of little head of radius,** f. capituli radii.
**malleolar f. of fibula, lateral,** facies articularis malleoli lateralis.
**f. of Morgagni,** fossa navicularis urethrae.
**f. oblon'ga cartila'ginis arytenoi'deae** [TA], oblong fovea of arytenoid cartilage: a depression on the anterolateral surface of the arytenoid cartilage, separated from the triangular pit above by the arcuate crest; called also *oblong pit of arytenoid cartilage.*
**f. pterygoi'dea mandi'bulae** [TA], **f. pterygoi'dea proces'sus condyloi'dei,** pterygoid fovea of mandible: a depression on the inner side of the neck of the condyloid process of the mandible, for attachment of the external pterygoid muscle; called also *f. of condyloid process,* and *pterygoid depression* or *pit.*
**f. sublingua'lis** [TA], sublingual fovea: a depression on the inner surface of the body of the mandible, lodging a portion of the sublingual gland. Called also *sublingual fossa.*
**f. submandibula'ris** [TA], **f. submaxilla'ris,** submandibular fovea: a depression on the medial aspect of the body of the mandible, lodging a small portion of the submandibular gland; called also *submandibular* or *submaxillary fossa.*
**f. supe'rior** [TA], superior fovea: an angular depression in the floor of the fourth ventricle produced by widening of the sulcus limitans at the level of the facial colliculus; called also *cranial f.* and *f. cranialis.*
**supratrochlear f., anterior,** fossa coronoidea humeri.
**supratrochlear f. of humerus,** fossa coronoidea humeri.
**f. supravesica'lis peritonae'i,** fossa supravesicalis.
**f. of talus,** sulcus tali.
**f. of tooth of atlas,** f. dentis atlantis.
**f. triangula'ris cartila'ginis arytenoi'deae** [TA], triangular pit of arytenoid cartilage: a depression on the anterolateral surface of the arytenoid cartilage, separated from the oblong pit below by the arcuate crest.
**f. trochlea'ris** [TA], trochlear fovea: a depression on the anteromedial part of the orbital surface of the frontal bone for the attachment of the trochlea of the superior oblique muscle; it is often replaced by the trochlear spine. Called also *trochlear fossa* and *fossa trochlearis.*

**fo·ve·ae** (fo've-e) genitive and plural of *fovea.*

**fo·ve·ate** (fo've-āt) [L. *foveatus*] pitted.

**fo·ve·a·tion** (fo″ve-a'shən) a pitted condition.

**fo·ve·o·la** (fo-ve'o-lə) gen. and pl. *fove'olae* [L., dim. of *fovea*] [TA] a small pit: a general term for an extremely small depression.
**f. coccy'gea** [TA], coccygeal foveola: a dermal pit near the tip of the coccyx, indicative of the site of attachment of the embryonic neural tube to the skin; called also *postanal dimple* or *pit.*
**fove'olae gas'tricae** [TA], gastric pits: the numerous pits in the gastric mucosa marking the openings of the gastric glands.
**fove'olae granula'res** [TA], **fove'olae granula'res [Pachio'ni],** granular foveolae: small pits on the internal surface of the cranial bones on either side of the sagittal sulcus; they are occupied by the arachnoidal granulations.
**fove'olae papil'lae,** foramina papillaria renis.
**f. re'tinae** [TA], foveola of retina: an extremely small depression in

the floor of the fovea centralis, which is devoid of rod cells but contains rodlike elongated cones.
**f. suprameata'lis,** TA alternative for *f. suprameatica.*
**f. suprame'a'tica** [TA], suprameatal pit: a small triangular depression at the junction of the posterior and superior borders of the external acoustic meatus, posterior to the suprameatal spine; called also *f. suprameatalis* [TA alternative], *mastoid* or *supramastoid fossa, Macewen's triangle,* and *suprameatal triangle.*

**fo·ve·o·lae** (fo-ve'o-le) [L.] genitive and plural of *foveola.*

**fo·ve·o·lar** (fo″ve-o'lər) pertaining to a foveola, such as the foveola retinae.

**fo·ve·o·late** (fo-ve'o-lāt) pitted.

**Fo·ville's syndrome** (fo-vēlz') [Achille Louis François *Foville,* French neurologist, 1799–1878] see under *syndrome.*

**Fow·ler's position** (fou'lərz) [George Ryerson *Fowler,* American surgeon, 1848–1906] see under *position.*

**Fow·ler's solution** (fou'lərz) [Thomas *Fowler,* English physician, 1736–1801] potassium arsenite solution.

**fowl·pox** (foul'poks) [MeSH: Fowlpox] a contagious disease of domestic poultry and birds due to a poxvirus; characteristics include epithelial nodules on unfeathered areas of skin, especially the wattles, comb, and legs, sometimes with membranous lesions in the respiratory passages.

**Fox-For·dyce disease** (foks-for'dīs) [G. H. *Fox,* American dermatologist, 1846–1937; John Addison *Fordyce,* American dermatologist, 1858–1925] [MeSH: Fox-Fordyce Disease] see under *disease.*

**fox·glove** (foks'glov) see *digitalis.*
**purple f.,** digitalis.

**F.p.** abbreviation for L. *fi'at po'tio,* let a potion be made; freezing point.

**fp** foot-pound.

**FPG** fasting plasma glucose.

**F.pil.** abbreviation for L. *fi'ant pil'ulae,* let pills be made.

**Fr** symbol for *francium.*

**Fra·cas·to·ri·us** (frah″kəs-to're-əs) [It. Girolamo *Fracastoro*] an Italian physician, born in Verona (1483–1553), a poet and geologist, who published in 1530 a medical poem, *Syphilis sive morbus gallicus,* in which the name syphilis was first given to the disease.

**Fract. dos.** abbreviation for L. *frac'ta do'si,* in divided doses.

**frac·tion** (frak'shən) 1. a portion of something larger; see also *fractionation* and *fractional dose,* under *dose.* 2. in chemistry, one of the separable constituents of a substance.
**attributable f.,** see under *risk.*
**ejection f.,** the proportion of the volume of blood in the ventricles at the end of diastole that is ejected during systole; it is the stroke volume divided by the end-diastolic volume, often expressed as a percentage. It is normally 65 ± 8 per cent; lower values indicate ventricular dysfunction.
**filtration f.,** the portion of the plasma that is filtered through the renal glomerular membranes, calculated as the fraction of total glomerular filtration rate divided by total renal blood flow.
**growth f.,** a fraction whose numerator is the number of cells in a population that are actively passing through the cell cycle and whose denominator is the total number in the population.
**human plasma protein f.,** plasma protein f.
**mole f.,** in a system, the ratio of the mass in moles of a component to the mass in moles of all components.
**plasma f's,** the various components separated from the blood plasma by electrophoresis or by other means.
**plasma protein f.** [USP], a sterile preparation of serum albumin and globulin obtained by fractionating material (source blood, plasma, or serum) from healthy human donors; used as a blood volume supporter.
**population attributable f.,** see under *risk.*
**recombination f.,** see under *frequency.*

**frac·tion·al** (frak'shən-əl) [L. *fractio* a breaking] pertaining to a fraction; see also *fractional dose,* under *dose.*

**frac·tion·ate** (frak'shən-āt) to break up into smaller, generally equal, parts, such as a dose of chemotherapy or radiotherapy; see also *fractionated dose.*

**frac·tion·a·tion** (frak″shən-a'shən) [MeSH: Fractionation] 1. in radiotherapy, division of the total dose of radiation into small doses administered at intervals, which usually causes less biological damage than the same total dose given at one time; see also *hyperfractionation.* Called also *dose fractionation.* 2. division of the total dosage of a drug into smaller doses *(fractional doses)* administered at frequent intervals. Called also *dose f.* 3. in chemistry, separation of a substance into components, as by distillation or crystallization. 4. in histology, isolation of components of living cells by differential centrifugation.
**dose f.,** see *fractionation* (defs. 1 and 2).
**plasma f.,** separation and removal of plasma fractions, using membrane filtration, specific sorption, or other physicochemical methods.

**frac·tog·ra·phy** (frak-tog'rə-fe) [*fractus* + *-graphy*] a technique of photography which permits observation of jagged surfaces at high magnification.

**frac·ture** (frak'chər) [L. *fractura,* from *frangere* to break] [MeSH: Fractures] 1. the breaking of a part, especially a bone. 2. a break or rupture in a bone.

## Fracture

**agenetic f.,** spontaneous fracture due to imperfect osteogenesis.
**apophyseal f.,** one in which a small smear fragment or a bony prominence is torn from the bone.
**articular f.,** a fracture of the joint surface of a bone; called also *joint f.*
**atrophic f.,** a spontaneous fracture resulting from atrophy of the bone.
**avulsion f.,** an indirect fracture caused by avulsion or pull of a ligament.
**axial compression f.,** fracture of a vertebra by excessive vertical force, so that pieces of it move out in horizontal directions, often injuring the spinal cord; it usually occurs in the thoracic or lumbar region as a result of flexion. Called also *burst f.*
**Barton's f.,** fracture of the distal end of the radius into the wrist joint.
**basal neck f.,** fracture of the neck of the femur at its junction with the trochanteric region.
**bending f.,** an indirect fracture caused by bending of the limb.
**Bennett's f.,** a fracture of the base of the first metacarpal bone running into the carpometacarpal joint and complicated by subluxation.
**blow-out f.,** fracture of the orbital floor caused by a sudden increase of intraorbital pressure due to traumatic force; the orbital contents herniate into the maxillary sinus so that the inferior rectus or inferior oblique muscle may become incarcerated in the fracture site, producing diplopia on looking up. In the pure type there is disruption of the orbital floor without involvement of the orbital rim; the impure type involves the rim, i.e., there is concomitant midfacial fracture.
**boxer's f.,** fracture of the metacarpal neck with volar displacement of the metacarpal head caused by striking a hard object with the closed fist.
**bucket-handle f.,** a tear in the semilunar cartilage, along the middle portion, leaving a loop of cartilage lying in the intercondylar notch.
**bumper f.,** fracture of one or both legs immediately below the knee caused by an automobile bumper, often involving the tibial plateau.
**burst f.,** axial compression f.
**bursting f.,** a comminuted fracture of the distal phalanx; called also *tuft f.*
**butterfly f.,** a comminuted fracture in which there are two fragments on each side of a main fragment, somewhat resembling the wings of a butterfly.
**buttonhole f.,** fracture in which the bone is perforated by a missile; called also *perforating f.*
**capillary f.,** a fracture that appears in the radiograph as a fine hairlike line, the segments of bone not being separated; sometimes seen in fractures of the skull.
**cemental f., cementum f.,** see under *tear.*
**Chance f.,** horizontal splitting of the neural arch and body of a vertebra, usually in the lumbar region, caused by a flexion-distraction force; called also *seat belt f.*
**chisel f.,** oblique detachment of a piece from the head of the radius.
**cleavage f.,** shelling off of cartilage with a small fragment of bone from the upper surface of the capitellum humeri.

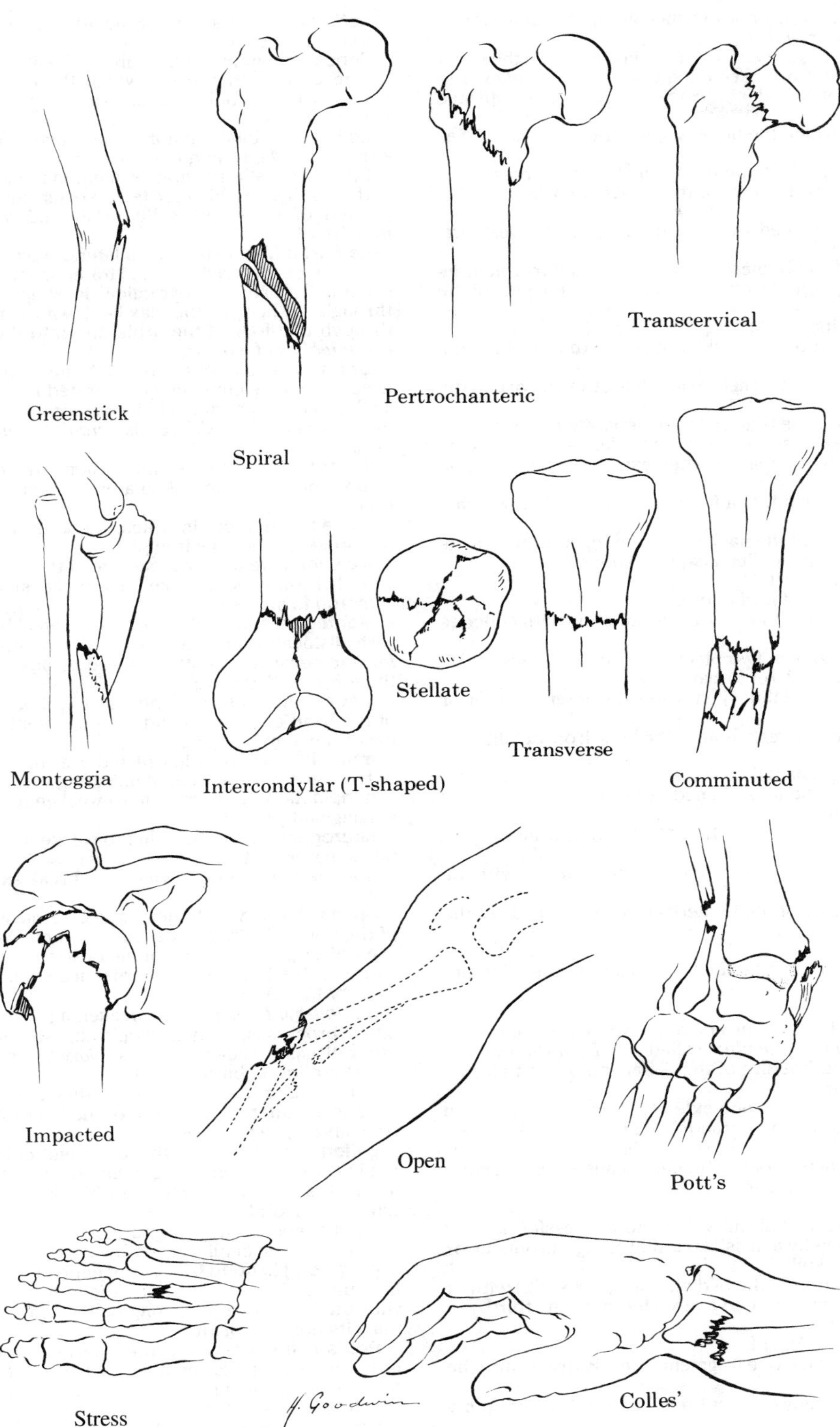


**PLATE 18**—VARIOUS TYPES OF FRACTURES

**closed f.**, a fracture that does not produce an open wound in the skin; cf. *open f.* Called also *simple f.*

**Colles' f.**, fracture of the lower end of the radius in which the lower fragment is displaced posteriorly (see Plate 18). A *reverse Colles' fracture* or *Smith's fracture* is one in which the lower fragment is displaced anteriorly.

**comminuted f.**, one in which the bone is splintered or crushed. See Plate 18.

**complete f.**, one in which the bone is entirely broken across.

**complicated f.**, fracture with injury of the adjacent parts.

**compound f.**, open f.

**compression f.**, one produced by compression, as of a vertebra; see also *axial compression f.*

**condylar f.**, fracture of the humerus in which a small fragment including the condyle is separated from the inner or outer aspect of the bone.

**congenital f.**, intrauterine f.

**f. by contrecoup**, a fracture of the skull opposite to the site of impact.

**crown-root f.**, an oblique tooth fracture involving the crown and the adjacent distal part of the root.

**deferred f.**, in the horse, one that does not separate at the time of injury because of the presence of powerful muscles or a strong covering of periosteum, but does separate when extra strain is put upon the injured part.

**depressed f., depressed skull f.**, a fracture of the skull in which a fragment is depressed.

**de Quervain's f.**, fracture of the navicular bone together with a volar luxation of the lunate bone. Called also *Quervain's f.*

**diacondylar f.**, transcondylar f.

**direct f.**, a fracture at the point of injury.

**dislocation f.**, fracture of a bone near an articulation with concomitant dislocation of that joint.

**double f.**, fracture of a bone in two places; called also *segmental f.*

**Dupuytren's f.**, 1. Pott's f. 2. (of forearm) Galeazzi's f.

**Duverney's f.**, fracture of the ilium just below the anterior superior spine.

**dyscrasic f.**, fracture due to weakening of the bone from debilitating disease.

**f. en coin** (ah kwă′), a V-shaped fracture.

**endocrine f.**, fracture of a bone weakened by an endocrine disorder such as hyperparathyroidism.

**f. en rave** (ah rahv′), a fracture in which the break is transverse at the surface, but not within.

**epiphyseal f.**, fracture at the point of union of an epiphysis with the shaft of a bone.

**extracapsular f.**, a fracture of the humerus or femur outside of the capsule.

**fatigue f.**, stress f.

**fissure f., fissured f.**, a crack extending from a surface into, but not through, a long bone.

**freeze f.**, see *freeze-fracturing.*

**Galeazzi's f.**, fracture of the radius above the wrist combined with dislocation of the distal end of the ulna; called also *Dupuytren's f.*

**Gosselin's f.**, a V-shaped fracture of the distal end of the tibia, extending into the ankle joint.

**greenstick f.**, fracture in which one side of a bone is broken, the other being bent (see Plate 18); an infraction; called also *hickory-stick* or *willow f.*

**grenade-thrower's f.**, fracture of the humerus caused by muscular contraction, as in throwing a grenade.

**Guérin's f.**, Le Fort I f.

**gutter f.**, a fracture of the skull in which the depression is long elliptic in form; often caused by a missile passing along the outside or grooving the inside of the skull.

**hangman's f.**, fracture through the pedicles of the axis (C2) with or without subluxation of the second cervical vertebra on the third.

**hickory-stick f.**, greenstick f.

**horizontal maxillary f.**, Le Fort I f.

**impacted f.**, fracture in which one fragment is firmly driven into the other. See Plate 18.

**incomplete f.**, one which does not entirely destroy the continuity of the bone.

**indirect f.**, a fracture at a point distant from the site of injury.

**inflammatory f.**, fracture of a bone weakened by inflammatory disease.

**insufficiency f.**, a stress fracture that occurs during normal stress on a bone of abnormally decreased density. Cf. *osteoporosis.*

**interperiosteal f.**, incomplete or greenstick fracture.

**intra-articular f.**, a fracture of the articular surface of a bone.

**intracapsular f.**, one within the capsule of a joint.

**intraperiosteal f.**, a fracture without rupture of the periosteum.

**intrauterine f.**, fracture of a fetal bone occurring *in utero;* called also *congenital f.*

**Jefferson's f.**, fracture of the atlas (first cervical vertebra).

**joint f.**, articular f..

**Jones f.**, diaphyseal fracture of the fifth metatarsal.

**lead pipe f.**, fracture in which the cortex of the bone is slightly compressed and bulges on one side with a slight crack on the opposite side of the bone.

**Le Fort's f.**, bilateral horizontal fracture of the maxilla, classified as either *Le Fort I, Le Fort II,* or *Le Fort III.*

**Le Fort I f.**, a horizontal segmented fracture of the alveolar process of the maxilla, in which the teeth are usually contained in the detached portion of the bone; called also *Guérin's fracture* and *horizontal maxillary f.*

**Le Fort II f.**, unilateral or bilateral fracture of the maxilla, in which the body of the maxilla is separated from the facial skeleton and the separated portion is pyramidal in shape; the fracture may extend through the body of the maxilla down the midline of the hard palate, through the floor of the orbit, and into the nasal cavity. Called also *pyramidal f. (of maxilla).*

**Le Fort III f.**, a fracture in which the entire maxilla and one or more facial bones are completely separated from the craniofacial skeleton; such fractures are almost always accompanied by multiple fractures of the facial bones. Called also *craniofacial disjunction* and *transverse facial f.*

**linear f.**, a fracture extending along the length of a bone.

**longitudinal f.**, a break in a bone extending in a longitudinal direction.

**loose f.**, a fracture in which the bone is completely broken so that the broken ends have free play.

**Maisonneuve f.**, spiral fracture of the neck of the fibula, associated with disruption of the tibiofibular syndesmosis.

**march f.**, stress f.

**Monteggia's f.**, fracture in the proximal half of the shaft of the ulna, with dislocation of the head of the radius. Sometimes called *parry fracture* because it is often caused by attempts to fend off blows with the forearm. See Plate 18.

**Moore's f.**, fracture of the lower end of the radius with dislocation of the head of the ulna and imprisonment of the styloid process beneath the annular ligaments.

**multiple f.**, a variety in which there are two or more lines of fracture of the same bone not communicating with each other.

**neoplastic f.**, fracture due to weakening of the bone as a result of a malignant process.

**neurogenic f.**, fracture due to weakening of the bone as a result of tabes, paresis, etc.

**oblique f.**, fracture in which the break extends in an oblique direction.

**open f.**, one in which there is an external wound leading to the break of the bone; cf. *closed f.* Called also *compound f.* See Plate 18.

**paratrooper f.**, fracture of the posterior articular margin of the tibia and/or of the internal or external malleolus.

**parry f.**, Monteggia's f.

**pathologic f.**, one due to weakening of the bone structure by pathologic processes, such as neoplasia, osteomalacia, osteomyelitis, and other diseases. Called also *secondary f.* and *spontaneous f.*

**perforating f.**, buttonhole f.

**periarticular f.**, a fracture extending close to, but not into, a joint.

**pertrochanteric f.**, fracture of the femur passing through the great trochanter. See Plate 18.

**pillion f.**, a fracture of the lower end of the femur occurring when the knee of a person riding pillion on a motorcycle is struck in a collision; it is a T-shaped fracture with displacement of the condyles behind the femoral shaft.

**pilon f.**, comminuted fracture of the inferior articular surface of the tibia and the malleoli, caused by axial compression of the ankle joint.

**ping-pong f., pond f.**, a type of depressed skull fracture usually seen in young children, resembling the indentation that can be produced with the finger in a ping-pong ball; when elevated it resumes and retains its normal position.

**Pott's f.**, fracture of the lower part of the fibula, with serious injury of the lower tibial articulation, usually a chipping off of a portion of the medial malleolus, or rupture of the medial ligament; called also *Dupuytren's f.* See Plate 18.

**pressure f.**, one caused by pressure on the bone from an adjoining tumor.

**pyramidal f., pyramidal f. of maxilla**, Le Fort II f.

**Quervain's f.**, de Quervain's f.

**resecting f.**, a fracture in which a piece of the bone is removed by violence, as by a bullet.

**sagittal slice f.**, fracture of a vertebra breaking it in an oblique direction; the spinal column above is displaced horizontally, usually causing paraplegia.

**Salter-Harris f.**, an epiphyseal fracture in children that involves the epiphyseal growth plate.

**seat belt f.**, Chance f.

**secondary f.,** pathologic f.
**segmental f.,** double f.
**Segond f.,** avulsion fracture of the tibial attachment of the iliotibial band.
**Shepherd's f.,** fracture of the astragalus, with detachment of the outer protecting edge.
**silver-fork f.,** a name sometimes given to Colles' fracture because of the shape of the deformity that it causes.
**simple f.,** closed f.
**simple f., complex,** a closed fracture in which there is considerable injury to adjacent soft tissues.
**Skillern's f.,** complete fracture of the lower third of the radius with greenstick fracture of the lower third of the ulna.
**Smith's f.,** a fracture of the lower end of the radius near its articular surface with forward displacement of the lower fragment; sometimes called *reverse Colles' fracture.*
**spiral f.,** one in which the bone has been twisted apart; called also *torsion f.* See Plate 18.
**splintered f.,** a type of comminuted fracture in which the bone is splintered into thin, sharp fragments.
**spontaneous f.,** pathologic f.
**sprain f.,** the separation of a tendon or ligament from its insertion, taking with it a piece of bone.
**sprinter's f.,** fracture of the anterior superior or of the anterior inferior spine of the ilium, a fragment of the bone being pulled off by muscular violence, as at the start of a sprint.
**stellate f.,** a fracture with a central point of injury, from which radiate numerous fissures. See Plate 18.
**Stieda's f.,** fracture of the internal condyle of the femur.
**stress f.,** a fracture caused by unusual or repeated stress on a bone, such as with soldiers or athletes. Called also *fatigue* or *march f.* See Plate 18.
**subcapital f.,** fracture of a bone just below its head, especially an intracapsular fracture of the neck of the femur at the junction of the head and neck.
**subcutaneous f.,** closed f.
**subperiosteal f.,** a crack through a bone without alteration in its alignment or contour, the supposition being that the periosteum is not broken.
**supracondylar f.,** fracture of the humerus in which the line of fracture is through the lower end of the shaft of the humerus.
**Tillaux f.,** vertical fracture of the distal lateral margin of the tibia.
**torsion f.,** spiral f.
**torus f.,** a fracture in which there is a localized expansion or torus of the cortex, with little or no displacement of the lower end of the bone.
**transcervical f.,** fracture through the neck of the femur. See Plate 18.
**transcondylar f.,** fracture of the humerus in which the line of fracture is at the level of the condyles, traverses the fossae, and is in part within the capsule of the joint; called also *diacondylar f.*
**transverse f.,** a fracture at right angles to the axis of the bone. See Plate 18.
**transverse facial f.,** Le Fort III f.
**transverse maxillary f.,** Le Fort I f.
**trimalleolar f.,** fracture of the medial and lateral malleoli and the posterior tip of the tibia.
**triplane f.,** fracture of the distal lateral tibia occurring in three planes: sagittally through the epiphysis, horizontally through the physis, and coronally through the metaphysis.
**trophic f.,** one due to a trophic (nutritional) disturbance.
**tuft f.,** bursting f.
**Wagstaffe's f.,** separation of the internal malleolus.
**wedge-compression f.,** compression fracture of only the anterior part of a vertebra, leaving a wedge-shaped vertebra.
**willow f.,** greenstick f.

**frac·ture-dis·lo·ca·tion** (frak′chər-dis″lo-ka′shən) a fracture of a bone near a joint, also involving dislocation.

**Fraenk·el** see *Fränkel.*

**frag·i·form** (fraj′ĭ-form) [L. *fraga* strawberry + *form*] shaped like a strawberry.

**fra·gil·i·tas** (frə-jil′ĭ-təs) [L., from *frangere* to break] fragility.
**f. cri′nium,** a brittle condition of the hair.
**f. os′sium,** osteogenesis imperfecta.
**f. un′guium,** abnormal brittleness of the nails.

**fra·gil·i·ty** (frə-jil′ĭ-te) susceptibility, or lack of resistance, to factors capable of causing disruption of continuity or integrity.
**f. of blood,** erythrocyte f.
**capillary f.,** unusual susceptibility of capillaries under stress to disruption with extravasation.
**erythrocyte f.,** the susceptibility, or lack of resistance, of erythrocytes to hemolysis under certain circumstances; see *mechanical f.* and *osmotic f.*
**hereditary f. of bone,** osteogenesis imperfecta.
**mechanical f.,** unusual susceptibility of erythrocytes to rupture from mechanical stress.
**osmotic f.,** susceptibility of erythrocytes to rupture when subjected to increasingly hypotonic saline solutions; seen in some forms of hemolytic anemia and spherocytosis. See also *osmotic fragility test,* under *test.*

**fra·gilo·cyte** (frə-jil′o-sīt) an erythrocyte characterized by osmotic fragility.

**fra·gilo·cy·to·sis** (frə-jil″o-si-to′sis) the presence of fragilocytes in the blood, as seen in some types of hemolytic anemia and spherocytosis.

**frag·ment** (frag′mənt) one of the small pieces into which a larger entity has been broken.
**Fab f.,** see *Fab.*
**F(ab′)$_2$ f.,** see F(ab′)$_2$.
**Fc f.,** see *Fc.*
**restriction f.,** a DNA fragment produced by a restriction endonuclease.
**Spengler's f's,** small round bodies seen in tuberculous sputum.

**frag·men·ta·tion** (frag″mən-ta′shən) 1. a division into fragments. 2. a form of reproduction seen in certain organisms, such as flatworms, in which the body of the parent may break into several pieces, each piece then regenerating the missing parts and developing into a whole animal.
**f. of myocardium,** transverse rupture of the muscle fibers of the heart.

**frag·men·tog·ra·phy, mass** (frag″mən-tog′rə-fe) combined gas chromatography and mass spectrometry in which quantitative analysis of the substance in question (e.g., a steroid) is based on a determination of the abundance of certain fragments characteristic of that substance.

**Frag·min** (frag′min) trademark for a preparation of dalteparin sodium.

**fraise** (frāz) [Fr. "strawberry"] a conical or hemispherical bur for cutting osteoplastic flaps or enlarging trephine openings.

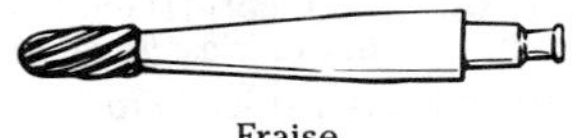

Fraise.

**fram·be·sia** (fram-be′zhə) [Fr. *framboise* raspberry] yaws.
**f. tro′pica,** yaws.

**fram·be·si·o·ma** (fram-be″ze-o′mə) mother yaw; see under *yaw.*

**fram·boe·sia** (fram-be′zhə) yaws.

**fram·boe·si·o·ma** (fram-be″ze-o′mə) mother yaw; see under *yaw.*

**frame** (frām) a structure, usually rigid, designed for giving support to or for immobilizing a part.
**Balkan f.,** a rectangular frame attached to and overhanging a bed; particularly useful in allowing bedridden patients to move more effectively and for attachment of splints. Called also *Balkan splint.*
**Bradford f.,** a rectangular frame of pipe to which is attached a sheet of heavy canvas; used as a bed frame for patients who must remain immobile.
**Deiters' terminal f.,** plates in the lamina reticularis uniting Deiters' phalanges with the cells of Hensen.
**Foster f.,** one similar to the Stryker frame.
**occluding f.,** a dental articulator.
**quadriplegic standing f.,** a device for supporting in the upright position a patient whose four limbs are paralyzed.
**reading f.,** one of the three possible ways of reading a nucleotide

sequence as a series of triplets. An open reading frame contains no termination codons and is thus potentially translatable into protein.
**Stryker f.**, one consisting of canvas stretched on anterior and posterior frames, on which the patient can be rotated around his longitudinal axis.
**trial f.**, a frame specially devised to permit easy insertion of different lenses used in correcting refractive errors of vision.
**Whitman's f.**, a frame similar to the Bradford frame except that it is curved.

**frame·work** (frām'wərk) 1. the basic structure about which something is formulated or built. 2. the metallic skeletal portion of a dental prosthesis to which are attached the resin flange and base components of the partial denture and the artificial teeth.
**implant f.**, see under *substructure.*
**scleral f.**, the larger and coarser part of the angle of the iris which is adjacent to the sclera.
**uveal f.**, ligamentum pectinatum anguli iridocornealis.

**Fran·ce·schet·ti's syndrome** (frahn″chĕ-sket'e) [Adolphe *Franceschetti,* Swiss ophthalmologist, 1896–1968] see under *syndrome.*

**Fran·ce·schet·ti-Jad·as·sohn syndrome** (frahn″chĕ-sket'e yah'dah-sōn) [A. *Franceschetti;* Josef *Jadassohn,* German dermatologist, 1863–1936] see under *syndrome.*

**Fran·cis' disease** (fran'sis) [Edward *Francis,* American bacteriologist, 1872–1957] tularemia.

**Fran·ci·sel·la** (fran-sĭ-sel'ə) [Edward *Francis*] [MeSH: Francisella] a genus of gram-negative, aerobic, coccoid or rod-shaped bacteria of uncertain affiliation, made up of very small, nonmotile organisms that are human pathogens, found in rabbits, voles, muskrats, beavers, squirrels, and sheep, and in waters frequented by these animals.
**F. novi'cida**, the etiologic agent of a disease resembling tularemia in guinea pigs, hamsters, and white mice; not known to infect man. Formerly called *Pasteurella novicida.*
**F. tularen'sis**, the etiologic agent of tularemia in man. It is transmitted from wild animals, usually rabbits, to man by contact with infected tissue, from the bites of blood-sucking insects, by inhalation, and by ingestion. It is also the cause of a severe form of conjunctivitis (oculoglandular tularemia). Called also *Brucella tularensis* and *Pasteurella tularensis.*

**fran·ci·um** (fran'se-um) [MeSH: Francium] the chemical element of atomic number 87, atomic weight 223, symbol Fr, all isotopes of which are radioactive.

**Fran·co's operation** (frahn'koz) [Pierre *Franco,* French surgeon, 1500–1561] suprapubic cystotomy.

**Fran·çois' syndrome** (frahn-swahz') [Jules *François,* Belgian ophthalmologist, born 1907] oculomandibulofacial syndrome.

**frange** (frahnzh) [Fr. "brush"] a fringe or band of cilia in the oral area of certain ciliate protozoa, made up of kinetofragments. Called also *hypostomial frange.* Cf. *pseudomembranelle.*

**Frank's operation** (frahngks) [Rudolf *Frank,* Austrian surgeon, 1862–1913] Ssabanejew-Frank operation; see under *operation.*

**Frank-Starling curve** (frahngk-stahr'ling) [Otto *Frank,* German physiologist, 1865–1944; Ernest Henry *Starling,* English physiologist, 1866–1927] see under *curve.*

**Fran·kel Classification** (frang'kəl) [Hans Ludwig *Frankel,* British physician, born 1932] see under *classification.*

**Frän·kel's sign** (freng'kelz) [Albert *Fränkel,* German physician, 1848–1916] see under *sign.*

**Frän·kel's speculum, test** (freng'kelz) [Bernhard *Fränkel,* German laryngologist, 1836–1911] see under *test.*

**Frank·en·häu·ser's ganglion** (frahngk'en-hoi″zərz) [Ferdinand *Frankenhäuser,* German gynecologist, 1832–1894] see under *ganglion.*

**Fra·ser syndrome** (fra'zer) [George Robert *Fraser,* Czechoslovakian-born American geneticist, born 1932] see under *syndrome.*

**F-ratio, test** [Sir Ronald Aylmer *Fisher,* British statistician, 1890–1962] see under *ratio* and *tests.*

**Frax·i·nus** (frak-si'nəs) the ashes, a genus of deciduous trees of the family Oleaceae. *F. or'nus* and other species are sources of mannitol, and the bark of many species is astringent and antiperiodic.

**Fra·zier-Spil·ler operation** (fra'zhər-spil'ər) [Charles Harrison *Frazier,* American surgeon, 1870–1936; William Gibson *Spiller,* American neurologist, 1863–1940] see under *operation.*

**FRC** functional residual capacity.

**FRCP** Fellow of the Royal College of Physicians.

**FRCP(C)** Fellow of the Royal College of Physicians of Canada.

**FRCPE** Fellow of the Royal College of Physicians of Edinburgh.

**FRCP(Glasg)** Fellow of the Royal College of Physicians and Surgeons of Glasgow *qua* Physician.

**FRCPI** Fellow of the Royal College of Physicians in Ireland.

**FRCS** Fellow of the Royal College of Surgeons.

**FRCS(C)** Fellow of the Royal College of Surgeons of Canada.

**FRCSE** Fellow of the Royal College of Surgeons of Edinburgh.

**FRCS(Glasg)** Fellow of the Royal College of Physicians and Surgeons of Glasgow *qua* Surgeon.

**FRCSI** Fellow of the Royal College of Surgeons in Ireland.

**FRCVS** Fellow of the Royal College of Veterinary Surgeons.

**Fre·Am·ine II** (fre-am'ēn) trademark for a crystalline amino acid solution for intravenous administration, containing a mixture of essential and nonessential amino acids but no peptides.

**freck·le** (frek'əl) [Middle English *frakel, frekel*] [MeSH: Melanosis] a benign, small, tan to brown macule occurring on sun-exposed skin, especially in children and tending to fade in adult life. Freckles resemble lentigines, but they darken after exposure to sunlight, whereas lentigines do not; and in freckles, the number of melanocytes is not increased. Called also *ephelis.*
**melanotic f. of Hutchinson**, see *lentigo maligna melanoma,* under *melanoma.*

**freck·ling** (frek'ling) the occurrence of freckles.

**Fre·det-Ram·stedt operation** (frĕ-da'rahm'shtet) [Pierre *Fredet,* French surgeon, 1870–1946; Conrad *Ramstedt,* German surgeon, 1867–1963] see under *operation.*

**Free·man-Shel·don syndrome** (fre'mən-shel'dən) [Ernest Arthur *Freeman,* British orthopedic surgeon, 1900–1975; Joseph Harold *Sheldon,* British physician, 1920–1964] craniocarpotarsal dystrophy; see under *dystrophy.*

**free·mar·tin** (fre'mahr-tin) a sexually maldeveloped female calf born as a twin to a normal male calf; it is commonly sterile and intersexual as the result of male hormone reaching it through anastomosed placental vessels.

**freeze-cleav·ing** (frēz-clēv'ing) freeze-etching.

**freeze-dry·ing** (frēz-dri'ing) a method of tissue preparation in which the tissue specimen is frozen and then dehydrated at low temperature in a high vacuum. See also *lyophilization.*

**freeze-etch·ing** (frēz-ech'ing) a method used to study unfixed cells by electron microscopy, in which the object to be studied is placed in 20 per cent glycerol, frozen at −100°C., and then mounted on a chilled holder.

**freeze-frac·tur·ing** (frēz-frak'chər-ing) a method of preparing cells for electron-microscopical examination: a tissue specimen is frozen at −150°C., inserted into a vacuum chamber, and fractured by a microtome; a platinum carbon replica of the exposed surfaces is made, freed of the underlying specimen, and then examined.

**freeze-sub·sti·tu·tion** (frēz-sub″stĭ-too'shən) a modification of freeze-drying in which the ice within the frozen tissue is replaced by alcohol or other solvents at a very low temperature.

**Frei's antigen, disease, test** (frīz) [Wilhelm Siegmund *Frei,* German dermatologist, 1885–1943] see *lymphogranuloma venereum,* and see under *antigen*

**Frei·berg's infraction (disease)** (fri'bərgz) [Albert Henry *Freiberg,* American surgeon, 1868–1940] see under *infraction.*

**Frej·ka pillow (pillow splint)** (frāj'kah) [Bedrich *Frejka,* Czechoslovakian orthopedic surgeon, born 1890] see under *pillow.*

**frem·i·tus** (frem'ĭ-təs) [L.] a vibration perceptible on palpation; cf. *thrill.*
**bronchial f.**, rhonchal f.
**friction f.**, rub.
**hydatid f.**, see under *thrill.*
**pectoral f.**, vocal f.
**pericardial f.**, a thrill of the chest wall due to the friction of the surfaces of the pericardium over each other.
**pleural f.**, a palpable vibration of the wall of the thorax due to a friction rub between the opposing surfaces of the pleura.
**rhonchal f.**, palpable vibrations produced by the passage of air through a large bronchial tube filled with mucus; see also *rhonchus.* Called also *bronchial f.*
**subjective f.**, one felt by the patient on humming with the mouth closed.
**tactile f.**, a strong vocal fremitus that can be felt by a hand on the thorax.
**tussive f.**, one felt on the chest when the patient coughs.
**vocal f. (VF)**, a thrill caused by speaking, perceived by the ear of the auscultator applied to the chest; called also *pectoral f.*

**fre·na** (fre'nə) [L.] plural of *frenum.*

**fre·nal** (fre'nəl) pertaining to a frenum.

**French** (french) see *French scale,* under *scale.*

**fre·nec·to·my** (fre-nek'tə-me) [*frenum* + *-ectomy*] excision of the frenum (frenulum).

**Fren·kel's movements (treatment)** (freng'kəlz) [Heinrich S. *Frenkel,* Swiss neurologist in Germany, 1860–1931] see under *movement.*

**fre·no·plas·ty** (fre″no-plas'te) the correction of an abnormally attached frenum by surgically repositioning it.

**fre·not·o·my** (fre-not'ə-me) [L. *frenum* + *-tomy*] cutting the frenum (frenulum), especially for release of ankyloglossia (tongue-tie).
**lingual f.,** incision of the lingual frenum; ankylotomy.

**fren·u·la** (fren'u-lə) [L.] plural of *frenulum.*

**fren·u·lum** (fren'u-ləm) pl. *fren'ula* [L., dim. of *frenum* bridle] [TA] a small bridle; a general term for a small fold of integument or mucous membrane that checks, curbs, or limits the movements of an organ or part; see also *frenum.*
**f. clito'ridis** [TA], the tissue fold on the under surface of the clitoris formed by union of the two medial parts of the labia minora; called also *crus glandis clitoridis.*
**f. of cranial medullary velum,** f. veli medullaris superioris.
**f. of ileocecal valve,** f. valvae ileocaecalis.
**f. la'bii inferio'ris** [TA], frenulum of lower lip: the fold of mucous membrane on the inside of the middle of the lower lip, connecting the lip with the gums.
**f. la'bii superio'ris** [TA], frenulum of upper lip: the fold of mucous membrane on the inside of the middle of the upper lip, connecting the lip with the gums.
**f. labio'rum puden'di** [TA], frenulum of pudendal labia: the posterior union of the labia minora, anterior to the posterior commissure; called also *f. pudendi, fourchette,* and *frenum of labia.*
**f. lin'guae** [TA], frenulum of tongue: the vertical fold of mucous membrane inferior to the tongue, attaching it to the floor of the mouth; called also frenum of tongue.

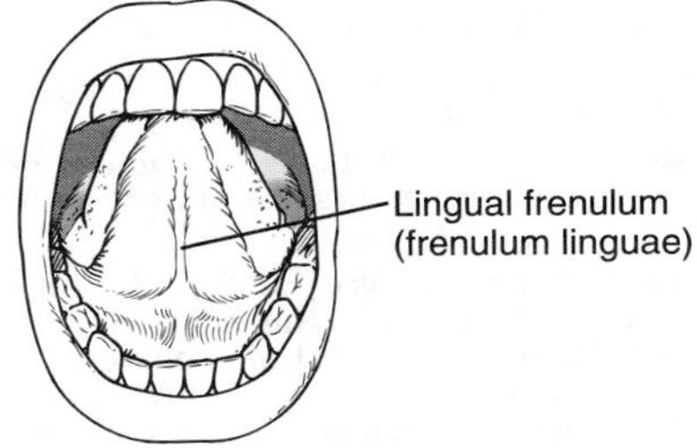


**f. prepu'tii pe'nis** [TA], frenulum of prepuce of penis: the fold on the lower surface of the glans penis that connects it with the prepuce.
**f. of pudendal labia, f. puden'di,** f. labiorum pudendi.
**f. of rostral medullary velum,** f. veli medullaris superioris.
**f. of superior lip,** f. labii superioris.
**f. of superior medullary velum,** f. veli medullaris superioris.
**f. of tongue,** f. linguae.
**f. val'vae ilea'lis,** f. valvae ileocaecalis.
**f. val'vae ileocaeca'lis,** frenulum of ileocecal valve: a fold formed by the joined extremities of the ileocecal valve, extending partly around the lumen of the colon; called also *f. valvae ilealis* and *frenum of Morgagni.*
**f. ve'li medulla'ris crania'lis, f. ve'li medulla'ris rostra'lis,** f. veli medullaris superioris.
**f. ve'li medulla'ris superio'ris** [TA], frenulum of superior medullary velum: a median ridge that descends upon the rostral medullary velum from between the inferior colliculi; called also *f. of cranial medullary velum, f. of rostral medullary velum, f. veli medullaris cranialis,* and *f. veli medullaris rostralis.*

**fre·num** (fre'nəm) pl. *fre'na* [L. "bridle"] a restraining structure or part; see *frenulum.*
**buccal f.,** a fold of mucous membrane connecting the alveolar ridge to the cheek and separating the labial vestibule from the buccal vestibule.
**f. of labia,** frenulum labiorum pudendi.
**lingual f.,** frenulum linguae.
**Macdowel's f.,** a group of fibers attached to the tendon of the pectoralis muscle and strengthening the intermuscular septum.
**f. of Morgagni,** frenulum valvae ileocaecalis.
**f. of tongue,** frenulum linguae.

**fre·quen·cy** (fre'kwən-se) 1. the number of occurrences of a periodic or recurrent process per unit time, e.g., the number of vibrations of a particle per second or the number of repetitions of a complete wave form (cycles) per second. Symbol $\nu$. 2. the number of occurrences of a particular event or the number of members of a population or statistical sample falling in a particular class. Symbol *f.* 3. relative f.
**audio f.,** any frequency corresponding to a normally audible sound wave. See also *audibility limit,* under *limit.*
**class f.,** in statistics, the number of variables contained in a class.
**critical flicker f., critical fusion f.,** the number of flashes per second at which a flickering light just appears to be continuous; see also *flicker.*
**fusion f.,** critical fusion frequency.
**gene f.,** the proportion of loci at which a given allele is found in a given population.
**high f.,** 1. an alternating current where frequency in cycles per second is high in reference to a certain standard. 2. a frequency of sound waves that is above a certain standard such as middle C. 3. the rate of oscillation in an alternating current exceeding the rate at which muscular contraction ceases, approximately 10,000 per second.
**infrasonic f.,** any frequency below the audio frequency range.
**low f.,** 1. an alternating current where frequency in cycles per second is low in reference to a certain standard. 2. a frequency of sound waves that is below a certain standard such as middle C.
**radio f.,** the range of frequencies of electromagnetic radiation between 10 kilohertz and 100 gigahertz, that used for radio communication; cf. *radio waves,* under *wave.*
**recombination f.,** the frequency with which new combinations of linked genes are formed because of crossing over occurring between their loci, i.e., the number of recombinants divided by the total number of progeny. Because an even number of crossovers does not result in recognizable recombination, the recombination frequency underestimates the crossover frequency unless the loci are very closely linked.
**recruitment f.,** in a recruitment pattern, the firing rate of one motor unit action potential at the time that a different potential first appears; cf. *recruitment interval.*
**relative f.,** the ratio of the number of occurrences of a specified phenomenon in a population to the total size of the population.
**subsonic f.,** infrasonic f.
**supersonic f.,** ultrasonic f.
**ultrasonic f.,** any frequency above the audio frequency range; see *ultrasonics.*
**urinary f.,** urination at short intervals without increase in daily volume of urinary output, due to reduced bladder capacity.

**Fres·nel lens** (fra-nel') [Augustin Jean *Fresnel,* French physicist and engineer, 1788–1827] see under *lens.*

**fress·re·flex** (fres're-fleks) [Ger. "eating reflex"] rhythmic sucking, chewing, and swallowing movements elicited by stroking of the lips and cheeks.

**fre·ta** (fre'tə) [L.] plural of *fretum.*

**fre·tum** (fre'təm) pl. *fre'ta* [L.] a constriction or isthmus.
**f. hal'leri,** a constriction between the atria and ventricles of the fetal heart; called also *Haller's isthmus.*

**Freud** (froid) Sigmund. German-born psychiatrist in Austria, 1856–1939; the founder of psychoanalysis. He developed such fundamental concepts as the unconscious, infantile sexuality, repression, sublimation, and superego, ego, and id formation and their applications to all human behavior.

**freud·i·an** (froi'de-ən) 1. pertaining to Sigmund Freud or his psychological theories and method of psychotherapy (psychoanalytic theory and technique). 2. an adherent or user of freudian theory or methods.

**Freund's adjuvant** (froindz) [Jules Thomas *Freund,* Hungarian-born bacteriologist in the United States, 1890–1960] [MeSH: Freund's Adjuvant] see under *adjuvant.*

**Freund's anomaly, operation** (froindz) [Wilhelm Alexander *Freund,* German surgeon, 1833–1918] see under *anomaly* and *operation.*

**Frey's hairs** (frīz) [Max Rupert Franz von *Frey,* Austrian physiologist, 1852–1932] see under *hair.*

**Frey's syndrome** (frīz) [Lucja *Frey,* Polish neurologist, 1889–1944] auriculotemporal syndrome; see under *syndrome.*

**Frey·er's operation** (fri'ərz) [Sir Peter Johnston *Freyer,* British surgeon, 1851–1921] see under *operation.*

**FRFPSG** Fellow of the Royal Faculty of Physicians and Surgeons of Glasgow.

**fri·a·ble** (fri'ə-bəl) [L. *friabilis*] easily pulverized or crumbled.

**fric·a·tive** (frik'ə-tiv) a speech sound produced by forcing an air stream through a narrow opening, such as *f* or *s.*

**fric·tion** (frik'shən) [L. *frictio*] [MeSH: Friction] the act of rubbing; attrition.

**Frid·er·ich·sen-Wa·ter·house syndrome** (frid″ər-ik'sən-wawt'ər-hous) [Carl *Friderichsen,* Danish pediatrician, born 1886; Rupert *Waterhouse,* British physician, 1873–1958] Waterhouse-Friderichsen syndrome.

**Fried·län·der's bacillus, disease, pneumobacillus, pneumonia** (frēd'len-dərz) [Karl *Friedländer,* German pathologist, 1847–1887] see *Klebsiella pneumoniae,* under *K.*; see *endarteritis obliterans,* under endarteritis; and see under *pneumonia.*

**Fried·mann's vasomotor syndrome** (frēd'mahnz) [Max *Friedmann,* German neurologist, 1858–1925] postconcussional syndrome.

**Fried·reich's ataxia,** etc. (frēd'rīks) [Nikolaus *Friedreich,* German physician, 1825–1882] see under *ataxia, foot,* and *sign,* and see *paramyoclonus multiplex.*

**fri·gid·i·ty** (frĭ-jid'ĭ-te) [MeSH: Frigidity] 1. coldness. 2. former name for *female sexual arousal disorder.*

**frigo·la·bile** (frig″o-la'bīl) [L. *frigor* cold + *labile*] easily affected or destroyed by cold.

**frigo·rif·ic** (frig″o-rif'ik) [L. *frigorificus*] producing coldness.

**frigo·sta·bile** (frig″o-sta'bīl) frigostable.

**frigo·sta·ble** (frig″o-sta'bəl) [L. *frigor* cold + *stable*] resistant to cold or low temperature.

**frig·o·ther·a·py** (frig″o-ther'ə-pe) cryotherapy.

**Frisch** (frish) Karl Ritter von. Austrian zoologist, 1886–1982; co-winner, with Konrad Lorenz and Nikolaas Tinbergen, of the Nobel prize for medicine or physiology in 1973 for his work on the behavior of bees.

**frit** (frit) a fused mass produced by firing a mixture of quartz, kaolin, pigments, opacifiers, a suitable flux, and other substances, which is ground to form a fine powder for use in fabricating dental porcelain restorations and artificial teeth.

**frog** (frog) 1. any of various tailless leaping amphibians of the order Anura, with a smooth skin and fully webbed feet, often used in laboratory experiments. Cf. *toad.* 2. the band of horny substance in the middle of the sole of a horse's foot, dividing into two branches and running toward the heel in the form of a fork.
**clawed f.,** *Xenopus laevis.*

**Fröh·lich's syndrome** (frer'liks) [Alfred *Fröhlich,* Austrian pharmacologist in the United States, 1871–1953] adiposogenital dystrophy.

**Froin's syndrome** (frwahnz) [Georges *Froin,* French physician, 1874–1932] see under *syndrome.*

**frole·ment** (frōl-maw') [Fr.] a rustling sound often heard in auscultation in disease of the pericardium.

**Fro·ment's paper sign** (fro-mawz') [Jules *Froment,* French physician, 1878–1946] see under *sign.*

**From·mann's lines** (from'ənz) [Carl *Frommann,* German anatomist, 1831–1892] see under *line.*

**From·mel's disease** (from'əlz) [Richard Julius Ernst *Frommel,* German gynecologist, 1854–1912] Chiari-Frommel syndrome; see under *syndrome.*

**From·mel-Chi·a·ri syndrome** (from'əl-ke-ah're) [R. J. Ernst *Frommel;* Johann Baptist *Chiari,* German obstetrician 1817–1854] Chiari-Frommel syndrome; see under *syndrome.*

**fron·dose** (fron'dōs) [L. *frondosus* leafy] bearing fronds, or villi, as the chorion frondosum.

**frons** (fronz) [L. "the front, forepart"] [TA] the forehead; the region of the face superior to the eyes. Called also *brow.*

**fron·tad** (frun'tad) toward a frontal aspect.

**fron·tal** (frun'təl) [L. *frontalis*] 1. pertaining to the forehead. 2. denoting a longitudinal plane of the body at right angles to the sagittal plane; see under *plane.*

**fron·ta·lis** (frən-tal'is) [L., from *frons,* forehead] [TA] frontal: a general term denoting a relationship to the frontal or coronal planes.

**fron·tip·e·tal** (frən-tip'ə-təl) [*frontalis* + *-petal*] directed to the front; moving in a frontal direction.

**fron·to·ma·lar** (frun″to-ma'lər) pertaining to the frontal and zygomatic (malar) bones; zygomaticofrontal.

**fron·to·max·il·lary** (frun″to- mak'sĭ-lar″e) pertaining to the frontal bone and the maxilla.

**fron·to·na·sal** (frun″to-na'zəl) nasofrontal.

**fron·to·oc·cip·i·tal** (frun″to-ok-sip'ĭ-təl) pertaining to the forehead and the occiput.

**fron·to·pa·ri·e·tal** (frun″to-pə-ri'ə-təl) pertaining to the frontal and parietal bones.

**fron·to·tem·por·al** (frun″to-tem'por-əl) pertaining to the frontal and temporal bones.

**fron·to·zy·go·mat·ic** (frun″to-zi″go-mat'ik) zygomaticofrontal.

**Fro·riep's ganglion** (fro'rēps) [August von *Froriep,* German anatomist, 1849–1917] see under *ganglion.*

**Fro·riep's induration** (fro'rēps) [Robert *Froriep,* Berlin surgeon, 1804–1861] myositis fibrosa.

**frost** (frost) a deposit resembling that of frozen dew or vapor.
**urea f.,** urhidrosis crystallina.

**frost·bite** (frost'bīt) [MeSH: Frostbite] damage to tissues as the result of exposure to low environmental temperatures; called also *congelation.*
**deep f.,** damage resulting from exposure to extremely low temperatures, involving not only the skin and subcutaneous tissue but also deeper tissues, sometimes leading to gangrene and loss of affected parts; it is marked by persistent ischemia, secondary thrombosis, and livid cyanosis.
**superficial f.,** damage resulting from exposure to low temperatures, involving only the skin or extending to the tissue immediately beneath it; it may be manifested as simple erythema, transient anesthesia, and superficial bullae.

**frot·tage** (fro-tahzh') [Fr. "rubbing"] frotteurism.

**frot·teur** (fro-toor') an individual who achieves sexual gratification by practicing frotteurism.

**frot·teur·ism** (frŏ-toor'iz-əm) [DSM-IV] a paraphilia in which sexual arousal or orgasm is achieved by rubbing up against another person, usually in a crowded place with an unsuspecting victim, or by fantasies of such actions. Sexual arousal achieved by real or fantasized touching or fondling may also be included or may be classified separately as *toucherism.* Called also *frottage.*

**FRS** Fellow of the Royal Society.

**fruc·tan** (frook'tan) fructosan.

**fruc·ti·fi·ca·tion** (frook″tĭ-fĭ-ka'shən) 1. the production of fruit. 2. a fruiting body. 3. a spore-bearing structure.

**fruc·tiv·o·rous** (frook-tiv'ə-rəs) [L. *fructus* fruit + *vorare* to eat] subsisting on or eating fruits.

**fruc·to·fu·ra·nose** (frook″to-fu'rə-nōs) fructose occurring in the cyclic furanose configuration; it is the more reactive form of fructose.

**fruc·to·ki·nase** (frook″to-ki'nās) [EC 2.7.1.3] an enzyme of the transferase class that catalyzes the ATP-dependent phosphorylation of fructose to form fructose 1-phosphate as an initial step in the utilization of fructose. The enzyme is present in the liver, intestine, and kidney cortex. Deficiency of the enzyme, an autosomal recessive trait, causes essential fructosuria.

**fruc·to·py·ra·nose** (frook″to-pi'rə-nōs) fructose occurring in the cyclic pyranose configuration; it is the more common form in solution.

**fruc·to·san** (frook'to-san) any polymer composed solely or mainly of fructose residues; e.g., inulin.

**fruc·to·sa·zone** (frook-tōs'ə-zōn) the osazone formed from fructose by reaction with phenylhydrazine; it is identical to glucosazone.

**fruc·tose** (frook'tōs) [L. *fructus* fruit] [MeSH: Fructose] 1. chemical name: D-fructose. A ketohexose, $C_6H_{12}O_6$, occurring in honey and many sweet fruits and a component of many di- and polysaccharides; it is obtainable by inversion of aqueous solutions of sucrose and subsequent separation of fructose from glucose. Called also *fructopyranose, fruit sugar,* and *levulose.* 2. [USP] the official preparation, administered intravenously in solution as a fluid and nutrient replenisher.
**f. 1,6-bisphosphate,** a key intermediate in the Embden-Meyerhof pathway (q.v.) and in gluconeogenesis.
**f. 2,6-bisphosphate,** an effector synthesized in small amounts in the liver to activate phosphofructokinase and inhibit fructose-1,6-bisphosphatase. Its formation is inhibited by catecholamines or glucagon, which thereby promote gluconeogenesis and diminish conversion of glucose to fatty acids.
**f. 1,6-diphosphate,** f. 1,6-bisphosphate.
**f. 1-phosphate,** an intermediate in fructose metabolism.
**f. 6-phosphate,** an intermediate in the Embden-Meyerhof pathway (q.v.) of glucose metabolism.

**fruc·tose-bis·phos·pha·tase** (frook'tōs bis-fos'fə-tās″) [EC 3.1.3.11] [MeSH: Fructose-Bisphosphatase] EC nomenclature for *fructose-1,6-bisphosphatase.*

**fruc·tose-1,6-bis·phos·pha·tase** (frook'tōs bis-fos'fə-tās″) an enzyme of the hydrolase class that catalyzes the hydrolysis of fructose 1,6-bisphosphate to form fructose 6-phosphate. The reaction is part of the route of gluconeogenesis in the liver and kidneys. In EC nomenclature, called *fructose-bisphosphatase.*

**fruc·tose-1,6-bis·phos·pha·tase de·fi·cien·cy** an autosomal recessive disorder marked by apnea, hyperventilation, hypoglycemia, ketosis, and lactic acidosis resulting from impaired gluconeogenesis due to deficiency of hepatic fructose-1,6-bisphosphatase; it may be fatal to newborns, but patients past early childhood develop normally.

**fruc·tose-2,6-bis·phos·pha·tase** (frook'tōs bis-fos'fə-tās) fructose-2,6-bisphosphate 2-phosphatase.

**fruc·tose bis·phos·phate al·do·lase** (frook'tōs bis-fos'fāt al'do-lās) [EC 4.1.2.13] an enzyme of the lyase class that catalyzes the cleavage of fructose 1,6-bisphosphate to form dihydroxyacetone phosphate and glyceraldehyde 3-phosphate, a reaction of the Embden-Meyerhof pathway (see illustration at *pathway*). The enzyme also catalyzes the conversion of fructose 1-phosphate to dihydroxyacetone phosphate and glyceraldehyde. Three isozymes are recognized: A (occurring primarily in skeletal muscle), B (in liver, kidney, small intestine, and leukocytes), and C (in brain). Isozyme B, often referred to as fructose 1-phosphate aldolase, has greater affinity for fructose 1-phosphate. Deficiency of this latter activity, an autosomal recessive trait, results in hereditary fructose intolerance. Called also *aldolase*.

**fruc·tose-2,6-bis·phos·phate 2-phos·pha·tase** (frook'tōs bis-fos'fāt fos'fə-tās) [EC 3.1.3.46] an enzyme activity that catalyzes the hydrolysis of fructose 2,6-bisphosphate to form fructose 6-phosphate; it occurs on the same polypeptide as the enzyme activity 6-phosphofructo-2-kinase (q.v.); in liver, the two activities form part of a mechanism for regulating carbohydrate metabolism. The liver enzyme activity is activated via phosphorylation by cyclic-AMP–dependent protein kinase, thus increasing the rate of removal of fructose 2,6-bisphosphate and slowing glycolysis. Called also *fructose-2,6-bisphosphatase*.

**fruc·tose 1,6-di·phos·pha·tase** (frook'tōs di-fos'-fə-tās") former name for *fructose-1,6-bisphosphatase*.

**fruc·to·se·mia** (frook"to-se'me-ə) the presence of fructose in the blood, as occurs in hereditary fructose intolerance and essential fructosuria.

**fruc·tose 1-phos·phate al·do·lase** (frook'tōs fos'fāt al'do-lās) fructose bisphosphate aldolase, isozyme B.

**fruc·to·side** (frook'to-sīd) a glycoside of fructose.

**fruc·to·suria** (frook"to-su're-ə) the presence of fructose in the urine, as occurs in hereditary fructose intolerance and essential fructosuria.
**essential f.**, a benign, asymptomatic, autosomal recessive disorder of carbohydrate metabolism due to deficiency of hepatic fructokinase; the only manifestations are fructosemia and fructosuria. See also *hereditary fructose intolerance*, under *intolerance*.

**fruc·to·syl** (frook'to-səl) a radical of fructose.

**fruc·to·veg·e·ta·tive** (frook"to-vej'ə-ta"tiv) composed of or pertaining to fruits and vegetables.

**fru·giv·o·rous** (froo-jiv'ə-rəs) [L. *frux*, gen. *frugis*, fruit + *vorare* to eat] fructivorous; eating or subsisting on fruit.

**fruit** (frōōt) [L. *fructus*] [MeSH: Fruit] the developed ovary of a plant, including the seed and its envelopes.

**fruit·ar·i·an** (froo-tar'e-ən) one who practices fruitarianism.

**fruit·ar·i·an·ism** (froo-tar'e-ən-izm) restriction of the diet to fruits, nuts, honey, and olive oil.

**fruit bro·me·lain** (frōōt bro'mə-lān) [EC 3.4.22.33] see *bromelain*.

**frus·e·mide** (frus'ə-mīd) BAN for furosemide.

**Frust.** abbreviation for L. *frustilla'tim*, in small pieces.

**frus·tra·tion** (frəs-tra'shən) [MeSH: Frustration] 1. the blocking or thwarting of purposes, desires, actions, or impulses. 2. a feeling of tension arising when such thwarting occurs.

**F.s.a.** abbreviation for L. *fi'at secun'dum ar'tem*, let it be made skillfully.

**FSF** [MeSH: Factor XIII] fibrin-stabilizing factor (factor XIII; see under *coagulation factors*, at *factor*).

**FSG** focal segmental glomerulosclerosis; see *focal glomerular sclerosis*.

**FSGS** focal segmental glomerulosclerosis; see *focal glomerular sclerosis*.

**FSH** [MeSH: FSH] follicle-stimulating hormone.

**FSH/LH-RH** follicle-stimulating hormone and luteinizing hormone releasing–hormone; see *gonadotropin-releasing hormone*, under *hormone*.

**FSH-RH** follicle-stimulating hormone–releasing hormone; see *gonadotropin-releasing hormone*, under *hormone*.

**ft.** abbreviation for L. *fi'at* or *fi'ant*, let there be made, and for *foot* and *feet*.

**Ft. mas. div. in pil.** abbreviation for L. *fi'at mas'sa dividen'da in pil'ulae*, let a mass be made and divided into pills.

**Ftor·a·fur** (ftor'ə-fur) trademark for preparations of tegafur.

**Ft. pulv.** abbreviation for L. *fi'at pul'vis*, let a powder be made.

**5-FU** 5-fluorouracil; see *fluorouracil*.

**Fu·a·din** (foo'ə-din) trademark for a preparation of stibophen.

**Fuchs' coloboma,** etc. (fūks) [Ernst *Fuchs*, Austrian ophthalmologist, 1851–1930] see under *coloboma, dimple, dystrophy*, and *syndrome*.

**fuch·sin** (fūk'sin) [from the pink, red, or purple flower *fuchsia*, after Leonard *Fuchs*, German botanist, 1501–1566] any of several red to purple triaminotriphenylmethane dyes.
**acid f.**, a mixture of sulfonated fuchsins used in Andrade's indicator and in various complex stains; called also *acid magenta*.
**basic f.** [USP], a triphenylmethane dye, a mixture of rosaniline and pararosaniline hydrochlorides and magenta II, used in the form of carbolfuchsin in the Gram and Ziehl-Neelsen stains, as an antifungal agent in Castellani's paint, as a germicide, and as a histologic stain. Called also *basic magenta*.
**new f.**, a basic dye with staining properties much like those of basic fuchsin; it is a tricyclic compound, trimethyl fuchsin.

**fuch·sin·o·phil** (fūk-sin'o-fil) [*fuchsin* + *-phil*] 1. any cell or other element readily stained with fuchsin. 2. fuchsinophilic.

**fuch·sin·o·phil·ia** (fūk"sin-o-fil'e-ə) the property of staining readily with fuchsin dyes; especially the affinity of infarcted areas of the heart for acid fuchsin.

**fuch·sin·o·phil·ic** (fūk"sin-o-fil'ik) readily stained by fuchsin; pertaining to or characterized by fuchsinophilia.

**fuch·sin·oph·i·lous** (fūk"sin-of'ĭ-ləs) fuchsinophilic.

**fu·co·san** (fu'ko-san) any of a group of pentosans composed of L-fucose residues; they are constituents of the cell walls of many seaweeds and occur in human milk.

**fu·cose** (fu'kōs) [MeSH: Fucose] a methylpentose structurally derived from galactose (6-deoxygalactose); the L-isomer occurs naturally in various oligo- and polysaccharides (fucosans) and fucosides and in the carbohydrate portion of some mucopolysaccharides and glycoproteins, including the A, B, and O blood group antigens.

**α-L-fu·co·si·dase** (fu-ko'sĭ-dās) [EC 3.2.1.51] an enzyme of the hydrolase class that catalyzes the cleavage of terminal α-linked L-fucose residues from fucosides. The reaction is important in the degradation of fucose-containing oligosaccharides and glycoproteins. Deficiency of the enzyme, an autosomal recessive trait, results in fucosidosis.

**fu·co·side** (fu'ko-sīd) a glycoside of fucose.

**fu·co·si·do·sis** (fu"ko-sĭ-do'sis) [MeSH: Fucosidosis] a lysosomal storage disease caused by defective α-L-fucosidase and accumulation of fucose-containing glycoconjugates. Clinical symptoms include psychomotor deterioration, growth retardation, hepatosplenomegaly, cardiomegaly, and seizures. There are two clinical types based on age of onset: *Type I*, the fatal infantile type, has age of onset by 18 months and causes death before six years of age. Marked increase of sodium chloride in sweat is an additional feature. *Type II*, the juvenile form, has age of onset by four years of age and slower psychomotor and neurologic deterioration; patients survive to their twenties.

**fu·co·xan·thin** (fu"ko-zan'thin) [L. *fucus* rock lichen + *xanthin*] the brown carotenoid found in diatoms, brown algae, and dinoflagellates.

**FUDR, FUdR** 5-fluorouracil deoxyribonucleoside; see *floxuridine*.

**Fuer·bring·er** (fər'bring-ər) see *Fürbringer*.

**fu·gac·i·ty** (fu-gas'ĭ-te) [L. *fugacitas*, from *fugere* to flee] a measure of the escaping tendency of a substance from one phase to another phase, or from one part of a phase to another part of the same phase. The logarithm of the fugacity is proportional to the chemical potential; measured by the correction for the deviation of the behavior of a gas from ideal.

**-fugal**[1] [L., *fugare* to put to flight] a word termination implying banishing, or driving away, affixed to a stem designating the object of banishment, as *culicifugal*, driving away mosquitoes and gnats (*Culex*), or *febrifugal*, relieving or dispelling fever.

**-fugal**[2] [L., *fugere* to flee from] a word termination implying traveling away from, affixed to a stem designating the object from which flight is made, as *centrifugal*, traveling away from a center, or *corticifugal*, directed away from the cortex.

**-fuge** [L. *fugare* to put to flight] a word termination denoting an agent that drives away or banishes, as *febrifuge,* that which drives away fever.

**fu·gi·tive** (fu'jĭ-tiv) [L. *fugitivus*] 1. wandering. 2. transient.

**Fugl-Mey·er assessment** (foo'gəl-mi'ər) [A.R. *Fugl-Meyer,* physiatrist, 20th century] see under *assessment.*

**Fu·gu** (foo'goo) [Jap.] a genus of Japanese marine puffer fish of the family Tetraodontidae. Their gonads and viscera contain tetrodotoxin, and when they are eaten without special cooking, fatal tetrodotoxism may result.

**fu·gu** (foo'goo) [Jap.] 1. a puffer fish of the genus *Fugu.* 2. the flesh of such fish, which contains tetrodotoxin.

**fugue** (fūg) [L. *fuga* a flight] a pathological state of altered consciousness in which an individual may act and wander around as though conscious but his behavior is not directed by his complete normal personality and is not remembered after the fugue ends. The term is often used to denote *dissociative f.* specifically.
**dissociative f.** [DSM-IV], a dissociative disorder characterized by an episode of sudden, unexpected travel away from home or business, with amnesia for the past and partial to total confusion about identity or assumption of a new identity; the disorder is usually related to emotional conflicts due to some traumatic, stressful, or overwhelming event, remits spontaneously, and rarely recurs.
**epileptic f.,** a fuguelike state of running or wandering that occasionally occurs as an ictal or postictal phenomenon in psychomotor (temporal lobe) epilepsy.
**psychogenic f.,** dissociative f.

**fu·gu·ism** (foo'goo-iz-əm) [*fugu* + *-ism*] tetrodotoxism (def. 1).

**fu·gu·is·mus** (foo"goo-iz'məs) [see *fuguism*] tetrodotoxism (def. 1).

**fu·gu·tox·in** (foo-goo-tok'sin) tetrodotoxin.

**Fu·ka·la's operation** (foo-kah'lahz) [Vincenz *Fukala,* Austrian ophthalmologist, 1847–1911] see under *operation.*

**Fu·ku·ya·ma type congenital muscular dystrophy (syndrome)** (foo"koo-yah'mah) [Yukio *Fukuyama,* Japanese physician, 20th century] see under *dystrophy.*

**ful·gu·rant** (ful'gu-rənt) [L. *fulgurans,* from *fulgur* lightning] coming and going like a flash of lightning.

**ful·gu·rate** (ful'gu-rāt) 1. to come and go like a flash of lightning. 2. to destroy by fulguration.

**ful·gu·ra·tion** (ful"gu-ra'shən) [L. *fulgur* lightning] destruction of living tissue by electric sparks generated by a high frequency current. See *electrocautery.*
**direct f.,** that in which an insulated electrode with a metal point is connected to the uniterminal and an electric spark is allowed to impinge on the area being treated.
**indirect f.,** that in which the patient is connected directly by a metal handle to the uniterminal and the operator uses an active electrode to complete an arc from the patient.

**fu·lig·i·nous** (ful-lij'ĭ-nəs) [L. *fuligo* soot] sooty in color or appearance.

**Fül·le·born's method** (fēl'ə-bornz) [Friedrich *Fülleborn,* German parasitologist, 1866–1933] see under *method.*

**Ful·ler's operation** (fool'ərz) [Eugene *Fuller,* American urologist, 1858–1930] see under *operation.*

**ful·mi·nant** (ful'mĭ-nənt) [L. *fulminare* to flare up] sudden, severe; occurring suddenly and with great intensity.

**ful·mi·nate** (ful'mĭ-nāt) to occur suddenly with great intensity.

**Ful·vi·cin** (ful'vĭ-sin) trademark for a preparation of griseofulvin.

**fu·ma·gil·lin** (fu"mə-jil'in) an antibiotic active against microsporidia, produced by certain strains of *Aspergillus fumigatus;* applied topically to the conjunctiva in the treatment of microsporidial keratoconjunctivitis.

**fu·ma·rase** (fu'mə-rās) fumarate hydratase.

**fu·ma·rate** (fu'mə-rāt) a salt or anionic form of fumaric acid.

**fu·ma·rate hy·dra·tase** (fu'mə-rāt hi'drə-tās) [EC 4.2.1.2] [MeSH: Fumarate Hydratase] an enzyme of the lyase class that catalyzes the hydration of fumarate to form L-malate in a reaction of the tricarboxylic acid cycle (see illustration at *cycle*). Called also *fumarase.*

**fu·mar·ic ac·id** (fu-mar'ik) *trans*-butanedioic acid, the trans isomer of maleic acid, an intermediate in the tricarboxylic acid cycle (q.v.).

**fu·mar·ic·ac·id·uria** (fu-mar"ik-as"ĭ-du're-ə) excretion of fumaric acid in the urine.

**fu·ma·ryl·ace·to·ac·e·tase** (fu"mə-ril"ə-se"to-as'ə-tās) [EC 3.7.1.2] an enzyme of the hydrolase class that catalyzes the cleavage of fumarylacetoacetate to form acetoacetate and fumarate; the reaction is a step in the tyrosine catabolic pathway. Deficiency of the enzyme, an autosomal recessive trait, causes tyrosinemia, type I.

**fu·ma·ryl·ac·e·to·ac·e·tate** (fu"mə-ril"ə-se"to-as'ə-tāt) a compound composed of fumarate linked to acetoacetate; it is an intermediate in the degradation of tyrosine and phenylalanine.

**fu·ma·ryl·ac·e·to·ac·e·tate hy·dro·lase** (fu"mə-ril"ə-se"to-as'ə-tāt hi'dro-lās) fumarylacetoacetase.

**fu·mi·gant** (fu'mĭ-gənt) a substance used in fumigation.

**fu·mi·ga·tion** (fu"mĭ-ga'shən) [L. *fumus* smoke, steam, vapor] [MeSH: Fumigation] exposure of an area or object to disinfecting fumes.

**fum·ing** (fūm'ing) [L. *fumus* smoke] smoking; emitting a visible vapor.

**Fum·i·ron** (fūm'i-ron) trademark for a preparation of ferrous fumarate.

**fu·mon·i·sin** (fu-mon'ĭ-sin) any of a group of toxic factors produced by *Fusarium moniliforme,* which contaminates corn; they cause moldy corn poisoning in livestock and are carcinogenic.

**func·tio** (funk'she-o) [L.] function.
**f. lae'sa,** loss of function, one of the cardinal signs of inflammation.

**func·tion** (funk'shən) [L. *functio,* from *fungi* to do] 1. the special, normal, or proper physiologic activity of an organ or part. 2. to perform such activity. 3. in chemistry, a characteristic behavior of a chemical compound due to the presence of a specific functional group (q.v.) 4. in mathematics, a rule that assigns to each member of one set (the domain) a value in another set (the range).
**cumulative distribution f. (cdf),** a mathematical function that defines the probability distribution of a random variable by giving for each random variable $X$ the probability of observing a value less than or equal to a specified value $x$.
**density f.,** probability density f.
**distribution f.,** cumulative distribution f.
**likelihood f.,** see *likelihood.*
**probability density f.,** in statistics, a mathematical function that describes the distribution of measurements for a population; a curve that describes a population. Its integral is the cumulative distribution function, so the probability that an individual measurement will fall between two numbers $a$ and $b$ is equal to the proportion of the area under the curve between points $a$ and $b$, with the entire area under the function being 1.
**ventricular f.,** ventricular performance (q.v.) as related to end-diastolic volume, dimension, or pressure; Starling curves (ventricular function curves) are used in the assessment of loading conditions and of cardiac contractility.

**func·tion·al** (funk'shən-əl) 1. of or pertaining to a function. 2. affecting the function but not the structure; see under *disorder.*

**func·ti·o·na·lis** (funk"she-o-na'lis) [L.] 1. functional. 2. stratum functionale.

**func·tion·ing** (funk'shən-ing) carrying out an activity.
**borderline intellectual f.** [DSM-IV], a classification of mental ability covering persons with I.Q. scores in the range of 71 to 84, with only slight impairments in adaptive behavior. Called also *borderline mental retardation.*

**fun·dal** (fun'dəl) pertaining to a fundus.

**fun·da·ment** (fun'də-mənt) [L. *fundamentum*] 1. a base or foundation, such as the breech or rump. 2. the anus and parts adjacent to it.

**fun·da·men·tal** (fun"də-men'təl) pertaining to a base or foundation.

**fun·dec·to·my** (fun-dek'tə-me) fundusectomy.

**fun·di** (fun'di) [L.] genitive and plural of *fundus.*

**fun·dic** (fun'dik) pertaining to a fundus.

**fun·di·form** (fun'dĭ-form) [L. *funda* sling + *form*] shaped like a sling.

**fun·do·pli·ca·tion** (fun"do-plĭ-ka'shən) [MeSH: Fundoplication] plication of the fundus of the stomach around the lower end of the esophagus, done as treatment for reflux esophagitis that may be associated with disorders such as hiatal hernia. Called also *fundic wrapping.*
**Belsey Mark IV f.,** see under *operation.*
**Nissen f.,** a type in which the fundus is wrapped completely around the distal esophagus. Called also *Nissen operation.*
**Toupet f.,** a type in which the fundus is wrapped 180° to 200° around the distal esophagus; done for patients with poor esophageal clearance and asymmetrical extrinsic pressure. Called also *Toupet's operation.*

**Fun·du·lus** (fun'du-ləs) the killifish, a genus of the order Cyprinodontidae. *F. heterocli'tus* is the common or green killifish, a species much used in biological research.

**fun·dus** (fun'dəs) gen. and pl. *fun'dus* [L.] 1. the bottom or base of

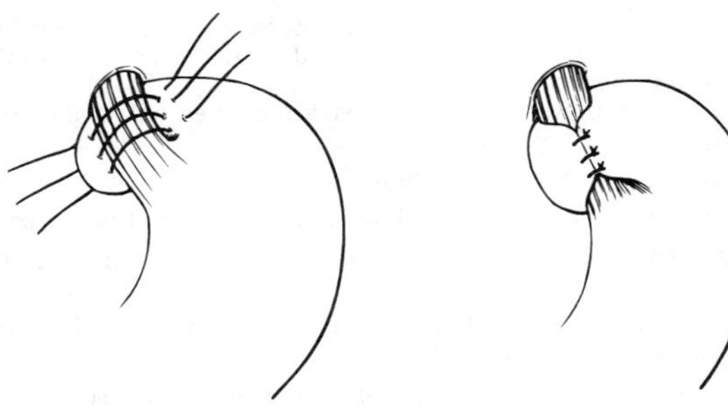

Nissen fundoplication for control of gastroesophageal reflux.

something. 2. [TA] in anatomical nomenclature, a general term for the bottom or base of an organ, or the part of a hollow organ farthest from its mouth.
**albinotic f.,** a fundus of the eye which permits clear visualization of the choroidal vasculature, owing to lack of pigment in the pigment epithelium and choroid.
**f. albipuncta'tus,** a disorder in which gray or white mottling of the fundus of the eye is associated with night blindness; called also *Lauber's disease.*
**f. of bladder,** 1. f. vesicae urinariae. 2. apex vesicae.
**f. diabe'ticus,** a fundus of the eye having dilated veins, a prodrome of diabetic retinopathy.
**f. of eye,** f. oculi.
**f. flavimacula'tus,** a condition characterized by the presence of yellow to white atrophic lesions in the midperiphery or perimacular region of the fundus of the eye.
**f. of gallbladder,** f. vesicae biliaris.
**f. gas'tricus** [TA], gastric fundus: that part of the stomach to the left and above the level of the entrance of the esophagus; called also *f. of stomach, f. ventricularis,* and *f. ventriculi.* See also *fornix gastricus.*
**f. of internal acoustic meatus,** f. mea'tus acus'tici inter'ni.
**leopard f.,** the mottled fundus of the eye seen in tapetoretinal degeneration; called also *leopard retina.*
**f. mea'tus acus'tici inter'ni** [TA], fundus of internal acoustic meatus: the laterally placed end or bottom of the internal acoustic meatus.
**f. o'culi,** fundus of the eye: the back portion of the interior of the eyeball, as seen by means of the ophthalmoscope.
**salt and pepper f.,** a fundus of the eye that is dusted with fine blue pigmented and orange depigmented spots, characteristic of hereditary syphilis; also seen in other disorders, e.g., rubella.
**f. of stomach,** f. gastricus.
**tessellated f., f. ti'gre, tigroid f.,** a normal, nonpathological fundus of the eye with marked exposure of the choroidal vessels due to scanty pigmentation; called also *tessellated* or *tigroid retina.*
**f. tym'pani,** paries jugularis cavi tympani.
**f. of urinary bladder,** 1. f. vesicae urinariae. 2. apex vesicae.
**f. u'teri** [TA], fundus of uterus: the part of the uterus above the orifices of the uterine tubes.
**f. of vagina, f. vagi'nae,** fornix vaginae.
**f. ventricula'ris, f. ventri'culi,** f. gastricus.
**f. vesi'cae bilia'ris** [TA], fundus of gallbladder: the inferior dilated portion of the gallbladder; called also *f. vesicae felleae* [TA alternative].
**f. vesi'cae fel'leae,** TA alternative for *f. vesicae biliaris.*
**f. vesi'cae urina'riae** [TA], fundus of urinary bladder: the base or posterior surface of the bladder; called also *f. of bladder* and *infundibulum of urinary bladder.*

**fun·du·scope** (fun'də-skōp) ophthalmoscope.

**fun·dus·co·py** (fən-dus'kə-pe) ophthalmoscopy.

**fun·du·sec·to·my** (fun"də-sek'tə-me) [*fundus* + *-ectomy*] excision of the fundus of an organ as of the fundus of the stomach or uterus.

**fun·gal** (fun'gəl) fungous.

**fun·gate** (fun'gāt) 1. to produce funguslike growths. 2. to grow rapidly, like a fungus.

**fun·ge·mia** (fən-je'me-ə) [MeSH: Fungemia] the presence of fungi in the blood stream; called also *mycethemia* and *mycohemia.*

**Fun·gi** (fun'ji) [L.] [MeSH: Fungi] a kingdom of eukaryotic, heterotrophic organisms that live as saprobes or parasites; it includes mushrooms, yeasts, and molds. They lack chlorophyll, have a cell wall composed of polysaccharides, sometimes polypeptides, and chitin, reproduce either sexually or asexually, and have a life cycle that ranges from simple to complex. The thallus is unicellular or mycelial; aseptate, partially septate, or septate; and nonmotile. Fruiting bodies range from microscopic hyphae in yeasts to large, complex structures showing limited and reversible tissue differentiation (as in mushrooms). In some systems of classification, the Fungi have been considered a subdivision of the plant kingdom. Several different classification systems for the Fungi have been devised; for example, some authorities use the term *phylum* and others use *division* for the level just below *kingdom.*
**F. Imperfec'ti,** Deuteromycota.

**fun·gi** (fun'ji) [L.] [MeSH: Fungi] plural of *fungus.*

**fun·gi·ci·dal** (fun"jĭ-si'dəl) [*fungus* + L. *caedere* to kill] destroying fungi.

**fun·gi·cide** (fun'jĭ-sīd) an agent that destroys fungi.

**fun·gi·ci·din** (fun"jĭ-si'din) nystatin.

**fun·gi·form** (fun'jĭ-form) shaped like a fungus; see also *fungoid.*

**fun·gi·sta·sis** (fun-jĭ-sta'sis) [*fungus* + *-stasis*] inhibition of growth of fungi. Called also *mycostasis.*

**fun·gi·stat** (fun'jĭ-stat) an agent that inhibits the growth of fungi. Called also *mycostat.*

**fun·gi·stat·ic** (fun"jĭ-stat'ik) inhibiting the growth of fungi.

**fun·gis·ter·ol** (fən-jis'tər-ol) a sterol, $C_{25}H_{44}O$, found in ergot and other fungi.

**fun·gi·tox·ic** (fun"jĭ-tok'sik) exerting a toxic effect upon fungi.

**fun·gi·tox·ic·i·ty** (fun"jĭ-tok-sis'ĭ-te) the quality of exerting a toxic effect upon fungi.

**Fun·gi·zone** (fun'jĭ-zōn) trademark for preparations of amphotericin B.

**fun·goid** (fun'goid) [*fungus* + *-oid*] resembling a fungus; see also *fungiform.*

**fun·go·ma** (fəng-go'mə) [*fungus* + *-oma*] fungus ball.

**fun·gos·i·ty** (fən-gos'ĭ-te) a fungoid growth or excrescence.

**fun·gous** (fun'gəs) [L. *fungosus*] 1. poertaining to or caused by a fungus. 2. resembling a fungus. Called also *fungal.*

**fun·gus** (fun'gəs) pl. *fun'gi* [L.] any organism belonging to the Fungi. See also *mycosis* and *mycotoxicosis.*
**f. of the brain,** hernia cerebri.
**cerebral f., f. cere'bri,** hernia cerebri.
**club fungi,** Basidiomycotina.
**dimorphic f.,** a fungus that lives as a yeast or a mold, depending on environmental conditions.
**foot f.,** a fungus, such as *Madurella mycetomi,* which produces maduromycosis, or other foot infection.
**imperfect f.,** one whose perfect (sexual) stage is unknown; all such fungi are classified in the phylum Deuteromycota.
**mosaic f.,** a mycelium-like intercellular deposit of cholesterol sometimes seen in scrapings from lesions thought to be fungal in origin.
**perfect f.,** a fungus for which both sexual and asexual types of spore formation are known; these fungi are classified in the subphyla Ascomycotina and Basidiomycotina, and the phylum Zygomycota.
**proper fungi,** Eumycota.
**ray f.,** *Actinomyces.*
**sac fungi,** Ascomycotina.
**slime f.,** see under *mold.*
**f. tes'tis,** protrusion from a scrotal sinus of a mass of granulation tissue in tuberculous epididymitis.
**true fungi,** Eumycota.

**fu·nic** (fu'nik) pertaining to a funis.

**fu·ni·cle** (fu'nĭ-kəl) funiculus.

**fu·nic·u·lar** (fu-nik'u-lər) pertaining to a funiculus.

**fu·nic·u·li** (fu-nik'u-li) genitive and plural of *funiculus.*

**fu·nic·u·li·tis** (fu-nik"u-li'tis) 1. inflammation of the spermatic cord. 2. inflammation of that portion of a spinal nerve root which lies within the intervertebral canal.

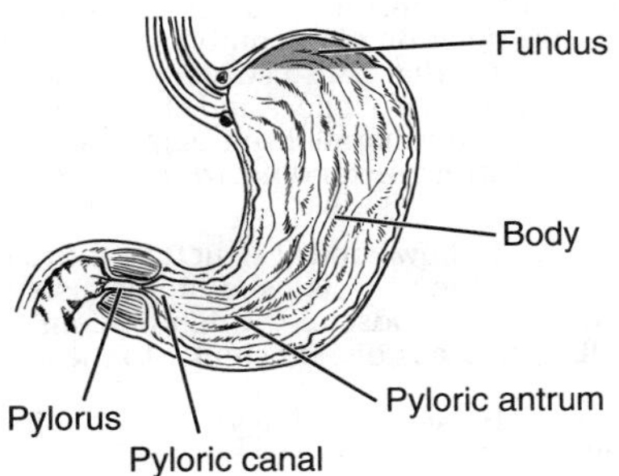


Fundus gastricus (gastric fundus).

**endemic f.**, a disease of unknown etiology occurring chiefly in Ceylon and southern India, marked by painful swelling of the spermatic cord, chills, nausea, and vomiting. The disease also occurs sporadically in temperate climates.
**filarial f.**, secondary involvement of the spermatic cord in lymphatic filariasis.

**fu·nic·u·lo·ep·i·did·y·mi·tis** (fu-nik″u-lo-ep″ĭ-did″ĭ-mi′tis) inflammation of the spermatic cord and the epididymis.

**fu·nic·u·lo·pexy** (fu-nik′u-lo-pek″se) [*funiculus* + *-pexy*] surgical fixation of the spermatic cord to the surrounding tissues in the correction of undescended testes.

**fu·nic·u·lus** (fu-nik′u-ləs) pl. *funic′uli* [L.] [TA] a cord: in anatomical nomenclature, a general term for a cordlike structure or part.
**f. am′nii,** a cord of tissue by which the amnion and chorion are temporarily united in certain ruminant animals.
**f. ante′rior medul′lae spina′lis** [TA], anterior funiculus of spinal cord: the white substance of the spinal cord lying on either side between the anterior median fissure and the anterior roots of the spinal nerves; called also *ventral f. of spinal cord* and *f. ventralis medullae spinalis.*
**cuneate f., f. cunea′tus [Burdachi],** fasciculus cuneatus medullae spinalis.
**f. cunea′tus latera′lis,** a longitudinal ridge on the medulla oblongata between the line of roots of the spinal accessory nerve and the fasciculus cuneatus.
**dorsal f. of spinal cord, f. dorsa′lis medul′lae spina′lis,** f. posterior medullae spinalis.
**hepatic f.,** ductus choledochus.
**lateral f. of medulla oblongata,** f. lateralis medullae oblongatae.
**lateral f. of spinal cord,** f. lateralis medullae spinalis.
**f. latera′lis medul′lae oblonga′tae** [TA], lateral funiculus of medulla oblongata: the continuation into the medulla oblongata of all the fiber tracts of the lateral funiculus of the spinal cord, with the exception of the lateral pyramidal tract.
**f. latera′lis medul′lae spina′lis** [TA], lateral funiculus of spinal cord: the white substance of the spinal cord that lies on either side between the dorsal and ventral roots of the spinal nerves; called also *anterolateral column.*
**ligamentous f.,** ligamentum collaterale carpi ulnare.
**funi′culi medul′lae spina′lis** [TA], funiculi of spinal cord: the large bundles of fiber tracts that make up the white substance of the spinal cord.
**f. poste′rior medul′lae spina′lis** [TA], posterior funiculus of spinal cord: the white substance of the spinal cord lying on either side between the posterior median sulcus and the posterior roots of the spinal nerves; called also *dorsal f. of spinal cord* and *f. dorsalis medullae spinalis.*
**f. se′parans** [TA], a narrow translucent ridge of thickened ependyma in the floor of the fourth ventricle that runs across the lower part of the trigone of the vagus nerve and separates it from the area postrema; the blood-brain barrier may be modified in this area. See also *circumventricular organs,* under *organ.*
**f. sperma′ticus** [TA], spermatic cord: a structure that extends from the abdominal inguinal ring to the testis, comprising the ductus deferens, testicular artery, pampiniform plexus, and nerves, as well as various other vessels, enclosed by its various coverings *(tunicae funiculi spermatici).* Called also *chorda spermatica.*
**funiculi of spinal cord,** funiculi medullae spinalis.
**f. umbilica′lis,** umbilical cord: the flexible structure connecting the umbilicus with the placenta and giving passage to the umbilical arteries and vein; called also *chorda umbilicalis* and *funis.* See *umbilical cord,* under *cord.*
**ventral f. of spinal cord, f. ventra′lis medul′lae spina′lis,** f. anterior medullae spinalis.

**fu·ni·form** (fu′nĭ-form) [*funis* + *form*] resembling a rope or cord.

**fu·nis** (fu′nis) [L. "cord"] 1. any cordlike structure; see *chorda* and *funiculus.* 2. funiculus umbilicalis.
**f. hippoc′ratis,** tendo calcaneus.

**fu·ni·si·tis** (fu″nĭ-si′tis) inflammation of the umbilical cord.
**necrotizing f.,** inflammation of the umbilical cord resulting from infection with organisms that cause sexually transmitted diseases or with normal lower genital tract flora and characterized by yellowish-white chalky stripes that parallel the umbilical vessels and an inflammatory cell infiltrate extending from the vascular intima to Wharton's jelly.

**fun·nel** (fun′əl) 1. a hollow conical structure with a narrow opening at the apex, such as the vessels used in chemistry and pharmacy for filtering and other purposes. 2. infundibulum.
**accessory müllerian f.,** a rudiment similar to the primordial uterine tube.
**mitral f.,** the cone-shaped mitral valve seen in mitral stenosis, the orifice being at the apex of the cone.
**muscular f.,** the funnel-shaped space bounded by the four rectus muscles of the eye.
**pial f.,** a sheath of adventitia, extended from the pia mater, loosely surrounding blood vessels as they enter the brain or spinal cord; see also *Virchow-Robin space.*
**vascular f.,** the light-colored depression at the center of the disk of the retina.

**FUO** fever of undetermined origin.

**Fu·ra·cin** (fu′rə-sin) trademark for preparations of nitrofurazone.

**Fur·a·dan·tin** (fūr″ə-dan′tin) trademark for preparations of nitrofurantoin.

**fu·ral·ta·done** (fu-ral′tə-dōn) a nitrofuran antibacterial and antiprotozoal used in poultry.

**fu·ran** (fu′ran) a heterocyclic compound, the ring structure that is the basis of the furanoses and furfural.

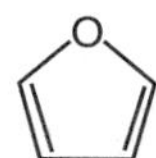


**fu·ra·nose** (fu′rə-nōs) any sugar containing a furan ring structure, a cyclic form that ketoses and aldoses may take in solution. See also individual sugars, e.g., *fructofuranose.*

**fu·ran·o·side** (fu-ran′o-sīd) a glycoside in which the sugar is in furanose configuration.

**fu·ra·zol·i·done** (fu″rə-zol′ĭ-dōn) [USP] [MeSH: Furazolidone] a nitrofuran antibacterial and antiprotozoal, effective against many gram-negative enteric organisms; used in humans and many species of domestic animals in the treatment of diarrhea and enteritis due to susceptible organisms, usually administered orally. Various combinations of furazolidone and nifuroxime are administered intravaginally in treatment of bacterial, candidal, and trichomonal vaginitis.

**fur·ca** (fur′kə) gen. and pl. *fur′cae* [L. "fork"] furcation.

**fur·cal** (fur′kəl) [L. *furca* fork] shaped like a fork; forked.

**fur·ca·tion** (fər-ka′shən) the area where the roots divide on a multirooted tooth. See also *bifurcation* and *trifurcation.*

**fur·co·cer·cous** (fur″ko-ser′kəs) [*furca* + *cerko-* + *-ous*] having a forked tail.

**fur·cu·la** (fur′ku-lə) [L. "little fork"] a horseshoe-shaped ridge in the embryonic larynx, bounding the pharyngeal aperture ventrally and laterally.

**fur·fu·ra·ceous** (fur″fu-ra′shəs) [L. *furfur* bran] fine and loose; said of scales resembling bran or dandruff.

**fur·fu·ral** (fur′fu-rəl) furan carrying a carbonyl substituent, an intermediate formed from pentosans of cereal straws and brans and used in a variety of industrial processes; it irritates mucous membranes and causes photosensitivity and headaches.

**fur·fu·ran** (fur′fu-rən) furan.

**fur·i·fos·min** (fu″rĭ-foz′min) a phosphine which when labeled with technetium 99m is used in myocardial perfusion imaging; see table at *technetium.*

**fu·ro·cou·ma·rin** (fu″ro-koo′mə-rin) any of a group of antifungal dyestuffs produced by certain species of plants (e.g., parsley and figs) which, on contact with skin, cause photosensitization.

**fu·ror** (fu′ror) [L.] fury; rage.
**f. epilep′ticus,** an attack of intense anger occasionally occurring in epilepsy.

**fu·ro·sem·ide** (fu-ro′sə-mīd) [USP] [MeSH: Furosemide] a loop diuretic used in the treatment of edema associated with congestive heart failure or hepatic or renal disease and in the treatment of hypertension, usually in combination with other drugs; administered orally, intramuscularly, or intravenously.

**Fur·ox·one** (fər-ok′sōn) trademark for preparations of furazolidone.

**fur·row** (fur′o) a groove or sulcus.
**atrioventricular f.,** sulcus coronarius cordis.
**digital f.,** any one of the transverse folds across the joints on the palmar surface of a finger.
**genital f.,** a groove that appears on the genital tubercle of the fetus at the end of the second month.
**gluteal f.,** 1. crena analis. 2. sulcus glutealis.
**Jadelot's f's,** see under *line.*
**Liebermeister's f's,** depressions sometimes seen on the upper surface of the liver from pressure of the ribs, generally caused by tight garments or tight lacing of a girdle or corset.
**mentolabial f.,** see under *sulcus.*
**nympholabial f.,** a groove separating the labium majus and labium minus on either side.

**primitive f.**, primitive groove.
**scleral f.**, sulcus sclerae.
**Sibson's f.**, the inferior border of the pectoralis major muscle.
**skin f's**, sulci cutis.

**fu·run·cle** (fu'rung-kəl) [L. *furunculus*] [MeSH: Furunculosis] a painful nodule formed in the skin by circumscribed inflammation of the corium and subcutaneous tissue, enclosing a central slough or "core." It is caused by staphylococci, which enter through the hair follicles, and its formation is favored by constitutional or digestive derangement and local irritation. Called also *boil* and *furunculus.*

**fu·run·cu·lar** (fu-rung'ku-lər) pertaining to or of the nature of a furuncle or boil.

**fu·run·cu·loid** (fu-rung'ku-loid) resembling a furuncle or boil.

**fu·run·cu·lo·sis** (fu-rung″ku-lo'sis) [MeSH: Furunculosis] 1. the persistent sequential occurrence of furuncles over a period of weeks or months. 2. the simultaneous occurrence of a number of furuncles.
**f. blastomyce'tica, f. cryptococ'cica,** any systemic fungous infection in which the lesions resemble furuncles.

**fu·run·cu·lus** (fu-rung'ku-ləs) pl. *furun'culi* [L.] furuncle.

**FUS** feline urological syndrome.

**fu·sar·io·tox·i·co·sis** (fu-sar″e-o-tok″sĭ-ko'sis) any of numerous types of mycotoxicosis in humans or other animals caused by fungi of the genus *Fusarium;* see also *alimentary toxic aleukia,* under *aleukia.*

**fu·sa·ri·um** (fu-sar'e-əm) pl. *fusa'ria* [MeSH: Fusarium] any fungus of the genus *Fusarium.*

**Fu·sa·ri·um** (fu-sar'e-əm) [MeSH: Fusarium] a genus of Fungi Imperfecti of the form-class Hyphomycetes, form-family Moniliaceae (sometimes classified in the small form-family Tuberculariaceae). Perfect stages of many species are included in the order Hypocreales. Some species are important pathogens of plants, some are opportunistic infectious agents of humans and other animals, some produce trichothecene mycotoxins, and some have been isolated from otomycosis externa and mycotic keratitis. See also *fusariotoxicosis.*
**F. graminea'rum,** *F. roseum.*
**F. monilifor'me,** a species that contains fumonisins and sometimes contaminates corn, causing moldy corn poisoning in domestic animals.
**F. oxyspo'rum,** a species causing banana wilt, and occasionally human eumycotic mycetoma.
**F. po'ae,** a species that contaminates grain and contains T-2 toxin, causing fusariotoxicosis in farm animals and alimentary toxic aleukia in humans.
**F. ro'seum,** a species that contaminates grain and produces the estrogenic mycotoxin zearalenone; farm animals that eat contaminated grain or flour products may develop fertility problems or vulvovaginitis. Called also *F. graminearum.*
**F. so'lani,** a species causing potato wilt and occasionally human eumycotic mycetoma or mycotic keratitis.
**F. sporotrichiel'la,** a species believed to be the etiologic agent of Kashin-Bek disease.
**F. sporotrichioi'des,** a species that sometimes contaminates grain and contains T-2 toxin, causing fusariotoxicosis in livestock and alimentary toxic aleukia in humans.
**F. tricinc'tum,** a species that contaminates corn and contains T-2 toxin, causing fusariotoxicosis in farm animals and alimentary toxic aleukia in humans.

**fus·cin** (fu'sin) [L. *fuscus* brown] a yellow to brown pigment of the retinal epithelium.

**fuse** (fūz) 1. a bar, strip, or wire of easily fusible metal inserted for safety in an electric circuit; when the current increases beyond a safe strength the metal melts, thus breaking the circuit and thereby saving an apparatus from overload. 2. to join together, as the abnormal coherence of adjacent body structures.

**fu·seau** (fu-zo') pl. *fuseaux'* [Fr.] a macroaleuriospore or macroconidium.

**fu·si** (fu'si) [L.] plural of *fusus.*

**fu·si·ble** (fu'zĭ-bəl) susceptible of being melted or fused.

**fu·si·cel·lu·lar** (fu″sĭ-sel'u-lər) fusocellular.

**fu·si·date** (fu'si-dāt) a salt of fusidic acid.

**fu·sid·ic ac·id** (fu-sid'ik) [MeSH: Fusidic Acid] a fermentation product of the fungus *Fusidium coccineum* used as an antibiotic.

**fu·si·form** (fu'zĭ-form) [*fusus* + *form*] spindle-shaped.

**Fu·si·form·is** (fu″sĭ-for'mis) a name formerly given to the genus *Fusobacterium.*
**F. necro'phorus,** *Fusobacterium necrophorum.*

**fu·si·mo·tor** (fu″sĭ-mo'tor) innervating intrafusal fibers of the muscle spindle; said of motor nerve fibers of gamma motoneurons.

**fu·sion** (fu'zhən) [L. *fusio*] 1. the act, process, or result of melting. 2. the merging or coherence of adjacent parts or bodies. 3. the coordination of the separate images of the same object in the two eyes into one. 4. the operative formation of an ankylosis or arthrodesis (*f. of joint*).
**anterior interbody f.,** spinal fusion in the lumbar region using a retroperitoneal approach, with immobilization by bone grafts on the anterior and lateral surfaces, primarily for patients in whom other types of fusion have failed.
**binocular f.,** see *fusion,* def. 3.
**centric f.,** robertsonian translocation.
**cervical spinal f.,** spinal fusion in the cervical region to correct instability when traumatic vertebral fractures do not heal with other techniques.
**diaphyseal-epiphyseal f.,** operative establishment of bony union between the diaphysis and epiphysis, to arrest growth in the length of a bone.
**midline f.,** the process of symmetrical union along the midline that forms the neural tube in the embryo; cf. *dysraphism.*
**f. of joint,** see *fusion,* def. 4.
**spinal f.,** operative immobilization or ankylosis of two or more vertebrae, often with diskectomy or laminectomy; types are named for the surface immobilized, such as *anterior spinal f., lateral spinal f., posterior spinal f.,* and *posterolateral spinal f.* Called also *spondylosyndesis.*

**fu·sion·al** (fu'zhən-əl) marked by fusion.

**Fu·so·bac·te·ri·um** (fu″zo-bak-ter'e-əm) [L. *fusus* spindle +*bacteria*] [MeSH: Fusobacterium] a genus of gram-negative, anaerobic, nonsporulating bacteria of the family Bacteroidaceae, consisting of slender cells with tapered ends that are normal inhabitants of the cavities of humans and animals. Some species are pathogenic, causing purulent or gangrenous infections. Formerly called *Fusiformis.*
**F. gonidiafor'mans,** a species isolated from human infections of the respiratory, urogenital, and gastrointestinal tracts. Called also *Actinomyces gonidiaformis.*
**F. morti'ferum,** a species isolated from normal sources and from abscesses, septicemia, pleurisy, and urinary tract infections.
**F. navifor'me,** a species isolated from human abscesses and other clinical specimens, and from the intestines of rats.
**F. necro'phorum,** a pleomorphic species found in normal body cavities, which is also the cause of foot rot in cattle, sheep, and pigs; interdigital dermatitis in sheep; calf diphtheria; and Schmorl's disease. Called also *Schmorl's bacillus.* Former names include *Actinomyces necrophorus* or *pseudonecrophorus, Bacteroides fundiliformis, Fusiformis necrophorus,* and *Sphaerophorus necrophorus.*
**F. nuclea'tum,** a species isolated from the normal mouth, the upper respiratory, genital, and gastrointestinal tracts, and infections of the mouth, lungs, and brain. It is the organism most commonly found, in association with spirochetes *(Treponema vincentii),* in acute necrotizing gingivitis. Called also *Bacillus fusiformis.*
**F. plau'ti-vincen'ti,** *Leptotrichia buccalis.*
**F. rus'sii,** a species isolated from perianal abscesses, and from human and animal feces.
**F. va'rium,** a species isolated from the intestinal cavities of humans and animals, and from human purulent infections.

**fu·so·bac·te·ri·um** (fu″zo-bak-tēr'e-əm) pl. *fusobacte'ria* [MeSH: Fusobacterium] 1. a rod-shaped bacterium in which the cell is thicker in the center and tapers toward the ends. 2. an organism of the genus *Fusobacterium.*

**fu·so·cel·lu·lar** (fu″so-sel'u-lər) [*fusus* + *cellular*] having spindle-shaped cells.

**fu·so·spi·ril·lary** (fu″so-spi'rĭ-lar″e) pertaining to or caused by fusiform bacilli and spirilla, as in acute necrotizing ulcerative gingivitis.

**fu·so·spi·ril·lo·sis** (fu″so-spi″rĭ-lo'sis) acute necrotizing ulcerative gingivitis.

**fu·so·spi·ro·che·tal** (fu″so-spi″ro-ke'təl) pertaining to or caused by fusobacteria and spirochetes.

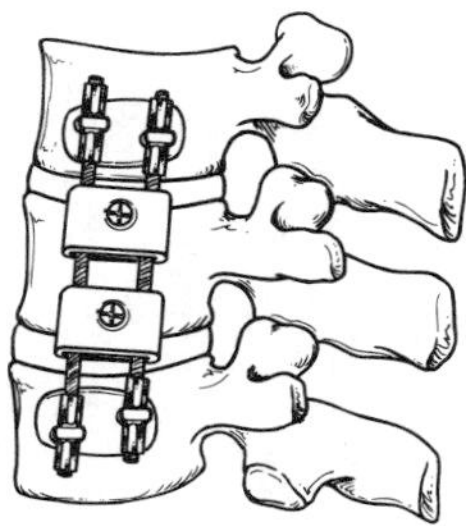

Spinal fusion.

**fu·so·spi·ro·che·to·sis** (fu″so-spi″ro-ke-to′sis) infection with fusobacteria and spirochetes.

**fu·sus** (fu′səs) pl. *fu′si* [L.] a spindlelike object; applied especially to minute air vesicles in a hair shaft.
**cortical fusi,** the delicate air spaces appearing among the cells of the cortex as a hair grows out, produced by drying out of the fluid which fills the spaces in the living portion of the hair root.
**fracture fusi,** minute rifts or ruptures observed between the keratinized cells of the cortex of a mature hair shaft which has been subjected to pressure sufficient to dissociate the cells of the particular region.

**Fut·cher's line** (fuch′ər) [Palmer Howard *Futcher,* American physician, born 1910] Voigt's line.

**FVC** forced vital capacity.

**F. vs.** abbreviation for L. *fi′at venaesec′tio,* let the patient be bled.

# G

**G** symbol for *gauss, giga-, gravida,* and *guanine* or *guanosine.*

***G*** symbol for *conductance, gravitational constant, Gibbs free energy,* and *G force.*

**g** symbol for *gram.*

***g*** symbol for *standard gravity.*

**γ** gamma, the third letter of the Greek alphabet; symbol for the heavy chain of IgG (see *immunoglobulin*) and the γ chains of fetal hemoglobin; former symbol for *microgram* (now *μg*).

**γ-** a prefix designating (1) the third carbon atom along a chain starting with that adjacent to the principal functional group, e.g., γ-aminobutyric acid (see *α-*); (2) a plasma protein migrating with the γ band in protein electrophoresis, a gamma globulin; (3) one in a series of related entities or chemical compounds, e.g., γ-carotene or γ-ray. For terms prefixed with the symbol γ-, see the unprefixed form.

**Ga** symbol for *gallium.*

**GABA** [MeSH: GABA] γ-aminobutyric acid.

**GABA·er·gic** (gab″ə-ər′jik) transmitting or secreting γ-aminobutyric acid; said of nerve fibers, synapses, and other neural structures.

**gab·a·pen·tin** (gab″ə-pen′tin) a substance chemically related to γ-aminobutyric acid (GABA), used as adjunctive therapy in the treatment of partial seizures; administered orally.

**GABA trans·am·i·nase** (gab″ə-trans-am′ĭ-nās) 1. 4-aminobutyrate transaminase. 2. a renal transaminase that catalyzes the transfer of an amino group from γ-aminobutyrate (GABA) to pyruvate, forming alanine and succinate semialdehyde; the reaction may play a role in chloride permeability in the nephron.

**Gab·i·tril** (gab′ĭ-tril) trademark for a preparation of tiagabine hydrochloride.

**G-ac·tin** see *actin.*

**GAD** generalized anxiety disorder.

**gad·fly** (gad′fli) tabanid.

**gad·o·lin·i·um** (gad″o-lin′e-əm) [MeSH: Gadolinium] a rare element of atomic number 64, atomic weight 157.25, symbol Gd; chelated gadolinium is used as a paramagnetic contrast agent in magnetic resonance imaging.
**g. 153,** an artificial isotope of gadolinium used in dual photon absorptiometry. It has a half-life of 241.6 days and decays by electron capture and emission of 0.070, 0.097, and 0.103 MeV gamma rays.

**gad·o·pen·te·tate di·meg·lu·mine** (gad″o-pen′tə-tāt) [USP] the dimeglumine salt of the gadolinium complex of pentetic acid; a paramagnetic agent used as a contrast agent in magnetic resonance imaging of intracranial lesions and lesions of the spine and associated tissues, administered intravenously.

**Ga·dus** (ga′dəs) [L.; Gr. *gados*] a genus of marine fishes of the family Gadidae. *G. mor′rhua* is the common cod, source of cod liver oil.

**Gaens·len's sign (test)** (genz′lənz) [Frederick Julius *Gaenslen,* American surgeon, 1877–1937] see under *sign.*

**Gaert·ner** see *Gärtner.*

**Gaff·ky scale (table)** (gahf′ke) [Georg Theodor August *Gaffky,* German bacteriologist, 1850–1918] see under *scale.*

**Gaff·kya** (gaf′ke-ə) [G.T.A. *Gaffky*] in former systems of classification, a genus of bacteria, species of which are now included in the genus *Aerococcus.*

**GAG** glycosaminoglycan.

**gag** (gag) 1. a surgical device for holding the mouth open. 2. to retch, or strive to vomit.

**gage** (gāj) gauge.

**Gai·ge·ria** (ga-je′re-ə) a genus of hookworms of the family Ancylostomatidae. *G. pachysce′lis* infests the intestines of sheep in India, Indonesia, Africa, and South America; it is a voracious blood sucker and often kills its host.

**Gail·lard-Arlt suture** (ga-yahr′ahrlt) [François Lucien *Gaillard,* French physician, 1805–1869; Carl Ferdinand Ritter von *Arlt,* Austrian ophthalmologist, 1812–1887] see under *suture.*

**gain** (gān) 1. an increase in amount or value; a benefit or advantage. 2. the increase achieved by amplification of a signal. 3. to acquire, obtain, or increase.
**antigen g.,** the acquisition by cells of new antigenic determinants not normally present or not normally accessible in the parent tissue.
**primary g.,** the direct alleviation of anxiety by a defense mechanism; the relief from emotional conflict or tension provided by neurotic symptoms or illness.
**secondary g.,** external and incidental advantage derived from an illness, such as rest, gifts, personal attention, release from responsibility, and disability benefits.

**Gais·böck's disease** (gīs′bərkz) [Felix *Gaisböck,* German physician, 1868–1955] stress polycythemia.

**gait** (gāt) [MeSH: Gait] the manner or style of walking. See also *gait cycle,* under *cycle.*
**antalgic g.,** a limp adopted so as to avoid pain on weight-bearing structures (as in hip injuries), characterized by a very short stance phase.
**ataxic g.,** an unsteady, uncoordinated walk, with a wide base and the feet thrown out, due to some form of ataxia; see *cerebellar g., Charcot's g.,* and *tabetic g.*
**calcaneus g.,** the gait resulting when the gastrocnemius-soleus muscles are paralyzed, with lack of push-off and shift of the tibia posteriorly over the talus at the end of the stance phase.
**cerebellar g.,** a staggering ataxic gait, sometimes with a tendency to fall to one side, indicative of cerebellar lesions.
**Charcot's g.,** the peculiar gait seen in Friedreich's ataxia.
**gluteus medius g., compensated,** the gait characteristic of paralysis of the gluteus medius muscle, marked by a listing of the trunk toward the affected side at each step. Called also *gluteal g.* and *Trendelenburg g.*; cf. *uncompensated gluteus medius g.*
**double step g.,** a gait in which the length and/or timing of alternate steps is noticeably different; see also *intermittent double-step g.*.
**drag-to g.,** a gait in which the feet are dragged (rather than lifted) toward the crutches.
**drop-foot g.,** steppage g.
**dystrophic g.,** myopathic g.
**equine g.,** steppage g.
**festinating g.,** a gait in which the patient involuntarily moves with short, accelerating steps, often on tiptoe, as seen in paralysis agitans and other nervous disorders; called also *propulsion g.* See also *festination.*
**four-point g.,** a gait in forward motion: first one crutch and then the opposite leg, followed by the other crutch and then the other leg, and so on.
**gluteal g.,** compensated gluteus medius g.
**gluteus medius g.,** see *compensated gluteus medius g.* and *uncompensated gluteus medius g.*
**heel-toe g.,** the normal, nonpathologic gait in which the heel touches down first and the toes last.
**helicopod g.,** a gait in which the feet describe half-circles, as in some cases of conversion disorder.
**hemiplegic g.,** a gait involving flexion of the hip because of drop-foot and circumduction of the leg.
**hip extensor g.,** an abnormal gait due to weakness or paralysis of the gluteus maximus and other hip extensor muscles; with each step on the affected side, after the heel strikes the floor the hip is thrown forward and the trunk and pelvis are thrown back.
**hysterical g.,** a bizarre gait pattern not due to a physical cause, such as *helicopod g.* or *stuttering g.*
**intermittent double-step g.,** a hemiplegic gait in which there is a pause after the short step of the normal foot, or in some cases after the step of the affected foot.
**maximus g.,** hip extensor g.
**myopathic g.,** exaggerated alternation of lateral trunk movements with an exaggerated elevation of the hip, suggesting the gait of a duck or penguin; characteristic of muscle diseases such as progressive muscular dystrophy, spinal muscular atrophy, and sometimes acute febrile polyneuropathy.
**paraplegic spastic g.,** a walk in which the legs are held together and move in a stiff manner, the toes seeming to drag and catch; caused by lesions of the central nervous system.
**point g.,** any of several gaits in which at least one foot and one crutch are on the ground at any given time; see *two-point g., three-point g.,* and *four-point g.*
**propulsive g.,** festinating g.
**quadriceps g.,** a gait seen when the quadriceps muscle is paralyzed or absent; with each step of the affected leg, the knee goes into hyperextension and the trunk tends to lurch forward.
**scissor g.,** a gait in which one foot is passed in front of the other, producing a cross-legged progression.
**spastic g.,** paraplegic spastic g.
**staggering g.,** a reeling, tottering, and tipping gait in which the individual appears as if he may fall backward or lose his balance; it is associated with alcohol or barbiturate intoxication.
**steppage g.,** the gait in drop foot in which the advancing leg is lifted high in order that the toes may clear the ground. It is due to paralysis of the anterior tibial and peroneal muscles and is seen in lesions

of the lower motor neuron, such as multiple neuritis, lesions of the anterior motor horn cells, and lesions of the cauda equina. Called also *drop-foot g.* and *equine g.*
**stuttering g.**, a walking disorder characterized by hesitancy that resembles stuttering; seen in some hysterical or schizophrenic patients as well as in patients with neurologic damage.
**swaying g.**, cerebellar g.
**swing g.**, a gait in which the lower body is swung between the crutches at each step; see *swing-through g.* and *swing-to g.*
**swing-through g.**, a gait in which the crutches are advanced and then the legs are swung past them.
**swing-to g.**, a gait in which the crutches are advanced and the legs are swung to the same point.
**tabetic g.**, an ataxic gait that accompanies tabes dorsalis.
**three-point g.**, a gait in which both crutches and the affected leg are advanced together and then the normal leg is moved forward.
**Trendelenburg g.**, compensated gluteus medius g.
**two-point g.**, a gait in which the right foot and left crutch (or cane) are advanced together, and then the left foot and right crutch.
**gluteus medius g., uncompensated,** a gait that occurs with moderate weakness of the gluteus medius muscle; with each step of the affected leg, the pelvis on the opposite side dips, causing protrusion of the stationary affected hip. Cf. *compensated gluteus medius g.*
**waddling g.**, myopathic g.

**Gaj·du·sek** (gi'doo-shek) Daniel Carleton. American pediatrician, born 1923; co-winner, with Baruch Samuel Blumberg, of the Nobel prize for medicine or physiology in 1976 for their discoveries of new mechanisms for the origin and dissemination of infectious diseases.

**ga·lac·ta·cra·sia** (gə-lak″tə-kra'zhə) [*galact-* + *a-*[1] + *-crasia*] abnormal condition of the breast milk.

**ga·lac·ta·gog·in** (gə-lak'tə-gog″in) old name for *human placental lactogen.*

**ga·lac·ta·gogue** (gə-lak'tə-gog) [*galact-* + *-agogue*] 1. promoting the flow of milk. 2. an agent that promotes the flow of milk.

**ga·lac·tan** (gə-lak'tən) any polymer composed of galactose residues and occurring in plants, e.g., agar.

**gal·ac·te·mia** (gal″ak-te'me-ə) [*galact-* + *-emia*] the presence of milk in the blood.

**ga·lac·tic** (gə-lak'tik) 1. pertaining to milk. 2. galactagogue.

**gal·ac·tis·chia** (gal″ak-tis'ke-ə) [*galact-* + *isch-* + *-ia*] suppression of the secretion of milk.

**ga·lac·ti·tol** (gə-lak'tĭ-tol) the alcohol obtained on reduction of galactose, occurring naturally in manna and other plant products. Galactitol is formed in excess in the lens of the eye in galactosemia caused by deficiency of galactokinase; the result is cataracts in infancy.

**galact(o)-** [Gr. *gala,* gen. *galaktos* milk] a combining form denoting relationship to milk.

**ga·lac·to·bol·ic** (gə-lak″to-bol'ik) of or relating to the action of neurohypophyseal peptides which contract the mammary myoepithelium and cause ejection of milk.

**ga·lac·to·cele** (gə-lak'to-sēl) [*galacto-* + *-cele*[1]] 1. a cystic enlargement of the mammary gland containing milk. 2. a hydrocele filled with a milky fluid. Called also *galactoma.*

**ga·lac·to·ce·re·bro·side** (gə-lak″to-sə-re'bro-sīd″) any of the cerebrosides in which the monosaccharide head group is galactose; they are abundant in the cell membranes of nervous tissue, particularly the myelin sheath, and in the kidney, and they accumulate abnormally in Krabbe's disease.

**ga·lac·to·cer·e·bro·side β-ga·lac·to·si·dase** (gə-lak″to-sə-re'bro-sīd″ gə-lak″to-si'dās) galactosylceramidase.

**ga·lac·to·chlo·ral** (gə-lak″to-klor'əl) a derivative of chloral hydrate and galactose in glossy scales; it is used as a hypnotic.

**ga·lac·to·cra·sia** (gə-lak″to-kra'zhə) galactacrasia.

**gal·ac·tog·e·nous** (gal″ak-toj'ə-nəs) [*galacto-* + *-genous*] favoring the production of milk.

**ga·lac·to·gogue** (gə-lak'to-gog) galactagogue.

**gal·ac·tog·ra·phy** (gal″ak-tog'rə-fe) [*galacto-* + *-graphy*] radiography of the mammary ducts after injection of a radiopaque substance into the duct system.

**ga·lac·to·ki·nase** (gə-lak″to-ki'nās) [MeSH: Galactokinase] [EC 2.7.1.6] an enzyme of the transferase class that catalyzes the reaction ATP + galactose = ADP + galactose 1-phosphate; the initial step of galactose utilization. Absence of enzyme activity, an autosomal recessive trait, results in galactokinase deficiency galactosemia.

**gal·ac·to·ma** (gal″ak-to'mə) [*galact-* + *-oma*] galactocele.

**ga·lac·to·me·tas·ta·sis** (gə-lak″to-mə-tas'tə-sis) galactoplania.

**gal·ac·tom·e·ter** (gal″ak-tom'ə-tər) [*galacto-* + *-meter*] an instrument for measuring the specific gravity of milk.

**ga·lac·to·pex·ic** (gə-lak″to-pek'sik) fixing or holding galactose.

**ga·lac·to·pexy** (gə-lak'to-pek″se) [*galacto-* + *-pexy*] the fixation of galactose by the liver.

**gal·ac·toph·a·gous** (gal″ak-tof'ə-gəs) lactivorous.

**ga·lac·to·phle·bi·tis** (gə-lak″to-flə-bi'tis) [*galacto-* + *phlebitis*] phlegmasia alba dolens.

**gal·ac·toph·ly·sis** (gal″ak-tof'lə-sis) [*galacto-* + Gr. *phlysis* eruption] a vesicular eruption containing a milky fluid.

**ga·lac·to·phore** (gə-lak'to-for) 1. galactophorous. 2. a milk duct.

**ga·lac·to·pho·ri·tis** (tə-lak″to-for-i'tis) [*galacto-* + Gr. *pherein* to carry + *-itis*] inflammation of the milk ducts.

**gal·ac·toph·o·rous** (gal'ak-tof'o-rəs) [*galacto-* + Gr. *pherein* to bear] conveying milk.

**gal·ac·toph·y·gous** (gal″ak-tof'ə-gəs) [*galacto-* + Gr. *phygē* flight] arresting the milk secretion.

**ga·lac·to·pla·nia** (gə-lak″to-pla'ne-ə) [*galacto-* + Gr. *planē* wandering] the secretion of milk in some abnormal part; the metastasis of milk. Called also *galactometastasis.*

**ga·lac·to·poi·e·sis** (gə-lak″to-poi-e'sis) [*galacto-* + *-poiesis*] the production of milk by the mammary glands; lactogenesis.

**ga·lac·to·poi·et·ic** (gə-lak″to-poi-et'ik) 1. pertaining to, characterized by, or promoting the production of milk. 2. an agent that promotes the secretion of milk.

**ga·lac·to·py·ra** (gə-lak″to-pi'rə) [*galacto-* + Gr. *pyr* fire] milk fever.

**ga·lac·to·py·ra·nose** (gə-lak″to-pir'ə-nōs) galactose occurring in the cyclic pyranose configuration.

**ga·lac·tor·rhea** (gə-lak″to-re'ə) [*galacto-* + *-rrhea*] [MeSH: Galactorrhea] excessive or spontaneous flow of milk irrespective of nursing; it is sometimes associated with hyperprolactinemia (q.v.).

**gal·ac·to·sa·mine** (gal″ak-to'sə-mēn) [MeSH: Galactosamine] the amino sugar derivative of galactose, substituted at the 2 position; it occurs in a variety of glycosaminoglycans and complex polysaccharides, such as blood group substances, and is generally acetylated.

**gal·ac·to·sa·mine-6-sul·fa·tase** (gal″ak-to'sə-mēn sul'fə-tās) *N*-acetylgalactosamine-6-sulfatase.

**ga·lac·to·san** (gə-lak'to-san) galactan.

**gal·ac·to·sa·zone** (gal″ak-to'sə-zōn) the osazone formed from galactose by reaction with phenylhydrazine; it has been used to identify galactose.

**gal·ac·tos·che·sis** (gal″ak-tos'kə-sis) [*galacto-* + Gr. *schesis* suppression] galactischia.

**ga·lac·tose** (gə-lak'tōs) [Gr. *gala,* gen. *galaktos* milk] [MeSH: Galactose] an aldohexose epimeric with glucose at the 4 carbon but less soluble and less sweet, occurring naturally in both D- and L- forms (the latter in plants); it is a component of lactose and other oligosaccharides, cerebrosides and gangliosides, and various glycolipids and glycoproteins.
**g. 1-phosphate,** galactose containing a phosphate substitution, an intermediate in carbohydrate metabolism.

**ga·lac·tos·e·mia** (gə-lak″to-se'me-ə) [*galactose* + *-emia*] [MeSH: Galactosemia] any of three genetic disorders resulting from defective galactose metabolism. *Classic galactosemia,* which is often fatal to neonates, is caused by deficient UDPglucose–hexose-1-phosphate uridylyltransferase, and is marked by accumulation of galactose 1-phosphate and galactose, with cataracts, cirrhosis of the liver, hepatomegaly, vomiting, diarrhea, jaundice, poor weight gain, and malnutrition in infancy, and mental retardation in survivors. *Galactokinase deficiency* results in accumulation of galactose in blood and tissues and of galactitol in the lens of the eye, and causes cataracts in infants and children. *Galactose epimerase deficiency* is caused by defective UDPglucose 4-epimerase, results in accumulation of galactose 1-phosphate in the red blood cells, and is nearly always benign.

**ga·lac·tose 1-phos·phate u·ri·dyl·trans·fer·ase** (gə-lak″tōs fos'fāt ur″ĭ-dəl-trans'fər-ās) UDPglucose–hexose-1-phosphate uridylyltransferase.

**ga·lac·tose 1-phos·phate uri·dyl·yl·trans·fer·ase** (gə-lak'tōs fos'fāt u″rĭ-dil″əl-trans'fər-ās) UTP–hexose-1-phosphate uridylyltransferase.

**ga·lac·to·si·al·i·do·sis** (gə-lak″to-si-al″ĭ-do'sis) an autosomal recessive disorder clinically almost indistinguishable from sialidosis, type II (q.v.), but due to deficiency of both sialidase and β-galactosidase. As in sialidosis, multiple variants occur, of increasing severity with decreasing age of onset; congenital, infantile, and juvenile forms have been identified. The defect appears to be in a protein necessary for activation or protection of the two enzymes.

**α-ga·lac·to·si·dase** (gə-lak″to-si′dās) [EC 3.2.1.22] 1. an enzyme of the hydrolase class that catalyzes the cleavage of terminal, nonreducing, α-linked galactose residues from galactosides. 2. α-g. A.
**α-g. A,** a lysosomal enzyme that catalyzes the cleavage of terminal galactose residues from glycosphingolipids, particularly ceramide trihexosides. Deficiency of the enzyme, an X-linked trait, causes accumulation of ceramide trihexosides and other glycosphingolipids in plasma and tissues and results in Fabry's disease. Called also *ceramide trihexosidase* and *α-g.*
**α-g. B,** α-*N*-acetylgalactosaminidase.

**β-ga·lac·to·si·dase** (gə-lak″to-si′dās) [EC 3.2.1.23] any of a group of enzymes of the hydrolase class that catalyze the cleavage of terminal, β-linked, nonreducing galactose residues from a variety of substrates, including ganglioside $GM_1$, lactosylceramides, lactose, and various glycoproteins and oligosaccharides. See also *lactase.* The lysosomal (acid) isozyme catalyzes the hydrolysis of β-galactosides in gangliosides and keratan sulfate, and its catalytic activity with these substrates is differentially impaired in several autosomal recessive disorders caused by allelic mutations. In $GM_1$ gangliosidosis, activity toward ganglioside $GM_1$ is particularly decreased or absent, while in Morquio's syndrome, type B, this activity is normal but activity toward keratan sulfate is decreased.

**ga·lac·to·side** (gə-lak′to-sīd) a glycoside containing galactose.

**gal·ac·to·sis** (gal″ak-to′sis) the formation of milk by the lacteal glands.

**ga·lac·to·sta·sia** (gə-lak″to-sta′shə) galactostasis.

**gal·ac·tos·ta·sis** (gal″ak-tos′tə-sis) [*galacto-* + *-stasis*] 1. cessation of milk secretion. 2. an abnormal collection of milk in the mammary glands.

**ga·lac·tos·uria** (gə-lak″to-su′re-ə) presence of galactose in the urine.

**gal·ac·to·syl** (gal″ak-to′səl) a radical of galactose.

**gal·ac·to·syl·ce·ram·i·dase** (gal″ak-tōs″əl-sə-ram′ĭ-dās) [EC 3.2.1.46] [MeSH: Galactosylceramidase] an enzyme of the hydrolase class that catalyzes the hydrolytic cleavage of galactose from galactocerebrosides to form ceramides, a reaction occurring in the lysosomal degradation of sphingolipids. Deficiency of the enzyme, an autosomal recessive trait, causes Krabbe's disease. Called also *galactocerebroside β-galactosidase.*

**gal·ac·to·syl·cer·a·mide** (gal″ak-tōs″əl-ser′ə-mīd) galactocerebroside.

**gal·ac·to·syl·cer·am·ide β-ga·lac·to·si·dase** (gal″ak-tōs″əl-ser′ə-mīd gə-lak″to-si′dās) galactosylceramidase.

**gal·ac·to·syl·hy·droxy·ly·syl glu·co·syl·trans·fer·ase** (gal″ak-tōs″əl-hi-drok″se-līs′əl gloo″ko-səl-trans′fər-ās) procollagen glucosyltransferase.

**ga·lac·to·syl·trans·fer·ase** (gal″ak-tos″əl-trans′fər-ās) a term used in the trivial and recommended names of some hexosyltransferases [EC 2.4.1] that catalyze the transfer of a galactosyl group from a donor to an acceptor compound.

**ga·lac·to·tox·in** (gə-lak′to-tok″sin) [*galacto-* + *toxin*] a basic substance formed in milk.

**ga·lac·to·tox·ism** (gə-lak′to-tok″siz-əm) poisoning by milk.

**gal·ac·tot·ro·phy** (gal″ak-tot′rə-fe) [*galacto-* + *-trophy*] feeding with milk.

**gal·ac·tox·ism** (gal″ak-tok′siz-əm) galactotoxism.

**ga·lac·tox·is·mus** (gə-lak″tok-siz′məs) galactotoxism.

**gal·ac·tu·ria** (gal″ak-tu′re-ə) [*galact-* + *-uria*] chyluria.

**ga·lac·tu·ron·ic ac·id** (gə-lak″tu-ron′ik) the uronic acid formed by the oxidation of C-6 of galactose to a carboxy group; it occurs in pectins.

**ga·lan·ta·mine hy·dro·bro·mide** (gə-lan′tə-mēn) galanthamine hydrobromide.

**ga·lan·tha·mine hy·dro·bro·mide** (gə-lan′thə-mēn) the hydrobromide salt of an alkaloid obtained in the Caucasus region from the Caucasian snowdrop *Galanthus woronowii* and closely related species. It is a cholinesterase inhibitor and is used in the former USSR in the treatment of myasthenia, myopathy, and sensory and motor dysfunction associated with disorders of the central nervous system and may be used as an antidote to nonpolarizing muscle relaxants. Called also *galantamine hydrobromide.*

**ga·lea** (ga′le-ə) [L. "helmet"] [TA] a general term for a helmetlike structure.
**g. aponeuro′tica** [TA], the aponeurotic structure of the scalp, connecting the frontal and occipital bellies of the occipitofrontalis muscle. Called also *aponeurosis epicranialis* [TA alternative] and *epicranial aponeurosis.*

**Ga·le·a·ti's glands** (gah-la-ah′tēz) [Domenico Gusmano *Galeati,* Italian physician, 1686–1775] glandulae duodenales.

**gal·e·a·tus** (gal″e-a′təs) [L., from *galea* helmet] born with a caul.

**Gal·e·az·zi's fracture, sign** (gah-la-aht′sēz) [Riccardo *Galeazzi,* Italian orthopedic surgeon, 1866–1952] see under *fracture* and *sign.*

**Ga·len** (ga′lən) (c. 129 to c. 200) a Greek physician and teacher, born in Pergamum (Asia Minor), author of 500 books on philosophy, philology, and medicine (83 medical books survive). He was court physician to Marcus Aurelius, a surgeon to gladiators, and a practicing anatomist (he performed vivisections and post mortems on the Barbary ape [*Macaca sylvana*], but not on humans). An eclectic Dogmatist, he revered Hippocrates and Plato and respected Aristotle, but also freely advanced his own findings and opinions. Galen was the great compiler and systemizer of Greco-Roman medicine, physiology, and anatomy. He accepted Aristotelian teleology and the theories of humoralism, the four qualities, and pneumatism, and he promulgated that of the four temperaments (cf. *temperament*). Galen's piety, half-Stoic, half-Christian, appealed strongly to late antiquity and the Middle Ages. By experiment he showed that arteries carried blood, believed the brain to be the seat of intelligence, and understood the diagnostic value of the pulse. His work was superseded by Vesalius in anatomy and by Harvey in physiology.

**Ga·len's nerve (anastomosis),** etc. (ga′lənz) [*Galen*] see *ramus communicans nervi laryngei superioris cum nervo laryngeo inferiore, venae cerebri interni, vena cerebri magna,* and *ventriculus laryngis.*

**ga·len·ic** (gə-len′ik) pertaining to the ancient system of medicine taught and practiced by Galen.

**ga·len·i·ca** (gə-len′ĭ-kə) galenicals.

**ga·len·i·cals** (gə-len′ĭ-kəlz) medicines prepared according to the formulas of Galen; the term is now used to denote standard preparations containing one or several organic ingredients, as contrasted with pure chemical substances.

**ga·len·ics** (gə-len′iks) galenicals.

**Gal·e·o·rhi·nus** (gal″e-o-ri′nəs) a genus of sharks. *G. zyop′terus* is the soupfin shark, whose fin is used by the Chinese for soup and whose liver is a source of shark liver oil.

**ga·leo·pho·bia** (ga″le-o-fo′be-ə) [Gr. *galeē* weasel, cat + *-phobia*] ailurophobia.

**Gal·er·i·na** (gal-ə-ri′nə) a genus of mushrooms of the family Cortinariaceae. They contain amatoxins but cause mushroom poisoning less frequently than *Amanita* species because of being considerably smaller in size.

**gal·er·o·pia** (gal″ər-o′pe-ə) [Gr. *galeros* cheerful + *-opia, -opsia*] abnormal clearness of vision due to a pathologic condition.

**gal·er·op·sia** (gal″ər-op′se-ə) galeropia.

**gall** (gawl) [L. *galla*] 1. bile. 2. nutgall. 3. a localized swelling or skin sore caused by friction.
**Aleppo g.,** nutgall.
**collar g.,** a wound or pressure ulcer on a horse caused by repeated trauma from an ill-fitting harness or collar.
**ox g.,** see *ox bile extract,* under *extract.*
**saddle g.,** a wound or pressure ulcer on a horse caused by repeated trauma from an ill-fitting saddle. Called also *saddle sore.*
**Smyrna g.,** nutgall.
**wind g.,** windgall.

**gal·la·mine tri·eth·io·dide** (gal′ə-mēn tri″ə-thi′o-dīd) [USP] [MeSH: Gallamine Triethiodide] a quaternary ammonium compound used to induce skeletal muscle relaxation during surgery and other procedures, such as endoscopy or intubation, administered intravenously. Called also *benzcurine iodide.*

**gal·late** (gal′āt) any salt of gallic acid.

**gall·blad·der** (gawl′blad″ər) [MeSH: Gallbladder] vesica biliaris.
**Courvoisier's g.,** a distended gallbladder resulting from biliary tract obstruction.
**fish-scale g.,** a gallbladder with a fish-scale–like appearance due to multiple small cysts of the mucosa.
**floating g.,** wandering g.
**folded fundus g.,** phrygian cap.
**hourglass g.,** a gallbladder in which there is an annular constriction dividing it into a wide upper and a narrower lower compartment; the anomaly may be congenital or acquired.
**mobile g.,** wandering g.
**porcelain g.,** diffuse or focal calcification of the gallbladder wall, arising in chronic cholecystitis and frequently associated with the development of carcinoma.
**sandpaper g.,** a rough state of the mucous membrane of the gallbladder caused by the presence of cholesterin crystals.

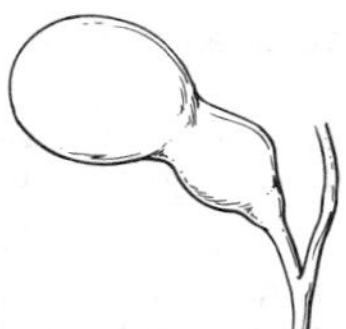
Hourglass gallbladder.

**stasis g.**, a gallbladder that contracts sluggishly in response to a fatty meal.
**strawberry g.**, a gallbladder with a strawberry-like appearance due to fine grains of cholesterin-fat material embedded in the mucosa, seen in cholesterolosis with inflammation.
**wandering g.**, abnormal mobility of the fundus and body of the gallbladder.

**gal·le·in** (gal'ēn) an aniline dye indicator that is changed in color by an alkali to red and by an acid to yellow.

**gal·lic ac·id** (gal'ik) [MeSH: Gallic Acid] 3,4,5-trihydroxybenzoic acid, obtained from nutgalls and formerly used as an astringent.

**gal·lid** (gal'id) [L. *gallus* cock] pertaining to fowl. Cf. *avian*.

**Gal·lie transplant** (gal'e) [William Edward *Gallie*, Canadian surgeon, 1882–1959] see under *transplant*.

**gal·li·um** (gal'e-əm) [L., from *Gallia* Gaul] [MeSH: Gallium] a rare metal liquid at room temperature; atomic number, 31, atomic weight, 69.72; symbol, Ga: some of its compounds are poisonous.
**g. 67,** a radioisotope of gallium, atomic mass 67, having a half-life of 3.26 days and decaying by electron capture and emission of 0.093, 0.184, 0.300, and 0.393 MeV gamma rays; used primarily chelated with citrate; see *g. Ga 67 citrate*.
**g. Ga 67 citrate,** a radiopharmaceutical imaging agent, the citrate salt of $^{67}$Ga; it binds initially to plasma proteins, then localizes primarily in the liver, spleen, bone marrow, and skeleton. It is used to image neoplasms, particularly of soft tissues, and sites of inflammation and abscess.
**g. nitrate,** a hydrated nitrate salt of gallium, a potent inhibitor of bone calcium resorption; administered intravenously to treat cancer-related hypercalcemia.

**gall·nut** (gawl'nət) nutgall.

**gal·lon** (gal'on) [L. *congius*] a measure of volume, four quarts (3785 mL); in the United States, 231 cubic inches.

**gal·lop** (gal'op) a disordered rhythm of the heart; see under *rhythm*.
**atrial g.**, $S_4$ g.
**diastolic g.**, $S_3$ g.
**fourth heart sound g.**, $S_4$ g.
**presystolic g.**, $S_4$ g.
**protodiastolic g.**, an older term for *$S_3$ g.*
**$S_3$ g.**, an accentuated third heart sound detected in patients with cardiac disease characterized by pathologic alterations in ventricular filling in early diastole.
**$S_4$ g.**, an accentuated, audible fourth heart sound usually associated with cardiac disease, often that characterized by altered ventricular compliance.
**summation g.**, a gallop rhythm in which the third and fourth sounds are superimposed, appearing as one loud sound; it may occur in some patients with tachycardia but is usually associated with cardiac disease.
**third heart sound g.**, $S_3$ g.
**ventricular g.**, $S_3$ g.

**gal·lo·tan·nic ac·id** (gal-o-tan'ik) tannic acid.

**gall·sick·ness** (gawl'sik-nəs) anaplasmosis.

**gall·stone** (gawl'stōn) [MeSH: Cholelithiasis] a concretion formed in the gallbladder or bile duct; the usual composition is cholesterol, a blood pigment liberated by hemolysis, or a calcium salt. Called also *biliary calculus* and *cholelith*. See also *cholelithiasis*.
**cholesterol g.**, a gallstone whose main component is cholesterol, most commonly found within the gallbladder.
**pigment g.**, a gallstone whose major component is a bile pigment. Black pigment stones are usually found in the gallbladder and are composed of calcium bilirubinate or pigment polymers, with or without calcium carbonate, calcium phosphate, and mucin; they are hard and often have spicules on the surface. Brown pigment stones are usually found in the common bile duct, are not as hard as black ones, and are composed of calcium bilirubinate and calcium salts of fatty acids, as well as more cholesterol than is found in the black type.

**GalNAc** *N*-acetylgalactosamine.

**GALT** gut-associated lymphoid tissue; see under *tissue*.

**Gal·ton's law of regression** (gawl'tənz) [Sir Francis *Galton*, English anthropologist and biologist, 1822–1911] see under *law*.

**Galv.** galvanic.

**gal·van·ic** (gal-van'ik) 1. named for or discovered by Luigi *Galvani*, Italian physicist and physiologist, 1737–1798. 2. pertaining to galvanism.

**gal·va·nism** (gal'və-niz-əm) [Luigi *Galvani*] 1. galvanic current: unidirectional electric current derived from a chemical battery. 2. the therapeutic use of direct current.
**dental g.**, production of galvanic current in the oral cavity due to the presence of two or more dissimilar metals in dental restorations that are bathed in saliva, or a single metal restoration and two electrolytes, saliva and pulp tissue fluid, thus producing an electrolytic cell and an electric current. When such restorations touch each other, the current may be high enough to irritate the dental pulp and cause sharp pain. The anodic restoration or areas of a restoration are subject to electrolytic corrosion.

**gal·va·ni·za·tion** (gal″və-nĭ-za'shən) treatment by galvanic current.

**gal·va·no·con·trac·til·i·ty** (gal″və-no-kon″trak-til'ĭ-te) contractility in response to a galvanic stimulus.

**gal·va·no·gus·tom·e·ter** (gal″və-no-gəs-tom'ə-tər) an apparatus for the clinical determination of taste thresholds by the use of a galvanic current.

**gal·va·nom·e·ter** (gal″və-nom'ə-tər) [*galvanism* + *-meter*] an instrument for measuring current by electromagnetic action.
**Einthoven's g., string g., thread g.,** *(obs.)*, a forerunner of the electrocardiograph, consisting of a delicate thread of silvered quartz or platinum stretched between the poles of a strong magnet; the thread is displaced by an electric current flowing through it in proportion to the strength of the current.

**gal·va·no·pal·pa·tion** (gal″və-no-pal-pa'shən) a method of testing the sensory and vasomotor nerves of the skin by applying a sharp-pointed anode electrode to the part of the skin to be tested, the cathode being applied to some other part of the body.

**gal·va·no·tax·is** (gal″və-no-tak'sis) the tendency of an organism to arrange itself in a medium so that its axis bears a certain relation to the direction of the current in the medium.

**gal·va·no·ther·a·py** (gal″və-no-ther'ə-pe) the therapeutic use of galvanic current.

**gal·va·not·rop·ism** (gal″və-not'ro-piz-əm) [*galvanism* + *-tropism*] the tendency of an organism to turn or move under the action of an electric current.

**Gam·a·stan** (gam'ə-stan″) trademark for a preparation of immune human serum globulin.

**Gam·bi·an horse sickness, trypanosomiasis (sleeping sickness)** (gam'be-ən) [*Gambia*, West Africa] see under *sickness* and *trypanosomiasis*.

**gam·bir** (gam'bēr) the dried aqueous, astringent extract from the leaves and twigs of the shrub *Uncaria gambier;* its main constituents are catechin, catechutannic acid, and quercetin. Formerly used as an antidiarrheal and as a gargle for sore throat. Called also *catechu* or *pale catechu*.

**gam·bling** (gam'bling) [MeSH: Gambling] betting money or other valuables on the outcome of a game or event.
**pathological g.** [DSM-IV], an impulse control disorder consisting of persistent failure to resist the urge to gamble, to such an extent that personal, family, and vocational life are seriously disrupted.

**Gam·bu·sia** (gam-boo'se-ə) a genus of fish effective in destroying mosquito larvae.
**G. affi'nis**, a top minnow that has been introduced into every major malarious region in the world; it feeds upon the larvae of *Anopheles* mosquitoes along the surface of the water.

**ga·me·far** (gah'mə-fahr) pamaquine.

**gam·e·tan·gi·um** (gam″ə-tan'je-əm) pl. *gametan'gia* [*gamet-* + Gr. *angeion* vessel] the structure in which zygospores are developed. See also*zygophore*.

**gam·ete** (gam'ēt) [Gr. *gametē* wife, *gametēs* husband] 1. a haploid reproductive cell (oocyte or spermatozoon), whose union is necessary in sexual reproduction to initiate the development of a new individual. 2. the malarial parasite in its sexual form in the gut of the mosquito vector, either male *(microgamete)* or female *(macrogamete)*; the latter fertilizes the former to develop into an ookinete.

**ga·met·ic** (gə-met'ik) pertaining to gametes or to primordial sexual elements.

**gamet(o)-** [Gr. *gametē* wife, *gametēs* husband] a combining form denoting relationship to a gamete.

**ga·me·to·ci·dal** (gə-me″to-si'dəl) capable of destroying gametes or gametocytes.

**ga·me·to·cide** (gə-me'to-sīd) [*gameto-* + *-cide*] an agent that destroys gametes or gametocytes.

**ga·me·to·cyte** (gə-me'to-sīt) [*gameto-* + *cyte*] 1. a cell capable of dividing to form gametes; an oocyte or spermatocyte. 2. gamont.

**ga·me·to·cy·te·mia** (gə-me"to-si-te'me-ə) the presence of malarial gametocytes in the blood.

**gam·e·to·gen·e·sis** (gam"ə-to-jen'ə-sis) [*gameto-* + *-genesis*] [MeSH: Gametogenesis] the development of the male and female sex cells, or gametes.

**gam·e·to·gen·ic** (gam"ə-to-jen'ik) producing or favoring the production of germ cells.

**gam·e·tog·o·ny** (gam"ə-tog'ə-ne) 1. the development of merozoites of malarial plasmodia and other sporozoa into male and female gametes, which later fuse to form a zygote; called also *gamogony.* 2. reproduction by means of gametes.

**gam·e·toid** (gam'ə-toid) resembling gametes or reproductive cells.

**gam·e·to·ki·net·ic** (gam"ə-to-kĭ-net'ik) [*gameto-* + *kinetic*] stimulating gamete action.

**gam·e·to·pha·gia** (gam"ə-to-fa'jə) gamophagia.

**gam·e·to·phyte** (gam'ə-to-fīt) [*gameto-* + *-phyte*] the haploid or sexual stage in organisms having alternation of generations (metagenesis); it may be female (megagametophyte) or male (microgametophyte).

**Gam·gee tissue** (gam'je) [Joseph Sampson *Gamgee,* British surgeon, 1828–1886] see under *tissue.*

**gam·ic** (gam'ik) sexual; applied to eggs that develop only after fertilization.

**Gam·i·mune N** (gam'ĭ-mūn) trademark for a preparation of immune globulin for intravenous use.

**gam·ma** (gam'ə) [Γ, γ] 1. the third letter of the Greek alphabet. See also *γ-*. 2. an obsolete equivalent for microgram.

**gam·ma-ami·no·bu·tyr·ic ac·id** (gam'ə-ə-me"no-bu-tir'ik) γ-aminobutyric acid; see under *A.*

**gam·ma ben·zene hex·a·chlo·ride** (gam"ə-ben'zēn hek"sə-klor'īd) [MeSH: Lindane] lindane.

**gam·ma·cism** (gam'ə-siz-əm) [*gamma* + *-ism*] a speech disorder involving deficient pronunciation of velar speech sounds such as *g* and *k.* Called also *paragammacism.*

**Gam·ma·gard** (gam'ə-gahrd) trademark for a preparation of immune globulin.

**gam·ma glob·u·lin** (gam"ə glob'u-lin) [MeSH: Gamma-Globulins] see under *globulin.*

**gam·ma·glob·u·li·nop·a·thy** (gam"ə-glob"u-lin-op'ə-the) any gammopathy.

**gam·ma·gram** (gam'ə-gram) a graphic record of the gamma rays emitted by an object or substance.

**Gam·ma·her·pes·vi·ri·nae** (gam"ə-hər"pēz-vir-i'ne) [MeSH: Gammaherpesvirinae] the lymphocyte-associated viruses: a subfamily of the Herpesviridae, members of which are specific for either B- or T-lymphocytes; it contains the genera *Lymphocryptovirus* and *Rhadinovirus* and a large number of unassigned species.

**gam·ma-lac·tone** (gam"ə-lak'tōn) a compound having a five-membered ring structure formed by internal reaction of a carboxylic acid group with a hydroxyl group on the gamma carbon of a carbon chain.

**Gam·mar-P** (gam'ahr) trademark for a preparation of human immune globulin.

**gam·ma-pip·ra·dol** (gam"ə-pip'rə-dol) azacyclonol.

**gam·mop·a·thy** (gam-op'ə-the) [*gamma* globulin + *-pathy*] a condition marked by disturbed immunoglobulin synthesis.
**monoclonal g's,** plasma cell dyscrasias.
**monoclonal g., benign,** the presence of a serum M component without signs or symptoms of multiple myeloma, Waldenström's macroglobulinemia, or other plasma cell neoplasms; it occurs in about 3 per cent of the population over age 70. A few patients eventually develop a malignant plasma cell dyscrasia.

**Gam·na's disease** (gahm'nəz) [Carlo *Gamna,* Italian physician, 1896–1950] see under *disease.*

**gam(o)-** [Gr. *gamos* marriage] a combining form denoting relationship to marriage or sexual union.

**gamo·gen·e·sis** (gam"o-jen'ə-sis) [*gamo-* + *-genesis*] sexual reproduction.

**gamo·ge·net·ic** (gam"o-jə-net'ik) pertaining to or exhibiting sexual reproduction.

**gam·og·o·ny** (gam-og'ə-ne) gametogony, def. 1.

**gam·one** (gam'ōn) 1. a sex hormone released by certain plants. 2. a hypothetical substance in animals presumed to be released by the ovum and spermatozoon to facilitate their fusion.

**gam·ont** (gam'ont) [*gam-* + Gr. *ōn* being] the sexual (gametic) stage in the sporozoan life cycle, produced by gamogony from a trophozoite or a merozoite. Called also *gametocyte.*

**gamo·pha·gia** (gam"o-fa'jə) [*gamo-* + *-phagia*] the disappearance of the male or female element in the conjugation of unicellular organisms.

**gamp·so·dac·ty·ly** (gamp"so-dak'tə-le) [Gr. *gampsos* crooked + *daktylos* digit] deformity of the toes marked by hyperextension of the first phalanx on the metatarsal and flexion of the other two phalanges; called also *clawfoot.*

**Gam·storp's disease** (gahm'storps) [Ingrid *Gamstorp,* Swedish pediatrician, born 1924] familial periodic paralysis II.

**Gam·u·lin Rh** (gam'u-lin) trademark for a preparation of $Rh_O$(D) immune serum globulin.

**gan·ci·clo·vir** (gan-si'klo-vir) [MeSH: Ganciclovir] 3,4-dihydroxyphenylglycol (DHPG), a derivative of acyclovir with in vitro activity against human herpesviruses; used for the treatment of cytomegalovirus infections; administered orally and by intravitreal implant.
**g. sodium,** the monosodium salt of ganciclovir, used for the treatment of cytomegalovirus retinitis in immunocompromised patients; administered intravenously.

**gan·glia** (gang'gle-ə) [Gr.] [MeSH: Ganglia] plural of *ganglion.*

**gan·gli·al** (gang'gle-əl) pertaining to a ganglion.

**gan·gli·at·ed** (gang'gle-āt"əd) ganglionated.

**gan·gli·ec·to·my** (gang"gle-ek'tə-me) ganglionectomy.

**gan·gli·form** (gang'glĭ-form) having the form of a ganglion.

**gan·gli·itis** (gang"gle-i'tis) ganglionitis.

**gangli(o)-** [Gr. *ganglion,* q.v.] a combining form denoting relationship to a ganglion.

**gan·glio·blast** (gang'gle-o-blast) [*ganglio-* + *-blast*] an embryonic cell of the cerebrospinal ganglia.

**gan·glio·cyte** (gang'gle-o-sīt) [*ganglio-* + *-cyte*] a ganglion cell.

**gan·glio·cy·to·ma** (gang"gle-o-si-to'mə) ganglioneuroma.

**gan·glio·form** (gang'gle-o-form") gangliform.

**gan·glio·gli·o·ma** (gang"gle-o-gli-o'mə) [MeSH: Ganglioglioma] a ganglioneuroma in the central nervous system; called also *ganglioglioneuroma* and *neuroglioma ganglionare.*

**gan·glio·glio·neu·ro·ma** (gang"gle-o-gli"o-noo͝-ro'mə) ganglioneuroma.

**gan·glio·lyt·ic** (gang"gle-o-lit'ik) ganglioplegic.

**gan·gli·o·ma** (gang"gle-o'mə) [*gangli-* + *-oma*] ganglioneuroma.

**gan·gli·on** (gang'gle-on) pl. *gang'lia* or *ganglions* [Gr. "knot"] 1. a knot, or knotlike mass. 2. [TA] a general term for a group of nerve cell bodies located outside the central nervous system; occasionally applied to certain nuclear groups within the brain or spinal cord, e.g., basal ganglia. 3. a benign cystic tumor occurring on an aponeurosis or tendon, as in the wrist or dorsum of the foot; it consists of a thin fibrous capsule enclosing a clear mucinous fluid.

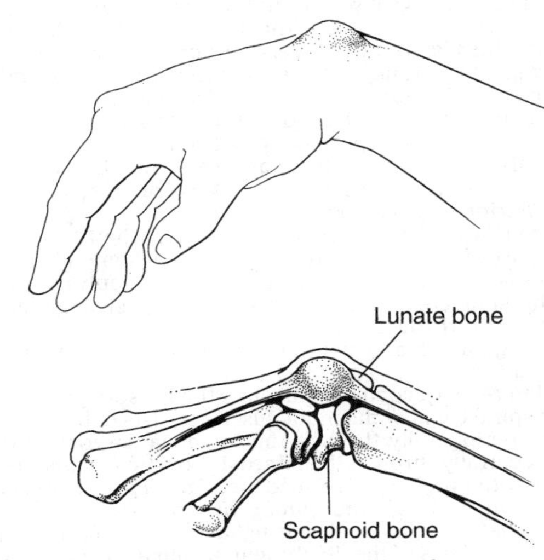

Ganglion of wrist arising from a tendon.

## Ganglion

Descriptions of specific anatomic structures are given on TA terms, and include anglicized names of specific ganglia.

**aberrant g.,** a small ganglion sometimes found on a dorsal cervical nerve root between the spinal ganglia and the spinal cord.

**accessory ganglia,** ganglia intermedia.

**acousticofacial g.,** a ganglion of early embryonic life, a portion of which persists as the geniculate ganglion.

**Acrel's g.,** a cystic tumor on an extensor tendon of the wrist.

**Andersch's g.,** g. caudalis nervi glossopharyngei.

**ganglia aorticorena'lia** [TA], aorticorenal ganglia: a more or less detached inferolateral extension of the celiac ganglion.

**auditory g.,** 1. g. cochleare. 2. (in pl.) nuclei cochleares.

**Auerbach's g.,** any of the small ganglia of Auerbach's plexus.

**g. autono'micum** [TA], autonomic ganglion: the ganglia found along the sympathetic trunks, on the peripheral plexuses, and within the walls of organs supplied by the autonomic nervous system; they are divided into two structurally similar groups, the sympathetic ganglia and the parasympathetic ganglia. Called also *visceral g.* and *g. viscerale.*

**ganglia of autonomic plexuses,** ganglia plexuum autonomicorum.

**basal ganglia,** see under *nucleus.*

**Bezold's g.,** a series of ganglion cells in the interatrial septum.

**Bidder's ganglia,** ganglia on the cardiac nerves, situated at the lower end of the atrial septum. Called also *ventricular ganglia.*

**Blandin's g.,** g. submandibulare.

**Bochdalek's g.,** plexus dentalis superior.

**Bock's g.,** carotid g.

**gan'glia cardi'aca** [TA], cardiac ganglia: ganglia of the cardiac plexus near the arterial ligament; called also *Wrisberg's ganglia.*

**carotid g.,** a ganglion of the internal carotid plexus in the cavernous sinus; called also *Bock's g.*

**caudal g. of glossopharyngeal nerve,** g. inferius nervi glossopharyngei.

**caudal g. of vagus nerve,** g. inferius nervi vagi.

**g. cauda'lis ner'vi glossopharyn'gei,** g. inferius nervi glossopharyngei.

**g. cauda'lis ner'vi va'gi,** g. inferius nervi vagi.

**celiac ganglia, gan'glia celi'aca,** ganglia coeliaca.

**cerebrospinal ganglia,** the ganglia associated with the cranial and spinal nerves.

**cervical g., inferior,** ganglion cervicale inferioris.

**cervical g., middle,** g. cervicale medium.

**cervical g., superior,** g. cervicale superius.

**cervical g. of uterus,** a ganglion situated near the cervix uteri; called also *Lee's g.* and *Frankenhäuser's g.*

**g. cervica'le inferio'ris** [TA], inferior cervical ganglion: an inconstant ganglion formed in place of the usual cervicothoracic ganglion by fusion of the lower two cervical ganglia in instances where the first thoracic ganglion remains separate.

**g. cervica'le me'dium** [TA], middle cervical ganglion: a variable ganglion, often fused with the vertebral ganglion, on the sympathetic trunk at about the level of the cricoid cartilage; its postganglionic fibers are distributed mainly to the heart, cervical region, and upper limb.

**g. cervica'le supe'rius** [TA], superior cervical ganglion: the uppermost ganglion on the sympathetic trunk, lying behind the internal carotid artery and in front of the second and third cervical vertebrae; it gives rise to postganglionic fibers to the heart via cervical cardiac nerves, to the pharyngeal plexus and thence to the larynx and pharynx, and to the head via the external and internal carotid plexuses.

**g. cervicothora'cicum** [TA], cervicothoracic ganglion: a ganglion on the sympathetic trunk at the level of the 7th cervical and 1st thoracic vertebrae, anterior to the 8th cervical and 1st thoracic nerves; it has two components, the inferior cervical and first thoracic ganglia, which are usually fused, partially or completely. Its postganglionic fibers are distributed to the head and neck, heart, and upper limb. Called also *stellate g.* and *g. stellatum* [TA alternative].

**cervicouterine g.,** cervical g. of uterus.

**g. cilia're** [TA], ciliary ganglion: a parasympathetic ganglion in the posterior part of the orbit; it receives preganglionic fibers from the oculomotor nerve, and its postganglionic fibers supply the ciliary muscle and the sphincter pupillae. Sensory and postganglionic sympathetic fibers pass through the ganglion.

**Cloquet's g.,** an enlargement of the nasopalatine nerve in the anterior palatine canal.

**g. cochlea're** [TA], cochlear ganglion: the sensory ganglion located within the spiral canal of the modiolus. It consists of bipolar cells that send fibers peripherally through the foramina nervosa to the spiral organ and centrally through the internal acoustic meatus to the cochlear nuclei of the brain stem. Called also *Corti's g., g. spirale cochleae* [TA alternative], *spiral g.,* and *spiral g. of cochlea.*

**gan'glia coelia'ca** [TA], celiac ganglia: two irregularly shaped ganglia, one on each crus of the diaphragm, within the celiac plexus; each contains sympathetic nerve cells and preganglionic sympathetic fibers from the greater and lesser splanchnic nerves: preganglionic parasympathetic and sensory fibers pass through the ganglia. Called also *ganglia celiaca.*

**collateral ganglia,** prevertebral ganglia.

**compound g.,** a cystic tumor of a tendon sheath that has been compressed into two parts by a ligament.

**Corti's g.,** g. cochleare.

**cranial sensory g.,** g. sensorium nervi cranialis.

**g. craniospina'le senso'rium** [TA], craniospinal sensory ganglion: the ganglia sensoria nervorum spinalium and the ganglia sensoria nervorum cranialium considered together.

**diffuse g.,** a swelling of several adjoining tendon sheaths due to inflammatory effusion.

**dorsal root g.,** g. sensorium nervi spinalis.

**Ehrenritter's g.,** g. superius nervi glossopharyngei.

**gan'glia encepha'lica,** g. sensorium nervi cranialis.

**encephalospinal g., g. encephalospina'le,** g.craniospinale sensorium.

**false g.,** an enlargement on a nerve that does not have a true ganglionic structure.

**first thoracic g.,** a portion of the ganglion cervicothoracicum, present sometimes as a separate ganglion.

**Frankenhäuser's g.,** cervical g. of uterus.

**Froriep's g.,** the ganglion of the lowest occipital segment in the human embryo.

**Gasser's g., gasserian g.,** g. trigeminale.

**geniculate g.,** g. geniculi nervi facialis.

**g. genicula'tum ner'vi facia'lis,** TA alternative for *g. geniculi nervi facialis.*

**g. geni'culi ner'vi facia'lis** [TA], the sensory ganglion of the facial nerve, situated on the geniculum nervi facialis. Called also *geniculate g.* and *g. geniculatum nervi facialis* [TA alternative].

**glossopharyngeal ganglia, ganglia of glossopharyngeal nerve,** see *g. inferius nervi glossopharyngei* and *g. superius nervi glossopharyngei.*

**hepatic g.,** a ganglion situated near the hepatic artery.

**hypogastric ganglia,** ganglia pelvica.

**hypoglossal g.,** a ganglion of the hypoglossal nerve; rarely found in humans except in the embryo.

**g. im'par** [TA], the ganglion commonly found in front of the coccyx, where the sympathetic trunks of the two sides unite.

**inferior g. of glossopharyngeal nerve,** g. inferius nervi glossopharyngei.

**inferior g. of vagus nerve,** g. inferius nervi vagi.

**g. infe'rius ner'vi glossopharyn'gei** [TA], inferior ganglion of glossopharyngeal nerve: the lower of two ganglia on the glossopharyngeal nerve as it passes through the jugular foramen; it contains cell bodies for some of the afferent fibers of the nerve. See also *g. superius nervi glossopharyngei.* Called also *g. caudalis nervi glossopharyngei, caudal g. of glossopharyngeal nerve, inferior petrosal g., petrosal g.,* and *petrous g.*

**g. infe'rius ner'vi va'gi** [TA], inferior ganglion of vagus nerve: a ganglion of the vagus nerve just below the jugular foramen, in front of the transverse processes of the first and second cervical vertebrae; it contains cell bodies for some of the afferent fibers of the nerve. Called also *caudal g. of vagus nerve, g. caudalis nervi vagi,* and *nodose g.* See also *g. superius nervi vagi.*

**inhibitory g.,** any ganglion performing an inhibitory function.

**gan'glia interme'dia** [TA], intermediate ganglia: small groups of sympathetic nerve cells present on spinal nerves and on rami communicantes, especially in the cervical, lower thoracic, and upper lumbar regions; called also *accessory ganglia.*

**jugular g. of glossopharyngeal nerve,** g. superius nervi glossopharyngei.

**jugular g. of vagus nerve,** g. superius nervi vagi.

**Küttner's g.,** nodus lymphoideus jugulodigastricus.

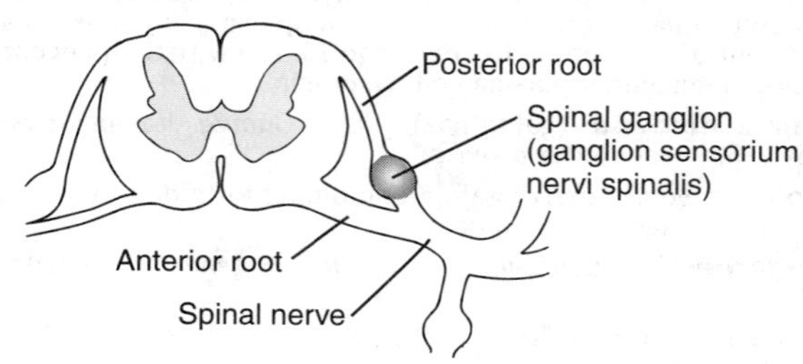


Ganglion sensorium nervi spinalis (spinal ganglion), seen in a cross-section of the spinal cord.

**Langley's g.,** a collection of nerve cells in the hilus of the submaxillary gland in some animals.
**Laumonier's g.,** carotid g.
**Lee's g.,** cervical g. of uterus.
**lesser g. of Meckel,** g. submandibulare.
**Lobstein's g.,** g. thoracicus splanchnicum.
**lower g. of glossopharyngeal nerve,** g. inferius nervi glossopharyngei.
**Ludwig's g.,** a ganglion connected with the cardiac plexus and situated near the right atrium of the heart.
**gan'glia lumba'lia** [TA], lumbar ganglia: the ganglia on the lumbar part of the sympathetic trunk, usually four or five on either side. Called also *ganglia lumbaria* [TA alternative].
**gan'glia lumba'ria,** ganglia lumbalia.
**gan'glia lympha'tica,** lymph nodes; see *nodus lymphoideus.*
**Meckel's g.,** g. pterygopalatinum.
**Meissner's g.,** one of the small groups of nerve cells in the submucosal (Meissner's) plexus.
**mesenteric g., inferior,** g. mesentericum inferius.
**mesenteric g., superior,** g. mesentericum superius.
**g. mesente'ricum infe'rius** [TA], inferior mesenteric ganglion: a sympathetic ganglion in the inferior mesenteric plexus near the beginning of the inferior mesenteric artery.
**g. mesente'ricum supe'rius** [TA], superior mesenteric ganglion: one or more sympathetic ganglia at the sides of, or just below, the superior mesenteric artery; commonly fused with the celiac ganglia.
**g. of Müller,** g. superius nervi glossopharyngei.
**nerve g.,** ganglion (def. 2).
**g. ner'vi splanch'nici,** g. thoracicus splanchnicum.
**neural g.,** ganglion (def. 2).
**nodose g.,** g. inferius nervi vagi.
**olfactory g.,** a mass of tissue in the embryo that develops into the olfactory nerves.
**g. o'ticum** [TA], otic ganglion: a parasympathetic ganglion in the infratemporal fossa, medial to the mandibular nerve and just inferior to the foramen ovale: its preganglionic fibers are derived from the glossopharyngeal nerve via the lesser petrosal nerve, and its postganglionic fibers supply the parotid gland. Sensory and postganglionic sympathetic fibers pass through the ganglion.
**parasympathetic g., g. parasympathe'ticum,** g. parasympathicum.
**g. parasympa'thicum** [TA], parasympathetic ganglion: one of the aggregations of cell bodies of primarily cholinergic neurons of the parasympathetic nervous system, located near to or within the wall of the organs being innervated; see also *cholinergic.*
**gan'glia pel'vica** [TA], pelvic ganglia: small sympathetic and parasympathetic ganglia located within the pelvic plexus.
**gan'glia pelvi'na,** ganglia pelvica.
**petrosal g., petrosal g., inferior, petrous g.,** g. inferius nervi glossopharyngei.
**gan'glia phre'nica** [TA], phrenic ganglia: any of various small sympathetic ganglia often found within the phrenic plexus at its junction with the celiac plexus.
**gan'glia plex'uum autonomico'rum,** ganglia of autonomic plexuses: groups of nerve cell bodies found in the autonomic plexuses, composed primarily of sympathetic postganglionic neurons; called also *ganglia of visceral plexuses.*
**gan'glia plex'uum viscera'lium,** ganglia plexuum autonomicorum.
**prevertebral ganglia,** sympathetic ganglia (other than those of the sympathetic trunk) in the prevertebral plexuses of the thorax and abdomen.
**primary g.,** a ganglion on a tendon or aponeurosis that does not follow a local inflammation.
**g. pterygopalati'num** [TA], pterygopalatine ganglion: a parasympathetic ganglion in the pterygopalatine fossa; its preganglionic fibers are derived from the facial nerve via the greater petrosal nerve and the nerve of the pterygopalatine canal. Its postganglionic fibers supply the lacrimal, nasal, and palatine glands; sensory and sympathetic fibers pass through the ganglion. Called also *Meckel's g., sphenomaxillary g.,* and *sphenopalatine g.*
**Remak's g.,** 1. a sympathetic ganglion in the heart wall near the superior vena cava; called also *sinoatrial g.* 2. one of the sympathetic ganglia in the diaphragmatic opening for the inferior vena cava. 3. one of the ganglia in the gastric plexus.
**gan'glia rena'lia** [TA], renal ganglia: small sympathetic ganglia within the renal plexus.
**Ribes' g.,** a small ganglion sometimes seen in the termination of the internal carotid plexus around the anterior communicating artery of the brain.
**rostral g. of glossopharyngeal nerve,** g. superius nervi glossopharyngei.
**rostral g. of vagus nerve,** g. superius nervi vagi.
**g. rostra'lis ner'vi glossopharyn'gei,** g. superius nervi glossopharyngei.
**g. rostra'lis ner'vi va'gi,** g. superius nervi vagi.
**gan'glia sacra'lia** [TA], sacral ganglia: the ganglia of the sacral part of the sympathetic trunk, usually three or four on either side.
**Scarpa's g.,** g. vestibulare.
**Schmiedel's g.,** carotid g.
**semilunar g.,** 1. ganglion trigeminale. 2. (in plural) ganglia coeliaca.
**g. sensoria'le,** sensory g.; see *g. craniospinale sensorium, g. sensorium nervi cranialis,* and *g. sensorium nervi spinalis.*
**g. senso'rium ner'vi crania'lis** [TA], sensory ganglion of cranial nerve: the ganglion found on the root of each cranial nerve, containing the cell bodies of afferent (sensory) neurons. Called also *cranial sensory g.*.
**g. senso'rium ner'vi spina'lis** [TA], spinal ganglion: the ganglion found on the posterior root of each spinal nerve, composed of the unipolar nerve cell bodies of the sensory neurons of the nerve. Called also *g spinale* and *dorsal root g.*
**sensory g.,** see *g. craniospinale sensorium, g. sensorium nervi cranialis,* and *g. sensorium nervi spinalis.*
**sensory g. of cranial nerve, sensory g. of encephalic nerve,** g. sensorium nervi cranialis.
**simple g.,** a cystic tumor in a tendon sheath.
**sinoatrial g.,** Remak's g., def. 1.
**sinus g.,** a group of nerve cells around the junction of the coronary sinus and the right atrium of the heart.
**sphenomaxillary g., sphenopalatine g.,** g. pterygopalatinum.
**spinal g., g. spina'le,** g. sensorium nervi spinalis.
**spiral g., spiral g. of cochlea, spiral g. of cochlear nerve,** g. cochleare.
**g. spira'le coch'leae,** TA alternative for *g. cochleare.*
**splanchnic g., splanchnic thoracic g., g. splanch'nicum,** g. thoracicum splanchnicum.
**stellate g.,** g. cervicothoracicum.
**g. stella'tum,** TA alternative for *g. cervicothoracicum.*
**g. sublingua'le** [TA], sublingual ganglion: a ganglion of nerve cells sometimes found on the fibers passing distally from the submandibular ganglion to the lingual nerve.
**g. submandibula're** [TA], submandibular ganglion: a parasympathetic ganglion located superior to the deep part of the submandibular gland, on the lateral surface of the hyoglossus muscle; its preganglionic fibers are derived from the facial nerve by way of the chorda tympani and lingual nerve, and its postganglionic fibers supply the submandibular and sublingual glands; sensory and postganglionic sympathetic fibers pass through the ganglion.
**superior g. of glossopharyngeal nerve,** g. superius nervi glossopharyngei.
**superior g. of vagus nerve,** g. superius nervi vagi.
**g. supe'rius ner'vi glossopharyn'gei** [TA], superior ganglion of glossopharyngeal nerve: the upper of two ganglia on the glossopharyngeal nerve as it passes through the jugular foramen; it contains cell bodies for some of the afferent fibers of the nerve. Called also *jugular g. of glossopharyngeal nerve, rostral g. of glossopharyngeal nerve,* and *g. rostralis nervi glossopharyngei.* See also *g. inferius nervi glossopharyngei.*
**g. supe'rius ner'vi va'gi** [TA], superior ganglion of vagus nerve: a small ganglion on the vagus nerve in the jugular foramen, giving off a meningeal and an auricular branch and containing cell bodies for some of the afferent fibers of the nerve. Called also *rostral g. of vagus nerve, g. rostralis nervi vagi,* and *jugular g. of vagus nerve.* See also *g. inferius nervi vagi.*
**suprarenal g.,** a small sympathetic ganglion in the suprarenal plexus.
**ganglia of sympathetic trunk,** ganglia trunci sympathetici.
**g. sympathe'ticum, g. sympa'thicum** [TA], sympathetic ganglion: any of the aggregations of cell bodies of primarily adrenergic neurons of the sympathetic nervous system, including the ganglia of the sympathetic trunks, the intermediate ganglia, the prevertebral ganglia, and some ganglionic cells in the autonomic plexuses. See also *adrenergic.*
**synovial g.,** myxoid cyst.
**g. termina'le** [TA], terminal ganglion: a group of nerve cells found along the terminal nerves, medial to the olfactory bulb.
**gan'glia thoraca'lia,** ganglia thoracica.
**gan'glia thora'cica** [TA], thoracic ganglia: the ganglia on the thoracic portion of the sympathetic trunk, about eleven or twelve on either side.
**g. thora'cicum splanch'nicum** [TA], splanchnic thoracic ganglion: a small ganglion formed on the greater thoracic splanchnic nerve near the twelfth thoracic vertebra; called also *ganglion splanchnicum* and *splanchnic g.*
**g. of trigeminal nerve, g. trigemina'le** [TA], trigeminal ganglion: a ganglion on the sensory root of the fifth cranial nerve, situated in a cleft within the dura mater (trigeminal cave) on the anterior surface of the petrous portion of the temporal bone, and giving off the ophthalmic and maxillary and part of the mandibular nerve; it contains

the cells of origin of most of the sensory fibers of the trigeminal nerve. Called also *Gasser's g., gasserian g.,* and *semilunar g.*
**Troisier's g.,** signal node.
**gan'glia trun'ci sympathe'tici, gan'glia trun'ci sympa'thici** [TA], ganglia of sympathetic trunk: sympathetic ganglia that are arranged in a chainlike fashion along each sympathetic trunk, about twenty to twenty-three on either side.
**tympanic g.,** intumescentia tympanica.
**tympanic g. of Valentin,** 1. a ganglion on a superior dental nerve. 2. intumescentia tympanica.
**g. tympa'nicum,** TA alternative for *intumescentia tympanica.*
**vagal g., inferior,** g. inferius nervi vagi.
**vagal g., superior,** g. superius nervi vagi.
**Valentin's g.,** 1. intumescentia tympanica. 2. a ganglion on a superior dental nerve.
**ventricular ganglia,** Bidder's ganglia.
**g. vertebra'le** [TA], vertebral ganglion: a small ganglion almost always present between the middle and inferior sympathetic ganglion, usually anterior to the vertebral artery; it contributes to the ansa subclavia and sends postganglionic fibers to the vertebral nerve and plexus and to the brachial plexus.
**g. vestibula're** [TA], vestibular ganglion: the sensory ganglion located in the upper part of the lateral end of the internal acoustic meatus, the bipolar nerve cells of which give rise to the fibers of the vestibular nerve.
**visceral g., g. viscera'le,** g. autonomicum.
**ganglia of visceral plexuses,** ganglia plexuum autonomicorum.
**Wrisberg's ganglia,** ganglia cardiaca.
**wrist g.,** cystic enlargement of a tendon sheath on the back of the wrist.

**gan·gli·on·at·ed** (gang'gle-ə-nāt″əd) provided with ganglia. Called also gangliated.

**gan·gli·on·ec·to·my** (gang″gle-ə-nek'tə-me) [*ganglion* + *-ectomy*] [MeSH: Ganglionectomy] excision of a ganglion. Called also *gangliectomy.*

**gan·glio·neu·ro·blas·to·ma** (gang″gle-o-noor″o-blas-to'mə) [MeSH: Ganglioneuroblastoma] a tumor with elements of both ganglioneuroma and neuroblastoma; regarded as a partially differentiated neuroblastoma.

**gan·glio·neu·ro·fi·bro·ma** (gang″gle-o-noor″o-fi-bro'mə) a ganglioneuroma outside of the central nervous system.

**gan·glio·neu·ro·ma** (gang″gle-o-noo͝-ro'mə) [MeSH: Ganglioneuroma] a benign neoplasm composed of nerve fibers and mature ganglion cells; regarded by many as a fully differentiated neuroblastoma. Called also *gangliocytoma, ganglioma, neurocytoma,* and *ganglionar, ganglionated,* or *ganglionic neuroma.* See also *ganglioglioma* and *ganglioneurofibroma.*

**gan·gli·on·ic** (gang″gle-on'ik) pertaining to a ganglion.

**gan·gli·on·itis** (gang″gle-ə-ni'tis) inflammation of a ganglion.
**acute posterior g.,** herpes zoster.
**gasserian g.,** herpes zoster ophthalmicus.

**gan·gli·ono·pleg·ic** (gang″gle-on″o-ple'jik) ganglioplegic.

**gan·gli·on·os·to·my** (gang″gle-ə-nos'tə-me) [*ganglion* + *-ostomy*] surgical creation of an opening into a cystic tumor on a tendon sheath or aponeurosis.

**gan·glio·pleg·ic** (gang″gle-o-ple'jik) [*ganglio-* + Gr. *plēgē* stroke] 1. referring to drugs or other agents that block transmission of impulses through the sympathetic and parasympathetic ganglia. 2. an agent with ganglioplegic activity.

**gan·glio·side** (gang'gle-o-sīd) any of a group of glycosphingolipids in which the polar head group on ceramide is a sialic acid–containing oligosaccharide linked via a glucose residue; they occur predominantly in tissues of the central nervous system. The most basic core structure is ceramide-glucose-galactose-*N*-acetylneuraminic acid.
**g. $G_{M1}$,** a ganglioside structurally similar to ganglioside $GM_2$ but with an additional galactose residue linked to the *N*-acetylgalactosamine residue of $GM_2$; it accumulates abnormally in tissues in $GM_1$ gangliosidoses.
**g. $G_{M2}$,** a ganglioside containing an *N*-acetylgalactosamine residue linked to the galactose of the core structure; it accumulates abnormally in tissues in $GM_2$ gangliosidoses.

**gan·glio·side si·al·i·dase** (gang'gle-o-sīd″ si-al'ĭ-dās) sialidase, def. 2.

**gan·gli·o·si·do·sis** (gang″gle-o-si-do'sis) pl. *gangliosido'ses.* Any of a group of lysosomal storage diseases generally characterized by abnormal accumulation of ganglioside $GM_1$ or $GM_2$ and related glycoconjugates due to a deficiency of specific lysosomal hydrolases, and by progressive psychomotor deterioration usually beginning in infancy or childhood and usually fatal. Two subgroups exist ($GM_1$ and $GM_2$), each having several forms of varying severity.
**generalized g.,** $GM_1$ g., usually specifically the infantile form.
**$GM_1$ g.,** an autosomal recessive disorder due to a deficiency of lysosomal *β*-galactosidase activity, with accumulation of ganglioside $GM_1$, glycoproteins, and keratan sulfate; it occurs as several forms, decreasing in severity with increasing age of onset. The *infantile,* or *type I,* form is characterized by onset at birth, severe retardation of mental and motor development, cerebral degeneration, dysostosis multiplex, hepatosplenomegaly, early blindness, coarse facies, edema, seizures, hypotonia, hyperacusis, dysarthria, and sometimes cherry-red macular spot; death occurs by the age of 2. The *juvenile,* or *type II,* form is characterized by onset between 6 and 20 months, accumulation of ganglioside $GM_1$ in brain but not viscera, seizures, late blindness, spasticity, and ataxia; death occurs between 3 and 10 years of age. The *adult,* or *type III,* form is characterized by onset in the teens, spasticity, and dysarthria, with little intellectual impairment and survival into the third decade.
**$GM_2$ g.,** 1. a lysosomal storage disease characterized by abnormal accumulation of ganglioside $GM_2$ and related glycoconjugates due to a deficiency of activity of specific hexosaminidase isozymes; it occurs as three clinically similar but biochemically distinct variants named for the isozyme still present in the tissues of those affected. 2. $GM_2$ g., variant B.
**$GM_2$ g., type I,** the infantile form of *$GM_2$ g., variant B.*
**$GM_2$ g., type II,** $GM_2$ g., variant 0 (Sandhoff's disease).
**$GM_2$ g., type III,** the juvenile form of *$GM_2$ g., variant B.*
**$GM_2$ g., variant 0,** the $GM_2$ gangliosidosis occurring when activity of both hexosaminidase A and B isozymes is decreased or absent, due to a defect in the *β* chain of the enzyme; it is generally called *Sandhoff's disease.*
**$GM_2$ g., variant AB,** the $GM_2$ gangliosidosis occurring when a sphingolipid activator protein, SAP-2, necessary for hexosaminidase A and B activity is absent; it is clinically identical to $GM_2$ gangliosidoses, variants B and 0.
**$GM_2$ g., variant B,** the $GM_2$ gangliosidosis occurring when hexosaminidase A activity is decreased or absent, due to a defect in the *α* chain of the enzyme, but hexosaminidase B activity is retained. Several forms exist, grouped by age of onset; at least some may be allelic. Tay-Sachs disease (q.v.) is the term usually used to denote the *infantile* (or *type I*) form; *juvenile* (or *type III*), *chronic,* and *adult* forms show progressively less neurologic and muscular involvement, greater heterogeneity, and longer survival time with later onset.

**gan·glio·spore** (gang'gle-o-spor″) [*ganglion* + *spore*] a type of aleuriospore developed from the swollen tip of a hypha.

**gan·glio·sym·pa·thec·to·my** (gang″le-o-sim″pə-thek'tə-me) excision of a sympathetic ganglion.

**gan·grene** (gang'grēn) [L. *gangraena;* Gr. *gangraina* an eating sore, which ends in mortification] [MeSH: Gangrene] death of tissue, usually in considerable mass and generally associated with loss of vascular (nutritive) supply and followed by bacterial invasion and putrefaction. Cf. *necrosis* and *necrobiosis.*
**atherosclerotic g.,** dry gangrene caused by vascular sclerosis.
**circumscribed g.,** gangrene that is clearly separated from normal tissue by a zone of inflammatory reaction.
**cold g.,** gangrene that is not preceded by inflammation.
**diabetic g.,** moist gangrene, usually of the feet, in persons with diabetes mellitus, due to neuropathy, angiopathy, and other complications. Cf. *diabetic ulcer.*
**dry g.,** necrosis occurring without subsequent bacterial decomposition, the tissues becoming dry and shriveled.
**embolic g.,** that which follows the blocking of the blood supply by an embolism.
**emphysematous g.,** gas g.
**epidemic g.,** ergotism.
**Fournier's g.,** an acute gangrenous type of necrotizing fasciitis of

the scrotum, penis, or perineum involving gram-positive organisms, enteric bacilli, or anaerobes; it may occur following local trauma, operative procedures, an underlying urinary tract disease, or a distant acute inflammatory process. Called also *Fournier's disease.*
**gas g., gaseous g.,** an acute, severe, and painful condition in humans and other animals, often resulting from dirty, lacerated wounds in which the muscles and subcutaneous tissues become filled with gas and a serosanguineous exudate. The condition is due to histotoxic infection by anaerobic bacteria, among which are *Clostridium perfringens, C. novyi, C. septicum, C. sporogenes,* and other species of *Clostridium.* Related conditions in domesticated animals are malignant edema, blackleg, and braxy. Called also *clostridial myonecrosis.*
**hot g.,** gangrene that follows an inflammation.
**humid g.,** moist g.
**inflammatory g.,** gangrene due to acute inflammation.
**Meleney's g.,** see under *ulcer.*
**Meleney's synergistic g.,** progressive synergistic g.
**mephitic g.,** gas g.
**moist g.,** necrosis of tissues, with proteolytic decomposition resulting from bacterial action.
**periosteal g.,** periostitis albuminosa.
**pressure g.,** gangrene due to pressure, as in decubitus ulcer.
**primary g.,** gangrene without preceding inflammation of the part.
**progressive g.,** gangrene in which an effective limiting zone of inflammatory reaction does not form.
**progressive bacterial synergistic g., progressive synergistic g., progressive synergistic bacterial g.,** gangrene of the skin due to a mixed synergistic infection by aerobic hemolytic *Staphylococcus aureus,* a microaerophilic nonhemolytic streptococcus, or gram-negative rods, seen as a complication of abdominal or thoracic surgery or a traumatic wound. The characteristic lesion is a wide area of pale red cellulitis that later ulcerates and enlarges to form an ulcerative plaque with central granulation surrounded by gangrenous skin that is in turn surrounded by an undermined, rolled, purplish border. See also *Meleney's ulcer* (def. 1). Called also *burrowing phagedenic ulcer, Meleney's ulcer, Meleney's synergistic g.,* and *undermining burrowing ulcer.*
**pulp g.,** gangrenous pulp necrosis.
**Raynaud's g.,** Raynaud's disease (def. 1).
**secondary g.,** a form that follows local inflammation.
**senile g.,** dry gangrene affecting the extremities of the elderly.
**static g.,** gangrene that results from stasis of blood in a part.
**symmetric g.,** gangrene of corresponding digits on both sides, due to vasomotor disturbances.
**sympathetic g.,** gangrene that results from some primary condition.
**thrombotic g.,** gangrene from thrombosis of an artery.
**traumatic g.,** gangrene that occurs as a consequence of accidental injury.
**trophic g.,** gangrene due to lesion of the trophic nerve supply of a part.
**venous g.,** static g.

**gan·gre·no·sis** (gang″rə-no′sis) the development of gangrene.

**gan·gre·nous** (gang′rə-nəs) pertaining to, characterized by, or of the nature of gangrene.

**Gan·ite** (gan′īt) trademark for a preparation of gallium nitrate.

**gan·o·blast** (gan′o-blast) ameloblast.

**Gan·ser's commissure, syndrome** (gahn′sərz) [Sigbert Joseph Maria *Ganser,* German psychiatrist, 1853–1931] see under *syndrome,* and see *supraoptic commissures,* under *commissure.*

**Gan·ta·nol** (gan′tə-nol) trademark for preparations of sulfamethoxazole.

**Gan·tri·sin** (gan′trĭ-sin) trademark for preparations of sulfisoxazole.

**gap** (gap) 1. hiatus. 2. an unoccupied interval in time.
**air-bone g.,** the lag between the audiographic curves for air- and bone-conducted stimuli, as an indication of a conductive hearing loss.
**anion g.,** the concentration of plasma anions not routinely measured by laboratory screening, accounting for the difference between the routinely measured anions and cations and equal to the plasma sodium − (chloride + bicarbonate); used in the evaluation of acid-base disorders.
**auscultatory g.,** time in which sound is not heard in the auscultatory method of sphygmomanometry, occurring particularly in hypertension and in aortic stenosis.
**Bochdalek's g.,** hiatus pleuroperitonealis.
**chromatid g.,** a nonstaining region in a chromatid, the portions of the chromatid immediately proximal and distal to the site remaining in alignment.
**excitable g.,** in cardiology, the area of repolarized, excitable tissue that can exist between the head of an approaching depolarizing wavefront and the tail of that preceding.
**interocclusal g.,** see under *distance.*
**isochromatid g.,** a nonstaining region of the same level in two sister chromatids, the distal segments remaining in alignment with the proximal portions.
**silent g.,** auscultatory g.
**urinary anion g.,** the amount of urinary anion not routinely measured by laboratory screening that accounts for the difference between the routinely measured anion and cation, equal to sodium + potassium − chloride; it is an indirect measure of ammonium excretion and is used in the evaluation of hyperchloremic metabolic acidosis.

**GAPD** glyceraldehyde-3-phosphate dehydrogenase.

**gapes** (gāps) infestation of the trachea in chickens, turkeys, or wild birds by the gapeworm *Syngamus trachea,* which causes gasping and choking.

**gape·worm** (gāp′wərm) *Syngamus trachea.*

**Ga·ra·my·cin** (gar″ə-mi′sin) trademark for preparations of gentamicin sulfate.

**gar·ban·zo** (gahr-bahn′zo) [Sp.] chickpea.

**Gar·cin's syndrome** (gahr-saz′) [Raymond *Garcin,* French physician, 1897–1971] see under *syndrome.*

**Gard·ner's syndrome**[1] (gahrd′nərz) [Eldon John *Gardner,* American geneticist, born 1909] see under *syndrome.*

**Gard·ner-Dia·mond syndrome** (gahrd′nər di′ah-mənd) [Frank H. *Gardner,* American physician, born 1919; Louis Klein *Diamond,* American physician, born 1902] painful bruising syndrome.

**Gard·ner·el·la** (gahrd″nər-el′ə) [H. L. *Gardner,* American bacteriologist] [MeSH: Gardnerella] a genus of small, pleomorphic, gram-negative, rod-shaped bacteria found in the normal female genital tract and also as a major cause of bacterial vaginitis. It comprises a single species, *G. vagina′lis.* Formerly called *Haemophilus vaginalis.*

**Garg.** abbreviation for L. *gargaris′ma,* gargle.

**gar·gal·an·es·the·sia** (gahr″gəl-an″əs-the′zhə) absence or loss of gargalesthesia.

**gar·gal·es·the·sia** (gahr″gəl-əs-the′zhə) [Gr. *gargalos* itching + *esthesia*] the perception of tickling (q.v.).

**gar·gal·es·thet·ic** (gahr″gəl-əs-thet′ik) pertaining to gargalesthesia.

**gar·get** (gahr′gət) bovine mastitis.

**gar·gle** (gahr′gəl) [L. *gargarisma*] 1. to agitate a solution in the throat by forcing air through it so as to rinse or medicate the mucous membranes. 2. a solution used for rinsing or medicating the mouth and throat.

**gar·goyl·ism** (gahr′goil-iz-əm) Hurler's syndrome.

**Gar·land's triangle** (gahr′ləndz) [George Minot *Garland,* American physician, 1848–1926] see under *triangle.*

**gar·lic** (gahr′lik) [NF] [MeSH: Garlic] 1. *Allium sativum,* a flowering plant with a bulbous stem base. 2. the bulbous stem base of *A. sativum;* it contains the antibacterial sulfur ester derivative allicin, and is a common home remedy as an antitussive, antiseptic, rubefacient, diaphoretic, toothache and earache remedy, vermifuge, and aid in nervous conditions.

**gar·ment** (gahr′mənt) an article of clothing.
**pneumatic antishock g.,** an inflatable garment used to combat shock, stabilize fractures, promote hemostasis, increase peripheral vascular resistance, and permit autotransfusion of small amounts of blood.
**pressure g.,** a garment that applies continual pressure over large areas of healing skin after burns, trauma, and surgical intervention; worn continually for several months to a year, it limits the hypertrophy and contraction of scar tissue.

**gar·net** (gahr′nət) a silicate of any combination of aluminum, cobalt, magnesium, iron, and manganese. Garnet particles are one of the abrasives commonly used on dental disks.

**Gar·ré's osteomyelitis (disease, osteitis)** (gah-rāz′) [Karl *Garré,* Swiss surgeon, 1857–1928] sclerosing nonsuppurative osteomyelitis; see under *osteomyelitis.*

**Gärt·ner's bacillus** (gart′nərz) [August Anton Hieronymus *Gärtner,* German bacteriologist, 1848–1934] *Salmonella enteritidis.*

**Gart·ner's cyst, duct (canal)** (gahrt′nərz) [Hermann Treschow *Gartner,* Danish surgeon and anatomist, 1785–1827] see under *cyst,* and see *ductus longitudinalis epoöphori.*

**Gärt·ner's phenomenon, tonometer** (gart′nərz) [Gustav *Gärtner,* Austrian pathologist, 1855–1937] see under *phenomenon* and *tonometer.*

**gas** (gas) any elastic aeriform fluid in which the molecules are separated from one another and so have free paths.

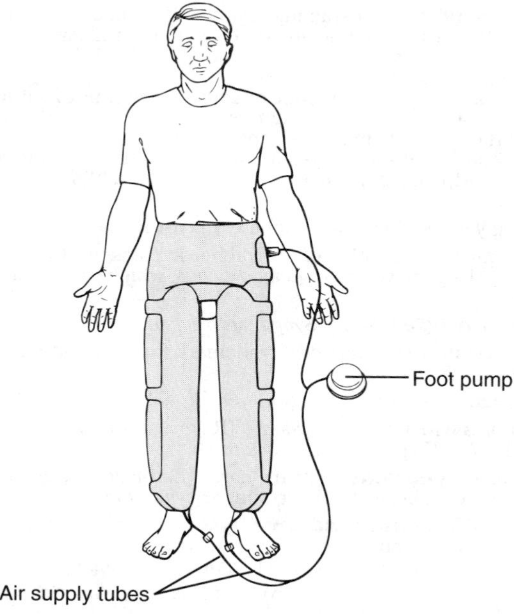


Pneumatic antishock garment.

**alveolar g.**, the gas in the alveoli of the lungs, where gaseous exchange with the capillary blood takes place; called also *alveolar air.*
**blood g's**, the partial pressures of oxygen and carbon dioxide in blood; see under *analysis.*
**coal g.**, a gas produced by the destructive distillation of coal and much used for domestic cooking; it is poisonous because it contains carbon monoxide.
**ethyl g.**, tetraethyl lead.
**expired g.**, gas expired from the lungs, especially a mixture of gas from the dead space and alveolar gas.
**hemolytic g.**, arsine.
**inert g.**, a gas that does not react chemically with the other constituents of a system, especially in reference to the noble gases, such as helium and argon.
**lacrimator g.**, tear g.
**laughing g.**, nitrous oxide.
**marsh g.**, a colorless, tasteless, odorless gas, predominantly methane, produced in swamps and marshes by decaying vegetation and organic matter.
**mustard g.**, dichlorodiethyl sulfide.
**noble g.**, the gas elements of group VIII of the periodic table, i.e., helium, neon, argon, krypton, xenon, and radon.
**sewer g.**, the mixture of gases and vapors from a sewer; often dangerous from the contained materials resulting from the decay of organic matter.
**sneezing g.**, diphenylchlorarsine.
**suffocating g.**, any of several war gases, e.g., phosgene, that causes intense irritation of the bronchial tubes and lungs, resulting in pulmonary edema.
**sweet g.**, old name for *carbon monoxide.*
**tear g.**, a gas that produces severe lacrimation by irritating the conjunctivae.
**vesicating g.**, dichlorodiethyl sulfide.
**war g.**, any noxious gas manufactured for possible use in warfare.

**gas·e·ous** (gash'əs) of the nature of a gas.

**gas·e·ous·ness** (gas'e-əs-nəs, gash'əs-nəs) burbulence.

**gas·i·form** (gas'ĭ-form) gaseous.

**gas·kin** (gas'kin) the part of the upper leg of the horse between the stifle joint and the hock, equivalent to the human calf.

**gas·o·gen·ic** (gas-o-jen'ik) producing gas.

**gas·om·e·ter** (gas-om'ə-tər) a calibrated container for measuring the volume of gases.

**gas·o·met·ric** (gas″o-met'rik) pertaining to gasometry.

**gas·om·e·try** (gas-om'ə-tre) [*gas* + *-metry*] the chemical determination of the amount of gas present in a mixture.

**Gas·ser** (gas'ər) Herbert Spencer. American physiologist, 1888–1963, noted for his work on the nervous system; co-winner, with E. Joseph Erlanger, of the Nobel prize for medicine or physiology in 1944.

**Gas·ser's ganglion** (gahs'ərz) [Johann Laurentius *Gasser,* Austrian professor, 1725–1765] ganglion trigeminale.

**Gas·ser's syndrome** (gahs'ərz) [Konrad Joseph *Gasser,* Swiss pediatrician, born 1912] hemolytic uremic syndrome; see under *syndrome.*

**gas·se·ri·an** (gə-se're-ən) named for Johann Laurentius *Gasser,* as gasserian (trigeminal) ganglion.

**gas·ter** (gas'tər) [Gr. *gastēr* the stomach] [TA] stomach: the musculomembranous expansion of the alimentary tract between the esophagus and the duodenum. The proximal portion is the *cardia;* the portion above the entrance of the esophagus is the *fundus;* the distal portion is the *pyloric part;* and the *body* is between the fundus and the pyloric part. The upper concave surface or edge is the *lesser curvature,* and the lower convex edge is the *greater curvature.* The coats of the stomach are four: an outer, peritoneal, or *serous coat;* a *muscular coat,* made up of longitudinal, oblique, and circular fibers; a *submucous coat;* and the *mucous coat* or membrane forming the inner lining. Gastric glands, which are in the mucous coat, secrete gastric juice containing hydrochloric acid, pepsin, and various other digestive enzymes into the cavity of the stomach. Food mixed with this secretion forms a semifluid substance (chyme) suitable for further digestion by the intestine. Called also *ventriculus.*

**Gas·tero·my·ce·tes** (gas″tər-o-mi-se'tēz) [*gaster* + Gr. *mykēs* fungus] in some systems of classification, a class of perfect fungi of the subphylum Basidiomycotina; it includes the order Lycoperdales. In other classifications its members are placed in the class Holobasidiomycetes.

**Gas·ter·oph·i·lus** (gas″tər-of'ĭ-ləs) [*gaster* + Gr. *philein* to love] a genus of botflies of the family Oestridae; the adults do not eat and die soon after laying their eggs on the hairs of the host. The eggs hatch into larvae that migrate through the skin and internal organs of the host.
**G. haemorrhoida'lis**, the nose botfly, a species with red orange terminal segments whose larvae usually infest the facial skin and pharynx of horses and migrate to the stomach; they sometimes attack humans.
**G. intestina'lis**, the most common species of *Gasterophilus;* its larvae usually infest the legs of horses. On their occasional human hosts, migration of their larvae beneath the skin causes larva migrans.
**G. nasa'lis**, the throat botfly, a species whose larvae infest horses and migrate from the mouth down to the duodenum.

**gas·trad·e·ni·tis** (gas″trad-ə-ni'tis) [*gastr-* + *adenitis*] inflammation of the stomach glands.

**gas·tral·gia** (gas-tral'jə) [*gastr-* + *-algia*] gastrodynia.

**gas·tral·go·ke·no·sis** (gas-tral″go-kə-no'sis) [*gastr-* + *algo-* + *keno-* + *-sis*] paroxysmal gastric pain when the stomach is empty, which is easily relieved by taking food.

**gas·tra·tro·phia** (gas″trə-tro-fe'ə) [*gastr-* + *atrophia*] atrophic gastritis.

**gas·trec·to·my** (gas-trek'tə-me) [*gastr-* + *-ectomy*] [MeSH: Gastrectomy] excision of all *(total g.)* or part *(subtotal* or *partial g.)* of the stomach. Called also *gastric resection.*
**Billroth g.**, Billroth's operation, def. 1.

**gas·tric** (gas'trik) [L. *gastricus;* Gr. *gastēr* stomach] pertaining to, affecting, or originating in the stomach.

**gas·tric·sin** (gas-trik'sin) [EC 3.4.23.3] EC nomenclature for *pepsin C.*

**gas·trin** (gas'trin) any of several polypeptide hormones released from peptidergic fibers in the vagus nerve and from G cells in the pyloric glands in the gastric antrum. Forms include little gastrins ($G_{17}$), with chain lengths of 17 amino acids, big gastrins ($G_{34}$), and minigastrins ($G_{14}$). Gastrin stimulates secretion of gastric acid (causing contraction of the lower esophageal sphincter and modifying gastric and esophageal motility), increases growth of acid-secreting mucosa cells, and weakly stimulates secretion of pancreatic enzymes and gallbladder contraction.

**gas·tri·no·ma** (gas″trĭ-no'mə) [MeSH: Gastrinoma] a tumor that secretes gastrin; most are islet cell tumors of non-beta cells in the pancreas, but some are found at sites such as the antrum of the stomach, the hilus of the spleen, or regional lymph nodes. This is the usual cause of Zollinger-Ellison syndrome.

**gas·trit·ic** (gas-trit'ik) pertaining to or affected with gastritis.

**gas·tri·tis** (gas-tri'tis) [*gastr-* + *-itis*] [MeSH: Gastritis] inflammation of the stomach.
**antral g., antrum g.**, inflammation affecting the antrum of the stomach.
**atrophic g.**, chronic gastritis with infiltration of the lamina propria by inflammatory cells as in superficial gastritis (q.v.), but involving the entire mucosa. Chief and parietal cell numbers decrease, lym-

phoid follicles may be present, the total thickness of the mucosa decreases, and intestinal metaplasia may develop.
**atrophic g., diffuse corporal,** autoimmune g.
**atrophic-hyperplastic g.,** a variant of atrophic gastritis in which the mucosa is of normal or even increased thickness.
**autoimmune g.,** an autoimmune disorder of the stomach resulting from the presence of circulating autoantibodies against the parietal cells, characterized by inflammation and atrophy of the mucosa of the body of the stomach, with replacement of normal mucosa by antral, pseudopyloric, and intestinal metaplasia. Destruction of the mucosal glands results in achlorhydria and a decrease in production of intrinsic factor, in severe cases leading to failure of vitamin $B_{12}$ absorption and pernicious anemia. Called also *diffuse corporal atrophic g.* and *type A g.*
**catarrhal g.,** inflammation of the mucous membrane of the stomach, with hypertrophy of the membrane, secretion of an excessive quantity of mucus, and alteration of the gastric juice. The condition is marked by loss of appetite, nausea, pain, vomiting, and tympanitic distention of the stomach.
**chemical g.,** inflammation caused by the ingestion of corrosive substances, with complete mucosal destruction in fatal cases; called also *corrosive g.*
**chronic cystic g.,** gastritis in which the gastric and pyloric glands are dilated and lined by flattened epithelium, suggestive of a degenerative rather than an inflammatory condition.
**chronic follicular g.,** an atrophic gastritis in which the size and number of lymphoid follicles in the mucosa and submucosa are greatly increased, with heavy infiltration of the entire mucosa by lymphocytes.
**cirrhotic g.,** linitis plastica.
**corrosive g.,** chemical g.
**eosinophilic g.,** gastritis in which there is considerable edema and a heavy infiltration of all coats of the wall of the pyloric antrum by eosinophils.
**erosive g.,** gastritis in which the surface epithelium is eroded, manifesting as a patchy or a diffuse lesion; exfoliative g.
**exfoliative g.,** chronic gastritis in which bits of the surface of the mucous membrane are shed; erosive g.
**follicular g.,** inflammation of the glands of the stomach.
**giant hypertrophic g.,** excessive proliferation of the gastric mucosa, producing diffuse thickening of the stomach wall; inflammatory changes may be associated. Called also *Ménétrier's disease.*
**hemorrhagic g.,** erosive gastritis with bleeding.
**hypertrophic g.,** gastritis with infiltration and enlargement of the glands.
**phlegmonous g.,** a variety with abscesses in the stomach walls.
**polypous g.,** hypertrophic gastritis with polypoid projections into the stomach.
**pseudomembranous g.,** a variety in which a false membrane occurs in patches within the stomach.
**radiation g.,** gastritis resulting from radiation injury.
**superficial g.,** chronic gastritis with infiltration of the lamina propria by neutrophils, lymphocytes, plasma cells, and a few eosinophils, with inflammation limited to the outer third of the mucosa in the foveolar area. Columnar cells of the surface epithelium are often morphologically abnormal. Cf. *atrophic g.*
**toxic g.,** gastritis caused by the action of a poison or a corrosive agent.
**type A g.,** autoimmune g.
**type B g.,** chronic gastritis without circulating autoantibodies (cf. *autoimmune g.*), affecting the gastric antrum; the most common type of chronic gastritis.
**zonal g.,** gastritis occurring in the vicinity of a gastric lesion, as that associated with peptic ulcer and gastric carcinoma.

**gastr(o)-** [Gr. *gastēr* stomach] a combining form denoting relationship to the stomach.

**gas·tro·aceph·a·lus** (gas″tro-ə-sef′ə-ləs) [*gastro-* + *acephalus*] asymmetrical conjoined twins in which the larger twin bears the smaller one as a headless parasite on its abdomen.

**gas·tro·ad·e·ni·tis** (gas″tro-ad″ə-ni′tis) gastradenitis.

**gas·tro·ady·nam·ic** (gas″tro-a″di-nam′ik) marked by an adynamic condition of the stomach.

**gas·tro·amor·phus** (gas″tro-a-mor′fəs) [*gastro-* + *amorphus*] asymmetrical conjoined twins in which the larger one has fetal parts of the smaller one concealed within its abdomen.

**gas·tro·anas·to·mo·sis** (gas″tro-ə-nas″to-mo′sis) gastrogastrostomy.

**gas·tro·cam·era** (gas″tro-kam′ə-rə) a small camera that can be swallowed or passed down the esophagus on an appropriate instrument to photograph the inside of the stomach; it is attached to an external control box by a hollow flexible tube, and fitted with a flash lamp and inflation bulb. After the camera is inserted into the stomach, the bulb is inflated and pictures are taken as the flash lamp is triggered.

**gas·tro·car·di·ac** (gas″tro-kahr′de-ak) pertaining to the stomach and heart.

**gas·tro·cele** (gas′tro-sēl) [*gastro-* + *-cele*[1]] hernial protrusion of the stomach or of a gastric pouch.

**gas·troc·ne·mi·us** (gas″tro-ne′me-əs) [*gastro-* + Gr. *knēmē* leg] see under *musculus.*

**gas·tro·coele** (gas′tro-sēl) [*gastro-* + *-coele*] archenteron.

**gas·tro·col·ic** (gas″tro-kol′ik) pertaining to or communicating with the stomach and colon, as a gastrocolic fistula.

**gas·tro·co·li·tis** (gas″tro-ko-li′tis) [*gastro-* + *colitis*] inflammation of the stomach and colon.

**gas·tro·co·los·to·my** (gas″tro-ko-los′tə-me) [*gastro-* + *colon* + *-stomy*] the creation of an artificial opening between the stomach and the colon; also, the opening so established.

**gas·tro·co·lot·o·my** (gas″tro-ko-lot′ə-me) [*gastro-* + *colon* + *-tomy*] incision into the stomach and colon.

**gas·tro·cu·ta·ne·ous** (gas″tro-ku-ta′ne-əs) pertaining to the stomach and skin, or communicating with the stomach and the cutaneous surface of the body, as a gastrocutaneous fistula.

**gas·tro·cys·to·plas·ty** (gas″tro-sis′to-plas″te) [*gastro-* + *cystoplasty*] cystoplasty in which a portion of the stomach is used to replace or increase the size of the urinary bladder.

**gas·tro·der·mis** (gas″tro-dər′mis) [*gastro-* + Gr. *derma* skin] the tissue lining the gut cavity of an invertebrate, which is responsible for digestion and absorption.

**gas·tro·di·a·phane** (gas″tro-di′ə-fān) [*gastro-* + *dia-* + *phainein* to show] a small electric lamp introduced into the stomach in gastrodiaphany.

**gas·tro·di·aph·a·nos·co·py** (gas″tro-di-af″ə-nos′kə-pe) [*gastro-* + *diaphanoscopy*] gastrodiaphany.

**gas·tro·di·aph·a·ny** (gas″tro-di-af′ə-ne) [*gastro-* + *dia-* + *phainein* to show] the exploration of the stomach by means of an electric lamp passed down the esophagus.

**gas·tro·did·y·mus** (gas″tro-did′ə-məs) [*gastro-* + *-didymus*] symmetrical conjoined twins joined in the abdominal region.

**gas·tro·dis·ci·a·sis** (gas″tro-dis-ki′ə-sis) infection caused by *Gastrodiscoides hominis.*

**Gas·tro·dis·coi·des** (gas″tro-dis-koi′dēz) [*gastro-* + Gr. *diskos* disk + *eidos* form] a genus of trematodes of the family Paramphistomatidae; many are parasitic in the intestinal tract, causing paramphistomiasis. Called also *Gastrodiscus. G. ho′minis* is found in the cecum and colon of pigs and occasionally humans in India, Indochina, and Malaysia.

**Gas·tro·dis·cus** (gas″tro-dis′kəs) *Gastrodiscoides.*

**gas·tro·disk** (gas′tro-disk) embryonic disc.

**gas·tro·du·o·de·nal** (gas″tro-doo″o-de′nəl) pertaining to or communicating with the stomach and duodenum, as a gastroduodenal fistula.

**gas·tro·du·o·de·nec·to·my** (gas″tro-doo″o-də-nek′tə-me) excision of stomach and duodenum.

**gas·tro·du·o·de·ni·tis** (gas″tro-doo-ad″ə-ni′tis) [*gastro-* + *duodenitis*] an inflammation of the stomach and duodenum.

**gas·tro·du·o·de·nos·co·py** (gas″tro-doo″o-də-nos′kə-pe) [*gastro-* + *duodeno-* + *-scopy*] examination of the stomach and duodenum, the gastroscope usually being passed through the mouth and esophagus; occasionally performed through incisions in the abdominal and gastric walls during laparotomy.

**gas·tro·du·o·de·nos·to·my** (gas″tro-doo″o-də-nos′tə-me) [*gastro-* + *duodeno-* + *-stomy*] surgical creation of an anastomosis between the stomach and the duodenum.

**gas·tro·dyn·ia** (gas″tro-din′e-ə) [*gastro-* + *-odynia*] a pain or ache in the stomach. Called also *gastralgia, stomachalgia,* and *stomachodynia.*

**gas·tro·en·ter·al·gia** (gas″tro-en″tər-al′jə) [*gastro-* + *entero-* + *-algia*] pain in the stomach and intestines.

**gas·tro·en·ter·ic** (gas″tro-ən-ter′ik) gastrointestinal.

**gas·tro·en·ter·i·tis** (gas″tro-en″tər-i′tis) [*gastro-* + *enteritis*] [MeSH: Gastroenteritis] an acute inflammation of the lining of the stomach and intestines, characterized by anorexia, nausea, diarrhea, abdominal pain, and weakness, which has various causes, including food poisoning due to infection with such organisms as *Escherichia coli, Staphylococcus aureus,* and *Salmonella* species; consumption of irritating food or drink; or psychological factors such as anger, stress, and fear. Called also *enterogastritis.*
**acute infectious g.,** gastritis with acute onset, caused by various bacteria and viruses.

**coliform g.**, a diarrheal disease of neonatal, nursing, and weanling pigs caused by enterotoxigenic strains of *Escherichia coli*, marked by profuse, watery diarrhea, dehydration, and acidosis, frequently leading to death; see also *edema disease*, under *disease*. Called also *enteric* or *enterotoxigenic colibacillosis*.
**canine coronaviral g.**, vomiting and diarrhea in dogs and other canines infected with coronaviruses; it has a sudden onset and can be fatal in puppies.
**canine hemorrhagic g.**, a syndrome of intestinal hemorrhage in dogs, of unknown etiology; characteristics include sudden onset, bloody diarrhea, dehydration, and hemoconcentration, often followed by collapse and death. Smaller dogs are most often affected.
**eosinophilic g.**, a disorder marked by infiltration of the mucosa of the small intestine by eosinophils, with edema but without vasculitis, and by eosinophilia of the peripheral blood. Symptoms, including abdominal pain, diarrhea, nausea, fever, and malabsorption, depend on the site and extent of the disorder. The stomach is also frequently involved. The disorder is commonly associated with intolerance to specific foods. See also *eosinophilic granuloma* (def. 2), under *granuloma*.
**Norwalk g.**, gastroenteritis caused by the Norwalk virus.
**transmissible g. of swine**, a viral disease of swine caused by the porcine transmissible gastroenteritis virus, occurring chiefly during the winter and characterized by severe diarrhea and acute inflammation of the gastric mucosa, which may lead to ulceration and hemorrhage. The mortality rate among piglets is very high.

**gas·tro·en·tero·anas·to·mo·sis** (gas″tro-en″tər-o-ə-nas″to-mo′sis) anastomosis between the stomach and small intestine in gastroenterostomy.

**gas·tro·en·tero·co·li·tis** (gas″tro-en″tər-o-ko-li′tis) inflammation of the stomach, small intestine, and colon.

**gas·tro·en·tero·co·los·to·my** (gas″tro-en″tər-o-ko-los′tə-me) [*gastro-* + *entero-* + *colon* + *-ostomy*] surgical creation of an opening between the stomach, intestine, and colon; also, the opening so established.

**gas·tro·ent·er·ol·o·gist** (gas″tro-en″tər-ol′ə-jist) a practitioner who specializes in diseases of the digestive tract.

**gas·tro·en·ter·ol·o·gy** (gas″tro-en″tər-ol′ə-je) [*gastro-* + *entero-* + *-logy*] [MeSH: Gastroenterology] the study of the stomach and intestines and their diseases.

**gas·tro·en·ter·op·a·thy** (gas″tro-en″tər-op′ə-the) any disease of the stomach and intestines.
**allergic g.**, eosinophilic gastritis of children with food allergies, particularly to cows' milk; signs of the disease include edema, malabsorption, eosinophilia, iron deficiency anemia, elevated levels of serum IgE, and protein-losing enteropathy.

**gas·tro·en·tero·plas·ty** (gas″tro-en″tər-o-plas′te) a plastic operation on the stomach and small intestine.

**gas·tro·en·ter·os·to·my** (gas″tro-en″tər-os′tə-me) [*gastro-* + *enter-* + *ostomy*] [MeSH: Gastroenterostomy] surgical creation of an artificial passage (anastomosis) between the stomach and intestines (usually the jejunum); see illustration.

**gas·tro·en·ter·ot·o·my** (gas″tro-en″tər-ot′ə-me) [*gastro-* + *entero-* + *-tomy*] surgical incision into the stomach and intestine.

**gas·tro·ep·i·plo·ic** (gas″tro-ep″ĭ-plo′ik) [*gastro-* + *epiploic*] pertaining to the stomach and epiploon (omentum).

**gas·tro·esoph·a·ge·al** (gas″tro-ĕ-sof″ə-je′əl) pertaining to the stomach and esophagus, as the gastroesophageal junction.

**gas·tro·esoph·a·gi·tis** (gas″tro-ə-sof″ə-ji′tis) inflammation of the stomach and esophagus.

**gas·tro·esoph·a·gos·to·my** (gas″tro-ə-sof″ə-gos′tə-me) surgical creation of an anastomosis between the stomach and the esophagus; done for stricture of the lower end of the esophagus.

**gas·tro·fi·ber·scope** (gas″tro-fi′bər-skōp) fiberoptic gastroscope.

**gas·tro·gas·tros·to·my** (gas″tro-gas-tros′tə-me) [*gastro-* + *gastro-* + *-stomy*] surgical creation of an anastomosis between the pyloric and cardiac ends of the stomach, usually performed because of hourglass contraction of the middle third of the stomach; also, the anastomosis so established.

**gas·tro·ga·vage** (gas″tro-gə-vahzh′) [*gastro-* + *gavage*] the introduction of nutriment into the stomach by means of a tube passed through the esophagus.

**gas·tro·gen·ic** (gas″tro-jen′ik) formed or originating in the stomach.

**Gas·tro·graf·in** (gas″tro-graf′in) trademark for a preparation of meglumine diatrizoate.

**gas·tro·graph** (gas′tro-graf) [*gastro-* + *-graph*] an apparatus for recording the motions of the stomach.

**gas·tro·he·pat·ic** (gas″tro-hə-pat′ik) [*gastro-* + *hepatic*] pertaining to the stomach and liver.

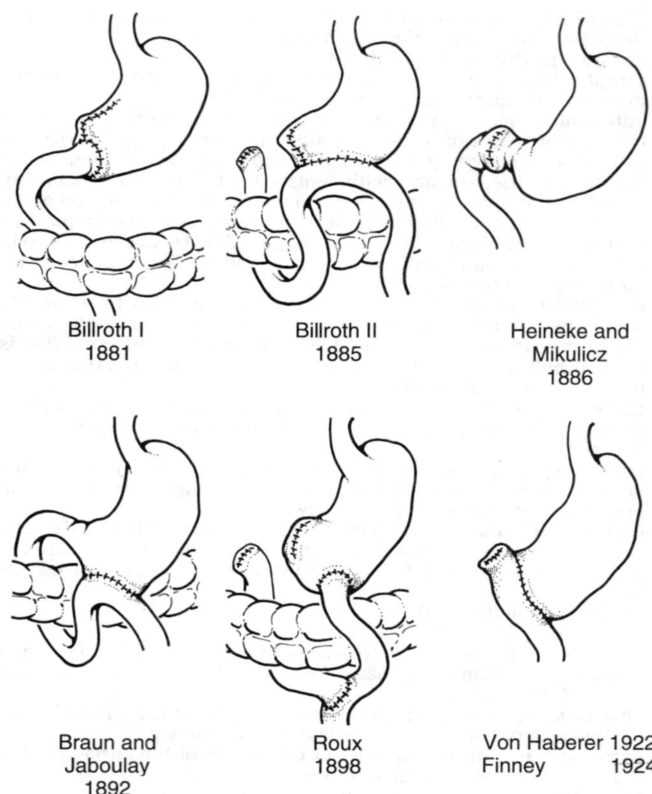

Types of gastroenterostomy.

**gas·tro·hep·a·ti·tis** (gas″tro-hep-ə-ti′tis) inflammation of the stomach and liver.

**gas·tro·il·e·ac** (gas″tro-il′e-ak) pertaining to stomach and ileum.

**gas·tro·il·e·itis** (gas″tro-il-e-i′tis) inflammation of the stomach and ileum.

**gas·tro·il·e·os·to·my** (gas″tro-il″e-os′tə-me) surgical creation of an anastomosis between the stomach and ileum; also, the anastomosis so established.

**gas·tro·in·tes·ti·nal** (gas″tro-in-tes′tĭ-nəl) [*gastro-* + *intestinal*] pertaining to or communicating with the stomach and intestine. Called also *enterogastric* and *gastroenteric*.

**gas·tro·je·ju·no·col·ic** (gas″tro-jə-joo″no-kol′ik) pertaining to or communicating with the stomach, jejunum, and colon, as a gastrojejunocolic fistula.

**gas·tro·je·ju·no·esoph·a·gos·to·my** (gas″tro-jə-joo″no-ə-sof″ə-gos′tə-me) esophagojejunogastrostomy.

**gas·tro·je·ju·nos·to·my** (gas″tro-jə-joo-nos′tə-me) [*gastro-* + *jejunostomy*] surgical creation of an anastomosis between the stomach and jejunum; also, the anastomosis so established.

**gas·tro·ki·neso·graph** (gas″tro-kĭ-nes′o-graf) [*gastro-* + *kinesis* + *-graph*] a device for recording the mechanical motions of the stomach.

**gas·tro·li·e·nal** (gas″tro-li′ən-əl) [*gastro-* + *lienal*] pertaining to the stomach and spleen.

**gas·tro·lith** (gas′tro-lith) [*gastro-* + *-lith*] a calcareous or other concretion formed in the stomach; called also *gastric* or *stomachic calculus*.

**gas·tro·li·thi·a·sis** (gas″tro-lĭ-thi′ə-sis) [*gastro-* + *lith-* + *-iasis*] the presence or formation of gastroliths.

**Gas·tro·lo·bi·um** (gas″tro-lo′be-um) a genus of leguminous plants found in Australia; most species contain fluoroacetate and can cause fatal fluoroacetate poisoning in ruminants.

**gas·trol·o·gist** (gas-trol′ə-jist) a specialist in diseases of the stomach.

**gas·trol·o·gy** (gas-trol′ə-je) [*gastro-* + *-logy*] the sum of knowledge regarding the stomach.

**gas·trol·y·sis** (gas-trol′ə-sis) [*gastro-* + *-lysis*] surgical division of perigastric adhesions in order to mobilize the stomach.

**gas·tro·ma·la·cia** (gas″tro-mə-la′shə) [*gastro-* + *malacia*] an abnormal softening or softness of the wall of the stomach; see *softening of the stomach.*

**gas·tro·meg·a·ly** (gas″tro-meg′ə-le) [*gastro-* + *-megaly*] enlargement of the stomach.

**gas·trom·e·lus** (gas-trom′ə-ləs) [*gastro-* + Gr. *melos* limb] a fetus with a supernumerary lower limb attached to the abdomen.

**gas·tro·my·co·sis** (gas″tro-mi-ko′sis) [*gastro-* + *mycosis*] a disease of the stomach caused by fungi.

**gas·tro·my·ot·o·my** (gas″tro-mi-ot′ə-me) [*gastro-* + *myotomy*] incision through the muscular coats of the stomach down to the mucosa.

**gas·tro·myx·or·rhea** (gas″tro-mik″so-re′ə) [*gastro-* + *myxo-* + *-rrhea*] excessive secretion of mucus by the stomach.

**gas·trone** (gas′trōn) a reputed hormonal inhibitor of gastric acid secretion, extracted from gastric mucosa.

**gas·tro·pan·cre·a·ti·tis** (gas″tro-pan″kre-ə-ti′tis) inflammation of the stomach and pancreas.

**gas·tro·pa·ral·y·sis** (gas″tro-pə-ral′ə-sis) gastroparesis.

**gas·tro·pa·re·sis** (gas″tro-pə-re′sis) [*gastro-* + *paresis*] [MeSH: Gastroparesis] paralysis of the stomach.

**gas·tro·pa·ri·e·tal** (gas″tro-pə-ri′ə-təl) pertaining to the stomach and the body wall.

**gas·tro·path·ic** (gas″tro-path′ik) pertaining to disease of the stomach.

**gas·trop·a·thy** (gas-trop′ə-the) [*gastro-* + *-pathy*] any disease of the stomach. Called also *gastrosis.*

**gas·tro·peri·odyn·ia** (gas″tro-per″e-o-din′e-ə) [*gastro-* + *period* + *-odynia*] periodic attacks of pain in the stomach.

**gas·tro·peri·to·ni·tis** (gas″tro-per″ĭ-to-ni′tis) inflammation of the stomach and peritoneum.

**gas·tro·pexy** (gas′tro-pek″se) [*gastro-* + *-pexy*] surgical fixation of the stomach to prevent displacement.
**Hill posterior g.,** an operation for gastroesophageal reflux in which the reduced gastroesophageal junction is anchored by sutures between the proximal lesser curvature and the preaortic fascia, and sutures are placed in the crura to narrow the hiatus.

**Gas·troph·i·lus** (gas-trof′ĭ-ləs) *Gasterophilus.*

**gas·tro·pho·tog·ra·phy** (gas″tro-fo-tog′rə-fe) photography of the interior of the stomach by means of a camera either built into the distal tip of the gastroscope, or attached to the eyepiece with light being transmitted to the stomach by a fiberoptic bundle system.

**gas·tro·phren·ic** (gas″tro-fren′ik) [*gastro-* + *phrenic*] pertaining to the stomach and diaphragm.

**gas·tro·phthis·is** (gas″tro-this′is) [*gastro-* + *phthisis* (def. 1)] 1. hyperplasia of the gastric mucosa and submucosa, leading to thickening of the stomach walls and diminution of its cavity. 2. emaciation due to abdominal disease.

**gas·tro·plas·ty** (gas′tro-plas″te) [*gastro-* + *-plasty*] [MeSH: Gastroplasty] plastic operation on the stomach.
**vertical banded g.,** the construction of a small pouch in the stomach, emptying through a narrow stoma into the distal stomach and duodenum; used in the treatment of morbid obesity.

**gas·tro·ple·gia** (gas″tro-ple′jə) [*gastro-* + *-plegia*] paralysis of the stomach.

**gas·tro·pli·ca·tion** (gas″tro-plĭ-ka′shən) [*gastro-* + *plication*] the surgical treatment of gastric dilatation by stitching a fold in the stomach.

**gas·tro·pneu·mon·ic** (gas″tro-noo-mon′ik) pertaining to the stomach and lungs.

**gas·tro·pod** (gas′tro-pod) a mollusk of the class Gastropoda.

**Gas·trop·o·da** (gas-trop′ə-də) [*gastro-* + Gr. *pous* foot] a class of mollusks embracing the snails, slugs, whelks, abalones, and others, including many species that serve as primary and intermediate hosts of pathogens.

**gas·trop·to·sis** (gas″trop-to′sis) [*gastro-* + *-ptosis*] downward displacement of the stomach; a term based on the outmoded concept that variation in position of abdominal organs is pathologic.

**gas·tro·pul·mo·nary** (gas″tro-pul′mo-nar-e) [*gastro-* + *pulmonary*] pertaining to the stomach and lungs.

**gas·tro·py·lo·rec·to·my** (gas″tro-pi″lə-rek′tə-me) [*gastro-* + *pylorectomy*] excision of the pyloric portion of the stomach.

**gas·tro·py·lor·ic** (gas″tro-pi-lor′ik) pertaining to the stomach in its entirety and to the pylorus.

**gas·tror·rha·gia** (gas″tro-ra′jə) [*gastro-* + *-rrhagia*] hemorrhage from the stomach.

**gas·tror·rha·phy** (gas-tror′ə-fe) [*gastro-* + *-rrhaphy*] suture of a wound of the stomach.

**gas·tror·rhea** (gas″tro-re′ə) [*gastro-* + *-rrhea*] excessive secretion by the stomach of gastric juice *(hyperchlorhydria)* or mucus.

**gas·tror·rhex·is** (gas″tro-rek′sis) [*gastro-* + *-rrhexis*] rupture of the stomach.

**gas·tros·chi·sis** (gas-tros′kĭ-sis) [*gastro-* + *-schisis*] a congenital fissure of the anterior abdominal wall not involving the site of insertion of the umbilical cord, and usually accompanied by protrusion of the small intestine and part of the large intestine.

**gas·tro·scope** (gas′tro-skōp) [*gastro-* + *-scope*] an endoscope for inspecting the interior of the stomach.
**fiberoptic g.,** a fiberscope for examining the stomach. Called also *gastrofiberscope.*

**gas·tro·scop·ic** (gas″tro-skop′ik) pertaining to gastroscopy or the gastroscope.

**gas·tros·co·py** (gas-tros′kə-pe) [*gastro-* + *-scopy*] [MeSH: Gastroscopy] inspection of the interior of the stomach by means of the gastroscope.

**gas·tro·se·lec·tive** (gas″tro-sə-lek′tiv) having an affinity for receptors involved in regulation of gastric activities.

**gas·tro·sis** (gas-tro′sis) gastropathy.

**gas·tro·spasm** (gas′tro-spaz″əm) [*gastro-* + *spasm*] spasm of the stomach.

**gas·tro·splen·ic** (gas″tro-splen′ik) pertaining to the stomach and spleen.

**gas·tro·stax·is** (gas″tro-stak′sis) [*gastro-* + *staxis*] the oozing of blood from the mucous membrane of the stomach; hemorrhagic gastritis.

**gas·tro·ste·no·sis** (gas″tro-stə-no′sis) [*gastro-* + *stenosis*] contraction or shrinkage of the stomach.

**gas·tros·to·ga·vage** (gas-tros″to-gə-vahzh′) introduction of nutriment into the stomach by means of a tube passed through a gastric fistula.

**gas·tros·to·la·vage** (gas-tros″to-lə-vahzh′) irrigation of the stomach through a gastric fistula.

**gas·tros·to·ma** (gas-tros′to-mə) [*gastro-* + *stoma*] a gastric fistula or a surgically created opening from the stomach through the abdominal wall.

**gas·tros·to·my** (gas-tros′tə-me) [*gastro-* + *-stomy*] [MeSH: Gastrostomy] surgical creation of an artificial opening into the stomach; also, the opening so established.
**Beck g.,** creation of a permanent gastric fistula by the formation of a tube from the greater curvature of the stomach to the surface of the abdominal wall.
**Glassman g.,** a permanent opening into the stomach created by forming a cone-shaped diverticulum from the anterior wall of the stomach.
**Janeway g.,** creation of a permanent gastric fistula by the formation of a tube from the anterior gastric wall to the surface of the abdominal wall.
**Stamm g.,** insertion of a tube into the gastric lumen, the tube exiting through a stab incision in the abdominal skin; the stomach is sutured to the peritoneum at the exit site.
**Witzel g.,** insertion of a tube into the gastric lumen, the tube being implanted so as to create a serosal tunnel of stomach as it enters the gastric lumen.

**gas·tro·suc·cor·rhea** (gas″tro-suk″o-re′ə) [*gastro-* + *succorrhea*] hyperchlorhydria.
**digestive g.,** a condition in which there is excessive secretion of gastric juice during digestion only.

**gas·tro·tho·ra·cop·a·gus** (gas″tro-thor″ə-kop′ə-gəs) [*gastro-* + *thoracopagus*] conjoined twins joined at the abdomen and thorax.
**g. dipy′gus,** asymmetrical conjoined twins in which there is attached to the abdomen of the larger twin a parasitic twin consisting of the pelvis and lower limbs only; called also *dipygus parasiticus.*

**gas·tro·tome** (gas′tro-tōm) a cutting instrument used in gastrotomy.

**gas·trot·o·my** (gas-trot′ə-me) [*gastro-* + *-tomy*] incision into the stomach.

**gas·tro·to·nom·e·ter** (gas″tro-to-nom′ə-tər) [*gastro-* + *tono-* + *-meter*] an instrument for measuring intragastric pressure.

**gas·tro·to·nom·e·try** (gas″tro-to-nom′ə-tre) the measurement of intragastric pressure.

**gas·tro·tox·in** (gas″tro-tok′sin) a substance that exerts a toxic effect on the stomach.

**Gas·tro·tricha** (gas″tro-trik′ə) [*gastro-* + Gr. *trichos* hair] a class of very small aquatic animals of the phylum Aschelminthes, which have cilia on the ventral surface and a triradiate esophagus. In some systems of classification, they are considered to be a separate phylum.

**gas·tro·trop·ic** (gas″tro-trop′ik) [*gastro-* + *-tropic*] having an affinity for or exerting a special effect upon the stomach.

**gas·tro·tym·pa·ni·tes** (gas″tro-tim″pə-ni′tēz) [*gastro-* + *tympanites*] tympanitic distention of the stomach.

**gas·tru·la** (gas′troo-lə) [MeSH: Gastrula] that early embryonic stage, which follows the blastula or blastocyst. The simplest type consists of two layers, the ectoderm and the mesentoderm, and of two cavities, one lying between the ectoderm and the endoderm; the other (the archenteron) formed by invagination so as to lie within the entoderm and having an opening (the blastopore). In human embryos the gastrula stage occurs during the third week, as the embryonic disc becomes trilaminar.

**gas·tru·la·tion** (gas″troo-la′shən) the process by which a blastula becomes a gastrula or, in forms without a true blastula, the process by which three germ cell layers are acquired.

**Gatch bed** (gach) [Willis Dew *Gatch,* American surgeon, 1878–1954] see under *bed.*

**gate** (gāt) 1. an electronic circuit that passes a pulse only when a signal (the gate pulse) is present at a second input; called also *gate circuit.* 2. a mechanism for opening or closing a protein channel in a cell membrane, regulated by a signal such as increased concentration of a neurotransmitter, change in electrical potential, or physical binding of a ligand molecule to the protein to cause a conformational change in the protein molecule. 3. to open and close selectively and function as a gate.

**gat·ing** (gāt′ing) 1. controlling access or passage through gates or channels. 2. selection of electrical signals by a gate, which passes signals only when a control signal, the gate pulse, is present, or which passes only signals with certain characteristics, such as a pulse height. 3. substrate- or ligand-binding induced opening and closing of a biologic membrane channel, believed to be due to conformational changes in proteins lining the channels. 4. sensory g.
**cardiac g.,** selective acquisition of cardiac function information at specific points in the cardiac cycle by using information from the electrocardiographic signal to time the cardiac cycle and control image sampling. It has been used in digital subtraction angiography, computed tomography, nuclear cardiology, and magnetic resonance imaging.
**sensory g.,** inhibition or blocking of incoming sensory stimuli or channels when attention is occupied by another channel or stimulus.

**ga·tism** (ga′tiz-əm) [Fr. *gâter* to spoil] rectal, vesical, or rectovesical incontinence.

**ga·to·pho·bia** (gat″-o-fo′be-ə) [Sp. *gato* from L. *catus* cat + *-phobia*] ailurophobia.

**gat·tine** (gat′ēn) a form of flacherie in which the cephalic end of a silkworm larva becomes swollen and almost translucent; thought to be caused by a mixed infection with an unidentified virus and an enterococcus related to *Streptococcus faecalis.*

**Gau·cher's cells, disease (splenomegaly)** (go-shāz′) [Phillippe Charles Ernest *Gaucher,* French physician, 1854–1918] see under *cell* and *disease.*

**gauge** (gāj) an instrument for determining physical properties of anything, including caliber, dimensions, or pressure.
**Boley g.,** a watchmaker's gauge used in dentistry for accurate measurement of arch, tooth, and facial dimensions.
**catheter g.,** a plate with graduated perforations for measuring the outside diameter of catheters.

**Gaul·the·ria** (gawl-the′re-ə) [Jean-François *Gaultier,* Quebec physician and botanist, 1708–1756] a genus of plants of the family Ericaceae. *G. procum′bens* is wintergreen, a North American species whose leaves contain methyl salicylate (see under *methyl*).

**gaunt·let** (gawnt′lət) [Fr. *gant* glove] a bandage that covers the hand and fingers like a glove.

**Gauss' sign** (gous) [Karl Johann *Gauss,* German obstetrician, 1875–1957] see under *sign.*

**gauss** (gous) [Karl Friedrich *Gauss,* German mathematician and physicist, 1777–1855] the cgs unit of magnetic flux density, equal to $10^{-4}$ tesla. Symbol, G.

**gauss·i·an curve, distribution** (gou′se-ən) [K.F. *Gauss*] see under *curve* and *distribution.*

**gauze** (gawz) a light, open-meshed fabric of muslin or similar material used in bandages, dressings, and surgical sponges. Before use in surgery, it is usually sterilized and frequently impregnated with various antiseptics.
**absorbable g.,** gauze made from oxidized cellulose.
**absorbent g.** [USP], a plain woven cloth of cotton or of a mixture of cotton and rayon; it is classified as Type I (the heaviest) to Type VIII (the lightest) on the basis of thread count and weight. It is supplied in various lengths and widths in the form of rolls and folds.
**absorbent g., sterile,** absorbent gauze that has been sterilized and subsequently protected from contamination.
**petrolatum g.** [USP], absorbent gauze saturated with white petrolatum; used as a protective covering for wounds.
**zinc gelatin impregnated g.,** absorbent gauze impregnated with zinc gelatin that may contain a small amount of ferric oxide as coloring matter; see also *Unna's boot,* under *boot.*

**ga·vage** (gə-vahzh′) [Fr. "cramming"] 1. forced feeding, especially through a tube passed into the stomach. 2. the therapeutic use of a very full diet; superalimentation.

**Ga·vard's muscle** (gə-vahrz′) [Hyacinthe *Gavard,* French anatomist, 1753–1802] see under *muscle.*

**Gav·is·con** (gav′is-kon) trademark for preparations of aluminum hydroxide and magnesium carbonate.

**Gay's glands** (gāz) [Alexander Heinrich *Gay,* Russian anatomist, 1842–1907] glandulae circumanales.

**Gay-Lus·sac's law** (ga′lu-sahks′) [Joseph Louis *Gay-Lussac,* French naturalist, 1778–1850] see under *law.*

**gaze** (gāz) [Middle English *gazen*] 1. to look steadily in one direction. 2. the act of looking steadily at something.
**conjugate g.,** the normal movement of the two eyes simultaneously in the same direction to bring something into view.

**GBG** glycine-rich $\beta$ glycoprotein, former name for *factor B.*

**GBM** glomerular basement membrane.

**GC** gas chromatography.

**g-cal.** gram calorie; see *small calorie,* under *calorie.*

**G-CSF** [MeSH: Granulocyte Colony-Stimulating Factor] granulocyte colony-stimulating factor.

**Gd** symbol for *gadolinium.*

**GDP** guanosine diphosphate.

**Ge** symbol for *germanium.*

**gear** (gēr) equipment.
**cervical g.,** an extraoral appliance by means of which the back of the neck is used for anchorage or as a base of traction in effecting tooth movement.
**head g.,** headgear.

**Gee's disease** (gēz) [Samuel Jones *Gee,* English physician, 1839–1911] the infantile form of celiac disease.

**Gee-Her·ter disease** (ge-hər′tər) [S.J. *Gee;* Christian Archibald *Herter,* American physician, 1865–1910] the infantile form of celiac disease.

**Gee-Her·ter-Heub·ner disease, syndrome** (ge-hər′tər-hoib′nər) [S.J. *Gee;* C.A. *Herter;* Johann Otto Leonard *Heubner,* German pediatrician, 1843–1926] the infantile form of celiac disease.

**Gee-Thay·sen disease** (ge-ti′sən) [S.J. *Gee;* Thorwald Einar Hess *Thaysen,* Danish physician, 1883–1936] the adult form of celiac disease.

**Ge·gen·baur's cell** (ga′gən-bou″ərz) [Carl *Gegenbaur,* German anatomist, 1826–1903] osteoblast.

**ge·gen·hal·ten** (ga″gən-hahlt′ən) [Ger. from *gegen* against + *halten* to hold] paratonia involving an involuntary resistance to passive movement, as may occur in cerebral cortical disorders.

**Gei·gel's reflex** (gi′gəlz) [Richard *Geigel,* German physician, 1859–1930] see under *reflex.*

**Gei·ger counter, Gei·ger-Mül·ler counter** (gi′gər, gi′gər-mūl′ər) [Hans Wilhelm *Geiger,* German physicist, 1882–1945; Walther Müller, German physicist, 20th century] see under *counter.*

**Geis·so·spe·rum** (gi″so-spe′rəm) a genus of plants of the family Apocynaceae. *G. lae′ve* and *G. vello′sii* Allem. are poisonous species that contain vellosine.

**gel** (jel) 1. a colloid in which the solid disperse phase forms a network in combination with the fluid continuous phase to produce a viscous semirigid sol. 2. to form a such a compound or any similar semi-solid material.
**aluminum carbonate g., basic** [USP], an aqueous suspension of a complex of aluminum hydroxide and aluminum carbonate, used as an antacid, for the treatment of hyperphosphatemia in renal insufficiency, and to prevent the formation of phosphate urinary calculi.
**aluminum hydroxide g.** [USP], a suspension of 5.5 to 6.7 per cent of aluminum hydroxide, in the form of amorphous aluminum hydroxide in which there is partial substitution of carbonate for hydroxide; used as a gastric antacid, especially in the treatment of peptic ulcer, and in the treatment of phosphate nephrolithiasis. Called also *colloidal aluminum hydroxide.*

**aluminum hydroxide g., dried** [USP], an amorphous form of aluminum hydroxide in which there is partial substitution of carbonate for hydroxide, prepared by drying aluminum hydroxide gel at low temperature; used as an antacid.
**aluminum phosphate g.** [USP], an aqueous suspension of aluminum phosphate, used as an antacid and to reduce excretion of phosphates in the feces.
**corticotropin g.,** repository corticotropin injection.
**silica g.,** a gel obtained by the reaction of sodium silicate with hydrochloric or sulfuric acid, and containing not less than 99 per cent of silica; used as a dispersing and suspending agent.
**sodium fluoride and orthophosphoric acid g., sodium fluoride and phosphoric acid g.** [USP], a fluoride-containing preparation, applied topically to the teeth as a dental caries prophylactic.

**ge·las·mus** (jə-las′məs) [G. *gelasma* a laugh] hysterical laughter.

**ge·las·tic** (jə-las′tik) [Gr. *gelastos* laughable] pertaining to gelasmus.

**gel·ate** (jel′āt) to form a gel.

**ge·lat·i·fi·ca·tion** (jə-lat″ĭ-fĭ-ka′shən) conversion into gelatin.

**gel·a·tig·e·nous** (jel″ə-tij′ə-nəs) producing or forming gelatin.

**gel·a·tin** (jel′ə-tin) [L. *gelatina,* from *gelare* to congeal] [NF] [MeSH: Gelatin] a product obtained by partial hydrolysis of collagen derived from the skin, white connective tissue, and bones of animals; used as a suspending agent. It is also used pharmaceutically in the manufacture of capsules and suppositories, has been suggested for intravenous use as a plasma substitute, and has been used as an adjuvant protein food.
**glycerinated g.,** a preparation of gelatin and glycerin.
**medicated g.,** gelatin mixed with medicated substances for local application.
**silk g.,** sericin.
**g. of Wharton,** Wharton's jelly.
**zinc g.,** a preparation of zinc oxide, gelatin, glycerin, and purified water, applied topically as a protective. See also *Unna's boot,* under *boot.*

**ge·lat·i·nase** (jə-lat′ĭ-nās) a nonspecific extracellular proteolytic enzyme, produced by certain microorganisms, that hydrolyzes gelatin.

**gel·a·ti·nif·er·ous** (jel″ə-tĭ-nif′ər-əs) [*gelatin* + *-ferous*] producing gelatin.

**ge·lat·i·nize** (jə-lat′ĭ-nīz) 1. to convert into gelatin. 2. to become converted into gelatin.

**ge·lat·i·noid** (jə-lat′ĭ-noid) resembling gelatin.

**gel·a·ti·no·lyt·ic** (jel″ə-tin-o-lit′ik) [*gelatin* + *-lytic*] dissolving or splitting up gelatin.

**gel·a·ti·no·sa** (jel″ə-tĭ-no′sə) [L.] gelatinous; see entries beginning *substantia gelatinosa,* under *substantia.*

**ge·lat·i·nous** (jə-lat′ĭ-nəs) [L. *gelatinosus*] like jelly or softened gelatin.

**gel·a·ti·num** (jel″ə-tin′əm) [L., from *gelare* to congeal] gelatin.
**g. glycerina′tum,** glycerinated gelatin.

**ge·la·tion** (jə-la′shən) the conversion of a sol into a gel.

**ge·la·tum** (jə-la′təm) [L., from *gelare* to congeal] jelly, or gel.

**geld** (geld) to castrate a male animal, especially a horse.

**geld·ing** (gel′ding) a castrated male animal, especially a horse.

**Gel·film** (jel′film) trademark for absorbable gelatin film (q.v., under *film*).

**Gel·foam** (jel′fōm) trademark for an absorbable gelatin sponge (q.v., under *sponge).*

**Gé·li·neau's syndrome** (zha-le-nōz′) [Jean Baptiste Edouard *Gélineau,* French neurologist, 1859–1906] narcolepsy.

**Gell and Coombs classification** (jel and ko͞omz) [Philip George Howthern *Gell,* British immunologist, born 1914; Robert Royston Amos *Coombs,* British immunologist, born 1921] see under *classification.*

**gel·om·e·ter** (gel-om′ə-tər) a device for determining the time required for a solution to gel.

**Gel. quav.** abbreviation for L. *gelati′na qua′vis,* in any kind of jelly.

**gel·se·mine** (jel′sə-mēn) an alkaloid toxic to both humans and animals, obtained from the roots and rhizomes of *Gelsemium sempervirens;* it acts as a central nervous system stimulant and also causes double vision, muscular weakness, and sometimes respiratory arrest.

**Gel·se·mi·um** (gel-sem′e-um sem″pər-vi′renz) a genus of woody vines of the family Loganaceae, native to Asia and the southeastern United States. *G. sempervi′rens* (L.) Alt. is the yellow jessamine, a flowering plant of North America that contains gelsemine and other toxic alkaloids. It causes weakness, incoordination, convulsions, and sometimes respiratory arrest in humans, cattle, and poultry.

**gel·sol·in** (jel-sol′in) [MeSH: Gelsolin] an actin-binding protein that nucleates actin polymerization at low calcium concentrations but causes severing of actin filaments at high concentrations. It also binds to phosphatidylinositol bisphosphate, linking actin organization and signal transduction. See also *profilin.*

**Gel·tabs** (jel′tabz) trademark for a preparation of ergocalciferol.

**Gé·ly's suture** (zha-lēz′) [Jules Aristide *Gély,* French surgeon, 1806–1861] see under *suture.*

**ge·mäs·te·te** (gə-mes′tə-tə) [Ger.] swollen or bloated: a term applied to enlarged astrocytes in the region of a degenerated area.

**gem·cit·a·bine hy·dro·chlo·ride** (jem-sit′ə-bēn) an antineoplastic agent used in chemotherapy for pancreatic carcinoma; administered by intravenous infusion.

**Ge·mel·la** (jə-mel′ə) [L., dim. of *gemellus* a twin] a genus of aerobic or facultatively anaerobic cocci of the family Streptococcaceae, occurring singly or in pairs with adjacent sides flattened; they are found as parasites of mammals.
**G. haemoly′sans,** a species found in bronchial secretions and slime from the respiratory tract.

**gem·el·lary** (jem′ə-lar″e) pertaining to twins.

**gem·el·lip·a·ra** (jem′ə-lip′ə-rə) [L. *gemelli* twins + *para*] a woman who has given birth to twins.

**gem·el·lol·o·gy** (jem″əl-ol′ə-je) [L. *gemellus* twin + *-logy*] the scientific study of twins and twinning.

**gem·fib·ro·zil** (jem-fib′ro-zil) [USP] [MeSH: Gemfibrozil] a hypolipidemic drug chemically and pharmacologically related to clofibrate that lowers elevated serum lipids by decreasing triglyceride levels; administered orally in the treatment of very high serum triglyceride levels that are not responsive to diet.

**gem·i·nate** (jem′ĭ-nāt) [L. *geminatus*] paired; occurring in pairs.

**gem·i·na·tion** (jem″ĭ-na′shən) a doubling; a form of fusion of two teeth that results in the formation of two teeth or of a double crown formed on a single root with a single pulp canal. The term is usually applied to fusion of two supernumerary teeth or union of one supernumerary with a regular tooth.

**gem·i·ni** (jem′ĭ-ni) [L.] plural of *geminus.*

**gem·i·nous** (jem′ĭ-nəs) geminate.

**gem·i·nus** (jem′ĭ-nəs) pl. *ge′mini* [L.] a twin.
**ge′mini aequa′les,** monozygotic twins.

**ge·mis·to·cyte** (jə-mis′to-sīt″) [Gr. *gemistos* laden, full + *-cyte*] a pathologic astrocyte in which the cell body swells considerably, the nucleus assumes an eccentric position, and the cytoplasm is clearly visible; seen particularly in demyelinating and neoplastic conditions. Called also *gemistocytic astrocyte.*

**ge·mis·to·cyt·ic** (jə-mis″to-sĭ′tik) composed of large round cells (gemistocytes) stuffed with fatty debris; a term applied to astrocytomas composed of such cells.

**gem·ma** (jem′ə) [L. "bud"] a budlike body or structure.
**g. gustato′ria,** TA alternative for *caliculus gustatorius.*

**gem·ma·tion** (jə-ma′shən) [L. *gemmare* to bud] reproduction by budding, a kind of reproduction in cells in which a portion of the cell body is thrust out and then becomes separated, forming a new individual; used particularly to describe the formation of chlamydospores in fungi. See *budding,* def. 1.

**Gem·min·ges** (jə-min′jēz) a genus of bacteria made up of gram-positive anaerobic cocci, occasionally isolated from human specimens.

**gem·mule** (jem′ūl) [L. *gemmula,* dim. of *gemma* bud] 1. a reproductive bud; the immediate product of gemmation. 2. any one of the many little excrescences upon the dendrites of a neuron; they are particularly common on Purkinje cells and pyramidal cells. Called also *dendritic spine.*

**Gem·o·nil** (jem′o-nil) trademark for a preparation of metharbital.

**Gem·zar** (jem′zahr) trademark for a preparation of gemcitabine hydrochloride.

**-gen** [Gr. *-genēs* born, with an alteration in meaning to "producing"] a word termination denoting an agent productive of the object or state indicated by the word stem to which it is affixed, as allergen (allergy), cryogen (cold), and pathogen (disease).

**ge·nal** (je′nəl) [L. *gena* cheek] pertaining to the cheek; buccal.

**gen·der** (jen′dər) 1. sex (def. 1). 2. see *gender identity,* under *identity.*

**gene** (jēn) [Gr. *gennan* to produce] [MeSH: Genes] a segment of a DNA molecule that contains all the information required for synthe-

sis of a product (polypeptide chain or RNA molecule), including both coding and noncoding sequences. It is the biologic unit of heredity, self-reproducing, and transmitted from parent to progeny. Each gene has a specific position (locus) on the chromosome map. From the standpoint of function, genes are conceived of as structural, operator, and regulatory genes (see subentries).
**allelic g's,** alleles.
**autosomal g.,** a gene located on any chromosome that is not a sex chromosome.
**cell interaction (CI) g's,** genes of the major histocompatibility complex that control cell-cell interactions between B cells, T cells, and macrophages and between cytotoxic T cells and target cells.
**chimeric g.,** an artificial gene constructed by juxtaposition of fragments of unrelated genes or other DNA, which may themselves have been altered in sequence.
**CI g's,** cell interaction g's.
**codominant g's,** alleles that are both fully expressed in the heterozygote; called also *codominance.*
**complementary g's,** two independent pairs of nonallelic genes, neither of which will produce its effect in the absence of the other; called also *reciprocal g's.*
**g. complex,** a DNA segment containing a number of genes coding for products with related functions, e.g. the human major histocompatibility complex (MHC).
**cumulative g's,** polygenes.
**derepressed g.,** in genetic theory, one that in response to an environmental demand for a particular enzyme functions to increase production of that enzyme; cf. *repressed g.*
**dominant g.,** one that is phenotypically expressed when present either in homozygous or heterozygous form. See *recessive g.*
**H g., histocompatibility g.,** a gene that determines a histocompatibility antigen.
**holandric g's,** genes in the nonhomologous region of the Y chromosome.
**housekeeping g.,** a gene that theoretically must be expressed in all cells because it encodes proteins needed for basic functioning.
**immune response (Ir) g's,** genes that govern the immune response to certain antigens. Animals carrying the gene are responders; those lacking the gene are nonresponders. In all species studied they are autosomal dominant genes that map with the genes for class II MHC antigens; thus the HLA-D/DR genes are probably immune response genes in humans.
**immune suppressor (Is) g's,** genes governing the ability of suppressor T cells to respond to certain antigens.
**immunoglobulin g's,** the genes coding for immunoglobulin heavy and light chains, which are organized in three loci coding for $\kappa$ light chains, $\lambda$ light chains, and heavy chains found on human chromosomes 2, 22, and 14, respectively. These genes undergo several DNA rearrangements during the differentiation of stem cells into B cells and plasma cells, permitting synthesis of the various immunoglobulin classes.
**Ir g's,** immune response g's.
**Is g's,** immune suppressor g's.
**leaky g.,** one in which a switch in the sequence of bases in a nucleotide results in the production of a mutant protein that, because of a single amino acid replacement, has only partial enzymatic activity; a hypomorph.
**lethal g.,** a gene the presence of which brings about the death of the organism, or permits its survival only under certain conditions; see also *lethal equivalent.*
**major g.,** a gene whose effect on the phenotype is always evident, regardless of how this effect is modified by other genes.
**mutant g.,** a gene in which the loss, gain, or exchange of material has resulted in a permanent transmissible change in function. Such a gene may have become practically inactive *(amorph),* may act to antagonize or inhibit normal activity *(antimorph),* may act to increase normal activity *(hypermorph),* or may show only a slight reduction in its effectiveness *(leaky gene* or *hypomorph).*
**operator g.,** in bacterial genetics, a gene that serves as a starting point for reading the genetic code and controls the activity of the structured genes by interacting with a repressor. Called also *operator* and *operator locus.*
**pleiotropic g.,** one producing many effects in the phenotype.
**recessive g.,** one that is phenotypically expressed only when homozygous or hemizygous. See *dominant g.*
**reciprocal g's,** complementary g's.
**regulator g., regulatory g.,** in genetic theory, a gene that synthesizes repressor, a substance which, through interaction with the operator gene, switches off the activity of the structural genes associated with it in the operon. More generally, a gene whose product affects the activity of other genes.
**repressed g.,** in genetic theory, one that under normal conditions does not always function to produce the maximum number of enzymes; cf. *derepressed g.*
**repressor g.,** regulator g.
**sex-conditioned g., sex-influenced g.,** a gene that is fully expressed in one sex only, e.g. human baldness.
**sex-limited g.,** a sex-linked or autosomal gene that will produce an effect in one sex only.
**sex-linked g.,** a gene carried on a sex chromosome (X or Y); only X linkage has clinical significance, and sex linkage is more correctly called X linkage.
**silent g.,** a mutant gene having no detectable phenotypic effect.
**split g.,** a gene containing multiple exons and at least one intron.
**structural g.,** a gene that specifies the amino acid sequence of a polypeptide chain. Messenger RNA is its primary product.
**sublethal g.,** a gene the presence of which handicaps or impairs the function of the organism.
**suicide g.,** a protein-coding sequence that produces an enzyme capable of converting a nontoxic prodrug to a cytotoxic compound; it is coupled to a promoter from a tumor-associated marker gene and introduced into tumor cells by a virus vector.
**supplementary g's,** two independent pairs of genes that interact in such a way that one dominant will produce its effect even in the absence of the other, but the second requires the presence of the first to be effective.
**suppressor g.,** see *suppression,* def. 3.
**syntenic g's,** genes located on the same chromosome.
**tumor suppressor g.,** a gene whose function is to limit cell proliferation and loss of whose function leads to cell transformation and tumor growth; called also *antioncogene.*
**wild-type g.,** the normal allele of a gene, sometimes symbolized by +.
**XIST g.** [*X-i*nactivation–*s*pecific *t*ranscript], a gene, expressed only from the inactive X chromosome (see *lyonization*), that is responsible for initiating the inactivation of genes on that chromosome. It does not encode a protein and is believed to function through an RNA transcription product by a mechanism that is not yet understood.
**X-linked g.,** a gene carried on the X chromosome; the corresponding trait, whether dominant or recessive, is always expressed in males, who have only one X chromosome. X linkage is used sometimes synonymously with sex linkage since no genetic disorders have as yet been associated with genes on the Y chromosome.
**Y-linked g.,** a gene located on the Y chromosome; the trait determined by it is therefore exhibited only by males and is transmitted by a father to all of his sons. Other than the genes that determine maleness, no clinically significant Y-linked genes have been identified in human beings.

**gen·era** (jen′ər-ə) [L.] plural of *genus.*

**gen·er·al** (jen′ər-əl) [L. *generalis*] affecting many parts or all parts of the organism; not local.

**gen·er·al·iza·tion** (jen″ər-əl-ĭ-za′shən) 1. act or process of generalizing. 2. a general principle or idea.
**stimulus g.,** exhibition of a conditioned response to stimuli similar but not identical to the conditioned stimulus.

**gen·er·al·ize** (jen′ər-əl-īz) 1. to spread throughout the body, as when local disease becomes systemic. 2. to form a general principle; to reason inductively.

**gen·er·a·tion** (jen″ər-a′shən) [L. *generatio*] 1. the act or process of reproduction. 2. a class composed of all individuals removed by the same number of successive ancestors from a common predecessor, or occupying positions on the same level in a genealogic chart.
**alternate g.,** the alternate reproduction by asexual and sexual means in an animal or plant species.
**asexual g.,** production of a new organism by budding, fission, or any method not requiring the union of sexual elements.
**direct g.,** asexual g.
**first filial g.,** all of the offspring produced by the mating of two individuals, as in a hybrid cross; symbol $F_1$.
**nonsexual g.,** asexual g.
**parental g.,** the generation with which a particular genetic study is begun; symbol $P_1$.
**second filial g.,** all of the offspring produced by the mating of two individuals of the first filial generation; symbol $F_2$.
**sexual g.,** production of a new individual (organism) by the union of male and female elements (gametes).
**spontaneous g.,** abiogenesis; the discredited concept of the development of living organisms from nonliving matter.

**gen·er·a·tive** (jen′ər-ə-tiv″) pertaining to the reproduction of the species.

**gen·er·a·tor** (jen′ər-a″tor) 1. something that produces or causes to exist. 2. a machine that converts mechanical to electrical energy.
**pattern g.,** a network of neurons, in vertebrates most often located in the central nervous system, that produces a stereotyped form of

complex movement, such as ambulation or chewing, that is almost invariable from one performance to the next.
**pulse g.**, the power source for a cardiac pacemaker system, usually fueled by lithium, supplying impulses to the implanted electrodes, either at a fixed rate or in some programmed pattern.

**ge•ner•ic** (jə-ner'ik) [L. *genus, generis* kind] 1. pertaining to a genus. 2. nonproprietary; denoting a drug name not protected by a trademark, usually descriptive of its chemical structure; sometimes called *public name.*

**ge•ne•si•al, ge•nes•ic** (jə-ne'zhəl, jə-nes'ik) pertaining to generation or to origin.

**ge•ne•si•ol•o•gy** (jə-ne"ze-ol'ə-je) [*genesis* + *-logy*] the scientific study of reproduction.

**gen•e•sis** (jən'ə-sis) [Gr. "production," "generation"] the coming into being of anything; the process of originating.

**-genesis** a word termination used to denote the production, formation, or development of the object or state indicated by the word stem to which it is affixed, as *biogenesis, gametogenesis,* and *pathogenesis.*

**gen•e•sis•ta•sis** (jen"ə-sis'tə-sis) [*genesis* + *-stasis*] interruption of the reproduction of organisms by chemotherapy so as to permit the body cells or fluids to dispose of them.

**gen•e•sta•tic** (jen"ə-stat'ik) tending to prevent sporulation.

**ge•net•ic** (jə-net'ik) 1. pertaining to reproduction, or to birth or origin. 2. determined by genes.

**ge•net•i•cist** (jə-net'ĭ-sist) a specialist in genetics.

**ge•net•ics** (jə-net'iks) [Gr. *gennan* to produce] [MeSH: Genetics] the study of genes and their heredity.
**bacterial g.**, the study of mechanisms of heredity in bacteria.
**biochemical g.**, the science concerned with the chemical and physical nature of genes and the mechanism by which they control the development and maintenance of the organism.
**clinical g.**, the study of the possible genetic factors influencing the occurrence of clinical disorders.
**mathematical g.**, the statistical analysis of probabilities of genetic transmission, genes in populations, and hypothesis testing.
**molecular g.**, that branch of genetics concerned with the molecular structure and activities of the genetic material, including the replication of DNA, its transcription into RNA, and the translation of RNA to form proteins.
**population g.**, the study of the distribution of genes in populations and of how genes and genotype frequencies are maintained or changed. See also *Hardy-Weinberg law,* under *law.*
**reverse g.**, the indirect exploration of a genetic disease by learning the location of the responsible gene, isolating and cloning its DNA, and translating the DNA to determine the protein product. By comparing this product with the product of the normal allele, one can also analyze the nature of the normal protein altered by the mutation. Called also *positional cloning.*

**ge•neto•troph•ic** (jə-net"o-trof'ik) pertaining to genetics and nutrition; relating to problems of nutrition that are hereditary in nature, or transmitted through the genes.

**gen•e•tous** (jen'ə-təs) dating from fetal life.

**Ge•ne•va Con•ven•tion** (jə-ne'və) an international agreement of 1864 whereby, among other pledges, the signatory nations pledged themselves to treat the wounded and the army medical and nursing staffs as neutrals on the field of battle.

**Gen•gou phenomenon** (zhaw-goo') [Octave *Gengou,* Belgian bacteriologist, 1875–1957] complement fixation.

**ge•ni•al, ge•ni•an** (jə-ni'əl, jə-ni'ən) [*geni-* + *-al*[1]] pertaining to the chin.

**gen•ic** (jen'ik) pertaining to or caused by genes.

**-genic** [Gr. *gennan* to produce] a word termination meaning producing, or productive of.

**ge•nic•u•la** (jə-nik'u-lə) [L.] plural of *geniculum.*

**ge•nic•u•lar** (jə-nik'u-lər) pertaining to the knee.

**ge•nic•u•late** (jə-nik'u-lāt) [L. *geniculatus*] bent, like a knee.

**ge•nic•u•lo•cal•car•ine** (jə-nik"u-lo-kal'kə-rīn) [*geniculum* + *calcarine*] pertaining to, or connecting, one of the geniculate bodies and the calcar avis or calcarine sulcus.

**ge•nic•u•lo•stri•ate** (jə-nik"u-lo-stri'āt) connecting one of the geniculate nuclei with the striate cortex.

**ge•nic•u•lum** (jə-nik'u-ləm) pl. *genic'ula* [L., dim. of *genu*] [TA] a general term designating a sharp, kneelike bend in a small structure or organ, such as a nerve.
**g. cana'lis facia'lis, g. cana'lis ner'vi facia'lis** [TA], geniculum of facial canal: the bend in the facial canal lodging the geniculum nervi facialis; called also *genu of facial canal.*
**g. ner'vi facia'lis** [TA], geniculum of facial nerve: the part of the facial nerve at the lateral end of the internal acoustic meatus, where the fibers turn sharply posteroinferiorly, and where the geniculate ganglion is found; called also *external genu of facial nerve.*

**gen•in** (jen'in) aglycon.

**geni(o)-** [Gr. *geneion* chin] a combining form denoting relationship to the chin. See also words beginning *ment(o)-.*

**ge•nio•chei•lo•plas•ty** (je"ne-o-ki'lo-plas"te) [*genio-* + *cheilo-* + *-plasty*] plastic surgery of the chin and lip.

**ge•nio•glos•sus** (je"ne-o-glos'əs) see under *musculus.*

**ge•nio•hyo•glos•sus** (je"ne-o-hi"o-glos'əs) musculus genioglossus.

**ge•nio•hy•oid** (je"ne-o-hi'oid) pertaining to the chin and hyoid bone.

**ge•nio•hy•oi•de•us** (je"ne-o-hi-oi'de-əs) see under *musculus.*

**ge•nio•plas•ty** (je'ne-o-plas"te) [*genio-* + *-plasty*] plastic surgery of the chin.

**gen•i•tal** (jen'ĭ-təl) [L. *genitalis* belonging to birth] 1. pertaining to reproduction or generation. 2. pertaining to the genitalia.

**gen•i•ta•lia** (jen"ĭ-tāl'e-ə) [L., pl.] [MeSH: Genitalia] the various external and internal organs concerned with reproduction; see *organa genitalia.*
**ambiguous g.**, genital organs with characteristics typical of both male and female, as seen in hermaphroditism and some types of pseudohermaphroditism.
**external g.**, see *organa genitalia feminina externa* and *organa genitalia masculina externa.*
**indifferent g.**, the reproductive organs of the embryo prior to the establishment of definitive sex. In human embryos this stage occurs during the fourth to seventh weeks.
**internal g.**, see *organa genitalia feminina interna* and *organa genitalia masculina interna.*

**gen•i•tal•oid** (jen'ĭ-tal-oid) [*genitalia* + *-oid*] pertaining to the primordial sex cells, before future sexuality is distinguishable.

**genit(o)-** [*genital,* q.v.] a combining form denoting relationship to the organs of reproduction.

**gen•i•to•cru•ral** (jen"ĭ-to-kroo'rəl) [*genital* + *crural*] pertaining to the genitalia and the leg.

**gen•i•to•fem•o•ral** (jen"ĭ-to-fem'or-əl) genitocrural.

**gen•i•tog•ra•phy** (jen"ĭ-tog'rə-fe) radiography of the urogenital sinus and internal duct structures after injection of a contrast medium through the opening of the sinus.

**gen•i•to•plas•ty** (jen'ĭ-to-plas"te) [*genital* + *-plasty*] plastic surgery on the genital organs.

**gen•i•to•uri•nary** (jen"ĭ-to-u'rĭ-nar-e) pertaining to the genital and urinary organs; called also *urinogenital* and *urogenital.*

**ge•nius** (jēn'yəs) 1. distinctive character or peculiar nature. 2. superlative aptitude or ability. 3. a person with superlative aptitude or ability.

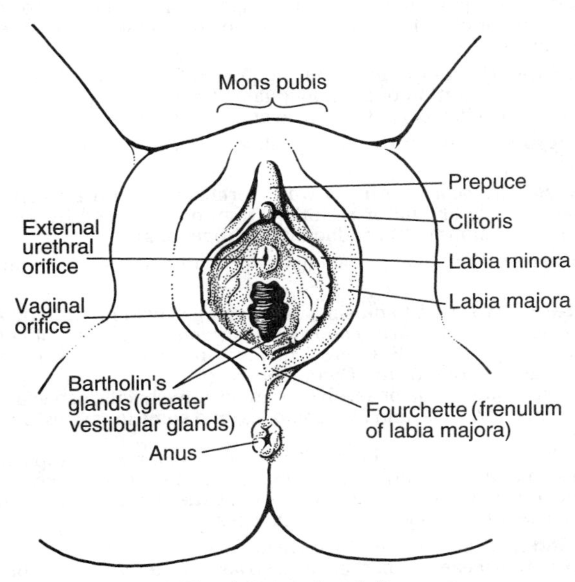


Female external genitalia.

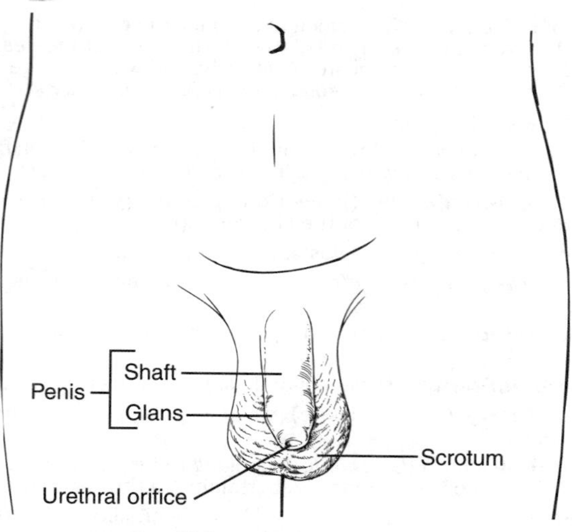

Male external genitalia.

**Gen·na·ri's line (band, stria, stripe)** (jĕ-nah'rēz) [Francesco *Gennari,* Italian anatomist, 1750–1796] see under *line.*

**gen(o)-** [Gr. *genos* offspring, race, kind] a combining form denoting relationship to (1) reproduction, (2) sex, (3) race or kind, or (4) a gene or genes.

**geno·blast** (jen'o-blast) [*geno-* + *-blast*[1]] 1. the nucleus of the fertilized oocyte. 2. a mature germ cell.

**geno·copy** (jen'o-kop"e) a genetic trait that is a phenotypic copy of another trait but caused by a different mechanism. See also *phenocopy.*

**geno·der·ma·tol·o·gy** (jen"o-dər"mə-tol'ə-je) that branch of dermatology that treats hereditary skin diseases.

**geno·der·ma·to·sis** (jen"o-dər"mə-to'sis) [*geno-* + *dermatosis*] a genetically determined disorder of the skin, usually generalized; if circumscribed, it is usually called *nevus.*

**ge·nome** (je'nōm) [*gene* + chromos*ome*] [MeSH: Genome] 1. the complete gene complement of an organism, contained in a set of chromosomes in eukaryotes, a single chromosome in bacteria, or a DNA or RNA molecule in viruses. 2. the full set of genes in an individual, either haploid (the set derived from one parent) or diploid (the double set, derived from both parents). In a human being the haploid set contains about 3 billion base pairs of DNA and 50,000–100,000 genes.

**ge·nom·ic** (je-nom'ik) pertaining to the genome.

**ge·no·spe·cies** (je'no-spe"shēz) a group of bacterial strains capable of genetic transfer and recombination.

**geno·tox·ic** (je"no-tok'sik) damaging to DNA: pertaining to agents (radiation or chemical substances) known to damage DNA, thereby causing mutations or cancer.

**geno·type** (jen'o-tīp) [*geno-* + *type*] [MeSH: Genotype] 1. the entire genetic constitution of an individual. 2. the alleles present at one or more specific loci. 3. the type species of a genus.

**geno·typ·ic** (jen"o-ti'pik) pertaining to or expressive of the genotype.

**-genous** [Gr. *-genēs* born] a word termination with two opposite meanings: (1) arising or resulting from, or produced by (endogenous, pyogenous); (2) producing (androgenous).

**Gen·ta·fair** (jen'tə-fār) trademark for a preparation of gentamicin sulfate.

**gen·ta·mi·cin** (jen"tə-mi'sin) an aminoglycoside antibiotic complex derived from *Micromonospora purpurea,* consisting of components designated A, B, C, etc. The form in clinical use is a mixture of three fractions of the C component ($C_1$, $C_{1A}$, $C_2$); it is effective against a wide range of aerobic gram-negative bacilli, especially the Enterobacteriaceae and *Pseudomonas,* and some gram-positive bacteria.
**g. sulfate** [USP], the sulfate salt of gentamicin, applied topically to the skin and conjunctiva and administered intramuscularly and intravenously in the treatment of a wide variety of infections caused by susceptible gram-negative organisms.

**gen·tian** (jen'shən) the dried rhizome and roots of *Gentiana lutea* L. (Gentianaceae); it has been used as a bitter tonic. It contains gentiin, gentiamarin, gentisin, gentisic acid, gentiopicrin, gentianose, and pectin. Also known as *yellow* or *pale gentian.*
**g. violet** [USP], a dye occurring as a dark green powder or greenish glistening pieces having a metallic luster, with antibacterial, antifungal, and anthelmintic properties, applied topically in the treatment of infections of the skin and mucous membranes associated with gram-positive bacteria and molds, and administered orally in pinworm and liver fluke infections. It has been given in strongyloidosis.

**gen·tian·o·phil** (jen'shən-o-fil) 1. an element staining readily with gentian violet. 2. gentianophilic.

**gen·tian·o·phil·ic** (jen'shən-o-fil'ik) [*gentian* + *-philic*] staining readily with gentian violet.

**gen·tian·oph·i·lous** (jen"shən-of'ĭ-ləs) gentianophilic.

**gen·tian·o·pho·bic** (jen"shən-o-fo'bik) not staining readily with gentian violet.

**gen·tian·oph·o·bous** (jen"shən-of'ə-bəs) gentianophobic.

**gen·tia·vern** (jen'shə-vərn) gentian violet.

**gen·tio·pic·rin** (jen"she-o-pik'rin) a bitter, crystalline glycoside found in gentian.

**gen·ti·sate** (jen'tĭ-sāt) a salt of gentisic acid.

**gen·tis·ic acid** (jen-tis'ik) trivial name for 2,5-dihydroxybenzoic acid.

**Gen·tran** (jen'tran) trademark for a preparation of dextran.

**gen·tro·gen·in** (jen"tro-jen'in) botogenin.

**ge·nu** (je'nu)gen. *ge'nus,* pl. *ge'nua* [L.] [TA] 1. the knee; the site of articulation between the thigh (femur) and leg. 2. a general term used to designate any anatomic structure bent like the knee.
**g. cap'sulae inter'nae** [TA], genu of internal capsule: the blunt angle formed by the union of the two limbs of the internal capsule, situated posterior to the caudate nucleus, anterior to the thalamus, and medial to the lentiform nucleus; called also *knee of internal capsule.*
**g. cor'poris callo'si** [TA], genu of corpus callosum: the sharp ventral curve at the anterior end of the trunk of the corpus callosum.
**g. extror'sum,** g. varum.
**g. of facial canal,** geniculum canalis facialis.
**g. of facial nerve,** 1. genu nervi facialis. 2. geniculum nervi facialis.
**g. of facial nerve, external,** geniculum nervi facialis.
**g. of facial nerve, internal,** g. nervi facialis.
**g. impres'sum,** a flattening and bending of the knee joint to one side, with consequent displacement of the patella up and to the same side.
**g. of internal capsule,** g. capsulae internae.
**g. intror'sum,** g. valgum.
**g. ner'vi facia'lis** [TA], genu of facial nerve: the bend in the fibers arising from the nucleus of the facial nerve, which produces the facial colliculus in the floor of the fourth ventricle; it is at this point that the fibers loop around the abducens nucleus.
**g. recurva'tum,** hyperextension of the knee; called also *back knee.*
**g. val'gum,** a deformity in which the knees are abnormally close together and the space between the ankles is increased; known also as *knock knee.*
**g. va'rum,** a deformity in which the knees are abnormally separated and the lower extremities are bowed inwardly; the deformity may be in the thigh or leg, or both. Known also as *bowleg.*

**gen·ua** (jen'u-ə) [L.] plural of *genu.*

**gen·u·al** (jen'u-əl) relating to or resembling a genu or knee.

**genu·cu·bi·tal** (jen"u-ku'bĭ-təl) [*genu* + *cubital*] pertaining to the knees and elbows; see under *position.*

**genu·fa·cial** (jen"u-fa'shəl) [*genu* + *facial*] pertaining to the knees and face; see under *position.*

**genu·pec·to·ral** (jen"u-pek'tor-əl) [*genu* + *pectoral*] pertaining to the knees and chest; see under *position.*

**ge·nus** (je'nəs) pl. *gen'era* [L.] a taxonomic category subordinate to a tribe (or subtribe) and superior to a species (or subgenus).

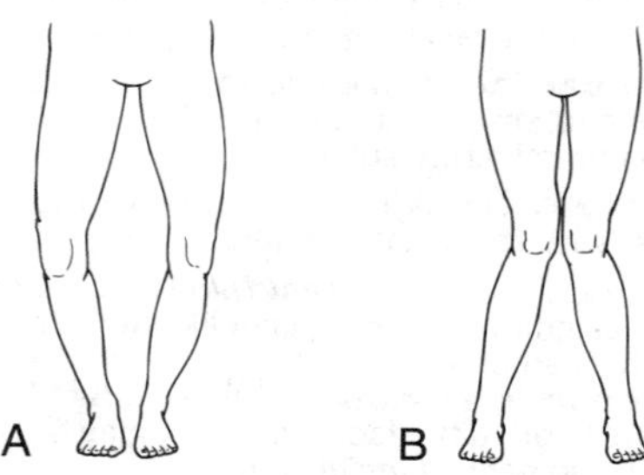

*(A),* Genu varum; *(B),* genu valgum.

**-geny** [Gr. *-geneia,* from *-genēs* born] a word termination denoting generation or origin.

**ge(o)-** [Gr. *gē* earth] a combining form denoting relationship to the earth, or to soil.

**geo·bi·ol·o·gy** (je″o-bi-ol′ə-je) [*geo-* + *biology*] the biology of terrestrial life.

**geo·chem·is·try** (je″o-kem′is-tre) [*geo-* + *chemistry*] the science concerned with study of the elements in the earth's crust and the chemical changes that occur therein.

**Geo·cil·lin** (je″o-sil′in) trademark for a preparation of carbenicillin indanyl sodium.

**ge·ode** (je′ōd) [Gr. *geōdes* earthlike: so called from a fancied resemblance to a mineral geode] a dilated lymph space.

**ge·o·gen** (je′o-jən) an aspect of the geography or geochemistry of an area that affects organisms in it, particularly with reference to disease.

**geo·med·i·cine** (je″o-med′ĭ-sin) [*geo-* + *medicine*] the branch of medicine dealing with the influence of geographic factors, such as climate and environmental conditions, on health and disease. Called also *nosogeography* and *geographic medicine.* See also *geographic pathology,* under *pathology.*

**geo·pa·thol·o·gy** (je″o-pə-thol′ə-je) [*geo-* + *pathology*] the study of the peculiarities of disease in relation to topography, climate, food habits, etc., of various regions of the earth.

**Ge·o·pen** (je′o-pən) trademark for a preparation of carbenicillin disodium.

**geo·pha·gia** (je-o-fa′jə) [*geo-* + *-phagia*] the habit of eating clay or earth; a form of pica.

**ge·oph·a·gism** (je-of′ə-jiz-əm) geophagia.

**ge·oph·a·gy** (je-of′ə-je) geophagia.

**geo·phil·ic** (je″o-fil′ik) [*geo-* + *-philic*] characterized by an affinity for soil; some geophilic organisms will infect humans or other animals when they are weak or immunocompromised. Cf. *anthropophilic* and *zoophilic.*

**geo·tac·tic** (je″o-tak′tik) pertaining to geotaxis.

**geo·tax·is** (je″o-tak′sis) [*geo-* + *taxis*] taxis of an animal in response to gravitational force.

**geo·tri·cho·sis** (je″o-trĭ-ko′sis) [MeSH: Geotrichosis] infection by *Geotrichum candidum,* which may attack the bronchi, lungs, mouth, or intestinal tract; its manifestations resemble those of candidiasis.

**Ge·ot·ri·chum** (je-ot′rĭ-kəm) [MeSH: Geotrichum] a genus of yeastlike imperfect fungi of the form-family Cryptococcaceae, closely related to *Trichosporon. G. can′didum,* found in the feces and in dairy products, is the etiologic agent of geotrichosis.

**ge·o·trop·ic** (je″o-trop′ik) influenced by gravity; pertaining to geotropism.

**ge·ot·ro·pism** (je-ot′ro-piz-əm) [*geo-* + *tropism*] tropism in an organism in response to gravitational force, as the downward growth of the roots of a plant *(positive g.),* while the stem grows upward *(negative g.).*

**ge·ra·ni·ol** (jə-ra′ne-ol) 1. a 10-carbon branched-chain alcohol occurring widely in essential oils of plants. 2. a pheromone of certain species of bees, being secreted by worker bees to signal the location of food.

**ge·rat·ic** (jə-rat′ik) [Gr. *gēras* old age] pertaining to old age.

**ger·a·tol·o·gy** (jer″ə-tol′ə-je) gereology.

**Ger·bich blood group** (gər′bich) [from the name of the American propositus first observed in 1960] see under *blood group.*

**ger·bil** (jər′bil) [MeSH: Gerbillinae] any of several species of small burrowing rodents of genus *Gerbillus* and related genera; they are native to the more arid parts of Africa and southwestern Asia. Some species serve as reservoirs for bubonic plague and others as reservoirs for Old World cutaneous leishmaniasis.
**great g.,** *Rhombomys opimus.*

**Ger·bil·lus** (jər-bil′əs) a genus of rodents of the family Muridae, including gerbils.

**GERD** gastroesophageal reflux disease.

**Ger·dy's fibers,** etc. (zher-dēz′) [Pierre Nicholas *Gerdy,* French surgeon, 1797–1856] see under *fiber, fontanelle, fossa, loop,* and *ligament.*

**ger·e·ol·o·gy** (jer″e-ol′ə-je) [*gero-* + *-logy*] the science that deals with old age and its phenomena.

**Ger·hardt's disease, sign (phenomenon), syndrome** (ger′hahrts) [Carl Adolf Christian Jacob *Gerhardt,* German physician, 1833–1902] see under *triangle* and see *erythromelalgia.*

**Ger·hardt's test** (zher-hahrts′) [Charles Frédéric *Gerhardt,* French chemist, 1816–1856] see under *test.*

**Ger·hardt-Se·mon law** (ger′harht-se′mon) [C.A.C.J. *Gerhardt;* Sir Felix *Semon,* German-born English laryngologist, 1849–1921] see under *law.*

**ger·i·at·ric** (jer″e-at′rik) 1. pertaining to elderly persons or to the aging process. 2. pertaining to geriatrics.

**ger·i·atri·cian** (jer″e-ə-trish′ən) a specialist in geriatrics.

**ger·i·at·rics** (jer″e-at′riks) [*ger-* + *-iatrics*] [MeSH: Geriatrics] that branch of medicine that treats all problems peculiar to old age and the aging, including the clinical problems of senescence and senility.
**dental g.,** gerodontics.

**geri·odon·tics** (jer″e-o-don′tiks) gerodontics.

**geri·odon·tist** (jer″e-o-don′tist) gerodontist.

**Ger·lach's valve** (ger′lahks) [Joseph von *Gerlach,* German anatomist, 1820–1896] see *valvula processus vermiformis.*

**Ger·lier's disease** (zher-le-āz′) [Felix *Gerlier,* Swiss physician, 1840–1914] see under *disease.*

**germ** (jərm) [L. *germen*] 1. a pathogenic microorganism. 2. living substance capable of developing into an organ, part, or organism as a whole; a primordium.
**dental g.,** tooth g.
**enamel g.,** the epithelial rudiment of the enamel organ.
**hair g.,** see *hair matrix,* under *matrix.*
**tooth g.,** a budlike thickening of the dental lamina that is the primordium of a tooth, and in which the enamel knot develops; the collective structures from which a tooth is formed, including the dental follicle, enamel organ, and dental papilla. Called also *dental g.* See also *tooth bud,* under *bud.*

**Ger·ma·nin** (jər′mə-nin) trademark for a preparation of suramin sodium.

**ger·ma·ni·um** (jər-ma′ne-əm) [MeSH: Germanium] a rare element, having the appearance of a bluish gray metalloid, atomic number 32, atomic weight 72.59; symbol, Ge.

**ger·mer·ine** (jər′mər-ēn) a crystalline alkaloid, $C_{36}H_{57}O_{11}N$, from *Veratrum senecio.*

**ger·mi·ci·dal** (gər″mĭ-si′dəl) [L. *germen* germ + *caedere* to kill] lethal to pathogenic microorganisms.

**ger·mi·cide** (jər′mĭ-sīd) an agent that kills pathogenic microorganisms.

**ger·mi·nal** (jər′mĭ-nəl) [L. *germinalis*] pertaining to or of the nature of a gamete (germ cell) or the primordial stage of development.

**ger·mi·na·tion** (jər″mĭ-na′shən) [L. *germinatio*] [MeSH: Germination] the sprouting of a seed or spore or of a plant embryo.

**ger·mi·na·tive** (jər′mĭ-na″tiv) [L. *germinativus*] pertaining to or causing germination.

**ger·mi·no·ma** (jər″mĭ-no′mə) [MeSH: Germinoma] a type of germ cell tumor consisting of large round cells with vesicular nuclei, usually found in the ovary, undescended testis, anterior mediastinum, or pineal gland; in males these are called *seminomas* and in females *dysgerminomas.*
**pineal g.,** a common type of pineal tumor, consisting of nests of large spherical germ cells that are surrounded by a network of reticular connective tissue and are histologically identical to the germ cells of the testes or ovaries.

**ger·mi·trine** (jər′mĭ-trēn) an antihypertensive alkaloid isolated from *Veratrum viride.*

**germ·line, germ line** (jərm′līn) the sequence of cells in the line of direct descent from zygote to gamete, as opposed to somatic cells (all other body cells). Mutations in germline cells are transmitted to progeny; those in somatic cells are not.

**ger(o)-** [Gr. *gēras* old age] combining form denoting relationship to old age or to the aged.

**ger·o·der·ma, gero·der·mia** (jer″o-dər′mə) [*gero-* + *derma*] dystrophy of the skin and genitals, producing the appearance of old age.
**g. osteodysplas′tica,** a condition believed to be transmitted as an autosomal recessive trait, in which geroderma is associated with osseous changes, including osteoporosis and lines in the bones somewhat resembling growth rings of a tree. Called also *Walt Disney dwarfism.*

**gero·der·mia** (jer″o-dər′me-ə) geroderma.

**ger·odon·tia** (jer-o-don′shə) gerodontics.

**ger·odon·tic** (jer″o-don′tik) [*gero-* + *odontic*] 1. pertaining to changes in the dental tissues with age. 2. pertaining to the practice of gerodontics.

**ger·odon·tics** (jer″o-don′tiks) [*gero-* + *odontic*] the delivery of dental care to aging persons; the diagnosis, prevention, and treatment of problems peculiar to advanced age. Called also *dental geriatrics* and *gerodontia.*

**ger·odon·tist** (jer″o-don′tist) a dentist who practices gerodontics.

**ger·odon·tol·o·gy** (jer″o-don-tol′ə-je) the study of the dentition and dental problems in the aged or aging.

**gero·ma·ras·mus** (jer″o-mə-raz′məs) [*gero-* + Gr. *marasmos* a wasting] the emaciation sometimes characteristic of old age.

**gero·mor·phism** (jer″o-mor′fiz-əm) [*gero-* + *morph-* + *-ism*] premature senility.
**cutaneous g.**, a condition in which the skin shows at a very early age the characteristics of old age.

**ger·on·tal** (jer-on′təl) senile.

**ger·on·tic** (jə-ron′tik) senile.

**geront(o)-** [Gr. *gerōn,* gen. *gerontos* old man] combining from denoting relationship to old age or to the aged.

**ger·on·tol·o·gist** (jer″on-tol′ə-jist) a specialist in gerontology.

**ger·on·tol·o·gy** (jer″on-tol′ə-je) [*geronto-* + *-logy*] the scientific study of the problems of aging in all their aspects—clinical, biologic, historical, and sociologic.

**ger·on·to·phil·ia** (jer″on-to-fil′e-ə) [*geronto-* + *-philia*] sexual attraction to old people.

**ger·on·to·pia** (ger″on-to′pe-ə) [*geronto-* + *-opsia*] senopia.

**ger·on·to·ther·a·peu·tics** (jer-on″to-ther″ə-pu′tiks) [*geronto-* + *therapeutics*] therapeutic management of aging persons designed to retard and prevent the development of many of the aspects of senescence.

**ger·on·to·ther·a·py** (jer-on′to-ther′ə-pe) gerontotherapeutics.

**ger·on·to·tox·on** (jer-on″to-tok′son, jer-on-tok′son) arcus corneae; see under *arcus.*
**g. len′tis,** equatorial couching of the lens in the aged; no longer done.

**ger·on·tox·on** (jer″on-tok′son) gerontotoxon.

**gero·psy·chi·a·try** (jer″o-si-ki′ə-tre) a subspecialty of psychiatry dealing with mental illness in the elderly.

**Ge·ro·ta's fascia (capsule), method** (ga-ro′tahz) [Dumitru *Gerota,* Romanian anatomist, 1867–1939] see under *method* and see *fascia renalis* under *fascia.*

**Gerst·mann's syndrome** (gerst′mahnz) [Josef *Gerstmann,* Austrian neurologist, 1887–1969] [MeSH: Gerstmann's Syndrome] see under *syndrome.*

**Gerst·mann-Sträus·sler syndrome** (gerst′mahn-shtrois′lər) [J. *Gerstmann; E. Sträussler,* Austrian physician, 20th century] Gerstmann-Strässler-Scheinker syndrome.

**Gerst·mann-Sträus·sler-Schein·ker syndome** (gerst′mahn-shtrois′lər-shīn′kər) [J. *Gerstmann;* E. *Sträussler;* I. *Scheinker,* Austrian physician, 20th century] see under *syndrome.*

**ge·rüst·mark** (gĕ-rūst′mahrk) [Ger., from *Gerüst* scaffolding + *Mark* marrow] a unique, collagen-poor zone of connective tissue lying across the bone marrow adjoining the growing ends of bones; observed in scurvy.

**Ge·sell developmental schedule** (gə-zel′) [Arnold Lucius *Gesell,* American pediatrician and psychologist, 1880–1961] see under *schedule.*

**ges·ta·gen** (jes′tə-jen) progestational agent.

**ge·stalt** (gə-stawlt′, gə-shtawlt′) [Ger.] form, shape; a whole perceptual configuration. See *gestaltism.*

**ge·stal·tism** (gə-stawl′tiz-əm, gə-shtawl′tiz-əm) [*gestalt* + *-ism*] that theory in psychology that claims that the objects of mind, as immediately presented to direct experience, come as complete, unanalyzable wholes or forms (Gestalten) that cannot be split up into parts; called also *gestalt theory.*

**ges·ta·tion** (jes-ta′shən) [L. *gestatio,* from *gestare* to bear] the period of development of the young in viviparous animals, from the time of fertilization of the oocyte (ovum) until birth; see also *pregnancy.*
**multiple g.,** multiple pregnancy.

**ges·to·sis** (jes-to′sis) pl. *gesto′ses* [L. *gestare* to bear] any manifestation of preeclampsia in pregnancy.

**ges·tri·none** (jes′trĭ-nōn) [MeSH: Gestrinone] a synthetic steroid hormone with androgenic, antiestrogenic, and antiprogestogenic properties, used in the treatment of endometriosis; administered orally.

**GeV, Gev** gigaelectron volt.

**GFAP** glial fibrillary acidic protein.

**GFR** glomerular filtration rate.

**GGT** γ-glutamyltransferase.

**GH** growth hormone.

**GHA** gluceptate (glucoheptonate).

**Ghon's complex, focus (primary lesion, tubercle)** (gonz) [Anton *Ghon,* Austrian-born pathologist in Czechoslovakia, 1866–1936] see *primary complex,* and see under *focus.*

**Ghon-Sachs bacillus** (gon-sahks) [A. *Ghon;* Anton *Sachs,* Austrian physician, 19th century] *Clostridium septicum.*

**ghost** (gōst) a faint or shadowy figure, lacking the customary substance of reality.
**red cell g.,** ghost cell (def. 2).

**GH-RH** growth hormone–releasing hormone.

**GI** gastrointestinal.

**Gia·co·mi·ni's band** (jah-ko-me′nēz) [Carlo *Giacomini,* Italian anatomist, 1841–1898] see under *band.*

**Gia·nel·li's sign** (jah-nel′ēz) [Giuseppe *Gianelli,* Italian physician, 1799–1871] Tournay's sign.

**Gian·nuz·zi's crescents (bodies, cells, demilunes)** (jah-nōōt′zēz) [Guiseppe *Giannuzzi,* Italian anatomist, 1839–1876] see under *crescent.*

**Gia·not·ti-Cros·ti syndrome** (jah-not′e-kros′te) [Fernando *Gianotti,* Italian dermatologist, born 1920; Agostino *Crosti,* Italian dermatologist, born 1896] see under *syndrome.*

**gi·ant** (ji′ənt) [Gr. *gigas*] a person or organism of very great size; see *gigantism.*

**gi·ant·ism** (ji′ənt-iz-əm) 1. gigantism. 2. excessive size, as of cells or nuclei.

**Gi·ar·dia** (e-ahr′de-ə) [Alfred *Giard,* biologist in Paris, 1846–1908] [MeSH: Giardia] a genus of usually nonpathogenic, flagellate intestinal protozoa (suborder Diplomonadina, order Diplomonadida) parasitic in various vertebrates, including humans, characterized by the presence of a large sucking disk on the ventral body surface, by means of which the organism adheres to the microvilli of the host's intestinal epithelium; two anterior nuclei; and eight flagella in four pairs.
**G. intestina′lis,** *G. lamblia.*
**G. lamb′lia,** a species that is the usual cause of giardiasis in humans; it may also infect domestic animals. Called also *Giardia intestinalis* and *Lamblia intestinalis.*

**Gib·ber·el·la** (jib″ə-rel′ə) [MeSH: Gibberella] a genus of fungi of the family Hypocreaceae. *G. fujiku′roi* is the perfect (sexual) stage of *Fusarium moniliforme* and causes a disease of rice plants; it was the original source of the gibberellins.

**gib·ber·el·lin** any in a group of plant growth hormones (auxins), originally isolated from the fungus *Gibberella fujikuroi.*

**gi·ar·di·a·sis** (je″ahr-di′ə-sis) [MeSH: Giardiasis] 1. a common infection of the human small intestine with the protozoan *Giardia lamblia,* spread via contaminated food or water or by direct person-to-person contact. Most of those infected are asymptomatic, but a small percentage present with symptoms ranging from nonspecific

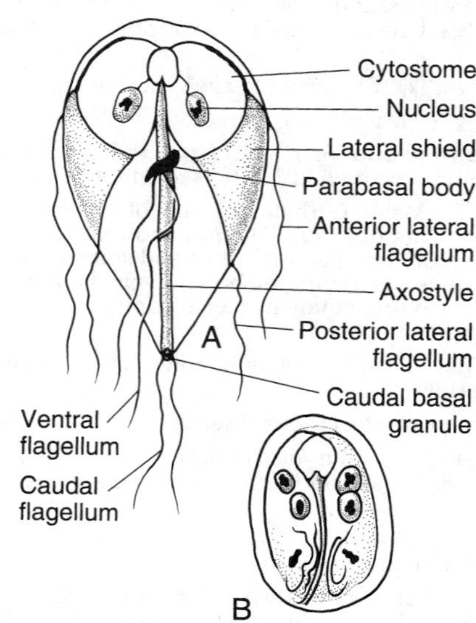


*Giardia lamblia: (A),* trophozoite; *(B),* cyst.

gastrointestinal discomfort to mild to profuse diarrhea, nausea, lassitude, anorexia, and weight loss. 2. infection of a dog or cat with *Giardia lamblia,* characterized by copious diarrhea and anorexia; it may be persistent or self-limiting. Called also *lambliasis* and *lambliosis.*

**Gib·bon-Lan·dis test** (gib'on-lan'dis) [John Heysham *Gibbon,* Jr., American physician, 1903–1973; Eugene Markley *Landis,* American physician, 1901–1987] see under *test.*

**gib·bos·i·ty** (gĭ-bos'ĭ-te) [L. *gibbosus* crooked] the condition of being humped; kyphosis.

**gib·bous** (gib'əs) [L. *gibbosus*] convex; humped; protuberant; humpbacked.

**Gibbs' free energy, theorem** (gibz) [Josiah Willard *Gibbs,* American physicist, 1839–1903] see under *theorem.*

**Gibbs-Don·nan equilibrium** (gibz-don'ən) [J. W. *Gibbs;* Frederick George *Donnan,* English chemist, 1870–1956] see under *equilibrium.*

**gib·bus** (gib'əs) [L.] a hump.

**Gib·ney's bandage (strapping), boot, perispondylitis (disease)** (gib'nēz) [Virgil Pendleton *Gibney,* New York surgeon, 1847–1927] see under *bandage* and *perispondylitis.*

**Gib·son's murmur, rule** (gib'sənz) [George Alexander *Gibson,* Scottish physician, 1854–1913] see under *murmur.*

**gid** (gid) a disease of the brain and spinal cord of sheep caused by the presence of *Coenurus cerebralis* (the larva of *Taenia multiceps*), and marked by unsteadiness of gait, which if untreated can progress to paralysis and blindness. Called also *coenurosis, coenuriasis, staggers, sturdy,* and *turnsickness.*

**gid·di·ness** (gid'e-nəs) dizziness.

**Giem·sa stain** (gēm'sə) [Gustav *Giemsa,* German chemist and bacteriologist, 1867–1948] see under *stain.*

**Gier·ke's corpuscles** (gēr'kez) [Hans Paul Bernhard *Gierke,* German anatomist, 1847–1886] see under *corpuscle.*

**Gie·son** see *van Gieson.*

**Gif·ford's operation, reflex** (gif'ərdz) [Harold *Gifford,* American oculist, 1858–1929] see under *operation* and see *orbicularis pupillary reflex,* under *reflex.*

**GIFT** gamete intrafallopian transfer.

**giga-** [Gr. *gigas* giant] a combining form designating gigantic size; used in naming units of measurement to indicate a quantity one billion ($10^9$) times the unit designated by the root with which it is combined. Symbol, G.

**gi·gan·tism** (ji-gan'tiz-əm, ji'gən-tiz-əm) [*gigant-* + *-ism*] [MeSH: Gigantism] abnormal overgrowth; excessive size and stature. Called also *giantism, hypersomia,* and *somatomegaly.*
**acromegalic g.,** pituitary gigantism in which the body also has the changes in the short and flat bones and in the distal parts that are characteristic of acromegaly.
**cerebral g.,** gigantism in the absence of increased levels of growth hormone, attributed to a cerebral defect; infants are large, and accelerated growth continues for the first four or five years, the rate being normal thereafter. The hands and feet are large, the head large and dolichocephalic, and the eyes have an antimongoloid slant with hypertelorism. The child is clumsy, and mental retardation of varying degree is usually present. Called also *Sotos' syndrome.*
**eunuchoid g.,** gigantism in which the body has eunuchoid features and hypogonadism.
**fetal g.,** see under *macrosomia.*
**hyperpituitary g.,** pituitary g.
**normal g.,** gigantism in which the body proportions and sexual development are normal.
**pituitary g.,** gigantism due to excessive pituitary secretion of growth hormone, occurring before puberty and before the epiphyses close; it is most often caused by eosinophilic cell hyperplasia or an eosinophilic adenoma, but sometimes results from a chromophobe adenoma. Called also *hyperpituitary g.* and *Launois' syndrome.*

**gigant(o)-** [Gr. *gigas,* gen. *gigantos* giant] a combining form meaning huge.

**gi·gan·to·cel·lu·lar** (ji-gan"to-sel'u-lər) pertaining to giant cells.

**gi·gan·to·mas·tia** (ji-gan"to-mas'te-ə) extreme macromastia.

**Gi·gar·ti·na** (ji"gahr-ti'nə) a genus of red algae. *G. mammillo'sa* (Goodenough & Woodward) J. Aghardt. is a source of carrageenan and chondrus.

**gi·gan·to·so·ma** (ji-gan"to-so'mə) gigantism.

**Gi·gli's operation, wire saw** (jēl'yēz) [Leonardo *Gigli,* Italian gynecologist, 1863–1908] see under *operation* and *saw.*

**gi·ki·ya·mi** (ge"ke-yah'me) nanukayami.

**Gil·bert's sign, syndrome (cholemia, disease)** (zhēl-bārz') [Nicolas Augustin *Gilbert,* French physician, 1858–1927] see under *sign* and *syndrome.*

**Gil·christ's disease, mycosis** (gil'krists) [Thomas Caspar *Gilchrist,* American dermatologist, 1862–1927] North American blastomycosis.

**gil·da·ble** (gil'də-bəl) susceptible of being colored with gold stains.

**gill** (gil) [MeSH: Gills] 1. the respiratory organ of aquatic animals, such as fish, mollusks, and many arthropods, usually a thin-walled projection from the body surface or from some part of the digestive tract whose surface is increased by filaments, lamellae, or other folds. 2. one of the thin perpendicular plates found on the underside of a mushroom cap and along which the basidia are produced. Called also *lamella.*

**Gilles de la Tou·rette's syndrome (disease)** (zhēl-də-lah-too-rets') [Georges Edouard Albert Brutus *Gilles de la Tourette,* French physician, 1857–1904] see under *syndrome.*

**Gil·les·pie's syndrome** (gĭ-les'pēz) [Frank David *Gillespie,* American ophthalmologist, born 1927] see under *syndrome.*

**Gil·lette's suspensory ligament** (zhe-lets') [Eugène Paulin *Gillette,* French surgeon, 1836–1886] tendo cricooesophageus.

**Gil·li·am's operation** (gil'e-əmz) [David Tod *Gilliam,* American gynecologist, 1844–1923] see under *operation.*

**Gil·lies' flap, operation** (gil'ēz) [Sir Harold Delf *Gillies,* British plastic surgeon, 1882–1960] see *tube flap,* under *flap,* and see under *operation.*

**Gil·man** (gil'mən) Alfred G. American pharmacologist, born 1941. Co-winner with Martin Rodbell of the Nobel prize for medicine or physiology in 1994 for his research into the role of G proteins in cell responses to environmental signals.

**Gil·mer's splint** (gil'mərz) [Thomas Lewis *Gilmer,* American oral surgeon, 1849–1931] see under *splint* and *wiring.*

**gilt** (gilt) a female pig that is intended for breeding but has not yet given birth.

**Gim·ber·nat's ligament, reflex ligament** (hēm-bār-nahts') [Antonio de *Gimbernat,* Spanish surgeon and anatomist, 1734–1817] see *ligamenta lacunare* and *ligamentum inguinale reflexum.*

**gin·ger** (jin'jər) [L. *zingiber;* Gr. *zingiberis*] [NF] 1. *Zingiber officinale.* 2. the dried rhizome of *Z. officinale,* used primarily as a flavoring agent. It has been used for the treatment of loss of appetite, flatulence, and colic and to prevent motion sickness in humans, and as a stimulant, carminative, and anticolic medication for horses.
**Indian g., wild g.,** *Asarum canadense.*

**gin·gi·va** (jin'jĭ-və, jin-ji'və) pl. *gin'givae* [L. "gum of the mouth"] [TA] [MeSH: Gingiva] gum: that part of the oral mucosa overlying the crowns of unerupted teeth and encircling the necks of those that have erupted, serving as the supporting structure for subadjacent tissues. It is formed by pale pink tissue immovably attached to the bone and the teeth, which joins the alveolar mucosa at the mucogingival junction.
**alveolar g.,** that part of the nonkeratinized oral mucosa that overlies the alveolar process.
**areolar g.,** the oral mucous membrane lying beyond the keratinized mucosa over the alveolar process, being continuous with the buccal and labial mucosa.
**attached g.,** periodontium protectionis.
**buccal g.,** that portion of the gingiva located on the buccal aspect of the teeth.
**cemental g.,** that portion of the attached gingiva adherent to the cementum.
**free g.,** periodontium insertionis.
**interdental g., interproximal g.,** the portion of the gingiva occupying the interproximal space beneath the area of tooth contact, consisting of two papillae and a depression (col) that connects the

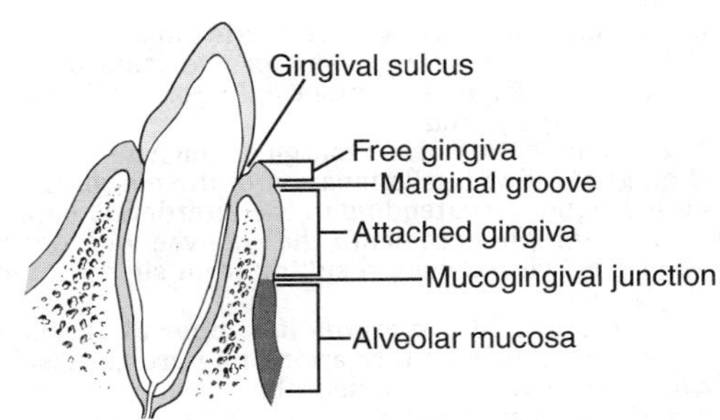


Gingiva of an incisor, in cross-section.

papillae and conforms to the shape of the interproximal contact area; called also *papillary g.* and *septal g.*
**labial g.**, that portion of the gingiva found on the labial aspect of the teeth.
**lingual g.**, that portion of the gingiva found on the lingual aspect of the teeth.
**marginal g.**, margo gingivalis.
**papillary g.**, interdental g.
**septal g.**, interdental g.
**unattached g.**, periodontium insertionis.

**gin·gi·vae** (jin′jĭ-ve, jin-ji′ve) [L., plural of *gingiva*] the gums; see under *gingiva.*

**gin·gi·val** (jin′jĭ-vəl) pertaining to the gingivae.

**gin·gi·val·gia** (jin″jĭ-val′jə) [*gingivo-* + *-algia*] pain in the gingivae.

**gin·gi·val·ly** (jin′jĭ-vəl″e) toward the gingivae.

**gin·gi·vec·to·my** (jin″gĭ-vek′tə-me) [*gingiv-* + *ectomy*] [MeSH: Gingivectomy] surgical excision of the gingiva at the level of its attachment, thus creating new marginal gingiva; used to eliminate gingival or periodontal pockets or to provide an approach for extensive surgical interventions, and to gain access necessary to remove calculus within the pocket.

**gin·gi·vi·tis** (jin″-jĭ-vi′tis) [*gingiv-* + *-itis*] [MeSH: Gingivitis] inflammation of the gingivae. Gingivitis associated with bony changes is referred to as *periodontitis.* Called also *oulitis* and *ulitis.*
**acute necrotizing ulcerative g. (ANUG)**, a progressive painful infection, also seen in subacute and recurrent forms, marked by crateriform lesions of interdental papillae with pseudomembranous slough circumscribed by linear erythema; fetid breath; increased salivation; and spontaneous gingival hemorrhage. The etiology is uncertain, but fusiform bacilli, spirochetes, and other microorganisms are present in the lesions; many postulate an etiology of a bacterial complex in the presence of predisposing factors such as gingival disease or nutritional deficiency. Although it often occurs in an epidemic pattern, it has not been shown to be contagious. Called also *fusospirillosis, fusospirochetal g., necrotizing ulcerative g., phagedenic g., trench mouth,* and *Vincent's g.* or *stomatitis.* When it spreads to nearby structures, it may be called *necrotizing ulcerative gingivostomatitis* or *Vincent's angina.*
**acute ulcerative g., acute ulceromembranous g.**, acute necrotizing ulcerative g.
**atrophic senile g.**, inflammation of the gingiva and oral mucosa in menopausal and postmenopausal women, characterized microscopically by atrophy of the germinal and prickle cell layers of the gingival epithelium and sometimes by areas of ulceration; considered to be caused by altered estrogen metabolism.
**bismuth g.**, see under *stomatitis.*
**catarrhal g.**, transitory gingivitis, sometimes associated with stomatitis, accompanied by erythema, swelling, and occasionally epithelial desquamation; believed to be caused by the oral bacterial flora.
**cotton-roll g.**, secondary infection of denuded areas of gingivae caused by adherence of epithelium to cotton rolls placed in the mouth during dental procedures.
**desquamative g.**, an inflammatory condition characterized by tendency of the surface epithelium of the gingivae to desquamate. Chronic desquamative gingivitis is called also *gingivosis.*
**Dilantin g.**, generalized hyperplasia of the gingivae, which may also rarely involve other areas of the oral mucosa, resulting from overgrowth of the fibrous tissue following anticonvulsant therapy with Dilantin (phenytoin). Called also *Dilantin hyperplasia.*
**eruptive g.**, gingivitis occurring at the time of tooth eruption, particularly the permanent teeth; food impaction and debris accumulation may be associated.
**fusospirochetal g.**, acute necrotizing ulcerative g.
**g. gravida′rum**, pregnancy g.
**hemorrhagic g.**, gingivitis characterized by profuse bleeding, as in ascorbic acid deficiency.
**herpetic g.**, that due to herpesvirus infection. See also under *gingivostomatitis.*
**hormonal g.**, that associated with endocrine imbalance.
**hyperplastic g.**, that associated with proliferation of the gingival cells. See *gingival enlargement,* under *enlargement,* and *gingival hyperplasia,* under *hyperplasia.*
**marginal g.**, inflammation of the marginal gingivae.
**marginal g., generalized**, inflammation of the marginal gingivae in all the teeth, frequently extending to the interdental papillae.
**marginal g., simple**, hyperemia of the gingivae with edema of the margins and gingival papillae, resulting from slight trauma or neglected dental hygiene.
**marginal g., suppurative, g. margina′lis suppurati′va**, inflammation of the gingival margins, with formation of a purulent discharge.
**necrotizing ulcerative g.**, acute necrotizing ulcerative g.
**papillary g.**, inflammation of the interdental papillae.
**phagedenic g.**, acute necrotizing ulcerative g.
**pregnancy g.**, any of various gingival changes during pregnancy, ranging from gingivitis to the so-called pregnancy tumor; called also *g. gravidarum.*
**scorbutic g.**, gingivitis associated with vitamin C deficiency (scurvy).
**streptococcal g.**, inflammation of the gingival margins caused by streptococcal infection.
**tuberculous g.**, tuberculous infection of the gingiva, characterized by diffuse, hyperemic, nodular or papillary proliferation of the gingival tissue. See also *oral tuberculosis,* under *tuberculosis.*
**Vincent's g.**, acute necrotizing ulcerative g.

**gingiv(o)-** [L. *gingiva* gum] a combining form denoting relationship to the gingivae.

**gin·gi·vo·buc·co·ax·i·al** (jin″jĭ-vo-buk″o-ak′se-əl) pertaining to or formed by the gingival, buccal, and axial walls of a tooth cavity preparation.

**gin·gi·vo·glos·si·tis** (jin″jĭ-vo-glos-i′tis) [*gingivo-* + *gloss-* + *-itis*] inflammation of gingivae and tongue.

**gin·gi·vo·la·bi·al** (jin″jĭ-vo-la′be-əl) pertaining to the gingivae and lips.

**gin·gi·vo·lin·guo·ax·i·al** (jin″jĭ-vo-ling″wo-ak′se-əl) pertaining to or formed by the gingival, lingual, and axial walls of a tooth cavity preparation.

**gin·gi·vo·peri·odon·ti·tis** (jin″jĭ-vo-per″e-o-don-ti′tis) inflammation involving the gingivae and periodontium.
**necrotizing ulcerative g.**, a severe form of periodontitis occurring after prolonged repeated bouts of acute necrotizing ulcerative gingivitis, manifested by generalized or localized destruction of interdental bone, and characterized by periods of exacerbation in which a gray pseudomembrane may be present in affected areas and by necrotic odor.

**gin·gi·vo·plas·ty** (jin′jĭ-vo-plas″te) [*gingivo-* + *-plasty*] [MeSH: Gingivoplasty] surgical reshaping of the gingivae and papillae for correction of deformities (particularly enlargements) and to provide the gingivae with a normal and functional form, the incision creating an external bevel.

**gin·gi·vo·sis** (jin″jĭ-vo′sis) [*gingiv-* + *-osis*] chronic desquamative gingivitis.

**gin·gi·vo·sto·ma·ti·tis** (jin″jĭ-vo-sto″mə-ti′tis) inflammation involving both the gingivae and the oral mucosa.
**herpetic g.**, an infection of the oral mucosa (including the gingivae) by the herpes simplex virus, characterized by redness of oral tissues, formation of multiple vesicles and painful ulcers, and fever.
**necrotizing ulcerative g.**, that caused by extension to the oral mucosa of necrotizing ulcerative gingivitis, characterized by ulceration, pseudomembrane, and odor, with lesions involving the palate or pharynx as well as the oral mucosa. Called also *fusospirochetal stomatitis* and *pseudomembranous angina.*

**gin·gly·form** (jin′glĭ-form) ginglymoid.

**gin·gly·mo·ar·thro·di·al** (jin″glə-mo-ahr-thro′de-əl) partly ginglymoid and partly arthrodial.

**gin·gly·moid** (jin′glə-moid) [*ginglymus* + *-oid*] resembling a ginglymus.

**gin·gly·mus** (jin′glĭ-məs) [L.; Gr. *ginglymos* hinge] [TA] a type of synovial joint that allows movement in but one plane, forward and backward, as the hinge of a door; called also *ginglymoid* or *hinge joint.*

**Gink·go** (ging′ko) a genus of deciduous, diecious trees with fan-shaped leaves and malodorous fleshy yellow fruit native to China, Japan, and Korea.
**G. bilo′ba**, the sole species of the genus; the leaves, and seeds are used medicinally. See *ginkgo.*

**gink·go** (ging′ko) [NF] the dried leaves of *Ginkgo biloba,* used for symptomatic relief of brain function, for intermittent claudication, and for tinnitus and vertigo of vascular origin.

**gin·seng** (jin′seng) [Chinese *jin-tsan* life of man] [MeSH: Ginseng] 1. any herb of the genus *Panax,* especially *P. ginseng* (Chinese ginseng) and *P. quinquefolius* (American ginseng). 2. the root of Chinese or American ginseng, used as a tonic and stimulant in fatigue and during convalescence.
**oriental g.** [NF], the dried roots of *Panax ginseng* (Chinese ginseng).

**Gior·da·no's sphincter** (jor-dah′nōz) [Davide *Giordano,* Italian surgeon, 1864–1954] musculus sphincter ductus choledochi.

**GIP** gastric inhibitory polypeptide.

**Gi·ral·dés' organ** (zhe-rahl-dāz′) [Joachim Albin Cardozo Cazado *Giraldés,* Portuguese surgeon in Paris, 1808–1875] paradidymis.

**Gi·rar·di·nus** (jĭ-rar′dĭ-nus) *Poecilia.*

**G. poeciloi'des,** *Poecilia reticulata.*

**gir·dle** (gər'dəl) 1. an encircling structure or part. 2. cingulum.
**Hitzig's g.,** an encircling zone of analgesia at the level of the breasts, in the area supplied by the third and sixth dorsal nerves, seen in the early stages of tabes dorsalis.
**limbus g.,** a corneal degeneration in the form of an opaque line concentric with the limbus; called also *white limbal g. of Vogt.*
**g. of lower limb,** cingulum pelvicum.
**pectoral g.,** cingulum pectorale.
**pelvic g.,** cingulum pelvicum.
**shoulder g., g. of upper limb,** cingulum pectorale.
**white limbal g. of Vogt,** limbus g.

**Gir·dle·stone resection (operation)** (ger'dəl-stōn) [Gathorne Robert *Girdlestone,* British orthopedic surgeon, 1881–1950] see under *resection.*

**git·a·lin** (jit'ə-lin) a mixture of the digitalis glycosides gitoxin, gitaloxin, and digitoxin, having the same actions and uses as digitalis; administered orally. Called also *amorphous g.*

**git·a·lox·in** (jit"ə-lok'sin) a cardiac glycoside from *Digitalis purpurea;* a component of gitalin.

**Git·el·man's syndrome** (git'əl-mənz) [H. J. *Gitelman,* American physician, 20th century] see under *syndrome.*

**gith·a·gism** (gith'ə-jiz-əm) poisoning as a result of seeds of *Agrostemma githago* that contaminate human or animal food; called also *corn cockle poisoning.*

**gi·tox·i·gen·in** (jĭ-tok'sĭ-jən-in) the steroid nucleus that is the aglycon of gitoxin.

**gi·tox·in** (jĭ-tok'sin) a cardiac glycoside, principally from *Digitalis purpurea* but also a constituent of *D. lanata,* consisting of gitoxigenin linked to three digitoxose molecules; a component of gitalin.

**Git·ter·fas·ern** (git'ər-fas"ərn) [Ger.] the reticular lattice fibers of the corium.

**Giuf·fri·da-Rug·gi·eri stigma** (joo-fre"də-roo"je-er'e) [Vincenzo *Giuffrida-Ruggieri,* Italian anthropologist, 1872–1922] see under *stigma.*

**Giv·ens' method** (giv'ənz) [Maurice Hope *Givens,* American biochemist, born 1888] see under *method.*

**GIX** an insecticidal compound, DFDT.

**giz·zard** (giz'ərd) [L. *gigeria* cooked entrails of poultry] [MeSH: Gizzard] 1. the highly modified posterior portion of the stomach in birds, characterized by muscular walls and glands that secrete a horny lining, in which food passed from the proventriculus is ground with the aid of ingested gravel. 2. a similar organ in the alimentary tract of certain invertebrates, such as insects.

**GL** abbreviation for *greatest length,* an axis of measurement or dimension used for small flexed embryos.

**gl.** abbreviation for L. *glan'dula* and *glan'dulae* (gland, glands).

**gla·bel·la** (glə-bel'ə) [L. *glabellus* smooth, dim. of *glaber*] 1. the smooth area on the frontal bone between the superciliary arches. 2. [TA] the most prominent point in the median plane between the eyebrows; used as an anthropometric landmark.

**gla·bel·lad** (glə-bel'əd) [*glabella* + *-ad*[1]] toward the glabella.

**gla·brous** (gla'brəs) [L. *glaber* smooth] smooth and bare.

**gla·cial** (gla'shəl) [L. *glacialis*] 1. resembling ice; vitreous; solid. 2. designating a highly pure state of certain acids, e.g., acetic or phosphoric acid, so called because the freezing point is only slightly below room temperature.

**gla·di·ate** (gla'de-āt) [L. *gladius* sword] sword-shaped; xiphoid.

**gla·di·o·lus** (glə-di'o-ləs) [L., dim. of *gladius* sword] corpus sterni.

**gla·dio·ma·nu·bri·al** (glad"e-o-mə-noo'bre-əl) pertaining to gladiolus (corpus sterni) and manubrium.

**glair·in** (glār'in) [L. *clarus* clear] a gelatinous substance of bacterial origin found on the surface of certain thermal and sulfur waters.

**glairy** (glār'e) resembling the white of an egg.

**gland** (gland) [L. *glans* acorn] glandula.

## Gland

For descriptions of specific glands not listed here, see under *glandula.*

**absorbent g.,** lymph node.
**accessory g.,** a minor mass of glandular tissue situated near or at some distance from a gland of similar structure.
**acid g's,** fundic g's.
**acinar g.,** acinous g.
**acinotubular g.,** tubuloacinar g.
**acinous g.,** a gland made up of one or more acini.
**admaxillary g.,** glandula parotidea accessoria.
**adrenal g.,** glandula suprarenalis.
**adrenal g's, accessory,** glandulae suprarenales accessoriae.
**aggregate g's, aggregated g's,** aggregated lymphoid nodules; see terms beginning *noduli lymphoidei aggregati,* under *nodulus.*
**Albarrán's g.,** that part of the median lobe of the prostate underneath the uvula vesicae.
**alveolar g.,** acinous g.
**anal g's,** glandulae circumanales.
**anteprostatic g.,** glandula bulbourethralis.
**apical g's of tongue,** glandulae linguales anteriores.
**apocrine g.,** a gland whose discharged secretion contains part of the secreting cells. Cf. *holocrine g.* and *merocrine g.*
**apocrine sweat g.,** a type of large, branched, specialized sudoriferous gland *(glandula sudorifera)* that empties into the upper portion of a hair follicle instead of directly onto the skin surface; found only on certain areas of the body, such as around the anus and in the axilla; after puberty they produce a viscous secretion that is acted on by bacteria to produce a characteristic acrid odor.
**areolar g's,** glandulae areolares.
**arteriococcygeal g.,** glomus coccygeum.
**arytenoid g's,** mucous glands in the posterior part of the larynx, near the aryepiglottic fold and the arytenoid cartilages; called also *posterior laryngeal g's.*
**Aselli's g's,** see under *pancreas.*
**axillary g's,** nodi lymphoidei axillares.
**Bartholin's g.,** glandula vestibularis major.
**Bauhin's g's,** glandulae linguales anteriores.
**g's of bile duct,** glandulae ductus choledochi.
**biliary g's, g's of biliary mucosa,** glandulae ductus choledochi.
**Blandin's g's, Blandin and Nuhn's g's,** glandulae linguales anteriores.
**Bowman's g's,** glandulae olfactoriae.
**brachial g's,** nodi lymphoidei cubitales.
**bronchial g's,** glandulae bronchiales.
**Bruch's g's,** the lymph follicles of the conjunctiva of the lower lid.
**Brunner's g's,** glandulae duodenales.
**buccal g's,** glandulae buccales.
**bulbocavernous g., bulbourethral g.,** glandula bulbourethralis.
**cardiac g's,** mucin-secreting glands at the cardiac end of the stomach surrounding the entrance of the esophagus into the stomach.
**carotid g.,** glomus caroticum.
**celiac g's,** lymph nodes anterior to the abdominal aorta.
**ceruminous g's,** glandulae ceruminosae.
**cervical g's of uterus,** glandulae cervicales uteri.
**cheek g's,** glandulae buccales.
**Ciaccio's g's,** glandulae lacrimales accessoriae.
**ciliary g's, ciliary g's of conjunctiva,** glandulae ciliares conjunctivales.
**circumanal g's,** glandulae circumanales.
**Cloquet's g.,** see under *node.*
**Cobelli's g's,** mucous glands in the mucosa of the esophagus just above the cardia.
**coccygeal g.,** glomus coccygeum.
**coil g.,** eccrine g.
**compound g.,** one made up of a number of smaller units whose excretory ducts combine to form ducts of progressively higher order.
**conglobate g.,** a lymph node.
**conjunctival g's,** glandulae conjunctivales.
**Cowper's g.,** glandula bulbourethralis.
**cutaneous g's,** glandulae cutis.
**ductless g's,** endocrine g's.
**duodenal g's,** glandulae duodenales.
**Duverney's g.,** glandula bulbourethralis.
**Ebner's g's,** serous secreting glands in the posterior part of the tongue near the vallate papillae; called also *gustatory g's.*
**eccrine g., eccrine sweat g.,** an ordinary, or simple, sweat gland

*(glandula sudorifera)*; they are of the merocrine type, unbranched, coiled, tubular glands that are distributed over almost all of the body surface, and promote cooling by evaporation of their secretion.

**endocrine g's,** ductless organs that secrete specific substances *(hormones)* that are released directly into the circulatory system and influence metabolism and other body processes. The endocrine glands include the hypothalamus, pituitary, thyroid, parathyroid, and adrenal glands, the pancreatic islets, the pineal body, and the gonads. See also under *system,* and see Plate 19. Called also *glandulae endocrinae* [TA] and *ductless g's.*

**endoepithelial g.,** intraepithelial g.

**esophageal g's,** glandulae oesophageae.

**excretory g.,** any gland that excretes waste products from the system.

**exocrine g.,** a gland that discharges its secretion through a duct opening on an internal or external surface of the body, as a lacrimal gland. Cf. *endocrine g's.*

**follicular g's of tongue,** noduli lymphoidei tonsillae lingualis.

**fundic g's, fundus g's,** numerous nearly straight tubular glands located in the mucosa of the fundus and body of the stomach; they contain the cells that produce acid and pepsin. Called also *gastric g's.*

**Galeati's g's,** glandulae duodenales.

**gastric g's,** the secreting glands of the stomach, including the fundic, cardiac, and pyloric glands; sometimes used specifically to denote the fundic glands.

**gastric g's, proper,** fundic g's.

**Gay's g's,** glandulae circumanales.

**genal g's,** glandulae buccales.

**genital g.,** 1. ovarium. 2. testis.

**gingival g's,** glandlike infoldings of epithelium at the junction of gingiva and tooth.

**Gley's g's,** parathyroid glands.

**glomiform g.,** anastomosis arteriovenosa glomeriformis.

**glossopalatine g's,** mucous glands at the posterior end of the smaller sublingual glands.

**Guérin's g's,** ductus paraurethrales urethrae femininae.

**gustatory g's,** Ebner's g's.

**g's of Haller,** glandulae preputiales.

**Harder's g's, harderian g's,** accessory lacrimal glands at the inner corner of the eye in animals that possess nictitating membranes; they excrete an unctuous fluid that facilitates the movement of the third eyelid. They are rudimentary in humans.

**haversian g's,** villi synoviales.

**hedonic g's,** glands in certain animals that function during the season of sexual activity. See also *scent g.*

**hemal g's, hemal lymph g's,** hemal nodes.

**hemolymph g's,** 1. hemal nodes. 2. hemolymph nodes, def. 2.

**Henle's g's,** tubular glands in the conjunctiva of the eyelids.

**hepatic g's,** glandulae ductus choledochi.

**heterocrine g.,** mixed g. (def. 2).

**holocrine g.,** a gland whose discharged secretion contains entire secreting cells.

**intercarotid g.,** glomus caroticum.

**intermediate g's,** according to some authorities, a fourth type of gastric gland (q.v.) found in a narrow region between the fundic and pyloric glands.

**interstitial g.,** 1. (pl.) the aggregations of Leydig cells of the testis; so called because of their occurrence in clusters and their endocrine function. 2. the interstitial cells of the ovary, collectively; so called because of their epithelioid appearance and presumed secretory function.

**intestinal g's,** glandulae intestinales.

**intraepithelial g.,** a gland situated in an epithelial layer.

**intramuscular g's of tongue,** glandulae linguales anteriores.

**jugular g.,** a lymph node behind the clavicular insertion of the sternomastoid muscle.

**Krause's g's,** glandulae conjunctivales.

**labial g's of mouth,** glandulae labiales oris.

**lacrimal g.,** glandula lacrimalis.

**lacrimal g's, accessory,** glandulae lacrimales accessoriae.

**lactiferous g.,** glandula mammaria.

**g's of large intestine,** see *glandulae intestinales.*

**large sweat g.,** an apocrine gland that usually produces an odoriferous secretion.

**laryngeal g's,** glandulae laryngeae.

**laryngeal g's, anterior,** mucous glands in the anterior part of the larynx.

**laryngeal g's, middle,** mucous glands located in the arytenoepiglottic fold.

**laryngeal g's, posterior,** arytenoid g's.

**lenticular g's of stomach,** folliculi lymphatici gastrici.

**lenticular g's of tongue,** noduli lymphoidei tonsillae lingualis.

**g's of Lieberkühn,** glandulae intestinales.

**lingual g's,** glandulae linguales.

**lingual g's, anterior (of Blandin and Nuhn),** glandulae linguales anteriores.

**Littre's g's,** 1. glandulae preputiales. 2. glandulae urethrales urethrae masculinae.

**Luschka's g.,** glomus coccygeum.

**lymph g., lymphatic g.,** see under *node.*

**lymph g's, extraparotid,** lymph nodes overlying the parotid gland, between the superficial and deep fasciae.

**malar g's,** glandulae buccales.

**mammary g.,** glandula mammaria.

**mammary g., accessory,** mamma accessoria.

**mandibular g.,** glandula submandibularis.

**Mehlis' g.,** gland cells surrounding the ootype of trematodes.

**meibomian g's,** glandulae tarsales.

**merocrine g.,** one in which the secretory cells maintain their integrity throughout the secretory cycle.

**mesenteric g's,** nodi lymphoidei mesenterici.

**mesocolic g's,** lymph nodes in the mesentery of the colon; see *nodi lymphatici colici nodi lymphatici ileocolici,* and *nodi lymphatici mesenterici inferiores.*

**mixed g.,** 1. one having both endocrine and exocrine portions. 2. a gland composed of both mucous and serous secreting cells, such as the labial glands. Called also *heterocrine g., seromucous g.,* and *glandula seromucosa.*

**molar g's,** glandulae molares.

**Moll's g's,** glandulae ciliares conjunctivales.

**monoptychic g.,** a gland in which the tubules or alveoli are lined with a single layer of secreting cells.

**Montgomery's g's,** glandulae areolares.

**Morgagni's g's,** glandulae urethrales urethrae masculinae.

**g's of mouth,** glandulae oris.

**mucilaginous g's,** villi synoviales.

**muciparous g., mucous g.,** a gland that secretes a slimy, chemically inert material.

**mucous g's, lingual,** glandulae linguales.

**mucous g's of auditory tube,** glandulae tubariae.

**mucous g's of duodenum,** glandulae duodenales.

**mucous g's of eustachian tube,** glandulae tubariae.

**multicellular g.,** one in which many cells cooperate to produce a gland complex, represented in its simplest form by a secretory sheet (q.v.) of epithelial cells.

**myometrial g.,** a tissue supposed to develop in the wall of the uterus at the site of implantation of the placenta and to last until the end of pregnancy.

**Naboth's g's, nabothian g's,** see under *follicle.*

**nasal g's,** glandulae nasales.

**Nuhn's g's,** glandulae linguales anteriores.

**odoriferous g's of prepuce,** glandulae preputiales.

**oil g.,** glandula sebacea.

**olfactory g's,** glandulae olfactoriae.

**oxyntic g's,** fundic g's.

**palatine g's,** glandulae palatinae.

**palpebral g's,** glandulae tarsales.

**parafrenal g's,** glands opening near the frenum of the prepuce.

**parathyroid g's,** small bodies apposed to the posterior surface of the thyroid gland, developed from the endoderm of the branchial clefts, occurring in a variable number of pairs, commonly two *(glandula parathyroidea inferior* and *glandula parathyroidea superior* [TA]) (see inset on Plate 19). The parenchyma comprises masses and cords of epithelial cells, which have been divided into two main types: chief cells and oxyphil cells, but intermediate forms exist. The chief cells secrete parathyroid hormone, a major regulator of calcium and phosphorus metabolism. Called also *Gley's glands, Sandström's bodies, parathyroids,* and *epithelial* or *parathyroid bodies.*

**paraurethral g's,** see *ductus paraurethrales urethrae femininae* and *ductus paraurethrales urethrae masculinae.*

**parotid g.,** glandula parotidea.

**parotid g., accessory,** glandula parotidea accessoria.

**pectoral g's,** see *nodi lymphoidei axillares.*

**peptic g's,** fundic g's.

**Peyer's g's,** noduli lymphoidei aggregati intestini tenuis.

**pharyngeal g's,** glandulae pharyngis.

**Philip's g's,** enlarged glands above the clavicle, seen in children with tuberculosis.

**pineal g.,** glandula pinealis.

**pituitary g.,** hypophysis.

**Poirier's g's,** lymph nodes on the conoid ligament at the upper border of the isthmus of the thyroid.

**polyptychic g.,** a gland in which the tubules or alveoli are lined with more than one layer of secreting cells.

**preen g.,** a large compound alveolar structure on the back of birds, above the base of the tail, which secretes an oily waterproof material that the bird applies to its feathers and skin by preening. Called also *uropygial g.*

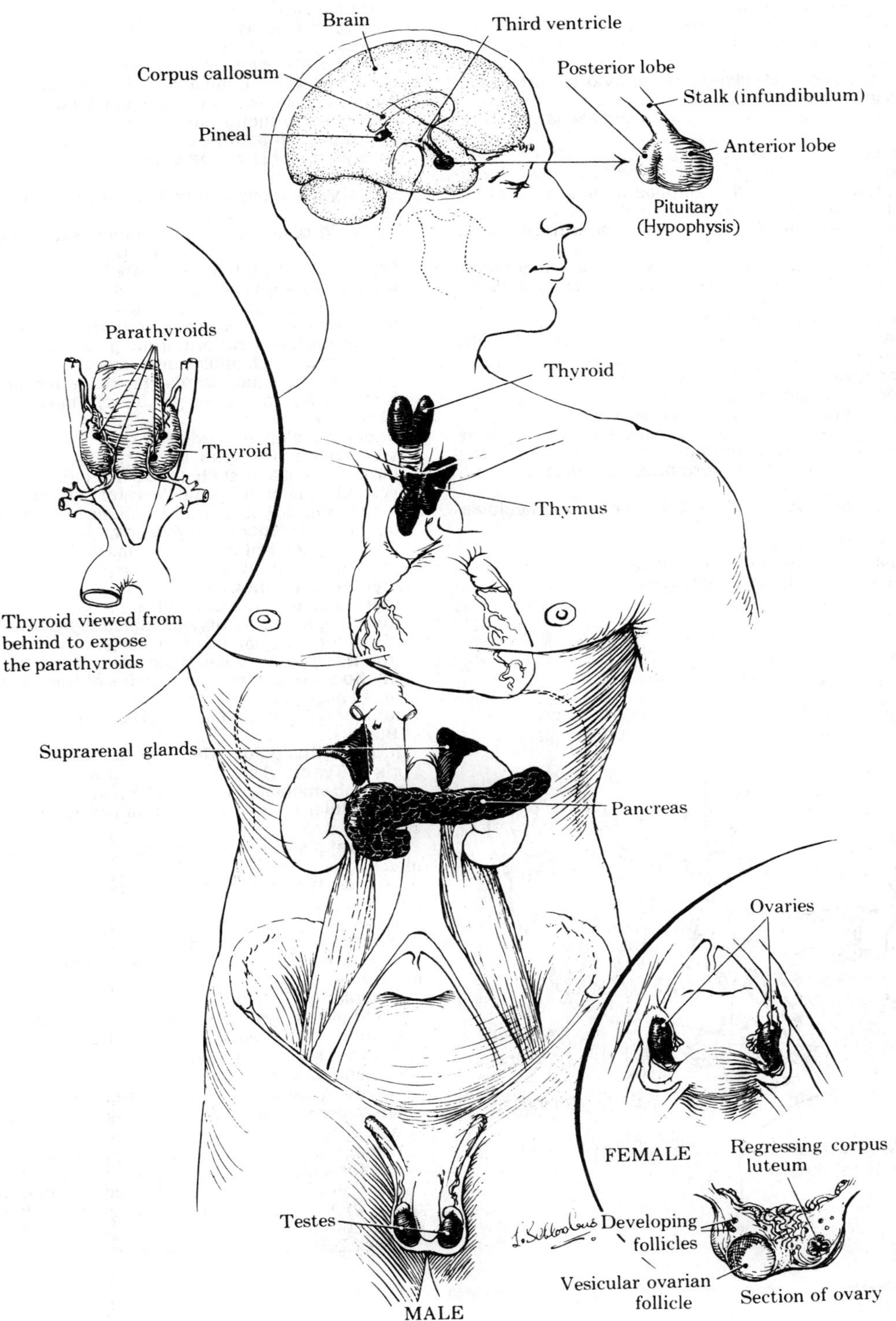


**PLATE 19**—THE ENDOCRINE GLANDS

**pregnancy g's,** the glands containing female genital hormone, that is, the ovarian follicle, corpus luteum, and placenta.
**prehyoid g's,** glandulae thyroidea accessoriae.
**preputial g's,** glandulae preputiales.
**prostate g.,** prostate.
**pyloric g's,** the mucin-secreting glands of the pyloric part of the stomach; called also *glandulae pyloricae.*
**racemose g's,** glands composed of acini arranged like grapes on a stem.
**retromolar g's,** glandulae molares.
**Rivinus g.,** glandula sublingualis.
**Rosenmüller's g.,** 1. pars palpebralis glandulae lacrimalis. 2. in the plural, nodi lymphoidei inguinales profundi.
**saccular g.,** a gland consisting of a sac or sacs, lined with glandular epithelium.
**salivary g's,** the glands of the oral cavity whose combined secretion constitutes the saliva; see *glandulae salivariae majores* and *glandulae salivariae minores.*
**salivary g., external,** glandula parotidea.
**salivary g., internal,** the glandula sublingualis and glandula submandibularis regarded as a unit.
**salivary g's, major,** glandulae salivariae majores.
**salivary g's, minor,** glandulae salivariae minores.
**Sandström's g's,** glandulae thyroideae accessoriae.
**scent g.,** any gland that secretes a pheromone, such as occurs in many animal species during mating season.
**Schüller's g's,** ductus paraurethrales urethrae femininae.
**sebaceous g.,** glandula sebacea.
**sebaceous g's of conjunctiva, sebaceous g's of eyelids,** glandulae sebaceae palpebrarum.
**seminal g.,** glandula vesiculosa.
**sentinel g.,** an enlarged lymph node, considered to be pathognomonic of some pathological condition elsewhere.

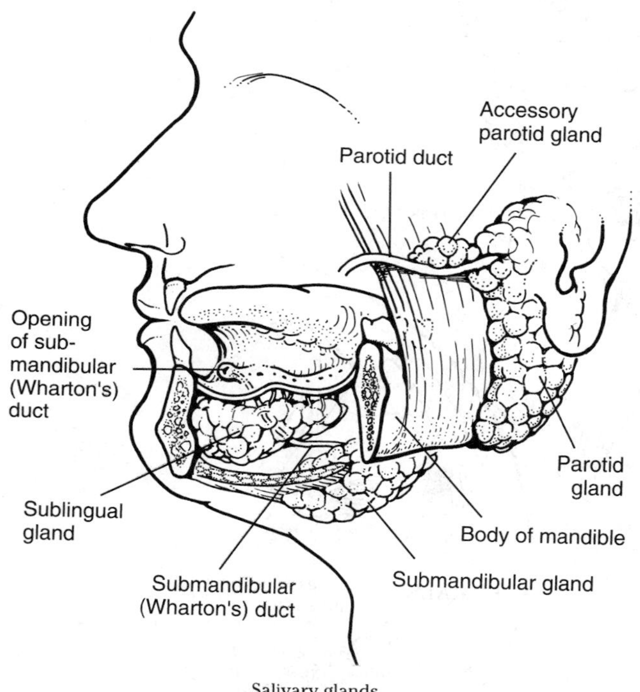


Salivary glands.

**seromucous g.,** mixed g. (def. 2).
**serous g.,** a gland that secretes a watery albuminous material, commonly but not always containing enzymes.
**Serres' g's,** Epstein's pearls.
**sexual g.,** 1. testis. 2. ovarium.
**Sigmund's g's,** nodi lymphoidei cubitales.
**simple g.,** one with a nonbranching duct.
**Skene's g's,** ductus paraurethrales urethrae femininae.
**g's of small intestine,** see *glandulae intestinales.*
**solitary g's of large intestine,** see *noduli lymphoidei solitarii,* under *nodulus.*
**solitary g's of small intestine,** see *noduli lymphoidei solitarii,* under *nodulus.*
**splenoid g.,** an apparently compensatory new growth that sometimes follows extirpation of the spleen.
**Stahr's g.,** a lymph node situated on the facial artery.
**subauricular g's,** nodi lymphoidei mastoidei.
**sublingual g.,** glandula sublingualis.
**submandibular g., submaxillary g.,** glandula submandibularis.
**sudoriferous g., sudoriparous g.,** glandula sudorifera.
**suprarenal g.,** glandula suprarenalis
**suprarenal g's, accessory,** glandulae suprarenales accessoriae.
**Suzanne's g.,** a mucous gland of the mouth, beneath the alveololingual groove.
**sweat g's,** glandula sudorifera.
**synovial g's,** villi synoviales.
**target g.,** a gland such as the thyroid, adrenal, or a gonad that is specifically affected by the secretory product of another gland; see also *releasing hormones* and *inhibiting hormones,* under *hormone.*
**tarsal g's, tarsoconjunctival g's,** glandulae tarsales.
**Theile's g's,** glandlike formations in the walls of the cystic duct and in the pelvis of the gallbladder.
**thymus g.,** thymus.
**thyroid g.,** glandula thyroidea.
**thyroid g's, accessory,** glandulae thyroideae accessoriae.
**g's of tongue,** glandulae linguales.
**tracheal g's,** glandulae tracheales.
**trachoma g's,** lymphoid follicles of the conjunctiva, found chiefly near the inner canthus of the eye.
**tubular g.,** any gland made up of or containing a tubule or a number of tubules.
**tubuloacinar g.,** one that is both tubular and acinous.
**g's of Tyson,** glandulae preputiales.
**ultimobranchial g's,** see under *body.*
**unicellular g.,** a single cell that functions as a gland, e.g., a goblet cell.
**urethral g's of female urethra,** glandulae urethrales urethrae femininae.
**urethral g's of male urethra,** glandulae urethrales urethrae masculinae.
**uropygial g.,** preen g.
**uterine g's, utricular g's,** glandulae uterinae.
**vaginal g.,** any gland occurring exceptionally in the vaginal mucous membrane.
**vascular g.,** 1. glomus. 2. a hemal node.
**vestibular g., greater,** glandula vestibularis major.
**vestibular g's, lesser,** glandulae vestibulares minores.
**Virchow's g.,** signal node.
**vitelline g.,** vitellarium.
**vulvovaginal g.,** glandula vestibularis major.
**Waldeyer's g's,** acinotubular glands in the inner skin of the attached edge of the eyelid.
**Weber's g's,** the tubular mucous glands of the tongue.
**Wölfler's g's,** glandulae thyroideae accessoriae.
**g's of Wolfring,** small tubuloalveolar glands in the subconjunctival tissue above the upper border of the tarsal plate, their ducts opening on the conjunctival surface.
**g's of Zeis,** glandulae sebaceae palpebrarum.

**glan·der·ous** (glan′dər-əs) of the nature of or affected with glanders.

**glan·ders** (glan′dərz) [MeSH: Glanders] a contagious disease of horses, communicable to humans, and caused by *Burkholderia mallei.* The acute form, which may be fatal, is marked by a purulent inflammation of mucous membranes and an eruption on the skin of nodules that coalesce and break down, forming deep ulcers that may end in necrosis of cartilages and bones. A chronic form known as *farcy* involves the lymphatic system. Called also *malleus.*
**African g., Japanese g.,** lymphangitis epizootica.

**glan·des** (glan′dēz) [L.] plural of *glans.*

**glan·di·lem·ma** (glan″dĭ-lem′ə) [*gland* + *-lemma*] the capsule or outer envelope of a gland.

**glan·du·la** (glan′du-lə) gen. and pl. *glan′dulae* [L.] [TA] a gland: an aggregation of cells, specialized to secrete or excrete materials not related to their ordinary metabolic needs.

Descriptions of glands are given on TA terms, and include anglicized names of specific glands.

**g. adrena'lis,** g. suprarenalis.

**glan'dulae areola'res** [TA], **glan'dulae areola'res [Montgome'rii],** areolar glands: sebaceous glands of the mammary areola; called also *Montgomery's glands.*

**glan'dulae bilia'res,** glandulae ductus choledochi.

**glan'dulae bronchia'les** [TA], bronchial glands: seromucous glands in the mucosa and submucosa of the bronchial walls.

**glan'dulae bucca'les** [TA], buccal glands: the serous and mucous glands on the inner surface of the cheeks.

**g. bulbourethra'lis** [TA], **g. bulbourethra'lis [Cow'peri],** bulbourethral gland: either of two glands embedded in the substance of the sphincter of the male urethra, just posterior to the membranous part of the urethra; they are homologues of the greater vestibular glands in the female. Called also *Cowper's gland.*

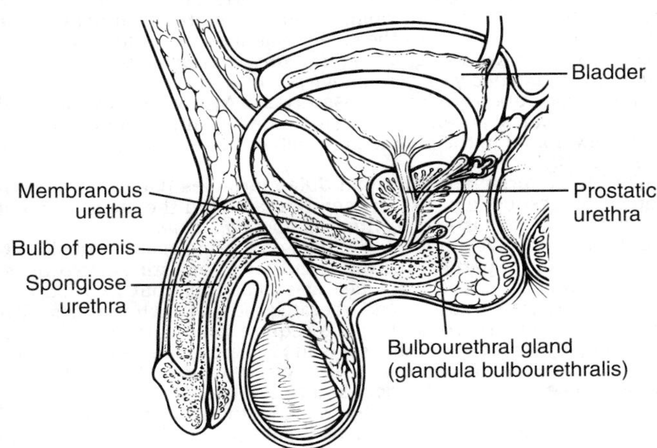


**glan'dulae cerumino'sae,** ceruminous glands: the glands in the skin of the external auditory canal that secrete the cerumen.

**glan'dulae cervica'les u'teri** [TA], cervical glands of uterus: mucus-secreting glands located in clefts in the wall of the uterine cervix.

**glan'dulae cilia'res conjunctiva'les** [TA], **glan'dulae cilia'res [Mol'li],** ciliary glands of conjunctiva: sweat glands that have become arrested in their development, situated obliquely in contact with and parallel to the bulbs of the eyelashes; called also *Moll's glands.*

**glan'dulae circumana'les,** circumanal glands: specialized sweat and sebaceous glands situated in an annular zone around the anus; called also *anal glands* and *Gay's glands.*

**glan'dulae conjunctiva'les** [TA], conjunctival glands: accessory lacrimal glands situated deep in the subconjunctival connective tissue, mainly in the upper fornix; called also *glandulae mucosae conjunctivae [Krausei]* and *Krause's glands.*

**glan'dulae cu'tis** [TA], cutaneous glands: the glands of the skin, including the sweat glands (see *glandula sudorifera*), sebaceous glands (see *glandula sebacea*), and the modified sweat glands that secrete cerumen (glandulae ceruminosae).

**glan'dulae duc'tus bilia'ris,** TA alternative for *glandulae ductus choledochi.*

**glan'dulae duc'tus chole'dochi** [TA], glands of bile duct: tubuloacinar glands in the mucosa of the bile ducts and the neck of the gallbladder; called also *biliary glands, glandulae biliaris, glandulae ductus biliaris* [TA alternative], *glandulae hepaticae, glandulae mucosae biliosae,* and *hepatic glands.*

**glan'dulae duodena'les** [TA], **glan'dulae duodena'les [Brun'neri],** duodenal glands: tubuloacinar glands in the submucous layer of the duodenum that open into the crypts of Lieberkühn; they secrete urogastrone. Called also *Brunner's glands.*

**glan'dulae endocri'nae** [TA], the endocrine glands (q.v.), including the thyroid, parathyroid, pituitary, and adrenal glands, and the gonads.

**glan'dulae esopha'geae,** glandulae oesophageae.

**g. glomifor'mis,** anastomosis arteriovenosa glomeriformis.

**glan'dulae hepa'ticae,** glandulae ductus choledochi.

**g. incisi'va,** a small intraoral gland in the median line of the upper jaw near the incisors.

**glan'dulae intestina'les** [TA], intestinal glands: simple tubular glands in the mucous membrane of either the small intestine *(glandulae intestinales intestini tenuis),* opening between the bases of the villi and containing argentaffin cells; the large intestine *(glandulae intestinales intestini crassi);* or of the rectum *(glandulae intestinales intestini recti).* Called also *crypts* or *glands of Lieberkühn,* and *Lieberkühn's* or *intestinal follicles.*

**glan'dulae labia'les o'ris** [TA], labial glands of the mouth: the serous and mucous glands on the inner part of the lips.

**g. lacrima'lis** [TA], lacrimal gland: either of a pair of glands, one at the upper outer angle of each orbit, secreting the tears; they are divided into two portions, the orbital and palpebral, by the orbital fascia.

**glan'dulae lacrima'les accesso'riae** [TA], accessory lacrimal glands: portions of the lacrimal gland sometimes found near the superior fornix of the conjunctiva.

**g. lacrima'lis infe'rior,** pars palpebralis glandulae lacrimalis.

**g. lacrima'lis supe'rior,** pars orbitalis glandulae lacrimalis.

**glan'dulae laryn'geae, glan'dulae laryngea'les** [TA], laryngeal glands: the mucous glands in the mucosa of the larynx.

**glan'dulae lingua'les** [TA], lingual glands: the mucous and serous glands on the surface of the tongue.

**glan'dulae lingua'les anterio'res,** anterior lingual glands: deeply placed mucoserous glands near the apex of the tongue.

**g. mamma'ria** [TA], mammary gland: the specialized accessory gland of the skin of female mammals that secretes milk. In the human female, it is a compound tubuloalveolar gland composed of 15 to 25 lobes arranged radially about the nipple and separated by connective and adipose tissue, each lobe having its own excretory (lactiferous) duct opening on the nipple. The lobes are subdivided into lobules, with the alveolar ducts and alveoli being the secretory portion of the gland. Called also *lactiferous gland.*

**glan'dulae mola'res** [TA], molar glands: the glands on the external aspect of the buccinator muscle, their ducts piercing it to open on the internal aspect of the cheek; called also *retromolar glands.*

**g. muco'sa,** mucous gland.

**glan'dulae muco'sae bilio'sae,** glandulae ductus choledochi.

**glan'dulae muco'sae conjuncti'vae [Kraus'ei],** glandulae conjunctivales.

**glan'dulae nasa'les** [TA], nasal glands: numerous large mucous and serous glands in the respiratory part of the nasal cavity.

**glan'dulae oesopha'geae** [TA], esophageal glands: the mucous glands in the submucosa of the esophagus. Written also *glandulae esophageae.*

**glan'dulae olfacto'riae** [TA], olfactory glands: small mucous glands in the olfactory mucosa; called also *Bowman's glands.*

**glan'dulae o'ris** [TA], the glands of the mouth; see *glandulae salivariae majores* and *glandulae salivariae minores.*

**glan'dulae palati'nae** [TA], palatine glands: the mucous glands on the soft palate and the posteromedial part of the hard palate.

**g. parathyroi'dea infe'rior** [TA], inferior parathyroid gland; see *parathyroid glands, under gland.*

**g. parathyroi'dea supe'rior** [TA], superior parathyroid gland; see *parathyroid glands,* under *gland.*

**g. paroti'dea** [TA], parotid gland: the largest of the three glands oc-

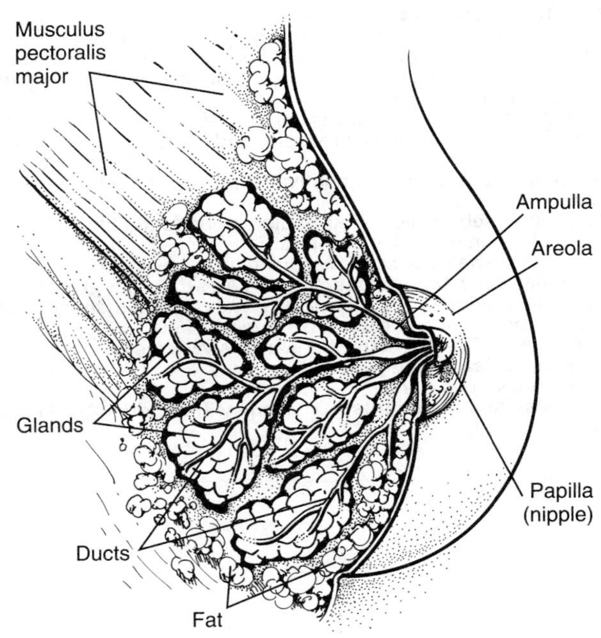


Glandula mammaria (mammary gland).

curring in pairs, which together with numerous small glands in the mouth constitute the salivary glands; it is located below the zygomatic arch, below and in front of the external acoustic meatus.

**g. paroti'dea accesso'ria** [TA], accessory parotid gland: a frequently present, more or less detached portion of the parotid gland.

**glan'dulae pel'vis rena'lis,** mucous glands in the wall of the kidney pelvis.

**glan'dulae pharyn'geae, glan'dulae pharyngea'les** [TA], **glan'dulae pharyn'gis,** pharyngeal glands: mucous glands beneath the tunica mucosa of the pharynx.

**g. pinea'lis** [TA], pineal gland: a small flattened cone-shaped body in the epithalamus, lying above the superior colliculi and below the splenium of the corpus callosum. Its hormonal function in human physiology is not firmly established; in response to norepinephrine it synthesizes and releases melatonin, whose rate of release declines when light activates retinal photoreceptors. Called also *epiphysis cerebri, corpus pineale* [TA alternative], and *pineal body.*

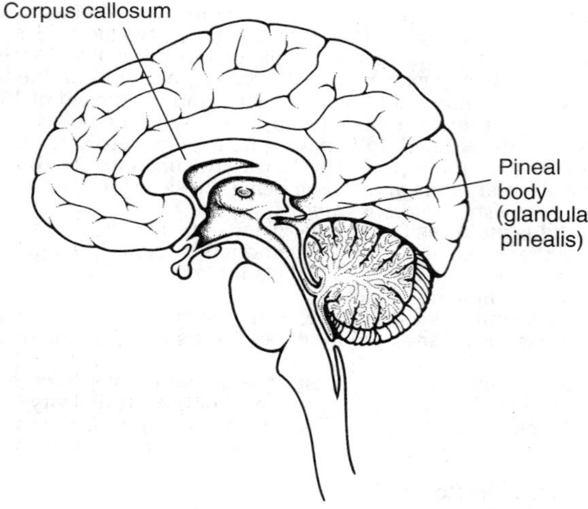


**g. pituita'ria,** TA alternative for *hypophysis.*

**glan'dulae preputia'les** [TA], preputial glands: small sebaceous glands of the corona of the penis and the inner surface of the prepuce, which secrete smegma; called also *crypts of Littre* or *Littre's glands.*

**g. prosta'tica,** prostate.

**glan'dulae pylo'ricae,** pyloric glands.

**glan'dulae saliva'riae majo'res** [TA], major salivary glands: the larger exocrine glands of the oral cavity, which together with the smaller salivary glands *(glandulae salivariae minores)* secrete saliva; the group includes the sublingual, submandibular, and parotid glands.

**glan'dulae saliva'riae mino'res** [TA], minor salivary glands: the smaller exocrine glands of the oral cavity, which together with the larger salivary glands *(glandulae salivariae majores)* secrete saliva; the group includes the labial, buccal, molar, palatine, and lingual glands, and the anterior lingual gland.

**g. seba'cea** [TA], sebaceous gland: one of the holocrine glands of the skin that secrete sebum and are situated in the corium. Called also *oil gland.*

**glan'dulae seba'ceae conjunctiva'les,** glandulae sebaceae palpebrarum.

**glan'dulae seba'ceae la'bii majo'ris pudenda'lis,** sebaceous glands in the skin of the labia majora.

**glan'dulae seba'ceae mam'mae,** glandulae areolares.

**glan'dulae seba'ceae palpebra'rum** [TA], sebaceous glands of eyelids: modified rudimentary sebaceous glands attached directly to the follicles of the eyelashes; called also *glands of Zeis.*

**g. semina'lis,** TA alternative for glandula vesiculosa.

**g. seromuco'sa,** mixed g. (def. 2).

**g. sero'sa,** serous gland..

**glan'dulae si'ne duc'tibus** [L. "glands without ducts"], glandulae endocrinae.

**g. sublingua'lis** [TA], sublingual gland: the smallest of the three salivary glands, occurring in pairs, predominantly mucous in type, and draining into the oral cavity through 10 to 30 sublingual ducts; called also *Rivinus gland.*

**g. submandibula'ris** [TA], **g. submaxilla'ris,** submandibular gland: one of the three chief, paired salivary glands, predominantly serous, lying partly above and partly below the posterior half of the base of the mandible.

**g. sudori'fera** [TA], sudoriferous or sweat gland: one of the glands that secrete sweat, situated in the corium or subcutaneous tissue, and opening by a duct on the surface of the body. There are two types: the ordinary or *eccrine sweat glands* and the *apocrine sweat glands.* Called also *sudoriparous gland.*

**g. suprarena'lis** [TA], suprarenal or adrenal gland: a flattened body found in the retroperitoneal tissues at the cranial pole of the kidney. In humans it consists of two components of different embryologic origin, the cortex and medulla. The adrenal cortex, under control of the pituitary hormone corticotropin, elaborates steroid hormones. The adrenal medulla elaborates the catecholamines epinephrine and norepinephrine. Called also *g. adrenalis, adrenal* or *suprarenal body, adrenal* or *suprarenal capsule,* and *epinephros.*

**glan'dulae suprarena'les accesso'riae** [TA], accessory suprarenal or adrenal glands: adrenal glandular tissue, usually either cortical or medullary, found in the abdomen or pelvis. Called also *adrenal* or *suprarenal rests.*

**glan'dulae tarsa'les** [TA], **glan'dulae tarsa'les [Meibo'mi],** tarsal glands: sebaceous follicles between the tarsi and the conjunctiva of the eyelids; called also *palpebral* or *meibomian glands.*

**g. thyroi'dea** [TA], thyroid gland: an endocrine gland normally situated in the lower part of the front of the neck, consisting of two lobes, one on either side of the trachea and joined in front by a narrow isthmus. It secretes, stores, and liberates the thyroid hormones (thyroxine and triiodothyronine), which require iodine for their elaboration and play major endocrine roles in regulating the metabolic rate. It also secretes thyrocalcitonin. Called also *thyroid* and *thyroid body.*

**glan'dulae thyroi'deae accesso'riae** [TA], accessory thyroid glands: small exclaves of the thyroid gland, found along the course of the thyroglossal duct and elsewhere; types (named for their locations) include *intrathoracic thyroid, lingual thyroid, suprahyoid thyroid,* and *retrosternal thyroid.* Called also *aberrant thyroids* and *prehyoid glands.*

**glan'dulae trachea'les** [TA], tracheal glands: mucous glands in the elastic submucous coat between the cartilaginous rings and on the posterior wall of the trachea.

**glan'dulae tuba'riae** [TA], mucous glands within the mucosa of the auditory tube, especially near its nasopharyngeal end; called also *mucous glands of auditory* or *eustachian tube.*

**glan'dulae urethra'les [Lit'trei],** glandulae urethrales urethrae masculinae.

**glan'dulae urethra'les ure'thrae femini'nae** [TA], urethral glands of female urethra: numerous small mucous glands in the mucosa of the female urethra, some of which on either side are drained by the inconstant paraurethral duct opening into the vestibule.

**glan'dulae urethra'les ure'thrae masculi'nae** [TA], urethral glands of male urethra: mucous glands in the wall of the male urethra; called also *Littre's glands.*

**glan'dulae urethra'les ure'thrae mulie'bris,** glandulae urethrales urethrae femininae.

**glan'dulae uteri'nae** [TA], uterine glands: simple tubular glands throughout the entire thickness and extent of the endometrium, which become enlarged during the premenstrual period.

**glan'dulae vesica'les ve'sicae urina'riae,** mucous glands in the wall of the urinary bladder.

**g. vesiculo'sa** [TA], seminal gland: either of the paired, sacculated pouches attached to the posterior part of the urinary bladder; the duct of each joins the ipsilateral ductus deferens to form the ejaculatory duct. Called also *seminal vesicle, vesicula seminalis* [TA alternative], and *g. seminalis* [TA alternative].

**g. vestibula'ris ma'jor** [TA], greater vestibular gland: either of two small reddish yellow bodies in the vestibular bulbs, one on each side of the vaginal orifice; they are homologues of the bulbourethral glands in the male. Called also *Bartholin's gland.*

**glan'dulae vestibula'res mino'res** [TA], lesser vestibular glands: small mucous glands opening upon the vestibular mucous membrane between the urethral and the vaginal orifice.

**glan·du·lae** (glan'du-le) [L.] genitive and plural of *glandula.*

**glan·du·lar** (glan'du-lər) 1. pertaining to or of the nature of a gland. Called also *adenic* and *adenous.* 2. pertaining to the glans penis or glans clitoridis.

**glan·dule** (glan'dūl) [L. *glandula*] a small gland.

**glan·du·lous** (glan'du-ləs) [L. *glandulosus*] abounding in kernels or small glands.

**glans** (glanz) pl. *glan'des* [L. "acorn"] [TA] a general term for a small rounded mass, or glandlike body.
**g. clito'ridis** [TA], glans of clitoris: erectile tissue at the end of the clitoris, which is continuous with the intermediate part of the vestibular bulbs.
**g. pe'nis** [TA], the cap-shaped expansion of the corpus spongiosum at the end of the penis; called also *balanus.*

**glan·u·lar** (glan'u-lər) pertaining to the glans penis or glans clitoris.

**glan·u·lo·plas·ty** (glan'u-lo-plas"te) plastic surgery on a glans, such as the glans penis to correct hypospadias.

**Glanz·mann's thrombasthenia (disease)** (glahnts'mənz) [Eduard *Glanzmann,* Swiss pediatrician, 1887–1959] see *thrombasthenia.*

**glare** (glār) [Middle English *glaren*] [MeSH: Glare] a condition of discomfort in the eye and of depression of central vision produced when a bright light enters the field of vision, especially when the eye is adapted to dark. The amount of glare is directly proportional to the candle power of the light and inversely proportional to the square of the distance of the light from the eye and to its angular distance from the visual axis.
**direct g.,** glare in which the image of the light falls on the fovea.
**indirect g.,** glare in which the image of the light falls outside the fovea.

**glar·om·e·ter** (glār-om'ə-tər) [*glare* + *-meter*] an instrument for measuring a person's resistance to glare from the lights of an approaching automobile.

**gla·se·ri·an fissure** (gla-se're-ən) [Johann Heinrich *Glaser* (Glaserius), Swiss anatomist, 1629–1675] fissura petrotympanica.

**Glas·gow Co·ma Scale, Out·come Scale** (glas'go) [*Glasgow,* Scotland, where the scales were developed] see under *scale.*

**Glas·gow's sign** (glas'gōz) [William Carr *Glasgow,* American physician, 1845–1907] see under *sign.*

**glass** (glas) [L. *vit'rum*] [MeSH: Glass] 1. a hard, brittle, and often transparent material, usually consisting of the fused amorphous silicates of potassium or sodium, and of calcium, with silica in excess. 2. a container, usually cylindrical, made from glass. 3. (pl.) lenses worn to aid or improve vision; see *glasses, lens,* and *spectacles.*
**cover g.,** a thin glass plate used to cover an object for microscopic examination. Spelled also *coverglass.*
**crown g.,** a glass of low refractive index (achieved by incorporating a considerable percentage of phosphorus pentoxide); used in combination with flint glass in multielement lenses.
**cupping g.,** a vessel of glass from which the air has been or can be exhausted, applied to the body for the purpose of drawing blood to the surface; currently used in some cultures to treat headaches, chills, fevers, back pain, and similar complaints.
**flint g.,** a highly refractive glass in which calcium has been replaced in large part by lead; used for lenses and prisms and in the manufacture of cut glass.
**object g.,** see *objective.*
**optical g.,** glass of high quality and controlled composition, used for lenses.
**quartz g.,** pure fused silica, used for prisms, lenses, and chemical vessels because its index of thermal expansion is so small that it does not crack when heated or cooled and because it transmits more ultraviolet radiation than does ordinary glass.
**test g.,** a small glass vessel, resembling a beaker, used in a chemical laboratory.
**Wood's g.,** see under *light.*

**glass·es** (glas'əz) spectacles; a pair of lenses arranged in a frame holding them in the proper position before the eyes, as an aid to vision. See also *lens* and *spectacles.*
**bifocal g.,** lenses which have two different refracting powers, one for distant and one for near vision.
**contact g.,** see *contact lens.*
**crutch g.,** glasses that will elevate and support the upper lid of patients with ptosis.
**Hallauer's g.,** glasses with grayish-green lenses that prevent the passage of blue and ultraviolet rays.
**safety g.,** see under *lens.*
**trifocal g.,** glasses with lenses that have three different refracting powers, one for distant, one for intermediate, and one for near vision.

**glassy** (glas'e) like glass; hyaline or vitreous.

**Glau·ber's salt** (glou'berz) [Johann Rudolf *Glauber,* German physician and chemist, 1604–1670] sodium sulfate.

**glau·co·ma** (glaw-ko'mə) [Gr. *glaukōma* opacity of the crystalline lens (from the dull gray gleam of the affected eye)] [MeSH: Glaucoma] a group of eye diseases characterized by an increase in intraocular pressure that causes pathologic changes in the optic disk and typical defects in the field of vision.
**absolute g.,** the final stage of glaucoma characterized by pain in the eye and blindness.
**acute congestive g.,** angle-closure g.
**air-block g.,** a form of postoperative glaucoma, resulting from blockage of the flow of aqueous by air injected behind the iris.
**angle-closure g.,** glaucoma caused by closure of the anterior angle by contact between the iris and the inner surface of the trabecular meshwork; called also *closed-angle g., narrow-angle g.,* and *pupillary block g.*
**angle-closure g., acute,** the third phase of angle-closure glaucoma and a grave medical emergency. Initially the symptoms resemble intermittent angle-closure glaucoma. Then, as the intraocular pressure continues increasing, the cornea becomes swollen and steamy; the iris fixes in mid-dilation; there is excruciating ocular pain radiating to the other areas of the trigeminal distribution, and there may be nausea and vomiting. Finally the eye may become red and congested; visual acuity fails rapidly as the cornea keeps swelling, and severe visual field loss or even blindness may result if the intraocular pressure is not lowered.
**angle-closure g., chronic,** the fourth, last stage of angle-closure glaucoma, it is an irreversible increase of intraocular pressure resulting from progressive damage to the angle structures and from permanent, at least partial closure of the anterior angle by synechiae.
**angle-closure g., intermittent,** the second phase of angle-closure glaucoma, usually lasting for several months, and characterized by intermittent, transient attacks of glaucoma with rapidly rising intraocular pressure, edematous cornea, and dull or throbbing pain in or around the eye.
**angle-closure g., latent,** the first phase of angle-closure glaucoma; patients may be free of symptoms or have minor attacks of varying severity, duration, and frequency for months or years before a crisis. Gonioscopy reveals narrow angles capable of closure. Called also *prodromal g.*
**angle-recession g.,** glaucoma secondary to contusion injury of the eye, in which the anterior chamber is deep and the angle recedes, with exposure of the ciliary body, as seen gonioscopically, with blocking of the trabecular spaces; called also *contusion g.*
**aphakic g.,** a general term referring to glaucoma in an eye from which the lens has been removed; the glaucoma may be related to the cataract extraction or to its sequelae, or it may have existed prior to the cataract extraction.
**apoplectic g.,** hemorrhagic g.
**auricular g.,** that associated with increased intralabyrinthine pressure.
**capsular g., g. capsulare,** an open-angle glaucoma associated with the exfoliation syndrome, and with particles of iris pigment scattered in the anterior angle.
**chronic g.,** open-angle g.
**chronic narrow-angle g.,** a form of narrow angle glaucoma without a severe congestive episode.
**chymotrypsin-induced g.,** enzyme g.
**closed-angle g.,** angle-closure g.
**congenital g.,** infantile g.
**congestive g.,** angle-closure g.
**g. consumma'tum,** absolute g.
**contusion g.,** angle-recession g.
**Donders' g.,** advanced open-angle g.
**enzyme g.,** a transient glaucoma developing postoperatively in patients in whom trypsin has been used in the lysis of the zonule during cataract surgery; it is usually self-limited, with no permanent damage.

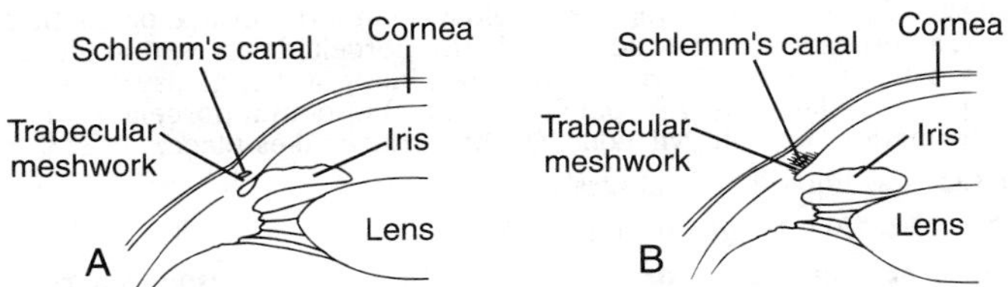

Glaucoma. Impairment of aqueous outflow is caused by closure of the anterior angle, with apposition of the iris and trabecular meshwork, in angle-closure glaucoma *(A),* and by other obstruction in open-angle glaucoma *(B).*

**ghost cell g.**, an open-angle glaucoma caused by erythroclasts obstructing aqueous outflow, occurring after vitreous hemorrhage caused by trauma or by retinal neovascularization or by cataract extraction.
**hemolytic g.**, an open-angle glaucoma caused by blood clots filling the anterior angle or by erythrocytes infiltrating the trabecular network.
**hemorrhagic g.**, that which is caused by pressure from retinal hemorrhage.
**infantile g.**, a form of congenital glaucoma that may be fully developed at birth, with characteristic signs (enlargement and hazing of the corneas), or it may develop at any time up to two or three years of age; these signs result from inability of the cornea and sclera to withstand the increased intraocular pressure. Called also *buphthalmos.* Cf. *juvenile g.*
**inflammatory g.**, a form attended with ciliary congestion, corneal opacity, and blindness, recurring in paroxysmal attacks.
**juvenile g.**, glaucoma differing from infantile glaucoma in that it occurs in older children and young adults up to 30 years of age, and there is no gross enlargement of the eyeball.
**lenticular g.**, glaucoma occurring in association with congenital or traumatic dislocation of the lens, or with swelling of the lens, usually due to mechanical obstruction at the peripheral angle of the anterior chamber.
**low-tension g.**, open-angle glaucoma without increased intraocular pressure.
**malignant g.**, glaucoma that grows rapidly worse in spite of iridectomy.
**melanomalytic g.**, glaucoma caused by mechanical blockage of the angle by macrophages in the eye with necrotic malignant melanoma.
**narrow-angle g.**, angle-closure g.
**neovascular g.**, a form of secondary glaucoma; glaucoma caused by neovascularization in the chamber angle.
**noncongestive g.**, open-angle g.
**obstructive g.**, angle-closure g.
**open-angle g.**, any glaucoma in which the angle of the anterior chamber remains open, but filtration is gradually diminished because of the tissues of the angle; called also *chronic g., simple g.,* and *wide-angle g.*
**phacogenic g., phacolytic g.**, an open-angle glaucoma secondary to leakage of lens protein into the aqueous from a mature or hypermature cataract with subsequent ingestion of the protein by macrophages, which swell and block the trabecular spaces.
**pigmentary g.**, a form of open-angle glaucoma associated with an abnormal amount of pigment dispersion in the anterior segment of the eye.
**primary g.**, increased intraocular pressure occurring in an eye without previous disease; see *angle-closure g.* and *open-angle g.*
**prodromal g.**, latent angle-closure g.
**pupillary block g.**, angle-closure g.
**secondary g.**, increased intraocular pressure resulting from a preexisting disease or injury.
**simple g.**, primary open-angle g.
**steroid g.**, a secondary open-angle glaucoma due to chronic use of topical or systemic corticosteroids.
**traumatic g.**, an increase in intraocular pressure due to a nonperforating injury of the globe, resulting in vascular congestion.
**vitreous-block g.**, postoperative glaucoma in which vitreous plugs the pupil, so that the aqueous, which is unable to move to the anterior chamber, forces the vitreous and iris forward, producing occlusion of the chamber angle and eventually peripheral anterior synechiae.
**wide-angle g.**, open-angle g.

**glau·co·ma·tous** (glaw-ko′mə-təs) pertaining to or of the nature of glaucoma.

**glau·co·sis** (glaw-ko′sis) blindness caused by glaucoma.

**glau·cos·uria** (glaw″ko-su′re-ə) [Gr. *glaukos* silvery + *uria*] indicanuria.

**glau·kom·fleck·en** (glou′kom-flek″ən) [Ger. "glaucoma spots"] glaucomatous cataract.

**glaze** (glāz) 1. to cover with a glossy, smooth surface or coating. 2. a ceramic veneer added to a dental porcelain restoration after it has been fired, to give a completely nonporous, glossy or semiglossy surface. 3. the final firing (in air) of dental porcelain, when formation of a thin, vitreous, glossy surface takes place.

**GLC** gas-liquid chromatography.

**GlcNAc** *N*-acetylglucosamine.

**Glea·son grade (score)** (gle′sən) [Donald F. *Gleason,* American pathologist, born 1920] see under *grade.*

**gleet** (glēt) 1. a chronic form of gonorrheal urethritis. 2. a urethral discharge, especially one that is mucous or purulent.
**vent g.**, cloacitis in domestic fowl.

**gleety** (glēt′e) pertaining to or of the nature of gleet.

**Glenn operation (anastomosis, shunt)** (glen) [William Wallace Lumpkin *Glenn,* American surgeon, born 1914] see under *operation.*

**gle·no·hu·mer·al** (gle″no-hu′mər-əl) pertaining to the glenoid cavity and to the humerus.

**gle·noid** (gle′noid) [Gr. *glēnē* socket + *-oid*] resembling a pit or socket; see *cavitas glenoidalis.*

**Gley's cells, glands** (glāz) [Marcel Eugène Émile *Gley,* French physiologist, 1857–1930] see under *cell* and see *glandulae thyroidea accessoriae.*

**GLI** glucagon-like immunoreactivity; see *enteroglucagon.*

**glia** (gli′ə) [Gr. "glue"] the neuroglia.
**ameboid g.**, degenerated neuroglial cells that are rich in pale protoplasm, possess few processes, and have densely staining nuclei.
**Bergmann's g.**, see under *cell.*
**cytoplasmic g.**, enlarged neuroglial cells, rich in cytoplasm, containing vacuoles and supplied with fibrils; seen in degeneration of the spinal cord.
**g. of Fañanás**, see under *cell.*
**fibrillary g.**, degenerated neuroglial cells containing an abundance of fibrils.
**radial g.**, a special type of glia in the developing central nervous system, whose cells have radial processes extending through the entire thickness from the ventricular surface to the exterior cortical surface; neurons formed on the ventricular surface are thought to migrate along these processes to their final positions in other parts of the cortex.

**-glia** [Gr. *glia* glue] a word termination denoting the neuroglia.

**glia·cyte** (gli′ə-sīt) [*glia* + *-cyte*] a neuroglia cell.

**Gli·a·del** (gli′ə-del) trademark for a preparation of polifeprosan 20 with a carmustine implant.

**gli·a·din** (gli′ə-din) [Gr. *glia* glue] [MeSH: Gliadin] a protein of the prolamin group, found in wheat and occurring in various forms ($\alpha$-, $\beta$-, $\gamma$-, and $\omega$-gliadins); it contains the toxic factor associated with celiac disease.

**gli·al** (gli′əl) neuroglial.

**gli·am·i·lide** (gli-am′ĭ-līd) $C_{23}H_{33}N_5O_5S$; a hypoglycemic, administered orally.

**gli·ben·cla·mide** (gli-ben′klə-mīd) glyburide.

**gli·born·ur·ide** (gli-born′ūr-īd) a sulfonylurea compound used as a hypoglycemic in the treatment of type 2 diabetes mellitus; administered orally.

**gli·cen·tin** (gli-sen′tin) a major form of enteroglucagon.

**gli·cet·a·nile so·di·um** (glĭ-set′ə-nīl) $C_{23}H_{24}ClN_4NaO_4S$; a hypoglycemic, administered orally. Called also *glydanile sodium.*

**glic·la·zide** (glik′lə-zīd) [MeSH: Gliclazide] a sulfonylurea compound used as a hypoglycemic in the treatment of type 2 diabetes mellitus; administered orally.

**glide** (glīd) 1. a smooth continuous movement. 2. a speech sound that is transitional between a vowel and a consonant.
**mandibular g.**, the side-to-side, protrusive, and intermediate movement of the mandible occurring when the teeth or other occluding surfaces are in contact.
**occlusal g.**, the movement induced by deflective tooth contact that diverts the mandible from a normal path of closure to a centric jaw relation.

**gli·flu·mide** (glĭ-floo′mīd) $C_{25}H_{29}FN_4O_4S$; a hypoglycemic, administered orally.

**gli·mep·i·ride** (gli-mep′ĭ-rīd) a sulfonylurea compound used as a hypoglycemic in the treatment of type 2 diabetes mellitus; administered orally.

**gli(o)-** [Gr. *glia* glue] a combining form denoting relationship to a gluey substance or, specifically, to the neuroglia.

**glio·bac·te·ria** (gli″o-bak-tēr′e-ə) [*glio-* + *bacteria*] bacteria that are surrounded by a gelatinous matrix.

**glio·blast** (gli′o-blast) spongioblast, def. 1.

**glio·blas·to·ma** (gli″o-blas-to′mə) [*glio-* + *blastoma*] [MeSH: Glioblastoma] a general term for malignant forms of astrocytoma.
**g. multifor′me**, the most malignant type of astrocytoma, usually classified as Grade IV, one of the most common primary tumors of the brain; it also occurs in the brain stem in children and occasionally in the spinal cord of an adult or child. It is a rapidly growing tumor, usually found in the cerebral hemispheres and composed of a mixture of spongioblasts, astroblasts, and astrocytes. Called also *spongioblastoma multiforme.*

**glio·coc·cus** (gli″o-kok′əs) [*glio-* + *coccus*] a micrococcus that forms gelatinous matter.

**glio·cyte** (gli'o-sīt) neuroglial cell.
**retinal g's,** Müller's fibers.

**glio·fi·bril·lary** (gli″o-fi'brĭ-lar-e) pertaining to fibrils of the neuroglia.

**gli·o·ma** (gli-o'mə) [*gli-* + *-oma*] [MeSH: Glioma] originally, a tumor composed of tissue representing neuroglia in any of its stages of development; the term has been extended to include all the primary intrinsic neoplasms of the brain and spinal cord, including astrocytomas, ependymomas, medulloblastomas, medulloepitheliomas, and others. Called also *neurogliocytoma, neuroglioma,* and *neurospongioma.*
**astrocytic g.,** astrocytoma.
**g. endo'phytum,** endophytic retinoblastoma.
**ependymal g.,** ependymoma.
**g. exo'phytum,** exophytic retinoblastoma.
**ganglionic g.,** ganglioglioma.
**mixed g.,** a glioma in which the cytologic components are of more than one cell type; the most common form consists of foci of oligodendroglioma in an otherwise typical astrocytoma.
**nasal g.,** a tumorlike mass composed of ectopic neural tissue in the nasal cavity.
**optic g.,** a slow-growing glioma of the optic nerve or optic chiasm heralded by visual loss, often with secondary strabismus, followed by proptosis and loss of ocular movement.
**peripheral g.,** schwannoma.
**g. re'tinae,** retinoblastoma.

**gli·o·ma·to·sis** (gli″o-mə-to'sis) diffuse formation of gliomas; called also *neurogliosis.*
**cerebral g., g. ce'rebri,** a rare variant of glioblastoma multiforme in which one hemisphere or the entire brain is infiltrated diffusely with anaplastic astrocytes.

**gli·o·ma·tous** (gli-o'mə-təs) affected with or of the nature of glioma.

**glio·neu·ro·ma** (gli″o-nŏŏ-ro'mə) ganglioglioma.

**glio·pha·gia** (gli″o-fa'jə) [*glio-* + *-phagia*] phagocytosis of neuroglial cells.

**glio·pil** (gli'o-pil) [*glio-* + Gr. *pilos* felt] a dense feltwork of glial processes, as in the subependymal tissue around the ventricles.

**glio·sar·co·ma** (gli″o-sahr-ko'mə) [*glio-* + *sarcoma*] [MeSH: Gliosarcoma] a glioma, usually a glioblastoma multiforme, that has sarcomatous components.

**gli·o·sis** (gli-o'sis) [MeSH: Gliosis] an excess of astroglia in damaged areas of the central nervous system; see also *astrocytosis.*
**diffuse g.,** gliosis affecting the whole of the cerebral tissue, or widely scattered through it.
**g. endome'trii,** g. uteri.
**hemispheric g.,** gliosis affecting one of the cerebral hemispheres.
**hypertrophic nodular g.,** a form of gliosis in which the brain is symmetrically enlarged because of hyperplasia of the neuroglial tissue.
**isomorphic g.,** gliosis in which there is a regular and parallel arrangement of glial fibers.
**perivascular g.,** a form of arteriosclerosis of the cerebral vessels, marked by an increase of neuroglia.
**unilateral g.,** hemispheric g.
**g. u'teri,** proliferation of neural tissue in the endometrium or endocervix.

**glio·some** (gli'o-sōm) [*glio-* + *-some*] one of the small cytoplasmic granules seen in neuroglial cells.

**glio·tox·in** (gli″o-tok'sin) [MeSH: Gliotoxin] an antibiotic obtained from several unrelated species of fungi, including species of *Trichoderma, Aspergillus,* and *Penicillium;* it is a neutral, nitrogen- and sulfur-containing compound.

**glip·i·zide** (glip'ĭ-zīd) [USP] [MeSH: Glipizide] a sulfonylurea compound used as a hypoglycemic in the treatment of type 2 diabetes mellitus; administered orally.

**Gli·ric·o·la** (gli-rik'o-lə) a genus of biting lice of the order Mallophaga; *G. porcel'li* infests guinea pigs.

**glis·chrin** (glis'krin) [Gr. *glischros* gluey] a mucin produced in urine by bacterial activity.

**glis·chru·ria** (glis-kroo're-ə) the presence of glischrin in the urine.

**glis·sade** (glĭ-säd') [Fr. "sliding"] a gliding involuntary movement of the eye in changing the point of fixation; it is a slower, smoother movement than is a saccade.

**glis·sad·ic** (glĭ-sad'ik) pertaining to a glissade.

**Glis·son's capsule, sling, sphincter** (glis'ənz) [Francis *Glisson,* English physician and anatomist, 1597–1677] see *capsula fibrosa perivascularis, musculus sphincter ampullae hepatopancreaticae,* and see under *sling.*

**glis·so·ni·tis** (glis″o-ni'tis) inflammation of Glisson's capsule (capsula fibrosa perivascularis [TA]).

**globe** 1. sphere. 2. bulbus oculi.

**glo·bi** (glo'bi) [L.] 1. genitive and plural of *globus.* 2. encapsulated globular masses containing bacilli, seen in smears of lepromatous leprosy lesions.

**glo·bid·i·o·sis** (glo-bid″e-o'sis) former name for *besnoitiosis.*

**Glo·bid·i·um** (glo-bid'e-əm) former name for *Besnoitia.*

**glo·bin** (glo'bin) [MeSH: Globin] 1. the protein constituent of hemoglobin; see also *globin chain,* under *chain.* 2. any member of a group of proteins similar to the typical globin.

**Glo·bo·ceph·a·lus** (glo″bo-sef'ə-lus) a genus of blood-sucking nematodes of the family Ancylostomatidae. *G. urosubula'tus* and other species infest the intestines of pigs, causing anemia.

**glo·boid** (glo'boid) globe-shaped; spheroid.

**glo·bose** (glo'bōs) [L. *globus* a ball] globe-shaped, spherical.

**glob·o·side** (glob'o-sīd) a glycosphingolipid containing acetylated amino sugars and simple hexoses of the general composition *N*-acetylgalactosamine-galactose-galactose-glucose-ceramide; it accumulates in tissues in Sandhoff's disease, but not in Tay-Sachs disease.

**globo·tri·a·o·syl·cer·a·mide** (glo″bo-tri-a″o-səl-ser'ə-mīd) ceramide trihexoside.

**glob·u·lar** (glob'u-lər) 1. like a globe or globule. 2. composed of globules.

**Glo·bu·la·ria** (glob″u-lar'e-ə) a genus of shrubs of the family Globulariaceae. *G. aly'pum* L. is a perennial herb indigenous to the Mediterranean region used as a purgative and for intermittent fevers.

**glob·ule** (glob'ūl) [L. *globulus* a globule] 1. a small spherical mass or body. 2. a small spherical drop of fluid or semifluid substance, e.g., a fat droplet in milk or a drop of water. 3. a little globe or pellet, as of medicine.
**dentin g's,** small spherical bodies in the peripheral dentin, created by beginning calcification of the matrix about discrete foci.
**Dobie's g.,** a minute stainable mass in the middle of the transparent disk of a muscle fibril.
**Marchi's g's,** fragments and particles of broken-up myelin that stain by Marchi's method, seen in degeneration of the spinal cord.
**Morgagni's g's,** round fragments of cells in the cortex of the lens; they are a sign of mature cataract.
**polar g's,** polar bodies (def. 1).

**glo·bu·li** (glob'u-li) genitive and plural of *globulus.*

**glob·u·lin** (glob'u-lin) [L. *globulus* globule] any member of a class of proteins, most of which are insoluble in water but soluble in saline solutions *(euglobulins),* but some of which *(pseudoglobulins)* are water soluble proteins whose other physical properties closely resemble those of the true globulins. See also *serum g's.*
**$\alpha$-g's,** the serum globulins with the most rapid electrophoretic migration, further subdivided into the faster $\alpha_1$-globulins and the slower $\alpha_2$-globulins. Written also *alpha g's.*
**AC g., accelerator g.,** factor V; see under *coagulation factors,* at *factor.*
**alpha g's,** $\alpha$-g's.
**antihemophilic g. (AHG),** factor VIII; see under *coagulation factors,* at *factor.*
**anti–human g. serum** [USP], monospecific or broad spectrum antiserum produced by immunizing a rabbit or other animal with human plasma proteins; used in the antiglobulin test (Coombs' test) and immunoelectrophoresis.
**antilymphocyte g. (ALG),** the gamma globulin fraction of antilymphocyte serum (q.v.), used an immunosuppressant in organ transplantation.
**antithymocyte g. (ATG),** the gamma globulin fraction of antiserum derived from animals that have been immunized against human thymocytes; an immunosuppressive agent that causes specific destruction of T lymphocytes, used in treatment of allograft rejection.
**$\beta$-g's,** globulins of plasma that have an electrophoretic mobility in neutral or alkaline solutions intermediate between that of the alpha and the gamma globulins.
**bacterial polysaccharide immune g. (BPIG),** a human hyperimmune globulin derived from the blood plasma of adult human donors immunized with *Haemophilus influenza* type b, pneumococcal, and meningococcal polysaccharide vaccines; used for passive immunization of infants under 18 months of age.
**beta g's,** $\beta$-g's.
**corticosteroid-binding g., cortisol-binding g. (CBG),** transcortin.
**$\gamma$-g's, gamma g's,** serum globulins having the least rapid electrophoretic migration. Since the gamma globulin fraction is composed almost entirely of immunoglobulin, gamma globulin came to be used as a synonym of "immunoglobulin" or "immune globulin." Because some immunoglobulins have $\alpha$ or $\beta$ electrophoretic mobility, this usage is imprecise and is in decline.

**hepatitis B immune g.** [USP], a specific immune globulin derived from plasma of human donors with high titers of antibodies against hepatitis B surface antigen ($HB_sAg$); used for postexposure prophylaxis following contact with $HB_sAg$-positive materials, also administered to infants of $HB_sAg$-positive mothers.
**human rabies immune g. (HRIG)** [USP], a specific immune globulin derived from plasma of human donors hyperimmunized with rabies vaccine; administered in conjunction with rabies vaccine in cases of bite or scratch exposure to animals known or suspected to be rabid.
**hyperimmune g.,** any of various immunoglobulin preparations that are especially high in antibodies against certain specific diseases.
**immune g.,** 1. immunoglobulin. 2. [USP] a concentrated preparation containing gamma globulins, predominantly IgG, from a large pool of human donors; used for prophylaxis of measles or hepatitis A and for treatment of hypogammaglobulinemia in immunodeficient patients. Formerly called *immune human serum g.* and *immune serum g.* Called also *gamma g.*
**immune human serum g., immune serum g.,** former names for *immune g.* (def. 2).
**intravenous immune g.,** a preparation of immune globulin suitable for intravenous administration; used in replacement therapy for antibody-deficiency disorders.
**lymphocyte immune g.,** antilymphocyte g.
**pertussis immune g.** [USP], a specific immune globulin derived from human donors immunized with pertussis vaccine; used for prophylaxis and treatment of pertussis. Formerly called *pertussis immune human g.*
**$Rh_0$(D) immune g.** [USP], a specific immune globulin derived from plasma of human donors immunized to produce high levels of antibodies against the $Rh_0$ antigen (D antigen); used to prevent Rh-sensitization of Rh-negative females and thus prevent erythroblastosis fetalis in subsequent pregnancies; administered within 72 hours after exposure to Rh-positive blood resulting from delivery of an Rh-positive child, abortion or miscarriage of an Rh-positive fetus, or transfusion of Rh-positive blood. It is also used as a platelet count stimulator in the treatment of idiopathic thrombocytopenic purpura. Formerly called *$Rh_0$(D) immune human g.*
**serum g's,** all plasma proteins except albumin, which is not a globulin, and fibrinogen, which is not in the serum. The serum globulins are subdivided into $\alpha$-, $\beta$-, and $\gamma$-globulins on the basis of their relative electrophoretic mobilities.
**sex hormone–binding g., sex steroid–binding g.,** a $\beta$-g. in plasma that binds to and transports testosterone, and to a lesser degree estrogens; it is formed in the liver. Called also *testosterone-estradiol–binding g.* and *testosterone-estrogen–binding g.*
**specific immune g.,** a preparation of immune globulin derived from a donor pool preselected for high antibody titer against a specific antigen, such as hepatitis B immune globulin.
**testosterone-estradiol–binding g. (TEBG), testosterone-estrogen–binding g.,** sex hormone–binding g.
**tetanus immune g.** [USP], a specific immune globulin derived from blood of human donors hyperimmunized with tetanus toxoid; used for prophylaxis and treatment of tetanus. Formerly called *tetanus immune human g.*
**thyronine-binding g. (TBG), thyroxine-binding g.,** an acidic glycoprotein that is the main binding protein in the blood for thyroxine (and less firmly, triiodothyronine); it is a serum globulin synthesized by the liver and has electrophoretic mobility intermediate between that of the $\alpha_1$- and $\alpha_2$-globulins.
**vaccinia immune g. (VIG)** [USP], a specific immune globulin derived from blood of human donors immunized with vaccinia virus smallpox vaccine; used for prophylaxis and treatment of vaccinia or smallpox. Formerly called *vaccinia immune human g.*
**varicella-zoster immune g. (VZIG),** a specific immune globulin derived from plasma of human donors with high titers of varicella-zoster antibodies; used for prevention or amelioration of varicella in immunodeficient or immunosuppressed patients exposed to the disease and in neonates whose mothers develop varicella in the perinatal period.

**glob·u·lin·uria** (glob″u-lĭ-nu′re-ə) the presence of globulin in the urine.

**glob·u·lose** (glob′u-lōs) a proteose produced by action of pepsin on the globulins; several varieties have been described.

**glo·bu·lus** (glob′u-ləs) gen. and pl. *glo′buli* [L.] a small spherical mass or body.
**glo′buli os′sei,** intrachondrial bone.

**glo·bus** (glo′bəs) gen. and pl. *glo′bi* [L.] 1. sphere. 2. [TA] a general term denoting a spherical structure. 3. bulbus oculi. 4. see *globi* (def. 2).
**g. of the heel,** that portion of the wall of a horse's hoof where it curves around the heel to form the bar.
**g. hyste′ricus,** the disturbing subjective sensation of a lump in the throat; seen in conversion disorder.
**g. ma′jor epididy′midis,** caput epididymidis.
**g. mi′nor epididy′midis,** cauda epididymidis.
**g. pal′lidus,** the smaller and more medial part of the lentiform nucleus of the brain, separated from the putamen by the lateral medullary lamina. In official anatomic nomenclature, it is divided by the medial medullary lamina into two parts, lateral and medial (see *g. pallidus lateralis* and *g. pallidus medialis*), both of which have extensive connections with the corpus striatum, thalamus, and mesencephalon. Called also *pallidum.* See also *paleostriatum.*
**g. pallidus external segment,** g. pallidus lateralis.
**g. pallidus internal segment,** g. pallidus medialis.
**g. pal′lidus latera′lis** [TA], globus pallidus lateral segment: the larger, lateral part of the globus pallidus, separated from the putamen by the lateral medullary lamina and from the smaller, medial part of the globus pallidus by the medial medullary lamina; called also *pallidum I.* See also *g. pallidus.*
**g. pal′lidus media′lis** [TA], globus pallidus medial segment: the smaller, medial part of the globus pallidus, separated from the larger, lateral part by the medial medullary lamina; called also *pallidum II.* See also *g. pallidus.*

**Gloe·o·trich·ia** (glo″e-o-trik′e-ə) a genus of cyanobacteria that sometimes contaminates water and can cause cyanobacteria poisoning.

**glo·man·gi·o·ma** (glo-man″je-o′mə) [*glomus* + *angioma*] glomus tumor, def. 1.

**glo·mec·to·my** (glo-mek′tə-me) excision of a glomus, especially one containing a glomus tumor.

**glom·era** (glom′ər-ə) [L.] plural of *glomus.*

**glom·er·ate** (glom′ər-āt) [L. *glomeratus* wound into a ball] crowded together into a ball.

**glo·mer·u·lar** (glo-mer′u-lər) pertaining to or of the nature of a glomerulus, especially a renal glomerulus.

**glo·mer·u·li** (glo-mer′u-li) [L.] genitive and plural of *glomerulus.*

**glo·mer·u·li·tis** (glo-mer″u-li′tis) inflammation of the glomeruli of the kidney, with proliferative or necrotizing changes of the endothelial or epithelial cells or thickening of the basement membrane.

**glomerul(o)-** [L. *glomerulus,* q.v.] combining form denoting relationship to the renal glomeruli.

**glo·mer·u·lo·ne·phri·tis** (glo-mer″u-lo-nə-fri′tis) [*glomerulo-* + *nephritis*] [MeSH: Glomerulonephritis] nephritis accompanied by inflammation of the capillary loops in the glomeruli of the kidney. It occurs in acute, subacute, and chronic forms and may be secondary to hemolytic streptococcal infection. Evidence also supports possible immune or autoimmune mechanisms.
**acute g.,** glomerulonephritis characterized by proteinuria, edema, hematuria, renal failure, and hypertension; it may be preceded by tonsillitis or febrile pharyngitis.
**chronic g.,** a slowly progressive glomerulonephritis generally leading to irreversible renal failure; it may be a primary disease, follow acute glomerulonephritis, or be secondary to systemic disease. Symptoms and course vary widely.
**chronic hypocomplementemic g.,** membranoproliferative g.
**crescentic g.,** 1. any glomerulonephritis in which epithelial crescents are present. 2. rapidly progressive g.
**diffuse g.,** a severe form of glomerulonephritis with proliferative changes in more than half the glomeruli, frequently with epithelial crescent formation and necrosis; it is often seen in cases of advanced systemic lupus erythematosus.
**fibrillary g.,** a rare lesion of the kidney characterized by infiltration of the glomeruli with fibrils that are slightly larger than amyloid fibrils and that do not stain with Congo red. Called also *immunotactoid* or *microtubular glomerulopathy.*
**focal g.,** a condition in which only some glomeruli show inflammatory changes, others appearing normal.
**focal embolic g.,** focal glomerulonephritis associated with bacterial endocarditis; see *Löhlein-Baehr lesion,* under *lesion.*
**IgA g.,** see under *nephropathy.*
**immune complex g.,** that due to formation of circulating immune complexes and their deposition in tissue, a type III hypersensitivity reaction, which causes activation of complement and an inflammatory response, leading to activation of leukocytes and damage to the glomerular basement membrane layer.
**lobular g.,** membranoproliferative g.
**lobulonodular g.,** membranoproliferative g.
**lupus g.,** see under *nephritis.*
**malignant g.,** rapidly progressive g.
**membranoproliferative g.,** a chronic glomerulonephritis characterized by mesangial cell proliferation and irregular thickening of the glomerular capillary wall. There are two subtypes: *Type I* is marked by subendothelial electron-dense deposits and classic complement pathway activation, and *Type II* (called also *dense deposit disease*) is marked by heavy electron-dense deposits in the glomerular basement membrane and alternative complement pathway activation involving C3 nephritic factor. Both types occur in older children and

young adults and follow a slowly progressive course with irregular remissions ultimately resulting in renal failure. Called also *chronic hypocomplementemic g., lobular g.,* and *mesangiocapillary g.*
**membranous g.,** a form characterized histologically by proteinaceous deposits on the glomerular capillary basement membrane or by thickening of the membrane. The clinical features are those of chronic glomerulonephritis, occasionally with transient nephrotic syndrome.
**mesangial proliferative g.,** a type of glomerulonephritis seen in patients with the nephrotic syndrome, characterized by diffuse glomerular proliferation of mesangial and endocapillary cells and mesangial matrix; IgM deposits and complement 3 are often found in the mesangium. Called also *IgM nephropathy.*
**mesangiocapillary g.,** membranoproliferative g.
**nodular g.,** membranoproliferative g.
**pauci-immune crescentic g., pauci-immune rapidly progressive g.,** rapidly progressive glomerulonephritis characterized by the presence of epithelial crescents and antineutrophil cytoplasmic antibodies, but few, if any, immune deposits.
**postinfectious g.,** glomerulonephritis following infection, usually by group A streptococci, seen mainly in children, adolescents, and young adults; characteristics include onset 10 days or more after the infection, oliguria, and hematuria, often with edema, hypertension, and circulatory congestion that can be resolved by diuresis. Serious cases sometimes lead to renal failure.
**poststreptococcal g.,** the most common type of postinfectious glomerulonephritis (q.v.), following infection by group A streptococci.
**rapidly progressive g.,** acute glomerulonephritis marked by a rapid progression to end-stage renal failure and, histologically, by profuse epithelial proliferation, often with epithelial crescents; principal signs are anuria, proteinuria, hematuria, and anemia. Called also *crescentic g.*
**segmental g.,** focal glomerulonephritis in which only limited segments of affected glomeruli are diseased.
**subacute g.,** persistence of acute glomerulonephritis, with or without periods of remission, which may develop into the lobular or malignant forms.

**glo·mer·u·lo·ne·phrop·a·thy** (glo-mer″u-lo-nə-frop′ə-the) any noninflammatory disease of the renal glomeruli.

**glo·mer·u·lop·a·thy** (glo-mer″u-lop′ə-the) any disease of the renal glomeruli.
**collapsing g.,** focal glomerular sclerosis with extensive collapse of glomerular capillaries and heavy proteinuria, usually progressing to end stage renal disease within two years.
**diabetic g.,** intercapillary glomerulosclerosis.
**immunotactoid g.,** fibrillary glomerulonephritis.
**microtubular g.,** fibrillary glomerulonephritis.
**minimal change g.,** see under *disease.*

**glo·mer·u·lo·scle·ro·sis** (glo-mer″u-lo-sklə-ro′sis) fibrosis and scarring which result in senescence of the renal glomeruli.
**diabetic g.,** intercapillary g.
**focal g.,** focal glomerular sclerosis.
**focal segmental g.,** focal glomerular sclerosis.
**intercapillary g.,** a degenerative complication of diabetes in which there is glomerular mesangial expansion with either diffuse or nodular lesions; the nodular lesions are known as *Kimmelstiel-Wilson lesions.* Symptoms include albuminuria, nephrotic edema, hypertension, renal insufficiency, and retinopathy. Called also *diabetic g.* The type with nodular lesions is also called *Kimmelstiel-Wilson syndrome.*

**glo·mer·u·lose** (glo-mer′u-lōs) glomerular.

**glo·mer·u·lus** (glo-mer′u-ləs) pl. *glomer′uli* [L., dim. of *glomus* ball] a tuft or cluster; used in anatomic nomenclature as a general term to designate such a structure, as one composed of blood vessels or nerve fibers. Often used alone to designate one of the glomeruli of the kidney (glomeruli renis [TA]).
**glome′ruli arterio′si coch′leae,** an arterial network surrounding the cochlea.
**glomeruli of kidney, malpighian glomeruli,** glomeruli renis.
**nonencapsulated nerve g.,** a type of free nerve ending in the connective tissue of various organs, with the terminal branches of the nerve forming spherical or elongated structures resembling glomeruli.
**olfactory g.,** one of the small globular masses of dense neuropil in the olfactory bulb; it contains the first synapse in the olfactory pathway and the axons of olfactory cells synapse here with dendrites primarily of mitral cells and tufted cells.
**renal glomeruli, glomer′uli re′nis** [TA], glomeruli of kidney: globular tufts of capillaries, one projecting into the expanded end or capsule of each of the uriniferous tubules, which together with its surrounding capsule *(glomerular capsule)* constitute the renal corpuscle. Called also *malpighian glomeruli.* See plate accompanying *kidney.*
**Ruysch's glomeruli,** glomeruli renis.
**synaptic g.,** a glomerulus formed by the coming together of a number of end-feet around a central dendrite, all enclosed by a layer of neuroglial cells; found in the sensory nuclei of the thalamus, in the olfactory bulbs, and in a few other locations in the brain. See also *olfactory g.*

**glo·mic** (glo′mik) pertaining to or affecting a glomus.

**glo·moid** (glo′moid) resembling a glomus.

**glo·mus** (glo′məs) pl. *glom′era* [L. "a ball"] 1. [TA] a small, histologically recognizable body, composed of fine arterioles connecting directly with veins, and possessing a rich nerve supply. 2. anastomosis arteriovenosa glomeriformis.
**glo′mera aor′tica,** corpora paraaortica.
**g. caro′ticum** [TA], carotid glomus: a small neurovascular structure lying in the bifurcation of the right and left carotid arteries, made up of richly innervated epithelioid glomus cells (type I) surrounded by type II cells. It functions as an arterial chemoreceptor (although which component is responsible is uncertain), with stimulation by hypoxia, hypercapnia, or elevated hydrogen ion concentration resulting in an increase in blood pressure, cardiac rate, and respiratory movements. Another function may be as an endocrine gland. Called also *carotid body.*
**g. choroi′deum** [TA], choroid glomus: an enlargement of the choroid plexus of the lateral ventricle where the inferior horn joins the central part. Called also *choroidal enlargement.*
**g. coccy′geum** [TA], coccygeal glomus: an oval structure consisting of irregular masses of spherical or polyhedral epithelioid cells grouped around a dilated, sinusoidal capillary vessel, occurring anterior to, or immediately inferior to, the apex of the coccyx, at the termination of the median sacral vessels. Called also *coccygeal body* or *gland, corpus coccygeum,* and *Luschka's body* or *gland.*
**jugular g., g. jugula′re,** tympanic body.
**g. tympa′nicum,** a tympanic body located adjacent to the middle ear. See also *g. tympanicum tumor,* under *tumor.*
**g. vaga′le,** a glomus along the vagus nerve. See also *glomus vagale tumor,* under *tumor.*

**glos·sa** (glos′ə) [Gr. *glōssa*] the tongue (lingua [TA]).

**glos·sa·gra** (glos-ag′rə) [*gloss-* + *-agra*] gouty pain of the tongue.

**glos·sal** (glos′əl) lingual.

**glos·sal·gia** (glos-al′jə) [*gloss-* + *-algia*] [MeSH: Glossalgia] pain in the tongue; called also *glossodynia.*

**glos·san·thrax** (glos-an′thraks) [*gloss-* + *anthrax*] carbuncle of the tongue.

**glos·sec·to·my** (glos-ek′tə-me) [*gloss-* + *-ectomy*] [MeSH: Glossectomy] partial or total surgical excision of the tongue.

**Glos·si·na** (glŏ-si′nə) the tsetse flies, a genus of biting flies of the family Muscidae. It is divided into three subgenera, *Nemorhina (palpalis* or riverine group), *Glossina (morsitans* or savannah group), and *Austenina (fusca* or forest group). The groups transmit by their bite trypanosomes pathogenic to humans and animals. The *palpalis* group transmits mainly *Trypanosoma brucei gambiense,* causing Gambian trypanosomiasis; the *morsitans* group transmits mainly *T. brucei rhodesiense,* causing Rhodesian trypanosomiasis; and the *fusca* group transmits trypanosomes pathogenic to livestock.
**G. fus′cipes,** a species in the *palpalis* group; its subspecies transmit Gambian trypanosomiasis in West and Central Africa, as well as Rhodesian trypanosomiasis in East Africa.
**G. mor′sitans,** a South African species that transmits *Trypanosoma brucei,* the cause of nagana in horses, and *T. rhodesiense,* the cause of Rhodesian trypanosomiasis.

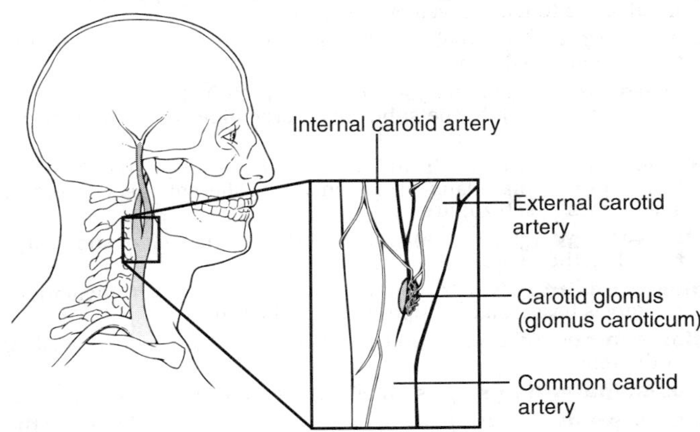

Glomus caroticum (carotid glomus), located deep to the carotid bifurcation and innervated by a plexus of glossopharyngeal, vagal, and sympathetic components.

**G. palli'dipes,** a species that transmits *Trypanosoma brucei.*
**G. palpa'lis,** a Central African species that transmits *Trypanosoma gambiense,* causing African trypanosomiasis.
**G. swynnerto'ni,** a species in the *morsitans* group; it transmits Rhodesian trypanosomiasis.
**G. tachinoi'des,** a species in the *palpalis* group; it transmits Gambian trypanosomiasis in West Africa and Rhodesian trypanosomiasis in Ethiopia.

**glos·si·tis** (glos-i'tis) [*gloss-* + *-itis*] [MeSH: Glossitis] inflammation of the tongue.
**g. area'ta exfoliati'va,** benign migratory g.
**atrophic g.,** Hunter's g.
**benign migratory g.,** a type with unknown etiology, characterized by annular areas of desquamation of the filiform papillae on the dorsal surface of the tongue, usually presenting pinkish-red central lesions outlined by thin, yellowish lines or bands that change patterns and shift location every few days. Called also *g. areata exfoliativa, g. migrans, erythema migrans, geographic tongue,* and *pityriasis linguae.*
**herpetic geometric g.,** painful longitudinal, crossed, or branched fissures on the dorsum of the tongue, occurring as a manifestation of herpes simplex virus type 1 infection in immunocompromised patients.
**Hunter's g.,** a chronic condition of the tongue seen in pernicious anemia, characterized by glossitis, glossodynia, glossopyrosis, and altered sense of taste; the pain and burning sensation are usually confined to the tongue but may also extend to other parts of the oral mucosa. Ultimately, the tongue becomes atrophic and assumes a beefy red color and a smooth shiny appearance, sometimes with small ulcers spreading over its surface. Called also *atrophic g.*
**idiopathic g.,** inflammation of the substance of the tongue and its mucous membrane.
**median rhomboid g.,** a congenital disorder of noninflammatory origin, characterized by a somewhat rhomboid reddish, smooth, and shiny lesion with some opalescent spots, occurring at about the middle third of the dorsal surface of the tongue, immediately anterior to the circumvallate papillae.
**g. mi'grans,** benign migratory g.
**Moeller's g.,** a chronic condition of the tongue characterized by superficial excoriation, principally of the tip and edges. The lesions are beefy red, well-defined, irregular patches, in which the filiform papillae are thinned or absent and the fungiform papillae are swollen. Called also *bald tongue* and *glossodynia exfoliativa.*
**g. rhomboi'dea media'na,** median rhomboid g.

**gloss(o)-** [Gr. *glōssa* tongue] a combining form denoting relationship to the tongue.

**glos·so·cele** (glos'o-sēl) [*glosso-* + *-cele*] swelling and protrusion of the tongue.

**glos·so·cin·es·thet·ic** (glos″o-sin-əs-thet'ik) glossokinesthetic.

**glos·soc·o·ma** (glos-ok'o-mə) retraction of the tongue.

**glos·so·dy·na·mom·e·ter** (glos″o-di″nə-mom'ə-tər) [*glosso-* + *dynamometer*] an instrument for recording the power of the tongue to resist pressure.

**glos·so·dyn·ia** (glos″o-din'e-ə) [*glosso-* + *-odynia*] glossalgia.
**g. exfoliati'va,** Moeller's glossitis.
**psychogenic g.,** glossopyrosis.

**glos·so·epi·glot·tic** (glos″o-ep-ĭ-glot'ik) glossoepiglottidean.

**glos·so·epi·glot·tid·e·an** (glos″o-ep-ĭ-glo-tid'e-ən) pertaining to the tongue and epiglottis.

**glos·so·graph** (glos'o-graf) [*glosso-* + *-graph*] an apparatus for recording the tongue movements in speech.

**glos·so·hy·al** (glos″o-hi'əl) [*glosso-* + *hyoid*] pertaining to the tongue and hyoid bone.

**glos·so·kin·es·thet·ic** (glos″o-kin″əs-thet'ik) [*glosso-* + *kinesthetic*] pertaining to the subjective perception of the movements of the tongue in speech.

**glos·so·la·lia** (glos″o-la'le-ə) [*glosso-* + *lal-* + *-ia*] speech in unknown or imaginary language, simulating coherent speech, seen in some types of schizophrenia.

**glos·sol·o·gy** (glos-ol'ə-je) [*glosso-* + *-logy*] the sum of knowledge regarding the tongue.

**glos·so·man·tia** (glos″o-man-ti'ə) [*glosso-* + Gr. *manteia* divination] prognosis based on the appearance of the tongue.

**glos·son·cus** (glos-ong'kəs) [*glosso-* + Gr. *onkos* mass] a swelling of the tongue.

**glos·so·pal·a·ti·nus** (glos″o-pal″ə-ti'nəs) musculus palatoglossus.

**glos·sop·a·thy** (glos-op'ə-the) [*glosso-* + *-pathy*] any disease of the tongue.

**glos·so·pexy** (glos″o-pek'se) lip-tongue adhesion.

**glos·so·pha·ryn·ge·al** (glos″o-fə-rin'je-əl) [*glosso-* + *pharynx*] pertaining to the tongue and pharynx.

**glos·so·pha·ryn·ge·um** (glos″o-fə-rin'je-əm) [*glosso-* + *pharynx*] the tongue and pharynx together.

**glos·so·pha·ryn·ge·us** (glos″o-fə-rin'je-əs) [L.] 1. pertaining to the tongue and pharynx. 2. musculus glossopharyngeus; see *pars glossopharyngea musculi constrictoris pharyngis superioris.*

**glos·so·pho·bia** (glos″o-fo'be-ə) [*glosso-* + *-phobia*] lalophobia.

**glos·so·phyt·ia** (glos″o-fit'e-ə) [*glosso-* + *phyt-* + *-ia*] black tongue.

**glos·so·plas·ty** (glos'o-plas″te) [*glosso-* + *-plasty*] plastic surgery of the tongue.

**glos·sop·to·sis** (glos″op-to'sis) [*glosso-* + *-ptosis*] downward displacement or retraction of the tongue.

**glos·so·py·ro·sis** (glos″o-pi-ro'sis) [*glosso-* + Gr. *pyrōsis* burning] a form of paresthesia characterized by pain, burning, itching, and stinging of the mucous membranes of the tongue without apparent lesions of the affected areas. Called also *burning tongue.*

**glos·sor·rha·phy** (glos-or'ə-fe) [*glosso-* + *-rrhaphy*] suture of the tongue.

**glos·sos·co·py** (glos-os'kə-pe) [*glosso-* + *-scopy*] examination of the tongue.

**glos·so·spasm** (glos'o-spaz-əm) [*glosso-* + *spasm*] spasm of the tongue muscles.

**glos·so·ster·e·sis** (glos″o-stə-re'sis) glossectomy.

**glos·sot·o·my** (glos-ot'ə-me) [*glosso-* + *-tomy*] incision of the tongue.

**glos·so·trich·ia** (glos″o-trik'e-ə) [*glosso-* + *trich-* + *-ia*] hairy tongue.

**glot·tal** (glot'əl) pertaining to the glottis.

**glot·tic** (glot'ik) glottal.

**glot·ti·des** (glot'ĭ-dēz) [Gr.] plural of *glottis.*

**glot·tis** (glot'is) pl. *glot'tides* [Gr. *glōttis*] [TA] [MeSH: Glottis] the vocal apparatus of the larynx, consisting of the true vocal cords (plica vocalis) and the opening between them (rima glottidis).
**false g.,** rima vestibuli.
**intercartilaginous g., g. respiratorius, respiratory g.,** pars intercartilaginea rimae glottidis.
**true g.,** rima glottidis.
**g. voca'lis,** pars intermembranacea rimae glottidis.

**glot·tog·ra·phy** (glŏ-tog'rə-fe) the recording of the movements of the vocal cords during respiration and phonation, usually measured as electrical potentials generated with movement.

**glot·tol·o·gy** (glot-ol'ə-je) glossology.

**glox·a·zone** (glok'sə-zōn) an anaplasmodastat used in cattle.

**Glu** glutamic acid.

**glu·ca·gon** (gloo'kə-gon) [MeSH: Glucagon] 1. a polypeptide hormone secreted by the alpha cells of the islets of Langerhans in response to hypoglycemia, acetylcholine, some amino acids, and growth hormone; it stimulates glycogenolysis in the liver by activating liver phosphorylase and promotes gluconeogenesis and ketogenesis and stimulates the release of insulin by the pancreatic islets. Called also *hyperglycemic-glycogenolytic factor.* 2. [USP] a preparation of this hormone obtained from the organs of slaughtered food animals; administered by injection.
**gut g.,** enteroglucagon.

**glu·ca·gon·o·ma** (gloo″kə-gon-o'mə) [MeSH: Glucagonoma] a type of islet cell tumor of the alpha cells that secretes glucagon; some are malignant. See also *glucagonoma syndrome,* under *syndrome.*

**glu·cal** (gloo'kal) a glycal of glucose.

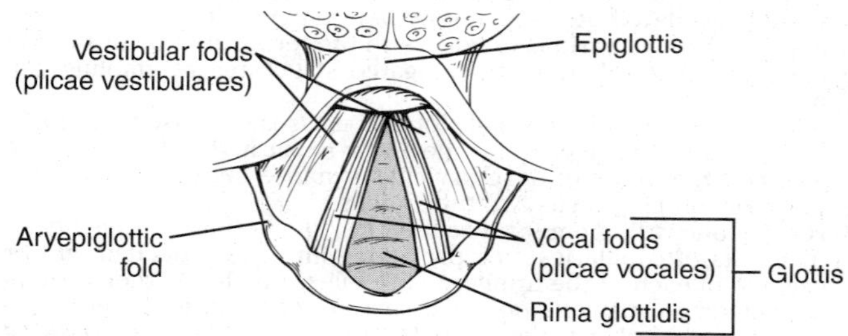


Glottis, comprising the vocal folds (cords) and rima glottidis, seen in a laryngoscopic view of the larynx. The trachea is visible through the rima glottidis.

**glu·can** (gloo'kan) any polysaccharide (e.g., glycogen, starch, and cellulose) composed only of recurring units of glucose; a homopolymer of glucose.

**1,4-α-glu·can branch·ing en·zyme** (gloo'kan branch'ing en'zīm) [EC 2.4.1.18] an enzyme of the transferase class that catalyzes the cleavage of internal α-1,4-glucoside linkages in glycogen (or, in plants, amylopectin) and transfer of the fragments into α-1,6 linkages, thus creating branches in the glycogen molecule. Deficiency of the enzyme, an autosomal recessive trait, results in glycogen storage disease, type IV. Called also *brancher* or *branching enzyme.*

**glu·can 1,4-α-glu·co·si·dase** (gloo'kan gloo-ko'sĭ-dās) [EC 3.2.1.3] a lysosomal enzyme of the hydrolase class that catalyzes the cleavage of glucose residues from polyglucoside chains by hydrolyzing terminal α-1,4 or α-1,6 bonds; the enzyme degrades glycogen to glucose in the lysosomes. Deficiency or absence of enzyme activity, an autosomal recessive trait, results in glycogen storage disease, type II. Called also *acid maltase* and *lysosomal α-glucosidase.*

**glu·can trans·fer·ase** (gloo'kan trans'fər-ās) an enzyme transferring glucosyl chains in glucans from one site to another, usually with specific conformations of donor and acceptor sites; see *oligo-1,4,-1,4-glucantransferase* and *1,4-α-glucan branching enzyme.*

**glu·car·ic ac·id** (gloo-kar'ik) [MeSH: Glucaric Acid] the aldaric acid resulting from oxidation of glucose.

**glu·cep·tate** (gloo-sep'tāt) USAN contraction for *glucoheptonate.* See also table at *technetium.*

**glu·ci·phore** (gloo'sĭ-for) glucophore.

**glu·ci·tol** (gloo'sĭ-tol) sorbitol.

**gluc(o)-** [Gr. *glykys* sweet] a combining form denoting relationship to sweetness, or to glucose. Cf. *glyc(o)-.*

**glu·co·am·y·lase** (gloo"ko-am'ə-lās) glucan 1,4-α-glucosidase.

**glu·co·ascor·bic ac·id** (gloo"ko-ə-skor'bik) a seven-carbon homologue of ascorbic acid having no vitamin C activity.

**glu·co·cer·e·bro·si·dase** (gloo"ko-ser"ə-bro-si'dās) glucosylceramidase.

**glu·co·cer·e·bro·side** (gloo"ko-ser'ə-bro-sīd") any of the cerebrosides in which the monosaccharide head group is glucose; they occur mostly in nonneuronal tissue and accumulate abnormally in Gaucher's disease. Called also *glucosylceramide.*

**glu·co·cin·in** (gloo"ko-sin'in) glucokinin.

**glu·co·cor·ti·coid** (gloo"ko-kor'tĭ-koid) 1. any of the corticosteroids (steroids produced by the adrenal cortex) that regulate carbohydrate, lipid, and protein metabolism and inhibit the release of adrenocorticotropic hormone. They also affect muscle tone and the microcirculation, participate in the maintenance of arterial blood pressure, increase gastric secretion, alter connective tissue response to injury, impede cartilage production, inhibit inflammatory, allergic, and immunologic responses, invoke shrinkage of lymphatic tissue, reduce the number of circulating lymphocytes, and affect the functions of the central nervous system. Some exert varying degrees of mineralocorticoid activity. In humans the most important ones are cortisol, cortisone, and corticosterone. Cf. *mineralocorticoid.* 2. of, pertaining to, having the properties or effects of, or resembling one of these substances.

**Glu·co-Fer·rum** (gloo"ko-fer'əm) trademark for preparations of ferrous gluconate.

**glu·co·fu·ra·nose** (gloo"ko-fu'rə-nōs) glucose occurring in the cyclic furanose configuration; it is a minor constituent of glucose solutions.

**glu·co·gen·e·sis** (gloo"ko-jen'ə-sis) [*gluco-* + *-genesis*] the formation of glucose from any of the products of glycolysis.

**glu·co·gen·ic** (gloo"ko-jen'ik) [*gluco-* + *-genic*] giving rise to or producing glucose.

**glu·co·he·mia** (gloo"ko-he'me-ə) glycemia.

**glu·co·hep·to·nate** (gloo"ko-hep'tə-nāt) GHA; a seven-carbon carbohydrate derivative; complexed with technetium 99m it is used in renal and brain imaging and in dynamic renal and cerebral perfusion studies. See table at *technetium.* Called also *gluceptate* (USAN contraction).

**glu·co·ki·nase** (gloo"ko-ki'nās) [MeSH: Glucokinase] 1. [EC 2.7.1.2] an enzyme of the transferase class that catalyzes the phosphorylation of D-glucose at the 6 carbon. The enzyme is found in invertebrates and microorganisms and is highly specific for glucose. 2. hexokinase, type IV (liver).

**glu·co·ki·net·ic** (gloo"ko-kĭ-net'ik) activating sugar so as to maintain the sugar level of the blood.

**glu·co·kin·in** (gloo"ko-kin'in) [*gluco-* + Gr. *kinein* to move] a hormonelike substance obtained from vegetable tissues and yeast, subcutaneous injection of which produces hypoglycemia in animals and acts on depancreatized dogs in a manner similar to insulin.

**glu·col·y·sis** (gloo-kol'ə-sis) glycolysis.

**glu·co·nate** (gloo'ko-nāt) a salt, ester, or anionic form of gluconic acid.

**glu·co·neo·gen·e·sis** (gloo"ko-ne"o-jen'ə-sis) [*gluco-* + *neo-* + *-genesis*] [MeSH: Gluconeogenesis] the formation of glucose from molecules that are not themselves carbohydrates, as from amino acids, lactate, and the glycerol portion of fats. Called also *glyconeogenesis.*

**glu·co·neo·ge·net·ic** (gloo"ko-ne"o-jə-net'ik) pertaining to or involved in gluconeogenesis.

**glu·con·ic ac·id** (gloo-kon'ik) the hexonic acid derived from glucose by oxidation of the aldehyde group at C-1 to a carboxyl group.

**Glu·co·no·bac·ter** (gloo"ko-no-bak'tər) [*gluconic acid* + Gr. *baktron* a rod] a genus of gram-negative, aerobic, rod-shaped bacteria of the family Acetobacteraceae. The organisms produce acetic acid from ethanol, and are found in soil, plants, fruits, and vegetables. The type species is *G. ox'ydans.*

**glu·co·no·lac·tone** (gloo"ko-no-lak'tōn) [USP] glucono delta-lactone; a chelating agent produced by the oxidation of glucose.

**glu·co·pe·nia** (gloo-ko-pe'ne-ə) glycopenia.

**Glu·co·phage** (gloo'ko-fāj") trademark for a preparation of metformin.

**glu·co·phore** (gloo'ko-for) [*gluco-* + *phore*] the group of atoms in a molecule of a compound that is responsible for its sweet taste.

**glu·co·pro·tein** (gloo"ko-pro'tēn) glycoprotein.

**glu·co·py·ra·nose** (gloo"ko-pir'ə-nōs) glucose occurring in the cyclic pyranose configuration; it is the major form in glucose solutions, polysaccharides, and glucosides.

**glu·co·reg·u·la·tion** (gloo"ko-reg"u-la'shən) regulation of glucose metabolism.

**glu·co·sa·mine** (gloo-ko'sə-mēn) [MeSH: Glucosamine] the amino sugar derivative of glucose, substituted at the 2 position, occurring in glycosaminoglycans and a variety of complex polysaccharides such as blood group substances. It is generally acetylated (*N*-acetylglucosamine).

**glu·co·sa·mine-phos·phate *N*-ac·e·tyl·trans·fer·ase** (gloo-ko'sə-mēn fos'fāt as"ə-tēl-trans'fər-ās) [EC 2.3.1.4] an enzyme of the transferase class that catalyzes the transfer of an acetyl group from acetyl coenzyme A to glucosamine 6-phosphate to form *N*-acetylglucosamine 6-phosphate, a step in the synthesis of UDP-*N*-acetylglucosamine.

**glu·co·san** (gloo'ko-san) glucan.

**glu·co·sa·zone** (gloo-ko'sə-zōn) the osazone formed from glucose by reaction with phenylhydrazine; it is a yellow crystalline substance that has been used to identify glucose. It is chemically identical to fructosazone and mannosazone.

**Glu·co·scan** (gloo'ko-skandprime;) trademark for a kit for the preparation of technetium Tc 99m gluceptate.

**glu·cose** (gloo'kōs) [Gr. *gleukos* sweetness] [MeSH: Glucose] 1. an aldohexose monosaccharide occurring naturally as the D-form in fruits and other plants and in the normal blood of all animals; it also is combined in glucosides and di-, oligo-, and polysaccharides. It is the end product of carbohydrate metabolism and is the chief source of energy for living organisms, its utilization being controlled by insulin. Excess glucose is converted to glycogen and stored in the liver and muscles for use as needed and, beyond that, is converted to fat and stored as adipose tissue. See also *hyperglycemia* and *hypoglycemia.* Called also *dextrose* and *blood sugar.* 2. liquid g.

**Brun's g.,** a histologic clearing solution composed of glucose, distilled water, camphor, and glycerin.

**fasting plasma g. (FPG),** a measurement of the concentration of glucose in the plasma after the patient has not eaten for at least 8 hours.

**liquid g.** [NF], an odorless, colorless or yellowish, thick syrupy liquid with a sweet taste, obtained by the incomplete hydrolysis of starch and consisting chiefly of dextrose, with dextrins, maltose, and water; used as a flavoring agent, tablet binder, and coating agent in pharmaceutical preparations. It may be used as a food, often administered rectally, and has been used in the treatment of dehydration. Sometimes simply called *glucose.*

**g. 1-phosphate,** an intermediate in carbohydrate metabolism. See also *Embden-Meyerhof pathway,* under *pathway.* Called also *Cori ester.*

**g. 6-phosphate,** an intermediate in carbohydrate metabolism. See also *Embden-Meyerhof pathway* and *pentose phosphate pathway,* under *pathway.* Called also *Robison ester.*

**glu·cose ox·i·dase** (gloo'kōs ok'sĭ-dās) [EC 1.1.3.4] [MeSH: Glucose Oxidase] an enzyme of the oxidoreductase class that catalyzes the oxidation of glucose, reducing oxygen to hydrogen peroxide. It is a flavoprotein, containing FAD, and is highly specific for β-D-glucose. The enzyme is produced by *Penicillium notatum* and other fungi and has antibacterial activity in the presence of glucose and oxygen because of the hydrogen peroxide produced. It is used to estimate glucose concentration in blood or urine samples through the formation of colored dyes by the hydrogen peroxide.

**glu·cose-6-phos·pha·tase** (gloo"kōs fos'fə-tās") [EC 3.1.3.9] [MeSH: Glucose-6-Phosphatase] an enzyme of the hydrolase class that catalyzes the dephosphorylation of glucose 6-phosphate. It occurs in the endoplasmic reticulum of liver, kidney, and intestinal mucosa, but not of muscle, and its reaction is the principal route for hepatic gluconeogenesis, controlling blood glucose concentrations. Deficiency of the enzyme, an autosomal recessive trait, results in glycogen storage disease, type I.

**glu·cose-6-phos·phate de·hy·dro·gen·ase (G6PD)** (gloo'kōs fos'fāt de-hi'dro-jən-ās) an enzyme of the oxidoreductase class that catalyzes the oxidation of glucose-6-phosphate to a lactone, reducing $NADP^+$ to NADPH. The reaction is the first step in the pentose phosphate pathway of glucose metabolism. Genetic deficiency of the enzyme causes severe hemolytic crises in affected individuals. In EC nomenclature, called *glucose-6-phosphate 1-dehydrogenase.*

**glu·cose-6-phos·phate de·hy·dro·gen·ase de·fi·cien·cy** the most common inborn error of metabolism, causing varying degrees of hemolytic anemia in many millions of people around the world. It can cause favism, some drug-induced hemolytic anemias, or chronic nonspherocytic hemolytic anemia. The G6PD gene is highly polymorphic, with over 300 variants known.

**glu·cose-6-phos·phate isom·er·ase** (gloo'kos fos'fāt i-som'ər-ās) [EC 5.3.1.9] an enzyme of the isomerase class that catalyzes the interconversion glucose 6-phosphate = fructose 6-phosphate. The forward reaction is a step in the Embden-Meyerhof pathway (see illustration at *pathway*), and the reverse is a step in gluconeogenesis. Deficiency of the enzyme, an autosomal recessive trait, results in hemolytic anemia.

**glu·cose 6-phos·phate trans·lo·case** (gloo'kōs fos'fāt trans-lo'kās) a transport system occurring in the endoplasmic reticulum of liver, kidney, and intestinal mucosa cells; it transports glucose 6-phosphate into the endoplasmic reticulum, where glucose-6-phosphatase is located. Deficiency of this system results in glycogen storage disease, type IB.

**α-glu·co·si·dase** (gloo-kō'sĭ-dās) [EC 3.2.1.20] any of a group of enzymes that catalyze the hydrolysis of terminal, nonreducing 1,4-linked α-D-glucose residues, primarily in oligosaccharides but also in polysaccharides, with release of α-D-glucose. Called also *maltase.*

**lysosomal α-g.,** glucan 1,4-α-glucosidase.

**α-1,4-glu·co·si·dase** (gloo-ko'sĭ-dās) 1. glucan 1,4-α-glucosidase. 2. the term can also mean any enzyme able to cleave α-1,4-glucosidic linkages (e.g., α-glucosidase).

**α-1,4-glu·co·si·dase deficiency** glycogen storage disease, type II.

**β-glu·co·si·dase** (gloo-ko'sĭ-dās) [EC 3.2.1.21] any of a group of enzymes of the hydrolase class that catalyze the hydrolysis of terminal, nonreducing, β-linked glucose residues from glycosides.

**glu·co·side** (gloo'ko-sīd) a glycoside in which the sugar constituent is glucose; originally the term glucoside was given to any of a variety of natural plant products containing a sugar, but it is now generally restricted to those in which the sugar is glucose. See *glycoside.*

**glu·co·si·do·lyt·ic** (gloo"ko-si"do-lit'ik) causing the splitting up of glucosides.

**glu·co·sul·fone so·di·um** (gloo"ko-sul'fōn) an antibacterial derivative of dapsone, having actions similar to those of the parent compound; used primarily as a leprostatic in the treatment of lepromatous and tuberculoid leprosy, administered intravenously.

**glu·cos·u·ria** (gloo"ko-su're-ə) glycosuria.

**glu·co·syl** (gloo'ko-səl) a glucose radical.

**glu·co·syl·cer·am·i·dase** (gloo"ko-səl-sər-am'ĭ-dās) [EC 3.2.1.45] [MeSH: Glucosylceramidase] an enzyme of the hydrolase class that catalyzes the hydrolytic cleavage of glucose from glucocerebrosides to form ceramides, a reaction occurring in the lysosomal degradation of sphingolipids. Deficiency of enzyme activity, an autosomal recessive trait, results in Gaucher disease. Called also *glucocerebrosidase.*

**glu·co·syl·cer·a·mide** (gloo-kos"əl-ser'ə-mīd) glucocerebroside.

**glu·co·syl·trans·fer·ase** (gloo"ko-səl-trans'fər-as) a term used in the trivial and recommended names of some hexosyltransferases [EC 2.4.1] that catalyze the transfer of a glucosyl group from a donor to an acceptor compound. Called also *transglucosylase.*

**Glu·co·trol** (gloo'ko-trōl") trademark for a preparation of glipizide.

**glu·cu·ro·nate** (gloo-ku'ro-nāt) a salt, ester, or anionic form of glucuronic acid.

**glu·cu·ron·ic ac·id** (gloo"ku-ron'ik) the uronic acid derived from glucose; it is a constituent of several glycosaminoglycans and also forms conjugates (glucuronides) with drugs and toxins in their biotransformation.

**β-glu·cu·ron·i·dase** (gloo"ku-ron'ĭ-dās) [EC 3.2.1.31] a lysosomal enzyme of the hydrolase class that catalyzes the cleavage of terminal glucuronic acid residues from a variety of β-glucuronides. It is important for the degradation of a variety of glycosaminoglycans, including dermatan sulfate, heparan sulfate, and the chondroitin sulfates. Deficiency of the enzyme, an autosomal recessive trait, results in Sly's syndrome (mucopolysaccharidosis VII).

**glu·cu·ron·ide** (gloo"ku-ron'īd) a glycoside of glucuronic acid; glucuronides are common soluble conjugates formed as a step in the metabolism and excretion of many toxins and drugs, such as phenols and alcohols.

**glu·cu·ron·o·syl·trans·fer·ase** (gloo"ku-ron"o-səl-trans'fər-ās) [EC 2.4.1.17] [MeSH: Glucuronosyltransferase] an enzyme of the transferase class that catalyzes the transfer of a glucuronate moiety from UDPglucuronate to an acceptor to form a glucuronide conjugate. The reaction occurs with a wide range of substrates and is important in the conversion of bilirubin to its more soluble glucuronide conjugates, which are then secreted into the bile. Deficiency of the enzyme, an autosomal recessive trait, results in Crigler-Najjar syndrome.

**glu·cu·ron·yl trans·fer·ase** (gloo"ku'ron-əl trans'fər-ās) a less accurate term for *glucuronosyltransferase.*

**glue** (gloo) [MeSH: Adhesives] an adhesive preparation in the form of impure gelatin derived from boiling certain animal substances, such as hoofs, in water.

**Gluge's corpuscles** (gloo'gəz) [Gottlieb *Gluge,* German pathologist, 1813–1899] see under *corpuscle.*

**Glu·gea** (gloo'je-ə) a genus of intracellular protozoa (suborder Apansporoblastina, order Microsporida) parasitic in fishes.

**glu·ta·mate** (gloo'tə-māt) a salt, ester, or anionic form of glutamic acid.

**g.-γ-semialdehyde,** glutamic-γ-semialdehyde.

**glu·ta·mate-am·mo·nia li·gase** (gloo'tə-māt ə-mōn'yə li'gās) [EC 6.3.1.2] [MeSH: Glutamate-Ammonia Ligase] an enzyme of the ligase class that catalyzes the ATP-dependent amination of glutamate by ammonium ions to form glutamine. Called also *glutamine synthetase.*

**glu·ta·mate-cys·te·ine li·gase** (gloo'tə-māt sis'te-ēn li'gās) [EC 6.3.2.2] an enzyme of the ligase class that catalyzes the ATP-dependent formation of a peptide bond between the γ-carboxyl group of glutamate and the amino group of cysteine to form γ-glutamylcysteine as a step in the synthesis of glutathione.

**glu·ta·mate de·car·box·y·lase** (gloo'tə-māt de-kahr-bok'sə-lās) [EC 4.1.1.15] [MeSH: Glutamate Decarboxylase] an enzyme of the lyase class that catalyzes the decarboxylation of glutamate to form γ-aminobutyrate (GABA). The enzyme is a pyridoxal phosphate protein, and the reaction occurs within the mitochondria in kidney, and outside the mitochondria in brain. Deficiency of the brain enzyme may be the cause of convulsions that begin in infancy and are responsive to pyridoxine therapy.

**glu·ta·mate de·hy·dro·gen·ase (NAD(P)⁺)** (gloo'tə-māt de-hi'dro-jən-ās) [EC 1.4.1.3] an enzyme of the oxidoreductase class that catalyzes the oxidative deamination of glutamate to form α-ketoglutarate, using either $NAD^+$ or $NADP^+$as an electron acceptor. The reversible reaction has a major function in both the synthesis and degradation of glutamic acid and, via transaminases, other amino acids as well.

**glu·ta·mate for·mim·i·no·trans·fer·ase** (gloo'tə-māt for-mim"ĭ-no-trans'fər-ās) [EC 2.1.2.5] an enzyme of the transferase class that catalyzes the transfer of a formimino group from formiminoglutamate to tetrahydrofolate, forming 5-formiminotetrahydrofolate. The reaction is a step in the degradation of histidine. The enzyme is bifunctional; it also contains a catalytic site with formiminotetrahydrofolate cyclodeaminase (q.v.) activity. Urinary excretion of formiminoglutamate and mental retardation have been associated with decreased enzyme activity, resulting from either a genetic disorder or a deficiency of tetrahydrofolate. Called also *formiminotransferase.*

**glu·tam·ic ac·id** (gloo-tam'ik) [MeSH: Glutamic Acid] a nonessential amino acid, α-aminoglutaric acid, occurring in proteins. It also serves as an excitatory neurotransmitter in all regions of the central nervous system. Symbols Glu and E. See also table at *amino acid.*

**g. a. hydrochloride,** a compound used as a gastric acidifier in replacement therapy for achlorhydria and hypochlorhydria.

**glu·tam·ic-ox·a·lo·ace·tic trans·am·i·nase (GOT)** (gloo-tam′ik oks″ə-lo-ə-se′tik trans-am′ĭ-nās) aspartate transaminase.

**glu·tam·ic-py·ru·vic trans·am·i·nase (GPT)** (gloo-tam′ik pi-roo′vik trans-am′ĭ-nās) alanine transaminase.

**glu·tam·i·nase** (gloo-tam′ĭ-nās) [MeSH: Glutaminase] [EC 3.5.1.2] an enzyme of the hydrolase class that catalyzes the deamination of glutamine to form glutamate and ammonium ions; most of the latter are converted to urea via the urea cycle.

**glu·ta·mine** (gloo′tə-mēn) [MeSH: Glutamine] the monoamide of glutamic acid, a nonessential amino acid occurring in the juices of many plants and in some animal tissues; it is an important carrier of urinary ammonia and is broken down in the kidney by the enzyme glutaminase. Symbols Gln and Q. See also table at *amino acid.*

**glu·ta·mine syn·the·tase** (gloo′tə-mēn sin′thə-tās) glutamate–ammonia ligase.

**glu·tam·i·nyl** (gloo-tam′ĭ-nəl) the acyl radical of glutamine.

**glu·ta·myl** (gloo′tə-məl) the acyl radical of glutamic acid.

**γ-glu·ta·myl·cy·clo·trans·fer·ase** (gloo″tə-məl-si″klo-trans′fər-ās) [EC 2.3.2.4] an enzyme of the transferase class that catalyzes the hydrolytic cyclization of glutamyl–amino acid to form 5-oxoproline and a free amino acid. The reaction is part of the γ-glutamyl cycle for transporting amino acids across the plasma membrane.

**γ-glu·ta·myl·cys·te·ine** (gloo″tə-məl-sis′te-ēn) glutamate linked via its γ-carboxyl group to the amino group of cysteine; it is an intermediate in the synthesis of glutathione.

**γ-glu·ta·myl·cys·te·ine syn·the·tase** (gloo″tə-məl-sis′te-ēn sin′thə-tās) glutamate–cysteine ligase.

**γ-glu·ta·myl·cys·te·ine syn·the·tase de·fi·cien·cy** a genetic aminoacidopathy of glutathione synthesis due to deficiency of glutamate–cysteine ligase and consisting of hemolytic anemia, spinocerebellar degeneration, peripheral neuropathy, myopathy, and aminoaciduria.

**γ-glu·ta·myl·trans·fer·ase (GGT)** (gloo″tə-məl-trans′fər-ās) an enzyme of the transferase class that catalyzes the transfer of the γ-glutamyl group from glutathione to an amino acid to form a glutamyl–amino acid and the dipeptide cysteinyl-glycine. The enzyme occurs on the outside of the plasma membrane, primarily in cells of the kidney and other sites involved in transport; the glutamyl–amino acids formed can cross the membrane and enter the cell as part of the glutamyl cycle. Deficiency of the enzyme, an autosomal recessive trait, results in γ-glutamyl transpeptidase deficiency.

**γ-glu·ta·myl trans·pep·ti·dase** (gloo′tə-məl trans-pep′tĭ-dās) γ-glutamyltransferase.

**γ-glu·ta·myl trans·pep·ti·dase de·fi·cien·cy** an autosomal recessive aminoacidopathy of glutathione synthesis, marked by mental retardation, behavioral disorders, glutathionemia, and urinary excretion of glutathione, γ-glutamylcysteine, and cysteine. Called also *glutathionuria.*

**glu·ta·ral** (gloo′tə-rəl) [MeSH: Glutaral] glutaraldehyde.
**g. concentrate** [USP], a solution of glutaraldehyde in purified water, used as a disinfectant.

**glu·ta·ral·de·hyde** (gloo″tə-ral′də-hīd) a disinfectant, $C_5H_8O_2$, effective against vegetative gram-positive, gram-negative, and acid-fast bacteria, bacterial spores, some fungi, and viruses; used in an aqueous solution for sterilization of endoscopic equipment, thermometers, and plastic, rubber, or other non–heat-resistant equipment. It is also used topically as an anhidrotic and may be used in the treatment of warts. Glutaraldehyde is also used as a tissue fixative for light and electron microscopy because of its preservation of fine structural detail and localization of enzyme activity. Called also *glutaral.*

**glu·tar·gin** (gloo′tər-jin) arginine glutamate.

**glu·tar·ic ac·id** (gloo-tar′ik) a dicarboxylic acid occurring at high levels in the blood and urine in glutaricaciduria.

**glu·tar·ic·ac·i·de·mia** (gloo-tar″ik-as″ĭ-de′me-ə) 1. glutaricaciduria, def. 1. 2. an excess of glutaric acid in the blood.

**glu·tar·ic·ac·id·uria** (gloo-tar″ik-as″ĭ-du′re-ə) 1. an autosomal recessive aminoacidopathy characterized by accumulation and excretion of glutaric acid and occurring in two types: *Type I* is due to deficiency of glutaryl-CoA dehydrogenase and is characterized by excretion also of 3-hydroxyglutaric acid, progressive dystonia and dyskinesia, hypoglycemia, mild ketosis and acidosis, opisthotonus, choreoathetosis, motor delay, mental retardation, hypotonia, and death within the first decade. *Type II* is due to deficiency of either electron transfer flavoprotein (α-subunit) or electron transfer flavoprotein:ubiquinone oxidoreductase and is characterized by accumulation and excretion of glutaric and 2-hydroxyglutaric acids as well as multiple organic acids normally oxidized by mitochondrial flavin-containing acyl-CoA dehydrogenases, which require both proteins for activity. Additional manifestations include hypoglycemia without ketosis, metabolic acidosis, and a spectrum of phenotypic manifestations varying with the particular defect. Increasing age of onset is correlated with decreasing severity; when of neonatal onset it may be accompanied by congenital anomalies and is rapidly fatal. Type II is called also *multiple acyl CoA dehydrogenation deficiency.* 2. excretion of glutaric acid in the urine.

**glu·ta·ryl** (gloo′tə-ril) the divalent radical of glutaric acid; as glutaryl CoA, a thioester formed with coenzyme A, it is an intermediate in the catabolism of lysine, hydroxylysine, and tryptophan.

**glu·ta·ryl-CoA de·hy·dro·gen·ase** (gloo′tə-rəl ko-a′ de-hi′dro-jən-ās) [EC 1.3.99.7] an enzyme of the oxidoreductase class that catalyzes the oxidative decarboxylation of glutaryl CoA, with sequential reduction of FAD and then electron transfer flavoprotein; the reaction is a step in the degradation of lysine, hydroxylysine, and tryptophan. Deficiency of the enzyme, an autosomal recessive trait, causes glutaricaciduria, type I.

**glu·ta·thi·one** (gloo″tə-thi′ōn) [MeSH: Glutathione] a tripeptide, γ-glutamyl-cysteinyl-glycine, that is widely distributed in animal and plant tissues; it exists in both the reduced thiol form (GSH) and the oxidized disulfide form (GSSG). It functions in various redox reactions, such as the destruction of peroxides and free radicals, the detoxification of harmful compounds, and activity as a cofactor for enzymes. In erythrocytes, these reactions prevent oxidative damage by reduction of methemoglobin and peroxides. Glutathione is also involved in the formation and maintenance of disulfide bonds in proteins and in transport of amino acids across cell membranes.

**glu·ta·thi·on·emia** (gloo″tə-thi″o-ne′me-ə) the presence of glutathione in the blood.

**glu·ta·thi·one per·ox·i·dase** (gloo″tə-thi′ōn pə-rok′sĭ-dās) [EC 1.11.1.9] [MeSH: Glutathione Peroxidase] an enzyme of the oxidoreductase class that catalyzes the detoxifying reduction of hydrogen peroxide and organic peroxides via oxidation of glutathione. The enzyme requires selenium at the active site; deficiency of enzyme activity may be linked to jaundice and hemolytic anemia in neonates.

**glu·ta·thi·one re·duc·tase (NADPH)** (gloo″tə-thi′ōn re-duk′tās) [EC 1.6.4.2] [MeSH: Glutathione Reductase] an enzyme of the oxidoreductase class that catalyzes the reduction of glutathione via oxidation of NADPH. It is a flavoprotein (FAD), occurring in erythrocytes, and is involved in many redox reactions. Deficiency of enzyme activity in erythrocytes usually results from nutritional or metabolic inadequacy of FAD and, except when severe, has not been linked to hemolysis. Diminished enzyme activity does decrease protection of cells from oxidative damage.

**glu·ta·thi·one syn·thase** (gloo″tə-thi′ōn sin′thās) [EC 6.3.2.3] glutathione synthetase.

**glu·ta·thi·one syn·the·tase** (gloo″tə-thi′ōn sin′thə-tās) [MeSH: Glutathione Synthetase] an enzyme of the ligase class that catalyzes the ATP-dependent formation of glutathione from glycine and γ-glutamylcysteine. Deficiency of the enzyme, an autosomal recessive trait, alters the γ-glutamyl cycle; γ′-glutamylcysteine synthesized futilely is converted to excess 5-oxoproline and cysteine. In EC nomenclature, called *glutathione synthase.*

**glu·ta·thi·one (GSH) syn·the·tase de·fi·cien·cy** an autosomal recessive aminoacidopathy due to decreased levels of GSH and increased levels of 5-oxoproline and cysteine, occurring in two phenotypes. Deficiency of glutathione synthetase confined to the erythrocytes results in a well-compensated hemolytic anemia; generalized deficiency of the enzyme causes high levels of 5-oxoproline in plasma and urine, metabolic acidosis, and often neurologic dysfunction, along with hemolytic anemia.

**glu·ta·thi·on·uria** (gloo″tə-thi″on-u′re-ə) 1. the excretion of excessive amounts of glutathione in the urine. 2. γ-glutamyl transpeptidase deficiency.

**glu·te·al** (gloo′te-əl) [Gr. *gloutos* buttock] pertaining to the buttocks. Called also *natal* and *pygal.*

**glu·ten** (gloo′tən) [L. "glue"] [MeSH: Gluten] the protein of wheat and other grains that gives to the dough its tough elastic character.

**glu·teo·fem·o·ral** (gloo″te-o-fem′or-əl) [*gluteal* + *femoral*] pertaining to the buttock and thigh.

**glu·teo·in·gui·nal** (gloo″te-o-in′gwĭ-nəl) pertaining to the buttock and groin.

**glu·teth·i·mide** (gloo-teth′ĭ-mīd) [MeSH: Glutethimide] a nonbarbiturate structurally related to phenobarbital occurring as a white, crystalline powder; used as a sedative and hypnotic, administered orally.

**glu·ti·nous** (gloo′tĭ-nəs) [L. *glutinosus*] sticky; adhesive; gluey; viscid.

**glu·ti·tis** (gloo-ti′tis) [Gr. *gloutos* buttock + *-itis*] inflammation of the buttock.

**Glu·tose** (gloo′tōs) trademark for preparations of glucose.

**Gly** glycine.

**gly·bur·ide** (gli′būr-īd) [USP] [MeSH: Glyburide] a sulfonylurea compound used as a hypoglycemic in the treatment of type 2 diabetes mellitus; administered orally. Called also *glibenclamide.*

**gly·cal** (gli′kal) an unsaturated derivative of a monosaccharide, in which a double bond between carbons 1 and 2 replaces their hydroxyl groups.

**gly·can** (gli′kan) polysaccharide.

**gly·cate** (gli′kāt) the product of glycation.

**gly·ca·tion** (gli-ka′shən) a nonenzymatic form of glycosylation in which glucose is incorporated into a protein when the environment has a high concentration of glucose.

**gly·ce·mia** (gli-se′me-ə) [*glyc-* + *-emia*] the presence of glucose in the blood; see also *hyperglycemia.* Called also *glucohemia, glycohemia,* and *glycosemia.*

**gly·cen·tin** (gli-sen′tin) glicentin.

**glyc·er·al·de·hyde** (glis″ər-al′də-hīd) [MeSH: Glyceraldehyde] an aldose, the aldehyde form of the triose derived by oxidation of glycerol; it is isomeric with dihydroxyacetone.
**g. 3-phosphate,** an intermediate in the metabolism of glucose, both in the Embden-Meyerhof pathway (see illustration at *pathway*) and in the pentose phosphate pathway.

**glyc·er·al·de·hyde-3-phos·phate de·hy·dro·gen·ase (phos·phor·y·lat·ing)** (glis″ər-al′də-hīd fos′fāt de-hi′dro-jən-ās fos-for′ə-lāt′ing) [EC 1.2.1.12] an enzyme of the oxidoreductase class that catalyzes the phosphorylation of glyceraldehyde 3-phosphate, one of two reactions by which high-energy phosphate is generated in the Embden-Meyerhof pathway. Abbreviated GAPD (See illustration at *pathway*). Called also *triosephosphate dehydrogenase.*

**glyc·er·ate** (glis′ər-āt) a salt or ester of glyceric acid.

**glyc·er·ate de·hy·dro·gen·ase** (glis′ər-āt de-hi′dro-jən-ās) [EC 1.1.1.29] an enzyme of the oxidoreductase class that catalyzes the reduction of hydroxypyruvate to form D-glycerate, using NADH as an electron donor. Deficiency of the enzyme is believed to be a cause of primary hyperoxaluria, type II, and of D-glycericacidemia.

**gly·cer·ic acid** (gli-sēr′ik) a hydroxy acid derived by oxidation of C1 of glycerol or glyceraldehyde to a carboxyl group; various phosphorylated derivatives are important intermediates in glucose metabolism. See also *1,3-* and *2,3-bisphosphoglycerate* and *phosphoglycerate.*

**D-gly·cer·ic·ac·i·de·mia** (gli-ser″ik-as″ĭ-de′me-ə) increased concentration of D-glyceric acid in the blood, believed to be due to a defect in glycerate dehydrogenase and characterized by hyperglycinemia without ketosis or acidosis; mental retardation may be associated.

**L-gly·cer·ic·ac·id·uria** (gli-ser″ik-as″ĭd-u′re-ə) primary hyperoxaluria, type II.

**glyc·er·i·dase** (glis′ər-ĭ-dās) any enzyme that catalyzes the cleavage of a glyceride, such as a lipase.

**glyc·er·ide** (glis′ər-īd) glycerol esterified with one or more organic acids, particularly with long chain fatty acids. Glycerides are classified as mono-, di-, or triglycerides as a function of the number of such substituents. Called also *acylglycerol.*

**glyc·er·in** (glis′ər-in) [L. *glycerinum*] [USP] [MeSH: Glycerin] a clear, colorless, syrupy liquid, $C_3H_8O_3$, obtained as a by-product of soap, by carbohydrate fermentation, and by propylene synthesis; administered rectally as a cathartic and orally as a diuretic to reduce intraocular pressure. It is also used as a solvent, humectant, and vehicle in various pharmaceutical preparations. See also *glycerol.*

**glyc·er·in·at·ed** (glis′ər-in-āt″əd) treated with or preserved in glycerin.

**glyc·er·i·num** (glis″ər-i′nəm) [L.] glycerin.

**glyc·er·ite** (glis′ər-īt) [L. *glyceritum*] a solution or mixture of a medicinal substance in glycerin; the glycerites for which official standards have been promulgated are starch and tannic acid glycerites.
**starch g.,** a preparation of starch, benzoic acid, glycerin, and purified water; used topically as an emollient.
**tannic acid g.,** a preparation of tannic acid, sodium citrate, exsiccated sodium sulfite, and glycerin, containing about 20 per cent of tannic acid; used as an astringent. Called also *glyceritum acidi tannici.*

**glyc·ero·gel** (glis′ər-o-jel) a gel in which glycerin is the dispersed medium.

**glyc·ero·gel·a·tin** (glis″ər-o-jel′ə-tin) glycerin jelly.

**glyc·er·ol** (glis′ər-ol) a trihydroxy sugar alcohol that is the backbone of many lipids and an important intermediate in carbohydrate and lipid metabolism. Pharmaceutical preparations are called glycerin (q.v.).
**iodinated g.,** an isomeric mixture of the iodinated dimers of glycerol used as an expectorant.
**g. phosphate, (L-)g. 3-phosphate,** an intermediate in the glycerol phosphate shuttle, in the utilization of glycerol, and in the biosynthesis of lipids.

**glyc·er·ol·ize** (glis′ər-ol-īz″) to treat with or preserve in glycerol, as in the treatment of red blood cells with a glycerol solution before they are frozen for preservation.

**glyc·er·ol ki·nase** (glis″ər-ol-ki′nās) [EC 2.7.1.30] [MeSH: Glycerol Kinase] an enzyme of the transferase class that catalyzes the phosphorylation of glycerol to form glycerol 3-phosphate. Deficiency of the enzyme, an X-linked trait, causes hyperglycerolemia.

**glyc·er·ol-3-phos·phate *O*-ac·yl·trans·fer·ase** (glis′ər-ol fos′fāt a″səl-trans′fər-ās) [EC 2.3.1.15] an enzyme of the transferase class that catalyzes the transfer of an acyl group to glycerol 3-phosphate from an acyl CoA with a chain longer than ten carbons, yielding a lysophosphatidate. The reaction is a step in the synthesis of triglycerides and phosphatidates, and the enzyme also catalyzes the addition of a second acyl group to the lysophosphatidate to form a phosphatidate.

**glyc·er·ol-3-phos·phate de·hy·dro·gen·ase** (glis′ər-ol fos′fāt de-hi′dro-jə-nās) [EC 1.1.99.5] an enzyme of the oxidoreductase class that catalyzes the oxidation of glycerol 3-phosphate to dihydroxyacetone phosphate. In mitochondria of striated muscle and of nervous tissue, the enzyme contains iron and the acceptor is FAD. The dihydroxyacetone phosphate formed can cross into the cytosol, where glycerol-3-phosphate dehydrogenase ($NAD^+$) catalyzes its reduction via electrons from NADH, regenerating glycerol 3-phosphate. See also *glycerol phosphate shuttle,* under *shuttle.*

**glyc·er·ol-3-phos·phate de·hy·dro·gen·ase ($NAD^+$)** (glis′ər-ol fos′fāt de-hi′dro-jən-ās) [EC 1.1.1.8] a cytosolic enzyme of the oxidoreductase class that catalyzes the oxidation of glycerol 3-phosphate to dihydroxyacetone phosphate, with $NAD^+$ as the electron acceptor. NADH formed from $NAD^+$ by other reactions displaces the equilibrium, producing glycerol 3-phosphate and the oxidized nucleotide $NAD^+$. The glycerol phosphate produced can cross into the mitochondria, where it is reoxidized by glycerol-3-phosphate dehydrogenase, regenerating dihydroxyacetone phosphate and donating electrons to FAD. See also *glycerol phosphate shuttle,* under *shuttle.*

**glyc·er·ol·uria** (glis″ər-ol-u′re-ə) excretion of glycerol in the urine.

**glyc·er·one** (glis′ər-ōn) [*glycerol* + *ketone*] formal, seldom used, term for *dihydroxyacetone.*

**glyc·er·yl** (glis′ər-əl) the mono-, di-, or trivalent radical formed by removal of a hydrogen from one, two, or three of the hydroxy groups of glycerol.
**g. guaiacolate,** guaifenesin.
**g. monostearate** [NF], a compound prepared from glycerin and stearic acid, occurring as a white, waxlike solid, or white, waxlike beads or flakes with a slight, pleasant, fatty odor and taste; used as an emulsifying agent.
**g. triacetate,** triacetin.
**g. trinitrate,** nitroglycerin.
**g. trioleate,** olein.
**g. tripalmitate,** palmitin.

**gly·cin·am·ide ri·bo·nu·cleo·tide** (gli-sin′ə-mīd ri″bo-noo′kle-o-tīd) an intermediate of purine biosynthesis in which glycine is linked to the amino group of phosphoribosylamine.

**gly·cin·ate** (gli′sin-āt) any salt of glycine (aminoacetic acid).

**gly·cine** (gli′sēn) [MeSH: Glycine] 1. chemical name: aminoacetic acid. The smallest of the amino acids, a nonessential amino acid occurring as a constituent of many proteins. It is glycogenic, participates in a variety of synthetic reactions such as purine formation, and is an inhibitory neurotransmitter in the central nervous system. Symbols Gly and G. See table at *amino acid.* 2. [USP] an official preparation used as a dietary supplement and gastric antacid, and as a bladder irrigation in transurethral prostatectomy.

**gly·cine am·i·di·no·trans·fer·ase** (gli′sēn am″ĭ-dēn″o-trans′fər-ās) [EC 2.1.4.1] an enzyme of the transferase class that catalyzes the transfer of an amidino group from arginine to glycine to form guanidinoacetate and ornithine. The reaction is a step in the synthesis of creatine.

**gly·cine hy·droxy·meth·yl·trans·fer·ase** (gli′sēn hi-drok″se-meth″əl-trans′fər-ās) [EC 2.1.2.1] an enzyme of the transferase class that catalyzes the reversible transfer of a methylene group from serine to tetrahydrofolate to form 5,10-methylenetetrahydrofolate and glycine. The enzyme is a pyridoxal phosphate protein. The reaction occurs in mitochondria and is a major source of one-carbon units for folate-mediated transfer reactions. Called also *serine hydroxymethyltransferase.*

**gly·cine trans·a·mid·in·ase** (gli'sēn trans"ə-mid'in-ās) glycine amidinotransferase.

**gly·cin·emia** (gli"sin-e'me-ə) hyperglycinemia.

**glyc·i·nin** (glis'ĭ-nin) a globulin which constitutes 90 to 95 per cent of the protein content of soybean.

**Gly·ciph·a·gus** (gli-sif'ə-gəs) *Glycyphagus.*

**glyc(o)-** [Gr. *glykys* sweet] a combining form denoting relationship to *(a)* sweetness, *(b)* sugar, sometimes specifically glucose, *(c)* glycerine, or *(d)* glycogen. Cf. *gluc(o)-.*

**gly·co·al·de·hyde** (gli"ko-al'də-hīd) glycolaldehyde.

**gly·co·bi·ar·sol** (gli"ko-bi-ahr'sol) a bismuth-containing pentavalent organic arsenical used as an antiamebic in the treatment of intestinal amebiasis; administered orally. Because of its toxicity, it has largely been replaced by other agents.

**gly·co·cal·ix, gly·co·cal·yx** (gli"ko-kal'iks) the glycoprotein and polysaccharide covering that surrounds many cells; in bacterial cells the glycocalyx forms masses of fibers that extend from the cell and by means of which the cell adheres to surfaces.

**gly·co·che·no·de·oxy·cho·late** (gli"ko-ke"no-de-ok"se-ko'lāt) chenodeoxycholylglycine.

**gly·co·che·no·de·oxy·cho·lic ac·id** (gli"ko-ke"no-de-ok"se-ko'lik) [MeSH: Glycochenodeoxycholic Acid] chenodeoxycholylglycine.

**gly·co·cho·late** (gli"ko-ko'lāt) cholylglycine.

**gly·co·cho·lic ac·id** (gli"ko-ko'lik) [MeSH: Glycocholic Acid] cholylglycine.

**gly·co·con·ju·gate** (gli"ko-kon'jə-gət) any of the complex molecules containing glycosidic linkages, such as glycolipids, glycopeptides, oligosaccharides, or glycosaminoglycans.

**gly·co·cy·amine** (gl"ko-si'ə-mēn) guanidinoacetic acid.

**gly·co·gel·a·tin** (gli"ko-jel'ə-tin) an ointment base containing glycerin and gelatin.

**gly·co·gen** (gli'ko-jən) [*glyco-* + *-gen*] [MeSH: Glycogen] a large polysaccharide similar to amylopectin but more highly branched, consisting of chains of glucose residues in α-(1,4) linkage with branches created by α-(1,6) linkages. It constitutes the major carbohydrate reserve of animals, stored primarily in liver and muscle, and is synthesized and degraded for energy as demanded.
**hepatic g.,** glycogen stored in the liver.
**tissue g.,** glycogen stored in tissues other than the liver, especially in muscle.

**gly·co·gen·e·sis** (gli"ko-jen'ə-sis) [*glyco-* + *-genesis*] 1. the formation or synthesis of glycogen. 2. older term for the production of glucose.

**gly·co·ge·net·ic** (gli"ko-jə-net'ik) pertaining to, characterized by, or promoting glycogenesis.

**gly·co·gen·ic** (gli"ko-jen'ik) [*glyco-* + *-genic*] 1. glycogenetic. 2. pertaining to or involving glycogen.

**gly·co·ge·nol·y·sis** (gli"ko-jə-nol'ə-sis) [*glycogen* + *-lysis*] the breakdown of glycogen to glucose by hydrolysis (as in digestion or within lysosomes) or phosphorolysis (as in mobilization of glycogen as a fuel).

**gly·co·geno·lyt·ic** (gli"ko-jen"o-lit'ik) pertaining to, characterized by, or promoting glycogenolysis.

**gly·co·ge·no·sis** (gli"ko-jə-no'sĭs) [*glycogen* + *-osis*] glycogen storage disease.
**brancher deficiency g.,** glycogen storage disease, type IV.
**generalized g.,** glycogen storage disease, type II.
**hepatophosphorylase deficiency g.,** glycogen storage disease, type VI.
**hepatorenal g.,** glycogen storage disease, type I.
**myophosphorylase deficiency g.,** glycogen storage disease, type V.

**gly·cog·e·nous** (gli-koj'ə-nəs) glycogenetic.

**gly·co·gen phos·phor·y·lase** (gli'ko-jən fos-for'ə-lās) [EC 2.4.1.1] [MeSH: Glycogen Phosphorylase] an enzyme of the transferase class that catalyzes the phosphorolysis of a terminal α-1,4-glycosidic bond at the non-reducing end of a glycogen molecule, releasing a glucose 1-phosphate residue. The inactive form of the enzyme (phosphorylase *b*) is converted to the active, phosphorylated form (phosphorylase *a*) by phosphorylase kinase, and phosphorylase *a* is deactivated by phosphorylase phosphatase; phosphorylase *b* can also be activated by AMP without being phosphorylated. Two isozymes exist: the liver isozyme replenishes blood glucose while the muscle isozyme mobilizes glycogen as fuel. Deficiency of glycogen phosphorylase, an autosomal recessive trait, causes glycogen storage disease. The muscle isozyme is absent in glycogen storage disease, type V; the liver isozyme is deficient in type VI. Called also *phosphorylase.*

**gly·co·gen phos·phor·y·lase ki·nase** (gli'ko-jən fos-for'ə-lās ki'nās) phosphorylase kinase.

**gly·co·gen starch syn·thase** (gli'ko-jən stahrch sin'thās) [EC 2.4.1.11] an enzyme of the transferase class that catalyzes the synthesis of glycogen by forming an α-1,4-glucoside linkage between the terminal hydroxyl group of glycogen chain and a glucosyl group donated by UDPglucose. The reaction is highly regulated by allosteric effectors, by kinases and phosphatases, and by insulin. The active form glycogen synthase *a* (formerly I) is not phosphorylated; the less active form glycogen synthase *b* (formerly D) is phosphorylated.

**gly·co·gen syn·thase** (gli'ko-jən sin'thās) see *glycogen starch synthase.*

**[gly·co·gen-syn·thase-D] phos·pha·tase** (gli'ko-jən sin'thās fos'fə-tās) [EC 3.1.3.42] an enzyme of the hydrolase class that catalyzes the cleavage of a phosphoryl group from (inactive) glycogen synthase *b* to form (active) glycogen synthase *a;* the reaction is part of the mechanism of regulation of glycogen metabolism. Recently, this enzyme has been considered by some to be an activity of the more general enzyme protein phosphatase 1 (q.v.).

**gly·co·geu·sia** (gli"ko-goo'zhə) [*glyco-* + Gr. *geusis* taste] a condition in which there is a sweet taste in the mouth.

**gly·co·he·mia** (gli"ko-he'me-ə) glycemia.

**gly·co·he·mo·glo·bin** (gli"ko-he"mo-glo'bin) glycated hemoglobin.

**gly·col** (gli'kol) any of a group of aliphatic dihydric alcohols having marked hygroscopic properties and useful as solvents and plasticizers.
**polyethylene g.,** see under P.

**gly·col·al·de·hyde** (gli"kol-al'də-hīd) a two-carbon aldehyde moiety that is the activated intermediate transferred to aldoses by transketolase and is the precursor of glycolic acid. Called also *glycoaldehyde.*

**gly·co·late** (gli'ko-lāt) a salt, anion, or ester of glycolic acid.

**gly·col·ic acid** (gli-kol'ik) hydroxyacetic acid, an intermediate in the conversion of serine to glycine; it is accumulated and excreted in primary hyperoxaluria, type I.

**gly·col·ic·ac·id·uria** (gli-kol"ik-as"ĭ-du're-ə) primary hyperoxaluria, type I.

**gly·co·lip·id** (gli"ko-lip'id) a lipid containing carbohydrate groups, usually galactose but also glucose, inositol, or others. While it can describe those lipids derived from either glycerol or sphingosine, with or without phosphate groups, the term is used almost exclusively to denote the sphingosine derivatives lacking phosphate groups (glycosphingolipids).

**gly·co·lyl** (gli'ko-ləl) the acyl radical of glycolic acid.

**gly·col·y·sis** (gli-kol'ə-sis) [*glyco-* &plus *-lysis*] [MeSH: Glycolysis] the anaerobic enzymatic conversion of glucose to the simpler compounds lactate or pyruvate, resulting in energy stored in the form of adenosine triphosphate (ATP), as occurs in muscle; it differs from respiration in that organic substances, rather than molecular oxygen, are used as electron acceptors. See *Embden-Meyerhof pathway,* under *pathway.*

**gly·co·lyt·ic** (gli"ko-lit'ik) pertaining to, characterized by, or promoting glycolysis.

**gly·cone** (gli'kōn) the sugar portion of a glycoside. Cf. *aglycon.*

**gly·co·neo·gen·e·sis** (gli"ko-ne"o-jen'ə-sis) [*glyco-* + *neo-* + *-genesis*] gluconeogenesis.

**gly·co·nu·cleo·pro·tein** (gli"ko-noo"kle-o-pro'tēn) a nucleoprotein bearing carbohydrate groups.

**gly·co·pe·nia** (gli"ko-pe'ne-ə) [*glyco-* + *-penia*] a deficiency of sugar in the tissues.

**gly·co·pep·tide** (gli"ko-pep'tīd) any of a class of peptides that contain carbohydrates, including those that contain amino sugars.

**gly·co·pex·ic** (gli"ko-pek'sik) pertaining to, characterized by, or promoting glycopexis.

**gly·co·pex·is** (gli"ko-pek'sis) [*glyco-* + *pexis*] the fixation or storing of sugar or glycogen.

**Gly·coph·a·gus** (gli-kof'ə-gəs) *Glycyphagus.*

**gly·co·phil·ia** (gli″ko-fil′e-ə) [*glyco-* + *-philia*] a condition in which a very small amount of glucose produces hyperglycemia.

**gly·co·phor·in** (gli″ko-for′in) [MeSH: Glycophorin] any of several related proteins that can project through the thickness of the cell membrane of erythrocytes; they attach to oligosaccharides at the outer cell membrane surface and to contractile proteins (spectrin and actin) at the cytoplasmic surface.

**gly·co·poly·uria** (gli″ko-pol″e-u′re-ə) [*glyco-* + *poly-* + *-uria*] polyuria due to glucosuria.

**gly·co·pri·val** (gli″ko-pri′vəl) [*glyco-* + L. *privus* deprived of] pertaining to or characterized by deprivation of carbohydrates.

**gly·co·pro·tein** (gli″ko-pro′tēn) a conjugated protein containing one or more covalently linked carbohydrate residues. While technically describing conjugates in which the carbohydrate is less than 4 per cent by weight, the term is often used generically to include the mucoproteins (q.v.) and proteoglycans (q.v.).
**α1-acid g.**, an acute phase protein found in blood plasma; its exact function is unclear. Called also *orosomucoid*.
**glycine-rich β g. (GBG)**, former name for *factor B*.
**g. Mac-1**, a $\beta_2$ integrin (CD11b/CD18) expressed on monocytes, macrophages, neutrophils, and NK cells that mediates leukocyte adhesion and serves as a receptor for inactivated complement fragment C3b (iC3b) and for some carbohydrates of certain bacteria and yeasts; it also plays a role in antibody-dependent cellular cytotoxicity. It comprises an α and a β chain; the latter is common also to CR4. Called also *Mac-1* and *complement receptor 3 (CR3)*.
**P-g. (Pgp)**, a 170-kilodalton cell-surface protein occurring normally in the colon, small intestine, adrenal glands, kidney, and liver, and also expressed by tumor cells. It is a modulator of multidrug resistance, mediating the transport of antineoplastic agents out of tumor cells.
**g. p150,95**, a $\beta_2$ integrin expressed on monocytes, macrophages, phagocytes, and NK cells that mediates leukocyte adhesion.
**variable surface g. (VSG)**, any of an array of glycoproteins that forms the antigenic protein coating of *Trypanosoma brucei*. The organisms contain numerous genes encoding hundreds of such glycoproteins and, by expressing individual ones successively, evade the immune system of the host.

**gly·co·pro·tein 4-β-ga·lac·to·syl·trans·fer·ase** (gli″ko-pro′tēn gə-lak″to-səl-trans′fər-ās) an enzyme of the transferase class that catalyzes the attachment of galactose moieties derived from UDPgalactose to *N*-acetylglucosamine residues of glycoproteins. The enzyme is present in many tissues; in secreting mammary gland cells it complexes with α-lactalbumin to form lactose synthase. In EC nomenclature, called *β-N-acetylglucosaminylglycopeptide β-1,4-galactosyltransferase*.

**gly·co·pro·tein si·al·i·dase** (gli″ko-pro′tēn si-al′ĭ-dās) sialidase, def. 1.

**gly·co·pty·al·ism** (gli″ko-ti′əl-iz-əm) [*glyco-* + *ptyal-* + *-ism*] glycosialia.

**gly·co·pyr·ro·late** (gli″ko-pir′o-lāt) [USP] [MeSH: Glycopyrrolate] a synthetic quaternary anticholinergic used in the treatment of peptic ulcer and other gastrointestinal disturbances in which hyperacidity, hypermotility, and/or spasm occur, administered orally, subcutaneously, intramuscularly, or intravenously. Called also *glycopyrronium bromide*.

**gly·co·pyr·ro·ni·um bro·mide** (gli″ko-pir-o′ne-əm) glycopyrrolate.

**gly·cor·rha·chia** (gli″ko-ra′ke-ə) [*glyco-* + *rhachi-* + *-ia*] presence of glucose in the cerebrospinal fluid.

**gly·cor·rhea** (gli″ko-re′ə) [*glyco-* + *-rrhea*] a sugary discharge, as with glycosuria.

**gly·co·sam·ine** (gli-ko′sə-mēn) an amino sugar, usually glucosamine.

**gly·cos·ami·no·gly·can** (gli″kōs-ə-me″no-gli′kan) any of several high molecular weight linear heteropolysaccharides having disaccharide repeating units containing an *N*-acetylhexosamine and a hexose or hexuronic acid; either or both residues may be sulfated. This class of compounds includes the chondroitin sulfates, dermatan sulfates, heparan sulfate and heparin, keratan sulfates, and hyaluronic acid. All except heparin occur in proteoglycans. One or more glycosaminoglycans are accumulated abnormally in the various mucopolysaccharidoses. Abbreviated GAG. Formerly called *mucopolysaccharide*.

**gly·co·se·cre·to·ry** (gli″ko-se-kre′to-re) causing or concerned in the deposition of glycogen.

**gly·co·se·mia** (gli″ko-se′me-ə) glycemia.

**gly·co·si·a·lia** (gli″ko-si-a′le-ə) [*glyco-* + *sial-* + *-ia*] presence of glucose in the saliva.

**gly·co·si·a·lor·rhea** (gli″ko-si″ə-lor′e-ə) [*glyco-* + *sialo-* + *-rrhea*] excessive flow of saliva containing glucose.

**gly·co·si·dase** (gli-ko′sĭ-dās) [EC 3.2] any of a large subclass of enzymes of the hydrolase class that catalyze the cleavage of hemiacetal bonds of glycosides; most are of broad specificity. See also *glucosidase*.
**β-g.**, 1. a glycosidase specifically cleaving β-linked sugar residues from glycosides. 2. see under *complex*.

**gly·co·side** (gli′ko-sīd) any compound that contains a carbohydrate molecule (sugar), particularly any such natural product in plants, convertible, by hydrolytic cleavage, into sugar and a nonsugar component (aglycone), and named specifically for the sugar contained, as glucoside (glucose), pentoside (pentose), fructoside (fructose), etc.
**cardiac g.**, any of a group of glycosides characterized by an aglycon consisting of a steroid nucleus with an α,β-unsaturated lactone ring attached at the C-17 position, occurring in certain plants (e.g., *Digitalis, Strophanthus, Urginea* ). Cardiac glycosides increase the force of contraction of cardiac muscle and some are used as cardiotonics and antiarrhythmics.
**digitalis g.**, any of a number of cardiotonic and antiarrhythmic glycosides derived from *Digitalis purpurea* and *D. lanata,* consisting of a steroid nucleus with an α, β-unsaturated lactone ring attached at the C-17 position and a digitoxose moiety attached at C-3. The term is often used to denote any drug chemically and pharmacologically related to these glycosides, although not all are derived from *Digitalis* (e.g., ouabain); in this case it is equivalent to *cardiac g.*

**gly·co·sphingo·lip·id** (gli″ko-sfing″o-lip′id) any sphingolipid in which the head group is a mono- or oligosaccharide unit; included are the cerebrosides, sulfatides, and gangliosides. See also *glycolipid*.

**gly·co·sphing·o·lip·i·do·sis** (gli″ko-sfing″o-lip″ĭ-do′sis) [*glyco-* + *sphingolipid* + *-osis*] Fabry's disease.

**gly·co·stat·ic** (gli″ko-stat′ik) [*glyco-* + *static*] tending to maintain a constant sugar level.

**gly·cos·uria** (gli″ko-su′re-ə) [*glycose,* older variant of *glucose* + *-uria*] [MeSH: Glycosuria] the presence of glucose in the urine, especially excretion of an abnormally large amount in the urine, such as more than 1 g in 24 hours. Called also *dextrosuria* and *glucosuria*.
**alimentary g.**, digestive g.
**benign g.**, renal g.
**digestive g.**, normal glycosuria following the ingestion of sugar; called also *alimentary g.*
**emotional g.**, glycosuria induced by violent emotion.
**epinephrine g.**, glycosuria following the injection of epinephrine.
**hyperglycemic g.**, glycosuria associated with hyperglycemia.
**magnesium g.**, glycosuria due to high concentration of magnesium in the blood.
**nondiabetic g., nonhyperglycemic g., normoglycemic g., orthoglycemic g.**, renal g.
**pathologic g.**, appearance of large amounts of sugar in the urine for a considerable period of time.
**phlorhizin g.**, glycosuria following the experimental administration of phlorhizin.
**renal g.**, glycosuria occurring when there is only the normal amount of sugar in the blood, due to inability of the renal tubules to reabsorb glucose completely. Called also *nondiabetic* or *normoglycemic g.* and *renal diabetes*.
**toxic g.**, glycosuria produced by poisons.

**gly·co·syl** (gli′ko-sil″) the radical formed from a saccharide by removal of the anomeric hydroxyl group.

**gly·co·syl·at·ed** (gli-ko′sə-lāt″əd) having formed a linkage with a glycosyl group.

**gly·co·syl·a·tion** (gli-ko″sə-la′shən) [MeSH: Glycosylation] the formation of linkages with glycosyl groups.
**nonenzymatic g.**, glycation.

**gly·co·syl·cer·am·i·dase** (gli-ko″səl-sə-ram′ĭ-dās) [EC 3.2.1.62] [MeSH: Glycosylceramidase] an enzyme of the hydrolase class that catalyzes the cleavage of a β-linked sugar residue from β-glycosides with large hydrophobic aglycons, such as galactosyl- and glycosylceramides and phlorizin. Such enzyme activity occurs as part of the β-glycosidase complex (q.v.), along with lactase, in the intestinal brush border membrane, where it is frequently referred to as *phlorhizin hydrolase* . In this context, it is sometimes described as a composite of glucosylceramidase [EC 3.2.1.45] and galactosylceramidase [3.2.1.46] activities and denoted *glycosylceramidase* [EC 3.2.1.45–6].

**gly·co·syl·trans·fer·ase** (gli″ko-səl-trans′fər-ās) [EC 2.4] any enzyme that catalyzes the transfer of glycosyl groups from one molecule to another; the glycosyltransferases include the hexosyltransferases (EC 2.4.1), the pentosyltransferases (EC 2.4.2), and those transferring other glycosyl groups (EC 2.4.99). Called also *transglycosylase*.

**gly·co·tax·is** (gli″ko-tak′sis) [*glyco-* + *-taxis*] the metabolic distribution of glucose to the body tissues.

**gly·co·trop·ic** (gli″ko-trop′ik) [*glyco-* + *-tropic*] having an affinity for or attracting sugar; antagonizing the effects of insulin, causing hyperglycemia.

**gly·cu·re·sis** (gli″ku-re′sis) [*glyc-* + *-uresis*] glycosuria.

**gly·cu·ron·ic ac·id** (gli″ku-ron′ik) uronic acid.

**gly·cu·ro·nide** (gli″ku-rōn′īd) a glycoside of a glycuronic (uronic) acid, often specifically a glucuronide.

**glyc·yl** (glis′əl) the acyl radical of glycine.

**glyc·yl·glyc·ine** (glis″əl-glis′in) [MeSH: Glycylglycine] the simplest dipeptide, $CH_2(NH_2){\cdot}CO{\cdot}NH{\cdot}CH_2{\cdot}CO_2{\cdot}H$.

**Gly·cyph·ag·i·dae** (gli″sĭ-faj′ĭ-de) a family of mites similar to Acaridae, free-living mites often found on organic material used by humans. It includes the genus *Glycyphagus* of medical interest.

**Gly·cyph·a·gus** (gli-sif′ə-gəs) [Gr. *glykys* sweet + *phagein* to eat] a genus of free-living mites of the family Glycyphagidae. *G. domes′ticus* is the food mite, a cause of grocers' itch in humans. Spelled also *Glyciphagus.*

**Glyc·yr·rhi·za** (glis″ə-ri′zə) [Gr. *glykys* sweet + *rhiza* root] [MeSH: Glycyrrhiza] a widely distributed genus of perennial herbs of the family Leguminosae. *G. glab′ra* is licorice, the species from which glycyrrhiza is derived.

**glyc·yr·rhi·za** (glis″ə-ri′zə) [MeSH: Glycyrrhiza] the dried rhizome and roots of various species of *Glycyrrhiza,* used as a flavoring and as a pharmaceutic necessity for the preparation of pure glycyrrhiza extract; see under *extract.* Called also *licorice, licorice root,* and *liquorice.*

**gly·da·nile so·di·um** (gli′də-nīl) glicetanile sodium.

**gly·ke·mia** (gli-ke′me-ə) glycemia.

**Gly·nase** (gli′nās) trademark for a preparation of glyburide.

**gly·ox·al** (gli-ok′səl) [MeSH: Glyoxal] a yellow crystalline compound prepared by the oxidation of acetaldehyde and used in organic synthesis, glues, and biocides; called also *biformyl, ethanedial,* and *oxalaldehyde.*

**gly·ox·a·lase** (gli-ok′sə-lās) a term used to describe the enzyme activity that converts methylglyoxal to lactic acid. It is composed of two enzymes: *lactoylglutathione lyase* (glyoxalase I) and *hydroxyacylglutathione hydrolase* (glyoxalase II).

**gly·ox·a·lin** (gli-ok′sə-lin) imidazole.

**gly·ox·i·some** (gli-ok′sĭ-sōm) glyoxosome.

**gly·ox·o·some** (gli-ok′so-sōm) any of the microbodies present in certain plants and microorganisms, resembling the peroxisomes of vertebrate animal cells, but having, in addition to catalase and oxidase enzymes, the enzymes of the glyoxylate cycle, a metabolic pathway involved in the conversion of fat to carbohydrate. Glyoxosomes, in association with chloroplasts, also participate in the process of photorespiration. Called also *glyoxisome.* See also *microbody* and *peroxisome,* def. 1.

**gly·ox·y·late** (gli-ok′sə-lāt) a salt, anion, or ester of glyoxylic acid.

**gly·ox·yl·ic ac·id** (gli-ok-sil′ik) an $\alpha$-keto acid occurring as an intermediate in the conversion of glycolic acid to glycine; it is also the primary precursor of oxalic acid in humans and is excreted in primary hyperoxaluria, type I. See also *glyoxylate cycle,* under *cycle.*

**Glyp·to·cra·ni·um** (glip″to-kra′ne-əm) *Mastophora.*

**Gly·the·o·nate** (gli-the′o-nāt) trademark for a preparation of theophylline sodium glycinate.

**Gm** See under *allotype.*

**gm** gram.

**GMC** General Medical Council (British).

**GM-CSF** [MeSH: Granulocyte-Macrophage Colony-Stimulating Factor] granulocyte-macrophage colony-stimulating factor.

**Gme·lin's test** (ma′linz) [Leopold *Gmelin,* German physiologist, 1788–1853] see under *test.*

**GMK** a preparation of green monkey kidney cells used as culture system for growing viruses, e.g., for recovering the rubella virus.

**GMP** guanosine monophosphate.
**3′,5′-GMP, cyclic GMP,** cyclic guanosine monophosphate.

**gnat** (nat) a small dipterous insect; see also *Diptera.* In England the term includes mosquitoes, but in North America it includes only members of *Diptera* smaller than mosquitoes.
**buffalo g.,** any of various insects of the family Simuliidae.
**eye g.,** *Hippelates pusio.*
**turkey g.,** any of various insects of the family Simuliidae.

**gnath·al·gia** (nath-al′jə) [*gnath-* + *-algia*] pain in the jaw.

**gnath·ic** (nath′ik) pertaining to the jaw or cheek.

**gnath·i·on** (nath′e-on) an anthropometric landmark indicating the lowest point on the median line of the mandible.

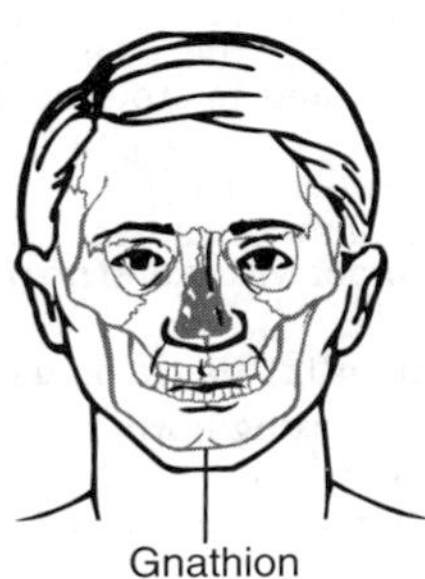
Gnathion

**gnath·itis** (nath-i′tis) [*gnath-* + *-itis*] inflammation of the jaw.

**gnath(o)-** [Gr. *gnathos* jaw] a combining form denoting relationship to the jaw.

**Gnath·ob·del·li·dae** (nath″ob-del′ĭ-de) a family of the Hirudinea, which includes leeches of the genera *Dinobdella, Haemadipsa, Haemopis, Hirudinaria, Hirudo, Limnatis, Macrobdella,* and *Theromyzon.*

**gnatho·ceph·a·lus** (nath″o-sef′ə-ləs) [*gnatho-* + *-cephalus*] a fetus with no head except the jaws.

**gnatho·dy·nam·ics** (nath″o-di-nam′iks) [*gnatho-* + *dynamics*] the study of the physical forces used in mastication.

**gnatho·dy·na·mom·e·ter** (nath″o-di″nə-mom′ə-tər) [*gnatho-* + *dynamometer*] an instrument for measuring the force exerted in closing the jaws; called also *occlusometer.*
**bimeter g.,** a gnathodynamometer equipped with a central-bearing point of adjustable height.

**gnath·odyn·ia** (nath″o-din′e-ə) [*gnatho-* + *-odynia*] gnathalgia.

**gnath·og·ra·phy** (nath-og′rə-fe) [*gnatho-* + *-graphy*] the recording of the strength of a patient's bite by a tracing of the changes in the flow of an electric current through a bite gauge.

**gnatho·log·ic** (nath″o-loj′ik) relating to gnathology.

**gnath·ol·o·gy** (nath-ol′ə-je) [*gnatho-* + *-logy*] the science that deals with the anatomy, histology, physiology, and pathology of the jaws and the masticatory system as a whole, including the applicable diagnostic, therapeutic, and rehabilitative procedures.

**gnatho·plas·ty** (nath′o-plas″te) [*gnatho-* + *-plasty*] plastic surgery of the jaw.

**gnath·os·chi·sis** (nath-os′kĭ-sis) [*gnatho-* + *-schisis*] cleft jaw.

**gnatho·so·ma** (nath″o-so′mə) [*gnatho-* + *soma*] the capitulum of an acarine.

**gnatho·stat** (nath′o-stat) a jaw-positioning device used in dental radiology, facial photography, cephalometry, and other procedures requiring exact positioning of the jaws. See also *cephalostat.*

**gnatho·stat·ics** (nath″o-stat′iks) [*gnatho-* + *-static*] a method of prosthodontic and orthodontic diagnosis based on determination of the basal and osteometric relationships between the teeth and their supporting structures.

**Gnath·os·to·ma** (nath-os′to-mə) [*gnatho-* + *stoma*] [MeSH: Gnathostoma] a genus of nematodes of the family Gnathostomatidae, which are parasitic in cats, swine, cattle, and sometimes humans. *G. spini′gerum* is parasitic in cats, dogs, and humans after they eat raw fish containing the larvae, causing gnathostomiasis.

**Gnatho·sto·mat·i·dae** (nath″o-sto-mat′ĭ-de) a family of nematodes parasitic in mammals, part of the superfamily Spiruroidea. It includes the genus *Gnathostoma.*

**gnatho·sto·mi·a·sis** (nath″o-sto-mi′ə-sis) infection with the nematode *Gnathostoma spinigerum,* occurring in humans or other animals when undercooked fish harboring the larvae are eaten. The larvae migrate, often in the subcutaneous tissue, causing a creeping eruption associated with intense eosinophilia; see *cutaneous larva migrans* (def. 2). Occasionally they migrate to deeper tissues and cause abscesses or to the central nervous system, where they cause eosinophilic myeloencephalitis.

**Gnath·os·to·mum** (nath-os′to-məm) *Gnathostoma.*

**gno·sia** (no′se-ə) [Gr. *gnosis* knowledge] the faculty of perceiving and recognizing.

**gno·to·bi·ol·o·gy** (no″to-bi-ol′ə-je) gnotobiotics.

**gno·to·bio·ta** (no″to-bi-o′tə) the specifically and entirely known microfauna and microflora of a specially reared laboratory animal.

**gno·to·bi·ote** (no″to-bi′ōt) a specially reared laboratory animal the microfauna and microflora of which are specifically known in their entirety.

**gno·to·bi·ot·ic** (no″to-bi-ot′ik) [MeSH: Germ-Free Life] pertaining to a gnotobiote or to gnotobiotics. Cf. *axenic.*

**gno·to·bi·ot·ics** (no″to-bi-ot′iks) [Gr. *gnotos* known + *biota* the fauna and flora of a region] the science of raising laboratory animals whose microfauna and microflora are specifically known in their entirety.

**gno·to·phor·e·sis** (no″to-for′ə-sis) [Gr. *gnotos* known + *-phoresis*] the state of existence of an organism bearing one or more known species in intimate contact with it and no other demonstrable viable microorganisms.

**gno·to·phor·ic** (no″to-for′ik) pertaining to gnotophoresis.

**Gn-RH** gonadotropin-releasing hormone; see *luteinizing hormone–releasing hormone,* under *hormone.*

**Goa powder** (go′ə) [*Goa,* a district in western India] see under *powder.*

**goat·pox** (gōt′poks) an acute, highly infectious disease of goats, caused by a poxvirus and less severe than sheep-pox; characteristics include vesicular eruption with catarrh of the respiratory mucous membranes. Called also *variola caprina.*

**Go·dé·lier's law** (go-da-lyāz′) [Charles Pierre *Godélier,* French physician, 1813–1877] see under *law.*

**Goeck·er·man treatment** (go′kər-mən) [William Henry *Goeckerman,* American dermatologist, 1884–1954] see under *treatment.*

**Gog·gia's sign** (go′jahz) [Carlo Paolo *Goggia,* Italian physician, 1871–1948] see under *sign.*

**goi·ter** (goi′tər) [L. *guttur* throat] [MeSH: Goiter] an enlargement of the thyroid gland, causing a swelling in the front part of the neck. Called also *struma.*
**aberrant g.,** enlargement of an ectopic or supernumerary thyroid gland.
**adenomatous g.,** goiter caused by hyperplasia of follicular cells or by multiple colloid nodules. See also *follicular adenoma,* under *adenoma.*
**Basedow's g.,** a colloid goiter that becomes hyperfunctional after administration of iodine.
**colloid g.,** a large soft type in which the follicles of the gland are greatly distended with colloid.
**congenital g.,** goiter present at birth, resulting from congenital absence of enzymes required for production of thyroxine and consequent overstimulation of the thyroid by thyrotropin.
**cystic g.,** one containing cysts formed by mucoid or colloid degeneration.
**diffuse g.,** one in which the gland is diffusely enlarged, as in Graves' disease.
**diving g.,** a movable goiter located sometimes above and sometimes below the sternal notch. Called also *plunging g.* and *wandering g.*
**endemic g.,** goiter that is endemic to a region, usually because the soil and hence the diet has a low iodide content; seen in mountainous areas around the world and various other regions.
**exophthalmic g.,** goiter accompanied by protrusion of the eyeballs, as in Graves' orbitopathy.
**fibrous g.,** goiter caused by hyperplasia of the capsule and stroma.
**follicular g.,** parenchymatous g.
**intrathoracic g.,** goiter in which a portion is in the thoracic cavity.
**iodide g.,** one that occurs in response to high concentrations of exogenous iodides, which inhibits iodide oxidation and incorporation into thyroglobulin *(Wolff-Chaikoff effect).*
**lingual g.,** an enlargement of the upper end of the original thyroglossal duct, forming a tumor at the posterior part of the dorsum of the tongue.
**lymphadenoid g.,** Hashimoto's disease.
**multinodular g.,** one containing circumscribed nodules within its substance.
**nodular g.,** multinodular g.

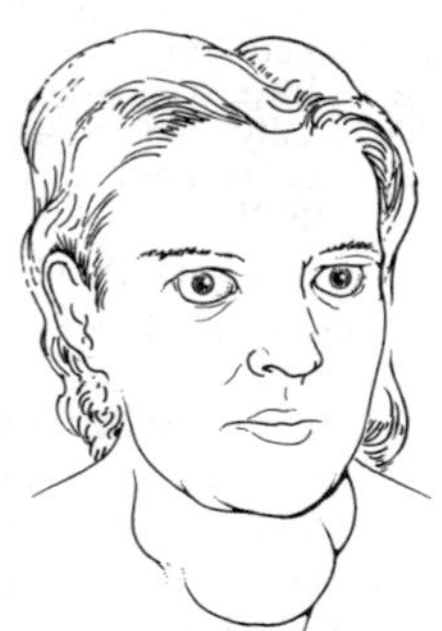
Exophthalmic goiter.

**nontoxic g.,** that occurring sporadically and not associated with hyperthyroidism; such goiters may be either diffuse or nodular.
**parenchymatous g.,** goiter marked by enlarged follicular cells and increased numbers of follicles.
**perivascular g.,** one that surrounds a large blood vessel.
**plunging g.,** diving g.
**retrovascular g.,** one with a portion behind a large blood vessel.
**simple g.,** simple hyperplasia of the thyroid gland.
**substernal g.,** one in which a portion is beneath the sternum.
**suffocative g.,** one that causes dyspnea by pressure on the trachea.
**toxic g., diffuse,** Graves' disease.
**toxic multinodular g.,** hyperthyroidism arising in a multinodular goiter, usually of long standing. Called also *toxic adenoma* and *Parry's* or *Plummer's disease.*
**vascular g.,** goiter due chiefly to dilatation of the blood vessels.
**wandering g.,** diving g.

**goi·tre** (goi′tər) [Fr.] goiter.

**goi·trin** (goi′trin) a goitrogenic substance isolated from rutabagas and turnips.

**goi·tro·gen** (goi′tro-jən) a goiter-producing compound.

**goi·tro·gen·ic** (goi-tro-jen′ik) producing goiter; called also *goitrogenous.*

**goi·tro·ge·nic·i·ty** (goi″tro-jə-nis′ĭ-te) the tendency to produce goiter.

**goi·trog·e·nous** (goi-troj′ə-nəs) goitrogenic.

**goi·trous** (goi′trəs) pertaining to or of the nature of goiter.

**gold** (gōld) [MeSH: Gold] a yellow metallic element occurring in masses or veins in rocks or in grains in the sand of rivers. Its symbol is Au (L. *au′rum*); atomic number, 79; atomic weight, 196.967; specific gravity, 19.32. When alloyed, in carats, pure gold has 24 parts (or carats). Gold compounds are used in medicine, chiefly in arthritis (see *chrysotherapy*). However, all the compounds are poisonous; see also *chrysiasis* and *chrysoderma.*
**g. Au 198,** the most common radioactive isotope of gold, atomic mass 198, used in solid form (seed) or colloidal solution. It has a half-life of 2.69 days and emits gamma (0.412 MeV) and beta particles (1.371, 0.962 MeV); it has been used by intracavitary or interstitial injection or implantation in the treatment of certain types of cancer and has also been used, in colloidal form, as a scintiscanning agent.
**cohesive g.,** cohesive gold foil.
**colloidal g.,** a purplish suspension of minute particles of metallic gold, used in medicine since alchemical times. The radioactive form, made by exposure to neutrons, has been used by intracavitary or interstitial injection in the treatment of certain types of cancer and also has been used as a scintiscanning agent.
**mat g.,** spongy strips of pure gold produced by the process of electroplating, which can be formed into ropes and cylinders and used in the base of dental restorations and as a direct filling material. See also under *foil.*
**g. sodium thiomalate** [USP], a monovalent gold salt used in the treatment of early active rheumatoid arthritis not controlled by nonsteroidal anti-inflammatory agents, rest, and physical therapy; administered intramuscularly. Called also *sodium aurothiomalate* [INN].
**g. thioglucose,** aurothioglucose.

**Gold·berg's syndrome** (gōld′bərgz) [Morton Falk *Goldberg,* American physician, born 1937] see under *syndrome.*

**Gold·blatt's clamp, hypertension, kidney** (gōld′blats) [Harry *Goldblatt,* American physician, 1891–1977] see under *clamp, hypertension,* and *kidney.*

**Gol·den·har's syndrome** (gōl′dən-hahrz) [Maurice *Goldenhar,* Swiss physician, 20th century] oculoauriculovertebral dysplasia; see under *dysplasia.*

**gol·den·seal** (gōl″dən-sēl′) *Hydrastis canadensis.*

**Gold·flam's disease** (gōlt′flahmz) [Samuel Vulfovich *Goldflam,* Polish neurologist, 1852–1932] myasthenia gravis.

**Gold·flam-Erb disease** (gōlt′flahm-erb′) [S. V. *Goldflam;* Wilhelm Heinrich *Erb,* German neurologist, 1840–1921] myasthenia gravis.

**Gold·schei·der's percussion, test** (gōlt′shi-dərz) [Johannes Karl August Eugen Alfred *Goldscheider,* Berlin physician, 1858–1935] see *threshold percussion,* under *percussion,* see *orthopercussion;* and see under *tests.*

**Gold·stein** (gōld′stīn) Joseph Leonard. American physician, born 1940; co-winner, with Michael Stuart Brown, of the Nobel prize for medicine or physiology in 1985 for their discoveries about the regulation of cholesterol metabolism and the treatment of diseases caused by abnormally high levels of cholesterol in the blood.

**Gold·stein's disease,** etc. (gōld′stīnz) [Hyman Isaac *Goldstein,* American physician, 1887–1954] see under *disease, hematemesis, hemoptysis,* and *sign.*

**Gold·thwait's brace, sign** (gōld'thwāts) [Joel Ernest *Goldthwait,* American orthopedic surgeon, 1866–1961] see under *brace* and *sign.*

**Gol·gi** (gol'je) Camillo. Italian neurologist and histologist, 1843–1926; co-winner, with Santiago Ramón y Cajal, of the Nobel prize for medicine or physiology in 1906 for their work on the structure of the nervous system.

**Gol·gi's complex,** etc. (gol'jēz) [Camillo *Golgi*] see under *complex, law, neuron, organ, stain,* and *theory.*

**gol·gio·some** (gol'je-o-sōm) one of the mitochondrion-sized, platelike structures that make up the Golgi complex of the cell; the platelike structure consists of stacks of flattened vessels (cisternae) more commonly known as dictyosomes.

**Goll's fasciculus (column, fibers, tract), nucleus** (golz) [Friedrich *Goll,* Swiss anatomist, 1829–1903] see *fasciculus gracilis medullae spinalis* and *nucleus gracilis,* and see under *fiber.*

**Goltz's experiment, theory** (golts'ez) [Friedrich Leopold *Goltz,* German physiologist, 1834–1902] see under *experiment* and *theory.*

**Goltz syndrome** (gōltz) [Robert William *Goltz,* American dermatologist, born 1923] focal dermal hypoplasia; see under *hypoplasia.*

**Gom·bault's degeneration, neuritis** (gom-bōz') [François Alexis Albert *Gombault,* French neurologist, 1844–1904] progressive hypertrophic neuropathy.

**Gom·bault-Phi·lippe triangle** (gom-bo'fe-lēp') [F. A. A. *Gombault;* Claudien *Philippe,* French pathologist, 1866–1903] see under *triangle.*

**go·mit·o·li** (go-mit'o-li) a network of capillaries in the upper infundibular stem (of the hypothalamus) that surround terminal arterioles of the superior hypophyseal arteries and that lead into portal veins to the adenohypophysis.

**Go·mo·ri's stains** (go-mo'rēz) [George *Gomori,* Hungarian histochemist in the United States, 1904–1957] see under *stain.*

**Gom·pertz' law (formula)** (gom'pərtz) [Benjamin *Gompertz,* British actuary, 1779–1865] see under *law.*

**gom·pho·sis** (gom-fo'sis) [Gr. *gomphōsis* a bolting together] 1. [TA] a type of fibrous joint in which a conical process is inserted into a socketlike portion, such as the styloid process in the temporal bone, or the teeth in the dental alveoli. Called also *socket.* 2. TA alternative for *syndesmosis dentoalveolaris.*

**gon·a·cra·tia** (gon″ə-kra'shə) [*gon-* + Gr. *akrateia* incontinence] spermatorrhea.

**go·nad** (go'nad) [L. *gonas,* from Gr. *gonos;* procreation] [MeSH: Gonads] a gamete-producing gland; an ovary, testis, or ovotestis.
**indifferent g.,** the sexually undifferentiated gonad of the early embryo. In human embryos this stage occurs during the fifth to seventh weeks.
**streak g's,** undeveloped gonadal structures found in the broad ligament below the fallopian tube and composed of whorled connective-tissue stroma with no germinal or secretory cells; seen most often in Turner's syndrome.

**go·nad·al** (go-nad'əl) pertaining to a gonad.

**go·nad·ar·che** (go″nə-dahr'ke) the onset of gonadal functioning.

**go·nad·ec·to·mize** (go″nə-dek'tə-mīz) to surgically remove one or both of the gonads; see also *castrate.*

**go·nad·ec·to·my** (go″nə-dek'tə-me) [*gonad-* + *-ectomy*] surgical removal of an ovary or testis. See also *castration.*

**go·nad(o)-** [L. *gonas,* gen. *gonadis* gonad, from Gr. *gonos* procreation] a combining form denoting relationship to the gonads.

**go·na·do·blas·to·ma** (go″nə-do-blas-to'mə) [MeSH: Gonadoblastoma] a rare benign type of germ cell tumor, usually arising in dysgenetic gonads, often bilaterally. It contains all gonadal elements, including germ cells, sex cord derivatives, and stromal derivatives and is frequently associated with an abnormal chromosomal karyotype. It may give rise to development of a dysgerminoma or other more malignant germ cell tumor.

**go·na·do·gen·e·sis** (go″nə-do-jen'ə-sis) [*gonado-* + *-genesis*] the development of the gonads in the embryo, especially the development of either ovaries or testes.

**go·na·do·in·hib·i·to·ry** (go″nə-do-in-hib'ĭ-tor-e) inhibiting or preventing gonadal activity.

**go·na·do·ki·net·ic** (go″nə-do-kĭ-net'ik) [*gonado-* + *kinetic*] gonadotropic.

**go·na·do·lib·er·in** (go″nə-do-lib'ər-in) [*gonado*tropin + *-liberin*] luteinizing hormone–releasing hormone.

**gon·a·dop·a·thy** (gon″ə-dop'ə-the) [*gonado-* + *-pathy*] any disease of the gonads.

**go·na·do·rel·in** (go″nə-do-rel'in) [MeSH: Gonadorelin] synthetic luteinizing hormone–releasing hormone, structurally identical to the natural hormone.
**g. hydrochloride** [USP], the mono- or dihydrochloride salt of gonadorelin or a mixture of these, used in the evaluation of the functional capacity and response of the anterior pituitary gonadotrophs in hypogonadism and in the treatment of delayed puberty and amenorrhea; administered subcutaneously or intravenously.

**go·nado·trope** (go-nad'o-trōp) 1. gonadotroph. 2. a gonadotropic substance.

**go·nado·troph** (go-nad'o-trōf) 1. a basophil of the adenohypophysis whose granules follicle-stimulating hormone and luteinizing hormone Called also *delta basophil, delta cell,* and *gonadotrope* or *gonadotropic cell.* 2. a substance that stimulates the gonads.

**go·na·do·troph·ic** (go″nə-do-trof'ik) gonadotropic.

**go·na·do·tro·phin** (go'nə-do-tro″fin) gonadotropin.

**go·na·do·trop·ic** (go″nə-do-trop'ik) [*gonado-* + *-tropic*] stimulating the gonads; applied to hormones of the anterior pituitary.

**go·nad·o·tro·pin** (go'nə-do-tro″pin) any hormone that stimulates the gonads, especially follicle-stimulating hormone and luteinizing hormone. See also *chorionic g.* Called also *gonadotropic hormone.*
**chorionic g.,** 1. a two-subunit glycopeptide hormone produced by syncytiotrophoblasts of the fetal placenta that maintains the function of the corpus luteum during the first few weeks of pregnancy, and is thought to promote steroidogenesis in the fetoplacental unit and to stimulate fetal testicular secretion of testosterone. The $\alpha$ subunit is identical to that of luteinizing hormone, follicle-stimulating hormone, and thyrotropin; the $\beta$ subunit shares homology with luteinizing hormone but is antigenically unique, containing an additional glycopeptide sequence. Chorionic gonadotropin can be detected by immunoassay in the maternal urine within days after fertilization and thus provides the basis for the most commonly used pregnancy tests. 2. [USP] the same principle obtained from the urine of pregnant women, used to treat certain cases of cryptorchidism and male hypogonadism, and to induce ovulation and pregnancy in anovulatory women in whom the anovulation is secondary and not due to ovarian failure, and to increase the numbers of oocytes for artificial insemination; administered intramuscularly. Called also *choriogonadotropin.*
**equine g.,** pregnant mare serum g.
**human chorionic g. (hCG),** see *chorionic g.*
**human menopausal g. (hMG),** menotropins.
**pregnant mare serum g.,** a preparation of the follicle-stimulating substance obtained from the blood serum of pregnant mares; it has been used in the treatment of cryptorchidism, sterility, pituitary dwarfism, and other conditions in both men and women. Called also *equine g.* Abbreviated PMSG.

**gon·a·duct** (gon'ə-dəkt) the duct of a gonad; an oviduct or seminal duct.

**gon·ag·ra** (gon-ag'rə) [Gr. *gony* knee + *-agra*] gout in the knee.

**go·nal·gia** (go-nal'jə) [Gr. *gony* knee + *-algia*] pain in the knee.

**gon·ar·thri·tis** (gon″ahr-thri'tis) [Gr. *gony* knee + *arthritis*] inflammation of a knee or knee joint.

**gon·ar·throc·a·ce** (gon″ahr-throk'ə-se) [Gr. *gony* knee + *arthro-* + Gr. *kakē* evil] white swelling of the knee, produced by tuberculous arthritis.

**gon·ar·thro·men·in·gi·tis** (gon-ahr″thro-men″in-ji'tis) [Gr. *gony* knee + *arthro-* + *mening-* + *-itis*] inflammation of the synovial membrane of the knee joint.

**gon·ar·thro·sis** (gon″ahr-thro'sis) arthritic affection of the knee joint, due to degeneration or trauma.

**gon·ar·throt·o·my** (gon″ahr-throt'ə-me) [Gr. *gony* knee + *arthrotomy*] surgical incision of the knee joint.

**go·nato·cele** (go-nat'o-sēl) [Gr. *gony* knee + *-cele*[1]] tumor of the knee.

**gon·e·cyst** (gon'ə-sist, gon″ə-sis'tis) [*gon-* + *cystis*] glandula vesiculosa.

**gon·e·cys·tis** (gon″ə-sis'tis) glandula vesiculosa.

**gon·e·cys·ti·tis** (gon″ə-sis-ti'tis) inflammation of a seminal vesicle.

**gon·e·cys·to·lith** (gon″ə-sis'to-lith) [*gonecyst* + *-lith*] a concretion in a seminal vesicle.

**gon·e·cys·to·py·o·sis** (gon″ə-sis″to-pi-o'sis) [*gonecyst* + *pyo-* + *-sis*] suppuration in a seminal vesicle.

**gon·e·itis** (gon″e-i'tis) [Gr. *gony* knee + *-itis*] gonitis, def. 1.

**gon·e·poi·e·sis** (gon″e-poi-e'sis) [*gon-* + *-poiesis*] the secretion or formation of the semen.

**gon·e·poi·et·ic** (gon″e-poi-et'ik) pertaining to, characterized by, or promoting gonepoiesis.

**Gon·gy·lo·ne·ma** (gon″jə-lo-ne'mə) [Gr. *gongylos* round + *nema*] a genus of nematodes of the superfamily Spiruroidea; infections cause only mild symptoms if any at all. *G. ingluvi'cola* infects chickens. *G. neoplas'ticum* infects rats and other laboratory rodents. *G. pul'chrum* (called also *G. scuta'tum*) infects the esophageal and oral mucous membranes of sheep, goats, cattle, pigs, and sometimes humans in the United States.

**gon·gy·lo·ne·mi·a·sis** (gon″je-lo-ne-mi'ə-sis) infection with *Gongylonema.*

**go·nia** (go'ne-ə) [Gr.] plural of *gonion.*

**go·ni·al** (go'ne-əl) pertaining to the gonion.

**gon·id·an·gi·um** (gon″id-an'je-əm) a cell within which gonidia are formed.

**go·nid·ia** (go-nid'e-ə) [L.] plural of *gonidium.*

**go·nid·i·um** (go-nid'e-əm) pl. *gonid'ia* [Gr. *gonē* seed] the algal cell part of the thallus of a lichen.

**Go·nin's operation** (go-naz') [Jules *Gonin,* Swiss ophthalmic surgeon, 1870–1935] see under *operation.*

**goni(o)-** [Gr. *gōnia* angle] a combining form denoting relationship to an angle, especially the angle of the anterior chamber of the eye.

**Go·nio·ba·sis** (go″ne-o-ba'sis) a genus of small fresh water snails of the family Pleuroceridae. *G. sili'cula* is a species found in the northwestern United States that acts as a host for the fluke *Troglotrema salmincola.*

**go·nio·dys·gen·e·sis** (go″ne-o-dis-jen'ə-sis) [*gonio-* + *dysgenesis*] defective development of the anterior ocular segment.

**go·ni·om·e·ter** (go″ne-om'ə-tər) [*gonio-* + *-meter*] 1. an instrument for measuring angles; used clinically to measure angles of joint motion. Called also *arthrometer.* 2. a plank, one end of which may be tilted to any height, used in testing for labyrinthine disease.
**finger g.,** an apparatus for measuring the limits of flexion and extension of the interphalangeal joints of the fingers.
**universal g.,** a goniometer consisting of a metal or plastic protractor in a full circle or half circle with two indicating arms that are several inches to a foot (10 to 30 cm) in length; the arms are held in place by a tight pivot at the center of the circle so that the instrument can be picked up and read; used to measure range of motion of a joint.

**go·ni·om·e·try** (go″ne-om'ə-tre) the measurement of angles, particularly those of range of motion of a joint.

**go·ni·on** (go'ne-on) pl. *go'nia* [Gr. *gōnia* angle] [TA] an anthropometric landmark located at the most inferior, posterior, and lateral point on the external angle of the mandible, being the apex of the maximum curvature of the mandible, where the ascending ramus becomes confluent with the corpus.

**go·nio·pho·tog·ra·phy** (go″ne-o-fo-tog'rə-fe) photography of the angle of the anterior chamber of the eye.

**Gon·i·ops** (gon'e-ops) a genus of biting flies of the family Tabanidae.

**go·nio·punc·ture** (go″ne-o-punk'chər) [*gonio-* + *puncture*] a rarely used filtering operation for glaucoma, done by inserting a knife blade through clear cornea just within the limbus, across the anterior chamber, and through the opposite corneoscleral wall.

**go·nio·scope** (go'ne-o-skōp″) [*gonio-* + *-scope*] an optical instrument for examining the angle of the anterior chamber and for demonstrating ocular motility and rotation.

**go·ni·os·co·py** (go″ne-os'kə-pe) [MeSH: Gonioscopy] examination of the angle of the anterior chamber of the eye with the gonioscope.

**go·nio·syn·ech·ia** (go'ne-o-sə-nek'e-ə) adhesion of the iris to the cornea at the angle of the anterior chamber of the eye.

**go·ni·ot·o·my** (go″ne-ot'ə-me) [*gonio-* + *-tomy*] an operation for glaucoma characterized by an open angle and normal depth of the anterior chamber; it consists of the opening of Schlemm's canal under direct vision secured by a contact glass.

**go·ni·tis** (go-ni'tis) [*gon-* + *-itis*] 1. inflammation of the knee; called also *goneitis.* 2. inflammation of the stifle joint in a horse.
**fungous g.,** inflammation of the knee joint in which the capsule is diffusely thickened.
**g. tuberculo'sa,** tuberculosis of the knee joint.

**gon(o)-**[1] [Gr. *gonē* offspring, seed, genitalia] a combining form meaning sexual or generative, or denoting relationship to semen or seed, or to the reproductive organs.

**gon(o)-**[2] [Gr. *gony* knee] combining form denoting relationship to the knee.

**gono·blen·nor·rhea** (gon″o-blen″o-re'ə) gonococcal conjunctivitis.

**gono·camp·sis** (gon″o-kamp'sis) [*gono-* + Gr. *kamptos* bent] permanent flexion of the knee.

**gono·cele** (gon'o-sēl) spermatocele.

**gon·och·o·rism** (gon-ok'ə-riz-əm) [*gono-* + Gr. *chōrizein* to separate] differentiation of the gonads with normal development of the reproductive organs appropriate to the sex; cf. *hermaphroditism.*

**gono·coc·cal** (gon″-o-kok'əl) pertaining to gonococci.

**gono·coc·ce·mia** (gon″o-kok-se'me-ə) [L. *gonococci* + *-emia*] the presence of gonococci in the blood.

**gono·coc·ci** (gon″o-kok'si) [L.] plural of *gonococcus.*

**gono·coc·cic** (gon″o-kok'sik) gonococcal.

**gono·coc·cide** (gon″o-kok'sīd) [*gonococcus* + *-cide*] an agent that kills gonococci.

**gono·coc·co·cide** (gon″o-kok'o-sīd) [*gonococcus* + *-cide*] gonococcide.

**gono·coc·cus** (gon″o-kok'əs) pl. *gonococ'ci* [*gono-* + *coccus*] an individual microorganism of the species *Neisseria gonorrhoeae,* the organism causing gonorrhea.

**gono·cyte** (gon'o-sīt) [*gono-* + *-cyte*] 1. the primitive reproductive cell of the embryo. 2. a secondary gamete-producing cell.

**gon·om·ery** (gon-om'ər-e) [*gono-* + Gr. *meros* part] the condition in which the paternal and the maternal chromosomes remain in separate groups and do not completely fuse, as occurs in certain hybrids.

**gono·neph·ro·tome** (gon″o-nef'rə-tōm) [*gono-* + *nephrotome*] that part of the mesoderm that develops into the reproductive and excretory organs of the embryo.

**gono·phage** (gon'o-fāj) a bacteriophage having the gonococcus as its natural host.

**gono·phore** (gon'o-for) [*gono-* + *-phore*] an accessory generative organ, such as the uterine tube and uterus in the female, or spermiduct and seminal vesicle in the male.

**gon·or·rhea** (gon″o-re'ə) [*gono-* + *-rrhea*] [MeSH: Gonorrhea] infection due to *Neisseria gonorrhoeae* transmitted sexually in most cases, but also by contact with infected exudates in neonatal children at birth, or by infants in households with infected inhabitants. It is marked in males by urethritis with pain and purulent discharge, but is commonly asymptomatic in females, although it may extend to produce suppurative salpingitis, oophoritis, tubo-ovarian abscess, and peritonitis. Bacteremia occurs in both sexes, resulting in cutaneous lesions, arthritis, and rarely meningitis or endocarditis. Formerly called *blennorrhagia* and *blennorrhea.*

**gon·or·rhe·al** (gon″o-re'əl) of or pertaining to gonorrhea.

**gono·to·kont** (gon″o-to'kont) auxocyte.

**gono·tome** (gon'o-tōm) [*gono-* + *-tome*] that part of the mesoderm that develops into the reproductive organs of the embryo.

**Gony·au·lax** (gon″e-aw'laks) [*gony-* + Gr. *aulakos* a furrow] a genus of plantlike marine protozoa (order Dinoflagellida, class Phytomastigophorea) having mainly brown to yellow chromatophores. Like other dinoflagellates, they produce discoloration of the water (red tide) when present in vast numbers, and certain species have been associated with a form of shellfish poisoning (q.v.). Representative species include *G. acatenella, G. catenella, G. polyedra,* and *G. tamarensis.*

**gony·camp·sis** (gon″ĭ-kamp'sis) [Gr. *gony* knee + Gr. *kampsis* bending] abnormal curvature of the knee.

**gony·cro·te·sis** (gon″e-kro-te'sis) [Gr. *gony* knee + *krotēsis* striking] genu valgum.

**gony·ec·ty·po·sis** (gon″e-ek″tĭ-po'sis) [Gr. *gony* knee + Gr. *ektypōsis* a modelling in relief] genu varum.

**gonyo·cele** (gon'e-o-sēl″) [Gr. *gony* knee + *-cele*[1]] synovitis or tuberculous arthritis of the knee.

**gony·on·cus** (gon″e-ong'kəs) [Gr. *gony* knee + *onkos* bulk] tumor of the knee.

**Good's syndrome** (goodz) [Robert Alan *Good,* American pediatrician, born 1922] immunodeficiency with thymoma.

**Goo·dell's sign (law)** (go͞o-delz') [William *Goodell,* American gynecologist, 1829–1894] see under *sign.*

**Good·man's syndrome** (good'mənz) [Richard M. *Goodman,* Israeli physician, 20th century] acrocephalosyndactyly, type IV.

**Good·pas·ture's stain, syndrome** (good'pas-chərz) [Ernest William *Goodpasture,* American pathologist, 1886–1960] see under *Table of Stains and Staining Methods* and under *syndrome.*

**Good·sall's rule** (good'sawlz) [David H. *Goodsall,* British surgeon, 1843–1906] see under *rule.*

**Goor·magh·tigh's apparatus (cells)** (go͞or'mah-tīz) [Norbert

*Goormaghtigh,* Belgian physician, 1890–1960] juxtaglomerular cells.

**Go·pa·lan's syndrome** (go'pah-lahnz) [Coluthur *Gopalan,* Indian biochemist, born 1918] see under *syndrome.*

**Gor·di·a·cea** (gor″de-a'se-ə) Nematomorpha.

**Gor·di·us** (gor'de-əs) [Gordian knot] a genus of worms of the class Nematomorpha, the hair snakes or horsehair worms.
**G. aqua'ticus,** a species occasionally found as a pseudoparasite of the intestinal tract of humans; its presence is the result of the accidental ingestion of infected insects.
**G. robus'tus,** a species that is generally a pseudoparasite of the intestinal tract (see *G. aquaticus*), but has also been reported as invading the periorbital tissues of humans.

**Gor·don** (gor'dən) Alexander (1752–1799). Scottish obstetrician who, in his *Treatise on the Epidemic Puerperal Fever of Aberdeen* (1795), first demonstrated the contagiousness of this disease.

**Gor·don's reflex, sign** (gor'dənz) [Alfred *Gordon,* American neurologist, 1874–1953] see *flexor reflex, paradoxical,* under *reflex,* and *finger phenomenon* (def. 1), under *phenomenon.*

**Gor·don's syndrome** (Gor'dənz) [Richard D. *Gordon,* Australian physician, 20th century] see under *syndrome.*

**gor·get** (gor'jet) a wide-grooved lithotome director.

**Gor·ham's disease** (gor'əmz) [Lemuel Whittington *Gorham,* American physician, 1885–1968] disappearing bone disease.

**Gor·lin formula** (gor'lin) [Richard *Gorlin,* American cardiologist, born 1926] see under *formula.*

**Gor·lin's sign, syndrome** (gor'linz) [Robert James *Gorlin,* American oral pathologist and geneticist, born 1923] see under *sign* and see *basal cell nevus syndrome,* under *syndrome.*

**Gor·lin-Goltz syndrome** (gor'lin gōltz) [R. J. *Gorlin;* Robert William *Goltz,* American physician, born 1923] basal cell nevus syndrome.

**go·se·rel·in** (go'sə-rel″in) [MeSH: Goserelin] an analogue of gonadorelin used to treat malignancies of the prostate and breast because of its testosterone-suppressing action.
**g. acetate,** the acetate salt of goserelin, used to treat carcinoma of the breast and prostate; administered by subcutaneous implant.

**Gos·lee tooth** (goz'le) [Hart John *Goslee,* American dentist, 1871–1930] see under *tooth.*

**Gosse·lin's fracture** (gos-laz') [Léon Athanase *Gosselin,* French surgeon, 1815–1887] see under *fracture.*

**Gos·syp·i·um** (gŏ-sip'e-əm) [L.] cotton; a genus of tropical and subtropical plants of the family Malvaceae. Three species, *G. barbaden'se, G. herba'ceum,* and *G. hirsu'tum* yield most of the commercial cotton and are also sources of cottonseed and cottonseed oil.

**gos·syp·i·um** (gŏ-sip'e-əm) gen. *gossy'pii* [L.] cotton.
**g. asep'ticum, g. depura'tum, g. purifica'tum,** purified cotton.

**gos·sy·pol** (gos'ə-pol) [*Gossypium* + *-ol*] [MeSH: Gossypol] a poisonous yellow pigment, found in cottonseed and detoxified by heating; it has male antifertility properties, apparently having its effects in the seminiferous tubules. Gossypol poisoning (q.v.) occurs when cottonseed cakes containing excessive gossypol are fed to pigs.

**GOT** glutamine-oxaloacetic transaminase, now known as aspartate transaminase.

**Gott·lieb's epithelial attachment** (got'lēbz) [Bernhard *Gottlieb,* Austrian dentist, 1885–1950] see under *attachment.*

**Gott·ron's papules, sign** (got'ronz) [Heinrich Adolf *Gottron,* German dermatologist, 1890–1974] see under *papule* and *sign.*

**gouge** (gouj) a hollow chisel used in cutting and removing bone.
**Kelley g.,** an instrument for removing cartilage grafts.

**Gou·ger·ot-Blum syndrome** (goo-zher-o' bloom) [Henri *Gougerot,* French physician, 1881–1955; Paul *Blum,* French physician, 1878–1933] pigmented purpuric lichenoid dermatitis.

**Gou·ger·ot-Car·teaud syndrome** (goo-zher-o' kahr-to') [H. *Gougerot;* Alexandre *Carteaud,* French physician, born 1897] confluent and reticulated papillomatosis.

**Gou·ger·ot-Nu·lock-Houw·er syndrome** (goo-zher-o' noo'lok how'ər) [H. *Gougerot, Nulock,* A.W.M. *Houwer,* Dutch physician, 20th century] Sjögren's syndrome.

**Gou·ley's catheter** (goo'lēz) [John Williams Severin *Gouley,* American surgeon, 1832–1920] see under *catheter.*

**goun·dou** (gōōn-doo') [West African] a late sequel of yaws and endemic syphilis manifested by massive periostitis of the nasal processes of the maxillae, characterized by the formation of bony hornlike exostoses at the sides of the nose, leading to distortion of the facial features and destruction of the nose and orbit. Called also *anakhré.*

**gou·siek·te** (goo-sēk'te) [Afrikaans "rapid disease"] a condition in sheep and cattle marked by myocarditis, dilatation, and heart failure, caused by eating any of several poisonous plants including species of *Pavetta* and the shrub *Vangueria pygmora.*

**gout** (gout) [L. *gutta* a drop, because of the ancient belief that the disease was due to a "noxa" falling drop by drop into the joint] [MeSH: Gout] a group of disorders of purine metabolism, manifested by various combinations of (1) hyperuricemia; (2) recurrent acute inflammatory arthritis induced by crystals of monosodium urate monohydrate; (3) tophaceous deposits of these crystals in and around the joints of the extremities, which may lead to crippling destruction of joints; and (4) uric acid urolithiasis.
**abarticular g.,** that which does not affect the joints.
**articular g.,** gout affecting the joints.
**chalky g.,** tophaceous g.
**idiopathic g.,** a gout of uncertain classification; primary or secondary gout.
**irregular g.,** abarticular g.
**latent g., masked g.,** lithemia without the typical features of gout.
**lead g.,** gout ascribed to lead poisoning.
**oxalic g.,** oxalism.
**polyarticular g.,** an atypical form that attacks many joints.
**primary g.,** gout that seems to be innate, not a consequence of an acquired disorder or condition such as use of thiazide diuretics, and not secondary to an inborn error of metabolism such as glycogen storage disease, type I; it afflicts almost entirely men from the fourth to sixth decades, as well as a few postmenopausal women.
**regular g.,** articular g.
**saturnine g.,** lead g.
**secondary g.,** that resulting from an acquired disorder such as polycythemia vera or chronic myelogenous leukemia, or from an inborn error of metabolism.
**tophaceous g.,** gout in which there are tophi or chalky deposits of sodium urate.
**visceral g.,** a disease of birds characterized by the deposition of sodium urates on the viscera.

**gou·ty** (gou'te) affected with or of the nature of gout.

**Gow·ers' tract (column, fasciculus),** etc. (gou'ərz) [Sir William Richard *Gowers,* English neurologist, 1845–1915] see under *sign* and *solution,* see *tractus spinocerebellaris anterior,* see *vasovagal attack,* under *attack,* and see *late distal hereditary myopathy,* under *myopathy.*

**GP** general practitioner; general paresis.

**G6PD** glucose-6-phosphate dehydrogenase.

**GPI** general paralysis of the insane.

**GPT** glutamic-pyruvic transaminase; see *alanine transaminase.*

**gr** grain.

**graaf·i·an follicle, vesicle** (grah'fe-ən) [Reijnier (Regner) de *Graaf,* Dutch physician and anatomist, 1641–1673] see *folliculi ovarici vesiculosi.*

**Grac·i·la·ria** (gras″ĭ-lar'e-ə) a genus of seaweeds. *G. lichenoi'des* (L.) Harv. is Ceylon moss, used as food, as a source of agar, and in China as an antidysenteric.

**grac·ile** (gras'il) [L. *gracilis*] slender or delicate.

**Grac·i·lic·u·tes** (gras″ĭ-lik'u-tēz, grah-sil'ĭ-ku″tēz) [L. *gracilis* thin + *cutis*] a division of the kingdom Procaryotae comprising bacteria with a gram-negative type of cell wall consisting of an outer membrane and a thin inner peptidoglycan layer containing muramic acid. It contains three classes: Scotobacteria, Anoxyphotobacteria, and Oxyphotobacteria.

**Grad.** abbreviation for L. *grada'tim,* by degrees.

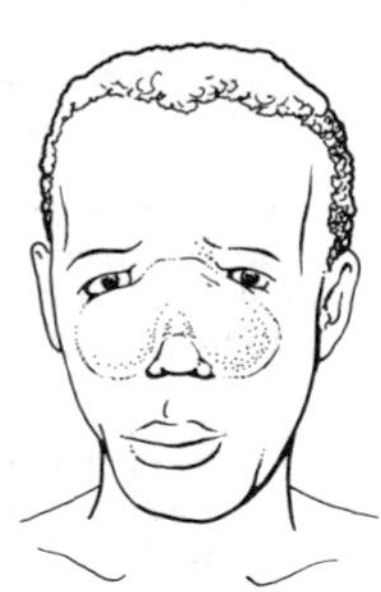

Goundou.

**gra·da·tim** (gra-da′tim) [L.] gradually; by degrees.

**grade** (grād) score.
**Gleason g.**, a rating of localized cancer of the prostate that assigns scores of 1 to 5 for degree of primary and secondary growth, with undifferentiated and destructive types having higher scores. Called also *Gleason score.*

**Gra·de·ni·go's syndrome** (grah-də-ne′gōz) [Giuseppe *Gradenigo,* Italian physician, 1859–1926] see under *syndrome.*

**gra·di·ent** (gra′de-ənt) 1. the increase or decrease of one variable expressed as a function of a second. 2. the graphic representation of such a change.
**density g.**, progressive variation in density over a distance; used particularly for that of a solute along the height or width of a confined solution; see also under *centrifugation.*
**electrochemical g.**, the difference in ion concentration and electrical potential from one point to another, so that ions tend to move passively along it.
**mitral g.**, the difference in pressure between the left atrium and the left ventricle in diastole.
**systolic g.**, the pressure difference between two communicating cardiac chambers or across a semilunar valve during systole.
**ventricular g.**, the net differences in ventricular electrical activity of varying duration, as determined by the algebraic sum of the electrocardiographic vectors representing the QRS and T-wave areas; as an index of duration of the excited state of the ventricles, it represents the local rate of repolarization.

**grad·u·ate** (graj′oo-ət) [L. *graduatus*] 1. a person who has received a degree from a university or college. 2. a measuring vessel marked by a series of lines.

**grad·u·at·ed** (graj′oo-āt″əd) [L. *gradus* step] marked by a succession of lines, steps, or degrees.

**Grae·fe's knife, operation, sign** (gra′fəz) [Albrecht Friedrich Wilhelm Ernst von *Graefe,* German ophthalmologist, 1828–1870] see under *knife,operation,* and *sign.*

**graft** (graft) 1. any tissue or organ for implantation or transplantation. 2. to implant or transplant such tissues. This term is preferred over *transplant* in the case of skin grafts. See also *implant.*
**accordion g.**, mesh g.
**activated g.**, a graft in which the nerves and blood supply have grown to nourish it, after a period of denervation and tenuous vascularity.
**allogeneic g.**, allograft.
**arteriovenous g.**, a means of arteriovenous access (q.v.) consisting of a venous autograft or xenograft or a synthetic tube, often made of polytef, grafted onto the artery and vein.
**autochthonous g.**, autograft.
**autodermic g., autoepidermic g.**, a skin graft taken from the patient's own body.
**autogenous g., autologous g., autoplastic g.**, autograft.
**avascular g.**, a graft of tissue in which not even transient vascularization is achieved.
**Blair-Brown g.**, a split-thickness skin graft of intermediate depth.
**bone g.**, bone transplanted from one site to another.
**brephoplastic g.**, the transplantation of tissue from an embryo or newborn to an adult animal.
**bypass g.**, an autograft consisting of a segment of vein or artery grafted into place in a bypass.
**cable g.**, a nerve graft made up of several sections of nerve in the manner of a cable.
**chorioallantoic g.**, the placing of cells, tissues, or parts on the chorioallantoic membrane of the embryonic chick.
**composite g.**, one that has more than one component, such as a bypass graft consisting of both a vein and a prosthesis.
**coronary artery bypass g. (CABG)**, see under *bypass.*
**cutis g.**, dermal g.
**Davis g.**, pinch g.
**delayed g.**, a skin graft which is sutured back into its bed and subsequently shifted to a new recipient bed.
**dermal g., dermic g.**, skin from which epidermis and subcutaneous fat have been removed; used instead of fascia in various plastic procedures. Called also *cutis g.*
**diced cartilage g's**, numerous small segments of cartilage that can be packed or molded into any desired contour like wet grains of sand; used to repair faulty cartilage or bone structure.
**epidermic g.**, a piece of epidermis implanted upon a raw surface; called also *Reverdin g.*
**Esser g.**, inlay g.
**fascia g.**, a graft taken from the fascia lata or from the lumbar fascia.
**fascicular g.**, a nerve graft in which the bundles of nerve fibers are approximated and sutured separately.
**fat g.**, a graft of fat completely freed from its bed; used in filling depressions.
**filler g.**, one used for the filling of defects, as the filling of depressions with fatty tissue or of a bony cyst cavity with bone chips or dried cartilage.
**free g.**, a graft of tissue completely freed from its bed, in contrast to a flap.
**full-thickness g.**, a skin graft consisting of the epidermis and the full depth of the dermis.
**heterodermic g.**, a skin graft taken from a donor of another species.
**heterologous g., heteroplastic g.**, xenograft.
**homologous g.**, allograft.
**homoplastic g.**, allograft.
**human umbilical vein g.**, a specially prepared umbilical vein used as an allograft.
**hyperplastic g.**, a skin graft that is in a state of active repair.
**inlay g.**, a skin or mucosal graft applied by spreading the graft over a stent and suturing the graft and mold into a prepared pocket; called also *Esser g.* and *Stent g.*
**island g.**, see under *flap.*
**isogeneic g., isologous g., isoplastic g.**, syngraft.
**jump g.**, see under *flap.*
**Kimura cartilage g.**, a split-thickness costal cartilage graft used in the management of tracheal stenosis.
**Krause-Wolfe g.**, a graft of full thickness of the skin.
**lamellar g.**, replacement of the superficial layers of an opaque cornea by a thin layer of clear cornea from a donor eye.
**mesh g.**, a thin split-thickness skin graft in which many tiny splits have been made to allow the graft to expand and be stretched to cover a large area.
**mucosal g.**, a graft of mucosal tissue, usually comprising the entire mucosal thickness.
**nerve g.**, replacement of an area of defective nerve with a segment from a sound one.
**Ollier-Thiersch g.**, a very thin skin graft consisting of epidermis and a thin layer of dermis, often cut in long, broad strips.
**omental g's**, free or attached segments of omentum used to cover suture lines following gastrointestinal or colonic surgery.
**onlay bone g.**, bone used as a graft that is laid on or over cortical bone of the recipient site(s).
**osseous g.**, bone g.
**outlay g.**, a modification of an inlay graft, used in ectropion of the eyelid.
**patch g.**, a graft of living tissue or prosthetic material used to repair a vascular incision in order to enlarge the lumen of the vessel.
**pedicle g.**, see under *flap.*
**penetrating g.**, a full-thickness corneal transplant.
**periosteal g.**, a piece of periosteum applied to a denuded area of a bone.
**Phemister g.**, a bone graft of cortical bone with cancellous bone chips to enhance callus formation.
**pinch g.**, a small split-thickness skin graft.
**Reverdin g.**, epidermic g.
**sieve g.**, a skin graft from which very small circular islands of skin are removed so that a larger denuded area can be covered, the sievelike portion being placed over one area, and the individual islands over surrounding or other denuded areas.
**skin g.**, skin transplanted to replace a lost portion of the body skin surface; it may be a full-thickness or split-thickness graft.
**sleeve g.**, a graft for repairing traumatic gaps in nerves by a sleevelike extension from the distal stump which is sutured to the central stump.
**split-skin g.**, a skin graft consisting of the epidermis and about one third of the dermis.
**split-thickness g.**, a skin graft consisting of the epidermis and a portion of dermis.
**Stent g.**, inlay g.
**syngeneic g.**, syngraft.
**thick-split g.**, a skin graft consisting of the epidermis and about two thirds of the dermis.
**Thiersch's g.**, Ollier-Thiersch g.
**thin-split g.**, Ollier-Thiersch g.
**tube g., tunnel g.**, tube flap.
**vein g.**, a bypass graft using a segment of vein, often the saphenous vein.
**white g.**, avascular g.
**Wolfe's g., Wolfe-Krause g.**, Krause-Wolfe g.
**xenogeneic g.**, xenograft.

**graft·ing** (graft′ing) transplantation; see also *graft.*
**skin g.**, implantation of patches of healthy skin on a denuded area to provide epithelial covering.

**Gra·ham's law** (gra′əmz) [Thomas *Graham,* British chemist, 1805–1869] see under *law.*

**Gra·ham's test** (gra′əmz) [Evarts Ambrose *Graham,* American surgeon, 1883–1957] see under *test.*

**Gra·ham Lit·tle syndrome** (gra′əm lit′əl) [Sir Ernest Gordon *Graham Little,* English physician, 1867–1950] see under *syndrome.*

**Gra·ham Steell murmur** (gra'əm stēl) [*Graham Steell,* English physician, 1851–1942] see under *murmur.*

**grain** (grān) [L. *gra'num*] 1. a seed, especially of a cereal plant. 2. the twentieth part of a scruple: 0.065 gram. Abbreviated gr. 3. an individual crystal of a metal or other crystalline structure.

**grain·age** (grān'əj) weight in grains or parts of a grain.

**Gram's method, stain, solution** (gramz) [Hans Christian Joachim *Gram,* Danish physician, 1853–1938] see under *stain,* and see *gram-negative* and *gram-positive.*

**gram** (gram) [Gr. *gramma* a small weight] the basic unit of mass of the CGS system; it is one thousandth of a kilogram and is equivalent to the weight of one milliliter of water at 4°C. Abbreviated gm. Symbol g.

**-gram** [Gr. *gramma* something drawn or written] a word termination meaning that which is drawn, written, or recorded.

**gram·i·ci·din** (gram"ĭ-si'din) [USP] [MeSH: Gramicidin] an antibiotic produced by *Bacillus brevis* that acts by damaging bacterial cell membranes. It is one of the two major components of tyrothricin, the other being tyrocidine. Gramicidin is applied topically in pyodermic, ocular, and other localized infections due to susceptible gram-positive organisms.

**gram·ine** (gram'ēn) a crystalline indole alkaloid found in barley; called also *donaxine.*

**Gra·min·eae** (grə-min'e-e) the grass family, a large family of plants that have hollow stems and slender leaves. Besides the plants popularly called *grass,* it includes food plants such as many grains and sugar cane.

**gram·i·niv·o·rous** (gram"ĭ- niv'ə-rəs) feeding or subsisting on grass or cereal grains.

**gram-neg·a·tive** (gram-neg'ə-tiv) losing the stain or decolorized by alcohol in Gram's method of staining, a primary characteristic of bacteria having a cell wall composed of a thin layer of peptidoglycan covered by an outer membrane of lipoprotein and lipopolysaccharide. Cf. *gram-positive.*

**gram-pos·i·tive** (gram-poz'ĭ-tiv) retaining the stain or resisting decolorization by alcohol in Gram's method of staining, a primary characteristic of bacteria whose cell wall is composed of a thick layer of peptidoglycan with attached teichoic acids. Cf. *gram-negative.*

**gra·na** (gra'nə) [pl. of L. *granum* grain] dense green, chlorophyll-containing bodies in chloroplasts consisting of numerous, closely packed lamellae which make them appear to be suspended in a matrix.

**gran·di·ose** (gran'de-ōs") in psychiatry, pertaining to exaggerated belief or claims of one's importance or identity, often manifested by delusions of great wealth, power, or fame.

**gran·di·os·i·ty** (gran"de-os'ĭ-te) the condition of being grandiose; an exaggerated belief of one's importance or identity.

**grand mal** (grahn mahl) [Fr.] see under *epilepsy.*

**Gran·ger line, sign** (grān'jər) [Amedee *Granger,* American radiologist, 1879–1939] see under *line* and *sign.*

**gran·i·se·tron** (grā-nĭ'sə-tron) an antiemetic used in conjunction with cancer chemotherapy; administered intravenously.

**Gran·it** (grahn'it) Ragnar Arthur. Finnish-born Swedish physiologist, 1900–1991; co-winner, with Haldan Keffer Hartline and George Wald, of the Nobel prize for medicine or physiology in 1967 for discoveries on the chemical and physiologic visual processes in the eye.

**Gra·nit's loop** (grahn'its) [R. A. *Granit*] gamma loop; see under *loop.*

**grano·plasm** (gran'o-plaz-əm) granular protoplasm.

**gran·u·la** (gran'u-lə) pl. *gran'ulae* [L.] 1. a small particle or grain. 2. granule, def. 2.
**g. iri'dica,** a black or brown outgrowth from the edge of the iris in cattle and horses; called also *nigroid body.*

**gran·u·lar** (gran'u-lər) [L. *granularis*] made up of or marked by presence of granules or grains.

**gran·u·la·tio** (gran"u-la'she-o) pl. *granulatio'nes* [L.] a general term denoting a granule, or granular mass.
**g.'nes arachnoi'deae** [TA], **g.'nes arachnoidea'les,** arachnoid granulations: small elevations, visible to the naked eye, thought by some to be enlargements of arachnoid villi, which project into the superior sagittal sinus and associated venous lacunae and create slight depressions on the inner surface of the cranium; these granulations are the structures through which cerebrospinal fluid is reabsorbed into the blood in the venous system. Called also *arachnoidal granulations* or *villi, cerebral granulations, meningeal granules,* and *pacchionian bodies, corpuscles,* or *granulations.*
**g.'nes cerebra'les,** granulationes arachnoideae.

**gran·u·la·tion** (gran"u-la'shən) [L. *granulatio*] 1. the process of forming granulation tissue. 2. the process of forming cytoplasmic granules. 3. granule (def. 1). 4. any granular material on the surface of a tissue, membrane, or organ. 5. the rendering of hard or metallic substances into granules or grains.
**arachnoid g's, arachnoidal g's,** granulationes arachnoideae.
**Bright's g's,** the granulations seen in chronic interstitial nephritis.
**cell g's,** small masses seen in the cytoplasm of certain cells that give the latter a characteristic appearance when stained; see the various granules, under *granule.*
**cerebral g's,** granulationes arachnoideae.
**exuberant g's,** excessive proliferation of granulation tissue in healing wounds.
**pacchionian g's,** granulationes arachnoideae.
**pyroninophilic g's,** structures seen in liver and other cells, which stain red with methyl green–pyronine by Pappenheim's stain; they are one of the early effects of carbon tetrachloride poisoning.
**Reilly g's,** large azurophilic granules in the cytoplasm of polymorphonuclear leukocytes and lymphocytes, occurring in Hurler's syndrome.
**Virchow's g's,** granulations containing ependymal and glial fibers, found in the walls of the cerebral ventricles in general paresis.

**gran·u·la·ti·o·nes** (gran"u-la"she-o'nēz) [L.] plural of *granulatio.*

**gran·ule** (gran'ūl) [L. *granulum*] 1. a small particle or grain, as the small beadlike masses of tissue formed on the surface of wounds, or the insoluble nonmembranous particles found in cytoplasm. 2. a small pill made from sucrose.
**acidophil g's,** 1. granules staining with acid dyes. 2. alpha g's (def. 3).
**acrosomal g.,** a large globule formed by the coalescence of proacrosomal granules, contained within a membrane-bounded *acrosomal vesicle,* which enlarges further to become the core of the acrosome of a spermatozoon.
**albuminous g's,** granules seen in the cytoplasm of many normal cells; they optically disappear on the addition of acetic acid, but are not affected by ether or chloroform; called also *cytoplasmic g's.*
**aleuronoid g's,** colorless myeloid colloidal bodies found in the base of pigment cells.
**alpha g's,** 1. the predominant type of granule found in platelets; they are round to oval in shape and contain fibrinogen, platelet factor 4, and various other proteins. 2. large granules in the alpha cells of the islets of Langerhans, which are insoluble in alcohol and contain glucagon. 3. the granules found in the acidophils (alpha cells) of the adenohypophysis. Called also *acidophil g's.*
**amphophil g's,** granules that stain with either acid or basic dyes.
**argentaffin g's,** granules that stain with silver.
**atrial g's,** specific atrial g's.
**azurophil g.,** 1. any granule that stains easily with azure dyes. See also *azurophilia.* 2. a type of azurophilic granule found in the promyelocyte; it contains numerous compounds that are antimicrobial, including myeloperoxidase. Called also *primary g.*
**Babès-Ernst g.,** metachromatic g.
**basal g.,** basal body.
**basophil g.,** 1. granules staining with basic dyes. 2. one of the coarse bluish-black granules found in basophils. 3. (in plural) beta granules (def. 2).
**beta g's,** 1. the granules in the beta cells of the islets of Langerhans, which contain insulin. 2. granules found in the basophils (beta cells) of the adenohypophysis; called also *basophil granules.*
**Birbeck g's,** membrane-bound, rod- or tennis racquet–shaped inclusions with a central linear, longitudinally striated nucleus, found in the cytoplasm of Langerhans' cells. Called also *Langerhans' g's* and *vermiform g's.*
**Bollinger's g's,** 1. small, yellowish white granules in mulberry-like masses, containing micrococci, seen in the granulation tissue of botryomycosis. 2. see under *body.*
**bull's eye g.,** dense body (def. 2).
**Bütschli's g's,** swellings on the bipolar rays of the amphiaster in the ovum.
**chromaffin g's,** organelles found in the chromaffin cells of the adrenal medulla, where epinephrine and norepinephrine are synthesized, stored, and released when needed.
**chromatic g's, chromophilic g's,** Nissl's bodies; see under *body.*
**cone g's,** the nuclei of the visual cells of the retina in its outer nuclear layer which are connected with the cones.
**cortical g's,** special structures in the cortex of the ovum of many animals, which break up during fertilization and supply the material for the development of the fertilization membrane.
**cytoplasmic g's,** albuminous g's.
**dense g.,** dense body (def. 2).
**Ehrlich's g's, Ehrlich-Heinz g's,** cell granules that stain with Ehrlich's triacid stain.
**elementary g's,** hemoconia.
**eosinophil g.,** one of the coarse round granules that stain with eosin and are found in eosinophils.

**fuchsinophil g's,** granules staining with fuchsin.
**Fordyce's g's,** ectopic sebaceous glands found on the lips and gums and in the mucosa of the cheeks, which present as yellowish white milia. Called also *Fordyce's disease* and *Fordyce's spots.*
**gamma g's,** a name applied to basophilic granules found in the blood, marrow, and in the tissues.
**gelatinase g.,** a type of neutrophil granule found primarily in mature cells and seen sedimenting out with specific granules in some fractionation techniques.
**Heinz g's,** Heinz-Ehrlich bodies.
**iodophil g's,** granules staining brown with iodine, seen in polymorphonuclear leukocytes in various acute infectious diseases.
**juxtaglomerular g's,** stainable osmophilic secretory granules present in the juxtaglomerular cells, closely resembling zymogen granules.
**kappa g.,** azurophil g. (def. 2).
**keratohyalin g's,** irregularly shaped granules, representing deposits of keratohyalin on tonofibrils in the stratum granulosum epidermidis. They stain with some acid dyes and with certain basic dyes. See also *keratohyalin,* def. 1.
**Kölliker's interstitial g's,** various sized granules seen in the sarcoplasm of muscle fibers.
**Kretz's g's,** granules found in the liver in cirrhosis.
**lamellar g.,** keratinosome.
**Langerhans' g's,** Birbeck g's.
**Langley's g's,** granules seen in secreting serous glands.
**membrane-coating g.,** keratinosome.
**meningeal g's,** granulationes arachnoideae.
**metachromatic g.,** a granular cell inclusion that stains a color different from that of the dye used. In certain bacteria, yeasts, yeastlike fungi, and protozoa, metachromatic granules appear red when stained with a blue dye. They are composed of complex polyphosphate, lipid, and nucleoprotein molecules (volutin) and serve as an intracellular phosphate reserve. Called also *Babès-Ernst body* or *granule.*
**monocytic g.,** one of the fine red azurophilic granules of a monocyte.
**Much's g's,** gram-positive, nonacid-fast granules and rods found in tuberculous sputum and thought to be modified tubercle bacilli.
**neutrophil g.,** any of the granules found in the cytoplasm of neutrophils; those in immature cells are called *primary* or *azurophil granules* and those in mature cells are called *secondary* or *specific granules.*
**Nissl's g's,** Nissl bodies.
**oxyphil g's,** acidophil g's.
**Paschen's g's,** see under *body.*
**perichromatin g's,** granules believed to contain nucleic acid, found near the masses of nuclear chromatin in the hepatic parenchymal cells.
**pigment g's,** small masses of coloring matter occurring in pigment cells.
**polar g's,** polar bodies, def. 2.
**primary g.,** azurophil g. (def. 2).
**proacrosomal g.,** any of the small, dense bodies found inside one of the vacuoles of the Golgi body, which fuse to form an acrosomal granule.
**protein g's,** microscopically observable particles of various proteins, some anabolic and others catabolic.
**rod g's,** the nuclei of rod visual cells in the outer nuclear layer of the retina that are connected with the rods.
**Schrön's g.,** a small body, of doubtful origin, seen in the germinal spot of the ovum.
**Schrön-Much g's,** Much's g's.
**Schüffner's g's,** see under *dot.*
**secondary g.,** specific g.
**secretory g's,** granules in secretory cells that apparently represent material that helps to form the secretion.
**seminal g's,** the small granular bodies seen in the spermatic fluid.
**specific g.,** a type of neutrophil granule found primarily in mature cells; most are released into the extracellular fluid. They contain lactoferrin, plasminogen activator, leukocyte alkaline activator, and collagenase, as well as membrane-bound molecules that they release onto the cell surface. Called also *secondary g.*
**specific atrial g's,** membrane-bound spherical granules with a dense homogeneous interior that are concentrated in the core of sarcoplasm of the atrial cardiac muscle, extending in either direction from the poles of the nucleus, usually near the Golgi complex; they also may be found in limited numbers in other regions of the cell. They are the storage site of atrial natriuretic peptide.
**sphere g.,** a large granular cell or corpuscle seen in serous exudation.
**sulfur g's,** peculiar granular bodies of a yellow color found in actinomycotic lesions and discharges.
**thread g's,** mitochondria.
**toxic g's,** dark-staining basophilic granules observed in neutrophils in infections and other toxic states; they are probably phagosomes or autophagic vacuoles.
**trichohyalin g's,** see *trichohyalin.*
**vermiform g's,** Birbeck g's.
**volutin g's,** see *volutin.*
**zymogen g's,** secretory granules in certain cells, containing the precursors of enzymes that become active after they have left the cell.

**gran·u·li·form** (gran'u-lĭ-form) in the form of, or resembling, small grains.

**gran·u·lo·ad·i·pose** (gran″u-lo-ad'ĭ-pōs) showing fatty degeneration that contains granules of fat.

**gran·u·lo·blast** (gran'u-lo-blast) former name for *myeloblast.*

**gran·u·lo·blas·to·sis** (gran″u-lo-blas-to'sis) myeloblastosis, def. 2.

**gran·u·lo·cor·pus·cle** (gran″u-lo-kor'pəs-əl) a small corpuscle observed in infected tissue in lymphogranuloma venereum.

**gran·u·lo·cyte** (gran'u-lo-sīt″) [*granulo-* + *-cyte*] [MeSH: Granulocytes] 1. any cell containing granules. 2. granular leukocyte.
**band-form g.,** band cell.
**segmented g.,** see under *cell.*

**gran·u·lo·cyt·ic** (gran″u-lo-sit'ik) 1. pertaining to, characterized by, or of the nature of granulocytes. 2. pertaining to the granulocytic series; see under *series.*

**gran·u·lo·cy·top·a·thy** (gran″u-lo-si-top'ə-the) any disorder of the granular leukocytes (granulocytes).

**gran·u·lo·cy·to·pe·nia** (gran″u-lo-si″to-pe'ne-ə) [*granulocyte* + *-penia*] reduction in the number of granular leukocytes in the blood. Cf. *agranulocytosis.* Called also *granulopenia* and *hypogranulocytosis.*

**gran·u·lo·cy·to·poi·e·sis** (gran″u-lo-si″to-poi-e'sis) granulopoiesis.

**gran·u·lo·cy·to·poi·et·ic** (gran″u-lo-si″to-poi-et'ik) granulopoietic.

**gran·u·lo·cy·to·sis** (gran″u-lo-si-to'sis) an abnormally large number of granulocytes in the blood.

**gran·u·lo·fat·ty** (gran″u-lo-fat'e) granuloadipose.

**gran·u·lo·ma** (gran″u-lo'mə) pl. *granulomas* or *granulo'mata* [*granul-* + *-oma*] [MeSH: Granuloma] an imprecise term applied to (1) any small nodular delimited aggregation of mononuclear inflammatory cells, or (2) such a collection of modified macrophages resembling epithelial cells *(epithelioid cells),* usually surrounded by a rim of lymphocytes, often with multinucleated giant cells. Some granulomas contain eosinophils and plasma cells, and fibrosis is commonly seen around the lesion. Granuloma formation represents a chronic inflammatory response initiated by various infectious and noninfectious agents. See also *granulomatosis.*
**acral lick g.,** see under *dermatitis.*
**actinic g.,** an annular lesion seen on skin chronically exposed to the sun; the border is raised and contains many histiocytes and giant cells, while the center may appear normal but is actually elastotic. See also *granulomatous cheilitis,* under *cheilitis.* Called also *Miescher's g.*
**amebic g.,** granulomatous lesions of the colon sometimes seen in amebiasis.
**g. annula're,** a benign, usually self-limited granulomatous disease of unknown etiology, chiefly involving the dermis, clinically characterized by annularly grouped, localized or disseminated, perforating papules or subcutaneous nodules, which predominantly affects female children. Histopathologic findings include the presence of palisading histiocytes surrounding foci of altered collagen (necrobiosis) in the mid and upper dermis.
**apical g.,** periapical g.
**beryllium g.,** a complication of chronic berylliosis, consisting of a chronic, local, noncaseating, sarcoidlike granulomatous reaction, usually in the lungs; it often progresses to fibrosis and hyalinization.
***Candida* g.,** candidal g.
**candidal g.,** a rare response to invasive candidiasis of the skin, usually seen in immunocompromised children; there are granulomatous lesions on the face, scalp, fingernails, trunk, legs, or pharynx, with primary vascularized papules covered with thick, adherent, yellow-brown crusts, sometimes developing into horns or protrusions. Called also *monilial g.*
**canine venereal g.,** canine transmissible venereal tumor.
**cholesterol g.,** a granulomatous lesion in which crystals of cholesterol esters are surrounded by foreign-body giant cells in a mass of fibrotic granulation tissue.
**coccidioidal g.,** secondary coccidioidomycosis.
**collagenolytic g.,** equine nodular necrobiosis.
**dental g.,** periapical g.
**eosinophilic g.,** 1. Langerhans cell histiocytosis. 2. a disorder similar to eosinophilic gastroenteritis and characterized by localized nodular or pedunculated lesions of the gastric submucosa and muscle walls, especially of the pyloric area of the stomach, caused by infiltration of eosinophils, but without peripheral eosinophilia and allergic symptoms. It may also affect the small intestine. 3. anisak-

iasis in humans. 4. see *eosinophilic granuloma complex,* under *complex.*

**g. fissura'tum,** a circumscribed, firm, reddish, fissured, fibrotic granuloma of the gum and buccal mucosa, occurring on an edentulous alveolar ridge and in the fold between the ridge and cheek; it is caused by an ill-fitting denture.

**foreign-body g.,** a localized histiocytic skin reaction to a foreign body in the tissue, such as starch, talc, or oil.

**g. fungoi'des,** mycosis fungoides.

**g. gangraenes'cens,** a condition beginning with the formation of proliferating granulations in the nasal mucous membrane which invade the adjacent tissues and soon become gangrenous.

**giant cell reparative g., central,** a lesion of the jaws considered by some authorities to be a giant cell tumor occurring in both benign and malignant forms, and by others as a form of osteogenic sarcoma, varying in degree of malignancy. Most consider it to be a central lesion of the bone of the jaws, presenting an inflammatory reaction to injury or hemorrhage, which is not regarded as a true neoplasm. It is composed of a spindle cell stroma punctuated by multinucleate giant cells.

**giant cell reparative g., peripheral,** giant cell epulis.

**g. glutea'le infan'tum,** a dermatosis occurring in the diaper area or buttocks of infants, characterized clinically by the development of oval, hemangioma-like or hematoma-like nodules, and histologically by hyperkeratosis and acanthosis, associated with a polymorphonuclear infiltrate mixed with plasma cells, histiocytes, and macrophages throughout the dermis. Spontaneous recovery usually occurs.

**Hodgkin's g.,** see under *disease.*

**infectious g.,** a granulomatous lesion due to an infectious agent, such as a bacterium or fungus.

**g. inguina'le,** a chronic, slowly progressive, ulcerative granulomatous disease, assumed to be sexually transmitted, caused by *Calymmatobacterium granulomatis,* and primarily involving the skin and lymphatics of the anogenital region but sometimes spreading to the perineum and perianal area or the inguinal region; it occurs principally in the tropics and is usually seen in dark-skinned people even in temperate areas, where it is rare. Called also *donovanosis, fourth venereal disease, g. pudendi, g. venereum,* and *pudendal ulcer.*

**laryngeal g.,** a firm nodule on the larynx due to trauma, particularly from endotracheal intubation or from excessive use of the voice.

**lethal midline g.,** a progressive, localized, destructive process occurring chiefly in males, predominantly involving the nose, paranasal sinuses, and palate, with erosion through contiguous structures such as the orbit and face and destruction of soft tissue, bone, and cartilage, and associated with nonspecific acute and chronic inflammation and necrosis with or without granuloma formation. Called also *midline g.*

**linear g.,** a skin lesion of young cats, consisting of circumscribed raised discolored linear plaques, usually on the posterior thigh but sometimes on the lips or in the mouth. It is part of the eosinophilic granuloma complex.

**lipoid g.,** a granuloma containing lipoid cells; xanthoma.

**lipophagic g.,** a granuloma attended by the loss of subcutaneous fat.

**Majocchi's g.,** trichophytic g.

**malarial g.,** a granulomatous lesion sometimes seen in the brain in fatal cases of cerebral malaria.

**midline g.,** lethal midline g.

**Miescher's g.,** actinic g.

**Mignon's eosinophilic g.,** a solitary destructive lesion affecting the skull and other bones of children and young adults.

**monilial g.,** candidal g.

**g. multifor'me,** a condition seen in Nigerian women, presumed to be an atypical form of granuloma annulare, characterized by the presence of multiple, sometimes very large, papulonodular circinate lesions, accompanied by plaques and nodules, which usually heal spontaneously without residual scarring but often with some hypopigmentation.

**paracoccidioidal g.,** paracoccidioidomycosis.

**periapical g.,** a slowly expanding, spherical, granulomatous lesion adjacent to the root apex of a tooth, usually occurring as a complication of pulpitis, which consists of a proliferating mass of chronic inflammatory tissue enclosed within a fibrous capsule that is an extension of the periodontal ligament. Called also apical g. and chronic apical periodontitis.

**plasma cell g.,** granuloma in which other inflammatory cells are very greatly outnumbered by plasma cells.

**pseudopyogenic g.,** a superficial variant of angiolymphoid hyperplasia.

**g. puden'di,** g. inguinale.

**g. pu'dens tro'picum,** g. inguinale.

**pyogenic g., g. pyoge'nicum,** a usually solitary polypoid capillary hemangioma often associated with trauma or local irritation, representing a vasoproliferative inflammatory response, found on the skin and gingival or oral mucosa, which presents as a small erythematous papule that enlarges and may become pedunculated and

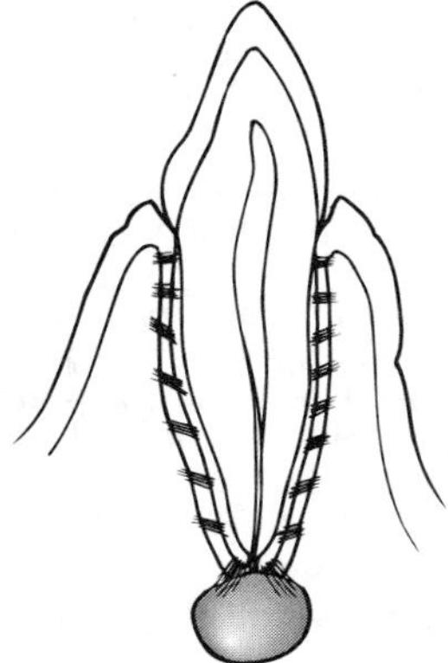

Periapical granuloma.

may become infected and ulcerate with accompanying purulent exudate. Called also *g. telangiectaticum.* See also *pregnancy tumor,* under *tumor.* Cf. *angiogranuloma.*

**reticulohistiocytic g.,** a solitary reticulohistiocytoma, seen mainly in men, which is not associated with systemic involvement, as in multicentric reticulohistiocytosis. Called also *reticulohistiocytoma.*

**rheumatic g's,** nodules occurring in various parts of the body in rheumatic fever.

**sarcoid g.,** the granuloma seen with sarcoidosis, consisting of multinucleated giant cells surrounded by macrophages and epithelioid cells derived from macrophages.

**silicotic g.,** granuloma induced by silica particles.

**swimming pool g.,** a chronic granulomatous bacterial infection caused by contamination of an abrasion sustained in a swimming pool by *Mycobacterium marinum,* which histologically and clinically resembles tuberculosis. It is characterized by the development of a reddish papule or pustule at the site of inoculation that enlarges and may break down and become covered by a brownish crust; it tends to heal spontaneously within a few months to 2 years.

**g. telangiecta'ticum,** pyogenic g.

**trichophytic g., g. trichophy'ticum,** a rare form of tinea corporis of the lower legs, also infecting the hairs, caused by *Trichophyton rubrum;* it is characterized by elevated, circumscribed, boggy red to blue granulomas, either disseminated or in chains; after persisting for several months the lesions are slowly absorbed or undergo necrosis, leaving depressed scars. Called also *Majocchi's g.* and *tinea profunda.*

**umbilical g.,** granulation tissue on the stem of the umbilical cord in newborn infants.

**g. vene'reum,** g. inguinale.

**xanthomatous g.,** eosinophilic g.

**zirconium g.,** a papular granulomatous eruption consisting of brownish red, dome-shaped, shiny lesions representing an allergic reaction to the zirconium ion or salts, which may be components of certain antiperspirants, deodorants, and lotions used in the treatment of poison ivy.

**gran·u·lo·ma·to·sis** (gran″u-lo″mə-to′sis) any condition characterized by the formation of multiple granulomas.

**allergic g.,** Churg-Strauss syndrome.

**bronchocentric g.,** a rare disorder consisting of necrosis of the walls of the lower airways, filling of the lumen with granular necrotic material, and eventually areas of lung consolidation; many cases are due to a hypersensitivity reaction to infection by fungi, such as with allergic bronchopulmonary aspergillosis.

**g. discifor'mis progressi'va et chro'nica,** a condition clinically resembling necrobiosis lipoidica in nondiabetics (and believed by some authorities to be a variant), characterized by the development on the dorsa of the hands, forearms, shins, and sometimes the face of yellowish red, sharply marginated, smooth, plaquelike granulomas with a tendency to enlarge peripherally.

**eosinophilic g.,** Langerhans cell histiocytosis.

**Langerhans cell g.,** see under *histiocytosis.*

**lipophagic intestinal g.,** Whipple's disease.

**lymphomatoid g.,** an immunoproliferative disorder that is angiogenic and characterized by tissue infiltration and nodular granulomatous inflammation with atypical lymphocytes and plasmacytoid cells; the organs involved are usually the lungs, skin, central nervous system, or kidneys. Presenting symptoms include cough, shortness of breath, and chest pain; extrapulmonary manifestations are common, such as skin nodules.

**necrotizing sarcoid g., necrotizing sarcoidal g.,** a rare lung condition characterized by focal areas of vasculitis with necrosis and confluent granulomas; it resembles sarcoidosis and usually has a benign course.

**g. sidero'tica,** a condition in which brownish nodules (Gamna nodules) are seen in the enlarged spleen.
**Wegener's g.,** a multisystem disease chiefly affecting males, characterized by necrotizing granulomatous vasculitis involving the upper and lower respiratory tracts, glomerulonephritis, and variable degrees of systemic, small vessel vasculitis; it is generally considered to be an aberrant hypersensitivity reaction to an unknown antigen.

**gran·u·lom·a·tous** (gran″u-lom'ə-təs) containing granulomas.

**gran·u·lo·mere** (gran'u-lo-mēr″) the center portion of a platelet, which in a dry, stained blood smear appears to be filled with fine purplish granules; it is surrounded by the hyalomere. Called also *chromomere.*

**gran·u·lo·pe·nia** (gran″u-lo-pe'ne-ə) granulocytopenia.

**gran·u·lo·plasm** (gran'u-lo-plaz'əm) endoplasm.

**gran·u·lo·plas·tic** (gran″u-lo-plas'tik) [*granule* + *plastic*] forming granules.

**gran·u·lo·poi·e·sis** (gran″u-lo-poi-e'sis) [*granulocyte* + *-poiesis*] the production or formation of granulocytes; see also *granulocytic series,* under *series.* Called also *granulocytopoiesis.*

**gran·u·lo·poi·et·ic** (gran″u-lo-poi-et'ik) pertaining to or concerned in the formation of granulocytes.

**gran·u·lo·poi·e·tin** (gran″u-lo-poi'ə-tin) a hypothesized substance, probably a colony-stimulating factor, that serves as the humoral regulator of granulopoiesis. Called also *leukopoietin.*

**gran·u·lo·po·tent** (gran″u-lo-po'tənt) capable of forming granules.

**Gran·u·lo·re·tic·u·lo·sea** (gran″u-lo-rə-tik″u-lo'se-ə) [*granulo-* + *reticular*] a class of ameboid protozoa (superclass Rhizopoda, subphylum Sarcodina), the organisms of which have delicate, finely granular or hyaline reticulopodia or, rarely, finely pointed, granular but nonanastomosing pseudopodia. It includes three orders: Athalamida, Monothalamida, and Foraminiferida.

**gran·u·lo·sa** (gran″u-lo'sə) cumulus oophorus; see also under *cell.*

**gran·u·lose** (gran'u-lōs) 1. a bacterial polysaccharide resembling amylopectin, occurring as cytoplasmic granules and staining red violet with iodine. 2. having a granular appearance.

**gran·u·lo·sis** (gran″u-lo'sis) the formation of a mass of granules.
**g. ru'bra na'si,** sweating and hyperhidrosis confined to the nose and surrounding area of the face and sometimes the chin, associated with red papules and sometimes many small vesicles; it occurs most often in children, usually clearing up at puberty. There is some evidence that an inheritable trait is involved in the etiology.

**gran·u·los·i·ty** (gran″u-los'ĭ-te) a mass of granulations.

**gran·u·lo·vac·u·o·lar** (gran″u-lo-vak'u-o-lər) characterized by granules and vacuoles.

**gra·num** (gra'nəm) pl. *gra'na* [L.] grain; see *grana.*

**grapes** (grāps) bovine tuberculosis.

**graph** (graf) [Gr. *graphein* to write, or record] a diagram or curve representing varying relationships between sets of data.

**-graph** a word termination denoting an instrument for writing or recording; also, the record made by such an instrument.

**graph·es·the·sia** (graf″əs-the'zhə) [*graph-* + *esthesia*] the sense by which figures or numbers are recognized when written on the skin with a dull-pointed object.

**graph·ic** (graf'ik) [*graph-* + *-ic*] written or drawn; pertaining to representation by diagrams.

**graph·ite** (graf'īt) [L. *graphites,* from Gr. *graphis* a writing instrument] [MeSH: Graphite] a form of native mineralized carbon; inhalation of its dust causes a form of pneumoconiosis. Called also *plumbago.*

**graph·i·to·sis** (graf″ĭ-to'sis) graphite pneumoconiosis.

**Graph·i·um** (graf'e-əm) a genus of imperfect fungi of the form-class Hyphomycetes that produce several cultural spore types; inhalation of sawdust containing the spores causes sequoiosis.

**graph(o)-** [Gr. *graphein* to write] a combining form denoting relationship to writing or to a record.

**grapho·anal·y·sis** (graf″o-ə-nal'ə-sis) analysis of personality based on handwriting.

**gra·phol·o·gy** (graf-ol'ə-je) [*grapho-* + *-logy*] the study of handwriting, applied to personal identification or psychological study of the writer.

**grapho·mo·tor** (graf″o-mo'tor) [*grapho-* + *motor*] pertaining to, or affecting, the movements required in writing.

**graph·or·rhea** (graf″o-re'ə) [*grapho-* + *-rrhea*] the writing of a long succession of meaningless and unconnected words.

**grapho·spasm** (graf'o-spaz-əm) [*grapho-* + *spasm*] writer's cramp.

**-graphy** [Gr. *-graphia,* from *graphein* to write] a word termination meaning the process of writing or recording, or a method of recording.

**grass** (gras) any plant of the family Gramineae; many are commonly used as fodder for cattle and horses, and the family also includes food plants such as grains and sugar cane. Grasses whose pollen is important as a cause of hay fever include Bermuda grass *(Cynodon dactylon);* Kentucky bluegrass or June grass *(Poa pratensis);* Johnson grass *(Sorghum halepense);* orchard grass *(Dactylis glomerata);* redtop grass *(Agrostis alba);* sweet vernal grass *(Anthoxanthum odoratum);* and timothy or timothy grass *(Phleum pratense).* Johnson grass, Sudan grass, and arrow grass (*Triglochin* species) contain cyanogenetic compounds; timothy sometimes contains the mold *Claviceps purpurea;* and sweet vernal grass contains dicumarol. Any of these, when eaten in large quantities, can be fatal to livestock.
**canary g.,** any of various species of grasses of the genus *Phalaris.* See also *P. staggers,* under *staggers.*
**couch g.,** the perennial grass *Agropyrum repens;* its long roots are diuretic, demulcent, and antitussive and have been used to treat cystitis.
**panic g.,** any of several members of the genus *Panicum.*
**scurvy g.,** *Cochlearia officinalis.*

**Gras·set's phenomenon (sign)** (grah-sāz') [Joseph *Grasset,* French physician, 1849–1918] see under *phenomenon.*

**Gras·set-Bychowski sign** (grah-sa' bi-kof'ske) [J. *Grasset;* Zygmunt *Bychowski,* Polish neurologist, 1860–1935] Grasset's phenomenon; see under *phenomenon.*

**Gras·set-Gaus·sel phenomenon** (grah-sa'go-sel') [J. *Grasset;* Amans *Gaussel,* French physician, 1871–1937] Grasset's phenomenon; see under *phenomenon.*

**Gras·set-Gaus·sel-Hoo·ver sign** (grah-sa'go-sel'hoo'vər) [J. *Grasset;* A. *Gaussel;* Charles Franklin *Hoover,* American physician, 1865–1927] see under *sign.*

**grat·ing** (gra'ting) a grill or grid, or something resembling such a structure.
**diffraction g.,** a surface, usually glass or polished metal, that is ruled closely with fine parallel lines, grooves, or slits; used to separate the wavelengths of light in spectroscopes.

**Gra·ti·o·la** (grə-ti'o-lə) a genus of small herbs of the family Scrophulaceae. *G. officina'lis* is the hedge hyssop, a European species used as a purgative, emetic, and diuretic.

**Gra·ti·o·let's radiating fibers, radiation** (grah-te″o-lāz') [Louis Pierre *Gratiolet,* French anatomist, 1815–1865] see under *fiber,* and see *radiatio optica.*

**grat·tage** (grah-tahzh') [Fr.] the removal of granulations (as in trachoma) by scraping or by friction with a stiff brush.

**grave** (grāv) [L. *gravis*] severe or serious.

**grav·el** (grav'əl) a term applied to fairly coarse concretions of mineral salts, as from the kidneys or bladder, of smaller size than the so-called stones.

**Graves' disease, orbitopathy (ophthalmopathy)** (grāvz) [Robert James *Graves,* Irish physician, 1796–1853] [MeSH: Graves' Disease] see under *disease* and *orbitopathy.*

**grave-wax** (grāv'waks) adipocere.

**grav·id** (grav'id) [L. *gravida* heavy, pregnant] pregnant.

**grav·i·da** (grav'ĭ-də) [L.] a pregnant woman. Called *gravida I* or *primigravida* during the first pregnancy, *gravida II* or *secundigravida* during the second pregnancy, *gravida III* or *tertigravida* during the third pregnancy, and so on. Symbol G. Cf. *para.*

**gra·vid·ic** (grə-vid'ik) occurring in pregnancy.

**grav·id·ism** (grav'id-iz-əm) pregnancy, or the sum of symptoms, signs, and conditions associated with it.

**gra·vid·i·tas** (grə-vid'ĭ-təs) [L.] pregnancy.
**g. examnia'lis,** pregnancy in which the amnion has burst and is retracted around the insertion of the umbilical cord, but the chorion is intact.
**g. exochoria'lis,** pregnancy in which the membranes have burst and shrunk, leaving the fetus in the uterus but outside of the chorion.

**gra·vid·i·ty** (grah-vid'ĭ-te) [L. *graviditas,* q.v.] pregnancy; the condition of being pregnant, without regard to the outcome. Cf. *parity.*

**grav·i·do·car·di·ac** (grav″ĭ-do-kahr'de-ak) [*gravida* + *cardiac*] pertaining to heart disease of pregnancy.

**grav·i·do·pu·er·per·al** (grav″ĭ-do-pu-er'pər-əl) [*gravida* + *puerperal*] pertaining to pregnancy and the puerperium.

**gra·vim·e·ter** (grə-vim'ə-tər) [L. *gravis* heavy + *-meter*] an instrument for determining specific gravities.

**grav·i·met·ric** (grav″ĭ-met'rik) pertaining to measurement by weight; performed by weight, as gravimetric method of drug assay.

**grav·i·ta·tion** (grav″ĭ-ta′shən) [MeSH: Gravitation] the phenomenon of attraction between massive bodies; see *law of gravitation.*

**grav·i·tom·e·ter** (grav″ĭ-tom′ə-tər) a balance for measuring specific gravity.

**grav·i·ty** (grav′ĭ-te) [L. *gravitas*] the force of gravitational attraction at the surface of the earth or other body.
**specific g.**, the ratio of the density of a substance to that of a reference substance at a specific temperature.
**standard g.**, the acceleration due to gravity at mean sea level, 9.80616 meters per second squared. Symbol *g.* Called also *acceleration of gravity.*

**Gra·witz's tumor** (grah′vits-əz) [Paul Albert *Grawitz,* German pathologist, 1850–1932] see under *tumor.*

**gray** (gra) 1. of a hue between white and black. 2. a unit of absorbed radiation dose equal to 100 rads. Abbreviated Gy.
**silver g., steel g.**, nigrosin.

**gray·a·no·tox·in** (gra′ə-no-tok″sin) andromedotoxin.

**grease** (grēs) greasy heel.

**grease-heel** (grēs-hēl′) greasy heel.

**green** (grēn) 1. having the color of fresh leaves or of grass. 2. a green coloring matter or dye.
**acid g.**, any of several green acid dyes, generally light g. SF.
**brilliant g.**, a basic dye having powerful bacteriostatic properties for gram-positive organisms.
**bromcresol g.**, an indicator, tetrabromo-*m*-cresolsulfonphthalein, used in the determination of hydrogen ion concentration, being yellow at pH 4.0 and blue at pH 5.4. Written also *bromocresol g.*
**diazin g. S,** Janus g. B.
**ethyl g.**, brilliant g.
**fast g. FCF,** a green acid dye used as a histologic stain for plasma and collagen.
**fast acid g. N,** light g. S F yellowish.
**Hoffman g.**, iodine g.
**indocyanine g.** [USP], a tricarbocyanine dye occurring as an olive-brown, dark green, dark blue, or black powder; used intravenously as a diagnostic aid in the determination of blood volume, cardiac output, and hepatic function.
**iodine g.**, a triphenylmethane dye used as a chromatin stain.
**Janus g. B,** an azo dye used supravitally for the demonstration of mitochondria.
**light g., 2 G or 2 GN,** light g. SF yellowish.
**light g. N,** malachite g.
**light g. SF,** see *acid g.*
**light g. SF yellowish,** an acid dye used as a plasma stain.
**malachite g.**, a triphenylmethane dye used as a stain for bacteria and as an antiseptic for wounds.
**malachite g. G,** brilliant g.
**methyl g.**, 1. a green basic triphenylmethane dye used as a histologic counterstain and as the DNA-staining component of methyl green–pyronin stain. 2. brilliant g.
**methylene g.**, a dye formed by nitrating methylene blue, interesting for its dark green metachromasia; it is a componenet of polychrome methylene blue.
**new solid g.**, malachite g.
**Paris g.**, copper acetoarsenite.
**Schweinfurt g.**, copper acetoarsenite.
**solid g.**, malachite g.
**Victoria g.**, malachite g.

**Green·field's disease** (grēn′fēldz) [Joseph Godwin *Greenfield,* British pathologist, 1884–1958] metachromatic leukodystrophy (infantile form); see under *leukodystrophy.*

**Green·field filter** (grēn′fēld) [Lazar J. *Greenfield,* American surgeon, 20th century] see under *filter.*

**greg·a·loid** (greg′ə-loid) [L. *grex* flock + *-oid*] see under *colony.*

**Greig's syndrome** (gregz) [David Middleton *Greig,* Scottish physician, 1864–1936] ocular hypertelorism; see under *hypertelorism.*

**grep·a·flox·a·cin hy·dro·chlo·ride** (grep″ə-flok′sə-sin) a fluoroquinolone antibacterial with activity against a wide variety of microorganisms, used in the treatment of bronchitis, pneumonia, cervicitis, urethritis, and gonorrhea due to susceptible organisms; administered orally.

**GRH** growth hormone–releasing hormone.

**grid** (grid) 1. an arrangement of thin lead strips separated by a radiolucent material; used to reduce the amount of scattered radiation reaching the x-ray film. 2. a chart with horizontal and perpendicular lines for plotting curves.
**baby g.**, a direct reading control chart on infant growth.
**crossed g.**, two parallel grids arranged so that the lead strips of one are at right angles to the lead strips of the other.
**focused g.**, a parallel grid in which the lead strips are angled so that they all point toward a focus at a specified distance.
**moving g.**, a parallel grid that is moved continuously or oscillated throughout the making of a radiograph; used to eliminate the grid lines that occur with the use of a stationary grid.
**parallel g.**, in radiography, one in which the lead strips are oriented parallel to each other; rather than angled as in a focused grid.
**Potter-Bucky g.**, a type of parallel grid that is an integral part of the x-ray table, located below the table top and above a cassette tray. It decreases the amount of secondary radiation reaching the film, thus increasing detail and contrast, and moves during exposure so that no grid lines appear in the radiograph.
**stationary g.**, a parallel grid placed in apposition to a radiographic film for its accentuation of detail; the grid lines will be visible on the resultant radiographs.
**Wetzel g.**, a direct reading chart for evaluating physical fitness in terms of body build, developmental level, and basal metabolism.

**grief** (grēf) [MeSH: Grief] the normal emotional response to an external and consciously recognized loss; it involves a period of mourning and generally is self-limited, gradually subsiding within a reasonable time. See also *mourning.*

**Grie·sin·ger's disease, sign** (gre′zing-erz) [Wilhelm *Griesinger,* German neurologist, 1817–1868] see *hookworm disease,* under *disease,* and see under *sign.*

**Grif·fith's sign** (grif′iths) [J. *Griffith,* English ophthalmologist, late 19th century] see under *sign.*

**Grig·nard's reagent (compound)** (grēn-yahrz′) [François Auguste Victor *Grignard,* French chemist, 1871–1935] see under *reagent.*

**Gri·ful·vin** (grĭ-ful′vin) trademark for a preparation of griseofulvin.

**grind·ing** (grīnd′ing) 1. rubbing together with force; wearing away or polishing by rubbing. 2. crushing of food by the posterior teeth in mastication, especially by molars. 3. bruxism. 4. shaping of a tooth contour through the use of abrasive tools. See also *occlusal adjustment,* under *adjustment.*
**selective g.**, modification of the occlusal forms of teeth by grinding at selected places.
**spot g.**, elimination of high places or occlusal interferences on natural dentitions or dentures by grinding.

**grind·ing-in** (grind′ing-in) the process of correcting errors in the centric and eccentric occlusions of natural or artificial teeth. See also *milling-in.*

**grip** (grip) 1. [Fr. *grippe*] influenza. 2. a grasping or seizing.
**devil's g.**, epidemic pleurodynia.
**hook g.**, a functional posture of the hand, as that usually assumed when grasping handles or straps or suspending or pulling upon an object: the fingers are flexed toward the palm, to a degree depending on the size of the grasped object.
**power g.**, a functional posture of the hand, as that usually assumed when holding a hammer or piece of rope: the fingers are flexed around an object, with counter pressure from the thumb, which is positioned to bring either its pad or its medial border firmly against the held object.
**precision g.**, a functional posture of the hand, as that usually assumed when holding a pen or pencil: the object is grasped between the tips of the thumb and fingers (most often the index, with the middle often involved).

**grip·pal** (grip′əl) influenzal.

**grippe** (grip; Fr. grēp) influenza.
**g. aurique** (o-rēk′), [Fr. "gold influenza"], a polyneuritis sometimes resulting from the therapeutic use of gold salts.

**Gris·ac·tin** (gris-ak′tin) trademark for a preparation of griseofulvin.

**Gris·cel·li syndrome** (grĭ-sel′e) [Claude *Griscelli,* French physician, born 1936] see under *syndrome.*

**Gri·sel's syndrome** (gre-zelz′) [P. *Grisel,* French physician, 20th century] see under *syndrome.*

**gris·eo·ful·vin** (gris″e-o-ful′vin) [USP] [MeSH: Griseofulvin] an antibiotic for humans and domestic animals, produced by *Penicillium griseofulvum* or by other means; used as an antifungal in the treatment of dermatophytic infections of the skin and nails. Adminis-

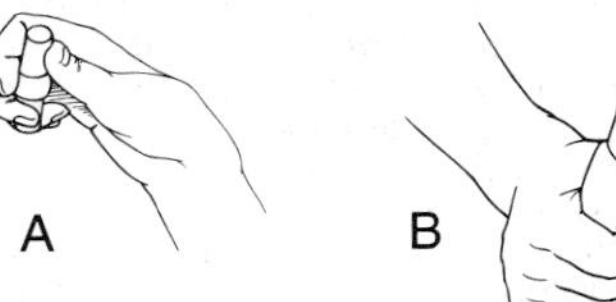

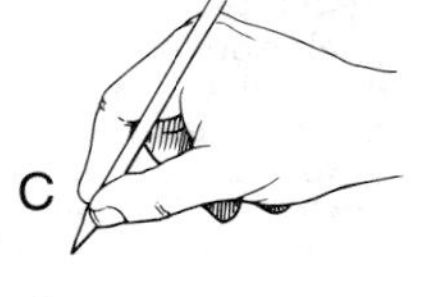


*(A),* Hook grip; *(B),* power grip; *(C),* precision grip.

tered orally to humans and small animals and as a feed additive to large animals.

**gris·eo·my·cin** (gris″e-o-mi′sin) proactinomycin B.

**Gris-PEG** (gris′peg) trademark for a preparation of griseofulvin.

**Grit·ti's amputation (operation)** (gre′tēz) [Rocco *Gritti,* Italian surgeon, 1828–1920] see under *amputation.*

**Grit·ti-Stokes amputation** (gre′te-stōks) [Rocco *Gritti;* Sir William Stokes, Irish surgeon, 1839–1900] see under *amputation.*

**Groc·co's sign (triangle, triangular dullness)** (grok′ōz) [Pietro *Grocco,* Italian physician, 1856–1916] see under *triangle.*

**Groe·nouw's type I corneal dystrophy, type II corneal dystrophy** (grer′nōz) [Arthur *Groenouw,* German ophthalmologist, 1862–1945] see *granular corneal dystrophy* and *macular corneal dystrophy,* under *dystrophy.*

**groin** (groin) [MeSH: Groin] inguen.

**Grön·blad-Strand·berg syndrome** (grern′blahd strahnd′berg) [Ester Elizabeth *Grönblad,* Swedish ophthalmologist, 1898–1942; James Victor *Strandberg,* Swedish dermatologist, 1883–1942] see under *syndrome.*

**groove** (grōōv) a shallow linear depression; see also *fissure* and *sulcus.*

**abomasal g.**, the part of the gastric groove that is located in the abomasum.
**alveolingual g.**, the groove between the lower jaw and the tongue.
**anal intersphincteric g.**, Hilton's white line.
**anterolateral g. of medulla oblongata**, sulcus anterolateralis medullae oblongatae.
**anterolateral g. of spinal cord**, sulcus anterolateralis medullae spinalis.
**anteromedian g. of medulla oblongata**, fissura mediana anterior medullae oblongatae.
**anteromedian g. of spinal cord**, fissura mediana anterior medullae spinalis.
**g. for aorta**, a longitudinal groove on the median surface of the left lung corresponding to the thoracic aorta. Called also *aortic sulcus.*
**arterial g's**, sulci arteriosi.
**atrioventricular g.**, sulcus coronarius cordis.
**g. for auditory tube**, sulcus tubae auditoriae.
**auriculoventricular g.**, sulcus coronarius cordis.
**basilar g.**, sulcus basilaris pontis.
**basilar g. of occipital bone**, clivus ossis occipitalis.
**basilar g. of sphenoid bone**, clivus ossis sphenoidalis.
**bicipital g., lateral**, sulcus bicipitalis lateralis.
**bicipital g., medial**, sulcus bicipitalis medialis.
**bicipital g., radial**, sulcus bicipitalis lateralis.
**bicipital g., ulnar**, sulcus bicipitalis medialis.
**bicipital g. of humerus**, sulcus intertubercularis humeri.
**Blessig's g.**, a trace in the eye of the developing embryo corresponding in position with the future ora serrata retinae.
**branchial g.**, pharyngeal g.
**buccal g., buccal developmental g.**, a groove on the buccal surface of a posterior tooth; see also *distobuccal g.* and *mesiobuccal g.*
**carotid g. of sphenoid bone, cavernous g. of sphenoid bone,** sulcus caroticus ossis sphenoidalis.
**central g., central developmental g.**, a groove in the central part of the occlusal surface of bicuspid and first molar teeth.
**costal g.**, sulcus costae.
**dental g., primitive**, a groove in the border of the jaws of the embryo.
**developmental g's**, fine grooves or lines marking the fusion area between adjacent cusps, named according to the portion of the crown which they connect. Called also *developmental lines* and *segmental lines.*

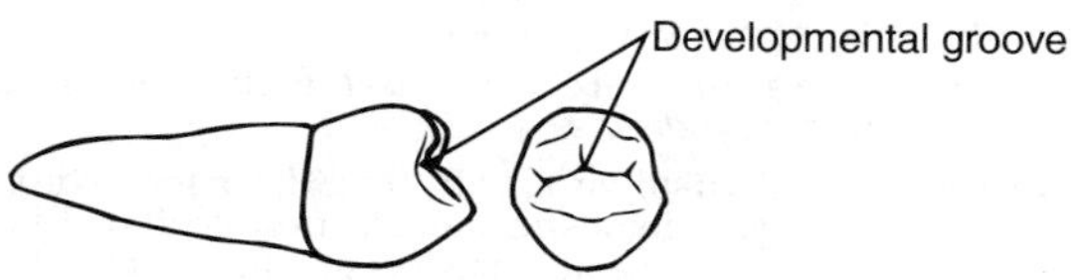


**digastric g.**, incisura mastoidea ossis temporalis.
**distobuccal g., distobuccal developmental g.**, the distal of the two buccal grooves ordinarily found on the mandibular first molar.
**distolingual g., distolingual developmental g.**, the distal of the lingual grooves of the bicuspid and maxillary molar teeth.
**enamel g's**, the grooves bounding the enamel knot.
**ethmoidal g.**, sulcus ethmoidalis ossis nasalis.
**g. for eustachian tube**, sulcus tubae auditoriae.
**gastric g.**, a groove or canal through the reticulum, omasum, and abomasum of a ruminant, analogous to the gastric canal of humans. It is subdivided into the *reticular, omasal,* and *abomasal grooves.*
**genital g.**, urethral g.
**gingival g., free**, a shallow groove on the facial surface of the gingiva, running parallel to the margin of the gingiva at a distance of 0.5 to 1.5 mm., and usually at the level of, or somewhat apical to, the bottom of the gingival sulcus.
**greater petrosal g., g. for greater petrosal nerve**, sulcus nervi petrosi majoris.
**hamular g.**, sulcus hamuli pterygoidei.
**Harrison's g.**, a horizontal depression along the lower border of the thorax, corresponding to the costal insertion of the diaphragm; seen in advanced rickets in children.
**infraorbital g. of maxilla**, sulcus infraorbitalis maxillae.
**interatrial g.**, a slight depression on the external surface of the heart, marking the separation of the atria.
**interdental g.**, a linear, vertical depression on the surface of the interdental papillae; it functions as a sluiceway for the egress of food from the interproximal areas.
**interosseous g. of calcaneus**, sulcus calcanei.
**intertubercular g. of humerus**, sulcus intertubercularis humeri.
**interventricular g., anterior**, sulcus interventricularis anterior.
**interventricular g., inferior**, sulcus interventricularis posterior.
**interventricular g., posterior**, sulcus interventricularis posterior.
**interventricular g. of heart**, interventricular sulcus of heart.
**labial g.**, an embryonic groove produced by degeneration of the central cells of the labial lamina, which later becomes the vestibule of the oral cavity.
**lacrimal g.**, fossa sacci lacrimalis.
**g. of lacrimal bone**, sulcus lacrimalis ossis lacrimalis.
**laryngotracheal g.**, a furrow at the caudal end of the floor of the embryonic pharynx that develops into the respiratory tract.
**lateral g. for lateral sinus of occipital bone**, sulcus sinus transversi.
**lateral g. for lateral sinus of parietal bone**, sulcus sinus sigmoidei ossis parietalis.
**lateral g. for sigmoidal part of lateral sinus**, sulcus sinus sigmoidei ossis temporalis.
**g. for lesser petrosal nerve**, sulcus nervi petrosi minoris.
**Liebermeister's g's**, developmental grooves on the surface of the liver.
**lingual g., lingual developmental g.**, a developmental groove on the lingual surface of a posterior tooth.
**major g.**, in DNA, the larger groove occurring between successive turns of the two antiparallel chains around the helical axis. See illustration at *deoxyribonucleic acid.* Cf. *minor g.*
**medullary g.**, neural g.
**mesiobuccal g., mesiobuccal developmental g.**, the mesial of the two buccal grooves ordinarily found on the mandibular first molar.
**mesiolingual g., mesiolingual developmental g.**, a groove marking the junction of the fifth cusp with the palatal surface on an upper molar tooth.
**g. for middle temporal artery**, sulcus arteriae temporalis mediae.
**minor g.**, in DNA, the smaller groove occurring between the two antiparallel chains as they wind around the helical axis. See illustration at *deoxyribonucleic acid.* Cf. *major g.*
**musculospiral g.**, sulcus nervi radialis.
**mylohyoid g. of inferior maxillary bone**, sulcus mylohyoideus mandibulae.
**nail g.**, a pathologic linear depression of the nail plate, running usually transversely but occasionally lengthwise.
**nasal g.**, sulcus ethmoidalis ossis nasalis.
**nasolacrimal g.**, an epithelial ingrowth parallel with but medial to the nasomaxillary groove of the embryo, which marks the site of later development of the nasolacrimal duct.
**nasomaxillary g.**, a furrow located between the maxillary and the lateral nasal prominences of the same side in the embryo.
**nasopalatine g.**, a furrow on the lateral surface of the vomer for the nasopalatine nerve and vessels.
**nasopharyngeal g.**, a faint line between the nasal cavity and the nasopharynx.
**neural g.**, the groove produced by the invagination of the neural plate of the embryo during the process of formation of the neural tube; called also *medullary g.*
**obturator g.**, sulcus obturatorius ossis pubis.
**occipital g.**, sulcus arteriae occipitalis.
**occlusal g.**, one of the developmental grooves on the occlusal surface of a posterior tooth.
**olfactory g.**, ethmoid fossa.
**omasal g.**, the part of the gastric groove that is located in the omasum.
**optic g.**, sulcus prechiasmaticus.
**palatine g's of maxilla**, sulci palatinae maxillae.
**palatine g. of palatine bone**, sulcus palatinus major ossis palatini.
**palatomaxillary g. of palatine bone**, sulcus palatinus major ossis palatini.
**paraglenoid g's of hip bone**, sulci paraglenoidales ossis coxae.
**pharyngeal g.**, the embryonic ectodermal cleft between successive pharyngeal arches; called also *branchial g., cleft,* or *fissure.*

**posterolateral g. of medulla oblongata,** sulcus posterolateralis medullae oblongatae.
**posterolateral g. of spinal cord,** sulcus posterolateralis medullae spinalis.
**preauricular g's of ilium,** sulci paraglenoidales ossis coxae.
**primitive g.,** a lengthwise median furrow in the primitive streak of the embryo. In human embryos it is clearly visible during the third week.
**radial g., g. for radial nerve,** sulcus nervi radialis.
**reticular g.,** the part of the gastric groove that is located in the reticulum.
**retroolivary g.,** sulcus retroolivaris.
**sagittal g.,** sulcus sinus sagittalis superioris.
**Sibson's g.,** a furrow sometimes seen at the lower border of the pectoralis major muscle.
**sigmoid g. of temporal bone,** sulcus sinus sigmoidei ossis temporalis.
**spiral g.,** sulcus nervi radialis.
**subclavian g.,** 1. see under *sulcus.* 2. sulcus musculi subclavii.
**g. for subclavian artery,** a broad, shallow, transverse groove across the top of each lung, lodging the subclavian artery. Called also *sulcus of subclavian artery, subclavian sulcus of lung,* and *sulcus subclavius pulmonis.*
**g. for subclavian vein,** sulcus venae subclaviae.
**subcostal g.,** sulcus costae.
**supplemental g's,** grooves on the surface of a tooth that do not mark (as do the developmental grooves) the junction of the primary lobes of the tooth.
**supra-acetabular g.,** sulcus supraacetabularis.
**g. for tibialis posticus muscle,** sulcus malleolaris tibiae.
**trigeminal g.,** the embryonic structure that develops into the trigeminal (gasserian) ganglion.
**ulnar g., g. of ulnar nerve,** sulcus nervi ulnaris.
**urethral g.,** the embryonic groove that becomes the penile urethra as the urogenital folds on each side fuse.
**venous g's,** venous sulci.
**Verga's lacrimal g.,** a groove running downward from the lower orifice of the nasal duct.
**vertebral g.,** the depression on each side of the spine between the spinous processes, laminae, and transverse processes; it lodges the deep back muscles.

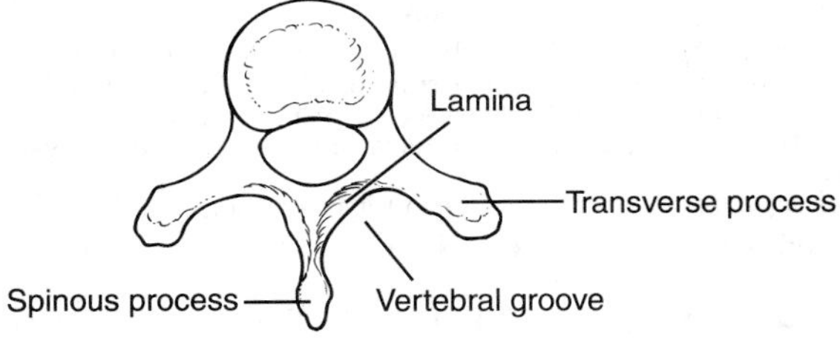


**vomeral g.,** sulcus vomeris.

**Gross disease** (grōs) [Samuel David *Gross,* American surgeon, 1805–1884] see under *disease.*

**gross** (grōs) [L. *grossus* rough] coarse or large; visible to the naked eye, as gross pathology; macroscopic; taking no account of minutiae.

**ground** (ground) 1. a path of conduction from an electrical circuit to the earth. 2. to connect an electrical circuit or electrical equipment to the earth.

**ground-glass** (ground-glas) having a filmy, hazy appearance, as in radiographs of a lung containing excess fluid.

**ground·hog** (ground'hog) woodchuck.

**group** (gro͞op) 1. an assemblage of objects or individuals having certain qualities in common; see also *population.* 2. a number of atoms forming a recognizable and usually a transferable portion of a molecule.
**alcohol g.,** a combination of carbon, hydrogen, and oxygen atoms in a molecule, which is characteristic of a chemical compound known as an alcohol. There are three: $—CH_2OH$, the primary, $=CHOH$, the secondary, and $\equiv COH$, the tertiary alcohol group.
**amide g.,** the monovalent radical $—CONH_2$, derived from an acid by the replacement of the OH of the carboxyl group with an amino group.
**azo g.,** a bivalent chemical group composed of two nitrogen atoms, $—N=N—$.
**blood g.,** see *blood group,* under *B.*
**CMN g.,** a group of bacteria composed of the genera *Clostridium, Mycobacterium,* and *Nocardia,* characterized by common peptidoglycan and mycolic acid constituents in the cell walls. Organisms of this group can be used as adjuvants in experimental immunization.
**coli-aerogenes g.,** coliform bacteria.
**colon-typhoid-dysentery g.,** a collective term referring to bacteria of the genera *Escherichia, Salmonella,* and *Shigella.*
**control g.,** see *control* (def. 3).
**coryneform g.,** see under *bacterium.*
**Diagnosis-Related G's,** groupings of diagnostic categories used as a basis for hospital payment schedules by Medicare and other third-party payment plans.
**dorsal respiratory g.,** part of the medullary respiratory center running the length of the medulla oblongata, largely within the nucleus of the solitary tract; its main function is to control the basic rhythm of respiration. Cf. *ventral respiratory g.*
**encounter g.,** a sensitivity group in which the members strive to gain emotional rather than intellectual insight with emphasis on the expression of interpersonal feelings in the group situation.
**functional g.,** a part of a molecule that gives it characteristic chemical properties, e.g., an aldehyde, alcohol, amine, carboxylic acid, ester, ether, or ketone group.
**glucophore g.,** see *glucophore.*
**hemorrhagic-septicemia g.,** a group of bacteria of which *Pasteurella multocida* is the type organism.
**methyl g.,** a monovalent chemical group, $—CH_3$.
**osmophore g.,** see *osmophore.*
**paratyphoid-enteritidis g.,** a group of organisms of the genus *Salmonella,* causing food poisoning in humans and various diseases in animals.
**peptide g.,** the bivalent radical, $—CO·NH—$, formed by reaction between the $NH_2$ and COOH groups of adjacent amino acids, and by such linkage building up compounds known as dipeptides, tripeptides, tetrapeptides, etc., depending on the number of amino acids making up the molecule.
**platelet g.,** that subset of platelets expressing a particular platelet-specific antigen, such as Pl(A1) antigen.
**PLT g.,** see *Chlamydia.*
**prosthetic g.,** a low molecular weight, nonprotein compound that binds with a protein component (apoprotein, specifically apoenzyme) to form a protein (e.g., holoenzyme) with biologic activity.
**Runyon g.,** one of four divisions of nontuberculous mycobacteria, classified according to pigmentation and rate of growth. See *nontuberculous mycobacteria,* under *mycobacterium.*
**sapophore g.,** see *sapophore.*
**sensitivity g., sensitivity training g.,** a nonclinical group not intended for persons with mental illnesses or substantial emotional problems, which, in an effort to develop the assets of leadership, management, counseling, or other roles, focuses on self-awareness and understanding and on interpersonal interactions. Called also *training g. (T-g.).*
**sulfonic g.,** a monovalent radical, $—SO_2OH$.
**T-g.,** sensitivity g.
**training g.,** sensitivity g.
**ventral respiratory g.,** part of the medullary respiratory center running the length of the medulla oblongata within and next to the nucleus ambiguus; these neurons mainly function during strong, active respiration, moving voluntary muscles in the control of inspiration and expiration or modifying the behavior of other respiratory motoneurons. Cf. *dorsal respiratory g.*

**group·ing** (gro͞op'ing) the classification of individual entities according to certain common characteristics.
**blood g.,** the classification of blood according to blood group, done to determine its suitability for transfusion in a given recipient, to settle cases of disputed paternity, and to trace substances in certain criminal cases. See *blood group,* under *B.*
**haptenic g.,** hapten.

**group-spe·cif·ic** (gro͞op"spə-sif'ik) specific for a given group; as a blood group or certain microorganisms; said of agglutinins.

**group-trans·fer** (gro͞op-trans'fər) denoting a chemical reaction, excluding oxidation and reduction, in which molecules exchange functional groups, a process catalyzed by enzymes called transferases.

**growth** (grōth) [MeSH: Growth] 1. a normal process of increase in size of an organism as a result of accretion of tissue similar to that originally present. Cf. *differentiation.* 2. an abnormal formation, such as a tumor. 3. the proliferation of cells, as in a bacterial culture.
**absolute g.,** an expression of the actual increase in size of an individual, or of a particular organ or part.
**accretionary g.,** increase in size resulting from increase in number of special cells by mitotic division, other more differentiated cells which perform various physiologic functions having lost the ability to proliferate.

**allometric g.,** the growth of different organs or parts of an organism at different rates.
**appositional g.,** growth by addition at the periphery of a particular structure or part. Cf. *interstitial g.*
**auxetic g.,** auxesis.
**balanced g.,** a steady state condition in which every component of the cell doubles in a cell generation (time between divisions).
**condylar g.,** the growth of the condyle of the temporomandibular joint, usually reflected in a downward and forward positioning of the mandible and teeth.
**differential g.,** an expression of the comparison of the increases in size of dissimilar organisms, organs, or parts.
**heterogonous g.,** growth of such a nature that, when it is plotted logarithmically, it gives a straight line.
**histiotypic g.,** uncontrolled growth of cells as occurs in tissue cultures.
**interstitial g.,** growth occurring in the interior of parts or structures already formed. Cf. *appositional g.*
**intussusceptive g.,** auxesis.
**isometric g.,** the growth of different organs or parts of an organism at the same rate.
**multiplicative g.,** increase in the size of an organism, organ, or part, resulting from increase in the number of cells brought about by their mitotic division, the average size of the cells remaining about the same.
**new g.,** a neoplasm, or tumor.
**organotypic g.,** controlled growth of cells as occurs normally in the production of organs and parts.
**relative g.,** an expression of the comparison of the increases in size of similar organisms, organs, or parts.

**grü·bel·sucht** (gre′bel-sookt) [Ger. *grübeln* to brood, ponder + *sucht* illness] the drawing of overly fine distinctions (hair-splitting); worrying over trifles. Seen particularly in obsessive-compulsive personalities.

**Gru·ber's fossa** (groo′berz) [Wenzel Leopoldovich *Gruber,* Russian anatomist, 1814–1890] see under *fossa.*

**Gru·ber's reaction** (groo′berz) [Maximilian Franz Maria von *Gruber,* Austrian bacteriologist in Germany, 1853–1927] Widal's test.

**Gru·ber's syndrome** (groo′berz) [Georg Benito Otto *Gruber,* German pathologist, 1884–1977] Meckel's syndrome.

**Gru·ber-Wi·dal reaction** (groo′ber-ve-dahl′) [M.F.M. von *Gruber;* George Fernand Isidore *Widal,* French physician, 1862–1929] Widal's test.

**Gru·by·el·la** (groo″be-el′ə) former name for the genus *Trichophyton.*

**Gruen·tzig balloon catheter** (grēn′tsig) [Andreas Roland *Gruentzig,* German radiologist, 1939–1985] see under *catheter.*

**gru·mose, gru·mous** (groo′mōs, groo′məs) [L. *grumus* heap] clotted or lumpy.

**grund·platte** (groont-plah′tə) [Ger.] lamina basalis.

**Gryn·feltt's hernia, triangle** (grin′felts) [Joseph Casimir *Grynfeltt,* French surgeon, 1840–1913] see under *hernia,* and see *Lesgaft's space,* under *space.*

**Gryn·feltt-Less·haft triangle** (grin′felt-les′hahft) [J. C. *Grynfeltt;* Peter Frantsevich *Lesshaft,* Russian physician, 1837–1909] Lesshaft's space.

**gryo·chrome** (gri′o-krōm) [Gr. *gry* morsel + *-chrome*] a nerve cell in which the stainable matter of the cell body appears as fine granules.

**gry·pho·sis** (grĭ-fo′sis) abnormal curvature; see *gryposis.*

**gry·po·sis** (grĭ-po′sis) [Gr. *grypōsis* a crooking, hooking] abnormal curvature, as of the nails.
**g. pe′nis,** chordee.

**GSC** gas-solid chromatography.

**GSH** reduced glutathione.

**GSS** Gerstmann-Sträussler-Scheinker syndrome.

**GSSG** oxidized glutathione.

**gt.** abbreviation for L. *gut′ta,* drop.

**GTH** gonadotropic hormone.

**GTN** gestational trophoblastic neoplasia.

**GTP** guanosine triphosphate.

**GTPase** enzyme activity that catalyzes the hydrolysis of guanosine triphosphate to guanosine diphosphate and orthophosphate. GTPase converts GTP-binding proteins (q.v.) from the active to the inactive form.

**GTP cy·clo·hy·dro·lase I** (si′klo-hi′dro-lās) [EC 3.5.4.16] an enzyme of the hydrolase class that catalyzes the first step in the biosynthesis of tetrahydrobiopterin from guanosine triphosphate. Deficiency of the enzyme, an autosomal recessive trait, causes malignant hyperphenylalaninemia.

**GTT** glucose tolerance test.

**gtt.** abbreviation for L. *gut′tae,* drops.

**GU** genitourinary.

**gua·co** (gwah′ko) [Spanish American] any of several plants, especially *Mikania guaco,* used in South America to treat asthma, dyspepsia, gout, rheumatism, skin diseases, and snakebite.

**guai·ac** (gwi′ək) [MeSH: Guaiac] a resin from the wood of the tropical trees *Guaiacum officinale* and *G. sanctum,* used as a reagent in tests for occult blood and formerly in the treatment of rheumatism.

**Guai·a·cum** (gwi′ə-kəm) a genus of trees and shrubs of the family Zygophyllaceae, native to tropical regions of the Americas. *G. officina′le* L. and *G. sanc′tum* L. are trees found in Haiti and the Dominican Republic whose wood yields the resin guaiac.

**guai·fen·e·sin** (gwi-fen′ə-sin) [USP] the glyceryl ester of guaiacol, used as an expectorant, administered orally. Called also *glyceryl guaiacolate, guaiphenesin,* and *methphenoxydiol.*

**guai·phen·e·sin** (gwi-fen′ə-sin) guaifenesin.

**guan·a·benz** (gwahn′ə-benz) [MeSH: Guanabenz] an $\alpha_2$-adrenergic agonist that stimulates the $\alpha_2$-adrenergic receptors of the central nervous system, resulting in a reduction of sympathetic outflow to the heart and peripheral vascular system; used as an antihypertensive.
**g. acetate** [USP], an antihypertensive agent having the same actions as the base, administered orally.

**guan·a·drel sul·fate** (gwahn′ə-drel) [USP] an adrenergic neuron blocking agent, used in the treatment of hypertension; administered orally.

**guan·ase** (gwahn′ās) guanine deaminase.

**guan·eth·i·dine mo·no·sul·fate** (gwahn-eth′ĭ-dēn) [USP] an adrenergic neuron blocking agent used as an antihypertensive; administered orally.

**guan·fa·cine hy·dro·chlo·ride** (gwahn′fə-sēn) [USP] an $\alpha_2$-adrenergic agonist that stimulates the $\alpha_2$-adrenergic receptors of the central nervous system, resulting in a reduction of sympathetic outflow to the heart and peripheral vascular system, used as an antihypertensive; administered orally.

**guan·i·dine** (gwahn′ĭ-dēn) the compound $NH{=}C(NH_2)_2$, a strong base found in the urine as a normal product of protein metabolism. It is used in laboratory research as a protein denaturant.
**g. hydrochloride,** a compound used in the treatment of myasthenia gravis.
**g. phosphate,** a less correct term for phosphoguanidine.

**guan·i·dine-acet·ic ac·id** (gwahn′ĭ-dēn-ə-se′tik) guanidinoacetic acid.

**guan·i·din·emia** (gwahn″ĭ-dĭ-ne′me-ə) the presence of guanidine in the blood.

**guan·i·din·i·um** (gwahn″ĭ-din′e-əm) the radical derived from guanidine; the guanidinium group is an important component of arginine and creatine.

**gua·ni·di·no** (gwahn″ĭ-de′no) guanidinium.

**gua·ni·di·no·ac·e·tate** (gwahn″ĭ-de″no-as′ə-tāt) a salt or anionic form of guanidinoacetic acid.

**gua·ni·di·no·ac·e·tate *N*-meth·yl·trans·fer·ase** (gwahn″ĭ-de″no-as′ə-tāt meth″əl-trans′fər-ās) [EC 2.1.1.2] a cytosolic enzyme of the transferase class that catalyzes the methylation of guanidinoacetate to form creatine, the final step in the biosynthesis of creatine. The methyl donor is *S*-adenosylmethionine, and the enzyme is concentrated in the kidney and pancreas.

**guan·i·di·no·a·ce·tic ac·id** (gwahn″ĭ-de″no-ə-se′tik) a nitrogenous compound formed enzymatically in the liver, pancreas, and kidney by a reaction transfering an amidino group between arginine and glycine, and *N*-methylated in the liver by *S*-adenosylmethionine to form creatine. Called also *glycocyamine, guanidine-acetic acid,* and *guanido-acetic acid.*

**guan·i·do** (gwahn′ĭ-do) guanidinium.

**guan·i·do-ace·tic ac·id** (gwahn″ĭ-do-ə-se′tik) guanidinoacetic acid.

**guan·ine** (gwahn′ēn) [MeSH: Guanine] a purine base, in animal and plant cells usually occurring condensed with ribose or deoxyribose to form the nucleosides guanosine and deoxyguanosine; these nucleosides are components of nucleic acids and of free nucleotides important in metabolism. Symbol G. See it also illustration at *purine base,* under *base.*
**g. nucleotide,** guanylic acid.

**guan·ine de·am·i·nase** (gwahn′ēn de-am′ĭ-nās) [EC 3.5.4.3]

[MeSH: Guanine Deaminase] an enzyme of the hydrolase class that catalyzes the deamination of guanine to form xanthine. The reaction is a step in the degradation of guanine to uric acid. The enzyme is present in liver, kidney, spleen, and other tissues. Called also *guanase.*

**guan·o·phore** (gwahn′o-for″) [*guanine* + *phore*] a cell filled with guanine crystals that produce interference in the light and thus give the cell a silvery or golden appearance; found in the skin of some cold-blooded vertebrates such as fishes.

**guan·o·sine** (gwahn′o-sin) [MeSH: Guanosine] a purine nucleoside, guanine linked by its N9 nitrogen to the C1 carbon of ribose. It is a component of ribonucleic acid and its nucleotides play important roles in metabolism. Symbol G.
**cyclic g. monophosphate,** a cyclic nucleotide, guanosine 3′,5′-cyclic monophosphate, an intracellular "second messenger" similar in action to cyclic adenosine monophosphate (q.v.); the two cyclic nucleotides activate different protein kinases and usually produce opposite effects on cell function. Abbreviated 3′,5′-GMP, cGMP, and cyclic GMP.
**g. diphosphate (GDP),** a nucleotide, the 5′-pyrophosphate of guanosine, which serves as a carrier for mannose residues in glycoprotein synthesis and as a substrate for a phosphorylation reaction of the tricarboxylic acid cycle.
**g. monophosphate (GMP),** a nucleotide, the 5′-phosphate of guanosine; it is a constituent of ribonucleic acid and a regulator of pyrimidine nucleotide biosynthesis.
**g. triphosphate (GTP),** a nucleotide, the 5′-triphosphate of guanosine; it is an activated precursor in the synthesis of ribonucleic acid and is also involved in energy metabolism, being produced from GDP by substrate level phosphorylation in the tricarboxylic acid (Krebs) cycle and serving as a source of free energy to drive protein synthesis. The ratio of GTP to ATP is maintained by the reversible transfer of phosphate catalyzed by GDP kinase.

**gua·nyl·ate** (gwah′nə-lāt) a dissociated form of guanylic acid.

**gua·nyl·ate cy·clase** (gwah′nə-lāt si′klās) [EC 4.6.1.2] [MeSH: Guanylate Cyclase] an enzyme of the lyase class that catalyzes the cyclization of guanosine triphosphate to form cyclic guanosine monophosphate and pyrophosphate.

**gua·nyl·ate ki·nase** (gwah′nə-lāt ki′nās) [EC 2.7.4.8] an enzyme of the transferase class that catalyzes the phosphorylation of GMP or dGMP to form the corresponding phosphate compound.

**gua·nyl·ic ac·id** (gwah-nil′ik) guanosine monophosphate.

**gua·nyl·yl** (gwah-nil′əl) the radical formed by removal of OH from the phosphate group of guanosine monophosphate.

**gua·ra·na** (gwə-rah′nə) [Tupi-Guarani] a dried paste prepared from the seeds of *Paullinia cupana,* a tree of Brazil; used as a stimulant and tonic in folk medicine.

**gua·ra·nine** (gwə-rah′nēn) caffeine.

**guard** (gahrd) a protective device.
**bite g.,** occlusal g.
**mouth g.,** a removable, soft plastic intraoral appliance that covers all occlusal surfaces and the palate and extends to the border of the attached gingiva on the vestibular surface of the teeth; used to protect the teeth, lips, and cheeks during contact sports.
**night g.,** occlusal g.
**occlusal g.,** a removable dental appliance, usually constructed of plastic, that covers one or both dental arches, designed to minimize the damaging effect of bruxism and other occlusal habits, being usually worn at night. Called also *bite g.* and *night g.*

**Gua·rea** (gwa′re-ə) a genus of tropical American trees and shrubs of the family Meliaceae. *G. rus′byi* (Britt.) has bark that is dried to yield the medicinal substance cocillana.

**Guar·ni·eri's bodies (corpuscles)** (gwahr″ne-er′ēz) [Giuseppi *Guarnieri,* Italian physician, 1856–1918] see under *body.*

**gu·ber·nac·u·la** (goo″bər-nak′u-lə) plural of *gubernaculum.*

**gu·ber·nac·u·lar** (goo″bər-nak′u-lər) pertaining to a gubernaculum.

**gu·ber·nac·u·lum** (goo″bər-nak′u-ləm) pl. *guberna′cula* [L. "helm, rudder"] a structure that guides.
**chorda g.,** a portion of the gubernaculum testis and round ligament that develops in the body wall of the embryo.
**Hunter's g.,** g. testis.
**g. tes′tis,** the fetal ligament attached to the inferior end of the epididymis and testis and, at its other end, to the bottom of the scrotum; it is present during, and is thought to guide, the descent of the testis into the scrotum and then atrophies. Called also *Hunter's g.*

**Gub·ler's hemiplegia, tumor** (goo-blāz′) [Adolphe Marie *Gubler,* French physician, 1821–1879] see under *tumor* and see *Millard-Gubler syndrome,* under *syndrome.*

**Gub·ler-Ro·bin typhus** (goo-bla′ ro-bă′) [A. M. *Gubler;* Albert Edouard Charles *Robin,* French physician, 1847–1928] see under *typhus.*

**Gud·den's commissure, law** (good′enz) [Bernhard Alloys von *Gudden,* German psychiatrist, 1824–1886] see *supraoptic commissures,* under *commissure,* and see under *law.*

**Guenz** (gints) see *Günz.*

**Guenz·burg** see *Günzburg.*

**Gué·rin's fold,** etc. (ga-raz′) [Alphonse François Marie *Guérin,* French surgeon, 1817–1895] see under *fold, gland, sinus,* and *valve* and see *Le Fort I fracture,* under *fracture.*

**guid·ance** (gi′dəns) 1. a guide. 2. an act of guiding.
**condylar g.,** the path that the horizontal rotation axis of the condyles travels during normal mandibular opening, measured in degrees as related to the Frankfort Horizontal plane. It also influences mandibular movements from the temporomandibular joint, articular guidance, or condylar elements. Called also *condylar guide.* See also under *inclination.*
**incisal g.,** the influence on mandibular movements by the contacting surfaces of the mandibular and maxillary anterior teeth.

**guide** (gīd) a device by which another object is led in its proper course, such as a grooved sound, or a filiform bougie over which a tunneled sound is passed, as in stricture of the urethra.
**adjustable anterior g.,** an anterior guide whose superior surface may be varied to provide desired separation of dental casts in various eccentric relationships.
**anterior g.,** that part of a dental articulator on which the anterior guide pin rests to maintain the vertical dimension of occlusion; it influences the degree of separation of the casts in eccentric relationships.
**condylar g.,** see under *guidance.*
**incisal g.,** that part of a dental articulator which maintains the incisal guide angle.

**guide·line** (gīd′līn) any line used as a marker or indicator.
**clasp g.,** survey line, def. 3.

**guide·wire** (gīd′wīr) a thin, usually flexible wire that can be inserted into a confined or tortuous space to act as a guide for subsequent insertion of a stiffer or bulkier instrument, such as a catheter.

**guil·lo·tine** (gē′o-tēn) [Fr.] an instrument for excising a tonsil or the uvula.

**Gui·di's canal** (gwe′dēz) [Guido *Guidi* (L. *Vidius*), Italian physician, 1508–1569] canalis pterygoideus.

**Guil·lain-Bar·ré syndrome** (ge-yă′ bə-ra′) [Georges *Guillain,* French neurologist, 1876–1951; Jean Alexander *Barré,* French neurologist, 1880–1967] acute idiopathic polyneuritis.

**Guil·le·min** (ge-ə-mă′) Roger Charles Louis. French-born American physician, born 1924; co-winner, with Andrew Victor Schally and Rosalyn Sussman Yalow, of the Nobel prize for medicine or physiology in 1977 for showing that the hypothalamus secretes hormones that control the pituitary gland and for developing methods for isolating peptide hormones.

**guin·ea pig** (gin′e pig) [MeSH: Guinea Pigs] *Cavia cobaya,* a rodent much used in laboratory experiments.

**Gui·non's disease** (ge-nawz′) [Georges *Guinon,* French physician, 1859–1929] Gilles de la Tourette's syndrome.

**gulf** (gulf) a large area of ocean or sea that is partially surrounded by land, or something resembling such an area.
**Lecat's g.,** the hollow of the bulbous portion of the urethra.

**Gull's disease** (gulz) [Sir William Withey *Gull,* English physician, 1816–1890] see under *disease.*

**gul·let** (gul′ət) the esophagus.

**Gull·strand** (gool′strahnd) Allvar. Swedish ophthalmologist, 1862–1930; winner of the Nobel prize for medicine or physiology in 1911 for elucidating the formation of optical images in the eye and incorporating it in the general laws governing optical image formation.

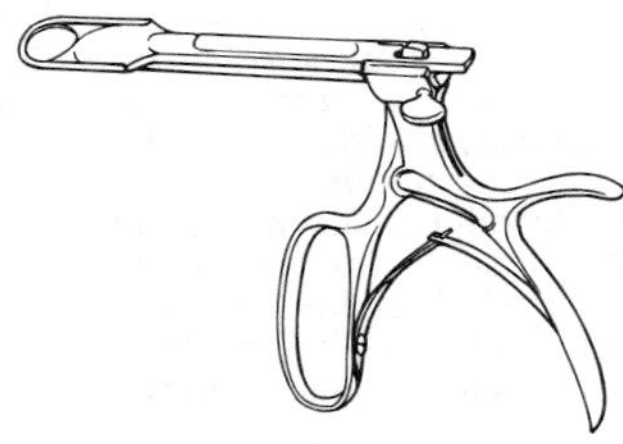

Guillotine.

**Gull·strand's slit lamp, law** (gool'strahndz) [Allvar *Gullstrand*] see *slit lamp* under *lamp*, and see under *law*.

**gu·lon·ic ac·id** (gu-lon'ik) the hexonic acid derived from glucose and formed by the reduction of the aldehyde group of glucuronic acid to an alcohol; it is an intermediate in the synthesis of ascorbic acid by many mammals.

**L-gu·lo·no·lac·tone** (gu"lo-no-lak'tōn) the immediate precursor of ascorbic acid in plants and in those animals capable of its biosynthesis; gulonolactone is itself formed from L-gulonic acid.

**gu·lose** (gu'lōs) an aldohexose isomeric with glucose but nonfermentable.

**gum** (gum) [L. *gummi*] [MeSH: Gingiva] 1. a mucilaginous excretion from various plants; on hydrolysis gums yield hexoses, pentoses, and uronic acids. 2. gingiva.
**g. arabic,** acacia (def. 2).
**Australian g.,** wattle g.
**g. benjamin, g. benzoin,** benzoin, def. 1.
**blue g.,** 1. *Eucalyptus globulus.* 2. the bluish discoloration of the gums seen in lead poisoning.
**British g.,** dextrin, particularly that prepared by dry heating of starch in the absence of acid.
**g. camphor,** camphor.
**Cape g.,** 1. *Acacia horrida.* 2. a type of acacia (gum arabic) from *A. horrida.*
**eucalyptus g.,** red g. (def. 2).
**free g.,** periodontium insertionis.
**ghatti g.,** a gum from *Anogeissus latifolia,* the dhava tree of India; used like acacia.
**guar g.** [NF], a gum obtained from the ground endosperms of the leguminous tree *Cyamopsis tetragonolobus;* used as a tablet binder and disintegrant in pharmaceutical preparations.
**Indian g.,** karaya g.
**karaya g.,** the dried gummy exudation from *Sterculia urens* or other species of *Sterculia,* which becomes gelatinous when moisture is added; used as a bulk laxative. Because of its adhesive properties, products containing karaya gum are used as dental adhesives and as skin adhesives and protective skin barriers in the fitting and care of colostomy appliances and in other conditions involving an artificial stoma. Called also *sterculia g.*
**Kordofan g.,** a superior type of acacia (gum arabic) from trees found in the Sudan.
**mesquite g.,** a gum from the mesquite plant, *Prosopis juliflora,* used as a substitute for acacia.
**g. opium,** opium.
**red g.,** 1. any of various trees of the genus *Eucalyptus,* especially *E. calophylla, E. camadulensis,* and *E. rostralis.* 2. an exudation from the bark of *Eucalyptus rostrata* and other species; used as an astringent in throat inflammation. See also *eucalyptus oil,* under *oil.* Called also *eucalyptus g.*
**sterculia g.,** karaya g.
**g. thus,** turpentine.
**g. tragacanth,** tragacanth.
**wattle g.,** the gum of several Australian species of *Acacia,* used as a substitute for acacia.
**xanthan g.** [NF], a dried, purified, high molecular weight polysaccharide gum produced by pure-culture fermentation of a carbohydrate with the bacterium *Xanthomonas campestris;* it contains D-glucose and D-mannose, along with D-glucuronic acid. It is used as the sodium, potassium, and calcium salts as a suspending agent in pharmaceutical preparations.

**gum·boil** (gum'boil) parulis.

**Gum·boro disease** (gum'bor-o) [*Gumboro,* Delaware, where the disease was first identified] see *infectious bursal disease,* under *disease.*

**gum·ma** (gum'ə) pl. *gummas* or *gum'mata* [L. *gummi* gum] 1. a chronic focal area of inflammatory destruction in tertiary syphilis thought to be due to localization of *Treponema pallidum* in a tissue, manifested by an indolent lesion with a center of rubbery, gray-white coagulation necrosis surrounded by epithelioid and fibroblastic cells and sometimes giant cells. Gummata, which vary in size from microscopic to large tumorous masses of necrotic material, may be single or multiple and may involve any organ or tissue, most commonly the mucocutaneous tissues, liver, bones, and testes. Those found in the skin resemble other chronic granulomatous lesions caused by tuberculosis, sarcoidosis, leprosy, and deep fungal infections. Called also *syphiloma.* 2. late benign syphilis.
**tuberculous g.,** a subcutaneous nodule(s) that becomes fluctuant and drains, with undermined ulceration and sinus formation; caused by hematogenous spread of tubercle bacilli from a primary focus of infection during a period of lowered resistance or immunodeficiency, especially in children. Called also *metastatic tuberculous abscess, tuberculosis colliquativa,* and *tuberculosis colliquativa cutis.* Cf. *scrofuloderma.*

**gum·ma·ta** (gum'ə-tə) [L.] plural of *gumma.*

**gum·ma·tous** (gum'ə-təs) of the nature of gumma.

**gum·mi** (gum'i) [L., from Gr. *kommi*] gum (def. 1).

**gum·my** (gum'e) 1. resembling a gum. 2. resembling a gumma.

**gum·res·in** (gum"rez'in) a dried exudation from various trees consisting of a principle soluble in water and insoluble in alcohol, combined with a volatile oil or resin soluble in alcohol, but not in water, such as myrrh and scammony.
**soluble g.-r.,** pyroxylin.

**gun·cot·ton** (gun-kot'ən) pyroxylin.

**Gunn's crossing sign, dots, pupil,** etc. (gunz) [Robert Marcus *Gunn,* English ophthalmologist, 1850–1909] see under *dot, sign,* and *syndrome;* see *Marcus Gunn pupil,* under *pupil;* and see *Marcus Gunn's pupillary phenomenon,* under *phenomenon.*

**Gun·ning's splint** (gun'ingz) [Thomas Brian *Gunning,* American dentist, 1813–1889] see under *splint.*

**Gün·ther disease** (gēn'ter) [Hans *Günther,* German physician, 1884–1956] congenital erythropoietic porphyria.

**Günz's ligament** (gēnts'əz) [Justus Gottfried *Günz,* German anatomist, 1714–1754] see under *ligament.*

**gur·ney** (gər'ne) a wheeled cot used in hospitals.

**gus·ta·tion** (gəs-ta'shən) [L. *gustatio,* from *gustare* to taste] taste.
**colored g.,** a pseudogeusia in which tastes are associated with colors; called also *color taste.*

**gus·ta·tism** (gus'tə-tiz-əm) pseudogeusia.

**gus·tin** (gus'tin) a polypeptide (molecular weight, 27,000) present in saliva and containing two zinc atoms; it is apparently necessary for normal development of the taste buds.

**gus·tom·e·ter** (gəs-tom'ə-tər) [L. *gustare* to taste + *-meter*] an apparatus used in the quantitative determination of taste thresholds; see also *electrogustometer.*

**gus·tom·e·try** (gəs-tom'ə-tre) the clinical determination of thresholds of the sense of taste.

**gut** (gut) 1. intestinum. 2. the primordial digestive tube, consisting of the foregut, midgut, and hindgut. 3. surgical g.
**blind g.,** caecum (def. 2).
**chromic g., chromicized g.,** surgical gut treated with a chromic salt to increase its resistance to absorption in tissues.
**postanal g.,** a temporary extension of the embryonic hindgut caudal to the cloaca.
**preoral g.,** Seessel's pouch.
**primitive g., primordial g.,** archenteron.
**ribbon g.,** an absorbable ribbon of the intestinal tissue of animals used for suturing where broad support is to be secured.
**surgical g.,** an absorbable sterile strand obtained from collagen derived from healthy mammals, originally prepared from the submucous layer of the intestines of sheep; used as a surgical ligature. See also *absorbable suture,* under *suture.* Called also *catgut.*
**tail g.,** postanal g.

**Guth·rie's muscle** (guth'rēz) [George James *Guthrie,* English surgeon, 1785–1856] musculus sphincter urethrae.

**Guth·rie test** (guth're) [Robert *Guthrie,* American microbiologist, born 1916] see under *test.*

**Gu·ti·er·re·zia** (goo"te-ə-re'ze-ə) the broomweeds or snakeweeds, a genus of herbs that have yellow flowers; several species, such as *G. diversifo'lia* and *G. saro'thrae,* may cause selenium poisoning in livestock when growing in selenium-rich soil. *G. microce'phala* causes abortion in pregnant female animals.

**gut·ta** (gut'ə) pl. *gut'tae* [L.] a drop.

**gut·tae** (gut'e) [L.] plural of *gutta.*

**gut·ta-per·cha** (gut"ə-pər'chə) [Malay *getah perca* sap of the percha tree] [USP] [MeSH: Gutta-Percha] the coagulated, dried, and purified latex of trees of the genera *Palaquium* and *Payena,* particularly *Palaquium gutta;* used in orthopedics for fracture splints, in surgery for temporary sealing of cavities, and in dentistry in the form of cones for filling the root canal and in the form of sticks for sealing cavities over treatment.

**Guttat.** abbreviation for L. *gutta'tim,* drop by drop.

**gut·tate** (gut'āt) characterized by lesions that are drop-shaped.

**gut·ta·tim** (gə-ta'tim) [L.] drop by drop.

**gut·tie** (gut'ti) 1. a hernia in cattle in which a loop of intestine passes through a tear in the peritoneum and is held there, producing obstruction of the bowels. 2. a twisting of the intestine in domestic animals.

**Gutt. quibusd.** abbreviation for L. *gut'tis quibus'dam,* with a few drops.

**gut·tur** (gut'ər) [L.] fauces.

**gut·tur·al** (gut'ər-əl) 1. pertaining to the throat; see also *pharyngeal.* Called also *faucial.* 2. velar, def. 2.

**gut·tur·oph·o·ny** (gut"ər-of'ə-ne) [*guttur* + Gr. *phōnē* voice] a throaty quality of the voice.

**gut·turo·tet·a·ny** (gut"ər-o-tet'ə-ne) [*guttur* + *tetany*] a guttural spasm, resulting in a kind of stutter.

**Gut·zeit's test** (goot'zītz) [Max Adolf *Gutzeit,* German chemist, 1847–1915] see under *test.*

**Guy de Chau·li·ac** see *Chauliac.*

**Gu·yon's amputation (operation), canal, sign** (ge-yonz') [Felix Jean Casimir *Guyon,* French surgeon, 1831–1920] see under *amputation, canal,* and *sign.*

**GVH** graft-versus-host (disease or reaction).

**GXT** graded exercise test.

**Gy** gray, def. 2.

**Gym·na·moe·bia** (jim"nə-me'be-ə) [*gymn-* + *ameba*] a subclass of free-living ameboid protozoa (class Lobosea, superclass Rhizopoda, subphylum Sarcodina), the organisms of which are "naked"; i.e., they lack a test. It comprises three orders: Amoebida, Schizopyrenida, and Pelobiontida.

**gym·nas·tics** (jəm-nas'tiks) [Gr. *gymnastikos* pertaining to athletics] [MeSH: Gymnastics] systematic muscular exercise.
**ocular g.,** systematic exercise of the eye muscles in order to secure proper movement, accommodation, or fixation.
**Swedish g.,** a system of exercise following a rigid pattern of carefully chosen free, active, deliberate movement, utilizing little equipment and stressing correct bodily posture.

**Gym·ne·ma** (jim-ne'mə) a genus of trees of the family Asclepiadaceae. *G. sylves'tre* R. Bv. is an African species whose leaves are used as a flavoring agent for medicines.

**gymn(o)-** [Gr. *gymnos* naked] a combining form meaning naked or denoting relationship to nakedness.

**Gym·no·as·ca·ceae** (jim"no-as-ka'se-e) a family of keratinophilic fungi of the order Onygenales in which the reproductive organs are in the form of naked asci. It includes the genera *Ajellomyces, Arthroderma,* and *Gymnoascus.*

**Gym·no·as·cus** (jim"no-as'kəs) a genus of fungi of the family Gymnoascaceae, some species of which are pathogenic. *G. gyp'seus* is a former name for *Microsporum gypseum.*

**gym·no·car·pous** (jim"no-kahr'pəs) [*gymno-* + Gr. *karpos* fruit] said of fungi that have the hymenium, or fertile layer, exposed during spore formation.

**gym·no·cyte** (jim'no-sīt) [*gymno-* + *-cyte*] a cell with no cell wall.

**Gym·no·din·i·um** (jim"no-din'e-əm) [*gymno-* + Gr. *dinein* to whirl] a genus of plantlike marine and freshwater protozoa (order Dinoflagellida, class Phytomastigophorea), most species of which have many colored (yellow, brown, green, or blue) chromatophores. Like other dinoflagellates, they produce discoloration of the water (red tide) when present in vast numbers, and certain species, especially *G. breve,* have been associated with a type of shellfish poisoning (q.v.).

**gym·no·plast** (jim'no-plast) [*gymno-* + *-plast*] gymnocyte.

**gym·no·sperm** (jim'no-spərm) [*gymno-* + *sperma*] a plant in which the seeds are not enclosed in an ovary.

**gym·no·spore** (jim'no-spor) a spore without any protective envelope.

**gym·no·the·ci·um** (jim"no-the'se-əm) a type of fruiting body (ascocarp) composed of a loose network of mycelia through which ascospores filter and are released at maturity; its reproductive organs are in the form of naked asci. Seen in fungi of the family Gymnoascaceae.

**gynaec(o)-** for words beginning thus, see those beginning *gynec(o)-.*

**gy·nan·der** (jə-nan'dər) [*gyn-* + Gr. *anēr, andros* man] 1. female pseudohermaphrodite. 2. hermaphrodite. 3. any female exhibiting masculinization.

**gy·nan·dria** (jə-nan'dre-ə) 1. female pseudohermaphroditism. 2. hermaphroditism. 3. masculinization (def. 1).

**gy·nan·drism** (jə-nan'driz-əm) [*gyn-* + *andr-* + *-ism*] 1. female pseudohermaphroditism. 2. hermaphroditism. 3. masculinization (def. 1).

**gy·nan·dro·blas·to·ma** (jə-nan"dro-blas-to'mə) [*gyn-* + *andro-* + *blastoma*] a rare ovarian tumor containing histologic features of both arrhenoblastoma and granulosa cell tumor.

**gy·nan·droid** (jə-nan'droid) [*gyn-* + *andr-* + *-oid*] 1. like a gynander. 2. hermaphrodite. 3. hermaphroditic.

**gy·nan·dro·morph** (jə-nan'dro-morf) 1. an individual exhibiting gynandromorphism. 2. hermaphrodite.

**gy·nan·dro·mor·phism** (jə-nan"dro-mor'fiz-əm) [*gyn-* + *andro-* + *morph-* + *-ism*] 1. the presence of chromosomes of both sexes in different tissues of the body, producing a mosaic of male and female characteristics; a condition common among bees and silkworms. 2. hermaphroditism.
**bilateral g.,** see under *hermaphroditism.*

**gy·nan·dro·mor·phous** (jə-nan"dro-mor'fəs) 1. pertaining to or characterized by gynandromorphism. 2. hermaphroditic.

**gy·nan·dry** (jī'nan-dre) 1. female pseudohermaphroditism. 2. hermaphroditism. 3. masculinization (def. 1).

**gyn·atre·sia** (jin"ə-tre'zhə) [*gyn-* + *atresia*] occlusion of some part of the female genital tract, especially of the vagina.

**gyne-** see *gynec(o)-.*

**gy·nec·ic** (jə-nes'ik) feminine.

**gy·ne·ci·um** (jə-ne'se-əm) [*gyn-* + Gr. *oikos* house] the female part of a flower; called also *pistil.*

**gynec(o)-** [Gr. *gynē,* gen. *gynaikos* woman] a combining form meaning female or denoting relationship to women or to the female reproductive organs. Also, *gynaec(o)-, gyne-,* and *gyn(o)-.*

**gyne·co·gen** (jin'ə-ko-jən) old term for *estrogen.*

**gyne·co·gen·ic** (jin"ə-ko-jen'ik) feminizing.

**gyne·cog·ra·phy** (jin"ə-kog'rə-fe) radiography of the female reproductive tract.

**gyn·e·coid** (jin'ə-koid) [*gynec-* + *oid*] womanlike; see also *feminine.*

**gy·ne·co·log·ic** (gi"nə-kə-loj'ik, jin"ə-) pertaining to or affecting the female reproductive tract.

**gy·ne·co·log·i·cal** (gi"nə-kə-loj'ĭ-kəl, jin"ə-) pertaining to gynecology.

**gy·ne·col·o·gist** (gi"nə-kol'ə-jist, jin"ə-) a person skilled in gynecology.

**gy·ne·col·o·gy** (gi"nə-kol'ə-je, jin"ə-) [*gyneco-* + *-logy*] [MeSH: Gynecology] that branch of medicine that treats of diseases of the genital tract in women.

**gyne·co·ma·nia** (jin"ə-ko-ma'ne-ə) [*gyneco-* + *-mania*] satyriasis.

**gyne·co·mas·tia** (jin"ə-ko-mas'te-ə) [*gyneco-* + *mast-* + *-ia*] [MeSH: Gynecomastia] excessive growth of the male mammary glands, in some cases including development to the stage at which milk is produced, usually associated with metabolic derangements that lead to estrogen accumulation, testosterone deficiency, and hyperprolactinemia. A mild form may develop transiently during normal puberty.
**nutritional g., refeeding g., rehabilitation g.,** transitory enlargement of the male breast developing during rehabilitation and recovery from a state of malnutrition or starvation.

**gyne·co·mas·tism** (jin"ə-ko-mas'tiz-əm) gynecomastia.

**gyne·co·mas·ty** (jin'ə-ko-mas"te) gynecomastia.

**gyne·cop·a·thy** (jin"ə-kop'ə-the) [*gyneco-* + *-pathy*] a disease peculiar to women.

**gyne·coph·o·ral** (jin"ə-kof'ə-rəl) see under *canal.*

**gyne·duct** (jin'ə-dəkt) [*gyne-* + *duct*] ductus paramesonephricus.

**Gyne-Lo·tri·min** (gi"nə-lo'trĭ-min) trademark for preparations of clotrimazole.

**gyne·pho·bia** (gi"nə-fo'be-ə, jin"ə-) [*gyne-* + *-phobia*] irrational fear of or aversion to women.

**gyne·plas·ty** (jin'ə-plas'te) gynoplasty.

**Gyn·er·gen** (jin'ər-jən) trademark for preparations of ergotamine tartrate.

**gyn·e·sin** (jin'ə-sin) trigonelline.

**gyn(o)-** see *gynec(o)-.*

**gyno·gen·e·sis** (jin"o-jen'ə-sis) [*gyno-* + *-genesis*] development of an ovum that is stimulated by a sperm in the absence of any participation of the sperm nucleus.

**gyno·mer·o·gon** (jin"o-mer'ə-gon) an organism developed from a fertilized oocyte that contains the female pronucleus only; as a result, the cells contain only the maternal set of chromosomes.

**gyno·mer·o·gone** (jin"o-mer'ə-gon) gynomerogon.

**gyno·me·rog·o·ny** (jin"o-mə-rog'ə-ne) [*gyno-* + *merogony*] development of a portion of a fertilized oocyte containing the female pronucleus only. Cf. *andromerogony* and *merogony.*

**gyno·path·ic** (jin"o-path'ik) [*gyno-* + *path-* + *-ic*] caused by or pertaining to disease of women.

**gyn·op·a·thy** (jin-op′ə-the) any disease of women.

**gyno·pho·bia** (gi″no-fo′be-ə, jin″o-) gynephobia.

**gyno·plas·tic** (jin′o-plas′tik) pertaining to gynoplasty.

**gyno·plas·tics** (jin″o-plas′tiks) gynoplasty.

**gyno·plas·ty** (ji′no-plas″te) plastic or reconstructive surgery of the female reproductive organs. Called also *gyneplasty* and *gynoplastics.*

**Gy·no·rest** (gi′no-rest) trademark for a preparation of dydrogesterone.

**gyp·sum** (jip′səm) [L.; Gr. *gypsos* chalk] native calcium sulfate dihydrate (see *calcium sulfate,* under *calcium*); when calcined, it becomes *plaster of Paris.*

**gy·rate** (ji′rāt) [L. *gyratus* turned round] twisted in a ring or spiral shape.

**gy·ra·tion** (ji-ra′shən) revolution in a circle or in circles.

**gy·rec·to·my** (ji-rek′tə-me) excision or resection of a cerebral gyrus, or of a portion of the cerebral cortex.
**frontal g.,** topectomy.

**Gy·ren·ceph·a·la** (ji″rən-sef′ə-lə) [*gyrus* + Gr. *enkephalos* brain] a group of higher mammals in which the cerebrum is characteristically marked by convolutions. Cf. *Lissencephala.*

**gy·ren·ce·phal·ic** (ji″rən-sə-fal′ik) 1. pertaining to the Gyrencephala. 2. having cerebral hemispheres marked by convolutions. Cf. *lissencephalic.*

**gy·ri** (ji′ri) [L.] genitive and plural of *gyrus.*

**gyr(o)-** [Gr. *gyros* circle] a combining form meaning round or denoting relationship to a gyrus.

**Gy·ro·dac·ty·lus** (ji″ro-dak′tĭ-lus) a genus of trematodes that infect the skin and gills of aquarium fish, causing hyperactivity and breathing problems that can be fatal.

**gy·rom·e·ter** (ji-rom′ə-tər) [*gyro-* + *-meter*] an instrument for measuring the cerebral gyri.

**Gy·ro·mi·tra** (ji′ro-mi′trə) a genus of mushrooms of the family Helvellaceae, found in North America and Europe; many species contain the toxin monomethylhydrazine.

**Gy·ro·pus** (gi′ro-pəs) a genus of biting lice of the order Mallophaga; *G. ova′lis* is found on guinea pigs.

**gy·rose** (ji′rōs) marked by curved lines or circles.

**gy·ro·spasm** (ji′ro-spaz-əm) [*gyro-* + *spasm*] rotatory spasm of the head.

**gy·rous** (ji′rəs) gyrose.

**gy·rus** (ji′rəs) gen. and pl. *gy′ri* [L., from Gr. *gyros* circle] [TA] one of the convolutions of the surface of the cerebral hemispheres caused by infolding of the cortex; see *gyri cerebri.*

## Gyrus

Descriptions of gyri are given on TA terms, and include anglicized names of specific gyri.

**g. angula′ris** [TA], angular gyrus: a convolution of the inferior parietal lobule, arching over the posterior end of the superior temporal sulcus and continuous with the middle temporal gyrus. Called also *pli courbe.*

**annectant gyri, annectent gyri, gy′ri annecten′tes,** gyri transitivi cerebri.

**ascending parietal g.,** g. postcentralis.

**gy′ri bre′ves in′sulae** [TA], short gyri of insula: the short, rostrally placed gyri on the surface of the insula; called also *preinsular gyri.*

**Broca′s g.,** see under *convolution.*

**callosal g., g. callo′sus,** g. cinguli.

**central g., anterior,** g. precentralis.

**central g., posterior,** g. postcentralis.

**g. cerebel′li,** folia cerebelli.

**cerebral gyri, gy′ri cerebra′les,** gyri cerebri.

**gy′ri ce′rebri** [TA], **gyri of cerebrum,** cerebral gyri: the tortuous convolutions of the surface of the cerebral hemispheres, caused by infolding of the cortex and separated by the fissures or sulci. Many are constant enough that they have been given special names.

**cingulate g., g. cingula′tus,** g. cinguli.

**g. cin′guli** [TA], cingulate gyrus: an arch-shaped convolution closely related to the surface of the corpus callosum, from which it is separated by the callosal sulcus; called also *callosal g., g. callosus,* and *g. cingulatus.*

**dentate g.,** 1. g. dentatus (def. 1). 2. g. fasciolaris.

**g. denta′tus,** 1. [TA] dentate gyrus: a serrated strip of gray matter under the medial border of the hippocampus and in its depths; it is an archaeocortex which develops along the edge of the hippocampal fissure and which consists of molecular, granular, and polymorphic layers. 2. g. fasciolaris.

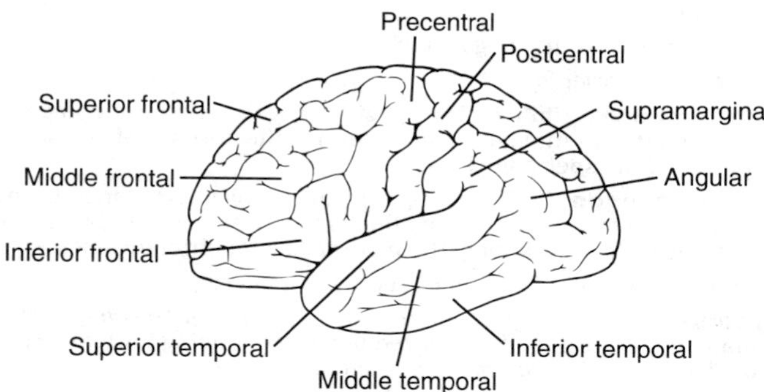


Gyri cerebri (cerebral gyri) in a lateral view of the left hemisphere.

**g. descen′dens,** the raised area posterior to the inferior and superior occipital gyri and anterior to the lunate sulcus when that is present.

**g. fasciola′ris** [TA], fasciolar gyrus: a posterior and upward extension of the dentate gyrus, forming a transitional area between the dentate gyrus and the indusium griseum; called also *fasciola cinerea.*

**g. fornica′tus,** the marginal portion of the cerebral cortex on the medial aspect of the hemisphere, including the gyrus cinguli, gyrus parahippocampalis, isthmus, and uncus; it forms a major part of the limbic system.

**frontal g., ascending,** g. precentralis.

**frontal g., inferior,** g. frontalis inferior.

**frontal g., medial,** g. frontalis medialis.

**frontal g., middle,** g. frontalis medius.

**frontal g., superior,** g. frontalis superior.

**g. fronta′lis infe′rior** [TA], inferior frontal gyrus: a convolution of the frontal lobe below the inferior frontal sulcus; it is divided by the anterior and ascending branches of the lateral sulcus into orbital, triangular, and opercular parts.

**g. fronta′lis media′lis** [TA], medial frontal gyrus: the medial surface of the frontal lobe, separated from the cingulate gyrus by the cingulate sulcus, and continuous with the superior frontal gyrus above and the gyrus rectus below.

**g. fronta′lis me′dius** [TA], middle frontal gyrus: a convolution of the frontal lobe between the superior and inferior frontal sulci, extending anteriorly from the precentral gyrus; a longitudinal sulcus is often present, dividing the gyrus into superior and inferior parts.

**g. fronta′lis supe′rior** [TA], superior frontal gyrus: a convolution of the frontal lobe above the superior frontal sulcus, extending anteriorly from the precentral gyrus.

**g. fusifor′mis,** fusiform gyrus: a gyrus of the temporal lobe on the inferior surface of the hemisphere between the inferior temporal gyrus and the parahippocampal gyrus. It consists of a lateral and a medial part, called *g. occipitotemporalis lateralis* [TA] and *g. occipitotemporalis medialis* [TA].

**g. geni′culi,** a vestigial gyrus at the anterior end of the corpus callosum.

**Heschl′s gyri,** gyri temporales transversi.

**hippocampal g., g. hippocam′pi,** g. parahippocampalis.

**infracalcarine g.,** g. lingualis.

**gy′ri in′sulae** [TA], insular gyri: the gyri that are found on the surface of the insula, including the *gyrus longus insulae* and the *gyri breves insulae.*

**interlocking gyri,** small gyri in the opposing walls of the central sulcus which interlock with each other like gears.

**intralimbic g.,** the posterior part of the inferior surface of the uncus, separated from the uncinate gyrus by Giacomini′s band.

**g. lingua′lis** [TA], lingual gyrus: a gyrus of the occipital lobe on the inferior surface of the hemisphere, forming the inferior lip of the calcarine sulcus and, with the cuneus, the visual cortex; it is continuous anteriorly with the parahippocampal gyrus.

**g. lon'gus in'sulae** [TA], long gyrus of insula: the long, occipitally directed gyrus on the surface of the insula.

**marginal g., marginal g. of Turner, g. margina'lis,** g. frontalis medialis.

**occipital g., inferior,** the lower of the two gyri separated by the lateral occipital sulcus on the lateral aspect of the occipital lobe.

**occipital gyri, lateral,** see *occipital g., inferior* and *occipital g., superior.*

**occipital g., superior,** the upper of the two gyri separated by the occipital lateral sulcus on the lateral aspect of the occipital lobe.

**occipitotemporal g., lateral,** g. occipitotemporalis lateralis.

**occipitotemporal g., medial,** g. occipitotemporalis medialis.

**g. occipitotempora'lis latera'lis** [TA], lateral occipitotemporal gyrus: the lateral portion of the gyrus fusiformis on the inferior surface of the cerebral hemisphere, separated from the medial portion by the occipitotemporal sulcus, and continuous laterally with the inferior temporal gyrus.

**g. occipitotempora'lis media'lis** [TA], medial occipitotemporal gyrus: the medial portion of the gyrus fusiformis on the inferior surface of the cerebral hemisphere, separated from the lateral portion by the occipitotemporal sulcus, and from the parahippocampal gyrus by the collateral sulcus.

**g. olfacto'rius latera'lis** [TA], lateral olfactory gyrus: the layer of gray substance covering the lateral olfactory stria.

**g. olfacto'rius media'lis** [TA], medial olfactory gyrus: the layer of gray substance covering the medial olfactory stria.

**olfactory g., lateral,** gyrus olfactorius lateralis.

**olfactory g., medial,** gyrus olfactorius medialis.

**gy'ri orbita'les** [TA], orbital gyri: the various irregular convolutions lateral to the olfactory sulcus on the orbital surface of the frontal lobe.

**paracentral g., g. paracentra'lis,** lobulus paracentralis.

**g. parahippocampa'lis** [TA], parahippocampal gyrus: a convolution on the inferior surface of each cerebral hemisphere, lying between the hippocampal and collateral sulci; called also *hippocampal g.* and *g. hippocampi.*

**g. paratermina'lis** [TA], paraterminal gyrus: a thin sheet of gray substance in front of and ventral to the genu of the corpus callosum; see also *septum precommissurale.*

**parietal g.,** any one of the convolutions into which the surface of the parietal lobe is divided.

**g. postcentra'lis** [TA], postcentral gyrus: the convolution of the parietal lobe lying between the central and postcentral sulci; the primary sensory area of the cerebral cortex. Called also *posterior central g.* and *ascending parietal g.*

**g. precentra'lis** [TA], precentral gyrus: the convolution of the frontal lobe lying between the precentral and central sulci; the primary motor area of the cerebral cortex. Called also *anterior central g.*

**preinsular gyri,** gyri breves insulae.

**g. rec'tus** [TA], straight gyrus: a convolution on the orbital surface of the frontal lobe, medial to the olfactory sulcus and continuous with the medial frontal gyrus on the medial surface.

**short gyri of insula,** gyri breves insulae.

**splenial g.,** g. fasciolaris.

**straight g.,** g. rectus.

**subcallosal g.,** area subcallosa.

**supracallosal g.,** indusium griseum.

**g. supramargina'lis** [TA], supramarginal gyrus: the convolution of the inferior parietal lobe that curves around the upper end of the posterior branch of the lateral fissure and is continuous behind it with the superior temporal gyrus.

**temporal g., anterior transverse,** gyrus temporalis transversus anterior.

**temporal g., inferior,** g. temporalis inferior.

**temporal g., middle,** g. temporalis medius.

**temporal g., posterior tranverse,** gyrus temporalis transversus posterior.

**temporal g., superior,** g. temporalis superior.

**temporal gyri, transverse,** gyri temporales transversi.

**g. tempora'lis infe'rior** [TA], inferior temporal gyrus: the convolution of the temporal lobe lying between the inferior temporal sulcus and the lateral occipitotemporal gyrus, the two gyri being continuous at the inferolateral margin of the temporal lobe.

**g. tempora'lis me'dius** [TA], middle temporal gyrus: the convolution of the temporal lobe lying between the superior and the inferior temporal sulci; it is continuous posteriorly with the angular gyrus.

**g. tempora'lis supe'rior** [TA], superior temporal gyrus: the convolution of the temporal lobe lying between the superior temporal sulcus and the lateral sulcus, continuous posteriorly with the supramarginal gyrus.

**gy'ri tempora'les transver'si** [TA], transverse temporal gyri: the transverse convolutions marking the posterior extremity of the superior temporal gyrus and lying mostly in the lateral sulcus; usually two, anterior and posterior, but sometimes single on one or both sides. Called also *Heschl's gyri* or *convolutions.*

**g. tempora'lis transver'sus ante'rior** [TA], anterior transverse temporal gyrus: the anterior, more marked, of the two transverse temporal gyri, where two exist; it represents the cortical center for hearing. See *gyri temporales transversi.*

**g. tempora'lis transver'sus poste'rior** [TA], posterior transverse temoral gyrus: the posterior of the two transverse temporal gyri, where two exist; see *gyri temporales transversi.*

**gy'ri transiti'vi ce'rebri,** various small folds on the cerebral surface that are too inconstant to bear special names; called also *annectant* or *annectent gyri.*

**uncinate g.,** the anterior part of the inferior surface of the uncus, separated from the intralimbic gyrus by Giacomini's band.

# H

**H** symbol for *hydrogen, Hauch, henry, Hounsfield unit,* and *hyperopia.*

***H*** symbol for *enthalpy* and *magnetic field strength.*

$H_0$ symbol for *null hypothesis.*

$H_1$ symbol for *alternative hypothesis.*

$H_a$ symbol for *alternative hypothesis.*

**h** symbol for *hecto-* and *hour.*

**h.** symbol for L. *ho'ra,* hour.

***h*** symbol for *Planck's constant* and *height.*

**HA** hemadsorbent.

**Ha** symbol for *hahnium* (element 105).

**HAA** hepatitis-associated antigen; see *hepatitis B surface antigen,* under *antigen.*

**Haab's magnet, reflex** (hahbz) [Otto *Haab,* Swiss ophthalmologist, 1850–1931] see under *magnet* and *reflex.*

**ha•be•na** (hə-be'nə) pl. *habe'nae* [L. "rein"] any straplike anatomic structure; cf. *habenula.*

**ha•ben•u•la** (hə-ben'u-lə) gen. and pl. *haben'ulae* [L., dim. of *habena,* q.v.] [MeSH: Habenula] 1. a frenulum, or reinlike structure, such as one of a set of such structures in the cochlea. 2. [TA] a component of the epithalamus, being the small eminence on the dorsomedial surface of the thalamus, just in front of the dorsal commissure on the lateral edge of the habenular trigone; called also *pineal peduncle.*
**h. cona'rii,** habenula (def. 2).
**Haller's h.,** vestigium processus vaginalis.
**habe'nulae perfora'tae,** foramina nervosa; see under *foramen.*
**h. urethra'lis,** either of two whitish lines extending from the urinary meatus to the clitoris in girls and young women.

**ha•ben•u•lae** (hə-ben'u-le) [L.] genitive and plural of *habenula.*

**ha•ben•u•lar** (hə-ben'u-lər) pertaining to a habenula.

**Ha•ber•mann's disease** (hah'ber-mahnz) [Rudolf *Habermann,* German dermatologist, 1884–1941] acute lichenoid pityriasis.

**hab•it** (hab'it) [L. *habitus,* from *habere* to hold] [MeSH: Habits] 1. a fixed or constant practice established by frequent repetition. 2. predisposition or bodily temperament; see also *type.*
**clamping h., clenching h.,** centric bruxism.
**endothelioid h.,** a condition in which the nucleus of a cell is relatively small as compared with the cytoplasm.
**glaucomatous h.,** shallowness of the anterior chamber of the eye with dilated pupil; seen in persons who have a predisposition to glaucoma.
**leukocytoid h.,** endothelioid h.
**oral h.,** one that causes changes in occlusal relationships, e.g., finger, thumb, and lip sucking, tongue thrusting, and the like. See also *habit-breaking appliance,* under *appliance.*

**hab•i•tat** (hab'ĭ-tat) the natural abode or home of an animal or plant species.

**ha•bit•u•a•tion** (hə-bich"u-a'shən) 1. the gradual adaptation to a stimulus or to the environment. 2. extinction or decrease of a conditioned reflex over time by repetition of the conditioned stimulus. 3. an older term used in describing habitual drug use, used sometimes to denote acquired drug tolerance (see *tolerance*) and other times to denote psychological but not physical dependence on a drug as a consequence of repeated consumption, with a desire to continue its use but with little or no tendency to increase the dose.

**hab•i•tus** (hab'ĭ-təs) [L. "habit"] 1. posture or position of the body. 2. physique; body build and constitution. See also entries under *type.*
**Buddha-like h.,** the froglike posture of the fetus.

**Hab•ro•ne•ma** (hab"ro-ne'mə) [Gr. *habros* graceful + *nema*] a genus of nematodes of the family Habronematidae. The larval forms are taken up from the feces of horses by flies and the flies, swallowed along with the feed, transmit the larvae to the horses' stomachs. The larvae may also be transmitted to the skin of horses where they produce cutaneous habronemiasis; in the conjunctiva they produce bungeye. The two most important species are *H. microsto'ma* (called also *H. ma'jus*) and *H. mus'cae. H. megasto'ma* has been reclassified as *Draschia megastoma.*

**Hab•ro•ne•mat•i•dae** (hab"ro-ne-mat'ĭ-de) a family of nematodes that includes the genera *Draschia* and *Habronema.* The adults are found in the stomachs of horses and the larvae cause habronemiasis.

**hab•ro•ne•mi•a•sis** (hab"ro-ne-mi'ə-sis) infection with a nematode of the family Habronematidae. *H. muscae* and *H. microstoma* in the stomach sometimes cause a mild catarrhal type of gastritis. *Draschia megastoma* causes gastric habronemiasis. Any of these species can also cause cutaneous habronemiasis.
**cutaneous h.,** a disease of horses in various parts of the world, including the southern United States, Brazil, India, and the Philippines, caused by skin infection with larvae of *Habronema* or *Draschia* species; cutaneous granulomas grow in size until the skin over and around them is destroyed, leaving a large raw surface. Because of the clinical similarity between cutaneous habronemiasis and pythiosis, the disorders are often confused. See also *swamp cancer,* under *cancer.* Called also *bursautee* and *summer sores.*
**gastric h.,** infestation of the stomach wall of a horse with larvae of *Draschia megastoma,* which form large nodules filled with worms and necrotic material. Many affected horses do not show clinical signs, but they may die if the stomach wall is perforated.

**ha•bu** (hah'boo) [native name in Ryukyu Islands] 1. *Trimeresurus flavoviridis,* an extremely venomous pit viper inhabiting the warmer parts of East Asia, especially the Ryukyu Islands. 2. *Trimeresurus mucrosquamatus* (also called the *Chinese habu*), a venomous pit viper found in Taiwan, southern China, and Southeast Asia.

**Had•field-Clarke syndrome** (had'fēld-klahrk) [Geoffrey *Hadfield,* British physician, 1889–1968; Cecil *Clarke,* British physician, 20th century] Clarke-Hadfield syndrome.

**hae-** for words beginning thus, see also those beginning *he-.*

**Haeck•el's law** (hek'əlz) [Ernst Heinrich Philipp August *Haeckel,* German naturalist, 1834–1919] see *recapitulation theory,* under *theory.*

**haem** (hēm) heme.

**hae•ma** (he'mə) [Gr. *haima, haimatos* blood] [TA] the blood (q.v.). Spelled also *hema.* Called also *sanguis* [TA alternative].

**haema-** see *hem(o)-*; for words beginning thus, see also those beginning *hema-.*

**Hae•mac•cel** (hē'mak-sel") trademark for a preparation of polygeline.

**Hae•ma•dip•sa** (he'mə-dip'sə) [*haema-* + *dipsia*] the land leeches, a genus of the family Gnathobdellidae.
**H. ceylo'nica,** a species common in Sri Lanka that has a painful bite and attacks humans and other animals.
**H. chilia'ni,** a species attacking horses and cattle in South America.
**H. japo'nica,** a species found in Japan.
**H. zeylan'dica,** a species attacking mammals in the tropical jungles of Asia.

**Hae•ma•gog•us** (hem"ə-gog'əs) [*haem-* + Gr. *agōgos* leading] a genus of mosquitoes of the tribe Aedini, family Culicinae, some of which transmit jungle yellow fever in tropical Central and South America.

**Hae•ma•phys•a•lis** (he"mə-fis'ə-lis) [*haema-* + *physallis* bubble] a large genus of ticks of the family Ixodidae; there are over 150 species.
**H. concin'na,** one of the vectors of *Rickettsia sibirica,* the etiologic agent of Siberian tick typhus.
**H. humero'sa,** the bandicoot tick, one of the vectors of *Coxiella burnetii.*
**H. lea'chi,** the common dog tick of South Africa; it transmits canine babesiosis.
**H. leporispalus'tris,** the rabbit tick, one of the vectors of Rocky Mountain spotted fever and tularemia among wild animals.
**H. longicor'nis,** a species that infests many types of mammals, including humans, in eastern Asia and the Pacific and transmits species of *Theileria* and *Babesia, Coxiella burnetii,* and Russian spring-summer encephalitis virus.
**H. oto'phila,** a species that parasitizes rodents and ruminants from southwestern Asia to southern Europe. Called also *H. parva.*
**H. par'va,** *H. otophila.*
**H. puncta'ta,** a species that infests ruminants and chickens from Central Asia across much of Europe, acting as a vector of babesiosis and possibly also as the cause of tick paralysis in chickens.
**H. spinige'ra,** a species occurring in the tropical forests of India that is a vector of Kyasanur Forest disease in forest workers.

**haemat(o)-** see *hemat(o)-.*

**Hae•ma•to•bia** (he"mə-to'be-ə) a genus of flies of the family Muscidae. *H. ir'ritans* is the horn fly, a small species that is very troublesome to cattle.

**Hae•ma•to•pi•nus** (he"mə-to-pi'nəs) [*haemato-* + Gr. *pinein* to drink] a genus of sucking lice (order Anoplura). *H. asi'ni* infests horses; *H. euryster'ni,* the short-nosed cattle louse, infests cattle; *H. quadrister'ni* infests cattle; and *H. su'is* is the most common louse of pigs.

**Hae·ma·top·o·ta** (he″mə-top′ə-tə) a genus of horse flies (family Tabanidae), large biting bloodsuckers that attack horses, cattle, and other mammals and cause anemia, mastitis, anthrax, anaplasmosis, and trypanosomiasis.

**Hae·ma·to·si·phon** (he″mə-to-si′fon) a genus of insects closely related to the genus *Cimex,* but having longer legs and a very long beak. *H. in′dorus,* a species of the southwestern United States and Mexico, may be a serious pest of poultry and sometimes attacks humans.

**Hae·ma·tox·y·lon** (he″mə-tok′sə-lon) [*haemato-* + Gr. *xylon* wood] a genus of trees of the family Leguminosae, native to Mexico, Central America and the West Indies. *H. campechia′num* L. is campechy or logwood, whose heartwood contains tannin, hematoxylin, and resin, and yields a purplish-red dye.

**Hae·men·te·ria** (he″mən-tēr′e-ə) a genus of leeches. *H. officina′lis* is used for medicinal purposes in Mexico and elsewhere in Latin America.

**haem(o)-** see *hem(o)-.*

**Hae·mo·bar·to·nel·la** (he″mo-bahr″to-nel′ə) [*haemo-* + *Bartonella*] a genus of bacteria of the family Anaplasmataceae, order Rickettsiales, occurring as parasites in various animals other than primates.

**H. ca′nis,** a nonpathogenic species found in dogs.

**H. fe′lis,** a species that causes feline infectious anemia and can be transmitted from cat to cat by biting during fights.

**H. mu′ris,** a common parasite of the laboratory rat, in which the infection is activated by splenectomy.

**hae·mo·bar·to·nel·lo·sis** (he″mo-bahr″tə-nə-lo′sis) feline infectious anemia.

**Hae·mo·dip·sus** (he″mo-dip′səs) a genus of lice. *H. ventrico′sus* is the common sucking louse of the rabbit and transmits the infective agent of tularemia from rabbit to rabbit.

**Hae·mo·greg·a·ri·na** (he″mo-greg″ə-ri′nə) [*hemo-* + L. *gregarius* crowding together] a genus of coccidian protozoa (suborder Adeleina, order Eucoccidiida) in which the life cycle involves two hosts, the vertebrate circulatory system (e.g., reptiles, amphibians, birds, certain mammals) and the invertebrate digestive system (e.g., blood-sucking invertebrates such as an insect or leech).

**hae·mon·cho·sis** (hēm″ong-ko′sis) infection of a ruminant with nematodes of the genus *Haemonchus,* especially *H. contortus,* characterized by weakness and anemia that can be fatal.

**Hae·mon·chus** (he-mon′kəs) [MeSH: Haemonchus] a genus of parasitic nematodes of the family Trichostrongylidae. *H. contor′tus* is the wireworm or barber's pole worm, a stomach worm that parasitizes the abomasum of ruminants, causing haemonchosis.

**Hae·moph·i·lus** (he-mof′ĭ-ləs) [*hemo-* + Gr. *philein* to love] [MeSH: Haemophilus] a genus of gram-negative, aerobic or facultatively anaerobic, rod-shaped or coccobacillary bacteria of the family Pasteurellaceae, made up of cells that sometimes form threads and filaments. The organisms require one or both growth factors (X factor, which can be replaced by hematin, or V factor, which can be replaced by nicotinamide adenine dinucleoside) present in blood. They are normal inhabitants of the upper respiratory tract but may become primary or secondary pathogens. Spelled also *Hemophilus.*

**H. aegyp′tius,** a species biovar of *H. influenzae* that produces infectious conjunctivitis in humans, especially in hot climates; formerly classified as a separate species.

**H. aphro′philus,** a species that is part of the normal oral microflora, and occasionally found as a cause of endocarditis.

**H. bronchisep′ticus,** *Bordetella bronchiseptica.*

**H. ducrey′i,** a species that causes soft chancres or chancroids on the genitals of humans. Called also *Ducrey's bacillus.*

**H. du′plex,** *Moraxella (Moraxella) lacunata.*

**H. equigenita′lis,** a species that causes contagious equine metritis in horses.

**H. haemoly′ticus,** a nonpathogenic species found as a normal inhabitant of the upper respiratory tract.

**H. influen′zae,** a species once thought to be the cause of epidemic influenza in humans. Noncapsulated strains are normal inhabitants of the human nasopharynx (biotypes II and III). In children, capsulated strains of biotype I are the major cause of bacterial meningitis, and may also cause potentially fatal acute epiglottitis (obstructive laryngitis). In both children and immunocompromised patients it can cause pneumonia (see *Haemophilus influenzae pneumonia*). Called also *Pfeiffer's bacillus.*

**H. paragallina′rum,** a species that causes infectious avian coryza in chickens.

**H. parainfluen′zae,** a species that is part of the normal oral flora and is occasionally associated with bacterial endocarditis.

**H. paraphro′philus,** a species that is part of the normal oral microflora. It has been associated with endocarditis and isolated from clinical specimens of abscessed internal organs.

**H. parasu′is,** a species found as a normal inhabitant of the upper respiratory tract of swine. It is a potential pathogen, causing respiratory tract infections and polyserositis; see also *Glasser's disease.* Called also *H. suis.*

**H. pertus′sis,** *Bordetella pertussis.*

**H. som′nus,** a species that causes thromboembolic meningoencephalitis and *Haemophilus* septicemia of cattle; its inclusion in the genus *Haemophilus* is sometimes disputed.

**H. su′is,** *H. parasuis.*

**H. vagina′lis,** *Gardnerella vaginalis.*

**Hae·mo·pho·ruc·tus** (he″mo-fə-ruk′təs) a genus of blood-sucking flies of the family Heleidae.

**Hae·mo·pis** (he-mo′pis) a genus of leeches, the horse leeches, of the family Gnathobdellidae. *H. paludum* is parasitic in the nose and throat in Sri Lanka. *H. sanguisuga* of Europe and North Africa infests the nasal passages.

**Hae·mo·pro·te·us** (he″mo-pro′te-əs) [*haemo-* + *Proteus*] a genus of coccidian protozoa (suborder Haemosporina, order Eucoccidiida) in which the vectors are blood-sucking insects other than mosquitoes and the vertebrate hosts are mammals, reptiles, and wild and domestic birds including ducks, pigeons, and turkeys. In these organisms merogony takes place not in erythrocytes but in the vascular endothelial cells, and the gametocytes are found only in the circulating erythrocytes.

**Hae·mo·spo·ri·na** (he″mo-spor-i′nə) [*hemo-* + *spore*] [MeSH: Haemosporina] a suborder of heteroxenous protozoa (subclass Coccidia, class Sporozoea) in which merogony takes place in a vertebrate, usually in the blood, and sporogony in the alimentary canal of a blood-sucking insect. Hemosporians are characterized by the independent development of macrogamete and microgamont; the absence of syzygy; the usual absence of a conoid; the production by the microgamont of eight flagellated microgametes; and the formation of a motile zygote (ookinete). Representative genera include *Haemoproteus, Hepatocystis, Leucocytozoon,* and *Plasmodium.*

**hae·mo·zo·in** (he″mo-zo′in) hemozoin.

**Hae·nel's symptom** (ha′nəlz) [Hans *Haenel,* German neurologist, 1874–1942] see under *symptom.*

**Hae·ser** see *Häser.*

**Haff disease** (hahf) [Ger. *Haff,* bay; named for Königsberg (or Frisches) *Haff,* a bay connected with the Baltic Sea, where epidemics occurred in 1924–5, 1932–3, and 1940] see under *disease.*

**Haf·nia** (haf′ne-ə) [L. *Hafnia* the old name for Copenhagen] a genus of gram-negative facultatively anaerobic rod-shaped bacteria of the family Enterobacteriaceae, made up of motile, peritrichously flagellated, unencapsulated organisms.

**H. al′vei,** a species found in feces, sewage, soil, water, and dairy products. Called also *Enterobacter hafnia.*

**haf·ni·um** (haf′ne-əm) [L. *Hafnia* Copenhagen] [MeSH: Hafnium] a chemical element of atomic number 72 and atomic weight 178.49; symbol Hf. Discovered in a zircon, in 1923, by Coster and Hevesy of Copenhagen.

**Hag·e·dorn's needles** (hahg′ə-dornz) [Werner *Hagedorn,* German surgeon, 1831–1894] see under *needle.*

**Hag·lund's disease** (hahg′loondz) [Sims Emil Patrik *Haglund,* Swedish orthopedist, 1870–1937] see under *disease.*

**Hag·ner bag** (hag′nər) [Francis Randall *Hagner,* American surgeon, 1873–1940] see under *bag.*

**Hag·ner's disease** (hahg′nərz) [name of the original propositus family studied in the 19th century] hypertrophic pulmonary osteoarthropathy; see under *osteoarthropathy.*

**Hahn's sign** (hahnz) [Eugen Heinrich *Hahn,* German physician, 1841–1902] see under *sign.*

**hah·ne·man·ni·an** (hahn″ə-man′e-ən) pertaining to Christian Friedrich Samuel *Hahnemann,* German physician, 1755–1843, founder of homeopathy.

**hah·ne·man·nism** (hahn′ə-mən″iz-əm) homeopathy.

**HAI** hemagglutination inhibition; see under *tests.*

**Hai·ding·er's brushes** (hi′ding-ərz) [Wilhelm von *Haidinger,* Austrian mineralogist, 1795–1871] see under *brush.*

**Hai·ley-Hai·ley disease** (ha′le ha′le) [Hugh *Hailey,* American dermatologist, born 1909; William Howard *Hailey,* American dermatologist, 1898–1967] benign familial pemphigus; see under *pemphigus.*

**hair** (hār) [L. *pilus;* Gr. *thrix*] [MeSH: Hair] a long slender filament. Applied especially to filamentous appendages of the skin, consisting of keratin (*pili* [TA]), or of the scalp (*capilli* [TA]). Each hair consists of a cylindrical *shaft* and a root, which is contained in a flasklike depression (*hair follicle*) in the corium and subcutaneous tissue. The base of the root is expanded into the *hair bulb,* which rests upon and encloses the *hair papilla.*

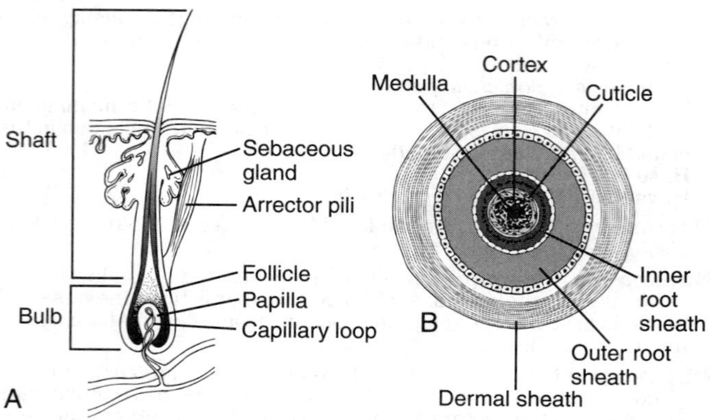


Hair in longitudinal section *(A)*, and in cross section *(B)*, showing the surrounding root and dermal sheaths.

**bamboo h.**, trichorrhexis nodosa.
**beaded h.**, hair marked with alternate swellings and constrictions, as seen in monilethrix. Called also *moniliform h.*
**burrowing h.**, one which does not emerge from the skin but grows horizontally beneath its surface, exciting a foreign body papule, which may become infected. Called also *pilus cuniculatus.* Cf. *ingrown h.*
**club h.**, a hair the root of which is surrounded by a bulbous enlargement composed of completely keratinized cells, preliminary to normal loss of the hair from the follicle; see *telogen.*
**exclamation point h.**, a hair which, when pulled out, shows atrophy and attenuation of the bulb; it is characteristic of alopecia areata.
**h's of eyebrow,** supercilia.
**Frey's h's,** stiff hairs of varying diameters, individually mounted in a handle; used for testing the sensitiveness of the pressure points of the skin.
**gustatory h's,** taste h's.
**ingrown h.**, one which emerges from the skin but curves and reenters it, exciting a foreign body papule, which may become infected. Called also *pilus incarnatus.* Cf. *burrowing h.*
**knotted h.**, trichonodosis.
**lanugo h.**, the fine, colorless hair growing on the body of the fetus, constituting the lanugo.
**moniliform h.**, beaded h.
**olfactory h's,** modified cilia that are extremely long and nonmotile, which project from the olfactory vesicle and function as sensory receptors. Called also *olfactory cilia.*
**pubic h.**, pubes, def. 1.
**resting h.**, see *telogen.*
**sensory h's,** hairlike projections on the cells of sensory epithelium; see also *olfactory h's,* and *taste h's.*
**stellate h.**, a hair split at the end in a starlike form.
**tactile h's,** hairs which are sensitive to touch, as the vibrissae of certain animals.
**taste h's,** clumps of microvilli that form short hairlike processes projecting into the lumen of a taste pore from the peripheral ends of the taste cells.
**terminal h.**, the coarse hair growing on various areas of the body during adult years.
**twisted h.**, a hair which at spaced intervals is twisted through an axis of 180 degrees, being abnormally flattened at the site of twisting. Called also *pilus tortus.*
**vellus h.**, the downy hair growing on the body during the prepubertal years, constituting the vellus.

**hair·ball** (hār'bawl) trichobezoar.

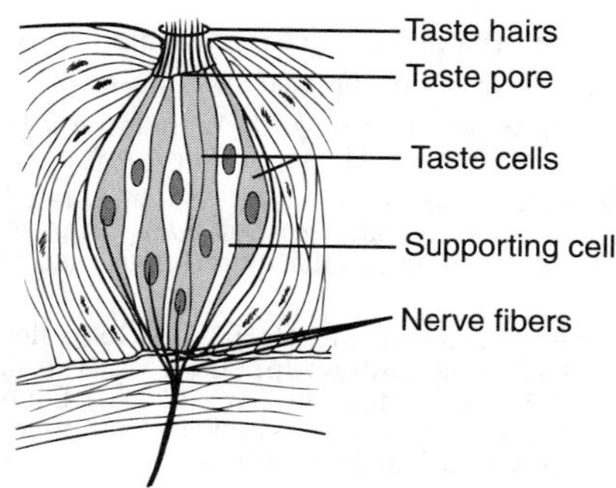


Taste hairs protruding from the pore of a taste bud.

**hair·cap** (hār'kap) *Polytrichum juniperinum.*

**hair·worm** (hār'wərm) threadworm.

**Ha·kim's syndrome** (hah-kēmz') [S. *Hakim,* American neurologist, 20th century] normal-pressure hydrocephalus; see under *hydrocephalus.*

**Ha·kim-Ad·ams syndrome** (hah-keem'ad'əmz) [S. *Hakim;* R.D. *Adams,* American physician, 20th century] normal-pressure hydrocephalus; see under *hydrocephalus.*

**Hal·a·rach·ni·dae** (hal"ə-rak'nĭ-de) a family of mites that parasitize monkeys and dogs; it includes the genera *Pneumonyssoides* and *Pneumonyssus.*

**hal·a·tion** (hal-a'shən) [Gr. *halōs* halo] indistinctness or blurring of the visual image by strong illumination coming from the same direction as the viewed object.

**hal·az·e·pam** (hal-az'ə-pam) a benzodiazepine used as an anxiolytic in the treatment of anxiety disorder and for short-term relief of anxiety symptoms; administered orally.

**hal·a·zone** (hal'ə-zōn) [USP] a white, crystalline powder, $C_7H_5Cl_2NO_4S$, having a chlorine-like odor; used as a disinfectant for water supplies.

**hal·cin·o·nide** (hal-sin'ə-nīd) [USP] [MeSH: Halcinonide] a synthetic corticosteroid used topically for the relief of inflammation and pruritus in corticosteroid-responsive dermatoses.

**Hal·ci·on** (hal'se-ən) trademark for a preparation of triazolam.

**Hal·dane chamber (apparatus), effect** (hawl'dān) [John Scott *Haldane,* Scottish physiologist, 1860–1936] see under *chamber* and *effect.*

**Hal·dol** (hal'dol) trademark for preparations of haloperidol.

**Hal·drone** (hal'drōn) trademark for a preparation of paramethasone acetate.

**Hales' piesimeter** (hālz) [Stephen *Hales,* English physiologist, 1677–1761] see under *piesimeter.*

**Hal·fan** (hal'fan) trademark for a preparation of halofantrine hydrochloride.

**half-ax·i·al** (haf-ak'se-əl) hemiaxial.

**half-life** (haf'līf) [MeSH: Half-Life] 1. the time required for the decay of half of a sample of particles of a radionuclide or elementary particle, equal to 0.693 divided by the decay constant; symbol $t_{1/2}$ or $T_{1/2}$. 2. half-time.
**antibody h.-l.**, a measure of the mean survival time of antibody molecules following their formation, usually expressed as the time required to eliminate 50 per cent of a known quantity of immunoglobulin from the animal body. Half-life varies from one immunoglobulin class to another.
**biological h.-l.**, the time required for a living tissue, organ, or organism to eliminate one half of a radioactive substance which has been introduced into it.
**drug h.-l.**, the time required for the plasma level of drug to fall to half of a certain measured level.
**effective h.-l.**, the time required for the radioactivity of a radioactive nuclide to be diminished 50 per cent through the combined action of radioactive decay and biological elimination.

**half-time** (haf'tīm) the time required for one half of a quantity of a substance to be eliminated from a system when the substance is eliminated at a rate proportional to its concentration (i.e., exhibits first-order kinetics); symbol $t_{1/2}$ or $T_{1/2}$.
**plasma iron clearance h.-t.**, the time required for half of the iron in the blood plasma at a given time to be removed, determined by administering radioactive iron-59 bound to the patient's own transferrin and calculating the slope of the best-fit line to a semilogarithmic plot of the amount of plasma radioactive iron over time.

**half-val·ue** (haf"val'u) see under *layer.*

**half·way house** (haf'wa hous) [MeSH: Halfway Houses] a residence for patients, such as mental patients, drug addicts, and alcoholics, who do not require complete hospitalization but who need an intermediate degree of care until they have again become established in the community.

**hal·i·but** (hal'ĭ-bət) any fish of the genus *Hippoglossus.*

**Hal·i·ceph·a·lo·bus** (hal"e-sef"ə-lo'bus) a genus of phasmid parasites of the order Rhabditoidea. *H. dele'trix* is a species that usually inhabits decaying organic matter and manure but sometimes infests horses, such as in nasal sinuses and the central nervous system. Called also *Micronema.*

**hal·ide** (hal'īd) 1. haloid. 2. a binary compound of one of the halogens (fluorine, chlorine, bromine, or iodine).

**ha·lis·te·re·sis** (hə-lis"tə-re'sis) [*hal-* + Gr. *sterēsis* privation] osteomalacia; a loss or lack of the lime salts (calcium) of bone.
**h. ce'rea,** waxy softening of the bones.

**ha·lis·te·ret·ic** (hə-lis″tə-ret′ik) affected with or of the nature of halisteresis.

**hal·i·to·sis** (hal″ĭ-to′sis) [L. *halitus* exhalation] [MeSH: Halitosis] offensive breath; bad breath. Called also *fetor ex ore, fetor oris,* and *stomatodysodia.*

**ha·lit·u·ous** (hə-lit′u-əs) [L. *halitus* exhalation] covered with moisture or vapor.

**hal·i·tus** (hal′ĭ-təs) [L.] exhalation (def. 3).

**Hall's sign** (hawlz) [Josiah Newhall *Hall,* American physician, 1859–1939] see under *sign.*

**hall·a·chrome** (hal′ə-krōm) a compound formed from dihydroxyphenylalanine by tyrosinase.

**Hal·lau·er's glasses** (hahl′ou-ərz) [Otto *Hallauer,* Swiss ophthalmologist, late 19th century] see under *glasses.*

**Hall·berg effect** (hawl′bərg) [Josef Hendrik *Hallberg,* American electrician, 20th century] see under *effect.*

**Hallé's point** (ah-lāz′) [Adrien Joseph Marie Noël *Hallé,* French physician, 1859–1947] see under *point.*

**Hal·ler's arch, duct,** etc. (hahl′erz) [Albrecht von *Haller,* Swiss physiologist, 1708–1777] see under *duct* and *layer,* and see *circulus vasculosus nervi optici, fretum halleri, glandulae preputiales, lamina vasculosa choroideae, ligamentum arcuatum laterale, ligamentum arcuatae mediale, lobuli epididymidis,* and *rete testis.*

**Hal·ler·mann-Streiff syndrome** (hah′lər-mahn-shtrīf) [Wilhelm *Hallermann,* German ophthalmologist, born 1901; Enrico Bernard *Streiff,* Swiss ophthalmologist, born 1908] oculomandibulofacial syndrome.

**Hal·ler·mann-Streiff-Fran·çois syndrome** (hah′lər-mahn-shtrīf-frahn-swah′) [W. *Hallermann;* E.B. *Streiff;* Jules *François,* Belgian ophthalmologist, 20th century] oculomandibulofacial syndrome.

**Hal·ler·vor·den-Spatz disease** (hah′lər-for″dən-shpahts) [Julius *Hallervorden,* German neurologist, 1882–1965; Hugo *Spatz,* German neurologist and psychiatrist, 1888–1969] see under *disease.*

**hal·lex** (hal′əks) pl. *hal′lices.* Hallux.

**Hal·lion's test** (al-yawz′) [Louis *Hallion,* French physiologist, 1862–1940] Tuffier's test.

**Hal·lo·peau's acrodermatitis** (ah-lo-pōz′) [François Henri *Hallopeau,* French dermatologist, 1842–1919] see *acrodermatitis continua.*

**Hall·pike's maneuver** (hawl′pīks) [Charles Skinner *Hallpike,* British otologist, 1900–1979] see under *maneuver.*

**hal·lu·cal** (hal′u-kəl) pertaining to the hallux, or great toe.

**hal·lu·ces** (hal′ə-sēz, hal′u-sēz) [L.] plural of *hallux.*

**hal·lu·ci·na·tion** (hə-loo″sĭ-na′shən) [L. *hallucinatio;* Gr. *alyein* to wander in the mind] [MeSH: Hallucinations] a sense perception without a source in the external world; a perception of an external stimulus object in the absence of such an object.
**auditory h.,** a hallucination involving the sense of hearing. Called also *paracusia* and *paracusis.*
**gustatory h.,** a hallucination involving the sense of taste.
**haptic h.,** tactile h.
**hypnagogic h.,** a vivid dreamlike hallucination occurring at sleep onset.
**hypnopompic h.,** a vivid dreamlike hallucination occurring on awakening.
**kinesthetic h.,** a hallucination involving the sense of bodily movement.
**lilliputian h.,** a visual hallucination in which the imagined objects, usually people or animals, seem smaller than they would be in reality. Cf. *micropsia.*
**olfactory h.,** a hallucination involving the sense of smell.
**somatic h.,** a hallucination involving the perception of a physical experience occurring with the body.
**stump h.,** phantom limb.
**tactile h.,** a hallucination involving the sense of touch.
**visual h.,** a hallucination involving the sense of sight.

**hal·lu·ci·na·tive** (hə-loo′sĭ-nə-tiv) characterized by hallucinations.

**hal·lu·ci·na·to·ry** (hə-loo′sĭ-nə-tor″e) hallucinative.

**hal·lu·ci·no·gen** (hə-loo′sĭ-no-jen″) [*hallucin*ation + *-gen*] an agent which induces hallucinations.

**hal·lu·ci·no·gen·e·sis** (hə-loo″sĭ-no-jen′ə-sis) the production of hallucinations.

**hal·lu·ci·no·ge·net·ic** (hə-loo″sĭ-no-jə-net′ik) hallucinogenic.

**hal·lu·ci·no·gen·ic** (hə-loo″sĭ-no-jen′ik) producing hallucinations.

**hal·lu·ci·no·sis** (hə-loo″sĭ-no′sis) a state characterized by the presence of hallucinations without other impairment of consciousness.
**alcoholic h.,** hallucinations occurring in a clear sensorium in alcoholics with a long history of dependence and heavy intake, usually following a bout of unusually heavy drinking.
**organic h.,** a term used in a former system of classification, denoting an organic mental syndrome characterized by the presence of hallucinations caused by a specific organic factor and not associated with delirium. Such disorders are now mainly classified as *substance-induced psychotic disorders* and *psychotic disorders due to general medical condition.*

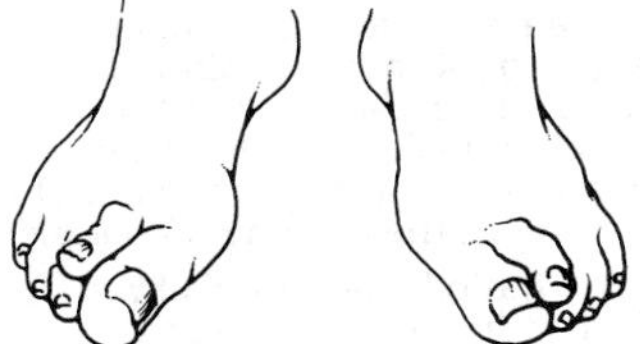
Hallux valgus.

**hal·lu·ci·not·ic** (hə-loo″sĭ-not′ik) pertaining to or characterized by hallucinosis.

**hal·lux** (hal′əks) gen. *hal′lucis,* pl. *hal′luces* [L.] [TA] [MeSH: Hallux] the great toe, or first digit of the foot; called also *digitus primus (I) pedis* [TA alternative].
**h. doloro′sus,** a painful condition of the great toe usually associated with flatfoot.
**h. flex′us,** h. rigidus.
**h. mal′leus,** hammer toe of the hallux.
**h. ri′gidus,** painful flexion deformity of the great toe in which there is limitation of motion at the metatarsophalangeal joint.
**h. val′gus,** angulation of the great toe away from the midline of the body, or toward the other toes; the great toe may ride under or over the other toes.
**h. va′rus,** angulation of the great toe toward the midline of the body, or away from the other toes.

**Hall·wachs effect** (hahl′vahks) [Wilhelm Ludwig Franz *Hallwachs,* German physiologist, 1859–1922] photoelectrical effect; see under *effect.*

**hal·ma·to·gen·e·sis** (hal″mə-to-jen′ə-sis) [Gr. *halma* a jump + *-genesis*] a sudden alteration of type from one generation to another; called also *saltatory variation.*

**ha·lo** (ha′lo) [L., from Gr. *halōs* disk of the sun or moon] 1. a luminous or colored circle, such as the colored circle seen around a light in glaucoma. 2. a ring seen around the macula luteae in ophthalmoscopical examination. 3. the imprint of the ciliary processes upon the vitreous body. 4. a metal or plastic band that encircles the head or neck, providing support and stability as part of a halo orthosis.

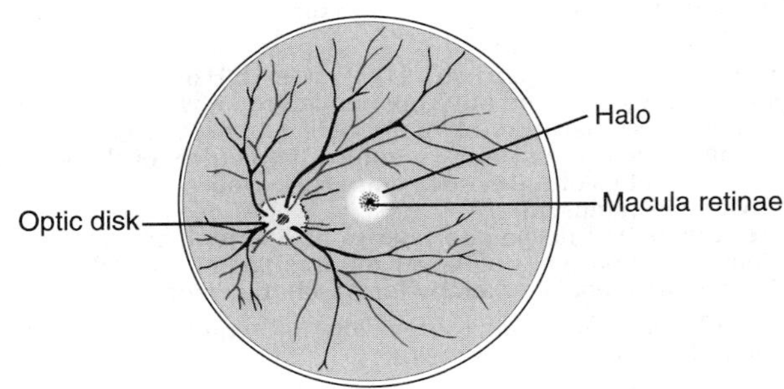


**Fick's h.,** a colored circle appearing around a light, caused by the wearing of contact lenses; see also *Fick's phenomenon.*
**h. glaucomato′sus, glaucomatous h.,** peripapillary atrophy seen in severe or chronic glaucoma.
**h. saturni′nus,** lead line.
**senile h.,** a zone of variable width surrounding the optic papilla, caused by exposure of various elements of the choroid as a result of senile atrophy of the pigmented epithelium.

**hal(o)-** [Gr. *hals,* gen. *halos* salt] a combining form denoting relationship to a salt.

**halo·bac·te·ria** (hal″o-bak-tēr′e-ə) plural of *halobacterium.*

**Halo·bac·te·ri·a·ceae** (hal″o-bak″te-re-a′se-e) [MeSH: Halobacteriaceae] a family of aerobic, rod-shaped and coccoid bacteria, made up of chemo-organotrophic organisms that require at least 8 per cent and in most cases 17 to 23 per cent sodium chloride for growth. These extremely halophilic bacteria, which belong to the archaeobacteria group, do not contain peptidoglycan in their cell walls and differ from other bacteria in ribosomal RNA and cell lipid structures. They contain carotenoid pigments, and they are found in pools of evaporating sea water and material preserved with sea salts. The family contains the genera *Halobacterium* and *Halococcus*.

**Halo·bac·te·ri·um** (hal″o-bak-tēr-e-əm) [*halo-* + *bacterium*] [MeSH: Halobacterium] a genus of gram-negative, aerobic, pleomorphic, rod-shaped bacteria of the family Halobacteriaceae that require a high concentration of sodium chloride (15 per cent or greater) for growth and are found in evaporating sea water, salt lakes, and heavily salted protein materials. They contain a purple pigment (bacteriorhodopsin), which powers a system of photosynthesis, and some contain a red carotenoid pigment (bacterioruberin). The type species is *H. salina′rium*.

**hal·o·bac·te·ri·um** (hal″o-bak-tēr-e-əm) pl. *halobacte′ria*. [MeSH: Halobacterium] Any member of the genus *Halobacterium*.

**Halo·coc·cus** (hal″o-kok′əs) [*halo-* + *coccus*] a genus of gram-negative aerobic bacteria of the family Halobacteriaceae, made up of coccoid cells that require a high concentration of sodium chloride (15 per cent or greater) for growth. They contain a red carotenoid pigment and are found in salted meats and fish. The type species is *H. morrhu′ae*.

**halo·der·mia** (hal″o-dər′me-ə) any skin eruption caused by a halide.

**halo·du·ric** (hal″o-du′rik) [*halo-* + L. *durare* to endure] capable of existing in a medium containing a high concentration of salt.

**ha·lo·fan·trine hy·dro·chlor·ide** (hal″o-fan′trēn) an antimalarial effective against the asexual forms of *Plasmodium* in the blood stream; used in the treatment of acute malaria caused by *P. falciparum* and *P. vivax*.

**Hal·og** (hal′og) trademark for preparations of halcinonide.

**hal·o·gen** (hal′ə-jən, ha′lə-jən) [*halo-* + *-gen*] an element of a closely related chemical family, all of which form similar (saltlike) compounds in combination with sodium and most other metals. The halogens are bromine, chlorine, fluorine, iodine, and astatine.

**hal·o·gen·a·tion** (hal″o-jə-na′shən) incorporation of a halogen into a chemical compound.

**hal·o·ge·ton** (hal-ə-ge′tən) a genus of small plants of the family Polygonaceae, which were introduced into the southwestern United States; they contain soluble oxalates that can be highly poisonous to grazing animals, causing respiratory difficulty, hemorrhage, and hypocalcemia. The major species is *H. glomera′tus* (Bieb.) C. A. Mey. See also *oxalate poisoning*, under *poisoning*.

**hal·oid** (hal′oid) [*halo-* + *-oid*] saltlike; derived from or resembling a halogen.

**ha·lom·e·ter** (hə-lom′ə-tər) [*halo* + *-meter*] 1. an instrument for measuring ocular halos; see *halo* (def. 1). 2. an instrument for estimating the size of erythrocytes by measuring the halos formed around them when a beam of light shines on them and is diffracted.

**ha·lom·e·try** (hə-lom′ə-tre) the measurement of halos with a halometer.

**hal·o·peri·dol** (hal″o-per′ĭ-dol) [USP] [MeSH: Haloperidol] an antipsychotic agent of the butyrophenone group, which also has antiemetic, hypotensive, and hypothermic actions; used especially in the management of psychoses and for the control of the vocal utterances and tics of Gilles de la Tourette's syndrome, administered orally and intramuscularly.
**h. decanoate,** the decanoate ester of haloperidol, having the same actions as the base but of longer duration; administered intramuscularly in maintenance therapy for psychotic disorders.

**hal·o·phil** (hal′o-fil) a microorganism that requires a high concentration of salt for optimal growth.

**hal·o·phile** (hal′o-fīl) 1. halophil. 2. halophilic.

**hal·o·phil·ic** (hal″o-fil′ik) [*halo-* + *-philic*] pertaining to or characterized by an affinity for salt; applied to microorganisms which require a high concentration of salt for optimal growth.

**hal·o·pro·gin** (hal″o-pro′jin) a synthetic topical antifungal used in the treatment of various forms of tinea.

**ha·los·te·re·sis** (hə-los″tə-re′sis) halisteresis.

**Hal·o·tes·tin** (hal″o-tes′tin) trademark for a preparation of fluoxymesterone.

**Hal·o·tex** (hal′o-teks) trademark for a preparation of haloprogin.

**hal·o·thane** (hal′o-thān) [USP] [MeSH: Halothane] a potent inhalational anesthetic, widely used for induction and maintenance of general anesthesia; it is nonflammable, induction and recovery are smooth and rapid, and the depth of anesthesia is rapidly altered.

**hal·quin·ol** (hal′kwin-ol) halquinols.

**hal·quin·ols** (hal′kwin-ols) a topical anti-infective compound, consisting of a mixture of 5,7-dichloro-8-quinolinol, 5-chloro-8-quinolinol, and 7-chloro-8-quinolinol in proportions resulting naturally from chlorination of 8-quinolinol; it has antiamebic, antifungal, and antibacterial actions.

**Hal·sted's operation, suture** (hal′stedz) [William Stewart *Halsted*, American surgeon, 1852–1922] see under *operation* and *suture* and see *radical mastectomy*, under *mastectomy*.

**Hal·tia-San·ta·vu·ori disease** (hahl′te-ah sahn″tah-vwo′re) [M. *Haltia*, Finnish physician, 20th century; Pirkko *Santavuori*, Finnish physician, 20th century] see under *disease*.

**Haly Ab·bas** see *Ali Abbas*.

**hal·zoun** (hal′zən) a pharyngeal form of fascioliasis occurring in the Middle East, caused by eating raw animal livers infected with *Fasciola*; young adult worms attach to the pharyngeal mucosa and produce pain, bleeding, and facial and neck edema.

**Ham's test** (hamz) [Thomas Hale *Ham*, American physician, born 1905] acidified serum test.

**Ham·a·me·lis** (ham″ə-me′lis) [Gr. *hama* together + *mēlon* apple] a genus of trees and shrubs of the family Hamamelidaceae. *H. virginia′na* is witch hazel; an extract of its twigs is made into the astringent liquid also called witch hazel.

**ham·a·me·lis** (ham″ə-me′lis) the dried leaves of *Hamamelis virginiana*, which have been used as an astringent; see also *witch hazel* (def. 2).

**ham·ar·tia** (ham-ahr′shə) [Gr. "defect"] a defect in tissue combination during development.

**ham·ar·ti·al** (ham-ahr′she-əl) pertaining to or exhibiting a hamartia.

**hamart(o)-** [Gr. *hamartia* fault] a combining form denoting relationship to a defect or to a hamartoma.

**ham·ar·to·blas·to·ma** (ham-ahr″to-blas-to′mə) [*hamarto-* + *blastoma*] a tumor developing from a hamartoma.

**ham·ar·to·ma** (ham″ahr-to′mə) [*hamart-* + *-oma*] [MeSH: Hamartoma] a benign tumor-like nodule composed of an overgrowth of mature cells and tissues that normally occur in the affected part, but with disorganization and often with one element predominating.
**pulmonary h.,** a benign tumor, usually a circumscribed nodule or coin lesion located in peripheral lung parenchyma or in a bronchus; tissue types and degree of calcification vary.
**sclerosing epithelial h.,** desmoplastic trichoepithelioma.

**ham·ar·to·ma·to·sis** (ham″ahr-to-mə-to′sis) the development of multiple hamartomas.

**ham·ar·to·ma·tous** (ham″ahr-to′mə-təs) pertaining to a disturbance in growth of a tissue in which the cells of a circumscribed area outstrip those of the surrounding areas.

**ham·ate** (ham′at) shaped like a hook. Cf. *uncinate*.

**ha·ma·tum** (hə-ma′təm) [L. "hooked"] 1. hamate. 2. os hamatum.

**Ham·bur·ger phenomenon (interchange)** (hahm′boor-gər) [Hartog Jakob *Hamburger*, Dutch physiologist, 1859–1924] chloride shift.

**Ham·il·ton's test** (ham′il-tonz) [Frank Hastings *Hamilton*, American surgeon, 1813–1886] see under *test*.

**Ham·man's disease, syndrome, sign** (ham′ənz) [Louis *Hamman*, American physician, 1877–1946] see *pneumomediastinum*, and see under *sign*.

**Ham·man-Rich syndrome** (ham′ən-rich) [L. *Hamman*; Arnold Rice *Rich*, American pathologist, 1893–1968] idiopathic pulmonary fibrosis.

**ham·mer** (ham′ər) 1. an instrument with a head designed for striking blows. 2. malleus.

**ham·ster** (ham′stər) [MeSH: Hamsters] any member of four genera of the rodent family Muridae; genera used as laboratory animals are *Cricetulus*, *Cricetus*, and *Mesocricetus*.
**Chinese h.,** *Cricetulus griseus*, a species that was formerly a common laboratory animal and is the source of the Chinese hamster ovary (CHO) cell line.
**European h.,** *Cricetus cricetus*, a species native to Europe and the Middle East, commonly used as a laboratory animal.
**golden h.,** *Mesocricetus auratus*, a species widely used as a laboratory animal and pet. Called also *Syrian h.*
**Syrian h.,** golden h.
**Syrian cardiomyopathic h.,** an inbred strain of Syrian hamster used as an animal model of hypertrophic cardiomyopathy.

**ham·string** (ham′string) 1. one of the tendons that bound the popliteal fossa laterally and medially. 2. pertaining to or related to these tendons; see under *muscle*.
**inner h.,** the tendons of the gracilis, sartorius, and two other muscles.
**outer h.,** the tendon of the biceps flexor femoris.

**ham·u·lar** (ham'u-lər) shaped like a hook.

**ham·u·lus** (ham'u-ləs) pl. *ham'uli* [L. "little hook"] [TA] a general term denoting a hook-shaped process.
**h. coch'leae,** h. laminae spiralis.
**h. of ethmoid bone,** processus uncinatus ossis ethmoidalis.
**frontal h., h. fronta'lis,** ala cristae galli.
**h. of hamate bone,** h. ossis hamati.
**h. lacrima'lis** [TA], lacrimal hamulus: the hooklike process on the anterior part of the inferolateral border of the lacrimal bone, articulating with the maxilla.
**h. la'minae spira'lis** [TA], hamulus of spiral lamina: the hooklike upper end of the osseous spiral lamina.
**h. os'sis hama'ti** [TA], hamulus of hamate bone: a hooklike process on the volar surface of the hamate bone, to which numerous structures are attached.
**h. pterygoi'deus** [TA], pterygoid hamulus: a hooklike process on the inferior extremity of the medial pterygoid plate of the sphenoid bone, around which the tendon of the tensor veli palatini muscle passes.
**h. of spiral lamina,** h. laminae spiralis.
**trochlear h.,** spina trochlearis.

**ha·my·cin** (hə-mi'sin) an antibiotic derived from *Streptomyces pimprina,* having antifungal, antitrichomonal, and anti-inflammatory actions; it has been used topically in various fungal infections of the skin.

**Han·cock's amputation (operation)** (han'koks) [Henry *Hancock,* English surgeon, 1809–1880] see under *amputation.*

**Ham·mond's disease** (ham'ondz) [William Alexander *Hammond,* American neurologist, 1828–1900] athetosis.

**Hand's disease** (handz) [Alfred *Hand,* Jr., American pediatrician, 1868–1949] Hand-Schüller-Christian disease; see under *disease.*

**Hand-Schül·ler-Chris·tian disease, syndrome** (hand-shēl'ər-kris'chən) [A. *Hand,* Jr.; Arthur *Schüller,* Austrian neurologist, 1874–1958; Henry Asbury *Christian,* American physician, 1876–1951] see under *disease* and *syndrome.*

**hand** (hand) [MeSH: Hand] the distal region of the upper limb, including the carpus, metacarpus, and digits. In offical terminology, called *manus.*
**ape h.,** a hand with the thumb permanently extended.
**benediction h.,** a hand in which the ring and little fingers are flexed; there is weakness of abduction and adduction of the index and middle fingers but they can be extended normally, and the thumb remains normal; seen in ulnar paralysis and syringomyelia.
**claw h.,** see *clawhand.*
**cleft h.,** a congenital anomaly of the hand in which the division between the fingers extends into the metacarpus; often there are just two large digits, one on either side of the cleft. Called also *lobster-claw h.* or *deformity, split h., split-hand deformity,* and *main fourchée.* See also *EEC syndrome,* under *syndrome.*

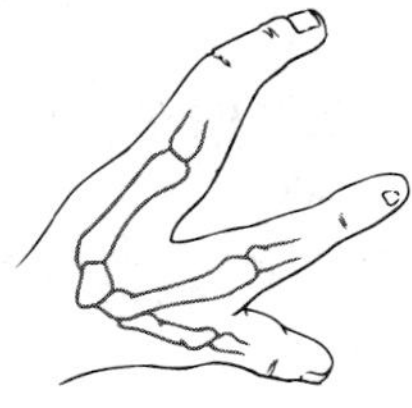

Cleft hand.

**club h.,** clubhand; see *talipomanus.*
**dead h.,** an occupational disorder seen sometimes in those who use vibratory tools, and apparently caused by the multitude of concussions. The hands are painful and dark blue in color, but blanch on exposure to cold.
**drop h.,** see *wristdrop.*
**flat h.,** manus plana.
**frozen h.,** stiffness of the hand resulting from edema accompanying trauma.
**lobster-claw h.,** cleft h.
**Marinesco's succulent h.,** a soft, swollen, cyanotic, and cold hand caused by thickening and edema of the subcutaneous tissues; seen in syringomyelia. Called also *main succulente* and *Marinesco's sign.* See also *Morvan's syndrome* (def. 2), under *syndrome.*
**mirror h's,** an anomaly in which there are two crude hands growing from a common wrist.
**mitten h.,** a hand in which several fingers are fused together and have a common nail.
**monkey h.,** a condition in which the thumb lies in adduction and extension and cannot be opposed so as to touch the tips of the other fingers, because of thenar muscle weakness, sometimes caused by lesions of the median nerve. Called also *main en singe* and *monkey paw.*
**obstetrician's h.,** the contraction of the hand in tetany, flexed at the wrist with fingers at the metacarpophalangeal joints but extended at the interphalangeal joints, the thumb being strongly flexed into the palm; so called because of a dubious resemblance to the position assumed by the hand of the obstetrician when examining the vagina.
**opera-glass h.,** a pawlike hand marked by telescoping of the fingers caused by absorption of the phalanges; occurs in chronic arthritis.
**phantom h.,** a paresthetic feeling as if the hand were still present after amputation.
**preacher's h.,** benediction h.
**skeleton h.,** a hand markedly atrophied and held in a position of extension: seen in progressive muscular atrophy; called also *main en squelette.*
**spade h.,** the thick square hand of myxedema and acromegaly.
**split h.,** cleft h.
**trench h.,** contracture or other incapacity of the hand from frostbite; so called from its occurrence in the trenches during World War I.
**trident h.,** the characteristic hand of achondroplasia: the fingers are relatively of the same length, and there is a peculiar separation of the second and third fingers at the second phalangeal joint, causing the fingers to spread out.
**writing h.,** a peculiar position of the hand in which the hand appears poised for writing; seen in paralysis agitans.

**H and E** hematoxylin and eosin (stain). See under *stain.*

**hand·ed·ness** (hand'əd-nəs) the preferential use in voluntary motor acts of the hand of one side.
**left h.,** the preferential use in voluntary motor acts of the left hand.
**right h.,** the preferential use in voluntary motor acts of the right hand.

**hand·i·cap** (han'dĭ-kap) any physical or mental defect or characteristic, congenital or acquired, preventing or restricting a person from participating in normal life or limiting his capacity to work.

**han·dle** (han'dəl) a part of a larger object enabling it to be grasped with the hand; see also *manubrium.*
**h. of malleus,** manubrium mallei.

**hand·piece** (hand'pēs) a hand-held device that engages rotary instruments used for removing tooth structures, cleaning teeth, and polishing dental restorations, connected to the dental engine by an adjustable arm in the case of a belt-driven instrument or by flexible tubing if air driven.

**HANE** hereditary angioneurotic edema; see *hereditary angioedema,* under *angioedema.*

**hang·nail** (hang'nāl) a shred of eponychium on a proximal or lateral nail fold.

**Han·hart's syndrome** (hahn'hahrts) [Ernst *Hanhart,* Swiss physician, 1891–1973] see under *syndrome.*

**Han·no·ver's canal** (hahn'o-vərz) [Adolph *Hannover,* Danish anatomist, 1814–1894] see under *canal.*

**Ha·not-Chauf·fard syndrome** (ahn-o' sho-fahr') [Victor Charles *Hanot,* French physician, 1844–1896; Anatole Marie Émile *Chauffard,* French physician, 1855–1932] see under *syndrome.*

**Han·sen's bacillus, disease** (hahn'sənz) [Gerhard Henrik Armauer *Hansen,* Norwegian physician, 1841–1912] see *Mycobacterium leprae* and *leprosy.*

**Han·sen·u·la** (hən-sen'u-lə) [MeSH: Hansenula] a genus of yeasts of the family Saccharomycetaceae, formerly called *Willia. H. ano 'mala* is a species commonly found in soil and as normal flora in the human respiratory and intestinal tracts.

**Han·ta·vi·rus** (han'tə-vi″rəs) [*Hantaan* River, Korea] [MeSH: Hantavirus] a genus of viruses of the family Bunyaviridae that cause epidemic hemorrhagic fever or pneumonia, comprising at least 20 species included in one serogroup and unclassified species. Each species appears to have a single rodent species as a host; transmission to humans is believed to be by contact, direct or indirect, with the excreta of infected rodents.

**Hap·a·lo·chlae·na** (hap″ə-lo-kle'nə) a genus of octopus. *H. maculo'sa* is the venomous blue-ringed octopus (q.v.).

**haph·al·ge·sia** (haf″al-je'ze-ə) [Gr. *haphē* touch + *algesia*] a type of tactile hyperesthesia in which normally painless touch sensations cause pain, as in Pitres' sign (def. 1) or certain mental disorders.

**haphe·pho·bia** (haf″e-fo'be-ə) [Gr. *haphē* touch + *-phobia*] irrational fear of being touched.

**hapl(o)-** [Gr. *haploos* simple, single] a combining form meaning simple or single.

**Hap·lo·chi·lus** (hap″lo-ki'ləs) a genus of small fish. *H. pan'chax,* called *ikan kapala timah* in Malay, is a species placed in fishponds in Indonesia to eat the larvae of *Anopheles* mosquitoes.

**hap·lo·dip·loi·dy** (hap″lo-dip′loi-de) [*haplo-* + *diploidy*] the state in which males develop from unfertilized eggs and are haploid, and females develop from fertilized eggs and are diploid, as in honeybees.

**hap·lo·dont** (hap′lo-dont) [*haplo-* + Gr. *odous* tooth] having molar teeth without cusps or ridges.

**hap·loid** (hap′loid) [*hapl-* + *-oid*] 1. having a single set of chromosomes, as normally carried by a gamete, or having one complete set of nonhomologous chromosomes. In man, the haploid number is 23. Symbol, n. Cf. *diploid* (def. 1). 2. an individual or cell having only one member of each pair of homologous chromosomes.

**hap·lo·iden·ti·cal** (hap″lo-i-den′tĭ-kəl) sharing a haplotype; having the same alleles at a set of closely linked genes on one chromosome.

**hap·lo·iden·ti·ty** (hap″lo-i-den′tĭ-te) the condition of being haploidentical.

**hap·loi·dy** (hap′loi-de) [MeSH: Haploidy] the state of having only one member of each pair of homologous chromosomes.

**hap·lo·my·co·sis** (hap″lo-mi-ko′sis) adiaspiromycosis.

**hap·lont** (hap′lont) [Gr. *haploun* to make single] a haploid individual.

**Hap·lo·pap·pus** (hap-lo-pap′əs) a genus of composite-flowered plants (family Compositae). Several species, such as *H. hetero′phyllus,* the rayless goldenrod, contain the toxin tremetol and cause trembles in cattle and sheep.

**hap·lop·a·thy** (hap-lop′ə-the) [*haplo-* + *-pathy*] an uncomplicated disease.

**hap·lo·phase** (hap′lo-fāz) that phase in the life history of germ cells when the nuclei are haploid.

**hap·lo·pia** (hap-lo′pe-ə) [*hapl-* + *-opia*] single vision; the condition in which an object looked at is seen single and not double.

**Hap·lor·chis** (hap-lor′kis) a genus of minute trematodes found in tropical areas; they are intestinal parasites of dogs, cats, and other vertebrates. *H. tai′chui* infects birds and mammals, occasionally including humans.

**hap·lo·scope** (hap′lo-skōp) [*haplo-* + *-scope*] an instrument that presents two separate views to the two eyes so that the views may be seen as one integrated view; it is used to measure, test, or stimulate various binocular functions.
**mirror h.,** a haploscope that uses mirrors to separate or displace the fields of vision of the two eyes.

**hap·lo·scop·ic** (hap-lo-skop′ik) pertaining to a haploscope; stereoscopic.

**hap·lo·spo·ran·gin** (hap″lo-spor-an′jin) an antigen derived from the fungus *Emmonsia parva.*

**Hap·lo·spo·ran·gi·um** (hap″lo-spor-an′je-əm) *Emmonsia.*

**hap·lo·type** (hap′lo-tīp) [*haplo-* + *type*] [MeSH: Haplotypes] 1. a set of alleles of a group of closely linked genes, such as the HLA complex, which is usually inherited as a unit. 2. the genetic constitution of an individual at a set of closely linked genes on a given chromosome.

**Haps·burg jaw, lip, disease** (haps′bərg) [*Hapsburg,* a German-Austrian royal family, including rulers of several European states, such as Austria (1278–1918) and Spain (1504–1700)] see under *jaw* and *lip,* and see *hemophilia.*

**hap·ten** (hap′tən) [Ger., from Gr. *haptein* to fasten] a small molecule, not antigenic by itself, that can react with antibodies of appropriate specificity and elicit the formation of such antibodies when conjugated to a larger antigenic molecule, usually a protein, called in this context the carrier or schlepper. Antibody production involves activation of B lymphocytes by the hapten and helper T lymphocytes by the carrier.

**hap·tene** (hap′tēn) hapten.

**hap·ten·ic** (hap-ten′ik) pertaining to or caused by haptens.

**hap·te·pho·bia** (hap″te-fo′be-ə) [*hapt-* + *-phobia*] haphephobia.

**hap·tic** (hap′tik) [Gr. *haptikos* able to lay hold of] tactile.

**hap·tics** (hap′tiks) the study of the sense of touch; see *touch.*

**hapt(o)-** [Gr. *haptein* to fasten, grasp, touch] a combining form denoting relationship to touch or to binding.

**hap·to·cor·rin** (hap″to-kor′in) R protein.

**hap·to·glo·bin** (hap″to-glo′bin) a 100,000-dalton plasma glycoprotein with alpha electrophoretic mobility that irreversibly binds free hemoglobin resulting in prompt removal of the hemoglobin-haptoglobin complex by the liver, preventing loss of free hemoglobin in the urine. Haptoglobin levels are decreased by hemolysis and increased owing to increased synthesis in conditions resulting in extensive tissue damage and necrosis. Haptoglobin has two major genetic variants, designated Hp 1 and Hp 2.

**hap·tom·e·ter** (hap-tom′ə-tər) [*hapto-* + *-meter*] an instrument for measuring sensitivity to touch.

**Ha·ra·da syndrome** (hah-rah′dah) [Einosuke *Harada,* Japanese ophthalmologist, 1892–1947] Vogt-Koyanagi-Harada syndrome; see under *syndrome.*

**ha·rara** (hə-rar′ə) 1. an allergic skin reaction caused by bites of the sand fly *Phlebotomus papatasii,* seen in the Middle East, and characterized by urticarial and inflammatory papules and blisters. Immunity usually follows the initial exposure. Called also *urticaria multiformis endemica.* 2. popular name for any of various other skin eruptions.

**Har·den-Young ester** (hahr′dən-yung) [Sir Arthur *Harden,* English biochemist, 1865–1940; William John *Young,* Australian biochemist, 20th century] see *fructose-1,6-diphosphate.*

**hard·en·ing** (hahr′dən-ing) 1. induration (def. 2). 2. sclerosis. 3. the procedure of rendering tissue firm, so that it may be more readily cut for purposes of microscopic examination.
**h. of arteries,** popular term for *arteriosclerosis.*

**Har·der's glands** (hahr′dərz) [Johann Jacob *Harder,* Swiss physician, 1656–1711] see under *gland.*

**hard·er·i·an** (hahr′dər-e-ən) named for J. J. *Harder,* as harderian *fossa* or *glands.*

**hard·ero·por·phy·ria** (hahr″dər-o-por-fīr′e-ə) a severe variant of hereditary coproporphyria differing in having earlier onset of attacks, excretion of harderoporphyrin in the feces, and virtual absence of coproporphyrinogen oxidase activity.

**hard·ero·por·phy·rin** (hahr″dər-o-por′fə-rin) an intermediate in heme biosynthesis, formed in the conversion of coproporphyrinogen to protoporphyrinogen and excreted excessively in the feces in harderoporphyria.

**hard·ness** (hahrd′nəs) [MeSH: Hardness] 1. a quality of water produced by soluble salts of calcium and magnesium or other substances which form an insoluble curd with soap and thus interfere with its cleansing power. 2. the quality of firmness produced by cohesion of the particles composing a substance, as evidenced by its inflexibility or resistance to indentation, distortion, or scratching. See also *hardness number,* under *number.* 3. the quality of x-rays that determines their penetrating power; hardness depends on wavelength: the shorter the wavelength the harder the rays and the greater their penetrating power. 4. the degree of refraction of the residual gas in a glass tube: the higher the vacuum the shorter the wavelength of the resulting x-rays.
**diamond pyramid h.,** Vickers hardness number.
**permanent h.,** hardness of water not removed by boiling; it is usually due to sulfates and chlorides.
**temporary h.,** hardness of water removed by boiling; it is due to soluble bicarbonates, which lose $CO_2$ on boiling and precipitate as normal carbonates.

**Har·dy-Wein·berg law** (hahr′de vīn′bərg) [Godfrey Harold *Hardy,* British mathematician, 1877–1947; Wilhelm *Weinberg,* German physician, 1862–1937] see under *law.*

**Hare's syndrome** (hārz) [Edward Selleck *Hare,* British surgeon, 1812–1838] Pancoast's syndrome, def. 1.

**hare·lip** (hār′lip) cleft lip.

**har·le·quin** (hahr′lə-kwin) [It. *arlecchino*] 1. a person or animal decorated like Harlequin, an old stock character in European comedies who wore colorful checkered clothing. 2. coral snake.

**har·ma·line** (hahr′mə-lēn) [MeSH: Harmaline] an alkaloid that has hallucinogenic properties, found in the seeds of African rue *(Peganum harmala)* and the South American vine *Banisteria caapi.*

**har·mine** (hahr′mēn) [MeSH: Harmine] an alkaloid that has hallucinogenic properties, found in the seeds of African rue *(Peganum harmala)* and the South American vine *Banisteria caapi.* Called also *banisterine.*

**har·mo·nia** (hahr-mo′ne-ə) [L.] sutura plana.

**har·mo·ny** (hahr′mo-ne) the state of working together smoothly.
**occlusal h.,** proper occlusion of the teeth occurring in various positions of the mandible.
**occlusal h., functional,** such occlusion of the teeth in all positions of the mandible during mastication as will provide the greatest masticatory efficiency without imposing undue strain or trauma on the supporting tissues.

**Har·mo·nyl** (hahr′mo-nəl) trademark for preparations of deserpidine.

**Har·pi·rhyn·chus** (hahr″pe-ring′kəs) [Gr. *harpē* bird of prey + Gr. *rhynchos* snout] a genus of mites parasitic on birds.

**har•poon** (hahr-po͞on′) [Gr. *harpazein* to seize] an instrument for removing small pieces of living tissue for diagnostic examination.

**Har•ring•ton instrumentation, rod** (har′ing-tən) [Paul R. *Harrington,* American orthopedic surgeon, born 1911] see under *instrumentation.*

**Har•ris lines** (har′is) [Henry Albert *Harris,* Welsh anatomist, 1886–1968] see under *line.*

**Har•ris' staining method** (har′is) [Downey Lamar *Harris,* American pathologist, 1875–1956] see under *stain.*

**Har•ris' syndrome** (har′is) [Seale *Harris,* American physician, 1870–1957] see under *syndrome.*

**Har•ri•son's groove (curve, sulcus)** (har′ĭ-sənz) [Edward *Harrison,* English physician, 1766–1838] see under *groove.*

**Har•tel's treatment** (hahr′telz) [Fritz *Hartel,* German surgeon, 20th century] see under *treatment.*

**Hart•ley-Krause operation** (hahrt′le-krou′zə) [Frank *Hartley,* American surgeon, 1857–1913; Fedor *Krause,* German surgeon, 1857–1937] see under *operation.*

**Hart•line** (hahrt′līn) Haldan Keffer. American physician and physiologist, 1903–1983; co-winner, with Ragnar Arthur Granit and George Wald, of the Nobel prize for medicine or physiology in 1967 for discoveries regarding the primary chemical and physiological visual processes in the eye.

**Hart•mann's curet, speculum** (hahrt′mənz) [Arthur *Hartmann,* German laryngologist, 1849–1931] see under *curet.*

**Hart•mann's pouch, procedure (operation, colostomy)** (hahrt′mahnz) [Henri *Hartmann,* French surgeon, 1860–1952] see under *pouch* and *procedure.*

**Hart•man•nel•la** (hahrt″mən-el′ə) [MeSH: Hartmannella] a genus of free-living protozoa (order Amoebida, class Rhizopoda) found in fresh water and soil, species of which, e.g., *H. hyali′na,* are capable of facultative parasitism, causing a primary amebic meningoencephalitis, especially in the immunocompromised host.

**hart•man•nel•li•a•sis** (hahrt″mə-nel-i′ə-sis) infection with *Hartmannella.*

**Hart•nup disease** (hahrt′nəp) [*Hartnup,* family of the propositus in Britain] [MeSH: Hartnup Disease] see under *disease.*

**harts•horn** (hahrts′horn) ammonium carbonate.

**har•vei•an** (hahr′ve-ən) named in honor of William *Harvey.*

**har•vest** (hahr′vəst) to remove tissues or cells from a donor and preserve for transplantation.

**Har•vey** (hahr′ve) William (1578–1657). English physician, student of Fabricius; he practiced in London and was physician to James I and Charles I. In his *Exercitatio anatomica de motu cordis et sanguinis* (1628), Harvey proved, among other things, that (1) contraction of the heart muscle coincides with the pulse as the ventricles pump blood into the aorta and pulmonary artery; (2) the pulse is produced by the arteries' filling with blood; (3) the septum is impervious; (4) venous and arterial blood are the same; and (5) the blood in the right ventricle goes through the arteries to the lungs and thence through the pulmonary veins to the left ventricle and thence through the arteries to the body whence it returns along the smaller veins to the venae cavae and then into the right ventricle—a complete circulation of the blood. Harvey's work was not fully substantiated until 1827.

**Ha•shi•mo•to's disease (thyroiditis, struma)** (hah″she-mo′tōz) [Hakaru *Hashimoto,* Japanese surgeon, 1881–1934] see under *disease.*

**hash•ish** (hă-shēsh′) [Arabic "herb"] a preparation of the unadulterated resin scraped from the flowering tops of cultivated female hemp plants, *Cannabis sativa* L. (Cannabaceae), which is smoked or chewed for its intoxicating effects. It is far more potent than marijuana. See *cannabis.*

**hash•i•tox•i•co•sis** (hash″ĭ-tok″sĭ-ko′sis) [*Hashimoto's disease* + *toxicosis*] hyperthyroidism in patients with Hashimoto's disease. Cf. *painless thyroiditis,* under *thyroiditis.*

**Has•ner's fold, valve** (hahs′nərz) [Joseph Ritter von Artha *Hasner,* Czech ophthalmologist, 1819–1892] see *plica lacrimalis.*

**Has•sall's corpuscles (bodies)** (has′əlz) [Arthur Hill *Hassall,* English chemist and physician, 1817–1894] see under *corpuscle.*

**HAT** hypoxanthine-aminopterin-thymidine (medium); see under *medium.*

**Ha•ta phenomenon** (hah′tah) [Sahachiro *Hata,* Japanese bacteriologist, 1872–1938] see under *phenomenon.*

**hatch•et** (hach′ət) a bibeveled or single beveled cutting dental instrument having its cutting edge in line with the axis of its blade; used for breaking down tooth structure undermined by caries, smoothing cavity walls, and sharpening line and point angles. Called also *hatchet excavator.*

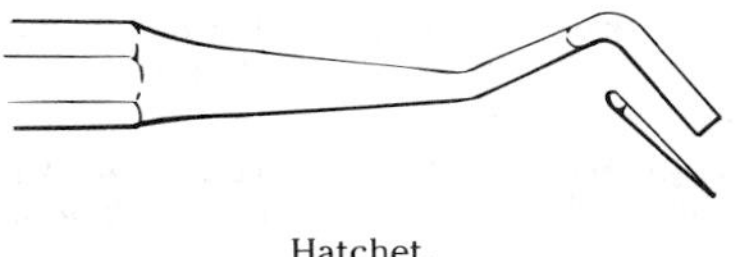

Hatchet.

**enamel h.,** one in which the broad side of the blade is parallel with the angle of the shank; used with a chipping or a lateral scraping stroke in developing an internal cavity form.

**H⁺-ATPase** H⁺-transporting ATP synthase.

**Hauch** (houk) [Ger. "breath" (because motile bacteria form a spreading film around colonies resembling that produced by breathing on glass)] used to describe certain bacterial colonies; see *H antigen* under *antigen* and *H colony* under *colony.* Symbol H.

**Hau•dek's sign (niche)** (hou′dəks) [Martin *Haudek,* Austrian radiologist, 1880–1931] see under *sign.*

**haunch** (hawnch) the hip and buttock.

**haupt•gan•gli•on of Kütt•ner** (houpt-gang′le-on) nodus lymphoideus jugulodigastricus.

**Haust.** abbreviation for L. *haus′tus,* a draft.

**haus•tel•lum** (haw-stel′əm) pl. *haustel′la* [L. from *haustus* draw up] a mouthpart of certain ectoparasites, such as bedbugs and lice, modified for piercing and sucking, consisting of a hollow tube with an eversible set of five stylets, by which the organism attaches itself to the host and through which the blood is drawn up.

**haus•tor•i•um** (haws-tor′e-əm) pl. *hausto′ria* [L. from *haustus* draw up] a structure of certain parasites adapted specially to penetrate the host's tissues and absorb nutrients and water.

**haus•tra** (haws′trə) [L.] plural of *haustrum.*

**haus•tral** (haws′trəl) pertaining to the haustra of the colon.

**haus•tra•tion** (haws-tra′shən) 1. the formation of a haustrum. 2. a haustrum.

**haus•trum** (haws′trəm) pl. *haus′tra* [L. *haustor* drawer] [TA] a general term denoting a recess or sacculation.
**haus′tra co′li** [TA], **haustra of colon,** sacculations in the wall of the colon produced by adaptation of its length to that of the tenia coli, or by the arrangement of the circular muscle fibers.

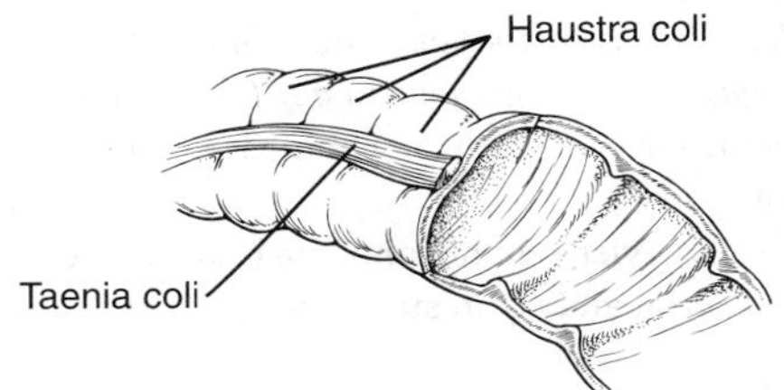


**haut-mal** (o-mahl′) [Fr.] grand mal; see under *epilepsy.*

**HAV** hepatitis A virus.

**Ha•ver•hill fever** (ha′vər-il) [*Haverhill,* Massachusetts, where an epidemic occurred in 1925] see under *fever.*

**Ha•ver•hil•lia mul•ti•for•mis** (ha″vər-il′e-ə mul″tĭ-for′mis) the name given to a slender gram-negative streptobacillus which was found in cases of Haverhill fever; now called *Streptobacillus moniliformis.*

**ha•ver•sian canal (space), glands, lamella, system** (ha-vərs′zhən) [Clopton *Havers,* English physician and anatomist, 1650–1702] see *canalis nutricius* and *villi synoviales,* and see under *lamella* and *system.*

**haw** (haw) 1. popular term for *nictitating membrane.* 2. haw syndrome.

**haw•kin•sin** (haw′kin-sin) a cyclic amino acid metabolite of tyrosine excreted in hawkinsinuria, a rare form of tyrosinemia. It is formed from an intermediate of the 4-hydroxyphenylpyruvate dioxygenase reaction combined with glutathione.

**haw•kin•sin•u•ria** (haw″kin-sin-u′re-ə) a rare autosomal dominant form of tyrosinemia associated with a defect of 4-hydroxyphenylpyruvate dioxygenase, manifested by the excretion of hawkinsin in the urine.

**Haw•ley retainer (appliance)** (haw′le) [C. A. *Hawley,* American dentist, early 20th century] see under *retainer.*

**Hay-Wells syndrome** (ha-welz) [R.J. *Hay,* British dermatologist, 20th century; Robert Stuart *Wells,* British dermatologist, 20th century] see under *syndrome.*

**Ha·yem's encephalitis, solution** (ah-yahnz') [Georges *Hayem,* French physician, 1841–1933] see under *solution.*

**Ha·yem-Wi·dal syndrome** (ah-yahn've-dahl') [G. *Hayem;* Georges Fernand Isidore *Widal,* French physician, 1862–1929] hemolytic anemia.

**Hay·flick's limit** (ha'fliks) [Leonard *Hayflick,* American microbiologist, born 1928] see under *limit.*

**HB** hepatitis B.

**$HB_c$** hepatitis B core (antigen).

**$HB_e$** hepatitis B e (antigen).

**$HB_s$** hepatitis B surface (antigen).

**Hb** symbol for *hemoglobin.*

**HBcAg** hepatitis B core antigen.

**HbCV** *Haemophilus influenzae* b conjugate vaccine.

**HBE** His bundle electrogram.

**HBeAg** hepatitis B e antigen.

**$HbO_2$** oxyhemoglobin.

**HbPV** *Haemophilus influenzae* b polysaccharide vaccine.

**HBsAg** hepatitis B surface antigen.

**HBV** hepatitis B virus.

**HC** hospital corps.

**HCFA** Health Care Financing Administration, part of the Department of Health and Human Services.

**HCG** human chorionic gonadotropin.

**hCG** human chorionic gonadotropin.

**HCM** hypertrophic cardiomyopathy.

**HCP** hereditary coproporphyria.

**Hct** hematocrit.

**HCV** hepatitis C virus.

**H.d.** abbreviation for L. *ho'ra decu'bitus,* at bedtime.

**HDCV** human diploid cell rabies vaccine.

**HDL** high-density lipoprotein.

**$HDL_1$** Lp(a) lipoprotein.

**$HDL_2$** see *high-density lipoprotein,* under *lipoprotein.*

**$HDL_3$** see *high-density lipoprotein,* under *lipoprotein.*

**HDN** hemolytic disease of the newborn; see *erythroblastosis fetalis.*

**HDV** hepatitis D virus.

**HDP** hydroxymethylene diphosphonate (oxidronate, q.v.).

**H & E** hematoxylin and eosin stain; see *Table of Stains and Staining Methods.*

**He** symbol for *helium.*

**he-** for words beginning thus, see also those beginning *hae-.*

**Head's zones** (hedz) [Sir Henry *Head,* British neurologist, 1861–1940] see under *zone.*

**head** (hed) [A.S. *hēafod*] [MeSH: Head] 1. caput (def. 1). 2. the upper, anterior, or proximal extremity of a structure or body. See also *caput.*
**angular h. of quadratus labii superioris muscle,** musculus levator labii superioris alaeque nasi.
**anterior h. of rectus femoris muscle,** caput rectum musculi recti femoris.
**articular h.,** an eminence on a bone by which it articulates with another bone.
**h. of astragalus,** caput tali.
**big h.,** bighead.
**h. of caudate nucleus,** caput nuclei caudati.
**h. of condyloid process of mandible,** caput mandibulae.
**coronoid h. of pronator teres muscle,** caput ulnare musculi pronatoris teretis.
**deep h. of triceps brachii muscle,** caput mediale musculi tricipitis brachii.
**deep h. of triceps extensor cubiti muscle,** caput mediale musculi tricipitis brachii.
**h. of dorsal horn of spinal cord,** caput cornus posterioris medullae spinalis.
**drum h.,** membrana tympanica.
**engaged h.,** the position of the fetal head when the biparietal plane has passed the pelvic inlet.
**h. of epididymis,** caput epididymidis.
**h. of femur,** caput femoris.
**h. of fibula,** caput fibulae.
**first h. of triceps brachii muscle,** caput longum musculi tricipitis brachii.
**first h. of triceps extensor cubiti muscle,** caput longum musculi tricipitis brachii.
**floating h.,** the head of the fetus when it is freely movable above the inlet of the birth canal.
**great h. of adductor hallucis muscle,** caput obliquum musculi adductoris hallucis.
**great h. of triceps brachii muscle,** caput laterale musculi tricipitis brachii.
**great h. of triceps extensor cubiti muscle,** caput laterale musculi tricipitis brachii.
**great h. of triceps femoris muscle,** musculus adductor magnus.
**hot cross bun h.,** former name for caput quadratum.
**hourglass h.,** a head in which the coronal suture is depressed.
**humeral h. of flexor carpi ulnaris muscle,** caput humerale musculi flexoris carpi ulnaris.
**humeral h. of flexor digitorum sublimis muscle,** caput humeroulnare musculi flexoris digitorum superficialis.
**humeral h. of pronator teres muscle,** caput humerale musculi pronatoris teretis.
**humeroulnar h. of flexor digitorum superficialis muscle,** caput humero-ulnare musculi flexoris digitorum superficialis.
**h. of humerus,** caput humeri.
**infraorbital h. of quadratus labii superioris muscle,** musculus levator labii superioris.
**lateral h. of abductor hallucis,** caput laterale abductoris hallucis.
**lateral h. of gastrocnemius muscle,** caput laterale musculi gastrocnemii.
**lateral h. of triceps brachii muscle,** caput laterale musculi tricipitis brachii.
**lateral h. of triceps extensor cubiti muscle,** caput laterale musculi tricipitis brachii.
**little h. of humerus,** capitulum humeri.
**little h. of mandible,** processus condylaris mandibulae.
**long h. of adductor hallucis muscle,** caput obliquum musculus adductoris hallucis.
**long h. of adductor triceps muscle,** musculus adductor longus.
**long h. of biceps brachii muscle,** caput longum musculi bicipitis brachii.
**long h. of biceps femoris muscle,** caput longum musculi bicipitis femoris.
**long h. of biceps flexor cruris muscle,** caput longum musculi bicipitis femoris.
**long h. of biceps flexor cubiti muscle,** caput longum musculi bicipitis brachii.
**long h. of triceps brachii muscle,** caput longum musculi tricipitis brachii.
**long h. of triceps extensor cubiti muscle,** caput longum musculi tricipitis brachii.
**long h. of triceps femoris muscle,** musculus adductor longus.
**h. of malleus,** caput mallei.
**h. of mandible,** 1. caput mandibulae. 2. processus condylaris mandibulae.
**medial h. of abductor hallucis,** caput mediale abductoris hallucis.
**medial h. of biceps brachii muscle,** caput breve musculi bicipitis brachii.
**medial h. of biceps flexor cubiti muscle,** caput breve musculi bicipitis brachii.
**medial h. of gastrocnemius muscle,** caput mediale musculi gastrocnemii.
**medial h. of triceps brachii muscle,** caput mediale musculi tricipitis brachii.
**medial h. of triceps extensor cubiti muscle,** caput mediale musculi tricipitis brachii.
**medusa h.,** caput medusae.
**h. of metacarpal,** caput metacarpalis.
**h. of metatarsal,** caput metatarsalis.
**middle h. of triceps brachii muscle,** caput longum musculi tricipitis brachii.
**middle h. of triceps extensor cubiti muscle,** caput longum musculi tricipitis brachii.
**h. of muscle,** the end of a muscle at the site of its attachment (origin) to a bone or other fixed structure; called also *caput musculi.*
**nasal h. of levator labii superioris alaeque nasi muscle,** musculus levator labii superioris alaeque nasi.
**oblique h. of adductor hallucis muscle,** caput obliquum musculus adductoris hallucis.
**oblique h. of adductor pollicis muscle,** caput obliquum musculi adductoris pollicis.
**overriding h.,** the condition of the fetal head when it overrides the symphysis pubis instead of sinking into the pelvic cavity.
**h. of pancreas,** caput pancreatis.
**h. of penis,** glans penis.

**h. of phalanx of fingers,** caput phalangis manus.
**h. of phalanx of toes,** caput phalangis pedis.
**plantar h. of flexor digitorum pedis longus muscle,** musculus quadratus plantae.
**h. of posterior horn of spinal cord,** caput cornus posterioris medullae spinalis.
**posterior h. of rectus femoris muscle,** caput reflexum musculi recti femoris.
**quadrate h. of flexor digitorum pedis longus muscle,** musculus quadratus plantae.
**radial h. of flexor digitorum sublimis muscle,** caput radiale musculi flexoris digitorum superficialis.
**radial h. of flexor digitorum superficialis muscle,** caput radiale musculi flexoris digitorum superficialis.
**radial h. of humerus,** capitulum humeri.
**h. of radius,** caput radii.
**reflected h. of rectus femoris muscle,** caput reflexum musculi recti femoris.
**h. of rib,** caput costae.
**saddle h.,** a head with a sunken crown.
**scapular h. of triceps brachii muscle,** caput longum musculi tricipitis brachii.
**scapular h. of triceps extensor cubiti muscle,** caput longum musculi tricipitis brachii.
**second h. of triceps brachii muscle,** caput laterale musculi tricipitis brachii.
**short h. of biceps brachii muscle,** caput breve musculi bicipitis brachii.
**short h. of biceps femoris muscle,** caput breve musculi bicipitis femoris.
**short h. of biceps flexor cruris muscle,** caput breve musculi bicipitis femoris.
**short h. of biceps flexor cubiti muscle,** caput breve musculi bicipitis brachii.
**short h. of coracoradialis muscle,** caput breve musculi bicipitis brachii.
**short h. of triceps brachii muscle,** caput mediale musculi tricipitis brachii.
**short h. of triceps extensor cubiti muscle,** caput mediale musculi tricipitis brachii.
**short h. of triceps femoris muscle,** musculus adductor brevis.
**h. of spleen,** extremitas posterior splenis.
**h. of stapes,** caput stapedis.
**steeple h.,** oxycephaly.
**straight h. of rectus femoris muscle,** caput rectum musculi recti femoris.
**swelled h.,** bighead, def. 2.
**h. of talus,** caput tali.
**tower h.,** oxycephaly.
**transverse h. of adductor hallucis muscle,** caput transversum musculi adductoris hallucis.
**transverse h. of adductor pollicis muscle,** caput transversum musculi adductoris pollicis.
**h. of ulna,** caput ulnae.
**ulnar h. of flexor carpi ulnaris muscle,** caput ulnare musculi flexoris carpi ulnaris.
**ulnar h. of pronator teres muscle,** caput ulnare musculi pronatoris teretis.
**white h.,** a South African term for *favus.*
**zygomatic h. of quadratus labii superioris muscle,** musculus zygomaticus minor.

**head·ache** (hed′āk) [MeSH: Headache] pain in the head; called also *cephalalgia, cephalgia,* and *cephalodynia.*
**anemic h.,** headache ascribed to anemia, local or general.
**bilious h.,** migraine.
**blind h.,** migraine.
**cluster h.,** a headache, possibly a type of migraine, characterized by attacks of unilateral excruciating pain over the eye and forehead, with temperature elevation, lacrimation, and rhinorrhea; attacks last from 15 minutes to about an hour and tend to occur in clusters, sometimes a few times a day for two to eight weeks followed by months or years without occurrence. Because attacks identical to the spontaneous attacks may be induced in sufferers by subcutaneous injection of histamine diphosphate, it is also known as *histamine cephalalgia* or *h.* See also *chronic paroxysmal hemicrania,* under *hemicrania.* Called also *Horton's disease* or *syndrome, migrainous neuralgia,* and *vasomotor h.*
**congestive h.,** headache ascribed to congestion or hyperemia.
**cough h.,** an exertional headache with stabbing pain produced by the traction on pain-sensitive structures resulting from coughing or straining.
**dynamite h.,** a severe headache occurring in persons handling high explosives.
**exertional h.,** headache after physical exercise; many are of short duration. Cf. *cough h.* and *postcoital h.*
**functional h.,** headache due to tension or other emotional upset.
**helmet h.,** pain involving the upper half of the head.
**histamine h., Horton's h.,** cluster h.
**hyperemic h.,** congestive h.
**lumbar puncture h.,** headache in the erect position, relieved by recumbency, after lumbar puncture; due to lowering of intracranial pressure by leakage of cerebrospinal fluid through the needle tract.
**migraine h.,** see *migraine.*
**organic h.,** headache due to intracranial disease or other organic disease.
**postcoital h.,** an exertional headache occurring during or after sexual activity, usually in males; one subtype lasts for hours.
**postspinal h.,** lumbar puncture h.
**post-traumatic h.,** any headache occurring after trauma to the head or neck; it may be either physical or psychogenic in origin and may resemble either a cluster or a tension headache. Physical causes include subdural hematoma, stretching or tearing of ligaments and muscles in the neck, and injury to cervical soft tissues.
**puncture h.,** lumbar puncture h.
**pyrexial h.,** that due to fever.
**reflex h.,** that associated with disease of some organ, as the stomach, eyes, etc.; called also *symptomatic h.*
**rhinogenous h.,** headache due to nasal disease.
**sick h.,** migraine.
**spinal h.,** lumbar puncture h.
**symptomatic h.,** reflex h.
**tension h., tension-type h.,** a type brought on by prolonged overwork or emotional strain, or both, affecting especially the occipital region; it is usually continuous for weeks or months. Some individuals are particularly susceptible, possibly because of a defect in neurologic pathways controlling pain. A distinction is made between episodic types, which abate within a few weeks to six months, and chronic types, which persist uninterrupted for six months or longer.
**toxic h.,** headache due to systemic poisoning.
**vacuum h.,** headache due to obstruction of the outlet of the frontal sinus.
**vasomotor h.,** cluster h.

**head·cap** (hed′kap) headgear.

**head·gear** (hed′gēr) a harnesslike device fitting over the top and back of the head, serving as a source of resistance for extraoral anchorage for an orthodontic appliance. Called also *headcap.*

**head·grit** (hed′grit) yellows, def. 2.

**head·gut** (hed′gət) foregut.

**Heaf test** (hēf) [Frederick Roland George *Heaf,* British physician, 1894–1973] Sterneedle tuberculin test; see under *test.*

**heal** (hēl) to restore wounded parts or to make healthy; to become well or healthy.

**heal·ing** (hēl′ing) a process of cure; the restoration of integrity to injured tissue.
**h. by first intention,** healing in which union or restoration of continuity occurs directly without the intervention of granulations.
**h. by granulation,** h. by second intention.
**h. by second intention,** union by closure of a wound with granulations which form from the base and both sides toward the surface of the wound.

**Heal·on** (heēl′on) trademark for a preparation of sodium hyaluronate.

**health** (helth) [MeSH: Health] a state of optimal physical, mental, and social well-being, and not merely the absence of disease and infirmity.
**holistic h.,** a system of preventive medicine that takes into account the whole individual, his own responsibility for his well-being and the total influences—social, psychological, environmental—that affect health, including nutrition, exercise, and mental relaxation.
**public h.,** the field of medicine concerned with safeguarding and improving the health of the community as a whole.

**health main·te·nance or·ga·ni·za·tion (HMO)** a broad term encompassing a variety of health care delivery systems utilizing group practice and providing alternatives to the fee-for-service private practice of medicine and allied health professions. They are essentially prepaid, organized systems for providing comprehensive health care within a geographic area to all persons under contract and they emphasize preventive medicine.

**healthy** (hel′the) pertaining to, characterized by, or promoting health.

**hear·ing** (hēr′ing) [L. *auditus*] [MeSH: Hearing] the sense by which sounds are perceived; capacity to perceive sound. Called also *audition.*
**color h.,** a form of chromesthesia in which sounds cause sensations of color.
**double disharmonic h.,** diplacusis.
**monaural h.,** hearing with one ear.
**visual h.,** lip reading.

**hear·ing loss** (hēr′ing los′) deafness.
**Alexander's h. l.,** See under *deafness.*
**conductive h. l.,** hearing loss due to a defect of the sound conducting apparatus, i.e., of the external auditory canal or middle ear. Called also *conduction deafness* and *transmission h. l.*
**functional h. l.,** hearing loss that lacks any organic lesion. Called also *functional* or *hysterical deafness* and *nonorganic h. l.*
**mixed h. l.,** deafness that is both conductive and sensorineural in nature.
**noise-induced h. l.,** sensorineural deafness caused either by a single very loud noise (acoustic trauma deafness) or by prolonged exposure to high levels of noise (socioacusis).
**nonorganic h. l.,** functional h. l.
**ototoxic h. l.,** hearing loss caused by ingestion of toxic substances. Called also *toxic deafness.*
**pagetoid h. l.,** see under *deafness.*
**paradoxic h. l.,** hearing loss in which the hearing is better during loud noise. Called also *paradoxic deafness, paracusis of Willis,* and *paracusia willisiana.*
**sensorineural h. l.,** see under *deafness.*
**transmission h. l.,** conductive h. l.

**heart** (hahrt) [L. *cor;* Gr. *kardia*] [MeSH: Heart] the viscus of cardiac muscle that maintains the circulation of the blood. Called also *cor* [TA]. It is divided into four cavities—two atria and two ventricles. The left atrium receives oxygenated blood from the lungs. From there the blood passes to the left ventricle, which forces it via the aorta through the arteries to supply the tissues of the body. The right atrium receives the blood after it has passed through the tissues and given up much of its oxygen. The blood then passes to the right ventricle, and then to the lungs, to be oxygenated. The major valves are four in number: the *left atrioventricular valve (mitral),* between the left atrium and ventricle; the *right atrioventricular valve (tricuspid),* between the right atrium and ventricle; the *aortic valve,* at the orifice of the aorta; and the *pulmonary valve,* at the orifice of the pulmonary trunk. The heart tissue itself is nourished by the blood in the coronary arteries. See Plate 20.
**armored h., armour h.,** a condition marked by calcareous deposits in the pericardium.
**artificial h.,** a pumping mechanism that duplicates the output, rate, and blood pressure of the natural heart. It may replace the function of the entire heart or a portion of it, and may be permanent or temporary, intracorporeal or extracorporeal.
**athletic h.,** hypertrophy or dilation of the heart with no disease of the valves or other disorder of the circulation, sometimes seen in athletes.
**beer h.,** beer-drinkers' cardiomyopathy.
**beriberi h.,** heart failure from thiamine deficiency.
**boat-shaped h.,** the radiologic appearance of the heart in aortic regurgitation, due to dilatation and hypertrophy of the left ventricle.
**bony h.,** a heart or pericardium containing calcareous deposits.
**booster h.,** auxiliary ventricle.
**bovine h.,** cor bovinum.
**chaotic h.,** a heart which exhibits frequent extrasystoles.
**dynamite h.,** a condition occurring in workers exposed to nitroglycerin, in which the blood vessels become dilated during exposure and then, when exposure is discontinued, contract and thus reduce the blood supply to heart.
**encased h.,** a heart affected with chronic constrictive pericarditis.
**extracorporeal h.,** an artificial heart located outside the body and usually performing a pumping and an oxygenating function.
**fat h., fatty h.,** 1. a heart affected with fatty degeneration. 2. a condition in which there is an excessive layer of fat deposited about and in the heart muscle. Called also *cor adiposum.*
**fibroid h.,** a heart in which fibrous tissue replaces portions of the myocardium, such as sometimes occurs in chronic myocarditis.
**flask-shaped h.,** the x-ray appearance of the heart in pericarditis with effusion.
**frosted h.,** a condition in which the pericardium is thickened, giving the heart the appearance of being frosted like a cake. Cf. *hyaloserositis.*
**hairy h.,** shaggy pericardium.
**horizontal h.,** a counterclockwise rotation of the electrical axis (deviation to the left) of the heart; a moderate deviation (0° to −20°) is normally observed in asthenic persons with a transversely situated heart, in the obese, and in pregnant women.
**hyperthyroid h.,** the heart in thyrotoxic heart disease.
**hypoplastic h.,** a heart of small size.
**icing h.,** frosted h.
**intracorporeal h.,** an artificial heart implanted in the body.
**irritable h.,** neurocirculatory asthenia.
**Jarvik-7 artificial h.,** Symbion Jarvik-7 artificial h.
**left h.,** the left atrium and ventricle; that portion of the heart which propels the blood in systemic circulation.
**lymph h.,** an organ in frogs and fishes concerned in the distribution of lymph.
**mechanical h.,** artificial h.
**myxedema h.,** an enlarged heart associated with hypothyroidism.
**ox h.,** cor bovinum.
**parchment h.,** the appearance of the right ventricle in Uhl's anomaly.
**pulmonary h.,** right h.
**right h.,** the right atrium and ventricle; that portion of the heart which propels the blood in the pulmonary circulation.
**sabot h.,** coeur en sabot.
**soldier's h.,** neurocirculatory asthenia.
**stone h.,** massive contraction band necrosis in an irreversibly noncompliant hypertrophied heart, occurring as a complication of cardiac surgery; it is believed due to a combination of low levels of adenosine triphosphate and calcium overload.
**Symbion Jarvik-7 artificial h.,** an air-driven artificial heart consisting of two smooth-surfaced, sac-like polyurethane pumps that replace the ventricles, with pyrolytic carbon disk valves and Dacron-covered prostheses connecting to the atria and great vessels; two pneumatic power units in the drive system regulate blood flow by pulsing air through polyurethane tubing drive lines.
**systemic h.,** left h.
**tabby cat h.,** a condition of the heart in which the inner surface of the ventricular wall and the papillary muscles are streaked and spotted; seen in marked cases of fatty degeneration. Called also *thrush breast h., tiger h.,* and *tiger lily h.*
**three-chambered h.,** a developmental anomaly in which the heart is missing the interventricular septum (cor triloculare biatriatum) or the interatrial septum (cor triloculare biventriculare) and so has only three compartments. Called also *cor triloculare* or *trilocular h.*
**thrush breast h., tiger h., tiger lily h.,** tabby cat h.
**triatrial h.,** cor triatriatum.
**trilocular h.,** three-chambered h.
**vertical h.,** a clockwise rotation of the electrical axis (deviation to the right) of the heart; a moderate deviation (90° to 100°) is normally observed in asthenic persons with a vertically situated heart and in early infancy.
**water-bottle h.,** a radiographic sign of pericardial effusion: the cardiopericardial silhouette is enlarged and assumes the shape of a flask or water bottle, with blurring of the left cardiac border and obscuring of the hilar vessels.

**heart·beat** (hahrt′bēt) a complete cardiac cycle, during which the electrical impulse is conducted and mechanical contraction occurs.

**heart block** (hahrt blok) [MeSH: Heart Block] impairment of conduction of an impulse in heart excitation; often applied specifically to atrioventricular block. For specific types of heart block, see under *block.*

**heart·burn** (hahrt′bərn) [MeSH: Heartburn] an esophageal symptom consisting of a retrosternal sensation of warmth or burning occurring in waves and tending to rise upward toward the neck; it may be accompanied by a reflux of fluid into the mouth (water brash). It is often associated with gastroesophageal reflux. Called also *pyrosis.*

**heart fail·ure** (hahrt fāl′yər) see under *failure.*

**heart·wa·ter** (hahrt′wah-tər) a fatal rickettsial disease of cattle, sheep, and goats in sub-Saharan Africa and on certain islands in the Indian Ocean, marked by fluid accumulation in the pleura, pericardium, and pleural cavity. It is caused by *Cowdria ruminantium,* which is transmitted by the ticks *Amblyomma hebraeum* and *A. variegata.* Called also *cowdriosis, veld* or *veldt disease,* and *veld* or *veldt sickness.*

**heart·worm** (hahrt′wərm) *Dirofilaria immitis.*

**heat** (hēt) [L. *calor*] [MeSH: Heat] 1. the sensation of an increase in temperature. 2. the energy which produces the sensation of heat. It exists in the form of molecular or atomic vibration (thermal agitation) and may be transferred, as a consequence of a gradient in temperature, by conduction through a substance, by convection by

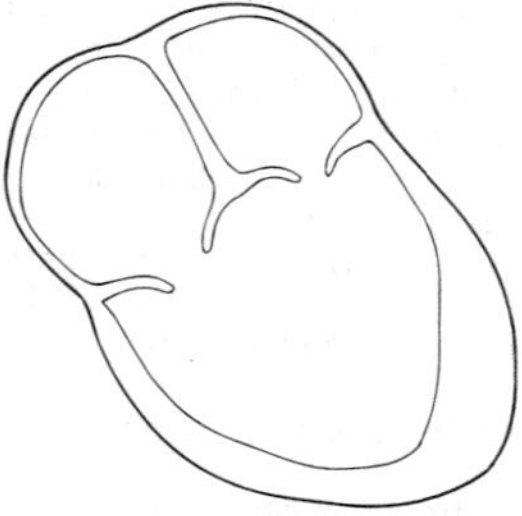

Three-chambered heart in which the interventricular septum is absent (cor triloculare biatriatum).

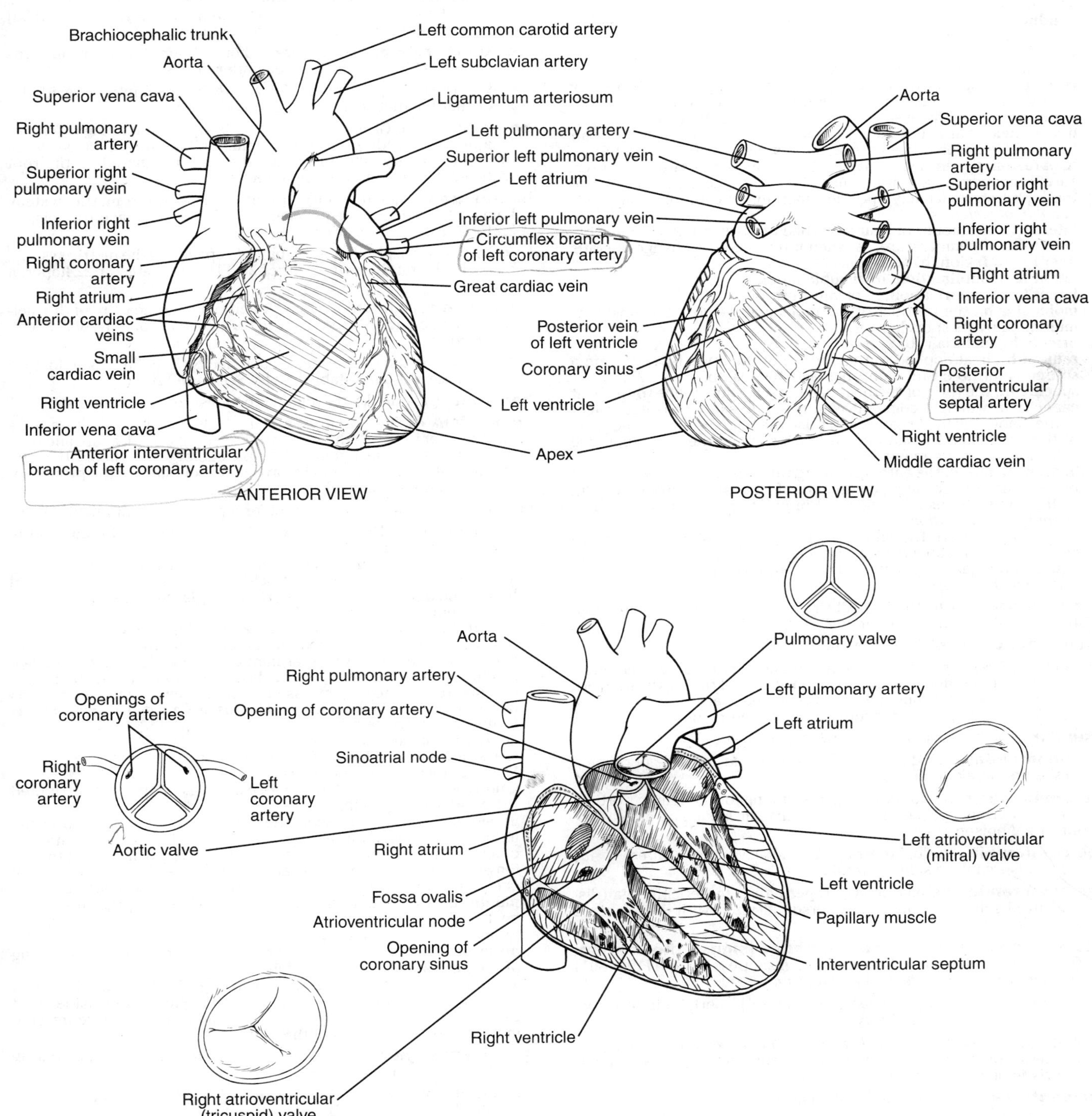


**PLATE 20—**STRUCTURES OF THE HEART

a substance, and by radiation as electromagnetic waves. Symbol *Q* or *q*. 3. estrus. 4. to become, or to cause to become, warm or hot.
**atomic h.,** the product of the atomic weight of an element and its specific heat.
**conductive h.,** heat transmitted to the body by contact with a heated object, such as a hot water bag.
**convective h.,** heat conveyed to the surface of the body from warm currents of water or air.
**conversive h.,** heat developed in the tissues by the resistance of the tissues to the passage of high-frequency electromagnetic radiation through them; used in various kinds of diathermy.
**dry h.,** heat that is not moist; usually produced by heated dry air that rapidly absorbs from the skin the moisture of perspiration.
**h. of fusion,** the enthalpy change at constant temperature and pressure in converting a unit amount of a substance from the solid to the liquid state, usually specified in cal/g or cal/mol. Called also *latent h. of fusion.*
**latent h.,** the amount of heat absorbed or given off by a body without changing temperature, as when it undergoes a change of state.
**latent h. of fusion,** h. of fusion.
**latent h. of sublimation,** h. of sublimation.
**latent h. of vaporization,** h. of vaporization.
**molecular h.,** the product of the molecular weight of a substance multiplied by its specific heat.
**prickly h.,** miliaria rubra.
**radiant h.,** heat applied to the surface of the body by rays from a source of infrared radiation, such as a heat lamp.
**specific h.,** the ratio of the heat capacity of a substance to the heat capacity of water at constant volume or pressure; it is equivalent to the amount of heat required to raise the temperature of one gram of the substance by one degree Celsius, since the corresponding value for water is defined as 1.0.
**h. of sublimation,** the enthalpy change at constant temperature and pressure in converting a unit amount of a substance from the solid to the gas state, usually specified in cal/g or cal/mol. Called also *latent h. of sublimation.*
**h. of vaporization,** the enthalpy change at constant temperature and pressure in converting a unit amount of a substance from the liquid to the gas state, usually specified in cal/g or cal/mol. Called also *latent h. of vaporization.*

**Heath's operation** (hēths) [Christopher *Heath,* English surgeon, 1835–1905] see under *operation.*

**heat·stroke** (hēt′strōk″) see under *stroke.*

**heaves** (hēvz) chronic obstructive pulmonary disease in equines, resulting from reduced elasticity and rupture of the elastic network of the respiratory bronchioles and pulmonary alveoli; characteristics include coughing, bronchitis, and labored respiration.

**Hebdom.** abbreviation for L. *hebdo′mada,* a week.

**heb·dom·a·dal** (heb-dom′ə-dəl) [L. *hebdomada* a week] pertaining to the first week of life.

**Heb·e·lo·ma** (heb″ə-lo′mə) a genus of fungi of the family Cortinariaceae. Certain species are called *asetake* in Japan and are gastrointestinal poisons.

**he·be·phre·nia** (he″bə-fre′ne-ə) [Gr. *hēbē* youth + *phren* + *-ia*] *(obs.)* disorganized schizophrenia.

**he·be·phren·ic** (he″bə-fren′ik) 1. pertaining to hebephrenia (disorganized schizophrenia). 2. a person affected with disorganized schizophrenia.

**He·ber·den's asthma, disease, nodes (signs), rheumatism** (he′bər-dənz) [William *Heberden,* English physician, 1710–1801] see under *disease, node,* and *rheumatism.*

**he·bet·ic** (hə-bet′ik) [Gr. *hēbētikos* youthful] pertaining to or occurring at the time of puberty.

**heb·e·tude** (heb′ə-to͞od) [L. *hebetudo* from *hebes,* dull] apathy or dullness from any cause; in psychiatry, emotional dullness, a characteristic of schizophrenia.

**he·bi·at·rics** (he″be-at′riks) ephebiatrics.

**He·bra's disease, prurigo** (ha′brahz) [Ferdinand Ritter von *Hebra,* Austrian dermatologist, 1816–1880] see *erythema multiforme minor,* and see under *prurigo.*

**hec·a·tom·er·al** (hek″ə-tom′ər-əl) hecatomeric.

**hec·a·to·mer·ic** (hek″ə-to-mer′ik) [Gr. *hekateron* each of two + *meros* part] having processes which divide into two, one going to each side of the spinal cord; said of certain neurons.

**Hecht's phenomenon** (hekts) [Adolf Franz *Hecht,* Austrian physician, 20th century] Rumpel-Leede phenomenon.

**Hecht syndrome** (hekt) [Frederick *Hecht,* American physician, born 1930] trismus-pseudocamptodactyly syndrome.

**Hecht-Beals syndrome** (hekt-bēlz) [F. *Hecht;* Rodney K. *Beals,* American orthopedic surgeon, 20th century] trismus-pseudocamptodactyly syndrome.

**Hecht-Beals-Wil·son syndrome** (hekt-bēlz-wil′sən) [F. *Hecht;* R. K. *Beals;* Ralph V. *Wilson,* American orthopedic surgeon, born 1938] trismus-pseudocamptodactyly syndrome.

**Heck·a·thorn's disease** (hek′ə-thōnz) [name of the propositus first observed in the 1970s] see under *disease.*

**hec·tic** (hek′tik) [L. *hecticus;* Gr. *hektikos* consumptive] said of a fever that fluctuates each day; see under *fever.*

**hecto-** [Fr., from Gr. *hekaton* one hundred] a combining form designating one hundred; used in naming units of measurement to indicate a quantity 100 ($10^2$) times the unit designated by the root with which it is combined. Symbol h.

**hec·to·gram** (hek′to-gram) a unit of mass of the metric system, being $10^2$ grams; the equivalent of 3.527 ounces avoirdupois, or 3.215 ounces apothecaries' weight.

**hec·to·li·ter** (hek′to-le′tər) a unit of capacity of the metric system, being $10^2$ liters; the equivalent of 26.4 United States or 22 Imperial gallons.

**hec·tom·e·ter** (hek-tom′ə-tər) a unit of linear measure of the metric system, being $10^2$ meters, or the equivalent, roughly, of 328 feet, one inch.

**HED** abbreviation for German *Haut-Einheits-Dosis* (unit skin dose), a unit of x-ray dosage established by Seitz and Wintz.

**he·don·ic** (he-don′ik) pertaining to pleasure or to hedonism.

**he·do·nism** (he′don-iz-əm) [Gr. *hēdonē* pleasure] 1. pleasure-seeking behavior. 2. the ethical doctrine that regards pleasure and happiness as the highest good. 3. in psychology, the theory that the attainment of pleasure and the avoidance of pain are the prime motivators of human behavior.

**Hed·u·lin** (hed′u-lin) trademark for a preparation of phenindione.

**heel** (hēl) [MeSH: Heel] 1. calx, def. 2. 2. the posterior part of the wall of a horse's hoof.
**anterior h.,** a triangular-shaped piece of leather fastened obliquely across the ball of the shoe just behind the heads of the metatarsal bones, the object being to support the heads, equalize the pressure, and support the anterior arch.
**basketball h.,** black heel (q.v.) in basketball players.
**black h.,** a benign condition characterized by the sudden appearance of unilateral or bilateral minute, blood-filled punctate black macules on the bottom of the heel and sometimes the distal toe(s); it is due to the shearing stress of certain athletic activities such as basketball, volleyball, tennis, and lacrosse. Called also *calcaneal petechiae* and *talon noir.*
**contracted h.,** see under *hoof.*
**cracked h's,** pitted keratolysis.
**Elso h.,** inherited spastic paresis.
**gonorrheal h.,** the development of exostoses on the heel, attributed to gonorrheal infection.
**greasy h.,** swelling and seborrheic dermatitis in the region of the fetlock and pastern on the back of a horse's leg, with formation of cracks in the skin and excretion of oily matter, usually due to prolonged standing in wet or unsanitary quarters. A similar condition occurs in cattle. Called also *grease, grease-heel,* and *scratches.*
**painful h.,** a condition in which pain is caused by pressure on the heel.
**policeman's h.,** calcanodynia in a policeman.
**prominent h.,** a swelling on the back of the heel due to thickening of the periosteum of the os calcis.
**Thomas h.,** a shoe correction consisting of a heel one half inch longer and an eighth to a sixth of an inch higher on the inside, used to bring the heel of the foot into varus and to prevent depression in the region of the head of the talus.

**Heer·fordt's syndrome (disease)** (hār′forts) [Christian Frederik *Heerfordt,* Danish oculist, 1872–1953] see under *syndrome.*

**he·fil·con** (hə-fil′kon) either of two hydrophilic contact lens materials, designated A or B.

**Hef·ke-Tur·ner sign** (hef′ke-tər′nər) [Hans William *Hefke,* American surgeon, born 1871; Vernon Charles *Turner,* American orthopedic surgeon, 20th century] see under *sign.*

**He·gar dilator, sign** (ha′gahrz) [Alfred *Hegar,* German gynecologist, 1830–1914] see under *dilator* and *sign.*

**Hegg·lin's anomaly** [Robert Marquand *Hegglin,* Swiss physician, born 1907] May-Hegglin anomaly.

**hEGF** human epidermal growth factor.

**Hei·den·hain's cells, demilunes,** etc. (hi′dən-hīnz) [Rudolf Peter *Heidenhain,* German physiologist, 1834–1897] see *chief cells* (def. 1) and *parietal cells,* under *cell,* and *crescents of Gianuzzi,* under *crescent,* and see under *law, rod,* and *stain.*

**Hei•den•hain's syndrome** (hi'dən-hīnz) [Adolf *Heidenhain,* German neurologist, 20th century] see under *syndrome.*

**height** (hīt) the vertical measurement of an object or body.

**h. of contour,** the line encircling a tooth at its greatest bulge with reference to a predetermined path of insertion for a removable partial denture.

**h. of contour, surveyed,** a line scribed or marked on a cast that designates the greatest bulge or diameter with respect to a selected path of denture placement or removal.

**cusp h.,** 1. the shortest distance between the tip of a cusp of a tooth and its base plane. 2. the shortest distance between the deepest part of the central fossa of a posterior tooth and a line connecting the points of the cusps of the tooth.

**facial h.,** the linear measurement of portions of the face, in the midline, using specified reference points, including *anterior, upper, lower,* and *posterior facial h.* See illustration.

**facial h., anterior,** the linear distance from the nasion to the bottom of the chin, the precise point variously specified as the pogonion, gnathion, or menton. It is subdivided into *upper* and *lower facial h.* See also illustration.

**facial h., lower,** the linear distance between the chin, specified as either the menton, gnathion, or pogonion, and the region of the teeth, usually the anterior nasal spine or the interdentale inferius. See illustration.

**facial h., posterior,** a quite variable measure of the linear height of the face in the region of the ear. The most common measure is between a point on the inferior border of the mandible, generally the gonion, and the condylare, sella, or a point defined as the center facial point. Other measurements of height exist, some involving lines of intersection drawn between major facial planes. See illustration.

**facial h., upper,** the linear distance between the nasion and a point in the region of the maxillary teeth, usually the anterior nasal spine but sometimes the interdentale superius or prosthion. See illustration.

**sitting h.,** sitting vertex h.

**sitting suprasternal h.,** the distance from the middle of the anterior-superior border of the manubrium sterni to the surface on which the subject is seated.

**sitting vertex h.,** the distance from the highest point of the head in the sagittal plane to the surface on which the subject is seated; commonly called *sitting h.* Cf. *crown-rump length.*

**standing h.,** the distance from the highest point of the head in the sagittal plane to the surface on which the individual is standing, measured when the subject is not wearing shoes. Cf. *crown-heel length.*

**Heil•bron•ner's thigh (sign)** (hīl'bron-ərz) [Karl *Heilbronner,* Dutch physician, 1869–1914] see under *thigh.*

**Heim-Krey•sig sign** (hīm-kri'sig) [Ernst Ludwig *Heim,* German physician, 1747–1834; Friedrich Ludwig *Kreysig,* German physician, 1770–1839] see under *sign.*

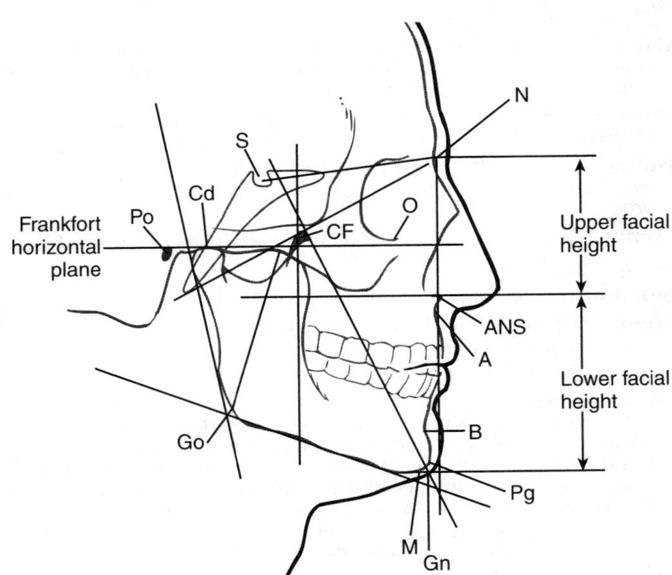


Facial height. Anterior facial height is the sum of upper and lower facial heights, the lower limit of the latter variously defined as the pogonion, gnathion or menton. Posterior facial height is often measured from the gonion to the condylare, sella, or center of face point. *A,* subspinale; *ANS,* anterior nasal spine; *B,* supramentale; *Cd,* condylare; *CF,* center of face; *Gn,* gnathion; *Go,* gonion; *M,* menton; *N,* nasion; *O,*orbitale; *Pg,* pogonion; *Po,* porion; *S,* sella.

**Heim•lich maneuver** (hīm'lik) [Henry Jay *Heimlich,* American surgeon, born 1920] see under *maneuver.*

**Heine's operation** (hi'nəz) [Leopold *Heine,* German oculist, 1870–1940] see under *operation.*

**Hei•ne-Med•in disease** (hi'nĕ-ma'din) [Jacob von *Heine,* German physician, 1800–1879; Karl Oskar *Medin,* Swedish physician, 1847–1927] see *poliomyelitis.*

**Hei•ne•ke-Mik•u•licz pyloroplasty (operation)** (hi'nĕ-ke-me-koo'lich) [Walter Hermann *Heineke,* German surgeon, 1834–1901; Johann von *Mikulicz*-Radecki, Romanian-born surgeon in Germany, 1850–1905] see under *pyloroplasty.*

**Hei•nig's projection** (hi'nigz) [C.F. *Heinig,* American radiologist, 20th century] see under *projection.*

**Heinz bodies (granules)** (hīnts) [Robert *Heinz,* German pathologist, 1865–1924] Heinz-Ehrlich bodies; see under *body.*

**Heinz-Ehr•lich bodies** (hīnts-er'lik) [Robert *Heinz;* Paul *Ehrlich,* German bacteriologist, 1854–1915] see under *body.*

**Heis•ter's diverticulum, fold, valve** (hīs'tərz) [Lorenz *Heister,* German anatomist, 1683–1758] see *bulbus superior venae jugularis* and *plica spiralis.*

**HEK** human embryo kidney (cell culture).

**Hek•toen phenomenon** (hek'tōn) [Ludvig *Hektoen,* American pathologist, 1863–1951] see under *phenomenon.*

**HEL** human embryo lung (cell culture).

**HeLa cells** (he'lə) [from the name of the patient from whose carcinoma of the cervix uteri the parent carcinoma cells were isolated in 1951] [MeSH: Hela Cells] see under *cell.*

**Hel•bing's sign** (hel'bingz) [Carl Ernst *Helbing,* German physician, 1842–1914] see under *sign.*

**hel•coid** (hel'koid) [Gr. *helkos* ulcer + *-oid*] resembling an ulcer.

**hel•col•o•gy** (hel-kol'ə-je) [Gr. *helkos* ulcer + *-logy*] the scientific study of ulcers.

**hel•co•ma** (hel-ko'mə) [Gr.] corneal ulcer.

**hel•co•sis** (hel-ko'sis) [Gr. *helkōsis*] ulceration.

**Held's end bulb, end foot** (heldz) [Hans *Held,* German anatomist, 1866–1942] see under *bulb* and see *end feet.*

**He•le•i•dae** (hə-le'ĭ-de) a family of flies of the suborder Nematocerca, order Diptera, containing, among others, the four genera *Culicoides, Haemophoructus, Lasiohelea,* and *Leptoconops,* various species of which suck the blood of man, and may serve as vectors of disease. Called also *Ceratopogonidae.*

**He•le•ni•um** [hə-le'ne-um] sneezeweed, a genus of composite plants found in North America that cause vomiting and neurological symptoms in sheep.

**he•li•an•thin** (he-le-an'thin) methyl orange; see under *orange.*

**hel•i•cal** (hel'ĭ-kəl) spiral (def. 2).

**He•li•cel•la** (he″lĭ-sel'ə) a genus of snails of the family Helicellidae; they serve as hosts of the liver fluke *Dicrocoelium dentriticum* in Europe.

**He•li•cel•li•dae** (he″lĭ-sel'ĭ-de) a family of snails of the suborder Stylommatophora that serve as hosts of trematodes infecting humans.

**He•lic•i•dae** (he-lis'ĭ-de) a family of terrestrial and fresh water snails of the order Pulmonata, suborder Stylommatophora. It includes the genera *Alocinma* and *Helix.*

**hel•i•cine** (hel'ĭ-sēn) spiral (def. 2).

**helic(o)-** [Gr. *helix* coil, gen. *helikos*] a combining form denoting relationship to a coil.

**He•li•co•bac•ter** (hel″ĭ-ko-bak'tər) [*helico-* + *-bacter*] [MeSH: Helicobacter] a genus of gram-negative, microaerophilic bacteria of the family Spirillaceae, consisting of motile, spiral organisms with multiple sheathed flagella; formerly classified in the genus *Campylobacter.*

**H. cinae'di,** a species, formerly *Campylobacter cinaedi,* that causes proctitis and colitis in homosexual men; it has also been implicated in septicemia in immunocompromised patients and as a cause of neonatal septicemia and meningitis.

**H. pylo'ri,** a species that causes gastritis and pyloric ulcers in humans; *H. pylori* infection is associated with gastric cancer. Formerly called *Campylobacter pylori.*

**hel•i•coid** (hel'ĭ-koid) [*helico-* + *-oid*] resembling a coil or helix.

**hel•i•co•pod** (hel'ĭ-ko-pod″) denoting a peculiar dragging gait; see under *gait.*

**hel·i·co·tre·ma** (hel″ĭ-ko-tre′mə) [*helico-* + Gr. *trēma* hole] [TA] the passage of the ear that connects the scala tympani and scala vestibuli at the apex of the cochlea; called also *Breschet's* or *Scarpa's hiatus.*

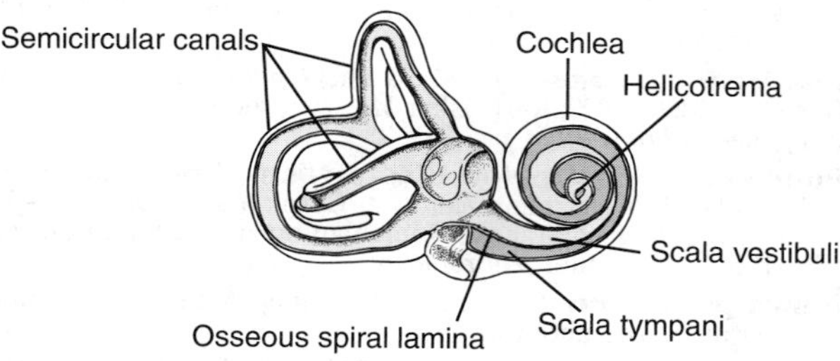


Helicotrema, shown in the interior of the right osseous labyrinth.

**heli(o)-** [Gr. *hēlios* sun] a combining form denoting relationship to the sun.

**he·lio·sin** (he″le-o′sin) a compound containing keratin and various inorganic salts.

**he·li·o·sis** (he″le-o′sis) [*helio-* + *-osis*] sunstroke.

**he·lio·tax·is** (he″le-o-tak′sis) [*helio-* + *taxis*] the movement of cells and microorganisms in response to either or both light and heat from the sun. The response may be toward *(positive h.)* or away *(negative h.)* from the source of stimulus. Cf. *heliotropism, phototaxis,* and *thermotaxis.*

**he·lio·ther·a·py** (he″le-o-ther′ə-pe) [*helio-* + *therapy*] [MeSH: Heliotherapy] the treatment of disease by exposing the body to the sun's rays; the therapeutic use of the sun bath.

**he·lio·trope B** (he′le-o-trōp″) amethyst violet; see under *violet.*

**he·li·ot·ro·pism** (he″le-ot′ro-piz-əm) [*helio-* + *tropism*] the turning of an organism, especially a plant, toward *(positive h.)* or away from *(negative h.)* the sun. Cf. *heliotaxis.*

**he·li·um** (he′le-əm) [Gr. *hēlios* sun] [MeSH: Helium] a colorless, odorless, tasteless gas, which is not combustible and does not support combustion. It is one of the inert gaseous elements, which was first detected in the sun and is now obtained from natural gas. Symbol, He; atomic number, 2; atomic weight, 4.003. Used in medicine [USP] as a diluent for other gases, being especially useful with oxygen in the treatment of certain cases of respiratory obstruction, and as a vehicle for general anesthetics.

**He·lix** (he′liks) a genus of snails of the family Helicidae, including some of the common garden snails.

**he·lix** (he′liks) pl. *helixes* or *he′lices* [Gr. "snail," "coil"] 1. a winding structure. See also *coil* and *spiral.* 2. [TA] the superior and posterior free margin of the pinna of the ear.
**α h., alpha h.,** a secondary structure occurring in many proteins; it is a right-handed helix with 3.6 amino acid residues per turn stabilized by hydrogen bonds between the imino hydrogen of each peptide bond and the carbonyl oxygen of the peptide bond four residues further along the polypeptide chain.
**double h., Watson-Crick h.,** a double helix, each chain of which contains information completely specifying the other chain, representing a structural formulation of the mechanism by which the genetic information in DNA reproduces itself; see illustration at *deoxyribonucleic acid.*

**hel·le·bore** (hel′ə-bor) [L. helleborus; Gr. helleboros] 1. any plant of the genus *Helleborus,* perennial herbs that were formerly used medicinally. See *black h.* 2. any of various plants of the genus *Veratrum,* used medicinally but sometimes toxic to livestock.
**American h.,** *Veratrum viride.*
**black h.,** 1. *Helleborus niger.* 2. the medicinal root of *H. niger.*
**European h.,** *Veratrum album.*
**green h.,** *Veratrum viride.*
**white h.,** *Veratrum album.*

**Hel·le·bo·rus** (hel″ə-bo′rəs) a genus of plants of the family Ranunculaceae, native to Europe and Asia. *H. ni′ger* is the black hellebore, a perennial herb whose root (also called *black hellebore*) contains a cardiac glycoside and was formerly used medicinally.

**Hel·ler's esophagomyotomy (myotomy, operation)** (hel′ərz) [Ernst *Heller,* German surgeon, 1877–1964] esophagocardiomyotomy.

**Hel·ler's plexus** (hel′ərz) [Arnold Ludwig Gotthilf *Heller,* German pathologist, 1840–1913] see under *plexus.*

**Hel·ler-Döh·le disease** (hel′ər-der′le) [A. L. G. *Heller;* Karl Gottfried Paul *Döhle,* German pathologist, 1855–1928] syphilitic aortitis.

**Hel·lin's law** (hel′inz) [Dyonizy *Hellin,* Polish pathologist, 1867–1935] see under *law.*

**Helm·holtz ligament, theory** (helm′holtz) [Hermann Ludwig Ferdinand von *Helmholtz,* German physiologist, inventor of the ophthalmoscope, 1821–1894] see under *ligament* and *theory.*

**hel·minth** (hel′minth) [Gr. *helmins* worm] a parasitic worm.

**hel·min·tha·gogue** (hel-min′thə-gog) anthelmintic (def. 2).

**hel·min·them·e·sis** (hel″min-them′ə-sis) [*helminth* + *emesis*] the vomiting of worms.

**hel·min·thi·a·sis** (hel″min-thi′ə-sis) [MeSH: Helminthiasis] vermination, def 1.

**hel·min·thic** (hel-min′thik) pertaining to or caused by parasitic worms.

**hel·min·thi·cide** (hel-min′thĭ-sīd) [*helminth* + *-cide*] anthelmintic (def. 2).

**hel·min·thism** (hel′min-thiz-əm) vermination, def. 1.

**hel·min·thoid** (hel-min′thoid) [*helminth* + *-oid*] wormlike.

**hel·min·thol·o·gy** (hel″min-thol′ə-je) [*helminth* + *-logy*] the scientific study of parasitic worms.

**hel·min·tho·ma** (hel″min-tho′mə) [*helminth* + *-oma*] a tumor caused by a parasitic worm.

**hel·min·thous** (hel-min′thəs) verminous, def. 1.

**hel(o)-** [Gr. *hēlos* nail, corn, callus] a combining form denoting relationship to a nail, or to a wart or callus.

**He·lo·der·ma** (he″lo-dər′mə) [*helo-* + *derma*] a genus of venomous lizards of the southwestern United States and Mexico. *H. hor′ridum* is the beaded lizard and *H. suspec′tum* is the Gila monster.

**he·lo·ma** (he-lo′mə) [*helo-* + *-oma*] a corn or callosity on the hand or foot.
**h. du′rum,** hard corn.
**h. mol′le,** soft corn.

**He·loph·i·lus** (hə-lof′ĭ-ləs) a genus of flies, hover flies, of the family Syrphidae, whose "rat-tail" maggots (larvae) may cause nasal and intestinal myiasis.

**he·lo·sis** (he-lo′sis) the condition of having corns.

**He·lo·ti·a·les** (he″lo-she-a′lēz) an order of fungi of the subphylum Ascomycotina, series Unitunicatae, having inoperculate asci; some species are saprobes and others are parasites of plants. It includes the genus *Sclerotinia.*

**he·lot·o·my** (he-lot′ə-me) [*helo-* + *-tomy*] the excision or, more often, the paring of corns or calluses.

**Hel·vel·la** (hel-vel′ə) the saddle fungi, a genus of the family Helvellaceae. Some species contain a heat-stable hemolysin. *H. esculen′ta* and other species cause mycetismus sanguinarius, a form of mushroom poisoning.

**Hel·vel·la·ceae** (hel″vəl-a′se-e) a family of fungi of the order Pezizales; some species are edible and others are poisonous. It includes the genera *Gyromitra* and *Helvella.*

**Hel·weg's bundle (tract)** (hel′vəgz) [Hans Kristian Saxtorph *Helweg,* Danish physician, 1847–1901] olivospinal tract.

**Hel·weg-Lar·sen's syndrome** (hel′veg-lahr′sənz) [Hans F. *Helweg-Larsen,* Danish dermatologist, 20th century] see under *syndrome.*

**he·ma** (he′mə) [Gr. *haima, haimatos* blood] haema; see also *blood.*

**hema-** see *hem(o)-.*

**hema·chro·ma·to·sis** (he″mə-kro″mə-to′sis) hemochromatosis.

**hema·chrome** (he′mə-krōm) an oxygen-carrying blood pigment, e.g., hemoglobin or hemocyanin.

**hema·cyte** (he′mə-sīt) blood cell.

**hema·cy·tom·e·ter** (he″mə-si-tom′ə-tər) a device used in manual blood counts, consisting of a microscopic slide with a depression whose base is marked in grids, and into which a measured volume of a sample of blood or bacterial culture is placed and covered with a cover glass. The number of cells and formed blood elements in the squares is counted under a microscope and used as a representative sample for calculating the unit volume. Called also *counting cell, counting chamber,* and *hemocytometer.*

**hema·cy·tom·e·try** (hēm″ə-si-tom′ə-tre) the counting of blood cells using a hemacytometer; called also *hemocytometry.*

**he·ma·do·ste·no·sis** (he″mə-do-, hem-ə-to-stə-no′sis) stenosis of a blood vessel; see also *angiostenosis.*

**he·mad·sor·bent** (he″mad-zor′bənt) inducing or characterized by hemadsorption.

**he·mad·sorp·tion** (he″mad-zorp′shən) [MeSH: Hemadsorption] the adherence of red cells to other cells, particles, or surfaces; see hemadsorption test, under *test.*

**he·ma·dy·na·mom·e·try** (he″mə-di″nə-mom′ə-tre) measurement of blood pressure.

**he·ma·fa·cient** (he″mə-fa′shənt) hematopoietic.

**he·mag·glu·ti·na·tion** (he″mə-gloo″tĭ-na′shən) [MeSH: Hemagglutination] agglutination of erythrocytes, which may be caused by antibodies such as hemagglutinins, by viruses such as those of influenza and mumps, or by other substances such as lectins.
**indirect h., passive h.,** agglutination of erythrocytes due to the reaction of specific antibody with antigen passively adsorbed on the surface or chemically coupled to the cells; the basis of many serologic tests.
**viral h.,** the agglutination of erythrocytes by viruses, either by intact virions or by viral products; the basis of hemagglutination or hemagglutination inhibition methods for viral titration.

**he·mag·glu·ti·na·tive** (he″mə-gloo′tĭ-na″tiv) pertaining to, characterized by, or causing agglutination of erythrocytes.

**he·mag·glu·ti·nin** (he″mə-gloo′tĭ-nin) [*hem-* + *agglutinin*] an agglutinin, e.g., an antibody or lectin, that agglutinates erythrocytes.
**cold h.,** a cold agglutinin (q.v.) that agglutinates red cells.
**warm h.,** a warm agglutinin (q.v.) that agglutinates red cells.

**he·mal** (he′məl) 1. ventral to the spinal axis, where the heart and great vessels are located, as, e.g., the hemal arches. Cf. *neural.* 2. hemic. 3. pertaining to the blood vessels; see *vascular.*

**hem·al·um** (he′mə-ləm) a mixture of hematoxylin and alum introduced by Mayer, widely used as a nuclear stain, especially in combination with eosin as a general oversight method. Also, any alum and hematoxylin stain. Called also *alum hematoxylin.*

**hem·a·nal·y·sis** (he″mə-nal′ə-sis) [*hem-* + *analysis*] analysis or examination of the blood.

**he·man·gi·ec·ta·sia** (he-man″je-ek-ta′shə) angiectasis.

**he·man·gi·ec·ta·sis** (he-man″je-ek′tə-sis) angiectasis.

**hemangi(o)-** [Gr. *haima* blood + *angeion* vessel] a combining form denoting relationship to the blood vessels.

**he·man·gio·amelo·blas·to·ma** (he-man″je-o-ə-mel″o-blas-to′mə) [*hemangio-* + *ameloblastoma*] a highly vascular ameloblastoma.

**he·man·gio·blast** (he-man′je-o-blast) [*hemangio-* + *-blast*] a mesodermal cell which gives rise to both vascular endothelium and hemocytoblasts.

**he·man·gio·blas·to·ma** (he-man″je-o-blas-to′mə) [*hem-* + *angioblast* + *-oma*] [MeSH: Hemangioblastoma] a benign blood vessel tumor of the cerebellum, spinal cord, or retina, consisting of proliferated blood vessel cells and angioblasts. Called also *angioblastoma* and *Lindau's tumor.*
**cerebellar h.,** hemangioblastoma of the cerebellum, often cystic; an autosomal dominant form is associated with von Hippel-Lindau disease.
**retinal h.,** von Hippel's disease.
**spinal h.,** a hemangioblastoma of the spinal cord, usually small and encapsulated and in an intramedullary location.

**he·man·gio·blas·to·ma·to·sis** (he-man″je-o-blas″to-mə-to′sis) multiple or widespread hemangioblastomas.

**he·man·gio·en·do·the·lio·blas·to·ma** (he-man″je-o-en″do-the″le-o-blas-to′mə) [*hemangioendothelioma* + *blastoma*] a hemangioendothelioma with embryonic elements of mesenchymal origin.

**he·man·gio·en·do·the·lio·ma** (he-man″je-o-en″do-the″le-o′mə) [*hemangioma* + *endothelioma*] [MeSH: Hemangioendothelioma] a true neoplasm of vascular origin, characterized by proliferation of endothelial cells in and about the vascular lumen; it is usually considered to be intermediate in grade between hemangioma and hemangiosarcoma but sometimes is used to denote the latter.
**benign h.,** a benign neoplasm of blood-vessel endothelium; the term is usually used to denote an infantile hemangioendothelioma.
**epithelioid h.,** a rare vascular neoplasm occurring in the medium to large veins of the distal extremities of adults, particularly young males; it may be benign or malignant and is characterized by proliferation of epithelioid or histiocytoid endothelial cells lining dilated vascular channels.
**infantile h.,** a rare, benign tumor of the liver in infants, generally multicentric, composed of anastomosing vascular channels lined with thick endothelial cells; it may be associated with disseminated hemangiomatosis, and death often occurs as the result of congestive heart failure.
**malignant h.,** hemangiosarcoma.
**vertebral h.,** a benign vascular tumor of the spine, seen primarily in middle-aged adults; usually asymptomatic, but in time it may expand or hemorrhage and compress the spinal canal and cord.

**he·man·gio·en·do·the·lio·sar·co·ma** (he-man″je-o-en″do-the″le-o-sahr-ko′mə) hemangiosarcoma.

**he·man·gio·fi·bro·ma** (he-man″je-o-fi-bro′mə) [*hemangio-* + *fibroma*] a hemangioma containing fibrous tissue.

**he·man·gi·o·ma** (he-man″je-o′mə) [*hem-* + *angioma*] [MeSH: Hemangioma] 1. an extremely common benign tumor, occurring most commonly in infancy and childhood, made up of newly formed blood vessels, and resulting from malformation of angioblastic tissue of fetal life. There are two main types: capillary and cavernous. 2. a general term denoting a benign or malignant vascular tumor that resembles the classic type of hemangioma but occurs at any age. Cf. *angioma* and *lymphangioma.*
**ameloblastic h.,** hemangioameloblastoma.
**capillary h.,** 1. the most common type of hemangioma; most are composed of closely packed aggregations of capillaries separated by scant connective stroma, which for the most part conform to the caliber of normal capillaries. According to one classification, *strawberry h., nevus flammeus, cherry angioma, and pyogenic granuloma* are all types of capillary hemangiomas. Cf. *cavernous h.* and *vascular nevus.* 2. strawberry h.
**cavernous h.,** a vascular tumor preponderantly composed of large dilated blood vessels, often containing large amounts of blood, occurring in the skin, subcutaneously, or both, and also in many viscera, particularly the liver, spleen, pancreas, and sometimes the brain. Most present in early life but are usually not present at birth. The typical superficial lesions are bright to dark red in color; deep lesions have a blue color. Called also *angioma cavernosum* and *strawberry mark* or *nevus.* See also *vascular nevus,* under *nevus.* Cf. *capillary h.*
**sclerosing h.,** a form of benign fibrous histiocytoma characterized not only by histiocytic and fibroblastic elements but also by numerous blood vessels and hemosiderin deposits. It is sometimes considered synonymous with or a variant of dermatofibroma.
**h. sim′plex,** strawberry h.
**strawberry h.,** 1. a firm red, dome-shaped hemangioma sharply demarcated from surrounding skin, usually on the head and neck, which grows rapidly and generally undergoes regression and involution without scarring. It is caused by proliferation of immature capillary vessels in active stroma, and is usually present at birth or within the first 2 or 3 months of life. See also *capillary h.* and *vascular nevus.* Called also *h. simplex, strawberry mark,* and *strawberry nevus.* 2. vascular nevus.
**venous h.,** a type of cavernous hemangioma in which the dilated vessels have thick, fibrous walls.

**he·man·gio·ma·to·sis** (he-man″je-o-mə-to′sis) a condition in which multiple hemangiomas are developed.

**he·man·gio·peri·cyte** (he-man″je-o-per′ĭ-sīt) pericyte.

**he·man·gio·peri·cy·to·ma** (he-man″je-o-per″ĭ-si-to′mə) [*hemangiopericyte* + *-oma*] [MeSH: Hemangiopericytoma] a tumor composed of spindle cells with a rich vascular network, which apparently arises from pericytes. It may be benign or malignant and usually occurs in the lower extremities or retroperitoneum.
**h. of kidney,** juxtaglomerular cell tumor.

**he·man·gio·sar·co·ma** (he-man″je-o-sahr-ko′mə) [*hemangio-* + *sarcoma*] [MeSH: Hemangiosarcoma] a rare malignant tumor of vascular origin, formed by proliferation of endothelial tissue lining irregular vascular channels; it usually occurs in the skin, soft tissues, breast, or liver. Called also *angiosarcoma* and *malignant hemangioendothelioma.* See also *lymphangiosarcoma.*

**he·ma·phe·ic** (he″mə-fe′ik) pertaining to or characterized by hemaphein.

**he·ma·phe·in** (he′mə-fēn″) [*hema-* + Gr. *phaios* dusky, gray] a brown coloring matter of the blood and urine.

**he·ma·phe·ism** (he″mə-fe′iz-əm) the presence of hemaphein in the urine.

**he·ma·phe·re·sis** (he″mə-fə-re′sis) [*hem-* + *apheresis*] apheresis.

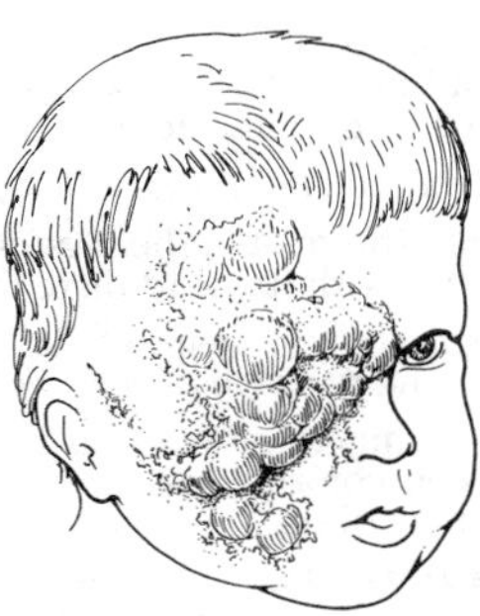

Cavernous hemangioma.

**he·ma·poi·e·sis** (he″mə-poi-e′sis) [*hema-* + *-poiesis*] hematopoiesis.

**he·ma·poi·et·ic** (he″mə-poi-et′ik) hematopoietic.

**he·ma·poph·y·sis** (he″mə-pof′ə-sis) [*hem-* + *apophysis*] a costal cartilage regarded as an apophysis of the hemal spine.

**he·mar·thros** (he-mahr′thros) hemarthrosis.

**he·mar·thro·sis** (he″mahr-thro′sis) [*hem-* + *arthrosis*] [MeSH: Hemarthrosis] extravasation of blood into a joint or its synovial cavity.

**he·ma·stron·ti·um** (he″mə-stron′she-əm) a tissue stain prepared by adding strontium chloride to a solution of hematein and aluminum chloride in alcohol and citric acid.

**he·ma·tal** (he′mə-təl) hemic.

**he·mat·apos·te·ma** (he″mat-ap″os-te′mə) [*hemat-* + Gr. *apostēma* abscess] an abscess containing effused blood.

**he·ma·te·in** (he′mə-tēn) [NF] a brownish-red, crystalline substance derived from hematoxylin by oxidation; used as an indicator and stain.

**he·ma·tem·e·sis** (he″mə-tem′ə-sis) [*hemat-* + *emesis*] [MeSH: Hematemesis] the vomiting of blood.
**Goldstein's h.,** hematemesis due to bleeding telangiectases in the stomach.

**he·mat·en·ceph·a·lon** (he″mat-, hem″at-en-sef′ə-lon) [*hemat-* + *encephalon*] cerebral hemorrhage.

**he·ma·ther·a·py** (he″mə-ther′ə-pe) hemotherapy.

**he·ma·ther·mal** (he″mə-thər′məl) homeothermic.

**he·ma·ther·mous** (he″mə-thər′məs) homeothermic.

**he·ma·tho·rax** (he″mə-thor′aks) hemothorax.

**he·mat·ic** (he-mat′ik) 1. hemic. 2. hematinic.

**he·ma·tid·ro·sis** (he″mə-, hem″ə-tid-ro′sis) [*hemat-* + Gr. *hidrōsis* sweating] the excretion of bloody sweat. Called also *hematohidrosis*.

**he·ma·tim·e·ter** (he″mə-, hem″ə-tim′ə-tər) hemacytometer.

**he·ma·tin** (he′mə-tin) 1. a porphyrin chelate of iron (III) formed by the oxidation of free heme; the hydroxide of heme. It stimulates the synthesis of globin and inhibits the synthesis of porphyrin by inactivation of 5-aminolevulinate synthase and is a component of the cytochromes and peroxidases. Hematin derived synthetically from hemin is used as a reagent. 2. hemin (def. 1).

**he·ma·tin·emia** (he″mə-, hem″ə-tĭ-ne′me-ə) the presence of hematin (heme) in the blood.

**he·ma·tin·ic** (he″mə-tin′ik) 1. pertaining to hematin. 2. an agent that increases the hemoglobin level and the number of erythrocytes in the blood.

**he·ma·tin·om·e·ter** (he″mə-, hem″ə-tin-om′ə-tər) old term for *hemoglobinometer*.

**he·ma·tin·uria** (he″mə-tĭ-nu′re-ə) the presence of hematin (heme) in the urine.

**he·ma·tite** (he′mə-tīt) a mineral made up of ferric oxide with a small amount of silica; inhalation of its dust can cause hematite pneumoconiosis.

**hemat(o)-** [Gr. *haima,* gen. *haimatos* blood] a combining form denoting relationship to the blood. Also, *haemat(o)-*.

**he·ma·to·bil·ia** (he″mə-to-, hem″ə-to-bil′e-ah) hemobilia.

**he·ma·to·blast** (he′mə-to-, he-mat′o-blast″) blast cell (def. 2).

**he·ma·to·cele** (he′mə-to-, hem′ə-to-sēl″) [*hemato-* + *-cele*[1]] [MeSH: Hematocele] an effusion of blood into a cavity, such as into the tunica vaginalis testis.
**parametric h., pelvic h.,** swelling caused by effusion of blood into Douglas' pouch.
**retrouterine h.,** parametric h.
**scrotal h.,** effusion of blood into the tissues of the scrotum.
**vaginal h.,** effusion of blood into the tunica vaginalis testis.

**he·ma·to·ce·lia** (he″mə-to-, hem″ə-to-se′le-ə) hematocoelia.

**he·ma·to·ceph·a·lus** (he″mə-to-, hem″ə-to-sef′ə-ləs) [*hemato-* + *-cephalus*] a fetus born with its head distended with blood.

**he·ma·to·che·zia** (he″mə-to-, hem″ə-to-ke′ze-ə) [*hemato-* + Gr. *chezein* to defecate] the passage of bloody feces.

**he·ma·to·chlo·rin** (he″mə-to-, hem″ə-to-klo′rin) [*hemato-* + Gr. *chlōros* green] a green coloring matter occurring in the placenta and derived from hemoglobin.

**he·ma·to·chro·ma·to·sis** (he″mə-to-, hem″ə-to-kro″mə-to′sis) [*hemato-* + *chromato-* + *-sis*] 1. staining of tissues with blood pigment. 2. hemochromatosis.

**he·ma·to·chy·lu·ria** (he″mə-to-, hem″ə-to-ki-lu′re-ə) [*hemato-* + *chyluria*] the discharge of blood and chyle with the urine, a symptom of *Wuchereria bancrofti* infection.

**he·ma·to·coe·lia** (he″mə-to-, hem″ə-to-se′le-ə) [*hemato-* + *coel-* + *-ia*] effusion of blood into the peritoneal cavity.

**he·ma·to·col·po·me·tra** (he″mə-to-, hem″ə-to-kol″po-me′trə) [*hemato-* + *colpo-* + *metra*] accumulation of menstrual blood in the vagina and uterus.

**he·ma·to·col·pos** (he″mə-to-, hem″ə-to-kol′pəs) [*hemato-* + Gr. *kolpos* vagina] [MeSH: Hematocolpos] an accumulation of menstrual blood in the vagina.

**he·mat·o·crit (Hct)** (he-mat′ə-krit) [*hemato-* + Gr. *krinein* to separate] [MeSH: Hematocrit] 1. the proportion of the volume of a blood sample that is red blood cells (packed red blood cells), measured in mL per dL of whole blood or as a per cent. 2. former name for a tube or other apparatus used in making this calculation, such as the Wintrobe hematocrit tube.
**large vessel h.,** the hematocrit of blood from a large vessel, usually a vein; cf. *total body h.*
**total body h., whole body h.,** the average hematocrit of the whole body, as determined by tracer dilution methods; it is normally about 0.92 times the large vessel hematocrit.

**he·ma·toc·ry·al** (he″mə-, hem″ə-tok′re-əl) [*hemato-* + *cryo-* + *-al*[1]] poikilothermic.

**he·ma·to·cy·a·nin** (he″mə-to-, hem″ə-to-si′ə-nin) [*hemato-* + Gr. *kyanos* blue] hemocyanin.

**he·ma·to·cyst** (he′mə-to-, he-mat′o-sist″) [*hemato-* + *cyst*] an effusion of blood into the bladder or into a cyst.

**he·ma·to·cys·tis** (he″mə-to-, hem″ə-to-sis′tis) hematocyst.

**he·ma·to·cyte** (he′mə-to-, he-mat′o-sīt″) blood cell.

**he·ma·to·cy·to·blast** (he″mə-to-, hem″ə-to-si′to-blast) blast cell (def. 2).

**he·ma·to·cy·tol·y·sis** (he″mə-to-, hem″ə-to-si-tol′ĭ-sis) hemolysis.

**he·ma·to·cy·tom·e·ter** (he″mə-to-, hem″ə-to-si-tom′ə-tər) hemacytometer.

**he·ma·to·cy·to·pe·nia** (he″mə-to-, hem″ə-to-si″to-pe′ne-ə) [*hematocyte* + *-penia*] cytopenia.

**he·ma·to·cy·tu·ria** (he″mə-to-, hem″ə-to-si-tu′re-ə) [*hematocyte* + *-uria*] the presence of red blood cells in the urine.

**he·ma·to·di·al·y·sis** (he″mə-to-, hem″ə-to-di-al′ə-sis) hemodialysis.

**he·ma·to·en·ce·phal·ic** (he″mə-to-, hem″ə-to-en″sə-fal′ik) [*hemato-* + *encephalic*] pertaining to the blood and the brain.

**he·ma·to·gen·e·sis** (he″mə-to-, hem″ə-to-jen′ə-sis) [*hemato-* + *genesis*] hematopoiesis.

**he·ma·to·gen·ic** (he″mə-to-, he-mat″o-jen′ik) 1. hematopoietic. 2. hematogenous.

**he·ma·tog·e·nous** (he″mə-toj′ĕ-nus) 1. produced by or derived from the blood. 2. disseminated by the circulation or through the blood stream.

**he·ma·to·gone** (he′mə-to-, he-mat′o-gōn) old name for *blast cell* (def. 2).

**he·ma·to·hid·ro·sis** (he′mə-to-, hem″ə-to-hid-ro′sis) hematidrosis.

**he·ma·to·his·tio·blast** (he″mə-to-, hem″ə-to-his′te-o-blast) old name for *blast cell* (def. 2).

**he·ma·to·hy·a·loid** (he″mə-to-, hem″ə-to-hi′ə-loid) [*hemato-* + *hyaloid*] said of a thrombus that undergoes hyaline degeneration.

**he·ma·toid** (he′mə-toid) [*hemato-* + *-oid*] resembling blood.

**he·ma·toid·in** (he-mə-toid′in) a yellow-brown or red pigment, apparently chemically identical with bilirubin but with a different site of origin, formed locally in the tissues from hemoglobin, particularly under conditions of reduced oxygen tension.

**he·ma·to·kol·pos** (he″mə-to-, hem″ə-to-kol′pəs) hematocolpos.

**he·ma·tol·o·gist** (he″mə-tol′ə-jist) a specialist in hematology.

**he·ma·tol·o·gy** (he″mə-tol′ə-je) [*hemato-* + *-logy*] [MeSH: Hematology] that branch of medical science that deals with the blood and blood-forming tissues.

**he·ma·to·lymph·an·gi·o·ma** (he″mə-to-, hem″ə-to-lim″fan-je-o′mə) [*hemato-* + *lymph-* + *angioma*] a benign tumor composed of blood vessels and lymph vessels. Called also *hemolymphangioma*.

**he·ma·tol·y·sis** (he″mə-tol′ə-sis) hemolysis.

**he·ma·to·lyt·ic** (he″mə-to-lit′ik) hemolytic.

**he·ma·to·ma** (he″mə-to′mə) pl. *hemato′mas* [*hemato-* + *-oma*]

[MeSH: Hematoma]a localized collection of blood, usually clotted, in an organ, space, or tissue, due to a break in the wall of a blood vessel.
**aneurysmal h.**, false aneurysm.
**auricular h., h. au'ris,** hematoma of the perichondrium of the auricle, a common precursor of cauliflower ear.
**dissecting h.**, dissecting aneurysm.
**epidural h.**, accumulation of blood in the epidural space, due to damage to and leakage of blood from the middle meningeal artery, producing compression of the dura mater and thus compression of the brain. Unless evacuated, it may result in herniation through the tentorium, and death.
**parenchymatous h.**, a mass of blood within the brain tissue itself, usually from rupture of an artery or vein within the brain.
**pelvic h.**, a collection of blood in the pelvic soft tissue.
**perianal h.**, a hematoma under the perianal skin, caused by rupture of a subcutaneous vessel, the blood being kept localized by fibroelastic septa and causing much pain.
**pulsating h.**, pseudoaneurysm.
**retrouterine h.**, an effusion of blood into the retrouterine connective tissue.
**subdural h.**, accumulation of blood in the subdural space. In the severe *acute* form, both blood and cerebrospinal fluid enter the space as a result of laceration of the brain and a tear in the arachnoid, adding subdural compression to the direct injury to the brain. In the *chronic* form, only blood effuses into the subdural space as a result of rupture of the bridging veins, usually due to closed head injury. The effusion is a gradual process resulting, weeks after the injury, in headache and progressive focal signs that reflect the location of the mass.
**subungual h.**, an accumulation of blood under the nail plate.

**he•ma•to•ma•nom•e•ter** (he″mə-to-, hem″ə-to-mə-nom′ə-tər) sphygmomanometer.

**he•ma•to•me•di•as•ti•num** (he″mə-to-, hem″ə-to-me″de-əs-ti′nəm) [*hemato-* + *mediastinum*] hemomediastinum.

**he•ma•tom•e•ter** (he″mə-, hem″ə-tom′ə-tər) old term for *hemoglobinometer.*

**he•ma•to•me•tra** (he″mə-to-, hem″ə-to-me′trə) [*hemato-* + *metra*] [MeSH: Hematometra] an accumulation of blood in the uterus.

**he•ma•tom•e•try** (he″mə-tom′ə-tre) [*hemato-* + *-metry*] measurement of various parameters of the blood, such as the complete blood count (see under *count*).

**he•ma•to•my•e•lia** (he″mə-to-, hem″ə-to-mi-e′le-ə) [*hemato-* + *myel-* + *-ia*] hemorrhage into the spinal cord, usually confined to the gray substance, most often due to trauma but also seen in arteriovenous malformations; marked by the sudden onset of flaccid paralysis with sensory disturbances.

**he•ma•to•my•eli•tis** (he″mə-to-, hem″ə-to-mi″ə-li′tis) [*hemato-* + *myelitis*] acute myelitis with bloody effusion within the spinal cord.

**he•ma•to•my•elo•pore** (he″mə-to-, hem″ə-to-mi′əl-o-por″) [*hemato-* + *myelo-* + *pore*] a disease marked by the formation of canals in the spinal cord, due to hemorrhage.

**he•ma•to•ne•phro•sis** (he″mə-to-, hem″ə-to-nə-fro′sis) presence of blood in the pelvis of the kidney.

**he•ma•to•pa•thol•o•gy** (he″mə-to-, hem″ə-to-pə-thol′ə-je) hemopathology.

**he•ma•to•pe•nia** (he″mə-to-, hem″ə-to-pe′ne-ə) [*hemato-* + *-penia*] deficiency of blood; see also *anemia.*

**he•ma•to•peri•car•di•um** (he″mə-to-, hem″ə-to-per″ĭ-kahr′de-əm) hemopericardium.

**he•ma•to•peri•to•ne•um** (he″mə-to-, hem″ə-to-per″ĭ-to-ne′əm) hemoperitoneum.

**he•ma•to•phage** (he′mə-to-, he′mə-to-fāj) hemophagocyte.

**he•ma•to•pha•gia** (he″mə-to-, hem″ə-to-fa′jə) 1. blood drinking. 2. subsisting on the blood of another animal.

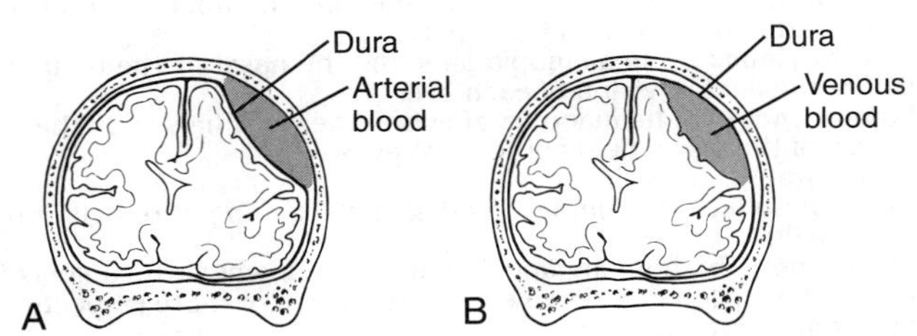


*(A),* Epidural hematoma, the dura separated from the skull; *(B),* subdural hematoma, the dura remaining attached to the skull.

**he•ma•to•phago•cyte** (he″mə-to-, hem″ə-to-fag′o-sīt) hemophagocyte.

**he•ma•toph•a•gous** (he″mə-, hem″ə-tof′ə-gəs) [*hemato-* + *phag-* + *-ous*] characterized by hematophagia.

**he•ma•toph•a•gy** (he″mə-, hem″ə-tof′ə-je) hematophagia.

**he•ma•to•phil•ia** (he″mə-to-, hem″ə-to-fil′e-ə) hemophilia.

**he•ma•to•pho•bia** (he″mə-to-, hem″ə-to-fo′be-ə) hemophobia.

**he•ma•to•plas•tic** (he″mə-to-, hem″ə-to-plas′tik) [*hemato-* + *plastic*] hematopoietic.

**he•ma•to•poi•e•sis** (he″mə-to-, hem″ə-to-poi-e′sis) [*hemato-* + *-poiesis*] [MeSH: Hematopoiesis] the formation and development of blood cells. In the embryo and fetus it takes place in a variety of sites including the liver, spleen, thymus, lymph nodes, and bone marrow; from birth throughout the rest of life it is mainly in the bone marrow with a small amount occurring in lymph nodes. See also *erythropoiesis, leukopoiesis,* and *thrombocytopoiesis.* Called also *hematogenesis, hemogenesis,* and *hemopoiesis.*
**cyclic h.**, see under *neutropenia.*
**extramedullary h.**, the formation and development of blood cells outside the bone marrow, as in the spleen, liver, and lymph nodes.

**he•ma•to•poi•et•ic** (he″mə-to-, hem″ə-to-poi-et′ik) 1. pertaining to or effecting hematopoiesis; called also *hemapoietic, hematogenic, hematoplastic, hemogenic,* and *hemopoietic.* 2. an agent that promotes hematopoiesis.

**he•ma•to•poi•e•tin** (he″mə-to-, hem″ə-to-poi′ə-tin) erythropoietin.

**he•ma•to•por•phy•rin** (he″mə-to-, hem″ə-to-por′fə-rin) a dark red to purple pigment, a porphyrin (q.v.) in which two pyrrole rings have one methyl and one propionate side chain and the other two pyrrole rings have one methyl and one 1-hydroxyethyl side chain.

**he•ma•to•por•phy•rin•emia** (he″mə-to-, hem″ə-to-por″fĭ-rin-e′me-ə) the presence of hematoporphyrin in the blood.

**he•ma•to•por•phy•rin•ism** (he″mə-to-, hem″ə-to-por′fĭ-rin-iz″əm) a state characterized by hematoporphyrinemia and a sensitivity to sunlight.

**he•ma•to•por•phy•rin•uria** (he″mə-to-, hem″ə-to-por″fĭ-rin-u′re-ə) the occurrence of hematoporphyrin in the urine.

**He•ma•top•o•ta** (he″mə-, hem″ə-top′o-tə) *Haematopota.*

**he•ma•tor•rha•chis** (he″mə-to-, hem″ə-tor′ə-kis) [*hemato-* + Gr. *rhachis* spine] hematomyelia.

**he•ma•to•sal•pinx** (he″mə-to-, hem″ə-to-sal′pinks) an accumulation of blood in the uterine tube.

**he•ma•tos•cheo•cele** (he″mə-, hem″ə-tos′ke-o-sēl″) [*hemato-* + *oscheo-* + *-cele*[1]] a collection of blood within the scrotum.

**he•ma•to•sep•sis** (he″mə-to-, hem″ə-to-sep′sis) septicemia.

**he•ma•to•spec•tro•scope** (he″mə-to-, hem″ə-to-spek′tro-skōp) [*hemato-* + *spectroscope*] a spectroscope for examining thin layers of blood.

**he•ma•to•spec•tros•co•py** (he″mə-to-, hem″ə-to-spek-tros′ko-pe) [*hemato-* + *spectroscopy*] spectroscopic examination of the blood.

**he•ma•to•sper•mato•cele** (he″mə-to-, hem″ə-to-spər-mat′o-sēl) [*hemato-* + *spermato-* + *-cele*[1]] a spermatocele containing blood.

**he•ma•to•sper•mia** (he″mə-to-, hem″ə-to-spər′me-ə) hemospermia.

**he•ma•to•stat•ic** (he″mə-to-, hem″ə-to-stat′ik) [*hemato-* + *-static*] hemostatic (def. 3).

**he•ma•tos•te•on** (he″mə-, hem″ə-tos′te-on) [*hemat-* + *osteon*] hemorrhage into the medullary cavity of a bone.

**he•ma•to•ther•a•py** (he″mə-to-, hem″ə-to-ther′ə-pe) hemotherapy.

**he•ma•to•ther•mal** (he″mə-to-, hem″ə-to-thər′məl) [*hemato-* + *thermal*] homeothermic.

**he•ma•to•tho•rax** (he″mə-to-, hem″ə-to-thor′aks) hemothorax.

**he•ma•to•tox•ic** (he″mə-to-, hem″ə-to-tok′sik) [*hemato-* + *toxic*] 1. pertaining to hematotoxicosis. 2. poisonous to the blood and hematopoietic system.

**he•ma•to•tox•i•co•sis** (he″mə-to-, hem″ə-to-tok″sĭ-ko′sis) toxic damage to the hematopoietic system.

**he•ma•to•tra•che•los** (he″mə-to-, hem″ə-to-trə-ke′ləs) [*hemato-* + Gr. *trachēlos* neck] distention of the cervix of the uterus with blood, owing to atresia of the external os or of the vagina.

**he•ma•to•trop•ic** (he″mə-to-, hem″ə-to-trop′ik) [*hemato-* + *-tropic*] having a special affinity for or exerting a specific effect on the blood or blood cells.

**he•ma•to•tym•pa•num** (he″mə-to-, hem″ə-to-tim′pə-nəm) [*hemato-* + *tympanum*] hemotympanum.

**he·ma·tox·ic** (he″mə-tok′sik) hematotoxic.

**he·ma·tox·y·lin** (he″mə-tok′sĭ-lin) [MeSH: Hematoxylin] a colorless crystalline compound obtained by extracting logwood *(Haematoxylon campechianum)* with ether. It may be used as an indicator with a pH range of 5–6, but is mainly used in oxidized form as a stain in microscopy. See also under *stain.*
**alum h.,** hemalum.
**Delafield's h.,** see under *stain.*
**iron h.,** see *iron hematoxylin method, Heidenhain's iron hematoxylin stain,* and *Weigert's iron hematoxylin stain,* all under *stain.*

**He·ma·tox·y·lon** (he″mə-tok′sĭ-lən) *Haematoxylon.*

**he·ma·to·ze·mia** (he″mə-to-, hem″ə-to-ze′me-ə) [*hemato-* + Gr. *zēmia* loss] a gradual loss of blood.

**he·ma·to·zoa** (he″mə-to-, hem″ə-to-zo′ə) plural of *hematozoon.*

**he·ma·to·zo·al** (he″mə-to-, he″mə-to-zo′əl) hematozoan, def. 1.

**he·ma·to·zo·an** (he″mə-to-, hem″ə-to-zo′ən) [*hemato-* + Gr. *zōon* animal] 1. pertaining to or caused by animal parasites living in the host's blood. Called also *hematozoal, hematozoic,* and *hemozoic.* 2. any animal parasite living in the host's blood. Called also *hematozoon* and *hemozoon.*

**he·ma·to·zo·ic** (he″mə-to-, hem″ə-to-zo′ik) hematozoan, def. 1.

**he·ma·to·zo·on** (he″mə-to-, hem″ə-to-zo′ən) pl. *hematozo′a..* Hematozoan, def. 2.

**he·ma·tu·re·sis** (he″mə-, hem″ə-tu-re′sis) hematuria.

**he·ma·tu·ria** (he″mə-, hem″ə-tu′re-ə) [*hemat-* + *-uria*] [MeSH: Hematuria] blood in the urine.
**benign familial h.,** thin basement membrane nephropathy.
**benign recurrent h.,** hematuria that does not progress to renal insufficiency, such as that seen with IgA nephropathy.
**endemic h.,** urinary schistosomiasis.
**enzootic bovine h.,** a disease of cattle marked by passing of blood in the urine, anemia, and debilitation; it is usually due to bracken poisoning.
**essential h.,** hematuria for which no cause has been determined; called also *primary h.* and *functional h.*
**false h.,** redness of the urine due to food or drugs containing pigment.
**functional h.,** essential h.
**gross h.,** redness of the urine due to blood in the urine; called also *macroscopic h.*
**macroscopic h.,** gross h.
**microscopic h.,** blood in the urine visible only with a microscope, defined as at least two or three red blood cells per high power field.
**persistent h.,** hematuria present in every specimen.
**primary h.,** essential h.
**renal h.,** hematuria in which the blood comes from the kidney.
**urethral h.,** hematuria in which the blood comes from the urethra.
**vesical h.,** hematuria in which the blood comes from the bladder.

**heme** (hēm) [MeSH: Heme] 1. any quadridentate chelate of iron with the four pyrrole groups of a porphyrin, further distinguished as ferroheme or ferriheme referring to the chelates of Fe(II) and Fe(III) respectively. The four porphyrin ligands form a square-planar complex; the fifth and sixth coordination positions of the iron atom are perpendicular to the plane of the porphyrin and both may be occupied by strong field ligands, such as a nitrogen atom of a histidine residue of a protein, as in cytochromes, or only one may be so occupied, as in hemoglobin where the sixth position reversibly binds oxygen. 2. ferroheme, the Fe(II) chelate; see also *hematin.* 3. protoheme IX, the heme of hemoglobin. See *protoheme.*

**hem·en·do·the·li·o·ma** (hēm″en-do-the″le-o′mə) hemangioendothelioma.

**heme oxy·gen·ase (de·cy·cliz·ing)** (hēm ok′sĭ-jən-ās de-si′kli-zing) [EC 1.14.99.3] an enzyme of the oxidoreductase class that catalyzes the cleavage of heme to form biliverdin, a step in heme catabolism.

**hem·er·al·ope** (hem′ər-əl-ōp) a person affected with hemeralopia.

**hem·er·a·lo·pia** (hem″ər-ə-lo′pe-ə) [Gr. *hēmera* day + *alaos* blind + *-opia*] day blindness; defective vision in a bright light.

**Hem·ero·cam·pa** (hem″ər-o-kam′pə) a genus of moths. *H. leukostig′ma* is the tussock moth, a species with white markings whose larval stage has venomous hairs that may produce severe urticaria. See also *insect dermatitis,* under *dermatitis.*

**hem·eryth·rin** (hēm″ə-rith′rin) [*hem-* + Gr. *erythros* red] [MeSH: Hemerythrin] the coloring matter of the blood of earthworms which is contained in the plasma.

**heme syn·thase** (hēm sin′thās) ferrochelatase.

**hemi-** [Gr. *hēmi-* half] a prefix meaning one half.

**hemi·acar·di·us** (hem″e-ə-kahr′de-əs) [*hemi-* + *acardius*] one of twin fetuses in which only a part of the circulation is accomplished by its own heart.

**hemi·aceph·a·lus** (hem″e-ə-sef′ə-ləs) [*hemi-* + *acephalus*] a fetus whose head lacks part of the brain and calvaria.

**hemi·ac·e·tal** (hem″e-as′ə-tal) a derivative formed by a combination of an aldehyde with an alcohol.

**hemi·achro·ma·top·sia** (hem″e-ə-kro″mə-top′se-ə) [*hemi-* + *achromatopsia*] color blindness in one half, or in corresponding halves, of the visual field.

**hemi·ac·i·drin** (hem″e-as′ĭ-drin) a solution containing citric and gluconic acids, magnesium hydroxycarbonate, magnesium acid citrate, and calcium carbonate; it is capable of dissolving struvite calculi.

**hemi·ageu·sia** (hem″e-ə-goo′zhə) [*hemi-* + *ageusia*] ageusia on one side of the tongue; called also *hemiageustia* and *hemigeusia.*

**hemi·ageus·tia** (hem″e-ə-gōōs′te-ə) hemiageusia.

**hemi·al·bu·min** (hem″e-al-bu′min) [*hemi-* + *albumin*] hemialbumose.

**hemi·al·bu·mose** (hem″e-al-bu′mōs) a crystallizable product of the digestion of certain proteins; normally found in bone marrow, and occurring in the urine of osteomalacia and diphtheria.

**hemi·al·bu·mos·uria** (hem″e-al-bu″mo-su′re-ə) the presence of hemialbumose in the urine.

**hemi·al·gia** (hem″e-al′jə) [*hemi-* + *-algia*] pain affecting one side of the body only.

**hemi·am·bly·o·pia** (hem″e-am″ble-o′pe-ə) hemianopia.

**hemi·amy·os·the·nia** (hem″e-ə-mi″os-the′ne-ə) [*hemi-* + *a-*[1] + *myo-* + *sthen-* + *-ia*] lack of muscular power on one side of the body.

**hemi·an·acu·sia** (hem″e-an″ə-koo′ze-ə) [*hemi-* + *an-*[1] + *acou-* + *-ia*] loss of hearing in one ear only.

**hemi·an·al·ge·sia** (hem″e-an″əl-je′ze-ə) [*hemi-* + *analgesia*] analgesia of one side of the body.

**hemi·an·en·ceph·a·ly** (hem″e-an″ən-sef′ə-le) [*hemi-* + *anencephaly*] congenital absence of one side of the brain.

**hemi·an·es·the·sia** (hem′e-an″əs-the′zhə) anesthesia affecting only one side of the body; called also *unilateral anesthesia.*
**alternate h.,** h. cruciata.
**cerebral h.,** that which is due to lesion of the internal capsule of the lenticular nucleus.
**crossed h.,** h. cruciata.
**h. crucia′ta,** loss of sensation on one side of the face with contralateral loss of pain and temperature sense on the body, resulting from a lateral lesion in the pons or medulla, affecting both the sensory root of the trigeminal nerve and the spinothalamic tract.
**mesocephalic h., pontile h.,** that which is due to disease of the pons.
**spinal h.,** that which is due to a lesion of the spinal cord.

**hemi·an·o·pia** (hem″e-ə-no′peə) [*hemi-* + *an-*[1] + *-opia*] defective vision or blindness in half of the visual field of one or both eyes; loosely, scotoma in less than half of the visual field of one or both eyes.
**absolute h.,** blindness to light, color, and form, in half of the visual field.
**altitudinal h.,** hemianopia in the upper or lower half of the visual field.
**bilateral h.,** hemianopia affecting both eyes.
**binasal h.,** heteronymous hemianopia in which the defects are in the nasal half of the field of vision in each eye.
**binocular h.,** bilateral h.
**bitemporal h.,** heteronymous hemianopia in which the defects are in the temporal half of the field of vision in each eye.
**complete h.,** hemianopia affecting an entire half of the visual field of each eye.
**congruous h.,** homonymous hemianopia in which the defects in the field of vision in each eye are symmetrical in position, shape, size, and degree.
**crossed h.,** altitudinal hemianopia affecting the upper field of one eye and the lower field of the other.
**heteronymous h.,** hemianopia affecting the nasal or the temporal half of the field of vision of each eye.
**homonymous h.,** hemianopia affecting the right halves or the left halves of the visual fields of the two eyes.
**horizontal h.,** altitudinal h.
**incomplete h.,** hemianopia affecting less than an entire half of the visual field.
**incongruous h.,** homonymous hemianopia in which the defects in the field of vision in the two eyes differ in one or more respects, as in extent or intensity.
**lateral h.,** homonymous h.

**nasal h.**, hemianopia in the nasal halves of the visual fields.
**quadrant h., quadrantic h.**, quadrantanopia.
**relative h.**, defective vision of or blindness to form or color in half of the visual field, the perception of light being retained.
**temporal h.**, hemianopia in the temporal halves of the visual fields.
**unilateral h.**, hemianopia in one eye only.

**hemi·an·op·ic** (hem″e-ə-nop′ik) pertaining to or characterized by hemianopia.

**hemi·an·op·sia** (hem″e-ən-op′se-ə) [MeSH: Hemianopsia] hemianopia.

**hemi·an·op·tic** (hem″e-ən-op′tik) hemianopic.

**hemi·an·os·mia** (hem″e-ən-oz′me-ə) [*hemi-* + *anosmia*] anosmia in one of the nostrils.

**hemi·aprax·ia** (hem″e-ə-prak′se-ə) [*hemi-* + *apraxia*] apraxia affecting one side of the body only.

**hemi·ar·thro·sis** (hem″e-ahr-thro′sis) [*hemi-* + *arthrosis*] a spurious synchondrosis.

**hemi·aso·ma·tog·no·sia** (hem″e-ə-so″mə-tog-no′zhə) defective or lack of awareness of the condition of one side of one's body.

**hemi·asyn·er·gia** (hem″e-as″ə-nər′jə) [*hemi-* + *asynergia*] asynergia affecting one side of the body only.

**hemi·atax·ia** (hem″e-ə-tak′se-ə) [*hemi-* + *ataxia*] ataxia affecting one side of the body only.

**hemi·ataxy** (hem″e-ə-tak′se) hemiataxia.

**hemi·ath·e·to·sis** (hem″e-ath″ə-to′sis) [*hemi-* + *athetosis*] athetosis affecting one side of the body only.

**hemi·at·ro·phy** (hem″e-at′ro-fe) [*hemi-* + *atrophy*] atrophy of one side of the body or of one half of an organ or part.
**facial h.**, progressive atrophy, of unknown etiology, of the tissues of one side of the face, frequently accompanied by pigmentation disorders and alopecia, jacksonian epilepsy, and trigeminal neuralgia; both sides of the face are occasionally affected and the ipsilateral trunk, viscera, and extremities are sometimes involved. Called also *hemifacial atrophy, Romberg's disease* or *trophoneurosis, facial trophoneurosis,* and *Parry-Romberg syndrome.*
**progressive lingual h.**, progressive atrophy of one lateral half of the tongue.

**hemi·ax·i·al** (hem″e-ak′se-əl) at any oblique angle to the long axis of the body or a part.

**hemi·bal·lism** (hem″e-bal′iz-əm) hemiballismus.

**hemi·bal·lis·mus** (hem″e-bə-liz′məs) [*hemi-* + *ballismus*] a violent form of dyskinesia involving only one side of the body and being most marked in the upper extremity, resulting from a destructive lesion of the nucleus subthalamicus (Luys' body). Cf. *hemichorea.* Called also *body of Luys syndrome.*

**hemi·blad·der** (hem′e-blad″ər) a half bladder; a developmental anomaly in which the bladder is formed as two physically separated parts, each with its own ureter.

**hemi·block** (hem′e-blok) failure in conduction of the cardiac impulse in either of the two main divisions of the left ventricular conducting system (bundle of His); it is called *left anterior hemiblock* when the anterior-superior division is interrupted and *left posterior hemiblock* when the posterior division is interrupted.

**he·mic** (he′mik, hem′ik) [Gr. *haima* blood] pertaining to the blood; called also *hemal, hematal, hematic,* and *sanguineous.*

**hemi·ca·nit·i·es** (hem″e-kə-nish′e-ēz) grayness of the hair on one side of the body.

**hemi·car·dia** (hem″e-kahr′de-ə) [*hemi-* + *cardia*] 1. a congenital anomaly characterized by the presence of only half of a four-chambered heart. 2. either lateral half of a normal heart.

**hemi·car·di·us** (hem″e-kahr′de-əs) a free twin fetus whose development is greatly reduced but whose body form and various parts are still recognizable.

**hemi·cel·lu·lose** (hem″e-sel′u-lōs) a general name for a group of high molecular weight polysaccharides, found in plant cell walls, similar to cellulose but smaller, alkali-soluble, and composed of various sugars, including aldopentoses, aldohexoses, and uronic acids; the most ubiquitous are the xylans.

**hemi·cen·trum** (hem″e-sen′trəm) [*hemi-* + *centrum*] either lateral half of a vertebral centrum.

**hemi·ce·pha·lia** (hem″e-sə-fa′le-ə) [*hemi-* + *cephal-* + *-ia*] congenital absence of the cerebrum.

**hemi·ceph·a·lus** (hem″e-sef′ə-ləs) a fetus exhibiting hemicephalia.

**hemi·cer·e·brum** (hem″e-ser′ə-brəm) [*hemi-* + *cerebrum*] a cerebral hemisphere.

**hemi·cho·rea** (hem″e-kə-re′ə) [*hemi-* + *chorea*] chorea which affects only one side; called also *chorea dimidiata* and *hemilateral chorea.* Cf. *hemiballismus.*

**hemi·chro·ma·top·sia** (hem″e-kro″mə-top′se-ə) hemiachromatopsia.

**he·mi·chrome** (he′mĭ-krōm) an oxidized derivative of methemoglobin in which a functional group of globin has replaced the normal water substituent of the heme; it precipitates readily, aggregating to form Heinz bodies and ultimately causing cell lysis.

**hemi·co·lec·to·my** (hem″ĭ-ko-lek′tə-me) [*hemi-* + *colectomy*] excision of approximately half of the colon.
**left h.**, surgical removal of the left colon.
**right h.**, surgical removal of the right colon.

**hemi·cor·por·ec·to·my** (hem″e-kor-por-ek′ tə-me) [*hemi-* + *corpus* + *-ectomy*] surgical removal of the lower part of the body through the lumbar region, including the bony pelvis, legs, genitalia, and pelvic contents such as the anus and lower rectum.

**hemi·cor·ti·cec·to·my** (hem″ĭ-kor″tĭ-sek′tə-me) excision of a cerebral hemisphere leaving the basal ganglia intact; done in intractable epilepsy.

**hemi·cra·nia** (hem″e-kra′ne-ə) [*hemi-* + Gr. *kranion* skull] 1. pain or aching in one side of the head. 2. incomplete anencephaly or meroanencephaly.
**chronic paroxysmal h.**, a type of one-sided headache resembling a cluster headache but occurring in paroxysms of half an hour or less, several times a day, sometimes daily for years.

**hemi·cra·ni·ec·to·my** (hem″ĭ-kra″ne-ek′tə-me) [*hemi-* + *craniectomy*] exposure of half of the brain by sectioning the vault of the skull from front to back near the median line and forcing the entire side outward.

**hemi·cra·ni·o·sis** (hem″e-kra″ne-o′sis) a condition marked by hyperostosis on one half of the cranium or face, with cerebral involvement. The condition is believed to be due to endothelioma of the dura.

**hemi·cra·ni·ot·o·my** (hem″e-kra″ne-ot′ə-me) [*hemi-* + *craniotomy*] hemicraniectomy.

**hemi·de·cor·ti·ca·tion** (hem″e-de-kor″tĭ-ka′shən) removal of one half of the cerebral cortex.

**hemi·des·mo·some** (hem″e-des′mo-sōm) [*hemi-* + *desmosome*] a structure similar to a desmosome but representing only half of it, found on the basal surface of some epithelial cells, forming the site of attachment between the basal surface of the cell and the basement membrane. Called also *half desmosome.*

**hemi·dia·pho·re·sis** (hem″e-di″ə-for-e′sis) [*hemi-* + *diaphoresis*] hemihyperidrosis.

**hemi·dia·phragm** (hem″e-di′ə-fram) one half of the diaphragm.

**hem·idro·sis** (hem″i-dro′sis) hemihidrosis.

**hemi·dys·er·gia** (hem″e-dis-er′je-ə) dysergia affecting one side of the body.

**hemi·dys·es·the·sia** (hem″e-dis″əs-the′zhə) [*hemi-* + *dysesthesia*] a dysesthesia affecting one side of the body only.

**hemi·dys·tro·phy** (hem″e-dis′tro-fe) unequal development of the two sides of the body.

**hemi·ec·tro·me·lia** (hem″e-ek-tro-me′le-ə) a developmental anomaly characterized by imperfect development of the limbs of one side of the body.

**hemi·elas·tin** (hem″e-ə-las′tin) a substance formed by the digestion or hydrolysis of elastin.

**hemi·en·ceph·a·lus** (hem″e-ən-sef′ə-ləs) [*hemi-* + Gr. *enkephalos* brain] a fetus that lacks one cerebral hemisphere.

**hemi·epi·lep·sy** (hem″e-ep′ĭ-lep-se) [*hemi-* + *epilepsy*] epilepsy affecting one side of the body only.

**hemi·fa·cial** (hem″ĭ-fa′shəl) pertaining to or affecting one half of the face.

**hemi·gas·trec·to·my** (hem″ĭ-gas-trek′tə-me) excision of half of the stomach.

**hemi·geu·sia** (hem″e-goo′zhə) [*hemi-* + Gr. *geusis* taste + *-ia*] hemiageusia.

**hemi·gi·gan·tism** (hem″ĭ-ji′gən-tiz-əm) overgrowth of one side of the entire body or of a portion of one side, as of the face.

**hemi·glos·sal** (hem″ĭ-glos′əl) [*hemi-* + *glossal*] affecting one side of the tongue; hemilingual.

**hemi·glos·sec·to·my** (hem″ĭ-glos-ek′tə-me) [*hemi-* + *glossectomy*] resection of one side of the tongue.

**hemi·glos·si·tis** (hem″ĭ-glos-i′tis) [*hemi-* + *glossitis*] inflammation involving only one side of the tongue.

**hemi·gna·thia** (hem″ĭ-na′the-ə) [*hemi-* + *gnath-* + *-ia*] a developmental anomaly characterized by partial to complete absence of the lower jaw on one side.

**hemi·hep·a·tec·to·my** (hem″ĭ-hep″ə-tek′tə-me) excision of half of the liver.

**hemi·hi·dro·sis** (hem″e-hi-dro′sis) [*hemi-* + Gr. *hidrōs* sweat] sweating on one side of the body only. Called also *hemidrosis.*

**hemi·hy·pal·ge·sia** (hem″e-hi″pəl-je′ze-ə) [*hemi-* + *hypalgesia*] hypalgesia on one side of the body.

**hemi·hy·per·es·the·sia** (hem″e-hi″pər-əs-the′zhə) [*hemi-* + *hyperesthesia*] hyperesthesia on one side of the body.

**hemi·hy·per·idro·sis** (hem″e-hi″pər-i-dro′sis) [*hemi-* + Gr. *hyper* over + *hidrōs* sweat] excessive sweating on one side of the body only; called also *hemidiaphoresis.*

**hemi·hy·per·me·tria** (hem″e-hi″pər-me′tre-ə) hypermetria affecting one side of the body.

**hemi·hy·per·pla·sia** (hem″e-hi″pər-pla′zhə) overdevelopment of one side of the body, or of one half of an organ or part, as of the cranium.

**hemi·hy·per·to·nia** (hem″e-hi″pər-to′ne-ə) [*hemi-* + *hypertonia*] increased tone of the muscles of one side, which may result in contractures; sometimes seen after a stroke. Called also *hemitonia.*

**hemi·hy·per·tro·phy** (hem″e-hi-pər′trə-fe) [*hemi-* + *hypertrophy*] 1. overgrowth of one half of the body or unilateral hypertrophy of a part. 2. Curtius' syndrome.
**facial h.,** hypertrophy of half of the face.

**hemi·hy·pes·the·sia** (hem″e-hi″pəs-the′zhə) hypoesthesia on one side of the body; called also *hemihypoesthesia.*

**hemi·hy·po·es·the·sia** (hem″e-hi″po-əs-the′zhə) hemihypesthesia.

**hemi·hy·po·me·tria** (hem″e-hi″po-me′tre-ə) hypometria affecting one side of the body.

**hemi·hy·po·pla·sia** (hem″e-hi″po-pla′zhə) underdevelopment of one side of the body, or of one half of a part or organ, as of the brain.

**hemi·hy·po·to·nia** (hem″e-hi″po-to′ne-ə) [*hemi-* + *hypotonia*] reduced muscle tone of one side of the body.

**hemi·in·at·ten·tion** (hem″e-in-ə-ten′shən) unilateral neglect.

**hemi·kary·on** (hem″ĭ-kar′e-on) [*hemi-* + *karyon*] a cell nucleus which contains the haploid number of chromosomes.

**hemi·ke·tal** (hem″ĭ-ke′təl) a derivative formed by a combination of a ketone group with an alcohol.

**hemi·lam·i·nec·to·my** (hem″ĭ-lam″ĭ-nek′tə-me) surgical removal of one side of the vertebral lamina.

**hemi·lar·yn·gec·to·my** (hem″ĭ-lar″in-jek′tə-me) excision of one lateral half of the larynx.

**hemi·lat·er·al** (hem″ĭ-lat′ər-əl) affecting one lateral half.

**hemi·lin·gual** (hem″ĭ-ling′wəl) [*hemi-* + *lingual*] affecting one side of the tongue; hemiglossal.

**hemi·ma·cro·glos·sia** (hem″ĭ-mak″ro-glos′e-ə) enlargement of one side of the tongue.

**hemi·man·dib·u·lec·to·my** (hem″ĭ-man-dib″u-lek′tə-me) surgical excision of half of the mandible.

**hemi·max·il·lec·to·my** (hem″i-mak″sil-ek′tə-me) [*hemi-* + *maxillectomy*] surgical excision of half or part of the maxilla.

**hemi·me·lia** (hem″ĭ-me′le-ə) [*hemi-* + *-melia*] a developmental anomaly characterized by absence of all or part of the distal half of a limb.
**fibular h.,** hemimelia of the lower limb in which the fibular side is absent.
**radial h.,** hemimelia of the upper limb in which the radial side is absent.
**tibial h.,** hemimelia of the lower limb in which the tibial side is absent.
**ulnar h.,** hemimelia of the upper limb in which the ulnar side is absent.

**hem·im·e·lus** (hem-im′ə-ləs) an individual exhibiting hemimelia.

**he·min** (he′min) [MeSH: Hemin] 1. a porphyrin chelate of iron (III), derived from red blood cells; the chloride of heme. It is used to ameliorate the symptoms of acute intermittent porphyria, porphyria variegata, and hereditary coproporphyria; administered intravenously. 2. hematin (def. 1).

**hemi·ne·phrec·to·my** (hem″ĭ-nə-frek′tə-me) excision of a portion of a kidney.

**hemi·neph·ro·ure·ter·ec·to·my** (hem″ĭ-nef″ro-u-re″tər-ek′tə-me) excision of a portion of a kidney and ureter.

**hemi·obe·si·ty** (hem″e-o-bēs′ĭ-te) [*hemi-* + *obesity*] obesity of one side of the body only.

**hemi·op·al·gia** (hem″e-op-al′jə) [*hemi-* + *opalgia*] pain in one side of the head and in one eye.

**hemi·opia** (hem″e-o′pe-ə) hemianopia.

**hemi·op·ic** (hem″e-op′ik) hemianopic.

**hem·ip·a·gus** (hem-ip′ə-gəs) [*hemi-* + *-pagus*] conjoined twins united laterally at the thorax.

**hemi·pa·ral·y·sis** (hem″ĭ-pə-ral′ə-sis) hemiplegia.

**hemi·par·a·ple·gia** (hem″ĭ-par″ə-ple′jə) [*hemi-* + *paraplegia*] paralysis of the lower half of one side of the body.

**hemi·pa·re·sis** (hem″ĭ-pə-re′sis) [*hemi-* + *paresis*] muscular weakness or partial paralysis affecting one side of the body.

**hemi·par·es·the·sia** (hem″ĭ-par″əs-the′zhə) [*hemi-* + *paresthesia*] perverted sensation on one side of the body.

**hemi·pa·ret·ic** (hem″ĭ-pə-ret′ik) 1. pertaining to hemiparesis. 2. one affected with hemiparesis.

**hemi·par·kin·son·ism** (hem″ĭ-pahr′kin-son-iz-əm) parkinsonism affecting only one side of the body.

**hemi·pel·vec·to·my** (hem″ĭ-pel-vek′tə-me) [MeSH: Hemipelvectomy] amputation of a lower limb through the sacroiliac joint. Called also *hindquarter* or *interpelviabdominal amputation* and *Jaboulay's amputation* or *operation.*

**hemi·pep·tone** (hem″ĭ-pep′tōn) [*hemi-* + *peptone*] one of the intermediate products of pepsin digestion of protein; it is formed along with antipeptone, and differs from the latter in being convertible into amino acids by trypsin.

**hemi·phal·an·gec·to·my** (hem″ĭ-fal″ən-jek′tə-me) the excision of part of a digital phalanx.

**hemi·pla·cen·ta** (hem″ĭ-plə-sen′tə) [*hemi-* + *placenta*] an organ, composed of the chorion, yolk sac, and, usually, allantois, which puts marsupial embryos into temporary relation with the maternal uterus.

**hemi·ple·gia** (hem″ĭ-ple′jə) [*hemi-* + *-plegia*] [MeSH: Hemiplegia] paralysis of one side of the body.
**h. al′ternans hypoglos′sica,** hemiplegia due to lesion of the hypoglossal nerve on the side opposite the paralyzed part.
**alternate h.,** that which affects a part on one side of the body and another part on the opposite side.
**alternating oculomotor h.,** Weber's syndrome.
**ascending h.,** ascending paralysis of one lateral half of the body.
**capsular h.,** hemiplegia due to lesion of the internal capsule.
**cerebral h.,** that which is due to a lesion of the brain.
**contralateral h.,** hemiplegia on the side of the body opposite the site of the brain lesion causing it.
**crossed h.,** alternate h.
**h. crucia′ta,** alternate h.
**facial h.,** paralysis of one side of the face, the body being unaffected.
**faciobrachial h.,** paralysis of one half of the face and of the arm on the same side.
**faciolingual h.,** paralysis of one side of the face and tongue.
**flaccid h.,** hemiplegia with loss of tone of the muscles of the paralyzed part and absence of tendon reflexes. Cf. *spastic h.*
**Gubler's h.,** Millard-Gubler syndrome.
**infantile h.,** hemiplegia due to cerebral thrombosis or hemorrhage at delivery or occurring before birth.
**laryngeal h.,** paralysis of one side of the larynx of a horse, which produces roaring (q.v.).
**puerperal h.,** hemiplegia of women occurring shortly after childbirth.
**spastic h.,** hemiplegia marked by spasticity of the muscles of the paralyzed part and increased tendon reflexes. Cf. *flaccid h.*
**spinal h.,** a form due to a lesion of the spinal cord.
**Wernicke-Mann h.,** partial hemiplegia of the extremities.

**hemi·ple·gic** (hem″ĭ-ple′jik) pertaining to or of the nature of hemiplegia.

**He·mip·tera** (he-mip′tər-ə) [*hemi-* + Gr. *pteron* wing] [MeSH: Hemiptera] an order of insects that may be winged or wingless and have mouth parts adapted to piercing or sucking; it includes ticks and lice. The families Cimicidae and Reduviidae (suborder Heteroptera) contain species of considerable medical importance. See also *bug.*

**he·mip·ter·ous** (he-mip′tər-əs) of or pertaining to insects of the order Hemiptera.

**hemi·py·lor·ec·to·my** (hem″ĭ-pi″lor-ek′tə-me) excision of half of the pylorus.

**hemi·pyo·cy·a·nin** (hem″ĭ-pi″o-si′ə-nin) an antibiotic produced by the growth of *Pseudomonas aeruginosa* which is active against *Trichophyton schoenleinii* and *Candida albicans.*

**hemi·pyo·ne·phro·sis** (hem″ĭ-pi″o-nə-fro′sis) a hydronephrotic sac in a portion of the kidney; or pyonephrosis of half of a double kidney.

**hemi·ra·chis·chi·sis** (hem″ĭ-rə-kis′kĭ-sis) rachischisis without prolapse of the spinal cord.

**hemi·sa·cral·iza·tion** (hem″ĭ-sa″krə-lĭ-za′shən) fusion of the fifth lumbar vertebra to the first segment of the sacrum on only one side.

**hemi·sco·to·sis** (hem″ĭ-sko-to′sis) hemianopia.

**hemi·sec·tion** (hem″ĭ-sek′shən) 1. division into two equal parts. 2. surgical division of a multiple rooted tooth from the crown to the furcation with removal of a root and part of the crown.

**hemi·sec·to·my** (hem″ĭ-sek′tə-me) [*hemi-* + *-ectomy*] amputation of one root of a two-rooted mandibular tooth. Cf. *apicoectomy.*

**hemi·sep·tum** (hem″ĭ-sep′təm) either half of a septum, especially the lamina of the septum pellucidum of the brain.
**h. ce′rebri,** the lateral half of the septum pellucidum of the brain.

**hemi·so·mus** (hem″ĭ-so′məs) [*hemi-* + Gr. *sōma* body] an imperfectly developed fetus.

**hem·iso·ton·ic** (hem″i-so-ton′ik) [*hem-* + *isotonic*] having the same osmotic pressure as the blood.

**hemi·spasm** (hem′ĭ-spaz″əm) spasm affecting one side only.

**hemi·sphae·ri·um** (hem″is-fe′re-əm) pl. *hemisphae′ria* [L.] hemispherium.

**hemi·sphere** (hem′is-fēr) [*hemi-* + *sphere*] half of any spherical or roughly spherical structure; see also *hemispherium.*
**animal h.,** the half of the mass of cells formed by cleavage of a fertilized telolecithal ovum that is nearest the animal pole.
**cerebellar h.,** hemispherium cerebelli.
**cerebral h.,** hemispherium cerebri.
**dominant h.,** that cerebral hemisphere which is more concerned than the other in the integration of sensations and the control of many functions, such as speech and language and the preferential use of one or the other of paired organs in voluntary movements. The hemisphere opposite to the handedness of the individual, i.e., the left cerebral hemisphere in right-handed persons, and vice versa, is the dominant one for many functions, but the left hemisphere is usually dominant for speech and language functions regardless of the handedness.
**nondominant h.,** the hemisphere opposite to the dominant one; it plays a far smaller role in speech and language but may play a far larger role in mediating spatial responses and emotional responses.
**vegetal h.,** the half of the mass of cells formed by cleavage of a fertilized telolecithal ovum that is nearest the vegetal pole.

**hemi·spher·ec·to·my** (hem″is-fēr-ek′tə-me) [*hemisphere* + *-ectomy*] resection of a cerebral hemisphere.

**hemi·sphe·ri·um** (hem″is-fe′re-əm) pl. *hemisphe′ria* [L.] [TA] hemisphere: a general term denoting half of a spherical or spheroid structure. Spelled also *hemisphaerium.*
**hemisphe′ria bul′bi ure′thrae,** the lateral halves of the bulb of the urethra.
**h. cerebel′li** [TA], cerebellar hemisphere: the part of the cerebellum lateral to the vermis. See also *cerebellum.*
**h. cerebra′lis,** h. cerebri.
**h. ce′rebri** [TA], cerebral hemisphere: either of the pair of structures, formed by evagination of the embryonic telencephalon, lying on either side of the midline, partly separated by the longitudinal cerebral fissure, containing a central cavity, the lateral ventricle, and covered by a layer of gray substance, the cerebral cortex; together they constitute the largest part of the brain in humans.

**hemi·sphyg·mia** (hem″ĭ-sfig′me-ə) [*hemi-* + *sphygm-* + *-ia*] a condition in which there appear to be twice as many pulse beats as heart beats, such as pulsus bisferiens.

**hemi·spore** (hem′ĭ-spor) a spore formed by the differentiation and division of the terminal portion of a hypha.

**hemi·syn·drome** (hem″ĭ-sin′drom) a syndrome that affects just one side of the body.

**hemi·ter·a·ta** (hem″ĭ-ter′ə-tə) [*hemi-* + *teras*] a grouping of congenitally deformed individuals whose anomalies are less severe than teratisms.

**hemi·ter·at·ic** (hem″ĭ-tər-at′ik) congenitally deformed, but not exhibiting teratism.

**hemi·tet·a·ny** (hem″ĭ-tet′ə-ne) tetany limited to one side of the body.

**hemi·ther·mo·an·es·the·sia** (hem″ĭ-thər″mo-an″əs-the′zhə) thermanesthesia on one side of the body.

**hemi·tho·rax** (hem″ĭ-thor′aks) [*hemi-* + *thorax*] one side of the chest.
**frozen h.,** prevention of a mediastinal shift away from the affected lung in diffuse pleural mesothelioma, caused by encasement of the lung by nodular thickening of the pleura.

**hemi·thy·roi·dec·to·my** (hem″ĭ-thi″roid-ek′tə-me) excision of one lobe of the thyroid gland.

**hemi·to·nia** (hem″ĭ-to′ne-ə) [*hemi-* + *ton-* + *-ia*] hemihypertonia.

**hemi·tox·in** (hem″ĭ-tok′sin) a toxin the toxicity of which has been reduced by one half.

**hemi·tre·mor** (hem″ĭ-trĕ′mor) tremor of one side of the body.

**hemi·va·got·o·ny** (hem″ĭ-və-got′o-ne) vagotonia on one side.

**hemi·ver·te·bra** (hem″ĭ-vər′tə-brə) 1. a developmental anomaly characterized by incomplete development of one half of a vertebra. 2. (pl., *hemiver′tebrae*) a vertebra which is incompletely developed on one side.

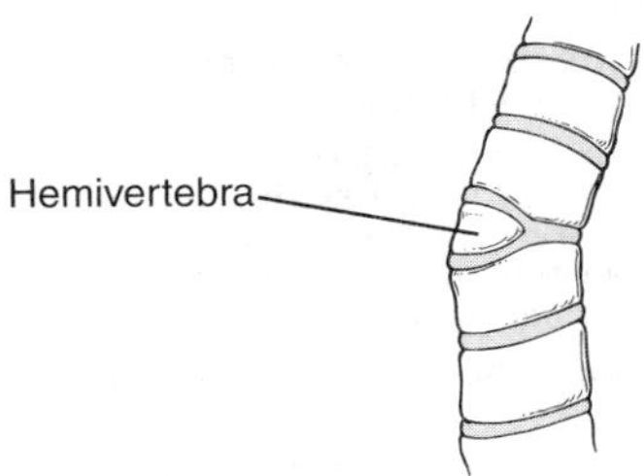


**hemi·zy·gos·i·ty** (hem″ĭ-zi-gos′ĭ-te) [*hemi-* + *zygosity*] possession of only one of a pair of alleles; refers particularly to the state of the male for X-linked genes, and also to abnormal conditions in which a segment of DNA has been deleted from one member of chromosome pair, so that the individual is *hemizygous* for the genes lost with that segment.

**hemi·zy·gote** (hem″ĭ-zi′gōt) an individual or cell exhibiting hemizygosity.

**hemi·zy·gous** (hem″ĭ-zi′gəs) possessing only one instead of a pair of genes of a particular kind; see *hemizygosity.*

**hem·lock** (hem′lok) [MeSH: Hemlock] 1. any fir tree of the genus *Tsuga.* 2. any of the plants of the genera *Cicuta* and *Conium.* 3. poison h.
**poison h.,** *Conium maculatum,* a large herb that contains the poisonous alkaloid coniine; in both humans and other animals it causes nausea and vomiting, followed by potentially fatal muscle paralysis and respiratory failure. The dried fully grown but unripe fruit has sedative, anodyne, and antispasmodic properties. Called also *hemlock.*
**water h.,** any tree of the genus *Cicuta.*

**hem(o)-** [Gr. *haima* blood] combining form denoting relationship to the blood; variant forms are *haema-, haem(o)-,* and *hema-.*

**he·mo·ac·cess** (he″mo-ak′səs) arteriovenous access.

**he·mo·ag·glu·ti·na·tion** (he″mo-ə-gloo″tĭ-na′shən) hemagglutination.

**he·mo·ag·glu·ti·nin** (he″mo-ə-gloo′tĭ-nin) hemagglutinin.

**he·mo·bil·ia** (he″mo-bil′e-ə) [MeSH: Hemobilia] bleeding into the biliary passages.

**he·mo·bi·lin·uria** (he″mo-bi-lĭ-nu′re-ə) [*hemo-* + *bilin* + *-uria*] the presence of urobilin in the blood and urine.

**he·mo·blast** (he′mo-blast) blast cell (def. 2).
**lymphoid h. of Pappenheim,** pronormoblast.

**he·mo·ca·ther·e·sis** (he″mo-kə-ther′ə-sis) hemolysis.

**He·moc·cult** (he′mo-kəlt) trademark for a modification of the guaiac test for occult blood, in which guaiac-impregnated filter paper is used; the test is positive if the specimen turns blue.

**he·mo·cele** (he′mo-sēl) hemocoelom.

**he·mo·ce·lom** (he″mo-se′lom) hemocoelom.

**he·mo·cho·le·cyst** (he″mo-ko′le-sist) nontraumatic hemorrhage of the gallbladder.

**he·mo·cho·le·cys·ti·tis** (he″mo-ko-le-sis-ti′tis) cholecystitis with hemorrhage into the gallbladder.

**he·mo·cho·ri·al** (he″mo-kor′e-əl) [*hemo-* + *chorion*] denoting a type of placenta in which maternal blood comes in direct contact with the chorion.

**he·mo·chro·ma·to·sis** (he″mo-kro″mə-to′sis) [*hemo-* + *chromatosis*] [MeSH: Hemochromatosis] a disorder due to deposition of hemosiderin in the parenchymal cells, causing tissue damage and dysfunction of the liver, pancreas, heart, and pituitary. Other clinical signs include bronze pigmentation of skin, arthropathy, diabetes,

cirrhosis, hepatosplenomegaly, hypogonadism, and loss of body hair. Full development of the disease among women is restricted by menstruation and pregnancy. Cf. *hemosiderosis* and *siderosis.*
**acquired h.,** hemochromatosis resulting from blood transfusions or excessive dietary iron, or secondary to other disease, e.g., thalassemia or sideroblastic anemia; called also *secondary h.*
**genetic h., hereditary h., idiopathic h.,** an autosomal recessive disorder of iron metabolism associated with a gene tightly linked to the A locus of the HLA complex on chromosome 6; iron accumulation is lifelong, with symptoms appearing usually in the fifth or sixth decades of life.
**neonatal h., perinatal h.,** a rare fulminant disease of the liver, of unknown cause, characterized by massive deposition of iron in the liver, pancreas, heart, and endocrine glands; symptoms are those of neonatal hepatitis and appear in utero or within the first week of life, with death usually occurring by 4 months of age.
**secondary h.,** acquired h.

**he·mo·chro·ma·tot·ic** (he″mo-kro″mə-tot′ik) pertaining to or characterized by hemochromatosis.

**he·mo·chrome** (he′mo-krōm) [*hemo-* + *-chrome*] a heme compound in which the fifth and sixth coordination positions of the central iron atom are occupied by strong field ligands, usually nitrogen atoms, as in cytochromes; originally a complex of 2 moles of a nitrogenous base per mole of heme. Called also *hemochromogen.*

**he·mo·chro·mo·gen** (he″mo-kro′mo-jən) [*hemo-* + *chromo-* + *-gen*] hemochrome.

**he·mo·cla·sis** (he-mok′lə-sis) [*hemo-* + Gr. *klasis* a breaking] hemolysis.

**he·mo·clas·tic** (he-mo-klas′tik) hemolytic.

**he·mo·clip** (he′mo-klip) a metal clip used to ligate blood vessels.

**he·mo·co·ag·u·lin** (he″mo-ko-ag′u-lin) a constituent of the venom of certain snakes which causes coagulation of the blood.

**he·mo·coe·lom** (he″mo-se′lom) [*hemo-* + *coelom*] 1. the part of the coelom in which the heart is developed. 2. collectively, the spaces between the cells and tissues of many invertebrates, such as most mollusks, arthropods, and tunicates, through which a bloodlike fluid (hemolymph) circulates. Sometimes spelled *hemocele* and *hemocoel.*

**he·mo·coe·lo·ma** (he″mo-se-lo′mə) [*hemo-* + *coeloma*] hemocoelom.

**he·mo·con·cen·tra·tion** (he″mo-kon″sən-tra′shən) decrease of the fluid content of the blood, with resulting increase in its concentration. Cf. *exemia.*

**he·mo·co·nia** (he″mo-ko′ne-ə) [*hemo-* + *coni-* + *-ia*] small, round or dumbbell-shaped particles demonstrating brownian movement, observed in blood platelets in a wet film of blood under darkfield microscopy. Called also *blood dust.*

**he·mo·co·ni·o·sis** (he″mo-ko″ne-o′sis) the presence in the blood of abnormal amounts of hemoconia.

**he·mo·cry·os·co·py** (he″mo-kri-os′kə-pe) [*hemo-* + *cryoscopy*] cryoscopy of the blood; the ascertaining of the freezing point of the blood.

**he·mo·cul·ture** (he″mo-kul′chər) [*hemo-* + *culture*] blood culture.

**he·mo·cu·pre·in** (he″mo-ku′pre-in) superoxide dismutase.

**he·mo·cy·a·nin** (he″mo-si′ə-nin) [MeSH: Hemocyanin] a nonheme blue respiratory pigment that is found in the blood plasma of many mollusks and arthropods and is composed of monomers each of which contains two atoms of $Cu^+$ and can bind one molecule of $O_2$.
**keyhole-limpet h. (KLH),** a hemocyanin from the keyhole limpet; it is a commonly used antigen in laboratory immunology.

**he·mo·cyte** (he′mo-sīt) [*hemo-* + *-cyte*] [MeSH: Hemocytes] blood cell.

**he·mo·cy·to·blast** (he″mo-si′to-blast) [*hemocyte* + *-blast*] blast cell (def. 2).

**he·mo·cy·to·ca·ther·e·sis** (he″mo-si″to-kə-ther′ə-sis) hemolysis.

**he·mo·cy·to·ma** (he′mo-si-to′mə) acute undifferentiated leukemia.

**he·mo·cy·tom·e·ter** (he″mo-si-tom′ə-tər) hemacytometer.

**he·mo·cy·tom·e·try** (he″mo-si-tom′ə-tre) [*hemo-* + *cytometry*] hemacytometry.

**he·mo·cy·to·pha·gia** (he″mo-si″to-fa′jə) [*hemocyte* + *-phagia*] hemophagocytosis.

**he·mo·cy·to·phag·ic** (he″mo-si″to-faj′ik) hemophagocytic.

**he·mo·cy·to·poi·e·sis** (he″mo-si″to-poi-e′sis) hematopoiesis.

**he·mo·cy·to·trip·sis** (he″mo-si″to-trip′sis) [*hemocyte* + *tripsis*] disintegration of the blood corpuscles by pressure.

**he·mo·di·a·fil·tra·tion** (he″mo-di″ə-fil-tra′shən) [MeSH: Hemodiafiltration]hemofiltration with a dialytic component added; blood flow is accelerated to twice that of conventional dialysis. Called also *high flux hemodiafiltration.*

**he·mo·di·ag·no·sis** (he″mo-di″əg-no′sis) [*hemo-* + *diagnosis*] diagnosis by examination of the blood.

**he·mo·di·al·y·sis** (he″mo-di-al′ə-sis) [MeSH: Hemodialysis] the removal of certain elements from the blood by virtue of the difference in the rates of their diffusion through a semipermeable membrane, e.g., by means of a hemodialyzer. Two distinct physical processes are involved, diffusion and ultrafiltration (qq.v.). See also *clearance.* Called also *dialysis.*
**high flux h.,** hemodialysis using a high flux membrane so that solutes composed of large molecules can be cleared rapidly; it filters slightly more rapidly than high efficiency hemodialysis.

**he·mo·di·a·lyz·er** (he″mo-di′ə-līz″ər) an apparatus by which hemodialysis may be performed, blood being separated by a semipermeable membrane from a solution of such composition as to secure diffusion of certain elements out of the blood. Popularly called *artificial kidney.*

**he·mo·di·a·pe·de·sis** (he″mo-di″ə-pə-de′sis) [*hemo-* + *diapedesis*] the extravasation of blood through the skin.

**he·mo·di·lu·tion** (he″mo-di-loo′shən) [MeSH: Hemodilution] increase of the fluid content of the blood with resulting decrease in concentration of its erythrocytes. See also *hypervolemia.*

**he·mo·dy·nam·ic** (he″mo-di-nam′ik) [MeSH: Hemodynamics] pertaining to the movements involved in the circulation of the blood.

**he·mo·dy·nam·ics** (he″mo-di-nam′iks) [MeSH: Hemodynamics] the study of the movements of the blood and of the forces concerned therein.

**he·mo·dy·na·mom·e·try** (he″mo-di″nə-mom′ə-tre) measurement of blood pressure.

**he·mo·dys·tro·phy** (he″mo-dis′tro-fe) [*hemo-* + *dystrophy*] any blood disease due to faulty blood nutrition.

**he·mo·en·do·the·li·al** (he″mo-en-do-the′le-əl) [*hemo-* + *endothelium*] denoting a type of placenta in which maternal blood comes in contact with the endothelium of chorionic vessels.

**He·mo·fil** (he′mo-fil) trademark for a highly concentrated preparation of coagulation factor VIII.

**he·mo·fil·ter** (he′mo-fil″tər) a filter used in hemofiltration.

**he·mo·fil·tra·tion** (he″mo-fil-tra′shən) [MeSH: Hemofiltration] the removal of waste products from the blood by passing the blood through extracorporeal filters. Cf. *hemoperfusion.*
**continuous arteriovenous h.,** a form of continuous renal replacement therapy consisting of hemofiltration via an arteriovenous pathway, using small-volume, low-resistance hemofilters powered by the patient's arterial pressure, without need for a mechanical pump; used as an alternative to conventional hemodialysis ultrafiltration.
**continuous venovenous h.,** a process similar to continuous arteriovenous hemofiltration but using a venovenous pathway and a mechanical pump.

**he·mo·flag·el·late** (he″mo-flaj′ə-lāt) [*hemo-* + *flagellate*] any flagellate microorganism parasitic in the blood, especially protozoa of the suborder Trypanosomatina.

**he·mo·fus·cin** (he″mo-fūs′in) [*hemo-* + *fuscus*] a brownish-yellow pigment that results from the decomposition of hemoglobin; it is sometimes seen in the urine.

**he·mo·gen·e·sis** (he″mo-jen′ə-sis) hematopoiesis.

**he·mo·gen·ic** (he″mo-jen′ik) 1. hematopoietic. 2. hematogenous.

**he·mo·glo·bin** (he′mo-glo″bin) the red oxygen-carrying pigment of erythrocytes, formed by developing erythrocytes in bone marrow. It is a type of hemoprotein that contains four heme groups and globin and has the property of reversible oxygenation. A molecule of hemoglobin contains four polypeptide globin chains, composed of between 141 and 146 amino acids; those most often found are $\alpha$ and $\beta$ chains, with $\gamma$ and $\delta$ chains seen somewhat less often. Different types of hemoglobins are determined by different combinations of chains, with the number of chains of each type in the molecule being indicated by a subscript. For example, *hemoglobin F (fetal h.),* the predominant type in the newborn, may be written $\alpha_2{}^A\gamma_2{}^F$., and *hemoglobin A (adult h.),* which is normally predominant in the adult, may be written $\alpha_2{}^A\beta_2{}^A$ or $\alpha_2\beta_2$. Another hemoglobin, *hemoglobin* $A_2$ (designated $\alpha_2{}^A\delta_2{}^{A2}$ or $\alpha_2{}^A\delta_2$), is usually present in limited minor concentrations. Hundreds of hemoglobins with differing electrophoretic mobilities and characteristics have been reported; the first ones were given capital letters, such as S, C, D, E, G, H, I, J, K, L, M, N, and Q. As refined biochemical techniques led to the discovery of many additional hemoglobins, newer standards for nomenclature were devised: those with electrophoretic mobility equal to one of the lettered hemoglobins could be named with that letter using the

place of discovery as a subscript, such as hemoglobin $M_{Saskatoon}$ or hemoglobin $M_{Milwaukee}$. New hemoglobins with unique electrophoretic mobilities are now often named simply for the laboratory, hospital, or town where they were discovered, such as hemoglobin Chesapeake or hemoglobin Gun Hill. When known, the number of each amino acid substituting in each polypeptide in the molecule should be indicated by the appropriate superscript numeral. Symbol *Hb*.
**h. A,** normal adult hemoglobin, composed of two $\alpha$ and two $\beta$ chains, $\alpha_2{}^A\beta_2{}^A$.
**h. A$_{1c}$,** a type of glycated hemoglobin A, having a hexose attached to the N terminal of its $\beta$ chain; its levels are increased in poorly controlled diabetics.
**h. A$_2$,** $\alpha_2{}^A\delta_2$, a type of normal adult hemoglobin present in small amounts, in which $\delta$ chains replace the $\beta$ chains.
**h. anti-Lepore,** an abnormal crossover hemoglobin similar to hemoglobin Lepore but whose non-$\alpha$ chains have fusion in the opposite configuration from those of hemoglobin Lepore ($\beta$ chain portions at the N terminus and $\delta$ chain portions at the C terminus); most individuals with this hemnoglobin have predominantly normal hemoglobin and do not suffer from anemia or thalassemia.
**h. Bart's,** an abnormal hemoglobin composed of four $\gamma$ chains having high oxygen affinity, seen in Southeast Asians and a few other groups; infants born with only this type of hemoglobin have hydrops fetalis and usually die within a few hours. Hemoglobin Bart's is often found mixed with hemoglobin H, resulting in $\alpha$-thalassemia.
**h. C,** a common abnormal hemoglobin in which lysine replaces glutamic acid at position six of the $\beta$ chains; it was one of the earliest hemoglobins to have its molecular abnormality defined. The homozygous state manifests as the anemic condition called *hemoglobin C disease,* and the asymptomatic heterozygous state is called *hemoglobin C trait.*
**h. Chesapeake,** an abnormal hemoglobin in which leucine is substituted for arginine in the $\alpha$ chain, resulting in high oxygen affinity so that the individual has polycythemia.
**h. Constant Spring,** an abnormal hemoglobin seen in Southeast Asians, characterized by 31 extra amino acid residues at the C terminus of the $\alpha$ chain, resulting in a form of $\alpha$-thalassemia.
**crossover h.,** an abnormal hemoglobin that has a globin chain formed from parts of two chains that have undergone crossover, such as hemoglobin Lepore, h. anti-Lepore, and h. Kenya.
**h. D,** any of several abnormal hemoglobins, all characterized by electrophoretic mobility equal to that of hemoglobin S on paper or cellulose acetate but unequal on acid agar gel. The most common one is *h. D Los Angeles* (also known as *h. D Punjab*), which has glycine substituted for glutamic acid at position 121 of the $\beta$ chain. In the homozygous state, hemoglobin D manifests as the anemic state called hemoglobin D disease; the heterozygous state is clinically silent.
**deoxygenated h.,** deoxyhemoglobin.
**h. E,** an abnormal hemoglobin with lysine substituted for glutamic acid at position 26 of the $\beta$ chain, seen most often in Southeast Asia, especially Thailand. The homozygous state may be asymptomatic or may be manifested as the anemic state called hemoglobin E disease, while the heterozygous state is clinically silent.
**h. F,** fetal h.
**fast h's,** those with greater mobility on electrophoresis (in an alkaline buffer) than normal hemoglobin A, such as hemoglobin K, J, or N.
**fetal h.,** the hemoglobin normally comprising more than half of that in the fetus, composed of two alpha and two gamma polypeptides ($\alpha_2{}^A\gamma_2{}^F$); it has higher affinity for oxygen under physiologic conditions than does hemoglobin A. It is present in minimal amounts in adulthood and is abnormally elevated in aplastic anemia, leukemia, and certain types of thalassemia. Called also *h. F.*
**h. G,** any of various abnormal hemoglobins with an amino acid substitution on the $\alpha$ chain; the most common one is *h. G Philadelphia,* which causes $\alpha$-thalassemia.
**glycated h., glycosylated h.,** any of various hemoglobins to which glucose is bound by glycation; the most common one is hemoglobin $A_{1c}$.
**Gower h., h. Gower,** a normal hemoglobin present in early embryonic life and disappearing before birth; it occasionally consists entirely of epsilon chains ($\epsilon_4$), but the usual forms are *h. Gower-1,* consisting of two zeta and two epsilon chains ($\zeta_2\epsilon_2$) and *h. Gower-2,* consisting of two alpha and two epsilon chains ($\alpha_2\epsilon_2$).
**h. Gun Hill,** an unstable hemoglobin with a segmental deletion of amino acids in the $\beta$ chain that causes inability to bind heme and mild hemolytic anemia.
**h. H,** a rapidly migrating abnormal hemoglobin composed of four $\beta$ chains, having a high oxygen affinity, found mainly in Southeast Asians, natives of the Mediterranean region, and a few other ethnic groups. Infants may be born with a mixture of hemoglobin H and hemoglobin Bart's. See *hemoglobin H disease,* under *disease.*
**h. I,** an abnormal hemoglobin resulting from an amino acid substitution in the $\alpha$ chain, causing $\alpha$-thalassemia.
**h. Kansas,** an abnormal hemoglobin with threonine substituted for asparagine at position 102 of the $\beta$ chain, resulting in decreased oxygen affinity and cyanosis.
**h. Kenya,** an abnormal type of crossover hemoglobin in which the non-$\alpha$ chain has a $\gamma$ chain portion at the N terminus and a $\beta$ chain portion at the C terminus, resulting in $\beta$-thalassemia.
**h. Köln,** an unstable hemoglobin that has methionine substituted for valine at position 95 of the $\beta$ chain, usually resulting in Heinz body anemia.
**h. Lepore,** any of several abnormal crossover hemoglobins having two normal $\alpha$ chains and two globin chains that have portions of a $\delta$ chain at the N terminus and portions of a $\beta$ chain at the C terminus. Homozygous individuals have about 90 per cent hemoglobin F, 10 per cent hemoglobin Lepore, and no Hemoglobin A or $A_2$, which results in thalassemia major; heterozygotes have varying amounts of hemoglobin Lepore and hemoglobin A and may have mild anemia.
**h. M,** any of several abnormal hemoglobins having amino acid substitutions in the $\alpha$ or $\beta$ chains and all associated with methemoglobinemia.
**mean corpuscular h. (MCH),** the average hemoglobin content of an erythrocyte, conventionally expressed in picograms per red cell, obtained by multiplying the blood hemoglobin concentration (in g/dL) by ten and dividing by the red cell count (in millions per $\mu$L): MCH = Hb/RBC.
**muscle h.,** myoglobin.
**oxidized h., oxygenated h.,** oxyhemoglobin.
**h. Portland,** a normal hemoglobin present in the fetus late in the first trimester of pregnancy, consisting of zeta and gamma chains ($\zeta_2\gamma_2$); it disappears in utero.
**h. Rainier,** an abnormal hemoglobin in which histidine replaces tyrosine at position 145 in the $\beta$ chain; it has increased oxygen affinity and is associated with polycythemia.
**reduced h.,** deoxyhemoglobin.
**h. S,** the most common abnormal hemoglobin, having valine substituted for glutamic acid at position six of the $\beta$ chain; the homozygous state results in sickle cell anemia, and the asymptomatic heterozygous state is called *sickle cell trait.* The delineation of the abnormality in molecular structure was a milestone in biochemical genetics, paving the way for other investigations demonstrating how substitutions of a single amino acid could produce significant clinical effects. anemia.
**h. Seattle,** an abnormal hemoglobin in which glutamic acid is substituted for alanine at position 76 of the $\beta$ chain; it has decreased oxygen affinity.
**slow h's,** those less mobile on electrophoresis (in an alkaline buffer) than normal hemoglobin A, such as hemoglobin S or D.
**unstable h's,** abnormal hemoglobins whose molecule is unstable, usually owing to substitution or deletion of at least one amino acid. Many have increased oxygen affinity and some have Heinz bodies; affected individuals often have Heinz body anemia or some other type of hemolytic anemia.
**h. Yakima,** an abnormal hemoglobin in which histidine is substituted for aspartic acid at position 99 of the $\beta$ chain; it has increased oxygen affinity and is associated with polycythemia.

**he·mo·glo·bin·at·ed** (he″mo-glo′bin-āt-əd) containing hemoglobin.

**he·mo·glo·bin·emia** (he″mo-glo′bin-e′me-ə) the presence of free hemoglobin in the blood plasma, an indication of significant intravascular hemolysis.

**he·mo·glo·bino·cho·lia** (he″mo-glo″bin-o-ko′le-ə) [*hemoglobin* + *chol-* + *-ia*] the occurrence of hemoglobin in the bile.

**he·mo·glo·bin·ol·y·sis** (he″mo-glo″bin-ol′ə-sis) [*hemoglobin* + *-lysis*] splitting up of hemoglobin.

**he·mo·glo·bin·om·e·ter** (he″mo-glo″bin-om′ə-tər) [*hemoglobin* + *-meter*] an instrument for measuring the hemoglobin of the blood.

**he·mo·glo·bin·om·e·try** (he″mo-glo″bin-om′ə-tre) [MeSH: Hemoglobinometry] the measurement of the hemoglobin of the blood.

**he·mo·glo·bin·op·a·thy** (he″mo-glo″bin-op′ə-the) [*hemoglobin* + *-pathy*] [MeSH: Hemoglobinopathies] 1. any inherited disorder caused by abnormalities of hemoglobin, resulting in conditions such as sickle cell anemia, hemolytic anemia, or thalassemia. 2. sometimes more specifically, a hemoglobin disorder involving a variation or variations of a globin chain such as changes or substitutions in the amino acid sequences, or moving of a chain from its usual place in the molecule. (In this case hemoglobinopathies are distinguished from *thalassemias,* which involve reduced or absent synthesis of normal polypeptide chains.) When the site of an aberration is known, the abnormality of the peptide chain, the number of the altered amino acid, and the nature of the replacement are indicated. For example, hemoglobin S is expressed as $\alpha_2{}^A\beta_2{}^S$, or $\alpha_2{}^A\beta_2{}^{6\ \mathrm{valine}}$, and hemoglobin $G_{Philadelphia}$ is expressed as $\alpha_2{}^G\beta_2{}^A$, or $\alpha_2{}^{6\ \mathrm{lysine}}\beta_2{}^A$. If more than one hemoglobin is present, the phenotype is designated by listing them in order of decreasing concentrations; for example, the phenotype for sickle cell trait is expressed as AS, for sickle cell anemia as SS, and for sickle cell–hemoglobin C disease as SC.

**he·mo·glo·bino·pep·sia** (he″mo-glo″bin-o-pep′se-ə) [*hemoglobin* + Gr. *pepsis* digestion] hemoglobinolysis.

**he·mo·glo·bi·nous** (he″mo-glo′bĭ-nəs) hemoglobinated.

**he·mo·glo·bin·uric** (he″mo-glo″bĭ-nu′rik) pertaining to or characterized by hemoglobinuria.

**he·mo·gram** (he′mo-gram) [*hemo-* + *-gram*] a written record or graphic representation of a detailed blood assessment such as the complete blood count or differential leukocyte count.

**he·mo·his·tio·blast** (he″mo-his′te-o-blast″) [*hemo-* + *histio-* + *-blast*] old name for *blast cell* (def. 2).

**he·mo·ki·ne·sis** (he″mo-kĭ-ne′sis) [*hemo-* + *-kinesis*] circulation.

**he·mo·ki·net·ic** (he″mo-kĭ-net′ik) circulatory.

**he·mol·o·gy** (he-mol′ə-je) hematology.

**he·mo·lymph** (he′mo-limf″) [*hemo-* + *lymph*] [MeSH: Hemolymph] 1. the blood and lymph. 2. the bloodlike fluid moving through the hemocoelom of those invertebrates (e.g., mollusks, arthropods, and tunicates) with open circulatory systems, which combines the properties of blood and lymphlike interstitial fluid.

**he·mo·lymph·an·gi·o·ma** (he″mo-lim-fan″je-o′mə) hematolymphangioma.

**he·mol·y·sate** (he-mol′ə-sāt) the product of hemolysis.

**he·mol·y·sin** (he-mol′ə-sin) [*hemo-* + *lysin*] a substance that causes hemolysis; called also *erythrocytolysin* and *erythrolysin.*
**alpha h.,** 1. one producing alpha hemolysis. 2. the hemolysin of the alpha toxin of *Staphylococcus aureus,* which hemolyzes rabbit, sheep, cow, and goat but not human erythrocytes. See also *staphylococcal toxin,* under *toxin.*
**bacterial h.,** a toxic hemolysin produced by bacteria.
**beta h.,** 1. one producing beta hemolysis. 2. the hemolysin of the beta toxin of *Staphylococcus aureus.* It is a sphingomyelinase that lyses human and sheep erythrocytes in the cold following a warm incubation. See also *staphylococcal toxins,* under *toxin.*
**heterophile h.,** a hemolysin that has affinity for erythrocytes of animal species in addition to the one for which it is specific.
**hot-cold h.,** one that lyses erythrocytes in the cold following preliminary warm incubation, such as the beta hemolysin of *Staphylococcus aureus.*
**immune h.,** a hemolysin produced by deliberate immunization of an animal with blood or blood cells foreign to it, such as the rabbit anti-sheep red blood cell serum (hemolysin) that is used in complement fixation tests.

**he·mol·y·sis** (he-mol′ə-sis) [*hemo-* + *-lysis*] [MeSH: Hemolysis] disruption of the integrity of the erythrocyte membrane causing release of hemoglobin; it may be caused by bacterial hemolysins, by antibodies that cause complement-dependent lysis, by placing erythrocytes in a hypotonic solution, or by defects in the cell membrane. Called also *erythrocytolysis, erythrolysis,* and *hematolysis.*
**alpha h.,** the production of a zone of greenish discoloration surrounding a bacterial colony on blood-agar medium, caused by partial decomposition of the hemoglobin of the erythrocytes; it is characteristic of pneumococci and certain streptococci.
**beta h.,** the production of a clear zone immediately surrounding a bacterial colony on blood-agar medium, which is characteristic of certain pathogenic bacteria.
**colloid osmotic h.,** hemolysis due to swelling of the erythrocyte when defective membrane permeability allows excessive sodium to enter followed by excessive water.
**contact h.,** the hastened hemolysis of erythrocytes in contact with a surface.
**gamma h.,** a term used to indicate absence of hemolysis around a bacterial colony on blood agar, which indicates that the bacteria is nonhemolytic.
**immune h.,** the lysis by complement of erythrocytes sensitized as a consequence of interaction with specific antibody to the erythrocytes.
**passive h.,** the lysis of erythrocytes on which antigen has been adsorbed in the presence of complement and antiserum to that antigen.
**venom h.,** hemolysis produced by snake venom.

**he·mo·lyt·ic** (he″mo-lit′ik) pertaining to, characterized by, or producing hemolysis.

**he·mo·lyz·a·ble** (he″mo-li′zə-bəl) capable of undergoing hemolysis.

**he·mo·ly·za·tion** (he″mo-li-za′shən) the production of hemolysis.

**he·mo·lyze** (he′mo-līz) 1. to subject to hemolysis. 2. to undergo hemolysis.

**he·mo·ma·nom·e·ter** (he″mo-mə-nom′ə-tər) a manometer for determining blood pressure.

**he·mo·me·di·as·ti·num** (he″mo-me″di-as-ti′nəm) an effusion of blood in the mediastinum.

**he·mom·e·ter** (he-mom′ə-tər) old term for *hemoglobinometer.*

**he·mo·me·tra** (he″mo-me′trə) hematometra.

**he·mom·e·try** (he-mom′ə-tre) hematometry.

**he·mo·ne·phro·sis** (he″mo-nə-fro′sis) hematonephrosis.

**he·mo·path·ic** (he″mo-path′ik) pertaining to disease of the blood; due to blood disorder.

**he·mo·pa·thol·o·gy** (he″mo-pə-thol′ə-je) [*hemo-* + *pathology*] the study of diseases of the blood; called also *hematopathology.*

**he·mop·a·thy** (he-mop′ə-the) [*hemo-* + *-pathy*] any disease of the blood.

**he·mo·per·fu·sion** (he″mo-pər-fu′zhən) [MeSH: Hemoperfusion] the passing of large volumes of blood over an extracorporeal adsorbent substance in order to remove toxic substances. Cf. *hemofiltration.*

**he·mo·peri·car·di·um** (he″mo-per″ĭ-kahr′de-əm) [*hemo-* + *pericardium*] an effusion of blood within the pericardium.

**he·mo·peri·to·ne·um** (he″mo-per″ĭ-to-ne′əm) [*hemo-* + *peritoneum*] [MeSH: Hemoperitoneum] an effusion of blood in the peritoneal cavity.

**he·mo·pex·in** (he″mo-pek′sin) [MeSH: Hemopexin] a plasma glycoprotein, mol. wt. 57,000, in the $\beta_1$-globulin band; it is produced by hepatocytes and its function is the binding of free heme in plasma; it has one binding site for hematin forming a tight complex that is taken up and degraded by hepatocytes.

**he·mo·phage** (he′mo-fāj) hemophagocyte.

**he·mo·phago·cyte** (he″mo-fag′o-sīt) [*hemo-* + *phagocyte*] a macrophage that destroys blood cells. Called also *hemophage* and *hematophage.*

**he·mo·phag·o·cyt·ic** 1. pertaining to hemophagocytes. 2. pertaining to or characterized by hemophagocytosis; called also *hemocytophagic.*

**he·mo·phago·cy·to·sis** (he″mo-fag″o-si-to′sis) [*hemo-* + *phagocytosis*] the ingestion and destruction of blood cells by macrophages. Called also *hemocytophagia.*

**he·mo·phil** (he′mo-fil) [*hemo-* + *-phil*] 1. an organism thriving on blood. 2. a microorganism which grows best in media containing hemoglobin.

**he·mo·phil·ia** (he″mo-fil′e-ə) [*hemo-* + *-philia*] [MeSH: Hemophilia] a hemorrhagic diathesis occurring in two main forms: *hemophilia A,* deficiency of coagulation factor VIII; and *hemophilia B,* deficiency of coagulation factor IX. Both forms are determined by a mutant gene near the telomere of the long arm of the X chromosome (Xq), but at different loci, and are characterized by subcutaneous and intramuscular hemorrhages; bleeding from the mouth, gums, lips, and tongue; hematuria; and hemarthroses.
**h. A,** the most common type of hemophilia (q.v.), an X-linked condition caused by deficiency of coagulation factor VIII. Called also *classical h.*
**h. B,** a common type of hemophilia (q.v.), an X-linked condition caused by deficiency of coagulation factor IX. Called also *Christmas disease.*
**h. B, Leyden,** a transient form in which there is a deficiency of coagulation factor IX, the bleeding tendency abating after puberty.
**h. C,** an autosomal disorder due to lack of coagulation factor XI; seen predominantly in persons of Ashkenazi Jewish ancestry and characterized by recurring episodes of minor bleeding and mild bruising, menorrhagia, severe prolonged postsurgical bleeding, and prolonged recalcification and partial thromboplastin times. Called also *plasma thromboplastin antecedent deficiency, PTA deficiency,* and *Rosenthal syndrome.*
**classical h.,** h. A.
**vascular h.,** von Willebrand's disease.

**he·mo·phil·i·ac** (he″mo-fil′e-ak) an individual exhibiting hemophilia.

**he·mo·phil·ic** (he-mo-fil′ik) 1. having an affinity for blood; living in blood. In bacteriology, growing especially well in culture media containing blood or having a nutritional affinity for constituents of fresh blood; said of bacteria of the genera *Haemophilus* and *Bordetella.* 2. pertaining to or characterized by hemophilia.

**he·mo·phil·i·oid** (he″mo-fil′e-oid) [*hemophilia* + *-oid*] resembling hemophilia but not due solely to a deficiency of factor VIII, such as any of the hemorrhagic disorders due to deficiencies of other coagulation factors.

**He·moph·i·lus** (he-mof′ĭ-ləs) *Haemophilus.*

**he·moph·i·lus** (he-mof′ĭ-ləs) any bacterium of the genus *Haemophilus.*

**he·mo·pho·bia** (he″mo-fo′be-ə) [*hemo-* + *-phobia*] irrational fear of blood.

**he·moph·thal·mia** (he″mof-thal′me-ə) hemophthalmos.

**he·moph·thal·mos** (he″mof-thal′mos) [*hemo-* + Gr. *ophthalmos* eye] an extravasation of blood within the eye.

**he·moph·thal·mus** (he″mof-thal′məs) hemophthalmos.

**he·moph·thi·sis** (he-mof′thĭ-sis) [*hemo-* + Gr. *phthisis* wasting] old term for any anemia due to insufficient nutrition of blood cells.

**he·mo·pi·ezom·e·ter** (he″mo-pi″ə-zom′ə-tər) [*hemo-* + Gr. *piesis* pressure + *meter*] any apparatus for measuring blood pressure.

**he·mo·plas·tic** (he″mo-plas′tik) hematopoietic.

**he·mo·pleu·ra** (he″mo-ploor′ə) hemothorax.

**he·mo·pneu·mo·peri·car·di·um** (he″mo-noo″mo-per″ĭ-kahr′de-əm) pneumohemopericardium.

**he·mo·pneu·mo·tho·rax** (he″mo-noo″mo-thor′aks) [MeSH: Hemopneumothorax] pneumothorax with hemorrhagic effusion; called also *pneumohemothorax.*

**he·mo·poi·e·sis** (he″mo-poi-e′sis) hematopoiesis.

**he·mo·poi·et·ic** (he″mo-poi-et′ik) hematopoietic.

**he·mo·poi·e·tin** (he″mo-poi-e′tin) [*hemo-* + Gr. *poein* to make] erythropoietin.

**he·mo·po·sia** (he″mo-po′zhə) [*hemo-* + *-posia*] hematophagia.

**he·mo·pre·cip·i·tin** (he″mo-pre-sip′ĭ-tin) a precipitin that precipitates leukoantigens.

**he·mo·proc·tia** (he″mo-prok′shə) [*hemo-* + *proct-* + *-ia*] hemorrhage from the rectum.

**he·mo·pro·tein** (he″mo-pro′tēn) a conjugated protein containing heme as the prosthetic group; examples include catalase, cytochrome, hemoglobin, and myoglobin.

**he·mop·so·nin** (he″mop-so′nin) [*hemo-* + *opsonin*] an opsonin that renders red blood cells more liable to phagocytosis.

**he·mop·tic, he·mop·to·ic** (he-mop-to′ik) hemoptysic.

**he·mop·ty·sic** (he″mop-ti′sik) pertaining to or marked by hemoptysis.

**he·mop·ty·sis** (he-mop′tĭ-sis) [*hemo-* + Gr. *ptyein* to spit] [MeSH: Hemoptysis] the expectoration of blood or of blood-stained sputum.
**cardiac h.,** hemoptysis due to heart disease and related pulmonary hypertension, as in mitral stenosis or Eisenmenger's syndrome.
**endemic h.,** parasitic h.
**Goldstein's h.,** hemoptysis due to bleeding telangiectases in the tracheobronchial tree.
**Manson's h.,** parasitic h.
**Oriental h.,** parasitic h.
**parasitic h.,** a type of paragonimiasis, usually infestation with *Paragonimus westermani;* symptoms include coughing, spitting of blood, and gradual deterioration of health. Called also *endemic, Manson's,* or *Oriental h.*
**vicarious h.,** that which occurs at the time of normal menstruation; see *vicarious menstruation.*

**he·mo·py·elec·ta·sis** (he″mo-pi-ə-lek′tə-sis) [*hemo-* + *pyelectasis*] dilatation of the renal pelvis with an accumulation of bloody fluid.

**he·mo·rhe·ol·o·gy** (he″mo-re-ol′ə-je) [*hemo-* + *rheology*] [MeSH: Hemorheology] the scientific study of the deformation and flow properties of cellular and plasmatic components of blood in macroscopic, microscopic, and submicroscopic dimensions, and the rheological properties of vessel structure with which the blood comes in direct contact. Also spelled *hemorrheology.*

**he·mor·rha·chis** (he-mor′ə-kis) hematomyelia.

**hem·or·rhage** (hem′ə-rəj) [*hemo-* + *-rrhage*] [MeSH: Hemorrhage] the escape of blood from the vessels; bleeding. Small hemorrhages are classified according to size as petechiae (very small), purpura (up to 1 cm), and ecchymoses (larger). A large accumulation of blood within a tissue is called a hematoma. See also *bleeding.*
**alveolar h.,** hemorrhage from a dental alveolus.
**arterial h.,** the escape of blood from an artery, e.g., ruptured aneurysm.
**brain h.,** cerebral h.
**capillary h.,** the oozing of blood from the minute vessels.
**capsuloganglionic h.,** hemorrhage into the basal ganglia and internal and external capsule of the brain.
**cerebral h.,** a hemorrhage into the cerebrum. See also *stroke syndrome,* under *syndrome.* Called also *intracerebral* or *parenchymatous h.*
**concealed h.,** internal h.
**Duret's h's,** small, linear hemorrhages in the midline of the brainstem and upper pons caused by traumatic downward displacement of the brainstem.
**expulsive h.,** hemorrhage of the eye, breaking through both the choroid and the retina and extruding the ocular contents before it; usually occurring during the course of intraocular surgical procedure.
**external h.,** one in which blood escapes from the body.
**extradural h.,** intracranial hemorrhage into the epidural space.
**fetomaternal h.,** the leakage of fetal red blood cells into the maternal circulation.
**fibrinolytic h.,** that due to abnormalities of fibrinolysis rather than hypofibrinogenemia.
**flame-shaped h's,** large hemorrhagic spots in the eyeground; called also *flame spots.*
**internal h.,** hemorrhage in which the extravasated blood remains within the body.
**intracerebral h.,** cerebral h.
**intracranial h.,** bleeding within the cranium, which may be extradural, subdural, subarachnoid, or cerebral (parenchymatous). See also *stroke syndrome,* under *syndrome.*
**intramedullary h.,** hematomyelia.
**intrapartum h.,** hemorrhage occurring during parturition.
**intraventricular h.,** cerebral hemorrhage into the ventricles.
**massive h.,** loss of blood so rapid and profuse that shock supervenes unless appropriate replacement is instituted promptly.
**nasal h.,** epistaxis.
**parenchymatous h.,** 1. hemorrhage into the parenchyma of an organ. 2. cerebral h.
**h. per rhexin,** hemorrhage from rupture of a blood vessel.
**petechial h.,** hemorrhage from capillary leakage at minute points beneath the skin; called also *punctate h.*
**postpartum h.,** that which occurs soon after labor or childbirth.
**pulmonary h.,** hemorrhage from the lungs; called also *pneumorrhagia.*
**punctate h.,** petechial h.
**renal h.,** hemorrhage from the kidney; nephrorrhagia.
**splinter h's,** linear hemorrhages beneath the nail; when located near the base of the nail they are characteristic of subacute bacterial endocarditis.
**spontaneous h.,** bleeding occurring without overt provocation.
**subarachnoid h.,** intracranial hemorrhage into the subarachnoid space.
**subdural h.,** cerebral hemorrhage into the subdural space; see also *subdural hematoma, under hematoma,* and *stroke syndrome,* under *syndrome.*
**venous h.,** the escape of blood from a vein.

**hem·or·rha·gen·ic** (hem″o-rə-jen′ik) [*hemorrhage* + *-genic*] causing hemorrhage.

**hem·or·rha·gic** (hem″ə-raj′ik) pertaining to or characterized by hemorrhage.

**hem·or·rha·gin** (hem″ə-ra′jin) a cytolysin existing in certain venoms and poisons, such as snake venom and ricin, which is destructive to endothelial cells and blood vessels. Cf. *endotheliotoxin.*

**he·mor·rhe·ol·o·gy** (he″mo-re-ol′ə-je) hemorheology.

**hem·or·rhoid** (hem′ə-roid) [Gr. *haimorrhois*] [MeSH: Hemorrhoids] a varicose dilatation of a vein of the superior or inferior hemorrhoidal plexus, resulting from a persistent increase in venous pressure.
**combined h.,** mixed h.
**external h.,** a varicose dilatation of a vein of the inferior hemorrhoidal plexus, situated distal to the pectinate line and covered with modified anal skin.
**internal h.,** a varicose dilatation of a vein of the superior hemorrhoidal plexus, originating above the pectinate line, and covered by mucous membrane.
**mixed h.,** a varicose dilatation of a vein connecting the superior and inferior hemorrhoidal plexuses, forming an external and an internal hemorrhoid in continuity.
**mucocutaneous h.,** mixed h.
**prolapsed h.,** an internal hemorrhoid which has descended below the pectinate line and protruded outside the anal sphincter.
**strangulated h.,** an internal hemorrhoid which has been prolapsed sufficiently and for long enough time for its blood supply to become occluded by the constricting action of the anal sphincter.
**thrombosed h.,** one containing clotted blood.

**hem·or·rhoi·dal** (hem″o-roi′dəl) 1. pertaining to, or of the nature of, hemorrhoids. 2. an old anatomical term now synonymous with *rectal.*

**hem·or·rhoid·ec·to·my** (hem″ə-roid-ek′tə-me) excision of hemorrhoids.

**he·mo·sal·pinx** (he″mo-sal′pinks) [*hemo-* + *salpinx*] hematosalpinx.

**he·mo·sid·er·in** (he″mo-sid′ər-in) [*hemo-* + Gr. *sidēros* iron] [MeSH: Hemosiderin] an intracellular storage form of iron, found in the form of pigmented yellow to brown granules consisting of a complex of ferric hydroxides, polysaccharides, and proteins with an iron content of about 33 per cent by weight.

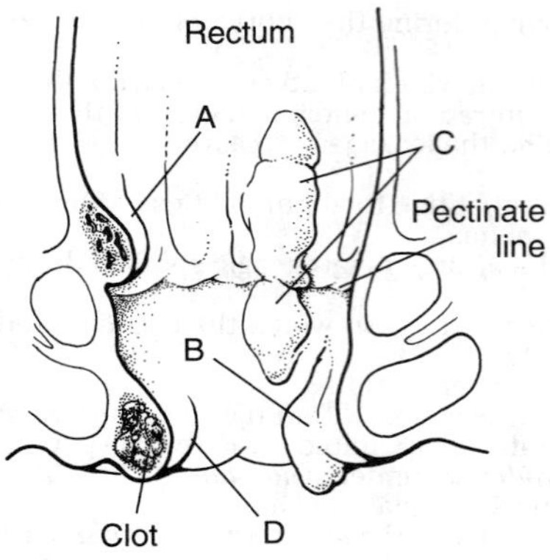

Hemorrhoids: *(A)*, internal; *(B)*, external; *(C)*, combined; *(D)*, thrombosed.

**he·mo·sid·er·in·uria** (he″mo-sid″ər-ĭ-nu′re-ə) the presence of hemosiderin in the urine.

**he·mo·sid·er·o·sis** (he″mo-sid″ər-o′sis) [MeSH: Hemosiderosis] a focal or general increase in tissue iron stores without associated tissue damage. Cf. *hemochromatosis.*
**hepatic h.,** the deposit of an abnormal quantity of hemosiderin in the liver, usually in Kupffer cells, which is not associated with cirrhosis, as is hemochromatosis.
**pulmonary h.,** the deposition of abnormal amounts of hemosiderin in the lungs, due to bleeding into the lung. The hemosiderin is found mainly in macrophages in the air spaces, but also in the interstitium. It is seen in any condition, such as severe congestive heart failure, in which repeated hemorrhages into the lungs occur.

**he·mo·sper·mia** (he″mo-spər′me-ə) [*hemo-* + *sperm* + *-ia*] the presence of blood in the semen.

**he·mo·spo·ri·an** (he″mo-spor′e-ən) 1. any protozoan of the suborder Haemosporina. 2. pertaining to protozoa of the suborder Haemosporina. Called also *hemosporidian.*

**he·mo·spo·rid·i·an** (he″mo-spor-id′e-ən) hemosporian.

**he·mo·sta·sia** (he″mo-sta′zhə) hemostasis.

**he·mo·sta·sis** (he″mo-sta′sis, he-mos′tə-sis) [*hemo-* + *stasis*] [MeSH: Hemostasis] 1. arrest of bleeding, either by the physiological properties of vasoconstriction and coagulation or by surgical means. 2. interruption of blood flow through a vessel or to a part.

**he·mo·stat** (he′mo-stat) 1. a small surgical clamp for constricting a blood vessel. 2. an agent that checks hemorrhage when properly applied to a bleeding point.

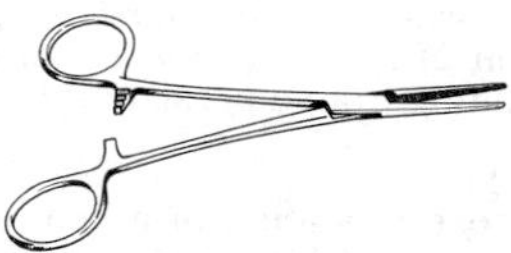
Hemostat.

**he·mo·stat·ic** (he″mo-stat′ik) [*hemo-* + *-static*] 1. causing hemostasis. 2. an agent that arrests the flow of blood. 3. due to or characterized by stasis of the blood; called also *hematostatic.*
**capillary h.,** an agent that reduces capillary bleeding time by increasing the contractility and resistance and decreasing the permeability of the capillary wall.

**he·mo·styp·tic** (he″mo-stip′tik) hemostatic.

**he·mo·ther·a·peu·tics** (he″mo-ther″ə-pu′tiks) hemotherapy.

**he·mo·ther·a·py** (he″mo-ther′ə-pe) [*hemo-* + *therapy*] treatment of disease by the administration of blood or blood products, such as blood plasma. Called also *hematherapy* and *hematotherapy.*

**he·mo·tho·rax** (he″mo-thor′aks) [*hemo-* + *thorax*] [MeSH: Hemothorax] a pleural effusion containing blood. Cf. *hemorrhagic pleurisy.* Called also *hemathorax, hematothorax,* and *hemopleura.*

**he·mo·tox·ic** (he″mo-tok′sik) hematotoxic.

**he·mo·tox·in** (he″mo-tok′sin) an exotoxin that causes hemolysis; see also *hemolysin.*
**cobra h.,** the constituent of cobra venom which is able to lyse red blood cells of man and of various other animals without the presence of blood serum.

**he·mo·troph** (he′mo-trof) [*hemo-* + Gr. *trophē* nourishment] the totality of the nutritive substances supplied to the embryo from the maternal blood during gestation. Cf. *histotroph.*

**he·mo·trophe** (he′mo-trof) hemotroph.

**he·mo·troph·ic** (he″mo-trof′ik) pertaining to or derived through hemotroph.

**he·mo·trop·ic** (he″mo-trop′ik) hematotropic.

**he·mo·tym·pa·num** (he″mo-tim′pə-nəm) a hemorrhagic exudation into the middle ear; called also *hematotympanum.*

**he·mo·zo·ic** (he″mo-zo′ik) hematozoan, def. 1.

**he·mo·zo·in** (he″mo-zo′in) [*hemo-* + Gr. *zōon* animal] a pigment produced by malarial parasites, derived from the hemoglobin in the host's cells, and consisting of insoluble ferriprotoporphyrin polymers that enable the parasites to sequester in benign form. In chronic cases of malaria, hemozoin collects in tissues, e.g., the spleen, giving the organ a grayish to dark brown or black color. Also written *haemozoin.*

**he·mo·zo·on** (he″mo-zo′on) [*hemo-* + Gr. *zōon* animal] hematozoan, def. 2.

**hem·pa** (hem′pə) [MeSH: Hempa] a colorless liquid with an ammonia-like odor, used as a de-icing additive in jet fuel, as a solvent, and as a chemosterilant for insect pests; it is carcinogenic. Called also *hexamethylphosphoramide* and abbreviated *HMPA.*

**HEM·PAS** (hem′pəs) [*h*ereditary *e*rythroblastic *m*ultinuclearity with *p*ositive *a*cidified *s*erum] the most common type of congenital dyserythropoietic anemia.

**hem·ure·sis** (hem″u-re′sis) [*hem-* + *uresis*] the voiding of bloody urine.

**hen·bane** (hen′bān) 1. *Hyoscyamus niger.* 2. hyoscyamus.

**Hench** (hench) Philip Showalter. American physician, 1896–1965; co-winner, with Edward Calvin Kendall and Tadeus Reichstein, of the Nobel prize for medicine or physiology in 1950 for his treatment of rheumatoid arthritis with ACTH and cortisone.

**Hench-Ro·sen·berg syndrome** (hench-ro′zən-bərg) [P.S. *Hench;* Edward Frank *Rosenberg,* American physician, born 1908] palindromic rheumatism; see under *rheumatism.*

**Hen·der·son-Has·sel·balch equation** (hen′dər-sən-has′əl-bawlk) [Lawrence Joseph *Henderson,* American chemist, 1878–1942; Karl A. *Hasselbalch,* Danish biochemist, 1874–1962] see under *equation.*

**Hen·der·son-Jones disease** (hen′dər-sən-jōz′) [Melvin Starkey *Henderson,* American orthopedic surgeon, 1883–1954; Hugh T. *Jones,* American orthopedic surgeon, 20th century] see under *disease.*

**Hen·der·son·u·la** (hen″dər-son′u-lə) a genus of Fungi Imperfecti of the form-class Coelomycetes. *H. toruloi′dea* has been isolated from numerous cases of dermatomycosis and phaeohyphomycosis; it is a synanamorph of *Scytalidium hyalinum.*

**Hen·der·son-Pat·er·son bodies** (hen′dər-sən pat′ər-sən) [William *Henderson,* Scottish pathologist, 1810–1872; Robert *Paterson,* Scottish physician, 1814–1889] molluscum bodies.

**Hen·ke's space, triangle (trigone)** (heng′kəz) [Philipp Jakob Wilhelm *Henke,* German anatomist, 1834–1896] see under *space* and *triangle.*

**Hen·le's loop,** etc. (hen′lēz) [Friedrich Gustav Jakob *Henle,* German anatomist, 1809–1885] see under *fiber, gland, layer, membrane, reaction,* and *sphincter,* and see *ampulla ductus deferentis, ansa nephroni, falx inguinalis,* and *spina suprameatica.*

**Henne·bert's sign** (en″ə-bārz′) [Camille *Hennebert,* Belgian otologist, 1867–1958] see under *sign.*

**Hen·ning's sign** (hen′ingz) [Wilhelm *Hennings,* German physician, 1716–1794] see under *sign.*

**He·noch's purpura** (hĕ″nawks) [Edouard Heinrich *Henoch,* German pediatrist, 1820–1910] see under *purpura.*

**He·noch-Schön·lein purpura (syndrome)** (hĕ′nawk-shern′līn) [E.H. *Henoch;* Johann Lukas *Schönlein,* German physician, 1793–1864] Schönlein-Henoch purpura.

**heno·gen·e·sis** (hen″o-jen′ə-sis) [Gr. *hen* one + *-genesis*] ontogeny.

**Hen·ry's law** (hen′rēz) [William *Henry,* English chemist, 1774–1836] see under *law.*

**hen·ry** (hen′re) [Joseph *Henry,* American physicist, 1797–1878] the unit of electric inductance, equivalent to one weber per ampere. Symbol H.

**Hen·sen's body,** etc. (hen′sənz) [Victor *Hensen,* German anatomist and physiologist, 1835–1924] see under *body, cell, knot,* and *node,* see *H band* and *M band,* under *band,* and see *ductus reuniens.*

**Hen·sing's ligament (fold)** (hen′singz) [Frederich Wilhelm *Hensing,* German anatomist, 1719–1745] see under *ligament.*

**HEP** hepatoerythropoietic porphyria.

**Hep·aci·vi·rus** (hep-as'ĭ-vi"rəs) [*hepatitis C* + *virus*] the hepatitis C–like viruses: a genus of viruses of the family Flaviviridae consisting of hepatitis C virus and related viruses.

**Hep·ad·na·vi·ri·dae** (hep-ad"nə-vir'ĭ-de) [*hepat-* + *DNA* + *virus*] [MeSH: Hepadnaviridae] the hepatitis B–like viruses: a family of DNA viruses having a virion 42 nm in diameter consisting of a lipid-containing envelope (containing hepatitis B surface antigen, HBsAg) surrounding an icosahedral nucleocapsid (containing hepatitis B core antigen, HBcAg). The genome consists of a single circular molecule of DNA that contains a large single-stranded gap (size of fully double-stranded molecule 3.2 kbp). Viruses contain two major polypeptides composing HBsAg, one composing HBcAg, and a number of others comprising the e antigen (HBeAg); they are resistant to heat and organic solvents. Replication occurs in the nuclei of hepatocytes. HBsAg occurs in the cytoplasm and shedding of 22-nm HBsAg particles into the bloodstream produces antigenemia. Persistent infection is common and is associated with chronic disease and neoplasia. There are two genera, one *(Orthohepadnavirus)* containing species infecting mammals and the other *(Avihepadnavirus)* containing species infecting birds.

**Hep·ad·na·vi·rus** (hep-ad'nə-vi"rəs) [MeSH: Hepadnaviridae] a former genus of the Hepadnaviridae; see *Avihepadnavirus* and *Orthohepadnavirus.*

**hep·ad·na·vi·rus** (hep-ad'nə-vi"rəs) [MeSH: Hepadnaviridae] any virus belonging to the family Hepadnaviridae.

**he·par** (he'par) [Gr. *hēpar* liver] 1. [TA] the liver (q.v.), a large gland of a dark red color situated in the upper part of the abdomen on the right side. 2. the liver of certain animals, used in pharmaceutical preparations.

**h. adipo'sum,** fatty liver.

**h. loba'tum,** a liver divided into numerous lobes by deep fissures produced by syphilis.

**h. sicca'tum,** the dried and powdered liver of pigs; used as a food and medicine in organic diseases of the liver.

**hep·a·ran-α-glu·co·sam·i·nide *N*-ac·e·tyl·trans·fer·ase** (hep'ə-ran gloo"ko-sam'ĭ-nīd as"ə-tēl-trans'fər-ās) [EC 2.3.1.78] a lysosomal enzyme of the transferase class that catalyzes the acetylation of the amino groups of terminal desulfated glucosamine residues in heparan sulfate chains, a step in the degradation of heparan sulfate. Acetyl coenzyme A is the acetyl donor. Deficiency of the enzyme, an autosomal recessive trait, results in Sanfilippo's syndrome, type C. Called also *acetyl CoA:α-glucosaminide* N-*acetyltransferase.*

**hep·a·ran *N*-sul·fa·tase** (hep'ə-ran sul'fə-tās) a lysosomal enzyme of the hydrolase class that catalyzes the removal of sulfate from terminal *N*-sulfated glucosamine residues of heparan sulfate chains. Deficiency of the enzyme, an autosomal recessive trait, causes Sanfilippo's syndrome, type A. See also N-*sulfoglucosamine sulfohydrolase.*

**hep·a·ran sul·fate** (hep'ə-ran) a glycosaminoglycan occurring in the cell membrane of most cells. It consists of repeating disaccharide units in specific linkage, each composed of a glucosamine residue linked to a uronic acid, either glucuronic acid or L-iduronic acid, which may be sulfated. The glucosamine residues frequently contain acetyl or sulfate group substituents. It is an accumulation product in several mucopolysaccharidoses.

**hep·a·ran sul·fate sul·fam·i·dase** (hep'ə-ran sul'fāt səl-fam'ĭ-dās) heparan *N*-sulfatase.

**hep·a·rin** (hep'ə-rin) [Gr. *hēpar* liver] [MeSH: Heparin] a sulfated glycosaminoglycan of mixed polysaccharide nature varying in molecular weights and composed of polymers of alternating derivatives of D-glycosamine and L-iduronic acid or D-glucuronic acid; it is released by mast cells and by basophils of the blood and is present in many tissues, especially the liver and lungs. Heparin is a mixture of active principles, some of which have potent anticoagulant properties that result from binding to and greatly enhancing the activity of antithrombin III and from inhibition of a number of coagulation factors, particularly activated factor X (factor Xa). Heparin also has lipotrophic properties, promoting transfer of fat from the blood to the fat depots by activation of lipoprotein lipase.

**h. calcium** [USP], the calcium salt of the mixture of active principles that compose heparin, usually obtained from the intestinal mucosa or other suitable tissues of domestic food animals; used in the prophylaxis and treatment of disorders in which there is undesirable or excessive clotting, such as deep venous thrombosis, thromboembolism, and disseminated intravascular coagulation and to prevent clotting during extracorporeal circulation, blood transfusion, and blood sampling. Administered intravenously or subcutaneously.

**h. sodium** [USP], the sodium salt of the mixture of active principles that compose heparin, usually obtained from the intestinal mucosa or other suitable tissues of domestic food animals, and having the same indications, uses, and routes of administration as the calcium salt.

**hep·a·rin·ate** (hep'ə-rin-āt) any salt of heparin.

**hep·a·rin·emia** (hep"ə-rĭ-ne'me-ə) the presence of heparin in the blood.

**hep·a·ri·nize** (hep'ə-rĭ-nīz") to treat with heparin in order to increase the clotting time of the blood.

**hep·a·ri·tin sul·fate** (hep'ə-rĭ-tin) [MeSH: Heparitin Sulfate] heparan sulfate.

**hep·a·tal·gia** (hep"ə-tal'jə) [*hepat-* + *-algia*] pain in the liver; called also *hepatodynia.*

**hep·a·ta·tro·phia** (hep"ə-tə-tro'fe-ə) [*hepat-* + *atrophia*] atrophy of the liver.

**hep·a·tat·ro·phy** (hep"ə-tat'rə-fe) hepatatrophia.

**hep·a·tec·to·mize** (hep"ə-tek'to-mīz) to deprive of the liver by surgical removal.

**hep·a·tec·to·my** (hep"ə-tek'tə-me) [*hepat-* + *-ectomy*] [MeSH: Hepatectomy] excision of all *(total h.)* or part *(partial* or *subtotal h.)* of the liver.

**he·pat·ic** (hə-pat'ik) [L. *hepaticus;* Gr. *hēpatikos*] pertaining to the liver.

**hepatic(o)-** [Gr. *hēpatikos* of the liver] a combining form denoting relationship to a hepatic duct, or, sometimes, to the liver.

**he·pat·ic li·pase** (hə-pat'ik li'pās) see under *lipase.*

**he·pat·i·co·cho·lan·gio·je·ju·nos·to·my** (hə-pat'ĭ-ko-ko-lan"je-o-je"joo-nos'to-me) surgical creation of a communication between the hepatic duct, another biliary duct, and the jejunum.

**he·pat·i·co·cho·led·o·chos·to·my** (hə-pat'ĭ-ko-ko-led"o-kos'tə-me) surgical anastomosis of the hepatic duct and the common bile duct.

**he·pat·i·co·do·chot·o·my** (hə-pat"ĭ-ko-do-kot'ə-me) surgical incision of the hepatic duct and the common bile duct.

**he·pat·i·co·du·o·de·nos·to·my** (hə-pat"ĭ-ko-doo"o-də-nos'tə-me) surgical creation of a communication between the hepatic duct and the duodenum.

**he·pat·i·co·en·ter·os·to·my** (hə-pat"ĭ-ko-en"tər-os'tə-me) [*hepatico-* + *enterostomy*] surgical creation of a communication between the hepatic duct and the intestine.

**he·pat·i·co·gas·tros·to·my** (hə-pat"ĭ-ko-gas-tros'tə-me) [*hepatico-* + *gastrostomy*] surgical creation of a communication between the hepatic duct and the stomach.

**he·pat·i·co·je·ju·nos·to·my** (hə-pat"ĭ-ko-jə-joo-nos'tə-me) [*hepatico-* + *jejunostomy*] surgical creation of a communication between the hepatic duct and the jejunum.

**Hep·a·tic·o·la** (hep"ə-tik'o-lə) *Capillaria.*

**he·pat·i·co·li·a·sis** (hə-pat"ĭ-ko-li'ə-sis) capillariasis.

**he·pat·i·co·li·thot·o·my** (hə-pat"ĭ-ko-lĭ-thot'ə-me) incision of the hepatic duct and removal of one or more calculi.

**he·pat·i·co·litho·trip·sy** (hə-pat"ĭ-ko-lith'o-trip-se) the operation of crushing a stone in the hepatic duct.

**he·pat·i·co·pul·mo·nary** (hə-pat"ĭ-ko-pul'mo-nar"e) hepatopneumonic.

**he·pat·i·cos·to·my** (hə-pat"ĭ-kos'tə-me) [*hepatico-* + *-stomy*] surgical creation of an artificial opening into the hepatic duct.

**he·pat·i·cot·o·my** (hə-pat"ŏ-kot'ə-me) [*hepatico-* + *-tomy*] incision of the hepatic duct.

**he·pat·ic phos·phor·y·lase** (hə-pat'ik fos-for'ə-lās) the liver isozyme of glycogen phosphorylase.

**he·pat·ic phos·phor·y·lase de·fi·cien·cy** glycogen storage disease, type VI.

**he·pat·ic phos·phor·y·lase ki·nase** (hə-pat'ik fos-for'ə-lās ki'nās) the liver isozyme of phosphorylase kinase.

**he·pat·ic phos·phor·y·lase ki·nase de·fi·cien·cy** phosphorylase *b* kinase deficiency.

**hep·a·tism** (hep'ə-tiz-əm) ill health due to liver disease.

**hep·a·tit·i·des** (hep"ə-tit'ĭ-dēz) [MeSH: Hepatitis] plural of *hepatitis.*

**hep·a·ti·tis** (hep"ə-ti'tis) pl. *hepatit'ides* [*hepat-* + *-itis*] [MeSH: Hepatitis] inflammation of the liver.

**h. A,** a self-limited viral disease of worldwide distribution caused by the hepatitis A virus, which is more prevalent in areas of poor hygiene and low socioeconomic standards, being transmitted almost exclusively by the fecal-oral route, although parenteral transmission is possible; there is no carrier state. The incubation period is about

30 days, with a range of 15 to 50 days. Most cases are clinically inapparent or have mild flulike symptoms; jaundice, if present, is usually mild. Massive hepatic necrosis (fulminant hepatitis) can occur but much less commonly than with hepatitis B or C. Formerly called *epidemic h.* or *jaundice, infectious h., MS-1 h.,* and *short-incubation h.*
**acute parenchymatous h.,** massive hepatic necrosis.
**alcoholic h.,** liver inflammation resulting from alcoholism, often a precursor of cirrhosis of the liver.
**amebic h.,** invasion of liver parenchyma by trophozoites of *Entamoeba histolytica,* leading to amebic abscess.
**anicteric h.,** viral hepatitis without jaundice.
**autoimmune h.,** an autoimmune disease of the liver, occurring chiefly in females, characterized by circulating autoantibodies and hypergammaglobulinemia and associated with extrahepatic complaints such as malaise, fever, and arthralgia. *Type 1* is characterized by antinuclear and anti–smooth muscle antibodies; *type 2* is less common and is characterized by antibodies against the microsomal antigen of liver and kidney.
**avian infectious h., avian vibrionic h.,** avian campylobacteriosis.
**h. B,** a viral disease caused by the hepatitis B virus that is endemic worldwide, the areas of highest endemicity being China and Southeast Asia, sub-Saharan Africa, most Pacific islands, and the Amazon basin. The virus is shed in all body fluids by individuals with acute or chronic infections and by asymptomatic carriers, and is transmitted primarily by parenteral routes, such as by blood transfusion or by sharing of needles among drug users; oral transmission can occur but has low efficiency, and it can be spread by intimate personal contact, especially sexual contact, and by vertical transmission from mother to neonate. The incubation period averages about 90 days, with a range of 40 to 180 days, and the clinical course is more variable than in hepatitis A. In the prodromal phase there may be fever, malaise, anorexia, nausea, and vomiting, which decline with the onset of clinical jaundice, and urticaria, angioedema, arthritis, or, rarely, glomerulonephritis or a serum sickness–like syndrome may occur. Most patients recover completely and become $HB_SAg$-negative in 3 to 4 months, but some remain chronic carriers or develop chronic active hepatitis or chronic persistent hepatitis. Massive hepatic necrosis (fulminant hepatitis) is an infrequent complication. In areas of high endemicity a relationship has been shown between hepatitis and virus infection, cirrhosis, and primary hepatocellular carcinoma, with the latter being one of the most common neoplasms. Formerly called *inoculation h., long-incubation h., MS-2 h., serum h.,* and *homologous serum h.* or *jaundice.* See also under *antigen.*
**h. C,** a viral disease caused by the hepatitis C virus, the most common form of post-transfusion hepatitis; it also follows parenteral drug abuse and is a common acute sporadic hepatitis, with approximately 50 per cent of acutely infected persons developing chronic hepatitis. Chronic infection is generally mild and asymptomatic, but cirrhosis may occur. See also *chronic active h.* and *non-A, non-B h.*
**canine virus h.,** infectious canine h.
**cholangiolitic h.,** cholestatic h. (def. 1).
**cholangitic h.,** cholestatic h. (def. 1).
**cholestatic h.,** 1. a rare form of viral hepatitis in which there is cholestasis with obstructive jaundice, pruritus, dark urine, light stools, and elevated alkaline phosphatase and conjugated bilirubin and in which the course is prolonged compared to that of other forms. Called also *cholangitic h.* and *cholangiolitic h.* 2. hepatic inflammation and cholestasis resulting from reaction to drugs such as estrogens, methyltestosterone, and chlorpromazine.
**chronic active h.,** a chronic inflammation of the liver occurring as a sequel to hepatitis B or non-A, non-B hepatitis. The same disease may occur in congenital or acquired hypogammaglobulinemia, or in association with the administration of certain drugs. It is characterized by infiltration of portal areas by plasma cells and macrophages, piecemeal necrosis (destruction of hepatocytes in the periphery of lobules), and fibrosis. The course is highly variable; there may be long asymptomatic periods interspersed with periods of symptomatic hepatitis with jaundice, malaise, anorexia, and fever; there may be extrahepatic manifestations, including amenorrhea, arthritis, skin rashes, vasculitis, thyroiditis, glomerulonephritis ulcerative colitis, and Sjögren's syndrome; or the disease may progress to cirrhosis and liver failure. An autoimmune pathogenesis is suspected. Called also *chronic aggressive h., lupoid h., autoimmune h., plasma cell h., subacute h.,* and *acute juvenile cirrhosis.*
**chronic aggressive h.,** chronic active h.
**chronic interstitial h.,** cirrhosis of the liver.
**chronic persisting h.,** a chronic, nonprogressive inflammatory process affecting primarily the portal areas without producing fibrosis, necrosis, or cirrhosis, an uncommon sequel of viral hepatitis; the disease may be asymptomatic or may produce symptoms of mild hepatitis; it does not progress to cirrhosis or liver failure but may persist for years.
**h. contagio'sa ca'nis,** infectious canine h.
**h. D,** infection with the hepatitis D virus, requiring antecedent or simultaneous infection with hepatitis B virus; manifestations are similar to those of hepatitis B, whose severity it may increase. Called also *delta h.*
**delta h.,** h. D.
**duck virus h.,** a highly fatal, rapidly spreading disease of waterfowl ducklings, caused by a virus of the genus *Avihepadnavirus,* characterized primarily by hepatitis marked by an enlarged, mottled, hemorrhagic liver.
**h. E,** a type of hepatitis caused by a calcicivirus and transmitted by the fecal-oral route, usually via contaminated water; chronic infection does not occur, but acute hepatitis may be fatal in pregnant women. Called also *enterically transmitted non-A, non-B h.*
**enterically transmitted non-A, non-B h. (ET-NANB),** h. E.
**epidemic h.,** h. A.
**familial h.,** Wilson's disease.
**fatty liver h.,** nonalcoholic steatohepatitis.
**fulminant h.,** massive hepatic necrosis (q.v.) resulting from viral hepatitis, usually hepatitis B or non-A, non-B hepatitis.
**h. G,** a posttransfusion disease caused by the hepatitis G virus, ranging in severity from asymptomatic infection to fulminant hepatitis.
**giant cell h.,** neonatal h.
**halothane h.,** the extremely rare cases of transient jaundice or massive hepatic necrosis associated with halothane anesthesia.
**homologous serum h.,** h. B.
**inclusion body h.,** a viral disease of young chickens, caused by an adenovirus and characterized by hemorrhage, jaundice, and anemia; hepatocytes have eosinophilic inclusion bodies. Mortality in a flock may reach 25 per cent.
**infectious h.,** h. A.
**infectious canine h.,** a highly contagious type of hepatitis in canines, caused by an adenovirus; symptoms may be mild to severe and range from fever, vomiting, and abdominal pain to convulsions, hemorrhage, and death. Called also *canine virus h., h. contagiosa canis,* and *Rubarth's disease.*
**infectious necrotic h.,** a usually fatal infectious disease of sheep, and occasionally cattle, pigs, and horses, caused by multiplication of *Clostridium novyi* in areas of hepatic necrosis from liver flukes, with resultant septicemia. Called also *black disease.*
**inoculation h.,** h. B.
**long-incubation h.,** h. B.
**lupoid h.,** chronic active hepatitis with autoimmune manifestations. Called also *Bearn-Kunkel-Slater syndrome* and *Kunkel syndrome.*
**MS-1 h.,** h. A.
**MS-2 h.,** h. B.
**neonatal h.,** hepatitis of unknown etiology with onset in the first few weeks of life; some cases are associated with viral or bacterial infection; a few are familial. It is characterized by the transformation of hepatocytes into multinucleated giant cells and by conjugated hyperbilirubinemia with jaundice. Most patients recover completely, some develop chronic disease or fatal cirrhosis. Cf. *neonatal hemochromatosis.* Called also *giant cell h.*
**neonatal giant cell h.,** neonatal h.
**non-A–E h.,** viral hepatitis occurring without the serotypic markers of hepatitis viruses A, B, C, D or E.
**non-A, non-B h.,** acute viral hepatitis occurring without the serologic markers of hepatitis A or B, including hepatitis C and hepatitis E.
**plasma cell h.,** chronic active h.
**post-transfusion h.,** viral hepatitis transmitted via transfusion of blood or blood products, especially multiple pooled donor products such as clotting factor concentrates. Originally limited to hepatitis B, this now primarily refers to hepatitis C. Called also *transfusion h.*
**serum h.,** h. B.
**short-incubation h.,** h. A.
**subacute h.,** chronic active h.
**syncytial giant-cell h.,** h. G.
**toxic h.,** hepatitis produced by hepatotoxins such as *Amanita phalloides toxin,* carbon tetrachloride, yellow phosphorus, and a variety of drugs. Cf. *drug-induced h.*
**transfusion h.,** post-transfusion h.
**vibrionic h.,** avian campylobacteriosis.
**viral h.,** see *h. A, h. B, h. C, h. D,* and *h. E.*

**hep·a·ti·za·tion** (hep″ə-tĭ-za′shən) consolidation of tissue into a liverlike mass, especially as seen in the lung in pneumococcal pneumonia.
**gray h.,** a usually late stage of hepatization in which the affected lung tissue is grayish.
**red h.,** a usually early stage of hepatization in which the solidified lung tissue is red from excess of blood.
**yellow h.,** hepatization in which lung tissue is yellowish from a purulent exudate.

**hep·a·tized** (hep′ə-tīzd) changed into a liver-like substance.

**hepat(o)-** [Gr. *hēpar,* gen. *hēpatos* liver] combining form denoting relationship to the liver.

**hep·a·to·bil·i·ary** (hep″ə-to-bil′e-ar″e) pertaining to the liver and the bile or the biliary ducts.

**hep·a·to·blas·to·ma** (hep″ə-to-blas-to′mə) [MeSH: Hepatoblastoma] a malignant intrahepatic tumor occurring in infants and young children and consisting chiefly of embryonic hepatic tissue.

**hep·a·to·bron·chi·al** (hep″ə-to-brong′ke-əl) pertaining to or communicating with the liver and a bronchus, as a hepatobronchial fistula.

**hep·a·to·car·ci·no·gen·e·sis** (hep″ə-to-kahr″sĭ-no-jen′ə-sis) the production of carcinoma of the liver.

**hep·a·to·car·cin·o·gen·ic** (hep″ə-to-kahr″sĭ-no-jen′ik) causing carcinoma of the liver.

**hep·a·to·car·ci·no·ma** (hep″ə-to-kahr″sĭ-no′mə) hepatocellular carcinoma.

**hep·a·to·cele** (hə-pat′o-sēl) [*hepato-* + *-cele*[1]] hernial protrusion of a part of the liver.

**hep·a·to·cel·lu·lar** (hep″ə-to-sel′u-lər) pertaining to or affecting liver cells.

**hep·a·to·cho·lan·ge·itis** (hep″ə-to-ko-lan″je-i′tis) inflammation of the liver and bile ducts.

**hep·a·to·cho·lan·gio·car·ci·no·ma** (hep″ə-to-ko-lan″je-o-kahr″sĭ-no′mə) cholangiohepatoma.

**hep·a·to·cho·lan·gio·du·o·de·nos·to·my** (hep″ə-to-ko-lan″je-o-doo″o-də-nos′tə-me) the operation of establishing drainage of the hepatic duct into the duodenum.

**hep·a·to·cho·lan·gio·ent·er·os·to·my** (hep″ə-to-ko-lan″je-o-en″tər-os′tə-me) [*hepato-* + *cholangio-* + *enterostomy*] surgical creation of a communication between the hepatic duct and the intestine.

**hep·a·to·cho·lan·gio·gas·tros·to·my** (hep″ə-to-ko-lan″je-o-gas-tros′tə-me) the operation of establishing drainage of the hepatic duct into the stomach.

**hep·a·to·cho·lan·gi·os·to·my** (hep″ə-to-ko-lan″je-os′tə-me) the operation of establishing drainage of the hepatic duct either through the abdominal wall *(external h.)* or into some part of the gastrointestinal tract *(internal h.)*.

**hep·a·to·cho·lan·gi·tis** (hep″ə-to-ko″lan-ji′tis) inflammation of the liver and bile ducts.

**hep·a·to·cir·rho·sis** (hep″ə-to-sĭ-ro′sis) [*hepato-* + *cirrhosis*] cirrhosis of the liver.

**hep·a·to·col·ic** (hep″ə-to-kol′ik) pertaining to the liver and the colon.

**hep·a·to·cu·prein** (hep″ə-to-koo′prēn) a soluble, bluish-green copper protein present in liver tissue; it contains about 0.34 per cent copper.

**hep·a·to·cys·tic** (hep″ə-to-sis′tik) pertaining to the liver and gallbladder.

**Hep·a·to·cys·tis** (hep″ə-to-sis′tis) [*hepato-* + *cyst*] a genus of coccidian protozoa (suborder Haemosporina, subclass Sporozoea) comprising parasites of Old World lower monkeys, fruit bats, and squirrels, in which merogony takes place in the hepatocytes, resulting in large glistening schizonts (merocysts) on the surface of the liver, from which merozoites are released to invade erythrocytes and develop into gametocytes.

**hep·a·to·cyte** (hep′ə-to-sīt) a hepatic cell.
**ground-glass h.,** see under *cell.*

**hep·a·to·du·o·de·nos·to·my** (hep″ə-to-doo″o-də-nos′tə-me) [*hepato-* + *duodenostomy*] the surgical creation of a communication between the liver and the duodenum.

**hep·a·to·dyn·ia** (hep″ə-to-din′e-ə) [*hepat-* + *-odynia*] hepatalgia.

**hep·a·to·en·ter·ic** (hep″ə-to-ən-ter′ik) pertaining to the liver and intestine.

**hep·a·to·en·ter·os·to·my** (hep″ə-to-en″tər-os′tə-me) surgical creation of a communication between the liver and the intestine.

**hep·a·tof·u·gal** (hep″ə-tof′u-gəl) [*hepato-* + *-fugal*[2]] directed or flowing away from the liver.

**hep·a·to·gas·tric** (hep″ə-to-gas′trik) pertaining to the liver and stomach.

**hep·a·to·gen·ic** (hep″ə-to-jen′ik) 1. giving rise to or forming liver tissue. 2. hepatogenous.

**hep·a·tog·e·nous** (hep″ə-toj′ə-nəs) 1. produced in or originating in the liver. 2. hepatogenic.

**hep·a·to·gram** (hep′ə-to-gram) a radiograph of the liver.

**hep·a·tog·ra·phy** (hep″ə-tog′rə-fe) [*hepato-* + *-graphy*] the making of a radiograph of the liver.

**He·pat·o·lite** (hep′ə-to-līt″) trademark for a kit for the preparation of technetium Tc 99m disofenin.

**hep·a·toid** (hep′ə-toid) [*hepat-* + *-oid*] resembling the liver in structure.

**hep·a·to·jug·u·lar** (hep″ə-to-jug′u-lər) pertaining to the liver and jugular vein; see under *reflux.*

**hep·a·to·len·tic·u·lar** (hep″ə-to-lən-tik′u-lər) pertaining to the liver and the lenticular nucleus.

**hep·a·to·li·e·nal** (hep″ə-to-li-e′nəl) pertaining to the liver and spleen.

**hep·a·to·li·e·nog·ra·phy** (hep″ə-to-li″ə-nog′rə-fe) [*hepato-* + *lieno-* + *-graphy*] radiography of the liver and spleen after intravenous injection of an opaque medium.

**hep·a·to·li·e·no·meg·a·ly** (hep″ə-to-li″ə-no-meg′ə-le) hepatosplenomegaly.

**hep·a·to·lith** (hep′ə-to-lith″) [*hepato-* + *-lith*] a gallstone, especially one within the liver.

**hep·a·to·li·thec·to·my** (hep″ə-to-lĭ-thek′tə-me) [*hepato-* + *lithectomy*] removal of a calculus from the liver.

**hep·a·to·li·thi·a·sis** (hep″ə-to-lĭ-thi′ə-sis) [*hepato-* + *lithiasis*] the formation or presence of calculi in the intrahepatic biliary ducts.

**hep·a·tol·o·gist** (hep″ə-tol′ə-jist) a specialist in hepatology.

**hep·a·tol·o·gy** (hep″ə-tol′ə-je) [*hepato-* + *-logy*] the study of the liver.

**hep·a·tol·y·sin** (hep″ə-tol′ĭ-sin) a cytolysin destructive to liver cells.

**hep·a·tol·y·sis** (hep″ə-tol′ĭ-sis) [*hepato-* + *-lysis*] destruction of the liver cells.

**hep·a·to·lyt·ic** (hep″ə-to-lit′ik) pertaining to, characterized by, or causing hepatolysis.

**hep·a·to·ma** (hep″ə-to′mə) 1. a tumor of the liver. 2. hepatocellular carcinoma.
**fibrolamellar h.,** see under *carcinoma.*
**malignant h.,** hepatocellular carcinoma.

**hep·a·to·ma·la·cia** (hep″ə-to-mə-la′shə) [*hepato-* + *-malacia*] softening of the liver.

**hep·a·to·me·ga·lia** (hep″ə-to-mə-ga′le-ə) hepatomegaly.

**hep·a·to·meg·a·ly** (hep″ə-to-meg′ə-le) [*hepato-* + *-megaly*] [MeSH: Hepatomegaly] enlargement of the liver.

**hep·a·to·mel·a·no·sis** (hep″ə-to-mel″ə-no′sis) melanosis of the liver.

**hep·a·tom·e·try** (hep″ə-tom′ə-tre) determination of the size of the liver.

**hep·a·tom·pha·lo·cele** (hep″ə-tom′fə-lo-sēl) omphalocele with the liver also being projected into the membranous sac outside the abdomen.

**hep·a·tom·pha·los** (hep″ə-tom′fə-los) [*hepat-* + Gr. *omphalos* navel] projection of the liver through the abdominal wall near the umbilicus.

**hep·a·to·neph·ric** (hep″ə-to-nef′rik) pertaining to the liver and kidney.

**hep·a·to·ne·phrit·ic** (hep″ə-to-nə-frit′ik) pertaining to or characterized by hepatonephritis.

**hep·a·to·ne·phri·tis** (hep″ə-to-nə-fri′tis) [*hepato-* + *nephritis*] a form of severe jaundice due to simultaneous inflammation of the liver and kidneys from the same cause, e.g., leptospiral infection.

**hep·a·to·neph·ro·meg·a·ly** (hep″ə-to-nef″ro-meg′ə-le) [*hepato-* + *nephro-* + *-megaly*] enlargement of the liver and kidney.

**hep·a·to·pan·cre·as** (hep″ə-to-pang′kre-əs) any of certain digestive glands of invertebrates, as the so-called liver of certain crustaceans, which secretes a fluid acting on both fats and proteins.

**hep·a·to·path** (hep′ə-to-path) a person with liver disease.

**hep·a·top·a·thy** (hep″ə-top′ə-the) [*hepato-* + *-pathy*] any disease of the liver.

**hep·a·to·peri·to·ni·tis** (hep″ə-to-per″ĭ-to-ni′tis) [*hepato-* + *peritonitis*] inflammation of the peritoneum covering the liver.

**hep·a·top·e·tal** (hep″ə-top′ə-təl) [*hepato-* + *-petal*] directed or flowing toward the liver.

**hep·a·to·pexy** (hep″ə-to-pek′se) [*hepato-* + *-pexy*] surgical fixation of the displaced liver.

**hep·a·to·phle·bi·tis** (hep″ə-to-flə-bi′tis) inflammation of the veins of the liver.

**hep·a·to·phle·bog·ra·phy** (hep″ə-to-flə-bog′rə-fe) radiologic visualization of the outflow of the venous network of the liver performed through retrograde injection of a radiopaque solution.

**hep·a·to·pleu·ral** (hep″ə-to-ploor′əl) pertaining to the liver and the pleura, or communicating with the liver and pleural cavity, as a hepatopleural fistula.

**hep·a·to·pneu·mon·ic** (hep″ə-to-noo-mon′ik) [*hepato-* + *pneumonic*] pertaining to, affecting, or communicating with the liver and lungs; called also *hepaticopulmonary* and *hepatopulmonary.*

**hep·a·to·poi·e·tin A (HPTA)** (hep″ə-to-poi′ə-tin) hepatocyte growth factor.

**hep·a·to·por·tal** (hep″ə-to-por′təl) pertaining to the portal system of the liver.

**hep·a·to·por·to·en·ter·os·to·my** (hep″ə-to-por″to-en″tər-os′tə-me) portoenterostomy.

**hep·a·top·to·sis** (hep″ə-top-to′sis) [*hepato-* + *-ptosis*] 1. displacement of the liver because of laxness of suspensory ligaments, diminished tone of abdominal muscles, emphysema, right pleural effusion or empyema, subphrenic abscess, or spinal deformity. 2. positioning of the colon between liver and diaphragm on x-ray.

**hep·a·to·pul·mo·nary** (hep″ə-to-pul′mo-nar-e) hepatopneumonic.

**hep·a·to·re·nal** (hep″ə-to-re′nəl) pertaining to the liver and kidneys.

**hep·a·tor·rha·gia** (hep″ə-to-ra′jə) [*hepato-* + *-rrhagia*] hemorrhage from the liver.

**hep·a·tor·rha·phy** (hep″ə-tor′ə-fe) [*hepato-* + *-rrhaphy*] operative repair of the liver.

**hep·a·tor·rhea** (hep″ə-to-re′ə) [*hepato-* + *-rrhea*] a morbidly excessive secretion of bile; any morbid flow from the liver.

**hep·a·tor·rhex·is** (hep″ə-to-rek′sis) [*hepato-* + *-rrhexis*] rupture of the liver.

**hep·a·to·scan** (hep′ə-to-skan) a surface scintiscan of the liver.

**hep·a·tos·co·py** (hep″ə-tos′kə-pe) [*hepato-* + *-scopy*] examination of the liver.

**hep·a·to·sis** (hep″ə-to′sis) any functional disorder of the liver.
**h. diete′tica,** a form of vitamin E–selenium deficiency syndrome (q.v.) in pigs, characterized by necrosis of the liver, edema, and often sudden death. Called also *dietary hepatic necrosis.*
**serous h.,** veno-occlusive disease of the liver; see under *disease.*

**hep·a·to·so·le·no·trop·ic** (hep″ə-to-so-le″no-trop′ik) [*hepato-* + *soleno-* + *-tropic*] having an affinity for or exerting a specific effect on the cholangioles and interlobular ducts of the liver.

**hep·a·to·sple·ni·tis** (hep″ə-to-splə-ni′tis) inflammation of the liver and spleen.

**hep·a·to·sple·nog·ra·phy** (hep″ə-to-splə-nog′rə-fe) radiography of the liver and spleen.

**hep·a·to·sple·no·meg·a·ly** (hep″ə-to-sple″no-meg′ə-le) [*hepato-* + *spleno-* + *-megaly*] enlargement of the liver and spleen.

**hep·a·to·sple·nom·e·try** (hep″ə-to-splə-nom′ə-tre) determination of the size of the liver and spleen.

**hep·a·to·sple·nop·a·thy** (hep″ə-to-splə-nop′ə-the) any combined disorder of the liver and spleen.

**hep·a·tos·to·my** (hep″ə-tos′tə-me) [*hepato-* + *-stomy*] surgical creation of an opening into the liver.

**hep·a·to·ther·a·py** (hep″ə-to-ther′ə-pe) [*hepato-* + *therapy*] treatment of disease by the administration of liver or liver extract.

**hep·a·tot·o·my** (hep″ə-tot′ə-me) [*hepato-* + *-tomy*] surgical incision of the liver.
**transthoracic h.,** incision of the liver by resecting a rib, opening the pleural sac, and incising the diaphragm; often performed in two or three stages.

**hep·a·to·tox·ic** (hep″ə-to-tok′sik) toxic to liver cells.

**hep·a·to·tox·i·ci·ty** (hep″ə-to-tok-sis′ĭ-te) the quality or property of exerting a destructive or poisonous effect upon liver cells.

**hep·a·to·tox·in** (hep″ə-to-tok′sin) [*hepato-* + *toxin*] a toxin that destroys liver cells.

**hep·a·to·trop·ic** (hep″ə-to-trop′ik) [*hepato-* + *-tropic*] having a special affinity for or exerting a specific effect on the liver.

**Hep·a·to·vi·rus** (hep′əto-vi″rəs) [*hepato-* + *virus*] a genus of viruses of the family Picornaviridae, comprising the hepatitis A viruses.

**hep·a·tox·ic** (hep″ə-tok′sik) hepatotoxic.

**Hep·a·to·zo·on** (hep″ə-to-zo′on) [*hepato-* + Gr. *zōon* animal] a genus of coccidian protozoa (suborder Adeleina, order Eucoccidiida) found in the red blood cells of birds and mammals. *Haemobartonella canis* is transmitted to canines by the tick *Rhipicephalus sanguineus* (see *hepatozoonosis*). *H. muris,* found in the liver cells of rats, and *H. perniciosum,* found in dogs, are transmitted by the mite *Echinolaelaps echidninus.*

**hep·a·to·zoo·no·sis** (hep″ə-to-zo″o-no′sis) an infectious, sometimes fatal disease of dogs caused by *Hepatozoon canis,* and characterized by intermittent fever, emaciation, mild anemia, muscular hyperesthesia, especially affecting the back, purulent ocular and nasal discharge, and sometimes diarrhea.

**Hep·i·ce·brin** (hep″ĭ-se′brin) trademark for a preparation of hexavitamin.

**hept(a)-** [Gr. *hepta* seven] a combining form meaning seven.

**hep·ta·bar·bi·tal** (hep″tə-bahr′bĭ-təl) a short-acting barbiturate, used as a sedative and hypnotic, administered orally.

**hep·ta·chro·mic** (hep″tə-kro′mik) [*hepta-* + *chrom-* + *-ic*] 1. pertaining to or exhibiting seven colors. 2. able to distinguish all seven colors of the spectrum; possessing full color vision.

**hep·tad** (hep′təd) any element having a valency of seven.

**hep·ta·dac·tyl·ia** (hep″tə-dak-til′e-ə) heptadactyly.

**hep·ta·dac·ty·lism** (hep″tə-dak′tə-liz-əm) heptadactyly.

**hep·ta·dac·ty·ly** (hep″tə-dak′tə-le) [*hepta-* + Gr. *daktylos* finger] the occurrence of seven digits on one hand or foot.

**hep·ta·ene** (hep′tə-ēn) a chemical compound in which there are seven conjugated double bonds.

**-hep·ta·ene** suffix denoting a chemical compound in which there are seven conjugated double bonds.

**hep·ta·nal** (hep′tə-nəl) a 7-carbon aldehyde occurring as an ether-soluble oil; used in pharmaceuticals.

**hep·ta·no·ate** (hep″tə-no′āt) enanthate.

**hep·ta·no·ic ac·id** (hep″tə-no′ik) systematic name for *enanthic acid.*

**hep·ta·pep·tide** (hep″tə-pep′tīd) a polypeptide containing seven amino acids.

**hep·ta·tom·ic** (hep″tə-tom′ik) septivalent.

**hep·ta·va·lent** (hep′tə-va″lənt) [*hepta-* + L. *valere* to be able] septivalent.

**Hep·ta·vax-B** (hep′tə-vaks) trademark for a preparation of hepatitis B vaccine.

**hep·to·glo·bin** (hep″to-glo′bin) a protein that is one of the fractions of blood plasma and may be increased in infections, malignancy, and certain endocrine disorders.

**hep·tose** (hep′tōs) [*hept-* + *-ose*] a monosaccharide containing seven carbon atoms in a molecule.

**hep·tos·uria** (hep″to-su′re-ə) presence of a heptose in the urine.

**herb** (ərb, hərb) [L. *herba*] [MeSH: Herbs] any leafy plant without a woody stem, especially one used medicinally or as a flavoring.
**death's h.,** belladonna (def. 1).

**her·ba·ceous** (ər-, hər-ba′shəs) having the characters of an herb.

**her·bal** (ər′-, hər′bəl) 1. pertaining to herbs. 2. a book on herbs.

**her·bal·ist** (ər′-, hər′bəl-ist) a person versed in the use of herbs, especially medicinal herbs.

**Her·bert's operation, pits** (hər′bərts) [Major Herbert *Herbert,* English ophthalmic surgeon in India, 1865–1942] see under *operation* and *pit.*

**her·bi·cide** (ər′-, hər′bĭ-sīd) [*herb* + *-cide*] an agent that is destructive to weeds or causes an alteration in their normal growth.

**her·bi·vore** (ər′-, hər′bĭ-vor) a herbivorous animal.

**her·biv·o·rous** (ər′-, hər-biv′ə-rəs) [L. *herba* herb + *vorare* to eat] subsisting upon plants.

**Herb. recent.** abbreviation for L. *herba′rium recen′tium,* of fresh herbs.

**Herbst's corpuscles** (hərbsts) [Ernst Friedrich Gustav *Herbst,* German physician, 1803–1893] see under *corpuscle.*

**he·red·i·tary** (hə-red′ĭ-tar-e) [L. *hereditarius*] genetically transmitted from parent to offspring.

**he·red·i·ty** (hə-red′ĭ-te) [L. *hereditas*] 1. the genetic transmission of a particular quality or trait from parent to offspring. 2. the genetic constitution of an individual.
**autosomal h.,** the transmission of a quality or trait by a gene located on an autosome.
**X-linked h.,** transmission of a quality or trait located on the X chromosome.
**Y-linked h.,** transmission of a quality or trait located on the Y chromosome.

**her•e•do•atax•ia** (her″ə-do-ə-tak′se-ə) hereditary ataxia, as in Friedreich's ataxia.

**her•e•do•de•gen•er•a•tion** (her″e-do-de-jen″ər-a′shən) hereditary degeneration due to disease or defect of the hyaloplasm; hereditary cerebellar ataxia.

**her•e•do•di•ath•e•sis** (her″ə-do-di-ath′ə-sis) [L. *heres* heir + *diathesis*] hereditary diathesis or predisposition.

**her•e•do•fa•mil•i•al** (her″ə-do-fə-mil′e-əl) occurring in certain families under circumstances that implicate a hereditary basis, as heredofamilial disease. The term is being discarded in favor of *familial, hereditary,* or *genetic,* whichever is more appropriate.

**her•e•do•in•fec•tion** (her″ə-do-in-fek′shən) germinal infection.

**her•e•do•lu•es** (her″ə-do-lu′ēz) congenital syphilis.

**her•e•do•lu•et•ic** (her″ə-do-lu-et′ik) pertaining to congenital syphilis.

**her•e•do•path•ia** (her″ə-do-path′e-ə) a hereditary disease.
**h. atac′tica polyneuritifor′mis,** Refsum's disease.

**her•e•do•ret•i•no•path•ia con•gen•i•ta** (her″ə-do-ret″ĭ-no-path′e-ə kən-jen′ĭtə) [L] hereditary retinopathy; see *amaurosis congenita,* under *amaurosis.*

**her•e•do•syph•i•lis** (her″ə-do-sif′ĭ-lis) congenital syphilis.

**her•e•do•syph•i•lit•ic** (her″ə-do-sif″ĭ-lit′ik) a person affected with congenital syphilis.

**her•e•do•syph•i•lol•o•gy** (her″ə-do-sif″ĭ-lol′ə-je) the study of congenital syphilis.

**He•relle** see *d'Herelle.*

**He•rel•lea** (hə-rel′e-ə) in former systems of classification, a genus of bacteria, species of which are now included in the genus *Acinetobacter.*
**H. vagini′cola,** *Acinetobacter calcoaceticus.*

**Her•ing's law, test, theory** (her′ingz) [Karl Ewald Constantin *Hering,* German physiologist, 1834–1918] see under *law, test,* and *theory.*

**Her•ing's nerve, phenomenon** (her′ingz) [Heinrich Ewald *Hering,* German physiologist, 1866–1948] see *ramus sinus carotici nervi glossopharyngei,* and see under *phenomenon.*

**Her•ing-Breu•er reflex** (her′ing-broi′ər) [H.E. *Hering;* Josef Robert *Breuer,* Austrian physician, 1842 –1925] see under *reflex.*

**her•i•ta•bil•i•ty** (her″ĭ-tə-bil′ĭ-te) 1. the quality of being heritable. 2. a measure of the extent to which a phenotype is influenced by the genotype.

**her•i•ta•ble** (her′ĭ-tə-bəl) capable of being inherited, as a genetic trait.

**Her•litz's disease** (her′litz) [Carl Gillis *Herlitz,* Swedish pediatrician, born 1902] junctional epidermolysis bullosa.

**Her•man•sky-Pud•lak syndrome** (hər-mahn′ske-pood′lahk) [F. *Hermansky,* Czechoslovakian internist, 20th century; P. *Pudlak,* Czechoslovakian internist, 20th century] see under *syndrome.*

**her•maph•ro•dism** (hər-maf′ro-diz-əm) hermaphroditism.

**her•maph•ro•dite** (hər-maf′ro-dīt) [Gr. *hermaphroditos*] an individual having hermaphroditism (q.v.).
**pseudo-h.,** see *pseudohermaphrodite.*
**true h.,** an individual with true hermaphroditism, having both testicular and ovarian tissue. Called also *true intersex.*

**her•maph•ro•dit•ic** (hər-maf″ro-dit′ik) pertaining to or characterized by hermaphroditism; called also *ambisexual, androgynous, bisexual, gynandroid,* and *gynandromorphous.*

**her•maph•ro•di•tism** (hər-maf′ro-di-tiz″əm) [Gr. *hermaphroditos* hermaphrodite] [MeSH: Hermaphroditism] the presence of both male and female gonadal tissue in the same individual. *True hermaphroditism* (q.v.) is distinguished from *male pseudohermaphroditism* and *female pseudohermaphroditism.* Called also *gynandrism, hermaphrodism,* and *intersexuality.*
**bilateral h.,** that in which gonadal tissue typical of both sexes occurs on each side of the body.
**false h.,** pseudohermaphroditism.
**lateral h.,** presence of gonadal tissue typical of one sex on one side of the body and tissue typical of the other sex on the opposite side.
**spurious h.,** pseudohermaphroditism.
**transverse h.,** a condition in which the external genital organs are characteristic of one sex and the gonads are typical of the other.
**true h.,** coexistence, in the same individual, of both ovarian and testicular tissue, caused by anomalous differentiation of the gonads; secondary sex characters of both genders may be present. Types include *lateral, bilateral, unilateral,* and *transverse hermaphroditism.*
**unilateral h.,** presence of gonadal tissue typical of both sexes on one side and of an ovary or testis on the other.

**her•maph•ro•di•tis•mus** (hər-maf″ro-di-tiz′məs) hermaphroditism.
**h. ve′rus,** true hermaphroditism.
**h. ve′rus bilatera′lis,** bilateral hermaphroditism.
**h. ve′rus latera′lis,** lateral hermaphroditism.
**h. ve′rus unilatera′lis,** unilateral hermaphroditism.

**Her•me•tia il•lu•cens** (hər-me′sh-e-ə il-u′sənz) the soldier fly, the larvae of which may cause intestinal myiasis or pseudomyiasis in man.

**her•met•ic** (hər-met′ik) [L. *hermeticus*] impervious to air; airtight.

**Her•mod•sson's projection** (her′mod-sənz) [I. *Hermodsson,* radiologist, 20th century] see under *projection.*

**her•nia** (hər′ne-ə) [L.] [MeSH: Hernia] the protrusion of a loop or knuckle of an organ or tissue through an abnormal opening. See also *herniation.*

## Hernia

**abdominal h.,** herniation of omentum, intestine, or some other internal body structure through the abdominal wall; called also *ventral h.* and *laparocele.*
**acquired h.,** one brought on by lifting or by a strain or other injury.
**h. adipo′sa,** fat h.
**axial hiatal h.,** sliding hiatal h.
**Barth's h.,** hernia of loops of intestine between the serosa of the abdominal wall and that of a persistent vitelline duct.
**Béclard's h.,** femoral hernia through the saphenous opening.
**Birkett's h.,** synovial h.
**Bochdalek's h.,** congenital diaphragmatic hernia due to failure of closure of the pleuroperitoneal hiatus (foramen of Bochdalek).
**cecal h.,** an intestinal hernia containing all or part of the cecum.
**cerebral h., h. ce′rebri,** protrusion of the brain substance through the skull, through either a cranium bifidum, the foramen magnum, or the tentorial notch. See *encephalocele* and see *tonsillar herniation* and *transtentorial herniation,* under *herniation.*
**Cloquet's h.,** pectineal h.
**complete h.,** one in which the sac and its contents have passed through the defect.
**concealed h.,** hernia not perceptible on palpation.
**congenital h.,** that which exists at birth, most commonly scrotal or umbilical.
**Cooper's h.,** a femoral hernia with additional tracts into the scrotum, toward the labium majus, and toward the obturator foramen.
**crural h.,** femoral h.
**diaphragmatic h.,** herniation of the abdominal or retroperitoneal structures into the thorax.
**diaphragmatic h., congenital,** congenital protrusion of the abdominal viscera into the thorax through an opening resulting from defective development of the pleuroperitoneal membrane, most often incomplete closure of the pleuroperitoneal hiatus (foramen of Bochdalek); it often leads to fatal pulmonary hypoplasia.
**direct h., direct inguinal h.,** see *inguinal h.*
**diverticular h.,** Littre's h.
**dry h.,** a hernia in which the sac and its contents have become intimately adherent to each other.
**duodenojejunal h.,** Treitz's h.
**encysted h.,** scrotal or oblique inguinal hernia in which the bowel, enveloped in its own proper sac, passes into the tunica vaginalis in such a way that the bowel has three coverings of peritoneum; called also *Hey's h.*
**epigastric h.,** an abdominal hernia through the linea alba above the navel.
**external h.,** indirect inguinal hernia; see *inguinal h.*
**extrasaccular h.,** sliding h.

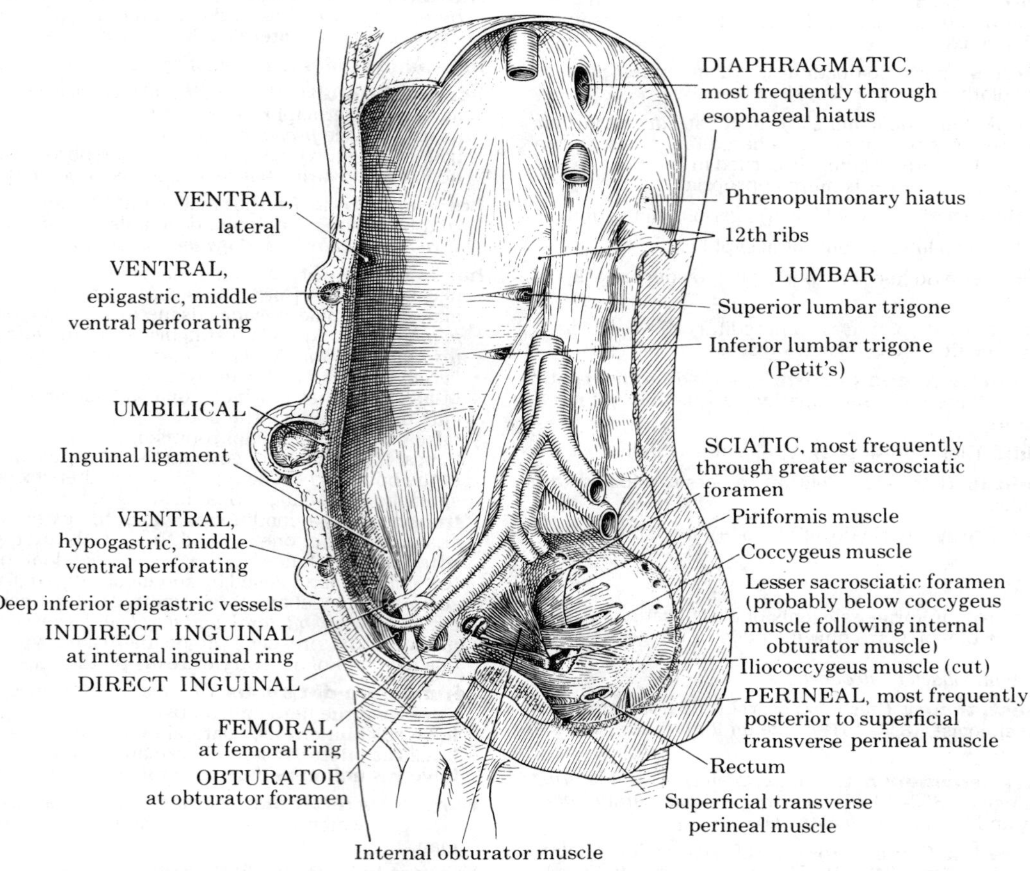


TYPES OF INTESTINAL HERNIA: ABDOMINAL AND PELVIC OPENINGS.

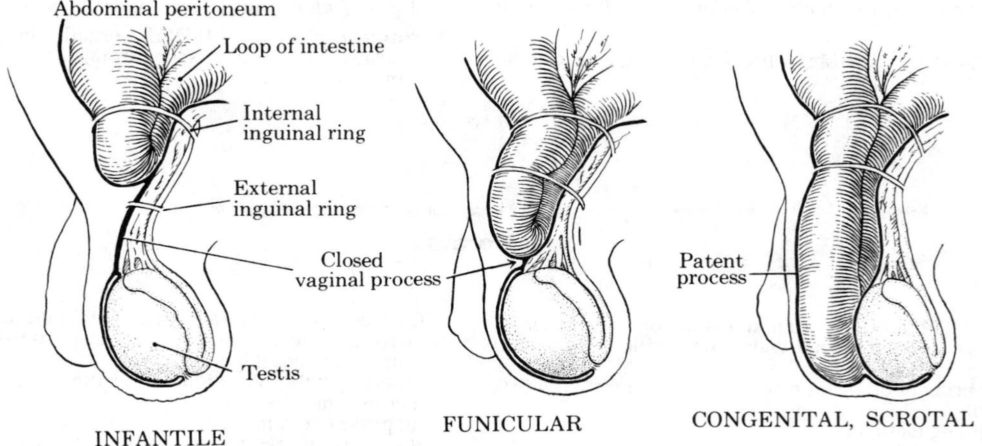


TYPES OF INDIRECT INGUINAL HERNIA

**PLATE 21**—INTESTINAL AND INGUINAL HERNIAS

**fat h.,** hernial protrusion of properitoneal fat through the abdominal wall; called also *h. adiposa.*

**femoral h.,** hernia of a loop of intestine into the femoral canal. Called also *crural h.* and *femorocele.*

**foraminal h.,** hernia through the epiploic foramen.

**gastroesophageal h.,** paraesophageal h.

**Grynfeltt h.,** lumbar hernia through Lesshaft's space (Grynfeltt's triangle).

**Hesselbach's h.,** hernia of a loop of intestine through the cribriform fascia.

**Hey's h.,** encysted h.

**hiatal h., hiatus h.,** herniation of an abdominal organ, usually the stomach, through the esophageal hiatus of the diaphragm. It occurs in two major anatomic patterns: the *sliding hiatal h.* (type I), which is the more common type, and the *paraesophageal h.* (type II).

**Holthouse's h.,** an inguinal hernia which has turned outward into the groin.

**incarcerated h.,** hernia of intestine that cannot be returned or reduced by manipulation; it may or may not become strangulated. Called also *irreducible h.*

**incisional h.,** an abdominal hernia at the site of a previously made incision.

**incomplete h.,** one which has not passed entirely through the defect.

**indirect h., indirect inguinal h.,** see *inguinal h.*

**infantile h.,** oblique inguinal hernia behind the funicular process of the peritoneum.

**inguinal h.,** hernia of an intestinal loop into the inguinal canal. An *indirect inguinal hernia* (*external* or *oblique hernia*) leaves the abdomen through the deep inguinal ring, and passes down obliquely through the inguinal canal, lateral to the inferior epigastric artery. A *direct inguinal hernia* (*internal hernia*) emerges between the inferior epigastric artery and the edge of the rectus muscle.

**inguinocrural h., inguinofemoral h.,** a combined inguinal and femoral hernia.

**inguinoproperitoneal h.,** hernia that is partly inguinal and partly properitoneal; called also *Krönlein's h.*

**inguinosuperficial h.,** interstitial hernia which passes through the internal inguinal ring, the inguinal canal, and the external inguinal ring, but at this point is deflected upward and outward so as to lie upon the aponeurosis of the external oblique muscle.

**intermuscular h.,** an interstitial hernia which lies between one or another of the fascial or muscular planes of the abdomen.

**internal h.,** direct inguinal hernia; see *inguinal h.*

**interparietal h.,** intermuscular h.

**intersigmoid h.,** hernia of the intestine through the intersigmoid fossa.

**interstitial h.,** an intestinal hernia in which a loop lies between two layers of the abdominal wall.

**intra-abdominal h., intraperitoneal h.,** a congenital anomaly of intestinal positioning, occurring within the abdomen, in which a portion of bowel protrudes through a defect in the peritoneum or, as a result of abnormal rotation of the intestine during embryonic development, becomes trapped in a sac of peritoneum.

**h. of the iris,** protrusion of a part of the iris.

**irreducible h.,** incarcerated h.

**ischiatic h.,** sciatic h.

**ischiorectal h.,** perineal h.

**Krönlein's h.,** inguinoproperitoneal h.

**labial h.,** herniation of intestine into a labium majus.

**labial h., posterior,** vaginolabial h.

**Laugier's h.,** a femoral hernia perforating Gimbernat's ligament.

**levator h.,** pudendal h.

**Littre's h.,** protrusion of a Meckel's diverticulum; called also *diverticular h.*

**lumbar h.,** herniation of omentum or intestine in the lumbar region, through Lesshaft's space *(Grynfeltt hernia)* or the trigonum lumbale *(Petit's hernia).*

**mesenteric h.,** herniation of intestine through an opening in the mesentery.

**mesentericoparietal h.,** mesocolic h.

**mesocolic h.,** an intra-abdominal hernia in which the small intestine rotates incompletely during development and becomes trapped within the mesentery of the colon. Called also *paraduodenal h.*

**Morgagni's h.,** congenital retrosternal diaphragmatic hernia, with extrusion of tissue into the thorax through the foramen of Morgagni.

**oblique h.,** indirect inguinal hernia; see *inguinal h.*

**obturator h.,** herniation of intestine or other abdominal organs through the obturator foramen.

**omental h.,** an abdominal hernia containing omentum.

**ovarian h.,** hernial protrusion of an ovary.

**pantaloon h.,** inguinal hernia in which there are both direct and indirect hernial sacs.

**paraduodenal h.,** mesocolic h.

**paraesophageal h.,** hiatal hernia in which part or almost all of the stomach protrudes through the hiatus into the thorax to the left of the esophagus, with the gastroesophageal junction remaining in place. Called also *type II hiatal hernia.*

**parahiatal h.,** paraesophageal h.

**paraperitoneal h.,** hernia of the bladder in which only a part of the protruded bladder is covered by the peritoneum of the sac.

**parasaccular h.,** sliding h.

**parietal h.,** Richter's h.

**pectineal h.,** a type of femoral hernia that enters the femoral canal and then perforates the aponeurosis of the pectineus muscle; called also *Cloquet's h.*

**perineal h.,** protrusion of abdominal viscera into the perineum.

**Petit's h.,** lumbar hernia through the trigonum lumbale (Petit's triangle).

**prevascular h.,** a hernia in the femoral sheath, anterior to the femoral vessels.

**properitoneal h.,** an interstitial hernia which is located between the parietal peritoneum and the transversalis fascia.

**pudendal h.,** herniation of intestine into the pudendum, having passed through a rent in the levator muscle and its fascia; called also *levator h.*

**pulsion h.,** a hernia produced by sudden increase of intra-abdominal pressure.

**rectovaginal h.,** rectocele.

**reducible h.,** one that may be returned by manipulation.

**retrocecal h.,** protrusion of the intestine into a pouch behind the cecum; called also *Rieux's h.*

**retrograde h.,** herniation of two loops of intestine, the portion of intestine between the two loops lying within the abdominal cavity. Called also *w h.*

**retroperitoneal h.,** Treitz's h.

**retrovascular h.,** a femoral hernia that passes within the femoral sheath but exits posterior to the femoral vessels; called also *Serafini's h.*

**Richter's h.,** an incarcerated or strangulated hernia in which only a portion of the circumference of the bowel wall is involved; called also *parietal h.*

**Rieux's h.,** retrocecal h.

**Rokitansky's h.,** protrusion of a sac of mucous membrane or of the peritoneum through separated muscular fibers of the intestine.

**rolling h.,** paraesophageal h.

**sciatic h.,** hernia through the greater or lesser sciatic foramen. Called also *ischiatic h.* and *ischiocele.*

**scrotal h.,** an inguinal hernia which has descended into the scrotum.

**Serafini's h.,** retrovascular h.

**sliding h.,** hernia of the cecum (on the right) or the sigmoid colon (on the left) in which the intestinal wall forms a portion of the hernial sac, the remainder of the sac being formed by the parietal peritoneum. Called also *slip h.* or *slipped h.*

**sliding hiatal h.,** hiatal hernia in which the upper stomach and the cardioesophageal junction protrude upward into the posterior mediastinum; the protrusion, which may be fixed or intermittent, is partially covered by a peritoneal sac. Called also *axial hiatal h.* and *type I hiatal h.*

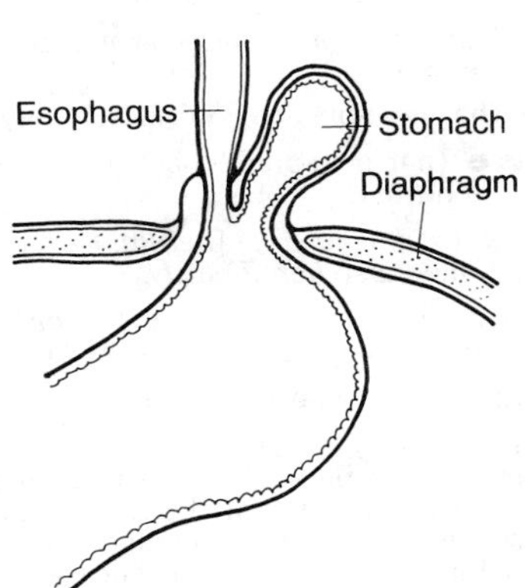


Paraesophageal hernia.

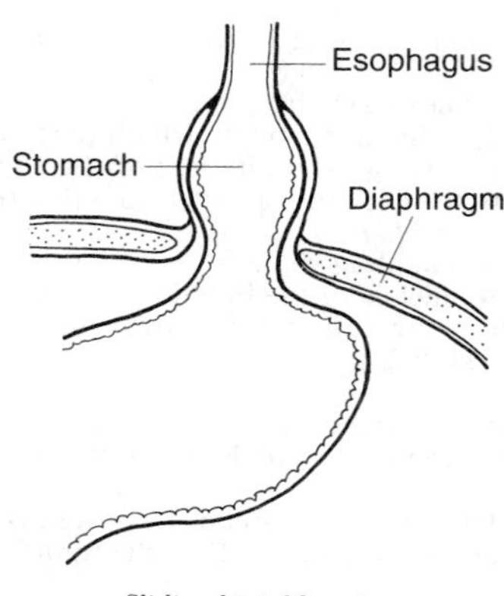

Sliding hiatal hernia.

**slip h., slipped h.,** sliding h.
**spigelian h.,** abdominal hernia through the linea semilunaris.
**strangulated h.,** an incarcerated hernia that is so tightly constricted as to compromise the blood supply of the contents of the hernial sac, leading to gangrene.
**synovial h.,** protrusion of the inner lining membrane through the stratum fibrosum of a joint capsule; called also *Birkett's h.*
**tonsillar h.,** tonsillar herniation.
**Treitz's h.,** hernia of the intestine through the superior duodenal recess; called also *duodenojejunal h.* and *retroperitoneal h.*
**umbilical h.,** a type of abdominal hernia in which part of the intestine protrudes at the umbilicus and is covered with skin and subcutaneous tissue; cf. *omphalocele.* Called also *exomphalos* and *exumbilication.*
**h. u'teri inguina'lis,** a common type of persistent müllerian duct syndrome.
**uterine h.,** hernial protrusion of the uterus.
**vaginal h.,** hernia into the vagina; called also *colpocele* and *vaginocele.*
**vaginal h., posterior,** downward protrusion of the pouch of Douglas, with its intestinal contents, between the posterior vaginal wall and the rectum; called also *enterocele.*
**vaginolabial h.,** hernia of a viscus into the posterior end of the labium majus.
**Velpeau's h.,** femoral hernia in front of the femoral vessels.
**ventral h.,** abdominal h.
**vesical h.,** protrusion of the bladder.
**w h.,** retrograde h.

**her•ni•al** (hər'ne-əl) pertaining to a hernia.

**her•ni•at•ed** (hər'ne-āt″əd) protruding like a hernia; enclosed in a hernia.

**her•ni•a•tion** (hər″ne-a'shən) the abnormal protrusion of an organ or other body structure through a defect or natural opening in a covering, membrane, muscle, or bone. See also *hernia.*
**caudal transtentorial h.,** tentorial h.
**disk h., h. of intervertebral disk,** protrusion of the nucleus pulposus or anulus fibrosus of an intervertebral disk, which may impinge on nerve roots; called also *herniated, protruded,* or *ruptured disk* and *herniated nucleus pulposus.*
**h. of nucleus pulposus,** see *h. of intervertebral disk.*
**painful fat h.,** piezogenic papules.
**tentorial h.,** downward displacement of the most medially-placed cerebral structures through the tentorial notch, caused by a supratentorial mass. Pressure is exerted on underlying structures, including the brain stem. Called also *caudal transtentorial h., transtentorial h.,* and *uncal h.*
**tonsillar h.,** protrusion of the cerebellar tonsils through the foramen magnum, exerting pressure on the medulla oblongata. Called also *tonsillar hernia.*
**transtentorial h.,** tentorial h.
**uncal h.,** tentorial h.

**her•nio•ap•pen•dec•to•my** (hər″ne-o-ap″ən-dek'tə-me) herniotomy combined with appendectomy.

**her•nio•en•ter•ot•o•my** (her″ne-o-en″tər-ot'ə-me) herniotomy conjoined with enterotomy.

**her•ni•oid** (hər'ne-oid) resembling hernia.

**her•nio•lap•a•rot•o•my** (hər″ne-o-lap″ə-rot'ə-me) laparotomy for the treatment of hernia.

**her•nio•plas•ty** (hər'ne-o-plas″te) herniorrhaphy.

**her•nio•punc•ture** (hər″ne-o-punk'chər) [*hernia* + *puncture*] surgical puncture of a hernia.

**her•ni•or•rha•phy** (hər″ne-or'ə-fe) [*hernia* + *-rrhaphy*] surgical repair of a hernia. Called also *hernioplasty.*

**her•ni•ot•o•my** (hə-r″ne-ot'ə-me) [*hernia* + *-tomy*] a surgical operation for the repair of hernia; called also *celotomy* and *kelotomy.*

**her•o•in** (her'o-in) diacetylmorphine.

**He•roph•i•lus** (hə-rof'ĭ-ləs) **of Chalcedon** [c. 300 B.C.] a Greek physician at Alexandria, a pupil of Praxagoras and an elder contemporary of Erasistratus. He performed public human post mortems and possibly also vivisection on condemned criminals. In his studies of the brain (for him the seat of intelligence and the organ of the soul) he distinguished the cerebrum from the cerebellum, described and named the meninges, calamus scriptorius, and the torcular Herophili. He studied the vascular and nervous systems and distinguished sensory from motor nerves, tendons from nerves, and veins from arteries. Herophilus recognized that the pulse derives from the heart and is not an innate function of the arteries, and he classified pulses by speed, regularity, etc., and furnished a mathematical law of systole and diastole. For *torcular Herophili,* see *confluens sinuum.*

**herp•an•gi•na** (hər″pən-ji'nə) [*herpes* + *angina*] [MeSH: Herpangina] an acute infectious disease caused by either group A or group B coxsackievirus or by echoviruses, chiefly affecting young children in the summer; characteristics include vesiculoulcerative lesions on the mucous membranes of the throat, dysphagia, vomiting, and fever. Called also *aphthous pharyngitis, vesicular pharyngitis, herpes angina,* and *Zahorsky's syndrome.*

**her•pes** (hər'pēz) [L.; Gr. *herpēs,* a spreading cutaneous eruption, from *herpein* to creep] any inflammatory skin disease caused by a herpesvirus and characterized by the formation of clusters of small vesicles. When used alone, the term may refer to *h. simplex* or to *h. zoster.*
**h. blat'tae,** a herpetiform contact dermatitis caused by a cockroach *(Blatta)* crawling on the skin of a susceptible person, usually in the region of the mouth.
**h. cor'neae,** herpetic inflammation involving the cornea.
**h. digita'lis,** herpes simplex of the fingers.
**h. facia'lis,** herpes simplex of the face.
**h. febri'lis,** herpes simplex caused by human herpesvirus 1, and primarily spread by oral secretions; it usually occurs as a concomitant of fever, but may develop in the absence of fever or prior illness, and commonly involves the facial region, especially the vermilion border of the lips *(h. labialis)* and the nares; the vesicular lesions are self-limited. Called also *cold sore* and *fever blister.*
**genital h., h. genita'lis,** herpes simplex due to human herpesvirus 2, primarily transmitted sexually via genital secretions, and contact with viroids, and involving the genital region in both sexes; although symptoms in the female are more severe than in the male, the vesicular lesions are self-limited. Genital herpes at term in the pregnant female may lead to infection of the neonate and result in disseminated or localized infection or progress from localized to disseminated disease. Called also *h. progenitalis.*
**h. gestatio'nis,** a rare, self-limited blistering cutaneous disorder of unknown origin (not due to herpesvirus); it usually begins on the abdomen during the second and third trimesters of pregnancy and spreads to other sites, and is characterized by the presence of an intensely pruritic polymorphous eruption, which may recur with subsequent pregnancies.
**h. gladiato'rum,** see *traumatic h.*
**h. labia'lis,** herpes febrilis affecting the vermilion border of the lips.
**ocular h.,** herpes of the eye and its adnexa; see *herpetic keratoconjunctivitis.*
**h. ophthal'micus,** h. zoster ophthalmicus.
**h. progenita'lis,** genital h.
**h. sim'plex,** a group of acute infections caused by human herpes-

viruses 1 and 2, characterized by the development of one or more small fluid-filled vesicles with a raised erythematous base on the skin or mucous membrane, and occurring as a primary infection or recurring because of reactivation of a latent infection. Type 1 infections usually involve nongenital regions of the body, whereas in type 2 infections the lesions are primarily seen on the genital and surrounding areas, although there is overlap between the two types. Precipitating factors include fever, exposure to cold temperature or to ultraviolet rays, sunburn, cutaneous or mucosal abrasions, emotional stress, and nerve injury.

**traumatic h.,** primary cutaneous herpes simplex acquired by direct exogenous infection of traumatized skin, usually associated with localization of lesions to the area of trauma and regional lymphadenopathy and often by symptoms of systemic illness such as fever and malaise. Such infections have been seen in wrestler's h. *(h. gladiatorum),* and are acquired from mats or body contact.

**wrestler's h.,** see *traumatic h.*

**h. zos'ter,** an acute infectious, usually self-limited, disease believed to represent activation of latent human herpesvirus 3 in those who have been rendered partially immune after a previous attack of chickenpox. It involves the sensory ganglia and their areas of innervation, is characterized by severe neuralgic pain along the distribution of the affected nerve and crops of clustered vesicles over the area of the corresponding dermatome, and is usually unilateral and confined to a single or adjacent dermatomes. Postherpetic neuralgia may be a complication. In immunocompromised patients it may disseminate and be fatal. Called also *acute posterior ganglionitis, shingles, zona,* and *zoster.*

**h. zos'ter auricula'ris,** Ramsay Hunt syndrome, def. 1.

**h. zos'ter ophthal'micus,** herpes zoster involving the ophthalmic division of the trigeminal nerve, characterized by a cutaneous vesicular rash on an erythematous base along the nerve path, preceded by lancinating pain, usually accompanied by conjunctivitis and sometimes by keratitis, scleritis, iridocyclitis, extraocular muscle palsies, ptosis, and mydriasis. Called also *gasserian ganglionitis, h. ophthalmicus,* and *ophthalmic zoster.*

**h. zos'ter o'ticus,** Ramsay Hunt syndrome, def. 1.

**her·pes·vi·ral** (hər'pēz-vi"rəl) pertaining to or caused by herpesviruses.

**Her·pes·vi·ri·dae** (hər"pēz-vi'rĭ-de) [MeSH: Herpesviridae] the herpesviruses: a family of DNA viruses having a virion 102–200 nm in diameter consisting of four components: a lipid bilayer envelope with surface projections, a tegument of amorphous material, an icosahedral nucleocapsid with 162 prismatic capsomers, and a protein spool on which the DNA is wrapped. The genome consists of a single molecule of linear double-stranded DNA (MW 70–150 $\times$ $10^6$, size 124–235 kbp). Viruses contain at least 20 structural polypeptides and are sensitive to lipid solvents, heat, and extremes of pH. Replication occurs in the nucleus and the envelope is acquired by budding through the inner lamella of the nuclear membrane; virions are released by transport via the endoplasmic reticulum to the cell membrane. Persistence for the lifetime of the host is common and some herpesviruses induce neoplasia. There are three subfamilies: Alphaherpesvirinae, Betaherpesvirinae, and Gammaherpesvirinae. A large number of herpesviruses have not yet been assigned to a subfamily or genus.

**her·pes·vi·rus** (hər'pēz-vi"rəs) [*herpes* + *virus*] [MeSH: Herpesviridae] any virus belonging to the family Herpesviridae.

**h. B,** a virus of the genus *Simplexvirus* that infects Asiatic macaques. Human infection, usually fatal, can result from monkey bites and may cause ascending myelopathy or acute meningitis. Called also *B virus* and *cercopithecine herpesvirus 1.*

**bovine h. 1,** a virus of the genus *Varicellovirus* that is the etiologic agent of infectious bovine rhinotracheitis. Called also *infectious bovine rhinotracheitis virus.*

**bovine h. 2,** a virus of the genus *Simplexvirus* that is the etiologic agent of bovine ulcerative mammillitis.

**cercopithecine h. 1,** h. B.

**equid h. 1,** a virus of the genus *Varicellovirus* that is an etiologic agent of equine viral rhinopneumonitis; see also *equid h. 4.* Called also *equine h. 1.*

**equid h. 3,** a virus of the subfamily *Alphaherpesvirinae* that is the etiologic agent of equine coital exanthema.

**equid h. 4,** a virus of the genus *Varicellovirus,* closely related to equid herpesvirus 1, that is an etiologic agent of equine viral rhinopneumonitis. Called also *equine h. 4.*

**equine h. 1,** equid h. 1.

**equine h. 3,** equid h. 3.

**equine h. 4,** equid h. 4.

**felid h. 1, feline h. 1,** a virus in the subfamily Alphaherpesvirinae (family Herpesviridae) that is the main cause of disease in the feline respiratory disease complex. See also *feline rhinotracheitis.* Called also *feline rhinotracheitis virus.*

**gallid h. 1,** a herpesvirus in the subfamily Alphaherpesvirinae, the cause of infectious laryngotracheitis in poultry. Called also *infectious laryngotracheitis virus.*

**gallid h. 2,** a species of viruses of the family Herpesviridae that is the etiologic agent of Marek's disease. Called also *Marek's disease h. 1.*

**gallid h. 3,** a species of viruses in the family Herpesviridae, antigenically related to gallid herpesvirus 2 and isolated from turkeys.

**human h. 1,** a virus of the genus *Simplexvirus* that is an etiologic agent of herpes simplex in humans, causing predominantly nongenital infections. Primary infection usually occurs in early childhood and is often asymptomatic, although gingivostomatitis and pharyngitis may occur. The virus can pass along nerves and remain latent in ganglia, from which it may be reactivated. Called also herpes simplex virus 1. See Plate 55.

**human h. 2,** a virus of the genus *Simplexvirus* that is an etiologic agent of herpes simplex, transmitted venereally and causing primarily genital infections. Called also *herpes simplex virus 2.* See Plate 55.

**human h. 3,** a virus of the genus *Varicellovirus* that is the etiologic agent of chickenpox and herpes zoster. Called also *varicella-zoster virus.*

**human h. 4,** Epstein-Barr virus.

**human h. 5,** the sole species of the genus *Cytomegalovirus;* it causes a widespread, usually asymptomatic infection in humans. Primary infection during pregnancy can result in infection and brain damage in the fetus. Infection of immunocompromised patients can cause fatal pneumonia or hepatitis. It also can cause mononucleosis.

**human h. 6,** a ubiquitous virus belonging to the subfamily Betaherpesvirinae that is the etiologic agent of exanthema subitum. Most healthy adults carry the virus and are asymptomatic; infection results in lifelong persistence.

**human h. 7,** a virus belonging to the subfamily Betaherpesvirinae, closely related to human herpesvirus 6, but not known to be associated with any disease.

**human h. 8,** a virus in the family Herpesviridae that has been implicated as the etiologic agent of Kaposi's sarcoma and primary effusion lymphoma. Called also *Kaposi's sarcoma–associated h.*

**Kaposi's sarcoma–associated h.,** human h. 8.

**Marek's disease h. 1,** gallid h. 2.

**Marek's disease h. 2,** gallid h. 3.

**suid h. 1,** pseudorabies virus.

**her·pet·ic** (hər-pet'ik) [L. *herpeticus*] pertaining to or of the nature of herpes; relating to or caused by herpesviruses.

**her·pet·i·form** (hər-pet'ĭ-form) [*herpet-* + *form*] resembling herpes; having grouped vesicles.

**herpet(o)-** [Gr. *herpeton* creeping thing, crawler, reptile, from *herpein* to creep] a combining form denoting a relationship to (1) herpes or (2) a snake or other reptile.

**her·pe·tol·o·gist** (hər"pə-tol'o-jist) a specialist in herpetology.

**her·pe·tol·o·gy** (hər"pə-tol'o-je) [*herpeto-* + *-logy*] the branch of zoology that specializes in the study of reptiles and amphibians.

**her·peto·pho·bia** (hər-pet"o-fo'be-ə) irrational fear of reptiles or amphibians.

**Her·pe·to·so·ma** (hər-pet"o-so'mə) [*herpeto-* + *soma*] in some systems of classification, a subgenus of stercorarian trypanosomes, including among others the species *Trypanosoma lewisi, T. duttoni,* and *T. rangeli.*

**Her·plex** (hər'pleks) trademark for a preparation of idoxuridine.

**Her·ring bodies** (her'ing) [Percy Theodore *Herring,* English physiologist, 1872–1967] see under *body.*

**Herr·mann's syndrome** (her'mənz) [Christian *Herrmann,* Jr., American physician, born 1921] see under *syndrome.*

**Hers' disease** (ārz) [Henri-Géry *Hers,* Belgian physiologist and biochemist, 20th century] glycogen storage disease (type VI); see under *disease.*

**her·sage** (ār-sahzh') [Fr. "combing"] surgical dissociation of the fibers in a scarred area of a peripheral nerve by splitting the sheath and separating the nerve into a ribbon of fine free fibers. Called also *endoneurolysis.*

**Her·shey** (hər'she) Alfred Day. American biologist, born 1908; co-winner, with Max Delbruck and Salvador E. Luria, of the Nobel Prize in medicine or physiology for 1969, for research on the mechanism and materials of inheritance of viruses.

**Her·ter's disease** (hər'tərz) [Christian Archibald *Herter,* American physician, 1865–1910] see under *disease.*

**Her·ter-Heub·ner disease** (hər'tər hoib'nər) [C.A. *Herter;* Johann Otto Leonhard *Heubner,* German pediatrician, 1843–1926] 1. see *celiac disease,* under *disease.* 2. see under *disease.*

**Her·tig-Rock ova** (hər'tig-rok) [Arthur Tremain *Hertig,* American pathologist, 1904–1990; John *Rock,* American gynecologist, 1890–1984] see under *ovum.*

**Hert·wig's sheath** (hərt'viks) [Richard Carl Wilhelm Theodor von *Hertwig,* German zoologist, 1850–1937] root sheath, def. 1.

**Hert·wig-Ma·gen·die phenomenon** (hərt′vik mah-zhahn-de′) [R.C.W.T. von *Hertwig;* François *Magendie,* French physiologist, 1783–1855] skew deviation.

**hertz** (hərtz) a unit of frequency equal to one cycle per second; abbreviated Hz.

**Herx·heim·er's fibers (spirals), reaction** (hərks′hīm-ərz) [Karl *Herxheimer,* German dermatologist, 1861–1944] see under *fiber,* and see *Jarisch-Herxheimer reaction,* under *reaction.*

**herz·tod** (herts′tōt) [Ger. "cardiac death"] porcine stress syndrome.

**Heschl's convolution, gyrus** (hesh′əlz) [Richard L. *Heschl,* Austrian pathologist, 1824–1881] see *gyri temporales transversi,* under *gyrus.*

**Hes·pan** (hes′pan) trademark for a preparation of hetastarch.

**hes·per·i·din** (hes-per′ĭ-din) [MeSH: Hesperidin] a bioflavonoid predominant in lemons and oranges.

**Hess** (hes) Walter Rudolf. Swiss physiologist, 1881–1973; co-winner, with Antonio Egas Moniz, of the Nobel prize for medicine or physiology for 1949, for his discovery of the functional organization of the interbrain as a coordinator of the activities of the internal organs.

**Hess capillary test** (hes) [Alfred Fabian *Hess,* American physician, 1875–1933] tourniquet test (def. 1); see under *test.*

**Hes·sel·bach's fascia, hernia, ligament, triangle** (hes′əl-bahks) [Franz Kaspar *Hesselbach,* German surgeon, 1759–1816] see under *hernia,* and see *ligamentum interfoveolare,* and *trigonum inguinale.*

**het·a·cil·lin** (het″ə-sil′in) a semisynthetic penicillin which itself has no antibacterial activity, but is converted in the body to ampicillin and has actions and uses similar to those of ampicillin (q.v.); administered orally.
**h. potassium,** the potassium salt of hetacillin, having antibacterial actions and uses similar to those of ampicillin; administered intravenously and intramuscularly.

**het·a·starch** (het′ə-stahrch) [MeSH: Hetastarch] a starch containing not more than 90 per cent of amylopectin, and that has been etherified so that an average of 7 to 8 of the OH groups in every 10-D-glucopyranose units of starch polymer have been converted into $OCH_2CH_2OH$ groups; used as a plasma volume expander, administered by infusion.

**HETE** hydroxyeicosatetraenoic acid.

**het·er·a·del·phus** (het″ər-ə-del′fəs) [*heter-* + *-adelphus*] asymmetrical conjoined twins; see under *twin.*

**Het·er·ak·i·dae** (het″ər-ak′ĭ-de) a family of nematodes some of which parasitize birds; it includes the genus *Heterakis.*

**Het·er·a·kis** (het″ər-a′kis) [*heter-* + Gr. *akis* pointed object] a genus of nonpathogenic nematodes of the family Heterakidae, parasitic in the ceca of chickens, turkeys, and other birds. *H. galli′nae* serves as a paratenic host for *Histomonas meleagridis,* the etiologic agent of histomoniasis.

**het·er·a·li·us** (het″ər-a′le-əs) [*heter-* + Gr. *halios* fruitless] an extreme example of heteradelphus.

**het·er·aux·e·sis** (het″ər-awk-ze′sis) [*heter-* + *auxesis*] disproportionate growth of a part in relation to another part.

**het·er·ax·i·al** (het″ər-ak′se-əl) [*heter-* + *axial*] having axes of unequal length.

**het·er·e·cious** (het″ər-e′shəs) [*heter-* + Gr. *oikos* house] living upon one host in one stage or generation and upon another in the next.

**het·er·e·cism** (het″ər-e′siz-əm) the state of being heterecious.

**het·er·er·gic** (het″ər-ər′jik) [*heter-* + Gr. *ergon* work] having different effects; said of two drugs one of which produces a particular effect and the other does not.

**het·er·es·the·sia** (het″ər-es-the′zhə) [*heter-* + *esthesia*] variation in the degree of cutaneous sensibility on adjoining areas of the body surface.

**heter(o)-** [Gr. *heteros* other, different] a combining form meaning other, different, or abnormal, or denoting relationship to another.

**het·ero·ag·glu·ti·na·tion** (het″ər-o-ə-gloo″tĭ-na′shən) agglutination of particulate antigens (on cells or adsorbed on inert carrier particles) of one species by agglutinins derived from organisms of another species.

**het·ero·ag·glu·ti·nin** (het″ər-o-ə-gloo′tĭ-nin) an agglutinin with reactive specificity for particulate antigen(s) in one or more species other than the species in which it originates.

**het·ero·al·bu·mose** (het″ər-o-al′bu-mōs) a form of hemialbumose that is not soluble in water but is soluble in hydrochloric acid and sodium chloride solutions.

**het·ero·al·bu·mos·uria** (het″ər-o-al″bu-mōs-u′re-ə) the presence of heteroalbumose in the urine.

**het·ero·an·ti·body** (het″ər-o-an″tĭ-bod′e) an antibody specific for antigens originating in a species other than that of the antibody producer.

**het·ero·an·ti·gen** (het″ər-o-an′tĭ-jən) an antigen originating in a species different from, and therefore foreign to, the antibody producer.

**het·er·o·at·om** (het″ər-o-at′om) any atom in an organic compound other than carbon or hydrogen.

**het·er·o·aux·in** (het″ər-o-awk′sin) indoleacetic acid.

**Het·ero·bil·har·zia** (het″ər-o-bil-hahr′zhə) a genus of trematodes of the family Schistosomatidae that parasitize mammals. *H. america′na* has cercariae that cause a nonpatent visceral schistosomiasis in humans.

**het·ero·blas·tic** (het″ər-o-blas′tik) [*hetero-* + *blast-* + *-ic*] having origin in different kinds of tissue.

**het·ero·cel·lu·lar** (het″ər-o-sel′u-lər) composed of cells of different kinds.

**het·ero·cen·tric** (het″ər-o-sen′trik) [*hetero-* + *centric*] 1. made up of rays of light that neither are parallel nor meet in one point. 2. allocentric.

**het·ero·ceph·a·lus** (het″ər-o-sef′ə-ləs) [*hetero-* + *-cephalus*] a fetus with two unequal heads.

**het·ero·chi·ral** (het″ər-o-ki′rəl) [*hetero-* + *chiral*] reversed as regards right and left, but otherwise the same in form and size, as the hands.

**het·ero·chro·ma·tin** (het″ər-o-kro′mə-tin) [*hetero-* + *chromatin*] [MeSH: Heterochromatin] that state of chromatin in which it is dark-staining and tightly coiled, forming irregular clumps (karyosomes) or Barr bodies in the nuclei of cells in interphase, or stains densely in certain areas of mitotic chromosomes. Cf. *euchromatin.*
**constitutive h.,** the chromatin in regions of the chromosomes that are invariably heterochromatic, located in secondary constrictions of chromosomes 1, 9, and 16, the distal end of the long arm of the Y chromosome, and the centromeric and telomeric regions; it contains highly repetitive sequences of DNA that are genetically inactive, and serves as a structural element of the chromosome. See also *C banding,* under *banding.*
**facultative h.,** the chromatin in regions of the chromosomes that become heterochromatic in certain cells and tissues; e.g., it makes up the inactive X chromosome in female somatic cells.

**het·ero·chro·ma·tin·iza·tion** (het″ər-o-kro″mə-tin-ĭ-za′shən) 1. the condensation of euchromatin into heterochromatin. Called also *heterochromatization.* 2. lyonization.

**het·ero·chro·ma·ti·za·tion** (het″ər-o-kro″mə-tĭ-za′shən) 1. heterochromatinization. 2. lyonization.

**het·ero·chro·ma·to·sis** (het″ər-o-kro″mə-to′sis) heterochromia.

**het·ero·chro·mia** (het″ər-o-kro′me-ə) [*hetero-* + *chrom-* + *-ia*] diversity of color in a part or parts that should normally be of one color.
**h. i′ridis,** difference of color in the two irides, or in different areas of the same iris.

**het·ero·chro·mo·some** (het″ər-o-kro′mo-sōm) [*hetero-* + *chromosome*] a sex chromosome.

**het·ero·chro·mous** (het″ər-o-kro′məs) marked by diversity of color; exhibiting heterochromia.

**het·ero·chro·nia** (het″ər-o-kro′ne-ə) [*hetero-* + *chron-* + *-ia*] 1. the formation of parts or tissues, or the occurrence of a phenomenon, at an unusual time. Cf. *synchronia* (def. 2). 2. a difference in the rate or time of occurrence between two processes.

**het·ero·chron·ic** (het″ər-o-kron′ik) [*hetero-* + *chron-* + *-ic*] 1. pertaining to or characterized by heterochronia. 2. denoting different ages or stages of development, as between the excised organ and the implanted organ in transplantation procedures.

**het·er·och·ro·nous** (het″ər-ok′ro-nəs) heterochronic.

**het·ero·chy·lia** (het″ər-o-ki′le-ə) the sudden varying of the gastric secretion from normal acidity to hyperacidity or anacidity.

**het·ero·clad·ic** (het″ər-o-klad′ik) [*hetero-* + Gr. *klados* branch] indicating an anastomosis between terminal branches from different arteries.

**het·ero·crine** (het′ər-o-krin) [*hetero-* + Gr. *krinein* to separate] secreting more than one kind of matter.

**het·er·oc·ri·sis** (het″ər-o-kri′sis) [*hetero-* + *crisis*] an abnormal crisis with unusual timing and symptoms.

**het·ero·cyc·lic** (het″ər-o-sīk′lik) having or pertaining to a closed chain or ring formation which includes atoms of different elements.

**het·ero·cy·to·trop·ic** (het″ər-o-si″to-trop′ik) [*hetero-* + *cyto-* + *-tropic*] having an affinity for cells of different species; see under *antibody.*

**Het·er·od·era rad·i·cic·o·la** (het″ər-od′ə-ra rad″ĭ-sik′o-lə) a nematode parasitic on the common root vegetables, such as radishes, carrots, turnips, potatoes, etc., as well as on celery. When infested vegetables are eaten, ova of the parasite may appear in the stools and must be distinguished from those of true parasites.

**het·ero·der·mic** (het″ər-o-dər′mik) [*hetero-* + *dermic*] denoting a skin graft taken from a member of another species. See *dermatoheteroplasty.*

**het·ero·des·mot·ic** (het″ər-o-des-mot′ik) [*hetero-* + *desmo-* + *-ic*] joining dissimilar parts of the central nervous system; see under *fiber.*

**het·ero·did·y·mus** (het″ər-o-did′ə-məs) heterodymus.

**het·ero·di·mer** (het″ər-o-di′mər) a dimer consisting of unlike subunits.

**het·ero·dont** (het′ər-o-dont) [*heter-* + Gr. *odous* tooth] having teeth of different types, such as incisors and molars.

**Het·ero·dox·us** (het″ər-o-dok′səs) a genus of parasitic biting lice (order Mallophaga). *H. longitar′sus* is parasitic on kangaroos, wallabies, and sometimes dogs in Australia. *H. spi′niger* is parasitic on coyotes, wolves, and sometimes dogs in North and South America.

**het·er·od·ro·mous** (het″ər-od′ro-məs) [*hetero-* + *drom-* + *-ous*] moving, acting, or arranged in the opposite direction.

**het·er·od·y·mus** (het″ər-od′ə-məs) [*hetero-* + *-didymus*] asymmetrical conjoined twins in which one fetus has a second head, neck, and thorax attached to its thorax.

**het·er·oe·cious** (het″ər-e′shəs) requiring two or more hosts to complete the life cycle; said of certain fungi and insects, as opposed to *autoecious.*

**het·ero·erot·ic** (het″er-o-ĕrot′ik) 1. pertaining to or characterized by heteroeroticism. 2. alloerotic.

**het·ero·erot·i·cism** (het″ər-o-ə-rot′ĭ-siz-əm) 1. sexual feeling directed toward someone of the opposite sex. 2. alloeroticism (def. 1). 3. a stage in the development of object relationships in which the erotic energy is directed toward objects other than oneself, specifically to those of the opposite sex. Cf. *alloeroticism, autoeroticism.*

**het·ero·er·o·tism** (het″ər-o-er′o-tiz-əm) heteroeroticism.

**het·ero·fer·men·ta·tion** (het″ər-o-fər″mən-ta′shən) fermentation producing more than one major product; the term is often used as a synonym of heterolactic fermentation (q.v.).

**het·ero·fer·ment·er** (het″ər-o-fər-men′tər) a microorganism that exhibits heterofermentation.

**het·ero·gam·ete** (het″ər-o-gam′ēt) a gamete of different size and structure than the one with which it unites.

**het·ero·ga·met·ic** (het″ər-o-gə-met′ik) pertaining to the sex that produces gametes of different kinds, in terms of their sex chromosomes. In human beings the male, who possesses X-bearing and Y-bearing sperm, is the heterogametic sex.

**het·ero·gam·e·ty** (het″ər-o-gam′ə-te) the production of unlike gametes by an individual of one sex, as the production of X- and Y-bearing gametes by the human male.

**het·er·og·a·mous** (het″ər-og′ə-məs) pertaining to heterogamy.

**het·er·og·a·my** (het″ər-og′ə-me) [*hetero-* + Gr. *gamōs* marriage] reproduction resulting from the union of two gametes that differ in size and structure; called also *oogamy.* See also *homogamy* and *isogamy.*

**het·ero·gan·gli·on·ic** (het″ər-o-gang″le-on′ik) [*hetero-* + *ganglion* + *-ic*] interganglionic.

**het·ero·ge·ne·i·ty** (het″ər-o-jə-ne′ĭ-te) the state or quality of being heterogeneous. In genetics, the production of identical or similar phenotypes by different genetic mechanisms. A phenotype resembling a known phenotype but determined by a different genetic mechanism is called a genocopy or genetic mimic.

**genetic h.**, the production of a specific clinical or biochemical phenotype by more than one genetic mechanism or by mutation at more than one gene.

**het·ero·ge·ne·ous** (het″ər-o-je′ne-əs) [*hetero-* + Gr. *genos* kind] 1. consisting of or composed of dissimilar elements or ingredients; not having a uniform quality throughout. 2. in genetics, the term denotes a trait that can be produced by different genes or combinations of genes.

**het·ero·gen·e·sis** (het″ər-o-gen′ə-sis) [*hetero-* + *-genesis*] 1. alternation of generations; reproduction that differs in character in successive generations. 2. asexual generation.

**het·ero·ge·net·ic** (het″ər-o-jə-net′ik) 1. pertaining to heterogenesis. 2. not arising within the organism.

**het·er·o·gen·ic** (het″ər-o-jen′ik) derived from a different source or species; see *xenograft.*

**het·ero·ge·nic·i·ty** (het″ər-o-jə-nis′ĭ-te) heterogeneity.

**het·ero·ge·note** (het′ər-o-je″nōt) [*hetero-* + *gene* (analogy with zygote)] in bacterial genetics, a merozygote in which the corresponding alleles at a specific locus of the diploid region of the genome are different. See also *homogenote* and *merozygote.*

**het·er·og·e·nous** (het″ər-oj′ə-nəs) 1. derived from a different source or species; see *xenograft.* 2. heterogeneous.

**het·ero·geu·sia** (het″ər-o-goo′zhə) [*hetero-* + Gr. *geusis* taste + *-ia*] any parageusia in which all gustatory stimuli are distorted in a similar way; Cf. *cacogeusia.*

**het·ero·glob·u·lose** (het″ər-o-glob′u-lōs) a heteroalbumose obtained from a globulin.

**het·er·og·o·ny** (het″ər-og′ə-ne) [*hetero-* + Gr. *gonos* procreation] heterogenesis.

**het·ero·graft** (het′ər-o-graft″) xenograft.

**het·ero·hem·ag·glu·ti·na·tion** (het″ər-o-hem″ə-gloo″tĭ-na′shən) agglutination of erythrocytes of one species by hemagglutinins derived from an individual of a different species.

**het·ero·hem·ag·glu·ti·nin** (het″ər-o-hem″ə-gloo′tĭ-nin) a hemagglutinin derived from one species that agglutinates erythrocytes of organisms of one or more other species.

**het·ero·he·mol·y·sin** (het″ər-o-he-mol′ə-sin) 1. a hemolysin occurring spontaneously in the blood of an untreated animal that will hemolyze the blood cells of an animal of another species. 2. hemolysin established in one species by deliberate immunization with blood cells of an animal of another species.

**het·ero·hex·o·san** (het″ər-o-hek′so-san) any one of a class of heterosaccharides in which the sugar components are hexoses.

**Het·er·o·hy·rax** (het″ə-ro-hi′raks) a genus of rock hyraxes. *H. bru′cei* is a species found in hilly regions of Ethiopia that is a common reservoir for *Leishmania aethiopica,* the cause of Ethiopian cutaneous leishmaniasis.

**het·ero·im·mune** (het″ər-o-ĭ-mūn′) pertaining to or characterized by heteroimmunity.

**het·ero·im·mu·ni·ty** (het″ə-ro-ĭ-mu′nĭ-te) 1. an immune state that results from the immunization of an animal belonging to one species with cells of an animal of a different species. 2. a state in which immunological response by the body to exogenous antigens, which include drugs and infectious agents, results in immunopathological changes.

**het·ero·kary·on** (het″ər-o-kar′e-on) [*hetero-* + *karyon*] a cell or hypha containing two or more nuclei of different genetic constitutions.

**het·ero·kary·o·sis** (het″ər-o-kar″e-o′sis) [*heterokaryon* + *-osis*] 1. the formation of heterokaryons. 2. the state of containing heterokaryons.

**het·ero·ker·a·to·plas·ty** (het″ər-o-ker′ə-to-plas″te) [*hetero-* + *keratoplasty*] grafting of corneal tissue from an individual of a species other than that of the recipient.

**het·ero·ki·ne·sis** (het″ər-o-kĭ-ne′sis) [*hetero-* + *kinesis*] the differential distribution of the sex chromosomes (X and Y in humans) in the developing gametes of a heterogametic organism.

**het·ero·lac·tic** (het″ər-o-lak′tik) bacterial fermentation which produces large quantities of lactic acid along with acetic acid, ethanol, and $CO_2$.

**het·ero·la·lia** (het″ər-o-la′le-ə) [*hetero-* + *lal-* + *-ia*] heterophasia.

**het·ero·lat·er·al** (het″ər-o-lat′ər-əl) [*hetero-* + *lateral*] relating to the opposite side; contralateral.

**het·ero·lit·er·al** (het″ər-o-lit′ər-əl) marked by the substitution of one letter for another in pronouncing words.

**het·ero·lith** (het′ər-o-lith) [*hetero-* + *-lith*] an intestinal concretion not formed of mineral matter.

**het·er·ol·o·gous** (het″ər-ol′ə-gəs) [*hetero-* + Gr. *logos* due relation, proportion] 1. made up of tissue not normal to the part. 2. xenogeneic. 3. pertaining to antigen and antibody that are not homologous, i.e., the antigen is not the one that elicited the production of the antibody.

**het·er·ol·o·gy** (het″ər-ol′ə-je) 1. abnormality in structure, arrangement, or manner of formation. 2. in chemistry, the relationship between substances of partial identity of structure but of different properties.

**het·er·ol·y·sin** (het″ər-ol′ĭ-sin) a lysin that dissolves cells of species other than the one in which it is formed, by leading to interruption of the integrity of the cell membranes; a lysin that is formed on the introduction of antigen from a different species.

**het·er·ol·y·sis** (het″ər-ol′ĭ-sis) [*hetero-* + *-lysis*] lysis of the cells of one species by lysin from a different species.

**het·ero·ly·so·some** (het″ər-o-li′so-sōm) a secondary lysosome containing exogenous substances with digestion in progress.

**het·ero·lyt·ic** (het″ər-o-lit′ik) pertaining to or caused by heterolysis or a heterolysin.

**het·ero·mas·ti·gote** (het″ər-o-mas′ti-gōt) [*hetero-* + *mastigote*] having one or more forward flagella together with at least one directed backward.

**het·er·om·er·al** (het″ər-om′ər-əl) heteromeric.

**het·ero·mer·ic** (het″ər-o-mer′ik) [*hetero-* + *mer-*[1] + *-ic*] sending processes through one of the commissures to the white matter of the other side of the spinal cord; said of spinal neurons.

**het·er·om·er·ous** (het″ər-om′ər-əs) heteromeric.

**het·ero·meta·pla·sia** (het″ər-o-met″ə-pla′shə) [*hetero-* + *metaplasia*] development of tissue into a variety foreign to the part where it is produced.

**het·ero·me·tro·pia** (het″ər-o-mə-tro′pe-ə) [*hetero-* + Gr. *metron* measure + *-opia*] the state in which there are differences in degree of refraction in the two eyes.

**het·ero·mor·phic** (het″ər-o-mor′fik) heteromorphous.

**het·ero·mor·pho·sis** (het″ər-o-mor-fo′sis) [*hetero-* + *morphosis*] the development, in regeneration, of an organ or structure different from the one that was lost.

**het·ero·mor·phous** (het″ər-o-mor′fəs) [*hetero-* + *-morphous*] 1. of abnormal shape or structure; differing from the type. 2. having synaptic chromosome mates which differ in size, form, or structure.

**het·er·on·o·mous** (het″ər-on′ə-məs) [*hetero-* + *nom-* + *-ous*] in biology, subject to different laws of growth; specialized along different lines.

**het·er·on·y·mous** (het″ər-on′ĭ-məs) [*heter-* + Gr. *onyma* name] in ophthalmology, pertaining to the noncorresponding vertical halves of the visual fields of both eyes, i.e., the nasal half of the left eye and the nasal of the right, or the temporal half of the left eye and the temporal of the right.

**het·ero·os·teo·plas·ty** (het″ər-o-os′te-o-plas″te) [*hetero-* + *osteoplasty*] the grafting of bone from an individual of one species to an individual of another.

**het·ero·ov·u·lar** (het″ər-o-ov′u-lər) pertaining to or derived from different ova; dizygotic.

**het·er·op·a·gus** (het″ər-op′ə-gəs) [*hetero-* + *-pagus*] asymmetrical conjoined twins; see under *twin.*

**het·ero·pan·cre·a·tism** (het″ər-o-pan′kre-ə-tiz-əm) an irregular condition of functioning on the part of the pancreas.

**het·er·op·a·thy** (het″ər-op′ə-the) [*hetero-* + *-pathy*] 1. hyperesthesia. 2. allopathy.

**het·ero·pen·to·san** (het″ər-o-pen′to-san) any of a class of heterosaccharides in which the sugar components are pentoses, e.g., gums, mucilages, and pectins.

**het·ero·phago·some** (het″ər-o-fag′o-sōm) [*hetero-* + *phagosome*] an intracytoplasmic vacuole formed by phagocytosis or pinocytosis, which becomes fused with a lysosome, subjecting its contents to enzymatic digestion. Called also *heterophagic vacuole.*

**het·er·oph·a·gy** (het″ər-of′ə-je) [*hetero-* + *-phagy*] the taking into a cell of exogenous material by phagocytosis or pinocytosis and the digestion of the ingested material after fusion of the newly formed vacuole with a lysosome. Cf. *autophagy.*

**het·er·oph·a·ny** (het″ər-of′ə-ne) [*hetero-* + Gr. *phainein* to appear] a difference in the manifestations of the same condition.

**het·ero·pha·sia** (het″ər-o-fa′zhə) [*hetero-* + *-phasia*] the uttering of words other than those intended by the speaker; called also *heterolalia, heterophasis,* and *heterophemia.*

**het·ero·pha·sis** (het″ər-o-fa′sis) heterophasia.

**het·ero·phe·mia** (het″ər-o-fe′me-ə) [*hetero-* + *-phemia*] heterophasia.

**het·ero·phil** (het′ər-o-fil″) [*hetero-* + *-philic*] 1. a type of granular leukocyte represented in humans by the neutrophil and in other mammals by cells whose granules have variable sizes and staining characteristics. Called also *heterophilic leukocyte.* 2. pertaining to any group of cross-reacting antigens *(heterophil antigens)* occurring in several species and having a species distribution that does not correspond to phylogenetic relationships or to antibody directed against such antigens.

**het·ero·phile** (het′ər-o-fīl″, fil″) heterophil.

**het·ero·phil·ic** (het″ər-o-fil′ik) 1. pertaining to or having heterophils. 2. heterophil (def. 2). 3. staining with a type of stain other than the usual one.

**het·ero·pho·ral·gia** (het″ər-o-fo-ral′jə) [*hetero-* + Gr. *phoros* bearing + *-algia*] heterophoria associated with pain.

**het·ero·pho·ria** (het″ər-o-for′e-ə) [*hetero-* + Gr. *phora* movement, range] failure of the visual axes to remain parallel after the visual fusional stimuli have been eliminated. The various forms of heterophoria are called *phorias,* their direction being indicated by the appropriate prefix. See *cyclophoria, esophoria, exophoria, hyperphoria, hypophoria,* and *latent deviation.*

**het·ero·phor·ic** (het″ər-o-for′ik) pertaining to or characterized by heterophoria.

**het·er·oph·thal·mia** (het″ər-of-thal′me-ə) [*hetero-* + *ophthalm-* + *-ia*] difference in the direction of the axes, or in the color, of the two eyes.

**het·er·oph·thal·mos** (het″ər-of-thal′mos) heterophthalmia.

**het·ero·phy·di·a·sis** (het″ər-o-fə-di′ə-sis) heterophyiasis.

**Het·er·oph·y·es** (het″ər-of′e-ēz) [*hetero-* + Gr. *phyē* stature] a genus of minute trematodes of the family Heterophyidae, found in the middle third of the small intestine of humans, dogs, cats, and other fish-eating mammals. *H. hetero′phyes* is found in Egypt, Asia, and Turkey. *H. katsura′dai* and *H. brevicae′ca* have been reported in humans in Japan and the Philippines.

**het·ero·phy·i·a·sis** (het″ər-o-fi-i′ə-sis) infection with trematodes of the genus *Heterophyes;* it is generally asymptomatic.

**Het·ero·phy·i·dae** (het″ər-o-fi′ĭ-de) [MeSH: Heterophyidae] a family of trematodes that includes the genera *Heterophyes* and *Metagonimus.*

**het·ero·pla·sia** (het″ər-o-pla′zhə) [*hetero-* + *-plasia*] the replacement of normal by abnormal tissue; malposition of normal cells.

**het·ero·plasm** (het′ər-o-plaz-əm) any heterologous tissue.

**het·ero·plas·tic** (het′ər-o-plas″tik) 1. pertaining to heteroplasia. 2. xenogeneic.

**het·ero·plas·tid** (het″ər-o-plas′tid) a xenograft.

**het·ero·plas·ty** (het′ər-o-plas″te) [*hetero-* + *-plasty*] heterotransplantation.

**het·ero·ploid** (het′ər-o-ploid″) 1. pertaining to or characterized by heteroploidy. 2. an individual or cell with an abnormal number of chromosomes.

**het·ero·ploi·dy** (het′ər-o-ploi″de) the state of having an abnormal number of chromosomes.

**Het·er·op·o·da** (het″ər-op′o-də) a genus of large spiders sometimes confused with tarantulas.
**H. venato′ria,** a large spider found in shipments of tropical fruit, particularly bananas; its bite is painful, but not serious.

**het·er·op·o·dal** (het″ər-op′o-dəl) [*hetero-* + *pod-* + *-al*[1]] having branches or processes of different kinds; said of nerve cells.

**het·ero·poly·mer·ic** (het″ər-o-pol″e-mer′ik) composed of dissimilar constituent building units, as a macromolecule, e.g., a protein.

**het·ero·poly·sac·cha·ride** (het″ər-o-pol″e-sak′ə-rīd) any polysaccharide macromolecule containing two or more different sugars, its function varying with the nature of its residues.

**het·ero·pro·so·pus** (het″ər-o-pro′so-pəs) [*hetero-* + Gr. *prosōpon* face] janiceps.

**het·ero·pro·te·ose** (het″ər-o-pro′te-ōs) a primary proteose that is insoluble in water but soluble in dilute salt solution.

**het·er·op·sia** (het″ər-op′se-ə) [*hetero-* + *-opsia*] unequal vision in the two eyes.

**Het·er·op·tera** (het″ər-op′tər-ə) [*hetero-* + Gr. *pteron* wing] a suborder of Hemiptera characterized by the possession of two pairs of wings, one horny, the other membranous; it includes the medically important families Cimicidae and Reduviidae.

**het·er·op·tics** (het″ər-op′tiks) [*hetero-* + *optics*] false or perverted vision; visual perception of objects not in the field of vision or misinterpretation of visual images.

**het·ero·pyk·no·sis** (het″ər-o-pik-no′sis) [*hetero-* + *pyknosis*] 1. the quality of showing variations in density throughout. 2. a state of differential condensation observed in comparison of different chromosomes, or of different regions of the same chromosome.
**negative h.,** attenuation of condensation observed in comparison of different chromosomes, or of different regions of the same chromosome.

**positive h.**, accentuation of condensation observed in comparison of different chromosomes, or of different regions of the same chromosome.

**het•ero•pyk•not•ic** (het″ər-o-pik-not′ik) pertaining to or characterized by heteropyknosis.
**negatively h.**, showing areas of lesser condensation than normal.
**positively h.**, showing areas of greater condensation than normal.

**het•ero•sac•cha•ride** (het″ər-o-sak′ə-rīd) a polysaccharide containing a carbohydrate and a noncarbohydrate unit. Cf. *holosaccharide.*

**het•ero•sce•das•tic•i•ty** (het″ər-o-skə-das-tis′ĭ-te) [*hetero-* + Gr. *skedastikos* tending to scatter] the property of having unequal variances.

**het•ero•scope** (het′ər-o-skōp) [*heterophoria* + *-scope*] a pair of fusion tubes so mounted as to subserve the observation of the progress of cases of heterophoria.

**het•er•os•co•py** (het″ər-os′kə-pe) 1. inequality of vision in the two eyes. 2. examination with a heteroscope.

**het•ero•sex•u•al** (het″ər-o-sek′shoo-əl) 1. pertaining to the opposite sex; directed toward a person of the opposite sex; the opposite of homosexual. 2. one who is sexually attracted to persons of the opposite sex. 3. contrasexual (def. 2).

**het•ero•sex•u•al•i•ty** (het″ər-o-sek″shoo-al′ĭ-te) [*hetero-* + *sexuality*] sexual orientation to or activity with those of the opposite sex, as distinguished from homosexuality.

**het•er•o•sis** (het″ər-o′sis) [Gr. *heterōsis* alteration] the condition in which the first generation hybrid shows more vigor, as measured by growth, survival, and fertility, than either of the parent strains; it is believed to be caused by the dominance (or interaction) of favorable alleles not common to both parental populations. Called also *hybrid vigor.*

**het•er•os•mia** (het″ər-os′me-ə) [*heter-* + *osm-*[1] + *-ia*] any parosmia in which all olfactory stimuli are distorted in a similar way; cf. *cacosmia.*

**het•ero•some** (het″ər-o-sōm) [*hetero-* + *-some*] a sex chromosome.

**het•er•os•po•rous** (het″ər-os′pə-rəs) having spores of two kinds (such as megaspores and microspores), which reproduce asexually.

**het•ero•sug•ges•tion** (het″ər-o-səg-jes′chən) [*hetero-* + *suggestion*] suggestion received from another person; opposed to *autosuggestion.*

**het•ero•tax•ia** (het″ər-o-tak′se-ə) [*hetero-* + Gr. *taxis* arrangement] anomalous placement or transposition of viscera or parts.

**het•ero•tax•ic** (het″ər-o-tak′sik) affected with heterotaxia.

**het•ero•tax•is** (het″ər-o-tak′sis) heterotaxia.

**het•ero•taxy** (het′ə-ro-tak″se) heterotaxia.

**het•ero•thal•lic** (het″ər-o-thal′ik) pertaining to or exhibiting heterothallism.

**het•ero•thal•lism** (het″ər-o-thal′iz-əm) a form of sexual reproduction in which the isogamete must fuse with a gamete formed by a cell of a different mating type, as in various algae and fungi.

**het•ero•ther•a•py** (het″ər-o-ther′ə-pe) [*hetero-* + *therapya*] treatment of disease by remedies which are antagonistic to the principal symptoms of the disease; nonspecific therapy.

**het•ero•therm** (het′ər-o-thərm″) an animal which exhibits heterothermy.

**het•ero•ther•mic** (het″ər-o-thər′mik) pertaining to or characterized by heterothermy.

**het•ero•ther•my** (het′ər-o-thər″me) [*hetero-* + Gr. *thermē* heat] the exhibition of widely different body temperatures at different times or under different conditions, as certain species of birds, marsupials, or hibernating species.

**het•ero•to•nia** (het″ər-o-to′ne-ə) [*hetero-* + *ton-* + *-ia*] a state characterized by variations in tension or tone.

**het•ero•ton•ic** (het″ər-o-ton′ik) pertaining to or characterized by heterotonia.

**het•ero•to•pia** (het″ər-o-to′pe-ə) [*hetero-* + Gr. *top-* + *-ia*] [MeSH: Choristoma] 1. malposition. 2. choristoma.

**het•ero•top•ic** (het″ər-o-top′ik) ectopic.

**het•er•ot•o•py** (het″ər-ot′ə-pe) ectopia.

**het•ero•trans•plant** (het″ər-o-trans′plant) xenograft.

**het•ero•trans•plan•ta•tion** (het″ər-o-trans″plan-ta′shən) xenogeneic transplantation.

**het•ero•tri•cho•sis** (het″ər-o-trĭ-ko′sis) [*hetero-* + *trichosis*] growth of hair of different colors on the body.

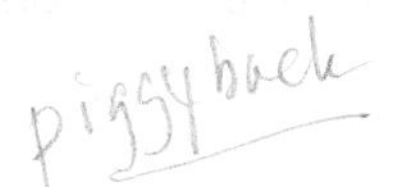

**h. supercilio′rum**, difference in color of the hairs of the two eyebrows.

**het•ero•tri•mer** (het″ər-o-tri′mər) a trimer having at least one subunit that differs from the others.

**het•ero•troph** (het′ər-o-trōf″) a heterotrophic organism.

**het•ero•tro•phia** (het″ər-o-tro′fe-ə) [*hetero-* + *troph-* + *-ia*] any disorder or fault of nutrition.

**het•ero•troph•ic** (het″ər-o-trof′ik) [*hetero-* + *-trophic*] not self-sustaining; said of a type of nutrition in which organisms derive energy from the oxidation of organic compounds either by consumption or absorption of other organisms. Called also *organotrophic.* Cf. *autotrophic.*

**het•er•ot•ro•phy** (het″ər-ot′rə-fe) 1. the state of being heterotrophic; heterotrophic nutrition. 2. heterotrophia.

**het•ero•tro•pia** (het″ər-o-tro′pe-ə) strabismus.

**het•ero•tro•pic** (het′ər-o-trōp″ik) [*hetero-* + *-tropic*] pertaining to an allosteric enzyme that is stimulated or inhibited by one or more effector molecules other than its substrate. Cf. *homotropic.*

**het•er•ot•ro•py** (het″ər-ot′rə-pe) strabismus.

**het•ero•typ•ic** (het″ə-ro-tip′ik) pertaining to, characteristic of, or belonging to a different type.

**het•ero•typ•i•cal** (het″ər-o-tip′ĭ-kəl) of a type differing from that usually or normally encountered; having characteristics peculiar to a different type; sometimes applied to the first meiotic division of the germ cells.

**het•ero•vac•cine** (het″ər-o-vak′sēn) a vaccine made from some microorganism other than the one causing the disease for which the vaccine is used; it is one form of nonspecific therapy.

**het•er•ox•e•nous** (het″ər-ok′sə-nəs) [*hetero-* + *xeno-* + *-ous*] requiring more than one host in the life cycle; said of certain parasites.

**het•ero•zo•ic** (het″ər-o-zo′ik) [*hetero-* + *zoic*] pertaining to another animal or species of animal.

**het•ero•zy•go•sis** (het″ər-o-zi-go′sis) the formation of a zygote by the union of gametes of unlike genetic constitution.

**het•ero•zy•gos•i•ty** (het″ər-o-zi-gos′ĭ-te) [*hetero-* + *zygosity*] the state of possessing different alleles at a given locus in regard to a given character.

**het•ero•zy•gote** (het″ər-o-zi′gōt) [*hetero-* + *zygote*] [MeSH: Heterozygote] an individual possessing different alleles in regard to a given character.
**manifesting h.**, a female heterozygous for an X-linked disorder in whom, because of unfavorable X inactivation, the trait is expressed clinically with about the same severity as in hemizygous affected males.

**het•ero•zy•gous** (het″ər-o-zi′gəs) pertaining to heterozygosity. *Doubly heterozygous:* having different alleles at each of two separate loci. See also *homozygous.*

**Het•ra•zan** (het′rə-zan) trademark for preparations of diethylcarbamazine citrate.

**Heub•lein method** (hoib′līn) [Arthur Carl *Heublein,* American radiologist, 1879–1932] see under *method.*

**Heub•ner's disease (endarteritis)** (hoib′nərz) [Johann Otto Leonhard *Heubner,* German pediatrician, 1843–1926] see under *disease.*

**Heub•ner-Her•ter disease** (hoib′nər-hər′tər) [J.O.L. *Heubner;* Christian Archibald *Herter,* American physician, 1865–1910] see under *disease.*

**heu•ris•tic** (hu-ris′tik) [Gr. *heuriskein* to find out, discover] encouraging or promoting investigation; conducive to discovery.

**Heu•ser's membrane** (hoi′zərz) [Chester *Heuser,* American embryologist, 1885–1965] see under *membrane.*

**He•vea** (he′ve-ə) the rubber trees, a genus of tropical trees of the family Euphorbiaceae, whose latex is the source of one kind of rubber. The most important species is *H. brasilien′sis.*

**HEW** Department of Health, Education, and Welfare; succeeded by the Department of Health and Human Services (HHS).

**hex(a)-** [Gr. *hex* six] a combining form meaning six.

**hexa•ba•sic** (hek″sə-ba′sik) [*hexa-* + *basic*] having six atoms replaceable by a base.

**Hexa-Be•ta•lin** (hek″sə-be′tə-lin) trademark for preparations of pyridoxine hydrochloride.

**hexa•chlo•ro•ben•zene** (hek″sə-klor″o-ben′zēn) [MeSH: Hexachlorobenzene] a compound used in organic synthesis and as a fungicide; it is toxic to humans and other animals, causing cutaneous porphyria and liver disease, and may be carcinogenic. Since it does not break down easily, when used to preserve livestock feeds it may build up in the tissues of the animals.

**hexa·chlo·ro·cy·clo·hex·ane** (hek″sə-klor″o-si″klo-hek′sān) benzene hexachloride.

**hexa·chlo·ro·eth·ane** (hek″sə-klor″o-eth′ān) a crystalline anthelmintic used to treat fascioliasis in cattle and sheep.

**hexa·chlo·ro·phene** (hek″sə-klor′o-fēn) [USP] [MeSH: Hexachlorophene] an antibacterial effective against gram-positive organisms; used as a topical anti-infective and detergent, mainly in soaps and dermatological preparations, and in veterinary medicine to combat flukes in poultry and ruminants.

**hex·a·co·sane** (hek″sə-ko′sān) [*hexa-* + Gr. *eikosi* twenty] an aliphatic hydrocarbon extracted from plant waxes.

**hex·ad** (hek′sad) 1. a group or combination of six similar or related entities. 2. any element having a valence of six.

**hexa·dac·tyl·ia** (hek″sə-dak-til′e-ə) hexadactyly.

**hexa·dac·ty·lism** (hek″sə-dak′tə-liz-əm) hexadactyly.

**hexa·dac·ty·ly** (hek″sə-dak′tə-le) [*hexa-* + *daktyl-* + *-ia*] the occurrence of six digits on one hand or foot.

**hexa·dec·a·no·ate** (hek″sə-dek″ə-no′āt) palmitate.

**hexa·dec·a·no·ic ac·id** (hek″sə-dek″ə-no′ik) systematic name for *palmitic acid;* see table at *fatty acid.*

**Hex·a·drol** (hek′sə-drol) trademark for preparations of dexamethasone.

**hex·a·ene** (hek′sə-ēn) a chemical compound in which there are six conjugated double bonds.

**-hex·a·ene** (hek′sə-ēn) a suffix denoting a chemical compound in which there are six conjugated double bonds.

**Hex·a·ge·nia** (hek″sə-je′ne-ə) a genus of mayflies (order Ephemeroptera). *H. bilinea′ta* is the lake fly, a species found on the shores of Lake Erie whose cast skins may cause asthma.

**hexa·hy·dric** (hek″sə-hi′drik) containing six atoms of hydrogen.

**Hex·a·len** (hek′sə-len) trademark for a preparation of altretamine.

**hex·a·mer** (hek′sə-mər) 1. a polymer molecule composed of six monomers. 2. a capsomer having six structural subunits.

**hex·a·meth·y·lat·ed** (hek″sə-məth′ə-lāt-əd) containing six methyl groups.

**hexa·meth·yl·en·amine** (hek″sə-meth″əl-ēn-am′ēn) methenamine.

**hexa·meth·yl·mel·amine (HMM)** (hek″sə-meth″əl-mel′ə-mēn) former name for altretamine.

**hexa·meth·yl·phos·phor·am·ide** (hek″sə-meth″əl-fos-for′ə-mīd) hempa.

**hex·a·mine** (hek″sə-mēn) methenamine.

**Hex·am·i·ta** (hek-sam′ĭ-tə) [*hexa-* + Gr. *mitos* thread] a genus of flagellate protozoa (suborder Diplomonadina, order Diplomonadida), characterized by the presence of two anterior nuclei and six anterior and two posterior flagella. It comprises free-living species as well as intestinal parasites. *H. melea′gridis* causes enteritis in wild and domestic fowl, including turkeys, chickens, quail, and partridges. *H. mu′ris* is found in rats, mice, hamsters, and various wild rodents, *H. salmo′nis* in trout and salmon, and *H. colum′bae* in pigeons.

**hex·am·i·ti·a·sis** (heks-am″ĭ-ti′ə-sis) infection with protozoa of the genus *Hexamita*; the most economically significant disease is an often fatal enteritis in turkeys caused by *H. meleagridis.*

**hex·ane** (hek′sān) n-hexane; an aliphatic hydrocarbon of the methane series, $C_6H_{14}$, obtained by distillation from petroleum, occurring as a colorless, volatile, highly flammable liquid with a characteristic odor; it is a constituent of petroleum benzin, and is used as a solvent and in spectrophotometry.

**Hex·a·nic·o·tol** (hek″sə-nik′o-tol) trademark for a preparation of inositol niacinate.

**hex·a·no·ate** (hek″sə-no′āt) caproate.

**hex·a·no·ic ac·id** (hek″sə-no′ik) systematic name for *caproic acid.*

**Hex·ap·o·da** (hek-sap′o-də) [*hexa-* + Gr. *pous* foot] Insecta.

**hex·atom·ic** (hek″sə-tom′ik) 1. containing six atoms of an element, or six replaceable univalent atoms.

**hexa·va·lent** (hek″sə-va′lənt) having a valence of six.

**Hexa·vi·bex** (hek″sə-vi′beks) trademark for a preparation of pyridoxine hydrochloride.

**hexa·vi·ta·min** (hek″sə-vi′tə-min) a preparation, in capsule or tablet form, containing vitamin A, vitamin D, ascorbic acid, thiamine hydrochloride, riboflavin, and niacinamide.

**hex·en·milch** (hek′sən-milk) [Ger. "witches' milk"] a milklike secretion from the breast of a newborn infant; called also *witch's milk.*

**hex·es·trol** (hek-ses′trol) [MeSH: Hexestrol] a diethylstilbestrol derivative having the uses of estrogen (q.v.); administered orally and parenterally.

**hex·e·thal so·di·um** (hek′sə-thal) a short-acting barbiturate used as a sedative and hypnotic.

**hex·et·i·dine** (hek-set′ĭ-dēn) [MeSH: Hexetidine] an antifungal, antiprotozoal, and antibacterial agent used mainly as a topical anti-infective in the treatment of vaginitis.

**hex·hy·dric** (heks-hi′drik) containing six atoms of replaceable hydrogen.

**hexo·bar·bi·tal** (hek″so-bahr′bĭ-təl) [MeSH: Hexobarbital] a short-acting barbiturate used as a sedative and hypnotic; administered orally.

**h. sodium,** the sodium salt of hexobarbital, which is a very short-acting barbiturate; used for pre- and postanesthesia sedation and hypnosis, administered orally.

**hexo·bar·bi·tone** (hek″so-bahr′bĭ-tōn) hexobarbital.

**hexo·ben·dine** (hek″so-ben′dēn) [MeSH: Hexobendine] a vasodilator which has been used in the treatment of coronary insufficiency and angina of effort.

**hexo·cy·cli·um meth·yl·sul·fate** (hek″so-si′kle-əm meth″əl-sul′fāt) a quaternary ammonium anticholinergic which inhibits gastric secretion and gastrointestinal motility; used especially as an adjunct in the treatment of peptic ulcer, administered orally.

**hexo·ki·nase** (hek″so-ki′nās) [EC 2.7.1.1] [MeSH: Hexokinase] an enzyme of the transferase class that catalyzes the phosphorylation of hexose at the 6 carbon, the initial step in the cellular utilization of free hexoses. The enzyme occurs in all tissues and exists as various isozymes. Those in brain and muscles are relatively nonspecific; glucose, fructose, and mannose are effective substrates at low concentrations. The liver isozyme, often designated type IV, is called also *glucokinase* because it is more specific for glucose.

**hex·one** (hek′sōn) see under *base.*

**hex·on·ic ac·id** (hek-son′ik) an aldonic acid formed specifically from an aldohexose, e.g., gluconic acid.

**hex·os·amine** (hek-sōs′ə-mēn) any of a class of amino sugars derived from hexoses.

**hex·os·amin·i·dase** (hek″sōs-ə-min′ĭ-dās) 1. any of the enzymes that cleave hexosamine or *N*-acetylhexosamine residues from gangliosides or other glycosides. Specific enzymes are named for the specific amino sugar and linkage that are potential substrates (e.g., *α-N*-acetylglucosaminidase). 2. *β-N*-acetylhexosaminidase.

**h. A,** *β-N*-acetylhexosaminidase, isozyme A.

**h. B,** *β-N*-acetylhexosaminidase, isozyme B.

**hex·o·san** (hek′so-san) any of the class of polysaccharides composed of hexose residues; included are fructosans, galactans, glucans, and mannans.

**hex·o·sa·zone** (hek-sōs′ə-zōn) any osazone formed from a hexose.

**hex·ose** (hek′sōs) a monosaccharide containing six carbon atoms in a molecule.

**h. monophosphate,** a general term used to describe any or all of the phosphorylated hexoses involved in carbohydrate metabolism.

**hex·ose 1-phos·phate uri·dyl·yl·trans·fer·ase** (hek″sōs fos′fāt u″rĭ-dil″əl-trans′fər-ās) UDPglucose–hexose-1-phosphate uridylyltransferase.

**hex·o·side** (hek′so-sīd) any glycoside in which the sugar component is a hexose.

**hex·o·syl·trans·fer·ase** (hek″so-səl-trans′fər-ās) [EC 2.4.1] one of a sub-subclass of enzymes of the transferase class that catalyze the transfer of a hexose group from one compound to another.

**hex·u·lose** (hek′su-lōs) ketohexose.

**hex·uron·ic ac·id** (hek″su-ron′ik) any uronic acid formed by oxidation of a hexose.

**hex·yl** (hek′səl) [*hex-* + *-yl*] a hydrocarbon, $C_6H_{13}$, in many isomeric forms.

**hex·yl·re·sor·ci·nol** (hek″səl-rə-sor′sĭ-nol) [USP] [MeSH: Hexylresorcinol] a substituted phenol with bactericidal properties used as an antiseptic in mouthwashes and skin wound cleansers; it has also been used as an anthelmintic but has largely been replaced by other drugs.

**Hey's amputation (operation),** etc. (hāz) [William *Hey,* English surgeon, 1736–1819] see under *amputation, derangement,* and *saw;* see *encysted hernia,* under *hernia;* and see *margo falciformis hiatus saphenus.*

**Hey·mann's nephritis** (ha′mahnz) [Walter *Heymann,* Belgian-born American physician, 1901–1985] see under *nephritis.*

**Hey·mans** (ha'mənz) Corneille. Belgian physiologist, 1892–1968; winner of the Nobel prize for medicine or physiology in 1938 for his discovery of the role played by the sinus and aortic mechanisms in the regulation of respiration.

**HF** [MeSH: Factor XII] Hageman factor (factor XII; see under *coagulation factors,* at *factor*); high frequency.

**Hf** symbol of *hafnium.*

**Hfr** high frequency of recombination; Hfr cells are the sexual or donor (male) stage of bacteria having the F (fertility) factor in the chromosome, which enables them to transfer chromosomal material to recipient (female) bacteria not having this factor.

**Hg** symbol for mercury (L. *hydrargyrum*).

**Hgb** hemoglobin.

**HGBV** hepatitis GB virus.

**HGE** human granulocytic ehrlichiosis.

**HGF** hyperglycemic-glycogenolytic factor (glucagon); hepatocyte growth factor.

**HGG** human gamma globulin.

**HGH, hGH** human (pituitary) growth hormone.

**hGHr** human growth hormone recombinant.

**HGPRT** hypoxanthine-guanine phosphoribosyltransferase, a common name for hypoxanthine phosphoribosyl transferase (HPRT).

**HGV** hepatitis G virus.

**HHS** Department of Health and Human Services; formerly Department of Health, Education, and Welfare (HEW).

**HHT** hydroxyheptadecatrienoic acid.

**HI** hemagglutination inhibition; see under *tests.*

**5-HIAA** 5-hydroxyindoleacetic acid.

**hi·a·tal** (hi-a'təl) pertaining to or affecting a hiatus.

**hi·a·tion** (hi-a'shən) yawning.

**hi·a·tus** (hi-a'təs) gen. and pl. *hia'tus* [L.] [TA] general term for a gap, cleft, or opening.

**h. adducto'rius** [TA], adductor hiatus: the opening between the long tendon of the adductor magnus and the femur, marking the distal end of the adductor canal; called also *h. tendineus.*

**h. aor'ticus** [TA], aortic hiatus: the opening in the diaphragm through which the aorta and thoracic duct pass.

**Breschet's h.,** helicotrema.

**h. of canal for greater petrosal nerve,** h. canalis nervi petrosi majoris.

**h. of canal for lesser petrosal nerve,** h. canalis nervi petrosi minoris.

**h. cana'lis facia'lis, h. cana'lis ner'vi petro'si majo'ris** [TA], hiatus for greater petrosal nerve: an opening in the petrous part of the temporal bone in the floor of the middle cranial fossa that transmits the greater petrosal nerve and a branch of the middle meningeal artery.

**h. cana'lis ner'vi petro'si mino'ris** [TA], hiatus for lesser petrosal nerve: the small, laterally placed opening on the anterior surface of the pyramid of the temporal bone that transmits the lesser petrosal nerve.

**esophageal h., h. esopha'geus,** h. oesophageus.

**h. of facial canal, h. of fallopian canal, h. fallo'pii, false h. of fallopian canal,** h. canalis nervi petrosi majoris.

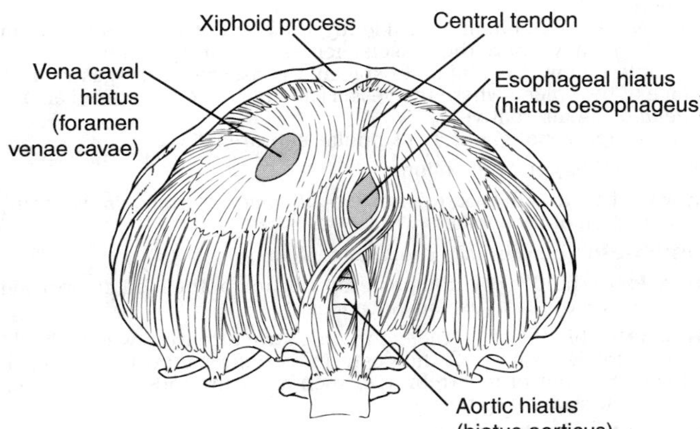


Inferior view of the diaphragm, showing the openings through which the aorta, esophagus, and vena cava pass.

**h. femora'lis,** anulus femoralis.

**h. fina'lis sacra'lis,** a cleft in the lowermost sacral vertebra.

**h. for greater petrosal nerve,** h. canalis nervi petrosi majoris.

**h. interme'dius lumbosacra'lis,** a cleft in the region of the first sacral vertebra, considered to represent a normally delayed ossification in young subjects.

**h. interos'seus,** the opening above the interosseous membrane of the forearm for the passage of the posterior interosseous vessels.

**h. for lesser petrosal nerve,** h. canalis nervi petrosi minor.

**h. leuke'micus,** a condition observed in acute myelogenous leukemia in which there are numerous myeloblasts and a number of mature neutrophils in the peripheral blood, with few or no intermediate forms; called also *h. leukemicus of Naegeli.*

**h. lumbosacra'lis,** the gap between the arches of the fifth lumbar and first sacral vertebrae, which is greater than the space between any vertebrae at a higher level.

**h. maxilla'ris** [TA], **h. of maxillary sinus,** maxillary hiatus: a small round or oval opening connecting the maxillary sinus and the middle nasal meatus; it is often indented so that the opening appears tubular. Called also *maxillary ostium* and *maxillary sinus ostium.*

**neural h.,** an opening in the neural tube during the process of closure.

**h. oesopha'geus** [TA], esophageal hiatus: the opening in the diaphragm for the passage of the esophagus and the vagus nerves.

**h. pleuroperitonea'lis,** a posterolateral opening in the fetal diaphragm; its failure to close leaves a congenital posterolateral defect which may become a site for congenital diaphragmatic hernia. Called also *foramen of Bochdalek.*

**h. sacra'lis** [TA], sacral hiatus: the opening at the inferior end of the sacral canal formed by failure of the laminae of the fifth and sometimes the fourth sacral vertebrae to meet in the midline.

**h. saphe'nus** [TA], saphenous hiatus: the depression in the fascia lata that is bridged by the cribriform fascia and perforated by the great saphenous vein; called also *fossa ovalis femoris* and *oval fossa of thigh.*

**Scarpa's h.,** helicotrema.

**h. semiluna'ris** [TA], semilunar hiatus: the deep semilunar groove anterior and inferior to the bulla of the ethmoid bone; the anterior ethmoidal (air) cells, the maxillary sinus, and sometimes the frontonasal duct drain through it via the ethmoid infundibulum.

**subarcuate h.,** fossa subarcuata ossis temporalis.

**h. tendi'neus,** h. adductorius.

**tentorial h.,** incisura tentorii cerebelli.

**h. tota'lis sacra'lis,** a cleft in all of the sacral vertebrae, sometimes also involving one or several of the contiguous lumbar vertebrae.

**vena caval h.,** foramen venae cavae.

**h. of Winslow,** foramen epiploicum.

**Hibbs' operation** (hibz) [Russell Aubra *Hibbs,* New York surgeon, 1869–1932] see under *operation.*

**hi·ber·na·tion** (hi″bər-na'shən) [L. *hibernare* to spend the winter] [MeSH: Hibernation] 1. the dormant state in which certain animal species pass the winter; it is characterized by narcosis and by sharp reduction in body temperature and metabolic activity. Cf. *estivation.* 2. an analogous temporary reduction in function, such as of an organ.

**artificial h.,** a state of reduced metabolism, muscle relaxation, and a twilight sleep resembling narcosis, produced pharmacodynamically by controlled inhibition of the sympathetic nervous system and reducing the level of the homeostatic reactions of the organism.

**myocardial h.,** chronic but potentially reversible cardiac dysfunction caused by chronic myocardial ischemia, persisting at least until blood flow is restored. Cf. *myocardial stunning.*

**hi·ber·no·ma** (hi″bər-no'mə) [L. *hibernus* pertaining to the winter + *-oma*] a rare, benign, encapsulated tumor of soft tissues, arising from vestiges of brown fat resembling that in certain hibernating animal species; it is a small, lobulated, nontender, tan to dark lesion occurring usually on the mediastinum or intrascapular region of female adults.

**Hib-Imune** (hib'ĭ-mūn″) trademark for a preparation of *Haemophilus influenzae* b polysaccharide vaccine.

**Hib·i·clens** (hi'bik-lens) trademark for a preparation of chlorhexidine gluconate.

**hic·cough** (hik'əp) hiccup.

**hic·cup** (hik'əp) [MeSH: Hiccup] an involuntary spasmodic contraction of the diaphragm, causing a beginning inspiration that is suddenly checked by closure of the glottis, causing a characteristic sound; called also *hiccough* and *singultus.*

**epidemic h's,** persistent hiccups sometimes seen with certain kinds of encephalitis.

**Hick·man catheter** (hik'mən) [R. O. *Hickman,* American surgeon, 20th century] see under *catheter.*

**Hicks' syndrome** (hiks) [Eric Perrin *Hicks,* British physician, 20th century] hereditary sensory radicular neuropathy; see under *neuropathy.*

**Hicks version** (hiks) [John Braxton *Hicks,* English gynecologist, 1825–1897] see *Braxton Hicks version,* under *version.*

**HIDA** hepatobiliary iminodiacetic acid; traditionally used to denote lidofenin (q.v.), but sometimes used more broadly for the class of radiolabeled ($^{99m}$Tc), substituted analogues of iminodiacetic acid used in hepatobiliary imaging, including disofenin, lidofenin, and mebrofenin.

**hide·bound** (hīd'bound) bound down tightly to the subcutaneous tissues, said of the skin in scleroderma.

**hi·drad·e·ni·tis** (hi″drad-ə-ni'tis) [*hidr-* + *aden-* + *-itis*] [MeSH: Hidradenitis] inflammation of a sweat gland, usually of the apocrine type. Called also *hidrosadenitis* and *hydradenitis.*
**h. axilla'ris,** h. suppurativa.
**h. suppurati'va,** a chronic suppurative and cicatricial disease of the apocrine gland–bearing areas, chiefly the axillae (especially in young women) and anogenital region (especially in men), which is caused by poral occlusion with secondary bacterial infection of apocrine sweat glands. It is characterized by the development of one or more tender red abscesses that enlarge and eventually break through the skin, yielding purulent or seropurulent drainage. Healing occurs with fibrosis, and recurrences lead to sinus tract formation and progressive scarring. Called also *apocrinitis* and *h. axillaris.*

**hi·drad·e·no·car·ci·no·ma** (hi-drad″ə-no-kahr″sĭ-no'mə) [*hidr-* + *adeno-* + *carcinoma*] carcinoma of the sweat glands.
**clear cell h.,** a very rare tumor occurring as an erythematous, sometimes ulcerated, nodule on the face or scalp; it histologically resembles a clear cell hidradenoma but displays cellular atypia and frequently deep invasion.

**hi·drad·e·noid** (hi-drad'ə-noid) resembling a sweat gland; having components resembling elements of a sweat gland.

**hi·drad·e·no·ma** (hi-drad″ə-no'mə) [*hidr-* + *adenoma*] a benign tumor originating in sweat gland epithelial cells; subtypes are variously designated according to histologic pattern and specific component from which the tumor appears to be derived.
**clear cell h.,** an epithelial tumor of the eccrine sweat glands usually occurring as a benign, solitary, well circumscribed, nodular, both solid and cystic skin lesion in middle-aged or older women; it is characterized histologically by large cuboidal or polyhedral glycogen-rich clear cells. Called also *eccrine acrospiroma, nodular h., solid-cystic h.,* and, incorrectly, *clear cell myoepithelioma.*
**h. erupti'vum,** an eruptive form of syringoma in which the lesions arise in large numbers in successive crops, usually on the anterior trunk or abdomen of a young person.
**nodular h.,** clear cell h.
**papillary h., h. papilli'ferum,** a benign tumor of apocrine glands, usually occurring as a solitary, firm, nodular, well-circumscribed, intradermal lesion in the vulva or anal region in adult women, and characterized by a central cystic space into which extend papilliferous projections.
**solid-cystic h.,** clear cell h.

**hidr(o)-** [Gr. *hidrōs* sweat] a combining form denoting relationship to sweat or to a sweat gland.

**hi·dro·ac·an·tho·ma** (hi″dro-ak″an-tho'mə) [*hidro-* + *acanthoma*] a benign tumor of an eccrine gland.
**h. sim'plex,** a slightly raised keratotic lesion sometimes described as the intraepidermal counterpart of an eccrine poroma.

**hi·dro·ad·e·no·ma** (hi″dro-ad″ə-no'mə) hidradenoma.

**hi·dro·cys·to·ma** (hi″dro-sis-to'mə) [*hidro-* + *cystoma*] [MeSH: Hidrocystoma] 1. a retention cyst of a sweat gland. 2. syringocystoma.
**apocrine h.,** a smooth, frequently bluish, firm, dome-shaped, translucent, usually solitary lesion occurring chiefly on the face; it is an adenomatous cystic proliferation of the apocrine glands. Called also *apocrine cystadenoma.*
**eccrine h.,** a small cystic lesion occurring singly or multiply, most often on the faces of older adults, particularly women, and frequently exacerbated by hot weather and perspiration.

**hi·dro·poi·e·sis** (hi″dro-poi-e'sis) [*hidro-* + *-poiesis*] the formation and secretion of sweat.

**hi·dro·poi·et·ic** (hi″dro-poi-et'ik) pertaining to, characterized by, or promoting hidropoiesis.

**hi·dros·ad·e·ni·tis** (hi″dros-ad″ə-ni'tis) [*hidro-* + *aden-* + *-itis*] hidradenitis.

**hi·dros·che·sis** (hi-dros'kə-sis) [*hidro-* + Gr. *schesis* holding] anhidrosis.

**hi·drot·ic** (hi-drot'ik) pertaining to, characterized by, or causing sweating.

**hi·e·mal** (hi'ə-məl) pertaining to or occurring in winter.

**hier(o)-** [Gr. *hieron* sacred, or sacrum] a combining form denoting relationship to the sacrum.

**High·more's antrum, body** (hi'morz) [Nathaniel *Highmore,* English anatomist, 1613–1685] see *sinus maxillaris* and *mediastinum testis.*

**high-grade** (hi'grād') occurring near the high end of a range, as of a malignancy.

**Hi·gou·mé·na·ki's sign** (he-goo-ma'nah-kēz) [G. *Higouménaki,* Polish physician, 20th century] clavicular sign; see under *sign.*

**hi·la** (hi'lə) [L.] plural of *hilum.*

**hi·lar** (hi'lər) pertaining to a hilum.

**hi·li** (hi'li) [L.] plural of *hilus.*

**Hill** (hil) Archibald Vivian. English biochemist, 1886–1977; co-winner, with Otto Fritz Meyerhof, of the Nobel prize for medicine or physiology in 1922 for his discovery relating to the production of heat in the muscle.

**Hill posterior gastropexy** (hil) [Lucius D. *Hill,* American surgeon, born 1921] see under *gastropexy.*

**Hill's sign** (hilz) [Sir Leonard Erskine *Hill,* English physiologist, 1866–1952] see under *sign.*

**Hill-Sachs lesion** (hill-saks) [Harold Arthur *Hill,* American radiologist, born 1901; Maurice D. *Sachs,* American radiologist, born 1909] see under *lesion.*

**hill·ock** (hil'ok) a small prominence or elevation.
**auricular h's,** embryonic tubercles adjoining the first pharyngeal (branchial) groove; they give rise to the auricle of the ear.
**axon h.,** the conical expansion of an axon at its point of attachment to the body of the nerve cell.
**seminal h.,** colliculus seminalis.

**Hil·ton's line, muscle, sac** (hil'tənz) [John *Hilton,* English surgeon, 1804–1878] see under *line* and see *musculus aryepiglotticus* and *sacculus laryngis.*

**hi·lum** (hi'ləm) pl. *hi'la* [L. "a small thing, a trifle"] [TA] a general term for a depression or pit at that part of an organ where the vessels and nerves enter. Formerly called *hilus.*
**h. of adrenal gland,** h. glandulae suprarenalis.
**h. of caudal olivary nucleus,** h. nuclei olivaris inferioris.
**h. of dentate nucleus,** h. nuclei dentati.
**h. glan'dulae suprare'nalis** [TA], hilum of adrenal or suprarenal gland: the depression on the anterior surface of the gland where the suprarenal vein enters it.
**h. he'patis,** porta hepatis.
**h. of inferior olivary nucleus,** h. nuclei olivaris inferioris.
**h. of kidney,** h. renale.
**h. liena'le,** TA alternative for *h. splenicum.*
**h. of lung,** h. pulmonis.
**h. of lymph node, h. lymphoglan'dulae,** h. nodi lymphoidei.
**h. no'di lympha'tici, h. no'di lymphoi'dei** [TA], hilum of lymph node: the indentation on a lymph node where the arteries enter and the veins and efferent lymphatic vessels leave.
**h. nu'clei denta'ti** [TA], hilum of dentate nucleus: the white core of the dentate nucleus of the cerebellum.
**h. nu'clei oliva'ris cauda'lis,** h. nuclei olivaris inferioris.
**h. nu'clei oliva'ris inferio'ris** [TA], hilum of inferior olivary nucleus: the white core of the inferior olivary nucleus of the medulla oblongata, most prominent medially. Called also *h. of caudal olivary nucleus* and *h. nuclei olivaris caudalis.*
**h. ova'rii** [TA], hilum of ovary: the point on the mesovarial border of the ovary where the vessels and nerves enter.
**h. pulmo'nis** [TA], hilum of lung: the depression on the mediastinal surface of the lung where the bronchus and the blood vessels and nerves enter.
**h. rena'le** [TA], hilum of the kidney: the point on the medial margin of the kidney where the vessels, nerves, and ureter enter.
**h. sple'nicum** [TA], hilum of spleen: the fissure on the gastric surface of the spleen where the vessels and nerves enter; called also *h. lienale* [TA alternative].
**h. of suprarenal gland,** h. glandulae suprarenalis.

**hi·lus** (hi'ləs) pl. *hi'li.* hilum.

**hi·man·to·sis** (hi″mən-to'sis) [Gr. *himantōsis,* from *himas* strap] elongation of the uvula.

**hind·brain** (hīnd'brān) rhombencephalon.

**hind·foot** (hīnd'foot) the posterior portion of the foot, comprising the region of the talus and calcaneus.

**hind·gut** (hīnd'gət) 1. the embryonic structure from which chiefly the colon is formed. 2. the posterior ectodermal portion of the alimentary tract of invertebrates, such as arthropods; it comprises an intestine and rectum.

**hind·kid·ney** (hīnd-kid'ne) metanephros.

**hind·quar·ter** (hīnd'kwor-tər) in a quadruped, the hind limb with the adjacent loin, pelvis, and musculature.

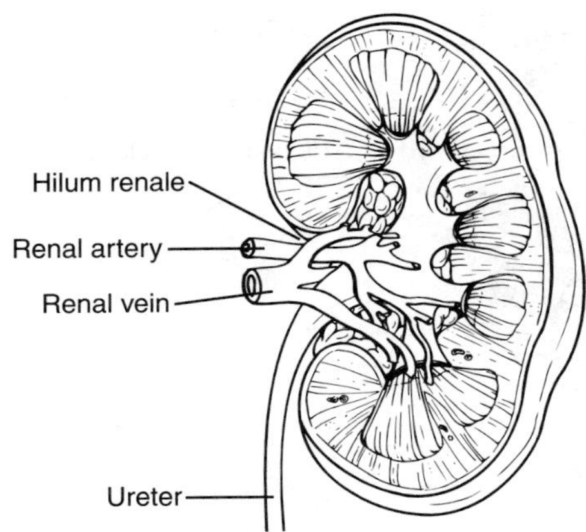


Longitudinal section through the kidney, showing the hilum renale.

**Hines-Ban·nick syndrome** (hīnz-ban′ik) [Edgar Alphonso *Hines,* Jr., American physician, born 1906; Edwin *Bannick,* American physician, born 1896] see under *syndrome.*

**Hines-Brown test** (hīnz-broun) [E. A. *Hines,* Jr.; George Elgie *Brown,* American physician, 1885–1935] see under *test.*

**hinge-bow** (hinj′bo) adjustable axis face-bow.

**Hin·man syndrome** (hin′mən) [Frank *Hinman* Jr., American urologist, born 1915] see under *syndrome.*

**hip** (hip) [MeSH: Hip] 1. the area of the body lateral to and including the hip joint; called also *coxa.* See also *regio glutealis.* 2. loosely, the hip joint (*articulatio coxae* [TA]).
**snapping h.,** a condition marked by a slipping around of the hip joint, sometimes with an audible snap, due to the slipping of a tendinous band over the greater trochanter; called also *Perrin-Ferraton disease.*

**Hip·pel's disease** (hip′əlz) [Eugen von *Hippel,* German ophthalmologist, 1867–1939] von Hippel's disease; see under *disease.*

**Hip·pel-Lin·dau disease** (hip′əl-lin′dou) [Eugen von *Hippel;* Arvid *Lindau,* Swedish pathologist, 1892–1958] [MeSH: Hippel-Lindau Disease] von Hippel-Lindau disease; see under *disease.*

**Hip·pe·la·tes** (hip″ə-la′tēz) a genus of small flies of the family Chloropidae. *H. fla′vipes* is thought to be a mechanical vector of yaws in Haiti, and *H. pal′lipes* is thought to be a mechanical vector of yaws in Jamaica. *H. pu′sio* is the eye gnat of the southern United States from Florida to California and is a mechanical vector of epidemic conjunctivitis, usually of a severe follicular type.

**Hip·peu·tis** (hi-pu′tis) a genus of fresh water snails of the family Planorbidae. *H. canto′ri* is a species found in eastern China that is one of the principal intermediate hosts of the trematode *Fasciolopsis buski.*

**hip·po** (hip′o) ipecac.

**hipp(o)-** [Gr. *hippos* horse] a combining form denoting relationship to a horse.

**Hip·po·bos·ca** (hip-o-bos′kə) [*hippo-* + Gr. *boskein* to feed] the typical genus of the family Hippoboscidae; the winged tick flies. They are pupiparous, dipterous, and parasitic to horses, cattle, and other animals. *H. ru′fipes* is a South American species whose bite transmits *Trypanosoma theileri.*

**hip·po·bos·cid** (hip″o-bos′kid) 1. pertaining to the family Hippoboscidae. 2. any fly of the family Hippoboscidae.

**Hip·po·bos·ci·dae** (hip″o-bos′kĭ-de) a family of parasitic flies found on bird and mammals; some have wings, others are wingless. It includes the genera *Hippobosca, Melophagus,* and *Pseudolynchia.*

**hip·po·cam·pal** (hip″o-kam′pəl) pertaining to the hippocampus.

**hip·po·cam·pus** (hip″o-kam′pəs) [Gr. *hippokampos* sea horse] [TA] [MeSH: Hippocampus] a curved elevation of gray matter extending the entire length of the floor of the temporal horn of the lateral ventricle. Starting on its ventricular aspect, the hippocampus is usually considered to comprise seven sublayers: ependyma, alveus, stratum oriens, stratum pyramidale, stratum radiatum, stratum lacunosum, and stratum moleculare.

**hip·po·co·pros·ter·ol** (hip″o-ko-pros′tər-ol) [*hippo-* + *copro-* + *sterol*] a sterol found in the feces of herbivorous animals and derived from the phytosterol of grass and other food plants; possibly related to coprostanol.

**Hip·poc·ra·tes** (hĭ-pok′rə-tēz) **of Cos** [c. 460–c. 375 B.C.] the Father of Medicine, a student and teacher, not founder, of the medical school on Cos. According to Plato and Aristotle, Hippocrates was a great physician. None of the works in the Hippocratic corpus can be surely ascribed to Hippocrates. His anatomy was vague: he knew only bones in detail, not being sure of the organs, muscles, nerves, tendons, or blood vessels. Hippocrates' physiology was based on humoralism; his diagnosis was directed toward general pathology; his prognosis, to foretell the stages, duration, and end of disease. Hippocrates closely observed fevers, skin, the tongue, eyes, sweat, urine, and feces. Malarial and pulmonary diseases, common in the ancient Mediterranean, provided Hippocrates with ample evidence of humors—hemorrhagic blood, black and yellow bile from fits of vomiting in remittent malaria, and phlegm in mucus and expectoration. Hippocrates' therapy was to restore the humoral equilibrium: rid the body of excess humors and replace the deficient humors. He relied on the healing power of nature and recommended diet and moderate exercise, but rejected drugs.

**hip·po·crat·ic** (hip″o-krat′ik) pertaining to or described by Hippocrates of Cos, or pertaining to his school of medicine.

**Hip·po·crat·ic Oath** (hip″o-krat′ik ōth) [MeSH: Hippocratic Oath] an oath of professional behavior sworn by physicians as they embark upon their medical careers; it is attributed to Hippocrates: "I swear by Apollo the physician, by Aesculapius, Hygeia, and Panacea, and I take to witness all the gods, all the goddesses, to keep according to my ability and my judgment the following Oath: To consider dear to me as my parents him who taught me this art; to live in common with him and if necessary to share my goods with him; to look upon his children as my own brothers, to teach them this art if they so desire without fee or written promise; to impart to my sons and the sons of the master who taught me and the disciples who have enrolled themselves and have agreed to the rules of the profession, but to these alone, the precepts and the instruction. I will prescribe regimen for the good of my patients according to my ability and my judgment and never do harm to anyone. To please no one will I prescribe a deadly drug, nor give advice which may cause his death. Nor will I give a woman a pessary to procure abortion. But I will preserve the purity of my life and my art. I will not cut for stone, even for patients in whom the disease is manifest; I will leave this operation to be performed by practitioners (specialists in this art). In every house where I come I will enter only for the good of my patients, keeping myself far from all intentional ill-doing and all seduction, and especially from the pleasures of love with women or with men, be they free or slaves. All that may come to my knowledge in the exercise of my profession or outside of my profession or in daily commerce with men, which ought not to be spread abroad, I will keep secret and will never reveal. If I keep this oath faithfully, may I enjoy my life and practice my art, respected by all men and in all times; but if I swerve from it or violate it, may the reverse be my lot."

**hip·poc·ra·tism** (hĭ-pok′rə-tiz-əm) the system of medicine attributed to Hippocrates and his school, based on imitating the processes of nature, and emphasizing treatment and prognosis.

**hip·poc·ra·tist** (hĭ-pok′rə-tist) a believer in or practitioner of the system of medicine attributed to Hippocrates and his school.

**Hip·po·glos·sus** (hip″o-glos′əs) the halibuts, a genus of large flat fish found in the northern Atlantic and Pacific oceans. They are eaten as food and their liver is the source of halibut liver oil.

**Hip·pom·a·ne** (hĭ-pom′ə-ne) a genus of tropical American trees of the family Euphorbiaceae. *H. mancinel′la* is the manchineel, a species with poisonous sap.

**hip·pom·a·ne** (hĭ-pom′ə-ne) small, rounded, flat, amber bodies found in the allantoic fluid of various animals, especially the ungulates and ruminants.

**hip·pu·rate** (hip′u-rāt) any salt of hippuric acid.

**hip·pu·ria** (hip-u′re-ə) [*hippo-* + *-uria*] excess of hippuric acid in the urine.

**hip·pu·ric ac·id** (hĭ-pūr′ik) a crystallizable acid, $C_6H_5$·CO·NH·$CH_2$·COOH, from the urine of domestic animals; more rarely found in human urine. Called also *benzoylglycine* and *urobenzoic acid.*

**hip·pu·ri·case** (hip-ūr′i-kās) aminoacylase.

**hip·pus** (hip′əs) [Gr. *hippos*] abnormally exaggerated rhythmic contraction and dilation of the pupil, independent of changes in illumination or in fixation of the eyes; called also *pupillary athetosis.*

**Hi·prex** (hi′preks) trademark for a preparation of methenamine hippurate.

**hir·ci** (hir′si) [L., plural of *hircus*] [TA] the hairs growing in the axilla.

**hir·cis·mus** (hir-siz′məs) [L. *hircus* goat] the strong odor of the axillae caused by bacterial decomposition of apocrine sweat, formed only in that site.

**hir·cus** (hir′kəs) pl. *hir′ci* [L. "a goat"] see *hirci.*

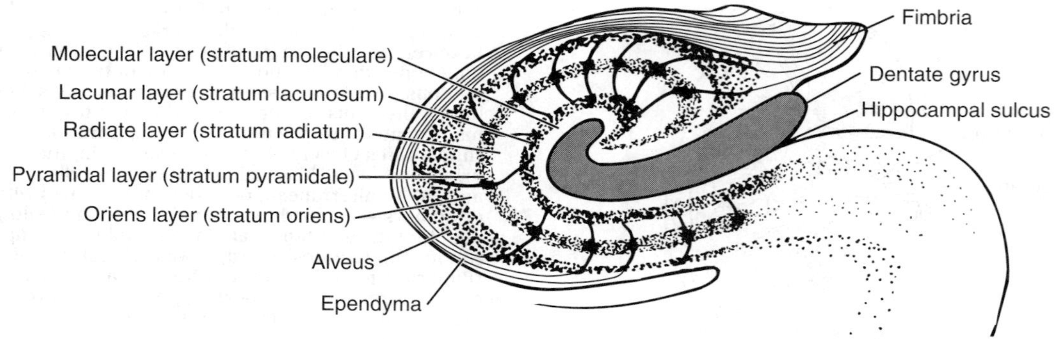


Transverse section through the hippocampus.

**Hirsch·berg's magnet, method** (hirsh'bərgz) [Julius *Hirschberg,* German ophthalmologist, 1843–1925] see under *magnet* and *method.*

**Hirsch·berg's sign** (hərsh'bərgz) [Leonard Keene *Hirschberg,* American physician, born 1877] see under *sign.*

**Hirsch·feld's canals** (hərsh'feldz) [Isador *Hirschfeld,* American dentist 1881–1965] interdental canals.

**Hirsch·sprung's disease** (hirsh'sproongz) [Harald *Hirschsprung,* Danish physician, 1830–1916] congenital megacolon.

**hir·sute** (hir'soot) [L. *hirsutus*] shaggy; having abundant or excessive hair.

**hir·su·ti·es** (hir-soo'she-ez) hirsutism.

**hir·sut·ism** (hir'soot-iz-əm) [MeSH: Hirsutism] abnormal hairiness, especially an adult male pattern of hair distribution in women. Cf. *hypertrichosis.*

**hi·ru·di·ci·dal** (hĭ-roo"dĭ-si'dəl) destructive to leeches.

**hi·ru·di·cide** (hĭ-roo'dĭ-sīd) an agent that is destructive to leeches.

**hi·ru·din** (hĭ-roo'din) [L. *hirudo* leech] [MeSH: Hirudin] the active principle of the secretion of the buccal glands of leeches, which prevents coagulation of the blood by acting as an antithrombin; hirudin prepared by recombinant technology is used as an anticoagulant.

**Hi·ru·di·na·ria** (hir"oo-dĭ-nar'e-ə) a genus of leeches of the family Gnathobdellidae.

**Hir·u·din·ea** (hir"oo-din'e-ə) the leeches, a class of the phylum Annelida; it includes the genera *Haementeria, Hirudo, Hirudinaria, Haemadipsa, Limnatis, Macrobdella,* and *Haemopis.* See also *leech.*

**hir·u·di·ni·a·sis** (hir"oo-dĭ-ni'ə-sis) infection or infestation by leeches, such as in the nose, mouth, pharynx, or larynx or on the skin.

**hir·u·di·ni·za·tion** (hĭ-roo"dĭ-nĭ-za'shən) [L. *hirudo* leech] 1. the process of rendering the blood noncoagulable by the injection of hirudin. 2. leeching.

**hi·ru·di·nize** (hĭ-roo'dĭ-nīz) to render the blood noncoagulable by the injection of hirudin.

**Hi·ru·do** (hĭ-roo'do) [L. "leech"] a genus of leeches of the family Gnathobdellidae. *H. japo'nica* and *H. medicina'lis* have been used medicinally (see *leeching*). Other species include *H. java'nica* of Indonesia and Burma, *H. quinquestria'ta* of Australia, and *H. trocti'na* of Europe.
**H. aegypti'aca,** *Limnatis nilotica.*

**hir·u·log** (hir'u-log) an analog of hirudin, used investigationally as an anticoagulant.

**His** histidine.

**His' bundle (band), disease, spindle** (hiz) [Wilhelm *His,* Jr., Swiss physician, 1863–1934] see under *bundle,* and see *trench fever,* under *fever,* and *aortic spindle* under *spindle.*

**His' bursa, canal, duct, space, zones** (hiz) [Wilhelm *His,* Swiss anatomist and embryologist in Germany, 1831–1904] see under *bursa, canal, space,* and *zone,* and see *ductus thyroglossalis.*

**His-Pur·kin·je system** (hiz-pər-kin'je) [Wilhelm *His,* Jr.; Johannes Evangelista *Purkinje,* Czech physiologist, 1787–1869] see under *system.*

**His·man·al** (his'man-al) trademark for a preparation of astemizole.

**His·pril** (his'pril) trademark for a preparation of diphenylpyraline hydrochloride.

**Hiss capsule stain** (his) [Philip Hanson *Hiss,* Jr., American bacteriologist, 1868–1913] see under *stain.*

**His-Wer·ner disease** (his-vər'nər) [Wilhelm *His,* Jr.; Heinrich *Werner,* German physician, 1874–1946] trench fever.

**His·ta·dyl** (his'tə-dəl) trademark for preparations of methapyrilene.

**his·tam·i·nase** (his-tam'ĭ-nās) amine oxidase (copper-containing).

**his·ta·mine** (his'tə-mēn) [MeSH: Histamine] chemical name: 1*H*-imidazole-4-ethanamine. A decarboxylation product of histidine, $C_5H_9N_3$, found in all body tissues, particularly in the mast cells and their related blood basophils, the highest concentration being in the lungs. It is also present in ergot and other plants and may be synthesized outside the body from histidine or citric acid. It has several functions, including (1) dilation of capillaries, which increases capillary permeability and results in a drop of blood pressure, (2) contraction of most smooth muscle tissue, including bronchial smooth muscle of the lung, (3) induction of increased gastric secretion, and (4) acceleration of the heart rate. It is also responsible for the triple response, and is implicated as a mediator of immediate hypersensitivity. On the basis of the antagonistic effects of antihistamines, it is postulated that cellular receptors of histamine are of two types: The $H_1$ receptors mediate the contraction of smooth muscle and the effects on capillaries; the $H_2$ receptors mediate the acceleration of heart rate and the promotion of gastric acid secretion. Both $H_1$ and $H_2$ receptors mediate the contraction of vascular smooth muscle. Histamine has also been postulated to be a neurotransmitter in the central nervous system.
**h.**$_1$, the cellular receptor site for histamine responsible for the dilation of blood vessels and the contraction of smooth muscle; abbreviated $H_1$.
**h.**$_2$, the cellular receptor site for histamine responsible for the stimulation of heart rate and gastric secretion; abbreviated $H_2$.
**h. hydrochloride,** the dihydrochloride salt of histamine, $C_5H_9N_3 \cdot 2HCl$, having the same actions as the base; used as an active ingredient of several analgesic dermatological preparations.
**h. phosphate** [USP], the phosphate salt of histamine, having the same actions as the base; used as a diagnostic aid in testing gastric secretion, administered subcutaneously. It is also used in the diagnosis of pheochromocytoma and has been used in treating various allergic manifestations, for desensitization in cases of hypersensitivity, and in the treatment of peripheral vascular diseases, Meniere's disease, and headache.

**his·tam·i·ne·mia** (his-tam"ĭ-ne'me-ə) the presence of histamine in the blood.

**his·ta·min·er·gic** (his"tə-min-ər'jik) denoting those responses by histamine receptors to histamine that are blocked by histamine antagonists (e.g., cimetidine).

**his·tan·ox·ia** (his"tan-ok'se-ə) [*hist-* + *anoxia*] oxygen deprivation of the tissues due to a lessening of the blood supply.

**His·ta·span** (his'tə-span) trademark for preparations of chlorpheniramine maleate.

**his·tic** (his'tik) pertaining to or of the nature of tissue.

**his·ti·dase** (his'tĭ-dās) [MeSH: Histidase] histidine ammonia-lyase.

**his·ti·dine** (his'tĭ-dēn, din) [MeSH: Histidine] an essential amino acid, α-amino-1H-imidazole-4-propanoic acid, first found as a decomposition product of the protamine of sturgeon testes (Kossel, 1896); it is obtainable from many proteins by the action of sulfuric acid and water. The decarboxylation of histidine results in the formation of histamine. Symbols His and H. See table at *amino acid.*

**his·ti·dine am·mo·nia-ly·ase** (his'tĭ-dēn ə-mo'ne-ə li'ās) [EC 4.3.1.3] an enzyme of the lyase class that catalyzes the deamination of histidine to urocanate, the initial step of histidine catabolism. Deficiency of the enzyme, an autosomal recessive trait, causes histidinemia. Called also *histidase.*

**his·ti·din·emia** (his″tĭ-dĭ-ne′me-ə) an autosomal recessive aminoacidopathy due to deficiency of histidine ammonia-lyase; it is characterized by accumulation of histidine in serum and urinary excretion of histidine and metabolites, but is usually benign. In some cases it may cause mild central nervous system dysfunction.

**his·ti·din·uria** (his″tĭ-dĭ-nu′re-ə) an excess of histidine in the urine, usually occurring in histidinemia or during pregnancy.

**his·ti·dyl** (his′tĭ-dəl) the acyl radical of histidine.

**histi(o)-** [Gr. *histion* web] a combining form denoting relationship to tissue.

**his·tio·blast** (his′te-o-blast″) a local histiocyte (macrophage).

**his·tio·cyte** (his′te-o-sīt″) [*histio-* + *-cyte*] [MeSH: Histiocytes] macrophage.
**cardiac h.**, Anichkov's cell.
**sea-blue h.**, an abnormal foamy, granulated histiocyte, sea-blue in color, containing ceroid material; seen in the sea-blue histiocyte syndrome, adult varieties of Niemann-Pick disease, and some forms of hemolytic anemia.
**wandering h.**, free macrophage.

**his·tio·cyt·ic** (his″te-o-sit′ik) pertaining to or containing histiocytes (macrophages).

**his·tio·cyt·oma** (his″te-o-si-to′mə) [*histiocyte* + *-oma*] a tumor containing histiocytes (macrophages).
**benign fibrous h.**, any of a group of benign neoplasms occurring in the dermis and characterized by histiocytes and fibroblasts. Classification of these tumors is variable; the term sometimes encompasses several types of neoplasms, such as dermatofibroma, nodular subepidermal fibrosis, and sclerosing hemangioma, but in other cases it is used synonymously with one or more of these terms.
**h. cu′tis**, dermatofibroma.
**fibrous h.**, dermatofibroma.
**lipoid h.**, fibroxanthoma.
**malignant fibrous h.**, any of a group of malignant neoplasms containing cells that resemble histiocytes and fibroblasts, occurring predominantly in soft tissues in middle-aged adults; depending on the tumor location and the classification system, the term is sometimes used synonymously with or as a general term including similar lesions such as atypical fibroxanthoma and dermatofibrosarcoma protuberans. The group is usually divided into five histological subtypes: *angiomatoid, giant cell, inflammatory, myxoid,* and *storiform-pleomorphic malignant fibrous histiocytomas.*

**his·tio·cy·to·ma·to·sis** (his″te-o-si″to-mə-to′sis) any generalized disorder of the reticuloendothelial system, such as xanthomatosis, Gaucher's disease, Niemann-Pick disease, or lymphogranulomatosis.

**his·tio·cy·to·sis** (his″te-o-si-to′sis) [MeSH: Histiocytosis] a condition marked by the abnormal appearance of histiocytes (macrophages) in the blood.
**Langerhans cell h.**, a generic term embracing a group of disorders characterized by proliferation of Langerhans' cells (q.v.); children are more often affected than adults. Lesions may be unifocal or multifocal and may involve the bone marrow, endocrine system, or lungs (the last being more common in adults than in children). Although the cause is uncertain, these disorders are believed to arise from disturbances in regulation of the immune system. Called also *eosinophilic granuloma* or *granulomatosis* and *Langerhans cell granulomatosis*. Formerly called *h. X.*
**Langerhans cell h., acute disseminated,** Letterer-Siwe disease.
**Langerhans cell h., multifocal,** Langerhans cell histiocytosis occurring as erosive accumulations of proliferating Langerhans' cells, commonly within the medullary cavities of bones, but also affecting the skin, gingiva, lungs, and stomach. It most commonly affects children and is accompanied by seborrheic eruptions, fever, frequent occurrences of otitis media, mastoiditis, and upper respiratory tract infection, often with lymphadenopathy and splenomegaly. When the triad of calvarial bone defects, exophthalmos, and diabetes insipidus is present, it is referred to as *Hand-Schüller-Christian disease.*
**Langerhans cell h., unifocal,** Langerhans cell histiocytosis occurring as a single osteolytic lesion, usually in a long or flat bone; it may be asymptomatic or may produce bone pain, tenderness, and swelling and, sometimes, pathologic fracture.
**malignant h.**, a rare type of histiocytosis found accompanying malignancies such as acute myelogenous leukemia; it may be a malignant transformation of stem cells of the monocyte series. It usually affects children or young adults and has a poor prognosis.
**sea-blue h.**, sea-blue histiocyte syndrome.
**sinus h.**, a disorder of the lymph nodes in which the distended sinuses are completely, or nearly completely, filled by histiocytes, as a result of active multiplication of the littoral cells.
**sinus h. with massive lymphadenopathy (SHML),** Rosai-Dorfman disease.
**h. X,** former name for *Langerhans cell h.*

**his·ti·o·gen·ic** (his″te-o-jen′ik) histogenous.

**his·ti·oid** (his′te-oid) histoid.

**his·ti·on·ic** (his″te-on′ik) pertaining to or derived from a tissue.

**hist(o)-** [Gr. *histos* web] a combining form denoting relationship to tissue.

**his·to·blast** (his′to-blast) [*histo-* + *-blast*] a tissue-forming cell.

**his·to·chem·i·cal** (his″to-kem′ĭ-kəl) pertaining to histochemistry or to the chemical components or activities of cells or tissues.

**his·to·chem·is·try** (his″to-kem′is-tre) that branch of histology which deals with the identification of chemical components in cells and tissues.

**his·to·che·mo·ther·a·py** (his″to-ke″mo-ther′ə-pe) see *chemotherapy.*

**his·to·clas·tic** (his″to-klas′tik) [*histo-* + *clastic*] breaking down tissue; said of certain cells.

**his·to·clin·i·cal** (his″to-klin′ĭ-kəl) combining histological and clinical evaluation.

**his·to·com·pa·ti·bil·i·ty** (his″to-kəm-pat″ĭ-bil′ĭ-te) [MeSH: Histocompatibility] 1. the quality or state of being histocompatible. 2. the degree to which two individuals are histocompatible.

**his·to·com·pat·i·ble** (his″to-kəm-pat′ĭ-bəl) pertaining to a donor and recipient who share a sufficient number of histocompatibility antigens (q.v.) so that a graft is accepted and remains functional.

**his·to·cyte** (his′to-sīt) macrophage.

**his·to·di·ag·no·sis** (his″to-di″əg-no′sis) [*histo-* + *diagnosis*] diagnosis by microscopic examination of the tissues.

**his·to·di·al·y·sis** (his″to-di-al′ə-sis) [*histo-* + *dialysis*] the disintegration or breaking down of tissues.

**his·to·dif·fer·en·ti·a·tion** (his″to-dif″ər-en″she-a′shən) the acquisition of tissue characteristics by cell groups.

**his·to·flu·o·res·cence** (his″to-flo͞o″-res′əns) fluorescence produced in the body by exposure to x-rays following the administration of a fluorescing drug.

**his·to·gen·e·sis** (his″to-jen′ə-sis) [*histo-* + *-genesis*] the formation or development of tissues from the undifferentiated cells of the germ layers of the embryo.

**his·to·ge·net·ic** (his″to-jə-net′ik) pertaining to histogenesis.

**his·tog·e·nous** (his-toj′ə-nəs) [*histo-* + *-genous*] formed by the tissues.

**his·tog·e·ny** (his-toj′ə-ne) histogenesis.

**his·to·gram** (his′to-gram) [Gr. *histos* mast + *-gram*] a graphic display of a frequency distribution, represented by a series of rectangles dividing the data into classes, the height of a rectangle indicating the number of values that are contained in that class (class frequency) and the width of each base being the size of the intervals into which the classes have been divided.

**his·tog·ra·phy** (his-tog′rə-fe) [*histo-* + *-graphy*] description of the tissues.

**his·to·hem·a·tog·e·nous** (his″to-hem″ə-toj′ə-nəs) [*histo-* + *hemato-* + *-genous*] formed from both the tissues and the blood.

**his·to·hy·dria** (his″to-hi′dre-ə) the presence of an excessive amount of water in body tissue.

**his·to·hy·pox·ia** (his″to-hi-pok′se-ə) an abnormally diminished concentration of oxygen in the tissues.

**his·toid** (his′toid) [*histo-* + *-oid*] 1. weblike. 2. developed from but one kind of tissue. 3. like one of the tissues of the body.

**his·to·in·com·pat·i·bil·i·ty** (his″to-in″kəm-pat″ĭ-bil′ĭ-te) the quality or state of being histoincompatible.

**his·to·in·com·pat·i·ble** (his″to-in″kəm-pat′ĭ bəl) pertaining to a donor and recipient who have sufficient differences in histocompatibility antigens to cause rejection of grafts.

**his·to·ki·ne·sis** (his″to-kĭ-ne′sis) [*histo-* + *-kinesis*] movement in the tissues of the body.

**his·to·log·ic, his·to·log·i·cal** (his″to-loj′ik, his″to-loj′ĭ-kəl) pertaining to histology.

**his·tol·o·gist** (his-tol′ə-jist) one who specializes in histology.

**his·tol·o·gy** (his-tol′ə-je) [*histo-* + *-logy*] [MeSH: Histology] that department of anatomy which deals with the minute structure, composition, and function of the tissues; called also *microscopical anatomy.*
**normal h.**, the histology of normal tissues.
**pathologic h.**, the histology of diseased tissues; histopathology.

**his·tol·y·sate** (his-tol′ə-zāt) a substance formed by histolysis.

**his·tol·y·sis** (his-tol′ə-sis) [*histo-* + *-lysis*] the dissolution or the breaking down of tissues.

**his·to·lyt·ic** (his″to-lit′ik) pertaining to, characterized by, or causing histolysis.

**his·to·meta·plas·tic** (his″to-met″ə-plas′tik) pertaining to, characterized by, or stimulating metaplasia of tissue.

**His·to·mo·nas** (his″to-mo′nəs) [*histo-* + Gr. *monas* unit, from *monos* single] a genus of ameboflagellate protozoa of the order Trichomonadida, parasitic in the cecum and liver of turkeys, chickens, pheasants, guinea fowl, and other wild and domestic fowl. *H. melea′gridis* is the only pathogenic species, being the etiologic agent of histomoniasis, which is especially severe in turkeys. It is usually transmitted in the eggs of the nematode coparasite *Heterakis gallinae.*

**his·to·mo·ni·a·sis** (his″to-mo-ni′ə-sis) an infectious protozoal disease caused by *Histomonas meleagridis,* which is especially lethal to turkeys although chickens and other fowl may also be affected. It is characterized by ulcerative and necrotic lesions of the cecum and liver, and the head may be cyanotic. Called also *blackhead* and *enterohepatitis.*
**h. of turkeys,** the lethal type of histomoniasis seen in turkeys; there are lesions of the intestine and liver and a dark discoloration of the comb.

**his·to·mor·phol·o·gy** (his″to-mor-fol′ə-je) the morphology of tissues; histology.

**his·to·mor·pho·met·ric** (his″to-mor″fo-met′rik) [*histo-* + *morpho-* + *metr-* + *ic*] pertaining to measurement of the histological organization of structures of organisms.

**his·tone** (his′tōn) a simple protein containing many basic groups, soluble in water and insoluble in dilute ammonia. The globin of hemoglobin is a histone. Combined with nucleic acids they form nucleohistone, and are associated with DNA in chromatin. Some are decidedly poisonous and contain a considerable amount of phosphorus. Blood treated with histone is altered so that it coagulates with difficulty. Histone has been found in the urine in leukemia and febrile conditions. Cf. *protamine.*
**h. nucleinate,** a compound of nucleic acid and histone, the characteristic constituent of lymph glands, spleen, and thymus.

**his·ton·o·my** (his-ton′ə-me) [*histo-* + Gr. *nomos* law] the scientific study of tissues based on the translation, into biological terms, of quantitative laws derived from histological measurement.

**his·ton·uria** (his-to-nu′re-ə) [*histone* + *-uria*] the presence of histone in the urine.

**his·to·pa·thol·o·gy** (his″to-pə-thol′ə-je) [*histo-* + *pathology*] pathologic histology.

**his·toph·a·gous** (his-tof′ə-gəs) [*histo-* + *phag-* + *-ous*] eating or subsisting on tissues; applied to certain protozoa, especially those ciliates ectoparasitic on or endoparasitic in nonvital tissues of their hosts.

**his·to·phys·i·ol·o·gy** (his″to-fiz″e-ol′ə-je) [*histo-* + *physiology*] the correlation of function with the microscopic structure of cells and tissues.

**His·to·plas·ma** (his″to-plaz′mə) [MeSH: Histoplasma] a genus of Fungi Imperfecti of the form-class Hyphomycetes, form-family Moniliaceae.
**H. capsula′tum,** the etiologic agent of classic histoplasmosis, occurring as small, oval, yeastlike cells which in tissue seem to be encapsulated but are not. It grows as a mycelial fungus in the soil and as a yeast at 37° C. on agar or in tissue. Its perfect (sexual) stage is *Ajellomyces capsulatus.* Former names include *H. pyriforme, Cryptococcus capsulatus,* and *Torulopsis capsulatus.*
**H. capsula′tum** var. **duboi′sii,** a variant form larger than other variants, the cause of the African form of histoplasmosis.
**H. capsula′tum** var. **farcimino′sum,** the etiologic agent of lymphangitis epizootica, differing from the other variants in having smooth macroaleuriospores in the saprobic stage. Called also *H. farciminosum.*
**H. farcimino′sum,** *H. capsulatum* var. *farciminosum.*
**H. pyrifor′me,** former name for *H. capsulatum.*

**his·to·plas·min** (his″to-plaz′min) [USP] [MeSH: Histoplasmin] a skin test antigen prepared from mycelial phase *Histoplasma capsulatum* organisms. Because positive skin tests are common in endemic areas and indicate only previous exposure, not necessarily active disease, histoplasmin is not useful in diagnosis of histoplasmosis. It is used primarily in epidemiologic surveys and in testing for cutaneous anergy in diagnosis of immunodeficiency.

**his·to·plas·mo·ma** (his″to-plaz-mo′mə) [*Histoplasma* + *-oma*] a rounded granuloma of the lung caused by infection with *Histoplasma capsulatum,* seen radiographically as a coin-shaped lesion.

**his·to·plas·mo·sis** (his″to-plaz-mo′sis) [MeSH: Histoplasmosis] infection resulting from inhalation, or sometimes ingestion, of spores of *Histoplasma capsulatum.* It is usually asymptomatic, but in a few cases it may cause acute pneumonia, disseminated reticuloendothelial hyperplasia with hepatosplenomegaly and anemia, or an influenzalike illness with joint effusion and erythema nodosum. Reactivated infection, such as in immunocompromised patients, involves the lungs, meninges, heart, peritoneum, and adrenals, in that order of frequency. Called also *Darling's disease.*
**African h., histoplasomosis duboi′sii,** a disease differentiated from the classic form of histoplasmosis by large yeast forms of *Histoplasma capsulatum* var. *duboisii* in the tissues.
**equine h.,** epizootic lymphangitis.
**ocular h.,** disseminated choroiditis resulting in scars in the periphery of the fundus near the optic nerve, and characteristic disciform macular lesions; *Histoplasma capsulatum* is strongly implicated as the causative agent.
**progressive disseminated h.,** a form, seen primarily in infants and in immunocompromised adults, caused by dissemination of *Histoplasma capsulatum* from the lungs to other areas of the body; in the oral, pharyngeal, and gastrointestinal tracts it may cause ulceration, bleeding, or obstruction and in the central nervous system it may present as focal cerebritis or diffuse meningitis.

**his·to·ra·di·og·ra·phy** (his″to-ra″de-og′rə-fe) [*histo-* + *radiography*] radiography of microscopic sections of tissue.

**his·to·re·ten·tion** (his″to-re-ten′shən) retention of matter by the tissues.

**his·tor·rhex·is** (his″to-rek′sis) [*histo-* + *rrhexis*] breaking up of tissue; Southard's term for focal destruction of nerve tissue of noninfectious nature.

**his·to·tel·i·o·sis** (his″to-tel″e-o′sis) [*histo-* + Gr. *tēle* + *-osis*] the final differentiation of cells whose fate has already been determined irreversibly.

**his·to·ther·a·py** (his″to-ther′ə-pe) [*histo-* + *therapy*] the treatment of disease by the administration of animal tissues.

**his·to·throm·bin** (his″to-throm′bin) thrombin from connective tissue.

**his·to·tome** (his′to-tōm) [*histo-* + *-tome* ] microtome.

**his·tot·o·my** (his-tot′ə-me) [*histo-* + *-tomy*] the dissection of the tissues; microtomy.

**his·to·tox·ic** (his″to-tok′sik) [*histo-* + *toxic*] poisonous to tissue or tissues.

**his·to·troph** (his′to-trōf) [*histo-* + Gr. *trophē* nourishment] in viviparous animals such as mammals, the totality of nutritive substances supplied to the embryo from sources other than the mother's blood. Cf. *hemotroph.*

**his·to·troph·ic** (his″to-trof′ik) 1. encouraging the formation of tissue. 2. pertaining to histotroph; with reference to nutrition through histotroph.

**his·to·trop·ic** (his″to-trop′ik) [*histo-* + *-tropic*] having special affinity for tissue cells.

**his·to·zo·ic** (his″to-zo′ik) [*histo-* + Gr. *zōē* life] living on or within the tissues; said of parasites.

**his·trel·in ace·tate** (his-trel′in) a synthetic preparation of gonadotropin-releasing hormone, used in the treatment of central precocious puberty; administered by injection.

**his·tri·on·ic** (his″tre-on′ik) of or relating to the behavioral characteristics of histrionic personality disorder; see under *personality.*

**hitch** (hich) a device that fastens one thing to another.
**psoas h.,** a type of ureteroneocystostomy in which the urinary bladder is raised within the abdominal cavity and sutured to the psoas minor muscle or tendon, in order for a ureter with a gap at the inferior end to be reimplanted.

**Hitch·ings** (hich′ingz) George Herbert. American pharmacologist, born 1905. Co-winner with Sir James W. Black and Gertrude B. Elion of the Nobel prize for medicine or physiology in 1988 for discoveries made with Elion about the structure and activity of normal and abnormal cells, facilitating the development of drugs active against specific disease states.

**Hit·torf's number** (hit′orfs) [Johann Wilhelm *Hittorf,* German physicist, 1824–1914] see under *number.*

**Hit·zig's girdle, test** (hits′igz) [Eduard *Hitzig,* German neurologist, 1838–1907] see under *girdle* and *test.*

**HIV** [MeSH: HIV] human immunodeficiency virus.

**hive** (hīv) wheal.

**hives** (hīvz) urticaria.

**Hiv·id** (hiv′id) trademark for a preparation of zalcitabine.

**HKAFO** hip-knee-ankle-foot orthosis.

**$H^+$,$K^+$-ATPase** (a-te-pe′ās) a membrane-bound enzyme occurring on the secretory surfaces of parietal cells; it uses the energy derived from the hydrolysis of ATP to drive the exchange of ions across the

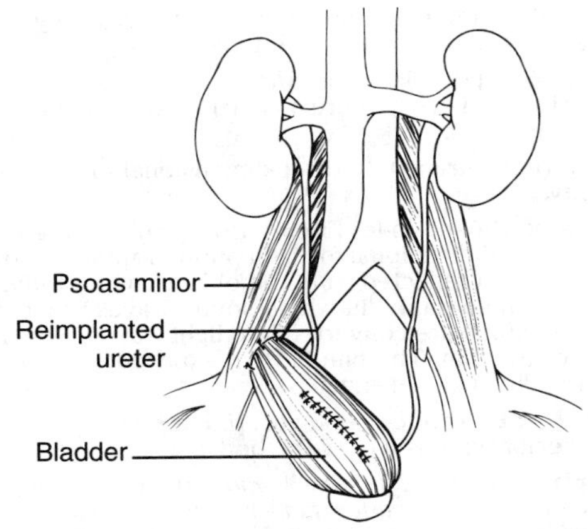

Psoas hitch in which the bladder has been opened by anterior cystotomy.

cell membrane, secreting acid into the gastric lumen. Protons and chloride ions are pumped against gradients across the apical membranes of activated parietal cells into the gastric lumen, in exchange for potassium ions. In EC nomenclature, called *$H^+$/$K^+$-exchanging ATPase.* See also *adenosinetriphosphatase.*

**H+/K+-ex·chang·ing ATP·ase** (eks-chanj'ing a-te-pe'ās) [EC 3.6.1.36] EC nomenclature for *$H^+$,$K^+$-ATPase.*

**H+/K+-trans·port·ing ATP·ase** (trans-port'ing a-te-pe'ās) $H^+$,$K^+$-ATPase.

**Hl** symbol for *latent hyperopia.*

**HLA** see under *antigen.*

**HLHS** hypoplastic left heart syndrome.

**Hm** symbol for *manifest hyperopia.*

**HMDP** hydroxymethylene diphosphonate (oxidronate, q.v.).

**HMG** 3-hydroxy-3-methylglutaryl.

**HMM** hexamethylmelamine.

**HMO** health maintenance organization.

**HMPA** hexamethylphosphoramide; see *hempa.*

**HMPAO** hexamethylpropyleneamine oxime (exametazime, q.v.).

**HMS** trademark for a preparation of medrysone.

**HMSN** hereditary motor and sensory neuropathy.

**HMWK** high-molecular-weight kininogen.

**HMW-NCF** high-molecular-weight neutrophil chemotactic factor.

**HN2** mechlorethamine.

**hnRNA** heterogeneous nuclear RNA; see under *RNA.*

**Ho** symbol for *holmium.*

**hoarse·ness** (hors'nəs) [MeSH: Hoarseness] a rough or noisy quality of voice. Called also *trachyphonia.*

**Ho·bo·ken's nodules, valves** (ho'bo-kənz) [Nicolas van *Hoboken,* Dutch anatomist and physician, 1632–1678] see under *nodule* and *valve.*

**Hoch·e·negg's operation** (hawk'ə-negz) [Julius von *Hochenegg,* Vienna surgeon, 1859–1940] see under *operation.*

**Hoch·sin·ger's phenomenon (sign)** (hawk'sing-ərz) [Karl *Hochsinger,* Austrian pediatrician, late 19th century] see under *phenomenon.*

**hock** (hok) the tarsal joint or region of the tarsus in the hind leg of a quadruped. Called also *ankle* and *hock joint.*
**capped h.,** a hygromalike cyst or a thickening of the skin over the point of the calcaneus in the horse. Cf. *capped elbow.*
**curby h.,** a hock affected with curb.
**spring h.,** stringhalt.

**HOCM** hypertrophic obstructive cardiomyopathy.

**Hodge's pessary, plane** (hoj'əz) [Hugh Lenox *Hodge,* American gynecologist, 1796–1873] see under *pessary* and *plane.*

**Hodg·en splint (apparatus)** (hoj'ən) [John Thompson *Hodgen,* American surgeon, 1826–1882] see under *splint.*

**Hodg·kin** (hoj'kin) Alan Lloyd. British physiologist, born 1914; co-winner, with Sir John Carew Eccles and Andrew Fielding Huxley, of the Nobel prize for medicine or physiology for 1963, for discoveries concerning the ionic mechanisms involved in excitation and inhibition in the peripheral and central portions of the nerve cell membrane.

**Hodg·kin's cells, disease (granuloma), sarcoma** (hoj'kinz) [Thomas *Hodgkin,* English physician, 1798–1866] see *Reed-Sternberg cells,* under *cell,* and see under *disease* and *sarcoma.*

**Hodg·kin cycle** (hoj'kin) [A. L. *Hodgkin*] see under *cycle.*

**Hodg·son's disease** (hoj'sonz) [Joseph *Hodgson,* English physician, 1788–1869] see under *disease.*

**ho·do·neu·ro·mere** (ho"do-noor'o-mēr) [Gr. *hodos* path + *neuro-* + *-mere*] a segment of the embryonic trunk with its pair of nerves and their branches.

**hoe** (ho) a cutting dental instrument having its cutting edge at a right angle to the axis of its blade and no constriction at the junction of its shank and blade; used for breaking down tooth structure undermined by caries, smoothing cavity walls, and sharpening line and point angles.

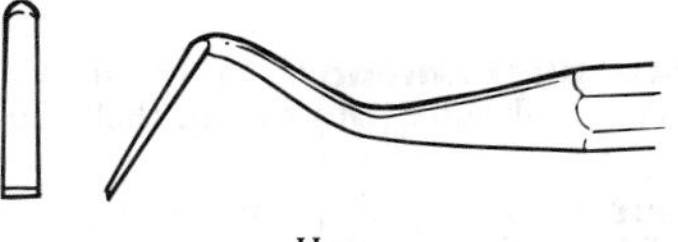
Hoe.

**Hoeh·ne's sign** (her'nəz) [Ottomar *Hoehne,* German gynecologist, 1871–1932] see under *sign.*

**hof** (hawf) [Ger. "court"] the area of the cytoplasm of a cell encircled by the concavity of the nucleus.

**Hof·bau·er cells** (hawf'bou-ər) [J. Isfred Isidore *Hofbauer,* American gynecologist, 1878–1961] see under *cell.*

**Hoff** see *van't Hoff.*

**Hof·fa's disease, operation** (hawf'əz) [Albert *Hoffa,* German surgeon, 1859–1907] see under *disease,* and see *Lorenz's operation,* under *operation.*

**Hof·fa-Lo·renz operation** (hawf'ə-lo'rənts) [A. *Hoffa;* Adolf *Lorenz,* Austrian surgeon, 1854–1946] Lorenz's operation.

**Hoff·mann's atrophy, phenomenon, sign (reflex)** (hawf'mahnz) [Johann *Hoffmann,* German neurologist, 1857–1919] see under *phenomenon* and *sign* and see *Werdnig-Hoffmann spinal muscular atrophy,* under *atrophy.*

**Hoff·mann's duct** (hawf'mahnz) [Moritz *Hoffmann,* German anatomist, 1622–1698] ductus pancreaticus.

**Hoff·mann-Werd·nig syndrome** (hawf'mahn-vərd'nig) [Johann *Hoffmann;* Guido *Werdnig,* Austrian neurologist, 1844–1919] Werdnig-Hoffmann paralysis.

**Hof·mann's bacillus** (hawf'mahnz) [Georg von *Hofmann*-Wellenhof, Austrian bacteriologist, 1843–1890] *Corynebacterium pseudodiphtheriticum.*

**Hof·mann's violet** (hawf'mahnz) [August Wilhelm von *Hofmann,* German chemist, 1818–1892] dahlia.

**Hof·meis·ter's test** (hawf'mi-stərz) [Franz *Hofmeister,* German physiologic chemist, 1850–1922] see under *test.*

**hol·an·dric** (hol-an'drik) [*hol-* + *andr-* + *-ic*] inherited exclusively through the male descent; transmitted through genes located on the Y chromosome.

**Hol·den's line** (hōl'dənz) [Luther *Holden,* English surgeon, 1815–1905] see under *line.*

**hold·fast** (hōld'fast) a mass of material secreted by a cell or organism by which it is attached to a substrate or surface; called also *holdfast organ* or *organelle.*

**hole** (hōl) an opening or perforation.
**bur h.,** one of a series of holes in the skull made with a bur in craniotomy.

**Hol·ger Niel·sen method** (hōl'gər nēl'sen) [*Holger Nielsen,* Danish army officer, 1866–1955] see *artificial respiration,* under *respiration.*

**hol·ism** (hōl'iz-əm) [*hol-* + *-ism*] the theory that the determining factors in nature are organisms, which are wholes and not mechanisms and are irreducible, autonomous, and functionally greater than the sums of their parts.

**ho·lis·tic** (ho-lis'tik) considering man as a functioning whole, or relating to the conception of man as a functioning whole; see also under *health.*

**Hol·len·horst plaques** (hol'ən-horst) [Robert W. *Hollenhorst,* American ophthalmologist, born 1913] see under *plaque.*

**Hol·ley** (hol'e) Robert William. American biochemist, born 1922; co-winner, with Har Gobind Khorana and Marshall Warren Nirenberg, of the Nobel prize for medicine or physiology in 1968 for their interpretation of the genetic code and its function in protein synthesis.

**hol·low** (hol'o) a depressed area or concavity.
**Sebileau's h.,** a depressed area beneath the tongue, formed by the oral mucosa and the sublingual glands.

**hol·low-back** (hol'o-bak) see *lordosis.*

**Holmes** (hōmz) Oliver Wendell (1809–1894). Noted American physician, anatomist, and writer, whose paper *On the Contagiousness of Puerperal Fever* (1843) antedated the work of Semmelweis in its appeal for surgical cleanliness to combat this disease.

**Holmes's degeneration, phenomenon (sign)** (hōmz) [Sir Gordon Morgan *Holmes,* English neurologist, 1876–1965] see under *degeneration,* and see *rebound phenomenon,* under *phenomenon.*

**Holmes-Adie syndrome** (hōmz-a'de) [G.M. *Holmes;* William John *Adie,* Australian neurologist in England, 1886–1935] Adie's syndrome.

**Holmes-Stew·art phenomenon** (hōmz-stoo'ərt) [G.M. *Holmes;* James Purves *Stewart,* English physician, 1869–1949] rebound phenomenon.

**Holm·gren's test** (hōm'grənz) [Alarik Frithiof *Holmgren,* Swedish physiologist, 1831–1897] see under *test.*

**hol·mi·um** (hōl'me-əm) [MeSH: Holmium] one of the rare earth elements; symbol, Ho; atomic number, 67; atomic weight, 164.930.

**hol(o)-** [Gr. *holos* entire] a combining form meaning entire, or denoting relationship to the whole.

**holo·acar·di·us** (hōl"o-ə-kahr'de-əs) [*holo-* + *acardius*] a separate, monozygotic twin represented by a more or less shapeless and unidentifiable mass; the vascular systems of the two fetuses are connected, and the circulation is accomplished solely by the heart of the more perfect twin.
**h. ace'phalus,** an imperfectly formed free twin fetus lacking the cranial part of the body.
**h. acor'mus,** an imperfectly formed free twin fetus lacking the caudal part of the body.
**h. amor'phus,** an imperfectly formed free twin fetus entirely without form and recognizable parts.

**holo·an·ti·gen** (hōl"o-an'tĭ-jən) complete antigen, as opposed to hapten.

**holo·ar·thric** (hōl"o-ahr'thrik) said of thallic-arthric conidiogenesis in which both of the cell walls form the conidia.

**Holo·ba·sid·io·my·ce·tes** (ho"lo-bə-sid"e-o-mi-se'tēz) [*holo-* + *basidium* + Gr. *mykēs* fungus] a class of perfect fungi of the subphylum Basidiomycotina, characterized by having an aseptate basidium; its orders include Agaricales, Aphyllophorales, Lycoperdales, and Phallales.

**Holo·ba·sid·io·my·ce·ti·dae** (ho"lo-bə-sid"e-o-mi-set'ĭ-de) name given to Holobasidiomycetes in some systems of classification, considering it a subclass.

**holo·blas·tic** (hōl"o-blas'tik) [*holo-* + *blast-* + *-ic*] 1. undergoing cleavage in which the entire oocyte (ovum) participates; dividing completely. 2. said of blastic conidiogenesis in which all of the cell wall is used to form the conidium.

**holo·car·boxy·lase syn·the·tase** (hōl"o-kahr-bok'sə-lās sin'thə-tās) an enzyme catalyzing the ATP-dependent biotinylation of the apoenzyme forms of the carboxylases acetyl-CoA carboxylase, methylcrotonoyl-CoA carboxylase, propionyl-CoA carboxylase, and pyruvate carboxylase, forming the active holoenzymes. Deficiency of the enzyme, probably an autosomal recessive trait, results in multiple carboxylase deficiency.

**holo·ce·phal·ic** (hōl"o-sə-fal'ik) [*holo-* + *cephalic*] said of a fetus that has a complete head but deficiencies in other parts of the body.

**holo·crine** (ho'lo-krin) [*holo-* + Gr. *krinein* to separate] wholly secretory: denoting that type of glandular secretion in which the entire secreting cell, along with its accumulated secretion, forms the secreted matter of the gland, as in the sebaceous glands. Cf. *merocrine* and *apocrine.*

**holo·di·a·stol·ic** (hōl"o-di"ə-stol'ik) [*holo-* + *diastole*] pertaining to the entire diastole.

**holo·en·dem·ic** (hōl"o-en-dem'ik) [*holo-* + *endemic*] endemic at a high level early in life in a population and leading to a state of equilibrium such that the adult population shows evidence of the disease less often than do the children. Cf. *hyperendemic.*

**holo·en·zyme** (hōl"o-en'zīm) the functional compound formed by the combination of an apoenzyme and its appropriate coenzyme.

**ho·log·a·my** (ho-log'ə-me) [*holo-* + Gr. *gamos* marriage] the condition in which the gametes are of the same size and structural type as the somatic cells.

**holo·gas·tros·chi·sis** (hōl"o-gas-tros'kĭ-sis) [*holo-* + *gastro-* + *-schisis*] a developmental anomaly characterized by a fissure extending the entire length of the abdomen.

**holo·gen·e·sis** (hōl"o-jen'ə-sis) [*holo-* + *-genesis*] the theory that humans originated everywhere on earth, instead of in a certain special region or regions.

**holo·gram** (hōl'o-gram") a three-dimensional image produced by holography.

**hol·og·ra·phy** (hōl-og'rə-fe) [MeSH: Holography] the recording of images in three-dimensional form on photographic film by exposing it to a laser beam reflected from the object under study.
**acoustical h.,** holography in which sound waves reflected from an object under study are converted into light waves, which act on the emulsion of the film. The film is then exposed to a laser beam to give a three-dimensional effect.

**holo·mas·ti·gote** (hōl"o-mas'tĭ-gōt) [*holo-* + *mastigote*] having numerous flagella scattered over the body.

**holo·morph** (hōl'o-morf") [*holo-* + *-morph*] a whole fungus in all of its forms and stages; a *perfect fungus* includes a *teleomorph* (sexual stage) and one or more *anamorphs* (asexual stages), whereas an *imperfect fungus* includes an anamorph only.

**holo·mor·pho·sis** (hōl"o-mor-fo'sis) [*holo-* + *morphosis*] the complete regeneration of a lost part.

**holo·phyt·ic** (hōl"o-fit'ik) [*holo-* + *phyt-* + *-ic*] having a type of nutrition or feeding resembling that of a plant; said of certain photosynthesizing protozoa. Cf. *holozoic.*

**holo·pros·en·ceph·a·ly** (hōl"o-pros"ən-sef'ə-le) [*holo-* + *prosencephalon*] [MeSH: Holoprosencephaly] failure of cleavage of the prosencephalon with a deficit in midline facial development. Cyclopia occurs in the severe form. In the form due to an extra chromosome 13 (trisomy 13, Patau syndrome), there are, characteristically, low-set ears, bilateral cleft lip and palate, microcephaly, ocular anomalies, hypotelorism, mental retardation, deafness, convulsions, and ventricular septal defects.
**familial alobar h.,** a form in which the chromosomes are normal but otherwise resembling that due to trisomy 13 (see *holoprosencephaly*).

**holo·ra·chis·chi·sis** (hōl"o-rə-kis'kĭ-sis) [*holo-* + *rhachischisis*] rachischisis totalis.

**holo·sac·cha·ride** (hōl"o-sak'ə-rīd) a polysaccharide composed of sugar units only. Cf. *heterosaccharide.*

**holo·schi·sis** (hōl"o-ski'sis) [*holo-* + *-schisis*] amitosis.

**holo·sys·tol·ic** (hōl"o-sis-tol'ik) [*holo-* + *systole*] pertaining to the entire systole.

**holo·thal·lik** (hōl"o-thal'ik) said of thallic conidiogenesis in which just one part of the parent cell disarticulates to form the conidium.

**holo·thu·rin** (hōl"o-thoo'rin) [MeSH: Holothurin] a hemotoxic mixture of steroid glycosides obtained from holothurians, or sea cucumbers.

**Holo·thy·rus** (hōl"o-thi'rəs) a genus of mites. *H. coccinel'la,* a species found in Mauritius, secretes toxic substances that may cause the death of ducks, geese, and chickens after ingestion; in humans it may produce a painful swelling of the tongue and throat.

**ho·lot·o·py** (ho-lot'ə-pe) [*holo-* + Gr. *topos* place] the position of an organ in relation to the whole body.

**ho·lot·ri·chous** (ho-lot'rĭ-kəs) [*holo-* + *trich-* + *-ous*] covered uniformly with cilia.

**holo·type** (hōl'o-tīp) the type culture of a species or subspecies of microorganisms, either because it was so designated in the original description or because the original description was based on only one strain.

**holo·xen·ic** (hōl"o-zen'ik) [*holo-* + *xen-* + *-ic*] raised under usual circumstances; said of an animal not raised under special laboratory conditions, as opposed to one raised in a germ-free environment. See also *axenic* and *gnotobiotic.*

**holo·zo·ic** (hōl"o-zo'ik) [*holo-* + *zoic*] having a type of nutrition or feeding resembling that of an animal; i.e., ingestion of whole organisms or relatively large particles. Called also *phagotrophic.* Cf. *holophytic* and *saprozoic.*

**Holt-Oram syndrome** (hōlt-o'rəm) [Mary Clayton *Holt,* British cardiologist, 20th century; Samuel *Oram,* English cardiologist, born 1913] see under *syndrome.*

**Hol·ter monitor** (hōl'tər) [Norman Jefferis *Holter,* American biophysicist, 1914–1983] see under *monitor.*

**Holth's operation** (holths) [Sören *Holth,* Norwegian ophthalmologist, 1863–1937] see under *operation.*

**Holt·house's hernia** (holt'houz-əs) [Carsten *Holthouse,* English surgeon, 1810–1901] see under *hernia.*

**Holz·knecht's space** (holts′knekts) [Guido *Holzknecht,* Austrian radiologist, 1872–1931] see under *space.*

**hom·a·lo·ceph·a·lus** (hom″ə-lo-sef′ə-ləs) [Gr. *homalos* level + *-cephalus*] a person with a flat head.

**hom·al·uria** (hom″ə-lu′re-ə) [Gr. *homalos* level, even + *-uria*] production and excretion of urine at a normal, even rate.

**Ho·mans' operation, sign** (ho′mənz) [John *Homans,* American surgeon, 1877–1954] see under *operation* and *sign.*

**Ho·ma·pin** (ho′mə-pin) trademark for preparations of homatropine methylbromide.

**hom·a·rine** (hom′ə-rēn) an organic nitrogen compound which is found in lobster muscle and tissues of other marine animals. It is the methyl betaine of picolinic acid, $C_5H_4N^+(CH_3)CO_2^-$.

**ho·mat·ro·pine** (ho-mat′ro-pēn) the tropine ester of mandelic acid, having anticholinergic effects similar to but weaker than those of atropine.
**h. hydrobromide** [USP], the hydrobromide salt of homatropine, used in ophthalmology as a cycloplegic and mydriatic, applied topically to the conjunctiva.
**h. methylbromide** [USP], the 8-methyl derivative of homatropine hydrobromide, used as an antispasmodic and inhibitor of secretions, especially in gastrointestinal disorders, administered orally.

**ho·max·i·al** (ho-mak′se-əl) having axes of the same length.

**Ho·mén's syndrome** (ho′mānz) [Ernst Alexander *Homén,* Finnish physician, 1851–1926] postconcussional syndrome.

**home(o)-** [Gr. *homoios* like, resembling] a combining form denoting sameness or similarity.

**ho·meo·box** (ho′me-o-boks″) any of a class of highly conserved DNA sequences, approximately 180 base pairs long, encoding a protein domain involved in binding to DNA; it was named for its initial discovery as a *Drosophila* locus important in homeotic mutation, but it also occurs in humans and is usually found in genes involved in the control of development.

**ho·meo·chrome** (ho′me-o-krōm″) [*homeo-* + *-chrome*] staining with mucin stains after formol-bichromate fixation; applied to certain serous cells of the salivary glands. Cf. *tropochrome.*

**ho·meo·ki·ne·sis** (ho″me-o-kĭ-ne′sis) [*homeo-* + *-kinesis*] the stage of meiosis in which the daughter cells receive equal amounts and kinds of chromatin.

**ho·meo·mor·phous** (ho″me-o-mor′fəs) [*homeo-* + *morph-* + *-ous*] of like form and structure.

**ho·meo·os·teo·plas·ty** (ho″me-o-os″te-o-plas′te) [*homeo-* + *osteo-* + *-plasty*] the grafting of bone from one individual to another within the same species.

**ho·meo·path** (ho′me-o-path) homeopathist.

**ho·meo·path·ic** (ho″me-o-path′ik) pertaining to homeopathy.

**ho·me·op·a·thist** (ho″me-op′ə-thist) one who practices homeopathy.

**ho·me·op·a·thy** (ho″me-op′ə-the) [*homeo-* + *-pathy*] [MeSH: Homeopathy] a system of therapeutics founded by Samuel Hahnemann (1755–1843), in which diseases are treated by drugs which are capable of producing in healthy persons symptoms like those of the disease to be treated, the drug being administered in minute doses. Cf. *allopathy.*

**ho·meo·pla·sia** (ho″me-o-pla′zhə) [*homeo-* + *-plasia*] the formation of new tissue like that adjacent to it and normal to the part.

**ho·meo·plas·tic** (ho″me-o-plas′tik) 1. resembling in structure the adjacent parts. 2. pertaining to, characterized by, or stimulating homeoplasia.

**ho·me·or·rhe·sis** (ho″me-o-re′sis) [*homeo-* + Gr. *rhein* to flow] the tendency to maintain a biological process, as a growth process, along a particular pathway despite the operation of factors tending to divert it.

**ho·me·o·sis** (ho″me-o′sis) [Gr. *homoiōsis* likeness, resemblance] the formation of a body part having the characteristics normally found in a related part at a different body site.

**ho·meo·sta·sis** (ho″me-o-sta′sis) [*homeo-* + *-stasis*] [MeSH: Homeostasis] a tendency to stability in the normal body states (internal environment) of the organism. It is achieved by a system of control mechanisms activated by negative feedback; e.g., a high level of carbon dioxide in extracellular fluid triggers increased pulmonary ventilation, which in turn causes a decrease in carbon dioxide concentration.

**ho·meo·stat·ic** (ho″me-o-stat′ik) pertaining to homeostasis.

**ho·meo·ther·a·py** (ho″me-o-ther′ə-pe) [*homeo-* + *therapy*] treatment or prevention of disease with a substance similar to but not the same as the causative agent of the disease.

**ho·meo·therm** (ho′me-o-thərm″) [*homeo-* + Gr. *thermē* heat] 1. an animal that exhibits homeothermy; a so-called warm-blooded animal, as opposed to a poikilotherm. 2. endotherm.

**ho·meo·ther·mal** (ho″me-o-thər′məl) [*homeo-* + *thermal*] homeothermic.

**ho·meo·ther·mic** (ho″me-o-thər′mik) 1. pertaining to or characterized by homeothermy. 2. endothermic (def. 2).

**ho·meo·ther·mism** (ho″me-o-thər′miz-əm) homeothermy.

**ho·meo·ther·my** (ho′me-o-thər″me) the maintenance of a constant body temperature despite changes in the environmental temperature. Cf. *poikilothermy* (defs. 1 and 2).

**ho·meo·typ·ic, ho·meo·typ·i·cal** (ho″me-o-tip′ik, ho″me-o-tip′ĭ-kəl) [*homeo-* + Gr. *typos* type] resembling the normal or usual type.

**ho·meo·typ·i·cal** (ho″me-o-tip′ĭ-kəl) homeotypic.

**hom·er·gic** (hōm-ər′jik) [*hom-* + Gr. *ergon* work] having the same effect; said of two drugs each of which produces the same overt effect.

**Ho·mer Wright rosette** (ho′mər rīt) [James *Homer Wright,* American pathologist, 1871–1928] see under *rosette.*

**hom·i·cide** (hom′ĭ-sīd) [L. "murderer," from *homo* man + *caedere* to kill] [MeSH: Homicide] the taking of the life of one person by another.

**ho·mid·i·um** (ho-mid′e-əm) a trypanosomicide used as the bromide and chloride salts in the treatment of infections with *Trypanosoma congolense* and *T. vivax* in cattle and horses. Its bromide salt is also used in biochemistry as a fluorochrome in the detection of double-stranded nucleic acids; in that context it is usually called *ethidium.*

**hom·i·nal** (hom′i-nəl) [L. *homo* man] 1. pertaining to human beings. 2. pertaining to male human beings.

**hom·ing** (ho′ming) any mechanism seen in cells causing them to migrate to a specific tissue, organ, or other location, such as that causing organ-specific metastasis or that mediating binding of particular lymphocytes to specific vascular endothelium.

**hom·i·nid** (hom′ĭ-nid) [MeSH: Hominidae] 1. pertaining to the family of humans (Hominidae). 2. a living or extinct human or humanlike type.

**Ho·min·i·dae** (ho-min′ĭ-de) [L. *homo* man + Gr. *eidos* resemblance] [MeSH: Hominidae] a family of primates (superfamily Hominoidea, suborder Anthropoidea), including both modern man *(Homo sapiens)* and fossil hominids.

**hom·i·noid** (hom′ĭ-noid)) 1. pertaining to the Hominoidea. 2. a member of the Hominoidea.

**Hom·i·noi·dea** (hom″ĭ-noi′de-ə) [L. *homo* man + Gr. *oeidos* likeness] a superfamily of primates, including the families Pongidae and Hominidae. Cf. *Anthropoidea.*

**homme** (um) [Fr.] man.
**h. rouge** (ro͞ozh) [Fr. "red man"], a stage in mycosis fungoides in which the red plaques become infiltrated and coalesce over a wide area of the body.

**Ho·mo** (ho′mo) [L. *man*] a genus of primates of the family Hominidae, including humans *(H. sa′piens)* and fossil hominids.

**hom(o)-** [Gr. *homos* same] 1. a combining form meaning the same. 2. a prefix in chemical names indicating the addition of one $CH_2$ group to the main compound.

**ho·mo·ar·te·re·nol hy·dro·chlo·ride** (ho″mo-ahr″tə-re′nol) nordefrin hydrochloride.

**ho·mo·bio·tin** (ho″mo-bi′o-tin) a homologue of biotin having an additional $CH_2$ group in the side chain and acting as a biotin antagonist.

**ho·mo·body** (ho′mo-bod″e) an antibody with an idiotypic determinant that is stereochemically similar to the epitope on the antigen against which the antibody was originally directed; it is therefore able to mimic the behavior of the antigen.

**ho·mo·car·no·sin·ase** (ho″mo-kahr′no-sĭ-nās) former name for an enzyme activity now believed to be part of the serum isozyme of X-His dipeptidase (carnosinase).

**ho·mo·car·no·sine** (ho″mo-kahr′no-sēn) a dipeptide consisting of γ-aminobutyric acid and histidine; in humans it is found in the brain but not in other tissues.

**ho·mo·car·no·sin·o·sis** (ho″mo-kahr-no″sĭ-no′sis) an inherited aminoacidopathy characterized by accumulation of homocarnosine in cerebrospinal fluid and the brain but not in plasma or urine, accompanied by carnosinuria. Progressive spastic paraplegia, mental deterioration, and retinal pigmentation may be sequelae. The disorder is due to deficiency of the serum isozyme of X-His dipeptidase, but its relationship to serum carnosinase deficiency (q.v.) has not been elucidated.

**ho·mo·cen·tric** (ho″mo-sen′trik) [*homo-* + *centric*] having the same center or focus.

**ho·moch·ro·nous** (ho-mok′ro-nəs) [*homo-* + *chron-* + *-ous*] occurring at the same age in successive generations.

**ho·mo·cin·cho·nine** (ho″mo-sin′ko-nin) an alkaloid, $C_{19}H_{22}ON_2$, from cinchona, isomeric with cinchonine.

**ho·mo·clad·ic** (ho″mo-klad′ik) [*homo-* + Gr. *klados* branch] formed between small branches of the same artery; said of such an anastomosis.

**ho·mo·cyc·lic** (ho″mo-sik′lik) having or pertaining to a closed chain or ring formation which includes only atoms of the same element.

**ho·mo·cys·te·ine** (ho″mo-sis′te-ēn) [MeSH: Homocysteine] a sulfur-containing amino acid homologous with cysteine and produced by demethylation of methionine. It can serve as an intermediate in the biosynthesis of cysteine from methionine via cystathionine or can be remethylated to methionine.

**ho·mo·cys·te·ine–tet·ra·hy·dro·fo·late meth·yl·trans·fer·ase** (ho″mo-sis′teēn tet″rə-hi″dro-fo′lāt meth″əl-trans′fər-ās) 5-methyltetrahydrofolate-homocysteine *S*-methyltransferase.

**ho·mo·cys·tine** (ho″mo-sis′tēn) [MeSH: Homocystine] a disulfide homologous with cystine and formed by oxidation and subsequent condensation of two molecules of homocysteine. It is a source of sulfur in the body.

**ho·mo·cys·tin·emia** (ho″mo-sis″tin-e′me-ə) an excess of homocystine in the blood; see *homocystinuria.*

**ho·mo·cys·tin·uria** (ho″mo-sis″tin-u′re-ə) [MeSH: Homocystinuria] excretion of excess homocystine in the urine, a biochemical abnormality with a variety of autosomal recessive genetic as well as nongenetic causes, characterized by developmental delay, failure to thrive, and neurologic abnormalities, with other features, such as hematologic abnormalities, varying with specific causes. Principal causes include deficiency of cystathionine $\beta$-synthase activity (q.v.), any of several genetic disorders causing deficiency of 5-methyltetrahydrofolate–homocysteine *S*-methyltransferase activity (q.v.), and nutritional vitamin $B_{12}$ or folate deficiency; certain drugs can also elevate urinary homocystine. In older literature, the term usually denotes the disorder caused by deficiency of cystathionine $\beta$-synthase activity.

**ho·mo·cy·to·trop·ic** (ho″mo-si″to-trop′ik) [*homo-* + *cyto-* + *-tropic*] having an affinity for cells from the same species; see under *antibody.*

**ho·mo·des·mot·ic** (ho″mo-dəs-mot′ik) [*homo-* + Gr. *desmos* bond] joining similar parts of the central nervous system; see under *fiber.*

**ho·mo·dont** (ho′mo-dont) [*hom-* + Gr. *odous* tooth] having teeth of only one type.

**ho·mod·ro·mous** (ho-mod′ro-məs) [*homo-* + *dromo-* + *-ous*] moving or acting in the same direction.

**homoe(o)-** see *home(o)-.*

**ho·moe·o·sis** (ho″me-o′sis) homeosis.

**ho·mo·erot·ic** (ho″mo-ə-rot′ik) pertaining to or characterized by homoeroticism.

**ho·mo·erot·i·cism** (ho″mo-ə-rot′ĭ-siz-əm) 1. sexual feeling directed toward a person of the same sex. 2. a stage in the development of object relationships characterized by suppression of libidinal energies and occurring between the Oedipal stage and adolescence; see also *latency stage,* under *latency.*

**ho·mo·er·o·tism** (ho″mo-er′o-tiz-əm) homoeroticism.

**ho·mo·fer·men·ta·tion** (ho″mo-fər″mən-ta′shən) fermentation that produces one major product; the term is often used as a synonym of homolactic fermentation (q.v.).

**ho·mo·fer·ment·er** (ho″mo-fər-ment′ər) a microorganism that exhibits homofermentation.

**ho·mo·gam·ete** (ho″mo-gam′ēt) one of two gametes of the same size and structure, as the X chromosome in the human female.

**ho·mo·ga·met·ic** (ho″mo-gə-met′ik) pertaining to the sex that produces gametes of only one kind, in terms of their sex chromosomes. In human beings, the female is the homogametic sex.

**ho·mog·a·mous** (ho-mog′ə-məs) characterized by or pertaining to homogamy.

**ho·mog·a·my** (ho-mog′ə-me) [*homo-* + Gr. *gamos* marriage] 1. inbreeding. 2. reproduction resulting from the union of two gametes that are identical in size and structure. 3. maturation of the male (stamens) and female (pistils) gametes of a flower at the same time. Cf. *heterogamy* and *isogamy.*

**ho·mog·e·nate** (ho-moj′ə-nāt) material subjected to homogenization, as tissue that is finely shredded and mixed.

**ho·mo·ge·ne·i·ty** (ho″mo-jə-ne′ĭ-te) the state or quality of being homogeneous.

**ho·mo·ge·ne·iza·tion** (ho″mo-je″ne″ĭ-za′shən) homogenization.

**ho·mo·ge·ne·ous** (ho″mo-je′ne-əs) [*homo-* + Gr. *genos* kind] consisting of or composed of similar elements or ingredients; of a uniform quality throughout.

**ho·mo·gen·e·sis** (ho″mo-jen′ə-sis) [*homo-* + *-genesis*] the reproduction by the same process in each generation, as contrasted with heterogenesis.

**ho·mo·ge·net·ic** (ho″mo-jə-net′ik) pertaining to or characterized by homogenesis.

**ho·mo·gen·ic** (ho″mo-jen′ik) homozygous.

**ho·mo·ge·nic·i·ty** (ho″mo-jə-nis′ĭ-te) homogeneity.

**ho·mog·e·ni·za·tion** (ho-moj″ə-nĭ-za′shən) the act or process of rendering homogeneous.

**ho·mog·e·nize** (ho-moj′ə-nīz) to render homogeneous, or of uniform quality or consistency throughout.

**ho·mo·ge·note** (ho″mo-je′nōt) in bacterial genetics, a merozygote in which the corresponding alleles at a specific locus of the diploid region of the genome are identical.

**ho·mog·e·nous** (ho-moj′ə-nəs) having a similarity of structure because of descent from a common ancestor.

**ho·mo·gen·tis·ate** (ho″mo-jən-tis′āt) the anionic form of homogentisic acid.

**ho·mo·gen·tis·ate 1,2-di·oxy·gen·ase** (ho″mo-jən-tis′āt di-ok′sə-jən-ās) [EC 1.13.11.5] an enzyme of the oxidoreductase class that catalyzes the oxidation of homogentisate to form 4-methylacetoacetate as a step in the degradation of tyrosine and phenylalanine. Deficiency of the enzyme, an autosomal recessive trait, causes alkaptonuria.

**ho·mo·gen·tis·ic ac·id** (ho″mo-jen-tis′ik) [MeSH: Homogentisic Acid] an aromatic hydrocarbon formed as an intermediate in the catabolism of tyrosine and phenylalanine. It is accumulated abnormally and excreted in the urine in alkaptonuria.

**ho·mo·gen·tis·ic ac·id ox·i·dase** (ho″mo-jen-tis′ik as′id ok′sĭ-dās) homogentisate 1,2-dioxygenase.

**ho·mo·gen·tis·ic ac·id ox·i·dase de·fi·cien·cy** alkaptonuria.

**ho·mo·gen·ti·su·ria** (ho″mo-jen″tĭ-su′re-ə) the excretion of homogentisic acid in the urine, as occurs in alkaptonuria.

**ho·mog·e·ny** (ho-moj′ə-ne) homogenesis.

**ho·mo·glan·du·lar** (ho″mo-glan′du-lər) pertaining to the same gland.

**ho·mo·graft** (ho′mo-graft) allograft.

**homoi(o)-** see *home(o)-.*

**ho·moi·op·o·dal** (ho″moi-op′o-dəl) [*homoio-* + Gr. *pous* foot] having processes of one kind only; said of nerve cells.

**ho·moi·os·ta·sis** (ho″moi-os′tə-sis) homeostasis.

**ho·moio·tox·in** (ho-moi′o-tok-sin) a toxin from one individual which is toxic for other individuals of the same species.

**ho·mo·ker·a·to·plas·ty** (ho″mo-ker′ə-to-plas″te) [*homo-* + *keratoplasty*] corneal grafting with tissue derived from another individual of the same species.

**ho·mo·lac·tic** (ho″mo-lak′tik) bacterial fermentation that produces lactic acid by way of the Embden-Meyerhof pathway.

**ho·mo·lat·er·al** (ho″mo-lat′ər-əl) situated on, pertaining to, or affecting the same side; ipsilateral.

**ho·mol·o·gen** (ho-mol′o-jən) homologue, def. 2.

**ho·mol·o·gous** (ho-mol′o-gəs) [Gr. *homologos* agreeing, correspondent] 1. corresponding in structure, position, origin, etc., as *(a)* the feathers of a bird and the scales of a fish, *(b)* antigen and its specific antibody, *(c)* allelic chromosomes. Cf. *analogous.* 2. allogeneic. 3. pertaining to an antibody and the antigen that elicited its production.

**ho·mo·logue** (ho′mo-log) 1. any homologous organ or part; an organ similar in structure, position, and origin to another organ, as the front flippers of a seal and human hands. See *analogue.* 2. in chemistry, one of a series of compounds, each of which is formed from the one before it by the addition of a constant element or a constant group of elements, as in the homologous series $CH_4$, $C_2H_6$, $C_3H_8$, etc.; called also *homologen.*

**ho·mol·o·gy** (ho-mol′ə-je) [Gr. *homologia* agreement] the quality of being homologous; the morphological identity of corresponding parts; structural similarity due to descent from a common form.

**ho·mol·y·sin** (ho-mol′ə-sin) a lysin (e.g., isohemolysin) produced

Propane Butane Pentane

Homologues.

by injection into the body of antigen derived from an individual of the same species.

**ho·mol·y·sis** (ho-mol'ə-sis) [*homo-* + *-lysis*] lysis of a cell by extracts of the same type of tissue.

**ho·mo·mor·phic** (ho-mo-mor'fik) [*homo-* + *morph-* + *-ic*] having chromosome mates of similar size and form during synapsis of the first meiotic division.

**ho·mo·mor·pho·sis** (ho″mo-mor-fo'sis) [*homo-* + *morphosis*] regenerative replacement of a lost part by a similar part.

**ho·mon·o·mous** (ho-mon'ə-məs) [*homo-* + Gr. *nomos* law] designating homologous serial parts, such as somites.

**ho·mon·y·mous** (ho-mon'ĭ-məs) [*hom-* + Gr. *onoma* name] 1. having the same or corresponding sound or name. 2. in ophthalmology, pertaining to the corresponding vertical halves of the visual fields of both eyes, i.e., the right visual field (the nasal half of the left eye, the temporal of the right) and the left visual field (the temporal half of the left eye, the nasal of the right).

**ho·mo·phil** (ho'mo-fil) pertaining to antibody that reacts only with its homologous antigen.

**ho·mo·phil·ic** (ho″mo-fil'ik) [*homo-* + *-philic*] having affinity for or reacting with a specific antigen; said of an antibody.

**ho·mo·plas·tic** (ho″mo-plas'tik) [*homo-* + *plastic*] 1. allogeneic. 2. denoting organs or parts, as the wings of birds and insects, that resemble one another in structure and function but not in origin or development.

**ho·mo·plas·ty** (ho'mo-plas″te) 1. allogeneic transplantation. 2. similarity between organs or parts not due to common ancestry.

**ho·mo·poly·mer** (ho″mo-pol'ĭ-mər) [*homo-* + *polymer*] a polymer containing the same repeating units of one amino acid in a molecule.

**ho·mo·poly·sac·cha·ride** (ho″mo-pol″e-sak'ə-rīd) a polysaccharide consisting of a single recurring monosaccharide unit, as glycogen is a polymer of glucose.

**hom·or·gan·ic** (hom″or-gan'ik) [*homo-* + *organic*] produced by the same or by homologous organs.

**ho·mo·sal·ate** (ho″mo-sal'āt) [USP] an ultraviolet sunscreen, applied topically to the skin.

**ho·mo·sce·das·tic·i·ty** (ho″mo-skə-das-tis'ĭ-te) [*homo-* + Gr. *skedastikos* tending to scatter] the property of having equal variances.

**ho·mo·sex·u·al** (ho″mo-sek'shoo-əl) [MeSH: Homosexuality] 1. pertaining to the same sex; directed toward a person of the same sex; the opposite of heterosexual. 2. one who is sexually attracted to persons of the same sex.

**ho·mo·sex·u·al·i·ty** (ho″mo-sek″shoo-al'ĭ-te) [*homo-* + *sexuality*] [MeSH: Homosexuality] sexual orientation toward or activity with those of the same sex, as distinguished from heterosexuality.

**ho·mo·spore** (ho'mo-spor) a homosporous organism.

**ho·mos·po·rous** (ho-mos'pə-rəs) [*homo-* + *spor-* + *-ous*] having spores of only one kind, which reproduce asexually.

**ho·mo·stim·u·lant** (ho″mo-stim'u-lənt) 1. stimulating the same organ from which it is derived. 2. an extract from an organ which, on injection into the body, stimulates the same organ from which it is derived.

**ho·mo·stim·u·la·tion** (ho″mo-stim″u-la'shən) treatment by a homostimulant.

**Ho·mo-Tet** (ho-mo-tet') trademark for a preparation of tetanus immune human globulin.

**ho·mo·thal·lic** (hom″o-thal'ik) pertaining to or exhibiting homothallism.

**ho·mo·thal·lism** (ho″mo-thal'iz-əm) a form of sexual reproduction in which the isogamete produced by one cell can fuse with another isogamete produced by the same cell, as in various algae and fungi. Cf. *heterothallism.*

**ho·mo·therm** (ho'mo-thərm) homeotherm.

**ho·mo·ther·mal** (ho″mo-thər'məl) homeothermic.

**ho·mo·ther·mic** (ho″mo-thər'mik) homeothermic.

**ho·mo·top·ic** (ho″mo-top'ik) [*homo-* + *top-* + *-ic*] occurring at the same place upon the body.

**ho·mo·trans·plant** (ho″mo-trans'plant) allograft.

**ho·mo·tro·pic** (ho'mo-trōp″ik) [*homo-* + *-tropic*] pertaining to an allosteric enzyme that is modulated by its usual substrate. Cf. *heterotropic.*

**ho·mot·ro·pism** (ho-mot'ro-piz-əm) [*homo-* + *tropism*] the property of cells to attract cells of a like order.

**ho·mo·type** (ho'mo-tīp) [*homo-* + Gr. *typos* type] a part that has a reversed symmetry with its fellow of the opposite side of the body, as the hand.

**ho·mo·typ·ic** (ho″mo-tip'ik) pertaining to or characteristic of a homotype.

**ho·mo·va·nil·lic ac·id** (ho″mo-və-nil'ik) [MeSH: Homovanillic Acid] a product of catecholamine metabolism; elevated urinary levels occur in patients with pheochromocytoma or other catecholamine-secreting tumors. Abbreviated HVA.

**ho·mox·e·nous** (ho-mok'sə-nəs) [*homo-* + *xen-* + *-ous*] requiring only one host in the life cycle; said of certain parasites. Called also *monoxenous.*

**ho·mo·zo·ic** (ho″mo-zo'ik) [*homo-* + *zoic*] pertaining to the same animal or the same species.

**ho·mo·zy·go·sis** (ho″mo-zi-go'sis) the formation of a zygote by the union of gametes that possess one or more identical alleles.

**ho·mo·zy·gos·i·ty** (ho″mo-zi-gos'ĭ-te) [*homo-* + *zygosity*] the state of possessing a pair of identical alleles at a given locus.

**ho·mo·zy·gote** (ho″mo-zi'gōt) [*homo-* + *zygote*] [MeSH: Homozygote] an individual possessing a pair of identical alleles at a given locus.

**ho·mo·zy·gous** (ho″mo-zi'gəs) possessing a pair of identical alleles at a given locus; called also *homogenic.* See also *heterozygous.*

**ho·mun·cu·lus** (ho-munk'u-ləs) [L. "a little man"] 1. the miniature human form once thought to be preformed in the sperm or ovum. 2. normal dwarf.

**hon·ey** (hun'e) [MeSH: Honey] a sweet-tasting substance deposited by the honeybee, which contains between 62 and 83 per cent glucose and fructose, and small amounts of sucrose, dextrin, and malic and acetic acids; its pH is 3.8 to 4.3.

**hon·ey·comb** (hun'e-kōm) 1. a network of hexagonal cells, made out of beeswax by honeybees. 2. something resembling this structure, such as a honeycomb lung. 3. reticulum, def. 3.

**hood** (hood) a flexible covering.
**tooth h.,** dental operculum.

**hoof** (hoof) [L. *ungula*] the hard, horny casing of the end of certain digits of a group of mammals that are, because of this feature, known as the *ungulates.* Called also *ungula.*
**contracted h.,** a condition in a horse's hoof in which it becomes dried out and reduced in size, which causes inadequate pressure on the frog and lameness. Called also *contracted foot* and *contracted heel.*
**ribbed h., ringed h.,** a condition in which the wall of a horse's hoof is marked by ridges running parallel with the coronary margin.

**hook** (hook) a curved instrument, usually with a sharp point, designed for holding, elevating, or exerting traction on a tissue.
**blunt h.,** an instrument for exercising traction on a dead fetus in breech presentation.
**Loughnane's h.,** a double-pronged hook for removing fragments of the prostate in transurethral prostatectomy.
**muscle h.,** a hook for securing and isolating an extraocular muscle; called also *squint h.*
**palate h.,** a hook for raising the palate in posterior rhinoscopy.
**squint h.,** muscle h.
**Tyrrell's h.,** a slender hook used in eye surgery.

**hook-up** (hook'əp) the method of arranging circuits, appliances, and electrodes for a particular diagnostic or therapeutic procedure.

**hook·worm** (hook'wərm) any nematode of the family Ancylostomatidae. See also *hookworm disease,* under *disease.*
**American h.,** *Necator americanus.*
**dog h.,** a hookworm infesting dogs, such as *Ancylostoma braziliense* or *A. caninum.*
**European h.,** *Ancylostoma duodenale.*
**New World h.,** *Necator americanus.*
**Old World h.,** *Ancylostoma duodenale.*
**rat h.,** *Nippostrongylus muris.*
**h. of ruminants,** *Bunostomum.*

**hoose** (hōōz) verminous bronchitis in sheep, cattle, goats, and swine, caused by the presence of nematodes of genera *Dictyocaulus, Metastrongylus, Muellerius,* and *Protostrongylus* in the bronchial tubes or lungs; it is marked by cough, dyspnea, anorexia, and constipation. Called also *husk.*

**Hoo·ver's sign** (hoo'vərz) [Charles Franklin *Hoover,* American physician, 1865–1927] see under *sign.*

**HOP** 1. high oxygen pressure. 2. a regimen of hydroxydaunomycin (doxorubicin), Oncovin (vincristine), and prednisone, used in cancer chemotherapy.

**Hope's sign** (hōps) [James *Hope,* English physician, 1801–1841] see under *sign.*

**Hop·kins** (hop'kinz) Sir Frederick Gowland. British biologist, 1861–1947; co-winner, with Christiaan Eijkmann, of the Nobel prize for medicine or physiology in 1929 for his discovery of the growth-stimulating vitamins.

**Hop·lop·syl·lus anom·a·lus** (hop″lo-sil'əs ə-nom'ə-ləs) a species of flea found in the ground squirrels of western United States and transmitting plague.

**Hop·pe-Sey·ler's test** (hawp″ə-si'lərz) [Ernst Felix Immanuel *Hoppe-Seyler,* German physiologic chemist, 1825–1895] see under *test.*

**Hor. decub.** abbreviation for L. *ho'ra decu'bitus,* at bedtime.

**hor·de·o·lum** (hor-de'o-ləm) [L. "barleycorn"] [MeSH: Hordeolum] a localized, purulent, inflammatory staphylococcal infection of one or more sebaceous glands (meibomian or zeisian) of the eyelids; called also *stye.*
**external h.,** one that occurs on the surface of the skin at the edge of the lid.
**internal h.,** one that is marked by swelling on the conjunctival surface of the lid.

**hore·hound** (hor'hound) 1. *Marrubium vulgare.* 2. the leaves and tops of *M. vulgare,* used as an expectorant, bitter tonic, vermifuge, and laxative.

**Hor. interm.** abbreviation for L. *ho'ris interme'diis,* at the intermediate hours.

**ho·ri·zon** (hor-i'zon) a numbered stage of human embryonic development defined by anatomical characteristics in order to circumvent individual uncertainties of age and variations of dimension from both natural and technical causes. Streeter outlined 23 horizons, each spanning 2 or 3 days, covering the 7-week period beginning with fertilization.
**Streeter's h's,** see *horizon.*

**hor·i·zon·tal** (hor″ĭ-zon'təl) 1. parallel to the plane of the horizon; see also *horizontalis.* 2. spreading from one individual to another; see under *transmission.*

**hor·i·zon·ta·lis** (hor″ĭ-zon-ta'lis) [TA] horizontal: a term denoting relationship to this orientation when the body is in the anatomical, i.e., the upright, position.

**hor·me·sis** (hor-me'sis) [Gr. *hormēsis* rapid motion] the stimulating effect of subinhibitory concentrations of any toxic substance on any organism.

**hor·mi·on** (hor'me-on) [Gr. *hormos* a wreath] the median anterior point of the spheno-occipital bones.

**Hor·mo·car·di·ol** (hor″mo-kahr'de-ol) [*hormone* + Gr. *kardia* heart] a commercial preparation of an extract from the sinus of the frog's heart that stimulates the contraction of the frog's ventricle; used as a coronary vasodilator.

**Hor·mo·den·drum** (hor″mo-den'drəm) a former genus of Fungi Imperfecti; many saprobic species have been placed in the genus *Cladosporium,* and human pathogens in *Fonsecaea. H. pedrosoi* is now called *F. pedrosoi.*

**hor·mon·a·gogue** (hor-mōn'ə-gog) [*hormone* + *-agogue*] an agent that stimulates the production of hormones.

**hor·mo·nal** (hor-mo'nəl) pertaining to or of the nature of a hormone; called also *endocrine.*

**hor·mone** (hor'mōn) [Gr. *hormaein* to set in motion, spur on] a chemical substance produced in the body by an organ, cells of an organ, or scattered cells, having a specific regulatory effect on the activity of an organ or organs. The term was originally applied to substances secreted by endocrine glands and transported in the bloodstream to distant target organs, but later it was applied to various substances having similar actions but not produced by special glands. See also *endocrine system,* under *system.*

## Hormone

**adaptive h.,** one secreted during the organism's adaptation to unusual circumstances, which contributes to the ability to cope; examples include the corticosteroids and adrenocorticotropic hormone.
**adenohypophysial h's,** anterior pituitary h's.
**adipokinetic h.,** 1. former name for $\beta$-lipotropin. 2. (in plural) lipolytic h's.
**adrenocortical h.,** 1. any of the corticosteroids elaborated by the adrenal cortex, the major ones being the glucocorticoids and mineralocorticoids, and including some androgens, progesterone, and perhaps estrogens. See also *corticosteroid.* 2. corticosteroid.
**adrenocorticotropic h. (ACTH),** a 39–amino-acid peptide hormone secreted by the adenohypophysis, one of the derivatives of pro-opiomelanocortin; it acts primarily on the adrenal cortex, stimulating its growth and the secretion of corticosteroids. Its production is increased during times of stress. Called also *adrenocorticotropin, adrenocorticotrophin, adrenotropin, adrenotrophin, corticotropin,* and *corticotrophin.*
**adrenomedullary h's,** substances secreted by the adrenal medulla, such as epinephrine and norepinephrine.
**androgenic h.,** androgen.
**anterior pituitary h's,** the hormones secreted by the adenohypophysis (anterior pituitary), including growth hormone, thyrotropin, prolactin, follicle-stimulating hormone, luteinizing hormone, $\beta$-lipotropin, and adrenocorticotropic hormone. Called also *adenohypophysial h's.*
**antidiuretic h.,** vasopressin.
**antimüllerian h.,** a glycoprotein produced by Sertoli's cells of the fetal testis that acts ipsilaterally in the male to suppress the müllerian ducts, consequently preventing development of the uterus and uterine tubes, thus influencing control of the formation of the male phenotype. Called also *müllerian inhibiting factor* or *substance, müllerian duct inhibitory factor,* and *müllerian regression factor.*
**chromaffin h.,** a hormone released from chromaffin cells; epinephrine is a major type.
**conjugated estrogen h's,** an amorphous preparation of naturally occurring, water-soluble, conjugated forms of mixed estrogens, chiefly sodium estrone sulfate, extracted from the urine of pregnant mares; used in estrogen hormone therapy.
**corpus luteum h.,** progesterone.
**cortical h.,** corticosteroid.
**corticotropin-releasing h. (CRH),** a neuropeptide elaborated by the median eminence of the hypothalamus, the pancreas, and the brain; it binds to specific receptors on the corticotrophs of the adenohypophysis and stimulates production of adrenocorticotropic hormone (corticotropin).
**diabetogenic h.,** a hormone such as hydrocortisone that causes gluconeogenesis. Called also *diabetogenic factor.*
**ectopic h.,** a hormone released from a neoplasm or cells outside the usual source of the hormone. Such hormones may be useful as tumor markers. Cf. *eutopic h.*
**estrogenic h.,** estrogen.
**eutopic h.,** a peptide hormone released from its usual site or from a neoplasm of that tissue; cf. *ectopic h.*
**fat-mobilizing h's,** lipolytic h's.
**fibroblast growth h.,** a peptide hormone secreted by the adenohypophysis, affecting many of the same cell types as platelet-derived growth factor; it is a potent mitogen of vascular endothelial cells and is a regulator of tissue vascularization.
**follicle-stimulating h. (FSH),** one of the gonadotropic hormones of the adenohypophysis, a glycopeptide of approximately 30,000 daltons that stimulates the growth and maturation of ovarian follicles, stimulates estrogen secretion, promotes the endometrial changes characteristic of the first portion (proliferative phase) of the mammalian menstrual cycle, and stimulates spermatogenesis in the male. See also *menotropins.* Called also *follitropin.*
**follicle-stimulating h., human,** 1. follicle-stimulating h. 2. menotropins.
**follicle-stimulating h.–releasing h. (FSH-RH),** luteinizing hormone–releasing h.
**galactopoietic h.,** prolactin.
**gastrointestinal h's,** hormones that originate in and regulate motor and secretory activity of the digestive organs, such as gastrin, secretin, and cholecystokinin.
**gonadotropic h.,** gonadotropin.
**gonadotropin-releasing h. (Gn-RH),** 1. luteinizing hormone–releasing h. 2. more generally, any hypothalamic factor that stimulates the release of both follicle-stimulating hormone and luteinizing hormone.
**growth h. (GH),** 1. any of several related hormones secreted epi-

sodically by the adenohypophysis that affect protein, carbohydrate, and lipid metabolism and control the rate of skeletal and visceral growth; their secretion is in part controlled by the hypothalamus. The major form of human growth hormone (hGH) is a single chain of 191 amino acids (about 21,500 daltons). Called also *somatotrophin, somatotropin,* and *somatotrophic* or *somatotropic h.* 2. hGHr; a preparation manufactured by recombinant technology, used to treat growth failure (dwarfism) in children with congenital deficiency of growth hormone. 3. any substance that stimulates growth, such as a growth factor (q.v.).

**growth hormone release–inhibiting h.,** somatostatin.

**growth hormone–releasing h. (GH-RH),** a neuropeptide elaborated in the hypothalamus that binds to specific receptors on the somatotrophs of the adenohypophysis and stimulates the secretion of growth hormone. Called also *somatocrinin, somatoliberin,* and *somatotropin-releasing h.*

**human growth h. (hGH), human pituitary growth h.,** see *growth h.*

**hypophysiotropic h's,** hormones produced by the hypothalamus, usually releasing hormones, which maintain the endocrine functions of cells of the adenohypophysis.

**inhibiting h's,** hormones elaborated by one structure that inhibit release of hormones from another structure, such as those from the hypothalamus that act on the adenohypophysis. Examples include folliculostatin, prolactin-inhibiting hormone (prolactostatin), and somatostatin. The term is applied to substances of established clinical identity, whereas substances of unknown chemical structure are called *inhibiting factors* (see under *factor*).

**interstitial cell–stimulating h.,** luteinizing h.

**juvenile h.,** the secretion of the corpora allata which prevents metamorphosis, keeping the insect in the larval state and ensuring that the larva will molt several times and reach large size before pupating.

**lactation h., lactogenic h.,** prolactin.

**lipolytic h's,** hormones that promote the degradation of triacylglycerols to diacylglycerols, monoacylglycerols, glycerols, and fatty acids; they include the catecholamines, glucagon, growth hormone, and (in high levels only) adrenocorticotropic hormone and thyroid-stimulating hormone. Called also *fat-mobilizing h's.*

**lipotropic h. (LPH),** lipotropin.

**local h.,** a substance with hormonelike properties that acts at an anatomically restricted site; most are rapidly degraded. Examples are histamine, serotonin, angiotensin, and the prostaglandins. Called also *autacoid* and *autocoid.*

**luteal h.,** progesterone.

**luteinizing h. (LH),** a glycoprotein gonadotropin (28,000 daltons) of the adenohypophysis that acts with follicle-stimulating hormone to promote ovulation as well as secretion of androgens and progesterone. It instigates and maintains the second (secretory) portion of the mammalian estrus and menstrual cycle. In females it is concerned with corpus luteum formation and in males it stimulates the development and functional activity of testicular Leydig's cells. Called also *interstitial cell–stimulating h.* and *lutropin.*

**luteinizing hormone–releasing h.,** 1. a decapeptide hormone elaborated by the median eminence of the hypothalamus that binds to specific receptor sites on gonadotrophs of the adenohypophysis and stimulates the release of follicle-stimulating hormone and luteinizing hormone. High levels continuously maintained desensitize gonadotrophs and terminate gonadotropin release. Long-acting analogs are used to inhibit gonadal steroid secretion in individuals with prostate cancer and some other hormone-responsive cancers. Called also *follicle-stimulating hormone–releasing h., gonadotropin-releasing h., gonadoliberin,* and *luliberin.* 2. a preparation of the acetate and hydrochloride salts of this hormone obtained from the brains of certain food animals, used in the differential diagnosis of hypothalamic, pituitary, and gonadal dysfunction and sometimes in treatment of types of male or female infertility or hypogonadism.

**luteotropic h.,** prolactin.

**melanocyte-stimulating h., melanophore-stimulating h. (MSH),** a melanotropic peptide secreted by the pituitary glands of certain other animals but not humans; it is derived from pro-opiomelanocortin. Types are designated $\alpha$, $\beta$, and $\gamma_1$ to $\gamma_3$; $\alpha$-MSH and $\beta$-MSH are released by the pars intermedia of the adenohypophysis in fish and amphibians. The acylated forms cause dispersion of pigment granules of melanocytes, producing a rapid change in skin coloration, while the nonacylated forms are neurotransmitters. $\alpha$-MSH is identical to the N-terminal 13 residues of adrenocorticotropic hormone, and $\beta$-MSH to the C-terminal 18 residues of $\gamma$-lipotropin. Immunoreactive "$\beta$-MSH" in humans consists of $\beta$- and $\gamma$-lipotropin. Administration of $\alpha$-MSH or elevation of adrenocorticotropic hormone in humans causes a slight increase in melanization. Called also *intermedin* and *melanotropin.*

**neurohypophysial h's,** posterior pituitary h's.

**ovarian h's,** those secreted by the ovary, such as estrogens and progestational agents.

**parathyroid h.,** a polypeptide hormone (84 amino acid residues) secreted by the parathyroid glands. It promotes release of calcium from bone to extracellular fluid by activating osteoclasts and inhibiting osteoblasts, indirectly promotes increased intestinal absorption of calcium, promotes renal tubular reabsorption of calcium and increased renal excretion of phosphates, and is a major regulator of bone metabolism. Secretion of parathyroid hormone increases when the level of calcium in the extracellular fluid is low. Its action is opposed by that of calcitonin. Called also *parathormone* and *parathyrin.*

**placental h's,** those produced by the placenta during pregnancy, including chorionic gonadotropin and certain other substances having estrogenic, progestational, or adrenocorticoid activity.

**placental growth h.,** human placental lactogen.

**plant h.,** phytohormone.

**posterior pituitary h's,** the hormones released from the neurohypophysis (posterior pituitary), which are formed in the neuronal cells of the hypothalamic nuclei and stored in nerve cell endings in the neurohypophysis. The principal ones are vasopressin and oxytocin. Called also *neurohypophysial h's.*

**progestational h.,** 1. progesterone. 2. see under *agent.*

**prolactin-inhibiting h.,** a hormone released by the hypothalamus that inhibits the secretion of prolactin by the anterior pituitary. Called also *prolactin-inhibiting factor* and *prolactostatin.*

**prolactin-releasing h.,** any of various hormones elaborated by the hypothalamus that stimulate the release of prolactin by the anterior pituitary. Most such activity is exerted by vasoactive intestinal peptide, although in humans thyrotropin-releasing h. can also have this action. Called also *prolactin-releasing factor* and *prolactoliberin.*

**proparathyroid h.,** an inactive biosynthetic precursor of parathyroid hormone; it is of larger molecular size than the active hormone.

**prothoracicotropic h.,** in the development of insects, the hormone that controls secretion of ecdysone by the prothoracic glands. It is secreted by a gland in the brain.

**releasing h's,** hormones elaborated in one structure that cause the release of hormones from another structure, such as those from the hypothalamus that act on the adenohypophysis. The term is applied to substances of established chemical identity, whereas substances of unknown chemical structure are called *releasing factors* (see under *factor*).

**sex h's,** the estrogens and androgens considered together.

**sex h., female,** estrogen.

**sex h., male,** androgen.

**somatotrophic h., somatotropic h.,** growth h.

**somatotropin release–inhibiting h.,** somatostatin.

**somatotropin-releasing h. (SRH),** growth hormone–releasing h.

**steroid h's,** hormones that are biologically active steroids; they are secreted by the adrenal cortex, testis, ovary, and placenta and include the progestogens, glucocorticoids, mineralocorticoids, androgens, and estrogens. They act by binding to specific receptors to form complexes, which then enhance or inhibit the expression of specific genes.

**testicular h., testis h.,** testosterone.

**thyroid h's,** the hormones produced by the thyroid gland, thyroxine, triiodothyronine, and calcitonin.

**thyroid-stimulating h. (TSH), thyrotropic h.,** thyrotropin.

**thyrotropin-releasing h. (TRH),** 1. a tripeptide hormone, elaborated by the median eminence of the hypothalamus, which stimulates release of thyrotropin from the adenohypophysis. In human subjects, it can also promote a prolactin-releasing factor. Called also *thyroliberin.* 2. a synthetic preparation of the hormone, used in diagnosis of mild hyperthyroidism and Graves' disease, and in differentiating among primary, secondary, and tertiary hypothyroidism. Called also *protirelin.*

**hor·mon·ic** (hor-mon'ik) hormonal.

**hor·mon·o·gen** (hor'mon-o-jen") prohormone.

**hor·mo·no·gen·e·sis** (hor-mo"no-jen'ə-sis) the production of hormones; called also *hormonopoiesis.*

**hor·mo·no·gen·ic** (hor-mo"no-jen'ik) pertaining to, characterized by, or stimulating hormonogenesis; called also *hormonopoietic.*

**hor·mo·nol·o·gy** (hor"mo-nol'ə-je) the study of hormones; see endocrinology.

**hor·mo·no·poi·e·sis** (hor-mo″no-poi-e′sis) [*hormone* + *-poiesis*] hormonogenesis.

**hor·mo·no·poi·et·ic** (hor-mo″no-poi-et′ik) hormonogenic.

**hor·mo·no·priv·ia** (hor-mo″no-priv′e-ə) [*hormone* + L. *privus* deprived of] a hormone deficiency.

**hor·mo·no·sis** (hor-mo-no′sis) a condition caused by excessive quantities of one or more hormones; cf. *endocrinopathy*.
**exogenous h.,** hormonosis caused by administration of pharmacologic amounts of a hormone as in cortisone therapy.

**hor·mo·no·ther·a·py** (hor-mo″no-ther′ə-pe) endocrine therapy.

**Horn's sign** (hornz) [C. ten *Horn*, Dutch surgeon, early 20th century] see under *sign*.

**horn** (horn) [L. *cornu*] [MeSH: Horns] 1. a pointed projection, often paired,, found on the heads of various animals. 2. any structure resembling the horn of an animal. Called also *cornu* [TA].
**h. of Ammon,** hippocampus.
**anterior h. of lateral ventricle,** cornu frontale ventriculi lateralis.
**anterior h. of spinal cord,** cornu anterius medullae spinalis.
**cicatricial h.,** a hard, dry outgrowth from a cicatrix, commonly scaly and very rarely osseous.
**coccygeal h.,** cornu coccygeum.
**cutaneous h.,** a horny excrescence of the skin, chiefly seen on the scalp and face; they often overlie premalignant keratoses or squamous or basal cell carcinomas.
**dorsal h. of spinal cord,** cornu posterius medullae spinalis.
**frontal h. of lateral ventricle,** cornu frontale ventriculi lateralis.
**gray h's of spinal cord,** see *columnae griseae*.
**greater h. of hyoid bone,** cornu majus ossis hyoidei.
**inferior h. of falciform margin,** cornu inferius marginis falciformis.
**inferior h. of lateral ventricle,** cornu temporale ventriculi lateralis.
**inferior h. of thyroid cartilage,** cornu inferius cartilaginis thyroideae.
**lateral h. of spinal cord,** cornu laterale medullae spinalis.
**lesser h. of hyoid bone,** cornu minus ossis hyoidei.
**occipital h. of lateral ventricle, posterior h. of lateral ventricle,** cornu occipitale ventriculi lateralis.
**posterior h. of spinal cord,** cornu posterius medullae spinalis.
**h. of pulp,** an extension of the pulp into an accentuation of the roof of the pulp chamber directly under a cusp or a developmental lobe of the tooth.

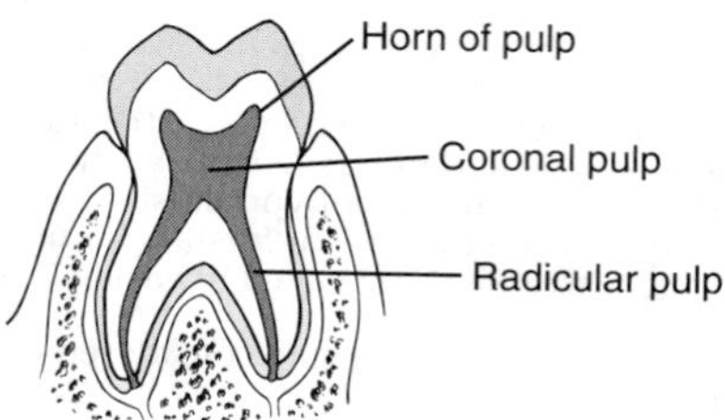


**sacral h.,** cornu sacrale.
**superior h. of falciform margin,** cornu superius marginis falciformis.
**superior h. of thyroid cartilage,** cornu superius cartilaginis thyroideae.
**temporal h. of lateral ventricle,** cornu temporale ventriculi lateralis.
**h. of uterus,** cornu uteri.
**ventral h. of spinal cord,** cornu anterius medullae spinalis.

**Hor·ner's law, syndrome (ptosis)** (hor′nərz) [Johann Friedrich *Horner*, Swiss ophthalmologist, 1831–1886] see under *law* and *syndrome*.

**Hor·ner's muscle** (hor′nərz) [William Edmonds *Horner*, American anatomist, 1793–1853] pars lacrimalis musculi orbicularis oculi.

**Horn·er's sign** (hor′nerz) [David Alfred *Horner*, American obstetrician and gynecologist born 1884] Spalding's sign; see under *sign*.

**hor·net** (hor′nət) [MeSH: Wasps] any of various wasps of the genera *Vespa* and *Vespula* that build papery nests.

**horn·i·fi·ca·tion** (hor″nĭ-fĭ-ka′shən) cornification.

**horny** (hor′ne) having the nature and appearance of horn.

**ho·rop·ter** (ho-rop′tər) [Gr. *horos* limit + *optēr* observer] the sum of all the spatial points whose images at a given distance fall on corresponding points of the retina. If the point of fixation is 2 meters, the horopter is a straight line across the observer's front (the *apparent frontoparallel plane h.*); if the point of fixation is less than 2 meters, the horopter is a curve concave to the observer *(concave h.)*; and if the point of fixation is more than 2 meters, the horopter is a curve convex to the observer *(convex h.)*.
**Vieth-Müller h.,** a circle which joins the fixation point with the nodal points of the two eyes; called also *Vieth-Müller circle*.

**hor·op·ter·ic** (hor″op-ter′ik) pertaining to a horopter.

**hor·rip·i·la·tion** (hor″ĭ-pĭ-la′shən) [L. *horrere* to bristle, to stand on end + *pilus* hair] erection of the fine hairs of the skin, as in cutis anserina.

**hor·ror** (hor′ər) [L.] dread; terror.
**h. autotox′icus,** [L. "fear of self poisoning"], a term coined by Ehrlich and Morgenroth in 1900 to express the refusal of a normal animal to form autoantibodies; it was believed that formation of such antibodies might result in self-destruction of the antibody producer as a result of the reaction between autoantibody and the corresponding antigen present in tissues. Now called *self tolerance*.

**horse·fly** (hōrs′fli) tabanid.

**horse·pox** (hors′poks) a mild form of poxvirus infection in horses, marked by a pustular eruption of the skin and sometimes of the oral and nasal mucosa.
**Canadian h.,** contagious acne of horses.

**horse·rad·ish** (hōrs′rad-ish) 1. *Armoracia lapathifolia*. 2. any of several other plants of the family Cruciferae resembling *A. lapathifolia*. 3. the pungent root of one of these plants, used as a condiment and appetite stimulant; in the past it was used as a rubefacient and plaster like mustard, because it contains sinigrin.

**horse·rad·ish per·ox·i·dase** (hors′rad-ish pər-ok′sĭ-dās″) [MeSH: Horseradish Peroxidase] peroxidase isolated from horseradish *(Armoracia lapathifolia)*; used as a reagent in biochemical assays. Abbreviated HRP.

**Hors·ley's operation, sign, wax** (hors′lēz) [Sir Victor Alexander Haden *Horsley*, English surgeon, 1857–1916] see under *operation, sign*, and *wax*.

**Hor·te·ga cell, method** (or-ta′gə) [Pío del Río *Hortega*, Spanish histologist in Argentina, 1882–1945] see *microglia* and see under *stain*.

**hor·to·be·zoar** (hor″to-be-zor′) phytobezoar.

**Hor·ton's arteritis (disease, syndrome), headache** (hor′tənz) [Bayard Taylor *Horton*, American physician, 1895–1980] see *giant cell arteritis*, under *arteritis*, and see *cluster headache* under *headache*.

**Hor. un. spatio** abbreviation for L. *ho′rae uni′us spa′tio*, at the end of one hour.

**Ho·sack·ia** (ho-sak′e-ə) [David *Hosack*, American biologist, 19th century] a genus of herbaceous plants found in the western United States, one of the groups called *locoweed*.

**hos·pice** (hos′pis) [MeSH: Hospices] a facility that provides palliative and supportive care for terminally ill patients and their families, either directly or on a consulting basis.

**hos·pi·tal** (hos′pĭ-təl) [L. *hospitalium*, from *hospes*, host, guest] [MeSH: Hospitals] an institution for the treatment of the sick. "An institution suitably located, constructed, organized, managed and personneled, to supply, scientifically, economically, efficiently and unhindered, all or any recognized part of the complex requirements for the prevention, diagnosis, and treatment of physical, mental, and the medical aspect of social ills; with functioning facilities for training new workers in the many special professional, technical and economic fields essential to the discharge of its proper functions; and with adequate contacts with physicians, other hospitals, medical schools and all accredited health agencies engaged in the better health program."—Council on Medical Education.
**base h.,** a hospital unit within the line of communication of a branch of the armed forces, usually in a permanent building, designed for the reception of wounded and other patients received via field hospitals from the battle front, and for cases originating within the line of communication itself.
**camp h.,** an immobile military unit organized and equipped for the care of the sick and wounded in camp in order to allow continued mobility of field hospitals or other mobile sanitary organizations.
**closed h., closed staff h.,** a hospital in which only members of the staff are permitted to treat patients.
**cottage h.,** a hospital consisting of a number of detached buildings.
**day h.,** see *partial hospitalization*, under *hospitalization*.
**evacuation h.,** a mobile advance hospital unit within the line of communication, designed to take over the functions of field hospitals when they move away with their divisions and to supplement base hospitals in their functions.
**field h.,** a portable military hospital, manned by noncommissioned officers and men, located beyond the zone of conflict, 3–4 miles beyond the dressing stations, designed to shelter and care for wounded brought in by ambulance companies until they can be transported to the line of communications.

**lying-in h., maternity h.**, an institution for the care of obstetric patients.
**night h.**, see *partial hospitalization*, under *hospitalization*.
**open h.**, 1. a mental hospital, or section of a hospital, without locked doors or other forms of physical restraint. 2. a hospital to which physicians who are not staff members may send their own patients and supervise their treatment.
**teaching h.**, one that allocates a substantial part of its resources to conduct, in its own name or in association with a college or university, formal educational programs or courses of instruction that lead to granting of recognized certificates, diplomas, degrees, or other documents required for professional certification or licensure.
**voluntary h.**, a private, not-for-profit hospital; one of the major purposes of voluntary hospitals is the provision of uncompensated care to the poor.
**weekend h.**, see *partial hospitalization*, under *hospitalization*.

**hos·pi·tal·ist** (hos'pĭ-təl-ist) a physician specializing in hospital inpatient care.

**hos·pi·tal·iza·tion** (hos"pĭ-təl-ĭ-za'shən) [MeSH: Hospitalization] the confinement of a patient in a hospital, or the period of such confinement.
**partial h.**, a psychiatric treatment program for patients who do not need full-time hospitalization, involving a special facility or an arrangement within a hospital setting to which the patient may come for treatment during the day and return home at night *(day hospital);* or return at night after a day in the community to receive treatment during the evening and to remain all night *(night hospital);* or return at the end of the week to receive treatment and remain all weekend, resuming his normal activities during the week *(weekend hospital).*

**hos·pi·tal·ize** (hos'pĭ-təl-īz) to place a patient in a hospital.

**host** (hōst) [L. *hospes*] 1. an animal or plant that harbors or nourishes another organism (parasite). 2. the recipient of an organ or tissue transplanted from another organism (the donor).
**accidental h.**, one that harbors an organism that is not ordinarily parasitic in the particular species.
**definitive h., final h.**, a host in which a parasite attains sexual maturity; called also *primary h.*
**intermediate h.**, a host in which a parasite passes one or more of its asexual (larval) stages; usually designated first and second, if there is more than one.
**paratenic h.**, a potential or substitute intermediate host that serves until the appropriate definitive host is reached, and in which no development of the parasite occurs; it may or may not be necessary to the completion of the parasite's life cycle. Called also *transfer h.* and *transport h.*
**h. of predilection**, the host preferred by a parasite.
**primary h.**, definitive h.
**reservoir h.**, reservoir, def. 3.
**secondary h.**, intermediate h.
**transfer h., transport h.**, paratenic h.

**hot** (hot) 1. characterized by high temperature. 2. radioactive; particularly used to denote the presence of significantly or dangerously high levels of radioactivity.

**hot line** (hot līn) telephone assistance for those in need of crisis intervention (q.v.), as in suicide prevention, usually available 24 hours a day, seven days a week, and staffed by nonprofessionals with mental health professionals serving as advisors or in a backup capacity.

**Houns·field** (hounz'fēld) Sir Godfrey Newbold. British research scientist, born 1919; co-winner, with Allan MacLeod Cormack, of the Nobel prize for medicine or physiology in 1979 for their development of computerized axial tomography.

**Houns·field unit** (hounz'fēld) [Sir G. N. *Hounsfield*] see under *unit*.

**Hous·say** (o-si') Bernardo Alberto. Argentine physiologist, 1887–1971; co-winner, with Carl Ferdinand Cori and Gerty Theresa Cori, of the Nobel prize for medicine or physiology in 1947 for his demonstrations that a hormone secreted by the pituitary gland prevents metabolism of sugar and that injections of pituitary extract induce diabetes symptoms.

**Hous·say animal, phenomenon** (o-si') [B. A. *Houssay*] see under *animal* and *phenomenon*.

**Hous·ton's muscle, valve** (hu'stonz) [John *Houston*, Irish surgeon, 1802–1845] see under *muscle* and see *plicae transversae recti*, under *plica*.

**ho·ven** (ho'vən) tympany of the stomach.

**Hov·er·bed** (hov'ər-bed) trademark for a bed used for burn victims in which the entire body of the victim is supported on a stream of warm sterile air flowing upward through openings along the length of the bed.

**Ho·vi·us' canal, circle, plexus** (ho've-əs) [Jacobus *Hovius*, Dutch ophthalmologist, born 1675] see under *canal, circle*, and *plexus*.

**How·el-Ev·ans' syndrome** (hov'əl-ev'ənz) [W. *Howel-Evans*, British physician, 20th century] see under *syndrome*.

**How·ell's bodies** (hou'əlz) [William Henry *Howell*, American physiologist, 1860–1945] see under *body*.

**How·ell-Jol·ly bodies** (hou'el-zho-le') [W. H. *Howell;* Justin Marie Jules *Jolly*, French histologist, 1870–1953] see under *body*.

**How·ship's lacuna** (hou'ships) [John *Howship*, English surgeon, 1781–1841] see *absorption lacuna*, under *lacuna*.

**How·ship-Rom·berg sign** (hou'ship-rom'berg) [J. *Howship;* Moritz Heinrich von *Romberg*, German neurologist, 1795–1873] see under *sign*.

**Hoyne's sign** (hoinz) [Archibald Lawrence *Hoyne*, American pediatrician, 1878–1963] see under *sign*.

**HP** house physician.

**Hp** haptoglobin.

**HPETE** hydroperoxyeicosatetraenoic acid.

**HPF** high-power field.

**HPL, hPL** human placental lactogen.

**HPLC** high-performance liquid chromatography.

**HPRT** hypoxanthine phosphoribosyltransferase.

**HPV** human papillomavirus.

**HRA** high right atrium.

**HRCT** high-resolution computed tomography.

**HRF** histamine-releasing factor; homologous restriction factor.

**HRIG** human rabies immune globulin.

**HRP** horseradish peroxidase.

**HRSA** Health Resources and Services Administration, an agency of the United States Public Health Service.

**HS** house surgeon.

**h.s.** abbreviation for L. *ho'ra som'ni*, at bedtime.

**HSA** human serum albumin.

**HSAN** hereditary sensory and autonomic neuropathy.

**HSAN-I** hereditary sensory and autonomic neuropathy (type I); see *hereditary sensory radicular neuropathy*, under *neuropathy*.

**HSAN-II** hereditary sensory and autonomic neuropathy (type II); see *hereditary sensory radicular neuropathy*, under *neuropathy*.

**HSAN-III** hereditary sensory and autonomic neuropathy (type III); see *dysautonomia*.

**HSF** hydrazine-sensitive factor, former name for alternative pathway complement factor *C3;* see under *complement*.

**HSR** homogeneously staining regions.

**HSV** herpes simplex virus.

**5-HT** 5-hydroxytryptamine (serotonin).

**Ht** symbol for *total hyperopia*.

**HTACS** human thyroid adenylate cyclase stimulators.

**HTC** homozygous typing cells.

**$^3$H-TdR** tritium-labeled thymidine.

**HTLV-1** human T-lymphotropic virus 1.

**HTLV-2** human T-lymphotropic virus 2.

**HTLV-III** human T-cell lymphotropic virus type III; see *human immunodeficiency virus*, under *virus*.

**$H^+$-trans·port·ing ATP syn·thase** (trans-port'ing sin'thās) [EC 3.6.1.34] an enzyme complex of the mitochondrial membrane that catalyzes the phosphorylation of ADP to form ATP. The energy for the synthesis of ATP is produced at three sites in the electron transport chain (see illustration at *chain*) and oxidative phosphorylation and electron transport are coupled via translocation of protons across the mitochondrial membrane. When removed from the membrane, the enzyme acts as an ATPase. Called also *ATP synthase*, *$H^+$-ATPase*, and *mitochondrial ATPase*.

**Hua** (hu'ə) a genus of fresh water snails of the family Thiaridae.
**H. ningpoen'sis**, a species of central and southern China that ingests eggs of the liver fluke *Opisthorchis sinensis*, which then hatch in its body.
**H. touchea'na**, a first intermediate host of the lung fluke *Paragonimus westermani*.

**Hubbard tank** (hub'ərd) [Carl *Hubbard*, American engineer, 20th century] see under *tank*.

**Hu·bel** (hu'bəl) David Hunter. Canadian-born American neurobiologist, born 1926; co-winner, with Tolsten Nils Wiesel and Roger Wolcott Sperry, of the Nobel prize for medicine or physiology for 1981 for their research on information processing in the visual system.

**Hu·chard's disease, sign (symptom)** (u-shahrz') [Henri *Huchard,* French physician, 1844–1910] see under *disease.*

**Hueck's ligament** (hēks) [Alexander Friedrich *Hueck,* German anatomist, 1802–1842] reticulum trabeculare anguli iridocornealis.

**Hue·ter's line, maneuver, sign** (he'tərz) [Karl *Hueter,* German surgeon, 1838–1882] see under *line, maneuver,* and *sign.*

**Hug·gins** (hug'inz) Charles Brenton. Canadian-born American surgeon, born 1901; co-winner, with Francis Peyton Rous, of the Nobel prize for medicine or physiology in 1966 for his discoveries in hormonal treatment of cancer of the prostate.

**Hug·gins operation** (hug'inz) [Charles Brenton *Huggins*] see under *operation.*

**Hughes' reflex** (hūz) [Charles Hamilton *Hughes,* American neurologist, 1839–1916] virile reflex (def. 2).

**Hughes-Sto·vin syndrome** (hūz-sto'vin) [John Patterson *Hughes,* British physician, 20th century; Peter George Ingle *Stovin,* British physician, 20th century] see under *syndrome.*

**Hugh·ston's projection** (hu'stənz) [J.C. *Hughston,* American radiologist, 20th century] see under *projection.*

**Hu·guier's canal, circle, sinus** (u-ge-āz') [Pierre Charles *Huguier,* French surgeon, 1804–1873] see under *circle* and *sinus* and see *iter chordae anterius.*

**Huh·ner test** (hōōn'ər) [Max *Huhner,* New York urologist, 1873–1947] see under *test.*

**HuIFN** human interferon.

**hum** (hum) an indistinct, low, prolonged sound.
**venous h.,** a continuous blowing, singing, or humming murmur heard on auscultation over the right jugular vein in the sitting or erect position; it is an innocent sign that is obliterated on assumption of the recumbent position or on exerting pressure over the vein. Called also *bruit de diable* and *humming-top murmur.*

**Hu·ma·log** (hu'mə-log) trademark for preparations of insulin lispro.

**Hu·ma·tin** (hu'mə-tin) trademark for preparations of paromomycin sulfate.

**hu·mec·tant** (hu-mek'tənt) [L. *humectus,* from *humectare* to be moist] 1. moistening. 2. a moistening or diluent substance.

**hu·mec·ta·tion** (hu″mək-ta'shən) the act of moistening.

**hu·mer·al** (hu'mər-əl) [L. *humeralis*] of or pertaining to the humerus.

**hu·meri** (hu'mər-i) [L.] genitive and plural of *humerus.*

**hu·mero·ra·di·al** (hu″mər-o-ra'de-əl) pertaining to the humerus and the radius.

**hu·mero·scap·u·lar** (hu″mər-o-skap'u-lər) pertaining to the humerus and the scapula.

**hu·mero·ul·nar** (hu″mər-o-ul'nər) pertaining to the humerus and the ulna.

**hu·mer·us** (hu'mər-əs) gen. and pl. *hu'meri* [L.] [TA] [MeSH: Humerus] the bone that extends from the shoulder to the elbow articulating proximally with the scapula and distally with the radius and ulna; see Plate 45.
**h. va'rus,** a bent humerus.

**hu·mid·i·fi·er** (hu-mid'ĭ-fi″ər) an apparatus for controlling humidity by adding moisture to the air of a room.

**hu·mid·i·ty** (hu-mid'ĭ-te) [L. *humiditas*] [MeSH: Humidity] the degree of moisture, especially of that in the air.
**absolute h.,** the actual amount of vapor in the atmosphere expressed in weight per unit volume.
**relative h.,** the percentage of moisture in the air as compared to the amount necessary to cause saturation, which is taken as 100.

**hu·mor** (hu'mər) pl. *humors, humo'res* [L. "a liquid"] 1. a fluid or semifluid substance; used in anatomical nomenclature to designate certain fluid materials in the body. 2. one of the four hypothetical fluids of humoralism.
**h. aquo'sus** [TA], aqueous humor: the fluid produced in the eye, occupying the anterior and posterior chambers, and diffusing out of the eye into the blood; regarded as the lymph of the eye, its composition varies from that of lymph in the body generally. Called also *aqueous* and *hydatoid.*
**h. cristalli'nus, crystalline h.,** 1. crystalline lens. 2. vitreous body.
**ocular h.,** one of the humors of the eye; see *h. aquosus* and *h. vitreus.*
**plasmoid h.,** aqueous or vitreous humor containing an abnormally high amount of protein; formed after trauma or inflammation, it has a cloudy appearance and the proteins tend to coalesce.

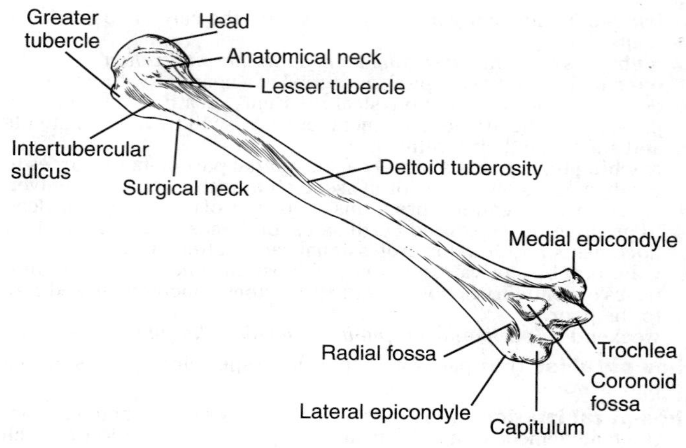

Anterior view of right humerus.

**vitreous h.,** 1. corpus vitreum. 2. h. vitreus.
**h. vi'treus** [TA], vitreous humor: the watery substance, resembling aqueous humor, contained within the interstices of the stroma in the vitreous body.

**hu·mor·al** (hu'mər-əl) 1. pertaining to elements dissolved in the blood or body fluids, e.g., humoral immunity from antibodies in the blood as opposed to cellular immunity. 2. pertaining to one of the humors of the body or to humoralism.

**hu·mor·al·ism** (hu'mər-əl-iz″əm) [MeSH: Humoralism] the ancient theory that health and illness result from a balance or imbalance of bodily liquids ("humors"). The theory is especially associated with Hippocratic writers, but it long antedates Hippocrates. Humoralism is a variant of Empedocles' theory of the four "roots" (earth, air, fire, water), later the four "elements," then the four qualities (hot, cold, moist, dry), then the four temperaments (cf. *temperament*). The four humors and the four qualities are (1) phlegm (water, or a watery substance), which is cold and moist; (2) blood, which is hot and moist; (3) black bile or gall, secreted from the kidneys and spleen, cold and dry; and (4) yellow bile or choler, secreted from the liver, hot and dry. Humoralism was decisively displaced only in 1858 by Rudolf Virchow's *Cellularpathologie.* Called also *humoral theory* and *humorism.*

**hu·mor·ism** (hu'mər-iz-əm) humoralism.

**Hu·mor·sol** (hu'mor-sol) trademark for a solution of demecarium bromide.

**hump** (hump) a rounded eminence.
**buffalo h.,** obesity confined to the neck, head, and trunk; seen in Cushing's syndrome. Called also *buffalo type.*
**dowager's h.,** popular name for dorsal kyphosis caused by multiple wedge fractures of the thoracic vertebrae seen in osteoporosis.
**Hampton's h.,** a homogeneous wedge-shaped density in the peripheral region of the lung, with a convex apex toward the hilum; seen on the radiograph after pulmonary infarction.

**hump·back** (hump'bak) kyphosis.

**Hum·phry's ligament** (hum'frēz) [Sir George Murray *Humphry,* English anatomist, 1820–1896] ligamenta meniscofemorale anterius.

**Hu·mu·lin** (hu'mu-lin) trademark for preparations of insulin human produced by recombinant DNA technology.

**hunch·back** (hunch'bak) 1. kyphosis. 2. an individual characterized by a rounded deformity of the back, or kyphosis.

**hun·ger** (hung'ər) [MeSH: Hunger] a craving, as for food.
**air h.,** Kussmaul's respiration.
**calcium h.,** a condition due to calcium defect, marked by severe headache during and after menstruation.

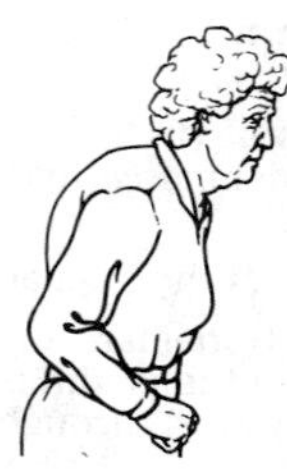
Dowager's hump.

**Hun·ner's ulcer** (hun'ərz) [Guy LeRoy *Hunner,* American surgeon, 1868–1957] see under *ulcer.*

**Hunt's atrophy, disease, phenomenon, syndrome** (huntz) [James Ramsay *Hunt,* American neurologist, 1872–1937] see under *atrophy* and *phenomenon;* see *dyssynergia cerebellaris myoclonica;* and see *Ramsay Hunt syndrome,* under *syndrome.*

**Hun·ter's canal, gubernaculum, operation** (hun'tərz) [John *Hunter,* Scottish anatomist and surgeon, 1728–1793] see *canalis adductorius* and *gubernaculum testis,* and see under *operation.*

**Hun·ter's glossitis** (hunt'ərz) [William *Hunter,* English physician, 1861–1937] see under *glossitis.*

**Hun·ter's ligament, line** (hunt'ərz) [William *Hunter,* Scottish anatomist, 1718–1783] see *ligamentum teres uteri* and *linea alba.*

**Hunter's syndrome** (hun'tərz) [Charles H. *Hunter,* Canadian physician, 1873–1955] see under *syndrome.*

**hun·ter·i·an** (hun-tēr'e-ən) named for or described by John Hunter, as hunterian chancre (hard chancre).

**Hun·ting·ton's chorea (disease), sign** (hunt'ing-tənz) [George Sumner *Huntington,* American physician, 1850–1916] see under *chorea* and *sign.*

**Hur·ler's syndrome (disease)** (hər'lərz) [Gertrud *Hurler,* Austrian pediatrician, 1889–1965] see under *syndrome.*

**Hurler-Scheie syndrome** (her'ler-sha) [G. *Hurler;* Harold G. *Scheie,* American ophthalmologist, 1909–1990] see under *syndrome.*

**Hürth·le cells, cell tumor** (hērt'lə) [Karl *Hürthle,* German histologist, 1860–1945] see *Askanazy cells,* under *cell,* and see under *tumor.*

**Husch·ke's foramen (canal), ligament,** etc. (hoosh'kəz) [Emil *Huschke,* German anatomist, 1797–1858] see under *foramen* and see *dentes acustici, plica gastropancreatica,* and *plica lacrimalis.*

**husk** (husk) hoose.

**Hutch·in·son's disease,** etc. (huch'in-sənz) [Sir Jonathan *Hutchinson,* English surgeon, 1828–1913] see under *disease, facies, mask, pupil, sign, tooth,* and *triad,* and see *salmon patch,* def. 1, under *patch.*

**Hutch·in·son-Gil·ford syndrome** (huch'in-sən-gil'ford) [Sir Jonathan *Hutchinson;* Hastings *Gilford,* English physician, 1861–1941] progeria.

**hutch·in·so·ni·an** (huch″in-so'ne-ən) named for or described by Sir Jonathan Hutchinson.

**Hutch·i·son syndrome** (huch'ĭ-sən) [Sir Robert *Hutchison,* English pediatrician, 1871–1960] see under *syndrome.*

**Hu-Tet** (hu'tet) trademark for a preparation of tetanus immune human globulin.

**Hu·tin·el's disease** (u-tin-elz') [Victor Henri *Hutinel,* pediatrician in Paris, 1849–1933] see under *disease.*

**Hux·ley** (huks'le) Andrew Fielding. British physiologist, born 1917; co-winner, with Sir John Carew Eccles and Alan Lloyd Hodgkin, of the Nobel prize for medicine or physiology for 1963, for discoveries concerning the ionic mechanism involved in excitation and inhibition in peripheral and central parts of the nerve cell membrane.

**Hux·ley's layer (membrane)** (huks'lēz) [Thomas Henry *Huxley,* English physiologist and naturalist, 1825–1895] see under *layer.*

**huy·gen·i·an** (hi-jen'e-ən) [Christiaan *Huygens* (or Huyghens), Dutch physicist, 1629–1695] see under *eyepiece.*

**HVA** homovanillic acid.

**HVL** half-value layer.

**hy·al** (hi'əl) hyoid.

**hy·a·lin** (hi'ə-lin) [Gr. *hyalos* glass] [MeSH: Hyalin] 1. a translucent albuminoid substance, one of the products of amyloid degeneration. 2. a substance composing the walls of hydatid cysts.

**hy·a·line** (hi'ə-lēn) [Gr. *hyalos* glass] glassy and transparent or nearly so; see also under *membrane.*

**hy·a·lin·iza·tion** (hi″ə-lin″ĭ-za'shən) conversion into a substance resembling glass.
**Crooke's h.,** degeneration of pituitary gland corticotrophs, with loss of specific granulation and progressive hyalinization, seen in the presence of elevated plasma corticosteroid levels of any cause. Called also *Crooke's* or *Crooke-Russell changes* and *Crooke's hyaline degeneration.*

**hy·a·li·no·sis** (hi″ə-lin-o'sis) hyaline degeneration.
**h. cu'tis et muco'sae,** lipoid proteinosis.

**hy·a·lin·u·ria** (hi″ə-lĭ-nu're-ə) the discharge of hyalin in the urine, usually in the form of casts composed of protein in an acid pH.

**hy·a·li·tis** (hi″ə-li'tis) [*hyal-* + *-itis* ] an inflammation of the hyaloid membrane of the eye or of the vitreous humor. Called also *hyaloiditis, vitritis,* and *vitreitis.*
**asteroid h.,** see under *hyalosis.*
**h. puncta'ta, punctate h.,** inflammation of the vitreous body marked by the formation of small opacities.
**h. suppurati'va, suppurative h.,** a purulent inflammation of the vitreous body.

**hyal(o)-** [Gr. *hyalos* glass] a combining form denoting a relationship to glass or to the vitreous body or vitreous humor, or denoting a resemblance to glass.

**hy·al·o·gen** (hi-al'o-jən) [*hyalo-* + *-gen*] an albuminous substance occurring in cartilage, the vitreous body, etc., and convertible into hyalin.

**hy·a·lo·hy·pho·my·co·sis** (hi″ə-lo-hi″fo-mi-ko'sis) [*hyalo-* + *hyphomycosis*] a hyphomycosis caused by mycelial fungi with colorless walls; most are opportunistic.

**hy·a·loid** (hi'ə-loid) [*hyal-* + *-oid*] resembling glass.

**hy·a·loid·itis** (hi″ə-loi-di'tis) hyalitis.

**hy·a·lo·mere** (hi'ə-lo-mēr″) [*hyalo-* + *-mere*] a zone of homogeneous or finely fibrillar pale blue cytoplasm surrounding the central granulomere of a platelet in a dry, stained blood smear.

**hy·a·lo·mit·ome** (hi″ə-lo-mit'ōm) hyaloplasm.

**Hy·a·lom·ma** (hi″ə-lom'ə) [*hyal-* + Gr. *omma* eye] a genus of ticks of the family Ixodidae. *H. anato'licum* is a cattle tick of Africa, India, and southern Europe, which may transmit hemorrhagic fever and a Middle Eastern variety of equine encephalomyelitis. *H. margina'tum* transmits Crimean-Congo hemorrhagic fever. *H. maurita'nicum* transmits *Theileria parva,* a protozoan parasite that causes many deaths in cattle in northern Africa. *H. trunca'tum* causes sweating sickness in African cattle.

**hy·a·lo·mu·coid** (hi″ə-lo-mu'koid) [*hyalo-* + *mucoid* (def. 1)] the mucoid of the vitreous body.

**hy·a·lo·nyx·is** (hi″ə-lo-nik'sis) [*hyalo-* + *nyxis*] the surgical puncturing of the vitreous body.

**hy·a·lo·pha·gia** (hi″ə-lo-fa'je-ə) [*hyalo-* + *-phagia*] the eating of glass.

**hy·a·loph·a·gy** (hi″ə-lof'ə-je) hyalophagia.

**hy·a·lo·plasm** (hi'ə-lo-plaz″əm) [*hyalo-* + *-plasm*] the more fluid, finely granular substance of the cytoplasm of cells; called also *paraplasm, interfilar mass, interfilar substance, interfibrillar substance of Flemming, paramitome, enchylema,* and *cytolymph.*
**nuclear h.,** karyolymph.

**hy·a·lo·se·ro·si·tis** (hi″ə-lo-se″ro-si'tis) [*hyalo-* + *serositis*] a form of inflammation of serous membranes marked by hyalinization of the serous exudate into a pearly investment of the organ concerned. Cf. *frosted heart* and *perihepatitis chronica hyperplastica.*
**progressive multiple h.,** Concato's disease.

**hy·a·lo·sis** (hi″ə-lo'sis) [*hyal-* + *-osis*] degenerative changes in the vitreous humor.
**asteroid h.,** a usually unilateral condition of the eye, most frequently seen in older men, characterized by the presence of spherical or star-shaped, calcium-containing opacities in the vitreous humor, which, when illuminated under an examining light, appear to sparkle; vision is usually unaffected. Called also *asteroid hyalitis* and *Benson's disease.*

**hy·al·o·some** (hi-al'o-sōm) [*hyalo-* + *-some*] a structure resembling the nucleolus of a cell, but staining only slightly.

**hy·al·o·tome** (hi-al'o-tōm) hyaloplasm.

**hy·al·uro·nate** (hi″ə-lo͞o'ro-nāt) a salt, anion, or ester of hyaluronic acid.

**hy·al·uron·ate ly·ase** (hi″ə-lo͞o-ron'āt li'ās) [EC 4.2.2.1] an enzyme of the lyase class that catalyzes the fragmentation of hyaluronic acid via an elimination reaction in which the bond from *N*-acetylglucosamine to glucuronate is broken and a double bond introduced into the latter. It is one of the enzymes called hyaluronidases; see also *hyaluronoglucosaminidase* and *hyaluronoglucuronidase.*

**hy·al·uron·ic ac·id** (hi″ə-lo͞o-ron'ik) [MeSH: Hyaluronic Acid] a glycosaminoglycan found in lubricating proteoglycans of synovial fluid, vitreous humor, cartilage, blood vessels, skin, and the umbilical cord. It is a linear chain of about 2500 repeating disaccharide units in specific linkage, each composed of an *N*-acetylglucosamine residue linked to one of glucuronic acid.

**hy·al·uron·i·dase** (hi″ə-lo͞o-ron'ĭ-dās) [MeSH: Hyaluronidase] 1. any of three enzymes (hyaluronate lyase, hyaluronoglucosaminidase, and hyaluronoglucuronidase) that catalyze the breakdown of hyaluronic acid. These enzymes are found in mammalian testicular and spleen tissue, in bee and snake venoms, and in certain species of *Clostridium, Staphylococcus,* and *Streptococcus.* Called also *Duran-Reynals factor, invasin,* and *diffusion* or *spreading factor.* 2. [USP] a preparation derived from mammalian testes and capable of hydrolyzing hyaluronic acid and similar glycosaminoglycans, used to aid absorption and dispersion of other injected drugs and fluids, for hypodermoclysis, and for improving resorption of radiopaque media; administered intramuscularly or subcutaneously.

**hy·al·urono·glu·co·sa·min·i·dase** (hi″ə-lo͞o-ron″o-gloo″kōs-ə-min′ĭ-dās) [EC 3.2.1.35] an enzyme of the hydrolase class that catalyzes the hydrolysis of random $\beta$-1,4 linkages between *N*-acetylglucosamine and D- glucuronic acid residues in hyaluronic acid. It also hydrolyzes chondroitin, chondroitin 4- and 6-sulfates, and dermatan sulfate. It is one of the enzymes called hyaluronidases; see also *hyaluronate lyase* and *hyaluronoglucuronidase.*

**hy·al·urono·glu·cu·ron·i·dase** (hi″ə-loo-ron″o-gloo″ku-ron′ĭ-dās) [EC 3.2.1.36] an enzyme of the hydrolase class that catalyzes the hydrolysis of $\beta$-1,3 linkages between glucuronic acid and *N*-acetylglucosamine residues in hyaluronic acid. It is one of the enzymes called hyaluronidases; see also *hyaluronate lyase* and *hyaluronoglucosaminidase.*

**Hy·ate:C** (hi′āt-se″) trademark for a preparation of antihemophilic factor (porcine).

**hy·bar·ox·ia** (hi″bar-ok′se-ə) inhalation therapy using hyperbaric oxygen, i.e., oxygen at pressures greater than 1 atmosphere.

**hy·ben·zate** (hi-ben′zāt) USAN contraction for *o*-(4-hydroxybenzoyl)benzoate.

**Hy·bo·mi·tra** (hi″bo-mi′trə) a genus of horse flies (family Tabanidae) that bite humans and other mammals in North America and can spread anaplasmosis, anthrax, equine infectious anemia, and tularemia.

**hy·brid** (hi′brid) [L. *hybrida* mongrel] [MeSH: Chimera] an animal or plant produced from parents different in kind, such as parents belonging to two different strains, varieties, or species.

**false h.,** an individual produced by a form of gynogenesis in which the foreign spermatozoon enters the ovum and activates it to cell division, but does not fuse with the egg nucleus.

**hy·brid·ism** (hi′brid-iz-əm) 1. the state of being a hybrid. 2. the production of hybrids.

**hy·brid·i·ty** (hi-brid′ĭ-te) the state of being a hybrid.

**hy·brid·iza·tion** (hi″brid-ĭ-za′shən) [MeSH: Hybridization] 1. the act or process of producing hybrids; called also *crossbreeding.* 2. molecular h. 3. somatic cell h. 4. in chemistry, a procedure whereby orbitals of intermediate energy and desired directional character are constructed by taking an appropriate linear combination of atomic orbitals, e.g., $sp^3$ hybrid orbitals are formed from one s and three p orbitals.

**colony h.,** a screening method for detecting the occurrence of a specific nucleic acid sequence in a heterogeneous population of bacterial colonies: a replica of a plate of colonies is prepared and all colonies are lysed with preservation of their relative positions; hybridization to the nucleic acid sequence of interest reveals the colonies carrying this sequence, and they can be retrieved from the master plate.

**dot blot h.,** see under *technique.*

**in situ h.,** molecular hybridization in which a known nucleic acid, single stranded and usually labeled with radioactivity or fluorescence, is applied to prepared cells or histologic sections and annealing occurs in situ; performed to analyze the intracellular or intrachromosomal distribution, transcription, or other characteristics of the nucleic acids.

**molecular h.,** in molecular biology, formation of a partially or wholly complementary nucleic acid duplex by association of single strands, usually between DNA and RNA strands or previously unassociated DNA strands, but also between RNA strands; used to detect and isolate specific sequences, measure homology, or define other characteristics of one or both strands.

**Northern blot h.,** see under *technique.*

**slot blot h.,** a variation on a dot blot hybridization with substitution of a slotted template for the usual one with circular holes; it increases sample capacity and maintains precision.

**somatic cell h.,** formation of a heterokaryon by fusion of two somatic cells, usually of different species.

**Southern blot h.,** see under *technique.*

**Southwestern blot h.,** see under *technique.*

**Western blot h.,** see under *technique.*

**hy·brid·o·ma** (hi″brid-o′mə) [*hybrid* + *-oma*] a somatic cell hybrid formed by fusion of normal lymphocytes and tumor cells; the resulting hybridoma cells will produce the same secretion as the normal parent cells and proliferate indefinitely in culture like the parent tumor cells.

**B cell h.,** a hybridoma formed by the fusion of antibody-secreting B lymphocytes and nonsecretory myeloma cells; used in the production of monoclonal antibodies.

**T cell h.,** a hybridoma formed by the fusion of T lymphocytes and myeloma cells, used particularly in the production of T lymphocyte–derived lymphokines.

**Hy·cam·tin** (hi-cam′tin) trademark for a preparation of topotecan hydrochloride.

**hy·can·thone mes·y·late** (hi-kan′thōn) an antischistosomal agent effective against *Schistosoma haematobium* and *S. mansoni.*

**hy·clate** (hi′klāt) USAN contraction for monohydrochloride hemiethanolate hemihydrate.

**Hy·co·dan** (hi′ko-dən) trademark for preparations of hydrocodone bitartrate.

**hy·dan·to·in** (hi-dan′to-in) 1. a crystalline base derivable from allantoin,

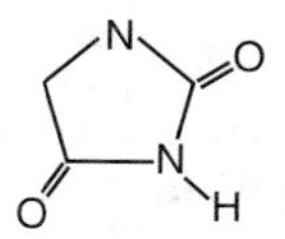

2. any of a group of anticonvulsants, including phenytoin, ethotoin, and methyphenytoin, containing such a ring structure.

**hy·dan·to·in·ate** (hi″dan-to′in-āt) any salt of hydantoin.

**hy·da·tid** (hi′də-tid) [L. *hydatis,* a drop of water] 1. a hydatid cyst. 2. any cystlike structure; see under *mole.*

**alveolar h's,** see *alveolar hydatid disease,* under *disease.*

**h. of Morgagni,** see *appendix testis* and *appendices vesiculosae epoophori.*

**sessile h.,** appendix testis.

**Virchow's h.,** alveolar hydatid disease.

**hy·da·tid·i·form** (hi″də-tid′ĭ-form) resembling a hydatid cyst; see under *mole.*

**hy·da·tid·o·sis** (hi″də-tĭ-do′sis) hydatid disease.

**hy·da·tid·os·to·my** (hi″də-tĭ-dos′tə-me) [*hydatid* + *-stomy*] incision and drainage of a hydatid cyst.

**hy·da·tid·uria** (hi″də-ti-du′re-ə) the excretion of hydatid material in the urine.

**Hy·da·tig·ena** (hi″də-tij′ə-nə) *Taenia.*

**hy·da·tism** (hi′də-tiz-əm) [Gr. *hydatis* water] the presence of fluid in a cavity.

**hy·da·toid** (hi′də-toid) [Gr. *hydōr* water + *-oid*] 1. the aqueous humor. 2. pertaining to the aqueous humor. 3. the hyaloid membrane (membrana vitrea [TA]).

**Hy·del·tra** (hi-del′trə) trademark for preparations of prednisolone.

**Hy·del·tra·sol** (hi-del′trə-sol) trademark for a preparation of prednisolone sodium phosphate.

**Hy·der·gine** (hi′dər-jēn) trademark for a mixture of equal parts of dihydroergocornine, dihydroergocristine, and dihydrocryptine, in the form of methansulfonate salts, used as a vasodilator for the treatment of peripheral vascular disease.

**hy·drad·e·ni·tis** (hi″drad-ə-ni′tis) hidradenitis.

**hy·drad·e·no·ma** (hi″drad-ə-no′mə) hidradenoma.

**hy·draero·peri·to·ne·um** (hi-drar″o-per″ĭ-to-ne′əm) [*hydr-* + *aero-* + *peritoneum*] a collection of watery fluid and gas in the peritoneal cavity.

**hy·dra·gogue** (hi′drə-gog) [*hydr-* + *-agogue*] 1. producing watery discharge, especially from the bowels. 2. a cathartic which causes watery purgation.

**hy·dral·a·zine** (hy-dral′ə-zēn) [MeSH: Hydralazine] a peripheral vasodilator used as an antihypertensive.

**h. hydrochloride** [USP], the monohydrochloride salt of hydralazine, used as an antihypertensive; administered orally, intramuscularly, or intravenously. It is also used in combination with nitrates, diuretics, or digitalis glycosides, or a combination of these, in the treatment of congestive heart failure.

**hy·dra·mine** (hi′drə-mēn) an amine derived from a glycol in which one hydroxyl is replaced by an amino group.

**hy·dram·ni·on** (hi-dram′ne-on) hydramnios.

**hy·dram·ni·os** (hi-dram′ne-os) [*hydr-* + *amnion*] excess of amniotic fluid.

**hy·dran·en·ceph·a·ly** (hi″dran-ən-sef′ə-le) [MeSH: Hydranencephaly] complete or almost complete absence of the cerebral hemispheres, the space they normally occupy being filled with cerebrospinal fluid.

**hy·drar·gy·rum** (hi-drahr′jə-rəm) gen. *hydrar′gyri* [L. "liquid silver"] mercury.

**hy·drar·thro·di·al** (hi″drahr-thro′de-əl) pertaining to hydrarthrosis.

**hy·drar·thro·sis** (hi″drahr-thro′sis) [*hydr-* + *arthro-* + *-osis*] [MeSH: Hydrarthrosis] an accumulation of watery fluid in the cavity of a joint.
**intermittent h.,** serous effusion into a joint occurring periodically.

**Hy·dras·tis** (hi-dras′tis) a genus of North American herbs of the family Ranunculaceae. *H. canaden′sis* L. is goldenseal, whose dried root contains berberine and is used as a folk remedy.

**hy·dra·tase** (hi′drə-tās) [EC 4.2.1] a term used in the recommended or trivial names of some enzymes of the sub-subclass hydro-lyase when the reaction equilibrium lies toward hydration.

**hy·drate** (hi′drāt) [L. *hydras*] 1. any compound of a radical with $H_2O$. 2. any salt or other compound that contains water of crystallization.

**hy·drat·ed** (hi′drāt-əd) [L. *hydratus*] combined with water; forming a hydrate or a hydroxide.

**hy·dra·tion** (hi-dra′shən) 1. the act of combining or causing to combine with water. 2. the condition of being combined with water.

**hy·drau·lics** (hi-draw′liks) [*hydr-* + Gr. *aulos* pipe] the branch of physics which treats of the action of liquids under physical laws.

**hy·dra·zine** (hi′drə-zēn) a toxic, irritant, carcinogenic, colorless, gaseous diamine, $H_2N·NH_2$; also any member of a group of its substitution derivatives.
**h. sulfate,** diamine, def. 2.

**hy·dra·zin·ol·y·sis** (hi″drə-zin-ol′ə-sis) cleavage of the peptide bonds of a peptide by hydrazine, with the C-terminal residue appearing as a free amino acid.

**hy·dra·zone** (hi′drə-zōn) a compound containing the group —NH·N:C—, formed from an aldehyde or ketone by the action of phenylhydrazine or other hydrazine.

**Hy·drea** (hi-dre′ə) trademark for a preparation of hydroxyurea.

**hy·dre·mia** (hi-dre′me-ə) [*hydr-* + Gr. *haima* blood] excessive dilution of the blood, so that the proportion of serum to corpuscles is excessive; seen in splenomegaly and other conditions. Called also *dilution anemia.*

**hy·dren·ceph·a·lo·cele** (hi″dren-sef′ə-lo-sēl″) hydroencephalocele.

**hy·dren·ceph·a·lo·me·nin·go·cele** (hi″drən-sef″ə-lo-mə-ning′o-sēl) hydroencephalocele.

**hy·dren·ceph·a·lus** (hi″drən-sef′ə-ləs) hydrocephalus.

**hy·dren·ceph·a·ly** (hi″drən-sef′ə-le) hydrocephalus.

**hy·drepi·gas·tri·um** (hi″drep-ĭ-gas′tre-əm) [*hydr-* + *epigastrium*] a collection of watery fluid between the peritoneum and the abdominal wall.

**Hy·drer·gine** (hi′drər-jēn) trademark for preparations of ergoloid mesylates.

**hy·dric** (hi′drik) pertaining to or combined with hydrogen; containing replaceable hydrogen.

**hy·dride** (hi′drīd) [Gr. *hydōr* water] any compound of hydrogen with an element or radical.

**hy·drin·di·cu·ria** (hi″drin-dĭ-ku′re-ə) the presence in the urine of indoles related to both tryptophan and phenylalanine.

**hy·dri·od·ic ac·id** (hi″dri-o′dik) a term applied to aqueous solutions of hydrogen iodide, HI, a strong mineral acid.

**hy·dri·on** (hi-dri′on) hydrogen ion.

**hydr(o)-** [Gr. *hydōr* water] a combining form denoting *(a)* relationship to water, *(b)* the accumulation of fluid in a body part, or *(c)* the presence of hydrogen in a chemical compound.

**hy·droa** (hi-dro′ə) [*hydro-* + Gr. *ōon* egg] a vesicular or bullous eruption.
**h. estiva′le,** h. vacciniforme.
**h. vaccinifor′me,** a vesicular and bullous eruption, which may be preceded by pruritus and burning sensation, having a tendency to recur each summer during childhood on sun-exposed areas of the skin; the lesions dry up with the formation of brown adherent crusts, and each lesion is surrounded by an erythematous zone, giving the appearance of a vaccination vesicle. Called also *h. estivale* and *summer prurigo of Hutchinson.*

**hy·dro·adip·sia** (hi″dro-ə-dip′se-ə) [*hydro-* + *a-*[1] + *dipsa*] absence of thirst for water.

**hy·dro·ap·pen·dix** (hi″dro-ə-pen′diks) distention of the vermiform appendix with a watery fluid.

**Hy·dro·bi·i·dae** (hi″dro-be′ĭ-de) a family of snails of the order Mesogastropoda, including the subfamilies Hydrobiinae and Bulimi-nae, which are intermediate hosts of various species of parasitic flukes.

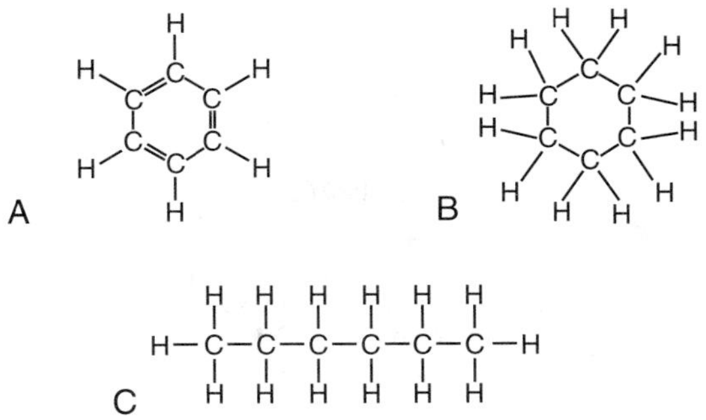

Hydrocarbons. *(A),* Benzene, $C_6H_6$, an aromatic hydrocarbon; *(B),* cyclohexane, $C_6H_{12}$, an alicyclic hydrocarbon; *(C), n*-hexane, $C_6H_{14}$, an aliphatic hydrocarbon.

**Hy·dro·bi·i·nae** (hi″dro-be′ĭ-ne) a subfamily of snails (family Hydrobiidae, order Mesogastropoda) that includes the genus *Oncomelania,* the intermediate host of *Schistosoma japonicum.*

**hy·dro·bil·i·ru·bin** (hi″dro-bil″ĭ-roo′bin) [*hydro-* + *bilirubin*] a brownish-red pigment derivable from bilirubin by reduction. It is believed to be identical with stercobilin and urobilin.

**hy·dro·bleph·a·ron** (hi″dro-blef′ə-ron) [*hydro-* + Gr. *blepharon* eyelid] edema of the eyelids.

**hy·dro·bro·mic ac·id** (hi-dro-bro′mik) [MeSH: Hydrobromic Acid] a term applied to aqueous solutions of hydrogen bromide, HBr, a strong mineral acid.

**hy·dro·bro·mide** (hi″dro-bro′mīd) an addition salt of hydrobromic acid. Cf. *hydrochloride.*

**hy·dro·ca·ly·co·sis** (hi″dro-ka″lĭ-ko′sis) [*hydro-* + *calyx* + *-osis*] a usually asymptomatic cystic dilatation of a major renal calix, lined by transitional epithelium and due to obstruction of the infundibulum.

**hy·dro·ca·lyx** (hi″dro-ka′līks) a cyst in the renal cortex caused by obstruction at the infundibulum; the entire calix dilates to form the cyst wall.

**hy·dro·car·bon** (hi″dro-kahr′bon) an organic compound that contains carbon and hydrogen only. The hydrocarbons are divided into *alicyclic, aliphatic,* and *aromatic* hydrocarbons, according to the arrangement of the atoms and the chemical properties of the compounds.
**alicyclic h.,** a hydrocarbon that has cyclic structure and aliphatic properties.
**aliphatic h.,** a hydrocarbon in which no carbon atoms are joined to form a ring.
**aromatic h.,** a hydrocarbon that has cyclic structure and a closed conjugated system of double bonds that gives it the characteristic chemical properties of the parent aromatic hydrocarbon, benzene ($C_6H_6$); other typical aromatic hydrocarbons are toluene ($C_7H_8$), naphthalene ($C_{10}H_8$), anthracene ($C_{14}H_{10}$), and phenanthrene ($C_{14}H_{10}$).
**chlorinated h.,** any of a group of hydrocarbons with chlorine substitution; they accumulate in body fat of humans and other animals and as such can build up to toxic levels to various degrees. They are used mainly as refrigerants, industrial solvents, insecticides, and dry cleaning fluids, and some have been used as anesthetics. See table at *organochlorine.* Called also *chlorohydrocarbon.*
**cyclic h.,** one of a series of hydrocarbons having the general formula $C_nH_{2n}$, the carbon atoms being thought of as having a closed ring structure.
**saturated h.,** a hydrocarbon that has the maximum number of hydrogen atoms for a given carbon structure, such as methane, ethane, propane, cyclopropane, and the butanes.
**unsaturated h.,** any hydrocarbon that has at least one double or triple bond between a pair of carbon atoms and thus has less than the maximum number of hydrogen atoms for a given structure.

**hy·dro·car·bon·ism** (hi″dro-kahr′bon-iz-əm) poisoning by hydrocarbons.

**hy·dro·cele** (hi′dro-sēl) [*hydro-* + *-cele*[1]] [MeSH: Hydrocele] a circumscribed collection of fluid, especially a collection of fluid in the tunica vaginalis of the testicle or along the spermatic cord.
**cervical h.,** a serous dilatation of a persistent cervical duct, or sometimes of a deep cervical lymph space; called also *h. colli* and *Maunoir's h.*
**chylous h.,** a form in which the fluid is milky in appearance.
**h. col′li,** cervical h.

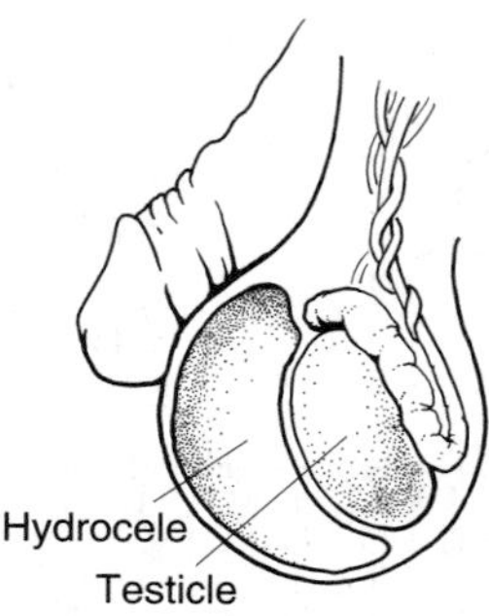


**communicating h.**, hydrocele in which the processus vaginalis testis is patent.
**congenital h.**, hydrocele in the unobliterated canal between the peritoneal cavity and that of the tunica vaginalis.
**diffused h.**, a collection of fluid diffused in the loose connective tissue of the spermatic cord.
**Dupuytren's h.**, bilocular hydrocele of the tunica vaginalis testis.
**encysted h.**, one which occurs in cysts outside the cavity of the tunica vaginalis testis.
**h. fe'minae**, an affection of the round ligament of the female resembling ordinary hydrocele.
**funicular h.**, hydrocele of the tunica vaginalis of the spermatic cord in a space closed toward the testis and open toward the peritoneal cavity.
**hernial h.**, distention of the hernial sac with a fluid.
**Maunoir's h., h. of neck**, cervical h.
**h. rena'lis**, a condition in which the renal capsule forms part of a cyst wall so that the kidney is partially or almost wholly surrounded by the cyst; although often found after trauma in adults, such a cyst is of congenital origin.
**scrotal h.**, a circumscribed collection of fluid in the scrotum.
**h. spina'lis**, spina bifida.

**hy·dro·ce·lec·to·my** (hi″dro-se-lek′tə-me) [*hydrocele* + *-ectomy*] excision of a hydrocele.

**hy·dro·ce·phal·ic** (hi″dro-sə-fal′ik) pertaining to or affected with hydrocephalus.

**hy·dro·ceph·a·lo·cele** (hi″dro-sef′ə-lo-sēl″) hydroencephalocele.

**hy·dro·ceph·a·loid** (hi″dro-sef′ə-loid) 1. resembling hydrocephalus. 2. see under *disease*.

**hy·dro·ceph·a·lus** (hi″dro-sef′ə-ləs) [*hydro-* + *-cephalus*] [MeSH: Hydrocephalus] a condition marked by dilatation of the cerebral ventricles, most often occurring secondarily to obstruction of the cerebrospinal fluid pathways (see *ventricular block*, under *block*), and accompanied by an accumulation of cerebrospinal fluid within the skull; the fluid is usually under increased pressure, but occasionally may be normal or nearly so. In children it may occur prior to closure of the skull sutures and is typically characterized by enlargement of the head, prominence of the forehead, brain atrophy, mental deterioration, and convulsions. In adults the syndrome includes incontinence, imbalance, and dementia. It may be congenital or acquired and may be of sudden onset *(acute h.)* or be slowly progressive *(chronic* or *primary h.)*. Called also *hydrocephaly, hydrencephaly,* and *hydrencephalus.*
**acquired h.**, hydrocephalus resulting from a disease process, such as meningitis, or from trauma. Called also *secondary h.*
**communicating h.**, hydrocephalus in which there is no obstruction in the ventricular system, and cerebrospinal fluid passes readily out of the brain into the spinal canal, but is not absorbed. Cf. *obstructive h. (noncommunicating h.).*
**congenital h.**, hydrocephalus resulting from a developmental obstruction of the cerebrospinal fluid pathways, called also *primary h.*
**h. ex va'cuo**, a compensatory replacement by cerebrospinal fluid of the volume of tissue lost in atrophy of the brain.
**noncommunicating h.**, obstructive h.
**normal-pressure h., normal-pressure occult h.**, dementia, ataxia, and urinary incontinence with hydrocephalus, i.e., with enlarged ventricles associated with inadequacy of the subarachnoid spaces, occurring in middle-aged and older persons. The cerebrospinal and spinal fluid pressures are at the upper end of normal, but with the excess spinal fluid volume, that pressure is actually abnormally high. Called also *occult normal-pressure h.*
**obstructive h.**, hydrocephalus due to ventricular block (q.v.); called also *noncommunicating h.* Cf. *communicating h.*
**occult normal-pressure h.**, normal-pressure h.
**otitic h.**, acute hydrocephalus caused by spread of the inflammation of otitis media to the cranial cavity.
**posthemorrhagic h.**, hydrocephalus in an infant following intracranial hemorrhage that has distended the ventricles and obstructed normal pathways for cerebrospinal fluid; in some infants it resolves spontaneously, but in others it leads to permanent neurodevelopmental deficits.
**primary h.**, 1. congenital h. 2. chronic h.; see *hydrocephalus.*
**secondary h.**, acquired h.
**tension h.**, obstructive h.

**hy·dro·ceph·a·ly** (hi″dro-sef′ə-le) hydrocephalus.

**Hy·dro-Chlor** (hi′dro-klor″) trademark for a preparation of hydrochlorothiazide.

**hy·dro·chlo·ric ac·id** (hi″dro-klor′ik) [MeSH: Hydrochloric Acid] a term applied to aqueous solutions of hydrogen chloride, HCl. It is a highly corrosive strong mineral acid commonly used as a laboratory reagent. HCl is secreted by the gastric parietal cells in response to gastrin, histamine, and vagal stimulation. This normally reduces the pH of the gastric content to below 2.0.

**hy·dro·chlo·ride** (hi″dro-klor′īd) a salt formed by addition of hydrochloric acid; chemically it is a chloride salt of the moiety formed by protonation of a neutral organic compound. The term *hydrochloride* is used primarily in drug names.

**hy·dro·chlo·ro·thi·a·zide** (hi″dro-klor″o-thi′ə-zīd) [USP] [MeSH: Hydrochlorothiazide] a thiazide diuretic, used for treatment of hypertension and edema; administered orally. It is often used in combination with a potassium-sparing diuretic.

**hy·dro·cho·le·cys·tis** (hi″dro-ko″le-sis′tis) [*hydro-* + *cholecystis*] distention of the gallbladder with watery fluid; hydrops of the gallbladder.

**hy·dro·cho·le·re·sis** (hi″dro-ko″lə-re′sis) [*hydro-* + *choleresis*] choleresis characterized by increase in water output, or induction of the excretion of bile relatively low in specific gravity, viscosity, and total solid content.

**hy·dro·cho·le·ret·ic** (hi″dro-ko″lə-re′tic) pertaining to, characterized by, or producing hydrocholeresis.

**hy·dro·cho·les·ter·ol** (hi″dro-kə-les′tər-ol) a reduced form of cholesterol.

**hy·dro·cin·chon·i·dine** (hi″dro-sin-kon′ĭ-din) an alkaloid, $C_{19}H_{24}ON_2$, isomeric with cinchonine.

**hy·dro·cir·so·cele** (hi″dro-sir′so-sēl) [*hydro-* + *cirsocele*] hydrocele combined with varicocele.

**hy·dro·co·done** (hi″dro-ko′dōn) [MeSH: Hydrocodone] a semisynthetic narcotic derivative of codeine having sedative and analgesic effects more powerful than those of codeine.
**h. bitartrate** [USP], a semisynthetic derivative of codeine used as an antitussive; administered orally.
**h. polistirex,** sulfonated styrene-divinylbenzene copolymer complex with dextromethorphan, administered orally as an extended-release antitussive.

**hy·dro·col·loid** (hi″dro-ko′loid) [*hydro-* + *colloid*] [MeSH: Colloids] a colloid system in which water is the dispersion medium.
**irreversible h.**, a hydrocolloid that can be converted from the sol to the gel condition but cannot be reverted to a sol by any simple means. Common examples are the soluble alginates (see *alginate*).
**reversible h.**, a hydrocolloid that can be reverted from the gel to the sol condition by increase in temperature; a common example is agar.

**hy·dro·col·pos** (hi″dro-kol′pos) [*hydro-* + Gr. *kolpos* vagina] a collection of watery fluid in the vagina.

**hy·dro·co·ni·on** (hi″dro-ko′ne-on) [*hydro-* + Gr. *konis* dust] an atomizer or vaporizer for throwing liquids in a fine spray.

**hy·dro·cor·ta·mate hy·dro·chlo·ride** (hi″dro-kor′tə-māt) a synthetic glucocorticoid, used topically as an anti-inflammatory in the treatment of steroid-responsive dermatoses.

**hy·dro·cor·ti·sone** (hi″dro-kor′tĭ-sōn) [USP] [MeSH: Hydrocortisone] the name given to cortisol when used as a pharmaceutical, applied to both the natural hormone and the same substance produced synthetically; it has life-maintaining and blood pressure–sustaining properties and also has limited mineralocorticoid activity. The official preparation and its salts are used in the treatment of inflammations, allergies, pruritus, collagen diseases such as rheumatoid arthritis and systemic lupus erythematosus, some neoplasms, acute or chronic adrenocortical insufficiency, severe status asthmaticus, and shock.
**h. acetate** [USP], an ester of hydrocortisone, having actions and uses similar to those of the base; administered by intra-articular, intralesional, or soft-tissue injection or applied topically to the skin, external acoustic canal, or conjunctiva.
**h. butyrate** [USP], an ester of hydrocortisone used topically for the relief of inflammation and pruritus in corticosteroid-responsive dermatoses.
**h. cypionate,** an ester of hydrocortisone used in replacement therapy for adrenal insufficiency and as an anti-inflammatory and im-

munosuppressant in a wide variety of disorders; administered orally.
**h. hemisuccinate** [USP], an ester of hydrocortisone, having actions and uses similar to those of the base.
**h. sodium phosphate** [USP], a water-soluble ester of hydrocortisone used in replacement therapy for adrenal insufficiency and as an anti-inflammatory and immunosuppressant in a wide variety of disorders; administered intramuscularly, intravenously, or subcutaneously.
**h. sodium succinate** [USP], a water-soluble ester of hydrocortisone used in replacement therapy for adrenal insufficiency and as an anti-inflammatory and immunosuppressant in a wide variety of disorders; administered intramuscularly or intravenously.
**h. valerate** [USP], an ester of hydrocortisone used topically for the relief of inflammation and pruritus in corticosteroid-responsive dermatoses.

**Hy·dro·cor·tone** (hi″dro-kor′tōn) trademark for preparations of hydrocortisone.

**hy·dro·cy·an·ic ac·id** (hi″dro-si-an′ik) hydrogen cyanide.

**hy·dro·cy·an·ism** (hi″dro-si′ən-iz-əm) cyanide poisoning (q.v.) caused by hydrogen cyanide.

**hy·dro·cyst** (hi′dro-sist) [*hydro-* + *cyst* (def. 2)] a cyst with watery contents.

**hy·dro·cyst·ad·e·no·ma** (hi″dro-sist″ad-ə-no′mə) syringocystadenoma.

**hy·dro·cy·to·sis** (hi″dro-si-to′sis) stomatocytosis.

**hy·dro·de·lin·e·a·tion** (hi″dro-de-lin″e-a′shən) the injection of fluid between the layers of the nucleus of the lens, using a blunt needle; done to delineate the nuclear zones during cataract surgery.

**hy·dro·dif·fu·sion** (hi″dro-dĭ-fu′zhən) diffusion in an aqueous medium.

**hy·dro·dip·so·ma·nia** (hi″dro-dip″so-ma′ne-ə) an epileptic condition characterized by attacks of insatiable thirst.

**hy·dro·dis·sec·tion** (hi″dro-di-sek′shən) [*hydro-* + *dissection*] injection of a small amount of fluid, usually an isotonic salt solution, into the capsule of the lens in order to dissect its anterior part from the cortex of the lens and allow maneuverability of the nucleus of the lens during extracapsular or phacoemulsification surgery.

**hy·dro·di·ure·sis** (hi″dro-di″u-re′sis) [*hydro-* + *diuresis*] copious secretion of urine of low specific gravity.

**Hy·dro·DI·U·RIL** (hi″dro-di′u-ril) trademark for a preparation of hydrochlorothiazide.

**hy·dro·dy·nam·ics** (hi″dro-di-nam′iks) [*hydro-* + *dynamics*] that branch of the science of mechanics which treats of the movement of fluids and of solids contained in fluids.

**hy·dro·elec·tric** (hi″dro-e-lek′trik) pertaining to water and electricity.

**hy·dro·en·ceph·a·lo·cele** (hi″dro-en-sef′ə-lo-sēl) [*hydro-* + *encephalocele*] encephalocele into a distended sac containing cerebrospinal fluid; called also *encephalocystocele, hydrencephalocele,* and *hydrocephalocele.*

**hy·dro·flu·me·thi·a·zide** (hi″dro-floo″mə-thi′ə-zīd) [USP] [MeSH: Hydroflumethiazide] a thiazide diuretic, used for treatment of hypertension and edema; administered orally.

**hy·dro·flu·o·ric ac·id** (hi″dro-flo͝or′ik) [MeSH: Hydrofluoric Acid] a term applied to aqueous solutions of hydrogen fluoride, an organic acid used in dilute solutions for cleaning and etching. It is extremely poisonous, as well as corrosive to the skin.

**hy·dro·gel** (hi′dro-jəl) a gel that has water as its dispersion medium.

**hy·dro·gen** (hi′dro-jən) [*hydro-* + Gr. *gennan* to produce] [MeSH: Hydrogen] the lightest element, an odorless, tasteless, colorless gas that is inflammable and explosive when mixed with air. It is found in water and in almost all organic compounds. Its ion is the active constituent of all acids in the water system. Its symbol is H; atomic number, 1; atomic weight, 1.00797; specific gravity, 0.069. Hydrogen exists in three isotopes: ordinary, or light, hydrogen is the mass 1 isotope, also called *protium;* heavy hydrogen is the mass 2 isotope, also called *deuterium;* the mass 3 isotope is *tritium.*
**arseniuretted h.,** see *arsine.*
**h. cyanide,** an extremely poisonous colorless liquid or gas, HCN, a decomposition product of various naturally occurring glycosides and a common cause of cyanide poisoning (q.v.) in humans and domestic animals. Inhalation of the gas can cause death within a minute. Called also *hydrocyanic acid* and *prussic acid.*
**h. disulfide,** an ill-smelling liquid, $H_2S_2$.
**h. fluoride,** a corrosive inorganic acid, HF; see *hydrofluoric acid.*
**heavy h.,** see *hydrogen.*
**light h.,** see *hydrogen.*
**ordinary h.,** see *hydrogen.*
**h. peroxide,** a strongly disinfectant cleansing and bleaching liquid, $H_2O_2$, used in dilute solution in water, mainly as a wash or spray.
**h. selenide,** a poisonous gas, $H_2Se$; its inhalation causes an obstinate coryza and destroys the sense of smell.
**h. sulfide,** a poisonous gas with an offensive smell, $H_2S$, used as a chemical reagent.
**sulfuretted h.,** h. sulfide.

**hy·dro·gen·ate** (hi′dro-jən-at″) to cause to combine with hydrogen; to reduce with hydrogen.

**hy·dro·gen·ize** (hi′dro-jən-īz) hydrogenate.

**hy·drog·e·noid** (hi-droj′ə-noid) a homeopathic term denoting a constitution or temperament that will not tolerate much moisture.

**hy·dro·gym·nas·tic** (hi″dro-jim-nas′tik) pertaining to exercises performed in the water.

**hy·dro·gym·nas·tics** (hi″dro-jim-nas′tiks) therapeutic exercise performed in water.

**hy·dro·hem·a·to·ne·phro·sis** (hi″dro-hēm″ə-to-nə-fro′sis) [*hydro-* + *hemato-* + *nephro-* + *-osis*] distention of the pelvis of the kidney with an accumulation of bloody urine.

**hy·dro·hy·men·itis** (hi″dro-hi″mən-i′tis) [*hydro-* + *hymen-* + *-itis*] inflammation of a serous membrane.

**hy·dro·ki·net·ic** (hi″dro-kĭ-net′ik) relating to the movement of water or other fluid, as in a whirlpool bath.

**hy·dro·ki·net·ics** (hi″dro-kĭ-net′iks) [*hydro-* + *kinet-* + *-ic*] that branch of mechanics which treats of fluids in motion.

**hy·dro·la·bile** (hi″dro-la′bil) having a tendency to lose weight under carbohydrate or salt restriction or following infections or gastrointestinal disease. Cf. *hydrostabile.*

**hy·dro·la·bil·i·ty** (hi″dro-lə-bil′ĭ-te) [*hydro-* + *lability*] a condition in which tissue fluids tend to vary in quantity.

**hy·dro·lase** (hi′dro-lās) [EC 3] any member of the class of enzymes that catalyze the cleavage of a chemical bond with the addition of water, e.g., esterases, glycosidases, lipases, nucleotidases, peptidases, and phosphatases.

**hy·drol·o·gy** (hi-drol′ə-je) [*hydro-* + *-logy*] the sum of knowledge regarding water and its uses.

**Hy·dro·lose** (hi′dro-lōs) trademark for a preparation of methylcellulose.

**hy·dro·ly·ase** (hi″dro-li′ās) [EC 4.2.1] a sub-subclass of enzymes of the lyase class. These enzymes catalyze the removal of water from a substrate by breakage of a carbon-oxygen bond, leading to formation of a double bond. The recommended name is usually dehydratase. The term synthase or hydratase is used when the reverse aspect of the reaction is dominant.

**hy·dro·lymph** (hi′dro-limf) [*hydro-* + *lymph*] the thin, watery nutritive fluid of certain of the lower animals.

**hy·drol·y·sate** (hi-drol′ə-zāt) a compound produced by hydrolysis.
**protein h.,** a mixture of amino acids prepared by splitting a protein with acid, alkali, or enzyme. Such preparations provide the nutritive equivalent of the original material (casein, lactalbumin, fibrin, etc.) in the form of its constituent amino acids; used as a fluid and nutrient replenisher.

**hy·drol·y·sis** (hi-drol′ə-sis) pl. *hydrol′yses* [*hydro-* + *-lysis*] [MeSH: Hydrolysis] the splitting of a compound into fragments by the addition of water, the hydroxyl group being incorporated in one fragment, and the hydrogen atom in the other.

**hy·dro·lyst** (hi′dro-list) an agent that promotes hydrolysis.

**hy·dro·lyte** (hi′dro-līt) a substance undergoing hydrolysis.

**hy·dro·lyt·ic** (hi-dro-lit′ik) pertaining to, characterized by, or promoting hydrolysis.

**hy·dro·lyze** (hi′dro-līz) to subject to hydrolysis.

**hy·dro·ma** (hi-dro′mə) hygroma.

**hy·dro·mas·sage** (hi″dro-mə-sahzh′) massage by means of moving water.

**hy·dro·men·in·gi·tis** (hi″dro-men″in-ji′tis) [*hydro-* + *meningitis*] meningitis with serous effusion.

**hy·dro·me·nin·go·cele** (hi″dro-mə-ning′go-sēl) [*hydro-* + *meningocele*] a meningocele forming a sac containing cerebrospinal fluid but no brain or spinal cord substance, in contrast to a myelomeningocele or an encephalocele.

**hy·drom·e·ter** (hi-drom′ə-tər) [*hydro-* + *-meter*] an instrument for determining the specific gravity of a fluid.

**hy·dro·me·tra** (hi″dro-me′trə) [*hydro-* + *metra*] a collection of watery fluid in the uterus.

**hy·dro·met·ric** (hi″dro-met′rik) pertaining to hydrometry.

**hy·dro·me·tro·col·pos** (hi″dro-me″tro-kol′pos) [*hydro-* + *metro-* + *kolpos* vagina] a collection of watery fluid in the uterus and vagina.

**hy·drom·e·try** (hi-drom′ə-tre) the measurement of the specific gravity of a fluid by means of the hydrometer.

**hy·dro·mi·cro·ceph·a·ly** (hi″dro-mi″kro-sef′ə-le) microcephaly with an abnormal amount of cerebrospinal fluid.

**hy·dro·mor·phone** (hi″dro-mor′fōn) [MeSH: Hydromorphone] a morphine alkaloid, having narcotic analgesic effects similar to but greater and of shorter duration than those of morphine; administered as the sulfate salt by subcutaneous injection.
**h. hydrochloride** [USP], the hydrochloride salt of hydromorphone, having the same actions as the base; administered orally and subcutaneously. Called also *dihydromorphinone hydrochloride.*

**Hy·dro·mox** (hi′dro-moks) trademark for preparations of quinethazone.

**hy·drom·pha·lus** (hi-drom′fə-ləs) [*hydro-* + *omphalus*] a cystic accumulation of watery fluid at the umbilicus.

**hy·dro·my·e·lia** (hi″dro-mi-e′le-ə) [*hydro-* + *myel-* + *-ia*] a pathological condition in which there is dilation of the central canal of the spinal cord with increased fluid accumulation. Cf. *syringobulbia* and *syringomyelia.*

**hy·dro·my·elo·cele** (hi″dro-mi′ə-lo-sēl) [*hydro-* + *myelocele*] hydromyelomeningocele.

**hy·dro·my·elo·me·nin·go·cele** (hi″dro-mi″ə-lo-mə-ning′go-sēl) [*hydro-* + myelomeningocele] a myelomeningocele that contains both cerebrospinal fluid and spinal cord tissue; cf. *hydromeningocele.*

**hy·dro·my·o·ma** (hi″dro-mi-o′mə) [*hydro-* + *myoma*] uterine leiomyoma with cystic degeneration.

**hy·dro·ne·phro·sis** (hi″dro-nə-fro′sis) [*hydro-* + *nephro-* + *-osis*] [MeSH: Hydronephrosis] distention of the pelvis and calices of the kidney with urine, as a result of obstruction of the ureter.
**closed h.**, a permanent condition, resulting from complete obstruction of the ureter.
**open h.**, an intermittent condition, resulting from sporadic or incomplete obstruction of the ureter.

**hy·dro·ne·phrot·ic** (hi″dro-nə-frot′ik) pertaining to or characterized by hydronephrosis.

**hy·dro·ni·um** (hi-dro′ne-əm) the hydrated proton, $H_3O^+$; it is the form in which the proton (hydrogen ion, $H^+$) exists in aqueous solution, a combination of $H^+$ and $H_2O$.

**hy·dro·par·o·ti·tis** (hi″dro-par″o-ti′tis) distention of the parotid gland with watery fluid.

**hy·dro·pe·nia** (hi″dro-pe′ne-ə) [*hydro-* + *-penia*] deficiency of water in the body.

**hy·dro·pe·nic** (hi′dro-pe″nik) relating to hydropenia.

**hy·dro·peri·car·di·tis** (hi″dro-per″ĭ-kahr-di′tis) [*hydro-* + *pericarditis*] pericarditis associated with a watery effusion in the pericardial sac.

**hy·dro·peri·car·di·um** (hi″dro-per″ĭ-kahr′de-əm) [*hydro-* + *pericardium*] abnormal accumulation of serous fluid in the pericardial cavity.

**hy·dro·peri·ne·phro·sis** (hi″dro-per″ĭ-nə-fro′sis) [*hydro-* + *peri-* + *nephro-* + *-osis*] a collection of fluid in the retroperitoneal connective tissue and opening into the pelvis of the kidney.

**hy·dro·per·i·on** (hi″dro-per′e-on) [*hydro-* + *peri-* + *ōon* egg] the fluid between the capsular and parietal decidua.

**hy·dro·peri·to·ne·um** (hi″dro-per″ĭ-to-ne′əm) [*hydro-* + *peritoneum*] ascites, or abnormal accumulation of fluid in the peritoneal cavity.

**hy·dro·peri·to·nia** (hi″dro-per″ĭ-to′ne-ə) ascites.

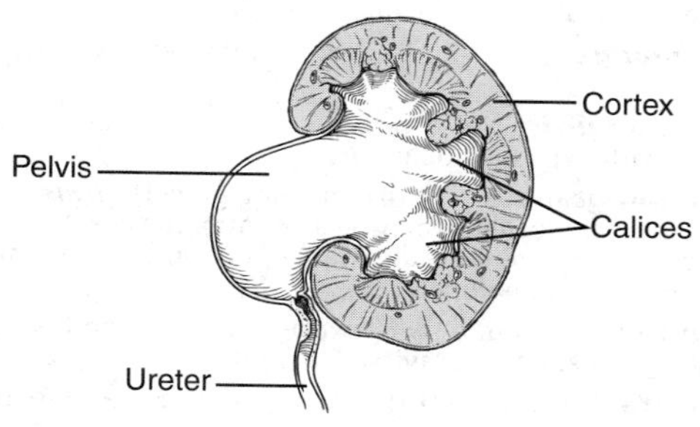

Hydronephrosis.

**hy·dro·per·ox·ide** (hi″dro-pər-ok′sīd) an organic peroxide in which one of the groups attached to the —O—O— is a hydrogen group; i.e., R—O—O—H.

**hy·dro·per·oxy·ei·co·sa·tet·ra·eno·ic acid (HPETE)** (hi″dro-pər-ok″se-i-ko″sə-tet″rə-e-no′ik) any of several arachidonic acid metabolites produced by the actions of lipoxygenases. 5-HPETE (5-hydroperoxy-6,8,11,14-eicosatetraenoic acid) is the precursor of the leukotrienes. 12-HPETE (12-hydroperoxy-5,8,10,14-eicosatetraenoic acid) is the precursor of 12-HETE, which is chemotactic for neutrophils and eosinophils. 15-HPETE is the precursor of 15-HETE and of lipoxins.

**hy·dro·pex·ia** (hi″dro-pek′se-ə) hydropexis.

**hy·dro·pex·ic** (hi″dro-pek′sik) [*hydro-* + *pexic*] fixing or holding water; pertaining to the holding of water.

**hy·dro·pex·is** (hi″dro-pek′sis) the fixation or holding of water.

**hy·dro·phago·cy·to·sis** (hi″dro-fag″o-si-to′sis) [*hydro-* + *phagocytosis*] the absorption by macrophages of plasma surrounding them; called also *Lewis' phenomenon.*

**Hy·dro·phi·idae** (hi″dro-fi′ĭ-de) the sea snakes, a family of venomous snakes adapted for living in the ocean, found in the Indian and Pacific Oceans and characterized by an oarlike tail and immovable hollow fangs. Genera include *Enhydrina, Kerilia,* and *Pelamis.* See table at *snake.*

**hy·dro·phil** (hi′dro-fil) hydrophilic.

**hy·dro·phil·ia** (hi-dro-fil′e-ə) [*hydro-* + *-philia*] the property of absorbing water.

**hy·dro·phil·ic** (hi″dro-fil′ik) readily absorbing moisture; hygroscopic; having strongly polar groups that readily interact with water.

**hy·droph·i·lism** (hi-drof′ĭ-liz-əm) hydrophilia.

**hy·droph·i·lous** (hi-drof′ĭ-ləs) hydrophilic.

**hy·dro·pho·bia** (hi″dro-fo′be-ə) [*hydro-* + *-phobia*] 1. irrational fear of water. 2. choking, gagging, and fear on attempts to drink in the acute neurologic phase of rabies, caused by pain from spasms of the pharynx or larynx. 3. former term for rabies.
**paralytic h.**, see under *rabies.*

**hy·dro·pho·bic** (hi″dro-fo′bik) 1. pertaining to or affected with hydrophobia (rabies). 2. not readily absorbing water, or being adversely affected by water, as a hydrophobic colloid. 3. lacking polar groups and, therefore, insoluble in water.

**hy·dro·pho·ro·graph** (hi″dro-for′ə-graf) [*hydro-* + Gr. *phora* a being borne, or carried along + *-graph*] an instrument for measuring and recording the pressure and/or flow of a fluid, especially the flow of urine or the pressure of the spinal fluid.

**hy·droph·thal·mia** (hi″drof-thal′me-ə) hydrophthalmos; buphthalmos.

**hy·droph·thal·mos** (hi″drof-thal′mos) [*hydro-* + Gr. *ophthalmos* eye] [MeSH: Hydrophthalmos] a form of glaucoma characterized by marked enlargement and distention of the fibrous coats of the eye; buphthalmos.
**h. ante′rior,** that which affects the anterior portion of the eyeball only.
**h. poste′rior,** that affecting the posterior part of the eyeball only.
**h. tota′lis,** that which affects the entire eyeball.

**hy·droph·thal·mus** (hi″drof-thal′məs) hydrophthalmos; buphthalmos.

**hy·dro·phy·so·me·tra** (hi″dro-fi″so-me′trə) [*hydro-* + *physometra*] physohydrometra.

**hy·dro·phyte** (hi′dro-fīt) [*hydro-* + *-phyte*] a plant adapted to grow in a very wet environment, either completely aquatic or rooted in water or mud but with stems and leaves above the water.

**hy·drop·ic** (hi-drop′ik) edematous.

**hy·dro·plas·ma** (hi″dro-plaz′mə) [*hydro-* + *plasma*] the watery or liquid part of the protoplasm.

**hy·dro·pneu·ma·to·sis** (hi″dro-noo″mə-to′sis) [*hydro-* + *pneumatosis*] a collection of fluid and gas within the tissues.

**hy·dro·pneu·mo·go·ny** (hi″dro-noo-mo′gə-ne) [*hydro-* + *pneumo-* + Gr. *gony* knee] the injection of air into a joint to detect effusion or other abnormality.

**hy·dro·pneu·mo·peri·car·di·um** (hi″dro-noo″mo-per″ĭ-kahr′de-əm) pneumohydropericardium.

**hy·dro·pneu·mo·peri·to·ne·um** (hi″dro-noo″mo-per″ĭ-to-ne′əm) [*hydro-* + *pneumo-* + *peritoneum*] a collection of watery fluid and gas in the peritoneal cavity.

**hy·dro·pneu·mo·tho·rax** (hi″dro-noo″mo-thor′aks) [*hydro-* + *pneumothorax*] [MeSH: Hydropneumothorax] a collection of fluid and gas within the pleural cavity. Called also *pneumohydrothorax, pneumoserothorax,* and *seropneumothorax.*

**Hy·dro·pres** (hi'dro-pres) trademark for preparations of hydrochlorothiazide with reserpine.

**hy·drops** (hi'drops) [L.; Gr. *hydrōps*] edema.
**h. ad ma'tulam,** polyuria.
**h. am'nii,** hydramnios.
**h. arti'culi,** hydrarthrosis.
**endolymphatic h.,** Meniere's disease.
**fetal h., h. feta'lis,** gross edema of the entire body of a fetus or newborn infant, associated with severe anemia, occurring in erythroblastosis fetalis.
**h. fetalis, immune,** hydrops fetalis caused by maternal sensitization to a fetal blood group antigen; see *erythroblastosis fetalis.*
**h. fetalis, nonimmune,** hydrops fetalis caused by any of a variety of nonimmunologic disorders, particularly cardiac defects.
**h. folli'culi,** accumulation of fluid in the graafian follicle, forming a large solitary follicular cyst.
**h. labyrin'thi, labyrinthine h.,** Meniere's disease.
**h. spu'rius,** pseudomyxoma peritonei.
**h. tu'bae,** hydrosalpinx.
**h. tu'bae pro'fluens,** a condition in which the abdominal opening of the uterine tube becomes closed, and the tube may reach enormous proportions as it fills with serum; peristaltic action of the tube causes colicky pain, until the fluid escapes through the uterine opening. Called also *intermittent hydrosalpinx.*

**hy·dro·pyo·ne·phro·sis** (hi"dro-pi"o-nə-fro'sis) [*hydro-* + *pyo-* + *nephro-* + *-osis*] the accumulation of urine and pus in the pelvis of the kidney.

**hy·dro·quin·one** (hi"dro-kwĭ-nōn') [USP] the reduced form of quinone, containing two hydroxyl groups; applied topically to bleach hyperpigmented skin.

**hy·dro·ra·chis** (hi"dro-ra'kis) [*hydro-* + *rhachis*] hydromyelia.

**hy·dror·rhea** (hi"dro-re'ə) [*hydro-* + *-rrhea*] a copious watery discharge.
**h. gravida'rum,** a periodic or intermittent discharge of clear, yellowish, or bloody fluid from the uterus, caused by escape of amniotic fluid or resulting from decidual metritis.

**hy·dro·sal·pinx** (hi"dro-sal'pinks) [*hydro-* + *salpinx*] a collection of watery fluid in a uterine tube, occurring as the end-stage of pyosalpinx.
**h. follicula'ris,** hydrosalpinx in which there is no central cystic cavity, the lumen being broken up into compartments as the result of fusion of the tubal plicae.
**intermittent h.,** hydrops tubae profluens.
**h. sim'plex,** hydrosalpinx characterized by excessive distention and thinning of the wall of the uterine tube, the plicae being few and widely separated.

**hy·dro·sar·co·cele** (hi"dro-sahr'ko-sēl) [*hydro-* + *sarcocele*] combined hydrocele and sarcocele.

**hy·dro·sol** (hi'dro-sol) a sol in which the dispersion medium is water.

**hy·dro·sol·u·ble** (hi"dro-sol'u-bəl) soluble in water.

**hy·dro·sphyg·mo·graph** (hi"dro-sfig'mo-graf) [*hydro-* + *sphygmograph*] a sphygmograph with water for an index.

**hy·dro·sta·bile** (hi"dro-sta'bil) preserving a stable weight under diet restrictions or gastrointestinal disease. Cf. *hydrolabile.*

**hy·dro·stat** (hi'dro-stat) [*hydro-* + *-stat*] a device by which the height of fluid in a container (column or reservoir) is regulated.

**hy·dro·stat·ic** (hi"dro-stat'ik) [*hydro-* + *-static*] pertaining to a liquid in a state of equilibrium; see under *pressure.*

**hy·dro·stat·ics** (hi"dro-stat'iks) the science of liquids in a state of rest or equilibrium and of the pressures they exert.

**hy·dro·syn·the·sis** (hi"dro-sin'thə-sis) a chemical reaction in which water is formed.

**hy·dro·sy·rin·go·my·e·lia** (hi"dro-sĭ-ring"go-mi-e'le-ə) syringomyelia.

**Hy·dro·taea** (hi"dro-te'ə) a genus of flies of the family Muscidae that do not bite but often cause irritation by landing in large numbers on animals. *H. ir'ritans* is the head fly, a common species of northern Europe that is attracted to any surface of an animal's body where there are secretions such as sweat, blood, saliva, or tears. *H. meteo'rica* is a species that gathers around the eyes and nostrils of humans and other animals.

**hy·dro·tax·is** (hi"dro-tak'sis) [*hydro-* + *-taxis*] an orientation movement of motile organisms or cells in response to stimulation by water or moisture.

**hy·dro·ther·a·py** (hi"dro-ther'ə-pe) [*hydro-* + *therapy*] [MeSH: Hydrotherapy] the application of water in any form, but usually externally, in the treatment of disease.

**hy·dro·ther·mal** (hi-dro-thər'məl) relating to the temperature effects of water, as in hot baths.

**hy·dro·ther·mic** (hi"dro-thər'mik) hydrothermal.

**hy·dro·thio·ne·mia** (hi"dro-thi"o-ne'me-ə) [*hydro-* + Gr. *theion* sulfur + *-emia*] the presence of hydrogen sulfide in the blood.

**hy·dro·thi·on·uria** (hi"dro-thi"o-nu're-ə) [*hydro-* + Gr. *theion* sulfur + *-uria*] the presence of hydrogen sulfide in the urine.

**hy·dro·tho·rax** (hi"dro-thor'aks) [*hydro-* + *thorax*] [MeSH: Hydrothorax] a pleural effusion containing serous fluid. See also *pleurisy with effusion.*
**chylous h.,** chylothorax.

**hy·drot·o·my** (hi-drot'ə-me) [*hydro-* + *-tomy*] the dissection or separation of parts by the forcible injection of water.

**hy·drot·ro·pism** (hi-drot'ro-piz-əm) [*hydro-* + *tropism*] a growth response of a nonmotile organism elicited by the presence of water or moisture.

**hy·dro·tu·ba·tion** (hi"dro-too-ba'shən) introduction of saline solution into the uterine tube; solution containing dye may be used to determine patency of the tube.

**hy·dro·ure·ter** (hi"dro-u-re'tər) abnormal distention of the ureter with urine or with a watery fluid, due to obstruction from any cause; cf. *megaloureter.*

**hy·dro·ure·tero·neph·ro·sis** (hi"dro-u-re"tər-o-nə-fro'sis) [*hydro-* + *uretero-* + *nephr-* + *-osis*] distention of both the ureter and the renal pelvis and calices with urine because of obstruction of the ureter.

**hy·dro·ure·ter·o·sis** (hi"dro-u-re"tər-o'sis) hydroureter.

**hy·dro·uria** (hi"dro-u're-ə) [*hydro-* + *-uria*] hydruria.

**hy·drous** (hi'drəs) containing water.

**hy·dro·va·ri·um** (hi"dro-var'e-əm) [*hydro-* + *ovarium*] a collection of serous fluid in an ovary.

**hy·drox·ide** (hi-drok'sīd) any compound of hydroxyl radical (OH), or of hydroxide ion, $OH^-$, with another radical or atom.

**hy·droxo·co·bal·a·min** (hi-drok"so-ko-bal'ə-min) [USP] [MeSH: Hydroxocobalamin] a cobalamin derivative in which the substituent is a hydroxyl group; it is the naturally occurring form of vitamin $B_{12}$ (cf. *cyanocobalamin*) and is sometimes used as a source of that vitamin. Abbreviated OH-Cbl.

**hydroxy-** a chemical prefix indicating presence of the univalent radical OH.

**hy·droxy·ac·yl CoA** (hi-drok"se-a'səl ko-a') hydroxyacyl coenzyme A.

**3-hy·droxy·ac·yl-CoA de·hy·dro·gen·ase** (hi-drok"se-a'səl ko-a' de-hi'dro-jən-ās) [EC 1.1.1.35] an enzyme of the oxidoreductase class that catalyzes the oxidation at the C-3 of L-hydroxyacyl coenzyme A to form ketoacyl coenzyme A, using $NAD^+$ as an electron acceptor. The reaction is one of the steps in fatty acid oxidation.

**3-hy·droxy·ac·yl-CoA epim·er·ase** (hi-drok"se-a'səl ko-a' ə-pim'ər-ās) 3-hydroxybutyryl-CoA epimerase.

**hy·droxy·ac·yl co·en·zyme A** (hi-drok"se-a'səl ko-en'zīm) a hydroxy derivative of acyl coenzyme A; the L- stereoisomer hydroxylated at C-3 is an intermediate in fatty acid oxidation.

**hy·droxy·ac·yl·glu·ta·thi·one hy·dro·lase** (hi-drok"se-as"əl-gloo"tə-thi'ōn hi'dro-lās) [EC 3.1.2.6] an enzyme of the hydrolase class that catalyzes the cleavage of a hydroxyacylglutathione compound to the corresponding hydroxy acid and glutathione, specifically converting lactoylglutathione to lactic acid as the last step in the conversion of methylglyoxal to lactic acid. The enzyme is found in red cells and other animal tissues. See also *glyoxalase.*

**hy·droxy·am·phet·amine hy·dro·bro·mide** (hi-drok"se-am-fet'ə-mēn) [USP] an adrenergic used as a mydriatic, applied topically to the conjunctiva. It is also used topically as a nasal decongestant and orally as a pressor agent in the treatment of heart block, carotid sinus syndrome, and postural hypotension.

**hy·droxy·an·thra·nil·ic ac·id** (hi-drok"se-an"thrə-nil'ik) a cyclic aromatic compound formed in the catabolism of tryptophan.

**hy·droxy·ap·a·tite** (hi-drok"se-ap'ə-tīt) an inorganic compound, $(Ca_3(PO_4)_2)_3 \cdot Ca(OH)_2$, found in the matrix of bone and the teeth, which gives rigidity to these structures. Compounds having this approximate chemical formula are synthesized for use as calcium supplements (see *tribasic calcium phosphate,* def. 2) and prosthetic aids (see *durapatite*). Called also *hydroxylapatite.*

**hy·droxy·ben·zene** (hi-drok"se-ben'zēn) phenol (def. 1).

**hy·droxy·bu·ty·rate** (hi-drok″se-bu′tĭ-rāt) a salt or anionic form of hydroxybutyric acid.

**3-hy·droxy·bu·ty·rate de·hy·dro·gen·ase** (hi-drok″se-bu′tə-rāt de-hi′dro-jən-ās) [EC 1.1.1.30] an enzyme of the oxidoreductase class that catalyzes the oxidation of D-3-hydroxybutyrate to form acetoacetate, using NAD$^+$ as an electron acceptor. The enzyme functions in nervous tissues and muscles, enabling use of circulating hydroxybutyrate as a fuel. In the liver mitochondrial matrix, the enzyme can also catalyze the reverse reaction, a step in ketogenesis. Written also *β-hydroxybutyrate dehydrogenase.*

**hy·droxy·bu·tyr·ic ac·id** (hi-drok″se-bu′tə-rik) any of several hydroxy derivatives of butyric acid, intermediates occurring at elevated levels in some metabolic disorders. Called also *oxybutyric acid.*
**3-h. a.,** β-h. a.
**4-h. a.,** γ-h. a.
**β-h. a.,** butyric acid substituted at the β, or 3, position, one of the ketone bodies produced in the liver and occurring at high levels in the blood and urine in ketosis. Called also *3-h. a.*
**γ-h. a.,** butyric acid substituted at the γ, or 4, position; it is an intermediate in the metabolism of γ-aminobutyric acid (GABA) and with GABA occurs at elevated levels in some body fluids in succinate semialdehyde dehydrogenase deficiency (q.v.). Called also *4-h. a.* and *succinate semialdehyde.*

**4-hy·droxy·bu·tyr·ic·ac·id·uria** (hi-drok″sə-bu-tir″ik-as″ĭ-du′re-ə) succinic semialdehyde dehydrogenase deficiency.

**γ-hy·droxy·bu·tyr·ic·ac·id·uria** (hi-drok″sə-bu-tir″ik-as″ĭ-du′re-ə) succinic semialdehyde dehydrogenase deficiency.

**hy·droxy·bu·ty·ryl** (hi-drok″se-bu′tə-rəl) the acyl radical of hydroxybutyric acid.

**3-hy·droxy·bu·ty·ryl-CoA epim·er·ase** (hi-drok″se-bu′tə-rəl ko-a′ ə-pim′ə-rās) [EC 5.1.2.3] an enzyme of the isomerase class that catalyzes the epimerization around C-3 of a D-3-hydroxyacyl coenzyme A to form the L isomer, a substrate for beta oxidation. The reaction is necessary for metabolism of some unsaturated fatty acids. Called also *3-hydroxyacyl CoA epimerase.*

**hy·droxy·chlo·ro·quine sul·fate** (hi-drok″se-klor′o-kwin) [USP] a 4-aminoquinoline compound with antiprotozoal and anti-inflammatory properties, used for the suppression and treatment of malaria, for the treatment of symptomatic giardiases, for suppression of lupus erythematosus, and as an anti-inflammatory in the treatment of rheumatoid arthritis; administered orally.

**25-hy·droxy·cho·le·cal·cif·e·rol** (hi-drok″se-ko″lə-kal-sif′ə-rol) the major metabolite synthesized from cholecalciferol (vitamin $D_3$) in the liver and occurring in the serum; it is the precursor of 1,25-dihydroxycholecalciferol. See also table at *cholecalciferol.* Called also *calcifediol, calcidiol,* and *25-hydroxyvitamin $D_3$.*

**hy·droxy·cho·les·ter·ol** (hi-drok″se-kə-les′-tə-rol) any of several hydroxylated derivatives of cholesterol. 7-α-hydroxycholesterol is an intermediate in the metabolism of cholesterol to bile acids.

**hy·droxy·cor·ti·co·ste·roid** (hi-drok″se-kor″tĭ-ko-ster′oid) a corticosteroid bearing a hydroxyl group on a designated carbon atom.
**17-h. (17-OHCS),** any steroid hydroxylated at carbon 17; some are intermediates in the biosynthesis of steroid hormones and are accumulated and excreted abnormally in various disorders of steroidogenesis. Those with dihydroxyacetone side chains *(Porter-Silber chromogens)* react positively in the Porter-Silber reaction.

**17β-hy·droxy·cor·ti·co·ster·one** (hi-drok″se-kor″tĭ-kos′tər-ōn) cortisol.

**hy·droxy·ei·co·sa·tet·ra·eno·ic acid (HETE)** (hi-drok″se-i-ko″sə-tet″rə-e-no′ik) any of several arachidonic acid metabolites produced by lipoxygenases from hydroperoxyeicosatetraenoic acid. 5-HETE is a byproduct of leukotriene metabolism. 12-HETE and 5,12-HETE are chemotactic for neutrophils and eosinophils and 12-HETE and 15-HETE may inhibit leukotriene production.

**hy·droxy·es·trin ben·zo·ate** (hi-drok″se-es′trin) estradiol benzoate.

**2-hy·droxy·eth·ane·sul·fo·nate** (hi-drok″se-eth″ān-sul′fə-nāt) any salt of 2-hydroxyethanesulfonic acid; see also *isethionate.*

**2-hy·droxy·eth·ane·sul·fon·ic ac·id** (hi-drok″se-eth″ān-sul-fon′ik) see *isethionic acid.*

**hy·droxy·for·mo·ben·zo·yl·ic ac·id** (hi-drok″se-for″mo-ben″zo-il′ik) a crystalline compound sometimes occurring in the urine in acute yellow atrophy of the liver.

**hy·droxy·glu·tar·ic ac·id** (hi-drok″sĭ-gloo-tar′ik) any of several hydroxylated derivatives of glutaric acid; 2-hydroxyglutaric acid is accumulated and excreted in glutaricaciduria, type II, and 3-hydroxyglutaric acid in glutaricaciduria, type I.

**hy·droxy·hep·ta·deca·tri·eno·ic ac·id (HHT)** (hi-drok″se-hep″tə-dek″ə-tri″e-no′ik) a prostaglandin metabolite that is a chemoattractant for neutrophils and eosinophils.

**5-hy·droxy·in·dole·ace·tic ac·id** (hi-drok″se-in″dōl-ə-se′tik) a product of serotonin metabolism excreted in large amounts by patients with carcinoid tumors. Abbreviated 5-HIAA.

**3-hy·droxy·iso·bu·ty·ryl** (hi-drok″se-i″so-bu′tə-rəl) the acyl radical of an isomer of 3-hydroxybutyric acid; the thioester formed with coenzyme A, 3-hydroxyisobutyryl CoA, is an intermediate in the catabolism of valine.

**3-hy·droxy·iso·bu·ty·ryl-CoA hy·dro·lase** (hi-drok″se-i″so-bu′tə-rəl ko-a′ hi′dro-lās) [EC 3.1.2.4] an enzyme of the hydrolase class that catalyzes the cleavage of the coenzyme A (CoA) moiety from 3-hydroxyisobutyryl CoA as a step in the use of valine as a fuel. Deficiency results in toxic tissue accumulation of the CoA thioester of methacrylic acid and its cysteine compound conjugates.

**3-hy·droxy·iso·va·ler·ic ac·id** (hi-drok″se-i″so-və-ler′ik) a methylated form of isovaleric acid accumulating abnormally and excreted in the urine in several disorders of leucine catabolism.

**hy·droxy·kyn·ure·nine** (hi-drok″se-kīn′u-rə-nēn″) a hydroxylated derivative of kynurenine, formed from kynurenine in the catabolism of tryptophan.

**hy·drox·yl** (hi-drok′səl) the univalent radical OH.

**hy·drox·yl·amine** (hi″drok-sil′ə-mēn) an unstable inorganic compound, $NH_2OH$, used as a reducing agent and in organic synthesis.

**hy·drox·yl·ap·a·tite** (hi-drok″səl-ap′ə-tīt) hydroxyapatite.

**hy·drox·y·lase** (hi-drok′sə-lās) a general term used to denote enzymes of the oxidoreductase class that catalyze the formation of a hydroxyl group on a substrate by incorporation of oxygen from $O_2$ [EC 1.13, 1.14]. Most are monooxygenases incorporating one atom of oxygen; more rarely the term is applied to a dioxygenase hydroxylating two substrates.
**11β-h.,** steroid 11β-monooxygenase.
**17α-h.,** steroid 17α-monooxygenase.
**18-h.,** corticosterone 18-monooxygenase; sometimes specifically the enzyme activity catalyzing the first (hydroxylation) reaction.
**21-h.,** steroid 21-monooxygenase.
**27-h.,** cholestanetriol 26-monooxygenase.

**11β-hy·drox·y·lase de·fi·cien·cy** an autosomal recessive disorder of steroidogenesis in which deficiency of steroid 11β-monooxygenase causes classic and nonclassic forms of one type of congenital adrenal hyperplasia (type IV). In the classic *(hypertensive)* form, the enzyme deficiency results in increased levels of cortisol precursors such as 11-deoxycortisol and the salt-retaining hormone 11-deoxycorticosterone, and decreased cortisol and aldosterone synthesis. Clinical manifestations include hypertension and, due to increased androgens, female pseudohermaphroditism and postnatal virilization of both sexes. The nonclassic *(late onset)* form is milder, and patients are frequently normotensive. See table at *hyperplasia.*

**17α-hy·drox·y·lase de·fi·cien·cy** an autosomal recessive disorder of steroidogenesis in which deficiency of steroid 17α-monooxygenase causes one type of congenital adrenal hyperplasia (type V). The disorder is characterized by decreased cortisol, androgens, estrogens, and aldosterone production and increases in 17-deoxysteroids such as corticosterone and deoxycorticosterone, resulting in hypertension, hypokalemia, and hypogonadism. Severe deficiency during fetal life can cause male pseudohermaphroditism; postnatally, it can impair sexual development in both males and females. See table at *hyperplasia* and see also *17,20 lyase deficiency.*

**18-hy·drox·y·lase de·fi·cien·cy** corticosterone methyl oxidase deficiency, sometimes used specifically to denote one of the two types.

**21-hy·drox·y·lase de·fi·cien·cy** an autosomal recessive disorder of steroidogenesis that can be lethal if not treated; deficiency of steroid 21-monooxygenase impairs the ability to produce all glucocorticoids. It causes several forms of the most common type of congenital adrenal hyperplasia (type III) and is divided into the more severe *classic forms* present at birth (*salt-losing* or *salt-wasting* and *simple virilizing* subtypes) and the less severe *nonclassic forms* of later onset (*late-onset* or *attenuated* and *cryptic* subtypes). The simple virilizing form is characterized clinically by female pseudohermaphroditism and postnatal virilization with advanced bodily development and biochemically by elevated androgens and decreased corticoids. The salt-losing form is additionally characterized by aldosterone deficiency and salt wasting. Patients with nonclassic forms display variable expression of androgen excess later in life, ranging from hirsutism and infertility *(late onset)* to absence of clinical signs *(cryptic).* See also table at *hyperplasia.*

**hy·droxy·ly·sine** (hi-drok″se-li′sēn) [MeSH: Hydroxylysine] a hydroxylated derivative of the amino acid lysine; it is a component of collagen, where its residues participate in the formation of cross-links and also act as attachment sites for disaccharide groups; it also occurs in complement C1q.

**hy·droxy·ly·syl ga·lac·to·syl·trans·fer·ase** (hi-drok″se-li′səl gal″ak-tōs″əl-trans′fər-ās) procollagen galactosyltransferase.

**hy·droxy·meth·yl** (hi-drok″se-meth′əl) the univalent radical $HOCH_2$— derived from methanol.

**hy·droxy·meth·yl·bil·ane syn·thase** (hi-drok″se-meth″əl-bil′ān sin′thās) [EC 4.3.1.8] an enzyme of the lyase class that catalyzes the deamination and condensation of four molecules of porphobilinogen to form a linear tetrapyrrole intermediate, hydroxymethylbilane, which cyclizes to form uroporphyrinogen. Alone, the enzyme produces uroporphyrinogen I; in the presence of uroporphyrinogen synthase it produces uroporphyrinogen III, the physiologically important isomer. Deficiency of the enzyme, an autosomal dominant trait, results in acute intermittent porphyria. Called also *porphobilinogen deaminase* and *uroporphyrinogen I synthase.*

**3-hy·droxy-3-meth·yl·glu·tar·ic ac·id** (hi-drok″sĭ-meth″əl-gloo-tar′ik) a dicarboxylic acid occurring at elevated levels in the urine in 3-hydroxy-3-methylglutaricaciduria.

**3-hy·droxy-3-meth·yl·glu·tar·ic·ac·id·uria** (hi-drok″sĭ-meth″əl-gloo-tar″ik-as″ə-du′re-ə) 1. an autosomal recessive aminoacidopathy characterized by excessive urinary excretion of 3-hydroxy-3-methylglutaric, 3-methylglutaconic, and related organic acids. Most cases are due to deficiency of hydroxymethylglutaryl-CoA lyase, are of neonatal or infantile onset, and are clinically similar to Reye's syndrome, with vomiting, lethargy, hypotonia, coma, nonketotic acidosis, hypoglycemia, and hyperammonemia. 2. urinary excretion of excess 3-hydroxy-3-methylglutaric acid. Written also *β-hydroxy-β-methylglutaricaciduria.*

**3-hy·droxy-3-meth·yl·glu·ta·ryl** (hi-drok″se-meth″əl-gloo′tə-rəl) a radical of 3-hydroxy-3-methylglutaric acid; the thioester it forms with coenzyme A, 3-hydroxy-3-methylglutaryl CoA, is an intermediate in the catabolism of leucine and in the synthesis of ketone bodies and cholesterol. Written also *β-hydroxy-β-methylglutaryl.*

**hy·droxy·meth·yl·glu·ta·ryl-CoA ly·ase** (hi-drok″se-meth″əl-gloo′tə-rəl ko-a′ li′ās) [EC 4.1.3.4] an enzyme of the lyase class that catalyzes the cleavage of 3-hydroxy-3-methylglutaryl CoA to form acetyl coenzyme A and acetoacetate. The reaction is a step in ketogenesis and in the catabolism of leucine. Deficiency of the enzyme, an autosomal recessive trait, causes 3-hydroxy-3-methylglutaricaciduria.

**hy·droxy·meth·yl·glu·ta·ryl-CoA re·duc·tase (NADPH)** (hi-drok″se-meth″əl-gloo′tə-rəl ko-a′ re-duk′tās) [EC 1.1.1.34] an enzyme of the oxidoreductase class that catalyzes the reduction of 3-hydroxy-3-methylglutaryl CoA to mevalonate, using NADPH as an electron donor. The reaction is a key rate-limiting step in the biosynthesis of cholesterol and the enzyme is inactivated by a specific kinase and reactivated by a specific phosphorylase.

**hy·droxy·meth·yl·glu·ta·ryl-CoA syn·thase** (hi-drok″se-meth″əl-gloo′tə-rəl ko-a′ sin′thās) [EC 4.1.3.5] [MeSH: Hydroxymethylglutaryl-CoA Synthase] an enzyme of the lyase class that catalyzes the condensation of acetyl coenzyme A and acetoacetyl coenzyme A to form 3-hydroxy-3-methylglutaryl CoA. A liver and kidney mitochondrial enzyme catalyzes the reaction as a step in ketogenesis; a cytosolic enzyme acts in the synthesis of cholesterol and other isoprenoids.

**hy·droxy·meth·yl·trans·fer·ase** (hi″-drok″se-meth″əl-trans′fər-ās) a term used in the names of some of the enzymes of the sub-subclass hydroxymethyl-, formyl-, and related transferases [EC 2.1.2] to denote those that catalyze the transfer of a hydroxymethyl group from a donor to an acceptor compound. Cf. *formyltransferase.*

**4-hy·droxy-2-oxo·glu·ta·rate al·do·lase** (hi-drok″se-ok″so-gloo′tə-rāt al′do-lās) [EC 4.1.3.16] an enzyme of the lyase class that catalyzes the cleavage of 4-hydroxy-α-ketoglutarate to form pyruvate and glyoxylate. The reaction is a step in the degradation of free hydroxyproline.

**hy·droxy·phen·a·mate** (hi-drok″se-fen′ə-māt) a minor tranquilizer formerly used in the treatment of anxiety and tension.

**hy·droxy·phen·yl·eth·yl·amine** (hi-drok″se-fen″əl-eth′əl-ə-mēn″) tyramine.

***p*-hy·droxy·phen·yl·py·ru·vate** (hi-drok″se-fen″əl-pi′roo-vāt) the anionic form of *p*-hydroxyphenylpyruvic acid. Written also *4-hydroxyphenylpyruvate.*

**4-hy·droxy·phen·yl·py·ru·vate di·oxy·gen·ase** (hi-drok″se-fen″əl-pi′roo-vāt di-ok′sə-jən-ās) [EC 1.13.11.27] [MeSH: 4-Hydroxyphenylpyruvate Dioxygenase] an enzyme of the oxidoreductase class that catalyzes the oxidation of *p*-hydroxyphenylpyruvate to homogentisate as a step in the use of tyrosine and phenylalanine as fuels. Deficiency of the enzyme, an autosomal dominant trait, causes hawkinsinuria.

***p*-hy·droxy·phen·yl·py·ru·vate ox·i·dase** (hi-drok″se-fen″əl-pi′roo-vāt ok′sĭ-dās) 4-hydroxyphenylpyruvate dioxygenase.

***p*-hy·droxy·phen·yl·py·ru·vic ac·id** (hi-drok″se-fen″əl-pi-roo′vik) the keto acid formed by transamination of tyrosine in the catabolism of tyrosine and phenylalanine; it occurs at elevated levels in the urine of patients with defects in tyrosine catabolism. Abbreviated PHPPA. Written also *4-hydroxyphenylpyruvic acid.*

**hy·droxy·preg·nen·o·lone** (hi-drok″se-preg-nēn′ə-lōn) [MeSH: Hydroxypregnenolone] pregnenolone bearing a hydroxyl; it is an intermediate in the biosynthesis of steroid hormones and is accumulated and excreted abnormally in some disorders of steroidogenesis.

**21-hy·droxy·pro·ges·ter·one** (hi-drok″se-pro-jes′tər-ōn) 11-deoxycorticosterone.

**17α-hy·droxy·pro·ges·ter·one al·do·lase** (hi-drok″se-pro-jes′tə-rōn al′do-lās) [EC 4.1.2.30] an enzyme of the lyase class that catalyzes the cleavage of the bond between carbons 17 and 20 in 17α-hydroxyprogesterone to form $\Delta^4$-androstenedione, an androgen. It also catalyzes the conversion of 17α-hydroxypregnenolone to dehydroepiandrosterone. The enzyme activity is part of the enzyme steroid 17α-monooxygenase. Deficiency of enzyme activity is called 17,20-lyase deficiency. Called also *17,20-lyase* and *17,20-desmolase.*

**hy·droxy·pro·ges·ter·one cap·ro·ate** (hi-drok″se-pro-jes′tər-ōn) [USP] a synthetic progestin used in the treatment of dysfunctional uterine bleeding, abnormalities of the menstrual cycle, endometriosis, and endometrial cancer, administered intramuscularly.

**hy·droxy·pro·line** (hi-drok″se-pro′lēn) [MeSH: Hydroxyproline] a hydroxylated form of the amino acid proline; it occurs in connective tissue proteins, particularly collagen. The majority is 4-hydroxyproline, but some of the 3-hydroxy form is also present.

**hy·droxy·pro·lin·e·mia** (hi-drok″sĭ-pro″lĭ-ne′meə) 1. excess of hydroxyproline in the blood. 2. an autosomal recessive aminoacidopathy characterized by an excess of free hydroxyproline in the plasma and urine, due to a defect in the enzyme hydroxyproline oxidase; it may be associated with mental retardation. Called also *hyperhydroxyprolinemia.*

**hy·droxy·pro·line ox·i·dase** (hi-drok″se-pro′lēn ok′sĭ-dās) an enzyme of the oxidoreductase class that catalyzes the oxidation of 4-hydroxyproline to form the 3-hydroxy analog of $\Delta^1$-pyrroline 5-carboxylate as part of the pathway of degradation of free hydroxyproline. Deficiency of the enzyme, an autosomal recessive trait, results in hydroxyprolinemia.

**hy·droxy·pro·pyl meth·yl·cel·lu·lose** (hi-drok″sə-pro′pəl meth″əl-sel′u-lōs) the propylene glycol ether of methylcellulose, supplied in differing degrees of viscosity; used as a suspending and viscosity-increasing agent and tablet excipient in pharmaceutical preparations, and applied topically to the conjunctiva to protect the cornea during certain ophthalmic procedures and to lubricate the cornea.

**hy·droxy·py·ru·vate** (hi-drok″sĭ-pi′roo-vāt) a carboxylic acid formed by the transamination of serine, serving as the primary source of D- and L-glyceric acid in plants and animals.

**8-hy·droxy·quin·o·line** (hi-drok″se-kwin′o-lēn) oxyquinoline.

**hy·droxy·ste·roid** (hi-drok″se-ster′oid) a steroid carrying a hydroxyl group, with the position and sometimes conformation of the group specified in the name of the compound.

**17-h.,** a steroid hydroxylated at the 17 carbon; usually used to denote a 17-hydroxycorticosteroid.

**3β-hy·droxy-Δ⁵-ste·roid de·hy·dro·gen·ase** (hi-drok″se-ster′oid de-hi′dro-jən-ās) [EC 1.1.1.145] an enzyme of the oxidoreductase class that catalyzes the dehydrogenation and isomerization of 3β-hydroxysteroids (e.g., pregnenolone) to 3-ketosteroids (e.g., progesterone), a step occurring in the biosynthetic pathways of all classes of corticosteroids.

**3β-hy·droxy·ste·roid de·hy·dro·gen·ase de·fi·cien·cy** an autosomal recessive disorder of steroidogenesis causing several forms of one type of congenital adrenal hyperplasia (type II): the classic forms are *salt-wasting* and the milder *non-salt-wasting,* and the nonclassic form is *late onset.* The enzyme deficiency is present in adrenals and gonads; pathways to cortisol, sex steroids, and aldosterone are blocked; and pregnenolone, 17α-hydroxypregnenolone, and dehydroepiandrosterone are elevated in plasma. Males affected during fetal life are pseudohermaphroditic; both sexes have slight postnatal virilization. Most common is the mildest form (late onset) but of the classic forms, salt-wasting is predominant. See also table at *hyperplasia.*

**11β-hy·droxy·ste·roid de·hy·dro·gen·ase** (hi-drok″se-ster′oid de-hi′dro-jən-ās) [EC 1.1.1.146] an enzyme of the oxidoreductase class that catalyzes the reversible hydrogenation-dehydrogenation reaction between cortisone and cortisol.

**11β-hy·droxy·ster·oid de·hy·dro·gen·ase de·fi·cien·cy** an enzyme deficiency resulting in excessive excretion of cortisol metabolites in the urine and an excess of mineralocorticoids in the kidneys, which causes potassium excretion (hypokalemia), sodium retention (hypernatremia), and hypertension.

**17β-hy·droxy·ste·roid de·hy·dro·gen·ase** (hi-drok″se-ster′oid de-hi′dro-jən-ās) testosterone 17β-dehydrogenase.

**17β-hy·droxy·ste·roid de·hy·dro·gen·ase de·fi·cien·cy** an autosomal recessive disorder of steroidogenesis due to deficiency of the testicular enzyme testosterone 17β-dehydrogenase. It is characterized by male pseudohermaphroditism with postpubertal virilization and sometimes gynecomastia. Plasma testosterone is decreased and androstenedione increased.

**18-hy·droxy·ste·roid de·hy·dro·gen·ase** (hi-drok″se-ster′oid de-hi′dro-jən-ās) the enzyme activity of corticosterone 18-monooxygenase specifically catalyzing the second (oxidation) reaction. Deficiency of this enzyme activity is called corticosterone methyl oxidase deficiency, type II.

**hy·droxy·stil·bam·i·dine is·eth·io·nate** (hi-drok″se-stil-bam′ĭ-dēn īs-ĕ-thi′ə-nāt) an antifungal and antiprotozoal used as an antileishmanial, administered by intramuscular or intravenous infusion. It has also been used in the treatment of some fungal infections, such as North American blastomycosis.

**5-hy·droxy·tryp·ta·mine (5-HT)** (hi-drok″se-trip′tə-mēn) serotonin.

**3-hy·droxy·ty·ra·mine** (hi-drok″se-ti′rə-mēn) dopamine.

**hy·droxy·urea** (hi-drok″se-u-re′ə) [USP] [MeSH: Hydroxyurea] an inhibitor of the enzyme ribonucleoside diphosphate reductase, which catalyzes the conversion of ribonucleotides to deoxyribonucleotides, an essential step in DNA synthesis. It is used as an antineoplastic agent primarily for treatment of busulfan-resistant chronic granulocytic leukemia, and also for the treatment of carcinoma of the head and neck, ovary, and cervix, malignant melanoma, and polycythemia vera; administered orally.

**hy·droxy·val·ine** (hi-drok″se-val′in) an amino acid obtained by protein hydrolysis.

**25-hy·droxy·vi·ta·min D** (hi-drok″se-vi′tə-min) either 25-hydroxycholecalciferol, the corresponding hydroxy- derivative of ergocalciferol, or both; assays evaluating stores of vitamin D by measuring serum levels of 25-hydroxyvitamin D usually reflect the total level of both compounds.

**25-hy·droxy·vi·ta·min $D_3$** (hi-drok″se-vi′tə-min) 25-hydroxycholecalciferol.

**hy·droxy·zine** (hi-drok′sə-zēn) [MeSH: Hydroxyzine] a synthetic drug with central nervous system depressant, antispasmodic, antihistaminic, and antifibrillatory actions.
**h. hydrochloride** [USP], the dihydrochloride salt of hydroxyzine used in the treatment of anxiety, tension, and agitation in conditions of emotional stress, in acute and chronic urticaria and other manifestations of allergic dermatoses, as an antiemetic, and as pre- and postoperative sedative, administered orally or intramuscularly.
**h. pamoate** [USP], the pamoate salt of hydroxyzine, having the actions and uses of the hydrochloride salt; administered orally.

**Hy·dro·zoa** (hi″dro-zo′ə) [Gr. *Hydra* a mythical nine-headed monster + *zoon* animal] a class of cnidarians that usually possess colonial branching polyps and small medusae (see *jellyfish*); it includes the poisonous genus *Physalia* (Portuguese man-of-war).

**hy·dro·zo·an** (hi″dro-zo′ən) an individual of the class Hydrozoa.

**hy·dru·ria** (hi-droo′re-ə) [*hydr-* + *-uria*] excretion of urine of low osmolality or specific gravity.

**hy·dru·ric** (hi-droo′rik) characterized by hydruria.

**Hy·ae·nan·che** (hi-ə-nang′ke) a genus of trees of the family Euphorbiaceae, native to southern Africa. *H. globo′sa* has poisonous fruit that contains the alkaloid hyenanchin.

**hy·e·nan·chin** (hi″ə-nan′kin) a poisonous alkaloid from the outer envelope of the fruit of *Hyaenanche globosa;* it somewhat resembles strychnine in its action.

**Hy·geia** (hi-je′ə) [Gr. *Hygieia*] the goddess of health, one of the daughters of Aesculapius.

**hy·gie·ist** (hi-je′ist) hygienist.

**hy·giene** (hi′jēn) [Gr. *hygieia* health] [MeSH: Hygiene] the science of health and of its preservation.
**dental h.,** oral h.
**industrial h.,** that branch of preventive medicine which is concerned with the protection of health of the industrial population.
**mouth h.,** oral h.
**oral h.,** the personal maintenance of cleanliness and hygiene of the teeth and oral structures by toothbrushing, tissue stimulation, gum massage, hydrotherapy, and other procedures recommended by the dentist or dental hygienist for the preservation of dental and oral health. Called also *dental h.* and *mouth h.*
**radiation h.,** the science of practices involved in human protection from radiation injury.

**hy·gien·ic** (hi-jen′ik) pertaining to hygiene, or conducive to health.

**hy·gien·ics** (hi-jen′iks) a system of principles for promoting health; hygiene.

**hy·gien·ist** (hi-jen′ist, hi″je-en′ist) a specialist in hygiene.
**dental h.,** a dental auxiliary specially trained in dental prophylaxis, who meets certain prescribed standards of education and clinical competence. Dental hygienists work under the direct supervision of the dentist; their functions include scaling and polishing the teeth, dental radiography, and teaching oral hygiene. Some states permit them to apply fluoride solution to the teeth.

**hy·gien·iza·tion** (hi-jen″ĭ-za′shən) the establishment of hygienic conditions.

**hy·gie·ol·o·gy** (hi″je-ol′ə-je) [Gr. *hygieia* health + *-logy*] the complete science upon which the arts of hygiene and sanitation are based.

**hy·gio·gen·e·sis** (hi″je-o-jen′ə-sis) [Gr. *hygiēs* healthy + *-genesis*] the mechanism of the processes which lead to maintenance of health.

**hy·gi·ol·o·gy** (hi″je-ol′ə-je) hygieology.

**hy·gre·che·ma** (hi″grə-ke′mə) an auscultation sound caused by the presence of water.

**hy·gric** (hi′grik) [*hygr-* + *-ic*] pertaining or relating to moisture.

**hygr(o)-** [Gr. *hygros* moist] a combining form meaning moist or denoting relationship to moisture.

**hy·gro·ble·phar·ic** (hi″gro-blə-far′ik) [*hygro-* + *blephar-* + *-ic*] 1. denoting an excessive watery condition of the eyelids. 2. pertaining to any gland bringing moisture to the eyelids.

**hy·gro·ma** (hi-gro′mə) pl. *hygromas* or *hygro′mata* [*hygro-* + *-oma*] a sac, cyst, or bursa distended with a fluid.
**h. col′li,** a watery tumor of the neck.
**cystic h., h. cys′ticum,** a lymphangioma, usually in the neck area, composed of large, multilocular, thin-walled cysts. It may become large and exert pressure on adjacent structures. Called also *cavernous* or *cystic lymphangioma.*
**h. praepatella′re,** housemaid's knee.
**subdural h.,** a collection of fluid in the subdural space resulting from liquefaction of a subdural hematoma; see under *hematoma.*

**hy·gro·ma·tous** (hi-gro′mə-təs) pertaining to or of the nature of hygroma.

**hy·grom·e·ter** (hi-grom′ə-tər) [*hygro-* + *-meter*] an instrument for measuring the moisture of the atmosphere.
**hair h., Saussure's h.,** a hygrometer whose action is determined by the elongation and contraction of a hair under the influence of moisture.

**hy·gro·met·ric** (hi″gro-met′rik) pertaining to hygrometry.

**hy·grom·e·try** (hi-grom′ə-tre) [*hygro-* + *-metry*] the measurement of the proportion of moisture in the air.

**hy·gro·my·cin** (hi″gro-mi′sin) an antibiotic produced by *Streptomyces hygroscopicus* and *S. noboritoensis;* called also *hygromycin A.*
**h. B,** an antibiotic unrelated to hygromycin but also produced by *Streptomyces hygroscopicus;* used as an anthelmintic in swine.

**hy·gro·scop·ic** (hi″gro-skop′ik) taking up and retaining moisture readily.

**Hy·gro·ton** (hi′gro-ton) trademark for a preparation of chlorthalidone.

**Hy·kin·one** (hi′kin-ōn) trademark for a preparation of menadione sodium bisulfite.

**hyle-** see *hyl(o)-.*

**Hy·le·my·ia** (hi″lə-mi′ə) a genus of flies, the larvae of which infest vegetables and may be swallowed if the latter are eaten raw. *H. anti′qua,* onion root maggot. *H. bras′sicae,* the cabbage root maggot.

**hyl(o)-** [Gr. *hylē* matter] a combining form denoting relationship to matter, material, or substance. Also *hyle-.*

**Hy·lo·rel** (hi′lo-rel″) trademark for a preparation of guanadrel sulfate.

**hy·lo·trop·ic** (hi″lo-trop′ik) pertaining to or characterized by hylotropy.

**hy·lot·ro·py** (hi-lot′rə-pe) [*hylo-* + *-tropy*] the ability of a substance to change from one physical form to another (e.g., solid to liquid, liquid to gas) without change in chemical composition; change of phase.

**hy·men** (hi′mən) [Gr. *hymēn* membrane] [TA] [MeSH: Hymen] the membranous fold which partially or wholly occludes the external orifice of the vagina.
**annular h.,** circular h.
**h. bifenestra′tus, h. bifo′ris,** a hymen with two openings side by side and a broad septum between them.

**circular h.**, a hymen with a circular opening.
**cribriform h.**, a hymen pierced by many small perforations.
**denticular h.**, a hymen with an opening which has serrate edges.
**falciform h.**, a sickle-shaped hymen.
**fenestrated h.**, cribriform h.
**imperforate h.**, one which completely closes the vaginal orifice.
**lunar h.**, a moon-shaped hymen.
**persistent h.**, white heifer disease.
**septate h., h. sep'tus**, a hymen in which the opening is divided by a narrow septum.
**h. subsep'tus**, a hymen in which the opening is partially filled by a septum growing out of one wall, but not reaching the other.

**hy·men·al** (hi'mən-əl) pertaining to the hymen.

**hy·men·ec·to·my** (hi"mən-ek'tə-me) [*hymen-* + *-ectomy*] excision of the hymen.

**hy·men·itis** (hi"mən-i'tis) [*hymen-* + *-itis*] inflammation of the hymen.

**hy·me·ni·um** (hi-me'ne-əm) [dim. of Gr. *hymēn* membrane] the fertile, or spore-forming, surface of a fungus, which is composed of hyphae lining the fruiting body.

**hymen(o)-** [Gr. *hymēn* membrane] a combining form denoting a relationship to a membrane or a membranous structure, or to the hymen.

**hy·me·no·lep·i·a·sis** (hi"mə-no-lep-i'ə-sis) [MeSH: Hymenolepiasis] infection with *Hymenolepis*.

**Hy·me·no·lep·i·di·dae** (hi"mən-o-lep'ĭ-di-de) a family of small to medium-sized tapeworms of the order Cyclophyllidea, subclass Cestoda, which parasitizes birds and mammals, including man. *Hymenolepis* is the genus of medical importance.

**Hy·me·nol·e·pis** (hi"mə-nol'ə-pis) [Gr. *hymēn* membrane + *lepis* rind] [MeSH: Hymenolepis] a genus of tapeworms of the family Hymenolepididae.
**H. diminu'ta**, a tapeworm of rats and mice, occasionally found in man.
**H. frater'na**, the rodent form of *H. nana;* often called *H. nana* var. *fraterna.*
**H. lanceola'ta**, a species that infects ducks and geese and has been reported in a human being.
**H. na'na**, the dwarf tapeworm, a species about 7 to 80 mm long that is parasitic in rats, mice, and man, especially children. Infected persons are usually asymptomatic, but in massive infection symptoms may include dizziness, abdominal pain, diarrhea, insomnia, convulsions, etc.
**H. na'na** var. **frater'na**, *H. fraterna.*

**hy·men·ol·o·gy** (hi"mən-ol'ə-je) [*hymeno-* + *-logy*] the sum of what is known regarding the membranes of the body.

**Hy·me·no·my·ce·tes** (hi"mə-no-mi-se'tēz) [*hymeno-* + Gr. *mykēs* fungus] in some classification systems, a category of perfect fungi at around the class level that would include the subclasses Phragmobasidiomycetidae and Holobasidiomycetidae.

**Hy·men·op·tera** (hi"mən-op'tər-ə) [*hymeno-* + Gr. *pteron* wing] [MeSH: Hymenoptera] an order of insects usually having two pairs of well-developed membranous wings. It includes the families Apidae (bees), Formicidae (ants), and Vespidae (wasps).

**hy·men·op·ter·an** (hi"mən-op'tər-ən) any insect of the order Hymenoptera.

**hy·men·op·ter·ism** (hi"mən-op'tər-iz-əm) poisoning by the stings or bites of insects of the order Hymenoptera, as of a bee or wasp.

**hy·men·or·rha·phy** (hi"mən-or'ə-fe) [*hymeno-* + *-rrhaphy*] the closure of the vagina by sutures at the hymen.

**Hy·me·no·sto·ma·tia** (hi"mə-no-sto-ma'she-ə) [*hymeno-* + Gr. *stoma* mouth] a subclass of chiefly freshwater, ciliate protozoa (class Oligohymenophorea, phylum Ciliophora) with uniform, heavy body ciliature and a ventral buccal cavity when one is present; if kinetodesmata are present, they are usually conspicuous. It comprises three orders: Hymenostomatida, Scuticociliatida, and Astomatida.

**Hy·me·no·sto·ma·ti·da** (hi"mə-no-sto-ma'tĭ-də) [MeSH: Hymenostomatida] an order of ciliate protozoa (subclass Hymenostomatia, class Oligohymenophorea) characterized by the presence of a well-defined buccal cavity containing membranelles or peniculi with infraciliary bases typically three to four rows of kinetosomes wide; and by a ventral oral area, usually in the anterior half of the body. It comprises three suborders: Tetrahymenina, Ophryoglenina, and Peniculina.

**hy·men·ot·o·my** (hi"mən-ot'ə-me) [*hymeno-* + *-tomy*] surgical incision of the hymen.

**hy·me·no·vin** (hi"mə-no'vin) a toxic lactone that is the active principle in species of *Hymenoxys* and causes gastroenteritis in cattle and sheep.

**Hy·men·ox·ys** (hi"mə-nok'sis) a genus of herbs found in North America; some species contain the lactone hymenovin, which causes gastroenteritis and vomiting in cattle and sheep. Two common poisonous species are *H. odora'ta,* the bitterweed, and *H. richardso'nii,* the pingue or rubberweed.

**hyo·epi·glot·tic** (hi"o-ep"ĭ-glot'ik) pertaining to the hyoid bone and the epiglottis.

**hyo·epi·glot·tid·e·an** (hi"o-ep"ĭ-glŏ-tid'e-ən) hyoepiglottic.

**hyo·glos·sal** (hi"o-glos'əl) [hyoid bone + *glossal*] pertaining to the hyoid bone and the tongue or to the hyoglossal muscle.

**hy·oid** (hi'oid) [Gr. *hyoeides* shaped like the Greek letter upsilon (υ)] 1. shaped like the lower case Greek letter upsilon (υ). Cf. *hypsiloid.* 2. shaped like a U. 3. pertaining to the hyoid bone.

**hyo·scine** (hi'o-sēn) [L. *hyoscina*] scopolamine.

**hyo·scy·amine** (hi"o-si'ə-mēn) [USP] an anticholinergic alkaloid derived from *Hyoscyamus niger, Atropa belladonna,* and other solanaceous plants; it is the levorotatory component of racemic atropine with actions and uses similar to those of atropine but with more potent central and peripheral effects. It is administered orally or parenterally.
**h. hydrobromide** [USP], a salt of hyoscyamine, having actions and uses similar to those of atropine, administered orally or parenterally.
**h. sulfate** [USP], a salt of hyoscyamine, having actions and uses similar to those of atropine, administered orally or parenterally.

**Hyo·scy·a·mus** (hi"o-si'ə-məs) [L.; Gr. *hys* swine + *kyamos* bean] a genus of annual or biennial plants of the family Solanaceae. *H. ni 'ger* L. is henbane, whose leaves, seeds, flowers, and tops contain the anticholinergic alkaloids hyoscyamine and scopolamine and cause neurotoxicity in livestock. See also *hyoscyamus.*

**hy·o·scy·a·mus** (hi"o-si'ə-məs) the dried leaf of *Hyoscyamus niger,* with or without its stem and top, which contains the anticholinergic alkaloids hyoscyamine and scopolamine; formerly used as a smooth muscle relaxant and to produce parasympathetic blockade. Called also *henbane* and *black henbane.*

**Hyo·stron·gy·lus** (hi"o-stron'jə-ləs) a genus of nematodes of the family Trichostrongylidae. *H. ru'bidus* is found in the stomachs of pigs.

**hyo·thy·roid** (hi"o-thi'roid) pertaining to the hyoid bone and the thyroid cartilage.

**hyp·acu·sia** (hi"pə-koo'zhə) hypoacusis.

**hyp·acu·sis** (hi"pə-koo'sis) hypoacusis.

**hyp·al·bu·min·emia** (hi"pal-bu"mĭn-e'me-ə) hypoalbuminemia.

**hyp·al·ge·sia** (hi"pal-je'ze-ə) [*hyp-* + *algesia*] decreased pain sense; called also *hypalgia* and *hypoalgesia.*

**hyp·al·ge·sic** (hi"pəl-je'sik) pertaining to, characterized by, or producing hypalgesia.

**hyp·al·get·ic** (hi"pəl-jet'ik) hypalgesic.

**hyp·al·gia** (hi-pal'jə) hypalgesia.

**hyp·am·ni·on** (hi-pam'ne-on) hypamnios.

**hyp·am·ni·os** (hi-pam'ne-os) [*hypo* + *amnion*] deficiency of the amniotic fluid.

**hyp·ana·ki·ne·sia** (hi-pan"ə-kĭ-ne'zhə) [Gr. *hypo* under + *anakinēsis* exercise + *-ia*] hypokinesia.

**hyp·ana·ki·ne·sis** (hi-pan"ə-kĭ-ne'sis) hypokinesia.

**hy·paph·o·rine** (hi-paf'o-rin) a crystalline alkaloid, obtained from *Erythrina americana* Mill., and other members of Leguminosae; it is a convulsive poisonous alkaloid.

**Hy·paque** (hi'pāk) trademark for preparations of diatrizoate meglumine and diatrizoate sodium.

**hyp·ar·te·ri·al** (hi"par-tēr-e-əl) [*hypo* + *arterial*] beneath an artery, applied especially to the bronchi which are so situated.

**hyp·ax·i·al** (hi-pak'se-əl) ventral to the long axis of the body.

**hyp·azo·tu·ria** (hĭ-paz"o-tu're-ə) hypoazoturia.

**hyp·en·chyme** (hi'pən-kīm) the primitive embryonic tissue formed in the cavity of the archenteron.

**hyper-** [Gr. *hyper* above] a prefix meaning above, beyond, more than normal, or excessive.

**hy·per·ab·sorp·tion** (hi"pər-ab-sorp'shən) increased intestinal absorption of a substance.

**hy·per·ac·an·tho·sis** (hi"pər-ak"ən-tho'sis) [*hyper-* + *acanth-* + *-osis*] acanthosis.

**hy·per·ac·id** (hi"pər-as'id) [*hyper-* + L. *acidus* sour] abnormally or excessively acid.

**hy·per·ac·id·am·in·uria** (hi″pər-as″id-am″ĭ-nu′re-ə) excess of amino acids in the urine.

**hy·per·ac·id·i·ty** (hi″pər-ə-sid′ĭ-te) an excessive degree of acidity.
**gastric h.**, hyperchlorhydria.

**hy·per·acou·sia** (hi″pər-ə-koo′zhə) hyperacusis.

**hy·per·ac·tive** (hi″pər-ak′tiv) pertaining to or characterized by hyperactivity.

**hy·per·ac·tiv·i·ty** (hi-pər-ak-tiv′ĭ-te) 1. excessive or abnormally increased muscular function or activity. 2. former name for, but now one of the signs of, *attention-deficit/hyperactivity disorder.*

**hy·per·acu·sia** (hi″pər-ə-koo′ze-ə) hyperacusis.

**hy·per·acu·sis** (hi″pər-ə-koo′sis) [*hyper-* + *acou-* + *-sis*] exceptionally acute hearing, the hearing threshold being unusually low. It may or may not be accompanied by pain. Called also *hyperacousia, hyperacusia, hyperakusis,* and *acoustic* or *auditory hyperesthesia.*

**hy·per·acute** (hi″pər-ə-kūt′) extremely acute.

**hy·per·ad·e·no·sis** (hi″pər-ad″ə-no′sis) [*hyper-* + *adenosis*] a condition characterized by enlargement of the glands.

**hy·per·ad·i·po·sis** (hi″pər-ad″ĭ-po′sis) [*hyper-* + *adiposis*] morbid obesity.

**hy·per·ad·i·pos·i·ty** (hi″pər-ad″ĭ-pos′ĭ-te) morbid obesity.

**hy·per·adre·nal·ism** (hi″pər-ə-dre′nəl-iz-əm) abnormally increased secretion of adrenal hormones.

**hy·per·adre·no·cor·ti·cism** (hi″pər-ə-dre″no-kor′tĭ-siz-əm) abnormally increased secretion of adrenocortical hormones, as in *Cushing's syndrome.* Called also *hypercorticalism, hypercorticism,* and *hypercortisolism.*

**hy·per·aku·sis** (hi″pər-ə-koo′sis) hyperacusis.

**hy·per-β-al·a·nin·emia** (hi″pər-ba″tə-al″ə-nĭ-ne′me-ə) a rare disorder of β-alanine metabolism, possibly an autosomal recessive trait, due to deficiency of β-alanine–α-ketoglutarate transaminase activity; β-alanine, β-aminoisobutyric acid, taurine, and γ-aminobutyric acid are accumulated and excreted at elevated levels and the disorder is characterized by lethargy, somnolence, and grand mal seizures. Called also *β-alaninemia.*

**hy·per·al·bu·min·emia** (hi″pər-al-bu″mĭ-ne′me-ə) an abnormally high albumin content of the blood.

**hy·per·al·bu·min·o·sis** (hi″pər-al-bu″mĭ-no′sis) a condition characterized by presence of an excess of albuminoids.

**hy·per·al·dos·ter·on·emia** (hi″pər-al-dos″tə-ro-ne′me-ə) abnormal increase in the level of aldosterone in the blood.

**hy·per·al·dos·ter·on·ism** (hi″pər-al-dos′tə-ro-niz″əm) [MeSH: Hyperaldosteronism] aldosteronism.

**hy·per·al·dos·ter·on·uria** (hi″pər-al-dos″tə-ro-nu′re-ə) the presence of excessive amounts of aldosterone in the urine. Called also *aldosteronuria.*

**hy·per·al·ge·sia** (hi″pər-al-je′ze-ə) [*hyper-* + Gr. *algesia*] [MeSH: Hyperalgesia] abnormally increased pain sense; called also *hyperalgia.*
**auditory h.**, the condition in which slight noises cause pain.
**muscular h.**, the condition in which slight exertion causes great pain.

**hy·per·al·ge·sic** (hi″pər-al-je′sik) pertaining to or characterized by hyperalgesia.

**hy·per·al·get·ic** (hi″pər-al-jet′ik) hyperalgesic.

**hy·per·al·gia** (hi-pər-al′jə) [*hyper-* + *-algia*] hyperalgesia.

**hy·per·al·i·men·ta·tion** (hi″pər-al″ĭ-men-ta′shən) 1. ingestion of excessive quantities; see also *bulimia* and *binge eating.* 2. administration of a greater than optimal amount of nutrients.
**parenteral h.**, see *total parenteral alimentation,* under *alimentation.*

**hy·per·al·i·men·to·sis** (hi″pər-al″ĭ-men-to′sis) disease due to hyperalimentation (q.v.).

**hy·per·al·ka·les·cence** (hi″pər-al″kə-les′əns) an excess of alkalinity.

**hy·per·al·ka·lin·i·ty** (hi″pər-al″kə-lin′ĭ-te) excessive alkalinity.

**hy·per·al·lan·to·in·uria** (hi″pər-ə-lan″to-ĭ-nu′re-ə) an excess of allantoin in the urine.

**hy·per·al·o·ne·mia** (hi″pər-al″o-ne′me-ə) [*hyper-* + Gr. *hals* salt + *-emia*] hypersalemia.

**hy·per·al·pha·lipo·pro·tein·emia** (hi″pər-al″fə-lip″o-pro″te-ne′me-ə) the presence of abnormally high levels of high-density lipoproteins in the serum.
**familial h.**, an inherited elevation of high-density lipoproteins and cholesterol; it is associated with longevity and decreased risk of myocardial infarction.

**hy·per·am·i·no·ac·i·de·mia** (hi″pər-ə-me″-no-as″ĭ-de′me-ə) presence of amino acids in the blood in excess of the normal amount.

**hy·per·ami·no·ac·id·uria** (hi″pər-ə-me″no-as″ĭ-du′re-ə) aminoaciduria.

**hy·per-β-ami·no·iso·bu·tyr·ic·ac·id·uria** (hi″pər-ə-me″no-i″so-bu-tir″ik-as″ĭ-du′re-ə) β-aminoisobutyricaciduria.

**hy·per·am·mo·ne·mia** (hi″pər-am″o-ne′me-ə) elevated levels of ammonia or its compounds in the blood. Called also *ammonemia.*
**cerebroatrophic h.**, Rett syndrome.

**hy·per·am·mo·nu·ria** (hi″pər-am″o-nu′re-ə) increased excretion of ammonia in the urine.

**hy·per·am·y·las·emia** (hi″pər-am″ə-la-se′me-ə) abnormally high elevation of amylase in the blood serum.

**hy·per·ana·ci·ne·sia** (hi″pər-an″ə-si-ne′zhə) hyperdynamia.

**hy·per·ana·ki·ne·sia** (hi″pər-an″ə-kĭ-ne′zhə) [*hyper-* + Gr. *anakinēsis* exercise + *-ia*] hyperdynamia.

**hy·per·an·dro·gen·ism** (hi″pər-an′dro-jən-iz-əm) [MeSH: Hyperandrogenism] the state of having excessive secretion of androgens, as seen in congenital adrenal hyperplasia, some types of precocious puberty, and other conditions.

**hy·per·aphia** (hi″pər-a′fe-ə) [*hyper-* + Gr. *haphē* touch] tactile hyperesthesia.

**hy·per·aph·ic** (hi″pər-af′ik) pertaining to or characterized by hyperaphia (tactile hyperesthesia).

**hy·per·ar·gin·in·emia** (hi″pər-ahr″jĭ-nĭ-ne′me-ə) 1. arginase deficiency. 2. excess of arginine in the blood.

**hy·per·arou·sal** (hi″pər-ə-rou′səl) a state of increased psychological and physiological tension marked by such effects as reduced tolerance to pain, anxiety, exaggerated startle responses, insomnia, fatigue, and accentuation of personality traits.

**hy·per·azo·te·mia** (hi″pər-az″o-te′me-ə) an excess of nitrogenous matter, usually urea, in the blood.

**hy·per·azo·tu·ria** (hi″pər-az″o-tu′re-ə) presence of an excessive amount of nitrogenous matter in the urine.

**hy·per·bar·ic** (hi″pər-bar′ik) [*hyper-* + *bar-* + *-ic*] having greater than normal pressure or weight; applied to gases under greater than atmospheric pressure, or to a solution of greater specific gravity than another taken as a standard of reference.

**hy·per·bar·ism** (hi″pər-bar′iz-əm) the condition resulting from exposure to ambient gas pressure or atmospheric pressures that exceed the pressure within body tissues, fluids, and cavities.

**hy·per·baso·phil·ic** (hi″pər-ba″so-fil′ik) staining intensely with basic dyes.

**hy·per·be·ta·lipo·pro·tein·emia** (hi″pər-ba″tə-lip″o-pro″te-ne′me-ə) increased accumulation of low-density lipoproteins in the blood.
**familial h.**, familial hypercholesterolemia.

**hy·per·bi·car·bo·nat·emia** (hi″pər-bi-kahr″bə-na-te′me-ə) the presence of an excessive amount of bicarbonate in the blood; see also *alkalosis.*

**hy·per·bil·i·ru·bin·emia** (hi″pər-bil″ĭ-roo″bĭ-ne′me-ə) [MeSH: Hyperbilirubinemia] excessive concentrations of bilirubin in the blood, which may lead to jaundice; the hyperbilirubinemias are classified as conjugated or unconjugated, according to the predominant form of bilirubin in the blood.
**h. I**, Gilbert syndrome.
**congenital h.**, Crigler-Najjar syndrome.
**conjugated h.**, that due to defective excretion of conjugated bilirubin by the liver cells or to anatomic obstruction to bile flow within the liver or in the extrahepatic bile duct system; it includes Dubin-Johnson syndrome and Rotor's syndrome.
**constitutional h.**, Gilbert syndrome.
**neonatal h.**, a mild, transient hyperbilirubinemia of the unconjugated type occurring in the normal neonate; a transient familial form also occurs, with onset of jaundice within four days after birth, which may lead to kernicterus.
**unconjugated h.**, that due to excessive bilirubin production (hemolysis), to defective clearance of bilirubin from the blood by the liver, or to defective conjugation by the liver; it includes hemolytic states, Crigler-Najjar syndrome, Gilbert syndrome, and neonatal hyperbilirubinemia.

**hy·per·brachy·ce·phal·ic** (hi″pər-brak″e-sə-fal′ik) having a cephalic index of 85.5 or more.

**hy·per·brachy·ceph·a·ly** (hi″pər-brak″e-sef′ə-le) the condition of being hyperbrachycephalic.

**hy·per·brady·ki·nin·emia** (hi″pər-brad″e-ki″nĭ-ne′me-ə) elevated levels of bradykinin in the blood, marked by a feeling of warmth, flushing, wheezing, or nausea.

**hy·per·brady·ki·nin·ism** (hi″pər-brad″e-ki′nĭ-niz-əm) a syndrome characterized by high plasma levels of bradykinin, in which standing produces a fall in systolic blood pressure, an increase in diastolic pressure and heart rate, and a purplish discoloration and ecchymoses over the legs.

**hy·per·cal·ce·mia** (hi″pər-kal-se′me-ə) [*hyper-* + *calci-* + *-emia*] [MeSH: Hypercalcemia] an excess of calcium in the blood; manifestations include fatigability, muscle weakness, depression, anorexia, nausea, and constipation. Called also *calcemia* and *hypercalcinemia.*
**familial hypocalciuric h.,** an autosomal dominant type of hypercalcemia with vague and mild symptoms.
**idiopathic h.,** a condition of infants, associated with vitamin D intoxication, and characterized by elevated serum calcium levels and increased density of the skeleton, with mental deterioration progressing to severe retardation, and nephrocalcinosis causing chronic uremia.

**hy·per·cal·ci·ne·mia** (hi″pər-kal″sĭ-ne′me-ə) hypercalcemia.

**hy·per·cal·ci·nu·ria** (hi″pər-kal″sĭ-nu′re-ə) hypercalciuria.

**hy·per·cal·ci·pexy** (hi″pər-kal′sĭ-pek″se) excessive fixation of calcium.

**hy·per·cal·ci·to·nin·emia** (hi″pər-kal″sĭ-to″nĭ-ne′me-ə) an excess of calcitonin in the blood.

**hy·per·cal·ci·uria** (hi″pər-kal″se-u′re-ə) excess of calcium in the urine.
**absorptive h.,** hypercalciuria due to hyperabsorption of calcium, with formation of calcium oxalate or calcium phosphate renal stones.

**hy·per·cap·nia** (hi″pər-kap′ne-ə) [*hyper-* + *capn-* + *-ia*] [MeSH: Hypercapnia] excess of carbon dioxide in the blood. Called also *hypercarbia.*
**permissive h.,** artificially induced hypercapnia in patients with acute respiratory distress syndrome or respiratory failure, done to lower the inspiratory pressure and tidal volume and thus the possibility of lung injury.

**hy·per·cap·nic** (hi″pər-kap′nik) pertaining to or characterized by hypercapnia.

**hy·per·car·bia** (hi″pər-kahr′be-ə) hypercapnia.

**hy·per·car·o·ten·emia** (hi″pər-kar″ə-tə-ne′me-ə) an elevated level of carotene in the blood, resulting from excessive ingestion of carotenoids or from decreased ability to convert carotenoids to vitamin A; it is often characterized by yellowing of the skin (see *carotenosis* ). Called also *carotenemia.*

**hy·per·cat·a·bol·ic** (hi″pər-kat″ə-bol′ik) pertaining to, characterized by, or causing hypercatabolism.

**hy·per·ca·tab·o·lism** (hi″pər-kə-tab′o-liz-əm) abnormally increased catabolism.

**hy·per·ca·thar·sis** (hi″pər-kə-thahr′sis) [*hyper-* + *catharsis*] excessive purgation.

**hy·per·ca·thar·tic** (hi″pər-kə-thahr′tik) excessively cathartic.

**hy·per·cel·lu·lar** (hi″pər-sel′u-lər) pertaining to or characterized by hypercellularity.

**hy·per·cel·lu·lar·i·ty** (hi″pər-sel″u-lar′ĭ-te) a state characterized by an abnormal increase in the number of cells present, as in bone marrow.

**hy·per·ce·men·to·sis** (hi″pər-se″mən-to′sis) [MeSH: Hypercementosis] a regressive change of teeth characterized by excessive development of secondary cementum on the tooth surface; it may occur on any part of the root, but the apical two-thirds are most commonly affected. Called also *cementosis* and *cementum hyperplasia.*

**hy·per·chlor·emia** (hi″pər-klor-e′me-ə) an excess of chloride in the blood.

**hy·per·chlor·emic** (hi″pər-klor-e′mik) pertaining to or characterized by hyperchloremia.

**hy·per·chlor·hy·dria** (hi″pər-klor-hi′dre-ə) excessive secretion of hydrochloric acid by the stomach cells. Called also *chlorhydria* and *hyperhydrochloria.*

**hy·per·chlor·ura·tion** (hi″pər-klor″u-ra′shən) an excess of chlorides in the body.

**hy·per·chlor·uria** (hi″pər-klor-u′re-ə) excess of chlorides in the urine.

**hy·per·cho·les·ter·emia** (hi″pər-kə-les″tər-e′me-ə) hypercholesterolemia.

**hy·per·cho·les·ter·ol·emia** (hi″pər-kə-les″tər-ol-e′me-ə) [MeSH: Hypercholesterolemia] excess of cholesterol in the blood.
**familial h.,** an inherited disorder of lipoprotein metabolism resulting from defects in the cellular receptor for plasma low-density lipoprotein (LDL) and inherited as an autosomal dominant trait with gene dosage effect. It is characterized by cutaneous and tendinous xanthomas, corneal arcus, and premature coronary atherosclerosis. The biochemical phenotype, elevated plasma LDL and cholesterol, is that of a type II-a hyperlipoproteinemia; rarely, plasma very-low-density lipoproteins and triglycerides may also be elevated, a type II-b phenotype. See table at *hyperlipoproteinemia.*
**polygenic h.,** any of a diverse group of disorders in which some combination of genetic, and frequently also environmental, factors interact to cause elevated plasma cholesterol (i.e., a hyperlipoproteinemia type II-a or II-b phenotype; see table at *hyperlipoproteinemia*). It is distinguished from familial hypercholesterolemia and familial combined hyperlipidemia.

**hy·per·cho·les·ter·ol·emic** (hi″pər-kə-les″tər-ol-e′mik) pertaining to, characterized by, or tending to produce hypercholesterolemia.

**hy·per·cho·les·ter·ol·ia** (hi″pər-kə-les″tər-ol′e-ə) abnormally high cholesterol content of the bile.

**hy·per·cho·lia** (hi″pər-ko′le-ə) [*hyper-* + *chol-* + *-ia*] excessive secretion of bile.

**hy·per·chon·dro·pla·sia** (hi″pər-kon″dro-pla′shə) excessive development of cartilage.

**hy·per·chro·maf·fin·ism** (hi″pər-kro-maf′ĭ-niz-əm) a condition caused by excessive release of biogenic amines from chromaffin cells, as in pheochromocytoma; the major symptom is arterial hypertension.

**hy·per·chro·ma·sia** (hi″pər-kro-ma′shə) hyperchromatism.

**hy·per·chro·mat·ic** (hi″pər-kro-mat′ik) 1. staining more intensely than is normal. 2. pertaining to or marked by hyperchromatism.

**hy·per·chro·ma·tin** (hi″pər-kro′mə-tin) the part of the chromatin that stains with blue aniline dyes.

**hy·per·chro·ma·tism** (hi″pər-kro′mə-tiz-əm) [*hyper-* + *chromato-* + *-ism*] excessive pigmentation in the form of a darkly staining cell nucleus, the consequence of an excess of chromatin. Called also *hyperchromasia, hyperchromatosis,* and *hyperchromia.*

**hy·per·chro·ma·to·sis** (hi″pər-kro″mə-to′sis) 1. increased staining capacity. 2. hyperchromatism.

**hy·per·chro·mia** (hi″pər-kro′me-ə) hyperchromatism.

**hy·per·chro·mic** (hi″pər-kro′mik) highly or excessively stained or colored.

**hy·per·chy·lia** (hi″pər-ki′le-ə) excessive secretion of gastric juice.

**hy·per·chy·lo·mi·cron·emia** (hi″pər-ki″lo-mi″kro-ne′me-ə) the presence in the blood of an excess of chylomicrons. Called also *chylomicronemia.*
**familial h.,** an inherited disorder of lipoprotein metabolism characterized by elevated plasma chylomicrons and triglycerides and manifest clinically by episodic abdominal pain and pancreatitis, cutaneous xanthomas, lipemia retinalis, and hepatosplenomegaly. It is usually due to deficiency of lipoprotein lipase (q.v.) or its cofactor apolipoprotein C-II (see under *deficiency* ), or to a combination of a familial hypertriglyceridemia with an exacerbating secondary factor. The biochemical phenotype is that of a type I or type V hyperlipoproteinemia, depending on whether very-low-density lipoprotein levels are normal or elevated, respectively; the latter case is sometimes called *hyperprebetalipoproteinemia.* See also table at *hyperlipoproteinemia.*
**familial h. with hyperprebetalipoproteinemia,** see *familial h.*

**hy·per·ci·ne·sia** (hi″pər-sĭ-ne′zhə) hyperkinesia.

**hy·per·co·ag·u·la·bil·i·ty** (hi″pər-ko-ag″u-lə-bil′ĭ-te) the state of being more readily coagulated than normal.

**hy·per·co·ag·u·la·ble** (hi″pər-ko-ag′u-lə-bəl) characterized by hypercoagulability.

**hy·per·co·ria** (hi″pər-kor′e-ə) hyperkoria.

**hy·per·cor·ti·cal·ism** (hi″pər-kor′tĭ-kəl-iz-əm) hyperadrenocorticism.

**hy·per·cor·ti·cism** (hi″pər-kor′tĭ-siz-əm) hyperadrenocorticism.

**hy·per·cor·ti·sol·ism** (hi″pər-kor′tĭ-sol″iz-əm) hyperadrenocorticism.

**hy·per·cre·a·tin·emia** (hi″pər-kre″ə-tĭ-ne′me-ə) an abnormality of creatine metabolism in skeletal muscle, a common feature of thyrotoxicosis.

**hy·per·cry·al·ge·sia** (hi″pər-kri″al-je′ze-ə) [*hyper-* + Gr. *cryo-* + *algesia*] hypercryesthesia.

**hy·per·cry·es·the·sia** (hi″pər-kri″es-the′ze-ə) [*hyper-* + *cryo-* + *esthesia*] particularly severe cryesthesia; called also *hypercryalgesia.*

**hy·per·cu·pre·mia** (hi″pər-ku-pre′me-ə) an excess of copper in the blood. See also *copper poisoning,* under *poisoning.*

**hy·per·cu·pri·uria** (hi″pər-ku-pre-u′re-ə) an excess of copper in the urine.

**hy·per·cy·a·not·ic** (hi″pər-si″ə-not′ik) extremely cyanotic.

**hy·per·cy·e·sis** (hi″pər-si-e′sis) [*hyper-* + Gr. *kyēsis* gestation] superfetation.

**hy·per·cy·the·mia** (hi″pər-si-the′me-ə) [*hyper-* + *cyt-* + *-emia*] polycythemia.

**hy·per·cy·to·chro·mia** (hi″pər-si″to-kro′me-ə) [*hyper-* + *cyto-* + *chrom-* + *-ia*] increased staining capacity of a blood cell.

**hy·per·cy·to·sis** (hi″pər-si-to′sis) [*hyper-* + *cyt-* + *-osis*] old term for *leukocytosis.*

**hy·per·dac·tyl·ia** (hi″pər-dak-til′e-ə) hyperdactyly.

**hy·per·dac·ty·lism** (hi″pər-dak′təl-iz-əm) hyperdactyly.

**hy·per·dac·ty·ly** (hi″pər-dak′tə-le) [*hyper-* + Gr. *daktylos* finger] the presence of more than the normal number of fingers or toes.

**hy·per·di·crot·ic** (hi″pər-di-krot′ik) [*hyper-* + *dicrotic*] exhibiting marked dicrotism.

**hy·per·di·cro·tism** (hi″pər-dik′rə-tiz-əm) [*hyper-* + *dicrotism*] the quality of being hyperdicrotic; extreme dicrotism.

**hy·per·dip·loid** (hi″pər-dip′loid) [*hyper-* + *diploid*] aneuploid with more than the diploid number of chromosomes (usually only a few more).

**hy·per·dip·sia** (hi″pər-dip′se-ə) [*hyper-* + *dipsia*] intense thirst of relatively brief duration.

**hy·per·dis·ten·tion** (hi″pər-dis-ten′shən) excessive distention.

**hy·per·di·ure·sis** (hi″pər-di″u-re′sis) [*hyper-* + *diuresis*] excessive excretion of urine.

**hy·per·don·tia** (hi″pər-don′shə) [*hyper-* + *odont-* + *-ia*] an anomaly characterized by the presence of an excessive number of teeth.

**hy·per·dy·na·mia** (hi″pər-di-na′me-ə) [*hyper-* + *dynam-* + *-ia*] hyperactivity, def. 1.
**h. u′teri,** excessive uterine contractions in labor.

**hy·per·dy·nam·ic** (hi″pər-di-nam′ik) pertaining to or characterized by hyperdynamia.

**hy·per·ec·cris·ia** (hi″pər-ə-kris′e-ə) [*hyper-* + *eccrisis* + *-ia*] a state characterized by abnormally increased excretion.

**hy·per·ec·cri·sis** (hi″pər-ək′rĭ-sis) hypereccrisia.

**hy·per·ec·crit·ic** (hi″pər-ə-krit′ik) pertaining to or exhibiting hypereccrisia.

**hy·per·echo·ic** (hi″pər-ə-ko′ik) in ultrasonography, giving off many echoes; said of tissues or structures that reflect relatively many of the ultrasound waves directed at them.

**hy·per·elec·tro·ly·te·mia** (hi″pər-e-lek″tro-li-te′me-ə) an abnormally high concentration of electrolytes in the blood.

**hy·per·em·e·sis** (hi″pər-em′ə-sis) [*hyper-* + *emesis*] excessive vomiting.
**h. gravida′rum,** pernicious vomiting of pregnancy.
**h. lacten′tium,** excessive vomiting of nursing babies.

**hy·per·emet·ic** (hi″pər-ə-met′ik) characterized by excessive vomiting.

**hy·per·emia** (hi″pər-e′me-ə) [*hyper-* + *-emia*] [MeSH: Hyperemia] an increase of blood in a part; cf. *congestion.* Called also *engorgement.*
**active h.,** increased blood in a part due to local or general relaxation of the arterioles. Called also *arterial h.* and *fluxionary h.*
**arterial h.,** active h.
**collateral h.,** increased flow of blood through collateral vessels when the flow through the main artery is arrested.
**exercise h.,** vasodilation of the capillaries in muscles in response to the onset of exercise; it is proportionate to the force of the muscular contractions.
**fluxionary h.,** active h.
**passive h.,** increased blood in a part resulting from obstruction to its outflow from the area. Called also *venous h.*
**reactive h.,** an excess of blood in a part following restoration of its temporarily arrested flow.
**venous h.,** passive h.

**hy·per·emic** (hi″pər-e′mik) marked by hyperemia.

**hy·per·emi·za·tion** (hi″pər-e″mĭ-za′shən) the production of hyperemia, especially when employed for therapeutic purposes.

**hy·per·en·ceph·a·lus** (hi″pər-ən-sef′ə-ləs) acranius.

**hy·per·en·dem·ic** (hi″pər-ən-dem′ik) [*hyper-* + *endemic*] equally endemic, at a high level, in all age groups of a population. Cf. *holoendemic.*

**hy·per·eo·sin·o·phil·ia** (hi″pər-e″o-sin″o-fil′e-ə) extreme eosinophilia.
**filarial h.,** tropical pulmonary eosinophilia.

**hy·per·epi·neph·rin·emia** (hi″pər-ep″ĭ-nef″rĭ-ne′me-ə) an excess of epinephrine in the blood, as in pheochromocytoma.

**hy·per·equi·lib·ri·um** (hi″pər-e′kwĭ-lib′re-əm) an excessive tendency to vertigo; see also *sense of equilibrium,* under *sense.*

**hy·per·er·gia** increased sensitivity in allergy.

**hy·per·eryth·ro·cy·the·mia** (hi″pər-ə-rith″ro-si-the′me-ə) polycythemia.

**hy·per·eso·pho·ria** (hi″pər-es″o-for′e-ə) [*hyper-* + *esophoria*] a tendency of the visual axis to deviate upward and inward.

**hy·per·es·the·sia** (hi″pər-es-the′zhə) [*hyper-* + *esthesia*] [MeSH: Hyperesthesia] a dysesthesia consisting of increased sensitivity, particularly a painful sensation from a normally painless touch stimulus. Cf. *hyperalgesia.*
**acoustic h., auditory h.,** hyperacusis.
**cerebral h.,** that due to a cerebral lesion.
**gustatory h.,** hypergeusia.
**muscular h.,** muscular oversensitivity to pain or fatigue.
**olfactory h.,** hyperosmia.
**oneiric h.,** increase of sensitivity or of pain during sleep and dreams.
**optic h.,** abnormal sensitivity of the eye to light.
**tactile h.,** a paraphia consisting of excessive sensitivity of the sense of touch; called also *hyperaphia* and *hyperpselaphesia.*

**hy·per·es·thet·ic** (hi″pər-əs-thet′ik) pertaining to or characterized by hyperesthesia.

**hy·per·es·tro·gen·emia** (hi″pər-es″tro-jə-ne′me-ə) excessively high blood estrogen levels; in men it may cause gynecomastia and similar changes.

**hy·per·es·tro·gen·ism** (hi″pər-es′tro-jən-iz-əm) excessive amounts of estrogens in the body.

**hy·per·es·tro·gen·o·sis** (hi″pər-es″tro-jə-no′sis) hyperestrogenism.

**hy·per·eu·ryo·pia** (hi″pər-u″re-o′pe-ə) euryopia.

**hy·per·evol·u·tism** (hi″pər-e-vol′u-tiz-əm) accelerated development.

**hy·per·ex·cre·to·ry** (hi″pər-eks′krə-tor-e) marked by excessive secretion.

**hy·per·exo·pho·ria** (hi″pər-ek″so-for′e-ə) [*hyper-* + *exophoria*] a tendency of the visual axis to deviate upward and outward.

**hy·per·ex·plex·ia** (hi″pər-eks-plek′se-ə) a congenital condition of exaggerated startle reactions. In infants it has been observed in a syndrome accompanied by hypertonia, hypokinesia, and brisk cerebral bulbar reflexes, and in adults it is similar to jumping disease. Called also *startle disease.*

**hy·per·ex·ten·sion** (hi″pər-ək-sten′shən) extreme or excessive extension of a limb or part.

**hy·per·fer·re·mia** (hi″pər-fer-e′me-ə) an excess of iron in the blood; see also *iron poisoning,* under *poisoning.* Called also *hyperferricemia* and *siderosis.*

**hy·per·fer·re·mic** (hi″pər-fer-e′mik) pertaining to or characterized by hyperferremia.

**hy·per·fer·ri·ce·mia** (hi″pər-fer″ĭ-se′me-ə) hyperferremia.

**hy·per·fi·bri·no·ge·ne·mia** (hi″pər-fi-brin″o-jə-ne′me-ə) an excess of fibrinogen in the blood; called also *fibrinogenemia.*

**hy·per·fil·tra·tion** (hi″pər-fil-tra′shən) an elevation in the glomerular filtration rate, often a sign of early insulin-dependent diabetes mellitus.

**hy·per·flex·ion** (hi″pər-flek′shən) forcible overflexion of a limb or part.

**hy·per·frac·tion·a·tion** (hi″pər-frak″shən-a′shən) the subdivision

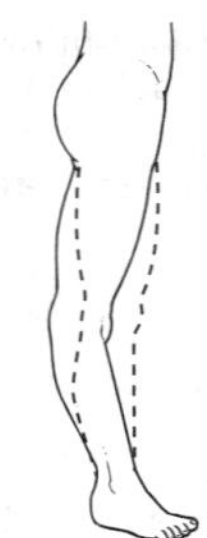
Hyperextension of the knee.

of a radiotherapy schedule with reduction of dose per exposure but no decrease in overall treatment span; done to decrease side effects while delivering an equivalent or greater total dose. Called also *hyperfractionated radiotherapy.*

**hy·per·func·tion** (hi″pər-funk′shən) excessive functioning of an organ.

**hy·per·ga·lac·tia** (hi″pər-gə-lak′she-ə) [*hyper-* + *galact-* + *-ia*] excessive secretion of milk.

**hy·per·gal·ac·to·sis** (hi″pər-gal″ak-to′sis) hypergalactia.

**hy·per·ga·lac·tous** (hi″pər-gə-lak′təs) pertaining to, characterized by, or causing hypergalactia.

**hy·per·gam·ma·glob·u·lin·emia** (hi″pər-gam″ə-glob″u-lĭ-ne′me-ə) [MeSH: Hypergammaglobulinemia] an excess of gamma globulins in the blood, seen frequently in chronic infectious diseases.
**monoclonal h's,** plasma cell dyscrasias.
**polyclonal h.,** that due to increased quantity of all immunoglobulin classes, rather than only one.

**hy·per·gas·trin·emia** (hi″pər-gas′trĭ-ne′me-ə) excessively high blood gastrin levels.

**hy·per·gen·e·sis** (hi″pər-jen′ə-sis) [*hyper-* + *-genesis*] excessive development, hypertrophy, or redundancy.

**hy·per·ge·net·ic** (hi″pər-jə-net′ik) pertaining to or characterized by hypergenesis.

**hy·per·gen·i·tal·ism** (hi″pər-jen′ĭ-təl-iz-əm) hypergonadism.

**hy·per·geus·es·the·sia** (hi″pər-go͞os″əs-the′zhə) hypergeusia.

**hy·per·geu·sia** (hi″pər-goo′zhə) [*hyper-* + Gr. *geusis* taste] a parageusia involving increased sensitivity of taste; called also *hypergeusesthesia* and *gustatory hyperesthesia.*

**hy·per·glan·du·lar** (hi″pər-glan′du-lər) marked by abnormally increased activity of any gland.

**hy·per·glob·u·lin·emia** (hi″pər-glob″u-lĭ-ne′me-ə) abnormally high content of any globulin in the blood; see also *hypergammaglobulinemia.*

**hy·per·glu·ca·gon·emia** (hi″pər-gloo″kə-gə-ne′me-ə) abnormally high levels of glucagon in the blood.

**hy·per·gly·ce·mia** (hi″pər-gli-se′me-ə) [*hyper-* + *glyc-* + *emia*] [MeSH: Hyperglycemia] abnormally increased glucose in the blood, such as in diabetes mellitus.
**rebound h.,** Somogyi phenomenon.

**hy·per·gly·ce·mic** (hi″pər-gli-se′mik) 1. pertaining to, characterized by, or causing hyperglycemia. 2. an agent that causes an increase in the level of glucose in the blood.

**hy·per·glyc·er·i·de·mia** (hi″pər-glis″ər-i-de′me-ə) an excess of glycerides, usually triglycerides, in the blood.

**hy·per·glyc·er·i·de·mic** (hi″pər-glis′ər-i-de″mik) pertaining to, characterized by, or producing hyperglyceridemia.

**hy·per·glyc·er·ol·emia** (hi″pər-glis″ər-ol-e′me-ə) 1. accumulation and excretion of glycerol caused by deficiency of glycerol kinase activity, an X-linked trait. The *infantile* or *microdeletion* form is caused by a chromosomal deletion that usually also involves one or both of the loci for Duchenne muscular dystrophy and congenital adrenal hypoplasia; resultant phenotypes include features characteristic to the defective locus or loci. The *juvenile* form is characterized by episodes of vomiting, metabolic acidosis, stupor, and coma and is caused by deficiency of glycerol kinase only, as is the *adult* form, which is generally symptomless. 2. excess of glycerol in the blood.

**hy·per·gly·cin·e·mia** (hi″pər-gli″sĭ-ne′me-ə) excess of glycine in the blood or other body fluids. Called also *glycinemia.*
**ketotic h.,** a term used to denote the elevated accumulation and excretion of glycine accompanied by ketosis that is secondary to methylmalonicacidemia, isovalericacidemia, and other organic acidemias, as distinguished from nonketotic hyperglycinemia.
**nonketotic h.,** a usually fatal autosomal recessive aminoacidopathy with accumulation of glycine in body fluids, particularly the blood, urine, and cerebrospinal fluid; it is characterized by neonatal onset, lethargy, absence of cerebral development, seizures, myoclonic jerks, and frequently coma and respiratory failure. It is caused by a defect in one or more enzymes of the glycine cleavage system.

**hy·per·gly·cin·uria** (hi″pər-gli″sĭ-nu′re-ə) an excess of glycine in the urine; see *hyperglycinemia.*

**hy·per·gly·cis·tia** (hi″pər-gli-sis′te-ə) [*hyper-* + *glyc-* + *hist-* + *-ia*] excess of sugar in the bodily tissues.

**hy·per·gly·co·gen·ol·y·sis** (hi″pər-gli″ko-jən-ol′ə-sis) excessive splitting up of glycogen, resulting in an excess of glucose in the body.

**hy·per·gly·cor·rha·chia** (hi″pər-gli″ko-ra′ke-ə) [*hyper-* + *glyco-* + *rhachi-* + *-ia*] the presence of a greater than normal concentration of glucose in the cerebrospinal fluid.

**hy·per·gly·co·se·mia** (hi″pər-gli″ko-se′me-ə) hyperglycemia.

**hy·per·gly·cos·uria** (hi″pər-gli″ko-su′re-ə) extreme glycosuria.

**hy·per·gly·cys·tia** (hi″pər-gli-sis′te-ə) hyperglycistia.

**hy·per·gno·sis** (hi″pər-no′sis) [*hyper-* + Gr. *gnōsis* knowledge] an exaggerated perception, e.g., expansion of an isolated idea into a complex philosophical system; seen in paranoia.

**hy·per·go·nad·ism** (hi″pər-go′nad-iz-əm) a condition caused by excessive secretion of gonadal hormones; manifestations include accelerated and precocious sexual development. See also *hyperorchidism* and *hyperovarianism.*

**hy·per·gon·a·do·trop·ic** (hi″pər-gon″ə-do-trop′ik) relating to or caused by excessive amounts of gonadotropins.

**hy·per·guan·i·din·emia** (hi″pər-gwan″ĭ-dĭ-ne′me-ə) the presence of an excess of guanidine in the blood.

**hy·per·he·mo·glo·bin·emia** (hi″pər-he″mo-glo″bĭ-ne′me-ə) the presence of an excessive amount of hemoglobin in the blood.

**hy·per·hep·a·rin·emia** (hi″pər-hep″ə-rĭ-ne′me-ə) excessive heparin in the blood, usually leading to increased clotting time and tendency to hemorrhage.

**hy·per·he·pat·ia** (hi″pər-hə-pat′e-ə) [*hyper-* + *hepat-* + *-ia*] hyperfunction of the liver.

**hy·per·hi·dro·sis** (hi″pər-hi-dro′sis) [*hyper-* + Gr. *hidrōsis* sweating] [MeSH: Hyperhidrosis] excessive perspiration. Called also *hyperidrosis, polyhidrosis,* and *polyidrosis.*
**axillary h.,** see *emotional h.*
**emotional h.,** an autosomal dominant disorder of the eccrine sweat glands, most often of the palms, soles, and axillae, in which emotional stimuli (e.g., anxiety) and sometimes mental or sensory stimuli elicit volar or axillary sweating (usually not both in the same individual); eccrine sweat glands in other areas of the body are affected less often and are less sensitive to such stimuli.
**h. unilatera′lis,** excessive sweating on one side of the body only.
**volar h.,** see *emotional h.*

**hy·per·hi·drot·ic** (hi″pər-hi-drot′ik) pertaining to, characterized by, or causing hyperhidrosis.

**hy·per·hy·dra·tion** (hi″pər-hi-dra′shən) a state of excessive water content of the body.

**hy·per·hy·dro·chlo·ria** (hi″pər-hi″dro-klor′e-ə) hyperchlorhydria.

**hy·per·hy·dro·chlo·rid·ia** (hi″pər-hi″dro-klor-id′e-ə) hyperchlorhydria.

**hy·per·hy·droxy·pro·lin·e·mia** (hi″pər-hi-drok″se-pro″lĭ-ne′me-ə) hydroxyprolinemia.

**Hy·per·i·cum** (hi-per′ĭ-kum) a genus of herbs with yellow flowers, including several types of St. John's wort; sheep and cattle that consume it suffer dermatitis and hepatogenous photosensitization.
**H. perfora′tum,** St. John's wort (q.v.); a species whose aboveground parts are used medicinally.

**hy·per·idro·sis** (hi″pər-i-dro′sis) hyperhidrosis.

**hy·per·im·ido·di·pep·tid·uria** (hi″pər-im″ĭ-do-di-pep″tĭ-du′re-ə) 1. prolidase deficiency. 2. imidodipeptiduria.

**hy·per·im·mune** (hi″pər-ĭ-mūn′) possessing very large quantities of specific antibodies in the serum.

**hy·per·im·mu·ni·ty** (hi″pər-ĭ-mu′nĭ-te) the high levels of specific antibody produced by hyperimmunization.

**hy·per·im·mu·ni·za·tion** (hi″pər-im″u-nĭ-za′shən) any process of immunization that produces very high levels of circulating antibodies, especially immunization of an animal or human donor with repeated doses of antigen for the production of therapeutic antisera or immune globulins.

**hy·per·im·mu·no·glob·u·lin·emia** (hi″pər-im″u-no-glob″u-lĭ-ne′me-ə) abnormally high levels of immunoglobulins in the serum.
**h. E,** extremely high levels of IgE in the serum, associated with cutaneous anergy and deficient antibody response, as occurs in Job's syndrome.

**hy·per·in·fla·tion** (hi″pər-in-fla′shən) excessive inflation or expansion, as of the lungs; called also *overinflation.*

**hy·per·in·ges·tion** (hi″pər-in-jes′chən) ingestion of a greater than optimal amount of nutrients.

**hy·per·in·su·lin·ar** (hi″pər-in′sə-lin-ər) pertaining to or characterized by excessive secretion of insulin.

**hy·per·in·su·lin·emia** (hi″pər-in″sə-lĭ-ne′me-ə) [MeSH: Hyperinsulinemia] excessively high blood insulin levels.

**hy·per·in·su·lin·ism** (hi″pər-in′sə-lin-iz″əm) [MeSH: Hyperinsulinism] 1. excessive secretion of insulin by the pancreatic islets, resulting in hypoglycemia. 2. insulin shock. 3. hyperinsulinemia.

**hy·per·in·vo·lu·tion** (hi″pər-in″vo-loo′shən) superinvolution.

**hy·per·io·de·mia** (hi″pər-i″o-de′me-ə) the presence of an excessive amount of iodine in the blood. See also *iodism.*

**hy·per·ir·ri·ta·bil·i·ty** (hi″pər-ir″ĭ-tə-bil′ĭ-te) excessive irritability.

**hy·per·iso·to·nia** (hi″pər-i″so-to′ne-ə) [*hyper-* + *isotonia*] marked equality of tone or of tonicity.

**hy·per·iso·ton·ic** (hi″pər-i″so-ton′ik) [*hyper-* + Gr. *isos* equal + *tonos* tension, or tone] hypertonic.

**hy·per·ka·le·mia** (hi″pər-kə-le′me-ə) [MeSH: Hyperkalemia] abnormally high potassium concentration in the blood, most often due to defective renal excretion. It is characterized clinically by electrocardiographic abnormalities (elevated T waves, depressed P waves, and wide QRS complexes, eventually with atrial asystole). In severe cases, weakness and flaccid paralysis may occur. Called also *potassemia* and *hyperpotassemia.*

**hy·per·kal·i·emia** (hi″pər-kal″e-e′me-ə) hyperkalemia.

**hy·per·ker·a·tin·iza·tion** (hi″pər-ker″ə-tin″ĭ-za′shən) [*hyper-* + *keratinization*] the excessive development or retention of keratin by the epidermis.

**hy·per·ker·a·to·sis** (hi″pər-ker″ə-to′sis) [*hyper-* + *keratosis*] 1. hypertrophy of the stratum corneum of the skin, or any disease characterized by it. See also *callus* and *keratosis* 2. hypertrophy of the cornea. 3. a skin disease of cattle marked by inflammation and thickening of the horny layer, and caused by the ingestion of feed containing chlorinated naphthalenes. It was once thought to be caused by a virus and was called *x disease.*
**epidermolytic h.,** a form of ichthyosis present at birth, inherited as an autosomal dominant trait, and characterized by generalized erythroderma and severe hyperkeratosis with small, hard verrucous scales over the entire body, accentuated in flexural areas, which may involve the palms and soles. Recurrent bullae usually localized to the lower limbs are characteristic in infancy and childhood. Formerly called *bullous congenital ichthyosiform erythroderma.* See also *ichthyosis hystrix.*
**follicular h.,** a skin condition characterized by hyperkeratosis of hair follicles, resulting in rough, cone-shaped, elevated papules, the openings of which are often closed with a white plug of encrusted sebum. Deficiencies of vitamins A and E, B complex vitamins, and essential fatty acids have all been implicated in the etiology. Called also *phrynoderma* and *toadskin.*
**h. follicula′ris in cu′tem pe′netrans, h. follicula′ris et parafollicula′ris in cu′tem pe′netrans,** Kyrle's disease.
**h. lacuna′ris,** keratosis pharyngea.
**h. lenticula′ris per′stans,** an autosomal dominant skin disorder, usually occurring in the third or fourth decade of life, characterized clinically by the presence of pink or reddish or yellowish brown hyperkeratotic scaly papules on the lower leg and dorsum of the foot, sometimes involving the trunk, thigh, arms, and dorsum of the hand, and usually associated with punctate keratoses on the palms and soles; and histologically by a lack of keratinosomes and a reduction of keratohyalin granules in the epidermis underlying the lesions. Called also *Flegel's disease.*
**h. of palms and soles,** palmoplantar keratoderma.
**h. pe′netrans,** h. follicularis in cutem penetrans.
**progressive dystrophic h.,** keratoma hereditarium mutilans.
**h. subungua′lis,** hyperkeratosis affecting the nail beds.

**hy·per·ke·ton·emia** (hi″pər-ke″to-ne′me-ə) ketonemia.

**hy·per·ke·ton·uria** (hi″pər-ke″to-nu′re-ə) ketonuria.

**hy·per·ke·to·sis** (hi″pər-ke-to′sis) ketosis.

**hy·per·ki·ne·mia** (hi″pər-kĭ-ne′me-ə) [*hyper-* + *kin-* + *-emia*] abnormally high cardiac output; increased rate of blood flow through the circulatory system.

**hy·per·ki·ne·mic** (hi″pər-kĭ-ne′mik) 1. increasing blood flow through a tissue. 2. an agent which increases the flow of blood through a tissue area.

**hy·per·ki·ne·sia** (hi″pər-kĭ-ne′zhə) hyperactivity.

**hy·per·ki·ne·sis** (hi″pər-kĭ-ne′sis) [*hyper-* + *-kinesis*] [MeSH: Hyperkinesis] hyperactivity.

**hy·per·ki·net·ic** (hi″pər-kĭ-net′ik) pertaining to or characterized by hyperactivity (hyperkinesis).

**hy·per·ko·ria** (hi″pər-kor′e-ə) [*hyper-* + Gr. *koros* satiety + *-ia* ] an early sense of satiety.

**hy·per·lact·ac·i·de·mia** (hi″pər-lak″tas-ĭ-de′me-ə) an excessive amount of lactic acid in the blood.

**hy·per·lac·ta·tion** (hi″pər-lak-ta′shən) lactation in greater than normal amount or for a longer than usual period.

**hy·per·lec·i·thin·emia** (hi″pər-les″ĭ-thĭ-ne′me-ə) excess of lecithin in the blood.

**hy·per·le·thal** (hi″pər-le′thəl) more than sufficient to cause death.

**hy·per·leu·ko·cy·to·sis** (hi″pər-loo″ko-si-to′sis) [*hyper-* + *leukocyte* + *-osis*] extreme leukocytosis, as seen in certain forms of leukemia.

**hy·per·ley·dig·ism** (hi″pər-li′dig-iz-əm) overactivity of Leydig's cells, resulting in hyperandrogenism.

**hy·per·li·pe·mia** (hi″pər-li-pe′me-ə) hyperlipidemia.
**carbohydrate-induced h.,** elevated blood lipids, particularly triglycerides, after carbohydrate ingestion; it is characteristic of disorders with type IV or type V hyperlipoproteinemia phenotypes and is sometimes used as a synonym for these phenotypes or for the genetic disorders causing them.
**combined fat- and carbohydrate-induced h.,** persistently elevated blood levels of very-low-density lipoproteins and chylomicrons after ingestion of fat or carbohydrates; it is characteristic of disorders with a type V hyperlipoproteinemia phenotype and is sometimes used as a synonym for this phenotype or for genetic disorders causing it.
**endogenous h.,** elevated plasma lipids derived from body stores rather than dietary sources (i.e., very-low-density lipoproteins); used as a generic descriptor of the type IV hyperlipoproteinemia phenotype. See table at *hyperlipoproteinemia.*
**essential familial h.,** a term used to describe an inherited disorder causing a type I hyperlipoproteinemia phenotype or the phenotype itself.
**exogenous h.,** elevated plasma levels of lipoproteins derived from dietary sources (i.e., chylomicrons); used as a generic descriptor of the type I hyperlipoproteinemia phenotype. See table at *hyperlipoproteinemia.*
**familial fat-induced h.,** persistently elevated blood chylomicrons after ingestion of fat; it is characteristic of disorders with a type I hyperlipoproteinemia phenotype and is sometimes used as a synonym for this phenotype or genetic disorders causing it.
**mixed h.,** generic designation for a hyperlipoproteinemia in which several classes of lipoproteins are elevated; usually used to denote a type V phenotype but sometimes used for a type II-b phenotype. See table at *hyperlipoproteinemia.*

**hy·per·lip·id·emia** (hi″pər-lip″ĭ-de′me-ə) [MeSH: Hyperlipidemia] a general term for elevated concentrations of any or all of the lipids in the plasma, including hypertriglyceridemia, hypercholesterolemia, etc. See also table at *hyperlipoproteinemia.* Called also *hyperlipemia, lipemia,* and *lipidemia.*
**combined h.,** a generic designation for a hyperlipidemia in which several classes of lipids are elevated; usually used to denote the phenotype of a type II-b hyperlipoproteinemia. See table at *hyperlipoproteinemia.*
**familial combined h.,** an autosomal dominant disorder of lipoprotein metabolism manifest in adulthood as hypercholesterolemia (type II-a hyperlipoproteinemia phenotype), hypertriglyceridemia (type IV hyperlipoproteinemia phenotype), or a combination (type II-b hyperlipoproteinemia phenotype); different phenotypes may succeed each other in a single individual. The disorder is characterized by greatly elevated plasma apolipoprotein B and premature coronary atherosclerosis, but only rarely by xanthomas. Called also *multiple lipoprotein–type h.* See also table at *hyperlipoproteinemia.*
**mixed h.,** see under *hyperlipemia.*
**multiple lipoprotein–type h.,** familial combined h.
**remnant h.,** a hyperlipoproteinemia in which the accumulated lipoproteins are normally transient intermediates, chylomicron remnants and intermediate density lipoproteins. See table at *hyperlipoproteinemia.*

**hy·per·lip·i·de·mic** (hi″pər-lip″ĭ-de′mik) pertaining to or characterized by hyperlipidemia.

**hy·per·lipo·pro·tein·emia** (hi″pər-lip″o-pro″te-ne′me-ə) [MeSH: Hyperlipoproteinemia] an excess of lipoproteins in the blood, due to a disorder of lipoprotein metabolism; it may be an acquired or familial condition or some combination. The disorder has been subdivided on the basis of biochemical phenotype, and each type has since been shown to have a variety of causes. See accompanying table for individual phenotypes as well as some primary genetic disorders that cause them. See also *familial h., hyperlipemia,* and *hyperlipidemia.*
**acquired h.,** hyperlipoproteinemia occurring secondarily to some other disorder, such as hypothyroidism, nephrotic syndrome, or hypoadrenocorticism, or as a result of environmental factors, including diet.
**familial h.,** an inherited hyperlipoproteinemia, classified on the basis of the type I–V phenotypes described in the accompanying table. For any given phenotype, the term is frequently used loosely to denote either the phenotype or any or all of the genetic disorders causing the phenotype. However, the latter usage is frequently imprecise or inaccurate because a single phenotype may have multiple causes and a single genetic disorder may result in multiple phenotypes.

**hy·per·li·po·sis** (hi″pər-lĭ-po′sis) an excess of fat in the blood serum or tissues.

**Hyperlipoproteinemias**

| Phenotype | Generic Designation | Elevated Lipoprotein Class | Elevated Lipid Class | Primary Genetic Disorders |
|---|---|---|---|---|
| I | Exogenous hyperlipemia | Chylomicrons | Triglycerides | Familial lipoprotein lipase deficiency<br>Familial apolipoprotein C-II deficiency<br>Unclassified |
| II-a | Hypercholesterolemia | LDL | Cholesterol | Familial hypercholesterolemia<br>Familial combined hyperlipidemia<br>Polygenic hypercholesterolemia |
| II-b | Combined hyperlipidemia | LDL, VLDL | Cholesterol, Triglycerides | Familial combined hyperlipidemia<br>Unclassified |
| III | Remnant hyperlipidemia | $\beta$-VLDL | Triglycerides, Cholesterol | Familial dysbetalipoproteinemia<br>Unclassified |
| IV | Endogenous hyperlipemia | VLDL | Triglycerides | Familial hypertriglyceridemia (mild)<br>Familial combined hyperlipidemia<br>Sporadic hypertriglyceridemia<br>Tangier disease |
| V | Mixed hyperlipemia | VLDL, Chylomicrons | Triglycerides, Cholesterol | Familial hypertriglyceridemia (severe)<br>Familial lipoprotein lipase deficiency<br>Familial apolipoprotein C-II deficiency |

LDL, Low-density lipoproteins; VLDL, very-low-density lipoproteins; $\beta$-VLDL, a class of abnormal VLDL.

**hy·per·li·the·mia** (hi″pər-lĭ-the′me-ə) presence in the blood of a high concentration of lithium.

**hy·per·lith·ic** (hi″pər-lith′ik) pertaining to or characterized by an excess of lithic (uric) acid.

**hy·per·li·thu·ria** (hi″pər-lith-u′re-ə) excess of lithic (uric) acid in the urine.

**hy·per·lo·gia** (hi″pər-lo′jə) [*hyper-* + *log-* + *-ia*] logorrhea.

**hy·per·lor·do·sis** (hi″pər-lor-do′sis) extremely marked lordosis.

**hy·per·lu·cen·cy** (hi″pər-loo′sən-se) increased radiolucency.

**hy·per·lu·te·in·iza·tion** (hi″pər-loo″te-in-ĭ-za′shən) excessive luteinization of the cystic follicles of the ovary.

**hy·per·ly·sin·e·mia** (hi″pər-li″se-ne′me-ə) 1. excess of lysine in the blood. 2. an autosomal recessive aminoacidopathy due to a deficiency of one or both activities of $\alpha$-aminoadipic semialdehyde synthase (q.v.), characterized by excess of lysine, and sometimes also of saccharopine, in the blood and urine. There is a possible association with mental retardation; a relationship to congenital lysine intolerance (q.v.) is unclear. See also *saccharopinuria*.

**hy·per·mag·ne·se·mia** (hi″pər-mag″nə-se′me-ə) an abnormally high magnesium content of the blood; manifestations include lethargy, weakness, electrocardiographic abnormalities and, as levels increase, loss of deep tendon reflexes, somnolence, and coma. Called also *magnesemia*.

**hy·per·ma·nia** (hi″pər-ma′ne-ə) intense mania with overwhelming tensions, marked disorientation, and incoherence.

**hy·per·mas·tia** (hi″pər-mas′te-ə) [*hyper-* + *mast-* + *-ia*] 1. the presence of one or more supernumerary mammary glands. 2. macromastia.

**hy·per·ma·ture** (hi″pər-mə-choor′) past the stage of maturity.

**hy·per·mel·a·not·ic** (hi″pər-mel″ə-not′ik) characterized by an excessive deposit of melanin.

**hy·per·men·or·rhea** (hi″pər-men″o-re′ə) [*hyper-* + *menorrhea*] excessive uterine bleeding occurring at regular intervals, the period of flow being of usual duration. Called also *menorrhagia*.

**hy·per·met·a·bol·ic** (hi″pər-met″ə-bol′ik) exhibiting an increased metabolic rate.

**hy·per·me·tab·o·lism** (hi″pər-mə-tab′o-liz-əm) abnormally increased utilization of oxygen, nutrients, and other materials by the body; increased metabolism.
**extrathyroidal h.**, abnormally elevated basal metabolism unassociated with thyroid disease.

**hy·per·meta·mor·pho·sis** (hi″pər-met″ə-mor′fə-sis) excessive attentiveness and reaction to visual stimuli, as in the Klüver-Bucy syndrome.

**hy·per·meta·pla·sia** (hi″pər-met″ə-pla′zhə) increased metaplasia.

**hy·per·me·thi·o·nin·emia** (hi″pər-mə-thi″o-nĭ-ne′me-ə) excess of methionine in the blood.

**hy·per·me·tria** (hi″pər-me′tre-ə) [Gr. "a passing all measure, overflow"] a condition in which voluntary muscular movement overreaches the intended goal.

**hy·per·met·rope** (hi″pər-me′trōp) hyperope.

**hy·per·me·tro·pia** (hi″pər-me-tro′pe-ə) hyperopia.

**hy·per·mim·ia** (hi″pər-mim′e-ə) [*hyper-* + Gr. *mimia* representation by means of art] excessive use of gestures when speaking.

**hy·per·min·er·al·iza·tion** (hi″pər-min″ər-əl-ĭ-za′shən) the presence of an excess of mineral elements in the body.

**hy·perm·ne·sia** (hi″pərm-ne′zhə) [*hyper-* + Gr. *mnēmē* memory] extreme retentiveness or unusual clarity of memory.

**hy·perm·ne·sic** (hi″pərm-ne′sik) pertaining to or characterized by hypermnesia.

**hy·per·mo·dal** (hi″pər-mo′dəl) in statistics, relating to the values or items falling above the mode of the frequency distribution.

**hy·per·morph** (hi′pər-morf) [*hyper-* + *-morph*] a mutant gene characterized by an increase in the activity it influences. Cf. *hypomorph*.

**hy·per·mo·til·i·ty** (hi″pər-mo-til′ĭ-te) excessive or abnormally increased motility, as of the gastrointestinal tract.

**hy·per·myo·to·nia** (hi″pər-mi″o-to′ne-ə) hypertonia.

**hy·per·my·ot·ro·phy** (hi″pər-mi-ot′rə-fe) [*hyper-* + *myotrophy*] excessive development of the muscular tissue.

**hy·per·na·sal·i·ty** (hi″pər-na-zal′ĭ-te) an excessively nasal quality of voice, which may result in unintelligible speech; the cause is velopharyngeal incompetence with emission of too much air through the nose. Called also *rhinolalia aperta* and *open rhinolalia*.

**hy·per·na·tre·mia** (hi″pər-nə-tre′me-ə) [*hyper-* + *natremia*] [MeSH: Hypernatremia] excessive amount of sodium in the blood.
**hypodipsic h.**, an uncommon syndrome of chronic or recurrent episodes of severe hypernatremia with dehydration and lack of thirst, seen in persons with various congenital or acquired diseases of the brain.

**hy·per·na·tre·mic** (hi″pər-nə-tre′mik) pertaining to, characterized by, or causing hypernatremia.

**hy·per·nat·ron·emia** (hi″pər-nat″ro-ne′me-ə) hypernatremia.

**hy·per·neo·cy·to·sis** (hi″pər-ne″o-si-to′sis) [*hyper-* + *neocytosis*] hyperleukocytosis in which an excessive number of immature forms of leukocytes are present.

**hy·per·neph·roid** (hi″pər-nef′roid) resembling the adrenal gland.

**hy·per·ne·phro·ma** (hi″pər-nə-fro′mə) [*hyper-* + Gr. *nephros* kidney + *-oma*] renal cell carcinoma.

**hy·per·ni·tre·mia** (hi″pər-ni-tre′me-ə) [*hyper-* + *nitrogen* + *-emia*] excessive nitrogen in the blood.

**hy·per·nom·ic** (hi″pər-nom′ik) [*hyper-* + *nom-* + *-ic*] above the law; unrestrained; excessive.

**hy·per·nor·mal** (hi″pər-nor′məl) in excess of what is normal.

**hy·per·nu·tri·tion** (hi″pər-noo-trish′ən) hyperalimentation (def. 1).

**hy·per·onych·ia** (hi″pər-o-nik′e-ə) [*hyper-* + *onych-* + *-ia*] onychauxis.

**hy·per·ope** (hi′pər-ōp) an individual exhibiting hyperopia.

**hy·per·opia** (hi″pər-o′pe-ə) [*hyper-* + *-opia*] [MeSH: Hyperopia] that error of refraction in which rays of light entering the eye parallel to the optic axis are brought to a focus behind the retina, as a result of the eyeball being too short from front to back. Symbol H. Called also *farsightedness* (because the near point is more distant than it is in emmetropia with an equal amplitude of accommodation) and *hypermetropia.*

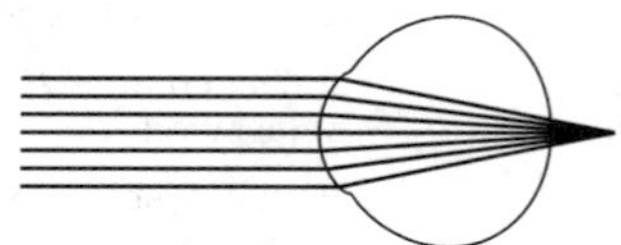

Hyperopia.

**absolute h.,** that amount of hyperopia which cannot be corrected by accommodation.
**axial h.,** that which is due to shortness of the anteroposterior axis of the eye.
**curvature h.,** hyperopia due to insufficient convexity of the refracting surfaces.
**facultative h.,** that amount of hyperopia which can be entirely corrected by the ciliary muscle, i.e., by the effort of accommodation.
**index h.,** hyperopia caused by deficient refractive power in the media of the eye.
**latent h.,** that part of the total hyperopia corrected by the physiologic tone of the ciliary muscle and revealed only when that muscle is paralyzed by the use of a drug, such as atropine.
**manifest h.,** that part of the total hyperopia not corrected by the physiologic tone of the ciliary muscle nor revealed with cycloplegic examination.
**relative h.,** facultative hyperopia allowing clear vision, but causing excessive convergence or convergent strabismus.
**total h.,** the sum of manifest and latent hyperopia; it can be determined only with mydriasis.

**hy·per·op·ic** (hi″pər-op′ik) pertaining to or exhibiting hyperopia; farsighted.

**hy·per·or·chi·dism** (hi″pər-or′kĭ-diz-əm) [*hyper-* + *orchid-* + *-ism*] abnormally increased testicular function; see also *hyperleydigism.*

**hy·per·orex·ia** (hi″pər-o-rek′se-ə) [*hyper-* + Gr. *orexis* appetite + *-ia*] an abnormally increased appetite. See also *hyperalimentation* (def. 1) and *bulimia.*

**hy·per·or·ni·thin·emia** (hi″pər-or″nĭ-thĭ-ne′me-ə) excess of ornithine in the plasma, such as occurs in the genetic disorders gyrate atrophy of choroid and retina and hyperornithinemia-hyperammonemia-homocitrullinuria syndrome.

**hy·per·or·tho·cy·to·sis** (hi″pər-or″tho-si-to′sis) [*hyper-* + *orthocytosis*] hyperleukocytosis in which the proportion of the various forms of leukocytes is normal.

**hy·per·os·mia** (hi″pər-oz′me-ə) [*hyper-* + *osm-*[1] + *-ia*] a parosmia involving increased sensitivity of smell; called also *hyperosphresia* and *olfactory hyperesthesia.*

**hy·per·os·mo·lal·i·ty** (hi″pər-oz″mo-lal′ĭ-te) an increase in the osmolality of the body fluids.

**hy·per·os·mo·lar·i·ty** (hi″pər-oz″mo-lar′ĭ-te) abnormally increased osmolar concentration.

**hy·per·os·mot·ic** (hi″pər-oz-mot′ik) 1. producing or caused by abnormally rapid osmosis. 2. containing a higher concentration of osmotically active components than a standard solution.

**hy·per·os·phre·sia** (hi″pər-os-fre′zhə) [*hyper-* + *osphresi-* + *-ia*] hyperosmia.

**hy·per·os·te·og·e·ny** (hi″pər-os″te-oj′ə-ne) [*hyper-* + *osteo-* + *-geny*] excessive development of bone.

**hy·per·os·to·sis** (hi″pər-os-to′sis) [*hyper-* + *osteo-* + *-osis*] [MeSH: Hyperostosis] hypertrophy of bone; exostosis.
**h. cortica′lis defor′mans juveni′lis,** an autosomal recessive disorder beginning in childhood and marked by multiple fractures and bowing of all extremities, by thickening of the frontal, parietal, and occipital bones, by osteoporosis, and by elevated concentrations of serum alkaline phosphatase and of urinary hydroxyproline. Called also *juvenile Paget disease, chronic congenital idiopathic hyperphosphatasemia,* and *familial osteoectasia.*
**h. cortica′lis generalisa′ta,** an autosomal recessive disorder, characterized principally by osteosclerosis of the skull, mandible, clavicles, ribs, and diaphyses of long bones, associated with elevated blood alkaline phosphatase; beginning during puberty, it sometimes leads to optic atrophy and perceptive deafness due to nerve pressure exerted by thickening of the base of the skull. Called also *hyperphosphatasemia tarda* and *van Buchem's syndrome.*
**h. cra′nii,** hyperostosis involving the cranial bones.
**flowing h.,** melorheostosis.
**h. fronta′lis inter′na,** thickening of the inner table of the frontal bone, which may be associated with hypertrichosis and obesity; it most commonly affects women near menopause. Called also *Morel's syndrome.*
**infantile cortical h.,** a disease of young infants characterized by soft tissue swellings over the affected bones, fever, and irritability, and marked by periods of remission and exacerbation; called also *Caffey's disease.*
**senile ankylosing h. of spine,** a disorder of the elderly characterized by large osteophytes that bridge vertebrae and, in association with calcified ligaments, may resemble ankylosing spondylitis.

**hy·per·os·tot·ic** (hi″pər-os-tot′ik) pertaining to or exhibiting hyperostosis.

**hy·per·ova·ri·an·ism** (hi″pər-o-var′e-ən-iz-əm) [*hyper-* + *ovarian* + *-ism*] sexual precocity in girls due to excessive and untimely ovarian secretion.

**hy·per·ova·rism** (hi″pər-o′və-riz-əm) hyperovarianism.

**hy·per·ox·al·uria** (hi″pər-ok″sə-lu′re-ə) [MeSH: Hyperoxaluria] the excretion of an excessive amount of oxalate in the urine; high concentrations of oxalates in the urine may lead to the formation of urinary calculi. Called also *oxaluria.*
**enteric h.,** a form occurring after extensive resection or disease of the ileum and resulting from excessive absorption of oxalate from the colon, with formation of calcium oxalate calculi in the urinary tract.
**primary h.,** a genetic disorder characterized by urinary excretion of large amounts of oxalate, with nephrolithiasis, nephrocalcinosis, early onset of renal failure, and often a generalized deposit of calcium oxalate (oxalosis), resulting from a defect in glyoxylate metabolism. The disorder occurs in two types: *type I,* an autosomal recessive disorder, is characterized by urinary excretion of oxalic, glyoxylic, and glycolic acids and is due to deficiency of alanine–glyoxylate transaminase. *Type II* is characterized by excretion of oxalic and L-glyceric acids and is due to a defect in the metabolism of hydroxypyruvate to D-glycerate, causing increased production of L-glycerate, probably an autosomal recessive defect in glycerate dehydrogenase.

**hy·per·ox·emia** (hi″pər-ok-se′me-ə) [*hyper-* + *ox-* + *-emia*] excessive acidity of the blood.

**hy·per·ox·ia** (hi″pər-ok′se-ə) [MeSH: Hyperoxia] an excess of oxygen in the system, resulting from exposure to high oxygen concentrations, especially to hyperbaric pressures of oxygen. See *oxygen toxicity,* under *toxicity.*

**hy·per·ox·ic** (hi″pər-ok′sik) pertaining to or characterized by hyperoxia.

**hy·per·ox·i·da·tion** (hi″pər-ok″sĭ-da′shən) excessive oxidation.

**hy·per·pal·les·the·sia** (hi″pər-pal″əs-the′zhə) [*hyper-* + *pallesthesia*] abnormally increased sensitivity of the vibration sense; see *pallesthesia.*

**hy·per·pan·cre·or·rhea** (hi″pər-pan″kre-o-re′ə) excessive secretion from the pancreas.

**hy·per·par·a·site** (hi″pər-par′ə-sīt) [*hyper-* + *parasite*] a parasite that preys on a parasite.
**second degree h.,** a parasite that preys on a hyperparasite.

**hy·per·par·a·sit·ic** (hi″pər-par″ə-sit′ik) living parasitically upon a parasite; biparasitic.

**hy·per·par·a·sit·ism** (hi″pər-par′ə-si″tiz-əm) infestation with a hyperparasite.

**hy·per·para·thy·roid·ism** (hi″pər-par″ə-thi′roid-iz-əm) [MeSH: Hyperparathyroidism] a condition caused by excessive amounts of parathyroid hormone, which invokes hypercalcemia and hypophosphatemia and affects the functions of many cell types. Manifestations include calcium deposits in the renal tubules, generalized decalcification of bone (osteoporosis), resulting in pain and tenderness of bones and spontaneous fractures or in localized bone cysts, hypercalcemia, leading to muscular weakness, gastrointestinal symptoms such as anorexia, nausea, vomiting, and abdominal pains, and drowsiness or obtundity.
**primary h.,** hyperparathyroidism due to excessive production of parathyroid hormone, either from hyperplasia of the parathyroid gland or from a neoplasm.
**secondary h.,** a type occurring when the serum calcium falls below normal levels, as in chronic disease or vitamin D deficiency.
**secondary h., nutritional,** secondary hyperparathyroidism in domestic animals due to an unbalanced diet; there may be insufficient calcium, excessive phosphorus that competes with calcium, or (in ruminants) oxalates that bind to calcium and form insoluble calcium

oxalate crystals. The most prominent symptoms are swelling of the mandible and maxilla, loosening of the teeth, and lameness. Called also *bran disease, miller's disease,* and *bighead.*
**tertiary h.,** a type in which parathyroid adenomas arise from secondary hyperplasia caused by chronic renal failure.

**hy·per·path·ia** (hi″pər-path′e-ə) abnormally exaggerated subjective response to painful stimuli; see also *hyperesthesia* and *hyperalgesia.*

**hy·per·pep·sia** (hi″pər-pep′se-ə) [*hyper-* + Gr. *pepsis* digestion] impairment of digestion, due to hyperchlorhydria.

**hy·per·pep·sin·emia** (hi″pər-pep″sĭ-ne′me-ə) an abnormally high level of pepsin in the blood.

**hy·per·pep·sin·ia** (hi″pər-pep-sin′e-ə) abnormally profuse secretion of pepsin in the stomach.

**hy·per·pep·sin·uria** (hi″pər-pep″sĭ-nu′re-ə) an abnormally high level of pepsin in the urine.

**hy·per·peri·stal·sis** (hi″pər-per″ĭ-stahl′sis) excessively active peristalsis.

**hy·per·per·me·a·bil·i·ty** (hi″pər-pər″me-ə-bil′ĭ-te) undue or abnormal permeability, as of a cell membrane or a vessel wall.

**hy·per·pex·ia** (hi″pər-pek′se-ə) [*hyper-* + *pexia*] fixation of an excessive amount of a substance by a tissue.

**hy·per·pexy** (hi″pər-pek′se) hyperpexia.

**hy·per·pha·gia** (hi″pər-fa′jə) [*hyper-* + *-phagia*] [MeSH: Hyperphagia] polyphagia.

**hy·per·pha·lan·gia** (hi″pər-fə-lan′je-ə) presence of more than the normal number of phalanges in the longitudinal axis of a digit.

**hy·per·pha·lan·gism** (hi″pər-fə-lan′jiz-əm) hyperphalangia.

**hy·per·phen·yl·al·a·nin·emia** (hi″pər-fen″əl-al″ə-nĭ-ne′me-ə) 1. any of several autosomal recessive defects in the hydroxylation of phenylalanine resulting in accumulation and excretion of dietary phenylalanine. Most commonly the defect is in the enzyme phenylalanine 4-monooxygenase; the most severe manifestation of this is classic phenylketonuria (q.v.), but two benign forms also occur (see *transient h.* and *persistent h.*). Rarely, the defect is one of tetrahydrobiopterin metabolism; see *malignant h.* 2. excess of phenylalanine in the blood.
**malignant h.,** any of several disorders in the synthesis or regeneration of the cofactor tetrahydrobiopterin; it is initially clinically similar to phenylketonuria but is unresponsive to dietary phenylalanine restriction, with cerebral dysfunction, muscular hypotonia, and rapid progression to death. Defects in dihydropteridine reductase, GTP cyclohydrolase I, or 6-pyruvoyltetrahydropterin synthase activity are known. Called also *atypical phenylketonuria.*
**maternal h.,** elevated serum phenylalanine in a conceiving or gravid woman; when levels are high enough, maternal phenylketonuria results.
**persistent h.,** minimally elevated plasma and urinary phenylalanine due to partial deficiency of phenylalanine 4-monooxygenase activity.
**transient h.,** a transitory neonatal disorder characterized by minimal elevation of plasma and urinary phenylalanine and usually due to delayed maturation of phenylalanine 4-monooxygenase. Cf. *neonatal tyrosinemia.*

**hy·per·pho·ne·sis** (hi″pər-fo-ne′sis) [*hyper-* + *phon-* + *-esis*] an increase in intensity of the vocal sound in auscultation, or of the percussion note.

**hy·per·pho·nia** (hi″pər-fo′ne-ə) [*hyper-* + *phon-* + *-ia*] a dysphonia with excessively energetic phonation, as in stuttering. Called also *superenergetic phonation.*

**hy·per·pho·ria** (hi′pər-for′e-ə) [*hyper-* + *phoria*] a form of heterophoria in which there is permanent upward deviation of the visual axis of an eye after the visual fusional stimulus has been eliminated.

**hy·per·phos·pha·ta·se·mia** (hi″pər-fos″fə-ta-se′me-ə) high levels of alkaline phosphatase in the blood.
**chronic congenital idiopathic h.,** hyperostosis corticalis deformans juvenilis.
**h. tar′da,** hyperostosis corticalis generalisata.

**hy·per·phos·pha·ta·sia** (hi″pər-fos″fə-ta′zhə) hyperphosphatasemia.

**hy·per·phos·pha·te·mia** (hi″pər-fos″fə-te′me-ə) an excessive amount of phosphates in the blood; it is usually asymptomatic.

**hy·per·phos·pha·tu·ria** (hi″pər-fos″fə-tu′re-ə) an excessive amount of phosphates in the urine.

**hy·per·phos·pho·re·mia** (hi″pər-fos″fə-re′me-ə) an excessive amount of phosphorus compounds in the blood.

**hy·per·phra·sia** (hi″pər-fra′zhə) logorrhea.

**hy·per·phre·nia** (hi″pər-fre′ne-ə) [*hyper-* + *phren-* + *-ia*] excessive mental activity.

**hy·per·pig·men·ta·tion** (hi″pər-pig″mən-ta′shən) [MeSH: Hyperpigmentation] abnormally increased pigmentation.

**hy·per·pi·ne·al·ism** (hi″pər-pin′e-əl-iz-əm) a presumed abnormal increase in secretion by the pineal body.

**hy·per·pip·e·co·la·te·mia** (hi″pər-pip″ə-kol″ə-te′me-ə) excess of pipecolic acid in the blood, usually associated with cerebrohepatorenal syndrome but also a consequence of hyperlysinemia.

**hy·per·pi·tu·i·ta·rism** (hi″pər-pĭ-too′ĭ-tə-riz″əm) [MeSH: Hyperpituitarism] a condition due to excessive secretion of pituitary hormones. Adenomas producing growth hormone can cause acromegaly and pituitary gigantism; those producing corticotropin can cause Cushing's disease; and those producing prolactin can cause galactorrhea-amenorrhea syndrome.

**hy·per·pla·sia** (hi″pər-pla′zhə) [*hyper-* + *-plasia*] [MeSH: Hyperplasia] abnormal multiplication or increase in the number of normal cells in normal arrangement in a tissue. See also *hypertrophy* and *proliferation.*
**adrenal h., congenital (CAH),** a group of inherited disorders in which deficiencies of enzymes that catalyze the biosynthesis of cortisol result in compensatory hypersecretion of adrenocorticotropic hormone and subsequent adrenal hyperplasia as well as excessive androgen production. There are several different forms, numbered

**Congenital Adrenal Hyperplasia**

| Type | Deficiency | Form | Ambiguous Genitalia | Postnatal Virilization | Salt Metabolism | Elevated Steriods | Decreased Steriods |
|---|---|---|---|---|---|---|---|
| I | Cholesterol desmolase | Lipoid hyperplasia | Males | No | Salt wasting | None | All |
| II | 3β-Hydroxysteroid dehydrogenase | Classic | | | | | |
| | | Salt-wasting | Males | Yes | Salt wasting | DHEA, 17-OH-Pregnenolone | Aldo, T, Cort, Estradiol |
| | | Non-salt-wasting | Males | Yes | Normal | DHEA, 17-OH-Pregnenolone | Aldo, T, Cort, Estradiol |
| | | Nonclassic | No | Yes | Normal | DHEA, 17-OH-Pregnenolone | — |
| III | 21-Hydroxylase | Classic | | | | | |
| | | Salt-wasting | Females | Yes | Salt wasting | 17-OHP, $\Delta^4$-A | Aldo, Cort |
| | | Simple virilizing | Females | Yes | Normal | 17-OHP, $\Delta^4$-A | Cort |
| | | Nonclassic | No | Yes | Normal | 17-OHP, $\Delta^4$-A | — |
| IV | 11 β-Hydroxylase | Classic | Females | Yes | Hypertension | DOC, 11-Deoxycortisol | Cort, Aldo |
| | | Nonclassic | No | Yes | Normal | 11-Deoxycortisol ± DOC | — |
| V | 17 α-Hydroxylase | — | Males | No | Hypertension | DOC, Corticosterone | Aldo, Andro, Cort, Estro |
| | 17,20-Lyase | — | Males | No | Normal | — | DHEA, T, $\Delta^4$-A |

Aldo = Aldosterone; T = Testosterone; Andro = Androgens; $\Delta^4$-A = $\Delta^4$-Androstenedione; Cort = Cortisol; DHEA = Dehydroepiandrosterone; DOC = (11-)Deoxycorticosterone; Estro = Estrogens; 17-OHP = 17α-Hydroxyprogesterone.

in order of increasing severity, of which the most common type is type III, or 21-hydroxylase deficiency (see accompanying table). They range from "classic" forms present at birth with severe salt wasting or hypertension and pseudohermaphroditism to less severe "nonclassic" forms of later onset. See also deficiency conditions at names of specific enzymes.
**adrenal h., lipoid,** an autosomal recessive disorder of steroidogenesis in which deficiency of cholesterol monooxygenase (side-chain-cleaving) causes a type of congenital adrenal hyperplasia (type I). The disorder is characterized by accumulation of lipids and cholesterol in the adrenal cortex, decreased or absent steroid hormones, severe salt wasting, sexual infantilism, and male pseudohermaphroditism; the adrenal insufficiency is usually lethal. See also accompanying table. Called also *cholesterol desmolase deficiency.*
**adrenal h., nodular,** uneven hyperplasia of the adrenal cortical tissue producing small nests or masses resembling adenomas between the columns of cortical cells. Called also *nodular adrenocortical h.*
**adrenal cortical h., adrenocortical h.,** hyperplasia of adrenal cortical cells, as in adrenogenital syndrome and Cushing's syndrome.
**adrenocortical h., nodular,** nodular adrenal hyperplasia.
**angiolymphoid h. with eosinophilia,** a type of erythematous dermal or subcutaneous nodule occurring singly or multiply, primarily on the head and neck of young adults, sometimes associated with lymphadenopathy, and characterized histologically by lymphoid hyperplasia, angioid proliferation, and tissue eosinophilia. The more superficial, usually larger, lesions have been called *pseudopyogenic granuloma.* See also *Kimura's disease,* under *disease.*
**C-cell h.,** a premalignant stage in the development of the familial forms of medullary thyroid carcinoma, characterized by multicentric patches of parafollicular cells (C cells).
**cementum h.,** hypercementosis.
**chronic perforating pulp h.,** internal tooth resorption (def. 1).
**cutaneous lymphoid h.,** a term for several benign cutaneous disorders with lesions clinically and histologically resembling those of malignant lymphoma. The lesions may be lymphoreticular, granulomatous, and follicular and include lymphocytes, histiocytes, eosinophils, plasma cells, and lymphoid follicles. The disorders may be of unknown etiology or be reactions to insect bites, allergy hyposensitization injections, light, trauma, and tattoo pigment. The term embraces lymphocytoma cutis, lymphocytic infiltration of the skin, and insect bite reactions.
**Dilantin h.,** see under *gingivitis.*
**endometrial h., h. endome'trii,** abnormal overgrowth of the endometrium.
**fibrous inflammatory h.,** masses of collagenized, fibrous connective tissue along the borders of ill-fitting dentures or in other areas where chronic irritation exists. Called also *epulis fissuratum.*
**follicular h.,** a form of chronic lymphadenitis, characterized by expansion of the germinal centers, which contain large numbers of rapidly proliferating lymphocytes in various stages of differentiation and histiocytes containing phagocytized debris; morphologically, it resembles follicular lymphoma.
**focal nodular h. (FNH),** a benign, usually asymptomatic tumor of the liver, occurring chiefly in women; it is a firm, nodular, highly vascular mass resembling cirrhosis, usually with a stellate fibrous core containing numerous small bile ducts, and having vessels lined by Kupffer cells.
**giant follicular h.,** a disorder of the lymph nodes, generally confined to the cervical lymph nodes, which may simulate follicular lymphoma, but cytologically the follicles contain both macrophages and lymphoblasts.
**giant lymph node h.,** Castleman's disease.
**gingival h.,** noninflammatory enlargement of the gingivae produced by factors other than local irritation. See also under *enlargement.*
**inflammatory h.,** hyperplasia brought about by inflammation.
**intimal h.,** thickening of the intima of a blood vessel as a complication of a reconstruction procedure or endarterectomy.
**intravascular papillary endothelial h.,** a benign vascular tumor usually occurring as a solitary nodule of the head, neck, or finger; it is characterized by papillary lobules of proliferating endothelial cells with an underlying fibrous stroma, and often resembles angiosarcoma.
**juxtaglomerular cell h.,** Bartter's syndrome.
**lipoid h.,** increased formation of lipoid-containing cells.
**lymphoid h.,** a form of chronic lymphadenitis occurring as an immunologic response, often induced by drugs, and characterized by transformation of T cells to lymphoblasts, endothelial cell hypertrophy, and the presence of a mixed leukocyte infiltrate.
**myofiber h.,** a hereditary condition of cattle characterized by increased muscle mass because of greater than average numbers of fibers in the muscles, with decreased fat and connective tissue. Called also *culard, doppellender,* and *double muscle.*
**neoplastic h.,** hyperplasia brought about by a new growth.
**nodular lymphoid h.,** a proliferation of small nodules of lymphoid tissue, seen in the terminal ileum and colon of children, in the small intestine and sometimes colon and stomach of adults with primary immunodeficiency disease, and, rarely, in adults with malignant lymphoma.
**nodular h. of the prostate,** benign prostatic hypertrophy.
**nodular regenerative h.,** a rare liver condition characterized by nodules of hyperplastic hepatocytes in the parenchyma that do not cause fibrosis or other major alterations in lobular architecture. Called also *nodular transformation of the liver.*
**ovarian stromal h.,** thecomatosis.
**polar h.,** excessive development at either extremity of the embryo, producing a fetus either with two heads or with three or more lower limbs.
**prostatic h., benign,** see under *hypertrophy.*
**prostatic h., cystic,** a usually benign type of hyperplasia of the prostate in dogs, with fluid-filled cysts, often due to obstruction of excretory ducts.
**pseudoepitheliomatous h.,** a benign proliferative epithelial hyperplasia, the cytoarchitectural features of which are suggestive of squamous cell carcinoma; occurring in certain diseases, especially granulomatous inflammatory reactions, ulcerations and certain tumors, e.g., granular cell tumors.
**sebaceous h.,** single or multiple yellowish, irregularly round lesions, usually occurring on the faces of older adults and representing enlargement and malformation of mature, well-organized sebaceous structures; they often mimic basal cell carcinoma in appearance.
**Swiss-cheese h.,** hyperplasia of a tissue which on section shows openings as in Swiss cheese.
**verrucous h.,** a superficial, typically white, hyperplastic lesion of the oral mucosa, usually occurring in older males; it is believed to be a precursor to verrucous carcinoma.

**hy·per·plas·mia** (hi″pər-plaz'me-ə) [*hyper-* + *plasma*] hypervolemia.

**hy·per·plas·tic** (hi″pər-plas'tik) pertaining to or characterized by hyperplasia.

**hy·per·ploid** (hi'pər-ploid) [*hyper-* + *-ploid*] 1. having more than the typical number of chromosomes in unbalanced sets, as in Down's syndrome. 2. an individual or cell having more than the typical number of chromosomes in unbalanced sets.

**hy·per·ploi·dy** (hi″pər-ploi'de) the state of being hyperploid. Cf. *aneuploidy.*

**hy·per·pnea** (hi″pər-ne'ə, hi″pərp-ne'ə) [*hyper-* + *-pnea*] abnormal increase in the depth and rate of breathing; see also *hyperventilation* (def. 1) and *tachypnea.* Called also *polypnea.*

**hy·per·pne·ic** (hi″pər-ne'ik, hi″pərp-ne'ik) pertaining to or characterized by hyperpnea. Called also *polypneic.*

**hy·per·po·lar·iza·tion** (hi″pər-po″lər-ĭ-za'shən) any increase in the amount of electrical charge separated by the cell membrane and hence in the strength of the transmembrane potential; thus it is a negative shift in the resting potential of the cell.

**hy·per·poly·pep·tid·emia** (hi″pər-pol″e-pep″tĭ-de'me-ə) excess of polypeptides in the blood.

**hy·per·po·ne·sis** (hi″pər-po-ne'sis) [*hyper-* + *pon-* + *-esis*] dysponesis in which there is excessive action-potential output from the motor and premotor areas of the cortex.

**hy·per·po·net·ic** (hi″pər-po-net'ik) pertaining to or characterized by hyperponesis.

**hy·per·po·sia** (hi″pər-po'zhə) [*hyper-* + *posia*] abnormally increased ingestion of fluids for relatively brief periods. Cf. *polyposia.*

**hy·per·po·tas·se·mia** (hi″pər-po″tə-se'me-ə) hyperkalemia.

**hy·per·pra·gia** (hi″pər-pra'je-ə) excessive mental activity.

**hy·per·prax·ia** (hi″pər-prak'she-ə) [*hyper-* + *praxis*] excessive activity; restlessness.

**hy·per·pre·be·ta·lipo·pro·tein·emia** (hi″pər-pre-ba″tə-lip″o-pro″te-ne'me-ə) an excess of pre-beta lipoproteins (very-low-density lipoproteins) in the blood.
**familial h.,** see under *hypertriglyceridemia.*

**hy·per·pres·by·opia** (hi″pər-pres″be-o'pe-ə) excessive presbyopia.

**hy·per·pro·in·su·lin·emia** (hi″pər-pro-in″sə-lĭ-ne'me-ə) elevated levels of proinsulin or proinsulin-like material in the blood.

**hy·per·pro·lac·tin·emia** (hi″pər-pro-lak″tĭ-ne'me-ə) [MeSH: Hyperprolactinemia] increased levels of prolactin in the blood; in women it is associated with amenorrhea and galactorrhea, and in men it has been reported to cause hypogonadism, impotence, and in some cases gynecomastia. It is often associated with microadenoma of the adenohypophysis.

**hy·per·pro·lac·tin·emic** (hi″pər-pro-lak″tĭ-ne'mik) pertaining to, characterized by, or affected by hyperprolactinemia.

**hy·per·pro·lin·emia** (hi″pər-pro″lĭ-ne'me-ə) 1. an autosomal recessive aminoacidopathy characterized by an excess of proline in the body fluids and occurring as two types, both of which are probably benign. *Type I* is caused by deficiency of proline oxidase; *type II* is due to deficiency of 1-pyrroline-5-carboxylate dehydrogenase and is characterized by accumulation of higher levels of proline and by urinary excretion of $\Delta^1$-pyrroline 5-carboxylate. 2. excess of proline in the blood.

**hy·per·pro·sex·ia** (hi″pər-pro-sek′se-ə) [*hyper-* + Gr. *prosechein* to heed] a condition in which the mind is occupied by one idea to the exclusion of others.

**hy·per·pros·o·dy** (hi″pər-pros′ə-de) dysprosody marked by exaggerated variations in stress, pitch, or rhythm.

**hy·per·pro·tein·emia** (hi″pər-pro″te-ne′me-ə) [*hyper-* + *protein* + *-emia*] the presence of an abnormally high amount of protein in the blood; see also *hyperlipoproteinemia.*

**hy·per·pro·te·o·sis** (hi″pər-pro″te-o′sis) a condition caused by an excess of protein in the diet.

**hy·perp·sel·a·phe·sia** (hi″pərp-sel″ə-fe′zhə) [*hyper-* + Gr. *psēlaphēsis* touch + *-ia*] tactile hyperesthesia.

**hy·per·pty·al·ism** (hi″pər-ti′əl-iz-əm) [*hyper-* + Gr. *ptyalon* spittle] ptyalism.

**hy·per·py·re·mia** (hi″pər-pi-re′me-ə) [*hyper-* + Gr. *pyreia* fuel + *emia*] excess of unoxidized carbonaceous matter in the blood.

**hy·per·py·ret·ic** (hi″pər-pi-ret′ik) pertaining to, exhibiting, or causing hyperpyrexia.

**hy·per·py·rex·ia** (hi″pər-pi-rek′se-ə) [*hyper-* + *pyrexia*] hyperthermia.
**malignant h.,** see under *hyperthermia.*

**hy·per·py·rex·i·al** (hi″pər-pi-rek′se-əl) pertaining to hyperpyrexia.

**hy·per·re·ac·tive** (hi″pər-re-ak′tiv) pertaining to or characterized by a greater than normal response to a stimulus or irritant. Cf. *irritability* and *reaction.*

**hy·per·re·ac·tiv·i·ty** (hi″pər-re-ak-tiv′ĭ-te) the quality of being hyperreactive. Cf. *irritability.* Called also *hyperresponsiveness.*

**hy·per·re·flex·ia** (hi″pər-re-flek′se-ə) [*hyper-* + *reflex* + *-ia*] dysreflexia characterized by exaggeration of reflexes.
**autonomic h.,** your paroxysmal hypertension, bradycardia, sweating of the forehead, severe headache, and gooseflesh due to distention of the bladder and rectum; it is associated with lesions above the outflow of the splanchnic nerves.
**detrusor h.,** increased contractile activity of the detrusor urinae muscle, resulting in urinary incontinence, seen in spinal neural disease, dementia, parkinsonism, and supraspinal neural and vascular disease. Cf. *detrusor instability,* under *instability.*

**hy·per·re·nin·emia** (hi″pər-re″nĭ-ne′me-ə) a condition of elevated levels of renin in the blood, which may lead to aldosteronism. See also *reninism.*

**hy·per·re·nin·emic** (hi″pər-re″nĭ-ne′mik) producing or characterized by hyperreninemia.

**hy·per·res·o·nance** (hi″pər-rez′o-nəns) an exaggerated resonance.

**hy·per·re·spon·sive** (hi″pər-rə-spon′siv) hyperreactive.

**hy·per·re·spon·sive·ness** (hi″pər-rə-spon′siv-nes) hyperreactivity.
**airway h.,** an abnormality of the airways in which there is an exaggerated bronchoconstrictor response to any of various physical or chemical stimuli; seen in conditions such as asthma and sometimes chronic obstructive pulmonary disease.

**hy·per·sal·emia** (hi″pər-sal-e′me-ə) abnormally increased salt in the blood. Called also *hyperalonemia.*

**hy·per·sa·line** (hi″pər-sa′lēn) excessively saline: a term applied to treatment by the administration of large doses of sodium chloride.

**hy·per·sal·i·va·tion** (hi″pər-sal″ĭ-va′shən) ptyalism.

**hy·per·sar·co·sin·e·mia** (hi″pər-sahr″ko-sĭ-ne′me-ə) sarcosinemia.

**hy·per·se·cre·tion** (hi″pər-se-kre′shən) excessive secretion.
**gastric h.,** hyperchlorhydria.

**hy·per·seg·men·ta·tion** (hi″pər-seg″mən-ta′shən) a condition of having more segments or lobes than usual.
**hereditary h. of neutrophils,** a hereditary condition in which the neutrophils are multilobed; called also *Undritz anomaly.*

**hy·per·sen·si·bil·i·ty** (hi″pər-sen″sĭ-bil′ĭ-te) excessive sensibility.

**hy·per·sen·si·tive** (hi″pər-sen′sĭ-tiv) 1. exhibiting abnormally increased sensitivity. 2. having the specific or general ability to react with characteristic signs and symptoms to the application or contact with certain substances (allergens) in amounts innocuous to normal (nonsensitized) individuals. See *hypersensitivity.*

**hy·per·sen·si·tiv·i·ty** (hi″pər-sen″sĭ-tiv′ĭ-te) [MeSH: Hypersensitivity] a state of altered reactivity in which the body reacts with an exaggerated or inappropriate immune response to what is perceived to be a foreign substance. The resulting hypersensitivity reactions are usually subclassified as types I–IV on the basis of the Gell and Coombs classification of immune responses; see individual types under *hypersensitivity reaction* at *reaction.*
**anaphylactic h.,** the most severe form of type I hypersensitivity, manifest as anaphylaxis. The term is sometimes used more loosely to describe any form of type I hypersensitivity, when contrasting this group with other types of hypersensitivity (e.g., types II–IV).
**antibody-mediated h.,** 1. type II h. 2. occasionally, any form of hypersensitivity in which antibodies are the primary mediators, as contrasted with that mediated by T lymphocytes; included are *types I, II,* and *III h.*
**antibody-mediated cytotoxic h.,** type II h.
**cell-mediated h.,** type IV h.
**contact h.,** a type IV hypersensitivity produced by contact of the skin with a chemical substance having the properties of an antigen or hapten, the resulting skin condition being allergic contact dermatitis.
***Culicoides* h.,** allergic dermatitis in horses as a reaction to the bites of various species of *Culicoides* flies, characterized by severe pruritus in the mane and tail region, alopecia or broken hairs from scratching, and a serous effusion with crusting. Called also *Queensland itch* and *sweet itch.*
**cutaneous basophil h.,** Jones-Mote reaction.
**cytotoxic h.,** type II h.
**delayed h. (DH), delayed-type h. (DTH),** the type of hypersensitivity which (as opposed to *immediate h.*) takes 24 to 72 hours to develop and is mediated by T lymphocytes rather than by antibodies; the term is usually used to denote the subset of type IV hypersensitivity involving cytokine release and macrophage activation, as opposed to direct cytolysis, but can be used more broadly, even sometimes being used synonymously with *type IV h.* (q.v.)
**immediate h.,** 1. type I h. 2. occasionally, any form of hypersensitivity mediated by antibodies and developing rapidly, generally in minutes to hours (i.e., *type I, II,* or *III h.*), as distinguished from that mediated by T lymphocytes and macrophages and generally requiring 24 to 72 hours to develop (*type IV h.,* sometimes called *delayed h.*).
**immune complex–mediated h.,** type III h.
**T cell–mediated h.,** type IV h.
**tuberculin-type h.,** older name for *delayed h.*
**type I h.,** that occurring rapidly, within several minutes, upon reexposure to an antigen, due to interaction of IgE and the antigen; see *type I hypersensitivity reaction,* under *hypersensitivity reaction,* at *reaction.*
**type II h.,** that resulting from antibody-antigen interactions on cell surfaces; see *type II hypersensitivity reaction,* under *hypersensitivity reaction,* at *reaction.* Called also *antibody-mediated h.*
**type III h.,** that due to formation of circulating antigen-antibody complexes and their deposition in tissues; see *type III hypersensitivity reaction,* under *hypersensitivity reaction,* at *reaction.* Called also *immune complex–mediated h.*
**type IV h.,** that initiated by antigen-specific T lymphocytes; unlike forms of hypersensitivity mediated by antibodies, it takes one or more days to develop and can be transferred by lymphocytes but not by serum. The term is often equated with *delayed hypersensitivity*, although the latter is sometimes restricted to hypersensitivity involving cytokine-mediated reactions (as contrasted with direct cytolysis). See *type IV hypersensitivity reaction,* under *hypersensitivity reaction,* at *reaction.* Called also *cell-* or *T cell–mediated h.*

**hy·per·sen·si·ti·za·tion** (hi″pər-sen″sĭ-tĭ-za′shən) the process of rendering or the condition of being abnormally sensitive. See *hypersensitivity.*

**hy·per·sero·to·ne·mia** (hi″pər-se″ro-to-ne′me-ə) an elevation of the serum serotonin level.

**hy·per·sex·u·al·i·ty** (hi″pər-sek″shoo-al′ĭ-te) abnormally increased sexual desire or activity; nymphomania; satyriasis.

**hy·per·so·mato·trop·ism** (hi″pər-so-mat″o-trop′iz-əm) excessive secretion of growth hormone, as seen in acromegaly and gigantism.

**hy·per·so·mia** (hi″pər-so′me-ə) [*hyper-* + *-somia*] gigantism.

**hy·per·som·nia** (hi″pər-som′ne-ə) [*hyper-* + *somn-* + *-ia*] [MeSH: Hypersomnia] excessive sleeping or sleepiness, as in any of a group of sleep disorders with a variety of physical and psychogenic causes.
**primary h.** [DSM-IV], a dyssomnia consisting of persistent excessive sleepiness and sleeping, with prolonged sleep episodes or regularly occurring voluntary or involuntary napping, and not due to any other psychological or physical condition.

**hy·per·som·no·lence** (hi″pər-som′no-lens) hypersomnia.

**hy·per·sphyx·ia** (hi″pər-sfik′se-ə) [*hyper-* + Gr. *sphyxis* pulse + *-ia*] increased activity of the circulation with increased blood pressure.

**hy·per·sple·nia** (hi″pər-sple′ne-ə) hypersplenism.

**hy·per·splen·ism** (hi″pər-splen′iz-əm) [MeSH: Hypersplenism] a condition characterized by exaggeration of the suggested inhibitory or destructive functions of the spleen, resulting in deficiency of the peripheral blood elements, singly or in combination, hypercellularity of the bone marrow, and usually, but not always, splenomegaly.

**hy·per·spon·gi·o·sis** (hi″pər-spon″je-o′sis) proliferation of the substantia spongiosa ossium.

**Hy·per·stat** (hi′pər-stat) trademark for a preparation of diazoxide.

**hy·per·ste·a·to·sis** (hi″pər-ste-ə-to′sis) [*hyper-* + *steatosis*] increased or excessive sebaceous secretion, as in seborrhea.

**hy·per·ster·eo·ra·di·og·ra·phy** (hi″pər-ste″re-o-ra″di-og′rə-fe) stereoradiography with great distance between the homologous points.

**hy·per·ster·eo·ski·ag·ra·phy** (hi″pər-ster″e-o-ski-ag′rə-fe) hyperstereoradiography.

**hy·per·sthe·nia** (hi″pər-sthe′ne-ə) [*hyper-* + *sthenia*] great strength or tonicity.

**hy·per·sthen·ic** (hi″pər-sthen′ik) pertaining to or characterized by hypersthenia.

**hy·per·sthen·uria** (hi″pər-sthə-nu′re-ə) [*hyper-* + *sthen-* + *-uria*] increased osmolality of the urine.

**hy·per·su·pra·re·nal·ism** (hi″pər-soo″prə-re′nəl-iz-əm) hyperadrenalism.

**hy·per·sus·cep·ti·bil·i·ty** (hi″pər-sə-sep″tĭ-bil′ĭ-te) a condition of abnormally increased susceptibility to poisons, infective agents, or agents to which the normal individual is less susceptible.

**hy·per·sym·path·i·co·to·nus** (hi″pər-sim-path″ĭ-ko-to′nəs) abnormally increased tone of the sympathetic nervous system; see also sympathicotonia.

**hy·per·ta·rach·ia** (hi″pər-tə-rak′e-ə) [*hyper-* + Gr. *tarachē* confusion + *-ia*] extreme irritability of the nervous system. See *nervous irritability* (def. 2), under *irritability*.

**hy·per·tau·ro·don·tism** (hi″pər-taw″ro-don′tiz-əm) [*hyper-* + *taurodontism*] taurodontism in which the tooth roots do not branch.

**hy·per·telo·rism** (hi″pər-te′lor-iz-əm) [*hyper-* + Gr. *tēlouros* distant] [MeSH: Hypertelorism] 1. abnormally increased distance between two organs or parts. 2. ocular h.
**ocular h., orbital h.,** a condition characterized by abnormal increase in the interorbital distance, often associated with cleidocranial or craniofacial dysostosis, and occasionally accompanied by mental deficiency.

**hy·per·ten·sion** (hi″pər-ten′shən) [*hyper-* + *tension*] [MeSH: Hypertension] high arterial blood pressure; various criteria for its threshold have been suggested, ranging from 140 mm Hg systolic and 90 mm Hg diastolic to as high as 200 mm Hg systolic and 110 mm Hg diastolic. Hypertension may have no known cause *(essential* or *idiopathic h.)* or be associated with other primary diseases *(secondary h.)*. See also *blood pressure*, under *pressure*.
**accelerated h.,** progressive hypertension marked by the funduscopic vascular changes of malignant hypertension but without papilledema.
**adrenal h.,** hypertension caused by an adrenal tumor that secretes mineralocorticoids, such as in hyperaldosteronism; in many cases it may be associated with excessive production of other adrenocortical hormones normally made in minute amounts.
**benign intracranial h.,** pseudotumor cerebri.
**borderline h.,** a condition in which the arterial blood pressure is sometimes within the normotensive range and sometimes within the hypertensive range; called also *labile h.*
**essential h.,** hypertension occurring without discoverable organic cause; called also *primary h.* and *idiopathic h.*
**familial dyslipidemic h.,** an inherited syndrome of seriously disordered blood lipid levels and essential hypertension.
**Goldblatt h.,** hypertension experimentally induced with clamping that causes a Goldblatt kidney; called also *Goldblatt phenomenon.*
**idiopathic h.,** essential h.
**intracranial h.,** increased intracranial pressure; if symmetrically distributed it may have few neurologic symptoms (see *pseudotumor cerebri*), but if it is asymmetrical, as with hydrocephalus, neurologic symptoms are often severe.
**labile h.,** borderline h.
**low-renin h.,** essential hypertension associated with low levels of plasma-renin concentration or low renin activity.
**malignant h.,** a severe hypertensive state with poor prognosis; it is characterized by papilledema of the ocular fundus with vascular exudative and hemorrhagic lesions, medial thickening of small arteries and arterioles, and left ventricular hypertrophy. Diastolic pressures as high as 130 mm Hg or more are commonly present.
**ocular h.,** persistently elevated intraocular pressure in the absence of any other signs of glaucoma; it may or may not progress to chronic simple glaucoma.
**portal h.,** abnormally increased blood pressure in the portal venous system, a frequent complication of cirrhosis of the liver.
**primary h.,** essential h.
**pulmonary h.,** increased pressure (above 30 mm Hg systolic and 12 mm Hg diastolic) within the pulmonary arterial circulation.
**renal h.,** hypertension due to or associated with renal disease with a factor of parenchymal ischemia.
**renovascular h.,** hypertension due to occlusive disease of the renal arteries.
**secondary h.,** hypertension due to or associated with a variety of primary diseases, such as renal disorders, disorders of the central nervous system, endocrine diseases, and vascular diseases.
**splenoportal h.,** obstruction of the splenic venous system resulting in enlargement of the liver and manifestation of ascites and other evidence of portal cirrhosis.
**symptomatic h.,** hypertension accompanied by symptoms such as dizziness or headache.
**systemic venous h.,** elevation of systemic venous pressure, usually detected by inspection of the jugular veins.
**vascular h.,** hypertension.

**hy·per·ten·sive** (hi″pər-ten′siv) 1. characterized by increased tension or pressure. 2. an agent that causes hypertension; called also *arteriopressor.* 3. a person with hypertension.

**hy·per·ten·sor** (hi″pər-ten′sor) a pressor agent.

**Hy·per-Tet** (hi′pər-tet″) trademark for a preparation of tetanus immune human globulin.

**hy·per·the·co·sis** (hi″pər-the-ko′sis) hyperplasia with excessive luteinization of the cells of the inner stromal layer, the theca interna, of the ovary; it may be associated with hirsutism and amenorrhea and is seen in most cases of Stein-Leventhal syndrome.

**hy·per·the·lia** (hi″pər-the′le-ə) [*hyper-* + *thel-* + *-ia*] the presence of supernumerary nipples.

**hy·per·ther·mal** (hi″pər-ther′məl) marked by abnormally high temperature.

**hy·per·ther·mal·ge·sia** (hi″pər-thər″məl-je′ze-ə) [*hyper-* + *thermalgesia*] abnormally increased sensitivity to heat; cf. *thermalgesia.* Called also *hyperthermesthesia* and *hyperthermoesthesia*.

**hy·per·ther·mes·the·sia** (hi″pər-ther″mes-the′zhə) [*hyper-* + *therm-* + *esthesia*] hyperthermalgesia.

**hy·per·ther·mia** (hi″pər-ther′me-ə) [*hyper-* + *therm-* + *-ia*] 1. elevation of core body temperature to above 37.2°C (99°F). 2. the raising of body temperature to between 42°C (107.6°F) and 45° C (113.0°F) for therapeutic purposes. Cf. *thermotherapy.*
**h. of anesthesia,** malignant h.
**malignant h.,** 1. an autosomal dominant disorder with multifactorial inheritance, occurring in patients undergoing general anesthesia, and causing a sudden, rapid rise in body temperature, associated with signs of increased muscle metabolism, such as tachycardia, tachypnea, sweating, cyanosis, increased carbon dioxide production, and usually muscle rigidity. Called also *h. of anesthesia* and *malignant hyperpyrexia.* 2. a similar condition in pigs, a type of porcine stress syndrome in reaction to drugs such as halothane or succinylcholine chloride.

**hy·per·ther·mo·es·the·sia** (hi″pər-thər″mo-əs-the′zhə) hyperthermalgesia.

**hy·per·ther·my** (hi″pər-thər′me) hyperthermia.

**hy·per·throm·bin·emia** (hi″pər-throm″bĭ-ne′me-ə) abnormally high thrombin content of the blood.

**hy·per·thy·mia** (hi″pər-thi′me-ə) [*hyper-* + *thymo-* + *-ia*] 1. excessive emotionalism. 2. excessive activity, verging on hypomania.

**hy·per·thy·mic** (hi″pər-thi′mik) marked by hyperthymia.

**hy·per·thy·mism** (hi″pər-thi′miz-əm) a condition attributed to excessive activity of the thymus gland.

**hy·per·thy·rea** (hi″pər-thi′re-ə) hyperthyroidism.

**hy·per·thy·roid** (hi″pər-thi′roid) marked by or due to hyperthyroidism.

**hy·per·thy·roid·ism** (hi″pər-thi′roid-iz-əm) [MeSH: Hyperthyroidism] a condition caused by excessive production of iodinated thyroid hormones; characteristics include goiter, tachycardia or atrial fibrillation, widened pulse pressure, palpitations, fatigability, nervousness and tremor, heat intolerance and excessive sweating, warm, smooth, moist skin, weight loss, muscular weakness, hyperdefecation, emotional lability, and ocular signs (stare, lid lag, photophobia, and sometimes exophthalmos). Called also *hyperthyrea* and *hyperthyroidosis.* See also *Graves' disease* and *thyrotoxicosis.*
**iodine-induced h.,** hyperthyroidism following administration of iodine or iodide, either as a dietary supplement or as contrast medium. Called also *jodbasedow.*

**masked h.**, hyperactivity of the thyroid gland in which the classic signs and symptoms are subtle, and predominance of cardiovascular symptoms leads to suspicion of heart disease rather than thyroid disease; it occurs chiefly in middle-aged or elderly persons.

**hy·per·thy·roid·osis** (hi″pər-thi″roid-o′sis) hyperthyroidism.

**hy·per·thy·rox·in·emia** (hi″pər-thi-rok″sĭ-ne′me-ə) [MeSH: Hyperthyroxinemia] excessively high blood levels of thyroxine.
**familial dysalbuminemic h.**, an autosomal dominant disorder in which an elevation in total serum thyroxine concentration suggests the presence of hyperthyroidism; however, patients are euthyroid by clinical evaluation and other tests because an excess of $T_4$-binding serum albumin results in normal free thyroxine concentration and triiodothyroxine resin uptake.

**hy·per·to·nia** (hi″pər-to′ne-ə) [*hyper-* + *ton-* + *-ia*] a condition of excessive tone of the skeletal muscles; increased resistance of muscle to passive stretching.
**h. polycythae′mica,** increased blood pressure associated with polycythemia.

**hy·per·ton·ic** (hi″pər-ton′ik) 1. denoting a solution which when bathing body cells causes a net flow of water across the semipermeable cell membrane out of the cell. 2. denoting a solution having a greater tonicity than another solution, e.g., the blood, with which it is compared. 3. exhibiting hypertonia.

**hy·per·to·nic·i·ty** (hi″pər-to-nis′ĭ-te) the state or quality of being hypertonic.

**hy·per·to·nus** (hi″pər-to′nəs) hypertonia.

**hy·per·tox·ic** (hi″pər-tok′sik) excessively toxic.

**hy·per·tox·ic·i·ty** (hi″pər-tok-sis′ĭ-te) the state or quality of being excessively toxic.

**hy·per·trans·fu·sion** (hi″pər-trans-fu′zhən) a regimen of regular transfusions, usually given to children with chronic conditions such as $\beta$-thalassemia or sickle cell disease to prevent anemia.

**hy·per·tri·cho·sis** (hi″pər-trĭ-ko′sis) [*hyper-* + *trich-* + *-osis*] [MeSH: Hypertrichosis] excessive growth of the hair. Called also *polytrichia* and *polytrichosis.* Cf. *hirsutism.*
**h. lanugino′sa,** persistent or acquired production of lanugo. It may be a congenital, autosomal dominant disorder in which there is excessive hair distributed over the entire body throughout life, usually in association with other congenital anomalies, called also *h. universalis;* or it may be acquired, with the degree of hairiness being variable, and usually involving the face, and in most cases associated with internal carcinoma.
**h. pin′nae au′ris,** hypertrichosis involving the pinna of the ear; it may be a Y-linked or an autosomal dominant trait. Called also *hairy ears.*
**h. universa′lis,** the congenital form of hypertrichosis lanuginosa.

**hy·per·tri·glyc·er·i·de·mia** (hi″pər-tri-glis′ə-ri-de′me-ə) [MeSH: Hypertriglyceridemia] an excess of triglycerides in the blood.
**familial h.**, an autosomal dominant disorder of lipoprotein metabolism characterized by mildly elevated triglycerides and very-low-density lipoproteins, thus having a type IV hyperlipoproteinemia phenotype but lacking other biochemical or clinical features. The disorder can interact with secondary factors to cause more severe elevation of triglycerides with hyperchylomicronemia, a type V phenotype; see *familial hyperchylomicronemia* and see also table at *hyperlipoproteinemia.*
**sporadic h.**, hypertriglyceridemia that appears to be identical to an inherited form but in which inheritance cannot be documented; used in classifying disorders of lipoprotein metabolism.

**hy·per·tro·phia** (hi″pər-tro′fe-ə) hypertrophy.

**hy·per·troph·ic** (hi″pər-trof′ik) pertaining to or marked by hypertrophy.

**hy·per·tro·phy** (hi-pər′tro-fe) [*hyper-* + *-trophy*] [MeSH: Hypertrophy] the enlargement or overgrowth of an organ or part due to an increase in size of its constituent cells. See also *hyperplasia* and *proliferation.*
**adaptive h.**, increase in size in response to changed conditions, as, for example, increased thickness of the walls of a hollow organ when the outflow is obstructed.
**asymmetrical septal h. (ASH),** hypertrophic cardiomyopathy; sometimes used specifically for cases in which the hypertrophy is localized to the interventricular septum. Cf. *hypertrophic obstructive cardiomyopathy.*
**Billroth h.**, idiopathic benign hypertrophy of the pylorus.
**compensatory h.**, that which results from an increased workload due to some physical defect, as occurs in one kidney when the other is absent or destroyed by disease.
**complementary h.**, increase in size of the remaining part of an organ to take the place of a portion which has been lost.
**concentric h.**, hypertrophy of a hollow organ in which there is increased thickness of the walls with no enlargement in external size, with diminished capacity.
**eccentric h.**, hypertrophy of a hollow organ in which there is dilatation of its cavity and enlargement of its external size.
**false h.**, enlargement due to an increase in only one constituent element of an organ or part, commonly the stroma.
**functional h.**, hypertrophy of an organ or part caused by its increased activity.
**hemifacial h.**, overgrowth of one side of the face.
**Marie's h.**, enlargement of the soft parts of the joints resulting from periostitis.
**numeric h.**, that which is due to an increased number of structural elements.
**physiologic h.**, temporary increase in the size of an organ produced by physiologic activity, as in the female breast during pregnancy and lactation.
**prostatic h., benign,** age-associated enlargement of the prostate resulting from proliferation of both glandular and stromal elements, beginning generally in the fifth decade of life; it may cause urethral compression and obstruction. Called also *benign prostatic hypertrophy* and *nodular hyperplasia of the prostate.*
**pseudomuscular h.**, pseudohypertrophic muscular dystrophy.
**simple h.**, that which is due to a simple increase of the number of structural elements.
**true h.**, enlargement due to an increase of all the component elements of an organ or part.
**unilateral h.**, overgrowth of one side of the entire body or of a portion of one side, as of the face.
**ventricular h.**, hypertrophy of the myocardium of a ventricle, due to chronic pressure overload; it is manifest electrocardiographically by increased QRS complex voltage, frequently accompanied by repolarization changes.
**vicarious h.**, hypertrophy of an organ in consequence of the failure of another organ of allied function. Cf. *compensatory h.*

**hy·per·tro·pia** (hi″pər-tro′pe-ə) [*hyper-* + *trop-* + *-ia*] strabismus in which there is permanent upward deviation of the visual axis of an eye.

**Hy·per·tus·sis** (hi″pər-tus′is) trademark for a preparation of pertussis immune human globulin.

**hy·per·ty·ro·sin·emia** (hi″pər-ti″ro-sĭ-ne′me-ə) 1. an elevated concentration of tyrosine in the blood, as occurs in a variety of disorders of tyrosine catabolism. 2. tyrosinemia.

**hy·per·ure·sis** (hi″pər-u-re′sis) polyuria.

**hy·per·u·ric·ac·i·de·mia** (hi″pər-u″rik-as″ĭ-de′me-ə) hyperuricemia.

**hy·per·u·ric·ac·i·du·ria** (hi″pər-u″rik-as″ĭ-du′re-ə) hyperuricuria.

**hy·per·uri·ce·mia** (hi″pər-u″rĭ-se′me-ə) excess of uric acid or urates in the blood; it is a prerequisite for the development of gout and may lead to renal disease. Called also *hyperuricacidemia, uricacidemia,* and *uricemia.*

**hy·per·uri·ce·mic** (hi″pər-u″rĭ-se′mik) pertaining to or characterized by hyperuricemia.

**hy·per·uri·co·su·ria** (hi″per-u″rĭ-ko-su′re-ə) hyperuricuria.

**hy·per·u·ric·uria** (hi″pər-u″rik-u′re-ə) excess of uric acid or urates in the urine. Called also *hyperuricaciduria, uricaciduria,* and *uricosuria.*

**hy·per·vac·ci·na·tion** (hi″pər-vak″sĭ-na′shən) the subsequent inoculation (one or more times) of a previously immunized animal with enough vaccine to enable it to afford a serum protective to other animals.

**hy·per·val·i·ne·mia** (hi″pər-val″ĭ-ne′me-ə) 1. an autosomal recessive aminoacidopathy, probably due to a defect in valine transaminase, characterized by elevated levels of valine in the plasma and urine and by failure to thrive. 2. elevated levels of valine in the plasma. Called also *valinemia.*

**hy·per·vas·cu·lar** (hi″pər-vas′ku-lər) extremely vascular.

**hy·per·ven·ti·la·tion** (hi″pər-ven″tĭ-la′shən) [MeSH: Hyperventilation] 1. a state in which there is an increased amount of air entering the pulmonary alveoli (increased *alveolar ventilation*; see under *ventilation*). This results in reduction of carbon dioxide tension, eventually leading to alkalosis. See also *hyperpnea, tachypnea,* and *hyperventilation syndrome.* 2. abnormally prolonged, rapid, and deep breathing (polypnea), frequently used as a test procedure in epilepsy and tetany.

**hy·per·vig·i·lance** (hi″pər-vij′ĭ-lans) abnormally increased arousal, responsiveness to stimuli, and scanning of the environment for threats; it is often associated with delusional or paranoid states.

**hy·per·vis·cos·i·ty** (hi″pər-vis-kos′ĭ-te) excessive viscosity, as of the blood; see also *hyperviscosity syndrome,* under *syndrome.*

**hy·per·vi·ta·min·o·sis** (hi″pər-vi″tə-mĭ-no′sis) a condition due to ingestion of an excess of one or more vitamins; called also *supervitaminosis.*

**h. A,** a symptom complex resulting from ingestion of excessive amounts of vitamin A, with hair loss, skin disorders, headache, bone and joint pain, anorexia, fatigue, irritability, hyperostosis, hepatosplenomegaly, papilledema, and pseudotumor cerebri.
**h. D,** a symptom complex resulting from ingestion of excessive amounts of vitamin D, with weakness, fatigue, loss of weight, and other symptoms.

**hy·per·vi·ta·min·ot·ic** (hi″pər-vi″tə-mĭ-not′ik) pertaining to or characterized by hypervitaminosis.

**hy·per·vo·le·mia** (hi″pər-vo-le′me-ə) [*hyper-* + *volume* + *-emia*] abnormal increase in the volume of circulating blood plasma; see also *hemodilution.*

**hy·per·vo·le·mic** (hi″pər-vo-le′mik) pertaining to or characterized by hypervolemia.

**hy·per·vo·lia** (hi″pər-vo′le-ə) augmented water content or volume of a given compartment, e.g., as of a cell.

**hyp·es·the·sia** (hīp″əs-the′zhə) [MeSH: Hypesthesia] hypoesthesia.

**hy·pha** (hi′fə) pl. *hy′phae* [L., from Gr. *hyphe* web] 1. one of the filaments or threads composing the mycelium of a fungus. 2. branching filamentous outgrowths produced by certain bacteria (e.g., *Actinomyces, Hyphomicrobium*), sometimes forming a mycelium.
**aerial h.,** one produced above the surface of a culture medium.
**racket h.,** one composed of racket cells, found in various kinds of dermatophytes.

**hy·phal** (hi′fəl) pertaining to a hypha.

**hyp·he·do·nia** (hīp″hə-do′ne-ə) [*hypo-* + Gr. *hēdonē* pleasure + *-ia*] pathologic diminution of the feeling of pleasure in acts that normally give pleasure.

**hy·phe·ma** (hi-fe′mə) [Gr. *hyphaimos* suffused with blood, bloodshot; especially of the eyes] [MeSH: Hyphema] hemorrhage within the anterior chamber of the eye. Called also *hyphemia.*

**hy·phe·mia** (hi-fe′me-ə) hyphema.

**hyp·hid·ro·sis** (hīp″hi-dro′sis) [*hypo-* + Gr. *hidrōs* sweat + *-osis*] hypohidrosis.

**Hy·pho·my·ce·ta·les** (hi″fo-mi″se-ta′lēz) name used for the form-order Moniales in some classifications of fungi.

**hy·pho·my·cete** (hi″fo-mi′sēt) any individual organism of the class Hyphomycetes.

**Hy·pho·my·ce·tes** (hi″fo-mi-se′tēz) [pl., Gr. *hyphē* web + Gr. *mykēs* fungus] [MeSH: Hyphomycetes] a form-class of Fungi Imperfecti (subphylum Deuteromycotina), consisting of the mycelial (hyphal) fungi, i.e., molds. It usually is considered to include the form-families Dematiaceae and Moniliaceae, and sometimes Cryptococcaceae.

**hy·pho·my·co·sis** (hi″fo-mi-ko′sis) any infection caused by an imperfect fungus of the form-class *Hyphomycetes*; the group has been divided into *hyalohyphomycosis* and *phaeohyphomycosis* based on the color of the mycelium and wall of the fungus.
**h. de′struens e′qui,** pythiosis.

**hyp·iso·ton·ic** (hīp″i-so-ton′ik) less than isotonic.

**hyp·na·gog·ic** (hip″nə-goj′ik) 1. producing sleep. 2. occurring just before sleep; applied to hallucinations occurring at sleep onset.

**hyp·na·gogue** (hip′nə-gog) [*hypno-* + *-agogue*] 1. hypnotic; pertaining to drowsiness. 2. an agent that induces sleep or drowsiness.

**hyp·nal·gia** (hip-nal′jə) [*hypno-* + *-algia*] pain that occurs during sleep.

**hyp·nic** (hip′nik) [Gr. *hypnikos*] inducing or pertaining to sleep.

**hypn(o)-** [Gr. *hypnos* sleep] a combining form denoting relationship to sleep or to hypnosis.

**hyp·no·anal·y·sis** (hip″no-ə-nal′ə-sis) [*hypno-* + *analysis*] a method of psychotherapy in which psychoanalysis is employed in conjunction with hypnosis.

**hyp·no·an·es·the·sia** (hip″no-an″əs-the′zhə) induction of the anesthetic state by hypnosis.

**hyp·no·cine·mato·graph** (hip″no-sin″ə-mat′o-graf) [*hypno-* + Gr. *kinēma* movement + *-graph*] somnocinematograph.

**hyp·no·cyst** (hip′no-sist) [*hypno-* + *cyst*] a quiescent cyst.

**hyp·no·don·tia** (hip″no-don′shə) hypnodontics.

**hyp·no·don·tics** (hip″no-don′tiks) [*hypno-* + *odont-* + *-ic*] the application of controlled suggestion and hypnosis in the practice of dentistry.

**hyp·no·gen·e·sis** (hip″no-jen′ĕ-sis) [*hypno-* + *-genesis*] the causing or entering a state of hypnosis or of sleep.

**hyp·no·ge·net·ic** (hip″no-jə-net′ik) hypnogenic.

**hyp·no·gen·ic** (hip″no-jen′ik) [*hypno-* + *-genic*] inducing sleep or a hypnotic state.

**hyp·nog·e·nous** (hip-noj′ə-nəs) hypnogenic.

**hyp·noid** (hip′noid) pertaining to or resembling hypnosis, the hypnotic state, or sleep.

**hyp·noi·dal** (hip-noi′dəl) pertaining to a state resembling hypnosis.

**hyp·nol·o·gy** (hip-nol′ə-je) [*hypno-* + *-logy*] the scientific study of sleep or hypnosis.

**hyp·no·pe·dia** (hip″no-pe′de-ə) [*hypno-* + *paideia* education] sleep learning; learning during sleep, as by listening to recordings.

**hyp·no·pom·pic** (hip″no-pom′pik) [*hypno-* + Gr. *pompē* a sending away, a sending home] persisting after sleep; applied to hallucinations occurring on awakening.

**hyp·no·sis** (hip-no′sis) [Gr. *hypnos* sleep] [MeSH: Hypnosis] a state of altered consciousness, usually artificially induced, characterized by focusing of attention, heightened responsiveness to suggestions and commands, suspension of disbelief with lowering of critical judgment, the potential of alteration in perceptions, motor control, or memory in response to suggestions, and the subjective experience of responding involuntarily.

**hyp·no·ther·a·py** (hip″no-ther′ə-pe) [*hypno-* + *therapy*] the use of hypnosis in the treatment of disease.

**hyp·not·ic** (hip-not′ik) 1. inducing sleep. 2. pertaining to or of the nature of hypnosis or hypnotism. 3. an agent that acts to induce sleep.

**hyp·no·tism** (hip′no-tiz-əm) the study of or the method or practice of inducing hypnosis.

**hyp·no·tist** (hip′no-tist) one who induces hypnosis.

**hyp·no·ti·za·tion** (hip″no-tĭ-za′shən) the induction of hypnosis.

**hyp·no·tize** (hip′no-tīz) to induce a state of hypnosis.

**hyp·no·tox·in** (hip″no-tok′sin) a toxic substance derived from the tentacles of *Physalia,* the Portuguese man-of-war, characteristically causing a central nervous system depression, affecting both motor and sensory elements.

**hyp·no·zo·ite** (hip″no-zo′īt) [*hypno-* + Gr. *zōon* animal] the round-to-ovoid, uninucleate, dormant intracellular (hepatic) stage of the malarial parasite, which succeeds the infecting sporozoite stage in *Plasmodium* species capable of producing malarial relapse; it is believed to be the true latent stage associated with relapse in malaria.

**hy·po** (hi′po) 1. a popular designation for a hypodermic inoculation or syringe. 2. a contraction for sodium thiosulfate, used as a photographic fixing agent.

**hyp(o)-** [Gr. *hypo* under] a prefix signifying beneath, under, below normal, or deficient. Cf. *sub-*. In chemistry, it denotes a compound, usually an acid or a salt, containing the lowest proportion of oxygen in a series of similar compounds, e.g., hypochlorous acid (HClO) or sodium hypochlorite (NaClO).

**hy·po·ac·id·i·ty** (hi″po-ə-sid′ĭ-te) deficiency of acid; lack of normal acidity.

**hy·po·ac·tive** (hi″po-ak′tiv) pertaining to or characterized by hypoactivity.

**hy·po·ac·tiv·i·ty** (hi″po-ak-tiv′ĭ-te) 1. abnormally diminished activity, as of peristalsis. 2. abnormally decreased motor and cognitive activity, with slowing of thought, speech, and movement.

**hy·po·acu·sis** (hi″po-ə-ku′sis) [*hypo-* + *acou-* + *-sis*] slightly diminished auditory sensitivity, with hearing threshold levels above the normal limit so that the impairment is measurable in decibels; called also *hypacusia, hypacusis,* and *acoustic* or *auditory hypoesthesia.*

**hy·po·adren·a·lism** (hi″po-ə-dre′nəl-iz-əm) adrenal insufficiency (def. 1).

**hy·po·adre·no·cor·ti·cism** (hi″po-ə-dre″no-kor′tĭ-siz-əm) adrenocortical insufficiency.

**hy·po·al·bu·min·emia** (hi″po-al-bu″min-e′me-ə) an abnormally low albumin content of the blood; called also *hypalbuminemia.*

**hy·po·al·bu·min·o·sis** (hi″po-al-bu″mĭ-no′sis) hypoalbuminemia.

**hy·po·al·dos·ter·on·emia** (hi″po-al-dos″tər-o-ne′me-ə) an abnormally low level of aldosterone in the blood.

**hy·po·al·dos·ter·on·ism** (hi″po-al-dos′tə-ro-niz″əm) [MeSH: Hypoaldosteronism] aldosterone deficiency, usually associated with hypoadrenalism, and characterized by hypotension, dehydration, and a tendency to excrete excessive amounts of sodium.
**hyporeninemic h.,** the most common type of isolated hypoaldosteronism, caused by decreased renin production by the kidney.

**isolated h.**, a rare endocrine disorder characterized by aldosterone deficiency, with normal production of cortisol and all other adrenocortical steroids.

**hy·po·al·dos·ter·on·uria** (hi″po-al-dos″tə-ro-nu′re-ə) presence of an abnormally low level of aldosterone in the urine.

**hy·po·al·ge·sia** (hi″po-al-je′ze-ə) hypalgesia.

**hy·po·al·i·men·ta·tion** (hi″po-al″ĭ-mən-ta′shən) insufficient nourishment.

**hy·po·al·ka·line** (hi″po-al′kə-lin) less alkaline than normal.

**hy·po·al·ka·lin·i·ty** (hi″po-al″kə-lin′ĭ-te) the state of being less alkaline than normal.

**hy·po·al·o·ne·mia** (hi″po-al″o-ne′me-ə) [*hypo-* + Gr. *hals* salt + *-emia*] hyposalemia.

**hy·po·al·pha·lipo·pro·tein·emia** (hi″po-al″fə-lip″o-pro″te-ne′me-ə) 1. deficiency of high-density (alpha) lipoproteins in the blood. 2. Tangier disease.

**hy·po·am·i·no·ac·i·de·mia** (hi″po-ə-me″no-as″ĭ-de′me-ə) the presence of less than the normal amount of amino acids in the blood.

**hy·po·an·dro·gen·ism** (hi″po-an-dro′jən-iz-əm) a state characterized or caused by deficiency of androgens.

**hy·po·azo·tu·ria** (hi″po-az″o-tu′re-ə) [*hypo-* + *azote* + *-uria*] diminished excretion of nitrogenous material in the urine.

**hy·po·bar·ic** (hi″po-bar′ik) [*hypo-* + *bar-* + *-ic*] characterized by less than normal pressure or weight; applied to gases under less than atmospheric pressure or to a solution of lower specific gravity than another taken as a standard of reference. See under *solution.*

**hy·po·bar·ism** (hi″po-bar′iz-əm) the condition resulting from exposure to ambient gas pressure or atmospheric pressures that are below those within body tissues, fluids, cavities.

**hy·po·bar·op·a·thy** (hi″po-bar-op′ə-the) [*hypo-* + *baro-* + *-pathy*] 1. the disturbances experienced in high altitudes due to reduced air pressure; see *high altitude sickness* and *mountain sickness,* under *sickness.* 2. hypobarism.

**hy·po·be·ta·lipo·pro·tein·emia** (hi″po-ba″tə-lip″o-pro″te-ne′me-ə) [MeSH: Hypobetalipoproteinemia] the presence of abnormally low levels of low-density (beta) lipoproteins in the serum, as in debilitating diseases and malabsorption syndromes.
**familial h.**, a disorder of lipid metabolism clinically similar to abetalipoproteinemia, but of autosomal dominant inheritance and usually milder; relationship between the two disorders is unclear.

**hy·po·bil·i·ru·bin·emia** (hi″po-bil″ĭ-roo″bĭ-ne′me-ə) abnormal diminution of bilirubin in the blood.

**hy·po·blast** (hi′po-blast) [*hypo-* + *-blast*] the lower layer of the bilaminar embryonic disc in a human embryo, present during the second week; it gives rise to the endoderm.

**hy·po·blas·tic** (hi″po-blas′tik) pertaining to the hypoblast.

**hy·po·bran·chi·al** (hi″po-brang′ke-əl) [*hypo-* + *branchial*] located beneath the branchial (pharyngeal) arches.

**hy·po·bro·mite** (hi″po-bro′mīt) any salt of hypobromous acid.

**hy·po·bro·mous ac·id** (hi′po-bro′məs) an unstable acid, HBrO; used as a disinfectant, bleaching agent, and in testing for urea.

**hy·po·cal·ce·mia** (hi″po-kal-se′me-ə) [*hypo-* + *calci-* + *-emia*] [MeSH: Hypocalcemia] reduction of the blood calcium below normal; manifestations include hyperactive deep tendon reflexes, Chvostek's sign, muscle and abdominal cramps, and carpopedal spasm.

**hy·po·cal·ce·mic** (hi″po-kal-se′mik) pertaining to or characterized by hypocalcemia.

**hy·po·cal·cia** (hi″po-kal′se-ə) calcipenia.

**hy·po·cal·ci·fi·ca·tion** (hi″po-kal″sĭ-fĭ-ka′shən) diminished calcification.
**enamel h.**, an autosomal dominant form of amelogenesis imperfecta due to faulty mineralization of enamel, characterized by a tooth crown that appears normal at eruption but soon assumes a white chalky appearance and gradually undergoes brown discoloration; the affected teeth are soft and rough.

**hy·po·cal·ci·pec·tic** (hi″po-kal″sĭ-pek′tik) pertaining to or characterized by hypocalcipexy.

**hy·po·cal·ci·pexy** (hi″po-kal′sĭ-pek″se) deficient calcium fixation.

**hy·po·cal·ci·uria** (hi″po-kal″se-u′re-ə) an abnormally diminished amount of calcium in the urine.

**hy·po·cap·nia** (hi″po-kap′ne-ə) [*hypo-* + *capn-* + *-ia*] [MeSH: Hypocapnia] deficiency of carbon dioxide in the blood, resulting from hyperventilation and eventually leading to alkalosis. Called also *hypocarbia.*

**hy·po·cap·nic** (hi″po-kap′nik) pertaining to or characterized by hypocapnia.

**hy·po·car·bia** (hi″po-kahr′be-ə) hypocapnia.

**hy·po·cat·a·la·sia** (hi″po-kat″ə-la′zhə) an asymptomatic variant of acatalasia in which some catalase activity is present; it occurs in some heterozygotes.

**hy·po·cel·lu·lar** (hi″po-sel′u-lər) pertaining to or characterized by hypocellularity.

**hy·po·cel·lu·lar·i·ty** (hi″po-sel″u-lar′ĭ-te) a state of abnormal decrease in the number of cells present, as in bone marrow.

**hy·po·ce·lom** (hi″po-se′lom) hypocoelom.

**hy·po·chlor·emia** (hi″po-klor-e′me-ə) an abnormally diminished level of chloride in the blood.

**hy·po·chlor·emic** (hi″po-klor-e′mik) pertaining to or characterized by hypochloremia.

**hy·po·chlor·hy·dria** (hi″po-klor-hi′dre-ə) [*hypo-* + *chloro-* + *hydr-* + *-ia*] deficiency of hydrochloric acid in the gastric juice. Cf. *achlorhydria.*

**hy·po·chlo·ri·da·tion** (hi″po-klor″ĭ-da′shən) chloride deficiency in the system.

**hy·po·chlo·rid·emia** (hi″po-klor″i-de′me-ə) hypochloremia.

**hy·po·chlo·rite** (hi″po-klor′īt) [*hypo-* + *chlorite*] any salt of hypochlorous acid; used as a medicinal agent, particularly as a diluted solution of sodium hypochlorite. See *diluted sodium hypochlorite solution,* under *solution.*

**hy·po·chlo·ri·za·tion** (hi″po-klor″ĭ-za′shən) reduction of the amount of sodium chloride in the diet.

**hy·po·chlo·rous ac·id** (hi″po-klor′əs) [MeSH: Hypochlorous Acid] an unstable compound, HClO, a disinfectant and bleaching agent; its salts (hypochlorites) are used as medicinal agents, particularly as surgical solution of chlorinated soda. See *diluted sodium hypochlorite solution,* under *solution.*

**hy·po·chlor·uria** (hi″po-klor-u′re-ə) [*hypo-* + *chlor-* + *-uria*] deficiency of chlorides in the urine.

**hy·po·cho·les·te·re·mia** (hi″po-kə-les″tə-re′me-ə) hypocholesterolemia.

**hy·po·cho·les·te·re·mic** (hi″po-kə-les″tə-re′mik) hypocholesterolemic.

**hy·po·cho·les·ter·ol·emia** (hi″po-kə-les″tər-ol-e′me-ə) an abnormally diminished amount of cholesterol in the blood.

**hy·po·cho·les·ter·ol·emic** (hi″po-kə-les″tər-ol-e′mik) pertaining to, characterized by, or producing hypocholesterolemia.

**hy·po·chol·uria** (hi″po-ko-lu′re-ə) abnormal reduction in the amount of bile in the urine.

**hy·po·chon·dria** (hi″po-kon′dre-ə) 1. plural of *hypochondrium.* 2. hypochondriasis.

**hy·po·chon·dri·ac** (hi″po-kon′dre-ak) 1. pertaining to the hypochondrium. 2. pertaining to hypochondriasis. 3. a person affected with hypochondriasis.

**hy·po·chon·dri·a·cal** (hi″po-kon-dri′ə-kəl) 1. pertaining to the hypochondrium. 2. pertaining to or affected with hypochondriasis.

**hy·po·chon·dri·a·sis** (hi″po-kon-dri′ə-sis) [so called because it was supposed by the ancients to be due to disturbed function of the organs of the upper abdomen; see also *regio hypochondriaca*] [MeSH: Hypochondriasis] [DSM-IV] a somatoform disorder characterized by a preoccupation with bodily functions and the interpretation of normal sensations (such as heart beats, sweating, peristaltic action, and bowel movements) or minor abnormalities (such as a runny nose, minor aches and pains, or slightly swollen lymph nodes) as indications of serious problems needing medical attention. Negative results of diagnostic evaluations and reassurance by physicians only increase the patient's anxious concern about his health, although the concern is not of delusional intensity. Called also *hypochondriacal neurosis.*

**hy·po·chon·dri·um** (hi″po-kon′dre-əm) pl. *hypochon′dria* [*hypo-* + Gr. *chondros* cartilage] [TA] either of the superolateral regions of the abdomen, lateral to the epigastric region, overlying the costal cartilages. Called also *regio hypochondriaca* [TA alternative] and *hypochondriac region.*

**hy·po·chon·dro·pla·sia** (hi″po-kon″dro-pla′zhə) a common chondrodystrophy resembling achondroplasia but with milder clinical features, which include short stature with a long trunk and short limbs, broad and short fingers, and a normal face; it is transmitted as an autosomal dominant trait.

**hy·po·chor·dal** (hi″po-kor′dəl) situated ventral to the notochord.

**hy·po·chro·ma·sia** (hi″po-kro-ma′zhə) [*hypo-* + Gr. *chrōma* color]

1. the condition of staining less intensely than normal. 2. hypochromia (def. 1).

**hy·po·chro·mat·ic** (hi″po-kro-mat′ik) 1. containing an abnormally small number of chromosomes; marked by hypochromatism. 2. characterized by hypochromatism.

**hy·po·chro·ma·tism** (hi″po-kro′mə-tiz-əm) [*hypo-* + *chromat-* + *-ism*] 1. abnormally deficient pigmentation, especially deficiency of the chromatin in a cell nucleus. 2. hypochromia (def. 1).

**hy·po·chro·ma·to·sis** (hi″po-kro′mə-to-sis) the gradual fading and disappearance of the nuclear chromatin of a cell.

**hy·po·chro·mia** (hi″po-kro′me-ə) [*hypo-* + *chrom-* + *-ia*] 1. abnormal decrease in the hemoglobin content of the erythrocytes. Called also *hypochromasia* and *hypochromatism.* 2. hypochromatism (def. 1).

**hy·po·chro·mic** (hi″po-kro′mik) pertaining to or marked by hypochromia.

**hy·po·chro·mo·trich·ia** (hi″po-kro″mo-trik′e-ə) achromotrichia.

**hy·po·chy·lia** (hi″po-ki′le-ə) [*hypo-* + *chyle* + *-ia*] deficiency of chyle.

**hy·po·ci·ne·sia** (hi″po-sĭ-ne′zhə) hypokinesia.

**hy·po·cist** (hi′po-sist) hypocistis.

**hy·po·cis·tis** (hi″po-sis′tis) the juice and extract of various species of the parasitic herb *Cytinus,* as of *C. hypocistis* of southern Europe; it is an astringent.

**hy·po·cit·ra·tu·ria** (hi″po-sĭ-tra-tu′re-ə) excretion of urine containing an abnormally small amount of citrate.

**hy·po·ci·tre·mia** (hi″po-sĭ-tre′me-ə) [*hypo-* + *citr*ic acid + *-emia*] abnormally low content of citric acid in the blood.

**hy·po·ci·tru·ria** (hi″po-sĭ-troo′re-ə) [*hypo-* + *citr*ic acid + *-uria*] excretion of urine containing an abnormally small amount of citric acid.

**hy·po·co·ag·u·la·bil·i·ty** (hi″po-ko-ag″u-lə-bil′ĭ-te) the state of being less readily coagulated than normal.

**hy·po·co·ag·u·la·ble** (hi″po-ko-ag′u-lə-bəl) characterized by abnormally decreased coagulability.

**hy·po·coe·lom** (hi″po-se′lom) [*hypo-* + *coelom*] the ventral portion of the coelom of any embryonic vertebrate.

**hy·po·com·ple·men·te·mia** (hi″po-kom″plə-men-te′me-ə) abnormally low levels of complement in the blood.

**hy·po·com·ple·men·te·mic** (hi″po-kom″plə-men-te′mik) denoting or involving lowered levels of complement in the blood.

**hy·po·con·dy·lar** (hi″po-kon′də-lər) below a condyle.

**hy·po·cone** (hi′po-kōn) [*hypo-* + Gr. *kōnos* cone] the distolingual cusp of an upper molar tooth.

**hy·po·con·id** (hi″po-ko′nid) the distobuccal cusp of a lower molar tooth.

**hy·po·con·u·lid** (hi″po-kon′u-lid) the distal, or fifth, cusp of a lower molar tooth; usually found on the mandibular first molar.

**hy·po·cor·ti·cal·ism** (hi″po-kor′tĭ-kəl-iz-əm) adrenocortical insufficiency.

**hy·po·cor·ti·cism** (hi″po-kor′ti-siz-əm) adrenocortical insufficiency.

**hy·po·cot·yl** (hi″po-kot′əl) [*hypo-* + *kotyle* hollow] [MeSH: Hypocotyl] the part of the axis of a plant embryo or seedling below the point of attachment of the cotyledon and from which the radicle, or primary root, grows.

**Hy·po·crea** (hi″po-kre′ə) a genus of fungi of the family Hypocreaceae, including the perfect (sexual) stage of some species of *Trichoderma.*

**Hy·po·cre·a·ceae** (hi″po-kre-a′se-e) a family of fungi of the order Hypocreales. It includes the genera *Gibberella, Hypocrea, Nectria,* and *Podostroma,* which contain the perfect (sexual) stages of several species of *Acremonium, Fusarium,* and *Trichoderma* and the etiologic agents of numerous types of plant wilt.

**Hy·po·cre·a·les** (hi″po-kre-a′ləs) [MeSH: Hypocreales] an order of perfect fungi of the subphylum Ascomycotina, series Unitunicatae, characterized by inoperculate asci; it includes the family Hypocreaceae.

**hy·po·cu·pre·mia** (hi″po-ku-pre′me-ə) an abnormally diminished concentration of copper in the blood.

**hy·po·cy·clo·sis** (hi″po-si-klo′sis) [*hypo-* + *cycl-* + *-osis*] insufficiency of accommodation due either to undue rigidity of the crystalline lens *(lenticular h.)* or to weakness of the ciliary muscle *(ciliary h.).*

**hy·po·cy·the·mia** (hi″po-si-the′me-ə) [*hypo-* + *cyt-* + *hem-* + *-ia*] deficiency in the number of erythrocytes in the blood.

**hy·po·cy·to·sis** (hi″po-si-to′sis) [*hypo-* + *-cyte* + *-osis*] cytopenia.

**hy·po·dac·ty·ly** (hi″po-dak′tə-le) the presence of less than the normal number of fingers or toes.

**hy·po·dense** (hi′po-dens) being less dense than some other objects; applied particularly to objects or areas that are less dense than others on radiographs.

**hy·po·derm** (hi′po-dərm) [*hypo-* + *-derm*] subcutaneous tissue.

**Hy·po·der·ma** (hi″po-dər′mə) [*hypo-* + Gr. *derma* skin] the ox-warble flies, a genus of insects of the family Oestridae whose larvae cause creeping eruptions in humans and warbles in cattle. Called also *heel flies.*

**H. bo′vis,** a species whose larvae cause warbles in cattle and a creeping eruption in humans; in cattle they prefer to migrate to the area near the spinal canal.

**H. linea′tum,** an ox-warble fly that prefers to migrate to the area near the esophagus.

**hy·po·der·mat·ic** (hi″po-dər-mat′ik) hypodermic.

**hy·po·der·mato·cly·sis** (hi″po-dər-mə-tok′lə-sis) hypodermoclysis.

**hy·po·der·mat·o·my** (hi″po-dər-mat′ə-me) [*hypo-* + *derma-* + *-tomy*] incision of the subcutaneous tissue.

**hy·po·der·mi·a·sis** (hi″po-dər-mi′ə-sis) infection by *Hypoderma,* particularly their larvae, which migrate through the host's body; see *cutaneous larva migrans* (def. 2).

**hy·po·der·mic** (hi″po-dər′mik) [*hypo-* + *dermic*] applied or administered beneath the skin.

**hy·po·der·mis** (hi″po-dər′mis) [*hypo-* + Gr. *derma* skin] 1. subcutaneous tissue. 2. the outer cellular layer of the body of invertebrates which secretes the cuticular exoskeleton.

**hy·po·der·mo·cly·sis** (hi″po-dər-mok′lə-sis) [*hypoderm* + *clysis*] introduction into the subcutaneous tissues of fluids, especially physiologic sodium chloride solution, to replace inadequate intake or loss of water and salt during illness or operation.

**hy·po·der·mo·li·thi·a·sis** (hi″po-dər″mo-lĭ-thi′ə-sis) [*hypo-* + *dermo-* + *lithiasis*] the formation or presence of subcutaneous calcareous nodes.

**hy·po·der·mo·sis** (hi″po-dər-mo′sis) hypodermiasis.

**hy·po·di·a·phrag·mat·ic** (hi″po-di″ə-frag-mat′ik) inferior to the diaphragm.

**hy·po·dip·loid** (hi″po-dip′loid) 1. pertaining to or characterized by hypodiploidy. 2. an individual or cell with less than the diploid number of chromosomes.

**hy·po·dip·loi·dy** (hi″po-dip′loi-de) the state of having less than the diploid number of chromosomes (<2n).

**hy·po·dip·sia** (hi″po-dip′se-ə) [*hypo-* + *dipsia*] abnormally diminished thirst. Cf. *subliminal thirst,* under *thirst.*

**hy·po·dip·sic** (hi″po-dip′sik) characterized by abnormally diminished thirst.

**hy·po·don·tia** (hi″po-don′shə) [*hypo-* + *odont-* + *-ia*] partial absence of the teeth. A relatively common congenital condition characterized by absence of one or more teeth because of absence of their anlage, which is seldom associated with other anomalies. Called also *partial anodontia.*

**hy·po·dy·na·mia** (hi″po-di-na′me-ə) [*hypo-* + *dynam-* + *-ia*] diminished power.

**h. cor′dis,** diminished cardiac power.

**hy·po·dy·nam·ic** (hi″po-di-nam′ik) marked by or exhibiting diminished power or strength; used particularly to describe poor ventricular contractility.

**hy·po·ec·cris·ia** (hi″po-ə-kris′e-ə) [*hypo-* + Gr. *ekkrisis* excretion + *-ia*] a state characterized by abnormally diminished excretion.

**hy·po·ec·cri·sis** (hi″po-ek′rĭ-sis) hypoeccrisia.

**hy·po·ec·crit·ic** (hi″po-ə-krit′ik) pertaining to or characterized by hypoeccrisia.

**hy·po·echo·ic** (hi″po-ə-ko′ik) in ultrasonography, giving off few echoes; said of tissues or structures that reflect relatively few of the ultrasound waves directed at them.

**hy·po·elec·tro·ly·te·mia** (hi″po-e-lek″tro-li-te′me-ə) abnormally decreased electrolyte content of the blood.

**hy·po·eo·sin·o·phil·ia** (hi″po-e″o-sin″o-fil′e-ə) eosinopenia.

**hy·po·ep·i·neph·rin·emia** (hi″po-ep″ĭ-nef″rĭ-ne′me-ə) an abnormally low level of epinephrine in the blood.

**hy·po·equi·lib·ri·um** (hi″po-e″kwĭ-lib′re-əm) decreased or absent reactions to changes in position; see also *sense of equilibrium,* under *sense.*

**hy·po·er·gia** (hi″po-ər′jə) hyposensitivity to allergens.

**hy·po·er·gic** (hi″po-ər′jik) 1. less energetic than normal. 2. pertaining to or characterized by hypoergia.

**hy·po·er·gy** (hi″po-ər′je) hypoergia.

**hy·po·eso·pho·ria** (hi″po-es″o-for′e-ə) a tendency of the visual axis to deviate downward and medially when fusion is prevented.

**hy·po·es·the·sia** (hi″po-es-the′zhə) [*hypo-* + *esthesia*] a dysesthesia consisting of abnormally decreased sensitivity, particularly to touch. Called also *hypesthesia*.
**acoustic h., auditory h.,** hypoacusis.
**gustatory h.,** hypogeusia.
**olfactory h.,** hyposmia.
**tactile h.,** a paraphia consisting of diminution or dullness of the sense of touch; called also *amblyaphia* and *hypopselaphesia*.

**hy·po·es·thet·ic** (hi″po-es-thet′ik) pertaining to or characterized by hypoesthesia.

**hy·po·es·tro·gen·emia** (hi″po-es″tro-jə-ne′me-ə) a diminished amount of estrogen in the blood, as after menopause.

**hy·po·evol·u·tism** (hi″po-e-vol′u-tiz-əm) retarded development.

**hy·po·exo·pho·ria** (hi″po-ek″so-for′e-ə) a tendency of the visual axis to deviate downward and laterally when fusion is prevented.

**hy·po·fer·re·mia** (hi″po-fə-re′me-ə) deficiency of iron in the blood; see also *iron deficiency,* under *deficiency*.

**hy·po·fer·rism** (hi″po-fer′iz-əm) [*hypo-* + *ferrum* + *-ism*] iron deficiency.

**hy·po·fer·tile** (hi″po-fər′til) having diminished reproductive capacity.

**hy·po·fer·til·i·ty** (hi″po-fər-til′ĭ-te) diminished reproductive capacity.

**hy·po·fi·brin·o·gen·emia** (hi″po-fi-brin″o-jə-ne′me-ə) abnormally low fibrinogen content of the blood; called also *fibrinogenopenia*.

**hy·po·func·tion** (hi″po-funk′shən) diminished function.

**hy·po·ga·lac·tia** (hi″po-gə-lak′she-ə) deficiency of milk secretion.

**hy·po·ga·lac·tous** (hi″po-gə-lak′təs) [*hypo-* + *galact-* + *-ous*] producing a deficient secretion of milk.

**hy·po·gam·ma·glob·u·lin·emia** (hi″po-gam″ə-glob″u-lĭ-ne′me-ə) abnormally low levels of all classes of immunoglobulins; see also *agammaglobulinemia, dysglobulinemia,* and *immunodeficiency*.
**acquired h.,** common variable immunodeficiency.
**common variable h.,** see under *immunodeficiency*.
**physiologic h.,** a normal period of hypogammaglobulinemia seen in all infants at about 5–6 months of age as the level of transplacentally acquired maternal immunoglobulins declines before endogenous immunoglobulin synthesis rises to normal levels.
**transient h. of infancy,** prolongation of the normal physiologic hypogammaglobulinemia of infancy caused by delayed development of endogenous immunoglobulin production and associated with increased susceptibility to infections.
**X-linked h., X-linked infantile h.,** see under *agammaglobulinemia*.

**hy·po·gan·gli·o·no·sis** (hi″po-gang″le-o-no′sis) deficiency in the number of myenteric ganglion cells in the distal segment of the large bowel, resulting in constipation; it is a variant of congenital megacolon.

**hy·po·gas·tric** (hi″po-gas′trik) [L. *hypogastricus*] 1. situated inferior the stomach. 2. pertaining to the hypogastrium. 3. pertaining to the internal iliac artery.

**hy·po·gas·tri·um** (hi″po-gas′tre-əm) [*hypo-* + Gr. *gastēr* stomach] [TA] the middle portion of the most inferior region of the abdomen, located inferior to the umbilical region and between the inguinal regions. Called also *regio hypogastrica, hypogastric region, regio pubica* [TA alternative], and *pubic region*.

**hy·po·gas·trop·a·gus** (hi″po-gəs-trop′ə-gəs) [*hypo-* + *gastro-* + *-pagus*] conjoined twins united at the hypogastric region.

**hy·po·gas·tros·chi·sis** (hi″po-gəs-tros′kĭ-sis) [*hypo-* + *gastro-* + *-schisis*] a developmental anomaly in which an abdominal fissure is restricted to the hypogastric region.

**hy·po·gen·e·sis** (hi″po-jen′ə-sis) [*hypo-* + *-genesis*] defective embryonic growth or development.
**polar h.,** defective development at either extremity of the embryo, resulting in deformity.

**hy·po·ge·net·ic** (hi″po-jə-net′ik) pertaining to or characterized by hypogenesis.

**hy·po·gen·i·tal·ism** (hi″po-jen′ĭ-təl-iz″əm) hypogonadism.

**hy·po·geus·es·the·sia** (hi″po-gōōs″əs-the′zhə) hypogeusia.

**hy·po·geu·sia** (hi″po-goo′zhə) [*hypo-* + Gr. *geusis* taste] a parageusia involving diminished sensitivity of taste. Called also *amblygeustia, hypogeusesthesia,* and *gustatory hypoesthesia*.

**hy·po·glan·du·lar** (hi″po-glan′du-lər) marked by abnormally decreased glandular activity.

**hy·po·glos·sal** (hi″po-glos′əl) [*hypo-* + Gr. *glōssa* tongue] sublingual.

**hy·po·glu·ca·gon·emia** (hi″po-gloo″kə-gon-e′me-ə) abnormally reduced levels of glucagon in the blood.

**hy·po·gly·ce·mia** (hi″po-gli-se′me-ə) [*hypo-* + *glyc-* + *-emia*] [MeSH: Hypoglycemia] an abnormally diminished concentration of glucose in the blood, which may lead to tremulousness, cold sweat, piloerection, hypothermia, and headache; when chronic and severe it may cause central nervous system manifestations that in rare cases can even be fatal (see *neuroglycopenia*).
**alimentary h.,** a type of reactive hypoglycemia seen in patients who have had surgical modification of the digestive tract so that ingested food moves too quickly past the stomach into the duodenum.
**autoimmune h.,** hypoglycemia caused by antibodies to insulin or occasionally by autoantibodies to insulin receptors.
**factitial h., factitious h.,** hypoglycemia that appears spontaneous but actually is not, such as in a diabetic or nondiabetic after surreptitious injection of insulin.
**fasting h.,** hypoglycemia occurring in the fasting state, i.e., after the glucose contents of the intestine have been absorbed; it occurs in such conditions as insulinoma, glycogen storage disease, severe hepatic failure, starvation, malabsorption, hypopituitarism, and adrenocortical insufficiency.
**insulin-induced h.,** factitial h.
**ketotic h.,** episodic hypoglycemia, ketonuria, convulsions, and vomiting occurring in young children in the early morning after carbohydrate deprivation.
**leucine-induced h.,** a familial type of neonatal hypoglycemia transmitted as an autosomal recessive trait; hypoglycemia is induced by ingestion of leucine-containing protein, which causes an exaggerated release of insulin in susceptible persons.
**mixed h.,** hypoglycemia occurring both during the fasting state and following the ingestion of carbohydrate; it occurs in hypoglycemia of infancy, anterior pituitary and adrenocortical insufficiency, and insulin-secreting tumors of the islet cells of the pancreas.
**neonatal h.,** 1. fasting hypoglycemia in a neonate; those most at risk have diabetic mothers or are premature or small for gestational age. Leucine-induced hypoglycemia is a type that is hereditary. 2. hypoglycemia during the first week of life of piglets, a common cause of death; it may result from inadequate nursing, such as when there is a large litter, or from hypothermia. Called also *h. of piglets*.
**h. of piglets,** neonatal h. (def. 2).
**postprandial h., reactive h.,** hypoglycemia occurring after the ingestion of carbohydrate, with a consequent excessive release of insulin.

**hy·po·gly·ce·mic** (hi″po-gli-se′mik) 1. pertaining to, characterized by, or producing hypoglycemia. 2. an agent that acts to lower the level of glucose in the blood.

**hy·po·gly·ce·mo·sis** (hi″po-gli″sə-mo′sis) an abnormally diminished content of glucose in the blood and tissues; see *hypoglycemia*.

**hy·po·gly·cin** (hi″po-gli′sin) either of two toxic amino acids, designated A and B, occurring in the seeds and arils of the unripe akee (q.v.); they induce hypoglycemia by inhibiting cofactors responsible for hepatic gluconeogenesis. Hypoglycin A, the more potent of the two, is sometimes referred to simply as hypoglycin.

**hy·po·gly·co·gen·ol·y·sis** (hi″po-gli″ko-jən-ol′ə-sis) depressed glycogenolysis.

**hy·po·gly·cor·rha·chia** (hi″po-gli″ko-ra′ke-ə) [*hypo-* + *glyco-* + *rhachi-* + *-ia*] less than the normal content of glucose in the cerebrospinal fluid; usually indicative of meningeal infection.

**hy·pog·na·thous** (hi-pog′nə-thəs) 1. having a protruding lower jaw. 2. of the nature of a hypognathus.

**hy·pog·na·thus** (hi-pog′nə-thəs) [*hypo-* + Gr. *gnathos* jaw] a parasitic twin attached to the lower jaw of the larger twin in asymmetrical conjoined twins. See also *polygnathus*.

**hy·po·go·nad·ism** (hi″po-go′nad-iz-əm) [MeSH: Hypogonadism] a condition resulting from abnormally decreased gonadal function, with retardation of growth, sexual development, and secondary sex characters; see *hypo-orchidism, hypo-ovarianism,* and *eunuchoidism*. Called also *hypogenitalism*.
**eugonadotropic h.,** that associated with normal levels of pituitary gonadotropins.
**hypergonadotropic h.,** that due to defective development or function of the gonads, with elevated levels of pituitary gonadotropins; usually there is some degree of androgen resistance (steroid hormone receptor defects). Klinefelter's syndrome is one type. Called also *primary h.*
**hypogonadotropic h.,** that due to lack of gonadotropin secretion; either luteinizing hormone or follicle-stimulating hormone or both may be deficient; it may also be caused by lack of secretion of go-

nadotropin-releasing hormone, as in Kallmann's syndrome. Called also *secondary h.* and *hypogonadotropic eunuchoidism.*
**primary h.,** hypergonadotropic h.
**secondary h.,** hypogonadotropic h.

**hy·po·gon·a·do·trop·ic** (hi″po-gon″ə-do-trop′ik) relating to or caused by deficiency of gonadotropin.

**hy·po·gran·u·lo·cy·to·sis** (hi″po-gran″u-lo-si-to′sis) granulocytopenia.

**hy·po·he·pat·ia** (hi″po-hə-pat′e-ə) [*hypo-* + *hepat-* + *-ia*] deficient functioning of the liver.

**hy·po·hi·dro·sis** (hi″po-hi-dro′sis) [*hypo-* + Gr. *hidrōsis* sweating] [MeSH: Hypohidrosis] abnormally diminished perspiration.

**hy·po·hi·drot·ic** (hi″po-hi-drot′ik) pertaining to, characterized by, or causing hypohidrosis; see also *anhidrosis.*

**hy·po·hy·dro·chlo·ria** (hi″po-hi″dro-klor′e-ə) hypochlorhydria.

**hy·po·hyp·not·ic** (hi″po-hip-not′ik) marked by light sleep.

**hy·po·idro·sis** (hi″po-id-ro′sis) hypohidrosis.

**hy·po·in·su·lin·emia** (hi″po-in″sə-lĭ-ne′me-ə) abnormally low insulin blood levels.

**hy·po·in·su·lin·ism** (hi″po-in′su-lin-iz″əm) deficient secretion of insulin by the pancreas, resulting in hyperglycemia.

**hy·po·in·tense** (hi″po-in-tens′) having a lower intensity than some other object.

**hy·po·io·di·dism** (hi″po-i-o′dĭ-diz-əm) [*hypo-* + *iodide* + *-ism*] deficiency of iodide in the body.

**hy·po·iso·ton·ic** (hi″po-i″so-ton′ik) less than isotonic; said of a solution having a lesser osmotic power than another.

**hy·po·ka·le·mia** (hi″po-kə-le′me-ə) [MeSH: Hypokalemia] abnormally low potassium concentration in the blood; it may result from excessive potassium loss by the renal or the gastrointestinal route, from decreased intake, or from transcellular shifts. It may be manifested clinically by neuromuscular disorders ranging from weakness to paralysis, by electrocardiographic abnormalities (depression of the T wave and elevation of the U wave), by renal disease, and by gastrointestinal disorders.

**hy·po·ka·le·mic** (hi″po-kə-le′mik) 1. pertaining to or characterized by hypokalemia. 2. an agent that acts to lower the potassium content of the blood.

**hy·po·kali·emia** (hi″po-kal″e-e′me-ə) hypokalemia.

**hy·po·ki·ne·mia** (hi″po-kĭ-ne′me-ə) [*hypo-* + *kin-* + *-emia*] subnormal cardiac output; decreased rate of blood flow through the circulatory system.

**hy·po·ki·ne·sia** (hi″po-kĭ-ne′zhə) [*hypo-* + *kinesi-* + *-ia*] [MeSH: Hypokinesia] abnormally decreased mobility; abnormally decreased motor function or activity. Cf. *dyskinesia.* Called also *hypanakinesia, hypanakinesis, hypocinesia,* and *hypokinesis.*

**hy·po·ki·ne·sis** (hi″po-kĭ-ne′sis) hypokinesia.

**hy·po·ki·net·ic** (hi″po-kĭ-net′ik) pertaining to or characterized by hypokinesia.

**hy·po·lac·ta·sia** (hi″po-lak-ta′zhə) deficiency of lactase activity in the intestines; see *lactose deficiency.*

**hy·po·lar·ynx** (hi″po-lar′inks) cavitas infraglottica.

**hy·po·lem·mal** (hi″po-lem′əl) [*hypo-* + Gr. *lemma* sheath] located beneath a sheath, as the end-plates of motor nerves under the sarcolemma of muscle.

**hy·po·le·thal** (hi″po-le′thəl) not sufficient to cause death.

**hy·po·ley·dig·ism** (hi″po-li′dig-iz-əm) abnormally diminished functional activity of Leydig's cells; resulting in hypoandrogenism.

**hy·po·li·pe·mia** (hi″po-lĭ-pe′me-ə) an abnormally decreased amount of fat in the blood.

**hy·po·lip·id·emic** (hi″po-lip″ĭ-de′mik) promoting the reduction of lipid concentrations in the serum.

**hy·po·lipo·pro·tein·emia** (hi″po-lip″o-pro″te-ne′me-ə) [MeSH: Hypolipoproteinemia] the presence of abnormally low levels of lipoproteins in the serum, as in hypobetalipoproteinemia and Tangier disease.

**hy·po·li·po·sis** (hi″po-lĭ-po′sis) a deficiency of lipids in the blood or tissues. Lipids are transported in the blood as lipoproteins; see *hypolipoproteinemia.*

**hy·po·lym·phe·mia** (hi″po-lim-fe′me-ə) [*hypo-* + *lymph* + *-emia*] lymphocytopenia.

**hy·po·mag·ne·se·mia** (hi″po-mag″nə-se′me-ə) an abnormally low magnesium content of the blood plasma, usually the result of malabsorption, dehydration, alcoholism, or renal disease; the chief manifestation is neuromuscular irritability.

**hy·po·ma·nia** (hi″po-ma′ne-ə) [*hypo-* + *-mania*] an abnormality of mood resembling mania (persistent elevated or expansive mood, hyperactivity, inflated self-esteem, etc.) but of lesser intensity.

**hy·po·man·ic** (hi″po-man′ik) pertaining to hypomania.

**hy·po·mas·tia** (hi″po-mas′te-ə) [*hypo-* + *mast-* + *-ia*] micromastia.

**hy·po·mel·an·cho·lia** (hi″po-mel″ən-ko′le-ə) [*hypo-* + *melancholia*] mild depression (melancholia).

**hy·po·mel·a·no·sis** (hi″po-mel″ə-no′sis) [*hypo-* + *melanosis*] a deficiency of melanin in the tissues, especially in the skin. Cf. *amelanosis, depigmentation,* and *hypopigmentation.*
**idiopathic guttate h.,** a common condition of unknown etiology manifested by small, sharply demarcated, irregular hypopigmented spots that appear chiefly on the sun-exposed areas of the extremities in individuals over the age of 30. Called also *leukopathia punctata reticularis symmetrica.*
**h. of Ito,** incontinentia pigmenti achromians.

**hy·po·men·or·rhea** (hi″po-men″o-re′ə) [*hypo-* + *meno-* + *-rrhea*] uterine bleeding of less than the normal amount occurring at regular intervals, the period of flow being of the same or less than usual duration.

**hy·po·mere** (hi′po-mēr) 1. the ventrolateral portion of a myotome, innervated by an anterior ramus of a spinal nerve. 2. the lateral plate of mesoderm that develops into the walls of the body cavities.

**hy·po·met·a·bol·ic** (hi″po-met″ə-bol′ik) pertaining to hypometabolism.

**hy·po·me·tab·o·lism** (hi″po-mə-tab′o-liz-əm) [*hypo-* + *metabolism*] abnormally decreased utilization of any substance by the body in metabolism; low metabolic rate.

**hy·po·me·thi·o·nin·emia** (hi″po-mə-thi″o-nĭ-ne′me-ə) decreased concentration of methionine in the blood.

**hy·po·me·tria** (hi″po-me′tre-ə) ["a deficiency"; by analogy with Gr. *eumetria, hypermetria*] dysmetria in which voluntary muscular movement falls short of reaching the intended goal.

**hy·po·min·er·al·iza·tion** (hi″po-min″ər-əl-ĭ-za′shən) deficiency of mineral elements in the body.

**hy·pom·ne·sia** (hi″pom-ne′zhə) [*hypo-* + Gr. *mnēmē* memory] defective memory.

**hy·po·mo·dal** (hi″po-mo′dəl) in statistics, relating to the values or items falling below the mode of the frequency distribution.

**hy·po·morph** (hi′po-morf) [*hypo-* + *-morph*] a mutant gene that shows only a partial reduction in the activity it influences. Cf. *hypermorph.*

**hy·po·mo·til·i·ty** (hi″po-mo-til′ĭ-te) deficient movement in any part.

**hy·po·myx·ia** (hi″po-mik′se-ə) [*hypo-* + *myx-* + *-ia*] decreased secretion of mucus.

**hy·po·na·sal·i·ty** (hi″po-na-zal′ĭ-te) a quality of voice in which there is a complete lack of nasal emission of air and nasal resonance, so that speakers sound as if they have a cold. Called also *denasality* and *rhinolalia clausa.*

**hy·po·na·tre·mia** (hi″po-nə-tre′me-ə) [MeSH: Hyponatremia] deficiency of sodium in the blood.
**depletional h.,** that in which there is a low plasma concentration of sodium associated with low total body sodium.
**dilutional h.,** that in which there is a low plasma concentration of sodium resulting from loss of sodium from the body with nonosmotic retention of water, such as that induced by antidiuretic hormone.

**hy·po·na·tru·ria** (hi″po-nə-troo′re-ə) an abnormally low level of sodium in the urine.

**hy·po·neo·cy·to·sis** (hi″po-ne″o-si-to′sis) [*hypo-* + *neocytosis*] leukopenia with immature forms of leukocytes present in the blood.

**hy·po·ni·tre·mia** (hi″po-ni-tre′me-ə) a low level of nitrogen in the blood, sometimes associated with protein malnutrition or overhydration.

**hy·po·noia** (hi″po-noi′ə) [*hypo-* + Gr. *noein* to think] sluggish mental activity.

**hy·po·nych·i·al** (hi″po-nik′e-əl) subungual; beneath a nail.

**hy·po·nych·i·um** (hi″po-nik′e-əm) [*hypo-* + Gr. *onyx* nail] [TA] the thickened epidermis underneath the free distal end of the nail.

**hy·pon·y·chon** (hi-pon′ə-kon) [*hypo-* + Gr. *onyx* nail] ecchymosis beneath the nail.

**hy·po·or·chi·dism** (hi″po-or′kĭ-diz-əm) defective activity of the testes; see also *hypoandrogenism.*

**hy·po-or·tho·cy·to·sis** (hi″po-or″tho-si-to′sis) [*hypo-* + *orthocytosis*] leukopenia in which the proportion of the various forms of leukocytes is normal.

**hy·po·os·mo·lal·i·ty** (hi″po-os″mo-lal′ĭ-te) a decrease in the osmolality of the body fluids.

**hy·po·ova·ri·an·ism** (hi″po-o-var′e-ən-iz-əm) deficient endocrine activity of the ovaries; see also *hypoestrogenemia.*

**hy·po·pal·les·the·sia** (hi″po-pal″es-the′zhə) [*hypo-* + *pallesthesia*] abnormally decreased sensibility of vibration sense (pallesthesia).

**hy·po·pan·cre·a·tism** (hi″po-pan′kre-ə-tiz″əm) pancreatic insufficiency; diminished pancreatic activity.

**hy·po·pan·cre·or·rhea** (hi″po-pan″kre-o-re′ə) abnormally diminished secretion from the pancreas.

**hy·po·para·thy·roid** (hi″po-par″ə-thi′roid) pertaining to or characterized by reduced function of the parathyroid glands; called also *parathyroprival.*

**hy·po·para·thy·roid·ism** (hi″po-par″ə-thi′roid-iz-əm) [MeSH: Hypoparathyroidism] the condition produced by greatly reduced function of the parathyroid glands; it may be due to autoimmune disease, genetic factors, or the removal of the glands. Lack of parathyroid hormone leads to a fall in plasma calcium level (hypocalcemia), which may result in increased neuromuscular excitability and ultimately tetany, as well as a rise in plasma phosphate level. Bone turnover is reduced; there may also be dermatologic, ophthalmologic (cataracts), psychiatric, and dental symptoms, and associated primary failure of other endocrine glands such as the adrenal cortex. See also *pseudohypoparathyroidism.* Called also *parathyroid insufficiency* and *parathyroprivia.*

**hy·po·pep·sia** (hi″po-pep′se-ə) [*hypo-* + Gr. *pepsis* digestion + *-ia*] impairment of digestion, due to hypochlorhydria.

**hy·po·pep·sin·ia** (hi″po-pep-sin′e-ə) deficiency in the pepsin secretion of the stomach.

**hy·po·per·fu·sion** (hi″po-pər-fu′zhən) decreased blood flow through an organ, as in circulatory shock; if prolonged it may result in permanent cellular dysfunction and death.

**hy·po·peri·stal·sis** (hi″po-per″ĭ-stal′sis) abnormally sluggish peristalsis.

**hy·po·pex·ia** (hi″po-pek′se-ə) [*hypo-* + *pexia*] the fixation by a tissue of a deficient amount of a substance.

**hy·po·pexy** (hi′po-pek″se) hypopexia.

**hy·po·pha·lan·gism** (hi″po-fə-lan′jiz-əm) less than the usual number of phalanges of a finger or toe.

**hy·po·pha·ryn·ge·al** (hi″po-fə-rin′je-əl) pertaining to the hypopharynx.

**hy·po·pha·ryn·go·scope** (hi″po-fə-ring′go-skōp) an instrument for inspecting the hypopharynx.

**hy·po·pha·ryn·gos·co·py** (hi″po-far″in-gos′kə-pe) examination of the hypopharynx.

**hy·po·phar·ynx** (hi″po-far′inks) [MeSH: Hypopharynx] pars laryngea pharyngis.

**hy·po·pho·ne·sis** (hi″po-fo-ne′sis) [*hypo-* + *phon-* + *-esis*] diminished intensity of the sound in auscultation or percussion.

**hy·po·pho·nia** (hi″po-fo′ne-ə) [*hypo-* + *phon-* + *-ia*] a dysphonia in which there is decreased phonation, resulting in whispering. Called also *leptophonia, microphonia,* and *subenergetic phonation.*

**hy·po·pho·ria** (hi″po-for′e-ə) [*hypo-* + *phoria*] heterophoria in which there is downward deviation of the visual axis of an eye when visual fusional stimuli are eliminated. When both eyes are affected, it is called *cataphoria.*

**hy·po·phos·pha·ta·sia** (hi″po-fos″fə-ta′zhə) [*hypo-* + *phosphatase* + *-ia*] [MeSH: Hypophosphatasia] a genetic metabolic disorder resulting from serum and bone alkaline phosphatase deficiency leading to hypercalcemia, ethanolamine phosphatemia, and ethanolamine phosphaturia. Clinical manifestations include severe skeletal defects resembling vitamin D–resistant rickets, failure of the calvarium to calcify, dyspnea, cyanosis, vomiting, constipation, renal calcinosis, failure to thrive, disorders of movement, beading of the costochondral junction, and rachitic bone changes (bowing). There are three clinical types based upon age of onset and the severity of the symptoms. Two are autosomal recessive: *infantile,* the severest, lethal in over 50 per cent of the cases; *childhood,* whose first symptom is usually the spontaneous loss of the deciduous teeth; and *adult,* the mildest form, is autosomal dominant. See *pseudohypophosphatasia.*

**hy·po·phos·pha·te·mia** (hi″po-fos″fə-te′me-ə) [*hypo-* + *phosphate* + *-emia*] [MeSH: Hypophosphatemia] an abnormally decreased amount of phosphates in the blood; manifestations include hemolysis, lassitude, weakness, and convulsions. It may be found in hyperparathyroidism, rickets, osteomalacia, and several renal tubular abnormalities, including the Fanconi syndrome.

**familial h.,** familial hypophosphatemic rickets; the term is sometimes used specifically for X-linked hypophosphatemia.

**X-linked h.,** a form of familial hypophosphatemic rickets inherited as an X-linked dominant trait; the bone disease is due to defects in the resorption of phosphate by the proximal renal tubule and in the regulation of renal 25-hydroxyvitamin D activation, and to decreased intestinal absorption of calcium with secondary hyperparathyroidism.

**hy·po·phos·pha·te·mic** (hi″po-fos″fə-te′mik) pertaining to or characterized by hypophosphatemia.

**hy·po·phos·pha·tu·ria** (hi″po-fos″fə-tu′re-ə) an abnormally decreased amount of phosphate in the urine.

**hy·po·phos·phite** (hi″po-fos′fīt) any salt of hypophosphorous acid.

**hy·po·phos·pho·re·mia** (hi″po-fos″fə-re′me-ə) hypophosphatemia.

**hy·po·phos·phor·ous ac·id** (hi″po-fos-for′əs) a strong monobasic acid, $H_3PO_2$, used as a reducing agent.

**hy·po·phren·ic** (hi″po-fren′ik) [*hypo-* + *phrenic*] inferior to the diaphragm.

**hy·po·phre·ni·um** (hi″po-fre′ne-əm) a peritoneal space between the diaphragm and the transverse colon.

**hy·po·phys·e·al** (hi″po-fiz′e-əl) hypophysial.

**hy·po·phys·ec·to·mize** (hi″po-fəz-ek′to-mīz) to remove the hypophysis (pituitary gland).

**hy·po·phys·ec·to·my** (hi-pof″ə-sek′tə-me) [*hypophysis* + *-ectomy*] [MeSH: Hypophysectomy] surgical removal or destruction of the hypophysis (pituitary gland). Called also *pituitectomy.*

**hy·po·phys·eo·por·tal** (hi″po-fiz″e-o-por′təl) hypophysioportal.

**hy·po·phys·eo·priv·ic** (hi″po-fiz″e-o-priv′ik) hypophysioprivic.

**hy·po·phys·eo·trop·ic** (hi″po-fiz″e-o-trop′ik) hypophysiotropic.

**hy·po·phys·i·al** (hi″po-fiz′e-əl) pertaining to the hypophysis; called also *pituitary.*

**hy·po·phys·io·por·tal** (hi″po-fiz″e-o-por′təl) pertaining to the venules and capillaries that connect the hypothalamus and the adenohypophysis. Also spelled *hypophyseoportal.*

**hy·po·phys·io·priv·ic** (hi″po-fiz″e-o-priv′ik) pertaining to deficiency of hormone secretion by the hypophysis (pituitary gland); see *hypopituitarism.*

**hy·po·phys·io·trop·ic** (hi″po-fiz″e-o-trop′ik) acting on the hypophysis (pituitary gland), as certain hormones.

**hy·poph·y·sis** (hi-pof′ə-sis) [*hypo-* + Gr. *phyein* to grow] [TA] the pituitary gland, an epithelial body located at the base of the brain in the sella turcica, attached by a stalk to the hypothalamus, from which it receives an important neural and vascular outflow. It consists of two lobes of differing embryonic origin, the *anterior lobe (adenohypophysis),* which secretes most of the hormones, and the *posterior lobe (neurohypophysis),* which stores and releases neurohormones that it receives from the hypothalamus. Called also *glandula pituitaria* [TA alternative], *pituitary body,* and *h. cerebri.*

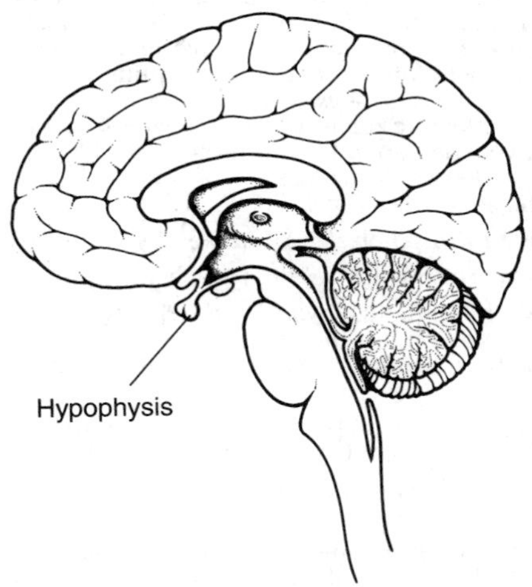


**h. ce′rebri,** hypophysis.

**pharyngeal h., h. pharyngea′lis** [TA], a small median residual collection of adenohypophysial glandular tissue in the mucoperiosteum of the roof of the nasopharynx; it develops from Rathke's pouch in the embryo. Called also *pars pharyngea lobi anterioris hypophyseos* and *pharyngeal pituitary.*

**hy·poph·y·si·tis** (hi-pof″ə-si′tis) inflammation of the hypophysis (pituitary gland).
**lymphocytic h.,** destruction of the normal parenchyma of the pituitary gland by infiltrating lymphocytes and plasma cells, with resultant hypopituitarism, usually seen during pregnancy and thought to be an autoimmune reaction.

**hy·po·pi·e·sia** (hi-po-pi-e′shə) [*hypo-* + *-piesia*] hypotension.

**hy·po·pi·e·sis** (hi″po-pi-e′sis) hypotension.

**hy·po·pi·et·ic** (hi″po-pi-et′ik) hypotensive.

**hy·po·pig·men·ta·tion** (hi″po-pig″mən-ta′shən) [*hypo-* + *pigmentation*] [MeSH: Hypopigmentation] abnormally diminished pigmentation, resulting from decreased melanin production. Cf. *amelanosis, depigmentation,* and *hypomelanosis.*

**hy·po·pig·men·ter** (hi″po-pig-men′tər) an agent that reduces pigmentation of the skin; a bleach.

**hy·po·pin·e·al·ism** (hi″po-pin′e-ə-liz″em) a presumed decrease in normal secretory activity of the pineal body.

**hy·po·pi·tu·i·ta·rism** (hi″po-pĭ-too′ĭ-tə-riz″əm) [MeSH: Hypopituitarism] diminution or cessation of function of the adenohypophysis due to surgical removal, to ablation by irradiation, or to spontaneous causes, as in chromophobe adenoma or postpartum necrosis (Sheehan's syndrome). There is variable deficiency of hormones, including: gonadotropins (causing *secondary hypogonadism*); somatotropin (causing *pituitary dwarfism* in children); thyrotropin (causing secondary *hypothyroidism*); and corticotropin (causing *secondary adrenocortical insufficiency*).

**hy·po·pla·sia** (hi″po-pla′zhə) [*hypo-* + *-plasia*] incomplete development or underdevelopment of an organ or tissue; it is less severe in degree than aplasia.
**cartilage-hair h.,** an autosomal recessive characterized by bone dysplasia with short-limbed dwarfism, fine sparse light-colored hair, and neutropenia with defective cell-mediated immunity. It was originally described in an Amish population but has subsequently been seen in other groups
**enamel h.,** a form of amelogenesis imperfecta characterized by incomplete formation of the dental enamel. It may be transmitted as an X-linked or autosomal dominant trait, or be associated with vitamin A, C, or D deficiency, measles, chickenpox, scarlet fever, congenital syphilis (Hutchinson's teeth), prematurity, birth injuries, Rh incompatibility, trauma, local infection, or Morquio's disease. Small grooves, pits, and fissures on the enamel surface may be seen in mild cases, deep horizontal rows of pits in severe cases; or absence of enamel in extreme cases; associated with yellow, reddish, or brown discoloration of the teeth. Called also *hypoplastic emphysema*
**focal dermal h.,** a hereditary disorder found exclusively in females, transmitted as an X-linked dominant trait, characterized typically by linear areas of dermal hypoplasia with herniation of underlying tissue through the defects, telangiectasia, linear or reticular areas of hyper- or hypopigmentation, localized superficial fatty deposits in the skin, papillomas of mucous membranes of periorificial skin, and anomalies of the extremities, including syndactyly, adactyly, and oligodactyly. Called also *Coltz's syndrome.*
**myofibrillar h.,** a congenital condition of piglets in which leg muscles are weak, usually in the rear legs, and the legs spread apart. Affected animals have difficulty moving and may starve or be crushed by their mothers. It can have many causes, including *in utero* poisoning or infection or perinatal injury. Called also *splayleg, splay legs,* and *spraddle legs.*
**oligomeganephronic renal h.,** oligomeganephronia.
**h. of right ventricle,** parchment heart.
**thymic h.,** DiGeorge syndrome.
**Turner's h.,** see under *tooth.*

**hy·po·plas·tic** (hi″po-plas′tik) marked by hypoplasia.

**hy·po·plas·ty** (hi″po-plas″te) hypoplasia.

**hy·po·ploid** (hi′po-ploid) [*hypo-* + *-ploid*] the aneuploid, almost always fatal condition in which there is less than the normal diploid number of chromosomes, e.g., 45 chromosomes in man, the $2n - 1$ state.

**hy·pop·nea** (hi-pop′ne-ə) [*hypo-* + *-pnea*] abnormal decrease in the depth and rate of breathing. Cf. *bradypnea* and *hypoventilation.*

**hy·pop·ne·ic** (hi″pop-ne′ik) pertaining to or characterized by hypopnea.

**hy·po·po·ne·sis** (hi″po-po-ne′sis) [*hypo-* + *pon-* + *-esis*] dysponesis in which there is insufficient action-potential output from the motor and premotor areas of the cortex.

**hy·po·po·ro·sis** (hi″po-po-ro′sis) [*hypo-* + *por-*[2] + *-osis*] deficient formation of callus after fracture.

**hy·po·po·sia** (hi″po-po′zhə) [*hypo-* + Gr. *posis* drinking + *-ia*] abnormally diminished ingestion of fluids.

**hy·po·po·tas·se·mia** (hi″po-po″tə-se′me-ə) hypokalemia.

**hy·po·po·tas·se·mic** (hi″po-po″tə-se′mik) hypokalemic (def. 1).

**hy·po·po·ten·tia** (hi″po-po-ten′shə) [*hypo-* + *potentia*] a condition of diminished power, especially of diminished electrical activity of the cerebral cortex.

**hy·po·prax·ia** (hi″po-prak′shə) [*hypo-* + Gr. *praxis* action + *-ia*] abnormally diminished activity.

**hy·po·pros·o·dy** (hi″po-pros′o-de) dysprosody marked by diminution of the normal variation of stress, pitch, and rhythm of speech.

**hy·po·pro·tein·emia** (hi″po-pro″te-ne′me-ə) [MeSH: Hypoproteinemia] abnormal decrease in the amount of protein in the blood, sometimes resulting in edema and fluid accumulation in serous cavities.
**prehepatic h.,** hypoproteinemia occurring as a result of prolonged ingestion of faulty low or incomplete protein diet.

**hy·po·pro·tein·ia** (hi″po-pro-tēn′e-ə) a subnormal protein status of the body.

**hy·po·pro·tein·ic** (hi″po-pro-tēn′ik) pertaining to or characterized by hypoproteinia.

**hy·po·pro·tein·o·sis** (hi″po-pro″tēn-o′sis) deficiency of proteins or protein foods.

**hy·po·pro·throm·bin·emia** (hi″po-pro-throm″bĭ-ne′me-ə) [MeSH: Hypoprothrombinemias] deficiency of prothrombin (coagulation factor II) in the blood; called also *prothrombinopenia.*

**hy·po·psel·a·phe·sia** (hi″pop-sel″ə-fe′zhə) [*hypo-* + Gr. *psēlaphēsis* touch + *-ia*] tactile hypoesthesia.

**hy·po·pty·al·ism** (hi″pop-ti′əl-iz-əm) [*hypo-* + *ptyal-* + *-ism*] abnormally decreased secretion of saliva, as in xerostomia. Called also *hyposalivation* and *hyposialosis.*

**hy·po·pus** (hi-po′pəs) a stage in the development of the grain mites (Acaridae) between the first and the second nymph stages.

**hy·po·py·on** (hi-po′pe-on) [*hypo-* + Gr. *pyon* pus] an accumulation of pus in the anterior chamber of the eye.

**hy·po·re·ac·tive** (hi″po-re-ak′tiv) pertaining to or characterized by a less than normal response to stimuli. Cf. *irritability* and *reaction.*

**hy·po·re·flex·ia** (hi″po-re-flek′se-ə) dysreflexia characterized by weakening of the reflexes.

**hy·po·re·nin·emia** (hi″po-re″nĭ-ne′me-ə) low levels of renin in the blood.

**hy·po·re·nin·emic** (hi″po-re″nĭ-ne′mik) characterized by low levels of renin in the blood.

**hy·po·sa·le·mia** (hi″po-sə-le′me-ə) [*hypo-* + *sal* + *-emia*] abnormally decreased concentration of salt in the blood; called also *hypoalonemia.*

**hy·po·sal·i·va·tion** (hi″po-sal″ĭ-va′shən) hypoptyalism.

**hy·po·sar·ca** (hi″po-sahr′kə) anasarca.

**hy·po·scle·ral** (hi″po-skler′əl) under the sclerotic coat of the eye.

**hy·po·se·cre·tion** (hi″po-sə-kre′shən) diminished secretion as of a gland.

**hy·po·sen·si·tive** (hi″po-sen′sĭ-tiv) 1. exhibiting abnormally decreased sensitivity. 2. having the specific or general ability to react to a specific allergen reduced by repeated and gradually increasing doses of the offending substance.

**hy·po·sen·si·tiv·i·ty** (hi″po-sen″sĭ-tiv′ĭ-te) the condition of being hyposensitive.

**hy·po·sen·si·ti·za·tion** (hi″po-sen″sĭ-tĭ-za′shən) the act or process of making hyposensitive; desensitization.

**hy·po·sex·u·al·i·ty** (hi″po-sek″shoo-al′ĭ-te) abnormally decreased sexual desire.

**hy·po·si·a·lo·sis** (hi″po-si″ə-lo′sis) hypoptyalism.

**hy·pos·mia** (hi-poz′me-ə) [*hypo-* + *osm-*[1] + *-ia*] a parosmia involving diminished sensitivity of smell; called also *olfactory hypoesthesia.*

**hy·pos·mo·lar·i·ty** (hi-poz″mo-lar′i-te) abnormally decreased osmolar concentration.

**hy·pos·mo·sis** (hi″pos-mo′sis) decreased speed of osmosis.

**hy·po·so·mato·tro·pism** (hi″po-so-mat″o-tro′piz-əm) pituitary dwarfism.

**hy·po·so·mia** (hi″po-so′me-ə) [*hypo-* + *-somia*] inadequate bodily development; see also *dwarfism.*

**hy·po·som·nia** (hi″po-som′ne-ə) reduced time of sleep; cf. *insomnia.*

**hy·po·spa·dia** (hi″po-spa′de-ə) [MeSH: Hypospadias] hypospadias.

**hy·po·spa·di·ac** (hi″po-spa′de-ək) a person affected with hypospadias.

**hy·po·spa·di·as** (hi″po-spa′de-əs) [*hypo-* + Gr. *spadōn* a rent] [MeSH: Hypospadias] a developmental anomaly in the male in which the urethra opens on the underside of the penis or on the perineum.
**balanic h., balanitic h.,** the most common type of hypospadias, in which the urethral orifice opens at the site of the frenum, which may be rudimentary or absent; the normal site of the urinary meatus is represented on the glans penis as a blind pit. Called also *glandular h.*
**female h.,** a developmental anomaly in the female in which the urethra opens into the vagina.
**glandular h.,** balanic h.
**penile h.,** hypospadias in which the urethral opening lies between the glandular sulcus and the junction of the penis and scrotum.
**penoscrotal h.,** hypospadias in which the urethral orifice is at the junction of the penis and scrotum; it may be associated with congenital chordee.
**perineal h.,** hypospadias with anomalous development of the genitalia, the rudimentary penis often being engulfed by an overlying bifid scrotum; seen in 5$\alpha$-reductase deficiency and other disorders. The extreme form is called *pseudovaginal h.*
**pseudovaginal h.,** see *perineal h.*

**hy·po·splen·ism** (hi″po-splen′iz-əm) a condition characterized by diminished functioning of the spleen.

**hy·pos·ta·sis** (hi-pos′tə-sis) [*hypo-* + *stasis*] poor or stagnant circulation in a dependent part of the body or organ, as in venous insufficiency.

**hy·po·stat·ic** (hi″po-stat′ik) 1. pertaining to, caused by, or associated with hypostasis. 2. abnormally static; said of certain inherited traits which are liable to be suppressed by other traits.

**hy·po·ste·a·tol·y·sis** (hi″po-ste″ə-tol′ə-sis) inadequate hydrolysis of fats during ingestion.

**hy·pos·the·nia** (hi″pos-the′ne-ə) [*hypo-* + *sthen-* + *-ia*] an enfeebled state; weakness.

**hy·pos·the·ni·ant** (hi″pos-the′ne-ənt) reducing the strength.

**hy·pos·then·ic** (hi″pos-then′ik) pertaining to or characterized by hyposthenia.

**hy·pos·then·uria** (hi″pos-thə-nu′re-ə) a condition characterized by inability to form urine of high osmolality.
**tubular h.,** hyposthenuria occurring as a result of injury to the epithelial cells of the renal tubules.

**hy·po·stome** (hi′po-stōm) [*hypo-* + *stoma*] any of several structures, parts, or organs found in association with the mouth in various organisms; e.g., the rodlike piercing mouth part, sometimes with spines or teeth, used by certain ticks and mites to thrust into and hold firmly onto the tissues of a prey or host.

**hy·po·sto·mia** (hi″po-sto′me-ə) [*hypo-* + *stom-* + *-ia*] a developmental anomaly characterized by abnormal smallness of the mouth, the slit being vertical instead of horizontal.

**hyp·os·to·sis** (hip″os-to′sis) [*hypo-* + *osteo-* + *-osis*] deficient development of bone.

**hy·po·styp·sis** (hi″po-stip′sis) [*hypo-* + *stypsis*] moderate astringency.

**hy·po·styp·tic** (hi″po-stip′tik) moderately or mildly styptic.

**hy·po·sul·fite** (hi″po-sul′fīt) thiosulfate.

**hy·po·su·pra·re·nal·ism** (hi″po-soo″prə-re′nəl-iz-əm) adrenal insufficiency.

**hy·po·sym·path·i·co·to·nus** (hi″po-sim-path″ĭ-ko-to′nəs) abnormally decreased tone of the sympathetic nervous system; see also *sympathicotonia.*

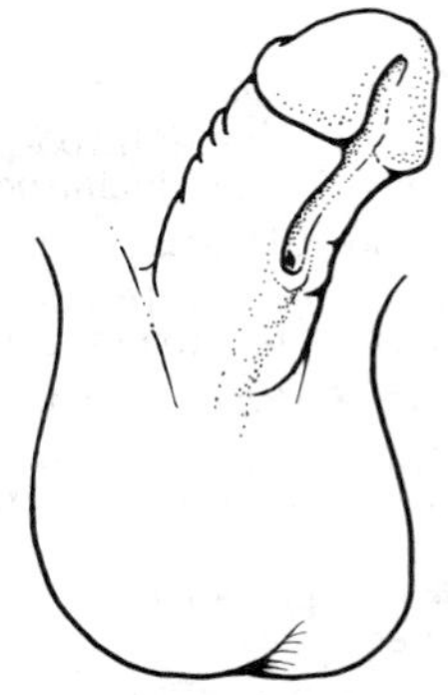
Hypospadias with chordee.

**hy·po·syn·er·gia** (hi″po-sĭ-nər′jə) [*hypo-* + *synergia*] dyssynergia.

**hy·po·telo·rism** (hi″po-tel′ə-riz-əm) [*hypo-* + *tele-*[2] + *-ism*] abnormally decreased distance between two organs or parts.
**ocular h., orbital h.,** a condition characterized by abnormal decrease in the intraorbital distance, consistently present in trigonocephaly.

**hy·po·ten·sion** (hi″po-ten′shən) [MeSH: Hypotension] abnormally low blood pressure; seen in shock but not necessarily indicative of it. See also *blood pressure,* under *pressure.*
**chronic orthostatic h., chronic idiopathic orthostatic h., idiopathic orthostatic h.,** 1. Shy-Drager syndrome. 2. Bradbury-Eggleston syndrome.
**orthostatic h.,** a fall in blood pressure associated with dizziness, blurred vision, and sometimes syncope, occurring upon standing or when standing motionless in a fixed position; it can be acquired or idiopathic, transient or chronic, and may occur alone or secondary to a disorder of the central nervous system such as the Shy-Drager syndrome. Called also *postural h.*
**postural h.,** orthostatic h.
**vascular h.,** severe hypotension from dilatation of the blood vessels.

**hy·po·ten·sive** (hi″po-ten′siv) 1. characterized by or causing diminished tension or pressure, as abnormally low blood pressure. 2. a person with abnormally low blood pressure.

**hy·po·ten·sor** (hi″po-ten′sor) a substance that lowers the blood pressure; a hypotensive agent.

**hy·po·tha·lam·ic** (hi″po-thə-lam′ik) of or involving the hypothalamus.

**hy·po·thal·a·mot·o·my** (hi″po-thal″ə-mot′ə-me) [*hypothalamus* + *-tomy*] production of lesions in the posterolateral part of the hypothalamus; performed in the treatment of psychotic disorders.

**hy·po·thal·a·mus** (hi″po-thal′ə-məs) [*hypo-* + *thalamus*] [TA] [MeSH: Hypothalamus] the ventral part of the diencephalon that forms the floor and part of the lateral wall of the third ventricle. Anatomically, it includes the preoptic area, optic tract, optic chiasm, mammillary bodies, tuber cinereum, infundibulum, and neurohypophysis, but for physiological purposes the neurohypophysis is considered a distinct structure. The hypothalamus may be divided into five regions or areas *(area hypothalamica rostralis, area hypothalamica dorsalis, area hypothalamica intermedia, area hypothalamica lateralis* and *area hypothalamica posterior)* or into three longitudinal zones *(periventricular zone, medial zone,* and *lateral zone).* The hypothalamic nuclei constitute that part of the corticodiencephalic mechanism that activates, controls and integrates the peripheral autonomic mechanisms, endocrine activity, and many somatic functions, e.g., a general regulation of water balance, body temperature, sleep, and food intake, and the development of secondary sex characteristics. The hypothalamus secretes vasopressin and oxytocin, which are stored in the pituitary, as well as many releasing factors (hypophysiotropic hormones), by means of which it exerts control over functions of the adenohypophysis.

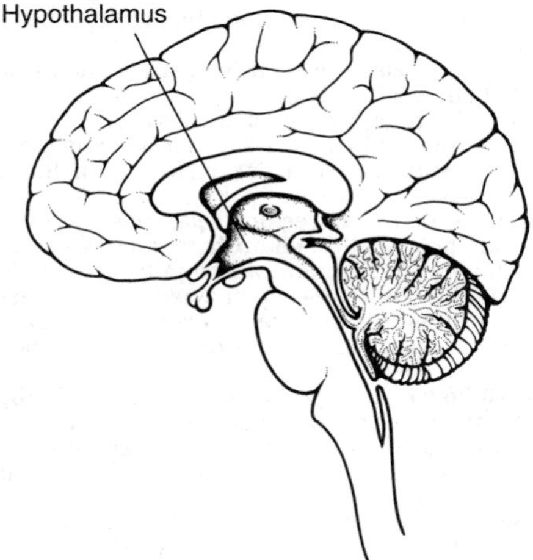


**hy·poth·e·nar** (hi-poth′ə-nər) [*hypo-* + *thenar*] [TA] 1. the fleshy eminence on the palm along the ulnar margin; called also *eminentia hypothenaris* [TA alternative] and *hypothenar eminence.* 2. relating to this eminence.

**hy·po·ther·mal** (hi″po-thər′məl) [*hypo-* + *thermal*] pertaining to or characterized by reduced body temperature.

**hy·po·ther·mia** (hi″po-thər′me-ə) [*hypo-* + *therm-* + *-ia*] [MeSH: Hypothermia] 1. a reduction of core body temperature to 32°C (89°F) or lower, as that due to exposure in cold weather or induced as a means of decreasing metabolism of tissues and thereby the need for oxygen, as used in various surgical procedures, especially on the heart. 2. a state of low temperature induced in an excised organ being preserved for transplantation.
**accidental h.,** unintentional reduction of the core body temperature, as in a cold environment, without primary disturbance of the thermoregulatory center.
**environmental h.,** accidental hyperthermia due to heat loss due to a combination of convection, conduction, and radiation to the surrounding ambient air.
**endogenous h.,** abnormally reduced body temperature resulting from physiologic causes, due to hypofunction of the central nervous system (diencephalon) or of the endocrine system, e.g., the thyroid gland.
**mild h.,** that in which core body temperature is between 33°C (91.4°F) and 35°C (95°F).
**moderate h.,** that in which core body temperature is between 28°C (82.4°F) and 33°C (91.4°F).
**severe h.,** that in which core body temperature is between 9°C (48.2°F) and 28°C (82.4°F).

**hy·po·ther·mic** (hi″po-thər′mik) pertaining to or exhibiting reduced body temperature, pertaining to hypothermia.

**hy·po·ther·my** (hi″po-thər′me) hypothermia.

**hy·poth·e·sis** (hi-poth′ə-sis) a supposition that appears to explain a group of phenomena and is advanced as a basis for further investigation; a proposition that is subject to proof or to an experimental or statistical test. See also *theory.*
**alternative h.,** the hypothesis that is compared with the null hypothesis in a statistical test. Symbol $H_1$ or $H_a$.
**biogenic amine h.,** the hypothesis that depression is associated with deficiency of biogenic amines (catecholamines and serotonin), especially norepinephrine, at functionally important receptor sites in the brain and that elation is associated with excess of such amines.
**Dreyer and Bennett h.,** see *recombinational germline theory,* under *theory.*
**gate h.,** gate theory.
**insular h.,** the hypothesis that diabetes mellitus is due to disordered function of the pancreatic islets.
**jelly roll h.,** a theory explaining the formation of nerve myelin, which states that it consists of successive layers of the plasma membrane of a Schwann cell wrapped spirally around the axon in a jelly roll fashion.
**lattice h.,** a theory of the nature of the antigen-antibody reaction which postulates reaction between multivalent antigen and divalent antibody to give an antigen-antibody complex of a lattice-like structure.
**Lyon h.,** in all mammalian somatic cells, all X chromosomes in excess of one are inactivated (in the form of sex chromatin) on a random basis at an early stage of embryogenesis. Thus the normal human female is in effect a mosaic for heterozygous X-linked genes, since the paternal X chromosome is inactivated in some cells and the maternal one in the others, and females heterozygous for an X-linked disorder often exhibit some stigmata for the condition. See also *lyonization.*
**Makeham's h.,** the assumption that death is due to two co-existing causes: (1) chance, which is constant; (2) inability to withstand destruction, which progresses geometrically.
**null h.,** the particular hypothesis under investigation; termed null because it frequently asserts a lack of effect or of difference. Symbol $H_0$. Cf. *alternative h.*
**one gene–one enzyme h.,** see *one gene–one polypeptide chain h.*
**one gene–one polypeptide chain h.,** a gene is the DNA sequence that codes for the production of one polypeptide chain; formerly referred to as the one gene–one enzyme or one gene–one protein hypothesis. Antibody genes are an exception; separate genes for variable and constant regions are rearranged to code for a single polypeptide.
**response-to-injury h.,** a hypothesis explaining atherogenesis as initiating with some injury to the endothelial cells lining the artery walls, which causes a variety of forms of endothelial dysfunction and leads to abnormal cellular interactions and initiation and progression of atherogenesis.
**sliding-filament h.,** the stretching of individual muscle fibers raises the number of tension-developing bridges that can be formed between the sliding contractile protein elements (actin and myosin) and thus augments the force of the next muscle contraction.
**Starling's h.,** the direction and rate of fluid transfer between blood plasma in the capillary and fluid in the tissue spaces depend on the hydrostatic pressure on each side of the capillary wall, on the osmotic pressure of protein in plasma and in tissue fluid, and on the properties of the capillary wall as a filtering membrane.
**unitarian h.,** the theory that antibody is a single species of modified serum globulin regardless of the overt consequences of its reaction with homologous antigen, e.g., agglutination, precipitation, complement fixation, etc.
**wobble h.,** a hypothesis proposed by F. H. C. Crick to explain how a specific transfer RNA (tRNA) molecule can translate different codons in a messenger RNA (mRNA) template. It states that the third base of the tRNA anticodon does not have to pair with a complementary codon (as do the first two bases) but can form base pairs with several mRNA codons.

**hy·po·threp·sia** (hi″po-threp′se-ə) malnutrition.

**hy·po·throm·bin·emia** (hi″po-throm″bĭ-ne′me-ə) a deficiency of thrombin in the blood.

**hy·po·thy·mia** (hi″po-thi′me-ə) [*hypo-* + *thymo-*[2] + *-ia*] abnormal diminution of emotional tone, as in depression.

**hy·po·thy·mic** (hi″po-thi′mik) marked by hypothymia.

**hy·po·thy·mism** (hi″po-thi′miz-əm) abnormally deficient thymus activity.

**hy·po·thy·rea** (hi″po-thi′re-ə) hypothyroidism.

**hy·po·thy·roid** (hi″po-thi′roid) marked by or due to hypothyroidism. Called also *athyrotic, thyroprival,* and *thyroprivic.*

**hy·po·thy·roid·ism** (hi″po-thi′roid-iz-əm) [MeSH: Hypothyroidism] deficiency of thyroid activity, characterized by decrease in basal metabolic rate, fatigue, and lethargy; if untreated, it progresses to myxedema. In adults it is more common in women than men, and in infants it can lead to cretinism. Called also *athyria, athyroidism, athyroidosis, hypothyrosis, thyroprivia,* and *thyroid insufficiency.*
**central h.,** secondary h.
**hypothalamic h.,** secondary hypothyroidism caused by a defect or lesion of the hypothalamus that interferes with its production of thyrotropin-releasing hormone. Called also *tertiary h.*
**infantile h.,** that first seen in infancy; when severe, it leads to cretinism.
**juvenile h.,** that first seen in childhood, with manifestations intermediate between those of the infantile and adult types, including slowed bone and dental growth and delayed sexual development; in children under age three it may cause mental retardation.
**juvenile acquired h.,** hypothyroidism with an insidious onset in childhood, caused by thyrotropin deficiency; it is marked by slowing and cessation of growth, thickening and yellowing of the skin, coarse facies, delayed pubertal development, and short stature at maturity.
**pituitary h.,** secondary hypothyroidism caused by a defect or lesion of the pituitary gland (usually a tumor) that interferes with production of thyrotropin.
**primary h.,** hypothyroidism due to a disease or lesion of the thyroid gland itself, usually accompanied by increased levels of thyrotropin.
**secondary h.,** that resulting from inadequate secretion of thyrotropin by the pituitary gland; see *hypothalamic h.* and *pituitary h.* Called also *central h.*
**tertiary h.,** hypothalamic h.

**hy·po·thy·ro·sis** (hi″po-thi-ro′sis) hypothyroidism.

**hy·po·to·nia** (hi″po-to′ne-ə) [*hypo-* + *ton-* + *-ia*] a condition of diminished tone of the skeletal muscles; diminished resistance of muscles to passive stretching.
**benign congenital h.,** a condition marked by signs of weakness and floppiness in babies, due to nonprogressive weakness of skeletal muscles from birth.
**h. o′culi,** low intraocular pressure.

**hy·po·ton·ic** (hi-po-ton′ik) 1. denoting a solution which, when bathing body cells, causes a net flow of water across the semipermeable cell membrane into the cell. 2. denoting a solution having less tonicity than another solution, e.g., the blood, with which it is compared. 3. exhibiting hypotonia.

**hy·po·to·nic·i·ty** (hi″po-to-nis′ĭ-te) the state or quality of being hypotonic.

**hy·pot·o·nus** (hi-pot′ə-nəs) hypotonia.

**hy·po·tox·ic·i·ty** (hi″po-tok-sis′ĭ-te) [*hypo-* + *toxicity*] the state or quality of possessing mitigated or diminished toxicity.

**hy·po·tri·chi·a·sis** (hi″po-trĭ-ki′ə-sis) congenital alopecia.

**hy·po·tri·cho·sis** (hi″po-trĭ-ko′sis) [*hypo-* + *trich-* + *-osis*] [MeSH: Hypotrichosis] presence of less than the normal amount of hair.

**hy·pot·ro·phy** (hi-pot′rə-fe) [*hypo-* + *-trophy*] abiotrophy.

**hy·po·tro·pia** (hi″po-tro′pe-ə) [*hypo-* + *trop-* + *-ia*] strabismus in which there is permanent downward deviation of the visual axis of an eye.

**hy·po·tryp·to·phan·ic** (hi″po-trip-to-fan′ik) caused by deficiency of tryptophan in the diet.

**hy·po·tym·pan·ic** (hi″po-tim-pan′ik) located below the sulcus tympanicus.

**hy·po·tym·pa·not·o·my** (hi″po-tim″pə-not′ə-me) surgical opening of the hypotympanum.

**hy·po·tym·pa·num** (hi″po-tim′pə-nəm) a space in the middle ear, below the lower edge of the sulcus tympanicus.

**hy·po·ure·mia** (hi″po-u-re′me-ə) an abnormally low level of urea in the blood.

**hy·po·ure·sis** (hi″po-u-re′sis) oliguria.

**hy·po·uri·ce·mia** (hi″po-u″rĭ-se′me-ə) deficiency of uric acid in the blood, along with xanthinuria, due to deficiency of xanthine oxidase, the enzyme required for conversion of hypoxanthine to xanthine and of xanthine to uric acid.

**hy·po·uri·cu·ria** (hi″po-u″rĭ-ku′re-ə) deficiency of uric acid in the urine.

**hy·po·uro·crin·ia** (hi″po-u″ro-krin′e-ə) deficient secretion of urine; cf. *oliguria.*

**hyp·ovar·i·an·ism** (hi″po-var′e-ən-iz-əm) hypo-ovarianism.

**hy·po·ve·nos·i·ty** (hi″po-ve-nos′ĭ-te) incomplete development of the venous system in any area.

**hy·po·ven·ti·la·tion** (hi″po-ven″tĭ-la′shən) [MeSH: Hypoventilation] a state in which there is a reduced amount of air entering the pulmonary alveoli (decreased *alveolar ventilation;* see under *ventilation*), resulting in increased carbon dioxide tension. Cf. *hypopnea* and *bradypnea.*
**primary alveolar h.,** impairment of automatic control of respiration, usually due to a spinal cord or brain stem lesion; voluntary control remains intact but apnea occurs during sleep. Called also *Ondine's curse.*

**hy·po·vi·ta·min·o·sis** (hi″po-vi″tə-min-o′sis) a condition due to a deficiency of one or more essential vitamins; see specific vitamins.

**hy·po·vo·le·mia** (hi″po-vo-le′me-ə) [*hypo-* + *volume* + *-emia*] abnormally decreased volume of circulating blood in the body; the most common cause is hemorrhage.

**hy·po·vo·le·mic** (hi″po-vo-le′mik) pertaining to or characterized by hypovolemia.

**hy·po·vo·lia** (hi″po-vo′le-ə) diminished water content or volume, as of extracellular fluid.

**hy·po·xan·thine** (hi″po-zan′thēn) [MeSH: Hypoxanthine] 6-oxypurine, a purine base formed as an intermediate in the degradation of purines and purine nucleosides to uric acid and in the salvage of free purines. It is found in some transfer RNA molecules and occurs complexed with ribose as the nucleoside inosine.

**hy·po·xan·thine-guan·ine phos·pho·ri·bo·syl·trans·fer·ase (HGPRT)** (hi″po-zan′thēn-gwahn′ēn fos″fo-ri″bo-səl-trans′fər-ās) hypoxanthine phosphoribosyltransferase.

**hy·po·xan·thine phos·pho·ri·bo·syl·trans·fer·ase (HPRT)** (hi″po-zan′thēn fos″fo-ri″bo-səl-trans′fər-ās) [MeSH: Hypoxanthine Phosphoribosyltransferase] an enzyme of the transferase class that catalyzes the phosphorylation of hypoxanthine or guanine to its corresponding nucleoside monophosphate, a salvage mechanism for recovery of preformed purines, especially in the central nervous system. Absence of enzyme activity, an X-linked trait, results in Lesch-Nyhan syndrome; partially decreased enzyme activity results in hyperuricemia and severe gouty arthritis, but the neurologic sequelae of Lesch-Nyhan syndrome do not occur. Called also *hypoxanthine-guanine phosphoribosyltransferase.*

**hy·pox·emia** (hi″pok-se′me-ə) [*hyp-* + *ox-* + *-emia*] deficient oxygenation of the blood; cf. *hypoxia.*

**hy·pox·ia** (hi-pok′se-ə) reduction of oxygen supply to tissue below physiological levels despite adequate perfusion of the tissue by blood. Cf. *anoxia.*
**anemic h.,** hypoxia due to reduction of the oxygen-carrying capacity of the blood as a result of a decrease in the total hemoglobin or an alteration of the hemoglobin constituents. Cf. *anemic anoxia.*
**fetal h.,** hypoxia in utero, caused by conditions such as inadequate placental function (often abruptio placentae), preeclamptic toxicity, prolapse of the umbilical cord, or complications from anesthetic administration. See also *fetal asphyxia* under *asphyxia* and *hypoxic-ischemic encephalopathy* under *encephalopathy.*
**histotoxic h.,** that due to impaired utilization of oxygen by tissues, as in cyanide poisoning.
**hypoxic h.,** that due to insufficient oxygen reaching the blood, as at decreased barometric pressures at high altitudes. Cf. *anoxic anoxia.*
**stagnant h.,** that due to failure to transport sufficient oxygen because of inadequate blood flow, as in heart failure.

**hy·pox·ia-is·che·mia** (hi-pok′se-ə-is-ke′me-ə) the changes occurring in tissues when the blood supply is cut off, particularly in a fetus or infant with asphyxia; see also *hypoxic-ischemic encephalopathy* under *encephalopathy.*

**hy·pox·ic** (hi-pok′sik) pertaining to or characterized by hypoxia.

**hy·pox·i·do·sis** (hi-pok″sĭ-do′sis) impaired cell function due to reduced supply of oxygen.

**hyp·oxy·phi·lia** (hi-pok″se-fil′e-ə) [*hyp-* + *oxy-* + *-philia*] a paraphilia in which sexual arousal or activity depends on oxygen deprivation.

**hy·pro·mel·lose phthal·ate** (hi″pro-mel′ōs) [NF] a phthalic acid ester of hydroxypropyl methylcellulose, used as a coating agent for tablets and granules.

**Hyp·Rho-D** (hi′pro-de) trademark for a preparation of $Rh_0$(D) immune serum globulin.

**hyp·sa·rhyth·mia** (hi″sə-rith′me-ə) see *hypsarrhythmia.*

**hyp·sar·rhyth·mia** (hi″sə-rith′me-ə) [*hyps-* + *arrhythmia*] an electroencephalographic abnormality sometimes observed in infants, with random, high-voltage slow waves and spikes that arise from multiple foci and spread to all cortical areas. It is seen most commonly in cases of jackknife seizures.

**hypsi-** [Gr. *hypsi* aloft] a combining form meaning high.

**hyp·si·brachy·ce·phal·ic** (hip″sĭ-brak″e-sə-fal′ik) [*hypsi-* + *brachycephalic*] having the head broad and high.

**hyp·si·ce·phal·ic** (hip″sĭ-sə-fal′ik) [*hypsi-* + *cephalic*] oxycephalic.

**hyp·si·ceph·a·ly** (hip″sĭ-sef′ə-le) oxycephaly.

**hyp·si·con·chous** (hip″sĭ-kong′kəs) [*hypsi-* + *concha* + *-ous*] having an orbital index over 85.

**hyp·si·loid** (hip′sĭ-loid) [Gr. *hypsiloeidēs*] shaped like a capital Greek letter upsilon (Υ). Cf. *hyoid.*

**hyp·si·sta·phyl·ia** (hip″sĭ-stə-fil′e-ə) [*hypsi-* + *staphyl-* + *-ia*] a condition characterized by an unusually high-arched, narrow palate.

**hyp·si·steno·ce·phal·ic** (hip″sĭ-sten″o-sə-fal′ik) [*hypsi-* + *steno-* + *cephalic*] having a high, curved vertex, cheek bones prominent, and jaws prognathic.

**hyps(o)-** [Gr. *hypsos* height] a combining form denoting relationship to height.

**hyp·so·ceph·a·lous** (hip″so-sef′ə-ləs) oxycephalic.

**hyp·so·chrome** (hip′so-krōm) [*hypso-* + *-chrome*] an atom or group whose introduction into a compound shifts the compound's absorption maximum to a shorter wavelength; cf. *bathochrome.*

**hyp·so·chro·my** (hip″so-kro′me) a shift of the absorption band toward higher frequencies (shorter wavelengths), with lightening of color.

**hyp·so·dont** (hip′so-dont) [*hypso-* + Gr. *odous* tooth] having prism-shaped teeth with high crowns, as in many herbivorous mammals.

**hyp·so·ki·ne·sis** (hip″so-kĭ-ne′sis) [*hypso-* + *kin-* + *-esis*] a backward swaying, retropulsion, or falling when in erect posture, seen in paralysis agitans, Wilson's disease, and similar conditions.

**hy·pur·gia** (hi-pur′je-ə) [L.; Gr. *hypourgiai* medical services] the sum of the minor or subsidiary factors that make for recovery in any particular case.

**hy·rax** (hi′raks) any of several species of rabbit-sized ungulates of the genera *Procavia, Dendrohyrax,* and *Heterohyrax,* found in Africa and the Middle East; they have fat furry bodies, short legs, small ears, and short tails. Some are reservoirs for *Leishmania aethiopica.* Called also *coney.*
**rock h.,** any of several ground-dwelling species of the genera *Procavia* and *Heterohyrax,* often reservoirs for *Leishmania aethiopica;* called also *dassie.*
**tree h.,** any of several tree-dwelling species of the genus *Dendrohyrax,* often reservoirs for *Leishmania aethiopica.*

**Hyrtl's loop (anastomosis), recess, sphincter** (hər′təlz) [Jozsef *Hyrtl,* Hungarian anatomist in Austria, 1810–1894] see under *loop* and *sphincter,* and see *recessus epitympanicus.*

**hys·ter·al·gia** (his″tər-al′jə) [*hystero-* + *-algia*] pain in the uterus. Called also *hysterodynia, metralgia, metrodynia,* and *uteralgia.*

**hys·ter·atre·sia** (his″tər-ə-tre′zhə) atresia of the opening into the uterus. Called also *atretometria.*

**hys·ter·ec·to·my** (his″tər-ek′tə-me) [*hystero-* + *-ectomy*] [MeSH: Hysterectomy] the operation of excising the entire uterus, performed either through the abdominal wall *(abdominal h.)* or through the vagina *(vaginal h.).*
**abdominal h.,** excision of the uterus through an incision in the abdominal wall. Called also *abdominohysterectomy, celiohysterectomy,* and *laparohysterectomy.*
**cesarean h.,** cesarean section followed by removal of the uterus.
**complete h.,** total h.
**partial h.,** subtotal h.
**radical h.,** hysterectomy with pelvic lymphadenectomy and wide

lateral excision of parametrial and paravaginal supporting structures; called also *Wertheim's operation* or, when done by the vaginal route, *Schauta's operation*.
**subtotal h., supracervical h., supravaginal h.,** hysterectomy in which the cervix is left in place.
**total h.,** hysterectomy in which the uterus and cervix are completely excised; called also *panhysterectomy*.
**vaginal h.,** excision of the uterus through the vagina.

**hys·te·re·sis** (his″tə-re′sis) [Gr. *hysterēsis* a lagging behind] 1. a time lag in the occurrence of two associated phenomena, as between cause and effect. 2. in cardiac pacemaker terminology, the number of pulses per minute below the programmed pacing rate that the heart must drop in order to cause initiation of pacing.
**protoplasmic h.,** a postulated cause of cell senescence: the colloidal state of the protoplasm is altered, becoming less dispersed, with loss of water and electrical charge.

**hys·ter·eu·ry·sis** (his″tər-u′rə-sis) dilation of the os uteri.

**hys·ter·ia** (his-ter′e-ə) [Gr. *hystera* womb, from the antiquated belief that wandering of the uterus caused mental disturbances] [MeSH: Hysteria] a now somewhat nebulous term formerly used widely in psychiatry. Its meanings have included (1) classic hysteria (now *somatization disorder*); (2) hysterical neurosis (now divided into *conversion disorder* and *dissociative disorders*); (3) anxiety hysteria; and (4) hysterical personality (now *histrionic personality*).
**anxiety h.,** Freud's term for phobias, reflecting his view that the same defense mechanisms, repression and displacement, and the same unconscious conflicts involving infantile sexuality are involved in both hysteria and phobias.
**conversion h.,** former name for a subtype of hysterical neurosis (see *hysteria*); currently classified as conversion disorder.
**dissociative h.,** former name for a subtype of hysterical neurosis (see *hysteria*); the current classification is *dissociative disorders*.
**farrowing h.,** a psychological abnormality seen in sows that have just given birth, usually for the first time, in which they attack their offspring when the piglets attempt to nurse; sometimes the piglets may die of their injuries.
**fixation h.,** a form of conversion disorder in which the symptoms are based on an existing or previous organic disease or injury, as the persistence of a nervous cough after pertussis.
**major h.,** 1. la grande hystérie of Charcot, hysteria with dramatic epileptiform attacks involving intense emotional display. 2. hysteroepilepsy.

**hys·ter·ic** (his-ter′ik) 1. pertaining to or characterized by hysteria. 2. a person affected with hysteria.

**hys·ter·i·cal** (his-ter′i-kəl) characterized by hysteria.

**hys·ter·i·cism** (his-ter′i-siz-əm) a tendency toward hysteria.

**hys·ter·ics** (his-ter′iks) popular term for an uncontrollable emotional outburst.

**hys·ter·i·form** (his-ter′ĭ-form) having the appearance of hysteria.

**hyster(o)-** [Gr. *hystera* uterus] a combining form denoting relationship to the uterus, or to hysteria; see also *metr(o)-*.

**hys·tero·bu·bono·cele** (his″tər-o-bu-bon′o-sēl) an inguinal hernia containing the uterus.

**hys·tero·cele** (his′tər-o-sēl″) [*hystero-* + *-cele*[1]] hernia of the uterus.

**hys·tero·clei·sis** (his″tər-o-kli′sis) [*hystero-* + Gr. *kleisis* closure] surgical closure of the ostium uteri.

**hys·tero·col·pec·to·my** (his″tər-o-kol-pek′tə-me) [*hystero-* + *colpo-* + *-ectomy*] surgical removal of the uterus and vagina.

**hys·tero·cys·tic** (his″tər-o-sis′tik) pertaining to the uterus and the bladder.

**hys·tero·cys·to·clei·sis** (his″tər-o-sis″to-kli′sis) [*hystero-* + *cysto-* + *kleisis* closure] the operation of turning the cervix uteri into the bladder and suturing it; done for the relief of vesicouterovaginal fistula or ureterouterine fistula. Called also *Bozeman's operation*.

**hys·ter·odyn·ia** (his″tər-o-din′e-ə) [*hystero-* + *-odynia*] hysteralgia.

**hys·tero·ep·i·lep·sy** (his″tər-o-ep′ĭ-lep″se) hysteria with attacks imitating epileptic seizures.

**hys·tero·gram** (his′tər-o-gram″) a radiograph of the uterus.

**hys·tero·graph** (his′tər-o-graf) [*hystero-* + *-graph*] an apparatus for measuring the strength of uterine contractions in labor.

**hys·ter·og·ra·phy** (his″tər-og′rə-fe) [*hystero-* + *-graphy*] 1. graphic recording of the strength of uterine contractions in labor. 2. radiography of the uterus after instillation of a contrast medium; see also *hysterosalpingography*. Called also *metrography* and *uterography*.

**hys·ter·oid** (his′tər-oid) [*hyster-* + *-oid*] resembling hysteria.

**hys·tero·lith** (his′tər-o-lith″) [*hystero-* + *-lith*] a uterine calculus.

**hys·ter·ol·y·sis** (his″tər-ol′ə-sis) [*hystero-* + *-lysis*] the operation of loosening the uterus from its attachments or adhesions.

**hys·te·rom·e·try** (his″tə-rom′ə-tre) [*hystero-* + *-metry*] the measurement of the dimensions of the uterus.

**hys·tero·myo·ma** (his″tər-o-mi-o′mə) uterine leiomyoma.

**hys·tero·myo·mec·to·my** (his″tər-o-mi″o-mek′tə-me) [*hystero-* + *myoma* + *-ectomy*] uterine myomectomy.

**hys·tero·my·ot·o·my** (his″tər-o-mi-ot′ə-me) [*hystero-* + *myotomy*] incision of the uterus.

**hys·te·rop·a·thy** (his″tə-rop′ə-the) [*hystero-* + *-pathy*] any uterine disease or disorder.

**hys·tero·pexy** (his′tər-o-pek-se) [*hystero-* + *-pexy*] the fixation of a displaced uterus by a surgical operation. It may be done by ventrofixation, shortening of the round ligaments, shortening of the sacrouterine ligaments, or shortening of the endopelvic fascia. It is called *abdominal* or *vaginal*, depending on whether the uterus is fastened to the abdominal wall or to the vagina.

**hys·ter·op·to·sia** (his″tər-op-to′zhə) uterine prolapse.

**hys·ter·op·to·sis** (his″tər-op-to′sis) uterine prolapse.

**hys·ter·or·rha·phy** (his-tər-or′ə-fe) [*hystero-* + *-rrhaphy*] 1. hysteropexy. 2. the operation of suturing of the lacerated uterus.

**hys·ter·or·rhex·is** (his″tər-o-rek′sis) metrorrhexis.

**hys·tero·sal·pin·gec·to·my** (his″tər-o-sal″pin-jek′tə-me) [*hystero-* + *salpingectomy*] excision of the uterus and uterine tubes.

**hys·tero·sal·pin·gog·ra·phy** (his″tər-o-sal″ping-gog′rə-fe) [*hystero-* + *salpingography*] [MeSH: Hysterosalpingography] radiography of the uterus and uterine tubes after the injection of opaque material. Called also *uterosalpingography, uterotubography, hysterotubography, metrosalpingography, metrotubography*.

**hys·tero·sal·pin·go·ooph·o·rec·to·my** (his″tər-o-sal-ping″go-o-of″ə-rek′tə-me) excision of the uterus, uterine tubes, and ovaries.

**hys·tero·sal·pin·gos·to·my** (his″tər-o-sal″ping-gos′tə-me) [*hystero-* + *salpingostomy*] the operation of forming an anastomosis between the uterus and the oviduct after excision of a strictured or obstructed portion of the tube.

**hys·tero·scope** (his′tər-o-skōp″) [*hystero-* + *-scope*] an endoscope used in direct visual examination of the canal of the uterine cervix and the cavity of the uterus.

**hys·ter·os·co·py** (his″tər-os′kə-pe) [MeSH: Hysteroscopy] inspection of the interior of the uterus with an endoscope.

**hys·tero·spasm** (his′tər-o-spaz″əm) spasm of the uterus.

**hys·tero·stat** (his′tər-o-stat) [*hystero-* + *-stat*] a mechanical intrauterine device for holding sealed sources of ionizing radiation (radium, cesium-137, etc.) in order to give planned patterns of irradiation.

**hys·tero·ther·mom·e·try** (his″tər-o-thər-mom′ə-tre) uterothermometry.

**hys·tero·tome** (his′tər-o-tōm″) [*hystero-* + *-tome*] an instrument for incising the uterus.

**hys·ter·ot·o·my** (his″tər-ot′ə-me) [*hystero-* + *-tomy*] incision of the uterus, usually for delivery of a fetus.
**abdominal h.,** incision of the uterus through the wall of the abdomen. Called also *abdominohysterotomy, abdominouterotomy,* and *laparohysterotomy*.
**vaginal h.,** incision of the uterus through the vagina.

**hys·tero·tra·chel·ec·ta·sia** (his″tər-o-tra″kəl-ek-ta′zhə) surgical dilation of the cervix and uterus.

**hys·ter·o·tra·chel·ec·to·my** (his″tər-o-tra″kəl-ek′tə-me) cervicectomy.

**hys·tero·tra·chelo·plas·ty** (his″tər-o-tra′kəl-o-plas″te) plastic repair of the cervix uteri; tracheloplasty.

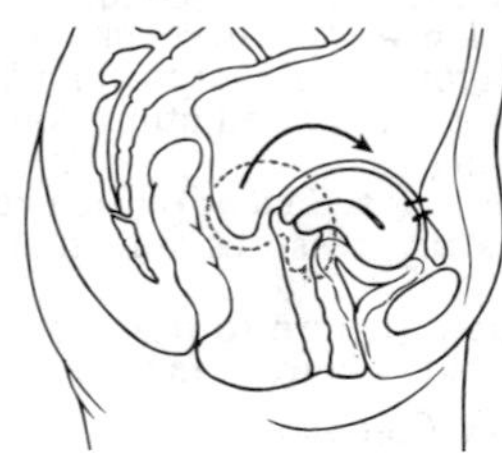

Hysteropexy, with fixation to the anterior abdominal wall.

**hys·tero·tra·chel·or·rha·phy** (his″tər-o-tra″kəl-or′ə-fe) [*hystero-* + *trachlo-* + *-rrhaphy*] suture of the cervix uteri.

**hys·tero·tra·chel·ot·o·my** (his″tər-o-tra″kəl-ot′ə-me) [*hystero-* + *trachelo-* + *-tomy*] incision of the cervix uteri.

**hys·tero·tu·bog·ra·phy** (his″tər-o-too-bog′rə-fe) hysterosalpingography.

**hys·tero·vag·i·no·en·tero·cele** (his″tər-o-vaj″ĭ-no-en′tər-o-sēl) [*hystero-* + *vagina* + *enterocele*] hernia containing the uterus, vagina, and intestine.

**Hy·tak·er·ol** (hi-tak′ər-ol) trademark for preparations of dihydrotachysterol.

**Hy·tone** (hi′tōn) trademark for preparations of hydrocortisone.

**Hy·trin** (hi′trin) trademark for a preparation of terazosin hydrochloride.

**Hy·zaar** (hi′zahr) trademark for a combination preparation of losartan potassium and hydrochlorothiazide.

**Hyz·yd** (hiz′id) trademark for a preparation of isoniazid.

**Hz** hertz.

# I

**I** symbol for *incisor, iodine,* and *inosine* (in nucleotides).

***I*** symbol for *electric current, intensity* (of radiant energy), and *ionic strength.*

**-ia** [L. and Gr. noun-forming suffix] a word termination denoting a state or condition.

**IAB** intra-aortic balloon; see under *counterpulsation.*

**IABP** intra-aortic balloon pump.

**IAEA** International Atomic Energy Agency.

**IAHA** immune adherence hemagglutination assay.

**IAPP** islet amyloid polypeptide; see *amylin.*

**-iasis** a word termination meaning a process or the condition resulting therefrom, particularly a morbid condition. See *-sis.*

**ia·tra·lip·tic** (i″ə-trə-lip′tik) [Gr. *iatreia* cure + *aleiphein* to anoint] pertaining to the application of remedies by inunction and friction.

**ia·tra·lip·tics** (i″ə-trə-lip′tiks) treatment by inunction and friction.

**iat·ric** (i-at′rik) [Gr. *iatrikos*] pertaining to medicine or to a physician.

**-iatric** [Gr. *iatrikos* pertaining to a physician, from *iatros* physician] a combining form denoting relationship to medical treatment.

**-iatrics** [*-iatric*] a combining form denoting medical treatment.

**iatr(o)-** [Gr. *iatros* physician] a combining form denoting relationship to a physician or to medicine.

**iat·ro·chem·i·cal** (i-at″ro-kem′ĭ-kəl) pertaining to iatrochemistry.

**iat·ro·chem·is·try** (i-at″ro-kem′is-tre) [*iatro-* + *chemistry*] a school of medicine active from 1525 to 1660; it theorized that life, health, and disease were the result of chemical balances, and that disease was to be treated chemically. Its most famous members were Paracelsus, J.B. van Helmont, and François de la Boë (see *Sylvius*).

**iat·ro·gen·e·sis** (i-at″ro-jen′ə-sis) [*iatro-* + *-genesis*] the creation of additional problems or complications resulting from treatment by a physician or surgeon.

**iat·ro·gen·ic** (i-at″ro-jen′ik) [*iatro-* + *-genic*] resulting from the activity of physicians. Originally applied to disorders induced in the patient by autosuggestion based on the physician's examination, manner, or discussion, the term is now applied to any adverse condition in a patient occurring as the result of treatment by a physician or surgeon, especially to infections acquired by the patient during the course of treatment. Cf. *nosocomial.*

**ia·trol·o·gy** (i″ə-trol′o-je) [*iatro-* + *-logy*] the science of medicine.

**iat·ro·math·e·mat·i·cal** (i-at″ro-math″ə-mat′ĭ-kəl) iatrophysical.

**iat·ro·me·chan·i·cal** (i-at″ro-mə-kan′ĭ-kəl) iatrophysical.

**iat·ro·phys·i·cal** (i-at″ro-fiz′ĭ-kəl) an Italian school of medicine active in the 17th century; the school opposed iatrochemistry and, inspired by the earlier experiments of Harvey and Sanctorius, combined medicine, physics, and mechanics. René Descartes was an early exponent of iatrophysics, and his posthumous *De homine* (1662) was the first modern textbook on physiology.

**iat·ro·phys·ics** (i-at″ro-fiz′iks) [*iatro-* + *physics*] the physics of medicine or of medical and surgical treatment.

**-iatry** [Gr. *iatreia* healing, from *iatros* physician] a word termination denoting medical treatment.

**IB** inclusion body.

**IBC** iron-binding capacity.

**IBF** immunoglobulin-binding factor.

**Ibn Rushd** see *Averroes.*

**Ibn Sinā** see *Avicenna.*

**Ibn Zuhr** see *Avenzoar.*

**ibo·ga·ine** (i-bo′gə-ēn) [MeSH: Ibogaine] an alkaloid from the root of *Tabernanthe iboga* Baill. (Apocynaceae) that has antidepressant and euphoric properties; it is isomeric with tabernanthine.

**ibo·ten·ic ac·id** (i″bo-ten′ik) [MeSH: Ibotenic Acid] an excitotoxin found in the mushroom *Amanita muscaria;* it is 3 to 10 times as potent as glutamic acid and is used to study the excitatory mechanisms of glutamate transmitters.

**ibu·fe·nac** (i-bu′fə-nak) an analgesic and anti-inflammatory formerly used in the treatment of rheumatic conditions.

**ibu·pro·fen** (i″bu-pro′fən) [USP] [MeSH: Ibuprofen] a nonsteroidal analgesic, antipyretic, and anti-inflammatory agent that is a propionic acid derivative; used for relief of pain, reduction of fever, and in the treatment of osteoarthritis and rheumatoid arthritis.

**ibu·ti·lide ace·tate** (ĭ-bu′tĭ-līd) a cardiac depressant used as an antiarrhythmic agent in the treatment of atrial arrhythmias; administered by intravenous infusion.

**IC** inspiratory capacity; irritable colon.

**-ic** [L. *-icus,* from Gr. *-ikos*] 1. a suffix meaning pertaining to or characteristic of, e.g., acidic. 2. in chemistry, a suffix used to indicate an ion or acid exhibiting the higher of two oxidation states, the other being indicated by the suffix *-ous.*

**ICAM-1** intercellular adhesion molecule 1.

**ICAM-2** intercellular adhesion molecule 2.

**ICD** International Classification of Diseases (of the World Health Organization); intrauterine contraceptive device.

**ice** (īs) [MeSH: Ice] any of the six solid forms of water; but usually the common low-density form melting at 0°C at 1 atmosphere. **dry i.,** carbon dioxide snow.

**Ice·land disease** (īs′lənd) [*Iceland,* island country in the North Atlantic, where an epidemic occurred in 1948] chronic fatigue syndrome.

**ich** (ik) white spot disease, def. 3.

**ich·no·gram** (ik′no-gram) [Gr. *ichnos* a footprint + *-gram*] a footprint, in ink on paper.

**ich·tham·mol** (ik′thəm-ol) [USP] a reddish brown to brownish black viscous fluid, with a strong, characteristic odor, obtained by the destructive distillation of certain bituminous schists, sulfonation of the distillate, and neutralization of the product with ammonia; used as a local skin anti-infective.

**ich·thy·ism** (ik′the-iz-əm) ichthyotoxism.

**ich·thy·is·mus** (ik″the-iz′məs) [Gr. *ichthys* fish] ichthyotoxism.

**ichthy(o)-** [Gr. *ichthys* fish] a combining form denoting relationship to fish.

**ich·thyo·acan·tho·tox·in** (ik″the-o-ə-kan″tho-tok′sin) [*ichthyo-* + *acantho-* + *toxin*] the venom secreted by venomous fishes, in connection with stings, spines, or "teeth."

**ich·thyo·acan·tho·tox·ism** (ik″the-o-ə-kan″tho-tok′siz-əm) intoxication resulting from injuries produced by the stings, spines, or "teeth" of venomous fishes.

**ich·thyo·col·la** (ik″the-o-kol′ə) [*ichthyo-* + Gr. *kolla* glue] isinglass.

**ich·thyo·he·mo·tox·in** (ik″the-o-he″mo-tok′sin) [*ichthyo-* + *hemo-* + *toxin*] a toxic substance found in the blood of certain fish.

**ich·thyo·he·mo·tox·ism** (ik″the-o-he″mo-tok′siz-əm) intoxication caused by the ingestion of ichthyohemotoxin, characterized by gastrointestinal and neurological disturbances.

**ich·thy·oid** (ik′the-oid) [*ichthyo-* + *-oid*] resembling a fish; shaped like a fish.

**Ich·thy·ol** (ik′the-ol) trademark for a preparation of ichthammol.

**ich·thy·ol·o·gy** (ik″the-ol′o-je) that branch of zoology specializing in the study of fishes.

**ich·thy·oo·tox·in** (ik″the-o″o-tok′sin) [*ichthyo-* + *oo-* + *toxin*] a toxic substance derived from the roe of certain fish; see also *ichthyootoxism.*

**ich·thy·oo·tox·ism** (ik″the-o″o-tok′siz-əm) intoxication caused by the ingestion of toxic fish roe, characterized by gastrointestinal and neurological disturbances.

**ich·thyo·pha·gia** (ik″the-o-fa′jə) [*ichthyo-* + *-phagia*] the practice of subsisting on fish.

**ich·thy·oph·a·gous** (ik″the-of′ə-gəs) eating or subsisting on fish.

**ich·thy·oph·thi·ri·a·sis** (ik″the-o-thi′re-ə-sis) [*Ichthyophthirius* + *-iasis*] white spot disease, def. 3.

**Ich·thy·oph·thi·ri·us** (ik″the-o-thi′re-əs) [*ichthyo-* + Gr. *phtheir* louse] a genus of histophagous protozoa of the order Hymenostomatida, suborder Ophryoglenina. *I. multifi′liis* causes white spot disease in marine and freshwater fishes.

**ich·thyo·sar·co·tox·in** (ik″the-o-sahr″ko-tok′sin) [*ichthyo-* + *sarco-* + *toxin*] the poison found in the flesh of poisonous fishes, excluding toxins which may result from bacterial contamination.

**ich·thyo·sar·co·tox·ism** (ik″the-o-sahr-ko-tok′siz-əm) intoxication characterized by various gastrointestinal and neurological disturbances, resulting from the ingestion of the flesh of poisonous fishes; the term excludes ordinary bacterial food poisoning. Some types are *elasmobranch, Gymnothorax, fugu* or *puffer fish,* and *scombroid poisoning* and *ciguatera.* Called also *fish poisoning.*

**ich·thyo·si·form** (ik″the-o′sĭ-form) resembling ichthyosis.

**ich·thy·o·sis** (ik″the-o′sis) [*ichthy-* + *-osis*] [MeSH: Ichthyosis] any in a group of cutaneous disorders characterized by increased or aberrant keratinization, resulting in noninflammatory scaling of the skin. Many different metaphors have been used to describe the appearance and texture of the skin in the various types and stages of ichthyosis, e.g., alligator, collodion, crocodile, fish, and porcupine skin. Most ichthyoses are genetically determined, while some may be acquired and develop in association with various systemic diseases or be a prominent feature in certain genetic syndromes. The term is commonly used alone to refer to *i. vulgaris.*
**i. conge′nita, congenital i.,** 1. in humans, ichthyosis present at birth. See also *collodion baby,* under *baby,* and *harlequin fetus,* under *fetus.* 2. in cattle, a lethal autosomal recessive condition in which most hair is lacking and the entire body is covered with thick horny plaques.
**harlequin i.,** the ichthyosis affecting a harlequin fetus.
**i. hys′trix,** a localized form of epidermolytic hyperkeratosis having the appearance of linear epidermal nevi.
**lamellar i.,** a congenital, chronic form of ichthyosis present at birth, inherited as an autosomal recessive trait, in which the affected infant is born encased in a collodionlike membrane (see *collodion baby,* under *baby)* that is soon shed, the skin then becoming covered with large, coarse scales with involvement of all of the flexures as well as the palms and soles. Universal erythroderma and pruritus are characteristic, and ectropion of variable degree is usually present. Formerly called *nonbullous congenital ichthyosiform erythroderma.*
**i. linea′ris circumflex′a,** a congenital autosomal recessive disorder present at birth, and characterized by the presence of generalized erythroderma and scaling associated with migratory, polycyclic lesions with a peripheral double-edged scale and hyperkeratosis of the flexural areas, and hyperhidrosis of the palms and soles.
**i. palma′ris et planta′ris,** palmoplantar keratoderma.
**i. sim′plex,** i. vulgaris.
**i. u′teri,** a condition marked by the transformation of the columnar epithelium of the endometrium into stratified squamous epithelium.
**i. vulga′ris,** the most common form of ichthyosis, inherited as an autosomal dominant trait, having an onset sometime after the first year of life, especially near puberty. It is characterized by the presence of prominent fine scaling principally on the extensor surfaces of the extremities and back, with the flexures being spared and the abdomen and face being relatively spared; accentuated marking and creases on the palms and soles; and, possibly, atopy. Called also *i. simplex.*
**X-linked i.,** a chronic form of ichthyosis affecting males, transmitted as an X-linked recessive trait and due to deficiency of the microsomal enzyme steryl-sulfatase; it may be present at birth or appear in early infancy. It is characterized by the presence of prominent, very adherent scales, often brown, especially on the neck, extremities, trunk, and buttocks. Corneal opacities that do not interfere with vision are a frequent associated finding; these may occur in minor form in heterozygotic female carriers.

**ich·thy·ot·ic** (ik″the-ot′ik) pertaining to or characterized by ichthyosis.

**ich·thyo·tox·ic** (ik″the-o-tok′sik) caused by the toxic principle of fish.

**ich·thyo·tox·i·col·o·gy** (ik″the-o-tok″sĭ-kol′o-je) [*ichthyo-* + *toxico-* + *-logy*] the science of poisons derived from certain fish, their cause, detection, and effects, and the treatment of conditions produced by them.

**ich·thyo·tox·in** (ik″the-o-tok′sin) [*ichthyo-* + *toxin*] a general term applied to any type of toxic substance derived from fish.

**ich·thyo·tox·ism** (ik″the-o-tok′siz-əm) [*ichthyo-* + *toxin* + *-ism*] a general term applied to intoxication caused by any toxic substance derived from fish.

**ick** (ik) white spot disease, def. 3.

**ICN** International Council of Nurses.

**icon** (i′kon) [Gr. *eikōn* likeness, image] 1. an image, model, or representation. 2. a brief sensory image in the mind, often pictorial, which may or may not become part of short-term memory.

**ico·sa·he·dral** (i″ko-sə-he′drəl) [Gr. *eikosi* twenty + *hedra* seat] pertaining to an icosahedron, a solid having 20 faces and 12 vertices.

**ico·sa·no·ic ac·id** (i″ko-sə-no′ik) arachidic acid.

**ICP** intracranial pressure.

**ICRP** International Commission on Radiological Protection.

**ICRU** International Commission on Radiological Units and Measurements.

**ICS** International College of Surgeons.

**ICSH** interstitial cell–stimulating hormone (luteinizing hormone).

**ICSI** intracytoplasmic sperm injection.

**ICT** insulin coma therapy.

**ic·tal** (ik′təl) [L. *ictus* stroke] pertaining to, characterized by, or caused by a stroke or an acute epileptic seizure.

**ic·ter·ic** (ik-ter′ik) pertaining to or affected with jaundice.

**ic·ter·i·tious** (ik″tər-ish′əs) icteric.

**icter(o)-** [L. *icterus,* q.v.] a combining form meaning affected with or pertaining to jaundice.

**ic·tero·ane·mia** (ik″tər-o-əne′me-ə) anemia with jaundice.

**ic·tero·gen·ic** (ik″tər-o-jen′ik) [*ictero-* + *-genic*] causing icterus.

**ic·tero·ge·nic·i·ty** (ik″tər-o-jə-nis′ĭ-te) ability to cause icterus.

**ic·tero·hem·a·tu·ria** (ik″tər-o-hem″ə-tu′re-ə) jaundice associated with hematuria.

**ic·tero·hem·a·tu·ric** (ik″tər-o-hem″ə-tu′rik) pertaining to icterohematuria; marked by jaundice and hematuria.

**ic·tero·he·mo·glob·in·uria** (ik″tər-o-he″mo-glo″bĭ-nu′re-ə) combined jaundice and hemoglobinuria.

**ic·tero·hep·a·ti·tis** (ik″tər-o-hep″ə-ti′tis) inflammation of the liver with marked jaundice.

**ic·ter·oid** (ik′tər-oid) [*ictero-* + *-oid*] resembling jaundice.

**ic·ter·us** (ik′tər-əs) [L.; Gr. *ikteros*] jaundice.
**chronic familial i., congenital familial i., congenital hemolytic i.,** hereditary spherocytosis.
**i. gra′vis neonato′rum,** severe jaundice in the newborn, usually a form of isoimmunization with Rh factor; called also *erythroleukoblastosis.* See also *kernicterus.*
**i. neonato′rum,** the jaundice sometimes seen in newborn children; called also *neonatal jaundice* and *jaundice of the newborn.*
**nuclear i.,** kernicterus.
**i. prae′ cox,** mild jaundice developing within the first 24 hours of life (before physiologic jaundice normally occurs), due to incompatibility of the ABO blood group system between mother and infant; it usually clears rapidly and spontaneously, only occasionally resulting in hemolytic disease.

**ic·tus** (ik′təs) pl. *ic′tus* [L. "stroke"] a seizure, stroke, blow, or sudden attack.
**i. epilep′ticus,** seizure (def. 2).
**i. paraly′ticus,** paralytic stroke.
**i. san′guinis,** stroke syndrome.
**i. so′lis,** sunstroke.

**ICU** intensive care unit.

**ID** intradermal; inside diameter.

**$ID_{50}$** median infective dose.

**Id.** abbreviation for L. *i′dem,* the same.

**id** (id) [L. *id,* it Ger. *es*] [MeSH: Id] in psychoanalytic theory, the innate, totally unconscious, primitive aspect of the personality dominated by the pleasure principle and harboring instinctive impulses that seek immediate personal pleasure, gratification, or satisfaction. Cf. *ego* and *superego.*

**-id** [Gr. *eidos* form, shape] a word termination denoting (1) having the shape of, or resembling or (2) an id reaction associated with the disorder specified by the root word.

**IDA** iminodiacetic acid.

**-idae** [Gr. *-idai,* pl. of *-ides* patronymic ending] in zoology, a word termination denoting a family.

**Ida·my·cin** (i″də-mi′sin) trademark for a preparation of idarubicin hydrochloride.

**ida·ru·bi·cin hy·dro·chlo·ride** (i″də-roo′bĭ-sin) [USP] an anthracycline antineoplastic used in the treatment of acute myelogenous leukemia; administered intravenously.

**IDD** insulin-dependent diabetes; see *type 1 diabetes,* under *diabetes.*

**-ide** a suffix signifying a binary chemical compound, such as a chloride, sulfide, or carbide.

**idea** (i-de′ə) [Gr. "form"] an impression, thought, or conception resulting from mental activity.
**autochthonous i.,** a persistent idea originating within the mind, usually from the unconscious, but seeming to have come from an outside source and often therefore felt to be of malevolent origin.
**dominant i.,** one that controls or colors every action and thought.
**fixed i.,** a morbid impression or belief which stays in the mind and cannot be changed by reason; called also *idée fixe.*
**overvalued i.,** a false or exaggerated belief sustained beyond reason or logic but with less rigidity than a delusion, also often being less patently unbelievable.
**i. of reference, referential i.,** the assumption by a patient that the

words and actions of others refer to himself or the projection of the causes of his own imaginary difficulties upon someone else; if frequent or intense, or if organized and systematized, called *delusion of reference.*

**ide·al** (i-de'əl) 1. having some relation to ideas, impressions, or imaginations. 2. a standard of perfection.
**ego i.,** the component of the superego comprising the internalized image of what one desires to become and toward the attainment of which the ego strives, formed through conscious or unconscious identification with or emulation of one who plays a significant role or has a place of esteem in the life of the developing child.

**ide·al·iza·tion** (i-de"əl-ĭ-za'shən) a conscious or unconscious mental mechanism in which the individual overestimates an admired aspect or attribute of another person.

**ide·a·tion** (i"de-a'shən) the formation of a mental concept, image, or thought.
**paranoid i.,** the persistent idea, not of delusional intensity, that one is being persecuted, harassed, or otherwise unfairly treated.

**ide·a·tion·al** (i"de-a'shən-əl) relating to or characterized by ideation.

**idée** (e-da') [Fr.] idea.
**i. fixe** (fēks), fixed idea.

**iden·ti·fi·ca·tion** (i-den"tĭ-fi-ka'shən) a largely unconscious process by which a person patterns himself after one or more other people, associating closely with them and assuming their viewpoints; sometimes used as a defense mechanism.
**cosmic i.,** identification of one's self with the universe, as in schizophrenic delusions of omnipotence.
**projective i.,** an unconscious defense mechanism in which unacceptable aspects of the self are falsely attributed to others; it differs from projection in that the target is transformed, unconsciously identifying and responding, and the aspects that are projected are not completely disavowed but rather are perceived as justifiable reactions to the other person's induced responses.

**iden·ti·ty** (i-den'tĭ-te) the aggregate of characteristics by which an individual is recognized by himself and others.
**core gender i.,** gender i.
**ego i.,** a sense of unity and continuity of oneself.
**gender i.,** a person's concept of himself as being male and masculine or female and feminine, or ambivalent, usually based on physical characteristics, parental attitudes and expectations, and psychological and social pressures. It is the private experience of gender role. Cf. *gender role,* under *role.*

**ideo·ge·net·ic** (i"de-o-jə-net'ik) related to mental processes in which images of sense impressions are used, rather than ideas that are ready for verbal expression.

**ideo·ki·net·ic** (i-de"o-ki-net'ik) ideomotor.

**ide·ol·o·gy** (i"de-ol'ə-je, id"e-ol'ə-je) [Gr. *idea* + *-logy*] 1. the science of the development of ideas. 2. the body of ideas characteristic of an individual or of a social unit.

**ideo·mo·tion** (i"de-o-mo'shən) motion or muscular action which is neither reflex nor volitional, but is induced by some dominant idea.

**ideo·mo·tor** (i"de-o-mo'tər) aroused by an idea or thought; said of involuntary motion so aroused.

**idi(o)-** [Gr. *idios* one's own, separate] a combining form meaning one's own, separate, or self-produced.

**id·io·ag·glu·ti·nin** (id"e-o-ə-gloo'tĭ-nin) [*idio-* + *agglutinin*] an agglutinin that originates independently of any transfer or artificial means in the animal in which it is formed.

**id·io·chro·mo·some** (id"e-o-kro'mə-sōm) any sex chromosome.

**id·i·o·cy** (id'e-ə-se) obsolete, offensive term for *profound mental retardation.*
**amaurotic i., amaurotic familial i.,** former name for *neuronal ceroid lipofuscinosis.*
**cretinoid i.,** former name for cretinism.
**microcephalic i.,** former term for profound mental retardation associated with microcephaly.
**mongolian i.,** a name formerly applied to the marked mental retardation associated with *Down syndrome* or to the syndrome itself; now considered offensive.
**moral i.,** *(obs.)* see under *insanity.*
**xerodermic i.,** former name for *De Sanctis-Cacchione syndrome.*

**id·io·gen·e·sis** (id"e-o-jen'ə-sis) [*idio-* + *-genesis*] the origin of disease without a known cause, as in an idiopathic disease.

**id·io·glos·sia** (id"e-o-glos'e-ə) [*idio-* + *gloss-* + *-ia*] extremely defective imperfect articulation, with the utterance of vocal sounds that are virtually unintelligible. Called also *idiolalia.*

**id·io·glot·tic** (id"e-o-glot'ik) pertaining to idioglossia.

**id·io·gram** (id'e-o-gram") [*idio-* + *-gram*] a diagrammatic representation of a chromosome complement, based on measurement of the chromosomes of a number of cells. Cf. *karyotype.*

**id·io·het·ero·ag·glu·ti·nin** (id"e-o-het"ər-o-ə-gloo'tĭ-nin) [*idio-* + *heteroagglutinin*] a heteroagglutinin normally present in the blood.

**id·io·het·er·ol·y·sin** (id"e-o-het"ər-ol'ə-sin) a heterolysin normally present in the blood.

**id·io·hyp·no·tism** (id"e-o-hip'no-tiz-əm) [*idio-* + *hypnotism*] spontaneous or self-induced hypnotism.

**id·io·iso·ag·glu·ti·nin** (id"e-o-i"so-ə-gloo'tĭ-nin) an isoagglutinin normally present in the blood, and not produced by artificial means.

**id·io·isol·y·sin** (id"e-o-i-sol'ə-sin) a lysin normally present which lyses the cells of other members of the same species as the animal in which it is formed.

**id·io·la·lia** (id"e-o-la'le-ə) idioglossia.

**id·i·ol·y·sin** (id"e-ol'ə-sin) [*idio-* + *lysin*] a lysin, normally present in the blood and not produced by artificial means, that lyses the cells of the animal in which it is formed.

**id·io·mere** (id'e-o-mēr) chromomere (def. 1).

**id·io·mus·cu·lar** (id"e-o-mus'ku-lər) [*idio-* + *muscular*] pertaining to the muscular tissue apart from any nerve stimulus; a term applied to certain muscular contractions which occur in degenerated muscles only.

**id·io·pa·thet·ic** (id"e-o-pə-thet'ik) idiopathic.

**id·io·path·ic** (id"e-o-path'ik) of unknown cause or spontaneous origin; of the nature of an idiopathy. Called also *agnogenic.*

**id·i·op·a·thy** (id"e-op'ə-the) [*idio-* + *-pathy*] a pathologic condition of unknown cause or spontaneous origin.

**id·io·re·flex** (id"e-o-re'fleks) [*idio-* + *reflex*] a reflex brought about by a cause within the same organ.

**id·io·ret·i·nal** (id"e-o-ret'ĭ-nəl) pertaining to the retina alone; a term applied to a visual sensation occurring without any visual stimulus.

**id·io·some** (id'e-o-sōm") [*idio-* + *-some*] the centrosome of a spermatocyte, together with surrounding Golgi apparatus and mitochondria.

**id·io·spasm** (id'e-o-spaz-əm) a spasm of a limited area or region.

**id·io·syn·cra·sy** (id"e-o-sin'krə-se) [*idio-* + Gr. *synkrasis* mixture] 1. a habit or quality of body or mind peculiar to any individual. 2. an abnormal susceptibility to some drug, protein, or other agent which is peculiar to the individual.

**id·io·syn·crat·ic** (id"e-o-sən-krat'ik) pertaining to or characterized by idiosyncrasy.

**id·i·ot** (id'e-ət) [Gr. *idiōtēs* a person not in public life, a nonexpert or layman] obsolete, offensive name for a person with profound mental retardation; see *mental retardation,* under *retardation.*
**mongolian i.,** former name for a person affected with Down syndrome; now considered offensive.
**i. savant** (e-dyo' sah-vahn') [Fr. "learned idiot"], a person who is severely mentally retarded in some respects, yet has a particular mental faculty that is developed to an unusually high degree, as memory, mathematics, or music.

**id·io·tope** (id'ĭ-o-tōp") idiotypic determinant; an antigenic determinant on a variable domain of an immunoglobulin molecule. Cf. *allotope.*

**id·io·topy** (id'e-o-top"e) [*idio-* + Gr. *topos* place] the position and relation of the parts of an organ among themselves.

**id·io·troph·ic** (id"e-o-trof'ik) [*idio-* + *-trophic*] capable of selecting its own nourishment.

**id·i·o·trop·ic** (id"e-o-trop'ik) [*idio-* + *-tropic*] introspective; egocentric.

**id·io·type** (id'e-o-tīp') a set of one or more idiotopes that distinguish a clone of immunoglobulin-producing cells from other clones. Idiotypes occur in the variable domains of immunoglobulin molecules and may be within, near to, or outside of the antigen-binding site; antibodies to idiotypes located within or near to the antigen-binding site will prevent the immunoglobulin from combining with antigen.

**id·io·typ·ic** (id"e-o-tip'ik) pertaining to idiotypes.

**id·io·var·i·a·tion** (id"e-o-var"e-a'shən) a mutation or change in the germ plasm, the cause of which is unknown.

**id·io·ven·tric·u·lar** (id"e-o-vən-trik'u-lər) relating to or affecting the cardiac ventricles alone, as idioventricular rhythm.

**idi·tol** (i'dĭ-tol) the alcohol formed by reduction of the aldehyde group of idose.

**L-idi·tol 2-de·hy·dro·ge·nase** (i'dĭ-tol de-hi'dro-jən-ās) [EC 1.1.1.14] an enzyme of the oxidoreductase class that catalyzes the oxidation of L-iditol to L-fructose, using $NAD^+$ as an electron acceptor; the enzyme also acts on some other sugar alcohols. The enzyme occurs in significant quantities only in the liver; increased activity in serum is used as an indicator of parenchymal liver damage. Called also *sorbitol dehydrogenase.*

**IDL** intermediate-density lipoprotein.

**idose** (i'dōs) an aldohexose; structurally, L-idose is an epimer of D-glucose.

**idox·ur·i·dine** (i-doks-ūr'ĭ-dēn) [USP] [MeSH: Idoxuridine] an analog of pyrimidine which inhibits viral DNA synthesis; used as an antiviral agent in the treatment of herpes simplex keratitis, applied topically to the conjunctiva. Abbreviated IDU.

**IDU** idoxuridine.

**iduron·ate** (i″du-ron'āt) a salt, ester, or anionic form of iduronic acid.

**idu·ron·ate-2-sul·fa·tase** (ĭ″du-ron'āt sul'fə-tās) [EC 3.1.6.13] a lysosomal enzyme of the hydrolase class that catalyzes the cleavage of sulfate groups from the L-iduronate residues of dermatan sulfate and heparan sulfate, a step in the degradation of these glycosaminoglycans. Deficiency of the enzyme, an X-linked recessive trait, results in Hunter's syndrome (mucopolysaccharidosis II ).

**idu·ron·ic ac·id** (i″du-ron'ik) [MeSH: Iduronic Acid] the uronic acid derived from idose; L- iduronic acid is an epimer of glucuronic acid and a constituent of dermatan sulfate, heparan sulfate, and heparin.

**L-idu·ron·i·dase** (ĭ″du-ron'ĭ-dās) [EC 3.2.1.76] an enzyme of the hydrolase class that catalyzes the hydrolysis of terminal desulfated α-L-iduronic acid residues of dermatan sulfate and heparan sulfate, a step in the degradation of these glycosaminoglycans. Deficiency of the enzyme, an autosomal recessive trait, leads to mucopolysaccharidosis I.

**IEP** immunoelectrophoresis.

**IF** intrinsic factor.

**IFA** immunofluorescence assay; see *fluorescence immunoassay,* under *immunoassay.*

**Ifex** (i'feks) trademark for a preparation of sterile ifosfamide.

**IFN** interferon.

**ifos·fa·mide** (i-fos'fə-mīd) [USP] [MeSH: Ifosfamide] a cytotoxic alkylating agent of the nitrogen mustard group, a structural analogue of and similar in action to cyclophosphamide; it is itself pharmacologically inert and must be activated by the microsomal enzyme system of the liver. Used in the treatment of solid tumors of the testis, ovary, and lung as well as sarcomas; administered intravenously.

**Ig** immunoglobulin. The five classes are designated IgM, IgG, IgA, IgD, IgE. Subclasses are designated by numerical suffixes, e.g., IgG1.

**IGF** insulin-like growth factor.

**ig·na·tia** (ig-na'she-ə) [L.] the poisonous dried ripe seed of *Strychnos ignatii;* it contains several alkaloids, the principal ones being strychnine and brucine, and has been used as a bitter tonic.

**ig·ni·punc·ture** (ig'nĭ-punk″chər) [*ignis* + *puncture*] therapeutic puncture with hot needles.

**ig·nis** (ig'nis) [L.] fire.
**i. inferna'lis,** ["infernal fire"], ergotism.

**ig·ni·sa·tion** (ig″nĭ-za'shən) [L. *ignis* fire] hyperthermia produced by exposure to artificial sources of heat.

**ig·no·tine** (ig'no-tēn) carnosine.

**IGT** impaired glucose tolerance.

**IH** infectious hepatitis.

**IHD** ischemic heart disease.

**IHS** Indian Health Service, an agency of the United States Public Health Service.

**IL** interleukin.

**il-** see *in-.*

**ILA** International Leprosy Association.

**Ile** isoleucine.

**il·e·ac** (il'e-ak) 1. of the nature of ileus. 2. pertaining to the ileum.

**ile·adel·phus** (il″e-ə-del'fəs) iliopagus.

**il·e·al** (il'e-əl) pertaining to the ileum.

**ile·ec·to·my** (il″e-ek'tə-me) [*ile-* + *-ectomy*] surgical removal of the ileum.

**il·e·itis** (il″e-i'tis) [MeSH: Ileitis] inflammation of the ileum.
**distal i.,** regional i.
**regional i., terminal i.,** Crohn's disease affecting the ileum.

**ile(o)-** [L. *ileum*] a combining form denoting relationship to the ileum.

**il·eo·ce·cal** (il″e-o-se'kəl) pertaining to the ileum and cecum.

**il·eo·ce·co·cys·to·plas·ty** (il″e-o-se″ko-sis'to-plas″te) cystoplasty in which a segment of ileum and cecum is used to reconstruct or augment the bladder.

**il·eo·ce·cos·to·my** (il″e-o-se-kos'tə-me) surgical creation of an opening between the ileum and the cecum; also, the opening so established.

**il·eo·ce·cum** (il″e-o-se'kəm) the ileum and cecum considered as one organ.

**il·eo·col·ic** (il″e-o-kol'ik) pertaining to the ileum and colon.

**il·eo·co·li·tis** (il″e-o-ko-li'tis) inflammation of the ileum and colon.
**tuberculous i.,** tuberculous inflammation of the ileum and colon.
**i. ulcero'sa chro'nica,** a chronic form characterized by fever, rapid pulse, anemia, diarrhea, and right iliac pain.

**il·eo·co·lon·ic** (il″e-o-ko-lon'ik) ileocolic.

**il·eo·co·los·to·my** (il″e-o-ko-los'tə-me) [*ileo-* + *colo-* + *-stomy*] surgical creation of an opening between the ileum and colon; also, the opening so established.

**il·eo·co·lot·o·my** (il″e-o-ko-lot'ə-me) [*ileo-* + *colo-* + *-tomy*] surgical incision of the ileum and colon.

**il·eo·cys·to·plas·ty** (il″e-o-sis'to-plas″te) [*ileo-* + *cystoplasty*] cystoplasty incorporating an isolated loop of the ileum as part of the bladder wall.

**il·eo·cys·tos·to·my** (il″e-o-sis-tos'tə-me) surgical creation of an opening between the urinary bladder and ileum.

**il·eo·ile·os·to·my** (il″e-o-il″e-os'tə-me) [*ileo-* + *ileo-* + *-stomy*] surgical creation of an opening between two parts of the ileum; also, the opening so established.

**il·eo·proc·tos·to·my** (il″e-o-prok-tos'tə-me) [*ileo-* + *procto-* + *-stomy*] anastomosis of the ileum and rectum.

**il·eo·rec·tal** (il″e-o-rek'təl) pertaining to or communicating with the ileum and rectum, as an ileorectal fistula.

**il·eo·rec·tos·to·my** (il″e-o-rek-tos'tə-me) ileoproctostomy.

**il·e·or·rha·phy** (il″e-or'ə-fe) [*ileo-* + *-rrhaphy*] operative repair of the ileum.

**il·eo·sig·moid** (il″e-o-sig'moid) pertaining to the ileum and the sigmoid.

**il·eo·sig·moi·dos·to·my** (il″e-o-sig″moi-dos'tə-me) [*ileo-* + *sigmoidostomy*] 1. surgical creation of an opening between the ileum and the sigmoid colon. 2. the opening created by such a procedure.

**il·e·os·to·my** (il″e-os'tə-me) [*ileo-* + *-stomy*] [MeSH: Ileostomy] surgical creation of an opening into the ileum, usually by establishing an ileal stoma on the abdominal wall.
**continent i.,** an ileostomy that maintains continence of feces, usually through construction of a continent ileal reservoir; now largely replaced by ileoanal anastomosis procedures.
**Kock i.,** the most common type of continent i., having a Kock pouch; now mostly of historic interest.

**il·e·ot·o·my** (il″e-ot'ə-me) [*ileo-* + *-tomy*] incision of the ileum.

**il·eo·trans·vers·os·to·my** (il″e-o-trans″vərs-os'tə-me) surgical creation of an opening between the ileum and the transverse colon.

**Il·e·tin** (il'ə-tin) trademark for preparations of insulin.
**Lente I.,** trademark for preparations of insulin zinc suspension.
**NPH I.,** trademark for preparations of insulin isophane suspension.
**Protamine, Zinc & I.,** trademark for preparations of protamine zinc insulin suspension.
**Regular I.,** trademark for preparations of insulin injection (regular insulin).
**Semilente I.,** trademark for preparations of prompt insulin zinc suspension.
**Ultralente I.,** trademark for preparations of extended zinc insulin suspension.

**il·e·um** (il'e-əm) [L.] [MeSH: Ileum] the distal portion of the small intestine, extending from the jejunum to the cecum; called also *intestinum ileum.*
**duplex i.,** congenital duplication of the ileum.

**il·e·us** (il'e-əs) [L.; Gr. *eileos,* from *eilein* to roll up] obstruction of the intestines.
**adynamic i.,** ileus resulting from inhibition of bowel motility, which may be produced by numerous causes, most frequently by peritonitis.

**dynamic i., hyperdynamic i.,** spastic i.
**mechanical i.,** ileus due to mechanical causes, such as hernia, adhesions, volvulus, etc.
**meconium i.,** ileus in the newborn due to blocking of the bowel with thick meconium; a manifestation of fibrocystic disease (mucoviscidosis).
**occlusive i.,** mechanical i.
**paralytic i., i. paraly'ticus,** adynamic i.
**spastic i.,** ileus due to persistent contracture of a bowel segment; see also *Ogilvie's syndrome,* under *syndrome.*
**i. subpar'ta,** ileus due to pressure of the gravid uterus on the pelvic colon.

**Ilex** (i'leks) the hollies, a genus of small trees and shrubs of the family Aquifoliaceae. *I. paraguayen'sis* St. Hil. is a South American species whose leaves are the herb maté (q.v.). *I. verticilla'ta* L. Gray, the black alder or winterberry, has a tonic and astringent bark.

**Il·he·us encephalitis, virus** (ēl-ya'o͞os) [*Ilheus,* Brazil, where the disease was first observed in 1944] see under *encephalitis* and *virus.*

**il·ia** (il'e-ə) [L.] plural of *ilium.*

**il·i·ac** (il'e-ak) [L. *iliacus*] pertaining to the ilium.

**ili·adel·phus** (il″e-ə-del'fəs) iliopagus.

**Il·i·dar** (il'ĭ-dahr) trademark for a preparation of azapetine phosphate.

**ili(o)-** [L. *ilium*] a combining form denoting relationship to the ilium or iliac region.

**il·io·coc·cyg·e·al** (il″e-o-kok-sij'e-əl) pertaining to the ilium and coccyx.

**ilio·coc·cy·ge·us** (il″e-o-kok-sij'e-us) [L., from *ilio-* + *coccygeus*] iliococcygeal; see under *musculus.*

**il·io·cos·tal** (il″e-o-kos'təl) [*ilio-* + *costal*] connecting or pertaining to the ilium and ribs.

**il·io·fem·or·al** (il″e-o-fem'or-əl) 1. pertaining to the ilium and femur. 2. pertaining to or connecting the iliac and femoral arteries.

**il·io·hy·po·gas·tric** (il″e-o-hi″po-gas'trik) pertaining to the ilium and hypogastrium.

**il·io·in·gui·nal** (il″e-o-in'gwĭ-nəl) pertaining to the iliac and inguinal regions.

**il·io·lum·bar** (il″e-o-lum'bər) pertaining to the iliac and lumbar regions, or to the flank and loin.

**il·io·lum·bo·cos·to·ab·dom·i·nal** (il″e-o-lum″bo-kos″to-ab-dom'ĭ-nəl) pertaining to the iliac, lumbar, costal, and abdominal regions.

**il·i·om·e·ter** (il″e-om'ə-tər) [*ilio-* + *-meter*] an instrument for determining the relative heights of the iliac spines and their relative distance from the center of the spinal column.

**il·i·op·a·gus** (il″e-op'ə-gəs) [*ilio-* + *-pagus*] symmetrical conjoined twins united in the iliac region.

**il·io·pec·tin·e·al** (il″e-o-pek-tin'e-al) pertaining to the ilium and pubic bone.

**il·io·pel·vic** (il″e-o-pel'vik) pertaining to the iliac region or muscle and to the pelvis.

**il·io·pso·as** (il″e-o-so'əs) see under *musculus.*

**il·io·pu·bic** (il″e-o-pu'bik) iliopectineal.

**il·io·sa·cral** (il″e-o-sa'krəl) pertaining to the ilium and the sacrum.

**il·io·sci·at·ic** (il″e-o-si-at'ik) pertaining to the ilium and the ischium.

**il·io·spi·nal** (il″e-o-spi'nəl) pertaining to the ilium and the spinal column.

**il·io·tho·ra·cop·a·gus** (il″e-o-thor″ə-kop'ə-gəs) [*ilio-* + *thoraco-* + *-pagus*] symmetrical conjoined twins fused from the pelvis to the thorax.

**il·io·tib·i·al** (il″e-o-tib'e-əl) pertaining to or extending between the ilium and tibia.

**il·io·tro·chan·ter·ic** (il″e-o-tro-kan-ter'ik) pertaining to the ilium and a trochanter.

**il·io·xi·phop·a·gus** (il″e-o-zi-fop'ə-gəs) symmetrical conjoined twins fused from the pelvis to the xiphoid process.

**il·i·um** (il'e-əm) pl. *il'ia* [L.] [MeSH: Ilium] TA alternative for *os ilium.*

**ill** (il) 1. not well; sick. 2. a disease or disorder.
**föhn i.,** headache, weariness, and depression felt during the föhn (a wind from the south in Central Europe).
**joint i.,** navel i.
**louping i.,** encephalomyelitis primarily affecting sheep in Great Britain and Ireland, caused by a flavivirus which is transmitted by the tick, *Ixodes ricinus.*
**navel i.,** generalized septicemia affecting foals, lambs, and calves, usually characterized by omphalophlebitis and the formation of abscesses in the joints resulting in polyarthritis; it is due to infection through the open navel by various organisms, including species of *Staphylococcus, Streptococcus, Shigella, Escherichia,* and *Pasteurella,* and has a high mortality rate. Called also *joint i.*
**quarter i.,** blackleg.

**il·lac·ri·ma·tion** (ĭ-lak″rĭ'ma'shən) epiphora.

**il·laq·ue·a·tion** (ĭ-lak″we-a'shən) [L. *illaqueare* to ensnare] the cure of an ingrowing eyelash by drawing it out with a loop.

**Il·lic·i·um** (ĭ-lis'e-əm) [L.] a genus of trees and shrubs of the family Magnoliaceae. *I. ve'rum* is an Asian tree whose fruit is Chinese or Indian anise (see under *anise*). *I. religio'sum* is the star anise or sikimi, a Japanese species whose leaves are poisonous, containing sikimin.

**il·li·ni·tion** (il″ĭ-nish'ən) [L. *illinire* to smear] the application of an ointment or liniment with rubbing.

**ill·ness** (il'nəs) disease.
**compressed-air i.,** decompression sickness.
**emotional i.,** a colloquialism roughly equivalent to "mental disorder," but not usually applied to those with a specific organic etiology or to mental retardation.
**manic-depressive i.,** older term for bipolar disorder; see *bipolar disorders* (def. 2), under *disorder.*
**mental i.,** see under *disorder.*
**psychosomatic i.,** see under *disorder.*
**radiation i.,** see under *sickness.*

**ill thrift** (il thrift) unthriftiness.

**il·lu·mi·na·tion** (ĭ-loo″mĭ-na'shən) [L. *illuminatio*] 1. the lighting up of a part, cavity, organ, or object for inspection. 2. the luminous flux per unit area of a given surface; its unit is the lux, the phot, or the foot-candle. Symbol *E.*
**axial i.,** the transmission or reflection of light along the axis of a microscope.
**central i.,** axial i.
**contact i.,** illumination of the eye by means of an instrument which is pressed directly to the cornea and conjunctiva.
**critical i.,** the focusing of light precisely upon an object inspected.
**darkfield i., dark-ground i.,** the throwing of peripheral rays of light upon a microscopical object from the side, the center rays being blocked out: the object appears bright upon a dark background. See under *microscope,* and see *ultramicroscope.*
**direct i.,** the throwing of light upon a microscopical object from above or from the direction of observation.
**focal i.,** 1. the throwing of light upon the focus of a lens or mirror. 2. illumination of an object by focusing a source of light on it through an optical system.
**Köhler i.,** an improved method of illumination by adjustment of the substage Abbe condenser, for obtaining the best image detail in microscopical work.
**lateral i., oblique i.,** illumination in which the object is illuminated by oblique light.
**through i.,** the transmission of light through an object, or from the direction opposite to that of observation.

**il·lu·mi·na·tor** (ĭ-loo″mĭ-na'tor) the source of light for viewing an object.
**Abbe's i.,** see under *condenser.*

**il·lu·min·ism** (ĭ-loo'min-iz-əm) a hallucinatory state characterized by conversations with imaginary, usually supernatural, beings.

**il·lu·sion** (ĭ-loo'zhən) [L. *illusio*] [MeSH: Illusions] a false or misinterpreted sensory impression; a false interpretation of a real sensory image. Cf. *delusion.*

**il·lu·sion·al** (ĭ-loo'zhən-əl) pertaining to or characterized by illusions.

**Il·o·pan** (il'o-pan) trademark for a preparation of dexpanthenol.

**Il·o·sone** (il'o-sōn) trademark for a preparation of erythromycin estolate.

**Ilo·ty·cin** (i″lo-ti'sin) trademark for preparations of erythromycin.

**Il·o·zyme** (il'o-zīm) trademark for a preparation of pancrelipase.

**ILT** infectious laryngotracheitis.

**IM** intramuscularly (by intramuscular injection).

**im-**[1] see *in-.*

**im-**[2] a prefix in chemical names indicating the bivalent group =NH.

**ima** (i'mə) [L.] lowest.

**im·age** (im'əj) [L. *imago*] a picture or conception with more or less likeness to an objective reality. See also *imaging.*
**accidental i.,** afterimage.
**body i.,** a three-dimensional concept of one's self, recorded in the

cortex by the perception of ever-changing postures of the body and constantly changing with them.
**direct i., erect i.,** virtual i.
**eidetic i.,** an unusually vivid, elaborate, and exact mental image of objects previously seen or imagined.
**false i.,** the one formed by the deviating eye in strabismus.
**heteronymous i.,** the two images seen when the eyes are focused on a point beyond the object; cf. *crossed diplopia.*
**homonymous i.,** the two images seen when the eyes are focused on a point nearer than the object; cf. *direct diplopia.*
**incidental i.,** the impression of an image which remains on the retina after the object has been removed.
**inverted i.,** real i.
**memory i.,** a sensation or sense perception as it is pictured in the memory.
**mental i.,** any concept corresponding to an object appreciated by the senses.
**mirror i.,** 1. the image of light made visible by the reflecting surface of the cornea and lens when illuminated through the slit lamp. 2. an identical reproduction of an object except for transposition of right and left relations, as appears in the reflection of an object in a mirror.
**motor i.,** the organized cerebral model of the possible movements of the body.
**negative i.,** afterimage.
**optical i.,** one formed by the reflection of refraction of rays of light.
**Purkinje-Sanson mirror i's,** reflected images formed on the anterior surface of the cornea and the anterior and posterior surfaces of the crystalline lens. The images on the two anterior surfaces are virtual and noninverted, and the image on the posterior surface is real and inverted. Useful in the study of the movement of the lens surfaces in accommodation and, formerly, in the evaluation of cataract.
**radioisotope i.,** a quasi-pictorial representation of the distribution of radioactive materials in the body.
**real i.,** one formed where the emanating rays are collected, in which the object is pictured as being inverted.
**retinal i.,** the representation formed upon the retina of an object seen.
**Sanson's i's,** Purkinje-Sanson mirror i's.
**sensory i.,** a representation formed by means of one or more of the sense organs.
**specular i.,** mirror i., def. 1.
**virtual i.,** a picture from projected light rays that are intercepted before focusing, as by a plane mirror; it cannot be received on a screen, and it has the same orientation as the object. Called also *direct* or *erect i.*

**Im·a·gent GI** (im'a-jənt) trademark for a preparation of perflubron.

**imag·i·nes** (ĭ-maj'ĭ-nēz) [L.] plural of *imago.*

**imag·ing** (im'ə-jing) the production of clarity, contrast, and detail in images, especially in radiological and ultrasound images.
**color flow Doppler i.,** a method for visualizing direction and velocity of movement, such as of blood flow within the cardiac chambers or blood vessels: color coded flow direction and velocity information gathered by Doppler ultrasonography at multiple sites across the imaging field are superimposed onto a black and white cross-sectional image. Direction and velocity are coded as colors and shades, respectively, and used to produce color maps depicting blood flow.
**echo planar i.,** a technique for obtaining a magnetic resonance image in less than 50 msec; a single radiofrequency pulse is recalled several times in a series of echoes that are each encoded differently and from which the image can be reconstructed.
**electrostatic i.,** a method of visualizing deep structures of the body, in which an electron beam, rather than x-rays, is passed through the patient and the emerging beam (unabsorbed electrons) strikes an electrostatically charged vacuum-packed plate, dissipating the charge according to the strength of the beam. A record (e.g., a film) is then made from the plate.
**gated cardiac blood pool i.,** equilibrium radionuclide angiocardiography.
**hot spot i.,** infarct avid scintigraphy.
**infarct avid i.,** see under *scintigraphy.*
**magnetic resonance i. (MRI),** a method of visualizing soft tissues of the body by applying an external magnetic field that makes it possible to distinguish between hydrogen atoms in different environments. This is an application of the principle of nuclear magnetic resonance (q.v.).
**magnetic resonance i., gated,** a method for magnetic resonance imaging in which motion or other artifacts are minimized by gating signal acquisition, such as by linking sampling to electrocardiographic information in cardiac studies.
**myocardial perfusion i.,** see under *scintigraphy.*
**pyrophosphate i.,** infarct avid scintigraphy.
**technetium Tc 99m pyrophosphate i.,** 1. infarct avid scintigraphy. 2. any type of imaging in which technetium Tc 99m pyrophosphate is the imaging agent.
**thallium i.,** see *thallium-201 myocardial perfusion scintigraphy,* under *scintigraphy* and *thallium stress test,* under *tests.*

**ima·go** (ĭ-ma'go) pl. *ima'goes,* or *imag'ines* [L.] 1. the final or adult stage of an insect. Cf. *larva, pupa.* 2. in psychoanalytic theory, a usually idealized, unconscious mental image of a key person in one's early life.

**ima·go·cide** (ĭ-ma'go-sīd) [*imago* + *-cide*] an agent that destroys adult insects, especially adult mosquitoes.

**im·a·pun·ga** (im-ə-pung'ə) a rare disease of African cattle, closely related in pathology to African horse sickness.

**im·bal·ance** (im-bal'əns) 1. dysequilibrium (def. 2). 2. inability to stand upright; lack of balance between muscles.
**autonomic i.,** autonomic ataxia; any disturbance of the autonomic nervous system.
**binocular i.,** inequality in some aspect of binocular vision, such as aniseikonia, anisometropia, heterophoria, or strabismus.
**sympathetic i.,** vagotonia.
**vasomotor i.,** autonomic i.

**im·be·cile** (im'bə-sil) [L. *imbecillus* weak, feeble] obsolete and offensive name for a person with an intermediate level of mental retardation, now split into *moderate* and *severe* mental retardation; see *mental retardation,* under *retardation.*

**im·be·cil·i·ty** (im"bə-sil'ĭ-te) obsolete, offensive term for moderate to severe mental retardation; see *mental retardation,* under *retardation.*
**moral i.,** *(obs.)* see under *insanity.*

**im·bed** (im-bed') embed; see *embedding.*

**im·bi·bi·tion** (im"bĭ-bish'ən) [L. *imbibere* to drink] 1. the absorption of a liquid. 2. insudation.

**im·bri·cat·ed** (im'brĭ-kāt"əd) [L. *imbricatus; imbrex* tile] overlapping like tiles or shingles.

**im·bri·ca·tion** (im"brĭ-ka'shən) the overlapping of apposing surfaces, like shingles on a roof.

**$ImD_{50}$** median immunizing dose.

**Imers·lund syndrome** (e'mər-slund) [Olga *Imerslund,* Norwegian physician, 20th century] see under *syndrome.*

**Imers·lund-Graes·beck syndrome** (e'mər-slund grās'bek) [Olga *Imerslund;* Ralph Gustav *Graesbeck,* Finnish biochemist, born 1930] see under *syndrome.*

**I-Meth·a·sone** (i-meth'ə-sōn") trademark for preparations of dexamethasone sodium phosphate.

**Im·fer·on** (im'fer-on) trademark for a preparation of iron dextran injection.

**Im·hoff tank** (im'hof) [Karl *Imhoff,* German engineer, 1876–1965] digestion tank; see under *tank.*

**im·id·amine** (im"id-am'in) antazoline.

**im·id·az·ole** (im"id-az'ōl) 1. a base, found combined with alanine in histidine.

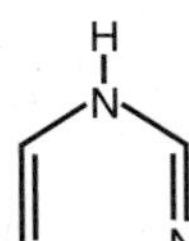


2. It is an antimetabolite and inhibitor of histamine and is used as an insecticide. 3. any of a class of imidazole-containing fungistatic compounds, effective against a wide range of fungi, which alter cell membrane permeability by inhibiting the biosynthesis of ergosterol.

**im·id·azo·lyl·eth·yl·amine** (im"id-az"o-ləl-eth"əl-am'in) histamine.

**im·ide** (im'id) any compound containing the bivalent group =NH, to which are attached only acid radicals.

**imido-** a prefix denoting the presence in a compound of the bivalent group =NH attached to two acid radicals.

**imid·o·carb hy·dro·chlo·ride** (im'ĭ-do-kahrb) a veterinary antiprotozoal used against *Babesia.*

**imi·do·di·pep·tide** (im"ĭ-do-di-pep'tīd) a dipeptide in which the C-terminal amino acid is an imino acid. Cf. *iminodipeptide.*

**imi·do·di·pep·ti·du·ria** (im"ĭ-do-di-pep"tĭ-du're-ə) excretion of imidodipeptides in the urine.

**imi·do·gen** (ĭ-mid'o-jən) the bivalent radical =NH.

**im·i·glu·cer·ase** (im"ĭgloo'sər-ās) an analogue of glucosylceramidase produced by recombinant DNA technology, used as an enzyme replenisher to replace glucosylceramidase (glucocerebrosidase) in type 1 Gaucher's disease; administered by intravenous infusion.

**im·in·az·ole** (im″in-az′ōl) imidazole.

**imine** (ĭ-mēn′) an organic compound containing an imino group; in a *substituted imine,* a nonacyl group replaces the imino hydrogen.

**imino-** a prefix used to denote the presence of the bivalent group =NH attached to nonacid radicals.

**im·i·no ac·id** (im′ə-no) an organic acid containing the bivalent group =NH, such as proline or hydroxyproline.

**imi·no·di·ace·tic ac·id** (im″ĭ-no-di″ə-se′tik) IDA; a simple dicarboxylic acid containing an imino group; radiolabeled ($^{99m}$Tc) analogues of iminodiacetic acid are used in hepatobiliary imaging.

**im·i·no·di·pep·tide** (im″ĭ-no-di-pep′tīd) a dipeptide in which the N-terminal amino acid is an imino acid. Cf. *imidodipeptide.*

**im·i·no·gly·cin·uria** (im″ĭ-no-gli″sin-u′re-ə) a benign hereditary disorder of renal tubular reabsorption of glycine and imino acids (proline and hydroxyproline), marked by excessive levels of all three substances in the urine.

**im·i·no·stil·bene** (im″ĭ-no-stil′bēn) a tricyclic tertiary amine similar in ring structure to the tricyclic antidepressants; the term is used to describe a class of anticonvulsants with such a structure that are employed in the treatment of epilepsy, e.g., carbamazepine.

**imi·no·urea** (im″ĭ-no-u′re-ə) guanidine.

**im·i·pen·em** (im″ĭ-pen′əm) [USP] [MeSH: Imipenem] a broad spectrum beta-lactam antibacterial derived from thienamycin with activity against a wide range of gram-positive and gram-negative organisms. Because it is hydrolyzed by a dipeptidase occurring in the proximal renal tubule, it is administered with the dipeptidase inhibitor cilastatin.

**imip·ra·mine** (im-ip′rə-mēn) [MeSH: Imipramine] a tricyclic antidepressant of the dibenzazepine class, the first of the tricyclic antidepressants to be used.
**i. hydrochloride** [USP], the monohydrochloride salt of imipramine, useful especially in endogenous depression; used also in the treatment of childhood enuresis, anxiety in panic syndrome, chronic pain, attention-deficit/hyperactivity disorder, cataplexy associated with narcolepsy, and bulimia.
**i. pamoate,** a tricyclic antidepressant with uses similar to those of imipramine hydrochloride, except that it is not used to treat enuresis.

**Im·i·trex** (im′ĭ-treks″) trademark for a preparation of sumatriptan succinate.

**Im·lach's fat plug** (im′laks) [Francis *Imlach,* Scottish physician, 1819–1891] see under *plug.*

**im·ma·ture** (im″ə-choor′) [*in-*[2] + *mature*] unripe or not fully developed.

**im·me·di·ate** (ĭ-me′de-ət) [*in-*[2] + *mediate*] direct; with nothing intervening; occurring without delay.

**im·med·i·ca·ble** (ĭ-med′ĭ-kə-bəl) beyond the hope of cure.

**im·mer·sion** (ĭ-mər′zhən) [L. *immersio*] [MeSH: Immersion] 1. the placing or plunging of a body into a liquid. 2. the use of the microscope with the object and object glass both covered with a liquid.
**homogeneous i.,** the employment in microscopy of a liquid of nearly the same refractive power as the cover glass.
**oil i.,** the covering of the microscopical objective and the object with oil.
**water i.,** the covering of the microscopical objective and the object with water.

**im·mis·ci·ble** (ĭ-mis′ĭ-bəl) not susceptible to being mixed.

**im·mit·tance** (ĭ-mit′əns) [*im*pedance + ad*mittance*] a term coined to express the effect of both admittance and impedance.
**acoustic i.,** measurement of energy flow through the middle ear by assessing acoustic admittance, acoustic impedance, or both.

**im·mo·bil·i·ty** (ĭ″mo-bil′ĭ-te) the state of being immovable.

**im·mo·bil·iza·tion** (ĭ-mo″bil-ĭ-za′shən) [MeSH: Immobilization] the act of rendering immovable, as by a cast or splint.

**im·mo·bi·lize** (ĭ-mo′bil-īz) [*in-*[2] + *mobilis* movable] to render incapable of being moved, as by a cast or splint.

**im·mo·bi·liz·er** (ĭ-mo′bĭ-li″zər) an object or apparatus that immobilizes.
**sternal-occipital-mandibular i. (SOMI),** any of a variety of cervical orthoses that have two or three posts running between head plates and a jacket or corset; called also *SOMI orthosis.*

**im·mor·tal·iza·tion** (ĭ-mor″tə-lə-za′shən) the gaining of immunity to normal limitations on growth or life span, sometimes achieved by animal cells in vitro or by tumor cells; causes may be spontaneous mutation, exposure to chemical carcinogens, or viral infection.

**im·mune** (ĭ-mūn′) [L. *immunis* free, exempt] 1. protected against infectious disease by either specific or nonspecific mechanisms. 2. pertaining to the immune system and immune responses.

**im·mu·ni·ty** (ĭ-mu′nĭ-te) [L. *immunitas*] [MeSH: Immunity] the condition of being immune; the protection against infectious disease conferred either by the immune response generated by immunization or previous infection or by other nonimmunologic factors.
**acquired i.,** immunity involving the functioning of the immune system acquired by natural infection or vaccination (active immunity) or transfer of antibody or lymphocytes from an immune donor (passive immunity). Cf. *innate i.*
**active i.,** acquired immunity developing in response to antigenic stimulus. Cf. *passive i.*
**adoptive i.,** passive immunity of the cell-mediated type conferred by the administration of sensitized lymphocytes from an immune donor.
**antibacterial i.,** immunity against the action of bacteria, i.e., the ability to resist infection by bacteria.
**antitoxic i.,** immunity against toxins, attributable to the presence of specific antitoxin(s) in the immune individual.
**antiviral i.,** immunity against viruses.
**artificial i.,** acquired (active or passive) immunity produced by deliberate exposure to an antigen, as in vaccination.
**cell-mediated i. (CMI), cellular i.,** immunity mediated by T lymphocytes either through release of lymphokines or through exertion of direct cytotoxicity, transmissible by transfer of lymphocytes but not serum; it includes type IV hypersensitivity reactions, such as contact dermatitis, granulomatous disease, allograft rejection, graft-versus-host disease, and systemic responses to viral or microbial infections or to tumor cells. Called also *T cell–mediated i.* Cf. *humoral i.*
**community i.,** herd i.
**concomitant i.,** infection i.
**cross i.,** immunity produced by inoculation with an agent (e.g., a bacterium or virus) that is different from, but closely related to, the agent causing the disease.
**familial i.,** innate i.
**genetic i.,** innate i.
**herd i.,** the resistance of a group to attack by a disease because of the immunity of a large proportion of the members and the consequent lessening of the likelihood of an affected individual coming into contact with a susceptible individual.
**humoral i.,** immunity mediated by antibodies. Cf. *cell-mediated i.*
**infection i.,** the development of resistance to reinfection even though the original infection persists, an apparent paradox. Called also *concomitant i.*
**inherent i.,** innate i.
**inherited i.,** innate i.
**innate i.,** immunity based on the genetic constitution of the individual, e.g., immunity of man to canine distemper. Called also *familial i., genetic i., inherent i., inherited i.,* and *native i.*
**intrauterine i.,** passive immunity acquired by the fetus as a consequence of the passage of maternal IgG antibodies from an immune mother through the placenta into the fetal circulation.
**local i.,** immunity confined to a particular tissue or organ.
**maternal i.,** passively transferred humoral immunity from the mother to the offspring, across the placenta before birth in primates, from the colostrum via the intestines in ungulates, and from the egg yolk in birds.
**native i.,** innate i.
**natural i.,** immunity mediated by cells capable of immune activity without being stimulated by immunization and without antigen specificity, e.g., the activity of NK cells against virus infection and tumor cells.
**nonspecific i.,** immunity that does not involve the recognition of antigen by lymphocytes and the mounting of a specific immune response; e.g., the protection afforded by lysozyme, interferon, the cells involved in natural immunity, and anatomical barriers to infection.
**passive i.,** immunity acquired by transfer of antibody or lymphocytes from an immune donor. Cf. *active i.*
**species i.,** resistance of members of a particular species to a disease; immunity enjoyed by members of a particular species and determined by their genetic constitution.
**specific i.,** immunity against a particular disease, e.g., scarlet fever, or against a particular antigen.
**T cell–mediated i. (TCMI),** cell-mediated i.
**tissue i.,** local i.

**im·mu·ni·za·tion** (im″u-nĭ-za′shən) [MeSH: Immunization] the induction of immunity; see *active i.* and *passive i.*
**active i.,** stimulation of the immune system to confer protection against disease, e.g., by administration of a vaccine or toxoid.
**adoptive i.,** passive immunization by transfer of sensitized lymphocytes from an immune donor to a previously nonimmune recipient.
**passive i.,** the conferring of specific immune reactivity on previously nonimmune individuals by the administration of sensitized lymphoid cells or serum from immune individuals.

**im·mu·nize** (im'u-nīz) to render immune.

**im·mu·no·ad·ju·vant** (im″u-no-aj'ə-vənt) a nonspecific stimulator of the immune response, e.g., BCG vaccine or Freund's complete and incomplete adjuvants.

**im·mu·no·ad·sor·bent** (im″u-no-ad-sor'bənt) a preparation of antigen or antibody in an insoluble form used to bind homologous antibody or antigen, respectively, and remove it from a mixture of substances.

**im·mu·no·ad·sorp·tion** (im″u-no-ad-sorp'shən) the use of an immunoadsorbent to effect a chemical separation of antigen or antibody, as in immunoassays or in affinity chromatography.

**im·mu·no·as·say** (im″u-no-as'a) [MeSH: Immunoassay] any of several methods for the quantitative determination of chemical substances that utilize the highly specific binding between an antigen or hapten and homologous antibodies, including radioimmunoassay, enzyme immunoassay, and fluoroimmunoassay.
**enzyme i. (EIA),** any of several immunoassay methods that use an enzyme covalently linked to an antigen or antibody as a label, the two most common being ELISA (enzyme-linked immunosorbent assay) and EMIT (enzyme multiplied immunoassay technique).
**fluorescence i. (FIA),** any immunoassay using fluorochrome-labeled antibody or antigen; classified as either *heterogeneous* or *homogeneous.* Called also *fluorescent i., fluoroimmunoassay,* and *immunofluorescence assay.*
**fluorescence i., heterogeneous,** a fluorescence immunoassay that has more than one phase, requiring separation of the bound label (antigen-antibody complex) from the free labeled immunoreactant by physiochemical methods.
**fluorescence i., homogeneous,** a fluorescence immunoassay that is single-phase and uses a change in fluorescence (such as quenching or increased polarization) accompanying antigen-antibody binding to measure the amount of bound label without separation.
**fluorescent i. (FIA),** fluorescence i.

**im·mu·no·bio·log·i·cal** (im″u-no-bi″o-loj'ĭ-kəl) an antigenic or antibody-containing preparation derived from a pool of human or animal donors, including vaccines, toxoids, immune globulins, and antitoxins; used for immunization and immune therapy.

**im·mu·no·bi·ol·o·gy** (im″u-no-bi-ol'o-je) that branch of biology dealing with immunologic effects on such phenomena as infectious disease, growth and development, recognition phenomena, hypersensitivity, heredity, aging, cancer, and transplantation.

**im·mu·no·blast** (im″u-no-blast') lymphoblast.

**im·mu·no·blas·tic** (im″u-no-blas'tik) pertaining to or involving immunoblasts (lymphoblasts).

**im·mu·no·blot** (im'u-no-blot″) a technique for, or the blot resulting from, analyzing or identifying proteins via antigen-antibody specific reactions, as in Western blot or dot blot techniques.

**im·mu·no·chem·i·cal** (im″u-no-kem'ĭ-kəl) pertaining to immunochemistry.

**im·mu·no·chem·is·try** (im″u-no-kem'is-tre) [MeSH: Immunochemistry] 1. the study of the chemical basis of immunological phenomena. 2. the application of antibodies as chemical reagents.

**im·mu·no·che·mo·ther·a·py** (im″u-no-ke″mo-ther'ə-pe) a combination of immunotherapy and chemotherapy.

**im·mu·no·com·pe·tence** (im″u-no-kom'pə-təns) [MeSH: Immunocompetence] the ability or capacity to develop an immune response (i.e., antibody production and/or cell-mediated immunity) following exposure to antigen; called also *immunoresponsiveness* and *immunologic competence.*

**im·mu·no·com·pe·tent** (im″u-no-kom'pə-tənt) exhibiting immunocompetence.

**im·mu·no·com·plex** (im″u-no-kom'pləks) antigen-antibody complex.

**im·mu·no·com·pro·mised** (im″u-no-kom'prə-mīzd) having the immune response attenuated (see *immunodeficiency*); it may be by administration of immunosuppressive drugs, by irradiation, by malnutrition, or by some disease processes (e.g., cancer or the acquired immune deficiency syndrome). Called also *immunodeficient.*

**im·mu·no·con·glu·ti·nin** (im″u-no-kən-gloo'tĭ-nin) an autoantibody, usually of the immunoglobulin M class, that is specific for activated C3 and C4 components of complement. It is found in low titer in most normal sera and in increased levels in certain infectious diseases, in autoimmune disease, and after immunization with many antigens. Not to be confused with *conglutinin.* Called also *immune conglutinin.*

**im·mu·no·cyte** (im″u-no-sīt') a cell of the lymphoid series which can react with antigen to produce antibody or to become active in cell-mediated immunity or delayed hypersensitivity reactions; called also *immunologically competent cell.*

**im·mu·no·cy·to·ad·her·ence** (im″u-no-si″to-ad-hēr'əns) the formation of rosettes by the binding of red cells bearing a homologous antigen to lymphocytes bearing surface immunoglobulin (B cells); used to identify B cells.

**im·mu·no·cy·to·chem·is·try** (im″u-no-si″to-kem'is-tre) the application of immunochemical techniques, e.g., immunoperoxidase staining, to cytochemistry.

**im·mu·no·de·fi·cien·cy** (im″u-no-də-fish'ən-se) a deficiency of immune response or a disorder characterized by deficient immune response; classified as *antibody* (B cell), *cellular* (T cell), or *combined immunodeficiency,* or *phagocytic dysfunction disorders.* See accompanying table. See also *acquired immunodeficiency syndrome,* under *syndrome.*
**antibody i.,** deficiency in immunity mediated by B lymphocytes, marked by hypo- or dysgammaglobulinemia and recurrent bacterial otitis media and sinopulmonary infections. For a list of disorders of this type, see table.
**cellular i.,** deficiency in cellular immunity (q.v.), marked by recurrent infections with low-grade or opportunistic pathogens, by graft-versus-host reactions following blood transfusions, and by severe disease following immunization with live vaccines. For a list of disorders of this type, see table.

**Primary Immunodeficiency Disorders, Diseases, and Syndromes**

*Antibody (B Cell) Deficiency Disorders*
- X-linked agammaglobulinemia (Bruton's disease)
- Common variable immunodeficiency
- Transient hypogammaglobulinemia of infancy
- Selective IgA deficiency
- Immunodeficiency with hyper-IgM
- Selective IgM deficiency
- Selective deficiency of IgG subclasses
- Kappa light chain deficiency
- Secretory component deficiency
- Specific antibody deficiency with normal immunoglobulins
- X-linked lymphoproliferative syndrome (Duncan's syndrome)

*Cellular (T Cell) Deficiency Disorders*
- Thymic hypoplasia (DiGeorge syndrome)
- Chronic mucocutaneous candidiasis
- Acquired immunodeficiency syndrome (AIDS)

*Combined (B Cell and T Cell) Deficiency Disorders*
- Severe combined immunodeficiency (SCID)*
  - Autosomal recessive SCID
  - SCID with adenosine deaminase deficiency
  - SCID with purine nucleoside phosphorylase deficiency
  - X-linked recessive SCID
  - Reticular dysgenesis
- Cellular immunodeficiency with immunoglobulins (Nezlof syndrome)
- Immunodeficiency with thrombocytopenia and eczema (Wiskott-Aldrich syndrome)
- Ataxia-telangiectasia
- Immunodeficiency with short-limbed dwarfism
- Immunodeficiency with thymoma
- Transcobalamin II deficiency
- Episodic lymphopenia with lymphotoxin

*Phagocytic Dysfunction Disorders*
- Chédiak-Higashi syndrome
- Chronic granulomatous disease
- Job syndrome
- Lazy leukocyte syndrome
- Deficiency disorders
  - Alkaline phosphatase deficiency
  - Glucose-6-phosphate dehydrogenase deficiency
  - Myeloperoxidase deficiency
  - Tuftsin deficiency
- Elevated IgE with defective chemotaxis, eczema, and recurrent infection
- Leukocyte movement disorders

* Some forms of SCID, although deficient in both antibody and cellular immunity, actually have normal numbers of B cells.

**combined i.,** deficiency of lymphoid cells that mediate both antibody (B-lymphocytes) and cellular (T-lymphocytes) immunity. See table. Called also *combined immunodeficiency disease.*
**common variable i. (CVID), common variable unclassifiable i.,** a heterogeneous group of disorders characterized by hypogammaglobulinemia, decreased antibody production in response to antigenic challenge, and recurrent pyogenic infections, and often associated with hematologic and autoimmune disorders. Most patients have normal numbers of circulating B cells, which can identify antigens and proliferate, but lack plasma cells and appear to have an intrinsic defect of B cell differentiation. However, two other forms are also recognized: that due to a disorder of T lymphocyte regulation and that due to production of autoantibodies against T and B lymphocytes. Called also *common variable agammaglobulinemia* or *hypogammaglobulinemia.*
**i. with elevated IgM, i. with hyper-IgM,** a rare syndrome characterized by elevated immunoglobulin M levels and decreased levels of G and A immunoglobulins, associated with recurrent pyogenic infections, and possibly caused by failure of IgM-producing cells to switch to production of IgC and IgA. Most cases appear to exhibit X-linked recessive inheritance. Called also *i. with elevated* (or *increased*) *IgM.*
**severe combined i. (SCID),** a group of rare congenital disorders characterized by gross impairment of both humoral and cell-mediated immunity and absence of T lymphocytes; some forms are also characterized by a lack of B lymphocytes. In most cases all classes of immunoglobulins are nearly or completely absent, and there is marked lymphocytopenia. Persistent diarrhea, chronic mucocutaneous candidiasis, and failure to thrive occur in infancy. Blood transfusions can result in graft-versus-host disease and routine vaccinations in fatal infection. Unless immune function is restored by a histocompatible bone marrow or fetal tissue transplant or the patient is kept in gnotobiotic isolation, death from opportunistic infection usually occurs before the first birthday. In approximately 50 per cent of cases, the disorder is X-linked and due to a defect in the $\gamma$ chain of the receptor for IL-2 and other interleukins. B lymphocyte numbers are usually normal. The remaining 50 per cent of cases are of autosomal recessive inheritance and have varying etiologies, with approximately half of these due to a defect in either adenosine deaminase or, rarely, purine-nucleoside phosphorylase activity. A rare type of the autosomal recessive form is called *reticular dysgenesis.*
**i. with short-limbed dwarfism,** short-limbed dwarfism marked by short, pudgy hands, redundant skin, and hyperextensible joints of the hands and feet associated with immunodeficiency, which may be either antibody or cellular or combined.
**i. with thymoma,** an immunodeficiency disorder in which thymoma, usually of the benign spindle-cell type, is associated with hypogammaglobulinemia; deficiencies of cell-mediated immunity, such as eosinopenia, hypoplastic or aplastic anemia, or autoimmune diseases, may occur also. Removal of the thymoma does not cure the immunodeficiency, and patients suffer from recurrent severe infections.

**im·mu·no·de·fi·cient** (im″u-no-də-fish′ənt) immunocompromised.

**im·mu·no·de·pres·sion** (im″u-no-də-presh′ən) immunosuppression.

**im·mu·no·de·pres·sive** (im″u-no-də-pres′iv) immunosuppressive.

**im·mu·no·der·ma·tol·o·gy** (im″u-no-dər″mə-tol′ə-je) the study of immunologic phenomena as they affect skin disorders and their treatment or prophylaxis.

**im·mu·no·de·tec·tion** (im″u-no-de-tek′shən) detection of a substance or reaction by means of the specific interaction of antibody with antigen.

**im·mu·no·de·vi·a·tion** (im″u-no-de″ve-a′shən) split tolerance, def. 2.

**im·mu·no·di·ag·no·sis** (im″u-no-di″əg-no′sis) diagnosis based on blood serum reactions to antigens; serodiagnosis.

**im·mu·no·dif·fu·sion** (im″u-no-dĭ-fu′zhən) [MeSH: Immunodiffusion] any technique involving diffusion of antigen or antibody through a semisolid medium, usually agar or agarose gel, resulting in a precipitin reaction. Precipitin lines or bands form where the concentrations of antigen and antibody are serologically equivalent.
**radial i. (RID),** single radial diffusion.

**im·mu·no·dom·i·nance** (im″u-no-dom′ĭ-nəns) the degree to which a subunit of an antigenic determinant is involved in binding or reacting with specific antibody.

**im·mu·no·dom·i·nant** (im″u-no-dom′ĭ-nənt) denoting the subunits of the antigenic determinant group that most influence the specificity of the induced antibodies.

**im·mu·no·elec·tro·pho·re·sis** (im″u-no-e-lek-tro-fo-re′sis) [MeSH: Immunoelectrophoresis] a technique combining protein electrophoresis and double immunodiffusion; proteins are separated by agarose gel electrophoresis; then specific antisera are placed in a trough cut parallel to the protein track, and the proteins and antibodies are allowed to diffuse through the gel, the proteins diffusing radially from their electrophoretic placement and the antibodies diffusing perpendicularly from the trough, resulting in a distinct elliptical precipitin arc for each protein detectable by the antisera. Abbreviated IEP.
**counter i.,** counterimmunoelectrophoresis.
**countercurrent i.,** counterimmunoelectrophoresis.
**crossed i.,** a combination of protein electrophoresis and rocket immunoelectrophoresis; protein antigens are separated by agarose gel electrophoresis; then a strip containing the separated antigens is cut out and placed in a trough in a gel containing antiserum, and an electric field perpendicular to the trough is applied, producing a "rocket" precipitin pattern for each antigen.
**rocket i.,** one-dimensional single electroimmunodiffusion; a technique in which antigen is placed in a row of wells in an agar plate containing antiserum and an electric field perpendicular to the line of wells is applied; this drives the antigen through the gel, forming a spike or "rocket" precipitin pattern trailing away from each well. The length of the rocket is proportional to the amount of antigen placed in the well. Called also *Laurell technique.*

**im·mu·no·fer·ri·tin** (im″u-no-fer′ĭ-tin) an antibody labeled with ferritin; when combined with antigen, the antigenic determinant sites are visible under the electron microscope.

**im·mu·no·fil·tra·tion** (im″u-no-fil-tra′shən) the purification of antigen or antibody using an immunoadsorbent.

**im·mu·no·flu·o·res·cence** (im″u-no-floo″o-res′əns) any immunohistochemical method using antibody labeled with a fluorescent dye; called *direct* if a specific antibody or antiserum is conjugated with a fluorochrome and used as a specific fluorescent stain and *indirect* if the fluorochrome is attached to an antiglobulin, and a tissue constituent is stained using an unlabeled specific antibody and the labeled antiglobulin, which binds the unlabeled antibody.

**im·mu·no·gen** (im′u-no-jən) a substance capable of inducing an immune response, in most contexts synonymous with antigen; in some contexts immunogen is used to draw a distinction with substances capable of reacting only with antibody (antigens or haptens) or to denote a form of an antigen that induces an immune response as opposed to a tolerogen, a form that induces tolerance.

**im·mu·no·ge·net·ic** (im″u-no-jə-net′ik) pertaining to immunogenetics.

**im·mu·no·ge·net·ics** (im″u-no-jə-net′iks) [*immuno-* + *genetics*] [MeSH: Immunogenetics] the study of the genetics of the immune response, e.g., the study of immune response genes, or the association of HLA antigens with disease susceptibility, or the generation of antibody diversity.

**im·mu·no·gen·ic** (im″u-no-jen′ik) producing immunity; evoking an immune response.

**im·mu·no·ge·nic·i·ty** (im″u-no-jə-nis′ĭ-te) the property that endows a substance with the capacity to provoke an immune response, or the degree to which a substance possesses this property.

**im·mu·no·glob·u·lin** (im″u-no-glob′u-lin) any of the structurally related glycoproteins that function as antibodies, divided into five classes (IgM, IgG, IgA, IgD, and IgE) on the basis of structure and biologic activity. The basic structural unit of the immunoglobulin molecule, referred to as a monomer, is a Y-shaped molecule composed of two heavy (H) chains and two light (L) chains (see accompanying illustration). IgD, IgG, and IgE occur only as monomers; IgM and IgA may occur as monomers or polymers. The polymeric forms contain an additional polypeptide called the J chain, and secretory IgA contains another structure called the secretory component (SC). Each chain consists of a variable region ($V_H$ or $V_L$) and a constant region ($C_H$ or $C_L$), which are coded for by different genes. Parts of the $V_H$ and $V_L$ regions make up the antigen-binding site, one on each "arm" (Fab region) of the monomer. An individual can make about $10^4$ different $V_H$ regions and $10^3$ $V_L$ regions, which combine to make about $10^7$ different antigen-binding sites, each with a distinct antigenic specificity. Parts of the $C_H$ regions make up the "body" (Fc region) of the monomer, which contains various sites responsible for the biological activity of the molecule. In any one immunoglobulin molecule, all of the H chains are identical, as are the L chains. The $C_H$ region determines both the heavy chain class to which the H chain belongs and the immunoglobulin class to which the molecule belongs. The H chain classes are denoted by the Greek letters ($\mu$, $\delta$, $\gamma$, $\epsilon$, and $\alpha$) corresponding to the Latin letters of the immunoglobulin classes, e.g., $\mu$ to IgM. There are two types of light chains (denoted $\kappa$ and $\lambda$), either of which may combine with any of the heavy chains and thus occur in any of the immunoglobulin classes. In human immunoglobulins, three of the classes (IgM, IgG, and IgA) have subclasses; i.e., there are several similar but distinct $C_H$ region genes in these classes. In addition, the λ light chain type has subtypes. The subclasses (subtypes) are denoted by numerical suffixes, e.g., IgG1 and γ1 subclasses and λ2 subtype. Immunoglobulins (monomeric IgM and IgD) first appear on the surface of B cells as antigen receptors. When a cell is activated by contact with antigen and differentiates into a plasma cell, the cell continues to produce the same L chain and $V_H$ region of the H chain, but gene rearrangement may occur to attach this $V_H$ region to a different $C_H$ region (class switching). Thus the secreted immunoglobulin may be of any class but has the same antigenic specificity as the antigen receptors of the parent B cell. In addition to the effects produced solely by the binding of antigen by antibody, e.g., viral neutralization or the inability of some bacteria to invade mucosal surfaces when coated by antibody, certain classes of antibodies can trigger other processes when bound to antigen: IgM and IgG activate the classic complement pathway, IgA and IgG activate the alternative pathway, and IgM, IgG1, and IgG3 act as opsonins, triggering phagocytosis of the bound antigens by macrophages and neutrophils. IgE has the unique function of mediating immediate hypersensitivity (q.v.) reactions; it binds to specific receptors on basophils and mast cells

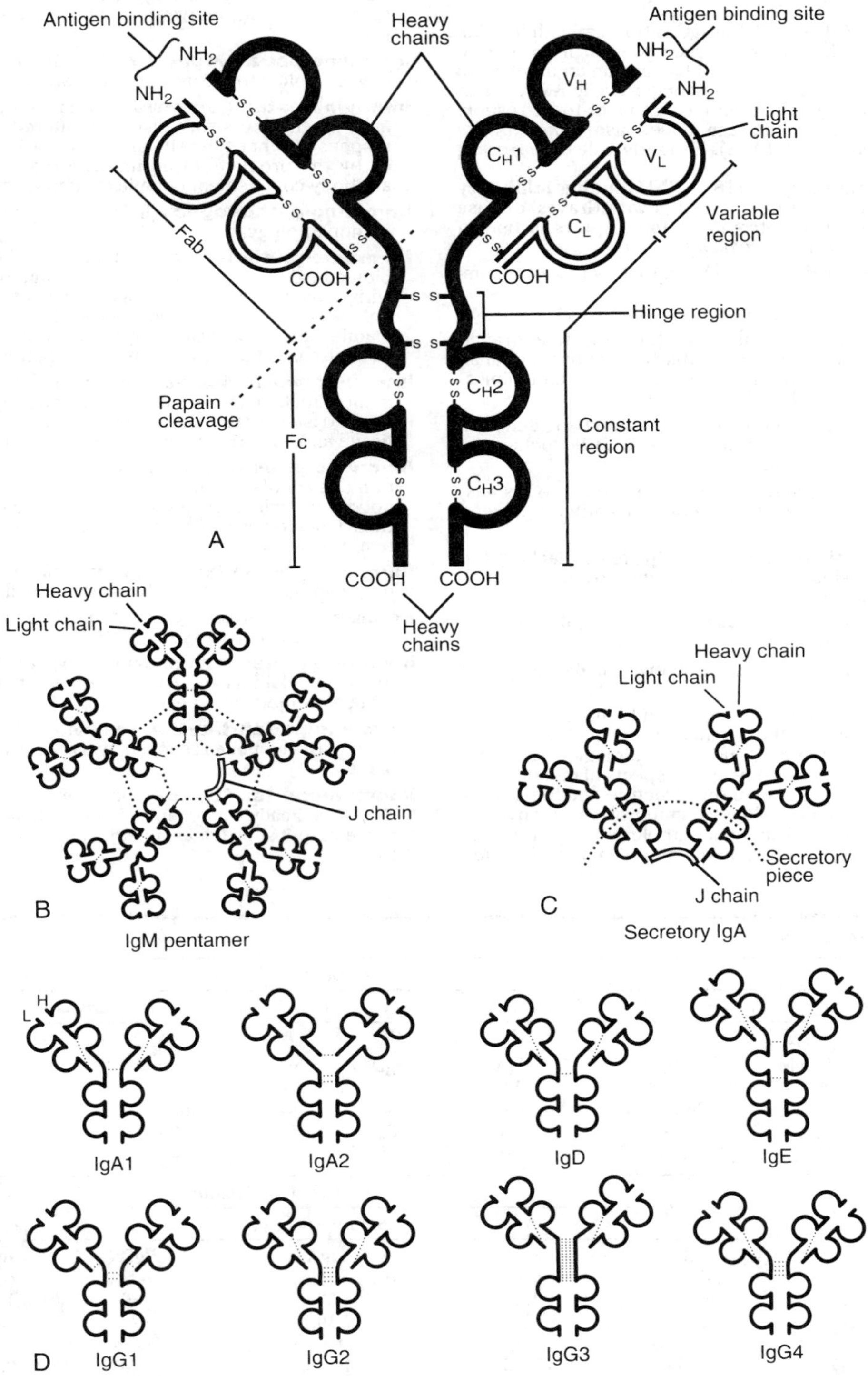


Molecular structure of the five classes of immunoglobulins. *(A)*, Schematic representation, using an IgG1 molecule, of the basic arrangement of heavy and light chains into the four-polypeptide chain unit, the antigen binding sites, the variable, constant, and hinge regions, and the site of papain cleavage generating the Fab and Fc fragments. Both intra- and interchain disulfide bonds are depicted (—SS—). *(B)*, IgM pentamer showing the arrangement of five four-chain monomers, interchain disulfide bonds *(dotted lines)*, and the J chain. *(C)*, Secretory IgA, here composed of IgA1 monomers, showing the position of the interchain disulfide bonds *(dotted lines)*, J chain, and secretory piece. *(D)*, Structure of IgA, IgD, IgE, and IgG subclasses, showing the interchain disulfide bonds *(dotted lines)*.

and triggers the release of mediators on contact with antigen. IgG is the only class transferred across the placenta, providing the fetus and neonate with protection against infection. See also *immunoglobulin genes,* under *gene, homology region,* under *region,* and *allotype, idiotype,* and *isotype.*

**antilymphocyte i.,** see under *globulin.*

**monoclonal i.,** see *M component.*

**secretory i. A,** secretory IgA; the predominant immunoglobulin in secretions (oral, nasal, bronchial, urogenital, and intestinal mucous secretions and tears, saliva, and milk), a dimer containing the J chain and the secretory component (SC).

**thyroid-binding inhibitory i's (TBII),** thyrotropin-binding inhibitory i's.

**thyroid-stimulating i's (TSI),** circulating IgG antibodies with the ability to mimic thyrotropin by binding to receptors for it on thyroid cells and activating adenylate cyclase, thus causing an increase in the level of the intracellular second messenger cyclic AMP, which results in the release of thyroid hormones; thought to be responsible for most cases of Graves' disease. Called also *human thyroid adenylate cyclase stimulators* (HTACS). Formerly called *long-acting thyroid stimulator.*

**thyrotropin-binding inhibitory i's (TBII), TSH-binding inhibitory i's,** proteins present in the serum of patients with Graves' disease that inhibit the binding of thyrotropin to its receptors in human thyroid tissues. Called also *TSH-displacing antibody.*

**im·mu·no·glob·u·lin·op·a·thy** (im″u-no-glob″u-lin-op′ə-the) gammopathy.

**monoclonal i's,** plasma cell dyscrasias.

**im·mu·no·hem·a·tol·o·gy** (im″u-no-hēm″ə-tol′o-je) that branch of hematology which studies antigen-antibody reactions and analogous phenomena as they relate to the pathogenesis and clinical manifestations of blood disorders.

**im·mu·no·his·to·chem·i·cal** (im″u-no-his″to-kem′ĭ-kəl) denoting the application of antigen-antibody interactions to histochemical techniques, as in the use of immunofluorescence.

**im·mu·no·his·to·flu·o·res·cence** (im″u-no-his-to-floo″o-res′əns) histofluorescence accomplished by injection of antibody labeled with fluorochrome.

**im·mu·no·in·com·pe·tent** (im″u-no-in-kom′pə-tent) lacking the ability or capacity to develop an immune response to antigenic challenge. See also *immunodeficiency.*

**im·mu·no·log·ic, im·mu·no·log·i·cal** (im″u-no-loj′ik, im″u-no-loj′ĭ-kəl) pertaining to immunology.

**im·mu·nol·o·gist** (im″u-nol′o-jist) a person who makes a special study of immunology.

**im·mu·nol·o·gy** (im″u-nol′o-je) that branch of biomedical science concerned with the response of the organism to antigenic challenge, the recognition of self and not self, and all the biological *(in vivo),* serological *(in vitro),* and physical chemical aspects of immune phenomena. It encompasses the study of the structure and function of the immune system (basic immunology); immunization, organ transplantation, blood banking, and immunopathology (clinical immunology); laboratory testing of cellular and humoral immune function (laboratory immunology); and the use of antigen-antibody reactions in other laboratory tests (serology and immunochemistry).

**im·mu·no·lym·pho·scin·tig·ra·phy** (im″u-no-lim″fo-sin-tig′rə-fe) scintigraphic detection of metastatic tumor in lymph nodes using radiolabeled monoclonal antibodies or antibody fragments specific for tumor-associated antigens.

**im·mu·no·mod·u·la·tion** (im″u-no-mod″u-la′shən) adjustment of the immune response to a desired level, as in immunopotentiation, immunosuppression, or induction of immunologic tolerance.

**im·mu·no·mod·u·la·tor** (im″u-no-mod′u-la″tor) an agent that specifically or nonspecifically augments or diminishes immune responses, i.e., an adjuvant, immunostimulant, or immunosuppressant.

**im·mu·no·par·a·si·tol·o·gy** (im″u-no-par″ə-si-tol′o-je) immunology as applied to the interaction of animal parasites and their hosts.

**im·mu·no·patho·gen·e·sis** (im″u-no-path″o-jen′ə-sis) a process in which the course of a disease is altered or affected by an immune response (either the cellular [T-cell] or humoral [B-cell] response) or by the products of an immune reaction, such as the antigen-antibody-complement complexes deposited in renal glomeruli.

**im·mu·no·patho·log·ic** (im″u-no-path″o-loj′ik) pertaining to immunopathology.

**im·mu·no·pa·thol·o·gy** (im″u-no-pə-thol′o-je) 1. that branch of biomedical science concerned with immune responses to disease, with immunodeficiency diseases, and with diseases with an immunological etiology or pathogenesis. 2. the structural and functional manifestations associated with immune responses to disease or with diseases having an immunologic etiology.

**im·mu·no·per·ox·i·dase** (im″u-no-pər-ok′sĭ-das) pertaining to immunocytochemical methods using antibody coupled to the enzyme peroxidase to stain tissue constituents; frequently used to identify tissue antigens to aid diagnosis in surgical pathology.

**im·mu·no·phe·no·type** (im″mu-no-fe′no-tīp) 1. the characterization of a set of cells according to the antigens expressed. 2. a phenotype of cells of hematopoietic neoplasms defined according to their resemblance to normal T cells and B cells of the immune system. See also listings under *leukemia* and *lymphoma.*

**im·mu·no·phe·no·typ·ing** [MeSH: Immunophenotyping] analysis of the antigens expressed by cells, as by flow cytometry.

**im·mu·no·phys·i·ol·o·gy** (im″u-no-fiz″e-ol′o-je) the physiology of immunological processes.

**im·mu·no·po·ten·cy** (im″u-no-po′tən-se) the immunogenic capacity of an individual antigenic determinant on an antigen molecule to initiate antibody synthesis.

**im·mu·no·po·ten·ti·a·tion** (im″u-no-po-ten″she-a′shən) enhancement of the immune response by use of an adjuvant or immunostimulant.

**im·mu·no·po·ten·ti·a·tor** (im″u-no-po-ten′she-a-tor) an agent that specifically or nonspecifically enhances or augments the immune response, such as an adjuvant, BCG vaccine, or transfer factor.

**The Human Immunoglobulins**

| | *Polypeptide Chains* | | | | | | | | |
|---|---|---|---|---|---|---|---|---|---|
| | *H Chains* | | | | | *L Chains* | | *Other* | |
| | $\mu$ | $\gamma$ | $\alpha$ | $\delta$ | $\epsilon$ | $\kappa$ | $\lambda$ | J | SC* |
| Immunoglobulin classes | IgM | IgG | IgA | IgD | IgE | all | all | IgM, IgA | IgA |
| Subclasses or subtypes | — | 1–4 | 1,2 | — | — | — | 1–4 | — | |
| Allotypes | — | Gm(1–25) | Am(1–2) | — | — | Km(1–3) | — | — | — |
| Mol. wt. *(kDa)* | 70 | 50 | 55 | 62 | 70 | 23 | 23 | 15 | 70 |
| Carbohydrate (%) | 15 | 4 | 10 | 18 | 18 | — | — | 8 | 16 |

| | *Immunoglobulins* | | | | | |
|---|---|---|---|---|---|---|
| | *Serum* | | | | | *Secretory* |
| | IgM | IgG | IgA | IgD | IgE | IgA |
| Molecular formula | $(\mu_2L_2)_5J$ | $\gamma_2L_2$ | $\alpha_2L_2$ or $(\alpha_2L_2)_nJ$† | $\delta_2L_2$ | $\epsilon_2L_2$ | $(\alpha_2L_2)_2J$, SC |
| Mol. wt. *(kDa)* | 900 | 150 | 153;325;580 | 180 | 190 | 400 |
| Sedimentation coefficient *(S)* | 19 | 7 | 7;10;14 | 7 | 8 | — |
| Electrophoretic mobility | fast $\gamma$ to $\beta$ | $\gamma$ | fast $\gamma$ to $\beta$ | fast $\gamma$ | fast $\gamma$ | — |
| Serum concentration *(mg/dl)* | 25–200 | 700–1500 | 40–350 | 1–40 | <0.06 | — |
| Serum half-life *(days)* | 5 | 23 | 6 | 3 | 2 | — |

* Secretory component.
† n = 2 or 3.

**im·mu·no·pre·cip·i·ta·tion** (im″u-no-pre-sip″ĭ-ta′shən) precipitation resulting from interaction of specific antibody and antigen. See *precipitin reaction,* under *reaction.*

**im·mu·no·pro·lif·er·a·tive** (im″u-no-pro-lif′ər-ə-tiv) a term used to refer to the uncontrolled proliferation of lymphoid cells, as in immunoproliferative disorders.

**im·mu·no·pro·phy·lax·is** (im″u-no-pro″fə-lak′sis) the prevention of disease by the use of vaccines or therapeutic antisera.

**im·mu·no·ra·dio·met·ric** (im″u-no-ra″de-o-met′rik) pertaining to immunoradiometry or to immunoradiometric assay.

**im·mu·no·ra·di·om·e·try** (im″u-no-ra″de-om′ə-tre) the use of radiolabeled antibody (in the place of radiolabeled antigen) in radioimmunoassay techniques.

**im·mu·no·re·ac·tant** (im″u-no-re-ak′tənt) a substance that participates in an immune reaction, e.g., an antigen or antibody.
**glucagon i.,** enteroglucagon.

**im·mu·no·re·ac·tion** (im″u-no-re-ak′shən) the reaction that takes place between an antigen and its antibody or between an antigen and an immunocyte sensitized to it.

**im·mu·no·re·ac·tive** (im″u-no-re-ak′tiv) exhibiting immunoreaction.

**im·mu·no·re·ac·tiv·i·ty** (im″u-no-re″ak-tiv′ĭ-te) the quality or state of being immunoreactive.
**glucagon-like i.,** enteroglucagon.

**im·mu·no·reg·u·la·tion** (im″u-no-reg″u-la′shən) control of the immune response by mechanisms such as suppressor and contrasuppressor lymphocyte circuits and the immunoglobulin idiotype–anti-idiotype network.

**im·mu·no·re·spon·sive·ness** (im″u-no-re-spon′siv-nəs) immunocompetence.

**im·mu·no·scin·tig·raphy** (im″u-no-sin-tig′rə-fe) scintigraphic imaging of a lesion using labeled monoclonal antibodies or antibody fragments specific for antigen associated with the lesion.

**im·mu·no·se·lec·tion** (im″u-no-sə-lek′shən) the survival of certain cell lines attributable to their having the least surface antigenicity and thus the least susceptibility to antibody and/or immune lymphoid cells.

**im·mu·no·sor·bent** (im″u-no-sor′bənt) immunoadsorbent.

**im·mu·no·stain·ing** (im″u-no-stān′ing) the use of antibody labeled with a compound visible by light, fluorescence, or electron microscopy to identify tissue or cellular constituents by the antigens (markers) expressed.
**double i.,** immunostaining using two antibodies in order to visualize two different antigens in the same smear.

**im·mu·no·stim·u·lant** (im″u-no-stim′u-lənt) an agent capable of stimulating immune responses, usually used to refer to agents other than adjuvants.

**im·mu·no·stim·u·la·tion** (im″u-no-stim″u-la′shən) stimulation of an immune response, e.g., by use of BCG vaccine.

**im·mu·no·sup·pres·sant** (im″u-no-sə-pres′ənt) an agent capable of suppressing immune responses. See also *immunodeficiency.*

**im·mu·no·sup·pres·sion** (im″u-no-sə-presh′ən) [MeSH: Immunosuppression] the prevention or diminution of the immune response, as by irradiation or by administration of antimetabolites, antilymphocyte serum, or specific antibody; see also *immunodeficiency.* Called also *immunodepression.*

**im·mu·no·sup·pres·sive** (im″u-no-sə-pres′iv) 1. pertaining to or inducing immunosuppression. 2. immunosuppressant.

**im·mu·no·sur·veil·lance** (im″u-no-sər-va′ləns) immune surveillance.

**im·mu·no·ther·a·py** (im″u-no-ther′ə-pe) [MeSH: Immunotherapy] a general term encompassing active and passive immunization, treatment with immunopotentiators and immunosuppressants, hyposensitization for allergic disorders, bone marrow transplantation, and thymus implantation.
**adoptive i., adoptive cellular i.,** the treatment of cancer by transferring cultured lymphocytes having antitumor activity into the tumor-bearing host.

**im·mu·no·tox·in** (im′u-no-tok″sin) a hybrid molecule formed by coupling an entire toxin or the A chain of a toxin to an antibody or antigen molecule; the resulting molecule has the specificity of the antibody or antigen and the toxicity of the toxin.

**im·mu·no·trans·fu·sion** (im″u-no-trans-fu′zhən) transfusion of blood from donors previously immunized by the bacteria infecting the patient, or from the specific infection or of blood from persons recently recovered from the specific infection.

**Imo·di·um** (i-mo′de-əm) trademark for a preparation of loperamide hydrochloride.

**IMPA** incisal mandibular plane angle.

**im·pact** (im′pakt) [L. *impactus*] a sudden and forcible collision.

**im·pact·ed** (im-pak′təd) [L. *impactus*] driven firmly in; closely or firmly lodged in position, as an impacted tooth or impacted twins.

**im·pac·tion** (im-pak′shən) [L. *impactio*] 1. the condition of being firmly lodged or wedged. 2. in obstetrics, the indentation of any fetal parts of one twin onto the surface of its co-twin, so that simultaneous partial engagement of both twins occurs. See *impacted twins,* under *twin.*
**ceruminal i.,** impacted cerumen.
**dental i.,** the blocking of a tooth by a physical barrier, usually other teeth, so that it cannot erupt. See also *impacted tooth,* under *tooth.*
**fecal i.,** a collection of putty-like or hardened feces in the rectum or sigmoid.
**food i.,** forceful wedging of food into the peridontium by occlusal forces, which may occur interproximally or in relation to the vestibular or oral tooth surfaces. It is a common contributing factor in gingival and periodontal disease.

**im·pal·pa·ble** (im-pal′pə-bəl) [*in-*[2] + *palpable*] impossible of being detected by touch; extremely fine, or small.

**im·par** (im′pahr) [L. "unequal"] a general anatomical term meaning unpaired; having no fellow; azygous.

**im·pari·dig·i·tate** (im-par″ĭ-dij′ĭ-tāt) [L. *impar* unequal + *digitus* finger] perissodactylous.

**im·pa·ten·cy** (im-pa′tən-se) the condition of being closed or obstructed.

**im·pa·tent** (im-pa′tənt) not open; closed or obstructed.

**im·ped·ance** (im-pe′dəns) 1. opposition to the flow of an alternating current, which is the vector sum of ohmic resistance plus any additional resistance due to induction, to capacity, or to both. Symbol *Z.* The resistance due to the inductive and condenser characteristics of a circuit is called *reactance.* 2. In mechanics, the resistance to an applied force.
**acoustic i.,** an expression of the opposition to passage of sound waves, such as through the middle ear, being a function of the density and elasticity of a substance.
**aortic i.,** the sum of the external factors that resist ventricular ejection, expressed as the ratio of pressure to flow in the aorta and determined by the physical properties of the blood and of the arterial walls.

**im·per·cep·tion** (im″pər-sep′shən) defective power of perception.

**im·per·fect** (im-pər′fəkt) said of a fungus that reproduces only by means of conidia (asexual spores). Cf. *perfect.*

**im·per·fo·rate** (im-pər′fə-rāt) [L. *imperforatus*] not open; abnormally closed, as imperforate anus.

**im·per·fo·ra·tion** (im-pər″fə-ra′shən) the state of being abnormally closed; see also *atresia.*

**im·pe·ri·al·ine** (im-pe′re-al″in) a toxic crystalline alkaloid, from the bulbs of the liliaceous plant *Fritillaria imperialis.*

**im·per·me·a·ble** (im-pər′me-ə-bəl) [*in-*[2] + *per-* + *meare* to move] not permitting passage, as of fluid.

**im·per·vi·ous** (im-pər′ve-əs) [L. *impervius*] impenetrable; not affording a passage.

**im·pe·tig·i·ni·za·tion** (im″pə-tij″ĭ-nĭ-za′shən) the development of impetigo upon an area previously affected with some other skin disease.

**im·pe·tig·i·nous** (im″pə-tij′ĭ-nəs) [L. *impetiginosus*] pertaining to or of the nature of impetigo.

**im·pe·ti·go** (im″pə-ti′go) [L.] [MeSH: Impetigo] 1. a contagious pyoderma caused by direct inoculation of group A streptococci or *Staphylococcus aureus* into superficial cutaneous abrasions or compromised skin. It is usually seen in children, usually on the face, especially near the nose and mouth, and is characterized by discrete fragile vesicles with an erythematous border that become pus-

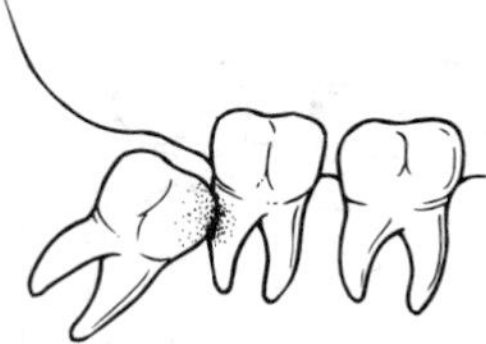

Impaction of the third molar.

tular and rupture to discharge a thin yellow seropurulent fluid that dries and forms a thick crust; the pustules may spread peripherally with central healing, evolving into annular, circinate, or gyrate patterns. Called also *i. contagiosa, i. vulgaris,* and *streptococcal i.* 2. i. bullosa.

**Bockhart's i.,** a superficial folliculitis, usually caused by *Staphylococcus aureus,* marked by the formation of small purulent pustules at the orifices of the pilosebaceous glands, and affecting especially the scalp and the extremities. Called also *superficial pustular perifolliculitis.*

**i. bullo'sa, bullous i.,** a highly contagious, usually localized pyoderma caused by *Staphylococcus aureus,* affecting usually newborns but sometimes older children or adults. Characteristics include eruption on the skin of flaccid bullae with erythematous rims containing a thin fluid; the lesions later rupture and form a thin varnishlike crust, and they sometimes spread to involve large areas of the skin. Called also *impetigo, i. contagiosa bullosa, i. neonatorum,* and *staphylococcal i.*

**i. contagio'sa,** impetigo, def. 1.

**i. contagio'sa bullo'sa,** i. bullosa.

**i. herpetifor'mis,** a rare, acute, severe dermatosis, generally considered to be a form of pustular psoriasis precipitated by pregnancy, associated with hypocalcemia and sometimes tetany and high fetal and maternal mortality, and characterized by the development of crops of pruritic sterile pustules that resolve with desquamation, each crop of lesions being accompanied by fever, lethargy, and prostration.

**i. neonato'rum,** i. bullosa.

**staphylococcal i.,** i. bullosa.

**streptococcal i.,** impetigo, def. 1.

**udder i.,** a staphylococcal infection of the udders of cows, with pustules near the teats that sometimes extend into boils. Cf. *staphylococcal mastitis.*

**i. vulga'ris,** impetigo, def. 1.

**im·pi·la·tion** (im″pĭ-la′shən) rouleau formation; see under *formation.*

**im·pinge·ment** (im-pinj′mənt) encroachment upon or collision with something; see *impingement syndrome,* under *syndrome.*

**Im·plac·en·ta·lia** (im″plas-ən-ta′le-ə) in former classifications, a division of the class Mammalia, comprising the mammals that do not have a placenta, such as the monotremes.

**im·plant**[1] (im-plant′) to insert or graft an object or material, such as an alloplastic or radioactive material, a drug capsule, or tissue, into the body of a recipient.

**im·plant**[2] (im′plant) an object or material, such as an alloplastic or radioactive material or tissue, partially or totally inserted or grafted into the body for prosthetic, therapeutic, diagnostic, or experimental purposes. See also *graft* and *insert.*

**Bosker i.,** a common type of transmandibular implant.

**Brånemark i.,** a type of osseointegrated implant consisting of a two-stage system of titanium screws.

**dental i.,** a prosthetic device of alloplastic material implanted into the oral tissues beneath the mucosal or periosteal layer or within the bone to provide support and retention to a partial or complete denture.

**endodontic i.,** a metallic implant extending through the root canal of a tooth into the periapical bone structure, thereby lengthening the root of a pulpless tooth.

**endometrial i's,** fragments of endometrial mucosa transferred through the oviducts and implanted on the uterus, ovaries, or pelvic peritoneum.

**endosseous i., endosteal i.,** a dental implant made of metal or sometimes ceramic or polymeric material, consisting of a blade, screw, pin, or vent, inserted into the jaw bone through the alveolar or basal bone, either directly or through the root canal and apex of a tooth, with a post protruding through the mucoperiosteum into the oral cavity to serve as an abutment for dentures or orthodontic appliances, or to serve in fracture fixation.

**intraperiosteal i.,** a frame that conforms to the shape of the jawbone and is implanted beneath the outer or fibrous layer of the periosteum so that it rests firmly on the bone, with a post protruding into the oral cavity to serve as an abutment for dentures; used most commonly for upper fixed partial dentures and in the treatment of cleft palate.

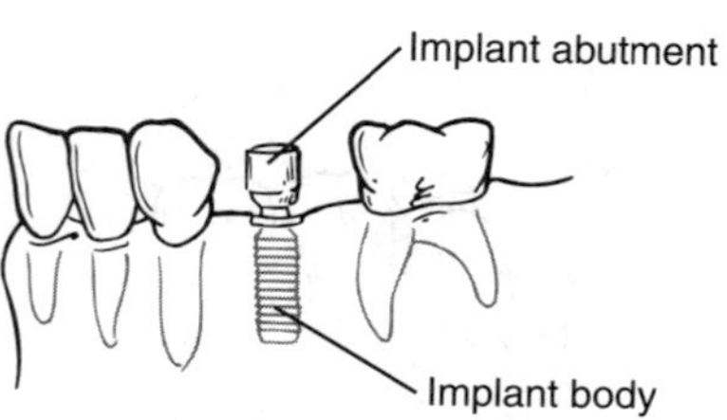

Endosseous implant.

**magnet i.,** denture magnet.

**osseointegrated i.,** an endosseous implant containing pores into which osteoblasts and supporting connective tissue can migrate. Metallic, ceramic, and polymeric materials have been used.

**penile i.,** see under *prosthesis.*

**subperiosteal i.,** a dental implant consisting of a metal frame implanted under the periosteum and firmly bound by the mucoperiosteum, resting on the jaw bone, with a post protruding into the oral cavity; used most commonly as an abutment for upper fixed partial dentures and in the treatment of cleft palate.

**transmandibular i.,** a dental implant consisting of baseplate, cortical screws, threaded posts, and a superstructure that attaches to a denture, inserted via submandibular incision and fixed to the symphyseal border. The implant transverses the mandible, bears the denture directly, and is designed for patients with severe mandibular alveolar atrophy.

**transosteal i.,** a dental implant consisting of a bolt that crosses the mandible and is secured in place by a nut; a post protrudes into the oral cavity and serves as an abutment for dentures or orthodontic appliances.

**im·plan·ta·tion** (im″plan-ta′shən) [*in-*[1] + *plantation*] 1. attachment of the blastocyst to the epithelial lining of the uterus, its penetration through the epithelium, and, in humans, its embedding in the compact layer of the endometrium, beginning six or seven days after fertilization of the ovum. 2. the insertion of an organ or tissue, such as skin, nerve, or tendon, in a new site in the body. 3. the insertion or grafting into the body of biological, living, inert, or radioactive material.

**central i., circumferential i.,** superficial i.

**eccentric i.,** embedding of the blastocyst within a recess of the uterine cavity.

**hypodermic i.,** the placing of a medicine in the subcutaneous tissue.

**interstitial i.,** complete embedding of a blastocyst within the endometrium, as in humans.

**LeDuc i.,** see under *technique.*

**nerve i.,** the operation of inserting and attaching a nerve into the sheath of another nerve.

**periosteal i.,** surgical insertion of a normal tendon into the periosteum of a bone at the insertion of a paralyzed tendon, to take its place.

**superficial i.,** embedding of the blastocyst so that the blastocyst, and later the chorionic sac, come to occupy the uterine cavity. Called also *central* or *circumferential i.*

**teratic i.,** the partial blending of an imperfect with a nearly perfect fetus.

**im·plan·to·don·tics** (im-plan″to-don′tiks) the branch of dentistry dealing with the implantation of artificial devices and materials into the oral hard and soft tissues for prosthetic, therapeutic, or diagnostic purposes. Called also *dental* or *oral implantology* and *implantodontology.*

**im·plan·to·don·tist** (im-plan″to-don′tist) a dentist who specializes in the practice of implantodontics; called also *implantologist.*

**im·plan·to·don·tol·o·gy** (im-plan″to-don-tol′ə-je) implantodontics.

**im·plan·tol·o·gist** (im″plan-tol′ə-jist) 1. a specialist in implantology. 2. implantodontist.

**im·plan·tol·o·gy** (im″plan-tol′ə-je) the science dealing with the study and practice of inserting implants into the body.

**dental i., oral i.,** implantodontics.

**im·plo·sion** (im-plo′zhən) see *flooding.*

**im·po·tence** (im′pə-təns) [*in-*[2] + *potentia*] [MeSH: Impotence] 1. lack of power. 2. specifically, lack of copulative power in the male due to failure to initiate an erection or to maintain an erection until ejaculation; usually classified as either *psychogenic i.* or *organic i.* Called also *erectile dysfunction.*

**diabetic i.,** impotence that commonly occurs in men with diabetes mellitus, resulting from a variety of organic effects of the disease.

**endocrinologic i.,** organic impotence resulting from an endocrine disorder, usually of either the gonads or the hypothalamus and pituitary gland.

**functional i.,** psychogenic i.

**neurogenic i.,** organic impotence resulting from a lesion in the nervous system, either in the central nervous system or along peripheral nerves such as the nervi erigentes.

**organic i.,** impotence caused by some physical disorder that affects the sexual apparatus, usually classified as either vasculogenic, neurogenic, or endocrinologic. It is sometimes caused by accidental or iatrogenic trauma or it may occur as a side effect of certain drugs. Cf. *psychogenic i.*

**primary i.,** impotence that is persistent throughout the patient's life; formerly thought to be entirely psychogenic, it is now known sometimes to have physical causes such as trauma at a young age or organic disorders.
**psychic i.,** psychogenic i.
**psychogenic i.,** impotence caused by some underlying psychological condition; in DSM-IV, called *male erectile disorder* (q.v.). Cf. *organic i.*
**secondary i.,** impotence occurring in men who previously had experienced normal penile function.
**vasculogenic i.,** organic impotence resulting from some disorder (usually insufficient flow) of penile arteries or veins.

**im·po·ten·cy** (im'pə-tən-se) impotence.

**im·preg·nate** (im-preg'nāt) [L. *impregnare*] 1. fertilize. 2. to saturate or charge with.

**im·preg·na·tion** (im″prəg-na'shən) [L. *impregnatio*] 1. fertilization. 2. the process or act of saturation; a saturated condition.

**im·pres·sio** (im-pres'e-o) pl. *impressio'nes* [L.] [TA] an impression, indentation, or concavity; a general term for an indentation produced in the surface of one organ by pressure exerted by another.
**i. cardi'aca he'patis** [TA], cardiac impression of the liver: a depression on the superior part of the mediastinal (medial) surface of the liver, corresponding to the position of the heart.
**i. cardi'aca pulmo'nis** [TA], cardiac impression of lung: the indentation on the medial surface of either lung produced by the heart and pericardium.
**i. co'lica he'patis** [TA], colic impression of liver: a variable concavity in the right lobe of the liver, where it is in contact with the right flexure of the colon.
**impressio'nes digita'tae,** TA alternative for *impressiones gyrorum.*
**i. duodena'lis he'patis** [TA], duodenal impression of liver: a concavity on the right lobe of the liver where it is in contact with the descending part of the duodenum.
**i. esopha'gea he'patis,** i. oesophagea hepatis.
**i. gas'trica he'patis** [TA], gastric impression of liver: a large concavity in the left lobe of the liver where it is in contact with the anterior surface of the stomach.
**i. gas'trica re'nis,** gastric impression of kidney: a concavity on the anterior surface of the left kidney where it is in contact with the stomach.
**impressio'nes gyro'rum** [TA], impressions of cerebral gyri: poorly defined depressions on the inner surface of the cranium, corresponding to the gyri of the brain. Called also *digital* or *digitate impressions, gyrate impressions, impressiones digitatae* [TA alternative] and *juga cerebralia* [TA alternative].
**i. hepa'tica re'nis,** hepatic impression of kidney: an impression on the anterior surface of the left kidney where it is in contact with the liver.
**i. ligamen'ti costoclavicula'ris** [TA], impression of costoclavicular ligament: the point on the inferior surface of the clavicle where the costoclavicular ligament is attached; called also *tuberositas costalis claviculae* and *costal tuberosity of clavicle.*
**i. meningea'lis,** see *foveolae granulares,* under *foveola.*
**i. muscula'ris re'nis,** muscular impression of kidney: a depression on the posterior surface of the kidney where it is in contact with the psoas muscle.
**i. oesopha'gea he'patis** [TA], esophageal impression of liver: a concavity on the left hepatic lobe corresponding to the position of the abdominal part of the esophagus.
**i. petro'sa pal'lii,** petrosal impression of pallium: a shallow groove on the base of the brain corresponding to the superior angle of the petrous portion of the temporal bone.
**i. rena'lis he'patis** [TA], renal impression of liver: the concavity on the right lobe of the liver where it is in contact with the right kidney.
**i. suprarena'lis he'patis** [TA], suprarenal impression of liver: a small concavity on the right lobe of the liver, superior to the renal impression, caused by contact with the right adrenal (suprarenal) gland.
**i. trigemina'lis os'sis tempora'lis** [TA], **i. trige'mini os'sis tempora'lis,** trigeminal impression of temporal bone: the shallow impression in the floor of the middle cranial fossa on the petrous part of the temporal bone, lodging the semilunar ganglion of the trigeminal nerve.

**im·pres·sion** (im-presh'ən) [L. *impressio*] 1. a slight indentation or depression; see *impressio.* 2. a negative copy or the impressed reverse of the surface of an object. 3. an effect produced upon the mind, body, or senses by some external stimulus or agent. 4. dental i.
**anatomic i.,** an impression of the form of a dental arch or portion thereof that records the structures in a passive or unstrained form, making possible a static relationship of a prosthesis produced from such an impression.
**basilar i.,** 1. platybasia. 2. basilar invagination.
**bridge i.,** an impression made for the purpose of constructing or assembling a fixed restoration, fixed partial denture, or bridge.
**cardiac i.,** an impression made by the heart on another organ; see *impressio cardiaca hepatis* and *impressio cardiaca pulmonis.*
**i's of cerebral gyri,** impressiones gyrorum.
**cleft palate i.,** an impression of the upper jaw made in patients with cleft palate, to be used in the prosthetic repair of the defect.
**colic i. of liver,** impressio colica hepatis.
**i. of costoclavicular ligament,** impressio ligamenti costoclavicularis.
**deltoid i. of humerus,** tuberositas deltoidea humeri.
**dental i.,** an imprint or negative likeness of the teeth and/or edentulous areas, made in plastic material that becomes hardened or set while in contact with the tissue; it is later filled with plaster of Paris or artificial stone to produce a facsimile of the oral structures present.
**denture i., complete,** 1. one made of the entire edentulous arch of the maxilla or mandible, for the purpose of construction of a complete denture. 2. a negative registration of the entire denture-bearing area of the maxilla or mandible. 3. a negative registration of the entire denture-bearing and border seal areas of the edentulous mouth.
**denture i., partial,** a negative copy of the partially edentulous dental arch or its section made for the purpose of constructing a partial denture.
**digastric i.,** fossa digastrica.
**digital i's, digitate i's,** impressiones gyrorum.
**direct bone i.,** an impression of denuded bone used in the construction of dental implants.
**duodenal i. of liver,** impressio duodenalis hepatis.
**esophageal i. of liver,** impressio oesophagea hepatis.
**final i.,** secondary i.
**gastric i.,** an impression made by the stomach on another organ; see *impressio gastrica hepatis* and *impressio gastrica renis.*
**gastric i. of liver,** impressio gastrica hepatis.
**gyrate i's, i's of gyri,** impressiones gyrorum.
**hydrocolloid i.,** a denture impression made of a hydrocolloid material.
**lower i.,** mandibular i.
**mandibular i.,** an impression of the mandibular jaw and related tissues and dental structures.
**maxillary i.,** an impression of the maxillary jaw and related tissues and dental structures; called also *upper i.*
**meningeal i.,** see *foveolae granulares,* under *foveola.*
**preliminary i.,** primary i.
**primary i.,** an impression of the edentulous mouth that usually lacks fine details of the tissue and is often used for construction of a secondary impression. Called also *preliminary i.*
**renal i. of liver,** impressio renalis hepatis.
**rhomboid i. of clavicle,** impressio ligamenti costoclavicularis.
**secondary i.,** an impression made by using an impression material in a tray, produced by the primary impression method for the reproduction of fine details of an edentulous mouth. Called also *final i.*
**sectional i.,** a dental impression that is made in sections.
**suprarenal i. of liver,** impressio suprarenalis hepatis.
**trigeminal i. of temporal bone,** impressio trigemini ossis temporalis.
**upper i.,** maxillary i.

**im·pres·sio·nes** (im-pres″e-o'nēz) [L.] plural of *impressio.*

**im·print·ing** (im-print'ing) rapid learning of species-specific behavior patterns that occurs with exposure to the proper stimulus at a sensitive period of early life.
**genomic i.,** differential expression of a gene or genes as a function of whether they were inherited from the male or the female parent, e.g., a deletion on chromosome 15 that causes Prader-Willi syndrome if inherited from the father causes instead Angelman's syndrome if inherited from the mother.

**im·pulse** (im'pəls) 1. a sudden pushing force. 2. a sudden uncontrollable determination to act. 3. nerve i.
**apex i., apical i.,** see under *beat.*
**cardiac i.,** the palpable or recorded movement of the chest wall caused by the heartbeat.
**ectopic i.,** 1. the impulse that causes an ectopic beat. 2. a pathologic nerve impulse that begins in the middle of an axon and proceeds simultaneously towards the cell body and the periphery; it may be connected to a paresthesia or some other disorder of transmission.
**irresistible i.,** an impulse to commit a criminal act that cannot be resisted because mental disease has destroyed the person's freedom of will and power to choose between right and wrong. The "irresistible impulse test" that a person is not criminally responsible if the act was due to an irresistible impulse is still used in some states.
**left parasternal i's,** cardiac impulses categorized according to their location along the upper, mid, or lower left sternal border. An *upper*

*left parasternal impulse* is usually caused by a systolic expansion of a dilated pulmonary artery; a *mid* to *lower left parasternal impulse* usually occurs as a result of a right ventricular contraction, and is characterized by an outward movement beginning synchronously with the first heart sound, but is sometimes caused by mitral incompetence.
**nerve i., neural i.,** the electrochemical process propagated along nerve fibers.
**right parasternal i's,** cardiac impulses categorized according to their location along the upper, mid, or lower right sternal border.

**im·pul·sion** (im-pul′shən) blind obedience to internal drives, without regard for acceptance by others or pressure from the superego; seen in children and in adults with weak defensive organization.

**im·pu·ta·tion** (im″pu-ta′shən) the use of statistical methods to estimate missing values from available values when data are missing, e.g., due to lack of response to a survey.

**Im·u·ran** (im′u-ran) trademark for preparations of azathioprine.

**IMV** intermittent mandatory ventilation; see under *ventilation.*

**IMViC, imvic** a mnemonic indicating the tests used in classifying coliform bacteria, namely indole, methyl red, Voges-Proskauer, and citrate.

**In** symbol for *indium.*

**in-**[1] [L. *in* in, into] a prefix meaning in or into; occurs as *il-* before *l, im-* before *b, m,* or *p,* and *ir-* before *r.*

**in-**[2] [L. *in-* not] a prefix meaning not; occurs as *il-* before *l, im-* before *b, m,* or *p,* and *ir-* before *r.*

**INA** International Neurological Association.

**in·acid·i·ty** (in″ə-sid′ĭ-te) anacidity.

**in·ac·ti·vate** (in-ak′tĭ-vāt) to render inactive; to destroy the activity of.

**in·ac·ti·va·tion** (in-ak″tĭ-va′shən) the destruction of biological activity, as of a virus or enzyme, by the action of heat or other physical or chemical means.
**complement i.,** any method of destroying the complement activity of serum, such as heat inactivation or treatment with hydrazine.
**heat i.,** any destruction of biological activity by heating, such as the destruction of complement activity in serum by heating to 56°C for 30 minutes.
**X-chromosome i., X-i.,** lyonization.

**in·ac·ti·va·tor** (in-ak′tĭ-va″tər) an agent that renders another inactive.
**anaphylatoxin i. (AI),** a serum carboxypeptidase that destroys the anaphylatoxin activity of C3a, C4a, and C5a by removing C-terminal arginyl or lysyl residues.
**C3b i. (C3b INA),** former name for complement *factor I.*
**electrocerebral i. (ECI),** see under *silence.*

**in·ad·e·qua·cy** (in-ad′ə-kwə-se) [*in-*[2] + *adaequare* to make equal] inability to perform an allotted function; insufficiency; incompetence.

**in·al·i·men·tal** (in″al-ĭ-men′təl) [*in-*[2] + *aliment* + *-al*[1]] not nutritious; not serviceable as food.

**in·an·i·mate** (in-an′ĭ-mət) [*in-*[2] + *animatus* alive] 1. without life. 2. lacking in animation.

**in·a·ni·tion** (in″ə-nish′ən) [L. *inanis* empty] marked weakness, extreme weight loss, and decreased metabolism due to prolonged severe insufficiency of food (starvation).

**in·ap·pe·tence** (in-ap′ə-təns) [*in-*[2] + *appetere* to desire] lack of desire or appetite.

**In·ap·sine** (in-ap′sēn) trademark for a preparation of droperidol.

**in·ar·tic·u·late** (in″ahr-tik′u-lət) [*in-*[2] + *articulate*[2]] not having joints; disjointed; not uttered like articulate speech.

**in ar·tic·u·lo mor·tis** (in ahr-tik′u-lo mor′tis) [L.] at the very point of death.

**in·as·sim·i·la·ble** (in″ə-sim′ĭ-lə-bəl) [*in-*[2] + *assimilable*] not susceptible of being utilized as nutriment.

**in·at·ten·tion** (in″ə-ten′shən) [*in-* + *attention*] lack of attention.
**selective i.,** 1. unilateral neglect. 2. the ignoring or otherwise screening out of stimuli that are threatening, anxiety-producing, or felt to be unimportant.

**in·born** (in′born) congenitally formed, genetically determined, or acquired during intrauterine life; see also *inborn error of metabolism,* under *metabolism.*

**in·breed·ing** (in′brēd-ing) [MeSH: Inbreeding] the mating of closely related individuals, or of individuals having closely similar genetic constitutions.

**in·can·des·cent** (in″cən-des′ənt) [L. *incandescens* glowing] glowing with heat and light; emitting light on being heated.

**in·car·cer·at·ed** (in-kahr′sər-āt″əd) [L. *incarceratus* imprisoned] imprisoned; constricted; subjected to incarceration.

**in·car·cer·a·tion** (in-kahr″sər-a′shən) [L. *in* in + *carcer* prison] unnatural retention or confinement of a part, as may occur in hernia.

**in·car·na·tio** (in″kahr-na′she-o) [L., from *in* in + *caro,* gen. *carnis* flesh] ingrowth.
**i. un′guis,** ingrown toenail.

**in·car·na·tive** (in-kahr′nə-tiv) [L. *incarnare* to invest in flesh] 1. promoting the formation of granulations. 2. an agent that promotes granulations.

**in·cer·tae se·dis** (in-ser′te se′dis) [L.] of uncertain position; said of taxa that are of uncertain classification.

**in·cest** (in′sest) [L. *incestus* impure] [MeSH: Incest] sexual intercourse or other sexual activity between persons so closely related that marriage between them is legally or culturally prohibited.

**inch** (inch) a unit of linear measure, one-twelfth of a foot, being the equivalent of 2.54 cm.

**in·ci·dence** (in′sĭ-dəns) [L. *incidere* to occur, to happen] [MeSH: Incidence] 1. the rate at which a certain event occurs, e.g., the number of new cases of a specific disease occurring during a certain period in a population at risk (see *incidence rate,* under *rate*). Cf. *prevalence.* 2. the arrival of radiant energy at a surface.
**cumulative i.,** cumulative incidence rate.

**in·ci·dent** (in′sĭ-dənt) [L. *incidere* to fall upon] falling or striking upon, as incident radiation.

**in·cin·e·ra·tion** (in-sin″ə-ra′shən) [*in-*[1] + *cineres* ashes] [MeSH: Incineration] the act of burning to ashes; cremation.

**in·cip·i·ent** (in-sip′e-ənt) beginning to exist; coming into existence.

**in·ci·sal** (in-si′zəl) 1. cutting. 2. pertaining to the cutting edge of an anterior tooth.

**in·cised** (in-sīzd′) [L. *incisus*] cut; made by cutting.

**in·ci·sion** (in-sizh′ən) [L. *incidere* to cut open, to cut through] 1. a cut, or a wound produced by cutting with a sharp instrument. 2. the act of cutting.
**Battle's i., Battle-Jalaguier-Kammerer i.,** Kammerer-Battle i.
**Bevan's i.,** one along the outer border of the rectus muscle, for operations in the upper abdominal quadrants.
**celiotomy i.,** an incision made through the abdominal wall to give access to the peritoneal cavity.
**Cherney i.,** an abdominal incision in the surgical approach to the female reproductive organs.
**Deaver's i.,** incision through the anterior sheath of the right rectus muscle, the muscle then being retracted medially.
**Dührssen's i's,** incisions made in the cervix uteri to facilitate delivery.
**epigastric i.,** see illustration.
**Fergusson's i.,** see under *operation.*
**gridiron i.,** McBurney's i.
**Kammerer-Battle i.,** a vertical abdominal incision through the skin and superficial fascia, vertical division of the anterior layer of the rectal sheath, with retraction of the rectus muscle medialward, and

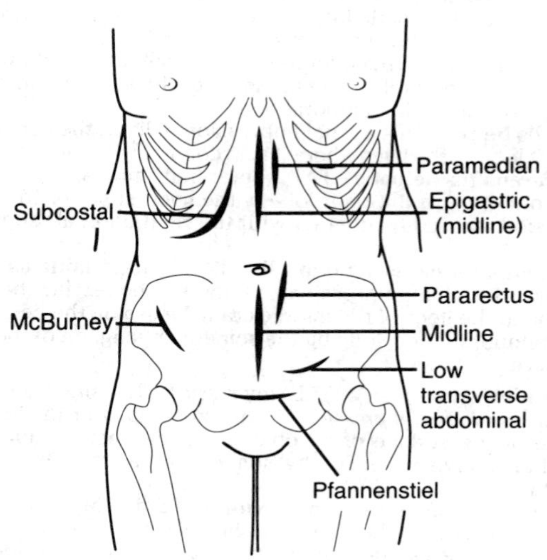


Various abdominal incisions.

vertical division of the posterior layer of the sheath nearer the median line, together with the subserous areolar tissue and peritoneum.
**Kocher's i.,** a subcostal incision that, when made on the right, provides exposure of the gallbladder and common bile duct and, when made on the left, provides exposure for splenectomy or splenorenal venous anastomosis.
**low transverse abdominal i.,** see illustration.
**McBurney's i.,** an abdominal incision parallel to the fibers of the external oblique muscle, about one-third the distance along a line from the anterior superior iliac spine to the umbilicus, half the incision being above and the remainder below this point. The skin and subcutaneous fat are incised down to the external oblique muscle, the fibers of which are split; the underlying internal oblique and transversus abdominalis are then split and separated.
**Maylard i.,** an abdominal incision in the surgical approach to the female reproductive organs.
**midline i.,** see illustration.
**Munro Kerr i.,** a transverse incision of the lower uterine segment for cesarean section.
**Nagamatsu i.,** in renal surgery, an extrapleural retroperitoneal dorsolumbar approach to the kidney that provides an osteoplastic flap of the lower rib cage.
**paramedian i.,** see illustration.
**pararectus i.,** see illustration.
**paravaginal i.,** incision of the vagina and perineum in order to secure enlargement of the vulvovaginal outlet, and thereby permit easy access to the vagina in cancer operations and, rarely, to facilitate childbirth; called also *Schuchardt's i.* and *vaginoperineotomy.*
**Pfannenstiel's i.,** a curved abdominal incision, the convexity being directed downward, just above the symphysis, passing through skin, superficial fascia, and aponeurosis, exposing the pyramidalis and rectus muscles, which are separated from each other in the midline, the peritoneum then being opened vertically. See illustration.
**relief i.,** one made to relieve tension in tissue.
**Rockey-Davis i.,** an incision similar to McBurney's incision, except that the skin incision is transverse rather than vertical.
**Schuchardt's i.,** paravaginal i.
**subcostal i.,** see illustration.
**Warren's i.,** an incision following the thoracomammary fold, permitting access to any part of the breast.

**in•ci•sive** (in-si'siv) [L. *incisivus*] 1. having the power or quality of cutting. 2. pertaining to the incisor teeth.

**in•ci•so•la•bi•al** (in-si″zo-la'be-əl) denoting the incisal and labial surfaces of an anterior tooth.

**in•ci•so•lin•gual** (in-si″zo-ling'gwəl) denoting the incisal and lingual surfaces of an anterior tooth.

**in•ci•so•prox•i•mal** (in-si″zo-prok'sĭ-məl) denoting the incisal and proximal surfaces of an anterior tooth.

**in•ci•sor** (in-si'zor) [L. *incidere* to cut into] [MeSH: Incisor] 1. adapted for cutting. 2. incisor tooth.
**central i., first i.,** the two incisor teeth (see under *tooth*) in each jaw which are located closer to the midline of the body.
**hawk-bill i's,** shovel-shaped i's.
**Hutchinson's i's,** see under *tooth.*
**lateral i.,** the second incisor tooth on either side of the midline of each jaw, located distal to the central incisor and mesial to the canine.
**medial i.,** central i.
**second i.,** lateral i.
**shovel-shaped i's,** large upper medial incisor teeth that are concave on the lingual side; called also *hawk-bill i's.*
**winged i.,** a rotation deformity of a maxillary incisor tooth in which the distal edge of the tooth protrudes labially.

**in•ci•su•ra** (in-si-su'rə) gen. and pl. *incisu'rae* [L., from *incidere* to cut into] [TA] a cut, notch, or incision; a general term for an indentation or depression, chiefly on the edge of a bone or other structure. Called also *incisure* and *notch.*

## Incisura

Descriptions of anatomic structures are given on TA terms, and include anglicized names of specific incisurae.

**i. acetabula'ris, i. aceta'buli** [TA], acetabular notch: a notch in the inferior portion of the lunate surface of the acetabulum.
**i. angula'ris gas'tris** [TA], **i. angula'ris ventri'culi,** angular incisure of stomach: the lowest point on the lesser curvature of the stomach, marking the junction of the cranial two-thirds and caudal one-third of the stomach. Called also *angular notch of stomach* and *gastric notch.*
**i. ante'rior auri'culae** [TA], anterior notch of auricle: a depression between the crus of the helix and the tragus; called also *auricular notch.*
**i. a'picis cor'dis** [TA], notch of cardiac apex: a slight notch found at the site where the anterior and posterior interventricular sulci become continuous and cross the right margin of the heart.
**i. cardi'aca gas'tris,** i. cardialis.
**i. cardi'aca pulmo'nis sinis'tri** [TA], cardiac notch of left lung: a notch in the anterior border of the left lung.
**i. cardi'aca ventri'culi,** i. cardialis.
**i. cardia'lis** [TA], cardial notch: a notch at the junction of the esophagus and the greater curvature of the stomach. Called also *cardiac notch of stomach* and *i. cardiaca gastris.*
**i. cartila'ginis mea'tus acus'tici** [TA], notch in cartilage of acoustic meatus: two vertical fissures in the anterior part of the cartilage of the external acoustic meatus.
**i. cerebel'li ante'rior,** a wide notch on the anterior surface of the cerebellum, occupied by the inferior colliculi and superior cerebellar peduncles; called also *anterior cerebellar notch.*
**i. cerebel'li poste'rior,** a notch between the cerebellar hemispheres posteriorly, containing the falx cerebelli; called also *posterior cerebellar notch.*
**i. clavicula'ris ster'ni** [TA], clavicular notch of sternum: an oval surface on each side of the cranial border of the manubrium of the sternum, where it articulates with the clavicle..
**incisu'rae costa'les ster'ni** [TA], costal notches of sternum: the facets on the sternum, seven on each lateral edge, for articulation with the costal cartilages.
**i. ethmoida'lis os'sis fronta'lis** [TA], ethmoidal notch of frontal bone: a space between the orbital parts of the frontal bone, in which the ethmoid bone is lodged.
**i. fasti'gii,** a transverse furrow on the ventricular surface of the cerebellar lamina of the developing cerebellum.
**i. fibula'ris ti'biae** [TA], fibular notch of tibia: a depression on the lateral surface of the lower end of the tibia, which articulates with the lower end of the fibula.
**i. fronta'lis** [TA], frontal notch: a notch located in the supraorbital margin of the frontal bone medial to the supraorbital notch or foramen, for transmission of branches of the supraorbital nerve and vessels; frequently converted into a foramen *(foramen frontale)* by a bridge of osseous tissue.
**i. interarytenoi'dea** [TA], interarytenoid notch: the posterior portion of the aditus laryngis between the two arytenoid cartilages.
**i. interloba'ris he'patis,** i. ligamenti teretis.
**i. intertra'gica** [TA], intertragic incisure: the notch at the lower part of the pinna of the ear between the tragus and the antitragus; called also *intertragic notch.*
**i. ischia'dica ma'jor** [TA], greater sciatic notch: the large notch on the posterior border of the hip bone, where the posterior borders of the ilium and the ischium become continuous. Called also *greater ischiadic notch,* and *greater notch of ischium.*
**i. ischia'dica mi'nor** [TA], lesser sciatic notch: the notch on the posterior border of the ischium just inferior to the ischiadic spine. Called also *lesser ischiadic notch* and *lesser notch of ischium.*
**i. ischia'lis ma'jor,** i. ischiadica major.
**i. ischia'lis mi'nor,** i. ischiadica minor.
**i. jugula'ris os'sis occipita'lis** [TA], jugular notch of occipital bone: a notch on the anterior surface of the jugular process of the occipital bone, forming the posterior wall of the jugular foramen.
**i. jugula'ris os'sis tempora'lis** [TA], jugular notch of temporal bone: a prominent depression on the inferior surface of the petrous part of the temporal bone. It forms the anterior and lateral wall of the jugular foramen and lodges the superior bulb of the internal jugular vein in its lateral part and the glossopharyngeal, vagus, and accessory nerves in its medial part.
**i. jugula'ris ster'ni** [TA], jugular notch of sternum: the notch on the upper border of the sternum between the clavicular notches; called also *interclavicular, presternal,* or *suprasternal notch.*
**i. lacrima'lis maxil'lae** [TA], lacrimal notch of maxilla: an indenta-

tion on the posterior border of the frontal process of the maxilla, that lodges the lacrimal sac.

**i. ligamen'ti te'retis** [TA], notch for ligamentum teres: a notch in the inferior border of the liver, occupied by the ligamentum teres in the adult; called also *i. umbilicalis* and *umbilical notch* or *incisure.*

**i. mandi'bulae** [TA], mandibular notch: a deep notch on the upper edge of the ramus of the mandible between the condyle and the coronoid process.

**i. mastoi'dea os'sis tempora'lis** [TA], mastoid notch: a deep groove on the medial surface of the mastoid process of the temporal bone, which gives origin to the posterior belly of the digastric muscle.

**i. nasa'lis maxil'lae** [TA], nasal notch of maxilla: the large notch in the anterior border of the maxilla that forms the lateral and inferior margins of the anterior nasal aperture.

**i. pancre'atis** [TA], pancreatic notch: a notch at the junction of the left half of the head of the pancreas and the neck of the pancreas.

**i. parieta'lis os'sis tempora'lis** [TA], parietal notch of temporal bone: the notch found on the upper margin of the temporal bone where the squamous and parietomastoid sutures meet.

**i. perone'a ti'biae,** i. fibularis tibiae.

**i. preoccipita'lis** [TA], preoccipital notch: a notch near the posterior end of the inferolateral border of the cerebral hemisphere. A line joining it to the parietooccipital sulcus serves to delineate the parietal and temporal lobes from the occipital lobe.

**i. pterygoi'dea** [TA], pterygoid notch: a notch on the inferior portion of the pterygoid processes of the sphenoid bone, where the pyramidal process of the palatine bone is inserted between the diverging medial and lateral pterygoid plates; called also *palatine notch, fissura pterygoidea,* and *pterygoid fissure.*

**i. radia'lis ul'nae** [TA], radial notch of ulna: the cavity on the outer side of the coronoid process, articulating with the rim of the head of the radius.

**i. Rivi'ni,** i. tympanica.

**i. Santori'ni,** 1. i. anterior auriculae. 2. i. cartilaginis meatus acustici.

**i. sca'pulae** [TA], **i. scapula'ris,** suprascapular notch: a notch, converted into a foramen by a ligament, on the upper border of the scapula at the base of the coracoid process; called also *scapular notch.*

**i. semiluna'ris ti'biae,** i. fibularis tibiae.

**i. semiluna'ris ul'nae,** i. trochlearis ulnae.

**i. sphenopalati'na os'sis palati'ni** [TA], sphenopalatine notch of palatine bone: a notch between the orbital and sphenoid processes of the palatine bone; it is converted into a foramen by the inferior surface of the sphenoid bone; called also *palatine notch.*

**i. supraorbita'lis** [TA], supraorbital notch: a palpable notch in the frontal bone at the junction of the medial one-third and lateral two-thirds of the supraorbital margin, for transmission of the supraorbital nerve and vessels to the forehead. In life it is bridged by fibrous tissue, which is sometimes ossified, forming a bony aperture *(foramen supraorbitale).*

**i. tento'rii cerebel'li** [TA], **i. of tentorium of cerebellum,** tentorial notch: an opening at the anterior part of the cerebellum, formed by the free, internal border of the tentorium and the dorsum sellae of the sphenoid, and occupied chiefly by the mesencephalon.

**i. termina'lis auricula'ris** [TA], **i. termina'lis au'ris,** terminal notch of auricle: a deep notch separating the lamina tragi and cartilage of the external acoustic meatus from the main auricular cartilage.

**i. thyroi'dea infe'rior** [TA], inferior thyroid notch: a notch at the lower part of the anterior border of the thyroid cartilage.

**i. thyroi'dea supe'rior** [TA], superior thyroid notch: a deep notch in the upper portion of the anterior border of the thyroid cartilage.

**i. tra'gica,** i. intertragica.

**i. trochlea'ris ul'nae** [TA], trochlear notch of ulna: a large concavity on the anterior surface at the proximal end of the ulna, formed by the olecranon and coronoid processes, for articulation with the trochlea of the humerus. Called also *i. semilunaris ulnae, greater semilunar incisure of ulna,* and *semilunar* or *sigmoid fossa of ulna.*

**i. tympa'nica** [TA], **i. tympa'nica [Rivi'ni],** tympanic notch: a defect in the upper portion of the tympanic part of the temporal bone, between the greater and lesser tympanic spines, which is filled in by the pars flaccida of the tympanic membrane. Called also *Rivinus' incisure* or *notch, rivinian incisure* or *notch,* and *tympanic incisure.*

**i. ulna'ris ra'dii** [TA], ulnar notch of radius: a concavity on the medial side of the distal extremity of the radius, articulating with the head of the ulna..

**i. umbilica'lis,** i. ligamenti teretis.

**i. vertebra'lis infe'rior** [TA], inferior vertebral notch: the indentation found below each pedicle of a vertebra which, with the indentation located above the pedicle of the vertebra below, forms the intervertebral foramen.

**i. vertebra'lis supe'rior** [TA], superior vertebral notch: the indentation found above each pedicle of a vertebra which, with the indentation located below the corresponding pedicle of the vertebra above, forms the intervertebral foramen.

**in·ci·su·rae** (in″si-su′re) [L.] genitive and plural of *incisura.*

**in·ci·sure** (in-si′zhər) a cut, notch, or incision; called also *incisura* [TA].

**i. of acetabulum,** incisura acetabuli.
**angular i. of stomach,** incisura angularis gastris.
**anterior i. of ear,** incisura anterior auriculae.
**i. of apex of heart,** incisura apicis cordis.
**i. of calcaneus,** sulcus tendinis musculi flexoris hallucis longi calcanei.
**cardiac i. of left lung,** incisura cardiaca pulmonis sinistri.
**cardiac i. of stomach,** incisura cardialis.
**i. of cartilage of acoustic meatus,** incisura cartilaginis meatus acustici.
**clavicular i. of sternum,** incisura clavicularis sterni.
**costal i's of sternum,** incisurae costales sterni.
**cotyloid i.,** incisura acetabuli.
**digastric i. of temporal bone,** incisura mastoidea ossis temporalis.
**ethmoidal i. of frontal bone,** incisura ethmoidalis ossis frontalis.
**falciform i. of fascia lata,** margo falciformis hiatus saphenus.
**fibular i. of tibia,** incisura fibularis tibiae.
**frontal i.,** incisura frontalis.
**greater i. of ischium,** incisura ischiadica major.
**humeral i. of ulna,** incisura trochlearis ulnae.
**iliac i., lesser,** incisura ischiadica minor.
**interarytenoid i.,** incisura interarytenoidea.
**interclavicular i.,** incisura jugularis sterni.
**intertragic i.,** incisura intertragica.
**ischiadic i., greater,** incisura ischiadica major.
**ischiadic i., lesser,** incisura ischiadica minor.
**ischial i., greater,** incisura ischiadica major.
**ischial i., lesser,** incisura ischiadica minor.
**jugular i. of occipital bone,** incisura jugularis ossis occipitalis.
**jugular i. of sternum,** incisura jugularis sterni.
**jugular i. of temporal bone,** incisura jugularis ossis temporalis.
**lacrimal i. of maxilla,** incisura lacrimalis maxillae.
**i's of Lanterman, Lanterman-Schmidt i's,** channels of cytoplasm in the myelin sheath of neurons that lead back to the Schwann cell body; they appear as oblique lines or slashes in the sheath. Called also *Lanterman's clefts* and *Schmidt-Lanterman i's.*
**lateral i. of sternum,** incisura clavicularis sterni.
**lesser i. of ischium,** incisura ischiadica minor.
**i. of mandible,** incisura mandibulae.
**mastoid i. of temporal bone,** incisura mastoidea ossis temporalis.
**nasal i. of frontal bone,** margo nasalis ossis frontalis.
**nasal i. of maxilla,** incisura nasalis maxillae.
**obturator i. of pubic bone,** sulcus obturatorius ossis pubis.
**palatine i., palatine i. of Henle,** 1. incisura pterygoidea. 2. incisura sphenopalatina ossis palatini.
**parietal i. of temporal bone,** incisura parietalis ossis temporalis.
**patellar i. of femur,** facies patellaris femoris.
**peroneal i. of tibia,** incisura fibularis tibiae.
**popliteal i.,** fossa intercondylaris femoris.
**preoccipital i.,** incisura preoccipitalis.
**pterygoid i.,** incisura pterygoidea.
**radial i. of ulna,** incisura radialis ulnae.
**rivinian i., Rivinus' i.,** incisura tympanica.
**i. of scapula, scapular i.,** incisura scapulae.
**Schmidt-Lanterman i's,** i's of Lanterman.
**semilunar i.,** incisura scapulae.
**semilunar i. of mandible,** incisura mandibulae.
**semilunar i. of radius,** incisura ulnaris radii.
**semilunar i. of scapula,** incisura scapulae.
**semilunar i. of sternum,** incisura clavicularis sterni.
**semilunar i. of sternum, superior,** incisura jugularis sterni.
**semilunar i. of tibia,** incisura fibularis tibiae.

**semilunar i. of ulna,** incisura trochlearis ulnae.
**semilunar i. of ulna, greater,** incisura trochlearis ulnae.
**semilunar i. of ulna, lesser,** incisura radialis ulnae.
**sigmoid i. of mandible,** incisura mandibulae.
**sigmoid i. of ulna,** incisura trochlearis ulnae.
**sphenopalatine i. of palatine bone,** incisura sphenopalatina ossis palatini.
**sternal i.,** incisura jugularis sterni.
**supraorbital i.,** incisura supraorbitalis.
**suprascapular i.,** incisura scapulae.
**i. of talus,** sulcus tendinis musculi flexoris hallucis longi tali.
**temporal i.,** a slight fissure between the uncus of the parahippocampal gyrus and the apex of the temporal lobe.
**i. of tentorium of cerebellum,** incisura tentorii cerebelli.
**terminal auricular i.,** incisura terminalis auricularis.
**terminal i. of ear,** incisura terminalis auris.
**thoracic i.,** angulus infrasternalis.
**thyroid i., inferior,** incisura thyroidea inferior.
**thyroid i., superior,** incisura thyroidea superior.
**trochlear i. of ulna,** incisura trochlearis ulnae.
**tympanic i.,** incisura tympanica.
**ulnar i. of radius,** incisura ulnaris radii.
**umbilical i.,** incisura ligamenti teretis.
**vertebral i., greater, vertebral i., inferior,** incisura vertebralis inferior.
**vertebral i., lesser, vertebral i., superior,** incisura vertebralis superior.

**in·cli·na·tio** (in″klĭ-na′she-o) pl. *inclinatio′nes* [L., from *inclinare* to lean] inclination.
**i. pel′vis** [TA], pelvic inclination: the angle between the plane of the superior aperture of the minor pelvis and the horizontal plane, when the body is in the erect position; called also *pelvic incline.*

**in·cli·na·tion** (in″klĭ-na′shən) [L. *inclinare* to lean] 1. a deviation from the horizontal or vertical; a sloping or leaning. 2. deviation of the long axis of a tooth from the perpendicular line. 3. deviation of a portion of the surface of a tooth from the general plane of that surface. 4. description of the angles with the surface of a tooth at which the walls of a cavity may be cut, or of the relation of the opposing walls to each other, as *outward inclination, inward inclination,* etc. 5. inclination of enamel rods from a line perpendicular to the surface of a tooth.
**condylar guidance i., condylar guide i.,** the angle of inclination of the condylar guidance to an accepted horizontal plane.
**lateral condylar i.,** the direction of the lateral condyle path.
**lingual i.,** deviation of a tooth from the vertical, in the direction of the tongue.
**pelvic i., i. of pelvis,** inclinatio pelvis.

**in·cli·na·ti·o·nes** (in″klĭ-na″she-o′nēz) [L.] plural of *inclinatio.*

**in·cline** (in′klīn) inclination.
**pelvic i., i. of pelvis,** inclinatio pelvis.

**in·cli·nom·e·ter** (in″klĭ-nom′ə-tər) [*inclination* + *-meter*] an instrument for determining ocular inclinations, angles, and directions of the visual axes.

**in·clu·sion** (in-kloo′zhən) [L. *inclusio*] 1. the act of enclosing or condition of being enclosed. 2. anything that is enclosed; often used alone to refer to cell inclusions.
**cell i.,** a usually lifeless, often temporary, constituent of the cytoplasm of a cell, such as an accumulation of proteins, fats, carbohydrates, pigments, secretory granules, crystals, or other insoluble components.
**dental i.,** 1. a tooth so surrounded with bony material that it is unable to erupt. 2. a cyst of oral soft tissue or bone.
**fetal i.,** endadelphos.
**Guarnieri's i's,** see under *body.*
**intranuclear i's,** inclusion bodies.
**leukocyte i's,** Döhle's bodies.
**Walthard's i's,** see under *islet.*

**in·co·ag·u·la·bil·i·ty** (in″ko-ag″u-lə-bil′ĭ-te) the state of being incoagulable.

**in·co·ag·u·la·ble** (in″ko-ag′u-lə-bəl) not susceptible to coagulation.

**in·co·her·ent** (in″ko-hēr′ənt) [*in-*[2] + *cohaerere* to cling together] without proper sequence; incongruous.

**in·com·pat·i·bil·i·ty** (in″kəm-pat″ĭ-bil′ĭ-te) the quality of being incompatible. See also *histoincompatibility.*
**chemical i.,** the quality of not being miscible with another given substance without a chemical change.
**physiologic i.,** the quality of not being administrable with another given remedy on account of their antagonistic pharmacologic effects.
**therapeutic i.,** opposition in therapeutic effect between two or more medicines.

**in·com·pat·i·ble** (in″kəm-pat′ĭ-bəl) [L. *incompatibilis*] not suitable for combination or simultaneous administration; mutually repellent. See also *histoincompatible.*

**in·com·pe·tence** (in-kom′pə-təns) [L. *in* not + *competens* sufficient] 1. insufficiency. 2. mental inadequacy. 3. the legal status of a person determined by the court to be unable to manage his own affairs.
**aortic i.,** see under *insufficiency.*
**congenital palatopharyngeal i.,** CPI; a congenital variety of velopharyngeal insufficiency.
**atrial chronotropic i.,** inability to increase the heart rate to levels capable of satisfying the needs of the body.
**ileocecal i.,** see under *insufficiency.*
**mitral i.,** see under *insufficiency.*
**primary valvular i.,** venous insufficiency.
**pulmonary i.,** see under *insufficiency.*
**tricuspid i.,** see under *insufficiency.*
**valvular i.,** see under *insufficiency.*
**velopharyngeal i.,** see under *insufficiency.*

**in·com·pe·ten·cy** (in-kom′pə-tən″se) incompetence.

**in·com·pe·tent** (in-kom′pə-tənt) 1. lacking competence; unable to perform the required functions. 2. an individual who is unable to perform the required functions of everyday living. 3. a person determined by the court to be unable to manage his own affairs.

**in·com·pres·si·ble** (in″kəm-pres′ĭ-bəl) not susceptible of being squeezed together.

**in·con·ti·nence** (in-kon′tĭ-nəns) [L. *incontinentia*] 1. inability to control excretory functions, such as defecation (fecal i.) or urination (urinary i.). 2. immoderation or excess.
**active i.,** urinary or fecal incontinence in which the bowels or bladder is emptied involuntarily, but at regular intervals and in the normal way.
**fecal i., i. of the feces,** failure of control of the anal sphincters, with involuntary passage of feces and flatus; it may be either psychogenic or organic in origin. See also *encopresis.*
**intermittent i.,** urinary i. upon sudden movement of or pressure on the bladder, due to interruption of the voluntary path above the lumbar center.
**melanin i., melanin pigment i.,** release of melanin from lysed keratinocytes with uptake by melanophages of the superficial epidermis, producing a slate-colored discoloration of the skin.
**overflow i.,** urinary i. due to pressure of retained urine in the bladder after the bladder has contracted to its limits, with dribbling of urine; called also *paradoxical i.*
**paradoxical i.,** overflow i.
**paralytic i.,** fecal or urinary i. caused by relaxation of the sphincters from destruction of the lumbar centers.
**passive i.,** urinary i. in which the bladder is full and cannot be emptied in the normal way, but the urine dribbles away from mere pressure.
**rectal i.,** fecal i.
**stress i.,** urinary i. due to anatomic displacement that exerts an opening pull on the bladder orifice, as in straining or coughing.
**urge i., urgency i.,** urinary i. preceded by a sudden, uncontrollable impulse to urinate.
**urinary i., i. of urine,** failure of voluntary control of the vesical and urethral sphincters, with constant or frequent involuntary urination. See also *enuresis.*

**in·con·ti·nent** (in-kon′tĭ-nənt) 1. unable to control excretory functions; see *incontinence.* 2. immoderate.

**in·con·ti·nen·tia** (in-kon″tĭ-nen′shə) [L.] incontinence.
**i. al′vi,** fecal incontinence.
**Bloch-Sulzberger i. pigmen′ti,** i. pigmenti.
**Naegeli's i. pigmen′ti,** Franceschetti-Jadassohn syndrome.
**i. pigmen′ti,** a male-lethal X-linked dominant syndrome with onset at birth or shortly thereafter, characterized by the presence of brown or slate-brown bands, whorls, swirls, or splatter-like hyperpigmented cutaneous lesions, preceded by vesiculobullous and verrucous inflammatory changes, often associated with developmental anomalies involving other structures, such as the hair, eyes, and skeletal and central nervous systems. Called also *Bloch-Sulzberger i. pigmenti* and *Bloch-Sulzberger syndrome.* Cf. *Franceschetti-Jadassohn syndrome.*
**i. pigmen′ti achro′mians,** a congenital neurocutaneous syndrome, not present at birth but appearing in early life, characterized by the presence of peculiar whorled, linear, and splatter-like patterns of hypopigmentation, and often associated with other abnormalities,

including hair loss and ocular, musculoskeletal, and mental disturbances. It is unrelated to incontinentia pigmenti. Called also *hypomelanosis of Ito.*

**i. uri'nae,** urinary incontinence.

**in·co·or·di·na·tion** (in″ko-or″dĭ-na'shən) [*in-*[2] + *coordination*] 1. ataxia. 2. failure of organs to work harmoniously.

**in·cor·po·ra·tion** (in-kor″por-a'shən) [L. *in* into + *corpus* body] 1. the union of one substance with another, or with others, in a composite mass. 2. in psychoanalytic theory, a primitive unconscious defense mechanism in which aspects of another person are assimilated into the self through a figurative process of symbolic oral ingestion; it is the earliest mechanism of identification and is a form of introjection.

**in·co·sta·pe·di·al** (ing″ko-sta-pe'de-əl) incudostapedial.

**in·cre·ment** (in'krə-mənt) [L. *incrementum*] addition, or increase; the amount by which a given quantity or value is increased.

**in·cre·tin** (in-kre'tin) any of various gastrointestinal hormones and factors that act as potent stimulators of insulin secretion, such as gastric inhibitory polypeptide.

**in·cre·tion** (in-kre'shən) internal secretion.

**in·cross** (in'kros) [*in-*[1] + *cross* (def. 2)] the mating of individuals homozygous for the same gene; cf. *intercross.*

**in·crus·ta·tion** (in″krəs-ta'shən) [L. *in* on + *crusta* crust] 1. the formation of a crust. 2. a crust, scale, or scab.

**in·cu·bate** (in'ku-bāt) [L. *incubare* to lie in or on; to watch over jealously] 1. to place in an optimal situation for development, as by provision of the proper temperature and humidity for the growth of living cells, such as ova, microorganisms, or tissue cells. 2. to maintain a culture or a reaction mixture at a fixed temperature. 3. material which has been incubated.

**in·cu·ba·tion** (in″ku-ba'shən) [L. *incubatio*] 1. the development of the embryo in the eggs of oviparous animals. 2. the maintenance of an environment with controlled temperature, humidity, and oxygen for the development of an infant, especially of a premature one. 3. the development of an infectious disease from the entrance of the pathogen to the appearance of clinical symptoms (see also under *period,* and cf. *decubation*). 4. the development of microorganisms or other cells in an appropriate medium under controlled environmental conditions, especially of temperature, to permit optimum growth. 5. the process of maintaining reaction mixtures at a given temperature for specified time periods for the development of chemical or enzymatic reactions.

**in·cu·ba·tor** (in'ku-ba-tor) [MeSH: Incubators] 1. an apparatus for maintaining a premature infant in an environment of proper temperature and humidity. 2. an apparatus for maintaining a constant and suitable temperature for the development of eggs, cultures of microorganisms, or other living cells.

**in·cu·dal** (ing'ku-dəl) [L. *incus* anvil] pertaining to the incus.

**in·cu·dec·to·my** (ing″ku-dek'tə-me) [*incus* + *-ectomy*] surgical removal of the incus.

**in·cu·di·form** (ing-ku'dĭ-form) anvil-shaped.

**in·cu·do·mal·le·al** (ing″ku-do-mal'e-əl) incudomalleolar.

**in·cu·do·mal·le·ar** (ing″ku-do-mal'e-ər) incudomalleolar.

**in·cu·do·mal·le·o·lar** (ing″ku-do-mal″e-o'lər) pertaining to the incus and the malleus, particularly to the articulation between them. Called also *incudomalleal* and *incudomallear.*

**in·cu·do·sta·pe·di·al** (ing″ku-do-sta-pe'de-əl) pertaining to the incus and stapes, particularly to the articulation between them.

**in·cur·a·ble** (in-ku'rə-bəl) not susceptible of being cured.

**in·cur·va·tion** (in″kər-va'shən) [L. *incurvare* to bend in] a condition of being bent in.

**in·cus** (ing'kəs) gen. *incu'dis* [L. "anvil"] [TA] [MeSH: Incus] the middle of the three ossicles of the ear, which, with the stapes and malleus, serves to conduct vibrations from the tympanic membrane to the inner ear. Called also *anvil.*

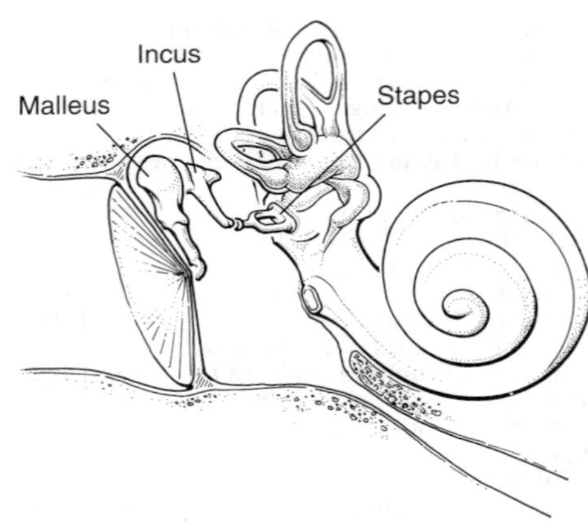


**in·cy·clo·pho·ria** (in-si″klo-for'e-ə) [L. *in* toward + *cyclophoria*] cyclophoria in which the upper pole of the vertical axis of the eye deviates toward the midline of the face, or toward the nose; called also *negative* or *minus cyclophoria.* Cf. *excyclophoria.*

**in·cy·clo·tro·pia** (in-si″klo-tro'pe-ə) [L. *in* toward + *cyclotropia*] cyclotropia in which the upper pole of the vertical axis of the eye deviates toward the midline of the face, or toward the nose; called also *negative* or *minus cyclotropia.*

**in d.** abbreviation for L. *in di'es,* daily.

**in·da·crin·ic ac·id** (in″də-krin'ik) INN for indacrinone.

**in·da·cri·none** (in″də-kri'nōn) a uricosuric diuretic.

**in·dane·di·one** (in″dān-di'ōn) any of a group of synthetic anticoagulants derived from 1,3-indanedione; they are chemically different from the coumarin (q.v.) drugs but similar to them in structure and actions, i.e., they impair the hepatic synthesis of the vitamin K–dependent coagulation factors (prothrombin, factors VII, IX, and X). It includes diphenadione and phenindione, used as anticoagulant drugs, and pindone and valone, used mainly as rodenticides.

**in·dap·amide** (in-dap'ə-mīd) [USP] [MeSH: Indapamide] an antihypertensive and diuretic with actions and uses similar to those of chlorothiazide; administered orally either alone or in combination with other antihypertensive agents.

**In·de·cid·ua** (in″də-sid'u-ə) a division of the class Mammalia, comprising the mammals without a decidua, including whales and ungulates.

**in·den·iza·tion** (in-den″ĭ-za'shən) innidiation.

**in·den·ta·tion** (in″dən-ta'shən) [L. *in* + *dens*] 1. a condition of being notched; a notch, pit, or depression. 2. the act of indenting, as with the finger.

**In·der·al** (in'dər-əl) trademark for a preparation of propranolol hydrochloride.

**In·der·ide** (in'der-īd) trademark for preparations of propranolol hydrochloride with hydrochlorothiazide.

**in·dex** (in'deks) pl. *indexes* or *indices* [L. "that which points out," from *indicare*] 1. [TA] the second digit of the hand, the finger adjacent to the thumb; called also *forefinger, index finger,* and *digitus secundus (II) manus* [TA alternative]. 2. a unitless quantity, usually a ratio of two measurable quantities having the same dimensions, or such a ratio multiplied by 100. 3. a core or mold used in dentistry to record or maintain the relative position of a tooth or teeth to one another and/or to a cast, to ensure reproduction in the dental prosthesis of their original position. 4. a directory, in particular an alphabetized list of terms, each term accompanied by page numbers or other notations telling where it appears in a given work or set of works. 5. a subscript, as in $x_i$, used to indicate that there is a collection of objects, one corresponding to each value of the subscript, with the sequence indexed by $i$. For example, the sequence $x_1$, $x_2$, $x_3$, . . . can be written $x_i$, $i = 1, 2, 3, \ldots$ .

## Index

**absorbancy i.,** absorptivity.

**ACH i.,** an index for nutritional condition of children based on measurements of arm girth, chest depth, and hip width.

**Addiction Severity I. (ASI),** a scale used in assessing alcoholism and substance abuse by measuring the severity of problems in six areas, comprising drug and alcohol abuse, medical, psychological, legal, family and social, and employment and support.

**altitudinal i.,** the relation of the cranial height to the cranial length; called also *height i.* and *length-height i.*

**alveolar i.,** gnathic i.

**Arneth i.,** a calculation formerly much used in reference to the Arneth count of lobes of neutrophil nuclei; in a normal population the percentages with one or two lobes plus half the percentage with three lobes should total 60 per cent.

**auricular i.,** the relation of the width to the height of the auricle of the ear.

**auriculoparietal i.,** the ratio of the breadth of the skull between the auricular points to its greatest breadth.

**auriculovertical i.,** the ratio of the height of the skull superior to the auricular point to its greatest height.

**baric i.,** 100 times the body weight in grams divided by the cube of the height in centimeters.

**Barthel i.,** a common method used for functional assessment (q.v.), using standardized classifications to measure skills such as activities of daily living and mobility.

**basilar i.,** the ratio of the distance between the basion and the alveolar point to the total length of the skull.

**Becker-Lennhoff i.,** Lennhoff's i.

**body build i.,** body weight in grams divided by the square of the height in centimeters.

**body mass i. (BMI),** the weight in kilograms divided by the square of the height in meters or, alternatively, 703.1 times the weight in pounds divided by the square of the height in inches.

**brachial i.,** 100 times the length of the arm from the head of the radius to the styloid process divided by the length of the arm from the acromion to the head of the radius.

**Broders' i.,** an index of malignancy based on the fact that the more undifferentiated or embryonic the cells of a tumor, the more malignant the tumor. Grade 1 contains one fourth undifferentiated cells; grade 2, one half undifferentiated cells; grade 3, three fourths undifferentiated cells; grade 4, all cells undifferentiated.

**Brugsch i.,** 100 times the chest circumference divided by body length.

**calcium i.,** the relative amount of calcium in the blood compared with that in a 1:6000 solution of calcium oxide.

**cardiac i. (CI),** cardiac output per unit time divided by body surface area; normally calculated in liters per minute per square meter.

**cardiothoracic i.,** the size of the heart in relation to the size of the chest, being the greatest transverse diameter of the heart shadow as compared with the greatest transverse diameter of the chest shadow on radioscopy.

**I.-Catalogue,** Index-Catalogue of the Library of the Surgeon General's Office, published from 1880 to 1950; replaced by Current List of Medical Literature published to 1959; in 1960 replaced by Index Medicus.

**centromeric i.,** the ratio of the length of the shorter arm of a mitotic chromosome to the total length of the chromosome.

**cephalic i.,** 100 times the maximal head breadth divided by the maximal head length.

**cephalo-orbital i.,** 100 times the capacity of the cranium divided by the capacity of the two orbits.

**cephalorachidian i., cephalorhachidian i.,** cerebrospinal i.

**cephalospinal i.,** the ratio of the area of the foramen magnum in square meters and the cranial capacity in cubic centimeters.

**cerebral i.,** the ratio of the greatest transverse to the greatest anteroposterior diameter of the cranial cavity.

**cerebrospinal i.,** the figure obtained by multiplying the final cerebrospinal pressure by the quantity of fluid withdrawn in spinal puncture and then dividing by the initial pressure.

**chemotherapeutic i.,** therapeutic i.

**Colour I.,** a publication of the Society of Dyers and Colourists and the American Association of Textile Chemists and Colorists containing an extensive list of dyes and dye intermediates. Each chemically distinct compound is identified by a specific number, the CI number, avoiding the confusion of trivial names used for dyes in the dye industry.

**coronofrontal i.,** the ratio of the greatest frontal to the greatest coronal breadth of the head.

**cranial i.,** 100 times the maximal breadth of the skull divided by its length.

**Cumulated I. Medicus,** an annual publication of the National Library of Medicine, comprising the twelve monthly issues of the Index Medicus.

**degenerative i.,** the percentage of neutrophils exhibiting toxic granulation (basophilic granules probably representing phagosomes or autophagic vacuoles).

**dental i.,** a craniometric index obtained by multiplying the dental length by 100 and dividing the product by the basinasal length. Called also *Flower's i.*

**dyspnea i.,** the ratio of peak exercise ventilation to maximal voluntary ventilation.

**effective temperature i.,** an index indicating the warmth due to air temperature, air movement, and humidity.

**endemic i.,** the percentage of persons in any locality affected with an endemic disease.

**erythrocyte indices,** the mean corpuscular volume, mean corpuscular hemoglobin, and mean corpuscular hemoglobin concentration. Called also *red blood cell indices* and *red cell indices.*

**facial i.,** the relation of the length of the face to its width, obtained by multiplying by 100 the bizygomatic width and dividing the product by the distance from the ophryon to the alveolar point.

**fatigue i.,** the ratio between the muscle tension after a period of intermittent tetanic stimulation and the tension present before stimulation was applied.

**femorohumeral i.,** 100 times the length of the humerus divided by the length of the femur.

**Flower's i.,** dental i.

**forearm-hand i.,** 100 times the length of the hand divided by the length of the forearm.

**Fourmentin's thoracic i.,** the number obtained by multiplying the transverse diameter of the thorax by 100 and dividing by the anteroposterior diameter.

**free thyroxine i.,** an estimate of the physiologically active free thyroxine in serum, obtained by multiplying the total serum thyroxine concentration by the thyroxine uptake.

**free triiodothyronine i.,** an estimate of the physiologically active free triiodothyronine in serum, obtained by multiplying the total serum triiodothyronine concentration by the triiodothyronine uptake.

**gnathic i.,** the degree of prominence of the upper jaw, expressed as a percentage of the distance from basion to nasion. Called also *alveolar i.*

**habitus i.,** 100 times the sum of the chest girth and the abdominal girth divided by the stature.

**hair i.,** the figure obtained by dividing the least diameter of the cross section of a hair by its greatest diameter and multiplying by 100; a high index indicates an approximately round shape; a low index indicates an ovoid cross section.

**hand i.,** 100 times the breadth of the hand divided by the length of the hand.

**height i.,** altitudinal i.

**intermembral i.,** 100 times the length of the humerus plus radius divided by the length of the femur plus tibia.

**juxtaglomerular i.,** semiquantitative estimation of the degree of granulation of juxtaglomerular cells, obtained by a counting method and expressed as a ratio to the number of glomeruli.

**length-breadth i.,** the breadth of the skull expressed as a percentage of its length.

**length-height i.,** the height of the skull expressed as a percentage of its length.

**Lennhoff's i.,** the number obtained by dividing 100 times the distance from the sternal notch to the symphysis pubis by the greatest circumference of the abdomen.

**lower leg–foot i.,** 100 times the length of the foot divided by the length of the lower leg.

**maxilloalveolar i.,** the distance between the two most lateral points on the external surface of the upper alveolar margin, usually opposite the middle of the second permanent molar teeth, divided by the maxilloalveolar length.

**I. Medicus,** a monthly publication of the National Library of Medicine in which the world's leading biomedical literature is indexed by author and subject; see also *Cumulated I. Medicus.*

**metacarpal i.,** the average of the figures obtained by dividing the lengths of the right second, third, fourth, and fifth metacarpal bones by their respective breadths at the exact midpoint; stated to range normally between 5.4 and 7.9. A value above 8.4 is diagnostic of arachnodactyly.

**mitotic i.,** the ratio of the number of cells in a population undergoing mitosis to the number not undergoing mitosis.

**morphologic face i.,** 100 times the distance from the nasion to the gnathion divided by the bizygomatic breadth.

**morphological i.,** the volume of the trunk divided by the length of the limbs.

**nasal i.,** 100 times the maximal breadth of the nasal aperture divided by the nasion-nasospinale height.

**nucleoplasmic i.,** the relation of the size of the nucleus of a cell to that of the cytoplasm, expressed numerically by the quotient of the nuclear volume divided by the difference between the volume of the cell and the nuclear volume.

**obesity i.,** body weight divided by body volume.
**opsonic i.,** a measure of opsonic activity determined by the ratio of the number of microorganisms phagocytized by normal leukocytes in the presence of serum from an individual infected by the microorganism, to the number phagocytized in serum from a normal individual.
**orbital i. (of Broca),** 100 times the height of the opening of the orbit, divided by its width.
**palatal i., palatine i., palatomaxillary i.,** a numerical expression of the ratio of various proportions of the palate obtained by multiplying the palatal breadth by 100 and dividing the product by the palatal length. See also *brachystaphyline* and *leptostaphyline.*
**parasite i.,** the percentage of individuals in a population whose blood smears show the presence of parasites.
**penile brachial i.,** the ratio of the penile systolic pressure to the radial systolic pressure; a ratio of less than 0.6 indicates impotence resulting from vascular incompetence.
**peripheral vascular resistance i.,** a measure of the total vascular resistance, normalized for body surface area.
**phagocytic i.,** any arbitrary measure of the ability of neutrophils to ingest native or opsonized particles determined by various assays; it reflects either the average number of particles ingested or the rate at which particles are cleared from the blood or culture medium.
**physiognomonic upper face i.,** 100 times the distance from the nasion to the stomion divided by the bizygomatic breadth.
**Pirquet's i.** (of nutritional status), multiply the weight in grams by 10, divide this product by the sitting height in centimeters and extract the cube root of this quotient. A result lower than 0.945 indicates faulty nutrition. See also *pelidisi.*
**ponderal i.,** an index of body mass equal to 100 times the weight in grams divided by the square of the height (or of the crown-heel length in newborns) in centimeters.
**Quarterly Cumulative I. Medicus,** a former publication of the American Medical Association, in which was indexed most of the medical literature in the world; replaced by Cumulated I. Medicus.
**radiohumeral i.,** 100 times the maximal length of the radius divided by the maximal length of the humerus.
**rapid shallow breathing i.,** the ratio of respiratory rate to tidal volume during spontaneous breathing; a higher value means less effective spontaneous breathing and greater likelihood of need for assisted ventilation.
**red blood cell indices, red cell indices,** erythrocyte indices.
**refractive i.,** the refractive power of a medium compared with that of air, which is assumed to be 1. Symbol n, *n,* or $n_D$.
**sacral i.,** 100 times the breadth of the sacrum divided by the length.
**short increment sensitivity i. (SISI),** tones of 1- to 5-decibel increments in intensity and lasting 0.5 second are superimposed on a continuous (carrier) tone of the same frequency at random intervals, the carrier tone being 20 decibels above the speech reception threshold; only patients with cochlear damage can detect these increments.
**spleen i., splenic i.,** the percentage of individuals in the population having enlarged spleens; used in malaria surveys.
**splenometric i.,** an index of the amount of malarial infection; obtained by multiplying the spleen rate by the size of the average enlarged spleen.
**stimulation i. (SI),** see *lymphocyte proliferation test,* under *tests.*
**stroke i.,** the stroke volume per heartbeat corrected for body surface area; usually expressed in mL per beat per square meter.
**therapeutic i.,** originally, the ratio of the maximum tolerated dose to the minimum curative dose; now defined, so as to account for variability of individual response, as the ratio of the median lethal dose ($LD_{50}$) to the median effective dose ($ED_{50}$). It is used in assessing the safety of a drug. Called also *chemotherapeutic i.*
**thoracic i.,** the ratio of the anteroposterior diameter of the thorax to the transverse diameter.
**tibiofemoral i.,** 100 times the length of the tibia divided by the length of the femur.
**tibioradial i.,** 100 times the length of the radius divided by the length of the tibia.
**trunk i.,** 100 times the bi-acromial breadth divided by the sitting suprasternal height.
**uricolytic i.,** the percentage of uric acid oxidized to allantoin before being secreted.
**venous filling i.,** a measure of the rate of refilling of the veins, usually in the legs, expressed in milliliters per second; calculated by dividing 0.9 of the functional venous volume by the time needed to go from minimum volume (after patient has been supine with legs elevated) to 0.9 of the venous volume (with patient standing up).
**vertical i.,** 100 times the height of the skull divided by the length of the skull.
**zygomaticoauricular i.,** the ratio between the zygomatic and auricular diameters of the skull.

**in·di·can** (in'dĭ-kən) [MeSH: Indican] 1. a yellow indoxyl glycoside from plants that yield indigo. On hydrolysis it yields glucose and indoxyl. 2. potassium indoxyl sulfate, formed by decomposition of tryptophan in the intestines, absorbed, conjugated, and excreted in the urine.

**in·di·can·emia** (in″dĭ-kə-ne'me-ə) the presence of indican in the blood.

**in·di·can·me·ter** (in″dĭ-kən-me'tər) an instrument for estimating the amount of indican in the urine.

**in·di·cano·ra·chia** (in″dĭ-kan-o-ra'ke-ə) the presence of indican in the spinal fluid.

**in·di·cant** (in'dĭ-kənt) 1. indicating. 2. a symptom which indicates the true diagnosis or treatment.

**in·di·can·uria** (in″dĭ-kə-nu're-ə) the presence in the urine of indican in excessive quantity.

**in·di·car·mine** (in″dĭ-kahr'mēn) indigotindisulfonate sodium.

**in·di·ca·tio** (in″dĭ-ka'she-o) [L., from *indicare* to point out] indication.
**i. causa'lis,** an indication as to the treatment of a disease afforded by its cause.
**i. curati'va, i. mor'bi,** an indication as to treatment afforded by the nature of the morbid processes observed.
**i. symptoma'tica,** an indication as to disease afforded by the symptoms that may arise.

**in·di·ca·tion** (in″dĭ-ka'shən) [L. *indicatio*] a sign or circumstance which points to or shows the cause, pathology, treatment, or issue of an attack of disease; that which points out; that which serves as a guide or warning.

**in·di·ca·tor** (in'dĭ-ka″tər) [L.] 1. the index finger (index [TA]). 2. the extensor muscle of the index finger (musculus extensor indicis [TA]). 3. a substance, usually a dye or intermediate, that shows the concentration of a substance, the completion of a reaction, or the attainment of a particular pH range by a change in color or other visible sign.
**anaerobic i.,** a dilute solution of methylene blue is decolorized in the absence of oxygen.
**biological i.,** a viable culture of specific microorganisms resistant to a given sterilization process, used to develop sterilization processes or monitor sterilization cycles; it may consist of spores added to paper, glass or plastic carrier or of spores added to representative units of the lot to be sterilized (or to similar units).
**dew point i.,** an instrument for measuring relative humidity or moisture content of a gas by measuring its dew point.
**radioactive i.,** see under *tracer.*
**redox i.,** a pigment which indicates by a change of color a change in the oxidation potential.
**Schneider's i.,** an index designed to reflect cardiovascular fitness, based mainly on heart rate during and after mild exercise.

**in·di·co·phose** (in'dĭ-ko″fōz) an indigo-colored phose.

**In·di·el·la** (in″de-el'ə) former name for the genus *Madurella.*

**in·dif·fé·rence** (ă-de″fa-rahns') [Fr.] indifference.
**la belle i.** [Fr. "beautiful indifference"], an inappropriately complacent attitude toward their condition and symptoms shown by individuals with conversion disorder.

**in·dif·fer·ent** (in-dif'ər-ənt) [L. *indifferens*] not tending one way or another; neutral; having no preponderating affinity.

**in·dig·e·nous** (in-dij'ə-nəs) [L. *indigenus*] native, or not exotic; native to a particular place or country.

**in·di·gest·i·ble** (in″di-jes'tĭ-bəl) [*in-*[2] + *digestible*] not susceptible of being digested.

**in·di·ges·tion** (in″dĭ-jes'chən) lack or failure of digestion; commonly used to denote vague abdominal discomfort after meals.
**acid i.,** hyperchlorhydria.
**fat i.,** inability to digest fat; steatorrhea.

**gastric i.**, indigestion taking place in or due to some disorder of the stomach.
**intestinal i.**, imperfect performance of the digestive function of the intestine.
**sugar i.**, defective ability to digest sugar, resulting in fermentative diarrhea.
**vagus i.**, a condition in cattle and sometimes sheep caused by damage to the vagus nerve, such as after traumatic reticuloperitonitis; characteristics include impaired motility through the stomachs and intestines, abdominal distention, chronic constipation, and anorexia.

**in·dig·i·ta·tion** (in-dij″ĭ-ta′shən) [L. *in* into + *digitus* finger] intussusception (def. 1).

**in·di·go** (in′dĭ-go) [Gr. *Indikon* Indian dye] 1. any of various plants of the genus *Indigofera.* 2. a blue dyeing material, the aglycon of indican, found in *I. tinctoria* and other plants, or made synthetically. It is sometimes found in the sweat and the urine, where it is derived from urinary indican (indoxyl sulfate).

**In·di·gof·e·ra** (in″dĭ-gof′ə-rə) a genus of leguminous herbs. *I. do′minii* (formerly called *I. ennea′phylla*) causes Birdsville disease among horses in Australia. *I. spica′ta* causes liver damage in horses. *I. tincto′ria* is a source of indigo.

**in·di·go·gen** (in′dĭ-go-jən) a crystalline principle from indigo.

**in·di·go·pur·pu·rine** (in″dĭ-go-pur′pu-rin) a purple pigment occasionally found in the urine.

**in·dig·o·tin** (in″dĭ-go′tin) a neutral, tasteless, dark blue powder, the principal ingredient of commercial indigo; called also *indigo blue.*

**in·di·go·tin·di·sul·fon·ate so·di·um** (in″dĭ-go″tin-di-sul′fo-nāt) [USP] a dye, occurring as a dusky, purplish blue powder or blue granules; used as a diagnostic aid for determining renal function, administered intravenously. Called also *indigo carmine, indicarmine,* and *soluble indigo blue.*

**in·di·na·vir sul·fate** (in-di′nə-vir) [MeSH: Indinavir] a protease inhibitor active against the human immunodeficiency virus, causing the formation of immature, noninfectious viral particles, used in the treatment of human immunodeficiency virus infection and acquired immunodeficiency syndrome; administered orally.

**in·di·rect** (in″di-rekt′) [L. *indirectus*] 1. not immediate or straight. 2. acting through an intermediary agent.

**in·di·ru·bin** (in″di-roo′bin) a red pigment occasionally found in the urine.

**in·di·ru·bin·uria** (in″di-roo″bĭ-nu′re-ə) the presence of indirubin in the urine.

**in·dis·crim·i·nate** (in″dis-krim′ĭ-nət) [L. *in* not + *discrimen* distinction] affecting various parts without distinction.

**in·dis·po·si·tion** (in″dis-pə-zish′ən) the condition of being slightly ill; a slight illness.

**in·di·um** (in′de-əm) [L. *indicum* indigo] [MeSH: Indium] a metallic element; atomic number, 49; atomic weight, 114.82; symbol, In; named from its blue line in the spectrum. It is used in semiconductor research and in bearing alloys.
**i. 111**, an artificial radioactive isotope of indium, having a half-life of 2.81 days; it decays by electron capture, emitting 0.172 and 0.247 MeV gamma rays, and is used as a tracer in nuclear medicine.
**i. 113m**, a radioactive isotope having a half-life of 1.66 hours, decaying by isomeric transition and emitting gamma rays of energy 0.393 MeV; used as a radioactive tracer in nuclear medicine.
**i. In 111 chloride,** see under *solution.*
**i. In 111 DTPA,** i. 111 pentetate.
**i. In 111 oxine,** i. In 111 oxyquinoline.
**i. In 111 oxyquinoline** [USP], a chelate of $^{111}$In with oxyquinoline, used to label platelets and leukocytes; labeled leukocytes are used for the diagnosis and localization of inflammatory lesions, as in abscesses, infections, or inflammatory bowel diseases, and labeled platelets are used in the detection of thrombi and studies of platelet survival.
**i. In 111 pentetate** [USP], a chelate of $^{111}$In with pentetic acid, administered intrathecally, intracisternally, or intraventricularly in radionuclide cisternography to evaluate disorders of the flow of cerebrospinal fluid.
**i. In 111 pentetreotide** [USP], a chelate of $^{111}$In with the somatostatin analogue pentetreotide, used in the imaging of neuroendocrine tumors with somatostatin receptors; administered intravenously.
**i. In 111 satumomab pentetide,** an indium 111–labeled monoclonal antibody used as a diagnostic imaging agent to determine the location and extent of extrahepatic malignant lesions in patients with colorectal or ovarian cancer.

**in·di·vid·u·a·tion** (in″dĭ-vid″u-a′shən) [MeSH: Individuation] 1. the process of developing individual characteristics. 2. differential regional activity in the embryo occurring in response to organizer influence.

**In·do·cin** (in′do-sin) trademark for a preparation of indomethacin.

**in·dol·ac·e·tu·ria** (in″dōl-as″ə-tu′re-ə) the presence of indoleacetic acid in the urine; excessive amounts of 5-OH-indoleacetic acid, the urinary metabolite of serotonin, may be excreted when carcinoid tumors are present.

**in·dol·amine** (in-dol′ə-mēn) an amine-substituted derivative of indole, e.g., serotonin or melatonin.

**in·dole** (in′dōl) a heterocyclic compound, obtained from coal tar, and produced by the decomposition of tryptophan in the intestine, being partly responsible for the peculiar odor of the feces. It is also found in cultures of *Vibrio cholerae* and other bacteria; a color test for its production is used in classifying enteric bacteria.

**in·dole·ace·tic acid** (in″dōl-ə-se′tik) a plant growth hormone (auxin) commonly found in higher plants. Called also *auxin B* and *heteroauxin.*

**in·do·lent** (in′do-lənt) [L. *in* not + *dolens* painful] 1. causing little pain, as an indolent lesion. 2. slow growing, as an indolent tumor.

**in·do·log·e·nous** (in″do-loj′ə-nəs) causing the formation of indole.

**in·dol·uria** (in″dōl-u′reə) the presence of indole in the urine.

**in·do·meth·a·cin** (in″do-meth′ə-sin) [USP] [MeSH: Indomethacin] a nonsteroidal anti-inflammatory agent; used in the treatment of rheumatoid arthritis, osteoarthritis, ankylosing spondylitis, and acute gouty arthritis.
**i. sodium** [USP], the trihydrated sodium salt of indomethacin, used to induce closure of a hemodynamically significant patent ductus arteriosus in premature infants weighing between 500 and 1750 g who do not respond to conservative treatment; administered intravenously.

**in·do·phe·nol** (in″do-fe′nol) [MeSH: Indophenol] any one of a series of dyes which are nitrogen derivatives of quinone.

**in·dor·a·min** (in-dor′ə-min) [MeSH: Indoramin] a selective antagonist of alpha$_1$-adrenergic receptors, used as an antihypertensive; administered orally.

**in·dox·yl** (in-dok′səl) [*indigo* + *ox-* + *-yl*] an oxidation product of indole, formed by decomposition from tryptophan and excreted in the urine as indican (potassium indoxyl sulfate).

**in·dox·yl·emia** (in-dok″sə-le′me-ə) the presence of indoxyl in the blood.

**in·dox·yl·uria** (in-dok″sə-lu′re-ə) the presence of an excess of indoxyl in the urine.

**in·duced** (in-do͞ost′) [L. *inducere* to lead in] 1. produced artificially. 2. produced by induction.

**in·duc·er** (in-do͞os′ər) in molecular genetics, a molecule that causes a cell or organism to accelerate synthesis of an enzyme or sequence of enzymes in response to an environmental signal. The inducer often acts by antagonizing the action of a corresponding repressor, and may be a substrate of the enzyme or may be some other molecule, such as a hormone.

**in·du·ci·ble** (in-doo′sĭ-bəl) produced because of stimulation by an inducer; cf. *constitutive.*

**in·duc·tance** (in-duk′təns) that property of a circuit whereby changing current generates an electromotive force (EMF) in the same or a neighboring circuit; the EMF is proportional to the rate of change of the current and inductance is quantitated as the ratio of these two, in SI units expressed as the henry. It is sometimes used to denote mutual inductance specifically. See also *self-inductance.*
**mutual i.**, that generated in a neighboring circuit. Symbol *M.* Called also *inductance.*

**in·duc·tion** (in-duk′shən) [L. *inductio*] 1. the act or process of inducing or causing to occur. See also under *chemotherapy.* 2. the production of a specific morphogenetic effect in the developing embryo through the influence of evocators or organizers. 3. the production of anesthesia or unconsciousness by use of appropriate agents. 4. the appearance of an electric current or of magnetic properties in a body because of the presence of another electric current or magnetic field nearby.
**autonomous i.**, induction in which the inductor forms no part of the portion produced.
**complementary i.**, induction in which the inductor forms a part of the portion produced.
**enzyme i.**, increased synthesis of an enzyme in response to an inducer or other stimulus.
**magnetic i.**, magnetic flux density.
**ovulation i.**, treatment of infertility in the female by administration of hormones that stimulate the ovaries.
**Spemann's i.**, the stimulating and directing effect shown by certain

tissues on neighboring tissues or parts in early development of the embryo.

**spinal i.,** that process by which one reflex lowers the threshold of another reflex which otherwise cannot be penetrated.

**in·duc·tor** (in-duk'tər) a tissue elaborating a chemical substance which acts to determine the growth and differentiation of embryonic parts. Cf. *activator* (def. 2) and *organizer.*

**in·duc·to·therm** (in-duk'to-thərm) an apparatus for producing high body temperature by electric induction.

**in·duc·to·ther·my** (in-duk'to-thər″me) the production of artificial fever by electric induction.

**in·du·lin** (in'du-lĭn) a coal tar dye, used as a histologic stain.

**in·du·lin·o·phil** (in″du-lin'o-fil) 1. an element easily stainable with indulin. 2. indulinophilic.

**in·du·lin·o·phil·ic** (in″du-lin-o-fil'ik) [*indulin* + *-philic*] stainable with indulin.

**in·du·rat·ed** (in'du-rāt″əd) [L. *indurare* to harden] hardened; rendered hard.

**in·du·ra·tion** (in″du-ra'shən) [L. *induratio*] 1. the quality of being hard. 2. the process of becoming hard; called also *hardening* and *sclerosis.* 3. an abnormally hard spot or place.

**black i.,** the hardening and pigmentation of lung tissue seen in coal workers' pneumoconiosis.

**brawny i.,** inflammatory hardening and thickening of tissues.

**brown i.,** 1. a deposit of altered blood pigment in the lung. 2. marked increase of the connective tissue of the lung and excessive pigmentation, due to long-continued congestion from heart disease. Cf. *gray i.*

**cyanotic i.,** a congested, dense, and purple state of the kidney in which the blood current is slowed and the transudation of fluid through the glomeruli is impeded.

**fibrous i.,** fibrous hardening of a tissue or organ induced by diffuse scarring.

**Froriep's i.,** myositis fibrosa.

**granular i.,** cirrhosis.

**gray i.,** an induration of lung tissue in or after pneumonia, without the pigmentation seen in brown induration.

**laminate i.,** a thin layer of round-cell infiltration of the corium in chancre.

**parchment i.,** laminate i.

**penile i.,** Peyronie's disease.

**phlebitic i.,** indurated cellulitis.

**plastic i.,** sclerosis of the corpora cavernosa of the penis.

**red i.,** red, congested lung tissue seen in idiopathic pulmonary fibrosis.

**in·du·ra·tive** (in'du-ra″tiv) pertaining to or marked by induration.

**in·du·si·um gris·e·um** (in-doo'ze-əm gris'e-əm) [L.] [TA] a thin layer of gray substance on the dorsal aspect of the corpus callosum; called also *supracallosal gyrus.*

**in·dwell·ing** (in'dwel-ing) pertaining to a catheter or other tube left within an organ or body passage for drainage, maintenance of patency, or administration of drugs or nutrients.

**-ine** a suffix indicating an alkaloid, an organic base, or a halogen.

**in·e·bri·ant** (in-e'bre-ənt) [L. *inebriare* to make drunk] 1. an inebriating agent. 2. inebriating.

**in·e·bri·ate** (in-e'bre-āt) to intoxicate with alcohol. See also *alcoholism.*

**in·e·bri·a·tion** (in-e″bre-a'shən) [L. *inebriare* to make drunk] 1. intoxication with alcohol; see also *alcoholism.* 2. a state resembling alcoholic intoxication. Called also *drunkenness.*

**in·e·bri·e·ty** (in″ə-bri'ə-te) [L. *in* intensive prefix + *ebriety*] inebriation.

**in·elas·tic** (in″e-las'tik) lacking elasticity.

**In·er·mi·cap·si·fer** (in-ər″mĭ-kap'sĭ-fər) a genus of tapeworms of the family Linstowiidae; some are parasitic in hyraxes and rodents in Africa. *I. arvican'thidis* has been found in humans in Cuba and Central America.

**in·ert** (in-ərt') having no action; not reacting with other elements, as inert gases.

**in·er·tia** (in-ər'shə) [L.] inactivity; inability to move spontaneously.

**colonic i.,** weak muscular activity of the colon, leading to distention of the organ and constipation.

**immunological i.,** specific depression of immunity in a mother toward the histocompatibility antigens of a fetus, or in a fetus toward those of the mother; it does not include immunologic tolerance.

**i. u'teri,** insufficiently strong or poorly coordinated uterine contractions during labor.

**in ex·tre·mis** (in ek-stre'mis) [L. "at the end"] at the point of death.

**Inf.** abbreviation for L. *infun'de,* pour in.

**in·fan·cy** (in'fən-se) the early period of life; see *infant.*

**in·fant** (in'fənt) [L. *infans; in* neg. + *fans* speaking] [MeSH: Infant] a young child; considered to designate the human young from birth (see *neonate*) to 12 months.

**dysmature i.,** an infant with dysmaturity syndrome. Called also *postmature i.*

**floppy i.,** see under *syndrome.*

**immature i.,** one usually weighing less than 2500 grams at birth and not physiologically fully developed.

**low birth weight (LBW) i.,** an infant weighing less than 2500 grams at birth.

**mature i.,** one weighing 2500 grams (5.5 pounds) or more at birth, usually at or near full term, physiologically fully developed, and having an optimum chance of survival.

**moderately low birth weight (MLBW) i.,** an infant weighing at least 1500 but less than 2500 grams at birth. See also *low birth weight i.*

**newborn i.,** the human young during the first four weeks after birth.

**postmature i., post-term i.,** 1. an infant born at any time after the beginning of the forty-second week (288 days) of gestation. 2. dysmature i.

**premature i.,** one usually born after the twentieth completed week and before full term, and arbitrarily defined as an infant weighing 500 to 2499 grams (2.2 to 5.5 lbs.) at birth, having poor to good chance of survival, depending on the weight. In countries where adults are smaller than in the United States, the upper limit may be lower. Other criteria such as crown-heel length (less than 47 cm) and occipitofrontal diameter (less than 11.5 cm) have also been used.

**preterm i.,** an infant born at any time before the thirty-seventh completed week (259 days) of gestation.

**term i.,** an infant born anytime from the beginning of the thirty-eighth week (260 days) to the end of the forty-first week (287 days) of gestation.

**very low birth weight (VLBW) i.,** an infant weighing less than 1500 grams at birth. See also *low birth weight i.*

**in·fan·ti·cide** (in-fan'tĭ-sīd) [*infant* + *-cide*] [MeSH: Infanticide] the taking of the life of an infant.

**in·fan·tile** (in'fən-tīl) [L. *infantilis*] pertaining to an infant or to infancy.

**in·fan·ti·lism** (in'fən-tĭ-liz″əm, in-fan'tĭ-liz″əm) persistence of the characteristics of childhood into adult life; it is marked by mental retardation, underdevelopment of the sexual organs, and often, but not always, by dwarfism. Cf. *progeria.*

**Brissaud's i.,** former name for *cretinism.*

**celiac i.,** infantilism accompanying the infantile form of celiac disease.

**dysthyroidal i.,** former name for *cretinism.*

**hepatic i.,** infantilism associated with hepatic cirrhosis.

**Herter's i.,** the infantile form of celiac disease.

**hypophysial i.,** a type of dwarfism with retention of infantile characteristics, due to undersecretion of growth hormone and gonadotropin deficiency. Called also *hypophysial dwarfism, Lévi-Lorain i.* or *dwarfism, Lorain-Lévi dwarfism,* and *pituitary i.* or *dwarfism.*

**intestinal i.,** the infantile form of celiac disease.

**Lévi-Lorain i., Lorain's i.,** hypophysial i.

**lymphatic i.,** infantilism associated with lymphatism.

**myxedematous i.,** former name for *cretinism.*

**pancreatic i.,** a form caused by inadequate secretion of pancreatic islet hormones, especially insulin.

**partial i.,** arrested development of a single part or tissue.

**pituitary i.,** hypophysial i.

**regressive i.,** reversion to an infantile state after body growth has been completed.

**renal i.,** renal osteodystrophy.

**sexual i.,** retardation of sexual development, as in adiposogenital dystrophy and hypophysial infantilism.

**symptomatic i.,** infantilism due to general defective development of tissues.

**universal i.,** short stature with undeveloped secondary sex characters, as in hypophysial infantilism.

**in·farct** (in'fahrkt) [L. *infarctus*] an area of coagulation necrosis in a tissue due to local ischemia resulting from obstruction of circulation to the area, most commonly by a thrombus or embolus. Called also *infarction.*

**anemic i.,** an area of necrosis in a tissue produced by sudden arrest of circulation in a vessel; called also *pale i.* and *white i.*

**bilirubin i's,** masses of crystals of bilirubin in the pyramids of the kidneys, especially in the newborn.

**bland i.,** an uninfected infarct.

**bone i.,** an area of bone tissue which has become necrotic as a result of loss of its arterial blood supply.

**Brewer's i's,** dark-red, wedge-shaped areas, resembling infarcts, seen on section of a kidney in pyelonephritis.

**calcareous i.,** a deposit of calcium salt in the tissues.

**cystic i.,** an infarct enclosed in a membrane.

**embolic i.**, one caused by an embolus.
**hemorrhagic i.**, an infarct that is red in color owing to the oozing of red corpuscles into the dead area; seen principally in the lung. Called also *red i.*
**lacunar i.**, lacune (def. 1).
**pale i.**, anemic i.
**red i.**, hemorrhagic i.
**septic i.**, one in which the tissues have been invaded by pathogenic organisms.
**thrombotic i.**, one caused by a thrombus.
**uric acid i.**, a deposit of uric acid crystals in the renal tubules of the newborn.
**white i.**, anemic i.
**i. of Zahn**, an area of reddish blue discoloration in the liver, with stasis and hepatocellular atrophy, seen following occlusion of an intrahepatic branch of the portal vein; not a true infarct, because there is no necrosis.

**in•farc•tec•to•my** (in″fahrk-tek′tə-me) surgical removal of an infarct.

**in•farc•tion** (in-fahrk′shən) [L. *infarcire* to stuff in] [MeSH: Infarction] 1. infarct. 2. the formation of an infarct.
**acute myocardial i. (AMI)**, that occurring during the period when circulation to a region of the heart is obstructed and necrosis is occurring; it is usually characterized by severe pain, frequently associated with pallor, perspiration, nausea, dyspnea, and dizziness; electrographic abnormalities may include Q wave, ST segment, and T wave alterations.
**anterior myocardial i.**, infarction localized to the left ventricular free wall between the interventricular groove and the lateral margin of the anterior papillary muscle.
**anteroinferior myocardial i.**, one involving features of both anterior and inferior myocardial infarction; it is characterized electrocardiographically by abnormal Q waves in leads II, III, and $aV_L$ and in one or more of leads $V_1$ to $V_4$.
**anterolateral myocardial i.**, one involving features of both anterior and lateral myocardial infarction; it is characterized electrocardiographically by abnormal Q waves in leads I, $aV_L$, and $V_3$ to $V_6$.
**anteroseptal myocardial i.**, one involving features of both anterior and septal myocardial infarction; it is characterized electrocardiographically by abnormal Q waves in leads $V_1$ to $V_4$.
**apical myocardial i.**, anteroinferior myocardial i.
**atrial i.**, the formation of an infarct in a cardiac atrium, which may be due to coronary artery occlusion, periarteritis nodosa, obliterating endarteritis of the small branches of coronary arteries, or other conditions.
**cardiac i.**, myocardial i.
**cerebral i.**, an ischemic condition of the brain, producing local tissue death and usually a persistent focal neurological deficit in the area of distribution of one of the cerebral arteries. See also *stroke syndrome*, under *syndrome, reversible ischemic neurologic deficit*, under *deficit*, and *transient ischemic attack*, under *attack*. Called also *cerebral ischemia*.
**diaphragmatic myocardial i.**, inferior myocardial i.
**extensive anterior myocardial i.**, infarction of the anterior region of the heart, with a more diffuse distribution than anterior myocardial infarction; it is characterized electrocardiographically by abnormal Q waves in leads I, $aV_L$, and $V_1$ to $V_6$.
**Freiberg's i.**, Köhler's bone disease, def. 2.
**high lateral myocardial i.**, infarction localized to the upper portion of the lateral region; it is characterized by abnormal Q waves in leads I and $aV_L$.
**inferior myocardial i.**, one localized in the region between the lateral border of the posterior papillary muscle and the posterior septum; it is characterized electrocardiographically by abnormal Q waves in leads II, III, and $aV_F$.
**inferolateral myocardial i.**, one involving features of both inferior and lateral myocardial infarction; it is characterized electrocardiographically by abnormal Q waves in leads II, III, $aV_F$, $V_5$, and $V_6$.
**intestinal i.**, occlusion of an artery or arteriole in the wall of the intestine, resulting in the formation of an area of coagulation necrosis.
**lateral myocardial i.**, infarction in the region between the lateral margin of the anterior papillary muscle and the lateral margin of the posterior papillary muscle; it is marked electrocardiographically by abnormal Q waves in leads I, $aV_L$, $V_5$, and $V_6$.
**maternal floor i.**, a disorder of the placenta resulting from decreased maternal blood flow and characterized by the deposition of fibrin in the decidua basalis with induration of the maternal surface of the placenta.
**mesenteric i.**, coagulation necrosis of the intestines due to a decrease in blood flow in the mesenteric vasculature; it may be caused by occlusion of the mesenteric arteries or by cardiogenic abnormalities or hypovolemia *(nonocclusive mesenteric i.)*.
**migrainous i.**, a focal neurologic deficit that constituted part of a migrainous aura but that has persisted for a long period and may be permanent. Called also *complicated migraine*.
**myocardial i. (MI)**, gross necrosis of the myocardium as a result of interruption of the blood supply to the area; it is almost always caused by atherosclerosis of the coronary arteries, upon which coronary thrombosis is usually superimposed.
**non–Q wave i.**, myocardial infarction not characterized by abnormal Q waves; cf. *Q wave i.*
**nonocclusive mesenteric i.**, see *mesenteric i.*
**nontransmural myocardial i.**, one involving less than the full thickness of the myocardial wall; sometimes used synonymously with *subendocardial myocardial infarction.*
**posterior myocardial i.**, one localized in the basal third of the posteroinferior heart wall; it is characterized electrocardiographically by abnormally large R waves in leads $V_1$ or $V_2$.
**pulmonary i.**, localized necrosis of lung tissue caused by obstruction of the arterial blood supply, most often due to pulmonary embolism. Clinical manifestations range from the subclinical to pleuritic chest pain, dyspnea, hemoptysis, and tachycardia.
**Q wave i.**, myocardial infarction characterized by Q waves that are abnormal either in character or number or both. Cf. *transmural myocardial i.*
**right ventricular i.**, one localized to the free wall of the right ventricle, usually associated with inferior myocardial infarctions of the left ventricle; it is characterized electrocardiographically by ST segment elevation in one or more right precordial leads.
**septal myocardial i.**, one localized to the interventricular septum and characterized electrocardiographically by abnormal Q waves in leads $V_1$ and $V_2$.
**silent myocardial i.**, infarction occurring without pain or other symptoms; it may be recognized by electrographic or postmortem examination.
**subendocardial myocardial i.**, infarction localized to the inner one third to one half of the myocardial wall; sometimes described as *nontransmural myocardial infarction*
**transmural myocardial i.**, one involving the entire thickness of the heart wall. The term is sometimes incorrectly used as a synonym of Q wave infarction.
**watershed i.**, cerebral infarction in a watershed area (q.v.) during a time of prolonged systemic hypotension.

**in•faust** (in′foust) [L. *infaustus* unlucky] unfavorable.

**in•fec•ti•ble** (in-fek′tĭ-bəl) capable of being infected.

**in•fec•tion** (in-fek′shən) [MeSH: Infection] 1. invasion and multiplication of microorganisms in body tissues, which may be clinically inapparent or result in local cellular injury due to competitive metabolism, toxins, intracellular replication, or antigen-antibody response. The infection may remain localized, subclinical, and temporary if the body's defense mechanisms are effective. A local infection may persist and spread by extension to become an acute, subacute, or chronic clinical infection or disease state. A local infection may also become systemic when the microorganisms gain access to the lymphatic or vascular system. 2. an infectious disease. Cf. *infestation*.
**airborne i.**, an infection that is contracted by inhalation of microorganisms or spores suspended in air on water droplets or dust particles. Microorganisms are often rendered airborne as a result of a sneeze or cough. Cf. *droplet i.*
**apical i.**, infection situated at the apex of the root of a tooth.
**ascending i.**, infection of the fetus by microorganisms that gain access to the uterus from the vagina, usually following rupture of membranes but sometimes acquired in utero while the membranes are intact; called also *transcervical i.*
**chronic Epstein-Barr virus i.**, chronic fatigue syndrome.
**colonization i.**, an infection characterized by the attachment and

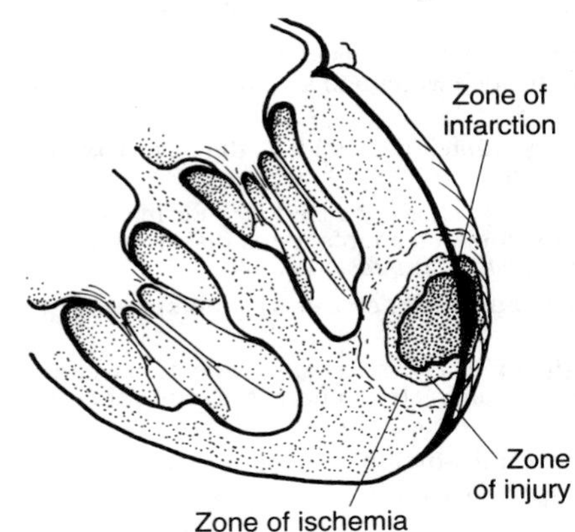

Myocardial infarction shown in cross-section of heart (ventricles only).

subsequent growth of the invading microorganism on or within tissue.
**cross i.**, infection transmitted between individuals infected with different pathogenic microorganisms.
**cryptogenic i.**, infection whose pathogenesis is unclear or undefinable, as salmonella arteritis with no preceding salmonella infection elsewhere.
**droplet i.**, that due to inhalation of droplet nuclei. Cf. *airborne i.*
**dust-borne i.**, airborne infection by pathogens that have become attached to particles of dust and are transmitted by that means.
**ectogenous i.**, exogenous i.
**endogenous i.**, infection due to reactivation of organisms present in a dormant focus, such as occurs in tuberculosis, histoplasmosis, and coccidioidomycosis.
**exit site i.**, infection in the area where an artificial tube exits from the body.
**exogenous i.**, infection caused by organisms not normally present in the body but which have gained entrance from the environment.
**germinal i.**, transmission of infection to the fetus or child by means of the oocyte or sperm of the parent.
**hematogenous i.**, transplacental i.
**iatrogenic i.**, see *iatrogenic.*
**inapparent i.**, an infection with no clinical symptoms that is unnoticed by the affected individual; cf. *subclinical i.*
**latent i.**, 1. a phase during the course of some established infections during which the pathogenic microorganisms are dormant and manifestations of disease that may have been recognizable earlier are no longer detectable, as in latent syphilis. 2. infection in which the etiologic agent has not yet produced or does not produce symptoms.
**mass i.**, infection produced by a large number of pathogenic organisms in the circulation.
**mixed i.**, infection of an organ or tissue by more than one microorganism, as in wound infections, abscesses, pneumonia, and rarely meningitis and endocarditis; mixtures of every type occur, e.g., bacterial and viral, bacterial and fungal, and protozoan and viral. Called also *polyinfection.*
**nosocomial i.**, see *nosocomial.*
**opportunistic i.**, infection by an organism that does not ordinarily cause disease but that, under certain circumstances (e.g., impaired immune responses), becomes pathogenic.
**perinatal i.**, infection in the newborn acquired shortly before or during delivery, due to ascending infection following rupture of the membranes or contact with microorganisms in the birth canal during delivery.
**pyogenic i.**, an infection caused by pus-producing microorganisms, commonly species of *Staphylococcus* and *Streptococcus.* The most numerous white blood cells responding immunologically to a pyogenic infection are the polymorphonuclear leukocytes.
**secondary i.**, infection by a microorganism following an infection by another kind of microorganism.
**subclinical i.**, infection in which symptoms and signs are not detectable by clinical examination or laboratory tests; this may occur in an early stage(s) of the infection, with symptoms and signs becoming manifest later during the course of the infection, or the symptoms and signs may never become apparent. Cf. *inapparent i.*
**TORCH i.**, see under *syndrome.*
**transcervical i.**, ascending i.
**transplacental i.**, infection acquired by the fetus in utero by the hematogenous spread of a maternal infection across the placenta via the chorionic villi; called also *hematogenous i.*
**tunnel i.**, subcutaneous infection of an artificial passage into the body that has been kept patent for continuous or repeated entry of a catheter or other tube.
**vector-borne i.**, infection caused by microorganisms transmitted from one host to another by a carrier, such as a mosquito, louse, fly, or tick.
**water-borne i.**, infection caused by microorganisms which may be transmitted through water and acquired through ingestion, bathing, or other means.

**in·fec·ti·os·i·ty** (in-fek″she-os′ĭ-te) the degree of infectiousness of a microorganism.

**in·fec·tious** (in-fek′shəs) caused by or capable of being communicated by infection, as an infectious disease; infective. Cf. *communicable, contagious,* and *infestation.*

**in·fec·tious·ness** (in-fek′shəs-nəs) the state or quality of being infectious.

**in·fec·tive** (in-fek′tiv) [L. *infectivus*] infectious; capable of producing infection; pertaining to or characterized by the presence of pathogens.

**in·fec·tiv·i·ty** (in″fek-tiv′ĭ-te) infectiousness.

**in·fe·cun·di·ty** (in″fe-kun′dĭ-te) [L. *infecunditas*] infertility.

**InFeD** (in′fed) trademark for a preparation of iron dextran injection.

**in·fer·ent** (in′fər-ənt) afferent.

**In·fer·gen** (in′fər-jen) trademark for a preparation of interferon alfacon-1.

**in·fe·ri·or** (in-fēr′e-ər) [L. "lower"] 1. situated below, or directed downward. 2. [TA] a term used in reference to the lower surface of an organ or other structure, or to the lower of two (or more) similar structures.

**in·fe·ro·lat·er·al** (in″fər-o-lat′ər-əl) [L. *inferus* low + *lateral*] situated inferiorly and to one side.

**in·fe·ro·me·di·an** (in″fər-o-me′de-ən) [L. *inferus* low + *median*] situated in the middle of the inferior side.

**in·fe·ro·na·sal** (in″fər-o-na′zəl) [L. *inferus* low + *nasal*] in ophthalmology, that quadrant of the eye or of the visual field inferior to the horizontal meridian of the eye and medial to the vertical meridian.

**in·fe·ro·pos·te·ri·or** (in″fər-o-pos-tēr′e-ər) situated inferiorly and posteriorly.

**in·fe·ro·tem·po·ral** (in″fər-o-tem′pər-əl) [L. *inferus* low + *temporal*] in ophthalmology, that quadrant of the eye or of the visual field inferior to the horizontal meridian of the eye and lateral to the vertical meridian.

**in·fer·tile** (in-fər′til) not fertile; exhibiting infertility.

**in·fer·til·i·tas** (in″fər-til′ĭ-təs) [L.] infertility.

**in·fer·til·i·ty** (in″fər-til′ĭ-te) [*in-*[2] + *fertility*] [MeSH: Infertility] diminished or absent capacity to produce offspring; the term does not denote complete inability to produce offspring as does *sterility.* Called also *relative sterility.*
**primary i.**, infertility occurring in patients who have never conceived.
**secondary i.**, infertility occurring in patients who have previously conceived.

**in·fes·ta·tion** (in-fes-ta′shən) parasitic attack or subsistence on the skin and its appendages by ectoparasites such as insects, mites, or ticks.

**in·fib·u·la·tion** (in-fib″u-la′shən) [L. *infibulare* to buckle together] the act of buckling, or fastening as if with buckles, especially the practice of fastening the prepuce or labia minora together with clasps, stitches, or other devices to prevent coitus. Cf. *female circumcision,* under *circumcision.*

**in·fil·trate** (in-fil′trāt) 1. to penetrate the interstices of a tissue or substance. 2. the material or solution so deposited; called also *infiltration.*
**Assmann's tuberculous i.**, see under *focus.*

**in·fil·tra·tion** (in″fil-tra′shən) [*in-*[1] + *filtration*] 1. the pathological accumulation in tissue or cells of substances not normal to it or in amounts in excess of the normal. 2. infiltrate, def. 2. 3. the deposition of a solution directly into tissue; see under *anesthesia.*
**adipose i.**, fatty i.; see *fatty change,* under *change.*
**calcareous i.**, a deposit of lime and magnesium salts in the tissues.
**calcium i.**, a deposit of calcium salts within the tissues of the body.
**cellular i.**, the migration and accumulation of cells within the tissues.
**epituberculous i.**, a collateral hyperemia and inflammatory infiltration surrounding a tuberculous focus.
**fatty i.**, 1. a deposit of fat in the tissues, especially between the cells; the term describes an older concept now included in *fatty change* (q.v.). 2. the presence of fat vacuoles in the cytoplasm of cells, as occurs in fatty change in the liver, myocardium, and kidneys.
**gelatinous i.**, gray i.
**glycogen i.**, abnormal accumulations of glycogen within the cytoplasm of cells, as occurs in diabetes mellitus and the glycogen storage diseases.
**gray i.**, a condition of the lungs in acute pulmonary tuberculosis in which they have large amounts of semisolid grayish exudate; seen primarily at autopsy. Called also *gelatinous i.*
**inflammatory i.**, that formed by an inflammatory exudation penetrating the interstices of a tissue.
**lymphocytic i. of skin**, a manifestation of cutaneous lymphoid hyperplasia, occurring most often in men, characterized by the appearance of asymptomatic, single or multiple, firm, reddish papules or plaques that expand peripherally to form circinate lesions, sometimes with central clearing; the lesions may be induced or aggravated by light exposure.
**paraneural i., perineural i.**, perineural anesthesia.
**pulmonary i. with eosinophilia**, infiltration of the pulmonary parenchyma by eosinophils; see *PIE syndrome,* under *syndrome.*
**sanguineous i.**, infiltration with extravasated blood.
**serous i.**, the abnormal presence of lymph in a tissue.
**tuberculous i.**, the formation of a group or of groups of tuberculous cells and bacilli in a tissue.
**urinous i.**, extravasation of urine into a tissue.

**in·firm** (in-firm') [L. *infirmis; in-*[2] + *firmus* strong] weak; feeble, as from disease or old age.

**in·fir·ma·ry** (in-fər'mə-re) [L. *infirmarium*] a hospital or place where sick or infirm persons are maintained or treated; commonly used to denote a space or a building set aside for the care of members of a group or community; a dispensary.

**in·fir·mi·ty** (in-fir'mĭ-te) [L. *infirmitas*] 1. a feeble or weak state of the body or mind. 2. a disease or condition producing weakness.

**In·fla·mase** (in'flə-mās") trademark for preparations of prednisolone sodium phosphate.

**in·flam·ma·gen** (in-flam'ə-jən) an irritant that elicits both edema and the cellular response of inflammation. Cf. *edemagen.*

**in·flam·ma·tion** (in"flə-ma'shən) [L. *inflammatio; inflammare* to set on fire] [MeSH: Inflammation] a localized protective response elicited by injury or destruction of tissues, which serves to destroy, dilute, or wall off (sequester) both the injurious agent and the injured tissue. It is characterized in the acute form by the classical signs of pain (dolor), heat (calor), redness (rubor), swelling (tumor), and loss of function (functio laesa). Histologically, it involves a complex series of events, including dilatation of arterioles, capillaries, and venules, with increased permeability and blood flow; exudation of fluids, including plasma proteins; and leukocytic migration into the inflammatory focus.
**acute i.**, inflammation, usually of sudden onset, characterized by the classical signs (see *inflammation*), in which the vascular and exudative processes predominate.
**adhesive i.**, that which promotes the adhesion of contiguous surfaces.
**atrophic i.**, a form which results in atrophy and deformity.
**catarrhal i.**, a form which affects principally a mucous surface, and which is marked by a copious discharge of mucus and epithelial debris.
**chronic i.**, inflammation of slow progress and marked chiefly by the formation of new connective tissue; it may be a continuation of an acute form or a prolonged low-grade form, and usually causes permanent tissue damage.
**cirrhotic i.**, atrophic i.
**diffuse i.**, one that is both interstitial and parenchymatous or is spread over a large area.
**disseminated i.**, one that has a number of distinct foci.
**exudative i.**, one in which the prominent feature is an exudate.
**fibrinous i.**, one that is characterized by an exudate of coagulated fibrin.
**fibrosing i.**, atrophic i.
**focal i.**, one that is confined to a single spot or to a few limited spots.
**granulomatous i.**, an inflammation, usually chronic, characterized by the formation of granulomas; see also *granuloma.*
**hyperplastic i.**, one which leads to the formation of new connective tissue fibers.
**hypertrophic i.**, inflammation marked by increase in the size of the elements composing the affected tissue.
**interstitial i.**, one that primarily affects the stroma of an organ.
**metastatic i.**, one that is reproduced in a distant part by the conveyance of infectious material through the blood vessels and lymph organs.
**necrotic i.**, inflammation attended by death of the affected tissue.
**obliterative i.**, inflammation of the lining membrane of a cavity or vessel, producing adhesions between the surfaces and consequent obliteration of the lumen.
**parenchymatous i.**, one that primarily affects the essential tissue elements of an organ.
**plastic i., productive i., proliferous i.**, hyperplastic i.
**pseudomembranous i.**, an acute inflammatory response to a powerful necrotizing toxin, such as the diphtheria toxin, characterized by the formation on a mucosal surface, most often in the pharynx, larynx, respiratory passages, and intestinal tract, of a false membrane composed of precipitated fibrin, necrotic epithelium, and inflammatory white cells.
**purulent i.**, suppurative i.
**sclerosing i.**, atrophic i.
**seroplastic i.**, inflammation accompanied by both serous and plastic exudation.
**serous i.**, one which produces an exudation of serum.
**simple i.**, that in which there is no flow of pus or other product of inflammation.
**specific i.**, one that is due to a particular microorganism.
**subacute i.**, a condition intermediate between chronic and acute inflammation, exhibiting some of the characteristics of each.
**suppurative i.**, one characterized by the formation of pus.
**toxic i.**, one that is caused by a poison, such as a bacterial product.
**traumatic i.**, one that is caused by an injury.
**ulcerative i.**, that in which necrosis on or near the surface leads to loss of tissue and creation of a local defect (ulcer).

**in·flam·ma·to·ry** (in-flam'ə-tor"e) pertaining to or characterized by inflammation.

**in·fla·tion** (in-fla'shən) [L. *in-*[1] + *flare* to blow] 1. distention with air, gas, or a fluid. 2. the act of distending with air or with a gas.

**in·fla·tor** (in-fla'tor) an instrument for inflating any organ for therapeutic or diagnostic purposes.

**in·flec·tion, in·flex·ion** (in-flek'shən) [L. *inflexio; in* in + *flectere* to bend] the act of bending inward or the state of being bent inward, as of a limb.

**in·flo·res·cence** (in"flo-res'əns) the structure or arrangement of the flowers of a plant.

**in·flu·en·za** (in"floo-en'zə) [Ital., from L. *influentia* influence, from the belief that the stars influenced epidemics] [MeSH: Influenza] an acute viral infection of the respiratory tract, occurring in isolated cases, in epidemics, or in pandemics; it is caused by serologically different strains of viruses (influenzaviruses) designated A, B, and C, has a 3-day incubation period, and usually lasts for 3 to 10 days. It is marked by inflammation of the nasal mucosa, pharynx, and conjunctiva; headache; myalgia; often fever, chills, and prostration; and occasionally involvement of the myocardium or central nervous system. A necrotizing bronchitis and interstitial pneumonia are features of severe cases, opening the way for secondary bacterial pneumonia due to *Streptococcus pneumoniae, Haemophilus influenzae,* or *Staphylococcus aureus.* Called also *flu* and *grippe.*
**i. A,** the most common variety of influenza caused by influenza virus A; epidemics of this form occur at two- to three-year intervals. The causative strain is subject to wide variations in antigenic type, called antigenic shift, and outbreaks of influenza A caused by such antigenic types have been called *Asian i., Spanish i., Russian i.,* and so on.
**Asian i.**, a pandemic of influenza A that occurred in 1957 and was thought to originate in China.
**avian i.**, 1. Newcastle disease. 2. fowl plague.
**i. B,** a variety of influenza caused by influenza virus B; epidemics of this form occur at four- to five-year intervals.
**i. C,** a variety of influenza occurring sporadically and caused by influenza virus C.
**endemic i.**, infection with influenza virus occurring continuously within a population, i.e., between epidemics, either sporadically and not recognized as influenza or as a clinically inapparent infection.
**equine i.**, a highly contagious febrile respiratory disease of horses caused by two immunologically distinct strains of influenza virus A. Called also *equine infectious bronchitis.*
**feline i.**, feline respiratory disease complex.
**goose i.**, 1. infectious avian serositis in geese. 2. a type of serositis in geese, caused by a parvovirus.
**Hong Kong i.**, a pandemic of influenza A that occurred in 1968 and was thought to have originated in Hong Kong.
**Russian i.**, a pandemic of influenza A that occurred in 1978 and was thought to have originated in Russia.
**Spanish i.**, an acute influenzalike disease that occurred in a pandemic in Europe and the Americas during the summer and autumn of 1918.
**swine i.**, an acute highly contagious respiratory disease of hogs caused by a type A influenza virus.

**in·flu·en·zal** (in"floo-en'zəl) pertaining to influenza; called also *grippal.*

**In·flu·en·za·vi·rus** (in"floo-en'zə-vi"rəs) [*influenza* + *virus*] a formerly used name comprising *Influenzavirus A* and *Influenzavirus B.*
**I. A,** influenza A virus; a genus of viruses of the family Orthomyxoviridae containing the agent of influenza A. See *influenza virus,* under *virus.*
**I. B,** influenza B virus; a genus of viruses of the family Orthomyxoviridae containing the agent of influenza B. See *influenza virus,* under *virus.*
**I. C,** influenza C virus; a genus of viruses of the family Orthomyxoviridae containing the agent of influenza C. See *influenza virus,* under *virus.*

**in·fold·ing** (in-fōl'ding) 1. the folding inward of a layer of tissue, as in the formation of the neural tube in the embryo. 2. the enclosing of redundant tissue by suturing together the walls of the organ on either side of it.

**infra-** [L. *infra* beneath] a prefix meaning inferior to, below, or beneath.

**in·fra·ax·il·la·ry** (in"frə-ak'sĭ-lar"e) inferior to the axilla.

**in·fra·bulge** (in'frə-bəlj) the surfaces of a tooth gingival to the height of contour, or sloping cervically; the surface of the crown of a tooth cervical to the clasp guideline or surveyed height of contour, being the retention area of a tooth. Cf. *suprabulge.*

**in·fra·cil·i·a·ture** (in"frə-sil'e-ə-chər) [*infra-* + *cilium*] the basal bodies and kinetodesmata of ciliate protozoa considered collectively.

**in·fra·class** (in'frə-klas) a taxonomic category sometimes established, subordinate to a subclass and superior to an order.

**in·fra·cla·vic·u·lar** (in"frə-klə-vik'u-lər) inferior to a clavicle.

**in·fra·clu·sion** (in″frə-kloo′zhən) malocclusion in which a tooth has failed to erupt fully and reach the line of occlusion and is out of contact with the opposing tooth. Called also *infraversion.*

**in·fra·col·ic** (in″frə-kol′ik) [*infra-* + *colon*] inferior to the colon.

**in·fra·con·stric·tor** (in″frə-kən-strik′tər) musculus constrictor pharyngis inferior.

**in·fra·cor·ti·cal** (in″frə-kor′tĭ-kəl) beneath a cortex, such as the cerebral cortex.

**in·fra·cos·tal** (in″frə-kos′təl) [*infra-* + *costal*] inferior to a rib or to all the ribs.

**in·fra·cot·y·loid** (in″frə-kot′ə-loid) inferior to the cotyloid cavity or acetabulum.

**in·frac·tion** (in-frak′shən) [L. *in* into + *frac′tio* break] incomplete fracture of a bone without displacement of the fragments.
**Freiberg's i.,** osteochondrosis of the head of the second metatarsal bone.

**in·fra·den·ta·le** (in″frə-dən-ta′le) an osteometric landmark, being the highest anterior point on the gingiva between the mandibular central incisors.

**in·fra·di·an** (in″frə-de′ən) [*infra-* + L. *dies* day] pertaining to the rhythmic repetition of certain phenomena in living organisms occurring in cycles of less frequency than circadian, that is, less frequently than once a day. Cf. *circadian* and *ultradian.*

**in·fra·di·a·phrag·mat·ic** (in″frə-di″ə-frag-mat′ik) subphrenic.

**in·fra·duc·tion** (in″frə-duk′shən) [*infra-* + *duction*] 1. the downward rotation of an eye around its horizontal axis. 2. the downward rotation of one eye independent of the other by a base-up prism in testing for vertical divergence. See also *infravergence* and *infraversion.* Called also *deorsumduction* and *subduction.*

**in·fra·gle·noid** (in″frə-gle′noid) inferior to the fossa of the glenoid cavity.

**in·fra·glot·tic** (in″frə-glot′ik) subglottic.

**in·fra·hy·oid** (in″frə-hi′oid) inferior to the hyoid bone.

**in·fra·in·gui·nal** (in″frə-ing′gwə-nəl) inferior to the inguinal ligament.

**in·fra·mal·le·o·lar** (in″frə-mal-e-o′lər) below one or both of the malleoli.

**in·fra·mam·ma·ry** (in″frə-mam′ə-re) submammary.

**in·fra·mam·mil·la·ry** (in″frə-mam′ĭ-lar″e) inferior to the nipple.

**in·fra·man·dib·u·lar** (in″frə-man-dib′u-lər) inferior to the lower jaw.

**in·fra·mar·gin·al** (in″frə-mahr′jĭ-nəl) situated inferior to a margin or border.

**in·fra·max·il·lary** (in″frə-mak′sĭ-lar″e) submaxillary.

**in·fra·nu·cle·ar** (in″frə-noo′kle-ər) inferior to a nucleus in the nervous system.

**in·fra·or·bi·tal** (in″frə-or′bĭ-təl) lying under, or on the inferior surface of, the orbit. Called also *suborbital.*

**in·fra·pa·tel·lar** (in″frə-pə-tel′ər) inferior to the patella. Called also *subpatellar.*

**in·fra·pop·lit·e·al** (in″frə-pop-lit′e-əl) below the back of the knee.

**in·fra·psy·chic** (in″frə-si′kik) below the conscious level; automatic.

**in·fra·red** (in-frə-red′) denoting thermal radiation of wavelength greater than that of the red end of the visible spectrum, between the red waves and the radio waves, having wavelengths between 0.75 and 1000 μm. Infrared rays emanating from tissues are the basis of thermography.
**far i., long-wave i.,** infrared radiation of the longest wavelength, i.e., furthest from the visible spectrum (wavelength about 3.0 to 1000 μm).
**near i., short-wave i.,** infrared radiation of the shortest wavelength, i.e., closest to the visible spectrum (wavelength about 0.75 to 3.0 μm).

**in·fra·scap·u·lar** (in″frə-skap′u-lər) inferior to the scapula.

**in·fra·son·ic** (in″frə-son′ik) below the frequency range of the waves normally perceived as sound by the human ear.

**in·fra·spi·nous** (in″frə-spi′nəs) inferior to the spine of the scapula.

**in·fra·ster·nal** (in″frə-stər′nəl) substernal.

**in·fra·struc·ture** (in″frə-struk′chər) substructure, def. 2.
**implant i.,** see under *substructure.*

**in·fra·tem·po·ral** (in″frə-tem′pər-əl) inferior to the temple or temporal fossa; called also *subtemporal.*

**in·fra·ten·to·ri·al** (in″frə-ten-tor′e-əl) inferior to the tentorium of the cerebellum.

**in·fra·ton·sil·lar** (in″frə-ton′sĭ-lər) inferior to the palatine tonsil.

**in·fra·tra·che·al** (in″frə-tra′ke-əl) inferior to the trachea.

**in·fra·troch·le·ar** (in″frə-trok′le-ər) subtrochlear.

**in·fra·tu·bal** (in″frə-too′bəl) inferior to a tube.

**in·fra·tym·pan·ic** (in″frə-tym-pan′ik) inferior to the tympanic membrane; called also *subtympanic.*

**in·fra·um·bil·i·cal** (in″frə-əm-bil′ĭ-kəl) inferior to the umbilicus.

**in·fra·ver·gence** (in″frə-vər′jəns) [*infra-* + *vergence*] disjunctive reciprocal movement of the eyes in which one eye rotates downward while the other one remains still; called also *deorsumvergence.*

**in·fra·ver·sion** (in″frə-vər′zhən) [*infra-* + *version*] 1. infraclusion. 2. the downward deviation of one eye. 3. conjugate downward rotation of both eyes; called also *deorsumversion.*

**in·fra·ves·i·cal** (in″frə-ves′ĭ-kəl) [*infra-* + *vesical*] situated or taking place below the urinary bladder.

**in·fric·tion** (in-frik′shən) [L. *in* on + *friction*] the rubbing of medicaments upon the skin.

**in·fun·dib·u·la** (in″fən-dib′u-lə) [L.] plural of *infundibulum.*

**in·fun·dib·u·lar** (in″fən-dib′u-lər) of the nature of or resembling an infundibulum or funnel.

**in·fun·dib·u·lec·to·my** (in″fən-dib″u-lek′tə-me) excision of the infundibulum of the heart.
**Brock's i.,** transventricular closed valvotomy.

**in·fun·dib·u·li·form** (in″fən-dib′u-lĭ-form) [*infundibulum* + *form*] shaped like a funnel.

**in·fun·dib·u·lo·ma** (in″fən-dib″u-lo′mə) a tumor of the infundibulum hypothalami.

**in·fun·dib·u·lo·pel·vic** (in″fən-dib″u-lo-pel′vik) pertaining to an infundibulum and a pelvis, as of the kidney.

**in·fun·dib·u·lum** (in″fən-dib′u-ləm) pl. *infundi′bula* [L. "funnel"] 1. a general anatomical term for a funnel-shaped structure. 2. i. neurohypophyseos. 3. conus arteriosus. 4. the deep, often tubular or funnel-shaped part of the buccal cavity seen in certain protozoa, especially peritrichous ciliates.
**crural i., i. crura′le,** canalis femoralis.
**ethmoidal i. of cavity of nose,** i. ethmoidale cavitatis nasi.
**ethmoidal i. of ethmoid bone,** i. ethmoidale ossis ethmoidalis.
**i. ethmoida′le cavita′tis na′si** [TA], ethmoidal infundibulum of nasal cavity: a passage connecting the cavity of the nose with the anterior ethmoidal cells and the frontal sinus.
**i. ethmoida′le os′sis ethmoida′lis** [TA], ethmoidal infundibulum of ethmoid bone: a variable sinuous passage extending upward from the middle nasal meatus through the ethmoidal labyrinth, communicating with the anterior ethmoidal cells and often with the frontal sinus.
**i. of fallopian tube,** i. tubae uterinae.
**i. of heart,** conus arteriosus.
**i. of hypophysis, i. hypotha′lami, i. of hypothalamus,** i. neurohypophyseos.
**infundibula of kidney,** calices renales minores.
**i. lo′bi posterio′ris hypophy′seos,** TA alternative for *i. neurohypophyseos.*
**i. na′si, i. of nose,** 1. i. ethmoidale cavi nasi. 2. i. ethmoidale ossis ethmoidalis.
**i. neurohypophy′seos** [TA], infundibulum of neurohypophysis: a hollow, funnel-shaped mass in front of the tuber cinereum, which extends to the neurohypophysis. Called also *i. of hypophysis* or *of hypothalamus, i. hypothalami, i. lobi posterioris hypophyseos* [TA alternative], and *hypophysial, infundibular, neural,* or *pituitary stalk.*
**infundi′bula re′num,** calices renales minores.
**i. tu′bae uteri′nae** [TA], infundibulum of uterine tube: the funnel-like dilation at the distal end of the uterine tube.
**i. of urinary bladder,** fundus vesicae.

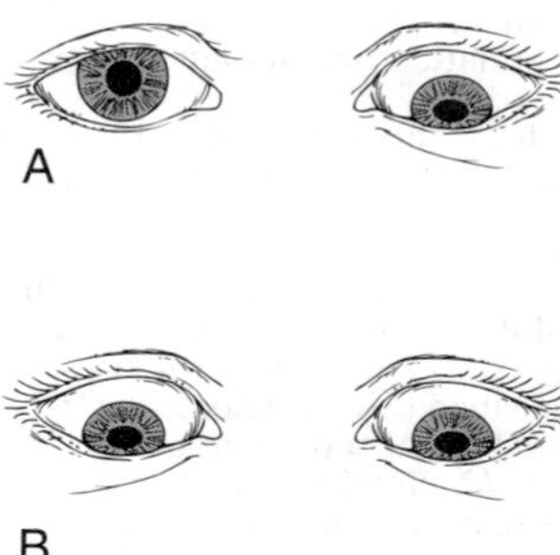

Infraversion of one *(A)* or both *(B)* eyes.

**i. of uterine tube,** i. tubae uterinae.

**in·fu·si·ble** (in-fu'zĭ-bəl) incapable of being melted.

**in·fu·sion** (in-fu'zhən) [L. *infusio;* from *in* + *fundere* to pour] 1. the steeping of a substance in water to obtain its medicinal principles. 2. the product of the process of steeping a drug for the extraction of its medicinal principles. 3. the therapeutic introduction of a fluid other than blood, as saline solution, into a vein. NOTE: An *infusion* flows in by gravity, an *injection* is forced in by a syringe, an *instillation* is dropped in, and an *insufflation* is blown in.
**cold i.,** the product of steeping a drug in cold water.
**continuous subcutaneous insulin i.,** CSII; insulin pump.
**meat i.** (for bacteriological use)**,** fresh lean meat free from fat is ground and extracted with water; the mixture is infused overnight in the refrigerator, gradually raised to the boiling point, and filtered.
**saline i.,** administration, either subcutaneously or intravenously, of saline solution.

**in·fu·so·de·coc·tion** (in-fu″so-de-kok'shən) a mixture of the infusion and the decoction of a substance.

**In·fu·so·ria** (in″fu-sor'e-ə) [L. pl., so called because found in *infusions,* after exposure to air] former name for Ciliophora.

**in·fu·sum** (in-fu'səm) [L.] infusion, def. 2.

**in·ges·ta** (in-jes'tə) [L. pl., *in* into + *gerere* to carry] food and drink taken into the stomach.

**in·ges·tant** (in-jes'tənt) a substance that is or may be taken into the body by way of the mouth, or through the digestive system.

**in·ges·tion** (in-jes'chən) the act of taking food, medicines, etc., into the body, by mouth.

**in·ges·tive** (in-jes'tiv) pertaining to or affecting an ingestion.

**in·glu·vi·es** (in-gloo've-ēz) [L.] 1. crop, def. 1. 2. rumen.

**In·gras·sia's wing (apophysis)** (in-grah'se-ahs) [Giovanni Filippo *Ingrassia,* Italian anatomist, 1510–1580] ala minor ossis sphenoidalis.

**in·gra·ves·cent** (in″grə-ves'ənt) [L. *in* upon + *gravesci* to grow heavy] gradually increasing in severity.

**in·growth** (in'grōth) an inward growth; something that grows inward or into.
**epithelial i.,** a complication of intraocular surgery, most often cataract extraction, or of penetrating wounds of the cornea where wound healing is poor, in which epithelium proliferates through the wound into the anterior chamber, causing obstruction of the trabecula, and sometimes pupillary block, resulting in glaucoma.
**stromal fatty i.,** the replacement of connective tissue stroma by adipose tissue, most often occurring in the pancreas and heart, usually without any alteration in the organ's function.

**in·guen** (ing'gwən) pl. *in'guina* [L.] [TA] [MeSH: Groin] groin: the junctional region between the abdomen and thigh. Called also *regio inguinalis* [TA alternative] and *iliac* or *inguinal region.*

**in·gui·na** (ing'gwĭ-nə) [L.] plural of *inguen.*

**in·gui·nal** (ing'gwĭ-nəl) [L. *inguinalis*] pertaining to the inguen, or groin.

**in·gui·no·ab·dom·i·nal** (ing″gwĭ-no-ab-dom'ĭ-nəl) pertaining to the groin and the abdomen.

**in·gui·no·cru·ral** (ing″gwĭ-no-kroo'rəl) pertaining to the groin and the thigh.

**in·gui·no·dyn·ia** (ing″gwĭ-no-din'e-ə) pain in the groin.

**in·gui·no·la·bi·al** (ing″gwĭ-no-la'be-əl) pertaining to the groin and labium.

**in·gui·no·scro·tal** (ing″gwĭ-no-skro'təl) pertaining to the groin and the scrotum.

**INH** trademark (from *iso*n*i*cotine *h*ydrazine) for preparations of isoniazid.

**in·hal·ant** (in-ha'lənt) 1. a substance that is or may be taken into the body by way of the nose and trachea, or through the respiratory system. 2. a class of psychoactive substances whose volatile vapors are subject to abuse; see *substance abuse,* under *abuse.*
**antifoaming i.,** an agent inhaled as a vapor to prevent the formation of foam in the respiratory passages of a patient with pulmonary edema.

**in·ha·la·tion** (in″hə-la'shən) [L. *inhalatio*] 1. the drawing of air or other substances into the lungs; called also *aspiration* and *inspiration.* 2. any drug or solution of drugs administered (as by means of nebulizers or aerosols) by the nasal or oral respiratory route for local or systemic effect.
**isoproterenol sulfate i.** [USP], a solution of isoproterenol hydrochloride in purified water made isotonic by the addition of sodium chloride; used as a bronchodilator, administered by inhalation as an aerosol.

**in·hale** (in-hāl') [L. *inhalare*] to take into the lungs by breathing; called also *inspire.*

**in·hal·er** (in-hāl'ər) [MeSH: Nebulizers and Vaporizers] 1. an apparatus for administering vapor or volatilized medications by inhalation. 2. ventilator (def. 2).
**dry powder i.,** an inhaler that disperses a cloud of dry powdered medication; most types are breath-activated.
**ether i.,** an apparatus for administering the vapor of ether as an anesthetic.
**metered dose i.,** an inhaler used to deliver aerosolized medications in fixed doses to patients with respiratory disease.

**in·her·ent** (in-her'ənt) [L. *inhaerens* sticking fast] implanted by nature; intrinsic; innate.

**in·her·i·tance** (in-her'ĭ-təns) [L. *inhereditare* to appoint an heir] 1. the acquisition of characters or qualities by transmission from parent to offspring. 2. that which is transmitted from parent to offspring. See also the entries of and subentries to *character* (def. 2) and *gene.*
**alternative i.,** inheritance in which the characters are inherited from one parent.
**codominant i.,** see under *gene.*
**complemental i.,** inheritance of characters dependent on the presence of two independent pairs of nonallelic genes (complementary genes), both of which must be present before a given character can be expressed.
**cytoplasmic i.,** mitochondrial i.
**dominant i.,** see under *gene.*
**extrachromosomal i.,** mitochondrial i.
**holandric i.,** inheritance carried only by males, as by genes on the Y chromosome.
**homochronous i.,** the inheritance of characteristics which appear in the offspring at the same age as they appeared in the parent.
**homotropic i.,** the alleged inheritance of acquired characteristics.
**intermediate i.,** inheritance in which the phenotype of the heterozygote is intermediate between that of the two homozygous types. Contrast *codominant gene.*
**maternal i.,** the transmission of characters that are dependent on peculiarities of the egg cytoplasm produced, in turn, by nuclear genes or by mitochondrial genes.
**mendelian i.,** see *Mendel's laws,* under *law.*
**mitochondrial i.,** the inheritance of traits controlled by genes on the DNA of mitochondria in the ooplasm; the genes are thus inherited entirely from the mother (maternal inheritance). Inheritance is nonmendelian, since mitochondria are randomly distributed to the daughter cells at meiosis or mitosis. Mutations of the mitochondrial DNA cause a number of maternally inherited disorders; phenotypic expression of these disorders is variable and depends on the proportions of normal and mutant DNA. Called also *cytoplasmic i.* and *extrachromosomal i.*
**monofactorial i.,** the acquisition of a characteristic or quality, the transmission of which depends on a single gene.
**multifactorial i.,** inheritance determined by multiple factors, genetic and possibly nongenetic (environmental), each with only a partial effect. See also *polygenic i.*
**polygenic i., quantitative i.,** inheritance determined by many genes at different loci, with small additive effects. See also *multifactorial i.*
**quasidominant i.,** inheritance in which there is direct transmission, generation to generation, of a recessive trait; thus, although it is produced by the mating of a recessive homozygote with a heterozygote, the proportion of affected offspring resembles that in dominant inheritance.
**recessive i.,** see under *gene.*
**sex-linked i.,** see under *gene.*

**in·hib·in** (in-hib'in) [MeSH: Inhibin] either of two glycoproteins (designated A and B), secreted by the gonads and present in seminal plasma and follicular fluid, that inhibit pituitary production of follicle-stimulating hormone. They also contribute to the control of gametogenesis, embryonic and fetal development, and hematopoiesis. Their actions are opposed by activins.

**in·hib·it** (in-hib'it) to retard, arrest, or restrain.

**in·hi·bi·tion** (in″hĭ-bish'ən) [L. *inhibēre* to restrain, from *in* in + *habēre* to hold] 1. arrest or restraint of a process. 2. in psychoanalytic theory, the conscious or unconscious restraining of an impulse or desire.
**allogenic i.,** injury to cells in vitro as a consequence of contact with lymphocytes that are of a different genotype.
**allosteric i.,** inhibition of an enzyme by binding of an inhibitor at an allosteric site that causes at the catalytic site either reduced binding affinity of the enzyme for the substrate or decreased rate of catalytic turnover.
**competitive i.,** inhibition of enzyme activity in which the inhibitor (substrate analogue) reversibly combines with catalytic sites, thus competing with the substrate for binding on the enzyme. The inhibition is reversible since it can be overcome by increasing the sub-

strate concentration. Similarly, the reversible binding of a physiologic antagonist to a receptor site for a hormone or neurotransmitter.
**contact i.,** the inhibition of cell division and cell motility in normal animal cells when in close contact with each other.
**endproduct i.,** feedback i.
**enzyme i.,** inhibition of enzyme activity, as in competitive or endproduct inhibition.
**feedback i.,** inhibition of the initial steps of a process by an endproduct of the reaction.
**hemagglutination i. (HI, HAI),** see under *test.*
**mixed i.,** inhibition of enzyme activity in a manner that has features of both competitive and noncompetitive inhibition, both substrate binding and rate of turnover of the enzyme being affected.
**noncompetitive i.,** inhibition of enzyme activity by a substance that combines with the enzyme at a site other than that utilized by the substrate, causing a change in enzyme configuration and a decrease in activity. Similarly, the inhibition of a hormone or neurotransmitter by binding of a physiologic antagonist to a receptor at a site other than the active center.
**proactive i.,** the interference of earlier learning in the retention of new learning; cf. *retroactive i.*
**reciprocal i.,** the inhibition of one group of muscles on excitation of their antagonists, a phenomenon resulting from reciprocal innervation (q.v.).
**retroactive i.,** the interference of new learning in the recall of earlier learning; cf. *proactive i.*
**uncompetitive i.,** inhibition of an enzyme by a substance that binds reversibly to the enzyme-substrate complex. The enzyme-substrate-inhibitor complex cannot yield the normal product until the inhibitor is released.
**Wedensky i.,** a partial block to conduction in a nerve may transmit impulses at low frequencies but not at higher frequencies.

**in·hib·i·tive** (in-hib'ĭ-tiv) inhibitory.

**in·hib·i·tor** (in-hib'ĭ-tor) 1. any substance that interferes with a chemical reaction, growth, or other biological activity. 2. a chemical substance that inhibits an enzyme reaction. See also *inhibition.*
**ACE i's,** angiotensin-converting enzyme i's.
**alpha$_1$-proteinase i.,** alpha$_1$-antitrypsin.
**alpha$_1$-proteinase i. (human),** a sterile, stable, lyophilized preparation of human alpha$_1$-proteinase inhibitor obtained from the pooled plasma of normal human donors; used in the treatment of congenital alpha$_1$-antitrypsin deficiency.
**angiotensin-converting enzyme i's,** competitive inhibitors of peptidyl-dipeptidase A (angiotensin-converting enzyme), used for treatment of hypertension, usually in conjunction with a diuretic. They are effective in both renovascular and essential low-renin hypertension. Called also *ACE i's.*
**C1 i. (C1 INH),** an $\alpha_2$-globulin that inhibits the complement component C1 (see under *complement*), binding the complex of C1r and C1s, removing it from C1q and preventing activation of the classical complement pathway. It also inhibits plasmin, thrombin, and kallikrein. Deficiency of or defect in the protein causes hereditary angioedema.
**carbonic anhydrase i.,** any of a class of agents that inhibit carbonic anhydrase activity, in the kidney decreasing the hydrogen ion concentration in the renal tubule resulting in increased excretion of bicarbonate, sodium, potassium, and water, and in the eye depressing the production of aqueous humor and lowering intraocular pressure. Originally used as diuretics but replaced by other agents because their diuretic effect is self-limiting; now used chiefly for the treatment of glaucoma, and also for the treatment of epilepsy, familial periodic paralysis, acute mountain sickness, and uric acid renal calculi.
**C1 esterase i.,** C1 i.
**cholesterol i.,** an agent that suppresses the production of cholesterol or decreases the level of cholesterol in the blood.
**cholinesterase i.,** a chemical compound that prevents the hydrolysis of acetylcholine by the enzyme acetylcholinesterase, thereby permitting high levels of acetylcholine to accumulate at reactive sites. Some are used as drugs, some are insecticides, and certain potent ones are nerve gases that can be deadly to humans or other animals. Called also *anticholinesterase.*
**gastric acid pump i.,** an agent that inhibits gastric acid secretion by blocking the action of $H^+,K^+$-ATPase at the secretory surface of gastric parietal cells; called also *proton pump i.*
**HIV protease i.,** any of a group of antiretroviral drugs active against the human immunodeficiency virus; they prevent cleavage of viral polyproteins, causing production of immature viral particles that are noninfective. Examples include indinavir sulfate, nelfinavir mesylate, ritonavir, and saquinavir mesylate.
**lupus i.,** see under *anticoagulant.*
**membrane attack complex i. (MAC INH),** former name for *S protein;* see *vitronectin.*
**membrane i. of reactive lysis (MIRL),** protectin.
**mitotic i.,** a substance that slows or arrests the process of mitosis, e.g., colchicine.
**monoamine oxidase i. (MAOI),** any of a group of antidepressant drugs that have the ability to block the oxidative deamination of monoamines. It is thought that by inhibiting monoamine oxidase activity the inhibitors increase the level of catecholamines in the central nervous system, which would have been otherwise neutralized by the enzyme, and that these increased concentrations are responsible for their antidepressant effects.
**phosphodiesterase i.,** any of a class of drugs that inhibit the activity of phosphodiesterases, each agent having a different effect because of differing affinities for the various phosphodiesterase fractions; included in this class are amrinone, dipyridamole, enoximone, milrinone, papaverine, piroximone, and theophylline.
**$\alpha_2$-plasmin i.,** $\alpha_2$-antiplasmin.
**plasminogen activator i. (PAI),** any of several regulators of the fibrinolytic system that act by binding to and inhibiting free plasminogen activator. The concentration in plasma of the inhibitors is normally low, but is altered in some disturbances of the hemostatic system. *PAI-1* is an important fast-reacting inhibitor of t-PA and u-PA. Its synthesis, activity, and release are highly regulated. Elevated levels of the inhibitor have been described in a number of disease states. *PAI-2* is a normally minor inhibitor that greatly increases in concentration during pregnancy and in certain disorders. *PAI-3* is *protein C inhibitor.*
**platelet i.,** any of a group of agents that inhibit the clotting activity of platelets; the most common ones are aspirin, dipyridamole, sulfinpyrazone, and ticlopidine hydrochloride. See also *antiplatelet therapy,* under *therapy.*
**protein C i.,** the primary inhibitor of activated anticoagulant protein C; it is a glycoprotein, $M_r$ 57,000, of the serpin superfamily of proteinase inhibitors and also inhibits several other proteins involved in coagulation and urokinase. Called also *plasminogen activator inhibitor 3.*
**proton pump i.,** gastric acid pump i.
**selective serotonin reuptake i. (SSRI),** any of a group of drugs that inhibit the inactivation of serotonin by blocking its absorption in the central nervous system; used as antidepressants.
**serine proteinase i.,** serpin.

**in·hib·i·to·ry** (in-hib'ĭ-tor″e) [L. *inhibere* to restrain] restraining or arresting any process; effecting a stay or arrest, partial or complete.

**in·ho·mo·ge·ne·i·ty** (in-ho″mo-jə-ne'ĭ-te) lack of normal homogeneity.

**in·ho·mo·ge·neous** (in-ho″mo-je'ne-əs) lacking homogeneity.

**in·i·ac** (in'e-ək) pertaining to the inion.

**in·i·ad** (in'e-əd) toward the inion.

**in·i·al** (in'e-əl) iniac.

**in·i·en·ceph·a·lus** (in″e-ən-sef'ə-ləs) a fetus exhibiting iniencephaly.

**in·i·en·ceph·a·ly** (in″e-ən-sef'ə-le) [*inion* + *enkephalos* brain] a developmental anomaly characterized by enlargement of the foramen magnum and absence of the laminal and spinous processes of the cervical, dorsal, and sometimes lumbar vertebrae, with vertebrae reduced in number and irregularly fused, the brain and much of the spinal cord occupying a single cavity.

**inio-** [Gr. *inion* occiput] a combining form denoting relationship to the occiput.

**in·i·od·y·mus** (in″e-od'ĭ-məs) [*inio-* + *-didymus*] iniopagus.

**in·i·on** (in'e-on) [Gr. "the back of the head"] [TA] the most prominent point of the external occipital protuberance.

**in·i·op·a·gus** (in″e-op'ə-gəs) [*inio-* + *-pagus*] symmetrical conjoined twins fused at the occiput.

**in·i·ops** (in'e-ops) [*inio-* +Gr. *ōps* eye] a double-faced fetus with the posterior face incomplete.

**ini·tial** (ĭ-nish'əl) [L. *initialis,* from *initium* beginning] pertaining to the very first stage of any process.

**ini·ti·a·tion** (ĭ-nĭ″she-a'shən) in toxicology, the creation of a small alteration in the genetic makeup of a cell by a low level of exposure to a carcinogen; the cell may later become neoplastic upon repeated exposure to the same carcinogen or exposure to a promoter.

**ini·ti·a·tor** (ĭ-nish'e-a″tər) an agent that initiates polymerization of a resin when mixed with the resin.

**in·i·tis** (in-i'tis) [Gr. *is, inos* fiber] myositis.

**in·ject·a·ble** (in-jek'tə-bəl) [MeSH: Injections] 1. capable of being injected. 2. a substance that may be injected.

**in·ject·ed** (in-jek'təd) 1. introduced by injection. 2. congested.

**in·jec·tion** (in-jek'shən) [L. *injectio,* from *inicere* to throw into] [MeSH: Injections] 1. the act of forcing a liquid into a part, as into the subcutaneous tissues, the vascular tree, or an organ. Cf. *infusion*

(def. 3). 2. a substance so forced or administered. Officially, in pharmacy, a solution of a medicament suitable for injection. See also under specific substances. 3. the condition of being injected; congestion.
**aminohippurate sodium i.** [USP], a sterile solution of aminohippuric acid in water for injection prepared with the aid of sodium hydroxide; administered by intravenous infusion for the measurement of effective renal plasma flow and determination of the functional capacity of the tubular excretory mechanism.
**aminophylline i.** [USP], a sterile solution of aminophylline in water for injection, or of theophylline in water for injection prepared with the aid of ethylenediamine.
**anatomical i.,** an injection into the vessels or organs of the cadaver, designed to facilitate dissection or demonstration.
**benzylpenicilloyl polylysine i.** [USP], a solution of benzylpenicilloyl polylysine having a molar concentration of the benzylpenicilloyl moiety of $5.4 \times 10^{-5}$ to $7.0 \times 10^{-5}$ *M,* with one or more suitable buffers; used as a diagnostic aid for penicillin sensitivity.
**caffeine and sodium benzoate i.** [USP], a sterile solution of caffeine and sodium benzoate in water for injection, used as a central nervous system stimulant; administered intramuscularly or intravenously.
**circumcorneal i.,** dilatation of the ciliary and conjunctival blood vessels close to the limbus, and diminishing toward the periphery.
**coarse i.,** an anatomical injection that fills only the larger vessels.
**depot i.,** injection of a medication that stays in a local area (a *depot*) and is distributed slowly into the body; absorption is often kept slow by mixing the medication with a suitable excipient.
**dextrose i.** [USP], a sterile solution of dextrose in water for injection; used as a fluid and nutrient replenisher.
**endermic i.,** intracutaneous i.
**epifascial i.,** one made upon the surface of a fascia, particularly the fascia lata.
**fine i.,** an anatomical injection that fills even the smallest vessels.
**fructose i.,** a sterile solution of fructose in water, used as a fluid and nutrient replenisher.
**gaseous i.,** injection of gas or air for therapeutic purposes as in collapse therapy; for diagnostic purposes, as in ventriculography; or for facilitating anatomical demonstrations.
**gelatin i.,** a preservative injection of which gelatin is the base.
**hypodermic i.,** an injection made into the subcutaneous tissues; called also *subcutaneous i.*
**intracutaneous i., intradermal i., intradermic i.,** one made into the corium or substance of the skin.
**intracytoplasmic sperm i. (ICSI),** insertion of a single spermatocyte into an oocyte by micropuncture; used in the treatment of male infertility.
**intramuscular i.,** an injection into the substance of a muscle.
**intrathecal i.,** injection of a substance through the theca of the spinal cord into the subarachnoid space.
**intravascular i.,** an injection made into a vessel.
**intravenous i.,** an injection made into a vein.
**invert sugar i.** [USP], a sterile aqueous solution prepared by mixing equal amounts of dextrose and fructose or by hydrolysis of an equivalent amount of sucrose; used as a fluid and nutrient replenisher.
**iobenguane I 123 i.** [USP], a sterile solution of iobenguane I 123 sulfate, used as a radioactive tracer in the diagnosis of neuroendocrine tumors and disorders of the adrenal medulla; administered intravenously.
**iodinated I 131 albumin aggregated i.** [USP], a sterile aqueous suspension of albumin human iodinated with $^{131}I$ and denatured to produce aggregates of controlled particle size; each mL contains 300 μg to 3.0 mg of aggregated albumin with specific activity of 200 microcuries to 1.2 millicuries per mg.
**iron dextran i.** [USP], a sterile colloidal solution of ferric hydroxide complexed with partially hydrolyzed low molecular weight dextran, in water for injection; used as a hematinic.
**iron sorbitex i.** [USP], a sterile solution of a complex of iron, sorbitol, and citric acid that is stabilized with the aid of dextrin and an excess of sorbitol; used as a hematinic.
**jet i.,** injection of a drug in solution through the intact skin by an extremely fine jet of the solution under high pressure.
**multiple electrolytes i.,** a sterile solution of electrolytes in water for injection to provide various combinations of ions; official preparations [USP] contain different combinations of salts and may also include carbohydrates (see table at electrolyte).
**opacifying i.,** the injection of a radiopaque substance into the vessels or into some body cavity for diagnostic radiological study.
**parenchymatous i.,** one made into the substance of an organ.
**posterior pituitary i.,** a sterile solution in water of the principles from the posterior lobe of the pituitary of domestic food animals; used as an oxytocic, in the treatment of diabetes insipidus, and to stimulate intestinal peristalsis.
**preservative i.,** an injection that serves to protect a cadaver or specimen from decay.
**protamine sulfate i.** [USP], a sterile isotonic solution prepared from the sperm or from the mature testes of fish belonging to the genus *Oncorhynchus, Salmo,* or *Trutta;* used to counteract the action of heparin.
**protein hydrolysate i.** [USP], a sterile solution of amino acids and short-chain peptides, used as a fluid and nutrient replenisher.
**repository corticotropin i.** [USP], corticotropin in a solution of partially hydrolyzed gelatin, having prolonged effects and used for diagnostic testing of adrenocortical function and to stimulate adrenal cortex activity; administered subcutaneously and intramuscularly.
**Ringer's i.** [USP], a sterile solution of sodium chloride, potassium chloride, and calcium chloride in water for injection, given as a fluid and electrolyte replenisher by intravenous infusion.
**Ringer's i., lactated** [USP], a sterile solution of calcium chloride, potassium chloride, sodium chloride, and sodium lactate in water for injection, given as a fluid and electrolyte replenisher by intravenous infusion; called also *lactated Ringer's solution.*
**sclerosing i.,** sclerotherapy.
**sodium chloride i.** [USP], a sterile isotonic solution of sodium chloride in water for injection, used as a fluid and electrolyte replenisher and as an irrigating solution. It is also used as a vehicle for the injection of medications.
**sodium radiochromate i.,** sodium chromate Cr 51 i.
**subcutaneous i.,** hypodermic i.
**vasopressin i.** [USP], a sterile solution of the water-soluble, pressor principle of the posterior lobe of the pituitary of domestic food animals in water for injection; used as an antidiuretic.

**in·jec·tor** (in-jek'tər) [L. *injicere* to inject] an instrument used in making injections.

**in·ju·ry** (in'jə-re) [L. *injuria; in* not + *jus* right] [MeSH: Wounds and Injuries] harm or hurt; usually applied to damage inflicted on the body by an external force. Called also *trauma* and *wound.*
**birth i.,** see under *trauma.*
**blast i.,** the injuries caused by an explosion (see *blast*[2]), most commonly blast chest (q.v.), laceration of other thoracic and abdominal viscera, ruptured ear drums, and minor effects on the central nervous system.
**deceleration i.,** an injury sustained by sudden deceleration in the movement of the body, as in a motor vehicle accident; the brain is especially liable to such trauma.
**Goyrand's i.,** pulled elbow.
**reperfusion i.,** adverse effects of the restoration of blood flow following an ischemic episode, including cellular swelling and necrosis, edema, hemorrhage, the no-reflow phenomenon, and tissue damage by free oxygen radicals.
**steering-wheel i.,** injury to the chest and sometimes contusion of the heart in motorists, caused by being thrown forward against the steering wheel.
**unintentional i.,** in public health, the cause of death when the death occurs under accidental circumstances.
**whiplash i.,** a popular nonspecific term applied to injury to the spine and spinal cord at the junction of the fourth and fifth cervical vertebrae, occurring as the result of rapid acceleration or deceleration of the body. Because of their greater mobility, the four upper vertebrae act as the lash, and the lower three act as the handle of the whip.

**in·lay** (in'la) [MeSH: Inlays] 1. material, such as bone or skin, inserted into a tissue defect. 2. a dental restoration made outside of a tooth to correspond with the form of a prepared cavity and then cemented into the tooth.
**epithelial i.,** a method of securing epithelialization of an unhealed deep wound. A mold of the wound cavity is taken and covered with a Thiersch graft of epidermis, the whole being inserted into the wound cavity, and the edges then approximated with sutures. The mold is removed after ten days, leaving the cavity completely epithelialized. Called also *Esser's operation.* See also under *onlay.*

**in·let** (in'lət) an avenue of ingress.
**pelvic i.,** apertura pelvis superior.
**thoracic i.,** apertura thoracis superior.

**INN** International Nonproprietary Names, the nonproprietary designation recommended by the World Health Organization for any pharmaceutical preparation. Such names are selected according to general principles set forth by the World Health Organization, and lists are published periodically in the *WHO Chronicle.*

**in·nate** (ĭ-nāt') [L. *in* in + *nasci* to be born] inborn; hereditary; congenital.

**in·ner·va·tion** (in"ər-va'shən) [*in-*[1] + *nervus*] 1. the distribution or supply of nerves to a part. 2. the supply of nervous energy or of nerve stimulus sent to a part.
**double i.,** innervation of a structure by two kinds of nerve fibers, e.g., sympathetic and parasympathetic.
**reciprocal i.,** the innervation of muscles around the joints, where the motor centers are so connected in pairs that when one is excited the center of the corresponding antagonist is inhibited.

**in·nid·i·a·tion** (ĭ-nid"e-a'shən) [*in-*[1] + *nidus*] the development of

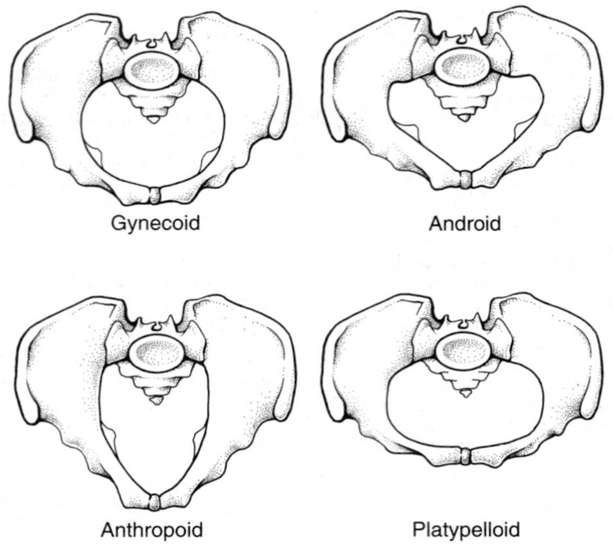


Various types of pelvic inlets.

cells in a part to which they have been carried by metastasis; called also *colonization* and *indenization*.

**in·no·cent** (in'o-sənt) [L. *innocens; in* not +*nocere* to harm] not malignant; benign; not tending of its own nature to a fatal issue. See *innocent bystander,* under *bystander.*

**in·noc·u·ous** (ĭ-nok'u-əs) harmless.

**in·nom·i·na·tal** (ĭ-nom"ĭ-na'təl) pertaining to the innominate (brachiocephalic) artery or to the innominate (hip) bone.

**in·nom·i·nate** (ĭ-nom'ĭ-nāt) [L. *innominatus* nameless; *in* not +*nomen* name] not having a name; nameless. The term has been applied to certain structures better identified by their descriptive names, as the innominate (brachiocephalic) artery and the innominate (hip) bone.

**In·no·var** (in'o-vahr) a trademark for a preparation of droperidol and fentanyl citrate in a 50:1 ratio; used as a neuroleptanalgesic.

**in·nox·ious** (ĭ-nok'shəs) [*in-*[2] + *noxius*] not injurious; not hurtful.

**in(o)-** [Gr. *is,* gen. *inos* fiber] a combining form denoting relationship to a fiber, or fibrous material.

**ino·blast** (in'o-blast) [*ino-* + *-blast*] any connective tissue cell in the formative stage.

**ino·chon·dri·tis** (in"o-kon-dri'tis) [*ino-* + *chondr-* + *-itis*] inflammation of a fibrocartilage.

**In·o·cor** (in'o-kor) trademark for a preparation of amrinone.

**in·oc·u·la** (ĭ-nok'u-lə) [L.] plural of *inoculum.*

**in·oc·u·la·bil·i·ty** (ĭ-nok"u-lə-bil'ĭ-te) the quality or state of being inoculable.

**in·oc·u·la·ble** (ĭ-nok'u-lə-bəl) 1. susceptible of being inoculated; transmissible by inoculation. 2. not immune against a disease transmissible by inoculation.

**in·oc·u·late** (ĭ-nok'u-lāt) to communicate a disease by inserting its etiologic agent; to implant microbes or infective materials in or on culture media; to introduce immune serum, vaccines of various kinds, and other antigenic materials for preventive, curative, or experimental purposes.

**in·oc·u·la·tion** (ĭ-nok"u-la'shən) [L. *inoculatio,* from *in* into + *oculus* bud] introduction of microorganisms, infective material, serum, and other substances into tissues of living plants and animals, or culture media; introduction of a disease agent, e.g., vaccine virus, into a healthy individual to produce a mild form of the disease followed by immunity.
**protective i.,** the injection of a biological preparation, e.g., a vaccine or an antiserum, to protect against a disease; vaccination against a disease.

**in·oc·u·lum** (ĭ-nok'u-ləm) pl. *inoc'ula* [L.] the substance used in inoculation.

**I·no·cy·be** (i-nos'ĭ-be) a genus of mushrooms (order Agaricales) that are common in North America; many species contain muscarine.

**ino·cyte** (in'o-sīt) [*ino-* + *-cyte*] a cell of fibrous tissue.

**ino·di·la·tor** (in"o-di'lāt-ər) an agent that has both positive inotropic and vasodilator effects.

**ino·gen·e·sis** (in"o-jen'ə-sis) the formation of fibrous tissue.

**in·og·e·nous** (in-oj'ə-nəs) produced from or producing fibrous tissue.

**in·og·lia** (in-og'le-ə) [*ino-* + *-glia*] fibroglia.

**ino·lith** (in'o-lith) [*ino-* + *-lith*] a fibrous concretion.

**ino·myo·si·tis** (in"o-mi"o-si'tis) fibromyositis.

**in·op·er·a·ble** (in-op'ər-ə-bəl) not suitable to be operated upon.

**in·o·per·cu·late** (in"o-pər'ku-lāt) not having an operculum; said of an ascus.

**ino·phrag·ma** (in"o-frag'mə) [*ino-* + Gr. *phragmos* a fencing in] ground membrane; a name given to the Z band and M band (q.v. under *band* ) because they continue uninterruptedly as transverse membranes through all the adjoining fibrils of a muscle fiber. See *mesophragma* and *telophragma.*

**in·or·gan·ic** (in"or-gan'ik) [*in-*[2] + *organic*] 1. having no organs. 2. not of organic origin. 3. pertaining to substances not of organic origin. 4. in chemistry, denoting substances not derived from hydrocarbons.

**in·or·gan·ic py·ro·phos·pha·tase** (in"or-gan'ik pi"ro-fos'fə-tās) [EC 3.6.1.1] an enzyme of the hydrolase class that catalyzes the cleavage of a pyrophosphate molecule to form two molecules of orthophosphate. The enzyme is present in all cells and regulates the concentration of endogenous pyrophosphate. Inorganic pyrophosphatase may be identical with alkaline phosphatase in some tissues.

**ino·scle·ro·sis** (in"o-sklə-ro'sis) [*ino-* + *sclerosis*] sclerosis or induration by increase of fibrous tissue.

**in·os·co·py** (in-os'ko-pe) [*ino-* + *-scopy*] the diagnosis of disease by artificial digestion and examination of the fibers or fibrinous matter of the sputum, blood, effusions, etc.

**in·os·cu·late** (in-os'ku-lāt) [*in-*[1] + *osculum*] to unite or communicate by means of small openings or anastomoses.

**in·os·cu·la·tion** (in-os"ku-la'shən) the establishment of communication, by means of small openings or anastomoses, applied especially to establishment of such communication between already existing blood vessels or other tubular structures that come in contact.

**in·ose** (in'ōs) inositol.

**in·o·se·mia** (in"o-se'me-ə) 1. the presence of inose (inositol) in the blood. 2. an excess of fibrin in the blood.

**in·o·si·nate** (in-o'sĭ-nāt) a salt, anion, or ester of inosinic acid (inosine monophosphate).

**in·o·sine** (in'o-sēn) [MeSH: Inosine] a purine nucleoside, hypoxanthine linked by its N9 nitrogen to the C1 carbon of ribose. It is an intermediate in the degradation of purines and purine nucleosides to uric acid and in pathways of purine salvage. It also occurs in the anticodon of certain transfer RNA molecules. Symbol I.
**i. monophosphate (IMP),** a nucleotide, the 5′-phosphate of inosine, formed by deamination of adenosine monophosphate (AMP); it is the precursor of AMP and GMP (guanosine monophosphate) in purine biosynthesis and an intermediate in the salvage of purines and the degradation of purines to uric acid.
**i. triphosphate (ITP),** a nucleotide, the 5′-triphosphate of inosine; it acts as a phosphate donor in certain carboxylation reactions.

**in·o·sin·ic acid** (in"o-sin'ik) inosine monophosphate.

**in·o·site** (in'o-sīt) inositol.

**ino·sit·ide** (in-o'sĭ-tīd) a compound containing inositol, particularly phosphatidylinositol and related lipids.

**in·o·si·tis** (in"o-si'tis) [*ino-* + *-itis*] inflammation of fibrous tissue.

**ino·si·tol** (ĭ-no'sĭ-tol) [MeSH: Inositol] a cyclic sugar alcohol, the fully hydroxylated derivative of cyclohexane, occurring naturally in a variety of stereoisomers, particularly the *myo*-isomer. Used alone, the term usually denotes this isomer.
***myo*-i.,** the *myo*-isomer of inositol, occurring in a variety of plant and animal tissues and microorganisms; it is often phosphorylated and is a component of phosphatidylinositols. It is a member of the vitamin B complex and can be obtained from vegetables, citrus fruits, cereal grains, and organ and other meats.
**i. niacinate,** a peripheral vasodilator, $C_{42}H_{30}N_6O_{12}$.
**i. 1,4,5-triphosphate (InsP$_3$, IP$_3$),** a second messenger generated by cleavage of phosphatidylinositol 4,5-bisphosphate in calcium-mediated hormonal responses; it causes the release of calcium from certain intracellular organelles.

**in·o·si·tol·uria** (in"o-sĭ"tol-u're-ə) inosituria.

**in·o·si·tu·ria** (in"o-sĭ-tu're-ə) the occurrence of inositol in the urine; called also *inosuria.*

**in·os·to·sis** (in″os-to′sis) the re-formation of bony tissue to replace such tissue which has been destroyed.

**in·os·uria** (in″o-su′re-ə) 1. an excess of fibrin in the urine. 2. inosituria.

**ino·tag·ma** (in″o-tag′mə) [*ino-* + Gr. *tagma* arrangement] a linear arrangement of the contractile structural elements of a muscle cell.

**in·o·trop·ic** (in″o-trop′ik) [*ino-* + *-tropic*] affecting the force or energy of muscular contractions.
**negatively i.,** weakening the force of muscular contraction.
**positively i.,** increasing the strength of muscular contraction.

**in·ot·ro·pism** (in-ot′rə-piz-əm) the quality of influencing the contractility of muscle fibers.

**in ovo** (in o′vo) [L.] in the egg; referring specifically to various experimental procedures involving the use of chick embryos.

**in·pa·tient** (in′pa-shənt) [MeSH: Inpatients] a patient who comes to a hospital or other health care facility for diagnosis or treatment that requires an overnight stay.

**in·quest** (in′kwest) [L. *in* into + *quaerere* to seek] a legal inquiry before a coroner or medical examiner, and usually a jury, into the manner of a death.

**in·qui·line** (in′kwĭ-līn) [L. *inquilinus* a lodger] an organism that lives within the body of another, but does not derive its nourishment from the host.

**in·sal·i·va·tion** (in″sal-ĭ-va′shən) [*in-*[1] + *salivation*] the saturation of the food with saliva in mastication.

**In·sall-Sal·va·ti ratio** (in′səl sahl-vah′te) [J.N. *Insall,* American orthopedist, 20th century; E. *Salvati,* American orthopedist, 20th century] see under *ratio.*

**in·sa·lu·bri·ous** (in″sə-loo′bre-əs) not salubrious; not conducive to health.

**in·sane** (in-sān′) [*in-*[2] + *sane*] pertaining to, exhibiting, or characterized by insanity.

**in·san·i·tary** (in-san′ĭ-tar-e) not in a good sanitary condition; not conducive to good health; unclean.

**in·san·i·ty** (in-san′ĭ-te) [L. *insanitas,* from *in* not + *sanus* sound] mental derangement or disorder, a legal rather than a medical term denoting a condition due to which a person lacks criminal responsibility for a crime and therefore cannot be convicted of it.
**moral i.,** *(obs.)* a 19th century concept corresponding roughly to antisocial personality disorder; a disorder of emotions and habits without impairment of the intellectual faculties in which the moral sense (concern for the rights and feelings of others) is stunted *(moral imbecility)* or absent *(moral idiocy.)*

**in·scrip·tio** (in-skrip′she-o) pl. *inscriptio′nes* [L., from *inscribere* to write on] 1. inscription. 2. intersectio.
**i. tendi′nea,** intersectio tendinea.
**inscriptio′nes tendin′eae mus′culi rec′ti abdom′inis,** intersectiones tendineae musculi recti abdominis.

**in·scrip·tion** (in-skrip′shən) [L. *inscriptio*] 1. a mark, or line. 2. that part of a prescription which contains the names and amounts of the ingredients.
**tendinous i.,** intersectio tendinea.
**tendinous i's of rectus abdominis muscle,** intersectiones tendineae musculi recti abdominis.

**in·scrip·ti·o·nes** (in-skrip″she-o′nēz) [L.] plural of *inscriptio.*

**in·sect** (in′sekt) [MeSH: Insects] any individual of the class Insecta.

**In·sec·ta** (in-sek′tə) [L. from *in* + *sectum* cut] a class of the Arthropoda whose members are characterized by division into three parts: head, thorax, and abdomen; there are three orders of medical interest, Hemiptera, Diptera, and Siphonaptera.

**in·sec·ta·ri·um** (in″sek-tar′e-əm) a place for breeding and raising insects.

**in·sec·ti·cide** (in-sek′tĭ-sīd) [*insect* + *-cide*] any substance selectively poisonous to insects.

**in·sec·ti·fuge** (in-sek′tĭ-fūj) [*insect* + *-fuge*] a preparation that repels insects.

**In·sec·tiv·o·ra** (in″sek-tiv′o-rə) [*insect* + L. *vorare* to devour] [MeSH: Insectivora] an order of small, terrestrial mammals, including the moles and shrews, which feed primarily on insects and other invertebrates.

**in·sec·ti·vore** (in-sek′tĭ-vor) an individual of the order Insectivora.

**in·sec·tiv·o·rous** (in″sek-tiv′ə-rəs) subsisting on insects.

**in·sem·i·na·tion** (in-sem″ĭ-na′shən) [L. *inseminatus* sown, from *in* into + *semen* seed] [MeSH: Insemination] the deposit of semen or seminal fluid within the vagina or cervix, as during sexual intercourse.
**artificial i.,** introduction of semen into the vagina or cervix by artificial means.
**donor i., heterologous i.,** artificial insemination in which the semen used is that of a man other than the woman's husband; called also AID.
**homologous i.,** artificial insemination in which the husband's semen is used; called also AIH.

**in·se·nes·cence** (in″sə-nes′əns) the process of growing old.

**in·sen·si·ble** (in-sen′sĭ-bəl) [*in-*[2] + *sensible*] 1. not appreciable by or perceptible to the senses. 2. devoid of consciousness or of sensibility.

**in·sert**[1] (in-sərt′) [L. *inserere* to graft, insert] to put in, introduce, or implant something into another thing.

**in·sert**[2] (in′sərt) something that is put in or introduced; cf. *implant*[2].
**intramucosal i., mucosal i.,** a nonreactive metal stud, consisting of a base, cervix, and head, attached to a prosthesis inserted into a pocket of oral mucosa just before fitting of a denture; most commonly used for added retention of complete upper dentures.

**in·ser·tio** (in-sər′she-o) [L.] [TA] insertion.
**i. velamento′sa,** velamentous insertion.

**in·ser·tion** (in-ser′shən) [L. *inserere* to join to] 1. the place of attachment, as of a muscle to the bone which it moves. 2. in genetics, a rare nonreciprocal translocation (q.v.) involving three breaks in which a segment is removed from one chromosome and then inserted into a broken region of a nonhomologous chromosome. See Plate 1.
**parasol i.,** insertion of the umbilical cord in the placenta, in which the vessels of the cord separate before they join the placenta and resemble the ribs of a parasol.
**velamentous i.,** attachment of the umbilical cord to the membranes, with the vessels coursing for a long or short distance between the amnion and the smooth chorion to reach the placenta.

**in·sheathed** (in-shēthd′) enclosed within a sheath.

**in·sid·i·ous** (in-sid′e-əs) [L. *insidiosus* deceitful, treacherous] coming on in a stealthy manner; of gradual and subtle development.

**in·sight** (in′sīt) 1. in psychiatry, the patient's awareness and understanding of the origins and meaning of his attitudes, feelings, and behavior and of his disturbing symptoms; self-understanding. 2. in problem solving, the sudden perception of the appropriate relationships of things that results in a solution.
**intellectual i.,** understanding of the objective reality of a situation without the ability to apply that knowledge in the future or without true feeling.
**true i.,** understanding of the objective reality of a situation coupled to true feeling and to the motivation and capability to use the understanding in the future.

**in si·tu** (in si′tu) [L.] in the natural or normal place; confined to the site of origin without invasion of neighboring tissues.

**in·so·la·tion** (in″so-la′shən) [L. *insolare* to expose to the sun; *in* in + *sol* sun] 1. heliotherapy. 2. sunstroke.
**asphyxial i.,** sunstroke with low temperature, cold skin, and feeble pulse.
**hyperpyrexial i.,** thermic fever with very high temperature, coma, and congested skin.

**in·sol·u·ble** (in-sol′u-bəl) [L. *insolubilis,* from *in* not + *solvere* to dissolve] not susceptible of being dissolved.

**in·som·nia** (in-som′ne-ə) [*in-*[2] + *somn-* + *-ia*] [MeSH: Insomnia] inability to sleep; abnormal wakefulness.
**fatal familial i.,** an inherited prion disease, transmitted as an autosomal dominant trait, affecting primarily the ventral and dorsomedial nuclei of the thalamus and characterized by progressive insomnia, hallucinations, stupor, and coma ending in death within 6 months to 3 years of onset; autonomic and motor disturbances are also present.
**initial i.,** that characterized by difficulty falling asleep, often due to anxiety, tension, or depression.
**middle i.,** that characterized by awakening during the sleep period, with difficulty in falling back to sleep.
**primary i.** [DSM-IV], a dyssomnia characterized by persistent difficulty initiating or maintaining sleep or by persistently nonrestorative sleep; it is not due to another sleep disorder or mental disorder or to a general medical condition or substance use.
**terminal i.,** that characterized by early awakening with difficulty in falling back to sleep, often occurring in depression, bereavement, chronic anxiety, and cerebral arteriosclerosis.

**in·som·ni·ac** (in-som′ne-ak) 1. pertaining to insomnia. 2. an individual exhibiting insomnia.

**in·som·nic** (in-som′nik) insomniac.

**in·so·nate** (in-so′nāt) to expose to ultrasound waves.

**in·sorp·tion** (in-sorp′shən) the movement of a substance into the blood; said of such movement from the contents of the gastrointestinal tract into the circulating blood.

**InsP$_3$** inositol 1,4,5-triphosphate.

**in·sper·sion** (in-spər'zhən) [L. *inspersio; in* upon + *spargere* to sprinkle] the act of sprinkling, as with a powder.

**in·spi·rate** (in'spĭ-rāt) inhaled air or other gas.

**in·spi·ra·tion** (in″spĭ-ra'shən) inhalation (def. 1).

**in·spi·ra·to·ry** (in-spi'rə-tor″e) pertaining to inhalation (inspiration).

**in·spire** (in-spīr') [L. *inspirare*] inhale.

**in·spi·rom·e·ter** (in″spi-rom'ə-tər) [*inspire* + *-meter*] an apparatus for measuring the amount of air inspired.

**in·spis·sat·ed** (in-spis'āt-əd) [L. *inspissatus,* from *in* intensive + *spissare* to thicken] being thickened, dried, or rendered less fluid.

**in·spis·sa·tion** (in″spis-a'shən) [L. *inspissatio*] 1. the act or process of rendering dry or thick by the evaporation of readily vaporizable parts. 2. the condition of being rendered less thin by evaporation.

**in·spis·sa·tor** (in-spis'a-tər) an apparatus for inspissating fluids, such as blood serum.

**in·sta·bil·i·ty** (in-stə-bil'ĭ-te) lack of steadiness or stability.
**detrusor i.,** involuntary contraction of the detrusor muscle of the bladder caused by nonneurological problems such as bladder outlet obstruction; cf. *detrusor hyperreflexia.*

**in·star** (in'stahr) [L. "a form"] any stage of an arthropod between molts.

**in·step** (in'step) the dorsal part of the arch of the foot.

**in·stil·la·tion** (in″stĭ-la'shən) [L. *instillatio,* from *in* into + *stillare* to drop] administration of a liquid drop by drop.

**in·stil·la·tor** (in'stĭ-la″tər) an instrument for performing instillations.

**in·stinct** (in'stinkt) [L. *instinctus; in* on +*stinguere* to prick] [MeSH: Instinct] a complex of unlearned responses that is characteristic of a species.
**aggressive i.,** death i.
**death i.,** Freud's concept of an unconscious drive toward dissolution and death, in opposition to the life instinct.
**ego i.,** one of the nonsexual, self-preservative instincts originally postulated by Freud; they were later subsumed under the life instinct.
**herd i.,** the instinct or urge to be one of a group and to conform to the standards of that group in conduct and opinion.
**life i.,** Freud's concept of all the constructive tendencies of the organism aimed at maintenance and perpetuation of the individual and species, in opposition to the death instinct.
**mother i.,** the complex behavior in a mother which accomplishes the care of the young; whether such an instinct exists in human females is questioned.
**sexual i.,** life i.

**in·stinc·tive** (in-stink'tiv) of the nature of, related to, or prompted by instinct; performed spontaneously, without thinking.

**in·sti·tu·tion·al·iza·tion** (in-stĭ-too″shən-əl-ĭ-za'shən) [MeSH: Institutionalization] 1. commitment of a patient to a health care facility for treatment, often psychiatric. 2. in patients hospitalized for a long period, the development of excessive dependency on the institution and its routines, with diminishing of the will to function independently.

**in·stru·ment** (in'strə-mənt) [L. *instrumentum; instruere* to furnish] any tool, appliance, or apparatus.

**in·stru·men·tal** (in″strə-men'təl) pertaining to or performed by instruments.

**in·stru·men·tar·i·um** (in″strə-mən-tar'e-əm) the instruments or equipment required for any particular operation or purpose; the physical adjuncts with which a physician combats disease.

**in·stru·men·ta·tion** (in″strə-mən-ta'shən) the use of instruments; work performed with instruments.
**Cotrel-Dubousset i.,** a system of rods, hooks, and screws used to treat scoliosis in the thoracic and lumbar regions with spinal fusion and also to set vertebral fractures.
**Dwyer i.,** a method to correct scoliosis by using rods, screws, and staples for anterior spinal fusion in the lumbar region; see also *Zielke i.*
**Harrington i.,** a system of metal hooks and rods inserted surgically in the posterior elements of the spine to provide distraction and compression in treatment of scoliosis and other deformities.
**Luque i.,** a method to correct scoliosis by using rods and wires for anterior spinal fusion in the lumbar region.
**Zielke i.,** a method to correct scoliosis by using rods and screws for anterior spinal fusion in the lumbar region; it has largely replaced Dwyer instrumentation because it provides more stable support.

**in·suc·ca·tion** (in″sə-ka'shən) [L. *insuccare* to soak in; *in* into + *succus* juice] the thorough soaking of a drug before preparing an extract from it.

**in·su·date** (in-soo'dāt) the substance accumulated in insudation.

**in·su·da·tion** (in″soo-da'shən) [*in-* + L. *sudare* to sweat] the accumulation, as in the kidney or the arterial (intimal) wall, of substances derived from the blood.

**in·suf·fi·cien·cy** (in″sə-fish'ən-se) [L. *insufficientia,* from *in* not + *sufficiens* sufficient] the condition of being insufficient or inadequate to the performance of the allotted function. Called also *incompetence.*
**active i.,** the inability of a muscle to act owing to the abnormal (or other) approximation of its insertion to its origin.
**adrenal i.,** 1. abnormally diminished activity of the adrenal gland; see also *adrenocortical i.* Called also *hypoadrenalism.* 2. adrenocortical i.
**adrenal i., primary,** Addison's disease.
**adrenal i., secondary,** secondary adrenocortical i.
**adrenocortical i.,** abnormally diminished secretion of corticosteroids by the adrenal cortex, as in Addison's disease. Called also *hypoadrenocorticism, hypocorticalism,* and *hypocorticism.*
**adrenocortical i., acute,** addisonian crisis.
**adrenocortical i., chronic, adrenocortical i., primary,** Addison's disease.
**adrenocortical i., secondary,** any type caused by dysfunction of the pituitary or hypothalamus, with low plasma levels of cortisol and often of adrenocorticotropic hormone. Called also *secondary adrenal i.*
**aortic i.,** defective functioning of the aortic valve, with incomplete closure resulting in aortic regurgitation.
**basilar i.,** vertebrobasilar i.
**cardiac i.,** insufficiency of the heart muscle or function; see also *heart failure.*
**coronary i.,** decrease in flow of blood through the coronary blood vessels.
**i. of the externi,** insufficient power in the externi muscles of the eye, so that they are overbalanced by the interni, producing esophoria.
**i. of the eyelids,** a condition in which the eyes are closed only by a conscious effort.
**gastric i., gastromotor i.,** inability of the stomach to empty itself; myasthenia gastrica.
**hepatic i.,** inability of the liver properly to perform its functions.
**ileocecal i.,** inability of the ileocecal valve to prevent backflow of contents from the cecum into the ileum.
**i. of the interni,** insufficient power in the interni muscles of the eye, so that they are overbalanced by the externi, producing exophoria.
**mitral i.,** defective functioning of the mitral valve, with incomplete closure causing mitral regurgitation.
**muscular i.,** the inability of a muscle to do its normal work by a normal contraction.
**myocardial i.,** functional insufficiency of the heart muscle; see also *heart failure.*
**parathyroid i.,** hypoparathyroidism.
**placental i.,** dysfunction of the placenta, with reduction in the area of exchange of nutrients; it often leads to fetal growth retardation.
**pulmonary i.,** 1. defective functioning of the pulmonary valve, with incomplete closure resulting in pulmonic regurgitation. 2. respiratory i.
**renal i.,** a state of disordered function of the kidneys verifiable by quantitative tests. See also *renal failure,* under *failure.*
**respiratory i.,** a condition in which the lungs cannot provide adequate oxygen intake or carbon dioxide expulsion to meet the needs of the body and its cells. See also *respiratory failure,* under *failure.*
**thyroid i.,** hypothyroidism.
**tricuspid i.,** incomplete closure of the tricuspid valve, resulting in tricuspid regurgitation; it is usually secondary to systolic overload in the right ventricle.
**uterine i.,** weakness of the contractile power of the uterus.
**i. of the valves, valvular i.,** 1. dysfunction of one of the cardiac valves, with incomplete valve closure resulting in valvular regurgitation; see *aortic i., mitral i., pulmonary i.,* and *tricuspid i.* 2. venous i.
**velopharyngeal i.,** inability to achieve velopharyngeal closure, due to muscular dysfunction, deficiency of the soft palate or superior constrictor muscle, cleft palate, or other disorders; it often results in a speech disorder. Called also *velopharyngeal incompetence.*
**venous i.,** inadequacy of the venous valves and impairment of venous return from the legs (venous stasis), often with edema and sometimes with stasis ulcers at the ankle. Called also *primary valvular incompetence* and *valvular incompetence.*
**vertebrobasilar i.,** transient or intermittent ischemia of the brain

stem and cerebellum due to stenosis, thrombosis, or other obstruction of the vertebral or basilar artery; this results in attacks of such symptoms as vertigo, diplopia, nystagmus, muscle weakness, and dysarthria. A more severe syndrome also exists, consisting of paralysis, coma, and death. Cf. *subclavian steal.* Called also *basilar i., basilar artery syndrome,* and *vertebrobasilar ischemia* or *syndrome.*

**in·suf·fla·tion** (in″sə-fla′shən) [L. *in* into + *sufflatio* a blowing up] [MeSH: Insufflation] 1. the act of blowing a powder, vapor, gas, or air into a body cavity. Cf. *infusion* (def. 3). 2. finely powdered or liquid drugs carried into the respiratory passages by such devices as aerosols.
**cranial i.,** the forcing of air into the subdural space and the cerebral ventricles.
**i. of the lungs,** the act of blowing air into the lungs for the purpose of artificial respiration.
**perirenal i.,** the injection of air around the kidneys for the purpose of radiographic visualization of the adrenal glands.
**presacral i.,** the injection of gas, usually carbon dioxide, around the kidneys through a needle inserted into the retrorectal space for the purpose of radiographic visualization of the entire retroperitioneal space, with delineation of renal and adrenal areas.
**tubal i.,** see *Rubin's test,* under *test.*

**in·suf·fla·tor** (in′sə-fla″tər) an instrument used in performing insufflation.

**in·su·la** (in′sə-lə) gen. and pl. *in′sulae* [L. "island"] 1. an islandlike structure. 2. [TA] the portion of the cerebral cortex lying deep in the lateral sulcus, almost surrounded by the circular sulcus, which is covered over and hidden from view by juxtaposition of the opercula; called also *lobus insularis* [TA alternative], *insular lobe,* and *insula of Reil.*
**insulae of Peyer,** noduli lymphoidei aggregati intestini tenuis.
**i. of Reil,** insula (def. 2).

**in·su·lar** (in′sə-lər) pertaining to an island, especially to the insula or to the pancreatic islets.

**In·su·la·tard NPH** (in′su-lə-tahrd) trademark for preparations of isophane insulin suspension.

**in·su·la·tion** (in″sə-la′shən) [L. *insulare* to make an island of] 1. the surrounding of a space or body with material designed to prevent the entrance or escape of radiant or electrical energy. 2. the material so used.

**in·su·la·tor** (in′sə-la″tər) any substance or appliance of such nonconducting properties that it can be used to secure insulation.

**in·su·lin** (in′sə-lin) [L. *insula* island + *-in*] [MeSH: Insulin] 1. a protein hormone secreted by the beta cells of the pancreatic islets, serving as a hormonal signal of the fed state; it is secreted in response to elevated blood levels of glucose and amino acids and promotes efficient storage and use of these fuel molecules by controlling transport of metabolites and ions across cell membranes and regulating intracellular biosynthetic pathways. It promotes entry of glucose, fatty acids, and amino acids into cells; promotes glycogen, protein, and lipid synthesis; and inhibits gluconeogenesis, glycogen degradation, protein degradation, and lipolysis. Its secretion is also influenced by gastrointestinal hormones and by autonomic nervous activity. It is formed from a single polypeptide chain *(proinsulin)* that is cleaved by proteases at two points; the end pieces *(A* and *B chains),* held together by disulfide bridges, make up insulin; the connecting *C peptide* is also secreted but has no physiologic activity. Relative insulin deficiency is the cause of most cases of diabetes mellitus. 2. [USP] preparation of the hormone, used in treatment of diabetes mellitus; it may be bovine or porcine in origin or a recombinant human type. Types vary in rapidity of onset, duration of action, and degree of purification (most containing some proinsulin and other antigenic components).
**extended i. human zinc suspension** [USP], a long-acting insuln consisting of insulin human reacted with a zinc salt to produce zinc-insulin crystals.
**extended i. zinc suspension** [USP], a long-acting insulin with time of onset about 7 hours after injection and duration of action of 36 hours, consisting of bovine or porcine insulin in the form of large zinc-insulin crystals.
**globin i.,** see *globin zinc i.*
**globin zinc i. injection,** an intermediate-acting insulin with an approximate time of onset of 2 hours and duration of action of 18 hours, consisting of bovine or porcine insulin reacted with zinc chloride and globin I (from bovine hemoglobin) to form a protein complex from which insulin is slowly released; now rarely used.
**i. human** [USP], a protein corresponding to insulin elaborated in the human pancreas, derived from pork insulin by enzymatic action that changes its amino acid sequence or produced synthetically by recombinant DNA techniques.
**i. injection** [USP], a rapid-acting insulin with an approximate time of onset of 1 hour and duration of action of 6–8 hours, consisting of crystalline bovine or porcine insulin dissolved in a clear fluid. Called also *regular i.*

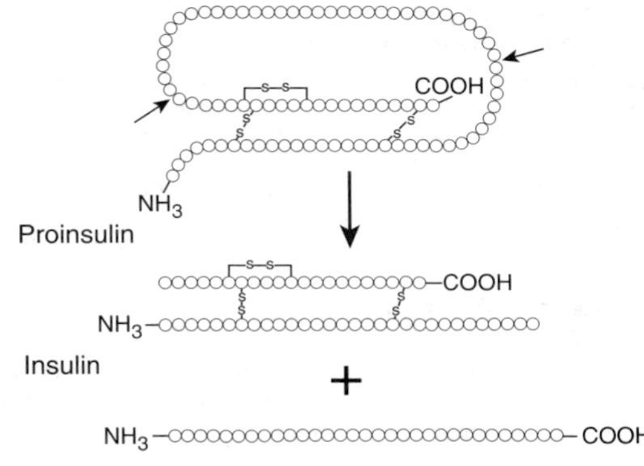


Insulin. The precursor proinsulin is cleaved internally at two sides *(arrows)* to yield insulin and C peptide.

**intermediate-acting i.,** an insulin preparation whose onset of action is from 1.5 to 3.0 hours after injection and peak of action is between about 6 and 12 hours after injection. Examples include globin zinc insulin injection, isophane insulin suspension, and insulin zinc suspension.
**isophane i. human suspension** [USP], an intermediate-acting insulin consisting of insulin human reacted with zinc protamine sulfate to form a protein complex consisting of insulin human, protamine, and zinc.
**isophane i. suspension** [USP], an intermediate-acting insulin with time of onset about 2 hours after injection and duration of action of 24 hours, consisting of bovine or porcine insulin reacted with zinc chloride and protamine to form a protein complex with a ratio of free and bound insulin. Called also *NPH i.*
**Lente i.,** trademark for preparations of insulin zinc suspension.
**i. lispro,** a rapid-acting analog of human insulin, created by reversing the lysine and proline at positions 28 and 29 on the insulin B chain, and produced by genetically altered *Escherichia coli;* used in the treatment of diabetes mellitus, administered subcutaneously.
**long-acting i.,** an insulin preparation whose onset of action is more than 3 hours after injection and peak of action is between 10 and 30 hours after injection. Examples include extended insulin zinc suspension and protamine zinc insulin suspension.
**NPH i.** [*N*eutral *P*rotamine *H*agedorn], isophane i. suspension.
**prompt i. zinc suspension** [USP], a rapid-acting insulin with an approximate time of onset of 1 hour and duration of action of 14 hours, consisting of bovine or porcine insulin modified by the addition of zinc chloride to produce a suspension of amorphous insulin.
**protamine zinc i. suspension,** a long-acting insulin with time of onset about 7 hours after injection and duration of action of 36 hours, consisting of bovine or porcine insulin reacted with zinc chloride and protamine to form a protein complex from which insulin is slowly released.
**rapid-acting i.,** an insulin preparation whose onset of action is from 0.5 to 1.5 hours after injection and peak of action about 2 to 4 hours after injection. Examples include insulin injection and prompt zinc insulin suspension. Called also *short-acting insulin zinc.*
**regular i.,** i. injection.
**Semilente i.,** trademark for preparations of prompt insulin zinc suspension.
**short-acting i.,** rapid-acting i.
**three-to-one i.,** a combination of regular insulin and protamine zinc insulin, having the activity of three parts of the former and one part of the latter.
**Ultralente i.,** trademark for preparations of extended insulin zinc suspension.
**i. zinc suspension** [USP], an intermediate-acting insulin with an approximate time of onset of 2 hours and duration of action of 24 hours, consisting of a stable mixture of prompt and extended insulin zinc suspensions yielding a 7:3 ratio of crystalline to amorphous insulin.

**in·su·lin·emia** (in″sə-lĭ-ne′me-ə) [*insulin* + *-emia*] 1. the presence of insulin in the blood. 2. hyperinsulinemia.

**in·su·lin·li·po·dys·tro·phy** (in″sə-lin-li″po-dis′tro-fe) the local disappearance of fat at the sites of injection in diabetic patients on insulin treatment.

**in·su·lin·o·gen·e·sis** (in″sə-lin-o-jen′ə-sis) the formation and release of insulin by the islands of Langerhans.

**in·su·lin·o·gen·ic** (in″sə-lin″o-jen′ik) pertaining to, characterized by, or promoting insulinogenesis.

**in·su·lin·oid** (in′sə-lin-oid″) 1. resembling insulin. 2. any substance with hypoglycemic properties like those of insulin.

**in·su·li·no·ma** (in″sə-lin-o′mə) [MeSH: Insulinoma] an islet cell tumor of pancreatic beta cells; although usually benign, such tumors secrete excessive amounts of insulin and are among the most important causes of hypoglycemia. Called also *insuloma.*

**in·su·lin·op·a·thy** (in″su-lin-op′ə-the) any defect in the genetically determined molecular structure of insulin, usually manifested as hyperinsulinemia and a mild syndrome similar to type 2 diabetes mellitus.

**in·su·lin·o·pe·nic** (in″sə-lin-o-pe′nik) pertaining to or characterized by hypoinsulinism.

**in·su·li·tis** (in″sə-li′tis) lymphocytic infiltration of the islets of Langerhans, suggesting an inflammatory or immunologic reaction.

**in·su·lo·gen·ic** (in″sə-lo-jen′ik) insulinogenic.

**in·su·lo·ma** (in″sə-lo′mə) insulinoma.

**in·sult** (in′səlt) [L. *insultus* attack] 1. injury. 2. attack.

**in·sus·cep·ti·bil·i·ty** (in″sə-sep″tĭ-bil′ĭ-te) the quality of not being susceptible; immunity.

**in·take** (in′tāk) the substances, or the quantities thereof, taken in and utilized by the body.
**caloric i.,** the food ingested or otherwise taken into the body.
**fluid i.,** the fluid taken into the body by drinking or parenterally.

**In·tal** (in′tal) trademark for a preparation of cromolyn sodium.

**in·te·gra·tion** (in″tə-gra′shən) 1. assimilation; anabolic action or activity. 2. the combining of different acts so that they cooperate toward a common end; coordination. 3. constructive assimilation into the personality of knowledge and experience. 4. in bacterial genetics, assimilation of genetic material from one bacterium (donor) into the chromosome of another (recipient).
**biological i.,** the acquisition of functional coordination during embryonic development through humoral and nervous influences.

**in·te·gra·tor** (in′tə-gra′tor) an instrument for measuring body surfaces.

**in·te·grin** (in′tə-grin) any of a family of heterodimeric cell-adhesion receptors, consisting of two noncovalently linked polypeptide chains, designated $\alpha$ and $\beta$, that mediate cell-to-cell and cell-to–extracellular matrix interactions.
**$\beta_1$ i.,** any integrin containing a $\beta_1$ chain; members of this group are variously expressed on leukocytes, platelets, and some non-blood cells and mediate cell-matrix adhesion. Heterodimers of this class were first identified on T cells 2 to 4 weeks after activation in vitro and were called very late activation (VLA) antigens; the designation VLA has been continued for other proteins of this group, with numbers designating individual members.
**$\beta_2$ i.,** any integrin containing a $\beta_2$ chain; members of this group (LFA-1, Mac-1, and p150,95) are expressed on leukocytes and mediate leukocyte adhesion and act as complement receptors; called also *leukocyte adhesion protein.*
**$\beta_3$ i.,** any integrin containing a $\beta_3$ chain; members of this group are expressed on nonlymphoid cells and serve as receptors for fibrinogen, fibronectin, thrombospondin, von Willebrand factor, and vitronectin.

**in·teg·u·ment** (in-teg′u-mənt) [L. *integumentum*] 1. a covering or investment. 2. integumentum commune.
**common i.,** integumentum commune.

**in·teg·u·men·ta·ry** (in-teg-u-men′tar-e) 1. pertaining to or composed of skin. 2. serving as a covering, like the skin.

**in·teg·u·men·tum** (in-teg″u-men′təm) [L., from *in* on + *tegere* to cover] [TA] 1. a covering or investment. 2. i. commune.
**i. commu′ne** [TA], common integument: the covering of the body, or skin, including its various layers and their appendages; in humans, it comprises the epidermis, dermis, subcutaneous tissue, hair, nails, cutaneous glands, the breast, and mammary glands. Called also *integument* and *integumentum.*

**in te·la** (in te′lə) [L.] in tissue; relating especially to stained histological preparations.

**in·tel·lect** (in′tə-lekt) [L. *intellectus,* from *intelligere* to understand] the mind, thinking faculty, or understanding.

**in·tel·lec·tu·al·iza·tion** (in″tə-lek″choo-əl-ĭ-za′shən) an unconscious defense mechanism in which reasoning is used to avoid confronting an objectionable impulse, emotional conflict, or other stressor and thus to defend against anxiety.

**in·tel·li·gence** (in-tel′ĭ-jəns) [L. *intelligere* to understand] [MeSH: Intelligence] the ability to comprehend or understand; see also under *quotient.*

**in·tem·per·ance** (in-tem′pər-əns) [L. *in* not + *temperare* to moderate] excess or lack of self-control in respect of food and drink, particularly in the use of alcoholic drinks.

**in·ten·si·fi·ca·tion** (in-ten″sĭ-fĭ-ka′shən) [L. *intensus* intense + *facere* to make] 1. the act of making anything intense. 2. the process of becoming intense.

**in·ten·sio·nom·e·ter** (in-ten″se-o-nom′ə-tər) an ionometric instrument for measuring the intensity of x-rays. Two series of plates, separated by an air gap that serves as the dielectric, are connected to opposite terminals in a closed chamber. An electric circuit is completed when the air becomes ionized by the x-rays, and the difference in electric potential is registered by deflection of a galvanometer needle.

**in·ten·si·ty** (in-ten′sĭ-te) [L. *intensus* intense; *in* on + *tendere* to stretch] the condition or quality of being intense; a high degree of tension, activity, or energy.
**electric i.,** the force exerted on a unit charge at a point in an electric field. Symbol *E.* Called also *electric field strength.*
**luminous i.,** the light-giving power of a source of light. Cf. *candle power.*
**i. of x-rays,** the x-ray energy passing per unit time through unit area normal to the direction of propagation.

**in·ten·sive** (in-ten′siv) [L. *in* on + *tendere* to stretch] of great force or intensity; see also *intensive care unit,* under *unit.*

**in·ten·siv·ist** (in-ten′sĭ-vist) a physician who specializes in the provision of care in the intensive care unit.

**in·ten·tion** (in-ten′shən) [L. *intentio,* from *in* upon + *tendere* to stretch] 1. a manner of healing; see under *healing.* 2. a goal or desired end; a term used to refer to neurogenic abnormalities that arise when a goal is consciously sought.
**paradoxical i.,** the hypothesis that struggling against one's mental symptoms only exacerbates them whereas invoking them deliberately may do the opposite; used as a form of psychotherapy in which the behavior or feelings to be avoided are commanded to be performed or felt.

**inter-** [L. *inter* between] a prefix meaning between or among.

**in·ter·ac·ces·so·ry** (in″tər-ak-ses′ər-e) connecting the accessory processes of the vertebrae.

**in·ter·ac·i·nar** (in″tər-as′ĭ-nər) situated between acini.

**in·ter·ac·i·nous** (in″tər-as′ĭ-nəs) interacinar.

**in·ter·ac·tion** (in″tər-ak′shən) the quality, state, or process of (two or more things) acting on each other.
**drug i.,** the action of one drug upon the effectiveness or toxicity of another (or others).

**in·ter·al·ve·o·lar** (in″tər-al-ve′o-lər) between alveoli.

**in·ter·an·gu·lar** (in″tər-ang′u-lər) situated or occurring between two or more angles.

**in·ter·an·nu·lar** (in″tər-an′u-lər) [*inter-* + *annular*] situated between two rings or constrictions.

**in·ter·ar·tic·u·lar** (in″tər-ahr-tik′u-lər) [*inter-* + *articular*] situated between articular surfaces.

**in·ter·ar·y·te·noid** (in″tər-ar″e-te′noid) between the arytenoid cartilages.

**in·ter·atri·al** (in″tər-a′tre-əl) situated between the atria of the heart.

**in·ter·au·ric·u·lar** (in″tər-aw-rik′u-lər) 1. interatrial. 2. situated between the auricles or pinnae. 3. situated between the auricles of the heart.

**in·ter·brain** (in′tər-brān″) diencephalon.

**in·ter·ca·lary** (in-tər′kə-lar″e) [L. *intercalarius; inter-* + *calare* to call] inserted or placed between; interposed.

**in·ter·ca·late** (in-tər′kə-lāt) [L. *intercalare*] to insert between.

**in·ter·can·a·lic·u·lar** (in″tər-kan″ə-lik′u-lər) between canaliculi.

**in·ter·cap·il·lary** (in″tər-kap′ĭ-lar-e) among or between capillaries.

**in·ter·ca·pit·u·lar** (in′tər-kə-pit′u-lər) passing between small heads; see under *vein.*

**in·ter·ca·rot·ic** (in″tər-kə-rot′ik) between the carotid arteries.

**in·ter·ca·rot·id** (in″tər-kə-rot′id) intercarotic.

**in·ter·car·pal** (in″tər-kahr′pəl) between the carpal bones.

**in·ter·car·ti·lag·i·nous** (in″tər-kahr″tĭ-laj′ĭ-nəs) connecting or situated between two or more cartilages.

**in·ter·cav·er·nous** (in″tər-kav′ər-nəs) between two cavities.

**in·ter·cel·lu·lar** (in″tər-sel′u-lər) situated between the cells of any structure.

**in·ter·cen·tral** (in″tər-sen′trəl) situated between or connecting two or more nerve centers.

**in·ter·cer·e·bral** (in″tər-ser′ə-brəl) connecting or situated between the two cerebral hemispheres.

**in·ter·change** (in′tər-chānj″) 1. translocation. 2. an exchange or trading.
**Hamburger i.**, chloride shift.

**in·ter·chon·dral** (in″tər-kon′drəl) intercartilaginous.

**in·ter·cil·i·um** (in″tər-sil′e-əm) [*inter-* + *cilium*] the space between the eyebrows.

**in·ter·cla·vic·u·lar** (in″tər-klə-vik′u-lər) [*inter-* + *clavicular*] situated between the clavicles.

**in·ter·cli·noid** (in″tər-kli′noid) pertaining to or passing between the clinoid processes.

**in·ter·coc·cyg·e·al** (in″tər-kok-sij′e-əl) situated between the segments of the coccyx.

**in·ter·co·lum·nar** (in″tər-kə-lum′nər) [*inter-* + *column*] situated between columns or pillars.

**in·ter·con·dy·lar** (in″tər-kon′də-lər) situated between two condyles.

**in·ter·con·dy·loid** (in″tər-kon′də-loid) intercondylar.

**in·ter·con·dy·lous** (in″tər-kon′də-ləs) intercondylar.

**in·ter·cos·tal** (in″tər-kos′təl) [*inter-* + *costal*] situated between the ribs.

**in·ter·cos·to·hu·mer·al** (in″tər-kos-to-hu′mər-əl) pertaining to an intercostal space and the humerus.

**in·ter·course** (in′tər-kors) [L. *intercursus* running between] 1. mutual exchange. 2. sexual i.
**sexual i.**, 1. coitus. 2. any physical contact between two individuals involving stimulation of the genital organs of at least one.

**in·ter·cri·co·thy·rot·o·my** (in″tər-kri″ko-thi-rot′o-me) [*inter-* + *cricothyroid* + Gr. *temnein* to cut] cricothyrotomy.

**in·ter·cris·tal** (in″tər-kris′təl) between two crests.

**in·ter·cri·ti·cal** (in″tər-krit′ĭ-kəl) denoting the period between attacks, as of gout.

**in·ter·cross** (in′tər-kros) [*inter-* + *cross* (def. 2)] the mating of individuals heterozygous for the same gene; cf. *incross.*

**in·ter·cru·ral** (in″tər-kroo′rəl) between two crura.

**in·ter·cur·rent** (in″tər-kur′ənt) [L. *intercurrens,* from *inter-* + *currere* to run] breaking into and modifying the course of an already existing disease.

**in·ter·cus·pa·tion** (in″tər-kəs-pa′shən) the fitting together of cusps of opposing teeth in occlusion; the cusp-to-fossa relationship of the upper and lower posterior teeth to each other.

**in·ter·cusp·ing** (in″tər-kusp′ing) the occlusion of the cusps of the teeth of one jaw with the depressions in the teeth of the other jaw.

**in·ter·def·er·en·tial** (in″tər-def″ər-en′shəl) between the two ductus deferentes.

**in·ter·den·tal** (in″tər-den′təl) [*inter-* + *dental*] situated between the proximal surfaces of adjacent teeth in the same dental arch. See also *interocclusal* and *interproximal.*

**in·ter·den·ta·le** (in″tər-dən-ta′le) a craniometric landmark located between the right and left central incisors, in the midline on the tip of the alveolar septum.

**in·ter·den·ti·um** (in″tər-den′she-əm) the interproximal space; see under *space.*

**in·ter·dia·lyt·ic** (in″tər-di″ə-lit′ik) pertaining to the time between hemodialysis treatments.

**in·ter·dig·it** (in″tər-dij′it) the space between any two contiguous fingers or toes.

**in·ter·dig·i·tal** (in″tər-dij′ĭ-təl) [*inter-* + *digital*] situated between two adjacent fingers or toes.

**in·ter·dig·i·tate** (in″tər-dij′ĭ-tāt) [*inter-* + *digitate*] to interlock and interrelate, as the fingers of clasped hands.

**in·ter·dig·i·ta·tion** (in″tər-dij″ĭ-ta′shən) [*inter-* + *digitation*] 1. an interlocking of parts by fingerlike processes. 2. any one of a set of fingerlike processes.

**in·ter·face** (in′tər-fās) in chemistry, the surface of separation or boundary between two phases of a heterogeneous system.
**dineric i.**, the interface between two immiscible liquids.

**in·ter·fa·cial** (in″tər-fa′shəl) pertaining to an interface.

**in·ter·fas·cic·u·lar** (in″tər-fə-sik′u-lər) [*inter-* + *fascicular*] situated between fasciculi.

**in·ter·fem·o·ral** (in″tər-fem′o-rəl) between the thighs.

**in·ter·fer·ence** (in″tər-fēr′əns) [*inter-* + L. *ferire* to strike] 1. opposition to or hampering of an action or procedure. 2. the process in which two or more light, sound, or electromagnetic waves of the same frequency combine to reinforce or cancel each other, the amplitude of the resulting wave being equal to the sum of the amplitudes of the combining waves. 3. impairment of cardiac impulse conduction due to refractoriness of the tissue where the refractoriness is a physiological response to passage of a preceding impulse. See also *interference dissociation,* under *dissociation.* 4. any premature contact point along the occlusal surface of the teeth that prevents maximum contact, function, and proper alignment in full occlusion. See also *deflective occlusal contact,* under *contact.*
**cuspal i.**, deflective occlusal contact.
**occlusal i's**, areas of interference on teeth that hamper smooth, gliding, harmonious jaw movements with the teeth maintaining contact.
**proactive i.**, see under *inhibition.*
**retroactive i.**, see under *inhibition.*

**in·ter·fer·ing** (in″tər-fēr′ing) the striking or rubbing of the fetlock of a horse by the opposite foot during locomotion.

**in·ter·fe·rom·e·ter** (in″tər-fēr-om′ə-tər) an instrument for measuring lengths or movements by means of the phenomena caused by the interference of two rays of light, or of sound (acoustic i.).

**in·ter·fe·rom·e·try** (in″tər-fēr-om′ə-tre) [MeSH: Interferometry] the use of the interferometer for measuring distances or movements.

**in·ter·fer·on** (in″tər-fēr′on) any of a family of glycoproteins that exert virus-nonspecific but host-specific antiviral activity by inducing the transcription of cellular genes coding for antiviral proteins that selectively inhibit the synthesis of viral RNA and proteins. Interferons also have immunoregulatory functions (inhibition of B cell activation and antibody production enhancement of T cell activity, and enhancement of NK cell cytotoxic activity) and can inhibit the growth of nonviral intracellular parasites. Production of interferon can be stimulated by viral infection, especially by the presence of double-stranded RNA, by intracellular parasites (chlamydiae, rickettsiae), by protozoa *(Toxoplasma),* and by bacteria (streptococci, staphylococci) and bacterial products (endotoxins). Interferons have been divided into three distinct types ($\alpha$, $\beta$, and $\gamma$) associated with specific producer cells and functions, but all animal cells are able to produce interferons, and certain producer cells (leukocytes and fibroblasts) produce more than one type (both interferon-$\alpha$ and interferon-$\beta$). Abbreviated IFN.
**i.-$\alpha$ (IFN-$\alpha$)**, the major interferon produced by virus-induced leukocyte cultures; the primary producer cells are null lymphocytes, and the major activities are antiviral activity and activation of NK cells. It is used in the experimental treatment of hairy cell leukemia and other selected neoplasias. Called also *leukocyte i.*
**i.-alfa**, i.-$\alpha$.
**i. alfa-2a**, a synthetic form of interferon-$\alpha$ produced by recombinant technology that acts as a biological response modifier, used as an antineoplastic in the treatment of hairy cell leukemia and AIDS-related Kaposi's sarcoma; administered intramuscularly or subcutaneously.
**i. alfa-2b**, a synthetic form of interferon-$\alpha$ produced by recombinant technology that acts as a biological response modifier, used in the treatment of condylomata acuminata, hepatitis B, and chronic hepatitis C and as an antineoplastic in the treatment of hairy cell leukemia, malignant melanoma, and AIDS-related Kaposi's sarcoma; administered intramuscularly, subcutaneously, or intralesionally.
**i. alfa-n3**, a highly purified mixture of natural human interferon proteins, manufactured from pooled human leukocytes that have been induced to produce interferon alfa-n3, that acts as a biologic response modifier; used in the treatment of condylomata acuminata, administered intralesionally.
**i. alfacon-1**, a synthetic interferon produced by recombinant DNA technology, consisting of 166 amino acids whose sequence was derived by comparing the sequences of several naturally occurring interferon subtypes and assigning the most commonly occurring amino acid at each position, with changes in four amino acids being made to facilitate construction of the molecule; used in the treatment of chronic hepatitis C virus infection, administered subcutaneously.
**i.-$\beta$ (IFN-$\beta$)**, the major interferon produced by double-stranded RNA–induced fibroblast cultures; the primary producer cells are fibroblasts, epithelial cells, and macrophages, and the major activity is antiviral activity. Called also *epithelial, fibroblast,* or *fibroepithelial i.*
**i. beta-2**, a cytokine derived from T cells that stimulate B cells to proliferate in vitro but (unlike B cell differentiation factors) do not stimulate antibody secretion. Called also B-cell growth factor.
**consensus i.**, i. alfacon-1.
**epithelial i., fibroblast i., fibroepithelial i.**, i.-$\beta$.
**i.-$\gamma$ (IFN-$\gamma$)**, the major interferon produced by immunologically stimulated (by mitogens or antigens) lymphocyte cultures; the primary

producer cells are T lymphocytes, and the major activity is immunoregulation. IFN-γ has been implicated in aberrant expression of class II histocompatibility antigens by tissue cells (such as thyroid cells) that do not normally express them, leading to autoimmune disease. Called also *immune i.*
**i. gamma-1b**, a synthetic form of interferon-γ produced by recombinant technology that acts as a biologic response modifier; used to enhance phagocytic function in order to reduce the frequency and severity of serious infections associated with chronic granulomatous disease, administered subcutaneously.
**immune i.**, i.-γ.
**leukocyte i.**, i.-α.
**type I i.**, i.-α and i.-β.
**type II i.**, i.-γ.

**in·ter·fi·bril·lar** (in″tər-fi′bril-ər) [*inter-* + *fibrillar*] between or among fibrils.

**in·ter·fi·bril·lary** (in″tər-fi′brĭ-lar″e) interfibrillar.

**in·ter·fi·brous** (in″tər-fi′brəs) between fibers.

**in·ter·fil·a·men·tous** (in″tər-fil″ə-men′təs) between filaments.

**in·ter·fi·lar** (in″tər-fi′lər) [*inter-* + *filar*] between or among the fibrils of a reticulum.

**in·ter·fron·tal** (in″tər-fron′təl) between the halves of the frontal bone.

**in·ter·fur·ca** (in″tər-fur′kə) pl. *interfur′cae* [*inter-* + L. *furca* fork] the area lying between and at the base of divided tooth roots.

**in·ter·fur·cae** (in″tər-fur′se) [L.] plural of *interfurca.*

**in·ter·gan·gli·on·ic** (in″tər-gang″gle-on′ik) [*inter-* + *ganglion*] between ganglia.

**in·ter·gem·mal** (in″tər-jem′əl) [*inter-* + *gemma*] between taste buds or other buds.

**in·ter·glob·u·lar** (in″tər-glob′u-lər) [*inter-* + *globular*] between or among globules, as of the dentin.

**in·ter·glu·te·al** (in″tər-gloo′te-əl) between the buttocks. Called also *internatal.*

**in·ter·go·ni·al** (in″tər-go′ne-əl) between the tips of the two angles of the mandible.

**in·ter·gra·da·tion** (in″tər-grə-da′shən) [*inter-* + L. *gradus* step] the interbreeding of two subspecies of the same species in the environmental area where they meet *(primary i.)* or of closely related species whose ranges overlap before isolating mechanisms are fully developed *(secondary i.).*

**in·ter·gran·u·lar** (in″tər-gran′u-lər) between the granule cells of the brain.

**in·ter·gy·ral** (in″tər-ji′rəl) between cerebral gyri or convolutions.

**in·ter·hemi·cer·e·bral** (in″tər-hem″e-ser′ə-brəl) intercerebral.

**in·ter·hemi·sphe·ric** (in″tər-hem″ĭ-sfĕr′ik) intercerebral.

**in·ter·ic·tal** (in″tər-ik′təl) occurring between attacks or paroxysms; called also *interparoxysmal.*

**in·te·ri·or** (in-tēr′e-ər) [L. "inner"; neut. *interius*] 1. situated inside; inward. 2. an inner part or cavity.

**in·ter·is·chi·ad·ic** (in″tər-is″ke-ad′ik) between the two ischia.

**in·ter·ki·ne·sis** (in″tər-ki-ne′sis) [*inter-* + Gr. *kinēsis* motion] a period intervening between the first and second divisions in meiosis, similar to the interphase in mitosis.

**in·ter·la·bi·al** (in″tər-la′be-əl) [*inter-* + *labial*] between the lips, or between any two labia.

**in·ter·la·mel·lar** (in″tər-lə-mel′ər) [*inter-* + *lamellar*] situated between lamellae.

**in·ter·leu·kin** (in″tər-loo′kin) [*inter-* + *leukocyte*] a generic term for a group of multifunctional cytokines that are produced by a variety of lymphoid and nonlymphoid cells and have effects at least partly within the lymphopoietic system; originally believed to be produced chiefly by and to act chiefly upon leukocytes.
**i.-1 (IL-1)**, a predominately macrophage-produced interleukin that mediates the host inflammatory response in innate immunity; two principal forms exist, designated α and β, with apparently identical biological activity. At low concentrations, IL-1 principally acts to mediate local inflammation, causing mononuclear phagocytes and endothelial cells to synthesize leukocyte-activating chemokines; at high concentrations IL-1 enters the blood stream and acts as an endocrine hormone, in some actions resembling tumor necrosis factor by its ability to cause fever, initiate hepatic synthesis of acute phase proteins, and induce cachexia.
**i.-2 (IL-2)**, an interleukin produced by T cells in response to antigenic or mitogenic stimulation, acting to regulate the immune response. It stimulates the proliferation of T cells and the synthesis of other T cell–derived cytokines, stimulates the growth and cytolytic function of NK cells to produce lymphokine-activated killer cells, is a growth factor for and stimulates antibody synthesis in B cells, and may promote apoptosis in antigen-activated T cells. IL-2 is used as an anticancer drug in the treatment of a wide variety of solid malignant tumors. Formerly called *T-cell growth factor.*
**i.-3 (IL-3)**, a lymphokine produced by antigen- or mitogen-activated T lymphocytes, which stimulates proliferation of hematopoietic as well as lymphoid stem cells; a colony-stimulating factor for all bone marrow progenitor cells. IL-3 supports the growth and differentiation of early hematopoietic and lymphoid stem cells as well as that of more mature hematopoietic cells, including granulocytes, macrophages, and mast cells.
**i.-4 (IL-4)**, a lymphokine produced by antigen- or mitogen-activated T cells; its principal role is regulation of IgE- and eosinophil-mediated immune reactions. It stimulates switching of B cells for production of IgE, is a growth and differentiation factor for T cells, particularly $T_H2$ cells, is a growth factor for mast cells, and stimulates the expression of some adhesion molecules on endothelial cells. Formerly called *B lymphocyte stimulatory factor 1.*
**i.-5 (IL-5)**, a lymphokine produced by antigen- or mitogen-activated T cells and by activated mast cells that stimulates the growth and differentiation of eosinophils and activates mature eosinophils to kill helminths. It may act as a cofactor in the growth and differentiation of B cells and may also be involved in increasing synthesis of IgA by mature B cells.
**i.-6 (IL-6)**, a lymphokine produced by antigen- or mitogen-activated T cells, fibroblasts, macrophages, and other cells that serves as a differentiation factor for B cells and thymocytes and stimulates immunoglobulin production by B cells; it also induces hepatocytes to synthesize various plasma proteins involved in the acute phase response and is a cofactor in initiation of the cell cycle in primitive hematopoietic cells in vitro.
**i.-7 (IL-7)**, an interleukin produced by epithelial and mesangial stromal cells that serves as a differentiation factor for B cells in the early stages of their development and also supports the growth of some thymocytes and T lymphocytes.
**i.-8 (IL-8)**, a chemokine produced by monocytes, endothelial cells, and other cells that acts as a chemotactic and activator for neutrophils and may play a role in the extravasation of neutrophils in inflammation.
**i.-9 (IL-9)**, a cytokine produced by T cells and macrophages that acts as a growth factor for some T cell populations and bone marrow–mast cell progenitors.
**i.-10 (IL-10)**, a cytokine produced by activated macrophages, certain lymphocytes, and other cells that decreases both innate and T cell–mediated immune inflammation; it inhibits the production of cytokines by activated T cells, plays a role in B cell activation, inhibits production of interferon-γ, and blocks antigen presentation and macrophage formation of IL-1, IL-6, and tumor necrosis factor.
**i.-11 (IL-11)**, a cytokine produced by bone marrow stromal cells that stimulates megakaryocyte proliferation and B cell differentiation.
**i.-12 (IL-12)**, a heterodimeric cytokine produced by phagocytic cells, B cells, and other antigen-presenting cell types; it is a potent inducer of cytokine production, causes T and NK cells to secrete interferon-γ, is a growth factor for preactivated T and NK cells, and enhances cytotoxic activity in $CD8^+$ T cells and NK cells. It also has a role in the generation of T-helper type 1 cells and in the differentiation of cytotoxic T lymphocytes.
**i.-13 (IL-13)**, a cytokine produced by activated T lymphocytes that has structural and functional similarities to IL-4; it inhibits inflammatory cytokine production by lipopolysaccharide in human peripheral blood monocytes and may be involved in promoting B cell division.
**i.-14 (IL-14)**, a cytokine produced by T lymphocytes and malignant B lymphocytes that induces B cell proliferation and inhibits immunoglobulin secretion.
**i.-15 (IL-15)**, a cytokine released by mononuclear phagocytes and some tissue cells in response to events triggering innate immunity; such as viral infection; its primary function appears to be promotion of NK cell proliferation

**in·ter·lig·a·men·ta·ry** (in″tər-lig″ə-men′tə-re) between or among ligaments.

**in·ter·lig·a·men·tous** (in″tər-lig″ə-men′təs) interligamentary.

**in·ter·lo·bar** (in″tər-lo′bər) [*inter-* + *lobar*] situated or occurring between lobes.

**in·ter·lo·bi·tis** (in″tər-lo-bi′tis) interlobular pleurisy.

**in·ter·lob·u·lar** (in″tər-lob′u-lər) [*inter-* + *lobular*] situated or occurring between lobules.

**in·ter·lock·ing** (in″tər-lok′ing) a complication of labor in twin births in which the inferior surface of the chin of one twin is hooked to that of its co-twin above or below the pelvic inlet. When this condition occurs in the true pelvis, it is called *compaction.*

**in·ter·mal·le·o·lar** (in″tər-mə-le′o-lər) between the malleoli.

**in·ter·mam·ma·ry** (in″tər-mam′ə-re) between the breasts.

**in·ter·mam·mil·la·ry** (in″tər-mam′ĭ-lar″e) between the nipples.

**in·ter·mar·riage** (in″tər-mar′əj) [*inter-* + L. *maritare* to wed] 1. the marriage of persons related by blood or consanguinity. 2. the marriage of persons of different racial, ethnic, social, or religious groups.

**in·ter·max·il·lary** (in″tər-mak′sĭ-lar″e) situated between the two maxillae.

**in·ter·me·di·ary** (in″tər-me′de-ar″e) [*inter-* + L. *medius* middle] 1. performed or occurring in a median stage; neither early nor late; intermediate. 2. an intermediate stage.

**in·ter·me·di·ate** (in″tər-me′de-ət) [*inter-* + L. *medius* middle] 1. placed between; see *medial* and *median.* 2. resembling, in part, each of two extremes. 3. a substance formed in a chemical process that is essential to the formation of the end product of the process.

**in·ter·me·din** (in″tər-me′din) melanocyte-stimulating hormone.

**in·ter·me·dio·lat·er·al** (in″tər-me″de-o-lat′ər-əl) both intermediate and lateral.

**in·ter·me·di·us** (in″tər-me′de-əs) [TA] intermediate: a term denoting the middle of three structures, one of which is situated closer to and the other farther from the median plane of the body or part.

**in·ter·mem·bra·nous** (in″tər-mem′brə-nəs) situated or occurring between membranes.

**in·ter·me·nin·ge·al** (in″tər-mə-nin′je-əl) situated or occurring between the meninges.

**in·ter·men·stru·al** (in″tər-men′stroo-əl) [*inter-* + *menstrual*] occurring between the menstrual periods.

**in·ter·men·stru·um** (in″tər-men′stroo-əm) the interval between two menstrual periods.

**in·ter·meta·car·pal** (in″tər-met″ə-kahr′pəl) [*inter-* + *metacarpal*] situated between the metacarpal bones.

**in·ter·meta·mer·ic** (in″tər-met″ə-mer′ik) between two metameres.

**in·ter·meta·tar·sal** (in″tər-met″ə-tahr′səl) situated or occurring between the metatarsal bones.

**in·ter·mis·sion** (in″tər-mish′ən) [L. *intermissio; inter* between + *mittere* to send] an interval; a period of temporary cessation, as between two occurrences or paroxysms.

**in·ter·mi·tot·ic** (in″tər-mi-tot′ik) pertaining to or occurring during the interval between successive mitoses.

**in·ter·mit·tent** (in″tər-mit′ənt) [L. *intermittens; inter* between + *mittere* to send] occurring at separated intervals; having periods of cessation of activity.

**in·ter·mo·lec·u·lar** (in″tər-mo-lek′u-lər) between molecules.

**in·ter·mu·ral** (in-tər-mu′rəl) [*inter-* + *mural*] situated between the walls of organs.

**in·ter·mus·cu·lar** (in″tər-mus′ku-lər) situated between muscles.

**in·tern** (in′tərn) 1. [Fr. *interne*] a graduate of a medical or dental school serving in a hospital preparatory to being licensed to practice medicine or dentistry. Cf. *resident.* 2. [Fr. *interner*] to confine within certain geographical or physical boundaries.

**in·ter·nal** (in-tər′nəl) [L. *internus*] situated or occurring within or on the inside; many anatomical structures formerly called internal are now correctly termed medial.

**in·ter·nal·iza·tion** (in-tər″nəl-ĭ-za′shən) the mental process whereby certain attributes, attitudes, or standards of others are unconsciously taken as one's own.

**in·ter·nar·i·al** (in″tər-nar′e-əl) [*inter-* + L. *nares* nostrils] situated between the nares.

**in·ter·na·sal** (in″tər-na′zəl) situated between the nasal bones.

**in·ter·na·tal** (in″tər-na′təl) [*inter-* + *natal*] intergluteal.

**In·ter·na·tion·al Non·pro·pri·e·tary Names** see *INN.*

**in·terne** (ă-tern′) [Fr.] intern.

**in·ter·neu·ron** (in″tər-noor′on) [MeSH: Interneurons] 1. any neuron in a chain of neurons that is situated between a primary sensory neuron and the final motoneuron. 2. any neuron whose processes are entirely confined within a specific area, as within the olfactory lobe, and which synapse with neurons extending into that area. Called also *intercalary, intercalated,* or *internuncial neuron.*

**in·tern·ist** (in-ter′nist) a physician who specializes in the diagnosis and medical, as opposed to surgical and obstetrical, treatment of diseases of adults.

**in·ter·no·dal** (in″tər-no′dəl) between two nodes.

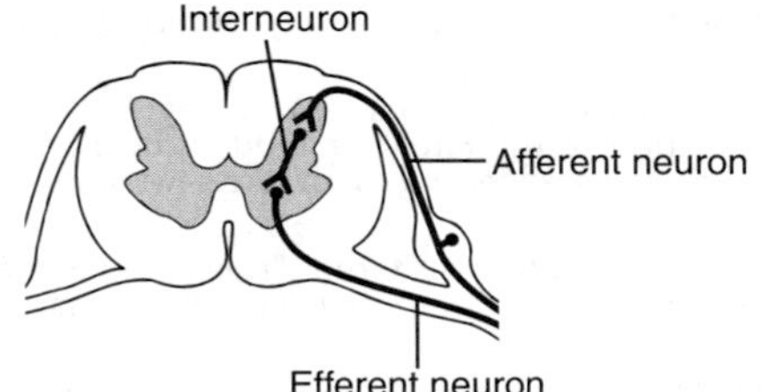

Interneuron as part of a three-neuron reflex arc in the spinal cord.

**in·ter·node** (in′tər-nōd) [*inter-* + *node*] internodal segment. **i. of Ranvier,** internodal segment.

**in·ter·nod·u·lar** (in″tər-nod′u-lər) between two nodules.

**in·tern·ship** (in′tərn-ship) the position or term of service of an intern in a hospital.

**in·ter·nu·cle·ar** (in″tər-noo′kle-ər) 1. pertaining to or affecting structures between nuclei, as internuclear ophthalmoplegia. 2. between the nuclear layers of the retina.

**in·ter·nun·ci·al** (in″tər-nun′she-əl) [L. *internuncius* a go-between] serving as a medium of communication between nerve cell bodies or neurons; see *interneuron.*

**in·ter·nus** (in-tər′nəs) [TA] internal: a term denoting something situated nearer to the center of an organ or a cavity.

**in·ter·oc·clu·sal** (in″tər-o-kloo′zəl) situated between the occlusal surfaces of opposing teeth of the mandibular and maxillary arches. See also *interdental* and *interproximal.*

**in·tero·cep·tive** (in″tər-o-sep′tiv) pertaining to interoceptors and the stimuli they receive.

**in·tero·cep·tor** (in″tər-o-sep′tor) any one of the sensory nerve terminals which are located in and transmit impulses from the viscera; see *receptor* (def. 3), *exteroceptor,* and *proprioceptor.*

**in·tero·in·fe·ri·or·ly** (in″tər-o-in-fēr′e-ər-le) inwardly and in a downward position or direction.

**in·ter·ol·i·vary** (in″tər-ol′ĭ-var″e) situated between the olivary bodies of the brain.

**in·ter·or·bi·tal** (in″tər-or′bĭ-təl) [*inter-* + *orbital*] situated between the orbits.

**in·ter·os·se·al** (in″tər-os′e-əl) [*inter-* + *osse-* + *-al*[1]] 1. situated between bones. 2. pertaining to the interossei muscles.

**in·ter·os·se·ous** (in″tər-os′e-əs) [L. *interosseus; inter* between + *os* bone] between bones.

**in·ter·pal·pe·bral** (in″tər-pal′pə-brəl) between the eyelids.

**in·ter·pa·ri·e·tal** (in″tər-pə-ri′ə-təl) [*inter-* + *parietal*] 1. intermural. 2. situated between the parietal bones.

**in·ter·par·ox·ys·mal** (in″tər-par″ok-siz′məl) interictal.

**in·ter·pe·dic·u·late** (in″tər-pə-dik′u-lāt) between the pedicles of a vertebra, as interpediculate distance.

**in·ter·pe·dun·cu·lar** (in″tər-pə-dunk′u-lər) [*inter-* + *peduncular*] situated between two peduncles, as between two cerebellar peduncles.

**in·ter·pha·lan·ge·al** (in″tər-fə-lan′je-əl) [*inter-* + *phalangeal*] situated between two contiguous phalanges.

**in·ter·phase** (in′tər-fāz) [MeSH: Interphase] the interval between two successive cell divisions, during which the chromosomes are not individually distinguishable and the normal physiological processes proceed. Formerly called *resting phase.*

**in·ter·phy·let·ic** (in″tər-fi-let′ik) [*inter-* + *phyletic*] intermediate in form between two types of cell.

**in·ter·pi·al** (in″tər-pi′əl) situated between the two layers of the pia mater.

**in·ter·plant** (in′tər-plant) [*inter-* + L. *plantare* to set] an embryonic part isolated by transference to an indifferent environment provided by another embryo.

**in·ter·pleu·ral** (in″tər-ploor′əl) between two layers of the pleura.

**in·ter·po·lar** (in″tər-po′lər) [*inter-* + *polar*] situated between two poles.

**in·ter·po·la·tion** (in-tər″po-la′shən) the determination of intermediate values in a series on the basis of observed values.

**in·ter·po·si·tion** (in″tər-pə-zish′ən) the act of placing between; the condition of being interposed.

**in·ter·pos·i·tum** (in″tər-poz′ĭ-təm) [L.] interposed; see under *velum.*

**in·ter·pre·ta·tion** (in-tər″prə-ta′shən) in psychotherapy, the therapist's explanation of the latent or hidden meanings of what the patient says, does, or experiences, in terms which are understandable to him.

**in·ter·pro·to·met·a·mere** (in″tər-pro″to-met′ə-mēr) [*inter-* + *proto* + *meta-* + *-mere*] the structure between the primary segments of the embryo.

**in·ter·prox·i·mal** (in″tər-prok′sĭ-məl) between adjoining surfaces, as the space between adjacent teeth. See also *interdental* and *interocclusal.*

**in·ter·pu·bic** (in″tər-pu′bik) [*inter-* + *pubic*] between the pubic bones.

**in·ter·pu·pil·lary** (in″tər-pu′pĭ-lar″e) between the pupils.

**in·ter·ra·di·al** (in″tə-ra′de-əl) situated between rays.

**in·ter·re·nal** (in″tə-re′nəl) [*inter-* + *renal*] between the kidneys.

**in·ter·rupt·ed** (in″tə-rup′təd) [L. *interruptus; inter* between + *ruptus* broken] not continuous; marked by intermissions or breaches of continuity.

**in·ter·rup·tion** (in″tər-rup′shən) an interference or blocking.
**vena caval i.,** interference with free flow of blood through the inferior vena cava by means of a filter to trap emboli and prevent pulmonary embolism; see also *vena cava filter,* under *filter.*

**in·ter·sca·pil·i·um** (in″tər-skə-pil′e-əm) [L.] the space between the scapulae.

**in·ter·scap·u·lar** (in″tər-skap′u lər) [*inter-* + *scapular*] situated between the scapulae.

**in·ter·scap·u·lum** (in″tər-skap′u-ləm) the interscapilium.

**in·ter·sci·at·ic** (in″tər-si-at′ik) between the two ischia.

**in·ter·sec·tio** (in″tər-sek′she-o) pl. *intersectio′nes* [L., from *inter* between + *secare* to cut] [TA] 1. a general term denoting a cutting across, or between. 2. a site at which one structure cuts across another.
**i. tendi′nea** [TA], tendinous intersection: a fibrous band that crosses the belly of a muscle and more or less completely divides it into two parts; called also *inscriptio tendinea.*
**intersec′tiones tendi′neae mus′culi rec′ti abdo′minis** [TA], tendinous intersections of rectus abdominis muscle: three or more fibrous bands that cross the front of the rectus abdominis muscle, fusing with the anterior layer of its sheath; called also *inscriptiones tendineae musculi recti abdominis.*

**in·ter·sec·tion** (in″tər-sek′shən) a site at which one structure cuts across another.
**tendinous i.,** intersectio tendinea.

**in·ter·sec·ti·o·nes** (in″tər-sek″she-o′nēz) [L.] plural of *intersectio.*

**in·ter·seg·ment** (in″tər-seg′mənt) 1. any one of a series of segments, like the angiotomes, etc. 2. a metamere.

**in·ter·seg·men·tal** (in″tər-seg-men′təl) between segments.

**in·ter·sep·tal** (in″tər-sep′təl) between two septa.

**in·ter·sep·tum** (in″tər-sep′təm) [L.] the diaphragm.

**in·ter·sex** (in′tər-seks) 1. hermaphrodite. 2. pseudohermaphrodite. 3. androgyne. 4. intersexuality.
**female i.,** female pseudohermaphrodite.
**male i.,** male pseudohermaphrodite.
**true i.,** true hermaphrodite.

**in·ter·sex·u·al** (in″tər-sek′shoo-əl) 1. hermaphroditic. 2. androgynous.

**in·ter·sex·u·al·i·ty** (in″tər-sek″shoo-al′ĭ-te) 1. hermaphroditism. 2. pseudohermaphroditism. 3. androgyny.

**in·ter·space** (in′tər-spās) a space between two similar structures.
**dineric i.,** the surface between two liquid phases.

**in·ter·sphinc·ter·ic** (in″tər-sfingk-ter′ik) between the internal and external anal sphincters.

**in·ter·spi·nal** (in″tər-spi′nəl) between two spinous processes.

**in·ter·spi·nous** (in″tər-spi′nəs) interspinal.

**in·ter·ster·nal** (in″tər-stər′nəl) between parts of the sternum.

**in·ter·stice** (in-ter′stis) [L. *interstitium*] a small interval, space, or gap in a tissue or structure.

**in·ter·sti·tial** (in″tər-stish′əl) pertaining to or situated between parts or in the interstices of a tissue.

**in·ter·sti·ti·um** (in″tər-stish′e-əm) [L.] 1. interstice. 2. interstitial tissue.

**in·ter·tar·sal** (in″tər-tahr′səl) situated between the tarsal bones.

**in·ter·trans·verse** (in″tər-trans-vərs′) [*inter-* + *transverse*] situated between or connecting the transverse processes of the vertebrae.

**in·ter·trig·i·nous** (in″tər-trij′ĭ-nəs) affected with or of the nature of intertrigo.

**in·ter·tri·go** (in″tər-tri′go) [*inter-* + L. *terere* to rub] [MeSH: Intertrigo] a superficial dermatitis occurring on apposed skin surfaces, such as the axillae, creases of the neck, intergluteal fold, groin, between the toes, and beneath pendulous breasts, with obesity being a predisposing factor, caused by moisture, friction, warmth, and sweat retention, and characterized by erythema, maceration, burning, itching, and sometimes erosions, fissures, and exudations and secondary infections. Called also *eczema intertrigo.*
**i. labia′lis,** perlèche.

**in·ter·tro·chan·ter·ic** (in″tər-tro″kan-ter′ik) [*inter-* + *trochanter*] situated in or pertaining to the space between the greater and the lesser trochanter.

**in·ter·tu·ber·cu·lar** (in″tər-too-bər′ku-lər) between tubercles.

**in·ter·tu·bu·lar** (in″tər-too′bu-lər) [*inter-* + *tubular*] situated between or among tubules.

**in·ter·ure·ter·al** (in″tər-u-re′tər-əl) interureteric.

**in·ter·ure·ter·ic** (in″tər-u″rə-ter′ik) [*inter-* + *ureter*] situated between the ureters.

**in·ter·vag·i·nal** (in″tər-vaj′ĭ-nəl) situated between sheaths.

**in·ter·val** (in′tər-vəl) [*inter-* + L. *vallum* rampart] the space between two objects or parts; the lapse of time between two recurrences or paroxysms.
**A–H i.,** the period between the onset of depolarization of the lower right atrium, measured as the A wave, and that of the bundle of His, measured as the His bundle deflection; approximates the time for impulse conduction across the atrioventricular node. See also illustration at *electrogram.*
**atrioventricular (AV) i.,** the time between the start of atrial and the start of ventricular systole; it is equivalent to the P–R interval of electrocardiography.
**cardioarterial i.,** the time between the apex beat and arterial pulsation; it measures the rate of propagation of the pulse wave.
**confidence i.,** a type of statistical interval estimate for an unknown parameter: a range of values believed to contain the parameter, with a predetermined degree of confidence. Its endpoints are the *confidence limits* and it has a stated probability (the *confidence coefficient*) of containing the parameter.
**conservative confidence i.,** a confidence interval having a confidence coefficient at least as great as a stated nominal value.
**coupling i.,** the length of time between an ectopic beat and the sinus beat preceding it; in an arrhythmia characterized by such beats, the intervals may be constant *(fixed coupling intervals)* or inconstant *(variable coupling intervals).*
**escape i.,** the interval between an escape beat and the normal beat preceding it.
**focal i.,** the distance from the anterior to the posterior focal point; called also *Sturm's i.*
**H–V i.,** the period between the onset of depolarization of the bundle of His, the H deflection in a His bundle electrogram, and the onset of ventricular activity, measured by surface or intracardiac leads; it approximates the time for conduction through the His-Purkinje system. See also illustration at *electrogram.*
**interdischarge i.,** the time between two discharges of the action potential of a single muscle fiber.
**interpotential i.,** the length of time between discharges of action potentials of two different fibers from the same motor unit.
**lucid i.,** 1. a brief period of remission of symptoms in a psychosis. 2. a brief return to consciousness after loss of consciousness in head injury.
**P–A i.,** the period from the onset of atrial activity, measured as the P wave in an electrocardiogram, and the onset of activity of the lower right atrial septum, measured as the A wave in a His bundle electrogram; it approximates the time for intra-atrial impulse conduction. See also illustration at *electrogram.*
**pacemaker escape i.,** the period between the last sensed spontaneous cardiac activity and the first beat stimulated by the pacemaker.
**P–P i.,** in electrocardiography, the time from the beginning of one P wave to that of the next P wave; it is the length of the cardiac cycle. See also illustration at *electrocardiogram.*
**PQ i.,** P–R i.
**P–R i.,** the portion of the electrocardiogram between the onset of the P wave (atrial depolarization) and the onset of the QRS complex (ventricular depolarization), lasting approximately 0.12 to 0.20 second in the adult. It is the time taken for an impulse to traverse the atrioventricular node, bundle of His, and bundle branches. See also illustration at *electrocardiogram.*
**QRS i.,** in electrocardiography, the interval from the beginning of

the Q wave to the termination of the S wave, representing the time for ventricular depolarization. See also illustration at *electrocardiogram.*
**QRST i., Q–T i.**, in electrocardiography, the time from the beginning of the Q wave to the end of the T wave; it represents the duration of ventricular electrical activity. See also illustration at *electrocardiogram.*
**Q–Tc i.**, the Q–T interval corrected for heart rate; see *Bazett's formula,* under *formula.*
**recruitment i.**, the inverse of the recruitment frequency; in a recruitment pattern, the length of time between two consecutive discharges of a given motor unit when an additional motor unit is recruited.
**reference i.**, see under *value.*
**ST i.**, the portion of the electrocardiogram from the end of the S wave to the end of the T wave, comprising the ST segment and the T wave.
**Sturm's i.**, focal i.
**systolic time i's (STI)**, any of several intervals measured for assessing left ventricular performance, particularly left ventricular ejection time (LVET), electromechanical systole ($QS_2$), and preejection period (PEP); electrocardiography, phonocardiography, and carotid pulse tracings are used to determine LVET and $QS_2$, and from them, PEP. See also individual intervals.
**V-A i.**, the time between a ventricular stimulus and the atrial stimulus following it.

**in·ter·val·vu·lar** (in″tər-val′vu-lər) between valves.

**in·ter·vas·cu·lar** (in″tər-vas′ku-lər) between blood vessels.

**in·ter·ven·tion** (in″tər-ven′shən) [L. *intervenire* to come between] 1. the act or fact of interfering so as to modify. 2. specifically, any measure whose purpose is to improve health or to alter the course of a disease.
**crisis i.**, 1. an immediate, short-term, psychotherapeutic approach, the goal of which is to help resolve a personal crisis within the individual's immediate environment. 2. the procedures involved in responding to an emergency.

**in·ter·ven·tric·u·lar** (in″tər-vən-trik′u-lər) [*inter-* + *ventricular*] situated between ventricles.

**in·ter·ver·te·bral** (in″tər-ver′tə-brəl) [*inter-* + *vertebra*] situated between two contiguous vertebrae; see under *disk.*

**in·ter·vil·lous** (in″tər-vil′əs) [*inter-* + L. *villus* tuft] situated between or among villi.

**in·tes·ti·nal** (in-tes′tĭ-nəl) [L. *intestinalis*] pertaining to the intestine.

**in·tes·tine** (in-tes′tin) [L. *intesti′nus* inward, internal; Gr. *enteron*] [MeSH: Intestines] intestinum.
**blind i.**, caecum (def. 2).
**empty i.**, jejunum.
**iced i.**, peritonitis chronica fibrosa encapsulans.
**jejunoileal i.**, intestinum tenue mesenteriale.
**large i.**, intestinum crassum.
**mesenterial i.**, intestinum tenue mesenteriale.
**segmented i.**, colon.
**small i.**, intestinum tenue.
**straight i.**, rectum.

**in·tes·ti·no·in·tes·ti·nal** (in-tes″tĭ-no-in-tes′tĭ-nəl) pertaining to two different portions of the intestine, as the intestino-intestinal reflex.

**in·tes·ti·num** (in″tes-ti′-nəm) pl. *intesti′na* [L., from *intestinus* inward, internal] intestine: the portion of the alimentary canal extending from the pyloric opening of the stomach to the anus: it is a membranous tube, comprising the intestinum tenue and the intestinum crassum, whose function is to complete the processes of digestion, to provide the body (through absorption) with water, electrolytes, and nutrients, and to move along and store fecal wastes until they are expelled. Called also *bowel* and *gut.*
**i. cae′cum**, caecum (def. 2).
**i. cras′sum** [TA], large intestine: the distal portion of the intestine, about five feet long, extending from its junction with the small intestine to the anus; it comprises the cecum, colon, rectum, and anal canal.
**i. i′leum**, ileum.
**i. jeju′num**, jejunum.
**i. rec′tum**, rectum.
**i. te′nue** [TA], small intestine: the proximal portion of the intestine, smaller in caliber than the large intestine, and about twenty feet long, extending from the pylorus to the cecum; it comprises the duodenum, jejunum, and ileum. Called also *enteron.*
**i. te′nue mesenteria′le**, the portion of the small intestine which has a mesentery, comprising the jejunum and ileum.

**in·ti·ma** (in′tĭ-mə) [L. "innermost"] 1. innermost. 2. tunica intima vasorum.

**in·ti·mal** (in′tĭ-məl) pertaining to the inner layer of the blood vessels (tunica intima vasorum).

**in·ti·mi·tis** (in″tĭ-mi′tis) endangitis.

**In·to·cos·trin** (in″to-kos′trin) trademark for a preparation of tubocurarine chloride.

**in·tol·er·ance** (in-tol′ər-əns) [*in-*[2] + *tolerance*] inability to withstand; sensitivity, as to a drug.
**carbohydrate i.**, inability to properly metabolize one or more carbohydrate(s), as in glucose intolerance, hereditary fructose intolerance, and the various types of disaccharide intolerance.
**disaccharide i.**, inability to properly metabolize one or more disaccharides, usually due to deficiency of the corresponding disaccharidase(s), although it may have other causes such as impaired absorption. The results are a complex of symptoms seen after ingestion of the disaccharide, particularly abdominal symptoms such as diarrhea, flatulence, borborygmus, distention, and pain. See also *lactose i.* and *congenital sucrose i.,* and see *sucrase-isomaltase deficiency* and *disaccharidase deficiency,* under *deficiency.*
**drug i.**, the state of reacting to the normal pharmacologic doses of a drug with the symptoms of overdosage.
**exercise i.**, limitation of ability to perform work or exercise at normally accepted levels; cf. *exercise tests,* under *test.*
**fructose i., hereditary**, an autosomal recessive type of carbohydrate intolerance due to deficiency of fructose bisphosphate aldolase, isozyme B, with onset in infancy; it is characterized by hypoglycemia, with variable manifestations of fructosuria, fructosemia, anorexia, vomiting, failure to thrive, jaundice, splenomegaly, and an aversion to fructose-containing foods. If untreated, it may be fatal. See also *essential fructosuria,* under *fructosuria.*
**glucose i.**, inability to properly metabolize glucose, a type of carbohydrate intolerance; see also *impaired glucose tolerance,* under *tolerance,* and *diabetes mellitus.*
**lactose i.**, a disaccharide intolerance specific for lactose, usually due to an inherited deficiency of lactase activity in the intestinal mucosa; see also *lactase deficiency.*
**lactose i., congenital**, 1. lactose intolerance present at birth, due to deficiency of lactase activity; see *lactase deficiency.* 2. a severe autosomal dominant disorder with vomiting, dehydration, failure to thrive, disacchariduria (including lactosuria and aminoaciduria), and cataracts; it is probably due to abnormal permeability of the gastric mucosa.
**lysine i., congenital**, an autosomal recessive disorder due to a defect in the degradation of lysine, characterized by high levels of ammonia, lysine, and arginine in the blood, with vomiting, rigidity, and coma. Cf. *hyperlysinemia.*
**lysinuric protein i.**, a hereditary disorder of metabolism transmitted as an autosomal recessive trait, involving a defect in dibasic amino acid transport and resulting in a lack of sufficient ornithine to support activity of ornithine transcarbamylase, an intramitochondrial urea cycle enzyme, in the liver. It is characterized by growth retardation, episodic hyperammonemia, seizures, mental retardation, hepatomegaly, muscle weakness, and osteopenia and is treated by citrulline supplementation.
**sucrose i., congenital**, a disaccharide intolerance specific for sucrose, usually due to a congenital defect in the sucrase-isomaltase enzyme complex; see *sucrase-isomaltase deficiency.*

**in·tor·sion** (in-tor′shən) [L. *in* toward + *torsio* twisting] inward rotation of the upper pole of the vertical meridian of each eye; called also *adtorsion* and *conclination.* Cf. *extorsion.*

**in·tort·or** (in′tor-tər) [L. *intorquēre* to twist] 1. an internal rotator. 2. an extraocular muscle that produces intorsion, i.e., the superior oblique or the superior rectus muscle. Cf. *extortor.*

**in·tox·i·ca·tion** (in-tok″sĭ-ka′shən) [L. *in* intensive + Gr. *toxikon* poison] 1. stimulation, excitement, or stupefaction produced by a chemical substance, or as if by one. 2. substance i., particularly that in which the substance is alcohol (see *alcohol i.*). 3. poisoning.
**alcohol i.** [DSM-IV], substance intoxication occurring during or shortly after ingestion of alcohol and characterized by maladaptive psychological or behavioral changes combined with physiologic responses such as slurred speech, incoordination, impaired memory or attention, unsteady gait, stupor, or coma.
**alcohol idiosyncratic i.**, a term previously used for maladaptive behavioral change, usually belligerence, produced by ingestion of amounts of alcohol insufficient to cause intoxication in most persons. It is no longer considered to be separate from alcohol intoxication because evidence for a distinction is lacking.
**bongkrek i.**, see under *poisoning.*
**pathological i.**, alcohol idiosyncratic i.
**roentgen i.**, radiation sickness.
**substance i.** [DSM-IV], a type of substance-induced disorder comprising reversible, substance-specific, maladaptive behavioral or psychological changes directly resulting from the physiologic effects on the central nervous system of recent ingestion of or exposure to a psychoactive substance. Specific cases are named on the

basis of etiology, e.g., alcohol intoxication. DSM-IV recognizes specific syndromes for these drugs: alcohol, amphetamines or related substances, caffeine, cannabis, cocaine, hallucinogens, inhalants, opioids, PCP or related substances, and sedatives, hypnotics, or anxiolytics.

**water i.**, the condition induced by the undue retention of water with decrease in sodium concentration; it is marked by lethargy, nausea, vomiting, and mild mental aberrations, and in severe cases by convulsions and coma.

**intra-** [L. *intra* within] a prefix meaning within, into, or during.

**in·tra·ab·dom·i·nal** (in″trə-ab-dom′ĭ-nəl) within the abdomen.

**in·tra·ac·i·nous** (in″trə-as′ĭ-nəs) within an acinus.

**in·tra·ap·pen·dic·u·lar** (in″trə-ap′ən-dik′u-lər) within the appendix.

**in·tra·arach·noid** (in″trə-ə-rak′noid) within or underneath the arachnoid.

**in·tra·ar·te·ri·al** (in″trə-ahr-tēr′e-əl) within an artery or arteries; called also *endarterial*.

**in·tra·ar·tic·u·lar** (in″trə-ahr-tik′u-lər) within a joint.

**in·tra·atri·al** (in″trə-a′tre-əl) within one or both atria of the heart.

**in·tra·au·ral** (in″trə-aw′rəl) within the ear.

**in·tra·au·ric·u·lar** (in″trə-aw-rik′u-lər) within an auricle of the ear.

**in·tra·bron·chi·al** (in″trə-brong′ke-əl) situated or occurring within a bronchus.

**in·tra·buc·cal** (in″trə-buk′əl) within the mouth or within the cheek.

**in·tra·can·a·lic·u·lar** (in″trə-kan″ə-lik′u-lər) within a canaliculus or canaliculi.

**in·tra·cap·su·lar** (in″trə-kap′su-lər) within a capsule.

**in·tra·car·di·ac** (in″trə-kahr′de-ak) within the heart.

**in·tra·car·pal** (in″trə-kahr′pəl) within the wrist.

**in·tra·car·ti·lag·i·nous** (in″trə-kahr″tĭ-laj′ĭ-nəs) within a cartilage; endochondral.

**in·tra·cav·er·no·sal** (in″trə-kav″ər-no′səl) within the corpus cavernosum.

**in·tra·cav·i·tary** (in″trə-kav′ĭ-tar″e) within a cavity, as that of the cervix or of the uterus.

**in·tra·ce·li·al** (in″trə-se′le-əl) within one of the body cavities.

**in·tra·cel·lu·lar** (in″trə-sel′u-lər) within a cell.

**in·tra·ce·phal·ic** (in″trə-sə-fal′ik) within the brain.

**in·tra·cer·e·bel·lar** (in″trə-ser″ə-bel′ər) situated within the cerebellum.

**in·tra·cer·e·bral** (in″trə-ser′ə-brəl) situated within the cerebrum.

**in·tra·cer·vi·cal** (in″trə-sər′vĭ-kəl) situated within the canal of the cervix uteri.

**in·tra·chon·dral** (in″trə-kon′drəl) endochondral.

**in·tra·chon·dri·al** (in″trə-kon′dre-əl) endochondral.

**in·tra·chor·dal** (in″trə-kor′dəl) within the notochord.

**in·tra·cis·ter·nal** (in″trə-sis-tər′nəl) within a cistern, especially the cisterna cerebellomedullaris.

**in·tra·col·ic** (in″trə-kol′ik) within the colon.

**in·tra·cor·po·ral** (in″trə-kor′por-əl) intracorporeal.

**in·tra·cor·po·re·al** (in″trə-kor-por′e-əl) situated or occurring within the body.

**in·tra·cor·pus·cu·lar** (in″trə-kor-pus′ku-lər) within a blood corpuscle. Called also *endocorpuscular, endoglobar, endoglobular,* and *intraglobular*.

**in·tra·cos·tal** (in″trə-kos′təl) on the inner surface of the rib.

**in·tra·cra·ni·al** (in″trə-kra′ne-əl) situated within the cranium.

**in·tra·crine** (in′trə-krin) denoting a type of hormone function in which a regulatory factor acts within the cell that synthesizes it by binding to intracellular receptors.

**in·tra·cru·re·us** (in″trə-kroo′re-əs) the internal part of the musculus vastus intermedius.

**in·trac·ta·ble** (in-trak′tə-bəl) resistant to cure, relief, or control.

**in·tra·cu·ta·ne·ous** (in″trə-ku-ta′ne-əs) within the skin; called also *intradermal*.

**in·tra·cys·tic** (in″trə-sis′tik) within a cyst.

**in·tra·cy·to·plas·mic** (in″trə-si″to-plaz′mik) within the cytoplasm of a cell.

**in·trad** (in′trad) [*intra-* + *-ad*[1]] inward in direction.

**in·tra·der·mal** (in″trə-dər′məl) 1. within the dermis. 2. intracutaneous.

**in·tra·di·a·lit·ic** taking place during dialysis.

**in·tra·duc·tal** (in″trə-duk′təl) situated or occurring within the duct of a gland.

**in·tra·du·o·de·nal** (in″trə-doo″o-de′nəl) within the duodenum.

**in·tra·du·ral** (in″trə-doo′rəl) within or beneath the dura.

**in·tra·epi·der·mal** (in″trə-ep″ĭ-dər′məl) within the epidermis.

**in·tra·ep·i·phys·e·al** (in″trə-ep″ĭ-fiz′e-əl) within an epiphysis.

**in·tra·ep·i·the·li·al** (in″trə-ep″ĭ-the′le-əl) situated among the cells of the epithelium.

**in·tra·eryth·ro·cyt·ic** (in″trə-ə-rith″ro-sit′ik) within an erythrocyte.

**in·tra·fas·cic·u·lar** (in″trə-fə-sik′u-lər) within a fascicle.

**in·tra·fat** (in″trə-fat′) situated in or introduced into fatty tissue, as the subcutaneous tissue.

**in·tra·fe·ta·tion** (in″trə-fe-ta′shən) the development of a fetus within another fetus; see *endadelphos*.

**in·tra·fi·lar** (in″trə-fi′lər) within a reticulum.

**in·tra·fis·su·ral** (in″trə-fish′ə-rəl) within a cerebral fissure.

**in·tra·fis·tu·lar** (in″trə-fis′tu-lər) within a fistula.

**in·tra·fol·lic·u·lar** (in″trə-fo-lik′u-lər) within a follicle.

**in·tra·fu·sal** (in″trə-fu′zəl) [*intra-* + *fusus*] pertaining to the striated fibers within a muscle spindle.

**in·tra·gas·tric** (in″trə-gas′trik) situated or occurring within the stomach.

**in·tra·gem·mal** (in″trə-jem′əl) within a bud, such as a taste bud.

**in·tra·gen·ic** (in″trə-jen′ik) within a gene.

**in·tra·glan·du·lar** (in″trə-glan′du-lər) within a gland.

**in·tra·glob·u·lar** (in″trə-glob′u-lər) 1. within a globe or globule. 2. intracorpuscular.

**in·tra·gy·ral** (in″trə-ji′rəl) within a cerebral gyrus.

**in·tra·he·pat·ic** (in″trə-hə-pat′ik) within the liver.

**in·tra·hy·oid** (in″trə-hi′oid) within the hyoid bone.

**in·tra·ic·tal** (in″trə-ik′təl) occurring during an attack or seizure.

**in·tra·in·tes·ti·nal** (in″trə-in-tes′tĭ-nəl) within the intestine.

**in·tra·jug·u·lar** (in″trə-jug′u-lər) within the jugular foramen, process, or vein.

**in·tra·la·mel·lar** (in″trə-lə-mel′ər) within lamellae.

**in·tra·la·ryn·ge·al** (in″trə-lə-rin′je-əl) endolaryngeal.

**in·tra·le·sion·al** (in″trə-le′zhən-əl) occurring in or introduced directly into a localized lesion.

**in·tra·leu·ko·cyt·ic** (in″trə-lu″ko-sit′ik) within a leukocyte.

**in·tra·lig·a·men·tous** (in″trə-lig″ə-men′təs) within a ligament.

**in·tra·lin·gual** (in″trə-ling′gwəl) within the tongue.

**in·tra·lo·bar** (in″trə-lo′bər) within a lobe.

**in·tra·lob·u·lar** (in″trə-lob′u-lər) within a lobule.

**in·tra·loc·u·lar** (in″trə-lok′u-lər) within the loculi of a structure.

**in·tra·lu·mi·nal** (in″trə-loo′mĭ-nəl) within the lumen of a tube, as of a blood vessel.

**in·tra·mam·ma·ry** (in″trə-mam′ə-re) within the breast.

**in·tra·mar·gin·al** (in″trə-mahr′jĭ-nəl) within a margin.

**in·tra·mat·ri·cal** (in″trə-mat′rĭ-kəl) within a matrix.

**in·tra·med·ul·lary** (in″trə-med′u-lar″e) 1. within the spinal cord. 2. within the medulla oblongata. 3. within the marrow cavity of a bone.

**in·tra·mem·bra·nous** (in″trə-mem′brə-nəs) within a membrane.

**in·tra·me·nin·ge·al** (in″trə-mə-nin′je-əl) within the meninges.

**in·tra·mo·lec·u·lar** (in″trə-mo-lek′u-lər) within the molecule.

**in·tra·mu·ral** (in″trə-mu′rəl) within the wall of an organ.

**in·tra·mus·cu·lar** (in″trə-mus′ku-lər) within the substance of a muscle.

**in·tra·myo·car·di·al** (in″trə-mi″o-kahr′de-əl) within the myocardium.

**in·tra·nar·i·al** (in″trə-nar′e-əl) within the nares.

**in·tra·na·sal** (in″trə-na′zəl) within the nose. Called also *endonasal*.

**in·tra·na·tal** (in″trə-na′təl) occurring during birth.

**in·tra·neu·ral** (in″trə-no͞or′əl) endoneural.

**in·tra·nu·cle·ar** (in″trə-noo′kle-ər) within a nucleus, as a cell nucleus.

**in·tra·oc·u·lar** (in″trə-ok′u-lər) within the eye.

**in·tra·op·er·a·tive** (in″trə-op′ər-ə-tiv) occurring during the course of a surgical operation.

**in·tra·oral** (in″trə-or′əl) within the mouth.

**in·tra·or·bi·tal** (in″trə-or′bĭ-təl) within the orbit.

**in·tra·os·se·ous** (in″trə-os′e-əs) within a bone.

**in·tra·os·te·al** (in″trə-os′te-əl) intraosseous.

**in·tra·ovar·i·an** (in″trə-o-var′e-ən) within the ovary.

**in·tra·ov·u·lar** (in″trə-ov′u-lər) within an oocyte or ovum.

**in·tra·pan·cre·at·ic** (in″trə-pan″kre-at′ik) within the pancreas.

**in·tra·par·en·chym·a·tous** (in″trə-par″ən-kim′ə-təs) within the parenchyma of an organ.

**in·tra·pa·ri·e·tal** (in″trə-pə-ri′ə-təl) [*intra-* + *parietal*] 1. intramural. 2. situated in the parietal region of the brain.

**in·tra·par·tal** (in″trə-pahr′təl) intrapartum.

**in·tra·par·tum** (in″trə-pahr′təm) occurring during childbirth, or during delivery.

**in·tra·pel·vic** (in″trə-pel′vik) within the pelvis.

**in·tra·peri·car·di·al** (in″trə-per″ĭ-kahr′de-əl) within the pericardium.

**in·tra·per·i·ne·al** (in″trə-per″ĭ-ne′əl) within the tissues of the perineum.

**in·tra·peri·to·ne·al** (in″trə-per″ĭ-to-ne′əl) within the peritoneal cavity.

**in·tra·pi·al** (in″trə-pe′əl) within or beneath the pia mater.

**in·tra·pla·cen·tal** (in″trə-plə-sen′təl) within the placenta.

**in·tra·pleu·ral** (in″trə-ploor′əl) within the pleura.

**in·tra·pon·tine** (in″trə-pon′tin) [*intra-* + *pontine*] within the substance of the pons.

**in·tra·pros·tat·ic** (in″trə-pros-tat′ik) within the prostate gland.

**in·tra·pro·to·plas·mic** (in″trə-pro″to-plaz′mik) within the protoplasm.

**in·tra·psy·chic** (in″trə-si′kik) arising, occurring, or situated within the mind.

**in·tra·pul·mo·nary** (in″trə-pul′mo-nar″e) within a lung.

**in·tra·py·ret·ic** (in″trə-pi-ret′ik) during the stage of fever.

**in·tra·ra·chid·i·an** (in″trə-rə-kid′e-ən) intraspinal.

**in·tra·rec·tal** (in″trə-rek′təl) within the rectum.

**in·tra·re·nal** (in″trə-re′nəl) within the kidney.

**in·tra·ret·i·nal** (in″trə-ret′ĭ-nəl) within the retina.

**in·tra·scle·ral** (in″trə-skler′əl) within the sclera.

**in·tra·scro·tal** (in″trə-skro′təl) within the scrotum.

**in·tra·seg·men·tal** (in″trə-seg-men′təl) within a single segment, such as a bronchopulmonary segment or spinal segment.

**in·tra·sel·lar** (in″trə-sel′ər) within the sella turcica.

**in·tra·spi·nal** (in″trə-spi′nəl) situated or occurring within the vertebral column.

**in·tra·sple·nic** (in″trə-sple′nik) within the spleen.

**in·tra·ster·nal** (in″trə-stər′nəl) within the sternum.

**in·tra·sti·tial** (in″trə-stish′əl) within the cells or fibers of a tissue.

**in·tra·stro·mal** (in″trə-stro′məl) within the stroma of an organ.

**in·tra·syno·vi·al** (in″trə-sĭ-no′ve-əl) within the synovial cavity of a joint.

**in·tra·tar·sal** (in″trə-tahr′səl) within or on the inner side of the tarsus.

**in·tra·ten·di·nous** (in″trə-ten′dĭ-nəs) within a tendon.

**in·tra·tes·tic·u·lar** (in″trə-tes-tik′u-lər) within the testis.

**in·tra·the·cal** (in″trə-the′kəl) within a sheath; see also under *injection.*

**in·tra·the·nar** (in″trə-the′nər) situated between the thenar and hypothenar eminences.

**in·tra·tho·rac·ic** (in″trə-tho-ras′ik) endothoracic.

**in·tra·ton·sil·lar** (in″trə-ton′sĭ-lər) within a tonsil.

**in·tra·tra·bec·u·lar** (in″trə-trə-bek′u-lər) within a trabecula.

**in·tra·tra·che·al** (in″trə-tra′ke-əl) endotracheal.

**in·tra·tu·bal** (in″trə-too′bəl) situated or occurring within a tube, especially within a uterine tube.

**in·tra·tu·bu·lar** (in″trə-too′bu-lər) within the tubules of an organ.

**in·tra·tym·pan·ic** (in″trə-tim-pan′ik) within the tympanic cavity.

**in·tra·ure·ter·al** (in″trə-u-re′tər-əl) within the ureter.

**in·tra·ure·thral** (in″trə-u-re′thrəl) within the urethra.

**in·tra·uter·ine** (in″trə-u′tər-in) within the uterus.

**in·tra·vag·i·nal** (in″trə-vaj′ĭ-nəl) within the vagina.

**in·trav·a·sa·tion** (in-trav″ə-za′shən) the entrance of foreign material into a blood vessel.

**in·tra·vas·cu·lar** (in″trə-vas′ku-lər) within a vessel.

**in·tra·ve·na·tion** (in″trə-ve-na′shən) the entrance or injection of foreign matter into a vein.

**in·tra·ve·nous** (in″trə-ve′nəs) within a vein or veins.

**in·tra·ven·tric·u·lar** (in″trə-ven-trik′u-lər) within a ventricle.

**in·tra·ver·sion** (in″trə-vər′zhən) in orthodontics, malocclusion in which the teeth or other maxillary structures are too near the median plane. Cf. *extroversion* (def. 3).

**in·tra·ver·te·bral** (in″trə-vər′tə-brəl) intraspinal.

**in·tra·ves·i·cal** (in″trə-ves′ĭ-kəl) within the bladder.

**in·tra·vil·lous** (in″trə-vil′əs) situated within a villus.

**in·tra·vi·tal** (in″trə-vi′təl) occurring during life.

**in·tra vi·tam** (in′trə vi′təm) [L.] during life.

**in·tra·vi·tel·line** (in″trə-vi-tel′in) within the vitellus or yolk.

**in·tra·vit·re·al** (in-trə-vit′re-əl) into or within the vitreous.

**in·tra·vit·re·ous** (in″trə-vit′re-əs) intravitreal.

**in·trin·sic** (in-trin′sik) [L. *intrinsecus* situated on the inside] situated entirely within or pertaining exclusively to a part.

**intro-** [L. *intro* within] a prefix meaning into or within.

**in·tro·duc·er** (in″trə-doo′sər) an intubator.

**in·tro·fi·er** (in′tro-fi″ər) a liquid which has the property of lowering the interfacial tension of emulsions.

**in·tro·flex·ion** (in″tro-flek′shən) a bending inward.

**in·tro·gas·tric** (in″tro-gas′trik) [*intro-* + *gastric*] conveyed or leading into the stomach.

**in·tro·gres·sion** (in″tro-gresh′ən) [*intro-* + L. *gressus* course] the incorporation of a gene from one complex into another as a result of hybridization.

**in·troi·tus** (in-tro′ĭ-təs) pl. *intro′itus* [L., from *intro* within + *ire* to go] a general term for the entrance to a cavity or space.
**i. pel′vis,** apertura pelvis superior.
**i. vagi′nae,** ostium vaginae.

**in·tro·jec·tion** (in″tro-jek′shən) [*intro-* + L. *jacēre* to throw] an immature unconscious defense mechanism in which loved or hated external objects are absorbed into the self; anxiety is diminished by reducing the possibility of loss in the case of a loved object, or by internally controlling aggression on the part of a hated object.

**in·tro·mis·sion** (in″tro-mish′ən) [*intro-* + L. *mittere* to send] the insertion of one part or instrument into another, as of the penis into the vagina.

**in·tron** (in′tron) [MeSH: Introns] a noncoding intervening sequence in a gene; almost all eukaryotic genes contain several introns separating the coding sequences (exons). After the 5′ cap and polyA tail are added to a primary mRNA transcript, the introns are removed and the exons spliced together by enzymes that recognize short sequences that identify exon-intron junctions, resulting in a mature mRNA that is ready for translation (protein synthesis). Called also *intervening sequence.*

**In·tron A** (in′tron) [MeSH: Interferon Alfa-2b] trademark for a preparation of interferon alfa-2b.

**In·tro·pin** (in′tro-pin) trademark for a preparation of dopamine hydrochloride.

**in·tro·spec·tion** (in″tro-spek′shən) [*intro-* + L. *spicere* to look] the contemplation or observation of one's own thoughts and feelings; self-analysis.

**in·tro·sus·cep·tion** (in″tro-sə-sep′shən) [*intro-* + L. *suscipere* to receive] intussusception.

**in·tro·ver·sion** (in″tro-vər′zhən) [*intro-* + *version*] 1. the turning outside in, more or less completely, of an organ, or the resulting condition. 2. the turning inward to the self of one's interest, with lack of interest in the external world. 3. intraversion.

**in·tro·vert** (in′tro-vərt) 1. a person whose interest is turned inward to the self. 2. to turn one's interest inward to the self. 3. a structure that can be turned or drawn inwards. 4. to turn a part or organ inward upon itself.

**in·tru·sion** (in-troo'zhən) in orthodontic therapy, a technique of depressing a tooth back into the occlusal plane or an effort to prevent its eruption or elongation during the correction of an excessive overbite. Called also *tooth depression.* Cf. *extrusion,* def. 3.

**in·tu·bate** (in'too-bāt) to treat by intubation.

**in·tu·ba·tion** (in″too-ba'shən) [L. *in* into + *tuba* tube] [MeSH: Intubation] the insertion of a tube into a body canal or cavity; see also *cannulation* and *catheterization.*
**endotracheal i.,** insertion of an endotracheal tube; see under *tube.*
**nasal i.,** insertion of a tube through the nose, such as a nasogastric or endotracheal tube.
**nasotracheal i.,** insertion of a nasotracheal tube.
**oral i.,** insertion of a tube through the mouth.
**orotracheal i.,** insertion of an orotracheal tube.

**in·tu·ba·tion·ist** (in-too-ba'shən-ist) one who performs an intubation.

**in·tu·ba·tor** (in'too-ba-tər) an instrument used in intubation.

**in·tu·mesce** (in-too-mes') to swell up.

**in·tu·mes·cence** (in-too-mes'əns) [L. *intumescentia*] 1. a swelling, normal or abnormal. 2. the process of swelling.

**in·tu·mes·cent** (in-too-mes'ənt) [L. *intumescens*] swelling or becoming swollen.

**in·tu·mes·cen·tia** (in-too-mə-sen'she-ə) pl. *intumescen'tiae* [L.] [TA] a general term for an enlargement or swelling.
**i. cervica'lis** [TA], cervical enlargement: the enlargement of the cervical spinal cord at the level of attachment of the nerves to the upper limbs.
**i. lumba'lis,** i. lumbosacralis.
**i. lumbosacra'lis** [TA], lumbosacral enlargement: the enlargement of the lumbar spinal cord at the level of attachment of the nerves to the lower limbs; called also *i. lumbalis.*
**i. tympa'nica** [TA], tympanic enlargement: a pseudoganglion on the tympanic branch (nerve) of the glossopharyngeal nerve; called also *ganglion tympanicum* [TA alternative], *tympanic ganglion, tympanic ganglion of Valentin,* and *Valentin's pseudoganglion.*

**in·tus·sus·cep·tion** (in″tə-sə-sep'shən) [L. *intus* within + *suscipere* to receive] [MeSH: Intussusception] 1. a receiving within. 2. the prolapse of one part of the intestine into the lumen of an immediately adjoining part. There are four varieties: *colic,* involving segments of the large intestine; *enteric,* involving only the small intestine; *ileocecal,* in which the ileocecal valve prolapses into the cecum, drawing the ileum along with it; and *ileocolic,* in which the ileum prolapses through the ileocecal valve into the colon. 3. in physiology, the reception into an organism of matter, such as food, and its transformation into new protoplasm.
**agonic i., postmortem i.,** intussusception occurring at the time of death.
**retrograde i.,** the invagination of a distal part of the bowel into a proximal part.

**in·tus·sus·cep·tum** (in″tə-sə-sep'təm) [L.] the portion of intestine that has been invaginated within another part in intussusception.

**in·tus·sus·cip·i·ens** (in″tə-sə-sip'e-əns) [L.] the portion of intestine into which another portion has invaginated in intussusception.

**In·u·la** (in'u-lə) [L.] a genus of composite-flowered plants (family Compositae), whose rhizomes contain inulin. The root has numerous uses in folk medicine.

**in·u·lase** (in'u-lās) inulinase.

**in·u·lin** (in'u-lin) [MeSH: Inulin] a vegetable starch, $(C_6H_{10}O_5)_4$, an indigestible polysaccharide occurring in the rhizome of certain plants (Compositae). It is a polymer of fructofuranose, yields fructose on hydrolysis, and is used in a test for determining glomerular filtration rate.

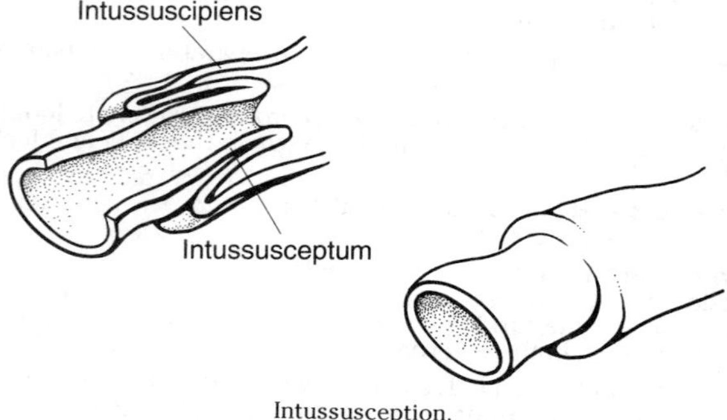

Intussusception.

**in·u·lin·ase** (in'u-lin-ās) [EC 3.2.1.7] an enzyme of the hydrolase class that catalyzes the cleavage of specific linkages between fructose residues in inulin, releasing fructose. The enzyme occurs in a variety of fungi and in higher plants.

**in·u·loid** (in'u-loid) a colorless compound, $C_6H_{10}O_5$, resembling inulin, but more soluble.

**in·unc·tion** (in-ungk'shən) [*in-*[1] + *unction*] 1. the act of anointing or of applying an ointment with friction. 2. an ointment made with lanolin as a menstruum.

**in·unc·tum** (in-ungk'təm) inunction, def. 2.
**i. men'tholis compo'situm,** compound menthol ointment.

**in utero** (in u'tər-o) [L.] within the uterus.

**Inv** [abbreviation of a patient's name] see *Km allotypes,* under *allotype.*

**in vac·uo** (in vak'u-o) [L.] in a vacuum.

**in·vag·i·nate** (in-vaj'ĭ-nāt) to infold one portion of a structure within another portion.

**in·vag·i·na·tion** (in-vaj″ĭ-na'shən) [L. *invaginatio,* from *in* within + *vagina* sheath] 1. the state of being or the process of becoming invaginated. 2. in embryology, a process by which *(a)* one region of a hollow, single-walled, spherical blastula caves in to form and line a new cavity in the now cup-shaped, double-walled gastrula, or *(b)* an ever-deepening pit develops into a diverticulum or tube from the surface into the tissues below. 3. intussusception.
**basilar i.,** a developmental deformity of the occipital bone and upper end of the cervical spine in which the latter appears to have pushed the floor of the occipital bone upward; see also *platybasia.* Called also *basilar impression.*

**in·va·lid** (in'və-lid) [L. *invalidus; in* not + *validus* strong] 1. not well and strong. 2. a person who is disabled by illness or infirmity.

**in·va·sin** (in-va'zin) hyaluronidase.

**in·va·sion** (in-va'shən) [L. *invasio; in* into + *vadere* to go] 1. the attack or onset of a disease. 2. the simple harmless entrance of bacteria into the body or their deposition in the tissues, as distinguished from infection. 3. the infiltration and active destruction of surrounding tissue, a characteristic of malignant tumors.

**in·va·sive** (in-va'siv) 1. having the quality of invasiveness. 2. involving puncture or incision of the skin or insertion of an instrument or foreign material into the body; said of diagnostic techniques.

**in·va·sive·ness** (in-va'siv-nəs) 1. the ability of a pathogenic microorganism to enter and spread throughout the tissues of the body. 2. the ability to infiltrate and actively destroy surrounding tissue; said of malignant tumors.

**in·ven·to·ry** (in'vən-tor″e) [MeSH: Equipment and Supplies] a comprehensive list of personality traits, aptitudes, and interests.
**Beck Depression I.,** a self-report questionnaire for measuring the symptoms of depression, focusing on the cognitive symptoms.
**California Personality I.,** CPI; a self-report, true-false test designed to measure aspects of personality style; generally used in counseling situations or for less than severe psychopathology.
**Millon Clinical Multiaxial I.,** MCMI; a self-report inventory designed to produce a profile of the personality style and structure underlying mental disorders.
**Minnesota Multiphasic Personality I.,** MMPI; a self-report, true-false test designed to evaluate personality and particularly to assess psychopathology.

**in·ver·mi·na·tion** (in-vər″mĭ-na'shən) infestation of the body by vermin.

**In·ver·sine** (in-vər'sēn) trademark for a preparation of mecamylamine hydrochloride.

**in·ver·sion** (in-vər'zhən) [L. *inversio; in* into + *vertere* to turn] 1. a turning inward, inside out, upside down, or other reversal of the normal relation of a part. 2. in psychiatry, a term used by Freud for homosexuality. 3. in genetics, a chromosomal aberration caused by the inverted reunion of a chromosome segment after breakage of a chromosome at two points, resulting in a change in sequence of genes or nucleotides; e.g., the sequence *abcdefg* may be inverted to *abfedcg.*
**carbohydrate i.,** hydrolysis of disaccharides or polysaccharides to monosaccharides.
**paracentric i.,** inversion in which the inverted chromosome segment is on one side of the centromere, i.e., both breaks occur in one arm. See Plate 1.
**pericentric i.,** inversion in which the inverted chromosome segment includes the centromere. See Plate 1.
**thermic i.,** the state in which the body temperature is highest in the morning.
**i. of uterus,** a turning of the uterus inside out, whereby the fundus

is forced through the cervix and protrudes into or outside of the vagina.
**visceral i.,** the more or less complete right and left transposition of the viscera; see *situs inversus viscerum.*

**in•ver•sus** (in-vər'səs) [L., past participle of *invertere* to invert] opposite to, or inverted from, the normal; see *situs inversus viscerum.*

**In•ver•te•bra•ta** (in-vər″tə-bra'tə) a former division of the animal kingdom, including all forms that have no spinal column.

**in•ver•te•brate** (in-vər'tə-brāt) [MeSH: Invertebrates] 1. any animal that has no spinal column; a nonvertebrate animal. 2. having no spinal column.

**in•ver•tor** (in-vər'tor) a muscle that turns a part inward.

**in•vest** (in-vest') 1. to envelop in or cover another tissue or part (as fascia). 2. to surround, envelop, or embed in an investment material.

**in•vest•ing** (in-vest'ing) 1. the act or process of covering or enveloping wholly or in part an object, such as a denture, tooth, wax form, or crown with a refractory investment material before curing, soldering, or casting. 2. the covering or enveloping of a tissue or part by another tissue, such as a fascia.
**i. the pattern,** surrounding the wax pattern with an investment material, such as a mix of a plaster, for low temperature casting, or a mix consisting of dental stone and a silica refractory for high temperature casting; the investment hardens to form a mold into which casting materials are poured.
**vacuum i.,** subjecting the water-investment mixture to a vacuum during the investing procedure in order to remove air bubbles from the mixture.

**in•vest•ment** (in-vest'mənt) [MeSH: Investments] 1. any tissue, such as fascia, that envelops or covers other tissues or parts. 2. a material applied as a soft paste to a pattern that hardens to form a mold for casting.
**gypsum-bonded i.,** an investment bonded by gypsum or one of its derivatives, used with metals or alloys that have low fusion temperatures.
**phosphate-bonded i.,** an investment bonded by phosphate and a metallic oxide, used with metals or alloys that have high fusion temperatures.
**silica-bonded i.,** an investment bonded by silica, used with metals or alloys that have high fusion temperatures.

**in•vet•er•ate** (in-vet'ər-ət) [L. *inverteratus; in* intensive + *vetus* old] chronic and confirmed; long established and of difficult cure.

**In•vi•rase** (in'vĭ-rās) trademark for a preparation of saquinavir mesylate.

**in•vis•ca•tion** (in″vis-ka'shən) [L. *in* among + *viscum* slime] the mixing of the food with the mucous secretion of the mouth in mastication.

**in vi•tro** (in ve'tro) [L.] [MeSH: In Vitro] within a glass; observable in a test tube; in an artificial environment.

**in vi•vo** (in ve'vo) [L.] within the living body.

**in•vo•lu•cre** (in'vo-loo″kər) an involucrum.

**in•vo•lu•crum** (in″vo-loo'krəm) pl. *involu'cra* [L.; *in* in + *volvere* to wrap] a covering or sheath, such as contains the sequestrum of a necrosed bone.

**in•vol•un•tary** (in-vol'ən-tar″e) [L. *involuntarius; in* against + *voluntas* will] performed independently of the will; contravolitional.

**in•vol•un•to•mo•to•ry** (in-vol″ən-to-mo'tor-e) pertaining to motion that is not voluntary.

**in•vo•lute** (in'vo-lo͞ot) [L. *in* into + *volvere* to roll] 1. to return to normal size after enlargement. 2. to regress; to change to an earlier or to a more primitive condition. See *involution.*

**in•vo•lu•tion** (in″vo-loo'shən) [L. *involutio; in* into +*volvere* to roll] 1. a rolling or turning inward. 2. one of the movements involved in the gastrulation of many animals. 3. a retrograde change of the entire body or in a particular organ, as the retrograde changes in the female genital organs that result in normal size after delivery. 4. the progressive degeneration occurring naturally with advancing age, resulting in a reduction in size or function of organs or tissues.
**senile i.,** the progressive degeneration that occurs naturally with advancing age, resulting in the shriveling of organs or tissues.

**in•vo•lu•tion•al** (in″vo-loo'shən-əl) pertaining to, due to, or occurring in involution.

**io•ben•guane** (i″o-ben'gwān) *m*-iodobenzylguanidine (mIBG), an analogue of norepinephrine with affinity for the sympathetic nervous system and related tumors; it is believed to share the same transport pathway with norepinephrine and displace norepinephrine from intraneuronal storage granules in adrenergic nerves.
**i. I 123,** iobenguane in which a portion of the molecules are labeled with $^{123}$I, used as a radioactive tracer for diagnostic imaging of neuroendocrine tumors and disorders of the adrenal medulla; administered intravenously as the sulfate (*iobenguane I 123 injection* [USP]).
**i. I 123 sulfate,** the sulfate salt of iobenguane I 123; see *i. I 123* and *iobenguane I 123 injection,* under *injection.*
**i. I 131,** iobenguane in which a portion of the molecules are labeled with $^{131}$I, used as a radioactive tracer for diagnostic imaging of neuroendocrine tumors and disorders of the adrenal medulla. It is also used for local radiation therapy in the treatment of carcinoid syndrome, pheochromocytoma, and neuroblastoma.

**io•ce•tam•ic ac•id** (i-o-se-tam'ik) a water-insoluble iodinated radiographic contrast medium that after oral administration is absorbed from the gastrointestinal tract, conjugated with glucuronic acid in the liver, and excreted in the bile; it is used for oral cholecystography.

**io•da•mide** (i-o'də-mide) [MeSH: Iodamide] a water-soluble iodinated radiopaque contrast medium, used for intravenous excretory urography and computed tomography of the brain.

**io•date** (i'o-dāt) any salt of iodic acid; the $IO_3^-$ anion.

**iod-Bas•e•dow** (i″ōd baz'ə-do) iodine-induced hyperthyroidism.

**io•de•mia** (i″o-de'me-ə) [*iodine* + *-emia*] the presence of iodides in the blood.

**iod•ic ac•id** (i-o'dik) a strong inorganic acid, $HIO_3$, which is a highly corrosive oxidizing agent.

**io•dide** (i'o-dīd) any binary compound of iodine; the $I^-$ anion. Dietary iodine is reduced to iodide, absorbed in the intestines, and later taken up from the bloodstream by the thyroid gland for incorporation into thyroid hormones.

**io•dide per•ox•i•dase** (i'o-dīd pər-ok'sĭ-dās) [EC 1.11.1.8] [MeSH: Iodide Peroxidase] an enzyme of the oxidoreductase class that catalyzes a series of reactions occurring in the synthesis of thyroxine; it catalyzes the oxidation of iodide to iodine, the iodination of tyrosyl residues of thyroglobulins, and the intramolecular condensation of such iodinated residues to form iodothyronines. Deficiency of the enzyme, an autosomal recessive disorder, results in congenital goiter. Called also *thyroid peroxidase* and *thyroperoxidase.*

**io•dim•e•try** (i″o-dim'ə-tre) [*iodine* + *-metry*] 1. the estimation of the quantity of iodine in a mixture or compound. 2. in quantitative analysis, the procedure used to determine an oxidizing agent consisting of the quantitative oxidation of potassium iodide to free iodine, and then titration with sodium thiosulfate.

**io•di•nate** (i-o'dĭ-nāt) to combine or compound with iodine.

**io•din•a•tion** (i″o-din-a'shən) the incorporation or addition of iodine in a compound.

**io•dine** (i'o-dīn) [Gr. *ioeides* violet-like, from the color of its vapor] [MeSH: Iodine] 1. a halogen element of a peculiar odor and acrid taste; symbol, I; atomic number, 53; atomic weight, 126.904. It is a nonmetallic element, occurring in heavy, grayish black plates or granules. Iodine is essential in nutrition, being especially necessary for the synthesis of thyroid hormones (thyroxine and triiodothyronine), which regulate the metabolic rate in all cells. 2. [USP] a preparation of iodine used as a topical anti-infective (see also under *solution*). Iodine, usually in the form of iodides, is used in the treatment of hyperthyroidism.
**i. 123,** a radioactive isotope of iodine, atomic mass 123, having a half-life of 13.2 hours; it decays by electron capture, emitting gamma rays (0.159 MeV) and x-rays. It is used as a tracer in diagnostic imaging and as a radiation source in radiation therapy.
**i. 125,** a radioisotope of iodine, atomic mass 125, having a half-life of 60.14 days and emitting gamma rays (0.035 MeV); used as a radioactive tracer, particularly as a label in radioimmunoassays and other *in vitro* tests, and also for thyroid imaging.
**i. 131,** a radioactive isotope of iodine, atomic mass 131, having a half-life of 8.04 days; it emits beta particles (0.607, 0.81, 0.336 MeV) and gamma rays (0.080, 0.284, 0.364, 0.637, 0.723 MeV) and is used as a tracer in diagnostic imaging and as a radiation source in radiation therapy.
**imidecyl i.,** a topical anti-infective compound, consisting of a mixture of 2-alkyl-($C_7H_{15}$ to $C_{17}H_{35}$)-1-(carboxymethyl)-1-(2-hydroxyethyl)-2-imidazolinium chloride; 3,6,9,12,15,18,21,24,27,30,33,36,39-tridecaoxadopentacontan–1-ol; and iodine.
**Lugol's i.,** a solution of potassium iodide and iodine in water, each 100 mL containing 10 g of potassium iodide and 5 g of iodine; used in Gram's method (see under *stain*) and as a stain for protozoa; see also *strong iodine solution,* under *solution.*
**povidone-i.,** see *povidone-iodine.*
**protein-bound i. (PBI),** iodine bound to protein in the blood serum, measured in the protein-bound iodine test.
**radioactive i.,** radioiodine.

**io•din•o•phil** (i″o-din'o-fil) [*iodine* + *-phil*] 1. any cell or other element readily stainable with iodine. 2. iodinophilous.

**io•din•oph•i•lous** (i″o-din-of'ĭ-ləs) readily stainable with iodine.

**io·dip·amide** (i″o-dip′ə-mīd) [USP] [MeSH: Iodipamide] a water-soluble iodinated radiographic contrast medium used for intravenous cholangiography and cholecystography.
**i. meglumine** [USP], **i. methylglucamine,** the meglumine salt of iodipamide, used as a radiopaque medium in cholangiography and cholecystography, administered intravenously.
**i. sodium,** the sodium salt of iodipamide, used as a radiopaque medium in cholangiography and cholecystography, administered intravenously.

**io·dism** (i′o-diz-əm) chronic poisoning by iodine or iodine compounds; it is marked by coryza, ptyalism, frontal headache, emaciation, weakness, and skin eruptions (iododerma). Called also *iodine poisoning.*

**io·dix·a·nol** (i″o-dik′sə-nol) a nonionic contrast medium used in angiography, computed tomography, and excretory urography.

**io·dize** (i′o-dīz) to impregnate with iodine or to incorporate iodine or one of its compounds.

**iod(o)-** [Fr. *iode* iodine] word element denoting a relationship to iodine.

**io·do·ace·tic ac·id** (i-o″do-ə-se′tik) a compound, used in biochemical studies; it alkylates free thiol groups but not disulfide bridges.

***m*-io·do·ben·zyl·gua·ni·dine** (i″o-do-ben″zəl-gwah′nĭ-dēn) iobenguane.

**io·do·chlor·hy·drox·y·quin** (i-o″do-klor″hi-drok′sə-kwin) clioquinol.

**io·do·cho·les·ter·ol I 131** (i-o″do-kə-les′tər-ol) a radiopharmaceutical, cholesterol iodinated with $^{131}I$, which has been used in radionuclide imaging of the adrenal cortex; now largely replaced by iodomethylnorcholesterol.

**io·do·der·ma** (i-o″do-dər′mə) [*iodo-* + *derma*] any skin eruption or lesion resulting from iodism.

**io·do·form** (i-o′do-form) [*iodo-* + *formyl*] chemical name: triiodomethane. A greenish yellow powder or crystals, $CHI_3$, having a strong, penetrating odor, containing about 96 per cent of iodine, and soluble in chloroform and ether and somewhat in alcohol and water: used as a topical anti-infective, applied to the skin.

**io·do·form·ism** (i-o″do-form′iz-əm) poisoning by iodoform.

**io·do·for·mum** (i-o″do-for′məm) iodoform.

**io·do·gen·ic** (i-o″do-jen′ik) [*iodine* + *genic*] yielding or producing iodine.

**io·do·glob·u·lin** (i-o″do-glob′u-lin) an iodine-containing globulin.

**io·do·gor·gor·ic ac·id** (i-o″do-gor′gər-ik) diiodotyrosine.

**io·do·hip·pu·rate so·di·um** (i-o″do-hip′u-rāt) an iodine-containing compound that has been used as a radiopaque medium in pyelography.
**i. s. I 123** [USP], that in which a portion of the molecules are labeled with $^{123}I$; administered intravenously in renography to determine renal function, urinary obstruction, and effective renal plasma flow and also in renal imaging.
**i. s. I 131** [USP], that in which a portion of the molecules are labeled with $^{131}I$; administered intravenously in renography to determine renal function, urinary obstruction, and effective renal plasma flow and also in renal imaging.

**io·do·log·ra·phy** (i-o″do-log′rə-fe) radiographic visualization of an organ or part after the injection into it of iodized oil.

**io·do·meth·ane** (i-o″do-meth′ān) methyl iodide.

**io·do·meth·yl·nor·cho·les·ter·ol** (i-o″do-meth″əl-nor″kə-les′tər-ol) norcholesterol, a cholesterol analogue, iodinated with $^{131}I$, used in radionuclide imaging of the adrenal cortex. Called also *NP-59.*

**io·do·met·ric** (i-o″do-met′rik) pertaining to iodometry.

**io·dom·e·try** (i″o-dom′ə-tre) [*iodo-* + *-metry*] estimation of the quantity of a chemical by titration with iodine.

**io·do·pa·no·ic ac·id** (i-o″do-pə-no′ik) iopanoic acid.

**io·do·phe·nol** (i-o″do-fe′nol) a preparation of iodine, phenol, and glycerin, used as an antiseptic.

**io·do·phil** (i-o′do-fil) iodinophil.

**io·do·phil·ia** (i-o″do-fil′e-ə) [*iodo-* + *-philia*] the reaction shown by leukocytes in certain conditions when treated with iodine or iodides. Normal leukocytes are colored bright yellow, but in certain pathologic conditions, as toxemia and severe anemia, the polymorphonuclears show diffuse brownish coloration. When the staining affects the leukocytes themselves, it is termed *intracellular;* when only the particles around the leukocytes are affected, it is *extracellular.*

**io·do·phor** (i-o′do-for) any of various compounds of iodine with carriers such as polyvinylpyrrolidone; used as surgical scrubs, surface disinfectants, and veterinary medicine skin disinfectants.

**io·do·phthal·ein so·di·um** (i-o″do-thal′ēn) the disodium salt of tetraiodophenolphthalein; used as a radiopaque medium in cholecystography.

**io·dop·sin** (i″o-dop′sin) [Gr. *iōdēs* violet colored + *opsis* vision] a photosensitive violet retinal pigment found in the retinal cones of some animals and important for color vision.

**io·do·pyr·a·cet** (i-o″do-pi′rə-set) [MeSH: Iodopyracet] a radiopaque medium, used especially in urography; administered intravenously or intramuscularly.

**io·do·quin·ol** (i-o″do-kwin′ol) [USP] [MeSH: Iodoquinol] an amebicide, used in the treatment of intestinal amebiasis, administered orally, and in *Trichomonas vaginalis* vaginitis, administered intravaginally. It has also been used topically in fungal and bacterial skin infections and in seborrheic dermatitis. Called also *diiodohydroxyquin.*

**io·do·sul·fate** (i-o″do-sul′fāt) a combination of a base with iodine and sulfuric acid.

**io·do·ther·a·py** (i-o″do-ther′ə-pe) [*iodo-* + *therapy*] treatment, usually of a goiter, with iodine or iodides.

**io·do·thy·ro·glob·u·lin** (i-o″do-thi″ro-glob′u-lin) iodinated thyroglobulin.

**io·do·thy·ro·nine** (i-o″do-thi′ro-nēn) an iodinated thyronine, such as the thyroid hormones triiodothyronine and tetraiodothyronine (thyroxine).

**io·do·ty·ro·sine** (i-o″do-ti′ro-sēn) [MeSH: Iodotyrosine] any iodinated derivative of tyrosine.

**io·do·ty·ro·sine de·hal·o·gen·ase** (i-o″do-ti′ro-sēn de-hal′o-jən-ās) iodotyrosine deiodinase.

**io·do·ty·ro·sine de·io·din·ase** (i″o-do-ti′ro-sēn de-i′o-dĭ-nās) an enzyme that catalyzes the removal of iodine from monoiodotyrosine and diiodotyrosine. The reaction is a step in the conservation of iodine by the thyroid. Congenital deficiency of the enzyme results in severe loss of iodine, resulting in hypothyroidism and goiter. Called also *iodotyrosine dehalogenase.*

**io·do·ven·tric·u·log·ra·phy** (i-o″do-vən-trik″u-log′rə-fe) ventriculography with iodine contrast medium.

**io·do·vol·a·til·iza·tion** (i-o″do-vol″ə-til-ĭ-za′shən) the liberation of free iodine by living epidermal cells in the iodogenic layer of certain brown algae or kelp. It accumulates in the algae as potassium iodide and has been used as a commercial source of iodine.

**io·dox·am·ic ac·id** (i-o″dok-sam′ik) an ionic dimeric radiopaque medium used in cholecystography.

**io·du·ria** (i″o-du′re-ə) the presence of iodides in the urine.

**io·fet·amine hy·dro·chlo·ride I 123** (i″o-fet′ə-mēn) an aromatic hydrocarbon iodinated with $^{123}I$; it is used as a brain imaging agent in the localization and evaluation of certain kinds of stroke.

**io·gly·cam·ic ac·id** (i″o-gli-kam″ik) [MeSH: Ioglycamic Acid] an acid, the meglumine and sodium salts of which are used as diagnostic radiopaque media in cholecystography.

**io·hex·ol** (i″o-hek′sol) [USP] [MeSH: Iohexol] a nonionic, water-soluble, low-osmolality radiopaque medium, administered by intrathecal or intravascular injection.

**ion** (i′on) [Gr. *iōn* going] an atom or radical having a charge of positive (cation) or negative (anion) electricity owing to the loss or gain of one or more electrons. Substances that form ions are called electrolytes. See *ionic theory,* under *theory.*
**dipolar i.,** zwitterion.
**hydrogen i.,** the nucleus of the hydrogen atom or a hydrogen atom that has lost its electron, $H^+$; it bears a positive charge equivalent to the negative charge of the electron and is called a proton.
**hydronium i.,** the hydrated form, $H_3O^+$, in which the proton (hydrogen ion, $H^+$) exists in aqueous solution; a combination of $H^+$ and $H_2O$.

**Io·na·min** (i-o′nə-min) trademark for a preparation of phentermine.

**ion·ic** (i-on′ik) pertaining to an ion or to ions.

**ion·iza·tion** (i″on-ĭ-za′shən) 1. any process by which a neutral atom or molecule gains or loses electrons, thus acquiring a net charge, as the dissociation of a substance in solution into ions or ion production by the passage of radioactive particles. 2. iontophoresis.
**avalanche i.,** the multiplicative process in which a single charged particle, accelerated by a strong electric field, produces additional charged particles through collision with neutral gas molecules; called also *Townsend i.*
**Townsend i.,** avalanche i.

**ion·ize** (i′on-īz) to separate into ions.

**ion·o·col·or·im·e·ter** (i″ŏ-no-kol″or-im′ə-tər) an apparatus for measuring the ionic acidity of a solution.

**ion·o·gen·ic** (i-on″o-jen′ik) forming or supplying ions.

**ion·o·mer** (i-on′ə-mər) a polymer having covalent bonds within the long-chain molecules and ionic bonds between the chains; see also *glass ionomer cement,* under *cement,* and *ionomer resin,* under *resin.*

**ion·om·e·ter** (i″ŏ-nom′ə-tər) an instrument for the measurement of the intensity or quantity of radiation from an ionizing radiation source.

**ion·o·phore** (i-on′ə-for″) any molecule, as of a drug, that increases the permeability of cell membranes to a specific ion.

**ion·o·phose** (i′ŏ-no-fōz″) [Gr. *ion* violet + *phose*] a violet phose.

**ion·o·scope** (i-on′o-skōp) an instrument for detecting alkaline or acid impurity in nitrous oxide.

**ion·o·ther·a·py** (i″o-no-ther′ə-pe) 1. [*ion* + *therapy*] iontophoresis. 2. [Gr. *ion* violet + *therapy*] treatment by means of ultraviolet rays.

**ion-pro·tein** (i-on-pro′tēn) a protein molecule combined with an inorganic ion.

**ion·ther·a·py** (i″on-ther′ə-pe) iontophoresis.

**ion·to·pho·re·sis** (i-on″to-fə-re′sis) [MeSH: Iontophoresis] the introduction by means of the electric current, of ions of soluble salts into the tissues of the body, often for therapeutic purposes; a form of electro-osmosis. Called also *iontherapy.*

**ion·to·pho·ret·ic** (i-on″to-fə-ret′ik) pertaining to iontophoresis.

**ion·to·quan·tim·e·ter** (i-on″to-kwahn-tim′ə-tər) [*ion* + *quantimeter*] ionometer.

**ion·to·ra·di·om·e·ter** (i-on″to-ra″de-om′ə-tər) ionometer.

**IOP** intraocular pressure.

**io·pam·i·dol** (i″o-pam′ĭ-dol) [MeSH: Iopamidol] a nonionic, water-soluble, low-osmolality radiopaque medium used in myelography; administered intravenously or orally.

**io·pa·no·ic ac·id** (i″o-pə-no′ik) [USP] [MeSH: Iopanoic Acid] an iodinated radiographic contrast medium that after oral administration is absorbed from the duodenum, conjugated with glucuronic acid in the liver, and secreted in the bile; it is used for oral cholecystography and cholangiography.

**io·phen·dy·late** (i″o-fen′də-lāt) [USP] [MeSH: Iophendylate] a radiopaque medium used in myelography, administered intrathecally or by special injection.

**io·phen·ox·ic ac·id** (i″o-fən-ok′sik) a radiopaque medium used in cholecystography. Called also *triiodoethionic acid.*

**Io·pi·dine** (i-o′pĭ-dēn) trademark for a preparation of apraclonidine hydrochloride.

**io·pro·mide** (i-o-pro′mīd) [USP] a nonionic, low-osmolality radiopaque medium used for imaging of the cardiovascular system, for excretory urology, and for contrast enhancement in computed tomography; administered intra-arterially or intravenously.

**io·ser·ic ac·id** (i″o-ser′ik) a radiopaque medium, $C_{15}H_{16}I_3N_3O_7$.

**io·sul·a·mide meg·lu·mine** (i″o-sul′ə-mīd) a compound used as a radiopaque medium, $C_{28}H_{28}I_6N_4O_{10}S{\cdot}C_7H_{17}NO_5$.

**io·ta** (i-o′tə) [I, ι] the ninth letter of the Greek alphabet.

**io·thal·a·mate** (i″o-thal′ə-māt) a water-soluble iodinated radiographic contrast medium used for angiography, angiocardiography, excretory urography, retrograde urography, and contrast enhancement of computed tomographic brain images. Available as *i. meglumine* [USP], *i. sodium* [USP], or as a mixture of the two salts.
**i. meglumine** [USP], a radiopaque medium consisting of iothalamic acid in water for injection, prepared with the aid of meglumine; used intra-arterially in cerebral angiography and peripheral arteriography and intravenously in excretory urography and peripheral pyelography.
**i. sodium** [USP], a radiopaque medium consisting of iothalamic acid in water for injection, prepared with the aid of sodium hydroxide; used intra-arterially or intravenously in angiocardiography and aortography.
**i. I 125 sodium** [USP], sodium iothalamate in which a portion of the molecules have been iodinated with $^{125}$I; used in the determination of the glomerular filtration rate.

**io·tha·lam·ic ac·id** (i″o-thal′ə-mik) [USP] [MeSH: Iothalamic Acid] the free acid of iothalamate, used in the preparation of certain radiopaque media.

**io·ver·sol** (i″o-vər′sol) [USP] a nonionic contrast medium used in angiography and urography and for contrast enhancement in computed tomography.

**iox·ag·late** (i″ok-sag′lāt) a salt or ester of ioxaglic acid.
**i. meglumine** [USP], a salt of ioxaglic acid used as a low-osmolality radiopaque medium.
**i. sodium** [USP], a salt of ioxaglic acid used as a low-osmolality radiopaque medium.

**iox·ag·lic ac·id** (i″ok-sag′lik) [USP] [MeSH: Ioxaglic Acid] a low-osmolality radiopaque medium.

**iox·i·lan** (i-ok′sĭ-lan) [USP] a low-viscosity, low-osmolality, nonionic contrast agent used in arteriography, excretory urography, and computed tomography.

**IP** intraperitoneally; isoelectric point.

**IP$_3$** inositol 1,4,5-triphosphate.

**IPAA** International Psychoanalytical Association.

**IPD** intermittent peritoneal dialysis.

**ip·e·cac** (ip′ə-kak) [USP] the dried rhizome and roots of *Cephaelis ipecacuanha* (Brotero) Rich. (Rubiaceae) (Rio or Brazilian i.) or of *C. acuminata* Karsten (Cartagena, Nicaragua, or Panama i.). Originally introduced as a remedy for dysentery, it has been replaced by its alkaloid emetine for that purpose, and is now used in syrup as an emetic, particularly in cases of poisoning. It also has expectorant properties.
**powdered i.** [USP], ipecac reduced to a very fine powder; used in the preparation of ipecac syrup.

**ipo·date** (i′po-dāt) [MeSH: Ipodate] $C_{12}H_{13}I_3N_2O_2$, a radiographic contrast agent usually given as the calcium or sodium salt.
**i. calcium,** the calcium salt of ipodate, used as a radiopaque medium in cholecystography, administered orally.
**i. sodium** [USP], the sodium salt of ipodate, used as a radiopaque medium in cholecystography, administered orally.

**ip·o·mea** (i″po-me′ə) the dried root of *Ipomoea orizabensis,* used as a cathartic; called also *Mexican scammony* and *orizaba jalap root.*

**Ip·o·moea** (i″po-me′ə) a large genus of herbs and shrubs of the family Convolvulaceae, including morning glories and sweet potatoes. Some species, such as *I. orizaben′sis,* contain cathartic resins; others, such as some morning glories, contain psychotomimetic indole alkaloids including lysergic acid amide and are classified as toxic for humans and other animals.
**I. calo′bra,** the weir plant, an Australian weed that is toxic to ruminants, causing neurological problems and blindness.
**I. muelle′ri,** the most common species of morning glory; it contains psychotomimetic alkaloids and is toxic to humans and other animals, sometimes causing fatal neurological disease in ruminants.
**I. viola′cea L.,** a species of morning glory that contains the psychotomimetic alkaloid lysergic acid amide and is toxic to humans and other animals.
**I. orizaben′sis Ledenois,** a Mexican species that is the source of the cathartic ipomea.

**IPPB** intermittent positive pressure breathing; see under *breathing.*

**Ip·ral** (ip′rəl) trademark for preparations of probarbital.

**ipra·tro·pi·um bro·mide** (ip″rə-tro′pe-əm) a synthetic congener of atropine that acts as an anticholinergic agent; used as a bronchodilator and administered intranasally for the relief of rhinorrhea.

**iprin·dole** (ĭ-prin′dōl) [MeSH: Iprindole] an antidepressant with actions and uses similar to those of amitriptyline hydrochloride; administered orally.

**ipro·nid·a·zole** (i-pro-nīd′ə-zōl) [MeSH: Ipronidazole] an antiprotozoal effective against *Histomonas.*

**ipro·pla·tin** (i′pro-plat″in) an antineoplastic analogue of cisplatin, administered intravenously; its actions are similar to those of cisplatin, but its toxicities are different and usually milder.

**ipsi-** [L. *ipse* self] a combining form meaning the same.

**ip·si·lat·er·al** (ip″sĭ-lat′ər-əl) [*ipsi-* + *lateral*] situated on, pertaining to, or affecting the same side, as opposed to contralateral.

**IPSP** inhibitory postsynaptic potential.

**IPV** poliovirus vaccine inactivated.

**IQ** intelligence quotient.

**Ir** symbol for *iridium.*

**ir-** see *in-.*

**IRC** inspiratory reserve capacity.

**Ir·con** (ir′kon) trademark for a preparation of ferrous fumarate.

**iri·dal** (i′rĭ-dəl) iridic.

**iri·dal·gia** (i″rĭ-dal′jə) [*irid-* + *-algia*] pain in the iris.

**ir·id·aux·e·sis** (ir″id-awk-se′sis) [*irid-* + *auxesis*] thickening of the iris.

**iri·dec·tome** (ir″ĭ-dek′tōm) [*irid-* + Gr. *ektemnein* to cut out] a cutting instrument for use in iridectomy.

**iri·dec·to·me·so·di·al·y·sis** (ir″ĭ-dek″to-me″so-di-al′ə-sis) [*irid-* + *-ectomy* + *meso-* + *dialysis*] surgical formation of an artificial iris by excision and separation of adhesions around the inner edge of the iris.

**iri·dec·to·mize** (ir″ĭ-dek′to-mīz) to remove part of the iris by excision.

**iri·dec·to·my** (ir″ĭ-dek′tə-me) [*irid-* + *-ectomy*] surgical excision of a full-thickness piece of the iris; called also *corectomy.*
**basal i.,** iridectomy at the base of the iris close to its attachment to the ciliary body.
**buttonhole i.,** peripheral i.
**complete i.,** surgical excision of a whole radial section of the iris from the root to, and including, the margin. Called also *sector i.* and *total i.*
**optic i., optical i.,** excision of part of the iris as a means of enlarging an abnormally small pupil and improving vision.
**peripheral i.,** a surgical treatment for narrow-angle glaucoma, and consisting of a full-thickness excision of a portion of the periphery or root of the iris, the pupillary border and sphincter muscle being left intact. Called also *basal i., buttonhole i.,* and *stenopeic i.*
**preliminary i., preparatory i.,** iridectomy performed before removal of the lens in cataract surgery.
**sector i.,** complete i.
**stenopeic i.,** peripheral i.
**therapeutic i.,** iridectomy performed for the cure of disease of the eye.
**total i.,** complete i.

**iri·dec·tro·pi·um** (ir″ĭ-dek-tro′pe-əm) ectropion uveae.

**iri·de·mia** (ir″ĭ-de′me-ə) [*irid-* + *-emia*] hemorrhage from the iris.

**iri·den·clei·sis** (ir″ĭ-dən-kli′sis) [*irid-* + Gr. *enklein* to lock in] the surgical creation of a permanent drain by incarceration of a slip of the iris within a corneal or limbal incision to act as a wick through which the aqueous is filtered from the anterior chamber to the subconjunctival tissues; done to reduce intraocular pressure.

**iri·den·tro·pi·um** (ir″ĭ-dən-tro′pe-əm) entropion uveae.

**iri·de·re·mia** (ir″ĭ-də-re′me-ə) [*irid-* + Gr. *erēmia* want of, absence] congenital absence of the iris.

**iri·des** (i′rĭ-dēz, ir′ĭ-dēz) [Gr.] plural of *iris.*

**iri·des·cence** (ir″ĭ-des′əns) [L. *iridescere* to gleam like a rainbow] the condition of gleaming with bright and changing colors.

**iri·des·cent** (ir″ĭ-des′ənt) [Gr. *iris* rainbow] having a rainbow-like display of colors in reflected light, as in mother-of-pearl; said of a colony of microorganisms.

**irid·e·sis** (i-rid′ə-sis) [*irid-* + *-desis*] the operation of repositioning the pupil by bringing a sector of the iris through a corneal or limbal incision and fixing the sector with a suture.

**iri·di·ag·no·sis** (i″rĭ-di-əg-no′sis) iridodiagnosis.

**irid·i·al** (i-rid′e-əl) iridic.

**irid·i·an** (i-rid′e-ən) iridic.

**irid·ic** (i-rid′ik) pertaining to the iris.

**irid·i·um** (ĭ-rid′e-əm) [L. *iris* rainbow, from the tints of its salts] [MeSH: Iridium] a very hard white metal; symbol, Ir; atomic number, 77; atomic weight, 192.2.
**i. Ir 192,** an artificial radioactive isotope of iridium, atomic mass 192, with a half-life of 73.83 days; it emits beta particles (0.67 MeV) and gamma rays (0.296, 0.308, 0.317, 0.468, 0.589, 0.604, 0.612 MeV) and is used in radiotherapy.

**iri·di·za·tion** (ir″ĭ-dĭ-za′shən) the subjective perception of iridescent halos about lights, occurring in glaucoma.

**irid(o)-** [Gr. *iris,* gen *iridos* rainbow] a combining form meaning iridescent, or denoting relationship to the iris.

**iri·do·avul·sion** (ir″ĭ-do-ə-vul′shən) complete tearing away of the iris from its periphery.

**iri·do·cap·su·li·tis** (ir″ĭ-do-kap-su-li′tis) inflammation of the iris and the capsule of the lens.

**iri·do·cele** (i-rid′o-sēl) [*irido-* + *-cele*] hernial protrusion of a part of the iris through the cornea.

**iri·do·cho·roi·di·tis** (ir″ĭ-do-ko″roi-di′tis) inflammation of the iris and the choroid.

**iri·do·col·o·bo·ma** (ir″ĭ-do-kol″o-bo′mə) [*irido-* + *coloboma*] congenital fissure or coloboma of the iris.

**iri·do·con·stric·tor** (ir″ĭ-do-kən-strik′tər) [*irido-* + *constrictor*] a muscle element or an agent that causes constriction of the pupil of the eye.

**iri·do·cor·neo·scle·rec·to·my** (ir″ĭ-do-kor″ne-o-sklə-rek′tə-me) surgical excision of a portion of the iris, cornea, and sclera for glaucoma.

**iri·do·cy·clec·to·my** (ir″ĭ-do-sə-klek′tə-me) [*irido-* + *cyclo-* + *ectomy*] surgical removal of a portion of the iris and of the ciliary body.

**iri·do·cy·cli·tis** (ir″ĭ-do-sə-kli′tis) [*irido-* + *cyclitis*] [MeSH: Iridocyclitis] inflammation of the iris and of the ciliary body; see also *anterior uveitis.*
**heterochromic i.,** unilateral low-grade iridocyclitis, leading to depigmentation of the iris of the affected eye; called also *heterochromic uveitis.*
**recurrent i.,** periodic ophthalmia.

**iri·do·cy·clo·cho·roi·di·tis** (ir″ĭ-do-si″klo-ko″roi-di′tis) [*irido-* + *cyclo-* + *choroiditis*] inflammation of the iris, ciliary body, and choroid coat.

**iri·do·cys·tec·to·my** (ir″ĭ-do-sis-tek′tə-me) [*irido-* + *cyst-* + *ectomy*] an operation to establish an artificial pupil in an eye in which the iris adheres to the residual lens capsule, accomplished by excising a portion of the iris and lens capsule through a corneal incision.

**iri·do·cyte** (i-rid′o-sīt) [*irido-* + *-cyte*] one of the cells in the scales of fishes that contains crystals of guanine capable of producing iridescence.

**iri·dod·e·sis** (ir″ĭ-dod′ə-sis) iridesis.

**iri·do·di·ag·no·sis** (ir″ĭ-do-di″əg-no′sis) [*irido-* + *diagnosis*] diagnosis of disease by the appearance of the iris, its color, markings, changes, etc.

**iri·do·di·al·y·sis** (ir″ĭ-do-di-al′ə-sis) [*irido-* + *dialysis*] separation or loosening of the iris from its root at the ciliary body, either from trauma or from surgical accident.

**iri·do·di·as·ta·sis** (ir″ĭ-do-di-as′tə-sis) [*irido-* + *diastasis*] a defect of the peripheral border of the iris, but not affecting the pupillary margin, producing the clinical appearance of more than one pupil.

**iri·do·di·la·tor** (ir″ĭ-do-di-la′tor) [*irido-* + *dilator*] 1. the dilator muscle of the pupil. 2. an agent that causes dilation of the pupil of the eye.

**iri·do·do·ne·sis** (ir″ĭ-do-do-ne′sis) [*irido-* + Gr. *donēsis* tremor] abnormal tremulousness of the iris on movements of the eye, occurring in subluxation of the lens, depriving the iris of this support.

**iri·do·ker·a·ti·tis** (ir″ĭ-do-ker″ə-ti′tis) [*irido-* + *keratitis*] inflammation of the iris and cornea.

**iri·do·ki·ne·sia** (ir″ĭ-do-kĭ-ne′zhə) iridokinesis.

**iri·do·ki·ne·sis** (ir″ĭ-do-kĭ-ne′sis) [*irido-* + *kinesis*] the contraction and expansion of the iris.

**iri·do·ki·net·ic** (ir″ĭ-do-kĭ-net′ik) pertaining to iridokinesis.

**iri·do·lep·tyn·sis** (ir″ĭ-do-ləp-tin′sis) [*iris* + Gr. *leptynsis* attenuation] thinning or atrophy of the iris.

**iri·dol·o·gy** (ir″ĭ-dol′ə-je) [*irido-* + *-logy*] the study of the iris, particularly of its color, markings, changes, etc., as associated with disease.

**iri·do·ma·la·cia** (ir″ĭ-do-mə-la′shə) [*irido-* + *malacia*] softening of the iris.

**iri·do·me·so·di·al·y·sis** (ir″ĭ-do-me″so-di-al′ə-sis) [*irido-* + *meso-* + *dialysis*] surgical loosening of adhesions around the inner edge of the iris.

**iri·do·mo·tor** (ir″ĭ-do-mo′tər) pertaining to movements of the iris; affecting contraction or dilation of the pupil of the eye.

**iri·don·cus** (ir″ĭ-dong′kəs) [*irid-* + Gr. *onkos* bulk] tumor or swelling of the iris.

**iri·do·pa·ral·y·sis** (ir″ĭ-do-pə-ral′ə-sis) iridoplegia.

**iri·dop·a·thy** (ir″ĭ-dop′ə-the) [*irido-* + *-pathy*] disease of the iris.

**iri·do·peri·pha·ki·tis** (ir″ĭ-do-per″e-fa-ki′tis) [*irido-* + *peri-* + *phakitis*] inflammation of the capsule of the crystalline lens.

**iri·do·ple·gia** (ir″ĭ-do-ple′jə) [*irido-* + *-plegia*] paralysis of the sphincter of the iris, with lack of contraction or dilation of the pupil.
**accommodation i.,** failure of the pupil to contract when an accommodative effort is made.
**complete i.,** paralysis of the sphincter of the pupil, with failure to react to any stimulus.
**reflex i.,** failure of the pupil to contract under the influence of light or when skin is stimulated.
**sympathetic i.,** failure of the pupil to dilate when the skin is stimulated.

**iri·dop·to·sis** (ir″ĭ-dop-to′sis) [*irido-* + *-ptosis*] prolapse of the iris.

**iri·do·pu·pil·lary** (ir″ĭ-do-pu′pĭ-lar″e) pertaining to the iris and the pupil.

**iri·do·rhex·is** (ir″ĭ-do-rek′sis) [*irido-* + *-rrhexis*] 1. rupture of the iris. 2. the tearing away of the iris.

**iri·dos·chi·sis** (ir″ĭ-dos′kĭ-sis) [*irido-* + *-schisis*] splitting of the mesodermal stroma of the iris into two layers so that the anterior section separates and disintegrates into fibrils, the unattached ends of which float freely in the anterior chamber.

**iri·do·scle·rot·o·my** (ir″ĭ-do-skle-rot′ə-me) [*irido-* + *sclero-* + *-tomy*] incision of the sclera and of the edge of the iris in treatment of glaucoma.

**iri·do·ste·re·sis** (ir″ĭ-do-stə-re′sis) [*irido-* + Gr. *sterēsis* loss] the absence or loss or removal of part or all of the iris.

**iri·dot·a·sis** (ir″ĭ-dot′ə-sis) [*irido-* + Gr. *tasis* stretching] the operation of stretching the iris in treatment of glaucoma.

**iri·dot·o·my** (ir″ĭ-dot′ə-me) [*irido-* + *-tomy*] incision of the iris, as in creating an artificial pupil.

**Iri·do·vi·ri·dae** (ir″ĭ-do-vir′ĭ-de) [MeSH: Iridoviridae] the iridoviruses: a family of DNA viruses having a virion 125–300 nm in diameter, consisting of a lipid envelope modified by protein subunits surrounding an icosahedral nucleocapsid. The genome consists of a single molecule of linear, double-stranded DNA (MW 100–250$\times10^6$, size 150–350 kbp). Viruses contain more than 20 structural proteins and are sensitive to ether, chloroform, deoxycholate, heat, and some disinfectants. Replication and assembly occur in the cytoplasm; virions are released by budding or cell destruction. Most species have a narrow host range; transmission may be horizontal or vertical. Most members are insect viruses (genera *Iridovirus, Chloriridovirus),* but some are pathogenic for fish *(Lymphocystivirus)* and frogs *(Ranavirus);* African swine fever virus was formerly assigned to this family.

**iri·do·vi·rus** (ir″ĭ-do-vi′rəs) [MeSH: Iridovirus] any virus belonging to the family Iridoviridae.

**iri·no·te·can hy·dro·chlo·ride** (i″rĭ-no-te′kan) a DNA topoisomerase inhibitor used as an antineoplastic in the treatment of colorectal carcinoma; administered by intravenous infusion.

**IRIS** [MeSH: Iris] International Research Information Service.

**Iris** (i′ris) [MeSH: Iris] a genus of perennial herbs of the family Iridaceae. The roots of several species, such as *I. florenti′na* L., *I. germa′nica* L., and *I. pal′lida* L., are the source of orris. *I. versi′color* L. (blue flag), a plant indigenous to the Americas, is the source of the medicinal substance *iris.* Some species, such as *I. missourien′sis* Nutt., have been reported to be poisonous to livestock due to an irritant principle in the leaves and rootstalks that causes gastroenteritis.

**iris** (i′ris) pl. *i′rides* [Gr. "rainbow, halo"] [MeSH: Iris] 1. [TA] the circular pigmented membrane behind the cornea, perforated by the pupil; the most anterior portion of the vascular tunic of the eye, it is made up of a flat bar of circular muscular fibers surrounding the pupil, a thin layer of smooth muscle fibers by which the pupil is dilated, thus regulating the amount of light entering the eye, and posteriorly two layers of pigmented epithelial cells. 2. the rhizome of *Iris versicolor,* formerly used as a purgative, emetic, and diuretic.

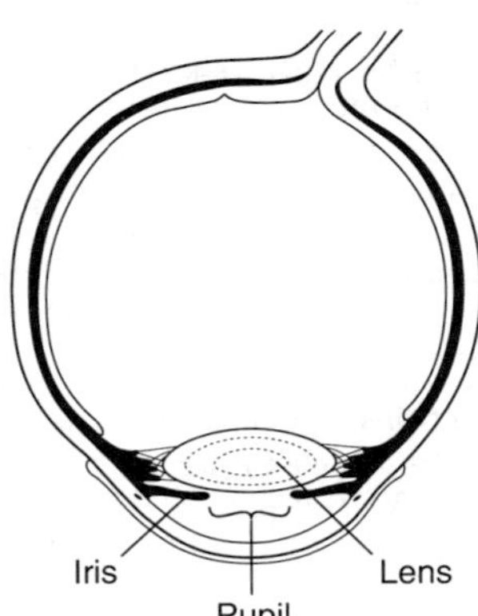


**i. bombé,** a condition in which the iris is bowed forward by the collection of aqueous humor between the iris and lens in total posterior synechia.
**detached i.,** iridodialysis.
**tremulous i.,** iridodonesis.
**umbrella i.,** i. bombé.

**iri·sin** (i′rĭ-sin) a fructose polysaccharide from *Iris pseudo-acorus;* it is an aperient and cholagogue.

**iris·op·sia** (i″ris-op′se-ə) [Gr. *iris* rainbow + *-opsia*] a visual defect in which objects appear surrounded by rings of colored light.

**iri·tic** (i-rit′ik) pertaining to or of the nature of iritis.

**iri·tis** (i-ri′tis) [*iris* + *-itis*] [MeSH: Iritis] inflammation of the iris, usually marked by pain, congestion in the ciliary region, photophobia, contraction of the pupil, and discoloration of the iris.
**i. catamenia′lis,** iritis recurring before each menstrual period.
**diabetic i.,** iritis marked by the deposit of glycogen in diabetic patients.
**follicular i.,** iritis marked by multiple small nodules the size of a pinhead.
**gouty i.,** painful iritis occurring in gouty patients; uratic iritis.
**i. papulo′sa,** iritis with papules in the iris; usually syphilitic.
**plastic i.,** a variety in which the exudate consists of fibrinous matter which forms new tissue.
**purulent i.,** iritis in which the exudate is purulent.
**serous i.,** iritis in which the exudate consists of serum.
**spongy i.,** iritis with a fibrinous exudate, forming a spongy mass in the anterior chamber.
**sympathetic i.,** iritis occurring in sympathetic ophthalmoplegia.
**uratic i.,** gouty i.

**iri·to·ec·to·my** (ir″ĭ-to-ek′tə-me) [*iris* + *-ectomy*] surgical excision of iritic deposits of after-cataract, together with iridectomy, to form an artificial pupil.

**irit·o·my** (i-rit′ə-me) iridotomy.

**ir·i·um** (ir′e-əm) sodium lauryl sulfate.

**IRMA** immunoradiometric assay.

**iron** (i′ərn) [A. S. *iren;* L. *ferrum*] [MeSH: Iron] a metallic element found in certain minerals, in nearly all soils, and in mineral waters: atomic number 26; atomic weight, 55.847; specific gravity, 7.85–7.88; symbol, Fe. Iron is an essential constituent of hemoglobin, cytochrome, and other components of respiratory enzyme systems; its chief functions are in the transport of oxygen to tissues (in hemoglobin) and in cellular oxidation mechanisms. Dietary sources include muscle meats, eggs, grains, and certain vegetables and fruits. Depletion of iron stores may result in iron-deficiency anemia (q.v.). Excessive consumption of iron causes iron poisoning (see under *poisoning*). See also *ferric* and *ferrous.*
**i. 55,** a radioactive isotope of iron, atomic mass 55, having a half-life of 2.73 years and decaying by electron capture.
**i. 59,** a radioactive isotope of iron, atomic mass 59, having a half-life of 44.50 days and emitting beta particles (0.273, 0.475 MeV) and gamma rays (1.095, 1.292 MeV); it is used in ferrokinetic studies to determine the rate at which iron is cleared from the plasma and incorporated in red cells.
**i. acetate,** a compound, $Fe(C_2H_3O_2)_3$, used as an astringent.
**i. and ammonium sulfate,** see *ferric ammonium sulfate,* under *ammonium.*
**available i.,** that portion of iron in the food which can be separated from the total iron content by digestive processes.
**i. chloride,** either of the binary compounds $FeCl_2$ or $FeCl_3$.
**i. choline citrate,** ferrocholinate.
**i. citrate,** ferric citrate.
**i. gluconate,** ferrous gluconate.
**i. protosulfate,** ferrous sulfate.
**Quevenne's i.,** reduced i.
**reduced i.,** finely powdered metallic iron obtained by precipitation with hydrogen from a solution of any soluble salt of iron.
**i. sorbitex,** a hematinic preparation consisting of a sterile colloidal solution of a complex of trivalent iron, sorbitol, and citric acid, stabilized with dextrin and sorbitol.
**i. sulfate,** ferrous sulfate.

**irot·o·my** (i-rot′o-me) iridotomy.

**ir·ra·di·ate** (ĭ-ra′de-āt) to apply ionizing radiation for therapeutic or diagnostic purposes; see *radiotherapy.*

**ir·ra·di·a·tion** (ĭ-ra″de-a′shən) [*ir-* + *radiation*] 1. radiotherapy. 2. the dispersion of nervous impulse beyond the normal path of conduction. 3. the application of rays, such as ultraviolet rays, to a substance to increase its vitamin efficiency and shelf life. 4. a phenomenon in which, owing to the difference in the illumination of the field of vision, objects appear to be much larger than they really are.
**extended field i.,** irradiation of an extended field (q.v.) in the treatment of malignant lymphomas; called also *extended field radiotherapy.*
**external beam i.,** see under *radiotherapy.*
**hemibody i.,** external beam radiotherapy involving exposure of half the body; called also *hemibody radiotherapy.*
**interstitial i.,** see under *radiotherapy.*
**inverted Y field i.,** irradiation of an inverted Y field (q.v.) in the treatment of malignant lymphoma; called also *inverted Y field radiotherapy.*
**involved field i.,** irradiation of only the involved field (q.v.) in the treatment of malignant lymphoma; called also *involved field radiotherapy.*
**mantle field i.,** irradiation of a mantle field (q.v.) as a treatment for malignant lymphoma; called also *mantle field radiotherapy.*
**radical i.,** external beam i.

**total body i.**, TBI; external beam radiotherapy involving exposure of the entire body; called also *whole-body i.* or *radiotherapy.*
**total lymphoid i. (TLI)**, irradiation of all the lymph node–bearing areas of the body, including the spleen, the thymus, and Waldeyer's tonsillar ring; used in the treatment of Hodgkin's disease and sometimes to induce immunosuppression prior to transplantation.
**ultraviolet blood i.**, a treatment involving removal of blood from a patient, exposing it to ultraviolet light, and returning it to the patient's circulation; abbreviated UBI.
**whole-body i.**, total body i.

**ir·re·duc·i·ble** (ir″e-do͞os′ĭ-bəl) not susceptible to reduction, as a fracture, dislocation, or chemical substance.

**ir·reg·u·lar** (ĭ-reg′u-lər) [*ir-* + *regular*] not in conformity with the rule of nature; not recurring at regular intervals.

**ir·reg·u·lar·i·ty** (ĭ-reg″u-lar′ĭ-te) the quality of not conforming with the rule of nature, or of not occurring at regular intervals.
**i. of pulse,** arrhythmia.

**ir·re·ver·si·ble** (ir″e-vər′sĭ-bəl) incapable of being reversed.

**ir·ri·gate** (ir′ĭ-gāt) to wash out, as a wound; lavage.

**ir·ri·ga·tion** (ir″ĭ-ga′shən) [L. *irrigatio; in* into + *rigare* to carry water] [MeSH: Irrigation] 1. washing by a stream of water or other fluid; see also *lavage.* 2. a liquid used for irrigation.
**acetic acid i.** [USP], a sterile aqueous solution of glacial acetic acid; used to irrigate the bladder in the treatment of urinary infections with cystitis.
**glycine i.** [USP], a sterile solution of glycine in water for injection, used to irrigate the bladder during urogenital surgical procedures.
**Ringer's i.** [USP], a sterile solution containing, in each 100 mL, 820–900 mg of sodium chloride, 25–35 mg of potassium chloride, and 30–36 mg of calcium chloride in water for injection; used as a topical physiological salt solution. Called also *Ringer's mixture* or *solution.*
**sodium chloride i.** [USP], a sterile aqueous solution of sodium chloride; used to irrigate wounds and body cavities and as an enema to flush the colon and promote evacuation. Called also *sodium chloride solution.*

**ir·ri·ga·tor** (ir′ĭ-ga″tər) [L. "waterer"] an apparatus for performing irrigation.

**ir·ri·go·ra·di·os·co·py** (ir″ĭ-go-ra″de-os′ko-pe) fluoroscopy of the intestines during the introduction of a contrast enema.

**ir·ri·gos·co·py** (ir″ĭ-gos′ko-pe) irrigoradioscopy.

**ir·ri·ta·bil·i·ty** (ir″ĭ-tə-bil′ĭ-te) [L. *irritabilitas,* from *irritare* to tease] 1. the quality or state of being irritable. 2. abnormal responsiveness to slight stimuli.
**i. of the bladder,** a condition in which the presence of a small amount of urine in the bladder produces a desire to urinate.
**chemical i.**, responsiveness to a chemical stimulus; see *chemoreceptor.*
**electric i.**, responsiveness of nerve or muscle to the stimulus of an electric current passed through it.
**mechanical i.**, responsiveness to a mechanical stimulus; see *mechanoreceptor.*
**muscular i.**, the normal contractile quality of muscular tissue.
**myotatic i.**, the power of a muscle to contract in response to stretching.
**nervous i.**, 1. the ability of a nerve to transmit impulses. 2. morbid excitability of the nervous system.
**specific i.**, see under *law.*
**i. of the stomach,** a condition of the stomach in which vomiting is caused by normal amounts of digestible food.
**tactile i.**, a condition of cells that repels foreign particles; negative chemotaxis.

**ir·ri·ta·ble** (ir′ĭ-tə-bəl) [L. *irritare* to tease] 1. capable of reacting to a stimulus. 2. abnormally sensitive to a stimulus. 3. prone to excessive anger, annoyance, or impatience.

**ir·ri·tant** (ir′ĭ-tənt) [L. *irritans*] 1. giving rise to irritation. 2. an agent that produces irritation.
**primary i.**, an agent that produces irritation, especially of the skin, on the first exposure to it.

**ir·ri·ta·tion** (ir″ĭ-ta′shən) [L. *irritatio*] 1. the act of stimulating. 2. a state of overexcitation and undue sensitivity.
**direct i.**, irritation due to direct stimulation of a part.
**functional i.**, that which is attended with functional derangement without organic lesion; also overexcitability due to excessive functional activity.

**ir·ri·ta·tive** (ir′ĭ-ta″tiv) dependent on or caused by irritation.

**Ir·u·kand·ji sting** (ir″u-kan′je) [*Irukandji,* an aboriginal tribe in the vicinity of Cairns, Queensland, Australia] see under *syndrome.*

**IRV** inspiratory reserve volume.

**IS** intercostal space.

**ISA** intrinsic sympathomimetic activity.

**I·saacs' syndrome** (i′zəks) [H. *Isaacs,* American neurologist, 20th century] see under *syndrome.*

**I·saacs-Mer·tens syndrome** (i′zəks mer′tenz) [H. *Isaacs;* H.G. *Mertens,* German neurologist, 20th century] see under *syndrome.*

**isa·tin** (i′sə-tin) [MeSH: Isatin] a crystalline compound, $C_8H_5O_2N$, in the form of yellowish red crystals, soluble in alcohol and ether, slightly soluble in water; used as a reagent.

**is·aux·e·sis** (is″awk-se′sis) [*iso-* + *auxesis*] growth of a part or parts at the same rate as the growth of the whole.

**is·che·mia** (is-ke′me-ə) [*isch-* + *emia*] [MeSH: Ischemia] deficiency of blood in a part, usually due to functional constriction or actual obstruction of a blood vessel.
**brachiocephalic i.**, Takayasu's arteritis.
**cerebral i.**, see under *infarction.*
**hypoxia-i.**, see under H.
**myocardial i.**, deficiency of blood supply to the heart muscle, due to obstruction or constriction of the coronary arteries.
**nonocclusive mesenteric i.**, ischemia of the intestine caused by a low rate of blood flow rather than by occlusion; risk of intestinal gangrene is high because the subtlety of clinical and radiological signs often delays diagnosis. See also *mesenteric infarction.*
**i. re′tinae,** anemia of the retina; it may occur after profuse hemorrhage in another part of the body or result from arterial embolism or poison.
**silent i.**, cardiac ischemia without pain or other symptoms.
**subendocardial i.**, deficiency of blood supply to the myocardium adjacent to the endocardium.
**vertebrobasilar i.**, see under *insufficiency.*

**is·che·mic** (is-kem′ik) pertaining to, or affected with, ischemia.

**is·che·sis** (is-ke′sis) [Gr. *ischein* to suppress] retention or suppression of a discharge.

**is·chia** (is′ke-ə) [L.] plural of *ischium.*

**is·chi·a·del·phus** (is″ke-ə-del′fəs) [*ischio-* + *-adelphus*] ischiodidymus.

**is·chi·ad·ic** (is″ke-ad′ik) 1. sciatic. 2. ischial.

**is·chi·al** (is′ke-əl) pertaining to the os ischii (ischium); ischiadic; ischiatic; sciatic.

**is·chi·al·gia** (is″ke-al′jə) [*ischio-* + *-algia*] pain in the os ischii (ischium); ischiodynia.

**is·chi·at·ic** (is″ke-at′ik) [L. *ischiaticus*] 1. sciatic. 2. ischial.

**is·chi·ec·to·my** (is″ke-ek′tə-me) surgical removal or excision of the ischium.

**ischi(o)-** [Gr. *ischion* hip] a combining form denoting relationship to the os ischii (ischium), or to the hip.

**is·chio·anal** (is″ke-o-a′nəl) [*ischio-* + *anus*] pertaining to the ischium and anus.

**is·chio·bul·bar** (is″ke-o-bul′bər) [*ischio-* + *bulbar*] pertaining to the os ischii (ischium) and the bulb of the urethra.

**is·chio·cap·su·lar** (is″ke-o-kap′su-lər) [*ischio-* + *capsular*] pertaining to the ischium and the capsular ligament of the hip joint.

**is·chio·cele** (is′ke-o-sēl″) [*ischio-* + Gr. *kēlē* hernia] sciatic hernia.

**is·chio·coc·cyg·e·al** (is″ke-o-kok-sij′e-əl) pertaining to the ischium and coccyx.

**is·chio·coc·cyg·e·us** (is″ke-o-kok-sij′e-əs) [*ischio-* + *coccygeus*] 1. musculus coccygeus. 2. the posterior part of the levator ani muscle.

**is·chio·did·y·mus** (is″ke-o-did′ĭ-məs) [*ischio-* + *-didymus*] symmetrical conjoined twins united at the pelvis.

**is·chio·dym·ia** (is″ke-o-dim′e-ə) [*ischio-* + Gr. *didymos* twin + *-ia*] the condition of symmetrical conjoined twins united at the pelvis.

**is·chio·dyn·ia** (is″ke-o-din′e-ə) [*ischio-* + *-odynia*] ischialgia.

**is·chio·fem·o·ral** (is″ke-o-fem′o-rəl) [*ischio-* + *femur*] pertaining to the ischium and femur.

**is·chio·fib·u·lar** (is″ke-o-fib′u-lər) pertaining to the ischium and the fibula.

**is·chi·om·e·lus** (is″ke-om′ə-ləs) [*ischio-* + Gr. *melos* limb] a fetus with an extra limb attached at the base of the vertebral column.

**is·chio·ni·tis** (is″ke-o-ni′tis) inflammation of the tuberosity of the ischium.

**is·chio·pa·gia** (is″ke-o-pa′jə) the condition exhibited by an ischiopagus.

**is·chi·op·a·gus** (is-ke-op′ə-gəs) [*ischio-* + *-pagus*] conjoined twins fused at the ischia, the axes of the two bodies extending in a straight line but in opposite directions; according to the number of lower limbs shared, classified as *bipus, tripus,* and *tetrapus.*

**is·chi·op·a·gy** (is″ke-op′ə-je) ischiopagia.

**is·chio·pu·bic** (is″ke-o-pu′bik) pertaining to the ischium and pubis.

**is·chio·rec·tal** (is″ke-o-rek′təl) pertaining to the ischium and rectum; see also *ischioanal.*

**is·chio·sa·cral** (is″ke-o-sa′krəl) pertaining to the ischium and sacrum.

**is·chio·tho·ra·cop·a·gus** (is″ke-o-tho″rə-kop′ə-gəs) iliothoracopagus.

**is·chio·vag·i·nal** (is″ke-o-vaj′ĭ-nəl) pertaining to the ischium and vagina.

**is·chio·ver·te·bral** (is″ke-o-ver′tə-brəl) pertaining to the ischium and the vertebral column.

**is·chi·um** (is′ke-əm) pl. *is′chia* [L.; Gr. *ischion* hip] [MeSH: Ischium] TA alternative for *os ischii.* See illustration at *skeleton.*

**isch(o)-** [Gr. *ischein* to suppress] a combining form denoting relationship to suppression or deficiency.

**is·cho·gy·ria** (is″ko-ji′re-ə) [*ischo-* + *gyrus*] a condition in which the cerebral convolutions have a jagged appearance, as in bulbar sclerosis.

**isch·uret·ic** (is″ku-ret′ik) pertaining to ischuria.

**isch·uria** (is-ku′re-ə) [*ischo-* + *-uria*] suppression or retention of the urine.
**i. paradox′a,** a condition in which the bladder is overdistended with urine, although the patient continues to urinate.
**i. spas′tica,** ischuria caused by spasm of the sphincter urinae.

**ISCP** International Society of Comparative Pathology.

**-ise** see *-ize.*

**is·ei·co·nia** (i″si-ko′ne-ə) isoiconia.

**is·ei·con·ic** (i″si-kon′ik) isoiconic.

**is·ei·ko·nia** (i″si-ko′ne-ə) isoiconia.

**is·eth·i·o·nate** (is″ə-thi′o-nāt) USAN contraction for 2-hydroxyethanesulfonate.

**is·eth·i·o·nic ac·id** (is″eth-i-on′ik) [MeSH: Isethionic Acid] trivial name for 2-hydroxyethanesulfonic acid; used in detergents and surfactants and in synthesis.

**ISGE** International Society of Gastro-Enterology.

**ISH** International Society of Hematology.

**Ish·i·ha·ra's plates, test** (ish″e-hah′rahz) [Shinobu *Ishihara,* Japanese ophthalmologist, 1879–1963] see under *plate* and *test.*

**isin·glass** (i′sin-glas) a form of gelatin prepared from the swimming bladders of the Russian sturgeon, *Acipenser huso*; used as an adhesive and clarifying agent. Called also *ichthyocolla.*

**is·land** (i′lənd) a cluster of cells or an isolated piece of tissue. See also *islet.*
**blood i's,** aggregations of mesenchyme cells in the angioblast of the early embryo, as in the wall of the yolk sac; they subsequently develop into vascular endothelium and blood corpuscles.
**bone i.,** a benign focus of mature cortical bone appearing within trabecular bone on a radiograph.
**i's of Calleja,** discrete collections of pyramidal and polymorphic cells in the caudal part of the anterior perforated substance (olfactory tubercle). Called also *olfactory i's* and *islets of Calleja.*
**cartilage i's,** see *intrachondrial bone,* under *bone.*
**i's of Langerhans,** see under *islet.*
**olfactory i's,** i's of Calleja.
**i's of pancreas,** pancreatic islets.
**Pander's i's,** reddish yellow cords of corpuscular matter in the splanchnopleure of the embryo which develop into blood and blood vessels.
**i. of Reil,** insula.

**is·let** (i′lət) a cluster of cells or an isolated piece of tissue; see also *island.*
**blood i's,** see under *island.*
**Calleja's i's,** see under *island.*
**i's of Langerhans, pancreatic i's,** irregular microscopic structures scattered throughout the pancreas and comprising its endocrine part (the *endocrine pancreas*). In humans, they are composed of at least four types of cells: the *alpha cells,* which secrete glucagon; the *beta cells,* which are the most abundant and secrete insulin; the *delta cells,* which secrete somatostatin; and the *PP cells,* which secrete pancreatic polypeptide. Degeneration of the beta cells, whose secretion (insulin) is important in carbohydrate metabolism, is the major cause of type I diabetes mellitus. Called also *islands of Langerhans* or *of pancreas.*
**Walthard's i's,** microscopic inclusions of the germinal epithelium of the ovary, found either in contact with the serosal covering or just below it; they have been implicated in the development of Brenner tumors. Called also *Walthard's cell rests* or *inclusions.*

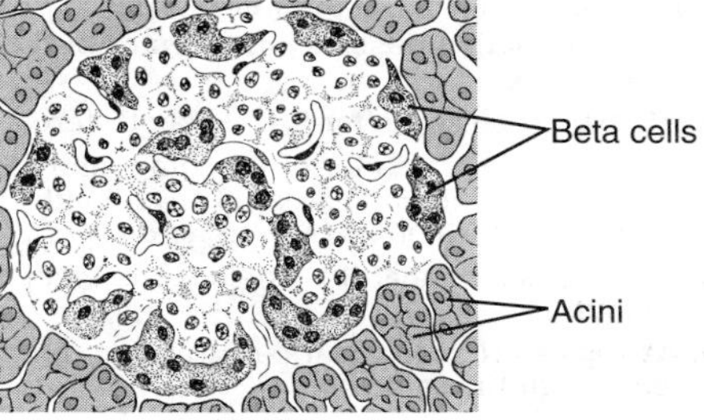


Pancreatic islet, surrounded by acini, stained with aldehyde-fuchsin to highlight the insulin-secreting beta cells.

**ISM** International Society of Microbiologists.

**-ism** [Gr. *-ismos* noun-forming suffix] a word termination denoting *(a)* a state or condition, particularly a disease state resulting from a specific cause, e.g., alcoholism, *(b)* a process, *(c)* the result of an action, or *(d)* a doctrine or principle, e.g., determinism.

**Is·me·lin** (is′mə-lin) trademark for a preparation of guanethidine monosulfate.

**ISO** International Standards Organization.

**iso-** [Gr. *isos* equal] a prefix or combining form meaning equal, alike, the same, or uniform. In immunology, it indicates *from* a genetically identical individual (as an isograft) or existing in alternate forms in the same species (as an isoantigen). In chemistry it denotes a structural isomer; used in trivial names of alkanes to indicate a one-carbon branch next to the end of the chain, e.g., isohexane is 2-methylpentane; an isoalkyl radical has its free valence at the end of the chain opposite the branch, i.e., isohexyl is 4-methylpentyl.

**iso·adre·no·cor·ti·cism** (i″so-ə-dre″no-kor′tĭ-siz-əm) euadrenocorticism.

**iso·ag·glu·ti·na·tion** (i″so-ə-gloo″tĭ-na′shən) agglutination of cells from members of a species by agglutinins originating in genetically dissimilar members of the same species.

**iso·ag·glu·ti·nin** (i″so-ə-gloo′tĭ-nin) an agglutinin from members of a species that agglutinates cells of genetically different members of the same species.

**iso·al·lele** (i″so-ə-lēl′) [*iso-* + *allele*] an allelic gene that is considered as being normal but can be distinguished from another allele by its differing phenotypic expression when in combination with a mutant allele.

**iso·al·le·lism** (i″so-ə-le′liz-əm) [*iso-* + *allele*] the presence of more than one kind of normal allele at a locus.

**iso·al·lox·a·zine** (i″so-ə-lok′sə-zēn) a tricyclic compound comprising a pyrazine ring flanked by a benzene ring and uracil; it is the parent compound of riboflavin and other flavins.

**iso·am·yl·eth·yl·bar·bi·tu·ric acid** (i″so-am″əl-eth″əl-bahr″bĭ-tu′rik) amobarbital.

**iso·am·yl ni·trite** (i″so-am′əl ni′trīt) amyl nitrite.

**iso·an·dro·ster·one** (i″so-an-dro′stər-ōn) epiandrosterone.

**iso·an·ti·body** (i-so-an′tĭ-bod″e) an antibody produced by one individual that reacts with antigens (isoantigens) of another individual of the same species; called also *alloantibody.*

**iso·an·ti·gen** (i″so-an′tĭ-jən) an antigen that induces an immune response when transferred (as by blood transfusion or tissue graft) to a genetically dissimilar individual of the same species.

**iso·bar** (i′so-bahr) [*iso-* + Gr. *baros* weight] one of two or more chemical species with the same atomic weight but different atomic numbers.

**iso·bar·ic** (i″so-bar′ik) [*iso-* + *bar-* + *-ic*] 1. having equal or constant pressure or weight across space or time; see also under *solution.* 2. pertaining to an isobar or isobars.

**iso·bu·caine hy·dro·chlo·ride** (i″so-bu′kān) a local anesthetic, used in combination with epinephrine in dentistry.

**iso·bu·tane** (i″so-bu′tān) a branched chain configuration of butane, $CH_3CH(CH_3)_2$; cf. *normal butane* and see illustration at *isomerism.*

**iso·ca·lo·ric** (i″so-kə-lor′ik) containing or providing the same number of calories; equicaloric.

**iso·car·box·a·zid** (i″so-kahr-bok′sə-zid) [MeSH: Isocarboxazid] a monoamine oxidase inhibitor, used as an antidepressant, administered orally.

**iso·cel·lu·lar** (i″so-sel′u-lər) [*iso-* + *cellular*] composed of cells of the same kind and size.

**iso·cen·ter** (i'so-sen'tər) a point at which there is a maximum or minimum of the radiation dose, i.e., the center of the surrounding isodose curves.

**iso·cho·les·ter·in** (i"so-kə-les'tər-in) isocholesterol.

**iso·cho·les·ter·ol** (i"so-kə-les'tər-ol) a compound found with cholesterol in wool; apparently a mixture of $C_{30}$ trimethyl cholestanes; a component of lanolin alcohols (see under *alcohol*).

**iso·chro·mat·ic** (i"so-kro-mat'ik) [*iso-* + *chromatic*] of the same color throughout.

**iso·chro·mat·o·phil** (i"so-kro-mat'o-fil) [*iso-* + *chromato-* + *-phil*] staining equally with the same dye.

**iso·chro·mo·some** (i"so-kro'mə-sōm) [*iso-* + *chromosome*] [MeSH: Isochromosomes] an abnormal chromosome having a median centromere and two identical arms, probably formed by the transverse, rather than the normal longitudinal separation of the centromere of the replicating chromosome. See Plate 1.

**isoch·ro·nal** (i-sok'rə-nəl) isochronous.

**iso·chro·nia** (i-so-kro'ne-ə) isochronism.

**iso·chron·ic** (i"so-kron'ik) isochronous.

**isoch·ro·nism** (i"sə-kro'niz-əm) [*iso-* + *chrono-* + *-ism*] a condition of correspondence between processes with respect to their time, rate, or frequency.

**isoch·ro·nous** (i-sok'rə-nəs) [*iso-* + *chrono-* + *-ous*] performed in equal times; said of motions and vibrations occurring at the same time and being equal in duration.

**isoch·ro·ous** (i-sok'ro-əs) [*iso-* + Gr. *chroa* color] isochromatic.

**iso·ci·trate** (i"so-sĭ'trāt) a fully dissociated (ionized) salt of isocitric acid.

**iso·ci·trate de·hy·dro·gen·ase (NAD⁺) (NAD⁺)** (i"so-sĭ'trāt de-hi'drə-jən-ās) [MeSH: Isocitrate Dehydrogenase] a mitochondrial enzyme that catalyzes the oxidative decarboxylation of isocitrate to form α-ketoglutarate, using $NAD^+$ as an electron acceptor; the reaction is the key rate-limiting step of the tricarboxylic acid cycle. The enzyme requires $Mg^{2+}$ or $Mn^{2+}$ and is activated by ADP, citrate, and $Ca^{2+}$ and inhibited by NADH, NADPH, and ATP.

**iso·ci·trate de·hy·dro·gen·ase (NADP⁺) (NADP⁺)** (i"so-sĭ'trāt de-hi'drə-jən-ās) [MeSH: Isocitrate Dehydrogenase] an enzyme of the oxidoreductase class that catalyzes the oxidative decarboxylation of isocitrate to form α-ketoglutarate, using $NADP^+$ as an electron acceptor. The enzyme exists as two isozymes, one cytoplasmic and one mitochondrial, requires $Mg^{2+}$ or $Mn^{2+}$, and occurs in all tissues. The reaction serves to maintain the level of reducing equivalents within the cell.

**iso·cit·ric ac·id** (i"so-sit'rik) a structural isomer of citric acid, that is an intermediate in the citric (tricarboxylic) acid cycle (q.v.).

**iso·co·na·zole** (i"so-ko'nə-zōl) an imidazole antifungal and antibacterial used in the treatment of vaginal candidiasis and of dermatophytes; administered topically or in pessary form.

**iso·co·ria** (i"so-kor'e-ə) [*iso-* + *cor-* + *-ia*] equality in size of the two pupils.

**iso·cor·tex** (i"so-kor'teks) [*iso-* + *cortex*] [TA] the neocortex as opposed to the allocortex, so called because histologically it consists of six layers and is much more uniform than the allocortex. Called also *homotypical cortex.*

**Iso·crin** (i'so-krin) trademark for a preparation of oxyphenisatin acetate.

**iso·cy·a·nate** (i"so-si'ə-nāt) the radical —NCO, often occurring as diisocyanate (q.v.). See also under *asthma.*

**iso·cy·a·nide** (i"so-si'ə-nīd) one of a class of organic compounds isomeric with the cyanide compounds, containing the N≡C group; and characterized by a disagreeable odor; called also *isonitrile.*

**iso·cy·clic** (i"so-sik'lik) [*iso-* + Gr. *kyklos* circle] homocyclic.

**iso·cy·tol·y·sin** (i"so-si-tol'ə-sin) [*iso-* + *cytolysin*] a cytolysin that acts on the cells of animals of the same species as that from which it is derived.

**iso·cy·to·sis** (i"so-si-to'sis) [*iso-* + *-cyte* + *-osis*] equality of the size of cells, especially red blood corpuscles.

**iso·dac·tyl·ism** (i-so-dak'təl-iz-əm) [*iso-* + *dactyl-* + *-ism*] a condition in which the fingers are of relatively even length.

**iso·des·mo·sine** (i"so-des'mo-sēn) [MeSH: Isodesmosine] one of two unusual amino acids found in elastin, the other being desmosine.

**iso·di·a·met·ric** (i"so-di"ə-met'rik) [*iso-* + *dia-* + *metron* measure] having the same diameter in all directions.

**iso·don·tic** (i"so-don'tik) [*iso-* + *odontic*] having all the teeth of the same size and shape.

**iso·dose** (i'so-dōs) a radiation dose of equal intensity to more than one body area; see also under *curve.*

**iso·dy·nam·ic** (i"so-di-nam'ik) [*iso-* + *dynamic*] exhibiting equal force or power.

**iso·dy·nam·o·gen·ic** (i"so-di-nam"o-jen'ik) [*iso-* + *dynamogenic*] producing equal force or power.

**iso·ef·fect** (i"so-ə-fekt') an effect midway between two reference points; see under *line.*

**iso·elec·tric** (i"so-e-lek'trik) [*iso-* + *electric*] showing no variation in electric potential.

**iso·en·er·get·ic** (i"so-en"ər-jet'ik) exhibiting equal energy.

**iso·en·zyme** (i"so-en'zīm) isozyme.
**Regan i.**, an isoenzyme of alkaline phosphatase, similar or identical to placental alkaline phosphatase and originating in a variety of tumors, particularly those of the lung. It is occasionally detectable in normal serum.

**iso·eth·a·rine** (i-so-eth'ə-rēn) [MeSH: Isoetharine] an adrenergic, used as a bronchodilator in the treatment of bronchial asthma and bronchospasm, administered by inhalation.
**i. hydrochloride** [USP], the hydrochloride salt of isoetharine, having the same actions and uses as the base.
**i. mesylate** [USP], the mesylate salt of isoetharine, having the same actions and uses as the base.

**iso·eu·gen·ol** (i"so-u'jən-ol) an aromatic compound used in fragrances and a significant cause of fragrance sensitization, characterized by contact dermatitis.

**iso·feb·ri·fu·gine** (i"so-feb"rĭ-fu'jēn) an antimalarial alkaloid found in the plant *Dichroa febrifuga* (ch'ang shan).

**iso·flu·rane** (i"so-floo'rān) [MeSH: Isoflurane] a potent inhalational anesthetic, an isomer of enflurane with similar properties, used for induction and maintenance of general anesthesia.

**iso·flu·ro·phate** (i"so-flo͝or'o-fāt) [USP] [MeSH: Isoflurophate] nonproprietary drug name for diisopropyl flurophosphate (DFP), a potent irreversible anticholinesterase agent; used topically to produce miosis, decrease intraocular pressure, and potentiate accommodation in treatment of open-angle glaucoma and accommodative convergent strabismus.

**iso·form** (i'so-form") any of a group of two or more different proteins that are produced by different genes and are specific to different tissues but have the same function and a similar sequence.

**isog·a·me** (i-sog'ə-me) isogamy.

**iso·gam·ete** (i"so-gam'ēt) [*iso-* + *gamete*] a gamete of the same size as the gamete with which it unites; cf. *heterogamete* and *homogamete.*

**iso·ga·met·ic** (i"so-gə-met'ik) characterized by the production of gametes of the same size.

**iso·gam·e·ty** (i"so-gam'ə-te) production by an individual of one sex of gametes identical with respect to the sex chromosome.

**isog·a·mous** (i-sog'ə-məs) pertaining to isogamy.

**isog·a·my** (i-sog'ə-me) [*iso-* + Gr. *gamos* marriage] reproduction resulting from the union of two cells (gametes) that are identical in size and structure, as occurs in protozoa. See also *heterogamy* and *homogamy.*

**iso·ge·ne·ic** (i"so-jə-ne'ik) syngeneic.

**iso·ge·ner·ic** (i"so-jə-ner'ik) of the same kind; pertaining to or obtained from individuals of the same genus.

**iso·gen·e·sis** (i"so-jen'ə-sis) [*iso-* + *-genesis*] similarity in the processes of development.

**iso·gen·ic** (i"so-jen'ik) syngeneic.

**isog·e·nous** (i-soj'ə-nəs) developed from the same cell.

**iso·graft** (i'so-graft) syngraft.

**iso·hem·ag·glu·ti·na·tion** (i"so-hem"ə-gloo"tĭ-na'shən) agglutination of erythrocytes caused by a hemagglutinin from another individual of the same species.

**iso·hem·ag·glu·ti·nin** (i"so-hem"ə-gloo'tĭ-nin) a hemagglutinin that agglutinates the erythrocytes of other individuals of the same species.

**iso·he·mol·y·sin** (i"so-he-mol'ə-sin) [*iso-* + *hemolysin*] a hemolysin that acts on the blood of animals of the same species as that from which it is derived.

**iso·he·mol·y·sis** (i"so-he-mol'ə-sis) hemolysis of the blood corpuscles of an animal by the lysins in serum from another animal of the same species.

**iso·he·mo·lyt·ic** (i"so-he"mo-lit'ik) pertaining to or characterized by isohemolysis.

**iso·hy·dric** (i″so-hi′drik) maintaining a steady pH (concentration of hydrogen ions); see *buffer.*

**iso·ico·nia** (i″so-i-ko′ne-ə) [*iso-* + *icon* + *-ia*] a condition in which the image of an object is the same in both eyes.

**iso·icon·ic** (i″so-i-kon′ik) marked by isoiconia.

**iso·im·mu·ni·za·tion** (i″so-im″u-nĭ-za′shən) development of antibodies against an antigen derived from a genetically dissimilar individual of the same species; see also *isoantigen.*
**Rh i.,** development of antibodies against Rh antigens, the antigen involved in almost all cases being the $Rh_0$ antigen (D antigen). Rh isoimmunization of Rh-negative women may occur after transfusion of Rh-positive blood or during pregnancy with an Rh-positive fetus, when the mother is exposed to fetal blood during delivery, amniocentesis, miscarriage, or abortion, and may result in the development of erythroblastosis fetalis in any subsequent pregnancy with an Rh-positive fetus. See also *$Rh_0$ (D) immune globulin,* under *globulin.*

**iso·in·tense** (i″so-in-tens′) having the same intensity as some other object.

**iso·ki·net·ic** (i″so-kə-net′ik) said of a type of exercise that maintains constant torque and tension as muscles shorten or lengthen.

**iso·late** (i′so-lāt) 1. to separate from other persons, materials, or objects. 2. in microbiology, to obtain from a source such as a clinical specimen a pure strain that may have been part of a mixed primary culture. 3. a population that has been obtained by isolation (such as bacteria or other cells obtained in pure culture), or a group of individuals prevented by geographic, ecologic, or social barriers from interbreeding with others of their kind, and thus differentiated by the accumulation of new characteristics.

**iso·la·tion** (i″so-la′shən) 1. the process of isolating, or the state of being isolated. 2. the physiologic separation of a part, as by tissue culture or by interposition of inert material. 3. the extraction and purification of a chemical substance of unknown structure from a natural source. 4. the separation of infected individuals from those uninfected for the period of communicability of a particular disease; cf. *quarantine* (def. 1). 5. the successive propagation of a growth of microorganisms until a pure culture is obtained. 6. in psychiatry, a defense mechanism in which emotions are separated from the ideas, impulses, or memories to which they usually connect, so that the idea or impulse enters consciousness detached from its unacceptable feeling. Called also *isolation of affect.*

**iso·la·tor** (i″so-la′tər) anything that isolates.
**surgical i.,** a large, clear, plastic bag with man-sized pockets that is attached to the patient's body during surgical procedures to prevent contamination by infective agents; the pockets, in which the nurses and surgeons stand, have plastic helmets, earphones and microphones for communication, and closed sleeves leading into the bag through which the surgeons work.

**iso·lec·i·thal** (i″so-les′ĭ-thəl) [*iso-* + *-lecithal*] having yolk evenly distributed throughout the cytoplasm of the ovum.

**iso·leu·cine** (i″so-loo′sēn) [MeSH: Isoleucine] an essential amino acid, α-amino-β-methylvaleric acid, produced by the hydrolysis of fibrin and other proteins; necessary for optimal growth in infants and for nitrogen equilibrium in human adults. Symbols Ile and I. See table at *amino acid.*

**iso·leu·cyl** (i″so-loo′səl) the acyl radical of isoleucine.

**iso·leu·ko·ag·glu·ti·nin** (i″so-loo″ko-ə-gloo′tĭ-nin) a leukocyte agglutinin.

**isol·o·gous** (i-sol′ə-gəs) characterized by an identical genotype; see *isograft.*

**iso·ly·ser·gic ac·id** (i″so-li-sur′jik) one of the main cleavage products of the alkaline hydrolysis of the alkaloids characteristic of ergot, and the parent compound of the ergotinine group of alkaloids.

**isol·y·sin** (i-sol′ə-sin) a lysin that acts on the cells of animals of the same species as that from which it is derived.

**isol·y·sis** (i-sol′ə-sis) lysis of cells by isolysins.

**iso·ly·tic** (i″so-lit′ik) pertaining to isolysis.

**iso·mal·tase** (i″so-mawl′tās) oligo-1,6-glucosidase; see *α-dextrinase.*

**iso·mal·tose** (i″so-mawl′tōs) [MeSH: Isomaltose] a reducing disaccharide isomeric with maltose, differing in having α-(1,6) rather than α-(1,4) glycosidic linkage; it occurs at branch points of polymers such as glycogen and amylopectin.

**iso·mas·ti·gote** (i″so-mas′tĭ-gōt) [*iso-* + *mastigote*] having two equal and similar flagella at the anterior pole.

**iso·mer** (i′so-mər) [*iso-* + Gr. *meros* part] any compound exhibiting, or capable of exhibiting, isomerism. An isomer may be structural or stereochemical; see *isomerism.*

**isom·er·ase** (i-som′ər-ās) [EC 5] a class of enzymes that catalyze geometric or structural changes within a molecule to form a single product. The reactions do not involve a net change in the concentration of compounds other than the substrate and the product. The class includes epimerases, isomerases, mutases, and racemases.

**iso·mer·ic** (i″so-mer′ik) pertaining to or exhibiting isomerism.

**isom·er·ide** (i-som′ər-īd) isomer.

**isom·e·rism** (i-som′ə-riz-əm) [*iso-* + Gr. *meros* part] [MeSH: Isomerism] the relationship that exists between two or more different chemical compounds that have the same molecular formula; it is divided into two broad classes: *structural i.* and *stereoisomerism* (q.v.).
**chain i.,** a type of structural isomerism in which the compounds differ in regard to the linkages in the basic chain of carbon atoms; see illustration.
***cis-trans* i.,** geometric i.
**configurational i.,** stereoisomerism.
**conformational i.,** the relationship between stereoisomers that differ only by rotations about single bonds (conformers).
**constitutional i.,** the relationship between two or more isomers that have different structures (the same atoms linked in different ways), in contrast to stereoisomerism in which the isomers have the same structure but different configurations (the same linkages but different spatial arrangements). Called also *structural i.*
**functional group i.,** a type of structural isomerism dependent upon the presence of different functional groups, such compounds being of distinct chemical types, e.g., ethyl alcohol, $C_2H_5OH$, and dimethyl ether, $CH_3OCH_3$.
**geometric i.,** an old division of stereoisomerism that contains isomers that differ in the arrangement of substituents of a rigid structure, such as double-bonded carbon atoms or a ring. The *cis* isomer has two referenced groups on the same side of the ring or double bond; the *trans* isomer on opposite sides. Geometric isomers are thus diastereomers. Called also *cis-trans i.*
**optical i.,** an old division of stereoisomerism that contains isomers that differ in the arrangement of substituents at one or more asymmetric carbon atoms; thus some but not necessarily all are optically active, e.g., *d-*, *l-*, and *meso-*tartaric acid. Some optical isomers are enantiomers (the *d* and *l* forms); some are diastereomers (the *d* and *meso* forms).
**position i.,** a type of structural isomerism in which the position occupied by an atom or group differs with reference to the same fundamental carbon chain; for example, *n*-propyl chloride, $CH_3CH_2CH_2Cl$, and isopropyl chloride, $CH_3CHClCH_3$.
**spatial i., stereochemical i.,** stereoisomerism.
**structural i.,** constitutional i.
**substitution i.,** position i.

**isom·er·iza·tion** (i-som″ər-ĭ-za′shən) the process whereby any isomer, whether structural or stereochemical, is converted into another, usually requiring special conditions of temperature, pressure, or catalysts.

**iso·meth·ep·tene mu·cate** (i″so-mə-thep′tēn mu′kāt) [USP] an indirect-acting sympathomimetic amine that reduces the stimuli that lead to vascular headaches by constricting dilated carotid and cerebral vessels, used in combination with dichloralphenazone and acetaminophen in the treatment of migraine and tension headache.

**iso·met·ric** (i″so-met′rik) [*iso-* + Gr. *metron* measure] 1. maintaining the same measurements; of equal dimensions. 2. maintaining uniform length; see under *contraction* and *exercise.*

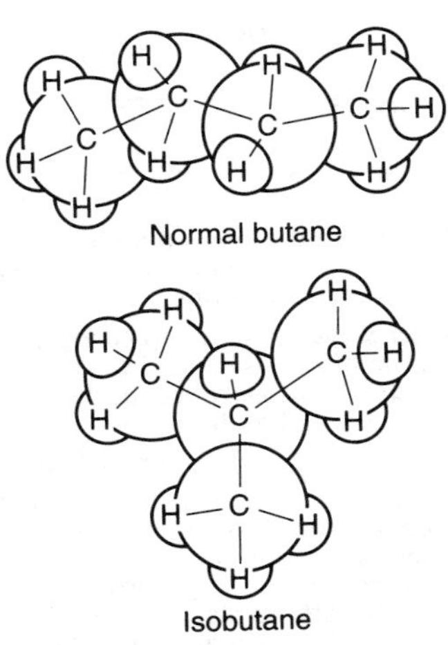


Chain isomerism.

**iso·me·tro·pia** (i″so-mə-tro′pe-ə) [*iso-* + Gr. *metron* measure + *-opia*] equality in the refraction of the two eyes.

**isom·e·try** (i-som′ə-tre) equality of dimension.

**iso·mor·phic** (i″so-mor′fik) isomorphous.

**iso·mor·phism** (i″so-mor′fiz-əm) the quality of being isomorphous.

**iso·mor·phous** (i″so-mor′fəs) [*iso-* + *-morphous*] having the same form. In genetics, denoting genotypes of polyploid organisms which produce similar gametes even though containing genes in different combinations on homologous chromosomes.

**iso·mus·ca·rine** (i″so-mus′kə-rēn) a basic substance formed by oxidizing choline; it is isomeric with muscarine, but has different physiologic properties.

**iso·naph·thol** (i″so-naf′thol) betanaphthol.

**iso·neph·ro·tox·in** (i″so-nef″ro-tok′sin) [*iso-* + *nephrotoxin*] a nephrotoxin which acts on cells of the animals of the same species from which it is derived.

**iso·ni·a·zid** (i″so-ni′ə-zid) [USP] [MeSH: Isoniazid] an antibacterial, used as a tuberculostatic, administered orally and intramuscularly.

**iso·nic·o·tin·o·yl·hy·dra·zine** (i″so-nik″o-tin″o-əl-hi′drə-zēn) isoniazid.

**iso·nic·o·tin·yl·hy·dra·zine** (i″so-nik″o-tin″əl-hi′drə-zēn) isoniazid.

**iso·ni·trile** (i″so-ni′trīl) isocyanide.

**iso·on·cot·ic** (i″so-on-kot′ik) having the same oncotic pressure.

**iso·os·mot·ic** (i″so-oz-mot′ik) isosmotic.

**Iso·paque** (i″so-pāk′) trademark for preparations of metrizoate sodium.

**Iso·par·or·chis tri·sim·i·li·tu·bis** (i″so-pər-or′kis tri-sim″ĭ-lĭ-too′bis) a fluke, commonly parasitic in the air bladder of fish in India and China and sometimes found in man.

**isop·a·thy** (i-sop′ə-the) [*iso-* + *-pathy*] the treatment of disease by means of products of the disease or with material from the organ affected, e.g., smallpox by giving minute doses of variolous matter, disease of the liver by giving extract of liver, etc.

**isoph·a·gy** (i-sof′ə-je) [*iso-* + *-phagy*] autolysis.

**iso·pho·ria** (i″so-for′e-ə) [*iso-* + *phoria*] equality in the tension of the vertical muscles of each eye; absence of hyperphoria and of hypophoria.

**Iso·phrin** (i′so-frin) trademark for a preparation of phenylephrine hydrochloride.

**iso·pia** (i-so′pe-ə) [*iso-* + *-opia*] equality of vision in the two eyes.

**iso·plas·tic** (i″so-plas′tik) [*iso-* + *plastic*] taken from another animal of the same species or from another inbred strain within the same species; said of tissue transplants or grafts.

**iso·pre·cip·i·tin** (i″so-pre-sip′ĭ-tin) a precipitin that is active against antigens of animals of the same species (but of dissimilar genetic makeup) as the animal in which it is formed.

**iso·preg·ne·none** (i″so-preg′nə-nōn) dydrogesterone.

**iso·pren·a·line** (i″so-pren′ə-lēn) isoproterenol.

**iso·prene** (i′so-prēn) an unsaturated branched chain five-carbon hydrocarbon that is the molecular unit of isoprenoid compounds.

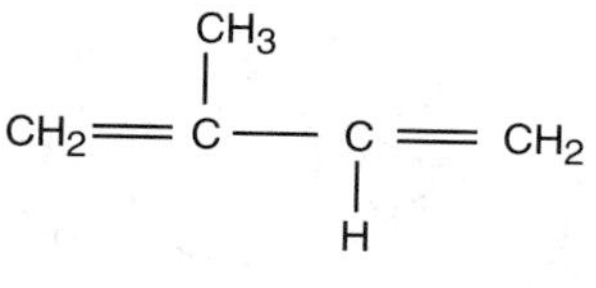

$$\begin{array}{ccccccc} & & CH_3 & & & & \\ & & | & & & & \\ CH_2 & = & C & - & C & = & CH_2 \\ & & & & | & & \\ & & & & H & & \end{array}$$

**iso·pre·noid** (i″so-pre′noid) any compound biosynthesized from or containing isoprene units, including terpenes, carotenoids, fat soluble vitamins, ubiquinone, rubber, and some steroids.

**iso·pro·pa·mide io·dide** (i″so-pro′pə-mīd) [USP] a long-acting quaternary anticholinergic, used in the treatment of peptic ulcer and other gastrointestinal disorders marked by hyperacidity and hypermotility, administered orally.

**iso·pro·pa·nol** (i″so-pro′pə-nol) isopropyl alcohol.

**iso·pro·pyl** (i″so-pro′pəl) the univalent radical, $(CH_3)_2CH$—.
**i. alcohol, i. rubbing alcohol,** see under *alcohol.*
**i. meprobamate,** carisoprodol.
**i. myristate** [NF], a compound of isopropyl alcohol and saturated high molecular weight fatty acids, principally myristic acid, occurring as a clear, oily liquid; used as an emollient in pharmaceutical preparations.

**iso·pro·pyl·ar·te·re·nol** (i″so-pro″pəl-ahr″tə-re′nol) isoproterenol.

**iso·pro·te·re·nol** (i″so-pro-ter′ə-nol) [MeSH: Isoproterenol] a synthetic adrenergic, derived from norepinephrine, having powerful bronchodilator and cardiac stimulant actions.
**i. hydrochloride** [USP], the hydrochloride salt of isoproterenol, used chiefly as a bronchodilator in the treatment of bronchial asthma, administered by oral inhalation, sublingually, and parenterally. It may also be used in the management of shock, treatment and prevention of cardiac standstill and arrhythmias, and treatment of bronchospasm during anesthesia.
**i. sulfate** [USP], the sulfate salt of isoproterenol, having the same actions and uses as the hydrochloride salt; administered by oral inhalation.

**isop·ter** (i-sop′tər) [*iso-* + Gr. *optēr* observer] a line depicting the area in the field of vision in which the visual acuity is the same.

**Isop·tin** (īs-op′tin) trademark for preparations of verapamil hydrochloride.

**Isop·to-Car·pine** (i-sop″to-kahr′pēn) trademark for a preparation of pilocarpine hydrochloride.

**iso·pyk·nic** (i″so-pik′nik) [*iso-* + *pykn-* + *-ic*] of equal density or thickness; see under *centrifugation.*

**iso·pyk·no·sis** (i″so-pik-no′sis) [*iso-* + *pyknosis*] the state of being of uniform density; applied especially to a state of uniform condensation observed in comparison of different chromosomes, or of different regions of the same chromosome.

**iso·pyk·not·ic** (i″so-pik-not′ik) pertaining to or characterized by isopyknosis.

**Isor·dil** (i′sor-dil) trademark for preparations of isosorbide dinitrate.

**iso·ri·bo·fla·vin** (i″so-ri′bo-fla″vin) an isomer of riboflavin that acts as an antimetabolite to riboflavin and can cause riboflavin deficiency in laboratory animals.

**isor·rhea** (i″so-re′ə) [*iso-* + *-rrhea*] the maintenance of a relatively constant body fluid volume and composition; water and solute intake is balanced by an equivalent output of the substances from the body.

**isor·rhe·ic** (i″so-re′ik) pertaining to or characterized by isorrhea.

**iso·ru·bin** (i″so-roo′bin) new fuchsin.

**iso·scope** (i′so-skōp) [*iso-* + *-scope*] an apparatus for observing the changes of position of the horizontal and vertical lines in the movements of the eyeball.

**iso·sen·si·ti·za·tion** (i″so-sen″sĭ-tĭ-za′shən) allosensitization.

**iso·se·rine** (i″so-se′rēn) a compound, isomeric with serine.

**iso·sex·u·al** (i″so-sek′shoo-əl) [*iso-* + *sexual*] pertaining to or characteristic of the same sex.

**isos·mot·ic** (i″sos-mot′ik) having the same osmotic pressure.

**isos·mo·tic·i·ty** (i″sos-mo-tis′ĭ-te) the state or quality of being isosmotic.

**iso·sor·bide** (i″so-sor′bīd) [MeSH: Isosorbide] a bicyclic ether derivative of glucitol; used as an osmotic diuretic to reduce intraocular pressure.
**i. dinitrate,** the dinitric acid ester of isosorbide, having coronary and peripheral vasodilating properties; used in the treatment of coronary insufficiency and angina pectoris, administered sublingually and orally.

**Isos·po·ra** (i-sos′pə-rə) [*iso-* + *spore*] [MeSH: Isospora] a genus of coccidian protozoa (suborder Eimeriina, order Eucoccidiida) characterized by the presence of two sporocysts in each oocyst and four sporozoites in each sporocyst; found in birds, amphibians, reptiles, and mammals, including humans.
**I. bel′li,** a species that parasitizes the small intestine of man; infection (coccidiosis) is usually asymptomatic but may result in a severe watery mucous diarrhea.
**I. bige′mina,** *Cystoisospora burrowsi.*
**I. fe′lis,** *Cystisospora felis.*
**I. ho′minis,** see *Sarcocystis bovihominis* and *S. suihominis.*
**I. laca′zei,** a species causing intestinal coccidiosis in passerine birds.
**I. rivol′ta,** *Cystisospora rivolta.*
**I. su′is,** a species that may cause coccidiosis in swine.

**iso·spore** (i′so-spor) [*iso-* + *spore*] 1. an isogamete of organisms that reproduce by spores. 2. an asexual spore produced by a homosporous organism.

**isos·po·ri·a·sis** (i-sos″pə-ri′ə-sis) infection with *Isospora.* See *coccidiosis.*

**isos·po·rous** (i-sos′pə-rəs) having isospores.

**iso·stere** (i′so-stēr) a compound resembling another compound in electron arrangement but differing in chemical structure.

**isos·then·uria** (i″sos-thə-nu′re-ə) [*iso-* + *sthen-* + *-uria*] the excretion of urine with the same osmolality as that of plasma.

**iso·the·ba·ine** (i″so-the′ba-in) an alkaloid from *Papaver orientalis.*

**iso·ther·a·py** (i″so-ther′ə-pe) [*iso-* + *therapy*] isopathy.

**iso·ther·mo·gno·sis** (i″so-ther″mo-no′sis) [*iso-* + *therm-* + *gnōsis* recognition] a dysesthesia in which pain, cold, and heat stimuli are all perceived as heat.

**iso·thi·a·zine hy·dro·chlo·ride** (i″so-thi′ə-zēn) ethopropazine hydrochloride.

**iso·thi·o·cy·a·nate** (i″so-thi″o-si′ə-nāt) an ester of isothiocyanic acid, R—N═C═S.
**allyl i.**, see under *allyl.*

**iso·thi·o·cy·an·ic ac·id** (i″so-thi″o-si-an′ik) the molecular species H—N═C═S, which occurs in equilibrium with thiocyanic acid.

**iso·throm·bo·ag·glu·ti·nin** (i″so-throm″bo-ə-gloo′tĭ-nin) a platelet isoagglutinin.

**iso·tone** (i′so-tōn) one of several nuclides having the same number of neutrons, but differing in the number of protons in their nuclei.

**iso·to·nia** (i″so-to′ne-ə) [*iso-* + *ton-* + *-ia*] 1. a condition of equal tone, tension, or activity. 2. equality of osmotic pressure between two elements of a solution or between two different solutions.

**iso·ton·ic** (i″so-ton′ik) [*iso-* + *tonic*] 1. denoting a solution in which body cells can be bathed without a net flow of water across the semipermeable cell membrane. 2. denoting a solution having the same tonicity as some other solution with which it is compared, such as physiologic salt solution and the blood serum. 3. maintaining uniform tonus; see under *contraction* and *exercise.*

**iso·to·nic·i·ty** (i″so-to-nis′ĭ-te) the quality of being isotonic.

**iso·tope** (i′so-tōp) [*iso-* + *-tope*] a chemical element having the same atomic number as another (i.e., the same number of nuclear protons) but possessing a different atomic mass (i.e., a different number of nuclear neutrons).
**radioactive i.**, radioisotope.
**stable i.**, an isotope that does not transmute into another element with emission of corpuscular or electromagnetic radiations.

**iso·to·pol·o·gy** (i″so-to-pol′ə-je) the scientific study of isotopes, and of their uses and applications.

**iso·tox·ic** (i″so-tok′sik) pertaining to an isotoxin.

**iso·tox·in** (i″so-tok′sin) [*iso-* +*toxin*] a toxin that is poisonous to other animals of the same species.

**iso·trans·plant** (i″so-trans′plant) [*iso-* + *transplant*] isograft.

**iso·trans·plan·ta·tion** (i″so-trans″plan-ta′shən) the transplanting of an isograft.

**iso·tret·i·noin** (i″so-tret′ĭ-noin) [MeSH: Isotretinoin] 13-*cis*-retinoic acid, used systemically for treatment of severe cystic and conglobulate acne; it inhibits the secretion of sebum and alters the lipid composition of the skin surface.

**Isot·ri·cha** (i-sot′rĭ-kə) [*iso-* + Gr. *thrix, trichos* hair] a genus of ciliate protozoa (suborder Trichostomatina, order Trichostomatida) found in the stomachs of ungulates, and characterized by the presence of an apical cytostome and by dense longitudinal rows of cilia over the entire body surface. Species include *I. prostoma* and *I. intestinalis.*

**iso·tri·mor·phism** (i″so-tri-mor′fiz-əm) [*iso-* + *tri-* + *morph-* + *-ism*] isomorphism between the three forms of two trimorphous substances.

**iso·tri·mor·phous** (i″so-tri-mor′fəs) pertaining to or characterized by isotrimorphism.

**iso·tron** (i′so-tron) an apparatus for separating isotopes electromagnetically.

**iso·trop·ic** (i″so-trop′ik) [*iso-* + *-tropic*] 1. similar in all directions with respect to a property, as in a cubic crystal or a piece of glass. 2. being singly refractive.

**isot·ro·py** (i-sot′ro-pe) the quality or condition of being isotropic.

**iso·type** (i′so-tīp) an immunoglobulin heavy or light chain class or subclass characterized by antigenic determinants (isotypic markers) in the constant region. Every normal individual expresses all of the isotypes of its species. Cf. *allotype* and *idiotype.*

**iso·typ·ic** (i″so-tip′ik) pertaining to isotypes.

**iso·typ·i·cal** (i″so-tip′ĭ-kəl) [*iso-* + *typical*] of the same type.

**iso·ure·tin** (i″so-u-re′tin) formamidoxim, a compound isomeric with urea.

**iso·va·ler·ic ac·id** (i″so-və-ler′ik) a carboxylic acid occurring in excess in the plasma and urine in isovalericacidemia.

**iso·va·ler·ic·ac·i·de·mia** (i″so-və-ler″ik-as″ĭ-de′me-ə) an autosomal recessive aminoacidopathy due to deficiency of isovaleryl-CoA dehydrogenase, with elevated plasma isovaleric acid and urinary isovaleric acid and isovalerylglycine, causing a characteristic odor of sweaty feet. Clinical signs include severe acidosis and ketosis, lethargy, convulsions, pernicious vomiting, thrombocytopenia, neutropenia, and pancytopenia. Two clinical forms, possibly allelic, exist: the *acute neonatal form* leads rapidly to coma and death; the *chronic intermittent form* is milder and usually of later onset, with acute episodic attacks and variable psychomotor dysfunction.

**iso·va·ler·yl** (i″so-və-ler′əl) the radical of isovaleric acid; the thioester formed with coenzyme A, isovaleryl CoA, is an intermediate in the catabolism of leucine.

**iso·val·er·yl-CoA de·hy·dro·gen·ase** (i″so-və-ler′əl-ko-a′ de-hi′dro-jən-ās) [EC 1.3.99.10] an enzyme of the oxidoreductase class that catalyzes the dehydrogenation of isovaleryl CoA to 3-methylcrotonyl CoA, using ubiquinone as an electron acceptor. The reaction is a step in the use of leucine as a fuel. Deficiency of the enzyme, an autosomal recessive trait, results in isovalericacidemia.

**iso·va·ler·yl·gly·cine** (i″so-və-ler″əl-gli′sēn) a conjugate of isovaleric acid and the amide group of glycine; high levels are formed and excreted in the urine in isovalericacidemia.

**iso·vo·lu·mic** (i″so-və-loo′mik) [*iso-* + *volume*] maintaining the same volume.

**Iso·vue** (i′so-vu) trademark for preparations of iopamidol.

**isox·su·prine hy·dro·chlo·ride** (i-sok′su-prēn) [USP] an adrenergic, used as a vasodilator in the treatment of cerebral vascular insufficiency and of peripheral vascular diseases such as arteriosclerosis obliterans, thromboangiitis obliterans, and Raynaud's disease. It is administered orally or intramuscularly.

**iso·zyme** (i′so-zīm) one of various structurally related forms of an enzyme, each having the same mechanism but with differing chemical, physical, or immunological characteristics. For example, lactate dehydrogenase, a tetramer, exists as five isozymes arising from different combinations of its two kinds of subunits. Called also *isoenzyme.*

**is·rad·i·pine** (is-rad′ĭ-pēn) [USP] [MeSH: Isradipine] a calcium channel blocking agent with actions similar to those of nifedipine, used alone or with a thiazide diuretic for the treatment of hypertension; administered orally.

**is·sue** (ish′oo) a discharge of pus, blood, or other matter; a suppurating lesion emitting such a discharge.

**isth·mec·to·my** (is-mek′tə-me) [*isthmus* + *-ectomy*] excision of an isthmus, particularly the isthmus of the thyroid gland affected with goiter.

**isth·mi** (is′mi) [L.] plural of *isthmus.*

**isth·mi·an** (is′me-ən) isthmic.

**isth·mic** (is-mik) pertaining to an isthmus.

**isth·mi·tis** (is-mi′tis) inflammation of the isthmus of the fauces.

**isth·mo·pa·ral·y·sis** (is″mo-pə-ral′ə-sis) isthmoplegia.

**isth·mo·ple·gia** (is″mo-ple′jə) [*isthmus* + *-plegia*] paralysis of the isthmus of the fauces.

**isth·mus** (is′məs) pl. *isth′mi* [L., from Gr *isthmos*] [TA] a narrow connection between two larger bodies or parts.
**anterior i. of fauces,** i. faucium.
**i. aor′tae** [TA], **aortic i.,** isthmus of aorta: a narrowed portion of the aorta, especially noticeable in the fetus, at the point where the ductus arteriosus is attached.
**i. of auditory tube,** i. tubae auditivae.
**i. cartila′ginis auricula′ris** [TA], **i. cartila′ginis au′ris,** isthmus of auricular cartilage: a bridge of cartilage connecting the cartilage of the external acoustic meatus with the main part of the cartilage of the auricle of the external ear.
**i. of cingulate gyrus,** i. gyri cinguli.
**i. of eustachian tube,** i. tubae auditivae.
**i. of external auditory meatus,** a narrowing in the osseous part of the meatus about 2 cm from the internal end of the concha.
**i. of fallopian tube,** i. tubae uterinae.
**i. fau′cium** [TA], isthmus of fauces: the constricted aperture between the cavity of the mouth and the pharynx.
**i. glan′dulae thyroi′deae** [TA], isthmus of thyroid gland: the band of tissue connecting the lobes of the thyroid gland.
**i. gy′ri cingula′tus, i. gy′ri cin′guli** [TA], isthmus of cingulate gyrus: the constricted portion of the cingulate gyrus, connecting with the parahippocampal gyrus in the region of the splenium of the corpus callosum.
**i. gy′ri fornica′ti,** i. gyri cinguli.

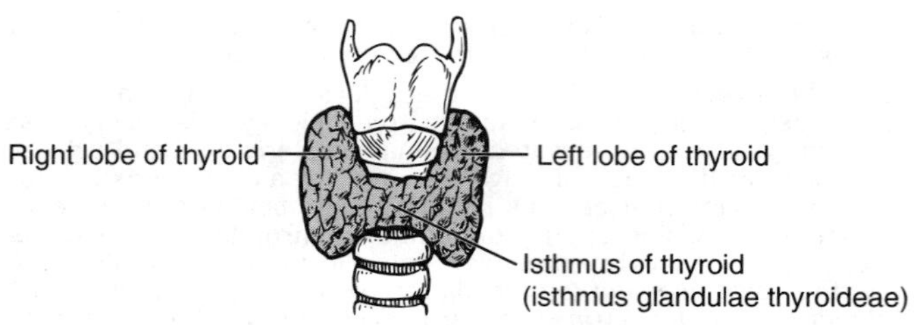


Isthmus glandulae thyroideae (isthmus of thyroid gland) connecting the two lobes.

**Haller's i.**, fretum halleri.
**i. of His**, i. rhombencephali.
**i. of limbic lobe**, i. gyri cinguli.
**oropharyngeal i., pharyngo-oral i.**, i. faucium.
**i. prosta'tae** [TA], isthmus of prostate: the commissure on the base of the prostate, between the right and the left lateral lobe.
**i. rhombence'phali** [TA], isthmus of rhombencephalon: a narrow segment of the brain in the fetus, forming the plane of separation between the rhombencephalon and the cerebrum; called also *i. of His*.
**i. of thyroid gland**, i. glandulae thyroideae.
**i. tu'bae auditi'vae** [TA], isthmus of auditory tube: the narrowest part of the auditory tube, at the junction of the pars ossea and the pars cartilaginea of the tube. Called also *i. tubae auditoriae* [TA alternative].
**i. tu'bae audito'riae**, TA alternative for *i. tubae auditivae*.
**i. tu'bae uteri'nae** [TA], isthmus of uterine tube: the narrow part of the uterine tube at its junction with the uterus.
**i. ure'thrae**, isthmus of urethra: a constricted part of the urethra, at the junction of the cavernous with the membranous urethra.
**i. u'teri** [TA], isthmus of uterus: the constricted part of the uterus between the cervix and the body.
**i. of Vieussens**, limbus fossae ovalis.

**ISU** International Society of Urology.

**Isu·prel** (i'su-prəl) trademark for a preparation of isoproterenol.

**isu·ria** (i-su're-ə) [*iso-* + *-uria*] excretion of urine at a uniform rate.

**ITA** International Tuberculosis Association.

**itch** (ich) 1. a skin sensation marked by pruritus. 2. any of various skin disorders in which pruritus is a characteristic. 3. scabies.
**Aujeszky's i.**, pseudorabies.
**bakers' i.**, any of several inflammatory dermatoses of the hands seen in bakers, especially chronic tinea unguium.
**barbers' i.**, 1. sycosis barbae. 2. tinea barbae. 3. pseudofolliculitis.
**barn i.**, sarcoptic mange.
**chorioptic i.**, see under *mange*.
**clam diggers' i.**, cercarial dermatitis.
**copra i.**, a dermatitis affecting those who unload coconuts, caused by the mite *Tyrophagus castellani*.
**Cuban i.**, old name for *variola minor*.
**dew i.**, ground i.
**dhobie i.**, 1. dhobie mark i. 2. tinea cruris
**dhobie mark i.**, allergic contact dermatitis seen in laundry workers (dhobies) in India, caused by oleoresins in a type of marking fluid, bhilawanol oil.
**grain i.**, a self-limited, wheal-like, pruritic eruption caused by the mite *Pyemotes ventricosus*, which parasitizes the larvae of various insects that infest straw, grain, and other plants, and affecting those coming in contact with host plants. Called also *acarodermatitis urticarioides, prairie i.*, and *straw i.*
**grocers' i.**, a vesicular dermatitis in grocers, caused by mites such as *Glycyphagus domesticus*, found in stored hides, dried fruits, and grain, or *Tyrophagus castellani* or *T. longior*, found in copra and cheese.
**ground i.**, an itching eruption caused by the entrance into the skin of hookworm larvae, such as *Necator americanus* or *Ancylostoma duodenale*. See also *hookworm disease*, under *disease*. Called also *uncinarial dermatitis*.
**jock i.**, tinea cruris.
**mad i.**, pseudorabies.
**prairie i.**, grain i.
**Queensland i.**, *Culicoides* hypersensitivity.
**seven-year i.**, scabies.
**straw i.**, grain i.
**sweet i.**, *Culicoides* hypersensitivity.
**swimmers' i.**, cercarial dermatitis.
**winter i.**, xerotic eczema.

**itch·ing** (ich'ing) pruritus.

**-ite**[1] [Gr. *-itēs* noun and adjective suffix] a suffix denoting a mineral or a rock, or a part of a body or of an organ.

**-ite**[2] [F., alteration of *-ate*] in chemistry, a suffix denoting a salt or ester of an acid with a name ending in *-ous*, e.g., phosphite. Cf. *-ate*[2].

**iter** (i'tər) [L.] a way or tubular passage.
**i. ad infundi'bulum**, the passage from the third ventricle of the brain to the infundibulum.
**i. chor'dae ante'rius**, an opening in the anterior part of the middle ear for exit of the chorda tympani nerve from the tympanic cavity; called also *Huguier's canal*.
**i. chor'dae poste'rius**, apertura tympanica canaliculi chordae tympani.
**i. den'tium**, the area through which a permanent tooth makes its appearance.
**i. e ter'tio ad quar'tum ventric'ulum**, aqueductus cerebri.
**i. of Sylvius**, aqueductus mesencephali.

**iter·al** (i'tər-əl) pertaining to an iter.

**it·ero·par·i·ty** (it″ər-o-par'ĭ-te) [L. *iterare* to repeat + *parity*[1]] the state, in an individual organism, of reproducing repeatedly, or more than once in a lifetime.

**it·er·op·a·rous** (it″ər-op'ə-rəs) reproducing more than once in a lifetime.

**-ites** [Gr. *-itēs*, a masculine adjectival termination agreeing with *hydrōps* dropsy (understood)—e.g., tympanites, the windy dropsy] a word termination indicating edema of the part denoted by the word stem to which it is attached.

**ith·y·cy·phos** (ith″e-si'fōs) ithyokyphosis.

**ith·y·lor·do·sis** (ith″e-lor-do'sis) [Gr. *ithys* straight + *lordosis*] lordosis without any lateral curvature.

**ith·yo·ky·pho·sis** (ith″e-o-ki-fo'sis) [Gr. *ithys* straight + *kyphosis*] backward projection of the spinal column.

**-itides** plural of *-itis*.

**-itis** pl. *-it'ides* [*-itis*, a feminine adjectival termination agreeing with Gr. *nosos* disease (understood)] a word termination denoting inflammation of the part indicated by the word stem to which it is attached.

**Ito nevus** (e'to) [Minor *Ito*, Japanese dermatologist, 20th century] see under *nevus*.

**ITP** idiopathic thrombocytopenic purpura; inosine triphosphate.

**it·ra·co·na·zole** (it″rə-ko'nə-zōl) [MeSH: Itraconazole] a synthetic triazole compound that inhibits the synthesis of ergosterol, a component of the fungal cell membrane, used as an antifungal agent; administered orally.

**IU** international unit.

**IUCD** intrauterine contraceptive device.

**IUD** intrauterine contraceptive device.

**IUGR** intrauterine growth restriction.

**IV** intravenously (by intravenous injection).

**IVC** inferior vena cava.

**Ive·mark's syndrome** (e'və-mahrks) [Björn Isaac Isaacson *Ivemark*, Swedish pathologist, born 1925] see under *syndrome*.

**iver·mec·tin** (i-vər-mek'tin) [MeSH: Ivermectin] a semisynthetic member of the avermectin group, most commonly used as an antiparasitic in domestic animals; it is sometimes used to treat human onchocerciasis.

**IVF** in vitro fertilization.

**IVIC syndrome** (e'vēk) [*I*nstituto *V*enezolano de *I*nvestigaciones *C*ientíficas, where it was first observed in 1980] see under *syndrome*.

**Ivo·mec** (i'vo-mek) trademark for a preparation of ivermectin.

**ivo·ry** (i'vo-re) 1. the bonelike substance (modified dentin) of the tusks of elephants and other large mammals. Called also *ebur*. 2. dentinum.

**IVP** intravenous pyelogram; intravenous pyelography.

**IVRT** isovolumic relaxation time.

**IVS** interventricular septum (of heart).

**Ivy loop wiring** (i've) [Robert Henry *Ivy*, English-born American maxillofacial surgeon, 1881–1974] see under *wiring*.

**Ivy's test (method)** (i'vēz) [Andrew Conway *Ivy*, American physiologist, 1893–1978] see under *test*.

**Iwan·off's (Iwan·ow's) cysts** (e-vahn'ofs) [Wladimir P. *Iwanoff* (or *Iwanow*), Russian ophthalmologist, late 19th century] see *Blessig's cysts*, under *cyst*.

**Ix·o·des** (iks-o'dēz) [Gr. *ixōdes* like bird-lime] [MeSH: Ixodes] a genus of ticks of the family Ixodidae; they are parasitic on humans and other animals.
**I. bicor'nis,** *Rhipicentor bicornis.*
**I. canisu'ga,** the British dog tick, a species commonly infesting dogs in Britain; also found in Western Europe and North America.
**I. cavipal'pus,** an African tick that infests monkeys and children.
**I. dam'mini,** former name for a species (the eastern deer tick) now included in *I. scapularis.*
**I. fre'quens,** a species that infests cattle, horses, and man in Japan.
**I. hexa'gonus,** a species that infests wild and domestic carnivores in Europe and Africa.
**I. holocy'clus,** a type particularly found on marsupials, but causing a tick paralysis in young cattle in southeastern Australia, and possibly acting as a vector of Queensland tick typhus.
**I. paci'ficus,** a common deer and cattle tick of California, which may bite humans; it is the vector of Lyme disease in the western United States and is a possible vector of tularemia.
**I. persulca'tus,** the taiga tick, sometimes a vector of Russian spring-summer encephalitis in humans and of louping ill in sheep.
**I. pilo'sus,** a species infesting many animals in South Africa; formerly thought to cause paralysis in sheep.
**I. pu'tus,** a species that infests the nests of many marine birds.
**I. ra'sus,** a species that attacks a variety of insectivores, rodents, ungulates, carnivores, and occasionally man and other primates in Africa.
**I. rici'nus,** the castor bean tick, which is parasitic on cattle, sheep, and wild animals, and transmits the agents of anaplasmosis, canine babesiosis, tularemia, louping ill, erythema chronicum migrans, acrodermatitis, chronica atrophicans, and Russian spring-summer encephalitis.
**I. rubicun'dus,** a species that may cause a tick paralysis in sheep, goats, and cattle in West Africa. A single human case has been reported.
**I. scapula'ris,** the eastern black-legged tick, the principal vector of Lyme disease in the eastern and north central United States and an occasional vector of tularemia; its usual reservoirs are mice of the genus *Peromyscus.* The species includes organisms formerly classified as *I. dammini.*
**I. spinipal'pus,** a species that infests rabbits and squirrels in western Canada, and may transmit Powassan virus.

**ix·o·di·a·sis** (ik″so-di'ə-sis) any disease or lesion due to the bite of ticks; infestation with ticks.

**ix·od·ic** (ik-sod'ik) caused by ticks.

**ix·o·did** (ik'so-did) 1. pertaining to ticks of the family Ixodidae. 2. a tick of the family Ixodidae; called also *hard tick* and *hard-bodied tick.* 3. pertaining to ticks of the genus *Ixodes.*

**Ix·od·i·dae** (ik-sod'ĭ-de) the hard ticks, a family of the superfamily Ixodoidea, distinguished from the soft ticks (Argasidae) by the presence of a scutum. It includes the genera *Amblyomma, Anocentor, Aponomma, Boophilus, Dermacentor, Haemaphysalis, Hyalomma, Ixodes, Margaropus, Rhipicentor,* and *Rhipicephalus.*

**Ix·od·i·des** (ik-sod'ĭ-dēz) the ticks, a suborder of Acarina, including the superfamily Ixodoidea, which comprises the families Ixodidae and Argasidae.

**Ix·o·diph·a·gus** (ik″so-dif'ə-gəs) a genus of hymenopteran insects. *I. caucur'tei* is a parasite of ticks of the family Ixodidae.

**ix·o·dism** (ik'so-diz-əm) ixodiasis.

**Ix·o·doi·dea** (ik″so-doi'de-ə) a superfamily of the suborder Ixodides, which embraces the families Argasidae and Ixodidae.

**-ize** [Gr. *-izein* verb-forming suffix] a word termination meaning *(a)* to cause to be, *(b)* to cause to acquire some quality, *(c)* to become, *(d)* to become similar to, *(e)* to subject to an action or treatment.

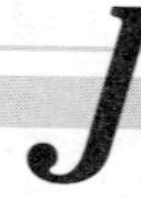

**J** symbol for *joule.*

**jaag·siek·te, jaag·ziek·te** (yahg-sēk'tə) pulmonary adenomatosis, def. 2.

**Ja·bou·lay's amputation (operation), button** (zhah"boo-lāz') [Mathieu *Jaboulay,* French surgeon, 1860–1913] see *hemipelvectomy,* and see under *button.*

**Jac·coud's syndrome (arthritis)** (zhah-ko͞oz') [Sigismond *Jaccoud,* French physician, 1830–1913] see under *syndrome.*

**jack·et** (jak'ət) 1. an enveloping structure or garment, especially a covering for the trunk or for the upper part of the body. 2. jacket crown; see under *crown.*
**Minerva j.,** a plaster-of-Paris jacket that includes both the trunk and the head, with the ears and face left free; used for fractures of the cervical spine and after operations for torticollis.
**plaster-of-Paris j.,** a casing of plaster of Paris enveloping the body for the purpose of correcting deformities.
**porcelain j.,** a jacket crown of porcelain.
**Risser j.,** a combination of plaster, turnbuckles, and hinges, extending from the chin and occiput to one knee, sometimes including one arm as far as the elbow; used in scoliosis.
**strait j.,** informal name for *camisole.*

**jack·screw** (jak'skroo) a threaded device used in orthodontic appliances for the separation or approximation of teeth or jaw segments.

**Jack·son appliance, crib** (jak'sən) [Victor Hugo *Jackson,* American dentist, 1850–1929] see under *appliance.*

**Jack·son's law (rule), syndrome** (jak'sənz) [John Hughlings *Jackson,* English neurologist, 1835–1911] see under *law* and *syndrome.*

**Jack·son's membrane (veil)** (jak'sənz) [Jabez North *Jackson,* American surgeon, 1868–1935] see under *membrane.*

**Jack·son's safety triangle, sign** (jak'sənz) [Chevalier *Jackson,* American laryngologist, 1865–1958] see under *triangle.*

**jack·so·ni·an epilepsy, march** (jak-so'ne-ən) [John Hughlings *Jackson*] see under *epilepsy* and *march.*

**Ja·cob** (zhah-kōb') François. French biologist, born 1920; co-winner, with André Michael Lwoff and Jacques Lucien Monod, of the Nobel prize in medicine and physiology for 1965, for discoveries concerning the genetic control of enzymes and virus synthesis.

**Ja·cob's membrane, ulcer** (ja'kobz) [Arthur *Jacob,* Irish ophthalmologist, 1790–1874] see *layer of rods and cones,* under *layer,* and see under *ulcer.*

**ja·co·bine** (ja'ko-bin) a poisonous pyrrolizidine alkaloid from the composite-flowered plant *Senecio jacobae;* it causes seneciosis in ruminants.

**Ja·cob·son's canal,** etc. (ja'kob-sənz) [Ludwig Levin *Jacobson,* Danish anatomist, 1783–1843] see under *canal, cartilage, nerve, organ,* and *sulcus,* and see *plexus tympanicus.*

**Ja·cob·son's retinitis** (yah'kəb-sənz) [Julius *Jacobson,* German ophthalmologist, 1828–1889] syphilitic retinitis.

**Ja·cod's syndrome (triad)** (zhah-kōz') [Maurice *Jacod,* French physician, born 1880] see under *syndrome.*

**Jac·quet's dermatitis (erythema)** (zhah-kāz') [Léonard Marie Lucien *Jacquet,* French dermatologist, 1860–1914] diaper dermatitis.

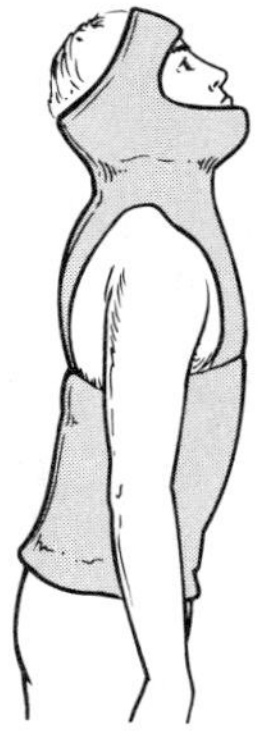

Minerva jacket.

**jac·ta·tio** (jak-ta'she-o) [L., from *jactare* to toss about] jactitation.
**j. ca'pitis noctur'na,** rhythmic rolling of the head of a child just before falling asleep.

**jac·ta·tion** (jak-ta'shən) jactitation.

**jac·ti·ta·tion** (jak"tĭ-ta'shən) [L. *jactitatio; jactitare* to toss] the tossing to and fro of a patient in acute disease.

**Jad·as·sohn's anetoderma, sebaceous nevus, test** (yah'dah-sōnz) [Josef *Jadassohn,* German dermatologist in Switzerland, 1863–1936] see under *anetoderma* and *nevus,* and see *irrigation test,* under *test.*

**Jad·as·sohn-Lew·an·dow·sky syndrome** (yah'dah-sōn-lev-ahn-dov'ske) [Josef *Jadassohn;* Felix *Lewandowsky,* German dermatologist, 1879–1921] pachyonychia congenita.

**Jad·as·sohn-Pel·li·za·ri anetoderma** (yah'dah-sōn-pel"ĭ-zah're) [Josef *Jadassohn;* Pietro *Pellizari,* Italian dermatologist, 1823–1892] see under *anetoderma.*

**Jade·lot's lines (furrows)** (zhah-də-lōz') [Jean François Nicolas *Jadelot,* physician in Paris, 1791–1830] see under *line.*

**Jae·ger's test type** (ya'gərz) [Edward *Jaeger* von Jastthal, Austrian oculist, 1818–1884] see under *test type.*

**Jaf·fe's reaction, test** (yah'fez) [Max *Jaffe,* German physiologic chemist, 1841–1911] see under *reaction* and *test.*

**Jaf·fe-Lich·ten·stein disease** (jaf'e-lik'tən-stīn) [Henry Lewis *Jaffe,* American pathologist, born 1896; Louis *Lichtenstein,* American physician, born 1906] see under *disease.*

**jag·siek·te** (yahg-sēk'tə) [Afrikaans *jag* hunt + *siekte* sickness] pulmonary adenomatosis, def. 2.

**jag·ziek·te** (yahg-zēk'tə) pulmonary adenomatosis, def. 2.

**Ja·kob's disease** (yah'kobz) [Alfons Maria *Jakob,* German psychiatrist, 1884–1931] Creutzfeldt-Jakob disease.

**Ja·kob-Creutz·feldt disease** (yah'kob-kroits'fəlt) [Alfons Maria *Jakob;* Hans Gerhard *Creutzfeldt,* German psychiatrist, 1885–1964] Creutzfeldt-Jakob disease.

**jal·ap** (jal'ap) [Sp. *jalapa,* from *Jalapa,* a city of Mexico] the dried tuberous root of *Exogonium purga* (Hayne) Lindl. Convolvulaceae; its resins possess cathartic properties.

**ja·mais vu** (zhah'ma voo) [Fr. "never seen"] the sensation that familiar surroundings are strangely unfamiliar; the illusion that one has never seen anything like that before.

**Ja·net's test** (zhah-nāz') [Pierre Marie Felix *Janet,* French physician, 1859–1947] see under *test.*

**Jane·way's lesion** (jān'wāz) [Edward Gamaliel *Janeway,* American physician, 1841–1911] see under *lesion.*

**jan·i·ceps** (jan'ĭ-seps) [L. *Janus* a two-faced god + *caput* head] conjoined twins with one head and two opposite faces.
**j. asym'metros,** conjoined twins with one imperfect and one more complete face.
**j. parasi'ticus,** conjoined twins in which there is partial duplication of the head in the frontal plane.

**Jan·i·mine** (jăn'ĭ-mīn) trademark for a preparation of imipramine hydrochloride.

**Jan·net·ta procedure** (jə-net'ə) [Peter Joseph *Jannetta,* American neurosurgeon, born 1932] see under *procedure.*

**Ja·no·šík's embryo** (yahn'o-siks) [Jan *Janošík,* Czechoslovakian anatomist, 1856–1927] see under *embryo.*

**Jan·sen's disease** (yahn'sənz) [W. Murk *Jansen,* Dutch orthopedic surgeon, 1867–1935] see *metaphyseal dysostosis,* under *dysostosis.*

**Jan·ský-Biels·chow·sky disease** (yahn'ske byels-chov'ske) [Jan *Janský,* Czech psychiatrist, 1873–1921; Alfred *Bielschowsky,* German ophthalmologist, 1871–1940] see under *disease.*

**Jan·thi·no·so·ma** (jan"thĭ-no-so'mə) a genus of mosquitoes, sometimes considered to be a subgenus of the genus *Psorophora. J. lut'zi* and *J. postica'ta* transport the eggs of botflies *(Dermatobia)* glued to their abdomens.

**Ja·quet's apparatus** (zhah-kāz') [Alfred *Jaquet,* Swiss pharmacologist, 1865–1937] see under *apparatus.*

**jar** (jahr) a wide-mouthed glass or earthenware container.
**bell j.,** a glass vessel, closed at top, open at bottom, used in laboratory vacuum experiments.
**Leyden j.,** a glass jar partially covered inside and out with tinfoil or other metal, used as a condenser or collector of electricity.

**ja·ra·ra·ca** (jah"rah-rah'kə) *Bothrops jararaca,* a venomous pit viper found throughout South America.

**Jar·cho's pressometer** (jahr'kōz) [Julius *Jarcho,* Russian-born obstetrician in United States, 1882–1963] see under *pressometer.*

**Jar·cho-Lev·in syndrome** (jahr'ko-lev'in) [Saul Wallenstein *Jarcho,* American physician, born 1906; Paul M. *Levin,* American physician, 20th century] see under *syndrome.*

**jar·gon** (jahr'gən) 1. the technical or specialized language used in a profession or other field of activity. 2. incoherent speech, consisting either of neologisms or of actual words placed in an incoherent order. See also *jargon aphasia,* under *aphasia.*

**jar·gon·a·pha·sia** (jahr"gon-ə-fa'zhə) jargon aphasia.

**Ja·risch-Herx·heim·er reaction** (yah'rish-herks'hi-mər) [Adolf *Jarisch,* Austrian dermatologist, 1850–1902; Karl *Herxheimer,* German dermatologist, 1861–1944] see under *reaction.*

**Jar·ja·vay's ligament, muscle** (zhahr-zhah-vāz') [Jean François *Jarjavay,* French physician, 1815–1868] see under *muscle* and see *uterosacral ligament,* under *ligament.*

**Jar·vik-7 artificial heart** (jahr'vik) [Robert Koffler *Jarvik,* American cardiologist, 20th century] see under *heart.*

**Jat·ro·pha** (jat'ro-fə) [Gr. *iatros* physician + *trophē* nourishment] a genus of plants of the family Euphorbiaceae, commonly found from Mexico to South America; various species have purgative, stomachic, febrifuge, and astringent properties. *J. cur'cas* L. and *J. multi'fida* L. (both called *physic nut* or *purging nut*) have seeds containing a purgative oil and a phytotoxin; when consumed by ruminants they cause diarrhea and damage to various internal organs.

**jaun·dice** (jawn'dis) [Fr. *jaunisse,* from *jaune* yellow] [MeSH: Jaundice] a syndrome characterized by hyperbilirubinemia and deposition of bile pigment in the skin, mucous membranes, and sclera, with resulting yellow appearance of the patient; called also *icterus.*
**acholuric j.,** jaundice without bilirubinuria, associated with elevated unconjugated bilirubin that is not excreted by the kidney; seen in hemolytic disease and other forms of unconjugated hyperbilirubinemia.
**acholuric familial j.,** hereditary spherocytosis.
**anhepatic j., anhepatogenous j.,** yellow appearance of the skin and mucous membranes not caused by liver disease.
**black j.,** Winckel's disease.
**breast milk j.,** elevated unconjugated bilirubin in some breast-fed infants due to the presence of 5-$\beta$-pregnane-3-$\alpha$-20-$\beta$-diol in breast milk, which inhibits glucuronyl transferase conjugating activity, or to dehydration.
**cholestatic j.,** jaundice resulting from an abnormality in the flow of bile, usually accompanied by elevation of serum alkaline phosphatase, retention of bile salts (with resulting pruritus), and varying hypercholesterolemia. The cholestasis may be *extrahepatic,* due to obstruction caused by a stone, stricture, or neoplasm, or *intrahepatic,* which may be due to liver cell disease (e.g., hepatitis), or altered permeability and/or obstruction of the intrahepatic biliary system (as in drug reactions or hepatic infiltrative disease).
**chronic acholuric j., congenital hemolytic j.,** hereditary spherocytosis.
**Crigler-Najjar j.,** see under *syndrome.*
**epidemic j.,** hepatitis A.
**familial acholuric j.,** hereditary spherocytosis.
**hemolytic j.,** jaundice caused by increased production of bilirubin from hemoglobin under conditions causing accelerated degradation of erythrocytes.
**hepatocellular j.,** jaundice caused by injury to or disease of the liver cells.
**hepatogenic j., hepatogenous j.,** that which is due to some disease or disorder of the liver.
**homologous serum j., human serum j.,** hepatitis B.
**infectious j., infective j.,** 1. infectious hepatitis. 2. Weil's syndrome.
**latent j.,** hyperbilirubinemia without yellow staining of the tissues.
**leptospiral j.,** Weil's syndrome.
**malignant j. of dogs,** canine babesiosis.
**mechanical j.,** obstructive j.
**neonatal j., j. of the newborn,** icterus neonatorum.
**nonhemolytic j.,** jaundice caused by an abnormality in the metabolism of bilirubin, and resulting in an excessive accumulation of unconjugated bilirubin in the blood. The various forms include *Crigler-Najjar syndrome, Dubin-Johnson syndrome, Gilbert syndrome, physiologic jaundice,* and *Rotor's syndrome.*
**nonhemolytic j., congenital,** Crigler-Najjar syndrome.
**nonhemolytic j., congenital familial,** Crigler-Najjar syndrome.
**nonhemolytic j., familial,** Gilbert syndrome.
**nuclear j.,** kernicterus.
**obstructive j.,** that which is due to an impediment to the flow of the bile from the liver cells to the duodenum.
**physiologic j.,** mild icterus neonatorum lasting the first few days after birth.
**picric acid j.,** jaundice due to picric acid poisoning; seen in munition workers and in malingering soldiers who deliberately ingest picric acid.
**regurgitation j.,** jaundice attributed to escape of bile from the bile canaliculi into the blood stream and marked by urobilinogen in the urine.
**retention j.,** a form of jaundice due to inability of the liver to dispose of the bilirubin provided by the circulating blood.
**Schmorl's j.,** kernicterus.
**spirochetal j.,** Weil's syndrome.
**toxemic j., toxic j.,** jaundice produced by poisons, such as phosphorus, arseniuretted hydrogen, picric acid, or carbon tetrachloride.

**jaw** (jaw) [MeSH: Jaw] either the mandible or the maxilla, the two bony structures in the head of vertebrates; in dentate species they bear the teeth, enabling carnivores to seize their prey and others to bite and chew food.
**bird-beak j.,** micrognathia (def. 1).
**big j.,** actinomycosis in cattle.
**bottle j.,** edema in the mandibular region of a grazing horse or cow, seen secondary to many different edematous conditions; it may clear up if the animal is switched to feeding from a trough.
**cleft j.,** a cleft between the median nasal and maxillary prominences through the alveolus. Called also *gnathoschisis.*
**crackling j.,** noise (crepitation) in the normal or diseased temporomandibular joint associated with jaw movement.
**drop j., dropped j.,** in paralytic rabies in dogs, dropping of the mandible and inability to close the mouth.
**Hapsburg j.,** a mandibular prognathous jaw, often accompanied by a thick overdeveloped lower lip (Hapsburg lip), as seen in many members of the Hapsburg family of European nobility.
**lower j.,** mandibula.
**lumpy j.,** actinomycosis in cattle.
**overshot j.,** veterinary term for *retrognathia.*
**parrot j.,** micrognathia (def. 1).
**phossy j.,** phosphorus necrosis.
**pipe j.,** a painful condition of the jaws caused by carrying a tobacco pipe in the mouth.
**rubber j.,** a type of osteoporosis in dogs and cats with softening of the jaws, resorption, and replacement of the bone by fibrous tissue, occurring in association with renal osteodystrophy.
**undershot j.,** veterinary term for *prognathism;* it is normal in animals such as boxers and bulldogs.
**upper j.,** maxilla.

**Ja·wor·ski's corpuscles (bodies), test** (yə-vor'skēz) [Walery *Jaworski,* Polish physician, 1849–1924] see under *corpuscle* and *tests.*

**JCV** JC virus.

**Jean·selme's nodules** (zhah-selmz') [Antoine Edouard *Jeanselme,* French dermatologist, 1858–1935] see under *nodule.*

**Jec·to·fer** (jek'to-fər) trademark for a preparation of iron sorbitex.

**Jef·fer·son's fracture, syndrome** (jef'ər-sənz) [Sir Geoffrey *Jefferson,* English neurosurgeon, 1886–1961] see under *fracture,* and see *cavernous sinus syndrome,* under *syndrome.*

**Jef·fer·so·nia** (jef"ər-so'ne-ə) [Thomas *Jefferson,* naturalist and third President of the United States, 1743–1826] a genus of American and Asian herbs of the family Berberidaceae. The root of *J. diphyl'la* (L.) Pers., of North America, is tonic, diuretic, and expectorant; emetic in large doses.

**Jef·ron** (jef'ron) trademark for a preparation of polyferose.

**jejun(o)-** [L. *jejunum,* q.v.] a combining form denoting relationship to the jejunum.

**je·ju·nal** (jə-joo'nəl) pertaining to the jejunum.

**je·ju·nec·to·my** (jə"joo-nek'tə-me) [*jejuno-* + *-ectomy*] excision of the jejunum.

**je·ju·ni·tis** (jə"joo-ni'tis) inflammation of the jejunum.

**je·ju·no·ce·cos·to·my** (jə-joo"no-se-kos'tə-me) [*jejuno-* + *ceco-* + *-stomy*] the formation of an anastomosis between the jejunum and cecum; also, the anastomosis so formed.

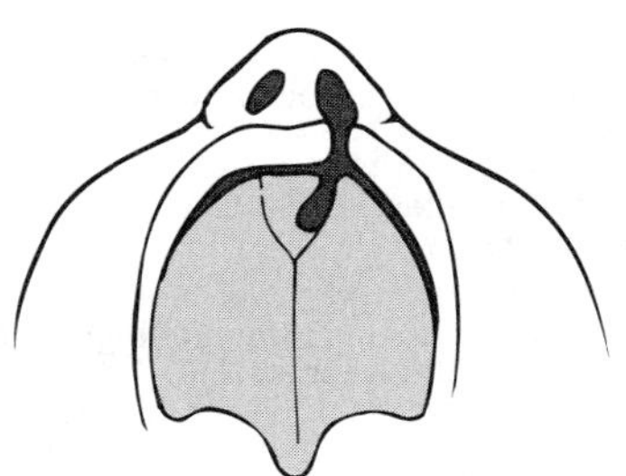

Unilateral cleft of the jaw and lip.

**je·ju·no·co·los·to·my** (jə-joo″no-ko-los′tə-me) [*jejuno-* + *colo-* + *-stomy*] the formation of an anastomosis between the jejunum and the colon; also, the anastomosis so formed.

**je·ju·no·il·e·al** (jə-joo″no-il′e-əl) pertaining to the jejunum and ileum; connecting the proximal jejunum with the distal ileum.

**je·ju·no·il·e·itis** (jə-joo″no-il″e-i′tis) inflammation of the jejunum and ileum together.

**je·ju·no·il·e·os·to·my** (jə-joo″no-il″e-os′tə-me) [*jejuno-* + *ileo-* + *-stomy*] the formation of an anastomosis between the proximal jejunum and the terminal ileum; also, the anastomosis so formed.

**je·ju·no·je·ju·nos·to·my** (jə-joo″no-jə″joo-nos′tə-me) the operative formation of an anastomosis between two portions of the jejunum; also, the anastomosis so formed.

**je·ju·nor·rha·phy** (jə″joo-nor′ə-fe) [*jejuno-* + *-rrhaphy*] operative repair of the jejunum.

**je·ju·nos·to·my** (jə″joo-nos′tə-me) [*jejuno-* + *-stomy*] [MeSH: Jejunostomy] the surgical creation of a permanent opening between the jejunum and the surface of the abdominal wall; also, the opening so established.

**je·ju·not·o·my** (jə″joo-not′ə-me) [*jejuno-* + *-tomy*] surgical incision of the jejunum.

**je·ju·num** (jə-joo′nəm) [L. "empty"] [TA] [MeSH: Jejunum] that portion of the small intestine which extends from the duodenum to the ileum; called also *intestinum jejunum*.

**jel·ly** (jel′e) [L. *gelatina*] a soft substance which is coherent, tremulous, and more or less translucent; generally, a colloidal semisolid mass.
**cardiac j.**, a gelatinous substance present between the endothelium and myocardium of the embryonic heart, which transforms into the connective tissue of the endocardium.
**contraceptive j.**, a nongreasy jelly or cream for introduction into the vagina or onto a diaphragm to prevent conception.
**glycerin j.**, a compound of gelatin, arsenic trioxide, and glycerin, used as a reagent; called also *glycerogelatin*.
**mineral j.**, petrolatum.
**petroleum j.**, petrolatum.
**Wharton's j.**, the soft, jellylike, homogeneous intercellular substance of the umbilical cord; it gives the reaction for mucin and contains thin collagenous fibers which increase in number with the age of the fetus.

**jel·ly·fish** (jel′e-fish) [MeSH: Jellyfish] any of various free-swimming umbrella-shaped cnidarians with transparent bodies varying from a few millimeters to two meters in diameter; this form represents just one stage in the life cycle. Genera that inflict poisonous stings include *Aurelia, Carukia, Chironex, Chiropsalmus,* and *Physalia*. Called also *medusa*.

**Jen·dras·sik's maneuver, sign** (yən-drah′siks) [Ernst *Jendrassik*, Hungarian physician, 1858–1921] see under *maneuver* and *sign*.

**Jen·ner** (jen′ər) Edward. An English physician (1749–1823), who developed the process of producing immunity to smallpox by inoculation (vaccination) with cowpox (vaccinia) vaccine.

**Jen·ner's method** (jen′ərz) [Louis Leopold *Jenner*, English physician, 1866–1904] see under *stain*.

**jen·ne·ri·an** (jen-e′re-ən) named for Edward *Jenner*.

**jen·ner·iza·tion** (jen″ər-ĭ-za′shən) production of immunity to a disease by inoculation of an attenuated form of the virus producing the disease.

**Jen·sen's disease** (yen′sənz) [Edmund *Jensen*, Danish ophthalmologist, 1861–1950] retinochoroiditis juxtapapillaris.

**Jen·sen's sarcoma (tumor)** (yen′sənz) [Carl Oluf *Jensen*, Danish veterinary pathologist, 1864–1934] see under *sarcoma*.

**jerk** (jərk) a sudden reflex or involuntary movement.
**Achilles j.**, **ankle j.**, triceps surae reflex.
**biceps j.**, biceps reflex.
**crossed adductor j.**, see under *reflex*.
**elbow j.**, triceps reflex.
**hypnic j's**, sudden brief contractions, usually of the legs but sometimes also of the head and arms, occurring during the onset of sleep.
**jaw j.**, jaw reflex.
**knee j.**, patellar reflex.
**quadriceps j.**, patellar reflex.
**tendon j.**, see under *reflex*.
**triceps surae j.**, see under *reflex*.

**Jerne** (yed′nĕ) Niels Kaj. Danish immunologist, born 1911; co-winner with Cesar Milstein and Georges J. F. Köhler of the Nobel prize for medicine or physiology in 1984 for his three theories: of the selective theory of antibody formation, of the T lymphocyte's distinction of "self" from "non-self," and of the functional network of interacting antibodies and lymphocytes.

**Jer·vell and Lange-Niel·sen syndrome** (yer-vel′-lahng′ə-nēl′sən) [Anton *Jervell*, Norwegian cardiologist, born 1901; Friedrik *Lange-Nielsen*, Norwegian cardiologist, 20th century] see under *syndrome*.

**jes·sur** (jes′ər) Bengalese name for *Russell's viper*.

**jet** (jet) [L. *iacere* to throw] 1. a stream of fluid projected at high velocity under pressure, or the device for producing such a stream. 2. a high-velocity stream of blood emerging from a stenotic lesion.
**water-j.**, see under *dissector*.

**Jeune's syndrome** (zhoonz) [Mathis *Jeune*, French pediatrician, born 1910] asphyxiating thoracic dystrophy; see under *dystrophy*.

**Jew·ett nail** (joo′ət) [Eugene Lyon *Jewett*, American surgeon, born 1900] see under *nail*.

**jig·ger** (jig′ər) chigoe.

**Jim·son weed** (jim′sən wēd) *Datura stramonium*.

**jit·ter** (jit′ər) in single fiber electromyography, the variability in interpotential interval as consecutive discharges occur; usually expressed as the mean of consecutive differences (q.v.).

**Job's syndrome** (jōbz) [*Job*, character in the Old Testament who suffered from skin disease and other misfortunes] [MeSH: Job's Syndrome] see under *syndrome*.

**Jo·bert's fossa** (zho-bārz′) [Antoine Joseph *Jobert* de Lamballe, French surgeon, 1799–1867] see under *fossa*.

**jod·bas·e·dow** (i″ōd-baz′ə-do) [Ger.] iodine-induced hyperthyroidism.

**Joest's bodies** (yersts) [Ernst *Joest*, German veterinary pathologist, 1873–1926] see under *body*.

**Jof·froy's reflex** (zhof-rwahz′) [Alexis *Joffroy*, French physician, 1844–1908] see under *reflex*.

**Joh·ne's bacillus, disease** (yo′nez) [Heinrich Albert *Johne*, German pathologist, 1839–1910] see *Mycobacterium paratuberculosis* and under *disease*.

**joh·nin** (yo′nin) a filtrate of cultures of *Mycobacterium paratuberculosis* (Johne's bacillus), similar to tuberculin, used to produce a skin reaction (johnin reaction) in testing cattle for Johne's disease.

**John·son-Ste·vens disease** (jon′sən-ste′vənz) [Frank Chambliss *Johnson*, American pediatrician 1894–1934; Albert Mason *Stevens*, American pediatrician 1884–1945] Stevens-Johnson syndrome.

**joint** (joint) [L. *junctio* a joining, connection] [MeSH: Joints] the place of union or junction between two or more bones of the skeleton. See *articulatio* [TA].
**acromioclavicular j.**, articulatio acromioclavicularis.
**amphidiarthrodial j.**, amphidiarthrosis.
**ankle j.**, articulatio talocruralis.
**arthrodial j.**, articulatio plana.
**atlantoaxial j., lateral**, articulatio atlanto-axialis lateralis.
**atlantoaxial j., medial**, articulatio atlanto-axialis medialis.
**atlanto-occipital j.**, articulatio atlanto-occipitalis.
**j's of auditory ossicles**, articulationes ossiculorum auditoriorum.
**ball-and-socket j.**, articulatio spheroidea.
**biaxial j.**, one permitting movement in two of the assumed three mutually perpendicular axes, or having two degrees of freedom, as the ellipsoidal joint.
**bicondylar j.**, articulatio bicondylaris.
**bilocular j.**, a joint in which the synovial cavity is divided into two compartments by an interarticular cartilage, as the temporomandibular joint.
**bleeder's j.**, hemophilic arthropathy.
**bony j's**, juncturae ossium.
**Budin's j.**, a band of cartilage seen at birth between the squamous and the two condylar portions of the occipital bone.
**calcaneocuboid j.**, articulatio calcaneocuboidea.
**carpal j's**, 1. articulationes carpi. 2. see *articulationes intercarpales*.
**carpometacarpal j's**, articulationes carpometacarpales.
**carpometacarpal j. of thumb**, articulatio carpometacarpalis pollicis.
**cartilaginous j.**, junctura cartilaginea.
**Charcot's j.**, neuropathic arthropathy.
**chondrosternal j's**, articulationes sternocostales.
**Chopart's j.**, articulatio tarsi transversa.
**Clutton's j.**, painless symmetrical hydrarthrosis, especially of the knee joints, seen in congenital syphilis.
**cochlear j.**, a form of hinge joint which permits some rotation or lateral motion, as the knee joint.
**coffin j.**, the second interphalangeal joint of the foot of a horse.
**composite j.**, **compound j.**, articulatio composita.
**condylar j.**, **condyloid j.**, articulatio ellipsoidea.
**costochondral j's**, articulationes costochondrales.
**costotransverse j.**, articulatio costotransversaria.
**costovertebral j's**, articulationes costovertebrales.
**coxal j.**, articulatio coxae.

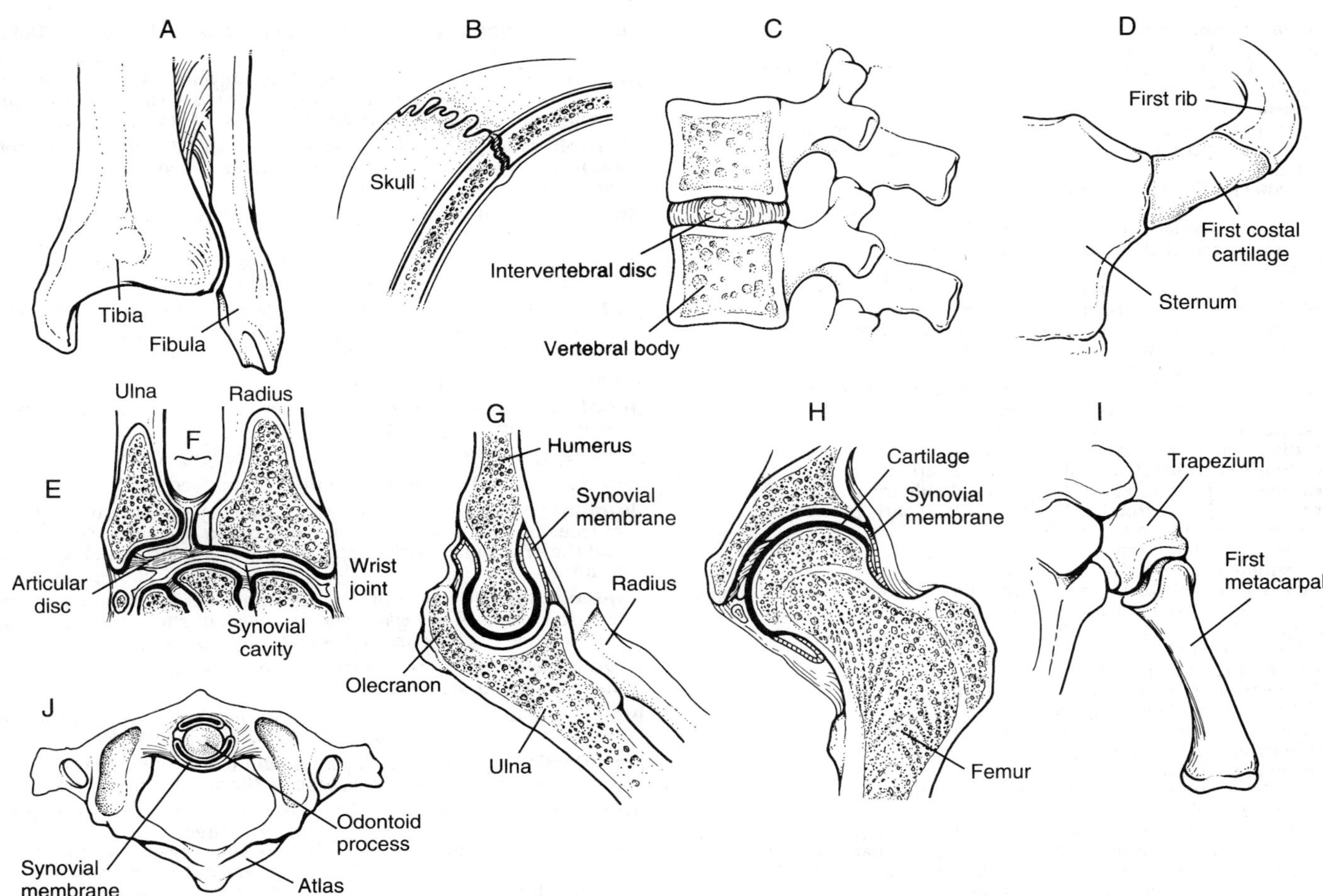


Various kinds of joints. *Fibrous: A,* syndesmosis (tibiofibular); *B,* suture (skull). *Cartilaginous: C,* symphysis (vertebral bodies); *D,* synchondrosis (first rib and sternum). *Synovial: E,* condyloid (wrist); *F,* gliding (radioulnar); *G,* hinge or ginglymus (elbow); *H,* ball and socket (hip); *I,* saddle (carpometacarpal of thumb); *J,* pivot (atlantoaxial).

**craniovertebral j.,** articulatio atlanto-occipitalis.
**cricoarytenoid j.,** articulatio crico-arytenoidea.
**cricothyroid j.,** articulatio cricothyroidea.
**Cruveilhier's j.,** articulatio atlanto-occipitalis.
**cubital j.,** articulatio cubiti.
**cuboideonavicular j.,** the articulation between the rounded lateral surface of the navicular bone and the posterior part of the medial surface of the cuboid bone; it is usually fibrous but is occasionally synovial.
**cuneocuboid j.,** articulatio cuneocuboidea.
**cuneonavicular j.,** articulatio cuneonavicularis.
**diarthrodial j.,** junctura synovialis.
**digital j's,** see *articulationes interphalangeales manus* and *articulationes interphalangeales pedis,* under *articulatio.*
**elbow j.,** articulatio cubiti.
**ellipsoidal j.,** a biaxial joint with the articulating surfaces much longer in one direction than in the direction at right angles; see *articulatio ellipsoidea* [TA].
**enarthrodial j.,** articulatio spheroidea.
**facet j's,** the articulations of the vertebral column.
**false j.,** pseudarthrosis.
**fetlock j.,** either the metacarpophalangeal joint or the metatarsophalangeal joint in an ungulate.
**fibrocartilaginous j.,** symphysis.
**fibrous j.,** junctura fibrosa.
**flail j.,** one showing abnormal mobility.
**freely movable j.,** junctura synovialis.
**fringe j.,** one affected with chronic villous arthritis.
**ginglymoid j.,** ginglymus.
**glenohumeral j.,** the articulation between the head of the humerus and the glenoid cavity.
**gliding j.,** articulatio plana.
**j. of head of rib,** articulatio capitis costae.
**hemophilic j.,** see under *arthropathy.*
**hinge j.,** ginglymus.
**hip j.,** articulatio coxae.
**hock j.,** hock.
**humeral j.,** articulatio humeri.
**humeroradial j.,** articulatio humeroradialis.
**humeroulnar j.,** articulatio humero-ulnaris.
**immovable j's,** articulationes fibrosae.
**incudomalleolar j.,** articulatio incudomallearis.
**incudostapedial j.,** articulatio incudostapedialis.
**intercarpal j's,** 1. articulationes intercarpales. 2. see *articulationes carpi.*
**interchondral j's,** articulationes interchondrales.
**intercuneiform j's,** articulationes intercuneiformes.
**intermetacarpal j's,** articulationes intermetacarpales.
**intermetatarsal j's,** articulationes intermetatarsales.
**interphalangeal j's of fingers,** articulationes interphalangeales manus.
**interphalangeal j's of foot,** articulationes interphalangeales pedis.
**interphalangeal j's of hand,** articulationes interphalangeales manus.
**interphalangeal j's of toes,** articulationes interphalangeales pedis.
**intertarsal j's,** articulationes intertarsales.
**irritable j.,** a joint subject to attacks of inflammation without discoverable cause.
**knee j.,** articulatio genus.
**ligamentous j.,** syndesmosis.
**Lisfranc's j.,** articulationes tarsometatarsales.
**lumbosacral j.,** articulatio lumbosacralis.
**j's of Luschka,** a series of jointlike structures at the lateral edges of the vertebral bodies from vertebra C3 to T1, forming small spurlike lips at the upper surface, covered with cartilage, and containing a capsule filled with fluid. They are considered by some to be true diarthrodial joints, and by others to be degenerative spaces of the intervertebral disks filled with extracellular fluid and lined by a membrane formed by fibrocytes. They are frequent sites of spur formation. Called also *uncovertebral j's.*
**mandibular j.,** articulatio temporomandibularis.
**manubriosternal j.,** see *symphysis manubriosternalis* and *synchondrosis manubriosternalis.*
**metacarpophalangeal j's,** articulationes metacarpophalangeales.

**metatarsophalangeal j's,** articulationes metatarsophalangeales.
**midcarpal j.,** articulatio mediocarpea.
**mixed j.,** one combining features of different types of joints.
**multiaxial j.,** articulatio spheroidea.
**neurocentral j.,** junctio neurocentralis.
**open j.,** a veterinary term for a joint in which the surface of the bones is exposed, as a result of inflammation and sloughing of the tissues.
**osseous j's,** juncturae ossium.
**pastern j.,** the joint between the short and long pastern bones of a horse, the second most distal of the leg joints.
**j's of pectoral girdle,** juncturae cinguli pectoralis.
**peg-and-socket j.,** gomphosis.
**j's of pelvic girdle,** juncturae cinguli pelvici.
**phalangeal j's,** see *articulationes interphalangeales manus* and *articulationes interphalangeales pedis,* under *articulatio.*
**pisotriquetral j.,** articulatio ossis pisiformis.
**pivot j.,** articulatio trochoidea.
**plane j.,** a type of synovial joint in which the opposed surfaces are flat or only slightly curved; see *articulatio plana* [TA].
**polyaxial j.,** articulatio spheroidea.
**radiocarpal j.,** articulatio radiocarpalis.
**radioulnar j., distal,** articulatio radio-ulnaris distalis.
**radioulnar j., middle,** syndesmosis radioulnaris.
**radioulnar j., proximal,** articulatio radio-ulnaris proximalis.
**rotary j.,** articulatio trochoidea.
**sacrococcygeal j.,** articulatio sacrococcygea.
**sacroiliac j.,** articulatio sacro-iliaca.
**saddle j.,** a joint having two saddle-shaped surfaces at right angles to each other; see *articulatio sellaris* [TA].
**scapuloclavicular j.,** articulatio acromioclavicularis.
**sellar j.,** articulatio sellaris.
**shoulder j.,** articulatio humeri.
**j's of shoulder girdle,** juncturae cinguli pectoralis.
**simple j.,** articulatio simplex.
**socket j. of tooth,** syndesmosis dentoalveolaris.
**spheroidal j.,** articulatio spheroidea.
**spiral j.,** cochlear j.
**sternoclavicular j.,** articulatio sternoclavicularis.
**sternocostal j's,** articulationes sternocostales.
**stifle j.,** a joint near the top of the hind leg of a quadruped, homologous to the knee joint of a human being; it actually consists of two joints, that between the femur and tibia, and that between the femur and patella. Called also *stifle* and *knee.*
**subtalar j.,** articulatio subtalaris.
**synarthrodial j.,** synarthrosis.
**synovial j.,** junctura synovialis.
**synovial j's of free lower limb,** articulationes membri inferioris liberi.
**synovial j's of free upper limb,** articulationes membri superioris liberi.
**talocalcaneal j.,** articulatio subtalaris.
**talocalcaneonavicular j.,** articulatio talocalcaneonavicularis.
**talocrural j.,** articulatio talocruralis.
**tarsal j's,** articulationes intertarseae.
**tarsal j., transverse,** articulatio tarsi transversa.
**tarsometatarsal j's,** articulationes tarsometatarsales.
**temporomandibular j.,** articulatio temporomandibularis.
**through j.,** junctura synovialis.
**tibiofibular j.,** 1. articulatio tibiofibularis (def. 1). 2. syndesmosis tibiofibularis.
**tibiofibular j., distal, tibiofibular j., inferior,** syndesmosis tibiofibularis.
**tibiofibular j., proximal, tibiofibular j., superior,** articulatio tibiofibularis.
**trochoid j.,** articulatio trochoidea.
**uncovertebral j's,** j's of Luschka.
**uniaxial j.,** one permitting movement in only one of the assumed three mutually perpendicular axes, or having only one degree of freedom, as a hinge joint and the interphalangeal joints.
**unilocular j.,** a synovial joint having only one cavity.
**von Gies j.,** a chronic syphilitic chondro-osteoarthritis.
**wedge-and-groove j.,** schindylesis.
**wrist j.,** articulatio radiocarpalis.
**xiphisternal j.,** synchondrosis xiphisternalis.
**zygapophyseal j's,** articulationes zygapophyseales.

**Jol·ly's bodies** (zho-lēz') [Justin Marie Jules *Jolly,* French histologist, 1870–1953] Howell-Jolly bodies; see under *body.*

**Jol·ly's reaction** (yol'ēz) [Friedrich *Jolly,* German neurologist, 1844–1904] see under *reaction.*

**Jones brace, fracture, position** (jōnz) [Sir Robert *Jones,* English orthopedic surgeon, 1858–1933] see under *brace, fracture,* and *position.*

**Jon·nes·co's fold, fossa** (jo-nes'kōz) [Thoma *Jonnesco,* Romanian surgeon, 1860–1926] see *parietoperitoneal fold,* under *fold,* and see *recessus duodenalis superior.*

**Jor·dans' anomaly** (yor'dənz) [Godefridus H. W. *Jordans,* Dutch physician, 1902–1979] see under *anomaly.*

**jo·sa·my·cin** (jo″sə-mi'sin) [MeSH: Josamycin] a macrolide antibiotic produced by *Streptomyces narbonensis* var. *josamyceticus,* having antibacterial activity similar to that of erythromycin.

**Jo·seph clamp, knife, rhinoplasty** (yo'səf) [Jacques *Joseph,* German surgeon, 1865–1934] see under *clamp, knife,* and *rhinoplasty.*

**Jo·seph disease** (jo-səf') [*Joseph,* an Azorean family affected by the disease] see *Azorean disease,* under *disease.*

**Jou·bert's syndrome** (zhoo-bārz') [Marie *Joubert,* Canadian neurologist, 20th century] see under *syndrome.*

**joule** (jo͞ol) [James Prescott *Joule,* English physicist, 1818–1889] the SI unit of energy and heat, being the work done by a force of 1 newton acting over a distance of 1 meter. Symbol, J.

**ju·ga** (joo'gə) [L.] plural of *jugum.*

**ju·gal** (joo'gəl) [L. *jugalis,* from *jugum* yoke] 1. connecting like a yoke. 2. pertaining to the cheek.

**ju·ga·le** (joo-ga'le) the jugal point; see under *point.*

**ju·gate** (joo'gāt) 1. locked together. 2. marked by ridges.

**Ju·glans** (joo'gləns) [L. "Jove's nut," walnut] the walnuts, a genus of trees of the family Juglandaceae. Certain species yield juglone, and the dried inner bark of *J. cine'rea* was formerly used as a mild laxative.

**jug·lone** (jug'lōn) an antibiotic substance derived from the leaves of certain species of *Juglans* and from walnut shells, which has antihemorrhagic properties and is active against certain fungi.

**ju·go·max·il·lary** (joo″go-mak'sĭ-lar″e) pertaining to the zygomatic bone and the maxilla.

**jug·u·lar** (jug'u-lər) [L. *jugularis,* from *jugulum* neck] 1. cervical (def. 1). 2. pertaining to a jugular vein. 3. a jugular vein.

**jug·u·la·tion** (jug″u-la'shən) [L. *jugulare* to cut the throat of] the sudden and rapid arrest of disease by therapeutic measures.

**ju·gum** (joo'gəm) pl. *ju'ga* [L. "a yoke"] [TA] a general term for a depression or ridge connecting two structures.
**ju'ga alveola'ria mandi'bulae** [TA], alveolar yokes of mandible: depressions on the anterior surface of the alveolar process of the mandible, between the ridges caused by the roots of the incisor teeth.
**ju'ga alveola'ria maxil'lae** [TA], alveolar yokes of maxilla: the depressions on the anterior surface of the alveolar process of the maxilla, between the ridges caused by the roots of the incisor teeth.
**ju'ga cerebra'lia,** TA alternative for *impressiones gyrorum.*
**j. sphenoida'le** [TA], sphenoidal yoke: the portion of the body of the sphenoid bone that connects its lesser wings.

**juice** (jo͞os) [L. *jus* broth] any fluid from an animal or plant tissue; see also *succus.*
**appetite j.,** gastric juice secreted during eating and varying in character with the appetite for the food which is being eaten.
**cherry j.,** liquid expressed from the fresh ripe fruit of *Prunus cerasus* L. (Rosaceae) used as an ingredient in preparing flavored vehicles for pharmaceuticals.
**gastric j.,** succus gastricus.
**intestinal j.,** succus entericus.
**pancreatic j.,** succus pancreaticus.
**press j.,** liquid obtained by submitting finely ground tissue to great pressure.
**raspberry j.,** the liquid expressed from the fresh ripe fruit of varieties of *Rubus idaeus* L. (European red raspberry) or *R. strigosus* Michx. (American red raspberry); used in a syrup as a flavored vehicle for drugs.

**Jukes** (jo͞oks) fictitious name of a New York family, described by the American sociologist R.L. Dugdale, exhibiting a high incidence of crime, immorality, disease, and poverty; used like the Kallikaks to advance the theory of genetic determinism.

**jump·ing** (jump'ing) 1. the skipping of several steps in a series; moving forward quickly. 2. see under *disease.*
**j. the bite,** correction of cross-bite. See also *Kingsley appliance,* under *appliance.*

**junc·tio** (junk'she-o) pl. *junctio'nes* [L., from *jungere* to join] 1. junction. 2. joint.
**j. anorecta'lis** [TA], anorectal junction: the site at which the rectum becomes continuous with the anal canal; called also *anorectal line.*
**j. neurocentra'lis,** neurocentral joint: a synchondrosis between the centrum of a vertebra and either half of the vertebral arch; it is obliterated by fusion of the vertebral arch and centrum during the third to sixth years of life.

**junc·tion** (junk'shən) the place of meeting or of coming together, as of two different organs or types of tissue; see also *articulatio* and *joint.* Called also *junctura.*

**adherent j.**, a type of intercellular junction that links cell membranes and cytoskeletal elements within and between cells, connecting adjacent cells mechanically. Examples include the zonula adherens of epithelial cells, fascia adherens of cardiac myocytes, and desmosomes.
**amelodentinal j.**, dentinoenamel j.
**anorectal j.**, junctio anorectalis.
**atrioventricular j., AV j.**, part or all of the entire region comprising the atrioventricular node and the bundle of His, with the bundle branches sometimes specifically excluded.
**cardioesophageal j.**, esophagogastric j.
**cementodentinal j.**, dentinocemental j.
**cementoenamel j.**, the line at which the cementum covering the root of a tooth and the enamel covering its crown meet, designated anatomically as the cervical line.
**communicating j.**, gap j.
**corneoscleral j.**, limbus corneae.
**craniovertebral j.**, articulatio atlanto-occipitalis.
**dentinocemental j.**, the plane of meeting between the dentin and cementum on the root of a tooth.
**dentinoenamel j.**, the plane of meeting between the dentin and enamel on the crown of a tooth.
**dentogingival j.**, the zone of meeting of the cementum and the gingiva, consisting of the epithelial attachment and the gingival fibers.
**dermoepidermal j.**, the plane of meeting between the dermis and epidermis.
**esophagogastric j.**, the site of transition from the stratified squamous epithelium of the esophagus to the simple columnar epithelium of the cardia of the stomach; see also *gastroesophageal sphincter,* under *sphincter.* Called also *cardioesophageal j.* and *gastroesophageal j.*
**fibromuscular j.**, a junction between the muscular elements of the wall of the corpus uteri and the fibrous tissue of the cervix.
**gap j.**, a type of intercellular junction comprising a narrowed portion (about 3 nm) of the intercellular space that contains channels or pores (about 2 nm) composed of hexagonal arrays of membrane-spanning proteins around a central lumen *(connexon)* through which pass ions and small molecules such as most sugars, amino acids, nucleotides, vitamins, hormones, and cyclic AMP. In electrically excitable tissues, these gap junctions serve to transmit electrical impulses via ionic currents and are known as *electrotonic synapses;* they are present in such tissues as myocardial tissue and the central nervous system. Called also *nexus.*
**gastroesophageal j.**, esophagogastric j.
**ileocecal j.**, the junction of the ileum and cecum, located at the lower right side of the abdomen and fixed to the posterior abdominal wall.
**intercellular j's**, specialized regions on the borders of cells that provide connections between adjacent cells; they are often divided into adherent, gap, and tight junctions, which are further divided on the basis of the shape and extent of the contact regions (e.g., macula, zonula, fascia).
**intermediate j.**, a type of adherent junction involving interactions with actin filaments. The term is sometimes used to denote the zonula adherens specifically or, rarely, the fascia adherens.
**lumbosacral j.**, articulatio lumbosacralis.
**manubriogladiolar j.**, synchondrosis sternalis.
**mucocutaneous j.**, the site of transition between skin and mucous membrane.
**mucogingival j.**, a sharply scalloped, generally indistinct line running parallel with the free margin, separating the gingival tissue from that of the oral mucosa; visible under the microscope. Called also *mucogingival line.*
**myoneural j.**, neuromuscular j.
**myotendinal j.**, the region where muscle fibers and the collagen of their associated tendons connect and interdigitate.
**neuromuscular j.**, the site of apposition of a motor end plate and the subneural cleft of the skeletal muscle fiber that it innervates. After the nerve is excited, the excitatory neurotransmitter acetylcholine is released from the axon terminal when the nerve is excited, diffuses across the synaptic cleft, and reversibly binds to receptor molecules on the muscle fiber surface, causing the initiation of an action potential that propagates along the muscle fiber and causes it to contract. Called also *myoneural j.*
**occluding j.**, tight j.
**osseous j's**, *articulationes.*

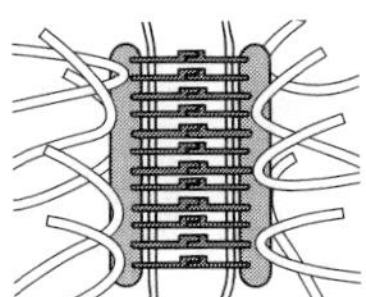

Adherent junction as exemplified by a desmosome.

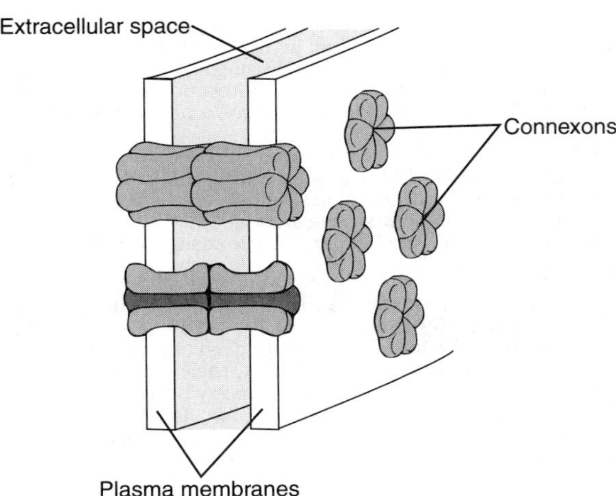


Gap junctions providing passageways between the interiors of adjacent cells.

**pharyngoesophageal j.**, the area where the esophagus and pharynx meet and the pharyngoesophageal sphincter is located.
**sclerocorneal j.**, limbus corneae.
**tendinous j's**, connexus intertendinei.
**tight j.**, 1. an intercellular junction at which adjacent plasma membranes are joined tightly together, separated by only 1 to 2 nm; these junctions variably occlude the intercellular space and limit or eliminate the intercellular passage of molecules. 2. zonula occludens.
**ureteropelvic j.**, junction of the ureter and the kidney at the pelvis of the kidney.
**ureterovesical j.**, the junction of the bladder and ureter; called also *ureterotrigonal complex.*

**junc·tion·al** (junk'shən-əl) pertaining to a junction.

**junc·tu·ra** (junk-too'rə) pl. *junctu'rae* [L. "a joining"] 1. junction. 2. (pl.) juncturae ossium.
**j. cartilagi'nea** [TA], cartilaginous joint: a type of synarthrosis in which the union of the bony elements is by intervening cartilage; the two types are *synchondrosis* and *symphysis.*
**junctu'rae cin'guli mem'bri inferio'ris**, articulationes cinguli membri inferioris.
**junctu'rae cin'guli mem'bri superio'ris**, articulationes cinguli membri superioris.
**junctu'rae cin'guli pectora'lis** [TA], joints of shoulder girdle: the acromioclavicular and sternoclavicular joints; called also *juncturae membri superioris* [TA alternative].
**junctu'rae cin'guli pel'vici** [TA], joints of pelvic girdle: the sacroiliac articulation and the symphysis pubica; called also *juncturae cinguli membri inferioris* [TA alternative].
**junctu'rae colum'nae vertebra'lis** [TA], the joints of the vertebral column, including the syndesmoses and the synovial joints *(articulationes columnae vertebrales).*
**junctu'rae cra'nii** [TA], joints of skull: junctions between bones of the skull or between skull bones and other bones. Most are sutures; there are a few syndesmoses; and the cranial synovial joints are the temporomandibular and atlanto-occipital joints.
**j. fibro'sa** [TA], fibrous joint: a type of synarthrosis in which the union of bony elements is by continuous intervening fibrous tissue, which makes little motion possible; the three types are the *sutura, syndesmosis,* and *gomphosis.*
**j. lumbosacra'lis**, articulatio lumbosacralis.
**junctu'rae mem'bri inferio'ris** [TA], joints of lower limb: the joints of the free lower limb and those of the pelvic girdle considered together.
**junctu'rae mem'bri inferio'ris li'beri** [TA], joints of free lower limb: the synovial joints and syndesmoses of the thigh, leg, and foot. See also *articulationes membri inferioris liberi,* under *articulatio.*
**junctu'rae mem'bri superio'ris** [TA], joints of upper limb: the joints of the free upper limb and those of the pectoral girdle considered together.
**junctu'rae mem'bri superio'ris li'beri,** joints of free upper limb: the synovial joints and syndesmoses of the arm, forearm, and hand. See also *articulationes membri superioris liberi,* under *articulatio.*
**j. os'sea** [TA], a union between adjacent bones or parts of a single bone formed by osseous material, such as ossified connecting cartilage or fibrous tissue. Called also *synostosis* [TA alternative].
**junctu'rae os'sium** [TA], bony joints: the places of junction between two or more bones of the skeleton. Called also *juncturae* and *osseous joints.*
**j. sacrococcy'gea,** articulatio sacrococcygea.

**j. synovia'lis,** synovial joint: a specialized joint permitting more or less free movement, the union of the bony elements being surrounded by an articular capsule enclosing a cavity lined by synovial membrane; called also *diarthrosis* [TA alternative], *diarthrodial joint, articulatio* [TA alternative], and *synovial articulations.* See illustration under *joint.*
**junctu'rae ten'dinum,** connexus intertendinei.
**junctu'rae tho'racis** [TA], thoracic joints: the joints of the thorax considered as a group, including syndesmoses, synchondroses, and the thoracic synovial joints *(articulationes thoracis).*
**junctu'rae zygapophysea'les,** articulationes zygapophyseales.

**junc·tu·rae** (junk-too're) [L.] genitive and plural of *junctura.*

**Jung** (yoong) Carl Gustav. Swiss psychiatrist and philosopher, 1875–1961. Originally a follower of Freud, Jung soon broke with Freud to become the founder of analytic psychology, hypothesizing two major aspects to the unconscious, the personal or individual and the collective. The striving for harmony between the conscious and the unconscious is seen to be an important lifelong task. Jung introduced new concepts such as *introvert, extrovert, anima,* and *animus,* and expanded ones that Freud had stressed, such as *libido* and *ego.*

**Jung's muscle** (yoongz) [Karl Gustav *Jung,* Swiss anatomist, 1794–1864] musculus pyramidalis auriculae.

**Jung·bluth's vasa propria (vessels)** (yoong'bl o͞o ts) [Hermann *Jungbluth,* German physician, 20th century] see *vasa propria of Jungbluth,* under *vas.*

**ju·ni·per** (joo'nĭ-pər) [MeSH: Juniper] any tree or shrub of the genus *Juniperus.*

**Ju·nip·er·us** (joo-nip'ər-əs) a genus of evergreen coniferous trees and shrubs of the family Cupressaceae. *J. commu'nis* L. is the juniper tree, which yields juniper oil. *J. oxyce'drus* is the cade tree, a European species that is the source of juniper tar. *J. sabi'na* L. is the shrub called savin, source of savin oil. *J. virginia'na* is the red cedar, source of cedarwood oil.

**jur·is·pru·dence** (jo͞or"is-proo'dəns) [L. *juris prudentia* knowledge of law] [MeSH: Jurisprudence] the scientific study or application of the principles of law and justice.
**dental j.,** the application of the principles of law and justice as they relate to the practice of dentistry, to the obligations of the practitioner to his patient, and to the relations of dentists to each other and to society in general. This term and *forensic dentistry* are sometimes used as synonyms, but some authorities consider the first a branch of law and the second a branch of dentistry. See also *medical j.* and *forensic dentistry.*
**medical j.,** the application of the principles of law as they relate to the practice of medicine, to the obligations of the practitioner to his patient, and to the relations of physicians to each other and to society in general. This term and *forensic medicine* are sometimes used as synonyms, but some authorities consider the first a branch of law and the second a branch of medicine.

**juscul.** abbreviation for L. *jus'culum,* soup or broth.

**jus·to ma·jor** (jus'to ma'jor) see *pelvis justo major.*

**jus·to mi·nor** (jus'to mi'nor) see *pelvis justo minor.*

**ju·ve·nile** (joo'və-nīl) 1. pertaining to youth or childhood; young or immature. 2. a youth or child; a young animal. 3. a cell or organism intermediate between the immature form and the mature form.

**juxta-** [L. *juxta* near, close by] a combining form meaning situated near or adjoining.

**jux·ta·ar·tic·u·lar** (juks"tə-ahr-tik'u-lər) periarticular.

**jux·ta·ep·i·phys·e·al** (juks"tə-ep-ĭ-fiz'e-əl) [*juxta-* + *epiphyseal*] near to or adjoining an epiphysis.

**jux·ta·glo·mer·u·lar** (juks"tə-glo-mer'u-lər) [*juxta-* + *glomerular*] near to or adjoining a glomerulus of the kidney, as juxtaglomerular cells.

**jux·tal·lo·cor·tex** (juk-stal"o-kor'teks) [*juxta-* + *allocortex*] mesocortex.

**jux·ta·po·si·tion** (juks"tə-pə-zish'ən) [*juxta-* + L. *positio* place] apposition.

**jux·ta·py·lor·ic** (juks"tə-pi-lor'ik) peripyloric.

**jux·ta·spi·nal** (juks-tə-spi'nəl) paravertebral.

**jux·ta·ves·i·cal** (juks"tə-ves'ĭ-kəl) perivesical.

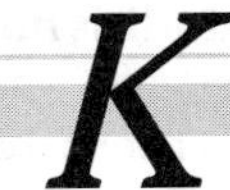

**K** symbol for *potassium* [L. *kalium*] and *kelvin*.

***K*** equilibrium constant (subscripts may be used to denote the method of measurement, e.g., $K_c$, $K_p$; see *equilibrium constant* under *constant*).

**$K_a$** symbol for *acid dissociation constant*.

**$K_b$** symbol for *base dissociation constant*.

**$K_d$** symbol for *dissociation constant*.

**$K_{eq}$** symbol for *equilibrium constant*.

**$K_M$, $K_m$** symbol for *Michaelis' constant*.

**$K_{sp}$** symbol for *solubility product constant*.

**$K_w$** symbol for the *ion product of water;* see *ion product* under *product*.

**k** symbol for *kilo-*.

***k*** symbol for *Boltzmann's constant* and *rate constant*.

**κ** kappa, the tenth letter of the Greek alphabet; symbol for *dielectric constant* and for one of the two types of immunoglobulin light chains (see *immunoglobulin*).

**Kab·i·ki·nase** (kab″ĭ-ki′nās) trademark for preparations of streptokinase.

**ka·bu·re** (kah-boo′re) a skin disease in Japan, probably caused by the burrowing of the cercariae of *Schistosoma japonica* in the skin.

**Ka·der's operation** (kah′dərz) [Bronislaw *Kader*, Polish surgeon, 1863–1937] see under *operation*.

**Ka·di·an** (ka′de-ən) trademark for a preparation of morphine sulfate.

**Kaes' feltwork (line)** (kāz) [Theodor *Kaes*, German neurologist, 1852–1913] Kaes-Bekhterev layer; see under *layer*.

**Kaes-Bekh·ter·ev layer** (kāz-bek-tār′yev) [Theodor *Kaes;* Vladimir Mikhailovich *Bekhterev*, Russian neurologist, 1857–1927] see under *layer*.

**KAFO** knee-ankle-foot orthosis.

**Ka·fo·cin** (ka-fo′sin) trademark for a preparation of cephaloglycin.

**Kah·ler's law** (kah′lərz) [Otto *Kahler*, German physician, 1849–1893] see under *law*.

**kain(o)-** see *cen(o)-* (def. 1).

**kain·ic ac·id** (kān′ik) [MeSH: Kainic Acid] an excitotoxin found in the seaweed *Diginea simplex;* it is 30 to 100 times as potent as glutamic acid and is used experimentally to study the excitatory mechanisms of glutamate transmitters.

**Kai·ser·ling's method, solution (fixative)** (ki′zər-lingz) [Karl *Kaiserling*, German pathologist, 1869–1942] see under *method* and *solution*.

**kai·ser·ling** (ki′zər-ling) 1. Kaiserling's solution. 2. a specimen preserved in Kaiserling's solution.

**Kai·ser·stuhl disease** (ki′zər-shto͞ol″) [*Kaiserstuhl* region in Germany, where the disease occurred] see under *disease*.

**kak-** for words beginning thus, see also those beginning *cac-*.

**kak·o·dyl** (kak′o-dil) cacodyl.

**kak·os·mia** (kak-oz′me-ə) cacosmia.

**kak·ot·ro·phy** (kak-ot′rə-fe) cacotrophy.

**ka·la-azar** (kah′lah-ah-zahr′) [Hindi, "black fever"] visceral leishmaniasis.

**kal·a·da·na** (kal″ə-da′nə) the dried seeds of *Ipomoea nil* L.; used in India and China for its purgative and anthelmintic properties.

**ka·la·fun·gin** (ka″lə-fun′jin) an antifungal antibiotic substance produced by *Streptomyces tanashiensis* strain *kala*.

**ka·la·gua** (kə-lah′gwə) a drug used in South America in the treatment of tuberculosis.

**ka·le·mia** (kə-le′me-ə) [*kalium* + *-emia*] the presence of potassium in the blood; see *hyperkalemia*.

**ka·li·e·mia** (ka″le-e′me-ə) kalemia.

**ka·lim·e·ter** (kə-lim′ə-tər) alkalimeter.

**ka·lio·pe·nia** (ka″le-o-pe′ne-ə) [*kalium* + *-penia*] hypokalemia.

**ka·lio·pe·nic** (ka″le-o-pe′nik) hypokalemic (def. 1).

**ka·li·um** (ka′le-əm) gen. *ka′lii* [L., from Ar. *gily* saltwort] potassium.

**ka·li·ure·sis** (ka″le-u-re′sis) [*kalium* + *-uresis*] the excretion of potassium in the urine.

**ka·li·uret·ic** (ka″le-u-ret′ik) 1. pertaining to, characterized by, or promoting kaliuresis. 2. an agent that promotes kaliuresis.

**kal·lak** (kal′ak) [Eskimo for disease of the skin] a pustular dermatitis occurring in the Eskimos.

**kal·li·din** (kal′ĭ-din) [MeSH: Kallidin] lysyl-bradykinin, a decapeptide kinin produced by the action of tissue and glandular kallikreins on low-molecular-weight (LMW) kininogen and having physiologic effects similar to those of bradykinin. Formerly the term was applied to both nona- and decapeptides; bradykinin was called *kallidin I* or *kallidin-9*, and lysyl-bradykinin was called *kallidin II* or *kallidin-10*.

**Kal·li·kak** (kal′ĭ-kak) [Gr. *kallos* beauty + *kakos* bad] fictitious name of a New Jersey family, described by the American sociologist H. H. Goddard, having two branches, one consisting of highly intelligent and successful individuals, the other exhibiting a high incidence of mental deficiency, immorality, and criminality; used to advance the theory that these traits are genetically determined.

**kal·li·kre·in** (kal″ĭ-kre′in) [MeSH: Kallikrein] any of several serine proteinases that cleave kininogens to form kinins (bradykinin, kallidin).

**plasma k.** [EC 3.4.21.34], a plasma enzyme of the hydrolase class that cleaves HMW kininogen to produce bradykinin; it also activates blood coagulation factors XII and VII and plasminogen. It is formed from prekallikrein by activated coagulation factor XII.

**tissue k.** [EC 3.4.21.35], an enzyme of the hydrolase class that cleaves LMW kininogen to produce kallidin. It and closely related forms are found in tissues and various glandular secretions including lymph, pancreatic juice, urine, and saliva.

**kal·li·kre·in·o·gen** (kal″ĭ-kre-in′ə-jən) prekallikrein.

**Kall·mann's syndrome** (kahl′mahnz) [Franz Josef *Kallmann*, German-born American psychiatrist, 1897–1965] hypogonadotropic eunuchoidism; see under *eunuchoidism*.

**Kal·mia** (kal′me-ə) a genus of shrubs of the family Ericaceae, whose leaves have been used to treat syphilis, diarrhea, and chronic inflammatory disorders, and are thought to possess cardiac and sedative properties. *K. latifo′lia* L. is mountain laurel; it and related species contain andromedotoxin and are poisonous to livestock.

**kal·ure·sis** (kal″u-re′sis) kaliuresis.

**kal·uret·ic** (kal″u-ret′ik) kaliuretic.

**ka·ma·la** (kah′mə-lə) 1. *Mallotus philippinensis*. 2. the glands and hairs of the capsules of *M. philippinensis*, used as a purgative and in veterinary medicine as a teniacide. Called also *rottlera*.

**Kam·bin's triangular working zone** (kam′binz) [Parviz *Kambin*, Iranian-born American orthopedist, born 1931] see under *zone*.

**Kam·mer·er-Bat·tle incision** (kam′ər-ər bat′əl) [Frederic *Kammerer*, American surgeon, 1856–1928; William Henry *Battle*, British surgeon, 1855–1936] see under *incision*.

**kan·a·my·cin** (kan″ə-mi′sin) [MeSH: Kanamycin] an aminoglycoside antibiotic complex derived from *Streptomyces kanamyceticus*, consisting of three components, designated A, B, and C. The form in clinical use is a mixture of kanamycins A and B; it is effective against aerobic gram-negative bacilli and some gram-positive bacteria, including mycobacteria, although its use is now limited because of the emergence of resistant strains.

**k. sulfate** [USP], the sulfate salt of kanamycin, administered intravenously, intramuscularly, and by inhalation and intraperitoneal infusion in the treatment of a wide variety of infections caused by susceptible gram-negative organisms and orally to suppress bowel flora in the adjunctive treatment of hepatic coma and in preoperative bowel preparation.

**Kan·a·vel's sign** (kə-na′vəlz) [Allen Buchner *Kanavel*, American surgeon, 1874–1938] see under *sign*.

**Kan·ner's syndrome** (kah′nərz) [Leo *Kanner*, Austrian-born American child psychiatrist, 1894–1981] autistic disorder.

**Kan·tor's sign** (kan′tərz) [John Leonard *Kantor*, American radiologist, 1890–1947] see under *sign*.

**Kan·trex** (kan′treks) trademark for preparations of kanamycin sulfate.

**kan·y·em·ba** (kan″e-em′bəh) an acute rectitis of unknown cause, reported from South America and Zambia.

**Ka·o·chlor** (ka′o-klor) trademark for a preparation of potassium chloride.

**ka·o·lin** (ka′o-lin) [*Kao-Ling* or *Gao-Ling*, city in southeastern China where it was first found] [MeSH: Kaolin] 1. a type of hydrated aluminum silicate, found in the form of clay and purified to form the medicinal product. Called also *argilla, bolus alba*, and *China clay*. 2. [USP] kaolin that has been purified and pulverized to form a white or light yellow powder with a claylike taste, used as an adsorbent and in *kaolin mixture with pectin* (see under *mixture*).

**ka·o·lin·o·sis** (ka″o-lin-o′sis) kaolin pneumoconiosis.

**Ka·on** (ka′on) trademark for preparations of potassium gluconate.

**Kap·lan-Mei·er survival curve, method** (kap′lən-mi′ər) [E. L. *Kaplan,* American statistician, 20th century; Paul *Meier,* American statistician, 20th century] see under *curve* and *method.*

**Ka·po·si's sarcoma, varicelliform eruption** (kah′po-shēz, kap′o-sēz) [Moritz *Kaposi* (Moritz Kaposi Kohn), Austrian dermatologist, 1837–1902] see under *eruption* and *sarcoma.*

**kap·pa** (kap′ə) [K, κ] 1. the tenth letter of the Greek alphabet. 2. a statistic calculated to quantify the extent to which agreement between observers exceeds that expected on the basis of chance alone.

**Kap·pa·di·one** (kap″ə-di′ōn) trademark for a preparation of menadiol sodium diphosphate.

**ka·ra·kurt** (kah′rah-koort″) *Latrodectus lugubris,* a venomous Russian spider.

**ka·ra·ya** (kah′rah-yə) see under *gum.*

**Kar·nof·sky scale** (kahr-nof′ske) [David A. *Karnofsky,* American clinical oncologist, 1914–1969] see under *scale.*

**Kar·plus' sign** (kahr′ploos) [Johann Paul *Karplus,* Austrian physician and physiologist, 1866–1936] see under *sign.*

**Kar·ta·gen·er's syndrome (triad)** (kahr-tag′ə-nərz) [Manes *Kartagener,* Swiss physician, 1897–1975] see under *syndrome.*

**Kar·win·skia** (kahr-win′ske-ə) a genus of shrubs of the family Rhamnaceae, found mostly in the southwestern United States and Mexico. *K. humboldtia′na* is the buckthorn or coyotillo, a shrub whose fruit causes buckthorn poisoning in humans and other animals.

**kary·ap·sis** (kar″e-ap′sis) [*karyo-* + Gr. *hapsis* joining] union of nuclei in a conjugating cell.

**kary·en·chy·ma** (kar″e-en′kə-mə) [*karyo-* + *enchyma*] karyolymph.

**kary(o)-** [Gr. *karyon* nut, kernel] a combining form denoting relationship to a nucleus; see also words beginning *cary(o)-.*

**karyo·chrome** (kar′e-o-krōm″) [*karyo-* + *-chrome*] a nerve cell whose nucleus is deeply stainable while its body is not; called also *karyochrome cell* and *caryochrome.*

**karyo·chy·le·ma** (kar″e-o-ki-le′mə) karyolymph.

**kary·oc·la·sis** (kar″e-ok′lə-sis) karyoklasis.

**karyo·clas·tic** (kar″e-o-klas′tik) karyoklastic.

**karyo·cyte** (kar′e-o-sīt) [*karyo-* + *-cyte*] a nucleated cell.

**karyo·gam·ic** (kar″e-o-gam′ik) [*karyo-* + Gr. *gamos* marriage] pertaining to or characterized by union of nuclei.

**kary·og·a·my** (kar″e-og′ə-me) [*karyo-* + Gr. *gamos* marriage] the union of the nuclei of cells following plasmogamy in fertilization.

**karyo·gen·e·sis** (kar″e-o-jen′ə-sis) [*karyo-* + *-genesis*] the development of the nucleus of a cell.

**kar·y·o·gen·ic** (kar″e-o-jen′ik) forming the nucleus of a cell; pertaining to karyogenesis.

**karyo·ki·ne·sis** (kar″e-o-kĭ-ne′sis) [*karyo-* + *-kinesis*] the phenomena involved in division of the nucleus, usually an early stage in the process of cell division, or mitosis.
**asymmetrical k.,** mitosis in which the chromosomes divide unequally and into dissimilar masses.
**hyperchromatic k.,** mitosis in which the number of chromosomes is abnormally large.
**hypochromatic k.,** mitosis in which the number of chromosomes is abnormally small.

**karyo·ki·net·ic** (kar″e-o-kĭ-net′ik) pertaining to or of the nature of karyokinesis.

**kary·ok·la·sis** (kar″e-ok′lə-sis) [*karyo-* + Gr. *klasis* breaking] the breaking down of the cell nucleus or nuclear membrane.

**karyo·klas·tic** (kar″e-o-klas′tik) 1. breaking down cell nuclei. 2. arresting mitosis.

**karyo·lymph** (kar′e-o-limf″) [*karyo-* + *lymph*] the liquid part of a cell nucleus, as contrasted with the chromatin and linin.

**kary·ol·y·sis** (kar″e-ol′ə-sis) [*karyo-* + *-lysis*] a form of necrobiosis in which the nucleus of a cell swells and gradually loses its chromatin.

**karyo·lyt·ic** (kar″e-o-lit′ik) 1. producing or pertaining to karyolysis. 2. destroying cell nuclei.

**karyo·mas·ti·gont** (kar″e-o-mas′tĭ-gont) [*karyo-* + *mastigont*] a condition characteristic of certain flagellate protozoa in which the mastigont system is associated with a nucleus. Cf. *akaryomastigont.*

**karyo·meg·a·ly** (kar″e-o-meg′ə-le) [*karyo-* + *-megaly*] abnormal enlargement of the nucleus of a cell, not caused by polyploidy.

**karyo·mere** (kar′e-o-mēr″) 1. chromomere (def. 1). 2. a vesicle containing only a small portion of the typical nucleus, usually following abnormal mitosis.

**kary·om·e·try** (kar″e-om′ə-tre) [*karyo-* + *-metry*] [MeSH: Karyometry] measurement of a cell nucleus.

**karyo·mi·cro·some** (kar″e-o-mi′kro-sōm) [*karyo-* + *microsome*] nucleomicrosome.

**karyo·mi·to·sis** (kar″e-o-mi-to′sis) division of the nucleus of a cell preceding mitosis.

**karyo·mi·tot·ic** (kar″e-o-mi-tot′ik) pertaining to karyomitosis.

**karyo·mor·phism** (kar″e-o-mor′fiz-əm) [*karyo-* + *morph-* + *-ism*] the shape of a cell nucleus.

**kary·on** (kar′e-on) [Gr. *karyon* nucleus] nucleus (def. 2).

**karyo·phage** (kar′e-o-fāj″) [*karyo-* + *-phage*] a protozoan that exercises phagocytic action on the nucleus of the cell it infects.

**karyo·plasm** (kar′e-o-plaz″əm) [*karyo-* + *-plasm*] the nucleoplasm, or protoplasm of the nucleus of a cell.

**karyo·plas·mic** (kar″e-o-plaz′mik) pertaining to karyoplasm.

**karyo·plast** (kar′e-o-plast) nucleus (def. 2).

**karyo·plas·tin** (kar″e-o-plas′tin) the substance of a mitotic spindle; the parachromatin.

**karyo·pyk·no·sis** (kar″e-o-pik-no′sis) shrinkage of a cell nucleus, with condensation of the chromatin into a solid, structureless mass or masses.

**karyo·pyk·not·ic** (kar″e-o-pik-not′ik) pertaining to, characterized by, or causing karyopyknosis.

**karyo·re·tic·u·lum** (kar″e-o-rə-tik′u-ləm) [*karyo-* + *reticulum*] the fibrillar part of the karyoplasm as distinguished from the fluid part of karyolymph.

**kary·or·rhec·tic** (kar″e-o-rek′tik) pertaining to, characterized by, or causing karyorrhexis.

**kary·or·rhex·is** (kar″e-o-rek′sis) [*karyo-* + *-rrhexis*] rupture of the cell nucleus in which the chromatin disintegrates into formless granules which are extruded from the cell.

**karyo·some** (kar′e-o-sōm″) [*karyo-* + *-some*] any of the condensed irregular clumps of chromatin dispersed in the chromatin network of a cell; called also *false nucleolus, chromatin nucleolus, chromatin reservoir,* and *chromocenter.*

**karyo·sta·sis** (kar″e-os′tə-sis) [*karyo-* + *-stasis*] the so-called resting stage of the nucleus between mitotic divisions.

**karyo·the·ca** (kar″e-o-the′kə) [*karyo-* + *theca*] nuclear membrane.

**karyo·tin** (kar′e-o-tin) chromatin.

**karyo·type** (kar′e-o-tīp) [*karyo-* + *type*] the full chromosome set of the nucleus of a cell; by extension, the photomicrograph of chromosomes arranged according to a standard classification. Cf. *idiogram,* and see illustration accompanying *chromosome.*

**karyo·typ·ic** (kar″e-o-tip′ik) pertaining to or representative of the karyotype.

**karyo·zo·ic** (kar″e-o-zo′ik) [*karyo-* + Gr. *zōon* animal] existing in or inhabiting the nuclei of cells, as do certain protozoa.

**Kas·a·bach-Mer·ritt syndrome** (kas′ə-bahk-mer′it) [Haig Haigouni *Kasabach,* American physician, 1898–1943; Katharine Krom *Merritt,* American pediatrician, 20th century] see under *syndrome.*

**Ka·sai operation** (kah-si′) [Morio *Kasai,* Japanese surgeon, 20th century] portoenterostomy.

**ka·sal** (ka′sal) chemical name: basic sodium aluminum phosphate; a food additive, with about 30 per cent dibasic sodium phosphate.

**Kas·chin-Beck disease** (kah′shēn-bek) see *Kashin-Bek disease.*

**Kash·in-Bek disease** (kah′shēn-bek) [Nikolai Ivanovich *Kashin* (or *Kaschin*), Russian orthopedist, 1825–1872; E. V. *Bek* (or *Beck*), Russian physician, early 20th century] see under *disease.*

**Kast's syndrome** (kahsts) [Alfred *Kast,* German physician, 1856–1903] Maffucci's syndrome.

**kat** symbol for *katal.*

**kat(a)-** [Gr. *kata* down] a prefix meaning down, lower, under, against, along with, very. For words beginning thus, see also those beginning *cat(a)-.*

**ka·ta** (kah′tə) peste des petits ruminants.

**kata·did·y·mus** (kat″ə-did′ə-məs) [*kata-* + *-didymus*] conjoined twins divided superiorly, but single toward the podalic pole. See also *dicephalus.*

**kat·al** (kat'əl) a unit of measurement proposed to express activities of all catalysts, including enzymes, being that amount of a catalyst, such as an enzyme, which catalyzes a reaction rate of 1 mole of substrate per second. Symbol kat.

**kata·ther·mom·e·ter** (kat″ə-thər-mom'ə-tər) a pair of alcoholic thermometers, one with a dry bulb and one with a wet bulb. They are heated to 110°F and exposed to the air, and the time is noted that it takes each bulb to fall from 100° to 90°F. From this the temperature as it affects the body can be deduced.

**Ka·ta·ya·ma** (kah-tah-yah'mə) *Oncomelania.*

**Ka·ta·ya·ma fever (disease)** (kah-tah-yah'mah) [*Katayama* River Valley, Japan, where it was first reported in the 19th century] see under *fever.*

**kath·a·rom·e·ter** (kath″ə-rom'ə-tər) an instrument for electrometric determination of basal metabolic rates.

**kath·iso·pho·bia** (kath″ĭ-so-fo'be-ə) intense, irrational fear of sitting down.

**Kath·on** (kath'on) trademark for preparations of methylisothiazolinone and methylchloroisothiazolinone.

**ka·tine** (ka'tin) an alkaloid from *Catha edulis* Forsk. (Celastraceae); but its actions on the nervous system are similar to those of cocaine, it has no local anesthetic properties, and is used as an appetite depressant and mild euphoriant. The leaves are used as tea and masticatory in Ethiopia, East and South Africa, and Yemen.

**ka·tol·y·sis** (kə-tol'ə-sis) [Gr. *katō* below + *-lysis*] the incomplete or intermediate conversion of complex chemical bodies into simpler compounds; applied especially to digestive processes.

**kato·pho·ria** (kat″ə-for'e-ə) cataphoria.

**kato·tro·pia** (kat″ə-tro'pe-ə) cataphoria.

**Katz** (kats) Sir Bernard. German-born British physiologist, born 1911; co-winner, with Julius Axelrod and Ulf Svante von Euler, of the Nobel prize for medicine or physiology in 1970 for his discovery of the manner of electrical impulse transmission from nerves to muscles.

**Kauff·mann-White classification** (kouf'mahn-hwīt) [Fritz *Kauffmann,* German microbiologist, 20th century; P.B. *White,* British microbiologist, 20th century] see under *classification.*

**Kauf·man-Mc·Ku·sick syndrome** (kouf'man-mə-ku'sik) [Robert Lionel *Kaufman,* American physician, born 1937; Victor Almon *McKusick,* American geneticist, born 1921] see under *syndrome.*

**Ka·wa·sa·ki disease** (kah″wah-sah'ke) [Tomisaku *Kawasaki,* Japanese pediatrician, 20th century] mucocutaneous lymph node syndrome.

**Kay Ciel** (ka'sē-el') trademark for preparations of potassium chloride.

**Kay·ex·a·late** (ka-ek'sə-lāt) trademark for a preparation of sodium polystyrene sulfonate.

**Kay·ser-Flei·scher ring** (ki'zər-fli'shər) [Bernhard *Kayser,* German ophthalmologist, 1869–1954; Bruno Richard *Fleischer,* German physician, 1848–1904] see under *ring.*

**Ka·zan·ji·an forceps, operation** (kah-zahn'je-ən) [Varaztad Hovhannes *Kazanjian,* Armenian-born plastic and maxillofacial surgeon in United States, 1879–1974] see under *forceps* and *operation.*

**kb** in genetics, kilobase (1000 bases); sometimes used incorrectly to denote kilobase pairs in double-stranded nucleic acid.

**kbp** in genetics, kilobase pairs (1000 base pairs in a nucleic acid).

**kcal** symbol for *kilocalorie.*

**kCi** kilocurie.

**kcps** kilocycles per second.

**kD, kDa** kilodalton.

**Ke** an antigenic marker distinguishing human immunoglobulin λ light chain subtypes. Called also *Kern.*

**Kearns-Sayre syndrome** (kernz-sār) [Thomas P. *Kearns,* American ophthalmologist, born 1922; George P. *Sayre,* American pathologist, born 1911] see under *syndrome.*

**kebo·ceph·a·ly** (keb″ə-sef'ə-le) cebocephaly.

**ked** (ked) the sheep tick, *Melophagus ovinus.*

**Keen's sign** (kēnz) [William Williams *Keen,* American surgeon, 1837–1932] see under *sign.*

**Kef·lex** (kef'leks) trademark for a preparation of cephalexin.

**Kef·lin** (kef'lin) trademark for a preparation of cephalothin sodium.

**Kef·tab** (kef'tab) trademark for a preparation of cephalexin hydrochloride monohydrate.

**Kef·ur·ox** (kef'oo-roks) trademark for a preparation of cefuroxime sodium.

**Kef·zol** (kef'zol) trademark for a preparation of cefazolin sodium.

**Kehr's sign** (kārz) [Hans *Kehr,* German surgeon, 1862–1916] see under *sign.*

**Kehr·er's reflex** (kār'ərz) [Ferdinand *Kehrer,* German neurologist, 1883–1966] see under *reflex.*

**Keith's node** (kēths) [Sir Arthur *Keith,* Scottish-born anatomist in England, 1866–1955] see *nodus sinuatrialis.*

**Keith-Flack node** (kēth-flak) [Sir Arthur *Keith;* Martin William *Flack,* British physiologist, 1882–1931] nodus sinuatrialis.

**Keith-Wag·en·er-Bar·ker classification** (kēth-wag'ə-nər-bahr'kər) [Norman Macdonnell *Keith,* Canadian physician in United States, born 1885; Henry Patrick *Wagener,* American physician, born 1890; N.W. *Barker,* American physician, 20th century] see under *classification.*

**ke·lec·tome** (ke'lek-tōm) [Gr. *kēlē* tumor + *-ectomy*] a device used in removing specimens of tissue from tumors.

**Kel·ene** (kel'ēn) trademark for a preparation of ethyl chloride.

**Kell blood group** (kel) [from the name of the propositus first observed in 1946] see under *blood group.*

**Kel·ler operation** (kel'ər) [Col. William Lordan *Keller,* American military surgeon, 1874–1959] see under *operation.*

**Kel·lock's sign** (kel'əks) [T.H. *Kellock,* American physician, late 19th century] see under *sign.*

**Kel·ly's operation, sign, speculum** (kel'ēz) [Howard Atwood *Kelly,* American surgeon, 1858–1943] see *Kelly's operation* (def. 1) and see under *sign* and *speculum.*

**ke·loid** (ke'loid) [Gr. *kēlis* blemish + *-oid*] [MeSH: Keloid] a sharply elevated, irregularly-shaped, progressively enlarging scar due to the formation of excessive amounts of collagen in the corium during connective tissue repair.

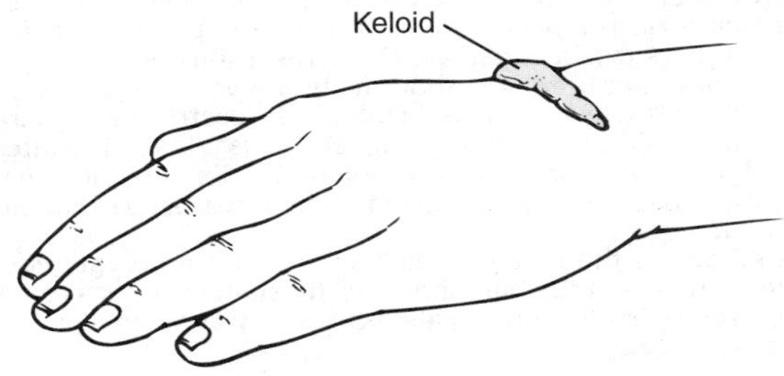


**acne k.,** dermatitis papillaris capillitii.
**k. of gums,** fibromatosis gingivae.

**ke·lo·so·mus** (ke″lo-so'məs) celosomus.

**ke·lot·o·my** (ke-lot'ə-me) [Gr. *kēlē* a rupture + *temnein* to cut] herniotomy.

**Kel·vin scale** (kel'vin) [William Thomson, Lord *Kelvin,* British physicist, 1824–1907] see under *scale.*

**kel·vin** (kel'vin) [after Lord *Kelvin*] the SI unit of thermodynamic temperature equal to 1/273.15 of the absolute temperature of the triple point of water. See also *absolute temperature,* under *temperature,* and *Kelvin scale,* under *scale.* Abbreviated K.

**Kem·a·drin** (kem'ə-drin) trademark for a preparation of procyclidine hydrochloride.

**Ken·a·cort** (ken'ə-kort) trademark for preparations of triamcinolone.

**Ken·a·log** (ken'ə-log) trademark for preparations of triamcinolone acetonide.

**Ken·dall** (ken'dəl) Edward Calvin. American biochemist, 1886–1972; co-winner, with Philip Showalter Hench and Tadeus Reichstein, of the Nobel prize for medicine or physiology in 1950 for his research on the hormones of the adrenal cortex.

**Ken·dall's rank correlation coefficient (tau)** (ken'dəlz) [Maurice George *Kendall,* British statistician, 1907–1983] see under *coefficient.*

**Ken·ne·dy classification** (ken'ə-de) [Edward *Kennedy,* American dentist, born 1883] see under *classification.*

**Ken·ne·dy's syndrome** (ken'ə-dēz) [Robert Foster *Kennedy,* American neurologist, 1884–1952] see under *syndrome.*

**Ken·ny's treatment** (ken'ēz) [Sister Elizabeth *Kenny,* Australian nurse, 1886–1952] see under *treatment.*

**ken(o)-** [Gr. *kenos* empty] a combining form denoting empty; see also words beginning *cen(o)-*.

**ke·no·tox·in** (ke'no-tok"sin) [*keno-* + *toxin*] a hypothetical toxin supposedly produced in muscle by muscular contractions, causing fatigue.

**Kent's bundle** (kents) [Albert Frank Stanley *Kent*, English physiologist, 1863–1958] see under *bundle*.

**Kent-His bundle** (kent-his) [A. F. S. *Kent;* Wilhelm *His,* Jr., Swiss-born physician in Germany, 1863–1934] bundle of His.

**Ke·pone** (ke'pōn) trademark for a preparation of chlordecone.

**Ker·an·del's sign** (ker"ahn-delz') [Jean François *Kerandel,* French physician in Africa, 1873–1934] see under *sign.*

**ker·a·phyl·lo·cele** (ker"ə-fil'o-sēl) [Gr. *keras* horn + *phyllo-* + *-cele*[1]] keratoma, def. 2.

**ker·a·sin** (ker'ə-sin) older name for a glucocerebroside in which the fatty acid is lignoceric acid.

**ker·a·tal·gia** (ker"ə-tal'jə) [*kerat-* + *-algia*] pain in the cornea.

**ker·a·tan sul·fate** (ker'ə-tan) [MeSH: Keratan Sulfate] a glycosaminoglycan found in the cornea, in cartilage, and in the nucleus pulposus and also as the accumulation product in Morquio's syndrome. It consists of repeating disaccharide units in specific linkage, each composed of a sulfated *N*-acetylglucosamine residue linked to one of galactose, which is usually sulfated. There are two forms, *keratan sulfate I* and *keratan sulfate II,* which differ in carbohydrate content and localization; the former occurs in the cornea and the latter in skeletal tissues. Called also *keratosulfate.*

**ker·a·tec·ta·sia** (ker"ə-tek-ta'zhə) [*kerat-* + *ectasia*] protrusion of a thinned, scarred cornea; called also *corneal ectasia.*

**ker·a·tec·to·my** (ker"ə-tek'tə-me) [*kerat-* + *ectomy*] excision of a portion of the cornea, usually done for anterior staphyloma.

**ker·at·ic** (ker-at'ik) 1. pertaining to keratin. 2. horny. 3. pertaining to the cornea.

**ker·a·tin** (ker'ə-tin) [MeSH: Keratin] any of a family of scleroproteins that form the primary constituents of epidermis, hair, nails, and horny tissues. Included are the cytokeratins of epithelial tissue and the hard keratins of ectodermally derived structures such as hair and nails. Because it is insoluble in gastric juice, keratin is sometimes used to coat pills designed to dissolve in the intestine.
**α-k., alpha k.,** keratin in the form of an $\alpha$ helix; it is the usual form for nail and hair keratins and thus is sometimes used synonymously with *hard k.*
**hard k.,** any of the family of high-sulfur keratin polypeptides that are constituents of the hair and nails. It usually occurs as an $\alpha$ helix and therefore is sometimes called *α-k. Cf. cytokeratin.*
**soft k.,** cytokeratin.

**ker·a·tin·ase** (ker'ə-tĭ-nās) an enzyme of the hydrolase class that catalyzes the cleavage keratin, such as occurs in the agent causing ringworm of the foot, *Trichophyton mentagrophytes,* and in *Streptomyces.*

**ker·a·tin·iza·tion** (ker"ə-tin"ĭ-za'shən) the development of or conversion into keratin.

**ker·a·tin·ize** (ker'ə-tin-īz) to make, or become, keratinous.

**ke·rat·i·no·cyte** (kə-rat'ĭ-no-sīt) [MeSH: Keratinocytes] the epidermal cell which synthesizes keratin; constituting 95 per cent of the epidermal cells and, with the melanocyte, forming the binary cell system of the epidermis. In its various successive stages it is known as basal cell, prickle cell, and granular cell. Called also *malpighian cell.*

**ker·a·tin·oid** (ker'ə-tin-oid) a form of keratin-coated tablet not soluble in the stomach, but readily soluble in the intestine.

**ke·rat·i·no·phil·ic** (kə-rat"in-o-fil'ik) keratin-seeking; using keratin as a substrate. Said of fungi.

**ke·rat·i·no·some** (kə-rat'ĭ-no-sōm") [*keratin* + *-some*] one of the spherical granules that are formed in the upper spinous and granula layers of the skin near the Golgi apparatus and migrate into the cytoplasm, ultimately fusing with the plasma membrane to discharge their contents (bipolar phospholipids, glycoproteins, and acid phosphates) into the intracellular space; this extruded material is thought to function as a barrier to penetration by foreign substances. Called also *lamellar granule* or *body, membrane-coating granule,* and *Odland body.*

**ke·rat·i·nous** (kə-rat'ĭ-nəs) containing or of the nature of keratin.

**ker·a·ti·tis** (ker"ə-ti'tis) [*kerat-* + *-itis*] [MeSH: Keratitis] inflammation of the cornea. Cf. *keratoconjunctivitis* and *keratopathy.*
***Acanthamoeba* k.,** keratitis due to infection by *Acanthamoeba* spp.; it is usually associated with soft contact lens wear, particularly overnight wear.
**acne rosacea k.,** rosacea k.
**actinic k.,** a form due to the action of ultraviolet light.
**aerosol k.,** keratitis following direct exposure of the eye to chemical sprays from aerosol cans.
**alphabet k.,** striate k.
**anaphylactic k.,** interstitial keratitis in one eye, caused by an antibody-antigen reaction to an intracorneal injection of protein in the eye after sensitization from intracorneal injection of protein into the other eye.
**annular k.,** marginal k.
**k. arbores'cens,** dendriform k.
**artificial silk k.,** keratitis occurring among workers in artificial silk manufacture; it is marked by blurring of vision with the appearance of haloes around lights.
**aspergillus k.,** keratitis due to infection from the *Aspergillus* fungus.
**band k., band-shaped k., k. bandelette,** ribbon-like k.
**k. bullo'sa,** the formation of large or small bullae or blebs upon the cornea.
**catarrhal ulcerative k.,** a mild form of keratitis secondary to conjunctivitis.
**chronic superficial k.,** bilateral cellular infiltration and vascularization of the corneas in dogs, usually beginning at the lateral corner and progressing towards the middle so that the cornea becomes pigmented. Since it is limited to German shepherds and a few other breeds, a genetic component is suspected. Called also *degenerative pannus* and *Uberreiter's syndrome.*
**deep k.,** interstitial k.
**deep pustular k.,** k. pustuliformis profunda.
**dendriform k., dendritic k.,** herpetic keratitis resulting in a branching ulceration of the cornea.
**desiccation k.,** lagophthalmic k.
**Dimmer's k.,** k. nummularis.
**disciform k., k. discifor'mis,** keratitis with the formation of a round or oval, disklike opacity of the cornea.
**eosinophilic k.,** neovascularization and cellular infiltration of the cornea of cats, with formation of an area of pink to white soft plaque beginning at a limbus and progressing towards the center.
**epithelial diffuse k.,** keratitis possibly due to vitamin $B_2$ deficiency, generally associated with uveitis, and characterized by minute gray epithelial flecks.
**epithelial punctate k.,** superficial punctate k.
**exfoliative k.,** keratitis that may occur with exfoliative dermatitis in a hypersensitive reaction to arsenic and marked by extensive denudation of the corneal epithelium.
**exposure k.,** lagophthalmic k.
**fascicular k.,** keratitis attended by the formation of a band of blood vessels.
**k. filamento'sa,** keratitis with twisted filaments of mucoid material on the surface of the cornea; called also *filamentary keratopathy.*
**furrow k.,** dendriform k.
**herpetic k.,** 1. keratitis, commonly with dendritic ulceration *(dendriform* or *dendritic k.),* due to infection with herpes simplex virus. 2. keratitis occurring in herpes zoster ophthalmicus.
**hypopyon k.,** suppurative keratitis associated with purulent infiltration and hypopyon; see *ulcus serpens corneae.*
**infectious bovine k.,** see under *keratoconjunctivitis.*
**interstitial k.,** chronic keratitis with deep deposits in the substance of the cornea, which becomes hazy with a ground-glass appearance. It usually occurs in children under age 15, associated with congenital syphilis. See also *nonsyphilitic interstitial k.* Called also *parenchymatous k., deep k.,* and *k. profunda.*
**interstitial k., nonsyphilitic,** interstitial keratitis not associated with congenital syphilis; see *Cogan's syndrome.*
**lagophthalmic k.,** that which accompanies lagophthalmos; it is due to exposure of the eyeball to the air.
**lattice k.,** bilateral hereditary dystrophy of the cornea with the formation of interwoven filamentous lesions.
**marginal k.,** phlyctenular keratitis in which the papules are arranged around the margin of the cornea; called also *annular k.*
**metaherpetic k.,** keratitis occurring as a result of recurrent herpesvirus infection of the cornea, characterized by shallow ulceration of an anesthetic cornea, accompanied by parenchymatous infiltration and often by persistent iridocyclitis and secondary glaucoma.
**microbial k.,** keratitis resulting from bacterial or fungal infection of the cornea; it is usually associated with soft contact lens wear.
**mycotic k.,** keratomycosis.
**neuroparalytic k.,** keratitis characterized by dryness and fissuring of the corneal epithelium as a result of an injury to the trifacial nerve which prevents proper closing of the eyelids; called also *trophic k.*
**neurotrophic k.,** keratitis due to loss of corneal sensation.
**k. nummula'ris,** a slowly developing benign type of keratitis marked by corneal deposits forming circular areas with sharply defined edges surrounded by a halo of less dense character; called also *Dimmer's k.*
**parenchymatous k.,** interstitial k.
**peripheral ulcerative k.,** a rare type of inflammation of the limbal part of the cornea and nearby sclera, which have cellular infiltration, vascular changes, and ulceration that may cause blindness; it

may be a complication of rheumatoid arthritis or a bacterial infection but sometimes is idiopathic.

**k. petri'ficans,** keratitis with calcareous changes.

**phlyctenular k.,** see under *keratoconjunctivitis.*

**k. profun'da,** interstitial k.

**k. puncta'ta, punctate k.,** an old term for the formation of cellular and fibrinous deposits (keratic precipitates) on the posterior surface of the cornea, occurring after injury or iridocyclitis and giving an appearance of fine drops of dew.

**k. puncta'ta lepro'sa,** a keratitis consisting of scattered, minute, white spots, occurring in leprosy.

**k. puncta'ta profun'da,** deep punctate k.

**k. puncta'ta subepithelia'lis,** a form with gray areas on the cornea under Bowman's membrane, with an intact superficial epithelium.

**punctate k., deep,** a rare keratitis occurring in hereditary or acquired syphilitic iritis and marked by sharply defined, pinhead-sized, grayish opacities in the substantia propria; called also *k. punctata profunda.*

**punctate k., superficial,** a keratitis often associated with epidemic keratoconjunctivitis and characterized by many small circular epithelial erosions.

**purulent k.,** severe keratitis characterized by a large ulcer with pus in the anterior chamber and purulent disintegration of the cornea.

**k. pustulifor'mis profun'da,** a painful keratitis marked by deep-seated yellow intracorneal spots, hypopyon, and purulent iritis; called also *deep pustular k.*

**reaper's k.,** suppurative k. due to the wounding of the cornea by husks or other fragments of grain.

**reticular k.,** familial degeneration of the cornea with reticular areas.

**ribbon-like k.,** the formation of a transverse film on the cornea.

**rosacea k.,** severe keratitis due to involvement of the cornea in rosacea, sometimes leading to ulceration; called also *acne rosacea k.*

**sclerosing k.,** keratitis associated with scleritis, leading to hyperplasia.

**scrofulous k.,** phlyctenular k.

**secondary k.,** keratitis due to disease of some other part of the eye.

**serpiginous k.,** ulcus serpens corneae.

**k. sic'ca,** keratoconjunctivitis sicca.

**striate k.,** keratitis marked by parallel and intersecting lines on the corneal epithelium; called also *alphabet k.* Cf. *striate keratopathy.*

**suppurative k.,** keratitis attended with, or associated with, suppuration.

**trachomatous k.,** pannus trachomatosus.

**trophic k.,** neuroparalytic k.

**ulcerative k.,** keratitis with ulceration of the corneal epithelium, frequently a result of microbial invasion of the cornea (see *microbial k.*). Called also *corneal ulcer.*

**vascular k.,** keratitis accompanied by the formation of blood vessels beneath the conjunctiva and outer layers of the cornea.

**vesicular k.,** keratitis with the development of small vesicles on the surface.

**xerotic k.,** dryness of the cornea; a condition that precedes keratomalacia.

**zonular k.,** ribbon-like k.

**kerat(o)-** [Gr. *keras,* gen. *keratos* horn] a combining form denoting relationship to horny tissue, or to the cornea.

**ker·a·to·ac·an·tho·ma** (ker″ə-to-ak″an-tho′mə) [*kerato-* + *acanthoma*] [MeSH: Keratoacanthoma] a benign, locally destructive epithelial tumor closely resembling squamous cell carcinoma clinically and histologically; exposure to sunlight is believed to play a role in its etiology.

**eruptive k.,** a form manifested by a generalized papular eruption of numerous dome-shaped, skin-colored papules, often sparing the palms and soles, and usually occurring in light-skinned, middle-aged adults.

**giant k.,** a solitary keratoacanthoma greater than two centimeters in diameter.

**multiple k.,** a form clinically and histologically identical to solitary keratoacanthoma, but differing in that it preferentially affects adolescents and young adults and occurs even on areas of skin unexposed to sunlight. See also *self-healing squamous epithelioma,* under *epithelioma.*

**solitary k.,** a form manifested by a firm, erythematous papule that enlarges rapidly to form a dome-shaped, skin-colored nodule with an umbilicated center, then slowly involutes and leaves a small focus of scarring; it occurs primarily on sunlight-exposed areas, particularly the face, neck, back of the hands, and arms of middle-aged to elderly persons, particularly white males.

**ker·a·to·cele** (ker′ə-to-sēl″) [*kerato-* + *-cele*] hernia of the innermost layer of the cornea (Descemet's membrane).

**ker·a·to·cen·te·sis** (ker″ə-to-sən-te′sis) [*kerato-* + *centesis*] aqueous paracentesis.

**ker·a·to·con·junc·ti·vi·tis** (ker″ə-to-kən-junk″tĭ-vi′tis) [*kerato-* + *conjunctivitis*] [MeSH: Keratoconjunctivitis] inflammation of the cornea and conjunctiva.

**epidemic k.,** a highly infectious disease characterized by scant ocular exudate, round subepithelial corneal opacities associated with the keratitis, and often swelling of regional lymph nodes; there may also be systemic symptoms, especially headache. Adenovirus type 8 has often been isolated from patients with the disease. Called also *shipyard k., viral k.,* and *Sanders' disease.*

**flash k.,** keratoconjunctivitis caused by exposure to a welding arc or other source of ultraviolet rays.

**infectious k.,** infectious keratitis with conjunctivitis in cattle, sheep, or goats, characterized by blepharospasm and sometimes corneal or conjunctival opacity. See also *infectious bovine k., infectious caprine k.,* and *infectious ovine k.* Called also *contagious* or *infectious ophthalmia.*

**infectious bovine k.,** infectious keratoconjunctivitis in cattle, usually caused by *Moraxella (Moraxella) bovis,* bovine herpesvirus 1, or *Mycoplasma* species. Called also *infectious bovine keratitis.*

**infectious caprine k.,** infectious keratoconjunctivitis in goats, usually caused by species of *Mycoplasma* or *Moraxella.*

**infectious ovine k.,** infectious keratoconjunctivitis in sheep, caused by *Mycoplasma* species, *Neisseria ovis,* and rickettsiae. Called also *heather blindness.*

**phlyctenular k.,** a form marked by the formation of a small, gray, circumscribed lesion, or phlyctenule, at the corneal limbus; it has been associated with malnutrition, tuberculosis, and staphylococcus sensitivity. Called also *phlyctenular keratitis, phlyctenular ophthalmia,* and *strumous ophthalmia.* See also *phlyctenulosis.*

**shipyard k.,** epidemic k.

**k. sic'ca,** a condition marked by hyperemia of the conjunctiva, lacrimal deficiency, thickening of the corneal epithelium, itching and burning of the eye, and often reduced visual acuity. Called also *dry eye.* Cf. *Sjögren syndrome.*

**viral k.,** epidemic k.

**ker·a·to·co·nus** (ker″ə-to-ko′nəs) [*kerato-* + *conus*] [MeSH: Keratoconus] a noninflammatory, usually bilateral protrusion of the cornea, the apex being displaced downward and nasally. It occurs most commonly in females at about puberty. The cause is unknown, but hereditary factors may play a role. Called also *conical cornea.*

**ker·a·to·cyst** (ker′ə-to-sist) [*kerato-* + *cyst*] [MeSH: Odontogenic Cysts] an odontogenic cyst lined with a layer of keratinized squamous epithelium and commonly associated with a primordial cyst.

**ker·a·to·cyte** (ker′ə-to-sīt″) [*kerato-* + *-cyte*] one of the flattened connective tissue cells between the lamellae of fibrous tissue composing the cornea.

**ker·a·to·der·ma** (ker″ə-to-der′mə) [*kerato-* + *derma*] 1. a horny skin or covering. 2. hypertrophy of the horny layer of the skin; see also *callus* and *hyperkeratosis* (def. 1). Called also *keratodermia.*

**k. blennorrha'gicum,** a cutaneous manifestation of Reiter's disease, most often involving the palms, soles, toes, and glans penis, and characterized by the presence of erythematous macules that vesiculate, become purulent, and develop thick keratotic coverings; the lesions are sometimes indistinguishable from those of pustular psoriasis. The disorder was formerly thought to be associated with gonorrhea. Called also *keratosis blennorrhagica.*

**k. climacte'ricum,** an acquired form of palmoplantar keratoderma occurring in women about the time of menopause, which may be associated with fissuring of the thickened patches.

**k. palma're et planta're,** palmoplantar k.

**palmoplantar k.,** a group of mostly inherited disorders characterized by the excessive formation of keratin, localized or diffuse, on the palms and soles, sometimes with painful lesions resulting from fissuring of the skin, which may occur alone or may accompany or be part of another disorder. Called also *hyperkeratosis of the palms and soles, ichthyosis palmaris et plantaris, k. palmare et plantare,* and *keratosis palmaris et plantaris.*

**palmoplantar k., diffuse,** an autosomal dominant disorder characterized by the presence of well-demarcated, usually bilateral and symmetrical, confluent areas of scaling on the palms and soles,

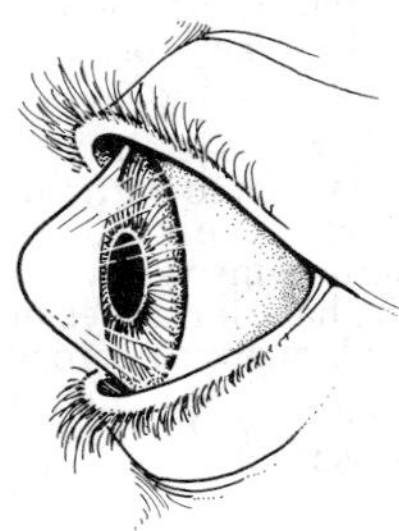

Keratoconus.

sometimes involving adjacent skin of the hands and feet, which is usually present early but may appear later in life. Striate and punctate variants have also been reported; the latter may be associated with focal gingival hyperkeratosis. Called also *Unna-Thost disease* or *syndrome.* See also *Howel-Evans' syndrome,* under *syndrome.*

**ker·a·to·der·ma·to·cele** (ker″ə-to-der′mə-to-sēl) [*kerato-* + *dermato-* + *-cele*[1]] keratocele.

**ker·a·to·der·mia** (ker″ə-to-der′me-ə) [*kerato-* + *derm-* + *-ia*] keratoderma, def. 2.

**ker·a·to·ec·ta·sia** (ker″ə-to-ek-ta′zhə) kerectasis.

**ker·a·to·gen·e·sis** (ker″ə-to-jen′ə-sis) the formation or production of horny material.

**ker·a·to·ge·net·ic** (ker″ə-to-jə-net′ik) pertaining to keratogenesis.

**ker·a·tog·e·nous** (ker″ə-toj′ə-nəs) [*kerato-* + *-genous*] giving rise to a growth of horny material.

**ker·a·to·glo·bus** (ker″ə-to-glo′bəs) megalocornea.

**ker·a·to·hel·co·sis** (ker″ə-to-həl-ko′sis) [*kerato-* + *helcosis*] ulceration of the cornea.

**ker·a·to·he·mia** (ker″ə-to-he′me-ə) [*kerato-* + *hem-* + *-ia*] the presence of deposits of blood in the cornea.

**ker·a·to·hy·a·lin** (ker″ə-to-hi′ə-lin) 1. a substance in the granules in the granular layer of the epidermis, the origin and chemistry of which is unclear, but which may be involved in the process of keratinization. See also *keratohyaline granules,* under *granule.* 2. a substance found in granules in the Hassall corpuscles of the thymus.

**ker·a·to·hy·a·line** (ker″ə-to-hi′ə-līn) 1. both horny and hyaline. 2. pertaining to keratohyalin or to the keratohyalin granules or the keratohyaline layer (stratum granulosum epidermidis). 3. keratohyalin.

**ker·a·toid** (ker′ə-toid) [*kerato-* + *-oid*] resembling horn or corneal tissue.

**ker·a·toi·di·tis** (ker″ə-toi-di′tis) keratitis.

**ker·a·to·ir·i·do·cyc·li·tis** (ker″ə-to-ir″ĭ-do-sik-li′tis) [*kerato-* + *irido-* + *cyclitis*] inflammation of the cornea, iris, and ciliary body.

**ker·a·to·i·rid·o·scope** (ker″ə-to-ĭ-rid′ə-skōp) [*kerato-* + *irido-* + *-scope*] a form of compound microscope for examining the eye.

**ker·a·to·i·ri·tis** (ker″ə-to-i-ri′tis) [*kerato-* + *iritis*] inflammation of the cornea and iris.
**hypopyon k.,** hypopyon keratitis.

**ker·a·to·lep·tyn·sis** (ker″ə-to-lep-tin′sis) [*kerato-* + Gr. *leptynsis* attenuation] removal of the anterior portion of the cornea and covering of the denuded area with bulbar conjunctiva.

**ker·a·to·leu·ko·ma** (ker″ə-to-loo-ko′mə) [*kerato-* + *leukoma*] a white opacity of the cornea.

**ker·a·tol·y·sis** (ker″ə-tol′ə-sis) [*kerato-* + *-lysis*] softening and dissolution or peeling of the horny layer of the epidermis.
**pitted k., k. planta′re sulca′tum,** a superficial bacterial infection of the skin of worldwide distribution usually involving the weight-bearing portions of the soles of the feet, and characterized by the formation of shallow asymptomatic discrete round pits, some of which become confluent and form fissures; the specific etiologic agent is unknown. Called also *cracked heels.*

**ker·a·to·lyt·ic** (ker″ə-to-lit′ik) 1. pertaining to, characterized by, or producing keratolysis. 2. an agent that promotes keratolysis.

**ker·a·to·ma** (ker″ə-to′mə) pl. *keratomas* or *kerato′mata* [*kerat-* + *-oma*] 1. callus. 2. a horny tumor on the inner surface of the wall of a horse's hoof. Called also *keraphyllocele.*
**k. heredita′rium mu′tilans,** an autosomal dominant, progressive, dystrophic form of palmoplantar keratoderma, beginning in childhood, characterized by a stellate pattern of hyperkeratosis on the backs of the hands and feet, linear keratoses on the elbows and knees, and annular ainhum-like constriction of the digits, and sometimes associated with scarring alopecia and deafness. Called also *progressive dystrophic hyperkeratosis* and *Vohwinkel's syndrome.*
**k. planta′re sulca′tum,** pitted keratolysis.
**k. seni′le,** older term for *actinic keratosis.*

**ker·a·to·ma·la·cia** (ker″ə-to-mə-la′shə) [*kerato-* + *malacia*] a usually bilateral condition associated with vitamin A deficiency. It begins with xerotic spots (Bitôt's spots) on the conjunctiva, while the cornea becomes xerotic and insensitive (xerotic keratitis); as the condition progresses, the haze increases until finally the entire cornea becomes soft, and colliquative necrosis occurs.

**ker·a·to·ma·ta** (ker″ə-to′mə-tə) plural of *keratoma.*

**ker·a·tome** (ker′ə-tōm) [*kerato-* + *-tome*] a knife for incising the cornea.

**ker·a·tom·e·ter** (ker″ə-tom′ə-tər) [*kerato-* + *-meter*] an instrument for measuring the curves of the cornea; called also *ophthalmometer.*

**ker·a·to·met·ric** (ker″ə-to-met′rik) pertaining to keratometry, or to measurements made with a keratometer.

**ker·a·tom·e·try** (ker″ə-tom′ə-tre) [*kerato-* + *-metry*] measurement of the anterior curvature of the cornea with a keratometer; called also *ophthalmometry.*

**ker·a·to·mi·leu·sis** (ker″ə-to-mĭ-lo͞o′sis) [*kerato-* + Gr. *smileusis* carving] keratoplasty in which a slice of the patient's cornea is removed, shaped to the desired curvature on a lathe after freezing, and then sutured back on the remaining cornea to correct optical error.
**laser-assisted in-situ k.,** keratoplasty in which the excimer laser and microkeratome are combined for vision correction; the microkeratome is used to shave a thin slice and create a hinged flap in the cornea, the flap is reflected back, the exposed cornea is reshaped by the laser, and the flap is replaced, without sutures, to heal back into position.

**ker·a·to·my·co·sis** (ker″ə-to-mi-ko′sis) [*kerato-* + *mycosis*] 1. a fungal infection of the cornea; called also *mycotic keratitis.* 2. a fungal infection of the horny layer of the epidermis.
**k. ni′gricans,** tinea nigra.

**ker·a·ton·o·sus** (ker″ə-ton′ə-səs) [*kerato-* + Gr. *nosos* disease] any disease of the cornea.

**ker·a·to·nyx·is** (kər″ə-to-nik′sis) [*kerato-* + *nyxis*] aqueous paracentesis.

**ker·a·top·a·thy** (ker″ə-top′ə-the) [*kerato-* + *-pathy*] a noninflammatory disease of the cornea.
**band k., band-shaped k.,** a degenerative condition in which a gray band develops axially from the limbus at the level of Bowman's membrane into the exposed part of the cornea in the palpebral aperture.
**bullous k.,** corneal degeneration marked by recurring epithelial blebs or bullae that rupture, expose corneal nerves, and cause great pain; it occurs in glaucoma, iridocyclitis, and Fuchs' epithelial dystrophy.
**climatic k.,** bilateral, symmetrical corneal degeneration due to extreme heat or cold; called also *Labrador k.*
**filamentary k.,** keratitis filamentosa.
**Labrador k.,** climatic k.
**lipid k.,** deposits of fat in an area of previous corneal vascularization.
**striate k.,** corneal stromal edema causing a network of lines, which is a common, temporary occurrence after cataract surgery. Cf. *striate keratitis.*
**vesicular k.,** corneal epithelial edema with formation of vacuoles. Cf. *vesicular keratitis.*

**ker·a·to·pha·kia** (ker″ə-to-fa′ke-ə) [*kerato-* + *phak-* + *-ia*] a form of keratoplasty in which a slice of donor's cornea is shaped to a desired curvature and inserted between layers of the recipient's cornea to change its curvature.

**ker·a·to·plas·ty** (ker′ə-to-plas″te) [*kerato-* + *-plasty*] plastic surgery of the cornea; corneal grafting.
**autogenous k.,** autokeratoplasty.
**lamellar k.,** a transplant of the anterior half of the cornea with the anterior chamber remaining intact.
**optic k.,** transplantation of corneal material to replace scar tissue which interferes with vision.
**penetrating k.,** a transplant of a section of full-thickness cornea.
**refractive k.,** that in which a section of cornea is removed from the patient or a donor, shaped to the desired curvature, and inserted either between (keratophakia) layers of or on (keratomileusis) the patient's cornea to change its curvature and correct optical errors.
**tectonic k.,** transplantation of corneal material to replace tissue which has been lost.

**ker·a·to·pro·tein** (ker″ə-to-pro′tēn) [*kerato-* + *protein*] the protein of the horny tissues of the body, such as the hair, nails, and epidermis.

**ker·a·to·rhex·is, ker·a·tor·rhex·is** (ker″ə-to-rek′sis) [*kerato-* + *rhexis*] rupture of the cornea.

**ker·a·to·scle·ri·tis** (ker″ə-to-sklə-ri′tis) inflammation of the cornea and sclera.

**ker·a·to·scope** (ker′ə-to-skōp″) [*kerato-* + *-scope*] a device consisting of alternate black or white concentric circles and used for examining corneal curvature; called also *Placido's disk.*

**ker·a·tos·co·py** (ker″ə-tos′kə-pe) the examination of the cornea; more especially the study of the reflections of light from its anterior surface.

**ker·a·to·sis** (ker″ə-to′sis) pl. *kerato′ses* [*kerato-* + *-osis*] [MeSH: Keratosis] any horny growth, such as a wart or callus; the most common types are actinic keratosis and seborrheic keratosis.
**actinic k.,** a sharply outlined, red or skin-colored, flat or elevated, verrucous or keratotic growth, which may develop into a cutaneous

horn, and may give rise to a squamous cell carcinoma; it usually affects the middle-aged or elderly, especially those of fair complexion, and is caused by excessive exposure to the sun. Called also *solar k.;* formerly called *keratoma senile* and *senile k.*

**arsenic k., arsenical k.,** a cutaneous manifestation of chronic arsenic poisoning, after use for medicinal purposes or other exposure, which may occur years after arsenic ingestion, characterized by the development of discrete hyperkeratotic papules, chiefly located on the palms and soles, and sometimes associated with premalignant and malignant epidermal lesions on other skin areas.

**k. blennorrha'gica,** keratoderma blennorrhagicum.

**equine linear k.,** ridges of hyperkeratotic hairless skin on the sides of the neck and chest of horses, with surface seborrhea; the etiology is unknown.

**k. follicula'ris,** a slowly progressive autosomal dominant disorder of keratinization characterized by pinkish to tan or skin-colored papules on the seborrheic areas of the body that coalesce to form plaques, which may become crusted and secondarily infected; over time, the lesions may become darker and may fuse to form papillomatous and warty malodorous growths. Called also *Darier's disease* and *Darier-White disease.*

**k. follicula'ris contagio'sa,** a widespread, symmetrical eruption of the skin resembling keratosis follicularis, most often involving the back of the neck, shoulders, and extensor surfaces of the extremities, which occurs in children, and is apparently an infectious disease. Called also *Brooke's disease* and *epidemic acne.*

**inverted follicular k.,** a benign, usually solitary epithelial tumor originating in a hair follicle; it occurs as a flesh-colored papule or nodule, usually on the face, and is characterized histologically by eddies of keratinizing squamous cells adjoining epidermis or follicular epithelium.

**k. lin'guae,** leukoplakia.

**k. obtu'rans,** obstruction of the external auditory meatus by a mass of desquamated epithelium and cerumen.

**k. palma'ris et planta'ris,** palmoplantar keratoderma.

**k. pharyn'gea,** projection of numerous white horny masses from the tonsils and from the orifices of the lymph follicles in the wall of the pharynx.

**k. pila'ris,** a condition in which hyperkeratosis is limited to the hair follicles, usually on the extensor surfaces of the thighs and arms, but occurring anywhere, with discrete follicular papules which reform after removal.

**k. puncta'ta,** a form of hyperkeratosis in which the lesions are localized in multiple points on the palms and soles; it is transmitted as an autosomal dominant trait.

**roentgen k.,** premalignant keratotic lesions occurring at the site of severe chronic radiodermatitis.

**seborrheic k., k. seborrhe'ica,** a common benign, noninvasive tumor composed of basaloid cells, usually occurring in middle life, sometimes rapidly in crops, commonly presenting as soft, friable plaques that show slight to marked pigmentation and are most often located on the face, trunk, and extremities. Called also *seborrheic wart* and *verruca seborrheica.* See also *Leser-Trélat sign,* under *sign.*

**senile k.,** older term for *actinic k.*

**solar k.,** actinic k.

**stucco k.,** a condition seen especially in men over the age of 40 who have dry skin, characterized by the presence of multiple superficial, gray to light brown, flat keratotic lesions with a "stuck-on" appearance on the dorsa of the feet and hands, ankles, instep, and forearms; thought by some authorities to be a variant of seborrheic keratosis.

**tar k.,** a keratosis caused by exposure to tar, in which keratotic foci develop, sometimes followed by the formation of keratoacanthomas or intraepidermal, squamous, or basal cell carcinoma.

**ker·a·to·sul·fate** (ker″ə-to-sul'fāt) keratan sulfate.

**ker·a·tot·ic** (ker″ə-tot'ik) pertaining to, characterized by, or promoting keratosis.

**ker·a·to·tome** (ker'ə-to-tōm″) keratome.

**ker·a·tot·o·my** (ker″ə-tot'ə-me) [*kerato-* + *-tomy*] surgical incision of the cornea.

**delimiting k.,** incision of the cornea in ulcus serpens by a cut tangential to the advancing border of the ulcer and made to emerge at a corresponding point in the other side.

**radial k.,** an operation in which a series of incisions is made in the cornea from its outer edge toward its center in spokelike fashion; done to flatten the cornea and thus to correct myopia.

**ker·a·to·to·rus** (ker″ə-to-to'rəs) [*kerato-* + *torus*] a vaultlike protrusion of the cornea.

**Kerck·ring's (Kerkring's) center (ossicle), folds (valves)** (kerk'ringz) [Theodorus *Kerckring* (or *Kerkring*), German-born anatomist in the Netherlands, 1640–1693] see under *center* and *fold.*

**ke·rec·ta·sis** (kə-rek'tə-sis) [Gr. *keras* cornea + *ectasis*] a uniform bulging or protrusion of the cornea.

**ke·rec·to·my** (kə-rek'tə-me) keratectomy.

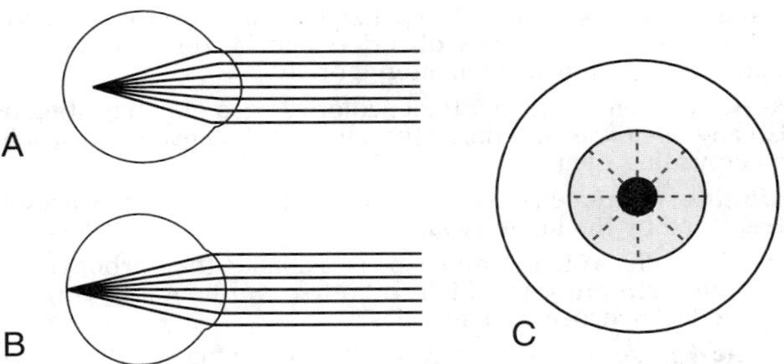


Radial keratotomy. *(A),* Presurgery, the myopic eye focusing in front of the retina; *(B),* postsurgery, the corneal flattening causing the light to focus on the retina; *(C),* anterior view of the eye, showing the lines of incision.

**Ker·ga·ra·dec's sign** (ker-gah-rah-deks') [Jean Alexandre le Jameau, Vicomte de *Kergaradec,* French obstetrician and gynecologist, 1788–1877] see *uterine souffle,* under *souffle.*

**Ke·ril·ia** (kə-ril'e-ə) a genus of poisonous sea snakes. *K. jerdo'ni* is the kerril, a species found in coastal areas of the Indian Ocean.

**ke·ri·on** (ke're-on) [Gr. *kērion* honeycomb] a nodular, boggy, exudative, circumscribed tumefaction which is covered with pustules, occurring in association with tinea infections, usually tinea barbae and tinea capitis.

**Kerk·ring** see *Kerckring.*

**Ker·ley's lines** (kər'lēz) [Peter J. *Kerley,* English radiologist, born 1900] see under *line.*

**Ker·lone** (kər'lōn) trademark for a preparation of betaxolol hydrochloride.

**ker·ma** (ker'mə) [*k*inetic *e*nergy *r*eleased in *ma*terial] a unit of quantity that represents the kinetic energy transferred to charged particles by the uncharged particles per unit mass of an irradiated medium.

**Kern** see *Ke.*

**ker·nic·ter·us** (kər-nik'tər-əs) [Ger. "nuclear jaundice"] [MeSH: Kernicterus] a condition associated with high levels of bilirubin in the blood, nearly always with severe neural symptoms, usually seen in infants as a sequela of icterus gravis neonatorum. It is characterized by deep yellow staining of the basal nuclei, globus pallidus, putamen, caudate nucleus, cerebellar nuclei, bulbar nuclei, and gray substance of the cerebrum, accompanied by widespread destructive changes. Called also *bilirubin encephalopathy.*

**Ker·nig's sign** (ker'nigz) [Vladimir Mikhailovich *Kernig,* Russian physician, 1840–1917] see under *sign.*

**Ker·no·han's notch** (kər'nə-hanz) [James Watson *Kernohan,* Irish-born American pathologist, born 1897] see under *notch.*

**ker·oid** (ker'oid) keratoid.

**ker·o·sene** (ker'o-sēn) a colorless volatile liquid distilled from petroleum; it is used as a reagent, engine fuel, and in insecticides, and is irritating to the skin and toxic by inhalation.

**ker·o·sine** (ker'o-sēn) [MeSH: Kerosine] kerosene.

**Kerr's sign** (kərz) [Henry Hyland *Kerr,* American surgeon, 1881–1963] see under *sign.*

**ker·ril** (ker'il) *Kerilia jerdoni.*

**Ker·tes·zia** (ker-te'ze-ə) a subgenus of mosquitoes of the genus *Anopheles; K. bella'tor* is a vector of malaria in Brazil.

**Ke·shan disease** (ke'shan) [*Keshan,* province in China where it is endemic] see under *disease.*

**Kes·ling appliance, spring** (kes'ling) [Harold D. *Kesling,* American orthodontist, born 1901] see under *appliance* and *spring.*

**Kes·ten·baum's sign** (kes'tən-boumz) [Alfred *Kestenbaum,* German physician, 20th century] see under *sign.*

**Ket·a·ject** (ket'ə-jekt) trademark for a preparation of ketamine hydrochloride.

**ke·tal** (ke'təl) [*ket*one + *al*cohol] an acetal derived by a combination of a ketone with two alcohols.

**Ke·ta·lar** (ke'tə-lər) trademark for a preparation of ketamine hydrochloride.

**keta·mine hy·dro·chlo·ride** (ke'tə-mēn) [USP] a rapid-acting general anesthetic, occurring as a white, crystalline powder; administered intramuscularly and intravenously.

**Ke·ta·set** (ke'tə-set) trademark for a preparation of ketamine hydrochloride.

**ke·ta·zo·lam** (ke-ta′zo-lam) a benzodiazepine used as an anxiolytic in the treatment of anxiety disorders and for the short-term relief of anxiety symptoms; administered orally.

**ke·tene** (ke′tēn) a highly toxic, colorless gas of penetrating odor; also any one of several derivatives from it. It is used industrially as an acetylating agent.

**ke·ti·mine** (ke′tĭ-mēn) a compound in which the oxygen of a ketone is replaced by the imino group.

**keto-** a prefix which denotes possession of the carbonyl group, C═O, in a structure in which the other two bonds to carbon are attached to hydrocarbon moieties.

**ke·to ac·id** (ke′to) a carboxylic acid containing a carbonyl group, e.g., α-ketoglutaric acid.
**branched-chain k. a.,** any of the keto acids formed by oxidative decarboxylation of branched-chain amino acids.

**3-ke·to·ac·id CoA trans·fer·ase** (ke″to-as′id ko-a′ trans′fər-ās) 3-oxoacid CoA-transferase.

**ke·to ac·id de·car·box·y·lase** (ke′to as′id de″kahr-bok′sə-lās) α-keto acid dehydrogenase.

**α-ke·to ac·id de·hy·dro·gen·ase** (ke′to as′id de-hi′dro-jən-ās) 1. see under *complex.* 2. the dehydrogenase component of any of the α-keto acid dehydrogenase complexes.

**α-ke·to ac·id de·hy·dro·gen·ase de·fi·cien·cy** 1. lipoamide dehydrogenase deficiency. 2. deficiency of any one of the α-keto acid dehydrogenase complexes.

**ke·to·ac·i·de·mia** (ke″to-as″id-e′me-ə) the presence of keto acids in the blood.

**ke·to·ac·i·do·sis** (ke″to-as″ĭ-do′sis) acidosis accompanied by the accumulation of ketone bodies (ketosis) in the body tissues and fluids, as in diabetic acidosis and starvation acidosis.
**diabetic k.,** see under *acidosis.*
**starvation k.,** see under *acidosis.*

**ke·to·ac·id·uria** (ke″to-as″ĭ-du′re-ə) the presence of keto acids in the urine.
**branched-chain k.,** maple syrup urine disease.

**ke·to·acyl** (ke″to-a′səl) the acyl radical of a keto acid; the coenzyme A thioesters of 3-keto acids, 3-ketoacyl CoA molecules, are intermediates in fatty acid oxidation.

**3-ke·to·ac·yl CoA thi·o·lase** (ke″to-a′səl ko′a- thi′o-lās) acetyl-CoA *C*-acyltransferase.

**α-ke·to·adip·ate** (ke″to-ə-dip′āt) the anionic form of α-ketoadipic acid.

**α-ke·to·adip·ate de·hy·dro·gen·ase** (ke″to-ə-dip′āt de-hi′dro-jən-ās) a mitochondrial enzyme activity that catalyzes the decarboxylation and esterification of α-ketoadipic acid, forming glutaryl CoA as a step in the degradation of lysine, hydroxylysine, and tryptophan. Deficiency of the enzyme results in α-ketoadipicacidemia.

**α-ke·to·adip·ic ac·id** (ke″to-ə-dip′ik) a dicarboxylic acid formed by transamination of α-aminoadipic acid in the degradation of lysine and hydroxylysine. Written also *2-ketoadipic acid.*

**α-ke·to·adip·ic·ac·i·de·mia** (ke″to-ə-dip″ik-as″ĭ-de′me-ə) 1. excess of α-ketoadipic acid in the blood. 2. deficiency of α-ketoadipate dehydrogenase activity, characterized by accumulation and excretion of α-ketoadipic, α-aminoadipic, and related acids, and possibly associated with mental retardation.

**α-ke·to·adip·ic·ac·id·uria** (ke″to-ə-dip″ik-as″ĭ-du′re-ə) excretion of α-ketoadipic acid in the urine.

**ke·to·a·mi·no·ac·i·de·mia** (ke″to-ə-me″no-as″ĭ-de′me-ə) maple syrup urine disease.

**β-ke·to·bu·tyr·ic ac·id** (ke″to-bu-tēr′ik) acetoacetic acid.

**ke·to·co·na·zole** (ke″to-ko′nə-zōl) [USP] [MeSH: Ketoconazole] an imidazole derivative used as a broad-spectrum antifungal agent, administered orally for a wide range of systemic and cutaneous fungal infections and applied topically to the skin in the treatment of various forms of tinea; also used investigationally in the treatment of prostatic carcinoma.

**Ke·to-Di·a·stix** (ke″to-di′ə-stiks) trademark for a reagent strip designed for the determination of ketones and glucose in urine.

**ke·to·gen·e·sis** (ke″to-jen′ə-sis) [*keto-* + *-genesis*] the production of ketone bodies.

**ke·to·ge·net·ic** (ke″to-jə-net′ik) ketogenic (def. 1).

**ke·to·gen·ic** (ke″to-jen′ik) 1. forming ketone bodies. 2. capable of being converted into ketone bodies.

**α-ke·to·glu·ta·rate** (ke″to-gloo′tə-rāt) an anionic form of α-ketoglutaric acid.

**α-ke·to·glu·ta·rate de·hy·dro·gen·ase** (ke″to-gloo′tə-rāt de-hi′dro-jən-ās) an enzyme of the oxidoreductase class that is a component of the multienzyme α-ketoglutarate dehydrogenase complex (q.v.). The enzyme catalyzes the decarboxylation and oxidation of α-ketoglutarate, forming succinyl bound to the cofactor thiamine pyrophosphate; the succinyl is subsequently transferred to lipoamide to form succinyldihydrolipoamide, an intermediate in the overall reaction catalyzed by the complex. Called *oxoglutarate dehydrogenase (lipoamide)* in EC nomenclature.

**α-ke·to·glu·tar·ic ac·id** (ke″to-gloo-tar′ik) 2-oxopentanedioic acid, 2-oxoglutaric acid, an intermediate in the tricarboxylic acid cycle (q.v.); α-ketoglutarate is also produced from glutamate in amino group transfer reactions and by oxidative deamination.

**ke·to·hep·tose** (ke″to-hep′tōs) any ketose containing seven carbon atoms.

**ke·to·hexo·ki·nase** (ke″to-hek″so-ki′nās) fructokinase.

**ke·to·hex·ose** (ke″to-hek′sōs) any ketose containing six carbon atoms, such as fructose. Cf. *aldohexose.*

**ke·to·hy·droxy·es·trin** (ke″to-hi-drok″se-es′trin) estrone.

**α-ke·to·iso·val·er·ate de·hy·dro·gen·ase** (ke″to-i″so-val′er-āt de-hi′dro-jən-ās) 3-methyl-2-oxobutanoate dehydrogenase (lipoamide).

**ke·tol** (ke′tol) a compound with both a ketone and an alcohol group.

**ke·tol-isom·er·ase** (ke″tol-i-som′ər-ās) a term used in the systematic names of that subset of the isomerases that catalyze the interconversion of aldoses and ketoses [EC 5.3.1].

**ke·tol·y·sis** (ke-tol′ə-sis) [*ketone* + *-lysis*] the cleavage of ketone bodies.

**ke·to·lyt·ic** (ke″to-lit′ik) pertaining to, characterized by, or promoting ketolysis.

**ke·tone** (ke′tōn) any of a large class of organic compounds containing the carbonyl group, C═O, whose carbon atom is joined to two other carbon atoms, that is, with the carbonyl group occurring within the carbon chain. See also under *body.*
**dimethyl k.,** acetone.

**ke·to·ne·mia** (ke″to-ne′me-ə) an excess of ketone bodies in the blood, as in starvation and diabetes mellitus. See also *ketosis.* Called also *hyperketonemia.*

**ke·ton·ic** (ke-to′nik) pertaining to or developed from a ketone.

**ke·to·ni·za·tion** (ke″to-nĭ-za′shən) conversion into a ketone.

**ke·ton·uria** (ke″to-nu′re-ə) ketone bodies in the urine, as in diabetes mellitus; called also *acetonuria* and *hyperketonuria.*

**ke·to·pen·tose** (ke″to-pen′tōs) any ketose containing five carbon atoms, such as ribulose or xylulose.

**ke·to·pla·sia** (ke″to-pla′zhə) ketogenesis.

**ke·to·plas·tic** (ke″to-plas′tik) [*ketone* + *-plastic*] ketogenic.

**ke·to·pro·fen** (ke″to-pro′fən) [USP] [MeSH: Ketoprofen] a propionic acid derivative used as a nonsteroidal anti-inflammatory drug; administered orally and rectally.

**9-ke·to·re·duc·tase** (ke″to-re-duk′tās) prostaglandin-$E_2$ 9-reductase.

**β-ke·to·re·duc·tase** (ke″to-re-duk′tās) 3-hydroxyacyl-CoA dehydrogenase.

**ke·to·ro·lac tro·meth·amine** (ke″to-ro′lak) [USP] a nonsteroidal anti-inflammatory agent used for short-term management of pain; administered intramuscularly and orally.

**ke·tose** (ke′tōs) one of two subgroups of monosaccharides, being those having a nonterminal carbonyl (keto) group. In all known natural ketoses, the position of the keto group is at the 2 carbon. The class is further divided on the basis of the number of carbon atoms in the sugar, e.g., ketopentose, ketohexose, ketoheptose, etc.

**ke·to·side** (ke′to-sīd) any glycoside formed from a ketose; e.g., a fructoside.

**ke·to·sis** (ke-to′sis) [MeSH: Ketosis] abnormally elevated concentration of ketone bodies in the body tissues and fluids when fatty acids are incompletely metabolized, a complication of diabetes mellitus, starvation, and alcoholism.
**k. of ruminants,** ketosis in cows and ewes during times of increased bodily mobilization of fat stores, usually just after they have given birth. See *fat cow syndrome* and *pregnancy toxemia in ewes.*

**ke·to·ster·oid** (ke″to-ster′oid) a steroid that possesses ketone groups on functional carbon atoms, which are designated in the name. Called also *oxosteroid.*
**17-k. (17-KS),** any of the $C_{19}$ steroids having a keto group on the 17 carbon, usually denoting the urinary metabolites of androgens secreted by the adrenal cortex and gonads. They are accumulated and

excreted abnormally in certain adrenal cortical and ovarian tumors and congenital adrenal hyperplasia.

**17β-ke·to·ster·oid re·duc·tase** (ke″to-ster′oid re-duk′tās) testosterone 17β-dehydrogenase.

**ke·tos·uria** (ke″tōs-u′re-ə) the presence of ketose in the urine.

**ke·to·tet·rose** (ke″to-tet′rōs) a ketose that contains four carbon atoms; see also *erythrulose.*

**3-ke·to·thi·o·lase** (ke″to-thi′o-lās) acetyl-CoA *C*-acyltransferase.

**β-ke·to·thi·o·lase** (ke″to-thi′o-lās) acetyl-CoA *C*-acyltransferase.

**β-ke·to·thi·o·lase de·fi·cien·cy** α-methylacetoaceticaciduria.

**ke·tot·ic** (ke-tot′ik) pertaining to, characterized by, or causing ketosis.

**ke·to·tri·ose** (ke″to-tri′ōs) a ketose containing three carbon atoms; see *dihydroxyacetone.*

**ke·tox·ime** (ke-tok′sīm) the oxime derivative of a ketone.

**Ke·ty-Schmidt method** (ke′te-shmit) [Seymour Solomon *Kety,* American physiologist, born 1915; Carl Frederic *Schmidt,* American physician, 1893–1988] see under *method.*

**keV, kev** kilo electron volt.

**key** (ke) 1. an instrument for opening a lock, or a device similar in appearance or function to such an instrument. 2. by extension, any tool for revealing specific information.
**torquing k.,** an orthodontic instrument used to facilitate the engaging of rectangular arch wires into the edgewise brackets.

**key·note** (ke′nōt) in homeopathy, the characteristic property of a drug which indicates its use in treating a similar symptom of disease.

**Key-Ret·zi·us sheath, foramen** (ke ret′ze-əs) [Ernst Axel Henrik *Key,* Swedish physician, 1832–1901; Magnus Gustaf *Retzius,* Swedish histologist, 1842–1919] see *sheath of Key and Retzius,* under *sheath,* and see *apertura lateralis ventriculi quarti* under *apertura.*

**keyway** (ke′wa) the slot into which the male portion of a precision attachment fits.

**kg** kilogram.

**Kho·ra·na** (ko-rah′nə) Har Gobind. Indian-born American chemist, born 1922; co-winner, with Robert William Holley and Marshall Warren Nirenberg, of the Nobel prize for medicine or physiology in 1968 for discovery of the process by which enzymes determine a cell's function in a genetic environment.

**kHz** symbol for *kilohertz.*

**ki·bis·i·tome** (ki-bis′ĭ-tōm) [Gr. *kibisis* pouch + *-tome*] cystitome.

**Kidd blood group** (kid) [from the name of the propositus first observed in 1951] see under *blood group.*

**kid·ney** (kid′ne) [L. *ren;* Gr. *nephros*] [MeSH: Kidney] either of the two organs in the lumbar region that filter the blood, excreting the end-products of body metabolism in the form of urine, and regulating the concentrations of hydrogen, sodium, potassium, phosphate, and other ions in the extracellular fluid. Called also *ren* [TA]. Each human kidney is about 11 cm long, 5–7.5 cm wide, and 2.5 cm thick, and weighs from 120–160 gm. The kidney is of characteristic shape, and presents a notch on the inner, concave, border, known as the *hilus,* which communicates with the cavity or sinus of the kidney and through which the vessels, nerves, and ureter pass. The kidney consists of a *cortex* and a *medulla.* The medullary substance forms pyramids, whose bases are in the cortex and whose apices, which are called *papillae,* project into the calices of the kidney. The renal pyramids number from 10 to 15. The parenchyma of each kidney is composed of about one million *renal tubules* (nephrons, the functional unit of the kidney), held together by a little connective tissue. Each tubule begins blindly in a renal corpuscle, consisting of a glomerulus and its capsule, situated within the cortex. After a neck or constriction below the capsule, it becomes the proximal convoluted tubule, Henle's loop, distal convoluted tubule, connecting tubule, and then the straight collecting tubule, which opens at the apex of a renal papilla. The straight collecting tubules converge as they descend, forming groups in the center, known as *medullary rays.* See also Plate 22.
**abdominal k.,** an ectopic kidney situated above the iliac crest with the hilus adjacent to the second lumbar vertebra.
**amyloid k.,** renal amyloidosis.
**Armanni-Ebstein k.,** a kidney that has Armanni-Ebstein lesions.
**arteriosclerotic k.,** one characterized by sclerotic changes of intrarenal arteries and large arterioles.
**artificial k.,** a popular name for an extracorporeal device employed to remove from the blood, while it is being circulated outside the body, elements which are usually excreted in the urine; see *hemodialyzer.*
**atrophic k.,** one that is diminished in size because of inadequate circulation and/or loss of nephrons.
**cake k.,** a solid, irregularly lobed organ of bizarre shape, usually situated in the pelvis toward the midline, developed as result of fusion of the two renal anlagen.
**cicatricial k.,** a shriveled, irregular, and scarred kidney, resulting from suppurative pyelonephritis.
**clump k.,** cake k.
**congested k.,** large red k.
**contracted k.,** an atrophic kidney which may be scarred and granular.
**crush k.,** lower nephron nephrosis.
**cyanotic k.,** passive congestion of the kidney.
**cystic k.,** a kidney containing one or more cysts.
**definite k., definitive k.,** metanephros.
**disk k.,** a disk-shaped organ produced by fusion of both poles of the contralateral kidney anlagen.
**doughnut k.,** an anomalous organ resulting from bipolar fusion of the renal anlagen before rotation begins, both kidneys being on the same level.
**fatty k.,** a kidney affected with fatty degeneration.
**flea-bitten k.,** a kidney which has small, randomly scattered petechiae on its surface, sometimes seen in bacterial endocarditis.
**floating k.,** hypermobile k.
**Formad's k.,** an enlarged and deformed kidney, sometimes seen in chronic alcoholism.
**fused k.,** a single anomalous organ developed as a result of fusion of the renal anlagen.
**Goldblatt k.,** one in which the blood flow is artificially obstructed by clamping (see *Goldblatt clamp,* under *clamp*), resulting in Goldblatt hypertension.
**head k.,** pronephros.
**hind k.,** metanephros.
**horseshoe k.,** a kidney anomaly in which the right and left kidneys are linked at one end by a band of tissue as a result of fusion of the corresponding poles of the renal anlagen.
**hypermobile k.,** one that is freely movable.
**lardaceous k.,** amyloid k.
**large red k.,** a congested, edematous kidney which may result from inflammation, impaired venous circulation, or urinary obstruction; called also *congested k.*
**lumbar k.,** an ectopic kidney situated opposite the sacral promontory in the iliac fossa, anterior to the iliac vessels.
**lump k.,** cake k.
**medullary sponge k.,** sponge k.
**middle k.,** mesonephros.
**mortar k.,** putty k.
**movable k.,** hypermobile k.
**mural k.,** a kidney located in a pocket of peritoneum in the abdominal wall.
**myelin k.,** a kidney infiltrated with myelin, producing minute whitish specks or streaks on its surface.
**myeloma k.,** renal changes occurring in multiple myeloma, due to filtration of large amounts of Bence Jones protein; they include tubular atrophy with the presence of intraluminal casts and multinucleated giant cells in tubular walls and interstitium, and they result in renal failure.
**pelvic k.,** an ectopic kidney situated opposite the sacrum and below the aortic bifurcation.
**polycystic k's,** see *polycystic disease of the kidneys,* under *disease.*
**primordial k.,** pronephros.
**putty k.,** one containing caseous material trapped by stricture of the ureter by tuberculous granulations in renal tuberculosis.
**Rose-Bradford k.,** a form of fibrotic kidney of inflammatory origin found in young subjects.
**sacciform k.,** a distended kidney; nephrectasia.
**sigmoid k.,** a deformed and fused kidney, the upper pole of one kidney being fused with the lower pole of the other.
**sponge k.,** a rare congenital condition, anatomically characterized by multiple small cystic dilatations of the collecting tubules of the medullary portion of the renal pyramids, giving the organ a spongy, porous feeling and appearance. It is usually asymptomatic, but there may be calculus formation within the cysts, hematuria, renal colic, or recurrent renal infection.
**supernumerary k.,** a kidney in addition to the two usually present, developed as the result of splitting of the nephrogenic blastema, or from separate metanephric blastemas into which partially or completely reduplicated ureteral stalks enter to form separate capsulated kidneys. In some cases the separation of the reduplicated organ is incomplete *(fused supernumerary k.).*
**thoracic k.,** an ectopic kidney that partially or completely protrudes above the diaphragm into the posterior mediastinum.
**wandering k.,** hypermobile k.
**waxy k.,** amyloid k.

**Kiel classification** (kēl) [*Kiel,* Germany, where it was developed] see under *classification.*

**Kiel·land's (Kjel·land's) forceps** (kyel′əndz) [Christian *Kielland*

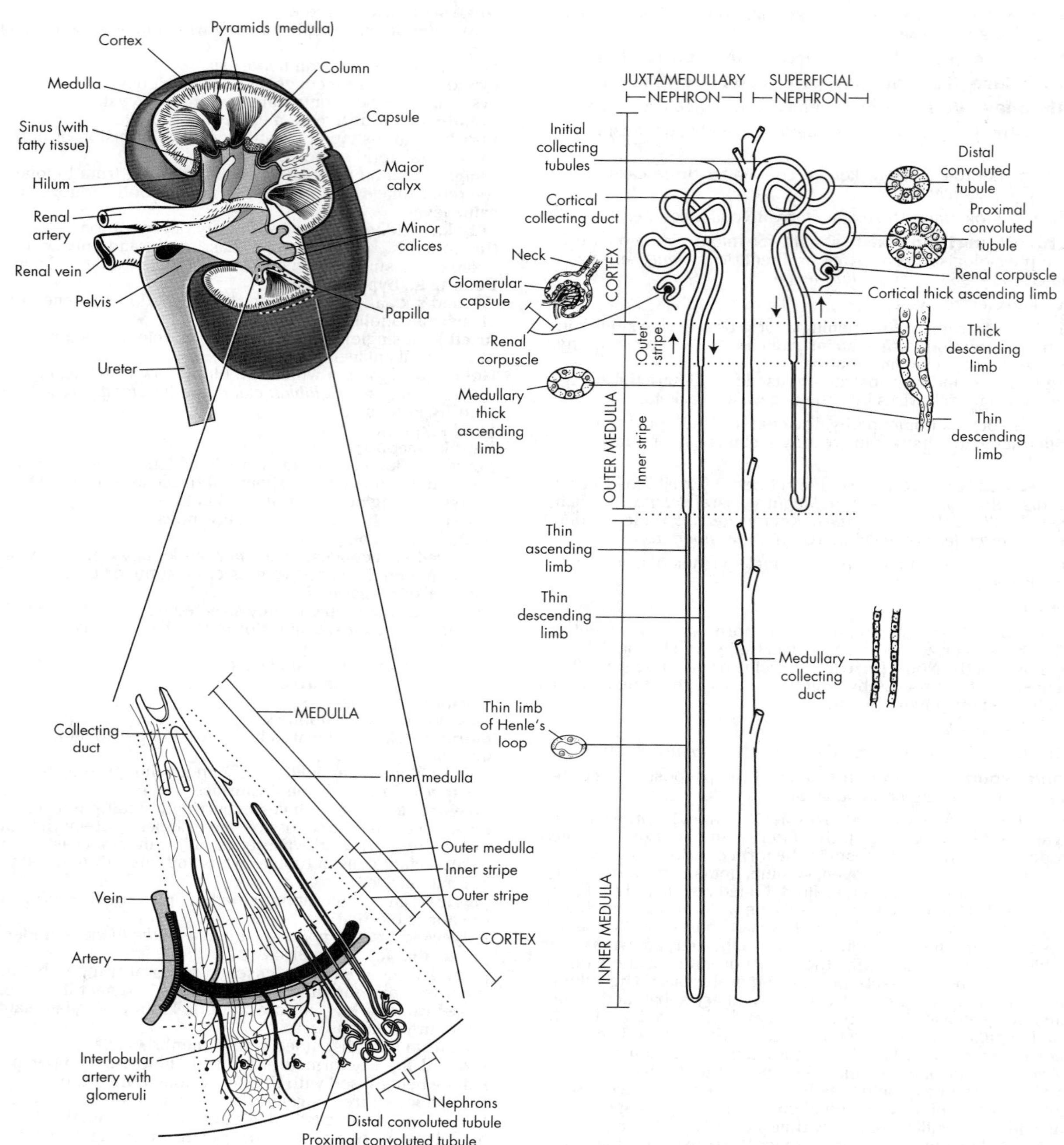


**PLATE 22**—STRUCTURE OF THE KIDNEY

(or *Kjelland*), Norwegian obstetrician and gynecologist, 1871–1941] see under *forceps*.

**Kien·böck disease,** etc. (kēn'berk) [Robert *Kienböck*, Austrian radiologist, 1871–1953] see under *disease, dislocation,* and *unit,* and see *paradoxical diaphragm phenomenon,* under *phenomenon*.

**Kien·böck-Ad·am·son points** (kēn'berk-ad'əm-sən) [Robert *Kienböck;* Horatio George *Adamson,* London dermatologist, 1865–1955] see under *point*.

**Kier·nan's spaces** (kēr'nənz) [Francis *Kiernan,* British physician, 1800–1874] see under *space*.

**Kies·sel·bach's area (space)** (ke'səl-bahks) [Wilhelm *Kiesselbach,* German laryngologist, 1839–1902] see under *area*.

**Ki·ku·chi's lymphadenitis (disease)** (ke-koo'chēz) [M. *Kikuchi,* Japanese pathologist, 20th century] see under *lymphadenitis*.

**kil** (kil) a white, sticky, soapy clay from the Black Sea region; when sterilized, it is employed as an ointment base for use in skin diseases.

**Kil·i·an's line** (kil'e-ənz) [Hermann Friedrich *Kilian,* German gynecologist, 1800–1863] see under *line*.

**kil·leen** (kil'ēn) 1. *Chondrus crispus*. 2. chondrus (def. 2).

**Kil·li·an's dehiscence (triangle), operation** (kil'e-ənz) [Gustav *Killian,* German laryngologist, 1860–1921] see under *dehiscence* and *operation*.

**Kil·li·an-Freer operation** (kil'e-ən-frēr) [Gustav *Killian;* Otto (Tiger) *Freer,* American laryngologist, 1857–1932] see under *operation*.

**kil·li·fish** (kil'e-fish) [MeSH: Killifish] a fish of the genus *Fundulus*.

**kilo-** [Fr., from Gr. *chilioi* thousand] a combining form used in naming units of measurement to indicate a quantity one thousand ($10^3$) times the unit designated by the root with which it is combined. Symbol, k.

**kilo·base** (kil'o-bās) a unit used in designating the length of a nucleic acid sequence; e.g., 7 kb indicates a sequence 7000 nucleotides long. Abbreviated kb.

**kilo·cal·o·rie** (kil'o-kal"o-re) large calorie; see under *calorie*.

**kilo·ku·rie** (kil"o-ku're) a unit of radioactivity, being one thousand ($10^3$) curies, or the quantity of radioactive material in which the number of nuclear disintegrations is $3.7 \times 10^{13}$ per second. Abbreviated kCi.

**kilo·dal·ton** (kil"o-dawl'ton) a unit of mass, being 1000 daltons. Abbreviated kD or kDa.

**kilo·gram** (kil'o-gram) the basic unit of mass of the SI system, being 1000 ($10^3$) grams, or one cubic decimeter of water; it is defined as the mass equivalent of an international prototype kilogram and is equivalent to 2.204623 pounds avoirdupois.

**kilo·hertz** (kil'o-hərtz) one thousand ($10^3$) hertz (cycles per second). Abbreviated kHz.

**Ki·loh-Nev·in syndrome** (ki'lo-nev'in) [Leslie Gordon *Kiloh,* Australian physician, 20th century; Samuel *Nevin,* English neurologist, born 1905] see under *syndrome*.

**ki·lom·e·ter** (kĭ-lom'ə-tər, kil'o-me"tər) [Fr. *kilométre* ] a unit of linear measurement of the metric system, being 1000 ($10^3$) meters, or the equivalent of 3280.83 feet, or about five-eighths of a mile. Abbreviated km.

**kilo·unit** (kil"o-u'nit) a quantity equivalent to one thousand ($10^3$) units.

**kilo·volt** (kil'o-vōlt) a unit of electrical pressure or electromotive force, being 1000 ($10^3$) volts. Symbol, kV.

**Kim·ber·ley horse disease** (kim'bər-le) [Kimberley, a district in northeastern Western Australia, where disease occurs] see under *disease*.

**Kim·mel·stiel-Wil·son lesion (nodule), syndrome** (kim'əl-stēl wil'sən) [Paul *Kimmelstiel,* German pathologist in the United States, 1900–1970; Clifford *Wilson,* English physician, born 1906] intercapillary glomerulosclerosis.

**Ki·mu·ra's disease** (ke-moo'rahz) [Tetsuji *Kimura,* Japanese pathologist, 20th century] angiolymphoid hyperplasia; see under *hyperplasia*.

**Ki·mu·ra cartilage graft** (ke-moo'rah) see under *graft*.

**kin·an·es·the·sia** (kin"an-es-the'zhə) akinesthesia.

**ki·nase** (ki'nās) 1. a term used in the recommended and trivial names of the phosphotransferases and diphosphotransferases of the transferase class [EC 2.7.1–6] that catalyze the transfer of a high-energy phosphate group from a donor compound (e.g., ATP or GTP) to an acceptor compound (alcohol, carboxyl, nitrogenous group, or another phosphate group). 2. a suffix used in the trivial names of some enzymes that convert an inactive or precursor form. See also *protein kinase*.

**kind·ling** (kind'ling) changes in brain physiology caused by repeated subthreshold electrical stimulation; the final result may be epileptogenic changes or less dramatic but chronic behavioral changes. It has been observed in reptiles, amphibians, and a variety of mammals but its occurrence in humans is controversial.

**kine-** [Gr. *kinein* to move] a combining form denoting relationship to movement. See also words beginning *cine-*.

**kine·mat·ics** (kin"ə-mat'iks) [Gr. *kinēma* motion] that phase of mechanics which deals with the possible motions of a material body.

**kine·plas·tics** (kin"ə-plas'tiks) kineplasty.

**kine·plas·ty** (kin'ə-plas"te) [*kine-* + *-plasty*] plastic amputation; amputation in which the stump is so formed as to be utilized for motor purposes.

**kine·sal·gia** (kin"ə-sal'jə) [*kinesio-* + *-algia*] pain on muscular exertion.

**kine·scope** (kin'ə-skōp) [*kine-* + *-scope*] an instrument for measuring ocular refraction, in which the patient observes a fixed object through a slit in a moving disk.

**ki·ne·sia** (kĭ-ne'zhə) kinetosis.

**ki·ne·si·al·gia** (kĭ-ne"se-al'jə) kinesalgia.

**ki·ne·si·at·rics** (ki-ne"se-at'riks) [*kinesio-* + *-iatrics*] kinesitherapy.

**ki·ne·sics** (ki-ne'siks) [MeSH: Kinesics] the study of body movement as a part of the process of communication.

**ki·ne·si·es·the·si·om·e·ter** (ki-ne"se-es-the"ze-om'ə-tər) kinesthesiometer.

**ki·ne·si·gen·ic** (ki-ne"sĭ-jen'ik) [*kinesi-* + *-genic*] caused by movement.

**kine·sim·e·ter** (kin"ə-sim'ə-tər) [*kinesio-* + *-meter*] an instrument for the quantitative measurement of movements.

**ki·ne·sin** (ki-ne'sin) [MeSH: Kinesin] a large, soluble, cytoplasmic protein that binds tightly to microtubules and transports vesicles and particles distally along them, using energy from ATP hydrolysis. Cf. *dynein*.

**kinesi(o)-** [Gr. *kinēsis* movement] a combining form denoting relationship to movement.

**ki·ne·si·ol·o·gy** (kĭ-ne"se-ol'ə-je) [*kinesio-* + *-logy*] the sum of what is known regarding human motion; the study of motion of the human body. Cf. *biomechanics*.

**ki·ne·si·om·e·ter** (kĭ-ne"se-om'ə-tər) kinesimeter.

**ki·ne·sio·neu·ro·sis** (kĭ-ne"se-o-noo͝-ro'sis) [*kinesio-* + *neurosis*] a functional nervous disorder characterized by motor disturbances, such as spasms or tics.

**ki·ne·sio·ther·a·py** (kĭ-ne"se-o-ther'ə-pe) kinesitherapy.

**ki·ne·sis** (ki-ne'sis) [Gr.] [MeSH: Kinesis] 1. movement. 2. stimulus-induced motion responsive only to the intensity of the stimulus, not the direction. Cf. *taxis*.

**-kinesis** a word termination denoting movement or activation, particularly in response to a stimulus specified by the root to which it is attached.

**ki·ne·si·ther·a·py** (kĭ-ne"sĭ-ther'ə-pe) [*kinesio-* + *therapy*] the treatment of disease by movements or exercise.

**kin·es·the·sia** (kin"es-the'zhə) [*kine-* + *esthesia*] 1. the awareness of movement, weight, tension, and position of body parts, which is dependent on input from joint and muscle receptors and hair cells. 2. movement sense.

**kin·es·the·si·om·e·ter** (kin"əs-the"ze-om'ə-tər) [*kinesthesia* + *-meter*] an instrument for testing kinesthesia.

**kin·es·the·sis** (kin"əs-the'sis) [MeSH: Kinesthesis] kinesthesia.

**kin·es·thet·ic** (kin"əs-thet'ik) pertaining to kinesthesia or the muscular sense.

**ki·ne·tia** (kĭ-ne'she-ə) plural of *kinety*.

**ki·net·ic** (kĭ-net'ik) [Gr. *kinētikos*] [MeSH: Kinetics] pertaining to or producing motion.

**ki·net·i·cist** (ki-net'ĭ-sist) a specialist in kinetics.

**ki·net·ics** (kĭ-net'iks, ki-net'iks) [Gr. *kinētikos* of or for putting in motion] [MeSH: Kinetics] the branch of dynamics that pertains to the turnover, or rate of change, of a specific factor (e.g., erythrocytes—erythrokinetics, leukocytes—leukokinetics, or iron—ferrokinetics), commonly expressed as units of amount per unit time.
**chemical k.,** the study of the rates and mechanisms of chemical reactions.
**urea k.,** the movement of urea in the body and its excretion through

the kidneys or dialysis apparatus; see also *urea clearance,* under *clearance.*

**ki·ne·tid** (kĭ-ne′tid) an elementary, repeating structural unit of ciliate protozoa, consisting of one or more kinetosomes together with various associated organelles.

**ki·ne·tin** (ki-ne′tin) a highly potent plant-growth factor; used to stimulate the growth of bacterial colonies.

**kine·tism** (kin′ə-tiz″əm) the ability to perform or initiate muscular action.

**kinet(o)-** [Gr. *kinētos* movable] a combining form denoting relationship to motion.

**ki·ne·to·car·dio·gram** (kĭ-ne″to-kahr′de-o-gram″) [*kineto-* + *cardiogram*] the graphic record obtained by kinetocardiography.

**ki·ne·to·car·di·og·ra·phy** (kĭ-ne″to-kahr″de-og′rə-fe) [*kineto-* + *cardiography*] [MeSH: Kinetocardiography] the technique of graphically recording the slow vibrations of the anterior chest wall in the region of the heart, the vibrations representing the absolute motion of the heart at a given point on the chest.

**ki·ne·to·chore** (ki-ne′to-kor) [*kineto-* + Gr. *chora* space] [MeSH: Kinetochores] a proteinaceous structure beside the centromere and to which the spindle fibers are attached.

**ki·ne·to·des·ma** (ki-ne″to-des′mə) pl. *kinetodesma′ta* [*kineto-* + Gr. *desmos* band, ligament] one of a bundle of fine, striated fibrils, each of which arises close to the base of a basal body and runs anteriorly parallel to and just beneath the surface of certain ciliate protozoa; the kinetodesmata serve to connect the basal bodies in longitudinal rows. Called also *kinetodesmos.*

**ki·ne·to·des·ma·ta** (kĭ-ne″to-dez-mah′tə) plural of *kinetodesma.*

**ki·ne·to·des·mos** (ki-ne″to-des′mos) kinetodesma.

**ki·ne·to·frag·ment** (kĭ-ne″to-frag′mənt) a group of somatic kinetids, not always completely covered with cilia, occurring in the region of the cytosome or oral area in certain ciliate protozoa, many of which are in the class Kinetofragminophorea. See also *frange* and *pseudomembranelle.*

**Ki·ne·to·frag·min·o·phor·ea** (ki-ne″to-frag″min-ə-for′e-ə) [*kineto-* + L. *fragmen* piece + Gr. *phōros* bearing] [MeSH: Kinetofragminophorea] a class of ciliate protozoa (phylum Ciliophora), characterized by the presence of isolated kineties in the oral region of the body (kinetofragments) bearing cilia but not compound ciliary organelles; a cytostome and cytopharyngeal apparatus are often present. It comprises four subclasses: Gymnostomatia, Vestibuliferia, Hypostomatia, and Suctoria.

**ki·ne·to·gen·ic** (kĭ-ne″to-jen′ik) [*kineto-* + *-genic*] causing or producing movement.

**ki·ne·to·nu·cle·us** (kĭ-ne″to-noo′kle-əs) [*kineto-* + *nucleus*] kinetoplast.

**ki·ne·to·plasm** (kĭ-ne′to-plaz″əm) [*kineto-* + *-plasm*] the most highly contractile portion of the cytoplasm of a cell.

**ki·ne·to·plast** (kĭ-ne′to-plast) [*kineto-* + *-plast*] a large rod-shaped or cylindrical, DNA-rich, independently replicating cytoplasmic organelle located in close association with the basal body (with which it may seem to be fused) and found within the elongated mitochondrion of protozoa of the order Kinetoplastida. Called also *kinetonucleus.*

**ki·ne·to·plas·tid** (kĭ-ne″to-plas′tid) pertaining or relating to protozoa of the order Kinetoplastida.

**Ki·ne·to·plas·ti·da** (kĭ-ne″to-plas′tĭ-də) [MeSH: Kinetoplastida] an order of flagellate protozoa (class Zoomastigophorea, subphylum Mastigophora), many species of which are free living, although most are parasites of plants, invertebrates, and vertebrates. Kinetoplastids have one or two flagella arising from a depression in the cell body and usually contain a conspicuous kinetoplast located near the flagellar basal bodies. The order comprises two suborders: Bodonina and Trypanosomatina. Called also *Protomastigida* and *Protomonadina.*

**ki·ne·to·scope** (kĭ-ne′tə-skōp) [*kineto-* + *-scope*] an apparatus designed to make serial photographs depicting body motions.

**ki·ne·tos·co·py** (kĭ″nə-tos′kə-pe) serial photography which exhibits the motions of the limbs or features; used in diagnosis of disorders of gait and in the study of muscle action.

**ki·ne·to·sis** (kĭ″nə-to′sis) pl. *kineto′ses* [*kineto-* + *-osis*] any disorder caused by unaccustomed motion; see *motion sickness.*

**ki·ne·to·some** (kĭ-ne′to-sōm) [*kineto-* + *-some*] basal body.

**ki·ne·to·ther·a·py** (kĭ-ne″to-ther′ə-pe) kinesitherapy.

**ki·ne·ty** (ki-ne′te) pl. *kine′tia, kineties* [Gr. *kinetos* movable] a longitudinal unit comprising cilia, basal bodies, and kinetodesmata in the infraciliature of ciliate protozoa. Called also *kinety system.*

**King syndrome** (king) [J.O. *King,* Australian physician, 20th century] see under *syndrome.*

**King unit** (king) [Earl Judson *King,* Canadian biochemist, 1901–1962] see under *unit.*

**king·dom** (king′dəm) [A.S. *cyningdom*] classically, one of the three categories into which natural objects are usually classified: the *animal kingdom,* including all animals; the *plant kingdom,* including all plants; and the *mineral kingdom,* including all objects and substance without life. A fourth kingdom, the *Protista,* has been added and includes all single-celled organisms.

**King·el·la** (king-el′ə) [Elizabeth O. *King,* American bacteriologist] [MeSH: Kingella] a genus of gram-negative, aerobic or facultatively anaerobic, rod-shaped bacteria of the family Neisseriaceae, found as natural inhabitants of the human oropharynx. The organisms are potential human pathogens.
**K. denitri′ficans,** a usually nonpathogenic species isolated from the upper respiratory tract and genital tract specimens.
**K. indolo′genes,** *Suttonella indologenes.*
**K. kin′gae,** a species that has been isolated from blood, bone, joint, and throat infections and from cultures of normal mucous membranes.

**Kings·ley appliance (plate), splint** (kingz′le) [Norman William *Kingsley,* American dentist, 1829–1913] see under *appliance* and *splint.*

**kin·ic ac·id** (kin′ik) quinic acid.

**ki·nin** (ki′nin) [Gr. *kinein* to move] any of a group of vasoactive straight-chain polypeptides formed by kallikrein-catalyzed cleavage of kininogens, e.g., bradykinin and kallidin; they cause vasodilation of most vessels but vasoconstriction of the pulmonary bed, and also alter vascular permeability.

**ki·nin·ase** (ki′nin-ās) an enzyme that destroys the activity of circulating kinins.
**k. I,** serine carboxypeptidase.
**k. II,** peptidyl-dipeptidase A.

**ki·nin·o·gen** (ki-nin′o-jen″) either of two plasma $\alpha_2$-globulins that are kinin precursors, called *high-molecular-weight k.* and *low-molecular-weight k.*
**high-molecular-weight k.,** HMWK; a kininogen of molecular weight 100,000–250,000 that is split by plasma kallikrein to produce bradykinin. Called also Fitzgerald factor.
**low-molecular-weight k.,** LMWK; a kininogen of molecular weight 50,000–75,000 that is split by tissue kallikrein to produce kallidin.

**Kin·ni·er Wil·son** (kin′e-ər-wil′sən) see *Wilson.*

**ki·no** (ki′no) the dried juice of *Pterocarpus marsupium* Roxb. (Leguminosae), of southern Asia, and of various other trees; it has been used as an astringent.

**kin(o)-** [Gr. *kinein* to move] see *kine-.*

**ki·no·cen·trum** (kĭ″no-sen′trəm) centrosome.

**ki·no·cil·i·um** (ki″no-sil′e-əm) pl. *kinocil′ia* [*kino-* + *cilium*] a motile, protoplasmic filament on the free surface of a cell. See also *hair cells,* under *cell,* and *stereocilium.*

**ki·no·hapt** (ki′no-hapt) [*kino-* + Gr. *haptein* to touch] an esthesiometer for making several tactile stimulations at definite intervals of time or space.

**ki·nol·o·gy** (kĭ-nol′ə-je) kinesiology.

**ki·no·mom·e·ter** (kĭ″no-mom′ə-ter) [*kino-* + *-meter*] goniometer.

**ki·no·sphere** (ki′no-sfēr) [*kino-* + *sphere*] aster.

**kin·ship** (kin′ship) [A.S. *cynscip*] a group of individuals of varying degrees of descent from a common ancestor.

**Kirch·ner's diverticulum** (kirk′nərz) [Wilhelm *Kirchner,* Austrian otologist, 1849–1936] see under *diverticulum.*

**Kirk's amputation** (kərks) [Norman Thomas *Kirk,* Surgeon General of U.S. Army, 1888–1960] see under *amputation.*

**Kirsch·ner wire** (kirsh′nər) [Martin *Kirschner,* German surgeon, 1879–1942] [MeSH: Bone Wires] see under *wire.*

**Kir·stein's method** (kir′shtīnz) [Alfred *Kirstein,* German physician, 1863–1922] see *direct laryngoscopy,* under *laryngoscopy.*

**Kisch's reflex** (kish′əz) [Bruno *Kisch,* German physiologist, 1890–1966] see under *reflex.*

**kit·a·sa·my·cin** (kit″ə-sə-mi′sin) [MeSH: Kitasamycin] a macrolide antibiotic produced by *Streptomyces kitasoensis,* active against most gram-positive and some gram-negative bacteria, as well as certain other pathogenic microorganisms. Called also *leucomycin.*

**ki·tol** (ki′tol) [Gr. *kētos* sea monster, big fish] a substance from whale oil which yields vitamin A on heating.

**kj** knee jerk.

**Kjel·dahl's method (test)** (kyel'dahlz) [Johan Gustav Christoffer *Kjeldahl,* Danish chemist, 1849–1900] see under *method.*

**Kjel·land** (kyel'ənd) see *Kielland.*

**kl** kiloliter.

**Klapp's creeping treatment** (klahps) [Rudolf *Klapp,* German surgeon, 1873–1949] see under *treatment.*

**Klats·kin's tumor** (klats'kinz) [Gerald *Klatskin,* American internist, born 1910] [MeSH: Klatskin's Tumor] hilar cholangiocarcinoma.

**Klebs' disease** (klebz) [Theodor Albrecht Edwin *Klebs,* German bacteriologist, 1834–1913] glomerulonephritis.

**Klebs-Löf·fler bacillus** (klebz-lerf'lər) [T. A. E. *Klebs;* Friederich A. J. *Löffler,* German bacteriologist, 1852–1915] *Corynebacterium diphtheriae.*

**Kleb·si·el·la** (kleb"se-el'ə) [T. A. E. *Klebs*] [MeSH: Klebsiella] a genus of bacteria of the family Enterobacteriaceae, made up of small, gram-negative, facultatively anaerobic, nonmotile rods, usually occurring singly; they are widely distributed in nature and are commonly found in the human intestinal tract. They are a frequent cause of nosocomial urinary and pulmonary infections and of wound infections.
**K. friedlän'deri,** *K. pneumoniae.*
**K. oxyto'ca,** a species similar to *K. pneumoniae* except that it is indole positive, is found in the mammalian intestinal tract and human clinical specimens, and is a cause of human urinary tract infections.
**K. ozae'nae,** *K. pneumoniae ozaenae.*
**K. planti'cola,** a species that is both indole positive and ornithine positive, found mainly in botanic, aquatic, and soil isolates.
**K. pneumo'niae,** an encapsulated species found in soil, water, and grain, in the intestinal tract of humans and animals, and in association with infections of the urinary and respiratory tracts. It is the etiologic agent of an acute bacterial pneumonia (see Klebsiella *pneumonia,* under *pneumonia*). Called also *K. friedländeri* and *Friedländer's bacillus* or *pneumobacillus.*
**K. pneumo'niae ozae'nae,** a species occurring in ozena and other chronic respiratory diseases.
**K. pneumo'niae rhinosclero'matis,** a species found in patients with rhinoscleroma and their contacts. Called also *Frisch bacillus.*
**K. rhinosclero'matis,** *K. pneumoniae rhinoscleromatis.*
**K. terrige'na,** a species similar to *K. pneumoniae* except that it ferments glucose at 5° C and 10° C; isolated from aquatic and soil samples.

**Kleb·si·el·leae** (kleb"se-el'e-e) in some systems of classification, a tribe of gram-negative, facultatively anaerobic, rod-shaped bacteria of the family Enterobacteriaceae, made up of the genera *Klebsiella, Enterobacter, Pectobacterium,* and *Serratia.*

**klee·blatt·schä·del** (kla"blaht-sha'dəl) [Ger.] cloverleaf skull; a congenital anomaly in which there is intrauterine synostosis of multiple or all cranial sutures. See *kleeblattschädel syndrome,* under *syndrome.*

**Klein-Waar·den·burg syndrome** (klīn-vahr'dən-bərg) [David *Klein,* Swiss physician, born 1908; Petrus Johannes *Waardenburg,* Dutch ophthalmologist, 1886–1979] Waardenburg's syndrome.

**Kleine-Lev·in syndrome** (klīn'ə-lev'in) [Willi *Kleine,* German psychiatrist, 20th century; Max *Levin,* American neurologist, born 1901] [MeSH: Kleine-Levin Syndrome] see under *syndrome.*

**Kleist's sign** (klīsts) [Karl *Kleist,* German neurologist, born 1879] see under *sign.*

**Klemm's sign** (klemz) [Paul *Klemm,* German surgeon, 1861–1921] see under *sign.*

**klept(o)-** [Gr. *kleptein* to steal] combining form denoting relationship to theft or stealing.

**klep·to·lag·nia** (klep"to-lag'ne-ə) [*klepto-* + Gr. *lagneia* lust] sexual gratification produced by theft.

**klep·to·ma·nia** (klep"to-ma'ne-ə) [*klepto-* + *-mania*] [DSM-IV] an uncontrollable impulse to steal objects unnecessary for personal use or monetary value, the act being preceded by tension and followed by pleasure or relief, and not caused by anger, delusion, vengeance, or hallucination.

**klep·to·ma·ni·ac** (klep"to-ma'ne-ak) an individual exhibiting kleptomania.

**Klieg eye** (klēg) [named from *Klieg,* the manufacturer of electric lamps used in motion picture making] see under *eye.*

**Kline·fel·ter's syndrome** (klīn'fel-tərz) [Harry Fitch *Klinefelter,* Jr., American physician, born 1912] [MeSH: Klinefelter's Syndrome] see under *syndrome.*

**Klip·pel-Feil syndrome** (klĭ-pel' fīl) [Maurice *Klippel,* French neurologist, 1858–1942; André *Feil,* French physician, 20th century] [MeSH: Klippel-Feil Syndrome] see under *syndrome.*

**Klip·pel-Tré·nau·nay syndrome** (klĭ-pel' tra-no-na') [Maurice *Klippel;* Paul *Trĕnaunay,* French physician, 20th century] see under *syndrome.*

**Klip·pel-Tré·nau·nay-We·ber syndrome** (klĭ-pel' tra-no-na' va'ber) [M. *Klippel;* P. *Trénaunay;* Frederick Parkes *Weber,* English physician, 1863–1962] see under *syndrome.*

**Klip·pel-Weil sign** (klĭ-pel' vīl) [Maurice *Klippel;* Mathieu Pierre *Weil,* French physician, 20th century] see under *sign.*

**klis·e·om·e·ter** (klis"e-om'ə-tər) cliseometer.

**klis·ma·phil·ia** (kliz"mə-fil'e-ə) love of enemas; a paraphilia in which sexual excitement depends on the use of enemas.

**Klon·o·pin** (klon'o-pin) trademark for a preparation of clonazepam.

**Klos·si·el·la** (klos"e-el'ə) a genus of coccidian protozoa (suborder Adeleina, order Eucoccidiida) parasitic in the renal cells of mammals, such as the mouse and guinea pig, characterized by the presence of an oocyst with many spores, each producing many sporozoites.

**Klump·ke's paralysis (palsy)** (kloomp'kəz) [Augusta Dejerine-*Klumpke,* French neurologist, 1859–1927] see under *paralysis.*

**Klump·ke-Dej·er·ine paralysis, syndrome** (kloomp'kə dĕ-zhĕ-rēn') [Augusta Dejerine-*Klumpke;* Joseph Jules *Dejerine,* French neurologist, 1849–1917] Klumpke's paralysis.

**Klü·ver-Bu·cy syndrome** (kle'vər-bu'se) [Heinrich *Klüver,* American psychologist and neurologist, 1897–1979; Paul Clancy *Bucy,* American neurologist, born 1904] see under *syndrome.*

**Kluy·vera** (kli'vər-ə) [A.J. *Kluyver,* Dutch microbiologist] a genus of gram-negative, facultatively anaerobic, rod-shaped bacteria of the family Enterobacteriaceae, occurring in human clinical specimens. It is an occasional opportunistic pathogen, causing respiratory and urinary infections. The type species is *K. ascorba'ta.*

**Km** see under *allotype.*

**km** kilometer.

**Knapp's operation, streaks (striae)** (knahps) [Herman Jakob *Knapp,* German-born ophthalmologist in United States, 1832–1911] see under *operation* and *streak.*

**knead·ing** (nēd'ing) pétrissage.

**knee** (ne) [MeSH: Knee] 1. genu, def. 1. 2. any structure bent like the knee. 3. in ungulates, the carpus of the foreleg or the stifle joint of the hind leg.
**back k.,** genu recurvatum.
**beat k.,** a subcutaneous cellulitis over the kneecap.
**big k.,** 1. in cattle, bursitis over the knee. 2. in horses, a tumor of the bony parts of the knee joint. 3. in goats, the adult form of caprine arthritis-encephalitis.
**Brodie's k.,** a chronic synovitis of the knee joint in which the affected parts acquire a soft and pulpy consistency.
**capped k.,** distention of the synovial bursa over the knee joint of horses or cattle.
**football k.,** a swollen, relaxed, somewhat tender condition of the knee seen in football players.
**housemaid's k.,** inflammation of the bursa in front of the patella, with fluid accumulating within it.
**in k.,** genu valgum.
**k. of internal capsule,** genu capsulae internae.
**jumper's k.,** pain and tenderness over the lower pole of the patella, similar to that occurring in Larsen-Johansson disease, without radiographic changes; so called because of its occurrence in athletes.
**knock k.,** genu valgum.
**locked k.,** inability to extend the leg fully as a result of tear of the medial semilunar cartilage.
**out k.,** genu varum.
**popped k.,** carpitis.
**rugby k.,** Osgood-Schlatter disease.
**septic k.,** a suppurating knee joint.
**sprung k.,** forward bending of the knee of a horse, due to shortening of the flexor tendons.
**trick k.,** popular term for a knee joint susceptible to locking in position, most often due to longitudinal splitting of the medial meniscus.

**knee-gall** (ne'gawl) thoroughpin.

**kneipp·ism** (nīp'iz-əm) [Rev. Sebastian *Kneipp,* German priest, 1821–1897, who introduced the practice] a system of hydrotherapy involving applications of cold water, including cold bathing and walking barefoot in the morning dew. etc.

**Kne·mi·do·kop·tes** (ne"mĭ-do-kop'tēz) a genus of mites. *K. galli'nae,* the depluming mite, causes depluming of fowls. *K. mu'tans* causes the disease called scaly leg in fowls and cage birds.

**Knies' sign** (knēz) [Max *Knies,* German ophthalmologist, 1851–1917] see under *sign.*

**knife** (nīf) a cutting instrument of various shapes and sizes.
**Blair k.**, a knife with a long sharp blade used to cut skin grafts.
**Buck k.**, a periodontal knife with spear-shaped cutting points, used for interdental incision during gingivectomy.
**button k.**, a small knife used for the cutting of cartilage.
**cataract k.**, a knife for cutting the cornea in operations for cataract.
**cautery k.**, a knife connected with an electric battery, so that the tissues may be seared while being cut, in order to prevent bleeding.
**electric k.**, a knife-shaped electrode or steel needle which cuts by causing dissolution of tissue when activated by a high-frequency current.
**gamma k.**, an apparatus for producing intracranial lesions by precisely aimed intersecting beams of gamma rays; used in stereotactic radiosurgery.
**Goldman-Fox k.**, any of a group of knives designed for incision and contouring of gingival tissues in periodontal surgery.
**Graefe's k.**, a slender knife used in linear extraction of cataract.
**Humby k.**, a knife with a roller attached, used for cutting skin grafts of varying thickness; the distance between the roller and the blade of the knife can be varied by means of a calibration device.
**Joseph k.**, a double-bladed knife used in corrective rhinoplasty.
**Kirkland k.**, a periodontal knife that consists of a thin, flattened blade attached to the handle by an angulated shank, the outer edge being elliptical and the inner straight; used for primary gingivectomy.
**Liston's k.**, a long-bladed amputation knife.
**Merrifield's k.**, a periodontal knife with a long narrow triangular blade; used in gingivectomy.

**Knight brace** (nīt) [James C. *Knight,* American physician, 1810–1887] see under *brace.*

**knis·mo·gen·ic** (nis″mo-jen′ik) [Gr. *knismos* tickling + *-genic*] producing a tickling sensation.

**knit·ting** (nit′ing) the physiological process of repair of a fractured bone.

**knob** (nob) a bulbous mass or protuberance.
**aortic k.**, the hump or knob formed by the aortic arch where it joins the descending thoracic aorta seen in radiographs in anteroposterior projections; called also *aortic knuckle.*
**olfactory k.**, olfactory vesicle (def. 2).
**surfers' k's**, see under *nodule.*
**synaptic k.**, bouton terminal; see under *bouton.*

**knock** (nok) a sound as of a blow against a firm surface.
**pericardial k.**, an early diastolic sound resembling an $S_3$ gallop but earlier and due to sudden deceleration of ventricular filling at capacity in cases of constrictive pericarditis.

**knock-knee** (nok′ne) genu valgum.

**Knops blood group** (nops) [from the name of the American propositus first reported on in 1970] see under *blood group.*

**knot** (not) 1. an intertwining of the ends or parts of one or more threads, sutures, or strips of cloth so they cannot easily be separated. 2. in anatomy, a knoblike swelling or protuberance, as a node.
**clove-hitch k.**, a knot consisting of two contiguous loops that are applied around an object, the ends of the cord being toward each other; used for making traction on a part for the reduction of dislocations.
**double k.**, a knot in which the ends of the cord are twisted around each other twice.
**enamel k.**, a small dense group of epithelial cells in the stellate reticulum of a developing tooth, which disappears before enamel formation begins.
**false k.**, 1. a local bulge on the umbilical cord caused by protuberant vessels. Cf. *true k.* 2. granny k.
**friction k.**, double k.

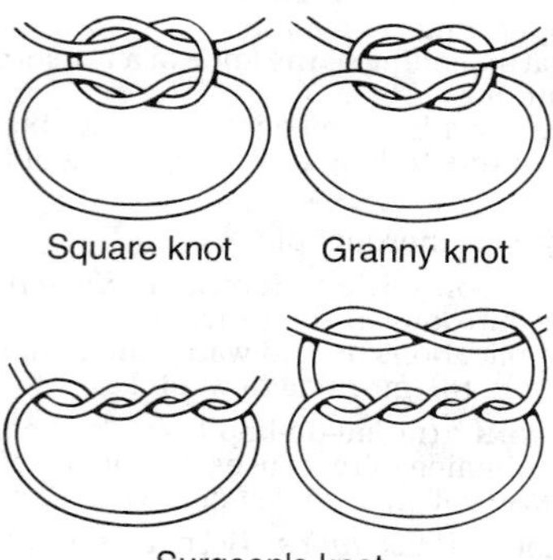


**granny k.**, a double knot in the second loop of which the end of one cord is over, and the other under, its fellow, so that the loops do not lie in the same line and the knot will not hold.
**Hensen's k.**, primitive k.
**primitive k.**, a mass of cells at the cranial end of the primitive streak, related to the organization of an embryo. Called also *primitive node.*
**protochordal k.**, primitive k.
**reef k.**, square k.
**square k.**, a double knot in which the free ends of the second knot lie in the same plane as the ends of the first knot.
**stay k.**, a knot made with two or more ligatures, each being tied with the first half of a square knot; then all the ends of one side are taken in one hand, and all the ends on the other side in the other hand, and tied as if they formed one single thread.
**surfers' k's**, see under *nodule.*
**surgeon's k., surgical k.**, a knot in which the thread is passed twice through the first loop to prevent slippage.
**syncytial k's**, protuberances of nuclei of the syncytiotrophoblast (syncytium) along the chorionic villi.
**true k.**, a simple knot produced in the looped umbilical cord during pregnancy. Cf. *false k.*

**knuck·le** (nuk′əl) the dorsal aspect of any phalangeal joint, especially of the metacarpophalangeal joints of the flexed fingers. By extension sometimes applied to any anatomical structure of similar appearance, such as an extruded loop of intestine in hernia.
**aortic k.**, see under *knob.*

**knuck·ling** (nuk′ling) a pushing forward and upward of the fetlock joint of a horse, due to shortening of the tendons behind.

**Ko·belt's tubes, tubules** (ko′bəlts) [George Ludwig *Kobelt,* German physician, 1804–1857] see under *tube* and *tubule.*

**Ko·ber's test** (ko′bərz) [Philip Adolph *Kober,* American chemist, born 1884] see under *test.*

**Koch** (kawk) Robert. German physician and bacteriologist, 1843–1910; winner of the Nobel prize for medicine or physiology in 1905 for his work and discoveries concerning tuberculosis.

**Koch's node** (kawks) [Walter *Koch,* German surgeon, born 1880] see *nodus atrioventricularis.*

**Koch's phenomenon (reaction), postulate, tuberculin** (kawks) [Robert *Koch*] see under *phenomenon, postulate,* and *tuberculin.*

**Koch-Weeks bacillus** (kawk-wēks) [Robert *Koch;* John Elmer *Weeks,* American ophthalmologist, 1853–1949] *Haemophilus aegyptius.*

**Ko·cher** (kō′kər) Emil Theodor. Swiss surgeon, 1841–1917; winner of the Nobel prize for medicine or physiology in 1909 for his work on the physiology and pathology of the thyroid gland and for thyroidectomy for treatment of goiter.

**Ko·cher's forceps,** etc. (kō′kərz) [Emil Theodor *Kocher*] see under *forceps, incision, maneuver, method, operation, reflex,* and *sign.*

**Ko·cher-De·bré-Sé·mé·laigne syndrome** (ko′kər də-bra′ sa-ma-len′yə) [Emil Theodor *Kocher;* Robert *Debré,* French pediatrician and bacteriologist, 1882–1978; Georges *Sémélaigne,* French pediatrician, 20th century] Debré-Sémélaigne syndrome.

**ko·cher·iza·tion** (ko″kər-ĭ-za′shən) Kocher maneuver.

**Ko·chia** (ko′ke-ə) a genus of herbs of the family Chenopodiaceae. *K. scopa′ria* is the summer cypress or fireweed, a shrub of Europe and Asia that has red foliage; when eaten by cattle it causes lacrimation, anorexia, liver damage, and photosensitization.

**Kock ileostomy (procedure), pouch** (kawk) [Nils G. *Kock,* Swedish surgeon, born 1924] see under *ileostomy* and *pouch.*

**Koe·ber·lé's forceps** (ko″ber-lāz′) [Eugène *Koeberlé,* French surgeon, 1828–1915] hemostatic forceps.

**Koeb·ner's phenomenon** (kərb′nərz) [Heinrich *Koebner,* German dermatologist, 1838–1904] see under *phenomenon.*

**Koer·ber-Sa·lus-Elsch·nig syndrome** (kər′bər sah′lo͞os elsh′nik) [Hermann *Koerber,* German ophthalmologist, born 1878; Robert *Salus,* Austrian ophthalmologist, 20th century; Anton *Elschnig,* Austrian ophthalmologist, 1863–1939] sylvian syndrome; see under *syndrome.*

**Ko·ge·nate** (ko′jə-nāt) trademark for a preparation of antihemophilic factor produced by recombinant technology.

**Ko·goj's pustule** (ko′goiz) [Franjo *Kogoj,* Yugoslavian physician, born 1894] see *spongiform pustule of Kogoj,* under *pustule.*

**Köhler** (kər′lər) Georges Jean Franz. German immunologist, born 1946. Co-winner with Niels Kaj Jerne and Cesar Milstein of the Nobel prize for medicine or physiology in 1984 for his and Milstein's production of monoclonal antibodies.

**Köh·ler's bone disease** (kər′lərz) [Alban *Köhler,* German physician, 1874–1947] see under *disease.*

**Köh·ler-Pel·le·gri·ni-Stie·da disease** (kər′lər pel-ə-gre′ne shte′dah) [Alban *Köhler;* Augusto *Pellegrini,* Italian physician, born 1877; Alfred *Stieda,* German physician, 1869–1945] see *Pellegrini's disease,* under *disease.*

**Kohl·rausch's folds (valves)** (kōl′roush-əz) [Otto Ludwig Bernhard *Kohlrausch,* German physician, 1811–1854] plicae transversae recti.

**Kohn·stamm's phenomenon** (kōn′shtahmz) [Oskar Felix *Kohnstamm,* German physician, 1871–1917] after-movement.

**koil(o)-** [Gr. *koilos* hollow] a combining form meaning hollow or concave.

**koi·lo·cyte** (koi′lo-sīt″) a concave or hollow cell, such as a normal red blood cell or one of the pyknotic vacuolated epithelial cells with clear cytoplasm seen in koilocytosis.

**koi·lo·cy·to·sis** (koi″lo-si-to′sis) [*koilo-* + *cyt-* + *-osis*] the presence of abnormal koilocytes that are vacuolated with clear cytoplasm or perinuclear halos and nuclear pyknosis. It is often seen in infections by human papillomavirus of epithelial layers of the uterine cervix or external anal or genital areas. See also *koilocytotic atypia,* under *atypia,* and *condyloma acuminatum.*

**koi·lo·cy·tot·ic** (koi-lo-si-tot′ik) pertaining to or resembling koilocytosis.

**koil·onych·ia** (koi″lo-nik′e-ə) [*koilo-* + *onychia*] dystrophy of the fingernails, sometimes associated with iron deficiency anemia, in which they are thin and concave, with the edges raised; called also *spoon nail.*

**koi·lor·rhach·ic** (koi″lo-rak′ik) [*koilo-* + *rhachi-* + *-ic*] having a vertebral column in which the lumbar curvature is concave anteriorly. Cf. *kyphosis, kyrtorrhachic,* and *orthorrhachic.*

**koi·lo·ster·nia** (koi″lo-stər′ne-ə) [*koilo-* + *stern-* + *-ia*] pectus excavatum.

**koin(o)-** see *cen(o)-*[3].

**ko·jic ac·id** (ko′jik) a pyrone formed from sugars by a variety of microorganisms, especially species of *Aspergillus;* it has antibiotic and antifungal properties.

**Ko·lan·tyl** (ko-lan′təl) trademark for a preparation of alumina and magnesia.

**Köl·li·ker's column, granule, membrane** (ker′lĭ-kərz) [Rudolf Abert von *Köllicker,* Swiss anatomist in Germany, 1817–1905] see under *granule,* and see *membrana reticularis organi spiralis, nucleus subparabrachialis,* and *sarcostyle.*

**Koll·mann's dilator** (kawl′mahnz) [Arthur *Kollmann,* German urologist, 19th century] see under *dilator.*

**Kol·mer test** (kōl′mər) [John A. *Kolmer,* American pathologist, 1886–1962] see under *test.*

**Kol·mo·go·rov-Smir·nov test** (kol-mog′ə-rov smēr′nov) [Andrei Nicolaievich *Kolmogorov,* Russian mathematician, 1903–1987; Nicolai Vasilievich *Smirnov,* Russian mathematician, born 1900] see under *test.*

**kolp-** for words beginning thus, see those beginning *colp-.*

**ko·ly·pep·tic** (ko″le-pep′tik) [Gr. *kōlyein* to hinder + *peptic*] hindering or checking digestion.

**Kon·a·ki·on** (kon″ə-ki′on) trademark for a preparation of phytonadione (vitamin $K_1$).

**Kon·do·le·on's operation** (kon-do′la-ənz) [Emmerich (Emmanuel) *Kondoleon,* Greek surgeon, 1879–1939] see under *operation.*

**Kö·nig's rods** (ker′nigz) [Charles Joseph *König,* German otologist, late 19th century] see under *rod.*

**Kö·nig's syndrome** (ker′nigz) [Franz *König,* German surgeon, 1832–1910] see under *syndrome.*

**ko·nim·e·ter** (ko-nim′ə-tər) an apparatus for counting the number of dust particles in the air. Called also *coniometer* and *konometer.*

**ko·nio·cor·tex** (ko″ne-o-kor′teks) [Gr. *konis* dust + *cortex,* so called because of the large number and small size of the granular cells] the cortex of the sensory areas of the brain that have particularly many prominent granule cells in layers II and IV; called also *granular cortex.*

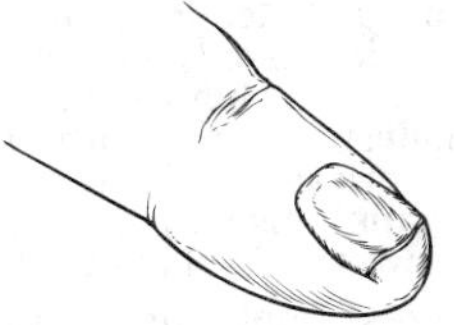

Koilonychia.

**ko·ni·ol·o·gy** (ko″ne-ol′ə-je) coniology.

**ko·nom·e·ter** (ko-nom′ə-tər) [Gr. *konis* dust + *metron* measure] konimeter.

**Kon·syl** (kon′səl) a brand of psyllium hydrophilic mucilloid.

**ko·pi·opia** (ko″pe-o′pe-ə) copiopia.

**Kop·lik's spots (sign)** (kop′liks) [Henry *Koplik,* American pediatrician, 1858–1927] see under *spot.*

**kopr-** for words beginning thus, see those beginning *copr-.*

**Ko·rán·yi's auscultation (percussion), sign** (ko-rahn′yēz) [Baron Friedrich von *Korányi,* Hungarian physician, 1828–1913] see under *auscultation.*

**Kor·do·fan gum** (kor′də-fan) [*Kordofan* province in the Sudan, where the trees are found] see under *gum.*

**Korn·berg** (korn′bərg) Arthur. American physician and biochemist, born 1918; co-winner, with Severo Ochoa, of the Nobel prize for medicine or physiology in 1959 for discovering the mechanisms in the biological synthesis of deoxyribonucleic acid and ribonucleic acid.

**ko·ro** (ko′ro) [MeSH: Koro] a culture-specific acute delusional syndrome occurring in south and east Asia in which the patient believes that the penis or the vulva and nipples are shrinking and may disappear into the abdomen, causing death.

**ko·ro·ni·on** (ko-ro′ne-on) pl. *koro′nia* [Gr. *korōnē* crow, crown] coronion.

**ko·ros·co·py** (ko-ros′kə-pe) retinoscopy.

**Ko·rot·koff's method, sounds, test** (kə-rot-kofs′) [Nicolai Sergeevich *Korotkoff,* Russian physician, 1874–1920] see under *method, sound,* and *test.*

**Kor·sa·koff's (Kor·sa·kov's) syndrome (psychosis)** (kor′sə-kəfs) [Sergei Sergeevich *Korsakoff* (or *Korsakov*), Russian neurologist, 1854–1900] see under *syndrome.*

**Kör·te-Bal·lance operation** (ker′tə bal′əns) [Werner *Körte,* German surgeon, 1853–1937; Sir Charles Alfred *Ballance,* British surgeon, 1856–1936] see under *operation.*

**ko·sam** (ko′səm) *Brucea sumatrana,* a small evergreen shrub whose seeds are sometimes used locally in the treatment of diarrhea, dysentery, and uterine hemorrhage.

**Ko·shev·ni·koff's (Ko·schew·ni·kow's, Ko·zhev·ni·kov's) disease, epilepsy** (ko-shev′nĭ-kofs) [Alexei Jakovlevich *Koshevnikoff* (or *Koschewnikow* or *Kozhevnikov*), Russian neurologist, 1836–1902] epilepsia partialis continua.

**Kos·sel** (kos′əl) Albrecht. German physiologist, 1853–1927; winner of the Nobel prize for medicine or physiology in 1910 for his contributions to cellular chemistry through his work on proteins, including nucleic substances.

**Kos·sel's test** (kos′əlz) [Albrecht *Kossel*] see under *test.*

**Kost·mann's neutropenia (syndrome)** (kost′mahnz) [Rolf *Kostmann,* Swedish physician, born 1909] infantile genetic agranulocytosis.

**Ko·va·lev·sky's canal** (ko″və-lev′skēz) [Alexander Onufrievich *Kovalevsky,* Russian embryologist, 1840–1901] neurenteric canal.

**Koy·ter's muscle** (koi′tərz) [Volcherus *Koyter,* Dutch anatomist, 1534–1600] musculus corrugator supercilii.

**KP** keratic precipitates; see *keratitis punctata.*

**K-Phos** (ka′fos) trademark for a preparation of monobasic potassium phosphate.

**Kr** symbol for *krypton.*

**Krabbe's disease (leukodystrophy)** (krah′bəz) [Knud H. *Krabbe,* Danish neurologist, 1885–1961] see under *disease.*

**Krae·pe·lin** (kra′pə-lin) Emil. German psychiatrist, 1856–1926; the father of descriptive psychiatry. He differentiated manic-depressive psychosis from dementia praecox (schizophrenia) and described the basic schizophrenic subtypes: catatonic, hebephrenic, and paranoid. Modern classifications of the psychoses are still essentially kraepelinian.

**krait** (krāt) any member of the genus *Bungarus,* extremely venomous crotalid snakes found from India across Southeast and East Asia. See table at *snake.*

**Kra·me·ria** (kra-me′re-ə) [J. G. H. and W. H. *Kramer,* German botanists] a genus of shrubs and herbs of the family Leguminosae. The dried roots of *K. trian′dra* R. et P., or Peruvian rhatany, and of *K. argen′tea* Mart., or Brazilian rhatany, were formerly used as an astringent.

**Kras·ke's operation** (krahs'kəz) [Paul *Kraske,* German surgeon, 1851–1930] see under *operation.*

**kra·tom·e·ter** (krə-tom'ə-tər) a prism-refracting instrument for use in orthoptic training.

**krau·ro·sis** (kraw-ro'sis) [Gr. *krauros* brittle] a dry, shriveled condition of a part, especially of the vulva (see *k. vulvae*).
**k. vul'vae,** *lichen sclerosus* in females; see under *lichen.*

**Krause's bulbs, corpuscle, line, membrane** (krou'zəz) [Wilhelm Johann Friedrich *Krause,* German anatomist, 1833–1910] see under *bulb, corpuscle, line,* and *membrane.*

**Krause's glands, ligament, valve** (krou'zəz) [Karl Friedrich Theodor *Krause,* German anatomist, 1797–1868] see *glandulae conjunctivales* and *ligamentum transversum perinei,* and see *Béraud's valve,* under *valve.*

**Krause's operation** (krou'zəz) [Fedor Victor *Krause,* German surgeon, 1857–1937] see under *operation.*

**Krause-Wolfe graft** (krou'zə-woolf) [F. V. *Krause;* John Reissberg *Wolfe,* Scottish ophthalmologist, 1824–1904] see under *graft.*

**kre·a·tin** (kre'ə-tin) creatine.

**kre·bi·o·zen** (krə-bi'o-zən) a substance identified as creatine by the Food and Drug Administration, isolated from the blood of horses injected with *Actinomyces bovis,* claimed to be effective in the treatment of cancer; its sale is banned in the United States.

**Krebs** (krebz) Edwin Gerhard. American biochemist, born 1918. Co-winner with Edmond Henri Fischer of the Nobel prize for medicine or physiology in 1992 for their work on protein kinases in cell metabolism.

**Krebs** (krebz) Sir Hans Adolf. German-born British biochemist, 1900–1981; co-winner, with Fritz Albert Lipmann, of the Nobel prize for medicine or physiology in 1953 for the discovery of the citric acid cycle.

**Krebs cycle** (krebz) [Sir Hans Adolf *Krebs*] tricarboxylic acid cycle; see under *cycle.*

**kre(o)-** for words beginning thus, see also those beginning *cre(o)-*

**kreo·tox·i·con** (kre″o-tok'sĭ-kon) the substance in poisonous meat that produces the toxic symptoms; see *meat poisoning,* under *poisoning.*

**kreo·tox·in** (kre″o-tok'sin) any basic poison generated in a flesh food by a plant microorganism; see *meat poisoning,* under *poisoning.*

**kreo·tox·ism** (kre″o-tok'siz-əm) [Gr. *kreas* meat + *toxi-* + *-ism*] meat poisoning; see under *poisoning.*

**kreso·fuch·sin** (kres″o-fo͝ok'sin) a blue-gray powder used as a stain in histology; its aqueous solution is red, the alcoholic solution blue.

**kres·ol** (kres'ol) cresol.

**Kretsch·mann's space** (krech'mahnz) [Friedrich *Kretschmann,* German otologist, 1858–1934] see under *space.*

**Kretsch·mer types** (krech'mər) [Ernst *Kretschmer,* German psychiatrist, 1888–1964] see under *type.*

**Kretz's granules** (krets'əz) [Richard *Kretz,* German pathologist, 1865–1920] see under *granule.*

**Krey·sig's sign** (kri'zigz) [Friedrich Ludwig *Kreysig,* German physician, 1770–1839] Heim-Kreysig sign.

**krimp·siek·te** (krimp-zēk'te) [Afrikaans] a disease of cattle in South Africa caused by poisoning with any of several plant species of the genus *Cotyledon,* which contain cotyledontoxin; symptoms include abdominal pain and convulsions that can be fatal.

**krin·gle** (kring'gəl) [MeSH: Kringles] see under *domain.*

**Kris·hab·er's disease** (krēs″hah-bārz') [Maurice *Krishaber,* Hungarian physician in France, 1836–1883] see under *disease.*

**Kri·sov·ski's sign** (krĭ-sov'skēz) [Max *Krisovski* (or *Krisowski*), German physician, late 19th century] see under *sign.*

**Kri·sow·ski** (krĭ-sov'ske) see *Krisovski.*

**Krogh** (krōg) Schack August Stenberg. Danish physiologist, 1874–1949; winner of the Nobel prize for medicine or physiology in 1920 for his discovery of the capillary motor regulating mechanism.

**Kro·may·er's lamp** (kro'mi-ərz) [Ernst Ludwig Franz *Kromayer,* German dermatologist, 1862–1933] see under *lamp.*

**Kro·neck·er's center, puncture** (kro'nek-ərz) [Karl Hugo *Kronecker,* German pathologist in Switzerland, 1839–1914] see *cardioinhibitory center,* under *center,* and see under *puncture.*

**Krön·lein's hernia, operation** (krərn'līnz) [Rudolf Ulrich *Krönlein,* Swiss surgeon, 1847–1910] see *inguinoproperitoneal hernia,* under *hernia,* and see under *operation.*

**Kru·ken·berg's spindle, tumor** (kroo'kən-bergz) [Friedrich Ernst *Krukenberg,* German pathologist, 1871–1946] see under *spindle* and *tumor.*

**Kru·ken·berg's veins** (kroo'kən-bergz) [Adolph *Krukenberg,* German anatomist, 1816–1877] venae centrales hepatis.

**krypt(o)-** for words beginning thus, see those beginning *crypt(o)-.*

**kryp·ton** (krip'ton) [Gr. *kryptos* hidden] [MeSH: Krypton] an inert gaseous chemical element found in the atmosphere; atomic number, 36; atomic weight, 83.80; symbol, Kr.
**k. Kr 81m** [USP], an unstable radioactive isotope of krypton, atomic mass 81, having a half-life of 13 seconds and emitting gamma rays (0.19 MeV); it is used in pulmonary ventilation studies to evaluate regional function.

**17-KS** 17-ketosteroid.

**Kt/v** an expression of the efficiency, or fractional urea clearance, of one hemodialysis session; *K* is the rate of clearance, *t* is the amount of time of the session, and *V* is the urea distribution volume after hemodialysis.

**KUB** kidney, ureter, and bladder.

**ku·bi·sa·ga·ri** (koo-be-sah-gah're) [Japanese] Japanese name for *vestibular neuronitis.*

**ku·bis·ga·ri** (koo'bēs-gah're) Japanese name for *vestibular neuronitis.*

**Kufs' disease** (koofs) [H. *Kufs,* German psychiatrist, 1871–1955] see under *disease.*

**Ku·gel·berg-Wel·an·der syndrome** (koo'gəl-berg vel'ən-dər) [Eric Klas Henrik *Kugelberg,* Swedish neurologist, born 1913; Lisa *Welander,* Swedish neurologist, born 1909] see under *syndrome.*

**Kuhl·mann's test** (ko͞ol'mənz) [Frederick *Kuhlmann,* American psychologist, 1876–1941] see under *test.*

**Küh·ne's muscular phenomenon, terminal plates** (ke'nez) [Wilhelm Friedrich (Willy) *Kühne,* German physiologist, 1837–1900] see *Porret's phenomenon,* under *phenomenon,* and see under *plate.*

**Kuhnt-Ju·ni·us disease** (ko͞ont-yoo'ne-es) [Hermann *Kuhnt,* German ophthalmologist, 1850–1925; Paul *Junius,* German ophthalmologist, born 1871] disciform macular degeneration; see under *degeneration.*

**Kul·chit·sky's cells** (ko͞ol-chit'skēz) [Nicolai K. *Kulchitsky,* Russian histologist, 1856–1925] see under *cell.*

**Külz's cast (cylinder), test** (kēlt-səz) [Rudolph Eduard *Külz,* German physician, 1845–1895] see *coma casts,* under *cast,* and see under *test.*

**Küm·mell's disease (spondylitis)** (kēm'əlz) [Hermann *Kümmell,* German surgeon, 1852–1937] see under *disease.*

**Küm·mell-Ver·neuil disease** (kēm'əl vār-nwe') [Hermann *Kümmell;* Aristide August Stanislas *Verneuil,* French surgeon, 1823–1895] Kümmell's disease.

**Kun·kel's syndrome** (kung'kəlz) [Henry George *Kunkel,* American physician, 1916–1983] lupoid hepatitis.

**Künt·scher nail** (kēnt'shər) [Gerhard *Küntscher,* German surgeon, 1902–1972] see under *nail.*

**Kupf·fer's cells** (koop'fərz) [Karl Wilhelm von *Kupffer,* German anatomist, 1829–1902] see under *cell.*

**ku·pra·mite** (koo'prə-mīt) a gas mask adsorbent for ammonia fumes.

**Kur·loff's (Kur·lov's) bodies** (ko͞or'lofs) [Mikhail Georgievich *Kurloff* (or *Kurlov*), Russian physician, 1859–1932] see under *body.*

**Kur·thia** (kər'the-ə) [Heinrich *Kurth,* German bacteriologist, 1860–1901] a genus of coryneform bacteria, consisting of gram-positive, regular, unbranched rods with rounded ends, occurring in chains and of pleomorphic forms. They have been isolated from human feces in mild cases of food poisoning and under normal conditions and from meats and meat products, and are found in the intestinal contents of chickens and in manure, stagnant water, and milk. It contains a single species, *K. zopfii.* Called also *Proteus zenkeri.*

**kur·to·sis** (kər-to'sis) [Gr. "convexity"] the degree of peakedness or flatness of a probability distribution, relative to the normal distribution with the same variance. See *leptokurtic* and *platykurtic.*

**ku·ru** (koo'roo) ["shivering" in language of the Fore people of New Guinea] [MeSH: Kuru] an infectious form of prion disease with a long incubation period, found only among the Fore and neighboring peoples of New Guinea and thought to be associated with ritual cannibalism. It is manifested by truncal and limb ataxia, a shivering-like tremor, and dysarthria and ends invariably in death; strabismus and extrapyramidal symptoms may also be found. Amyloid plaques are present in about two thirds of affected individuals.

**Küss' experiment** (kēs) [Emil *Küss,* German physiologist, 1815–1871] see under *experiment.*

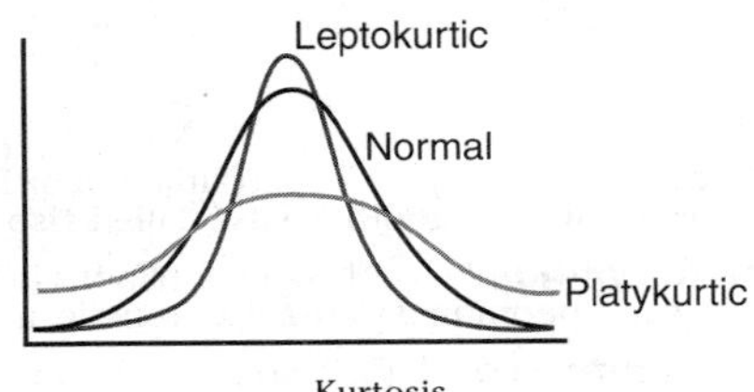

Kurtosis.

**Kuss·maul's disease, pulse,** etc. (koos'moulz) [Adolf *Kussmaul,* German physician, 1822–1902] see *polyarteritis nodosa;* see *paradoxical pulse,* under *pulse* and *diabetic coma,* under *coma;* and see under *respiration* and *sign.*

**Kuss·maul-Kien respiration** (koos'moul-kēn) [Adolf *Kussmaul;* Alphonse Marie Joseph *Kien,* German physician, late 19th century] see under *respiration.*

**Kuss·maul-Lan·dry paralysis** (koos'moul-lahn-dre') [Adolf *Kussmaul;* Jean Baptiste Octave *Landry,* French physician, 1826–1865] acute idiopathic polyneuritis.

**Kuss·maul-Mai·er disease** (koos'moul-mi'ər) [Adolf *Kussmaul;* Rudolf *Maier,* German physician, 1824–1888] polyarteritis nodosa.

**Küst·ner's law, sign** (kēst'nərz) [Otto Ernst *Küstner,* German gynecologist, 1849–1931] see under *law* and *sign.*

**Ku·trol** (ku'trol) trademark for a preparation of urogastrone.

**kV** kilovolt.

**Kveim test** (kvīm) [Morten Ansgar *Kveim,* Norwegian pathologist in Denmark, 20th century] [MeSH: Kveim Test] see under *test.*

**kVp** kilovolts peak.

**kW** kilowatt.

**kwash·i·or·kor** (kwahsh"e-or'kor) ["condition seen in the displaced child" in the language of the Ga people of Ghana] [MeSH: Kwashiorkor] a form of protein-energy malnutrition produced by severe protein deficiency; caloric intake may be adequate but is usually also deficient. It is characterized by retarded growth, changes in skin and hair pigment, edema, enlarged abdomen, immunodeficiency, and pathologic changes in the liver, including fatty infiltration, necrosis, and fibrosis. Other findings are mental apathy, atrophy of the pancreas, gastrointestinal disorders, anemia, low serum albumin, and dermatoses. The skin of the limbs and back may have dark thickened patches, which may desquamate, leaving pink, almost raw surfaces. Cf. *marasmus.*
**marasmic k.,** a condition in which there is deficiency of both calories and protein, with severe tissue wasting, loss of subcutaneous fat, and usually dehydration.

**kwa·ski** (kwah'ske) see under *shakes.*

**kW-hr** kilowatt-hour.

**kyan(o)-** for words beginning thus, see those beginning *cyano-.*

**Ky·a·sa·nur For·est disease** (ki-as'ə-noor) [*Kyasanur Forest,* in Mysore State, India, where the first cases were reported among forest workers and monkeys in 1957] [MeSH: Kyasanur Forest Disease] see under *disease.*

**kyl·lo·sis** (kə-lo'sis) [Gr. *kyllōsis* a crippling] clubfoot, or other deformity of the foot.

**ky·ma·tism** (ki'mə-tiz"əm) myokymia.

**ky·mo·cy·clo·graph** (ki"mo-si'klo-graf) kymograph.

**ky·mo·gram** (ki'mo-gram) a tracing or other graphic record made by a kymograph.

**ky·mo·graph** (ki'mo-graf) [Gr. *kyma* wave + *-graph*] an instrument for recording variations or undulations, arterial or other.

**ky·mog·ra·phy** (ki-mog'rə-fe) [MeSH: Kymography] the use of the kymograph.
**roentgen k.,** radiokymography.

**Ky·nex** (ki'neks) trademark for preparations of sulfamethoxypyridazine.

**ky·no·ceph·a·lus** (ki"no-sef'ə-ləs) [Gr. *kyōn* dog + *-cephalus*] a human fetus with a head resembling that of a dog.

**kyn·uren·ic ac·id** (kin"u-ren'ik) [MeSH: Kynurenic Acid] a bicyclic aromatic compound formed from kynurenine via a transamination reaction and cyclization as a step in one pathway of tryptophan catabolism. It is excreted in the urine in several disorders of tryptophan catabolism.

**kyn·ure·nin** (kīn"u-re'nin) kynurenine.

**kyn·u·ren·in·ase** (kīn"u-ren'ĭ-nās) [EC 3.7.1.3] an enzyme of the hydrolase class that catalyzes the cleavage of hydroxykynurenine to hydroxyanthranilic acid and alanine as a step in the metabolism of tryptophan; kynurenine is also a substrate. The enzyme is a pyridoxal phosphate protein, so enzyme activity is reduced in vitamin $B_6$ deficiency.

**kyn·ure·nine** (kin-u'rə-nēn") [Gr. *kyōn* dog + L. *ren* kidney] [MeSH: Kynurenine] an aromatic amino acid, first isolated from dog urine; it is formed as an intermediate in the metabolism of tryptophan.

**kyn·ure·nine for·mam·i·dase** (kīn-u'rə-nēn" for-mam'ĭ-dās) arylformamidase.

**kyn·ure·nine 3-hy·drox·y·lase** (kīn-u'rə-nēn" hi-drok'sĭ-lās) kynurenine 3-monooxygenase.

**kyn·ure·nine 3-mono·oxy·gen·ase** (kīn-u'rə-nēn" mon"o-ok'sĭ-jən-ās) [EC 1.14.13.9] an enzyme of the oxidoreductase class that catalyzes the hydroxylation of kynurenine as a step in the metabolism of tryptophan. The enzyme is a flavoprotein, containing FAD, and the reaction requires NADPH.

**ky·phos** (ki'fos) [Gr. "a hump"] the convex prominence of the spine in kyphosis.

**ky·pho·sco·li·o·sis** (ki"fo-sko"le-o'sis) [*kyphosis* + *scoliosis*] backward and lateral curvature of the spinal column, as in vertebral osteochondrosis (Scheuermann's disease).

**ky·pho·sis** (ki-fo'sis) [Gr. *kyphōsis* humpback] [MeSH: Kyphosis] abnormally increased convexity in the curvature of the thoracic spine as viewed from the side; hunchback. Cf. *lordosis* and *scoliosis.*
**k. dorsa'lis juveni'lis, juvenile k., Scheuermann's k.,** see *osteochondrosis.*

**ky·phot·ic** (ki-fot'ik) affected with or pertaining to kyphosis.

**Kyrle's disease** (kir'ləs) [Joseph *Kyrle,* Austrian dermatologist, 1880–1926] see under *disease.*

**kyr·tor·rhach·ic** (kir"to-rak'ik) [Gr. *kyrtos* curved, convex + *rhachis* spine] having a vertebral column in which the lumbar curvature is convex anteriorly. Cf. *koilorrhachic* and *orthorrhachic.*

**kysth(o)-** [Gr. *kysthos* vagina] a combining form formerly used to denote relationship to the vagina; for words beginning thus, see those beginning colp(o)-.

**kyt(o)-** [Gr. *kytos* hollow vessel] for words beginning thus, see those beginning *cyt(o)-.*

**Ky·tril** (ki'tril) trademark for a preparation of granisetron hydrochloride.

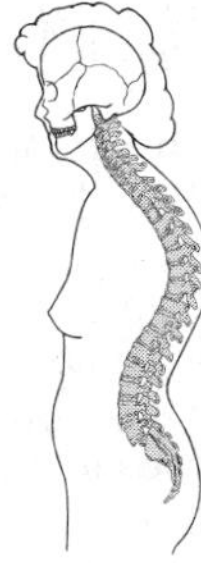
Kyphosis.

# L

**L** symbol for *lambert, left, liter, lung, light chain* (see *immunoglobulin*), and *lumbar vertebra* (L1 through L5).

**L.** symbol for L. *libra* pound.

***L*** symbol for *self-inductance* and *luminance.*

**$L_0$** symbol for *limes nul;* see *L0 dose,* under *dose.*

**L+, $L_+$** symbol for *limes tod;* see *L+ dose,* under *dose.*

**L-** a chemical prefix (small capital L) that specifies the relative configuration of an enantiomer, the mirror image being specified as D-. Carbohydrates having the same configuration as L-glyceraldehyde at the asymmetric carbon atom most distant from the carbonyl functional group are designated as L (or $L_g$). Amino acids having the same configuration as L-serine at the $\alpha$ carbon are designated as L (or $L_s$). See D- for further explanation.

**l** SI symbol for *liter.*

**l.** symbol for L. *ligamen'tum,* ligament.

***l*** symbol for *length.*

***l-*** [abbreviation for *levo* (left or counterclockwise)] a chemical prefix indicating an enantiomer that rotates the plane of polarization of a beam of light in the counterclockwise direction (levorotatory), the other enantiomer being specified as *d-* (for *dextro*). Largely replaced by (−)-; see note at *d-.*

**λ** lambda, the eleventh letter of the Greek alphabet; symbol for *wavelength, decay constant,* and one of the two types of immunoglobulin light chains; former symbol for *microliter.*

**L0** symbol for *limes nul;* see *L0 dose,* under *dose.*

**L & A** light and accommodation (reaction of pupils).

**La** symbol for *lanthanum.*

**La·bar·raque's solution** (lah-bah-rahks') [Antoine Germain *Labarraque,* French chemist, 1777–1850] see under *solution.*

**Lab·bé's triangle, vein** (lah-bāz') [Léon *Labbé,* French surgeon, 1832–1916] see under *triangle,* and see *vena anastomotica superior.*

**la·bel** (la'bəl) 1. a mark, tag, or other characteristic that identifies something. 2. to provide something with such a characteristic.
**radioactive l.,** a radioisotope that is incorporated into a compound to mark it.

**la·bet·a·lol** (lə-bet'ə-lol) [MeSH: Labetalol] a beta-adrenergic blocking agent with some alpha-adrenergic blocking activity; used as an antihypertensive.
**l. hydrochloride,** the hydrochloride salt of labetalol, used in the treatment of hypertension; administered orally or intravenously.

**la·bia** (la'be-ə) [L.] plural of *labium.*

**la·bi·al** (la'be-əl) [L. *labialis*] 1. pertaining to a lip or labium. 2. in dental anatomy, pertaining to the tooth surface that faces the lip; see under *surface.* 3. bilabial.

**la·bi·a·lism** (la'be-əl-iz"əm) a speech disorder involving excessive use of labial speech sounds.

**la·bi·al·ly** (la'be-əl-e) toward the lips.

**Lab·i·dog·na·tha** (lab"ĭ-dog'nə-thə) a suborder of spiders (order Araneae), including the medically important families, Theridiidae and Loxoscelidae.

**la·bile** (la'bīl) [L. *labilis* unstable, from *labi* to glide] 1. gliding; moving from point to point over the surface; unstable; fluctuating. 2. chemically unstable.
**heat l.,** thermolabile.

**la·bil·i·ty** (lə-bil'ə-te) 1. the quality of being labile. 2. in psychiatry, emotional instability; rapidly changing emotions.

**labio-** [L. *labium* lip] a combining form denoting relationship to a lip, especially to the lips of the mouth.

**la·bio·al·ve·o·lar** (la"be-o-al-ve'o-lər) 1. pertaining to the lip and dental alveoli. 2. pertaining to the labial side of a dental alveolus.

**la·bio·ax·io·gin·gi·val** (la"be-o-ak"se-o-jin'jĭ-vəl) pertaining to or formed by the labial, axial, and gingival walls of a tooth cavity preparation.

**la·bio·cer·vi·cal** (la"be-o-sər'vĭ-kəl) 1. pertaining to the labial surface of the neck of an anterior tooth. 2. labiogingival.

**la·bio·cho·rea** (la"be-o-kə-re'ə) [*labio-* + *chorea*] a choreic stiffening of the lips in speech, with stammering.

**la·bio·cli·na·tion** (la"be-o-klĭ-na'shən) deviation of an anterior tooth from the vertical, in the direction of the lips.

**la·bio·den·tal** (la"be-o-den'təl) 1. pertaining to the lips and teeth. 2. a speech sound produced by the contact of the lips and teeth, such as *f* and *v.*

**la·bio·gin·gi·val** (la"be-o-jin'jĭ-vəl) pertaining to or formed by the labial and gingival walls of a tooth cavity. Called also *labiocervical.*

**la·bio·glos·so·la·ryn·ge·al** (la"be-o-glos"o-lə-rin'je-əl) [*labio-* + *glosso-* + *laryngeal*] pertaining to the lips, tongue, and larynx.

**la·bio·glos·so·pha·ryn·ge·al** (la"be-o-glos"o-fə-rin'je-əl) pertaining to the lips, tongue, and pharynx.

**la·bio·graph** (la'be-o-graf") [*labio-* + *-graph*] an instrument for recording the motions of the lips in speaking.

**la·bio·in·ci·sal** (la"be-o-in-si'zəl) pertaining to or formed by the labial and incisal surfaces of a tooth.

**la·bio·lin·gual** (la"be-o-ling'gwəl) 1. pertaining to the lips and the tongue. 2. pertaining to the labial and lingual surfaces of an anterior tooth.

**la·bi·o·log·ic** (la"be-o-loj'ik) pertaining to labiology.

**la·bi·ol·o·gy** (la"be-ol'ə-je) the study of the movements of the lips.

**la·bio·men·tal** (la"be-o-men'təl) pertaining to the lip and chin.

**la·bio·my·co·sis** (la"be-o-mi-ko'sis) [*labio-* + *mycosis*] any disease of the lips due to a fungus, such as thrush.

**la·bio·na·sal** (la"be-o-na'zəl) pertaining to the lip and nose.

**la·bio·pal·a·tine** (la"be-o-pal'ə-tin) pertaining to the lip and palate.

**la·bio·place·ment** (la"be-o-plās'mənt) displacement of a tooth toward the lip.

**la·bio·plas·ty** (la'be-o-plas"te) [*labio-* + *-plasty*] cheiloplasty.

**la·bio·te·nac·u·lum** (la"be-o-tə-nak'u-ləm) [*labio-* + *tenaculum*] an instrument for holding the lip.

**la·bio·ver·sion** (la"be-o-vər'zhən) displacement of a tooth labially from the line of occlusion.

**la·bi·um** (la'be-əm) pl. *la'bia* [L.] 1. lip. 2. a term used in anatomical nomenclature for a liplike structure. In the plural, often used alone to designate the *labia majora* and *minora pudendi.* See also *limbus* and *margo.*
**l. ante'rius orifi'cii exter'ni u'teri,** l. anterius ostii uteri.
**l. ante'rius os'tii u'teri** [TA], anterior lip of ostium of uterus: the anterior projection of the cervix into the vagina; it is shorter and thicker than the posterior lip. Called also *l. anterius orificii externi uteri.*
**l. ce'rebri,** an edge of a deep sulcus, e.g., the lips of the calcarine sulcus.
**l. exter'num cris'tae ili'acae** [TA], the outer margin or external lip of the iliac crest.
**l. infe'rius o'ris** [TA], lower lip: the fleshy margin of the inferior border of the mouth.
**l. infe'rius val'vulae co'li,** the inferior lip of the valve between the ileum and cecum.
**l. inter'num cris'tae ili'acae** [TA], the inner margin or internal lip of the iliac crest.
**l. latera'le li'neae as'perae fe'moris** [TA], lateral lip of rough line of femur: the distinct outer part of the linea aspera that becomes continuous with the gluteal tuberosity and ends at the greater trochanter above and with the lateral supracondylar line below.
**l. lim'bi tympa'nicum** [TA], tympanic lip of limbus: the lower border of the internal spiral sulcus, formed by the lower extremity of the limbus laminae spiralis.
**l. lim'bi vestibula're** [TA], vestibular lip of limbus: the upper border of the internal spiral sulcus, formed by the upper extremity of the limbus laminae spiralis; called also *crista spiralis* and *spiral crest.*
**l. ma'jus puden'di** [TA] pl. *la'bia majo'ra puden'di,* greater lip of pudendum: an elongated fold running downward and backward from the mons pubis in the female, one on either side of the median pudendal cleft.
**l. mandibula're,** l. inferius oris.
**l. maxilla're,** l. superius oris.
**l. media'lis li'neae as'perae fe'moris** [TA], medial lip of rough line of femur: the distinct inner part of the linea aspera that becomes continuous with the intertrochanteric line above and the medial supracondylar line below.
**l. mi'nus puden'di** [TA] pl. *la'bia mino'ra puden'di,* lesser lip of pudendum: a small fold of skin located on either side, between the labium majus and the opening of the vagina.
**la'bia o'ris** [TA], the lips: the fleshy upper and lower margins of the mouth.
**l. poste'rius orifi'cii exter'ni u'teri,** l. posterius ostii uteri.
**l. poste'rius os'tii u'teri** [TA], posterior lip of ostium of uterus: the posterior projection of the cervix into the vagina; called also *l. posterius orificii externi uteri.*

**l. supe′rius o′ris** [TA], upper lip: the fleshy margin of the superior border of the mouth.
**l. supe′rius val′vulae co′li,** the superior lip of the valve between the ileum and cecum.
**l. ure′thrae,** either lateral margin of the external urinary meatus.
**l. voca′le,** plica vocalis.

**la·bor** (la′bər) [L. "work"] [MeSH: Labor] the function of the female organism by which the product of conception is expelled from the uterus through the vagina to the outside world. Labor may be divided into four stages: The first (the stage of cervical dilatation) begins with the onset of regular uterine contractions and ends when the os is completely dilated. The second stage (stage of expulsion) extends from the end of the first stage until the expulsion of the infant is completed. The third stage (placental stage) extends from the expulsion of the child until the placenta and membranes are expelled. The fourth stage denotes the hour or two after delivery, when uterine tone is established. Called also *childbirth, delivery,* and *parturition.* See also *labor pains,* under *pain.*
**artificial l.,** induced l.
**atonic l.,** labor protracted because of atony of the uterus.
**complicated l.,** labor in which cephalopelvic disproportion, hemorrhage, or some other untoward event occurs.
**delayed l.,** postponed l.
**dry l.,** labor in which the amniotic fluid escapes before the onset of uterine contractions.
**false l.,** see *false pains,* under *pain.*
**induced l.,** labor brought on by mechanical or other extraneous means, usually by the intravenous infusion of oxytocin.
**instrumental l.,** labor in which birth of the baby is facilitated by the use of instruments.
**mimetic l.,** see *false pains,* under *pain.*
**missed l.,** retention of a dead fetus in the uterus beyond the period of normal gestation.
**multiple l.,** labor in which two or more infants are born.
**obstructed l.,** labor hindered by some mechanical obstruction, such as a contraction in some region of the parturient canal or a tumor.
**postmature l., postponed l.,** labor occurring two weeks or more after the expected date of confinement. See also *postmature pregnancy,* under *pregnancy.*
**precipitate l.,** labor which occurs with undue rapidity.
**premature l.,** expulsion of a viable infant before the normal end of gestation, usually applied to interruption of pregnancy between the twentieth and the thirty-seventh completed weeks after the onset of the last menstrual period.
**premature l., habitual,** delivery occurring in at least three successive pregnancies at about the same stage of development and prior to completion of the full gestation period.
**prolonged l., protracted l.,** labor prolonged beyond the ordinary 18-hour limit.
**spontaneous l.,** labor in which no artificial aid is required.

**lab·o·ra·to·ri·an** (lab″rə-tor′e-ən) a person who devotes himself to laboratory work, as distinguished from a clinician.

**lab·o·ra·to·ry** (lab′rə-tor″e) [L. *laboratorium*] [MeSH: Laboratories] a place equipped for performing experimental work or investigative procedures, for the preparation of drugs, chemicals, etc.
**clinical l.,** a laboratory for measurement and examination of materials derived from the human body (e.g., fluids, tissues, cells) for the purpose of providing information on diagnosis, prognosis, prevention, or treatment of disease.

**La·borde's forceps, method, sign (test)** (lah-bordz′) [Jean Baptiste Vincent *Laborde,* French physician, 1830–1903] see under *method.*

**la·bra** (la′brə) [L.] plural of *labrum.*

**la·bra·le** (lə-bra′le) an anthropometric landmark on the border of the lip.
**l. infe′rius,** the lowest point, in the median plane, on the vermilion border of the lower lip.
**l. supe′rius,** the highest point, in the median plane, on the vermilion border of the upper lip.

**lab·ro·cyte** (lab′ro-sīt) [Gr. *labros* greedy + *-cyte*] a mast cell.

**la·brum** (la′brəm) pl. *la′bra* [L.] 1. [TA] a general term for an edge, brim, or lip. 2. any liplike part or structure, such as the shelflike projection of the head that anteriorly covers the mandibles of and forms the roof of the mouth of arthropods.
**l. acetabula′re, l. aceta′buli** [TA], acetabular lip: a ring of fibrocartilage attached to the rim of the acetabulum of the hip bone, increasing the depth of the cavity; called also *l. glenoidale articulationis coxae.*
**l. articula′re** [TA], articular lip: a prominent fibrocartilaginous rim around the periphery of certain joints, such as the acetabulum of the hip bone and the glenoid cavity of the scapula; see also *l. acetabuli* and *l. glenoidale.*
**l. glenoida′le** [TA], glenoid lip: a ring of fibrocartilage attached to the rim of the glenoid cavity of the scapula, increasing the depth of the cavity; called also *l. glenoidale articulationis humeri.*
**l. glenoida′le articulatio′nis cox′ae,** l. acetabulare.
**l. glenoida′le articulatio′nis hu′meri,** l. glenoidale.

**La·bur·num** (lə-bər′nəm) a genus of ornamental shrubs with yellow flowers, found in Europe and Asia; its flowers, pods, and seeds contain cystine and cause cysticism in humans and animals that ingest them. The most common species is *L. anagyroi′des.*

**la·bur·num** (lə-bər′nəm) 1. any member of the genus *Laburnum.* 2. *Cytisus laburnum.*

**lab·y·rinth** (lab′ə-rinth) [Gr. *labyrinthos*] [MeSH: Labyrinth] labyrinthus.
**bony l.,** labyrinthus osseus.
**cochlear l.,** labyrinthus cochlearis.
**cortical l.,** a network of tubules and blood vessels in the cortex of the kidney.
**endolymphatic l.,** labyrinthus membranaceus.
**l. of ethmoid, ethmoidal l.,** labyrinthus ethmoidalis.
**Ludwig's l's,** spaces between Bertin's columns and the cortical arches.
**membranous l.,** labyrinthus membranaceus.
**olfactory l.,** labyrinthus ethmoidalis.
**osseous l.,** labyrinthus osseus.
**perilymphatic l.,** spatium perilymphaticum.
**vestibular l.,** labyrinthus vestibularis.

**lab·y·rin·thec·to·my** (lab″ə-rin-thek′tə-me) [*labyrinth* + *-ectomy*] excision of the labyrinth of the ear, done for implacable vestibular dysfunction when severe hearing loss is already present.
**transcanal l.,** labyrinthectomy done through the auditory canals, with removal of the ossicles.
**transmastoid l.,** labyrinthectomy done through the mastoid bone.

**lab·y·rin·thi** (lab″ə-rin′thi) [L.] genitive and plural of *labyrinthus.*

**lab·y·rin·thine** (lab″ə-rin′thēn) pertaining to a labyrinth.

**lab·y·rin·thi·tis** (lab″ə-rin-thi′tis) [MeSH: Labyrinthitis] inflammation of the labyrinth; it may be accompanied by hearing loss or vertigo. Called also *otitis interna.*
**bacterial l.,** acute suppurative l.
**circumscribed l.,** acute serous labyrinthitis in a discrete area, due to erosion of the bony wall of a semicircular canal with exposure of the membranous labyrinth. Called also *labyrinthine fistula* and *perilabyrinthitis.*
**hematogenic l.,** acute suppurative labyrinthitis that results from invasion by bacteria from septicemia.
**meningogenic l.,** acute suppurative labyrinthitis that results from invasion of meningitis through an erosion of the temporal bone.
**l. ossi′ficans,** abnormal ossification in the labyrinth after a trauma or an infection with inflammation.
**purulent l.,** acute suppurative l.
**serous l., acute,** a type caused by chemical or toxic irritants that invade the labyrinth, usually from the middle ear. Called also *sterile l.* and *toxic l.*
**sterile l.,** acute serous l.
**suppurative l., acute,** labyrinthitis in which pus enters the labyrinth, usually either through a fistula after infection of the middle ear (tympanogenic labyrinthitis) or through temporal bone erosion from meningitis (meningogenic labyrinthitis). Occasionally it may be the result of septicemia (hematogenic labyrinthitis). It results in severe and often permanent vertigo and hearing loss. Called also *bacterial l.* and *purulent l.*
**toxic l.,** acute serous l.
**tympanogenic l.,** acute suppurative labyrinthitis that results from invasion from the tympanic cavity.

**lab·y·rin·thot·o·my** (lab″ə-rin-thot′ə-me) [*labyrinth* + Gr. *temnein* to cut] surgical incision into the labyrinth.

**lab·y·rin·thus** (lab″ərin′thəs) gen. and pl. *labyrin′thi* [L., from Gr. *labyrinthos*] 1. [TA] a general term for a system of intercommunicating cavities or canals. Called also *labyrinth.* 2. auris interna.
**l. cochlea′ris** [TA], cochlear labyrinth: the part of the membranous labyrinth that includes the perilymphatic space and the cochlear duct.
**l. ethmoida′lis** [TA], ethmoidal labyrinth: either of the paired lateral masses of the ethmoid bone, consisting of numerous thin-walled cellular cavities, the ethmoid cells. Called also *ectethmoid, ectethmoid bone, olfactory labyrinth, lateral mass of ethmoid bone,* and *massa lateralis ossis ethmoidalis.*
**l. membrana′ceus** [TA], the membranous labyrinth: a system of communicating epithelial sacs and ducts, including the endolymphatic duct, cochlear duct, utricle, saccule, and semicircular ducts, lodged within and attached at certain points to the wall of the osseous labyrinth but separated from the major portion of the bony labyrinth by the perilymphatic space, and containing endolymph; it is divided into vestibular and cochlear parts (see *l. vestibularis* and *l. cochlearis*).

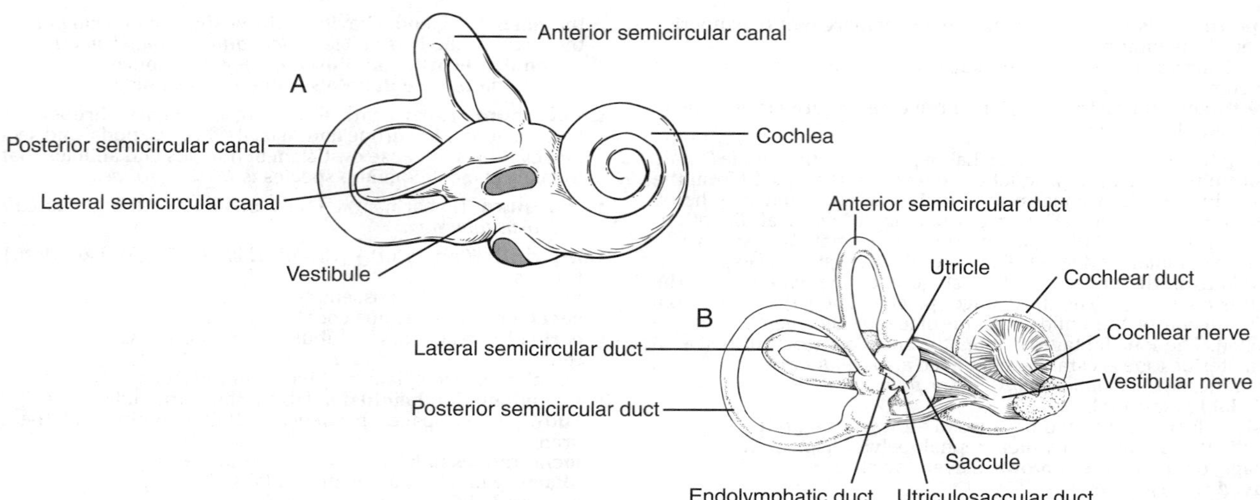


Labyrinthus. *(A),* Anterior view of the labyrinthus osseus (bony labyrinth). *(B),* Posterior view of the labyrinthus membranaceus (membranous labyrinth), which is contained within the bony labyrinth.

**l. os'seus** [TA], bony or osseous labyrinth: a layer of dense bone in the petrous portion of the temporal bone, in which the membranous labyrinth, the vestibular aqueduct, and the cochlear aqueduct are lodged; it consists of three parts: the vestibule, the semicircular canals, and the cochlea.
**l. vestibula'ris** [TA], vestibular labyrinth: the part of the membranous labyrinth that includes the utricle and saccule lodged within the vestibule and the semicircular ducts lodged eccentrically in the corresponding canals.

**lac** (lak) gen. *lac'tis* [L.] 1. milk. 2. any milklike medicinal preparation. 3. a resinous material collected from various tropical trees, secreted by an insect, *Laccifer lacca,* and used in the preparation of shellac.
**l. femini'num,** the secretion of the human mammary gland.
**l. vacci'num,** cow's milk.

**Lac·ci·fer** (lak'sĭ-fər) a genus of insects of the family Coccidae, order Hemiptera. *L. lac'ca* Kerr (Coccidae) is a source of lac and shellac.

**lac·er·a·ble** (las'ər-ə-bəl) capable of becoming lacerated.

**lac·er·at·ed** (las'ər-āt″əd) [L. *lacerare* to tear] torn; mangled; wounded by a jagged instrument.

**lac·er·a·tion** (las″ər-a'shən) [L. *laceratio*] 1. the act of tearing. 2. a torn, ragged, mangled wound.

**la·cer·tus** (lə-sər'təs) [L., "lizard," because of a fancied resemblance] [TA] a general term for certain fibrous attachments of muscles.
**l. cor'dis,** any one of the trabeculae carneae cordis.
**l. fibro'sus mus'culi bici'pitis bra'chii,** TA alternative for *aponeurosis musculi bicipitis brachii.*
**l. me'dius Weitbrech'tii, l. me'dius Wrisber'gii,** ligamentum longitudinale anterius.
**l. mus'culi rec'ti latera'lis bul'bi** [TA], the check ligament of the lateral rectus muscle, which is attached to the lateral palpebral ligament.

**Lach·e·sis** (lak'ə-sis) [L.; Gr. *Lachesis* one of the three Fates] a genus of venomous pit vipers of the family Crotalidae, found in Central and South America. *L. mu'tus* is the bushmaster or suruçucu.

**Lach·no·spi·ra** (lak″no-spi'rə) [Gr. *lachnos* woolly hair + Gr. *speira* coil] a genus of gram-negative anaerobic bacteria of the family Bacteroidaceae, made up of curved, rod-shaped cells found in the rumen of cattle. The type species is *L. multipa'ris.*

**lachry-** for words beginning thus, see those beginning *lacri-.*

**la·cis** (la'sis) [Fr. "network"] polkissen.

**lac·ri·ma** (lak'rĭ-mə) pl. *lac'rimae* [L.] see *tears.*

**lac·ri·mae** (lak'rĭ-me) [L.] plural of *lacrima;* the watery secretion of the lacrimal glands. See *tears.*

**lac·ri·mal** (lak'rĭ-məl) pertaining to the tears.

**lac·ri·ma·tion** (lak″rĭ-ma'shən) [L. *lacrimatio*] the secretion and discharge of tears.

**lac·ri·ma·tor** (lak'rĭ-ma″tər) a substance that increases the flow of tears, such as tear gas.

**lac·ri·ma·to·ry** (lak'rĭ-mə-tor″e) causing a flow of tears.

**lac·ri·mo·na·sal** (lak″rĭ-mo-na'zəl) pertaining to the lacrimal sac and the nose.

**lac·ri·mo·tome** (lak'rĭ-mo-tōm) [*lacrima* + *-tome*] a knife for incising the lacrimal sac or duct.

**lac·ri·mot·o·my** (lak″rĭ-mot'ə-me) [*lacrima* + *-tomy*] incision of the lacrimal sac or duct.

**lac·ta** (lak'tə) [L.] plural of *lac.*

**lac·tac·i·din** (lak-tas'ĭ-din) a food preservative composed of lactic and salicylic acids.

**lac·ta·cid·o·gen** (lak″tə-sid'o-jən) [*lactic acid* + *-gen*] a term used by Embden to designate the hexose phosphate precursor of lactic acid in muscle contraction.

**lac·tac·id·uria** (lak-tas″ĭ-du're-ə) [*lactic acid* + *-uria*] the presence of lactic acid in the urine.

**lac·ta·gogue** (lak'tə-gog) [*lact-* + *-agogue*] galactagogue.

**lac·tal·bu·min** (lak″tal-bu'min) [MeSH: Lactalbumin] any of a group of proteins occurring in milk; the lactalbumins and lactoglobulins constitute the bulk of the proteins in the whey of human milk.
**α-l.,** a milk protein that is a component of lactose synthase; it has no catalytic activity but alters the specificity of the catalytic subunit (glycoprotein 4-β-galactosyltransferase) so that glucose becomes the preferred acceptor substrate and lactose is synthesized.

**lac·tam** (lak'təm) a cyclic amide formed from aminocarboxylic acids by the elimination of water. They are isomeric with lactims, which are enol forms of lactams.

—C=O | —NH (Lactam)    —C—OH ‖ —N (Lactim)

**β-lac·ta·mase** (lak'tə-mās) [EC 3.5.2.6] any of a group of bacterial enzymes of the hydrolase class, produced by almost all gram-negative species, that catalyze the cleavage of β-lactam rings; such rings occur in penicillins and cephalosporins so that these antibiotics are inactivated by β-lactamases. Individual enzymes are produced by different bacterial species and are called also *penicillinases* or *cephalosporinases* on the basis of their specificities. The enzymes may occur bound to membranes, extracellularly, or in the periplasmic space, may be encoded on the chromosome or on a plasmid, and may be constitutive or inducible.

**lac·ta·mide** (lak'tə-mīd) the amide of lactic acid.

**Lac·ta·ri·us** (lak-ta're-əs) a genus of fungi of the order Agaricales having white spores; it includes both edible and poisonous species. When they are cut or broken, a white or milklike substance is discharged.

**lac·tase** (lak'tās) [USP] a β-galactosidase [EC 3.2.1.23] occurring in the brush border membrane of the intestinal mucosa; together with glycosylceramidase (phlorizin hydrolase), it forms the β-glycosidase complex (q.v.). The enzyme catalyzes the hydrolytic cleavage of lactose to galactose and glucose and also cleaves terminal nonreducing galactose residues from $\beta$-glycosides with large hydrophilic aglycons. Reduced or absent enzyme activity (lactase deficiency) may result in symptoms of lactose intolerance.

**lac·tase de·fi·cien·cy** the most common disaccharidase deficiency, reduced or absent lactase activity in the intestinal mucosa, usually due to an inherited defect in the enzyme but sometimes secondary to disorders involving the small intestinal mucosa. The hereditary adult form, an autosomal recessive trait, is the normal state in most populations other than white Northern Europeans and may be characterized by abdominal pain, flatulence, and diarrhea after ingestion of milk *(lactose intolerance);* the rare hereditary congenital form, an autosomal recessive trait, is characterized by diarrhea, vomiting, and failure to thrive *(congenital lactose intolerance).*

**lac·tate** (lak'tāt) 1. the anionic form of lactic acid; a salt of lactic acid. 2. to secrete milk.
**ferrous l.,** greenish white crystals or powder, $Fe(C_3H_5O_3)_2$, used orally as a hematinic.
**lactic acid l.,** a substance formed by concentration by the boiling of lactic acid; used in the preparation of sodium lactate.

**L-lac·tate de·hy·dro·gen·ase (LDH)** (lak'tāt de-hi'dro-jən-ās) [EC 1.1.1.27] an enzyme of the oxidoreductase class that catalyzes the reduction of pyruvate to *(S)*-lactate, using NADH as an electron donor. The reaction is the final step in glycolysis (white fibers). The reverse reaction is the first step in the combustion of lactate (heart, red fibers) or its conversion to glucose (liver). The enzyme occurs in the cytoplasm of nearly all cells. It is a tetramer containing M (muscle) and H (heart) subunits; it exists as five distinct isozymes ($M_4$, $M_3H$, $M_2H_2$, $MH_3$, $H_4$). Identification of isozyme types in serum is used for clinical diagnosis.

**lac·ta·tion** (lak-ta'shən) [L. *lactatio,* from *lactare* to suckle] [MeSH: Lactation] 1. the secretion of milk. 2. the period of the secretion of milk. 3. suckling.

**lac·ta·tion·al** (lak-ta'shən-əl) pertaining to lactation.

**lac·te·al** (lak'te-əl) [L. *lacteus* milky] 1. pertaining to milk. 2. any of the intestinal lymphatics that transport chyle; so called because during absorption they are white from absorbed fat. Called also *chyliferous vessel* and *lacteal vessel.*

**lac·te·nin** (lak'tə-nin) a bacteriostatic substance in milk.

**lac·tes·cence** (lak-tes'əns) [L. *lactescere* to become milky] resemblance to milk; milkiness.

**lac·tic** (lak'tik) pertaining to milk.

**lac·tic ac·id** (lak'tik) [MeSH: Lactic Acid] a metabolic intermediate involved in many biochemical processes; it is the end product of glycolysis, which provides energy anaerobically in skeletal muscle during heavy exercise, and it can be oxidized aerobically in the heart for energy production or can be converted back to glucose (gluconeogenesis) in the liver. Moderate elevations of blood lactate occur during heavy exercise; severe elevations (lactic acidosis) can occur in diabetes mellitus and in genetic deficiencies of enzymes involved in gluconeogenesis. Lactate is also the end product of fermentation in several bacterial species.

**lac·tic·ac·i·de·mia** (lak"tik-as"ĭ-de'me-ə) excess of lactic acid in the blood.

**Lac·ti·Care** (lak'tĭ-kār") trademark for preparations of hydrocortisone.

**lac·ti·ce·mia** (lak"tĭ-se'me-ə) lacticacidemia.

**lac·tif·er·ous** (lak-tif'ər-əs) [L. *lacto-* + *ferre* to bear] producing or conveying milk.

**lac·ti·fuge** (lak'tĭ-fūj) [*lact-* + *-fuge*] 1. checking or stopping the secretion of milk. 2. an agent that checks the secretion of milk.

**lac·tig·e·nous** (lak-tij'ə-nəs) [*lacto-* + *-genous*] producing or secreting milk.

**lac·tig·er·ous** (lak-tij'ər-əs) [L. *lac* milk + *gerere* to carry] lactiferous.

**lac·tim** (lak'tim) see under *lactam.*

**lac·ti·nat·ed** (lak'tĭ-nāt"əd) prepared with lactose.

**lac·ti·tol** (lak'tĭ-tol) [NF] a disaccharide analogue of lactulose having an intense sweet taste and used as a bulk sweetener; it also has laxative properties and is used in the management of constipation.

**lac·tiv·o·rous** (lak-tiv'ə-rəs) [*lact-* + L. *vorare* to devour] feeding or subsisting upon milk.

**lact(o)-** [L. *lac,* gen. *lactis* milk] a combining form denoting relationship to milk or to lactic acid.

**Lac·to·bac·il·la·ceae** (lak"to-bas"ĭ-la'se-e) [MeSH: Lactobacillaceae] a family of bacteria made up of gram-positive, asporogenous, straight or curved rods occurring singly or in chains. Formerly called *Lactobacteriaceae.*

**Lac·to·bac·il·leae** (lak"to-bə-sil'e-e) in former systems of classification, a tribe of bacteria of the family Lactobacillaceae, made up of straight or curved rods occurring singly or in chains, the organisms of which have been assigned to the genera *Lactobacillus* and *Eubacterium.*

**lac·to·bac·il·li** (lak"to-bə-sil'i) [L.] plural of *lactobacillus.*

**Lac·to·bac·il·lus** (lak"to-bə-sil'əs) [*lacto-* + L. *bacillus* small rod] [MeSH: Lactobacillus] a genus of bacteria of the family Lactobacillaceae, occurring as large, gram-positive, asporogenous, rod-shaped organisms. They are anaerobic or microaerophilic and occur widely in nature and in the human mouth, vagina, and intestinal tract. In the oral cavity, they are found associated with dental caries but have no known etiologic role. They are separable into two groups, the homofermentative group producing only lactic acid, and the heterofermentative group producing other end products of fermentation.
**L. acido'philus,** a homofermentative lactobacillus producing the fermented product, acidophilus milk.
**L. bi'fidus,** *Bifidobacterium bifidum.*
**L. bulga'ricus,** a homofermentative lactobacillus producing the fermented product known as Bulgarian or bulgaricus milk.

**lac·to·bac·il·lus** (lak"to-bə-sil'əs) pl. *lactobacil'li* [MeSH: Lactobacillus] An organism of the genus *Lactobacillus.*
**l. of Boas-Oppler,** Boas-Oppler bacillus.

**Lac·to·bac·te·ri·a·ceae** (lak"to-bak-te"re-a'se-e) a former name of a family of bacteria now called *Lactobacillaceae.*

**lac·to·cele** (lak'to-sēl) galactocele.

**lac·to·crit** (lak'to-krit) [*lacto-* + Gr. *kritēs* judge] an instrument for estimating the amount of fat in milk.

**lac·to·den·sim·e·ter** (lak"to-den-sim'ə-tər) lactometer.

**lac·to·fer·rin** (lak'to-fer"in) [MeSH: Lactoferrin] an iron-binding protein found in the specific granules of neutrophils where it apparently exerts an antimicrobial activity by withholding iron from ingested bacteria and fungi; it also occurs in many secretions and exudates, such as milk, tears, mucus, saliva, and bile.

**lac·to·gen** (lak'to-jən) [*lacto-* + *-gen*] any substance that enhances milk production, the principal one being prolactin.
**human placental l. (hPL),** a polypeptide hormone secreted by the placenta that enters the maternal circulation and disappears from the circulation immediately after delivery. It has growth-promoting activity, is immunologically similar to growth hormone, and inhibits maternal insulin activity during pregnancy. By inhibiting glucose oxidation it can increase the glucose supply to a fetus developing in a malnourished mother. Called also *choriomammotropin, chorionic somatomammotropin,* and *placental growth hormone.*

**lac·to·gen·e·sis** (lak'to-jen'ə-sis) [*lacto-* + *-genesis*] the secretion of milk by the mammary glands.

**lac·to·gen·ic** (lak"to-jen'ik) stimulating the production of milk.

**lac·to·glob·u·lin** (lak"to-glob'u-lin) a globulin occurring in milk.

**lac·tom·e·ter** (lak-tom'ə-tər) [*lacto-* + *meter*] an instrument for ascertaining the specific gravity of milk.

**lac·tone** (lak'tōn) a cyclic organic compound in which the chain is closed by ester formation between a carboxyl and a hydroxyl group in the same molecule.

**lac·to·ovo·ve·ge·ta·ri·an** (lak"to-o"vo-vej"ə-ter'e-ən) ovolacto-vegetarian.

**lac·to·pro·tein** (lak"to-pro'tēn) a protein derived from milk.

**lac·tor·rhea** (lak"to-re'ə) galactorrhea.

**lac·to·scope** (lak'to-skōp) [*lacto-* + *-scope*] a device showing the proportion of cream in milk.

**lac·tose** (lak'tōs) [L. *lac,* gen. *lactis* milk] [MeSH: Lactose] a reducing disaccharide occurring as the D-isomer, in both $\alpha$- and $\beta$-configurations, as a major constituent of mammalian milk; on hydrolysis by acids or intestinal lactase, it forms one residue each of galactose and glucose. Cf. *lactose intolerance,* under *intolerance.* Lactose is used as a tablet and capsule diluent, a powder bulking agent, in infant feeding formulas, and as a nutritional supplement.
**anhydrous l.** [NF], lactose without water of hydration, which may be primarily $\beta$-lactose or a mixture of $\alpha$-lactose and $\beta$-lactose.
**$\beta$-l.,** anhydrous D-lactose in the $\beta$-1 configuration, prepared by crystallizing a heated solution of lactose; sometimes used in pharmaceutical preparations because it is sweeter and more soluble in this configuration.
**l. monohydrate** [NF], a natural disaccharide obtained from milk and consisting of one glucose and one galactose moiety; it is monohydrated $\alpha$-lactose.

**lac·tose syn·thase** (lak'tōs sin'thās) [EC 2.4.1.22] [MeSH: Lactose Synthase] an enzyme of the transferase class that catalyzes the transfer of galactose from UDPgalactose to glucose, forming lactose.

The enzyme is a complex of the enzyme glycoprotein 4-β-galactosyltransferase (q.v.) and α-lactalbumin; the latter protein is present in lactating mammary gland cells where it alters the usual specificity of the former to make lactose synthesis the preferred reaction.

**lac·to·side** (lak'to-sīd) a glycoside whose sugar constituent is lactose.

**lac·tos·uria** (lak″to-su're-ə) the presence of lactose in the urine, observed frequently during lactation.

**lac·to·syl·cer·a·mide** (lak-to″səl-ser'ə-mīd) any of the glycosphingolipids in which the head group on the ceramide is lactose; they occur at low concentrations in all tissues.

**lac·to·tox·in** (lak″to-tok'sin) a toxic substance formed in milk.

**lac·to·trope** (lak'to-trōp) lactotroph.

**lac·to·troph** (lak'to-trōf) an acidophil of the adenohypophysis that stains with an affinity for azocarmine and erythrosin and secretes prolactin. Called also *lactotrope, mammatroph, mammotroph, epsilon acidophil, prolactin cell,* and *lactotroph* or *lactotropic cell.*

**lac·to·tro·phin** (lak'to-tro″fin) prolactin.

**lac·to·tro·pin** (lak'to-tro″pin) prolactin.

**lac·to·ve·ge·tar·i·an** (lak″to-vej″ə-ter'e-ən) one who practices lactovegetarianism.

**lac·to·veg·e·tar·i·an·ism** (lak″to-vej″ə-ter'e-ə-niz″əm) restriction of the diet to vegetables and dairy products, eschewing other foods of animal origin.

**lac·to·yl** (lak'to-əl) the radical of lactic acid; $CH_3CH(OH)CO$.

**lac·to·yl·glu·ta·thi·one** (lak″to-əl-gloo″tə-thi'ōn) glutathione linked to lactic acid; it is an intermediate formed in the conversion of methylglyoxal to lactic acid by glyoxalase.

**lac·to·yl·glu·ta·thi·one ly·ase** (lak″to-əl-gloo″tə-thi'ōn li'ās) [EC 4.4.1.5] an enzyme of the lyase class that catalyzes the condensation of methylglyoxal and glutathione to form lactoylglutathione as a step in the conversion of methylglyoxal to lactic acid. See also *glyoxalase.*

**lac·tu·lose** (lak'tu-lōs) [MeSH: Lactulose] a synthetic disaccharide used as a cathartic and to enhance excretion or formation of ammonia in the treatment of portosystemic encephalopathy, including the stages of hepatic precoma and coma.

**la·cu·na** (lə-ku'nə) gen. and pl. *lacu'nae* [L.] 1. [TA] a small pit or hollow cavity; a general term for such a compartment within or between other body structures. 2. a defect or gap, as in the field of vision (scotoma).
**absorption l.,** resorption l.
**Blessig's lacunae,** see *Blessig's cysts.*
**blood l.,** any one of the blood-filled spaces in the syncytiotrophoblast of the embryo that serve hemotrophic nutrition.
**bone l.,** a small cavity within the bone matrix containing an osteocyte and from which slender canaliculi radiate and penetrate the adjacent lamellae to anastomose with the canaliculi of neighboring lacunae, thus forming a system of cavities interconnected by minute canals. Called also *osseous l.*

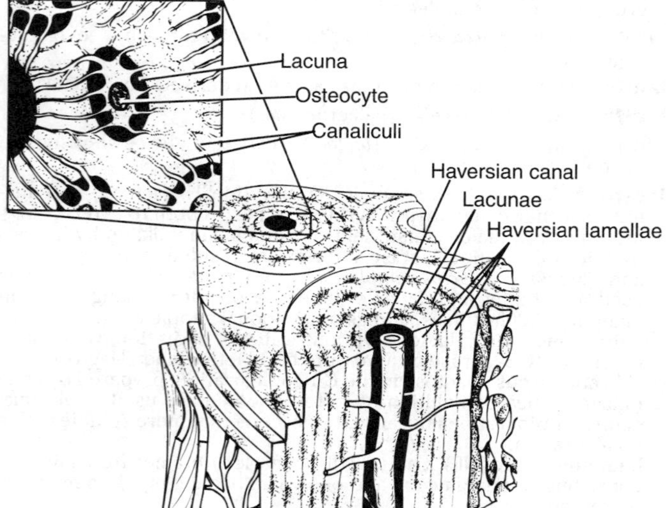


Bone lacunae in a section of the shaft of a long bone.

**cartilage l.,** any of the small cavities within the cartilage matrix, containing a chondrocyte, or cartilage cell.
**cerebral lacunae,** small areas of cerebral ischemic infarction resulting from occlusion of deep, small end-arterial branches of the middle cerebral, posterior cerebral, and basilar arteries; seen in association with hypertension and arteriosclerosis.
**great l. of urethra,** fossa navicularis urethrae.
**Howship's l.,** resorption l.
**intervillous l.,** one of the blood spaces of the placenta in which the fetal villi are found; called also *trophoblastic l.*
**lacu'nae latera'les** [TA], lateral lacunae: venous meshworks within the dura mater on either side of the superior sagittal sinus; arachnoidal granulations project into them. Called also *parasinusoidal lacunae, sinuses,* or *spaces.*
**l. mag'na,** fossa navicularis urethrae.
**lacunae of Morgagni,** lacunae urethrales in the male urethra.
**lacu'nae Morgag'nii ure'thrae mulie'bris,** glandulae urethrales urethrae femininae.
**l. of muscles, muscular l., l. musculo'rum** [TA], a compartment beneath the inguinal ligament for the passage of the iliopsoas muscle and femoral nerve, separated from the lacuna vasorum by the iliopectineal arch. Called also *muscular compartment* and *iliac canal.*
**osseous l.,** bone l.
**parasinusoidal lacunae,** lacunae laterales.
**l. pharyn'gis,** a depression at the pharyngeal end of the auditory tube.
**resorption l.,** a pit or concavity found in bones undergoing resorption, frequently containing osteoclasts. Similar lacunae also may be found in eroding surfaces of cementum, in which cementoclasts may or may not be located. Called also *absorption l.* and *Howship's l.*
**trophoblastic l.,** intervillous l.
**lacunae of urethra, urethral lacunae,** lacunae urethrales.
**urethral lacunae of Morgagni,** lacunae urethrales in the male urethra.
**lacu'nae urethra'les** [TA], urethral lacunae: numerous small depressions or pits in the mucous membrane of the urethra, with their openings usually directed distally. Some contain openings of ducts of the urethral glands.
**vascular l., l. vaso'rum** [TA], a space for the passage of the femoral vessels into the thigh, separated from the lacuna musculorum by the iliopectineal arch. Called also *vascular compartment.*

**la·cu·nae** (lə-ku'ne) [L.] genitive and plural of *lacuna.*

**la·cu·nar** (lə-ku'nər) pertaining to or containing lacunae; of the nature of a lacuna.

**la·cune** (lə-kūn') 1. lacuna. 2. a small (less than 1.5 cm) infarct occurring in the basal ganglia, internal capsule, pons, and white matter of the brain, usually in older hypertensive patients and diabetics; depending on their location, lacunes may be asymptomatic or cause significant impairment. The presence of multiple lacunes is known as *status lacunaris.*

**la·cu·nule** (lə-ku'nūl) [L. *lacunula*] a small lacuna.

**la·cus** (la'kəs) pl. *la'cus* [L.] lake.
**l. lacrima'lis** [TA], lacrimal lake: the triangular space at the medial angle of the eye, where the tears collect; called also *lacrimal bay* and *lake.*

**LAD** 1. left anterior descending (coronary artery); see *ramus interventricularis anterior arteriae coronariae sinistrae.* 2. left axis deviation.

**Ladd's bands, procedure, syndrome** (ladz) [William Edwards *Ladd,* American physician, 1880–1967] see under *band, procedure,* and *syndrome.*

**Ladd-Frank·lin theory** (lad-frangk'lin) [Christine *Ladd-Franklin,* American physician, 1847–1930] see under *theory.*

**lad·der·gram** ladder diagram.

**LAE** left atrial enlargement; see *atrial enlargement,* under *enlargement.*

**lae-** for words beginning thus, see also those beginning *le-.*

**Lae·laps** (le'laps) *Echinolaelaps.*

**Laën·nec's catarrh,** etc. (lah″ə-neks') [René Théophile Hyacinthe *Laënnec,* French physician and inventor of the stethoscope, 1781–1826] see under *cirrhosis, disease,* and *pearl.*

**La·e·trile** (la'ə-tril) trademark for *l*-mandelonitrile-β-glucuronic acid, derived by hydrolysis of amygdalin and oxidation of the resulting *l*-mandelonitrile-β-glucoside; it is alleged to have antineoplastic properties.

**lae·ve** (le'və) [L. *levis* smooth] nonvillous, as the *chorion laeve.*

**laev(o)-** for words beginning thus, see those beginning *lev(o)-.*

**La·fo·ra's bodies, myoclonic epilepsy (disease), sign** (lahfo'rahz) [Gonzalo Rodríguez *Lafora,* Spanish neurologist, 1887–1971] see under *body, epilepsy,* and *sign.*

**Lag.** abbreviation for L. *lage'na,* a flask.

**lag** (lag) 1. the period of time elapsing between the application of a stimulus and the resulting reaction. 2. see *lag phase,* under *phase.*
**anaphase l.,** delayed movement during anaphase of one homologous chromosome in mitosis or of one chromatid in meiosis, so that the chromosome is not incorporated into the nucleus of one of the daughter cells; the result is one normal cell and one cell with monosomy.
**nitrogen l.,** the time that elapses after the administration of a protein before there appears in the urine an amount of nitrogen equivalent to that administered.

**la·ge·na** (lə-je'nə) [L. "flask"] 1. a part of the upper extremity of the ductus cochlearis. 2. the curved, flask-shaped organ of hearing in vertebrates lower than mammals.

**la·gen·i·form** (lə-jen'ĭ-form) [*lagena* + *form*] flask-shaped.

**Lag·o·chi·las·ca·ris mi·nor** (lag"o-kĭ-la'kə-ris mi'nər) a nematode worm found in subcutaneous abscesses of humans in Trinidad and Surinam.

**lag·oph·thal·mos** (lag"of-thal'məs) [Gr. *lagōs* hare + *ophthalmos* eye] a condition in which the eye cannot be completely closed.

**lag·oph·thal·mus** (lag"of-thal'məs) lagophthalmos.

**La·grange's operation** (lah-grahn'zhəz) [Pierre Félix *Lagrange,* French ophthalmologist, 1857–1928] sclerectoiridectomy.

**LAH** left anterior hemiblock.

**lai·ose** (li'ōs) a pale yellow substance, found in the urine in diabetes mellitus; it is nonfermentable and levorotatory.

**lake** (lāk) [L. *lacus*] 1. to undergo separation of hemoglobin from the erythrocytes, a phenomenon sometimes occurring in blood. 2. a circumscribed collection of fluid in a hollow or depressed area.
**lacrimal l.,** lacus lacrimalis.
**marginal l's,** discontinuous venous lacunae, relatively free of villi, near the edge of the placenta, formed by merging of the marginal portions of the intervillous space with the subchorial lake. Called also *marginal sinus,* because it was thought to be circumferentially continuous and important for placental drainage.
**subchorial l.,** the portion of the placenta, relatively free of villi, just beneath the chorionic plate; at the edge of the placenta it becomes continuous with irregular channels to form the marginal lakes. Called also *subchorial space.*
**venous l.,** small blue-purple sessile, compressible papules or blebs seen most often on the lips, ears, and face of elderly persons, which histologically represent dilated capillaries filled with red blood cells and lined with flattened endothelial cells.

**lal·la·tion** (lə-la'shən) [L. *lallare* to sing a lullaby] a babbling, infantile form of speech.

**Lal·le·mand's bodies** (lahl-ə-mahnz') [Claude François *Lallemand,* French surgeon, 1790–1854] Bence Jones cylinders.

**lalo-** [Gr. *lalein* to babble, speak] a combining form denoting relationship to speech.

**lal·og·no·sis** (lal"og-no'sis) [*lalo-* + Gr. *gnōsis* knowledge] the understanding of speech.

**la·lop·a·thy** (lə-lop'ə-the) [*lalo-* + *-pathy*] speech disorder.

**lalo·pho·bia** (lal"ə-fo'be-ə) [*lalo-* + *-phobia*] irrational fear of speaking.

**lalo·ple·gia** (lal"ə-ple'jə) [*lalo-* + *-plegia*] logoplegia.

**lal·or·rhea** (lal"ə-re'ə) [*lalo-* + *-rrhea*] logorrhea.

**La·lou·ette's pyramid** (lah-loo-ets') [Pierre *Lalouette,* French physician, 1711–1792] see under *pyramid.*

**La·marck's theory** (lah-mahrks') [Jean Baptiste Pierre Antoine Monet de *Lamarck,* French naturalist, 1744–1829] see under *theory.*

**La·maze method** (lə-mahz') [Fernand *Lamaze,* French obstetrician, 1890–1957] see under *method.*

**lamb·da** (lam'də) [the eleventh letter of the Greek alphabet, Λ or λ] [TA] the point at the site of the posterior fontanel where the lambdoid and sagittal sutures meet; used as a craniometric landmark.

**lamb·da·cism, lamb·da·cis·mus** (lam'də-siz-əm, lam"də-siz'məs) [Gr. *lambdakismos*] 1. a speech disorder consisting of the substitution of *l* for *r.* 2. a speech disorder involving faulty pronunciation of *l.* Called also *paralambdacism.*

**lamb·doid** (lam'doid) [Gr. *lambda* + *-oid*] shaped like the Greek letter Λ or λ.

**Lam·bert's cosine law** (lahm'bərts) [Johann Heinrich *Lambert,* German mathematician and physicist, 1728–1777] see under *law.*

**Lam·bert-Ea·ton syndrome** (lam'bərt-e'tən) [Edward Howard *Lambert,* American physiologist, born 1915; Lealdes McKendree *Eaton,* American neurologist, 1905–1958] Eaton-Lambert syndrome.

**lam·bert** (lam'bərt) [J. H. *Lambert*] a unit of luminance, being the luminous intensity of a perfect diffuser emitting one lumen per square centimeter. Symbol L. The unit generally used is one one-thousandth of this and is called a *millilambert.* When the area chosen is one square foot, the unit is called a *foot lambert.*

**Lam·blia** (lam'ble-ə) [Vilem Dusan *Lambl,* Czechoslovakian physician, 1824–1895] *Giardia.*
**L. intestina'lis,** *Giardia lamblia.*

**lam·bli·a·sis** (lam-bli'ə-sis) giardiasis.

**lam·bli·o·sis** (lam"ble-o'sis) giardiasis.

**lame** (lām) incapable of normal locomotion; deviating from the normal gait. See also *claudication.*

**lame fo·li·a·cée** (lahm fōl-yah-sa') [Fr. "foliaceous plate"] the whorled or concentrically laminated connective tissue structures contained in some nevi; called also *foliate lamina.*

**lam·el** (lam'əl) lamella, def. 2.

**la·mel·la** (lə-mel'ə) gen. and pl. *lamel'lae* [L., dim. of *lamina*] 1. a thin leaf or plate, as of bone. 2. a medicated disk or wafer prepared from gelatin, glycerin, and distilled water, and containing a small quantity of an alkaloid, to be inserted under the eyelid. 3. gill (def. 2).
**annulate lamellae,** cytoplasmic organelles which consist of parallel arrays of cisternae exhibiting small annuli or circular fenestrae at very regular intervals along their length.
**articular l.,** the layer of bone to which an articular cartilage is attached.
**basic l.,** circumferential l.
**circumferential l.,** one of the layers of bone that underlie the periosteum *(external circumferential l.)* and endosteum *(internal circumferential l.);* called also *basic l.*
**concentric l.,** haversian l.
**cornoid l.,** a thick column of parakeratotic cells extending outward from a notch in the malpighian layer of the epidermis, and forming the raised border of a lesion of porokeratosis.
**enamel lamellae,** imperfectly calcified areas of enamel located generally in the cervical enamel but also found in the interdigitating surface of the premolars and molars; they are foliaceous structures visible only under the microscope and may extend from the surface to the dentinoenamel junctions and beyond.
**endosteal l.,** one of the bony plates lying beneath the endosteum.
**ground l.,** interstitial l.
**haversian l.,** one of the concentric bony plates surrounding a haversian canal.
**intermediate l.,** interstitial l.
**interstitial l.,** one of the bony plates that fill in between the haversian systems; called also *ground l.* or *intermediate l.*
**osseous l.,** any one of the thin plates into which bone can be divided.
**periosteal l., peripheral l.,** the layer of bone lying next to the periosteum.
**posterior border l. of Fuchs,** the fibrillar layer of the dilator muscle of the iris; called also *Henle's membrane.*
**triangular l.,** tela choroidea ventriculi tertii.
**vitreous l.,** lamina basalis.

**la·mel·lae** (lə-mel'e) [L.] genitive and plural of *lamella.*

**la·mel·lar** (lə-mel'ər) pertaining to or resembling lamellae.

**la·mel·li·form** (lə-mel'ĭ-form) resembling lamellae.

**la·mel·li·po·dia** (lə-mel"ĭ-po'de-ə) sing. *lamellipo'dium* [*lamella* + *pod-* + *-ia*] delicate sheetlike extensions of cytoplasm which form transient adhesions with the cell substrate and wave gently, enabling the cell to move along the substrate.

**la·mel·li·po·di·um** (lə-mel"ĭ-po'de-əm) singular of *lamellipodia.*

**lame·ness** (lām'nes) the condition of being lame; see also *gait.*
**fescue l., tall fescue l.,** fescue foot.

**La·mic·tal** (ləmik'tal) trademark for a preparation of lamotrigine.

**lam·in** (lam'in) any of a group of intermediate filaments that enmesh to form the nuclear lamina. They are structurally similar to keratin filaments.

**lam·i·na** (lam'ĭ-nə) gen. and pl. *la'minae* [L.] [TA] layer: a thin flat plate or stratum of a composite structure. The term is often used alone to mean the lamina arcus vertebrae.

## Lamina

Descriptions of anatomic structures are given on TA terms, and include anglicized names of specific layers.

**l. affix'a** [TA], the narrow strip of ependyma overlying the thalamostriate vein and stria terminalis in the central part of the lateral ventricle.

**l. ala'ris,** alar lamina: either of the pair of longitudinal zones of the embryonic neural tube dorsal to the sulcus limitans, from which are developed the dorsal gray columns of the spinal cord and the sensory centers of the brain; called also *alar plate.*

**la'minae al'bae cerebel'li,** white laminae of the cerebellum: the core of white substance that supports a folium of the cerebellar cortex.

**anterior limiting l.,** l. limitans anterior corneae.

**l. ante'rior vagi'nae mus'culi rec'ti abdo'minis** [TA], anterior lamina of sheath of rectus abdominis muscle: the portion of the muscle sheath lying anterior to the rectus abdominis muscle, formed by aponeuroses of the internal and external oblique muscles superior to the arcuate line and by the aponeuroses of the internal oblique and transversus muscles inferior to the arcuate line.

**l. ar'cus ver'tebrae** [TA], lamina of the vertebral arch: either of the pair of broad plates of bone flaring out from the pedicles of the vertebral arches and fusing together at the midline to complete the dorsal part of the arch and provide a base for the spinous process.

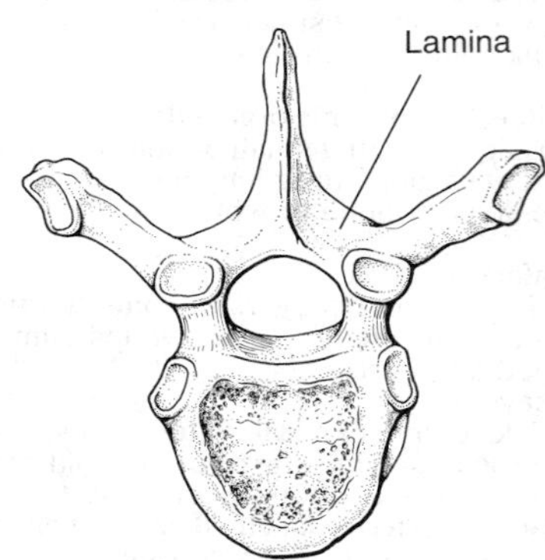


**basal l.,** 1. the layer of the basement membrane lying next to the basal surface of the adjoining cell layer, composed of an electron-dense lamina densa and an electron-lucent lamina lucida; sometimes used to denote the lamina densa alone. Cf. *reticular l.* 2. sometimes, the entire basement membrane. 3. l. basalis.

**basal l. of choroid,** lamina basalis choroideae.

**basal l. of ciliary body,** l. basalis corporis ciliaris.

**l. basa'lis,** 1. basal lamina: either of the pair of longitudinal zones of the embryonic neural tube ventral to the sulcus limitans, from which are developed the ventral gray columns of the spinal cord and the motor centers of the brain; called also *basal plate.* 2. basal l. (def. 1).

**l. basa'lis choroi'deae** [TA], basal lamina of choroid: the transparent inner layer of the choroid, which is in contact with the pigmented layer of the retina. Called also *Bruch's layer* or *membrane, basal lamina of choroid, complexus basalis choroideae,* and *vitreal* or *vitreous lamina.*

**l. basa'lis cor'poris cilia'ris** [TA], basal lamina of the ciliary body: the innermost layer of the ciliary body, continuous with the basal lamina of the choroid.

**l. basila'ris duc'tus cochlea'ris** [TA], basilar lamina of cochlear duct: the wall of the cochlear duct, which separates it from the scala tympani; the spiral organ lies against it.

**Bowman's l.,** l. limitans anterior corneae.

**l. cartila'ginis cricoi'deae** [TA], lamina of cricoid cartilage: the broad posterior part of the cricoid cartilage.

**l. cartila'ginis latera'lis tu'bae auditi'vae,** l. lateralis cartilaginis tubae auditivae.

**l. cartila'ginis media'lis tu'bae auditi'vae,** l. medialis cartilaginis tubae auditivae.

**l. cartila'ginis thyroi'deae dex'tra/sinis'tra** [TA], right/left lamina of thyroid cartilage: either of the broad plates that form the right and left sides of the cartilage, converging anteriorly to meet at the midline.

**l. choriocapilla'ris,** l. choroidocapillaris.

**l. choroidocapilla'ris** [TA], choriocapillary layer: the inner layer of the choroid, composed of a single-layered network of small capillaries; called also *l. choriocapillaris.*

**la'minae cor'ticis ce'rebri,** layers of cerebral cortex.

**l. I,** l. molecularis.
**l. II,** l. granularis externa.
**l. III,** l. pyramidalis externa.
**l. IV,** l. granularis interna
**l. V,** l. pyramidalis interna.
**l. VI,** l. multiformis.

**cribriform l.,** fascia cribrosa.

**cribriform l. of ethmoid bone,** l. cribrosa ossis ethmoidalis.

**cribriform l. of transverse fascia,** septum femorale.

**l. cribro'sa os'sis ethmoida'lis** [TA], cribriform lamina of ethmoid bone: the horizontal plate of the ethmoid bone that forms the roof of the nasal cavity; it is perforated by many foramina (foramina cribrosa ossis ethmoidalis) for the passage of the olfactory nerves. On its superior surface is a projection called the crista galli. Called also *cribriform plate of ethmoid bone.*

**l. cribro'sa scle'rae** [TA], the perforated portion of the sclera through which pass the axons of the ganglion cells of the retina; called also *optic foramen of sclera.*

**l. of cricoid cartilage,** l. cartilaginis cricoideae.

**l. den'sa,** an electron-dense layer of the basal lamina, consisting mainly of Type IV collagen fibrils and heparan sulfate proteoglycans, that closely follows the plasma membrane of the basal aspect of the adjacent cell layer, from which it is separated by the lamina lucida. In the renal glomeruli and the pulmonary alveoli, it is bounded by the lamina rara externa and the lamina rara interna.

**dental l.,** a horizontal band projecting perpendicularly from the vestibular lamina and extending into the substance of the embryonic gum, assuming a horseshoe-like shape to conform with the dental arches. Called also *l. dentalis* and *dentogingival l.*

**dental l., lateral,** a lateral band of cells believed to be functionally and structurally similar to the parent dental lamina, which connects the developing tooth germ to the dental lamina. Called also *lateral enamel strand.*

**l. denta'lis,** dental l.

**l. denta'ta,** labium limbi vestibulare.

**dentogingival l.,** dental l.

**l. du'ra,** see *bundle bone,* under *bone.*

**elastic l., external,** external elastic membrane.

**elastic l., internal,** internal elastic membrane.

**l. elas'tica ante'rior [Bow'mani],** l. limitans anterior corneae.

**l. elas'tica poste'rior [Demour'si], l. elas'tica poste'rior [Desce'meti],** l. limitans posterior corneae.

**l. episclera'lis** [TA], episcleral lamina: loose connective and elastic tissue covering the sclera and anteriorly connecting it with the conjunctiva.

**l. epithelia'lis,** epithelial lamina: the layer of ependymal cells covering the choroid plexus.

**l. exter'na calva'riae** [TA], external table of calvarium: the outer compact layer of bone of the flat bones of the skull. Called also *lamina externa cranii, lamina externa ossium cranii,* and *outer table of skull.*

**l. exter'na cra'nii, l. exter'na os'sium cra'nii,** l. externa calvariae.

**external l. of peritoneum,** peritoneum parietale.

**external l. of pterygoid process,** l. lateralis processus pterygoidei.

**l. fibrocartilagi'nea interpu'bica,** discus interpubicus.

**l. fibroreticula'ris,** reticular l. (def. 1).

**l. fibro'sa,** a fibrous layer, as occurs in the cusps of the semilunar valves.

**fibrous nuclear l.,** nuclear l.

**foliate l.,** lame foliacée.

**l. fus'ca scle'rae** [TA], a thin layer of loose, pigmented connective tissue on the inner surface of the sclera, connecting it with the choroid.

**l. granula'ris exter'na** [TA], external granular layer: layer II of the cerebral cortex, composed of many small pyramidal cells and granule cells with short axons.

**l. granula'ris inter'na** [TA], internal granular layer: layer IV of the cerebral cortex, composed of many densely packed granule cells with short axons and some small pyramidal cells, and traversed by a stria of horizontally arranged fibers (external or outer band or line of Baillarger); it contains neurites derived from cells of other layers and areas of the cerebral cortex and subcortical areas.

**l. horizonta'lis os'sis palati'ni** [TA], horizontal plate of palatine bone: the horizontal part of the palatine bone, forming the posterior part of the hard palate.

**l. inter'na calva'riae** [TA], internal table of calvaria: the inner compact layer of bone of the flat bones of the skull. Called also *lamina interna cranii, lamina interna ossium cranii,* and *inner table of skull.*

**l. inter'na cra'nii, l. inter'na os'sium cra'nii,** lamina interna calvariae.

**internal l. of pterygoid process,** l. medialis processus pterygoidei.

**interpubic l., fibrocartilaginous,** discus interpubicus.

**labial l.,** the ectodermal plate that on splitting separates lip from gum, thus forming the labial groove.

**labiodental l.,** the thickened ectodermal band from which the dental and labial laminae develop.

**labiogingival l.,** labial l.

**lateral l. of cartilage of auditory tube,** l. lateralis cartilaginis tubae auditivae.

**lateral l. of pterygoid process,** l. lateralis processus pterygoidei.

**l. latera'lis cartila'ginis tu'bae auditi'vae** [TA], lateral lamina of cartilage of auditory tube: the smaller of the two laminae that compose the tubal cartilage; it lies in the lateral wall of the auditory tube. Called also *l. lateralis cartilaginis tubae auditoriae* [TA alternative].

**l. latera'lis cartila'ginis tu'bae audito'riae,** TA alternative for *l. lateralis cartilaginis tubae auditivae.*

**l. latera'lis proces'sus pterygoi'dei** [TA], lateral lamina of pterygoid process: either of a pair of bony plates projecting downward from the roots of the greater wings of the sphenoid bone and forming the medial wall of the ipsilateral infratemporal fossa; called also *lateral pterygoid plate.*

**l. li'mitans ante'rior cor'neae** [TA], anterior limiting lamina: a thin layer of the cornea beneath the outer layer of stratified epithelium, composed of condensed stroma, between it and the substantia propria; called also *l. elastica anterior [Bowmani] and Bowman's membrane.*

**l. li'mitans poste'rior cor'neae** [TA], posterior limiting lamina: a thin hyaline membrane between the substantia propria and the endothelial layer of the cornea; called also *l. elastica posterior [Demoursi]* and *l. elastica posterior [Descemeti].*

**limiting l., anterior,** l. limitans anterior corneae.

**limiting l., posterior,** l. limitans posterior corneae.

**l. lu'cida,** an electron-lucent layer of the basal lamina, composed of laminin, fibronectin, and proteoglycans and lying between the lamina densa and the adjoining cell layer; in the pulmonary alveoli and renal glomeruli, there is a lamina lucida, termed the lamina rara interna and lamina rara externa, on either side of the lamina densa.

**medial l. of cartilage of auditory tube,** l. medialis cartilaginis tubae auditivae.

**medial l. of pterygoid process,** l. medialis processus pterygoidei.

**l. media'lis cartila'ginis tu'bae auditi'vae** [TA], medial lamina of cartilage of auditory tube: the larger of the two laminae that compose the tubal cartilage; it lies in the medial wall of the auditory tube. Called also *l. medialis cartilaginis tubae auditoriae* [TA alternative].

**l. media'lis cartila'ginis tu'bae audito'riae,** TA alternative for *l. medialis cartilaginis tubae auditivae.*

**l. media'lis proces'sus pterygoi'dei** [TA], medial lamina of pterygoid process: either of a pair of bony plates projecting inferiorly from the roots of the greater wings of the sphenoid bone and forming the lateral boundary of the ipsilateral posterior aperture of the nasal cavity and the most posterior part of the lateral wall of the nasal cavity. Called also *medial pterygoid plate.*

**l. medul'laris exter'na cor'poris stria'ti,** TA alternative for *l. medullaris lateralis corporis striati.*

**l. medulla'ris inter'na cor'poris stria'ti,** TA alternative for *l. medullaris medialis corporis striati.*

**l. medulla'ris latera'lis cor'poris stria'ti** [TA], lateral medullary lamina of corpus striatum: a layer of white substance that separates the lateral globus pallidus from the putamen; called also *external medullary l. of corpus striatum, lateral medullary stria of corpus striatum,* and *l. medullaris externa corporis striati* [TA alternative].

**l. medulla'ris latera'lis tha'lami** [TA], external medullary layer of thalamus: one of two layers of myelinated nerve fibers in the dorsal thalami; it covers the lateral surface of the dorsal thalamus and separates it from the internal capsule.

**l. medulla'ris media'lis cor'poris stria'ti** [TA], medial lamina of corpus striatum: a layer of white substance that divides the medial portion of the lentiform nucleus (globus pallidus) into a larger, lateral, and a smaller, medial part; called also *internal medullary l. of corpus striatum, medial medullary stria of corpus striatum,* and *l. medullaris interna corporis striati* [TA alternative].

**l. medulla'ris media'lis tha'lami** [TA], internal medullary layer of thalamus: one of two layers of myelinated nerve fibers in the dorsal thalami; it is a vertical sheet of white substance which partially splits anterosuperiorly and separates the medial and lateral nuclei. It contains the intralaminar nuclei.

**l. medulla'ris tha'lami exter'na,** l. medullaris lateralis thalami.

**l. medulla'ris tha'lami inter'na,** l. medullaris medialis thalami.

**medullary l. of corpus striatum, external,** l. medullaris lateralis corporis striati.

**medullary l. of corpus striatum, internal,** l. medullaris medialis corporis striati.

**medullary l. of corpus striatum, lateral,** l. medullaris lateralis corporis striati.

**medullary l. of corpus striatum, medial,** l. medullaris medialis corporis striati.

**medullary l. of thalamus, external,** l. medullaris lateralis thalami.

**medullary l. of thalamus, internal,** l. medullaris medialis thalami.

**l. membrana'cea tu'bae auditi'vae** [TA], membranous lamina of auditory tube: the connective tissue lamina that supports the medial and lateral parts of the auditory tube.

**l. membrana'cea tu'bae audito'riae,** TA alternative for *l. membranacea tubae auditivae.*

**l. modi'oli** [TA], lamina of modiolus: a bony plate extending upward toward the cupula as a continuation of the modiolus and of the bony spiral lamina of the cochlea.

**l. molecula'ris** [TA], molecular layer: layer I of the cerebral cortex, the most superficial of the six layers, composed chiefly of a stria of tangentially oriented myelinated nerve fibers; this layer also contains dendritic terminals from cells of deeper layers, some cortical afferent fibers, sparsely scattered horizontal cells of Cajal, and various other cell types. Called also *l. plexiformis corticis cerebri* and *plexiform* or *zonal layer of cerebral cortex.*

**l. multifor'mis** [TA], multiform layer: layer VI of the cerebral cortex, composed of various cell types, chiefly containing irregular fusiform cells, the axons of which project into the white substance of the cerebral cortex hemisphere. Called also *fusiform* or *polymorphic layer of cerebral cortex.*

**l. muscula'ris muco'sae,** muscular layer of tunica mucosa: the thin layer of smooth muscle fibers usually found as a part of the tunica mucosa deep to the lamina propria mucosae.

**l. muscula'ris muco'sae co'li,** the muscular layer of the tunica mucosa of the colon.

**l. muscula'ris muco'sae eso'phagi,** l. muscularis mucosae oesophagi.

**l. muscula'ris muco'sae gas'tris** [TA], the muscular layer of the tunica mucosa of the stomach.

**l. muscula'ris muco'sae intesti'ni cras'si** [TA], the muscular layer of the tunica mucosa of the large intestine.

**l. muscula'ris muco'sae intesti'ni rec'ti,** l. muscularis mucosae recti.

**l. muscula'ris muco'sae intesti'ni te'nuis** [TA], the muscular layer of the tunica mucosa of the small intestine.

**l. muscula'ris muco'sae oeso'phagi** [TA], the muscular layer of the tunica mucosa of the esophagus. Written also *l. muscularis mucosae esophagi.*

**l. muscula'ris muco'sae rec'ti,** the muscular layer of the tunica mucosa of the rectum.

**l. muscula'ris muco'sae ventri'culi,** l. muscularis mucosae gastris.

**nuclear l.,** a tightly woven meshwork composed of lamins that lines the nuclear side of the inner nuclear membrane; it is believed to control the shape of the nucleus.

**l. orbita'lis os'sis ethmoida'lis** [TA], orbital lamina of ethmoid bone: a thin plate of bone laterally bounding the ethmoid labyrinth on either side and forming part of the medial wall of the orbit; called also *l. papyracea.*

**palatine l. of maxilla,** processus palatinus maxillae.

**l. papyra'cea,** l. orbitalis ossis ethmoidalis.

**l. parieta'lis pericar'dii sero'si** [TA], parietal layer of serous pericardium: the outer of the two layers of the serous pericardium, lining the fibrous pericardium. Called also *parietal pericardium* and *parietal layer of pericardium.*

**l. parieta'lis tu'nicae vagina'lis pro'priae tes'tis, l. parieta'lis tu'nicae vagina'lis tes'tis** [TA], parietal layer of tunica vaginalis of testis: the outer layer of the tunica vaginalis of the testis, separated from the visceral layer by a cavity.

**periclaustral l.,** capsula extrema.

**l. perpendicula'ris os'sis ethmoida'lis** [TA], perpendicular lamina of ethmoid bone: a thin bony plate that descends from the inferior surface of the cribriform plate of the ethmoid bone and participates in forming the nasal septum; called also *perpendicular plate of ethmoid bone.*

**l. perpendicula'ris os'sis palati'ni** [TA], perpendicular plate of palatine bone: the flat, vertical, bony plate that extends superiorly on either side from the palatine bone; it is surmounted by the orbital and sphenoidal processes.

**l. plexifor'mis cor'ticis ce'rebri,** l. molecularis.

**posterior limiting l.,** l. limitans posterior corneae.

**l. poste'rior vagi'nae mus'culi rec'ti abdo'minis** [TA], posterior lamina of sheath of rectus abdominis muscle: the portion of the muscle sheath lying posterior to the rectus abdominis muscle, formed by the transversus abdominis muscle and its aponeurosis at the level of the xiphoid process; inferior to the xiphoid process, as far as the arcuate line, it is formed by the aponeuroses of the internal oblique and the transversus muscles.

**l. pretrachea'lis fas'ciae cervica'lis** [TA], pretracheal layer of cervical fascia: the layer of deep cervical fascia that is anterior to the trachea and surrounds the thyroid gland; see also *anterior visceral space.* Called also *pretracheal fascia* and *middle layer of deep cervical fascia.*

**l. prevertebra'lis fas'ciae cervica'lis** [TA], prevertebral layer of cervical fascia: the layer of deep cervical fascia that is anterior to the vertebrae and posterior to the trachea and esophagus; it invests the scalene and levator scapulae muscles and is continuous laterally with the membrana suprapleuralis. Called also *prevertebral fascia.*

**l. profun′da fas′ciae tempora′lis** [TA], deep layer of temporal fascia: the deep portion of the fascia investing the temporal muscle.
**l. profun′da mus′culi levato′ris pal′pebrae superio′ris** [TA], the deeper of the two layers of the levator palpebrae superioris muscle, the fibers of which are attached to the tarsus superior palpebrae.
**l. pro′pria membra′nae tympa′nicae,** fibrous stratum of tympanic membrane.
**l. pro′pria muco′sae,** proper mucous membrane: the connective tissue coat of a mucous membrane just deep to the epithelium and basement membrane.
**l. pyramida′lis exter′na** [TA], external pyramidal layer: layer III of the cerebral cortex, composed of an inner zone of medium-sized pyramidal cells and an outer zone of larger pyramidal cells and other cells whose dendrites and axons extend beyond this layer.
**l. pyramida′lis gangliona′ris, l. pyramida′lis inter′na** [TA], internal pyramidal layer: layer V of the cerebral cortex, composed of the largest pyramidal cells, Martinotti's cells, and Betz's cells, and traversed by a stria of horizontally arranged fibers (inner or internal line or band of Baillarger); the axons of the pyramidal cells leave this layer as either association, projection, or commissural fibers. Called also *ganglionic layer of cerebral cortex.*
**l. quadrige′mina,** TA alternative for *l. tecti mesencephali.*
**l. ra′ra,** 1. l. lucida. 2. see *l. rara externa* and *l. rara interna.*
**l. ra′ra exter′na,** the lamina lucida on the epithelial side of the lamina densa in renal glomeruli and pulmonary alveoli.
**l. ra′ra inter′na,** the lamina lucida on the endothelial side of the lamina densa in renal glomeruli and pulmonary alveoli.
**reticular l., l. reticula′ris,** 1. a layer of the basement membrane, adjacent to the connective tissue, seen in some epithelia; it is of variable thickness and is composed of condensed connective tissue with a reticulum of collagen fibers. Cf. *basal l.* 2. membrana reticularis organi spiralis.
**Rexed's laminae,** an architectural scheme used to classify the structure of the spinal cord, based on the cytological features of the neurons in different regions of the gray substance. It consists of nine laminae (I–IX) that extend throughout the cord, roughly paralleling the dorsal and ventral columns of the gray substance, and a tenth region (lamina X) that surrounds the central canal and consists of the dorsal and ventral commissures and the central gelatinous substance.

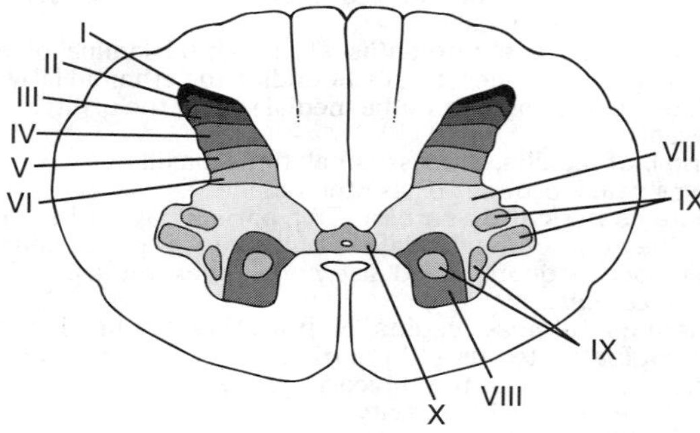

Rexed's laminae in a cross section of the spinal cord at approximately the level of the seventh cervical vertebra (C7).

**l. rostra′lis,** rostral lamina: the thin terminal part of the rostrum of the corpus callosum passing down in front of the anterior commissure to the anterior perforated substance and the paraterminal gyrus.
**l. sep′ti pellu′cidi** [TA], lamina of septum pellucidum: either of the thin, vertical sheets, separated by a cleftlike space, which constitute the septum pellucidum.
**spinal laminae, lami′nae spina′lis,** Rexed's laminae.
**spiral l., bony, spiral l., osseous,** l. spiralis ossea.
**spiral l., secondary,** l. spiralis secundaria.
**l. spira′lis os′sea** [TA], bony spiral lamina: a double plate of bone winding spirally around the modiolus and dividing the spiral canal of the cochlea incompletely into two parts, the scala tympani and the scala vestibuli; called also *spiral plate.*
**l. spira′lis secunda′ria** [TA], secondary spiral lamina: a bony projection on the outer wall of the osseous spiral lamina in the lower part of the first turn of the cochlea.
**submucous l. of stomach,** tela submucosa gastris.
**l. superficia′lis fas′ciae cervica′lis** [TA], superficial layer of cervical fascia: the most superficial of the deep layers of cervical fascia, surrounding the neck superficial to the pretracheal layer; it invests the trapezius and sternocleidomastoid muscles and is attached posteriorly to the vertebrae. Called also *superficial cervical fascia, superficial layer of deep cervical fascia,* and *investing layer of cervical fascia* or *of deep cervical fascia.*
**l. superficia′lis fas′ciae tempora′lis** [TA], superficial layer of temporal fascia: the superficial portion of the fascia investing the temporal muscle.
**l. superficia′lis mus′culi levato′ris pal′pebrae superio′ris** [TA], the superficial of the two layers of the levator palpebrae superioris muscle.
**l. suprachorioi′dea,** lamina suprachoroidea.
**l. suprachoroi′dea** [TA], suprachoroid lamina: the outermost layer of the choroid, which connects it with the sclera; called also *suprachoroid layer.*
**l. supraneuropo′rica,** the part of lamina terminalis caudal to the anterior neuropore of the embryo; it cannot be delimited accurately in human embryos.
**l. tecta′lis mesence′phali, l. tec′ti mesence′phali** [TA], tectal plate: the layer of mingled gray and white substance in the tectum of the mesencephalon, from which arise the superior and inferior colliculi. Called also *l. quadrigemina* and *quadrigeminal plate.*
**l. termina′lis hypotha′lami** [TA], terminal lamina of hypothalamus: a thin plate derived from the telencephalon extending upward from the optic chiasm and preoptic recess, and forming the anterior wall of the third ventricle of the cerebrum; called also *terminal plate.*
**l. of thyroid cartilage, right and left,** l. cartilaginis thyroideae [dextra/sinistra].
**l. tra′gi** [TA], **l. tra′gica,** lamina of tragus: the longitudinal curved lamina of cartilage in the tragus of the auricle, at the beginning of the cartilaginous portion of the external acoustic meatus.
**vascular l. of choroid,** l. vasculosa choroideae.
**vascular l. of stomach,** tela submucosa gastris.
**l. vasculo′sa chorioi′deae, l. vasculo′sa choroi′deae** [TA], vascular lamina of choroid: the layer of the choroid between the suprachoroid and choriocapillary layers, containing the largest blood vessels; called also *Haller's membrane.*
**l. of vertebra, l. of vertebral arch,** l. arcus vertebrae.
**l. viscera′lis pericar′dii sero′si** [TA], visceral layer of pericardium: the inner layer of the serous pericardium; it is in contact with the heart and the roots of the great vessels; called also *epicardium, visceral pericardium,* and *visceral layer of serous pericardium.*
**l. viscera′lis tu′nicae vagina′lis pro′priae tes′tis, l. viscera′lis tu′nicae vagina′lis tes′tis** [TA], tunica serosa testis.
**l. vi′trea, vitreal l., vitreous l.,** lamina basalis choroideae.
**white laminae of cerebellum,** laminae albae cerebelli.

**lam·i·nae** (lam′ĭ-ne) [L.] genitive and plural of *lamina.*

**lam·i·na·gram** (lam′ĭ-nə-gram) tomogram.

**lam·i·na·graph** (lam′ĭ-nə-graf) an x-ray machine for making radiographs of a layer of tissue at a selected depth.

**lam·i·nag·ra·phy** (lam″ĭ-nag′rə-fe) [*lamina* + *-graphy*] tomography.

**lam·i·na·plas·ty** (lam′ĭ-nə-plas″te) [*lamina* + *-plasty*] incision completely through one lamina of a vertebral arch with creation of a trough in the contralateral lamina; the vertebral arch is then opened like a door, with the trough acting as a hinge; performed to relieve compression of the spinal cord or nerve roots. Spelled also *laminoplasty.* Called also *open-door l.*

**lam·i·nar** (lam′ĭ-nər) [L. *laminaris*] made up of, or arranged in, layers or laminae.

**La·mi·na·ria** (lam″ĭ-nar′e-ə) [MeSH: Laminaria] a genus of seaweeds (kelps), various species of which are used as sources of alginates; see *laminarin. L. digita′ta* yields dry stems that are hydrophilic and gradually swell in moist environments, so that they can be used to dilate the uterine cervix in induced abortion.

**lam·i·na·rin** (lam″ĭ-na′rin) a polysaccharide from seaweed of the genus *Laminaria,* consisting essentially of β-D-glucose residues.
**l. sulfate,** the sulfated form, having antilipemic and anticoagulant properties.

**lam·i·nec·to·my** (lam″ĭ-nek′tə-me) [*lamina* + *-ectomy*] [MeSH: Laminectomy] excision of the posterior arch of a vertebra.

**lam·i·nin** (lam′ĭ-nin) [MeSH: Laminin] an adhesive glycoprotein component of the basement membrane; it binds to heparan sulfate, type IV collagen, and specific cell-surface receptors and is involved in the attachment of epithelial cells to underlying connective tissue.

**lam·i·ni·tis** (lam″ĭ-ni′tis) 1. inflammation of a lamina. 2. inflammation, congestion, and ischemia of the laminae of a hoof, with breakdown of the union between the horny and sensitive layers; it usually occurs in overweight, overfed animals. Called also *founder.*

**lam·i·no·gram** (lam′ĭ-no-gram) tomogram.

**lam·i·nog·ra·phy** (lam″ĭ-nog′rə-fe) tomography.

**lam·i·no·plas·ty** (lam′in-o-plas′te) laminaplasty.

**Lam·i·no·si·op·tes** (lam″ĭ-no-se-op′tēz) a genus of mites of the family Laminosioptidae. *L. cysti′cola* forms nodules in the subcutaneous tissue of chickens and other birds.

**Lam·i·no·si·op·ti·dae** (lam″ĭ-no-se-op′tĭ-de) a family of mites, some of which infest birds. It includes the genus *Laminosioptes.*

**lam·i·not·o·my** (lam″ĭ-not′ə-me) [*lamina* + *-tomy*] division of the lamina of a vertebra.

**La·mi·sil** (ləmi′sil) trademark for preparation of terbinafine hydrochloride.

**la·miv·u·dine** (lə-miv′u-dēn) [MeSH: Lamivudine] an inhibitor of reverse transcriptase used as an antiviral agent in combination with zidovudine in the management of human immunodeficiency virus infection and acquired immunodeficiency syndrome; administered orally.

**la·mo·tri·gine** (ləmo′trĭgēn) an anticonvulsant used as an adjunct in the treatment of partial seizures in adults with epilepsy; administered orally.

**lamp** (lamp) an apparatus for furnishing heat or light.
**annealing l.,** an alcohol lamp for heating and purifying gold foil to be used for filling tooth cavities.
**arc l.,** a source of light consisting of gaseous particles from the electrodes of an electric arc which are raised to a temperature of incandescence by an electric current.
**carbon arc l.,** a lamp that produces an intense white light from an electric arc between carbon rods; formerly used in artificial light therapy.
**cold quartz l.,** low pressure mercury arc l.
**diagnostic l.,** a light used for observing subtle shadings in weak fluorescence, for external body examinations, observations of tissue fluorescence, identification of vulvar fluorescence, chromatography, etc.
**Eldridge-Green l.,** an arrangement of lights for testing color vision.
**Finsen-Reya l.,** a modification of the Finsen lamp in which the electrodes are placed at right angles to each other.
**Gullstrand's slit l.,** slit l.
**heat l.,** a lamp held at a distance from the body and used for superficial heating of a part.
**high pressure mercury arc l.,** an ultraviolet radiation lamp having a high vapor pressure with high intensity light because of linear spectral emissions in many wavelength ranges; used as a source of ultraviolet B for treating dermatologic disorders. See also *Goeckerman treatment,* under *treatment.*
**hot quartz l.,** high pressure mercury arc l.
**Kromayer's l.,** a high pressure mercury arc lamp with a small field of irradiation, used to treat dermatologic disorders in small surface areas of the skin.
**low pressure mercury arc l.,** an ultraviolet radiation lamp having a low vapor pressure, low amperage, high voltage, and a glow discharge; more than 95 per cent of its emission is ultraviolet C in the mercury vapor resonance emission line at 254 nm. In the treatment of skin disorders such as acne, the radiation causes acute erythema followed by desquamation of the affected skin.
**mercury arc l., mercury vapor l.,** a lamp in which the arc is struck in mercury and is enclosed in a quartz burner; used in light therapy. The two most common types are the low pressure or cold quartz type and the high pressure or hot quartz type.
**quartz l.,** mercury arc l.
**slit l.,** one embodying a diaphragm containing a slitlike opening, by means of which a narrow flat beam of intense light may be projected into the eye. It gives intense illumination so that microscopic study may be made of the conjunctivae, cornea, iris, lens, and vitreous, the special feature being that it illuminates a section through the substance of these structures. Called also *Gullstrand's slit l.* and *slit-lamp biomicroscope.*
**sun l.,** a lamp that gives off radiation, especially ultraviolet, in ranges similar to those of the sun's rays.
**ultraviolet l.,** one which produces ultraviolet rays.
**Wood's l.,** a medium-pressure mercury arc lamp used in the diagnosis of erythrasma and fungus infections as well as for revealing the presence of porphyrins and fluorescent minerals of the skin, scalp, and hair. See also *Wood's light.*
**xenon arc l.,** a lamp that produces light of high intensity in a wide continuum of wavelengths; used with optical filters as the most common source of solar-simulating radiation; clinical uses include tests of photosensitivity.

**lam·pas** (lam′pəs) [Fr.] a swelling and hardening of the mucosa of the hard palate, immediately behind the upper incisors in horses; called also *palatitis.*

**La·mus** (la′məs) a former genus name of predatory insects of the family Reduviidae now placed under the genera *Panstrongylus* and *Triatoma.*

**lam·ziek·te** (lam′zēk-te) [Afrikaans "lame-sickness"] a type of botulism seen in cattle in South Africa after they chew on infected or putrefying bones in an effort to compensate for a phosphorus deficiency.

**la·na** (lan′ə) gen. and pl. *la′nae* [L.] wool.

**la·nat·o·side C** (lə-nat′o-sīd) an easily absorbed and stable glycoside obtained from the leaves of *Digitalis lanata,* having the same actions and uses as digitalis; administered orally.

**lance** (lans) [L. *lancea*] 1. lancet. 2. to cut or incise with a lancet.

**Lance·field classification** (lans′fēld) [Rebecca Craighill *Lancefield,* American bacteriologist, 1895–1981] see under *classification.*

**lan·ce·o·late** (lan′se-o-lāt) shaped like a lance.

**Lan·ce·reaux-Ma·thieu disease** (lahn-sə-ro′-mah-tyoo′) [Etienne *Lancereaux,* French physician, 1829–1910; Albert *Mathieu,* French physician, 1855–1917] Weil's syndrome.

**lan·cet** (lan′sət) [L. *lancea* lance] a small pointed and two-edged surgical knife.

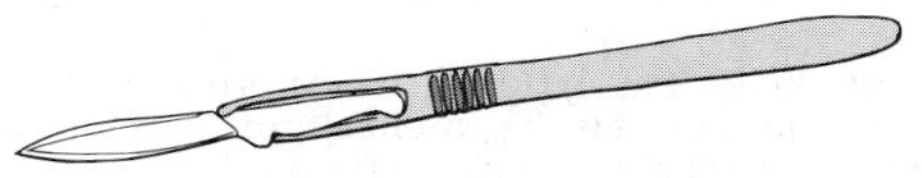

Lancet.

**abscess l.,** a wide-bladed lancet with one convex and one concave edge.
**acne l.,** a form with a narrow blade for puncturing the papules of acne.
**gingival l., gum l.,** a knife for incising the gingivae.
**spring l.,** one the blade of which is held by a spring.

**Lan·cet coefficient** (lan′sət) [*The Lancet,* a British medical periodical] see under *coefficient.*

**lan·ci·nat·ing** (lan′sĭ-nāt″ing) [L. *lancinas*] tearing, darting, or sharply cutting; see under *pain.*

**Lan·ci·si's nerves, stria** (lahn-che′zēz) [Giovanni Maria *Lancisi,* Italian physician, 1654–1720] see *stria longitudinalis lateralis corporis callosi* and *stria longitudinalis medialis corporis callosi.*

**Lan·dau-Kleff·ner syndrome** (lahn′dou klef′nər) [William M. *Landau,* American neurologist, 20th century; F. R. *Kleffner,* American neurologist, 20th century] [MeSH: Landau-Kleffner Syndrome] see under *syndrome.*

**land·mark** (land′mark) a readily recognizable anatomical structure used as a point of reference in establishing the location of another structure or in determining certain measurements.

**Lan·dolt's operation** (lahn-dōz′) [Edmond *Landolt,* French ophthalmologist, 1846–1926] see under *operation.*

**Lan·dou·zy's disease, dystrophy (type)** (lah-doo-zēz′) [Louis Théophile Joseph *Landouzy,* French physician, 1845–1917] see *Weil's syndrome,* under *syndrome,* and see *facioscapulohumeral muscular dystrophy,* under *dystrophy.*

**Lan·dou·zy-De·je·rine dystrophy (atrophy)** (lah-doo-ze′dĕ-zhĕ-rēn′) [L. T. J. *Landouzy;* Joseph Jules *Dejerine,* French neurologist, 1849–1917] facioscapulohumeral muscular dystrophy.

**Lan·dry's paralysis (syndrome)** (lah-drēz′) [Jean Baptiste Octave *Landry,* French physician, 1826–1865] acute idiopathic polyneuritis.

**Land·stei·ner** (lahnd′shti-nər) Karl. Austrian pathologist and immunologist, 1868–1943; winner of the Nobel prize for physiology or medicine in 1930 for his discovery of the human blood groups in 1901.

**Land·ström's muscle** (lahnd′strəmz) [John *Landström,* Swedish surgeon, 1869–1910] see under *muscle.*

**Lane's bands, disease, operation, plate** (lānz) [Sir William Arbuthnot *Lane,* British surgeon, 1856–1943] see under *band, disease, operation,* and *plate.*

**Lange's solution, test** (lahng′əz) [Carl *Lange,* German physician, 1883–1953] see under *solution* and *test.*

**Lan·gen·beck's amputation, flap, triangle** (lahng′ən-beks)

[Bernhard Rudolf Konrad von *Langenbeck,* German surgeon, 1810–1887] see under *amputation, flap,* and *triangle.*

**Lan·ger's axillary arch, lines, muscle** (lahng'ərz) [Carl Ritter von Edenberg von *Langer,* Austrian anatomist, 1819–1887] see under *arch, line,* and *muscle.*

**Lan·ger·hans' cells, granules, islets, (islands)** (lahng'ər-hahnz) [Paul *Langerhans,* German pathologist, 1847–1888] see under *cell* and *islet* and see *Birbeck's granules,* under *granule.*

**Lang·hans' cells, layer (stria)** (lahng'hahnz) [Theodor *Langhans,* German pathologist, 1839–1915] see under *cell,* and see *cytotrophoblast.*

**Lang·ley's ganglion, granules, nerves** (lang'lēz) [John Newport *Langley,* English physiologist, 1852–1925] see under *ganglion* and *granule,* and see *pilonidal nerves,* under *nerve.*

**lan·i·ary** (lan'e-ar″e) [L. *laniare* to tear to pieces] suitable for lacerating, or tearing to pieces; said of canine teeth.

**Lan·ne·longue's foramina** (lah-nə-lawgz') [Odilon Marc *Lannelongue,* French surgeon, 1840–1911] foramina venarum minimarum cordis.

**Lan·nois-Gra·de·ni·go syndrome** (lah-nwah'grah-də-ne'go) [Maurice *Lannois,* French physician, late 19th century; Giuseppe *Gradenigo,* Italian physician, 1859–1926] Gradenigo's syndrome.

**lan·o·lin** (lan'o-lin) [*lana* + *oleum*] [USP] [MeSH: Lanolin] the purified waxlike substance from the wool of sheep, cleaned, deodorized, and decolorized; mixed with 25 to 30 per cent water, it is used as a water-in-oil ointment base.
**modified l.** [USP], lanolin that has been processed to reduce the amount of free lanolin alcohols and detergent and pesticide residues.

**la·nos·ter·ol** (lə-nos'tər-ol) [MeSH: Lanosterol] a tetracyclic sterol formed from squalene; it is the parent steroid in animals, being itself converted in several steps to cholesterol.

**La·nox·in** (lə-nok'sin) trademark for preparations of digoxin.

**lan·so·pra·zole** (lan-so'prə'-zōl) a substituted benzimidazole that inhibits the secretion of gastric acid, used for the symptomatic treatment of duodenal ulcer and esophagitis and for the long-term treatment of hyperchlorhydria; administered orally.

**Lan·ter·man's incisures (clefts)** (lahn'tər-mahnz) [A. J. *Lanterman,* American anatomist in Germany, late 19th century] see under *incisure.*

**Lan·ter·man-Schmidt incisures** (lahn'tər-mahn-shmit) [A. J. *Lanterman;* Henry D. *Schmidt,* American anatomist, 1823–1888] incisures of Lanterman.

**lan·than·ic** (lan'thən-ik) [Gr. *lanthanein* to escape notice, to be concealed] symptom-free; said of a symptomless disease that is undetected, or detected by accident.

**lan·tha·nin** (lan'thə-nin) oxychromatin.

**lan·tha·num** (lan'thə-nəm) [Gr. *lanthanein* to be concealed] [MeSH: Lanthanum] a rare metallic element; symbol, La; atomic number, 57; atomic weight, 138.91.

**la·nu·gi·nous** (lə-noo'jĭ-nəs) [L. *lanuginosus*] covered with lanugo.

**la·nu·go** (lə-noo'go) [L.] [TA] the fine hair on the body of the fetus; called also *down* and *lanugo hair.*

**Lanz's point** (lahnts'əz) [Otto *Lanz,* Swiss surgeon in the Netherlands, 1865–1935] see under *point.*

**LAO** left anterior oblique.

**LAP** 1. leukocyte alkaline phosphatase; see under *alkaline phosphatase.* 2. leukocyte adhesion protein; see *$\beta_2$ integrin,* under *integrin.*

**la·pac·tic** (lə-pak'tik) [Gr. *lapaktikos, lapassein* to discharge] pertaining to or effecting a removal; purgative; laxative.

**lapar(o)-** [Gr. *lapara* flank] a combining form denoting relationship to the loin or flank. Sometimes used loosely in reference to the abdomen.

**lap·a·ro·cele** (lap'ə-ro-sēl″) abdominal hernia.

**lap·a·ro·cho·le·cys·tot·o·my** (lap″ə-ro-ko″le-sis-tot'ə-me) [*laparo-* + *cholecystotomy*] cholecystectomy.

**lap·a·ro·co·lec·to·my** (lap″ə-ro-ko-lek'tə-me) [*laparo-* + *colectomy*] colectomy.

**lap·a·ro·co·los·to·my** (lap″ə-ro-ko-los'tə-me) [*laparo-* + *colostomy*] surgical creation of a permanent opening into the colon through an incision in the anterolateral wall of the abdomen; colostomy.

**lap·a·ro·co·lot·o·my** (lap″ə-ro-ko-lot'ə-me) [*laparo-* + *colotomy*] colotomy.

**lap·a·ro·cys·tec·to·my** (lap″ə-ro-sis-tek'tə-me) [*laparo-* + *cystectomy*] removal of a cyst by an abdominal incision.

**lap·a·ro·cys·ti·dot·o·my** (lap″ə-ro-sis″tĭ-dot'ə-me) [*laparo-* + *cystido-* + *-tomy*] suprapubic cystotomy.

**lap·a·ro·cys·tot·o·my** (lap″ə-ro-sis-tot'ə-me) [*laparo-* + *cystotomy*] laparotomy with removal of the contents of a cyst.

**lap·a·ro·en·ter·os·to·my** (lap″ə-ro-en″tər-os'tə-me) [*laparo-* + *enterostomy*] surgical creation of an artificial opening into the intestine through the abdominal wall.

**lap·a·ro·en·ter·ot·o·my** (lap″ə-ro-en″tər-ot'ə-me) [*laparo-* + *enterotomy*] laparotomy with incision into the intestine.

**lap·a·ro·gas·tros·co·py** (lap″ə-ro-gas-tros'kə-pe) [*laparo-* + *gastroscopy*] examination of the interior of the stomach through an abdominal incision.

**lap·a·ro·gas·tros·to·my** (lap″ə-ro-gas-tros'tə-me) [*laparo-* + *gastrostomy*] surgical creation of a permanent gastric fistula through the abdominal wall.

**lap·a·ro·gas·trot·o·my** (lap″ə-ro-gas-trot'ə-me) [*laparo-* + *gastrotomy*] incision into the stomach through the abdominal wall. Called also *celiogastrotomy.*

**lap·a·ro·hep·a·tot·o·my** (lap″ə-ro-hep″ə-tot'ə-me) [*laparo-* + *hepatotomy*] incision of the liver through the abdominal wall.

**lap·a·ro·hys·ter·ec·to·my** (lap″ə-ro-his″tə-rek'tə-me) [*laparo-* + *hysterectomy*] abdominal hysterectomy.

**lap·a·ro·hys·tero·ooph·o·rec·to·my** (lap″ə-ro-his″tər-o-o″of-ə-rek'tə-me) [*laparo-* + *hystero-* + *oophorectomy*] laparotomy with removal of the uterus and ovaries.

**lap·a·ro·hys·tero·sal·pin·go-ooph·o·rec·to·my** (lap″ə-ro-his″tər-o-sal-ping″go-o″of-ə-rek'tə-me) removal of the uterus, uterine tubes, and ovaries through an abdominal incision.

**lap·a·ro·hys·ter·ot·o·my** (lap″ə-ro-his″tər-ot'ə-me) [*laparo-* + *hysterotomy*] abdominal hysterotomy.

**lap·a·ro·il·e·ot·o·my** (lap″ə-ro-il″e-ot'ə-me) [*laparo-* + *ileotomy*] laparotomy with incision of the ileum.

**lap·a·ro·mono·did·y·mus** (lap″ə-ro-mon″o-did'ə-məs) [*laparo-* + *mono-* + *-didymus*] conjoined twins that are double superiorly but single inferior to the pelvis.

**lap·a·ro·my·itis** (lap″ə-ro-mi-i'tis) [*laparo-* + *my-* + *-itis*] inflammation of the abdominal or lumbar muscles.

**lap·a·ro·myo·mec·to·my** (lap″ə-ro-mi″o-mek'tə-me) [*laparo-* + *myomectomy*] uterine myomectomy through an abdominal incision.

**lap·a·ro·ne·phrec·to·my** (lap″ə-ro-nə-frek'tə-me) [*laparo-* + *nephrectomy*] removal of a kidney by an incision in the loin.

**lap·a·ror·rha·phy** (lap″ə-ror'ə-fe) [*laparo-* + *-rrhaphy*] suture or repair of the abdominal wall. Called also *celiorrhaphy.*

**lap·a·ro·sal·pin·gec·to·my** (lap″ə-ro-sal″pin-jek'tə-me) [*laparo-* + *salpingectomy*] removal of a uterine tube through an abdominal incision. Called also *celiosalpingectomy.*

**lap·a·ro·sal·pin·go-ooph·o·rec·to·my** (lap″ə-ro-sal-ping″go-o″of-ə-rek'tə-me) removal of a uterine tube and ovary through an abdominal incision.

**lap·a·ro·sal·pin·gos·to·my** (lap″ə-ro-sal″ping-gos'tə-me) formation of an opening in the oviduct through an abdominal incision.

**lap·a·ro·sal·pin·got·o·my** (lap″ə-ro-sal″ping-got'ə-me) [*laparo-* + *salpingotomy*] incision of a uterine tube through an abdominal incision. Called also *celiosalpingotomy.*

**lap·a·ro·scope** (lap'ə-ro-skōp″) an instrument, comparable to an endoscope, that is inserted into the peritoneal cavity to inspect it. Called also *celioscope* and *peritoneoscope.*

**lap·a·ro·scop·ic** (lap″ə-ro-skop'ik) 1. pertaining to a laparoscope. 2. performed using a laparoscope.

**lap·a·ros·co·py** (lap″ə-ros'kə-pe) [*laparo-* + *-scopy*] [MeSH: Laparoscopy] examination of the interior of the abdomen by means of a laparoscope. Called also *abdominoscopy, celioscopy,* and *peritoneoscopy.*
**laser l.,** introduction of a laser beam into the abdomen through a laparoscope, done to vaporize tissue, as in treating endometriosis or to lyse adhesions. See also *pelvioscopy* and *videolaseroscopy.*

**lap·a·ro·sple·nec·to·my** (lap″ə-ro-sple-nek'tə-me) [*laparo-* + *splenectomy*] laparotomy with excision of the spleen.

**lap·a·ro·sple·not·o·my** (lap″ə-ro-sple-not'ə-me) [*laparo-* + *splenotomy*] laparotomy to gain access to the spleen, usually for the purpose of draining a cyst or abscess of the spleen.

**lap·a·rot·o·ma·phil·ia** (lap″ə-rot″o-mə-fil'e-ə) [*laparotomy* + *-philia*] Munchausen syndrome (q.v.) in which the patient desires abdominal surgery.

**lap·a·ro·tome** (lap'ə-rə-tōm) a knife used in laparotomy.

**lap·a·rot·o·my** (lap″ə-rot′ə-me) [*laparo-* + *-tomy*] [MeSH: Laparotomy] 1. surgical incision through the flank. 2. celiotomy.
**staging l.**, laparotomy for pathologic staging of subdiaphragmatic Hodgkin's disease. It always includes splenectomy, wedge and deep needle biopsies of liver lobes, and biopsies of multiple lymph nodes, and it may be accompanied by appendectomy and ovariopexy.

**lap·a·ro·typh·lot·o·my** (lap″ə-ro-tif-lot′ə-me) [*laparo-* + *typhlotomy*] incision into the cecum through the flank.

**La·picque's constant** (lah-pēks′) [Louis *Lapicque*, French physiologist, 1866–1952] see under *constant.*

**Lap·i·dus operation** (lap′ĭ-dəs) [Paul W. *Lapidus*, American orthopedic surgeon, born 1893] see under *operation.*

**lap·in·iza·tion** (lap″in-ĭ-za′shən) [Fr. *lapin* rabbit] passage of a virus through rabbits as a means of modifying its characteristics.

**lap·in·ize** (lap′in-īz) to attenuate (as a virus or vaccine) by serial passage through rabbits.

**La·place's law** (lah-plahs′əz) [Pierre Simon de *Laplace*, French mathematician and physicist, 1749–1827] see under *law.*

**lap·sus** (lap′səs) [L., from *labi* to slip or fall] an error, or slip, thought to be revealing of an unconscious wish or association.
**l. ca′lami**, an unconsciously motivated slip of the pen.
**l. lin′guae**, an unconsciously motivated slip of the tongue.
**l. memo′riae**, an unconsciously motivated lapse of memory.

**la·pyr·i·um chlo·ride** (lə-pēr′e-əm) a surfactant used in pharmaceutic preparations.

**lard** (lahrd) [L. *lardum*] the purified internal fat of the abdomen of the hog.
**benzoinated l.**, a preparation of lard containing 1 per cent benzoin; used as a vehicle for medicinal agents and in ointments. Called also *adeps benzoinatus.*

**lar·da·ceous** (lahr-da′shəs) 1. resembling lard. 2. containing lardacein.

**Lar·gon** (lahr′gon) trademark for a preparation of propiomazine hydrochloride.

**Lar·i·am** (lar′e-am) trademark for a preparation of mefloquine hydrochloride.

**la·rith·mics** (lə-rith′miks) [Gr. *laos* people + *arithmos* number] the study which deals with population in its quantitative aspects.

**lark·spur** (lahrk′spər) 1. any of various species of *Delphinium*, which are highly toxic; see *larkspur poisoning*, under *poisoning.* 2. the dried ripe seeds of *Delphinium ajacis*, used medically as a pediculicide.

**Lar·o·do·pa** (lar″o-do′pə) trademark for preparations of levodopa.

**La·ron dwarf, syndrome (dwarfism)** (lah-ron′) [Zvi *Laron*, Israeli endocrinologist, born 1927] see under *dwarf* and *syndrome.*

**Lar·o·tid** (lar′o-tid) trademark for preparations of amoxicillin.

**Lar·rey's amputation (operation), cleft, spaces** (lah-rāz′) [Dominique Jean (Baron de) *Larrey*, French military surgeon, 1766–1842] see under *amputation* and *space*, and see *trigonum sternocostale.*

**Lar·sen's disease** (lahr′sənz) [Christian Magnus Falsen Sinding *Larsen*, Norwegian physician, 1866–1930] see under *disease.*

**Lar·sen's syndrome** (lahr′sənz) [Loren Joseph *Larsen*, American orthopedic surgeon, born 1914] see under *syndrome.*

**Lar·sen-Jo·hans·son disease** (lahr′sən-yo-hahn′sən) [C.M.F. Sinding *Larsen;* Sven Christian *Johansson*, Swedish surgeon, born 1880] see *Larsen's disease*, under *disease.*

**lar·va** (lahr′və) gen. and pl. *lar′vae* [L. "ghost"] [MeSH: Larva] an independent, motile, sometimes feeding, developmental stage in the life history of an animal. Cf. *imago* (def. 1) and *pupa.*
**l. cur′rens**, a rapidly progressive creeping eruption manifested by an urticarial perianal band, representing autoinoculation of the larvae of *Strongyloides stercoralis* that migrate to and mature at the anus in intestinal infections with the parasite.
**l. mi′grans, l. migrans, cutaneous**, 1. a skin disease of humans or other animals marked by thin, curving, pruritic lines corresponding to the subcutaneous movements of parasitic larvae, usually those of the cat and dog hookworm, *Ancylostoma braziliense*, which burrow beneath the skin but cannot complete their migration to the gut. Called also *ox-warble* or *sandworm disease* and *creeping eruption.* 2. a similar condition caused by other parasites, such as those seen in gnathostomiasis or hypodermiasis; see also *myiasis linearis.*
**l. migrans, ocular**, infection of the eye with larvae of roundworms (*Toxocara canis* or *T. cati*), which may lodge in the choroid or retina or migrate to the vitreous; on the death of the larvae, a granulomatous inflammation occurs, the lesion varying from a translucent elevation of the retina, to massive retinal detachment and pseudoglioma.
**l. migrans, visceral**, a condition caused by prolonged migration of larvae of nematodes in human tissues other than skin, characterized by persistent hypereosinophilia, hepatomegaly, and frequently by pneumonitis; commonly caused by *Toxocara canis* or *T. cati*, which do not complete their life cycle in humans. See also *l. migrans, ocular.*
**rat-tailed l.**, see *Eristalis tenax.*

**lar·va·ceous** (lahr-va′shəs) larvate.

**lar·vae** (lahr′ve) [L.] plural of *larva.*

**lar·val** (lahr′vəl) 1. pertaining to larvae. 2. larvate.

**lar·vate** (lahr′vāt) [L. *larva* mask] masked; concealed: said of a disease or a symptom of disease.

**lar·vi·cide** (lahr′vĭ-sīd) [*larva* + *-cide*] an agent destructive to insect larvae.

**lar·vi·pha·gic** (lahr″vĭ-fa′jik) larvivorous.

**lar·vi·po·si·tion** (lahr″vĭ-pə-zish′ən) the act of depositing larvae (living maggots) in the tissues of a host.

**lar·viv·o·rous** (lahr-viv′ə-rəs) [*larva* + L. *vorare* to eat] feeding on or consuming larvae; said especially of fish which ingest mosquito larvae.

**lar·yn·gal·gia** (lar″in-gal′jə) [*laryng-* + *-algia*] pain in the larynx.

**lar·yn·ge·al** (lə-rin′je-əl) of or pertaining to the larynx.

**lar·yn·gec·to·mee** (lar″in-jek′tə-me) a person whose larynx has been removed.

**lar·yn·gec·to·my** (lar″in-jek′tə-me) [*laryng-* + *-ectomy*] [MeSH: Laryngectomy] surgical removal of the larynx.

**la·ryn·ges** (lə-rin′jēz) [L.] plural of *larynx.*

**lar·yn·gis·mus** (lar″in-jiz′məs) [L.; Gr. *laryngismos* a whooping] [MeSH: Laryngismus] laryngospasm.
**l. paraly′ticus**, laryngeal hemiplegia.
**l. stri′dulus**, sudden laryngeal spasm with a crowing inspiration and cyanosis, usually occurring in children at night. Called also *false croup, spasmodic croup, pseudocroup*, and *laryngitis stridulosa.*

**lar·yn·git·ic** (lar″in-jit′ik) pertaining to laryngitis.

**lar·yn·gi·tis** (lar″in-ji′tis) [MeSH: Laryngitis] inflammation of the larynx, usually with dryness and soreness of the throat, hoarseness, cough, and dysphagia.
**croupous l.**, a condition seen mainly in infants or small children and characterized by a resonant barking cough, hoarseness, and stridor. Infection, allergy, a foreign body, or a tumor may be the cause. Laryngeal diphtheria was once a common cause but is now rare.
**diphtheritic l.**, laryngeal diphtheria.
**membranous l.**, laryngitis attended with the formation of a false membrane.
**necrotic l.**, calf diphtheria in the larynx.
**l. stridulo′sa**, laryngismus stridulus.
**subglottic l.**, inflammation of the undersurface of the vocal cords. Called also *chorditis vocalis inferior.*
**syphilitic l.**, a chronic form due to syphilitic involvement of the larynx.
**tuberculous l.**, laryngitis due to tuberculosis of the larynx (q.v.).
**vestibular l.**, viral laryngitis in which edema forms a ring outlining the vestibule of the larynx.

**laryng(o)-** [L. *larynx*, q.v.] a combining form denoting relationship to the larynx.

**la·ryn·go·cele** (lə-ring′go-sēl) [*laryngo-* + *-cele*[2]] congenital anomalous filling of the laryngeal saccule with air, sometimes visible as an enlargement on the outside of the neck. There are *internal* and *external* types and mixtures of the two.
**external l.**, one that penetrates the thyrohyoid membrane and may be visible as a tumorlike enlargement on the neck, becoming larger with increased intralaryngeal pressure, as from coughing.
**internal l.**, one confined within the larynx and not visible on the surface of the neck. Called also *ventricular l.*
**ventricular l., l. ventricula′ris**, internal l.

**la·ryn·go·cen·te·sis** (lə-ring″go-sən-te′sis) [*laryngo-* + *-centesis*] surgical puncture of the larynx.

**la·ryn·go·fis·sure** (lə-ring″go-fish′ər) median laryngotomy.

**la·ryn·go·gram** (lə-ring′go-gram) a radiograph of the larynx.

**lar·yn·gog·ra·phy** (lar″ing-gog′rə-fe) [*laryngo-* + *-graphy*] radiography of the larynx after instillation of a radiopaque substance into it.

**lar·yn·gol·o·gy** (lar″ing-gol′ə-je) [*laryngo-* + *-logy*] that branch of medicine which has to do with the throat, pharynx, larynx, nasopharynx, and tracheobronchial tree.

**la·ryn·go·ma·la·cia** (lə-ring″go-mə-la′shə) [*laryngo-* + *malacia*] flaccidity of the epiglottis and aryepiglottic folds, as in congenital laryngeal stridor.

**lar·yn·gom·e·try** (lar″ing-gom′ə-tre) [*laryngo-* + *-metry*] measurement of the larynx.

**la·ryn·go·pa·ral·y·sis** (lə-ring″go-pə-ral′ə-sis) laryngeal paralysis.

**lar·yn·gop·a·thy** (lar-ing-gop′ə-the) [*laryngo-* + *-pathy*] any disorder of the larynx.

**la·ryn·go·pha·ryn·ge·al** (lə-ring″go-fə-rin′je-əl) pertaining to the larynx and pharynx.

**la·ryn·go·phar·yn·gec·to·my** (lə-ring″go-far″ən-jek′tə-me) excision of the larynx and pharynx.

**la·ryn·go·pha·ryn·ge·us** (lə-ring″go-fə-rin′je-əs) musculus constrictor pharyngis inferior.

**la·ryn·go·phar·yn·gi·tis** (lə-ring″go-far″ən-ji′tis) inflammation of the larynx and pharynx.

**la·ryn·go·phar·ynx** (lə-ring″go-far′ənks) [*laryngo-* + *pharynx*] pars laryngea pharyngis.

**lar·yn·goph·o·ny** (lar″ing-gof′ə-ne) [*laryngo-* + Gr. *phōnē* voice] a voice sound heard over the larynx.

**lar·yn·goph·thi·sis** (lar″ing-gof′thĭ-sis) [*laryngo-* + *phthisis*] laryngeal tuberculosis.

**la·ryn·go·plas·ty** (lə-ring′go-plas″te) [*laryngo-* + *-plasty*] reconstruction of the larynx.

**la·ryn·go·ple·gia** (lə-ring″go-ple′je-ə) [*laryngo-* + *-plegia*] laryngeal paralysis.

**la·ryn·go·pto·sis** (lə-ring″go-to′sis) [*laryngo-* + *ptosis*] a lowering and mobilization of the larynx, occurring either congenitally or as part of the aging process.

**la·ryn·go·pyo·cele** (lə-ring″go-pi′o-sēl) a laryngocele containing pus.

**lar·yn·gor·rha·gia** (lar″ing-go-ra′jə) [*laryngo-* + *-rrhagia*] hemorrhage from the larynx.

**lar·yn·gor·rha·phy** (lar″ing-gor′ə-fe) [*laryngo-* + *-rrhaphy*] the operation of suturing the larynx.

**la·ryn·gor·rhea** (la″ring-go-re′ə) [*laryngo-* + *-rrhea*] excessive secretion of mucus whenever the voice is used.

**la·ryn·go·scle·ro·ma** (lə-ring″go-sklər-o′mə) [*laryngo-* + *scleroma*] scleroma of the larynx.

**la·ryn·go·scope** (lə-ring′gə-skōp) [*laryngo-* + *-scope*] an endoscope for use in direct visual examination of the larynx.

**la·ryn·go·scop·ic** (lə-ring″go-skop′ik) pertaining to laryngoscopy.

**lar·yn·gos·co·pist** (lar″ing-gos′kə-pist) an expert in laryngoscopy.

**lar·yn·gos·co·py** (lar″ing-gos′kə-pe) [*laryngo-* + *-scopy*] [MeSH: Laryngoscopy] examination of the interior of the larynx, especially that performed with the laryngoscope *(direct laryngoscopy).*
**direct l.,** direct visual examination of the interior of the larynx performed with a speculum or with a laryngoscope.
**indirect l.,** examination of the interior of the larynx by observation of the reflection of it in a laryngeal mirror.
**mirror l.,** indirect l.
**suspension l.,** examination of the larynx performed with a direct laryngoscope suspended so as to leave both hands of the examiner free.

**la·ryn·go·spasm** (lə-ring′go-spaz″əm) [*laryngo-* + *spasm*] spasmodic closure of the larynx. Called also *laryngismus* and *glottic spasm.*

**la·ryn·go·stat** (lə-ring′go-stat) an appliance for holding a source of radioactive material within the larynx.

**la·ryn·go·ste·no·sis** (lə-ring″go-stə-no′sis) [*laryngo-* + *stenosis*] [MeSH: Laryngostenosis] narrowing or stricture of the larynx.

**lar·yn·gos·to·my** (lar″in-gos′tə-me) [*laryngo-* + *-stomy*] surgical creation of an artificial opening into the larynx.

**la·ryn·go·stro·bo·scope** (lə-ring″go-stro′bo-skōp″) [*laryngo-* + *stroboscope*] an apparatus for observing the intralaryngeal phenomena with a stroboscopic light.

**la·ryn·go·tome** (lə-ring′go-tōm) an instrument used in incising the larynx.

**lar·yn·got·o·my** (lar″ing-got′ə-me) [*laryngo-* + *-tomy*] surgical incision of the larynx.
**inferior l.,** cricothyrotomy.
**median l.,** incision of the larynx through the thyroid cartilage; called also *laryngofissure, thyrofissure,* and *thyrotomy.*
**subhyoid l., superior l.,** incision of the larynx through the thyrohyoid membrane; called also *thyrohyoid l.*
**thyrohyoid l.,** subhyoid l.

**la·ryn·go·tra·che·al** (lə-ring″go-tra′ke-əl) pertaining to the larynx and trachea.

**la·ryn·go·tra·che·itis** (lə-ring″go-tra″ke-i′tis) inflammation of the larynx and trachea.
**avian l., infectious avian l., infectious l. (ILT),** a viral disease of poultry caused by a herpesvirus and characterized by respiratory distress, an exudate or bleeding, and often death.

**la·ryn·go·tra·cheo·bron·chi·tis** (lə-ring″go-tra″ke-o-brong-ki′tis) inflammation of the larynx, trachea, and bronchi; an acute form is the most common cause of croup.

**la·ryn·go·tra·cheo·bron·chos·co·py** (lə-ring″go-tra″ke-o-brong-kos′kə-pe) endoscopic examination of the larynx, trachea, and bronchi.

**la·ryn·go·tra·che·os·co·py** (lə-ring″go-tra″ke-os′kə-pe) peroral laryngoscopy and tracheoscopy.

**la·ryn·go·tra·che·ot·o·my** (lə-ring″go-tra″ke-ot′o-me) [*laryngo-* + *tracheotomy*] incision of the larynx and trachea.

**lar·ynx** (lar′inks) gen. *laryn′gis,* pl. *laryn′ges* [L., from Gr.] [TA] [MeSH: Larynx] the musculocartilaginous structure, lined with mucous membrane, connected to the superior part of the trachea and to the pharynx inferior to the tongue and the hyoid bone; the essential sphincter guarding the entrance into the trachea and functioning secondarily as the organ of voice. It is formed by nine cartilages connected by ligaments and eight muscles.
**artificial l.,** an electromechanical device that enables a laryngectomized person to speak. When it is placed against the region of the laryngectomy a buzzing sound is produced, which is converted into simulated speech by movements of the organs of articulation (lips, tongue, glottis).

**la·sal·o·cid** (lə-sal′o-sid) [MeSH: Lasalocid] an antibiotic produced by *Streptomyces lasaliensis;* used as a coccidiostat in poultry.

**La·san** (la′san) trademark for a preparation of anthralin.

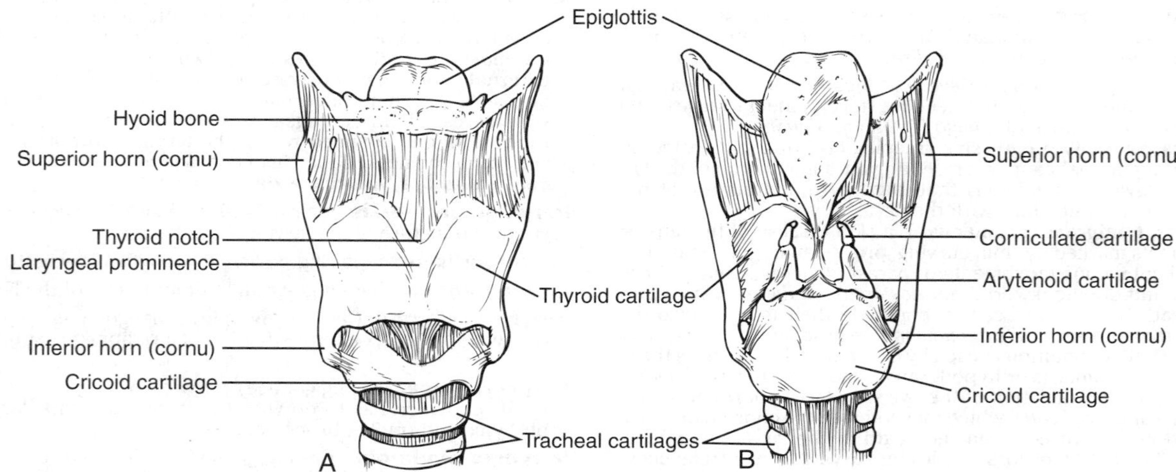


Anterior *(A)* and posterior *(B)* views of the larynx, showing the thyroid, epiglottic, cricoid, arytenoid, and corniculate cartilages. The cuneiform cartilages, not shown here, lie one on each side, in the aryepiglottic fold, anterosuperior to the corniculate cartilages.

**La·sègue's sign** (lah-segz′) [Ernest Charles *Lasègue,* French physician, 1816–1883] see under *sign.*

**la·ser** (la′zər) [*l*ight *a*mplification by *s*timulated *e*mission of *r*adiation] a device which transforms light of various frequencies into an extremely intense, small, and nearly nondivergent beam of monochromatic radiation in the visible region with all the waves in phase. Capable of mobilizing immense heat and power when focused at close range, it is used as a tool in surgical procedures, in diagnosis, and in physiologic studies.
**argon l.,** a laser with ionized argon as the active medium whose beam is in the blue and green visible light spectrum, with two energy peaks, at 488 and 514 nm; used for photocoagulation.
**carbon-dioxide l.,** a laser with carbon dioxide gas as the active medium that produces infrared radiation at 10,600 nm; used to excise and incise tissue and to vaporize.
**dye l.,** a laser with organic dye dissolved in a solvent as the active medium whose beam is in the visible light spectrum; used in photodynamic therapy.
**excimer l.,** [*exci*ted di*mer*], a laser with rare gas halides as the active medium whose beam is in the ultraviolet spectrum and penetrates tissues only a small distance; the beam breaks chemical bonds instead of generating heat to destroy tissue. Used in ophthalmological procedures and laser angioplasty.
**helium-neon l.,** a laser with a mixture of ionized helium and neon gases as the active medium whose beam is in the red visible light spectrum at 633 nm; used as a guiding beam for lasers operating at nonvisible wavelengths.
**holmium:YAG l.,** a laser whose active medium is a crystal of yttrium, aluminum, and garnet doped with holmium ions, and whose beam is in the near infrared spectrum at 2100 nm; used for photocoagulation and photoablation.
**ion l.,** a laser that uses one of the inert gases (argon, helium, neon, or krypton) as the active medium.
**krypton l.,** a laser with krypton ionized by electric current as the active medium whose beam is in the yellow-red visible light spectrum; used for photocoagulation.
**KTP l.,** a laser in which a beam generated from a neodymium:YAG crystal is directed through a potassium titanyl phosphate crystal to produce a beam in the green visible spectrum at 532 nm; its properties are similar to those of the argon laser and it is used for photoablation and photocoagulation.
**neodymium:yttrium-aluminum-garnet (Nd:YAG) l.,** a laser whose active medium is a crystal of yttrium, aluminum, and garnet doped with neodymium ions, and whose beam is in the near infrared spectrum at 1060 nm; used for photocoagulation and photoablation.
**potassium titanyl phosphate l.,** KTP l.
**pulsed dye l.,** a dye laser in which excitation of the dye by pulses of intense light from a flashlamp produces a beam in the yellow visible light spectrum with a wavelength of 577 or 585 nm, with alternating on and off phases of a few microseconds each; used to decolorize pigmented lesions.
**tunable dye l.,** a dye laser whose active medium can be altered so that the beam has any of several wavelengths.

**LASIK** laser-assisted in-situ keratomileusis.

**Las·io·he·lea** (las″e-o-he′le-ə) a genus of blood-sucking flies of the family Heleidae.

**La·six** (la′siks) trademark for preparations of furosemide.

**Lassa fever, virus** (lah′sə) [*Lassa,* town in Nigeria where the fever was first reported in 1959] see under *fever* and *virus.*

**Las·sar's paste, betanaphthol paste, plain zinc paste** (lahs′ərz) [Oskar *Lassar,* German dermatologist, 1849–1908] see under *paste.*

**las·si·tude** (las′i-to͞od) [L. *lassitudo* weariness] weakness; exhaustion.

**la·tah** (lah′tah) a culture-specific type of jumping disease seen chiefly among the Malays and other people of Southeast Asia, characterized by hypersuggestibility, echolalia, echopraxis, coprolalia, disorganization, and automatic obedience. It may be identical to myriachit.

**la·tan·o·prost** (lə-tan′o-prost″) an antiglaucoma agent applied topically to the conjunctiva in the treatment of open-angle glaucoma and ocular hypertension.

**Lat·ar·jet's nerve** (lah-tahr-zhāz′) [André *Latarjet,* French anatomist, 1877–1947] see under *nerve.*

**Lat. dol.** abbreviation for L. *lat′eri dolen′ti,* to the painful side.

**lat·e·bra** (lat′ə-brə) [L. "hiding place"] a flask-shaped mass of white yolk extending from the blastodisc to the center of eggs such as those of birds.

**la·ten·cy** (la′tən-se) 1. a state of seeming inactivity or being latent. 2. the time between the instant of stimulation and the beginning of a response; called also *latent period* and *conduction time.* 3. see under *stage.*
**l. of activation,** the time between initiation of an electrical stimulus and depolarization of a nerve fiber to begin conduction along the axon; called also *utilization time.*
**distal l.,** the motor or sensory latency measured from a site of stimulation as near as possible to the recording electrodes, i.e., to the terminal end of the nerve. Called also *terminal l.*
**motor l.,** the time between initiation of a stimulus and onset of a resultant compound muscle action potential; see also *distal l., proximal l.,* and *residual l.*
**proximal l.,** the motor or sensory latency measured from a site of stimulation as far as possible from the recording electrodes, i.e., from the terminal end of the nerve.
**REM l.,** a 70- to 100-minute period of NREM sleep that precedes the first period of REM sleep.
**residual l.,** the time difference between the observed distal latency of a motor nerve and the distal latency that was predicted based on conduction velocity measured in a segment of nerve near the stimulating electrode; it is due to factors slowing conduction such as decreased diameter of fine terminal axon branches, synaptic delay at the neuromuscular junction, and presence of unmyelinated segments.
**sensory l.,** the time between initiation of a stimulus and onset of a resultant compound sensory nerve action potential; see also *distal l.* and *proximal l.*
**sleep l.,** the period between the time a person lies down to rest and the onset of sleep.
**terminal l.,** distal l.

**la·tent** (la′tənt) [L. *latens* hidden] concealed; not manifest; potential; dormant; quiescent.

**la·ten·ti·a·tion** (la-ten″she-a′shən) the process of making latent; in pharmacology, the chemical modification of a biologically active compound to affect its absorption, distribution, etc., the modified compound being transformed after administration to the active compound by biological processes.

**lat·er·ad** (lat′ər-ad) toward a side or a lateral aspect.

**lat·er·al** (lat′ər-əl) [L. *lateralis*] 1. denoting a position farther from the median plane or midline of the body or of a structure. 2. pertaining to a side.

**lat·er·a·lis** (lat″ər-a′lis) [TA] lateral: a term denoting a structure situated farther from the median plane of the body.

**lat·er·al·i·ty** (lat″ər-al′ĭ-te) [MeSH: Laterality] a relationship to one side; see also *cerebral dominance* and *lateral dominance,* under *dominance.*
**crossed l.,** the preferential use, in voluntary motor acts, of contra-

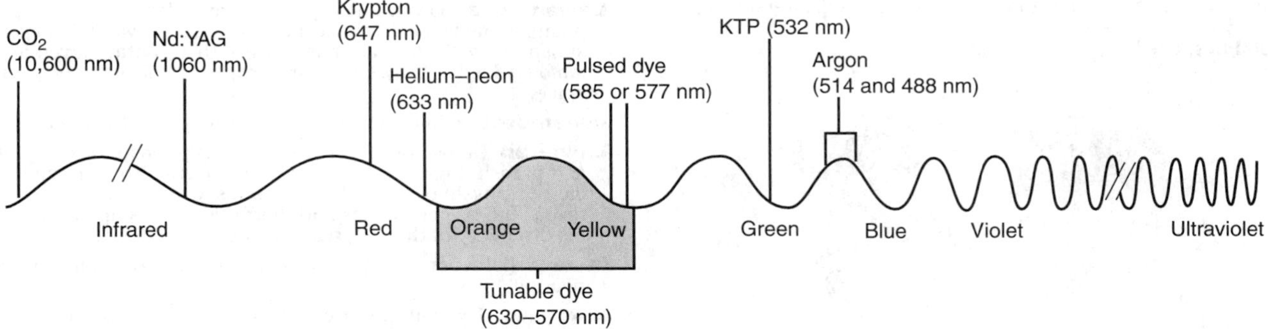

Relative positions of various types of lasers on the electromagnetic spectrum.

lateral members of the different pairs of organs, as the right eye and the left hand.
**dominant l.**, lateral dominance.

**lat·er·i·ceous** (lat″ər-ĭ′shəs) lateritious.

**lat·er·i·tious** (lat″ər-ĭ′shəs) [L. *lateritius; later* brick] resembling brick dust.

**latero-** [L. *latus,* gen. *lateris* side] a combining form denoting relationship to the side.

**lat·ero·ab·do·mi·nal** (lat″ər-o-ab-dom′ĭ-nəl) pertaining to the side of the abdomen.

**lat·ero·de·vi·a·tion** (lat″ər-o-de″ve-a′shən) deviation or slight displacement to one side.

**lat·ero·duc·tion** (lat″ər-o-duk′shən) [*latero-* + *duction*] movement of an eye to one side.

**lat·ero·flex·ion** (lat″ər-o-flek′shən) flexion to either side.

**lat·ero·po·si·tion** (lat″ər-o-pə-zish′ən) displacement to one side.

**lat·ero·pul·sion** (lat″ər-o-pul′shən) [*latero-* + *pulsion*] an involuntary tendency to go to one side while walking.

**lat·ero·tor·sion** (lat″ər-o-tor′shən) [*latero-* + *torsion*] turning the eyeball to the left or right on its anteroposterior axis.

**lat·ero·ver·sion** (lat″ər-o-vər′zhən) [*latero-* + *version*] a turning to one side, as of the uterus.

**la·tex** (la′teks) [L. "fluid"] [MeSH: Latex] 1. any of various white viscid fluids secreted by certain plants; the variety from rubber trees was formerly the main source of commercial rubber. 2. any of several synthetic fluids resembling natural latex, including polystyrene and polyvinyl chloride; see also *latex agglutination test* under *tests.* Allergic reactions to latex are an important cause of type IV hypersensitivity reactions.

**La·tham's circle** (la′thəmz) [Peter Mere *Latham,* English physician, 1789–1875] see under *circle.*

**lath·y·rism** (lath′ə-riz-əm) [MeSH: Lathyrism] a morbid condition seen in humans and other animals after excessive ingestion of seeds of the genus *Lathyrus,* which contain β-aminopropionitrile, an inhibitor of the enzyme lysyl oxidase. The disease is characterized by spastic paraplegia, pain, hyperesthesia, and paresthesia. Cf. *lupinosis* and *osteolathyrism.*

**lath·y·rit·ic** (lath″ə-rit′ik) pertaining to or characterized by lathyrism.

**lath·y·ro·gen** (lath′ə-ro-jən) any agent that causes lathyrism.

**lath·y·ro·gen·ic** (lath″ə-ro-jen′ik) capable of producing the symptoms characteristic of lathyrism.

**Lath·y·rus** (lath′ə-rəs) [Gr. *lathyros* chickling vetch] a genus of plants of the family Leguminosae. It includes varieties of peas consumed by humans and herbs used as forage for livestock; excessive consumption of some species causes lathyrism.

**la·tis·si·mus** (lə-tis′ĭ-məs) 1. widest. 2. widest: a general term denoting a broad structure, as a muscle.

**lat·ro·dec·tism** (lat″ro-dek′tiz-əm) [*Latrodectus* + *-ism*] intoxication caused by venom of spiders of the genus *Latrodectus.*

**Lat·ro·dec·tus** (lat″ro-dek′təs) [L. *latro* robber + Gr. *daknein* to bite] a genus of poisonous spiders. *L. mac′tans* is the black widow spider of the United States; *L. bisho′pi* is found in southern Florida; *L. curarien′sis* in Brazil and Argentina; *L. geomet′ricus* in California and southern Florida; *L. hassel′tii* in New Zealand; *L. lugu′bris* is the kara-kurt of Russia; *L. macula′tus* is found in South Africa; *L. malmigniat′tus* in Europe; and *L. tredecimgutta′tus* in southern Europe and Asiatic Russia.

**LATS** long-acting thyroid stimulator.

**LATS-p** LATS protector.

**lat·tice** (lat′is) 1. a framework of regularly placed, intersecting narrow strips. 2. space l.
**crystal l.**, space l.

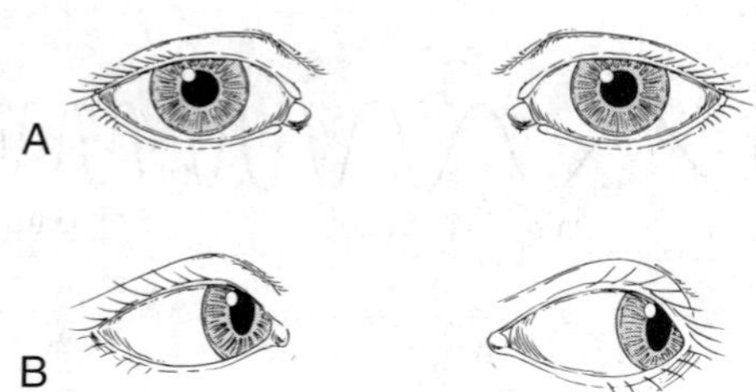

Forward gaze *(A)* contrasted with laterotorsion *(B).*

**space l.**, the regular, three-dimensional geometrical arrangement of atoms in a crystal; called also *lattice* and *crystal l.*

**la·tus**[1] (la′təs) [L.] broad, wide.

**la·tus**[2] (la′təs) pl. *la′tera* [L.] [TA] flank: the side of the body between the ribs and the pelvis. Called also *regio lateralis* [TA alternative].

**Latz·ko's cesarean section** (lahts′kōz) [Wilhelm *Latzko,* Austrian obstetrician, 1863–1945] see *cesarean section,* under *section.*

**Lau·ber's disease** (lou′bərz) [Hans *Lauber,* Swiss-born ophthalmologist in Austria, born 1876] fundus albipunctatus; see under *fundus.*

**laud·a·ble** (lawd′ə-bəl) [L. *laudabilis*] commendable; healthy; see under *pus.*

**lau·da·num** (law′də-nəm) opium tincture.

**laugh** (laf) 1. an act or paroxysm of laughter. 2. to indulge in laughter.
**canine l., sardonic l.**, risus sardonicus.

**laugh·ter** (laf′tər) [MeSH: Laughter] a series of spasmodic and partly involuntary expirations with inarticulate vocalization, normally indicative of merriment; it may also be a hysteric manifestation or a reflex result of tickling. See also *gelasmus* and *risus.*

**Lau·gier's hernia, sign** (lo″zhe-āz′) [Stanislas *Laugier,* French surgeon, 1799–1872] see under *hernia* and *sign.*

**Lau·mo·nier's ganglion** (lo-mon″e-āz′) [Jean Baptiste Philippe Nicolas René *Laumonier,* French surgeon, 1749–1818] carotid ganglion.

**Lau·nois syndrome** (lo-nwah′) [Pierre-Emile *Launois,* French physician, 1856–1914] see under *syndrome.*

**lau·rate** (law′rāt) a salt, ester, or anionic form of lauric acid.

**Lau·rence-Moon syndrome** (law′rəns-mo͞on) [John Zachariah *Laurence,* British ophthalmologist, 1830–1874; Robert C. *Moon,* American ophthalmologist, 1844–1914] see under *syndrome.*

**lau·reth 9** (law′rəth) a spermicide and surfactant consisting of a mixture of polyethylene glycol monododecyl ethers averaging about 9 ethylene oxide groups per molecule; it has also been used as a sclerosing agent in treatment of varicose veins. Called also *polidocanol.*

**lau·ric ac·id** (law′rik) a twelve-carbon saturated fatty acid occurring in many vegetable fats, particularly in coconut and palm kernel oils. See also table accompanying *fatty acid.*

**Lauth's canal, sinus** (lōts) [Ernst Alexander *Lauth,* French physiologist, 1803–1837] sinus venosus sclerae.

**Lauth's ligament** (lōts) [Thomas *Lauth,* French anatomist and surgeon, 1758–1826] ligamentum transversum atlantis.

**Lauth's violet** (lawths) [Charles *Lauth,* English chemist, 1836–1913] thionin.

**LAV** lymphadenopathy-associated virus; see *human immunodeficiency virus,* under *virus.*

**la·vage** (lah-vahzh′) [Fr.] 1. the irrigation or washing out of an organ, such as the stomach or bowel. 2. to wash out, or irrigate.
**bronchoalveolar l.**, a technique by which cells and fluid from bronchioles and lung alveoli are removed for diagnosis of disease or evaluation of treatment; a bronchoscope is wedged into a bronchus and sterile saline is pumped in and then removed along with the fluid and cells to be analyzed.
**peritoneal l.**, dialysis by instillation into the peritoneal cavity and subsequent withdrawal of dialysis fluid, for the removal of elements not being excreted by the kidneys.
**pleural l.**, irrigation of the pleural cavity to assess for presence of malignant or otherwise abnormal cells.

**La·van·du·la** (lə-van′du-lə) [L.] the lavenders, a genus of Eurasian plants of the family Labiatae, having spicate flowers. *L. angustifo′lia,* subsp. *angustifo′lia* Mill. has flowers that contain lavender oil. *L. latifo′lia* Medic. grows wild in Europe and is the source of oil of spike.

**lav·en·der** (lav′ən-dər) any plant of the genus *Lavandula.*

**La·ve·ran** (lah-vĕ-rah′) Charles Louis Alphonse. French physician and parasitologist, 1845–1922; winner of the Nobel prize for medicine or physiology in 1907 for his discoveries of hematozoa, protozoa, and trypanosomes and their role in causing disease, and for his discovery of the malarial parasite *Plasmodium.*

**la·veur** (lah-voor′) [Fr.] an instrument for performing lavage or irrigation.

**law** (law) 1. a uniform or constant fact or principle. Cf. *rule.* 2. in statistics, a synonym for *distribution;* for entries not found here, see under *distribution.*

**Allen's paradoxic l.**, whereas in normal individuals the more sugar is given the more is utilized, the reverse is true in diabetics.
**all-or-none l.**, see *all or none.*
**Ångström's l.**, the wavelengths of the light absorbed by a substance are the same as those given off by it when luminous.
**Aran's l.**, fractures of the base of the skull (except those by contrecoup) result from injuries to the vault, the fractures extending by radiation along the line of shortest circle.
**Arndt's l., Arndt-Schulz l.**, weak stimuli increase physiologic activity and very strong stimuli inhibit or abolish activity.
**l's of articulation,** a set of rules to be followed in arranging teeth to produce a balanced articulation.
**Avogadro's l.**, equal volumes of all perfect gases at the same temperature and pressure contain the same number of molecules or, in the case of monatomic gases, of atoms.
**Baer's l.**, those more general features that are common to all the members of a group of animals are developed in the embryo earlier than the more special features that distinguish the various members of the group. This concept is the predecessor of the recapitulation theory.
**Barfurth's l.**, the axis of the tissue in a regenerating structure is at first perpendicular to the cut.
**Bastian's l., Bastian-Bruns l.**, if there is a complete transverse lesion in the spinal cord cephalad to the lumbar enlargement, the tendon reflexes of the lower extremities are abolished.
**Beer's l., Beer-Lambert l.**, the absorbance *(A)* of a solution is directly proportional to the length of the light path *(b)* and the concentration *(c)*; the proportionality constant is the molar absorptivity $(\epsilon)$ thus $A = \epsilon bc$. The absorptivity is independent of the concentration and is thus a property of the solute and solvent. Beer's law generally holds only up to a certain concentration, above which the relation between concentration and absorbance becomes nonlinear.
**Behring's l.**, the blood and serum of an immunized person, when transferred to another subject, will render the latter immune.
**Bergonié-Tribondeau l.**, the sensitivity of cells to radiation varies directly with the reproductive capacity of the cells and inversely with their degree of differentiation.
**biogenetic l.**, recapitulation theory.
**Bowditch's l.**, all-or-none l.; see *all-or-none.*
**Boyle's l.**, at a constant temperature the volume of a perfect gas varies inversely as the pressure, and the pressure varies inversely as the volume.
**Bunsen-Roscoe l.**, the photochemical effect produced is equal to the product of the intensity of the illumination and the duration of exposure.
**Camerer's l.**, children of the same weight have the same food requirements regardless of their ages.
**Charles' l.**, at a constant pressure the volume of a given mass of perfect gas varies directly with the absolute temperature.
**l. of conservation of energy,** in any given system the amount of energy is constant; energy is neither created nor destroyed, but only transformed from one form to another.
**l. of conservation of mass,** mass (or matter) can be neither created nor destroyed; this law can be violated on the microscopic level.
**Cope's l.**, genera with little specialization originate many types of organisms; highly specialized genera produce but few biological variations.
**Coulomb's l.**, the force of attraction or repulsion between two electrified bodies is proportional directly to the quantities of electric charge, and inversely as the square of their distance apart.
**Courvoisier's l.**, when the common bile duct is obstructed by a stone, dilatation of the gallbladder is rare; when the duct is obstructed in some other way, dilatation is common.
**Coutard's l.**, in radiotherapy, the point of origin of a mucous membrane tumor is the last site to heal following irradiation.
**Curie's l.**, all substances may be rendered radioactive by the influence of the emanations of radium, and substances thus influenced hold their radioactivity longer when enclosed in some material through which the emanations cannot pass.
**Dalton's l.**, the pressure exerted by a mixture of nonreacting gases is equal to the sum of the partial pressures of the separate components; it holds true only at very low pressures.
**Dalton-Henry l.**, when a fluid absorbs a mixture of gases, it will absorb as much of each gas as it would have absorbed if the gas were present alone.
**l. of definite proportions,** any compound always contains the same kind of elements in the same proportions; called also *Proust's l.*
**Descartes' l.**, the sine of the angle of incidence bears a constant relation to the sine of the angle of refraction for two given media. Called also *l. of sines* and *Snell's l.*
**Desmarres' l.**, when the visual axes are crossed the images are uncrossed; when the axes are uncrossed (diverging) the images are crossed. Useful in determining presence of esophoria and exophoria, and esotropia and exotropia. See also *direct* and *crossed diplopia.*
**Dollo's l.**, phyletic development is irreversible, i.e., reversion to an ancestral peculiarity (atavism) is impossible.
**Donders' l.**, the rotation of the eye around the line of sight is not voluntary; when attention is fixed upon a remote object, the amount of rotation is determined entirely by the angular distance of the object from the median plane and from the horizon.
**Draper's l.**, only the rays that are absorbed by a photochemical substance will produce a chemical change in it.
**Dulong and Petit's l.**, the atomic heat capacity, the product of the atomic weight and the specific heat per gram, is constant for most elements; boron, carbon, and silicon are notable exceptions at normal temperatures.
**Einthoven's l.**, if electrocardiograms are taken simultaneously with the three leads, at any given instant the potential in lead II is equal to the sum of the potentials in leads I and III.
**Ewald's l.**, vestibular nystagmus resulting from endolymph currents in a semicircular canal is in a direction parallel with the plane of that canal and opposite to the current; vestibular nystagmus caused by currents in horizontal canals is primarily from canals whose hair cells are bent towards the utricle.
**Fajans' l.**, the product left after the emission of alpha rays has a valence less by two than that of the parent radioactive substance; the product left after the emission of beta rays has a valence greater by one than that of the parent radioactive substance.
**Faraday's l.**, 1. the amount of a chemical reaction produced by an electric current passed through a cell is proportional to the amount of charge passed. 2. the extent of dissolution or decomposition of electrolytes produced by the same electric current is proportional to their equivalent weights.
**Farr's l.**, "subsidence is a property of all zymotic diseases": the curve that represents the incidence of new cases in an epidemic ascends rapidly at first, then gradually levels off to a maximum, and finally descends more rapidly than it ascended, thus approximating a bell-shaped curve.
**l. of fatigue (Houghton's),** when the same muscle or group of muscles is kept in constant action until fatigue sets in, the total work done, multiplied by the rate of work, is constant.
**Ferry-Porter l.**, critical fusion frequency is directly proportional to the logarithm of the light intensity.
**Fick's first l. of diffusion,** a substance will diffuse through an area at a rate which is dependent upon the difference in concentration of the substance at two given points.
**first l. of thermodynamics,** see *l's of thermodynamics.*
**Flatau's l.**, the greater the length of the fibers of the spinal cord, the closer are they situated to the periphery.
**Flint's l.**, the ontogeny of an organ is the phylogeny of its blood supply.
**Flourens' l.**, stimulation of the semicircular canal causes nystagmus in the plane of that canal.
**Frank-Starling l.**, Starling's l.
**Froriep's l.**, the skull is developed by the annexation of true vertebrae, the head growing at the expense of the neck.
**Galton's l.**, each parent contributes, on an average, one half, or (0.5), of an individual's heritage, each grandparent one fourth, or $(0.5)^2$, each greatgrandparent one eighth, or $(0.5)^3$, etc.
**Galton's l. of regression,** average parents tend to produce average children, but the offspring of extreme parents inherit the parental peculiarities in a less marked degree than the latter were manifested in the parents themselves.
**gas l.**, ideal gas l.
**Gay-Lussac's l.**, 1. a modification of Charles' law, adding that, at constant temperature and pressure, the ratio of the volumes of two gases that react with each other is always a small whole number. 2. sometimes used synonymously with *Charles' l.*
**Gerhardt-Semon l.**, various peripheral and central lesions affecting the recurrent laryngeal nerve cause the vocal cord to assume a position between abduction and adduction, the paralysis of the parts being incomplete.
**Giraud-Teulon l.**, binocular retinal images are formed at the intersection of the primary and secondary axes of projection.
**Godélier's l.**, tuberculosis of the peritoneum is invariably associated with tuberculosis of the pleura.
**Golgi's l.**, the severity of a malarial attack depends upon the number of parasites in the blood.
**Gompertz's l.**, at advanced ages the risk of dying increases geometrically with age: the death rate at age *x* may be computed by the formula $q_x = q_0 \cdot e \cdot a^x$, where $q_x$ is the death rate at age *x*, $q_0$ is the death rate at age 0, and *a* is a constant. From middle age on, actual death rates closely approximate the curve that corresponds to this formula.
**Goodell's l.**, see under *sign.*
**Graham's l.**, the rate of diffusion of a gas through porous membranes is in inverse ratio to the square root of their density.
**l. of gravitation,** all bodies attract each other with a force that is

directly proportional to their masses and inversely proportional to the square of their distance apart; called also *Newton's l.*

**Grotthus' l., Grotthus-Draper l.,** only those rays of ultraviolet light that are absorbed produce a chemical effect upon the absorbing substance.

**Gudden's l.,** the degeneration of the proximal end of a divided nerve is cellulipetal.

**Guldberg and Waage's l.,** l. of mass action.

**Gull-Toynbee l.,** in otitis media, the lateral sinus and cerebellum are liable to involvement in mastoid disease, and the cerebrum may be attacked when the roof of the tympanum becomes carious. Called also *Toynbee's d.*

**Gullstrand's l.,** in strabismus, if the patient is made to turn his head while fixing a distant object and the corneal reflex of either eye moves in the direction in which the head is turning, then the movement is toward the weaker muscle.

**Haeckel's l.,** recapitulation theory.

**Hanau's l's of articulation,** a set of purely physical laws that must be observed in the formation of the masticatory surfaces of natural dentition or dentures, to assure establishment or production of balanced articulation.

**Hardy-Weinberg l.,** the proportions of the three genotypes determined by two alleles *(A* and *a)* occurring with a frequency of $p$ and $q$, respectively, in a randomly mating population will remain constant from one generation to the next: $AA = p^2$, $Aa = 2pq$, $aa = q^2$. Mutation, selection, non-random mating, migration, and genetic drift can disturb this equilibrium.

**l. of the heart,** Starling's l. of the heart.

**Heidenhain's l.,** glandular secretion always involves change in the structure of the gland.

**Hellin's l., Hellin-Zeleny l.,** one in about 89 pregnancies ends in the birth of twins; one in 89 × 89, or 7921, of triplets; one in 89 × 89 × 89, or 704,969, of quadruplets.

**Henry's l.,** the solubility of a gas in a liquid solution at constant temperature is proportional to the partial pressure of the gas above the solution.

**Hering's l.,** 1. the principle of bilateral ocular innervation; equal innervation is sent to the muscles of the two eyes so that one eye is never moved independently of the other. 2. the clearness or purity of any sensation depends on the proportion between its intensity and the total of the intensities of all the simultaneous sensations.

**Hoff's l.,** van't Hoff's l.

**Horner's l.,** ordinary color blindness is transmitted from males to males through normal females.

**ideal gas l.,** the equation of state for an ideal gas: $PV = nRT$, where $P$ is pressure, $V$ volume, $n$ the number of moles of gas, $R$ the gas constant, and $T$ the absolute temperature. It holds approximately for real gases at low pressures and high temperatures.

**l. of independent assortment,** see *Mendel's l's.*

**inverse square l.,** the intensity of radiation is inversely proportional to the square of the distance between a point source and the irradiated surface.

**isodynamic l.,** in the production of heat in the body the different foodstuffs are interchangeable in accordance with their heat-producing values.

**Jackson's l.,** the nerve functions that are latest developed are the first to be lost when the brain is damaged by disease; called also *Jackson's rule.*

**Kahler's l.,** the ascending branches of the posterior roots of the spinal nerves pass within the cord in succession from the root zone toward the mesial plane.

**Knapp's l.,** there should be no difference in retinal image size in the correction of spherical axial anisometropia, provided that the lenses are placed at the anterior focal point of the eye.

**Koch's l.,** see *Koch's postulates,* under *postulate.*

**Küstner's l.,** if an ovarian tumor is left-sided, torsion of its pedicle takes place toward the right; if right-sided, toward the left.

**Lambert's cosine l.,** the intensity of radiation on an absorbing surface varies as the cosine of the angle of incidence for parallel rays.

**Laplace's l.,** tension or stress on the cardiac ventricular walls is proportional to the intraventricular pressure and internal radius and inversely proportional to the wall thickness; for a sphere it is most simply expressed as: average circumferential wall stress = (pressure × radius of curvature of the wall) ÷ (2 × wall thickness); more complex equations describe ellipsoidal or other shapes.

**l. of large numbers,** any of several theorems dealing with the convergence of the sample average to the population mean as the sample size is increased.

**Listing's l.,** when the eyeball is moved from a resting position, the rotational angle in the second position is the same as if the eye were turned about a fixed axis perpendicular to the previous and new positions of the visual line (axis opticus; see under *axis*).

**Lossen's l.,** see under *rule.*

**Louis' l.,** 1. pulmonary tuberculosis generally begins in the left lung. 2. tuberculosis of any part is attended by localization in the lungs.

**malthusian l.,** the hypothesis that population tends to outrun the means available to sustain it.

**Marey's l.,** as the blood pressure rises, the pulse rate slows. See also *baroreceptor.*

**Mariotte's l.,** Boyle's l.

**mass l., l. of mass action,** the rate of a chemical reaction at constant temperature is proportional to the concentrations of the reacting substances; called also *Guldberg and Waage's l.*

**Maxwell-Boltzmann distribution l.,** a method for calculating the relative number of molecules in a given population which possess a given amount of velocity or energy.

**Mendel's l's,** the laws of inheritance of single-gene traits that form the basis of the science of genetics, first described by Gregor Mendel in 1865. From experimental crosses of pea plants differing in one or more characteristics determined by single genes, and counting the types of progeny in successive generations, Mendel derived two laws now usually expressed as the *law of segregation* (the members of a pair of allelic genes segregate from one another and pass to different gametes) and the *law of independent assortment* (genes that are not alleles are distributed to the gametes independently of one another).

**Mendeleev's (Mendeléef's, Mendeléeff's) l.,** periodic l.

**mendelian l's,** Mendel's l's.

**Meyer's l.,** the internal structure of fully developed normal bone represents the lines of greatest pressure or traction and affords the greatest possible resistance with the least possible amount of material.

**Minot's l.,** organisms age fastest when young.

**Müller-Haeckel l.,** recapitulation theory.

**l. of multiple proportions,** when two elements combine to form two or more different compounds, the weights of one compound that can combine with a given weight of the second compound form small whole number ratios.

**l. of multiple variants,** any variation from the normal in the bones of the hand or foot is always multiple.

**Nernst's l.,** the current required to stimulate muscle action varies as the square root of its frequency.

**Neumann's l.,** the molecular heat in compounds of analogous constitution is always the same.

**Newland's l.,** a forerunner of the periodic law, in which the chemical elements, arranged in order of their atomic weights, showed a repetition of properties in octaves.

**Newton's l.,** l. of gravitation.

**Nysten's l.,** rigor mortis affects first the muscles of mastication, next those of the face and neck, then those of the upper trunk and arms, and last of all those of the legs and feet.

**Ohm's l.,** the strength of an electric current varies directly as the electromotive force, and inversely as the resistance.

**Ollier's l.,** in the case of two parallel bones which are joined at their extremities by ligaments, arrest of growth in one of them involves growth disturbance in the other.

**Pajot's l.,** a solid body contained within another body having smooth walls will tend to conform to the shape of those walls; this law governs the rotating movements of the fetus during labor.

**Pascal's l.,** pressure applied to a liquid at any point is transmitted equally in all directions.

**periodic l.,** if the elements are arranged in the sequence of their atomic numbers, they fall into distinctive periods of 2, 8, 8, 18, 18, and 32 elements; see also *periodic table,* under *table.* Called also *Mendeleev's l.*

**Petit's l.,** Dulong and Petit's l.

**Pitres' l.,** in acquired aphasia with a multilingual patient, recovery comes first and most completely in the language most used just before the injury, whether or not it is the patient's mother tongue. See also *Ribot's l.* Called also *Pitres' rule.*

**Poiseuille's l.,** an equation describing the volume flow rate *(F)* of a liquid through a capillary tube:

$$F = \frac{P\pi R^4}{8\eta L},$$

where $P$ is the pressure drop along the tube, $R$ is the radius and $L$ the length of the tube, and $\eta$ is the viscosity of the fluid.

**Prévost's l.,** in a lateral cerebral lesion the head is turned toward the side involved.

**Proust's l.,** l. of definite proportions.

**Raoult's l.,** the partial pressure of a volatile component of an ideal solution is equal to the mole fraction of that substance in solution times its vapor pressure in the pure state at the temperature of the solution; it is true only for ideal solutions and ideal gases.

**l. of reciprocal innervation,** Sherrington's l. (def. 2).

**l. of reciprocal proportions,** two chemical elements that unite with a third element do so in proportions that are multiples of those in which they unite with each other.

**l. of referred pain,** referred pain only arises from irritation of nerves which are sensitive to those stimuli that produce pain when applied to the surface of the body.

**l. of refraction,** rays of light passing from a rarer to a denser medium are deflected toward a perpendicular to the surface of incidence, whereas rays passing from a denser to a rarer medium are deflected away from the perpendicular. Cf. *Descartes' l.*

**l. of regression,** Galton's l. of regression.

**Ribot's l.,** a law stating that in a multilingual patient with aphasia, recovery comes first in the person's mother tongue. This has been found to be true only in patients who are not truly fluent in the subsequently acquired language or languages. See also *Pitres' l.*

**Ricco's l.,** the relation between intensity and area of illumination: intensity times area equals constant.

**Rosa's l.,** the possibilities of phyletic variation in an organism decrease in proportion to the extent of its development.

**Rubner's l.,** 1. *(law of constant energy consumption)* the rapidity of growth is proportional to the intensity of the metabolic process. 2. *(law of constant growth quotient)* the same fractional part of the entire energy is utilized for growth; this fractional part is called the *growth quotient.*

**Schroeder van der Kolk's l.,** the sensory fibers of a mixed nerve are distributed to the parts moved by muscles which are stimulated by the motor fibers of the same nerve.

**second l. of thermodynamics,** see *l's of thermodynamics.*

**l. of segregation,** see *Mendel's l's.*

**Sherrington's l.,** 1. every posterior spinal nerve root supplies a special region of the skin, although fibers from adjacent spinal segments may invade such a region. 2. when a muscle receives a nerve impulse to contract, its antagonist receives simultaneously an impulse to relax; see *reciprocal innervation,* under *innervation.*

**l. of similars,** see *homeopathy.*

**l. of sines,** Descartes' l.

**Snell's l.,** Descartes' l.

**Spallanzani's l.,** the law that regeneration is more complete in younger individuals than in older ones.

**Starling's l., Starling's l. of the heart,** the energy liberated with each contraction of the heart is a function of the length of the fibers composing its muscular walls; increased preload causes increased end-diastolic volume (or pressure), which increases the force of ventricular contraction. Called also *Frank-Starling l.* or *mechanism.*

**Stokes' l.,** a muscle situated above an inflamed membrane is often affected with paralysis.

**surface l.,** at constant temperature, the heat production, heat loss, and oxygen consumption in an animal are inversely proportional to the free surface or to the square of a linear dimension.

**Talbot's l.,** when complete fusion occurs and the sensation is uniform, the intensity is the same as would occur were the same amount of light spread uniformly over the disk.

**Teevan's l.,** fractures of bones occur in the line of extension, and not in the line of compression.

**l's of thermodynamics,** *Zeroth law:* two systems in thermal equilibrium with a third system are in thermal equilibrium with each other. *First law:* energy is conserved in any process; i.e., the energy gained (or lost) by a system is exactly equal to the energy lost (or gained) by the surroundings. *Second law:* there is always an increase in entropy in any naturally occurring (spontaneous) process. *Third law:* absolute zero is unattainable.

**third l. of thermodynamics,** see *l's of thermodynamics.*

**Toynbee's l.,** Gull-Toynbee l.

**van der Kolk's l.,** Schroeder van der Kolk's l.

**van't Hoff's l.,** 1. a substance in solution exerts an osmotic pressure equal to the gas pressure that it would exert if its molecules were in a gaseous state and occupied a volume equal to that of the solution under the same conditions of temperature and pressure. 2. van't Hoff's rule.

**Virchow's l.,** the cell elements of tumors are derived from normal and preexisting tissue cells.

**Walton's l.,** l. of reciprocal proportions.

**Weigert's l.,** loss or destruction of elements in the organic world is apt to be followed by overproduction of such elements in the reparative process.

**Wolff's l.,** a bone, normal or abnormal, develops the structure most suited to resist the forces acting upon it.

**Wundt-Lamansky l.,** the line of vision in moving through a vertical plane parallel to the frontal plane moves in straight lines in the vertical and horizontal directions, but in curved paths in all other movements.

**Yerkes-Dodson l.,** as anxiety level increases, task performance is enhanced at first, but after a given point is reached, further anxiety causes declining performance.

**zeroth l. of thermodynamics,** see *l's of thermodynamics.*

**lawn** (lawn, lahn) an area sown with a thick growth of a living substance.

**bacterial l.,** the confluent blanket of merged colonies resulting from plating a concentrated bacterial solution.

**Law·rence-Seip syndrome** (law'rəns-sīp) [Robert Daniel *Lawrence,* English physician, 1912–1964; Martin Fredrik *Seip,* Norwegian pediatrician, born 1921] lipoatrophic diabetes.

**law·ren·ci·um** (law-ren'se-əm) [Ernest Orlando *Lawrence,* American physicist, 1901–1958; builder of the first cyclotron for the production of high-energy particles, and winner of the Nobel prize for physics in 1939] [MeSH: Lawrencium] the chemical element of atomic number 103, atomic weight 257, symbol Lw; produced in 1961 by bombardment of californium isotopes of mass 250, 251, and 252.

**law·sone** (law'sōn) a dye isolated from the leaves of *Lawsonia inermis,* used as a topical sunscreen agent.

**Law·so·nia** (law-so'ne-ə) a genus of tropical Old World shrubs of the family Lythraceae. *L. iner'mis* is the source of lawsone and henna.

**lax·a·tion** (lak-sa'shən) defecation.

**lax·a·tive** (lak'sə-tiv) [L. *laxativus*] 1. mildly cathartic. 2. an agent that acts to promote evacuation of the bowel; see also *cathartic* and *purgative.* Called also *aperient* and *aperitive.*

**bulk l., bulk-forming l.,** a hydrophilic agent that promotes evacuation of the bowel by absorbing water and expanding, thus increasing the volume of the feces.

**contact l.,** a laxative that increases the motor activity of the intestinal tract; the precise mechanism of action of contact laxatives is unknown, but they produce an accumulation of fluid and electrolytes in the colon and are thought to increase peristalsis by stimulating intramural nerve plexuses. Called also *stimulant l.*

**lubricant l.,** an agent, immiscible with water, that promotes softening of the stool and facilitates the passage of feces through the intestines by its lubricant effect.

**saline l.,** a salt, of which one or both ions are poorly absorbed, administered in hypertonic solution to draw water into the intestinal lumen by osmosis; the resulting distention promotes increased peristalsis and evacuation.

**stimulant l.,** contact l.

**lax·i·ty** (lak'sĭ-te) [L. *laxare* to loosen] slackness or displacement (whether normal or abnormal) in the motion of a joint. Cf. *hypermobility.*

**lay·er** (la'ər) 1. a stratum or lamina. 2. a female bird of the age when it is laying eggs; in chickens this is after about five months old.

# Layer

For descriptions of specific anatomic structures not listed here, see under *lamina* and *stratum.*

**adamantine l.,** dental enamel.
**alar l. of deep cervical fascia,** alar fascia.
**ameloblastic l.,** the inner layer of cells of the enamel organ, created by its invagination, which forms the enamel prisms.
**bacillary l.,** l. of rods and cones.
**basal l.,** 1. lamina basalis choroideae. 2. stratum basale epidermidis.
**basal l. of epidermis,** stratum basale epidermidis.
**basement l.,** see under *membrane.*
**Bechterew's l., Bekhterev's l.,** Kaes-Bekhterev l.
**Bernard's glandular l.,** a layer of cells lining the acini of the pancreas.
**blastodermic l.,** germ l.
**Bowman's l.,** lamina limitans anterior corneae.
**Bruch's l.,** lamina basalis choroideae.
**capillary l. of choroid,** lamina choroidocapillaris.
**cerebral l. of retina,** pars nervosa retinae.
**l's of cerebral cortex,** six anatomical divisions of the cerebral cortex (specifically, the *neocortex*), distinguished according to the types of cells and fibers they contain; called *laminae* in the official nomenclature. Numbered from the surface inward, they are: I, molecular layer *(lamina molecularis)*; II, external granular layer *(lamina granularis externa)*; III, external pyramidal layer *(lamina pyramidalis externa)*; IV, internal granular layer *(lamina granularis interna)*; V, internal pyramidal layer *(lamina pyramidalis interna)*; and VI, multiform layer *(lamina multiformis)*. See illustration at *neocortex.*
**Chievitz l.,** a transient fiber layer separating the inner and outer neuroblastic layers of the optic cup.
**choriocapillary l.,** lamina choroidocapillaris.
**circular l. of muscular coat of colon,** stratum circulare tunicae muscularis coli.
**circular l. of muscular coat of rectum,** stratum circulare tunicae muscularis recti.
**circular l. of muscular coat of small intestine,** stratum circulare tunicae muscularis intestini tenuis.
**circular l. of muscular coat of stomach,** stratum circulare tunicae muscularis gastris.
**circular l. of tympanic membrane,** stratum circulare membranae tympanicae.
**clear l. of epidermis,** stratum lucidum epidermidis.
**columnar l.,** mantle l.
**compact l.,** stratum compactum.
**cortical l.,** the cortex of an organ, as of the brain or kidney.
**cutaneous l. of tympanic membrane,** stratum cutaneum membranae tympanicae.
**cuticular l.,** a striate border of modified cytoplasm at the free end of some columnar cells.
**deep l's of cervical fascia, l's of deep cervical fascia,** the three internal layers of cervical fascia (superficial, pretracheal, and prevertebral) and the carotid sheath, considered as one unit.
**deep l. of temporal fascia,** lamina profunda fasciae temporalis.
**deep l. of triangular ligament,** diaphragma urogenitale.
**Dobie's l.,** Z band; see under *band.*
**enamel l., inner,** the inner, concave wall of the enamel organ.
**enamel l., outer,** the outer, convex wall of the enamel organ.
**ependymal l.,** the innermost layer of the wall of the primordial neural tube, bounding the central canal, which differentiates regionally into the roof plate and the floor plate.
**epitrichial l.,** the most superficial layer of the epidermis of the embryo.
**false l.,** a hen that behaves like a normal layer but does not lay eggs because of defective oviducts.
**fibrous l. of articular capsule,** membrana fibrosa capsulae articularis.
**fibrous l. of eyeball,** tunica fibrosa bulbi.
**fibrous l. of pharynx,** fascia pharyngobasilaris.
**fibrous l. of tympanic membrane,** see under *stratum.*
**Floegel's l.,** a granular layer in each transparent lateral disk of a muscle fibril.
**functional l.,** stratum functionale.
**fusiform l. of cerebral cortex,** lamina multiformis.
**ganglion cell l.,** a layer of the pars nervosa retinae, situated between the inner molecular layer and the stratum opticum, or nerve fiber layer, consisting essentially of the ganglion cells of the retina, and containing also the fibers of Müller, neuroglia, and branches of the retinal vessels.
**ganglionic l. of cerebellum,** stratum purkinjense cerebelli.
**ganglionic l. of cerebral cortex,** lamina pyramidalis interna.
**ganglionic l. of optic nerve,** the layer of the nervous part of the retina that contains the multipolar neurons, the axons of which form the fibers of the optic nerve; see also *retina.* Called also *stratum ganglionare nervi optici* and *ganglionic stratum of retina.*
**ganglionic l. of retina,** stratum ganglionicum retinae.
**gel l.,** the more gelatinous part of the tunica mucosa of the airways, overlying the sol layer.
**germ l.,** one of the three primary layers of cells of the embryo (ectoderm, endoderm, or mesoderm), from which the tissues and organs develop.
**germinative l., germinative l. of epidermis,** 1. stratum germinativum epidermidis [Malpighii]. 2. stratum basale epidermidis.
**germinative l. of nail,** stratum germinativum unguis.
**glomerular l.,** the layer of the olfactory bulb between the olfactory nerve fiber layer and the external granular layer, containing the olfactory glomeruli.
**granular l. of cerebellum,** stratum granulosum cerebelli.
**granular l. of cerebral cortex, external,** lamina granularis externa.
**granular l. of cerebral cortex, internal,** lamina granularis interna.
**granular l. of epidermis,** stratum granulosum epidermidis.
**granular l. of follicle of ovary,** stratum granulosum folliculi ovarici vesiculosi.
**granular l. of olfactory bulb, external,** a thin layer between the glomerular layer and the molecular layer, containing periglomerular cells.
**granular l. of olfactory bulb, internal,** the innermost layer of the olfactory bulb, adjacent to the beginning of the olfactory tract; it consists of rows of axons from mitral and tufted cells alternating with rows of cell bodies and dendrites of granule cells.
**granular l. of Tomes,** a layer of imperfectly calcified dentin made of small interglobular spaces immediately beneath the dentinocemental junction in the root of a tooth. Called also *Tomes' granular l.*
**granule l. of cerebellum,** stratum granulosum cerebelli.
**gray and white l's of rostral colliculus,** strata grisea et alba colliculi superioris.
**gray l. of superior colliculus, deep,** stratum griseum profundum colliculi superioris.
**gray l. of superior colliculus, intermediate,** stratum griseum intermedium colliculi superioris.
**gray l. of superior colliculus, superficial,** stratum griseum superficiale colliculi superioris.
**gray and white l's of superior colliculus,** strata grisea et alba colliculi superioris.
**half-value l.,** the thickness of a given substance that will reduce the intensity of a beam of radiation to one half of its initial value; called also *half-value thickness.* Abbreviated *HVL.*
**Haller's l.,** that portion of the vascular layer of the choroid which is made up of large vessels.
**Henle's l.,** the outer layer of cells of the inner root sheath of a hair follicle, lying between the outer root sheath and Huxley's layer.
**Henle's fiber l.,** the outer plexiform layer in the region of the macula retinae; see also *entoretina.*
**horny l. of epidermis,** stratum corneum epidermidis.
**horny l. of nail,** stratum corneum unguis.
**Huxley's l.,** a layer of the inner root sheath of a hair follicle, lying between Henle's layer and the inner sheath cuticle.
**inferior l. of pelvic diaphragm,** fascia inferior diaphragmatis pelvis.
**internal l.,** a hen whose eggs, usually deformed, are deposited into the abdominal cavity.
**internal l. of eyeball,** tunica interna bulbi.
**investing l. of cervical fascia, investing l. of deep cervical fascia,** lamina superficialis fasciae cervicalis.
**Kaes-Bekhterev l.,** a thin layer of fibers on the border between the external granular layer and the external pyramidal layer of the cerebral cortex; called also *Bekhterev's l., Kaes' feltwork, line,* or *stria, Kaes-Bekhterev stria,* and *Vicq d'Azyr's band* or *stripe.*
**Langhans' l.,** cytotrophoblast.
**limiting l., internal,** the basal lamina of the Müller cells in the retina, separating the inner, conical ends of the cells from the vitreous body. Called also *inner* or *internal limiting membrane.*
**longitudinal l. of muscular coat of colon,** stratum longitudinale tunicae muscularis coli.
**longitudinal l. of muscular coat of rectum,** stratum longitudinale tunicae muscularis recti.
**longitudinal l. of muscular coat of small intestine,** stratum longitudinale tunicae muscularis intestini tenuis.
**longitudinal l. of muscular coat of stomach,** stratum longitudinale tunicae muscularis gastris.
**malpighian l.,** stratum germinativum.
**mantle l.,** the middle layer of the wall of the primordial neural tube, containing primitive nerve cells and later forming the gray matter of the central nervous system.
**marginal l.,** the outermost layer of the wall of the primordial neural tube, a fibrous mesh into which the nerve fibers later grow, forming the white matter of the central nervous system.
**medullary l. of thalamus, external,** l. medullaris lateralis thalami.
**medullary l. of thalamus, internal,** lamina medullaris medialis thalami.

**Meynert's l.,** lamina pyramidalis externa.
**middle l. of deep cervical fascia,** lamina pretrachealis fasciae cervicalis.
**mitral cell l.,** a thin layer in the olfactory bulb between the molecular layer and the internal granular layer, containing the bodies of the mitral cells.
**molecular l., external,** external plexiform l.
**molecular l., inner, molecular l., internal,** internal plexiform l.
**molecular l., outer,** external plexiform l.
**molecular l. of cerebellum,** stratum moleculare cerebelli.
**molecular l. of cerebral cortex,** lamina molecularis.
**molecular l. of olfactory bulb,** a wide layer between the external granular layer and the mitral cell layer, primarily containing dendrites from mitral and tufted cells.
**mucous l.,** stratum germinativum.
**mucous l. of pharynx,** tunica mucosa pharyngis.
**mucous l. of tympanic membrane,** stratum mucosum membranae tympanicae.
**multiform l. of cerebral cortex,** lamina multiformis.
**muscular l. of fallopian tube,** tunica muscularis tubae uterinae.
**muscular l. of pharynx,** tunica muscularis pharyngis.
**nerve fiber l.,** a layer of the retina, situated between the ganglion cell layer and the internal limiting membrane, consisting essentially of the axons of the ganglion cells which pass through the lamina cribrosa to form the optic nerve.
**nervous l. of retina,** pars nervosa retinae.
**neuroepidermal l.,** ectoderm.
**neuroepithelial l. of retina,** l. of rods and cones.
**Nitabuch's l.,** an interrupted sheet of fibrinoid in the placenta at the junction of trophoblast and decidua; called also *Nitabuch's stria* or *zone.*
**nuclear l., external,** the layer of the pars nervosa retinae, situated between the external limiting membrane and the external plexiform layer, consisting essentially of the rod and cone granules (nuclei).
**nuclear l., inner, nuclear l., internal,** the layer of the pars nervosa retinae, situated between the inner and outer plexiform layers, consisting essentially of the visual cells.
**nuclear l., outer,** external nuclear l.
**nuclear l. of cerebellum,** stratum granulosum cerebelli.
**odontoblastic l.,** the epithelioid odontoblastic zone, one to five layers thick, which forms the outer surface of the dental pulp adjacent to the dentin, resting on Weil's basal zone. It produces and maintains the dentin.
**olfactory nerve fiber l.,** the outermost layer of the olfactory bulb, composed of axons of the olfactory cells before they terminate in the adjacent glomerular layer.
**Ollier's l.,** osteogenetic l.
**optic l. of superior colliculus,** stratum opticum colliculi superioris.
**oriens l. of hippocampus,** stratum oriens hippocampi.
**osteogenetic l.,** the innermost layer of the periosteum; called also *Ollier's l.*
**Pander's l.,** the splanchnopleural layer of the mesoblast.
**papillary l. of corium, papillary l. of dermis,** stratum papillare dermidis.
**parietal l. of pelvic fascia,** fascia superior diaphragmatis pelvis.
**parietal l. of pericardium, parietal l. of serous pericardium,** lamina parietalis pericardii serosi.
**parietal l. of tunica vaginalis of testis,** lamina parietalis tunicae vaginalis testis.
**peripheral l. of cerebral cortex,** lamina molecularis.
**perpendicular l. of ethmoid bone,** lamina perpendicularis ossis ethmoidalis.
**pigmented l. of ciliary body,** the part of the pigmented layer of the retina that rests on the ciliary body; see also *retina.* Called also *pigmented stratum of ciliary body* and *stratum pigmenti corporis ciliaris.*
**pigmented l. of eyeball,** stratum pigmenti bulbi oculi.
**pigmented l. of iris,** the part of the pigmented layer of the retina that rests on the posterior surface of the iris; see also *retina.* Called also *pigmented stratum of iris* and *stratum pigmenti iridis.*
**pigmented l. of retina,** pars pigmentosa retinae.
**piriform neuronal l.,** stratum purkinjense cerebelli.
**plexiform l., external,** the layer of the pars nervosa retinae, situated between the outer nuclear layer and the inner nuclear layer, consisting essentially of the arborizations of the axons of the rod and cone granules with the dendrites of the bipolar cells. Called also *external* or *outer molecular layer.*
**plexiform l., inner, plexiform l., internal,** the layer of the pars nervosa retinae situated between the inner nuclear layer and the ganglion cell layer, consisting primarily of the arborization of the axons of the bipolar cells with the dendrites of the ganglion cells. Called also *inner* or *internal molecular layer.*
**plexiform l., outer,** external plexiform l.
**plexiform l. of cerebellum,** stratum moleculare cerebelli.
**plexiform l. of cerebral cortex,** lamina molecularis.
**polymorphic l. of cerebral cortex,** lamina multiformis.
**pretracheal l. of cervical fascia,** lamina pretrachealis fasciae cervicalis.
**prevertebral l. of cervical fascia,** lamina prevertebralis fasciae cervicalis.
**prickle cell l.,** stratum spinosum epidermidis.
**Purkinje l., Purkinje cell l.,** stratum purkinjense cerebelli.
**pyramidal l. of cerebral cortex, external,** lamina pyramidalis externa.
**pyramidal l. of cerebral cortex, internal,** lamina pyramidalis interna.
**pyramidal l. of hippocampus,** stratum pyramidale hippocampi.
**radiate l. of hippocampus,** stratum radiatum hippocampi.
**radiate l. of tympanic membrane,** stratum radiatum membranae tympanicae.
**Rauber's l.,** the most external of the three layers of cells which form the blastodisc or embryonic disk in the young embryo; called also *blastodermic ectoderm* and *primitive ectoderm.*
**reticular l. of corium, reticular l. of dermis,** stratum reticulare dermidis.
**l. of rods and cones,** the layer of the nervous part of the retina, situated between the pigmented part and the external limiting membrane, comprising the sensitive elements of the retina, the cones, containing a visual pigment, iodopsin, and the rods, containing visual purple, or rhodopsin; see also *retina.* Called also *neuroepithelial l.* or *stratum of retina* and *stratum neuroepitheliale retinae.*
**Rohr's l.,** see under *stria.*
**Sattler's l.,** that portion of the vascular layer of the choroid which is made up of medium-sized vessels.
**sclerotogenous l.,** the layer of mesoderm cells surrounding the notochord of the embryo and developing into the axial skeleton.
**second half-value l.,** the additional thickness of material needed to reduce the intensity of a radiation beam from one half to one fourth of its original value. Cf. *half-value l.*
**skeletogenous l.,** sclerotogenous l.
**sol l.,** a thin layer of the tunica mucosa of the respiratory tract, underlying the gel layer.
**somatic l.,** the external layer of the lateral mesoderm after the coelomic split occurs; the inner component of somatopleure of the embryo.
**spinous l. of epidermis,** stratum spinosum epidermidis.
**splanchnic l.,** the internal layer of the lateral mesoderm after the coelomic split occurs; the component of splanchnopleure outside the entoderm of the embryo.
**spongy l.,** stratum spongiosum.
**subcallosal l.,** the layer of nerve fibers on the lower side of the corpus callosum.
**subendocardial l.,** the layer of loose fibrous tissue uniting the endocardium and myocardium; it also contains blood vessels, nerves, and some fibers of the conducting system of the heart.
**subendothelial l.,** a middle, fibrous layer of the tunica intima of typical blood vessels, located between the endothelium and internal elastic membrane; it also comprises the bulk of the endocardium, where it lies deep to the lining endothelium. It is composed of varying amounts of collagen and elastic fibers and smooth muscle cells.
**subepicardial l.,** a thin collagenous layer of loose connective tissue uniting the epicardium and myocardium; besides collagen and elastic fibers, it also contains fat cells, nerves, and lymphatic and blood vessels.
**submantle l.,** a layer of interglobular dentin usually situated just below the cover (mantle) dentin.
**submucous l.,** tela submucosa.
**submucous l. of bladder,** tela submucosa vesicae urinariae.
**submucous l. of bronchi,** tela submucosa bronchiorum.
**submucous l. of colon,** tela submucosa intestini crassi.
**submucous l. of esophagus,** tela submucosa oesophagi.
**submucous l. of pharynx,** tela submucosa pharyngis.
**submucous l. of small intestine,** tela submucosa intestini tenuis.
**submucous l. of stomach,** tela submucosa gastris.
**submucous l. of urinary bladder,** tela submucosa vesicae urinariae.
**submucous l. of uterine tube,** tela submucosa tubae uterinae.
**subodontoblastic l.,** Weil's basal l.
**subserous l.,** tela subserosa.
**subserous l. of gallbladder,** tela subserosa vesicae biliaris.
**subserous l. of liver,** tela subserosa hepatis.
**subserous l. of peritoneum,** tela subserosa peritonei.
**subserous l. of small intestine,** tela subserosa intestini tenuis.
**subserous l. of stomach,** tela subserosa gastris.
**subserous l. of urinary bladder,** tela subserosa vesicae urinariae.
**subserous l. of uterine tube,** tela subserosa tubae uterinae.
**subserous l. of uterus,** tela subserosa uteri.
**superficial l. of cervical fascia,** 1. lamina superficialis fasciae cervicalis. 2. superficial cervical fascia (def. 1).

**superficial l. of deep cervical fascia,** lamina superficialis fasciae cervicalis.
**superficial l. of fascia of perineum,** fascia perinei superficialis.
**superficial investing l. of cervical fascia,** lamina superficialis fasciae cervicalis.
**superficial l. of temporal fascia,** lamina superficialis fasciae temporalis.
**superficial l. of triangular ligament,** membrana perinei.
**l's of superior colliculus,** the seven layers forming the superior colliculus, from outer to inner being the stratum zonale (Layer I), stratum griseum superficiale (Layer II), stratum opticum (Layer III), stratum griseum intermedium (Layer IV), stratum medullare intermedium (Layer V), stratum griseum profundum (Layer VI), and stratum medullare profundum (Layer VII).
**superior l. of pelvic diaphragm,** fascia superior diaphragmatis pelvis.
**suprachoroid l.,** lamina suprachoroidea.
**synovial l. of articular capsule,** membrana synovialis capsulae articularis.
**Tomes' granular l.,** granular l. of Tomes.
**trophic l.,** endoderm.
**vascular l. of eyeball,** tunica vasculosa bulbi.
**vegetative l.,** endoderm.
**vertical l. of ethmoid bone,** lamina perpendicularis ossis ethmoidalis.
**visceral l. of pelvic fascia,** fascia pelvis visceralis.
**visceral l. of pericardium, visceral l. of serous pericardium,** lamina visceralis pericardii serosi.
**visceral l. of tunica vaginalis of testis,** lamina visceralis tunicae vaginalis testis.
**Waldeyer's l.,** the vascular layer of the ovary.
**Weil's basal l.,** a clear, relatively cell-free layer, located just inside the odontoblastic layer and overlying the cell-rich zone of the dental pulp, which is visible during the inactive phase of dentinogenesis. It is made up of delicate fibrils embedded in the ground substance; in dentinogenesis the fibrils are incorporated into the matrix. Called also *subodontoblastic l.* and *Weil's basal zone.*
**white l's of cerebellum,** laminae albae cerebelli.
**white l. of superior colliculus, deep,** stratum medullare profundum colliculi superioris.
**white l. of superior colliculus, intermediate,** stratum medullare intermedium colliculi superioris.
**Zeissel's l.,** a layer in the stomach wall between the tunica muscularis mucosae and the tela submucosa.
**zonal l. of cerebral cortex,** lamina molecularis.
**zonal l. of superior colliculus,** stratum zonale colliculi superioris.
**zonal l. of thalamus,** stratum zonale thalami.

**laz·a·ret·to** (laz″ə-ret′o) 1. a hospital for contagious diseases. 2. a quarantine station.

**lb** abbreviation for L. *li′bra,* pound.

**LBBB** left bundle branch block; see *bundle branch block,* under *block.*

**LBP** low back pain.

**LBW** low birth weight; see under *infant.*

**LCA** left coronary artery; leukocyte common antigen.

**LCAD de·fi·cien·cy** long-chain acyl-CoA dehydrogenase deficiency; see under *acyl-CoA dehydrogenase.*

**LCAT** lecithin-cholesterol acyltransferase; see *phosphatidylcholine–sterol O-acyltransferase.*

**LCAT deficiency** lecithin–cholesterol acyltransferase deficiency.

**LCIS** lobular carcinoma in situ.

**LD** lethal dose; light difference.

**$LD_{50}$** median lethal dose.

**LDA** left dorsoanterior (position of the fetus); left displacement of the abomasum.

**LDH** lactate dehydrogenase.

**LDL** low-density lipoproteins.

**L-dopa** see *dopa.*

**LDP** left dorsoposterior (position of the fetus).

**LE** 1. left eye. 2. lupus erythematosus; see also under *cell.*

**leach·ing** (lēch′ing) lixiviation.

**lead**[1] (led) [L. *plumbum*] [MeSH: Lead] a soft, grayish blue metal with poisonous salts; symbol, Pb; atomic number, 82; atomic weight, 207.19. Excessive ingestion causes lead poisoning; see under *poisoning.*
**l. acetate** [USP], colorless crystals, masses, or granules used as a reagent and astringent.
**black l.,** graphite.
**l. chloride,** a compound, $PbCl_2$, used as a reagent and pigment.
**l. dioxide,** a highly flammable oxidizing agent used as an analytical reagent.
**l. monoxide,** a binary compound, PbO, called *litharge* when crystalline and *massicot* when amorphous; used as a reagent.
**l. nitrate,** a sweetish crystalline agent, $Pb(NO_3)_2$, used as a reagent.
**l. oxide,** see *l. dioxide* and *l. monoxide.*
**l. subacetate,** a basic acetate of lead.
**tetra-ethyl l.,** a highly poisonous organic lead compound used as an antiknock agent in internal combustion motors; it can be absorbed through the skin and may cause mental symptoms and death. Called also *ethyl gas.*

**lead**[2] (lēd) [MeSH: Lead] any of the conductors connected to the electrocardiograph, each comprising two or more electrodes that are attached to specific sites on the body and used to examine electrical activity by monitoring changes in electrical potential between them. See also *electrocardiogram.*
**l. I,** the standard bipolar limb lead attached to the right and left arms.
**l. II,** the standard bipolar limb lead attached to the right arm and left leg.
**l. III,** the standard bipolar limb lead attached to the left arm and left leg.
**active fixation l.,** a pacing lead that attaches to the heart by pins, screws, claws, needles, or similar devices.
**augmented unipolar limb l.,** a unipolar limb lead that has been modified by disconnecting the input of the limb to the central terminal, increasing the voltage output; the three standard leads are designated $aV_F$, $aV_L$, and $aV_R$.
**$aV_F$ l.,** an augmented unipolar limb lead in which the positive (exploratory) electrode is on the left leg.
**$aV_L$ l.,** an augmented unipolar limb lead in which the positive (exploratory) electrode is on the left arm.
**$aV_R$ l.,** an augmented unipolar limb lead in which the positive (exploratory) electrode terminal is on the right arm.
**bipolar l.,** an array involving two electrodes, each of which makes significant contribution to the record, placed at different body sites.
**bipolar limb l.,** any bipolar array in which both electrodes are attached to limbs; usually used to denote one of the three standard limb leads, i.e., lead I, II, or III.
**bipolar precordial l.,** a bipolar array in which both electrodes are attached to the chest; it is often a modification of a standard limb lead.
**chest l's,** precordial l's.
**esophageal l.,** one attached to an electrode inserted within the esophagus.
**Frank XYZ l's,** XYZ l's.
**limb l.,** an array in which any registering electrodes are attached to limbs; it may be unipolar or bipolar.
**pacemaker l., pacing l.,** the connection between the heart and the power source of an artificial cardiac pacemaker, comprising an electrode to contact the heart, a conductor coil, and a terminal pin to connect to the generator.
**passive fixation l.,** a pacing lead that is attached to the heart by flanged areas or tines lodged under trabeculae.
**precordial l's,** leads in which the exploring electrode is placed on the chest and the other is connected to one or more extremities. The term is usually used to denote the V leads (q.v.).
**standard l's,** the 12 leads used in a standard electrocardiogram, comprising the standard bipolar limb leads (I, II and III), the augmented unipolar limb leads ($aV_F$, $aV_L$, and $aV_R$), and the standard precordial leads ($V_1$ to $V_6$).
**unipolar l.,** an array of two electrodes, one of which is an exploring electrode attached either to a limb *(unipolar limb l.)* or to the chest *(V l's)* while the other, an indifferent electrode contributing no input, uses a central terminal as reference point.
**unipolar limb l.,** any unipolar array in which the exploring electrode is placed on a limb; designated $V_F$, $V_L$, and $V_R$. In practice, it is usually modified; see *augmented unipolar limb l.*

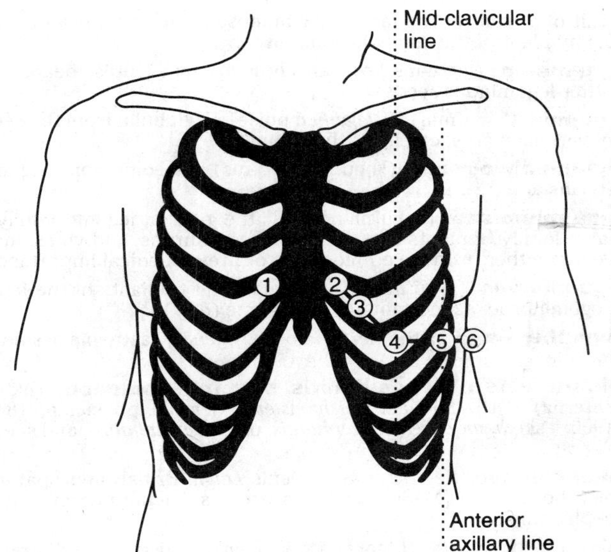

Positioning of V leads.

**unipolar precordial l's,** V l's.
**V l's,** the series of six standard unipolar leads in which the exploring electrode is attached to the chest; their positions are designated $V_1$ to $V_6$.
**Wilson's l's,** V l's.
**XYZ l's,** leads used in the Frank lead system (q.v.) in spatial vectorcardiography.

**leaf** (lēf) [A. S. *lēf*] a flattened structure of vascular plants, attached to the plant by a stem and usually green in color, that is the primary site of photosynthesis and transpiration.
**belladonna l.** [USP], the dried leaves and fruiting tops of *Atropa belladonna* or *A. belladonna* var. *acuminata,* used in the preparation of standardized dosage forms; see under *extract* and *tincture.*

**leaf·let** (lēf'lət) a structure resembling a small leaf, especially a cusp of a heart valve.

**Leão's spreading depression** (la-ahz') [A.A.P. *Leão,* Brazilian physiologist, born 1914] see under *depression.*

**learn·ing** (lər'ning) [MeSH: Learning] a relatively long-lasting adaptive behavioral change occurring as a result of experience.
**insight l.,** the highest form of learning, characterized by the ability to evaluate and combine previous experiences to solve a problem or achieve a desired goal.
**latent l.,** that which occurs without reinforcement, becoming apparent only when a reinforcement or reward is introduced.
**observational l.,** that in which new behaviors are learned through watching the actions and outcomes of others.

**leash** (lēsh) a bundle or fasciculus.

**Le·ber's congenital amaurosis,** etc. (la'bərz) [Theodor *Leber,* German ophthalmologist, 1840–1917] see *amaurosis congenita,* under *amaurosis, Hassall's corpuscles,* under *corpuscle,* and *Hovius' plexus,* under *plexus;* and see under *neuropathy.*

**Le·bis·tes** (lə-bis'tēz) a genus of small fish, the guppy.
**L. reticula'tus,** a species of top-feeding minnows, commonly known as "millions," cultivated in Barbados to eliminate mosquito larvae.

**Le·boy·er method (technique)** (lə-bwah-ya') [Frédérick *Leboyer,* French obstetrician, born 1918] see under *method.*

**lec·an·op·a·gus** (lek"ən-op'ə-gəs) [Gr. *lekanē* basin + *-pagus*] ischiodidymus.

**Le·cat's gulf** (lə-kahz') [Claude Nicolas *Lecat,* French surgeon, 1700–1768] see under *gulf.*

**le·che de hi·gue·rón** (la'cha da e-ga-rōn') [Sp. "milk of fig"] the sap or latex of the wild fig tree *Ficus anthelmintica,* used as a vermifuge.

**lech·o·py·ra** (lek"o-pi'rə) [Gr. *lechō* parturient woman + *pyr* fever] puerperal fever.

**le·chu·gui·lla** (la-choo-ge'yə) [Sp. "little lettuce"] *Agave lecheguilla.*

**lec·i·thal** (les'i-thəl) [*lecith-* + *-al*[1]] having a yolk or pertaining to a yolk.

**-lecithal** [Gr. *lekithos* yolk] a word termination denoting yolk, affixed to a word stem descriptive of the state of the yolk substance, as *centrolecithal, isolecithal,* etc. See also entries under *ovum.*

**lec·i·thid** (les'ĭ-thid) a compound of lecithin with venom hemolysin.
**cobra l.,** a hemolytic compound formed by cobra toxin and the lecithin of the blood.

**lec·i·thin** (les'ĭ-thin) phosphatidylcholine.

**lec·i·thin–cho·les·ter·ol ac·yl·trans·fer·ase (LCAT)** (les'i-thin kə-les'tər-ol a"səl-trans'fər-ās) phosphatidylcholine–sterol *O*-acyltransferase.

**le·ci·thin·cho·les·ter·ol ac·yl·trans·fer·ase (LCAT) de·fi·cien·cy** an autosomal recessive disorder due to failure of LCAT to esterify plasma cholesterol; cholesterol and phosphatidylcholine accumulate in the plasma and tissues, causing corneal opacities, anemia, and often proteinuria. All classes of lipoproteins show abnormalities. See also *fish eye disease* under *disease.*

**lec·i·thin·emia** (les"-ĭ-thĭ-ne'me-ə) the presence of lecithin in the blood.

**lecith(o)-** [Gr. *lekithos* yolk] a combining form denoting relationship to the yolk of an egg or ovum.

**lec·i·tho·blast** (les'ĭ-tho-blast") [*lecitho-* + *-blast*] the primordial endoderm of a two-layered blastodisc.

**lec·i·tho·pro·tein** (les"ĭ-tho-pro'tēn) a compound of the protein molecule with a molecule of lecithin; lecithoproteins occur in all cells.

**lec·i·tho·vi·tel·lin** (les"ĭ-tho-vi-tel'in) a saline extract of egg yolks used in egg-yolk agar to test for bacterial lecithinase.

**lec·tin** (lek'tin) any of a group of hemagglutinating proteins found primarily in plant seeds, which bind specifically to the branching sugar molecules of glycoproteins and glycolipids on the surface of cells. Certain lectins selectively cause agglutination of erythrocytes of certain blood groups and of malignant cells but not their normal counterparts; others stimulate the proliferation of lymphocytes.

**lec·to·type** (lek'to-tīp) in bacteriology, a culture taken from the original material to serve as a type culture when the original investigator did not designate a type.

**Lec·y·thoph·o·ra** (les"ĭ-thof'ə-rə) a genus of Fungi Imperfecti of the form-family Dematiaceae, formerly considered part of the genus *Phialophora. L. hoffman'nii* occasionally causes hyalohyphomycosis and *L. muta'bilis* has been found in cases of encocarditis, some fatal.

**Led·bän·der** (led'bān-der) [Ger.] Büngner's bands; see under *band.*

**Le Den·tu's suture** (lə-dahn-tūz') [Jean François-Auguste *Le Dentu,* Paris surgeon, 1841–1926] see under *suture.*

**Led·er·berg** (led'ər-bərg) Joshua. American biochemist, born 1925; co-winner, with George Wells Beadle and Edward Lawrie Tatum, of the Nobel prize for medicine or physiology in 1958 for discoveries concerning genetic recombination and the organization of the genetic material of bacteria.

**Led·er·cil·lin** (led"ər-sil'in) trademark for preparations of penicillin G procaine.

**Le·Duc technique (implantation)** (lədo͞ok) [A. *LeDuc,* French urologist, 20th century] see under *technique.*

**Lee's ganglion** (lēz) [Robert *Lee,* English obstetrician and gynecologist, 1793–1877] cervical ganglion of the uterus; see under *ganglion.*

**leech** (lēch) [L. *hirudo*] 1. any of the annelids of the class Hirudinea. Some species are bloodsuckers and may become temporarily parasitic upon animals, including humans. Leeches were formerly used extensively for drawing blood (see *leeching*). 2. to apply leeches.
**American l.,** *Macrobdella decora.*
**artificial l.,** an apparatus for drawing blood by artificial suction.
**horse l.,** see *Limnatis* and *Haemopis.*
**land l.,** *Haemadipsa.*
**medicinal l.,** *Hirudo medicinalis.*

**leeches** (lēch'əz) [pl. of *leech,* from the appearance of the lesions] [MeSH: Leeches] pythiosis.

**leech·ing** (lēch'ing) the application of a leech for the withdrawal of blood; formerly used extensively in the treatment of various disorders; called also *hirudinization.*

**Leeu·wen·hoe·kia** (la"wen-hoo'ke-ə) [Anton (Anthony, Antony) van *Leeuwenhoek,* Dutch microscopist, 1632–1723] a genus of mites. *L. australien'sis* is a species found in Australia that causes great irritation by burrowing in the skin.

**Le Fort fracture,** etc. (lə-for') [Léon-Clément *Le Fort,* French surgeon, 1829–1893] see under *amputation, fracture, operation, sound,* and *suture.*

**left-hand·ed** (left-hand'əd) using the left hand preferentially, or more skillfully than the right, in voluntary motor acts. See also *handedness* and *laterality*.

**leg** (leg) [MeSH: Leg] 1. that section of the lower limb between the knee and ankle; called also *crus* and *shank*. 2. in common usage, the entire lower limb (in which case, the part below the knee is called the *lower leg*). 3. any of the four limbs of a quadruped.
**badger l.**, inequality in the length of the legs.
**baker l.**, genu valgum.
**bandy l.**, genu varum.
**bayonet l.**, uncorrected backward displacement of the bones of the leg at the knee, followed by ankylosis at the joint.
**black l.**, blackleg.
**bow l.**, genu varum.
**hind l.**, the back leg (pelvic limb) of a quadruped. Cf. *foreleg*.
**milk l.**, phlegmasia alba dolens.
**red l.**, a fatal septicemia in frogs caused by *Aeromonas hydrophila*.
**restless l's**, see under *syndrome*.
**rider's l.**, strain of the adductor muscles of the thigh in horseback riders.
**scaly l.**, a type of mange in fowls in which the legs become enlarged and encrusted due to infestation by species of *Knemidokoptes*.
**scissor l.**, deformity with crossing of the legs in walking, due to spasticity of adductor muscles of the thighs.
**splay l's, spraddle l's**, myofibrillar hypoplasia.
**tennis l.**, a sudden tear at the musculotendinous junction of the medial belly of the gastrocnemius muscle, usually seen in older persons participating in tennis and other sports.
**white l.**, phlegmasia alba dolens.

**Legg's disease** (legz) [Arthur Thornton *Legg*, American surgeon, 1874–1939] see under *disease*.

**Legg-Cal·vé-Per·thes disease** (leg-kahl-va'per'təz) [Arthur T. *Legg*; Jacques *Calvé*, French orthopedist, 1875–1954; Georg Clemens *Perthes*, German surgeon, 1869–1927] see under *disease*.

**Le·gion·el·la** (le″jə-nel'ə) [from *legionnaires' disease*] [MeSH: Legionella] a genus of gram-negative, aerobic, rod-shaped bacteria of the family Legionellaceae, made up of motile, pleomorphic organisms that require cysteine and iron for growth. Their normal habitat is lakes, streams, and moist soil, but they have also been found as contaminants in human habitations. Human infection causes legionellosis, a pneumonialike disease; the mode of spread is the airborne route. The type species is *L. pneumo'phila*.
**L. bozema'nii**, a species isolated from human lung tissue that has been associated with pneumonia.
**L. dumof'fii**, a species isolated from human lung tissue and from cooling-tower water that has been associated with pneumonia.
**L. fee'leii**, a species isolated from coolant-system waters that has been associated with Pontiac fever.
**L. gorma'nii**, a species isolated from riparian soil that has been associated with pneumonia.
**L. jorda'nis**, a species isolated from riparian soil and treated sewage.
**L. long-beach'ae**, a species isolated from human lung tissue and respiratory secretions that has been associated with pneumonia.
**L. micda'dei**, a species isolated from human lung tissue, respiratory secretions, and pleural fluid and from cooling-tower water, shower heads, tap water, and nebulizers of respiratory therapy equipment. It is the causative agent of Pittsburgh pneumonia. Called also *L. pittsburgensis* and *Pittsburgh pneumonia agent*.
**L. pittsburgen'sis**, *L. micdadei*.
**L. pneumo'phila**, the causative agent of legionnaires' disease and Pontiac fever. It was the first species of the genus isolated and characterized, and it has been found in human lung tissue, respiratory secretions, pleural fluid, and blood and in numerous environmental sites such as riparian and other soil, and in cooling-tower water, tap water, shower heads, construction and excavation sites, and aerosolized droplets from heat-exchange systems.
**L. wadswor'thii**, a species isolated from pleural tissue, a cause of human pneumonia.

**le·gion·el·la** (le″jə-nel'ə) pl. *legionel'lae* [MeSH: Legionella] Any microorganism of the genus *Legionella*.

**Le·gion·el·la·ceae** (le″jə-nel-a'se-e) [MeSH: Legionellaceae] a family of bacteria that contains the single genus *Legionella*.

**le·gion·el·lae** (le″jə-nel'e) plural of *legionella*.

**le·gion·el·lo·sis** (le″jə-nel-o'sis) [MeSH: Legionellosis] any of several illnesses caused by infection with species of *Legionella*; see *legionnaires' disease, Pittsburgh pneumonia*, and *Pontiac fever*. Called also Legionella *pneumonia*.

**le·gion·naires' disease** (le-jən-ārz') [*legionnaires*, members of the American Legion, whose convention in Philadelphia in 1976 was the scene of a highly publicized epidemic] [MeSH: Legionnaires' Disease] see under *disease*.

**le·gume** (leg'ūm, lə-gūm') [MeSH: Legumes] 1. the pod, seed, or fruit of a plant of the family Leguminosae, such as a pea or bean. 2. any plant of the family Leguminosae.

**leg·u·me·lin** (leg″u-me'lin) an albumin from lentils, beans, and other leguminous seeds.

**le·gu·min** (lə-gu'min) [L. *legumen* pulse] a globulin from the seeds of various plants, chiefly of the legumes.

**le·gu·mi·niv·o·rous** (lə-gu″mĭ-niv'ə-rəs) feeding on legumes (beans and peas).

**Le·gu·mi·no·sae** (lə-gu″mĭ-noəse) the pea or legume family, a large family of plants that includes trees, shrubs, and vines; many genera either produce edible seeds or are of medical importance.

**le·gu·mi·nous** (lə-gu'mĭ-nəs) 1. pertaining to plants of the family Leguminosae. 2. pertaining to a legume (def. 2).

**lei·as·the·nia** (li″əs-the'ne-ə) [*leio-* + *asthenia*] asthenia of smooth muscle.

**Leich·ten·stern's encephalitis, sign (phenomenon)** (līk'tən-shternz) [Otto Michael *Leichtenstern*, German physician, 1845–1900] see *hemorrhagic encephalitis*, under *encephalitis*, and see under *sign*.

**Leigh disease** (le) [Archibald Denis *Leigh*, British neuropathologist, born 1915] [MeSH: Leigh Disease] subacute necrotizing encephalomyelopathy.

**Lei·ner's disease** (li'nərz) [Karl *Leiner*, Austrian pediatrician, 1871–1930] see under *disease*.

**leio-** [Gr. *leios* smooth] a combining form meaning smooth.

**leio·der·mia** (li″o-dər'me-ə) [*leio-* + *derm-* + *-ia*] abnormal glossiness and smoothness of the skin.

**leio·dys·to·nia** (li″o-dis-to'ne-ə) [*leio-* + *dystonia*] dystonia of smooth muscle.

**Lei·og·na·thus ba·co·ti** (li-og'nə-thəs bə-ko'te) *Ornithonyssus bacoti*.

**leio·myo·blas·to·ma** (li″o-mi″o-blas-to'mə) epithelioid leiomyoma.

**leio·myo·fi·bro·ma** (li″o-mi″o-fi-bro'mə) leiomyoma.

**leio·myo·ma** (li″o-mi-o'mə) [*leio-* + *myoma*] [MeSH: Leiomyoma] a benign tumor derived from smooth muscle, most commonly of the uterus; called also *fibroid* and *fibroid tumor*.
**bizarre l.**, epithelioid l.
**l. cu'tis**, one arising from cutaneous or subcutaneous smooth muscle fibers, occurring singly or multiply, usually in the form of lesions arising from arrectores pilorum muscles (piloleiomyoma); it may also occur as a solitary genital lesion arising from dartoic, vulvar, or mammillary muscle or as a solitary angioleiomyoma (q.v.) arising from the muscle of veins. Lesions present as smooth, firm, painful, often translucent or waxy nodules and are characterized by interlacing bundles of elongated rod- or spindle-shaped cells with finely fibrillar cytoplasm.
**epithelioid l.**, a relatively rare smooth muscle tumor, usually of the stomach, in which the cells are polygonal rather than spindle-shaped; called also *bizarre l.* and *leiomyoblastoma*.
**intraligamentous l.**, a uterine leiomyoma with lateral growth that extends outward between the folds of the broad ligament.
**intramural l.**, a uterine leiomyoma located within the substance of the myometrium in the uterine corpus.
**parasitic l.**, a pedunculated leiomyoma that has partially or completely detached from its site of origin and is attached to the omentum, which now has extended blood vessels into it.
**pedunculated l.**, a submucosal leiomyoma that protrudes into the uterine cavity, forming a bulbous polyp with a firm, round head.
**submucosal l.**, a uterine leiomyoma located next to the endometrium in the corpus of the uterus; this type frequently protrudes into the endometrial cavity, forming a pedunculated leiomyoma.
**subserosal l.**, a uterine leiomyoma located just beneath the tunica serosa of the corpus of the uterus.
**l. u'teri, uterine l.**, a leiomyoma of the uterus, usually occurring in the third and fourth decades, characterized by the development of multiple, sharply circumscribed, unencapsulated, gray-white tumors, which are firm, usually round, and show a whorled pattern on cut section. The majority are within the myometrium of the corpus of the uterus, but they may also occur in the cervix, usually in its posterior wall. Those in the corpus are distinguished by location as either *intramural, submucosal*, or *subserosal leiomyomas*. Called also *fibromyoma uteri, uterine myoma*, and, colloquially, *fibroids*.
**vascular l.**, angioleiomyoma.

**leio·my·o·ma·to·sis** (li″o-mi″o-mə-to'sis) [MeSH: Leiomyomatosis] a condition in which multiple leiomyomas occur throughout the body.
**l. peritonea'lis dissemina'ta**, abdominal smooth muscle tumors arising as small nodules scattered throughout the peritoneal surfaces, occurring exclusively in women of reproductive age and ap-

pearing very similar to low-grade leiomyosarcoma or metastatic carcinoma but usually regressing spontaneously following menopause.

**leio·myo·sar·co·ma** (li″o-mi″-o-sahr-ko′mə) [*leio-* + *myosarcoma*] [MeSH: Leiomyosarcoma] a sarcoma containing large spindle cells of smooth muscle, most commonly of the uterus, retroperitoneal region, or extremities.
**renal l.**, a rare leiomyosarcoma in the kidney, usually in the capsule; it occurs more often in women.

**leip(o)-** for words beginning thus, see those beginning *lip(o)-*.

**Leish·man's cells, stain** (lēsh′mənz) [Sir William Boog *Leishman*, English army surgeon and bacteriologist, 1865–1926] see under *cell* and see *stain*.

**Leish·man-Don·o·van body** (lēsh′mən don′ə-vən) [Sir William B. *Leishman;* Charles *Donovan*, Irish physician in India, 1863–1951] amastigote.

**Leish·ma·nia** (lēsh-ma′ne-ə) [Sir William B. *Leishman*] [MeSH: Leishmania] a genus of flagellate protozoa (suborder Trypanosomatina, order Kinetoplastida) comprising parasites of worldwide distribution, several species of which are pathogenic for humans. The organisms have two morphologic stages in their life cycle: amastigote (Leishman-Donovan body), found intracellularly in the vertebrate (i.e., human) host; and promastigote (leptomonad), found in the digestive tract of the invertebrate host (i.e., phlebotomine sandfly) and in cultures. Because all species are morphologically indistinguishable, the organisms have usually been assigned to species and subspecies according to their geographic origin, the clinical syndrome they produce, and their ecologic characteristics, or they have been separated on the basis of their tendency to cause visceral, cutaneous, or mucocutaneous leishmaniasis. In some classifications, leishmanias are placed in four complexes comprising species and subspecies: *L. donovani, L. tropica, L. mexicana,* and *L. viannia* (formerly *L. brasiliensis*).
**L. aethio′pica**, a species of the *L. tropica* complex causing Ethiopian cutaneous leishmaniasis; animal reservoirs are rock and tree hyraxes in the highlands of Ethiopia and Kenya; the vector in Ethiopia is *Phlebotomus longipes* and in Kenya it is *P. pedifer.* Called also *L. tropica aethiopica.*
**L. brasilien′sis**, 1. *L. viannia.* 2. *L. viannia braziliensis.*
**L. brazilien′sis**, 1. *L. viannia.* 2. *L. viannia braziliensis.*
**L. brazilien′sis brazilien′sis**, *L. viannia braziliensis.*
**L. brazilien′sis guyanen′sis**, *L. viannia guyanensis.*
**L. brazilien′sis panamen′sis**, *L. viannia panamensis.*
**L. donova′ni**, 1. a taxonomic complex comprising the subspecies causing varieties of visceral leishmaniasis: *L. d. donovani, L. d. infantum,* and *L. d. chagasi,* all of which multiply in the reticuloendothelial cells and spread to the lymph nodes and then hematogenously throughout the body. The subspecies can be distinguished only by differences in the epidemiology, clinical features, and response to treatment. 2. *L. d. donovani.*
**L. donova′ni chaga′si**, a subspecies of the *L. donovani* complex causing American visceral leishmaniasis, usually transmitted by the sandfly *Lutzomyia longipalpis.*
**L. donova′ni donova′ni**, a subspecies of the *L. donovani* complex causing Indian visceral leishmaniasis. It is transmitted by the sandfly *Phlebotomus argentipes,* with humans being the only major reservoir hosts. Called also *L. donovani.*
**L. donova′ni infan′tum**, a subspecies of the *L. donovani* complex causing infantile visceral leishmaniasis in the Mediterranean littoral (usual vectors *Phlebotomus perniciosus* and *P. major*), Middle East (usual vectors *P. papatasi* and *P. caucasicus*), sub-Saharan and East Africa (usual vectors *P. orientalis* and *P. martini*), and China (usual vectors *P. chinensis* and *P. sergenti*). Called also *L. infantum.*
**L. garnha′mi**, a species similar to (or identical with) *L. mexicana amazonensis* isolated from cases of cutaneous leishmaniasis in the region of the Venezuelan Andes.
**L. infan′tum**, *L. donovani infantum.*
**L. ma′jor**, a species of the *L. tropica* complex, transmitted by *Phlebotomus papatasi,* usually causing rural cutaneous leishmaniasis and sometimes causing viscerotropic cutaneous leishmaniasis. Called also *L. tropica major.*
**L. mexica′na**, a taxonomic complex comprising the species and subspecies causing New World cutaneous leishmaniasis in humans: *L. m. mexicana, L. m. amazonensis,* and *L. pifanoi,* which infect chiefly forest rodents and opossums. They develop only in the midgut and foregut of their sandfly vectors.
**L. mexica′na amazonen′sis**, a subspecies of the *L. mexicana* complex, transmitted by *Lutzomyia flaviscutellata,* and causing a form of New World cutaneous leishmaniasis in the Amazon region of Brazil and neighboring countries and in Trinidad. A single lesion is usually present but a few cases of diffuse cutaneous leishmaniasis caused by *L. m. mexicana* have been reported.
**L. mexica′na mexica′na**, a subspecies of the *L. mexicana* complex transmitted by *Lutzomyia olmeca* and causing chiclero ulcer.
**L. mexica′na pi′fanoi**, *L. pifanoi.*
**L. nilo′tica**, *L. tropica,* def. 2.
**L. peruvia′na**, *L. viannia peruviana.*
**L. pi′fanoi**, a species of the *L. mexicana* complex causing diffuse cutaneous leishmaniasis in Venezuela and certain areas of Brazil. Called also *L. mexicana pifanoi.*
**L. tro′pica**, 1. a taxonomic complex comprising the species causing Old World cutaneous leishmaniasis: *L. tropica, L. major,* and *L. aethiopica.* The species can be differentiated on ecologic, biochemical, and serologic grounds. 2. a species of the *L. tropica* complex causing dry cutaneous leishmaniasis. It is found in Iran, Iraq, and India, transmitted by *Phlebotomus sergenti;* and in southern France, Italy, and certain Mediterranean islands, transmitted by *P. papatasi.* Human to human transmission may also occur. Called also *L. nilotica, L. tropica minor,* and *L. tropica tropica.*
**L. tro′pica aethio′pica**, *L. aethiopica.*
**L. tro′pica ma′jor**, *L. major.*
**L. tro′pica mi′nor**, *L. tropica,* def. 2.
**L. tro′pica tro′pica**, *L. tropica,* def. 2.
**L. vian′nia**, a taxonomic complex comprising the subspecies that cause mucocutaneous leishmaniasis in its various forms; all of the subspecies develop in the midgut, foregut, and hindgut of their sandfly vectors. Formerly called *L. brasiliensis* or *L. braziliensis.*
**L. vian′nia brazilien′sis**, a subspecies of the *L. viannia* complex, transmitted by species of *Lutzomyia* and *Psychodopygus,* and causing cutaneous and mucocutaneous leishmaniasis in Brazil, Peru, Ecuador, Bolivia, Venezuela, Paraguay, and Columbia. Called also *L. braziliensis.*
**L. vian′nia guyanen′sis**, a subspecies of the *L. viannia* complex, transmitted chiefly by *Lutzomyia umbratilis* and causing pian bois (forest yaws).
**L. vian′nia panamen′sis**, a subspecies of the *L. viannia* complex, transmitted chiefly by *Lutzomyia trapidoi* and causing New World cutaneous leishmaniasis in Panama and adjacent areas of Central America and Colombia.
**L. vian′nia peruvia′na**, a subspecies of the *L. viannia* complex, found in the Peruvian Andes only at altitudes of 900 to 3000 meters, probably transmitted by *Lutzomyia verrucarum* and *L. peruensis* and causing uta in humans. Called also *L. peruviana.*

**leish·ma·nia** (lēsh-ma′ne-ə) [MeSH: Leishmania] 1. any protozoan of the genus *Leishmania.* 2. see *amastigote.*

**leish·ma·ni·al** (lēsh-ma′ne-əl) 1. pertaining to or caused by leishmanias. 2. denoting a morphologic stage in the life cycle of trypanosomatid protozoa; see *amastigote.*

**leish·ma·ni·a·sis** (lēsh″mə-ni′ə-sis) [MeSH: Leishmaniasis] infection caused by *Leishmania;* the principal classification is into cutaneous, mucocutaneous, and visceral types.
**American l.**, see *New World cutaneous l.* and *American visceral l.*
**anergic l.**, diffuse cutaneous l.
**canine l.**, infantile visceral l.
**cutaneous l.**, an endemic disease characterized by the development of a cutaneous papule that evolves into a nodule, breaks down to form an indolent ulcer, and heals, leaving a depressed scar. A distinction is made between varieties found in Asia and Africa that are caused by *Leishmania major, L. tropica,* or *L. aethiopica* (see *Old World cutaneous leishmaniasis*) and varieties found in Central and South America that are caused by *L. mexicana* or *L. viannia* (see *New World cutaneous leishmaniasis*).
**cutaneous l., anergic**, diffuse cutaneous l.
**cutaneous l., diffuse**, a rare chronic form of cutaneous leishmaniasis caused by *Leishmania aethiopica* in Ethiopia and Kenya, by *L. pifanoi* in Venezuela, and by protozoa of the *L. viannia* and *L. mexicana* complexes in South and Central America, respectively. It is characterized by the local and hematogenous spread from a primary lesion to produce generalized nodular lesions resembling those of lepromatous leprosy in the skin and sometimes involving the nasal mucosa and laryngopharynx. Individuals with this form of the disease do not develop an effective immune response to the infection. Called also *anergic l.* and *anergic cutaneous l.*
**cutaneous l., dry**, a type of Old World cutaneous leishmaniasis found mainly in large urban areas in the Middle East, the Mediterranean region, and the Indian subcontinent, caused by *Leishmania tropica* and transmitted by the vectors *Phlebotomus sergenti* and *P. papatasi.* The reservoir may be either human or canine. A slowly developing single lesion that persists for a year or more is typical. Called also *urban cutaneous l.*
**cutaneous l., Ethiopian**, a form of Old World cutaneous leishmaniasis seen in the highlands of Kenya and Ethiopia, caused by *Leishmania aethiopica;* reservoirs are hyraxes of the genera *Procavia, Heterohyrax,* and the vectors are *Phlebotomus pedifer* and *P. longipes.* Lesions are less inflamed and more chronic than those of other Old World forms, and generally last for several years; the condition is usually self-limited but may develop into diffuse cutaneous leishmaniasis.
**cutaneous l., New World**, any of the types of cutaneous leishmaniasis occurring in South America, Central America, or Mexico, zoonoses caused by species or subspecies of the *Leishmania mexicana* or *L. viannia* groups. Their lesions develop and heal similarly

to those of the Old World forms but tend to be less nodular and more ulcerative and destructive. Many varieties exist, differing as to animal reservoir, vector, geographical distribution, and clinical and other characteristics; some common forms are mucocutaneous leishmaniasis, chicle or chiclero ulcer, uta, and pian bois. Called also *American cutaneous l.*

**cutaneous l., Old World,** any of the types of cutaneous leishmaniasis occurring in Asia, Africa, or the Mediterranean basin; three separate types are distinguished according to the causative organism: *dry* or *urban cutaneous leishmaniasis* is caused by *Leishmania tropica; wet* or *rural cutaneous leishmaniasis* is caused by *L. major;* and *Ethiopian cutaneous leishmaniasis* is caused by *L. aethiopica.* It has received many names, often according to the locality of its occurrence (see under *boil*).

**cutaneous l., rural,** wet cutaneous l.

**cutaneous l., urban,** dry cutaneous l.

**cutaneous l., viscerotropic,** a rare type of infection found in northeastern Saudi Arabia; after infection with *Leishmania major,* instead of the usual cutaneous symptoms, fever and other systemic symptoms are seen and *Leishmania* can be detected in internal organs.

**cutaneous l., wet,** a type of Old World cutaneous leishmaniasis found mainly in rural areas in parts of the Middle East, central Asia, and the Indian subcontinent, caused by *Leishmania major;* its reservoirs are desert rodents such as ground squirrels and gerbils (particularly *Rhombomys opimus* and *Meriones* species) and it spreads to humans via the vector *Phlebotomus papatasi.* Infection is acute, rapidly evolving, and characterized by multiple sores with inflammation, ulceration, and crusting. Called also *rural cutaneous l.*

**mucocutaneous l.,** chronic, progressive metastatic spread of the lesions of New World cutaneous leishmaniasis caused by *Leishmania viannia braziliensis* to the nasal, pharyngeal, and buccal mucosa months to years after the appearance of the initial cutaneous lesion, which has usually healed. It is often associated with mutilating destruction of the nasal septum, palate, lips, pharynx, and larynx. Called also *espundia.*

**post–kala-azar dermal l.,** a condition associated with visceral leishmaniasis, commonly characterized by the appearance of hypopigmented or erythematous macules on the face and sometimes on the extremities and trunk; the facial lesions gradually progress to papules or nodules that resemble those of lepromatous leprosy. It is seen in about 20% of Indian patients, usually occurring years after the treatment of or spontaneous recovery from visceral leishmaniasis, and it may last for as long as 20 years. When the condition affects patients in East Africa (2%) and China (rare), it usually occurs shortly after or during treatment and usually does not persist. Called also *dermal leishmanoid, leishmanoid,* and *post–kala-azar dermal leishmanoid.*

**l. reci'divans,** a relapsing form of either wet or dry cutaneous leishmaniasis, resembling tuberculosis of the skin, in which the ulcer heals incompletely, scarring centrally but spreading peripherally, or heals and recrudesces at the edge of the scar; it may last for many years.

**rural l.,** wet cutaneous l.

**urban l.,** dry cutaneous l.

**visceral l.,** a chronic infectious disease, highly fatal if untreated, caused by *Leishmania donovani donovani, L. d. infantum,* and *L. d. chagasi,* found in various tropical and subtropical regions of the world; parasites are found in the cells of the reticuloendothelial system throughout the body, especially in the liver, spleen, bone marrow, lymph nodes, and skin. It is commonly characterized by hepatosplenomegaly, irregular fever, chills, vomiting, emaciation, anemia, leukopenia, hypergammaglobulinemia, and an earth-gray color of the skin. It has traditionally been divided into three different forms according to geographical distribution, vector, and other factors, but such a distinction may prove to be invalid. See *American visceral l., infantile visceral l.,* and *Indian visceral l.* Called also *kala-azar, tropical splenomegaly,* and *black, cachectic, cachexial,* or *Dumdum fever.*

**visceral l., American,** a variety seen in South America, Central America, and Mexico, caused by *Leishmania donovani chagasi,* and affecting humans of any age. Its major reservoirs are dogs and the usual vector is the sandfly *Lutzomyia longipalpis.*

**visceral l., Indian,** a form caused by *Leishmania donovani donovani,* usually affecting older children or young adults; humans are the only reservoir hosts and it is transmitted by the sandfly *Phlebotomus argentipes.* It occurs primarily in eastern India and Bangladesh. Called also *classic visceral l.*

**visceral l., infantile,** a form caused by *Leishmania donovani infantum,* usually affecting children between ages 1 and 4; reservoirs are dogs, foxes, jackals, and rodents, and vectors are species of *Phlebotomus* sandflies. It occurs in the Mediterranean region, sub-Saharan and East Africa, the Middle East, and China. Called also *Mediterranean visceral l.*

**visceral l., Mediterranean,** infantile visceral l.

**leish·man·i·ci·dal** (lēsh″mən-ī-si′dəl) destructive to *Leishmania.*

**leish·man·id** (lēsh′mən-īd) the early cutaneous nodule of cutaneous leishmaniasis.

**leish·ma·nin** (lēsh′mə-nin) a suspension of killed leishmania promastigotes; used in a skin test for cutaneous leishmaniasis (see *leishmanin test,* under *tests*).

**leish·ma·noid** (lēsh′mə-noid) 1. like or resembling leishmaniasis. 2. a lesion of post-kala-azar dermal leishmaniasis.

**dermal l., post–kala-azar dermal l.,** post–kala-azar dermal leishmaniasis.

**Lek·sell apparatus, technique** (lek′səl) [Lars *Leksell,* Swedish neurosurgeon, 20th century] see under *apparatus* and *technique.*

**Le·laps** (le′laps) *Echinolaelaps.*

**le·ma** (le′mə) [Gr. *lēmē*] sebum palpebrale.

**Lem·bert's suture** (lahm-bārz′) [Antoine *Lembert,* French surgeon, 1802–1851] see under *suture.*

**Le·mierre syndrome** (lə-myer′) [André *Lemierre,* French physician, born 1875] see under *syndrome.*

**Le·mi·eux-Nee·meh syndrome** (lə-myoo͞′ na′ma) [Guy *Lemieux,* Canadian physician, 20th century; Jean A. *Neemeh,* Canadian physician, 20th century] see under *syndrome.*

**lem·ma** (lem′ə) [Gr. "rind," "husk"] a collective term for the three egg membranes.

**-lemma** a word termination denoting a sheath around another structure.

**lem·mo·blast** (lem′o-blast) a primordial or immature lemmocyte.

**lem·mo·blas·tic** (lem″o-blas′tik) forming or developing into neurilemma tissue.

**lem·mo·cyte** (lem′o-sīt) [*lemma* + *-cyte*] a cell derived from the neural crest and developing into a cell of the neurilemma.

**lem·nis·ci** (lem-nis′i) plural of *lemniscus.*

**lem·nis·cus** (lem-nis′kəs) gen. and pl. *lemnis′ci* [L., from Gr. *lēmniskos* ribbon] 1. a ribbon or band. 2. [TA] a band or bundle of sensory fibers in the central nervous system; called also *fillet.* See also *bundle, fasciculus, tract,* and *tractus.*

**l. latera′lis** [TA], lateral lemniscus: a tract of longitudinal fibers extending upward through the lateral part of the tegmental substance of the pons, formed chiefly by fibers arising from the opposite cochlear nuclei and the trapezoid body, and ascending to terminate in the inferior colliculus and medial geniculate body.

**l. media′lis** [TA], medial lemniscus: a tract arising from the internal arcuate fibers of the nuclei gracilis and cuneatus, and crossing to the opposite side in the lower part of medulla oblongata to ascend, first between the two olives, and then through the pars dorsalis pontis just dorsal to the pontine nuclei; it continues through the tegmentum of the midbrain and ends in the ventral posterior part of the thalamus. Each lemniscus carries sensory impulses from the opposite side of the body. Called also *sensory l.*

**sensory l.,** l. medialis.

**l. spina′lis** [TA], spinal lemniscus: the part of each spinothalamic tract within the pons and mesencephalon, forming a diffuse bundle between the medial and lateral lemnisci. It carries pain, temperature, and tactile impulses from the opposite side of the body and ends in the ventral posterior part of the thalamus. Called also *tractus anterolaterales, anterolateral tracts,* and *anterolateral system.*

**l. trigemina′lis** [TA], trigeminal lemniscus: a group of fibers conveying sensory impulses from the trigeminal nuclei to the ventral posterior part of the opposite thalamus; it ascends intermingled with the spinal lemniscus and adjacent medial lemniscus. Called also *tractus trigeminothalamicus* [TA alternative] and *trigeminothalamic tract.*

**lem·on** (lem′ən) 1. *Citrus limon.* 2. the fruit of *C. limon,* which contains citric and ascorbic acids and whose peel contains lemon oil, a volatile oil used as a flavoring agent.

**Lem·pert's fenestration operation** (lem′pərts) [Julius *Lempert,* American otologist, 1890–1968] see under *operation.*

**LEMS** Lambert-Eaton myasthenic syndrome; see *Eaton-Lambert syndrome,* under *syndrome.*

**lem′ur** (lem′ər) [MeSH: Lemur] any member of the family Lemuridae.

**Le·mu·ri·dae** (lĕ-mu′rĭ-de) [MeSH: Lemuridae] the lemurs, a family of small, arboreal, usually nocturnal primates native to Madagascar and nearby islands; they resemble monkeys but have a sharp, foxlike muzzle and a tail that is long, furry, and never prehensile.

**Le·nè·gre's disease** (lə-neg′rəz) [Jean *Lenègre,* French cardiologist, born 1904] see under *disease.*

**length** (length) an expression of the longest dimension of an object, or of the measurement between the two ends. Symbol *l.*

**arch l.,** the length of a line segment within the median plane perpendicular to and extending from the line connecting the first premolars to the most labial point on the anterior arch, usually to the point between the maxillary central incisors. Called also *anterior arch l.*
**basialveolar l.,** the distance from the basion to the lower end of the intermaxillary suture.
**basinasal l.,** the distance from basion to nasion.
**crown-heel l. (CHL),** the length of an embryo, fetus, or infant from the crown of the head to the heel; used in estimating the age of the embryos during the eighth week and of fetuses. It is the equivalent of *standing height* in older individuals.
**crown-rump l. (CRL),** the length of an embryo, fetus, or infant from the crown of the head to the breech; used in estimating the age of embryos from the fourth to the eighth week. It is the equivalent of *sitting vertex height* in older individuals.
**focal l.,** the distance between a lens and an object from which all rays of light are brought to a focus. Symbol f.
**foot l.,** a heel-toe measurement useful in estimating the age of fetuses because the foot dimensions are less subject to artifacts of curvature and shrinkage than is the fetus as a whole.
**greatest l.,** a dimension used to express the size of very young embryos that have not yet developed the structures permitting measurement of crown-rump length, as during the third and early fourth weeks.
**sitting l.,** the distance from the crown of the head to the coccyx.
**stem l.,** the distance from the vertex to a line joining the ischial tuberosities.
**wave l.,** see *wavelength.*

**len·i·quin·sin** (len″ĭ-kwin′sin) chemical name: *N*-[(3,4-dimethoxyphenyl) methylene]-6,7-dimethoxy-4-quinolinamine; an antihypertensive, $C_{20}H_{20}N_2O_4$.

**len·i·tive** (len′ĭ-tiv) [L. *lenire* to soothe] 1. demulcent or soothing. 2. a demulcent remedy.

**Len·nert's classification, lymphoma** (len′ərts) [K. *Lennert,* German pathologist, 20th century] see *Kiel Classification* under *classification* and see under *lymphoma.*

**Lenn·hoff's index, sign** (len′hofs) [Rudolf *Lennhoff,* German physician, 1866–1933] see under *index* and *sign.*

**Len·nox syndrome** (len′əks) [William Gordon *Lennox,* American neurologist, 1884–1960] Lennox-Gastaut syndrome.

**Len·nox-Gas·taut syndrome** (len′əks-gahs-to′) [W. G. *Lennox;* Henri Jean Pascal *Gastaut,* French biologist, born 1915] see under *syndrome.*

**lens** (lenz) [L. "lentil"] 1. a piece of glass or other transparent substance so shaped as to converge or scatter the rays of light, especially the glass used in appropriate frames or other instruments to increase the visual acuity of the human eye. See also *glasses* and *spectacles.* 2. [TA] the transparent biconvex body of the eye situated between the posterior chamber and the vitreous body, constituting part of the refracting mechanism of the eye. Called also *l. crystallina* or *crystalline l.*

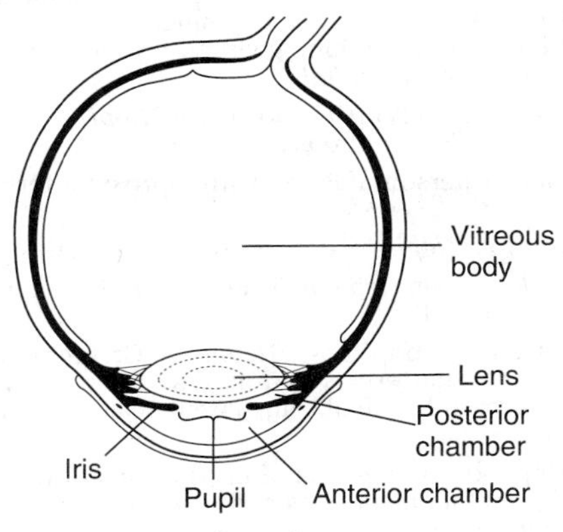

Lens of eye.

**achromatic l.,** one corrected for chromatic aberration.
**acrylic l.,** a plastic lens used to replace the crystalline lens after cataract surgery.
**adherent l.,** contact l.
**anastigmatic l.,** a lens with spherical surfaces only and no cylindrical ones; called also *stigmatic l.*
**aniseikonic l.,** iseikonic l.
**aplanatic l.,** one that serves to correct spherical aberration and coma.
**apochromatic l.,** one corrected for chromatic and spherical aberration.
**astigmatic l.,** cylindrical l.
**bandage l.,** a soft contact lens worn on a diseased or injured cornea to protect or treat it.
**biconcave l.,** a flat lens that has both surfaces concave; called also *concavoconcave l.*
**biconvex l.,** a flat lens that has both surfaces convex.
**bicylindrical l.,** one that has both surfaces cylindrical or toroidal.
**bifocal l.,** a lens made up of two segments with different refractive powers, ordinarily with the upper for far and the lower segment for near vision; see under *glasses.*
**bispherical l.,** one that is spherical on both sides.
**Brücke l.,** a combination of a double convex and double concave lens so arranged as to give considerable working distance.
**cataract l.,** a powerful lens for glasses to be used after cataract operation.
**compound l.,** a lens made up of two or more segments.
**concave l.,** a lens with one or both (biconcave) surfaces curved like a section of the interior of a hollow sphere; it diverges the rays of light. Called also *diverging l.* and *minus l.*
**concavoconcave l.,** biconcave l.
**concavoconvex l.,** one that has one concave surface and one convex; the concave surface is of greater curvature than the convex. Called also *periscopic convex l., converging meniscus l.,* and *positive meniscus l.*
**condensing l.,** a large, powerful convex spherical lens to focus available light upon the eye for examination.
**contact l.,** a curved shell of glass or plastic applied directly over the globe or cornea to correct refractive errors; called also *adherent l.*
**contact l., corneal,** one that rests on the cornea, not on the sclera, and requires no auxiliary liquid; called also *corneal l.*
**contact l., gas permeable,** any contact lens that transmits oxygen and carbon dioxide.
**contact l., hard,** a contact lens that maintains its shape without support and absorbs little or no water; it may be gas permeable or non–gas permeable. Called also *hydrophobic contact l.* or *rigid contact l.*
**contact l., hydrophilic,** soft contact l.
**contact l., hydrophobic, contact l., rigid,** hard contact l.
**contact l., non–gas permeable hard,** a contact lens, generally formed of polymethyl methacrylate, that transmits little to no oxygen and carbon dioxide to the cornea. Called also *PMMA contact l.*
**contact l., PMMA,** a contact lens made of polymethyl methacrylate; see *non–gas permeable contact l.*
**contact l., scleral,** a contact lens covering the cornea and resting on the sclera, with or without an auxiliary liquid between the lens and the cornea.
**contact l., soft,** a contact lens that when worn is soft, flexible, and water absorbent; called also *hydrophilic contact l.*
**converging l., convex l.,** a lens curved like a section of the exterior of a hollow sphere; it brings light to a focus. Called also *plus l.*
**convexoconcave l.,** one that has one convex and one concave surface; the convex surface is of greater curvature than the concave. Called also *periscopic concave l., diverging meniscus l.,* and *negative meniscus l.*
**corneal l.,** corneal contact l.
**Crookes' l.,** one made from glass rendered opaque to ultraviolet and infrared rays but transparent to visible light.
**crossed l.,** a converging lens with minimal spherical aberration.
**l. crystalli′na, crystalline l.,** the lens of the eye; see *lens,* def. 2.
**cylindrical l.,** a lens used to correct astigmatism, having one plane surface and one cylindrical, or one spherical surface and one toroidal. The meridian along the lens axis has no refractive power, but the meridian at right angles to the axis has maximum refractive power; thus the principal focus is a straight line, not a point. Symbol C. Abbreviated cyl. Called also *astigmatic l.*
**decentered l.,** one in which the optical axis does not pass through the geometric center.
**dispersing l.,** an incorrect name for *concave l.* (diverging l.).
**diverging l.,** concave l.
**flat l.,** a lens with equal curvature on both sides, as opposed to a meniscus lens.
**Fresnel l.,** a thin lens made up of a number of stepped setbacks concentrically arranged; it has the optical properties of a much thicker lens.
**honey bee l.,** a magnifying eyeglass lens designed to resemble the multifaceted eye of the honeybee. It consists of three or six small telescopes mounted in the upper portion of the spectacles and directed toward the center and right and left visual fields. Prisms are included to provide a continuous, unbroken magnified field of view.
**immersion l.,** see under *objective.*
**iseikonic l.,** a lens that magnifies but does not refract; it is used to treat aniseikonia because it changes the sizes of the images on the retinas of the eyes. Called also *aniseikonic l.* and *size l.*
**meniscus l.,** a crescent-shaped lens with one concave surface and

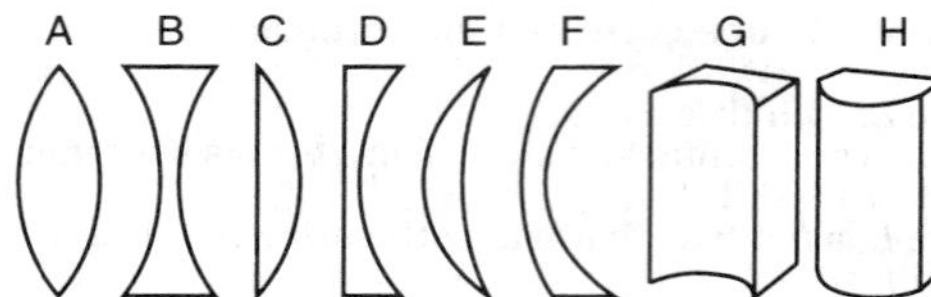


Lenses: *(A–F),* Spherical lenses: *(A),* biconvex; *(B),* biconcave; *(C),* planoconvex; *(D),* planoconcave; *(E),* concavoconvex, periscopic convex, converging meniscus; *(F),* convexoconcave, periscopic concave, diverging meniscus; *(G, H),* cylindrical lenses, concave and convex.

one convex; the surfaces have different degrees of curvature. See *concavoconvex l.* and *convexoconcave l.*
**meniscus l., converging,** concavoconvex l.
**meniscus l., diverging,** convexoconcave l.
**meniscus l., negative,** convexoconcave l.
**meniscus l., positive,** concavoconvex l.
**meter l.,** a converging lens with a focal length of one meter and a refracting power of one diopter.
**minus l.,** concave l.
**omnifocal l.,** a lens the power of which increases continuously and regularly in a downward direction, thereby avoiding the discontinuity in field and power which is apparent in bifocal and trifocal lenses.
**orthoscopic l.,** one that gives a very flat and undistorted field of vision, especially at the periphery.
**periscopic l.,** one with a 1.25D base curve.
**periscopic concave l.,** convexoconcave l.
**periscopic convex l.,** concavoconvex l.
**photochromic l., photosensitive l.,** a light-sensitive lens that darkens in full light and clears in reduced light.
**plane l., plano l.,** a lens with no curve and no refracting power; light rays enter and leave parallel.
**planoconcave l.,** a lens with one plane and one concave side.
**planoconvex l.,** a lens with one plane and one convex side.
**plus l.,** convex l.
**punktal l.,** a toric lens which is corrected for astigmatism over the entire field of vision.
**safety l.,** one that protects the eyes from injury, especially from impact. Impact-resistant lenses may be made by tempering or by using plastic or laminated lenses. Called also *safety glasses.*
**size l.,** iseikonic l.
**spherical l.,** one that is a segment of a sphere. Abbreviated S or Sph. See illustration.
**spherocylindrical l.,** a lens with one spherical and one cylindrical surface, and functioning as both a simple spherical lens and a simple cylindrical one.
**stigmatic l.,** anastigmatic l.
**toric l.,** a meniscus lens with a cylindrical curve ground on the outer, convex, surface.
**trial l.,** any one of a set of lenses used in testing the vision.
**trifocal l.,** a lens made up of three segments with different refractive powers, ordinarily with the upper for distant, the middle for intermediate, and the lower for near vision; see *trifocal glasses,* under *glasses.*

**lens·om·e·ter** (lenz-om′ə-tər) [*lens* + *-meter*] a device for measuring the optical characteristics of lenses; called also *phacometer.*

**Len·tard** (len′tərd) trademark for preparations of insulin zinc suspension.

**len·ti·cel** (len′tĭ-sel) a lens-shaped gland, especially one of those at the base of the tongue.

**len·ti·co·nus** (len″ti-ko′nəs) [*lens* + *conus*] a conical protrusion of the substance of the crystalline lens, covered by capsule or connective tissue, occurring more frequently on the posterior surface, and usually affecting only one eye.

**len·tic·u·la** (len-tik′u-lə) [L.] nucleus lentiformis.

**len·tic·u·lar** (len-tik′u-lər) [L. *lenticularis*] 1. pertaining to or shaped like a lens. 2. pertaining to the crystalline lens. 3. pertaining to the lenticular nucleus.

**len·tic·u·lo·op·tic** (len-tik″u-lo-op′tik) pertaining to the lenticular nucleus and the optic thalamus.

**len·tic·u·lo·stri·ate** (len-tik″u-lo-stri′āt) pertaining to the lenticular nucleus and the corpus striatum.

**len·tic·u·lo·tha·lam·ic** (len-tik″u-lo-thə-lam′ik) relating to the lenticular nucleus and the thalamus.

**len·ti·form** (len′tĭ-form) shaped like a lens; see under *bone* and *nucleus.*

**len·tig·i·nes** (len-tij′ĭ-nēz) [L.] plural of *lentigo.*

**len·tig·i·no·sis** (len-tij″ĭ-no′sis) the presence of multiple lentigines.
**progressive cardiomyopathic l.,** Moynahan's syndrome, def. 1.

**len·tig·i·nous** (len-tij′ĭ-nəs) characterized by multiple lentigines; pertaining to or of the nature of a lentigo.

**len·ti·glo·bus** (len″tĭ-glo′bəs) [*lens* + *globus*] an exaggerated curvation of the crystalline lens, producing a spherical bulging on its anterior surface.

**len·ti·go** (len-ti′go) pl. *lentig′ines* [L. "freckle"] [MeSH: Lentigo] a small, flat, tan to dark brown or black, macular melanosis on the skin resembling a freckle clinically but histologically distinct because of the presence of an increased number of normal-appearing melanocytes along the dermoepidermal junction. Lentigines do not darken on exposure to sunlight, as do freckles. Called also *l. simplex.*
**l. malig′na,** see under *melanoma.*
**nevoid l.,** a congenital lentigo involving the mucous membranes as well as the skin, occurring in association with various hereditary disorders, including the LEOPARD syndrome and Moynihan's syndrome, and characterized histologically by elongation of rete pegs, an increase in the number of melanocytes with formation of nests, an increase of melanin in both the melanocytes and basal keratinocytes, and melanophages in the upper dermis. Single or multiple lesions may occur, and size and configuration vary widely. Called also *l. simplex.*
**senile l., l. seni′lis,** a benign, discrete, hyperpigmented macule occurring on chronically sun-exposed skin in adults, especially on the back of the hands and on the forehead. Called also *liver spot* and *solar l.*
**l. sim′plex,** 1. lentigo. 2. nevoid l.
**solar l.,** senile l.

**Len·ti·vi·ri·nae** (len″tĭ-vir-i′ne) the HIV-like viruses: a former subfamily of viruses of the family Retroviridae, containing the genus *Lentivirus.*

**Len·ti·vi·rus** (len′tĭ-vi″rəs) [L. *lentus* slow + *virus*] [MeSH: Lentivirus] a genus of viruses of the family Retroviridae that cause persistent infection that typically results in chronic, progressive, usually fatal disease. It includes the human immunodeficiency viruses, simian immunodeficiency virus, feline immunodeficiency virus, maedi/visna virus, caprine arthritis-encephalitis virus, and equine infectious anemia virus.

**len·ti·vi·rus** (len′tĭ-vi″rəs) [MeSH: Lentivirus] any virus of the subfamily Lentivirinae.

**len·tu·la** (len′chu-lə) lentulo.

**len·tu·lo** (len′chu-lo, len-too′lo) in root canal therapy, a flexible, spiral, rotating instrument made of stainless steel wire attached to a handpiece, used to place cement into the prepared canal. Called also *lentula, lentulo paste carrier,* and *paste carrier.*

**Lenz's syndrome** (lent′səz) [Widukind D. *Lenz,* German physician, born 1919] see under *syndrome.*

**Leo's test** (la′ōz) [Hans *Leo,* German physician, 1854–1927] see under *test.*

**le·on·ti·a·sis** (le″on-ti′ə-sis) [Gr. *leōn* lion + *-iasis*] the leonine facies of lepromatous leprosy, due to nodular invasion of the subcutaneous tissue of the face, giving it a vaguely leonine appearance.
**l. os′sea, l. os′sium,** bilateral and symmetrical hypertrophy of the bones of the face and cranium, giving it a vaguely leonine appearance; called also *megalocephaly.*

**le·o·trop·ic** (le″o-trop′ik) [Gr. *laios* left + *-tropic*] running spirally from right to left. Cf. *dexiotropic.*

**lep·er** (lep′ər) a person afflicted with leprosy; a term now in disfavor.

**le·pid·ic** (lə-pid′ik) [*lepid-* + *-ic*] pertaining to scales.

**lepid(o)-** [Gr. *lepis,* gen. *lepidos* flake or scale] a combining form meaning scale or scaly.

**Lep·i·dop·tera** (lep″ĭ-dop′tər -ə) [*lepido-* + Gr. *pteron* wing] [MeSH: Lepidoptera] the butterflies and moths, an order of insects with large wings covered by small transparent scales. The larval form is the caterpillar.

**Lep·i·o·ta** (lep″e-o′tə) a genus of mushrooms of the family Agaricaceae. They contain amatoxins and can cause mushroom poisoning (see under *poisoning*).

**lepo·cyte** (lep′o-sīt) [Gr. *lepos* rind + *-cyte*] any nucleated cell having a cell wall.

**Lep·o·ri·pox·vi·rus** (lep″ə-rĭ-poks′vi-rəs) [L. *lepus,* gen. *leporis* hare + *poxvirus*] [MeSH: Leporipoxvirus] a genus of viruses of the subfamily Chordopoxvirinae (family Poxviridae) with serologic cross-reactivity that infect squirrels and rabbits, including myxoma virus and rabbit fibroma virus.

**lep·ra** (lep′rə) [Gr. *lepra* leprosy, which makes the skin scaly] leprosy; (prior to the mid 19th century) psoriasis. See also under *reaction.*

**lep·re·chaun·ism** (lep′rə-kon″iz-əm) a rare lethal familial condition marked by slow physical and mental development, the elfin facies suggested by the name (wide-set eyes, low-set ears, and hirsutism), and severe endocrine disorders such as enlargement of the clitoris and breasts in females and of the phallus in males. Called also *Donohue's syndrome.*

**lep·rid** (lep′rid) cutaneous lesion or lesions of tuberculoid leprosy, being hypopigmented or erythematous macules or plaques showing no evidence of *Mycobacterium leprae* by ordinary methods of examination. Cf. *leproma.*

**lep·ride** (lep′rēd) leprid.

**lep·rol·o·gist** (lep-rol′ə-jist) a physician experienced in the study and treatment of leprosy.

**lep·rol·o·gy** (lep-rol′ə-je) the study of leprosy.

**lep·ro·ma** (ləp-ro′mə) a superficial granulomatous nodule rich in *Mycobacterium leprae,* and the characteristic lesion of lepromatous leprosy. Cf. *leprid.*

**lep·ro·ma·tous** (ləp-ro′mə-təs) pertaining to lepromas; see *lepromatous leprosy,* under *leprosy.*

**lep·ro·min** (lep′ro-min) [MeSH: Lepromin] a purified homogenate of lepromatous skin nodules containing heat-killed *Mycobacterium leprae;* used in a skin test of immune status in leprosy (see *lepromin test,* under *tests*). Called also *Mitsuda antigen.*

**le·pro·sa·ri·um** (lep″ro-sar′e-əm) [L.] a hospital or colony for the treatment and isolation of leprosy patients.

**lep·ro·sary** (lep′ro-sar″e) [L. *leprosa′rium*] leprosarium.

**lep·ro·stat·ic** (lep″ro-stat′ik) 1. inhibiting the growth of *Mycobacterium leprae.* 2. an agent that inhibits the growth of *Mycobacterium leprae.*

**lep·ro·sy** (lep′rə-se) [Gr. *lepros* scaly, scabby, rough] [MeSH: Leprosy] a slowly progressive, chronic infectious disease caused by *Mycobacterium leprae* and characterized by the development of granulomatous or neurotrophic lesions in the skin, mucous membranes, nerves, bones, and viscera. It is manifested by a broad spectrum of clinical symptoms, consisting of two principal types, with the *lepromatous* type at one end of the spectrum and the *tuberculoid* type at the other; between these two polar types is the *borderline* type, with two subtypes, *borderline tuberculoid* and *borderline lepromatous.* See also *lepra reaction,* under *reaction,* and *lepromin test,* under *test.* Called also *Hansen's disease.*
**borderline l.,** an immunologically unstable form of leprosy transitional between the tuberculoid and lepromatous forms and having clinical and histological features of both types, which may evolve toward the former by reversal reactions or toward the latter by a downgrading reaction. Called also *dimorphous l.* and *intermediate l.*
**borderline lepromatous l.,** see *borderline l.*
**borderline tuberculoid l.,** see *borderline l.*
**bovine l.,** Johne's disease.
**diffuse l. of Lucio,** Lucio's l.
**dimorphous l.,** borderline l.
**feline l.,** a granulomatous skin condition in cats, characterized by nodules that ulcerate and drain, usually on the legs or head; it may be associated with infection by *Mycobacterium lepraemurium,* such as from contact with infected rodents.
**indeterminate l.,** a frequent early manifestation of leprosy, consisting of a single or few poorly defined anesthetic or hypoanesthetic, hypopigmented or erythematous, histologically uncharacteristic macules in exposed areas of the skin, which may heal spontaneously or progress and evolve into one of the more definitive forms.
**intermediate l.,** borderline l.
**lazarine l.,** Lucio's l.
**lepromatous l.,** the most malignant and infectious polar type of leprosy, characterized principally by widespread dissemination of leprosy bacilli in the tissues, reflecting the poor immune response to infection, and by cutaneous lesions mainly consisting of numerous pale, diffusely and symmetrically distributed macules that if untreated gradually progress to form plaques, nodules (lepromas), and infiltrations, resulting in destructive lesions and deformities; nerve involvement is seen in advanced disease.
**Lucio's l.,** a form characterized by diffuse lepromatous infiltration of the skin occurring especially in Latin America, particularly in Costa Rica and Mexico. Advanced cases may be complicated by a reactional state *(Lucio's phenomenon)* in which multiple areas of obstructive vasculitis cause dermal necrosis with resultant ulcers that heal with scarring. Called also *diffuse l. of Lucio* and *lazarine l.*
**murine l.,** rat l.
**rat l.,** a chronic epizootic disease of wild rats caused by *Mycobacterium lepraemurium,* characterized by lesions containing enormous numbers of acid-fast bacilli closely resembling *M. leprae* in size and shape, which may be transmitted to white rats, mice, and guinea pigs by inoculation of infected tissue; a relationship with human leprosy has not been established. Called also *murine l.*
**reactional l.,** see *lepra reaction,* under *reaction.*
**tuberculoid l.,** the relatively benign, least infectious, and usually self-limited polar type of leprosy in which, as a result of well-developed cell-mediated immunity to *Mycobacterium leprae,* acid-fast bacilli usually cannot be identified in the lesions. It is characterized by early severe damage to the nerves and by the presence of one to a few typically asymmetric, sharply defined, anesthetic, hypopigmented or erythematous macules or plaques with elevated borders and dry, rough surfaces (leprids).
**uncharacteristic l.,** indeterminate l.

**lep·rot·ic** (ləp-rot′ik) pertaining to or affected with leprosy.

**lep·rous** (lep′rəs) [L. *leprosus*] afflicted with leprosy.

**lep·ta·zol** (lep′tə-zol) (Brit.) pentylenetetrazol.

**lep·tin** (lep′tin) a hormone secreted by adipocytes in laboratory animals and humans, thought to be an appetite suppressant.

**lept(o)-** [Gr. *leptos* slender] a combining form meaning slender, thin, or delicate.

**lep·to·ce·phal·ic** (lep″to-sə-fal′ik) characterized by leptocephaly.

**lep·to·ceph·a·lous** (lep″to-sef′ə-ləs) leptocephalic.

**lep·to·ceph·a·lus** (lep″to-sef′ə-ləs) [*lepto-* + *-cephalus*] a person with an abnormally tall, narrow skull.

**lep·to·ceph·a·ly** (lep″to-sef′ə-le) abnormal tallness and narrowness of the skull.

**lep·to·chro·mat·ic** (lep″to-kro-mat′ik) [*lepto-* + *chromatin*] having a fine chromatin network.

**Lep·to·ci·mex** (lep″to-si′meks) *Cimex.*

**Lep·to·co·nops** (lep″to-ko′nops) a genus of blood-sucking flies of the family Heleidae.

**lep·to·cyte** (lep′to-sīt) [*lepto-* + *-cyte*] target cell (def. 1).

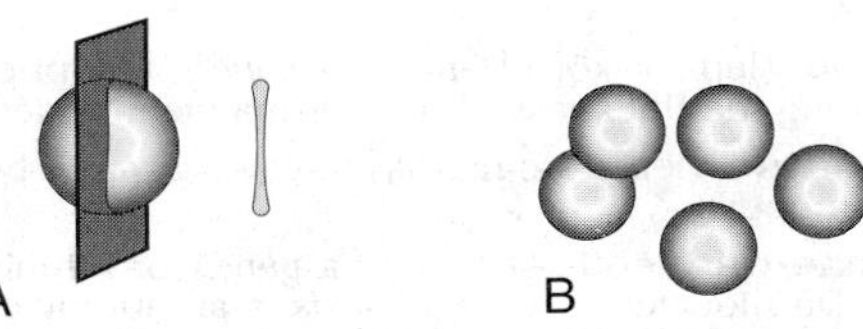


*(A),* Cross-section through a leptocyte, showing its thinness; *(B),* leptocytes.

**lep·to·cy·to·sis** (lep″to-si-to′sis) the presence of target cells (leptocytes) in the blood.

**lep·to·dac·ty·lous** (lep″to-dak′tə-ləs) [*lepto-* + *dactyl* + *-ous*] possessing slender digits.

**lep·to·dac·ty·ly** (lep″to-dak′tə-le) abnormal slenderness of the digits.

**lep·to·don·tous** (lep″to-don′təs) [*lepto-* + *odont-* + *-ous*] having slender teeth.

**lep·to·kur·tic** (lep″to-kər′tik) [*lepto-* + Gr. *kurtos* convex] pertaining to a probability distribution more heavily concentrated around the mean, i.e., having a sharper, narrower peak, than the normal distribution with the same variance. Cf. *platykurtic.*

**lep·to·me·nin·ge·al** (lep″to-mə-nin′je-əl) pertaining to the leptomeninges.

**lep·to·me·nin·ges** (lep″to-mə-nin′jēz) sing. *leptome′ninx* [*lepto-* + *meninges*] [TA] the pia mater and arachnoid considered together as one functional unit; the pia-arachnoid.

**lep·to·me·nin·gi·o·ma** (lep″to-mə-nin″je-o′mə) a tumor of the leptomeninges.

**lep·to·me·nin·gi·tis** (lep″to-men″in-ji′tis) [*leptomeninges* + *-itis*] inflammation of the leptomeninges.
**sarcomatous l.,** diffuse sarcomatous infiltration of the pia mater.

**lep·to·men·in·gop·a·thy** (lep″to-men″in-gop′ə-the) [*leptomeninges* + *-pathy*] any disease of the leptomeninges.

**lep·to·men·inx** (lep″to-men′inks) [*lepto-* + *meninx*] [TA] singular of leptomeninges. NOTE: In official nomenclature, this term is used as the preferred term when contrasting this structure (arachnoidea mater et pia mater) with the pachymeninx, which is equivalent to the dura mater.

**lep·to·mo·nad** (lep″to-mo′nad) [*lepto-* + *monad*] 1. pertaining to the genus *Leptomonas.* 2. denoting a morphologic stage in the development of certain trypanosomatid protozoa; see *promastigote.* 3. leptomonas.

**Lep·to·mo·nas** (lep″to-mo′nəs) [*lepto-* + Gr. *monas* unit, from *monos* single] a genus of parasitic protozoa (suborder Trypanosomatina, order Kinetoplastida) found in the digestive tract of various insects, and characterized by having an elongate body with a relatively large nucleus near the center and a long thin flagellum arising from a blepharoplast and a kinetoplast near the anterior end. During their life cycle the organisms pass through promastigote and amastigote stages.

**lep·to·mo·nas** (lep″to-mo′nəs) 1. any protozoan of the genus *Leptomonas.* 2. see *promastigote.*

**Lep·to·myx·i·da** (lep″to-mik′si-də) [*lepto-* + Gr. *myxa* mucus] an order of ameboid protozoa (class Acarpomyxea, superclass Rhizopoda) typically occurring in thin protoplasmic sheets that are sometimes polyaxial and sometimes cylindrical. Representative genera include *Leptomyxa* and *Rhizamoeba.*

**lep·to·ne·ma** (lep″to-ne′mə) [*lepto-* + Gr. *nēma* thread] a presynaptic stage of meiosis in which the chromatin is in the form of fine spireme threads.

**lep·to·no·mor·phol·o·gy** (lep″to-no-mor-fol′ə-je) the morphology of membranes.

**lep·to·pel·lic** (lep″to-pel′ik) [*lepto-* + Gr. *pella* bowl] having a narrow pelvis.

**lep·to·pho·nia** (lep″to-fo′ne-ə) [*lepto-* + *phon-* + *-ia*] hypophonia.

**lep·top·ro·sope** (lep-top′ro-sōp) an individual exhibiting leptoprosopia.

**lep·to·pro·so·pia** (lep″to-pro-so′pe-ə) [*lepto-* + *prosop-* + *-ia*] narrowness of the face, with slender features, round, open orbits, long nose, narrow nostrils, and small mouth.

**lep·to·pro·so·pic** (lep″to-pro-so′pik) pertaining to or characterized by leptoprosopia.

**Lep·to·psyl·la** (lep″to-səl′ə) a genus of fleas. *L. seg′nis* (also called *L. mus′culi*) is a common flea of the mouse and rat and a vector of plague.

**lep·tor·rhine** (lep′to-rīn) [*lepto-* + Gr. *rhis* nose] having a nasal index below 48.

**lep·to·scope** (lep′to-skōp) [*lepto-* + *-scope*] an optical apparatus for measuring the thickness of the plasma membrane of a cell.

**lep·to·so·mat·ic** (lep″to-so-mat′ik) [*lepto-* + *somatic* body] having a light, thin body.

**Lep·to·sphae·ria** (lep″to-sfe′re-ə) a genus of bitunicate fungi of the order Dothideales. *L. senegalen′sis* is an etiologic agent of eumycotic mycetoma in West Africa.

**Lep·to·spi·ra** (lep″to-spi′rə) [*lepto-* + Gr. *speira* coil] [MeSH: Leptospira] a genus of bacteria of the family Leptospiraceae, order Spirochaetales, consisting of single, finely coiled, motile, aerobic cells with hooked ends that are visible by darkfield microscopy.
**L. austra′lis,** *L. interrogans* serovar *australis.*
**L. autumna′lis,** *L. interrogans* serovar *autumnalis.*
**L. bata′viae,** *L. interrogans* serovar *bataviae.*
**L. biflex′a,** a species that contains saprophytic nonpathogenic strains of the genus found in fresh surface water and seawater, occasionally associated with mammalian infections.
**L. cani′cola,** *L. interrogans* serovar *canicola.*
**L. grippotypho′sa,** *L. interrogans* serovar *grippotyphosa.*
**L. hard′jo,** *L. interrogans* serovar *hardjo.*
**L. hebdo′madis,** *L. interrogans* serovar *hebdomadis.*
**L. hy′os,** former name for *L. interrogans* serovar *tarassovi.*
**L. icterohaemorrha′giae,** *L. interrogans* serovar *icterohaemorrhagiae.*
**L. inter′rogans,** the species containing all the pathogenic strains of the genus, i.e., those causing leptospirosis (q.v.), which are divided into serological groups that are in turn separated into serotypes. A wide range of wild and domestic animals serve as animal reservoirs, which shed the organism via the urine. Human infection occurs as a result of direct contact with urine or tissue of an infected animal or indirectly by contact with water, soil, or vegetation contaminated by the urine of an infected animal.
**L. inter′rogans** serovar **austra′lis,** a serovar carried by rodents and causing human leptospirosis (formerly believed to specifically cause cane-field fever). Type A, found in Australia, the United States, Europe, Southeast Asia, and Japan, also causes infection in dogs, cattle, raccoons, opossums, and hedgehogs. Type B, found in Australia, Southeast Asia, and Europe, is not known to cause infection in animals other than humans.
**L. inter′rogans** serovar **autumna′lis,** a serovar carried by rodents causing human leptospirosis (formerly believed to specifically cause Hasami fever and pretibial fever) and infection in dogs, opossums, raccoons, and cattle in Southeast Asia, Japan, and the United States.
**L. inter′rogans** serovar **bata′viae,** a serovar carried by rodents and causing human leptospirosis (formerly believed to specifically cause Weil's syndrome and rice-field fever) and infection in dogs and cats in Southeast Asia, Europe, Africa, and Japan.
**L. inter′rogans** serovar **cani′cola,** a serovar carried by dogs, causing Stuttgart disease; it may also cause leptospirosis in humans, pigs, and cattle in a worldwide distribution.
**L. inter′rogans** serovar **grippotypho′sa,** a serovar carried by rodents and causing human leptospirosis (formerly believed to specifically cause mud fever) and infection in cattle, horses, dogs, raccoons, and goats in worldwide distribution.
**L. inter′rogans** serovar **hard′jo,** a serovar carried by rodents and infecting cattle, sheep, and horses worldwide, causing fever, mastitis, and abortion.
**L. inter′rogans** serovar **hebdo′madis,** a serovar carried by field voles and causing human leptospirosis (formerly believed to specifically cause nanukayami) and infections in dogs and cattle in Japan.
**L. inter′rogans** serovar **hy′os,** former name for *L. interrogans* serovar *tarassovi.*
**L. inter′rogans** serovar **icterohaemorrha′giae,** a serovar of worldwide distribution that is carried by rodents and is the major cause of Weil's syndrome (leptospiral jaundice) in humans and of yellows in dogs, and also infects pigs, cattle, and horses.
**L. inter′rogans** serovar **pomo′na,** a serovar carried by pigs, cattle, and rodents; the primary cause of Pomona fever and swineherd's disease in humans and infection in various animals, e.g., dogs, horses, and skunks; it occurs worldwide.
**L. inter′rogans** serovar **pyro′genes,** a serovar carried by rodents and causing human leptospirosis in Japan and Southeast Asia.
**L. inter′rogans** serovar **taras′sovi,** a serovar found in swine and a primary cause of swineherd's disease.
**L. pomo′na,** *L. interrogans* serovar *pomona.*
**L. pyro′genes,** *L. interrogans* serovar *pyrogenes.*
**L. taras′sovi,** *L. inter′rogans* serovar *tarassovi.*

**lep·to·spi·ra** (lep″to-spi′rə) [MeSH: Leptospira] an individual organism belonging to the genus *Leptospira.* Called also *leptospire.*

**Lep·to·spi·ra·ceae** (lep″to-spi-ra′se-e) [MeSH: Leptospiraceae] a family of bacteria of the order Spirochaetales, consisting of flexible helical cells that are aerobic and utilize long-chain fatty acids or alcohols for growth. It consists of the single genus *Leptospira.*

**lep·to·spi·ral** (lep″to-spi′rəl) of, pertaining to, or caused by leptospiras.

**lep·to·spire** (lep′to-spīr) leptospira.

**lep·to·spi·ro·sis** (lep″to-spi-ro′sis) [MeSH: Leptospirosis] any of a group of febrile illnesses in humans and other animals caused by infection with one of the serovars of *Leptospira interrogans.* A wide variety of animals, including opossums, skunks, raccoons, foxes, pigs, and dogs, shed the infective organisms in the urine, and human infection is due to direct contact with the urine or tissue of such animals or to contact with contaminated water, soil, or vegetation. All serovars of *L. interrogans* are believed to be capable of causing any of the clinical syndromes, which vary from a mild carrier state to a fatal disease. Severe forms, such as Weil's syndrome, usually are characterized by jaundice. Different forms of the disease have often each been given different names, depending upon such factors as clinical features, which serovar of *L. interrogans* was originally believed to be causative, geographic distribution, occupation of those infected, and host.
**anicteric l.,** benign l.
**benign l.,** leptospirosis characterized by the absence of jaundice and by a milder course and symptoms than those in the more severe forms. Marked meningism may occur, and a skin rash may be an outstanding feature. Called also *anicteric l.* and *seven-day fever.*
**bovine l.,** a disease of cattle caused primarily by *Leptospira interrogans* serovar *pomona* and marked by fever, icterus, and anemia, especially in calves. Pregnant animals may abort, and lactating animals may develop mastitis.
**canine l.,** leptospirosis in canines; the most common types are Stuttgart disease and yellows (def.1).
**l. of cattle,** bovine l.
**equine l.,** a disease of horses caused by *Leptospira interrogans* and characterized by fever, icterus, and depression. Recurrent iridocyclitis and abortion are also associated.
**l. icterohaemorrha′gica,** Weil's syndrome.
**swine l.,** a disease of pigs, usually caused by *Leptospira interrogans* serovar *pomona.* The acute form, occurring in young pigs, is marked by fever, icterus, hemorrhages, and death. A nonacute form causes abortion in pregnant sows. Transmitted to humans, it causes swineherd's disease.

**lep·to·spir·uria** (lep″to-spir-u′re-ə) excretion of *Leptospira* in the urine, due to their invasion of the renal tubules.

**lep·to·staph·y·line** (lep″to-staf′ə-lēn) [*lepto-* + *staphyline* (def. 2)] pertaining to or characterized by a narrow palate, with a palatal index of 79.9 or less.

**lep·to·tene** (lep′to-tēn) [*lepto-* + Gr. *tainia* ribbon] the stage of meiosis in which the chromosomes are slender, like threads. See *meiosis.*

**lep·to·thri·co·sis** (lep″to-thri-ko′sis) leptotrichosis.

**Lep·to·thrix** (lep′to-thriks) [*lepto-* + Gr. *thrix* hair] a genus of sheathed bacteria, found in fresh or polluted waters and in sludge, made up of gram-negative, rod-shaped cells occurring singly, in pairs, or in chains. The chains are enclosed in sheaths often containing hydrated ferric or manganic oxides. The type species is *L. ochra'cea.*

**lep·to·thrix** (lep'to-thriks) any microorganism of the genus *Leptothrix.*

**Lep·to·trich·ia** (lep"to-trik'e-ə) [*lepto-* + Gr. *thrix,* gen. *trichos* hair] a genus of gram-negative, anaerobic bacteria of the family Bacteroidaceae, found in the human oral cavity, consisting of straight or slightly curved, nonmotile rods with one or both ends rounded or pointed, arranged frequently in pairs or long filaments.
**L. bucca'lis,** the single species, isolated frequently from the normal oral cavity and occasionally from the vagina and intestinal tract. It is sometimes associated with oral or urogenital infections. Called also *Fusobacterium plauti-vincenti.*

**lep·to·tri·cho·sis** (lep"to-trĭ-ko'sis) infection with any species of *Leptothrix.*
**l. conjuncti'vae,** Parinaud's oculoglandular syndrome caused by a leptothrix.

**Lep·to·trom·bid·i·um** (lep"to-trom-bid'e-əm) a subgenus of the mite genus *Trombicula.*

**Lep·tus** (lep'təs) [L.] a genus of chiggers, the larval form of mites of the genus *Trombicula.*

**Lerch's percussion** (lərch'əz) [Otto *Lerch,* American physician, born 1894] drop percussion.

**Le·redde's syndrome** (lə-redz') [Emile *Leredde,* French dermatologist, late 19th century] see under *syndrome.*

**Lé·ri's sign** (la-rēz') [André *Léri,* French physician, 1875–1930] see under *sign.*

**Le·riche's disease, syndrome** (lə-rēsh'əz) [René *Leriche,* French surgeon, 1879–1955] see *post-traumatic osteoporosis,* under *osteoporosis,* and see under *syndrome.*

**Ler·i·tine** (ler'ĭ-tīn) trademark for preparations of anileridine.

**Ler·mo·yez's syndrome** (ler"mwah-yāz') [Marcel *Lermoyez,* French otolaryngologist, 1858–1929] see under *syndrome.*

**les** local excitatory state.

**les·bi·an** (lez'be-ən) [Gr. *Lesbios* of Lesbos, a Greek island in the Aegean Sea, home of the poetess Sappho and her followers] [MeSH: Homosexuality, Female] 1. pertaining to homosexuality between females. 2. a female homosexual.

**les·bi·an·ism** (lez'be-ən-iz"əm) homosexuality between women; called also *sapphism.*

**Lesch-Ny·han syndrome** (lesh-ni'ən) [Michael *Lesch,* American cardiologist, born 1939; William L. *Nyhan,* Jr., American physician, born 1926] [MeSH: Lesch-Nyhan Syndrome] see under *syndrome.*

**Le·ser-Tré·lat sign** (la'zār-tra-lah') [Edmund *Leser,* German surgeon, 1853–1916; Ulysse *Trélat,* Jr., French surgeon, 1828–1890] see under *sign.*

**le·sion** (le'zhən) [L. *laesio; laedere* to hurt] any pathological or traumatic discontinuity of tissue or loss of function of a part.
**angiocentric immunoproliferative l.,** a multisystem disease with adult onset, consisting of invasion and destruction of body structures and tissue by atypical lymphocytoid and plasmacytoid cells resembling a lymphoma; many affected patients develop frank lymphoma. Two subtypes are *lymphomatoid granulomatosis* (involving the lungs, skin, kidneys, nervous system, and gastrointestinal tract) and *polymorphic reticulosis* (involving structures of the nose and face).
**Armanni-Ebstein l.,** vacuolization of epithelial cells in the proximal straight renal tubules (Armanni-Ebstein cells) due to glycogen deposition, a condition seen in untreated diabetes mellitus.
**Baehr-Löhlein l.,** Löhlein-Baehr l.
**Bankart l.,** avulsion of the anterior glenoid labrum following anterior dislocation of the shoulder.
**benign lymphoepithelial l.,** enlargement of the salivary glands, which sometimes become tender, with infiltration of the parenchyma by polyclonal B cells and T cells, atrophy of acini, and formation of lymphoepithelial islands; usually seen in middle-aged women associated with Sjögren syndrome, but also seen in a number of collagen disorders. The lesion is usually benign but may be associated with non-Hodgkin lymphoma. Called also *Mikulicz disease* (particularly when there is lacrimal gland enlargement) and *benign lymphoepithelial sialadenopathy.*
**birds' nest l's,** endocardial pockets.
**Blumenthal l.,** a proliferative vascular lesion in the smaller arteries in diabetics.
**Bracht-Wächter l.,** see under *body.*
**bull's-eye l.,** a round shadow seen on a radiogram, with a dark circle surrounding a central light circle, thus resembling a bull's eye or target; it is found most often on a view of the duodenal wall and represents tumor metastasis that forms a mass with central ulceration. Called also *target l.*
**central l.,** any lesion of the central nervous system.
**coin l.,** a round or nodular shadow seen on a chest x-ray, due to some disease process.
**Councilman's l.,** see under *body.*
**Ebstein's l.,** hyaline degeneration and insular necrosis of epithelial cells of the renal tubules in diabetes mellitus.
**Ghon's primary l.,** Ghon focus.
**gross l.,** a lesion that is visible to the naked eye.
**Hill-Sachs l.,** compression fracture of the posteromedial humeral head, sometimes occurring with anterior dislocation of the shoulder, caused by impaction of the humeral head on the anterior rim of the glenoid fossa.
**histologic l.,** a microscopic lesion.
**impaction l.,** an osteopathic term for a lesion of any spinal joint in which there is present abnormal thickening of the intervertebral disk with approximation of all the bony parts.
**indiscriminate l.,** a lesion affecting different distinct parts or systems of the body.
**irritative l.,** one that stimulates the functions of the part where it is situated.
**Janeway l.,** a small erythematous or hemorrhagic lesion, usually on the palms or soles, in subacute bacterial endocarditis.
**jet l.,** arterial dilatation distal to a stenosis, caused by the turbulence accompanying a poststenotic jet.
**Kimmelstiel-Wilson l.,** a microscopic spherical hyaline mass surrounded by capillaries, found in the kidney glomerulus in the nodular form of intercapillary glomerulosclerosis; called also *Kimmelstiel-Wilson nodule.*
**local l.,** one in the nervous system giving origin to distinctive local symptoms.
**Löhlein-Baehr l.,** a focal glomerular lesion of necrosis and hyalinization occurring in bacterial endocarditis; the process has been described as focal embolic glomerulonephritis.
**molecular l.,** a lesion not visible even with the aid of a microscope.
**onionskin l.,** 1. the concentric circumvascular fibrosis often found in the spleen and lymph nodes in systemic lupus erythematosus. 2. concentric layers of myointimal cells and collagen, causing luminal narrowing, seen in the interlobular arteries and arterioles of the kidney in malignant hypertension, microangiopathies, and scleroderma. Called also *hyperplastic arteriolitis.*
**organic l.,** structural l.
**partial l.,** one that involves only a part of an organ or of the diameter of a conducting tract.
**peripheral l.,** a lesion of the nerve endings.
**precancerous l.,** a lesion in a tissue in which the cells are likely to become malignant.
**primary l.,** the original lesion manifesting a disease, such as chancre in syphilis or tuberculous chancre.
**ring-wall l.,** a small ring hemorrhage in the brain that resembles a ring of glia; seen in pernicious anemia.
**structural l.,** one that produces an obvious change in a tissue.
**systemic l.,** one limited to a system or set of organs with a common function.
**target l.,** 1. bull's-eye l. 2. a small, sharply delineated focus of necrosis, seen in the lungs in invasive aspergillosis, consisting of a rounded gray center surrounded by a hemorrhagic border.
**total l.,** one involving the whole of an organ or of the diameter of a conducting tract.
**trophic l.,** a lesion manifested by a disturbance in the nutrition of a part.
**wire-loop l.,** thickened capillary walls of some parts of a glomerular tuft in disseminated lupus erythematosus.

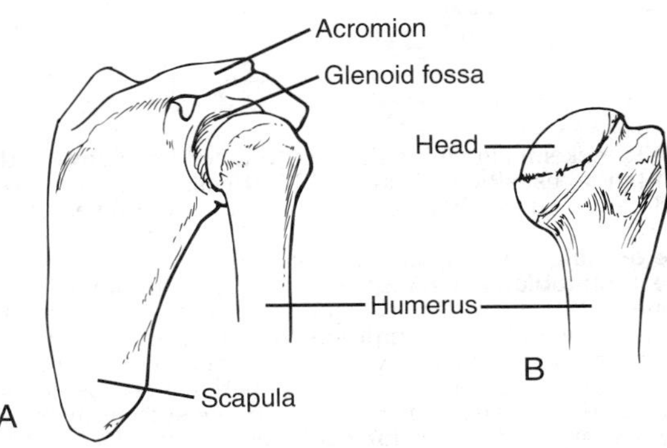


Hill-Sachs lesion due to anterior dislocation of the shoulder and impaction of the humeral head. *(A)* Posterolateral view of the shoulder. *(B)* Posterior view of the impacted humeral head.

**le·sion·ec·to·my** (le″zhən-ek′tə-me) [*lesion* + *-ectomy*] the surgical removal of a discrete lesion within the cerebral cortex while sparing the surrounding tissue; used in the treatment of epilepsy.

**Less·haft's space (triangle)** (les′hahfts) [Peter Frantsevich *Lesshaft,* Russian physician, 1836–1909] see under *space.*

**LET** linear energy transfer.

**let-down** (let′doun) the transport of milk from the alveoli of the breast to the ducts; called also *milk leg.* See also under *reflex.*

**le·thal** (le′thəl) [L. *lethalis*] fatal.

**le·thal·i·ty** (le-thal′ĭ-te) the capability of an agent or disease of causing death.

**leth·ar·gy** (leth′ər-je) [Gr. *lēthargia* drowsiness] 1. a lowered level of consciousness marked by listlessness, drowsiness, and apathy; see also *consciousness.* 2. a condition of indifference.

**Let·ter** (let′ər) trademark for a preparation of levothyroxine sodium.

**Let·ter·er-Si·we disease** (let′ər-ər-se′və) [Erich *Letterer,* German physician, 20th century; Sture August *Siwe,* Swedish pediatrician, 1897–1966] [MeSH: Letterer-Siwe Disease] see under *disease.*

**Leu** leucine.

**leu·ce·mia** (loo-se′me-ə) leukemia.

**leu·cine** (loo′sēn) [Gr. *leukos* white] [MeSH: Leucine] an essential amino acid, 2-amino-4-methylpentanoic acid, necessary for optimal growth in infants and for nitrogen equilibrium in human adults. It is obtained by the digestion or hydrolytic cleavage of protein. Symbols Leu and L. See table at *amino acid.*

**leu·cine ami·no·pep·ti·dase (LAP)** (loo′sēn ə-me″no-pep′tĭ-dās) [MeSH: Leucine Aminopeptidase] leucyl aminopeptidase.

**leu·cin·im·ide** (loo-sin′ĭ-mīd″) the anhydride of leucine, a diketopiperazine; it may be produced by evaporation of leucine solutions.

**leu·ci·no·sis** (loo″sĭ-no′sis) any condition in which leucine appears in the urine.

**leu·cin·uria** (loo″sĭ-nu′re-ə) excretion of leucine in the urine.

**leu·ci·tis** (loo-si′tis) scleritis.

**leuc(o)-** see *leuk(o)-.*

**leu·co·cyte** (loo′ko-sīt) leukocyte.

**leu·co·cy·to·sis** (loo″ko-si-to′sis) leukocytosis.

**Leu·co·cy·to·zo·on** (loo″ko-si″to-zo′on) [*leuco-* + *cyte* + Gr. *zōon* animal] a genus of coccidian protozoa (suborder Haemosporina, order Eucoccidiida) parasitic in wild and domestic birds, sometimes causing fatal leucocytozoonosis. Merogony occurs in the hepatocytes and vascular endothelial cells of the host, producing merozoites that invade erythroblasts, erythrocytes, lymphocytes, and monocytes and then develop into gametocytes. Species infecting domestic fowl include *L. simon′di* (called also *L. an′seris*) in ducks and geese; *L. smi′thi* in turkeys; and *L. caulle′ryi, L. andrew′si,* and *L. sabraze′si* in chickens. All are transmitted by black flies (*Simulium* spp.) except *L. caulleryi,* which is transmitted by biting midges (*Culicoides* spp.). Written also *Leukocytozoon.*

**leu·co·cy·to·zoo·no·sis** (loo″ko-si″to-zo″o-no′sis) an acute malaria-like protozoal disease of domestic fowl, including chickens, ducks, geese, and turkeys, caused by heavy infection with species of *Leucocytozoon,* and characterized by anemia, leukocytosis, and hepatosplenomegaly, which may result in death.

**leu·co·flu·o·res·ce·in** (loo″ko-floo″o-res′e-in) fluorescin, produced from fluorescein by reduction with zinc powder in an acid medium.

**Leu·co·i·um** (loo-ko′e-əm) [L.; Gr. *leukos* white + *ion* violet] a genus of Old World plants of the family Amaryllidaceae. *L. aesti′vum* and *L. ver′num,* both called snowflake, are common garden plants that are emetic and poisonous.

**leu·co·my·cin** (loo″ko-mi′sin) kitasamycin.

**Leu·co·nos·toc** (loo″ko-nos′tok) [*leuko-* + *Nostoc* a genus of blue-green algae] [MeSH: Leuconostoc] a genus of nonpathogenic, gram-positive, saprophytic, facultative anaerobes of the family Streptococcaceae. They are spherical but often lenticular, nonmotile cells, some species of which form dextran.
**L. citro′vorum,** *L. cremoris.*
**L. cremo′ris,** a species found in milk and dairy products; called also *L. citrovorum.*
**L. dextra′nicum,** a dextran-forming species found on fruit and vegetables and in milk and dairy products.
**L. lac′tis,** a species found in milk and dairy products.
**L. mesenteroi′des,** a dextran-forming species found in slimy sugar solutions, on fruit and vegetables, and in milk and dairy products.
**L. oenos′,** a species found in wine.

**leu·co·sin** (loo′ko-sin) an albumin found in the cereal grains.

**Leu·co·thrix** (loo′ko-thriks) [*leuko-* + Gr. *thrix* hair] a genus of gliding bacteria of the family Leucotrichaceae, order Cytophagales, found in water, and made up of short colorless cells growing in long filaments attached to solid substrates. The type species is *L. mu′cor.*

**leu·cot·o·my** (loo-kot′ə-me) prefrontal lobotomy.

**leu·co·vo·rin** (loo″ko-vo′rin) [MeSH: Leucovorin] folinic acid.
**l. calcium** [USP], the calcium salt of folinic acid, used as an antidote for folic acid antagonists, e.g., methotrexate, when there is need to reverse the toxic effects of the latter and in the treatment of megaloblastic anemias due to folic acid deficiency, administered intramuscularly.

**leu·cyl** (loo′səl) the acyl radical of leucine.

**leu·cyl ami·no·pep·ti·dase** (loo′səl ə-me″no-pep′tĭ-dās) [EC 3.4.11.1] a zinc containing enzyme of the hydrolase class that catalyzes the removal of the N-terminal amino acid from most L-peptides, particularly those with N-terminal leucine residues but not those with N-terminal lysine or arginine residues. It occurs in tissue cell cytosol, with high activity in the duodenum, liver, and kidney. Abbreviated LAP. Called also *cytosol aminopeptidase.*

**Leud·et's tinnitus** (loo͝-dāz′) [Théodor Emile *Leudet,* French physician, 1825–1887] see under *tinnitus.*

**leu-en·keph·a·lin** (loo″ən-kef′ə-lin) see *enkephalin.*

**leu·ka·phe·re·sis** (loo″kə-fə-re′sis) [*leuko*cyte + *apheresis*] [MeSH: Leukapheresis] the selective separation and removal of leukocytes from withdrawn blood, the remainder of the blood then being retransfused into the donor.

**leu·ke·mia** (loo-ke′me-ə) [*leuk-* + *-emia*] [MeSH: Leukemia] a progressive, malignant disease of the blood-forming organs, characterized by distorted proliferation and development of leukocytes and their precursors in the blood and bone marrow. It is classified according to degree of cell differentiation as *acute* or *chronic* (terms no longer referring to duration of disease), and according to predominant type of cell involved as *myelogenous* or *lymphocytic.*

## Leukemia

**acute l.,** leukemia in which the involved cell line shows little or no differentiation, usually consisting of blast cells; two types are distinguished, acute lymphoblastic leukemia and acute myelogenous leukemia.

**acute granulocytic l.,** acute myelogenous l.

**acute lymphoblastic l. (ALL),** acute leukemia of the lymphoblastic type, one of the two major categories of acute leukemia, primarily affecting young children. Symptoms include anemia, fatigue, weight loss, easy bruising, thrombocytopenia, granulocytopenia with bacterial infections, bone pain, lymphadenopathy, hepatosplenomegaly, and sometimes spread to the central nervous system (meningismus) or to other organs. The major subtypes are *pre–B-cell, B-cell,* and *T-cell acute lymphoblastic l.* Called also *acute lymphocytic l.*

**acute lymphoblastic l., B-cell type,** a rare subtype consisting of lymphoblasts that express surface immunoglobulins and have a chromosomal translocation similar to that of Burkitt's lymphoma. Called also *Burkitt-like acute lymphoblastic l.*

**acute lymphoblastic l., Burkitt-like,** acute lymphoblastic l., B-cell type.

**acute lymphoblastic l., common type,** a subclassification of the pre–B-cell type that refers to those showing expression of the common acute lymphoblastic leukemia antigen.

**acute lymphoblastic l., null cell type,** a subtype whose cells do not express surface antigens of either T cells or B cells; it is now considered a subgroup of the pre–B-cell type.

**acute lymphoblastic l., pre–B-cell type,** the most common subtype, consisting of small uniform lymphoblasts that do not synthesize complete functional immunoglobulins. The term has sometimes been restricted to the minority of the larger group that synthesize heavy chains of immunoglobulins.

**acute lymphoblastic l., T-cell type,** a type whose cells express surface antigens characteristic of T cells; it is more common in males than in females and affects adults and children equally.

**acute lymphocytic l.,** acute lymphoblastic l.

**acute megakaryoblastic l., acute megakaryocytic l.,** a form of acute myelogenous leukemia in which megakaryocytes are predominant and platelets are increased in the blood, often with fibrosis consisting of reticulin; it can occur at any age. Called also *megakaryoblastic l.* and *megakaryocytic l.*

**acute monocytic l.,** an uncommon form of acute myelogenous leukemia in which the predominating cells are identified as monocytes; it can affect any age group. A few myelocytes may be present, but not as many as in acute myelomonocytic leukemia. Called also *monocytic l.* and *Schilling's l.*

**acute myeloblastic l.,** 1. a common kind of acute myelogenous leukemia, in which myeloblasts predominate; it usually occurs in infants and middle-aged to older adults. Two types are distinguished; those that have minimal cell differentiation or maturation and those that have more advanced differentiation. Called also *myeloblastic l.,* and *acute myeloid l.* 2. acute myelogenous l.

**acute myelocytic l.,** acute myelogenous l.

**acute myelogenous l. (AML),** acute leukemia of the myelogenous type, one of the two major categories of acute leukemia; most types affect primarily middle-aged to elderly people. Symptoms include anemia, fatigue, weight loss, easy bruising, thrombocytopenia, and granulocytopenia that leads to persistent bacterial infections. Several types are distinguished, named according to the stage in which abnormal proliferation begins: *acute undifferentiated l., acute myeloblastic l., acute promyelocytic l., acute myelomonocytic l., acute monocytic l., acute erythroleukemia,* and *acute megakaryocytic l.* Called also *acute myelocytic l.* and *acute nonlymphocytic l.*

**acute myeloid l.,** 1. acute myeloblastic l. (def. 1). 2. acute myelogenous l.

**acute myelomonocytic l.,** one of the more common types of acute myelogenous leukemia, characterized by both malignant monocytes and myeloblasts; it usually affects middle aged to older adults. See also *chronic myelomonocytic l.* Called also *myelomonocytic* or *Naegeli's l.*

**acute nonlymphocytic l.,** acute myelogenous l.

**acute promyelocytic l.,** acute myelogenous leukemia in which more than half the cells are malignant promyelocytes, often associated with abnormal bleeding secondary to thrombocytopenia, hypofibrinogenemia, and decreased levels of coagulation factor V; it usually occurs in young adults. Called also *promyelocytic l.*

**acute undifferentiated l. (AUL),** acute myelogenous leukemia in which the predominating cell is so immature and primitive that it cannot be classified. Called also *stem cell l.* and *undifferentiated cell l.*

**adult T-cell l.,** adult T-cell l./lymphoma.

**adult T-cell l./lymphoma (ATL),** a malignancy of mature T lymphocytes with onset in adulthood, believed to be caused by human T-lymphotropic virus 1 and characterized by circulating pleomorphic malignant lymphocytes, skin lesions, lymphadenopathy, hepatosplenomegaly, hypercalcemia, and lytic bone lesions; its course may be subacute or chronic. Called also *adult T-cell l.* and *adult T-cell lymphoma.*

**aleukemic l., aleukocythemic l.,** leukemia in which the total white blood cell count in the peripheral blood is either normal or below normal; it may be lymphocytic, monocytic, or myelogenous.

**basophilic l.,** a rare type of leukemia in which basophils predominate; both acute and chronic varieties have been observed.

**blast cell l.,** acute undifferentiated l.

**bovine l.,** enzootic bovine leukosis.

**chronic l.,** leukemia in which the involved cell line is well-differentiated, usually B lymphocytes, but immunologically incompetent; types distinguished include chronic granulocytic, chronic lymphocytic, chronic myelomonocytic, eosinophilic, and hairy cell leukemia.

**chronic granulocytic l.,** chronic leukemia of the myelogenous type, occurring mainly between the age of 25 and 60, usually associated with a unique chromosomal abnormality. The major clinical manifestations of malaise, hepatosplenomegaly, anemia, and leukocytosis are related to abnormal, excessive, unrestrained overgrowth of granulocytes in the bone marrow. Called also *chronic myelocytic l.,* and *chronic myeloid l.*

**chronic lymphocytic l. (CLL),** chronic leukemia of the lymphocytic type, a common form mainly seen in the elderly; symptoms include lymphadenopathy, fatigue, renal involvement, and pulmonary leukemic infiltrates. Circulating malignant cells are usually differentiated B lymphocytes; a minority of cases have mixed T and B lymphocytes or entirely T lymphocytes.

**chronic myelocytic l., chronic myelogenous l., chronic myeloid l.,** chronic granulocytic l.

**chronic myelomonocytic l.,** a slowly progressing form of chronic leukemia that is myelomonocytic in nature and usually affects the elderly; sometimes it progresses to acute myelomonocytic leukemia. Symptoms include splenomegaly, monocytosis with granulocytosis, and thrombocytopenia.

**l. cu'tis,** a cutaneous manifestation of leukemia resulting from infiltration of the skin by malignant leukocytes and occurring as specific or nonspecific lesions, or both coexisting. See also *leukemid.*

**eosinophilic l.,** a form of leukemia in which the eosinophil is the predominating cell. Although resembling chronic myelocytic leukemia in many ways, this form may follow an acute course despite the absence of predominantly blast forms in the peripheral blood.

**feline l.,** a nonspecific term for any of various lymphoid leukemias seen in domestic cats that are infected with the feline leukemia virus; sites most often involved are the gastrointestinal tract, liver, spleen, and thymus.

**granulocytic l.,** myelogenous l.

**Gross' l.,** a transmissible murine leukemia, first transmitted to newborn C3H mice by inoculation of filtrate of leukemic tissue from AK2 mice, thus demonstrating its viral etiology.

**hairy cell l.,** a form of chronic leukemia marked by splenomegaly and by an abundance of abnormal large mononuclear cells covered by hairlike villi *(hairy cells)* in the bone marrow, spleen, liver, and peripheral blood. Called also *leukemic reticuloendotheliosis.*

**hand mirror–cell l.,** a rare form characterized by excessive numbers of abnormal, hand mirror–shaped mononuclear cells, usually occurring in females and relatively resistant to treatment. High blast cell counts and central nervous system involvement are common.

**hemoblastic l., hemocytoblastic l.,** acute undifferentiated l.

**histiocytic l.,** acute monocytic l.

**leukopenic l.,** aleukemic l.

**lymphatic l.,** lymphoblastic l.

**lymphoblastic l.,** leukemia associated with hyperplasia and overactivity of the lymphoid tissue; there are increased numbers of circulating malignant lymphocytes and lymphoblasts. See also *acute lymphoblastic l.* and *chronic lymphocytic l.* Called also *lymphatic, lymphocytic, lymphogenous,* and *lymphoid l.*

**lymphocytic l., lymphogenous l., lymphoid l.,** lymphoblastic l.

**lymphosarcoma cell l.,** B-cell type acute lymphoblastic l.

**mast cell l.,** a rare type of leukemia characterized by the presence of overwhelming numbers of tissue mast cells in the peripheral blood.

**megakaryoblastic l.,** acute megakaryocytic l.

**megakaryocytic l.,** acute megakaryocytic l.

**micromyeloblastic l.,** a form of myelogenous leukemia in which the immature, nucleoli-containing cells are small and are distinguishable from lymphocytes only by supravital staining.

**monocytic l.,** acute monocytic l.

**myeloblastic l.,** 1. myelogenous l. 2. acute myeloblastic l.

**myelocytic l.,** myelogenous l.

**myelogenous l., myeloid granulocytic l.,** leukemia arising from myeloid tissue in which the granular, polymorphonuclear leukocytes and their precursors predominate; see also *acute myelogenous l.* and *chronic granulocytic l.* Called also *granulocytic, myeloblastic,* or *myelocytic l.*

**myelomonocytic l.,** acute myelomonocytic l.

**Naegeli's l.,** acute myelomonocytic l.

**plasma cell l.,** a rare type of acute leukemia in which the predominating cell in the peripheral blood is the plasma cell; it is often seen in conjunction with multiple myeloma and may be a variant form of that disease.

**plasmacytic l.,** plasma cell l.

**prolymphocytic l.,** a chronic variety marked by large numbers of circulating lymphocytes, predominantly prolymphocytes, with massive splenomegaly and only rarely lymphadenopathy; prognosis is often poor.

**promyelocytic l.,** acute promyelocytic l.

**Rieder's cell l.,** a form of acute myelogenous leukemia in which the blood contains *Rieder's cells,* asynchronously developed lymphocytes that have immature cytoplasm and a lobulated, indented, comparatively more mature nucleus.

**Schilling's l.,** acute monocytic l.

**stem cell l.,** acute undifferentiated l.

**subleukemic l.,** aleukemic l.

**undifferentiated cell l.,** acute undifferentiated l.

**leu·ke·mic** (loo-ke′mik) pertaining to or affected with leukemia.

**leu·ke·mid** (loo-ke′mid) [*leukemia* + *-id*] any of the polymorphic skin eruptions associated with leukemia; clinically, they may be nonspecific, i.e., papular, macular, purpuric, etc., but histopathologically they may represent true leukemic infiltrations. Cf. *leukemia cutis.*

**leu·ke·mo·gen** (loo-ke′mo-gən) any substance that causes or produces leukemia.

**leu·ke·mo·gen·e·sis** (loo-ke″mo-gen′ə-sis) the induction of or development of leukemia.

**leu·ke·mo·gen·ic** (loo-ke″mo-jen′ik) causing leukemia.

**leu·ke·moid** (loo-ke′moid) [*leukemia* + *-oid*] having blood and sometimes clinical findings resembling those of leukemia; see under reaction.

**leuk·en·ceph·a·li·tis** (lo͝ok″ən-sef″ə-li′tis) [*leuko-* + *encephalitis*] inflammation of the white matter of the brain.

**Leu·ker·an** (loo′kər-ən) trademark for a preparation of chlorambucil.

**leu·kin** (loo′kin) a thermostable, bactericidal substance extracted from polymorphonuclear leukocytes. See *cationic proteins,* under *protein.*

**Leu·kine** (loo′kīn) trademark for a preparation of sargramostim.

**leuk(o)-** [Gr. *leukos* white] a combining form meaning white, or denoting relationship to a leukocyte. Also, *leuc(o)-.*

**leu·ko·ag·glu·ti·nin** (loo″ko-ə-gloo′tĭ-nin) leukocyte agglutinin.

**leu·ko·blast** (loo′ko-blast) old term for a precursor of a leukocyte; the term was not adopted by any classification scheme of cell development.

**leu·ko·blas·to·sis** (loo″ko-blas-to′sis) a general term for abnormal proliferation of leukocytes, as seen in certain types of leukemia.

**leu·ko·ci·din** (loo″ko-si′din) [*leuko-* + L. *caedere* to kill] a substance that is toxic to leukocytes; specifically, an exotoxin produced by some pathogenic staphylococci and streptococci that destroys leukocytes by lysis of the cytoplasmic granules and is partially responsible for the pathogenicity of the organisms.
**Neisser-Wechsberg l.,** a leukocidin produced by staphylococci that destroys rabbit but not human leukocytes; it is identical with alpha hemolysin.
**Panton-Valentine (P-V) l.,** a leukocidin produced by staphylococci that destroys human and rabbit leukocytes by injuring the cell membrane with subsequent cell degranulation; it is nonhemolytic.

**leu·ko·co·ria** (loo″ko-kor′e-ə) leukokoria.

**leu·ko·cy·tal** (loo″ko-si′təl) leukocytic.

**leu·ko·cyte** (loo′ko-sīt) [*leuko-* + *-cyte*] [MeSH: Leukocytes] a colorless blood cell capable of ameboid movement; there are several different types, classified into the two large groups *granular l's* (basophils, eosinophils, and neutrophils) and *nongranular l's* (lymphocytes and monocytes). Called also *white blood cell* or *corpuscle* and *white cell* or *corpuscle.*
**agranular l.,** nongranular l.
**basophilic l.,** basophil, def. 2.
**endothelial l.,** old term for *macrophage.*
**eosinophilic l.,** eosinophil.
**granular l.,** any leukocyte with abundant granules in the cytoplasm; there are three groups, the basophils, eosinophils, and neutrophils. See also *granulocytic series,* under *series.* Called also *granulocyte.*
**heterophilic l.,** heterophil, def. 1.
**mast l.,** basophil.
**motile l.,** a leukocyte that has the power of ameboid movement.
**neutrophilic l.,** neutrophil, def. 1.
**nongranular l.,** a leukocyte without specific granules in the cytoplasm, such as a lymphocyte or monocyte. Called also *agranular l.*
**nonmotile l.,** a leukocyte without the power of ameboid movement.
**polymorphonuclear l.,** any fully developed granular leukocyte whose nucleus contains multiple lobes joined by filamentous connections, especially a neutrophil.
**polynuclear neutrophilic l.,** neutrophil, def. 1.
**Türk's irritation l.,** Türk's cell.

**leu·ko·cyte elas·tase** (loo′ko-sīt e-las′tās) [EC 3.4.21.37] a serine endopeptidase secreted by certain leukocytes that catalyzes the hydrolysis of proteins, including elastin, and is inhibited by alpha$_1$-antitrypsin. Emphysema resulting from damage to lung tissue by leukocyte elastase occurs in alpha$_1$-antitrypsin deficiency. Called also *neutrophil elastase.*

**leu·ko·cy·the·mia** (loo″ko-si-the′me-ə) [*leukocyte* + *hem-* + *-ia*] old term for *leukemia.*

**leu·ko·cyt·ic** (loo″ko-sit′ik) pertaining to leukocytes.

**leu·ko·cy·to·gen·e·sis** (loo″ko-si″to-jen′ə-sis) [*leukocyte* + *-genesis*] leukopoiesis.

**leu·ko·cy·toid** (loo′ko-si″toid) [*leukocyte* + *-oid*] resembling a leukocyte.

**leu·ko·cy·tol·o·gy** (loo″ko-si-tol′ə-je) the study of leukocytes.

**leu·ko·cy·tol·y·sin** (loo″ko-si-tol′ə-sin) a lysin that leads to disruption of leukocytes.

**leu·ko·cy·tol·y·sis** (loo″ko-si-tol′ə-sis) [*leukocyte* + *-lysis*] the breaking down or destruction of leukocytes; called also *leukolysis.*
**venom l.,** destruction of leukocytes by a leukotoxin in snake venom.

**leu·ko·cy·to·lyt·ic** (loo″ko-si″to-lit′ik) 1. pertaining to, characterized by, or causing leukocytolysis. 2. an agent that causes leukocytolysis. Called also *antileukocytic* and *leukolytic.*

**leu·ko·cy·to·ma** (loo″ko-si-to′mə) [*leukocyte* + *-oma*] a tumorlike mass of leukocytes.

**leu·ko·cy·to·pe·nia** (loo″ko-si″to-pe′ne-ə) [*leukocyte* + *-penia*] leukopenia.

**leu·ko·cy·toph·a·gy** (loo″ko-si-tof′ə-je) [*leukocyte* + *-phagy*] the ingestion and destruction of leukocytes by histiocytes of the reticuloendothelial system.

**leu·ko·cy·to·pla·nia** (loo″ko-si″to-pla′ne-ə) [*leukocyte* + Gr. *planē* wandering] the wandering of leukocytes, such as their passage through a membrane.

**leu·ko·cy·to·poi·e·sis** (loo″ko-si″to-poi-e′sis) [*leukocyte* + *-poiesis*] leukopoiesis.

**leu·ko·cy·to·sis** (loo″ko-si-to′sis) [MeSH: Leukocytosis] a transient increase in the number of leukocytes in the blood; seen normally with strenuous exercise and pathologically accompanying hemorrhage, fever, infection, or inflammation. Cf. *hyperleukocytosis.*
**absolute l.,** increase in the total number of leukocytes in the blood.
**agonal l.,** leukocytosis occurring just before death; called also *terminal l.*
**basophilic l.,** basophilia (def. 1).
**eosinophilic l.,** eosinophilia (def. 1).
**mononuclear l.,** mononucleosis (def. 1).
**neutrophilic l.,** neutrophilia.
**pathologic l.,** that occurring as the result of some morbid condition, such as infection or trauma; cf. *physiologic l.*
**physiologic l.,** that caused by nonpathologic factors such as strenuous exercise; cf. *pathologic l.*
**pure l.,** increase of only the polymorphonuclear leukocytes of the blood.
**relative l.,** increase in the proportion of just one type of leukocyte in the blood, without increase of the total number of leukocytes.
**terminal l.,** agonal l.
**toxic l.,** leukocytosis occurring in septicemia and other toxic conditions.

**leu·ko·cy·to·tac·tic** (loo″ko-si″to-tak′tik) leukotactic.

**leu·ko·cy·to·tax·is** (loo″ko-si″to-tak′sis) leukotaxis.

**leu·ko·cy·to·ther·a·py** (loo″ko-si″to-ther′ə-pe) treatment by the administration of leukocytes.

**leu·ko·cy·to·tox·ic·i·ty** (loo″ko-si″to-tok-sis′ĭ-te) the quality or capability of leukocytolysis; see also *lymphocytotoxicity.*

**leu·ko·cy·to·trop·ic** (loo″ko-si″to-trop′ik) having a selective affinity for leukocytes.

**Leu·ko·cy·to·zo·on** (loo″ko-si″to-zo′on) *Leucocytozoon.*

**leu·ko·cy·tu·ria** (loo″ko-si-tu′re-ə) [*leukocyte* + *-uria*] the discharge of leukocytes in the urine.

**leu·ko·der·ma** (loo″ko-dər′mə) [*leuko-* + *derma*] an acquired type of cutaneous depigmentation produced by a specific substance or dermatosis. Called also *leukodermia, leukopathia,* and *leukopathy.* Cf. *piebaldism* and *vitiligo.*
**l. acquisi′tum centri′fugum,** halo nevus.
**l. col′li,** syphilitic l.
**occupational l.,** leukoderma resulting from contact with or ingestion or inhalation of certain chemicals, e.g., monobenzyl ether of hydroquinone and phenol-containing compounds, in the work place.
**postinflammatory l.,** leukoderma occurring after healing of various inflammatory dermatoses or infections, burns, or wounds; it may also be seen after dermabrasion or intralesional steroid injections.
**syphilitic l.,** round or oval, ill-defined, depigmented spots surrounded by hyperpigmentation occurring on the anterior region and sides of the neck and on the chest in secondary syphilis. Called also *collar of pearls, collar of Venus, l. colli, melanoleukoderma colli,* and *venereal collar.*

**leu·ko·der·ma·tous** (loo″ko-dər′mə-təs) pertaining to or characterized by leukoderma.

**leu·ko·der·mia** (loo″ko-dər′me-ə) leukoderma.

**leu·ko·der·mic** (loo″ko-dər′mik) leukodermatous.

**leu·ko·dex·trin** (loo″ko-deks′trin) an intermediate compound formed in the transformation of starch into sugar; achroodextrin.

**leu·ko·dys·tro·phy** (loo″ko-dis′trə-fe) disturbance of the white substance of the brain. See also *adrenoleukodystrophy* and *leukoencephalopathy.*
**globoid cell l.,** Krabbe's disease.
**hereditary adult-onset l.,** an autosomal dominant leukoencephalopathy characterized by degeneration of the white matter, beginning at the frontal lobes and extending to the centrum semiovale and cerebellum. Symptoms first appear in the fourth, fifth, or sixth decade and include motor disturbances, bowel and bladder incontinence, and orthostatic hypotension; mental acuity is often retained. Death occurs about 20 years after the appearance of symptoms.
**hereditary cerebral l.,** Pelizaeus-Merzbacher disease.
**Krabbe's l.,** see under *disease.*
**metachromatic l.,** an autosomal recessive disorder due to deficiency of cerebroside sulfatase or sphingolipid activator protein–1, characterized by accumulation of sulfatide in neural and nonneural tissues, with a diffuse loss of myelin in the central nervous system. There are three forms due to deficiency of cerebroside sulfatase, with variable age of onset, all initially presenting as mental regression and motor disturbances. The *infantile* form usually begins in the second year of life and is additionally characterized by developmental delay, seizures, optic atrophy, ataxia, weakness, loss of speech, and progressive spastic quadriparesis. The *juvenile* form is clinically similar, but presents between the ages of 4 and 12 and progresses more slowly; a variant of the juvenile form is caused by deficiency of sphingolipid activator protein–1. The *adult* form begins after 16 years of age, generally presenting initially as dementia and disturbances in behavior and progressing more slowly to motor and posture disturbances. Called also *sulfatide lipidosis.*
**spongiform l.,** spongy degeneration of the central nervous system; see under *degeneration.*
**sudanophilic l.,** a heterogeneous group of diseases, including adrenoleukodystrophy and Pelizaeus-Merzbacher disease, characterized by myelin destruction, with resulting breakdown products that stain bright red with fat stains.

**leu·ko·ede·ma** (loo″ko-ə-de′mə) [*leuko-* + *edema*] a disorder of the buccal mucosa resembling early leukoplakia, characterized by the presence of a filmy opalescence of the mucosa in the early stages to a whitish gray cast with a coarsely wrinkled surface in the later stages, associated with intracellular edema of the spinous or malpighian layer.

**leu·ko·en·ceph·a·li·tis** (loo″ko-ən-sef″ə-li′tis) [*leuko-* + *encephalitis*] 1. inflammation of the white substance of the brain. Cf. *leukoencephalomalacia.* 2. forage poisoning.
**acute hemorrhagic l., acute hemorrhagic l. of Weston Hurst,** acute necrotizing hemorrhagic encephalomyelitis.
**l. periaxia′lis concen′trica,** Baló's disease.
**van Bogaert's sclerosing l.,** subacute sclerosing panencephalitis.

**leu·ko·en·ceph·a·lo·ma·la·cia** (loo″ko-en-sef′ə-lo-mə-la′shə) [*leuko-* + *encephalomalacia*] 1. encephalomalacia affecting primarily the white matter. 2. forage poisoning.
**mycotoxic l.,** forage poisoning.

**leu·ko·en·ceph·a·lop·a·thy** (loo″ko-ən-sef″ə-lop′ə-the) any of a group of diseases affecting the white matter of the brain, especially of the cerebral hemispheres, and occurring as a rule in infants and children. The term *leukodystrophy* is used to denote such disorders due to defect in the formation and maintenance of myelin in infants and children.
**metachromatic l.,** see under *leukodystrophy.*
**necrotizing l.,** a complication sometimes seen after injection of methotrexate intrathecally to treat childhood leukemia of the central nervous system; symptoms include necrosis of white matter of the brain, sometimes with stupor and quadriplegia, and frequently with permanent learning disabilities.
**progressive multifocal l.,** an opportunistic infection of the central nervous system by the JC virus, seen in immunocompromised persons and sometimes secondary to neoplastic conditions such as lymphosarcoma, lymphoblastic leukemia, or myelogenous leukemia. The demyelination is usually found in the white matter of the cerebral hemispheres but may rarely be seen in the brain stem and cerebellum.
**subacute sclerosing l.,** subacute sclerosing panencephalitis.

**leu·ko·en·ceph·a·ly** (loo″ko-ən-sef′ə-le) leukoencephalopathy.

**leu·ko·eryth·ro·blas·tic** (loo″ko-ə-rith″ro-blas′tik) characterized by the presence of nucleated red cells and immature neutrophils.

**leu·ko·eryth·ro·blas·to·sis** (loo″ko-ə-rith″ro-blas-to′sis) anemia with space-occupying lesions of the bone marrow that cause bone marrow suppression with immature cells of the erythrocytic and granulocytic series in the circulation. Called also *leukoerythroblastic anemia, myelopathic anemia,* and *myelophthisic anemia.*

**leu·ko·ker·a·to·sis** (loo″ko-kər″ə-to′sis) [*leuko-* + *keratosis*] oral leukoplakia.

**leu·ko·ki·ne·sis** (loo″ko-kĭ-ne′sis) the movement of the leukocytes within the circulatory system.

**leu·ko·ki·net·ic** (loo″ko-kĭ-net′ik) pertaining to leukokinesis.

**leu·ko·ki·net·ics** (loo″ko-kĭ-net′iks) [*leuko*cyte + *kinetics*] the quantitative, dynamic study of *in vivo* production, circulation, and destruction of leukocytes.

**leu·ko·ki·nin** (loo″ko-ki′nin) the parent immunoglobulin molecule from which tuftsin is cleaved.

**leu·ko·ko·ria** (loo″ko-kor′e-ə) [*leuko-* + Gr. *korē* pupil + *-ia*] a condition characterized by appearance of a whitish reflex or mass in the pupillary area behind the lens; called also *cat's eye reflex.*

**leu·ko·krau·ro·sis** (loo″ko-kraw-ro′sis) lichen sclerosus in females; see under *lichen.*

**leu·ko·lym·pho·sar·co·ma** (loo″ko-lim″fo-sahr-ko′mə) leukosarcoma.

**leu·kol·y·sin** (loo-kol′ə-sin) leukocytolysin.

**leu·kol·y·sis** (loo-kol′ə-sis) leukocytolysis.

**leu·ko·lyt·ic** (loo″ko-lit′ik) leukocytolytic.

**leu·ko·ma** (loo-ko′mə) pl. *leuko′mata* [Gr. *leukōma* whiteness] a dense white opacity of the cornea.
**adherent l.,** a white tumor of the cornea enclosing a prolapsed adherent iris.

**leu·ko·maine** (loo′ko-mān) [Gr. *leukōma* whiteness] any one of a large group of basic substances resembling alkaloids, normally present in the tissues, which are products of metabolism and are probably excrementitious. Some of them may become toxic, and many are physiologically active.

**leu·ko·main·ic** (loo″ko-mān′ik) pertaining to, caused by, or characterized by a leukomaine.

**leu·ko·ma·la·cia** (loo″ko-məla′shə) softening of the white matter of the brain.
**periventricular l. (PVL),** bilateral necrosis of the white matter of the brain adjacent to the lateral ventricles, seen in the neonatal period, especially in premature newborns, and manifested by chalky, yellowish-white plaques in the white matter, with proliferation of astrocytes and microglia; cyst formation may lead to multicystic encephalopathy.

**leu·ko·ma·ta** (loo-ko′mə-tə) plural of *leukoma.*

**leu·ko·ma·tous** (loo-ko′mə-təs) affected with or of the nature of leukoma.

**leu·ko·my·eli·tis** (loo″ko-mi″ə-li′tis) [*leuko-* + *myelitis*] inflammation of the white substance of the spinal cord.

**leu·ko·my·elop·a·thy** (loo″ko-mi″ə-lop′ə-the) [*leuko-* + *myelopathy* disease] any disease of the white substance of the spinal cord.

**leu·kon** (loo′kon) the circulating leukocytes and the cells from which they arise; it is the counterpart of *erythron* and *thrombon.*

**leu·ko·ne·cro·sis** (loo″ko-nə-kro′sis) [*leuko-* + *necrosis*] gangrene resulting in the formation of a white slough.

**leu·ko·nych·ia** (loo″ko-nik′e-ə) [*leuko-* + *onych-* + *-ia*] a whitish discoloration of the nails, usually partial although occasionally it is total; very rarely it may occur in transverse streaks *(l. striata),* in bands, or in spots. There are several different causes. Called also *leukopathia unguium.*

**leu·ko·path·ia** (loo″ko-path′e-ə) [*leuko-* + *path-* + *-ia*] leukoderma.
**l. puncta′ta reticula′ris symmet′rica,** idiopathic guttate hypomelanosis.
**l. un′guium,** leukonychia.

**leu·kop·a·thy** (loo-kop′ə-the) leukoderma.

**leu·ko·pe·de·sis** (loo″ko-pə-de′sis) [*leuko*cyte + Gr. *pēdan* to leap] the outward passage *(diapedesis)* of leukocytes through intact vessel walls; called also *migration of leukocytes.*

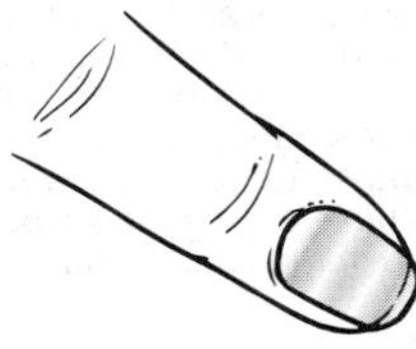

Leukonychia.

**leu·ko·pe·nia** (loo″ko-pe′ne-ə) [*leuko*cyte + *-penia*] [MeSH: Leukopenia] reduction in the number of leukocytes in the blood below about 5000 per cu. mm. Types are named for the type of cell, such as *agranulocytosis* and *neutropenia;* see also *pancytopenia.* Called also *aleukia, aleukocytosis,* and *leukocytopenia.*
**basophil l., basophilic l.,** basophilopenia.
**congenital l.,** old name for *infantile genetic agranulocytosis.*
**malignant l., pernicious l.,** agranulocytosis.

**leu·ko·pe·nic** (loo″ko-pe′nik) pertaining to, characterized by, or causing leukopenia.

**leu·ko·phago·cy·to·sis** (loo″ko-fag″o-si-to′sis) leukocytophagy.

**leu·ko·pla·kia** (loo″ko-pla′ke-ə) [*leuko-* + Gr. *plax* plate + *-ia*] [MeSH: Leukoplakia] 1. a white patch on a mucous membrane that will not rub off. 2. oral l.
**atrophic l.,** lichen sclerosus in females; see under *lichen.*
**l. bucca′lis,** the presence of white thickened patches on the mucous membrane of the cheeks. See *oral l.*
**hairy l.,** a white filiform to flat patch (see *oral l.*) occurring on the tongue or, rarely, on the buccal mucosa, caused by infection with Epstein-Barr virus and associated with human immunodeficiency virus infection; it is a predictor of the subsequent development of acquired immunodeficiency syndrome. Called also *oral hairy leukoplakia.*
**l. lingua′lis,** the presence of white thickened patches on the mucous membrane of the tongue. See *oral l.*
**oral l.,** white, thick patches on the oral mucosa produced by hyperkeratosis of the epithelium, with thickening of stratified squamous epithelium, hyperkeratosis, hyperplasia, inflammatory infiltration, and degeneration of epithelial cells. It is a benign condition but may predispose to development of epidermoid carcinoma. The etiology is unknown, but tobacco use has been implicated (see *stomatitis nicotina*). Called also *keratosis linguae, leukokeratosis, psoriasis buccalis,* and *psoriasis linguae.*
**oral hairy l.,** hairy l.
**speckled l.,** see under *erythroplakia.*
**l. vul′vae,** 1. lichen sclerosus in females; see under *lichen.* 2. any white-appearing lesion of the vulva.

**leu·ko·poi·e·sis** (loo″ko-poi-e′sis) the production of leukocytes; called also *leukocytogenesis* and *leukocytopoiesis.*

**leu·ko·poi·et·ic** (loo″ ko-poi-et′ ik) [*leuko*cyte + Gr. *poiein* to make] forming or producing leukocytes.

**leu·ko·poi·e·tin** (loo″ko-poi-e′tin) granulopoietin.

**leu·ko·pre·cip·i·tin** (loo″ko-pre-sip′ĭ-tin) a precipitin specific for leukocyte antigens.

**leu·kop·sin** (loo-kop′sin) [*leuko-* + *opsin*] visual white; the colorless matter into which rhodopsin is changed by exposure to white light. It is reconvertible into rhodopsin under proper conditions.

**leu·kor·rha·gia** (loo″ko-ra′je-ə) [*leuko-* + *-rrhagia*] profuse leukorrhea.

**leu·kor·rhea** (loo″ko-re′ə) [*leuko-* + *-rrhea*] [MeSH: Leukorrhea] a whitish, viscid discharge from the vagina and uterine cavity.
**menstrual l., periodic l.,** leukorrhea in place of or along with the menses.

**leu·kor·rhe·al** (loo″ko-re′əl) pertaining to or marked by leukorrhea.

**leu·ko·sar·co·ma** (loo″ko-sahr-ko′mə) [*leuko-* + *sarcoma*] the development of a leukemic blood picture in patients originally having a well-differentiated, lymphocytic type of malignant lymphoma. The circulating cells contain an ovoid nucleus and nucleoli, and are morphologically different from the mature-type lymphocyte seen in chronic lymphocytic leukemia. Called also *leukolymphosarcoma* and *leukocytic sarcoma.*

**leu·ko·scope** (loo′ko-skōp) [*leuko-* + *-scope*] an instrument that mixes colors to produce white for testing for color blindness.

**leu·ko·sis** (loo-ko′sis) pl. *leuko′ses.* proliferation of leukocyte-forming tissue; see *lymphoproliferative disorders, lymphoreticular disorders,* and *myeloproliferative disorders,* under *disorder.*
**acute l.,** see *Marek's disease,* under *disease.*
**avian l.,** a group of viral diseases of chickens, transmitted by related oncoviruses and characterized by proliferation of immature erythroid, myeloid, or lymphoid cells. Leukemic forms include erythroblastosis and myeloblastosis and, rarely, lymphoblastic leukemia. Solid tumors in visceral organs are seen in cases of lymphoid leukosis, erythroblastosis, and myelocytomatosis. Some of the causative viruses induce related neoplasms such as sarcomas, hemangiomas, nephroblastomas, hepatocarcinomas, and osteopetrosis gallinarum, which are now classified as belonging to the leukosis sarcoma group. See also *avian lymphomatosis* and *visceral lymphomatosis.*
**bovine l.,** enzootic bovine l.
**bovine l., enzootic,** a progressive fatal lymphosarcoma affecting adult cattle, caused by the bovine leukemia virus, and characterized by infiltration of lymphoid tissue throughout the body by malignant lymphocytes, with enlargement of lymph nodes and spleen. Called also *bovine malignant lymphoma, malignant lymphoma of cattle,* and *bovine leukemia.*
**bovine l., sporadic,** a disease similar to enzootic bovine leukosis, with malignant proliferation of lymphoid tissues but no culturable infectious agent; it occurs in three forms that vary in the age of the animal and organ affected: *calf,* seen in animals under six months of age and marked by generalized lymphadenopathy and widespread metastasis; *thymic,* seen in animals 6 to 18 months of age and confined mainly to the thymus; and *cutaneous* or *skin,* the only nonlethal form, affecting young adults and marked by cutaneous tumors that regress spontaneously.
**erythroid l.,** erythroblastosis, def. 2.
**fowl l.,** avian l.
**lymphoid l.,** one of the avian leukosis complex of tumors, involving transformation of B lymphocytes; symptoms include anorexia, emaciation, and an enlarged liver.
**myeloblastic l.,** avian myeloblastosis.
**myelocytic l.,** myelocytomatosis.
**skin l.,** Marek's disease primarily affecting the skin.

**leu·ko·sta·sis** (loo″ko-sta′sis) increased blood viscosity and hypercoagulability, seen in leukemia that is accompanied by hyperleukocytosis.

**leu·ko·tac·tic** (loo″ko-tak′tik) 1. able to attract leukocytes. 2. pertaining to leukotaxis; called also *leukocytotactic.*

**leu·ko·tax·is** (loo″ko-tak′sis) [*leuko-* + *-taxis*] the cytotaxis of leukocytes, tending to collect in regions of injury or inflammation. Called also *leukocytotaxis.*

**Leu·ko·thrix** (loo′ko-thriks) *Leucothrix.*

**leu·ko·throm·bin** (loo″ko-throm′bin) a fibrin factor formed by leukocytes in the blood.

**leu·ko·tome** (loo′ko-tōm) [*leuko-* + *-tome*] a cannula through which a loop of wire is passed to perform the operation of leukotomy or lobotomy.

**leu·kot·o·my** (loo-kot′ə-me) prefrontal lobotomy.
**transorbital l.,** see under *lobotomy.*

**leu·ko·tox·ic** (loo″ko-tok′sik) destructive to leukocytes.

**leu·ko·tox·ic·i·ty** (loo″ko-tok-sis′ĭ-te) the quality of having a toxic or deleterious effect on leukocytes.

**leu·ko·tox·in** (loo″ko-tok′sin) [*leuko*cyte + *toxin*] a cytotoxin destructive to the leukocytes.

**leu·ko·trich·ia** (loo″ko-trik′e-ə) [*leuko-* + *trich-* + *-ia*] whiteness of the hair in a circumscribed area; cf. *poliosis.*

**leu·ko·tri·ene** (loo″ko-tri′ēn) [from *leuko*cytes + *triene* indicating three double bonds] one of a group of biologically active compounds consisting of straight chain, 20-carbon carboxylic acids with one or two oxygen substituents and three or more conjugated double bonds. They are formed from arachidonic acid by the lipoxygenase pathway, and function as regulators of allergic and inflammatory reactions. Leukotrienes are identified by letters A, B, C, D, and E with subscripts indicating the number of double bonds in the molecule. Some (e.g., $LTB_4$) stimulate the movement of leukocytes; three others ($LTC_4$, $LTD_4$, and $LTE_4$) together constitute slow-reacting substance of anaphylaxis, which causes bronchial constriction and other allergic reactions.

**leu·ko·uro·bi·lin** (loo″ko-u-ro-bi′lin) [*leuko-* + *urobilin*] a colorless decomposition product of urobilin.

**leu·ko·vi·rus** (loo′ko-vi″rəs) [*leukemia* + *virus*] [MeSH: Retroviridae] former name for the subfamily Oncovirinae (family Retroviridae).

**leu·pro·lide ace·tate** (loo-pro′līd) a synthetic gonadotropin-releasing hormone analogue used as an antineoplastic in the palliative treatment of advanced prostatic cancer; it is also used in the treatment of endometriosis and central precocious puberty. Administered subcutaneously and intramuscularly.

**Leu·stat·in** (loo-stat′in) trademark for a preparation of cladribine.

**Lev's disease** (levz) [Maurice *Lev,* American pathologist, born 1908] see under *disease.*

**Lev·a·di·ti's method** (lev″ə-de′tēz) [Constantin *Levaditi,* Romanian-born bacteriologist in Paris, 1874–1953] see under *stain.*

**lev·al·lor·phan tar·trate** (lev″ə-lor′fan) an analogue of levorphanol that acts as a narcotic agonist-antagonist, used parenterally for its antagonistic effect in the treatment of respiratory depression caused by narcotic analgesics; in the absence of narcotic-induced respiratory depression it can itself cause respiratory depression.

**le·vam·i·sole hy·dro·chlo·ride** (le-vam′ĭ-sōl) [USP] an oral imidazole used as an anthelmintic, chiefly in the treatment of ascariasis and hookworm infections. It is also an immunopotentiator used as an adjunct with fluorouracil in the treatment of Dukes' stage C colon cancer following surgical resection of the primary tumor.

**lev•an** (lev'an) a homopolysaccharide containing fructose residues in 2,6-glycosidic linkage. Formed from sucrose by the enzyme levansucrase, levan, which is produced by certain species of *Bacillus* and *Leuconostoc,* increases the adhesion of bacteria to surfaces of the teeth and promotes the formation of dental plaque.

**lev•an•su•crase** (lev″an-soo'krās) [EC 2.4.1.10] an enzyme of the transferase class produced by certain species of *Bacillus* and *Leuconostoc;* it catalyzes the transfer of fructose residues from sucrose to a growing levan polymer, a constituent of dental plaque.

**Le•va•quin** (le'və-kwin) trademark for a preparation of levofloxacin.

**lev•ar•te•re•nol** (lev″ər-tə-re'nol) the levorotatory isomer of norepinephrine, a much more potent pressor agent than the natural dextrorotatory isomer.
**l. bitartrate,** norepinephrine bitartrate.

**Lev•a•tol** (lev'ə-tol) trademark for a preparation of penbutolol sulfate.

**le•va•tor** (le-va'tor) pl. *levato'res* [L. *levare* to raise] 1. [TA] a muscle for elevating the organ or structure into which it is inserted; see entries beginning *musculus levator,* under *musculus.* 2. a surgical instrument used to raise depressed osseous fragments in fractures of the skull and other bones.

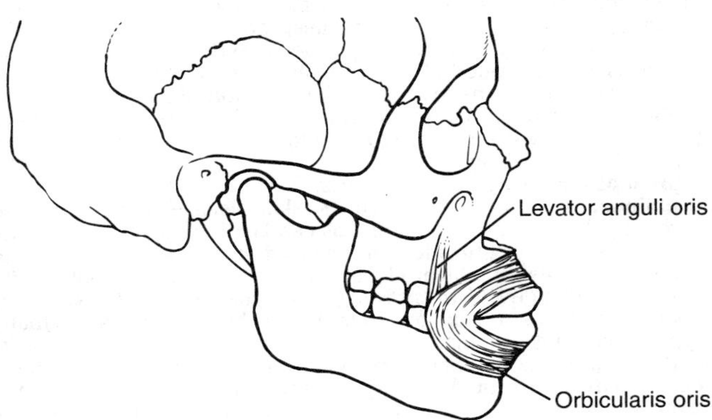

Musculus levator anguli oris.

**l. a'ni,** see under *musculus.*

**lev•a•to•res** (lev″ə-to'rēz) [L.] plural of *levator.*

**Lev•bid** (lev'bid) trademark for a preparation of hyoscyamine sulfate.

**lev•el** (lev'əl) relative position, rank, or concentration.
**$\alpha$ l.,** significance l.
**confidence l.,** one minus the confidence coefficient; the probability that a confidence interval does not contain the population parameter. Denoted $\alpha$. See also *Type I error,* under *error.*
**l's of consciousness,** clinically differentiable degrees of awareness and alertness such as alert wakefulness, lethargy, clouding of consciousness, stupor, and coma.
**isoelectric l.,** 1. the level of recorded resting potential of a cell. 2. see under line.
**lowest observed adverse effect l. (LOAEL), lowest observed effect l. (LOEL),** in studies of the toxicity of chemicals, the lowest dosage level at which chronic exposure to the substance shows adverse effects; usually calculated for laboratory animals.
**no observed adverse effect l. (NOAEL), no observed effect l. (NOEL),** in studies of the toxicity of chemicals, the highest dosage level at which chronic exposure to the substance shows no adverse effects; usually calculated for laboratory animals.
**significance l., l. of significance,** the probability of incorrectly rejecting the null hypothesis when such a hypothesis is tested. Denoted $\alpha$. See also *Type I error,* under *error.*

**Lé•vi-Lo•rain dwarf, infantilism (syndrome)** (la-ve'lo-rǎ') [E. Léopold *Lévi,* French endocrinologist, 1868–1933; Paul Joseph *Lorain,* French physician, 1827–1875] see *pituitary dwarf,* under *dwarf,* and *hypophysial infantilism,* under *infantilism.*

**lev•i•cel•lu•lar** (lev″i-sel'u-lər) [L. *levis* smooth + *cellular*] smooth celled.

**lev•i•ga•tion** (lev″i-ga'shən) [L. *levigare* to render smooth] the grinding to a powder of a hard or moistened substance.

**Le•vi-Mon•tal•ci•ni** (la've mōn-tahl-che'ne) Rita. Italian neurobiologist, born 1909. Co-winner with Stanley Cohen of the Nobel prize for medicine or physiology in 1986 for discoveries regarding the mechanisms by which growth factors regulate cell and organ growth.

**Le•vin's tube** (lə-vinz') [Abraham Louis *Levin,* American physician, 1880–1940] see under *tube.*

**lev•i•ta•tion** (lev″ĭ-ta'shən) [L. *levis* light] 1. a hallucinatory sensation of floating or rising in the air. 2. a support system for severe burn victims, consisting of a bed in the form of an inflatable chamber containing numerous outlets through which humidified, warm, sterile air is released at a pressure sufficient to raise the patient so that he is supported in a sterile air environment.

**lev(o)-** [L. *laevus* left] 1. a combining form meaning left, to the left. 2. chemical prefix used to designate the levorotatory enantiomorph of a substance; opposed to *dextro-.* Symbol (−)- (formerly *l-;* sometimes $\Lambda$).

**le•vo•car•dia** (le″vo-kahr'de-ə) [*levo-* + *cardia*] [MeSH: Levocardia] a term denoting the normal position of the heart, used when other viscera are transposed; cf. *dextrocardia.*
**isolated l.,** levocardia associated with transposition (situs inversus) of the abdominal viscera, congenital structural anomaly of the heart, and sometimes with absence of the spleen.
**mixed l.,** corrected transposition of the great vessels; see under *transposition.*

**le•vo•car•ni•tine** (le″vo-kahr'nĭ-tēn) [USP] a preparation of the biologically active L-isomer of carnitine, used to treat primary systemic carnitine deficiency; administered orally.

**le•vo•cli•na•tion** (le″vo-klĭ-na'shən) [*levo-* + L. *clinatus* leaning] rotation of the upper poles of the vertical meridians of the two eyes to the left. Cf. *dextroclination.*

**le•vo•cy•clo•duc•tion** (le″vo-si″klo-dək'shən) levoduction.

**le•vo•do•pa** (le″vo-do'pə) [USP] [MeSH: Levodopa] the levorotatory isomer of dopa, used in the treatment of parkinsonism; administered orally.

**Le•vo-Dro•mo•ran** (le″vo-dro'mə-ran) trademark for preparations of levorphanol tartrate.

**le•vo•duc•tion** (le″vo-dək'shən) movement of either eye to the left.

**le•vo•flox•a•cin** (le″vo-flok'sə-sin) a broad-spectrum quinolone antibacterial agent, administered orally or by injection.

**le•vo•gy•ral** (le″vo-ji'rəl) [*levo-* + L. *gyrare* to turn] levorotatory.

**le•vo•gy•ra•tion** (le″vo-ji-ra'shən) levorotation.

**Le•void** (le'void) trademark for a preparation of levothyroxine sodium.

**le•vo•me•pro•ma•zine** (le″vo-mə-pro'mə-zēn) methotrimeprazine.

**le•vo•meth•a•dyl ac•e•tate** (le″vo-meth'ə-dəl) a narcotic analgesic chemically related to oxymorphone and naloxone, used as an in adjunct in the treatment of heroin addiction; administered orally.

**le•vo•nor•de•frin** (le″vo-nor'də-frin) [USP] an adrenergic, the levo isomer of nordefrin, used as a vasoconstrictor in solutions of local anesthetics, especially in dentistry.

**le•vo•nor•ges•trel** (le'vo-nor-jes'trel) [USP] [MeSH: Levonorgestrel] the levorotatory form of norgestrel, used in combination with an estrogen component as an oral contraceptive.

**Lev•o•phed** (lev'o-fed) trademark for a preparation of norepinephrine bitartrate.

**Le•vo•prome** (le'vo-prōm) trademark for a preparation of methotrimeprazine.

**le•vo•pro•poxy•phene nap•sy•late** (le″vo-pro-pok'sə-fēn) the napsylate salt of the levo isomer of propoxyphene, used as an antitussive, administered orally.

**le•vo•pro•pyl•cil•lin po•tas•si•um** (le″vo-pro″pəl-sil'in) an antibacterial effective against gram-positive organisms. Called also *propicillin.*

**le•vo•ro•ta•ry** (le″vo-ro'tə-re) levorotatory.

**le•vo•ro•ta•tion** (le″vo-ro-ta'shən) a turning to the left.

**le•vo•ro•ta•to•ry** (le″vo-ro'tə-tor″e) [*levo-* + *rotatory*] turning the plane of polarization of polarized light to the left (counterclockwise).

**le•vor•pha•nol tar•trate** (le-vor'fə-nol) [USP] a synthetic narcotic analgesic with properties and actions similar to those of morphine; administered orally and subcutaneously.

**le•vo•sin** (le'vo-sin) a starch occurring in wheat flour, rye, bran, and stubble.

**le•vo•thy•rox•ine so•di•um** (le″vo-thi-rok'sēn) [USP] the monosodium salt of the levo isomer of thyroxine, used as replacement therapy for hypothyroidism; administered orally.

**le·vo·tor·sion** (le″vo-tor′shən) levoclination.

**le·vo·ver·sion** (le″vo-vər′zhən) an act of turning to the left; in ophthalmology, movement of the eyes to the left.

**Lev·ret's forceps** (ləv-räz′) [André *Levret,* French obstetrician, 1703–1780] see under *forceps.*

**Lev·u·gen** (lev′u-jən) trademark for a preparation of fructose.

**lev·u·lose** (lev′u-lōs) [L. *laevus* left + *-ose*] older name for *fructose.*

**Lé·vy-Rous·sy syndrome** (la-ve′roo-se′) [Gabrielle *Lévy,* French neurologist, 1886–1935; Gustave *Roussy,* French pathologist, 1874–1948] Roussy-Lévy syndrome.

**Le·wan·dow·sky's nevus elasticus** (lev-ahn-dov′skēz) [Felix *Lewandowsky,* German dermatologist, 1879–1921] nevus elasticus of Lewandowsky.

**Le·wan·dow·sky-Lutz disease** (lev-ahn-dov′ske-lo͞ots) [F. *Lewandowsky;* Wilhelm *Lutz,* Swiss dermatologist, 1888–1958] epidermodysplasia verruciformis.

**Lew·is blood group** (loo′is) [from the name of the English propositus first reported on in 1946] see under *blood group.*

**Lew·is-Pic·ker·ing test** (loo′is-pik′ər-ing) [Sir T. *Lewis;* Sir George White *Pickering,* English scientist, 1904–1980] see under *test.*

**lew·i·site** (loo′i-sīt) [named for W. Lee *Lewis,* American chemist, 1879–1943] a lethal war gas; it is a vesicant, lacrimator, and lung irritant.

**Le·wy bodies** (la′ve) [Frederic H. *Lewy,* German-born neurologist in United States, 1885–1950] [MeSH: Lewy Bodies] see under *body.*

**Ley·den's disease** (li′dənz) [Ernst Victor von *Leyden,* German physician, 1832–1910] see under *disease.*

**Ley·den jar** (li′dən) [*Leyden,* The Netherlands, where it was invented] see under *jar.*

**Ley·den-Mö·bi·us muscular dystrophy syndrome** (li′dən-mer′be-əs) [E. V. von *Leyden;* Paul Julius *Möbius,* German neurologist, 1853–1907] limb-girdle muscular dystrophy.

**Ley·dig's cells, cylinders, duct** (li′digz) [Franz von *Leydig,* German anatomist, 1821–1908] see under *cell* and *cylinder,* and see *ductus mesonephricus.*

**Lf** symbol for *limes flocculating;* see *Lf dose,* under *dose.*

**LFA** left frontoanterior (left mentoanterior, a position of the fetus).

**LFA-1** leukocyte function–associated antigen 1.

**LFA-2** leukocyte function–associated antigen 2.

**LFA-3** leukocyte function–associated antigen 3.

**L-form** L-phase variant; see under *variant.*

**LFP** left frontoposterior (left mentoposterior, a position of the fetus).

**LFT** left frontotransverse (left mentotransverse, a position of the fetus).

**LH** [MeSH: LH] luteinizing hormone.

**Lher·mitte's sign** (lār-mēts′) [Jean *Lhermitte,* Paris neurologist, 1877–1959] see under *sign.*

**LH-RH** luteinizing hormone–releasing hormone.

**Li** symbol for *lithium.*

**LIA** leukemia-associated inhibitory activity; see under *activity.*

**-liberin** [L. *liber* free] a word termination denoting a freeing or releasing; used in names of hormones.

**li·bid·i·nal** (lĭ-bid′ĭ-nəl) 1. pertaining to or of the nature of libido. 2. erotic.

**li·bid·i·nous** (lĭ-bid′ĭ-nəs) erotic.

**li·bi·do** (lĭ-be′do, lĭ-bi′do) pl. *libid′ines* [L.] [MeSH: Libido] 1. sexual desire. 2. the psychic energy derived from instinctive biological drives; in early freudian theory it was restricted to the sexual drive, then expanded to include all expressions of love and pleasure, but the concept has evolved to include also the death instinct.

**Lib·man-Sacks disease (endocarditis)** (lib′mən-saks) [E. *Libman;* Benjamin *Sacks,* New York physician, 1873–1939] atypical verrucous endocarditis.

**li·bra** (le′brə, li′brə) pl. *li′brae* [L.] pound. Symbol L.

**li·brary** (li′brer″e) [L. *libraria*] [MeSH: Libraries] in genetics, a set of cloned DNA fragments that together represent the entire genome, or the genes transcribed by a particular tissue. Called also *DNA l.*

**Lib·ri·tabs** (lib′rĭ-tabz) trademark for a preparation of chlordiazepoxide.

**Lib·ri·um** (lib′re-əm) trademark for preparations of chlordiazepoxide hydrochloride.

**lice** (līs) [MeSH: Lice] plural of *louse.*

**li·cense** (li′səns) [L. *licere* to be permitted] [MeSH: Licensure] a permit to perform acts which without it would be illegal.

**li·cen·ti·ate** (li-sen′she-āt) [L. *licentia* license] one holding a license from an authorized agency entitling him to practice a particular profession.

**Lich technique** (lik) see under *technique.*

**li·chen** (li′kən) [Gr. *leichēn* a tree-moss] 1. any of the many thallophytic plants formed by mutualistic combination of an alga and a fungus, the algal component being a green or blue-green alga, and the fungal usually an ascomycete. 2. any of a number of papular skin diseases in which the lesions are small, firm papules set close together; the specific type is indicated by a modifying term.

**l. amyloido′sus,** see under *amyloidosis.*

**l. cor′neus hypertro′phicus,** a papular skin eruption of thickened and horny lesions.

**l. fibromucinoido′sus,** l. myxedematosus.

**l. myxedemato′sus,** a condition resembling myxedema but not associated with thyroid dysfunction, characterized by a fibrocystic proliferation, increased deposition of acid mucopolysaccharides in the skin, and the presence of a circulating paraprotein, usually an immunoglobulin G, which presents as either discrete or generalized lichenoid papules with or without diffuse scleroderma, or as urticaria-like plaques and nodules. Called also *l. fibromucinoidosus, papular mucinosis, papular myxedema,* and *scleromyxedema.*

**l. ni′tidus,** a usually asymptomatic chronic inflammatory eruption consisting of numerous glistening, flat-topped, discrete, smooth, commonly skin-colored micropapules, located most often on the penis, lower abdomen, inner thighs, flexor aspects of the wrists and forearms, breasts, and buttocks. Widespread involvement may produce confluence of the lesions, with formation of scaly plaques.

**l. obtu′sus cor′neus,** a papular eruption of thickened, blunt lesions; probably identical with prurigo nodularis.

**l. pila′ris,** l. spinulosus.

**l. planopila′ris,** l. planus follicularis.

**l. pla′nus,** an inflammatory, pruritic skin disease, sometimes also involving the oral and genital mucosa and nails, which may be acute and widespread or chronic and localized. It is characterized by an eruption of violet umbilicated, flat-topped, scaly papules with white lines or puncta *(Wickham's striae),* which may either be discrete or coalesce to form plaques or other shapes. Lichen planus has many types, including vesicular, hypertrophic, atrophic, follicular, erosive and ulcerative, actinic, and erythematous; most resolve spontaneously, leaving residual hyperpigmentation and atrophy. Lichen planus–like lesions may also be caused by drugs or chemical substances. Called also *l. ruber planus.*

**l. planus, bullous,** see *vesiculobullous l. planus.*

**l. planus, vesiculobullous,** a variant in which small vesicles and bullae may occur as part of the general papular eruption, or present de novo or on uninvolved skin.

**l. pla′nus acti′nicus,** l. planus tropicum.

**l. pla′nus annula′ris,** a variant in which groups of papules form annular configurations, especially on the genitals, lower trunk, and lips, and in the mouth.

**l. pla′nus atro′phicus,** a variant characterized by atrophy in the center of preexisting lesions of lichen planus, ultimately leading to atrophic white spots on the skin, which aggregate to form small ivory- or violet-colored patches that may have an erythematous border.

**l. pla′nus erythemato′sus,** an unusual variant characterized by the presence of soft, nonpruritic, slightly erythematous or purpuric papules.

**l. pla′nus follicula′ris,** a variant characterized by the presence of acuminate, keratotic, patchy follicular lesions of the scalp, often leading to local atrophy or alopecia. Called also *l. planopilaris.*

**l. pla′nus hypertro′phicus,** a variant characterized by the presence of verrucous plaques covered with scales, which are most often located on the shins but may be found anywhere on the body. Called also *l. planus verrucosus.*

**l. pla′nus subtro′picum,** l. planus tropicum.

**l. pla′nus tro′picum,** a variant occurring in the tropics or subtropics, especially on sun-exposed areas of the skin of children and young adults of East Asian extraction, and characterized by papular lesions that may be pigmented, dyschromic, or granuloma annulare–like. Called also *l. planus actinicus* and *l. planus subtropicum.*

**l. pla′nus verruco′sus,** l. planus hypertrophicus.

**l. ru′ber monilifor′mis,** a generalized or localized eruption presenting as either round, dome-shaped, waxy, dark or bright red papules, or as waxy yellow, milia-like papules with a keloidal consistency, often forming a moniliform pattern, sometimes arranged in keloidal bands. Some authorities consider the condition to be a variant of lichen simplex chronicus. Called also *morbus moniliformis.*

**l. ru′ber pla′nus,** l. planus.

**l. sclero′sus,** a chronic, atrophic skin disease characterized by flat white indurated papules with erythematous halos and black follicular keratotic plugs; it is usually around the external genitalia or in the perianal region. In females it is seen in older women or the very young and results in destruction of vulvar architecture, scarring, and shrinkage of the labia with itching, dyspareunia, and dysuria. In males it affects the prepuce and glans penis and may result in stricture of the urethral meatus. Occasionally it may precede squamous cell carcinoma. Called also *l. sclerosus et atrophicus*. In females, called also *atrophic leukoplakia, atrophic* or *leukoplakic vulvitis, leukokraurosis,* and *kraurosis vulvae*. In males, called also *balanitis xerotica obliterans*.

**l. sclero'sus et atro'phicus,** l. sclerosus.

**l. scrofuloso'rum, l. scrofulo'sus,** a form of tuberculid manifested as an eruption of clusters of lichenoid papules on the trunk of children with tuberculous disease. Called also *tuberculosis cutis lichenoides* and *tuberculosis lichenoides*.

**l. sim'plex chro'nicus,** an eczematous dermatitis due to repeated itching and rubbing or scratching of the skin, arising spontaneously or initiated by or coexisting with other dermatoses, characterized by sharply demarcated, circumscribed, scaling patches of thickened, furrowed skin, located most commonly on the face, nuchal region, extremities, scrotum, vulva, and perianal region. Called also *circumscribed* or *localized neurodermatitis*.

**l. spinulo'sus,** a cutaneous disorder seen chiefly in children, characterized by the presence of discrete groups of minute, filiform, horny spines protruding from acuminate follicular openings, occurring in crops and located especially on the neck, buttocks, abdominal wall, popliteal spaces, and extensor surfaces of the arms.

**l. stria'tus,** a self-limited, usually unilateral eruption most commonly seen in children, predominantly located on the extremities and sides of the neck, and typically presenting as discrete, pink, papular or lichenoid lesions with an inconspicuous scale that tend to coalesce and form a continuous or interrupted linear patch.

**l. syphil'iticus,** a skin lesion seen in secondary syphilis, consisting of groups of small follicular papules. Called also *follicular syphilid*.

**l. tro'picus,** miliaria rubra.

**l. urtica'tus,** papular urticaria.

**li·chen·i·fi·ca·tion** (li-ken″ĭ-fi-ka'shən) hypertrophy of the epidermis, resulting in thickening of the skin with exaggeration of the normal skin markings, giving the skin a leathery barklike appearance, which is caused by prolonged rubbing or scratching. It may arise on seemingly normal skin, or it may develop at the site of another pruritic cutaneous disorder.

**li·chen·i·form·in** (li-ken″ĭ-form'in) a group of antibiotic substances (licheniformin A, B, and C) isolated from *Bacillus subtilis*, resembling subtilin in their properties.

**li·chen·oid** (li'kən-oid) [*lichen* + *-oid*] resembling the skin lesions designated as lichen.

**Licht·heim's aphasia,** etc. (likt'hīmz) [Ludwig *Lichtheim*, German physician, 1845–1928] see under *plaque, sign,* and *test,* and see *subacute combined degeneration of spinal cord,* under *degeneration*.

**lic·o·rice** (lik'o-ris) 1. *Glycyrrhiza glabra*. 2. glycyrrhiza.

**lid** (lid) [A.S. *hlid*] an eyelid.

**granular l's,** trachoma.

**tucked l. of Collier,** a retraction of the upper eyelid in cases of ophthalmoplegia due to a supranuclear lesion in the brain stem.

**li·dam·i·dine** (li-dam'ĭ-dēn) an amidinourea with antisecretory and antimotility action in animals that has been investigated as an antidiarrheal.

**li·da·mine** (li'də-mēn) an amidinourea that has been used as an antidiarrheal.

**Lid·dell and Sher·ring·ton reflex** (lĭ-del', sher'ing-tən) [Edward George Tandy *Liddell*, English physiologist, 1895–1981; Sir Charles Scott *Sherrington*, English physiologist, 1857–1952] stretch reflex.

**Lid·dle's syndrome** (lid'əlz) [Grant Winder *Liddle*, American physician, born 1921] see under *syndrome*.

**Li·dex** (li'deks) trademark for preparations of fluocinonide.

**li·do·caine** (li'do-kān) [USP] [MeSH: Lidocaine] a drug having anesthetic, sedative, analgesic, anticonvulsant, and cardiac depressant activities, used as a local anesthetic, applied topically to the skin and mucous membranes.

**l. hydrochloride** [USP], the monohydrated monohydrochloride salt of lidocaine, occurring as a white, crystalline powder; administered intravenously for use as a cardiac antiarrhythmic, and to produce local anesthesia by infiltration injection and epidural and peripheral nerve block.

**li·do·fen·in** (li″do-fen'in) HIDA; a dimethyl-substituted analogue of iminodiacetic acid (IDA); complexed with technetium 99m it is used for hepatobiliary imaging. See also table at *technetium*.

**li·do·fil·con** (li″do-fil'kon) either of two hydrophilic contact lens materials, one of which contains 70 per cent water *(lidofilcon A)*, and the other 79 per cent water *(lidofilcon B)*.

**lie** (li) the relation of the long axis of the fetus to that of the mother; see *presentation*.

**oblique l.,** the situation of the fetus when the long axis of its body crosses the long axis of the maternal body at an angle close to 45 degrees; the shoulder usually presents first, but the arm or part of the trunk may also present first.

**transverse l.,** the situation of the fetus when the long axis of its body crosses the long axis of the maternal body. The shoulder usually presents first, but the arm or any part of the trunk may be the first to appear. Called also *torso, transverse,* or *trunk presentation*. See table at *position*.

**Lie·ber·kühn's ampulla, crypts, follicles, glands** (le'ber-kēnz) [Johann Nathaniel *Lieberkühn*, German anatomist, 1711–1756] see under *ampulla*, and see *glandulae intestinales*.

**Lie·ber·mann-Bur·chard reaction, test** (le'bər-mahn-bərk'hahrd) [Carl Theodore *Liebermann*, German chemist, 1842–1914; H. *Burchard*, German chemist, 19th century] see under *test*.

**Lie·ber·meis·ter's furrows, grooves, rule** (le'bər-mīs″tərz) [Carl von *Liebermeister*, German physician, 1833–1901] see under *furrow, groove,* and *rule*.

**Lie·big's test, theory** (le'bigz) [Baron Justus von *Liebig*, German chemist, 1803–1873] see under *test* and *theory*.

**li·en** (li'ən) [L.] TA alternative for *splen*.

**l. accesso'rius,** splen accessorius.

**l. mo'bilis,** floating spleen.

**li·enal** (li-e'nəl) pertaining to the spleen; splenic.

**li·en·cu·lus** (li-en'ku-ləs) splen accessorius.

**li·en·ec·to·my** (li″ə-nek'tə-me) splenectomy.

**li·eni·tis** (li″ə-ni'tis) splenitis.

**lien(o)-** [L. *lien* spleen] a combining form denoting relationship to the spleen.

**li·eno·cele** (li-e'no-sēl) splenocele.

**li·en·og·ra·phy** (li″ə-nog'rə-fe) splenography.

**li·eno·ma·la·cia** (li-e″no-mə-la'shə) splenomalacia.

**li·eno·med·ul·lary** (li-e″no-med'u-lar″e) splenomedullary.

**li·eno·my·elog·e·nous** (li-e″no-mi″ə-loj'ə-nəs) splenomyelogenous.

**li·eno·my·elo·ma·la·cia** (le-e″no-mi″ə-lo-mə-la'shə) splenomyelomalacia.

**li·eno·pan·cre·at·ic** (li-e″no-pan″kre-at'ik) splenopancreatic.

**li·en·op·a·thy** (li″ə-nop'ə-the) splenopathy.

**li·eno·re·nal** (li-e″no-re'nəl) pertaining to the spleen and the kidney.

**li·eno·tox·in** (li-e″no-tok'sin) [*lieno-* + *toxin*] splenotoxin.

**li·en·ter·ic** (li″ən-ter'ik) affected by or of the nature of a lientery.

**li·en·tery** (li'ən-ter″e) [Gr. *leienteria; leios* smooth + *enteron* intestine] diarrhea in which the stools contain undigested food.

**li·en·un·cu·lus** (li″ən-ung'ku-ləs) splen accessorius.

**Liep·mann's apraxia** (lēp'mahnz) [Hugo Carl *Liepmann*, German neurologist, 1863–1925] see under *apraxia*.

**Lie·se·gang's phenomenon (striae, waves)** (le'zə-gahngz) [Raphael Eduard *Liesegang*, German chemist, 1869–1947] see under *phenomenon*.

**Lieu·taud's triangle (body), uvula** (lyoo-toz') [Joseph *Lieutaud*, French physician, 1703–1780] see *trigonum vesicae* and *uvula vesicae*.

**LIF** left iliac fossa; leukocyte inhibitory factor.

**life** (līf) [MeSH: Life] the aggregate of vital phenomena; a certain peculiar stimulated condition of organized matter; that obscure principle whereby organized beings are peculiarly endowed with certain powers and functions not associated with inorganic matter. Generally, living things share, in varying degrees, the following characteristics: organization, irritability, movement, growth, reproduction, and adaptation.

**animal l.,** vegetative life conjoined with the employment of the senses and with spontaneous movements.

**intrauterine l., uterine l.,** the period of life spent in the uterus; i.e., embryonic and fetal life.

**mean l.,** the average time until decay for a sample of particles of a radionuclide or elementary particle, equal to the reciprocal of the decay constant or 1.443 times the half-life; symbol $\tau$. Called also *lifetime*.

**vegetative l.,** that which is manifested in automatic acts requisite for the maintenance of the individual and the propagation of the species.

**life·time** (līf'tīm) mean life.

**lig.** ligament; ligamentum.

**lig·a·ment** (lig′ə-mənt) [MeSH: Ligaments] 1. a band of tissue that connects bones or supports viscera. Some ligaments are distinct fibrous structures; some are folds of fascia or of indurated peritoneum; still others are relics of fetal vessels or organs. 2. a double layer of peritoneum extending from one visceral organ to another. 3. cordlike remnants of fetal tubular structures that are nonfunctional after birth.

## Ligament

For names of specific anatomic structures, see under *ligamentum.*

**accessory l.,** any ligament that strengthens or supports another.
**accessory l's, palmar,** see *ligamenta palmaria articulationum metacarpophalangealium* and *ligamenta palmaria articulationum interphalangealium manus.*
**accessory l's, plantar,** see *ligamenta plantaria articulationum metatarsophalangealium* and *ligamenta plantaria articulationum interphalangealium pedis.*
**accessory l's, volar,** see *ligamenta palmaria articulationum metacarpophalangealium* and *ligamenta palmaria articulationum interphalangealium manus.*
**accessory l. of Henle, lateral,** ligamentum laterale articulationis temporomandibularis.
**accessory l. of Henle, medial,** ligamentum sphenomandibulare.
**accessory l. of humerus,** ligamentum coracohumerale.
**accessory l's of metacarpophalangeal joints,** ligamenta collateralia articulationum metacarpophalangealium.
**acromioclavicular l.,** ligamentum acromioclaviculare.
**acromiocoracoid l.,** ligamentum coraco-acromiale.
**adipose l. of knee (of Cruveilhier),** plica synovialis infrapatellaris.
**alar l's,** ligamenta alaria.
**alar l's of knee,** plicae alares.
**alveolodental l.,** periodontal l.
**annular l., dorsal common,** retinaculum musculorum extensorum manus.
**annular l., inferior,** ligamentum pubicum inferius.
**annular l., internal,** retinaculum musculorum flexorum pedis.
**annular l. of ankle, external,** retinaculum musculorum peroneorum superius.
**annular l. of ankle, internal,** retinaculum musculorum flexorum pedis.
**annular l. of base of stapes,** ligamentum anulare stapediale.
**annular l. of carpus, posterior,** retinaculum musculorum extensorum manus.
**annular l's of digits of foot,** see *pars anularis vaginae fibrosae digitorum pedis.*
**annular l's of digits of hand,** see *pars anularis vaginae fibrosae digitorum manus.*
**annular l. of femur,** zona orbicularis articulationis coxae.
**annular l's of fingers,** pars anularis vaginae fibrosae digitorum manus.
**annular l. of malleolus, external,** retinaculum musculorum extensorum inferius pedis.
**annular l. of malleolus, internal,** retinaculum musculorum flexorum pedis.
**annular l. of radius,** ligamentum anulare radii.
**annular stapedial l.,** ligamentum anulare stapedis.
**annular l. of tarsus, anterior,** retinaculum musculorum extensorum inferius pedis.
**annular l's of tendon sheaths of fingers,** see *pars anularis vaginae fibrosae digitorum manus.*
**annular l's of toes,** pars anularis vaginae fibrosae digitorum pedis.
**annular l's of trachea,** ligamenta anularia tracheae.
**annular l. of wrist, dorsal posterior,** retinaculum musculorum extensorum manus.
**anococcygeal l.,** corpus anococcygeum.
**anterior l. of colon,** taenia omentalis.
**anterior l. of head of fibula,** ligamentum capitis fibulae anterius.
**anterior l. of head of rib,** ligamentum capitis costae radiatum.
**anterior l. of malleus,** ligamentum mallei anterius.
**anterior l. of neck of rib,** the anterior portion of the ligamentum costotransversarium superius.
**anterior l. of radiocarpal joint,** ligamentum radiocarpale palmare.
**l. of antebrachium (of Weitbrecht),** chorda obliqua membranae interosseae antebrachii.
**l. of apex dentis, apical l. of dens, apical dental l.,** ligamentum apicis dentis.
**appendiculo-ovarian l.,** a fold of peritoneum extending between the appendix and the broad ligament of the uterus.
**Arantius' l.,** ligamentum venosum.
**arcuate l's,** ligamenta flava.
**arcuate l., lateral,** ligamentum arcuatum laterale.
**arcuate l., medial,** ligamentum arcuatum mediale.
**arcuate l., median,** ligamentum arcuatum medianum.
**arcuate l. of diaphragm, external,** ligamentum arcuatum laterale.
**arcuate l. of diaphragm, internal,** ligamentum arcuatum mediale.
**arcuate l. of diaphragm, lateral,** ligamentum arcuatum laterale.
**arcuate l. of knee,** ligamentum popliteum arcuatum.
**arcuate pubic l., arcuate l. of pubis, inferior,** ligamentum pubicum inferius.
**articular l. of vertebrae,** capsula articularis articulationum vertebrarum.
**arytenoepiglottic l.,** plica aryepiglottica.
**atlanto-occipital l., anterior, atlanto-occipital l., deep,** membrana atlanto-occipitalis anterior.
**atlanto-occipital l., lateral,** ligamentum atlanto-occipitale laterale.
**atlanto-occipital l., posterior,** membrana atlanto-occipitalis posterior.
**l's of auditory ossicles,** ligamenta ossiculorum auditoriorum.
**l's of auricle, auricular l's,** ligamenta auricularia.
**auricular l., anterior,** ligamentum auriculare anterius.
**auricular l., posterior,** ligamentum auriculare posterius.
**auricular l., superior,** ligamentum auriculare superius.
**Barkow's l.,** the anterior and posterior parts of the elbow joint capsule.
**Bellini's l.,** a band passing as part of the capsule of the hip joint to the greater trochanter.
**Bérard's l.,** the suspensory ligament of the pericardium, extending to the third and fourth thoracic vertebrae.
**Berry's l.,** ligamentum thyrohyoideum laterale.
**Bertin's l.,** ligamentum iliofemorale.
**Bichat's l.,** the lower bundle of the dorsal sacroiliac ligament.
**bifurcate l.,** ligamentum bifurcatum.
**bifurcate l's, deep,** ligamenta metatarsalia plantaria.
**bifurcate l's of Arnold, deep,** ligamenta tarsometatarsalia plantaria.
**bifurcated l.,** ligamentum bifurcatum.
**Bigelow's l.,** ligamentum iliofemorale.
**bigeminate l's of Arnold,** ligamenta tarsometatarsalia dorsalia.
**l. of Botallo,** ligamentum arteriosum.
**Bourgery's l.,** ligamentum popliteum obliquum.
**brachiocubital l.,** ligamentum collaterale ulnare.
**brachioradial l.,** ligamentum collaterale radiale.
**broad l. of liver,** ligamentum falciforme hepatis.
**broad l. of uterus,** ligamentum latum uteri.
**Brodie's l.,** transverse humeral ligament.
**Burns' l.,** margo falciformis hiatus saphenus.
**calcaneocuboid l.,** ligamentum calcaneocuboideum.
**calcaneocuboid l., plantar,** ligamentum calcaneocuboideum plantare.
**calcaneofibular l.,** ligamentum calcaneofibulare.
**calcaneonavicular l.,** ligamentum calcaneonaviculare.
**calcaneonavicular l., plantar,** ligamentum calcaneonaviculare plantare.
**calcaneotibial l.,** pars tibiocalcanea ligamenti medialis.
**Caldani's l.,** a band passing from the inner border of the coracoid process to the lower border of the clavicle, the first rib, and the tendon of the subclavius.
**Campbell's l.,** suspensory l. of axilla.
**Camper's l.,** diaphragma urogenitale.
**canthal l's,** see *ligamentum palpebrale mediale* and *ligamentum palpebrale laterale.*
**capitular l., volar,** deep transverse metacarpal l.
**capsular l's,** ligamenta capsularia.
**capsular l., internal,** ligamentum capitis femoris.
**capsular l., pelviprostatic,** fascia prostatae.
**Carcassonne's l.,** ligamentum puboprostaticum.
**cardinal l.,** part of a thickening of the visceral pelvic fascia beside the cervix and vagina, passing laterally to merge with the upper fascia of the pelvic diaphragm; called also *lateral cervical l.*
**carpal l., dorsal,** ligamenta intercarpalia dorsalia.
**carpal l., radiate,** ligamentum carpi radiatum.
**carpometacarpal l's, anterior,** ligamenta carpometacarpalia palmaria.
**carpometacarpal l's, dorsal,** ligamenta carpometacarpalia dorsalia.

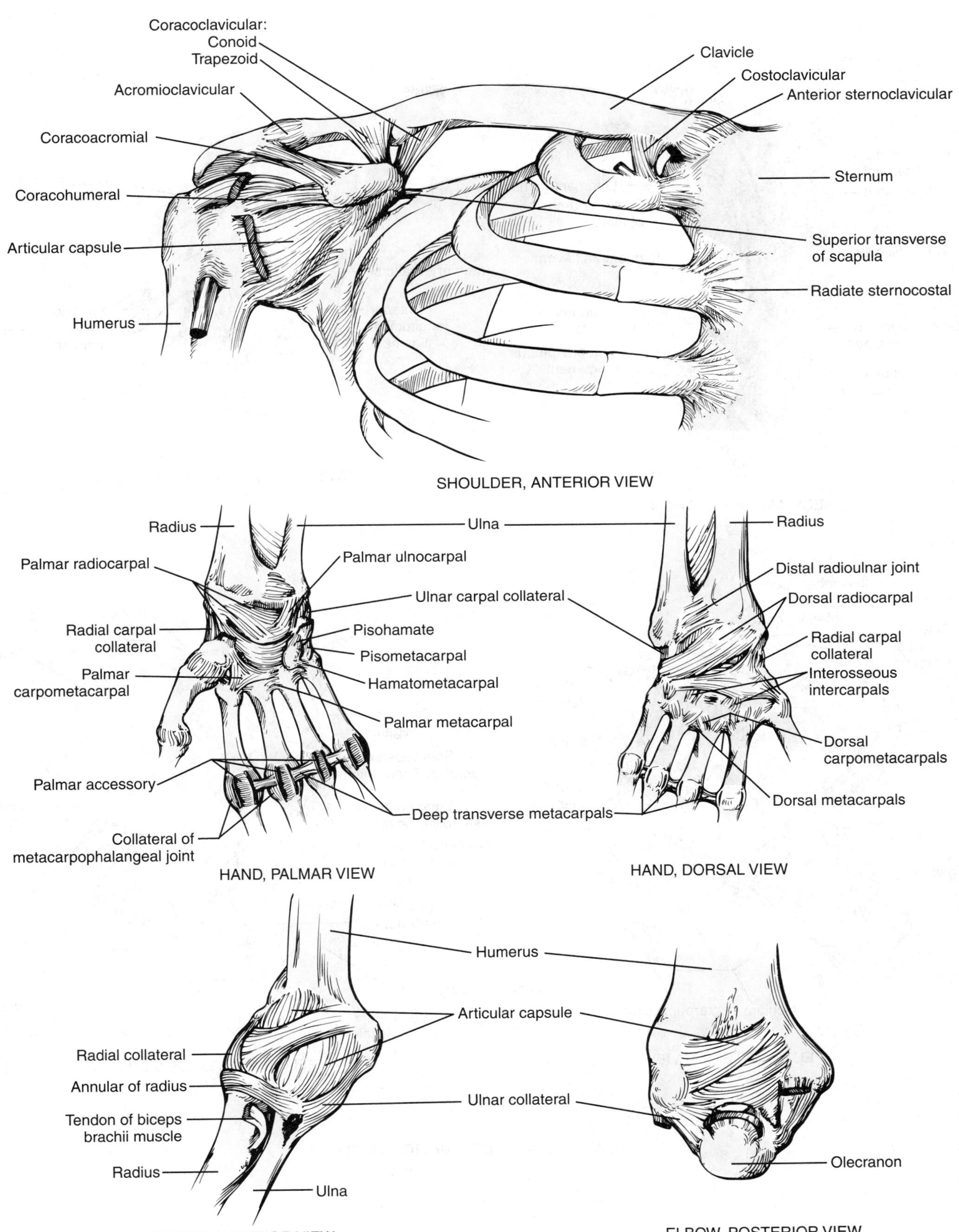


**PLATE 23**—ARTICULAR LIGAMENTS

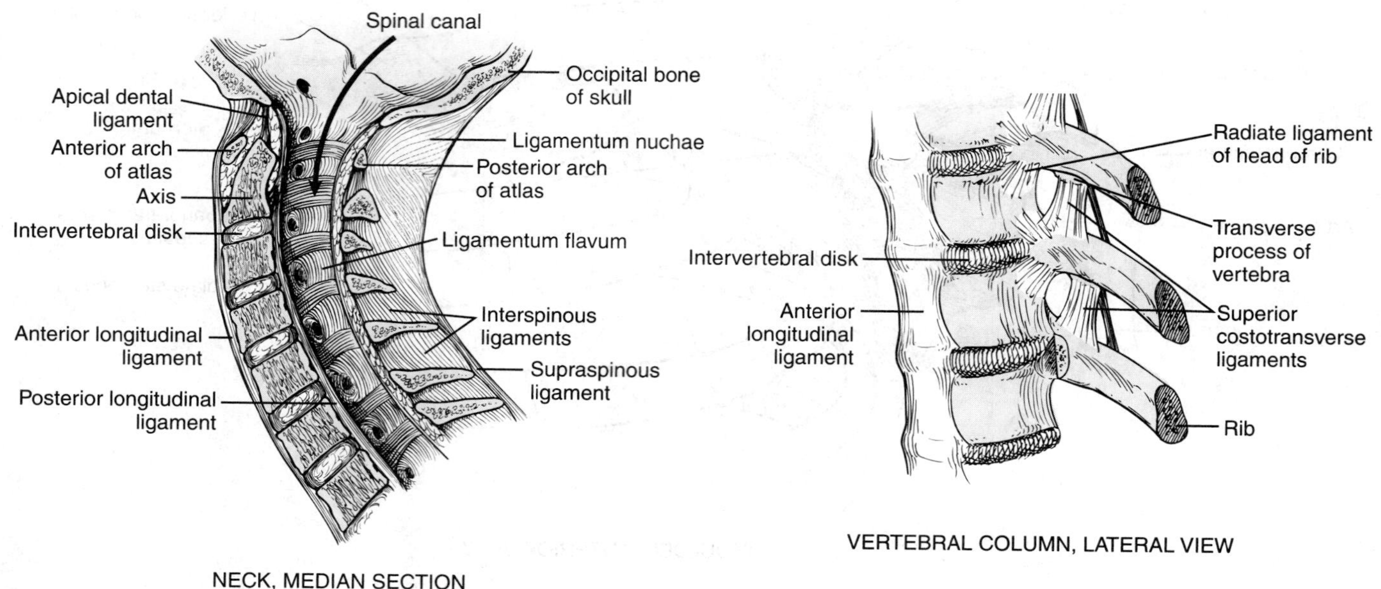


NECK, MEDIAN SECTION

VERTEBRAL COLUMN, LATERAL VIEW

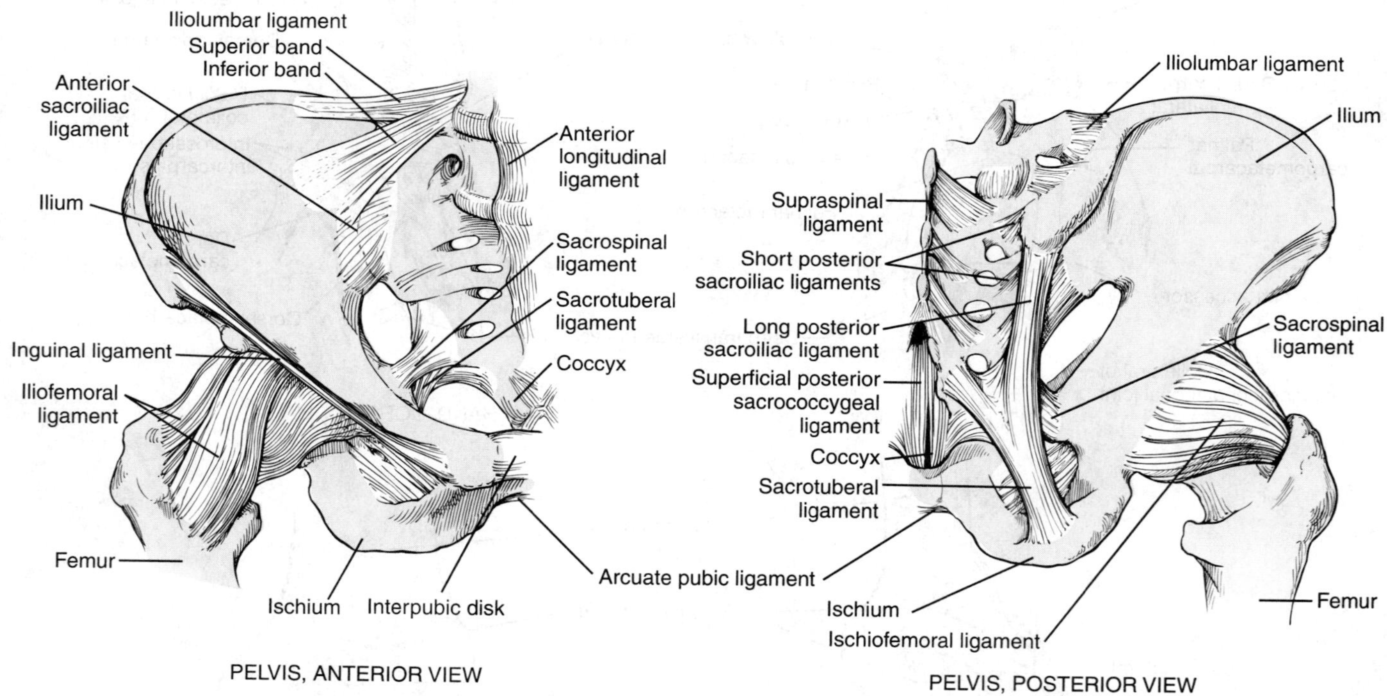


PELVIS, ANTERIOR VIEW

PELVIS, POSTERIOR VIEW

**PLATE 24**—ARTICULAR LIGAMENTS

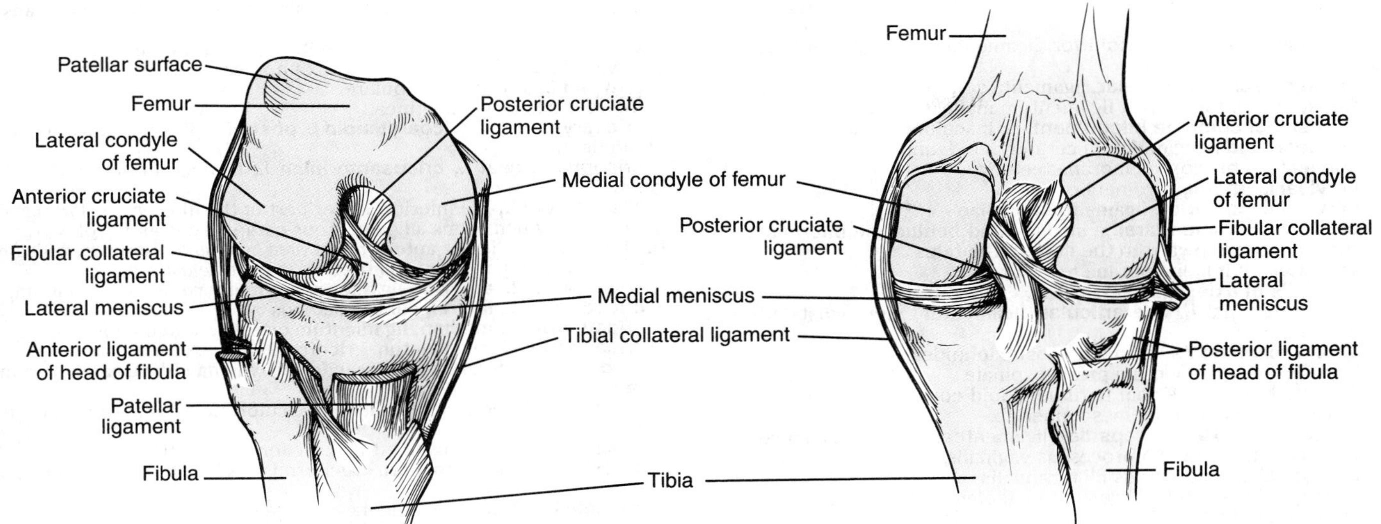


RIGHT KNEE, ANTERIOR VIEW

RIGHT KNEE, POSTERIOR VIEW

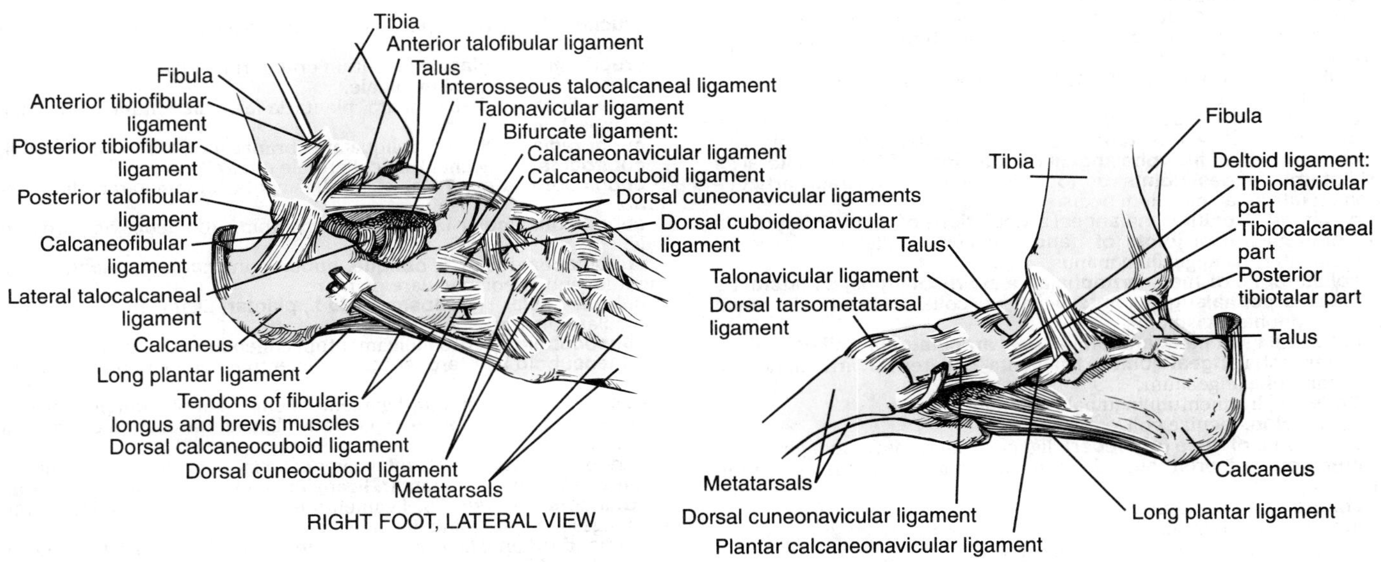


RIGHT FOOT, LATERAL VIEW

RIGHT FOOT, MEDIAL VIEW

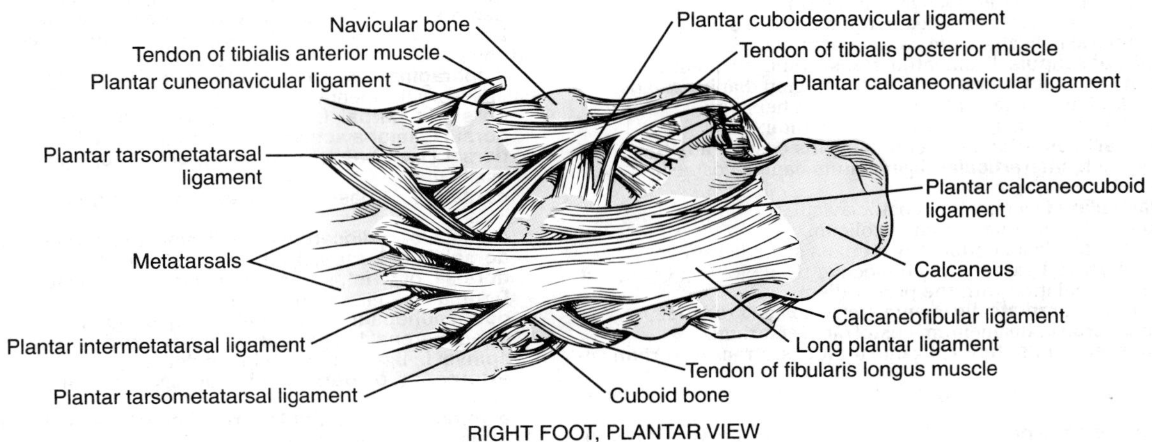


RIGHT FOOT, PLANTAR VIEW

**PLATE 25**—ARTICULAR LIGAMENTS

**carpometacarpal l's, palmar,** ligamenta carpometacarpalia palmaria.
**carpometacarpal l's, posterior,** ligamenta carpometacarpalia dorsalia.
**carpometacarpal l's, volar,** ligamenta carpometacarpalia palmaria.
**Casser's l., casserian l.,** ligamentum mallei laterale.
**caudal l. of common integument,** retinaculum caudale.
**ceratocricoid l.,** ligamentum ceratocricoideum.
**cervical l., anterior,** membrana tectoria.
**cervical l., lateral,** cardinal l.
**cervical l., posterior,** ligamentum nuchae.
**cervical l. of sinus tarsi,** a strong band behind the bifurcate ligament, extending upward to the neck of the talus.
**cervicobasilar l.,** membrana tectoria.
**check l's of axis,** ligamenta alaria.
**chondrosternal l., interarticular,** ligamentum sternocostale intraarticulare.
**chondroxiphoid l's,** ligamenta costoxiphoidea.
**l. of Civinini,** ligamentum pterygospinale.
**Clado's l.,** an occasional peritoneal fold connecting the infundibulopelvic ligament and the mesoappendix.
**clavicular l., external capsular,** ligamentum acromioclaviculare.
**Cloquet's l.,** vestigium processus vaginalis.
**coccygeal l.,** pars duralis fili terminalis.
**coccygeal l., superior,** ligamentum iliofemorale.
**collateral l., fibular,** ligamentum collaterale fibulare.
**collateral l., radial,** ligamentum collaterale radiale.
**collateral l., radial carpal,** ligamentum collaterale carpi radiale.
**collateral l., tibial,** ligamentum collaterale tibiale.
**collateral l., ulnar,** ligamentum collaterale ulnare.
**collateral l., ulnar carpal,** ligamentum collaterale carpi ulnare.
**collateral l. of ankle joint, lateral,** ligamentum collaterale laterale articulationis talocruralis.
**collateral l. of ankle joint, medial,** ligamentum collaterale mediale articulationis talocruralis.
**collateral l. of carpus, radial,** ligamentum collaterale carpi radiale.
**collateral l. of carpus, ulnar,** ligamentum collaterale carpi ulnare.
**collateral l's of interphalangeal articulations of foot, collateral l's of interphalangeal joints of foot,** ligamenta collateralia articulationum interphalangealium pedis.
**collateral l's of interphalangeal articulations of hand, collateral l's of interphalangeal joints of hand,** ligamenta collateralia articulationum interphalangealium manus.
**collateral l's of metacarpophalangeal articulations, collateral l's of metacarpophalangeal joints,** ligamenta collateralia articulationum metacarpophalangealium.
**collateral l's of metatarsophalangeal articulations, collateral l's of metatarsophalangeal joints,** ligamenta collateralia articulationum metatarsophalangealium.
**Colles' l.,** ligamentum inguinale reflexum.
**l's of colon,** taeniae coli.
**common l. of knee (of Weber),** ligamentum transversum genus.
**common l. of wrist joint, deep,** ligamentum collaterale carpi radiale.
**conoid l.,** ligamentum conoideum.
**conus l.,** tendo infundibuli.
**Cooper's l.,** ligamentum pectineum.
**Cooper's suspensory l's,** ligamenta suspensoria mammaria.
**coracoacromial l.,** ligamentum coraco-acromiale.
**coracoclavicular l.,** ligamentum coracoclaviculare.
**coracoclavicular l., external,** ligamentum trapezoideum.
**coracoclavicular l., internal,** ligamentum conoideum.
**coracohumeral l.,** ligamentum coracohumerale.
**coracoid l. of scapula,** ligamentum transversum scapulae superius.
**cordiform l. of diaphragm,** centrum tendineum diaphragmatis.
**coronary l. of liver,** ligamentum coronarium hepatis.
**coronary l. of radius,** ligamentum anulare radii.
**costocentral l., anterior,** ligamentum capitis costae radiatum.
**costocentral l., interarticular,** ligamentum capitis costae intra-articulare.
**costoclavicular l.,** ligamentum costoclaviculare.
**costocolic l.,** ligamentum phrenicocolicum.
**costocoracoid l.,** ligamentum transversum scapulae superius.
**costopericardiac l.,** a band of connective tissue joining the upper costosternal articulation with the pericardium.
**costosternal l's, radiate,** ligamenta sternocostalia radiata.
**costotransverse l.,** ligamentum costotransversarium.
**costotransverse l., anterior,** ligamentum costotransversarium superius.
**costotransverse l., lateral,** ligamentum costotransversarium laterale.
**costotransverse l., posterior,** ligamentum costotransversarium superius.
**costotransverse l., superior,** ligamentum costotransversarium superius.
**costotransverse l. of Krause, posterior,** ligamentum costotransversarium laterale.
**costovertebral l.,** ligamentum capitis costae radiatum.
**costoxiphoid l's,** ligamenta costoxiphoidea.
**cotyloid l.,** labrum acetabulare.
**Cowper's l.,** fascia pectinea.
**cricoarytenoid l., cricoarytenoid l., posterior,** ligamentum crico-arytenoideum.
**cricopharyngeal l., cricosantorinian l.,** ligamentum cricopharyngeum.
**cricothyroid l.,** the inferior, larger part of the fibroelastic laryngeal membrane, which forms a ligamentous complex consisting of two distinct parts: a median or anterior part (see *ligamentum cricothyroideum medianum)* and paired lateral parts (see *conus elasticus*).
**cricothyroid l., anterior,** ligamentum cricothyroideum medianum.
**cricothyroid l., lateral,** conus elasticus.
**cricothyroid l., median,** ligamentum cricothyroideum medianum.
**cricotracheal l.,** ligamentum cricotracheale.
**crucial l's of fingers,** pars cruciformis vaginae fibrosae digitorum manus.
**crucial l. of foot,** retinaculum musculorum extensorum inferius pedis.
**cruciate l. of atlas,** ligamentum cruciforme atlantis.
**cruciate l's of fingers,** pars cruciformis vaginae fibrosae digitorum manus.
**cruciate l's of knee,** ligamenta cruciata genus.
**cruciate l. of knee, anterior,** ligamentum cruciatum anterius genus.
**cruciate l. of knee, posterior,** ligamentum cruciatum posterius genus.
**cruciate l. of leg,** retinaculum musculorum extensorum inferius pedis.
**cruciate l's of toes,** pars cruciformis vaginae fibrosae digitorum pedis.
**cruciform l. of atlas,** ligamentum cruciforme atlantis.
**crural l.,** ligamentum inguinale.
**Cruveilhier's l's,** ligamenta plantaria articulationum metatarsophalangealium.
**cubitoradial l.,** chorda obliqua membranae interosseae antibrachii.
**cubitoulnar l.,** ligamentum collaterale ulnare.
**cuboideometatarsal l's, short,** ligamenta tarsometatarsalia plantaria.
**cuboideonavicular l., dorsal,** ligamentum cuboideonaviculare dorsale.
**cuboideonavicular l., oblique, cuboideonavicular l., plantar,** ligamentum cuboideonaviculare plantare.
**cubonavicular l., cuboscaphoid l., plantar,** ligamentum cuboideonaviculare plantare.
**cuneocuboid l., dorsal,** ligamentum cuneocuboideum dorsale.
**cuneocuboid l., interosseous,** ligamentum cuneocuboideum interosseum.
**cuneocuboid l., plantar,** ligamentum cuneocuboideum plantare.
**cuneometatarsal l's, interosseous,** ligamenta cuneometatarsalia interossea.
**cuneonavicular l's, dorsal,** ligamenta cuneonavicularia dorsalia.
**cuneonavicular l's, plantar,** ligamenta cuneonavicularia plantaria.
**cutaneophalangeal l's,** ligamentous fibers from the sides of the phalanges near the joints to the skin.
**cysticoduodenal l.,** an anomalous fold of peritoneum extending between the gallbladder and the duodenum.
**deltoid l. of ankle, deltoid l. of ankle joint,** ligamentum collaterale mediale articulationis talocruralis.
**deltoid l. of elbow,** ligamentum collaterale ulnare.
**dentate l. of spinal cord, denticulate l.,** ligamentum denticulatum.
**Denucé's l.,** a short, wide band connecting the radius and the ulna at the wrist.
**diaphragmatic l.,** the involuting urogenital ridge that becomes the suspensory ligament of the ovary.
**dorsal l's, carpal,** ligamenta intercarpalia dorsalia.
**dorsal l., talonavicular,** ligamentum talonaviculare.
**dorsal l's of bases of metacarpal bones,** ligamenta metacarpalia dorsalia.
**dorsal l's of bases of metatarsal bones,** ligamenta metatarsalia dorsalia.
**dorsal l. of radiocarpal joint,** ligamentum radiocarpale dorsale.
**dorsal l's of tarsus,** ligamenta tarsi dorsalia.
**dorsal l. of wrist,** retinaculum musculorum extensorum manus.
**Douglas' l.,** plica recto-uterina.
**duodenohepatic l.,** ligamentum hepatoduodenale.
**duodenorenal l.,** ligamentum duodenorenale.
**epihyal l.,** ligamentum stylohyoideum.
**external l's of Barkow, plantar,** ligamenta intercuneiformia plantaria.
**external l. of mandibular articulation,** ligamentum laterale articulationis temporomandibularis.
**fabellofibular l.,** an occasional ligament apparently replacing the short lateral ligament when the fabella is present; it originates directly from the fabella, passes between the condylar portions of the plantaris

and lateral gastrocnemius muscles, and is attached to the apex of the fibula.

**falciform l.,** processus falciformis ligamenti sacrotuberosi.

**falciform l. of liver,** ligamentum falciforme hepatis.

**fallopian l., l. of Fallopius,** ligamentum inguinale.

**false l.,** 1. any suspensory ligament that is a peritoneal fold and not of true ligamentous structure. 2. a peritoneal connection between the vertex and sides of the bladder and the walls of the pelvis.

**Ferrein's l.,** the thick external part of the capsule of the temporomandibular joint.

**fibrous l., anterior,** ligamentum sternoclaviculare anterius.

**fibrous l., posterior,** ligamentum sternoclaviculare posterius.

**flaval l's,** ligamenta flava.

**Flood's l.,** the superior glenohumeral ligament; see *ligamenta glenohumeralia.*

**fundiform l. of penis,** ligamentum fundiforme penis.

**gastrocolic l.,** ligamentum gastrocolicum.

**gastrohepatic l.,** ligamentum hepatogastricum.

**gastrolienal l.,** ligamentum gastrosplenicum.

**gastropancreatic l's of Huschke,** plica gastropancreatica.

**gastrophrenic l.,** ligamentum gastrophrenicum.

**gastrosplenic l.,** ligamentum gastrosplenicum.

**genitoinguinal l.,** ligamentum genitoinguinale.

**Gerdy's l.,** suspensory l. of axilla.

**Gillette's suspensory l.,** tendo crico-oesophageus.

**Gimbernat's l.,** ligamentum lacunare.

**glenohumeral l's,** ligamenta glenohumeralia.

**glenoid l's of Cruveilhier,** ligamenta plantaria articulationum metatarsophalangealium.

**glenoid l. of humerus, glenoid l. of Macalister,** labrum glenoidale.

**Günz's l.,** part of the obturator membrane.

**hamatometacarpal l.,** fibers connecting the hamulus of the hamate bone with the base of the fifth metacarpal bone.

**l. of head of femoral bone, l. of head of femur,** ligamentum capitis femoris.

**Helmholtz l.,** that part of the anterior ligament of the malleus which is attached to the greater tympanic spine.

**l's of Helvetius,** ligamenta pylori.

**Henle's l.,** falx inguinalis.

**Hensing's l.,** a small serous fold from the upper end of the descending colon to the abdominal wall.

**hepatic l's,** ligamenta hepatis.

**hepatocolic l.,** ligamentum hepatocolicum.

**hepatocystocolic l.,** a hepatocolic ligament arising from the gallbladder.

**hepatoduodenal l.,** ligamentum hepatoduodenale.

**hepatogastric l.,** ligamentum hepatogastricum.

**hepatogastroduodenal l.,** omentum minus.

**hepatorenal l.,** ligamentum hepatorenale.

**hepatoumbilical l.,** ligamentum teres hepatis.

**Hesselbach's l.,** ligamentum interfoveolare.

**Hey's l.,** margo falciformis hiatus saphenus.

**Hueck's l.,** reticulum trabeculare.

**Humphry's l.,** ligamentum meniscofemorale anterius.

**Hunter's l.,** ligamentum teres uteri.

**Huschke's l.,** plica gastropancreatica.

**hyaloideocapsular l.,** the tissue connecting the vitreous body to the peripheral zone of the lens capsule.

**hyoepiglottic l.,** ligamentum hyo-epiglotticum.

**iliocostal l.,** ligamentum lumbocostale.

**iliofemoral l.,** ligamentum iliofemorale.

**iliolumbar l.,** ligamentum iliolumbale.

**iliopectineal l.,** arcus iliopectineus.

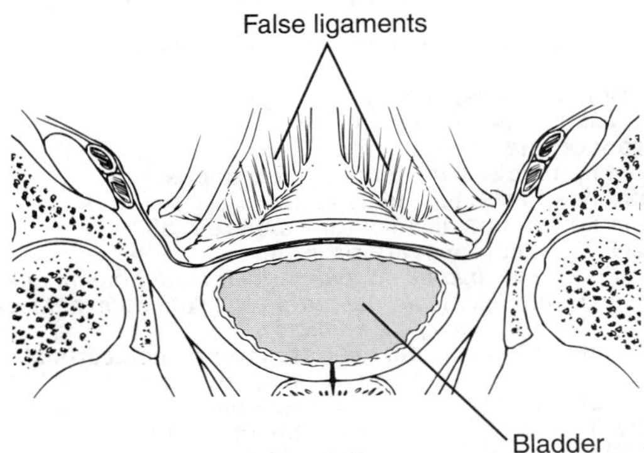


False ligaments (peritoneal folds) connecting the bladder to the pelvic walls; shown in frontal section.

**iliopubic l.,** ligamentum inguinale.

**iliosacral l., anterior,** ligamentum sacroiliacum anterius.

**iliosacral l., interosseous,** ligamentum sacroiliacum interosseum.

**iliosacral l., long,** ligamentum sacroiliacum posterius.

**iliotibial l. of Maissiat,** tractus iliotibialis.

**iliotrochanteric l.,** a portion of the articular capsule of the hip joint.

**inferior l. of epididymis,** ligamentum epididymidis inferius.

**inferior l. of neck of rib of Henle,** ligamentum costotransversarium.

**inferior l. of tubercle of rib,** ligamentum costotransversarium laterale.

**infundibulopelvic l.,** ligamentum suspensorium ovarii.

**inguinal l.,** ligamentum inguinale.

**inguinal l., anterior,** crus mediale annuli inguinalis superficialis.

**inguinal l., external,** ligamentum inguinale.

**inguinal l., internal,** 1. ligamentum inguinale reflexum. 2. crus mediale annuli inguinalis superficialis.

**inguinal l., posterior,** ligamentum interfoveolare.

**inguinal l., reflex,** ligamentum inguinale reflexum.

**inguinal l. of Blumberg,** ligamentum interfoveolare.

**inguinal l. of Cooper,** ligamentum pectineum.

**interarticular l.,** any ligament situated within the capsule of a joint.

**interarticular l. of articulation of humerus,** caput longum musculi bicipitis brachii.

**interarticular l. of head of rib,** ligamentum capitis costae intra-articulare.

**interarticular l. of hip joint,** ligamentum capitis femoris.

**intercarpal l's, dorsal,** ligamenta intercarpalia dorsalia.

**intercarpal l's, interosseous,** ligamenta intercarpalia interossea.

**intercarpal l's, palmar, intercarpal l's, volar,** ligamenta intercarpalia palmaria.

**interclavicular l.,** ligamentum interclaviculare.

**intercuneiform l's, dorsal,** ligamenta intercuneiformia dorsalia.

**intercuneiform l's, interosseous,** ligamenta intercuneiformia interossea.

**intercuneiform l's, plantar,** ligamenta intercuneiformia plantaria.

**interfoveolar l.,** ligamentum interfoveolare.

**intermetacarpal l's, anterior proximal,** ligamenta metacarpalia palmaria.

**intermetacarpal l., distal,** deep transverse metacarpal l.

**intermetacarpal l's, dorsal, intermetacarpal l's, dorsal transverse,** ligamenta metacarpalia dorsalia.

**intermetacarpal l's, interosseous,** ligamenta metacarpalia interossea.

**intermetacarpal l's, palmar,** ligamenta metacarpalia palmaria.

**intermetacarpal l's, posterior proximal,** ligamenta metacarpalia dorsalia.

**intermetacarpal l's, volar transverse,** ligamenta metacarpalia palmaria.

**intermetatarsal l., distal plantar,** deep transverse metatarsal l.

**intermetatarsal l's, dorsal proximal, intermetatarsal l's, dorsal transverse,** ligamenta metatarsalia dorsalia.

**intermetatarsal l's, interosseous,** ligamenta metatarsalia interossea.

**intermetatarsal l's, plantar proximal, intermetatarsal l's, plantar transverse,** ligamenta metatarsalia plantaria.

**intermuscular l., fibular,** septum intermusculare cruris anterius.

**intermuscular l. of arm, external,** septum intermusculare brachii laterale.

**intermuscular l. of arm, internal,** septum intermusculare brachii mediale.

**intermuscular l. of arm, lateral,** septum intermusculare brachii laterale.

**intermuscular l. of arm, medial,** septum intermusculare brachii mediale.

**intermuscular l. of thigh, external, intermuscular l. of thigh, lateral,** septum intermusculare femoris laterale.

**intermuscular l. of thigh, medial,** septum intermusculare femoris mediale.

**internal l. of neck of rib,** ligamentum costotransversarium superius.

**interosseous l., radioulnar,** membrana interossea antebrachii.

**interosseous l's, transverse metacarpal,** ligamenta metacarpalia interossea.

**interosseous l's of Barkow, internal,** ligamenta intercuneiformia plantaria.

**interosseous l's of bases of metacarpal bones,** ligamenta metacarpalia interossea.

**interosseous l's of bases of metatarsal bones,** ligamenta metatarsalia interossea.

**interosseous l. of Cruveilhier, costovertebral,** ligamentum capitis costae intra-articulare.

**interosseous l. of Cruveilhier, transversocostal,** ligamentum costotransversarium.

**interosseous l's of knee,** ligamenta cruciata genus.

**interosseous l. of leg,** membrana interossea cruris.

**interosseous l. of pubis,** discus interpubicus.

**interosseous l. of pubis (of Winslow),** ligamentum transversum perinei.
**interosseous l's of tarsus,** ligamenta tarsi interossea.
**l's of interphalangeal articulations of foot, plantar,** ligamenta plantaria articulationum interphalangealium pedis.
**l's of interphalangeal articulations of hand, palmar,** ligamenta palmaria articulationum interphalangealium manus.
**interprocess l.,** a ligament that connects two processes on the same bone.
**interpubic l.,** discus interpubicus.
**interspinal l's, interspinous l's,** ligamenta interspinalia.
**intertarsal l's, dorsal,** ligamenta tarsi dorsalia.
**intertarsal l's, interosseous,** ligamenta tarsi interossea.
**intertarsal l's, plantar,** ligamenta tarsi plantaria.
**intertransverse l's,** ligamenta intertransversaria.
**interureteral l.,** plica interureterica.
**intervertebral l.,** 1. either of the two longitudinal ligaments of the vertebrae (ligamentum longitudinale anterius and ligamentum longitudinale posterius). 2. one of the disci intervertebrales.
**intraarticular l. of head of rib,** ligamentum capitis costae intra-articulare.
**ischiocapsular l., ischiofemoral l.,** ligamentum ischiofemorale.
**ischioprostatic l.,** diaphragma urogenitale.
**ischiosacral l's,** see *ligamentum sacrospinale* and *ligamentum sacrotuberale.*
**Jarjavay's l.,** uterosacral l.
**Krause's l.,** ligamentum transversum perinei.
**laciniate l.,** retinaculum musculorum flexorum pedis.
**laciniate l., external,** retinaculum musculorum peroneorum superius.
**lacunar l., lacunar l. of Gimbernat,** ligamentum lacunare.
**lambdoid l.,** retinaculum musculorum extensorum inferius pedis.
**laryngeal l's, extrinsic,** the ligaments in and around the thyrohyoid membrane, including the lateral and median thyrohyoid, hyoepiglottic, thyroepiglottic, and cricotracheal ligaments.
**laryngeal l's, intrinsic,** the ligaments in and around the fibroelastic membrane of the larynx, including the conus elasticus, the median cricothyroid ligament, and the vocal ligament.
**lateral l., short,** a knee ligament attached to the lowest part of the lateral femoral condyle and extending beyond the dorsum of the semilunar cartilage to the apex of the fibula. See also *fabellofibular l.*
**lateral l. of ankle joint,** ligamentum collaterale laterale articulationis talocruralis.
**lateral l. of carpus, radial,** ligamentum collaterale carpi radiale.
**lateral l. of carpus, ulnar,** ligamentum collaterale carpi ulnare.
**lateral l. of colon,** taenia omentalis.
**lateral l's of joints of fingers,** ligamenta collateralia articulationum interphalangealium manus.
**lateral l's of joints of toes,** ligamenta collateralia articulationum interphalangealium pedis.
**lateral l. of knee,** ligamentum collaterale fibulare.
**lateral l's of liver,** see *ligamentum triangulare dextrum hepatis* and *ligamentum triangulare sinistrum hepatis.*
**lateral l. of malleus,** ligamentum mallei laterale.
**lateral meniscofemoral l.,** ligamentum meniscofemorale posterius.
**lateral l's of metacarpophalangeal joints,** ligamenta collateralia articulationum metacarpophalangealium.
**lateral l's of metatarsophalangeal joints,** ligamenta collateralia articulationum metatarsophalangealium.
**lateral l. of temporomandibular articulation, lateral l. of temporomandibular joint,** ligamentum laterale articulationis temporomandibularis.
**lateral l. of temporomandibular joint, external,** ligamentum laterale articulationis temporomandibularis.
**lateral l. of temporomandibular joint, internal,** ligamentum sphenomandibulare.
**lateral l. of wrist joint, external,** ligamentum collaterale carpi radiale.
**lateral l. of wrist joint, internal,** ligamentum collaterale carpi ulnare.
**Lauth's l.,** ligamentum transversum atlantis.
**l. of left vena cava,** ligamentum venae cavae sinistrae.
**lienophrenic l.,** ligamentum splenorenale.
**lienorenal l.,** a fold of peritoneum connecting the spleen and the left kidney.
**Lisfranc's l.,** a fibrous band running from the lower external surface of the medial cuneiform bone to the internal surface of the base of the second metatarsal bone.
**Lockwood's l.,** the thickened area of contact between Tenon's capsule and the sheaths of the inferior rectus and inferior oblique muscles.
**longitudinal l., anterior,** ligamentum longitudinale anterius.
**longitudinal l., posterior,** ligamentum longitudinale posterius.
**longitudinal l. of abdomen,** linea alba.
**lumbocostal l.,** ligamentum lumbocostale.
**lumbosacral l.,** the inferior portion of the iliolumbar ligament.
**l's of Luschka,** ligamenta sternopericardiaca.
**Mackenrodt's l.,** plica recto-uterina.
**l. of Maissiat,** tractus iliotibialis.
**Mauchart's l's,** ligamenta alaria.
**maxillary l., lateral,** ligamentum laterale articulationis temporomandibularis.
**l. of Mayer,** ligamentum carpi radiatum.
**Meckel's l.,** see under *band.*
**medial l. of ankle,** ligamentum collaterale mediale articulationis talocruralis.
**medial l. of elbow joint,** ligamentum collaterale ulnare.
**medial l. of temporomandibular articulation, medial l. of temporomandibular joint,** ligamentum mediale articulationis temporomandibularis.
**medial l. of wrist,** ligamentum collaterale carpi ulnare.
**meniscofemoral l., anterior,** ligamentum meniscofemorale anterius.
**meniscofemoral l., posterior,** ligamentum meniscofemorale posterius.
**mesocolic l. of colon,** taenia mesocolica.
**metacarpal l., deep transverse,** ligamentum metacarpeum transversum profundum. NOTE: the term may be used to denote any one of the series of bands connecting two adjacent metacarpal bones or may describe the entire series of three bands collectively.
**metacarpal l's, dorsal,** ligamenta metacarpalia dorsalia.
**metacarpal l's, interosseous,** ligamenta metacarpalia interossea.
**metacarpal l's, palmar,** ligamenta metacarpalia palmaria.
**metacarpal l., superficial transverse,** ligamentum metacarpale transversum superficiale.
**metacarpophalangeal l's, anterior, metacarpophalangeal l's, palmar,** ligamenta palmaria articulationum metacarpophalanealium.
**l's of metacarpophalangeal articulations, palmar,** ligamenta palmaria articulationum metacarpophalangealium.
**metatarsal l., anterior,** deep transverse metatarsal l.
**metatarsal l., deep transverse,** ligamentum metatarsale transversum profundum. NOTE: the term may be used to denote any of the series of bands connecting two adjacent metatarsal bones or may describe the entire series of four bands collectively.
**metatarsal l's, dorsal,** ligamenta metatarsalia dorsalia.
**metatarsal l's, interosseus, metatarsal l's, interosseous transverse,** ligamenta metatarsalia interossea.
**metatarsal l's, lateral,** ligamenta metatarsalia interossea.
**metatarsal l's, lateral proper (of Weber), metatarsal l's, lateral (of Weitbrecht),** ligamenta metatarsalia interossea.
**metatarsal l's, plantar,** ligamenta metatarsalia plantaria.
**metatarsal l., superficial transverse,** ligamentum metatarsale transversum superficiale.
**metatarsophalangeal l's, inferior, l's of metatarsophalangeal articulations, plantar,** ligamenta plantaria articulationum metatarsophalangealium.
**middle l. of neck of rib,** ligamentum costotransversarium.
**mucous l.,** plica synovialis.
**l. of nape,** ligamentum nuchae.
**navicularicuneiform l's, plantar,** ligamenta cuneonavicularia plantaria.
**nephrocolic l.,** fasciculi from the fatty capsule of the kidney passing inferiorly on the right side to the posterior wall of the ascending colon and on the left side to the posterior wall of the descending colon.
**nuchal l.,** ligamentum nuchae.
**oblique l. of Cooper, oblique l. of forearm,** chorda obliqua membranae interosseae antebrachii.
**oblique l's of knee,** ligamenta cruciata genus.
**oblique l. of knee, posterior,** ligamentum popliteum obliquum.
**oblique l. of scapula,** ligamentum transversum scapulae superius.
**oblique l. of superior radioulnar joint,** chorda obliqua membranae interosseae antebrachii.
**obturator l., atlantooccipital,** membrana atlanto-occipitalis anterior.
**obturator l. of atlas,** see *membrana atlanto-occipitalis anterior* and *posterior.*
**obturator l. of pelvis,** membrana obturatoria.
**occipitoaxial l.,** membrana tectoria.
**occipitoodontoid l's,** ligamenta alaria.
**odontoid l., middle,** ligamentum apicis dentis.
**odontoid l's of axis,** ligamenta alaria.
**orbicular l. of radius,** ligamentum anulare radii.
**ovarian l.,** ligamentum ovarii proprium.
**palmar l's,** 1. see *ligamenta palmaria articulationum interphalangealium manus* and *ligamenta palmaria articulationum metacarpophalangealium.* 2. see *aponeurosis palmaria.*
**palmar l., deep transverse,** deep transverse metacarpal l.
**palmar l. of carpus,** ligamentum carpi radiatum.
**palmar l. of radiocarpal joint,** ligamentum radiocarpale palmare.
**palpebral l., lateral,** ligamentum palpebrale laterale.
**palpebral l., medial,** ligamentum palpebrale mediale.
**patellar l.,** ligamentum patellae.
**patellar l., internal,** retinaculum patellae mediale.

**patellar l., lateral,** retinaculum patellae laterale.
**pectinate l., pectinate l. of iris,** reticulum trabeculare.
**pectineal l.,** ligamentum pectineum.
**pelvic l., great posterior,** ligamentum sacrotuberale.
**pelvic l., short posterior,** ligamentum sacrospinale.
**pelvic l., transverse,** ligamentum transversum perinei.
**pelviprostatic l., basal,** fascia prostatae.
**pericardiosternal l's,** ligamenta sternopericardiaca.
**perineal l., transverse, perineal l. of Carcassone,** ligamentum transversum perinei.
**periodontal l.,** the fibrous connective tissue that surrounds the root of a tooth, separating it from and attaching it to the alveolar bone. It extends from the base of the gingival mucosa to the fundus of the bony socket, and its main function is to hold the tooth in its socket. Called also *alveolodental l.* or *membrane, desmodontium,* and *peridental* or *periodontal membrane.* See also *periodontium.*
**Petit's l.,** uterosacral l.
**petrosphenoid l.,** 1. synchondrosis sphenopetrosa. 2. synchondrosis spheno-occipitalis.
**petrosphenoid l., anterior,** synchondrosis sphenopetrosa.
**phrenicocolic l.,** ligamentum phrenicocolicum.
**phrenicolienal l., phrenicosplenic l.,** ligamentum splenorenale.
**phrenocolic l.,** ligamentum phrenicocolicum.
**pisimetacarpal l.,** ligamentum pisometacarpeum.
**pisohamate l.,** ligamentum pisohamatum.
**pisometacarpal l.,** ligamentum pisometacarpeum.
**pisounciform l., pisouncinate l.,** ligamentum pisohamatum.
**plantar l's,** see *ligamenta plantaria articulationum metatarsophalangealium* and *ligamenta plantaria articulationum interphalangealium pedis.*
**plantar l., long,** ligamentum plantare longum.
**plantar l., short,** ligamentum calcaneocuboideum plantare.
**plantar l. of second metatarsal bone,** see *ligamenta tarsometatarsalia plantaria.*
**plantar l's of tarsus,** ligamenta tarsi plantaria.
**popliteal l., arcuate,** ligamentum popliteum arcuatum.
**popliteal l., external,** retinaculum ligamenti arcuati.
**popliteal l., oblique,** ligamentum popliteum obliquum.
**posterior l. of head of fibula,** ligamentum capitis fibulae posterius.
**posterior l. of incus,** ligamentum incudis posterius.
**posterior l. of pinna,** ligamentum auriculare posterius.
**posterior l. of radiocarpal joint,** ligamentum radiocarpale dorsale.
**Poupart's l.,** ligamentum inguinale.
**preurethral l. of Waldeyer,** ligamentum transversum perinei.
**prismatic l. of Weitbrecht,** ligamentum capitis femoris.
**proper l's of costal cartilages,** see *membrana intercostalis externa.*
**pterygomandibular l.,** raphe pterygomandibularis.
**pterygospinal l.,** ligamentum pterygospinale.
**pubic l., inferior,** 1. ligamentum pubicum inferius. 2. ligamentum suspensorium ovarii.
**pubic l., superior,** ligamentum pubicum superius.
**pubic l. of Cowper,** ligamentum inguinale.
**pubic l. of Cruveilhier, anterior,** discus interpubicus.
**pubocapsular l., pubofemoral l.,** ligamentum pubofemorale.
**puboischiadic l. of prostate gland,** diaphragma urogenitale.
**puboprostatic l.,** ligamentum puboprostaticum.
**puborectal l.,** 1. ligamentum puboprostaticum. 2. ligamentum pubovesicale.
**pubovesical l.,** ligamentum pubovesicale.
**pulmonary l.,** ligamentum pulmonale.
**quadrate l.,** ligamentum quadratum.
**radial l., lateral, radial l. of cubitocarpal articulation,** ligamentum collaterale carpi radiale.
**radiate l.,** ligamentum capitis costae radiatum.
**radiate l., lateral,** ligamentum collaterale carpi ulnare.
**radiate l. of carpus,** ligamentum carpi radiatum.
**radiate l. of head of rib,** ligamentum capitis costae radiatum.
**radiate l. of Mayer,** ligamentum carpi radiatum.
**radiocarpal l., anterior,** ligamentum radiocarpale palmare.
**radiocarpal l., dorsal,** ligamentum radiocarpale dorsale.
**radiocarpal l., palmar, radiocarpal l., volar,** ligamentum radiocarpale palmare.
**rectouterine l.,** musculus recto-uterinus.
**reflex l. of Gimbernat,** ligamentum inguinale reflexum.
**reinforcing l's,** ligaments that serve to reinforce joint capsules.
**rhomboid l. of clavicle,** ligamentum costoclaviculare.
**rhomboid l. of wrist,** ligamentum radiocarpale dorsale.
**ring l. of hip joint,** zona orbicularis articulationis coxae.
**Robert's l.,** ligamentum meniscofemorale posterius.
**round l. of acetabulum,** ligamentum capitis femoris.
**round l. of Cloquet,** ligamentum capitis costae intra-articulare.
**round l. of femur,** ligamentum capitis femoris.
**round l. of forearm,** chorda obliqua membranae interosseae antebrachii.
**round l. of uterus,** ligamentum teres uteri.
**sacciform l.,** capsula articularis radioulnaris distalis.
**sacrococcygeal l., anterior,** ligamentum sacrococcygeum anterius.
**sacrococcygeal l., deep dorsal, sacrococcygeal l., deep posterior,** ligamentum sacrococcygeum posterius profundum.
**sacrococcygeal l., lateral,** ligamentum sacrococcygeum laterale.
**sacrococcygeal l., superficial dorsal, sacrococcygeal l., superficial posterior,** ligamentum sacrococcygeum posterius superficiale.
**sacrococcygeal l., ventral,** ligamentum sacrococcygeum anterius.
**sacroiliac l., anterior,** ligamentum sacroiliacum anterius.
**sacroiliac l., dorsal,** ligamentum sacroiliacum posterius.
**sacroiliac l., interosseous,** ligamentum sacroiliacum interosseum.
**sacroiliac l., long posterior,** see *ligamentum sacroiliacum posterius.*
**sacroiliac l., posterior,** ligamentum sacroiliacum posterius.
**sacroiliac l., short posterior,** see *ligamentum sacroiliacum posterius.*
**sacroiliac l., ventral,** ligamentum sacroiliacum anterius.
**sacrosciatic l., anterior,** ligamentum sacrospinale.
**sacrosciatic l., great,** ligamentum sacrotuberale.
**sacrosciatic l., internal, sacrosciatic l., least,** ligamentum sacrospinale.
**sacrospinal l., sacrospinous l.,** ligamentum sacrospinale.
**sacrotuberal l., sacrotuberous l.,** ligamentum sacrotuberale.
**Santorini's l.,** ligamentum cricopharyngeum.
**Sappey's l.,** the thicker posterior part of the capsule of the temporomandibular joint.
**scaphocuneiform l's, plantar,** ligamenta cuneonavicularia plantaria.
**l. of Scarpa,** cornu superius marginis falciformis.
**Schlemm's l's,** two ligamentous bands strengthening the capsule of the shoulder joint.
**scrotal l. of testis,** gubernaculum testis.
**serous l.,** ligamentum serosum.
**sphenoidal l., external,** ligamenta intercuneiformia plantaria.
**sphenoideotarsal l's,** ligamenta tarsometatarsalia plantaria.
**sphenomandibular l.,** ligamentum sphenomandibulare.
**spinoglenoid l.,** ligamentum transversum scapulae inferius.
**spinosacral l.,** ligamentum sacrospinale.
**spiral l. of cochlea,** crista basilaris ductus cochlearis.
**splenogastric l.,** ligamentum gastrosplenicum.
**splenophrenic l.,** ligamentum splenorenale.
**splenorenal l.,** ligamentum splenorenale.
**spring l.,** ligamentum calcaneonaviculare plantare.
**stapedial l.,** ligamentum anulare stapediale.
**stellate l., anterior,** ligamentum capitis costae radiatum.
**sternoclavicular l., anterior,** ligamentum sternoclaviculare anterius.
**sternoclavicular l., posterior,** ligamentum sternoclaviculare posterius.
**sternocostal l's,** ligamenta sternocostalia radiata.
**sternocostal l., interarticular, sternocostal l., intra-articular,** ligamentum sternocostale intra-articulare.
**sternocostal l's, radiate,** ligamenta sternocostalia radiata.
**sternopericardiac l's,** ligamenta sternopericardiaca.
**l. of Struthers,** a fibrous band that sometimes extends from the supracondylar process of the humerus to the median epicondyle, enclosing the median nerve and usually the brachial artery and providing an anomalous attachment for the coracobrachialis and part of the pronator teres muscles.
**stylohyoid l.,** ligamentum stylohyoideum.
**stylomandibular l., stylomaxillary l.,** ligamentum stylomandibulare.
**subflaval l's,** ligamenta flava.
**subpubic l.,** ligamentum pubicum inferius.
**superficial l. of carpus,** 1. ligamentum radiocarpale dorsale. 2. ligamentum radiocarpale palmare.
**superior l. of epididymis,** ligamentum epididymidis superius.
**superior l. of hip,** ligamentum iliofemorale.
**superior l. of incus,** ligamentum incudis superius.
**superior l. of malleus,** ligamentum mallei superius.
**superior l. of neck of rib, anterior,** the anterior part of the superior costotransverse ligament.
**superior l. of neck of rib, external,** the posterior part of the superior costotransverse ligament.
**superior l. of pinna,** ligamentum auriculare superius.
**suprascapular l.,** ligamentum transversum scapulae superius.
**supraspinal l., supraspinous l.,** ligamentum supraspinale.
**suspensory l., marsupial,** plica synovialis infrapatellaris.
**suspensory l. of axilla,** a layer ascending from the axillary fascia and ensheathing the pectoralis minor muscle; so called because traction by it, when the arm is abducted, produces the hollow of the armpit. Called also *Campbell's l.* and *Gerdy's l.*
**suspensory l. of axis,** ligamentum apicis dentis.
**suspensory l. of bladder,** plica umbilicalis mediana.
**suspensory l's of breast,** ligamenta suspensoria mammaria.
**suspensory l. of clitoris,** ligamentum suspensorium clitoridis.
**suspensory l. of humerus,** ligamentum coracohumerale.
**suspensory l. of lens,** zonula ciliaris.

**suspensory l. of liver,** ligamentum falciforme hepatis.
**suspensory l's of mammary gland,** ligamenta suspensoria mammaria.
**suspensory l. of ovary,** ligamentum suspensorium ovarii.
**suspensory l. of penis,** ligamentum suspensorium penis.
**suspensory l. of spleen,** ligamentum splenorenale.
**sutural l.,** a band of fibrous tissue between the opposed bones of a suture or immovable joint.
**synovial l.,** a large synovial fold.
**synovial l. of hip,** ligamentum capitis femoris.
**talocalcaneal l., interosseous,** ligamentum talocalcaneum interosseum.
**talocalcaneal l., lateral,** ligamentum talocalcaneum laterale.
**talocalcaneal l., medial,** ligamentum talocalcaneum mediale.
**l. of talocrural joint, lateral,** the anterior and posterior talofibular ligaments and the calcaneofibular ligament considered together.
**talofibular l., anterior,** ligamentum talofibulare anterius.
**talofibular l., posterior,** ligamentum talofibulare posterius.
**talonavicular l.,** ligamentum talonaviculare.
**talotibial l., anterior,** pars tibiotalaris anterior ligamenti medialis.
**talotibial l., posterior,** pars tibiotalaris posterior ligamenti medialis.
**tarsal l., anterior,** retinaculum musculorum extensorum inferius pedis.
**tarsometatarsal l's, dorsal,** ligamenta tarsometatarsalia dorsalia.
**tarsometatarsal l's, plantar,** ligamenta tarsometatarsalia plantaria.
**l's of tarsus,** ligamenta tarsi.
**temporomandibular l.,** ligamentum laterale articulationis temporomandibularis.
**tendinotrochanteric l.,** a portion of the capsule of the hip joint.
**Teutleben's l.,** ligamentum pulmonale.
**thyroepiglottic l.,** ligamentum thyro-epiglotticum.
**thyrohyoid l.,** ligamentum thyrohyoideum laterale.
**thyrohyoid l., median,** ligamentum thyrohyoideum medianum.
**tibiocalcaneal l., tibiocalcanean l.,** pars tibiocalcanea ligamenti medialis.
**tibiofibular l.,** syndesmosis tibiofibularis.
**tibiofibular l., anterior,** ligamentum tibiofibulare anterius.
**tibiofibular l., posterior,** ligamentum tibiofibulare posterius.
**tibionavicular l.,** pars tibionavicularis ligamenti medialis.
**tracheal l's,** ligamenta anularia tracheae.
**transverse l.,** ligamentum costotransversarium.
**transverse l. of acetabulum,** ligamentum transversum acetabuli.
**transverse l. of atlas,** ligamentum transversum atlantis.
**transverse l. of carpus,** retinaculum musculorum flexorum manus.
**transverse humeral l.,** a band of fibers bridging the intertubercular groove of the humerus and holding the tendon of the biceps muscle in the groove; called also *Brodie's l.*
**transverse l. of knee,** ligamentum transversum genus.
**transverse l. of leg,** retinaculum musculorum extensorum superius pedis.
**transverse l. of little head of rib,** ligamentum capitis costae intraarticulare.
**transverse l. of pelvis,** ligamentum transversum perinei.
**transverse l. of scapula, inferior,** ligamentum transversum scapulae inferius.
**transverse l. of scapula, superior,** ligamentum transversum scapulae superius.
**transverse l. of tibia,** retinaculum musculorum extensorum superius pedis.
**transverse l. of wrist,** retinaculum musculorum flexorum manus.
**transverse l's of wrist, dorsal,** ligamenta intercarpalia dorsalia.
**transversocostal l., superior,** ligamentum costotransversarium superius.
**trapezoid l.,** ligamentum trapezoideum.
**l. of Treitz,** musculus suspensorius duodeni.
**triangular l. of abdomen,** ligamentum inguinale reflexum.
**triangular l. of Colles,** diaphragma urogenitale.
**triangular l. of linea alba,** adminiculum lineae albae.
**triangular l. of liver, left,** ligamentum triangulare sinistrum hepatis.
**triangular l. of liver, right,** ligamentum triangulare dextrum hepatis.
**triangular l. of pubis, anterior,** ligamentum pubicum inferius.
**triangular l. of scapula,** ligamentum transversum scapulae inferius.
**triangular l. of thigh,** ligamentum inguinale reflexum.
**triangular l. of urethra,** ligamentum puboprostaticum.
**trigeminate l's of Arnold,** ligamenta tarsometatarsalia dorsalia.
**triquetral l. of foot,** ligamentum calcaneofibulare.
**triquetral l. of scapula,** ligamentum transversum scapulae inferius.
**trochlear l.,** deep transverse metacarpal l.
**trochlear l's of foot,** ligamenta plantaria articulationum metatarsophalangealium.
**trochlear l's of hand,** ligamenta palmaria articulationum metacarpophalangealium.
**trochlear l. of little heads of metacarpal bones,** deep transverse metacarpal l.
**true l. of bladder, anterior,** 1. ligamentum puboprostaticum. 2. ligamentum pubovesicale.
**tuberosacral l.,** ligamentum sacrotuberale.
**tubopharyngeal l. of Rauber,** plica salpingopharyngea.
**Tuffier's inferior l.,** that part of the mesentery which is connected with the wall of the iliac fossa.
**ulnar l., lateral, ulnar l. of carpus,** ligamentum collaterale carpi ulnare.
**ulnocarpal l., palmar,** ligamentum ulnocarpale palmare.
**umbilical l., lateral, umbilical l., median, umbilical l., middle,** ligamentum umbilicale medianum.
**utero-ovarian l.,** ligamentum ovarii proprium.
**uteropelvic l's,** expansions of muscular tissue in the broad ligament of the uterus, radiating from the fascia over the obturator internus to the side of the uterus and the vagina.
**uterosacral l.,** a part of the thickening of the visceral pelvic fascia beside the cervix and vagina, passing posteriorly in the rectouterine fold to attach to the front of the sacrum; called also *Jarjavay's l.* and *Petit's l.*
**vaginal l's of fingers, l's of vaginal sheaths of fingers,** vaginae fibrosae digitorum manus.
**vaginal l's of toes, l's of vaginal sheaths of toes,** vaginae fibrosae digitorum pedis.
**l's of Valsalva,** ligamenta auricularia.
**venous l. of liver,** ligamentum venosum.
**ventricular l.,** ligamentum vestibulare.
**vertebropleural l.,** membrana suprapleuralis.
**l. of Vesalius,** ligamentum inguinale.
**vesical l., lateral,** ligamentum umbilicale medianum.
**vesicopubic l.,** ligamentum pubovesicale.
**vesicoumbilical l.,** ligamentum umbilicale medianum.
**vesicouterine l.,** a ligament that extends from the anterior aspect of the uterus to the bladder.
**vestibular l.,** ligamentum vestibulare.
**vocal l.,** ligamentum vocale.
**volar l. of carpus, proper, volar l. of wrist, anterior,** retinaculum musculorum flexorum manus.
**Walther's oblique l.,** ligamentum talofibulare posterius.
**Weitbrecht's l.,** chorda obliqua membranae interosseae antebrachii.
**Winslow's l.,** ligamentum popliteum obliquum.
**Wrisberg's l.,** ligamentum meniscofemorale posterius.
**xiphicostal l's of Macalister, xiphoid l's,** ligamenta costoxiphoidea.
**Y l.,** ligamentum iliofemorale.
**yellow l's,** ligamenta flava.
**Zinn's l.,** anulus tendineus communis.
**zonal l. of thigh,** zona orbicularis articulationis coxae.

**lig·a·men·ta** (lig″ə-men′tə) [L.] plural of *ligamentum.*

**lig·a·men·to·pexy** (lig″ə-men″to-pek′se) ventrosuspension by shortening or suturing the round ligaments of the uterus.

**lig·a·men·tous** (lig″ə-men′təs) pertaining to or of the nature of a ligament.

**lig·a·men·tum** (lig″ə-men′təm) pl. *ligamen′ta* [L. "a bandage," from *ligare* to bind] [TA] ligament.

## Ligamentum

Descriptions are given on TA terms, and include anglicized names of specific ligaments.

**l. acromioclavicula're** [TA], acromioclavicular ligament: a dense band that joins the superior surface of the acromion and the acromial extremity of the clavicle together, and strengthens the superior part of the articular capsule.

**ligamen'ta ala'ria** [TA], alar ligaments: two strong bands that pass from the posterolateral part of the tip of the dens of the axis upward and laterally to the condyles of the occipital bone; they limit rotation of the head.

**l. anococcy'geum,** corpus anococcygeum.

**ligamen'ta anula'ria digito'rum ma'nus,** pars anularis vaginae fibrosae digitorum manus.

**ligamen'ta anula'ria digito'rum pe'dis,** pars anularis vaginae fibrosae digitorum pedis.

**l. anula're ra'dii** [TA], annular ligament of radius: a strong fibrous band that encircles the head of the radius and holds it in position; it is attached to the anterior and posterior margins of the radial notch of the ulna, forming, with the notch, a complete ring.

**l. anula're stapedia'le** [TA], annular stapedial ligament: a ring of fibrous tissue that attaches the base of the stapes to the fenestra vestibuli of the inner ear; called also *l. anulare stapedis* and *annular ligament of base of stapes.*

**l. anula're stape'dis,** l. anulare stapediale.

**ligamen'ta anula'ria tra'cheae** [TA], annular ligaments of trachea: circular horizontal ligaments that join the tracheal cartilages together; called also *ligamenta trachealia* and *tracheal ligaments.*

**l. a'picis den'tis** [TA], ligament of apex dentis: a cord of tissue extending from the tip of the dens of the axis to the occipital bone, near the anterior margin of the foramen magnum; it is usually delicate, but is sometimes well developed. Called also *apical dental ligament* and *l. apicis dentis epistrophei.*

**l. a'picis den'tis epistro'phei,** l. apicis dentis axis.

**l. arcua'tum latera'le** [TA], lateral arcuate ligament: the ligamentous arch, formed by the fascia of the quadratus lumborum muscle, constituting part of the lumbar portion of the diaphragm; called also *external lumbocostal arch of diaphragm* and *lateral lumbocostal arch of Haller.*

**l. arcua'tum media'le** [TA], medial arcuate ligament: the ligamentous arch, formed by the fascia of the psoas muscle, constituting part of the lumbar portion of the diaphragm; called also *internal lumbocostal arch of diaphragm* and *medial lumbocostal arch of Haller.*

**l. arcua'tum media'num** [TA], median arcuate ligament: the ligamentous arch across the anterior surface of the aorta, interconnecting the crura of the diaphragm; called also *median arcuate ligament.*

**l. arterio'sum** [TA], a short, thick, strong fibromuscular cord extending from the pulmonary artery to the arch of the aorta; it is the remains of the ductus arteriosus. Called also *ligament of Botallo.*

**l. atlantooccipita'le ante'rius,** membrana atlantooccipitalis anterior.

**l. atlantooccipita'le latera'le** [TA], lateral atlantooccipital ligament: a thickened portion of the articular capsule of the atlantooccipital joint attached to the jugular processes of the occipital bone and to the base of the transverse process of the atlas.

**ligamen'ta auricula'ria** [TA], ligaments of auricle: the three ligaments (anterior, superior, and posterior) that help attach the auricle to the side of the head. Called also *ligaments of Valsalva.*

**l. auricula're ante'rius** [TA], anterior auricular ligament: the auricular ligament that passes from the eminence of the concha to the mastoid part of the temporal bone.

**l. auricula're poste'rius** [TA], posterior auricular ligament: the auricular ligament that passes from the eminence of the concha to the mastoid part of the temporal bone.

**l. auricula're supe'rius** [TA], superior auricular ligament: the auricular ligament that passes from the spine of the helix to the superior margin of the bony external acoustic meatus.

**l. bifurca'tum** [TA], bifurcate ligament: a Y-shaped ligament on the dorsum of the foot, comprising the calcaneonavicular and calcaneocuboid ligaments.

**l. calcaneocuboi'deum** [TA], calcaneocuboid ligament: the band of fibers connecting the superior surface of the calcaneus and the dorsal surface of the cuboid bone; called also *pars calcaneocuboidea ligamenti bifurcati.*

**l. calcaneocuboi'deum planta're** [TA], plantar calcaneocuboid ligament: a short, wide, strong band connecting the plantar surfaces of the calcaneus and the cuboid bone; called also *short plantar ligament.*

**l. calcaneofibula're** [TA], calcaneofibular ligament: a band of fibers arising from the lateral surface of the lateral malleolus of the fibula just anterior to the apex and passing inferiorly and posteriorly to be attached to the lateral surface of the calcaneus.

**l. calcaneonavicula're** [TA], calcaneonavicular ligament: the band of fibers connecting the superior surface of the calcaneus and the lateral surface of the navicular bone, together with the calcaneocuboid ligament constituting the bifurcate ligament. Called also *pars calcaneonavicularis ligamenti bifurcati.*

**l. calcaneonavicula're planta're** [TA], plantar calcaneonavicular ligament: a broad, thick band passing from the anterior margin of the sustentaculum tali to the plantar surface of the navicular bone; it bears on its deep surface a fibrocartilage that helps to support the head of the talus. Called also *spring ligament.*

**l. calcaneotibia'le,** pars tibiocalcanea ligamenti medialis.

**l. ca'pitis cos'tae intraarticula're** [TA], interarticular ligament of head of rib: a horizontal band of fibers attached to the crest separating the two articular facets on the head of the rib, and to the intervertebral disk, thus dividing the joint of the head of the rib into two cavities. It is lacking in the joints of the first, tenth, eleventh, and twelfth ribs. Called also *l. capituli costae interarticulare.*

**l. ca'pitis cos'tae radia'tum** [TA], radiate ligament of head of rib: fibers that from their attachment on the ventral surface of the head of a rib radiate medially, in a fanlike manner, to attach to the two adjacent vertebrae and to the intervertebral disk between them; called also *l. capituli costae radiatum.*

**l. ca'pitis fe'moris** [TA], ligament of head of femur: a curved triangular or V-shaped fibrous band, attached by its apex to the anterosuperior part of the fovea of the head of the femur and by its base to the sides of the acetabular notch and the intervening transverse ligament of the acetabulum. Called also *l. teres femoris* and *round ligament of femur.*

**l. ca'pitis fib'ulae ante'rius** [TA], anterior ligament of head of fibula: a band of fibers that passes obliquely superiorly from the anterior part of the head of the fibula to the lateral condyle of the tibia.

**l. ca'pitis fib'ulae poste'rius** [TA], posterior ligament of head of fibula: a band of fibers that passes obliquely superiorly from the posterior part of the head of the fibula to the lateral condyle of the tibia.

**l. capi'tuli cos'tae interarticula're,** l. capitis costae intraarticulare.

**l. ca'pituli cos'tae radia'tum,** l. capitis costae radiatum.

**ligamen'ta capi'tuli fi'bulae,** see *l. capitis fibulae anterius* and *l. capitis fibulae posterius.*

**ligamen'ta capsula'ria** [TA], capsular ligaments: thickenings of the fibrous membrane of a joint capsule.

**l. car'pi dorsa'le,** retinaculum musculorum extensorum manus.

**l. car'pi radia'tum** [TA], radiate carpal ligament: a group of about seven fibrous bands which diverge in all directions on the palmar surface of the mediocarpal joint; the majority radiate from the capitate to the scaphoid, lunate, and triquetral bones.

**l. car'pi transver'sum,** retinaculum musculorum flexorum manus.

**l. car'pi vola're,** transverse reinforcing fibers in the antebrachial fascia over the palmar surface of the wrist.

**ligamen'ta carpometacarpa'lia dorsa'lia** [TA], **ligamen'ta carpometacar'pea dorsa'lia,** dorsal carpometacarpal ligaments: a series of bands on the dorsal surface of the carpometacarpal articulations, joining the carpal bones to the bases of the second to fifth metacarpals. The second metacarpal bone is thus joined to the trapezium, trapezoid, and capitate, the third to the capitate, the fourth to the capitate and hamate, and the fifth to the hamate. Called also *posterior carpometacarpal ligaments.*

**ligamen'ta carpometacarpa'lia palma'ria** [TA], **ligamen'ta carpometacar'pea palma'ria,** palmar carpometacarpal ligaments: a series of bands on the palmar surface of the carpometacarpal articulations, joining the carpal bones to the second to fifth metacarpals. The second metacarpal bone is thus joined to the trapezium, the third to the trapezium, capitate, and hamate, the fourth to the hamate, and the fifth to the hamate. Called also *anterior* or *volar carpometacarpal ligaments.*

**l. cauda'le integumen'ti commu'nis,** retinaculum caudale.

**l. ceratocricoi'deum** [TA], ceratocricoid ligament: any of the three (anterior, lateral, or posterior) fibrous bands that serve to attach the capsule of the cricothyroid joint on either side.

**ligamen'ta collatera'lia articulatio'num digito'rum ma'nus,** ligamenta collateralia articulationum interphalangealium manus.

**ligamen'ta collatera'lia articulatio'num digito'rum pe'dis,** ligamenta collateralia articulationum interphalangealium pedis.

**ligamen'ta collatera'lia articulatio'num interphalangea'lium ma'nus** [TA], **ligamen'ta collatera'lia articulatio'num interphalangea'rum ma'nus,** collateral ligaments of interphalangeal articulations of hand: massive fibrous bands on each side of the interphalangeal joints of the fingers; they are placed diagonally, the proximal ends being near the dorsal, and the distal ends near the palmar margins of the digits. Called also *ligamenta collateralia articulationum digitorum manus.*

**ligamen'ta collatera'lia articulatio'num interphalangea'lium pe'dis** [TA], **ligamen'ta collatera'lia articulatio'num interphalangea'rum pe'dis,** collateral ligaments of interphalangeal articulations of foot: fibrous bands, one on either side of each of the interphalangeal joints of the toes. Called also *ligamenta collateralia articulationum digitorum pedis.*

**ligamen'ta collatera'lia articulatio'num metacarpophalangea'lium** [TA], **ligamen'ta collatera'lia articulatio'num metacarpophalangea'rum,** collateral ligaments of metacarpophalangeal articulations: massive, strong fibrous bands on either side of each metacarpophalangeal joint, holding the two bones involved in each joint firmly together.

**ligamen'ta collatera'lia articulatio'num metatarsophalangea'lium** [TA], **ligamen'ta collatera'lia articulatio'num metatarsophalangea'rum,** collateral ligaments of metatarsophalangeal articulations: strong fibrous bands on either side of each metatarsophalangeal joint, holding the two bones involved in each joint firmly together.

**l. collatera'le car'pi radia'le** [TA], radial carpal collateral ligament: a short, thick band that passes from the tip of the styloid process of the radius to attach to the scaphoid bone.

**l. collatera'le car'pi ulna're** [TA], ulnar carpal collateral ligament: a strong fibrous band that passes from the tip of the styloid process of the ulna and is attached to the triquetral and pisiform bones.

**l. collatera'le fibula're** [TA], collateral fibular ligament: a strong, round fibrous cord on the lateral side of the knee joint, entirely independent of the capsule of the knee joint; it is attached superiorly to the posterior part of the lateral epicondyle of the femur and inferiorly to the lateral side of the head of the fibula just in front of the styloid process.

**l. collatera'le latera'le articulatio'nis talocrura'lis** [TA], lateral collateral ligament of ankle joint: the three ligamentous fasciculi present on the lateral side of the ankle joint (i.e., the *l. calcaneofibulare, l. talofibulare anterius,* and *l. talofibulare posterius*) considered collectively. Called also *lateral ligament of ankle joint* and *l. laterale articulationis talocruralis.*

**l. collatera'le media'le articulatio'nis talocrura'lis** [TA], medial ligament of talocrural joint: a large fan-shaped ligament on the medial side of the ankle, passing from the medial malleolus of the tibia down onto the tarsal bones. It comprises four parts: *pars tibionavicularis, pars tibiocalcanea, pars tibiotalaris anterior,* and *pars tibiotalaris posterior.* Called also *l. deltoideum articulationis talocruralis* [TA alternative], *l. mediale articulationis talocruralis, deltoid ligament of ankle,* and *medial ligament of ankle.*

**l. collatera'le radia'le** [TA], collateral radial ligament: a large bundle of fibers arising from the lateral epicondyle of the humerus and fanning out to be attached to the lateral side of the annular ligament of the radius.

**l. collatera'le tibia'le** [TA], collateral tibial ligament: a broad, flat, longitudinal band on the medial side of the knee joint; it is attached superiorly to the medial epicondyle of the femur, inferiorly to the medial surface of the body of the tibia, and in between to the medial meniscus.

**l. collatera'le ulna're** [TA], collateral ulnar ligament: a triangular bundle of fibers attached proximally to the medial epicondyle of the humerus, distally to the coronoid process of the ulna and the medial surface of the olecranon, and to a ridge running between the two.

**l. col'li cos'tae,** l. costotransversarium.

**l. conoi'deum** [TA], conoid ligament: the conical, posteromedial portion of the coracoclavicular ligament, attached inferiorly by its tip to the base of the coracoid process of the scapula and superiorly by its base to the inferior surface of the clavicle.

**l. coracoacromia'le** [TA], coracoacromial ligament: one of three intrinsic ligaments of the scapula, a strong broad triangular band that is attached by its base to the lateral border of the coracoid process and by its tip to the summit of the acromion just in front of the articular facet for the clavicle.

**l. coracoclavicula're** [TA], coracoclavicular ligament: a strong band that joins the coracoid process of the scapula and the acromial extremity of the clavicle; it is divided into two parts, the trapezoid and conoid ligaments.

**l. coracohumera'le** [TA], coracohumeral ligament: a broad band that arises from the lateral border of the coracoid process of the scapula and passes downward and laterally to be attached to the major tubercle of the humerus.

**l. corona'rium he'patis** [TA], coronary ligament of the liver: the line of reflection of the peritoneum from the diaphragmatic surface of the liver to the under surface of the diaphragm.

**l. costoclavicula're** [TA], costoclavicular ligament: a short, powerful ligament that extends from the superior margin of the first costal cartilage to the inferior surface at the sternal end of the clavicle.

**l. costotransversa'rium** [TA], costotransverse ligament: short fibers that connect the dorsal surface of the neck of a rib with the anterior surface of the transverse process of the corresponding vertebra; called also *l. colli costae* and *l. transversum.*

**l. costotransversa'rium latera'le** [TA], lateral costotransverse ligament: a fibrous band that passes transversely from the posterior surface of the tip of a transverse process of a vertebra to the nonarticular part of the tubercle of the corresponding rib; called also *l. tuberculi costae.*

**l. costotransversa'rium supe'rius** [TA], superior costotransverse ligament: a strong band of fibers ascending from the crest of the neck of a rib to the transverse process of the vertebra above; it may be divided into a stronger anterior portion and a weaker posterior portion. It is lacking for the first rib.

**ligamen'ta costoxiphoi'dea** [TA], costoxiphoid ligaments: inconstant strandlike bands that pass obliquely from the anterior surface of the seventh and sometimes from the sixth costal cartilage to the anterior surface of the xiphoid process of the sternum. Some bands may also be present on the posterior surface.

**l. cricoarytenoi'deum** [TA], **l. crico-arytenoi'deum poste'rius,** cricoarytenoid ligament: the ligament extending from the lamina of the cricoid cartilage to the medial surface of the base and muscular process of the arytenoid cartilage.

**l. cricopharyn'geum** [TA], cricopharyngeal ligament: a ligament extending from the cricoid lamina to the midline of the pharynx.

**l. cricothyroi'deum media'num** [TA], median cricothyroid ligament: the median or anterior part of the inferior, larger part of the fibroelastic laryngeal membrane, occurring as a flat band of white tissue continuous medially with the conus elasticus and cranially with the plica vocalis and ligamentum vocale, and connecting the cricoid and thyroid cartilages; called also *anterior cricothyroid ligament.* See also *cricothyroid ligament,* under *ligament.*

**l. cricotrachea'le** [TA], cricotracheal ligament: a narrow fibrous ring that connects the lower margin of the cricoid cartilage with the upper tracheal cartilage; it is continuous posteriorly with the membranous wall of the trachea.

**l. crucia'tum ante'rius ge'nus** [TA], anterior cruciate ligament of knee: a strong band that arises from the posteromedial portion of the lateral condyle of the femur, passes anteriorly and inferiorly between the condyles, and is attached to the depression in front of the intercondylar eminence of the tibia.

**l. crucia'tum atlan'tis,** l. cruciforme atlantis.

**l. crucia'tum cru'ris,** retinaculum musculorum extensorum inferius pedis.

**ligamen'ta crucia'ta digito'rum ma'nus,** pars cruciformis vaginae fibrosae digitorum manus.

**ligamen'ta crucia'ta digito'rum pe'dis,** pars cruciformis vaginae fibrosae digitorum pedis.

**ligamen'ta crucia'ta genua'lia, ligamen'ta crucia'ta ge'nus,** cruciate ligaments of knee: strong, thick bundles situated in the knee joint between the condyles of the femur, which together form a somewhat cross-shaped structure. See *l. cruciatum anterius genus* and *l. cruciatum posterius genus.*

**l. crucia'tum poste'rius ge'nus** [TA], posterior cruciate ligament of knee: a strong band that arises from the anterolateral surface of the medial condyle of the femur, passes posteriorly and inferiorly between the condyles, and is inserted into the posterior intercondylar area of the tibia.

**l. crucifor'me atlan'tis** [TA], cruciform ligament of atlas: a ligament in the form of a cross, of which the transverse ligament of the atlas forms the horizontal bar, and the longitudinal fascicles the vertical bar of the cross; called also *l. cruciatum atlantis.*

**l. cuboideonavicula're dorsa'le** [TA], dorsal cuboideonavicular ligament: a fibrous bundle connecting the dorsal surfaces of the cuboid and navicular bones.

**l. cuboideonavicula're planta're** [TA], plantar cuboideonavicular ligament: a fibrous band connecting the plantar surfaces of the cuboid and navicular bones.

**l. cuneocuboi'deum dorsa'le** [TA], dorsal cuneocuboid ligament: fibers connecting the dorsal surfaces of the cuboid and lateral cuneiform bones.

**l. cuneocuboi'deum interos'seum** [TA], interosseous cuneocuboid ligament: fibers connecting the central portions of the adjacent surfaces of the cuboid and lateral cuneiform bones, between the articular surfaces.

**l. cuneocuboi'deum planta're** [TA], plantar cuneocuboid ligament: a band of fibers connecting the plantar surfaces of the cuboid and lateral cuneiform bones.

**ligamen'ta cuneometatarsa'lia interos'sea** [TA], **ligamen'ta cuneometatarsea interos'sea,** interosseous cuneometatarsal ligaments: fibrous bands that join the adjacent surfaces of the cuneiform and the metatarsal bones.

**ligamen'ta cuneonavicula'ria dorsa'lia** [TA], dorsal cuneonavicular ligaments: bands that join the dorsal surface of the navicular bone to the dorsal surfaces of the three cuneiform bones; called also *ligamenta navicularicuneiformia dorsalia.*

**ligamen'ta cuneonavicula'ria planta'ria** [TA], plantar cuneonavicular ligaments: bands that join the plantar surface of the navicular bone to the adjacent plantar surfaces of the three cuneiform bones; called also *ligamenta navicularicuneiformia plantaria.*

**l. deltoi'deum articulatio'nis talocrura'lis,** TA alternative for *l. collaterale mediale articulationis talocruralis.*

**l. denticula'tum** [TA], denticulate ligament: either of two symmetrical folds of pia mater of the spinal cord, each beginning in a longitudinal line between the lines of attachment of the anterior and posterior roots. The lateral edge is scalloped and has about 21 pointed processes that extend laterally and fuse with the arachnoid and dura mater. Called also *dentate ligament of spinal cord.*

**l. duodenorena'le,** duodenorenal ligament: a fold of peritoneum that passes from the duodenum to the right kidney.

**l. epididy'midis infe'rius** [TA], inferior ligament of epididymis: a strand of fibrous tissue, covered with a reflection of the tunica vaginalis, which connects the lower end of the body of the epididymis with the testis.

**l. epididy'midis supe'rius** [TA], superior ligament of epididymis: a strand of fibrous tissue, covered with a reflection of the tunica vaginalis, which connects the upper end of the body of the epididymis with the testis.

**ligamen'ta extracapsula'ria** [TA], ligaments of a joint capsule that are outside the capsule.

**l. falcifor'me he'patis** [TA], falciform ligament of the liver: a sickle-shaped sagittal fold of peritoneum that helps to attach the liver to the diaphragm, separates the right and left lobes of the liver, and extends from the coronary ligament of the liver behind to the umbilicus in front; called also *broad ligament of liver.*

**ligamen'ta fla'va** [TA], yellow ligaments: a series of bands of yellow elastic tissue attached to and extending between the ventral portions of the laminae of two adjacent vertebrae, from the junction of the axis and the third cervical vertebra to the junction of the fifth lumbar vertebra and the sacrum. They assist in maintaining or regaining the erect position and serve to close in the spaces between the arches. Called also *arcuate* or *flaval ligaments.*

**l. fundifor'me pe'nis** [TA], fundiform ligament of penis: a broad elastic band of fascial fibers that arises from the linea alba and from the fibrae intercrurales just above the symphysis pubis and then passes down to the penis, where it divides and passes around the penis and on into the scrotum.

**l. gastroco'licum** [TA], gastrocolic ligament: a peritoneal fold, part of the greater omentum, that extends from the greater curvature of the stomach to the transverse colon.

**l. gastroliena'le,** TA alternative for *l. gastrosplenicum.*

**l. gastrophre'nicum** [TA], gastrophrenic ligament: a fold of peritoneum continuous with the gastrosplenic ligament, extending from the right undersurface of the diaphragm to the cardiac part of the stomach.

**l. gastrosple'nicum** [TA], gastrosplenic ligament: a peritoneal fold extending from the greater curvature of the stomach to the hilum of the spleen; called also *l. gastrolienale* [TA alternative] and *gastrolienal* or *splenogastric ligament.*

**l. genitoinguina'le,** genitoinguinal ligament: the embryonic precursor of the gubernaculum testis.

**ligamen'ta glenohumera'lia** [TA], glenohumeral ligaments: bands, usually three in number, on the inner surface of the articular capsule of the humerus, attached to the margin of the glenoid cavity and to the anatomical neck of the humerus.

**ligamen'ta he'patis** [TA], hepatic ligaments: the ligaments of the liver, including the ligamenta coronarium hepatis, falciforme hepatis, triangulare dextrum hepatis, triangulare sinistrum hepatis, and hepatorenale.

**l. hepatoco'licum** [TA], hepatocolic ligament: an occasional fold of peritoneum, an extension of the lesser omentum to the right, passing from the lower surface of the liver near the gallbladder to the right colic flexure.

**l. hepatoduodena'le** [TA], hepatoduodenal ligament: a peritoneal fold that passes from the porta hepatis to the superior portion of the duodenum. It is continuous on the left with the gastrohepatic ligament, and on the right it forms one of the borders of the epiploic foramen. It contains the hepatic artery, portal vein, bile duct, nerves, and lymphatics.

**l. hepatogas'tricum** [TA], hepatogastric ligament: a peritoneal fold, part of the lesser omentum, that passes from the under surface of the liver to the lesser curvature of the stomach.

**l. hepatorena'le** [TA], hepatorenal ligament: a fold of peritoneum that passes from the back part of the lower surface of the liver to the front of the right kidney and forms the right margin of the epiploic foramen.

**l. hyoepiglot'ticum** [TA], hyoepiglottic ligament: a triangular elastic band with its base attached to the upper border of the body of the hyoid bone and its tip to the anterosuperior surface of the epiglottis.

**l. iliofemora'le** [TA], iliofemoral ligament: a very strong triangular or inverted Y-shaped band that covers the anterior and superior portions of the hip joint. It arises by its apex from the lower part of the anterior inferior iliac spine and is inserted by its base into the intertrochanteric line of the femur.

**l. iliolumba'le** [TA], iliolumbar ligament: a strong band that passes from the transverse processes of the fourth and fifth lumbar vertebrae to the internal lip of the adjacent portion of the iliac crest.

**l. incu'dis poste'rius** [TA], posterior ligament of incus: a fibrous band by which the tip of the short crus of the incus is fixed to the fossa incudis.

**l. incu'dis supe'rius** [TA], superior ligament of incus: a fibrous band that passes from the body of the incus to the roof of the tympanic cavity just back of the superior ligament of the malleus.

**l. inguina'le** [TA], inguinal ligament: a fibrous band running from the anterior superior spine of the ilium to the spine of the pubis. Called also *inguinal arch* and *arcus inguinalis* [TA alternative].

**l. inguina'le [Poupar'ti],** l. inguinale.

**l. inguina'le reflex'um** [TA], reflex inguinal ligament: a triangular band of fibers arising from the lacunar ligament and the pubic bone and passing diagonally upward and medially behind the superficial abdominal ring and in front of the inguinal aponeurotic falx to the linea alba.

**l. inguina'le reflex'um [Colle'si],** l. inguinale reflexum.

**ligamen'ta intercarpa'lia dorsa'lia** [TA], dorsal intercarpal ligaments: several bands that extend transversely across the dorsal surfaces of the carpal bones, connecting various ones together.

**ligamen'ta intercarpa'lia interos'sea** [TA], interosseous intercarpal ligaments: short fibrous bands that join the adjacent surfaces of the various carpal bones.

**ligamen'ta intercarpa'lia palma'ria** [TA], palmar intercarpal ligaments: several bands that extend transversely across the palmar surfaces of the carpal bones, connecting various ones together; called also *volar intercarpal ligaments.*

**l. interclavicula're** [TA], interclavicular ligament: a flattened band that passes from the superior surface of the sternal end of one clavicle across the superior margin of the sternum to the same position on the other clavicle.

**ligamen'ta intercuneifor'mia dorsa'lia** [TA], dorsal intercuneiform ligaments: fibrous bands connecting the dorsal surfaces of the three cuneiform bones.

**ligamen'ta intercuneifor'mia interos'sea** [TA], interosseous intercuneiform ligaments: short fibrous bands that join the adjacent surfaces of the medial and intermediate, and the intermediate and lateral, cuneiform bones.

**ligamen'ta intercuneifor'mia planta'ria** [TA], plantar intercuneiform ligaments: fibrous bands that join the plantar surfaces of the cuneiform bones.

**l. interfoveola're** [TA], interfoveolar ligament: a thickening in the transversalis fascia on the medial side of the deep inguinal ring; it is connected above to the transversus muscle and below to the inguinal ligament.

**l. interfoveola're [Hesselba'chi],** l. interfoveolare.

**ligamenta interspina'lia** [TA], interspinal ligaments: several fine fibrous membranes that extend from one vertebral spinous process to the next. They extend obliquely from the yellow ligaments ventrally to the supraspinous ligament dorsally, and contain white fibrous and yellow elastic tissue. They are poorly developed or lacking in the cervical region. Called also *interspinous ligaments.*

**ligamenta intertransversa'ria** [TA], intertransverse ligaments: several poorly developed fibrous bands that extend from one vertebral transverse process to the next. They consist of fine membranes in the lumbar region and of small cords in the thoracic region, and are lacking in the cervical region.

**ligamen'ta intracapsula'ria** [TA], intracapsular ligaments: ligaments within a joint capsule.

**l. ischiocapsula're,** l. ischiofemorale.

**l. ischiofemora'le** [TA], ischiofemoral ligament: a broad triangular band on the posterior surface of the hip joint. Its base is attached to the ischium posterior and inferior to the acetabulum; its fibers pass superiorly, laterally, and anteriorly across the capsule, bend over the neck, and in part are inserted into the inner side of the trochanteric fossa of the femur and in part blend into the zona orbicularis. Called also *l. ischiocapsulare* and *ischiocapsular ligament.*

**l. lacinia'tum,** retinaculum musculorum flexorum pedis.

**l. lacuna're** [TA], lacunar ligament: a small triangular membrane with its base just medial to the femoral ring; one side is attached to the inguinal ligament and the other to the pectineal line of the pubis.

**l. lacuna're [Gimberna'ti],** l. lacunare.

**l. later'ale articulatio'nis talocrura'lis,** l. collaterale laterale articulationis talocruralis.

**l. latera'le articulatio'nis temporomandibula'ris** [TA], lateral ligament of temporomandibular articulation: a strong triangular fibrous band that is attached superiorly by its base to the zygomatic process of the temporal bone, passes down on the lateral side of the joint in contact with the capsule, and is inserted by its apex into the lateral and posterior surfaces of the neck of the condyloid process of the mandible. Called also *l. temporomandibulare* and *temporomandibular ligament.*

**l. la'tum u'teri** [TA], broad ligament of uterus: a broad fold of peritoneum extending from the side of the uterus to the wall of the pelvis; it is divided into the mesometrium, mesosalpinx, and mesovarium.

**l. lienorena'le,** TA alternative for *l. splenorenale.*

**l. longitudina'le ante'rius** [TA], anterior longitudinal ligament: a single long, fibrous band in the midline, attached to the ventral surfaces

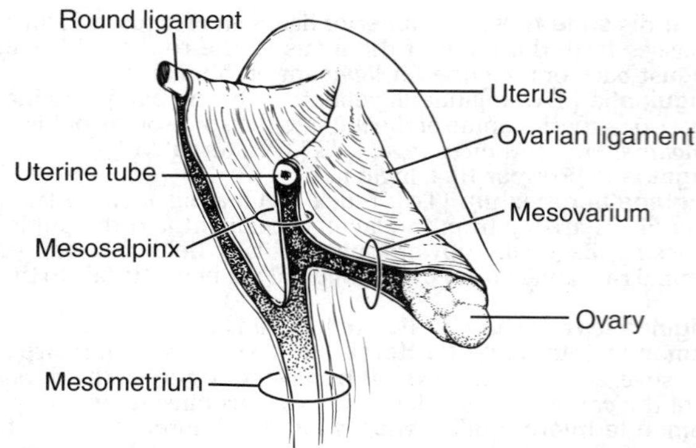


Ligamentum latum uteri (broad ligament of uterus), comprising the mesovarium, mesometrium, and mesosalpinx; shown in side view, with the anterior surface of the uterine body facing left.

of the bodies of the vertebrae; it extends from the occipital bone and the anterior tubercle of the atlas down to the sacrum.

**l. longitudina'le poste'rius** [TA], posterior longitudinal ligament: a single midline fibrous band attached to the dorsal surfaces of the bodies of the vertebrae, extending from the occipital bone to the coccyx.

**l. lumbocosta'le** [TA], lumbocostal ligament: a strong fascial band that passes from the twelfth rib to the tips of the transverse processes of the first and second lumbar vertebrae.

**l. mal'lei ante'rius** [TA], anterior ligament of malleus: a fibrous band that extends from the neck of the malleus just above the anterior process to the anterior wall of the tympanic cavity close to the petrotympanic fissure. Some of the fibers pass through the fissure to the spina angulares of the sphenoid bone.

**l. mal'lei latera'le** [TA], lateral ligament of malleus: a triangular fibrous band that passes from the posterior portion of the incisura tympanica to the head or neck of the malleus.

**l. mal'lei supe'rius** [TA], superior ligament of malleus: a delicate fibrous strand passing from the roof of the tympanic cavity to the head of the malleus.

**l. malle'oli latera'lis ante'rius,** l. tibiofibulare anterius.

**l. malle'oli latera'lis poste'rius,** l. tibiofibulare posterius.

**l. media'le articulatio'nis talocrura'lis,** l. collaterale mediale articulationis talocruralis.

**l. media'le articulatio'nis temporomandibula'ris** [TA], medial ligament of temporomandibular articulation.

**l. meniscofemora'le ante'rius** [TA], anterior meniscofemoral ligament: a small fibrous band of the knee joint, attached to the posterior area of the lateral meniscus and passing superiorly and medially, anterior to the posterior cruciate ligament, to attach to the anterior cruciate ligament.

**l. meniscofemora'le poste'rius** [TA], posterior meniscofemoral ligament: a small fibrous band of the knee joint, attached to the posterior area of the lateral meniscus and passing superiorly and medially, posterior to the posterior cruciate ligament, to the medial condyle of the femur.

**ligamen'ta metacarpa'lia dorsa'lia** [TA], **ligamen'ta metacar'pea dorsa'lia,** dorsal metacarpal ligaments: bands that interconnect the bases of the second to fifth metacarpal bones by passing transversely from bone to bone on their dorsal surfaces.

**ligamen'ta metacarpa'lia interos'sea** [TA], **ligamen'ta metacar'pea interos'sea,** interosseous metacarpal ligaments: short, strong fibrous bands situated between the adjacent surfaces of the bases of the second to fifth metacarpal bones, just distal to the articular surfaces.

**ligamen'ta metacarpa'lia palma'ria** [TA], **ligamen'ta metacar'pea palma'ria,** palmar metacarpal ligaments: bands that interconnect the bases of the second to fifth metacarpal bones by passing transversely from bone to bone on their palmar surfaces.

**l. metacarpa'le transver'sum profun'dum** [TA], deep transverse metacarpal ligament: a narrow fibrous band that extends across and is attached to the palmar surfaces of the heads of the second to fifth metacarpal bones, joining them together.

**l. metacarpa'le transver'sum superficia'le** [TA], superficial transverse metacarpal ligament: transverse fibers occupying the intervals between the diverging longitudinal bands of the palmar aponeurosis.

**l. metacar'peum transver'sum profun'dum,** ligamentum metacarpale transversum profundum.

**l. metacar'peum transver'sum superficia'le,** ligamentum metacarpale transversum superficiale.

**ligamen'ta metatarsa'lia dorsa'lia** [TA], **ligamen'ta metatar'sea dorsa'lia,** dorsal metatarsal ligaments: light transverse bands on the dorsal surfaces of the bases of the second to fifth metatarsal bones, similar to the corresponding ligaments on the metacarpal bones.

**ligamen'ta metatarsa'lia interos'sea** [TA], **ligamen'ta metatar'sea interos'sea,** interosseous metatarsal ligaments: bands between the bases of the second to fifth metatarsal bones, similar to the corresponding ligaments of the hand.

**ligamen'ta metatarsa'lia planta'ria** [TA], **ligamen'ta metatar'sea planta'ria,** plantar metatarsal ligaments: strong transverse bands on the plantar surfaces of the bases of the second to fifth metatarsal bones.

**l. metatarsa'le transver'sum profundum** [TA], **l. metatar'seum transver'sum profun'dum,** deep transverse metatarsal ligament: a narrow fibrous band that extends across, is attached to the plantar surfaces of, and thus joins together the heads of all the metatarsal bones.

**l. metatarsa'le transver'sum superficia'le** [TA], **l. metatar'seum transver'sum superficia'le,** superficial transverse metatarsal ligament: fibers that lie in the superficial fascia of the sole of the foot beneath the heads of the metatarsal bones.

**l. muco'sum,** plica synovialis infrapatellaris.

**ligamen'ta navicularicuneifor'mia dorsa'lia,** ligamenta cuneonavicularia dorsalia.

**ligamen'ta navicularicuneifor'mia planta'ria,** ligamenta cuneonavicularia plantaria.

**l. nu'chae** [TA], nuchal ligament: a broad, fibrous, roughly triangular sagittal septum in the back of the neck, separating the right and left sides. It extends from the tips of the spinous processes of all the cervical vertebrae to attach to the entire length of the external occipital crest. Caudally it is continuous with the supraspinous ligament.

**ligamen'ta ossiculo'rum auditorio'rum,** TA alternative for *ligamenta ossiculorum auditus.*

**ligamen'ta ossiculo'rum audi'tus** [TA], ligaments of auditory ossicles: the ligaments of the auditory ossicles, comprising the anterior, lateral, and superior ligaments of the malleus, the posterior and superior ligaments of the incus, and the annular ligament of the stapes.

**l. ova'rii pro'prium** [TA], ovarian ligament: a musculofibrous cord in the broad ligament, joining the ovary to the upper part of the lateral margin of the uterus just below the attachment of the uterine tube; called also *utero-ovarian ligament.*

**ligamen'ta palma'ria articulatio'num interphalangea'lium ma'nus** [TA], **ligamen'ta palma'ria articulatio'num interphalangea'rum ma'nus,** palmar ligaments of interphalangeal articulations of hand: thick, dense fibrocartilaginous plates on the palmar surfaces of the interphalangeal articulations of the hand, between the collateral ligaments.

**ligamen'ta palma'ria articulatio'num metacarpophalangea'lium** [TA], **ligamen'ta palma'ria articulatio'num metacarpophalangea'rum,** palmar ligaments of metacarpophalangeal articulations: thick dense fibrocartilaginous plates on the palmar surfaces of the metacarpophalangeal articulation, between the collateral ligaments. Called also *anterior* or *palmar metacarpophalangeal ligaments.*

**l. palpebra'le latera'le** [TA], lateral palpebral ligament: a ligament that anchors the lateral end of the superior and inferior tarsal plates to the margin of the orbit.

**l. palpebra'le media'le** [TA], medial palpebral ligament: fibrous bands that connect the medial ends of the tarsi to the bones of the orbit, an anterior bundle passing in front of the lacrimal sac and being attached to the frontal process of the maxilla, and a posterior bundle passing behind the lacrimal sac and being attached to the posterior crest of the lacrimal bone.

**l. patel'lae** [TA], patellar ligament: the continuation of the central portion of the tendon of the quadriceps femoris muscle distal to the patella; it extends from the patella to the tuberosity of the tibia.

**l. pectina'tum an'guli iridocornea'lis,** reticulum trabeculare.

**l. pectinea'le, l. pecti'neum** [TA], pectineal ligament: a strong aponeurotic lateral continuation of the lacunar ligament along the pectineal line of the pubis; called also *Cooper's ligament* and *inguinal ligament of Cooper.*

**l. phrenicoco'licum** [TA], phrenicocolic ligament: a peritoneal fold that passes from the left colic flexure to the adjacent costal portion of the diaphragm.

**l. phrenicoliena'le, l. phrenicosple'nicum,** l. splenorenale.

**l. pisohama'tum** [TA], pisohamate ligament: a fibrous band extending from the pisiform bone to the hook of the hamate bone.

**l. pisometacar'peum** [TA], pisometacarpal ligament: a fibrous band extending from the pisiform bone to the bases of the fifth, usually the fourth, and sometimes the third metacarpal bone.

**ligamen'ta planta'ria articulatio'num interphalangea'lium pe'dis** [TA], **ligamen'ta planta'ria articulatio'num interphalangea'rum pe'dis,** plantar ligaments of interphalangeal articulations of foot: thick, dense bands on the plantar surfaces of the interphalangeal articulations of the foot, between the collateral ligaments.

**ligamen'ta planta'ria articulatio'num metatarsophalangea'lium** [TA], **ligamenta planta'ria articulatio'num metatarsophalangea'rum,** plantar ligaments of metatarsophalangeal articulations:

thick, dense bands on the plantar surface of the metatarsophalangeal articulations, between the collateral ligaments. Called also *inferior metatarsophalangeal ligaments.*

**l. planta're lon'gum** [TA], long plantar ligament: the longest ligament of the foot, arising from the lower surface of the calcaneus as far back as the lateral and the medial processes, passing forward over the tendon of the peroneus longus, and inserting into the bases of the second through fifth metatarsal bones.

**l. popli'teum arcua'tum** [TA], arcuate popliteal ligament: a band of variable and ill-defined fibers at the posterolateral part of the knee joint; it is attached inferiorly to the apex of the head of the fibula, arches superiorly and medially over the popliteal tendon, and merges with the articular capsule. Called also *popliteal arch* and *arcuate ligament of knee.*

**l. popli'teum obli'quum** [TA], oblique popliteal ligament: a broad band of fibers that arises from the medial condyle of the tibia, merges more or less with the tendon of the semimembranosus, and passes obliquely across the back of the knee joint to the lateral epicondyle of the femur. It contains large openings for the passage of vessels and nerves.

**l. pterygospina'le** [TA], pterygospinal ligament: a band of fibers extending from the superior part of the superior border of the lateral pterygoid plate to the spine of the sphenoid bone.

**l. pu'bicum infe'rius** [TA], inferior pubic ligament: a thick archlike band of fibers situated along the inferior margin of the symphysis pubis. Its fibers are attached to the medial borders of the inferior rami of the pubic bones and thus it rounds out and forms the summit of the pubic arch. Called also *inferior pubic ligament.*

**l. pu'bicum supe'rius** [TA], superior pubic ligament: fibers that pass transversely across the superior margin of the symphysis pubis; attached to the bones and to the interpubic disk, they extend laterally as far as the pubic tubercle.

**l. pubocapsula're,** l. pubofemorale.

**l. pubofemora'le** [TA], pubofemoral ligament: a band that arises from the entire length of the obturator crest of the pubic bone and passes laterally and inferiorly to merge into the capsule of the hip joint, some fibers reaching to the lower part of the neck of the femur. Called also *l. pubocapsulare.*

**l. puboprosta'ticum** [TA], puboprostatic ligament: a thickening of the superior fascia of the pelvic diaphragm in the male that, laterally, extends from the prostate to the tendinous arch of the pelvic fascia and, medially, is a forward continuation of the tendinous arch to the pubis.

**l. pubovesica'le** [TA], pubovesical ligament: a thickening of the superior fascia of the pelvic diaphragm in the female that, laterally, extends from the neck of the bladder to the tendinous arch of the pelvic fascia and, medially, is a forward continuation of the tendinous arch to the pubis.

**l. pubovesica'le latera'le,** lateral extension of ligamentum pubovesicale.

**l. pubovesica'le me'dium,** medial extension of ligamentum pubovesicale.

**l. pulmona'le** [TA], pulmonary ligament: a vertical pleural fold associated with the lung, extending from the hilus down to the base on the medial surface of the lung; on the left it forms the posterior boundary of the impressio cardiaca.

**ligamen'ta pylo'ri,** thickened bands of the longitudinal muscular layer of the stomach situated on the anterior and the posterior surfaces of the antrum pyloricum. Called also *ligaments of Helvetius.*

**l. quadra'tum** [TA], quadrate ligament: a fibrous bundle connecting the distal margin of the radial notch of the ulna to the neck of the radius.

**l. radiocarpa'le dorsa'le** [TA], **l. radiocar'peum dorsa'le,** dorsal radiocarpal ligament: a fibrous band that passes obliquely from the posterior border of the distal extremity of the radius to the dorsal surfaces of the proximal row of carpal bones, especially the triquetral and lunate, and to the dorsal intercarpal ligaments.

**l. radiocarpa'le palma're** [TA], **l. radiocar'peum palma're,** palmar radiocarpal ligament: several bundles of fibers that pass obliquely from the styloid process and the distal anterior margin of the radius to the lunate, triquetral, capitate, and hamate bones; called also *volar radiocarpal ligament.*

**l. sacrococcy'geum ante'rius** [TA], anterior sacrococcygeal ligament: a flat band, homologous with the anterior longitudinal ligament of the vertebral column, that passes from the lower part of the sacrum over onto the anterior part of the coccyx. Called also *l. sacrococcygeum ventrale* [TA alternative] and *ventral sacrococcygeal ligament.*

**l. sacrococcy'geum dorsa'le profun'dum,** TA alternative for *l. sacrococcygeum posterius profundum.*

**l. sacrococcy'geum dorsa'le superficia'le,** TA alternative for *l. sacrococcygeum posterius superficiale.*

**l. sacrococcy'geum latera'le** [TA], lateral sacrococcygeal ligament: a fibrous band, homologous with the intertransverse ligaments, that passes from the transverse process of the first coccygeal vertebra to the lower lateral angle of the sacrum, thus helping to complete the foramen of the fifth sacral nerve.

**l. sacrococcy'geum poste'rius profun'dum** [TA], deep posterior sacrococcygeal ligament: the terminal portion of the posterior longitudinal ligament of the vertebral column; it helps to unite the dorsal surfaces of the fifth sacral and the coccygeal vertebrae. Called also *deep dorsal sacrococcygeal ligament* and *l. sacrococcygeum dorsale profundum* [TA alternative].

**l. sacrococcy'geum poste'rius superficia'le** [TA], superficial posterior sacrococcygeal ligament: a fibrous band continuous with the supraspinous ligament of the vertebral column; attached cranially to the margin of the sacral hiatus, and diverging as it passes caudally to attach to the dorsal surface of the coccyx. Called also *l. sacrococcygeum dorsale superficiale* [TA alternative] and *superficial dorsal sacrococcygeal ligament.*

**l. sacrococcy'geum ventra'le,** TA alternative for *l. sacrococcygeum anterius.*

**l. sacroili'acum ante'rius** [TA], anterior sacroiliac ligament: any of numerous thin fibrous bands passing from the ventral margin of the auricular surface of the sacrum to the adjacent portions of the ilium; called also *l. sacroiliacum ventralis* and *ventral sacroiliac ligaments.*

**l. sacroili'acum dorsa'lis,** l. sacroiliacum posterius.

**l. sacroili'acum interos'seum** [TA], interosseous sacroiliac ligament: any of numerous short, strong bundles connecting the tuberosities and adjacent surfaces of the sacrum and the ilium.

**l. sacroili'acum poste'rius** [TA], posterior sacroiliac ligament: any of numerous strong bands that pass from the ilium to the sacrum. The *long posterior sacroiliac ligament* is more superficial and connects the posterior superior iliac spine with the second, third, and fourth articular tubercles of the sacrum. The *short posterior sacroiliac ligament* is deeper and more nearly horizontal and connects the tuberosity of the ilium with the first and second tubercles on the dorsum of the sacrum. Called also *l. sacroiliacum dorsalis* and *dorsal sacroiliac ligament.*

**l. sacroili'acum ventra'lis,** l. sacroiliacum anterius.

**l. sacrospina'le** [TA], sacrospinal ligament: one of the long vertical fibrous bands attached by the apex to the spine of the ischium and by the base to the lateral margins of the sacrum. Called also *sacrospinous ligament.*

**l. sacrospino'sum,** l. sacrospinale.

**l. sacrotubera'le** [TA], sacrotuberal ligament: a large, flat band that is attached below to the ischial tuberosity, spreads out as it ascends, and is attached to the lateral margins of the sacrum and the coccyx and to the posterior inferior iliac spine; called also *l. sacrotuberosum.*

**l. sacrotubero'sum,** l. sacrotuberale.

**l. sero'sum,** serous ligament: a fold of peritoneum or other serous membrane that helps to hold an organ or part in position and transmits blood vessels and nerves.

**l. sphenomandibula're** [TA], sphenomandibular ligament: a thin aponeurotic band that extends from the angular spine of the sphenoid bone downward medial to the temporomandibular articulation and attaches to the lingula of the mandible.

**l. spira'le coch'leae, l. spira'le duc'tus cochlea'ris** [TA], spiral ligament of cochlea: a band of thickened periosteum in the bony cochlea. Cf. *crista basilaris ductus cochlearis.*

**l. splenorena'le** [TA], splenorenal ligament: a peritoneal fold that passes from the diaphragm to the concave surface of the spleen; called also *l. lienorenale* [TA alternative], *l. phrenicolienale, l. phrenicosplenicum,* and *lienophrenic, phrenicosplenic,* or *splenophrenic ligament.*

**l. sternoclavicula're,** see *l. sternoclaviculare anterius* and *l. sternoclaviculare posterius.*

**l. sternoclavicula're ante'rius** [TA], anterior sternoclavicular ligament: a thick reinforcing band on the anterior portion of the articular capsule of the sternoclavicular articulation. It is attached superiorly to the anterior and superior parts of the sternal extremity of the clavicle and inferiorly to the anterior surface of the manubrium of the sternum.

**l. sternoclavicula're poste'rius** [TA], posterior sternoclavicular ligament: a thick reinforcing band on the posterior portion of the articular capsule of the sternoclavicular articulation. It is attached superiorly to the posterior and superior parts of the sternal extremity of the clavicle and inferiorly to the posterior surface of the manubrium of the sternum.

**l. sternocosta'le interarticula're,** l. sternocostale intraarticulare.

**l. sternocosta'le intraarticula're** [TA], intra-articular sternocostal ligament: a horizontal fibrocartilaginous plate in the center of the second sternocostal joint, which joins the tip of the costal cartilage to the fibrous junction between the manubrium and the body of the sternum, and thus divides the joint into two parts. Called also *interarticular sternocostal ligament* and *l. sternocostale interarticulare.*

**ligamen'ta sternocosta'lia radia'ta** [TA], radiate sternocostal ligaments: fibrous bands attached to the sternal end of a costal cartilage, radiating from there out onto the ventral part of the sternum.

**ligamen'ta sternopericardi'aca** [TA], sternopericardiac ligaments:

two (superior and inferior) or more fibrous bands that attach the pericardium to the dorsal surface of the sternum.

**l. stylohyoi'deum** [TA], stylohyoid ligament: a vertical fibroelastic aponeurotic cord attached superiorly to the tip of the styloid process of the temporal bone and inferiorly to the lesser horn of the hyoid bone.

**l. stylomandibula're** [TA], stylomandibular ligament: an aponeurotic band attached superiorly to the tip of the styloid process of the temporal bone and inferiorly to the angle and posterior margin of the ramus of the mandible.

**l. supraspina'le** [TA], supraspinal ligament: a single long, vertical fibrous band passing over and attached to the tips of the spinous processes of the vertebrae from the seventh cervical to the sacrum; it is continuous above with the ligamentum nuchae.

**l. suspenso'rium clitor'idis** [TA], suspensory ligament of clitoris: a strong fibrous band that comes from the external deep investing fascia and attaches the root of the clitoris to the linea alba, symphysis pubis, and arcuate pubic ligament.

**ligamen'ta suspenso'ria mam'mae, ligamen'ta suspenso'ria mamma'ria** [TA], suspensory ligaments of mammary gland: fibrous processes, extending from the corpus mammae to the corium, homologous with the retinacula cutis of other regions of the body.

**l. suspenso'rium ova'rii** [TA], suspensory ligament of ovary: the portion of the broad ligament lateral to and above the ovary; it contains the ovarian vessels and nerves and passes upward over the iliac vessels.

**l. suspenso'rium pe'nis** [TA], suspensory ligament of penis: a strong fibrous band that comes from the external deep investing fascia and attaches the root of the penis to the linea alba, symphysis pubis, and arcuate pubic ligament.

**l. talocalcanea're interos'seum,** l. talocalcaneum interosseum.

**l. talocalcanea're latera'le,** l. talocalcaneum laterale.

**l. talocalcanea're media'le,** l. talocalcaneum mediale.

**l. talocalca'neum interos'seum** [TA], interosseous talocalcaneal ligament: fibrous bands in the sinus tarsi, passing between the opposed surfaces of the calcaneus and the talus; called also *l. talocalcaneare interosseum.*

**l. talocalca'neum latera'le** [TA], lateral talocalcaneal ligament: a fibrous band passing from the lateral surface of the talus to that of the calcaneus. Called also *l. talocalcaneare laterale.*

**l. talocalca'neum media'le** [TA], medial talocalcaneal ligament: a fibrous band connecting the medial tubercle of the talus with the sustentaculum tali of the calcaneus. Called also *l. talocalcaneare mediale.*

**l. talofibula're ante'rius** [TA], anterior talofibular ligament: one or more fibrous bands that pass from the anterior surface of the lateral malleolus of the fibula to the anterior margin of the lateral articular surface of the talus.

**l. talofibula're poste'rius** [TA], posterior talofibular ligament: a strong fibrous horizontal band passing from the posteromedial face of the lateral malleolus of the fibula to the area of the posterior process of the talus.

**l. talonavicula're** [TA], talonavicular ligament: a broad, thin fibrous band passing from the dorsal and lateral surfaces of the neck of the talus to the dorsal surface of the navicular bone; called also *l. talonaviculare [dorsale]* and *talonavicular dorsal ligament.*

**l. talonavicula're [dorsa'le],** l. talonaviculare.

**l. talotibia'le ante'rius,** pars tibiotalaris anterior ligamenti medialis.

**l. talotibia'le poste'rius,** pars tibiotalaris posterior ligamenti medialis.

**ligamen'ta tar'si** [TA], ligaments of tarsus: a general term encompassing the ligaments that connect the bones of the tarsus.

**ligamen'ta tar'si dorsa'lia** [TA], dorsal ligaments of tarsus: including the bifurcate, the dorsal cuboideonavicular, cuneocuboid, cuneonavicular, and intercuneiform, and the talonavicular ligaments; called also *dorsal intertarsal ligaments.*

**ligamen'ta tar'si interos'sea** [TA], interosseous ligaments of the tarsus, including the interosseous cuneocuboid, intercuneiform, and talocalcaneal ligaments.

**ligamen'ta tar'si planta'ria** [TA], plantar ligaments of tarsus: the inferior ligaments of the foot, comprising the long plantar and the plantar calcaneocuboid, calcaneonavicular, cuneonavicular, cuboideonavicular, intercuneiform, and cuneocuboid ligaments.

**ligamen'ta tarsometarsa'lia dorsa'lia** [TA], **ligamen'ta tarsometatar'sea dorsa'lia,** dorsal tarsometatarsal ligaments: fibrous bands passing from the dorsal surfaces of the bases of the metatarsal bones to the dorsal surfaces of the cuboid and the three cuneiform bones.

**ligamen'ta tarsometatarsa'lia planta'ria** [TA], **ligamen'ta tarsometatar'sea planta'ria,** plantar tarsometatarsal ligaments: fibrous bands passing from the plantar surfaces of the bases of the metatarsal bones to the plantar surfaces of the cuboid and the three cuneiform bones.

**l. temporomandibula're,** l. laterale articulationis temporomandibularis.

**l. te'res fe'moris,** l. capitis femoris.

**l. te'res he'patis** [TA], a fibrous cord, the remains of the left umbilical vein, extending from the porta hepatis, where it is attached to the left branch of the portal vein, out through the fissure of the ligamentum teres and the falciform ligament to the umbilicus.

**l. te'res u'teri** [TA], round ligament of uterus: a fibromuscular band in the female that is attached to the uterus near the attachment of the uterine tube, passing then along the broad ligament, out through the inguinal ring, and into the labium majus.

**l. thyroepiglot'ticum** [TA], thyroepiglottic ligament: a fibrous band that attaches the petiolus of the epiglottis to the thyroid cartilage just below the superior notch.

**l. thyrohyoi'deum latera'le** [TA], lateral thyrohyoid ligament: a round elastic cord that forms the posterior margin of the thyrohyoid membrane; it extends from the tip of the superior horn of the thyroid cartilage upward to the tip of the greater horn of the hyoid bone.

**l. thyrohyoi'deum media'num** [TA], median thyrohyoid ligament: the central, thicker portion of the thyrohyoid membrane; its broader upper part is attached to the body of the hyoid bone and its narrow lower end to the superior incisure of the thyroid cartilage.

**l. tibiofibula're ante'rius** [TA], anterior tibiofibular ligament: a flat triangular band that passes diagonally, inferiorly, and laterally from the anterior portion of the lateral surface of the distal end of the tibia to the anterior surface of the distal end of the fibula; called also *l. malleoli lateralis anterius.*

**l. tibiofibula're poste'rius** [TA], posterior tibiofibular ligament: a fibrous band that passes diagonally, inferiorly, and laterally from the posterior surface of the distal end of the tibia to the adjacent posterior surface of the distal end of the fibula; called also *l. malleoli lateralis posterius.*

**l. tibionavicula're,** pars tibionavicularis ligamenti medialis.

**ligamen'ta trachea'lia,** TA alternative for *ligamenta anularia tracheae.*

**l. transver'sum,** l. costotransversarium.

**l. transver'sum aceta'buli** [TA], transverse ligament of acetabulum: a fibrous band continuous with the acetabular lip of the hip joint, which bridges the acetabular notch and converts it into a foramen.

**l. transver'sum atlan'tis** [TA], transverse ligament of atlas: the strong horizontal portion of the cruciform ligament of the atlas. It is attached at each end to the lateral masses of the atlas and curves posteriorly around the dens of the axis. It thus divides the atlantal ring into a smaller anterior division for the dens and a larger posterior division for the spinal cord and related structures. Called also *Lauth's ligament.*

**l. transver'sum cru'ris,** retinaculum musculorum extensorum superius pedis.

**l. transver'sum genua'le,** l. transversum genus.

**l. transver'sum ge'nus** [TA], transverse ligament of knee: a more or less distinct bundle of fibers in the knee joint, joining together the anterior convex margin of the lateral meniscus and the anterior concave margin or anterior end of the medial meniscus; called also *l. transversum genuale.*

**l. transver'sum pel'vis,** l. transversum perinei.

**l. transver'sum perine'i** [TA], transverse perineal ligament: a fibrous band that spans the subpubic angle just behind the deep dorsal vein of the penis, formed by thickening of the anterior boundary of the perineal membrane.

**l. transver'sum sca'pulae infe'rius** [TA], inferior transverse ligament of scapula: one of three intrinsic ligaments of the scapula, composed of more or less distinct fascial fibers that pass from the lateral border of the spine of the scapula to the adjacent margin of the glenoid cavity, thus converting the notch at the base of the spine into a foramen for the passage of the suprascapular vessels and nerves to the infraspinous fossa.

**l. transver'sum sca'pulae supe'rius** [TA], superior transverse ligament of scapula: one of three intrinsic ligaments of the scapula, a band of fibers that bridges the scapular notch, thus forming a foramen for the passage of the suprascapular nerve. One end is attached to the base of the coracoid process, the other end to the medial border of the scapular notch.

**l. trapezoi'deum** [TA], trapezoid ligament: a broad, flat band forming the anterolateral portion of the coracoclavicular ligament; it is attached inferiorly to the superior surface of the coracoid process of the scapula and superiorly to the oblique ridge on the inferior surface of the clavicle.

**l. triangula're dex'trum he'patis** [TA], right triangular ligament of liver: the pointed right extremity of the coronary ligament of the liver where the superior and the inferior layer join in their attachment to the diaphragm.

**l. triangula're sinis'trum he'patis** [TA], left triangular ligament of liver: a triangular extension of the left extremity of the coronary ligament, which helps to attach the left lobe of the liver to the diaphragm.

**l. tuber'culi cos'tae,** l. costotransversarium laterale.

**l. ulnocarpa'le palma're** [TA], **l. ulnocar'peum palma're,** palmar

ulnocarpal ligament: bundles of fibers that pass from the styloid process of the ulna to the carpal bones.
**l. umbilica'le latera'le, l. umbilica'le media'le,** l. umbilicale medianum.
**l. umbilica'le media'num** [TA], median umbilical ligament: a fibrous cord, the remains of the partially obliterated urachus, extending from the urinary bladder to the umbilicus; it is situated in and produces the median umbilical fold. Called also *lateral,* or *middle umbilical ligament, l. umbilicale laterale,* and *l. umbilicale mediale.*
**ligamen'ta vagina'lia digito'rum ma'nus,** vaginae fibrosae digitorum manus.
**ligamen'ta vagina'lia digito'rum pe'dis,** vaginae fibrosae digitorum pedis.
**l. ve'nae ca'vae sinis'trae** [TA], ligament of left vena cava: a remnant of the embryonic left duct of Cuvier, extending from the left intercostal vein to the oblique vein of left atrium; it is enclosed by the fold of left vena cava.
**l. veno'sum** [TA], venous ligament of liver: a fibrous cord, the remains of the fetal ductus venosus, lying in the fissura ligamenti venosi.
**l. veno'sum [Aran'tii],** l. venosum.
**l. ventricula're,** l. vestibulare.
**l. vestibula're** [TA], vestibular ligament: the membrane that extends from the thyroid cartilage in front to the anterolateral surface of the arytenoid cartilage behind; it lies within the vestibular fold, above the vocal ligament. Called also *l. ventriculare* and *ventricular ligament.*
**l. voca'le** [TA], vocal ligament: the elastic tissue membrane that extends from the thyroid cartilage in front to the vocal process of the arytenoid cartilage behind; it lies within the vocal fold, below the vestibular ligament.

**li·gand** (li'gand; lig'and) [L. *ligare* to tie or bind] 1. a molecule that binds to another molecule, used especially to refer to a small molecule that binds specifically to a larger molecule, e.g., an antigen binding to an antibody, a hormone or neurotransmitter binding to a receptor, or a substrate or allosteric effector binding to an enzyme. 2. a molecule that donates or accepts a pair of electrons to form a coordinate covalent bond with the central metal atom of a coordination complex.

**li·gase** (li'gās) [EC 6] a class of enzymes that catalyze the formation of a bond between two substrate molecules, coupled with the hydrolysis of a pyrophosphate bond in ATP or a similar energy donor. See also *synthetase.*

**li·gate** (li'gāt) to tie or bind with a ligature.

**li·ga·tion** (lĭ-ga'shən) [L. *ligatio*] [MeSH: Ligation] the application of a ligature.
**Barron l.,** treatment of hemorrhoids by binding them at the base with rubber ligatures so that the distal portion sloughs away within several days.
**rubber band l.,** Barron l.
**teeth l.,** the binding together of teeth with wire, thread, or other material for their stabilization and immobilization as a method of tooth movement in orthodontic therapy or following traumatic injury.
**tubal l.,** sterilization of the female by constricting, severing, or crushing the uterine tubes; constriction may be with an encircling plastic ring or other ligature.

**lig·a·ture** (lig'ə-chər) [L. *ligatura*] 1. any substance, such as surgical gut, cotton, silk, or wire, used to tie a vessel or strangulate a part. 2. see under *wire.*
**elastic l.,** a band of rubber used to strangulate hemorrhoids and pedunculated growths.
**interlacing l., interlocking l.,** a continuous suture in which the loops interlock.
**lateral l.,** a ligature so applied as to check, but not to interrupt, the distal blood flow.
**occluding l.,** a ligature that occludes the blood supply to distal tissue.
**provisional l.,** one applied at the beginning of an operation, but removed before its termination.
**soluble l.,** a ligature of prepared animal membrane which is subsequently absorbed, the time of absorption depending upon the method of preparation and the size of the ligature.
**suboccluding l.,** a ligature that obstructs the main blood supply, but leaves unimpaired a portion of tissue capable of establishing capillary anastomosis.
**terminal l.,** a ligature applied to the transected end of a vessel.

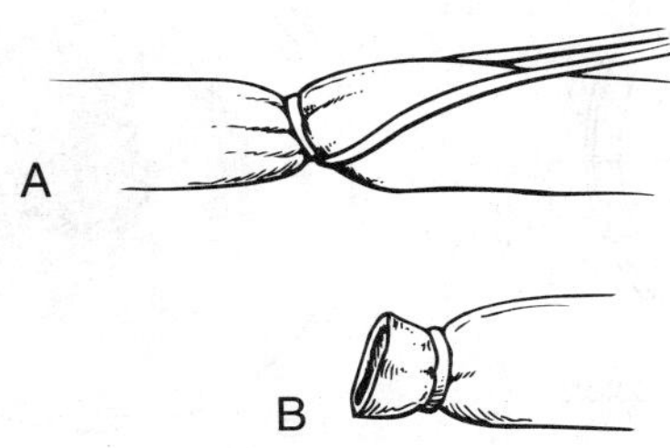

*(A),* Occluding ligature; *(B),* terminal ligature.

**thread-elastic l.,** an elastic thread used for various forms of orthodontic therapy, such as assisting in eruption of impacted teeth, closing spaces, and rotating teeth.

**ligg.** ligaments, or ligamenta.

**light** (līt) [MeSH: Light] the electromagnetic radiation having a velocity of about $3 \times 10^{10}$ cm (186,284 miles) per second, and the vibrations in space being at right angles to the direction of transmission. Frequently construed as limited to the range of wavelength between 390 and 770 nanometers, which provides the stimulus for the subjective sensation of sight, but sometimes considered as including part of the ultraviolet and infrared ranges as well.
**actinic l.,** the portion of the spectrum comprising the light rays capable of producing chemical effects.
**axial l., central l.,** light whose rays are parallel to each other and to the optic axis.
**coherent l.,** light of a single wavelength, phase, and frequency that travels in intense, nearly perfect, parallel rays without appreciable divergence.
**l. difference,** the difference between the two eyes in their sensitivity to light; often abbreviated LD.
**diffused l.,** that which has been scattered by reflection and refraction.
**idioretinal l.,** sensation of light that occurs in the complete absence of the electromagnetic waves that ordinarily stimulate the sensation.
**infrared l.,** see under *ray.*
**intrinsic l.** (of the retina), the dim light always present in the visual field.
**l. minimum,** the smallest degree of light perceived by the eye; often abbreviated LM.
**monochromatic l.,** one of the colors of the spectrum into which light is divided by a prism; it is light of a single wavelength or a narrow range of wavelengths.
**neon l.,** light from neon gas that has been excited by a high voltage discharge.
**oblique l.,** the light that falls obliquely on a surface.
**polarized l.,** light the vibrations of which are made over one plane or in circles or ellipses.
**reflected l.,** light whose rays have been turned back from an illuminated surface.
**refracted l.,** light whose rays have been bent out of their original course by passing through a transparent membrane.
**transmitted l.,** light the rays of which have passed through an object.
**Tyndall l.,** the light that is reflected or dispersed by particles suspended in a gas or liquid; see *Tyndall phenomenon,* under *phenomenon.*
**ultraviolet l.,** see under *ray.*
**white l.,** that produced by a mixture of all wavelengths of electromagnetic energy perceptible as light.
**Wood's l.,** ultraviolet radiation from a mercury-vapor source, transmitted through a nickel-oxide filter (Wood's filter or glass), which holds back all but a few violet rays of the visible spectrum and passes ultraviolet wavelengths of about 365 nm.

**light·en·ing** (līt'ən-ing) the sensation of decreased abdominal distention produced by the descent of the uterus into the pelvic cavity, usually occurring from two to three weeks before labor begins.

**Light·wood's syndrome** (līt'woodz) [Reginald *Lightwood,* English pediatrician, 20th century] see under *syndrome.*

**Lig·nac's syndrome** (le-nyahks') [George Otto Emil *Lignac,* Dutch pediatrician 1891–1954] 1. Fanconi's syndrome (def. 2). 2. cystinosis.

**Lig·nac-Fan·co·ni syndrome** (le-nyahk'fahng-ko'ne) [G.O.E. *Lignac*; Guido *Fanconi*, Swiss pediatrician, 1882–1979] 1. Fanconi's syndrome (def. 2). 2. cystinosis.

**lig·ne·ous** (lig'ne-əs) woody; having a wooden feeling.

**lig·no·caine** (lig'no-kān) lidocaine.

**lig·no·ce·rate** (lig"no-sēr'āt) a salt, ester, or anionic form of lignoceric acid.

**lig·no·cer·ic ac·id** (lig"no-sēr'ik) a saturated 24-carbon fatty acid occurring in sphingomyelin and as a minor constituent of many plant fats. See also table accompanying *fatty acid.*

**lig·num** (lig'nəm) gen. *lig'ni* [L.] wood.
**l. sanc'tum, l. vi'tae,** the heartwood of *Guaiacum officinale* Linne or of *G. sanctum* Linne.

**lig·ro·in, lig·ro·ine** (lig'ro-in) a saturated, volatile, flammable fraction from petroleum distillation, used as an organic solvent; it is sometimes described as encompassing a large range of fractions (boiling range 20–135°C), inclusive of a special grade that is called petroleum benzin (boiling range 30–80°C) but other times is described as similar to petroleum benzin but having a higher density, boiling range, and flash point.

**like·li·hood** (līk'le-hood) a function of data that specifies, for each value of an unknown parameter describing a population distribution, the probability of observing the values sampled. See also *maximum likelihood estimate,* under *estimate.*

**Lil·ey** (lil'ey) [Sir (Albert) William *Liley,* New Zealand perinatologist, 1929–1983] see under *chart.*

**limb** (lim) [MeSH: Extremities] 1. one of the paired appendages of the body used in locomotion or grasping; an arm or leg. Called also *membrum* [TA] and, formerly, *extremitas.* In embryology, the skeleton of each limb is divided into four main parts: the *zonoskeleton,* comprising the scapula and clavicle (as a unit) and the hip bone; the *stylopodium,* comprising the humerus and femur; the *zygopodium,* comprising the radius and ulna and the tibia and fibula; and the *autopodium,* comprising the hand and the foot. 2. a structure or part resembling an arm or leg.
**anacrotic l.,** ascending l. (def. 2).
**anterior l. of internal capsule,** crus anterius capsulae internae.
**anterior l. of stapes,** crus anterius stapedis.
**l's of anthelix,** crura anthelicis; see under *crus.*
**ascending l.,** 1. the distal part of the loop of Henle (ansa nephroni); see under *ansa.* 2. the ascending portion of a tracing of the pulse wave obtained by the manometer or the sphygmograph; called also *anacrotic l.*
**ascending l., thick,** tubulus rectus distalis.
**ascending l., thin,** any part of the distal end of the thin tubule that is within the ascending limb.
**catacrotic l.,** descending l. (def. 2).
**descending l.,** 1. the proximal part of the loop of Henle (ansa nephroni); see under *ansa.* 2. the descending portion of a tracing of the pulse wave obtained by the manometer or the sphygmograph. Called also *catacrotic l.*
**hind l.,** the back leg (pelvic limb) of a quadruped. Cf. *forelimb.*
**inferior l. of ansa cervicalis,** radix inferior ansae cervicalis.
**long l. of incus,** crus longum incudis.
**lower l.,** membrum inferius.
**lower l., free,** the freely movable lower limb from the hip joint to the foot.
**pectoral l.,** thoracic l.
**pelvic l.,** the limb attached to the pelvic girdle; the lower limb of a human or a homologous structure such as a hind limb (q.v.) on another animal.
**phantom l.,** a pseudesthesia after amputation of a limb, consisting of the sensation that the absent part is still present; there may also be paresthesias, transient aches, and intermittent or continuous pain perceived as originating in the absent limb. Called also *pseudomelia* and *stump hallucination.*
**posterior l. of internal capsule,** 1. crus posterius capsulae internae. 2. pars thalamolenticularis capsulae internae.
**posterior l. of stapes,** crus posterius stapedis.
**retrolenticular l. of internal capsule, retrolentiform l. of internal capsule,** pars retrolentiformis capsulae internae.
**short l. of incus,** crus breve incudis.
**sublenticular l. of internal capsule, sublentiform l. of internal capsule,** pars sublentiformis capsulae internae.
**superior l. of ansa cervicalis,** radix superior ansae cervicalis.
**thoracic l.,** the limb attached to the thoracic girdle; the upper limb of a human or a homologous structure (wing, foreleg, etc.) in another animal.
**upper l.,** membrum superius.
**upper l., free,** the freely movable upper limb from the acromioclavicular joint to the hand.

**lim·bal** (lim'bəl) 1. limbic. 2. occurring at the junction of the cornea and conjunctiva.

**lim·ber·neck** (lim'bər-nek) a type of botulism in birds, accompanied by flaccid paralysis.

**lim·bi** (lim'bi) [L.] genitive and plural of *limbus.*

**lim·bic** (lim'bik) 1. pertaining to a limbus, or margin; forming a border around. Called also *limbal.* 2. pertaining to a certain region of the rhinencephalon; see *limbic system,* under *system.*

**Lim·bi·trol** (lim'bĭ-trol) trademark for a combination of amitriptyline hydrochloride and chlordiazepoxide.

**lim·bus** (lim'bəs) gen. and pl. *lim'bi* [L.] a hem or fringe; used in anatomical nomenclature as a general term for such a structure. See also *border, labium,* and *margo.*
**l. aceta'buli** [TA], margin of acetabulum: the peripheral margin of the acetabulum to which the labrum acetabulare is attached; called also *border of acetabulum, margo acetabularis,* and *margo acetabuli* [TA alternative].
**alveolar l. of mandible,** arcus alveolaris mandibulae.
**alveolar l. of maxilla,** arcus alveolaris maxillae.
**l. alveola'ris mandi'bulae,** arcus alveolaris mandibulae.
**l. alveola'ris maxil'lae,** arcus alveolaris maxillae.
**l. ante'rior pal'pebrae** [TA], anterior palpebral margins: the rounded anterior edges of the free margin of the eyelids, from which the eyelashes arise.
**l. of bony spiral lamina,** l. spiralis.
**l. conjuncti'vae,** anulus conjunctivae.
**l. cor'neae** [TA], corneal limbus: the junctional region between the cornea and the sclera, marked on the outer surface of the eyeball by a slight furrow, the sulcus sclerae; called also *corneoscleral* or *sclerocorneal junction.*
**l. fora'minis ova'lis,** the border of the foramen ovale cordis.
**l. fos'sae ova'lis** [TA], limbus of fossa ovalis: the prominent rounded margin of the fossa ovalis cordis; it represents the edge of the fetal septum secundum. Called also *annulus ovalis, Vieussens' annulus,* and *isthmus, l.,* or *ring of Vieussens.*
**l. la'minae spira'lis os'seae,** l. spiralis.
**l. lu'teus re'tinae,** macula luteae.
**l. membra'nae tym'pani,** 1. the thickened margin of the tympanic membrane attached to the tympanic sulcus. 2. anulus fibrocartilagineus membranae tympani.
**l. palpebra'lis ante'rior,** limbus anterior palpebrae.
**l. palpebra'lis poste'rior,** limbus posterior palpebrae.
**l. poste'rior pal'pebrae** [TA], posterior palpebral margins: the sharp posterior edges of the free margin of the eyelids, closely applied to the eyeball.
**l. of sclera,** see *limbus* (def. 2).
**spiral l.,** 1. labium limbi vestibulare. 2. l. spiralis.
**l. spira'lis** [TA], spiral limbus: the thickened periosteum of the osseous spiral lamina at the attachment of the vestibular membrane. Called also *l. laminae spiralis osseae* and *l. of bony spiral lamina.*
**l. of Vieussens,** l. fossae ovalis.

**lime** (līm) [L. *calx*] 1. calcium oxide. 2. [USP] a pharmaceutical preparation of calcium oxide; used as a pharmaceutical necessity. 3. *Citrus aurantifolia.* 4. the acid fruit of *C. aurantifolia,* whose juice contains ascorbic acid; used as an antiscorbutic and refrigerant.
**barium hydroxide l.** [USP], a mixture of barium hydroxide octahydrate and calcium hydroxide used as a carbon dioxide absorbent in the administration of anesthetic gases and oxygen.
**chlorinated l.,** a white or grayish white powder used as a bleaching agent and disinfectant and, formerly, as a topical germicide.
**slaked l.,** calcium hydroxide.
**soda l.** [NF], a mixture of calcium oxide and sodium or potassium hydroxide or both; a reagent used to absorb carbon dioxide in anesthesia machines, in oxygen therapy, and in the determination of the basal metabolic rate.

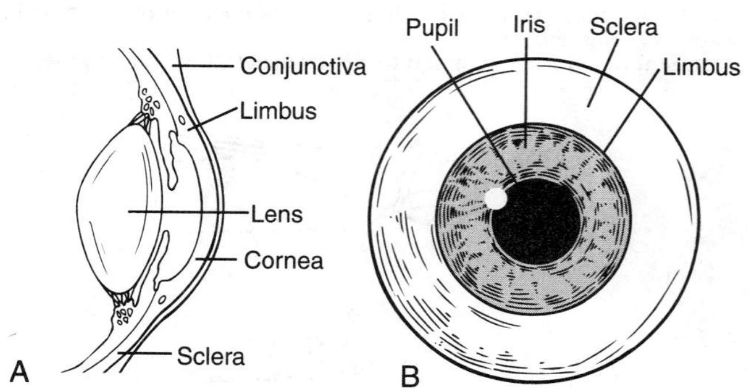


Limbus, in a horizontal section *(A)* and anterior view *(B)* of the eyeball.

**li•men** (li'mən) pl. *li'mina* [L.] 1. threshold, as of a stimulus. 2. [TA] a general term for the beginning point, boundary, or threshold of a structure.
**l. in'sulae** [TA], limen of insula: the point at which the cortex of the insula is continuous, on the inferior surface of the cerebral hemisphere, with the cortex of the frontal lobe. Called also *insular threshold.*
**l. na'si** [TA], the ridge at the junction of the lateral nasal cartilage and the lateral crus of the greater alar cartilage, marking the boundary between the vestibule of the nose and the nasal cavity proper. Called also *nasal valve.*
**l. of twoness,** double point threshold.

**li•mes** (li'mēz) [L. "boundary"] limit; boundary.
**l. dose,** see *L+ dose, L0 d., Lf d.,* and *Lr dose,* under *dose.*

**lim•i•na** (lim'ĭ-nə) [L.] plural of *limen.*

**lim•i•nal** (lim'ĭ-nəl) [L. *limen* threshold] barely appreciable to the senses; pertaining to a threshold.

**lim•i•nom•e•ter** (lim"ĭ-nom'ə-tər) [*limen* + *-meter*] an instrument for measuring the strength of a stimulus applied over a tendon and determining the reflex threshold.

**lim•it** (lim'it) [L. *limes* boundary] a boundary, as one that confines.
**assimilation l.,** saturation l.
**audibility l's,** the extremes of frequency beyond which the human ear perceives no sound: lower limit, 8 Hz; upper, 20,000 Hz. Called also *range of audibility.*
**confidence l's,** the endpoints or boundaries of a confidence interval, delineating the minimum and maximum values of the range expected to contain the parameter.
**elastic l.,** the extent to which elastic material may be deformed without impairing its ability to return to original dimensions. Cf. *proportional l.*
**l. of flocculation,** a term used in expressing the strength of toxin, toxoid, and antitoxin; see *Lf dose,* under *dose.*
**Hayflick's l.,** the maximum number of divisions a cell can undergo before cell death, between 50 and 60 in most human cells. Some malignant cell lines escape the limit and undergo immortalization (q.v.).
**l. of perception,** the minimum visual angle below which perception is impossible: an object to be perceived must subtend a visual angle of four or five minutes, thus making its image on the retina about the size of a retinal cone of 3.3–3.6 micrometers in diameter.
**proportional l.,** the highest amount of stress put on a material at which the proportion between stress and strain is linear; beyond this limit, deformation increases more rapidly and is permanent. Cf. *elastic l.*
**quantum l.,** minimum wavelength.
**saturation l.,** the amount of carbohydrate that an organism can metabolize without causing glycosuria; called also *assimilation l.*

**lim•i•tans** (lim'ĭ-tanz) [L.] limiting; see *membrana limitans.*

**lim•i•ta•tion** (lim"ĭ-ta'shən) circumscription; the act of limiting, or state of being limited.
**eccentric l.,** a circumscribed condition of the visual field, more pronounced at some parts of the periphery than at others.

**lim•it dex•trin•ase** (lim'it deks'trin-ās) oligo-1,6-glucosidase. See *α-dextrinase.*

**lim•i•troph•ic** (lim"ĭ-trof'ik) controlling nutrition.

**Lim•na•tis** (lim-na'tis) the land leeches, a genus of the family Gnathobdellidae, class Hirudinea.
**L. nilo'tica,** a species of North Africa, Central Europe, and the Middle East, commonly used for drawing blood; if large numbers become lodged in the nasal passages, larynx or pharynx of mammals, they may cause anemia and asphyxia (see also *hirudiniasis*). Called also *Hirudo aegyptiaca.*

**lim•o•nene** (lim'o-nēn) an essential oil, a monocyclic terpene, found in the peel of oranges and lemons.

**li•moph•thi•sis** (li-mof'thĭ-sis) [Gr. *limos* hunger + *phthisis*] inanition.

**li•mo•sis** (li-mo'sis) [Gr. *limos* hunger] abnormal hunger.

**limp** (limp) any gait that avoids weight bearing by one leg. Cf. *gait.*

**lim•pet** (lim'pət) any of various snaillike marine gastropods with cone-shaped shells, of the order Aspidobranchia, subclass Streptoneura.
**keyhole l.,** any member of the genus *Fissurella,* marine gastropods.

**Lin•a•cre** (lin'ə-kər) Thomas (1460–1524). A noted English physician and classicist, who was physician to Henry VIII and the first president of the Royal College of Physicians of London. He was also renowned for his translations of Greek classics (e.g., Galen) into Latin.

**lin•a•ma•rin** (lin"ə-mah'rin) a toxic cyanogenetic glycoside found in flax *(Linum usitatissimum)* and lima beans *(Phaseolus limensis),* which can cause cyanide poisoning in animals that eat linseed, beans, or the plants in large quantities. Called also *phaseolunatin.*

**Lin•co•cin** (lin-ko'sin) trademark for a preparation of lincomycin hydrochloride.

**lin•co•my•cin** (lin"ko-mi'sin) [MeSH: Lincomycin] an antibiotic, primarily a gram-positive specific antibacterial, produced by a variant of *Streptomyces lincolnesis.*
**l. hydrochloride** [USP], the monohydrated monohydrochloride salt of lincomycin, used as an antibacterial, mainly in the treatment of infections due to susceptible strains of streptococci, pneumococci, and staphylococci; administered intramuscularly and intravenously.

**linc•ture** (lingk'chər) an electuary.

**linc•tus** (lingk'təs) [L. "a licking"] an electuary.

**lin•dane** (lin'dān) [USP] [MeSH: Lindane] the gamma isomer of benzene hexachloride, an insecticide more potent than chlorophenothane (DDT), it is used as a pediculicide and scabicide, applied topically to the skin. Called also *gamma benzene hexachloride.*

**Lin•dau's disease, tumor** (lin'douz) [Arvid *Lindau,* Swedish pathologist, 1892–1958] see *von Hippel-Lindau disease,* under *disease,* and see *hemangioblastoma.*

**Lin•dau-von Hip•pel disease** (lin'dou-fōn-hip'əl) [Arvid *Lindau;* Eugen *von Hippel,* German ophthalmologist, 1867–1939] von Hippel-Lindau disease.

**Lind•bergh pump** (lind'bərg) [Charles A. *Lindbergh,* American aviator, 1902–1974] see under *pump.*

**lin•den** (lin'dən) any tree of the genus *Tilia.* Called also *basswood.*

**line** (līn) [L. *linea*] 1. a stripe, streak, mark, or narrow ridge. 2. in anthropometry, often an imaginary line connecting different anatomical landmarks. See also *axis* and *plane* (def. 1).

## Line

For descriptions of anatomical terms, see also under *linea.*

**abdominal l.,** any imaginary line projected upon the surface of the abdomen, such as one indicating the boundary of a region.
**absorption l's,** dark lines in the spectrum due to absorption of light by the substance (usually an incandescent gas or vapor) through which the light has passed. Cf. *absorption bands,* under *band.*
**accretion l's,** incremental l's.
**adrenal l.,** Sergent's white adrenal l.
**Aldrich-Mees l's,** Mees' l's.
**alveolobasilar l.,** a line from the basion to the upper alveolar limit.
**l. of Amici,** Z band.
**angular l.,** collarette.
**anococcygeal l., white,** corpus anococcygeum.
**anocutaneous l.,** linea anocutanea.
**anorectal l.,** junctio anorectalis.
**anterior humeral l.,** on a lateral radiograph of the elbow, a line paralleling the anterior cortex of the humerus; in the normal elbow, it intersects the middle third or the junction of the anterior and middle thirds of the capitellum.
**arcuate l. of ilium,** linea arcuata ossis ilii.
**arcuate l. of occipital bone, external superior,** linea nuchalis superior.
**arcuate l. of occipital bone, highest,** linea nuchalis suprema.
**arcuate l. of occipital bone, inferior,** linea nuchalis inferior.
**arcuate l. of occipital bone, superior,** linea nuchalis superior.
**arcuate l. of occipital bone, supreme,** linea nuchalis suprema.
**arcuate l. of pelvis,** linea terminalis pelvis.
**arcuate l. of sheath of rectus abdominis muscle,** linea arcuata vaginae musculi recti abdominis.
**atropic l.,** one normal to the place of the axes of rotation of the eye.
**auriculobregmatic l.,** a line from the auricular point to the bregma.

**axillary l.,** linea axillaris anterior.
**axillary l., median,** linea axillaris media.
**axillary l., posterior,** linea axillaris posterior.
**Baillarger's external l.,** stria laminae granularis internae.
**Baillarger's inner l., Baillarger's internal l.,** stria laminae pyramidalis internae.
**Baillarger's outer l.,** stria laminae granularis internae.
**base l.,** 1. one from the infraorbital ridge to the external acoustic meatus and the middle line of the occiput. 2. baseline.
**base-apex l.,** a line perpendicular to the edge of a prism and bisecting the refracting angle of the prism.
**basinasal l.,** a line from the basion to the nasion. Called also *nasobasal l.*
**basiobregmatic l.,** a line from the basion to the bregma.
**Baudelocque's l.,** conjugata externa pelvis.
**Beau's l's,** transverse lines or grooves in the nail plate caused by various systemic and local traumatic factors.
**biauricular l.,** a line passing over the vertex from one acoustic meatus to the other.
**bi-iliac l.,** one joining the most prominent points of the two iliac crests.
**bismuth l.,** a thin blue-black line in the marginal gingiva around the teeth, sometimes confined to the gingival papilla, observed in bismuth poisoning. See also *bismuth stomatitis,* under *stomatitis.*
**Blaschko's l's,** a developmental pattern of skin growth seen in functional x-chromosome mosaicism.
**blood l.,** a line of direct descent through several generations.
**blue l.,** see *bismuth l.* and *lead l.*
**Blumensaat's l.,** a linear shadow on the lateral radiograph of the knee, representing tangential bone in the intercondylar space.
**Borsieri's l.,** see under *sign.*
**Brödel's white l.,** a longitudinal white line on the anterior surface of the kidney near the convex border.
**Brücke's l's,** broad bands alternating with Z bands in the fibrils of the striated muscles.
**Bryant's l.,** 1. the vertical side of the iliofemoral triangle. 2. a test line for detecting shortening of the femur.
**Burton's l.,** lead l.
**calcification l's,** incremental l's.
**cell l.,** a group of animal cells derived from a primary culture at the time of first subculture; it is considered to be an *established cell l.* when it demonstrates the potential for indefinite subculture *in vitro.*
**cement l.,** a name applied to a line, visible in microscopic examination of bone in cross section, marking the boundary of an osteon (haversian system).
**cervical l.,** an anatomical landmark determined by the junction of the enamel- and the cementum-covered portions of a tooth (the cementoenamel junction); the dividing line between the crown and root portions of a tooth.
**choroid l.,** taenia choroidea.
**Clapton's l.,** a green line on the gums seen in copper poisoning.
**clavicular l.,** one following the course of the clavicles.
**cleavage l's,** Langer's l's.
**Conradi's l.,** a line from the base of the xiphoid process to the point on the chest at which the apex beat is felt, indicating the upper limit of percussion dullness of the left lobe of the liver.
**contour l's,** l's of Owen.
**copper l.,** a greenish or red line at the border of the gums seen in copper poisoning.
**Correra's l.,** a line in the radiograph of the chest, around the outline of the thorax, and bounding the lung fields.
**Corrigan's l.,** a purplish line observed on the gums in copper poisoning.
**costoarticular l.,** a line from the sternoclavicular joint to a point on the eleventh rib.
**costoclavicular l.,** linea parasternalis.
**costophrenic septal l's,** see *Kerley's l's.*
**cricoclavicular l.,** a line from the cricoid cartilage of the larynx to the point at which the superior projection of the anterior axillary line intersects the clavicle.
**cruciate l.,** eminentia cruciformis.
**curved l. of ilium,** linea arcuata ossis ilii.
**curved l. of ilium, inferior,** linea glutealis inferior.
**curved l. of ilium, middle,** linea glutealis anterior.
**curved l. of ilium, superior,** linea glutealis posterior.
**curved l. of occipital bone, highest,** linea nuchalis suprema.
**curved l. of occipital bone, inferior,** linea nuchalis inferior.
**curved l. of occipital bone, superior,** linea nuchalis superior.
**curved l. of occipital bone, supreme,** linea nuchalis suprema.
**Czermak's l's,** spatia interglobularia; see under *spatium.*
**Daubenton's l.,** see under *plane.*
**dentate l.,** linea anocutanea.
**De Salle's l.,** nasal l.
**developmental l's,** see under *groove.*
**Dobie's l.,** Z band; see under *band.*
**Donaldson's l.,** an imaginary line drawn longitudinally through the lateral semicircular canal and bisecting the perpendicular dimension of the posterior canal; in most individuals it will pass just above the endolymphatic sac.
**l. of Douglas,** linea arcuata vaginae musculi recti abdominis.
**Duhot's l.,** a line from the superior iliac spine to the apex of the sacrum.
**dynamic l's,** lines on the face, e.g., laugh lines and frown lines, which develop as a result of repetitious right-angled pull on the skin by the muscles of expression; they are considered a sign of aging.
**Eberth's l's,** microscopic broken or scalariform lines at the junction of the cardiac muscle cells.
**l's of Ebner,** delicate lines indicating periods of rest between daily increments of dentin, which are visible on ground sections of a tooth. Called also *incremental l's of Ebner.*
**ectental l.,** the line of junction between the ectoderm and endoderm.
**embryonic l.,** the primitive streak in the center of the germinal area.
**epiphyseal l.,** 1. linea epiphysialis. 2. a strip of lesser density apparent in the radiograph of a long bone, representing the linea epiphysialis.
**established cell l.,** see *cell l.*
**l's of expression,** relaxed skin tension l's.
**external l. of Baillarger,** stria laminae granularis internae.
**facial l.,** a line connecting the nasion with the pogonion, gnathion, or menton. See also under *height.*
**Farre's white l.,** the boundary of the insertion of the mesovarium at the hilus of the ovary.
**Feiss' l.,** a line from the medial malleolus to the plantar surface of the first metatarsophalangeal joint.
**l. of fixation,** a straight line extending through the center of rotation of the eye to the object of vision.
**focal l., anterior,** a line whose direction is perpendicular to the meridian of greatest curvature of a refracting surface.
**focal l., posterior,** a line whose direction is perpendicular to the meridian of least curvature of a refracting surface.
**Frommann's l's,** transverse marks on the axon of a medullated nerve fiber, rendered visible by silver nitrate.
**fulcrum l.,** an axis that extends from one abutment tooth to another, about which a partial denture can rotate during function.
**fulcrum l., retentive,** an imaginary line connecting the retentive points of clasp arms on retaining teeth adjacent to mucosa-borne denture bases, around which a denture tends to rotate when subjected to such forces as the pull of sticky foods.
**fulcrum l., stabilizing,** an imaginary line connecting occlusal rests, around which a denture will rotate under masticatory forces.
**Futcher's l.,** Voigt's l.
**genal l.,** one of Jadelot's lines, extending from the nasal line near the mouth toward the malar bone.
**l. of Gennari,** the name given to the prominent external band of Baillarger *(stria laminae granularis internae)* in the region of the calcarine sulcus; because it is so highly visible the region is called the *striate cortex.* Called also *band, stria,* or *stripe of Gennari.*
**gingival l.,** 1. a line determined by the level to which the gingiva extends on a tooth; although it tends to follow the curvature of the cervical line, the two rarely coincide. 2. any linear mark visible on the surface of the gingiva, such as the discoloration resulting from the ingestion of lead (lead l.).
**gluteal l., anterior,** linea glutealis anterior.
**gluteal l., inferior,** linea glutealis inferior.
**gluteal l., posterior,** linea glutealis posterior.
**Granger l.,** a curved line seen in radiographs of skulls, indicating the position of the optic groove.

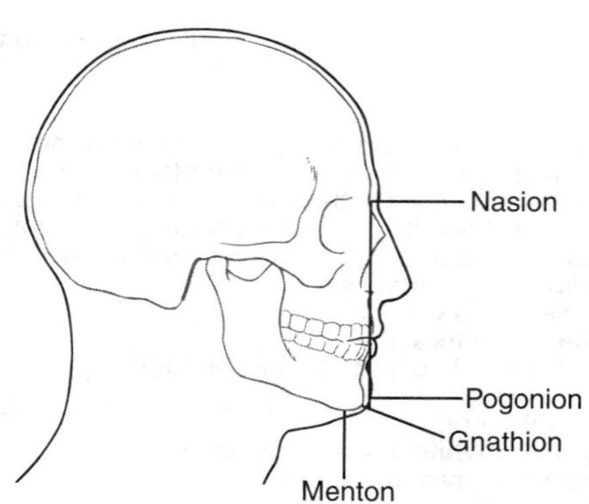

Facial line, shown as extending from nasion to gnathion.

**gum l.,** gingival l. (def. 1).

**Hampton l.,** a significant radiographic characteristic associated with the niche of the typical benign gastric ulcer in profile.

**Harris l's,** lines of retarded growth seen radiographically at the epiphyses of long bones.

**heave l.,** in an animal with heaves, a groove that appears along the costal arch during the forced contraction of abdominal muscles that follows the normal passive expiratory movement.

**Helmholtz l.,** a line perpendicular to the plane of the axis of rotation of the eyes.

**Hensen's l.,** M band; see under *band.*

**Hilton's white l.,** a narrow wavy zone, usually not visible macroscopically but palpable on digital examination, that forms the lower border of the pecten, at the level of the interval between the subcutaneous part of the external anal sphincter and the lower border of the internal sphincter; called also *anal intersphincteric groove.*

**Holden's l.,** a sulcus below the inguinal fold, crossing the capsule of the hip joint.

**hot l.,** see under *H.*

**Hudson's l., Hudson-Stähli l.,** a linear horizontal brown mark located at about the junction of the middle and lower thirds of the cornea but not reaching the limbus, seen in the normal corneas of 16 per cent of aged individuals. Called also *pigmented l. of the cornea, Stähli's pigment l.* and *superficial l. of the cornea.*

**Hueter's l.,** a straight line connecting the medial epicondyle of the humerus with the top of the olecranon when the arm is extended.

**Hunter's l.,** linea alba.

**iliopectineal l.,** linea arcuata ossis ilii.

**imbrication l's of cementum,** incremental l's of cementum.

**imbrication l's of Pickerill,** lines formed by ends of rod bundles that overlie one another and are arranged in scalariform fashion on the surface of the crown of a tooth; seen on longitudinal sections of a tooth together with the incremental lines, but forming areas not completely contained in the enamel. Called also *Pickerill's imbrication l's.* See also *incremental l's.*

**incremental l's,** lines showing the successive layers deposited in a tissue. In the enamel, they are brown striations visible under transmitted light and colorless in reflected light. They may be observed under the microscope in longitudinal sections as oblique lines running inward from the surface and toward the root and in cross sections as rings similar to those in a tree trunk. Dry dentin often shows a series of somewhat parallel lines caused by imperfectly calcified dentin arranged in layers. Called also *accretion l's, calcification l's, Retzius' l's,* and *Retzius' parallel striae.* See also *l's of Ebner, imbrication l's of Pickerill,* and *neonatal l.*

**incremental l's of cementum,** very fine dark lines present in longitudinal sections of a tooth, which follow the contour of the root and border with wider light bands, revealing the cyclic activity of cementogenesis. Called also *imbrication l's of cementum.*

**incremental l's of Ebner,** l's of Ebner.

**infracostal l.,** planum subcostale.

**infrascapular l.,** a horizontal line at the level of the inferior angles of the scapulae.

**inner l. of Baillarger,** stria laminae pyramidalis internae.

**intercondylar l., intercondyloid l.,** linea intercondylaris.

**intermediate l. of iliac crest,** linea intermedia cristae iliacae.

**internal l. of Baillarger,** stria laminae pyramidalis internae.

**interspinal l.,** planum interspinale.

**intertrochanteric l., intertrochanteric l., anterior,** linea intertrochanterica.

**intertrochanteric l., posterior,** crista intertrochanterica.

**intertuberal l.,** a line drawn between the prominences of the frontal bone.

**intertubercular l.,** planum intertuberculare.

**intraperiod l's,** see *period l's.*

**isoeffect l's,** in radiotherapy, lines on a rectangular graph representing doses of radiation having tumoricidal effects and those having complicating necrotic effects in normal tissues.

**isoelectric l.,** the baseline of the electrocardiogram.

**Jadelot's l's,** the genal, labial, nasal, and oculozygomatic lines, lines of the face in young children, formerly thought to indicate specific types of disease. Called also *Jadelot's furrows.*

**l. of Kaes,** Kaes-Bekhterev layer.

**Kerley's l's,** horizontal linear densities 1 to 2.5 cm long on chest radiograms; they are arranged in stepladder fashion and are believed to represent widening of the interlobular septa, as by edema (in mitral stenosis) or fibrosis (in silicosis). When peripherally situated, particularly at the base of the lungs, they are called *Kerley's B l's,* or *costophrenic septal l's.* When centrally situated, they are called *Kerley's A l's.*

**Kilian's l.,** a prominent line on the promontory of the sacrum.

**Krause's l.,** Z band; see under *band.*

**labial l.,** one of Jadelot's lines, extending laterally from the angle of the mouth, thought to indicate disease of the lungs.

**Langer's l's,** linear clefts in the skin indicative of direction of the fibers. The lines, which correspond closely to the crease lines in the skin, assume a characteristic pattern in each part of the body but vary with body configuration. Called also *cleavage l's.*

**lead l.,** a gray or bluish black line at the gingival margin in lead poisoning, seen especially in patients with poor oral hygiene; it is similar to the bismuth line, but is somewhat more diffuse. Called also *blue l.* and *Burton's l.* or *sign.*

**lip l.,** a line at the level to which the margin of either lip extends on the teeth.

**lip l., high,** the greatest height to which the maxillary lip is raised.

**lip l., low,** the lowest position of the lower lip during the act of smiling or voluntary retraction.

**lower lung l.,** a horizontal line in radiographs of the upper part of the abdomen, running from the lateral chest wall toward the first lumbar vertebra on each side, and representing the lower posterior boundary of the pleural cavity.

**magnetic l's of force,** lines indicating direction of force in a magnetic field.

**major dense l's, major period l's,** see *period l's.*

**mammary l.,** milk l.

**mammillary l.,** linea mammillaris.

**median l.,** an imaginary vertical line on the body surface, dividing the surface equally into right and left sides.

**median l., anterior,** linea mediana anterior.

**median l., posterior,** linea mediana posterior.

**medioclavicular l.,** linea medioclavicularis.

**Mees' l's,** single or multiple transverse white bands on the fingernails; they occur especially in association with arsenic poisoning and in other trace element intoxications, and have been reported in leprosy, septicemia, dissecting aortic aneurysm, and acute and chronic renal failure. Called *Aldrich-Mees l's.*

**mesenteric l.,** see *mesenteric triangle,* under *triangle.*

**Meyer's l.,** the axial line of the big toe which if extended passes through the center of the heel if shoes have never been worn.

**midaxillary l.,** linea axillaris media.

**midclavicular l.,** linea medioclavicularis.

**middle l. of scrotum,** raphe scroti.

**midspinal l.,** a perpendicular line down the middle of the vertebral column.

**midsternal l.,** a line passing through the middle of the sternum from the cricoid cartilage to the xiphoid.

**milk l.,** a ridge of thickened epithelium from axilla to groin in the mammalian embryo along which nipples and mammary glands develop, all but one usually disappearing in the human. Called also *mammary l.* and *mammary ridge.*

**l's of minimal tension,** relaxed skin tension l's.

**Monro's l.,** one from the umbilicus to the anterior superior iliac spine.

**Monro-Richter l.,** one from the umbilicus to the left anterior superior iliac spine.

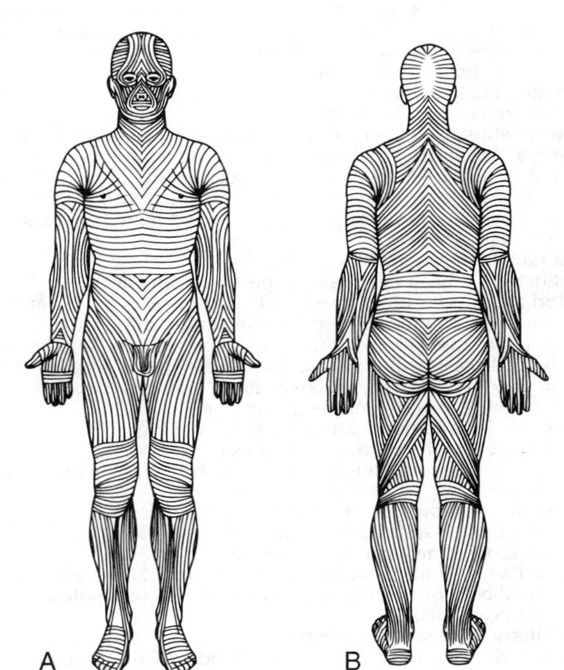


Anterior *(A)* and posterior *(B)* views of Langer's lines of skin cleavage.

**Morgan's l.**, a secondary crease in the lower eyelids in atopic dermatitis; called also *Dennie's sign.*
**Moyer's l.**, a line from the middle of the body of the third sacral vertebra to a point midway between the anterior superior iliac spines.
**mucogingival l.**, see under *junction.*
**muscular l's of scapula**, lineae musculares scapulae.
**mylohyoid l. of mandible, mylohyoidean l.**, linea mylohyoidea mandibulae.
**nasal l.**, one of Jadelot's lines, extending from the ala nasi in a semicircle around the mouth.
**nasobasal l.**, basinasal l.
**nasobasilar l.**, a line through the basion and nasal point.
**nasolabial l.**, a line extending from the ala nasi to the angle of the mouth; see also *sulcus nasolabialis.*
**Nélaton's l.**, a line from the anterior superior iliac spine to the most prominent part of the ischial tuberosity.
**neonatal l.**, a line seen on longitudinal sections of a tooth, showing a demarcation between the structures present at birth and those deposited postnatally; in cross sections, the lines are seen as rings (neonatal rings), and their variations indicate adaptational changes in tooth formation. See also *l's of Owen.*
**nigra l.**, linea nigra.
**nipple l.**, linea mammillaris.
**nuchal l., highest**, linea nuchalis suprema.
**nuchal l., inferior**, linea nuchalis inferior.
**nuchal l., median, nuchal l., middle**, crista occipitalis externa.
**nuchal l., superior**, linea nuchalis superior.
**nuchal l., supreme**, linea nuchalis suprema.
**oblique l.**, one which follows an oblique course; see terms beginning *linea obliqua.*
**oblique l. of femur**, linea intertrochanterica.
**oblique l. of fibula**, 1. crista medialis fibulae. 2. margo anterior fibulae.
**oblique l. of mandible**, linea obliqua mandibulae.
**oblique l. of mandible, internal**, linea mylohyoidea mandibulae.
**oblique l. of thyroid cartilage**, linea obliqua cartilaginis thyroideae.
**oblique l. of tibia**, linea musculi solei.
**l. of occlusion**, the alignment of the occluding surfaces of the teeth in a horizontal plane.
**oculozygomatic l.**, one of Jadelot's lines, extending outward from the medial canthus toward the zygoma; thought to indicate a disorder of the nervous system.
**omphalospinous l.**, a line on the abdomen connecting the umbilicus and the anterior superior iliac spine; a guide to the location of McBurney's point.
**orthostatic l's**, natural furrows on the neck, due to physiologic skin excess required at certain areas for the purpose of flexion and extension.
**outer l. of Baillarger**, stria laminae granularis internae.
**l's of Owen**, the sweeping bands seen on longitudinal section that outline the growth of the coronal or radicular dentin, representing a lag of several days between calcification phases, each lasting about 4 days. Called also *contour l's* and *Salter's l's*
**papillary l.**, linea mammillaris.
**pararectal l.**, linea pararectalis.
**parasternal l.**, linea parasternalis.
**paravertebral l.**, 1. linea paravertebralis. 2. linea vertebralis.
**Pastia's l's**, linear striations of hyperpigmentation produced by confluent petechiae in body creases, such as the antecubital fossae and inguinal regions, that occur at the onset of the rash of scarlet fever and persist after desquamation. Called also *Pastia's sign* and *Thomson's sign.*
**pectinate l.**, linea anocutanea.
**pectineal l.**, 1. linea pectinea. 2. pecten ossis pubis.
**period l's**, a series of light and dark lines occurring in a concentric, repeating pattern in mature myelin: the darker lines *(major dense l's)* represent the apposition of the inner, cytoplasmic surfaces of the Schwann cell plasma membrane; the lighter lines *(intraperiod l's)* bisect the spaces between the darker lines, and represent the apposition of the outer surfaces of the membrane.
**Pickerill's imbrication l's**, imbrication l's of Pickerill.
**pigmented l. of the cornea**, Hudson's l.
**Poirier's l.**, a line running from the nasofrontal angle to a point just above the lambda.
**popliteal l. of femur**, linea intercondylaris femoris.
**popliteal l. of tibia**, linea musculi solei.
**postaxillary l.**, linea axillaris posterior.
**Poupart's l.**, an imaginary line on the surface of the abdomen, passing perpendicularly through the midpoint of the inguinal ligament (Poupart's ligament).
**preaxillary l.**, linea axillaris anterior.
**precentral l.**, a line on the head, extending from a point midway between the inion and glabella downward and forward.
**primitive l.**, primitive streak.
**pupillary l.**, pupillary axis.
**quadrate l.**, a slight ridge sometimes seen passing vertically downward from the middle of the intertrochanteric crest on the posterior surface of the femur.
**radiocapitellar l.**, a line extending through the axis of the radial head and neck and normally intersecting the middle third of the capitellum in all radiographic views of the elbow.
**recessional l's**, lines or markings on the teeth due to the recession, in the formative period of the teeth, of the soft tissue which gives place to the dentin.
**regression l.**, a regression curve that is a straight line, indicating that two variables are in a simple direct or inverse arithmetic relationship. See also *regression* (def. 5).
**Reid's base l.**, base l. (def. 1).
**relaxed skin tension l's**, the natural skin lines and creases of the face and neck, which are the preferred lines of incision in facial and cervical surgery; called also *l's of expression* and *l's of minimal tension.*
**Retzius' l's**, incremental l's.
**Richter-Monro l.**, Monro-Richter l.
**Robson's l.**, an imaginary line drawn from the nipple to the umbilicus.
**Rolando's l.**, a line on the head marking the position of the central cerebral sulcus (fissure of Rolando) beneath.
**Roser's l.**, Nélaton's l.
**rough l.**, linea aspera.
**Salter's l's**, l's of Owen.
**Sampaolesis's wavy l.**, a pigmented line seen on the cornea in early stages of exfoliation syndrome.
**scapular l.**, linea scapularis.
**Schoemaker's l.**, one connecting the point of the trochanter with the anterior superior iliac spine; the extension of this line normally runs superior to the umbilicus, but runs inferior to it when the trochanter is higher than normal.
**l's of Schreger**, the dark and light lines visible under reflected light in a ground section of a tooth, which terminate at the dentinoenamel junctions, coinciding with the enamel prism curvatures. The dark bands are known as *diazones,* and the light ones as *parazones.* Called also *Hunter-Schreger bands, Schreger's bands* or *striae,* and *zones of Schreger.*
**segmental l's**, developmental grooves.
**semicircular l's, supreme**, linea nuchalis suprema.
**semicircular l. of Douglas**, linea arcuata vaginae musculi recti abdominis.
**semicircular l. of frontal bone**, linea temporalis ossis frontalis.
**semicircular l. of occipital bone, highest**, linea nuchalis suprema.
**semicircular l. of occipital bone, middle**, linea nuchalis superior.
**semicircular l. of occipital bone, superior**, linea nuchalis superior.
**semicircular l. of parietal bone, inferior**, linea temporalis inferior ossis parietalis.
**semicircular l. of parietal bone, superior**, linea temporalis superior ossis parietalis.
**semilunar l.**, linea semilunaris.
**Sergent's white adrenal l.**, a white line on the abdomen invoked by drawing the fingernail across it; seen in cases of adrenocortical insufficiency; called also *adrenal l.* and *white adrenal l.*
**Shenton's l.**, a curved line seen in the radiograph of the normal hip joint, formed by the top of the obturator foramen.
**l. of sight**, a straight line from the center of the pupil to the object viewed.
**simian l.**, see under *crease.*
**Skinner's l.**, Shenton's l.
**soleal l. of tibia**, linea musculi solei.
**Spieghel's l., spigelian l., Spigelius' l.**, linea semilunaris.
**spiral l. of femur**, linea intertrochanterica.
**Stähli's l., Stähli's pigment l.**, Hudson's l.
**sternal l., sternal l., lateral**, linea sternalis.
**subcostal l.**, a transverse line on the surface of the abdomen at the level of the inferior edge of the tenth costal cartilage.
**subscapular l's**, lineae musculares scapulae.
**superficial l. of the cornea**, Hudson's l.
**supracondylar l., lateral**, linea supracondylaris lateralis.
**supracondylar l., medial**, linea supracondylaris medialis.
**supracrestal l., supracristal l.**, planum supracristale.
**supraorbital l.**, a line across the forehead, just superior to the root of the external angular process of the frontal bone.
**survey l.**, 1. the line indicating the height of a tooth after the cast has been positioned according to the chosen path of insertion. 2. a line produced on a cast of a tooth by a surveyor scriber, marking the greatest height of contour in relation to the chosen path of insertion of the restoration. 3. a line drawn on a tooth or teeth by means of a surveyor for the purpose of determining the positions of the various parts of a clasp or clasps. Called also *clasp guideline.*
**suture l.**, 1. a line of juncture where parts of the body, internal or external, interface or converge. 2. système sécant.

## Line *Continued*

**Sydney l.**, a palmar crease correlated with an increased risk for leukemia and other malignancies in children; like the closely related simian crease, it appears in patients with Down syndrome.

**sylvian l.**, a line on the head extending from the external angular process of the frontal bone to a point three fourths of an inch inferior to the most prominent point of the parietal bone. It coincides with the direction of the lateral cerebral sulcus (fissure of Sylvius).

**temporal l., inferior,** linea temporalis inferior ossis parietalis.

**temporal l., superior,** linea temporalis superior ossis parietalis.

**temporal l. of frontal bone,** linea temporalis ossis frontalis.

**temporal l. of parietal bone, inferior,** linea temporalis inferior ossis parietalis.

**temporal l. of parietal bone, superior,** linea temporalis superior ossis parietalis.

**terminal l. of pelvis,** linea terminalis pelvis.

**Topinard's l.**, a line from the glabella to the pogonion.

**transverse l's of sacral bone, transverse l. of sacrum,** lineae transversae ossis sacri.

**trapezoid l.**, linea trapezoidea.

**Trümmerfeld l.**, a zone of metaphyseal degeneration sometimes seen in the bones in infantile scurvy.

**Ullmann's l.**, in cases of spondylolisthesis, a line extended upward at a right angle from the anterior edge of the first sacral vertebra to the superior surface of the sacrum will pass through the last lumbar vertebra.

**umbilicoiliac l.**, a line from the umbilicus to the anterior superior iliac spine.

**vertebral l.**, linea vertebralis.

**vibrating l.**, an imaginary line across the palate that separates its immovable portion, the hard palate, from its movable portion, the soft palate.

**Virchow's l.**, a line from the nasion to the lambda.

**visual l.**, see under axis.

**Voigt's l.**, a dorsoventral pigmented line of demarcation on the skin, usually bilateral, along the lateral edge of the biceps muscle; seen in over 20 per cent of black-skinned people but only occasionally in others. Called also *Futcher's l.*

**Wagner's l.**, a thin whitish line at the junction of the epiphysis and diaphysis of a bone, formed by preliminary calcification.

**white l.**, linea alba.

**white adrenal l.**, Sergent's white adrenal l.

**white l. of ischiococcygeal muscle,** corpus anococcygeum.

**white l. of pelvic fascia,** arcus tendineus fasciae pelvis.

**white l. of pelvis,** arcus tendineus musculi levatoris ani.

**white l. of pharynx,** raphe pharyngis.

**Z l.**, Z band.

**l's of Zahn,** laminations visible in antemortem blood clots, caused by alternating layers of gray-white fibrin interspersed with narrow zones of apparent red-blue clot.

**Zöllner's l's.**, an optical illusion in which long parallel lines seem to converge or diverge owing to their being crossed by a series of short lines parallel to one another but oblique to the long lines and at reverse oblique angles to both adjacent series of intersecting lines, as in a herringbone pattern.

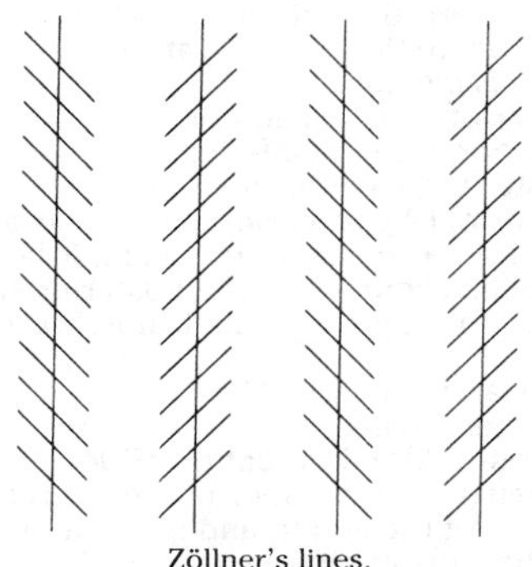

Zöllner's lines.

**li•nea** (lin'e-ə) gen. and pl. *li'neae* [L.] 1. a stripe, streak, mark, or narrow ridge. 2. [TA] a general term for a streak or narrow ridge on the surface of some structure. Called also *line.*

## Linea

Descriptions are given on TA terms, and include anglicized names of specific lines.

**l. al'ba** [TA], **l. al'ba abdo'minis**, white line: the tendinous median line on the anterior abdominal wall between the two rectus muscles, formed by the decussating fibers of the aponeuroses of the three flat abdominal muscles.

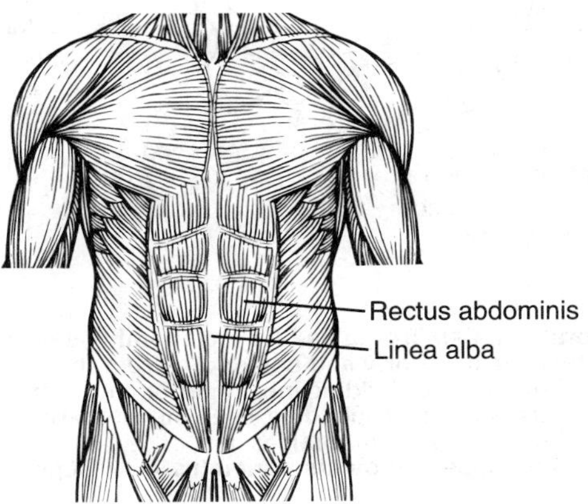


**l. al'ba cervica'lis,** the blending of the fascial sheaths of the sternothyroid and sternohyoid muscles in the median plane of the neck.

**li'neae albican'tes,** see *striae atrophicae.*

**l. anocuta'nea** [TA], anocutaneous line: the sinuous line following the level of the anal valves and crossing the bases between them, marking the junction of the zone of the anal canal lined with stratified squamous epithelium and that lined with columnar epithelium; called also *dentate line* or *margin* and *pectinate line.*

**l. anorecta'lis,** junctio anorectalis.

**l. arcua'ta os'sis i'lii** [TA], arcuate line of ilium: the iliac portion of the terminal line, limiting the ala of the ilium inferiorly on its medial surface.

**l. arcua'ta vagi'nae mus'culi rec'ti abdo'minis** [TA], arcuate line of sheath of rectus abdominis muscle: a crescentic line marking the termination of the posterior layer of the sheath of the rectus abdominis muscle, just inferior to the level of the iliac crest; called also *l. semicircularis* [*Douglasi*] and *semicircular line of Douglas.*

**l. as'pera** [TA], rough line: the broad, thickened ridge that forms the posterior border of the femur and has distinct lateral and medial lips.

**li'neae atro'phicae,** striae atrophicae.

**l. axilla'ris,** axillary line: an imaginary vertical line passing through the middle of the axilla, dividing the body into an anterior and a posterior portion.

**l. axilla'ris ante'rior** [TA], anterior axillary line: an imaginary vertical line continuing the line of the anterior axillary fold with the upper limb in the anatomical position; called also *l. preaxillaris* and *preaxillary line.*

**l. axilla'ris me'dia** [TA], middle axillary line: an imaginary line halfway between the anterior axillary line and the posterior axillary line, passing through the apex of the axilla; called also *l. medio-axillaris* and *midaxillary line.*

**l. axilla'ris poste'rior** [TA], posterior axillary line: an imaginary vertical line continuing the line of the posterior axillary fold with the upper limb in the anatomical position; called also *l. postaxillaris* and *postaxillary line.*

**l. epiphysia'lis** [TA], epiphyseal line: a plane or plate on a long bone, visible as a line, marking the junction of the epiphysis and diaphysis.

**l. glu'tea ante'rior** [TA], anterior gluteal line: the middle of three rough curved lines on the gluteal surface of the ala of the ilium; it begins from the iliac crest about an inch posterior to the anterior superior iliac spine and arches more or less posteriorly to the greater sciatic notch. Called also *l. gluteali s anterior.*

**l. glu'tea infe'rior** [TA], inferior gluteal line: a rough curved line, often indistinct, on the gluteal surface of the ala of the ilium; it runs from the notch between the anterior superior and anterior inferior iliac spines posteriorly to the anterior part of the greater sciatic notch. Called also *l. gluteali s inferior.*

**l. glutea'lis ante'rior,** l. glutea anterior.

**l. glutea'lis infe'rior,** l. glutea inferior.

**l. glutea'lis poste'rior,** l. glutea posterior.

**l. glu'tea poste'rior** [TA], posterior gluteal line: a rough curved line on the gluteal surface of the ala of the ilium; it begins from the iliac crest about two inches anterior to the posterior superior iliac spine and runs downward to the greater sciatic notch. Called also *l. glutealis posterior.*

**l. iliopecti'nea,** l. arcuata ossis ilii.

**l. innomina'ta,** l. terminalis pelvis.

**l. intercondyla'ris** [TA], **l. intercondyloi'dea,** intercondylar line: a transverse ridge separating the floor of the intercondylar fossa from the popliteal surface of the femur, and giving attachment to the posterior portion of the capsular ligament of the knee.

**l. interme'dia cris'tae ili'acae** [TA], intermediate line of iliac crest: the area between the inner and outer lips of the iliac crest.

**l. intertrochante'rica** [TA], intertrochanteric line: a line running obliquely downward and medially from the tubercle of the femur, winding around the medial side of the body of the bone.

**l. intertrochante'rica poste'rior,** crista intertrochanterica.

**l. mammilla'ris** [TA], mammillary line: an imaginary vertical line on the anterior surface of the body, passing through the center of the nipple.

**l. media'na ante'rior** [TA], anterior median line: an imaginary vertical line on the anterior surface of the body, dividing the surface equally into right and left sides.

**l. media'na poste'rior** [TA], posterior median line: an imaginary vertical line on the posterior surface of the body, dividing the surface equally into right and left sides.

**l. medio-axilla'ris,** l. axillaris media.

**l. medioclavicula'ris** [TA], midclavicular line: an imaginary vertical line on the anterior surface of the body, passing through the midpoint of the clavicle; called also *midclavicular plane.*

**li'neae muscula'res sca'pulae,** muscular lines of scapula: low ridges on the costal surface of the scapula, marking the site of attachment of muscle fibers.

**l. mus'culi so'lei** [TA], soleal line of tibia: a line extending from the fibular facet downward and inward across the posterior surface of the tibia, giving attachment to fibers of the soleus muscle; called also *l. poplitea tibiae* and *popliteal line of tibia.*

**l. mylohyoi'dea mandi'bulae** [TA], mylohyoid line of mandible: a ridge on the inner surface of the mandible from the base of the symphysis to the ascending ramus behind the last molar tooth; it affords attachment to the mylohyoid muscle and superior constrictor of the pharynx.

**l. ni'gra,** a name given the tendinous mesial line of the abdomen (l. alba) when it has become pigmented in pregnancy.

**l. nu'chae infe'rior,** linea nuchalis inferior.

**l. nu'chae supe'rior,** linea nuchalis superior.

**l. nu'chae supre'ma,** linea nuchalis suprema.

**l. nucha'lis infe'rior** [TA], inferior nuchal line: the most inferior of the three nuchal lines found on the outer surface of the occipital bone, extending laterally from the middle of the external occipital crest to the jugular process.

**l. nucha'lis supe'rior** [TA], superior nuchal line: a curved line on the outer surface of the occipital bone, extending from the external occipital protuberance toward the lateral angle, and giving attachment medially to the trapezius muscle and laterally to the sternocleidomastoid muscle.

**l. nucha'lis supre'ma** [TA], highest nuchal line: a sometimes indistinct line arching superiorly from the external occipital protuberance and running toward the lateral angle of the occipital bone: the epicranial aponeurosis attaches to it.

**l. obli'qua cartila'ginis thyroi'deae** [TA], oblique line of thyroid cartilage: a line on the external surface of the lamina of the thyroid cartilage, extending between the two thyroid tubercles.

**l. obli'qua fi'bulae,** crista medialis fibulae.

**l. obli'qua mandi'bulae** [TA], oblique line of mandible: a ridge on the external surface of the body of the mandible extending from the mental tubercle to the anterior border of the ascending ramus on either side.

**l. obli'qua ti'biae,** l. musculi solei.

**l. pararecta'lis,** pararectal line: an imaginary line corresponding to the lateral margin of the rectus abdominis muscle.

**l. parasterna'lis** [TA], parasternal line: an imaginary line on the anterior surface of the body midway between the mammillary line and the border of the sternum.

**l. paravertebra'lis** [TA], 1. paravertebral line; an imaginary line corresponding to the transverse vertebral processes. 2. l. vertebralis.

**l. pecti'nea** [TA], pectineal line: a line running down the posterior surface of the shaft of the femur, giving attachment to the pectineus muscle.

**l. popli'tea ti'biae,** l. musculi solei.

**l. postaxilla'ris,** l. axillaris posterior.

**l. preaxilla'ris,** l. axillaris anterior.

**l. scapula'ris** [TA], scapular line: an imaginary vertical line on the posterior surface of the body, passing through the inferior angle of the scapula when it is in the anatomical position, i.e., at rest.

**l. semicircula'ris [Doug'lasi],** l. arcuata vaginae musculi recti abdominis.

**l. semiluna'ris** [TA], **l. semiluna'ris [Spige'li],** semilunar line: a curved line along the lateral border of each rectus abdominis muscle, corresponding to the meeting of the aponeuroses of the internal oblique and transverse abdominal muscles; called also *Spieghel's line* and *Spigelius' line.*

**l. spira'lis,** l. intertrochanterica.

**l. splen'dens,** the sheath for the anterior spinal artery formed by the pia mater in the fissura mediana anterior medullae spinalis.

**l. sterna'lis** [TA], sternal line: an imaginary vertical line on the anterior surface of the body, corresponding to the lateral border of the sternum.

**l. supracondyla'ris latera'lis** [TA], lateral supracondylar line: a slight ridge on the lower third of the posterior surface of the femur that is continuous above with the lateral lip of the linea aspera and descends to the lateral epicondyle.

**l. supracondyla'ris media'lis** [TA], medial supracondylar line: an indistinct ridge on the lower third of the posterior surface of the femur that is continuous above with the medial lip of the linea aspera, being interrupted at its upper end to allow passage of the femoral artery, and descends to the adductor tubercle.

**l. tempora'lis infe'rior os'sis parieta'lis** [TA], inferior temporal line of parietal bone: a curved line on the external surface of the parietal bone, marking the limit of attachment of the temporal muscle.

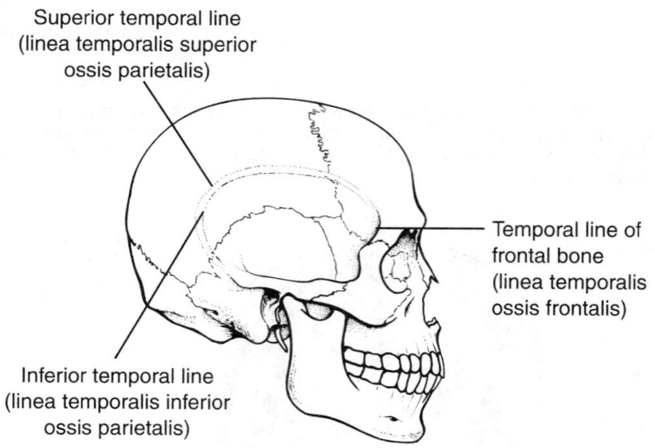

Superior temporal line (linea temporalis superior ossis parietalis)

Temporal line of frontal bone (linea temporalis ossis frontalis)

Inferior temporal line (linea temporalis inferior ossis parietalis)

**l. tempora'lis os'sis fronta'lis** [TA], temporal line of frontal bone: a ridge extending superiorly and posteriorly from the zygomatic process of the frontal bone, dividing into superior and inferior parts that are continuous with corresponding lines on the parietal bone, and giving attachment to the temporal fascia.

**l. tempora'lis supe'rior os'sis parieta'lis** [TA], superior temporal line of parietal bone: a curved line on the external surface of the parietal bone, superior and parallel to the inferior temporal line, giving attachment to the temporal fascia.

**l. termina'lis pel'vis** [TA], terminal line of pelvis: a line on the inner surface of either pelvic bone, extending from the sacroiliac joint to the iliopubic eminence anteriorly, and marking the plane separating the false from the true pelvis.

**li'neae transver'sae os'sis sa'cri** [TA], transverse lines of sacrum: four transverse ridges on the pelvic surface of the sacrum, running between the pairs of pelvic sacral foramina, marking the positions of the former intervertebral disks.

**l. trapezoi'dea** [TA], trapezoid line: a ridge extending anterolaterally from the conoid tubercle on the inferior surface of the clavicle, giving attachment to the trapezoid portion of the coracoclavicular ligament.

**l. vertebra'lis,** vertebral line: an imaginary vertical line halfway between the scapular and posterior median lines; called also *l. paravertebralis* and *paravertebral line.*

**lin·eae** (lin'e-e) [L.] genitive and plural of *linea.*

**lin·e·age** (lin'e-əj) [L. *linea* line] descent traced down from or back to a common ancestor.

**cell l.,** the developmental history of cells as traced from the first division of the original cell or cells.

**lin·e·ar** (lin'e-ər) [L. *linearis*] pertaining to or resembling a line.

**Lin·e·o·la** (lin″e-o'lə) formerly, a genus of spore-forming bacteria now classified in the genus *Bacillus.*

**lin·er** (līn'ər) material applied to the inside of the walls of a cavity or container, for protection or insulation of the surface.

**cavity l.,** an agent used to line a tooth cavity for protection of the pulp from irritation and for neutralization of the free acids of zinc phosphate or silicate cements.

**Line·weav·er-Burk equation, plot** (līn'wēv-ər-bərk) [Hans *Lineweaver,* American chemist, born 1907; Dean *Burk,* American biochemist, 1904–1988] see under *equation.*

**lin·gua** (ling'gwə) gen. and pl. *lin'guae* [L.] [TA] the tongue: the movable, muscular organ on the floor of the mouth, subserving the special sense of taste and aiding in mastication, deglutition, and the articulation of sound; called also *glossa.* See *tongue.*

**l. frena'ta,** ankyloglossia.

**l. geogra'phica,** benign migratory glossitis.

**l. ni'gra,** black tongue.

**l. plica'ta,** fissured tongue.

**l. villo'sa ni'gra,** black tongue.

**lin·guae** (ling'gwe) [L.] genitive and plural of *lingua.*

**lin·gual** (ling'gwəl) [L. *lingualis*] pertaining to or toward the tongue; glossal. In dental anatomy, used to refer to the tooth surface directed toward the tongue (oral cavity); see *facies lingualis dentis.*

**lin·gua·le** (ling-gwa'le) the point at the upper end of the symphysis of the lower jaw on its lingual surface.

**lin·gua·lis** (ling-gwa'lis) [L., from *lingua*] relating to the tongue.

**lin·gual·ly** (ling'gwə-le) toward the tongue.

**Lin·guat·u·la** (ling-gwat'u-lə) a genus of tongue worms, arthropods of the family Linguatulidae whose adult form inhabits the frontal, nasal, and maxillary sinuses of animals, sometimes including humans, and whose larval form (known as *Pentastoma* and *Porocephalus*) infests the digestive organs and lungs. See *halzoun.*

**L. rhina'ria,** *L. serrata.*

**L. serra'ta,** a species whose adult forms are found in the frontal sinuses and nasal passages of canines and felines. Eggs, passed in the nasal discharges of infected animals, may be ingested by cattle, sheep, rabbits, or occasionally humans, and on hatching, bore through the intestinal wall and finally become encysted in the viscera.

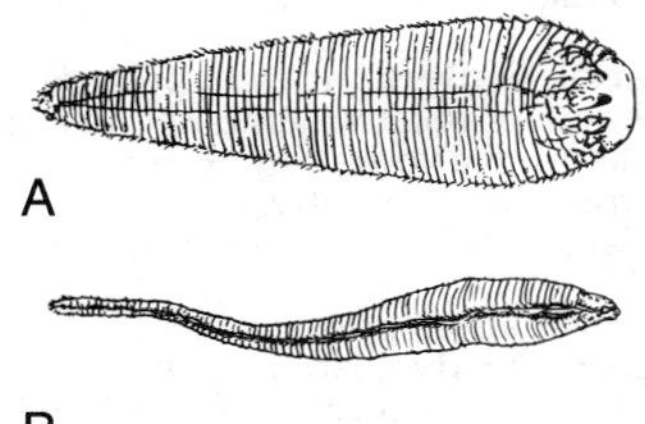


*Linguatula serrata. (A),* nymph (enlarged); *(B),* adult.

**lin·guat·u·li·a·sis** (ling-gwat″u-li'ə-sis) invasion of the body by *Linguatula.*

**lin·guat·u·lid** (ling-gwat'u-lid) any member of the family Linguatulidae.

**Lin·gua·tu·li·dae** (ling-gwə-tu'lĭ-de) a family of endoparasitic wormlike arthropods of the order Porocephalida that have flattened bodies. Adults are usually found in the nasal passages of felines and canines, and the larvae are found in the viscera of a variety of mammals, including humans. It includes the genus *Linguatula.*

**lin·guat·u·lo·sis** (ling-gwat″u-lo'sis) linguatuliasis.

**lin·gui·form** (ling'gwĭ-form) tongue-shaped.

**lin·gu·la** (ling'gu-lə) gen. and pl. *lin'gulae* [L., dim. of *lingua*] [TA] a general term for a small tonguelike structure.

**l. cerebel'li** [TA], lingula of cerebellum: the most ventral part of the anterior lobe of the cerebellum, where the superior medullary velum attaches.

**l. of left lung,** l. pulmonis sinistri.

**l. of lower jaw,** l. mandibulae.

**l. mandi'bulae** [TA], lingula of mandible: the sharp medial boundary of the mandibular foramen, to which is attached the sphenomandibular ligament.

**l. pulmo'nis sinis'tri** [TA], lingula of left lung: a projection from the lower portion of the upper lobe of the left lung, just beneath the cardiac notch, between the cardiac impression and the inferior margin. See also *culmen pulmonis sinistri.*

**l. of sphenoid, l. sphenoida'lis** [TA], sphenoidal lingula: a slender ridge of bone on the lateral margin of the carotid sulcus, projecting posteriorly between the body and greater wing of the sphenoid bone.

**lin·gu·lae** (ling'gu-le) [L.] genitive and plural of *lingula.*

**lin·gu·lar** (ling'gu-lər) pertaining to a lingula.

**lin·gu·lec·to·my** (ling″gu-lek'tə-me) excision of the lingula of the upper lobe of the left lung.

**lingu(o)-** [L. *lingua* tongue] a combining form denoting relationship to the tongue.

**lin·guo·ax·i·al** (ling″gwo-ak'se-əl) pertaining to or formed by the lingual and axial walls of a tooth cavity.

**lin·guo·ax·io·gin·gi·val** (ling″gwo-ak″se-o-jin'jĭ-vəl) pertaining to or formed by the lingual, axial, and gingival walls of a tooth cavity preparation.

**lin·guo·cer·vi·cal** (ling″gwo-sər'vĭ-kəl) 1. pertaining to the lingual surface of the neck of a tooth. 2. linguogingival.

**lin·guo·cli·na·tion** (ling″gwo-klĭ-na'shən) lingual inclination.

**lin·guo·clu·sion** (ling″gwo-kloo'zhən) lingual occlusion.

**lin·guo·den·tal** (ling″gwo-den'təl) 1. pertaining to the tongue and teeth. 2. dental, def. 2.

**lin·guo·dis·tal** (ling″gwo-dis'təl) pertaining to or formed by the lingual and distal surfaces of a tooth, or the lingual and distal walls of a tooth cavity.

**lin·guo·gin·gi·val** (ling″gwo-jin'ji-vəl) pertaining to the tongue and gingiva; pertaining to or formed by the lingual and gingival walls of a tooth cavity.

**lin·guo·in·ci·sal** (ling″gwo-in-si'zəl) pertaining to or formed by the lingual and incisal surfaces of a tooth.

**lin·guo·me·si·al** (ling″gwo-me'ze-əl) pertaining to or formed by the lingual and mesial surfaces of a tooth, or the lingual and mesial walls of a tooth cavity.

**lin·guo·oc·clu·sal** (ling″gwo-o-kloo'zəl) pertaining to or formed by the lingual and occlusal surfaces of a tooth.

**lin·guo·pap·il·li·tis** (ling″gwo-pap″ĭ-li'tis) [*linguo-* + *papillitis*] inflammation or ulceration of the papillae of the edges of the tongue.

**lin·guo·place·ment** (ling″gwo-plās'mənt) lingual placement.

**lin·guo·pul·pal** (ling″gwo-pul'pəl) pertaining to or formed by the lingual and pulpal walls of a tooth cavity.

**lin·guo·ver·sion** (ling″gwo-vər′zhən) displacement of a tooth lingually from the line of occlusion.

**lin·i·ment** (lin′ĭ-mənt) [L. *linimentum; linere* to smear] an oily liquid preparation to be used on the skin.
**camphor l.,** a preparation of camphor and cottonseed oil used as a local irritant to the skin.
**medicinal soft soap l.,** green soap tincture.

**lin·i·men·tum** (lin″ĭ-men′təm) [L.] liniment.
**l. cam′phorae,** camphor liniment.
**l. sapo′nis mol′lis,** green soap tincture.

**li·nin** (li′nin) [L. *linum* thread] the faintly staining substance composing the fine, netlike threads found in the nucleus of a cell, where it bears the chromatin in the form of granules. Cf. *achromatin.*

**li·ni·tis** (lĭ-ni′tis) [Gr. *linon* thread + *-itis*] inflammation of the gastric cellular tissue.
**l. plas′tica,** diffuse fibrous proliferation of the submucous connective tissue of the stomach, resulting in thickening and fibrosis so that the organ is constricted, inelastic, and rigid (like a leather bottle). It is almost always a manifestation of gastric adenocarcinoma but is occasionally seen in certain benign conditions. Called also *Brinton's disease, gastric sclerosis, cirrhotic gastritis,* and *leather bottle stomach.*

**link·age** (lingk′əj) 1. the connection between different atoms in a chemical compound, or the symbol representing it in structural formulas; see also *bond.* 2. in genetics, the association of genes having loci on the same chromosome, which results in the tendency of a group of such nonallelic genes to be associated in inheritance.

**linked** (linkt) in genetics, pertaining to linkage (def. 2); see also *X-linked,* under *gene.*

**link·er** (link′ər) any small fragment of DNA that contains one or more restriction sites and is used to splice together unrelated nucleic acid sequences in the production of recombinant DNA molecules. Called also *DNA linker.*

**lin·nae·an** (lĭ-ne′ən) [Carolus *Linnaeus* latinized form of Carl von Linné, Swedish botanist, 1707–1778] pertaining to Linnaeus or to the system of taxonomic classification of living organisms, which was originated by Linnaeus. Written also *linnean.*

**lin·ne·an** (lĭ-ne′ən) linnaean.

**Lin·o·dil** (lin′o-dil) trademark for a preparation of inositol niacinate.

**Lin·og·na·thus** (lin-og′nə-thəs) a genus of sucking lice (order Anoplura). *L. peda′lis,* the foot louse, and *L. ovil′lus* infest sheep; *L. seto′sus* infests dogs and foxes; *L. stenop′sis,* the goat sucking louse, infests goats; *L. africa′nus* infests either sheep or goats; and *L. vitu′li,* the long-nosed cattle louse, infests cattle.

**li·no·le·ate** (lĭ-no′le-āt) a salt (soap), ester, or anionic form of linoleic acid.
**ethyl l.,** a lipid occurring on the skin of warm-blooded animals and responsible for its passive water-holding capacity.

**lin·o·le·ic ac·id** (lin″o-le′ik) a polyunsaturated 18-carbon fatty acid occurring as a major constituent in many vegetable oils. It is an essential fatty acid used in the biosynthesis of prostaglandins and cell membranes. See also table at *fatty acid.*

**lin·o·le·in** (lin-o′lēn) [*linum* + *oleum*] a neutral fat from linseed oil; the triglyceride of linoleic acid.

**li·no·le·nate** (lĭ-no′lə-nāt) a salt, ester, or anionic form of linolenic acid.

**lin·o·len·ic ac·id** (lin″o-len′ik) a polyunsaturated 18-carbon fatty acid occurring in some fish oils (herring, menhaden) and many seed-derived oils. It is an essential fatty acid that cannot be synthesized by animal tissues and must be obtained in the diet. It is used in the formation of prostaglandins.

**lin·o·lic acid** (lin-o′lik) linoleic acid.

**lin·seed** (lin′sēd) the dried ripe seed of *Linum usitatissimum,* used as a topical demulcent and emollient and as a source of linseed oil; it contains the cyanogen linamarin, and animals eating large quantities of it may get cyanide poisoning. Called also *flaxseed* and *linum.*

**Lin·sto·wi·i·dae** (lin-sto-wi′ĭ-de) a family of medium-sized or small tapeworms of the order Cyclophyllidea, subclass Cestoda, which parasitize birds, reptiles, and mammals, including humans; medically important genera are *Oochoristica* and *Inermicapsifer.*

**lint** (lint) [L. *linteum,* from *linum,* flax] an absorbent surgical dressing material once made by scraping or picking apart old woven linen, but now a specially finished fabric woven in sheets; called also *patent l.* or *sheet l.*

**lin·tin** (lin′tin) a loose fabric of prepared absorbent cotton used in dressing wounds.

**Lin·ton shunt** (lin′ton) [Robert Ritchie *Linton,* Scottish-born American surgeon, born 1900] see under *shunt.*

**Li·num** (li′num) a genus of flowering plants of the family Linaceae. *L. usitatis′simum* L. is the common flax plant, the source of linseed and linseed oil; it also contains the cyanogenetic compound linamarin, which can cause fatal cyanide poisoning in livestock.

**li·num** (li′nəm) gen. *li′ni* [L. "flax"] linseed.

**lio-** for words beginning thus, see also those beginning *leio-.*

**Li·or·e·sal** (li-or′ə-sal) trademark for a preparation of baclofen.

**li·o·thy·ro·nine** (li″o-thi′ro-nēn) the synthetic levo isomer of triiodothyronine; it is more potent and has a more rapid action than thyroxine.
**l. I 125,** liothyronine iodinated with $^{125}$I; used for the in vitro determination of thyroid function.
**l. sodium** [USP], the monosodium salt of liothyronine, used for thyroid replacement or supplementation in hypothyroidism and simple (nontoxic) goiter, administered orally.

**li·o·trix** (li′o-triks) a mixture of liothyronine sodium and levothyroxine sodium in a ratio of 1:4 in terms of weight; used for replacement therapy in conditions in which there is deficient production of thyroid hormones, administered orally.

**lip** (lip) [MeSH: Lip] 1. either the upper or lower fleshy margin of the mouth, together called *labia oris* [TA]. 2. a marginal part; called also *labium.*
**acetabular l.,** labrum acetabulare.
**anterior l. of cervix of uterus,** labium anterius ostii uteri.
**anterior l. of ostium of uterus,** labium anterius ostii uteri.
**articular l.,** labrum articularis.
**cleft l.,** a congenital cleft or defect in the upper lip, usually due to complete or partial failure of migration and deposit of mesoderm around or over the head in the embryo, with consequent failure of the maxillary prominence to merge with the merged medial nasal prominences. It may be unilateral, bilateral, or median (the true harelip), and may be accompanied by maxillary and palatal defects. Called also *cheiloschisis, harelip,* and *stomatoschisis.*

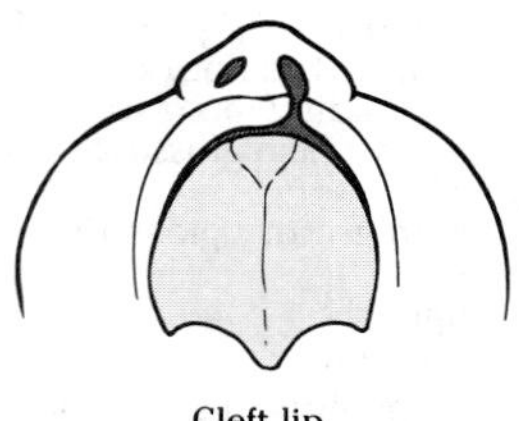

Cleft lip.

**double l.,** redundancy of the submucous tissue and mucous membrane of the lip on either side of the median line.
**external l. of iliac crest,** labium externum cristae iliacae.
**external l. of linea aspera of femur,** labium laterale lineae asperae femoris.
**fibrocartilaginous l. of acetabulum,** labrum acetabulare.
**glenoid l.,** labrum glenoidale.
**glenoid l. of articulation of hip,** labrum acetabulare.
**glenoid l. of articulation of humerus,** labrum glenoidale.
**greater l. of pudendum,** labium majus pudendi.
**Hapsburg l.,** a thick overdeveloped lower lip that often accompanies a Hapsburg jaw.
**inferior l.,** labium inferius oris.
**inferior l. of ileocecal valve,** labium inferius valvulae coli.
**internal l. of iliac crest,** labium internum cristae iliacae.
**lateral l. of linea aspera of femur,** labium laterale lineae asperae femoris.
**lesser l. of pudendum,** labium minus pudendi.
**lower l.,** labium inferius oris.
**medial l. of linea aspera of femur,** labium mediale lineae asperae femoris.
**posterior l. of cervix of uterus,** labium posterius ostii uteri.
**posterior l. of ostium of uterus,** labium posterius ostii uteri.
**posterior l. of pharyngeal opening of auditory tube,** labium posterius ostii pharyngei tubae auditivae.
**rhombic l.,** the lateral boundary of the rhombencephalon during embryonic life.
**superior l.,** labium superius oris.
**superior l. of ileocecal valve,** labium superius valvulae coli.
**tympanic l. of limbus,** labium tympanicum limbi.
**upper l.,** labium superius oris.
**vestibular l. of limbus,** labium vestibulare limbi.

**lip·ac·i·de·mia** (lip″as-ĭ-de′me-ə) [*lip-* + *acid* + *-emia*] the presence of excess of fatty acids in the blood, as in diabetes mellitus.

**lip·ac·i·du·ria** (lip″as-ĭ-du′re-ə) [*lip-* + *acid* + *-uria*] the presence of fatty acids in the urine.

**lip·aro·cele** (lip-ar′o-sēl) [Gr. *liparos* oily + *kēlē* tumor] adipocele.

**lip·a·ro·dysp·nea** (lip″ə-ro-disp′ne-ə) the dyspnea of the obese.

**lip·ase** (lip′ās, li′pās) [MeSH: Lipase] 1. triacylglycerol lipase. 2. any enzyme that hydrolytically cleaves a fatty acid anion from a triglyceride or phospholipid.
**acid l.**, see *acid lipase,* under *A.*
**hepatic l.**, a lipase acting at the endothelial surfaces of hepatic tissues (cf. *lipoprotein lipase*) to regulate the levels of plasma lipids. It participates in lipolysis of very-low-density and intermediate-density lipoproteins in the end stages of low-density lipoprotein formation and also in hydrolysis of phospholipids and triglycerides in the metabolism of high-density lipoproteins.
**lingual l.**, a lipase secreted in the mouth and most active in the stomach; it degrades medium- to short-chain triglycerides and appears to prepare ingested lipids for intestinal digestion by facilitating their solubilization.
**pancreatic l.**, the triacylglycerol lipase secreted by the pancreas; it is the major intestinal lipase, digesting ingested fats to fatty acids and monoglycerides. The enzyme requires bile salts and colipase for activity.

**lip·as·uria** (lip″ās-u′re-ə) the presence of lipase in the urine.

**li·pec·to·my** (lĭ-pek′tə-me) [*lip-* + *-ectomy*] [MeSH: Lipectomy] the excision of a mass of subcutaneous adipose tissue, as from the abdominal wall; called also *adipectomy.*
**suction l.**, liposuction.

**lip·ede·ma** (lip″ə-de′mə) [*lip-* + *edema*] an accumulation of excess fat and fluid in subcutaneous tissues.

**lip·emia** (lĭ-pe′me-ə) hyperlipidemia.
**alimentary l.**, hyperlipidemia after eating, such as carbohydrate-induced, familial fat-induced, and combined fat- and carbohydrate-induced hyperlipemia.
**diabetic l.**, a rare complication of uncontrolled diabetes mellitus consisting of massive increases in plasma triglyceride levels after ingestion of lipid-rich foods, due to deficient metabolism of low-density lipoproteins.
**l. retina′lis**, a milky appearance of the veins and arteries of the retina, occurring when the lipids of the blood exceed 5%, as in diabetes mellitus and leukemia.

**lip·emic** (lĭ-pe′mik) hyperlipidemic.

**lip·id** (lip′id) any of a heterogeneous group of fats and fatlike substances characterized by being water-insoluble and being extractable by nonpolar (or fat) solvents such as alcohol, ether, chloroform, benzene, etc. All contain as a major constituent aliphatic hydrocarbons. The lipids, which are easily stored in the body, serve as a source of fuel, are an important constituent of cell structure, and serve other biological functions. Lipids may be considered to include fatty acids, neutral fats, waxes, and steroids. *Compound lipids* comprise the glycolipids, lipoproteins, and phospholipids.
**l. A**, the glycolipid component of lipopolysaccharide (q.v.) that is responsible for its endotoxic activity.

**lip·i·de·mia** (lip″ĭ-de′me-ə) hyperlipidemia.

**lip·id·ic** (lip-id′ik) pertaining to or containing lipids.

**lip·i·dol·y·sis** (lip″ĭ-dol′ĭ-sis) the splitting of lipids.

**lip·i·do·lyt·ic** (lip″ĭ-do-lit′ik) pertaining to, characterized by, or causing lipidolysis.

**lip·i·do·sis** (lip″ĭ-do′sis) pl. *lipido′ses.* A term for several of the lysosomal storage diseases in which there is an abnormal accumulation of lipids in the reticuloendothelial cells. Called also *lipid storage disease.*
**galactosylceramide l.**, Krabbe's disease.
**glucosylceramide l.**, Gaucher's disease.
**sphingomyelin l.**, Niemann-Pick disease.
**sulfatide l.**, metachromatic leukodystrophy.

**lip·i·du·ria** (lip″ĭ-du′re-ə) the presence of lipids in the urine.

**Lip·io·dol** (lip-i′o-dol) trademark for iodized oil used as a contrast medium.

**Lip·i·tor** (lip′ĭ-tor) trademark for a preparation of atorvastatin calcium.

**Lip·mann** (lip′mən) Fritz Albert. German-born American biochemist, 1899–1986; co-winner, with Hans Adolph Krebs, of the Nobel prize for medicine or physiology for 1953 for his discovery of coenzyme A and its importance in intermediary metabolism.

**lip(o)-** [Gr. *lipos* fat] a combining form denoting relationship to fat or to lipids.

**lipo·ad·e·no·ma** (lip″o-ad″ə-no′mə) a fatty parenchymal cell tumor, especially the parathyroid.

**lipo·am·ide** (lip″o-am′īd) lipoic acid in amide linkage with lysine side chains of enzymes of the α-ketoglutarate dehydrogenase, branched-chain α-keto acid dehydrogenase, and pyruvate dehydrogenase complexes (q.v.). Its reactive disulfide group and long, flexible chain enable it to transfer intermediates among the enzymes of each complex.

**lipo·am·ide de·hy·dro·gen·ase** (lip″o-am′īd de-hi′dro-jən″ās) [MeSH: Lipoamide Dehydrogenase] erroneous name for *dihydrolipoamide dehydrogenase.*

**lipo·am·ide de·hy·dro·gen·ase de·fi·cien·cy** an autosomal recessive aminoacidopathy in which deficiency of dihydrolipoamide dehydrogenase activity causes combined deficiency of the branched-chain α-keto acid dehydrogenase complex, α-ketoglutarate dehydrogenase complex, and pyruvate dehydrogenase complex; it is characterized by neonatal onset, accumulation and excretion of lactic, pyruvic, α-ketoglutaric, and branched-chain keto acids, hypotonia with progressive nervous system impairment, and death in early childhood.

**lipo·ar·thri·tis** (lip″o-ahr-thri′tis) [*lipo-* + *arthritis*] inflammation of the fatty tissue of a joint.

**lipo·at·ro·phy** (lip″o-at′ro-fe) [*lipo-* + *atrophy*] 1. atrophy of subcutaneous fat. 2. lipodystrophy.
**insulin l.**, localized lipoatrophy occurring at the site of repeated insulin injections.

**lipo·blast** (lip′o-blast) [*lipo-* + *-blast*] a specialized connective tissue cell which develops into a fat cell.

**lipo·blas·tic** (lip″o-blas′tik) pertaining to or containing lipoblasts.

**lipo·blas·to·ma** (lip″o-blas-to′mə) [*lipo-* + *blastoma*] a benign fatty tumor composed of a mixture of embryonal lipoblastic cells in a myxoid stroma and mature fat cells; the tumor cells are arranged in lobules and occur most often in children.

**lipo·blas·to·ma·to·sis** (lip″o-blas-to″mə-to′sis) the occurrence of multiple lipoblastomas locally diffused but without a tendency to metastasize.

**lipo·car·di·ac** (lip″o-kahr′de-ak) [*lipo-* + *cardiac*] relating to a fatty heart.

**lipo·cata·bol·ic** (lip″o-cat″ə-bol′ik) pertaining to or effecting the destructive metabolism of fat.

**lipo·cele** (lip′o-sēl) adipocele.

**lipo·cer·a·tous** (lip″o-ser′ə-təs) adipoceratous.

**lipo·cere** (lip′o-sēr) [*lipo-* + *cera*] adipocere.

**lipo·chon·dro·ma** (lip″o-kon-dro′mə) [*lipo-* + *chondroma*] chondrolipoma.

**lipo·chrome** (lip′o-krōm) [*lipo-* + *-chrome*] any of a group of fat-soluble pigments, including carotene, lutein, lycopene, and xanthophyll, that are synthesized in plants and on ingestion impart a yellow, yellow-orange, or orange-red color to lipid-containing tissues. Called also *carotenoid, chromolipoid, lipochrome pigment, lipofuscin,* and *wear and tear pigment.*

**lipo·chro·me·mia** (lip″o-kro-me′me-ə) the presence of an excess of lipochrome in the blood.

**lip·o·chro·mo·gen** (lip″o-kro′mə-jən) a substance that becomes converted into lipochrome.

**lip·oc·la·sis** (lĭ-pok′lə-sis) [*lipo-* + Gr. *klasis* breaking] lipolysis.

**lipo·clas·tic** (lip″o-klas′tik) lipolytic.

**lip·o·cor·tin** (lip″o-kor′tin) annexin.

**lipo·cy·a·nine** (lip″o-si′ə-nēn) [*lipo-* + Gr. *kyanos* blue] a blue pigment resulting from the action of strong sulfuric acid on lipochrome.

**lipo·cyte** (lip′o-sīt) [*lipo-* + *-cyte*] [MeSH: Adipocytes] 1. a fat cell. 2. a fat-storing cell of the liver.

**lip·o·di·er·e·sis** (lip″o-di-er′ə-sis) [*lipo-* + *dieresis*] lipolysis.

**lip·o·di·er·et·ic** (lip″o-di-ər-et′ik) lipolytic.

**lipo·dys·tro·phia** (lip″o-dis-tro′fe-ə) lipodystrophy.
**l. intestina′lis**, former name for *Whipple's disease.*
**l. progressi′va**, partial lipodystrophy.

**lipo·dys·tro·phy** (lip″o-dis′tro-fe) [*lipo-* + *dystrophy*] [MeSH: Lipodystrophy] 1. any disturbance of fat metabolism. 2. a group of conditions due to defective metabolism of fat, resulting in the absence of subcutaneous fat, which may be congenital or acquired and partial or total. Called also *lipoatrophy* and *lipodystrophia.*
**congenital generalized l., congenital progressive l.**, total l.
**generalized l.**, total l.
**intestinal l.**, older name for *Whipple's disease.*
**partial l.**, a condition occurring especially in females in the first decade of life, characterized by a symmetrical loss of subcutaneous fat, usually beginning on the face and gradually extending to the chest, neck, back, and upper extremities, giving the lower part of the body an apparent, and possibly real, adiposity of the buttocks, thighs, and legs. Some affected patients develop insulin-resistant diabetes mellitus, hypertriglyceridemia, and renal disease. Called

also *Barraquer's* or *Simons' disease, lipodystrophia progressiva, progressive l.,* and *progressive partial l.*
**progressive l.,** partial l.
**progressive congenital l.,** total l.
**progressive partial l.,** partial l.
**total l.,** a rare autosomal recessive disorder seen mainly in females in infancy, characterized by generalized loss of subcutaneous and extracutaneous adipose tissue associated with hepatomegaly, hypoglycemia and insulin-resistant nonketotic diabetes, hyperlipemia, elevation of the basal metabolic rate, accelerated somatic growth, advanced bone age, acanthosis nigricans, and hirsutism. Called also *congenital generalized, congenital progressive,* or *generalized l., Berardinelli-Seip* or *Lawrence-Seip syndrome,* and *lipoatrophic diabetes.*

**lipo·fec·tion** (lip′o-fek″shən) transfection in which cationic liposomes are the vector for delivery of the nucleic acid, protein, or other negatively charged molecule into the cytoplasm of the foreign cell.

**li·pof·er·ous** (lĭ-pof′ər-əs) [*lipo-* + *-ferous*] 1. carrying fat. 2. sudanophil.

**lipo·fi·bro·ma** (lip″o-fi-bro′mə) fibrolipoma.

**lipo·fus·cin** (lip″o-fu′sin) [MeSH: Lipofuscin] 1. a yellow to brown, granular, iron-negative lipid pigment found particularly in muscle, heart, liver, and nerve cells undergoing slow, regressive change and accumulating in lysosomes with age, being the product of oxidation and polymerization of the membrane lipids of autophagocytosed organelles. 2. lipochrome.

**lipo·fus·cin·o·sis** (lip″o-fu″sin-o′sis) any disorder due to abnormal storage of lipofuscins.
**ceroid-l., neuronal ceroid-l.,** a term for several genetic lipidoses of diverse biochemical and clinical characteristics, all characterized by progressive neurodegeneration, loss of vision, and a fatal course; the *infantile type* is Haltia-Santavuori disease; the *late infantile type* is Jansky-Bielschowsky disease; the *juvenile type* is Vogt-Spielmeyer disease; and the *adult type* is Kufs' disease. Formerly called also *amaurotic familial idiocy.*

**lipo·gen·e·sis** (lip″o-gen′ə-sis) [*lipo-* + *genesis*] the formation of fat; the transformation of nonfat food materials into body fat.

**lipo·ge·net·ic** (lip″o-jə-net′ik) lipogenic.

**lip·o·gen·ic** (lip″o-jen′ik) forming, producing, or caused by fat.

**li·pog·e·nous** (li-poj′ə-nəs) lipogenic.

**lipo·gran·u·lo·ma** (lip″o-gran″u-lo′mə) [*lipo-* + *granuloma*] a nodule of lipoid material; a foreign body inflammation of adipose tissue containing granulation tissue and oil cysts.

**lipo·gran·u·lo·ma·to·sis** (lip″o-gran″u-lo-mə-to′sis) a condition of faulty lipid metabolism in which yellow nodules of lipoid matter are deposited in the skin and mucosae, giving rise to granulomatous reactions.
**Farber's l.,** see under *disease.*

**lipo·hem·ar·thro·sis** (lip″o-hem″ahr-thro′sis) [*lipo-* + *hemarthrosis*] the presence of fat-containing blood in a joint, with intra-articular fracture.

**Lipo-Hep·in** (lip″o-hep′in) trademark for a preparation of heparin sodium.

**lipo·his·tio·di·er·e·sis** (lip″o-his″te-o-di-er′ə-sis) [*lipo-* + *histio-* + *dieresis*] disappearance of stored fat from body tissue.

**lipo·hy·a·lin** (lip″o-hi′ə-lin) the lipid deposited in the beta cells of the pancreas in association with hyalinization in diabetes.

**lipo·hy·per·tro·phy** (lip″o-hi-pər′tro-fe) hypertrophy of subcutaneous fat.
**insulin l.,** localized hypertrophy of subcutaneous fat at insulin injection sites caused by the lipogenic effect of insulin.

**lipo·ic ac·id** (lip-o′ik) a necessary cofactor of the pyruvate dehydrogenase, branched-chain α-keto acid dehydrogenase, and α-ketoglutarate dehydrogenase complexes; it contains a reactive disulfide group that can bind and transfer reaction intermediates. In the enzyme complexes it occurs as lipoamide (q.v.).

**lip·oid** (lip′oid) [*lipo-* + Gr. *eidos* form] 1. fatlike; resembling fat; adipoid. 2. former name for *lipid.*

**lipo·lip·oi·do·sis** (lip″o-lip″oi-do′sis) the presence of lipids and neutral fats in the cells.

**Lipo-Lu·tin** (li″po-lu′tin) trademark for preparations of progesterone.

**li·pol·y·sis** (lĭ-pol′ə-sis) [*lipo-* + *-lysis*] [MeSH: Lipolysis] the decomposition or splitting up of fat.

**lip·o·lyt·ic** (lip″o-lit′ik) pertaining to, characterized by, or causing lipolysis.

**lip·o·ma** (lip-o′mə) [*lip-* + *-oma*] [MeSH: Lipoma] a benign, soft, rubbery, encapsulated tumor of adipose tissue, usually composed of mature fat cells; it generally occurs as a solitary lesion in the subcutaneous tissue of the trunk, nucha, or forearms but may occur in deeper soft tissues.
**l. annula′re col′li,** Madelung's neck.
**l. arbores′cens,** an intraarticular tumor usually occurring as a solitary lesion in the knee; it is characterized by numerous swollen treelike synovial villous projections of fatty tissue, and may arise de novo or be associated with disorders such as degenerative joint disease, chronic rheumatoid arthritis, or previous traumatic injury.
**l. capsula′re,** a fatty tumor due to increase of the fat in the capsule of an organ.
**l. caverno′sum,** angiolipoma.
**diffuse l.,** diffuse lipomatosis.
**l. doloro′sa,** see *nodular circumscribed lipomatosis,* under *lipomatosis.*
**epidural l.,** an intraspinal lipoma on or outside the spinal dura mater in the thoracic or lumbar region, often causing spinal cord compression; Cushing's disease and administration of steroids are common causes.
**l. fibro′sum,** fibrolipoma.
**intermuscular l.,** a slow-growing, infiltrating lesion composed of mature fat cells, occurring in the deeper soft tissues between large muscle groups, predominantly those of the thighs, shoulders, or arms of middle-aged to older adults.
**intradural l.,** an intraspinal lipoma with components within or beneath the dura mater of the spine or sacrum.
**intramedullary l.,** an intraspinal lipoma within the spinal cord.
**intramuscular l.,** a lesion similar to intermuscular lipoma, but occurring within muscle.
**intraspinal l.,** a lipoma within the spinal canal; it may exist entirely within the canal or it may protrude and form part of a lipomyelomeningocele.
**l. myxomato′des,** myxolipoma.
**l. ossi′ficans,** an ossified lipoma.
**l. sarcomato′des,** liposarcoma.
**spindle cell l.,** a rare, benign, circumscribed, painless lesion occurring in the dermis or subcutaneous tissue of the posterior neck or shoulder, particularly in middle-aged or older males; it is characterized by lipocytes, spindle cells, bundles of birefringent collagen, and a myxoid stroma.
**telangiectatic l., l. telangiecto′des,** angiolipoma.

**li·po·ma·toid** (lĭ-po′mə-toid) resembling a lipoma.

**li·po·ma·to·sis** (lip″o-mə-to′sis) [MeSH: Lipomatosis] a condition characterized by abnormal localized, or tumor-like, accumulations of fat in the tissues.
**l. atro′phicans,** localized accumulations of fat in certain tissues, associated with emaciation of the rest of the body; see also *lipodystrophia progressiva.*
**congenital l. of pancreas,** Shwachman-Diamond syndrome.
**diffuse l.,** abnormal increase of subcutaneous fat in the parts above the pelvis, usually in males.
**l. doloro′sa,** lipomatosis in which the adipose deposits are tender or painful.
**l. gigan′tea,** a form in which the adipose deposits form large masses.
**nodular circumscribed l.,** the formation of multiple circumscribed or encapsulated lipomas which may be distributed symmetrically (symmetrical lipomatosis) or haphazardly or which may form a collar around the neck (Madelung's neck). At times they may be painful (lipoma, or lipomatosis, dolorosa).
**renal l., l. re′nis,** fatty masses within the kidney.
**symmetrical l.,** see *nodular circumscribed l.*

**li·po·ma·tous** (lĭpo′mə-təs) affected with, or of the nature of, lipoma.

**lipo·me·nin·go·cele** (lip″o-mə-ning′go-sēl) meningocele associated with an overlying lipoma, in spina bifida.

**li·po·me·ria** (li″po-me′re-ə) [Gr. *leipein* to leave + *mer-* + *-ia*] amelia.

**lipo·meta·bol·ic** (lip″o-met″ə-bol′ik) pertaining to metabolism of fat.

**lipo·me·tab·o·lism** (lip″o-mə-tab′o-liz-əm) [*lipo-* + *metabolism*] the metabolism of fat; utilization of fat.

**lipo·my·e·lo·me·nin·go·cele** (lip″o-mi″ə-lo-mə-ning′go-sēl) [*lipoma* + *myelomeningocele*] myelomeningocele with an overlying lipoma.

**lipo·myo·he·man·gi·o·ma** (lip″o-mi″o-he-man″je-o′mə) [*lipo-* + *myo-* + *hemangioma*] angiomyolipoma.

**lipo·my·o·ma** (lip″o-mi-o′mə) [*lipo-* + *myoma*] myolipoma.

**lipo·myx·o·ma** (lip″o-mik-so′mə) [*lipo-* + *myxoma*] myxolipoma.

**lipo·ne·phro·sis** (lip″o-nə-fro′sis) lipid nephrosis.

**Lipo·nys·sus** (lip″o-nis′əs) [*lipo-* + Gr. *nyssein* to pierce] former name for *Ornithonyssus.*

**li·pop·a·thy** (lĭ-pop′ə-the) [*lipo-* + *-pathy*] any disorder of lipid metabolism.

**lipo·pec·tic** (lip″o-pek′tik) pertaining to, characterized by, or causing lipopexia.

**lipo·pe·nia** (lip″o-pe′ne-ə) [*lipo-* + *-penia*] deficiency of lipids in the body.

**lipo·pe·nic** (lip″o-pe′nik) pertaining to, characterized by, or causing lipopenia.

**lipo·pex·ia** (lip″o-pek′se-ə) [*lipo-* + *pexia*] the accumulation of fat in the tissues.

**lipo·pex·ic** (lip″o-pek′sik) lipopectic.

**lipo·phage** (lip′o-fāj) [*lipo-* + *-phage*] a cell that ingests or absorbs fat.

**lipo·pha·gia** (lip″o-fa′je-ə) lipophagy.
**l. granulomato′sis,** former name for *Whipple's disease.*

**lipo·pha·gic** (lip″o-fa′jik) pertaining to, characterized by, or causing lipophagy; lipolytic.

**li·poph·a·gy** (li-pof′ə-je) [*lipo-* + *-phagy*] the absorption of fat; lipolysis.

**lipo·phan·e·ro·sis** (lip″o-fan″ə-ro′sis) [*lipo-* + *phanerosis*] the process by which invisible fat in certain cells becomes detectable as small droplets.

**lipo·phil** (lip′o-fil) [*lipo-* + *-phil*] a substance that has an affinity for lipids.

**lipo·phil·ia** (lip″o-fil′e-ə) [*lipo-* + *-philia*] 1. affinity for fat. 2. solubility in lipids. 3. a tendency of the obese for fat fixation.

**lip·o·phil·ic** (lip″o-fil′ik) 1. having an affinity for fat; pertaining to or characterized by lipophilia. 2. absorbing, dissolving, or being dissolved in lipids; used particularly of certain stains or dyes.

**lip·o·phil·in** (lip″o-fil′in) proteolipid protein.

**lip·o·phore** (lip′o-for″) [*lipo-* + *-phore*] a pigment cell containing a lipochrome pigment.

**lipo·plas·ty** (lip″o-plas′te) liposuction.

**lipo·poly·sac·cha·ride** (lip″o-pol″e-sak′ə-rīd) 1. a complex of lipid and polysaccharide. 2. a major component of the cell wall of gram-negative bacteria; lipopolysaccharides are endotoxins and important group-specific antigens (O antigens). The lipopolysaccharide molecule consists of three parts. Lipid A, a glycolipid responsible for the endotoxic activity, is covalently linked to a heteropolysaccharide chain having two parts, the core polysaccharide, which is constant within related strains, and the O-specific chain, which is highly variable. Lipopolysaccharide from *Escherichia coli* is a commonly used B-cell mitogen (polyclonal activator) in laboratory immunology. Abbreviated LPS.

**lipo·pro·tein** (lip″o-, li″po-pro′tēn) any of the lipid-protein complexes in which lipids are transported in the blood; lipoprotein particles consist of a spherical hydrophobic core of triglycerides or cholesteryl esters surrounded by an amphipathic monolayer of phospholipids, cholesterol, and apolipoproteins; the four principal classes are high-density, low-density, and very-low-density lipoproteins and chylomicrons.
**α-l., alpha l.,** a lipoprotein with electrophoretic mobility equivalent to that of the $\alpha_1$-globulins; see *high-density l.*
**l. (a),** Lp(a) l.
**β-l., beta l.,** a lipoprotein with electrophoretic mobility equivalent to that of the β-globulins; see *low-density l.*
**Braun's l.,** in gram-negative bacteria, lipoprotein attached to the peptidoglycan and extending into the lipid bilayer of the outer membrane, anchoring it to the cell wall.
**floating beta l's,** β-VLDL; so called for the abnormally low density of these lipoproteins relative to their electrophoretic mobility.
**high-density l. (HDL),** a class of lipoproteins frequently divided into $HDL_2$ and $HDL_3$ (see table) and the minor variant $HDL_1$ (see *Lp(a) l.*). HDL promotes transport of cholesterol from extrahepatic tissue to the liver for excretion in the bile; synthesized by the liver as discoid "nascent HDL" particles lacking a lipid core, it accumulates a core of cholesteryl esters during reverse cholesterol transport (q.v.) and transfers them to the liver directly or indirectly via other lipoproteins. HDL also shuttles apolipoproteins C-II and E to and from triglyceride-rich lipoproteins during catabolism of the lipoproteins. Serum HDL cholesterol has been negatively correlated with premature coronary heart disease. Called also (referring to its electrophoretic mobility) *α-l.*
**intermediate-density l. (IDL),** a class of lipoproteins formed in the degradation of very-low-density lipoproteins; approximately half are cleared rapidly from the plasma into the liver by receptor-mediated endocytosis; the other half are further degraded to form low-density lipoproteins.
**low-density l. (LDL),** a class of lipoproteins responsible for transport of cholesterol to extrahepatic tissues. It is formed in the circulation when very-low-density lipoproteins are degraded first to intermediate-density lipoproteins and then to LDL by the gain and loss of specific apolipoproteins and the loss of most of their triglycerides. It is taken up and catabolized by both the liver and extrahepatic tissues by specific receptor-mediated endocytosis (see *LDL receptors,* under *receptor*). Called also (referring to its electrophoretic mobility) *β-l.*
**Lp(a) l.,** a lipoprotein particle with a density of 1.05–1.10 g/mL, containing apolipoprotein B-100 as well as an antigenically unique apolipoprotein. It is normally a minor plasma constituent but occurs at vastly elevated levels in some individuals, apparently as an autosomal dominant trait; such elevations have been correlated with increased risk of heart disease. Called also *sinking pre-β-l.* and *$HDL_1$.*
**pre-β-l., pre-beta l.,** very-low-density l.
**sinking pre-β-l.,** Lp(a) l.
**very-high-density l. (VHDL),** a class of lipoproteins with density greater than 1.210 g/mL and diameter 15–30 nm; they are composed predominantly of proteins and also contain a high concentration of free fatty acids.
**very-low-density l. (VLDL),** a class of lipoproteins that transport triglycerides from the intestine and liver to adipose and muscle tissues. Synthesized by the liver, they contain primarily triglycerides in their lipid cores, with some cholesteryl esters; as their triglycerides are cleaved by endothelial lipoprotein lipase and transferred to extrahepatic tissues, the VLDL particles lose most of their apolipoprotein C and become intermediate-density lipoproteins. Called also (referring to electrophoretic mobility) *pre-β-l.*
**l. X,** an abnormal low-density lipoprotein with a high content of free cholesterol and abnormal protein content that occurs in patients with cholestasis.

**lipo·pro·tein·emia** (lip″o-pro″te-ne′me-ə) the presence of excessive lipoproteins in the blood.

**lipo·pro·tein li·pase** (lip″o-pro′tēn li′pās) [EC 3.1.1.34] [MeSH: Lipoprotein Lipase] an enzyme of the hydrolase class that catalyzes the hydrolytic cleavage of fatty acyl groups from triglycerides (or di- or monoglycerides) in chylomicrons, very-low-density lipoproteins, and low-density lipoproteins. It occurs on capillary endothelial surfaces, especially in mammary, muscle, and adipose tissue and requires apolipoprotein C-II as a cofactor.

**lipo·pro·tein·o·sis** (lip″o-pro″tēn-o′sis) lipoid proteinosis.

**lipo·sar·co·ma** (lip″o-sahr-ko′mə) [*lipo-* + *sarcoma*] [MeSH: Liposarcoma] a malignant mesenchymal tumor usually arising from the

**Common Plasma Lipoprotein Classes**

| Class | Density *g/ml* | Diameter *nm* | Electrophorectic Mobility | Major Apolipoproteins | Predominant Core Lipids |
|---|---|---|---|---|---|
| Chylomicrons | 0.93 | 75–1200 | Origin | A-I, A-II, B-48, C | Dietary triglycerides |
| VLDL | 0.93–1.006 | 30–80 | Pre-β | B-100, C, E | Endogenous triglycerides |
| IDL | 1.006–1.019 | 25–35 | Slow pre-β | B-100, E | Endogenous triglycerides, Cholesteryl esters |
| LDL | 1.019–1.063 | 18–25 | β | B-100 | Endogenous cholesteryl esters |
| $HDL_2$<br>$HDL_3$ | 1.063–1.125<br>1.125–1.210 | 9–12<br>5–9 | α | A-I, A-II | Endogenous cholesteryl esters |

VLDL, Very-low-density lipoproteins; IDL, intermediate-density lipoproteins; LDL, low-density lipoproteins; HDL, high-density lipoproteins.

intermuscular fascia, particularly in the upper thigh, and occurring predominantly in male adults. It is derived from primitive or embryonal lipoblastic cells which exhibit varying degrees of lipoblastic and/or lipomatous differentiation, and is divided into several variant forms.
**dedifferentiated l.,** a highly malignant form in which areas of well-differentiated liposarcoma coexist with areas of specific or undifferentiated spindle cell sarcoma.
**myxoid l.,** the most common form of liposarcoma, characterized by primitive mesenchymal cells in a mucopolysaccharide-rich ground substance and a plexiform capillary network; lipoblasts may be scarce. It metastasizes late, if at all.
**pleomorphic l.,** a highly undifferentiated and anaplastic form with a high metastatic potential; it is characterized by many large tumor giant cells and unusual lipoblasts with frequent, abnormal mitotic figures.
**round cell l.,** a highly vascular form characterized by small round to oval cells with fine vacuolated cytoplasm and dark central nuclei and by occasional lipoblasts, which are commonly without mitotic figures; it frequently metastasizes.
**well-differentiated l.,** a form resembling lipoma, having adult type fat cells and sometimes bizarre, atypical lipoblasts, with infrequent mitoses and tumor giant cells; it may be locally aggressive but rarely metastasizes.

**li·po·sis** (lĭ-po'sis) [*lipo-* + *-osis*] lipomatosis.

**lipo·sol·u·ble** (lip″o-sol'u-bəl) [*lipo-* + *soluble*] soluble in fats.

**lipo·some** (lip'o-sōm) [*lipo-* + *-some*] [MeSH: Liposomes] a spherical particle in an aqueous medium, formed by a lipid bilayer enclosing an aqueous compartment.

**lipo·suc·tion** (lip″o-suk'shən) surgical removal of localized fat deposits via high pressure vacuum, which is applied by means of a cannula inserted subdermally through a small incision.

**lipo·tei·cho·ic ac·id** (lip″o-ti-ko'ik) any of various teichoic acids (q.v.) that are covalently linked to glycolipids of the plasma membrane of gram-positive bacteria. In certain bacteria, they are major antigenic determinants. Cf. *wall teichoic acid.*

**lipo·troph** (lip'o-trof) any of the acidophilic cells of the anterior lobe of the pituitary gland that contain β-lipotropin; see *corticotroph.*

**lipo·troph·ic** (lip″o-trof'ik) pertaining to, characterized by, or causing lipotrophy.

**li·pot·ro·phy** (lĭ-pot'rə-fe) [*lipo-* + *-trophy*] increase of bodily fat.

**lipo·trop·ic** (lip″o-trop'ik) [*lipo-* + *-tropic*] 1. acting on fat metabolism by hastening the removal of or decreasing the deposit of fat in the liver. 2. an agent that has such effects.

**lip·o·tro·pin** (lip'o-tro″pin) any of several polypeptide hormones produced in the adenohypophysis, derivatives of pro-opiomelanocortin, which promote lipolysis; the most important one in humans is *β-lipotropin.* Called also lipotropic hormone.
**β-l.,** a 91-amino acid polypeptide synthesized by cells of the adenohypophysis, which exerts a mild lipolytic action and promotes darkening of the skin by stimulation of melanocytes; it is the precursor molecule of endorphins and melanocyte-stimulating hormones.

**li·pot·ro·pism** (lĭ-pot'ro-piz″əm) the condition of being lipotropic.

**li·pot·ro·py** (lĭ-pot'rə-pe) lipotropism.

**lipo·vac·cine** (lip″o-vak'sēn) [*lipo-* + *vaccine*] a vaccine prepared by suspending microorganisms in vegetable oil for the purpose of delaying absorption of the antigenic substances.

**lipo·vi·tel·lin** (lip″o-vi-tel'in) [*lipo-* + *vitelline*] a lipoprotein found in the yolk of eggs.

**lipo·xan·thine** (lip″o-zan'thin) [*lipo-* + Gr. *xanthos* yellow] a yellow lipochrome.

**li·pox·i·dase** (lĭ-pok'sĭ-dās) lipoxygenase.

**lip·ox·in** (lĭ-pok'sin) any of several conjugated tetraene derivatives of arachidonic acid that oppose the actions of leukotrienes, have potent vasodilating effects, and appear to be toxic to natural killer cells.

**li·poxy·ge·nase** (lĭ-pok'se-jen-ās) [EC 1.13.11.12] [MeSH: Lipoxygenase] an enzyme of the oxidoreductase class that catalyzes the oxidation of linoleate and related polyunsaturated fatty acids to their hydroperoxide forms. Called also *lipoxidase.*
**5-l.,** arachidonate 5-lipoxygenase.
**12-l.,** arachidonate 12-lipoxygenase.
**15-l.,** arachidonate 15-lipoxygenase.

**lip·ox·ysm** (lip-oks'iz-əm) [*lipo-* + *oxys* sharp, acid] poisoning by oleic acid.

**lipo·yl** (lip'o-əl) the acyl radical of lipoic acid.

**lip·pa** (lip'ə) blepharitis ciliaris.

**lip·ping** (lip'ing) 1. a wedge-shaped shadow in the radiograph of chondrosarcoma between the cortex and the elevated periosteum. 2. the development of a bony overgrowth in osteoarthritis.

**lip·pi·tude** (lip'ĭ-tōōd) [L. *lippitudo; lippus* bleareyed] blepharitis ciliaris.

**Lip·schütz bodies, ulcer (disease)** (lip'shēs) [Benjamin *Lipschütz,* Austrian dermatologist, 1878–1931] see under *body,* and see *ulcus vulvae acutum.*

**li·pu·ria** (lĭ-pu're-ə) [*lip-* + *uria*] the presence of oil or fat in the urine.

**li·pu·ric** (lĭ-pu'rik) pertaining to or characterized by lipuria.

**Liq.** abbreviation for *liquor.*

**Li·qua·mar** (lik'wə-mahr) trademark for a preparation of phenprocoumon.

**liq·ue·fa·cient** (lik″wə-fa'shənt) 1. having the quality to convert a material into its liquid form; producing liquefaction. 2. an agent that produces liquefaction.

**liq·ue·fac·tion** (lik″wə-fak'shən) [L. *liquefactio,* from *liquere* to flow + *facere* to make] the conversion of a material into a liquid form.
**gas l.,** the conversion of gas into a liquid form, brought about by cooling and compression, resulting in a decrease of the average kinetic energy of the molecules sufficiently to allow intermolecular forces of attraction to pull the molecules together. Called also *condensation.*

**liq·ue·fac·tive** (lik″wə-fak'tiv) pertaining to, characterized by, or causing liquefaction.

**li·ques·cent** (lik-wes'ənt) [L. *liquescere* to become liquid] tending to become liquid; becoming liquid.

**liq·uid** (lik'wid) [L. *liquidus; liquere* to flow] 1. a substance that flows readily in its natural state. See also *fluid, liquor, mixture,* and *solution.* 2. flowing readily; neither solid nor gaseous. 3. a consonant sound articulated without friction, such as *l* or *r.*
**Müller's l.,** see under *fluid.*

**liq·ui·form** (lik'wĭ-form) resembling a liquid.

**li·quor** (lik'er, li'kwor) pl. *liquors, liquo'res* [L.] 1. a liquid, especially an aqueous solution containing a medicinal substance. 2. a general term used in anatomical nomenclature for certain fluids of the body. See also *fluid, liquid,* and *solution.*
**l. am'nii,** amniotic fluid.
**l. cerebrospina'lis** [TA], cerebrospinal fluid: the fluid contained within the four ventricles of the brain, the subarachnoid space, and the central canal of the spinal cord; formed by choroid plexuses and brain parenchyma, it circulates through the ventricles into the subarachnoid space and is absorbed into the venous system.
**l. cho'rii,** a fluid which separates the amnion from the chorion in the early stages of gestation.
**l. ente'ricus,** succus entericus.
**l. folli'culi,** follicular fluid: an albuminous fluid in the vesicular ovarian follicle surrounding the ovum.
**l. gas'tricus,** succus gastricus.
**mother l.,** the liquid from which any substance has been separated by crystallization.
**l. pancrea'ticus,** succus pancreaticus.
**l. prosta'ticus,** succus prostaticus.
**l. pu'ris,** the fluid portion of pus.
**l. of Scarpa,** endolympha.
**l. se'minis,** seminal plasma.

**li·quo·res** (li-kwo'rēz) [L.] plural of *liquor.*

**li·quor·ice** (lik'ər-is) 1. *Glycyrrhiza glabra.* 2. glycyrrhiza.

**Lisch nodules** (lish) [Karl *Lisch,* Austrian ophthalmologist, born 1907] see under *nodule.*

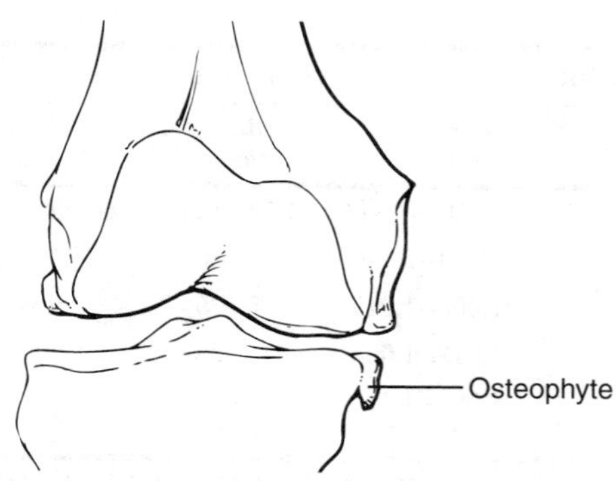

Lipping manifest as an osteophyte on the medial condyle of the right tibia.

**Lis·franc's amputation,** etc. (lis-frahngks') [Jacques *Lisfranc,* French surgeon, 1790–1847] see under *amputation, joint, ligament,* and *tubercle.*

**li·sin·o·pril** (li-sin'o-pril) [USP] [MeSH: Lisinopril] the lysine derivative of the active form of enalapril; an angiotensin-converting enzyme inhibitor used in the treatment of hypertension, congestive heart failure, and acute myocardial infarction, administered orally.

**lisp·ing** (lisp'ing) a form of sigmatism in which *th* sounds are substituted for *s* and *z.*

**Lis·sau·er's paralysis, tract (column, marginal zone)** (lis'ou-ərz) [Heinrich *Lissauer,* German neurologist, 1861–1891] see under *paralysis* and see *tractus posterolateralis.*

**Lis·sen·ceph·a·la** (lis"ən-sef'ə-lə) [Gr. *lissos* smooth + *enkephalos* brain] a group of placental mammals in which the cerebral hemispheres are characteristically smooth or marked by few convolutions; it includes bats, rodents, and others. Cf. *Gyrencephala.*

**lis·sen·ce·pha·lia** (lis"ən-sə-fa'le-ə) agyria.

**lis·sen·ce·phal·ic** (lis"ən-sə-fal'ik) 1. pertaining to the Lissencephala. 2. having cerebral hemispheres without or with only shallow convolutions, the normal appearance of the brain of many animals (e.g., bats, rodents). Cf. *gyrencephalic.* 3. agyric.

**lis·sen·ceph·a·ly** (lis"ən-sef'ə-le) agyria.
**Walker's l.,** Walker-Warburg syndrome.

**lis·sive** (lis'iv) [Gr. *lissos* smooth] relieving muscle spasm without interfering with function.

**Lis·ter** (lis'tər) Baron Joseph (1827–1912). English surgeon who, following Pasteur's theory that bacteria cause infection, introduced to surgery the principle of antisepsis. In 1865 Lister, using carbolic acid as his antiseptic agent together with heat-sterilized instruments, greatly reduced postoperative mortality.

**Lis·ter's tubercle** (lis'tərz) [Baron Joseph *Lister*] tuberculum dorsale radii.

**Lis·ter·el·la** (lis"tər-el'ə) *Listeria.*

**lis·ter·el·lo·sis** (lis"tər-ə-lo'sis) listeriosis.

**Lis·te·ria** (lis-te're-ə) [Baron Joseph *Lister*] [MeSH: Listeria] a genus of bacteria of uncertain affiliation, closely resembling those of the family Corynebacteriaceae, made up of small, coccoid, gram-positive rods that have a tendency to form chains and palisades; they are found in the feces of humans and other animals, on vegetation, and in silage.
**L. monocyto'genes,** a species widely distributed in nature, which has a striking monocytic action in blood and causes listeriosis in humans and ruminants. Called also *Corynebacterium infantisepticum* and *C. parvulum.*

**lis·te·ri·al** (lis-ter'e-əl) pertaining to or caused by organisms of the genus *Listeria.*

**lis·ter·i·o·sis** (lis-ter"e-o'sis) 1. human infection caused by *Listeria monocytogenes.* In utero infection occurs transplacentally and results in abortion, stillbirth, or premature birth. Infection acquired during birth causes cardiorespiratory distress, diarrhea, vomiting, and meningitis. In adults it produces meningitis, endocarditis, and disseminated granulomatous lesions. 2. infection of domestic animals by *L. monocytogenes.* In cattle and sheep this causes abortion, encephalitis, and other nervous signs; nonruminants may suffer from necrosis of the liver. Because affected animals tend to move in circles, it is also known as *circling disease.*

**lis·ter·ism** (lis'tər-iz"əm) the principles and practice of antiseptic and aseptic surgery.

**Lis·ting's law, plane** (lis'tingz) [Johann Benedict *Listing,* German physiologist, 1808–1882] see under *law* and *plane.*

**Lis·ton's knife, operation, splint** (lis'tənz) [Robert *Liston,* English surgeon, 1794–1847] see under *knife* and *splint.*

**Lis·tro·phor·i·dae** (lis"tro-for'ĭ-de) a family of mites often found clinging to the hair of mammals. Genera of veterinary interest include *Lynxacarus* and *Myocoptes.*

**li·ter** (le'tər, li'tər) [Fr. *litre*] a unit of volume in the metric system, equal to 1000 cubic centimeters, or 1 cubic decimeter, or to 1.0567 quarts liquid measure. Abbreviated L or l.

**-lith** [Gr. *lithos* stone] a word termination denoting a stone or calculus.

**lith·a·gogue** (lith'ə-gog) [*litho-* + *-agogue*] 1. expelling calculi. 2. a remedy that promotes the expulsion of calculi.

**Lith·ane** (lith'ān) trademark for a preparation of lithium carbonate.

**lith·an·gi·uria** (lith"an-je-u're-ə) [*litho-* + *angio-* + *-uria*] calculous disease of the urinary tract.

**lith·arge** (lith'ahrj) [Gr. *lithargyros; lithos* stone + *argyros* silver] see *lead monoxide.*

**lith·ate** (lith'āt) urate.

**li·thec·bo·le** (lĭ-thek'bo-le) [*litho-* + Gr. *ekbolē* expulsion] expulsion of a calculus.

**li·thec·ta·sy** (lĭ-thek'tə-se) [*litho-* + *ectasy*] the extraction of calculi through the mechanically dilated urethra.

**li·thec·to·my** (lĭ-thek'tə-me) lithotomy.

**lith·ia** (lith'e-ə) see *lithium.*

**lith·i·as·ic** (lith"e-as'ik) pertaining to lithiasis.

**li·thi·a·sis** (lĭ-thi'ə-sis) [*lith-* + *-iasis*] 1. the formation or presence of abnormal calculi or other concretions. 2. sometimes used as a synonym for one of the specific types of lithiasis, especially urolithiasis, nephrolithiasis, or cholelithiasis.
**appendicular l.,** appendicolithiasis.
**l. conjuncti'vae,** a condition marked by the formation of white, calcareous concretions in the acini of the meibomian glands.
**pancreatic l.,** pancreatolithiasis.
**uric acid l.,** urolithiasis in which the stones contain uric acid.
**urinary l.,** urolithiasis.

**lith·ic** (lith'ik) 1. pertaining to calculus. 2. pertaining to lithium.

**lith·ic ac·id** (lith'ic) uric acid.

**lith·i·um** (lith'e-əm) [Gr. *lithos* stone] [MeSH: Lithium] a white metal; atomic number, 3; atomic weight, 6.939; symbol, Li; its oxide, lithia, $Li_2O$, is alkaline; its salts are solvents of uric acid to a certain extent in vitro: based on this, it was formerly erroneously thought to be indicated in gout and rheumatic conditions.
**l. carbonate** [USP], a lithium salt used in the treatment of acute manic states and in the prophylaxis of recurrent affective disorders manifested by depression or mania only, or those in which both mania and depression occur occasionally; administered orally.
**l. citrate** [USP], the citrate salt of lithium, used to treat the manic phase of bipolar disorder.

**lith(o)-** [Gr. *lithos* stone] a combining form denoting relationship to stone or to a calculus.

**litho·ce·no·sis** (lith"o-sə-no'sis) [*litho-* + *ceno-*[2] + *-sis*] the removal from the bladder of the fragments of calculi that have been crushed.

**litho·cho·late** (lith"o-ko'lāt) a salt, ester, or anionic form of lithocholic acid.

**litho·cho·lic ac·id** (lith"o-ko'lik) [MeSH: Lithocholic Acid] a secondary bile acid formed by dehydroxylation of chenodeoxycholic acid in the intestine; some is reabsorbed and forms conjugates with glycine and taurine.

**litho·cho·lyl·gly·cine** (lith"o-ko"ləl-gli'sēn) a bile salt, the glycine conjugate of lithocholic acid.

**litho·cho·lyl·tau·rine** (lith"o-ko"ləl-taw'rēn) a bile salt, the taurine conjugate of lithocholic acid.

**litho·clast** (lith'o-klast) [*litho-* + *-clast*] a lithotrite, or stone-crushing forceps.

**litho·cys·tot·o·my** (lith"o-sis-tot'ə-me) [*litho-* + *cystotomy*] an operation for removing a stone from the bladder.

**litho·di·al·y·sis** (lith"o-di-al'ĭ-sis) [*litho-* + *dialysis*] 1. the dissolution of calculi in the bladder by injected solvents. 2. the crushing of a calculus in the bladder.

**litho·gen·e·sis** (lith"o-gen'ə-sis) [*litho-* + *-genesis*] the formation of calculi; called also *calculogenesis.*

**lith·o·gen·ic** (lith"o-jen'ik) promoting the formation of calculi.

**li·thog·e·nous** (lĭ-thoj'ə-nəs) producing or causing the formation of calculi.

**litho·kel·y·pho·pe·di·on** (lith"o-kel"ĭ-fo-pe'de-on) [*litho-* + Gr. *kelyphos* sheath + *paidion* child] a lithopedion in which both the fetus and the membranes are petrified.

**litho·kel·y·phos** (lith"o-kel'ĭ-fos) [*litho-* + Gr. *kelyphos* sheath] a dead fetus in which the fetal membranes are calcified.

**litho·labe** (lith'o-lab) [*litho-* + Gr. *lambanein* to hold] an instrument for holding a vesical calculus in the operation for its removal.

**li·thol·a·paxy** (lĭ-thol'ə-pak"se) [*litho-* + Gr. *lapaxis* evacuation] lithotripsy.

**li·thol·o·gy** (lĭ-thol'ə-je) [*litho-* + *-logy*] the sum of what is known regarding calculi and their treatment.

**li·thol·y·sis** (lĭ-thol'ĭ-sis) [*litho-* + *-lysis*] the dissolution of calculi.

**litho·lyte** (lith'o-līt) [*litho-* + Gr. *lysis* dissolution] an instrument used to inject calculi solvents into the bladder.

**litho·lyt·ic** (lith"o-lit'ik) 1. dissolving stones or calculi. 2. an agent that dissolves calculi.

**li·thom·e·ter** (lĭ-thom'ə-tər) [*litho-* + *-meter*] an instrument for measuring calculi.

**litho·myl** (lith'o-məl) [*litho-* + Gr. *mylē* mill] an instrument for crushing a stone in the bladder.

**litho·ne·phri·tis** (lith″o-nə-fri'tis) [*litho-* + *nephritis*] inflammation of the kidney due to irritation by calculi.

**litho·ne·phrot·o·my** (lith″o-nə-frot'ə-me) [*litho-* + *nephrotomy*] the operative removal of a renal calculus.

**litho·pe·di·on** (lith″o-pe'de-on) [L. *lithopaedium;* from Gr. *lithos* stone + *paidion* child] a dead fetus that has become stony or petrified in utero; called also *calcified fetus.*

**litho·scope** (lith'o-skōp) [*litho-* + *-scope*] an instrument for examining calculi in the bladder; cystoscope.

**Lith·o·stat** (lith'o-stat) trademark for a preparation of acetohydroxamic acid.

**litho·tome** (lith'o-tōm) a knife for performing lithotomy.

**li·thot·o·mist** (lĭ-thot'ə-mist) one who performs a lithotomy.

**li·thot·o·my** (lĭ-thot'ə-me) [*litho-* + *-tomy*] incision of a duct or organ, especially of the bladder, for removal of stone.
**bilateral l.,** one performed by a transverse incision across the perineum.
**high l.,** suprapubic l.
**lateral l.,** one in which the incision is before the rectum and to one side of the raphe.
**median l.,** one in which the incision is made on the raphe of the perineum anterior to the anus.
**mediolateral l.,** a combination of the median and lateral operations.
**perineal l.,** that in which the incision is made in the perineum.
**prerectal l.,** median l.
**rectal l., rectovesical l.,** one performed by an incision within the dilated rectum.
**suprapubic l.,** one performed by an incision above the pubes.
**vaginal l., vesicovaginal l.,** one performed by an incision within the vagina.

**li·thot·o·ny** (lĭ-thot'ə-ne) [*litho-* + Gr. *teinein* to stretch] the creation of an artificial bladder fistula which is dilated to allow the extraction of a stone.

**litho·tre·sis** (lith″o-tre'sis) [*litho-* + Gr. *trēsis* a boring] the drilling or boring of holes in a calculus.

**litho·trip·sy** (lith'o-trip″se) [*litho-* + *-tripsy*] [MeSH: Lithotripsy] the crushing of a calculus within the urinary system or gallbladder, followed at once by the washing out of the fragments; it may be done either surgically or by several different noninvasive methods. Called also *litholapaxy.*
**electrohydraulic l.,** a method used for large calculi in the upper urinary tract or gallbladder: a high-capacity condenser creates a high-voltage spark between two electrodes at the tip of a probe; in a fluid-filled organ this creates a hydraulic shock wave that can be directed toward a calculus, causing it to cavitate and fragment.
**extracorporeal shock wave l.,** a procedure for treating upper urinary tract stones and gallstones: the patient is immersed in a large tub of water or placed in contact with a water cushion; a high-energy shock wave generated by a high-voltage spark, electromagnetic impulse, or piezoelectric generator is focused by an ellipsoid reflector on the stone, which disintegrates into particles small enough to be expelled from the organ.
**laser l.,** lithotripsy of calculi in the urinary bladder or ureter using a pulsed dye laser.

**litho·trip·ter** (lith'o-trip″tər) lithotriptor.

**litho·trip·tic** (lith″o-trip'tik) pertaining to or producing lithotripsy.

**litho·trip·tor** (lith'o-trip″tor) an instrument for crushing calculi in the urinary tract.

**litho·trip·to·scope** (lith″o-trip'to-skōp) an instrument for performing lithotriptoscopy.

**litho·trip·tos·co·py** (lith″o-trip-tos'kə-pe) [*litho-* + Gr. *tripsis* a crushing + *-scopy*] the crushing of a vesical calculus under direct visual control.

**litho·trite** (lith'o-trīt) [*litho-* + Gr. *tribein* to rub] an instrument for crushing a stone in the bladder.

**li·thot·ri·ty** (lĭ-thot'rĭ-te) the crushing of a vesical calculus within the bladder by means of the lithotrite.

**litho·troph** (lith'o-trōf) [*litho-* + Gr. *trophē* nutrition] autotroph.

**lith·ous** (lith'əs) [*lith-* + *-ous*] pertaining to or of the nature of a calculus.

**lith·ox·i·du·ria** (lith″ok-sĭ-du're-ə) [*litho-* + *oxide* + *-uria*] xanthinuria.

**lith·ure·sis** (lith″u-re'sis) [*litho-* + *-uresis*] the passage of gravel through the urethra with the urine.

**lith·ure·te·ria** (lith″u-rə-tēr-eə) [*litho-* + *ureter-* + *-ia*] calculous disease of the ureter.

**lit·mus** (lit'məs) a pigment prepared from *Roccella tinctoria* and other lichens, used as a test for acidity and alkalinity. It has a pH range of 4.5 to 8.3. Crude fractions are *azolitmin, erythrolitmin* and *erythrolein.*

**Lit·o·mo·soi·des** (lit″o-mo-soi'dēz) a genus of filarial nematodes. *L. cari'nii* is found in the pleural and peritoneal cavities of the cotton rat, *Sigmodon hispidus,* and is widely used in studies of filariasis.

**li·tre** (le'tər) [Fr.] liter.

**lit·ter** (lit'ər) 1. stretcher. 2. the offspring produced at one birth by a multiparous animal.

**Lit·tle's area** (lit'əlz) [James Laurence *Little,* American surgeon, 1836–1885] see *Kiesselbach's area* under *area.*

**Lit·tle's disease** (lit'əlz) [William John *Little,* English physician, 1810–1894] see under *disease.*

**lit·to·ral** (lit'ə-rəl) pertaining to the shore of a large body of water.

**Lit·tre's crypts, glands, hernia** (le'trəz) [Alexis *Littre,* French surgeon, 1658–1725] see *glandulae preputiales* and *glandulae urethrales urethrae masculinae,* and see under *hernia.*

**lit·tri·tis** (lĭ-tri'tis) inflammation of the urethral (Littre's) glands.

**Litz·mann's obliquity** (litz'mənz) [Karl Konrad Theodor *Litzmann,* German gynecologist, 1815–1890] see under *obliquity.*

**li·ve·do** (lĭ-ve'do) [L.] a discolored spot or patch on the skin, commonly due to passive congestion; commonly used alone to refer to *l. reticularis.*
**l. racemo'sa,** l. reticularis.
**l. reticula'ris,** a vascular response to various disorders caused by dilation of the subpapillary venous plexus as a result of increased viscosity of the blood and changes in the blood vessels themselves that delay blood flow away from the skin. Clinical characteristics include a reticular cyanotic cutaneous discoloration surrounding pale central areas on the extremities and trunk, which becomes more intense on exposure to cold and may disappear on warming. The condition has been classified in three groups: (1) cutis marmorata, (2) idiopathic with or without ulceration, and (3) symptomatic, i.e., that associated with other disorders. Called also *l. racemosa.*
**l. reticularis, idiopathic,** a persistent form usually seen in women, characterized by symmetrical diffuse lesions. Greater changes occur in winter, with some patients developing ulcerations on the legs. Others develop edema of the feet and ankles in the spring and summer, followed by ulcerations.
**l. reticularis, symptomatic,** a variety that occurs in an asymmetrical, patchy distribution and is associated with various other disorders, most of which involve changes in the blood viscosity, embolization, or disease of the blood vessel wall. Associated conditions include vascular diseases such as arteriosclerosis, vascular calcification with hyperparathyroidism, and arteritis; intravascular occlusive conditions such as thrombocytopenia, cryoglobulinemia, emboli, and caisson disease; and miscellaneous others such as tuberculosis, syphilis, and rheumatic fever.
**l. telangiecta'tica,** permanent mottling of the skin due to anomaly of the capillaries of the skin.

**liv·e·doid** (liv'ə-doid) pertaining to or resembling livedo.

**liv·er** (liv'ər) [L. *jecur;* Gr. *hēpar*] [MeSH: Liver] 1. a large gland of a dark-red color situated in the upper part of the abdomen on the right side. Called also *hepar* [TA]. Its domed upper surface fits closely against and is adherent to the inferior surface of the right diaphragmatic dome, and it has a double blood supply from the hepatic artery and the portal vein. It comprises thousands of minute lobules (lobuli hepatitis), the functional units of the liver (see also *liver acinus,* under *acinus,* and *portal lobule,* under *lobule*). Its manifold functions include the storage and filtration of blood, the secretion of bile, the excretion of bilirubin and other substances formed elsewhere in the body, and numerous metabolic functions, including the conversion of sugars into glycogen, which it stores. 2. the same gland of certain animals sometimes used as food or from which pharmaceutical products are prepared.
**albuminoid l., amyloid l.,** a liver which is the seat of an albuminoid or amyloid degeneration; called also *waxy l.*
**biliary cirrhotic l.,** one in which the bile ducts are clogged and distended, the substance of the organ being inflamed; due to biliary cirrhosis.
**brimstone l.,** an enlarged liver of a deep-yellow color, seen in some cases of congenital syphilis.
**bronze l.,** the bronze-colored liver seen in malaria, which results from deposition of malarial pigment (q.v.).
**cirrhotic l.,** one that is the site of cirrhosis.
**degraded l.,** a human liver divided into many lobes.
**fatty l.,** one affected with fatty infiltration, usually from alcohol abuse, jejunoileal bypass surgery, or occasionally diabetes mellitus; fat is in large droplets and the liver is enlarged but of normal consistency; patients are often asymptomatic but the condition can pro-

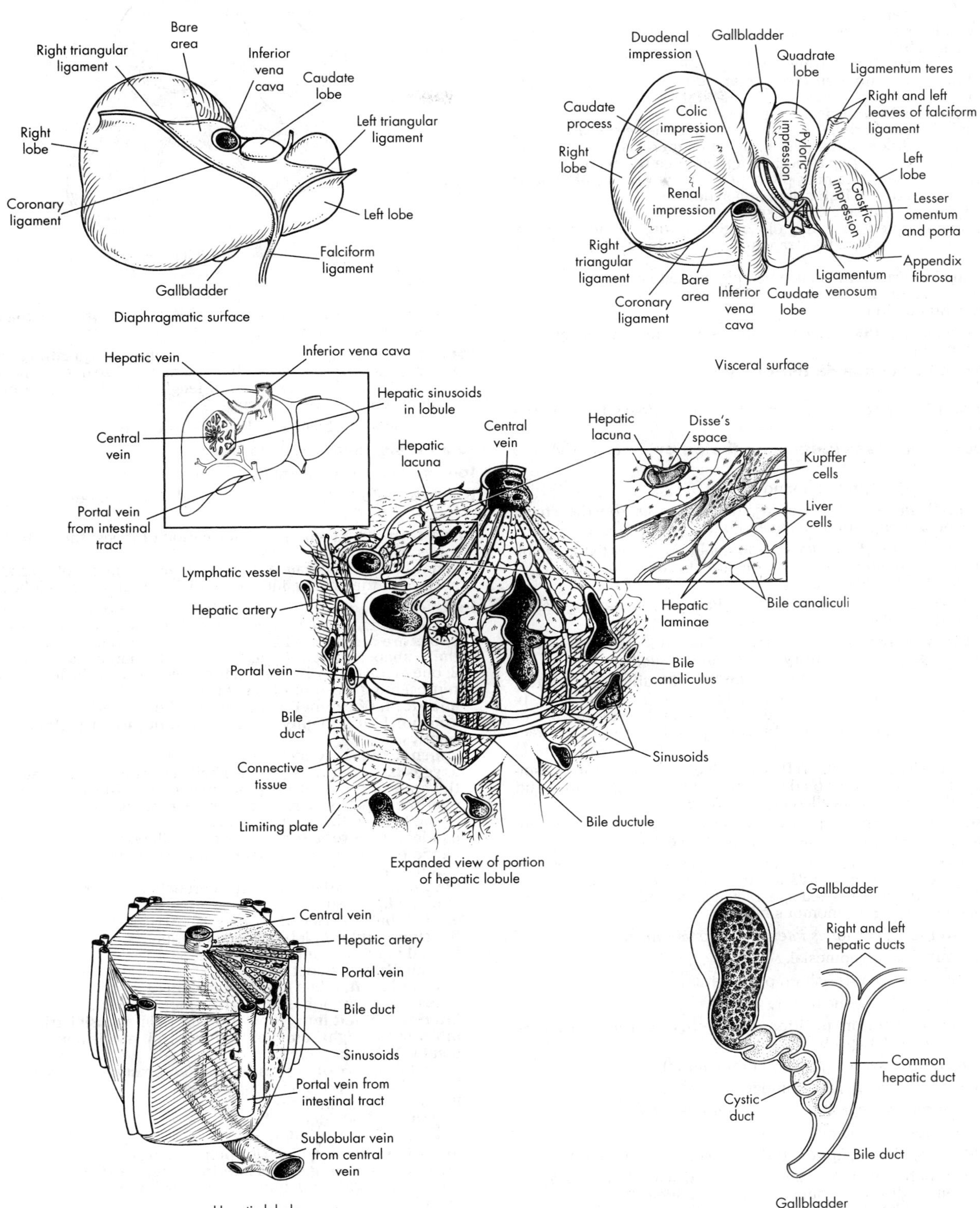


**PLATE 26—**STRUCTURE OF THE LIVER

gress to hepatitis or cirrhosis if the underlying cause is not removed.
**floating l.**, wandering l.
**foamy l.**, a liver seen post mortem, marked by the presence of numerous gas bubbles.
**frosted l.**, perihepatitis chronica hyperplastica.
**hobnail l.**, a liver whose surface is marked by nail-like points from cirrhosis.
**icing l.**, perihepatitis chronica hyperplastica.
**infantile l.**, biliary cirrhosis of children; see under *cirrhosis.*
**iron l.**, the condition of the liver in hepatic siderosis.
**nutmeg l.**, one presenting a mottled appearance when cut.
**pigmented l.**, one containing pigment, usually a result of malaria and melanemia, or the Dubin-Johnson syndrome.
**polycystic l.**, congenital cystic disease of the liver.
**sago l.**, one affected with amyloid degeneration, the acini resembling boiled sago grains, i.e., translucent granules 2 or 3 mm in diameter.
**sugar-icing l.**, perihepatitis chronica hyperplastica.
**wandering l.**, a displaced and movable liver.
**waxy l.**, albuminoid l.

**liv·er phos·phor·y·lase** (liv′ər fos-for′ə-lās) the liver isozyme of glycogen phosphorylase.

**liv·er phos·phor·y·lase de·fi·cien·cy** glycogen storage disease, type VI.

**liv·er phos·phor·y·lase ki·nase** (liv′ər fos-for′ə-lās ki′nās) the liver isozyme of phosphorylase kinase.

**liv·er phos·phor·y·lase ki·nase de·fi·cien·cy** phosphorylase *b* kinase deficiency.

**li·ve·tin** (li′və-tin) a protein found in yolk of egg.

**liv·id** (liv′id) [L. *lividus,* lead-colored] discolored, as from the effects of contusion or congestion; black and blue.

**li·vid·i·ty** (lĭ-vid′ĭ-te) [L. *lividitas*] the quality of being livid; discoloration, as of dependent parts, by the gravitation of the blood.
**postmortem l.**, livor mortis.

**Li·vi·e·ra·to's sign** (le″ve-ə-rah′tōz) [Panagino *Livierato,* Italian physician, 1860–1936] see under *sign.*

**Liv·ing·ston's triangle** (liv′ing-stənz) [Edward Meakin *Livingston,* American surgeon, 20th century] see under *triangle.*

**li·vor** (li′vor) pl. *livo′res* [L. "bluish color"] 1. lividity. 2. l. mortis.
**l. mor′tis,** discoloration appearing on dependent parts of the body after death, as a result of cessation of circulation, stagnation of blood, and settling of the blood by gravity; called also *postmortem lividity.*

**lix·iv·i·a·tion** (lik-siv″e-a′shən) [L. *lixivia* lye] the separation of soluble from insoluble matter by dissolving out the soluble matter and drawing off the solution; called also *leaching.*

**lix·iv·i·um** (lik-siv′e-əm) [L.] any alkaline filtrate obtained by leaching ashes or other similar powdered substance; lye.

**liz·ard** (liz′ərd) [MeSH: Lizards] any of numerous crawling reptiles with long bodies. One genus, *Heloderma,* has a venomous bite.
**beaded l.**, *Heloderma horridum,* a Mexican species related to the Gila monster, having a venomous bite.

**LLL** left lower lobe; see *lobus inferior pulmonis sinistri.*

**LM** light minimum; linguomesial.

**LMA** left mentoanterior (position of the fetus).

**LMF** lymphocyte mitogenic factor.

**LMP** left mentoposterior (position of the fetus); last menstrual period; latent membrane protein.

**LMT** left mentotransverse (position of the fetus).

**LMWK** low-molecular-weight kininogen.

**ln** symbol for natural logarithm; see under *logarithm.*

**LNPF** lymph node permeability factor.

**LOA** [MeSH: Loa] left occipitoanterior (position of the fetus).

**Loa** (lo′ə) [a native word in Angola, West Africa] [MeSH: Loa] a genus of nematodes of the superfamily Filarioidea.
**L. lo′a,** a threadlike species 1 to 2 inches (2.5 to 5 cm) long found in West Africa, which inhabits the subcutaneous connective tissue of the human body; it is seen especially as an eye worm about the orbit and under the conjunctiva. It causes itching and occasionally edematous swellings (Calabar swellings). The immature forms or microfilariae are diurnal, being found in the peripheral circulation in greatest concentrations during the day. Flies of the genus *Chrysops* are the intermediate hosts and vectors. Formerly called *Filaria loa.*

**load** (lōd) 1. the quantity of a measurable entity borne by an object or organism. 2. the body content, as of water, salt, or heat, especially as it varies from normal.

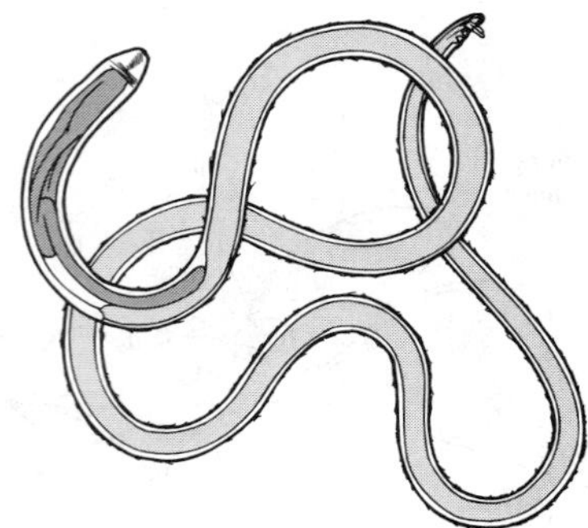

*Loa loa* adult male.

**occlusal l.**, the total force exerted on the teeth through the occlusal surfaces during mastication.

**load·ing** (lōd′ing) 1. administering sufficient quantities of a substance to test the subject's ability to metabolize it, as in the histidine loading test. 2. the exertion of lengthening force on a body part such as a muscle or ligament.

**LOAEL** lowest observed adverse effect level.

**lo·a·i·a·sis** (lo″ə-i′ə-sis) loiasis.

**lo·bar** (lo′bər) of, pertaining to, or affecting a lobe.

**lo·bate** (lo′bāt) [L. *lobatus*] provided with lobes, or disposed in lobes.

**lo·ba·tion** (lo-ba′shən) the formation of lobes; the state of having lobes.
**renal l.**, the appearance on x-ray films of small notches along the surface of the kidney, indicating the location of renal lobes.

**lobe** (lōb) [L. *lobus,* from Gr. *lobos*] 1. a more or less well-defined portion of any organ, especially of the brain, the lungs, or a gland. Lobes are demarcated by fissures, sulci, connective tissue, and by their shape. Called lobus in official anatomical nomenclature. 2. one of the main divisions of the crown of a tooth, developmentally representing a center of calcification.
**anterior l. of cerebellum,** lobus cerebelli anterior.
**anterior l. of hypophysis, anterior l. of pituitary gland,** adenohypophysis.
**appendicular l.**, Riedel's l.
**azygos l., l. of azygos vein,** a small accessory or anomalous lobe at the apex of the right lung, produced when the azygos vein arches over the superior part of the lung and presses deeply into the lung tissue to form the azygos fissure.
**caudal l. of cerebellum,** lobus cerebelli posterior.
**caudate l., caudate l. of liver,** lobus caudatus.
**cerebral l's,** lobi cerebri.
**cranial l. of cerebellum,** lobus cerebelli anterior.
**cuneate l.**, cuneus.
**ear l.**, lobulus auricularis.
**flocculonodular l.**, lobus flocculonodularis.
**frontal l.**, lobus frontalis.
**hepatic l's,** lobi hepatis.
**inferior l., left,** lobus inferior pulmonis sinistri.
**inferior l., right,** lobus inferior pulmonis dextri.
**inferior l. of left lung,** lobus inferior pulmonis sinistri.
**inferior l. of right lung,** lobus inferior pulmonis dextri.
**insular l.**, insula (def. 2).
**lateral l's of prostate gland,** see *lobus prostatae* [*dexter et sinister*].
**left l. of liver,** lobus hepatis sinister.
**limbic l.**, lobus limbicus.
**linguiform l.**, Riedel's l.
**lower l., left,** lobus inferior pulmonis sinistri.
**lower l., right,** lobus inferior pulmonis dextri.
**lower l. of left lung,** lobus inferior pulmonis sinistri.
**lower l. of right lung,** lobus inferior pulmonis dextri.
**l's of lung,** see *lung.*
**l's of mammary gland,** lobi glandulae mammariae.
**median l. of prostate,** lobus medius prostatae.
**middle l., right,** lobus medius pulmonis dextri.
**middle l. of cerebellum,** lobus cerebelli posterior.
**middle l. of right lung,** lobus medius pulmonis dextri.
**neural l., neural l. of neurohypophysis, neural l. of pituitary gland,** lobus nervosus neurohypophysis.
**occipital l.**, the posterior portion of the cerebral hemisphere; see *lobus occipitalis.*
**olfactory l.**, a term applied to the olfactory apparatus on the lower surface of the frontal lobe of the brain. It consists of the olfactory bulb, tract, and trigone.

**optic l's,** corpora bigemina; see under *corpus.*
**parietal l.,** the upper central lobe of the pallium; see *lobus parietalis.*
**piriform l.,** 1. piriform area. 2. in lower mammals, the lateral exposed portion of the olfactory cerebral cortex.
**polyalveolar l.,** a congenital disorder characterized in early infancy by the presence of far more than the normal number of alveoli in a lobe of the lungs; thereafter, normal multiplication of alveoli does not take place and they become enlarged, i.e., emphysematous.
**posterior l. of cerebellum,** lobus cerebelli posterior.
**posterior l. of hypophysis, posterior l. of pituitary gland,** neurohypophysis.
**l's of prostate,** see *lobus prostatae* [*dexter et sinister*].
**pulmonary l's,** see *lung.*
**pyramidal l. of thyroid gland,** lobus pyramidalis glandulae thyroideae.
**pyriform l.,** piriform l.
**quadrate l. of cerebral hemisphere,** precuneus.
**quadrate l. of liver,** lobus quadratus hepatis.
**renal l's,** lobi renales.
**Riedel's l.,** an anomalous tongue-shaped mass of tissue projecting from the right lobe of the liver.
**right l. of liver,** lobus hepatis dexter.
**rostral l. of cerebellum,** lobus cerebelli anterior.
**semilunar l., inferior,** lobulus semilunaris inferior.
**semilunar l., superior,** lobulus semilunaris superior.
**spigelian l.,** lobus caudatus.
**superior l., left,** lobus superior pulmonis sinistri.
**superior l., right,** lobus superior pulmonis dextri.
**superior l. of left lung,** lobus superior pulmonis sinistri.
**superior l. of right lung,** lobus superior pulmonis dextri.
**temporal l.,** lobus temporalis.
**l's of thymus,** see *lobus thymi* [*dexter/sinister*].
**l's of thyroid gland,** see *lobus glandulae thyroideae* [*dexter/sinister*].
**upper l., left,** lobus superior pulmonis sinistri.
**upper l., right,** lobus superior pulmonis dextri.
**upper l. of left lung,** lobus superior pulmonis sinistri.
**upper l. of right lung,** lobus superior pulmonis dextri.
**vagal l.,** visceral l.
**visceral l.,** the visceral sensory area of fishes.

**lo•bec•to•my** (lo-bek'tə-me) [*lobe* + *-ectomy*] excision of a lobe, as of the thyroid, liver, brain, or lung. See also *lobotomy.*
**occipital l.,** removal of the occipital lobe, to treat brain cancer or occasionally epilepsy with a focus in the occipital lobe.
**sleeve l.,** excision of a lobe of the lung with removal of a portion of the bronchus and reanastomosis of the resulting ends. Called also *sleeve resection.*
**temporal l.,** excision of part or all of a temporal lobe in the treatment of temporal lobe epilepsy.
**thyroid l.,** removal of all or part of a lobe of the thyroid gland.

**Lo•be•lia** (lo-be'le-ə) a genus of herbs of the family Campanulaceae; they contain lobeline and other toxic alkaloids and cause mouth ulcerations and diarrhea in ruminants. *L. berlandie'ri* grows in Mexico. *L. infla'ta* is Indian tobacco, which grows in the eastern United States and Canada.

**lo•be•lia** (lo-be'le-ə) 1. any plant of the genus *Lobelia.* 2. the dried leaves and tops of *Lobelia inflata,* an herb with properties resembling those of nicotine.

**lob•e•line** (lob'ə-lēn) [MeSH: Lobeline] alpha-lobeline, the principal alkaloid found in plants of the genus *Lobelia;* it is used in certain anti-smoking preparations and is responsible for the toxic effects seen in ruminants.

**lo•ben•da•zole** (lo-ben'də-zōl) a veterinary anthelmintic.

**lo•bi** (lo'bi) [L.] genitive and plural of *lobus.*

**lo•bite** (lo'bīt) limited to a definite lobe.

**lo•bi•tis** (lo-bi'tis) inflammation of a lobe, especially of a lobe of the lung.

**Lo•bo's disease** (lo'bōz) [Jorge *Lobo,* Brazilian physician, 20th century] keloidal blastomycosis; see under *blastomycosis.*

**Lo•boa** (lo-bo'ə) [Jorge *Lobo*] a proposed genus of fungi that would probably be in the family Moniliaceae. *L. lo'boi,* the causative agent of keloidal blastomycosis, has never been cultured successfully and is believed by some authorities to be a strain of *Paracoccidioides brasiliensis.*

**lo•bo•my•co•sis** (lo″bo-mi-ko'sis) keloidal blastomycosis.

**lo•bo•po•di•um** (lo″bo-po'de-əm) pl. *lobopo'dia* [*lobe* + *pous* foot] a wide, blunt pseudopodium composed of both ectoplasm and endoplasm. Cf. *axopodium, filopodium,* and *reticulopodium.*

**Lo•bo•sea** (lo-bo'se-ə) [Gr. *lobos* lobe] [MeSH: Lobosea] a class of ameboid protozoa (superclass Rhizopoda, subphylum Sarcodina) typically characterized by the presence of lobopodia, although filopodia or reticulopodia sometimes occur. It comprises two subclasses: Gymnamoebia and Testacealobosia.

**lo•bot•o•my** (lo-bot'ə-me) incision into a lobe; in psychosurgery, surgical incision of all the fibers of a lobe of the brain.
**frontal l.,** prefrontal l.
**prefrontal l.,** an operation in which, through holes drilled in the skull, the white matter of the frontal lobe is incised with a leukotome passed through a cannula; called also *leukotomy.*
**transorbital l.,** prefrontal lobotomy performed by way of the orbital plate; called also *transorbital leukotomy.*

**Lob•stein's disease (syndrome), ganglion** (lōb'shtīnz) [Johann Friedrich Georg Christian Martin *Lobstein,* German surgeon, 1777–1835] see *osteogenesis imperfecta,* and see under *ganglion.*

**lob•u•lar** (lob'u-lər) [L. *lobularis*] of or pertaining to a lobule.

**lob•u•lat•ed** (lob'u-lāt″əd) made up of or divided into lobules.

**lob•u•la•tion** (lob″u-la'shən) the process of becoming or the state of being lobulated.
**portal l.,** the pattern in the liver produced by bands of fibrous tissue interconnecting portal areas.

**lob•ule** (lob'ūl) a small lobe; see *lobulus.*
**ansiform l.,** lobuli semilunares.
**l. of auricle,** lobulus auricularis.
**biventral l.,** lobulus biventer.
**central l. of cerebellum,** lobulus centralis cerebelli.
**cortical l's of kidney,** lobuli corticales renis.
**l's of epididymis,** lobuli epididymidis.
**gracile l. of cerebellum,** lobulus gracilis cerebelli.
**hepatic l's,** lobuli hepatis.
**l's of liver,** lobuli hepatis.
**l's of mammary gland,** lobuli glandulae mammariae.
**l. of pancreas,** one of the distinct lobules into which the pancreas is divided by extension of septa of the capsule into the gland.
**paracentral l.,** lobulus paracentralis.
**paramedian l.,** lobulus gracilis cerebelli.
**parietal l., inferior,** lobulus parietalis inferior.
**parietal l., superior,** lobulus parietalis superior.
**portal l.,** a polygonal mass of liver tissue, larger than a liver acinus, containing portions of three adjacent hepatic lobules, and having a portal vein at its center and a central vein peripherally at each corner. See illustration.
**primary l. of lung,** terminal respiratory unit.
**quadrangular l. of cerebellum, anterior,** lobulus quadrangularis anterior cerebelli.
**quadrangular l. of cerebellum, posterior,** lobulus quadrangularis posterior cerebelli.
**respiratory l.,** terminal respiratory unit.
**secondary l. of lung,** an anatomical subdivision of a pulmonary segment, consisting of several branching primary lobules.
**semilunar l., caudal,** lobulus semilunaris inferior.
**semilunar l., cranial,** lobulus semilunaris superior.
**semilunar l., inferior,** lobulus semilunaris inferior.
**semilunar l., rostral, semilunar l., superior,** lobulus semilunaris superior.
**simple l. of cerebellum,** lobulus simplex cerebelli.
**l's of testis,** lobuli testis.
**l's of thymus,** lobuli thymi.
**l's of thyroid gland,** lobuli glandulae thyroideae.

**lob•u•li** (lob'u-li) [L.] genitive and plural of *lobulus.*

**lob•u•lose** (lob'u-lōs) divided into lobules.

**lob•u•lous** (lob'u-ləs) lobulose.

**lob•u•lus** (lob'u-ləs) gen. and pl. *lo'buli* [L., dim of *lobus*] [TA] lob-

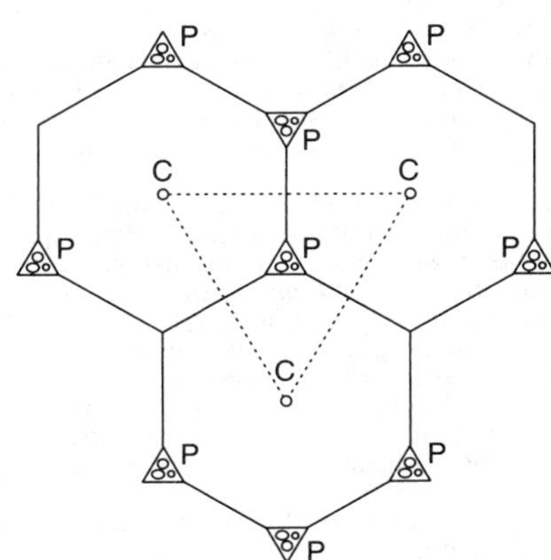


Diagram of hepatic *(solid lines)* and portal *(dotted lines)* lobules, showing the portal areas *(P)* and central veins *(C)*.

ule; a general term for a small lobe or one of the primary divisions of a lobe.
**l. ansifor'mis,** TA alternative for *lobuli semilunares.*
**l. auri'culae** [TA], **l. auricula'ris,** lobule of auricle: the inferior, dependent part of the auricle below the antitragus, which contains fibrous and fatty tissue but no cartilage. Called also *ear lobe.*
**l. biven'ter** [TA], biventral lobule: the part of the posterior lobe of the cerebellum that is between the tonsilla and the inferior semilunar lobule.
**l. centra'lis cerebel'li** [TA], central lobule of cerebellum: the portion of the anterior lobe of the cerebellum between the lingula and the culmen, resting on the lingula and the anterior medullary velum.
**lo'buli cortica'les re'nis,** cortical lobules of kidney: more or less distinctly marked small polygonal areas on the surface of a kidney; each area corresponds to a medullary ray together with its attached renal corpuscles and tubules.
**lo'buli epididy'midis** [TA], lobules of epididymis: the wedge-shaped parts of the head of the epididymis, each comprising a single efferent ductule of the testis; called also *coni epididymidis* [TA alternative].
**lo'buli glan'dulae mamma'riae** [TA], lobules of mammary gland: the smaller subdivisions that make up a lobe of the mammary gland, each drained by a single branch of a lactiferous duct. Called also *lobuli mammae.* See also *glandula mammaria.*
**lo'buli glan'dulae thyroi'deae** [TA], lobules of thyroid gland: irregular areas on the surface of the thyroid gland produced by entrance into the gland of fibrous trabeculae from the sheath.
**l. gra'cilis cerebel'li** [TA], gracile lobule of cerebellum: the portion of the posterior lobe of the hemisphere of the cerebellum between the lobulus simplex and the semilunar and biventral lobules; called also *l. paramedianus cerebelli* [TA alternative] and *paramedian lobule.*
**lo'buli he'patis** [TA], hepatic lobules: the small vascular units comprising the substance of the liver, each of which is polygonal in shape with a central vein at its center and portal canals peripherally at the corners. See also *liver acinus,* under *acinus,* and see illustration at *lobule.*
**lo'buli mam'mae,** lobuli glandulae mammariae.
**l. paracentra'lis** [TA], paracentral lobule: a lobe on the medial surface of the cerebral hemisphere, continuous with the precentral and postcentral gyri of the frontal and parietal lobes, and limited below by the cingulate sulcus; it is composed of sensorimotor cortex, chiefly for the lower limb and genitalia.
**l. paramedia'nus cerebel'li,** TA alternative for *l. gracilis cerebelli.*
**l. parieta'lis infe'rior** [TA], inferior parietal lobule: the lobule that forms the posterior part of the lateral portion of the parietal lobe of the cerebrum. It lies below the intraparietal sulcus, above the posterior ramus of the lateral cerebral fissure, and behind the postcentral sulcus. It includes the supramarginal and the angular gyri. In the dominant hemisphere, it is concerned with language mechanisms.
**l. parieta'lis supe'rior** [TA], superior parietal lobule: the posterior part of the upper portion of the parietal lobe of the brain; it lies behind the postcentral sulcus, in front of the parietooccipital fissure, and above the intraparietal sulcus. It comprises association areas concerned with general sensory functions.
**l. quadrangula'ris ante'rior cerebel'li** [TA], anterior quadrangular lobule of cerebellum: the portion of the cranial lobe of the hemisphere of the cerebellum lying between the postcentral and primary fissures, continuous with the culmen.
**l. quadrangula'ris poste'rior cerebel'li** [TA], posterior quadrangular lobule of cerebellum: the portion of the posterior lobe of the hemisphere of the cerebellum continuous with the declive.
**lo'buli semiluna'res** [TA], semilunar lobules: the lobulus semilunaris inferior and lobulus semilunaris superior considered together. Called also *l. ansiformis* [TA alternative].
**l. semiluna'ris cauda'lis, l. semiluna'ris infe'rior** [TA], inferior semilunar lobule: that portion of the posterior lobe of the cerebellum that is continuous with the tuber vermis; called also *caudal semilunar lobule* and *crus secundum lobuli ansiformis* [TA alternative].
**l. semiluna'ris rostra'lis, l. semiluna'ris supe'rior** [TA], superior semilunar lobule: that part of the cerebellar hemisphere that is continuous with the folium vermis; called also *cranial* or *rostral semilunar lobule* and *crus primum lobuli ansiformis* [TA alternative].
**l. sim'plex cerebel'li** [TA], simple lobule of cerebellum: the large anterior division of the posterior cerebellar lobe, comprising the lobulus quadrangularis cerebelli anterior and declive.
**lo'buli tes'tis** [TA], lobules of testis: the pyramidal subdivisions of the testicular substance, each with its base against the albuginea and its apex at the mediastinum, and composed largely of tubuli seminiferi.
**lo'buli thy'mi** [TA], lobules of thymus: the smaller subdivisions of the lobes of the thymus (q.v.), separated by fibrous trabeculae.

**lo·bus** (lo'bəs) gen. and pl. *lo'bi* [L.] 1. lobe: a more or less well-defined portion of an organ. 2. [TA] a general term for such a subdivision, especially of the brain, the lungs, or a gland, demarcated by fissures, sulci, or connective tissue septa.
**l. ante'rior cerebel'li,** l. cerebelli anterior.
**l. ante'rior hypophy'seos,** TA alternative for *adenohypophysis.*
**l. cauda'lis cerebel'li,** l. cerebelli posterior.
**l. cauda'tus he'patis** [TA], **l. cauda'tus [Spige'li],** caudate lobe of liver: a small lobe bounded on the right by the inferior vena cava, which separates it from the right lobe, and on the left by the attachment of the gastrohepatic ligament, which separates it from the left lobe.
**l. cerebel'li ante'rior** [TA], anterior lobe of cerebellum: the portion of the cerebellum lying in front of the primary fissure, comprising the lingula, central lobule, culmen, alae of central lobules, and quadrangular lobules; called also *cranial* or *rostral lobe of cerebellum, l. cranialis cerebelli,* and *l. rostralis cerebelli.*
**l. cerebel'li poste'rior** [TA], posterior lobe of cerebellum: the portion of the cerebellum separated from the anterior lobe by the primary fissure and from the flocculonodular lobe by the dorsolateral fissure; it comprises the declive, folium vermis, tuber vermis, pyramid, uvula, simple lobule, inferior and superior semilunar lobules, and tonsils. Called also *caudal* or *middle lobe of cerebellum* and *l. caudalis cerebelli.*
**lo'bi cerebra'les, lo'bi ce'rebri** [TA], cerebral lobes: the well defined areas of the cerebral cortex, demarcated by fissures, sulci, and arbitrary lines, including the frontal, temporal, parietal, and occipital lobes. See illustration.
**l. crania'lis cerebel'li,** l. cerebelli anterior.
**l. flocculonodula'ris** [TA], flocculonodular lobe: a fundamental subdivision of the cerebellum, located inferiorly, consisting of paired lateral flocculi, their pedunculi, and the nodulus.
**l. fronta'lis** [TA], frontal lobe: the anterior portion of the cerebral hemisphere, extending from the frontal pole to the sulcus centralis.
**lo'bi glan'dulae mamma'riae** [TA], lobes of mammary gland: the major subdivisions of the secreting portion of the mammary gland, each drained by a single lactiferous duct and further subdivided into lobules (lobuli glandulae mammariae). Called also *lobi mammae.* See also *glandula mammaria.*
**l. glan'dulae thyroi'deae** [TA], lobe of thyroid gland: either of the lobes (right or left) of the thyroid gland, located adjacent to either side of the trachea, cricoid cartilage, and thyroid cartilage.
**l. glandula'ris hypophy'seos,** adenohypophysis.
**l. he'patis dex'ter** [TA], right lobe of liver: the largest of the four lobes of the liver. Anteriorly, it is separated from the left lobe by the falciform ligament. Posteroinferiorly, it is separated from the caudate lobe by the inferior vena cava and from the quadrate lobe by the gallbladder. Used in the broad sense, the term includes the caudate and quadrate lobes.
**l. he'patis sinis'ter** [TA], left lobe of liver: the smaller of the two main lobes of the liver. Anteriorly, it is separated from the right lobe by the falciform ligament. Posteroinferiorly, it is separated from the caudate and quadrate lobes by the attachment of the gastrohepatic ligament and the ligamentum teres.
**l. infe'rior pulmo'nis dex'tri** [TA], lower lobe of right lung; see *lung.* It has five bronchopulmonary segments (see under *segmentum*). Called also *right lower lobe* and *inferior lobe of right lung.*
**l. infe'rior pulmo'nis sinis'tri** [TA], lower lobe of left lung; see *lung.* It has four or five bronchopulmonary segments (see under *segmentum*). Called also *left lower lobe* and *inferior lobe of left lung.*
**l. insula'ris,** TA alternative for *insula* (def. 2).
**l. lim'bicus** [TA], limbic lobe: the component parts and connections of the limbic system (q.v.).
**lo'bi mam'mae,** lobi glandulae mammariae.

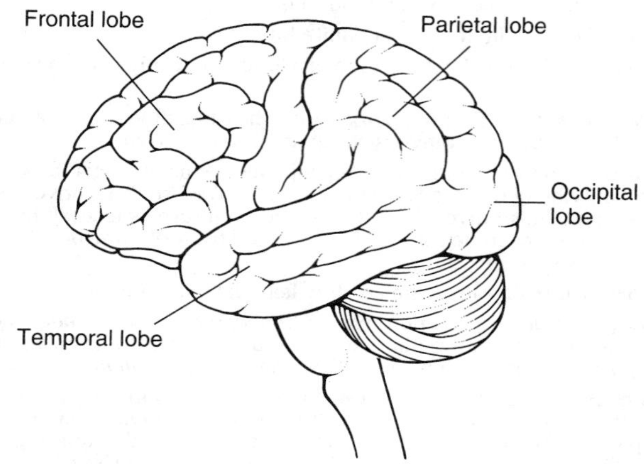

Lobes of the cerebrum.

**l. me'dius prosta'tae** [TA], median lobe of prostate: a normal enlargement of the isthmus of the prostate that sometimes occurs.
**l. me'dius pulmo'nis dex'tri** [TA], middle lobe of right lung; see *lung*. It has two bronchopulmonary segments (see under *segmentum*). Called also *right middle lobe*.
**l. nervo'sus neurohypophy'seos** [TA], neural lobe of neurohypophysis: the major portion of the neurohypophysis; called also *neural lobe of hypophysis* or *pituitary gland* and *pars nervosa neurohypophyseos* [TA alternative].
**l. occipita'lis** [TA], occipital lobe: the posterior portion of the cerebral hemisphere, on the medial surface extending from the posterior pole to the parietooccipital fissure but on the lateral surface continuous with the parietal lobe superiorly and with the temporal lobe inferiorly.
**l. parieta'lis** [TA], parietal lobe: the upper central lobe of the cerebral hemisphere, separated from the temporal lobe below by the lateral sulcus, but continuous at the posterior end of that sulcus, and separated from the frontal lobe by the central sulcus. Behind, it is continuous with the occipital lobe on the lateral surface, but separated from it by the parietooccipital sulcus on the medial surface.
**lo'bi placen'tae,** distinct areas on the uterine surface of the placenta, demarcated by the connective tissue septa.
**l. poste'rior cerebel'li,** l. cerebelli posterior.
**l. poste'rior hypo'physis,** TA alternative for *neurohypophysis*.
**lo'bi prosta'tae dex'ter et sinis'ter** [TA], lobe of prostate: either of the paired halves (right and left) of the prostate, separated by a more or less distinct median sulcus; called also *lateral lobes of prostate gland*.
**l. pyramida'lis glan'dulae thyroi'deae** [TA], pyramidal lobe of thyroid gland: an occasional third lobe that extends upward from the isthmus of the gland across the thyroid cartilage to the hyoid bone; it is the residuum of the thyroid stalk of the fetus.
**l. quadra'tus he'patis** [TA], quadrate lobe of liver: a small lobe of the liver bounded on the right by the gallbladder, which separates it from the right lobe, and on the left by the ligamentum teres, which separates it from the left lobe.
**lo'bi rena'les** [TA], renal lobes: the units of the kidney, each consisting of a pyramid and its surrounding cortical substance; the division of the kidney into lobes is more distinctly marked in some animals and in infants than in the human adult.
**l. rostra'lis cerebel'li,** l. cerebelli anterior.
**l. spige'lii,** l. caudatus hepatis.
**l. supe'rior pulmo'nis dex'tri** [TA], upper lobe of right lung; see *lung*. It has three bronchopulmonary segments (see under *segmentum*). Called also *right upper lobe* and *superior lobe of right lung*.
**l. supe'rior pulmo'nis sinis'tri** [TA], upper lobe of left lung; see *lung*. It has four bronchopulmonary segments (see under *segmentum*). Called also *left upper lobe* and *superior lobe of left lung*.
**l. tempora'lis** [TA], temporal lobe: the lower lateral lobe of the cerebral hemisphere, lying below the posterior ramus of the lateral sulcus, lateral to the collateral sulcus, and merging behind with the occipital lobe on the lateral and inferior surfaces.
**l. thy'mi** [TA], lobe of thymus: either of the two chief parts (right or left) of the thymus, which meet in the midline.
**l. va'gi,** visceral lobe.

**lo·cal** (lo'kəl) [L. *localis*] restricted to or pertaining to one spot or part; not general.

**lo·cal·iza·tion** (lo″kəl-ĭ-za'shən) 1. the determination of the site or place of any process or lesion. 2. restriction to a circumscribed or limited area. 3. prelocalization.
**cerebral l.,** the determination of the situation of the various centers of the brain; also the limitation of the various cerebral faculties to a particular center or organ of the brain.
**germinal l.,** the location on a blastoderm of prospective organs; see *fate map*, under *map*.

**lo·cal·ized** (lo'kəl-īzd) not general; restricted to a limited region or to one or more spots.

**lo·cal·iz·er** (lo'kəl-īz″ər) 1. an instrument for locating solid particles in the eyeball by radiography. 2. a visual training instrument for establishing correct spatial localization in treating amblyopia ex anopsia.

**lo·ca·tor** (lo'ka-tər) an instrument or apparatus by which the site of an object is determined.
**abutment l.,** a thin resin base made on a diagnostic denture cast into which holes have been cut to predetermine locations of the cuspid teeth and molar teeth on a subperiosteal implant.
**apex l.,** in root canal therapy, an electronic device used to determine the working length of a canal that has been cleaned out and when a file has reached the apical foramen.
**Berman-Moorhead l.,** an instrument for locating metallic fragments embedded in body tissues.
**electroacoustic l.,** an apparatus that amplifies into an audible click the contact of a probe with a solid object; used in locating foreign objects within the body.
**Moorhead foreign body l.,** Berman-Moorhead l.

**Loc. dol.** abbreviation for L. *lo'co dolen'ti*, to the painful spot.

**lo·chia** (lo'ke-ə) [Gr. *lochia*] the vaginal discharge that takes place during the first week or two after childbirth.
**l. al'ba,** the final vaginal discharge after childbirth, when the amount of blood is decreased and the leukocytes are increased.
**l. cruen'ta,** l. rubra.
**l. ru'bra,** the vaginal discharge of almost pure blood immediately after childbirth.
**l. sanguinolen'ta,** the thick, maroon-colored vaginal discharge occurring a few days after childbirth.
**l. sero'sa,** the serous vaginal discharge occurring about four or five days after childbirth.

**lo·chi·al** (lo'ke-əl) pertaining to the lochia.

**lo·chio·col·pos** (lo″ke-o-kol'pos) [*lochia* + Gr. *kolpos* vagina] distention of the vagina by retained lochia.

**lo·chio·me·tra** (lo″ke-o-me'trə) [*lochia* + *metra*] distention of the uterus by retained lochia.

**lo·chio·me·tri·tis** (lo″ke-o-me-tri'tis) [*lochia* + *metritis*] puerperal metritis.

**lo·chi·or·rha·gia** (lo″ke-o-ra'jə) [*lochia* + *-rrhagia*] lochiorrhea.

**lo·chi·or·rhea** (lo″ke-o-re'ə) [*lochia* + *-rrhea*] an abnormally profuse discharge of lochia.

**lo·chi·os·che·sis** (lo″ke-os'kə-sis) [*lochia* + Gr. *schesis* retention] retention of the lochia; lochiostasis.

**lo·chi·os·ta·sis** (lo″ke-os'tə-sis) [*lochia* + *-stasis*] retention of the lochia; lochioschesis.

**lo·cho·me·tri·tis** (lo″ko-me-tri'tis) [Gr. *lochos* childbirth + *metritis*] puerperal metritis.

**lo·ci** (lo'si) [L.] genitive and plural of *locus*.

**Locke's solution (fluid)** (loks) [Frank Spiller *Locke*, British physiologist, 1871–1949] see under *solution*.

**lock·jaw** (lok'jaw) trismus.

**Lock·wood's ligament** (lok'woodz) [Charles Barrett *Lockwood*, English surgeon, 1856–1914] see under *ligament*.

**lo·co** (lo'ko) [Sp. "insane"] 1. locoweed. 2. locoism. 3. an animal affected with locoism.

**Lo·coid** (lo'koid) trademark for preparations of hydrocortisone butyrate.

**lo·co·ism** (lo'ko-iz″əm) a disease of horses, cattle, and sheep caused by poisoning by any of the plants called *locoweed*; it is marked by locomotor disturbances, trembling, depression, and, in pregnant animals, absorption. Called also *loco disease* and *loco poisoning*.

**lo·co·mo·tion** (lo″ko-mo'shən) [*locus* + *motion*] [MeSH: Locomotion] movement or the ability to move from one place to another.
**brachial l.,** brachiation.

**lo·co·mo·tive** (lo″ko-mo'tiv) pertaining to locomotion.

**lo·co·mo·tor** (lo″ko-mo'tər) 1. of or pertaining to locomotion. 2. pertaining to or affecting a locomotor system; see under *system*.

**lo·co·mo·to·ri·al** (lo″ko-mo-tor'e-əl) pertaining to the locomotorium (locomotor system).

**lo·co·mo·to·ri·um** (lo″ko-mo-tor'e-əm) the structures of an organism concerned with locomotion; in humans, the bones, joints, and muscles of the lower limb, together with their vascular and nerve supplies.

**lo·co·mo·to·ry** (lo″ko-mo'tə-re) pertaining to locomotion.

**lo·co·re·gion·al** (lo″ko-re'jən-əl) limited to a localized area, as contrasted to *systemic* or *metastatic*, such as pertaining to spread of a pathological change beyond the site of origin but only into the nearby region.

**lo·co·weed** (lo'ko-wēd) [Sp. *loco* insane] any of numerous leguminous plants that grow in arid regions of North America, primarily members of the genera *Astragalus, Hosackia, Oxytropis,* and *Sophora;* they contain a variety of toxins and cause locoism in horses, cattle, and sheep.

**loc·u·lar** (lok'u-lər) pertaining to a loculus.

**loc·u·late** (lok'u-lāt) divided into loculi.

**loc·u·li** (lok'u-li) [L.] plural of *loculus*.

**loc·u·lus** (lok'u-ləs) pl. *lo'culi* [L., dim. of *locus*] 1. a small space or cavity. 2. a local enlargement of the uterus in some mammals, containing an embryo.

**lo·cum** (lo'kəm) [L., accusative of *locus*] place.
**l. te'nens, l. te'nent,** a practitioner who temporarily takes the place of another.

**lo·cus** (lo'kəs) gen. *lo'ci*, pl. *lo'ci* [L. "a place"] 1. [TA] a general anatomical term for a site in the body. 2. in genetics, the position of a gene on a chromosome, different forms of genes (alleles) being found at the same position on homologous chromosomes.
**l. caeru'leus** [TA], **l. ceru'leus,** a pigmented eminence in the superior angle of the floor of the brain. Called also *l. cinereus* and *l. coeruleus.*
**l. cine'reus, l. coeru'leus,** l. caeruleus.
**complex l.,** gene complex; see under *gene.*
**l. ferrugi'neus,** l. caeruleus.
**heteromorphic l.,** a locus that exists in two or more allelic forms.
**l. mino'ris resisten'tiae,** a site of lessened resistance; an area, structure, or organ offering little resistance to invasion by microorganisms and/or their toxins.
**operator l.,** operator gene.

**Lo·dine** (lo'dēn) trademark for preparations of etodolac.

**lo·dox·a·mide tro·meth·amine** (lo-dok'sə-mīd) a mast cell stabilizer that inhibits immediate (type I) hypersensitivity; applied topically to the eye for the treatment of vernal conjunctivitis, vernal keratitis, and vernal keratoconjunctivitis.

**Loeb's deciduoma, reaction** (lōb) [Leo *Loeb*, American pathologist, 1869–1959] see under *deciduoma* and *reaction.*

**Loef·fler** see *Löffler.*

**Loef·fler·el·la** (lef"lər-el'ə) in former systems of classification, a genus of bacteria, species of which are now assigned to *Pseudomonas.*

**LOEL** lowest observed effect level.

**Loe·wi** (lər've) Otto. German-born American physiologist and pharmacologist, 1873–1961; co-winner, with Sir Henry Hallett Dale, of the Nobel prize for medicine or physiology in 1936 for their study of the chemical transmission of nerve impulses.

**Löff·ler's coagulated serum medium, alkaline methylene blue stain** (lərf'lərz) [Friederich August Johannes *Löffler*, German bacteriologist, 1852–1915] see under *stain.*

**Löff·ler's endocarditis, syndrome (eosinophilia, pneumonia)** (lərf'lərz) [Wilhelm *Löffler*, Swiss physician, 1887–1972] see under *endocarditis* and *syndrome.*

**Löf·gren's syndrome** (lerf'grənz) [Sven Halvar *Löfgren*, Swedish physician, 20th century] see under *syndrome.*

**log·a·dec·to·my** (log"ə-dek'tə-me) [Gr. *logades* the whites of the eyes + *-ectomy*] excision of a portion of the conjunctiva.

**log·a·graph·ia** (log"ə-graf'e-ə) [*log-* + *agraphia*] agraphia.

**log·am·ne·sia** (log"am-ne'zhə) [*log-* + *amnesia*] 1. receptive aphasia. 2. any condition in which a person cannot remember words.

**log·a·pha·sia** (log"ə-fa'zhə) [*log-* + *aphasia*] motor aphasia.

**log·a·rithm** (log'ə-rith-əm) the power to which a number, fixed for a given system and usually called the base number, must be raised to obtain a second number. Logarithms are usually computed in the natural base *e*, and are denoted $\log_e$ (also expressed ln). For example, if $\log_e(y) = x$ then $e^x = y$. See also *e.*

**loge** (lōzh) [Fr.] a hut, box, or booth.
**l. de Guyon,** Guyon's canal.

**log(o)-** [Gr. *logos* word, reason] a combining form denoting relationship to words or speech.

**logo·clo·nia** (log"o-klo'ne-ə) [*logo-* + *clonus* + *-ia*] spasmodic repetition of words or parts of words, particularly the end syllables; often occurring in Alzheimer's disease. Cf. *stuttering.* Called also *logospasm.*

**logo·gram** (log'o-gram) the graphic record of the symptoms and signs exhibited by a specific patient, charted by means of the logoscope.

**logo·klony** (log'o-klon"e) logoclonia.

**logo·ma·nia** (log"o-ma'ne-ə) [*logo-* + *-mania*] logorrhea.

**log·op·a·thy** (log-op'ə-the) [*logo-* + *-pathy*] speech disorder.

**logo·pe·dia** (log"o-pe'de-ə) logopedics.

**logo·pe·dics** (log-o-pe'diks) [*logo-* + ortho*pedics*] the study and treatment of speech defects. See also *speech pathology.* Called also *logopedia.*

**logo·ple·gia** (log"o-ple'jə) [*logo-* + *-plegia*] paralysis of the speech organs.

**log·or·rhea** (log"o-re'ə) [*logo-* + *-rrhea*] excessive volubility, with rapid, pressured speech; as seen in manic episodes of bipolar disorder and in some types of schizophrenia. Called also *agitolalia, agitophasia, pressured speech, tachylalia, tachyphasia,* and *verbomania.*

**logo·spasm** (log'o-spaz-əm) 1. logoclonia. 2. stuttering.

**log·wood** (log'wood) *Haematoxylon campechianum.*

**-logy** [Gr. *logos* word, reason] a word termination meaning the science or study of, or a treatise on, the subject designated by the stem to which it is affixed.

**lo·i·a·sis** (lo-i'ə-sis) [MeSH: Loiasis] infection with nematodes of the genus *Loa;* called also *loaiasis.*

**loin** (loin) lumbus.

**Lo·li·um** (lo'le-əm) [MeSH: Lolium] the rye grasses, a genus of plants commonly found in pastures and consumed by livestock.
**L. peren'ne,** perennial rye grass, a variety that sometimes carries the fungus *Acremonium loliae,* which causes a type of rye grass staggers in ruminants. See *rye grass staggers,* def. 2, under *staggers.*
**L. ri'gidum,** Wimmera rye grass, a variety whose seed galls sometimes carry nematodes infected with species of *Corynebacterium,* causing a type of rye grass staggers in ruminants. See *rye grass staggers,* def. 1, under *staggers.*
**L. temulen'tum,** L. (Gram.), darnel, a rye grass whose seeds contain a narcotic; poisoning of humans and other animals can occur when they ingest moldy seeds. See *darnel poisoning,* under *poisoning.*

**lo·met·ra·line hy·dro·chlo·ride** (lo-met'rə-lēn) a tranquilizer and antiparkinsonian agent, $C_{13}H_{18}ClNO \cdot HCl$.

**lo·mo·fun·gin** (lo-mo-fun'jin) an antifungal antibiotic derived from *Streptomyces lomondensis* var. *lomondensis.*

**lo·mo·some** (lo'mo-sōm) [Gr. *lōma* hem, fringe + *-some*] a sponge-like structure in fungi contiguous with the hyphal wall.

**Lo·mo·til** (lo'mo-til) trademark for preparations of diphenoxylate hydrochloride and atropine.

**lo·mus·tine** (lo-mus'tēn) [MeSH: Lomustine] a cytotoxic alkylating agent of the nitrosourea (q.v.) group, used as an antineoplastic primarily for treatment of brain tumors, bronchogenic carcinoma, and Hodgkin's disease; administered orally. Called also *CCNU.*

**Lon·cho·car·pus** (lon"ko-kahr'pəs) a genus of tropical American woody plants of the family Leguminosae. *L. u'tilis* is the cubé, which yields the toxic insecticide rotenone.

**long-chain-fat·ty-ac·id–CoA li·gase** (long chān fat'e as'id ko-a' li'gās) [EC 6.2.1.3] an enzyme of the ligase class that catalyzes the formation of acyl coenzyme A from long chain fatty acids (12 or more carbons) and coenzyme A, using energy derived from ATP hydrolysis. The enzyme occurs in the mitochondrial outer membrane, endoplasmic reticulum, and peroxisome membrane, and it acts on saturated and unsaturated fatty acids as well as some hydroxy acids. Called also *acyl CoA synthetase.*

**lon·gev·i·ty** (lon-jev'ĭ-te) [L. *longus* long + *aevum* age] [MeSH: Longevity] the condition or quality of being long lived.

**lon·gi·lin·e·al** (lon"jĭ-lin'e-əl) built along long, narrow lines; dolichomorphic.

**lon·gi·man·ous** (lon"ji-man'əs) [*longus* + *manus*] having long hands.

**lon·gi·pe·date** (lon"jĭ-pe'dāt) [*longus* + *ped-*[2] + *-ate*] having long feet.

**lon·gis·si·mus** (lon-jis'ĭ-məs) [L. "longest, very long"] a general term denoting a long structure, as a muscle.

**lon·gi·tu·di·nal** (lon"jĭ-too'di-nəl) [L. *longitudo* length] lengthwise; parallel to the long axis of the body or an organ.

**lon·gi·tu·di·na·lis** (lon"ji-too"di-na'lis) [L.] [TA] lengthwise; a term denoting a structure that is parallel to the long axis of the body or an organ.

**lon·gi·typ·i·cal** (lon"ji-tip'ĭ-kəl) longilineal; dolichomorphic.

**long·sight·ed·ness** (long-sīt'əd -nəs) hyperopia.

**lon·gus** (long'gəs) [L.] [TA] long; a general term denoting a long structure, as a muscle.

**loop** (lo͞op) 1. a turn or sharp curve in a cordlike structure; see also *ansa.* 2. something, such as a figure or course, having such a curved or circular shape. 3. an instrument used in microbiology, consisting of a rod-shaped metal handle holding a firm wire, usually platinum or nichrome, formed into a loop at the free end. The standard loop has an inside diameter of 4 mm. It is used for the inoculation of cultures of bacteria and fungi.
**amplification l.,** in positive feedback, the loop through which increased output subsequently increases input and so increases output.
**bulboventricular l.,** ventricular l.
**capillary l's,** minute endothelial tubes that carry blood in the papillae of the skin.
**cervical l.,** peripheral cuboidal cells of the enamel organ that encircle the edge of a developing tooth.
**closed l.,** a type of feedback in which the input to one or more of the subsystems is affected by its own output.

**feedback l.**, the circular path seen in a system that has feedback, such that the output of the system participates in the control of the system.
**gamma l.**, a three-part reflex arc consisting of gamma motoneurons that send impulses along the gamma fibers to the intrafusal fibers, causing the muscle spindle to contract; that in turn excites afferent impulses, which pass through the posterior root to alpha motoneurons in the anterior horn, causing a stretch reflex. Called also *Granit l.*
**Gerdy's interatrial l.**, a small muscular bundle in the interatrial septum of the heart.
**Granit l.**, gamma l.
**l. of Henle, Henle's l.**, ansa nephroni.
**l. of hypoglossal nerve,** ansa cervicalis.
**Hyrtl's l.**, an occasional looplike anastomosis between the right and left hypoglossal nerves in the geniohyoid muscle.
**Ivy l.**, see under *wiring*.
**lenticular l.**, ansa lenticularis.
**Meyer's l.**, one formed by some of the fibers of the optic radiation as they loop around the inferior horn of the lateral ventricle before turning posteriorly.
**Meyer-Archambault l.**, Meyer's l.
**open l.**, a system in which an input alters the output, but the output has no effect on the input. See also *feedback*.
**peduncular l.**, ansa peduncularis.
**pressure-volume l's,** graphic representations of the pressure within cardiac ventricles as a function of their volumes, recorded over the course of the cardiac cycle under various conditions, such as increased preload or afterload; and used to assess cardiac contractility.
**sentinel l.**, a distended loop of small intestine near the pancreas seen on plain films of the abdomen in acute pancreatitis.
**l's of spinal nerves,** ansae nervorum spinalium.
**Storck's l.**, the primitive loop in the embryonic uriniferous tubule which develops into a Henle loop and a portion of the proximal convoluted tubule.
**subclavian l.**, ansa subclavia.
**ventricular l.**, the early U-shaped loop of the embryonic heart; called also *bulboventricular l.*
**l. of Vieussens,** ansa subclavia.

**loop·ful** (lo͞op'fəl) the quantity of liquid that can be held within the loop of wire used in transferring microorganisms to other culture media.

**loo·sen·ing** (loo'sən-ing) freeing from restraint or strictness.
**l. of associations,** in psychiatry, a disorder of thinking in which associations of ideas become so shortened, fragmented, and disturbed as to lack logical relationship; often seen in schizophrenia.

**Loo·ser's transformation zones** (lo'zərz) [Emil *Looser,* Swiss surgeon, 1877–1936] see under *zone*.

**Loo·ser-Milk·man syndrome** (lo'zər milk'man) [Emil *Looser;* Louis Arthur *Milkman,* American radiologist, 1895–1951] Milkman's syndrome.

**LOP** left occipitoposterior (position of the fetus).

**lo·per·amide hy·dro·chlo·ride** (lo-per'ə-mīd) an antiperistaltic which exerts a direct effect on the muscles of the intestinal wall; used in the treatment of acute nonspecific diarrhea and chronic diarrhea associated with inflammatory bowel disease and to reduce the volume of discharge from ileostomies. It is administered orally.

**loph(o)-** [Gr. *lophos* ridge, tuft] a combining form denoting a relationship to a ridge or to a tuft.

**loph·odont** (lof'o-dont) [*lopho-* + Gr. *odous* tooth] having cheek teeth on which the cusps have become connected to form ridges, as in elephants and some rodents.

**Lo·phoph·o·ra** (lo-fof'ə-rə) [*lopho-* + Gr. *phoros* bearing] a genus of Mexican cacti (family Cactaceae). *L. william'sii* (Lemaire) Coult. is mescal, the source of mescal buttons, which contain peyote and mescaline.

**lo·phoph·o·rine** (lo-fof'ə-rēn) a poisonous alkaloid from *Lophophora williamsii,* having effects similar to those of mescaline.

**lo·phot·ri·chous** (lo-fot'rĭ-kəs) [*lopho-* + Gr. *thrix* hair] having two or more flagella at one or both ends; said of a bacterial cell. See *flagellum*.

**Lo·pid** (lo'pid) trademark for a preparation of gemfibrozil.

**Lo·pres·sor** (lo-pres'or) trademark for preparations of metoprolol tartrate.

**Lo·prox** (lo'proks) trademark for a preparation of ciclopirox olamine.

**Lo·pur·in** (lo-pūr'in) trademark for preparations of allopurinol.

**Lor·a·bid** (lor'ə-bid) trademark for a preparation of loracarbef.

**lor·a·car·bef** (lor"ə-kahr'bef) [USP] a carbacephem antibiotic closely related to cefaclor and having similar antibacterial activity, used in the treatment of infections of the urinary and respiratory tracts and of the skin and soft tissues; administered orally.

**Lo·rain's infantilism (disease)** (lo-raz') [Paul Joseph *Lorain,* Paris physician, 1827–1875] hypophysial infantilism.

**Lo·rain-Lévi dwarfism (syndrome)** (lo-ră' la-ve') [P.J. *Lorain;* E. Léopold *Lévi,* French endocrinologist, 1868–1933] hypophysial infantilism.

**Lor·an·tha·ceae** the mistletoes, a family of parasitic plants found in Europe, Asia, and North America. It includes the genera *Phoradendron* and *Viscum*.

**lor·at·a·dine** (lə-rat'ə-dēn) [MeSH: Loratadine] an $H_1$ receptor antagonist used for the treatment of hay fever and chronic idiopathic urticaria and as a treatment adjunct in asthma; administered orally.

**lor·a·ze·pam** (lor-az'ə-pam) [USP] [MeSH: Lorazepam] a benzodiazepine with anxiolytic and sedative effects, administered orally in the treatment of anxiety disorders and short-term relief of anxiety symptoms and as a sedative-hypnotic agent, and intravenously or intramuscularly for preanesthetic medication; used also intravenously to control status epilepticus and as an antiemetic in cancer chemotherapy.

**lor·do·sco·li·o·sis** (lor"do-sko"le-o'sis) [*lordosis* + *scoliosis*] lordosis complicated with scoliosis.

**lor·do·sis** (lor-do'sis) [Gr. *lōrdosis*] [MeSH: Lordosis] 1. the anterior concavity in the curvature of the lumbar and cervical spine as viewed from the side. 2. abnormal increase in this curvature; called also *hollow back, saddle back,* and *swayback.* Cf. *kyphosis* and *scoliosis*.

**lor·dot·ic** (lor-dot'ik) pertaining to or characterized by lordosis.

**Lo·rel·co** (lo-rel'ko) trademark for a preparation of probucol.

**Lor·enz** (lor'ənts) Konrad Zacharias. Austrian zoologist born 1903; co-winner, with Karl von Frisch and Nikolaas Tinbergen, of the Nobel prize for medicine or physiology for 1973, for his pioneer work in ethology, particularly on imprinting and aggression.

**Lor·enz's operation, osteotomy** (lor'ənts-əz) [Adolf *Lorenz,* Austrian surgeon, 1854–1946] see under *operation* and *osteotomy*.

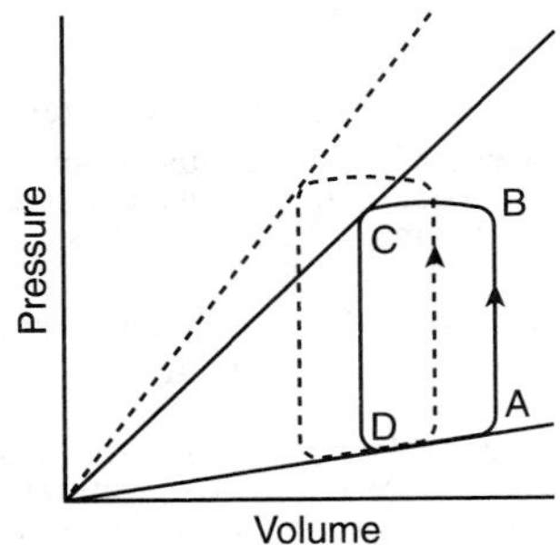

Pressure-volume loops comparing a control state *(solid line)* and a positive inotropic state *(dotted line),* such as that due to adrenergic stimulation, assuming constant stroke volume. Beginning with *A,* end-diastole, the period from *A* to *B* represents isovolumetric left ventricular contraction. Ejection occurs from *B,* opening of the aortic valve to *C,* end-systole. The period from *C* to *D,* opening of the mitral valve, represents isovolumetric relaxation, and is followed by ventricular filling in the period from *D* to *A*.

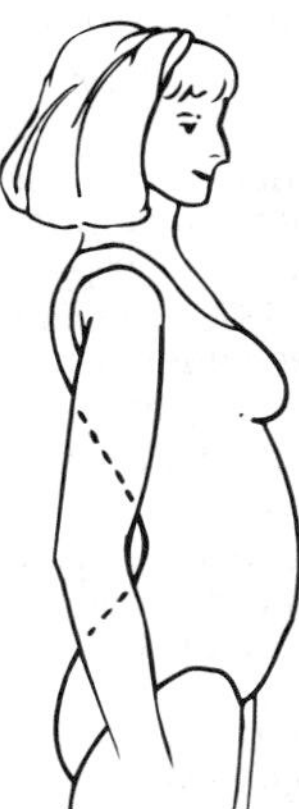
Abnormally increased curvature of the lower spine characteristic of lordosis.

**Lor·fan** (lor′fan) trademark for preparations of levallorphan tartrate.

**lo·ri·ca** (lo-ri′kə) pl. *lori′cae* [L. "leather cuirass"] a protective rigid encasement or shell, secreted or created by cementing together of various materials, as seen in some invertebrates such as certain protozoa and many rotifers.

**lor·i·cate** (lor′ĭ-kāt) enclosed in a lorica.

**Lor·i·dine** (lor′ĭ-dēn) trademark for a preparation of cephaloridine.

**Lor·tab** (lor′tab) trademark for a preparation of hydrocodone bitartrate.

**lo·sar·tan po·tas·si·um** (lo-sahr′tan) an angiotensin II receptor antagonist, used as an antihypertensive; administered orally.

**loss** (laws) escape of something from its proper place.
**hearing l.**, see under H.

**Los·sen's rule (law)** (los′ənz) [Herman Friedrich *Lossen,* German surgeon, 1842–1909] see under *rule.*

**LOT** left occipitotransverse (position of the fetus).

**Lot.** abbreviation for L. *lo′tio,* lotion.

**Lo·ten·sin** (lo-ten′sin) trademark for a preparation of benazepril hydrochloride.

**lo·tio** (lo′she-o) [L., from *lotus,* past participle of *lavare* to wash] lotion.
**l. al′ba, l. sulfura′ta,** white lotion.

**Lo·tio·blanc** (lo″she-o-blangk′) trademark for a preparation of white lotion.

**lo·tion** (lo′shən) [L. *lotio*] a liquid suspension or dispersion for external application to the body.
**benzyl benzoate l.** [USP], a watery solution of benzyl benzoate, triethanolamine, and oleic acid; used as a topical scabicide.
**benzyl benzoate-chlorophenothane-benzocaine l.,** a watery solution of benzyl benzoate, chlorophenothane, benzocaine, and polysorbate 80; used as a scabicide and pediculicide, applied topically.
**calamine l.** [USP], a preparation of calamine with zinc oxide, glycerin, bentonite magma, and calcium hydroxide solution, used topically as a protectant.
**calamine l., phenolated** [USP], a mixture of calamine lotion and liquefied phenol, used topically as a protectant.
**gamma benzene hexachloride l.,** lindane l.
**Goulard's l.,** diluted lead subacetate solution.
**lindane l.** [USP], a preparation of gamma benzene hexachloride in an aqueous vehicle, used as a pediculicide and scabicide; applied topically to the skin. Called also *gamma benzene hexachloride l.*
**methylbenzethonium chloride l.** [USP], an emulsion containing 0.067 per cent methylbenzethonium chloride; used as a local anti-infective, applied topically to the genitalia, rectum, thighs, and intertriginous areas in the treatment of ammonia dermatitis and in the treatment and prevention of dermatoses caused by contact with urine, feces, and perspiration.
**white l.** [USP], a preparation of zinc sulfate, sulfurated potash, and purified water, used as a topical astringent and protectant; called also *lotio alba.*

**Lo·trel** (lo′trel) trademark for a preparation of amlodipine besylate combined with benazepril hydrochloride.

**Lo·trim·in** (lo′trĭ-min) trademark for preparation of clotrimazole.

**Lo·tri·sone** (lo′trĭ-sōn″) trademark for a combination preparation of betamethasone dipropionate and clotrimazole.

**Lo·tus** (lo′tus) a genus of plants of the family Leguminosae, often found in pastures and used for animal feed. *L. america′nus* and *L. cornicula′tus,* both called bird's foot trefoil, contain a cyanogenetic compound that can cause cyanide poisoning in livestock.

**Lo·tu·sate** (lo′tə-sāt) trademark for a preparation of talbutal.

**Lou Geh·rig disease** (loo′ ger′ig) [Lou *Gehrig,* American baseball player, 1903–1941, who died of the disease] [MeSH: Amyotrophic Lateral Sclerosis] see *amyotrophic lateral sclerosis,* under *sclerosis.*

**Lou·is's angle, law** (loo-ēz′) [Pierre Charles Alexandre *Louis,* French physician, 1787–1872; the founder of medical statistics] see *angulus sterni,* and see under *law.*

**Lou·is-Bar's syndrome** (loo-e′bahrz) [Denise *Louis-Bar,* Belgian neuropathologist, 20th century] ataxia-telangiectasia; see under *ataxia.*

**loupe** (lo͞op) [Fr. "magnifying glass"] a convex lens for low magnification of minute objects at very close range; it may be monocular or binocular, held in the hand, set in a headband, or mounted on spectacles.

**louse** (lous) pl. *lice* [L. *pediculus*] any of various wingless insects parasitic on birds and mammals, including humans; they are classified into two orders, Anoplura (the sucking lice) and Mallophaga (the bird lice or biting lice). The causal organisms of typhus, relapsing fever, trench fever, and other diseases are transmitted by the bite of lice.
**bird l.,** 1. a biting louse of birds. 2. any biting louse.
**biting l.,** any member of the order Mallophaga.
**body l.,** *Pediculus humanus corporis.*
**chicken l.,** any of the various types of biting lice that infest chickens.
**clothes l.,** *Pediculus humanus corporis.*
**crab l.,** *Phthirus pubis.*
**foot l. of sheep,** *Linognathus pedalis.*
**goat sucking l.,** *Linognathus stenopis.*
**head l.,** *Pediculus humanus capitis.*
**long-nosed cattle l.,** *Linognathus vituli.*
**pubic l.,** *Phthirus pubis.*
**short-nosed cattle l.,** *Haematopinus eurysterni.*
**sucking l.,** any member of the order Anoplura.

**louse·wort** (lows′wort) *Delphinium staphisagria.*

**lous·i·cide** (lous′i-sīd) pediculicide.

**lov·a·sta·tin** (lo′və-stat″in) [USP] [MeSH: Lovastatin] an inhibitor of cholesterol biosynthesis used in the treatment of hypercholesterolemia; administered orally.

**Lo·ve·nox** (lo-ve′noks) trademark for a preparation of enoxaparin.

**Lö·we's ring** (lər′vəz) [Karl Friedrich *Löwe,* German optician, 1874–1955] see under *ring.*

**Lowe's syndrome (disease)** (lōz) [Charles Upton *Lowe,* American pediatrician, born 1921] oculocerebrorenal syndrome.

**Lowe-Ter·rey-Mac·Lach·lan syndrome** (lo-tar′e-mək-lahk′lən) [C. U. *Lowe; Mary Terrey,* American physician, 20th century; Elsie A. *MacLachlan,* American physician, 20th century] oculocerebrorenal syndrome.

**Lö·wen·berg's canal (scala), forceps** (lər′vən-bərgz) [Benjamin Benno *Löwenberg,* German otologist in Vienna and Paris, 1836–1905] see under *forceps* and see *ductus cochlearis.*

**Lö·wen·thal's tract** (lər′vən-tahlz) [Wilhelm *Löwenthal,* German physician, 1850–1894] tractus tectospinalis.

**Low·er's rings, tubercle** (lo′ərz) [Richard *Lower,* English anatomist, 1631–1691] see *anulus fibrosus dexter/sinister cordis* and *tuberculum intervenosum.*

**low·er·ing** (lo′ər-ing) a decrease.
**vapor pressure l.,** the decrease of the vapor pressure of a solution below that of the pure solvent; the percentage change in vapor pressure is equal to the mole fraction of the solute (osmoles of solute per osmoles of solute plus solvent) and is proportional to the osmolality.

**low-grade** (lo′grād′) occurring near the low end of a range, as of a fever or malignancy.

**Lown-Gan·ong-Le·vine syndrome** (loun-gan′ong-lə-vīn′) [Bernard *Lown,* American cardiologist, born 1921; William F. *Ganong,* American physiologist, born 1924; Samuel Albert *Levine,* Polish-born American cardiologist, 1891–1966] [MeSH: Lown-Ganong-Levine Syndrome] see under *syndrome.*

**lox·a·pine** (lok′sə-pēn) [MeSH: Loxapine] a tricyclic dibenzoxazepine derivative with antiemetic, sedative, anticholinergic, and α-antiadrenergic actions; used as an antipsychotic.
**l. hydrochloride,** the hydrochloride salt of loxapine, used as an antipsychotic; administered intramuscularly.
**l. succinate** [USP], the succinate salt of loxapine, used as an antipsychotic; administered orally.

**lox·ar·thron** (loks-ahr′thron) [Gr. *loxos* oblique + *arthron* joint] an oblique deformity of a joint without luxation.

**lox·ar·thro·sis** (loks″ahr-thro′sis) loxarthron.

**lox·ia** (lok′se-ə) torticollis.

**Lox·i·tane** (lok′sĭ-tān) trademark for preparations of loxapine.

**Lox·os·ce·les** (lok-sos′ə-lēz) a genus of six-eyed spiders of the family Loxoscelidae, whose bite causes loxoscelism. *L. lae′ta* is the brown spider of South America and *L. reclu′sa* is the brown recluse spider of North America.

**Lox·os·cel·i·dae** (lok″so-sel′ĭ-de) a family of spiders (suborder Labidognatha), the false hackled band spinners, which includes the genus *Loxosceles.*

**lox·os·ce·lism** (lok-sos′ə-liz-əm) a form of arachnidism caused by the bite of *Loxosceles laeta* (the brown spider) or *L. reclusa* (the brown recluse spider), seen from South America to southern North America; it begins with a painful erythematous vesicle and progresses to a gangrenous slough of the affected area.
**viscerocutaneous l.,** a sometimes fatal condition resulting from the bite of the brown spider, with fever and hematuria in addition to the local reaction.

**lox·ot·o·my** (lok-sot′ə-me) [Gr. *loxos* oblique + *-tomy*] oval amputation.

**Lox·o·tre·ma ova·tum** (lok″so-tre′mə o-va′təm) *Metagonimus yokogawai.*

**loz·enge** (loz′ənj) [Fr.] 1. a medicated tablet or disk; a troche. 2. a triangular area of tissue marked for excision in plastic surgery.

**Lo·zol** (lo′zol) trademark for a preparation of indapamide.

**Lp(a)** see under *lipoprotein.*

**LPF** low-power field.

**LPH** left posterior hemiblock; lipotropic hormone.

**LPN** Licensed Practical Nurse.

**LPS** lipopolysaccharide (def. 2).

**LPV** lymphotropic papovavirus.

**Lr** symbol for *limes reacting;* see *Lr dose,* under *dose.*

**LRD** living related donor.

**LSA** left sacroanterior (position of the fetus); Licentiate of Society of Apothecaries.

**LScA** left scapuloanterior (position of the fetus).

**LScP** left scapuloposterior (position of the fetus).

**LSD** lysergic acid diethylamide.

**LSO** lumbosacral orthosis.

**LSP** left sacroposterior (position of the fetus).

**LST** left sacrotransverse (position of the fetus).

**LT** lymphotoxin.

**$LTB_4$, $LTC_4$,** etc. symbols for various leukotrienes; see *leukotriene.*

**LTF** lymphocyte-transforming factor.

**LTR** long terminal repeat.

**Lu** symbol for *lutetium.*

**Lu·barsch's crystals** (loo′bahrsh-əz) [Otto *Lubarsch,* German pathologist, 1860–1933] see under *crystal.*

**lubb** (lub) a syllable used to represent, or mimic, the first sound of the heart in auscultation. See *lubb-dupp.*

**lubb-dupp** (ləb-dup′) syllables used to represent the combination of the first and second heart sounds. See *lubb* and *dupp.*

**lu·bri·cant** (loo′brĭ-kənt) [MeSH: Lubrication] a substance that is applied as a surface film to reduce friction between moving parts; see also under *laxative.*

**Luc's operation** (lūks) [Henri *Luc,* French laryngologist, 1855–1925] Caldwell-Luc operation.

**Lu·cas' sign** (loo′kəs) [Richard Clement *Lucas,* English surgeon, 1846–1915] see under *sign.*

**Lu·ci·bac·te·ri·um** (loo″si-bak-te′re-əm) [L. *lux* light + *bacterium*] a genus formerly comprising the vibrios, now assigned to the species *Vibrio harveyi.*

**lu·cid** (loo′sid) [L. *lucidus* clear] clear; not obscure; as, *lucid* interval.

**lu·cid·i·ty** (loo-sid′ĭ-te) the quality or state of having a clear mind; clearness of the mind.

**lu·cif·er·ase** (loo-sif′ər-ās) [MeSH: Luciferase] trivial name for a variety of monooxygenases that catalyze a reaction producing bioluminescence in certain marine crustaceans, fish, bacteria, and insects [EC 1.13.12.5–8, 1.14.14.3, 1.14.99.21]. The enzyme is a flavoprotein that oxidizes luciferin to an electronically excited compound that emits energy in the form of light. The color of light emitted varies with the organism. The firefly enzyme is a valuable reagent for measurement of ATP concentration.

**lu·cif·er·in** (loo-sif′ər-in) [MeSH: Luciferin] a heterocyclic phenol which can be reduced and oxidized. It exists in many forms and is present in certain animals capable of bioluminescence; when acted upon by luciferase, in the presence of ATP and molecular oxygen, it produces light.

**lu·cif·u·gal** (loo-sif′u-gəl) [*lux* + *-fugal*] avoiding, or being repelled by, bright light.

**Lu·cil·ia** (loo-sil′e-ə) *Phaenicia.*

**Lu·cio's leprosy, phenomenon** (loo′syōz) [Rafael *Lucio* Nájera, Mexican physician, 1819–1886] see under *leprosy* and *phenomenon.*

**lu·cip·e·tal** (loo-sip′ĭ-təl) [*lux* + *-petal*] seeking, or being attracted to, bright light.

**Lücke's test** (lēk′əz) [George Albert *Lücke,* German surgeon, 1829–1894] see under *test.*

**lück·en·schä·del** (lēk′en-sha″dəl) [Ger. "skull (with) gaps"] craniolacunia.

**lu·co·ther·a·py** (loo″ko-ther′ə-pe) [L. *lux,* gen. *lucis* light + *therapy*] phototherapy.

**Lu·di·o·mil** (loo′de-o-mil) trademark for a preparation of maprotiline hydrochloride.

**Lud·loff's sign** (lood′lawfs) [Karl *Ludloff,* German surgeon, 1864–1945] see under *sign.*

**Lud·wig's angina** (lood′vigz) [Wilhelm Friedrich von *Ludwig,* German surgeon, 1790–1865] [MeSH: Ludwig's Angina] see under *angina.*

**Lud·wig's angle** (lood′vigz) [Daniel *Ludwig,* German anatomist, 1625–1680] angulus sterni.

**Lud·wig's ganglion, nerve** (lood′vigz) [Karl Friedrich Wilhelm *Ludwig,* German physiologist, 1816–1895] see under *ganglion,* and see *Cyon's nerve* under *nerve.*

**Lu·er's syringe** (loo′ərz) [*Luer,* a German instrument maker in France, 19th century] see under *syringe.*

**lu·es** (loo′ēz) [L. "a plague"] syphilis.

**lu·et·ic** (loo-et′ik) syphilitic.

**Luft's disease** (loofts) [Rolf *Luft,* Swedish endocrinologist, born 1914] see under *disease.*

**lug** (lug) 1. a projecting part that holds or supports something. 2. the part of a dental casting that projects.
**retention l.,** a piece of metal soldered either to an orthodontic band or to an artificial crown to create greater undercut for retention of a dental prosthesis.

**Lu·gol's caustic,** etc. (loo-golz′) [Jean Guillaume Auguste *Lugol,* French physician, 1786–1851] see under *caustic, iodine,* and *stain,* and see *strong iodine solution,* under *solution.*

**Lukes-Col·lins Classification** (lo͝oks-kol′ənz) [L. J. *Lukes,* American pathologist, 20th century; R. D. *Collins,* American pathologist, 20th century] see under *classification.*

**LUL** left upper lobe; see *lobus superior pulmonis sinistri.*

**lu·lib·er·in** (loo-lib′ər-in) [*lu*tropin + *-liberin*] luteinizing hormone–releasing hormone.

**lum·ba·go** (ləm-ba′go) [L. *lumbus* loin] pain in the lumbar region.
**ischemic l.,** pain in the lower back and buttock(s) due to vascular insufficiency, as in terminal aortic occlusion.

**lum·bar** (lum′bahr) pertaining to the loins, the parts of the sides of the back between the thorax and the pelvis.

**lum·bar·iza·tion** (lum″bər-ĭ-za′shən) a condition in which the first segment of the sacrum is not fused with the second, so that there is one additional articulated vertebra and the sacrum consists of only four segments.

**lumb(o)-** [L. *lumbus* loin] a combining form denoting relationship to the loins.

**lum·bo·ab·dom·i·nal** (lum″bo-ab-dom′i-nəl) pertaining to the loins and abdomen; pertaining to the sides and the front of the abdomen.

**lum·bo·co·los·to·my** (lum″bo-ko-los′tə-me) [*lumbo-* + *colostomy*] the operation of forming a permanent opening into the colon by an incision through the lumbar region.

**lum·bo·co·lot·o·my** (lum″bo-ko-lot′ə-me) [*lumbo-* + *colotomy*] an incision into the colon through the loin.

**lum·bo·cos·tal** (lum″bo-kos′təl) pertaining to the loin and ribs.

**lum·bo·cru·ral** (lum″bo-kroo′rəl) pertaining to, affecting or extending between the lumbar and crural regions.

**lum·bo·dor·sal** (lum″bo-dor′səl) pertaining to the lumbar and thoracic (formerly called dorsal) regions.

**lum·bo·dyn·ia** (lum″bo-din′e-ə) [*lumbo-* + *-odynia*] lumbago.

**lum·bo·il·i·ac** (lum″bo-il′e-ak) pertaining to the loin and ilium.

**lum·bo·in·gui·nal** (lum″bo-ing′gwĭ-nəl) pertaining to the loins and the groin.

**lum·bo·sa·cral** (lum″bo-sa′krəl) pertaining to the loins and sacrum.

**lum·bri·cal** (lum′bri-kəl) 1. lumbricoid (def. 1). 2. a muscle of the hand; see *musculi lumbricales.*

**lum·bri·ci** (ləm-bri′si) [L.] plural of *lumbricus.*

**lum·bri·cide** (lum′brĭ-sīd) [*lumbricus* + *-cide*] ascaricide.

**lum·bri·coid** (lum′brĭ-koid) [*lumbricus* + *-oid*] 1. pertaining to or resembling an earthworm, especially *Ascaris lumbricoides;* called also lumbrical. 2. *Ascaris lumbricoides.*

**lum·bri·co·sis** (lum″brĭ-ko′sis) ascariasis.

**Lum·bri·cus** (ləm-bri′kəs) [L. "earthworm"] a genus of annelids. *L. terres′tris* is the common earthworm, which may act as a host of the nematode *Metastrongylus elongatus,* the intermediate host of the swine influenza virus.

**lum·bri·cus** (ləm-bri′kəs) pl. *lumbri′ci* [L.] 1. ascaris. 2. any member of the genus *Lumbricus;* an earthworm.

**lum·bus** (lum′bəs) [L.] loin: the part of the back between the thorax and the pelvis; see also *regio lumbaris.*

**lu·men** (loo′mən) pl. *lu′mina, lumens* [L. "light"] 1. the cavity or channel within a tube or tubular organ. 2. the unit of luminous flux: it is the flux emitted in a solid angle of one steradian by a uniform point source with luminous intensity of one candela.

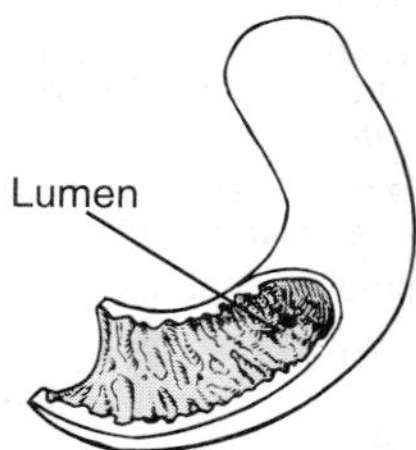


Lumen of the intestine in a cutaway view.

**residual l.,** the remains of the hypophyseal pouch *(Rathke's pouch),* located between the pars distalis and pars intermedia of the pituitary gland.

**lu·mi·chrome** (loo′mĭ-krōm) chemical name: 7,8-dimethylalloxazine; a product of the irradiation decomposition of riboflavin.

**lu·mi·fla·vin** (loo″mĭ-fla′vin) chemical name: 7,8,10-trimethylisoalloxazine; a product of the luminiferous decomposition of riboflavin.

**lu·mi·na** (loo′mĭ-nə) [L.] plural of *lumen.*

**Lu·mi·nal** (loo′mĭ-nəl) trademark for preparations of phenobarbital.

**lu·mi·nal** (loo′mĭ-nəl) pertaining to the lumen of a tubular structure.

**lu·mi·na·lis** (loo″mĭ-na′lis) [TA] luminal.

**lu·mi·nance** (loo′mĭ-nəns) the luminous intensity per unit of projected area of a surface as viewed in a given direction. Symbol *L.*

**lu·mi·nes·cence** (loo″mĭ-nes′əns) [MeSH: Luminescence] the property of giving off light without showing a corresponding degree of heat.

**lu·mi·nif·er·ous** (loo″mĭ-nif′ər-əs) [*lumen* + *-ferous*] conveying light or propagating those vibrations which constitute light.

**lu·mi·no·phor** (loo′mĭ-no-for″) [L. *lumen* light + Gr. *phoros* bearing] a chemical group that gives the property of luminescence to organic compounds.

**lu·mi·nous** (loo′mi-nəs) emitting or reflecting light; glowing with light.

**lu·mi·rho·dop·sin** (loo″mĭ-ro-dop′sin) a transient intermediate produced upon irradiation of rhodopsin in the visual cycle; see illustration at *visual cycle,* under *cycle.*

**lum·pec·to·my** (ləm-pek′tə-me) 1. surgical excision of only the palpable lesion in carcinoma of the breast; called also *tylectomy.* 2. surgical removal of a mass. Cf. *excisional biopsy.*

**Lums·den's center** (lumz′dənz) [Thomas William *Lumsden,* British physician, 1874–1953] pneumotaxic center.

**lu·na·cy** (loo′nə-se) [L. *luna* moon] *(obs.)* insanity; so named because it was supposed to be sometimes due to or affected by the influence of the moon.

**lu·nar** (loo′nər) [L. *luna* moon; in alchemy, silver, for which the moon was the symbol] pertaining to or containing silver, as lunar caustic (silver nitrate).

**lu·na·re** (loo-na′re) the lunate bone (os lunatum [TA]).

**lu·nate** (loo′nāt) [L. *luna* moon] moon-shaped, or crescentic; see *os lunatum.*

**lu·na·tic** (loo′nə-tik) [L. *lunaticus;* from *luna* moon] *(obs.)* a mentally deranged person.

**lu·na·to·ma·la·cia** (loo-na″to-mə-la′shə) osteochondrosis of the semilunar (carpal lunate) bone; see *Kienböck's disease,* under *disease.*

**Lund-Brow·der classification** (lund-brou′der) [C. C. *Lund,* American surgeon, 1895–1972; N.C. *Browder,* American pediatrician, 20th century] see under *classification.*

**lung** (lung) [L. *pulmo;* Gr. *pneumōn* or *pleumōn*] [MeSH: Lung] either of the pair of organs of respiration, one on the right and one on the left of the thorax (*pulmo dexter* [TA] and *pulmo sinister* [TA]), which are separated from each other by the heart and mediastinal structures. The right lung is composed of upper, middle, and lower lobes, and the left, of upper and lower lobes (see under *lobus*). Pulmonary disorders may be confined to, or localized in, one or more of the segments of the lobes. Each lung consists of an external serous coat (the visceral layer of the pleura), subserous areolar tissue, and lung parenchyma. The latter is made up of lobules, which are bound together by connective tissue. A primary lobule or *terminal respiratory unit* consists of a terminal bronchiole, respiratory bronchioles, and alveolar ducts, which communicate with many alveoli, each alveolus being surrounded by a network of capillary blood vessels. It is between the alveoli and capillaries that gas exchange takes place. See Plates 27 and 49.

**accessory l.,** pulmonary sequestration.

**air conditioner l.,** humidifier l.

**arc welder's l.,** welder's l.

**artificial l.,** oxygenator.

**bauxite l.,** see under *pneumoconiosis.*

**bird breeder's l., bird fancier's l., bird handler's l.,** pigeon breeder's l.

**black l.,** coal workers' pneumoconiosis.

**book l., book-l.,** a lunglike invagination that functions as a gas exchange organ, found on the underside of the abdomen of many arachnids, which opens to the surface by means of a spiracle and contains numerous thin membranous lamellae arranged like book leaves.

**brown l.,** byssinosis.

**cadmium l.,** an occupational disease similar to metal fume fever, caused by inhalation of cadmium dust or fumes; severe cases can be fatal. Cf. *cadmiosis.*

**cardiac l.,** chronic congestion of the lung due to mitral stenosis or left ventricular failure.

**cheese handler's l., cheese washer's l.,** hypersensitivity pneumonitis occurring in workers who wash the mold from cheeses during the aging process, caused by inhalation of spores of *Penicillium* from moldy cheese casings.

**coal miner's l.,** coal workers' pneumoconiosis.

**cobalt l.,** hard metal disease.

**corundum smelter's l.,** bauxite pneumoconiosis.

**epoxy resin l.,** a type of hypersensitivity pneumonitis caused by inhalation of the fumes of heated epoxy resin that contains phthalic anhydride.

**farmer's l.,** a type of hypersensitivity pneumonitis caused by inhalation of moldy hay dust, characterized by breathlessness with cyanosis or with a dry cough, anorexia, and weight loss. It is most often associated with inhalation of spores of *Micropolyspora faeni* or *Thermoactinomyces vulgaris.* Called also *thresher's l.* and *harvester's l.* See also *farmer's lung disease of cattle.*

**fibroid l.,** a lung affected with chronic fibrosis.

**grain handler's l.,** a type of hypersensitivity pneumonitis occurring in those exposed to grain, probably caused by fungal contaminants. See also *grain fever,* under *fever.*

**harvester's l.,** farmer's l.

**honeycomb l.,** the appearance of multiple small radiolucent shadows on the lung x-ray, representing dilatations of the lung parenchyma, such as in idiopathic pulmonary fibrosis; it is also seen with multiple small cysts or cavities.

**humidifier l.,** hypersensitivity pneumonitis caused by inhalation of air that has been passed through humidifiers, dehumidifiers, or air conditioners contaminated by any of a variety of fungi, amebas, or thermophilic actinomycetes. See also *humidifier fever,* under *fever.*

**hyperlucent l.,** unilateral emphysema.

**iron l.,** a popular name for the Drinker respirator.

**Labrador l.,** a type of mixed dust pneumoconiosis occurring in iron miners in western Labrador, caused by a mixture of particles of iron, silica, and some anthophyllite (a variety of amphibole asbestos); see also *siderosilicosis.*

**left l.,** see *lung.*

**malt worker's l.,** hypersensitivity pneumonitis in brewery and distillery workers, a form of allergic aspergillosis caused by inhalation of barley dust containing spores of *Aspergillus clavatus* and *A. fumigatus* during the malting process.

**mason's l.,** pneumoconiosis (usually silicosis) in stone masons due to the inhalation of stone dusts.

**meat wrapper's l.,** a type of hypersensitivity pneumonitis seen in meat wrappers, caused by inhalation of fumes of phthalic anhydride contained in the label or in the polyvinylchloride wrapping.

**miller's l.,** a type of hypersensitivity pneumonitis seen in those who work with grains or flours contaminated with the wheat weevil *Sitophilus granarius.*

**miner's l.,** coal workers' pneumoconiosis.

**mushroom worker's l.,** a type of farmer's lung seen in those working on mushroom farms, due to inhalation of mold spores from mushroom beds.

**pigeon breeder's l.,** a type of hypersensitivity pneumonitis caused by an acquired sensitivity to bird feces following intimate contact

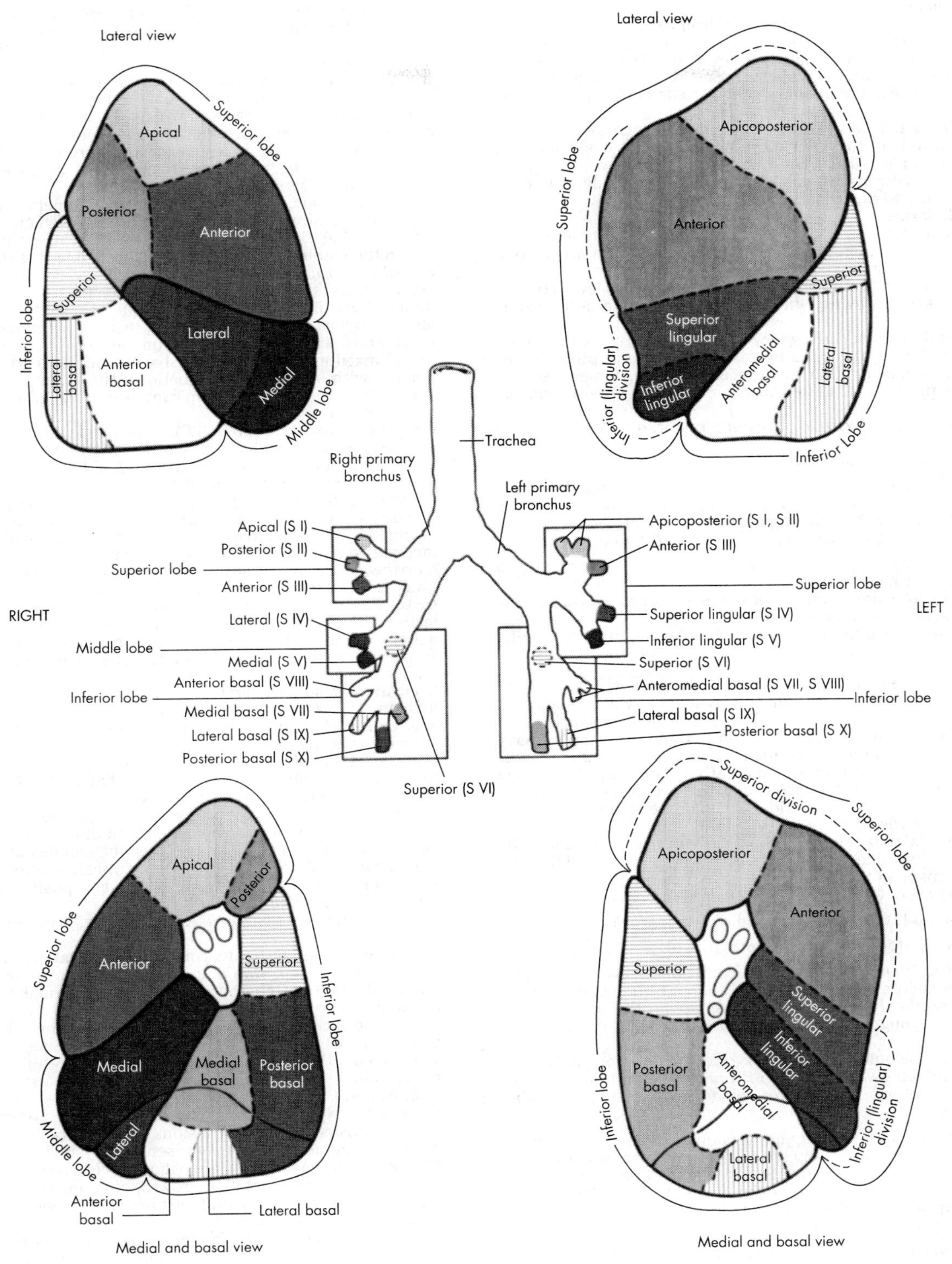


**PLATE 27**—PULMONARY SEGMENTS. TRACHEOBRONCHIAL BRANCHING CORRELATED WITH SUBDIVISION OF THE LUNGS.

with birds; symptoms include chills, fever, and cough. Pulmonary fibrosis may result. Called also *bird breeder's, bird fancier's,* or *bird handler's l.*

**right l.,** see *lung.*

**shock l.,** acute respiratory distress syndrome.

**silo filler's l.,** a rare type of acute bronchiolitis fibrosa obliterans affecting individuals who inhale high levels of nitrogen oxides, particularly nitrogen dioxide, while working in recently filled silos; death may occur from pulmonary edema. Called also *silo filler's disease.*

**silver finisher's l., silver polisher's l.,** siderosis occurring in silver finishers, caused by the inhalation of iron oxide (from jeweler's rouge) and silver particles. The iron oxide particles are phagocytized and the elastic tissue is stained black by the silver; fibrosis does not occur and pulmonary function is unimpaired.

**thresher's l.,** farmer's l.

**vanishing l.,** in emphysema, conversion of the lungs into a delicate, fine network of remaining blood vessels among which no alveolar walls survive.

**vineyard sprayer's l.,** hypersensitivity pneumonitis occurring in vineyard workers spraying vines with a copper sulfate–lime solution.

**welder's l.,** siderosis occurring in welders, caused by the inhalation of iron oxide fumes; the condition is generally asymptomatic, although the presence of other substances in welding fumes may lead to fibrotic lung disease. Called also *arc welder's disease* and *arc welder's l.*

**wet l.,** 1. pulmonary edema. 2. acute respiratory distress syndrome.

**white l.,** pneumonia alba.

**lung·worm** (lung'wərm) a parasitic worm that invades the lungs, such as the trematode *Paragonimus westermani* in humans, or nematodes of the family Protostrongylidae in other animals. See also *verminous bronchitis, verminous pneumonia,* and *hoose.*

**lu·nu·la** (loo'nu-lə) gen. and pl. *lu'nulae* [L., dim. of *luna* moon] a small crescent or moon-shaped area.

**lunulae of aortic valve, lunulae of cusps of aortic valve,** lunulae valvularum semilunarium valvae aortae.

**lunulae of cusps of pulmonary valve,** lunulae valvularum semilunarium valvae trunci pulmonalis.

**l. of nail,** l. unguis.

**l. of scapula,** incisura scapulae.

**l. un'guis** [TA], lunula of the nail: the crescentic white area at the base of the nail on a finger or toe. Called also *selene unguium.*

**lunulae of valves of pulmonary trunk, lunulae of pulmonary valves,** lunulae valvularum semilunarium valvae trunci pulmonalis.

**lu'nulae valvula'rum semiluna'rium val'vae aor'tae** [TA], lunulae of semilunar cusps of aortic valve: small thinned areas in the cusps of the aortic valve, one on each side of the nodule of the cusp. Called also *lunulae of aortic valve.*

**lu'nulae valvula'rum semiluna'rium val'vae trun'ci pulmona'lis** [TA], lunulae of semilunar cusps of pulmonary valve: small thinned areas in the cusps of the pulmonary valve, one on each side of the nodule of the cusp. Called also *lunulae of pulmonary valve.*

**lu·nu·lae** (loo'nu-le) [L.] genitive and plural of *lunula.*

**lu·pi·form** (loo'pĭ-form) [*lupus* + *form*] lupoid.

**lu·pin·o·sis** (loo"pĭ-no'sis) 1. acute atrophy of the liver, often fatal, in ruminants such as cattle, sheep, goats, and horses, due to the ingestion of seeds of plants of the genus *Lupinus* that are contaminated with the fungus *Phomopsis leptostromiformis.* Cf. *lathyrism.* 2. mycotoxic l.

**mycotoxic l.,** poisoning of livestock due to ingestion of *Lupinus* plants contaminated with the fungi *Phomopsis leptostromiformis* or *P. rossiana;* symptoms include liver damage with jaundice and photosensitization.

**Lu·pi·nus** (loo'pin-us) the lupins, a genus of leguminous herbs. Seeds of mature plants of many species contain toxic alkaloids that cause convulsions in ruminants. Seeds may also be contaminated with a fungus and cause mycotoxic lupinosis. Two species found in western North America, when eaten by pregnant cows, may cause crooked calf disease in fetuses.

**lu·poid** (loo'poid) [*lupus* + *-oid*] pertaining to or resembling lupus. Called also *lupiform.*

**Lu·pron** (loo'pron) trademark for preparations of leuprolide acetate.

**lu·pus** (loo'pəs) [L. "wolf" or "pike"] [MeSH: Lupus] a name originally given to localized destruction or degeneration of the skin caused by various cutaneous diseases. Although the term was formerly used to designate lupus vulgaris and now lupus erythematosus, without a modifier it has no specific meaning.

**chilblain l.,** chilblain l. erythematosus.

**drug-induced l.,** a syndrome similar to systemic lupus erythematosus, caused by any of various drugs, such as hydralazine, procainamide, isoniazid, D-penicillamine, and chlorpromazine; it usually resolves following withdrawal of the offending drug.

**l. erythemato'sus (LE),** a group of connective tissue disorders primarily affecting women aged 20 to 40 years, comprising a spectrum of clinical forms in which cutaneous disease may occur with or without systemic involvement. See *cutaneous lupus erythematosus* and *systemic lupus erythematosus.*

**l. erythematosus, chilblain,** a chronic unremitting form of lupus erythematosus, usually involving the fingertips, nose, face, ears, hands, calves, and heels, and caused by microvascular injury secondary to cold exposure. Initially the lesions resemble chilblains and may mimic those of lupus pernio in sarcoidosis, but they eventually assume the appearance of discoid lupus erythematosus. Called also *chilblain l.* and *l. pernio.*

**l. erythematosus, cutaneous,** a form that sometimes involves only the skin and sometimes precedes the involvement of other body systems One classification divides it into three clinically distinct types: the *chronic type,* in which the basic lesion is discoid *(discoid l. erythematosus)*; the *subacute type,* characterized by widespread symmetrical, superficial, nonscarring lesions that may leave self-limited hypopigmentation and telangiectases after resolution *(systemic l. erythematosus)*; and the *acute type,* characterized by an acute edematous, erythematous eruption, either a malar rash in a "butterfly" distribution, or an extensive morbilliform eruption often occurring with systemic exacerbations; the latter is sometimes the presenting symptom of systemic lupus erythematosus, such as after sun exposure.

**l. erythematosus, discoid (DLE),** a chronic form of cutaneous lupus erythematosus in which the skin lesions mimic those of the systemic form but systemic signs are rare, although multisystem manifestations may develop after many years. It is characterized by the presence of discoid skin plaques showing varying degrees of edema, erythema, scaliness, follicular plugging, and skin atrophy surrounded by an elevated erythematous border typically involving the face and scalp, but widespread dissemination may occur. See also *l. erythematosus profundus* and *hypertrophic l. erythematosus.*

**l. erythematosus, hypertrophic,** a form of discoid lupus erythematosus characterized by the presence of verrucous hyperkeratotic lesions that can be mistaken for keratoacanthoma or hypertrophic lichen planus, which may occur in association with cutaneous lesions with features clinically and histologically suggestive of lichen planus. Called also *l. hypertrophicus.*

**l. erythematosus, systemic (SLE),** a chronic, remitting, relapsing, inflammatory, often febrile multisystemic disorder of connective tissue, acute or insidious in onset, characterized principally by involvement of the skin *(cutaneous l. erythematosus),* joints, kidneys, and serosal membranes. It is of unknown etiology, but it is thought to represent a failure of regulatory mechanisms of the autoimmune system, as suggested by the high level of numerous autoantibodies against nuclear and cytoplasmic cellular components. It is marked by a wide variety of abnormalities, including arthritis and arthralgias, nephritis, central nervous system manifestations, pleurisy, pericarditis, leukopenia or thrombocytopenia, hemolytic anemia, elevated erythrocyte sedimentation rate, and positive LE-cell preparations. See also *drug-induced l.*

**l. erythematosus, systemic, ANA-negative,** antiphospholipid-antibody syndrome.

**l. erythematosus, systemic, transient neonatal,** neonatal l.

**l. erythemato'sus profun'dus,** a rare chronic form of cutaneous lupus erythematosus characterized by deep dermal and subcutaneous inflammatory involvement, producing deep, firm nodules, often without surface change, on the head, upper arms, chest, buttocks, and thighs, which heal and leave deeply depressed areas. The typical lesions of discoid lupus erythematosus are often present, and mild systemic involvement often occurs. Called also *LE* or *lupus panniculitis* and *l. profundus.*

**l. erythemato'sus tu'midus,** a variant of discoid or systemic lupus erythematosus in which the lesions consist of raised reddish purple or brown plaques, which may resemble erysipelas or cellulitis.

**l. hypertro'phicus,** 1. a variant of lupus vulgaris in which the lesions consist of a warty vegetative growth, often crusted or slightly exudative, usually occurring on moist areas near body orifices. 2. hypertrophic l. erythematosus.

**l. milia'ris dissemina'tus fa'ciei,** a papular eruption involving the central part of the face of adults that heals spontaneously with scarring. It has been variously considered to be a tuberculid, as a variant of granulomatous rosacea, and as a papular eruption of unknown etiology.

**neonatal l.,** a condition that sometimes affects infants born to mothers with systemic lupus erythematosus, characterized most commonly by a rash similar to that seen in discoid lupus and by transiently elevated levels of antinuclear antibodies and LE cells, less commonly by heart block or other cardiac conduction disturbances, hematologic abnormalities, hepatosplenomegaly, and pericarditis. It is usually benign and self-limited, but the discoid skin lesions may rarely persist. Called also *transient neonatal systemic l. erythematosus.*

# HEMATOPOIESIS

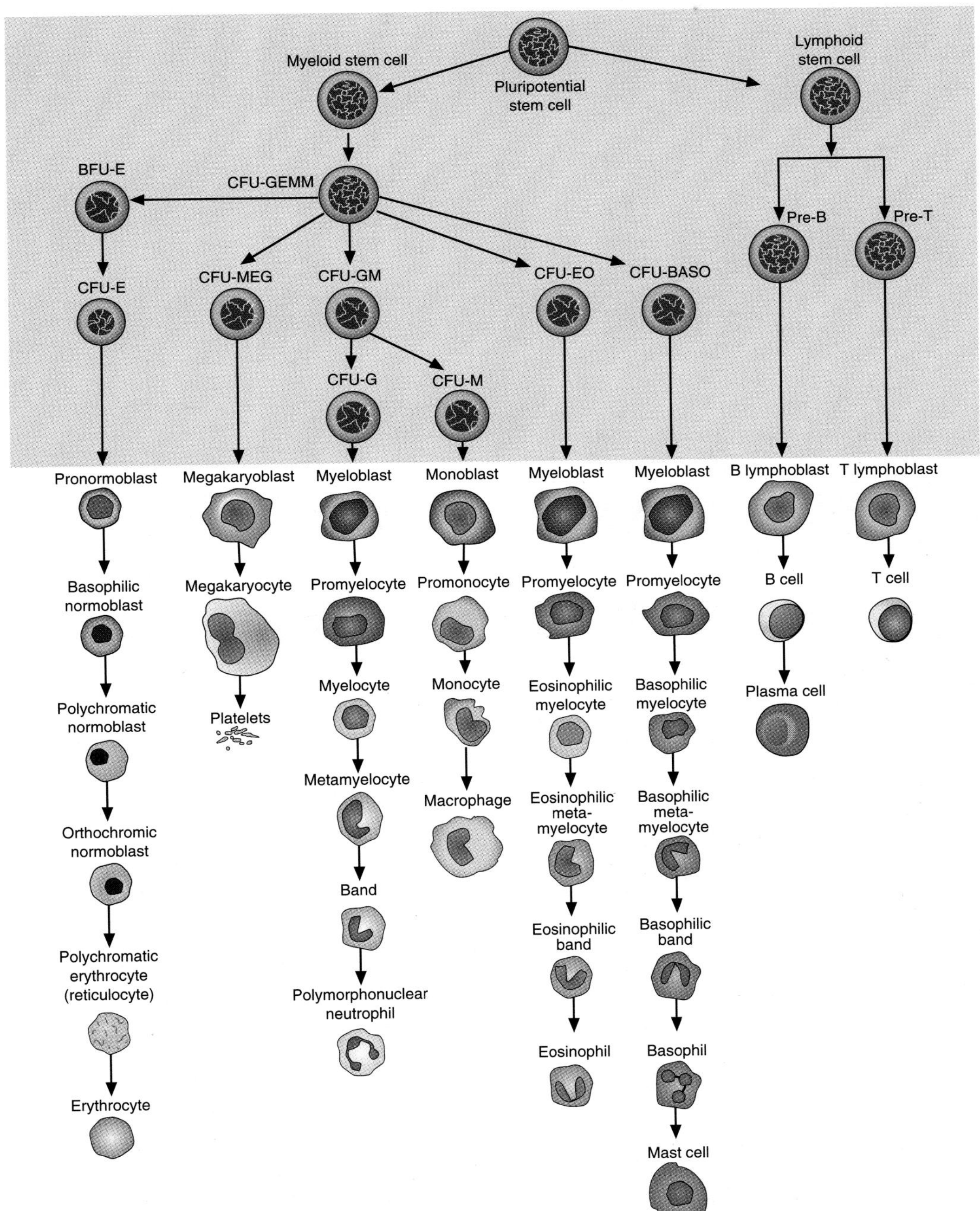


CFU-GEMM: colony-forming unit–granulocyte, erythrocyte, monocyte, megakaryocyte. BFU-E: burst-forming unit–erythroid. CFU-E: colony-forming unit–erythroid. CFU-MEG: colony-forming unit–megakaryocytic. CFU-GM: colony-forming unit–granulocyte-macrophage. CFU-EO: colony-forming unit–eosinophilic. CFU-BASO): colony-forming unit–basophilic. CFU-G: colony-forming unit–granulocytic. CFU-M: colony-forming unit–macrophage.

## ERYTHROCYTE ABNORMALITIES

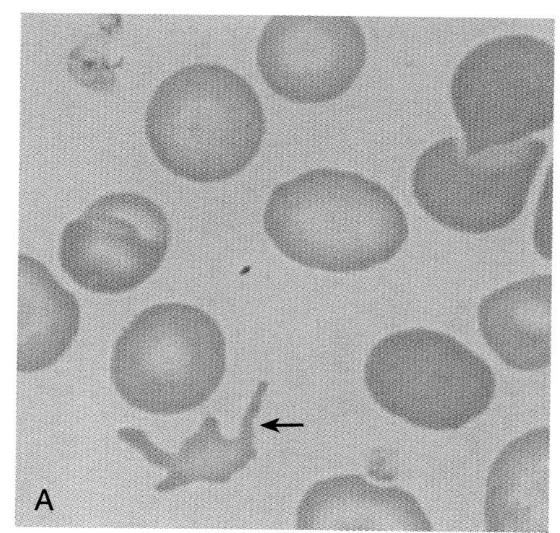


Acanthocyte

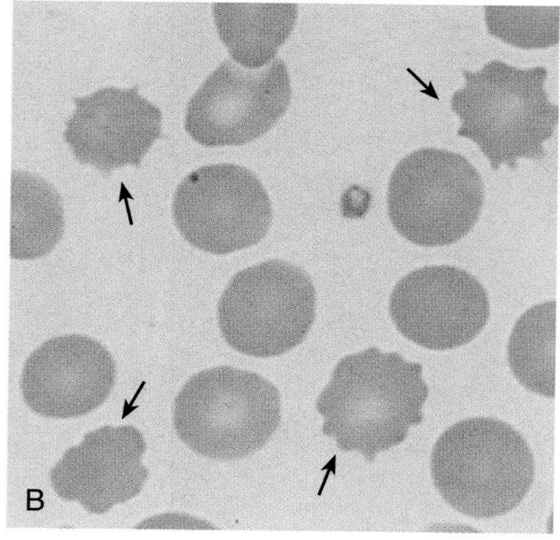


Burr cells

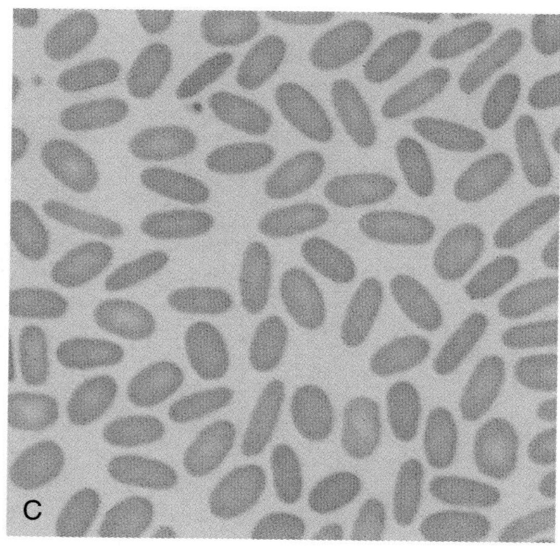


Elliptocytes

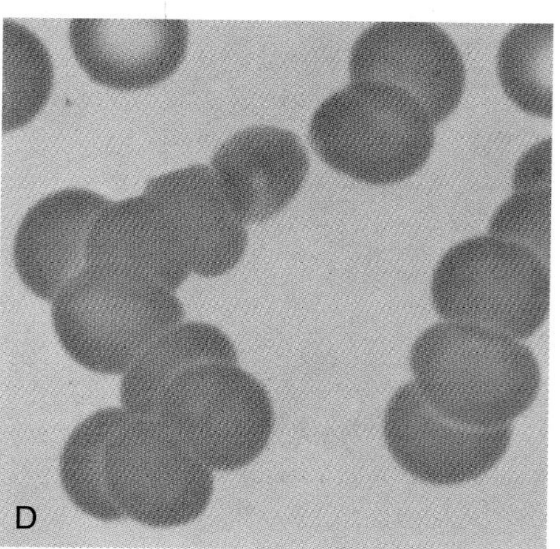


Rouleaux

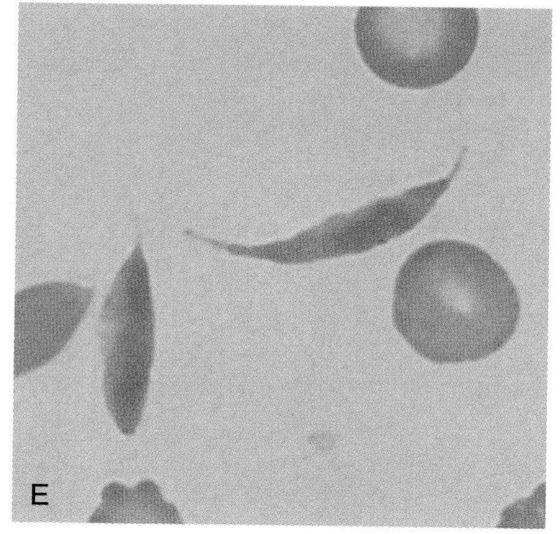


Sickle cell

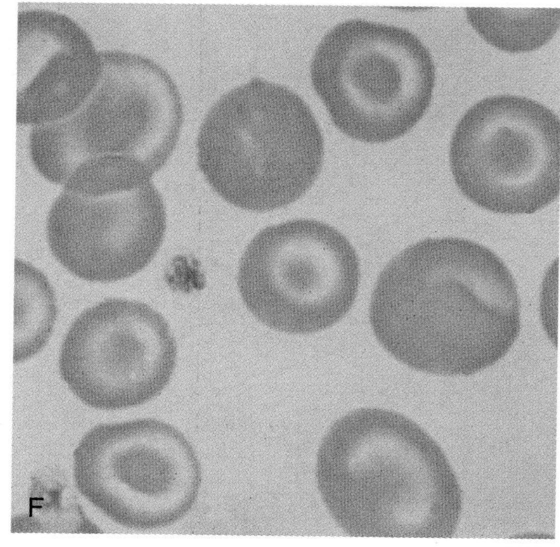


Target cells

## STAINS I

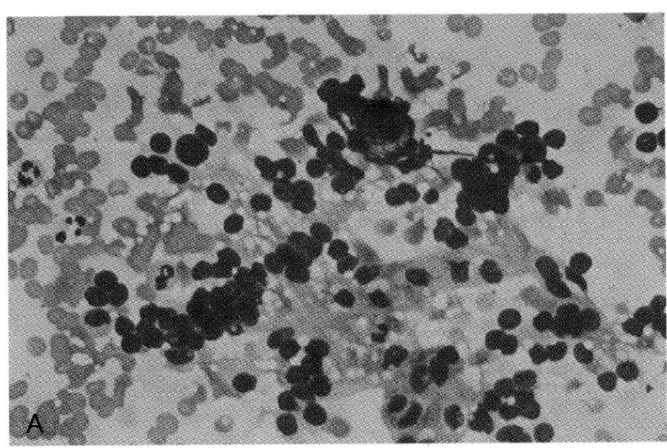


Diff-Quik
Benign cortical nodule mimicking oat cell carcinoma.

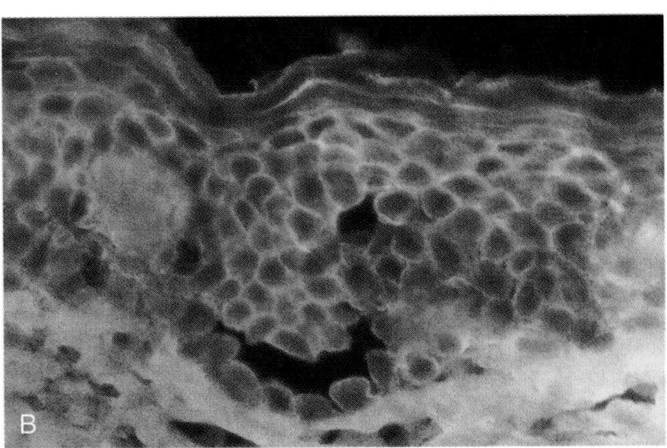


Direct immunofluorescence
Pemphigus vulgaris.

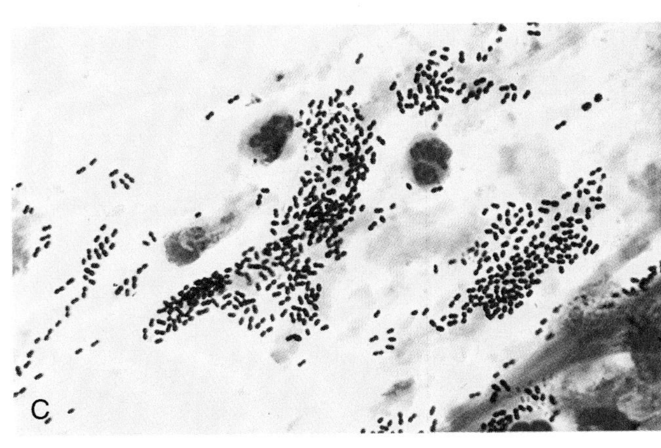


Gram's stain
Gram-positive diplococci in sputum smear.

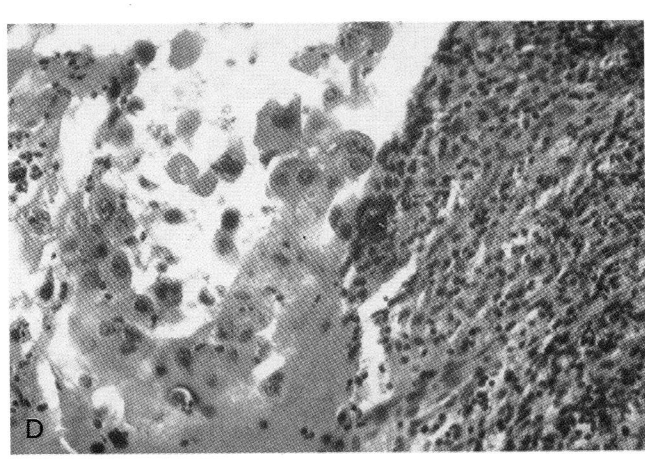


Hematoxylin and eosin
Malignant cells in cystic medullary carcinoma.

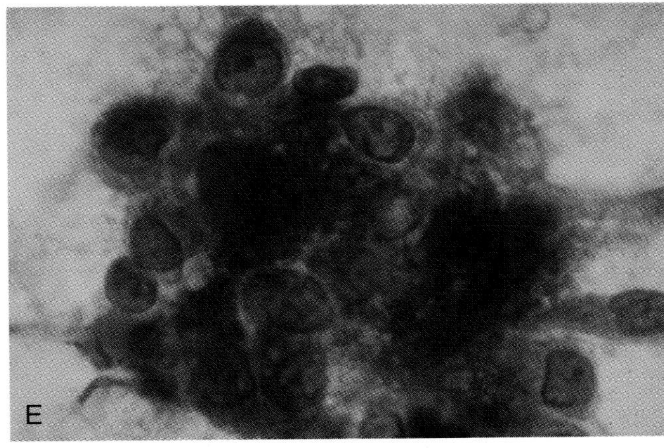


Immunoperoxidase staining
Positive staining for prostatic acid phosphatase in metastatic carcinoma.

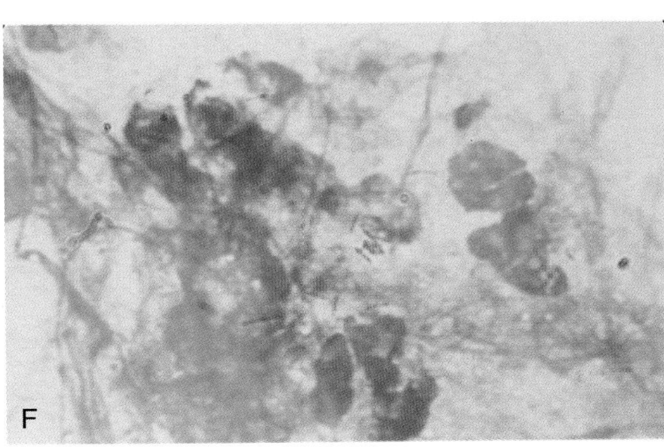


Kinyoun carbolfuchsin stain
Acid-fast bacilli *(Mycobacterium tuberculosis)* in sputum smear.

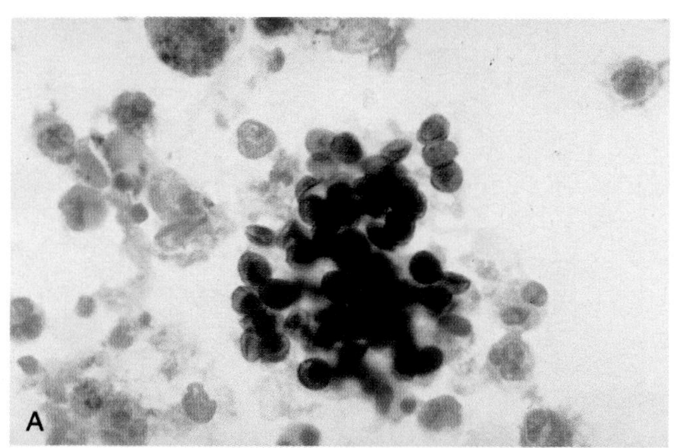


Methenamine silver stain
*Pneumocystis carinii* in alveolar cast.

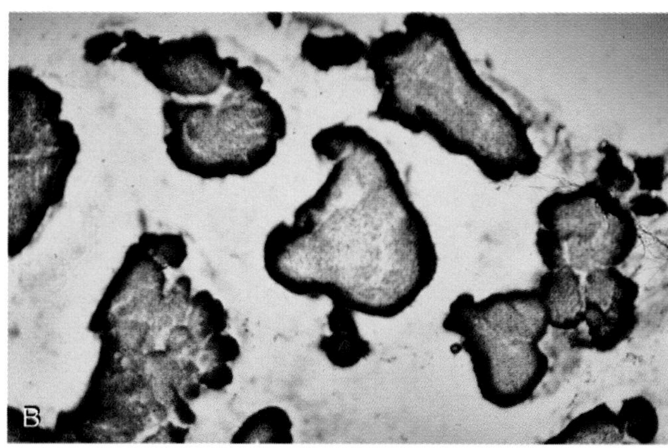


Methylene blue
Basal cell carcinoma.

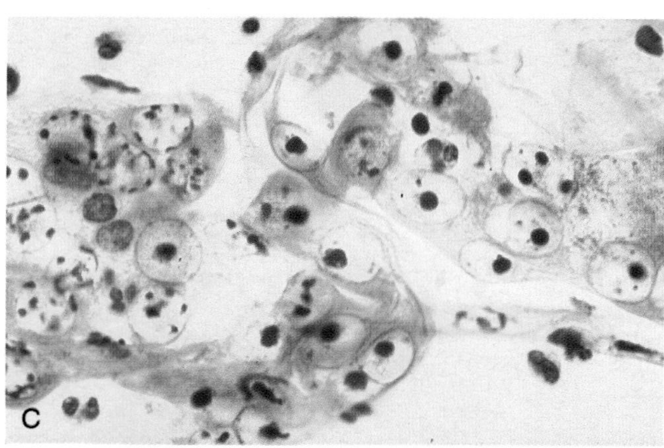


Papanicolaou's stain
Basophilic intranuclear inclusions in adenovirus infection.

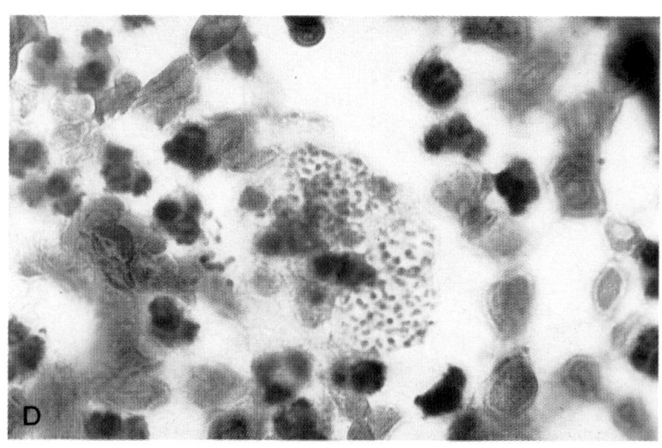


Papanicolaou's stain
Macrophage containing Donovan bodies.

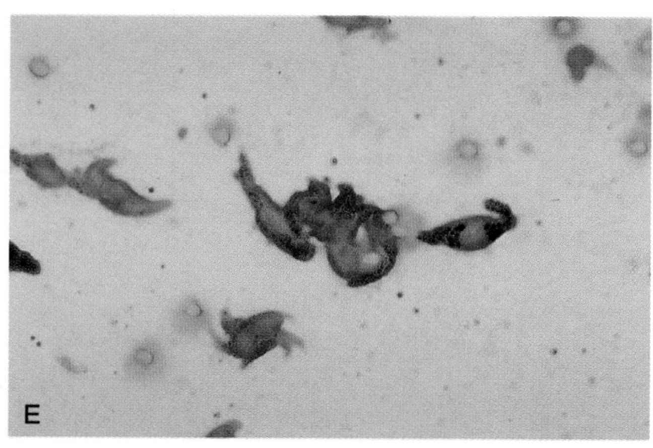


Streptavidin peroxidase
Tumor cells stained by monoclonal antibody to S-100 protein in metastatic malignant melanoma.

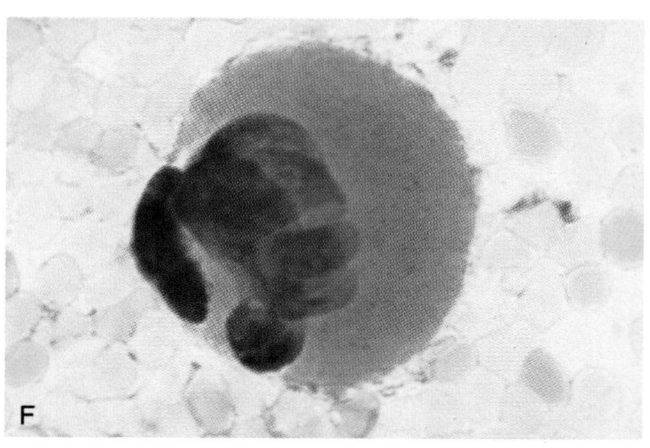


Toluidine blue
Normal megakaryocyte.

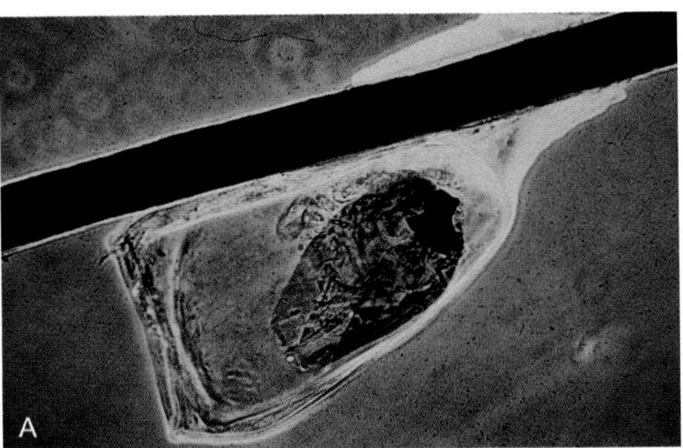


Pediculosis
Egg case attached to hair shaft.

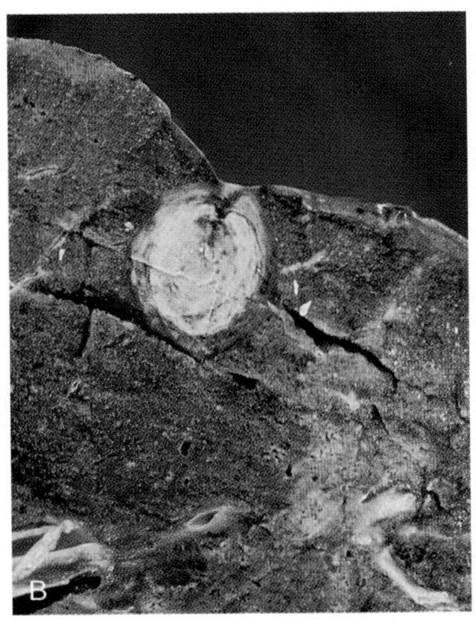


*Histoplasma*
Laminated granuloma of lung.

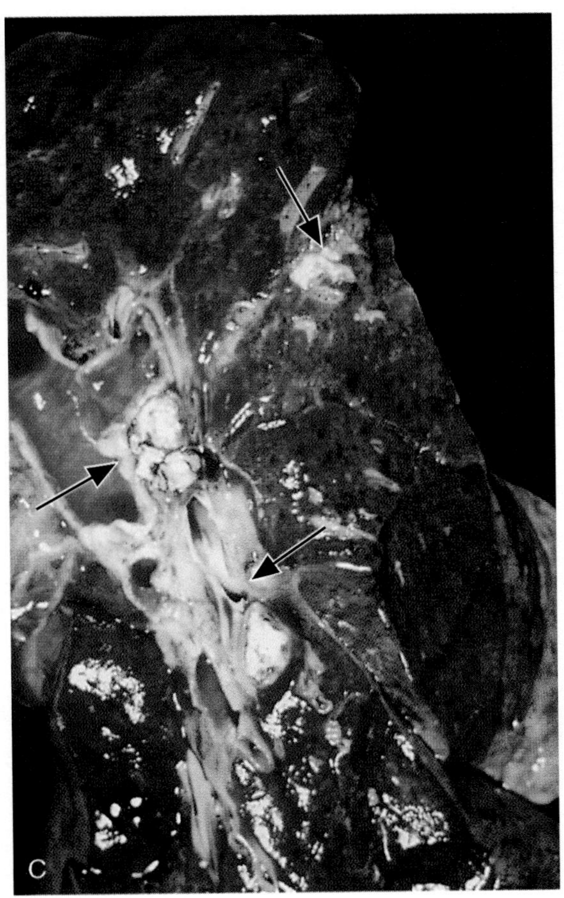


Ghon focus
Ghon focus *(upper arrow)* in pulmonary tuberculosis.

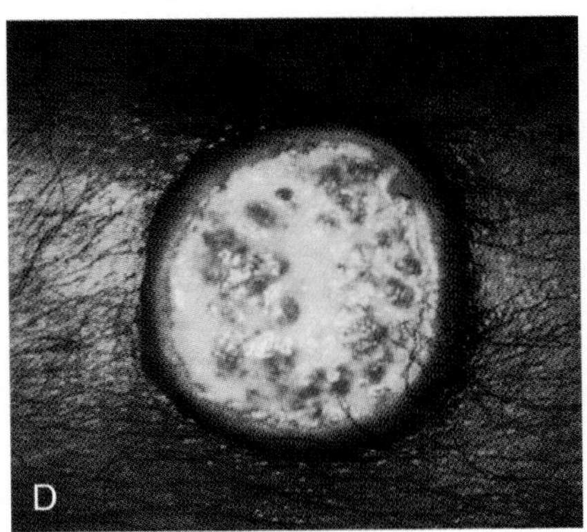


Cutaneous leishmaniasis

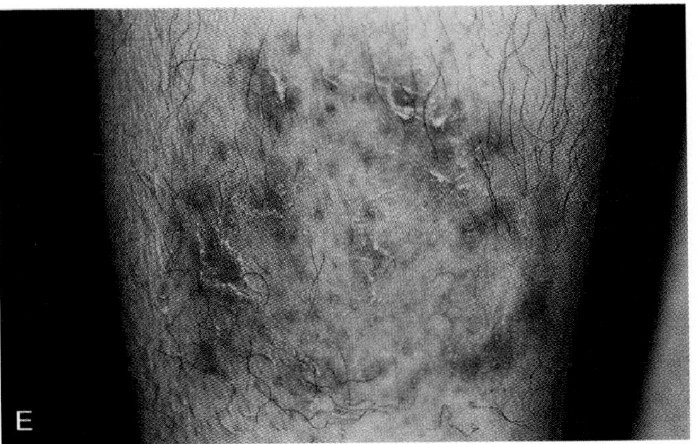


Tinea corporis

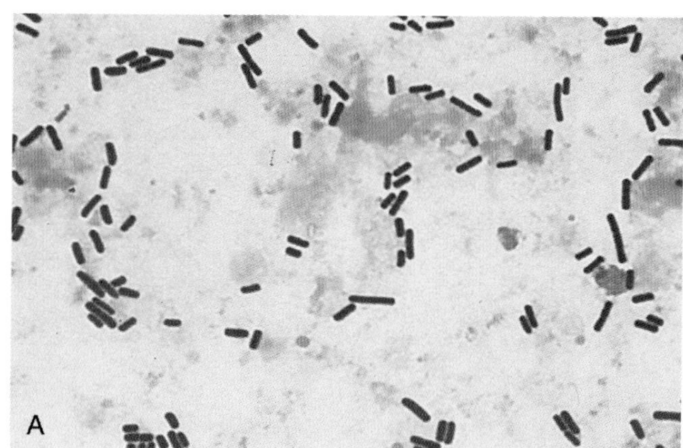


*Clostridium perfringens*

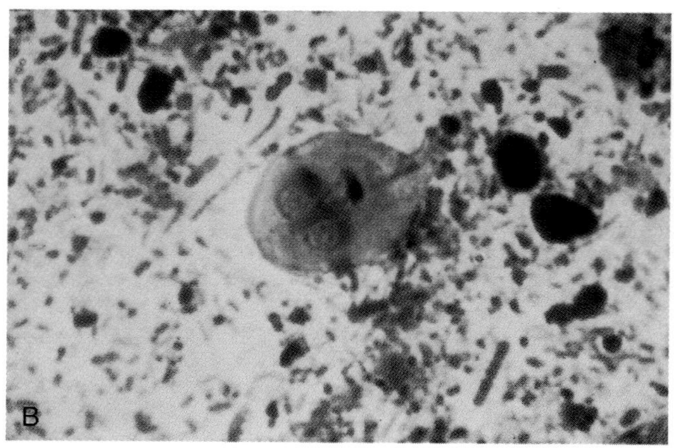


*Giardia lamblia*
Trophozoite in stool.

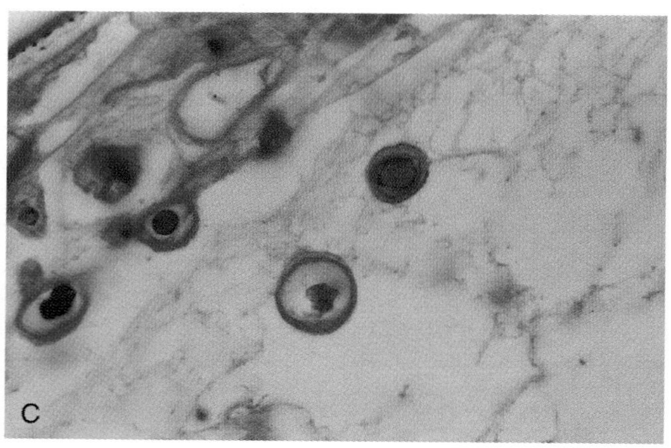


Herpes simplex
Glassy inclusion bodies from blister of herpes stomatitis.

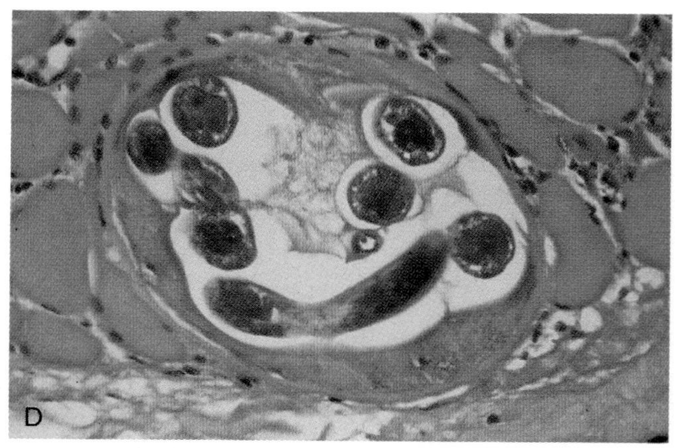


*Trichinella spiralis*
larva in a skeletal muscle cell.

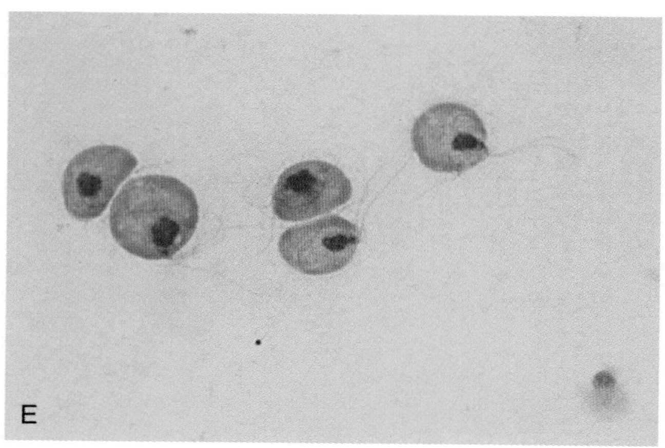


*Trichomonas vaginalis*
Flagellated trophozoites.

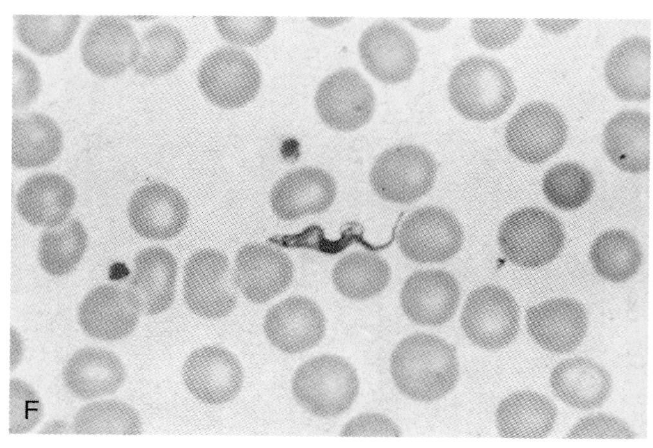


*Trypanosoma rhodesiense*
Organism in peripheral blood.

SKIN LESIONS I

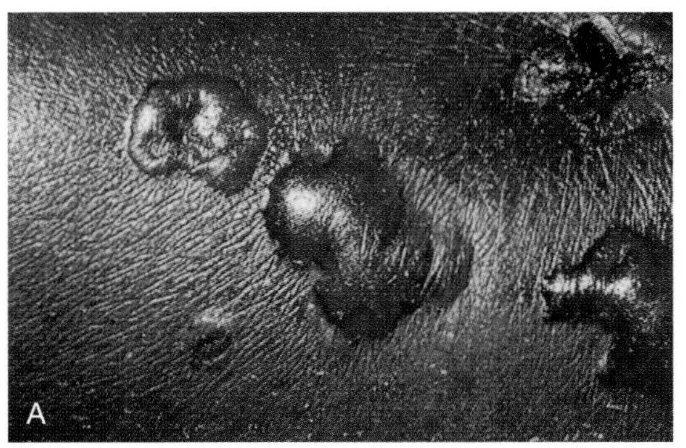


Bullae

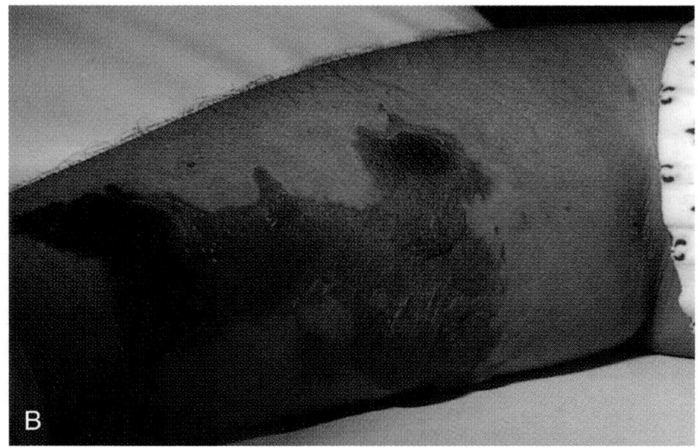


Macule

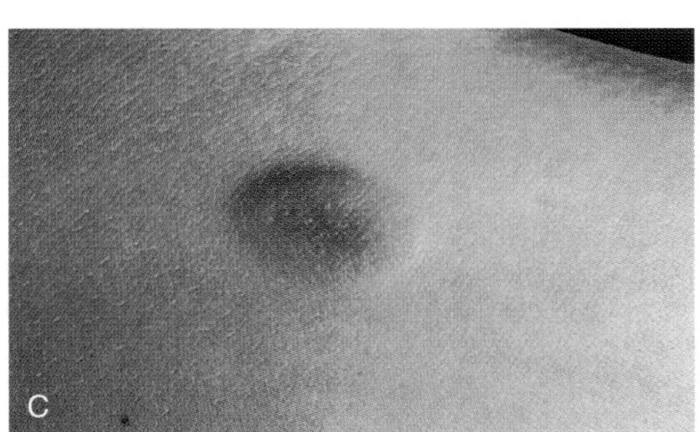


Papule

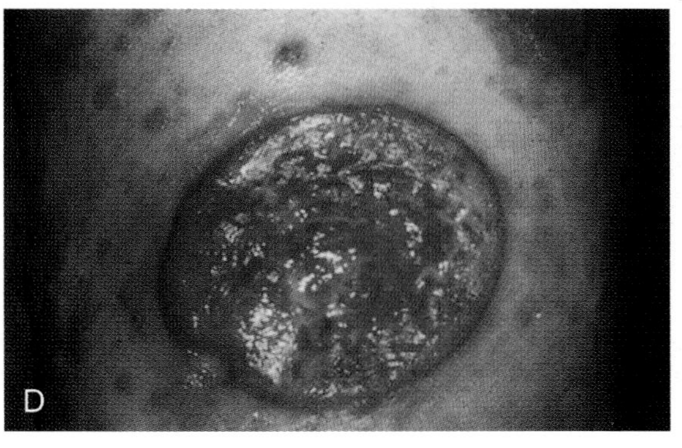


Plaque

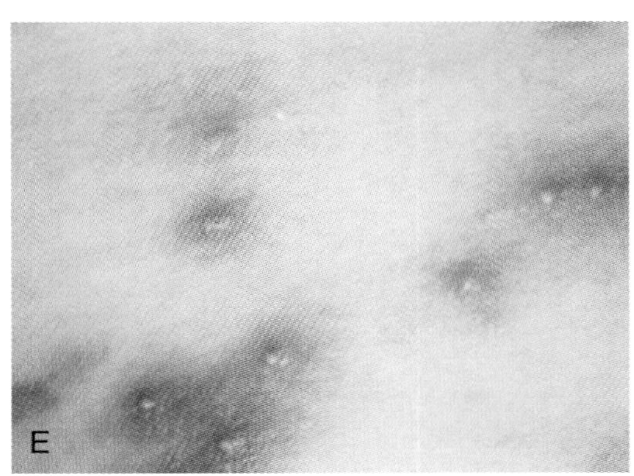


Pustules

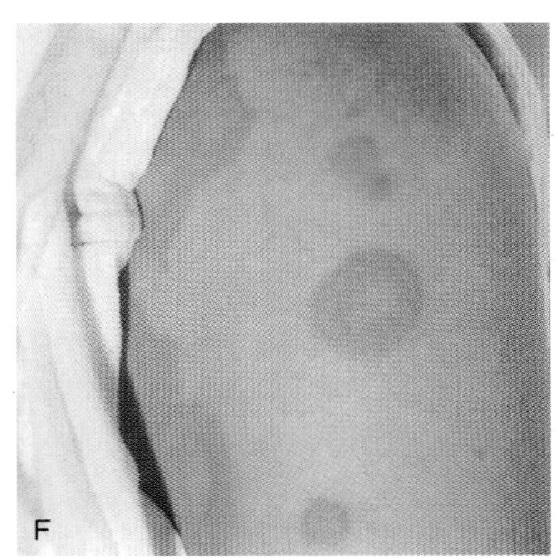


Wheals

# SKIN LESIONS II

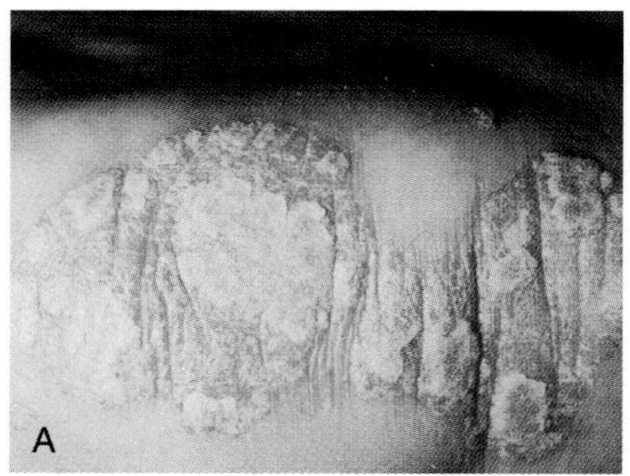


Psoriasis.

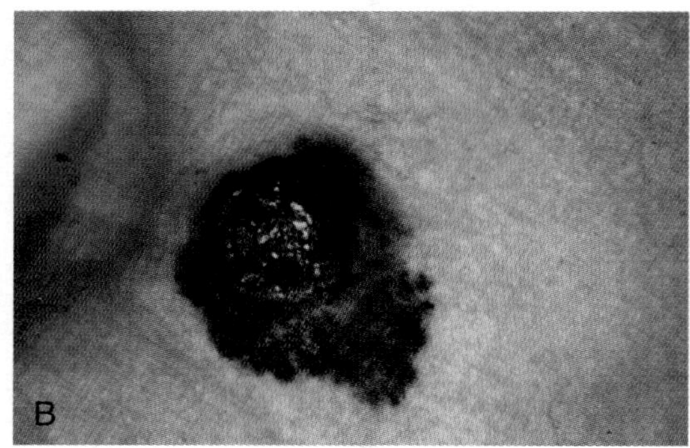


Malignant melanoma.

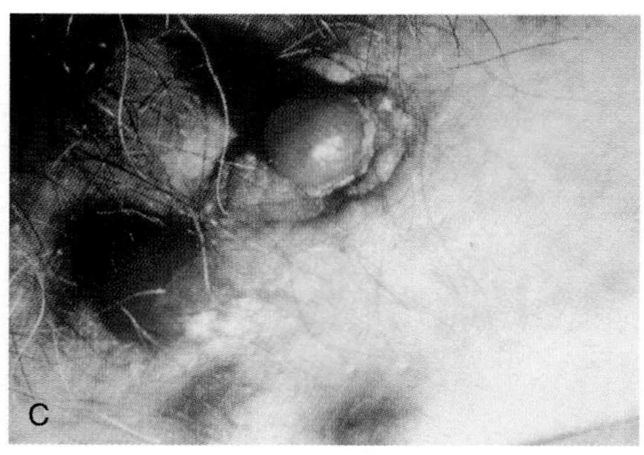


Nodules
Skin metastases.

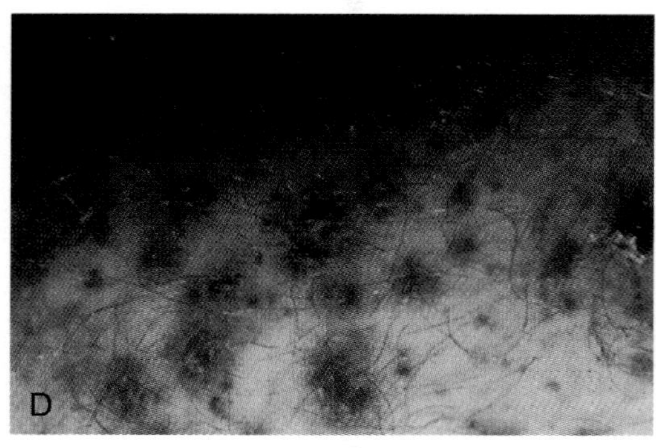


Purpura
Palpable purpura in hypersensitivity vasculitis.

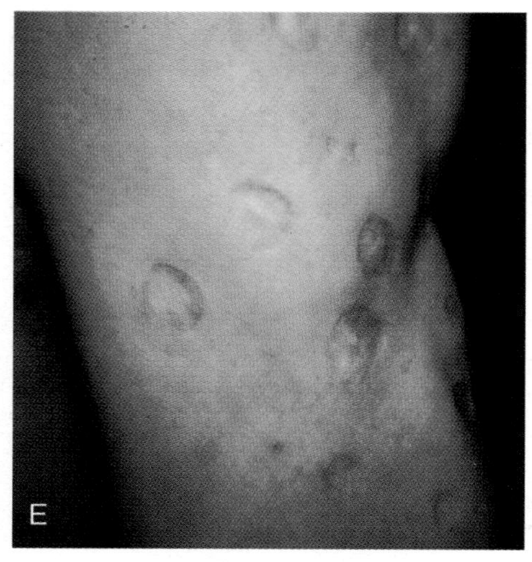


Scars
Healed diabetic ulcers.

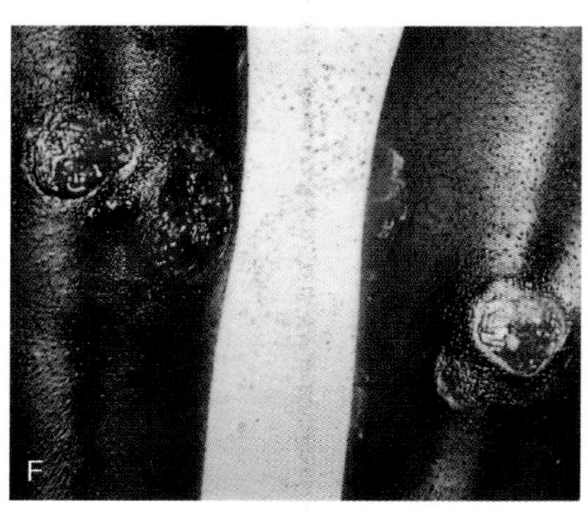


Ulcers
Caused by ischemia in sickle cell anemia.

**l. nephritis,** see under *nephritis.*
**l. per'nio,** 1. a cutaneous manifestation of sarcoidosis consisting of violaceous, smooth, shiny plaques on the ears, forehead, nose, fingers, and toes, which is frequently associated with bone cysts. 2. chilblain lupus erythematosus.
**l. profun'dus,** l. erythematosus profundus.
**l. tu'midus,** a variant of lupus vulgaris in which the lesions consist of localized, soft edematous patches somewhat resembling keloids.
**l. vulga'ris,** the most common, severe, and variable, but rare, form of tuberculosis of the skin, usually of the face, especially the nasal, buccal, and conjunctival mucosa, predominantly in women. Usual characteristics include the appearance in normal-appearing skin of a reddish brown plaque with deeply embedded peripheral nodules, characterized by extensive atrophy and progressive destruction of cartilage in involved sites, resulting in disfiguring scars, keloids, lymphedema, and functional impairment from contractures. The lesions may also present in other morphological forms, e.g., see *l. hypertrophicus* (def. 1) and *l. tumidus.*

**Luque instrumentation, rod** (loo'ka) [Eduardo Roberto *Luque,* Mexican orthopedic surgeon, 20th century] see under *instrumentation* and *rod.*

**Lur·ia** (loo're-ə) Salvador Edward. Italian-born American biologist, 1912–1991; co-winner, with Max Delbrück and Alfred Day Hershey, of the Nobel prize for medicine or physiology in 1969 for research on the mechanisms and materials of inheritance of viruses.

**Lu·ride** (loo'rīd) trademark for a preparation of sodium fluoride.

**Lusch·ka's crypts,** etc. (lo͝osh'kahz) [Hubert von *Luschka,* German anatomist, 1820–1875] see under *crypt, duct,* and *joint,* and see *apertura lateralis ventriculi quarti, bursa pharyngealis, carina urethralis vaginae, cartilago sesamoidea ligamenti vocalis, glomus coccygeum,* and *tonsilla pharyngea.*

**Lust's phenomenon (sign)** (lo͞osts) [Franz Alexander *Lust,* German pediatrician, 20th century] see under *phenomenon.*

**lute** (lo͞ot) [L. *lutum* mud] 1. a substance such as cement, wax, or clay that coats a surface or joint area to make a tight seal. Called also *luting agent.* 2. to coat or seal with such a substance.

**lu·te·al** (loo'te-əl) pertaining to or having the properties of the corpus luteum or its active principle.

**lu·te·ec·to·my** (loo″te-ek'tə-me) excision of the corpus luteum.

**lu·te·in** (loo'te-in) [L. *luteus* yellow] 1. a yellow pigment, or lipochrome from the corpus luteum, from fat cells, and from the yolk of eggs. It is closely related to xanthophyll. 2. any lipochrome.

**lu·te·in·ic** (loo″te-in'ik) 1. pertaining to lutein or to the corpus luteum. 2. pertaining to luteinization.

**lu·te·in·iza·tion** (loo″te-in″ĭ-za'shən) the process by which a postovulatory ovarian follicle transforms into a corpus luteum through vascularization, follicular cell hypertrophy, and lipid accumulation, the latter in some species giving the yellow color indicated by the term.

**Lu·tem·bach·er's syndrome (complex)** (loo'təm-bahk″ərz) [René *Lutembacher,* French cardiologist, 1884–1968] see under *syndrome.*

**lu·te·ol·y·sin** (loo″te-ol'ə-sin) a substance that causes degeneration of corpus luteum.
**uterine l.,** dinoprost.

**lu·te·ol·y·sis** (loo″te-ol'ə-sis) degeneration of corpus luteum.

**lu·te·o·ma** (loo″te-o'mə) [MeSH: Luteoma] 1. a granulosa-theca cell tumor in which there has been luteinization of the cells. Called also *luteinized granulosa-theca cell tumor.* 2. nodular hyperplasia of ovarian lutein cells sometimes occurring in the last trimester of pregnancy; it may be unilateral or bilateral. Called also *l. of pregnancy* or *pregnancy l.*

**lu·teo·trop·ic** (loo″te-o-trop'ik) stimulating the formation of the corpus luteum.

**lu·te·o·tro·pin** (loo'te-o-tro″pin) prolactin.

**lu·te·ti·um** (loo-te'she-əm) [MeSH: Lutetium] the chemical element, atomic number 71, atomic weight 174.97, symbol Lu.

**Lu·ther·an blood group** (loo'thər-ən) [from the name of the propositus first described in 1945] see under *blood group.*

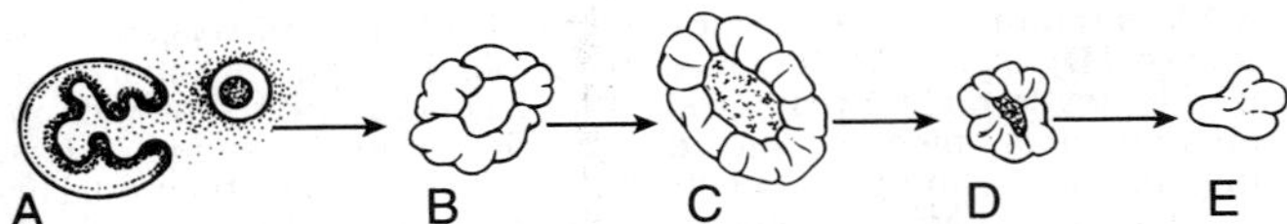

Luteinization, beginning after rupture of the ovarian follicle in ovulation *(A)* and progressing through vascularization and hypertrophy of the maturing corpus luteum *(B, C)*; it is followed by regression *(D)* to the corpus albicans *(E).*

**Lu·trex·in** (loo-trek'sin) trademark for a preparation of lututrin.

**Lu·tro·mone** (loo'tro-mōn) trademark for a preparation of progesterone.

**lu·tro·pin** (loo-tro'pin) luteinizing hormone.

**lu·tu·trin** (loo'tu-trin) a protein or polypeptide substance obtained from the corpus luteum of sow ovaries by a process of salting out followed by dialysis; used as a uterine relaxant in treatment of functional dysmenorrhea.

**Lutz-Splen·do·re-Al·mei·da disease** (lo͞ots-splen-do'ra-ahl-ma'dah) [Adolfo *Lutz,* Brazilian physician, 1855–1940; Alfonso *Splendore,* Italian physician in Brazil, 1871–1953; Floriano Paulo de *Almeida,* Brazilian physician, born 1898] paracoccidioidomycosis.

**Lut·zo·my·ia** (lo͞ot-zo-mi'ə) a genus of sandflies of the family Psychodidae, the females of which suck blood.
**L. flaviscutella'ta,** the vector of *Leishmania mexicana amazonensis,* the etiologic agent of cutaneous leishmaniasis in Brazil.
**L. longipal'pis,** the vector of *Leishmania donovani chagasi,* the etiologic agent of American visceral leishmaniasis.
**L. nogu'chi,** *Phlebotomus noguchii.*
**L. olme'ca,** the vector of *Leishmania mexicana mexicana,* the etiologic agent of chiclero ulcer.
**L. peruen'sis,** a probable vector of *Leishmania viannia peruviana,* the etiologic agent of uta.
**L. tra'pidoi,** a vector of *Leishmania viannia panamensis,* the etiologic agent of one form of New World cutaneous leishmaniasis.
**L. umbrati'lis,** the major vector of *Leishmania viannia guyanensis,* the etiologic agent of pian bois (forest yaws).
**L. verruca'rum,** a probable vector of *Leishmania peruviana,* the etiologic agent of uta.

**Lu·vox** (loo'voks) trademark for a preparation of fluvoxamine.

**lux** (luks) [L. "light"] in SI, the metric unit of illumination, being one lumen per square meter; called also *meter candle.* Cf. *foot-candle.*

**lux·a·tio** (lək-sa'she-o) [L.] dislocation.
**l. cox'ae conge'nita,** congenital dislocation of the hip.
**l. erec'ta,** dislocation of the shoulder so that the arm stands straight up above the head.
**l. imperfec'ta,** a sprain.
**l. perinea'lis,** a form of dislocation of the hip in which the head of the femur lies in the perineum.

**lux·a·tion** (lək-sa'shən) [L. *luxatio*] dislocation.
**Malgaigne's l.,** pulled elbow.

**lux·u·ri·ant** (ləg-zhoor'e-ənt) growing freely or excessively.

**Luys' body syndrome, nucleus** (loo-ēz') [Jules Bernard *Luys,* French neurologist, 1828–1895] see *hemiballismus* and *nucleus subthalamicus.*

**LVAD** left ventricular assist device.

**LVEDP** left ventricular end-diastolic pressure.

**LVEDV** left ventricular end-diastolic volume.

**LVET** left ventricular ejection time.

**LVH** left ventricular hypertrophy; see *ventricular hypertrophy,* under *hypertrophy.*

**LVN** licensed vocational nurse.

**Lw** symbol for lawrencium.

**Lwoff** (lvawf) André Michael. French microbiologist and virologist, born 1902; co-winner with François Jacob and Jacques Lucien Monod, of the Nobel prize for medicine or physiology for 1965, for discoveries concerning the genetic control of enzymes and virus synthesis.

**ly·ase** (li'ās) [EC 4] a class of enzymes that catalyze the cleavage of C—C, C—O, C—N, or other bonds without hydrolysis or oxidation to form two molecules, at least one of which contains a double bond. The reverse reaction occurs by the addition of a group to a molecule at a double bond. The class includes aldolases, deaminases, decarboxylases, hydratases or dehydratases, and other cleavage or cyclase enzymes. See also *synthase.*
**17,20-l.,** 17$\alpha$-hydroxyprogesterone aldolase.

**17,20-ly·ase de·fi·cien·cy** a disorder of steroidogenesis due to deficiency of 17$\alpha$-hydroxyprogesterone aldolase, an enzyme activity normally catalyzing the conversion of $C_{21}$ to $C_9$ steroid hormones (androgens and estrogens); the result is a type of congenital adrenal hyperplasia (type V). Males are pseudohermaphroditic and both sexes remain sexually infantile. The enzyme activity is part of the enzyme steroid 17$\alpha$-monooxygenase; see also *17$\alpha$-hydroxylase deficiency* and see table at *hyperplasia.*

**ly·can·thro·py** (li-kan'thrə-pe) [Gr. *lykos* wolf + *anthrōpos* man] a delusion in which the patient believes that he is a wolf or other animal or that he is able to change into one.

**Lych·nis gi·tha·go** (lik'nis gĭ-tha'go) *Agrostemma githago.*

**ly·cine** (li'sēn) betaine.

**ly·co·pene** (li'ko-pēn) the red carotenoid pigment of tomatoes and various berries and fruits.

**ly·co·pe·ne·mia** (li"ko-pə-ne'me-ə) a variant of carotenemia resulting from the prolonged and excessive ingestion of tomato juice, which contains lycopene.

**Ly·co·per·da·ceae** (li"ko-pər-da'se-e) a family of puffballs, fungi of the order Lycoperdales; it includes the genus *Lycoperdon.*

**Ly·co·per·da·les** (li"ko-pər-da'lēs) the puffballs, an order of perfect fungi of the class Holobasidiomycetes; it includes the family Lycoperdaceae.

**Ly·co·per·don** (li"ko-per'don) [Gr. *lykos* wolf + *perdesthai* to break wind] a genus of puffballs, fungi of the family Lycoperdaceae; in folk medicine their dust (spores) is inhaled to treat nosebleeds. See also *lycoperdonosis.*

**ly·co·per·do·no·sis** (li"ko-per"do-no'sis) a rare type of hypersensitivity pneumonitis caused by the inhalation of spores from mature *Lycoperdon* mushrooms.

**Ly·co·po·di·um** (li"ko-po'de-əm) [Gr. *lykos* wolf + *pous* foot] the club mosses, a genus of mosses. *L. clava'tum* and other species are sources of lycopodium.

**ly·co·po·di·um** (li"ko-po'de-əm) a light dry powder consisting of the spores of species of *Lycopodium,* especially *L. clavatum,* formerly used as a dusting and absorbent powder, and as a coating for pills. Since the spores are uniform in size, they can be used as a measuring unit in microscopy.

**lyco·rine** (lik'o-rin) a toxic crystalline alkaloid found in the bulbs of species of *Lycoris* and *Narcissus;* it causes vomiting, diarrhea, convulsions, and sometimes death in humans and other animals. Called also *narcissine.*

**Lyco·ris** (lik'ŏ-ris) a genus of poisonous plants of the family Amaryllidaceae, native to China and Japan, whose bulbs contain the toxin lycorine. *L. radia'ta* Herb. is the source of tazettine, and its bulbs are used in Chinese medicine as an expectorant and emetic.

**Ly·co·sa ta·ren·tu·la** (li-ko'sə) a genus of wolf spiders (family Lycosidae). *L. taren'tula* is the European tarantula.

**Ly·co·si·dae** (li-ko'sĭ-de) the wolf spiders, a family of venomous ground spiders that chase their prey. Genera include *Lycosa* and *Scaptocosa.*

**lyd·i·my·cin** (lid"ĭ-mi'sin) an antifungal antibiotic produced by *Streptomyces lydicus,* $C_{10}H_{14}N_2O_3S$.

**lye** (li) [MeSH: Lye] an alkaline percolate from wood ashes; lixivium. Household lye is a crude mixture of sodium hydroxide with some sodium carbonate.

**Ly·ell's disease, syndrome** (li'əlz) [Alan *Lyell,* English dermatologist, 20th century] toxic epidermal necrolysis.

**ly·ing-in** (li"ing-in') 1. puerperal. 2. the puerperium.

**Lyme disease (arthritis), borreliosis** (līm) [from Old *Lyme,* Connecticut, where the disease was first reported in 1975] see under *disease* and *borreliosis.*

**LYME·rix** (līm'riks) trademark for Lyme disease vaccine (recombinant OspA).

**Lym·naea** (lim-ne'ə) [MeSH: Lymnaea] a genus of pond snails of the order Lymneidae. *L. ollu'la* and *L. bulimoi'des* serve as first intermediate hosts of the liver fluke *Fasciola hepatica;* other species are the hosts of schistosome flukes that cause schistosome dermatitis.

**Lym·ne·i·dae** (lim-ne'ĭ-de) a family of fresh water snails of the suborder Basommatophora. It includes the genus *Lymnaea.*

**lymph** (limf) [L. *lympha* water] [MeSH: Lymph] 1. a transparent, slightly yellow liquid of alkaline reaction, found in the lymphatic vessels and derived from the tissue fluids. It is occasionally of a light-rose color from the presence of red blood corpuscles, and is often opalescent from particles of fat. Under the microscope, lymph is seen to consist of a liquid portion and of cells, most of which are lymphocytes. Lymph is collected from all parts of the body and returned to the blood via the lymphatic system. Called also *lympha* [TA]. See Plate 28. 2. any clear, watery fluid resembling true lymph.
**aplastic l.,** lymph that contains an excess of leukocytes and does not tend to become organized; called also *corpuscular l.*
**corpuscular l.,** aplastic l.
**croupous l.,** inflammatory lymph that tends to the formation of a false membrane.
**euplastic l., fibrinous l.,** that which tends to coagulate and become organized.
**inflammatory l.,** the lymph produced by inflammation, as in a wound.
**intercellular l.,** lymph occupying the intercellular spaces of tissues.
**intravascular l.,** the lymph of the lymph vessels.
**tissue l.,** lymph derived from the tissues and not from the blood.

**lym·pha** (lim'fə) [L. "water"] [TA] the fluid found in the lymphatic vessels; see *lymph.*

**lym·pha·den** (lim'fə-dən) [*lymph-* + Gr. *adēn* gland] a lymph node.

**lym·phad·e·nec·to·my** (lim-fad"ə-nek'tə-me) [*lymphaden* + *-ectomy*] surgical excision of a lymph node or nodes; often accompanied by an adjective referring to which node is removed, such as *axillary l., cervical l.,* or *inguinal l.* Called also *lymph node dissection.*
**retroperitoneal l.,** surgical removal of lymph nodes in the retroperitoneal space, usually because of cancer metastasis, such as from carcinomas of the genital organs in men. Called also *retroperitoneal lymph node dissection (RPLND).*

**lym·phad·e·ni·tis** (lim-fad"ə-ni'tis) [*lymphaden* + *-itis*] [MeSH: Lymphadenitis] inflammation of one or more lymph nodes, usually caused by a primary focus of infection elsewhere in the body.
**caseous l.,** a chronic disease of sheep and goats caused by *Corynebacterium pseudotuberculosis,* characterized by the formation in various lymph nodes of abscesses containing caseous material, sometimes associated with chronic pneumonia and pleurisy. Called also *pseudotuberculosis.*
**cervical l.,** see under *adenitis.*
**cervical l., tuberculous,** tuberculosis of the cervical lymph nodes; see *tuberculous l.* Called also *tuberculous cervical adenitis.* Formerly called *scrofula.*
**histiocytic necrotizing l.,** Kikuchi's l.
**Kikuchi's l.,** a benign, self-limited syndrome of lymphadenopathy, usually in the neck, with a female predominance; characteristics include patchy necrotizing lesions of the paracortex and proliferation of distinctive histiocytes, plasmacytoid monocytes, and immunoblasts surrounded by karyorrhectic debris. Some consider it a self-limited form of systemic lupus erythematosus. Called also *Kikuchi's disease, histiocytic necrotizing l.,* and *subacute necrotizing l.*
**mesenteric l.,** a condition clinically resembling acute appendicitis, in which there is inflammation of the mesenteric lymph nodes receiving lymph from the intestine. A septal form, which is frequently fatal, and a milder form, which is self-limited, are caused by *Yersinia (Pasteurella) pseudotuberculosis.* Called also *mesenteric adenitis.*
**paratuberculous l.,** caseous l.
**regional l.,** cat-scratch disease.
**streptococcal l. of swine,** streptococcal infection with abscesses in lymph nodes in the necks of pigs; it is often subclinical and discovered when the animal is slaughtered, whereupon the meat may have to be condemned. Called also *jowl abscess* and *cervical abscess.*
**subacute necrotizing l.,** Kikuchi's l.
**tuberculoid l.,** inflammation of the lymph nodes similar to that in tuberculous lymphadenitis; it may be caused by such disorders as sarcoidosis, regional enteritis, leprosy, syphilis, and several fungal infections.
**tuberculous l.,** tuberculosis of the lymph nodes, involving most often the cervical (see *tuberculous cervical l.*) or mediastinal nodes; it may occur as a primary infection or be caused by lymphatic or hematogenous spread from a primary focus of infection elsewhere in the body. Called also *tuberculous lymphadenopathy.* See also *scrofuloderma.*

**lym·phad·e·no·cele** (lim-fad'ə-no-sēl") a cyst of a lymph node; called also *adenolymphocele.*

**lym·phad·e·no·cyst** (lim-fad'ə-no-sist") a degenerated lymph node caused by occlusion of its incoming lymph vessels. By dilatation of the lymph sinuses it becomes a fine-meshed network.

**lym·phad·e·no·gram** (lim-fad'ə-no-gram") a radiograph of lymph nodes.

**lym·phad·e·nog·ra·phy** (lim-fad"ə-nog'rə-fe) radiographic visualization of the lymph nodes, following injection of radiopaque material into a lymphatic vessel.

**lym·phad·e·noid** (lim-fad'ə-noid) [*lymphaden* + *-oid*] resembling the tissue of lymph nodes; lymphadenoid tissue includes the spleen, bone marrow, tonsils, and the lymphatic tissue of the organs and mucous membranes.

**lym·phad·e·no·leu·ko·poi·e·sis** (lim-fad"ə-no-loo"ko-poi-e'sis) the production of leukocytes by the lymphadenoid tissue.

**lym·phad·e·no·ma** (lim-fad"ə-no'mə) lymphoma.

**lym·phad·e·nop·a·thy** (lim-fad"ə-nop'ə-the) [*lymphaden* + *-pathy*] disease of the lymph nodes.
**angioimmunoblastic l., angioimmunoblastic l. with dysproteinemia (AILD),** a systemic disorder resembling lymphoma, characterized by fever, night sweats, weight loss, generalized lymphadenopathy with a pleomorphic cellular infiltrate of lymphocytes, immunoblasts, and plasma cells that alters or effaces the nodal architecture, hepatosplenomegaly, maculopapular rash, polyclonal hypergammaglobulinemia, and Coombs-positive hemolytic anemia. It is considered to be a nonmalignant hyperimmune reaction to chronic antigenic stimulation; there is proliferation of B cells accom-

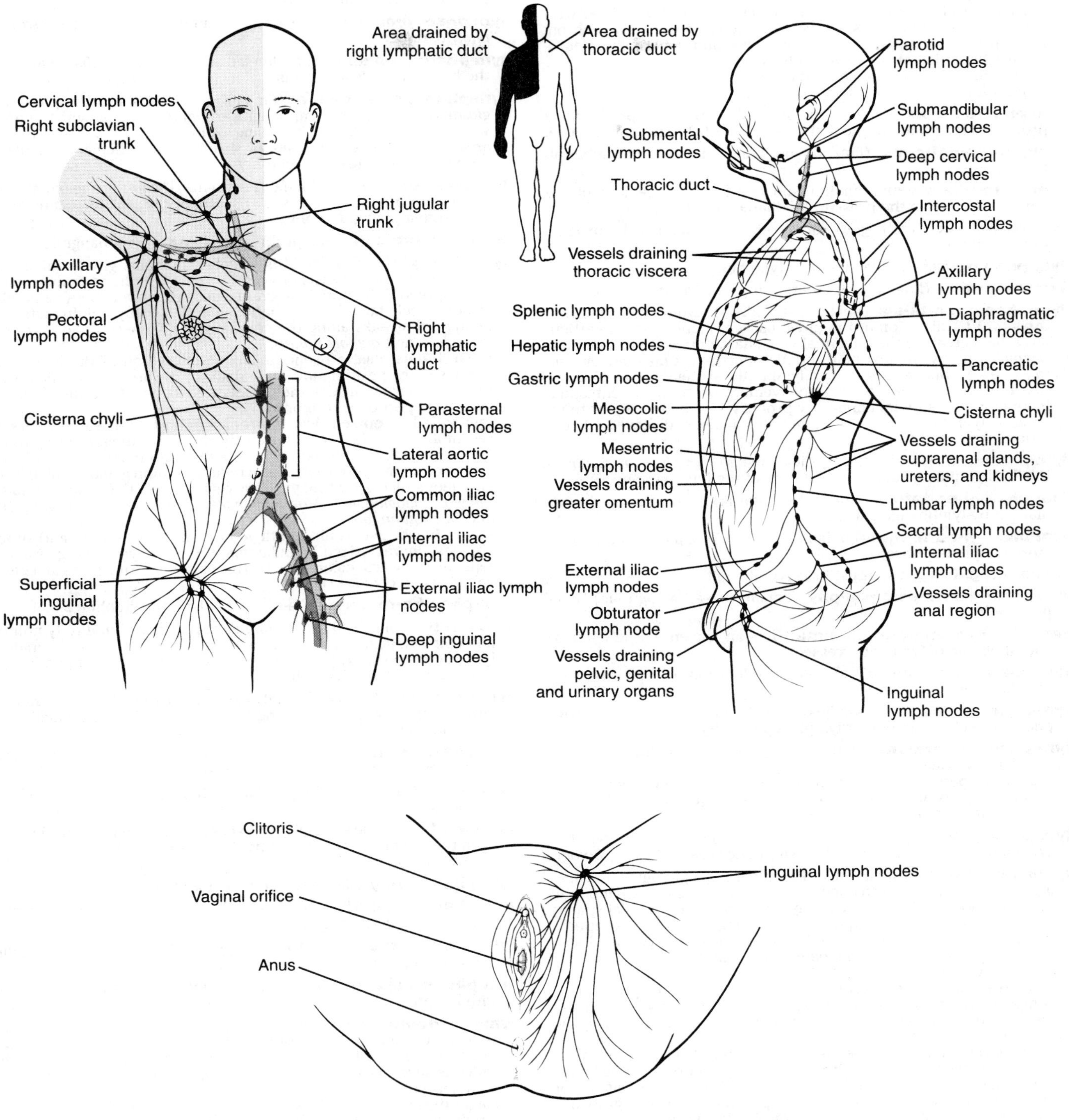

Area drained by right lymphatic duct
Area drained by thoracic duct

Cervical lymph nodes
Right subclavian trunk
Right jugular trunk
Axillary lymph nodes
Pectoral lymph nodes
Right lymphatic duct
Cisterna chyli
Parasternal lymph nodes
Lateral aortic lymph nodes
Common iliac lymph nodes
Internal iliac lymph nodes
Superficial inguinal lymph nodes
External iliac lymph nodes
Deep inguinal lymph nodes

Parotid lymph nodes
Submandibular lymph nodes
Submental lymph nodes
Deep cervical lymph nodes
Thoracic duct
Intercostal lymph nodes
Vessels draining thoracic viscera
Axillary lymph nodes
Splenic lymph nodes
Diaphragmatic lymph nodes
Hepatic lymph nodes
Pancreatic lymph nodes
Gastric lymph nodes
Cisterna chyli
Mesocolic lymph nodes
Vessels draining suprarenal glands, ureters, and kidneys
Mesentric lymph nodes
Vessels draining greater omentum
Lumbar lymph nodes
Sacral lymph nodes
Internal iliac lymph nodes
External iliac lymph nodes
Vessels draining anal region
Obturator lymph node
Vessels draining pelvic, genital and urinary organs
Inguinal lymph nodes

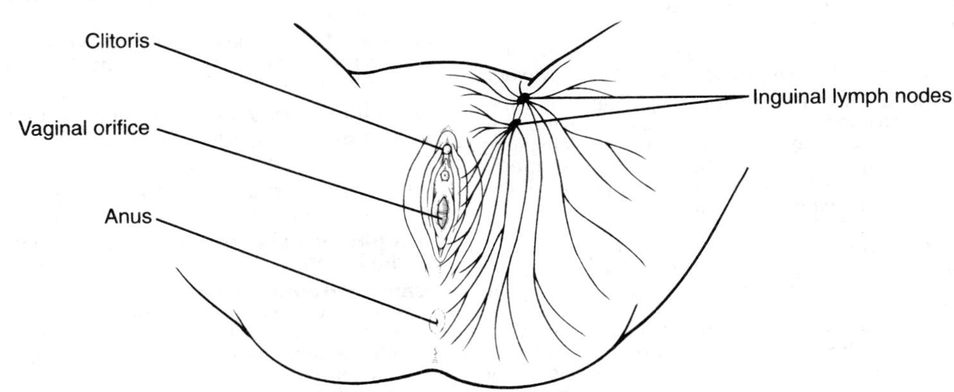


**PLATE 28**—DIAGRAMMATIC REPRESENTATION OF LYMPHATIC DRAINAGE OF VARIOUS PARTS OF THE BODY

panied by profound deficiency of T cells. The disease follows a progressive but extremely variable course; some patients have long survival without chemotherapy, whereas others have a rapid course with death due to overwhelming infections. Called also *immunoblastic l.*
**dermatopathic l.**, regional lymph node enlargement associated with melanoderma and various diseases in which erythroderma is chronically present, e.g., exfoliative dermatitis and generalized neurodermatitis; called also *lipomelanotic reticulosis.*
**immunoblastic l.**, angioimmunoblastic l.
**tuberculous l.**, see under *lymphadenitis.*

**lym·phad·e·no·sis** (lim-fad″ə-no′sis) old term for a proliferative process of lymphatic tissue that precedes certain types of leukemia.

**lym·phad·e·not·o·my** (lim-fad″ə-not′ə-me) incision into a lymph node.

**lym·phad·e·no·va·rix** (lim-fad″ə-no-va′riks) enlargement of the lymph nodes from the pressure of dilated lymph vessels.

**lym·pha·gogue** (lim′fə-gog) an agent that promotes the production of lymph.

**lym·phan·ge·itis** (lim″fan-je-i′tis) lymphangitis.

**lym·phan·gi·al** (lim-fan′je-əl) pertaining to a lymphatic vessel.

**lym·phan·gi·ec·ta·sia** (lim-fan″je-ək-ta′zhə) lymphangiectasis.
**intestinal l.**, dilatation of the intestinal lymphatic system, particularly the lacteals in the intestinal villi, characterized by protein-losing enteropathy, steatorrhea, and lymphopenia. It may be congenital, due to abnormality of the lymphatic system (as in Milroy's disease), or acquired, due to involvement of the major intestinal lymphatic ducts by inflammatory processes or neoplasm, or to increased lymphatic pressure, as in valvular heart disease and constrictive pericarditis.

**lym·phan·gi·ec·ta·sis** (lim-fan″je-ek′tə-sis) [*lymph-* + *angiectasis*] [MeSH: Lymphangiectasis] dilatation of the lymphatic vessels.

**lym·phan·gi·ec·tat·ic** (lim-fan″je-ək-tat′ik) pertaining to or marked by lymphangiectasis.

**lym·phan·gi·ec·to·my** (lim-fan″je-ek′tə-me) excision of one or more lymphatic vessels.

**lym·phan·gi·itis** (lim-fan″je-i′tis) lymphangitis.

**lym·phan·gio·ad·e·nog·ra·phy** (lim-fan″je-o-ad″ə-nog′rə-fe) lymphography.

**lym·phan·gio·en·do·the·li·o·ma** (lim-fan″je-o-en″do-the″le-o′mə) endothelioma of lymphatic vessels.

**lym·phan·gio·fi·bro·ma** (lim-fan″je-o-fi-bro′mə) a fibrosing lymphangioma.

**lym·phan·gio·gram** (lim-fan′je-o-gram″) a radiograph of the lymphatic vessels taken during lymphangiography.

**lym·phan·gi·og·ra·phy** (lim-fan″je-og′rə-fe) angiography of the lymphatic vessels.
**bipedal l., pedal l.**, radiography of the lymphatic channels of the lower extremity after injection of contrast medium into the first and second interdigital spaces of the foot.

**lym·phan·gi·ol·o·gy** (lim-fan″je-ol′ə-je) [*lymph-* + *angiology*] the branch of anatomy relating to the lymphatic vessels. Cf. *lymphology.*

**lym·phan·gi·o·ma** (lim-fan″je-o′mə) [MeSH: Lymphangioma] a benign tumor representing a congenital malformation of the lymphatic system, made up of newly formed lymph-containing vascular spaces and channels. The main types are lymphangioma circumscriptum, cavernous lymphangioma, and simple lymphangioma. Called also *angioma lymphaticum.* Cf. *angioma* and *hemangioma.*
**capillary l.**, simple l.
**l. caverno′sum, cavernous l.**, 1. a deeply situated lymphangioma, composed of cavernous lymphatic spaces, and always occurring in the neck or axilla. See also *vascular nevus,* under *nevus.* 2. cystic hygroma.
**l. circumscrip′tum**, a cutaneous and more superficial type of lymphangioma, usually occurring either on the upper portion of the limbs, in the axillary or inguinal folds (usually localized to one region), or on the oral mucosa, especially the tongue; it consists of a grapelike group of thin walled translucent lymph-filled vesicles that sometimes have a verrucous surface. Some lesions have a deeper component of lymphatic obstruction and lymphedema with localized swelling. See also *vascular nevus,* under *nevus.*
**cystic l., l. cys′ticum**, see under *hygroma.*
**fissural l.**, simple or cavernous lymphangiomas at the site of fetal fissures.
**simple l., l. sim′plex**, a lymphangioma composed of small lymphatic channels that tends to occur subcutaneously in the head and neck region or axilla and sometimes in internal organs. Superficial lesions present as slightly raised or sometimes nodular lesions; deeper lesions are sharply circumscribed, compressible, and gray to pink in color. Called also *capillary l.*

**lym·phan·gio·my·o·ma·to·sis** (lim-fan″je-o-mi″o-mə-to′sis) [MeSH: Lymphangiomyomatosis] a progressive disorder of women of child-bearing age, marked by proliferation of atypical smooth muscle cells in the walls of lymphatics of the lower respiratory tract, pleura, mediastinum, and retroperitoneum.

**lym·phan·gi·on** (lim-fan′je-on) a lymphatic vessel; see *vasa lymphatica,* under *vas.*

**lym·phan·gio·phle·bi·tis** (lim-fan″je-o-flə-bi′tis) inflammation of the lymph vessels and veins.

**lym·phan·gio·sar·co·ma** (lim-fan″je-o-sahr-ko′mə) [*lymph-* + *angiosarcoma*] [MeSH: Lymphangiosarcoma] a malignant tumor of vascular endothelial cells arising from lymphatic vessels; it may arise in a limb that is the site of chronic lymphedema, particularly secondary to radical mastectomy.

**lym·phan·gi·ot·o·my** (lim-fan″je-ot′ə-me) [*lymph-* + *angiotomy*] incision into a lymphatic vessel, usually performed for cannulation prior to lymphangiography.

**lym·phan·git·ic** (lim″fan-jit′ik) pertaining to lymphangitis.

**lym·phan·gi·tis** (lim″fan-ji′tis) [MeSH: Lymphangitis] inflammation of a lymphatic vessel or vessels. Acute lymphangitis may result from spread of bacterial infection (most commonly beta-hemolytic streptococci) into the lymphatics, manifested by painful subcutaneous red streaks along the course of the vessels. Called also *angioleukitis* and *angiolymphitis.*
**l. carcinomato′sa**, a pseudoinflammatory lesion of the lymphatic vessels of the peritoneum, with edema of the area and proliferation of fibrous tissues around the vessels, due to the infiltration of cancer cells from peritoneal tumors.
**epizootic l., l. epizoo′tica**, a chronic contagious disease of horses, resembling glanders but caused by the yeast fungus *Histoplasma farciminosus;* characteristics include purulent inflammation of subcutaneous lymphatic vessels and regional lymph glands, which form cutaneous ulcers that may take a year to heal. Called also *pseudofarcy, pseudoglanders, African glanders, Japanese farcy* or *glanders,* and *Neapolitan farcy.*
**ulcerative l.**, a chronic contagious disease of horses and other equines, characterized by inflammation of the lymph vessels and a tendency toward ulceration of the skin over the parts affected; called also *ulcerative cellulitis.*

**lym·pha·phe·re·sis** (lim″fə-fə-re′sis) lymphocytapheresis.

**lym·phat·ic** (lim-fat′ik) [L. *lymphaticus*] 1. pertaining to lymph or a lymph vessel; by extension, the term is used alone to designate a lymphatic vessel or, in the plural, to designate the lymphatic system. 2. of a sluggish or phlegmatic temperament.

**lym·phat·i·cos·to·my** (lim-fat″ĭ-kos′tə-me) [*lymphatic* + *-ostomy*] surgical creation of an opening into a lymphatic duct, usually the thoracic duct.

**lym·pha·tism** (lim′fə-tiz″əm) 1. status lymphaticus. 2. the lymphatic temperament; a slow or sluggish habit.

**lym·pha·ti·tis** (lim″fə-ti′tis) inflammation of some part of the lymphatic system.

**lym·pha·tog·e·nous** (lim″fə-toj′ə-nəs) produced by or derived from the lymph; disseminated by the lymph circulation or through the lymph channels.

**lym·pha·tol·o·gy** (lim″fə-tol′ə-je) lymphology.

**lym·pha·tol·y·sis** (lim″fə-tol′ə-sis) [*lymphatic* + *-lysis*] the destruction or solution of lymphatic tissue.

**lym·pha·to·lyt·ic** (lim″fə-to-lit′ik) [*lymphatic* + *-lytic*] destroying lymphatic tissue.

**lym·phec·ta·sia** (lim″fek-ta′zhə) [*lymph-* + *ectasia*] distention with lymph.

**lym·phe·de·ma** (lim″fə-de′mə) [*lymph-* + *edema*] [MeSH: Lymphedema] chronic unilateral or bilateral edema of the extremities due to accumulation of interstitial fluid as a result of stasis of lymph, which is secondary to obstruction of lymph vessels or disorders of the lymph nodes.
**congenital l.**, Milroy's disease.
**l. prae′cox**, lymphedema characterized by puffiness and swelling of the lower limbs, occurring at or near puberty, usually in young women.

**lym·phen·ter·itis** (lim″fən-tər-i′tis) enteritis with serous infiltration.

**lymph·epi·the·li·o·ma** (limf″ep-i-the″le-o′mə) lymphoepithelioma.

**lym·phi·za·tion** (lim″fĭ-za′shən) the formation of lymph.

**lymph·no·di·tis** (limf″no-di′tis) lymphadenitis.

**lymph(o)-** [L. *lympha* water] a combining form denoting relationship to lymph, lymphoid tissue, lymphatics, or lymphocytes.

**lym·pho·blast** (lim′fo-blast) [*lympho-* + *-blast*] a morphologically immature lymphocyte, once thought to represent an early stage in lymphocyte development but now known to be an activated lymphocyte that has been transformed in response to antigenic stimulation.

**lym·pho·blas·tic** (lim″fo-blas′tik) pertaining to a lymphoblast.

**lym·pho·blas·to·ma** (lim″fo-blas-to′mə) [*lymphoblast* + *-oma*] lymphoblastic lymphoma.

**lym·pho·blas·to·sis** (lim″fo-blas-to′sis) excess of lymphoblasts in the blood, as seen in lymphoblastic leukemia.

**lym·pho·cele** (lim′fo-sēl) [MeSH: Lymphocele] a cyst containing lymph.

**lym·pho·ce·ras·tism** (lim″fo-sə-ras′tiz-əm) [*lympho-* + Gr. *kerastos* mixed] the formation of cells of the lymphocytic series.

**lym·pho·ci·ne·sia** (lim″fo-si-ne′zhə) [*lympho-* + *cinesi-* + *-ia*] lymphokinesis.

**Lym·pho·cryp·to·vi·rus** (lim″fo-krip′to-vi″rəs) [*lympho-* + *crypto-* + *virus*] [MeSH: Lymphocryptovirus] Epstein-Barr–like viruses; a genus of viruses of the subfamily Gammaherpesvirinae (family Herpesviridae) containing both human and animal pathogens, including Epstein-Barr virus, Marek's disease virus, and species infecting nonhuman primates.

**lym·pho·cys·tis** (lim″fo-sis′tis) [*lympho-* + *cystis*] a common, chronic, nonfatal disease of marine and freshwater fish, caused by *Lymphocystivirus* and characterized by tumorlike nodules, generally on the skin and fins, consisting of hypertrophied connective tissue cells. Called also *lymphocystis disease.*

**Lym·pho·cys·ti·vi·rus** (lim″fo-sis′tĭ-vi″rəs) [*lymphocystis* + *virus*] lymphocystis viruses; a genus of viruses of the family Iridoviridae that cause lymphocystis in marine and freshwater fish.

**lym·pho·cy·ta·phe·re·sis** (lim″fo-si″tə-fə-re′sis) [*lymphocyte* + *apheresis*] the selective removal of lymphocytes from withdrawn blood, which is then retransfused into the donor. Called also *lymphapheresis.*

**lym·pho·cyte** (lim′fo-sīt) [*lympho-* + *-cyte*] [MeSH: Lymphocytes] any of the mononuclear, nonphagocytic leukocytes, found in the blood, lymph, and lymphoid tissues, that are the body's immunologically competent cells and their precursors. They are divided on the basis of ontogeny and function into two classes, B and T lymphocytes, responsible for humoral and cellular immunity, respectively. Most are *small lymphocytes,* 7–10 $\mu$m in diameter with a round or slightly indented heterochromatic nucleus that almost fills the cell and a thin rim of basophilic cytoplasm that contains few granules. When activated by contact with antigen, small lymphocytes begin macromolecular synthesis, the cytoplasm enlarges until the cells are 10–30 $\mu$m in diameter, and the nucleus becomes less completely heterochromatic; they are then referred to as *large lymphocytes* or *lymphoblasts.* These cells then proliferate and differentiate into B and T memory cells and into the various effector cell types, B cells into plasma cells and T cells into helper, cytotoxic, and suppressor cells. Surface markers identifying the lymphocyte types are shown in the accompanying table. See subentries here and under *cell.*
**amplifier T l.,** a T lymphocyte that modifies a developing immune response by releasing nonspecific signals to which other T lymphocytes (either effector or suppressor cells) respond.
**B l's,** B cells; bursa-dependent lymphocytes and their counterparts in nonavian vertebrates, the cells primarily responsible for humoral immunity, the precursors of antibody-producing cells (plasma cells). In birds B cell maturation takes place in the bursa of Fabricius; the hypothesized analogous tissue in other vertebrates was termed the "bursa-equivalent" tissue. It now appears that B cell maturation occurs primarily in the bone marrow in mammals. B cells are characterized by the presence of surface immunoglobulin, monomeric IgM or IgD, which constitutes the B-cell antigen receptors. When stimulated by antigen, a process that requires the cooperation of helper T cells and macrophages, B cells proliferate and differentiate into plasma cells and memory B cells. The entire clone of cells descended from a single activated B cell produces immunoglobulins having the same antigen combining site as that in the antigen receptors of the original cell; thus all of the antibody produced and all of the memory cells are specific for the antigen that induced their formation.
**cytotoxic T l's (CTL),** killer cells, killer T cells; differentiated T lymphocytes that can recognize and lyse target cells bearing specific antigens recognized by their antigen receptors. Recognition is MHC restricted; the foreign antigen is recognized only in association with self MHC antigens. The cytotoxic activity requires firm binding of the killer cell to the target cell and involves the production of holes in the plasma membrane of the target cell, loss of cell content, and osmotic lysis. CTL are important in graft rejection and killing of tumor cells and virus-infected host cells. Murine killer T cells are marked by the Ly-2 and Ly-3 antigens, human cells by the CD4 and CD8 antigens.
**large l.,** see *lymphocyte.*
**large granular l's,** lymphocytes marked by the presence of large granules visible by light microscopy, responsible for most natural killer cell activity.
**plasmacytoid l.,** a cell morphologically resembling a small lymphocyte but having a well-developed rough endoplasmic reticulum like that of a plasma cell; frequently observed in the blood of patients with plasma cell dyscrasias or hypergammaglobulinemia.
**Rieder's l.,** Rieder's cell.
**small l.,** see *lymphocyte.*
**T l's,** T cells; thymus-dependent lymphocytes; the cells primarily responsible for cell-mediated immunity; they originate from lymphoid stem cells that migrate from the bone marrow to the thymus and differentiate under the influence of the thymic hormones thymopoietin and thymosin. They are characterized by specific surface antigens: the pan-T antigens Thy-1 (murine) and CD3 (human) are found on all mature T cells; other markers characterize T cell subsets. T cell antigen receptors are triggered by antigen only when associated with self MHC antigens, e.g., by antigens processed and presented by macrophages, viral antigens on the surface of host cells, and tumor neoantigens. When activated by antigen, T cells proliferate and differentiate into T memory cells and the various types of regulatory and effector T cells; see *cytotoxic T l's* and *helper, suppressor, contrasuppressor,* and $T_{DTH}$ cells under *cell.* See accompanying table.
**thymus-dependent l's,** T l's.
**thymus-independent l's,** B l's.
**tumor-infiltrating l's (TIL),** lymphocytes isolated from the inflammatory infiltrate present in solid tumors and cultured in interleukin-2 (IL-2); they have specific activity against the tumor from which they are derived.

**lym·pho·cyt·ic** (lim″fo-sit′ik) pertaining to, characterized by, or of the nature of lymphocytes.

**lym·pho·cy·to·blast** (lim″fo-si′to-blast) lymphoblast.

**lym·pho·cy·to·ma** (lim″fo-si-to′mə) [*lymphocyte* + *-oma*] 1. pseudolymphoma. 2. well-differentiated lymphocytic lymphoma.
**l. cu′tis,** a manifestation of cutaneous lymphoid hyperplasia, seen especially in women, characterized by skin lesions ranging from a solitary plaque or nodule to several in a group or more widespread lesions; they are usually found on the face, ears, extremities, or areolae of the breasts. When multiple, they may resemble malignant lymphoma, although some may regress, sometimes with recur-

**Surface Markers of Lymphocytes**

| | mIg | T1 | T3 Thy-1 | T4 Ly-1 | T5, T8 Ly-2, 3 | FcR | CR |
|---|---|---|---|---|---|---|---|
| B cells | + | – | – | – | – | ± | ± |
| T cells | | | | | | | |
| Helper | – | + | + | + | – | ± | – |
| Killer | – | + | + | – | + | ± | – |
| Suppressor | – | + | + | – | + | ± | – |
| Null cells | | | | | | | |
| K cells | – | – | – | – | – | + | – |
| NK cells | – | – | – | – | – | + | – |

mIg = membrane immunoglobulin; Thy-1, Ly-1, Ly-2, Ly-3 = mouse T-cell surface antigens; T1, T3, T4, T5, T8 = human T-cell surface antigens; FcR = Fc receptors; CR = complement receptors; ± indicates present only on a subset of cells or on cells of certain maturities.

**Human T Lymphocyte Cell-Surface Markers**

| Developmental Stage | T Antigens | |
|---|---|---|
| Early thymocyte | T10, T9 | |
| Common thymocyte | T10, T6, T4, T5, T8 | |
| | Helper subset | Killer-suppressor subset |
| Mature thymocyte | T10, T1, T3, T4 | T10, T1, T3, T5, T8 |
| Circulating T cell | T1, T3, T4 | T1, T3, T5, T8 |

rences. Exposure to sunlight, insect bites, and mechanical trauma have been implicated as causative factors. Called also *Bäfverstedt's syndrome, cutaneous lymphoplasia,* and *Spiegler-Fendt pseudolymphoma* or *sarcoid.*

**lym·pho·cy·to·pe·nia** (lim″fo-si″to-pe′ne-ə) [*lymphocyte* + *-penia*] reduction in the number of lymphocytes in the blood; called also *lymphopenia, hypolymphemia,* and *sublymphemia.*

**lym·pho·cy·to·phe·re·sis** (lim″fo-si″to-fə-re′sis) lymphocytapheresis.

**lym·pho·cy·to·poi·e·sis** (lim″fo-si″to-poi-e′sis) [*lymphocyte* + *poiesis*] the development of lymphocytes.

**lym·pho·cy·to·poi·et·ic** (lim″fo-si″to-poi-et′ik) pertaining to or characterized by lymphocytopoiesis.

**lym·pho·cy·tor·rhex·is** (lim″fo-si″to-rek′sis) the rupturing or bursting of lymphocytes.

**lym·pho·cy·to·sis** (lim″fo-si-to′sis) [MeSH: Lymphocytosis] excess of normal lymphocytes in the blood or in any effusion.
**acute infectious l.,** an acute, benign infectious disease of children characterized by an excess of normal small lymphocytes in the blood without lymphadenopathy or splenomegaly, and with varying degrees of clinical expression and constitutional response.

**lym·pho·cy·tot·ic** (lim″fo-si-tot′ik) pertaining to lymphocytosis.

**lym·pho·cy·to·tox·ic·i·ty** (lim″fo-si″to-tok-sis′ĭ-te) the quality or capability of lysing lymphocytes, as that of cytotoxic antibodies in the presence of complement or that of primed histoincompatible cytotoxic T lymphocytes.

**lym·pho·cy·to·tox·in** (lim″fo-si″to-tok′sin) a toxin that has a specific destructive action on lymphocytes.

**lym·pho·duct** (lim′fo-dəkt) a lymphatic vessel.

**lym·pho·epi·the·li·o·ma** (lim″fo-ep″ĭ-the″le-o′mə) a pleomorphic, poorly differentiated (transitional cell) carcinoma arising from modified epithelium overlying the lymphoid tissue of the nasopharynx; it has a high frequency among young adults of East Asian extraction. Called also *lymphoepithelial carcinoma, Schmincke's tumor,* and *Regaud's tumor.*

**lym·pho·gen·e·sis** (lim″fo-jen′ə-sis) the production of lymph.

**lym·phog·e·nous** (lim-foj′ə-nəs) [*lympho-* + *-genous*] 1. producing lymph. 2. produced from lymph or in the lymphatics.

**lym·pho·glan·du·la** (lim″fo-glan′du-lə) pl. *lymphoglan′dulae.* nodus lymphoideus.

**lym·pho·gram** (lim′fo-gram) a radiograph of the lymphatic vessels and lymph nodes.

**lym·pho·gran·u·lo·ma** (lim″fo-gran″u-lo′mə) Hodgkin's disease.
**l. inguina′le,** l. venereum.
**l. malig′num,** Hodgkin's disease.
**l. vene′reum,** a sexually transmitted infection usually seen in warm climates, due to strains of *Chlamydia trachomatis,* characterized by a primary cutaneous or mucosal lesion at the site of infection, which may be a papular, ulcerative, herpetiform, or erosive lesion or urethritis or endocervicitis that heals spontaneously and may go unnoticed, followed by acute unilateral or bilateral lymphadenopathy. The site of the initial infection or lesion determines the later manifestations: in men, the primary lesion is usually on the prepuce, glans, and shaft of the penis, associated with inguinal lymphadenitis, often with draining buboes *(the inguinal syndrome);* in women, the primary lesion usually involves the posterior vagina, cervix, and labia, associated with hemorrhagic proctocolitis *(the anogenitorectal syndrome).* Late complications in untreated cases, chiefly in women, include locally destructive ulcerations, rectal strictures, rectovaginal fistulas, and genital elephantiasis. Called also *l. inguinale; climatic* or *tropical bubo; Durand-Nicolas-Favre, Favre-Durand-Nicolas,* or *Nicolas-Favre disease; lymphopathia venerea;* and *subacute inguinal poradenitis.*

**lym·pho·gran·u·lo·ma·to·sis** (lim″fo-gran″u-lo-mə-to′sis) European synonym for Hodgkin's disease.
**benign l.,** sarcoidosis.
**l. cu′tis,** the cutaneous manifestation of Hodgkin's disease.
**l. inguina′lis,** lymphogranuloma venereum.

**lym·phog·ra·phy** (lim-fog′rə-fe) [MeSH: Lymphography] radiography of the lymphatic channels and lymph nodes, following injection of radiopaque material in a lymphatic vessel.

**lym·pho·his·tio·cyt·ic** (lim″fo-his″te-o-sit′ik) involving lymphocytes and histiocytes.

**lym·pho·his·tio·cy·to·sis** (lim″fo-his″te-o-si-to′sis) lymphocytosis with histiocytosis.
**erythrophagocytic l., hemophagocytic l.,** any of several closely related disorders involving both lymphocytosis and histiocytosis, with excessive hemophagocytosis in the lymphoreticular system or the central nervous system, usually seen in children secondary to an infection that may be bacterial, viral, fungal, or parasitic and often fatal. A few cases seem to be passed by autosomal recessive inheritance. Called also *hemophagocytic syndrome.*

**lym·pho·his·tio·plas·ma·cyt·ic** (lim″fo-his″te-o-plaz″mə-sit′ik) involving lymphocytes, histiocytes, and plasmacytes.

**lym·phoid** (lim′foid) [*lymph* + Gr. *eidos* form] resembling or pertaining to lymph or tissue of the lymphoid system.

**lym·phoi·dec·to·my** (lim″foi-dek′tə-me) excision of lymphoid tissue, such as adenoids and tonsils.

**lym·phoi·do·cyte** (lim-foi′do-sīt) old name for *hemocytoblast.*

**lym·pho·ken·tric** (lim″fo-ken′trik) [*lympho-* + Gr. *kentron* a stimulant] stimulating lymphocytopoiesis.

**lym·pho·kine** (lim′fo-kīn) [*lympho-* + Gr. *kinēsis* movement] a soluble cytokine that mediates immune responses; it is not an antibody or a complement component and is released by sensitized lymphocytes on contact with antigen. Cf. *monokine.*

**lym·pho·ki·ne·sis** (lim″fo-kĭ-ne′sis) [*lympho-* + *kinesis*] 1. the movement of the endolymph in the semicircular canals. 2. the circulation of lymph in the body.

**lym·phol·o·gy** (lim-fol′ə-je) [*lympho-* + *-logy*] the study of the lymphatic system. Cf. *lymphangiology.*

**lym·phol·y·sis** (lym-fol′ĭ-sis) lysis of lymphocytes.
**cell-mediated l. (CML),** a variation of the mixed lymphocyte culture (MLC) technique that is a functional test of the ability of cytotoxic lymphocytes (CTL) to kill target cells. Lymphocytes from two individuals are cultured together for several days, one population having been prevented from proliferating by treatment with radiation or mitomycin (a "one-way" MLC); they are then cultured for several hours with $^{51}$Cr-labeled target cells that are HLA-identical to the stimulator cells. Cytotoxicity is measured as percentage of $^{51}$Cr released from specific target cells compared to percentage of $^{51}$Cr released from control (nonspecific target) cells.

**lym·pho·lyt·ic** (lim″fo-lit′ik) causing destruction of lymphocytes.

**lym·pho·ma** (lim-fo′mə) [*lymph-* + *-oma*] [MeSH: Lymphoma] 1. any neoplastic disorder of the lymphoid tissue. 2. malignant l.

## Lymphoma

**adult T-cell l., adult T-cell leukemia/l.,** see under *leukemia.*
**African l.,** Burkitt's l.
**B-cell l.,** any in a large group of non-Hodgkin's lymphomas characterized by malignant transformation of the B lymphocytes; among the many B-cell lymphomas are *Burkitt's l., l. cutis, follicular center cell l.,* and *small B-cell l.*
**B-cell monocytoid l.,** a low-grade marginal zone lymphoma in which cells resemble those of hairy cell leukemia.
**bovine malignant l.,** enzootic bovine leukosis.
**Burkitt's l.,** a form of small noncleaved-cell lymphoma, usually found in central Africa, but also reported from other areas, and manifested most often as a large osteolytic lesion in the jaw or as an abdominal mass. The Epstein-Barr virus, a herpesvirus, has been isolated from Burkitt's lymphoma, and has been implicated as a causative agent. Called also *Burkitt's tumor* and *African l.*
**centrocytic l.,** mantle cell l.
**l. cu′tis,** primary skin involvement by B-cell lymphoma without demonstrable systemic disease, most often presenting as a solitary, purple to pink nodule, especially on the head, neck, and face, and usually associated with dissemination to regional lymph nodes and distant hematogenous spread, leading to widespread involvement.
**diffuse l.,** malignant lymphoma in which the neoplastic cells diffusely infiltrate the entire lymph node, without any definite organized pattern. This category from the Rappaport Classification was replaced by some of the cleaved-cell lymphomas in the Lukes-Collins Classification, by the three subtypes of diffuse lymphomas in the Working

Formulation of Non-Hodgkin's Lymphomas, and by a variety of specific B- and T-cell neoplasms in the Revised European American Lymphoma Classification. Called also *lymphatic sarcoma* and *lymphosarcoma.*

**diffuse, large cell l.,** a type of non-Hodgkin's lymphoma composed of large cleaved and noncleaved cells in a diffuse pattern of infiltration; it is similar to the diffuse mixed variety and has an intermediate grade of malignancy.

**diffuse, mixed small and large cell l.,** a type of lymphoma that mixes the small cleaved cell and large cell varieties; it is similar to the diffuse, large cell type and has an intermediate grade of malignancy.

**diffuse, small cleaved cell l.,** small cleaved cell lymphoma with a diffuse infiltrate of small lymphocytes that have round nuclei and clumped chromatin; this type has an intermediate grade of malignancy.

**follicular l.,** any of several types of non-Hodgkin's lymphoma in which the lymphomatous cells are clustered into identifiable nodules or follicles. The cells may be either small cleaved or large (cleaved or uncleaved) cells; tumors in which most or all of the cells are small and cleaved have a better prognosis than those with large cells. Called also *Brill-Symmers disease, Symmers' disease, giant follicle l.,* and *nodular l.*

**follicular center cell l.,** any of a large group of B-cell lymphomas, comprising four subtypes classified on the basis of the predominant cell type (resembling small cleaved, large cleaved, small noncleaved, and large noncleaved follicular center cells). Because of the wide variety of prognostic levels and the existence of tumors with several types of cells, the original four categories have now been divided up and scattered among several new categories of follicular and diffuse lymphomas.

**follicular, mixed small cleaved and large cell l.,** a type of non-Hodgkin's lymphoma with a mixture of small cleaved, large cleaved, and large uncleaved cells; the percentage of large cells is noticeable but less than 50 per cent of the tumor. It has a low grade of malignancy.

**follicular, predominantly large cell l.,** a rare type of follicular lymphoma with large cells that are either cleaved or noncleaved; it has a poorer prognosis than other follicular lymphomas.

**follicular, predominantly small cleaved cell l.,** the most common type of follicular lymphoma; it has a low grade of malignancy and is characterized by the formation of malignant small cleaved follicular center cells. See also *small cleaved cell l.*

**giant follicle l., giant follicular l.,** follicular l.

**granulomatous l.,** Hodgkin's disease.

**histiocytic l.,** a rare type of non-Hodgkin's lymphoma of intermediate to high malignancy, characterized by the presence of large tumor cells that resemble histiocytes morphologically but are considered to be of lymphoid origin. Many tumors formerly placed in this category are now considered to belong in one of the large cell lymphoma groups.

**Hodgkin's l.,** see under *disease.*

**large cell l.,** any of several types of lymphoma characterized by the formation of malignant large lymphocytes in a diffuse pattern; some varieties contain exclusively one type of cell, such as lymphoblasts or cleaved or uncleaved follicular center cells, and others have a mixture of cells, sometimes including ones that cannot be characterized as to lineage. Cf. *large cleaved cell l., large noncleaved cell l.,* and *large cell, immunoblastic l.*

**large cell, immunoblastic l.,** a type of non-Hodgkin's lymphoma characterized by large lymphoblasts (immunoblasts) that resemble histiocytes rather than follicular center cells, and have a diffuse pattern of infiltration; the cell population may be exclusively B or T lymphoblasts or a mixture. It has a high degree of malignancy and often grows rapidly. Tumors of predominantly B cells are often associated with a preexisting immunologic disorder such as Sjögren's syndrome, systemic lupus erythematosus, or Hashimoto's thyroiditis, or with an immunosuppressed state.

**large cleaved cell l.,** a type of non-Hodgkin's lymphoma characterized by the formation of malignant large cleaved follicular center cells; there are both follicular and diffuse varieties. Because of the wide variety of prognostic levels and the existence of tumors with several types of cells, these tumors have been divided among several different groups of follicular and diffuse lymphomas.

**large noncleaved cell l.,** a type of non-Hodgkin's lymphoma characterized by the formation of malignant large noncleaved follicular center cells. Because of the wide variety of prognostic levels and the existence of tumors with several types of cells, these tumors have been divided among several different groups of follicular and diffuse lymphomas.

**Lennert's l.,** a type of non-Hodgkin's lymphoma with a high content of epithelioid histiocytes; bone marrow involvement is common and response to chemotherapy is often poor.

**lymphoblastic l.,** a highly malignant type of non-Hodgkin's lymphoma composed of a diffuse, relatively uniform proliferation of cells with round or convoluted nuclei and scanty cytoplasm, which are cytologically similar to the lymphoblasts seen in acute lymphocytic leukemia. See also *convoluted T-cell l.*

**lymphocytic l., intermediate, lymphocytic l., intermediately differentiated,** mantle cell l.

**lymphocytic l., plasmacytoid,** a rare variety of small lymphocytic lymphoma in which the predominant cell type is the plasma cell; it may be the manifestation in lymphoid tissue of Waldenström's macroglobulinemia in the blood.

**lymphocytic l., poorly differentiated,** follicular, predominantly small cleaved cell l.

**lymphocytic l., small,** a diffuse form of non-Hodgkin's lymphoma with a low grade of malignancy; it represents the neoplastic proliferation of well-differentiated B lymphocytes and may present with either focal lymph node enlargement or generalized lymphadenopathy and splenomegaly. The predominant cell type is a compact, small, normal-appearing lymphocyte with a dark-staining round nucleus, scanty cytoplasm, and little size variation. It nearly always involves the bone marrow, and often malignant cells are found in the blood, so that its clinical picture is similar to that of chronic lymphocytic leukemia. Called also *well-differentiated lymphocytic l.*

**lymphocytic l., well differentiated,** small lymphocytic l.

**malignant l.,** any of a group of malignant neoplasms characterized by the proliferation of cells native to the lymphoid tissues, i.e., lymphocytes, histiocytes, and their precursors and derivatives. The group is divided into two major clinicopathologic categories: *Hodgkin's disease* and *non-Hodgkin's lymphoma.*

**malignant l. of cattle,** enzootic bovine leukosis.

**MALT l.,** MALToma.

**mantle cell l., mantle zone l.,** a rare form of non-Hodgkin's lymphoma having a usually diffuse pattern with both small lymphocytes and small cleaved cells; it may be a subgroup of diffuse, small cleaved cell lymphoma. It mainly affects people over 50 years of age and runs an indolent course although it may metastasize to the spleen or liver.

**marginal zone l.,** a group of related B-cell neoplasms that involve the lymphoid tissues in the marginal zone, the patchy area outside the follicular mantle zone; included are MALTomas and B-cell monocytoid lymphomas.

**Mediterranean l.,** immunoproliferative small intestine disease.

**mixed lymphocytic-histiocytic l.,** non-Hodgkin's lymphoma characterized by the presence of a mixed population of cells, with the smaller cells resembling lymphocytes and the larger ones histiocytes. When predominantly follicular it is called *follicular, mixed small cleaved and large cell l.,* and when predominantly diffuse it is called *diffuse, mixed small and large cell l.*

**nodular l.,** follicular l.

**non-Hodgkin's l.,** a heterogeneous group of malignant lymphomas, the only common feature being an absence of the giant Reed-Sternberg cells characteristic of Hodgkin's disease. They arise from the lymphoid components of the immune system, and present a clinical picture broadly similar to that of Hodgkin's disease except the disease is initially more widespread, with the most common manifestation being painless enlargement of one or more peripheral lymph nodes. There have been numerous classifications of the non-Hodgkin's lymphomas; the most recent system is the Revised European American Lymphoma (REAL) Classification (see under *classification*).

**plasmacytoid l.,** a heterogeneous group of low-grade B-cell lymphomas characterized by a mixture of small lymphocytes and plasmacytoid lymphocytes; it is sometimes associated with Waldenström's macroglobulinemia and can involve a number of tissues, including the lymph nodes, spleen, bone marrow, and gastrointestinal tract. Many patients have abnormal local or systemic immune reactions.

**pleomorphic l.,** small non-cleaved cell l.

**primary central nervous system l.,** a large cell lymphoma originating in the central nervous system, with solitary or multifocal foci; their frequency is sharply increased in immunodeficient patients. Formerly called also *microglioma and reticulum cell sarcoma of the brain.*

**primary effusion l.,** a B-cell lymphoma associated with human herpesvirus 8 infection, characterized by the occurrence of lymphomatous effusions in body cavities without the presence of a solid tumor.

**small B-cell l.,** the usual type of small lymphocytic lymphoma, having predominantly B lymphocytes.

**small cleaved cell l.,** a group of non-Hodgkin's lymphomas characterized by the formation of malignant small cleaved follicular center cells; it may have either a follicular or a diffuse pattern. One type, called *follicular, predominantly small cleaved cell lymphoma,* is particularly common. Because of the wide variety of prognostic levels and the existence of tumors with several types of cells, these tumors have now been divided among several different groups of follicular and diffuse lymphomas.

**small noncleaved cell l.,** a highly malignant type of non-Hodgkin's lymphoma characterized by the formation of small noncleaved follicular center cells, usually in a diffuse pattern; Burkitt's lymphoma is the most common variety. The incidence of all types increases sharply among immunocompromised patients.

**T-cell l's,** a heterogeneous group of lymphoid tumors representing malignant transformation of the T lymphocytes. The category includes *convoluted T-cell lymphoma, cutaneous T-cell lymphoma, adult T-cell leukemia,* and certain other conditions. Some types of tumors formerly included in this group have been found to be mixtures of T cells and B cell precursors.

**T-cell l., convoluted,** lymphoblastic lymphoma with markedly convoluted nuclei.

**T-cell l., cutaneous,** a group of lymphomas including a spectrum of disorders, all of which exhibit (1) clonal expansion of malignant T lymphocytes arrested at varying stages of differentiation of cells committed to the series of helper T cells, and (2) malignant infiltration of the skin, which may be the chief or only manifestation of disease. Mycosis fungoides and Sézary syndrome are the best characterized of these disorders. See also *Sézary cell,* under *cell.*

**T-cell l., small lymphocytic,** small lymphocytic lymphoma that has predominantly T lymphocytes.

**U-cell l., undefined l.,** a category of non-Hodgkin's lymphomas comprising those tumors that cannot be classified into a definite type by either morphologic or currently available immunocytochemical markers.

**undifferentiated l.,** small noncleaved cell l.

---

**lym·pho·ma·toid** (lim-fo'mə-toid) resembling lymphoma.

**lym·pho·ma·to·sis** (lim″fo-mə-to'sis) the development of multiple lymphomas in various parts of the body.
**avian l.,** avian leukosis involving chiefly the lymphocytes. Called also *fowl l.*
**bovine l.,** enzootic bovine leukosis.
**fowl l., l. of fowls,** avian l.
**neural l.,** Marek's disease in which neurological symptoms are dominant.
**ocular l.,** Marek's disease with ocular symptoms.
**visceral l.,** avian leukosis with solid tumors of the viscera.

**lym·pho·ma·tous** (lim-fo'mə-təs) pertaining to or of the nature of lymphoma.

**lym·pho·myx·o·ma** (lim″fo-mik-so'mə) any benign growth consisting of adenoid tissue.

**lym·pho·no·di** (lim″fo-no'di) [L.] plural of *lymphonodus.*

**lym·pho·nod·u·li** (lim″fo-nod'u-li) [L.] plural of *lymphonodulus.*

**lym·pho·nod·u·lus** (lim″fo-nod'u-ləs) pl. *lymphono'duli* [*lympho-* + *nodulus*] nodulus lymphoideus.
**lymphono'duli sple'nici,** noduli lymphoidei splenici; see under *nodulus.*

**lym·pho·no·dus** (lim″fo-no'dəs) pl. *lymphono'di* [*lympho-* + *nodus*] TA alternative for *nodus lymphoideus.*

**lym·pho·path·ia** (lim″fo-path'e-ə) lymphopathy.
**l. vene'rea,** lymphogranuloma venereum.

**lym·phop·a·thy** (lim-fop'ə-the) [*lympho-* + *-pathy*] any disease of the lymphatic system.
**ataxic l.,** a sudden swelling of the lymph nodes sometimes accompanying the pain crises of locomotor ataxia.

**lym·pho·pe·nia** (lim″fo-pe'ne-ə) [MeSH: Lymphopenia] lymphocytopenia.

**lym·pho·pla·sia** (lim″fo-pla'zhə) [*lympho-* + *-plasia*] the accumulation of lymphoreticular cells in the tissues.
**cutaneous l.,** lymphocytoma cutis.

**lym·pho·plasm** (lim'fo-plaz″əm) spongioplasm, def. 1.

**lym·pho·plas·ma·phe·re·sis** (lim″fo-plaz″mə-fə-re'sis) the selective separation and removal of plasma and lymphocytes from withdrawn blood, the remainder of the blood then being retransfused into the donor.

**lym·pho·poi·e·sis** (lim″fo-poi-e'sis) [*lympho-* + *-poiesis*] 1. the development of lymphatic tissue. 2. lymphocytopoiesis.

**lym·pho·poi·et·ic** (lim″fo-poi-et'ik) pertaining to, characterized by, or causing lymphopoiesis.

**lym·pho·pro·lif·er·a·tive** (lim″fo-pro-lif'ər-ə-tiv) pertaining to or characterized by proliferation of the cells of the lymphoreticular system; used to refer to a group of malignant neoplasms. See under *disorder* and see also *lymphoreticular* and *myeloproliferative.*

**lym·pho·re·tic·u·lar** (lim″fo-rə-tik'u-lər) pertaining to the cells or tissues of both the lymphoid and reticuloendothelial systems; see under *system* and *disorder.*

**lym·pho·re·tic·u·lo·sis** (lim″fo-rə-tik″u-lo'sis) proliferation of the reticuloendothelial cells of the lymph nodes.
**benign l.,** cat-scratch disease.

**lym·phor·rhage** (lim'fo-rəj) an accumulation of lymphocytes in a muscle.

**lym·phor·rha·gia** (lim″fo-ra'jə) [*lympho-* + *-rrhagia*] lymphorrhea.

**lym·phor·rhea** (lim″fo-re'ə) [*lympho-* + *-rrhea*] a flow of lymph from cut or ruptured lymph vessels.

**lym·phor·rhoid** (lim'fə-roid) a localized dilatation of a perianal lymph channel, resembling a hemorrhoid; sometimes occurring in lymphogranuloma venereum.

**lym·pho·sar·co·ma** (lim″fo-sahr-ko'mə) [*lympho-* + *sarcoma*] a diffuse lymphoma.

**lym·pho·scin·tig·ra·phy** (lim″fo-sin-tig'rə-fe) scintigraphic detection of metastatic tumor in radioactively labeled lymph nodes, particularly *radiocolloid l.* See also *immunolymphoscintigraphy.*
**radiocolloid l.,** scintigraphy of the lymph nodes following the administration of radiocolloid, usually labeled with technetium 99m, which migrates to the lymph nodes, where it is retained by phagocytosis; uptake of the tracer is decreased in nodes containing metastatic tumor.

**lym·phos·ta·sis** (lim-fos'tə-sis) [*lympho-* + *-stasis*] stoppage of the lymph flow.

**lym·pho·tax·is** (lim″fo-tak'sis) [*lympho-* + *-taxis*] the property of attracting or repulsing lymphocytes.

**lym·pho·tism** (lim'fo-tiz″əm) a disordered state associated with the development of adenoid tissue.

**lym·pho·tox·in (LT)** (lim″fo-tok'sin) [MeSH: Lymphotoxin] a lymphokine with some homology to tumor necrosis factor; it is produced by activated T lymphocytes and inhibits the growth of tumors, causing lysis or stasis of sensitive cells, and also blocks transformation of cells.

**lym·phot·ro·phy** (lim-fot'rə-fe) [*lympho-* + *-trophy*] nourishment of cells by lymph in tissues lacking sufficient blood supply.

**lym·pho·trop·ic** (lim″fo-trop'ik) [*lympho-* + *tropic*] having an affinity for lymphatic tissue.

**lym·phous** (lim'fəs) pertaining to or containing lymph.

**Lynch's incision, operation** (linch'əz) [Robert Clyde *Lynch,* American otologist, born 1880] see under *incision* and *operation.*

**Lyn·chia mau·ra** (lin'ke-ə maw'rə) *Pseudolynchia canariensis.*

**Ly·nen** (le'nən) Feodor. German biochemist, 1911–1979; co-winner, with Konrad Bloch, of the Nobel prize for medicine or physiology in 1964, for investigations in biosynthesis of fatty acids and cholesterol.

**lyn·es·tre·nol** (lin-es'trə-nol) [MeSH: Lynestrenol] a progestational agent used as a component of oral contraceptives.

**Lyn·or·al** (lin'or-əl) trademark for a preparation of ethinyl estradiol.

**Lynx·ac·a·rus** (lingk-sak'ə-rəs) a genus of mites of the family Listrophoridae. *L. radov'skyi* is found clinging to the hair of domestic cats in Florida, Puerto Rico, and various Pacific islands, causing pruritus and skin lesions.

**lyo-** [Gr. *lyein* to dissolve] combining form meaning dissolved or dispersed.

**lyo·chrome** (li'o-krōm) [*lyo-* + *-chrome*] flavin.

**lyo·gel** (li'o-jel) [*lyo-* + *gel*] a gel containing much liquid. Cf. *xerogel.*

**Ly·on hypothesis** (li'on) [Mary Frances *Lyon,* English geneticist, born 1925] see under *hypothesis.*

**ly·on·iza·tion** (li″on-ĭ-za'shən) [after Mary F. *Lyon*] the process by which or the condition in which all X chromosomes of the cells in excess of one are inactivated on a random basis. Called also *heterochromatinization, heterochromatization,* and *X-inactivation.* See also *Lyon hypothesis,* under *hypothesis.*

**ly·on·ized** (li'o-nīzd) [after Mary F. *Lyon*] denoting the inactivated X chromosome in a cell, according to the Lyon hypothesis.

**lyo·phil** (li'o-fil) a lyophilic substance; a material that readily goes into solution.

**lyo·phile** (li'o-fīl) lyophil.

**lyo·phil·ic** (li″o-fil'ik) [*lyo-* + *-philic*] having an affinity for, or stable in, solution; denoting a tendency of atoms or groups of atoms to be wetted by a solvent. See also under *colloid*.

**ly·oph·i·li·za·tion** (li-of″ĭ-lĭ-za'shən) the creation of a stable preparation of a biological substance (blood plasma, serum, etc.), by rapid freezing and dehydration of the frozen product under high vacuum. See also *freeze-drying*.

**ly·oph·i·lize** (li-of'ĭ-līz) to subject to lyophilization.

**lyo·phobe** (li'o-fōb) a lyophobic substance; a material that does not readily go into or tends to separate out from solution.

**lyo·pho·bic** (li″o-fo'bik) [*lyo-* + Gr. *phobein* to fear] not having an affinity for, or unstable in, solution; denoting a tendency of atoms or groups of atoms to avoid being wetted by a solvent. See also under *colloid*.

**lyo·sorp·tion** (li″o-sorp'shən) the selective adsorption of the solvent portion of a solution.

**lyo·trop·ic** (li″o-trop'ik) [*lyo-* + *-tropic*] lyophilic; see also under *series*.

**Ly·per·o·sia ir·ri·tans** (li″pər-o'se-ə ir'ĭ-təns) *Haematobia irritans*.

**Ly·po·nys·sus** (li″po-nis'əs) former name for *Ornithonyssus*.

**ly·pres·sin** (li-pres'in) [MeSH: Lypressin] lysine vasopressin.

**ly·ra** (li'rə) [L., from Gr. "a stringed instrument resembling the lute"] a name applied to certain anatomical structures because of their fancied resemblance to a lute.
**l. Da'vidis,** *(obs.)* commissura fornicis.

**lyre** (līr) lyra.

**Lys** lysine.

**ly·sate** (li'sāt) 1. the material formed by the lysis of cells. 2. a medicinal preparation obtained from an animal organ by means of artificial digestion.

**lyse** (līz) 1. to cause or produce disintegration of a compound, substance, or cell. 2. to undergo lysis.

**ly·ser·gic ac·id** (li-sər'jik) [MeSH: Lysergic Acid] a constituent of the ergot alkaloids obtained by hydrolysis.
**l. a. diethylamide (LSD),** a synthetic ergot alkaloid with psychotomimetic properties and both sympathomimetic and serotoninergic blocking effects; it counteracts barbiturates and is counteracted by suppressants like chlorpromazine. Objective effects include ataxia, fever, hyperreflexia, mydriasis, piloerection, tremor, and sometimes nausea and vomiting. Subjective effects include visual perception disorders and varying degrees of depersonalization, synesthesia, delusions, hallucinations, distortions of thought, sense, time, mood, and body image (which may be extreme). Anxiety may develop into acute panic reactions, and a persistent toxic psychotic state may result. Physical or psychological dependence is rare. Called also *lysergide*.

**ly·ser·gide** (li-sər'jīd) nonproprietary drug name for lysergic acid diethylamide (LSD).

**lys·i·din** (lis'ĭ-din) a red crystalline body, methylglyoxalidin, or its yellowish or pinkish, soapy, 50 per cent solution: used as a solvent for uric acid.
**l. bitartrate,** a soluble, white, crystalline powder, of one third the solvent power of pure lysidin.

**ly·sin** (li'sin) [Gr. *lyein* to dissolve] 1. any substance that causes cell lysis. 2. immune lysin, immune cytolysin, an antibody that causes complement-dependent lysis of cells; often used with a prefix indicating the target cells, e.g., hemolysin or bacteriolysin.
**beta l.,** beta-lysin.
**sperm l.,** a general term for the enzymatic substances of spermatozoa which dissolve egg membranes and permit penetration; these lysins are thought to be produced by the acrosome.

**ly·sine** (li'sēn) [MeSH: Lysine] an essential amino acid, α,ε-diaminocaproic acid, a hydrolytic product of protein first isolated from casein (Drechsel, 1889); necessary for optimal growth in infants and for maintenance of nitrogen equilibrium in human adults. Symbols Lys and K. See table at *amino acid*.
**l. acetate** [USP], the monoacetate of L-lysine, used as a dietary supplement.
**l. hydrochloride** [USP], the monohydrochloride salt of L-lysine, used as a dietary supplement and for the treatment of severe metabolic alkalosis refractory to other treatment.

**ly·sine car·boxy·pep·ti·dase** (li'sēn kahr-bok″se-pep'tĭ-dās) [EC 3.4.17.3] [MeSH: Lysine Carboxypeptidase] an enzyme of the hydrolase class that catalyzes the removal of C-terminal basic amino acids from peptides, preferentially removing lysine residues but also removing arginine residues from kinins, inactivating them. The enzyme is found in plasma. Called also *arginine carboxypeptidase* and *kininase I*.

**ly·sine de·hy·dro·gen·ase** (li'sēn de-hi'dro-jən-ās) an enzyme of the oxidoreductase class that catalyzes the oxidative deamination of lysine, removing the α-amino acid as the first step in a minor pathway of lysine degradation (see also *α-aminoadipic semialdehyde synthase*). Deficiency of the enzyme, an autosomal recessive trait, causes congenital lysine intolerance.

**ly·sine ke·to·glu·ta·rate re·duc·tase** (li'sēn ke″to-gloo'tə-rāt re-duk'tās) saccharopine dehydrogenase (NADP$^+$, L-lysine-forming).

**ly·sine-ke·to·glu·ta·rate re·duc·tase de·fi·cien·cy** hyperlysinemia.

**L-ly·sine:NAD ox·i·do·re·duc·tase** (li'sēn ok″sĭ-do-re-duk'tās) lysine dehydrogenase.

**L-ly·sine:NAD ox·i·do·re·duc·tase de·fi·cien·cy** congenital lysine intolerance.

**ly·sin·o·gen** (li-sin'ə-jən) [*lysin* + Gr. *gennan* to produce] an antigenic substance capable of inducing the formation of lysins.

**ly·sin·uria** (li″sĭ-nu're-ə) excretion of lysine in the urine.

**ly·sis** (li'sis) [Gr. "dissolution; a loosing, setting free, releasing"] 1. destruction, as of cells by a specific lysin. 2. decomposition, as of a chemical compound by a specific agent. Cf. *degradation*. 3. mobilization of an organ by division of restraining adhesions. 4. the gradual abatement of the symptoms of a disease; cf. *crisis*, def. 1.
**hot-cold l.,** lysis that occurs only if the material is incubated as usual and then allowed to stand overnight at room temperature.

**-lysis** [Gr. "dissolution; a loosing, setting free, releasing"] a word termination denoting dissolution, decomposition, disintegration, or destruction; relief, reduction, or abatement; loosening or setting free.

**lys(o)-** [Gr. *lysis* dissolution] a combining form denoting relationship to lysis or dissolution.

**ly·so·cy·thin** (li″so-si'thin) a substance formed by combination between an animal poison and the body tissues and having a cytolytic action.

**Ly·so·dren** (li'so-drən) trademark for a preparation of mitotane.

**ly·so·gen** (li'so-jən) [*lyso-* + *-gen*] 1. an agent that induces lysis. 2. lysinogen. 3. a lysogenized bacterium.

**ly·so·gen·e·sis** (li″so-jen'ə-sis) the production of lysis or lysins.

**ly·so·gen·ic** (li-so-jen'ik) [*lyso-* + *-genic*] 1. producing lysins or causing lysis. 2. pertaining to lysogeny.

**ly·so·ge·nic·i·ty** (li″so-jə-nis'ĭ-te) [*lyso-* + Gr. *gennan* to produce + *-ity* condition] 1. the ability to produce lysins or cause lysis. 2. the potentiality of a bacterium to produce phage. 3. the specific association of the phage genome, the prophage, with the bacterial genome in such a way that only a few, if any, phage genes are transcribed.

**ly·sog·e·ny** (li-soj'ə-ne) [MeSH: Lysogeny] the phenomenon in which a bacterium is infected by a temperate bacteriophage, the viral DNA is integrated in the chromosome of the host cell and replicated along with the host chromosome for many generations (the lysogenic cycle), and then production of virions and lysis of host cells (the lytic cycle) begins again. The lytic cycle is initiated spontaneously about once in 10,000 cell divisions or may be induced by ultraviolet light or chemical agents.

**ly·so·ki·nase** (li″so-ki'nās) a substance that activates a proactivator in the fibrinolytic system.

**ly·so·phos·pha·ti·date** (li″so-fos″fə-ti'dāt) 1. the anionic form of lysophosphatidic acid. 2. any phosphatidic acid–containing phospholipid that lacks one of its fatty acyl groups; the compounds are present as minor constituents of cell membranes as a result of phospholipid metabolism and are so named for their membranolytic qualities at high concentrations.

**ly·so·phos·pha·tid·ic ac·id** (li″so-fos″fə-tid'ik) phosphatidic acid lacking one of its fatty acyl chains; an intermediate in the synthesis of phosphatidic acid and a component of the lysophosphatidates (def. 2).

**ly·so·phos·pho·li·pase** (li″so-fos″fo-li'pās) [EC 3.1.1.5] [MeSH: Lysophospholipase] an enzyme of the hydrolase class that catalyzes the hydrolysis of the acyl group from a 2-lysophospholipid, a step in the degradation of dietary and intracellular phospholipids.

**ly·so·phos·pho·lip·id** (li″so-fos″fo-lip'id) a phospholipid that lacks one of its fatty acyl chains; an intermediate formed during digestion of dietary and biliary phospholipids. The terms lysophospholipid and lysophosphatidate are sometimes used synonymously to denote the monoacyl derivatives of phosphatidic acid–containing compounds.

**ly·so·so·mal** (li″so-so′məl) of or pertaining to a lysosome.

**ly·so·so·mal α-glu·co·si·dase** (li″so-sōm′əl gloo-ko′sĭ-dās) glucan 1,4-α-glucosidase.

**ly·so·so·mal α-glu·co·si·dase de·fi·cien·cy** glycogen storage disease, type II.

**ly·so·some** (li′so-sōm) [*lyso-* + *-some*] one of the minute bodies seen with the electron microscope in many types of cells, containing various hydrolytic enzymes and normally involved in the process of localized intracellular digestion. Injury to a lysosome is followed by release into the cell of the enzymes, which may damage the cell and give rise to wasting and other pathologic aspects of certain diseases, as in muscular dystrophy. See Plate 13.
**primary l.**, one that has not yet been engaged in digestive activities.
**secondary l.**, a primary (or another secondary) lysosome that has fused with a phagosome (or pinosome), bringing hydrolases in contact with the ingested material and resulting in digestion of the material. See also *autophagy* (def. 2) and *heterophagy.*

**ly·so·staph·in** (li-so-staf′in) [MeSH: Lysostaphin] an antibacterial enzyme produced by *Staphylococcus staphylolyticus;* it is specifically active against staphylococci.

**ly·so·zyme** (li′so-zīm) [EC 3.2.1.17] an enzyme of the hydrolase class that catalyzes the hydrolysis of specific glycosidic linkages in peptidoglycans and in chitin. The enzyme occurs in saliva, tears, egg white, and many animal fluids and catalyzes the breakdown of some bacterial cell walls.

**ly·so·zy·mu·ria** (li″so-zi-mu′re-ə) urinary excretion of elevated levels of lysozyme.

**lys·sa** (lis′ə) [Gr. "frenzy"; "*the worm* under the tongue of dogs, removed because of the belief that it caused rabies"] former name for rabies.

**Lys·sa·vi·rus** (lis′ə-vi″rəs) [*lyssa* + *virus*] [MeSH: Lyssavirus] rabies-like viruses; a genus of viruses of the family Rhabdoviridae comprising the rabies virus and other related viruses that infect mammals and arthropods.

**lys·sic** (lis′ik) pertaining to rabies.

**lyss(o)-** [Gr. *lyssa* rabies] a combining form denoting relationship to rabies.

**lys·soid** (lis′oid) [*lysso-* + *-oid*] rabiform.

**lys·so·pho·bia** (lis″o-fo′be-ə) [Gr. *lyssa* rabies + *-phobia*] irrational fear of rabies.

**ly·syl** (li′səl) the acyl radical of lysine.

**ly·syl hy·drox·y·lase** (li′səl hi-drok′sə-lās) an enzyme of the oxidoreductase class that catalyzes the hydroxylation of specific lysine residues in nascent procollagen chains; the hydroxylysine residues act as sites of attachment for disaccharide prosthetic groups and are involved in the formation of strong interchain crosslinks in collagen. The enzyme requires $Fe^{2+}$, ascorbate, and α-ketoglutarate for activity. Deficiency of enzyme activity, an autosomal recessive trait, results in Ehlers-Danlos syndrome, type VI. In EC nomenclature, called *procollagen-lysine 5-dioxygenase.*

**ly·syl ox·i·dase** (li′səl ok′sĭ-dās) an enzyme of the oxidoreductase class that catalyzes the oxidative deamination of lysine and hydroxylysine residues to the corresponding aldehydes, a step in the formation of covalent crosslinks in collagens and elastins. The reaction requires pyridoxal phosphate and $Cu^{2+}$; the deficiency of enzyme activity and attendant physiological consequences occurring in Ehlers-Danlos syndrome, type IX (X-linked cutis laxa) and Menkes′ syndrome appear to be secondary to deficiencies in copper metabolism or transport.

**ly·te·ri·an** (li-te′re-ən) indicative of lysis of an attack of disease.

**lyt·ic** (lit′ik) [Gr. *lyticos* dissolving, from *lysis* dissolution] 1. pertaining to lysis or to a lysin. 2. producing lysis.

**-lytic** a word termination denoting lysis of the substance indicated by the stem to which it is affixed.

**Lyt·ta** (lit′ə) a genus of blister beetles (family Meloidae) that secrete cantharidin and can cause cantharidin poisoning in ruminants. Called also *Russian fly.*
**L. vesicato′ria,** a species whose dried bodies are the source of cantharidin. Called also *Cantharis vesicatoria, blister bug,* and *Spanish fly.*

**lyx·ose** (lik′sōs) an aldopentose isomeric with ribose at carbons 2 and 3.

**lyze** (līz) lyse.

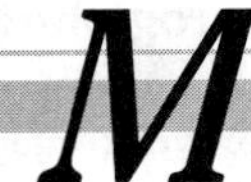

**M** symbol for *mega-*, *molar*[1](used with a number designating the strength of the solution relative to one molar, e.g., M/2 or 0.5M for half-molar), *molar*[2], *morgan*, *mucoid* (colony), *myopia*, and for the low frequency component of the first heart sound; see under *sound*.

**M.** symbol for *mis'ce* and *mistu'ra*.

***M*** symbol for *mutual inductance*, *molar mass*, and *molar*[1] (see M).

**$M_1$** symbol for *mitral valve closure;* see *first heart sound*, under *sound*.

**$M_r$** symbol for *relative molecular mass;* see *molecular weight*, under *weight*.

**m** symbol for *median*, *meter*, and *milli-*.

**m.** symbol for *minim* and for L. *mus'culus*, muscle.

***m*** symbol for *mass* and *molal* (used with a number designating the strength of the solution relative to one molal).

***m-*** chemical symbol for *meta-* (def. 2).

**$\mu$** mu, the twelfth letter of the Greek alphabet; symbol for *linear attenuation coefficient*, *population mean*, *micro-*, *micron*, *electrophoretic mobility*, and the heavy chain of IgM (see *immunoglobulin*).

**MA** mental age; meter angle; Master of Arts.

**mA** symbol for *milliampere*.

**$\mu$A** symbol for *microampere*.

**MAA** macroaggregated albumin; see *aggregated albumin*, under *albumin*. See also table at *technetium*.

**MAC** membrane attack complex; minimal alveolar concentration; *Mycobacterium avium* complex (see under *disease*).

**Mac.** abbreviation for L. *macerare*, macerate.

**Mac-1** see under *glycoprotein*.

**Ma·ca·ca** (mə-kah'kə) [MeSH: Macaca] the macaques, a genus of monkeys of the family Cercopithecidae. *M. fascicula'ris* is the cynomolgus monkey and *M. mulat'ta* is the rhesus monkey, both used in laboratory research.

**ma·caque** (mə-kahk') a member of the genus *Macaca*, short-tailed monkeys; most are native to southern Asia, with one species found in Northwestern Africa and another in South America.
**crab-eating m.**, cynomolgus monkey.
**rhesus m.**, see under *monkey*.

**Mc·Ar·dle's disease (syndrome)** (mə-kahr'dəlz) [Brian *McArdle*, English neurologist, born 1911] see *glycogen storage disease, type V*, under *disease*.

**Mc·Bride operation** (mək-brīd') [Earl D. *McBride*, American orthopedic surgeon, born 1891] see under *operation*.

**Mc·Bur·ney's incision,** etc. (mək-ber'nēz) [Charles *McBurney*, New York surgeon, 1845–1913] see under *incision, operation, point,* and *sign*.

**Mac·Cal·lum's patch, plaques** (mə-kal'əmz) [William George *MacCallum*, Canadian-born pathologist in the United States, 1874–1944] see under *patch* and *plaque*.

**Mc·Car·thy's reflex** (mə-kahr'thēz) [Daniel J. *McCarthy*, American neurologist, 1874–1958] see under *reflex*.

**Mc·Clin·tock** (mə-klin'tok) Barbara. American botanist and geneticist, 1902–1992; winner of the Nobel prize for medicine or physiology in 1983 for her discovery that genes of a corn plant move from one place to another and thus alter future plants.

**Mac·Con·key's agar** (mə-kong'kēz) [Alfred Theodore *MacConkey*, English bacteriologist, 1861–1931] see under *culture medium*.

**Mc·Cune-Al·bright syndrome** (mə-kūn' awl'brīt) [Donovan James *McCune*, American pediatrician, 1902–1976; Fuller *Albright*, American physician, 1900–1969] Albright's syndrome.

**Mc·Don·ald's maneuver, rule** (mək-don'əldz) [Ellice *McDonald*, Canadian gynecologist and pathologist in United States, 1876–1955] see under *maneuver* and *rule*.

**Mace** (mās) trademark for an aerosol mixture of chloroacetophenone.

**mac·er·ate** (mas'ər-āt) to soften by wetting or soaking; see *maceration*.

**mac·er·a·tion** (mas″ər-a'shən) [L. *maceratio*] 1. the softening of a solid by soaking. 2. in histology, the softening of a tissue by soaking, especially in acids, until the connective tissue fibers are so dissolved that the tissue components can be teased apart. 3. in obstetrics, the degenerative changes with discoloration and softening of tissues, and eventual disintegration, of a fetus retained in the uterus after its death.

**mac·er·a·tive** (mas'ər-ə″tiv) characterized by maceration.

**Mac·ew·en's operation, sign, triangle** (mə-ku'ənz) [Sir William *Macewen*, Scottish surgeon, 1848–1924] see under *operation* and *sign*, and see *foveola suprameatica*.

**Mc·Ginn-White sign** (mək-gin' hwīt) [Sylvester *McGinn*, American cardiologist, born 1904; Paul Dudley *White*, American cardiologist, 1886–1973] see under *sign*.

**Ma·cha·do-Jo·seph disease** (mah-chah'do-jo'səf) [*Machado* and *Joseph*, afflicted families] [MeSH: Machado-Joseph Disease] see under *disease*.

**ma·chine** (mə-shēn') [L. *machina*] a contrivance or apparatus for the production, conversion, or transmission of some form of energy or force.
**heart-lung m.**, a combination blood pump (artificial heart) and blood oxygenator (artificial lung) used in cardiopulmonary bypass for cardiac surgery.
**Holtz m.**, an apparatus for developing static electricity.
**Van de Graaff m.**, an electrostatic generator of high voltage.
**Wimshurst m.**, a machine for the development of static current.

**MAC INH** membrane attack complex inhibitor, former name for *S protein;* see *vitronectin*.

**Mac·Kay-Marg electronic tonometer** (mə-ka'mahrg) [Ralph Stuart *MacKay*, American biophysicist, born 1924; Elwin *Marg*, American physicist, born 1918] see under *tonometer*.

**Mack·en·rodt's ligament** (mahk'en-rots) [Alwin Karl *Mackenrodt*, German gynecologist, 1859–1925] see *plica rectouterina*.

**Mac·ken·zie's syndrome** (mə-ken'zēz) [Sir Stephen *Mackenzie*, London physician, 1844–1909] Jackson's syndrome.

**Mc·Ku·sick-Kauf·man syndrome** (mə-ku'sik-kawf'mən) [Victor Almon *McKusick*, American geneticist, born 1921; Robert L. *Kaufman*, American physician, born 1937] Kaufman-McKusick syndrome.

**Mac·Lean-Max·well disease** (mə-klān' maks'wəl) [Charles Murray *MacLean*, English physician in West Africa, 1788–1824; James Laidlaw *Maxwell*, Sr., English physician in Formosa, 1836–1921] see under *disease*.

**Mac·leod** (mə-kloud') John James Rickard. Scottish physiologist, 1876–1935; co-winner, with Sir Frederick Grant Banting, of the Nobel prize for medicine and physiology in 1923, for their discovery of insulin.

**Mc·Leod phenotype, syndrome** (mə-kloud') [from the name of the propositus first observed in 1961] see under *phenotype* and *syndrome*.

**Mac·leod's syndrome** (mə-kloudz') [William Mathieson *Macleod*, British physician, 1911–1977] see *Swyer-James syndrome*, under *syndrome*.

**McMurray's test (sign)** (mək-mur'ēz) [Thomas Porter *McMurray*, British orthopedic surgeon, 1887–1949] see under *test*.

**Mc·Naugh·ten** (mək-naw'tən) see *M'Naghten*.

**Mc·Phee·ters' treatment** (mək-fe'tərz) [Herman Oscar *McPheeters*, American surgeon, 20th century] see under *treatment*.

**Mac·ra·can·tho·rhyn·chus** (mak″rə-kan″tho-ring'kəs) a genus of acanthocephalans. *M. hirudina'ceus* is parasitic in swine in the United States.

**mac·rad·e·nous** (mak-rad'ə-nəs) [*macro-* + *adenous*] having large glands.

**mac·ren·ce·pha·lia** (mak-ren'sə-fa'le-ə) macrencephaly.

**mac·ren·ceph·a·ly** (mak″rən-sef'ə-le) [*macro-* + Gr. *enkephalos* brain] overgrowth of the brain.

**macr(o)-** [Gr. *makros* large, long] a combining form meaning large, or of abnormal size or length.

**mac·ro·abra·sion** (mak'ro-ə-bra″zhən) the removal of minute amounts of enamel with a high-speed carbide bur in order to correct tooth discoloration.

**mac·ro·ad·e·no·ma** (mak″ro-ad″ə-no'mə) a pituitary adenoma over 10 mm in diameter, large enough to be easily visualized by usual radiologic techniques; most are null-cell adenomas and are detected because they exert pressure on surrounding structures. Cf. *microadenoma*.

**mac·ro·ag·gre·gate** (mak″ro-ag'rə-gāt) an unusually large aggregate of a substance.

**mac·ro·aleu·rio·spore** (mak″ro-ə-lo͝or'e-o-spor) a large, usually multicellular, aleuriospore; the term is sometimes used interchangeably with *macroconidium*.

**mac·ro·am·y·lase** (mac″ro-am′ə-lās) serum amylase bound to a globulin. Because the complex formed (M.W. 200,000) is too large for renal clearance, its formation results in elevated levels of plasma amylase.

**mac·ro·am·yl·a·se·mia** (mak″ro-am″əl-ə-se′me-ə) a type of hyperamylasemia due to presence of macroamylase in the blood.

**mac·ro·am·yl·a·se·mic** (mak″ro-am″əl-ə-se′mik) pertaining to or characterized by macroamylasemia.

**mac·ro·anal·y·sis** (mak″ro-ə-nal′ə-sis) chemical analysis using 0.1 to 0.2 g of the substance under study.

**Mac·rob·del·la** (mak″ro-del′ə) a genus of leeches of the family Gnathobdellidae. *M. deco′ra* is a small species widely distributed in the United States and Canada that is sometimes used medicinally.

**mac·ro·bi·o·ta** (mak″ro-bi-o′tə) the macroscopic living organisms of a region; the combined macroflora and macrofauna of a region.

**mac·ro·bi·ot·ic** (mak″ro-bi-ot′ik) pertaining to the macrobiota, or to macroscopic living organisms.

**mac·ro·blast** (mak′ro-blast) [*macro-* + *-blast*] a large erythroblast resembling a megaloblast. Called also *macroerythroblast* and *macronormoblast.*

**mac·ro·ble·pha·ria** (mak″ro-blə-far′e-ə) [*macro-* + *blephar-* + *-ia*] abnormal largeness of the eyelid.

**mac·ro·bra·chia** (mak″ro-bra′ke-ə) [*macro-* + *brachia*] abnormal size or length of the arms.

**mac·ro·car·di·us** (mak″ro-kahr′de-əs) [*macro-* + Gr. *kardia* heart] a fetus with an extremely large heart.

**mac·ro·ce·pha·lia** (mak″ro-sə-fa′le-ə) macrocephaly.

**mac·ro·ce·phal·ic** (mac″ro-sə-fal′ik) macrocephalous.

**mac·ro·ceph·a·lous** (mak″ro-sef′ə-ləs) having an excessively large head.

**mac·ro·ceph·a·lus** (mak″ro-sef′ə-ləs) megalocephaly.

**mac·ro·ceph·a·ly** (mak″ro-sef′ə-le) [*macro-* + *-cephaly*] excessive size of the head.

**mac·ro·chei·lia** (mak″ro-ki′le-ə) [*macro-* + *cheil-* + *-ia*] excessive size of the lips.

**mac·ro·chei·ria** (mak″ro-ki′re-ə) [*macro-* + *cheir-* + *-ia*] excessive size of the hands.

**mac·ro·chem·i·cal** (mak″ro-kem′ĭ-kəl) pertaining to macrochemistry.

**mac·ro·chem·is·try** (mak″ro-kem′is-tre) [*macro-* + *chemistry*] chemistry in which the reactions may be seen with the naked eye. Cf. *microchemistry.*

**mac·ro·chi·lia** (mak″ro-ki′le-ə) macrocheilia.

**mac·ro·chi·ria** (mak″ro-ki′re-ə) macrocheiria.

**mac·ro·clit·o·ris** (mak″ro-klit′o-ris) hypertrophy of the clitoris.

**mac·ro·cne·mia** (mak″ro-ne′me-ə) [*macro-* + Gr. *knēmē* shin + *-ia*] a condition in which the lower limbs are abnormally large below the knees.

**mac·ro·co·lon** (mak′ro-ko″lən) megacolon.

**mac·ro·co·nid·i·um** (mak″ro-ko-nid′e-əm) pl. *macroconid′ia* [*macro-* + *conidium*] a large, frequently multicelled conidium or exospore of a fungus that also produces microconidia; the term is sometimes used interchangeably with *macroaleuriospore.*

**mac·ro·cor·nea** (mak′ro-kor′ne-ə) [*macro-* + *cornea*] megalocornea.

**mac·ro·cra·nia** (mak″ro-kra′ne-ə) abnormal increase in the size of the skull, the facial area being disproportionately small in comparison, such as with hydrocephalus.

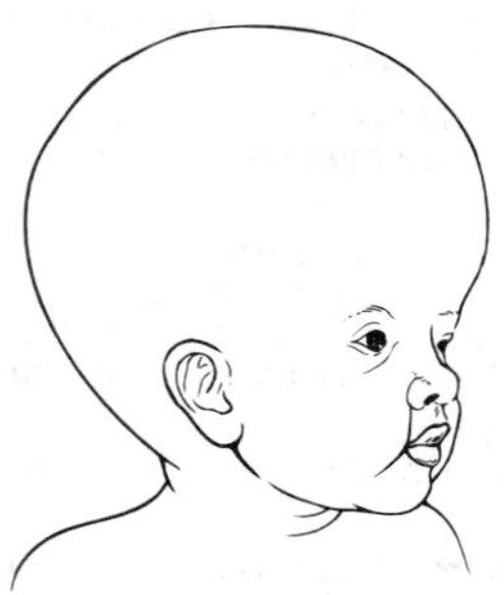

Macrocrania.

**mac·ro·cyc·lic** (mak″ro-sik′lik) pertaining to a large cyclic organic compound, usually one containing more than 15 atoms.

**mac·ro·cyst** (mak′ro-sist) [*macro-* + *cyst*] 1. a large cyst. 2. in mycology, an encysted reproductive cell of certain slime molds. Cf. *microcyst.*

**mac·ro·cyte** (mak′ro-sīt) [*macro-* + *-cyte*] an abnormally large erythrocyte, such as those seen in macrocytic anemia. Called also *megalocyte.*

**mac·ro·cy·the·mia** (mak″ro-si-the′me-ə) [*macrocyte* + *hem-* + *-ia*] a condition in which the erythrocytes are larger than normal, such as in macrocytic anemia and some types of liver disease. Called also *macrocytosis* and *megalocytosis.*

**mac·ro·cyt·ic** (mak″ro-sit′ik) pertaining to or characterized by macrocytes.

**mac·ro·cy·to·sis** (mak″ro-si-to′sis) macrocythemia.

**mac·ro·dac·tyl·ia** (mak″ro-dak-til′e-ə) megalodactyly.

**mac·ro·dac·ty·ly** (mak″ro-dak′tə-le) [*macro-* + Gr. *daktylos* finger] megalodactyly.

**Mac·ro·dan·tin** (mak″ro-dan′tin) trademark for a preparation of nitrofurantoin.

**mac·ro·dont** (mak′ro-dont) having large teeth; characterized by macrodontia. Called also *megadont.*

**mac·ro·don·tia** (mak″ro-don′shə) [*macro-* + *odont* + *-ia*] a developmental disorder characterized by increase in the size of the teeth; it may affect a single tooth or all of the teeth, or teeth of normal size may appear to be abnormally large in proportion to abnormally small jaws. Called also *macrodontism, megadontia,* and *megalodontia.*

**mac·ro·don·tic** (mak″ro-don′tik) pertaining to or characterized by macrodontia.

**mac·ro·don·tism** (mak″ro-don′tiz-əm) macrodontia.

**mac·ro·dys·tro·phia** (mak″ro-dis-tro′fe-ə) [*macro-* + *dys-* + *troph-* + *-ia*] overgrowth of a part.
**m. lipomato′sa progressi′va,** partial gigantism associated with tumor-like overgrowth of adipose tissue.

**mac·ro·el·e·ment** (mak″ro-el′ə-ment) any of the macronutrients that are chemical elements, including calcium, chloride, magnesium, phosphorus, potassium, sodium, and sulfur. Cf. *trace element.*

**mac·ro·en·ceph·a·ly** (mak″ro-ən-sef′ə-le) macrencephaly.

**mac·ro·e·ryth·ro·blast** (mak″ro-ə-rith′ro-blast) macroblast.

**mac·ro·es·the·sia** (mak″ro-əs-the′zhə) [*macro-* + *esthesia*] a dysesthesia in which all things touched seem larger than they really are.

**mac·ro·fau·na** (mak″ro-faw′nə) the animal life, visible to the naked eye, which is present in or characteristic of a special location.

**mac·ro·flo·ra** (mak″ro-flor′ə) the plant life, visible to the naked eye, which is present in or characteristic of a special location.

**mac·ro·gam·ete** (mak″ro-gam′ēt) [*macro-* + *gamete*] the larger, less active female anisogamete.

**mac·ro·ga·me·to·cyte** (mak″ro-gə-me′to-sīt) [*macro-* + *gametocyte*] macrogamont.

**mac·ro·gam·ont** (mak″ro-gam′ont) [*macro-* + *gamont*] a gamont that will produce or become a macrogamete. Called also *macrogametocyte.*

**mac·ro·gen·ia** (mak″ro-jen′e-ə) [*macro-* + *geni-* + *-ia*] enlargement of the jaw, especially the chin, which may involve only the osseous or soft-tissue components or both the bony and soft tissues.

**mac·ro·gen·i·to·so·mia** (mak″ro-jen″ĭ-to-so′me-ə) [*macro-* + *genito-* + *soma* + *-ia*] excessive somatic growth, with unusual enlargement of the genital organs.
**m. prae′cox,** epiphyseal syndrome.

**mac·ro·gin·gi·vae** (mak″ro-jin′jĭ-ve) fibromatosis gingivae.

**mac·rog·lia** (mak-rog′le-ə) neuroglial cells of ectodermal origin, i.e., the astrocytes and oligodendrocytes considered together. Originally, the term was used for the astrocytes alone.

**mac·ro·glob·u·lin** (mak″ro-glob′u-lin) [*macro-* + *globulin*] a plasma globulin with high molecular weight; alpha$_2$-macroglobulin or the IgM M component of Waldenström's macroglobulinemia.
**$\alpha_2$-m.,** a plasma protein that inhibits a wide variety of proteolytic enzymes including trypsin, plasmin, thrombin, kallikrein, and chymotrypsin. It is a tetramer of four identical subunits, $M_r$ between 650,000 and 735,000, and acts by means of a bait region that can entrap proteinases of very different substrate specificities as well as catalytic mechanisms, reducing the accessibility of the protein-ase functional sites, particularly to large molecules, but not completely inactivating them. Also written *alpha$_2$-macroglobulin.*

**mac·ro·glob·u·lin·emia** (mak″ro-glob″u-lĭ-ne′me-ə) [*macroglobulin* + *-emia*] a condition characterized by increase in macroglobulins in the blood.
**Waldenström's m.**, a plasma cell dyscrasia resembling leukemia, with cells of lymphocytic, plasmacytic, or intermediate morphology, that secrete an IgM M component. There is diffuse infiltration of bone marrow and in many cases also of the spleen, liver, lymph nodes, or central nervous system (Bing-Neel syndrome). The circulating macroglobulin produces symptoms of hyperviscosity syndrome: weakness, fatigue, bleeding disorders, and visual disturbances; peak incidence is in the sixth and seventh decades.

**mac·ro·glos·sia** (mak″ro-glos′e-ə) [*macro-* + *gloss-* + *-ia*] [MeSH: Macroglossia] excessive size of the tongue.

**mac·ro·gna·thia** (mak″ro-na′the-ə) [*macro-* + *gnath-* + *-ia*] a condition characterized by abnormally large jaws. See also *prognathism* and *maxillary protrusion,* under *protrusion.*

**mac·ro·gol** (mak′ro-gol) polyethylene glycol.

**mac·ro·gra·phia** (mak″ro-gra′fe-ə) macrography.

**mac·rog·ra·phy** (mak-rog′rə-fe) [*macro-* + *-graphy*] a form of dysgraphia in which written letters are larger than the normal writing of the individual. Called also *macrographia, megalographia,* and *megalography.*

**mac·ro·gy·ria** (mak″ro-ji′re-ə) [*macro-* + *gyrus*] moderate reduction in the number of sulci of the cerebrum, sometimes with increase in the brain substance, resulting in excessive size of the gyri.

**mac·ro·la·bia** (mak″ro-la′be-ə) [*macro-* + *labia*] macrocheilia.

**mac·ro·lec·i·thal** (mak″ro-les′ĭ-thəl) [*macro-* + *-lecithal*] having a large amount of yolk; see under *ovum.*

**mac·ro·lide** (mak′ro-līd) 1. a chemical compound characterized by a large lactone ring containing multiple keto and hydroxyl groups. 2. any of a large group of antibacterial antibiotics containing a macrolide ring linked glycosidically to one or more sugars; they are produced by certain species of *Streptomyces* and inhibit protein synthesis by binding to the 50S subunits of 70S ribosomes. Examples include erythromycin, azithromycin, and clarithromycin.

**mac·ro·lym·pho·cyte** (mak″ro-lim′fo-sīt) an abnormally large lymphocyte.

**mac·ro·mas·tia** (mak″ro-mas′te-ə) [*macro-* + *mast-* + *-ia*] oversize of the breasts or mammae.

**mac·ro·ma·zia** (mak″ro-ma′zhə) macromastia.

**mac·ro·me·lia** (mak″ro-me′le-ə) megalomelia.

**mac·rom·e·lus** (mak-rom′ə-ləs) [*macro-* + Gr. *melos* limb] a fetus with abnormally large or long limbs.

**mac·ro·mere** (mak′ro-mēr) [*macro-* + *-mere*] one of the large blastomeres formed by unequal cleavage of a fertilized ovum, located in the vegetal hemisphere and dividing less rapidly than the micromeres of the animal hemisphere.

**mac·ro·meth·od** (mak′ro-meth″əd) a chemical method in which the substance to be analyzed is used in customary (not minute) quantity. Cf. *micromethod.*

**mac·ro·min·er·al** (mak″ro-min′ər-əl) macroelement.

**mac·ro·mo·lec·u·lar** (mak″ro-mo-lek′u-lər) having large molecules; pertaining to macromolecules.

**mac·ro·mol·e·cule** (mak″ro-mol′ə-kūl) a very large molecule having a polymeric chain structure, as in proteins, polysaccharides, and other natural and synthetic polymers.

**mac·ro·mono·cyte** (mak″ro-mon′o-sīt) an abnormally large monocyte.

**mac·ro·my·elo·blast** (mak″ro-mi′ə-lo-blast) an abnormally large myeloblast.

**mac·ro·nem·a·tous** (mak″ro-nem′ə-təs) [*macro-* + Gr. *nēma* thread] pertaining to a conidiophore that is noticeably different morphologically from its hypha.

**mac·ro·nod·u·lar** (mak″ro-nod′u-lər) characterized by large nodules.

**mac·ro·nor·mo·blast** (mak″ro-nor′mo-blast) macroblast.

**mac·ro·nu·cle·us** (mak″ro-noo′kle-əs) [*macro-* + *nucleus*] 1. the larger of two types of nuclei when more than one is present in a cell. 2. in ciliate protozoa, the transcriptively active, polyploid nucleus, much larger than the micronucleus, that governs the organism's vegetative processes and is responsible for its phenotype. Called also *trophic nucleus* and *trophonucleus.*

**mac·ro·nu·tri·ent** (mak″ro-noo′tre-ent) an essential nutrient required in a relatively large amount, including carbohydrates, fats, proteins, and water. Minerals necessary in relatively large amounts (calcium, chloride, magnesium, phosphorus, potassium, sodium, and sulfur) are sometimes included and sometimes excluded from the definition.

**mac·ro·nych·ia** (mak″ro-nik′e-ə) [*macro-* + *onych-* + *-ia*] megalonychia.

**mac·ro·or·chi·dism** (mak″ro-or′kĭ-diz-əm) [*macro-* + *orchid-* + *-ism*] abnormal enlargement of the testis.

**mac·ro·ovalo·cyte** (mak″ro-o′və-lo-sīt) an enlarged, oval erythrocyte having a mean corpuscular volume greater than 100 $\mu m^3$, seen in megaloblastic anemia.

**mac·ro·pa·thol·o·gy** (mak″ro-pə-thol′ə-je) [*macro-* + *pathology*] the nonmicroscopical pathologic account of any disease or organ.

**mac·ro·phage** (mak′ro-fāj) [*macro-* + *-phage*] [MeSH: Macrophages] any of the many forms of mononuclear phagocytes found in tissues. They arise from hematopoietic stem cells in the bone marrow, which develop according to the stages of the monocytic series until they are monocytes; these then enter the blood, circulate for about 40 hours, and subsequently enter tissues, where they increase in size, phagocytic activity, and lysosomal enzyme content to become macrophages. Two types, *fixed macrophages* and *free macrophages* (qq. v.) are distinguished. Their morphology varies among different tissues and between normal and pathologic states, and not all macrophages can be identified by morphology alone. However, most are large cells with a round or indented nucleus, a well-developed Golgi apparatus, abundant endocytotic vacuoles, lysosomes, and phagolysosomes, and a plasma membrane covered with ruffles or microvilli. Their functions include nonspecific phagocytosis and pinocytosis, specific phagocytosis of opsonized microorganisms (mediated by Fc receptors and complement receptors); killing of ingested microorganisms; digestion and presentation of antigens to T and B lymphocytes; and secretion of many different products, including enzymes (lysozyme, collagenases, elastase), acid hydrolases, several complement components and coagulation factors, prostaglandins and leukotrienes, and regulatory molecules such as interferon and interleukin-1. Cells now recognized as macrophages include (in normal tissue) interdigitating cells, Kupffer's cells, Langerhans' cells, microglial cells, osteoclasts, and type A synovial cells, and (in inflamed tissues) epithelioid cells and Langerhans-type and foreign-body–type giant cells. Called also *histiocyte* and *macrophagocyte.*
**alveolar m.**, a rounded granular type, found within the alveoli of the lungs and serving to ingest inhaled particulate matter. Called also *alveolar phagocyte* and *dust cell.*
**armed m's**, those capable of inducing cytotoxicity as a consequence of antigen-binding by cytophilic antibodies on their surfaces or by factors derived from T lymphocytes.
**fixed m.**, a quiescent, sessile macrophage similar to a fibroblast in morphology, found in the lymph nodes, spleen, bone marrow, and connective tissue (where it is called a histiocyte).
**free m.**, an actively motile macrophage, usually having an ameboid shape and highly ruffled surface, found at sites of inflammation.
**inflammatory m.**, free m.

**mac·ro·phago·cyte** (mak″ro-fag′o-sīt) macrophage.

**mac·ro·phal·lus** (mak″ro-fal′əs) [*macro-* + *phallus*] abnormal largeness of the penis.

**mac·roph·thal·mia** (mak″rof-thal′me-ə) [*macro-* + *ophthalm-* + *-ia*] abnormal enlargement of the eyeball.

**mac·roph·thal·mous** (mak″rof-thal′məs) having abnormally large eyes.

**mac·ro·pla·sia** (mak″ro-pla′zhə) [*macro-* + *-plasia*] excessive growth of a part or tissue.

**mac·ro·plas·tia** (mak″ro-plas′te-ə) macroplasia.

**mac·ro·po·dia** (mak″ro-po′de-ə) [*macro-* + *pod-* + *-ia*] excessive size of the feet; called also *megalopodia.*

**mac·ro·poly·cyte** (mak″ro-pol′e-sīt) a large polymorphonuclear leukocyte with 6 to 14 lobes in the nucleus, seen in conditions such as pancytopenia, vitamin $B_{12}$ or folic acid deficiency, and intoxications involving neutrophilic leukocytosis. Cf. *polycyte.*

**mac·ro·pro·lac·ti·no·ma** (mak″ro-pro-lak″tĭ-no′mə) a prolactinoma more than 10 mm in diameter, usually associated with serum prolactin levels above 500 ng per ml.

**mac·ro·pro·my·elo·cyte** (mak″ro-pro-mi′ə-lo-sīt) an abnormally large promyelocyte.

**mac·ro·pro·so·pia** (mak″ro-pro-so′pe-ə) [*macro-* + *prosop* + *-ia*] excessive size of the face.

**ma·crop·sia** (mə-krop′se-ə) [*macro-* + *-opsia*] an illusion in which objects are seen as larger than they actually are.

**mac·ro·rhin·ia** (mak″ro-rin′e-ə) [*macro-* + *rhin-* + *-ia*] excessive size of the nose.

**mac·ro·sce·lia** (mak″ro-se′le-ə) [*macro-* + Gr. *skelos* leg + *-ia*] excessive size of the legs.

**mac·ro·scop·ic** (mak″ro-skop′ik) [*macro-* + Gr. *skopein* to examine] visible with the unaided eye or without the microscope.

**mac·ro·scop·i·cal** (mak″ro-skop′ĭ-kəl) 1. pertaining to macroscopy. 2. macroscopic.

**ma·cros·co·py** (mə-kros′kə-pe) examination with the naked eye.

**mac·ro·shock** (mak′ro-shok″) a term used in cardiology to denote a moderate to high level of electric current passing across two areas of intact skin; approximately 100 mA can cause ventricular fibrillation. Cf. *microshock.*

**mac·ro·sig·moid** (mak″ro-sig′moid) [*macro-* + *sigmoid*] abnormal enlargement of the sigmoid.

**mac·ro·sis** (mə-kro′sis) [*macro-* + *-osis*] increase in size.

**mac·ros·mat·ic** (mak″roz-mat′ik) [*macr-* + *osmatic*] having the sense of smell strongly or acutely developed.

**mac·ro·so·ma·tia** (mak″ro-so-ma′she-ə) [*macro-* + *somat-* + *-ia*] macrosomia.
**m. adipo′sa conge′nita,** premature development associated with obesity, attributed to hyperfunction of the adrenal cortex.

**mac·ro·so·mia** (mak″ro-so′me-ə) [*macro-* + *-somia*] abnormally large size; see also *gigantism* and *megasoma.* Called also *macrosomatia.*
**fetal m., neonatal m.,** excessive birth weight in a neonate, seen most often in children of diabetic mothers or those with cerebral gigantism.

**mac·ro·spore** (mak′ro-spor) [*macro-* + *spore*] 1. the larger spore form when spores of two sizes are present, as in certain fungi and protozoa. 2. megaspore.

**mac·ro·ste·a·to·sis** (mak″ro-ste″ə-to′sis) [*macro-* + *steatosis*] fatty change in which a single large droplet occupies most of the cell, displacing the cytoplasm and nucleus to a ring around the droplet. Cf. *microsteatosis.*

**mac·ro·ste·reo·gno·sia** (mak″ro-ste″re-o-no′zhə) [*macro-* + *stereo-* + *gnosia*] macroesthesia.

**mac·ro·sto·mia** (mak″ro-sto′me-ə) [*macro-* + *stom-* + *-ia*] [MeSH: Macrostomia] greatly exaggerated width of the mouth, resulting from failure of union of the maxillary and mandibular prominences, with extension of the oral orifice toward the ear. The defect may be unilateral or bilateral. See also *lateral facial cleft* and *oblique facial cleft,* under *cleft.*

**mac·ro·struc·tur·al** (mak″ro-struk′chər-əl) pertaining to gross structure.

**Mac·ro·tec** (mak′ro-tek) trademark for a kit for the preparation of technetium Tc 99m albumin aggregated.

**mac·ro·tia** (mak-ro′shə) [*macro-* + *ot-* + *-ia*] abnormal enlargement of the pinna of the ear.

**mac·ro·tome** (mak′ro-tōm) [*macro-* + *-tome*] an apparatus for cutting large sections of tissue for anatomical study.

**mac·ro·tooth** (mak′ro-tōōth) pl. *macroteeth.* An abnormally large tooth.

**Mac·ro·za·mia** (mak″ro-zam′e-ə) a genus of zamia palms that contain macrozamin and other toxic glycosides, causing hepatotoxicity, spinal cord degeneration, and cancer in humans and other animals. See also *zamia staggers,* under *staggers.*

**mac·ro·zam·in** (mak″ro-zam′in) a toxic principle from the seeds and leaves of species of the zamia family of palms. In humans it is neoplastic to the liver, kidneys, intestine, and lungs after hydrolysis by intestinal bacteria and yields the breakdown product methylazoxymethanol; in cattle it causes fatal gastrointestinal and liver damage.

**mac·u·la** (mak′u-lə) gen. and pl. *ma′culae* [L.] 1. [TA] a stain, spot, or thickening; a general term for an area distinguishable by color or otherwise from its surroundings. 2. m. luteae. 3. a discolored spot on the skin that is not elevated above the surface; called also *macule.* 4. a moderately dense scar of the cornea that can be seen without special optical aids, appreciated as a gray spot intermediate between a nebula and a leukoma.
**acoustic maculae, maculae acus′ticae,** the macula sacculi and macula utriculi considered together.
**m. adhe′rens,** desmosome.
**ma′culae al′bidae,** white spots sometimes seen after death on the serous layer of the peritoneum.
**ma′culae atro′phicae,** white patches resembling scars formed on the skin by atrophy.
**cerebral m.,** tache cérébrale.
**ma′culae ceru′leae,** small grayish blue stainlike, nonpruritic macules located chiefly on the chest, abdomen, thighs, and upper arms in pediculosis pubis, which are especially noticeable in light-skinned individuals. They are probably due to altered blood pigments in infested individuals, or to an excretion product in the louse's saliva that converts bilirubin to biliverdin. Called also *taches bleuâtres.*
**m. commu′nicans,** gap junction.
**m. commu′nis,** a thickened area on the wall of the otic vesicle; it later divides into the macula sacculi and macula utriculi.
**ma′culae cribro′sae** [TA], see *m. cribrosa inferior, m. cribrosa media,* and *m. cribrosa superior.*
**m. cribro′sa infe′rior** [TA], the perforated area on the wall of the vestibule through which branches of the vestibulocochlear nerve pass to the crista ampullaris and the posterior semicircular canal.
**m. cribro′sa me′dia** [TA], the perforated area on the vestibular wall through which branches of the vestibulocochlear nerve pass to the macula of the saccule.
**m. cribro′sa supe′rior** [TA], the perforated area on the vestibular wall through which branches of the vestibulocochlear nerve pass to the macula of the utricle and to the crista ampullaris of the anterior and lateral semicircular canals.
**m. den′sa,** a zone of compact, heavily nucleated cells, located in the distal renal tubule where it makes contact with the vascular pole of the glomerulus, and closely associated anatomically with the juxtaglomerular cells of the afferent arteriole.
**false m.,** the extramacular point on the retina of a squinting eye which receives the same light stimulus as the macula of the fixing eye.
**m. fla′va laryn′gis,** a yellowish nodule visible at one end of a vocal cord.
**m. fla′va re′tinae,** m. luteae.
**m. folli′culi,** follicular stigma.
**m. germinati′va,** embryonic disc.
**m. gonorrhoe′ica,** the red, inflamed orifice of the duct of Bartholin's gland in gonorrheal vulvitis; called also *Saenger's m.*
**ma′culae lac′teae,** maculae albidae.
**m. lu′teae** [TA], **m. lu′tea re′tinae,** an irregular yellowish depression on the retina, about 3 degrees wide, lateral to and slightly below the optic disk; it is the site of absorption of short wavelengths of light, and it is thought that its variation in size, shape, and coloring may be related to variant types of color vision. Called also *m. flava retinae.*
**maculae of membranous labyrinth,** acoustic maculae.
**mongolian m.,** see under *spot.*
**m. re′tinae,** m. luteae.
**m. sac′culi** [TA], macula of saccule: a thickening in the wall of the saccule where the epithelium contains hair cells that are stimulated by linear acceleration and deceleration and gravity. This and the macula utriculi together are called *acoustic maculae.*

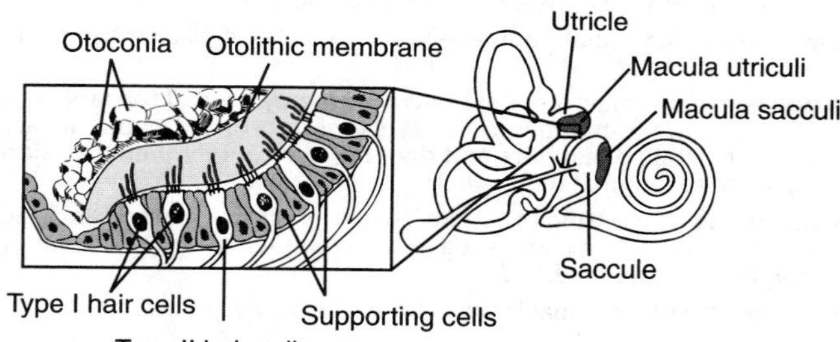


**Saenger's m.,** m. gonorrhoeica.
**ma′culae tendi′neae,** maculae albidae.
**m. utri′culi** [TA], macula of utricle: a thickening in the wall of the utricle where the epithelium contains hair cells that are stimulated by linear acceleration and deceleration and gravity. This and the macula utriculi together are called *acoustic maculae.*

**mac·u·lae** (mak′u-le) [L.] genitive and plural of *macula.*

**mac·u·lar** (mak′u-lər) 1. pertaining to or characterized by macules. 2. pertaining to the macula of the retina (macula lutea [TA]).

**mac·u·late** (mak′u-lāt) [L. *maculatus* spotted] macular.

**mac·ule** (mak′ūl) a macula.
**ash-leaf m.,** a hypopigmented lesion of the skin occurring in tuberous sclerosis, usually 1 to 3 cm in size and having the general shape of an ash leaf, round at one end and pointed at the other. Called also *lance-ovate macule* and *ash-leaf spot* or *patch.*
**coal m.,** a dark spot seen on the lung in coal workers' pneumoconiosis, representing an aggregation of dust, dust-filled macrophages, and fibroblasts.
**lance-ovate m.,** ash-leaf m.

**mac·u·lo·cer·e·bral** (mak″u-lo-ser′ə-brəl) pertaining to the macula retinae and the cerebrum; called also *cerebromacular.*

**mac·u·lo·pap·u·lar** (mak″u-lo-pap′u-lər) both macular and papular, as an eruption consisting of both macules and papules; sometimes erroneously used to designate a papule that is only slightly elevated.

**mac·u·lop·a·thy** (mak″u-lop′ə-the) [*macula* + *-pathy*] any pathological condition of the macula retinae. Cf. *retinopathy*.
**bull's eye m.**, increase in pigment of a circular area of the macula retinae, accompanying degeneration; seen in certain toxic states, macular corneal dystrophy, Stargardt's disease, and other conditions.

**mac·u·lo·ve·sic·u·lar** (mak″u-lo-və-sik′u-lər) both macular and vesicular.

**Mac·Wil·liam's test** (mək-wil′yəmz) [John Alexander *MacWilliam*, British physician, 1857–1937] see under *test*.

**mad** (mad) 1. insane. 2. rabid.

**mad·a·ro·sis** (mad″ə-ro′sis) [Gr. *madaros* bald] loss of the eyelashes or eyebrows. Cf. *milphosis*.

**MADD** multiple acyl CoA dehydrogenation deficiency; see *glutaricaciduria, type II*.

**mad·der** (mad′ər) the root of *Rubia tinctoria* L. (Rubiaceae) affording a red dye, mainly alizarin and purpurin.

**Mad·dox prism, rods** (mad′əks) [Ernest Edmund *Maddox*, English ophthalmologist, 1860–1933] see under *prism* and *rod*.

**Ma·de·lung's deformity, neck (disease)** (mah′dĕ-loongz) [Otto Wilhelm *Madelung*, German surgeon, 1846–1926] see under *deformity* and *neck*.

**Ma·du·ra foot** (mə-doo′rə) [*Madura*, India, where it was observed in the 1850s] see under *foot*.

**Mad·u·rel·la** (mad″u-rel′ə) a genus of Fungi Imperfecti of the form-class Hyphomycetes, form-family Dematiaceae. *M. gri′sea* and *M. myceto′matis* (called also *M. myceto′mi*) are etiologic agents of eumycotic mycetoma.

**ma·du·ro·my·co·sis** (mə-du″ro-mi-ko′sis) [MeSH: Maduromycosis] mycetoma.

**mae·di** (mi′the) [Icelandic "dyspnea"] the respiratory form of ovine progressive pneumonia.
**m.-visna**, ovine progressive pneumonia.

**MAF** macrophage activating factor; see *interferon-γ*, under *interferon*.

**maf·en·ide** (maf′ən-īd) [MeSH: Mafenide] an antibacterial homologue of sulfanilamide active against many gram-positive and gram-negative organisms.
**m. acetate** [USP], the monoacetate salt of mafenide, having the same antibacterial activity as the base; used as a topical anti-infective for adjunctive therapy of patients with second- and third-degree burns.
**m. hydrochloride**, the hydrochloride salt of mafenide, having antibacterial activity similar to that of the acetate salt; used as a topical anti-infective.

**Maf·fuc·ci's syndrome** (mə-foo′chēz) [Angelo *Maffucci*, Italian physician, 1847–1903] see under *syndrome*.

**ma·fil·con A** (mə-fil′kon) a hydrophilic contact lens material.

**MAG3** mertiatide.

**Mag.** abbreviation for L. *mag′nus*, large.

**mag·al·drate** (mag′əl-drāt) [USP] a chemical combination of aluminum hydroxide and magnesium hydroxide; used as an oral antacid.

**Mag·an** (mag′ən) trademark for magnesium salicylate.

**ma·gen·bla·se** (mah″gən-blah′zə) [Ger. "stomach bubble"] in the radiograph of the stomach, a dark area above the light shadow of the opaque meal, marking a collection of gas in the upper part of the stomach.

**Ma·gen·die's foramen, solution, space, symptom** (mah-zhah-dēz′) [François *Magendie*, French physiologist, 1783–1855] see under *solution* and *space;* see *apertura mediana ventriculi quarti;* and see *skew deviation*, under *deviation*.

**Ma·gen·die-Hert·wig sign** (mah-zhah-de′ hert′vig) [François *Magendie;* Richard Carl Wilhelm Theodor von *Hertwig*, German zoologist, 1850–1937] skew deviation.

**ma·gen·stras·se** (mah″gən-strahs′ə) [Ger. "stomach street"] canalis gastricus.

**ma·gen·ta** (mə-jen′tə) basic fuchsin.
**m. 0**, pararosaniline.
**m. I**, rosaniline.
**m. II**, triaminoditoylphenylmethane chloride, a component of basic fuchsin.
**m. III**, new fuchsin.
**acid m.**, acid fuchsin.
**basic m.**, basic fuchsin.

**mag·got** (mag′ot) a soft-bodied larva of an insect, especially a form living in decaying flesh; sometimes they infest wounds of live animals, including humans (see *myiasis*). Families of particular importance are Calliphoridae and Sarcophagidae. The living maggots of *Phaenicia sericata* and *Phormia regina* have been used in the treatment of osteomyelitis and other suppurative infections to clear away dead tissue and promote healing because their secretions contain allantoin.
**Congo floor m.**, the maggot of *Auchmeromyia luteola*.
**foot m.**, the larva of *Booponus intonsus*.
**rat-tail m.**, a maggot of one of the hover-flies (genera *Eristalis* and *Helophilus);* they cause intestinal and nasal myiasis.
**sheep m., wool m.**, the maggot of any of several species of the family Calliphoridae, which invade the tissues of sheep, causing cutaneous myiasis.

**mag·is·tral** (maj′is-trəl) [L. *magister* master] pertaining to a master; applied to medicines that are prepared in accordance with a physician's prescription. Cf. *officinal*.

**mag·ma** (mag′mə) [Gr. *massein* to knead] 1. a suspension of finely divided material in a small amount of water. 2. a thin, pastelike substance composed of organic material.
**bismuth m.**, milk of bismuth.
**magnesia m.**, milk of magnesia; see under *milk*.
**m. reticula′re**, a mesenchymal reticulum within the early chorionic sac.

**Mag·na·cort** (mag′nə-kort) trademark for a preparation of hydrocortamate hydrochloride.

**Mag·nan's movement, symptom (sign)** (mah-nyahz′) [Valentin Jacques Joseph *Magnan*, French psychiatrist, 1835–1916] see under *movement* and see *formication*.

**mag·nes·emia** (mag″nəs-e′me-ə) hypermagnesemia.

**mag·ne·sia** (mag-ne′zhə) [the name of a district in ancient Lydia] magnesium oxide.
**m. al′ba**, magnesium carbonate.
**m. calcina′ta**, magnesium oxide.
**m. carbonata′da**, magnesium carbonate.
**citrate of m.**, magnesium citrate.
**milk of m.**, see under *milk*.
**m. us′ta**, magnesium oxide.

**mag·ne·si·um** (mag-ne′ze-əm) gen. *magne′sii* [L.] [MeSH: Magnesium] a light, silvery, metallic element; symbol, Mg; atomic number, 12; atomic weight, 24.312; specific gravity, 1.74. Its salts are essential in nutrition, being required for the activity of many enzymes, especially those concerned with oxidative phosphorylation. It is a component of both intra- and extracellular fluids and is excreted in the urine and feces. The serum level is approximately 2 mEq/liter. Deficiency causes irritability of the nervous system with tetany, vasodilation, convulsions, tremors, depression, and psychotic behavior. Excessive amounts can be toxic; see *hypermagnesemia*.
**m. aluminum silicate** [NF], a colloid used as a suspending agent for pharmaceuticals, available in Types IA, IB, IC, IIA, IIIA, and IIIB, which differ in viscosity and ratio of aluminum content to magnesium content.
**m. carbonate** [USP], basic hydrated magnesium carbonate containing the equivalent of 40 to 43.5 per cent of magnesium oxide, used as an antacid.
**m. chloride** [USP], an electrolyte replenisher and a pharmaceutic necessity for hemodialysis and peritoneal dialysis fluids.
**m. citrate** [USP], a saline laxative used for bowel evacuation before diagnostic procedures or surgery of the colon; administered orally.
**dibasic m. phosphate**, a salt, $MgHPO_4 \cdot 3H_2O$, that has been used as a mild saline laxative.
**m. hydroxide** [USP], a bulky white powder, $Mg(OH)_2$, used as an antacid and cathartic.
**m. lactate**, a salt of magnesium used as an electrolyte replenisher.
**m. oxide** [USP], a bulky *(light m. oxide)* or relatively dense *(heavy m. oxide)* white powder, MgO; used as a sorbent in pharmaceutical preparations, and as an antacid and laxative.
**m. peroxide**, a white powder, $MgO_2$, insoluble in water, but gradually decomposed with the liberation of oxygen; used as an antacid.
**m. phosphate** [USP], tribasic magnesium phosphate: a bulky, white powder, $Mg_3(PO_4)_2 \cdot 5H_2O$, used as an antacid.
**m. salicylate**, the magnesium salt of salicylic acid, used as an antiarthritic.
**m. silicate**, $MgSiO_3$, a silicate salt of magnesium; the most common hydrated forms occurring in nature are asbestos and talc. See also *silicatosis*.
**m. stearate** [NF], a compound of magnesium with varying proportions of stearic and palmitic acids, used as a tablet lubricant in pharmaceutical preparations.
**m. sulfate** [USP], an anticonvulsant and electrolyte replenisher, $MgSO_4 \cdot xH_2O$, administered intramuscularly and intravenously. It is also used as a cathartic and as a local anti-inflammatory. Called also *Epsom salt*.

**m. sulfate, exsiccated,** hydrated magnesium sulfate the weight of which has been reduced 25 per cent by drying at 100°C: an aperient.
**tribasic m. phosphate,** see *m. phosphate.*
**m. trisilicate** [USP], a compound of magnesium oxide and silicon dioxide with varying proportions of water, used as a pharmaceutic necessity and antacid.

**mag•net** (mag′nət) [L. *magnes;* Gr. *magnēs* magnet] a lodestone; native iron oxide that attracts iron; also a bar of steel or iron that attracts iron and has magnetic polarity.
**denture m.,** a magnet made of a nonreactogenic platinum-cobalt alloy or a rare earth element, used for additional retention of dentures. One magnet is implanted into the mandible under the periosteum and the other is attached to the denture, its poles being opposite of those in the mandible. Called also *magnetic implant.*
**Grüning's m.,** one made up of a number of steel rods; used in removing metal particles from the eye.
**Haab's m.,** a powerful magnet for extracting foreign metallic bodies from the eye.
**Hirschberg's m.,** an electromagnet for removing particles of iron from the eye.
**permanent m.,** one with permanent magnetic qualities.
**temporary m.,** a substance that possesses magnetic properties only during the passage of an electric current or when a permanent magnet is near it.

**mag•net•ic** (mag-net′ik) [MeSH: Magnetics] pertaining to, derived from, or having the properties of a magnet.

**mag•ne•tism** (mag′nə-tiz-əm) magnetic attraction or repulsion.
**animal m.,** a hypothetical force or power alleged by Mesmer to be transmitted to his subjects undergoing therapeutic hypnosis. Cf. *mesmerism.*

**mag•ne•ti•za•tion** (mag″nət-ĭ-za′shən) the act or process of rendering an object or substance magnetic.
**longitudinal m.,** the component of a magnetization vector that is parallel to the direction of the magnetic field.
**transverse m.,** the components of a magnetization vector that are in a plane perpendicular to the direction of the magnetic field.

**mag•ne•to•car•dio•graph** (mag-ne″to-kahr′de-o-graf) a cardiograph that generates electrical signals proportional to magnetic pulses emanating from electrical activity in the heart.

**mag•ne•to•elec•tric•i•ty** (mag-ne″to-e″lek-tris′ĭ-te) electricity induced by means of a magnet.

**mag•ne•to•en•ceph•a•lo•graph** (mag-ne″to-ən-sef′ə-lo-graf) an instrument for recording magnetic signals proportional to electroencephalographic waves emanating from electrical activity in the brain.

**mag•ne•tol•o•gy** (mag″nə-tol′ə-je) that branch of physics which treats of magnetics.

**mag•ne•tom•e•ter** (mag″nə-tom′ə-tər) [*magnetic* + *-meter*] 1. an apparatus for measuring magnetic forces. 2. a device that uses an array of superconductors to detect changes in the magnetic field of the brain, used to diagnose epilepsy, stroke, and deafness.

**mag•ne•tron** (mag′nə-tron) an electric vacuum tube for generating extremely short electromagnetic waves (microwaves).

**mag•net•ro•pism** (mag-net′ro-piz-əm) [*magnet* + *tropism*] a growth response in a nonmotile organism under the influence of a magnet.

**Mag•ne•vist** (mag′nə-vist) trademark for a preparation of gadopentetate dimeglumine.

**mag•ni•cel•lu•lar** (mag″nĭ-sel′u-lər) composed of large cells, as opposed to parvicellular.

**mag•ni•fi•ca•tion** (mag″nĭ-fĭ-ka′shən) [L. *magnificatio; magnus* great + *facere* to make] 1. apparent increase in size as under the microscope. 2. the process of making something appear larger, as by use of lenses. 3. the ratio of apparent (image) size to real size.

**mag•ni•fy** (mag′nĭ-fi) to cause to appear larger by the use of lenses or suitable mirrors.

**mag•no•cel•lu•lar** (mag″no-sel′u-lər) magnicellular.

**Mag•no•lia** (mag-no′le-ə) [Pierre *Magnol,* French botanist, 1638–1715] a genus of deciduous trees of the family Magnoliaceae. *M. acumina′ta* L., *M. glau′ca* L., and *M. tripeta′la* L. are sources of the medicinal bark called magnolia.

**mag•no•lia** (mag-no′le-ə) 1. any member of the genus *Magnolia.* 2. the bitter aromatic bark of several species of *Magnolia,* formerly used as a diaphoretic and antifebrile in the southern United States.

**mag•num** (mag′nəm) [L.] 1. large; great. 2. the os magnum (os capitatum [TA]).

**Mag-Tab** (mag′tab) trademark for a preparation of magnesium lactate.

**Mah•ler's sign** (mah′lerz) [Richter A. *Mahler,* German obstetrician, 1863–1941] see under *sign.*

**ma huang** (mah hwəng′) [Chinese] any of various species of *Ephedra* used as herbs in Chinese medicine.

**Mai•er's sinus** (mi′erz) [Rudolf *Maier,* German physician, 1824–1888] see under *sinus.*

**maim** (mām) 1. to disable by a wound; to dismember by violence. 2. a dismemberment or disablement effected by violence.

**Mai•mon•i•des** (mi-mon′ĭ-dēz) [Moses ben Maimon, 1135–1204] rabbi, physician, and the greatest of the Jewish philosophers, born in Cordoba, Spain. He was the physician to Saladin in Egypt, during which time he wrote many medical works in Arabic, among them a commentary on the aphorisms of Hippocrates and treatises on asthma, diet, poisons, and hygiene. A prayer attributed to him is considered to rank beside the oath of Hippocrates as an ethical guide to the medical profession.

**main** (mă) [Fr.] hand.
**m. d'accoucheur** (dah-koo-shoor′), obstetrician's hand.
**m. en crochet** (ah-kro-sha′) [hooked hand], a permanently flexed condition of the third and fourth fingers.
**m. fourchée** (fōōr-sha′), cleft hand.
**m. en griffe** (ah-grēf′), clawhand.
**m. en lorgnette** (ah-lor-nyet′), opera-glass hand.
**m. en pince** (ah-pas′), cleft hand.
**m. en singe** (ah-sazh′), monkey hand.
**m. en squelette** (ah-skə-let′), skeleton hand.
**m. succulente** (su-ku-laht′), Marinesco's succulent hand.

**Mai•ni•ni** (mi-ne′ne) see *Galli Mainini.*

**main•tain•er** (mān-tān′ər) something that keeps or maintains in another thing existence or continuancy.
**space m.,** 1. an orthodontic appliance, fixed or removable, that maintains the space left by a prematurely lost tooth or the space to be filled by a tooth not yet erupted. See also under *regainer* and *retainer.* 2. separator, def. 2.

**main•te•nance** (mān′tə-nans) [MeSH: Maintenance] providing a stable state over a long period as distinguished from a short-term remedial or prophylactic effect; said of a drug or treatment. Also, the stable state so provided.

**mai•sin** (ma′zin) a protein found in the seeds of maize.

**Mai•son•neuve's amputation, sign, urethrotome** (ma″zo-noovz′) [Jules Germain François *Maisonneuve,* French surgeon, 1809–1897] see under *amputation, sign,* and *urethrotome.*

**Mais•siat's band (ligament, tract)** (ma″se-ahz′) [Jacques Henri *Maissiat,* French anatomist, 1805–1878] tractus iliotibialis.

**maize** (māz) [Sp. *maíz*] *Zea mays.*

**Ma•joc•chi's disease (purpura)** (mah-yok′ēz) [Domenico *Majocchi,* Italian physician, 1849–1929] purpura annularis telangiectodes.

**makr(o)-** for words thus beginning, see those beginning *macr(o)-.*

**mal** (mahl) [Fr. and Sp., from L. *malum* a bad thing] disease.
**m. de caderas** (da kah-da′rahs) [Sp. "illness of the hips"], 1. a fatal wasting trypanosomiasis associated with weakness, especially of the hindquarters, affecting chiefly South American horses, which is caused by *Trypanosoma equinum,* and transmitted by tabanid flies. 2. South American name for derriengue.
**grand m.** (grahn) [Fr.], see under *epilepsy.*
**haut m.** (o) [Fr.], grand mal epilepsy.
**m. de Meleda** (də mel′ə-dah) [Fr. "Meleda sickness"], a chronic, autosomal recessive form of palmoplantar keratoderma in which the hyperkeratosis spreads to involve the dorsal aspects of the hands and feet and other areas of the body, with erythematous, scaling, malodorous cutaneous lesions that may cause deep fissuring. Called also *Meleda disease.*
**m. de mer** (də mār) [Fr.], seasickness.
**m. morado** (mo-rah′do) [Sp. "purple sickness"], a cutaneous manifestation of onchocerciasis seen in Central America in which the skin has a blue or reddish mauve discoloration, especially on the trunk and upper limbs.

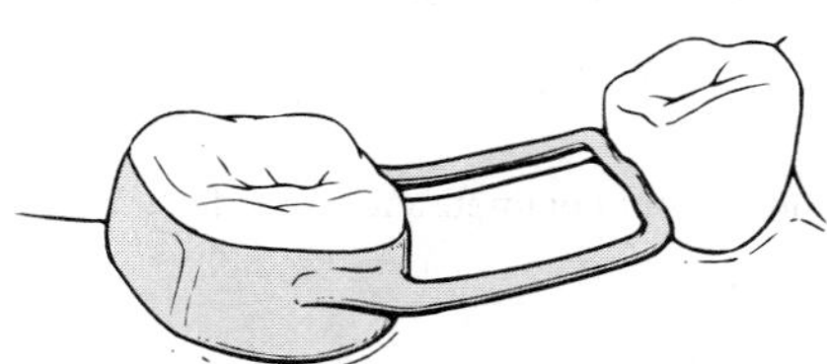

Band and loop space maintainer.

**m. perforant du pied** (per-fo-rahn′ du pya) [Fr. "penetrating disease of the foot"], plantar ulcer.
**petit m.** (pə-te′) [Fr.], absence epilepsy.
**m. rouge** (ro͞ozh) [Fr. "red sickness"], a syndrome occurring after inhalation or ingestion of calcium cyanamide followed by drinking an alcoholic beverage, marked by intense flushing, rapid pulse and pounding heart, panting respiration, and perception of the taste and smell of acetaldehyde in the exhaled breath, which may be followed by nausea, vomiting, and a precipitous fall in blood pressure; the extent and severity of the symptoms depend on the amount of calcium cyanamide and alcohol in the system. The reactions are due to the inhibition by calcium cyanamide of one or more of the enzymes required for oxidation of acetaldehyde formed from alcohol, resulting in the accumulation of acetaldehyde and the altered vascular reaction to it. A similar syndrome, also due to accumulation of acetaldehyde, occurs on ingestion of disulfiram followed by drinking an alcoholic beverage, but in addition there are impaired taste, unpleasant breath and perspiration, and lessened sexual potency.

**ma•la** (ma′lə) [L.] 1. bucca. 2. os zygomaticum.

**mal•ab•sorp•tion** (mal″əb-sorp′shən) impaired intestinal absorption of nutrients; see also *malabsorption syndrome,* under *syndrome.*
**congenital lactose m.,** disaccharide intolerance II.
**glucose-galactose m.,** a disorder of transport clinically characterized by neonatal onset of profuse, acidic, watery diarrhea leading to severe dehydration and death if untreated, due to a selective defect in the intestinal transport of glucose and galactose; it can be treated by a glucose- and galactose-free diet.
**sucrose-isomaltose m., congenital,** disaccharide intolerance due to deficient absorption of sucrose and isomaltose, usually caused by a defect in the sucrase-isomaltase complex.

**Ma•la•car•ne's pyramid** (mah″lah-kahr′nāz) [Michele Vincenzo Giacintos *Malacarne,* Italian surgeon, 1744–1816] see under *pyramid.*

**ma•la•cia** (mə-la′shə) [Gr. *malakia*] the morbid softening or softness of a part or tissue.
**metaplastic m.,** osteitis fibrosa cystica.
**myeloplastic m.,** osteogenesis imperfecta.
**porotic m.,** softening accompanied by proliferation of connective tissue.
**m. trauma′tica,** syringomyelia.

**-malacia** a word termination denoting abnormal softness or softening in the system designated by the root to which the term is affixed, as *osteomalacia.*

**ma•la•cic** (mə-la′sik) marked by malacia or morbid softness.

**malac(o)-** [Gr. *malakos* soft] a combining form denoting a condition of abnormal softness.

**mal•a•co•ma** (mal″ə-ko′mə) [*malaco-* + *-oma*] a morbidly soft part or spot.

**mal•a•co•pla•kia** (mal″ə-ko-pla′ke-ə) [*malaco-* + Gr. *plax* plaque] [MeSH: Malacoplakia] the formation of soft patches on the mucous membrane of a hollow organ.
**renal m.,** malacoplakia with infection of the renal parenchyma, a condition closely resembling xanthogranulomatous pyelonephritis, usually occurring secondary to urinary tract infections or immunocompromised conditions.
**m. vesi′cae,** soft, yellowish raised plaques on the mucous membrane of the bladder and ureters, containing von Hansemann cells with Michaelis-Gutmann bodies, resulting from infection.

**mal•a•co•sis** (mal″ə-ko′sis) malacia.

**mal•a•cos•te•on** (mal″ə-kos′te-on) [*malaco-* + *osteon*] osteomalacia.

**mal•a•cot•ic** (mal″ə-kot′ik) inclined to malacia; soft; said of teeth.

**ma•lac•tic** (mə-lak′tik) emollient (defs. 1 and 2).

**mal•a•die** (mahl″ah-de′) [Fr.] disease.
**m. des jambes** (da-zhahb′) ["disease of the legs"], a disease of rice growers in Louisiana, probably beriberi.
**m. de plongeurs** (də-plaw-zhoor′) ["divers' disease"], inflammation and ulceration in divers in the Mediterranean caused by the stings of sea anemones.
**m. de Roger** (də ro-ja′), Roger's disease.
**m. du sommeil** (du so-ma′) [sleeping sickness], African trypanosomiasis.
**m. des tics** (da-tēk′) ["disease of tics"], Gilles de la Tourette's syndrome.

**mal•ad•just•ment** (mal″ə-just′mənt) in psychiatry, failure to fit one's inner needs to the environment; inability to meet the challenges of daily life.

**mal•a•dy** (mal′ə-de) [Fr. *maladie*] disease.

**ma•lag•ma** (mə-lag′mə) [Gr.] an emollient or cataplasm.

**mal•aise** (mah-lāz′) [Fr.] a vague feeling of bodily discomfort and fatigue.

**mal•a•ko•pla•kia** (mal″ə-ko-pla′ke-ə) malacoplakia.

**mal•align•ment** (mal″ə-līn′mənt) displacement out of line, especially displacement of the teeth from their normal relation to the line of the dental arch. Spelled also *malalinement.* See *malocclusion.*

**mal•aline•ment** (mal″ə-līn′mənt) malalignment.

**ma•lar** (ma′lər) [L. *mala* cheek] 1. buccal. 2. zygomatic (def. 2).

**ma•la•ria** (mə-lar′e-ə) [It. "bad air"] [MeSH: Malaria] an infectious disease endemic in many warm regions of the world, caused by obligate intracellular protozoa of the genus *Plasmodium,* usually transmitted by the bites of infected anopheline mosquitoes. It is characterized by prostration with paroxysms of high fever, shaking chills, sweating, anemia, and splenomegaly, which may lead to death, often from its most severe complications, cerebral malaria and anemia. Intervals between the attacks are sometimes periodic, being determined by the time required for development of a new generation of parasites in the body. After the initial illness, it may follow a chronic or relapsing course. Called also *paludism.* Old names include *ague* and *jungle, malarial, marsh,* or *swamp fever.*
**algid m.,** a severe complication of falciparum malaria caused by a collapse of the vascular system and manifested by shock, syncope, peripheral vascular failure, hypotension, cold, clammy skin, and gastrointestinal symptoms, diarrhea, and vomiting, which is sometimes followed by coma and death.
**benign tertian m.,** vivax m.
**bilious remittent m.,** a complication of falciparum malaria mainly involving the liver, characterized by continuous vomiting, epigastric and hepatic tenderness, marked jaundice, and high remittent fever.
**cerebral m.,** a severe and often fatal complication of falciparum malaria mainly involving the brain, characterized either by the gradual onset of headache, confusion, and psychotic manifestations lapsing into delirium, convulsions, and coma, or by an abrupt rise in temperature sustained at high levels with convulsions and coma.
**congenital m.,** malaria in newborn infants that have been infected transplacentally, usually by *Plasmodium vivax* or *P. malariae.*
**falciparum m.,** malaria due to *Plasmodium falciparum,* in which the febrile paroxysms recur irregularly. It is associated with the highest levels of parasites in the blood and is the most severe form of malaria, sometimes fatal. It is the one most likely to be associated with pernicious symptoms, which occur as a result of sludging and formation of microinfarctions in the capillaries consisting of erythrocytes infected with later stages of *P. falciparum.* This may occur in the brain, liver, adrenal gland, gastrointestinal tract, kidneys, lungs, or other organs. Called also *malignant tertian m.* and *pernicious m.* See also *blackwater fever,* under *fever.*
**malignant tertian m.,** falciparum m.
**ovale m.,** malaria caused by *Plasmodium ovale* that is clinically similar to but milder than vivax malaria, and is frequently found in conjunction with infection due to *P. falciparum.* The infected erythrocytes assume an oblong or oval shape on a stained blood film. It most commonly occurs in sub-Saharan Africa.
**pernicious m.,** falciparum m.
**quartan m.,** that in which the febrile paroxysms occur every 72 hours, or every fourth day counting the day of occurrence as the first day of each cycle; it is caused by *Plasmodium malariae,* which requires 72 hours for completion of each asexual cycle in the erythrocyte. It is the mildest and most chronic of all human malarial infections.
**quotidian m.,** that in which the febrile paroxysms occur daily, thought to be due to simultaneous infection with two broods of *Plasmodium vivax* or *P. falciparum* that complete their cycles on alternate days. See also *vivax m.*
**subtertian m.,** falciparum m.
**tertian m.,** that in which the febrile paroxysms occur every third day counting the day of occurrence as the first day of the cycle, because of a synchronized infection with a single brood of *Plasmodium vivax* or *P. ovale.* See *ovale m.* and *vivax m.*
**transfusion m.,** infection with *Plasmodium falciparum, P. malariae, P. ovale,* or *P. vivax* transmitted directly from a blood donor, by accidental infection of a contaminated needle, or by intravenous drug users sharing needles.
**vivax m.,** malaria caused by *Plasmodium vivax;* although it is less severe than falciparum malaria, it does cause severe symptoms, including anemia, and is the one in which relapses are most likely to occur because of hypnozoite (or latent) forms that persist in the liver following cure of the blood stages of the parasite. In vivax malaria the febrile paroxysms often recur every other day (see *tertian m.*), but they may recur daily (see *quotidian m.*). The infected red cells often appear enlarged on a stained blood film since the parasite tends to infect younger erythrocytes. Called also *benign tertian m.*

**ma•lar•ia•ci•dal** (mə-lar″e-ə-si′dəl) destructive to malarial plasmodia; plasmodicidal.

**ma·lar·i·al** (mə-lar′e-əl) pertaining or due to malaria.

**ma·lar·i·ol·o·gist** (mə-lar″e-ol′o-jist) a person versed in or engaged in the study of malaria.

**ma·lar·i·ol·o·gy** (mə-lar″e-ol′o-je) [*malaria* + *-logy*] the study of malaria.

**ma·lar·io·ther·a·py** (mə-lar″e-o-ther′ə-pe) an obsolete method of treating neurosyphilis by infecting the patient with malarial parasites, generally *Plasmodium vivax* or *P. falciparum;* malariotherapy using *P. vivax* has been suggested for the treatment of the neurologic manifestations of Lyme disease.

**ma·lar·i·ous** (mə-lar′e-əs) malarial.

**ma·la·ris** (mə-la′ris) [L.] 1. buccal. 2. zygomatic (def. 2).

**Mal·as·sez's disease, rest** (mahl″ah-sāz′) [Louis Charles *Malassez,* French physiologist, 1842–1909] see under *disease* and *rest.*

**Mal·as·se·zia** (mal″ə-se′zhə) [Louis Charles *Malassez*] [MeSH: Malassezia] a genus of Fungi Imperfecti of the form-family Cryptococcaceae, consisting of yeast-like organisms that produce no mycelium; called also *Pityrosporum.*

**M. fur′fur,** a lipophilic species that forms a part of the normal flora of the human skin and causes tinea versicolor in susceptible individuals. Called also *Cladosporium mansonii* and *Pityrosporum orbiculare.*

**M. ova′lis,** a cultural variant of *M. furfur.*

**M. pachyder′matis,** a nonlipophilic species that forms a part of the normal flora of humans and animals and causes otitis externa associated with seborrheic dermatitis in dogs.

**mal·as·sim·i·la·tion** (mal″ə-sim″ĭ-la′shən) [L. *malus* ill + *assimilation*] 1. imperfect, faulty, or disordered assimilation. 2. the inability of the gastrointestinal tract to transport to the body fluids one or more ingested nutrients, whether due to faulty digestion (maldigestion) or to impaired intestinal mucosal transport (malabsorption).

**ma·late** (ma′lāt, mal′āt) an ionic form of malic acid.

**ma·late de·hy·dro·gen·ase** (ma′lāt de-hi′dro-jən-ās) [EC 1.1.1.37] [MeSH: Malate Dehydrogenase] an enzyme of the oxidoreductase class that catalyzes the oxidation of L-malate to oxaloacetate, reducing $NAD^+$. The enzyme occurs both in the mitochondria and in the cytosol. The reaction is important in the tricarboxylic acid cycle and in the malate-aspartate electron shuttle. See illustration at *tricarboxylic acid cycle,* under *cycle.*

**ma·late de·hy·dro·gen·ase (ox·alo·ac·e·tate-de·car·box·y·lat·ing) ($NADP^+$)** (ma′lāt de-hi′dro-jən-ās ok-sal″o-as′ə-tāt de-kahr-bok′sə-lāt″ing) an enzyme of the oxidoreductase class that catalyzes the oxidative decarboxylation of L-malate to form pyruvate, reducing $NADP^+$. The cytosolic and mitochondrial forms are isozymes; the cytosolic enzyme is a major source of NADPH for fatty acid synthesis.

**mal·a·thi·on** (mal″ə-thi′on) [MeSH: Malathion] an organophosphorus insecticide and veterinary topical parasiticide.

**mal·ax·ate** (mal′ək-sāt) to knead, as in making pills.

**mal·ax·a·tion** (mal″ək-sa′shən) [Gr. *malaxis* a softening] an act of kneading.

**Mal·co·tran** (mal′ko-trən) trademark for a preparation of homatropine methylbromide.

**mal·de·vel·op·ment** (mal″də-vel′əp-mənt) abnormal growth or development.

**mal·di·ges·tion** (mal″di-jes′chən) impaired digestion.

**male** (māl) [MeSH: Male] 1. an organism of the sex that begets young or that produces spermatozoa. 2. masculine.

**mal·e·ate** (mal′e-āt) any salt or ester of maleic acid.

**ma·le·ic ac·id** (mə-le′ik) trivial name for *cis*-butanedioic acid; the *cis* isomer of fumaric acid.

**mal·emis·sion** (mal″e-mish′ən) failure of the semen to be discharged from the urinary meatus in coitus.

**mal·erup·tion** (mal″ə-rup′shən) faulty eruption of a tooth, so that it is out of its normal position.

**mal·eth·a·mer** (məl-eth′ə-mər) a high weight copolymer of ethylene with maleic anhydride, cross-linked with 1 to 2 per cent, by weight, of vinyl crotonate; an antiperistaltic agent.

**4-ma·leyl·ac·e·to·ac·e·tate** (ma″le-əl-ə-se″to-as′ə-tāt) an isomer of fumarylacetoacetate, formed by oxidation of homogentisate in the degradation of tyrosine and phenylalanine.

**ma·le·yl·ace·to·ac·e·tate isom·er·ase** (ma′le-əl-ə-se″to-as′ə-tāt i-som′ər-ās) [EC 5.2.1.2] an enzyme of the isomerase class that catalyzes the interconversion of the isomers 4-maleylacetoacetate and 4-fumarylacetoacetate. The reaction is a step in the use of phenylalanine and tyrosine as fuel.

**mal·for·ma·tion** (mal″for-ma′shən) [L. *malus* evil + *formation*] 1. a type of anomaly. 2. a morphologic defect of an organ or larger region of the body, resulting from an intrinsically abnormal developmental process.

**Arnold-Chiari m.,** Chiari's malformation type II; herniation of the cerebellar tonsils and vermis through the foramen magnum into the spinal canal. It is always associated with lumbosacral myelomeningocele, and hydrocephalus and mental defects are common. Called also Arnold-Chiari deformity or syndrome

**cerebral arteriovenous m.,** a congenital anomaly of the brain vasculature composed of arterial and venous channels with many interconnecting shunts without a capillary bed; clinical characteristics include hemorrhage, headache, and focal epileptic seizures. Large malformations may have cranial bruits. Called also *arteriovenous angioma of brain.*

**Chiari's m.,** 1. Arnold-Chiari deformity. 2. a congenital anomaly in which the cerebellum and medulla oblongata, which is elongated and flattened, protrude into the spinal canal through the foramen magnum; it is classified into three types according to severity, ranging from prolapse of the cerebellar tonsils into the spinal canal without elongation of the brainstem (type I) to complete herniation of the cerebellum to form an occipital encephalocele (type III). It may be accompanied by hydrocephalus, spina bifida, syringomyelia, and mental defects. The classic form is Type II, Arnold-Chiari malformation (q.v.). Called also *Chiari's deformity.*

**cystic adenomatoid m.,** a rare variant of congenital cystic lung disease, characterized by a mass of interconnecting cysts lined with cuboidal or bronchial epithelium; respiratory distress usually occurs soon after birth and results from compression of normal lung tissue by the cystic lesion.

**Dandy-Walker m.,** a congenital anomaly caused by failure of the roof of the fourth ventricle to develop during embryogenesis, characterized by cystic dilatation of the fourth ventricle, absence or hypoplasia of the vermis, and enlargement of the posterior fossa; hydrocephalus is usually present. Called also *Dandy-Walker deformity* or *syndrome.*

**Dieulafoy's vascular m.,** a rare defect of the gastrointestinal mucosa, usually occurring near the gastroesophageal junction, although it may occur in the small intestine or colon, in which a submucosal artery in abnormally close contact with the mucosa causes pressure erosion of the epithelium and eventually ruptures into the stomach.

**Mondini's m.,** see under *deformity.*

**mal·func·tion** (mal-funk′shən) dysfunction.

**Mal·gaigne's amputation, luxation, triangle** (mahl-gen′yəz) [Joseph François *Malgaigne,* French surgeon, 1806–1865] see *subastragalar amputation,* under *amputation, pulled elbow,* under *elbow,* and *trigonum caroticum.*

**Mal·herbe's calcifying epithelioma** (mahl-ārbz′) [Albert *Malherbe,* French surgeon, 1845–1915] pilomatricoma.

**mal·ic ac·id** (ma′lik, mal′ik) an intermediate in the tricarboxylic acid (Krebs) cycle, formed from fumaric acid and itself oxidized to form oxaloacetic acid; found in apples, pears, and many other fruits; its action is similar to that of tartaric acid, and it is a permitted food additive.

**mal·ic en·zyme** (ma′lik, mal′ik en′zīm) malate dehydrogenase (oxaloacetate-decarboxylating) ($NADP^+$).

**ma·lig·nan·cy** (mə-lig′nən-se) [L. *malignare* to act maliciously] 1. a tendency to progress in virulence. 2. the quality of being malignant. 3. a cancer, especially one with the potential to cause death.

**ma·lig·nant** (mə-lig′nənt) [L. *malignans* acting maliciously] 1. tending to become progressively worse and to result in death. 2. having the properties of anaplasia, invasion, and metastasis; said of tumors.

**ma·lin·ger·er** (mə-ling′ər-ər) [Fr. *malingre* sickly] an individual who is guilty of malingering.

**ma·lin·ger·ing** (mə-ling′ər-ing) [MeSH: Malingering] the willful, deliberate, and fraudulent feigning or exaggeration of the symptoms of illness or injury, done for the purpose of a consciously desired end.

**mal·in·ter·dig·i·ta·tion** (mal″in-tər-dij″ĭ-ta′shən) failure of interdigitation of parts which are normally so related.

**mal·le·a·bil·i·ty** (mal″e-ə-bil′ĭ-te) the quality of being malleable.

**mal·le·a·ble** (mal′e-ə-bəl) [L. *malleare* to hammer] susceptible of being beaten out into a thin plate.

**mal·le·al** (mal′e-əl) mallear.

**mal·le·ar** (mal′e-ər) pertaining to the malleus (def. 1); called also *malleal* and *malleolar.*

**mal·le·a·tion** (mal″e-a′shən) [L. *malleare* to hammer] sharp and swift muscular twitching of the hands.

**mal·le·in** (mal′ēn) [L. *malleus* glanders] a concentrate prepared

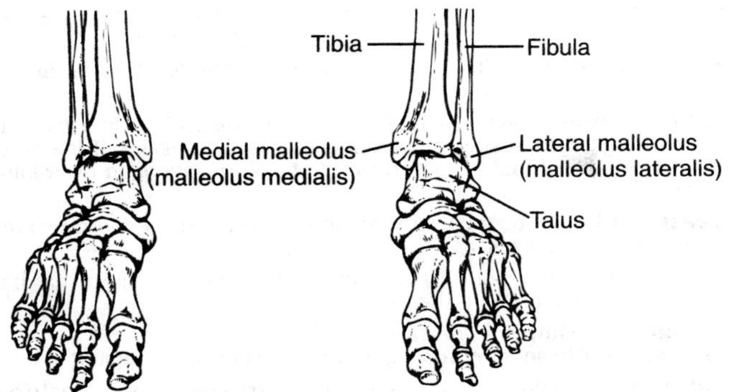


Malleolus lateralis (lateral malleolus) and malleolus medialis (medial malleolus), articulating with the talus in the ankle joint.

from cultures or extracts of the glanders bacillus, *Pseudomonas mallei,* used in a skin test analogous to the tuberculin test for the diagnosis of glanders.

**mal·leo·in·cu·dal** (mal″e-o-ing′ku-dəl) incudomalleolar.

**mal·le·o·lar** (mə-le′o-lər) 1. pertaining to a malleolus. 2. mallear.

**mal·le·o·li** (mə-le′o-li) [L.] genitive and plural of *malleolus.*

**mal·le·o·lus** (mə-le′o-ləs) gen. and pl. *malle′oli* [L., dim. of *malleus* hammer] [TA] a general term for a rounded process, such as the protuberance on either side of the ankle joint.
**external m., m. exter′nus,** m. lateralis.
**m. fi′bulae, fibular m.,** m. lateralis.
**inner m., internal m., m. inter′nus,** m. medialis.
**m. latera′lis** [TA], lateral malleolus: the process on the lateral side of the distal end of the fibula, forming, with the malleolus medialis, the mortise in which the talus articulates.
**m. media′lis** [TA], medial malleolus: the process on the medial side of the distal end of the tibia, forming, with the malleolus lateralis, the mortise in which the talus articulates.
**outer m.,** m. lateralis.
**radial m., m. radia′lis,** processus styloideus radii.
**m. ti′biae, tibial m.,** m. medialis.
**ulnar m., m. ulna′ris,** processus styloideus ulnae.

**Mal·leo·my·ces** (mal″e-o-mi′sēz) [L. *malleus* glanders + Gr. *mykēs* fungus] in former systems of classification, a genus of bacteria, species of which have been assigned to the genus *Pseudomonas.*

**mal·le·ot·o·my** (mal″e-ot′ə-me) [*malleus* + Gr. *tomē* a cutting] 1. surgical division of the malleus in cases of ankylosis of the ossicles. 2. surgical separation of the malleoli by division of the ligaments holding them together.

**mal·let** (mal′ət) a hammerlike tool, usually with a nonmetallic head, for striking something without leaving a mark.

**mal·le·us** (mal′e-əs) [L. "hammer"] [MeSH: Malleus] 1. [TA] the outermost of the auditory ossicles, and the one attached to the membrana tympani; its club-shaped head articulates with the incus. Called also *hammer.* See illustration. 2. glanders.

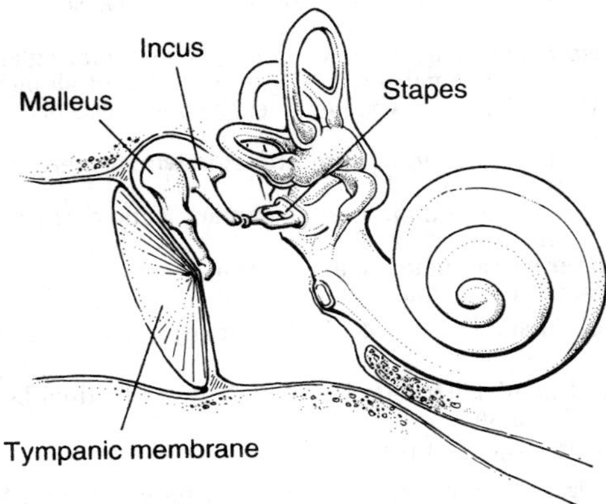


**mal·lo·cho·ri·on** (mal″o-kor′e-on) [Gr. *mallos* wool + *chorion*] the primordial chorion; so called because of its villi.

**Mal·loph·a·ga** (mal-of′ə-gə) [Gr. *mallos* wool + *phagein* to eat] [MeSH: Mallophaga] the biting lice (also called *bird lice*), a large order of insects that feed on the feathers and hair of birds and that sometimes attack mammals, including humans. Genera include *Damalinia, Felicola, Heterodoxus, Menacanthus,* and *Trichodectes.*

**Mal·lo·ry's bodies, stain** (mal′ə-rēz) [Frank Burr *Mallory,* American pathologist, 1862–1941] see under *body,* and see *stain.*

**Mal·lory-Weiss syndrome** (mal′ə-re-wīs) [G. Kenneth *Mallory,* American pathologist, born 1900; Soma *Weiss,* American physician, 1898–1942] [MeSH: Mallory-Weiss Syndrome] see under *syndrome.*

**mal·lo·tox·in** (mal′o-tok″sin) rottlerin.

**Mal·lo·tus** (mə-lo′təs) a genus of trees of the family Euphorbiaceae, native to southern and eastern Asia, the East Indies, and Australia. *M. philippinen′sis* (Lam.) Muell. Arg. is the kamala, source of the medicinal substance also called kamala and of the anthelmintic rottlerin.

**mal·low** (mal′o) [L. *malva*] any plant of the genus *Malva.*

**mal·nu·tri·tion** (mal″noo-trish′ən) any disorder of nutrition; it may be due to unbalanced or insufficient diet or to defective assimilation or utilization of foods.
**malignant m., protein m.,** kwashiorkor.
**protein-energy m. (PEM),** a class of disorders caused by varying degrees of protein and calorie deficiency, alone or in combination, frequently aggravated by accompanying physiologic and environmental stresses. It may be primary, including such disorders as marasmus, kwashiorkor, and marasmic kwashiorkor, or secondary to other diseases.

**mal·oc·clu·sion** (mal″o-kloo′zhən) [MeSH: Malocclusion] such malposition and contact of the maxillary and mandibular teeth as to interfere with the highest efficiency during the excursive movements of the jaw that are essential for mastication; originally classified by Angle into four major groups, depending on the anteroposterior jaw relationship as indicated by interdigitation of the first molar teeth, but Class IV is not used (see table).
**closed-bite m.,** closed bite.
**open-bite m.,** open bite.

**mal·o·nate-semi·al·de·hyde de·hy·dro·gen·ase (acet·y·lat·ing)** (mal′ə-nāt sem″e-al′də-hīd de-hi′dro-jən-ās ə-set′ə-lāt″ing) [EC 1.2.1.18] an enzyme of the oxidoreductase class that catalyzes the decarboxylation of malonate semialdehyde, linking it to coenzyme A to form acetyl coenzyme A; it uses $NAD(P)^+$ as an electron acceptor.

**ma·lon·ic ac·id** (mə-lon′ik) propanedioic acid, $HOOC\text{-}CH_2COOH$; malonyl coenzyme A is the source of 2-carbon groups transferred to the growing hydrocarbon chain in fatty acid synthesis.

**mal·o·nyl** (mal′ə-nəl) an acyl radical of malonic acid.

**Angle's Classification of Malocclusion**

| | |
|---|---|
| *Class I (Neutroclusion)* | Normal anteroposterior relationship of the jaws, as indicated by correct interdigitation of maxillary and mandibular molars, but with crowding and rotation of teeth elsewhere, i.e., a dental dysplasia or an arch length deficiency. |
| *Class II (Distoclusion)* | The lower dental arch is posterior to the upper in one or both lateral segments; the lower first molar is distal to the upper first molar. |
| Division 1 | Bilaterally distal with narrow maxillary arch and protruding upper incisors. |
| Subdivision | Unilaterally distal with other characteristics the same. |
| Division 2 | Bilaterally distal with normal or square-shaped maxillary arch, retruded maxillary central incisors, labially malposed maxillary lateral incisors, and an excessive overbite. |
| Subdivision | Unilaterally distal with other characteristics the same. |
| *Class III (Mesioclusion)* | The lower arch is anterior to the upper in one or both lateral segments; lower first molar is mesial to upper first molar. |
| Division | Mandibular incisors are usually in anterior crossbite. |
| Subdivision | Unilaterally mesial, with other characteristics the same. |
| *Class IV* | The dental arches are in distal occlusion upon one lateral half, and in mesial occlusion upon the other half of the mouth. |

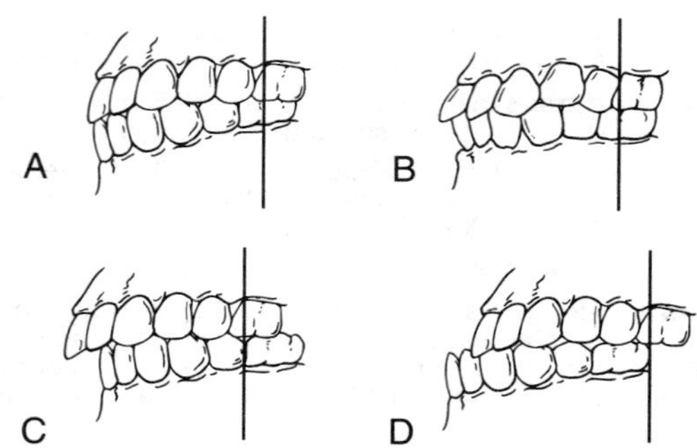

*(A),* Normal occlusion; *(B),* Class I malocclusion; *(C),* Class II malocclusion; *(D),* Class III malocclusion. Note the position of the mesial cusp of the maxillary molar relative to the mandibular molar in each type of occlusion.

**mal·o·nyl CoA** (mal′ə-nəl ko-a′) malonyl coenzyme A.

**mal·o·nyl co·en·zyme A** (mal′ə-nəl ko-en′zīm) [MeSH: Malonyl Coenzyme A] the coenzyme A thioester of malonic acid, formed from acetyl coenzyme A by acetyl-CoA carboxylase. It is an intermediate in fatty acid synthesis.

**mal·per·fu·sion** (mal″pər-fu′zhən) abnormal perfusion.

**Mal·pigh·ia** (mal-pig′e-ə) [Marcello *Malpighi*] a genus of tropical American fruit-bearing shrubs and trees of the family Malpighiaceae. *M. glab′ra, M. punicifo′lia,* and *M. u′rens* are all called acerola or Barbados cherry and their fruit is rich in vitamin C.

**mal·pigh·i·an bodies, corpuscles** etc. (mahl-pig′e-ən) [M. *Malpighi*] see under *stigma* and *tubule;* see *keratinocyte* and see *capsula glomeruli, corpuscula renis, noduli lymphoidei splenici, glomeruli renis,* and *stratum germinativum.*

**mal·posed** (mal-pōzd′) not in the normal position.

**mal·po·si·tion** (mal″pə-zish′ən) [L. *malus* bad + *positio* placement] abnormal or anomalous position of an organ or part; cf. *ectopia.* Called also *allotopia, displacement, dystopia,* and *heterotopia.*

**mal·prac·tice** (mal-prak′tis) [L. *mal* bad + *practice*] [MeSH: Malpractice] improper or injurious practice; unskillful and faulty medical or surgical treatment.

**mal·pres·en·ta·tion** (mal″prez-ən-ta′shən) a faulty or abnormal fetal presentation.

**mal·ro·ta·tion** (mal″ro-ta′shən) 1. abnormal or pathologic rotation, as of the vertebral column. 2. failure of normal rotation of an organ, such as the midgut, during embryological development.

**MALT** mucosa-associated lymphoid tissue.

**malt** (mawlt) grain, for the most part barley, which has been soaked, made to germinate, and then dried; it contains dextrin, maltose, and diastase.

**mal·tase** (mawl′tās) 1. α-glucosidase. 2. any enzyme with similar glycolytic activity, cleaving α-1,4 or sometimes α-1,6 linked glucose residues from nonreducing termini; in humans there are considered to be four such enzymes. Two are the heat-stable enzymes usually called maltases, constituting the glucoamylase complex (q.v.); the other two are the heat-labile enzymes more commonly called sucrase and α-dextrinase that constitute the *sucrase-isomaltase* complex (q.v.).

**mal·thu·si·an law** (mal-thoo′se-ən) [Rev. Thomas Robert *Malthus,* English economist, 1766–1834] see under *law.*

**mal·ti·tol** (mawl′tĭ-lol) [NF] a hydrogenated, partially hydrolyzed starch used as a bulk sweetener.

**mal·to·bi·ose** (mawl″to-bi′ōs) maltose.

**mal·to·dex·trin** (mawl″to-dek′strin) [NF] any polysaccharide of glucose residues in β-(1,4) linkage, such as are formed in incomplete hydrolysis of starch to maltose; used as an excipient in pharmaceutical preparations and a source of carbohydrates in oral dietary supplements and tube feeding.

**MALT·oma** (mawl-to′mə) a form of extranodal marginal zone B-cell lymphoma originating in mucosa-associated lymphoid tissue, particularly that of the gastrointestinal tract, as well as other organs including larynx, salivary gland, thyroid, and lung. It is characterized by small lymphocytes, marginal zone B cells, monocytoid B cells, and plasma cells. Tumors are generally localized and indolent, but may spread or become more aggressive.

**mal·tose** (mawl′tōs) [MeSH: Maltose] a reducing disaccharide composed of two glucose residues in α-(1,4)-glycosidic linkage; it is the fundamental structural unit of glycogen and starch and is used as a nutrient and sweetener.

**mal·to·side** (mawl′to-sīd) a glycoside composed of maltose residues.

**mal·tos·uria** (mawl″to-su′re-ə) the presence of maltose in the urine.

**mal·to·tri·ose** (mawl″to-tri′ōs) a reducing disaccharide consisting of three glucose residues in α-(1,4)-glycosidic linkage; it is one of the products of limited digestion of starch or glycogen by α-amylase.

**mal·turned** (mal-turnd′) turned abnormally; said of teeth twisted on their central axes.

**Mal·u·ci·din** (mal″u-si′din) trademark for a yeast extract that has abortifacient activity in the dog, cat, and sheep.

**ma·lum** (ma′ləm) [L.] disease.
**m. vertebra′le suboccipita′le,** tuberculosis of the atlas and axis.

**mal·un·ion** (mal-ūn′yon) union of the fragments of a fractured bone in a faulty position.

**Ma·lus** (ma′ləs) a genus of flowering trees of the family Rosaceae. *M. sylves′tris* Mill. is the apple (q.v.).

**Mal·va** (mal′və) [L.] the mallows, a genus of flowering plants of the family Malvaceae. The flowers and leaves of *M. sylves′tris* L. and *M. rotundifo′lia* L. are demulcent and emollient, and are used medicinally in India and other parts of Asia.

**mam·ba** (mahm′bə) [Zulu *im-amba*] any member of the genus *Dendroaspis,* extremely venomous elapid snakes.
**black m.,** *Dendroaspis polylepis,* a large black African tree snake whose venom is deadly.
**green m.,** *Dendroaspis angusticeps,* a large green or black tree snake of eastern and southern Africa whose venom is deadly.

**mam·e·lon** (mam′ə-lon) [Fr. "nipple"] 1. one of three tubercles sometimes present on the cutting edge of an incisor tooth. 2. the nipple-like elevation in the umbilicus, considered to be the remains of the solid proximal part of the umbilical cord which contained the umbilical arteries and urachus.

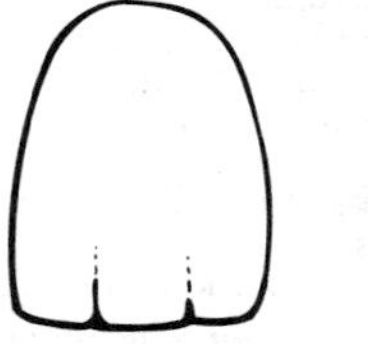
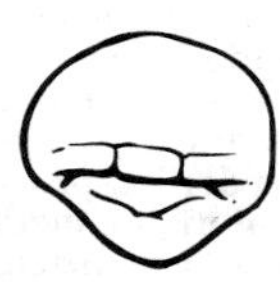
Incisor with mamelons.

**ma·mil·la** (mə-mil′ə) mammilla.

**mam·il·lary** (mam′ĭ-lar″e) mammillary.

**mam·il·lat·ed** (mam″ĭ-lāt′əd) mammillated.

**mam·il·la·tion** (mam″ĭ-la′shən) mammillation.

**ma·mil·li·form** (mə-mil′ĭ-form) mammilliform.

**mam·il·li·tis** (mam″ĭ-li′tis) mammillitis.

**mam·ma** (mam′ə) gen. and pl. *mam′mae* [L.] [TA] [MeSH: Mammae] the breast: the modified cutaneous, glandular structure on the anterior aspect of the thorax that contains, in the female, the elements that secrete milk for nourishment of the young. See also *glandula mammaria.*
**m. accesso′ria** [TA], accessory mamma: a mammary gland present in excess of the normal number, generally found along the line of the embryonic mammary ridge (crest); called also *accessory mammary gland.*
**m. areola′ta,** a condition of the breast in which there is bulging of the areola of the nipple.
**m. masculi′na,** the rudimentary mammary gland of the male breast; called also *m. virilis.*
**supernumerary m.,** mamma accessoria.
**m. vi′rilis,** m. masculina.

**mam·mae** (mam′e) [L.] [MeSH: Mammae] genitive and plural of *mamma.*

**mam·mal** (mam′əl) [MeSH: Mammals] an individual belonging to the class Mammalia.

**mam·mal·gia** (mə-mal′jə) mastalgia.

**Mam·ma·lia** (mə-mal′e-ə) a class of warm-blooded vertebrate animals, including all that possess hair and suckle their young. It includes three major groups: placentals and marsupials, which are viviparous, and monotremes, which are oviparous.

**mam·mal·o·gy** (mə-mal′ə-je) [*mammal* + *-logy*] the study of mammals.

**mam·ma·plas·ty** (mam′ə-plas″te) [*mamma* + *-plasty*] [MeSH: Mam-

maplasty] plastic reconstruction of the breast, as may be performed to augment or reduce its size. Called also *mammoplasty* and *mastoplasty*.
**Aries-Pitanguy m.**, an operation to reduce mild to moderate macromastia.
**augmentation m.**, plastic reconstruction of the breast, with increase of its volume by insertion of an autogenous or prosthetic material.
**Biesenberger m.**, a reduction mammaplasty using transposition of the nipple, consisting in excision of the lateral portion of the mammary gland, with rotation of the remaining glandular pedicle attached to the nipple and formation of a skin brassiere.
**Conway m.**, a method of correcting severe macromastia, consisting in partial breast amputation and free transplantation of the nipples and areolae.
**reduction m.**, plastic reconstruction of the breast with decrease in its volume by excision of tissue.
**Strömbeck m.**, a one-stage breast reduction operation that includes transposition of the nipple in a medial and lateral pedicle.

**mam·ma·ry** (mam'ər-e) [L. *mammarius*] pertaining to the mamma, or breast.

**mam·ma·troph** (mam'ə-trof) lactotroph.

**mam·mec·to·my** (mə-mek'to-me) [*mamm-* + *-ectomy*] mastectomy.

**mam·mi·form** (mam'ĭ-form) [*mammo-* + *form*] shaped like a breast.

**mam·mil·la** (mə-mil'ə) gen. and pl. *mammil'lae* [L., dim. of *mamma*, a breast, teat] 1. the nipple (papilla mamma'ria [TA]). 2. any nipple-like structure; spelled also *mamilla*.

**mam·mil·lary** (mam'ĭ-lar"e) [L. *mammilla*, dim. of *mamma*, a breast, teat] pertaining to or resembling a nipple; spelled also *mamillary*.

**mam·mil·lat·ed** (mam'ĭ-lāt"əd) having nipple-like projections.

**mam·mil·la·tion** (mam"ĭ-la'shən) 1. the condition of being mammillated. 2. a nipple-like elevation or projection.

**mam·mil·li·form** (mə-mil'ĭ-form) [*mammilla* + *form*] shaped like a nipple.

**mam·mil·li·plas·ty** (mə-mil'ĭ-plas"te) theleplasty.

**mam·mil·li·tis** (mam"ĭ-li'tis) [*mammilla* + *-itis*] inflammation of the mammilla, or nipple; spelled also *mamillitis*. Called also *thelitis*.
**bovine ulcerative m.**, a herpesviral disease affecting milking cows, characterized by ulcerative lesions on the teats and, less frequently, on the udders.

**mam·mi·pla·sia** (mam"ĭ-pla'zhə) mammoplasia.

**mam·mi·tis** (mam-i'tis) mastitis.

**mamm(o)-** [L. *mamma*, q.v.] a combining form denoting relationship to the breast, or to a mammary gland; see also words beginning *mast(o)-* and *maz(o)-*.

**mam·mo·gen** (mam'o-jən) any substance or influence that promotes breast development.

**mam·mo·gen·e·sis** (mam"o-jen'ə-sis) the development of the mammary glands to the functional state.

**mam·mo·gram** (mam'ə-gram) a radiograph of the breast.

**mam·mog·ra·phy** (mə-mog'rə-fe) [MeSH: Mammography] radiography of the mammary gland.

**Mam·mo·mo·nog·a·mus** (mam"o-mon"o-ga'mus) a genus of nematodes of the family Syngamidae. Various species infest the pharynx, larynx, and trachea of cats and other mammals.

**mam·mo·pla·sia** (mam"o-pla'zhə) [*mammo-* + *-plasia*] the development of breast tissue; called also *mastoplasia*.
**adolescent m.**, the development of breast tissue at adolescence, applied especially to the development and later regression which occurs in males during puberty.

**mam·mo·plas·ty** (mam'o-plas"te) mammaplasty.

**mam·mose** (mam'ōs) [L. *mammosus*] 1. having large breasts, or mammae. 2. mammillated.

**mam·mo·so·mat·o·trope** (mam"o-so-mat'o-trōp) mammosomatotroph.

**mam·mo·so·mat·o·troph** (mam"o-so-mat'o-trōf) an acidophilic cell of the adenohypophysis that secretes both growth hormone and prolactin.

**mam·mot·o·my** (mə-mot'o-me) mastotomy.

**mam·mo·troph** (mam'o-trōf) lactotroph.

**mam·mo·troph·ic** (mam"o-trof'ik) mammotropic.

**mam·mo·trop·ic** (mam"o-trop'ik) [*mammo-* + *-tropic*] having affinity for or a stimulating effect on the mammary gland. Called also *mammotrophic*.

**mam·mo·tro·pin** (mam'-o-tro"pin) prolactin.

**Man.** abbreviation for L. *mani'pulus*, a handful.

**Man·ches·ter operation** (man'chəs-tər) [*Manchester*, England, where it was developed] see under *operation*.

**man·chette** (man-shet') [Fr. "a cuff"] a temporary band around the neck of a spermatozoon.

**man·chi·neel** (man"kĭ-nēl') *Hippomane mancinella*, a tree of tropical America that has a caustic poisonous sap.

**Man·del·amine** (man"dəl-ah'mēn) trademark for a preparation of methenamine mandelate.

**man·del·ic acid** (man-del'ik, man-de'lik) [USP] an acid with active bacteriostatic properties, used in urinary tract infections, usually as the ammonium or calcium salt. Called also *amygdalic acid* and *phenylglycolic acid*.

**man·di·ble** (man'dĭ-bəl) [MeSH: Mandible] the bone of the lower jaw; see *mandibula*.

**man·dib·u·la** (man-dib'u-lə) gen. and pl. *mandib'ulae* [L., from *mandere* to chew] [TA] the mandible: the horseshoe-shaped bone forming the lower jaw; the largest and strongest bone of the face, presenting a body and a pair of rami, which articulate with the skull at the temporomandibular joints.

**man·dib·u·lae** (man-dib'u-le) [L.] genitive and plural of *mandibula*.

**man·dib·u·lar** (man-dib'u-lər) pertaining to the lower jaw bone, or mandible.

**man·dib·u·lec·to·my** (man-dib"u-lek'tə-me) surgical removal of the mandible.

**man·dib·u·lo·pha·ryn·ge·al** (man-dib"u-lo-fə-rin'je-əl) pertaining to the mandible and the pharynx.

**Man·drag·o·ra** (man-drag'o-rə) [L.] a genus of plants of the family Solanaceae. *M. officina'rum* L. is the true European or oriental mandrake, which has the general properties of belladonna and was formerly used as a narcotic and sedative. It contains the alkaloids mandragorine, hyoscyamine, and scopolamine.

**man·drake** (man'drāk) any plant of the genus *Mandragora*.

**man·drel** (man'drəl) a shaft in a handpiece that holds a disk, stone, or cup used for grinding or polishing. Called also *mandril*.

**man·dril** (man'dril) mandrel.

**man·drin** (man'drin) a stylet or guide for a catheter.

**ma·neu·ver** (mə-noo'vər) any dexterous procedure. See also entries under *method, operation, procedure, surgery,* and *technique*.
**Adson's m.**, a test for thoracic outlet syndrome: with the patient in a sitting position, hands resting on thighs, the examiner palpates both radial pulses as the patient rapidly fills the lungs by deep inspiration and, with breath held, hyperextends the neck and turns the head toward the affected side. If the radial pulse on that side is decidedly or completely obliterated, the result is considered positive. Called also *Adson's test*.
**Allen's m.**, with the forearm flexed at a right angle, the arm is extended horizontally and rotated externally at the shoulder, the head being rotated to the contralateral shoulder; obliteration of the radial pulse suggests scalenus anterior syndrome.
**Barlow m.**, a dislocation maneuver used together with the Ortolani maneuver in diagnosing congenital hip dislocation.
**Bracht's m.**, (for breech presentation), the breech is allowed to spontaneously deliver up to the umbilicus. The body and extended legs are held together with both hands maintaining the upward and anterior rotation of the fetal body. When the anterior rotation is nearly complete, the fetal body is held against the mother's sym-

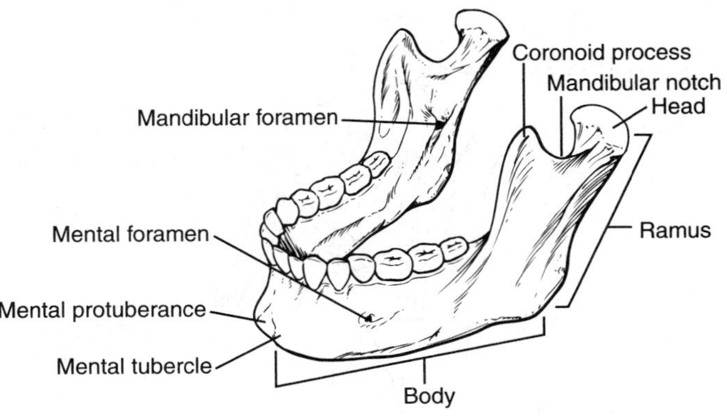


Mandibula (mandible).

physis. Maintenance of this position can lead to spontaneous completion of delivery.
**Brandt-Andrews m.**, a method of expressing the placenta from the uterus in the third stage of labor: the left hand grasps the umbilical cord while the right is placed on the maternal abdomen with the fingers over the anterior uterine surface. The right hand is gently pressed backward and slightly upward as the left applies gentle traction on the cord.
**Catell m.**, mobilization and reflection superiorly to the left of the right colon, root of the small bowel mesentery, duodenum, and head of the pancreas to expose the retroperitoneal vascular structures.
**Credé's m.**, see under *method.*
**forward-bending m.**, a method of detecting retraction signs in neoplastic changes in the mammae; the patient bends forward from the waist with chin held up and arms extended toward the examiner. If retraction is present, an asymmetry in the breast is seen.
**Gowers' m.**, Gowers' sign (def. 2).
**Hallpike's m.**, a test for benign positional vertigo: the examiner turns the head of the seated patient to one side and pulls the patient backwards into a supine position with the head hanging over the edge of the examining table; the patient then looks straight ahead and the examiner observes for positional nystagmus, which is indicative of benign positional vertigo.
**Heimlich m.**, a method of dislodging food or other material from the throat of a choking victim: after wrapping the arms around the victim at the belt line and allowing his upper torso to hang forward, make a fist with one hand and grasp it with the other; with both hands placed against the victim's abdomen slightly above the navel and below the rib cage, forcefully press into the abdomen with a quick upward thrust. If the victim is sitting, stand behind him and perform the same procedure; if he is prone, turn him on his back, kneel astride the torso, place both hands at the location on the victim's abdomen as described above and press forcefully with a sharp upward thrust. The maneuver may be repeated several times if necessary.
**Hoguet's m.**, in hernioplasty, conversion of the direct hernial sac to an indirect one by withdrawing the sac from beneath the deep epigastric vessels.
**Hueter's m.**, downward and forward pressure on the patient's tongue by the left forefinger of the physician during introduction of a stomach tube.
**Jendrassik's m.**, a procedure for emphasizing the patellar reflex: the patient hooks his hands together by the flexed fingers and pulls apart as hard as he can.
**Kocher m.**, operative mobilization of the duodenum for exposure of the retroduodenal, intrapancreatic, and intraduodenal portions of the common bile duct.
**Leopold's m's**, four maneuvers in palpating the abdomen for ascertaining the position and presentation of the fetus.
**McDonald m.**, measurement of the contour of the abdomen to calculate the duration of pregnancy; see also under *rule.*
**Mattox m.**, mobilization and medial reflection of the abdominal viscera to expose the suprarenal aorta for repair of traumatic injury.
**Mauriceau m.**, a method of delivering the aftercoming head in cases of breech presentation: the infant's body rests on the physician's palm and forearm with the index and middle fingers over the maxilla to flex the head while the other hand is placed on the infant's shoulders to apply traction. Called also *Mauriceau-Smellie-Veit m.* and *Smellie's method.*
**Mauriceau-Smellie-Veit m.**, Mauriceau m.
**Müller's m.**, an inspiratory effort with a closed glottis after expiration, used during fluoroscopic examination to cause a negative intrathoracic pressure with engorgement of intrathoracic vascular structures, which is helpful in recognizing esophageal varices, and distinguishing vascular from nonvascular structures.

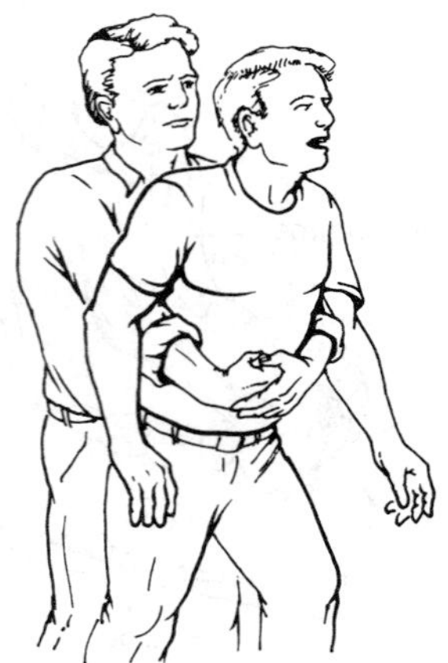

Heimlich maneuver.

**Ortolani m.**, a reduction maneuver used together with the Barlow maneuver in diagnosing congenital hip dislocation.
**Osler's m.**, a technique for identifying pseudohypertension: the sphygmomanometer cuff is inflated above systolic blood pressure; if the pulseless radial or brachial artery remains palpable, pseudohypertension may be present.
**Pajot's m.**, for forceps traction along the axis of superior strait; one hand over the lock of the forceps pulls downward towards the floor, while the other hand applies horizontal traction.
**Phalen's m.**, (for detection of carpal tunnel syndrome), the size of the carpal tunnel is reduced by holding the affected hand with the wrist fully flexed or extended for 30 to 60 seconds, or by placing a sphygmomanometer cuff on the involved arm and inflating to a point between diastolic and systolic pressure for 30 to 60 seconds.
**Pinard's m.**, a method of bringing down the foot in breech extraction.
**Prague m.**, a method in breech presentation of delivering the head when the fetal back is posterior, by bringing down the breech and making traction on the head with the finger, which is hooked over the nape of the neck.
**Ritgen m.**, delivery of the fetal head by extending it upward and forward through the vulva, between contractions, by pressing with the tips of the fingers upon the perineum behind the anus.
**Scanzoni m.**, a method of forceps rotation of the fetal head when it is in the posterior position of the occiput.
**Schreiber's m.**, rubbing of the inner side of the upper part of the thigh while testing for patellar reflex.
**Sellick m.**, the application of pressure to the cricoid cartilage in order to compress the esophagus and prevent passive regurgitation during endotracheal intubation.
**Toynbee m.**, pinching the nostrils and swallowing; if the auditory tube is patent, the tympanic membrane will retract medially. See also *Toynbee's test,* under *test.* Called also *Toynbee's experiment.*
**Valsalva's m.**, 1. forcible exhalation effort against a closed glottis; the resultant increase in intrathoracic pressure interferes with venous return to the heart. Called also *Valsalva's experiment.* 2. forcible exhalation effort against occluded nostrils and a closed mouth causes increased pressure in the eustachian tube and middle ear, so that the tympanic membrane moves outward. Formerly used as a test of patency of the auditory tube. Called also *Valsalva's method* or *test.*
**Wigand's m.**, see under *version.*

**man·ga·nese** (mang′gə-nēs) [L. *manganum, manganesium*] [MeSH: Manganese] a metal resembling iron; symbol, Mn; atomic number, 25; atomic weight, 54.938; specific gravity, 7.2. It occurs normally throughout the body, concentrated in the mitochondria, chiefly in the pituitary, liver, pancreas, kidney, and bone; it is necessary for the synthesis of mucopolysaccharides and activates a number of enzymes. Clinical deficiency is unknown in humans but may occur in other animals and causes perosis in poultry. Excessive inhalation of manganese dust can cause toxicity; see under *poisoning* and *pneumonitis.*
**m. chloride** [USP], the tetrahydrated chloride salt of manganese, $MnCl_2 \cdot 4H_2O$, used as a nutritional supplement; administered orally and intravenously as a component of total parenteral nutrition solutions.
**m. gluconate** [USP], the gluconate salt of manganese, having the same indications and uses as the chloride salt.
**m. sulfate** [USP], the tetrahydrated sulfate salt of manganese, $MnSO_4 \cdot 4H_2O$, used as a nutritional supplement; administered orally and intravenously as a component of total parenteral nutrition solutions. In veterinary medicine, administered to poultry as a source of manganese to prevent perosis.

**man·gan·ic** (mang-gan′ik) pertaining to manganese as a trivalent element.

**man·ga·nism** (mang′gə-niz-əm) manganese poisoning; see under *poisoning.*

**man·ga·nous** (mang′gə-nəs) pertaining to manganese as a divalent element.

**mange** (mānj) any of several contagious forms of dermatitis caused by the mange mites (q.v.) and affecting many different species of mammals and birds. Although the distribution, manner of spread, and clinical presentation vary with the host and parasite species, mange is typically characterized by cutaneous burrows produced by the mites; scratching associated with deeper lesions, producing crusts and scabs; alopecia; and epidermal hyperplasia with desquamation. Bacterial infection may occur.
**chorioptic m.**, mange caused by infestation with species of *Chorioptes;* it usually occurs on the posterior body of cattle or horses, from the udder and perineum to the hind legs. Called also *chorioptic acariasis* or *itch.*
**demodectic m.**, mange caused by infestation with species of *Demodex,* characterized by folliculitis with pustule formation, usually

on the head, neck, or shoulders; it is common in dogs and cattle and occurs sporadically in other species. Called also *demodectic acariasis, demodicosis,* and *follicular m.*
**follicular m.,** demodectic m.
**notoedric m.,** infestation of the ears, head, or neck of a cat by a species of *Notoedres;* it is intensely irritating and serious cases can be fatal.
**otodectic m.,** mange in the ear region from infestation by species of *Otodectes;* see also *otoacariasis.*
**psoroptic m.,** infestation by species of *Psoroptes. P. cuniculi* infests the ears of rabbits and goats, sometimes causing secondary infections of the inner ear or central nervous system. *P. ovis* causes sheep scab, the most common type of mange in sheep, as well as scabies in cattle and horses. *P. equi* infests sheltered areas on horses, such as those covered by hair.
**red m.,** demodectic mange in canines.
**sarcoptic m.,** scabies in animals other than humans.

**ma·nia** (ma'ne-ə) [Gr. "madness"] a phase of bipolar disorder characterized by expansiveness, elation, agitation, hyperexcitability, hyperactivity, and increased speed of thought and speech (flight of ideas); called also *manic syndrome.*
**delirious m.,** hypermania.
**unproductive m.,** a manic episode with some signs and symptoms of depression, such as repression of thought and speech.

**-mania** a word termination denoting excessive preoccupation with something, as in *dipsomania, erotomania, pyromania,* etc.

**ma·ni·ac** (ma'ne-ak) [L. *maniacus*] one who is affected with mania.

**ma·ni·a·cal** (mə-ni'ə-kəl) affected with mania.

**man·ic** (man'ik) pertaining to or affected with mania.

**man·ic-de·pres·sive** (man'ik-de-pres'iv) alternating between attacks of mania and depression, as in bipolar disorder.

**man·i·fold** (man'ĭ-fold) a tube fitting with several outlets on its sides for connecting to other tubes.

**Man·i·hot** (man'e-hot) [Tupi *manioca*] a genus of herbs and shrubs originally native to tropical regions of the Americas but now also grown in many other tropical regions. *M. esculen'ta* Crantz (Euphorbiaceae) is cassava (q.v.), an important food plant whose root causes cyanide poisoning to humans or livestock if eaten raw.

**man·i·kin** (man'ĭ-kin) [MeSH: Manikins] a model of the body, usually with movable or removable members and parts; uses include illustrating anatomy; teaching nursing and obstetrics; teaching certain surgical procedures, such as the removal of foreign bodies by bronchoscopy; and teaching cardiopulmonary resuscitation.

**ma·nil·o·quism** (mə-nil'o-kwiz-əm) [L. *manus* hand + *loqui* speak] dactylology.

**man·i·oc** (man'e-ok) [Fr., from Tupi *manioca*] cassava.

**Manip.** abbreviation for L. *mani'pulus,* a handful.

**man·i·pha·lanx** (man"ĭ-fa'lənks) [*manus* + *phalanx*] a phalanx of the hand.

**ma·nip·u·la·tion** (mə-nip"u-la'shən) [L. *manipulare* to handle] 1. skillful or dextrous treatment, as by the hand. 2. in physical therapy, the forceful passive movement of a joint beyond its active limit of motion.
**conjoined m.,** an obstetric maneuver done with both hands.
**endocrine m.,** see under *therapy.*
**hormonal m.,** endocrine therapy.

**Mann's sign** (manz) [John Dixon *Mann,* English physician, 1840–1912] see under *sign.*

**Mann-Boll·man fistula** (man-bol'mən) [Frank Charles *Mann,* American physiologist and surgeon, 1887–1962; Jesse Louis *Bollman,* American physiologist, 20th century] see under *fistula.*

**Mann-Whit·ney test** (man-hwit'ne) [Henry Berthold *Mann,* American mathematician, born 1905; Donald Ransom *Whitney,* American statistician, born 1915] rank sum test; see under *test.*

**Mann-Wil·liam·son ulcer** (man-wil'yəm-son) [Frank C. *Mann;* Carl S. *Williamson,* American surgeon, 1896–1952] see under *ulcer.*

**man·na** (man'ə) [L.] the dried saccharine exudation from the flowering ash tree, *Fraxinus ornus;* its chief constituents are mannitol, mucilage, and sugar, and it has been used as a laxative.

**man·nan** (man'an) any polymer consisting solely or mostly of mannose residues, occurring in a variety of plants and as a cell wall constituent of some fungi.

**man·ner** (man'ər) a way of acting or doing; method.
**m. of death,** the circumstances under which a death occurs, e.g., suicide or accident; cf. *cause of death,* under *cause.*

**man·ner·ism** (man'ər-iz-əm) a stereotyped movement or habit peculiar to a given individual.

**man·nite** (man'īt) mannitol.

**man·ni·tol** (man'ĭ-tol) [USP] [MeSH: Mannitol] a 6-carbon sugar alcohol formed by reduction of mannose or fructose and widely distributed in plants and fungi. Official preparations, administered intravenously, are used as an osmotic diuretic in the prophylaxis of acute renal failure, in the evaluation of acute oliguria, and for reducing intraocular and cerebrospinal fluid pressure and volume.
**m. hexanitrate,** a compound formed by the nitration of mannitol; used as a vasodilator, mainly in urinary insufficiency.

**Mann·kopf's sign** (mahn'kopfs) [Emil Wilhelm *Mannkopf,* German physician, 1836–1918] see under *sign.*

**man·no·py·ra·nose** (man"o-pir'ə-nōs) mannose occurring in the cyclic pyranose configuration.

**man·no·sa·mine** (mə-no'sə-mēn) the amino sugar derivative of mannose at the 2 carbon; it is a component of neuraminic acid.

**man·no·san** (man'o-sən) mannan.

**man·no·sa·zone** (mə-no'sə-zōn) the osazone formed from mannose by reaction with phenylhydrazine; it is identical to glucosazone.

**man·nose** (man'ōs) [MeSH: Mannose] an aldohexose epimeric with glucose at the 2 carbon; it occurs in oligosaccharides of many glycoproteins and glycolipids.
**m. 6-phosphate,** mannose phosphorylated at the 6 carbon; it is added to lysosomal enzymes during their biosynthesis and, via specific receptors, it serves as a recognition marker to target the enzymes to the lysosomes.

**man·nose-1-phos·phate gua·nyl·yl·trans·fer·ase (GDP)** (man'ōs fos'fāt gwah"nəl-əl-trans'fər-ās) [EC 2.7.7.22] an enzyme of the transferase class that catalyzes the synthesis of GDPmannose from GDP and mannose 1-phosphate.

**man·nose-6-phos·phate isom·er·ase** (man'ōs fos'fāt i-som'ər-ās) [EC 5.3.1.8] an enzyme of the isomerase class that catalyzes the interconversion between mannose 6-phosphate and fructose 6-phosphate, a step in the utilization of mannose. Called also *phosphomannose isomerase.*

**α-man·no·si·dase** (man'o-sĭ-dās) [EC 3.2.1.24] an enzyme of the hydrolase class that catalyzes the hydrolysis of terminal, nonreducing, α-linked mannose residues from mannosides, a step in the metabolism of *N*-linked oligosaccharides in glycoproteins. Deficiency of the lysosomal form of the enzyme, an autosomal recessive trait, results in mannosidosis.

**β-man·no·si·dase** (mə-nōs'ĭ-dās) [EC 3.2.1.25] an enzyme of the hydrolase class that catalyzes the cleavage of terminal, nonreducing, β-linked mannose residues from mannosides, a step in the metabolism of *N*-linked oligosaccharides of glycoproteins.

**man·no·side** (man'o-sīd) a glycoside of mannose.

**man·no·si·do·sis** (man"o-sĭ-do'sis) [MeSH: Mannosidosis] a lysosomal storage disease due to defective α-mannosidase with resultant oligosaccharide accumulation. Characteristics include coarse facies, upper respiratory congestion and infections, profound mental retardation, hepatosplenomegaly, cataracts, radiographic signs of dysostosis multiplex, and gibbus deformity. Mannosidosis is divided into type I (infantile onset) and type II (juvenile-adult onset).

**ma·nom·e·ter** (mə-nom'ə-tər) [Gr. *manos* thin + *-meter*] an instrument for measuring the pressure or tension of liquids or gases, as of the blood.
**aneroid m.,** a true total-pressure measuring device, which measures pressure by means of an elastic container as compared to that of a vacuum.
**mercury m.,** one that uses changes of height of a column of mercury to measure pressure.
**water m.,** one that uses changes of height of a column of water to measure pressure.

**mano·met·ric** (man"o-met'rik) 1. pertaining to or ascertained by the manometer. 2. varying with the pressure.

**ma·nom·e·try** (mə-nom'ə-tre) [MeSH: Manometry] the measurement of pressure by means of a manometer.
**anal m.,** the measurement of the pressure generated by the anal sphincter; used in the evaluation of fecal incontinence.

**man·op·to·scope** (mə-nop'to-skōp) [*manus* + *opto-* + *-scope*] an apparatus for detecting ocular dominance.

**Man. pr.** abbreviation for L. *ma'ne pri'mo,* early in the morning.

**man·quea** (mahn-ka'ah) [Sp.] actinobacillosis of young cattle in South America, marked by formation of abscesses on the legs.

**man·sa** (man'sə) [Sp.] the root or rhizome of *Anemonopsis californica,* used as a folk remedy in the southwestern United States and northern Mexico to relieve colds and indigestion, and to purify the blood.

**Man·sil** (man'sil) trademark for preparations of oxamniquine.

**Man·son's hemoptysis, schistosomiasis (disease)**

(man'sənz) [Sir Patrick *Manson,* British physician, 1844–1922] see *parasitic hemoptysis,* under *hemoptysis,* and see *schistosomiasis.*

**Man·son·el·la** (man″sən-el'ə) [MeSH: Mansonella] a genus of nematodes of the superfamily *Filarioidea,* characterized by a rounded, enlarged anterior end and a smooth cuticle, found in Central and South America and Africa.
**M. ozzar'di,** a filarial nematode parasite of Central and South America and the Caribbean, the cause of mansonellosis in man; transmitted by *Culicoides furens* and *Simulium amazonicum.*
**M. per'stans,** a species up to 8 cm long that infects humans in the tropical regions of Central and South America and Africa, transmitted by bites of the small flies of the genus *Culicoides.* The adults inhabit the pleural and peritoneal tissues, while the larval forms (microfilariae) are found in the peripheral blood. Although considered to be nonpathogenic, they have been implicated as the cause of such symptoms as eosinophilia, abdominal and pectoral pain, enlargement of the spleen and liver, and fever followed by urticaria and edema of the lower limbs and scrotum. Called also *Acanthocheilonema perstans, Dipetalonema perstans,* and *Filaria perstans.*
**M. streptocer'ca,** a species found in man and chimpanzees in western and central Africa, transmitted by the bite of small flies of the genus *Culicoides.* The microfilariae, which may be found in scarification smears, are sometimes confused with those of *Onchocerca volvulus.* It produces a pruritic rash resembling that of onchocerciasis. Called also *Acanthocheilonema streptocerca* and *Dipetalonema streptocerca.*

**man·so·nel·li·a·sis** (man″so-nəl-i'ə-sis) [MeSH: Mansonelliasis] mansonellosis.

**man·so·nel·lo·sis** (man″so-nəl-o'sis) infection with organisms of the genus *Mansonella;* an ill-defined syndrome of headache, coldness of the legs, pruritus, and articular swelling.

**Man·so·nia** (mən-so'ne-ə) a genus of mosquitoes of the tribe Mansoniini, subfamily Culicinae, several species of which transmit *Brugia malayi.* Some species may also transmit viruses such as those causing equine encephalomyelitis.

**Man·so·ni·i·ni** (man″sə-ne-i'ni) a tribe of mosquitoes of the subfamily Culicinae, including the genera *Coquillettidia* and *Mansonia.*

**Man·so·ni·oi·des** (man″so-ne-oi'dēz) a subgenus of mosquitoes of the genus *Mansonia. M. annuli'fera* is the chief vector of *Wuchereria malayi* in India.

**man·tle** (man'təl) [L. *mantellum* cloak] 1. an enveloping cover or layer. 2. cortex cerebri.
**brain m.,** cortex cerebri.
**chordomesodermal m.,** a continuous epithelial sheet composed of notochordal and mesodermal material during gastrulation.
**myoepicardial m.,** a layer of visceral mesoderm in the early embryo, surrounding the endocardial tube and developing into the myocardium and epicardium.

**Man·toux test (reaction)** (mahn-too') [Charles *Mantoux,* French physician, 1877–1947] see under *test.*

**man·u·al** (man'u-əl) [L. *manualis; manus* hand] of or pertaining to the hand; performed by the hand or hands.

**ma·nu·bria** (mə-noo'bre-ə) [L.] plural of *manubrium.*

**ma·nu·bri·um** (mə-noo'bre-əm) pl. *manu'bria* [L.] [TA] [MeSH: Manubrium] a general term for a handlelike structure or part; often used alone to designate the manubrium sterni.
**m. mal'lei** [TA], **m. of malleus,** the largest process of the malleus; it is attached to the middle layer of the tympanic membrane and has the tendon of the tensor tympani muscle attached to it.
**m. ster'ni** [TA], **m. of sternum,** the cranial portion of the sternum, which articulates with the clavicles and the first two pairs of ribs; called also *presternum.*

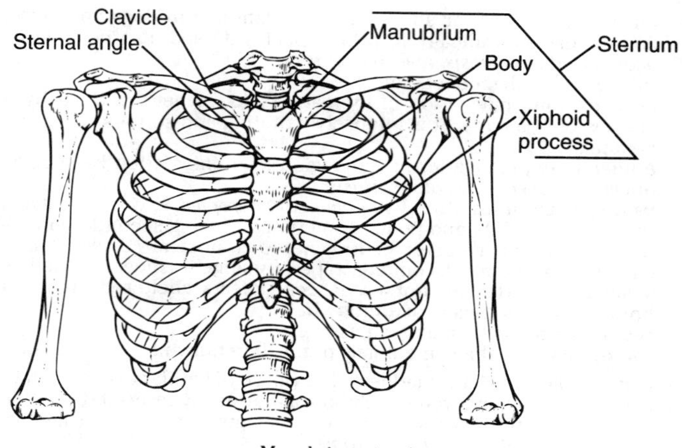

Manubrium sterni.

**manu·dy·na·mom·e·ter** (man″u-di″nə-mom'ə-tər) [*manus* + *dynamo-* + *-meter*] an apparatus for measuring the force of the thrust of an instrument.

**ma·nus** (ma'nəs) pl. *ma'nus* [L.] [TA] hand: the distal region of the upper limb, including the carpus, metacarpus, and digits.
**m. ca'va,** a hand deformed by a deep hollowing of the palm.
**m. exten'sa,** backward deviation of the hand.
**m. flex'a,** forward deviation of the hand.
**m. pla'na,** flattening of the arch formed normally by the proximal row of the carpal bones; flat hand.
**m. superexten'sa,** m. extensa.
**m. val'ga,** see *radial clubhand* and *ulnar clubhand,* under *clubhand.*
**m. va'ra,** see *radial clubhand* and *ulnar clubhand,* under *clubhand.*

**many·plies** (men'ĭ-plīz″) omasum.

**man·za·ni·ta** (man″zə-ne'ta) [Sp., dim. of *manzana* apple] *Arctostaphylos manzanita.*

**MAO** monoamine oxidase. See *amine oxidase (flavin-containing).*

**MAOI** monoamine oxidase inhibitor.

**Ma·o·late** (ma'o-lāt) trademark for a preparation of chlorphenesin carbamate.

**MAP** mean arterial pressure.

**map** (map) a two-dimensional graphic representation of arrangement in space.
**conjugation m.,** a gene map used in bacterial genetics, giving the distances between loci based on the time in minutes required to transfer DNA between loci in conjugation.
**contig m.,** a type of physical map composed of overlapping smaller DNA fragments whose order is determined by matching landmarks on the smaller fragments.
**cytogenetic m., cytologic m.,** a gene map giving the position of gene loci relative to chromosome bands.
**fate m.,** a plan of a blastula or early gastrula stage of an embryo showing areas of prospective significance in normal development.
**gene m.,** a map showing the positions of genetic loci on the chromosomes and usually giving some indication of the distance between loci.
**genetic m.,** a gene map giving the relative locations of genetic markers, based on recombination frequencies; the unit of measurement is the centimorgan. Called also *linkage m.*
**linkage m.,** genetic m.
**physical m.,** a gene map showing the locations of genetic markers

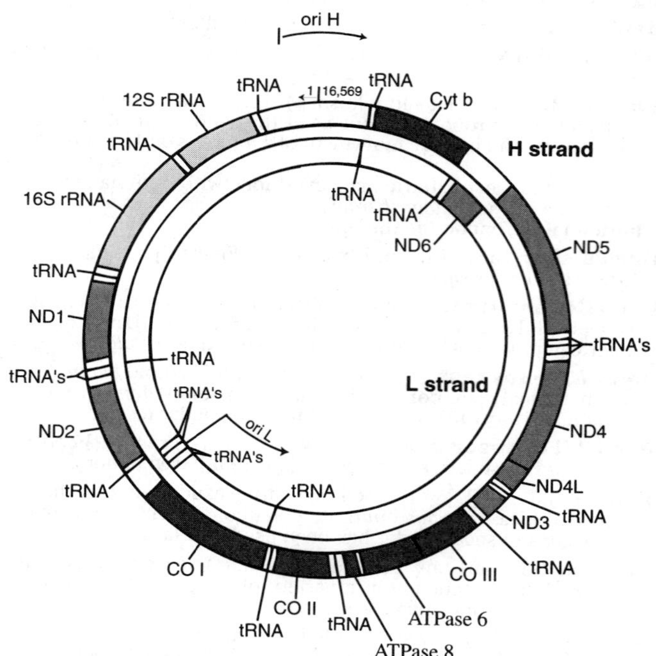

Gene map of human mitochondrial DNA, showing the genes transcribed from the heavy (H) and light (L) strands, transcription proceeding counterclockwise on H and clockwise on L. *Ori H, Ori L,* origins of replication; *ND1–6,* NADH dehydrogenase subunits; *Cyt b,* cytochrome b; *COI–III,* cytochrome oxidase subunits; *tRNA,* transfer RNA; *rRNA,* ribosomal RNA.

along with the physical distances between them, measured in kilobase pairs or megabase pairs.
**restriction m.**, a physical map indicating restriction enzyme cleavage sites.
**STS (sequence-tagged site) m.**, a physical map indicating the relative order of and distance between sequence-tagged sites (q.v.) within a DNA region.
**transduction m.**, a gene map used in bacterial genetics, giving distances between loci based on relative cotransduction frequencies.

**ma·ple** (ma'pəl) any plant of the genus *Acer.*

**map·ping** (map'ing) 1. the creation on a flat surface of a representation of an area, showing the relative positions of various features. 2. locating the relative position of genes on chromosomes. Called also *gene map*
**body surface m.**, creation of maps that use contour lines to delineate the isopotential areas of the body surface as determined by electrocardiography, with the potential distributions updated continually during the recording period.
**cardiac m.**, an electrophysiological procedure in which electrical potentials recorded by electrodes placed directly on the heart are processed to give a two-dimensional display of the origin and path of an electrical impulse as it depolarizes the heart.

**ma·pro·ti·line** (mə-pro'tĭ-lēn) [MeSH: Maprotiline] a tetracyclic antidepressant having pharmacological effects similar to those of the tricyclic antidepressants.
**m. hydrochloride** [USP], the hydrochloride salt of maprotiline, administered orally in the treatment of major depressive disorder; dysthymic disorder; the depressed phase of bipolar disorder; and anxiety associated with depression. It is also used to treat some types of chronic pain.

**ma·ran·tic** (mə-ran'tik) [Gr. *marantikos* wasting away] marasmic.

**mar·as·mat·ic** (mar″az-mat'ik) marasmic.

**ma·ras·mic** (mə-raz'mik) pertaining to or characterized by marasmus.

**ma·ras·moid** (mə-raz'moid) resembling marasmus.

**ma·ras·mus** (mə-raz'məs) [Gr. *marasmos* a dying away] a form of protein-energy malnutrition predominantly due to prolonged severe caloric deficit, chiefly occurring during the first year of life, characterized by growth retardation and progressive wasting of subcutaneous fat and muscle, but usually with retention of the appetite and mental alertness. Infectious diseases may be precipitating factors. Called also *infantile atrophy, athrepsia,* and *pedatrophia.* Cf. *kwashiorkor.*
**enzootic m.**, a condition of malnutrition in herbivorous animals due to a deficiency of one or more trace elements, especially cobalt or copper. It is marked by progressive emaciation, severe anemia, and finally prostration. See also *bush sickness* and *salt sickness,* under *sickness,* and *pining.*
**nutritional m.**, marasmic kwashiorkor.

**mar·ble·iza·tion** (mahr″bəl-ĭ-za'shən) the state of being veined like marble.

**Mar·burg disease (hemorrhagic fever), virus** (mahr'boork) [*Marburg,* Germany, where the disease was first recognized in 1967] see under *disease* and *virus.*

**marc** (mahrk) [Fr.] the residue left after maceration of substances used in the preparation of various drugs.

**Mar·caine** (mahr-kān') trademark for a preparation of bupivacaine hydrochloride.

**march** (mahrch) the progression of electrical activity through the motor cortex.
**cortical m., epileptic m.**, jacksonian m.
**jacksonian m.**, the spread of abnormal electrical activity from one area of the cerebral cortex to adjacent areas, characteristic of jacksonian epilepsy. Called also *cortical m.* and *epileptic m.*

**Mar·chand's adrenals (organs)** (mahr'shahndz) [Felix Jacob *Marchand,* German pathologist, 1846–1928] see under *adrenal,* and see *adventitial cell,* under *cell.*

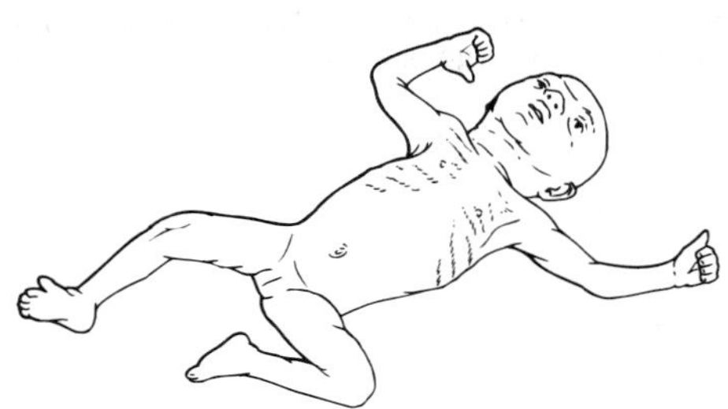

Marasmus.

**marche** (marsh) [Fr.] gait.
**m. à petits pas** (ah-pəte' pah') ["gait with little steps"], an abnormal gait in which the patient takes very short steps: seen in some forms of parkinsonism and cerebral arteriosclerosis.

**Mar·che·sa·ni's syndrome** (mahr″kə-sah'nēz) [Oswald *Marchesani,* German ophthalmologist, 1900–1952] Weill-Marchesani syndrome.

**Mar·chi's balls,** etc. (mahr'kēz) [Vittorio *Marchi,* Italian physician, 1851–1908] see under *ball, globule,reaction,* and *stain,* and see *tractus tectospinalis.*

**Mar·chi·a·fa·va-Bi·gna·mi disease** (mahr″ke-ə-fah'vah-bēn-yah'me) [Ettore *Marchiafava,* Italian pathologist, 1847–1935; Amico *Bignami,* Italian pathologist, 1862–1929] see under *disease.*

**Mar·chi·a·fa·va-Mi·che·li disease (syndrome)** (mahr″ke-ə-fah'vah-me-ka'le) [Ettore *Marchiafava;* Ferdinando *Micheli,* Italian physician, 1847–1935] paroxysmal nocturnal hemoglobinuria.

**Mar·cus Gunn** (mahr'kəs gun) see *Gunn.*

**Ma·rek's disease** (mah'reks) [Josef *Marek,* Hungarian veterinarian, 1867–1952] [MeSH: Marek's Disease] see under *disease.*

**ma·ren·nin** (mə-ren'in) [*Marennes,* France, where the oysters are found] a green pigment found in certain oysters, derived from the chlorophyll of a microorganism infesting them.

**Ma·rey's law** (mah-rāz') [Etienne Jules *Marey,* French physiologist, 1830–1904] see under *law.*

**Mar·e·zine** (mar'ə-zēn) trademark for a preparation of cyclizine hydrochloride.

**Mar·fan's sign, syndrome** (mahr-fahnz') [Antonin Bernard Jean *Marfan,* French pediatrician, 1858–1942] see under *sign* and *syndrome.*

**mar·fan·oid** (mahr'fən-oid) having the characteristic symptoms of Marfan's syndrome.

**mar·gar·i·to·ma** (mahr″gər-ĭ-to'mə) cholesteatoma.

**Mar·gar·o·pus** (mahr-gahr'ə-pəs) a genus of ticks of the family Ixodidae.
**M. annula'tus,** *Boophilus annulatus.*
**M. winthe'mi,** the beady-legged winter horse tick, a species found on horses and other large herbivores in South Africa.

**mar·gin** (mahr'jin) a boundary or edge, such as the boundary of an organ or tumor. Called also *border* and *margo* [TA].
**m. of acetabulum,** limbus acetabuli.
**alveolar m. of mandible,** arcus alveolaris mandibulae.
**alveolar m. of maxilla,** arcus alveolaris maxillae.
**anterior m. of fibula,** margo anterior fibulae.
**anterior m. of lung,** margo anterior pulmonis.
**anterior m. of parietal bone,** margo frontalis ossis parietalis.
**anterior m. of radius,** margo anterior radii.
**anterior m. of scapula,** margo lateralis scapulae.
**anterior m. of spleen,** margo superior splenis.
**anterior m. of testis,** margo anterior testis.
**anterior m. of tibia,** margo anterior tibiae.
**anterior m. of ulna,** margo anterior ulnae.
**arcuate m. of saphenous hiatus,** margo falciformis hiatus sapheni.
**axillary m. of scapula,** margo lateralis scapulae.
**cartilaginous m. of acetabulum,** labrum acetabulare.
**ciliary m. of iris,** margo ciliaris iridis.
**convex m. of testis,** margo anterior testis.
**coronal m. of frontal bone,** margo parietalis ossis frontalis.
**coronal m. of parietal bone,** margo frontalis ossis parietalis.
**crenate m. of spleen, cristate m. of spleen,** margo superior splenis.
**dentate m.,** linea anocutanea.
**dorsal m. of radius,** margo posterior radii.
**dorsal m. of ulna,** margo posterior ulnae.
**m. of exposure,** a term proposed to replace the term *m. of safety.*
**external m. of scapula,** margo lateralis scapulae.
**external m. of testis,** margo anterior testis.
**falciform m. of fascia lata, falciform m. of saphenus hiatus,** margo falciformis hiatus saphenus.
**falciform m. of white line of pelvic fascia,** arcus tendineus fasciae pelvis.
**fibular m. of foot,** margo lateralis pedis.
**free m. of eyelid,** the conjunctival-lined portion of each eyelid, about 1 mm broad, overlying the eyeball; the anterior border of each bears the eyelashes, and the posterior border is closely applied to the eyeball.
**free gingival m., free gum m.,** margo gingivalis.
**free m. of nail,** margo liber unguis.
**free m. of ovary,** margo liber ovarii.
**frontal m. of parietal bone,** margo frontalis ossis parietalis.
**gingival m., gum m.,** margo gingivalis.

**hidden m. of nail,** margo occultus unguis.
**m. of heart, acute,** margo dexter cordis.
**m. of heart, left,** the rounded margin separating the sternocostal and left surfaces of the heart, formed mainly by the left ventricle but also including a small part of the left atrium and extending obliquely from the left atrium to the apex of the heart in a curve that is convex to the left. Called also *obtuse m. of heart.*
**m. of heart, obtuse,** left m. of heart.
**m. of heart, right,** margo dexter cordis.
**incisal m.,** margo incisalis.
**inferior m. of lung,** margo inferior pulmonis.
**inferior m. of spleen,** margo inferior splenis.
**inferior m. of suprarenal gland,** facies renalis glandulae suprarenalis.
**inferolateral m. of cerebral hemisphere,** margo inferolateralis hemispherii cerebri.
**inferomedial m. of cerebral hemisphere,** margo inferomedialis hemispherii cerebri.
**infraorbital m. of body of maxilla,** margo infraorbitalis corporis maxillae.
**infraorbital m. of orbit,** margo infraorbitalis orbitae.
**internal m. of testis,** margo posterior testis.
**interosseous m. of fibula,** margo interosseus fibulae.
**interosseous m. of radius,** margo interosseus radii.
**interosseous m. of tibia,** margo interosseus tibiae.
**interosseous m. of ulna,** margo interosseus ulnae.
**lacrimal m. of maxilla,** margo lacrimalis maxillae.
**lambdoid m. of occipital bone,** margo lambdoideus ossis occipitalis.
**lambdoid m. of parietal bone,** margo occipitalis ossis parietalis.
**lateral m. of foot,** margo lateralis pedis.
**lateral m. of humerus,** margo lateralis humeri.
**lateral m. of kidney,** margo lateralis renis.
**lateral m. of nail,** margo lateralis unguis.
**lateral m. of orbit,** margo lateralis orbitae.
**lateral m. of scapula,** margo lateralis scapulae.
**lateral m. of tongue,** margo linguae.
**lateral m. of uterus,** margo uteri.
**malar m. of greater wing,** margo zygomaticus alae majoris.
**mammillary m.,** margo mastoideus ossis occipitalis.
**mastoid m. of occipital bone,** margo mastoideus ossis occipitalis.
**mastoid m. of parietal bone,** angulus mastoideus ossis parietalis.
**medial m. of adrenal gland,** margo medialis glandulae suprarenalis.
**medial m. of foot,** margo medialis pedis.
**medial m. of humerus,** margo medialis humeri.
**medial m. of kidney,** margo medialis renis.
**medial m. of orbit,** margo medialis orbitae.
**medial m. of scapula,** margo medialis scapulae.
**medial m. of suprarenal gland,** margo medialis glandulae suprarenalis.
**medial m. of tibia,** margo medialis tibiae.
**mesovarial m. of ovary,** margo mesovaricus ovarii.
**nasal m. of frontal bone,** margo nasalis ossis frontalis.
**obtuse m. of spleen,** margo inferior splenis.
**occipital m. of parietal bone,** margo occipitalis ossis parietalis.
**occipital m. of temporal bone,** margo occipitalis ossis temporalis.

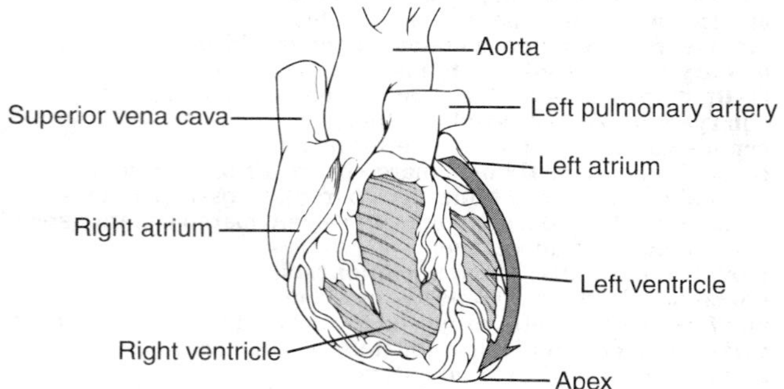


Left margin of heart. Anterior view of the heart, the arrow delineating the left margin.

**orbital m.,** margo orbitalis.
**palpebral m's, anterior,** limbi palpebrales anteriores.
**palpebral m's, posterior,** limbi palpebrales posteriores.
**parietal m. of frontal bone,** margo parietalis ossis frontalis.
**parietal m. of greater wing of sphenoid bone,** margo parietalis alae majoris.
**parietal m. of occipital bone,** margo lambdoideus ossis occipitalis.
**parietal m. of parietal bone,** margo sagittalis ossis parietalis.
**parietal m. of squamous part of temporal bone,** margo parietalis partis squamosae ossis temporalis.
**parietofrontal m. of greater wing of sphenoid bone,** margo frontalis alae majoris.
**peroneal m. of foot,** margo lateralis pedis.
**posterior m. of fibula,** margo posterior fibulae.
**posterior m. of petrous part of temporal bone,** margo posterior partis petrosae ossis temporalis.
**posterior m. of radius,** margo posterior radii.
**posterior m. of spleen,** margo inferior splenis.
**posterior m. of testis,** margo posterior testis.
**posterior m. of ulna,** margo posterior ulnae.
**pupillary m. of iris,** margo pupillaris iridis.
**radial m. of forearm,** margo radialis antebrachii.
**right/left m. of uterus,** margo uteri dexter/sinister.
**sagittal m. of parietal bone,** margo sagittalis ossis parietalis.
**m. of safety,** a calculation that takes the highest animal no observed adverse effect level (q.v.) and estimates a maximum safe level of exposure for humans. It is now generally superseded by the reference dose.
**sphenoidal m. of parietal bone,** angulus sphenoidalis ossis parietalis.
**sphenoidal m. of squamous part of temporal bone,** margo sphenoidalis partis squamosae ossis temporalis.
**sphenotemporal m. of parietal bone,** margo squamosus ossis parietalis.
**squamous m. of greater wing of sphenoid bone,** margo squamosus alae majoris.
**squamous m. of parietal bone,** margo squamosus ossis parietalis.
**straight m. of testis,** margo posterior testis.
**superior m. of adrenal gland,** margo superior glandulae suprarenalis.
**superior m. of cerebral hemisphere,** margo superior hemispherii cerebri.
**superior m. of pancreas,** margo superior corporis pancreatis.
**superior m. of parietal bone,** margo sagittalis ossis parietalis.
**superior m. of petrous part of temporal bone,** margo superior partis petrosae ossis temporalis.
**superior m. of scapula,** margo superior scapulae.
**superior m. of spleen,** margo superior splenis.
**superior m. of suprarenal gland,** margo superior glandulae suprarenalis.
**superomedial m. of cerebral hemisphere,** margo superior hemispherii cerebri.
**supraorbital m. of frontal bone,** margo supraorbitalis ossis frontalis.
**supraorbital m. of orbit,** margo supraorbitalis orbitae.
**temporal m. of parietal bone,** margo squamosus ossis parietalis.
**tibial m. of foot,** margo medialis pedis.
**m. of tongue,** margo linguae.
**ulnar m. of forearm,** margo ulnaris antebrachii.
**vertebral m. of scapula,** margo medialis scapulae.
**volar m. of radius,** margo anterior radii.
**volar m. of ulna,** margo anterior ulnae.
**zygomatic m. of greater wing of sphenoid bone,** margo zygomaticus alae majoris.

**mar·gi·nal** (mahr′jĭ-nəl) [L. *marginalis*] pertaining to a margin.

**mar·gi·na·tion** (mahr″jĭ-na′shən) accumulation and adhesion of leukocytes to the epithelial cells of blood vessel walls at the site of injury in the early stages of inflammation.

**mar·gi·nes** (mahr′jĭ-nēs) [L.] plural of *margo.*

**mar·gino·plas·ty** (mahr-jin′ə-plas-te) [*margin* + *-plasty*] surgical restoration of a border, as of the eyelid.

**mar·go** (mahr′go) pl. *mar′gines* [L.] [TA] a border, edge, or margin; a general term for the edge of a structure. See also *labium* and *limbus.*

## Margo

Descriptions are given on TA terms, and include anglicized names of specific borders.

**m. acetabula'ris,** limbus acetabuli.

**m. aceta'buli,** TA alternative for *limbus acetabuli.*

**m. alveola'ris,** see *arcus alveolaris mandibulae* and *arcus alveolaris maxillae.*

**m. ante'rior cor'poris pancre'atis** [TA], anterior border of body of pancreas: the pancreatic border that bounds the anterosuperior and anteroinferior surfaces.

**m. ante'rior fi'bulae** [TA], anterior margin of fibula: the anterolateral border of the body of the fibula; called also *crista anterior fibulae* and *anterior crest of fibula.*

**m. ante'rior he'patis,** m. inferior hepatis.

**m. ante'rior pulmo'nis** [TA], anterior margin of lung: the ventral border of either lung, which descends from behind the sternum, slightly lateral to the midline, and curves laterally to meet the inferior margin. Called also *anterior border of lung.*

**m. ante'rior ra'dii** [TA], anterior margin of radius: the edge of the radius that runs obliquely between the radial tuberosity and the styloid process; called also *m. volaris radii* and *volar margin of radius.*

**m. ante'rior sple'nis,** m. superior splenis.

**m. ante'rior tes'tis** [TA], anterior margin of testis: the rounded free border of the testis.

**m. ante'rior ti'biae** [TA], anterior margin of tibia: the prominent anteromedial margin of the body of the tibia, separating the medial and lateral surfaces; called also *crista anterior tibiae.*

**m. ante'rior ul'nae** [TA], anterior margin of ulna: the volar border of the ulna, separating the medial and posterior surfaces; called also *m. volaris ulnae* and *volar margin of ulna.*

**m. arcua'tus hia'tus saphe'ni,** TA alternative for *margo falciformis hiatus sapheni.*

**m. axilla'ris sca'pulae,** m. lateralis scapulae.

**m. cilia'ris i'ridis** [TA], ciliary margin of iris: the outer border of the iris, where it is continuous with the ciliary body.

**m. dex'ter cor'dis** [TA], right border of heart: the margin of the heart formed by the wall of the profile of the right atrium, running from the apex to the right, and marking the junction of the sternocostal and diaphragmatic cardiac surfaces; seen as a surface except in radiograms and two-dimensional illustrations. Called also *acute margin, inferior border,* or *right surface of heart.*

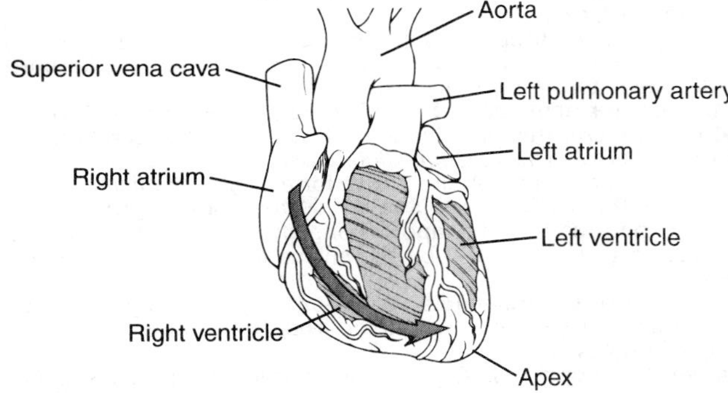


Margo dexter cordis (right margin of heart). Anterior view of the heart, the arrow delineating the right margin.

**m. dorsa'lis ra'dii,** m. posterior radii.

**m. dorsa'lis ul'nae,** m. posterior ulnae.

**m. falcifor'mis fas'ciae la'tae,** m. falciformis hiatus saphenus.

**m. falcifor'mis hia'tus saphe'ni** [TA], falciform margin of saphenous hiatus: the lateral margin of the saphenous hiatus; called also *m. arcuatus hiatus sapheni* [TA alternative] *arcuate margin of saphenous hiatus,* and *m. falciformis fasciae latae.*

**m. fibula'ris pe'dis,** TA alternative for *m. lateralis pedis.*

**m. fronta'lis a'lae mag'nae, m. fronta'lis a'lae majo'ris** [TA], frontal margin of greater wing of sphenoid bone: a roughened area on the greater wing where it articulates with the frontal bone; it is at the superolateral margin of the orbital surface of the greater wing at its junction with the cerebral and temporal surfaces.

**m. fronta'lis os'sis parieta'lis** [TA], frontal border of parietal bone: the edge of the parietal bone that articulates with the frontal bone along the coronal suture.

**m. gingiva'lis** [TA], gingival margin: the crest of the free gingiva that surrounds the teeth in a collarlike fashion, separated from the adjacent periodontium protectoris by the free gingival groove; it forms the wall of the gingival sulcus. Called also *free gum margin, gum margin,* and *marginal gingiva.*

**m. incisa'lis** [TA], incisal margin: the crest of the biting edge of an incisor tooth.

**m. infe'rior ce'rebri,** m. inferolateralis cerebri.

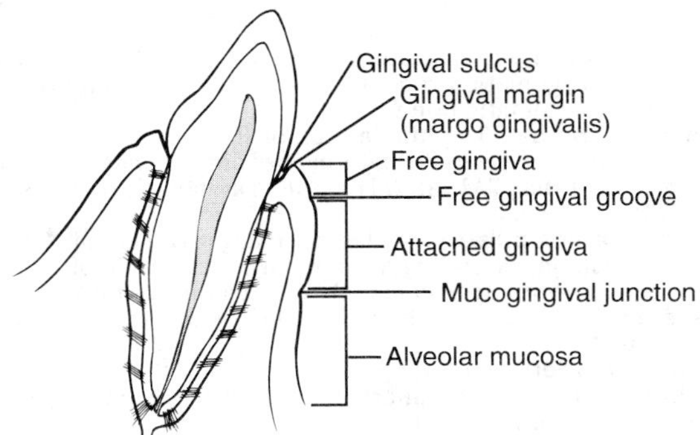


**m. infe'rior cor'poris pancre'atis,** inferior border of body of pancreas: the pancreatic border that bounds the anteroinferior and posterior surfaces; called also *m. posterior pancreatis.*

**m. infe'rior he'patis** [TA], inferior border of liver: the anteroinferior edge of the liver, separating the anterior and the visceral surface; called also *m. anterior hepatis.*

**m. infe'rior lie'nis,** TA alternative for *m. inferior splenis.*

**m. infe'rior pulmo'nis** [TA], inferior margin of lung: the border of the lung that extends in a curve behind the sixth costal cartilage, the upper margin of the eighth rib in the axillary line, the ninth or tenth rib in the scapular line, and passes medially to the eleventh costovertebral joint. Called also *inferior border of lung.*

**m. infe'rior sple'nis** [TA], inferior margin of spleen: a straight margin of the spleen somewhat less prominent than the superior margin, separating the renal surface from the diaphragmatic surface; called also *m. posterior splenis, m. inferior lienis* [TA alternative], and *obtuse* or *posterior margin of spleen.*

**m. inferolatera'lis hemisphe'rii ce'rebri** [TA], inferolateral margin of cerebral hemisphere: the inferior lateral border of the cerebral hemisphere.

**m. inferomedia'lis hemisphe'rii ce'rebri** [TA], inferomedial margin of cerebral hemisphere: the inferior medial margin of the cerebral hemisphere.

**m. infraglenoida'lis ti'biae,** the margin of bone that forms the circumference of the condyles of the tibia just inferior to the facies articularis superior.

**m. infraorbita'lis cor'poris maxil'lae** [TA], infraorbital margin of body of maxilla: the short rounded edge of the maxilla where the orbital surface becomes continuous with the anterior surface.

**m. infraorbita'lis or'bitae** [TA], infraorbital margin of orbit: the inferior edge of the entrance to the orbit, formed by the infraorbital process of the zygomatic bone and the infraorbital margin of the maxilla.

**m. interos'seus fi'bulae** [TA], interosseous margin of fibula: a prominent ridge medial to the anterior border of the fibula, connected with a similar ridge on the tibia by a strong, wide fibrous sheet, the interosseous membrane; called also *crista interossea fibulae* and *interosseous crest* or *ridge of fibula.*

**m. interos'seus ra'dii** [TA], interosseous margin of radius: the prominent medial border of the radius, connected with a similar ridge on the ulna by a strong, wide fibrous sheet, the interosseous membrane; called also *crista interossea radii* and *interosseous crest* or *ridge of radius.*

**m. interos'seus ti'biae** [TA], interosseous margin of tibia: the prominent lateral border of the body of the tibia, which separates the posterior and lateral surfaces and gives attachment to the interosseous membrane; called also *crista interossea tibiae* and *interosseous crest* or *ridge of tibia.*

**m. interos'seus ul'nae** [TA], interosseous margin of ulna: the prominent lateral border of the ulna, connected with a similar ridge on the radius by the interosseous membrane; called also *crista interossea ulnae* and *interosseous crest* or *ridge of ulna.*

**m. lacrima'lis maxil'lae** [TA], lacrimal margin of maxilla: the posterior border of the frontal process of the maxilla where it articulates with the lacrimal bone.

**m. lambdoi'deus os'sis occipita'lis** [TA], lambdoid margin of occipital bone: the edge of the occipital bone that extends from the lateral angle to the superior angle, articulating with the parietal bone to help form the lambdoid suture; called also *parietal margin of occipital bone.*

**m. latera'lis antebra'chii,** TA alternative for *m. radialis antebrachii.*

**mar'gines latera'les digito'rum pe'dis,** facies digitales laterales pedis.

**m. latera'lis hu'meri** [TA], lateral margin of humerus: the edge of the humerus that extends from posteroinferior part of the greater tubercle to the lateral epicondyle; called also *lateral angle of humerus*.

**m. latera'lis lin'guae,** m. linguae.

**m. latera'lis or'bitae** [TA], lateral margin of orbit: the orbital border formed by the zygomatic process of the frontal bone and the frontal process of the zygomatic bone.

**m. latera'lis pe'dis** [TA], the lateral, or fibular, border of the foot; called also *m. fibularis pedis* [TA alternative] and *peroneal border of foot.*

**m. latera'lis re'nis** [TA], lateral margin of kidney: the convex narrow border of the kidney.

**m. latera'lis sca'pulae** [TA], lateral margin of scapula: the thick edge of the scapula, extending from the inferior margin of the glenoid cavity to the inferior angle; called also *m. axillaris scapulae*.

**m. latera'lis un'guis** [TA], lateral margin of nail: the edge on either side of the nail.

**m. latera'lis u'teri,** m. uteri.

**m. li'ber ova'rii** [TA], free margin of ovary: the broad, convex border of the ovary, opposite the mesovarial margin.

**m. li'ber un'guis** [TA], free margin of nail: the distal overhanging edge of a nail.

**m. lin'guae** [TA], margin of tongue: the lateral border of the body of the tongue; called also *m. lateralis linguae*.

**m. mastoi'deus os'sis occipita'lis** [TA], mastoid margin of occipital bone: the edge of the occipital bone that extends from the jugular process to the lateral angle, articulating with the part of the temporal bone that bears the mastoid process.

**m. media'lis antebra'chii,** TA alternative for *m. ulnaris antebrachii.*

**m. media'lis ce'rebri,** m. inferomedialis cerebri.

**mar'gines media'les digito'rum pe'dis,** facies digitales mediales pedis.

**m. media'lis glan'dulae suprarena'lis** [TA], medial border of suprarenal gland: the border that with the superior border divides the anterior from the posterior surface.

**m. media'lis hu'meri** [TA], medial margin of humerus: the edge of the humerus that begins at the lesser tubercle above and continues downward to the medial epicondyle; called also *medial angle of humerus.*

**m. media'lis or'bitae** [TA], medial margin of orbit: the orbital border formed above by the bone and below by the lacrimal crest of the frontal process of the maxilla.

**m. media'lis pe'dis** [TA], the medial, or tibial, border of the foot; called also *m. tibialis pedis* [TA alternative].

**m. media'lis re'nis** [TA], medial margin of kidney: the concave border of the kidney, which contains the hilus.

**m. media'lis sca'pulae** [TA], medial margin of scapula: the thin edge of the scapula extending from the superior to the inferior angle; called also *m. vertebralis scapulae* and *vertebral margin of scapula.*

**m. media'lis ti'biae** [TA], medial margin of tibia: the border that extends between the medial condyle and medial malleolus of the tibia, separating the medial and posterior surfaces; called also *medial angle of tibia.*

**m. mesova'ricus ova'rii** [TA], mesovarial margin of ovary: the border of the ovary that is attached to the broad ligament by means of the mesovarium.

**m. nasa'lis os'sis fronta'lis** [TA], nasal margin of frontal bone: the articular surface, on each nasal part of the frontal bone, that articulates with the nasal bones and with the frontal processes of the maxilla.

**m. occipita'lis os'sis parieta'lis** [TA], occipital margin of parietal bone: the edge of the parietal bone that articulates with the occipital bone at the lambdoid suture.

**m. occipita'lis os'sis tempora'lis** [TA], occipital margin of temporal bone: the border of the petrous part of the temporal bone that articulates with the occipital bone along the occipitomastoid suture.

**m. occul'tus un'guis** [TA], hidden margin of nail: the proximal buried edge of a nail.

**m. orbita'lis** [TA], orbital margin: the edge of the entrance to the orbit, formed mainly by the frontal and zygomatic bones and the maxilla. See also *m. infraorbitalis orbitae* and *m. supraorbitalis orbitae.*

**m. pal'pebrae,** see *free margin of eyelid.*

**m. parieta'lis a'lae mag'nae, m. parieta'lis a'lae majo'ris** [TA], parietal margin of greater wing of sphenoid bone: the superior extremity of the squamous portion of the greater wing, where it articulates with the parietal bone. Called also *parietal angle of sphenoid bone.*

**m. parieta'lis os'sis fronta'lis** [TA], parietal margin of frontal bone: the posterior border of the frontal bone, semicircular in shape, which articulates with the parietal bones.

**m. parieta'lis par'tis squamo'sae os'sis tempora'lis** [TA], parietal border of squamous part of temporal bone: the superior border of the squamous part of the temporal bone where it articulates with the parietal bone; called also *m. parietalis squamae temporalis.*

**m. parieta'lis squa'mae tempora'lis,** m. parietalis ossis temporalis.

**m. poste'rior cor'poris pancre'atis,** m. inferior corporis pancreatis.

**m. poste'rior fi'bulae** [TA], posterior margin of fibula: the posterolateral margin of the body of the fibula; called also *crista lateralis fibulae*.

**m. poste'rior par'tis petro'sae os'sis tempora'lis** [TA], posterior margin of petrous part of temporal bone: the border of the petrous part extending from the apex to the jugular notch and articulating with part of the occipital bone. Called also *posterior border of petrous part of temporal bone.*

**m. poste'rior ra'dii** [TA], posterior margin of radius: the edge of the radius that extends from the posterior part of the radial tuberosity to the middle tubercle; called also *m. dorsalis radii* and *dorsal margin of radius.*

**m. poste'rior sple'nis,** m. inferior splenis.

**m. poste'rior tes'tis** [TA], posterior margin of testis: the border of the testis that is attached to the epididymis and the lower end of the ductus deferens; called also *dorsum of testis.*

**m. poste'rior ul'nae** [TA], posterior margin of ulna: the dorsal border of the ulna, separating the posterior and medial surfaces; called also *m. dorsalis ulnae.*

**m. pupilla'ris i'ridis** [TA], pupillary margin of iris: the inner edge of the iris, surrounding the pupil.

**m. radia'lis antebra'chii** [TA], the radial, or lateral, border of the forearm; called also *m. lateralis antebrachii* [TA alternative].

**m. radia'lis hu'meri,** m. lateralis humeri.

**m. sagitta'lis os'sis parieta'lis** [TA], sagittal border of parietal bone: the edge of the parietal bone that articulates with the other parietal bone along the sagittal suture; called also *parietal* or *superior margin of parietal bone.*

**m. sphenoida'lis par'tis squamo'sae os'sis tempora'lis** [TA], **m. sphenoida'lis squa'mae tempora'lis,** sphenoidal margin of squamous part of temporal bone: the anterior border of the temporal bone, articulating with the greater wing of the sphenoid bone.

**m. squamo'sus a'lae mag'nae, m. squamo'sus a'lae majo'ris** [TA], squamous margin of great wing of sphenoid bone: the border of the greater wing of the sphenoid bone that articulates with the squama of the temporal bone; called also *m. squamosus alae magnae.*

**m. squamo'sus os'sis parieta'lis** [TA], squamous border of parietal bone: the inferior edge of the parietal bone, which articulates with the sphenoid and temporal bones along the squamous suture.

**m. supe'rior cor'poris pancre'atis** [TA], superior border of body of pancreas: the pancreatic edge that bounds the anterosuperior and posterior surfaces.

**m. supe'rior glan'dulae suprarena'lis** [TA], superior margin of suprarenal gland: the superior border, which with the medial border divides the anterior from the posterior surface.

**m. supe'rior hemisphe'rii cer'ebri** [TA], superior margin of cerebral hemisphere: the superior medial margin of the cerebral hemisphere; called also *m. superomedialis cerebri.*

**m. supe'rior lie'nis,** TA alternative for *m. superior splenis.*

**m. supe'rior par'tis petro'sae os'sis tempora'lis** [TA], superior border of petrous part of temporal bone: the long upper border of the petrosal part; it is grooved by the sulcus for the superior petrosal sinus.

**m. supe'rior sca'pulae** [TA], superior margin of scapula: the thin, short edge of the scapula, extending from the superior angle to the coracoid process.

**m. supe'rior sple'nis** [TA], superior margin of spleen: a somewhat sharp, convex line, sometimes serrated, between the gastric and diaphragmatic surfaces of the spleen; called also *m. anterior splenis, m. superior lienis* [TA alternative], and *anterior* or *crenate margin of spleen.*

**m. superomedia'lis cer'ebri,** m. superior hemispherii cerebri.

**m. supraorbita'lis or'bitae** [TA], supraorbital margin of orbit: the superior edge of the entrance to the orbit, formed by the supraorbital margin of the frontal bone.

**m. supraorbita'lis os'sis fronta'lis** [TA], supraorbital margin of frontal bone: the antero-inferior edge of the frontal bone, bending down laterally to the zygomatic bone and medially to the frontal process of the maxilla; it marks the junction between the squama and the orbital portion of the bone.

**m. tibia'lis pe'dis,** TA alternative for *m. medialis pedis.*

**m. ulna'ris antebra'chii** [TA], the ulnar, or medial, border of the forearm; called also *m. medialis antebrachii* [TA alternative].

**m. ulna'ris hu'meri,** m. medialis humeri.

**m. u'teri** [TA], margin of uterus: either border of the uterus (right or left), at the upper portion of which the uterine tube is attached; called also *lateral margin of uterus* and *m. lateralis uteri.*

**m. vertebra'lis sca'pulae,** m. medialis scapulae.

**m. vola'ris ra'dii,** m. anterior radii.

**m. vola'ris ul'nae,** m. anterior ulnae.

**m. zygoma'ticus a'lae mag'nae, m. zygoma'ticus a'lae majo'ris** [TA], zygomatic margin of greater wing of sphenoid bone: the border on the greater wing separating its temporal and orbital surfaces and articulating with the zygomatic bone.

**Ma•rie's hypertrophy, sign** (mah-rēz') [Pierre *Marie,* French physician, 1853–1940] see under *hypertrophy* and *sign.*

**Ma•rie-Bam•ber•ger disease** (mah-re' bahm'bər-gər) [Pierre *Marie;* Eugen *Bamberger,* Austrian physician, 1858–1921] hypertrophic pulmonary osteoarthropathy.

**Ma•rie-Foix sign** (mah-re' fwah) [Pierre *Marie;* Charles *Foix,* French neurologist, 1882–1927] see under *sign.*

**Ma•rie-Strüm•pell disease, syndrome** (mah-re' strēm'pel) [Pierre *Marie;* Adolf von *Strümpell,* German physician, 1853–1925] rheumatoid spondylitis.

**Ma•rie-Tooth disease** (mah-re' to͞oth) [Pierre *Marie;* Howard Henry *Tooth,* English physician, 1856–1925] Charcot-Marie-Tooth disease.

**mar•i•hua•na** (mar"ĭ-hwah'nə) [Mexican Sp.] marijuana.

**mar•i•jua•na** (mar"ĭ-hwah'nə) [Mexican Sp.] 1. *Cannabis sativa.* 2. a crude preparation of the leaves and flowering tops of *C. sativa,* usually employed in cigarettes and inhaled as smoke for its euphoric properties. See *cannabis.*

**Ma•ri•nes•co's sign, succulent hand** (mah-re-nes'kōz) [Georges *Marinesco,* Romanian neurologist, 1863–1938] main succulente.

**Ma•ri•nes•co-Sjö•gren syndrome** (mah-re-nes'ko-shər'gren) [G. *Marinesco;* Karl Gustav Torsten *Sjögren,* Swedish physician, born 1896] see under *syndrome.*

**mar•i•no•bu•fa•gin** (mar"ĭ-no-bu'fə-jin) a cardiac poison from the skin of the toad, *Bufo marinus.*

**Mar•i•nol** (ma'rĭ-nol) trademark for a preparation of dronabinol.

**Ma•ri•on's disease** (mah-re-awz') [Jean Baptiste Camille Georges *Marion,* French urologist, 1869–1960] see under *disease.*

**Ma•ri•otte's experiment, law, spot** (mah-re-ots') [Edme *Mariotte,* French physicist, 1620–1684] see under *experiment,* and see *Boyle's law,* under *law,* and *blind spot,* under *spot.*

**mar•i•to•nu•cle•us** (mar"ĭ-to-noo'kle-əs) [L. *maritus* married + *nucleus*] the nucleus of the oocyte after the sperm cell has entered it.

**Mar•jo•lin's ulcer** (mahr"zho-laz') [Jean Nicolas *Marjolin,* French surgeon, 1780–1850] see under *ulcer.*

**mark** (mahrk) a spot, blemish, or other circumscribed area visible on a surface, particularly on the skin or mucous membrane.
**beauty m.,** a small pigmented nevus, particularly on the cheek, said to enhance the appearance.
**birth m.,** see *birthmark.*
**pock m.,** see *pockmark.*
**Pohl's m., Pohl-Pinkus m.,** a limited thinning of the shaft of a hair, usually accompanied by interruption of the medulla; it is usually a sign of systemic disease, but may be due to trauma, coronary occlusion, skin disease, or the therapeutic administration of a single substantial dose of an antimetabolite, such as methotrexate or cyclophosphamide.
**port-wine m.,** see under *stain.*
**strawberry m.,** 1. see under *hemangioma.* 2. cavernous hemangioma. 3. vascular nevus.

**mark•er** (mahrk'ər) something that identifies or that is used to identify; cf. *determinant.*
**Amsler's m.,** a form of caliper compass used for marking the point for the application of cautery in Gonin's operation.
**cell-surface m.,** an antigenic determinant occurring on the surface of a specific type of cell.
**genetic m.,** a genetic polymorphism with a simple mode of inheritance occurring with multiple alleles, and therefore useful in family studies, studies of the distribution of genes in populations, and linkage analysis.
**surrogate m.,** a phenomenon whose presence provides indirect evidence for the presence of another phenomenon, for example, the viral load as an indicator of the state of the immune system in HIV infection
**tumor m.,** a circulating biochemical substance indicative of neoplasia; the most useful being specific, sensitive, and proportional to tumor load. Tumor markers may be used to screen, diagnose, assess prognosis, follow response to treatment, and monitor for recurrence.

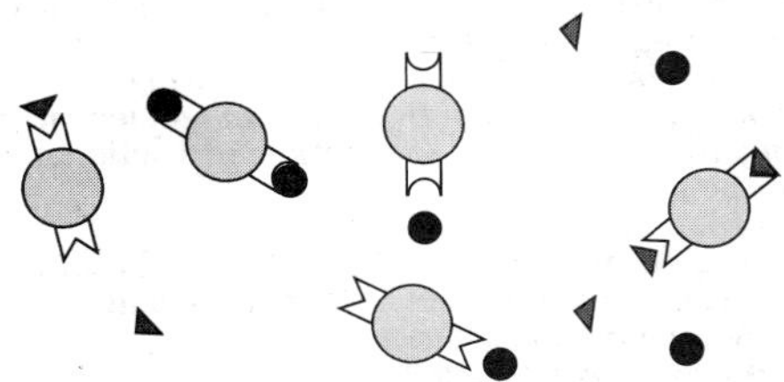

Schematic drawing of two different cell-surface markers on the surface of various cell types, each marker specific for a different antigen.

**Mar•low's test** (mahr'lōz) [Frank William *Marlow,* American ophthalmologist, 1858–1942] see under *test.*

**mar•mo•ra•tion** (mahr"mo-ra'shən) [L. *marmor* marble] marbleization.

**mar•mo•re•al** (mahr-mo're-əl) resembling marble, as bone in osteopetrosis.

**mar•mot** (mahr'mot) [MeSH: Marmota] any member of the genus *Marmota,* such as the hoary marmot, the yellow-bellied marmot, the woodchuck of North America, and the tarbagan of Asia; several are natural reservoirs of the plague.

**Mar•mo•ta** (mahr-mo'tə) [MeSH: Marmota] the marmots, a genus of the family Sciwiidae, terrestrial rodents of North America, Europe, and Asia that are sometimes reservoirs of plague. *M. bo'bak* is the tarbagan of Europe and Asia. *M. mo'max* is the woodchuck of northeastern North America.

**Mar•o•gen** (mar'ə-jen) trademark for a preparation of epoetin beta.

**Ma•ro•teaux-La•my syndrome** (mah-ro-to' lah-me') [Pierre *Maroteaux,* French physician, born 1926; Maurice Emile Joseph *Lamy,* French physician, 1895–1975] see under *syndrome.*

**Mar•plan** (mahr'plan) trademark for a preparation of isocarboxazid.

**mar•row** (mar'o) 1. medulla ossium. 2. any of various soft substances resembling bone marrow (medulla ossium).
**bone m.,** medulla ossium.
**bone m., red,** medulla ossium rubra.
**bone m., yellow,** medulla ossium flava.
**depressed m.,** bone marrow exhibiting decreased hematopoietic activity. See *myelosuppression.*
**fat m.,** medulla ossium flava.
**gelatinous m.,** bone marrow that has lost its blood cells and its fat and has acquired a gelatinous appearance.
**red m.,** medulla ossium rubra.
**spinal m.,** medulla spinalis.
**yellow m.,** medulla ossium flava.

**mar•ru•bi•in** (mə-roo'be-in) a lactone principle, the active ingredient of horehound.

**Mar•ru•bi•um** (mə-roo'be-əm) a genus of mints of the family Labiatae, native to Europe and Asia. *M. vulga're* (Tourn.) L. is horehound, whose leaves and tops (also called *horehound*) contain marrubiin and are used medicinally.

**Mars•de•nia** (mahrz-de'ne-ə) a genus of woody vines of the family Asclepiadaceae. *M. conduran'go* Reichb. f. is condurango, a South American species whose bark (also called condurango) is usually poisonous but in small amounts is medicinal.

**Marsh's disease** (mahrsh'əz) [Sir Henry *Marsh,* Irish physician, 1790–1860] Graves' disease.

**Mar•shall's fold, vein** (mahr'shəlz) [John *Marshall,* English anatomist, 1818–1891] see *plica venae cavae sinistrae* and *vena obliqua atrii sinistri.*

**mar•su•pia** (mahr-soo'pe-ə) [L.] plural of *marsupium.*

**mar•su•pi•al** (mahr-soo'pe-əl) [L. *marsupium* a pouch] a member of the order Marsupialia.

**Mar•su•pi•a•lia** (mahr-soo"pe-a'le-ə) [MeSH: Marsupialia] an order of the class Mammalia characterized by possession of a marsupium where the young, which are born in an underdeveloped state, are carried and nourished until their development is complete. In some systems of classification, it is considered to be an order of the infraclass or subclass Metatheria. It includes the opossums, kangaroos, wallabies, koalas, and wombats.

**mar•su•pi•al•iza•tion** (mahr-soo"pe-əl-ĭ-za'shən) [L. *marsupium* pouch] the creation of a pouch; applied especially to surgical exteriorization of a cyst by resection of the anterior wall and suture of the cut edges of the remaining cyst to the adjacent edges of the skin, thereby establishing a pouch of what was formerly an enclosed cyst.

**mar•su•pi•um** (mahr-soo'pe-əm) pl. *marsu'pia* [L. "a pouch"] 1. scrotum. 2. an external abdominal pouch or fold of skin for carrying the young; it contains the mammary glands and occurs in marsupials and the spiny anteaters. 3. a similar structure for carrying eggs or the young, as in the male sea horse.
**marsu'pia patella'ris,** plicae alares.

**mar•tial** (mahr'shəl) [L. *martialis* of Mars, the god of war] ferruginous.

**Mar·tin's bandage** (mahr'tinz) [Henry Austin *Martin,* American surgeon, 1824–1884] see under *bandage.*

**Mar·tin-Bell syndrome** (mahr'tin bel) [J. Purdon *Martin,* British physician, 20th century; Julia *Bell,* British physician, 20th century] fragile X syndrome.

**Mar·ti·not·ti's cells** (mahr"tĭ-not'ēz) [Giovanni *Martinotti,* Italian pathologist, 1857–1928] see under *cell.*

**Mar·tor·ell's syndrome** (mahr-to-relz') [Fernando *Martorell* Otzet, Spanish cardiologist, born 1906] see *Takayasu's arteritis,* under *arteritis.*

**masc** mass concentration.

**mas·chal·ad·e·ni·tis** (mas"kəl-ad"ə-ni'tis) [Gr. *maschalē* armpit + *aden-* + *-itis*] inflammation of the glands of the axilla.

**mas·cu·line** (mas'ku-lin) [L. *masculinus*] pertaining to or possessing qualities normally characteristic of the male sex; called also *male* and *virile.*

**mas·cu·lin·i·ty** (mas"ku-lin'ĭ-te) the possession of masculine qualities. Called also *virility.*

**mas·cu·lin·iza·tion** (mas"ku-lin-ĭ-za'shən) 1. the induction or development of male secondary sex characters in the female, such as enlargement of the clitoris, growth of facial and body hair, and deepening of the voice. Called also *gynandrism.* 2. the normal development of primary or secondary sex characters in the male. 3. the condition of having such sex characters. Called also *androgenization, virilescence, virilism,* and *virilization.*

**mas·cu·li·nize** (mas'ku-lĭ-nīz") 1. to produce normal sex-specific characteristics in a male. 2. to produce masculine characteristics in a female; see *masculinization.*

**mas·cu·lin·iz·ing** (mas'ku-lin-iz"ing) producing masculinization; called also *androgenic* and *virilizing.*

**ma·ser** (ma'zər) [*m*icrowave *a*mplification by *s*timulated *e*mission of *r*adiation] a device which produces an extremely intense, small, and nearly nondivergent beam of monochromatic radiation in the microwave region with all waves in phase.

**mask** (mask) [Fr. *masque*] [MeSH: Masks] 1. to cover or conceal, as the masking of the nature of a disorder by the presence of unrelated signs, symptoms, or organisms. 2. in audiometry, to obscure or diminish a sound by the presence of another sound of different frequency. 3. a covering for the face, as a bandage, an apparatus for administering oxygen, or a cloth that prevents droplets from the nose and mouth from spreading in the air. 4. in dentistry, to camouflage metal parts of a prosthesis by covering with opaque material.
**BLB m.,** a face mask that has a combined inspiratory and expiratory valve and a bag for rebreathing, used mainly with oxygen delivery systems at high altitudes, and occasionally for clinical administration of oxygen.
**death m.,** a plaster cast of the face of a dead person.
**ecchymotic m.,** cyanotic discoloration of the head and neck as a result of traumatic asphyxia.
**full-face m.,** a device used in anesthesia to confine the gas to be delivered through the mask into the respiratory tract through the nose or mouth.
**Hutchinson's m.,** a sensation as if the skin of the face were compressed by a mask; often a symptom of tabes dorsalis.
**meter m.,** a face mask used with oxygen delivery systems, designed to provide fixed percentage admixtures of air and oxygen.
**Parkinson's m.,** see under *facies.*
**m. of pregnancy,** see *melasma.*
**tabetic m.,** Hutchinson's m.
**Venturi m.,** a face mask used in oxygen therapy, delivering a controlled mixture of oxygen and air.

**masked** (maskt) 1. concealed from view; hidden. 2. not presenting or producing the usual symptoms. 3. blind (def. 2).

**maso·chism** (mas'o-kiz-əm) [Leopold von Sacher-*Masoch,* an Austrian novelist, 1836–1895] [MeSH: Masochism] the act or instance of gaining pleasure from experiencing physical or psychological pain; the term is usually used to denote *sexual m.*
**sexual m.** [DSM-IV], a paraphilia in which sexual gratification is derived from being hurt, humiliated, or otherwise made to suffer physically or psychologically.

**maso·chist** (mas'o-kist) one given to masochism.

**maso·chis·tic** (mas"o-kis'tik) pertaining to or characterized by masochism.

**ma·so·pro·col** (mə-so'prə-kol) an arachidonate 5-lipoxygenase inhibitor applied topically as an antineoplastic in the treatment of actinic keratoses.

**Mas. pil.** abbreviation for L. *mas'sa pilula'rum,* pill mass.

**mass** (mas) [L. *massa*] 1. a lump or body made up of cohering particles; see also *massa.* 2. a cohesive mixture suitable for being made up into pills. 3. that characteristic of matter which gives it inertia. The SI unit for mass is the kilogram. Atomic masses are generally expressed in terms of the unified atomic mass unit: u = $1.6605 \times 10^{-27}$ kg, and the mass of any other atom may be found by multiplying this number by the atomic weight of the atom. Symbol *m.*
**achromatic m.,** the nonstaining portion of the karyokinetic figure.
**appendiceal m., appendix m.,** a palpable mass in the right iliac fossa or right loin due to acute appendicitis, usually with abscess secondary to rupture; occasionally caused by adherent omentum and intestine.
**atomic m.,** atomic weight; used particularly when describing a single isotope of a nuclide.
**body cell m.,** the total weight of the cells of the body, including the cell nucleus, cytoplasm, water, salt, protein, and surrounding membrane, but excluding extracellular water and extracellular solids such as collagen, elastin, and bone matrix, constituting in essence the total mass of oxygen-utilizing, carbohydrate-burning, and energy-exchanging cells of the body; regarded as proportional to total exchangeable potassium in the body.
**fibrillar m. of Flemming,** spongioplasm, def. 1.
**injection m.,** a suspension or solution, usually colored, injected into blood vessels or other tissue spaces to permit their demonstration on dissection or sectioning.
**inner cell m.,** an aggregation of cells at the embryonic pole of the blastocyst, which is destined to form the embryo proper. Called also *embryoblast.*
**intermediate cell m.,** nephrotome.
**lateral m. of atlas,** massa lateralis atlantis.
**lateral m. of ethmoid bone,** labyrinthus ethmoidalis.
**lateral m. of sacrum,** pars lateralis ossis sacri.
**lateral m. of vertebrae,** pediculus arcus vertebrae.
**lean body m.,** that part of the body including all its components except neutral storage lipid; in essence, the fat-free mass of the body.
**molar m.,** the mass of a molecule in grams (or kilograms) per mole, derived by addition of the sum of the component atomic masses. Its dimensionless equivalent is molecular weight. Symbol *M.*
**molecular m.,** the mass of a molecule in daltons, derived by addition of the sum of the component atomic masses. Its dimensionless equivalent is molecular weight.
**pill m., pilular m.,** a drug mass of the proper consistency for being made into pills.
**relative molecular m.,** technically preferable term for *molecular weight;* symbol $M_r$.
**Stent's m.,** a plastic resinous material which sets into a very hard substance; used in surgery for making molds shaped to keep grafts in place. See also *stent.*
**tigroid m's,** Nissl's bodies.
**ventrolateral m.,** that portion of the primordial lateral mass of the embryo from which are developed the abdominal, thoracic, and anterior cervical muscles.

**mas·sa** (mas'ə) gen. and pl. *mas'sae* [L.] 1. mass; a cohesive lump of material. 2. [TA] a general term for an accumulation of cells or cohesive tissue.
**m. innomina'ta,** paradidymis.
**m. interme'dia,** adhesio interthalamica.
**m. latera'lis atlan'tis** [TA], lateral mass of atlas: the thickened lateral portion of the atlas to which the arches are attached and which bears the articulating surfaces and the transverse process.
**m. latera'lis os'sis ethmoida'lis,** labyrinthus ethmoidalis.
**m. latera'lis os'sis sa'cri,** pars lateralis ossis sacri.
**m. latera'lis ver'tebrae,** pediculus arcus vertebrae.

**mas·sae** (mas'e) [L.] genitive and plural of *massa.*

**mas·sage** (mə-sahzh') [Fr. from Gr. *massein* to knead] [MeSH: Massage] the systematic therapeutic friction, stroking, and kneading of the body.
**cardiac m.,** rhythmic compression of the heart by pressure applied manually over the sternum *(closed cardiac massage)* or directly to the heart through an opening in the chest wall *(open cardiac massage);* done to reinstate and maintain circulation.
**carotid sinus m.,** firm rotatory pressure applied to one side of the neck over the carotid sinus of the supine patient; it causes vagal stimulation, increasing vagal inhibition of sinus and atrioventricular nodes, and it can slow or terminate tachycardia.
**electrovibratory m.,** massage by means of an electric vibrator.
**gingival m.,** the systematic application of frictional rubbing and stroking to the gingiva.
**heart m.,** cardiac m.
**ice m.,** massage in which ice is rubbed over the body surface for local analgesic effects and relief of muscle spasms.
**pneumatic m.,** pneumomassage.
**vibratory m.,** electrovibratory m.

**mas·sa·sau·ga** [corruption of *Missisauga,* a river in Ontario, Canada] *Sistrurus catenatus,* a small venomous rattlesnake found from

New York State to the southwestern United States and northern Mexico. Called also *Massasauga rattlesnake.*

**Mas·se·lon's spectacles** (mahs″ə-lawz′) [Michel Julien *Masselon,* French ophthalmologist, 1844–1917] see under *spectacles.*

**mas·se·ter** (mə-se′tər) [Gr. *masētēr* chewer] see *musculus masseter.*

**mas·se·ter·ic** (mas″ə-ter′ik) pertaining to the masseter muscle.

**mas·seur** (mah-soor′) [Fr.] 1. a man who performs massage. 2. an instrument for performing massage.

**mas·seuse** (mah-sooz′) [Fr.] a woman who performs massage.

**mas·si·cot** (mas′ĭ-kot) lead monoxide, PbO.

**mas·sive** (mas′iv) having a solid bulky form; heavy; in a mass; complete.

**Mas·son stain** (mah-saw′) [Claude Laurent *Masson,* French-born pathologist in Canada, 1880–1959] see under *stain.*

**mas·so·ther·a·py** (mas″o-ther′ə-pe) [Gr. *massein* to knead + *therapy*] the treatment of disease by massage.

**MAST** [acronym for *m*ilitary or *m*edical *a*nti-*s*hock *t*rousers] see *pneumatic antishock garment,* under *garment.*

**mas·tad·e·ni·tis** (mas″tad-ə-ni′tis) [*mast-* + *aden-* + *-itis*] inflammation of the mammary gland; mastitis.

**Mas·tad·e·no·vi·rus** (mast-ad′ə-no-vi″rəs) [*mast-* + *adenovirus*] [MeSH: Mastadenovirus] mammalian adenoviruses; a genus of viruses of the family Adenoviridae that infect mammals, causing disease of the respiratory tract, gastrointestinal tract, conjunctiva, central nervous system, and urinary tract; infection may be asymptomatic. Many species induce malignancy. Human viruses are grouped into seven subgenera (A–G) on the basis of structural, immunological, biological, and chemical characteristics. (See accompanying table.)

**mas·tal·gia** (mas-tal′jə) [*mast-* + *-algia*] pain in the breast; called also *mammalgia* and *mastodynia.*

**mas·ta·tro·phia** (mas″tə-tro′fe-ə) mastatrophy.

**mas·tat·ro·phy** (mas-tat′rə-fe) [*mast-* + *atrophy*] atrophy of the mammary gland.

**mas·tauxe** (mas-tawk′se) [*mast-* + Gr. *auxē* increase] enlargement of the breast.

**mas·tec·to·my** (mas-tek′tə-me) [*mast-* + *-ectomy*] [MeSH: Mastectomy] excision of the breast; mammectomy.
**Halsted m.,** radical m.
**Meyer m.,** radical m.
**partial m.,** removal of only enough breast tissue to ensure that the margins of the resected surgical specimen are free of tumor; called also *segmental m.*
**radical m.,** removal of the breast, pectoral muscles, axillary lymph nodes, and associated skin and subcutaneous tissue in treatment of breast cancer.
**radical m., extended,** radical mastectomy with removal of the ipsilateral half of the sternum and a portion of ribs two through five with the underlying pleura and the internal mammary lymph nodes.
**radical m., modified,** total mastectomy with axillary lymphadenectomy, but with preservation of the pectoral muscles.
**segmental m.,** partial m.
**simple m.,** removal of only the breast tissue and nipple and a small portion of the overlying skin.
**subcutaneous m.,** excision of breast tissue with preservation of overlying skin, nipple, and areola so that breast form may be reconstructed.
**total m.,** simple m.

**Mas·ter "2-step" exercise test** (mas′tər) [Arthur Matthew *Master,* American physician, 1895–1973] see under *test.*

**mast·hel·co·sis** (mast″həl-ko′sis) [*mast-* + *helcosis*] ulceration of the breast or mammary gland.

**mas·tic** (mas′tik) [L. *mastiche;* Gr. *mastichē*] 1. *Pistacia lentiscus.* 2. a resinous exudation obtained from *P. lentiscus,* used as a flavored chewing gum base, in plasters, lacquers, and incense, and pharmaceutically in enteric coatings for tablets.

**Human Adenoviruses**

| Subgenus | Species |
|---|---|
| A | HAdV 12, 18, 31 |
| B | HAdV 3, 7, 11, 14, 16, 21, 34, 35 |
| C | HAdV 1, 2, 5, 6 |
| D | HAdV 8, 9, 10, 13, 15, 17, 19, 20, 22–30, 32, 33, 36, 37, 38, 39, 42, 43, 44, 45, 46, 47 |
| E | HAdV 4 |
| F–G | HAdV 40, 41 |

**mas·ti·ca·tion** (mas″tĭ-ka′shən) [L. *masticare* to chew] [MeSH: Mastication] the process of chewing food in preparation for swallowing and digestion.

**mas·ti·ca·to·ry** (mas′tĭ-kə-tor″e) 1. subserving or pertaining to mastication; affecting the muscles of mastication. 2. a remedy to be chewed but not swallowed.

**Mas·ti·go·my·co·ti·na** (mas″tĭ-go-mi″ko-ti′nə) [Gr. *mastix* whip + *mykēs* fungus] [MeSH: Mastigomycotina] a grouping of organisms usually considered a subphylum of fungi under the phylum Eumycota; they have a unicellular or mycelial thallus and motile reproductive cells. Animal pathogens are included in the class Oomycetes. In some systems of classification, they are assigned to the Protista rather than the Fungi.

**mas·ti·gont** (mas′tĭ-gont) [Gr. *mastigoun* to whip] a flagellum; see under *system.*

**Mas·ti·goph·o·ra** (mas″tĭ-gof′ə-rə) [Gr. *mastix* whip + *phoros* bearing] [MeSH: Mastigophora] a subphylum of protozoa (phylum Sarcomastigophora) comprising the flagellates, i.e., all those with one or more flagella in the trophozoite. Mastigophorans have a simple, centrally placed nucleus and reproduce by longitudinal binary fission, and most are free-living but many are parasitic in both invertebrates and vertebrates, including humans. The subphylum comprises two classes; Phytomastigophorea (plantlike protozoa, or phytoflagellates) and Zoomastigophorea (animal-like protozoa, or zooflagellates). Formerly called *Euflagellata* and *Flagellata.*

**mas·ti·goph·o·ran** (mas″tĭ-gof′ə-rən) any protozoan of the subphylum Mastigophora; a flagellate; a mastigote.

**mas·ti·goph·o·rous** (mas″tĭ-gof′ə-rəs) of or pertaining to the subphylum Mastigophora.

**Mas·ti·go·proc·tus** (mas″tĭ-go-prok′təs) a genus of whip scorpions (order Pedipalpa). *M. gigan′teus* is the vinegaroon, a species with irritating secretions.

**mas·ti·gote** (mas′tĭ-gōt) any protozoan of the subphylum Mastigophora; a flagellate; a mastigophoran.

**mas·ti·tis** (mas-ti′tis) [*mast-* + *-itis*] [MeSH: Mastitis] inflammation of the mammary gland, or breast.
**bovine m.,** inflammation of the mammary gland of a cow, usually due to an infectious agent such as a bacteria or fungus. Common bacterial pathogens are *Staphylococcus aureus* (see *staphylococcal m.*), *Streptococcus agalactiae,* other species of streptococci, and coliform bacteria (see *coliform m.*). The milk from infected cows may be watery or serous with clots or flakes and clear or brownish in color. Called also *garget.*
**chronic cystic m.,** fibrocystic disease of breast; see under *disease.*
**coliform m.,** bovine mastitis caused by *Escherichia coli, Klebsiella* species, or *Enterobacter aerogenes.* The udder becomes inflamed and slightly enlarged and the milk is thin, serous, and brown with flakes. Affected cows may suffer from anorexia, fever, and fatal toxemia.
**gargantuan m.,** pathologic enlargement of the breasts to a tremendous size.
**glandular m.,** parenchymatous m.
**interstitial m.,** inflammation of the stroma of the mammary gland.
**m.-metritis-agalactia,** lactation failure in swine (see under *failure*).
**m. neonato′rum,** a general term applied to an abnormal condition of the breast of the newborn, such as hypertrophy, engorgement and secretion, or inflammation, with or without suppuration.
**nocardial m.,** mastitis in cattle caused by an infection with *Nocardia asteroides* or *N. farcinica.* Characteristics include granulomatous lesions of the udder with fibrosis, inflammation, abscesses, and fever; damage to the udder and milk supply is usually permanent.
**parenchymatous m.,** inflammation of the secreting elements of the mammary gland.
**periductal m.,** inflammation of tissues about the ducts of the mammary gland.
**phlegmonous m.,** inflammation of the breast leading to abscess formation.
**plasma cell m.,** a condition of the breast characterized by infiltration of the breast stroma with plasma cells and proliferation of the cells lining the ducts, possibly related to mammary duct ectasia.
**puerperal m.,** a form of mastitis occurring after delivery.
**retromammary m., submammary m.,** paramastitis.
**stagnation m.,** a local engorgement affecting one or more lobules of the breast and forming a painful lump in the organ; it occurs during early lactation. Called also *caked breast.*
**staphylococcal m.,** bovine mastitis caused by infection with *Staphylococcus aureus;* it may be either subclinical or acute. The acute forms sometimes result in skin sloughing, gangrene, and death. Cf. *udder impetigo.*
**suppurative m.,** pyogenic infection of the breast.

**mast(o)-** [Gr. *mastos* breast] a combining form denoting relationship to the breast or to the mastoid process; see also words beginning *mamm(o)-* and *maz(o)-*.

**mas·toc·cip·i·tal** (mas″tok-sip′ĭ-təl) masto-occipital.

**mas·to·cyte** (mas′to-sīt) [Ger. *Mast* food + *-cyte*] a mast cell.

**mas·to·cy·to·ma** (mas″to-si-to′mə) [*masto-* + *cytoma*] a nodular cutaneous mast cell infiltrate, which is usually present at birth or soon after as a solitary nodule, although three to four lesions may occur. Lesions typical of urticaria pigmentosa may occur later. Called also *mast cell tumor.*

**mas·to·cy·to·sis** (mas″to-si-to′sis) [*masto-* + *cytosis*] [MeSH: Mastocytosis] a group of rare diseases characterized by infiltrates of mast cells in the tissues and sometimes other organs. The group includes *diffuse* and *systemic m., mastocytoma, urticaria pigmentosa,* and *telangiectasia perstans.*
**diffuse m., diffuse cutaneous m.,** a condition in which the entire skin is thickened, lichenified, and leathery in appearance and accompanied by generalized erythroderma and intense pruritus as a result of widespread infiltration with mast cells. In children, it is often associated with systemic mastocytosis.
**systemic m.,** a condition in which there are mast cell infiltrates in noncutaneous tissues, occurring with or without cutaneous lesions, and usually involving the liver, spleen, bone, lymph nodes, and gastrointestinal tract. See also *mastocytosis syndrome,* under *syndrome.*

**mas·to·dyn·ia** (mas″to-din′e-ə) [*masto-* + *-odynia*] mastalgia.

**mas·toid** (mas′toid) [*masto-* + *-oid*] [MeSH: Mastoid] 1. breast shaped. 2. the mastoid process of the temporal bone. 3. pertaining to the mastoid process.

**mas·toid·al** (mas-toid′əl) pertaining to the mastoid process of the temporal bone.

**mas·toi·da·le** (mas″toi-da′le) the lowest point of the mastoid process.

**mas·toid·al·gia** (mas″toid-al′jə) [*mastoid* + *-algia*] pain in the mastoid region.

**mas·toid·ec·to·my** (mas″toid-ek′tə-me) [*mastoid* + *-ectomy*] excision of the mastoid cells or the mastoid process of the temporal bone.
**Bondy's m.,** modified radical m.
**canal wall down m.,** open-cavity tympanomastoidectomy.
**canal wall up m.,** closed-cavity tympanomastoidectomy.
**closed-cavity m.,** see under *tympanomastoidectomy.*
**cortical m.,** complete simple m.
**intact canal wall m.,** closed-cavity tympanomastoidectomy.
**open-cavity m.,** see under *tympanomastoidectomy.*
**radical m.,** mastoidectomy with exenteration of air cells, removal of the entire posterior wall of the ear canal, and removal of the tympanic membrane, malleus, and incus, resulting in permanent hearing loss.
**radical m., modified,** mastoidectomy with exenteration of air cells and removal of part of the posterior wall of the ear canal but with preservation of some or all of the ossicles; hearing may be preserved.
**simple m.,** mastoidectomy with exenteration of air cells but no involvement of the wall of the ear canal.
**simple m., complete,** mastoidectomy with exenteration of the air cells and epitympanum but no involvement of the wall of the ear canal. Called also *cortical m.*

**mas·toi·deo·cen·te·sis** (mas-toi″de-o-sən-te′sis) [*mastoid* + *-centesis*] surgical puncture of the mastoid antrum.

**mas·toid·itis** (mas″toid-i′tis) [MeSH: Mastoiditis] inflammation of the mastoid antrum and cells, sometimes as a result of otitis media.
**Bezold's m.,** a form in which the pus has escaped and formed tracts into the neck; see *Bezold's abscess,* under *abscess.*
**coalescent m.,** a form in which the bony partitions between the air cells erode so that air cells coalesce into large cavities; further erosion of the temporal bone runs the risk of intracranial abscess.
**sclerosing m.,** mastoiditis attended with hardening and condensation of the bone.
**silent m.,** a progressive destructive mastoiditis with mild systemic and local manifestations.

**mas·toid·ot·o·my** (mas″toi-dot′ə-me) [*mastoid* + *-tomy*] surgical incision of the mastoid process of the temporal bone, usually into the antrum.

**mas·to·me·nia** (mas″to-me′ne-ə) [*masto-* + *men-* + *-ia*] vicarious menstruation from the breast.

**Mas·to·mys** a genus of small African rodents. *M. natalen′sis* is the multimammate mouse.

**mas·to·oc·cip·i·tal** (mas″to-ok-sip′ĭ-təl) pertaining to the mastoid process and the occipital bone.

**mas·to·pa·ri·e·tal** (mas″to-pə-ri′ə-təl) [*masto-* + *parietal*] pertaining to the mastoid process and the parietal bone.

**mas·to·path·ia** (mas″to-path′e-ə) mastopathy.
**m. cys′tica,** a morbid condition of the mammary gland, with the formation of cysts.

**mas·top·a·thy** (mas-top′ə-the) [*masto-* + *-pathy*] disease of the mammary gland.
**cystic m.,** mastopathia cystica.

**mas·to·pexy** (mas′to-pek-se) [*masto-* + *-pexy*] mammaplasty performed to correct a pendulous breast.

**Mas·toph·o·ra** (mas-tof′ə-rə) a genus of spiders; called also *Glyptocranium. M. gasteracanthoi′des* is the cat-headed spider of South America.

**mas·to·pla·sia** (mas″to-pla′zhə) mammoplasia.

**mas·to·plas·ty** (mas′to-plas″te) mammaplasty.

**mas·to·pto·sis** (mas″to-to′sis) [*masto-* + *-ptosis*] pendulous breasts.

**mas·tor·rha·gia** (mas″to-ra′je-ə) [*masto-* + *-rrhagia*] hemorrhage from the mammary gland.

**mas·to·scir·rhus** (mas″to-skir′əs) [*masto-* + Gr. *skirros* hardness] hardening, or scirrhus, of the mammary gland.

**mas·to·squa·mous** (mas-to-skwah′məs) pertaining to or affecting the mastoid and squama of the temporal bone.

**mas·tos·to·my** (mas-tos′tə-me) [*masto-* + *-stomy*] incision of the breast for drainage.

**mas·tot·o·my** (mas-tot′ə-me) [*masto-* + *-tomy*] surgical incision of a breast.

**mas·tur·ba·tion** (mas″tər-ba′shən) [L. *manus* hand + *stuprare* to rape] [MeSH: Masturbation] self-stimulation of the genitals for sexual pleasure.

**Ma·su·gi's nephritis** (mah-soo′gēz) [Matazo *Masugi,* Japanese pathologist, 20th century] see *nephrotoxic serum nephritis,* under *nephritis.*

**MAT** multifocal atrial tachycardia; see *chaotic atrial tachycardia,* under *tachycardia.*

**Mat·as' operation, test** (mat′əs) [Rudolph *Matas,* American surgeon, 1860–1957] see *endoaneurysmorrhaphy,* and see *tourniquet test* (def. 2), under *test.*

**match·ing** (mach′ing) 1. comparison and selection of objects having similar or identical characteristics. 2. the selection of compatible donors and recipients for transfusion or transplantation. See also *typing.* 3. the selection of subjects for clinical trials or other studies so that the different groups being compared are similar in specified characteristics, e.g., age, sex, or race, in order to reduce bias and error caused by comparison of dissimilar groups. Matching may be on an individual (matched pairs) or a group-wide basis.
**cross m.,** crossmatching.

**ma·té** (mah-ta′) [Fr., from Sp. *mate*] the dried leaves of *Ilex paraguensis,* used as a source of tea in South America; it contains caffeine and tannins, and has been used as a tonic, diuretic, stomachic, stimulant, and laxative (large doses).

**ma·ter** (ma′tər) [L.] mother.
**arachnoi′dea m.,** see *arachnoidea mater,* under *A.*
**dura m.,** see *dura mater,* under *D.*
**pi′a m.,** see *pia mater,* under *P.*

**ma·te·ria** (mə-ter′e-ə) [L.] matter.
**m. al′ba,** a whitish or cream-colored cheesy mass deposited around the necks of the teeth, composed of food debris, mucin, and dead epithelial cells.
**m. me′dica,** that branch of medical study which deals with drugs, their sources, preparations, and uses; pharmacology.

**ma·te·ri·al** (mə-tēr′e-əl) substance or elements from which a concept may be formulated, or an object constructed.
**baseplate m.,** any dental material used in the construction of a baseplate, including silver, gold, aluminum, platinum, alloys, and plastics.
**cross-reacting m. (CRM),** a functionally inactive protein, produced by a mutant structural gene, that reacts with antibody to the normal protein.
**dental m.,** any material used in dental practice, particularly a material used in the production of dental bases, restorations, impressions, or prostheses.
**genetic m.,** material transmitted from an organism to those of succeeding generations and responsible for the features characteristic of the species, as well as for the heritable difference between individuals of the species.
**impression m.,** any material used for making impressions of the teeth and oral structures for the purpose of producing restorations, prostheses, and dentures, including elastomeric materials, dental plasters, metallic oxide pastes, impression compounds, reversible and irreversible hydrocolloids, silicone base materials, polyethers, polysulfide rubber, and duplicating compounds.

**tissue equivalent m.**, a material whose absorbing and scattering properties for a given radiation simulate as closely as possible those of a given biological tissue, such as bone, fat, or muscle. Water, for example, is usually the best tissue equivalent material for muscle and soft tissue.

**ma·ter·nal** (mə-ter′nəl) [L. *maternus; mater* mother] pertaining to the mother.

**ma·ter·ni·ty** (mə-ter′nĭ-te) [L. *mater* mother] 1. motherhood. 2. a lying-in hospital.

**mat·ing** (māt′ing) [from Middle low Ger. *mate* companion] pairing of individuals of the opposite sex, especially for reproduction.
**assortative m., assorted m., assortive m.**, a nonrandom system of mating in which choice of a mate is influenced by phenotype. Among human beings, *positive assortative mating* occurs, for example, when tall men choose tall women; or short women, short men. *Negative assortative mating* occurs when phenotypically dissimilar mates are chosen, e.g., tall men and short women, or tall women and short men. Nonrandom mating can affect Hardy-Weinberg equilibrium (q.v.) in a population.
**backcross m.**, the mating of a heterozygote and a recessive homozygote; useful in revealing, through the phenotypes of the offspring, the genotype of the heterozygous parent.
**nonrandom m.**, assortative m.
**random m.**, mating in which any sperm (or any pollen grain) has an equal chance of fertilizing any egg; thus for any one genotype at any one locus there is a purely random probability of combining with any other genotype at that locus. Called also *panmixis.*

**mat·rass** (mat′rəs) a glass vessel with a long neck used for treating dry substances in chemical procedures.

**mat·ri·cal** (mat′rĭ-kəl) of or relating to a matrix.

**Ma·tri·ca·ria** (mat″rĭ-kar′e-ə) [L.] a genus of flowering herbs of the family Compositae, native to Europe and Asia. *M. chamomil′la* L. is one of two plants called chamomile, whose dried flower heads are used medicinally. *M. nigellaefo′lia* L. is a type of feverfew and causes hepatic encephalopathy in cattle.

**mat·ri·ca·ria** (mat″rĭ-kar′e-ə) any plant of the genus *Matricaria*; see also *chamomile.*

**ma·tri·ces** (ma′trĭ-sēz) plural of *matrix.*

**ma·tri·cial** (mə-trish′əl) matrical.

**mat·ri·cli·nous** (mat″rĭ-kli′nəs) matroclinous.

**ma·tri·lin·e·al** (ma″trĭ-lin′e-əl) [*mater* + *linea*] descended through the female line.

**ma·trix** (ma′triks) pl. *ma′trices* [L.] 1. the intracellular substance of a tissue or the tissue from which a structure develops. 2. the groundwork on which anything is cast, or that basic material from which a thing develops. 3. a mold or a form for casting. 4. a plastic or metal strip used to support and shape a plastic restorative material. 5. a piece of gold or platinum foil fitted against the sides and bottom of a cavity, used as a mold in which porcelain for an inlay is baked. 6. resin m. 7. in dental porcelain, feldspar, which provides a glassy matrix in which quartz particles are dispersed.
**amalgam m.**, matrix band.
**bone m.**, the intercellular substance of bone, consisting of osteocollagenous fibers embedded in an amorphous ground substance and inorganic salts.

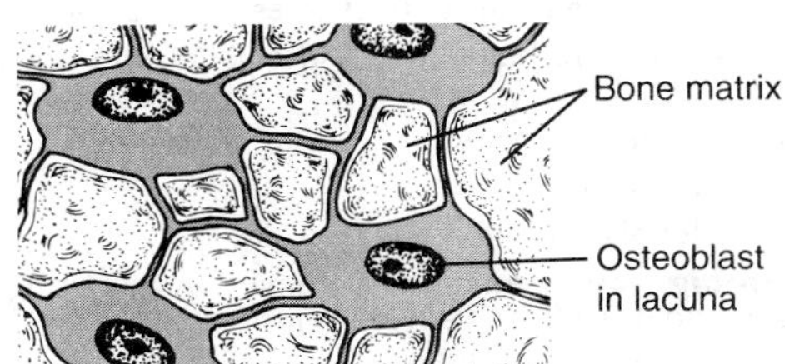


**capsular m.**, territorial m.
**cartilage m.**, the intercellular substance of cartilage, consisting of cells and extracellular fibers embedded in an amorphous ground substance; see also *interterritorial m.* and *territorial m.*
**cytoplasmic m.**, the aggregating factor of the basic molecular fabric which ties together the ribosomes, RNA, proteins, small molecules, and water in the cytoplasm.
**extracellular m. (ECM)**, any material produced by cells and excreted to the extracellular space within the tissues. It takes the form of both ground substance and fibers and is composed chiefly of fibrous elements, proteins involved in cell adhesion, and glycosaminoglycans and other space-filling molecules. It serves as a scaffolding holding tissues together and its form and composition help determine tissue characteristics. In epithelia, it includes the basement membrane.
**functional m.**, the contiguous and motivating soft tissue organs and tissues in the growth of the craniofacial complex.
**hair m.**, the epidermic root of the hair follicle.
**interterritorial m.**, a paler-staining region located among the darker territorial matrices.
**mitochondrial m.**, the dense substance, generally homogeneous but sometimes finely filamentous or granulated, found in the inner chamber (intercristal space) of mitochondria.
**nail m.**, m. unguis.
**resin m.**, in a resin matrix composite, the continuous phase (an organic polymer) in which the discrete particles of filler are dispersed. Called also *matrix.*
**sarcoplasmic m.**, the liquid substance which fills muscle cells; it contains the soluble enzymes of the cell.
**territorial m.**, basophilic material surrounding groups of cartilage cells.
**m. un′guis** [TA], nail matrix: the tissue upon which the deep aspect of the nail rests; called also *nail bed.* The term is also used to denote the proximal portion of the nail bed from which growth chiefly proceeds.

**mat·ro·cli·nous** (mat″ro-kli′nəs) [Gr. *mētēr* mother + *klinein* to incline] inheriting or inherited from the mother; possessing characters inherited from the mother. Cf. *patrocliny.*

**mat·ro·cli·ny** (mat″ro-kli′ne) the state of being matroclinous.

**matt, matte** (mat) a term applied to a macroscopic morphology of bacterial colonies that are dull and slightly granular, i.e., neither smooth and glistening nor rough.

**mat·ter** (mat′ər) 1. anything that occupies space. 2. substance; see anatomical terms under *substantia.* 3. pus.
**gray m. of nervous system,** substantia grisea.
**white m. of nervous system,** substantia alba.

**Mat·tox maneuver** (mat′əks) [Kenneth L. *Mattox,* American surgeon, born 1938] see under *maneuver.*

**Mat·u·lane** (mat′u-lān) trademark for a preparation of procarbazine hydrochloride.

**mat·u·rant** (mach′u-rənt) an agent that promotes suppuration.

**mat·u·rate** (mach′u-rāt) 1. to mature. 2. to suppurate.

**mat·u·ra·tion** (mach″u-ra′shən) [L. *maturatio; maturus* ripe] 1. the stage or process of becoming mature or fully developed. 2. the attainment of emotional and intellectual maturity. 3. in biology, a process of cell division during which the number of chromosomes in the germ cells is reduced to one half the number characteristic of the species. 4. suppuration.
**affinity m.**, the progressive increase in the affinity of antigen for antibody occurring during the immune response, due to selection of B lymphocytes with receptors having high affinity for the antigen.

**ma·ture** (mə-chōōr′) [L. *maturus*] 1. to develop to maturity; to ripen. 2. fully developed; ripe.

**ma·tur·i·ty** (mə-chōōr′ĭ-te) the period of attainment of maximal development.

**Matut.** abbreviation for L. *matuti′nus,* in the morning.

**ma·tu·ti·nal** (mə-too′tĭ-nəl) [L. *matutinalis*] pertaining to or occurring in the morning.

**Mau·chart's ligament** (mou′kahrts) [Burkhard David *Mauchart,* German anatomist, 1696–1751] ligamenta alaria.

**Mau·noir's hy·dro·cele** (mo-nwahrz′) [Jean Pierre *Maunoir,* Swiss surgeon, 1768–1861] cervical hydrocele.

**Mau·rer's dots (clefts, spots, stippling)** (mou′rerz) [Georg *Maurer,* German physician, born 1909] see under *dot.*

**Mau·ri·ac's syndrome** (mo″re-ahks′) [Pierre *Mauriac,* French physician, 1832–1905] see under *syndrome.*

**Mau·ri·ceau's maneuver** (mo″re-sōz′) [François *Mauriceau,* French obstetrician, 1637–1709] see under *maneuver.*

**Mauth·ner's cell, fiber, membrane (sheath)** (mout′nerz) [Ludwig *Mauthner,* Czech-born Austrian ophthalmologist, 1840–1894] see under *cell* and *fiber,* and see *axolemma.*

**mau·ve·in** (mo′ve-in) aniline purple, a violet dye used as an indicator, with a pH range of −0.1 to 2.9, being yellow at −0.1 and crimson at 2.9.

**Max·air** (mak-sār′) trademark for a preparation of pirbuterol acetate.

**MaxEPA** (max-e″pe-a′) trademark for a preparation of eicosapentaenoic acid and docosahexaenoic acid.

**Max·ib·o·lin** (mak-sib′o-lin) trademark for a preparation of ethylestrenol.

**Max·i·flor** (mak′sĭ-flor″) trademark for preparations of diflorasone diacetate.

**max·il·la** (mak-sil'ə) pl. *maxillas,* gen. and pl. *maxil'lae* [L.] [TA] [MeSH: Maxilla] the irregularly shaped bone that with its fellow forms the upper jaw; it assists in the formation of the orbit, the nasal cavity, and the palate, and lodges the upper teeth.

**max·il·lae** (mak-sil'e) [L.] genitive and plural of *maxilla.*

**max·il·lary** (mak'sĭ-lar"e) [L. *maxillaris*] pertaining to the maxilla.

**max·il·lec·to·my** (mak"sĭ-lek'tə-me) surgical removal of the maxilla.

**max·il·li·tis** (mak"sĭ-li'tis) inflammation of the maxilla.

**max·il·lo·den·tal** (mak-sil"o-den'təl) pertaining to the maxilla and the maxillary teeth.

**max·il·lo·eth·moi·dec·to·my** (mak"sil-o-eth"moi-dek'tə-me) excision of the portion of the maxilla surrounding the maxillary sinus and of the cribriform plate and anterior ethmoid cells.

**max·il·lo·fa·cial** (mak-sil"o-fa'shəl) pertaining to the maxilla and the face.

**max·il·lo·ju·gal** (mak-sil"o-joo'gəl) jugomaxillary.

**max·il·lo·la·bi·al** (mak-sil"o-la'be-əl) pertaining to the maxilla and the lip.

**max·il·lo·man·dib·u·lar** (mak-sil"o-man-dib'u-lər) pertaining to the maxilla and the mandible.

**max·il·lo·pal·a·tine** (mak-sil"o-pal'ə-tēn) palatomaxillary.

**max·il·lo·pha·ryn·ge·al** (mak-sil"o-fə-rin'je-əl) pharyngomaxillary.

**max·il·lot·o·my** (mak"sĭ-lot'ə-me) surgical sectioning of the maxilla which allows movement of all or a part of the maxilla into the desired position.

**max·i·ma** (mak'sĭ-mə) [L.] plural of *maximum.*

**max·i·mal** (mak'sĭ-məl) the greatest possible, allowable, or appreciable; the reverse of *minimal.*

**max·i·mum** (mak'sĭ-məm) pl. *max'ima* [L. "greatest"] 1. the greatest possible or actual effect or quantity. 2. the acme of a disease or process. 3. largest; utmost. 4. Pirquet's term for the greatest quantity of food which the organism can digest.
**transport m. for glucose,** renal threshold for glucose.
**tubular m.,** the highest rate in milligrams per minute at which the renal tubules can transfer a substance either from the tubular luminal fluid to the interstitial fluid or from the interstitial fluid to the tubular luminal fluid. Abbreviated $T_m$.

**Max·i·pen** (mak'sĭ-pən) trademark for a preparation of phenethicillin potassium.

**Max·i·tate** (mak'sĭ-tāt) trademark for preparations of mannitol hexanitrate.

**Max·i·vate** (mak'sĭ-vāt) trademark for preparations of betamethasone dipropionate.

**Max·on** (mak'son) trademark for polyglyconate.

**Max·well's ring, spot** (maks'wəlz) [Patrick William *Maxwell,* Irish ophthalmologist, 1856–1917] see under *ring,* and see *macula lutea.*

**max·well** (maks'wəl) [James Clerk *Maxwell,* British physicist, 1831–1879] the unit of magnetic flux; replaced in SI by the *weber.*

**May-Hegg·lin anomaly** (mi heg'lin) [Richard *May,* German physician, 1863–1936; Robert Marquard *Hegglin,* Swiss physician, born 1907] see under *anomaly.*

**May-White syndrome** (ma-hwīt) [Duane L. *May,* American physician, 20th century; Harry H. *White,* American physician, born 1934] see under *syndrome.*

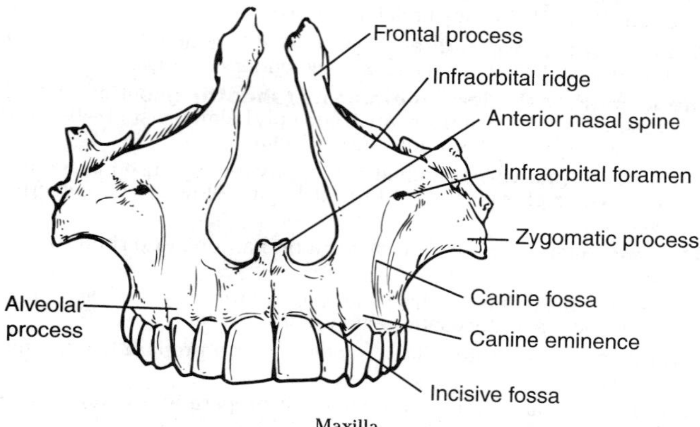


Maxilla.

**May·dl's operation** (mi'dəlz) [Karel *Maydl,* Czech surgeon, 1853–1903] see under *operation.*

**May·er's hemalum, mucihematein** (mi'erz) [Paul *Mayer,* German-Italian chemist, 1848–1923] see under *stain.*

**May·er's test** (ma'yərz) [Ferdinand F. *Mayer,* American pharmaceutical chemist, late 19th century] see under *test.*

**May·er-Ro·ki·tan·sky-Kü·ster-Hau·ser syndrome** (mi'er-ro-kĭ-tahn'ske-kē'ster-hou'zer) [August Franz Josef Karl *Mayer,* German physician, 1787–1865; Karl Freiherr von *Rokitansky,* Austrian pathologist, 1804 –1878; Hermann *Küster,* German gynecologist, early 20th century; G.A. *Hauser,* Swiss physician, 20th century] see under *syndrome.*

**may·er** (ma'yər) [Julius Robert von *Mayer,* German physicist, 1814–1878] a unit of heat capacity; it is the capacity of a body that is warmed one degree centigrade by one joule. Abbreviated my.

**may·fly** (ma'flī) any insect of the order Ephemeroptera.

**Ma·yo's operation** (ma'yōz) [William James *Mayo,* American surgeon, 1861–1939; Charles Horace *Mayo,* American surgeon, 1865–1939] see under *operation.*

**Ma·yo's vein** (ma'ōz) [William J. *Mayo*] vena prepylorica.

**Ma·yo Rob·son** see *Robson.*

**may·tan·sine** (ma-tan'sēn) [MeSH: Maytansine] an antineoplastic derived from species of *Maytenus,* a genus of tropical American shrubs and trees.

**may·weed** (ma'wēd) *Anthemis cotula.*

**maze** (māz) a complicated system of intersecting paths used in intelligence tests and in demonstrating learning in experimental animals.

**ma·zin·dol** (ma'zin-dol) [MeSH: Mazindol] an adrenergic having amphetamine-like actions; used as an anorexic in the short-term treatment of exogenous obesity, administered orally.

**maz(o)-** [Gr. *mazos* breast] a combining form denoting relationship to the breast; see also words beginning *mamm(o)-* and *mast(o)-.*

**ma·zo·dyn·ia** (ma"zo-din'e-ə) mastodynia.

**ma·zo·pexy** (ma'zo-pek"se) mastopexy.

**ma·zo·pla·sia** (ma"zo-pla'zhə) [*mazo-* + *-plasia*] degenerative epithelial hyperplasia of the mammary acini.

**Maz·zo·ni's corpuscle** (mad-zo'nēz) [Vittorio *Mazzoni,* Italian physiologist, 1880–1940] see under *corpuscle.*

**Maz·zot·ti test** (mə-zot'e) [Luis *Mazzotti,* Mexican parasitologist, 1900–1971] see under *reaction* and *test.*

**MB** abbreviation for L. *Medici'nae Baccalau'reus,* Bachelor of Medicine.

**Mb** symbol for *megabase.*

**m.b.** abbreviation for L. *mis'ce be'ne,* mix well.

**MBP** major basic protein; myelin basic protein.

**MBq** symbol for *megabecquerel.*

**mbun·du** (əm-boon'doo) [Umbundu language of Angola] a poison used in Angola, made from roots of trees of genus *Strychnos.*

**MC** abbreviation for L. *Magis'ter Chirur'giae,* Master of Surgery, and for *Medical Corps.*

**mC** symbol for *millicoulomb.*

**μC** symbol for *microcoulomb.*

**MCA** 3-methylcholanthrene.

**MCAD de·fi·cien·cy** medium-chain acyl-CoA dehydrogenase deficiency; see under *acyl-CoA dehydrogenase.*

**MCD** mean of consecutive differences.

**MCF** macrophage chemotactic factor.

**Mcg** an antigenic marker distinguishing human immunoglobulin λ light chain subtypes.

**mcg** symbol for *microgram.*

**MCH** mean corpuscular hemoglobin.

**MCHB** Maternal and Child Health Bureau, an agency of the Health Resources and Services Administration.

**MCHC** mean corpuscular hemoglobin concentration.

**MCi** symbol for *megacurie.*

**mCi** symbol for *millicurie.*

**μCi** symbol for *microcurie.*

**mCi-hr** millicurie-hour.

**MCI/MI** abbreviation for a mixture of methylchloroisothiazolinone and methylisothiazolinone; see *methylisothiazolinone.*

**MCMI** Millon Clinical Multiaxial Inventory.

**MCP** membrane cofactor protein.

**Mcps** megacycles per second.

**M-CSF** macrophage colony-stimulating factor.

**MCT** mean circulation time.

**MCV** mean corpuscular volume.

**MD** abbreviation for L. *Medici'nae Doc'tor,* Doctor of Medicine.

**Md** chemical symbol for *mendelevium.*

**MDA** methylenedioxyamphetamine; abbreviation for Latin *mento-dextro anterior* (right mentoanterior, a position of the fetus).

**MDF** myocardial depressant factor.

**MDMA** 3,4-methylenedioxymethamphetamine.

**MDP** [abbreviation for Latin] *mento-dextra posterior* (right mento-posterior, a position of the fetus); methylene diphosphonate (medronate, q.v.).

**MDS** myelodysplasia.

**MDT** [abbreviation for Latin] *mento-dextra transversa* (right mento-transverse, a position of the fetus).

**2-ME** 2-mercaptoethanol.

**Me** chemical symbol for *methyl,* or $CH_3$.

**meal** (mēl) a portion of food or foods taken at some particular and usually stated or fixed time. Often given with the specific purpose of aiding diagnostic examination. See also *test m.* (under *T*).
**Boyden m.,** see under *test m.*
**opaque m.,** a light meal that contains some substance opaque to x-rays, so that the outline of the stomach and the intestinal tract can be determined.
**retention m.,** a form of test meal which is retained, a specimen of the stomach contents being removed from time to time for analysis.
**test m.,** see under *T.*

**meal·worm** (mēl'wərm) 1. the larva of any of various grain beetles of the genus *Tenebrio,* which eat and contaminate grain products such as flour and are also raised as food for insectivorous domestic animals such as birds. Spelled also *meal worm.* 2. the larva of *Asopia farinalis.*

**mean** (mēn) [Old French *meien,* from L. *medianus* middle] 1. an average; a number that in some sense represents the central value of a set of numbers. 2. arithmetic m. 3. in probability and statistics, the expected value (mathematical expectation) of a random variable, the limiting value to which the sample mean converges as the sample size is increased indefinitely (if the limit exists).
**arithmetic m.,** the sum of *n* numbers divided by *n.*
**m. of consecutive differences (MCD),** the mean value of interpotential intervals when many readings are performed consecutively on the same pair of muscle fibers; see also *jitter.*
**geometric m.,** the *n*th root of the product of *n* numbers, e.g., the geometric mean of [2,8,32] is $(2 \times 8 \times 32)^{1/3} = 8$.
**harmonic m.,** reciprocal of the mean of the reciprocals of the individual values in a given set; e.g., for the set [10, 40, 60] the harmonic mean is $1 \div [\frac{1}{3}(\frac{1}{10} + \frac{1}{40} + \frac{1}{60})] = 21.2$.
**population m.,** the mean of the probability distribution characterizing a specified population; for a finite population, the arithmetic mean of the population values. Symbol $\mu$.
**sample m.,** the arithmetic mean of the observed values of a random sample, conventionally denoted by a barred variable, e.g., $\bar{X}$; (read "X bar").

**Mean's sign** (mēnz) [James Howard *Mean,* American endocrinologist, 1885–1967] Kocher's sign.

**mea·sles** (me'zəlz) [MeSH: Measles] 1. a highly contagious viral disease caused by a paramyxovirus, common among children but also seen in the nonimmune of any age. The virus enters the respiratory tract via droplet nuclei, multiplies in the epithelial cells, and spreads throughout the reticuloendothelial system, producing lymphoid hyperplasia, often with characteristic Warthin-Finkeldey giant cells. The skin eruption is usually preceded by coryza, cervical lymphadenitis, Koplik's spots, palpebral conjunctivitis, photophobia, myalgia, malaise, cough, and steadily mounting fever. The typical rash consists of generalized maculopapular lesions that are at first discrete but gradually become confluent, starting behind the ears and on the face and progressing rapidly down the trunk and onto the extremities. Although measles is usually benign, complications may sometimes occur, including secondary bacterial infections such as otitis media, pneumonia, or laryngitis; a rare, fatal giant cell pneumonia, often without a rash, in immunocompromised children; and rarely, subacute sclerosing panencephalitis that may develop years after an initial measles infection. Called also *morbilli* and *rubeola.* 2. cysticercal disease of domestic animals.
**atypical m.,** a severe form of measles occurring after exposure to wild measles virus in those who previously received inactivated (killed) measles vaccine, which was only available in the United States from 1963 to 1967, and in some cases live attenuated measles vaccine. It is characterized by fever, headache, myalgia, abdominal symptoms, and cough, followed by an atypical rash, which may be urticarial, vesicular, petechial, or maculopapular, on the wrists and ankles, and spreading to the palms, soles, and trunk before fading, and may be associated with peripheral edema, interstitial pulmonary infiltrates, and pleural effusion. Koplik spots are absent.
**beef m.,** cysticercosis in cattle.
**black m.,** a rare, severe, often fatal, form of measles in which hemorrhage into the skin lesions and mucous membranes is associated with a sudden rise in temperature, convulsions, delirium, stupor, coma, and marked respiratory distress. Called also *hemorrhagic m.*
**German m.,** rubella.
**hemorrhagic m.,** black m.
**pork m.,** cysticercosis in pigs.
**sheep m.,** cysticercosis in sheep.
**three-day m.,** rubella.

**mea·sly** (me'zle) said of meat that contains cysticerci, because of its speckled appearance.

**meas·ure** (mezh'ər) [L. *mensurare*] [MeSH: Weights and Measures] 1. to determine the extent or quantity of a substance. 2. a specific extent or quantity of a substance. 3. a graduated scale by which the dimensions or mass of an object or substance may be determined. See tables of weights and measures (Appendix 11).

**me·a·tal** (me-a'təl) pertaining to a meatus.

**me·a·tome** (me'ə-tōm) meatotome.

**me·a·tom·e·ter** (me″ə-tom'ə-tər) [L. *meatus* passage + *metrum* measure] an instrument for measuring the urinary meatus.

**me·a·to·plas·ty** (me-at'o-plas″te) plastic surgery of a meatus, such as an acoustic meatus.

**me·a·tor·rha·phy** (me″ə-tor'ə-fe) [L. *meatus* + Gr. *rhaphē* suture] suture of the cut end of the urethra to the glans penis after incision for enlarging the meatus.

**me·ato·scope** (me-at'ə-skōp) [L. *meatus* meatus + Gr. *skopein* to examine] a speculum for examining the urinary meatus.

**me·a·tos·co·py** (me″ə-tos'kə-pe) the inspection of any meatus, especially the urinary meatus.
**ureteral m.,** cystoscopic inspection of the vesical orifice of a ureter.

**me·ato·tome** (me-at'ə-tōm) an instrument for performing meatotomy.

**me·a·tot·o·my** (me″ə-tot'ə-me) [L. *meatus* passage + Gr. *temnein* to cut] incision of the urinary meatus in order to enlarge it.

**me·a·tus** (me-a'təs) pl. *mea'tus* [L., "a way, path, course"] [TA] a general term for an opening or passageway in the body.
**acoustic m., bony external,** m. acusticus externus osseus.
**acoustic m., bony internal,** m. acusticus internus.
**acoustic m., cartilaginous external,** m. acusticus externus cartilagineus.
**acoustic m., external,** m. acusticus externus.
**acoustic m., internal,** m. acusticus internus.
**m. acus'ticus exter'nus** [TA], external acoustic meatus: the passage of the external ear leading to the tympanic membrane, divided into an outer cartilaginous meatus and an inner bony meatus. Called also *external auditory m.* or *canal* and *m. auditorius externus.*
**m. acus'ticus exter'nus cartilagi'neus** [TA], cartilaginous external acoustic meatus: the cartilaginous part of the external acoustic meatus, found lateral to the bony part.

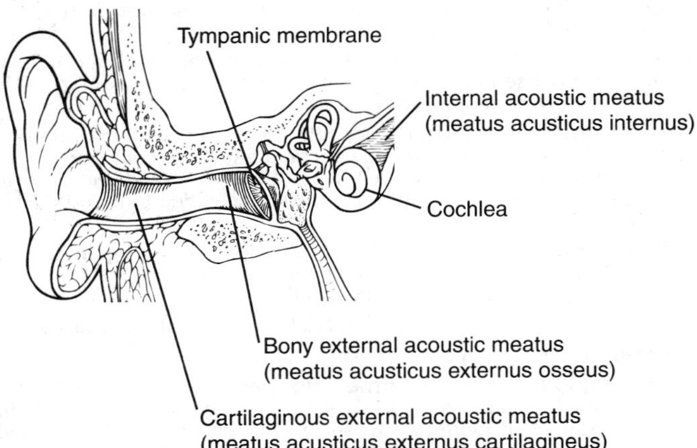

**m. acus'ticus exter'nus os'seus,** bony external acoustic meatus: the opening in the external surface of the temporal bone, posterior to the condyle of the mandible and anterior to the mastoid air cells.
**m. acus'ticus inter'nus** [TA], internal acoustic meatus: the passage in the petrous portion of the temporal bone through which the facial, intermediate, and vestibulocochlear nerves and the labyrinthine artery pass. Called also *internal auditory m.* or *canal* and *m. auditorius internus.*
**m. acus'ticus inter'nus os'seus,** m. acusticus internus.
**m. audito'rius exter'nus,** m. acusticus externus.
**m. audito'rius exter'nus cartilagi'neus,** m. acusticus externus cartilagineus.
**m. audito'rius exter'nus os'seus,** m. acusticus externus osseus.
**m. audito'rius inter'nus,** m. acusticus internus.
**auditory m., bony external,** m. acusticus externus osseus.
**auditory m., bony internal,** m. acusticus internus.
**auditory m., cartilaginous external,** m. acusticus externus cartilagineus.
**auditory m., external,** m. acusticus externus.
**auditory m., internal,** m. acusticus internus.
**fish-mouth m.,** a red, swollen, and everted urinary meatus seen in the first stage of acute gonorrhea.
**inferior m. of nose,** m. nasi inferior.
**middle m. of nose,** m. nasi medius.
**nasal m., inferior,** m. nasi inferior.
**nasal m., middle,** m. nasi medius.
**nasal m., superior,** m. nasi superior.
**m. na'si infe'rior** [TA], inferior meatus of nose: the space beneath the inferior nasal concha, into which the nasolacrimal duct opens.

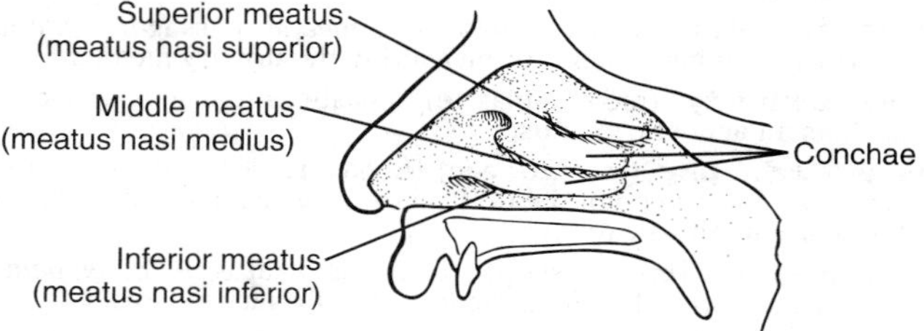


**m. na'si me'dius** [TA], middle meatus of nose: the space beneath the middle nasal concha, with which the anterior ethmoidal cells and frontal and maxillary sinuses communicate.
**m. na'si supe'rior** [TA], superior meatus of nose: the narrow cavity below the superior nasal concha, with which the posterior ethmoidal cells communicate.
**m. nasopharyn'geus** [TA], nasopharyngeal meatus: the part of the nasal cavity coinciding with the bony nasopharyngeal cavity.
**m. of nose,** see *m. nasi inferior, m. nasi medius,* and *m. nasi superior.*
**superior m. of nose,** m. nasi superior.
**m. urina'rius,** urinary meatus: the external urethral orifice; the opening of the urethra on the body surface through which urine is discharged. See *ostium urethrae externum feminina* and *ostium urethrae externum masculinae.*

**Me·ban** (me'ban) trademark for a preparation of dehydroemetine.

**Meb·a·ral** (meb'ə-rəl) trademark for a preparation of mephobarbital.

**me·ben·da·zole** (mə-ben'də-zōl) [USP] [MeSH: Mebendazole] a versatile benzimidazole anthelmintic agent that irreversibly inhibits glucose uptake in the parasite, causing immobilization and death; used in the treatment of infections in humans and dogs by *Ascaris lumbricoides, Enterobius vermicularis, Trichuris trichiura,* hookworm species, and *Capillaria philippinensis.*

**me·bev·er·ine hy·dro·chlo·ride** (mə-bev'ər-ēn) a smooth muscle relaxant, used as an antispasmodic in the treatment of irritable bowel syndrome; administered orally.

**me·bro·fen·in** (me'bro-fen"in) [USP] BrIDA; a trimethyl-bromine–substituted analogue of iminodiacetic acid (IDA); complexed with technetium 99m it is used for hepatobiliary imaging and hepatic function studies; administered intravenously. See table at *technetium.*

**me·bu·ta·mate** (mə-bu'tə-māt) a mildly tranquilizing antihypertensive agent used alone or in conjunction with diuretics and other hypotensive drugs, administered orally.

**Mec·a·dox** (mek'ə-doks) trademark for a preparation of carbadox.

**mec·amine** (mek'ə-mēn) mecamylamine.

**mec·a·myl·amine hy·dro·chlo·ride** (mek"ə-mil'ə-mēn) [USP] a ganglionic-blocking agent used as an antihypertensive, usually in the treatment of moderate to severe hypertension; administered orally.

**MeCbl** methylcobalamin.

**meCCNU** semustine.

**me·chan·i·cal** (mə-kan'ĭ-kəl) [Gr. *mēchanikos*] 1. pertaining to or accomplished by mechanical or physical forces. 2. performed by means of some artificial mechanism.

**me·chan·i·co·re·cep·tor** (mə-kan"ĭ-ko-re-sep'tor) mechanoreceptor.

**me·chan·i·co·ther·a·peu·tics, me·chan·i·co·ther·a·py** (mə-kan"ĭ-ko-ther"ə-pu'tiks, mə-kan"ĭ-ko-ther'ə-pe) mechanotherapy.

**me·chan·ics** (mə-kan'iks) [MeSH: Mechanics] the science dealing with the motions of material bodies, including kinematics, dynamics, and statics.
**animal m.,** biomechanics.
**body m.,** the application of kinesiology to use of the body in daily life activities and to the prevention and correction of problems related to posture.
**developmental m.,** embryological mechanisms as revealed mainly by experimentation.

**mech·a·nism** (mek'ə-niz-əm) [Gr. *mēchanē* machine] 1. a machine or machine-like structure. 2. the manner of combination of parts, processes, etc., which subserve a common function. 3. the theory that the phenomena of life are based on the same physical and chemical laws which operate in the inorganic world; opposed to *vitalism.*
**countercurrent m.,** the renal mechanism by which urine is concentrated; it is dependent upon unique solute transport processes and a specific anatomical arrangement of the loops of Henle and the vasa recta.
**defense m.,** a usually unconscious mental process that serves to relieve conflict and anxiety arising from one's impulses and drives, e.g., compensation, conversion, denial, rationalization, repression.
**double-displacement m.,** ping-pong m.
**Duncan m.,** expulsion of the placenta with the maternal, or rough, surface appearing at the vulva.
**escape m.,** in the heart, the mechanism of impulse initiation by lower centers, such as the atrioventricular node, in response to lack of impulse propagation by the sinoatrial node.
**Frank-Starling m.,** Starling's law of the heart.
**m. of labor,** the factors involved in the expulsion of the fetus, placenta, and membranes through the birth canal in labor.
**leading circle m.,** see under *model.*
**mental m.,** an unconscious process, such as a defense mechanism, memory, perception, or thinking, that is a function of the ego and determines behavior.
**oculogyric m.,** the series of nerve centers concerned in movements of the eye.
**ping-pong m.,** in an enzyme-catalyzed reaction, the dissociation of one or more products from the enzyme complex before all substrates have been bound; binding may occur in a fixed order or may be random. Cf. *sequential m.*
**reentrant m.,** the mechanism by which a locus of unidirectional block to conduction in cardiac muscle can result in ectopic beats or tachyarrhythmias. In addition to the block, also required are at least areas of slow conduction and refractoriness of the tissue to stimulation. Conduction of a normally initiated impulse is delayed by the block long enough for normal surrounding tissue to repolarize and to be reexcited by the delayed impulse; this may begin a self-perpetuating series of abnormal conduction cycles. See also *ring model, leading circle model,* and *figure-of-eight model,* under *model,* and *reentry.*
**Schultze m.,** expulsion of the placenta with the smooth, glistening, fetal surface appearing at the vulva; this is considered normal and is more common than the Duncan mechanism.
**sequential m.,** in an enzyme-catalyzed reaction, the binding of the enzyme by all substrates, forming a complex, prior to the release of any products; binding may occur in a fixed order or may be random. Cf. *ping-pong m.*
**Starling m.,** see under *law.*

**mech·a·nist** (mek'ə-nist) one who believes that all phenomena relating to life are based on physical and chemical properties only.

**mechan(o)-** [Gr. *mēchanē* machine] a combining form meaning mechanical, or denoting relationship to a machine, to physical forces, or to mechanics.

**mech·a·no·cyte** (mek'ə-no-sīt") [*mechano-* + *-cyte*] fibroblast.

**mech·a·nol·o·gy** (mek"ə-nol'ə-je) [*mechano-* + *-logy*] the science of mechanics.

**mech·a·no·re·cep·tor** (mek"ə-no-re-sep'tor) [MeSH: Mechanoreceptors] a receptor that is excited by mechanical pressures or distortions, as those responding to sound, touch, and muscular contractions. Specific types are variously called *corpuscles, nerve endings,* and *receptors.* See also *rapidly-adapting receptor, slowly-adapting receptor,* and *nonadapting receptor,* under *receptor.*
**high-threshold m.,** mechanical nociceptor.

**me·cha·no·sen·so·ry** (mek″ə-no-sen′sə-re) pertaining to sensory activation in response to mechanical pressures or distortions; cf. *mechanoreceptor.*

**mech·a·no·ther·a·py** (mek″ə-no-ther′ə-pe) [*mechano-* + *-therapy*] the use of mechanical apparatus in the treatment of disease or its results, especially as an aid in performing therapeutic exercises.

**mech·a·no·ther·my** (mek″ə-no-ther′me) [*mechano-* + Gr. *thermē* heat] therapeutic heat produced by massage, exercise, etc.

**mech·lor·eth·amine hy·dro·chlo·ride** (mek″lor-eth′ə-mēn) [USP] a cytotoxic alkylating agent of the nitrogen mustard group, used primarily for the treatment of disseminated Hodgkin's disease, especially in the MOPP (q.v.) treatment regimen, administered intravenously; it is also used in the treatment of chronic lymphocytic and chronic myelocytic leukemia, non-Hodgkin's lymphoma, mycosis fungoides, polycythemia vera, and bronchogenic carcinoma. Mechlorethamine is also administered intraperitoneally, intrapericardially, and intrapleurally for the palliative treatment of malignant effusion and has been applied topically in the treatment of mycosis fungoides. Called also *HN2* and *nitrogen mustard.*

**Mech·ni·kov** (mech′nĭ-kov″) see *Metchnikoff.*

**me·cil·li·nam** (mə-sil′ĭ-nəm) amdinocillin.

**me·cism** (me′siz-əm) [Gr. *mēkos* length] abnormal lengthening of a part.

**me·cis·to·ce·phal·ic** (me-sis″to-sə-fal′ik) [Gr. *mēkistos* tallest + *cephalic*] having a cephalic index less than 71.

**me·cis·to·ceph·a·lous** (me-sis″to-sef′ə-ləs) mecistocephalic.

**Me·cis·to·cir·rus** (me-sis″to-sir′əs) a genus of nematodes of the family Trichostrongylidae. *M. digita′lis* is a parasite found in the abomasum of various ruminants, in the stomach of pigs, and occasionally in the stomach of humans.

**Meck·el's band (ligament), ganglion, space** (mek′elz) [Johann Friedrich *Meckel* (the elder), German anatomist, 1724–1774] see under *band,* and see *cavum trigeminale, ganglion pterygopalatinum,* and *ganglion submandibulare.*

**Meck·el's cartilage (rod), diverticulum, plane, syndrome** (mek′elz) [Johann Friedrich *Meckel* (the younger) (grandson of J. F. Meckel, the elder), German anatomist, 1781–1833] see under *cartilage, diverticulum, plane,* and *syndrome.*

**Mec·lan** (mek′lan) trademark for a preparation of meclocycline sulfosalicylate.

**mec·li·zine hy·dro·chlo·ride** (mek′lĭ-zēn) [USP] an antihistamine used as an antiemetic in the management of nausea, vomiting, and dizziness associated with motion sickness, administered orally.

**mec·lo·cy·cline sul·fo·sal·i·cyl·ate** (mek″lo-si′klēn) [USP] a tetracycline antibiotic used for the treatment of acne vulgaris; applied topically.

**me·clo·fen·am·ate** (mə-klo″fən-am′āt) the conjugate base of meclofenamic acid; used as *meclofenamate sodium* for treatment of osteoarthritis and rheumatoid arthritis.

**me·clo·fen·am·ic ac·id** (mə-klo″fən-am′ik) [MeSH: Meclofenamic Acid] a nonsteroidal anti-inflammatory agent of the fenamate class.

**me·clo·fen·ox·ate** (mə-klo″fən-oks′āt) [MeSH: Meclofenoxate] a drug claimed to aid cellular metabolism in the presence of diminished oxygen concentrations.

**Me·clo·men** (mə-klo′mən) trademark for preparations of meclofenamate sodium.

**me·co·bal·amine** (me″ko-bal′ə-mēn) a naturally occurring hematopoietic vitamin found in the blood, closely related to cyanocobalamin, in which the cyano radical has been replaced by a methyl radical.

**me·co·ce·phal·ic** (me″ko-sə-fal′ik) [Gr. *mēkos* length + *cephalic*] dolichocephalic.

**meco·nate** (mek′o-nāt) [Gr. *mēkōn* poppy + *-ate*] any salt of meconic acid.

**me·con·ic ac·id** (mə-kon′ik) an acid occurring in opium that forms soluble salts with the opiates.

**me·co·ni·or·rhea** (mə-ko″ne-o-re′ə) [*meconium* + *-rrhea*] excessive discharge of meconium.

**me·co·ni·um** (mə-ko′ne-əm) [L.; Gr. *mēkōnion*] [MeSH: Meconium] a dark green mucilaginous material in the intestine of the full-term fetus, being a mixture of the secretions of the liver, intestinal glands, and some amniotic fluid.

**me·cryl·ate** (mə-kril′-āt) a type of cyanoacrylate adhesive used in surgery.

**me·cys·ta·sis** (mə-sis′tə-sis) [Gr. *mēkynein* to lengthen + *stasis*] a state in which a muscle fiber is relatively increased in length, resists stretch, contracts, and relaxes, and manifests the same tension as before elongation.

**MED** minimal effective dose; minimal erythema dose.

**Med·a·war** (med′ə-wər) Peter Brian. Brazilian-born British biologist, 1915–1987; co-winner, with Sir Frank Macfarlane Burnet, of the Nobel prize for medicine or physiology in 1960 for his discovery of the mechanism of acquired immunological tolerance.

**Med·ex** (med′eks) [Fr. *médecin extension* extension of the physician] a program that recruits former military medics for training and practice as physician assistants; abbreviated Mx.

**me·dia** (me′de-ə) [L.] 1. plural of *medium.* 2. middle. 3. tunica media vasorum.

**me·di·ad** (me′de-əd) [*medium* + *-ad*[1]] toward a median line or plane.

**me·di·al** (me′de-əl) [L. *medialis*] 1. pertaining to the middle; closer to the median plane or the midline of a body or structure. 2. pertaining to the middle layer of structures.

**me·di·a·lec·i·thal** (me″de-ə-les′ĭ-thəl) [*media-* + *-lecithal*] possessing a medium amount of yolk; see under *ovum.*

**me·di·a·lis** (me″de-a′lis) [TA] medial; a general term denoting a structure situated nearer to the median plane or the midline of a body or structure.

**me·di·an** (me′de-ən) [L. *medianus*] 1. situated in the median plane or in the midline of a body or structure. 2. any value that divides the probability distribution of a random variable in half, i.e., the probability of observing a value above the median and the probability of observing a value below the median are both less than or equal to one half. For a finite population or sample, the median is the middle value of an odd number of values (arranged in ascending order) or any value between the two middle values of an even number of values; in the latter case it is conventional to use the average of the two middle values.

**me·di·a·nus** (me″de-a′nəs) [L.] [TA] median, or situated in the middle; a general term denoting structures lying in the median plane.

**me·di·a·om·e·ter** (me″de-ə-om′ə-tər) [*media* + *-meter*] an instrument for detecting and measuring refractive errors of the dioptric media.

**me·di·as·ti·na** (me″de-əs-ti′nə) [L.] plural of *mediastinum.*

**me·di·as·ti·nal** (me″de-əs-ti′nəl) [L. *mediastinalis*] of or pertaining to the mediastinum.

**me·di·as·ti·ni·tis** (me″de-as″tĭ-ni′tis) [MeSH: Mediastinitis] inflammation of the mediastinum.
**acute m.,** an often fatal inflammation of the mediastinum, with sudden onset of chills, fever, and prostration. Other symptoms are severe chest pain and sometimes tachypnea, tachycardia, pneumomediastinum, and hemomediastinum. It is usually secondary to perforation of the esophagus by forceful vomiting or trauma; less often it may be caused by spread of an infectious process from some adjacent organ or area. There may be obstruction of structures in the area, such as the superior vena cava or the tracheobronchial tree.
**chronic m.,** any of numerous inflammatory conditions of the mediastinum, often secondary to a fungal or tuberculous infection; symptoms may be minimal or the result of obstruction of structures in the area. The most common specific condition is mediastinal fibrosis.
**fibrosing m., fibrous m.,** mediastinal fibrosis.
**granulomatous m.,** mediastinal fibrosis with granulomas.
**indurative m.,** mediastinal fibrosis.

**me·di·as·ti·no·gram** (me″de-əs-tĭ′no-gram) a radiograph of the mediastinum.

**me·di·as·ti·nog·ra·phy** (me″de-as″tĭ-nog′rə-fe) radiography of the mediastinum.

**me·di·as·ti·no·peri·car·di·tis** (me″de-as″tĭ-no-per″e-kahr-di′tis) adhesive pericarditis in which the adhesions extend from the pericardium to the mediastinum. See also *adhesive pericarditis,* under *pericarditis.*
**adhesive m.,** mediastinopericarditis.

**me·di·a·sti·no·scope** (me″de-ə-sti′no-skōp) a specially designed endoscope used in mediastinoscopy.

**me·di·as·ti·no·scop·ic** (me″de-as″tĭ-no-skop′ik) pertaining to the mediastinoscope or to mediastinoscopy.

**me·di·as·ti·nos·co·py** (me″de-as″tĭ-nos′kə-pe) [MeSH: Mediastinoscopy] examination of the mediastinum by means of an endoscope inserted through an anterior incision in the suprasternal notch, permitting direct inspection and biopsy of tissue in the anterior superior mediastinum.

**me·di·as·ti·not·o·my** (me″de-as″tĭ-not′ə-me) [*mediastinum* +

-*tomy*] the operation of cutting into the mediastinum. Performed from the front, it is *anterior* or *cervical mediastinotomy;* from the back, *posterior* or *dorsal mediastinotomy.*

**me·di·as·ti·num** (me″de-ə-s-ti′nəm) pl. *mediasti′na* [L.] [MeSH: Mediastinum] 1. a median septum or partition. 2. [TA] the mass of tissues and organs separating the two pleural sacs, between the sternum anteriorly and the vertebral column posteriorly and from the thoracic inlet superiorly to the diaphragm inferiorly. It contains the heart and pericardium, the bases of the great vessels, the trachea and bronchi, esophagus, thymus, lymph nodes, thoracic duct, phrenic and vagus nerves, and other structures and tissues. The mediastinum is divided into a superior region and an inferior region that comprises anterior, middle, and posterior parts.
**m. ante′rius** [TA], anterior mediastinum: the division of the mediastinum bounded posteriorly by the pericardium, anteriorly by the sternum, and on each side by the pleura. It contains loose areolar tissue and lymphatic vessels. Called also *anterior mediastinal cavity.*
**m. infe′rius** [TA], inferior mediastinum: the three inferior portions of the mediastinum, comprising the *m. anterius, m. medium,* and *m. posterius;* see also *mediastinum* (def. 2).
**m. me′dium** [TA], middle mediastinum: the division of the mediastinum containing the heart enclosed in its pericardium, the ascending aorta, the superior vena cava, the bifurcation of the trachea into bronchi, the pulmonary arteries and veins, the phrenic nerves, a large portion of the roots of the lungs, and the arch of the azygos vein. Called also *middle mediastinal cavity.*
**m. poste′rius** [TA], posterior mediastinum: the division of the mediastinum bounded posteriorly by the vertebral column, anteriorly by the pericardium, and on each side by the pleurae. It contains the descending aorta, parts of the greater and lesser azygos and superior intercostal veins, the thoracic duct, the esophagus, the vagus nerves, and the greater splanchnic nerves. Called also *posterior mediastinal cavity.*
**m. supe′rius** [TA], superior mediastinum: the division of the mediastinum extending from the pericardium to the root of the neck, and containing the esophagus and the trachea posteriorly, the thymus or its remains anteriorly, and the great vessels related to the heart and pericardium, the thoracic duct, and the vagus nerves in between. Called also *superior mediastinal cavity.*
**m. tes′tis** [TA], the partial septum of the testis, formed near its posterior border by fibrous tissue which is continuous with the tunica albuginea; called also *body of Highmore.*

**me·di·ate** (me′de-ət, me′de-āt) indirect; accomplished by the aid of an intervening medium.

**me·di·a·tion** (me″de-a′shən) the act of interposing or serving as an intermediary.
**chemical m.**, in neurophysiology, the intervention by a chemical substance (neurotransmitter) in the passing of an action potential from a presynaptic to a postsynaptic element.

**me·di·a·tor** (me′de-a″tor) an object or substance by which something is mediated, such as (1) a structure of the nervous system that transmits impulses eliciting a specific response; (2) a chemical substance (neurotransmitter) that induces activity in an excitable tissue, such as nerve or muscle; or (3) a substance released from cells as the result of the interaction of antigen with antibody or by the action of antigen with a sensitized lymphocyte.

**med·i·ca·ble** (med′ĭ-kə-bəl) subject to treatment with reasonable expectation of cure.

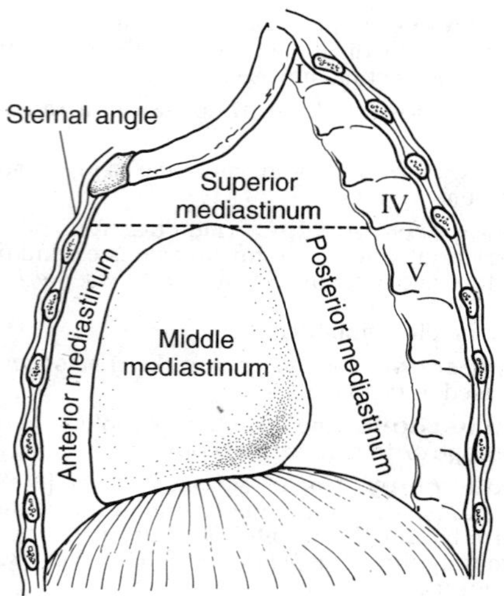

Subdivisions of the mediastinum.

**Med·i·ca·go** (med″ĭ-ka′go) a genus of grasses of the family Leguminosae. *M. polymor′pha* (also called *M. denticula′ta*) is the burr trefoil, which is often used as hay for livestock but sometimes causes the condition called trefoil dermatitis. *M. sati′va* is alfalfa, which is commonly used as hay for livestock; certain strains of it can cause photosensitization, primary ruminal tympany (frothy bloat), or other conditions.

**med·i·cal** (med′ĭ-kəl) pertaining to medicine or to the treatment of diseases; pertaining to medicine as opposed to surgery.

**med·i·ca·ment** (med′ĭ-kə-mənt, mə-dik′ə-mənt) [L. *medicamentum*] a medicinal substance or agent.

**med·i·ca·men·to·sus** (med″ĭ-kə-mən-to′səs) [L.] medicamentous.

**med·i·ca·men·tous** (med″ĭ-kə-men′təs) pertaining to, used in, or caused by a drug or drugs.

**Med·i·care** (med′ĭ-kār) [MeSH: Medicare] a program administered by the Social Security Administration which provides medical care for the aged.

**med·i·cate** (med′ĭ-kāt) [L. *medicatus*] to impregnate or imbue with a medicinal substance.

**med·i·cat·ed** (med′ĭ-kāt″əd) imbued with a medicinal substance.

**med·i·ca·tion** (med″ĭ-ka′shən) [L. *medicatio*] 1. a drug or medicine. 2. impregnation with a medicine. 3. the administration of remedies.
**conservative m.**, treatment not considered to be aggressive in nature.
**dialytic m.**, treatment by the internal use of artificial mineral waters, i.e., dilute aqueous solutions of salts.
**hypodermic m.**, the introduction of remedial agents beneath the skin.
**ionic m.**, iontophoresis.
**sublingual m.**, the administration of medicine by placing it beneath the tongue.
**substitutive m.**, medication for the purpose of causing an acute nonspecific inflammation to overcome a specific one.
**transduodenal m.**, the administration of medicine through a duodenal tube into the intestines without soiling the stomach.

**med·i·ca·tor** (med′ĭ-ka″tor) an instrument for carrying medicines into a cavity of the body; an applicator.

**me·dic·i·nal** (mə-dis′ĭ-nəl) [L. *medicinalis*] 1. having healing qualities. 2. pertaining to a medicine or to healing.

**med·i·cine** (med′ĭ-sin) [L. *medicina*] [MeSH: Medicine] 1. any drug or remedy. 2. the art and science of the diagnosis and treatment of disease and the maintenance of health. 3. the treatment of disease by nonsurgical means.
**aviation m.**, that branch of medicine which has to do with the physiological, medical, psychological, and epidemiological problems involved in aviation.
**behavioral m.**, a segment of psychosomatic medicine focussed on psychological means of influencing physical symptoms, such as biofeedback or relaxation.
**clinical m.**, 1. the study of disease by direct examination of the living patient. 2. the last two years of the usual curriculum in a medical college.
**comparative m.**, the study of phenomena basic to the diseases of all species.
**compound m.**, a medicine containing a mixture of several drugs.
**dosimetric m.**, the practice of administering medicines by an exact and determinate system of doses.
**emergency m.**, that specialty which deals with acutely ill or injured patients who require immediate medical treatment.
**environmental m.**, that which considers the effects of the environment on human beings, including such factors as rapid population growth, changes and extremes in temperature, alterations in atmospheric pressure, water pollution, air pollution, radiation, and travel.
**emporiac m.**, the subspecialty of tropical medicine consisting of the diagnosis and treatment or prevention of diseases of travelers. Called also *travelers′ m.*
**experimental m.**, the study of disease based on experimentation in animals.
**family m.**, see under *practice.*
**folk m.**, the use of home remedies and procedures as handed down by tradition.
**forensic m.**, that branch of medicine dealing with the application of medical knowledge to the purposes of law. This term and medical jurisprudence are sometimes used as synonyms, but some authorities consider the first as a branch of medicine and the second as a branch of law. Called also *legal m.*
**galenic m.**, an absolute system of practice based upon the teachings of Galen.
**geographic m.**, 1. geomedicine. 2. tropical m.
**geriatric m.**, geriatrics.
**group m.**, the practice of medicine by a group of physicians, usually

representing various specialties, who are associated together for the cooperative diagnosis, treatment, and prevention of disease. Called also *group practice.*
**hermetic m.,** see *spagyric m.*
**holistic m.,** a system of medicine which considers man as an integrated whole, or as a functioning unit.
**hyperbaric m.,** the treatment of disease in an environment of higher than atmospheric pressure.
**internal m.,** the medical specialty dealing especially with the diagnosis and medical treatment of diseases and disorders of the internal structures of the human body.
**ionic m.,** treatment by electrochemical means, as by cataphoresis and iontophoresis.
**laboratory animal m.,** a specialty of veterinary medicine that deals with the diagnosis, treatment, and prevention of disease in animals used as subjects in biomedical activities.
**legal m.,** forensic m.
**neo-hippocratic m.,** neo-hippocratism.
**nuclear m.,** that branch of medicine concerned with the use of radionuclides in the diagnosis and treatment of disease.
**occupational m.,** that branch of medicine dealing with the study, prevention, and treatment of workplace injuries and occupational diseases and with the promotion of optimal health and safety in the workplace.
**oral m.,** dentistry.
**patent m.,** a drug or remedy protected by a trademark, available without prescription.
**physical m.,** physiatry.
**preclinical m.,** 1. the first two years of the usual curriculum in a medical college. 2. preventive m.
**preventive m.,** that branch of study and practice which aims at the prevention of disease and the promotion of health.
**proprietary m.,** a drug or remedy to which the manufacturing pharmaceutical house has exclusive (proprietary) rights, and which is marketed usually under a name that is registered as a trademark.
**psychosomatic m.,** a system of medicine which aims at discovering the nature of the relationship of the emotions and bodily function, affirming the principle that the mind and body are one, as well as emphasizing psychosocial aspects of medical care.
**rational m.,** practice of medicine based upon actual knowledge; opposed to *empiricism.*
**rehabilitation m.,** the branch of physiatrics concerned with restoration of form and function after injury or illness.
**social m.,** phases of preventive medicine and the care of the sick which concern the community as a whole or large groups of persons rather than the individual.
**socialized m.,** a system of medical care regulated and controlled by the government, in which the government assumes responsibility for providing for the health needs and hospital care of the entire population, at no direct cost or at a nominal fee to the individual, by means of subsidies obtained by taxation. Called also *state m.*
**space m.,** that branch of aviation medicine concerned solely with conditions to be encountered by man in space.
**spagyric m.,** *(obs.),* semialchemistic system of practice established by Paracelsus (1493–1541).
**sports m.,** the field of medicine concerned with injuries sustained in athletic endeavors, including their prevention, diagnosis, and treatment.
**state m.,** socialized m.
**travelers' m.,** emporiac m.
**tropical m.,** medical science as applied to diseases occurring primarily in tropical and subtropical countries. Sometimes called *geographic m.* because diseases of interest to tropical medicine specialists may also occur in developing countries or areas in the temperate climate zones.
**veterinary m.,** a medical specialty consisting of the diagnosis and treatment of diseases of animals other than humans.

**med·i·co·chi·rur·gic** (med″ĭ-ko-ki-rur′jik) pertaining to medicine and surgery.

**med·i·co·den·tal** (med″ĭ-ko-den′təl) pertaining to both medicine and dentistry.

**med·i·co·le·gal** (med″ĭ-ko-le′gəl) pertaining to medicine and law, or to forensic medicine.

**med·i·co·me·chan·i·cal** (med″ĭ-ko-mə-kan′ĭ-kəl) both medicinal and mechanical.

**med·i·co·so·cial** (med″ĭ-ko-so′shəl) having both medical and social aspects, as, for example, the prevention and treatment of venereal disease.

**med·i·co·topo·graph·i·cal** (med″ĭ-ko-top″o-graf′ĭ-kəl) pertaining to topography in its relation to disease.

**med·i·co·zoo·log·i·cal** (med″ĭ-ko-zo-o-loj′ĭ-kəl) pertaining to zoology in its relation to medicine.

**me·di·fron·tal** (me″dĭ-fron′təl) median and frontal; pertaining to the middle of the forehead.

**Me·din's disease** (ma′dēnz) [Oskar *Medin,* Swedish pediatrician, 1847–1927] see *poliomyelitis.*

**me·dio·car·pal** (me″de-o-kahr′pəl) midcarpal.

**me·di·oc·cip·i·tal** (me″de-ok-sip′ĭ-təl) midoccipital.

**me·dio·lat·er·al** (me″de-o-lat′ər-əl) [L. *medius* middle + *lateral*] pertaining to the middle and to one side.

**me·dio·ne·cro·sis** (me″de-o-nə-kro′sis) necrosis of the tunica media of a blood vessel, often leading to its rupture.
**m. of aorta,** cystic medial necrosis.

**me·dio·tar·sal** (me″de-o-tahr′səl) [L. *medius* middle + *tarsal*] pertaining to the middle of the tarsus.

**Med·i·pren** (med′ĭ-pren″) trademark for a preparation of ibuprofen.

**me·di·sca·le·nus** (me″de-skə-le′nəs) musculus scalenus medius.

**me·di·sect** (me′dĭ-sekt) [L. *medius* middle + *secare* to cut] to divide or dissect medially.

**med·i·ta·tion** (med″ĭ-ta′shən) [MeSH: Meditation] the act of reflecting upon or contemplating; an exercise in contemplation.
**transcendental m.,** a technique for attaining a state of physical relaxation and psychological calm by the regular practice of a relaxation procedure which entails the repetition of a mantra.

**me·di·um** (me′de-əm) pl. *mediums* or *me′dia* [L. "middle"] 1. means. 2. a substance which transmits impulses. 3. a substance used in the culture of bacteria; see *culture medium,* under *C.* 4. a preparation used in treating histologic specimens.
**active m.,** the aggregated atoms, ions, or molecules, contained in a laser's optical cavity, in which stimulated emission will occur under the proper excitation.
**Bruns' glucose m.,** a mixture of distilled water, glucose, glycerin, and camphorated spirit, used for mounting fresh tissue specimens.
**clearing m.,** a substance used for rendering histologic specimens transparent.
**contrast m.,** a substance that is introduced into or around a structure and, because of the difference in absorption of x-rays by the contrast medium and the surrounding tissues, allows radiographic visualization of the structure.
**culture m.,** a substance used to support the growth of microorganisms or other cells; see *culture medium,* under *C.*
**dioptric media,** refracting media.
**disperse m., dispersion m., dispersive m.,** the continuous or external portion of a colloid system in which the particles of the disperse phase are distributed; it is analogous to the solvent in a true solution. Cf. *disperse phase.*
**HAT m.,** a tissue culture medium containing hypoxanthine, aminopterin, and thymidine, used in somatic cell fusion experiments. Aminopterin (an antifolate) blocks *de novo* synthesis of purine and thymine nucleotides, but these compounds can be produced from hypoxanthine and thymidine by normal cells possessing the enzymes hypoxanthine phosphoribosyltransferase (HPRT) and thymidine kinase (TK).
**mounting m.,** mountant.
**nutrient m.,** see *nutrient culture* under *culture medium.*
**radiolucent m.,** a contrast medium that permits the passage of x-rays.
**radiopaque m.,** a contrast medium that blocks the passage of x-rays.
**refracting media,** the transparent tissues and fluids in the eye through which light rays pass and by which they are refracted and brought to a focus on the retina; the structures include the cornea, aqueous humor, crystalline lens, and vitreous body. Called also *dioptric media.*
**separating m.,** any substance which facilitates separation, such as a coating used upon a surface that serves to prevent adherence to it of another surface; in dentistry, a substance applied to the investment surface of a denture flask to protect the resin from the surfaces in the mold space to avoid incorporation of water in the resin from the gypsum and to prevent adherence of the investing material and the resin.
**Wickersheimer's m.,** see under *fluid.*

**me·di·us** (me′de-əs) [L.] [TA] in the middle; a term used in reference to a structure lying between two other structures that are anterior and posterior, superior and inferior, or internal and external in position.

**MEDLARS** (med′lahrz) [*MED*ical *L*iterature *A*nalysis and *R*etrieval *S*ystem] [MeSH: MEDLARS] a computerized bibliographic system of the National Library of Medicine, from which the *Index Medicus* is produced.

**MEDLINE** (med′līn) [from *MED*LARS on-*line*] [MeSH: MEDLINE] a computerized bibliographic retrieval system, an on-line segment of MEDLARS.

**med·or·rhea** (med″o-re′ə) [Gr. *mēdea* genitals + *-rrhea*] urethrorrhea.

**med·ro·ges·tone** (med-ro-jes'tōn) [MeSH: Medrogestone] a progestational agent, used in the treatment of menstrual disorders and for the prevention of postmenopausal endometrial hyperplasia; administered orally.

**Med·rol** (med'rol) trademark for preparations of methylprednisolone.

**med·ro·nate** (med'ro-nāt) MDP; a methylene-substituted diphosphonate compound with an affinity for sites of osteoid mineralization; complexed with technetium 99m it is used in bone imaging. Called also *methylene diphosphonate.* See table at *technetium.*

**med·roxy·pro·ges·ter·one ac·e·tate** (med-rok"se-pro-jes'tər-ōn) [USP] a progestin administered orally in the treatment of secondary amenorrhea and functional uterine bleeding and intramuscularly as an antineoplastic in the treatment of metastatic endometrial and renal carcinoma and as a contraceptive.

**med·ry·sone** (med'rĭ-sōn") a synthetic glucocorticoid used topically in the treatment of corticosteroid-responsive allergic and inflammatory conditions of the eye.

**me·dul·la** (mə-dul'ə) gen. and pl. *medul'lae* [L.] 1. [TA] a general term for the most interior portion of an organ or structure. 2. m. oblongata. 3. m. ossium.
**adrenal m., m. of adrenal gland,** m. glandulae suprarenalis.
**m. of bone,** m. ossium.
**m. glan'dulae suprarena'lis** [TA], medulla of suprarenal or adrenal gland: the inner, reddish brown, soft part of the adrenal gland; it synthesizes, stores, and releases catecholamines. Called also *adrenal m.* and *suprarenal m.*
**inner m. of kidney,** inner zone of renal medulla.
**m. of kidney,** m. renalis.
**m. of lymph node,** m. nodi lymphoidei.
**m. ne'phrica,** m. renalis.
**m. no'di lympha'tici,** TA alternative for *m. nodi lymphoidei.*
**m. no'di lymphoi'dei** [TA], medulla of lymph node: the central part of a lymph node, comprising cords and sinuses; called also *m. nodi lymphatici* [TA alternative] and *medullary substance of lymph node.*
**m. oblonga'ta,** TA alternative for *myelencephalon;* the truncated cone of nerve tissue continuous above with the pons and below with the spinal cord. It lies anterior to the cerebellum, and the upper part of its posterior surface forms the floor of the lower part of the fourth ventricle; it contains ascending and descending tracts, and important collections of nerve cells that deal with vital functions, such as respiration, circulation, and special senses. Called also *bulb,* and *bulbus encephali* [TA alternative]. See also *brainstem.*

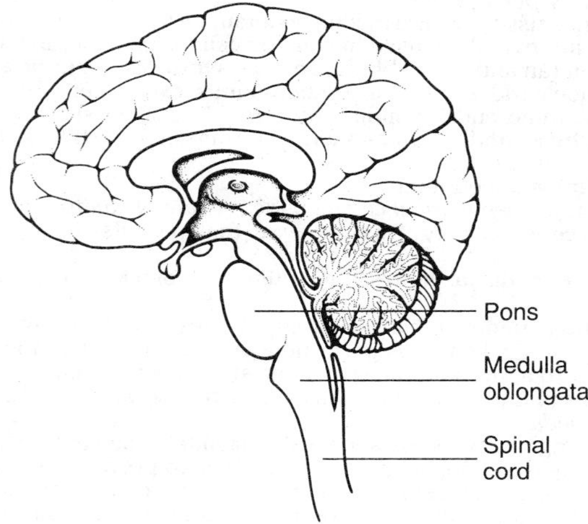


**m. os'sium** [TA], bone marrow: the soft material filling the cavities of the bones, made up of a meshwork of connective tissue containing branching fibers, the meshes being filled with marrow cells, which consist variously of fat cells, large nucleated cells or myelocytes, and giant cells called megakaryocytes. See also *m. ossium flava* and *m. ossium rubra.*
**m. os'sium fla'va** [TA], yellow bone marrow: ordinary bone marrow of the kind in which the fat cells predominate.
**m. os'sium ru'bra** [TA], red bone marrow: marrow of developing bone, of the ribs, vertebrae, and many of the smaller bones; it is the site of production of erythrocytes and granular leukocytes.
**outer m. of kidney,** outer zone of renal medulla.
**m. ova'rii** [TA], medulla of ovary: the loose fibroelastic tissue and mass of contorted blood vessels that forms the core of the ovary.
**renal m., m. rena'lis** [TA], **m. re'nis,** the inner part of the substance of the kidney, composed chiefly of collecting tubule elements, loops of Henle, and vasa recta, organized grossly into pyramids; called also *medullary substance of kidney.*
**m. spina'lis** [TA], spinal cord: that part of the central nervous system that is lodged in the vertebral canal. It extends from the foramen magnum, where it is continuous with the medulla oblongata, to the upper part of the lumbar region, ending between the twelfth thoracic and third lumbar vertebrae, often at or near the first and second lumbar vertebrae. It is composed of an inner core of *gray substance,* in which nerve cells predominate, and an outer layer of *white substance,* in which myelinated nerve fibers predominate, and is enclosed in three protective membranes, or *meninges*: the *dura mater, arachnoid,* and *pia mater.* Thirty-one *spinal nerves* originate from the spinal cord: 8 cervical, 12 thoracic, 5 lumbar, 5 sacral, and 1 coccygeal. It conducts impulses to and from the brain, and controls many automatic muscular activities (reflexes). See also *Rexed's laminae,* under *lamina,* and Plates 11 and 48.
**suprarenal m., m. of suprarenal gland,** m. glandulae suprarenalis.
**m. thy'mi** [TA], medulla of thymus: the central portion of each lobule of the thymus; it contains many more reticular cells and far fewer lymphocytes than does the surrounding cortex.

**me·dul·lae** (mə-dul'e) [L.] genitive and plural of *medulla.*

**med·ul·lary** (med'u-lar"e) [L. *medullaris*] 1. pertaining to a medulla. 2. pertaining to bone marrow. 3. pertaining to the spinal cord. Defs 2 and 3 called also *myeloid.*

**med·ul·lat·ed** (med'u-lāt"əd) myelinated.

**med·ul·la·tion** (med"u-la'shən) 1. myelinization. 2. myelopoiesis. 3. the formation of a medulla.

**med·ul·lec·to·my** (med"u-lek'tə-me) [*medull-* + *-ectomy*] excision of a medulla, such as the adrenal medulla.

**med·ul·li·tis** (med"u-li'tis) 1. osteomyelitis. 2. myelitis.

**med·ul·li·za·tion** (med"u-lĭ-za'shən) 1. the enlargement of the haversian canals in rarefying osteitis, followed by their conversion into marrow channels. 2. replacement of bone by marrow cells.

**medull(o)-** combining form denoting relationship to marrow or to a medulla.

**me·dul·lo·adre·nal** (mə-dul"o-ə-dre'nəl) adrenomedullary.

**me·dul·lo·ar·thri·tis** (mə-dul"o-ahr-thri'tis) [*medullo-* + *arthritis*] inflammation of the marrow spaces of the articular extremities of bones.

**me·dul·lo·blast** (mə-dul'o-blast) an undifferentiated cell of the embryonic medullary or neural tube which may develop into either a neuroblast or a spongioblast.

**me·dul·lo·blas·to·ma** (mə-dul"o-blas-to'mə) [MeSH: Medulloblastoma] a malignant, highly radiosensitive cerebellar tumor composed of undifferentiated neuroglial cells and usually considered a type of primitive neuroectodermal tumor. Most medulloblastomas occur in children and arise in or adjacent to the roof of the fourth ventricle.

**me·dul·lo·epi·the·li·o·ma** (mə-dul"o-ep"i-the"le-o'-mə) a rare type of neuroepithelial tumor, usually found in the brain or retina, composed of primitive neuroepithelial cells lining the tubular spaces; called also *neurocytoma* and *neuroepithelioma.* Cf. *diktyoma.*

**me·dul·lo·ther·a·py** (mə-dul"o-ther'ə-pe) Pasteur's preventive treatment of rabies with emulsions of fixed virus in rabbit spinal cord.

**me·du·sa** (mə-doo'sə) [Gr. *Medusa* one of the three mythological gorgons] jellyfish.

**Mees' lines** (māz) [R. A. *Mees,* Dutch scientist, 20th century] see under *line.*

**me·fe·nam·ic ac·id** (mef"ə-nam'ik) [USP] [MeSH: Mefenamic Acid] an analgesic, anti-inflammatory, and antipyretic used to relieve mild to moderate pain from rheumatoid arthritis and dysmenorrhea.

**mef·lo·quine hy·dro·chlo·ride** (mef'lo-kwin) a synthetic 4-quinolone methanol compound effective against chloroquine-resistant strains of *Plasmodium falciparum* and *P. vivax;* administered orally for the treatment of *P. falciparum* and *P. vivax* malaria and for the prophylaxis of chloroquine-resistant *P. falciparum* malaria.

**Me·fox·in** (mə-fok'sin) trademark for a preparation of cefoxitin sodium.

**MEG** see *magnetoencephalograph.*

**mega-** [Gr. *megas* big, great] a combining form meaning large, enlarged, or abnormally large size; see also words beginning *megal(o)-.* Used in naming units of measurement to indicate a quantity one million ($10^6$) times the unit designated by the root with which it is combined. Symbol, M.

**mega·base** (meg'ə-bās) a unit of length corresponding to one million bases of DNA. Abbreviated Mb.

**mega·bec·que·rel** (meg″ə-bək-ə-rel′) a unit of radioactivity, being one million ($10^6$) becquerels; abbreviated MBq.

**mega·blad·der** (meg″ə-blad′ər) a condition marked by permanent overdistention of the bladder.

**mega·cal·y·co·sis** (meg″ə-kal″ĭ-ko′sis) [*mega-* +*calyx* + *-osis*] nonobstructive dilatation of the renal calices due to malformation of the renal papillae.

**mega·caryo·blast** (meg″ə-kar′e-o-blast) megakaryoblast.

**mega·caryo·cyte** (meg″ə-kar′e-o-sīt″) megakaryocyte.

**Me·gace** (mə-gās′) trademark for a preparation of megestrol acetate.

**mega·ce·cum** (meg″ə-se′kəm) [*mega-* + *cecum*] a cecum which is abnormally large.

**mega·ce·phal·ic** (meg″ə-sə-fal′ik) megalocephalic.

**mega·ceph·a·lous** (meg″ə-sef′ə-ləs) megalocephalic.

**mega·ceph·a·ly** (meg″ə-sef′ə-le) megalocephaly.

**mega·cho·led·o·chus** (meg″ə-ko-led′o-kəs) abnormal dilatation of the common bile duct.

**mega·co·lon** (meg″ə-ko′lon) [MeSH: Megacolon] an abnormally large or dilated colon; the condition may be congenital or acquired, acute or chronic.
**acquired m., acquired functional m.,** colonic enlargement associated with chronic constipation; it may be due to faulty bowel habits and is particularly common in mentally retarded children and adults with chronic mental illness. Called also *idiopathic m.*
**acute m.,** toxic m.
**aganglionic m.,** congenital m.
**congenital m., m. conge′nitum,** megacolon due to congenital absence of myenteric ganglion cells in a distal segment of the large intestine. Loss of motor function in this segment causes massive hypertrophic dilatation of the normal proximal colon; the aganglionic segment usually remains narrowed, but may dilate passively. The condition appears soon after birth, is more common in males, and causes extreme constipation, abdominal distention, sometimes vomiting, and, when severe, growth retardation. Called also *Hirschsprung's disease, aganglionic m.,* and *pelvirectal achalasia.*
**idiopathic m.,** acquired m.
**toxic m.,** acute dilatation of the colon associated with amebic or ulcerative colitis; the dilatation may precede perforation of the colon. Called also *acute m.*

**mega·cu·rie** (meg″ə-ku′re) a unit of radioactivity, being one million ($10^6$) curies, or the quantity of radioactive material in which the number of nuclear disintegrations is $3.7 \times 10^{16}$ per second. Abbreviated MCi.

**mega·cys·tis** (meg″ə-sis′tis) megalocystis.

**mega·dont** (meg′ə-dont) [*mega-* + Gr. *odous* tooth] macrodont.

**mega·don·tia** (meg″ə-don′shə) macrodontia.

**mega·du·o·de·num** (meg″ə-doo″o-de′nəm) an abnormally large or dilated duodenum; it may be congenital or acquired, as in intestinal scleroderma, and is usually due to a disorder of motor function.

**mega·dyne** (meg′ə-dīn″) [*mega-* + *dyne*] one million ($10^6$) dynes.

**mega·esoph·a·gus** (meg″ə-ə-sof′ə-gəs) see *achalasia.*

**mega·ga·me·to·phyte** (meg″ə-gə-me′to-fīt) [*mega-* + *gameto-* + *-phyte*] the female gametophyte in heterosporous plants, developed from the megaspore.

**mega·hertz** (meg′ə-hərtz) a frequency unit indicating one million ($10^6$) cycles per second or one million Hertz, typically applied to the frequency of electromagnetic waves. Abbreviated MHz.

**mega·karyo·blast** (meg″ə-kar′e-o-blast) the earliest cytologically identifiable precursor in the thrombocytic series, a large cell that matures to form a promegakaryocyte. Spelled also *megacaryoblast.*

**mega·karyo·cyte** (meg″ə-kar′e-o-sīt) [*mega-* + *karyo-* + *-cyte*] [MeSH: Megakaryocytes] a giant cell 50 to 100 $\mu$ in diameter, with a greatly lobulated nucleus, found in the bone marrow; mature blood platelets are released from its cytoplasm. Called also *megalokaryocyte;* spelled also *megacaryocyte.*

**mega·karyo·cy·to·poi·e·sis** (meg″ə-kar″e-o-si′to-poi-e′sis) [*megakaryocyte* + *-poiesis*] the production of megakaryocytes.

**mega·karyo·cy·to·sis** (meg″ə-kar″e-o-si-to′sis) the presence of megakaryocytes in the blood or of excessive numbers in the bone marrow, as in polycythemia vera.

**mega·lec·i·thal** (meg″ə-les′ĭ-thəl) [*mega-* + *-lecithal*] macrolecithal.

**meg·al·en·ceph·a·lon** (meg″əl-ən-sef′ə-lon) [*megalo-* + *encephalon*] an abnormally large brain.

**meg·al·en·ceph·a·ly** (meg″əl-ən-sef′ə-le) macrencephaly.

**meg·al·gia** (məg-al′jə) [*mega-* + *-algia*] severe pain, as in muscular rheumatism.

**megal(o)-** [Gr. *megas,* gen. *megalou* big, great] a combining form meaning large, enlarged, or of abnormally large size; see also words beginning *mega-.*

**meg·a·lo·blast** (meg′ə-lo-blast″) [*megalo-* + *-blast*] [MeSH: Megaloblasts] a large, nucleated, immature progenitor of an abnormal red blood cell series seen in some types of anemia; it follows the promegaloblast in development and retains some of its features. Megaloblasts correspond to normoblasts (see *erythroblast*) of the normal red cell maturation series and are correspondingly classified as basophilic, polychromatophilic, and orthochromatic. See also *megaloblastic anemia,* under *anemia.*

**meg·a·lo·blas·toid** (meg″ə-lo-blas′toid) resembling a megaloblast.

**meg·a·lo·bul·bus** (meg″ə-lo-bul′bəs) enlargement of the duodenal cap in the radiograph.

**meg·a·lo·ce·pha·lia** (meg″ə-lo-sə-fa′le-ə) megalocephaly.

**meg·a·lo·ce·phal·ic** (meg″ə-lo-sə-fal′ik) pertaining to or characterized by megalocephaly.

**meg·a·lo·ceph·a·ly** (meg″ə-lo-sef′ə-le) [*megalo-* + *-cephaly*] 1. unusually large size of the head. 2. leontiasis ossium. Called also *megacephaly* and *megalocephalia.*

**meg·a·loc·e·ros** (meg″ə-los′ə-rəs) [*megalo-* + *keras* horn] a fetus having projections from the forehead resembling horns.

**meg·a·lo·chei·ria** (meg″ə-lo-ki′re-ə) [*megalo-* + *cheir-* + *-ia*] abnormal largeness of the hands.

**meg·a·lo·clit·o·ris** (meg″ə-lo-klit′o-ris) clitoromegaly.

**meg·a·lo·cor·nea** (meg″ə-lo-kor′ne-ə) [*megalo-* + *cornea*] a usually bilateral developmental anomaly of the cornea, which is of abnormal size at birth, sometimes reaching a diameter of more than 18 mm in the adult. It may be inherited as an X-linked recessive or as an autosomal dominant trait. Called also *macrocornea.*

**meg·a·lo·cys·tis** (meg″ə-lo-sis′tis) [*megalo-* + *cystis*] an abnormally enlarged bladder.

**meg·a·lo·cyte** (meg′ə-lo-sīt″) [*megalo-* + *-cyte*] macrocyte.

**meg·a·lo·cy·to·sis** (meg″ə-lo-si-to′sis) macrocythemia.

**meg·a·lo·dac·tyl·ia** (meg″ə-lo-dak-til′e-ə) megalodactyly.

**meg·a·lo·dac·ty·lism** (meg″ə-lo-dak′tə-liz-əm) megalodactyly.

**meg·a·lo·dac·ty·lous** (meg″ə-lo-dak′tə-ləs) exhibiting megalodactyly.

**meg·a·lo·dac·ty·ly** (meg″ə-lo-dak′tə-le) [*megalo-* + Gr. *daktylos* finger] abnormal largeness of fingers or toes.

**meg·a·lo·don·tia** (meg″ə-lo-don′shə) macrodontia.

**meg·a·lo·esoph·a·gus** (meg″ə-lo-ə-sof′ə-gəs) see *achalasia.*

**meg·a·lo·gas·tria** (meg″ə-lo-gas′tre-ə) [*megalo-* + *gastr-* + *-ia*] enlargement or abnormally large size of the stomach.

**meg·a·lo·glos·sia** (meg″ə-lo-glos′e-ə) [*megalo-* + *gloss-* + *-ia*] macroglossia.

**meg·a·lo·gra·phia, meg·a·log·ra·phy** (meg″ə-lo-gra′fe-ə, meg″ə-log′rə-fe) macrography.

**meg·a·lo·he·pat·ia** (meg″ə-lo-he-pat′e-ə) [*megalo-* + *hepat-* + *-ia*] hepatomegaly.

**meg·a·lo·kar·y·o·cyte** (meg″ə-lo-kar′e-o-sīt″) megakaryocyte.

**meg·a·lo·ma·nia** (meg″ə-lo-ma′ne-ə) [*megalo-* + *-mania*] unreasonable conviction of one's own extreme greatness, goodness, or power; the ideas in megalomania are known as *delusions of grandeur.*

**meg·a·lo·ma·ni·ac** (meg″ə-lo-ma′ne-ak) an individual exhibiting megalomania.

**meg·a·lo·me·lia** (meg″ə-lo-me′le-ə) [*megalo-* + *-melia*] abnormal largeness of a limb or limbs; called also *macromelia.*

**meg·a·lo·nych·ia** (meg″ə-lo-nik′e-ə) the condition of having unusually large nails. Called also *macronychia.*

**meg·a·lo·pe·nis** (meg″ə-lo-pe′nis) excessive size of the penis.

**meg·a·loph·thal·mos** (meg″ə-lof-thal′mos) [*megalo-* + Gr. *ophthalmos* eye] abnormally large size of the eyes.
**anterior m.,** megalocornea.

**meg·a·loph·thal·mus** (meg″ə-lof-thal′məs) megalophthalmos.

**meg·a·lo·pia** (meg″ə-lo′pe-ə) macropsia.

**meg·a·lo·po·dia** (meg″ə-lo-po′de-ə) [*megalo-* + *pod-* + *-ia*] macropodia.

**meg·a·lop·sia** (meg″ə-lop′se-ə) macropsia.

**Meg·a·lo·pyge** (meg″ə-lo-pij′e) a genus of hairy moths. *M. opercula′ris* is the flannel moth, whose caterpillar has stinging hairs that cause a form of insect dermatitis.

**meg·a·lo·sple·nia** (meg″ə-lo-sple′ne-ə) [*megalo-* + *splen-* + *-ia*] splenomegaly.

**meg·a·lo·spore** (meg′ə-lo-spor″) a macrospore.

**Meg·a·los·po·ron** (meg″ə-los′pə-ron) [*megalo-* + Gr. *sporos* seed] a former genus of fungi now included in *Trichophyton.*

**meg·a·lo·syn·dac·ty·ly** (meg″ə-lo-sin-dak′tə-le) [*megalo-* + *syndactyly*] a condition in which the digits are very large and more or less completely grown together.

**meg·a·lo·thy·mus** (meg″ə-lo-thi′məs) an enlarged thymus.

**meg·a·lo·ure·ter** (meg″ə-lo-u-re′tər) [*megalo-* + *ureter*] congenital ureteral dilatation without demonstrable cause; called also *congenital* or *primary megaloureter, megaureter, primary ureteral atony,* and *ureteral neuromuscular dysplasia.* Cf. *hydroureter.*
**congenital m., primary m.,** megaloureter.
**reflux m.,** dilatation of the ureter associated with vesicoureteral reflux.

**-megaly** [Gr. *megas,* gen. *megalou* big, great] a word termination denoting abnormal enlargement of the structure signified by the root to which it is attached, as splenomegaly.

**mega·pros·o·pous** (meg″ə-pros′o-pəs) [*mega-* + *prosopo-* + *-ous*] having a large face.

**mega·rec·tum** (meg″ə-rek′təm) a greatly dilated rectum.

**Mega·rhi·ni·ni** (meg″ə-ri′nī-ne) in some systems of classification, a tribe of tropical non-bloodsucking mosquitoes; they fly by day, feed on flowers, and are usually highly colored. Their large larvae are predaceous and have been used to control the breeding of bloodsucking mosquitoes.

**Mega·rhi·nus** (meg″ə-ri′nəs) a genus of large, showy, but harmless mosquitoes of tropical and subtropical countries.

**mega·seme** (meg′ə-sēm) [*mega-* + Gr. *sēma* sign] having an orbital index of 89 or more.

**mega·sig·moid** (meg″ə-sig′moid) [*mega-* + *sigmoid*] an enormously dilated sigmoid.

**mega·so·ma** (meg″ə-so′mə) [*mega-* + *soma*] great size and stature, not amounting to gigantism.

**Mega·sphae·ra** (meg″ə-sfe′rə) [*mega-* + Gr. *sphaira* ball] a genus of bacteria of the family Veillonellaceae, found in the rumen of cattle and sheep and in human feces, made up of gram-negative anaerobic cocci. The type species is *M. elsde′nii.*

**mega·spo·ran·gi·um** (meg″ə-spə-ran′je-əm) pl. *megasporan′gia* [*mega-* + *sporangium*] the sporangium in which megaspores develop.

**mega·spore** (meg′ə-spor) [*mega-* + *spore*] 1. macrospore. 2. macroconidium. 3. one of four haploid spores, usually larger than the microspore, formed in the megasporangium from a megaspore mother cell, and from which the megagametophyte, or female gametophyte, develops.

**mega·throm·bo·cyte** (meg″ə-throm′bo-sīt) an abnormally large platelet, usually newly formed; seen in greater numbers during an increase in platelet production.

**Mega·tri·choph·y·ton** (meg″ə-tri″kof′ĭ-ton) former name for *Trichophyton.*

**Mega·tryp·a·num** (meg″ə-trip′ə-nəm) [*mega-* + Gr. *trypanon* borer] in some systems of classification, a subgenus of stercorarian trypanosomes, including among others the species *Trypanosoma melophagium* and *T. theileri.*

**mega·unit** (meg′ə-u″nit) a quantity one million ($10^6$) times that of a standard unit.

**mega·ure·ter** (meg″ə-u-re′tər) megaloureter.

**mega·vi·ta·min** (meg″ə-vi′tə-min) a dose of vitamin(s) vastly exceeding the amount recommended for nutritional balance.

**mega·volt** (meg′ə-vōlt) [*mega-* + *volt*] a million ($10^6$) volts.

**mega·vol·tage** (meg′ə-vōl″təj) in radiotherapy, voltage greater than 1 megavolt. Cf. *orthovoltage* and *supervoltage.*

**me·ges·trol ac·e·tate** (mə-jes′trol) [USP] [MeSH: Megestrol Acetate] a synthetic progestin used as an antineoplastic in the palliative treatment of recurrent, inoperable, or metastatic carcinoma of the breast or endometrium and for the treatment of anorexia, cachexia, and significant weight loss in patients with acquired immunodeficiency syndrome; administered orally.

**Mé·glin's point** (ma-glaz′) [J. A. *Méglin,* French physician, 1756–1824] see under *point.*

**meg·lu·mine** (meg′lu-mēn) [USP] [MeSH: Meglumine] a crystalline base used in the preparation of certain radiopaque media. Called also *methylglucamine.* See also under *diatrizoate* and *iodipamide.*

**meg·ohm** (meg′ōm) [*mega-* + *ohm*] a million ($10^6$) ohms.

**meg·oph·thal·mos** (meg-of-thal′mos) [*mega-* + Gr. *ophthalmos* eye] buphthalmos; hydrophthalmos.

**MEGX** monoethylglycinexylidide.

**mehl·nähr·scha·den** (māl″nār-shah′dən) [Ger.] a nutritional deficiency syndrome similar to kwashiorkor, due to inadequate protein intake and overabundance of carbohydrate; the clinical characteristics include growth failure, preservation of subcutaneous fat with wasting of muscle, edema, and psychomotor abnormalities.

**mei·bo·mi·an cyst, glands, stye** (mi-bo′me-ən) [Heinrich *Meibom,* German anatomist, 1638–1700] see *chalazion* and *glandulae tarsales,* and see under *stye.*

**mei·bo·mi·a·ni·tis** (mi-bo″me-ə-ni′tis) inflammation of the meibomian (tarsal) glands; cf. *tarsadenitis.*

**mei·bo·mi·tis** (mi″bo-mi′tis) meibomianitis.

**Meige's disease, syndrome** (mezh′əz) [Henri *Meige,* French physician, 1866–1940] see under *syndrome* and see *Milroy's disease* under *disease.*

**Meigs' capillaries** (megz) [Arthur V. *Meigs,* American physician, 1850–1912] see under *capillary.*

**Meigs' syndrome** (megz) [Joe Vincent *Meigs,* American surgeon, 1892–1963] [MeSH: Meigs' Syndrome] see under *syndrome.*

**Meigs-Sal·mon syndrome** (megz să′mən) [J. V. *Meigs;* Udall J. *Salmon,* American obstetrician, born 1904] see under *syndrome.*

**meio-** see *mi(o)-.*

**mei·o·gen·ic** (mi″o-jen′ik) [*meio-* + *-genic*] promoting or causing meiosis.

**mei·o·sis** (mi-o′sis) [Gr. *meiōsis* diminution] [MeSH: Meiosis] a special method of cell division, occurring in maturation of the sex cells, by means of which each daughter nucleus receives half the number of chromosomes characteristic of the somatic cells of the species. See illustration. Cf. *mitosis.*

**mei·ot·ic** (mi-ot′ik) pertaining to, characteristic of, or characterized by meiosis.

**Mei·row·sky phenomenon** (mi-rof′ske) [Emil *Meirowsky,* German-American dermatologist, 1876–1960] see under *phenomenon.*

**Meiss·ner's corpuscles, ganglion, plexus** (mīs′nerz) [Georg *Meissner,* German physiologist, 1829–1905] see *corpusculum tactus, plexus submucosus,* and see under *ganglion.*

**mel** (mel) [L.] 1. honey. 2. a compound of honey with some medicinal agent.

**mel·ag·ra** (məl-ag′rə) [*mel-* + *-agra*] muscular pain in the extremities.

**Mel·a·leu·ca** (mel″ə-loo′kə) a genus of trees of the family Myrtaceae, native to Australia and the East Indies. *M. leucaden′dron* L. is the cajeput or cajuput tree, whose fresh leaves and twigs yield cajeput oil.

**mel·al·gia** (məl-al′jə) [*mel-* + *-algia*] pain in the limbs.

**mel·an·cho·lia** (mel″an-ko′le-ə) [*melan-* + *chol-* + *-ia*] a word used through the years to refer to what is now called depression. In the humoral theory of the ancient Greeks it was the temperament caused by an excess of black bile. In modern psychiatric terminology melancholia is used to refer to especially severe forms of major depressive disorder.
**m. agita′ta, agitated m.,** agitated depression.
**involutional m.,** former name for a mood disorder now subsumed under the category of major depressive disorder.

**mel·an·chol·ic** (mel″ən-kol′ik) characterized by melancholia.

**mel·an·choly** (mel′ən-kol″e) melancholia.

**mel·a·nem·e·sis** (mel″ə-nem′ə-sis) [*melano-* + *-emesis*] black vomit.

**mel·a·ne·mia** (mel″ə-ne′me-ə) [*melan-* + *-emia*] the presence of black, pigmentary masses in the blood, as in hemochromatosis.

**Me·la·nia** (mə-la′ne-ə) *Thiara.*

**mel·a·nic·ter·us** (mel″ə-nik′tər-əs) Winckel's disease.

**mel·a·nif·er·ous** (mel″ə-nif′ər-əs) [*melanin* + *-ferous*] containing melanin or other black pigment.

**mel·a·nin** (mel′ə-nin) [Gr. *melas* black] the dark amorphous pigment of the skin, hair, and various tumors, of the choroid coat of the eye and the substantia nigra of the brain. It is produced by polymerization of oxidation products of tyrosine and dihydroxyphenyl compounds, and contains carbon, hydrogen, nitrogen, oxygen, and often sulfur.

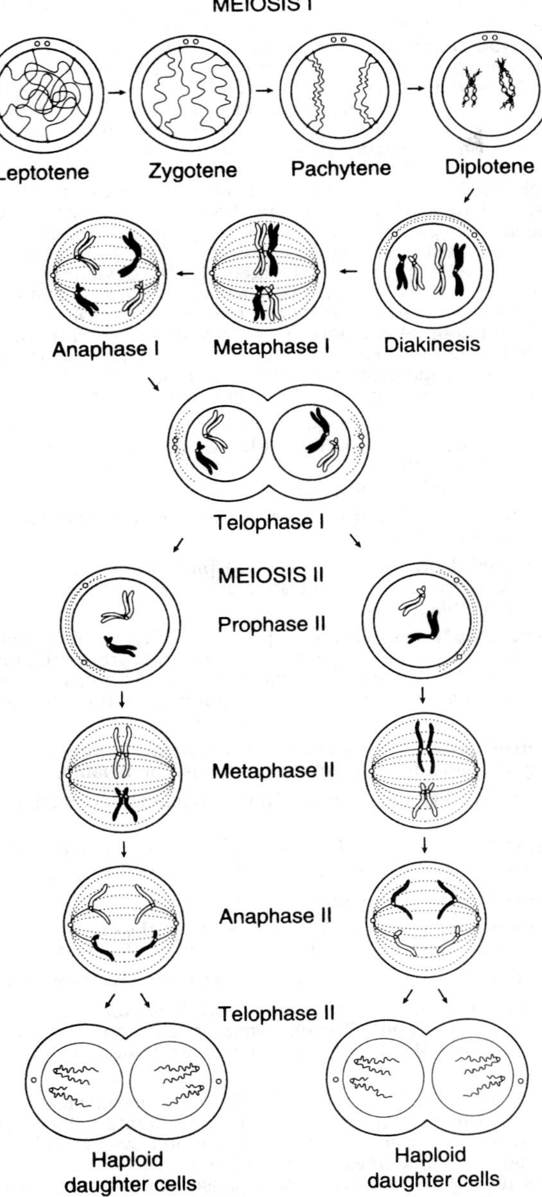


Meiosis (only two of the 23 human chromosome pairs are shown, the chromosomes from one parent in black, those from the other parent in outline).

**artificial m., factitious m.,** a compound resembling melanin, formed when a protein is heated in strong hydrochloric acid; called also *melanoid.*

**mel·a·nism** (mel'ə-niz-əm) excessive pigmentation or blackening of the integuments or tissues, usually of genetic origin; melanosis.
**industrial m.,** the gradual darkening of populations of organisms living in soot-darkened habitats due to the selective pressure of predators, the darker individuals tending to survive as the conspicuous individuals are eaten, thus favoring the genotype that darkens their color. The peppered moth, *Biston betularia,* has undergone this change.
**metallic m.,** argyria.

**mel·a·nis·tic** (mel″ə-nis'tik) characterized by melanism.

**melan(o)-** [Gr. *melas,* gen. *melanos* black] a combining form meaning black, or denoting relationship to melanin.

**mel·a·no·ac·an·tho·ma** (mel″ə-no-ak″ən-tho'mə) [*melano-* + *acanthoma*] a rare, benign epidermal neoplasm composed of keratinocytes pervaded with large dendritic, deeply pigmented melanocytes; it occurs on the head, predominantly in older white males.

**mel·a·no·a·melo·blas·to·ma** (mel″ə-no-ə-mel″o-blas-to'mə) [*melano-* + *ameloblastoma*] melanotic neuroectodermal tumor.

**mel·a·no·blast** (mel'ə-no-blast″, mə-lan'o-blast) [*melano-* + *-blast*] a cell that originates from the neural crest and differentiates into a melanocyte.

**mel·a·no·blas·to·ma** (mel″ə-no-blas-to'mə) [*melano-* + *blastoma*] malignant melanoma.

**mel·a·no·blas·to·sis** (mel″ə-no-blas-to'sis) a condition characterized by the presence of melanoblasts.

**mel·a·no·car·ci·no·ma** (mel″ə-no-kahr″sĭ-no'mə) [*melano-* + *carcinoma*] malignant melanoma.

**mel·a·no·cyte** (mel'ə-no-sīt, mə-lan'o-sīt) [*melano-* + *-cyte*] [MeSH: Melanocytes] any of the dendritic clear cells of the epidermis that synthesize tyrosinase and, within their melanosomes, the pigment melanin; the melanosomes are then transferred from melanocytes to keratinocytes.
**dendritic m.,** those having cytoplasmic projections laden with melanosomes to be transferred to keratinocytes.

**mel·a·no·cyt·ic** (mel″ə-no-sit'ik) pertaining to or composed of melanocytes.

**mel·a·no·cy·to·ma** (mel″ə-no-si-to'mə) [*melanocyte* + *-oma*] a neoplasm or hamartoma composed of melanocytes.
**compound m.,** spindle and epithelioid cell nevus.
**dermal m.,** 1. blue n. 2. cellular blue nevus.
**m. of optic disk,** a nonmalignant pigmented tumor of the optic disk, usually asymptomatic but sometimes causing blurred vision.

**mel·a·no·cy·to·sis** (mel″ə-no″si-to'sis) [*melanocyte* + *-osis*] a condition characterized by an excessive number of melanocytes in the tissues.
**oculodermal m.,** nevus of Ota.

**mel·a·no·der·ma** (mel″ə-no-der'mə) [*melano-* + *derma*] an abnormally increased amount of melanin in the skin, due either to an increase in the production of melanin by the melanocytes normally present or to an increase in the number of melanocytes, with production of hyperpigmented patches.
**parasitic m.,** vagabonds' disease.
**senile m.,** pigmentation of the skin in the aged.

**mel·a·no·der·ma·ti·tis** (mel″ə-no-der″mə-ti'tis) [*melano-* + *dermatitis*] dermatitis associated with an increased deposit of melanin in the skin.
**m. tox'ica lichenoi'des,** tar melanosis.

**me·lan·o·gen** (mə-lan'o-jən) [*melano-* + *-gen*] a colorless chromogen, convertible into melanin, which may occur in the urine in certain diseases, e.g., malignant melanoma..

**mel·a·no·gen·e·sis** (mel″ə-no-jen'ə-sis) [*melano-* + *-genesis*] the production of melanin.

**mel·a·no·gen·ic** (mel″ə-no-jen'ik) causing the production of melanin.

**mel·a·no·glos·sia** (mel″ə-no-glos'e-ə) [*melano-* + *gloss-* + *-ia*] black tongue.

**mel·a·noid** (mel'ə-noid) [*melan-* + *-oid*] 1. resembling melanin; of a dark color. 2. a material resembling melanin. See *artificial melanin,* under *melanin.*

**Mel·a·no·les·tes** (mel″ə-no-les'tēz) the corsairs, a genus of biting insects of the family Reduviidae.
**M. pi'cipes,** the "black corsair" or "kissing bug"; its bite much resembles the sting of a wasp, but it is often much more serious.

**mel·a·no·leu·ko·der·ma** (mel″ə-no-loo″ko-der'mə) [*melano-* + *leukoderma*] a mottled appearance of the skin, as in chronic arsenic poisoning.
**m. col'li,** syphilitic leukoderma.

**mel·a·no·ma** (mel″ə-no'mə) [*melan-* + *-oma*] [MeSH: Melanoma] a tumor arising from the melanocytic system of the skin and other organs. When used alone, the term refers to malignant melanoma.
**acral-lentiginous m.,** an uncommon type of melanoma, although it is the most common type seen in nonwhite individuals, occurring chiefly on the palms and soles, especially on the distal phalanges of the fingers and toes, often on the tip of the digit or nail fold or bed *(subungual m.),* and sometimes involving mucosal surfaces, such as the vulva or vagina. It typically presents as an irregular, enlarging black macule, which has a prolonged noninvasive stage.
**amelanotic m.,** an unpigmented malignant melanoma.
**benign juvenile m.,** spindle and epithelioid nevus.
**benign uveal m.,** uveal nevus.
**Cloudman's m. S91,** a firm, black subcutaneous tumor originally found at the base of the tail of a female DBA mouse, and proven to be transplantable to, and invariably metastatic in, other DBA mice and BALB/c mice.
**Harding-Passey m.,** a transplantable, nonmetastasizing melanoma originally found on the ear of a brown mouse.
**intraocular m.,** ocular m.
**juvenile m.,** spindle and epithelioid cell nevus.

**lenti'go malig'na m.,** a cutaneous malignant melanoma found most often on the sun-exposed areas of the skin, especially the face, which begins as a circumscribed macular patch of mottled pigmentation, showing shades of dark brown, tan, or black *(lentigo maligna* or *melanotic freckle of Hutchinson),* and enlarges by lateral growth before dermal invasion occurs. This type is the slowest growing, has the least tendency to metastasize, and seems to be the least aggressive form of malignant melanoma. Called also *circumscribed precancerous melanosis of Dubreuilh.*
**malignant m.,** a malignant neoplasm of melanocytes, arising *de novo* or from a preexisting benign nevus or lentigo maligna, which occurs most often in the skin but also may involve the oral cavity, esophagus, anal canal, vagina, leptomeninges, conjunctivae, or eye. The tumor is classified into four clinical types: *superficial spreading m., lentigo maligna m., acral-lentiginous m.,* and *nodular m.* Called also *melanotic carcinoma, melanoblastoma,* and *melanocarcinoma.*
**mucosal m.,** that occurring on a mucous membrane, chiefly the palate but also elsewhere on the head and neck, genitalia, and esophagus, usually in older women; most are lentiginous, but nodular and superficial spreading melanomas also occur.
**nodular m.,** a type of malignant melanoma arising without a perceptible radial growth phase, most often occurring on the head, neck, and trunk, typically presenting as a uniformly pigmented, elevated, bizarrely colored nodule that enlarges rather rapidly and commonly ulcerates, which may arise *de novo* or from a preexisting malignant melanoma of a different type.
**nontumorigenic m.,** melanoma in the stage of radial growth, when the risk of metastasis is slight; cf. *tumorigenic m.*
**ocular m., ocular malignant m.,** malignant melanoma arising from the structures of the eye, usually the choroid, ciliary body, or iris, and occurring most often in the fifth and sixth decades of life; the most common site of metastasis is the liver, hepatic metastasis being followed rapidly by death.
**subungual m.,** acral-lentiginous melanoma occurring in the nail fold or bed; called also *melanotic whitlow.*
**superficial spreading m.,** the most common type of malignant melanoma, characterized by a period of radial growth atypical of melanocytes in the epidermis, usually associated with a lymphocytic cellular host response that is sometimes accompanied by partial or complete regression of the radial growth phase; deeply invasive growth (vertical growth) is superimposed on the radial phase. It occurs most often on the lower leg or back, usually presenting as a small pigmented macule to a slightly palpable flat lesion that assumes an irregular outline on enlargement.
**tumorigenic m.,** melanoma in the stage of vertical growth, when the risk of metastasis becomes significant; cf. *nontumorigenic m.*
**uveal m., uveal malignant m.,** the most common type of ocular malignant melanoma, consisting of overgrowth of uveal melanocytes and often preceded by a uveal nevus.

**mel·a·no·ma·to·sis** (mel″ə-no″mə-to′sis) the formation of melanomas in various parts of the body.

**mel·a·no·ma·tous** (mel″ə-no′mə-təs) characterized by or pertaining to melanoma.

**mel·a·no·nych·ia** (mel″ə-no-nik′e-ə) [*melan-* + *onychia*] blackening of the nail by melanin pigmentation.

**mel·a·no·phage** (mel′ə-no-fāj″) [*melano-* + *-phage*] a histiocyte laden with phagocytosed melanin.

**mel·a·no·phore** (mel′ə-no-for″) [*melano-* + *-phore*] [MeSH: Melanophores] a dermal chromatophore containing melanin, especially such a cell in fishes, amphibians, and reptiles.

**mel·a·noph·o·rin** (mel″ə-nof′ə-rin) a principle thought to stimulate melanophores.

**mel·a·no·pla·kia** (mel″ə-no-pla′ke-ə) [*melano-* + Gr. *plax* plate + *-ia*] the presence of pigmented patches on the oral mucosa.

**mel·a·nop·ty·sis** (mel″ə-nop′tĭ- sis) [*melano-* + Gr. *ptyein* to spit] the expectoration of black sputum, as in coal workers' pneumoconiosis.

**mel·a·no·sis** (mel″ə-no′sis) [*melan-* + *-osis*] [MeSH: Melanosis] a disorder caused by a disturbance in melanin pigmentation; melanism.
**m. bul′bi,** m. oculi.
**circumscribed precancerous m. of Dubreuilh,** lentigo maligna melanoma.
**m. co′li,** a condition in which the mucous membrane of the colon is black or dark brown due to the presence of pigment-laden macrophages within the lamina propria. The pigment is not true melanin.
**m. i′ridis, m. of the iris,** abnormal pigmentation of the iris by infiltration of melanoblasts.
**neurocutaneous m.,** giant hairy nevus accompanied by malignant melanomas of the meninges.
**m. o′culi,** a usually congenital condition in which there is a diffuse increase in pigmentation of the uveal tract and often of the more superficial ocular tissues. Called also *m. bulbi.*
**oculocutaneous m.,** see *nevus of Ota,* under *nevus.*
**Riehl's m.,** a patchy melanoderma manifested as a light to dark brown pigmentation, which is most intense on the forehead, on the malar regions, behind the ears, on the sides of the neck, and on other sun-exposed areas. It is seen most often in women and may involve an inflammatory photosensitivity, perhaps phototoxic, reaction.
**m. scle′rae,** congenital flecks of pigmentation in the sclera.
**tar m.,** a dermatosis representing photosensitivity or phototoxicity induced by exposure to tar or other hydrocarbons, usually occupationally, most often involving the face or back of the hands, and characterized by pruritus associated with the development of reticular pigmentation, telangiectases, and small, dark, lichenoid, follicular papules. Called also *melanodermatitis toxica lichenoides.*
**transient neonatal pustular m.,** a congenital skin condition usually seen in babies of African descent, characterized by pigmented macules and vesicopustules that may rupture and leave a scaly collar. It usually resolves completely within a few weeks to two years.

**mel·a·no·some** (mel′ə-no-sōm″) [*melano-* + *-some*] [MeSH: Melanocytes] any of the granules within the melanocytes that contain tyrosinase and synthesize melanin; they are transferred from the melanocytes to keratinocytes.

**mel·a·not·ic** (mel″ə-not′ik) pertaining to or characterized by the presence of melanin.

**mel·a·no·trich·ia** (mel″ə-no-trik′e-ə) [*melano-* + *trich-* + *-ia*] abnormal hyperpigmentation of the hair.
**m. lin′guae,** black tongue.

**mel·a·no·troph** (mel′ə-no-trōf″) [*melano-* + Gr. *trophē* nourishment] a pituitary cell type that elaborates melanocyte-stimulating hormone and β-endorphins. Melanotrophs are abundant in animals that have a pars intermedia adenohypophyseos; humans have very few.

**mel·a·no·trop·ic** (mel″ə-no-trop′ik) [*melano-* + *-tropic*] having an affinity for melanin; influencing the deposit of melanin.

**mel·a·no·tro·pin** (mel′ə-no-tro″pin) melanocyte-stimulating hormone.

**me·lan·thin** (mə-lan′thin) an amorphous and poisonous glycoside or saponin from the seeds of *Nigella sativa.*

**mel·an·u·re·sis** (mel″ən-u-re′sis) melanuria.

**mel·an·uria** (mel″ə-nu′re-ə) [*melan-* + *uria*] the excretion of darkly stained urine or of urine which turns dark on standing.

**mel·an·uric** (mel″ən-u′rik) pertaining to or marked by melanuria.

**me·lar·so·prol** (mə-lahr′so-prol) [MeSH: Melarsoprol] an antiprotozoal effective against *Trypanosoma,* used in the treatment of advanced cases of African trypanosomiasis, administered intravenously.

**me·las·ma** (mə-laz′mə) [Gr. *melas* black] hypermelanosis characterized by the development of sharply demarcated blotchy, brown macules usually in a symmetric distribution over the cheeks and forehead and sometimes on the upper lip and neck. It frequently occurs during pregnancy, at menopause, and in those taking oral contraceptives. It is seen occasionally in nonpregnant women who are not taking oral contraceptives and sometimes in men. A similar pattern of facial hyperpigmentation may be associated with chronic liver disease. Called also *chloasma* and *mask of pregnancy.*

**mel·a·to·nin** (mel″ə-to′nin) [MeSH: Melatonin] a hormone synthesized by the pineal gland in many species of animals; its secretion increases during exposure to light. In adult amphibians it produces

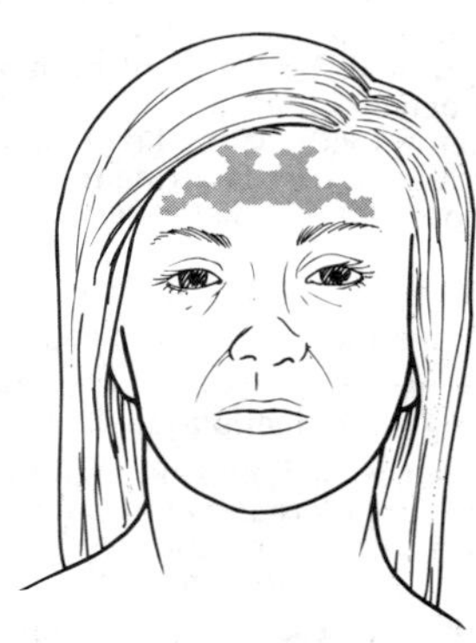

Melasma.

lightening of the dermal pigmentation by promoting aggregation of melanosomes. In mammals it influences hormone production and in many species it regulates seasonal changes such as reproductive pattern and fur color. In humans it is implicated in the regulation of sleep, mood, puberty, and ovarian cycles.

**Me·le·da disease** (mel'ə-dah) [*Meleda,* a small island in the eastern Adriatic Sea, where the condition is prevalent because of intermarriage] mal de Meleda.

**me·le·na** (mə-le'nə) [Gr. *melaina,* feminine of Gr. *melas* black] [MeSH: Melena] 1. the passage of dark and pitchy stools stained with blood pigments or with altered blood. 2. black vomit.
**m. neonato'rum,** melena of the newborn, due to the extravasation of blood into the alimentary canal.
**m. spu'ria,** melena in a nursing infant in which the blood comes from the fissured nipple of the mother.
**m. ve'ra,** true melena.

**Me·le·ney's ulcer (gangrene), synergistic gangrene** (mə-le'nēz) [Frank Lamont *Meleney,* American surgeon, 1889–1963] see under *ulcer,* and see *progressive synergistic gangrene,* under *gangrene.*

**mel·en·ges·trol ac·e·tate** (mel-ən-jes'trol) [MeSH: Melengestrol Acetate] a progestin and antineoplastic, commonly administered as a feed additive to cattle to suppress estrus and promote growth.

**me·le·nic** (mə-le'nik) marked by melena.

**me·lez·i·tose** (mə-lez'ĭ-tōs) a reducing trisaccharide composed of glucose and turanose, an isomer of sucrose. It occurs in poplars and conifers, and in the honey produced by bees that have collected from these trees.

**meli-** [Gr. *meli,* gen. *melitos* honey] a combining form meaning sweet, or denoting relationship to honey or to sugar.

**-melia** [Gr. *melos* limb + *-ia*] word termination denoting a limb.

**Me·lia** (mel'e-ə) a genus of deciduous trees of the family Meliaceae, native to Indonesia and Australia. *M. aze'darach* is the azedarach, chinaberry, or umbrella tree, a common shade tree whose seeds are used as beads, whose root bark is an anthelmintic, and whose leaf juice is a diuretic and emmenagogue. Its fruit is poisonous to humans and other animals, causing severe local irritation, neurological symptoms, cardiotoxicity, and dyspnea.

**meli·bi·ase** (mel''ĭ-bi'ās) $\alpha$-galactosidase.

**meli·bi·ose** (mel''ĭ-bi'ōs) [MeSH: Melibiose] a disaccharide composed of galactose in $\alpha$-(1,6) linkage with glucose; it is a constituent of the trisaccharide raffinose.

**meli·ce·ra, meli·ce·ris** (mel''i-se'rə, mel''ĭ-se'ris) [*meli-* + *cera*] 1. a cyst filled with honey-like substance. 2. viscid, syrupy.

**mel·i·lo·tox·in** (mel''ĭ-lo-tok'sin) dicumarol (def. 1).

**Mel·i·lo·tus** (mel''ĭ-lo'tus) the sweet clovers, a genus of leguminous herbs with trifoliate leaves; they are commonly consumed by livestock, but because they contain dicumarol, when they spoil they are the cause of the hemorrhagic condition called *sweet clover disease.*

**me·li·oi·do·sis** (me''le-oi-do'sis) [Gr. *mēlis* a distemper of asses + *-oid* + *-osis*] [MeSH: Melioidosis] an infection, usually of rodents, which can spread to other animals including humans, and is caused by *Burkholderia pseudomallei;* most cases are seen in Southeast Asia, but it has also been seen in temperate regions. Human disease, usually acquired through contamination of a break in the skin with soil or water, may range from a dormant infection to localized abscesses, benign pneumonia, or fatal septicemia; late activation of inapparent disease or recrudescence of previous symptoms may also occur. In other animals the syndrome varies considerably and usually involves caseous or suppurative lesions of the lymph nodes or viscera. Called also *pseudoglanders;* formerly called *Whitmore's disease.*

**mel·is·so·pho·bia** (mə-lis''o-fo'be-ə) [Gr. *melissa* bee + *-phobia*] apiphobia.

**Me·lis·sa** (mə-lis'ə) [Gr. "bee"] a genus of plants of the family Labiatae. The tops and leaves of *M. officina'lis,* containing tannin and an essential oil, are a cooling stimulant and diaphoretic. Called also *blue, lemon,* or *sweet balm.*

**me·lis·so·ther·a·py** (mə-lis''o-ther'ə-pe) [Gr. *melissa* bee + *therapy*] treatment with bee venom; called also *apiotherapy.*

**me·li·tis** (mə-li'tis) [Gr. *mēlon* cheek + *-itis*] inflammation of the cheek.

**melit(o)-** see *meli-.*

**mel·i·tose** (mel'ĭ-tōs) former name for *raffinose.*

**mel·i·tu·ria** (mel''ĭ-tu're-ə) [*melit-* + *-uria*] sugar in the urine; specific types are named for the sugar in question, such as *fructosuria, galactosuria, glycosuria, lactosuria, maltosuria, pentosuria, sucrosuria,* and so on.

**Mel·kers·son's syndrome** (mel'kər-sonz) [Ernst Gustaf *Melkersson,* Swedish physician, 1898–1932] see under *syndrome.*

**Mel·kers·son-Ro·sen·thal syndrome** (mel'ker-son ro'zen-tahl) [E. G. *Melkersson;* Curt *Rosenthal,* German psychiatrist, 20th century] [MeSH: Melkersson-Rosenthal Syndrome] Melkersson's syndrome.

**Mel·la·ril** (mel'ə-ril) trademark for preparations of thioridazine hydrochloride.

**mel·li·tum** (mə-li'təm) pl. *melli'ta* [L.] a pharmaceutical preparation made with honey.

**mel(o)-**[1] [Gr. *melos* limb] combining form denoting limb.

**mel(o)-**[2] [Gr. *mēlon* cheek] combining form denoting cheek.

**Me·lo·chia py·ram·i·da·ta** (mə-lo'ke-ə pĭ-ram''ĭ-da'tə) a shrub found in Central America; ingestion by cattle causes derrengue.

**melo·did·y·mus** (mel''ə-did'ə-məs) [*melo-*[1] + *-didymus*] an individual with a supernumerary limb.

**Me·lo·i·dae** (məlo'ĭ-de) the blister beetles, a family of beetles whose dried bodies raise blisters when rubbed on human skin and are sometimes used as counterirritants. Genera include *Epicauta* and *Lytta* (which contain cantharidin), *Paederus* (which contains pederin), *Psalydolytta,* and *Sessinia.* See also *cantharidin poisoning,* under *poisoning.*

**me·lom·e·lus** (mə-lom'ə-ləs) [*melo-*[1] + *melos* limb] a fetus with normal limbs and rudimentary supernumerary limbs.

**me·lono·plas·ty** (mə-lon'o-plas''te) meloplasty.

**Me·loph·a·gus** (mə-lof'ə-gəs) a genus of wingless flies of the family Hippoboscidae. *M. ovi'nus,* the sheep ked, is a common ectoparasite of sheep and goats.

**melo·plas·ty** (mel'o-plas''te) [*melo-*[2] + *-plasty*] plastic surgery of the cheek.

**Mel·o·psit·ta·cus** (mel''o-sit'ə-kəs) a genus of psittacine birds. *M. undula'tus* is the budgerigar (q.v.).

**melo·rhe·os·to·sis** (mel''o-re''os-to'sis) [*melo-*[1] + *rheo-* + *ostosis*] [MeSH: Melorheostosis] a form of osteosclerosis or hyperostosis extending in a linear track through one of the long bones of an extremity, and consisting of proliferated ivory-like new bone. See *rheostosis.*

**melo·sal·gia** (mel''o-sal'jə) [*melo-*[1] + *-algia*] pain in the lower limbs.

**me·los·chi·sis** (mə-los'kĭ-sis) [*melo-*[2] + *-schisis*] oblique facial cleft.

**me·lo·tia** (mə-lo'shə) [*mel-*[2] + *ot-* + *-ia*] a developmental anomaly characterized by displacement of the ear onto the cheek.

**mel·pha·lan** (mel'fə-lan) [USP] [MeSH: Melphalan] a cytotoxic alkylating agent that is the L-phenylalanine derivative of mechlorethamine, used as an antineoplastic, primarily for treatment of multiple myeloma, but also for carcinoma of the breast and ovarian and testicular carcinoma, administered orally; it is also used in regional limb perfusion for carcinoma of the extremity, administered by injection. Called also L-*sarcolysin* and L-phenylalanine mustard (L-PAM).

**melt·ing** (mel'ting) 1. undergoing or causing to undergo the transition from solid to liquid, as by the application of heat or pressure. 2. in molecular biology, the disruption of secondary structure in molecules or parts of molecules, such as the heat-induced general or localized separation of a double-stranded nucleic acid to form a single-stranded molecule or region.

**Melt·zer's sign** (melt'sərz) [Samuel James *Meltzer,* American physiologist, 1851–1920] see under *sign.*

**mem·ber** (mem'bər) [L. *membrum*] 1. a part of the body distinct from the rest in function or position. 2. a limb (see *membrum,* def. 2 [TA]).

**mem·ber·ment** (mem'bər-mənt) the manner of arrangement of parts in a body.

**mem·bra** (mem'brə) [L.] plural of *membrum.*

**mem·bra·na** (mem-bra'nə) gen. and pl. *membra'nae* [L.] [TA] a membrane, or thin skin; a general term for a thin layer of tissue covering a surface, lining a cavity, or dividing a space or organ.

## Membrana

Descriptions are given on TA terms, and include anglicized names of specific membranes.

**m. abdo'minis,** peritoneum.
**m. adamanti'na,** cuticula dentis.
**m. adventi'tia,** 1. tunica adventitia. 2. decidua capsularis.
**m. agni'na,** amnion.
**m. atlantooccipita'lis ante'rior** [TA], anterior atlanto-occipital membrane: a single midline ligamentous structure that passes from the anterior arch of the atlas to the anterior margin of the foramen magnum, and corresponds in position with the anterior longitudinal ligament of the vertebral column. Called also *anterior* or *deep atlanto-occipital ligament* and *ligamentum atlanto-occipitale anterius.*
**m. atlantooccipita'lis poste'rior** [TA], posterior atlanto-occipital membrane: a single midline ligamentous structure that passes from the posterior arch of the atlas to the posterior margin of the foramen magnum, and corresponds in position with the ligamenta flava.
**m. basa'lis,** basement membrane.
**m. basa'lis duc'tus semicircula'ris,** basal membrane of semicircular duct: the basement membrane underlying the epithelium of a semicircular duct.
**membra'nae cadu'cae,** membranae deciduae.
**m. capsula'ris,** 1. capsula articularis. 2. capsular membrane (def. 2).
**m. choriocapilla'ris,** lamina choroidocapillaris.
**m. cricovoca'lis,** conus elasticus.
**membra'nae decid'uae,** decidual or deciduous membranes: the endometrium of the pregnant uterus, all of which, except the deepest layer, is shed at parturition. See subentries under *decidua.*
**m. epipapilla'ris,** an abnormal fibrous membrane on the optic disk.
**m. fibroelas'tica laryn'gis** [TA], fibroelastic membrane of larynx: the fibroelastic layer beneath the mucous coat of the larynx, comprising the quadrangular membrane and the conus elasticus. See also *intrinsic laryngeal ligaments,* under *ligament.*
**m. fibro'sa cap'sulae articula'ris** [TA], fibrous membrane of articular capsule: the outer of the two layers of the articular capsule of a synovial joint, composed of dense white fibrous tissue; called also *stratum fibrosum capsulae articularis* [TA alternative].
**m. flac'cida,** pars flaccida membranae tympani.
**m. fus'ca,** lamina fusca sclerae.
**m. germinati'va,** blastoderm.
**m. granulo'sa,** layers of cuboidal epithelial cells at the periphery of an ovarian follicle and surrounding the antrum or fluid-filled cavity.
**m. granulo'sa exter'na,** the external granular layer of the retina.
**m. granulo'sa inter'na,** the internal granular layer of the retina.
**m. hyaloi'dea,** m. vitrea.
**m. intercosta'lis exter'na** [TA], external intercostal membrane: any of the aponeurotic bands parallel with, and perhaps replacing, the fibers of the external intercostal muscles in the spaces between the costal cartilages, from the ventral tips of the ribs medially to the sternum.
**m. intercosta'lis inter'na** [TA], internal intercostal membrane: any of the aponeurotic bands parallel with, and perhaps replacing, the fibers of the internal intercostal muscles in the spaces between the ribs, from the angles of the ribs medially to the vertebral column.
**m. interos'sea antebra'chii** [TA], **m. interos'sea antibra'chii,** interosseous membrane of forearm: a thin fibrous sheet that connects the bodies of the radius and ulna, passing from the interosseous margin of the radius to that of the ulna.
**m. interos'sea cru'ris** [TA], interosseous membrane of leg: a thin aponeurotic lamina attached to the interosseous margins of the tibia and fibula, deficient for a short distance at the proximal end of the bones; it separates the muscles on the anterior and posterior parts of the leg.
**m. li'mitans,** 1. one of the limiting membranes of the retina; see *external* and *internal limiting membrane* (def. 1), under *membrane.* 2. the limiting membrane of glia fibrils and perivascular feet separating the parenchyma of the central nervous system from the pia and blood vessels. It is sometimes considered together with the pia mater as the *pia-glia.*
**m. muco'sa vesi'cae fel'leae,** tunica mucosa vesicae biliaris.
**m. nic'titans,** 1. plica semilunaris conjunctivae. 2. nictitating membrane.
**m. obturato'ria** [TA], obturator membrane: a strong membrane that fills the obturator foramen except superiorly at the obturator groove, where a deficiency is left, the obturator canal.
**m. obtura'trix,** m. obturatoria.
**m. perfora'ta,** a term sometimes used to designate the first appearance of dentin in the fetus, manifested as a thick limiting line between the ameloblasts and odontoblasts.
**m. perine'i** [TA], membrane of perineum: the triangular fibrous membrane stretched horizontally between the ischiopubic rami, which is attached at its base to the perineal body, its apex thickening to form the transverse perineal ligament; called also *fascia diaphragmatis urogenitalis inferior, inferior fascia of urogenital diaphragm,* and *perineal membrane.* See also *diaphragma urogenitale.*
**m. pituito'sa,** tunica mucosa nasi.
**m. pro'pria,** lamina propria mucosae.
**m. pro'pria duc'tus semicircula'ris,** proper membrane of semicircular duct: the outer, loose, connective tissue layer of a semicircular duct.
**m. pupilla'ris** [TA], pupillary membrane: the portion of the tunica vasculosa lentis that is in front of the pupil; it is a mesodermal layer attached to the rim or front of the iris during embryonic development, sometimes persisting in the adult. Called also *Wachendorf's membrane.*
**m. quadrangula'ris** [TA], quadrangular membrane: the upper part of the fibroelastic membrane of the larynx.
**m. reticula'ris or'gani spira'lis** [TA], **m. reticula'ta,** reticular membrane of spiral organ: a netlike membrane over the spiral organ; the free ends of the outer hair cells pass through its apertures. Called also *reticular lamina.*
**m. ruyschia'na,** Ruysch's membrane.
**m. saccifor'mis,** the synovial membrane of the inferior radioulnar articulation.
**m. sero'sa,** 1. tunica serosa. 2. chorion.
**m. seroti'na,** decidua basalis.
**m. spira'lis duc'tus cochlea'ris,** TA alternative for *paries tympanicus ductus cochlearis.*
**m. stapedia'lis** [TA], **m. stape'dis,** stapedial membrane: a membrane filling the arch formed by the crura and base of the stapes.
**m. statoconio'rum macula'rum** [TA], statoconic membrane of maculae: the gelatinous membrane surmounting the maculae, containing the statoconia, and having special sensory hairs projecting into it.
**m. ster'ni** [TA], sternal membrane: the thick fibrous membrane that envelopes the sternum; it is formed by the intermingling of fibers of the radiate sternocostal ligaments, the periosteum, and the tendinous origin of the pectoralis major.
**m. suprapleura'lis** [TA], suprapleural membrane: the strengthened portion of the endothoracic fascia attached to the inner part of the first rib and the transverse process of the seventh cervical vertebra.
**m. synovia'lis cap'sulae articula'ris** [TA], synovial membrane of articular capsule: the inner of the two layers of the articular capsule of a synovial joint, composed of loose connective tissue and having a free smooth surface that lines the joint cavity. It secretes the synovial fluid. Called also *stratum synoviale capsulae articularis* [TA alternative].
**m. synovia'lis infe'rior articulatio'nis temporomandibula'ris** [TA], inferior synovial membrane of temporomandibular joint: the synovial membrane that lines the articular capsule of the joint below the articular disk.
**m. synovia'lis supe'rior articulatio'nis temporomandibula'ris** [TA], superior synovial membrane of temporomandibular joint: the synovial membrane that lines the articular capsule of the joint above the articular disk.

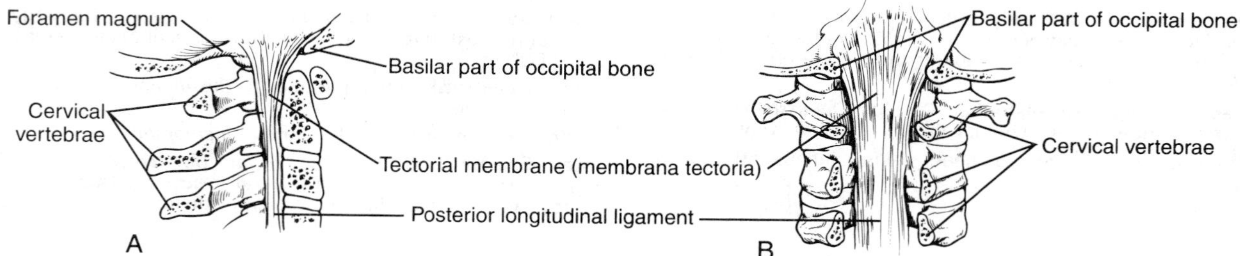


Membrana tectoria (tectorial membrane) in a median section *(A)* and posterior cross-section *(B)* of the upper cervical vertebrae and basilar part of occipital bone.

**m. tecto'ria** [TA], tectorial membrane: a strong fibrous band connected cranially with the basilar part of the occipital bone and caudally with the dorsal surface of the bodies of the second and third cervical vertebrae. It is actually the cranial prolongation of the deeper portion of the posterior longitudinal ligament of the vertebral column.

**m. tecto'ria duc'tus cochlea'ris** [TA], tectorial membrane of cochlear duct: a delicate gelatinous mass extending from the limbus and resting on the spiral organ of the ear and connected with the hairs of the hair cells; called also *Corti's membrane.*

**m. ten'sa,** pars tensa membranae tympanicae.

**m. thyrohyoi'dea** [TA], thyrohyoid membrane: a broad fibroelastic sheet attached above to the upper margin of the posterior surface of the hyoid bone and below to the upper border of the thyroid cartilage. See also *extrinsic laryngeal ligaments,* under *ligament.*

**m. tym'pani, m. tympa'nica** [TA], tympanic membrane: the obliquely placed, thin membranous partition between the external acoustic meatus and the tympanic cavity. The greater portion, the pars tensa, is attached by a fibrocartilaginous ring to the tympanic plate of the temporal bone; the much smaller, triangular portion, the pars flaccida, is situated anterosuperiorly between the two mallear folds. Called also *drumhead, drum, eardrum,* and *tympanum.*

**m. tym'pani secunda'ria** [TA], secondary tympanic membrane: the membrane that closes in the fenestra cochlearis; called also *Scarpa's membrane* and *membrane of round window.*

**m. vestibula'ris duc'tus cochlea'ris,** TA alternative for *paries vestibularis ductus cochlearis.*

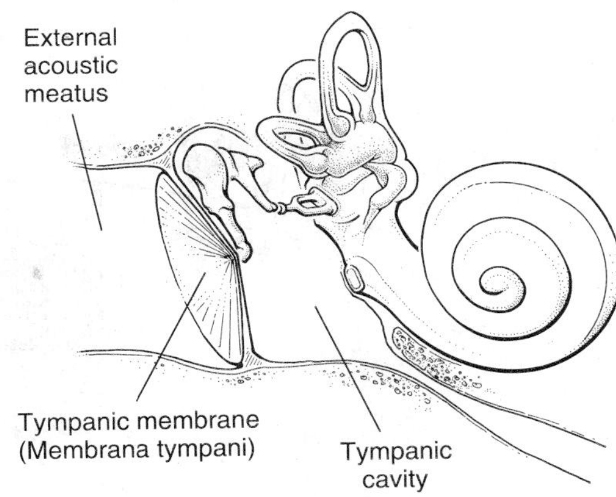


**m. vi'brans,** pars tensa membranae tympanicae.

**m. vitelli'na,** vitelline membrane.

**m. vi'trea** [TA], vitreous membrane: a delicate boundary layer investing the vitreous body of the eye; called also *m. hyaloidea* or *hyaloid membrane.*

**mem·bra·na·ceous** (mem"brə-na'shəs) [L. *membranaceus*] membranous.

**mem·bra·nae** (mem-bra'ne) [L.] genitive and plural of *membrana.*

**mem·bra·nate** (mem'brə-nāt) having the character of a membrane.

**mem·brane** (mem'brān) [MeSH: Membranes] a thin layer of tissue which covers a surface, lines a cavity, or divides a space or organ; see also *membrana.*

## Membrane

For names of specific anatomic structures not found here, see under *membrana.*

**abdominal m.,** peritoneum.

**accidental m.,** false m.

**adamantine m.,** cuticula dentis.

**alveolar-capillary m., alveolocapillary m.,** a thin tissue barrier between pulmonary alveoli and adjacent capillaries, the site of gas exchange between alveolar air and capillary blood. Called also *alveolar-capillary* or *alveolocapillary barrier* and *blood-air* or *blood-gas barrier.*

**alveolodental m.,** periodontal ligament.

**anal m.,** the dorsal part of the cloacal membrane after its division by the urorectal septum.

**animal m.,** a thin membranous diaphragm, as of bladder, used in dialysis or diffusion.

**antral m.,** a congenital abnormal membrane in the pyloric antrum, partially or completely blocking the gastric outlet. See also *prepyloric atresia.* Called also *antral diaphragm* and *antral web.*

**aponeurotic m.,** aponeurosis.

**arachnoid m.,** arachnoidea.

**Ascherson's m.,** the covering of casein enclosing the milk globules.

**asphyxial m.,** hyaline m. (def. 2); so called because of its interference with gaseous exchange in the lungs.

**atlanto-occipital m., anterior,** membrana atlanto-occipitalis anterior.

**atlanto-occipital m., posterior,** membrana atlanto-occipitalis posterior.

**basal m. of semicircular duct,** membrana basalis ductus semicircularis.

**basement m.,** a sheet of amorphous extracellular material upon which the basal surfaces of epithelial cells rest; it is also associated with muscle cells, Schwann cells, fat cells, and capillaries, interposed between the cellular elements and the underlying connective tissue. It comprises two layers, the basal lamina and the reticular lamina, and is composed of Type IV collagen (which is unique to basement membranes), laminin, fibronectin, and heparan sulfate proteoglycans.

**basilar m. of cochlear duct,** lamina basilaris ductus cochlearis.

**Bichat's m.,** fenestrated m.

**birth m's,** the amnion and chorion.

**Bowman's m.,** lamina limitans anterior corneae.

**Bruch's m.,** lamina basalis choroideae.

**Brunn's m.,** the epithelium of the olfactory region of the nose.

**bucconasal m.,** oronasal m.

**buccopharyngeal m.,** oropharyngeal m.

**capsular m.,** 1. capsula articularis. 2. the portion of the tunica vasculosa lentis that lies posterior to the lens.

**capsulopupillary m.,** the part of the tunica vasculosa lentis that is around the edges of the lens.

**cell m.,** plasma m.

**chorioallantoic m.,** chorioallantois.

**chromatic m.,** a continuous layer of chromatin substance situated on the internal surface of a nuclear membrane.

**cloacal m.,** the thin, temporary barrier between the hindgut and the exterior, formed by the endoderm of the hindgut and the ectoderm of the cloaca of the embryo; its dorsal part forms the *anal membrane.*

**complex m.,** a membrane made up of several layers differing in structure.

**compound m.,** a membrane, like that of the tympanum, made up of two distinct layers.

**Corti's m.,** membrana tectoria ductus cochlearis.

**costocoracoid m.,** fascia clavipectoralis.

**cribriform m.,** fascia cribrosa.

**cricothyroid m., cricovocal m.,** conus elasticus.

**croupous m.,** false m.

**cyclitic m.,** a false membrane which sometimes covers the vitreous body in cyclitis.

**cytoplasmic m.,** plasma m.

**Debove's m.,** the delicate layer between the epithelium and the tunica propria of the bronchial, tracheal, and intestinal mucous membranes.

**decidual m's, deciduous m's,** membranae deciduae.

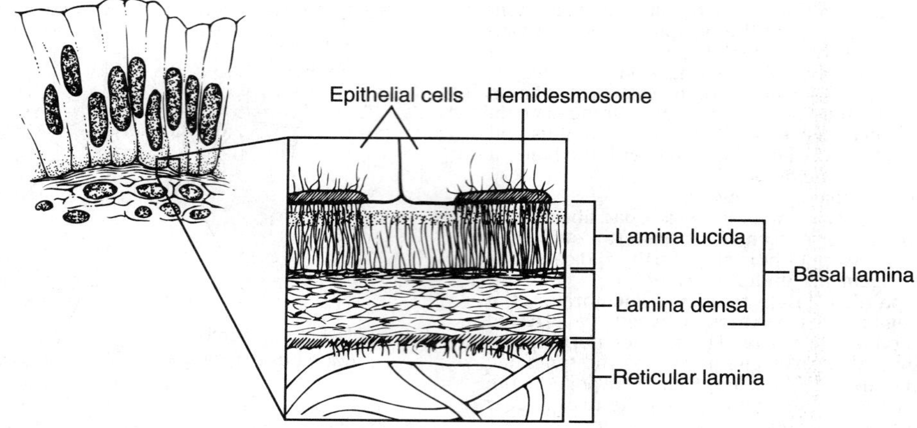


Basement membrane, comprising the basal lamina and reticular lamina, in a diagram of a section through epithelial tissue.

**dentinoenamel m.,** a continuous thin membrane laid down by ameloblasts adjoining the basement membrane separating them from the dentin in an early developing tooth.

**Descemet's m.,** lamina limitans posterior corneae.

**diphtheritic m.,** a false membrane characteristic of diphtheria and resulting from coagulation necrosis.

**drum m.,** membrana tympani.

**egg m.,** any of several investments surrounding the oocyte (ovum or egg): if derived from the oocyte itself, as the vitelline membrane, it is called *primary;* if from the follicular cells, as the zona pellucida, it is called *secondary;* if from the oviduct, as the albumen around rabbit's egg or the albumen and shell of hen's egg, it is called *tertiary.* Called also *egg envelope* and, collectively, *lemma.*

**elastic m.,** 1. a membrane composed largely of elastic fibers. 2. see *external elastic m.* and *internal elastic m.*

**elastic m., external,** a fenestrated elastic membrane that constitutes the innermost component of the tunica adventitia of arteries. Called also *external elastic lamina.*

**elastic m., internal,** a fenestrated elastic membrane that constitutes the outermost component of the tunica intima of arteries. Called also *internal elastic lamina.*

**enamel m.,** 1. cuticula dentis. 2. the inner layer of cells within the enamel organ of the dental germ in the fetus; called also *Hannover's intermediate m.*

**endoneural m.,** neurilemma.

**endoral m.,** paroral m.

**excitable m.,** the membrane of an excitable cell.

**exocoelomic m.,** Heuser's m.

**extraembryonic m's,** the trophoblastic parts of the conceptus that provide for the support of the embryo or fetus by attachment, mechanical protection, endocrine action, and the mediation of chemical exchange with the maternal circulation. They include the yolk sac, allantois, amnion, umbilical cord, and chorion, including the placenta. Called also *fetal m's.*

**false m.,** a layer resembling an organized and living membrane, but made up of coagulated fibrin with bacteria and leukocytes, such as may be formed on mucous membranes in diphtheria or in the gut with *Clostridium difficile* infection. Called also *neomembrane* and *pseudomembrane.*

**fenestrated m.,** either of the elastic membranes of arteries; see *internal elastic m.* and *external elastic m.*

**fertilization m.,** a strong membrane formed around the fertilized ovum in some species of animals by adhesion of part of the contents of the cortical granules to the inner surface of the vitelline membrane; it prevents the entry of additional spermatozoa.

**fetal m's,** extraembryonic m's.

**fibroelastic m. of larynx,** membrana fibroelastica laryngis.

**fibrous m. of articular capsule,** membrana fibrosa capsulae articularis.

**germinal m.,** blastoderm.

**glassy m.,** 1. the basement membrane of a vesicular ovarian follicle which in cross-section appears as a distinct brilliant line and which persists in the ovary long after its follicle has degenerated. Called also *m. of Slavianski.* 2. lamina basalis choroideae. 3. hyaline m., def. 1.

**glomerular m.,** the membrane covering a glomerular capillary.

**gradocol m's,** thin membranes made of collodion or similar substances and graded as to porosity; used in ultrafiltration and sometimes to estimate the diameters of viruses or other small particles.

**ground m.,** inophragma.

**Haller's m.,** lamina vasculosa choroideae.

**Hannover's intermediate m.,** enamel m., def. 2.

**hemodialyzer m.,** the semipermeable membrane that filters the blood in a hemodialyzer, commonly made of cuprophane, cellulose acetate, polyacrylonitrile, or polymethyl methacrylate.

**Henle's m.,** posterior border lamella of Fuchs; see under *lamella.*

**Henle's elastic m.,** external elastic m.

**Henle's fenestrated m.,** fenestrated m.

**Heuser's m.,** a delicate sac of mesoblastic tissue that develops as a lining of the blastocyst or chorionic cavity just after implantation, forms the exocoelomic cavity, and quickly disappears; called also *exocoelomic m..*

**high efficiency m.,** a hemodialyzer membrane that has clearance characteristics that increase progressively with increases in dialysis blood flow rates; this usually implies that the membrane is not a high flux membrane.

**high flux m.,** a hemodialyzer membrane that has a high permeability to fluids and solutes and thus a high rate of clearance of fluids and solutes composed of large molecules.

**Huxley's m.,** see under *layer.*

**hyaline m.,** 1. the membrane between the outer root sheath and the inner fibrous layer of a hair follicle. 2. a layer of eosinophilic hyaline material lining the alveoli, alveolar ducts, and bronchioles, found at autopsy in infants who have died of respiratory distress syndrome of the newborn (see under *syndrome*). Similar changes may be seen in adults who have died of viral respiratory infections. Called also *asphyxial m.* and *vernix m.*

**hyaloid m.,** membrana vitrea.

**hymenal m.,** hymen.

**hyoglossal m.,** a fibrous lamina connecting the under surface of the tongue with the hyoid bone.

**hyothyroid m.,** membrana thyrohyoidea.

**intercostal m., external,** membrana intercostalis externa.

**intercostal m., internal,** membrana intercostalis interna.

**interosseous m., radioulnar,** membrana interossea antebrachii.

**interosseous m. of leg,** membrana interossea cruris.

**interspinal m's,** see *ligamenta interspinalia.*

**intersutural m.,** the pericranium lying between the cranial sutures.

**ion-selective m.,** a membrane that is more permeable to particular types of ions than to other types, e.g., $K^+$-selective glass membrane. Many biological membranes exhibit ion-selective behavior.

**Jackson's m.,** a delicate curtain or web of adhesions (regarded by some as a sheet of peritoneum) which may extend from the lateral abdominal wall to the cecum, covering the cecum and producing obstruction of the bowel; called also *Jackson's veil.*

**Jacob's m.,** layer of rods and cones.

**keratogenous m.,** matrix unguis.

**Kölliker's m.,** membrana reticularis organi spiralis.

**Krause's m.,** Z band; see under *band.*

**ligamentous m.,** membrana tectoria.

**limiting m.,** a membrane which constitutes the border of some tissue or structure.

**limiting m., external,** 1. a thin fenestrated layer of the pars nervosa retinae adjacent to the outer nuclear layer and through which extend the visual rods and cones. 2. a membrane investing the external surface of the embryonic neural tube. Called also *outer limiting m.*

**limiting m., inner, limiting m., internal,** 1. internal limiting layer. 2. a membrane lining the internal surface of the embryonic neural tube.

**limiting m., outer,** external limiting m.

**Mauthner's m.,** axolemma.
**medullary m.,** endosteum.
**mucocutaneous m.,** a membrane that is partly mucous and partly cutaneous, like that of the tympanum.
**mucous m.,** tunica mucosa.
**mucous m., proper,** lamina propria mucosae.
**mucous m. of esophagus,** tunica mucosa oesophagi.
**mucous m. of gallbladder,** tunica mucosa vesicae biliaris.
**mucous m. of large intestine,** tunica mucosa intestini crassi.
**mucous m. of mouth,** tunica mucosa oris.
**mucous m. of pharynx,** tunica mucosa pharyngis.
**mucous m. of rectum,** tunica mucosa recti.
**mucous m. of small intestine,** tunica mucosa intestini tenuis.
**mucous m. of stomach,** tunica mucosa gastris.
**mucous m. of tongue,** tunica mucosa linguae.
**mucous m. of ureter,** tunica mucosa ureteris.
**mucous m. of urinary bladder,** tunica mucosa vesicae urinariae.
**Nasmyth's m.,** primary (enamel) cuticle.
**nictitating m.,** a transparent fold of skin lying deep to the other eyelids at the mesial side, which may be drawn over the front of the eyeball; found in reptiles and birds generally and in many mammals. See also *haw.* Called also *third eyelid* and *membrana nictitans.*
**nuclear m.,** 1. either of the membranes, inner and outer, comprising the nuclear envelope. 2. nuclear envelope.
**oblique m. of forearm,** chorda obliqua membranae interosseae antebrachii.
**obturator m.,** membrana obturatoria.
**obturator m. of atlas, anterior,** membrana atlanto-occipitalis anterior.
**obturator m. of atlas, posterior,** membrana atlanto-occipitalis posterior.
**occipitoaxial m., long,** membrana tectoria.
**olfactory m.,** the olfactory portion of the mucous membrane lining the nasal fossa.
**oral m.,** oropharyngeal m.
**oronasal m.,** a thin epithelial plate separating the nasal pits from the oral cavity of the embryo. Called also *bucconasal m.*
**oropharyngeal m.,** a transient embryonic septum at the cranial limit of the foregut, in the depths of the stomodeum; called also *buccopharyngeal m.*
**otolithic m.,** membrana statoconiorum macularum.
**ovular m.,** vitelline m.
**palatine m.,** the membrane covering the roof of the mouth.
**pansporoblastic m.,** a surface membrane surrounding the sporoblasts in a pansporoblast; characteristic of microsporidian protozoa of the suborder Pansporoblastina.
**paroral m.,** in certain ciliate protozoa, a movable membrane-like sheet(s) formed by fusion of the bases of a longitudinal row of cilia that borders the right side of the buccal cavity; it serves to gather food and push it toward the cytostome. Called also *endoral m.* and *undulating m.* Cf. *membranelle.*
**pericolic m.,** occasional bands of peritoneum extending between the abdominal wall and the serosa of the colon.
**peridental m.,** periodontal ligament.
**perineal m.,** membrana perinei.
**periodontal m.,** see under *ligament.*
**periorbital m.,** periorbita.
**peritrophic m.,** a delicate, cylindrical sheath of chitin continuously secreted from the posterior edge of the foregut of insects and millipedes that ingest solid food, which surrounds the food as it passes through the midgut.
**pharyngeal m.,** fascia pharyngobasilaris.
**pituitary m. of nose,** tunica mucosa nasi.
**placental m.,** the semipermeable membrane that separates the fetal from the maternal blood in the placenta. In the human (hemochorial) placenta, it is composed of fetal vascular endothelium, connective tissue, trophoblast, and syncytium, and it becomes thinner as pregnancy progresses. Sometimes inappropriately called the *placental barrier;* there are only a few substances that cannot pass through the membrane.
**plasma m.,** the structure enveloping a cell, enclosing the cytoplasm, and forming a selective permeability barrier; it consists of lipids, proteins, and some carbohydrates, the lipids thought to form a bilayer in which integral proteins are embedded to varying degrees. Called also *cell m., cytoplasmic m.,* and *plasmalemma.*
**platelet demarcation m.,** a more or less tridimensional system of paired membranes that serve to partition the megakaryocyte cytoplasm, each partition containing azurophilic granules and representing a future blood platelet.
**pleuropericardial m.,** a membrane in the embryo separating the pericardial cavity from the pleural cavity.
**pleuroperitoneal m.,** a membrane in the embryo separating the pleural cavity from the peritoneal cavity and developing into the posterolateral part of the diaphragm.

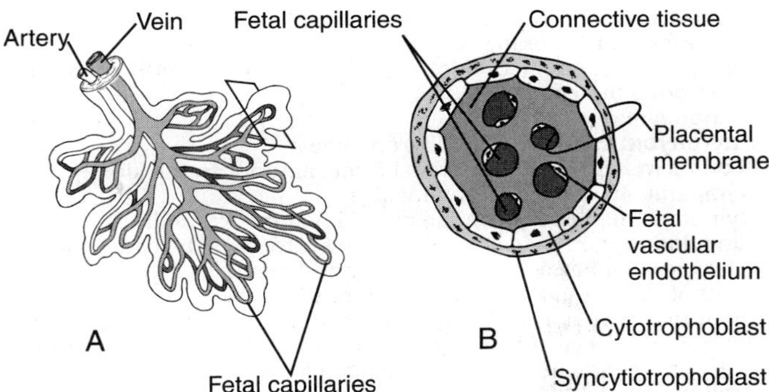


Placental membrane separating the blood in the fetal capillaries from the maternal blood in the intervillous space. *(A),* chorionic villus containing the fetal vessels and surrounded by maternal blood in the intervillous space; *(B),* cross-section through a villus, showing the layers of the placental membrane separating the fetal blood from the maternal blood surrounding the villus.

**postsynaptic m.,** the area of plasma membrane of a postsynaptic cell, either a muscle fiber or a neuron, that is within the synapse and has areas especially adapted for receiving neurotransmitters.
**presynaptic m.,** the area of plasma membrane of a presynaptic axon that is within the synapse and has sites (active zones) especially adapted for the release of neurotransmitters.
**proper m. of semicircular duct,** membrana propria ductus semicircularis.
**prophylactic m.,** pyophylactic m.
**pseudoserous m.,** a membrane resembling serous membrane, but differing from it in structure.
**pupillary m.,** membrana pupillaris.
**pupillary m., persistent,** a congenital defect in dogs in which remnants of the tunica vasculosa lentis are found on the surface of the iris or cornea, sometimes with a corneal opacity.
**pyloric m.,** a congenital abnormal membrane in the pylorus, partially or completely blocking the gastric outlet. See also *prepyloric atresia.* Called also *pyloric diaphragm* and *pyloric web.*
**pyogenic m.,** a membrane which produces pus.
**pyophylactic m.,** a fibrinous membrane lining a pus cavity and tending to prevent reabsorption of injurious materials.
**quadrangular m.,** membrana quadrangularis.
**Reissner's m.,** paries vestibularis ductus cochlearis.
**reticular m.,** membrana reticularis organi spiralis.
**Rivinus' m.,** pars flaccida membranae tympanicae.
**m. of round window,** membrana tympani secundaria.
**Ruysch's m., ruyschian m.,** the capillary layer of the choroid in addition to the pigmented layer of the retina and Bruch's membrane (the basal complex of the choroid). Called also *membrana ruyschiana, tunica ruyschiana,* and *Ruysch's tunic.*
**Scarpa's m.,** membrana tympani secundaria.
**schneiderian m.,** tunica mucosa nasi.
**Schwann's m.,** neurilemma.
**semipermeable m.,** a membrane that is freely traversed by solvent, such as water, but which permits the passage of only certain solutes.
**serous m.,** tunica serosa.
**shell m.,** a double fibrous layer lining the shell of the egg of some animals, such as birds.
**Shrapnell's m.,** pars flaccida membranae tympanicae.
**m. of Slavianski,** glassy m., def. 1.
**slit m.,** one of the exceedingly thin membranes that bridge the slit pores between adjacent pedicels of the podocytes of the renal glomerulus, and close the pores at their bases.
**spiral m. of cochlear duct,** paries tympanicus ductus cochlearis.
**stapedial m.,** membrana stapedialis.
**statoconic m. of maculae,** membrana statoconiorum macularum.
**sternal m.,** membrana sterni.
**striated m.,** see *zona pellucida,* def. 1.
**subepithelial m.,** basement m.
**submucous m.,** tela submucosa.
**submucous m. of stomach,** tela submucosa gastris.
**suprapleural m.,** membrana suprapleuralis.
**synaptic m.,** the part of the plasma membrane of a neuron that is within a synapse; see *postsynaptic m.* and *presynaptic m.*
**synovial m.,** membrana synovialis capsulae articularis.
**synovial m. of articular capsule,** membrana synovialis capsulae articularis.
**synovial m. of temporomandibular joint, inferior,** membrana synovialis inferior articulationis temporomandibularis.
**synovial m. of temporomandibular joint, superior,** membrana synovialis superior articulationis temporomandibularis.

**tarsal m.,** orbital septum.
**tectorial m.,** membrana tectoria.
**tectorial m. of cochlear duct,** membrana tectoria ductus cochlearis.
**tendinous m.,** aponeurosis.
**Tenon's m.,** vagina bulbi.
**thyrohyoid m.,** membrana thyrohyoidea.
**Toldt's m.,** the part of the renal fascia anterior to the kidney.
**tympanic m.,** membrana tympanica.
**tympanic m., secondary,** membrana tympani secundaria.
**undulating m.,** 1. in certain flagellate protozoa, a delicate finlike cytoplasmic membrane extending from and running along the lateral aspect of the body, the outer margin of which being formed by a flagellum that may continue free beyond the end of the body and the membrane. It serves a locomotor function; vibration of the membrane produces a characteristic undulating movement. 2. paroral m.
**unit m.,** the trilaminar structure of the plasma membrane as seen under the electron microscope and postulated to be the same for the membranes of all cells, the cell nucleus, and organelles (mitochondria, etc.).
**vascular m. of viscera,** tela submucosa.
**vernix m.,** hyaline m. (def. 2); so called because it was originally thought to be the result of aspiration of vernix by the fetus *in utero.*
**vestibular m. of cochlear duct,** paries vestibularis ductus cochlearis.
**virginal m.,** hymen.
**vitelline m.,** the cytoplasmic, noncellular membrane surrounding the eggs of various animals, especially the membrane enveloping the yolk of telolecithal eggs.
**vitreous m.,** 1. membrana vitrea. 2. lamina basalis choroideae. 3. lamina limitans posterior corneae. 4. hyaline membrane (def. 1).
**Volkmann's m.,** a thin, yellowish membrane, studded with miliary tubercles, lining the fibrous wall of a tubercular abscess.
**Wachendorf's m.,** 1. membrana pupillaris. 2. plasma m.
**yolk m.,** vitelline m.
**Zinn's m.,** zonula ciliaris.

**mem·bra·nec·to·my** (mem″brə-nek′tə-me) excision of a membrane.

**mem·bra·nelle** (mem″brə-nel′) a triangular or fan-shaped organelle bordering the left side of the buccal cavity or peristomial area in certain ciliate protozoa, formed by fusion of the bases of short, transverse rows (up to three) of cilia; it serves in locomotion and to gather and push food toward the cytostome. Cf. *paroral membrane.*

**mem·bra·ni·form** (məm-bra′nĭ-form) resembling a membrane.

**mem·bra·no·car·ti·lag·i·nous** (mem″brə-no-kahr″tĭ-laj′ĭ-nəs) 1. developed in both membrane and cartilage. 2. partly cartilaginous and partly membranous.

**mem·bra·noid** (mem′brə-noid) resembling a membrane.

**mem·bran·ol·y·sis** (mem″brān-ol′ĭ-sis) disruption of a cell membrane.

**mem·bra·nous** (mem′brə-nəs) [L. *membranosus*] pertaining to or of the nature of a membrane.

**mem·brum** (mem′brəm) pl. *mem′bra* [L.] [TA] a member or limb.
**m. infe′rius** [TA], lower limb: the limb extending from the gluteal region to the foot; see also *leg,* and see *regiones membrum inferioris,* under *regio.* It is specialized for weight-bearing and locomotion. Called also *extremitas inferior.*
**m. mulie′bre,** clitoris.
**m. supe′rius** [TA], upper limb: the limb of the body extending from the deltoid region to the hand; see also *arm,* and see *regiones membrum superioris,* under *regio.* It is specialized for functions requiring great mobility, such as grasping and manipulating. Called also *extremitas superior.*
**m. viri′le,** penis.

**mem·o·ry** (mem′ə-re) [L. *memoria*] [MeSH: Memory] that mental faculty by which sensations, impressions, and ideas are recalled.
**anterograde m.,** remote m.
**echoic m.,** that part of the sensory storage system that holds auditory stimuli.
**eye m.,** visual m.
**iconic m.,** that part of the sensory storage system that holds visual stimuli.
**immediate m.,** short-term m.
**immunologic m.,** the capacity of the immune system to respond more rapidly and strongly to subsequent antigenic challenge than to the first exposure. Called also *anamnesis.* See *memory cells,* under *cell,* and *primary* and *secondary immune response,* under *response.*
**kinesthetic m.,** motor m.
**long-term m.,** memory that is retained over long periods of time.
**motor m.,** the memory of movements in the limbs and other parts of the body.
**physiological m.,** the physical storage of engrams in the brain by means of RNA.
**remote m.,** a memory serviceable for events long past, but not able to acquire new recollections; called also *anterograde m.* and *palinmnesis.*
**replacement m.,** the replacing of one memory with a different one; cf. *screen m.*
**screen m.,** a consciously tolerable memory serving to "screen" or conceal another memory that might be disturbing or emotionally painful if recalled.
**short-term m.,** memory that is lost within a brief period (from a few seconds to a maximum of about 30 minutes) unless reinforced.
**visual m.,** memory for visual impressions.

**MEN** [MeSH: Men] multiple endocrine neoplasia.

**Mena·can·thus** (men″ə-kan′thus) a genus of parasitic biting lice (order Mallophaga). *M. palli′dulus* and *M. strami′neus* attack chickens and turkeys.

**me·nac·me** (mə-nak′me) [*men-* + Gr. *akmē* highest point] 1. the height of menstrual activity. 2. that period of a woman's life which is marked by menstrual activity.

**men·a·di·ol** (men″ə-di′ol) the reduced, dihydro form of menadione.
**m. sodium diphosphate** [USP], a synthetic, water-soluble derivative of menadione (vitamin $K_3$), to which it is converted in the body; used as a prothrombinogenic vitamin for the same purposes as menadione (q.v.); administered orally, intravenously, and subcutaneously.

**men·a·di·one** (men″ə-di′ōn) 1. [USP] a synthetic fat-soluble provitamin that can be chemically converted in the body to active vitamin K by addition of a long side chain; used as a source of vitamin K in the treatment of hemorrhagic conditions associated with hypoprothrombinemia, such as obstructive jaundice, biliary fistula, sprue, celiac disease, and ulcerative colitis, and after prolonged use of salicylates, administered orally and intramuscularly. 2. the basic double ring quinone structure that is the parent structure of the related compounds with vitamin K activity, which can be formed by addition of long side chain substituents. Called also *menaphthone* and *vitamin* $K_3$.
**m. sodium bisulfite,** a water-soluble derivative of menadione having the same actions and uses; administered intravenously and subcutaneously, and sometimes orally and intramuscularly.

**Men·a·gen** (men′ə-jən) trademark for a preparation of estrone.

**men·al·gia** (mən-al′jə) [*men-* + *-algia*] pain accompanying menstruation.

**men·aph·thone** (mən-af′thōn) menadione.

**men·a·quin·one** (men″ə-kwin′ōn) any of a series of compounds in which the phytyl side chain of phytonadione (vitamin $K_1$) is replaced by a side chain of prenyl units and which have vitamin K activity. This form of the vitamin is usually available to the human body even in cases of dietary deficiency because menaquinones are synthesized by the intestinal flora. Called also *vitamin* $K_2$.

**me·nar·chal** (mə-nahr′kəl) pertaining to menarche.

**me·nar·che** (mə-nahr′ke) [*men-* + Gr. *archē* beginning] [MeSH: Menarche] the establishment or beginning of the menstrual function.

**me·nar·che·al, me·nar·chi·al** (mə-nahr′ke-əl) pertaining to or characterized by the establishment of the menstrual function (menarche).

**Men·del's laws** (men′delz) [Gregor Johann *Mendel,* Austrian monk and naturalist, 1822–1884] see under *law.*

**Men·del's reflex** (men′delz) [Kurt *Mendel,* German neurologist, 1874–1946] see under *reflex.*

**Men·del's test** (men′delz) [Felix *Mendel,* German physician, 1862–1912] Mantoux test; see under *test.*

**Men·del-Bekh·ter·ev reflex, sign** (men′del-bek-ter′yev) [Kurt *Mendel;* V. M. *Bekhterev,* Russian neurologist, 1857–1927] see under *reflex* and *sign.*

**Men·de·lé·eff's (Men·de·le·ev's) law** (men″də-la′əfs) [Dimitri Ivanovich *Mendeléeff,* Russian chemist, 1834–1907] see *periodic law,* under *law.*

**Men·de·le·ev's law, table** (men″də-la′əfs) [Dimitri Ivanovich *Mendeleev* (or *Mendeléef* or *Mendeléeff*), Russian chemist, 1834–1907] see *periodic law,* under *law* and *periodic table,* under *table.*

**men·de·le·vi·um** (men″də-le′ve-əm) [Dimitri Ivanovich *Mendeléeff*] [MeSH: Mendelevium] the radioactive chemical element of atomic number 101, atomic weight 256, symbol Md, originally discovered in debris from a thermonuclear explosion in 1952.

**men·de·li·an** (mən-de′le-ən) named for Gregor Johann *Mendel;* see under *law.*

**men·del·ism** (men′dəl-iz -əm) the principles of heredity derived from Mendel's laws.

**men·del·iz·ing** (men′dəl-iz″ing) exhibiting the simple patterns of inheritance of various contrasting traits elaborated by Gregor Mendel; see *Mendel's laws,* under *law.*

**Men·del·son's syndrome** (men′dəl-sənz) [Curtis Lester *Mendelson,* American obstetrician and gynecologist, born 1913] see under *syndrome.*

**Men·doc·u·tes** (mən-dok′u-tēz, men″do-ku′tēz) Mendosicutes.

**Men·do·sic·u·tes** (men″do-sik′u-tēz, men″do-sĭ-ku′tēz) [L. *mendosus* having faults + *cutis* skin] a division of bacteria of the kingdom Procaryotae made up of organisms that usually have a cell wall, although it is lacking in muramic acid, and that have other evidences of an earlier phylogenetic origin (based on ribosomal RNA oligonucleotide analysis). These organisms (the Archaeobacteria) include methanogens, strict halophiles, and thermoacidophiles.

**Men·est** (men′əst) trademark for a preparation of esterified estrogens.

**Mé·né·trier's disease** (ma-na″tre-ārz′) [Pierre *Ménétrier,* French physician, 1859–1935] giant hypertrophic gastritis.

**Men·for·mon** (men′for-mon) trademark for a preparation of estrone.

**Menge's pessary** (meng′gəz) [Karl *Menge,* German gynecologist, 1864–1945] see under *pessary.*

**Men·go encephalomyelitis, virus** (men′go) [*Mengo* district in Uganda, where the disease was first seen in 1948] see under *encephalomyelitis* and *virus.*

**men·hi·dro·sis** (men″hi-dro′sis) [*men-* + *hidro-* + *-sis*] a form of vicarious menstruation consisting of monthly discharge of sweat, sometimes bloody.

**men·id·ro·sis** (men″id-ro′sis) menhidrosis.

**Men·i·ere's disease (syndrome)** (men″e-ārz′) [Prosper *Meniere,* French physician, 1799–1862. The spelling *Meniere* appears on his birth certificate, *Menière* and *Ménière* on his works. Ménière was the choice of his son] see under *disease.*

**me·nin·ge·al** (mə-nin′je-əl) of or pertaining to the meninges.

**me·nin·gem·a·to·ma** (mə-nin″jem-ə-to′mə) epidural hematoma.

**me·nin·geo·cor·ti·cal** (mə-nin″je-o-kor′tĭ-kəl) meningocortical.

**me·nin·ge·o·ma** (mə-nin″je-o′mə) meningioma.

**me·nin·ge·or·rha·phy** (mə-nin″je-or′ə-fe) [*meningo-* + *-rrhaphy*] suture of the meninges.

**me·nin·ges** (mə-nin′jēz) [Gr., pl. of *mēninx* membrane] [TA] [MeSH: Meninges] the three membranes that envelop the brain and spinal cord: the dura mater, pia mater, and arachnoid.

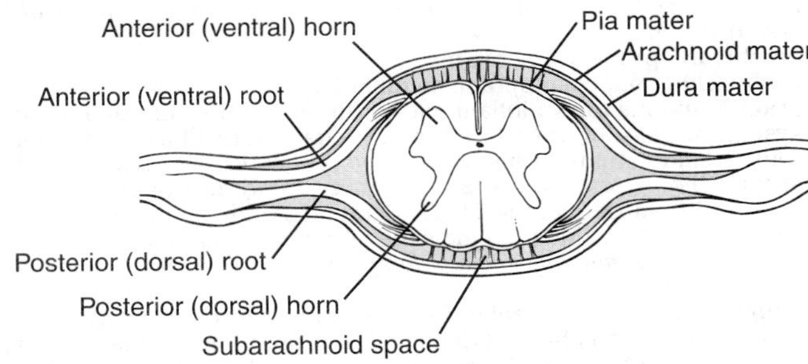


Meninges, comprising the dura mater, arachnoid mater, and pia mater; shown in a cross-section of the spinal cord.

**me·ning·hem·a·to·ma** (mə-ninj″hem-ə-to′mə) epidural hematoma.

**me·nin·gi·o·ma** (mə-nin″je-o′mə) [*meninges* + *-oma*] [MeSH: Meningioma] a benign, slow-growing tumor of the meninges, usually next to the dura mater, probably arising from cells associated with arachnoid villi. It may erode the skull or cause hyperostosis, and increased intracranial pressure is common. Meningiomas are now usually classified according to anatomic location; an older classification by histologic features exists, but histologic features have not been shown to influence clinical behavior.
**angioblastic m.,** a meningioma with many blood vessels, which may vary in size from capillary to cavernous; called also *angioblastoma.*
**cerebellopontine angle m.,** a posterior fossa meningioma located in the cerebellopontine angle; it may cause symptoms like those of an acoustic neuroma or may compress any of the first five cranial nerves.
**clival m.,** a posterior fossa meningioma located over the middle or rostral part of the clivus; symptoms include palsy of the fifth, seventh, or eighth cranial nerve and gait ataxia.
**convexity m's,** a diverse group of meningiomas located within the sulci of the brain, usually anterior to the rolandic fissure; they may be silent for long periods. Symptoms include seizures, weakness of the arm and face, and personality changes.
**cystic m.,** a meningioma containing or adjacent to cysts.
**falcine m., falx m.,** a meningioma in or near the falx cerebri; symptoms are similar to those of a parasagittal meningioma.
**fibroblastic m.,** a meningioma characterized by fibrous tissue with bundles of spindle cells; called also *fibrous m.* and *meningofibroblastoma.*
**fibrous m.,** fibroblastic m.
**meningotheliomatous m.,** a meningioma characterized by plump cells with poorly defined boundaries, sometimes in whorls or lobules; called also *syncytial m.* and *meningothelioma.*
**m. of the olfactory groove,** a meningioma located in the ethmoid fossa (olfactory groove); symptoms include anosmia, visual defects including Kennedy's syndrome, and psychic disturbances.
**parasagittal m.,** a meningioma located next to the superior sagittal sinus, often growing into the sinus; symptoms are variable according to location and may include seizures, leg weakness or paresthesias, and visual field defects. See also *falx m.*
**posterior fossa m.,** a meningioma in the posterior cranial fossa; these include tentorial, clival, and cerebellopontine angle meningiomas.
**psammomatous m.,** a transitional meningioma that contains many psammoma bodies; called also *psammoma.*
**m. of the sphenoid ridge,** a meningioma located along the sphenoid ridge; symptoms commonly include trigeminal neuralgia, unilateral exophthalmos progressing to blindness, Kennedy's syndrome, and Tolosa-Hunt syndrome.
**suprasellar m.,** a meningioma located above the sella turcica near its tuberculum; because of its proximity to the optic chiasm, it pushes against the optic nerve and causes bitemporal hemianopia and other visual deficits. Called also *m. of the tuberculum sellae.*
**syncytial m.,** meningotheliomatous m.
**tentorial m.,** a posterior fossa meningioma located on the tentorium cerebelli; it may cause seizures, visual hallucinations, and visual field deficits.
**transitional m.,** a meningioma histologically intermediate between the meningotheliomatous and fibroblastic types; calcification of whorls of cells often causes psammoma bodies. See also *psammomatous m.*
**m. of the tuberculum sellae,** suprasellar m.

**me·nin·gi·o·ma·to·sis** (mə-nin″je-o″mə-to′sis) a condition characterized by the formation of multiple meningiomas.

**me·nin·gism** (mə-nin′jiz-əm) [MeSH: Meningism] the symptoms and signs of meningeal irritation associated with acute febrile illness or dehydration without actual infection of the meninges. Called also *meningismus* and *pseudomeningitis.*

**men·in·gis·mus** (men″in-jis′məs) meningism.

**men·in·git·ic** (men″in-jit′ik) pertaining to or of the nature of meningitis.

**men·in·git·i·des** (men″in-jit′ĭ-dēz) [MeSH: Meningitis] plural of *meningitis.*

**men·in·gi·tis** (men″in-ji′tis) pl. *meningit′ides* [*mening-* + *-itis*] [MeSH: Meningitis] inflammation of the meninges, usually by either a bacterium *(bacterial m.)* or a virus *(viral m.).*
**acute aseptic m.,** aseptic m.
**aseptic m.,** any of several mild types of meningitis, most of which are caused by viruses; see *viral m.* Called also *acute aseptic m.* and *sterile m.*
**bacterial m.,** meningitis caused by bacteria; common pathogens are *Haemophilus influenzae* (see *Haemophilus influenzae m.*), *Neisseria meningitidis* (see *meningococcal m.*), *Streptococcus pneumoniae* (see

*pneumococcal m.*), and *Mycobacterium tuberculosis* (see *tuberculous m.*). Called also *purulent* or *pyogenic m.* Cf. *viral m.*

**basilar m.**, that which affects the meninges at the base of the brain.

**benign lymphocytic m.**, lymphocytic choriomeningitis.

**m. carcinomato'sa, carcinomatous m.**, a misnomer for meningeal carcinoma, a condition that is not inflammatory.

**cerebral m.**, inflammation of the meninges of the brain.

**cerebrospinal m.**, any inflammation of the membranes of the brain and spinal cord; see *bacterial m.* and *viral m.*

**chronic m.**, a variable syndrome of fever, headache, lethargy, stiff neck, confusion, nausea, and vomiting, with pleocytosis and with or without hypoglycorrachia, which fails to improve over a period of 4 weeks; it may be produced by any of a large number of infectious agents and noninfectious conditions.

**cryptococcal m.**, cryptococcosis in which the meninges are invaded by *Cryptococcus;* it has both a subacute chronic form and a more serious acute form and is increased in immunocompromised patients.

**eosinophilic m.**, meningitis characterized by an increase in lymphocytes and a high percentage of eosinophils in the cerebrospinal fluid; it usually results from infection with *Angiostrongylus cantonensis.* Called also *eosinophilic meningoencephalitis.*

**epidemic cerebrospinal m.**, meningococcal m.

**external m.**, external pachymeningitis.

**gummatous m.**, meningitis during the tertiary stage of syphilis in which there are many small gummata in the membranes.

***Haemophilus influenzae* m.**, bacterial meningitis caused by infection with *Haemophilus influenzae,* seen most often in young children and the elderly.

**internal m.**, internal pachymeningitis.

**lymphocytic m.**, see under *choriomeningitis.*

**meningococcal m.**, bacterial meningitis caused by infection with *Neisseria meningitidis*, an acute infectious disease with seropurulent meningeal inflammation. It usually appears in epidemics, and symptoms are those of acute cerebral and spinal meningitis, usually with an eruption of cutaneous erythematous, herpetic, or hemorrhagic spots. The fulminating or malignant form is known as *Waterhouse-Friderichsen syndrome.* Called also *cerebrospinal fever* and *epidemic cerebrospinal m.*

**Mollaret's m.**, recurrent febrile attacks, malaise, headache, and meningeal signs accompanied by a marked polymorphonuclear inflammatory reaction in the cerebrospinal fluid.

**mumps m.**, an aseptic meningitis secondary to mumps; see also *mumps meningoencephalitis.*

**neoplastic m.**, meningitis resulting from cancer metastasis to the leptomeninges or subarachnoid space.

**occlusive m.**, leptomeningitis of children which leads to the closure of the lateral and median apertures of the fourth ventricle.

**m. ossi'ficans**, ossification of the cerebral meninges.

**otitic m.**, a form that sometimes complicates an attack of otitis media.

**plague m.**, meningitis occurring as a rare complication of bubonic plague as a result of hematogenous spread of the infection from a bubo to involve the meninges, or less often as a primary infection without antecedent bubo formation. Called also *meningeal plague.*

**pneumococcal m.**, bacterial meningitis caused by a pneumococcus *(Streptococcus pneumoniae),* usually seen in young children or the elderly. Up to half the cases are secondary to other infections, such as those of the lungs, ears, or paranasal sinuses, and reinfection may occur. The incidence is increased in asplenic or immunocompromised patients, such as those with sickle cell disease or lymphocytic leukemia.

**purulent m., pyogenic m.**, bacterial m.

**m. sero'sa circumscrip'ta**, chronic adhesive arachnoiditis.

**spinal m.**, inflammation of the meninges of the spinal cord.

**sterile m.**, aseptic m.

**streptococcal m.**, meningitis in piglets caused by *streptococcus suis*; characteristics include incoordination, tremors, convulsions, and sometimes paralysis that can be fatal.

**m. sympa'thica**, a condition of the cerebrospinal fluid caused by inflammation in the neighborhood of the meninges. It is marked by increase in the pressure of the fluid and increase in its albumin and cellular content. The fluid is sterile and there may be symptoms of meningitis.

**syphilitic m.**, general paresis.

**tubercular m., tuberculous m.**, a severe bacterial meningitis caused by *Mycobacterium tuberculosis,* usually spreading from a primary infection in the lungs.

**viral m.**, meningitis due to various viruses, such as the coxsackieviruses, mumps virus, and the virus of lymphocytic choriomeningitis, characterized by malaise, fever, headache, nausea, cerebrospinal fluid pleocytosis (principally lymphocytic), abdominal pain, stiffness of the neck and back, and a short uncomplicated course. See also *aseptic m.*

**mening(o)-** [Gr. *mēninx,* gen. *mēningos* membrane] a combining form denoting relationship to a membrane, especially relationship to the meninges.

**me•nin•go•ar•ter•i•tis** (mə-ning″go-ahr″tər-i′tis) inflammation of the meningeal arteries.

**me•nin•go•cele** (mə-ning′go-sēl″) [*meningo-* + *-cele*[1]] [MeSH: Meningocele] hernial protrusion of the meninges through a bony defect; the two types are *cranial m.* and *spinal m.* See also *spina bifida cystica,* under *spina.*

**anterior m.**, a rare type of meningocele that protrudes anteriorly from the vertebral column, usually in the sacral region; symptoms often are mild and go unnoticed.

**cranial m.**, hernial protrusion of the meninges through a cranium bifidum, usually forming a fluid-filled sac; called also *craniomeningocele.* See also *encephalocele.*

**sacral m.**, a meningocele in the sacral region; symptoms may remain occult until adulthood and include neurologic deficits and abdominal masses with pressure. Both posterior and anterior types have been observed; see also *anterior m.*

**spinal m.**, hernial protrusion of the meninges through a defect in the vertebral column (spina bifida), usually posteriorly, forming a fluid-filled sac; locations are almost always in the thoracic or lumbar region although cervical and sacral ones do occur. See also *myelomeningocele.*

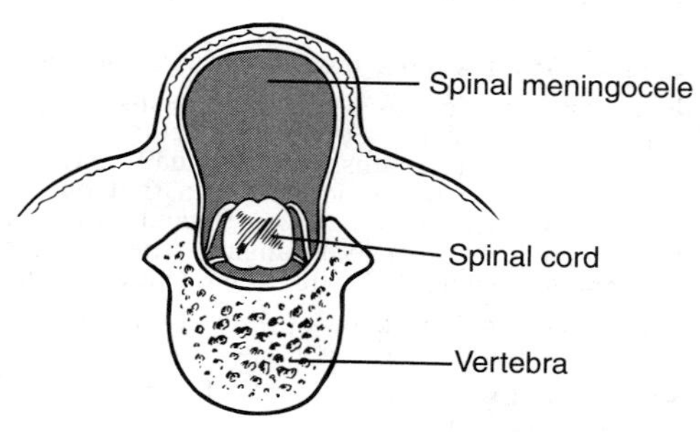


**spurious m., traumatic m.**, a condition resembling cranial meningocele, but caused by trauma; meninges herniate through a skull defect after tearing of the arachnoid. Called also *Billroth's disease* and *cephalhydrocele traumatica.*

**me•nin•go•ceph•a•li•tis** (mə-ning″go-sef″ə-li′tis) meningoencephalitis.

**me•nin•go•cer•e•bri•tis** (mə-ning″go-ser″ə-bri′tis) [*meningo-* + *cerebritis*] meningoencephalitis.

**me•nin•go•coc•ce•mia** (mə-ning″go-kok-se′me-ə) invasion of the blood stream by meningococci.

**acute fulminating m.**, Waterhouse-Friderichsen syndrome.

**me•nin•go•coc•ci** (mə-ning″go-kok′si) plural of *meningococcus.*

**me•nin•go•coc•cin** (mə-ning″go-kok′sin) an antigenic material precipitated from saline suspensions of the meningococcus by means of alcohol. It is applied as a skin test (intradermal) in the detection of meningococcus carriers.

**me•nin•go•coc•co•sis** (mə-ning″go-kŏ-ko′sis) infection caused by meningococci.

**me•nin•go•coc•cus** (mə-ning″go-kok′əs) pl. *meningococ′ci* [*meningo-* + *coccus*] an individual organism of the species *Neisseria meningitidis.*

**me•nin•go•cor•ti•cal** (mə-ning″go-kor′tĭ-kəl) pertaining to or affecting the meninges and cortex of the brain.

**me•nin•go•cyte** (mə-ning′go-sīt″) a histiocyte of the meninges.

**me•nin•go•en•ceph•a•li•tis** (mə-ning″go-ən-sef″ə-li′tis) [*meningo-* + *encephalo-* + *-itis*] [MeSH: Meningoencephalitis] inflammation of the brain and meninges. Called also *cerebromeningitis, encephalomeningitis,* and *meningocerebritis.*

**amebic m.**, primary amebic m.

**eosinophilic m.**, eosinophilic meningitis.

**granulomatous m.**, an inflammatory disease of the central nervous system of dogs, of unknown etiology, characterized by granulomatous accumulations of histiocytes, lymphocytes, and plasma cells around blood vessels in the white matter and meninges. Onset is acute, with subsequent seizures, dementia, and sometimes paralysis and blindness. Most animals die within two months. Called also *granulomatous meningoencephalomyelitis* and *inflammatory reticulosis.*

**mumps m.**, a usually benign form seen in children, caused by the mumps virus, and characterized by fever, vomiting, nuchal rigidity, lethargy, parotitis, headache, convulsions, abdominal pain, diarrhea, and delirium.

**primary amebic m.**, a rare and often fatal acute, febrile, purulent

meningoencephalitis caused by usually free-living soil and water amebas of the genera *Naegleria, Acanthamoeba,* or *Hartmannella.* Infection caused by *Naegleria* is generally seen in young persons who swim or bathe in contaminated fresh water, the pathogens gaining access to the central nervous system by penetrating the nasal mucosa and cribriform plate and then following the olfactory bulbs and nerves to the brain and meninges. By contrast, *Acanthamoeba* and *Hartmannella* infections tend to be more benign, are more often seen in older or immunocompromised persons, and are sometimes associated with spontaneous recovery; the mode of transmission of these infections is not known, but hematogenous spread from amebic infection at distant sites has been reported.
**thromboembolic m.,** an acute type of septicemia of cattle, characterized by fever, ataxia, blindness, coma, and death within hours, caused by infection with *Haemophilus somnus.* Called also *sleeper syndrome.* See also *Haemophilus septicemia of cattle.*
**toxoplasmic m.,** the meningoencephalitis that sometimes occurs in toxoplasmosis, characterized by seizures and mental confusion followed by coma. Pathologically, the brain may contain cysts and necrotic areas, with occasional hydrocephalus caused by blockage of aqueducts by sloughed material. It is often fatal if untreated. A sharply increased rate of infections, which may be recurrent, is seen in immunocompromised patients. Called also *toxoplasmic encephalitis* or *encephalomyelitis.*
**syphilitic m.,** general paresis.

**me·nin·go·en·ceph·a·lo·cele** (mə-ning″go-en-sef′ə-lo-sēl″) encephalocele.

**me·nin·go·en·ceph·a·lo·my·eli·tis** (mə-ning″go-en-sef″ə-lo-mi″ə-li′tis) [*meningo-* + *encephalo-*+ *myelo-* + *-itis*] inflammation of the meninges, brain, and spinal cord.
**granulomatous m.,** see under *meningoencephalitis.*

**me·nin·go·en·ceph·a·lo·my·elop·a·thy** (mə-ning″go-ən-sef″ə-lo-mi″ə-lop′ə-the) disease involving the meninges, brain, and spinal cord.

**me·nin·go·en·ceph·a·lop·a·thy** (mə-ning″go-ən-sef″ə-lop′ə-the) noninflammatory disease of the cerebral meninges and the brain. Called also *encephalomeningopathy.*

**me·nin·go·fi·bro·blas·to·ma** (mə-ning″go-fi″bro-blas-to′mə) fibroblastic meningioma.

**me·nin·go·gen·ic** (mə-ning″go-jen′ik) [*meningo-* + *-genic*] arising in the meninges.

**men·in·go·ma** (men″in-go′mə) meningioma.

**me·nin·go·ma·la·cia** (mə-ning″go-mə-la′shə) [*meningo-* + *-malacia*] softening of a membrane.

**me·nin·go·my·eli·tis** (mə-ning″go-mi″ə-li′tis) [*meningo-* + *myelo-* + *-itis*] inflammation of the spinal cord and its membranes. Called also *myelomeningitis.*
**syphilitic m.,** Erb's spastic paraplegia.

**me·nin·go·my·elo·cele** (mə-ning″go-mi′ə-lo-sēl″) [MeSH: Meningomyelocele] myelomeningocele.

**me·nin·go·my·elo·en·ceph·a·li·tis** (mə-ning″go-mi″ə-lo-en-sef″ə-li′tis) meningoencephalomyelitis.

**me·nin·go·my·elo·ra·dic·u·li·tis** (mə-ning″go-mi″ə-lo-rə-dik″u-li′tis) [*meningo-* + *myelo-* + *radiculitis*] inflammation of the meninges, spinal cord, and roots of the spinal nerves. Called also *rhizomeningomyelitis.*

**me·nin·go-os·teo·phle·bi·tis** (mə-ning″go-os″te-o-flə-bi′tis) [*meningo-* + *osteo-* bone + *phleb-* + *-itis*] periostitis with inflammation of the veins of a bone.

**men·in·gop·a·thy** (men″in-gop′ə-the) [*meningo-* + *-pathy*] any disease of the meninges.

**me·nin·go·pneu·mo·ni·tis** (mə-ning″go-noo-mo-ni′tis) a disease produced in experimental animals by the injection of the etiologic agent of psittacosis *(Chlamydia psittaci),* and marked by acute meningitis and pneumonitis.

**me·nin·go·poly·neu·ri·tis** (mə-ning″go-pol″e-no͞o-ri′tis) the triad of radiculoneuritis, aseptic meningitis, and cranial neuritis.

**me·nin·go·ra·chid·i·an** (mə-ning″go-rə-kid′e-ən) [*meningo-* + *rachidian*] pertaining to the spinal cord and its membranes.

**me·nin·go·ra·dic·u·lar** (mə-ning″go-rə-dik′u-lər) [*meningo-* + *radicular*] pertaining to the meninges and the roots of the cranial and spinal nerves.

**me·nin·go·ra·dic·u·li·tis** (mə-ning″go-rə-dik″u-li′tis) inflammation of the meninges and roots of the spinal nerves.

**me·nin·go·re·cur·rence** (mə-ning″go-re-kur′əns) syphilitic meningitis induced in a syphilitic patient by antisyphilitic treatment.

**me·nin·gor·rha·gia** (mə-ning″go-ra′je-ə) [*meningo-* + *-rrhagia*] hemorrhage from the cerebral or spinal membranes; see *subarachnoid hemorrhage* and *subdural hemorrhage.* Called also *meningorrhea.*

**me·nin·gor·rhea** (mĕ-ning″go-re′ə) [*meningo-* + *-rrhea*] meningorrhagia.

**men·in·go·sis** (men″in-go′sis) the membranous attachment of bones to each other.

**me·nin·go·the·li·o·ma** (mə-ning″go-the″le-o′mə) meningotheliomatous meningioma.

**me·nin·go·vas·cu·lar** (mə-ning″go-vas′ku-lər) pertaining to the meninges and blood vessels.

**me·ninx** (me′ninks) [Gr. *mēninx* membrane] singular of *meninges* (q.v.).

**me·nis·cal** (mə-nis′kəl) of or pertaining to a meniscus.

**men·is·cec·to·my** (men″ĭ-sek′tə-me) excision of an intra-articular meniscus, as in the knee joint.

**men·is·che·sis** (men″is-ke′sis) menoschesis.

**me·nis·ci** (mə-nis′i) [L.] genitive and plural of *meniscus.*

**men·is·ci·tis** (men″ĭ-si′tis) inflammation of a meniscus of the knee joint.

**me·nis·co·cyte** (mə-nis′ko-sīt) [Gr. *mēniskos* crescent + *-cyte*] sickle cell.

**me·nis·co·cy·to·sis** (mə-nis″ko-si-to′sis) old name for *sickle cell anemia.*

**me·nis·co·syn·o·vi·al** (mə-nis″ko-sə-no′ve-əl) pertaining to a meniscus and the synovial membrane.

**me·nis·cus** (mə-nis′kəs) gen. and pl. *menis′ci* [L., from Gr. *mēniskos,* crescent] 1. a crescent-shaped structure appearing at the surface of a liquid column, as in a pipet or buret, made concave or convex by the influence of capillarity. 2. [TA] a general term for a crescent-shaped structure of the body. Often used alone to designate one of the crescent-shaped disks of fibrocartilage attached to the superior articular surface of the tibia.
**m. of acromioclavicular joint,** discus articularis articulationis acromioclavicularis.
**m. articula′ris** [TA], articular meniscus: a pad, commonly a wedge-shaped crescent of fibrocartilage or dense fibrous tissue, found in some synovial joints; one side forms a marginal attachment at the articular capsule and the other two sides extend into the joint, ending in a free edge.
**converging m.,** a concavoconvex lens.
**discoid m., discoid lateral m.,** a semilunar lateral meniscus of the knee that has been transformed into a thickened, irregular discoid mass as a result of excess motion of the meniscus, which in turn results from congenital absence of attachment of the posterior horn of the meniscus to the tibial plateau. The excess motion also causes a clicking sound on flexion and extension of the knee. Occasionally, a discoid medial meniscus is observed. Called also *congenital discoid meniscus.*
**diverging m.,** a convexoconcave lens.
**m. of inferior radioulnar joint,** discus articularis articulationis radioulnaris distalis.

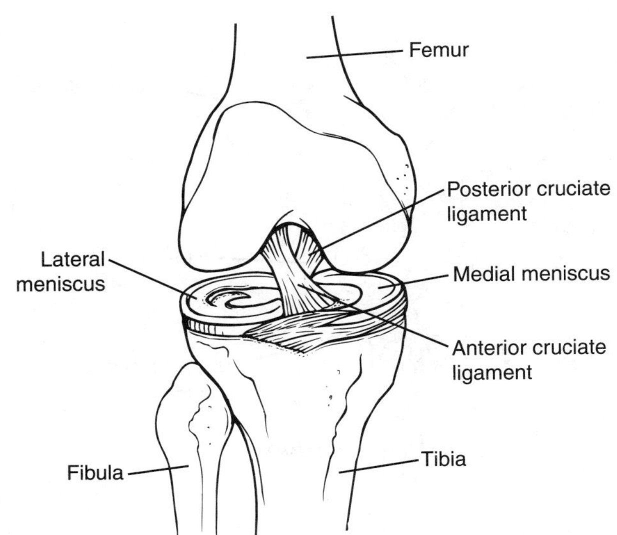


Articular menisci, exemplified by the lateral and medial menisci of the knee joint; shown in an anterior view of the right knee.

joint m., articular m.
**Kuhnt's m.,** the lining of the physiologic cup of the optic disk, composed of a thick accumulation of neuroglia.
**m. latera'lis articulatio'nis ge'nus** [TA], lateral meniscus of knee joint: a crescent-shaped disk of fibrocartilage, but nearly circular in form, attached to the lateral margin of the superior articular surface of the tibia; called also *malleolus lateralis articulationis genu.*
**m. media'lis articulatio'nis ge'nus** [TA], medial meniscus of knee joint: a crescent-shaped disk of fibrocartilage attached to the medial margin of the superior articular surface of the tibia; called also *malleolus medialis articulationis genu.*
**negative m.,** a convexoconcave lens.
**positive m.,** a concavoconvex lens.
**m. of sternoclavicular joint,** discus articularis articulationis sternoclavicularis.
**m. tac'tus,** tactile meniscus: one of the small, cup-shaped, tactile nerve endings within the skin; many of them are formed by branches of a single nerve fiber, and each one is in contact with a single, modified epithelial cell (Merkel cell); they are found in the deep epidermis, in hair follicles, and in the hard palate, and function as touch receptors. Called also *tactile disk.*
**m. of temporomandibular joint,** discus articularis articulationis temporomandibularis.

**Men·i·sper·mum** (men″ĭ-sper′məm) [Gr. *mēnē* moon + *sperma* seed] a genus of plants of the family Menispermaceae. *M. canaden'se* L. is the moonseed or yellow parilla, whose root was formerly used medicinally; the plant and its fruit resemble a grapevine and grapes and have been the cause of poisoning of children, sometimes fatal.

**Men·kes' syndrome** (meng′kəz) [John H. *Menkes,* American physician, born 1928] see under *syndrome.*

**Men·nell's sign** (men′əlz) [James Beaver *Mennell,* English physician, 1880–1957] see under *sign.*

**men(o)-** [Gr. *mēn* month] a combining form denoting relationship to the menses.

**meno·lip·sis** (men″o-lip′sis) temporary cessation of the menses.

**meno·met·ror·rha·gia** (men″o-met″ro-ra′jə) excessive uterine bleeding occurring both during the menses and at irregular intervals.

**meno·pau·sal** (men″o-paw′zəl) pertaining to or associated with the menopause.

**meno·pause** (men′o-pawz) [*meno-* + *pause*] [MeSH: Menopause] cessation of menstruation in the human female, occurring usually around the age of 50. See also *climacteric.*
**artificial m.,** cessation of menstruation produced by artificial means, such as surgical operation or irradiation.
**m. prae'cox,** premature failure of ovulation, possibly due to primary germ cell deficiency, acquired refractoriness to pituitary gonadotropin, or autoimmunization.

**meno·pla·nia** (men″o-pla′ne-ə) [*meno-* + Gr. *planē* deviation] metastasis or aberration of the menses; vicarious menstruation.

**men·or·rha·gia** (men″o-ra′jə) [*meno-* + *-rrhagia*] [MeSH: Menorrhagia] hypermenorrhea.

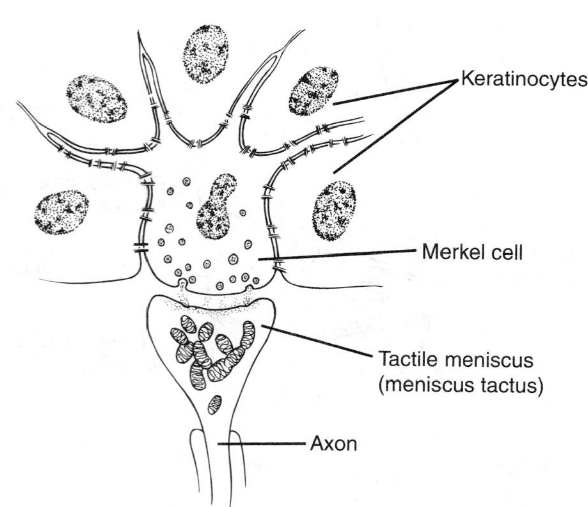


Schematic diagram of the meniscus tactus (tactile meniscus) of a nerve fiber in contact with a Merkel cell of the epithelium.

**men·or·rhal·gia** (men″o-ral′jə) [*menorrhea* + *-algia*] dysmenorrhea.

**men·or·rhea** (men″o-re′ə) [*meno-* + *-rrhea*] 1. the normal discharge of the menses. 2. profuse menstruation.

**men·or·rhe·al** (men″o-re′əl) pertaining to menorrhea.

**me·nos·che·sis** (mə-nos′kə-sis) [*meno-* + Gr. *schesis* retention] retention of the menses.

**meno·sta·sia, meno·sta·sis** (men″o-sta′zhə, men″o-sta′sis) amenorrhea.

**meno·stax·is** (men″o-stak′sis) [*meno-* + *staxis*] excessively prolonged menstruation.

**meno·tro·pins** (men′o-tro″pins) [USP] [MeSH: Menotropins] an extract of human postmenopausal urine containing both follicle-stimulating hormone and luteinizing hormone. In females, it has the property of stimulating growth and maturation of ovarian follicles. In males, it has the properties of maintaining and stimulating testicular Leydig's cells related to testosterone production and of being responsible for full development and maturation of spermatozoa in the seminiferous tubules. Called also *human follicle-stimulating hormone* and *human menopausal gonadotropin.*

**meno·uria** (men″o-u′re-ə) [*meno-* + *-uria*] the flowing of menstrual blood through a fistula into the bladder.

**Men·ri·um** (men′re-əm) trademark for preparations of chlordiazepoxide and water-soluble esterified estrogens.

**men·ses** (men′sēz) [L., pl. of *mensis* month] the monthly flow of blood from the genital tract of women; see *menstruation.*

**men·stru·al** (men′stroo-əl) [L. *menstrualis*] pertaining to the menses or to menstruation; called also *catamenial* and *emmenic.*

**men·stru·ant** (men′stroo-ənt) a person who is menstruating or is capable of menstruating.

**men·stru·ate** (men′stroo-āt) [L. *menstruare*] to undergo the monthly changes of menstruation (q.v.).

**men·stru·a·tion** (men″stroo-a′shən) [MeSH: Menstruation] the cyclic, physiologic discharge through the vagina of blood and mucosal tissues from the nonpregnant uterus; it is under hormonal control and normally recurs, usually at approximately four-week intervals, in the absence of pregnancy during the reproductive period (puberty through menopause) of the female of the human and a few species of primates. It is the culmination of the menstrual cycle; see illustration accompanying *cycle.*
**anovular m., anovulatory m.,** periodic uterine bleeding without preceding ovulation.
**delayed m.,** menstruation the first appearance of which is delayed beyond the sixteenth year.
**difficult m.,** dysmenorrhea.
**infrequent m.,** menstruation occurring less frequently than normal.
**nonovulational m.,** anovular m.
**profuse m.,** menstruation marked by excessive flow.
**regurgitant m.,** a back flow through the uterine tubes by which epithelial cells and other materials may be discharged through the tubal ostia and deposited on the ovaries and adjacent organs, as in endometriosis.
**retrograde m.,** regurgitant m.
**scanty m.,** menstruation marked by abnormally slight flow.
**supplementary m.,** menstrual discharge from the uterus and also from some other part.
**suppressed m.,** failure of the menstrual flow to appear.
**vicarious m.,** discharge of blood from an extragenital source at the time a menstrual period is normally expected; thought to result from generally increased capillary permeability related to the menstrual cycle.

**men·stru·ous** (men′stroo-əs) menstrual.

**men·stru·um** (men′stroo-əm) [L. *menstruus* menstruous: it was long believed that the menstrual fluid had a peculiar solvent quality] a solvent medium.
**Pitkin m.,** a medium for the administration of heparin, consisting of a mixture of gelatin, dextrose, glacial acetic acid, and water.

**men·su·al** (men′su-əl) [L. *mensis* month] monthly.

**men·su·ra·tion** (men″su-ra′shən) [L. *mensuratio; mensura* measure] the act or process of measuring.

**men·tal**[1] (men′təl) [L. *mens* mind] pertaining to the mind; psychic.

**men·tal**[2] (men′təl) [L. *mentum* chin] pertaining to the chin; called also *genial* and *genian.*

**men·ta·lis** (men-ta′lis) [L.] relating to the chin; see under *musculus.*

**men·tal·i·ty** (men-tal′ĭ-te) 1. mental power or capacity. 2. way of thought; mental set.

**men·ta·tion** (men-ta′shən) mental activity.

**Men·tha** (men'thə) [L.] the mints, a widely distributed genus of aromatic perennial herbs of the family Labiatae. *M. canaden'sis* L. is wild mint. *M. cardi'aca* (Scotch spearmint) and *M. spica'ta* L. (common spearmint) are sources of spearmint oil. *M. piperi'ta* is peppermint, the source of peppermint oil. *M. pule'gium* is European pennyroyal (see *pennyroyal*).

**men·thol** (men'thol) [USP] [MeSH: Menthol] an alcohol obtained from various mint oils or prepared synthetically, used as a topical antipruritic, and in inhalers for treatment of upper respiratory disorders or added to water for inhalation in acute bronchitis. Called also *peppermint camphor*.

**men·thyl** (men'thəl) the monovalent radical, $C_{10}H_{19}$.

**men·ti·cide** (men'tĭ-sīd) [*mental*[1] + *-cide*] brainwashing.

**ment(o)-** [L. *mentum* chin] a combining form denoting relationship to the chin. See also words beginning *geni(o)-*.

**men·to·an·te·ri·or** (men″to-an-tēr'e-or) [*mento-* + *anterior*] see under *position*.

**men·to·la·bi·al** (men″to-la'be-əl) [*mento-* + *labial*] pertaining to the chin and lip.

**men·ton** (men'ton) a cranial osteometric landmark, being the lowest point of the mandibular symphysis on the lateral jaw projection as seen on x-ray films.

**men·to·plas·ty** (men'to-plas″te) [*mento-* + *-plasty*] plastic surgery of the chin; surgical correction of deformities and defects of the chin.

**men·to·pos·te·ri·or** (men″to-pos-tēr'e-or) [*mento-* + *posterior*] see under *position*.

**men·to·trans·verse** (men″to-trans-vərs') [*mento-* + *transverse*] see under *position*.

**men·tum** (men'təm) [L.] [TA] the chin.

**Men·y·an·thes** (men″e-an'thēz) [perhaps from Gr. *mēn* month + *anthos* flower] a genus of plants of the family Gentianaceae. *M. trifolia'ta* L., or buckbean, is a bitter tonic and has febrifuge properties.

**Men·zel's ataxia** (Ment'selz) [P. *Menzel*, German physician, 19th century] see under *ataxia*.

**MEP** maximum expiratory pressure.

**mep·a·crine hy·dro·chlo·ride** (mep'ə-krēn) quinacrine hydrochloride.

**me·par·tri·cin** (mə-pahr'trĭ-sin) [MeSH: Mepartricin] an antifungal and antiprotozoal; it is a methyl ester of partricin (q.v.), used chiefly in the treatment of vaginal and cutaneous candidiasis, applied topically.

**mep·a·zine ac·e·tate** (mep'ə-zēn) a tranquilizer used mainly in the treatment of tension and anxiety states, but also used as a pre- or postoperative sedative; administered orally or intramuscularly.

**me·pen·zo·late bro·mide** (mə-pen'zo-lāt) a quaternary ammonium compound with antimuscarinic effects, used as an adjunct in the treatment of peptic ulcers and in the treatment of disorders in which hypermotility of the colon is a feature; administered orally.

**me·per·i·dine hy·dro·chlo·ride** (mə-per'ĭ-dēn) [USP] a synthetic narcotic analgesic, used as a preanesthetic medication and obstetric analgesic, and when a relatively short duration of analgesia is desired; administered orally, intramuscularly, subcutaneously, or intravenously. Abuse of this drug may lead to dependence. Called also *pethidine hydrochloride*.

**Meph·a·quin** (mef'ə-kwin) trademark for a preparation of mefloquine hydrochloride.

**me·phen·amine** (mə-fen'ə-mēn) orphenadrine.

**me·phen·e·sin** (mə-fen'ə-sin) [MeSH: Mephenesin] a centrally acting skeletal muscle relaxant, used for the treatment of painful muscle spasm; administered orally.

**me·phen·ter·mine sul·fate** (mə-fen'tər-mēn) an adrenergic, used for its vasopressor effects in the treatment of certain hypotensive states, administered orally, intramuscularly, and intravenously. It is also applied topically to the nasal mucosa as a decongestant.

**me·phen·y·to·in** (mə-fen'ə-to-in) [MeSH: Mephenytoin] an anticonvulsant, used for the control of grand mal, focal, jacksonian, and psychomotor epileptic seizures that are refractory to other drugs, administered orally.

**me·phit·ic** (mə-fit'ik) [L. *mephiticus; mephitis* foul exhalation] emitting a foul odor.

**me·phi·tis** (mə-fi'tis) [L.] a foul exhalation.

**meph·o·bar·bi·tal** (mef″o-bahr'bĭ-təl) [MeSH: Mephobarbital] a long-acting barbiturate, used as a sedative in the treatment of anxiety, tension, and apprehension and as an anticonvulsant in grand mal and petit mal epilepsy, administered orally.

**Meph·y·ton** (mef'ĭ-ton) trademark for preparations of phytonadione (vitamin $K_1$).

**me·piv·a·caine hy·dro·chlo·ride** (mə-piv'ə-kān) [USP] an analogue of lidocaine, used to produce local anesthesia by infiltration injection, peripheral nerve block, and epidural block.

**Me·prane** (me'prān) trademark for preparations of promethestrol dipropionate.

**me·pred·ni·sone** (mə-pred'nĭ-sōn) [USP] a synthetic glucocorticoid used in the treatment of inflammatory, allergic, rheumatic, and other corticosteroid-responsive diseases, such as certain endocrine, respiratory, neoplastic, and collagen diseases, administered orally.

**me·pro·ba·mate** (mə-pro'bə-māt, mep″ro-bam'āt) [USP] [MeSH: Meprobamate] a carbamate derivative, having tranquilizing, muscle relaxant, and anticonvulsant actions. It is used as an oral sedative for the relief of anxiety and tension, as an adjunct in the treatment of conditions in which anxiety and tension are manifested, and to promote sleep in anxious tense patients; it is also used in musculoskeletal disorders and as an anticonvulsant in petit mal epilepsy. An intramuscular injection is used as adjunctive therapy in tetanus.
**isopropyl m.**, carisoprodol.

**Me·pro·span** (mə-pro'spən) trademark for a preparation of meprobamate.

**Me·pro·tabs** (mə-pro'tabs) trademark for a preparation of meprobamate.

**me·pyr·amine** (mə-pir'ə-mēn) pyrilamine.

**me·py·ra·pone** (mə-pi'rə-pōn) metyrapone.

**mEq** milliequivalent.

**meq** milliequivalent.

**MER** the methanol extraction residue of BCG; used in cancer immunotherapy.

**me·ral·gia** (mə-ral'jə) [*mero-*[2] + *-algia*] pain in the thigh.
**m. paresthe'tica**, a type of entrapment neuropathy caused by entrapment of the lateral femoral cutaneous nerve at the inguinal ligament, causing paresthesia, pain, and numbness in the outer surface of the thigh in the region supplied by the nerve. Called also *Bernhardt's, Bernhardt-Roth, Roth's,* or *Roth-Bernhardt disease*.

**me·ral·lu·ride** (mə-ral'u-rīd) a mercurial diuretic; also used as *meralluride sodium*.

**mer·bro·min** (mər-bro'min) [MeSH: Merbromin] a mercurial antiseptic that has been used topically for the disinfection of skin and wounds.

**mer·cap·tan** (mər-kap'tən) [L. *mercurium captans* seizing or combining with mercury] thiol (def. 2).

**2-mer·cap·to·eth·a·nol (2-ME)** (mər-kap″to-eth'ə-nol) a foul-smelling sulfhydryl compound that acts as a reducing agent; used to differentiate between IgG and IgM in a mixture by disrupting the disulfide bonds of IgM so that only IgG is measurable. See also under *tests*.

**$\beta$-mer·cap·to·eth·yl·amine** (mər-kap″to-eth'əl-ə-mēn″) an amine, $NH_2—CH_2—CH_2—SH$, that is part of coenzyme A; its reactive thiol group is responsible for the biological activity of the molecule, carrying activated acyl groups.

**mer·cap·tol** (mər-kap'tol) a compound formed from a ketone by introducing two thio-alkyl (—SR) groups in place of the bivalent oxygen.

**mer·cap·to·mer·in sul·fate** (mər-kap″to-mer'in) [USP] a mercurial diuretic.

**mer·cap·to·pur·ine** (mər-kap″to-pūr'ēn) [USP] 6-MP, a purine analogue in which sulfur replaces the oxygen atom of purine and which can be incorporated into the nucleotide 6-thiolMP, an analogue of inosine monophosphate (IMP); 6-thiolMP inhibits *de novo* purine synthesis in two places, by serving as a pseudofeedback inhibitor of the first step in the pathway and also by inhibiting the conversion of IMP to adenine and guanine nucleotides; 6-MP is used as an antineoplastic for the treatment of acute lymphoblastic, acute lymphocytic, and acute myelogenous leukemia, administered orally. It is also used as an immunosuppressive in the treatment of Crohn's disease, ulcerative colitis, severe psoriatic arthritis, and polycythemia vera. Called also *6-mercaptopurine*.

**mer·cap·tur·ic ac·id** (mər-kap-tūr'ik) a cysteine conjugate of an aromatic compound formed initially as a glutathione conjugate in the liver and excreted in the urine.

**Mer·chant's projection** (mer'chənts) [A.C. *Merchant*, American radiologist, 20th century] see under *projection*.

**Mer·cier's bar (valve)** (mer-se-āz′) [Louis Auguste *Mercier,* French urologist, 1811–1882] plica interureterica.

**mer·co·cre·sols** (mer″ko-kre′solz) a combination of cresol derivatives and an organic mercury, used for its germicidal, fungicidal, and bacteriostatic properties.

**mer·cu·pu·rin** (mər-ku′pu-rin) former name for mercurophylline.

**mer·cu·ra·mide** (mər-kūr′ə-mīd) mersalyl.

**mer·cu·ram·mo·ni·um** (mər-kūr″ə-mo′ne-əm) a precipitate produced when ammonium hydroxide is added to a solution of a mercuric salt.
**m. chloride,** ammoniated mercury.

**mer·cu·ri·al** (mər-kūr′e-əl) [L. *mercurialis*] 1. pertaining to mercury. 2. a preparation of mercury.

**mer·cu·ri·al·ism** (mər-kūr′e-əl-iz″əm) mercury poisoning; see under *poisoning.*

**mer·cur·ic** (mər-kūr′ik) pertaining to mercury as a bivalent element.
**m. chloride,** mercury bichloride.
**m. oxide, yellow,** a yellow to orange-yellow, heavy, impalpable powder, HgO, used as a local anti-infective in ophthalmology. Called also *Pagenstecher's ointment.*

**Mer·cu·ro·chrome** (mər-kū′rə-krōm) trademark for preparations of merbromin.

**mer·cu·ro·phyl·line** (mer″kūr-o-fil′in) a mixture of the sodium salt of 3-[[3-(hydroxymercuri)-2-methoxypropyl]-carbamoyl]-1,2,2-trimethyl(±)cyclopentane carboxylic acid and theophylline in molecular proportions, used as a mercurial diuretic. Formerly called *mercupurin.*

**mer·cu·rous** (mer′kur-əs) pertaining to mercury as a monovalent element.
**m. chloride,** calomel.

**mer·cu·ry** (mer′kūr-e) [L. *mercurius,* or *hydrargyrum*] [MeSH: Mercury] a metallic element, liquid at ordinary temperatures; its chemical symbol is Hg; atomic number, 80; atomic weight, 200.59; specific gravity, 13.546. It is insoluble in ordinary solvents, partially soluble in boiling hydrochloric acid, and soluble in nitric acid. It forms two sets of compounds: *mercurous,* in which a single atom of mercury combines with a monovalent radical, and *mercuric,* in which a single atom of mercury combines with a bivalent radical. The mercuric salts are more soluble and irritant than the mercurous ones. Mercury and its salts have been used medicinally, but because of the risk of mercury poisoning (see under *poisoning*) their use is diminishing. Called also *quicksilver* and *hydrargyrum.*
**m. 197,** a radioactive isotope of mercury, atomic mass 197, having a half-life of 2.67 years and decaying by electron capture with emission of gamma rays (0.077 MeV); it has been used in renal imaging.
**m. 203,** a radioactive isotope of mercury, atomic mass 203, having a half-life of 46.60 days and emitting beta particles (0.214 MeV) and gamma rays (0.279 MeV); it has been used in renal imaging.
**ammoniated m.** [USP], a topical anti-infective, $HgNH_2Cl$, occurring in white, pulverulent pieces or as a white amorphous powder.
**m. bichloride,** an extremely poisonous compound, $HgCl_2$, occurring as odorless, heavy, colorless crystals, as crystalline masses, or as a white powder: formerly used in the treatment of syphilis and now as a disinfectant. Called also *mercuric chloride.*
**m. with chalk,** metallic mercury rubbed up with chalk and honey until the particles are very small; used in pediculosis pubis.
**m. chloride, mild,** calomel.
**m. oleate,** a mixture of yellow mercuric oxide and oleic acid: applied locally in parasitic skin diseases.
**m. perchloride,** m. bichloride.

**Mer·cu·zan·thin** (mer″ku-zan′thin) trademark for a preparation of mercurophylline.

**-mere** [Gr. *meros* part] a word termination denoting a segment or a part.

**mer·e·thox·yl·line pro·caine** (mer″ə-thok′sə-lēn) a combination of the organomercurial merethoxylline (dehydro-2-[*N*-(3′-hydroxymercuri-2′-methoxyethoxy)propylcarbamy]phenoxyacetic acid) with theophylline and procaine; used in the treatment of edema secondary to such conditions as congestive heart failure and nephrotic syndrome, administered intramuscularly and subcutaneously.

**Me·re·to·ja type familial amyloid polyneuropathy (syndrome)** (ma-ra-to′yah) [J. *Meretoja,* Finnish physician, 20th century] Finnish type familial amyloid polyneuropathy; see under *polyneuropathy.*

**me·rid·i·an** (mə-rid′e-ən) [MeSH: Meridians] an imaginary line on the surface of a spherical body; see also *meridianus.*
**m. of cornea,** an imaginary line marking the intersection with its surface of an anteroposterior plane passing through the apex of the cornea.
**m's of eyeball,** meridiani bulbi oculi.

**me·rid·i·a·ni** (mə-rid″e-a′ne) [L.] plural of *meridianus.*

**me·rid·i·a·nus** (mə-rid″e-a′nəs) pl. *meridia′ni* [L., from *medius* middle + *dies* day] an imaginary line on the surface of a spherical body, marking the intersection with the surface of a plane passing through its axis. Called also *meridian.*
**meridia′ni bul′bi o′culi** [TA], meridians of eyeball: imaginary lines encircling the eyeball, marking the intersection with its surface of planes passing through its anteroposterior axis.

**me·rid·i·o·nal** (mə-rid′e-o-nəl) pertaining to a meridian or made along a meridian; as *meridional section.*

**Mer·i·o·nes** (mer-e-o′nēz) a genus of gerbil-like rodents found in desert areas of Central Asia; several species are common reservoirs for *Leishmania major,* the cause of wet cutaneous leishmaniasis.

**mer·i·sis** (mer′ĭ-sis) growth in size due to cell division.

**mer·ism** (mer′iz-əm) [Gr. *meros* a part] the repetition of parts in an organism so as to form a regular pattern.

**mer·i·stem** (mer′ĭ-stem) [Gr. *merizein* to divide] [MeSH: Meristem] the undifferentiated embryonic tissue of plants.

**mer·i·ste·mat·ic** (mer″ĭ-stə-mat′ik) pertaining to or composed of meristem.

**mer·is·tic** (mər-is′tik) [Gr. *meristikos* fit for dividing] pertaining to or possessing merism; symmetrical; having symmetrically arranged parts.

**Mer·kel cell (corpuscle, disk, tactile cell)** (mer′kel) [Friedrich Sigmund *Merkel,* German anatomist, 1845–1919] see under *cell.*

**Mer·kel's filtrum, muscle** (mer′kelz) [Karl Ludwig *Merkel,* German anatomist, 1812–1876] see *filtrum ventriculi* and *musculus ceratocricoideus.*

**Mer·kel-Ran·vier cells** (mer′kel-rahn-vya′) [F. S. *Merkel;* Louis Antoine *Ranvier,* French pathologist, 1835–1922] see under *cell.*

**mer·lin** (mər′lin) a cytoskeletal protein that acts as a tumor suppressor; a defect in the gene that codes for this protein is the cause of neurofibromatosis 2. Called also *schwannomin.*

**mer·mi·thid** (mer′mĭ-thid) pertaining to or of the family Mermithidae.

**Mer·mith·i·dae** (mər-mith′ĭ-de) a family of nematodes of the superfamily Mermithoidea; the cabbage snakes.

**Mer·mith·oi·dea** (mer″mith-oi′de-ə) [MeSH: Mermithoidea] a superfamily of aphasmids including the cabbage snakes (family Mermithidae), the larvae of which may accidentally occur in the human digestive tract as contaminants of food or water.

**mer(o)-**[1] [Gr. *meros* part] a combining form meaning part.

**mer(o)-**[2] [Gr. *mēros* thigh] a combining form denoting relationship to the thigh.

**mero·acra·nia** (mer″o-ə-kra′ne-ə) [*mero-*[1] + *a-*[1] + Gr. *kranion* skull] congenital absence of part of the cranium.

**mero·an·en·ceph·a·ly** (mer″o-an″ən-sef′ə-le) [*mero-*[1] + *anencephaly*] congenital absence of part of the brain, usually the forebrain and midbrain. Cf. *anencephaly.*

**mero·blas·tic** (mer″o-blas′tik) [*mero-*[1] + *blast-* + *-ic*] undergoing cleavage in which only part of the ovum participates; partially dividing.

**mero·cox·al·gia** (me″ro-kok-sal′jə) [*mero-*[2] + *coxalgia*] pain in the thigh and hip.

**mero·crine** (mer′o-krin) [*mero-*[1] + Gr. *krinein* to separate] partly secreting; denoting that type of glandular secretion in which the secreting cell remains intact throughout the process of formation and discharge of the secretory products; as in the salivary and pancreatic glands. Cf. *apocrine* and *holocrine.*

**mero·cyst** (mer′o-sist) [*mero-*[1] + *cyst*] a large schizont seen in cer-

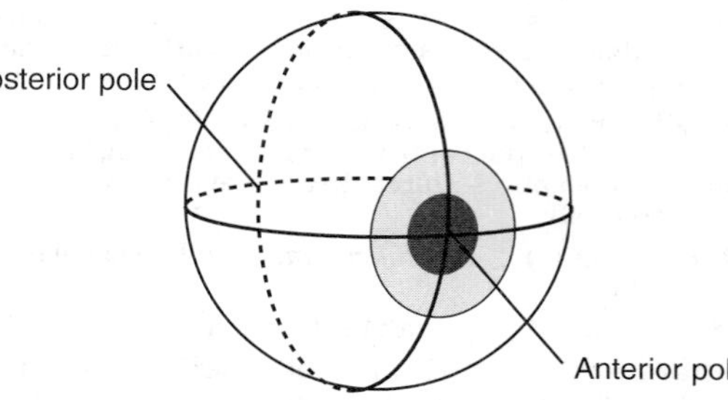

Meridiani bulbi oculi (meridians of eyeball).

tain hemosporidian protozoa from which merozoites are released to invade the host's erythrocytes, where they develop into gametocytes.

**mero•cyte** (mer'o-sīt) [*mero-*[1] + *-cyte*] supernumerary sperm nucleus in the ovum in cases of polyspermy.

**me•rog•a•my** (mə-rog'ə-me) microgamy.

**mero•gas•tru•la** (mer″o-gas'troo-lə) the gastrula of a meroblastic ovum.

**mero•gen•e•sis** (mer″o-jen'ə-sis) [*mero-*[1] + *-genesis*] cleavage of a zygote.

**mero•ge•net•ic** (mer″o-jə-net'ik) pertaining to merogenesis.

**mero•gen•ic** (mer″o-jen'ik) merogenetic.

**mero•gon•ic** (mer″o-gon'ik) pertaining to or resulting from merogony.

**me•rog•o•ny** (mə-rog'ə-ne) [*mero-*[1] + Gr. *gonos* procreation] 1. the development of a portion only of an ovum; see *andromerogony* and *gynomerogony.* 2. schizogony resulting in the production of merozoites.
**diploid m.,** development of a portion of an ovum containing the fused male and female pronuclei.
**parthenogenetic m.,** development, as a result of artificial stimulation, of a part of an ovum containing the nucleus.

**mero•me•lia** (mer″o-me'le-ə) [*mero-*[1] + *-melia*] congenital absence of any part of a limb, as in adactyly, hemimelia, or phocomelia; cf. *amelia.*

**mero•mi•cro•so•mia** (mer″o-mi″kro-so'me-ə) [*mero-*[1] + *microsomia*] unusual smallness of some part of the body.

**mero•mor•pho•sis** (mer″o-mor-fo'sis) [*mero-*[1] + *morphosis*] incomplete restoration or regeneration of a lost part.

**mero•my•ar•i•an** (mer″o-mi-ar'e-ən) [*mero-*[1] + Gr. *mys* muscle] designating a type of nematode musculature in which there are only a few muscle cells in a given area, the cells being platymyarian in type.

**mero•myo•sin** (mer″o-mi'o-sin) a fragment of the myosin molecule isolated by treatment with proteolytic enzymes; there are two types, heavy (H-meromyosin) and light (L-meromyosin). *L-meromyosin* makes up the major part of the rodlike backbone of the molecule; *H-meromyosin* contains the subfragment responsible for the ATPase activity of myosin. See Plate 35 at *muscle.*

**mer•ont** (mer'ont) [*mero*[1]*-* + *ontos* being] the asexual stage in the development of certain protozoa, especially nonsporozoa, that gives rise to merozoites. See also *schizont* and *segmenter.*

**mer•o•pen•em** (mer″o-pen'əm) a broad-spectrum beta-lactam antibacterial derived from thienamycin, similar to imipenem in structure and activity and used in the treatment of intra-abdominal infections and bacterial meningitis; administered intravenously. It is not as susceptible to metabolism in the kidneys as imipenem and need not be administered with cilastatin.

**me•ro•pia** (mə-ro'pe-ə) [*mero-*[1] + *-opia*] partial blindness.

**mero•ra•chis•chi•sis** (me″ro-rə-kis'kĭ-sis) [*mero-*[1] + *rachi-* + *schisis*] fissure of a part of the vertebral column; called also *mesorachischisis* and *rachischisis partialis.* Cf. *spina bifida.*

**me•ros•mia** (mə-ros'me-ə) [*mero-*[1] + *osm-*[1] + *-ia*] partial anosmia, with certain odors not being perceived.

**mero•spo•ran•gi•um** (mer″o-spə-ran'je-əm) a small sporangium, usually cylindrical, containing a few spores in a chain or row.

**mer•os•tot•ic** (mer″os-tot'ik) [*mero-*[1] + L. *os* bone] pertaining to or affecting only a part of a bone.

**me•rot•o•my** (mə-rot'ə-me) [*mero-*[1] + *-tomy*] dissection into segments, especially the dissection of a cell.

**mero•zo•ite** (mer″o-zo'īt) [*mero-*[1] + *zo-* + *-ite*[1]] a stage in the life cycle of certain sporozoan protozoa resulting from merogony. Called also *schizozoite.*

**mero•zy•gote** (mer″o-zi'gōt) [*mero-*[1] + *zygote*] the partially diploid bacterial zygote that results from the transfer of a portion of the genetic information of a donor cell to the total genetic information of the recipient. See also *heterogenote* and *homogenote.*

**Mer•phen•yl** (mer'fən-əl) trademark for preparations of phenylmercuric compounds.

**Mer•rem** (Mer'əm) trademark for a preparation of meropenem.

**mer•sa•lyl** (mer'sə-ləl) [MeSH: Mersalyl] a mercurial diuretic, used in combination with theophylline in the treatment of edema secondary to such conditions as cardiorenal diseases, nephrosis, and hepatic cirrhosis, administered intramuscularly and intravenously.

**mer•ti•a•tide** (mər'te-ə-tīd″) a carboxylated, diamido-, disulfur-containing compound; complexed with technetium Tc 99m it is used in functional and anatomical renal imaging. See table at *technetium.*

**Mer•thi•o•late** (mər-thi'o-lāt) trademark for preparations of thimerosal.

**Merz•bach•er-Pel•i•zae•us disease** (merts'bahk-er-pa″le-tsa'oos) [Ludwig *Merzbacher,* German physician 1875–1942; Friedrich *Pelizaeus,* German neurologist, 1850–1917] familial centrolobar sclerosis.

**me•sad** (me'sad) toward the median line or plane; mesiad.

**me•sal** (me'səl) [Gr. *mesos* middle] mesial.

**me•sal•amine** (mə-sal'ə-mēn) [USP] 5-aminosalicylic acid; an active metabolite of sulfasalazine, used in the treatment of mild to moderate distal ulcerative colitis, proctosigmoiditis, and proctitis.

**me•sal•a•zine** (mə-sal'ə-zēn) mesalamine.

**mes•an•gi•al** (mes-an'je-əl) of or pertaining to the mesangium.

**mes•an•gio•cap•il•lary** (mes-an″je-o-kap'ĭ-lar″e) pertaining to or affecting the mesangium and the associated capillaries.

**mes•an•gi•ol•y•sis** (mes-an″je-ol'ĭ-sis) degenerative changes to the mesangium, starting with loosening and detachment of its matrix and progressing to dissolution with degeneration of mesangial cells.

**mes•an•gi•um** (mes-an'je-əm) the thin membrane which helps to support the capillary loops in a renal glomerulus.
**extraglomerular m.,** collective term for the lacis cells.

**Me•san•to•in** (mə-san'toin) trademark for a preparation of mephenytoin.

**mes•a•ra•ic** (mes″ə-ra'ik) [Gr. *mesaraion* mesentery] mesenteric.

**mes•ar•ter•itis** (mes″ahr-tər-i'tis) [*mes-* + *arteritis*] inflammation of the tunica media of an artery.
**Mönckeberg's m.,** see under *arteriosclerosis.*

**me•sati•ce•phal•ic** (mə-sat″ĭ-sə-fal'ik) [Gr. *mesatos* medium + *cephal-* + *-ic*] mesocephalic.

**me•sati•ker•kic** (mə-sat″ĭ-ker'kik) [Gr. *mesatos* medium + *kerkis* the radius of the arm] having a radiohumeral index of 75 to 80.

**me•sati•pel•lic** (mə-sat″ĭ-pel'ik) [Gr. *mesatos* medium + *pella* bowl] having a transverse diameter of the pelvic inlet almost the same as that of the true conjugated diameter.

**me•sati•pel•vic** (mə-sat″ĭ-pel'vik) mesatipellic.

**mes•ax•on** (mes-ak'son) a pair of parallel membranes marking the line of edge-to-edge contact of the Schwann cell encircling the axon.

**mes•cal** (mes-kahl') [Nahuatl *metl ixcalli* concoction or stew of the maguey plant] 1. *Lophophora williamsii.* 2. a Mexican alcoholic beverage made from the maguey plant.

**mes•ca•line** (mes'kə-lēn) [MeSH: Mescaline] a poisonous hallucinogenic alkaloid found in mescal buttons; it produces an intoxication with delusions of color and music.

**mes•cal•ism** (mes'kə-liz″əm) intoxication caused by mescal buttons or mescaline.

**mes•ec•to•blast** (mez-ek'to-blast) ectomesoblast.

**mes•ec•to•derm** (mez-ek'to-dərm) embryonic migratory cells, derived from the neural crest of the head, that contribute to the formation of the meninges and become pigment cells.

**mes•en•ce•phal•ic** (mez-en″sə-fal'ik) pertaining to the mesencephalon.

**mes•en•ceph•a•li•tis** (mez″en-sef″ə-li'tis) inflammation of the mesencephalon.

**mes•en•ceph•a•lo•hy•po•phys•e•al** (mez″en-sef″ə-lo-hi″po-fiz'e-əl) pertaining to the mesencephalon and the pituitary gland (hypophysis).

**mes•en•ceph•a•lon** (mez″en-sef'ə-lon) [*meso-* + *encephalon*] [MeSH: Mesencephalon] 1. [TA] the part of the brain developed from the middle of the three primary vesicles of the embryonic neural tube; it comprises the tectum and the cerebral peduncles; see Plate 11. See also *brainstem.* 2. the middle of the three primary brain vesicles in the embryo, lying between the prosencephalon and the rhombencephalon. Called also *midbrain.*

**mes•en•ceph•a•lot•o•my** (mez″en-sef″ə-lot'ə-me) [*mesencephalon* + Gr. *tomē* a cutting] production of lesions in the midbrain, especially in the pain-conducting pathways for the relief of intractable pain. Formerly performed directly with a surgical incision, it is now done stereotactically with current from inserted electrodes.

**mes•en•chy•ma** (mez-eng'kĭ-mə) [*meso-* + Gr. *enchyma* infusion] mesenchyme: the meshwork of loosely organized embryonic connective tissue in the mesoderm from which are formed the connective tissues of the body, and also the blood vessels and lymphatic vessels.

**mes•en•chy•mal** (mez-eng'kĭ-məl) pertaining to the mesenchyma.

**mes•en•chyme** (mez'əng-kīm) mesenchyma.

**mes·en·chy·mo·ma** (mez″ən-ki-mo′mə) [MeSH: Mesenchymoma] a mixed mesenchymal tumor composed of two or more cellular elements not commonly associated, not counting fibrous tissue as one of the elements.
**benign m.**, a benign tumor composed of two or more clearly recognizable mesenchymal elements in addition to fibrous tissue.
**malignant m.**, a sarcoma composed of two or more cellular elements (excluding fibrous tissue); called also *mixed cell sarcoma.*

**mes·en·ter·ec·to·my** (mez″ən-tə-rek′tə-me) [*mesentery* + *-ectomy*] resection of mesentery.

**mes·en·ter·ic** (mez″ən-ter′ik) [Gr. *mesenterikos*] pertaining to the mesentery.

**mes·en·ter·i·o·lum** (mes″ən-tər-i′o-ləm) a small mesentery.
**m. appen′dicis vermifor′mis, m. proces′sus vermifor′mis,** meso-appendix.

**mes·en·ter·io·pexy** (mez″ən-ter′e-o-pek″se) [*mesentery* + *-pexy*] fixation or suspension of the mesentery.

**mes·en·ter·i·or·rha·phy** (mez″ən-ter″e-or′ə-fe) [*mesentery* + *-rrhaphy*] suture or repair of the mesentery.

**mes·en·ter·i·pli·ca·tion** (mez″ən-ter″ĭ-plĭ-ka′shən) [*mesentery* + *plication*] shortening the mesentery by plication.

**mes·en·ter·itis** (mez″en-tə-ri′tis) inflammation of the mesentery.
**retractile m.**, inflammation of the mesentery producing thickening, sclerosis, and retraction, and occasionally resulting in distortion of intestinal loops.

**mes·en·ter·i·um** (mes″ən-ter′e-əm) [TA] mesentery: the peritoneal fold attaching the small intestine to the posterior abdominal wall.
**m. commu′ne, m. dorsa′le commu′ne,** dorsal common mesentery: the primordial embryonic mesentery, a double-layered median partition formed by association of the splanchnic mesoderm with the endoderm, extending from the roof of the coelom toward the midventral wall, and dividing the coelom into halves; it contains the primitive gut, and encloses the heart, lungs, and liver as they develop.

**mes·en·ter·on** (mes-en′tər-on) [*meso-* + *enteron*] midgut.

**mes·en·tery** (mez′ən-ter″e) [MeSH: Mesentery] 1. mesenterium. 2. a membranous fold attaching any of various organs to the body wall.
**m. of ascending part of colon,** mesocolon ascendens.
**caval m.**, a ridge, at the right of the embryonic mesogastrium, in which develops a hepatic segment of the inferior vena cava.
**common m., common m., dorsal,** mesenterium dorsale commune.
**m. of descending part of colon,** mesocolon descendens.
**dorsal m.**, mesenterium dorsale commune.
**primitive m., primordial m.**, mesenterium dorsale commune.
**m. of rectum,** mesorectum.
**m. of sigmoid colon,** mesocolon sigmoideum.
**m. of transverse part of colon,** mesocolon transversum.
**ventral m.**, the embryonic mesentery attaching the stomach and the proximal duodenal region of the primordial intestine to the ventral body wall.
**m. of vermiform appendix,** meso-appendix.

**mes·en·to·derm** (mez-en′to-dərm) the inner layer of an amphibian gastrula not yet separated into mesoderm and entoderm.

**mes·en·to·mere** (mez-en′to-mēr) a blastomere not yet divided into mesomeres and entomeres.

**mes·en·tor·rha·phy** (mez″ən-tor′ə-fe) [*mesentery* + Gr. *rhaphē* suture] mesenteriorrhaphy.

**mes·epi·the·li·um** (mes″ep-ĭ-the′le-əm) mesothelium.

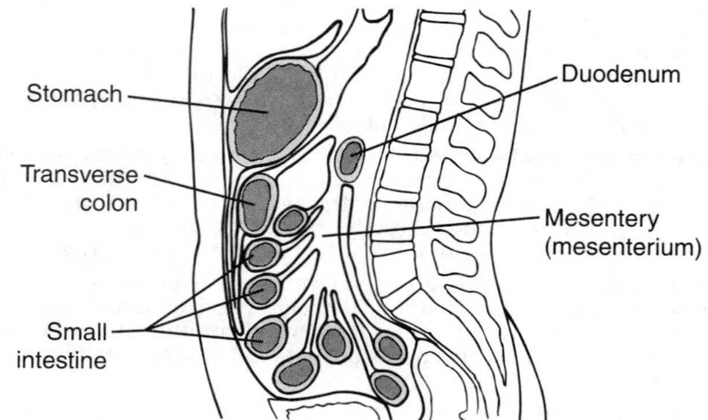

Mesenterium (mesentery) in a median sagittal section.

**MeSH** (mesh) *Me*dical *S*ubject *H*eadings, a thesaurus published by the National Library of Medicine for use in MEDLARS.

**mesh·work** (mesh′wərk) network; rete; reticulum.
**trabecular m.**, reticulum trabeculare.

**me·si·ad** (me′ze-ad) toward the middle; mesad.

**me·si·al** (me′ze-əl) nearer the center line of the dental arch.

**me·si·al·ly** (me′ze-al″e) toward the median line.

**me·si·en** (me′ze-ən) pertaining to the mesion.

**mesi(o)-** [Gr. *mesos* in the middle] in dentistry, a combining form denoting relationship to the middle; specifically, the mesial surface of a tooth or the mesial wall of a tooth cavity.

**me·sio·buc·cal** (me″ze-o-buk′əl) pertaining to or formed by the mesial and buccal surfaces of a tooth, or the mesial and buccal walls of a tooth cavity preparation.

**me·sio·buc·co·oc·clu·sal** (me″ze-o-buk″o-ŏ-kloo′zəl) pertaining to or formed by the mesial, buccal, and occlusal surfaces of a tooth.

**me·sio·buc·co·pul·pal** (me″ze-o-buk″o-pul′pəl) pertaining to or formed by the mesial, buccal, and pulpal walls of a tooth cavity.

**me·sio·cer·vi·cal** (me″ze-o-sər′vi-kəl) 1. pertaining to the mesial surface of the neck of a tooth. 2. mesiogingival.

**me·sio·cli·na·tion** (me″ze-o-klĭ-na′shən) deviation of a tooth from the vertical, in the direction of the tooth next mesial (anterior) to it in the dental arch.

**me·sio·clu·sion** (me″ze-o-kloo′zhən) malocclusion in which the mandibular arch is in an anterior position in relation to the maxillary arch (prognathism). Generally considered as identical with Class III in Angle's classification of malocclusion (see *malocclusion*). Called also *anterior occlusion, anteroclusion,* and *protrusive occlusion.*

**me·sio·dens** (me′ze-o-denz) pl. *mesioden′tes* [*mesio-* + *dens*] the most common supernumerary tooth, appearing singly or in pairs as a small tooth with a cone-shaped crown and a short root between the maxillary central incisors; it may be erupted, impacted, or even inverted.

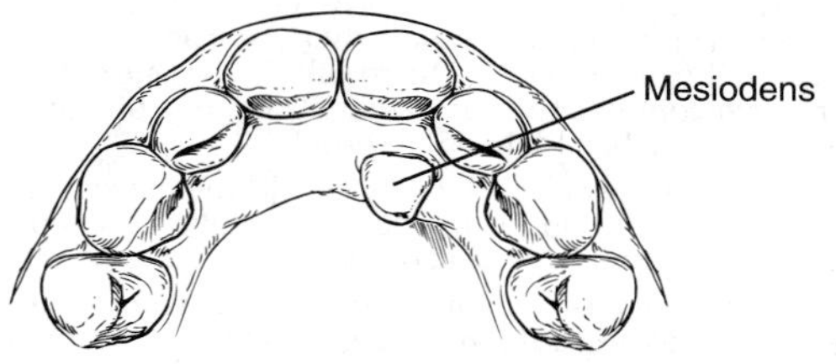


**me·sio·den·tes** (me″ze-o-den′tēz) plural of *mesiodens.*

**me·sio·dis·tal** (me″ze-o-dis′təl) pertaining to the mesial and distal surfaces of a tooth.

**me·sio·gin·gi·val** (me″ze-o-jin′jĭ-vəl) pertaining to or formed by the mesial and gingival walls of a tooth cavity.

**me·sio·in·ci·so·dis·tal** (me″ze-o-in-si″zo-dis′təl) pertaining to the mesial, incisal, and distal surfaces of an anterior tooth.

**me·sio·la·bi·al** (me″ze-o-la′be-əl) pertaining to or formed by the mesial and labial surfaces of a tooth, or the mesial and labial walls of a tooth cavity preparation.

**me·sio·la·bio·in·ci·sal** (me″ze-o-la″be-o-in-si′zəl) pertaining to or formed by the mesial, labial, and incisal surfaces of a tooth.

**me·sio·lin·gual** (me″ze-o-ling′gwəl) pertaining to or formed by the mesial and lingual surfaces of a tooth, or the mesial and lingual walls of a tooth cavity preparation.

**me·sio·lin·guo·in·ci·sal** (me″ze-o-ling″gwo-in-si′zəl) pertaining to or formed by the mesial, lingual, and incisal surfaces of a tooth.

**me·sio·lin·guo·oc·clu·sal** (me″ze-o-ling″gwo-ŏ-kloo′zəl) pertaining to or formed by the mesial, lingual, and occlusal surfaces of a tooth.

**me·sio·lin·guo·pul·pal** (me″ze-o-ling″gwo-pul′pəl) pertaining to or formed by the mesial, lingual, and pulpal walls of a tooth cavity preparation.

**me·si·on** (me′se-on) [Gr. *mesos* middle] the plane that divides the body into right and left symmetric halves.

**me·si·o·oc·clu·sal** (me″ze-o-ŏ-kloo′zəl) pertaining to or formed by the mesial and occlusal surfaces of a tooth, or the mesial and occlusal walls of a tooth cavity.

**me·si·o·oc·clu·sion** (me″ze-o-ŏ-kloo′zhən) mesioclusion.

**me·si·o·oc·clu·so·dis·tal** (me″ze-o-ŏ-kloo″zo-dis′təl) pertaining to the mesial, occlusal, and distal surfaces of a posterior tooth.

**me·sio·pul·pal** (me″ze-o-pul′pəl) pertaining to or formed by the mesial and pulpal walls of a tooth cavity preparation.

**me·sio·pul·po·la·bi·al** (me″ze-o-pul″po-la′be-əl) pertaining to or formed by the mesial, pulpal, and labial walls of a tooth cavity preparation.

**me·sio·pul·po·lin·gual** (me″ze-o-pul″po-ling′gwəl) pertaining to or formed by the mesial, pulpal, and lingual walls of a tooth cavity preparation.

**me·sio·ver·sion** (me″ze-o-vər′zhən) deviation of a tooth from the vertical, in the direction of the tooth next mesial (anterior) to it in the dental arch.

**me·sit·y·lene** (mə-sit′ə-lēn) a triply methylated derivative of benzene occurring in petroleum and coal tar or synthesized from acetone; used as a solvent.

**Mes·mer** (mez′mer) Franz (Friedrich) Anton. German physician in France and Switzerland (1734–1815); his theory of animal magnetism was a precursor of modern hypnotism and suggestion therapy. See *animal magnetism,* under *magnetism,* and *suggestion therapy,* under *therapy;* see also *mesmerism.*

**mes·mer·ism** (mez′mər-iz″əm) [Franz A. *Mesmer*] 1. the use of animal magnetism and hypnotism as practiced by Mesmer. 2. hypnotism.

**mes·na** (mez′nə) [MeSH: Mesna] a sulfhydryl compound given orally or intravenously together with a urotoxic antineoplastic agent such as ifosfamide or cyclophosphamide because it inactivates some of their metabolites and thus lessens damage to the bladder.

**mes(o)-** [Gr. *mesos* middle] 1. a prefix meaning in the middle, intermediate, or moderate. 2. (always in the form *meso-*) in chemistry, a prefix signifying inactive or without effect on polarized light even though the molecule has asymmetric carbon atoms, because the two halves are mirror images.

**meso·aor·ti·tis** (mez″o-a″or-ti′tis) inflammation of the tunica media of the aorta.
**m.-a. syphili′tica,** inflammation of the middle coat of the aorta due to syphilis.

**meso·ap·pen·di·ci·tis** (mez″o-ə-pen″dĭ-si′tis) inflammation of the mesoappendix.

**meso·ap·pen·dix** (mez″o-ə-pen′dix) [*meso-* + *appendix*] [TA] the peritoneal fold attaching the appendix to the mesentery of the ileum. Called also *mesenteriolum processus vermiformis.*

**meso·ar·i·al** (mez″o-ar′e-əl) pertaining to the mesovarium.

**meso·a·ri·um** (mez″o-ar′e-əm) mesovarium.

**meso·bi·lin** (mez″o-bi′lin) a compound occurring in the urine as a derivative of bilirubin via enterohepatic circulation.

**meso·bil·i·ru·bin** (mez″o-bil″ĭ-roo′bin) a compound formed by the reduction of bilirubin.

**meso·bil·i·ru·bin·o·gen** (mez″o-bil″ĭ-roo-bin′o-jən) a reduced form of bilirubin, formed in the intestine, which on oxidation forms stercobilin.

**meso·bil·i·vi·o·lin** (mez″o-bil″ĭ-vi′o-lin) an oxidation product of mesobilirubinogen and of stercobilinogen.

**meso·blast** (mez′o-blast) [*meso-* + *-blast*] mesoderm, especially in the early undifferentiated stages.

**meso·blas·te·ma** (mez″o-blas-te′mə) the cells composing the mesoblast.

**meso·blas·tic** (mez″o-blas′tik) pertaining to or derived from the mesoblast.

**meso·car·dia** (mez″o-kahr′de-ə) [*meso-* + *cardia*] atypical location of the heart with the apex in the middle line of the thorax.

**meso·car·di·um** (mez″o-kahr′de-əm) [*meso-* + Gr. *kardia* heart] that part of the embryonic mesentery which connects the embryonic heart with the body wall ventrally and the foregut dorsally.
**arterial m.,** that part of the lamina visceralis pericardii serosi (visceral pericardium) that encloses the aorta and pulmonary artery.
**dorsal m.,** the temporary dorsal mesentery of the heart in the embryo; its site in adults is represented by the transverse sinus of the pericardium.
**lateral m.,** pulmonary ridge.
**venous m.,** that part of the lamina visceralis pericardii serosi (visceral pericardium) that encloses the venae cavae and pulmonary veins.
**ventral m.,** a mesentery attaching the heart to the ventral body wall; it is scarcely represented in human development.

**meso·car·pal** (mez″o-kahr′pəl) midcarpal.

**meso·ca·val** (mez″o-ka′vəl) pertaining to or connecting the superior mesenteric vein and inferior vena cava.

**meso·ce·cal** (mez″o-se′kəl) pertaining to the mesocecum.

**meso·ce·cum** (mez″o-se′kəm) [*meso-* + *cecum*] the occasionally occurring mesentery of the cecum.

**meso·ce·phal·ic** (mez″o-sĕ-fal′ik) [*meso-* + *cephalic*] characterized by or pertaining to a skull having an average breadth-length index, with a cephalic index of 75.0 to 79.9.

**Meso·ces·toi·des** (mez″o-ses-toi′dēz) [MeSH: Mesocestoides] a genus of tapeworms of the family Mesocestoididae, whose larvae are often found in the coelom or peritoneum of dogs, cats, mice, snakes, and other vertebrates; the adult form is found in the intestines of carnivorous animals, including man, dogs, cats, racoons, and meat-eating birds.

**Meso·ces·toi·di·dae** (mez″o-ses-toi′dĭ-de) a family of medium-sized to large tapeworms of the order Cyclophyllidea, subclass Cestoda, which parasitize carnivorous birds and mammals. *Mesocestoides* is the type genus.

**meso·chon·dri·um** (mez″o-kon′dre-əm) [*meso-* + Gr. *chondros* cartilage] the matrix in which are embedded the cellular elements of hyaline cartilage.

**meso·cho·roi·dea** (mez″o-ko-roi′de-ə) the middle coat of the choroid.

**meso·col·ic** (mez″o-kol′ik) pertaining to the mesocolon.

**meso·co·lon** (mez′o-ko″lon) [*meso-* + *colon*] [TA] [MeSH: Mesocolon] the process of the peritoneum by which the colon is attached to the posterior abdominal wall. It is divided into ascending, transverse, descending, and sigmoid or pelvic portions, according to the segment of the colon to which it gives attachment.
**m. ascen′dens** [TA], ascending mesocolon: the peritoneum attaching the ascending colon to the posterior abdominal wall, usually obliterated when the ascending colon becomes retroperitoneal.
**m. descen′dens** [TA], descending mesocolon: the peritoneum attaching the descending colon to the posterior abdominal wall; it is usually absent because the descending colon is ordinarily retroperitoneal.
**iliac m.,** m. sigmoideum.
**left m.,** m. descendens.
**pelvic m.,** m. sigmoideum.
**right m.,** m. ascendens.
**m. sigmoi′deum** [TA], sigmoid mesocolon: the peritoneum attaching the sigmoid colon to the posterior abdominal wall; called also *pelvic m.*
**m. transver′sum** [TA], transverse mesocolon: the peritoneum attaching the transverse colon to the posterior abdominal wall.

**meso·co·lo·pexy** (mez″o-ko′lo-pek″se) [*mesocolon* + *-pexy*] suspension or fixation of the mesocolon.

**meso·co·lo·pli·ca·tion** (mez″o-ko″lo-pli-ka′shən) [*mesocolon* + *plication*] plication of the mesocolon to limit its mobility.

**meso·cord** (mez′o-kord) an umbilical cord adherent to the placenta by a connecting fold of the amnion; more correctly, the connecting fold itself.

**meso·cor·nea** (mez″o-kor′ne-ə) substantia propria corneae.

**meso·cor·tex** (mez″o-kor′teks) [*meso-* + *cortex*] [TA] the cortex of the cingulate gyrus, which is intermediate in form between the allocortex and the isocortex and has four or five distinct layers; called also *juxtallocortex.*

**meso·cra·nic** (mez″o-kra′nik) having a cranial index between 75.0 and 79.9.

**Meso·cri·ce·tus** (mes″o-kri-se′təs) [MeSH: Mesocricetus] a genus

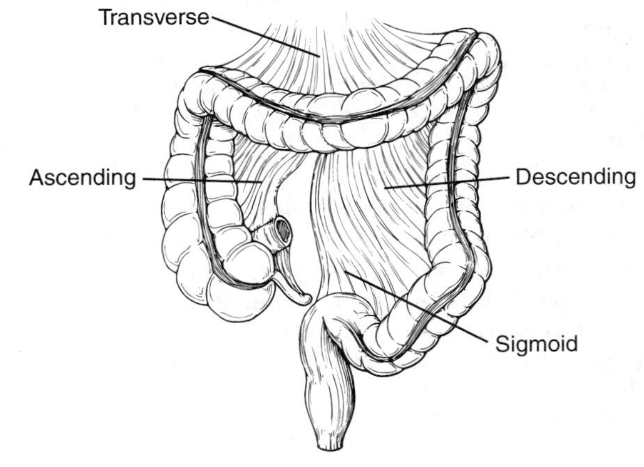

Mesocolon.

of rodents of the family Muridae, one of several genera of hamsters; *M. aura'tus* is the Syrian or golden hamster.

**meso·cu·nei·form** (mez″o-ku′ne-ĭ-form) os cuneiforme intermedius.

**meso·cyst** (mez′o-sist) [*meso-* + *cyst*] the layer of peritoneum attaching the gallbladder to the liver.

**meso·derm** (mez′o-dərm) [*meso-* + *-derm*] [MeSH: Mesoderm] the middle layer of the three primary germ layers of the embryo, lying between the ectoderm and the endoderm. From it are derived the connective tissue, bone and cartilage, muscle, blood and blood vessels, lymphatics and lymphoid organs, notochord, pleura, pericardium, peritoneum, kidney, and gonads. Cf. *ectoderm* and *endoderm*.
**extraembryonic m.,** that located outside the embryo and belonging to fetal accessory organs, covering for example the amnion and yolk sac.
**gastral m.,** that infolded with the endoderm during gastrulation.
**head m.,** loose mesoderm, cranial to the somites.
**lateral m.,** the lateral sheets of mesoderm within which the embryonic coelom arises.
**paraxial m.,** that lying alongside the notochord and neural tube.
**peristomal m.,** that derived from the ventral lip of the blastopore or from the primitive streak.
**somatic m.,** the outer of the two layers into which the embryonic mesoderm divides; associated with ectoderm to constitute the somatopleure.
**splanchnic m.,** the inner of the two layers into which the embryonic mesoderm divides; associated with endoderm to constitute splanchnopleure.

**meso·der·mal** (mez″o-dər′məl) pertaining to or derived from the mesoderm.

**meso·der·mic** (mez″o-dər′mik) pertaining to the mesoderm.

**mes·odont** (mez′o-dont) [*meso-* + Gr. *odous* tooth] having a dental index between 42 and 44.

**mes·odon·tic** (mez″o-don′tik) having medium sized teeth.

**mes·odon·tism** (mez″o-don′tiz-əm) the state of having medium sized teeth, or a dental index between 42 and 44.

**meso·du·o·de·nal** (mez″o-doo″o-de′nəl) pertaining to the mesoduodenum.

**meso·du·o·de·num** (mez″o-doo″o-de′nəm) [*meso-* + *duodenum*] the mesenteric fold which in early fetal life encloses the duodenum.

**meso·epi·did·y·mis** (mez″o-ep″ĭ-did′ĭ-mis) a fold of tunica vaginalis that sometimes connects the epididymis with the testicle.

**meso·esoph·a·gus** (mez″o-ə-sof′ə-gəs) the portion of the primordial mesentery that encloses the developing esophagus.

**meso·gas·ter** (mez″o-gas′tər) [*meso-* + *gaster*] mesogastrium.

**meso·gas·tric** (mez″o-gas′trik) pertaining to the mesogastrium.

**meso·gas·tri·um** (mez″o-gas′tre-əm) [*meso-* + Gr. *gastēr* belly] the portion of the primordial mesentery that encloses the stomach, and from which the greater omentum is developed.

**Meso·gas·trop·o·da** (mez″o-gas″trop″ə-də) an order of marine and fresh water snails of the subclass Streptoneura; it includes a number of intermediate hosts of parasitic trematodes, such as the families Hydrobiidae, Pilidae, and Pleuroceridae.

**meso·glea** (mez″o-gle′ə) [*meso-* + Gr. *gloia* glue] the layer between the epidermis and gastrodermis of coelenterates.

**meso·glu·te·al** (mez″o-gloo′te-əl) pertaining to the gluteus medius muscle.

**meso·glu·te·us** (mez″o-gloo′te-əs) musculus gluteus medius.

**mes·og·nath·ic** (mez″og-na′thik) mesognathous.

**me·sog·na·thous** (mə-sog′nə-thəs) [*meso-* + *gnath-* + *-ous*] pertaining to or characterized by moderate protrusion of the jaw, with a gnathic index of 98 to 103. Called also *mesognathic*.

**Meso·gon·i·mus** (mez″o-gon′ĭ-məs) a former name for a genus of flukes, certain species of which are now included in the genera *Paragonimus* and *Heterophyes*.
**M. hetero′phyes,** *Heterophyes heterophyes*.

**meso·hy·po·blast** (mez″o-hi′po-blast) mesentoderm.

**meso·ile·um** (mez″o-il′e-əm) the mesentery of the ileum.

***meso*-ino·si·tol** (mes″o-in-o′sĭ-tol) inositol, def. 2.

**meso·je·ju·num** (mez″o-je-ju′nəm) the mesentery of the jejunum.

**meso·lec·i·thal** (mez″o-les′ĭ-thəl) [*meso-* + *-lecithal*] possessing a moderate amount of yolk.

**meso·mel·ic** (mez″o-mel′ik) [*meso-* + *mel-* + *-ic*] pertaining to the midportion of the upper or lower limb.

**meso·mere** (mez′o-mēr) [*meso-* + *-mere*] 1. a blastomere of size intermediate between a macromere and a micromere. 2. a midzone of the mesoderm between the epimere and hypomere.

**meso·mer·ic** (mez″o-mer′ik) exhibiting mesomerism.

**me·som·er·ism** (mə-som′ər-iz″əm) the existence of organic chemical structures that can not be accurately represented by a single structural formula, the actual formula lying intermediate between several possible representations that differ only in the position of electrons.

**meso·me·tri·um** (mez″o-me′tre-əm) [*meso-* + Gr. *mētra* uterus] 1. [TA] the portion of the broad ligament below the mesovarium, composed of the layers of peritoneum that separate to enclose the uterus. 2. tunica muscularis uteri.

**meso·morph** (mez′o-morf) an individual having a type of body build in which tissues derived from the mesoderm predominate: there is a relative preponderance of muscle, bone, and connective tissue, usually with heavy, hard physique of rectangular outline, a somatotype classified between ectomorph and endomorph.

**meso·mor·phic** (mez″o-mor′fik) pertaining to or characteristic of a mesomorph.

**meso·mor·phy** (mez′o-mor″fe) [*meso*derm + Gr. *morphē* form] the condition of being a mesomorph.

**me·som·u·la** (mə-som′u-lə) an early stage of the embryo, when it consists of an epithelial ectoderm and endoderm enclosing a mass of mesenchyma.

**mes·on** (mes′on, me′zon) [Gr. *mesos* middle] [MeSH: Mesons] 1. mesion. 2. a short-lived subatomic particle of a mass usually less than that of a proton but more than that of an electron; it may carry either a positive, a negative, or a neutral electric charge.

**meso·na·sal** (mez″o-na′zəl) situated in the middle of the nose.

**meso·neph·ric** (mez″o-nef′rik) pertaining to the mesonephros.

**meso·neph·roi** (mez″o-nef′roi) plural of *mesonephros*.

**mes·o·ne·phro·ma** (mez″o-nə-fro′mə) [MeSH: Mesonephroma] clear cell adenocarcinoma.

**meso·neph·ron** (mez″o-nef′ron) mesonephros.

**meso·neph·ros** (mez″o-nef′ros) pl. *mesoneph′roi* [*meso-* + Gr. *nephros* kidney] [MeSH: Mesonephros] the excretory organ of the embryo, arising caudad to the pronephros or pronephric rudiments and using its duct; it consists of a long tube in the lower part of the body cavity, running parallel with the vertebral axis and joined at right angles by a row of twisting tubes. See also *metanephros*. Called also *corpus Wolffi, mesonephron, middle kidney,* and *wolffian body*.

**meso·omen·tum** (mez″o-o-men′təm) the fold by which the omentum is attached to the abdominal wall.

**meso·pexy** (mez′o-pek″se) mesenteriopexy.

**meso·phile** (mez′o-fīl) an organism which grows best at temperatures between 20° and 45° C.

**meso·phil·ic** (mez″o-fil′ik) [*meso-* + *-philic*] fond of moderate temperature; said of bacteria which develop best at temperatures between 20° and 45° C. Cf. *psychrophilic* and *thermophilic*.

**meso·phle·bi·tis** (mez″o-flə-bi′tis) inflammation of the tunica media of a vein.

**meso·phrag·ma** (mez″o-frag′mə) [*meso-* + Gr. *phragmos* a fencing in] a name given to the M band. Cf. *inophragma,* and *Z band,* under *band*.

**me·soph·ry·on** (mə-sof′re-on) [*meso-* + *ophryon*] the glabella or its central point.

**meso·phyll** (mez′o-fil) [*meso-* + Gr. *phyllon* leaf] the tissue of the inner part of a leaf.

**me·so·pia** (mə-so′pe-ə) the condition of having mesopic vision.

**me·sop·ic** (mə-sop′ik) [*meso-* + Gr. *ōpsis* sight] pertaining to vision at intermediate levels of illumination, e.g., at twilight.

**Mes·o·pin** (mes′o-pin) trademark for a preparation of homatropine methylbromide.

**meso·pneu·mon** (mez″o-noo′mon) [*meso-* + Gr. *pneumon* lung] the union of the two layers of the pleura at the hilus of the lung.

**meso·por·phy·rin** (mez″o-por′fĭ-rin) a porphyrin (q.v.) in which two pyrrole rings each have one methyl and one propionate side chain and the other two pyrrole rings each have one methyl and one ethyl side chain.

**meso·pro·sop·ic** (mez″o-pro-sop′ik) [*meso-* + *prosop-* + *-ic*] having a face of moderate width.

**meso·pul·mo·num** (mez″o-pəl-mo′nəm) the portion of the embryonic mesentery that encloses the laterally expanding lung.

**meso·ra·chis·chi·sis** (mez″o-rə-kis′kĭ-sis) merorachischisis.

**me·sor·chi·al** (mə-sor′ke-əl) pertaining to the mesorchium.

**me·sor·chi·um** (mə-sor'ke-əm) [*meso-* + Gr. *orchis* testis] the portion of the primordial mesentery that encloses the fetal testis, represented in the adult by a fold between the testis and epididymis.

**meso·rec·tum** (mez″o-rek'təm) [*meso-* + *rectum*] the fold of peritoneum connecting the upper portion of the rectum with the sacrum.

**meso·rid·a·zine** (mes″o-rid'ə-zēn) [MeSH: Mesoridazine] a phenothiazine that is a metabolite of thioridazine, having properties similar to those of chlorpromazine.
**m. besylate** [USP], **m. benzenesulfonate,** the besylate salt of mesoridazine; an antipsychotic agent used in the treatment of alcoholism, schizophrenia, psychoneurotic manifestations, and behavioral problems in mental deficiency and chronic brain syndrome, administered orally and intramuscularly.

**meso·rop·ter** (mez″o-rop'tər) [*meso-* + *horopter*] the normal position of the eyes with their muscles at rest.

**mes·or·rha·phy** (mez-or'ə-fe) mesenteriorrhaphy.

**mes·or·rhine** (mez'o-rin) [*meso-* + Gr. *rhis* nose] having a nasal index between 48 and 53.

**meso·sal·pinx** (mez″o-sal'pinks) [*meso-* + *salpinx*] [TA] the part of the broad ligament of the uterus above the mesovarium, composed of layers that enclose the uterine tube.

**meso·scap·u·la** (mez″o-skap'u-lə) spina scapulae.

**meso·seme** (mez'o-sēm) [*meso-* + Gr. *sēma* sign] having an orbital index between 83 and 89.

**meso·sig·moid** (mez″o-sig'moid) the peritoneal fold by which the sigmoid flexure is attached to the posterior abdominal wall.

**meso·sig·moi·di·tis** (mez″o-sig″moi-di'tis) inflammation of the mesosigmoid.

**meso·sig·moido·pexy** (mez″o-sig-moi'do-pek″se) [*mesosigmoid* + *-pexy*] suspension or fixation of the mesosigmoid in the treatment of prolapse of the rectum.

**meso·some** (mez'o-sōm) [*meso-* + *-some*] an invagination of the cell membrane occurring in certain bacteria. Various mesosomes are associated with DNA replication, with cell secretion, and with electron transport of the organism.

**meso·staph·y·line** (mez″o-staf'ə-lēn) [*meso-* + *staphyline* (def. 2)] pertaining to or characterized by a palate with a moderate width, with a palatal index of 80.0 to 84.9.

**meso·ste·ni·um** (mez″o-ste'ne-əm) mesenterium.

**meso·ster·num** (mez'o-ster″nəm) [*meso-* + *sternum*] the corpus sterni.

**meso·stro·ma** (mez″o-stro'mə) the embryonic fibrillar tissue analogous to the vitreous, which develops into Bowman's and Descemet's membranes.

**meso·tar·sal** (mez″o-tahr'səl) midtarsal.

**meso·tau·ro·don·tism** (mez″o-taw″ro-don'tiz-əm) [*meso-* + *taurodontism*] taurodontism in which the tooth roots branch only in the middle.

**meso·ten·din·e·um** (mez″o-tən-din'e-əm) [L.] [TA] the delicate connective tissue sheath attaching a tendon to its fibrous sheath.

**meso·ten·don** (mez″o-ten'don) mesotendineum.

**meso·ten·on** (mez″o-ten'on) mesotendineum.

**meso·the·li·al** (mez″o-the'le-əl) pertaining to the mesothelium.

**meso·the·li·o·ma** (mez″o-the'le-o'mə) [MeSH: Mesothelioma] a tumor derived from mesothelial tissue (peritoneum, pleura, pericardium); both benign and malignant varieties exist. Malignant varieties are often the result of excessive exposure to asbestos.
**benign fibrous m.,** a localized tumor of the pleura, firm and encapsulated and sometimes vascular; size ranges from small to enormous. It has not been linked to asbestos exposure. Called also *localized fibrous m.*
**diffuse m.,** malignant m.
**localized fibrous m.,** solitary fibrous tumor.
**malignant m.,** a malignant tumor of the pleura, peritoneum, or pericardium, appearing as broad sheets of cells; some regions contain spindle-shaped, sarcoma-like cells and others show adenomatous patterns. Many of these tumors, particularly in the pleura and peritoneum, have been linked to excessive exposure to asbestos. Called also *diffuse m.*
**peritoneal m.,** a malignant mesothelioma in the peritoneum, a form linked to heavy asbestos exposure and sometimes accompanying the pleural variety; it may spread to involve the intestines and cause obstruction. Symptoms include ascites, pain, and a mass in the abdomen.
**pleural m.,** a malignant mesothelioma of the pleural space, often spreading widely and invading other thoracic structures; patients are often older men who present with dyspnea, chest pain, and extensive pleural effusions. It is usually fatal within one year.
**m. of testis, m. of tunica vaginalis,** a malignant mesothelioma of the tunica vaginalis testis, usually first manifesting as a hydrocele; sometimes it is metastatic from the lungs, but not all cases have been linked to asbestos exposure. It often follows a more indolent course than the pleural or peritoneal varieties.

**meso·the·li·um** (mez″o-the'le-əm) [*meso-* + *epithelium*] the layer of flat cells, derived from the mesoderm, which lines the coelom or body cavity of the embryo. In the adult, it forms the simple squamous epithelium which covers all true serous membranes (peritoneum, pericardium, pleura).

**meso·the·nar** (məz-o-the'nər) [*meso-* + *thenar*] musculus adductor pollicis.

**mes·o·trop·ic** (mez″o-trop'ik) situated in the middle of a cavity, as the abdomen.

**meso·tym·pa·num** (mez″o-tim'pə-nəm) the portion of the middle ear medial to the tympanic membrane.

**meso·va·ri·um** (mez″o-var'e-əm) [L.] [TA] the portion of the broad ligament of the uterus between the mesometrium and mesosalpinx, which is drawn out to enclose and hold the ovary in place.

**me·squite** (mə-skēt') [Nahuatl *mizquitl*] any plant of the genus *Prosopis.* Called also *algaroba* or *algarroba.*

**mes·sen·ger** (mes'ən-jər) an information carrier such as a hormone or an electrical impulse.
**first m.,** a factor or hormone that binds to a receptor on the external surface of a cell and sets off a series of reactions that eventually convert a precursor into a second messenger.
**second m.,** any of several classes of intracellular signals acting at or situated within the plasma membrane that translate electrical or chemical messages from the environment (first messengers) into cellular responses; such messengers include changes in membrane potential, calcium ions, cyclic nucleotides, and products of phosphatidylinositol turnover.

**mes·ter·o·lone** (məs-ter'ə-lōn) [MeSH: Mesterolone] an androgen with actions and uses similar to those of testosterone.

**Mes·ti·non** (mes'tĭ-non) trademark for preparations of pyridostigmine bromide.

**mes·tra·nol** (mes'trə-nol) [USP] [MeSH: Mestranol] the 3-methyl ether of ethinyl estradiol, used as the estrogen component of several progestin-estrogen oral contraceptives.

**mes·u·prine hy·dro·chlo·ride** (mes'ə-prēn) a vasodilator and smooth muscle relaxant, $C_{19}H_{26}N_2O_5S{\cdot}HCl$.

**mes·uran·ic** (mez″u-ran'ik) [*meso-* + *uran-* + *-ic*] having a maxilloalveolar index between 110.0 and 114.9.

**mes·y·late** (mes'ə-lāt) USAN contraction for methanesulfonate.

**Met** methionine.

**met(a)-** [Gr. *meta* after, beyond, over] 1. a prefix indicating *(a)* change, transformation, or exchange or *(b)* after or next. 2. symbol *m-*; in organic chemistry, a prefix indicating a 1,3-substituted benzene ring, e.g., *m*-xylene (1,3-dimethylbenzene) or *m*-nitrophenol (3-nitrophenol). 3. in organic chemistry, a prefix indicating a polymeric acid anhydride, e.g., metaphosphoric acid.

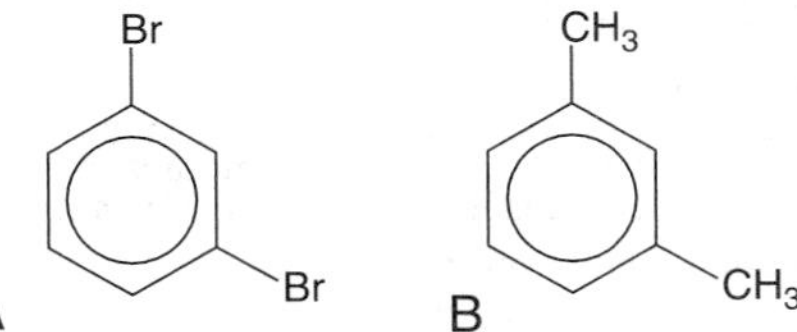


Two examples of disubstituted benzene derivatives with substituents in the *meta*-position. *(A),* 1,3-dibromobenzene; *(B), meta*-xylene (1,3-dimethylbenzene).

**meta-anal·y·sis** (met″ə-ə-nal'ĭ-sis) [*meta-* + *analysis*] [MeSH: Meta-Analysis] any systematic method that uses statistical analysis to integrate the data from a number of independent studies.

**me·tab·a·sis** (mə-tab'ə-sis) [*meta-* + Gr. *bainein* to go] 1. a change in the manifestations or course of a disease. 2. metastasis, or change in the site of a morbid process from one region of the body to another.

**meta·bi·o·sis** (met″ə-bi-o'sis) [*meta-* + *biosis*] the dependence of one organism upon another for its existence; commensalism.

**met·a·bol·ic** (met″ə-bol'ik) pertaining to or of the nature of metabolism.

**met·a·bo·lim·e·ter** (met″ə-bo-lim'ə-tər) [*metabolism* + *-meter*] an apparatus for measuring basal metabolism.

**met·a·bo·lim·e·try** (met″ə-bə-lim′ə-tre) the measurement of basal metabolism.

**me·tab·o·lism** (mə-tab′ə-liz″əm) [Gr. *metaballein* to turn about, change, alter] [MeSH: Metabolism] 1. the sum of all the physical and chemical processes by which living organized substance is produced and maintained (anabolism), and also the transformation by which energy is made available for the uses of the organism (catabolism). 2. biotransformation.
**ammonotelic m.,** that in which ammonia is the final product of nitrogen metabolism.
**basal m.,** the minimal energy expended for the maintenance of respiration, circulation, peristalsis, muscle tonus, body temperature, glandular activity, and the other vegetative functions of the body. The rate of basal metabolism (basal metabolic rate) is measured by means of a calorimeter, in a subject at absolute rest, 14 to 18 hours after eating, and is expressed in calories per hour per square meter of body surface.
**drug m.,** biotransformation of drugs.
**endogenous m.,** metabolism of the proteins of the body tissues.
**energy m.,** the metabolic processes by which energy is released.
**excess m. of exercise,** the amount by which the oxygen consumed or the carbon dioxide eliminated during exercise and recovery exceeds the corresponding amounts during sleep.
**exogenous m.,** metabolism of ingested foodstuffs.
**inborn error of m.,** a genetically determined biochemical disorder in which a specific enzyme defect produces a metabolic block that may have pathologic consequences at birth (e.g., phenylketonuria) or in later life (e.g., diabetes mellitus); called also *enzymopathy* and *genetotrophic disease.*
**intermediary m.,** the various chemical reactions involved in the transformation of food molecules into essential cellular building blocks.
**ureotelic m.,** that in which urea is the final product of nitrogen metabolism.
**uricotelic m.,** that in which uric acid is the final product of nitrogen metabolism.

**me·tab·o·lite** (mə-tab′o-līt) any substance produced by metabolism or by a metabolic process.
**essential m.,** a necessary constituent of normal metabolic processes.

**me·tab·o·liz·a·ble** (mə-tab′o-līz″ə-bəl) capable of being transformed by metabolism.

**me·tabo·re·cep·tor** (mətab″o-re-sep′tər) receptors found in skeletal muscle that respond to an increase in metabolic products and stimulate an increase in circulation in response to exercise.

**meta·brom·sa·lan** (met″ə-brom′sə-lən) a bromsalan disinfectant with antibacterial and antifungal activities used mainly in medicated soaps.

**meta·bu·teth·amine hy·dro·chlo·ride** (met″ə-bu-teth′ə-mēn) a local anesthetic used in dentistry to produce infiltration and nerve block anesthesia.

**meta·car·pal** (met″ə-kahr′pəl) 1. pertaining to the metacarpus. 2. (pl.) ossa metacarpi.

**meta·car·pec·to·my** (met″ə-kahr-pek′tə-me) excision or resection of a metacarpal bone.

**meta·car·po·pha·lan·ge·al** (met″ə-kahr″po-fə-lan′je-əl) pertaining to the metacarpus and phalanges.

**meta·car·pus** (met″ə-kahr′pəs) [*meta-* + *carpus*] [TA] [MeSH: Metacarpus] the part of the hand between the wrist and the fingers, its skeleton being five cylindric bones (metacarpals) extending from the carpus to the phalanges. See also *ossa metacarpi,* under *os*[2].

**met·a·cele** (met′ə-sēl) metacoeloma.

**meta·cen·tric** (met″ə-sen′trik) [*meta-* + *center* (def. 1)] having the centromere near the middle, so that the arms of the chromosome are approximately equal in length. Cf. *acrocentric* and *submetacentric.*

**meta·cer·ca·ria** (met″ə-sər-kar′e-ə) pl. *metacerca′riae.* The encysted resting or maturing stage of a trematode parasite in the tissues of an intermediate host (mollusks, aquatic arthropods, fishes, or amphibia) or on vegetation. The metacercaria may be the infective or transfer stage to man and other animals.

**meta·chro·ma·sia** (met″ə-kro-ma′zhə) [*meta-* + Gr. *chrōma* color] 1. a condition in which tissues do not stain true with a given stain. 2. staining in which the same stain colors different tissues in different tints. 3. the change of color produced by staining.

**meta·chro·mat·ic** (met″ə-kro-mat′ik) [*meta-* + *chromatic*] staining differently with the same dye; said of tissues in which different elements take on different colors when a certain dye is applied. By extension, said of dyes by which different tissues are stained differently.

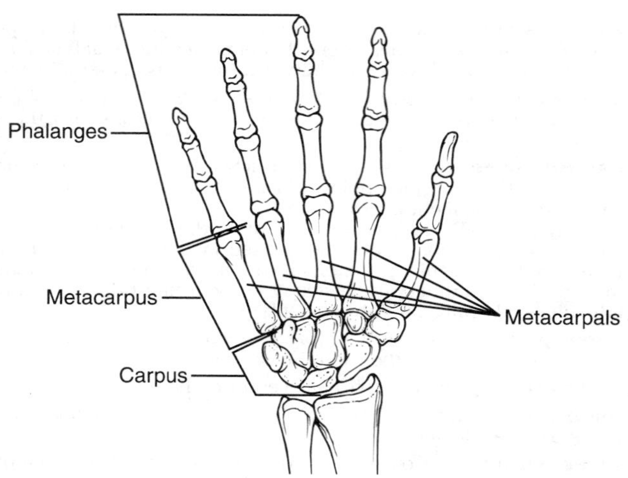


Metacarpus, comprising the metacarpal bones, which extend between the carpus and phalanges and are numbered lateromedially.

**meta·chro·ma·tin** (met″ə-kro′mə-tin) the basophil element in chromatin.

**meta·chro·ma·tism** (met″ə-kro′mə-tiz″əm) metachromasia.

**meta·chro·mato·phil** (met″ə-kro-mat′o-fil) a cell that does not stain in the usual manner with a given stain.

**meta·chro·mia** (met″ə-kro′me-ə) metachromasia.

**meta·chro·mic** (met″ə-kro′mik) metachromatic.

**meta·chro·mo·phil** (met″ə-kro′mo-fil) [*meta-* + *chromo-* + *-phil*] staining in an abnormal manner with a given stain.

**meta·chro·mo·phile** (met″ə-kro′mo-fīl) metachromophil.

**meta·chro·mo·some** (met″ə-kro′mo-sōm) one of two small chromosomes which conjugate only in the last phase of the spermatocyte division.

**me·tach·ro·nous** (mə-tak′rə-nəs) [*meta-* + *chrono-* + *-ous*] occurring at different times; cf. *synchronous.*

**meta·chro·sis** (met″ə-kro′sis) [*meta-* + Gr. *chrōsis* coloring] change of color in animals.

**meta·coele** (met′ə-sēl) [*meta-* + *-coele*] metacoeloma.

**meta·coe·lo·ma** (met″ə-se-lo′mə) that part of the embryonic coelom which develops into the pleuroperitoneal cavity; called also *metacele* and *metacoele.*

**meta·cone** (met′ə-kōn) [*meta-* + *cone*] the distobuccal cusp of an upper molar tooth.

**meta·con·id** (met″ə-kon′id) the mesiolingual cusp of a lower molar tooth.

**meta·con·ule** (met″ə-kon′ūl) the small intermediate cusp between the metacone and the protocone of the upper molar teeth of mammals, sometimes also present in man.

**meta·cor·tan·dra·lone** (met″ə-kor-tan′drə-lōn) prednisolone.

**meta·cre·sol** (met″ə-kre′sol) [USP] *m*-cresol; one of the three isomeric forms of cresol, and the most strongly antiseptic of the group; used as a disinfectant.
**m. purple, m. sulfonphthalein,** a triphenylmethane compound which is a brilliant indicator, being red at pH 1.2, blue at pH 2.8, yellow at pH 7.4, and purple at pH 9.0.

**meta·cy·e·sis** (met″ə-si-e′sis) [*meta-* + *cyesis*] extrauterine pregnancy.

**meta·du·o·den·um** (met″ə-doo″o-de′nəm) the portion of the duodenum distal to the duodenal papilla, developed embryonically from the midgut.

**meta·fe·male** (met″ə-fe′māl) [*meta-* + *female*] a sex chromosome abnormality, XXX karyotype, among females; called also *triple-X.*

**meta·gas·ter** (met″ə-gas′tər) [*meta-* + *gaster*] the permanent intestinal canal of the embryo.

**meta·gas·tru·la** (met″ə-gas′troo-lə) [*meta-* + *gastrula*] a gastrula with a cleavage differing from that of the standard type.

**meta·gel·a·tin** (met″ə-jel′ə-tin) a substance produced by treating gelatin with oxalic acid.

**meta·gen·e·sis** (met″ə-jen′ə-sis) [*meta-* + *-genesis*] alternation of generations; alternation in regular sequence of asexual with sexual methods of reproduction in the same species, as in certain fungi.

**meta·go·ni·mi·a·sis** (met″ə-go″nĭ-mi′ə-sis) infection with *Metagonimus.*

**Meta·gon·i·mus** (met″ə-gon′ĭ-məs) [*meta-* + Gr. *gonimos* productive] a genus of trematodes of the family Heterophyidae. *M. yokoga′wai (M. ova′tus)* is found in the small intestines of humans and other mammals in East Asia, Indonesia, Israel, and the Balkans.

**meta·he·mo·glo·bin** (met″ə-he″mo-glo′bin) methemoglobin.

**Meta·hy·drin** (met″ə-hi′drin) trademark for a preparation of trichlormethiazide.

**meta·ic·ter·ic** (met″ə-ik-ter′ik) occurring after jaundice.

**meta·in·fec·tive** (met″ə-in-fek′tiv) occurring after an infection; a term applied to a febrile state occurring during convalescence from an infectious disease.

**meta·iodo·ben·zyl·guan·i·dine (MIBG)** (met″ə-i″o-do-ben″zəl-gwahn′ĭ-dēn) iobenguane.

**meta·ki·ne·sis** (met″ə-kĭ-ne′sis) prometaphase.

**met·al** (met′əl) [L. *metallum;* Gr. *metallon*] [MeSH: Metals] any element marked by luster, malleability, ductility, and conductivity of electricity and heat and which will ionize positively in solution.
**alkali m.**, one of a group of monovalent metals including lithium, sodium, potassium, rubidium, and cesium.
**alkaline earth m's**, a group of grayish white, malleable metals that are easily oxidized in air, comprising beryllium, magnesium, calcium, strontium, barium, and radium.
**base m.**, a metal that oxidizes or corrodes relatively easily; cf. *noble m.*
**colloidal m.**, a colloidal solution of a metal; see *electrosol.*
**fusible m.**, an alloy that melts at a relatively low temperature, as at or around the boiling point of water. Bismuth, lead, and tin are usually the principal constituents.
**noble m.**, a metal that is highly resistant to oxidation and corrosion; cf. *base m.*

**met·al·de·hyde** (met-al′də-hīd) a molluscacide commonly used in gardens, mixed with bran to form flakes or pellets; animals eating it suffer neurotoxicity with tremors, dyspnea, and sometimes convulsions that can be fatal.

**me·tal·lic** (mə-tal′ik) 1. pertaining to, consisting of, or of the nature of metal. 2. made of metal.

**met·al·lized** (met′əl-īzd) treated with metals.

**met·al·liz·ing** (met′əl-īz-ing) making something metallic, as when treating the surface of impression material with metals so that it will conduct electricity before electroplating.

**me·tal·lo·car·boxy·pep·ti·dase** (mə-tal″o-kahr-bok″se-pep′tĭ-dās) [EC 3.4.17] any of a group of carboxypeptidases containing a tightly bound metal or metal ion that participates in catalysis.

**me·tal·lo·cy·a·nide** (mə-tal″o-si′ə-nīd) a compound of cyanogen with a metal.

**me·tal·lo·en·do·pep·ti·dase** (mə-tal″o-en″do-pep′tĭ-dās) [EC 3.4.24] any of a group of endopeptidases containing a tightly bound metal or metal ion that participates in catalysis.

**me·tal·lo·en·zyme** (mə-tal″o-en′zīm) an enzyme containing a tightly bound metal atom (e.g., cobalt, copper, iron, molybdenum, or zinc) as an integral part of its structure.

**me·tal·lo·fla·vo·pro·tein** (mə-tal″o-fla″vo-pro′tēn) a flavoprotein that contains a bound metal ion as part of its structure, e.g., xanthine oxidase.

**met·al·loid** (met′əl-oid) [*metal* + *-oid*] 1. any element with both metallic and nonmetallic properties, as silicon, boron, or arsenic. 2. any metallic element that has not all the characters of a typical metal. 3. resembling a metal.

**me·tal·lo·phil·ic** (mə-tal″o-fil′ik) having an affinity for metal-containing stains; said of cells.

**me·tal·lo·por·phy·rin** (mə-tal″o-por′fə-rin) a combination of a metal with porphyrin, e.g., heme (iron).

**me·tal·lo·pro·tein** (mĕ-tal″o-pro′tēn) a protein that has one or more tightly bound metal ions forming part of its structure.

**met·al·los·co·py** (met″əl-os′kə-pe) [*metal* + *-scopy*] observation of the effects of applying metal to the body.

**me·tal·lo·ther·a·py** (mə-tal″o-ther′ə-pe) [*metal* + *therapy*] the treatment of disease by applying metals to the skin.

**met·al·lur·gy** (met′əl-ur″je) [*metal* + Gr. *ergon* work] [MeSH: Metallurgy] the science and art of using metals.

**meta·mer** (met′ə-mər) a compound exhibiting, or capable of exhibiting, metamerism.

**meta·mere** (met′ə-mēr) [*meta-* + *-mere*] 1. one of a series of homologous segments of the body of an animal. 2. in genetic theory, one of a varying number of common repeating units that make up the repressor segment of a chromosomal locus, the actual number of metameres in a given locus being proportional to the degree of repression of the trait in question.

**meta·mer·ic** (met″ə-mer′ik) pertaining to or characterized by metamerism.

**me·tam·er·ism** (mə-tam′ər-is″əm) 1. isomerism, particularly a type of structural isomerism in which different radicals of the same chemical type are attached to the same polyvalent element and yet give rise to compounds possessing identical molecular formulas, for example, diethylamine, $(C_2H_5)_2NH$, and methyl propylamine, $CH_3NHC_3H_7$. 2. arrangement into metameres by the serial repetition of a structural pattern. Cf. *antimere.*

**Met·a·mine** (met′ə-mēn) trademark for preparations of trolnitrate phosphate.

**meta·mo·nad** (met″ə-mo′nad) [*meta-* + *monad*] a group of protozoa comprising all the zooflagellates except those in the orders Choanoflagellida and Kinetoplastida, most of which are symbionts in the insect gut.

**meta·mor·phop·sia** (met″ə-mor-fop′se-ə) [*meta-* + *morph-* + *-opsia*] a disturbance of vision in which objects are seen as distorted in shape.

**meta·mor·pho·sis** (met″ə-mor′fə-sis) [*meta-* + *morphosis*] change of shape or structure, particularly a transition from one developmental stage to another, as from larva to adult form.
**fatty m.**, fatty change.
**retrograde m., retrogressive m.**, degeneration; usually, a retrograde metabolic change.
**revisionary m.**, cataplasia.
**tissue m.**, any change in tissues, either normal or pathologic.

**meta·mor·phot·ic** (met″ə-mor-fot′ik) pertaining to or characterized by metamorphosis.

**Met·a·mu·cil** (met″ə-mu′sil) trademark for a preparation of psyllium hydrophilic mucilloid.

**meta·my·elo·cyte** (met″ə-mi′ə-lo-sīt″) a precursor in the granulocytic series, being a cell intermediate in development between a promyelocyte and the mature segmented and granular polymorphonuclear leukocyte. The protein synthesis seen in earlier stages decreases or stops; the nucleus becomes indented and its chromatin becomes coarse and clumped; and the cytoplasm becomes pink like that of a mature granulocyte. Called also *juvenile neutrophil, cell,* or *form.*

**Me·tan·dren** (mə-tan′drən) trademark for preparations of methyltestosterone.

**meta·neph·ric** (met″ə-nef′rik) of or pertaining to the metanephros.

**meta·neph·rine** (met″ə-nef′rin) [MeSH: Metanephrine] a methylated metabolite of epinephrine excreted in the urine and found in certain tissues.

**met·a·neph·ro·gen·ic** (met″ə-nef″ro-jen′ik) [*metanephros* + *-genic*] capable of giving rise to the metanephros.

**meta·neph·roi** (met″ə-nef′roi) plural of *metanephros.*

**meta·neph·ron** (met″ə-nef′ron) metanephros.

**meta·neph·ros** (met″ə-nef′ros) pl. *metaneph′roi* [*meta-* + Gr. *nephros* kidney] the primordium of the permanent kidney, which develops later than and caudal to the mesonephros, from the mesonephric duct and nephrogenic cord. Called also *definite, definitive,* or *hind kidney.*

**meta·neu·tro·phil** (met″ə-noo′tro-fil) [*meta-* + *neutrophil*] staining abnormally with neutral stains.

**meta·nu·cle·us** (met″ə-noo′kle-əs) [*meta-* + *nucleus*] the egg nucleus during the maturative period.

**meta·phase** (met′ə-fāz) [*meta-* + *phase*] [MeSH: Metaphase] the second stage of cell division (mitosis or meiosis), during which the contracted chromosomes, each consisting of two chromatids, are arranged in the equatorial plane of the spindle prior to separation. See *meiosis* and *mitosis.*

**Met·a·phed·rin** (met″ə-fed′rin) trademark for a preparation of nitromersol and ephedrine.

**Met·a·phen** (met′ə-fən) trademark for preparations of nitromersol.

**meta·phos·phor·ic ac·id** (met″ə-fos-for′ik) a glassy solid polymer of phosphoric acid, soluble in water; used as a reagent for chemical analysis and as a test for albumin in the urine. Called also *glacial phosphoric acid.*

**meta·phys·e·al** (met″ə-fiz′e-əl) pertaining to or of the nature of a metaphysis.

**me·taph·y·ses** (mə-taf′ə-sēz) plural of *metaphysis.*

**meta·phys·i·al** (met″ə-fiz′e-əl) metaphyseal.

**me·taph·y·sis** (mə-taf′ə-sis) pl. *metaph′yses* [*meta-* + *physis*] [TA] the wider part at the extremity of the shaft of a long bone, adjacent to the epiphyseal disk. During development it contains the growth zone and consists of spongy bone; in the adult it is continuous with the epiphysis.

**meta·phys·itis** (met″ə-fis-i′tis) inflammation of the metaphysis of a long bone.

**meta·pla·sia** (met″ə-pla′zhə) [*meta-* + *-plasia*] [MeSH: Metaplasia] the change in the type of adult cells in a tissue to another form of adult cells that are not normal for that tissue.
**myeloid m.,** a syndrome characterized by myeloid tissue in extramedullary sites with nucleated erythrocytes and immature granulocytes in the circulating blood and extramedullary hematopoiesis in the liver and spleen, as well as anemia and splenomegaly. Both a primary form *(agnogenic myeloid m.)* and secondary forms are known.
**myeloid m., agnogenic,** the primary or idiopathic form of myeloid metaplasia, which is often accompanied by myelofibrosis; it is considered one of the myeloproliferative disorders. Called also *aleukemic* or *nonleukemic myelosis* and *leukoerythroblastic anemia.*
**myeloid m., primary,** agnogenic myeloid m.
**myeloid m., secondary,** myeloid metaplasia secondary to some other condition, such as carcinoma, tuberculosis, leukemia, leukoerythroblastosis, or polycythemia vera.
**nephrogenic m.,** a rare benign neoplasm of the mucosa of the urinary bladder or the urethra, consisting of tubular structures resembling those of the nephron; called also *nephrogenic adenoma.*
**pseudopyloric m.,** gastric metaplasia in which the gastric glands disappear and are replaced by tubules that closely resemble normal pyloric glands.
**m. of pulp,** transformation of the usual types of cells normally found in the pulp tissue into entirely different types.
**squamous m.,** the transformation of pseudostratified ciliated epithelium into stratified squamous epithelium, as occurs in certain pathologic conditions or may be produced experimentally.

**me·tap·la·sis** (mə-tap′lə-sis) the stage in which the organism has attained completed growth.

**meta·plasm** (met′ə-plaz″əm) [*meta-* + *plasm*] deuteroplasm.

**meta·plas·tic** (met″ə-plas′tik) 1. pertaining to or characterized by metaplasia. 2. formed by or of the nature of metaplasm (deuteroplasm).

**meta·pneu·mon·ic** (met″ə-noo-mon′ik) [*meta-* + *pneumonic*] succeeding or following pneumonia.

**meta·po·di·a·lia** (met″ə-po″de-a′le-ə) [*meta-* + Gr. *pous* foot] a collective term for the bones of the metacarpus and metatarsus.

**meta·poph·y·sis** (met″ə-pof′ə-sis) [*meta-* + *apophysis*] the mammillary process on the superior articular or prearticular processes of certain vertebrae.

**Met·a·prel** (met′ə-prəl) trademark for preparations of metaproterenol sulfate.

**meta·pro·ter·e·nol sul·fate** (met″ə-pro-ter′ə-nol) a $\beta$-adrenergic, similar in chemical structure to isoproterenol but having longer lasting effects; used as a bronchodilator in the treatment of bronchial asthma and for reversible bronchospasm associated with bronchitis and emphysema, administered orally and by inhalation.

**meta·psy·chol·o·gy** (met″ə-si-kol′ə-je) a term applied to various philosophical theories about mental functions and mental "structures" which are justifiable on logical grounds but not verifiable by experiment or observation; in psychoanalysis such theories concern the topography (id, ego, superego) and economics (quantities of psychic energy or excitation) of mental processes.

**meta·py·rone** (met″ə-pi′rōn) metyrapone.

**meta·ram·i·nol bi·tar·trate** (met″ə-ram′ĭ-nol) [USP] a sympathomimetic agent acting mainly as an $\alpha$-adrenergic agonist but also stimulating the $\beta_1$-adrenergic receptors of the heart and having potent vasopressor activity, used especially for the prevention and treatment of acute hypotensive states occurring with spinal anesthesia and for adjunctive therapy of hypotension due to hemorrhage, reactions to medications, surgical complication, and shock associated with brain damage due to trauma or tumor; administered intramuscularly and intravenously.

**met·ar·chon** (mət-ahr′kon) an agent which, without being toxic, so changes the behavior of a pest that its persistence is diminished, e.g., a confusing sex attractant.

**meta·rho·dop·sin** (met″ə-ro-dop′sin) a transient intermediate produced upon irradiation of rhodopsin in the visual cycle and existing in two forms, metarhodopsins I and II. The latter dissociates to form opsin and all-*trans* retinal. See illustration at *visual cycle,* under *cycle.*

**met·ar·te·ri·ole** (met″ahr-tēr′e-ōl) arterial capillary.

**meta·ru·bri·cyte** (met″ə-roo′brĭ-sīt) orthochromatic erythroblast.

**meta·so·ma·tome** (met″ə-so′mə-tōm) one of the constrictions between successive protovertebrae.

**meta·sta·ble** (met′ə-sta″bəl) 1. a condition differing from stable in that, although the substance is stable in small perturbations, it can be transformed to a more stable condition by relatively large perturbations. 2. subject to inevitable change or destruction eventually, but apparently stable owing to slowness of change.

**me·tas·ta·sec·to·my** (mə-tas″tə-sek′tə-me) [*metastasis* + *-ectomy*] excision of one or more metastases.

**me·tas·ta·ses** (mə-tas′tə-sēz) [MeSH: Neoplasm Metastasis] plural of *metastasis* (def. 2).

**me·tas·ta·sis** (mə-tas′tə-sis) [*meta-* + Gr. *stasis* stand] 1. the transfer of disease from one organ or part to another not directly connected with it. It may be due either to the transfer of pathogenic microorganisms (e.g., tubercle bacilli) or to transfer of cells, as in malignant tumors. The capacity to metastasize is a characteristic of all malignant tumors. 2. pl. *metastases.* A growth of pathogenic microorganisms or of abnormal cells distant from the site primarily involved by the morbid process.
**biochemical m.,** the transportation from the point of production and the deposition in previously normal tissues of abnormal or pathologically produced biochemical substances which bring about immunological or other changes in the tissues.
**calcareous m.,** the formation of bone salts in the kidneys and elsewhere in softening of bone.
**contact m.,** transfer from one surface to another with which the former is in contact.
**crossed m.,** passage of material from the venous to the arterial circulation without going through the lungs.
**direct m.,** metastasis in the direction of the blood or lymph stream.
**paradoxical m., retrograde m.,** metastasis taking place in a direction opposite to that of the blood stream.

**me·tas·ta·size** (mə-tas′tə-sīz) to form new foci of disease in a distant part by metastasis.

**meta·stat·ic** (met″ə-stat′ik) pertaining to or of the nature of metastasis.

**meta·ster·num** (met″ə-stər′nəm) [*meta-* + *sternum*] processus xiphoideus.

**Meta·stron** (met′ə-stron) trademark for a preparation of strontium chloride Sr 89.

**Meta·stron·gyl·i·dae** (met″ə-stron-jəl′ĭ-de) a family of nematodes of the superfamily Strongyloidea, consisting of lungworms; it includes the genus *Metastrongylus.*

**Meta·stron·gy·lus** (met″ə-stron′jə-ləs) a genus of nematodes of the family Metastrongylidae, usually found as lungworms in pigs and sometimes causing verminous bronchitis. *M. elonga′tus* is a species that may also infect humans and ruminants but has little pathogenic effect.

**meta·sy·nap·sis** (met″ə-sĭ-nap′sis) end-to-end union of the chromosomes in synapsis.

**meta·syn·cri·sis** (met″ə-sin′krĭ-sis) the elimination of waste or morbid matter.

**meta·syn·de·sis** (met″ə-sin-de′sis) metasynapsis.

**meta·tar·sal** (met″ə-tahr′səl) [MeSH: Metatarsal Bones] 1. pertaining to the metatarsus. 2. a bone of the metatarsus.

**meta·tar·sal·gia** (met″ə-tahr-sal′jə) [*meta-* + *tars-* + *-algia*] pain and tenderness in the metatarsal region.
**Morton's m.,** see under *neuralgia.*

**meta·tar·sec·to·my** (met″ə-tahr-sek′tə-me) excision or resection of the metatarsus.

**meta·tar·so·pha·lan·ge·al** (met″ə-tahr″so-fə-lan′je-əl) pertaining to the metatarsus and the phalanges of the toes.

**meta·tar·sus** (met″ə-tahr′səs) [*meta-* + Gr. *tarsos* tarsus] [TA] [MeSH: Metatarsus] the part of the foot between the tarsus and the toes, its skeleton being the five long bones (the metatarsals) extending from the tarsus to the phalanges. See also *ossa metatarsi,* under *os*[2].
**m. adductoca′vus,** a deformity of the foot in which metatarsus adductus is associated with pes cavus.
**m. adductova′rus,** a deformity of the foot in which metatarsus adductus is associated with metatarsus varus.
**m. adduc′tus,** a congenital deformity of the foot in which the fore part of the foot deviates toward the midline.
**m. ata′vicus,** abnormal shortness of the first metatarsal bone.

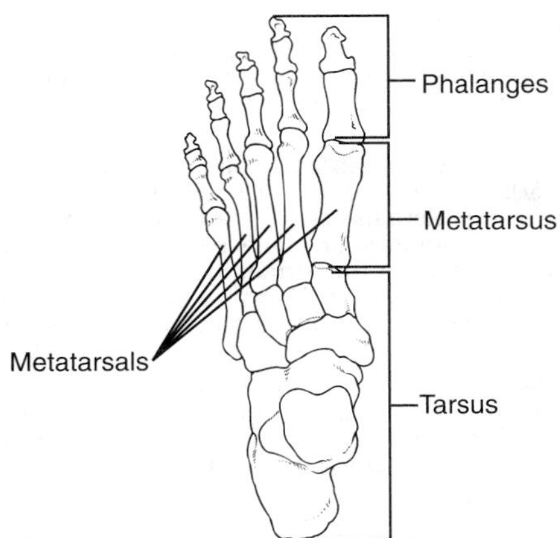


Metatarsus, comprising the metatarsal bones, which extend between the tarsus and phalanges and are numbered mediolaterally.

**m. bre'vis,** a condition in which the first metatarsal bone is shorter than normal and often abducted.
**m. la'tus,** a broadened foot due to spreading of the anterior part of the foot resulting from separation of the heads of the metatarsal bones from each other; called also *broad foot* and *spread foot.*
**m. pri'mus va'rus,** angulation of the first metatarsal bone toward the midline of the body, producing an angle sometimes of 20 degrees or more between its base and that of the second metatarsal bone.
**m. va'rus,** a congenital deformity of the foot in which its inner border is off the ground with the sole turned inward, the patient walking on the outer border of the foot.

**Met·a·ten·sin** (met″ə-ten'sin) trademark for preparations of trichlormethiazide with reserpine.

**meta·thal·a·mus** (met″ə-thal'ə-məs) [*meta-* + *thalamus*] [TA] the part of the diencephalon inferior to the caudal end of the dorsal thalamus, comprising the lateral and medial geniculate bodies.

**Meta·the·ria** (met″ə-the're-ə) [*meta-* + Gr. *thērion* beast, animal] in some systems of classification a subclass of the Mammalia, and in others an infraclass of the subclass Theria, including the pouched mammals or marsupials.

**meta·the·ri·an** (met″ə-the're-ən) any member of the Metatheria.

**me·tath·e·sis** (mə-tath'ə-sis) [*meta-* + Gr. *thesis* placement] 1. the artificial transfer of a morbid process. 2. a chemical reaction in which an element or radical in one compound exchanges places with another element or radical in another compound.

**meta·thet·ic** (met″ə-thet'ik) pertaining to or of the nature of metathesis.

**meta·throm·bin** (met″ə-throm'bin) [*meta-* + *thrombin*] the inactive combination of thrombin and antithrombin.

**meta·troph** (met'ə-trof) a metatrophic organism.

**meta·tro·phia** (met″ə-tro'fe-ə) 1. atrophy from malnutrition. 2. a change in diet.

**meta·troph·ic** (met″ə-trof'ik) utilizing organic matter for food. Cf. *paratrophic.*

**me·tat·ro·phy** (mə-tat'rə-fe) [*meta-* + *-trophy*] 1. the state of being metatrophic; metatrophic nutrition. 2. metatrophia.

**meta·typ·ic** (met″ə-tip'ik) metatypical.

**meta·typ·i·cal** (met″ə-tip'ĭ-kəl) composed of the elements of the tissue on which it develops, but having those elements arranged in an atypical manner; said of tumors.

**meta·van·a·date** (met″ə-van'ə-dāt) any salt of vanadic acid.
**sodium m.,** a highly poisonous salt having a variety of industrial applications.

**me·tax·a·lone** (mə-taks'ə-lōn) a smooth muscle relaxant used in the treatment of painful musculoskeletal conditions, administered orally.

**meta·xe·nia** (met″ə-ze'ne-ə) old, incorrect term for *ectogony.*

**me·tax·e·ny** (mə-tak'sə-ne) metoxeny.

**Meta·zoa** (met″ə-zo'ə) [*meta-* + Gr. *zōon* animal] that division of the animal kingdom which embraces all multicellular animals whose cells become differentiated to form tissues. It includes all animals except Protozoa.

**met·a·zoa** (met″ə-zo'ə) plural of *metazoon.*

**meta·zo·al** (met″ə-zo'əl) 1. belonging to the Metazoa. 2. pertaining to or caused by metazoa.

**meta·zo·an** (met″ə-zo'ən) 1. pertaining to metazoa; metazoal. 2. a metazoon.

**meta·zo·nal** (met″ə-zo'nəl) situated after or below a sclerozone.

**meta·zo·on** (met″ə-zo'on) pl. *metazo'a.* An individual of the Metazoa.

**Metch·ni·koff** (mech'nĭ-kof) Elie [Ilia Ilich *Mechnikov*] Russian zoologist in Paris, 1845–1916; co-winner, with Paul Ehrlich, of the Nobel prize for medicine or physiology in 1908 for his discovery of phagocytes and phagocytosis.

**Metch·ni·koff's theory** (mech'nĭ-kofs) [Elie *Metchnikoff*] see under *theory.*

**Metch·ni·ko·vel·li·da** (mech″nĭ-ko-vel'ĭ-də) an order of parasitic protozoa (class Rudimicrosporea, phylum Microspora) having characters of the class.

**me·te·cious** (mə-te'shəs) [*meta-* + Gr. *oikos* house] heterecious.

**met·en·ce·phal·ic** (met″ən-sə-fal'ik) pertaining to the metencephalon.

**met·en·ceph·a·lon** (met″en-sef'ə-lon) [*met-* + *encephalon*] 1. [TA] the anterior portion of the rhombencephalon, comprising the cerebellum and the pons. See Plate 11. 2. the anterior of the two brain vesicles formed by specialization of the rhombencephalon in the developing embryo. Called also *afterbrain.*

**met·en·ceph·a·lo·spi·nal** (met″ən-sef″ə-lo-spi'nəl) pertaining to the metencephalon (cerebellum and pons) and the spinal cord.

**met·en·keph·a·lin** (met″ən-kef'ə-lin) see *enkephalin.*

**me·te·or·ism** (me'te-ə-riz″əm) [Gr. *meteōrizein* to raise up] tympanites; the presence of gas in the abdomen or intestine.

**me·te·oro·pa·thol·o·gy** (me″te-ə-ro-pə-thol'ə-je) the pathology of conditions caused by atmospheric conditions.

**me·te·orop·a·thy** (me″te-ə-rop'ə-the) [Gr. *meteōros* high in the air + *pathos* disease] any disorder due to conditions of climate.

**me·te·oro·re·sis·tant** (me″te-ə-ro-re-zis'tənt) comparatively insensitive to weather conditions.

**me·te·oro·sen·si·tive** (me″te-ə-ro-sen'si-tiv) abnormally sensitive to weather conditions.

**me·te·oro·trop·ic** (me″te-ə-ro-trop'ik) responding to influence by meteorological factors; pertaining to or characterized by meteorotropism.

**me·te·orot·ro·pism** (me″te-ə-rot'rə-piz″əm) the response to influence by meteorological factors noted in certain biological events, such as sudden death, attacks of angina, joint pain, insomnia, and traffic accidents.

**me·ter** (me'tər) [Gr. *metron* measure; Fr. *mètre*] 1. the basic unit of linear measure in the metric system, approximately equivalent to 39.37 inches; formerly established as the length of a bar of an alloy of platinum and iridium preserved in a vault at the International Bureau of Weights and Measures, near Paris. Although its dimension is unchanged, it is now defined in terms of the wavelength of a certain line in the spectrum of krypton. Abbreviated m. 2. an apparatus devised to measure the quantity of anything passing through it, such as of a gas, amperes of electric current, etc.
**dosage m.,** dosimeter.
**light m.,** an instrument for measuring light in foot candles.
**peak flow m.,** an instrument for measuring the flow of air in the early part of forced expiration.
**rate m.,** a radiation detector whose output is proportional to instantaneous radiation intensity (rate of radioactive emissions).

**-meter** [Gr. *metron* measure] a word termination denoting an instrument used in measuring.

**met·er·ga·sis** (met″ər-ga'sis) [*meta-* + *erg-* + *-asis*] change of function.

**me·tes·trum** (mə-tes'trəm) metestrus.

**me·tes·trus** (mə-tes'trəs) [*meta-* + *estrus*] [MeSH: Metestrus] in female mammals that have estrous cycles, the period of subsiding follicular function or rest following estrus. Called also *metestrum.*

**met·for·min** (mət-for'min) [MeSH: Metformin] an antihyperglycemic agent related to buformin that potentiates the action of insulin, used in the treatment of type 2 diabetes mellitus; administered orally.

**meth·a·cho·line** (meth″ə-ko'lēn) a cholinergic agonist, having a longer duration of action than acetylcholine and predominantly muscarinic effects; it has vasodilator and cardiac vagomimetic effects but has largely been replaced by other drugs.
**m. bromide,** the bromide salt of methacholine, having actions and uses similar to those of the chloride salt; administered orally.

**m. chloride** [USP], the chloride salt of methacholine, used as a cholinergic, especially in the treatment of Raynaud's disease, scleroderma, vascular spasm due to cold, and chronic varicose ulcers, administered orally, subcutaneously, and by iontophoresis.

**meth·ac·ry·late** (meth-ak'rə-lāt) an ester of methacrylic acid, or the resin derived from polymerization of the ester. See also *acrylic resins,* under *resin.*
**methyl m.,** the methyl ester of methacrylic acid; it is an acrylic resin monomer easily polymerized and extensively used in medicine and dentistry.
**polymethyl m.,** a thermoplastic acrylic resin formed by polymerization of methyl methacrylate; it is used extensively in medicine and dentistry. Abbreviated PMMA. Written also *polymethylmethacrylate.*

**meth·a·cryl·ic ac·id** (meth"ə-kril'ik) an organic acid, 2-methylpropenoic acid, that polymerizes easily to form a ceramic-like mass. Its esters, methyl and polymethyl methacrylate, are used in the manufacture of acrylic resins and plastics.

**meth·a·cy·cline** (meth"ə-si'klēn) [MeSH: Methacycline] a semisynthetic broad-spectrum antibiotic of the tetracycline group, derived from oxytetracycline.
**m. hydrochloride** [USP], the monohydrochloride salt of methacycline, used as an antibacterial, administered orally.

**meth·a·done hy·dro·chlo·ride** (meth'ə-dōn) [USP] a synthetic narcotic, possessing pharmacologic actions similar to those of morphine and heroin and almost equal addiction liability; used as an analgesic and as a narcotic abstinence syndrome suppressant in the treatment of heroin addiction (see also *narcotic blockade,* under *blockade*), administered orally, intramuscularly, and subcutaneously.

**meth·al·le·nes·tril** (meth"əl-ə-nes'tril) a synthetic, nonsteroidal, orally effective, estrogenic drug, having uses similar to those of estrogen (q.v.).

**meth·al·li·bure** (məth-al'ĭ-būr) [MeSH: Methallibure] an anterior pituitary activator used to prevent estrus in swine.

**meth·am·phet·amine** (meth"am-fet'ə-mēn) [MeSH: Methamphetamine] a sympathomimetic amine closely related chemically to both amphetamine and ephedrine, having actions similar to those of amphetamine. Abuse of this drug may lead to dependence; see *amphetamine,* def. 1.
**m. hydrochloride** [USP], the sulfate salt of the dextrorotatory isomer of methamphetamine, having the same actions as the base; used orally in the treatment of attention-deficit/hyperactivity disorder. It has been used as an anorexiant in the treatment of obesity but is no longer recommended for this purpose.

**meth·a·nal** (meth'ə-nal) formaldehyde.

**meth·an·dro·sten·o·lone** (məth-an"dro-sten'ə-lōn) [MeSH: Methandrostenolone] an androgen, used especially in the adjunctive treatment of senile and postmenopausal osteoporosis and in selected cases of pituitary dwarfism, administered orally.

**meth·ane** (meth'ān) [MeSH: Methane] a colorless, odorless, inflammable gas, $CH_4$, produced by decomposition of organic matter, which may explode when mixed with air or oxygen; it is the first member of a homologous series of saturated hydrocarbons, including butane, ethane, hexane, pentane, and propane. Called also *marsh gas.*

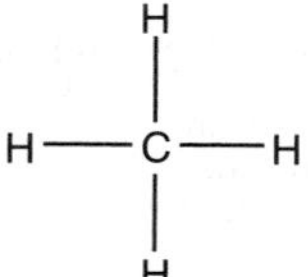


Methane.

**meth·ane·sul·fo·nate** (meth"ān-sul'fo-nāt) any salt or ester of methanesulfonic acid.

**meth·ane·sul·fon·ic ac·id** (meth"ān-səl-fon'ik) a corrosive, toxic acid, used as a catalyst and as a solvent.

**Meth·a·no·bac·te·ri·a·ceae** (meth"ə-no-bak-tēr"e-a'se-e) [MeSH: Methanobacteriaceae] a family of methane-producing bacteria, made up of coccoid or rod-shaped, strictly anaerobic cells that obtain energy by the formation of methane. The Methanobacteriaceae are grouped with the archaeobacteria because they lack muramic acid in their cell walls and differ from other bacteria in ribosomal RNA and cell lipid structures. They are found in sewage sludge, mud, and the rumens of cattle and sheep. The family contains the genera *Methanobacterium, Methanococcus,* and *Methanosarcina.*

**Meth·a·no·bac·te·ri·um** (meth"ə-no-bak-tēr-e-əm) [*methane* + Gr. *baktērion* little rod] [MeSH: Methanobacterium] a genus of methane-producing bacteria of the family Methanobacteriaceae, made up of nonspore-forming, coccoid, rod-shaped organisms that are strictly anaerobic and derive energy by the reduction of carbon dioxide to methane. They are widely distributed, occurring in mud, sewage, and the digestive tracts of animals. The type species is *M. soehnge'nii.*

**Meth·a·no·coc·cus** (meth"ə-no-kok'əs) [*methane* + Gr. *kokkos* berry] [MeSH: Methanococcus] a genus of methane-producing bacteria of the family Methanobacteriaceae, made up of spherical cells occurring singly, in pairs, or in masses. They are strict anaerobes that derive energy from the formation of methane from hydrogen, carbon dioxide, and formate. They are found in soils, mud, sewage sludge, and the intestinal tract of animals. The type species is *M. ma'zei.*

**meth·a·no·gen** (meth'ə-no-jen") an anaerobic microorganism that grows in the presence of carbon dioxide and produces methane gas. Methanogens are found in the stomach of cows, in swamp mud, and other environments in which oxygen is not present.

**meth·a·no·gen·ic** (meth"ə-no-jen'ik) producing methane.

**meth·a·nol** (meth'ə-nol) [USP] a clear, colorless, flammable liquid, $CH_3OH$, with characteristic odor, miscible with alcohol, ether, and water; used as a solvent.

**meth·a·nol·y·sis** (meth"ə-nol'ə-sis) alcoholysis of methyl alcohol.

**Meth·a·no·sar·ci·na** (meth"ə-no-sahr-si'nə) [*methane* + L. *sarcina* bundle] [MeSH: Methanosarcina] a genus of methane-producing bacteria of the family Methanobacteriaceae, made up of large, spherical, strictly anaerobic cells that derive energy by the formation of methane from acetate and sometimes methanol. They are found in mud and sewage. The type species is *M. metha'nica.*

**me·than·the·line bro·mide** (mə-than'thə-lēn) a quaternary ammonium anticholinergic, used in conditions requiring inhibition of gastrointestinal and genitourinary motility, in hyperhidrosis, or in control of normal sweating.

**meth·a·pyr·i·lene** (meth"ə-pēr'ĭ-lēn) [MeSH: Methapyrilene] an antihistaminic, which also has moderate sedative action.
**m. fumarate,** the fumarate salt of methapyrilene, having actions and uses similar to those of the hydrochloride salt; administered orally.
**m. hydrochloride,** the monohydrochloride salt of methapyrilene, having the same actions as the base; used in the treatment of allergic manifestations, nausea and vomiting of pregnancy, and insomnia; administered orally.

**me·thaq·ua·lone** (mə-thak'wə-lōn) [MeSH: Methaqualone] a nonbarbiturate compound formerly used as a sedative and hypnotic; abuse of this drug may lead to dependence.

**me·thar·bi·tal** (mə-thahr'bĭ-təl) a barbital derivative, used as an anticonvulsant for the control of grand mal, petit mal, myoclonic, and mixed types of epileptic seizures, administered orally.

**meth·a·zo·la·mide** (meth"ə-zo'lə-mīd) [USP] [MeSH: Methazolamide] a carbonic anhydrase inhibitor used as an adjunct to reduce intraocular pressure in the treatment of glaucoma; administered orally.

**meth·di·la·zine** (məth-di'lə-zēn) an antihistaminic, used as an antipruritic in dermatoses of various origins, administered in chewable tablets.
**m. hydrochloride** [USP], the monohydrochloride salt of methdilazine, having the same actions and uses as the base; administered orally.

**met·hem·al·bu·min** (met"he-mal-bu'min) [MeSH: Methemalbumin] a brown pigment formed by the binding of albumin with heme; this occurs only when the serum has been depleted of unsaturated haptoglobin and is indicative of intravascular hemolysis. Formerly called *pseudomethemoglobin.*

**met·hem·al·bu·min·emia** (met"hēm-al-bu"min-e'me-ə) the presence of methemalbumin in the blood.

**met·heme** (met'hēm) [*met-* + *heme*] heme in which the iron is in the ferric ($Fe^{3+}$) state.

**met·he·mo·glo·bin** (met-he'mo-glo"bin) [*met-* + *hemoglobin*] [MeSH: Methemoglobin] a brown pigment formed from hemoglobin by oxidation of the ferrous to the ferric state with essentially ionic bonds. A small amount is present in the blood normally, but injury or toxic agents convert a larger proportion of hemoglobin into methemoglobin, which does not function reversibly as an oxygen carrier.

**met·he·mo·glo·bin·emia** (met"he-mo-glo"bĭ-ne'me-ə) [*methemoglobin* + *-emia*] [MeSH: Methemoglobinemia] the presence of excessive methemoglobin in the blood, resulting in cyanosis and headache, dizziness, fatigue, ataxia, dyspnea, tachycardia, nausea, vomiting, and drowsiness, which can progress to stupor, coma, and occasionally death. It may be either chemical- or drug-induced *(acquired* or *toxic m.)* or hereditary *(congenital* or *hereditary m.).*
**acquired m.,** that caused by exposure to a toxic chemical or drug;

many different agents have been implicated, including nitrate and nitrite compounds, sulfonamides, and aniline dyes. Called also *toxic m.*
**congenital m., hereditary m.**, any of several rare types caused by inherited conditions. Deficiency of cytochrome-$b_5$ reductase is an autosomal recessive condition that may be either confined to the erythrocytes and relatively symptom-free or generalized to the leukocytes and sometimes the brain, muscle, and fibroblasts, in which case the individual may be mentally retarded. Abnormalities of hemoglobin M are autosomal dominant conditions that cause cyanosis in infancy but usually few other symptoms.
**toxic m.**, acquired m.

**met·he·mo·glo·bin·emic** (met″he-mo-glo″bĭ-ne′mik) 1. pertaining to or causing methemoglobinemia. 2. an agent that causes methemoglobinemia.

**met·he·mo·glo·bin re·duc·tase (NADH)** (met-he″mə-glo′bin re-duk′tās) [MeSH: Methemoglobin Reductase] cytochrome-$b_5$ reductase.

**met·he·mo·glo·bin re·duc·tase (NADPH)** (met-he″mo-glo′bin re-duk′tās) [MeSH: Methemoglobin Reductase] NADPH methemoglobin reductase.

**met·he·mo·glo·bin·uria** (met″he-mo-glo-bĭ-nu′re-ə) the occurrence of methemoglobin in the urine.

**meth·en·amine** (meth-en′ə-mēn) [USP] [MeSH: Methenamine] a compound that hydrolyzes formaldehyde in acidic urine to provide mild antiseptic activity, used as a urinary antibacterial; administered orally.
**m. hippurate** [USP], a compound of methenamine and hippuric acid, used orally as a urinary antibacterial.
**m. mandelate** [USP], a salt of methenamine and mandelic acid, used orally as a urinary antibacterial.
**m. silver,** a solution of methenamine and silver nitrate, used as a histopathological stain to demonstrate fungal cell walls, Donovan bodies, and *Klebsiella pneumoniae rhinoscleromatis.*

**meth·ene** (meth′ēn) methylene.

**5,10-meth·e·nyl·tet·ra·hy·dro·fo·late** (meth″ə-nəl-tet′rə-hi″dro-fo′lāt) a substituted derivative of tetrahydrofolate, carrying a methylidyne group; it is formed in histidine degradation and in the interconversion of various folates, linking the flow of activated one-carbon units from serine and thymidylate synthesis with purine synthesis and the liver enzyme system for discarding excess single carbons.

**meth·e·nyl·tet·ra·hy·dro·fo·late cy·clo·hy·dro·lase** (meth″ə-nəl-tet″rə-hi″dro-fo′lāt si″klo-hi′drə-lās) [EC 3.5.4.9] an enzyme activity of the hydrolase class that catalyzes the cleavage of 5,10-methenyltetrahydrofolate to 10-formyltetrahydrofolate, a step in the system of folate-mediated one-carbon transfer reactions. The enzyme activity is part of a trifunctional enzyme that also includes methylenetetrahydrofolate dehydrogenase ($NADP^+$) and formate–tetrahydrofolate ligase activities.

**5,10-meth·e·nyl·tet·ra·hy·dro·fo·late syn·the·tase** (meth″ə-nəl-tet″rə-hi″dro-fo′lāt sin′thə-tās) 5-formyltetrahydrofolate cyclo-ligase.

**Meth·er·gine** (meth′ər-jin) trademark for preparations of methylergonovine maleate.

**meth·es·trol di·pro·pi·o·nate** (meth′əs-trol) promethestrol dipropionate.

**me·thet·o·in** (mə-thet′o-in) an anticonvulsant which has been used in the treatment of epilepsy.

**meth·i·cil·lin so·di·um** (meth″ĭ-sil″in) [USP] a semisynthetic penicillin, used intravenously or intramuscularly as an antibacterial in resistant staphylococcal infections. Called also *dimethoxyphenyl penicillin sodium.*

**meth·im·a·zole** (meth-im′ə-zōl) [USP] [MeSH: Methimazole] a thyroid inhibitor, used in the treatment of hyperthyroidism, administered orally. Called also *thiamazole.*

**meth·ine** (meth′īn) methylidyne.

**me·thi·o·carb** (məthi′o-kahrb) [MeSH: Methiocarb] an organophosphorus molluscacide; larger animals that ingest it may suffer diarrhea, ataxia, and pulmonary edema that can be fatal.

**meth·io·dal so·di·um** (meth-i′o-dəl) an iodine-containing compound used as a radiopaque medium in urography, administered intravenously.

**me·thi·o·nine** (mə-thi′o-nēn) [MeSH: Methionine] chemical name: $\alpha$-amino-$\gamma$-methylmercaptobutyric acid; a naturally occurring essential amino acid furnishing both methyl groups and sulfur necessary for normal metabolism. Symbols Met and M. See table at *amino acid.*
**m. C 11** [USP], L-methionine in which a portion of the molecules have been labeled with carbon 11, used as a tracer in positron emission tomography for the detection of malignant neoplasms; administered intravenously.

**me·thi·o·nine ad·eno·syl·trans·fer·ase** (mə-thi′o-nēn ə-den″o-səl-trans′fər-ās) [EC 2.5.1.6] [MeSH: Methionine Adenosyltransferase] an enzyme of the transferase class that catalyzes the formation of *S*-adenosylmethionine from methionine and ATP, occurring in several isozymes. Deficiency of the hepatic isozyme causes hypermethioninemia, but is otherwise benign.

**me·thi·o·nine syn·thase** (mə-thi′o-nēn syn′thās) 5-methyltetrahydrofolate–homocysteine *S*-methyltransferase.

**me·thi·o·nyl** (mə-thi′o-nəl) the acyl radical of methionine.

**me·this·a·zone** (mə-this′ə-zōn) [MeSH: Methisazone] an antiviral agent; it has been used to provide short-term protection against smallpox and the severe complications of vaccination.

**me·thix·ene hy·dro·chlo·ride** (mə-thik′sēn) an anticholinergic having a direct spasmolytic effect on smooth muscle; used in the treatment of gastrointestinal hypermotility and spasm associated with functional bowel disease, administered orally.

**meth·o·car·ba·mol** (meth″o-kahr′bə-mol) [USP] [MeSH: Methocarbamol] a skeletal muscle relaxant, administered orally, intramuscularly, and intravenously.

**Meth·o·cel** (meth′o-sel) trademark for a preparation of methylcellulose.

**meth·od** (meth′əd) [Gr. *methodos*] the manner of performing any act or operation. See also under *maneuver, operation, procedure, technique, treatment, stain, test,* etc.

## Method

**Abbott's m.**, treatment of scoliosis by lateral pulling and counterpulling on the spinal column by means of wide bandages and pads until the deformity is overcorrected, and then applying a plaster jacket to produce pressure, counterpressure, and fixation of the spine in its corrected position.

**A.B.C. (alum, blood, clay) m.**, a method of deodorizing and precipitating sludge by the addition of alum, charcoal (or some other material), and clay to the raw sewage.

**absorption m.**, the separate and selective removal of agglutinins from specific immune sera by the addition of homologous particulate antigen(s) (e.g., bacterial cells or red blood cells) to the immune sera, or by the passage of specific immune sera through columns containing antigen on an insoluble support (immunosorbent) with which the homologous antibody combines and is thereby removed from the serum.

**acid hematin m.**, a formerly common method of estimating hemoglobin: the hemoglobin was converted into acid hematin by adding hydrochloric acid and the resulting color was compared to a standard color scale.

**Altmann-Gersh m.**, a method of preparing tissue for histologic study by freeze drying.

**autoclave m.**, see *Clark-Collip m.* (def. 2).

**back pressure–arm lift m.**, Holger Nielsen m.

**Barger's m.**, a method for determining osmotic pressure from vapor pressure.

**Barraquer's m.**, phacoerysis.

**Bethea's m.**, see under *sign.*

**Bivine's m.**, treatment of strychnine poisoning by administration of chloral hydrate.

**Bobath m.**, a system of therapeutic exercise designed to inhibit spasticity and to aid in the development of new reflex responses and equilibrium reactions by modifying postures that progress from simple movements to more complex ones in a sequence based on the neurological development of an infant.

**Brandt-Andrews m.**, see under *maneuver.*

**brine flotation m.**, *(for concentration of ova),* suspend a portion of the stool in a saturated solution of sodium chloride; let it stand for a time and collect the ova from the surface.

**Brunnstrom m.,** a system of therapeutic exercise designed to inhibit spasticity through the sensory stimulation of synergetic movements; to the degree that the synergies subside, the voluntary isolated movements that remain can be emphasized so that motor control is gradually increased.
**calcium, m's for,** see specific methods, including *Clark-Collip m.* (def. 1).
**caliper m.,** a method for approximating fat content in the body by measuring the thickness of folds of the skin at stated areas of the body by means of specially designed calipers.
**Callahan m.,** 1. in root canal therapy, a filling method in which the canal is first flooded with a chloroform-rosin solution and then gutta-percha is dissolved in the solution. 2. a method of tracing and opening up a root canal by destroying the pulp tissue with a 50 per cent sulfuric acid solution.
**Carrel's m.,** 1. a method of end-to-end suture of blood vessels. 2. see under *treatment.* 3. a method of determining when to make secondary closure of wounds. A loop of material is taken from the wound, spread on a slide, stained, and the number of bacteria counted.
**Castaneda's m.,** *(for rickettsiae in smears),* a thin smear is made in a phosphate buffer (pH 7.6) and air-dried, stained with methylene blue solution for 3 minutes, counterstained with safranine solution, and washed, blotted, and dried. Rickettsiae appear pale blue; cell nuclei and protoplasm are red.
**chest pressure–arm lift m.,** Silvester m.
**Chick-Martin m.,** a method for testing the bactericidal value of disinfectants for water supplies in the presence of organic matter. The procedure originally incorporated 3 per cent human feces. In the revised method, serial dilutions of disinfectant are incubated with a specified quantity of yeast and *Salmonella typhi* for a period of 30 minutes. The effectiveness is expressed by the ratio: effective concentration of phenol divided by effective concentration of test disinfectant (Chick-Martin coefficient).
**chloropercha m.,** in root canal therapy, a method of filling the canal with gutta-percha dissolved in a chloroform-rosin solution; see *Callahan m.* (def. 1) and *Johnson m.*
**Ciaccio's m.,** treatment of tissue for the purpose of rendering visible the intracellular lipids; they are fixed with acid chromate solution and stained with Sudan III.
**Clark-Collip m.,** 1. *(for calcium in serum)* dilute the serum and add ammonium oxalate; wash the precipitate, dissolve with sulfuric acid, and titrate with potassium permanganate. 2. *(for urea in blood)* to 5 mL of blood filtrate add 1 mL of $NH_4Cl$ and heat in autoclave at 150°C for ten minutes. Make alkaline, distill into acid, and titrate, using methyl red as indicator.
**Clauss m.,** a type of fibrinogen assay similar to the test for thrombin time, estimating the functional fibrinogen level by adding fibrin reagent to plasma and noting the time until fibrinogen converts to fibrin; it differs from the thrombin time by using plasma diluted with Owren's buffer and using a much stronger concentration of thrombin reagent. Called also *Clauss assay.*
**closed-plaster m.,** treatment of wounds, compound fractures, and osteomyelitis by enclosing the limb in an immobilizing plaster cast. See *Orr treatment* and *Trueta treatment,* under *treatment.*
**Converse m.,** reconstruction of the ear lobe by raising a flap of skin below the auricle with a superior base about one third larger than the proposed lobe; a full-thickness skin graft covers the defect at the site of the flap except for the last third of the medial aspect of the pedicle.
**Couette m.,** a method for measuring viscosity by calculating the rate of movement of an inner cylinder separated from an outer cylinder by a thin layer of the fluid whose viscosity is being tested.

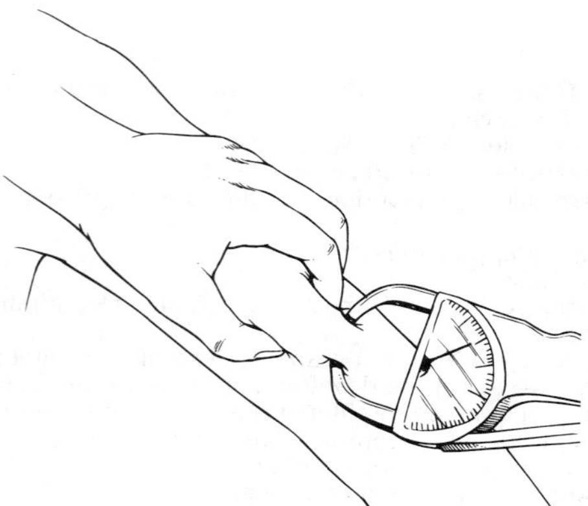

Caliper method being used to measure the thickness of the skinfold over the triceps muscle.

**Coutard's m.,** a method of x-ray irradiation by protracted and fractionated dosage.
**creatine, m's for,** see specific methods, including *Folin's m.* (defs. 4,5) and *Folin and Wu's m.* (def. 2).
**creatinine, m's for,** see specific methods, including *Folin's m.* (def. 6) and *Folin and Wu's m.* (defs. 1,2), and see under *test.*
**Credé's m.,** 1. method of expressing the placenta by forcing the uterus down into the pelvis and at the same time squeezing the uterus from all sides so that its contents are expelled. 2. a similar method for expressing urine from the bladder, especially in paralytic bladder. 3. the placing of a drop of 2 per cent solution of silver nitrate in each eye of a newborn child for the prevention of ophthalmia neonatorum.
**Cronin m.,** an operation to correct a flat nasal tip with short columella by using bilateral flaps of skin elevated in the floor of the nostrils.
**Cuignet's m.,** retinoscopy.
**cup plate m.,** see *ring test* (def. 1), under *tests.*
**Dakin-Carrel m.,** Carrel's treatment; see under *treatment.*
**Denis and Leche's m.,** *(for total sulfate),* add acid and autoclave to decompose protein, then precipitate with barium chloride, dry, and weigh.
**Denman's m.,** see under *evolution.*
**Dickinson m.,** a method of controlling postpartum hemorrhage: the entire uterus is grasped through the abdominal wall, lifted out of the pelvis, and compressed against the spinal column.
**direct m.,** in ophthalmoscopy, that in which the ophthalmoscope is held close to the eye examined and an erect virtual image is obtained of the fundus.
**direct centrifugal flotation m.,** Lane m.
**disk diffusion m.,** see *disk diffusion test,* under *test.*
**Domagk's m.,** *(for demonstration of reticuloendothelial cells),* a culture of gram-positive staphylococci in physiologic salt solution is injected into the femoral vein of a rat which is then killed in fifteen to thirty minutes. In formalin-fixed sections stained by cresyl violet or by Gram's stain followed by alum-carmine, Kupffer's cells and other cells of the reticuloendothelial system stand out strikingly.
**Duke's m.,** see under *test.*
**dye dilution m.,** a type of indicator dilution method for assessing flow through the circulatory system; the indicator is a dye, usually indocyanine green.
**Eicken's m.,** examination of the hypopharynx, with the cricoid cartilage drawn forward.
**Ellinger's m.,** *(for indican),* precipitate the urine with basic lead acetate and filter. To the filtrate add Obermayer's reagent. Shake out the indigo with chloroform, evaporate off the chloroform, and titrate the residue with potassium permanganate.
**Eskimo m.,** a closed reduction of anterior shoulder dislocation by having the patient lie on the unaffected side and applying traction against gravity by lifting the patient by the affected arm.
**external rotation m.,** closed reduction of anterior shoulder dislocation by adducting the arm to the patient's side with the elbow flexed to 90 degrees as the patient lies supine, then rotating the arm externally using the forearm as a lever.
**Fahraeus m.,** the original (1918) method that was used to determine the erythrocyte sedimentation rate.
**Faust's m.,** a method of diagnosing helminth and protozoan infections by centrifugation of washed feces with zinc sulfate of a specific gravity of 1.180, after which eggs and protozoan cysts may be removed from the supernatant layer.
**Fay m.,** a system of therapeutic exercise for overcoming spasticity; the central nervous system is reeducated according to a theory of hierarchical development starting with the performance of simple reflex movements and progressing to more advanced patterns of coordination.
**fibrinogen, m. for,** see *fibrinogen assay,* under *assay.*
**Fick m.,** a method for measuring cardiac output based on the Fick principle applied to pulmonary blood flow: the rate of oxygen consumption by the lungs, when divided by the arteriovenous oxygen difference (the difference in oxygen concentration between the arterial and venous systems), gives the rate of blood flow across the pulmonary capillaries and the cardiac output. See also *indicator dilution m.*
**Fishberg's m.,** one for determining specific gravity of the urine, which serves as a concentration test of renal function.
**Fiske's m.,** *(for total fixed base),* remove phosphates with ferric chloride, convert fixed bases into sulfates by heating in sulfuric acid, ignite, take up in water, precipitate sulfates as benzidine sulfate, and titrate with alkali.
**Fiske and Subbarow's m.,** 1. *(for acid-soluble phosphorus in blood)* destroy organic matter by heating with sulfuric and nitric acids, precipitate the phosphates as magnesium ammonium phosphate, and reduce the precipitate with para-amino-naphthol-sulfonic acid. Compare the blue color with a standard phosphate solution. 2. *(for inorganic phosphates)* the phosphates are precipitated as ammonium phos-

phomolybdate. This is then reduced by para-amino-naphthol-sulfonic acid and the blue color compared colorimetrically with a standard solution.

**fixed base, m. for,** see *Fiske's m.*

**flash m.,** see *pasteurization.*

**flotation m.,** any method for separating cysts and ova from the heavier component of the stool and which depends upon the use of a solution intermediate in density between the parasitic material (which floats) and the bulk of the feces (which remains as sediment after centrifugation).

**Folin's m.,** 1. *(for acetone)* micromethod. Aerate the acetone over into a solution of sodium bisulfite and then determine the amount of nephelometric comparison with a standard acetone solution using Scott and Wilson's reagent. 2. *(for amino acids in blood)* make 10 mL of protein-free blood filtrate slightly alkaline to phenolphthalein. Add 2 mL of beta-naphthaquinone solution and place in the dark. The next day add 2 mL of acetic acid-acetate solution and 2 mL of 4 per cent thiosulfate solution. Dilute to 25 mL and compare the blue color with a standard amino-acid solution similarly treated. 3. *(for ammonia nitrogen)* sodium carbonate is added to the urine to free the ammonia, which is aerated into standard acid and titrated. 4. *(for creatine)* precipitate the proteins of the blood with picric acid and filter. To the filtrate add sodium hydroxide and compare color with a standard solution of creatine. 5. *(for creatine in urine)* change creatine into creatinine by heating at 90°C for three hours in the presence of third normal HCl. Determine creatinine by picric acid and alkali and deduct the preformed creatinine. 6. *(for creatinine in urine)* to the urine add picric acid and sodium hydroxide and compare the red color with a half normal solution of potassium bichromate. 7. *(for ethereal sulfates)* remove the inorganic sulfates with barium chloride and then the conjugated sulfates after hydrolyzing with boiling dilute hydrochloric acid. 8. *(for inorganic sulfates)* acidify the urine with hydrochloric acid, precipitate with barium chloride, filter, dry, ignite, and weigh. 9. *(for protein in urine)* add acetic acid and heat, wash, dry, and weigh the precipitate. 10. *(for total acidity)* add potassium oxalate to the urine to precipitate the calcium which should otherwise precipitate at the neutral point, and titrate with tenth normal sodium hydroxide, using phenolphthalein as an indicator. 11. *(for total sulfates)* boil the urine for thirty minutes with dilute hydrochloric acid, precipitate with barium chloride, filter, dry, ignite, and weigh. 12. *(for urea and allantoin)* decompose the urea by heating with magnesium chloride and hydrochloric acid, distill off the ammonia, and titrate.

**Folin and Wu's m.,** 1. *(for creatinine)* the color produced by the unknown (protein-free blood filtrate or urine) in an alkaline solution of picric acid is compared in a colorimeter with the color produced by a known solution of creatinine or with a standard solution of potassium bichromate. 2. *(for creatine plus creatinine)* the creatine of a protein-free blood filtrate is changed to creatinine by heating with dilute hydrochloric acid in an autoclave, and the creatinine thus produced together with the preformed is determined colorimetrically after adding an alkaline picrate solution. 3. *(nonprotein nitrogen)* the total nonprotein nitrogen in the protein-free blood filtrate is determined by setting free the nitrogen as ammonia by the Kjeldahl process, nesslerizing this ammonia, and comparing with a standard. 4. *(for protein-free blood filtrate)* lake the blood with distilled water, add sodium tungstate and sulfuric acid, and filter. 5. *(for urea)* change the urea to ammonia by means of urease, and nesslerize. 6. *(for uric acid)* uric acid is precipitated from the protein-free blood filtrate or from urine by silver lactate, treated with phosphotungstic acid, and the blue color compared with the color produced by known amounts of uric acid.

**Fülleborn's m.,** *(for ova in stools),* grind 1 g of stool and mix with 20 mL of a saturated solution of sodium chloride. Allow to stand one hour or more, then float coverglasses on the surface and transfer them, without draining, to slides.

**Gerota's m.,** injection of the lymphatics with a dye, such as Prussian blue, which is soluble in chloroform or ether, but not in water.

**Givens' m.,** *(for peptic activity),* varying amounts of diluted gastric juice are added to a series of tubes containing pea globulin, the mixtures are incubated, and the amount of digestion noted.

**glucose, m's for,** See *glucose test,* under *test.*

**Gram's m.,** see under *stain.*

**Hamilton's m.,** *(in postpartum hemorrhage),* compress the uterus between a fist in the vagina and a hand pressing down the abdominal wall.

**Heublein m.,** ionizing irradiation of the whole body with low-dose increments protracted for ten to twenty hours per day over several days.

**hippocratic m.,** closed reduction of anterior shoulder dislocation by abduction of the arm with longitudinal traction and gentle external rotation; countertraction is provided by the placing of the physician's foot against the chest wall.

**Hirschberg's m.,** measurement of the deviation of a strabismic eye by observing the reflection of a candle from the cornea.

**holding m.,** see *pasteurization.*

**Holger Nielsen m.,** a nonmechanical method of emergency artificial respiration: with victim prone, rescuer alternately extends victim's arms to aid inspiration and presses down on victim's scapulae to aid expiration. Called also *Nielsen m.* and *back pressure–arm lift m.*

**indican, m's for,** see specific methods, including *Ellinger's m.,* and see under *test.*

**indicator dilution m.,** any of several methods for assessing flow through the circulatory system by injection of a known quantity of an indicator, such as a dye, radionuclide, or chilled liquid, into the system and monitoring its concentration over time at a specific point in the system. See also *dye dilution m.* and *thermodilution.*

**indole, m's for,** see under *test.*

**inorganic phosphates, m. for,** see *phosphates, inorganic, m. for.*

**iodine, m's for,** see under *test.*

**Ivy's m.,** see under *test.*

**Jendrassik-Grof m.,** 1. *(for conjugated bilirubin)* a fasting sample of serum or plasma is collected and acidified by the addition of hydrochloric acid. Ehrlich's diazo reagent is added so that the conjugated bilirubin begins forming blue azobilirubin. After 10 minutes the reaction is stopped and the amount of azobilirubin in the sample is measured. 2. *(for total bilirubin)* to an acidified fasting sample as in the previous method, caffeine benzoate is added as an accelerator for the unconjugated bilirubin to form azobilirubin. When the reaction is stopped, the azobilirubin in the sample thus represents the total of both conjugated and unconjugated bilirubin.

**Johnson m.,** a modification of the Callahan method (def. 1) of root canal therapy; the canal is first flooded with alcohol, allowing diffusion of the chloroform component of the chloroform-rosin solution; alcohol deep in the dentin facilitates rosin dissolved in the chloroform to be diffused into the dentin.

**Kaiserling's m.,** a procedure for preserving the natural colors in museum preparations, employing formaldehyde and potassium acetate.

**Kaplan-Meier m.,** that used in the analysis of survival data to create a Kaplan-Meier survival curve (q.v.). Called also *product-limit m.* or *estimate.*

**Kety-Schmidt m.,** a method of measuring perfusion flow of blood through brain tissue.

**Kirstein's m.,** direct laryngoscopy.

**Kjeldahl's m.,** (1883), a method of determining the amount of nitrogen in an organic compound. It consists in heating the material to be analyzed with strong sulfuric acid. The nitrogen is thereby converted to ammonia, which is distilled off and caught in tenth normal solution of sulfuric acid. By titration the amount of ammonia is determined, and from this the amount of nitrogen is estimated.

**Klüver-Barrera m.,** a histologic staining method in which myelin sheaths are stained blue-green and the cells purple.

**Kocher's m.,** closed reduction of anterior shoulder dislocation by applying traction and external rotation of the arm, then bringing the arm across the patient's chest to effect reduction, and finally internally rotating the arm.

**Korotkoff's m.,** the auscultatory method of determining blood pressure.

**Laborde's m.,** the making of rhythmic traction movements on the tongue in order to stimulate the respiratory center in asphyxiation.

**Lamaze m.,** a psychoprophylactic method of preparing for delivery, involving education of the prospective mother in the physiology of pregnancy and parturition and in techniques (e.g., breathing exercises and bearing down) to ease delivery.

**Lane m.,** a method of diagnosing hookworm infection by centrifugation of 1 mL of washed feces mixed with brine, the tube being covered with a cover slip on which the eggs can be counted. Called also *direct centrifugal flotation m.,* or *DCF.*

**lateral condensation m.,** a method of root canal therapy in which the main portion of the canal is filled with a primary gutta-percha cone or silver point and sealer cement or paste and the remaining space is packed with auxiliary gutta-percha cones. Spreader sites and pluggers are used to force gutta-percha into the canal laterally and sometimes vertically. Called also *multiple cone m.*

**Leboyer m.,** a method of delivery of the infant based upon the theory that the violence associated with birth causes emotional trauma to the infant and that this trauma will affect the child's personality throughout his life. The concepts of this method emphasize that the delivery should be gentle and controlled, without unnecessary intervention; the infant should be handled gently, with the head, neck, and sacrum supported; the infant should not be overstimulated and should be allowed to breathe spontaneously, without painful stimuli, such as spanking. Called also *Leboyer technique.*

**Milch's m.,** closed reduction of anterior shoulder dislocation by traction on the arm, which is abducted overhead with the patient in the supine position, external rotation, and pressure on the head of the humerus; in some modifications of this technique the patient lies prone.

**Monte Carlo m.,** artificial replication, usually by computer, of a sampling experiment; used to estimate a probability.

**mouth-to-mouth m.,** the most effective nonmechanical technique for emergency artificial respiration. With victim supine, the rescuer places one hand under the nape of the victim's neck and the other hand on the victim's forehead and presses the victim's nostrils closed; rescuer takes a deep breath and breathes out directly between victim's lips (two pairs of lips must form an airtight seal); repeat four times quickly to inflate victim's lungs before allowing the first exhalation.

**multiple cone m.,** lateral condensation m.

**Nielsen m.,** Holger Nielsen m.

**Nikiforoff's m.,** a method of fixing blood films by placing them for from five to fifteen minutes in absolute alcohol, pure ether, or equal parts of alcohol and ether.

**Ogino-Knaus m.,** the rhythm method of birth control.

**optical density m.,** the measuring of growth rates of cells by taking the optical density or turbidity of a dense population and comparing this with optical densities of known dilutions of the sample.

**Orr m.,** see under *treatment.*

**Orsi-Grocco m.,** palpatory percussion of the heart.

**ova concentration, m. for,** see *brine flotation m.*

**panoptic m.,** see *Giemsa stain,* under *stain.*

**Pap's silver m.,** a method for demonstrating reticulum.

**peptic activity, m's for,** see specific methods, including *Givens' m.*

**point source m.,** a method of intracavitary irradiation of the bladder wall utilizing a small point source of radiation at the center of a Foley catheter bag inflated with a radiopaque solution containing methylene blue or indigo carmine.

**Politzer's m.,** an imprecise test for patency of the auditory tube: with the mouth closed and one nostril occluded, air is forced into the other nostril through a rubber tube; this should cause positive pressure in the middle ear so that the tympanic membrane bulges outward. Called also *Politzer's test.*

**product-limit m.,** Kaplan-Meier m.

**proprioceptive neuromuscular facilitation m.,** see under *facilitation.*

**radioactive balloon m.,** a method of intracavitary irradiation of the bladder wall utilizing a Foley catheter bag filled with a radioactive solution.

**retrofilling m.,** see *retrofilling.*

**rhythm m.,** a method of preventing conception by restricting coitus to the so-called safe period, avoiding the days just before and after the expected time of ovulation.

**Rideal-Walker m.,** a method for testing the bactericidal activity of a disinfectant as compared with that of phenol. Cultures of *Salmonella typhi* are incubated with serial dilutions of the test compound, with dilutions of phenol as standards. Samples are removed at intervals, transferred to sterile broth, and the resulting cultures incubated and examined for bacterial growth. Activity is expressed as the ratio of effective concentration of test compound divided by that of phenol (phenol coefficient).

**Ritchie's formalin-ether m.,** a technique for detecting parasites in the feces, involving the centrifugation of diluted feces, the addition of formalin and ether to the sample, recentrifugation, and examination of the final sediment as a wet mount. Called also *Ritchie's formalin-ether sedimentation.*

**Ritgen's m.,** see under *maneuver.*

**Romanovsky's (Romanowsky's) m.,** see *stain.*

**Rood m.,** a technique for overcoming spasticity, based on the theory that stimulation of a specific area of the skin will promote the contraction of underlying muscles and lead to the reciprocal relaxation of related antagonistic muscles; stimulation is done by stroking with a special brush or with ice.

**Sahli's m.,** acid hematin m.

**Schafer m.,** a nonmechanical method of emergency artificial respiration: patient is prone with forehead on one arm; rescuer's knees are on either side of patient's hips; pressure is exerted on patient's back using two hands over the lower ribs; rescuer rises up slowly and simultaneously relaxes the pressure on patient's back; procedure is repeated every 5 seconds.

**sectional m.,** in root canal therapy, filling of the canal by packing in 2- to 3-mm cut sections of gutta-percha cones until it is filled.

**Sheather's sugar flotation m., modified,** a method for detecting oocysts of *Cryptosporidium* in a stool sample; a fecal suspension is mixed with a boiled sugar solution, phenol, and sugar flotation solution and then examined on a slide.

**Siffert m.,** a method for computing the volume of the gallbladder by tracing the gallbladder shadow on transparent paper and comparing it with a standard.

**silver cone m., silver point m.,** in root canal therapy, a method of filling the canal in which a prefitted silver point is sealed into the canal apex and irregularities in the canal that are not sealed with the point are obliterated by gutta-percha through lateral condensation or segmentation, or by a root canal paste or sealer.

**Silvester m.,** a nonmechanical method of emergency artificial respiration: with patient supine, rescuer pulls patient's arms firmly over head to raise the ribs and aid inspiration; the arms are then brought down and pressed against the chest to aid expiration; procedure is repeated 16 times per minute. Called also *chest pressure–arm lift m.*

**single cone m.,** in root canal therapy, a method of filling the canal with a single well-fitting gutta-percha cone or silver point in conjunction with a sealer cement or paste.

**Sluder m.,** a method formerly used for tonsillectomy; the tonsils were removed with a small guillotine-like apparatus.

**Smellie's m.,** Mauriceau maneuver.

**Somogyi m.,** *(for amylase activity)* a method based on the disappearance of the blue color given by iodine and amylose (linear fraction of starch) after amylase in serum, urine, etc., is allowed to act on starch.

**split cast m.,** 1. a procedure for placing indexed casts on a dental articulator to facilitate their removal and replacement on the instrument. 2. the procedure of checking the ability of a dental articulator to receive or be adjusted to a maxillomandibular relation record. Called also *split cast mounting.*

**Stimson's m.,** closed reduction of anterior shoulder dislocation by using a small weight to exert traction on the affected arm, which hangs over the edge of the table with the patient in the prone position.

**sugar, m's for,** see *sugar test,* under *test.*

**sulfosalicylic acid m.,** *(for proteinuria),* sulfosalicylic acid is added to urine and the mixture is left standing for 10 minutes; the degree of turbidity is then compared to a known scale to estimate the amount of protein in the urine.

**sulfur, total, m's for,** see specific methods, including *Denis and Leche's m.* and *Folin's m.* (def. 11).

**Sumner's m.,** *(for glucose in urine),* heat 1 mL of urine and 3 mL of Sumner's dinitrosalicylic acid reagent, dilute to 25 mL and compare the color with that of a standard glucose solution similarly treated.

**suspension m.,** a method of intracavitary irradiation of the bladder wall by instilling a radioactive solution or suspension directly into the bladder by means of a catheter.

**template m.,** a bleeding time test in which a template with a standard-sized slit is laid on the patient's forearm and an incision is made through the slit with a standard-sized knife.

**Thane's m.,** a method of locating the fissure of Rolando. Its upper end is about one-half inch behind the middle of a line uniting the inion and the glabella, and its lower end about one-quarter inch above and one and one-quarter inches behind the external angular process of the frontal bone.

**thermal dilution m.,** thermodilution.

**thyroid activity, m. for,** thyroid function test; see under *test.*

**traction-countertraction m.,** closed reduction of anterior shoulder dislocation by longitudinal traction on the arm with external rotation; countertraction is provided by a sheet passed around the chest under the axilla of the affected shoulder and held by an assistant.

**Trueta m.,** see under *treatment.*

**urea, m's for,** see specific methods, including *Clark-Collip m.* (def. 2), *Folin's m.* (def. 12), and *Folin and Wu's m.* (def. 5). See also *urea test,* under *test.*

**urease, m. for,** urease test; see under *test.*

**uric acid, m's for,** see specific methods, including *Folin and Wu's m.* (def. 6). See also *uric acid test,* under *test.*

**Valsalva's m.,** Valsalva's maneuver (def. 2).

**van Gehuchten's m.,** fixing of a histologic tissue in a mixture of glacial acetic acid 10 parts, chloroform 30 parts, and alcohol 60 parts.

**Van Slyke's m.,** see under *test.*

**vertical condensation m.,** in root canal therapy, a method of filling the canal by alternately heating and vertically condensing gutta-per-

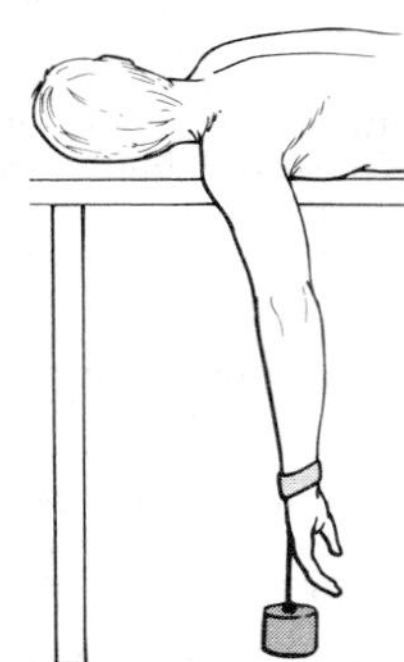

Stimson's method for reduction of anterior shoulder dislocation.

cha until the apical third of the canal is filled; the coronal portion of the canal is then filled with warmed 2- to 4-mm sections of gutta-percha cones.

**Waring's m.**, a method of sewage disposal by subsurface irrigation; called also *Waring's system*.

**Welcker's m.**, determination of the total blood volume by bleeding and then washing out the blood vessels.

**Westergren m.**, the most common method for testing the erythrocyte sedimentation rate; four volumes of whole blood are mixed with one volume of sodium citrate anticoagulant-diluent solution and placed in a Westergren tube graduated in millimeters from 0 to 200, filling to the 0 mark; the tube is placed in a vertical position for 1 hour and the fall of the level of red cells is recorded in mm/hr.

**Whipple's m.**, the use of liver in pernicious anemia.

**Wintrobe m.**, *(for erythrocyte sedimentation rate)*, EDTA-anticoagulated whole blood is placed in a Wintrobe hematocrit tube, the tube is left standing undisturbed in a vertical position, and the fall of the level of red cells in one hour is recorded in mm/hr. The volume of packed red cells can then be determined using the same tube.

**Wynn m.**, a procedure for repair of bilateral cleft lips by means of a long, narrow triangular flap.

**Yuzpe m.**, a regimen for postcoital contraception, consisting of a combination of 200 μg ethinyl estradiol and 2 mg norgestrel in two divided doses12 hours apart.

**Ziehl-Neelsen m.**, see under *stain*.

---

**meth·od·ism** (meth'ə-diz"əm) the system of the Methodist school of medicine.

**Meth·od·ist** (meth'ə-dist) an ancient Roman medical sect, influenced by Asclepiades, founded (c. 50 B.C.) by Themison, and perfected by Thessalus of Tralles; its most distinguished member was Soranus. Methodists believed in both atomism and solidism.

**meth·od·ol·o·gy** (meth"ədol'o-je) the science of method; the science which deals with the principles of procedure in research and study.

**meth·o·hex·i·tal** (meth"o-hek'si-təl) [USP] [MeSH: Methohexital] an ultrashort-acting barbiturate used as a pharmaceutic necessary in the preparation of the sodium salt for injection.

**m. sodium** [USP], the monosodium salt of methohexital, used as a general anesthetic; administered intravenously.

**meth·o·trex·ate** (meth"o-trek'sāt) [USP] [MeSH: Methotrexate] a folic acid antagonist that acts by inhibiting the synthesis of DNA, RNA, thymidylate, and protein; used as an antineoplastic in the treatment of a wide variety of malignancies, including acute lymphocytic, meningeal, and acute myelocytic leukemia; gestational choriocarcinoma; chorioadenoma destruens; hydatidiform mole; carcinoma of the breast, lung, and head and neck; non-Hodgkin's lymphoma; mycosis fungoides; and osteosarcoma; administered orally. It is also used as an antipsoriatic and antirheumatic in the treatment of severe, recalcitrant, disabling psoriasis, severe rheumatoid and psoriatic arthritis, and dermatomyositis.

**m. sodium** [USP], the sodium salt of methotrexate, having the same actions and uses as the base; administered orally, intrathecally, intramuscularly, intravenously, and intra-arterially.

**meth·o·tri·mep·ra·zine** (meth"o-tri-mep'rə-zēn) [USP] [MeSH: Methotrimeprazine] a phenothiazine derivative having analgesic activity, used as an antipsychotic, for the relief of pain, and as a preoperative sedative; administered orally and intramuscularly. Called also *levomepromazine*.

**me·thox·amine hy·dro·chlo·ride** (mə-thok'sə-mēn) an adrenergic used for its vasopressor effect to support, restore, or maintain blood pressure during anesthesia and in the treatment of paroxysmal supraventricular tachycardia, administered intramuscularly and intravenously.

**me·thox·sa·len** (mə-thok'sə-lən) [USP] [MeSH: Methoxsalen] a psoralen occurring in *Amni majus* and other plants; used orally and topically in conjunction with exposure to ultraviolet light to facilitate repigmentation in idiopathic vitiligo, and to produce a phototoxic reaction in psoriasis. It is also used as a suntan accelerator and sun protectant.

**me·thoxy·chlor** (mə-thok'sə-klor) [MeSH: Methoxychlor] a chlorinated hydrocarbon insecticide effective against mosquito larvae and houseflies.

**meth·oxy·flu·rane** (meth-ok"se-floo'rān) [USP] [MeSH: Methoxyflurane] a highly potent inhalational anesthetic agent, used primarily to produce analgesia during the first stage of labor; its use in surgery is limited by a dose-related nephrotoxicity to procedures of short duration; it produces profound analgesia and good muscle relaxation; induction and recovery are slower than with halothane or enflurane.

**me·thox·yl** (mə-thok'səl) the chemical group, $CH_3O$—.

**me·thoxy·phen·amine hy·dro·chlo·ride** (mə-thok"sĭ-fen'ə-mēn) [USP] an adrenergic used mainly as a bronchodilator in the treatment of bronchial asthma, administered orally.

**8-me·thoxy·psor·a·len** (mə-thok'se-sor'ə-lən) methoxsalen.

**meth·phen·oxy·di·ol** (meth"fən-ok"sĭ-di'ol) guaifenesin.

**meth·sco·pol·amine bro·mide** (meth"sko-pol'ə-mēn) an anticholinergic, the quaternary ammonium derivative of scopolamine hydrobromide; it has an inhibitory effect on gastric secretion and gastrointestinal motility and is used as an adjunct for the treatment of peptic ulcer and gastric disorders associated with spasm, hyperacidity, and hypermotility; administered orally, subcutaneously, and intramuscularly. Called also *scopolamine methylbromide*.

**meth·sux·i·mide** (meth-suk'sĭ-mīd) [USP] an anticonvulsant used in the treatment of petit mal and psychomotor epilepsy, administered orally.

**meth·y·clo·thi·a·zide** (meth"ĭ-klo-thi'ə-zīd) [USP] [MeSH: Methyclothiazide] a thiazide diuretic used for treatment of hypertension and edema; administered orally.

**meth·yl** (meth'əl) [Gr. *methy* wine + *hylē* wood] the chemical group or radical $CH_3$—, sometimes abbreviated Me.

**m. anthranilate**, a volatile oil, the odoriferous constituent of orange flower oil, bergamot, jasmine, and other essential oils.

**m. benzene**, toluene.

**m. bromide**, a colorless gas soluble in alcohol and benzene, used in ionization chambers and fire extinguishers and as a reagent and fumigant; it is also found in automobile exhaust. If inhaled in excessive amounts it is neurotoxic, and if a solution touches the skin it causes blistering.

**m. ethyl-pyrrole**, a substituted pyrrole obtained from, and probably a constituent of, bilirubin.

**m. hydride**, methane.

**m. hydroxy-furfural**, the furfural produced from the hexose in Molisch's test and which produces the color.

**m. iodide**, a colorless liquid that turns brown on exposure to light, used in microscopy and in testing for pyridine. It is irritating to skin and mucous membranes and is a suspected carcinogen. Called also *iodomethane*.

**m. isobutyl ketone** [NF], a transparent, colorless, mobile, volatile liquid used as an alcohol denaturant in pharmaceutical preparations.

**m. methacrylate**, a methyl ester of methacrylic acid, which polymerizes to form polymethyl methacrylate; used in the manufacture of acrylic resins (q.v.) and plastics.

**m. salicylate** [NF], a volatile oil with a characteristic wintergreen odor and taste; used as a counterirritant in ointments or liniments for muscle pain and also as a flavoring agent. Called also *betula oil, gaultheria oil, sweet birch oil,* and *wintergreen oil*.

**m. sulfonate**, a crystalline, noncaustic, and nonpoisonous antiseptic.

**m. *tert*-butyl ether**, a solvent used to dissolve cholesterol stones in the gallbladder; administered as a continuous infusion via catheter.

**meth·yl·ace·tic ac·id** (meth"əl-ə-se'tik) propionic acid.

**α-meth·yl·ac·e·to·ace·tic ac·id** (meth"əl-ə-se"to-ə-se'tik) acetoacetic acid methylated at the second carbon; attached to coenzyme A, it is an intermediate in isoleucine degradation. It is excreted in excess in the urine in α-methylacetoaceticaciduria.

**α-meth·yl·ac·e·to·ace·tic·ac·id·uria** (meth"əl-ə-se"to-ə-se"tik-as"ĭ-du're-ə) an autosomal recessive aminoacidopathy due to deficiency of α-methylacetoacetyl CoA thiolase, the β-ketothiolase catalyzing the final step in isoleucine catabolism; it is characterized by episodes of severe metabolic ketoacidosis and urinary excretion of several intermediates of isoleucine catabolism, including α-methylacetoacetic acid.

**α-meth·yl·ac·e·to·ac·e·tyl** (meth"əl-ə-se"to-as'ə-tēl") the acyl radical of α-methylacetoacetic acid; the thioester formed with coenzyme A, $\alpha$-methylacetoacetyl CoA, is an intermediate in the catabolism of isoleucine.

**$\alpha$-meth·yl·ac·e·to·ac·e·tyl CoA thi·o·lase** (meth″əl-ə-se″to-as′ə-tēl ko-a′ thi′o-lās) an acetyl-CoA *C*-acyltransferase ($\beta$-ketothiolase) specifically catalyzing the final step in isoleucine catabolism, the cleavage of $\alpha$-methylacetoacetyl CoA to form acetyl CoA and propionyl CoA. Deficiency of the enzyme, an autosomal recessive trait, results in $\alpha$-methylacetoaceticaciduria.

**meth·yl·amine** (meth′əl-ə-mēn″) a flammable, explosive gas, $CH_3NH_2$, used in tanning and in organic synthesis and produced naturally in some decaying fish, certain plants, and crude methanol; it is irritating to the eyes.

***N*-meth·yl-D-as·par·tate (NMDA)** (meth′əl as′pahr-tāt) a neurotransmitter similar to glutamate, found in the central nervous system; a synthetic preparation is used experimentally to study the excitatory mechanisms of glutamate transmitters.

**meth·yl·ate** (meth′əl-āt) 1. a compound of methyl alcohol and a base. 2. to add a methyl group to a substance.

**meth·yl·at·ed** (meth′əl-āt″əd) containing or combined with a methyl group.

**meth·yl·a·tion** (meth″əl-a′shən) [MeSH: Methylation] treatment with reagent to add a methyl group to a compound.

**meth·yl·at·ro·pine ni·trate** (meth″əl-at′tro-pēn) a quaternary ammonium derivative of atropine, having the same actions and uses as atropine (q.v.), but with much less effect on the central nervous system and with strong ganglionic blocking activity. Called also *atropine methonitrate* and *atropine methylnitrate.*

**meth·yl·az·oxy·meth·a·nol** (meth″əl-əz-ok″se-meth′ə-nol) a substance carcinogenic to the liver, kidneys, intestine, and lungs in humans and other animals; it is formed after hydrolysis of cycasin or macrozamin by intestinal bacteria.

**meth·yl·ben·ze·tho·ni·um chlo·ride** (meth″əl-ben″zə-tho′ne-əm) [USP] a disinfectant quaternary compound which is bacteriostatic for urea-splitting organisms that may cause ammonia dermatitis. It is applied topically to areas of the skin coming in contact with urine, feces, or perspiration, and is used in a rinse for diapers, bed linen, and undergarments of incontinent adults and children.

**meth·yl·cel·lu·lose** (meth″əl-sel′u-lōs) [USP] [MeSH: Methylcellulose] a methyl ether of cellulose, occurring as a white, fibrous powder or granules, supplied in differing degrees of viscosity; used as a suspending and viscosity-increasing agent and tablet excipient in pharmaceutical preparations, administered orally as a cathartic, and applied topically to the conjunctiva to protect the cornea during certain ophthalmic procedures and to lubricate the cornea.
**hydroxypropyl m.,** see under *H.*

**meth·yl·chlo·ro·for·mate** (meth″əl-klor″o-for′māt) a lacrimatory gas used as a warning agent in fumigations with hydrogen cyanide.

**meth·yl·chlo·ro·iso·thi·a·zo·li·none** (meth″əl-klor″o-i″so-thi-ə-zōl′ĭ-nōn) see *methylisothiazolinone.*

**3-meth·yl·cho·lan·threne** (meth″əl-ko-lan′thrēn) a highly carcinogenic polycyclic aromatic hydrocarbon synthesized by pyrolytic degradation of cholic acid, deoxycholic acid, or cholesterol. It is a procarcinogen that requires metabolic activation to exert a mutagenic effect and is widely used in laboratory studies of chemical carcinogenesis. Abbreviated MCA.

**meth·yl·co·bal·a·min** (meth″əl-ko-bal′ə-min) a cobalamin derivative in which the substituent is a methyl group. It is one of two metabolically active forms synthesized upon ingestion of vitamin $B_{12}$ and is the predominant form in the serum; it acts as a coenzyme in the reaction catalyzed by 5-methyltetrahydrofolate-homocysteine methyltransferase. Abbreviated MeCbl.

**3-meth·yl·cro·ton·ic ac·id** (meth″əl-kro-ton′ik) crotonic acid methylated at the 3 carbon; it is excreted at elevated levels in urine when 3-methylcrotonoyl-CoA carboxylase activity is impaired.

**meth·yl·cro·ton·o·yl-CoA car·box·y·lase** (meth″əl-kro-ton′o-əl ko-a′ kahr-bok′sə-lās) [EC 6.4.1.4] a biotin-containing enzyme of the ligase class that catalyzes the ATP-driven carboxylation of 3-methylcrotonyl CoA to form 3-methylglutaconyl CoA as a step in the use of leucine as a fuel. Deficiency of the enzyme, an autosomal recessive trait, results in 3-methylcrotonyl carboxylase deficiency; enzyme activity is also absent in multiple carboxylase deficiency (q.v.). Written also *methylcrotonyl CoA carboxylase.*

**3-meth·yl·cro·ton·yl** (meth″əl-kro′tə-nil″) the radical of 3-methylcrotonic acid; the thioester formed with coenzyme A, 3-methylcrotonyl CoA, is an intermediate in the degradation of leucine.

**3-meth·yl·cro·to·nyl CoA car·box·y·lase de·fi·cien·cy** (meth″əl-kro′tə-nil″ ko-a′ kahr-bok′sə-lās) an autosomal recessive aminoacidopathy due to deficiency of methylcrotonoyl-CoA carboxylase, characterized by increased urine levels of 3-methylcrotonylglycine, 3-methylcrotonic acid, and 3-hydroxyisovaleric acid and variable presentation of mental retardation, central nervous system dysfunction, and muscular atrophy. Written also *$\beta$-methylcrotonyl CoA carboxylase deficiency.*

**3-meth·yl·cro·ton·yl·gly·cine** (meth″əl-kro″to-nəl-gli′sēn) a conjugate of 3-methylcrotonic acid and glycine, formed and excreted in excess in the urine when 3-methylcrotonoyl-CoA carboxylase activity is impaired.

**$\beta$-meth·yl·cro·to·nyl·gly·cin·u·ria** (meth″əl-kro″to-nəl-gli″sĭ-nu′re-ə) 1. 3-methylcrotonyl CoA carboxylase deficiency. 2. excretion of 3-methylcrotonylglycine in the urine, as occurs in 3-methylcrotonyl CoA carboxylase deficiency or multiple carboxylase deficiency.

**meth·yl·cy·to·sine** (meth″əl-si′to-sēn) a pyrimidine occurring in deoxyribonucleic acid.

**meth·yl·di·chlor·ar·sin** (meth″əl-di″klor-ahr′sin) a lethal and vesicating war gas.

**meth·yl·di·hy·dro·mor·phi·none** (meth″əl-di-hi″dro-mor′fi-nōn) metopon (def. 2).

**meth·yl·do·pa** (meth″əl-do′pə) [USP] [MeSH: Methyldopa] a phenylalanine derivative administered orally in the treatment of hypertension, including that caused by renal disease.

**meth·yl·do·pate hy·dro·chlo·ride** (meth″əl-do′pāt) [USP] the ethyl ester hydrochloride of methyldopa, used as an antihypertensive, administered by intravenous infusion.

**meth·y·lene** (meth′ə-lēn) the bivalent hydrocarbon radical $—CH_2—$ or $CH_2=$. Called also *methene.*
**m. bichloride,** magnesium chloride.
**m. blue,** see under *blue.*

**meth·y·lene·di·oxy·am·phet·amine (MDA)** (meth″ə-lēn-di-ok″se-am-fet′ə-mēn) a compound chemically related to amphetamine and mescaline that has hallucinogenic properties; it is widely abused and causes dependence.

**3,4-meth·y·lene·di·oxy·meth·am·phet·amine** (meth″ə-lēn″di-ok″-se-meth″am-fet′ə-mēn) MDMA; a compound chemically related to amphetamine and having hallucinogenic properties; it is widely abused. Popularly called *Ecstasy.*

**5,10-meth·y·lene·tet·ra·hy·dro·fo·late** (meth″ə-lēn-tet″rə-hi″dro-fo′lāt) a doubly methylated, reduced derivative of folic acid occurring as an intermediate in the transfer of methyl groups to methionine, receiving them from formaldehyde, serine, and glycine.

**meth·yl·ene·tet·ra·hy·dro·fo·late de·hy·dro·gen·ase ($NADP^+$)** (meth″ə-lēn-tet″rə-hi″dro-fo′lāt de-hi′dro-jən-ās) [EC 1.5.1.5] [MeSH: Methylenetetrahydrofolate Dehydrogenase] an enzyme activity of the oxidoreductase class that catalyzes the oxidation of 5,10-methylenetetrahydrofolate to 5,10-methenyltetrahydrofolate, using $NADP^+$ as an electron acceptor. The reaction occurs in the system of folate-mediated one-carbon transfer reactions. The enzyme activity is part of a trifunctional enzyme that also includes methenyltetrahydrofolate cyclohydrolase and formate–tetrahydrofolate ligase activities.

**5,10-meth·y·lene·tet·ra·hy·dro·fo·late re·duc·tase ($FADH_2$)** (meth″ə-lēn-tet″rə-hi″dro-fo′lāt re-duk′tās) [EC 1.7.99.5] an enzyme of the oxidoreductase class that catalyzes the reduction of 5,10-methylenetetrahydrofolate to 5-methyltetrahdyrofolate, using $FADH_2$ and NADH as primary and secondary electron donors, respectively. The reaction is the means by which methyl groups are generated *de novo* for methylation reactions. Deficiency of the enzyme, an autosomal recessive trait, results in homocystinuria due to deficiency of 5-methyltetrahydrofolate–homocysteine *S*-methyltransferase; hypomethioninemia and neurologic abnormalities are present but megaloblastic anemia is absent.

**meth·y·lene·tet·ra·hy·dro·fo·late (THF) re·duc·tase deficiency** the most common genetic aminoacidopathy of folate metabolism; the chief biochemical finding is homocystinuria with normal levels of plasma methionine; the chief clinical sign is CNS damage.

**meth·y·len·o·phil** (meth″ə-len′o-fil) 1. an element easily stainable with methylene blue. 2. methylenophilous.

**meth·y·len·oph·i·lous** (meth″ə-lən-of′ĭ-ləs) [*methylene* + Gr. *philein* to love] stainable with methylene blue.

**meth·yl·er·go·no·vine mal·e·ate** (meth″əl-er″go-no′vēn) [USP] an oxytocic used especially to prevent or combat postpartum hemorrhage and atony; administered orally, intramuscularly, and intravenously.

**meth·yl·glu·ca·mine** (meth″əl-gloo′kə-mēn) 1. a compound prepared from D-glucose and methylamine, used in the synthesis of pharmaceuticals. 2. meglumine.

**3-meth·yl·glu·ta·con·ic ac·id** (meth″əl-gloo″tə-kon′ik) a dicarboxylic acid occurring at elevated levels in 3-methylglutaconicaciduria and 3-hydroxy-3-methylglutaricaciduria.

**3-meth·yl·glu·ta·con·ic·ac·id·uria** (meth″əl-gloo″tə-kon″ik-as″ĭ-du′re-ə) an aminoacidopathy characterized by excessive urinary excretion of 3-methylglutaconic acid and occurring in two forms. A mild form caused by deficiency of methylglutaconyl-CoA hydratase is characterized by speech retardation; a more severe form, of unknown etiology, is characterized by urinary excretion also of 3-methylglutaric acid and by progressive neurologic deterioration with hypotonia and optic atrophy.

**3-meth·yl·glu·ta·con·yl** (meth″əl-gloo″tə-kon′əl) a radical of 3-methylglutaconic acid; the thioester formed with coenzyme A, 3-methylglutaconyl CoA, is an intermediate in the catabolism of leucine.

**meth·yl·glu·ta·con·yl-CoA hy·dra·tase** (meth″əl-gloo″tə-kon′əl ko-a′ hi′drə-tās) [EC 4.2.1.18] an enzyme of the lyase class that catalyzes the hydration of 3-methylglutaconyl CoA to form 3-hydroxy-3-methylglutaryl CoA, a step in the catabolism of leucine. Deficiency of the enzyme, an autosomal recessive trait, causes 3-methylglutaconicaciduria.

**3-meth·yl·glu·tar·ic ac·id** (meth″əl-gloo-tar′ik) a dicarboxylic acid occurring at elevated levels in the urine in one form of 3-methylglutaconicaciduria and in 3-hydroxy-3-methylglutaricaciduria.

**meth·yl·gly·ox·al** (meth″əl-gli-ok′səl) the compound $CH_3$—CO—CHO, the aldehyde of pyruvic acid; it is formed from dihydroxyacetone phosphate in the liver and is a substrate for glyoxalase.

**meth·yl·gly·ox·a·lase** (meth″əl-gli-ok′sə-lās) lactoylglutathione lyase.

**meth·yl·gly·ox·al·i·din** (meth″əl-gli″ok-sal′ĭ-din) lysidin.

**3-meth·yl·his·ti·dine** an amino acid occurring in myofibrillar proteins that is released by catabolism and excreted in the urine; the rate of urinary excretion has been proposed as an indicator of muscle protein breakdown. Abbreviated 3MH.

**meth·yl·hy·dan·to·in** (meth″əl-hi-dan′to-in) a crystalline compound found in fresh meat and formed by the decomposition of creatine.

**me·thyl·ic** (mə-thil′ik) containing methyl.

**me·thyl·i·dyne** (mə-thil′ĭ-dīn) the trivalent hydrocarbon radical —CH= or CH≡. Called also *methine.*

**meth·yl·in·dol** (meth″əl-in′dol) skatole.

**meth·yl·iso·thi·a·zo·li·none** (meth″əl-i″so-thi-ə-zo′lĭ-nōn) a preservative used in conjunction with methylchloroisothiazolinone as a broad-spectrum antifungal and antibiotic agent in cosmetics, in swimming pool biocides, and in various industrial preparations. It is a common cause of contact allergy and can cause chemical burn at high concentrations.

**meth·yl·ma·lon·ic ac·id** (meth″əl-mə-lon′ik) [MeSH: Methylmalonic Acid] a carboxylic acid occurring in excess in the blood and other body fluids in methylmalonicacidemia.

**meth·yl·ma·lon·ic·ac·i·de·mia** (meth″əl-mə-lon″ik-as″ĭ-de′me-ə) 1. an autosomal recessive aminoacidopathy characterized by an excess of methylmalonic acid in the blood and urine, with metabolic ketoacidosis, hyperglycinemia, hyperglycinuria, and hyperammonemia, and presenting in infancy as failure to thrive, persistent vomiting and dehydration, respiratory distress, and hypotonia. It results from any of several defects that cause deficiency of methylmalonyl-CoA mutase (q.v.) activity, including defects in the apoenzyme, in the biosynthesis of adenosylcobalamin (see *cob(I)alamin adenosyltransferase* and *cobalamin reductase*), in the transport of cobalamin, or in the pathway of biosynthesis common to both cobalamin-containing coenzymes; the last two defects also cause homocystinuria due to deficiency of 5-methyltetrahydrofolate–homocysteine *S*-methyltransferase (q.v.). Called also *methylmalonicaciduria.* 2. excess of methylmalonic acid in the blood.

**meth·yl·ma·lon·ic·ac·id·uria** (meth″əl-mə-lon″ik-as″ĭ-du′re-ə) 1. excess of methylmalonic acid in the urine. 2. methylmalonicacidemia.

**meth·yl·mal·o·nyl** (meth″əl-mal′ə-nəl) the radical of methylmalonic acid; the thioester it forms with coenzyme A, methylmalonyl CoA, is an intermediate in the catabolism of certain amino acids and odd-number chain-length fatty acids.

**meth·yl·mal·o·nyl-CoA epim·er·ase** (meth″əl-mal′ə-nəl ko-a′ ə-pim′ər-ās) [EC 5.1.99.1] an enzyme of the isomerase class that catalyzes the equilibration of the D- and L- isomers of methylmalonyl CoA. The reaction is part of the route by which three-carbon compounds from some amino acids and from odd number chain length fatty acids are used as fuels. Called also *methylmalonyl-CoA racemase.*

**meth·yl·mal·o·nyl-CoA mu·tase** (meth″əl-mal′ə-nəl ko-a′ mu′tās) [EC 5.4.99.2] [MeSH: Methylmalonyl-CoA Mutase] an enzyme of the isomerase class that catalyzes the isomerization of L-methylmalonyl coenzyme A to succinyl coenzyme A, requiring adenosylcobalamin as a coenzyme. The reaction is a step in the use of isoleucine, threonine, valine, propionate, and other odd number chain length fatty acids as fuels. Deficiency of enzyme activity, which may be caused by defects in the apoenzyme, in the coenzyme, or in cobalamin metabolism, results in methylmalonicacidemia.

**meth·yl·mal·o·nyl-CoA ra·ce·mase** (meth″əl-mal′ə-nəl ko-a′ ra′sə-mās) methylmalonyl-CoA epimerase.

**meth·yl·mer·cap·tan** (meth″əl-mər-kap′tən) a gas formed in the intestines by the decomposition of proteins; said to impart to the urine the odor noticed after eating asparagus, and to the breath the characteristic odor of fetor hepatis.

**meth·yl·meth·ac·ry·late** (meth″əl-meth-ak′rə-lāt) see under *methyl.*

**meth·yl·mor·phine** (meth″əl-mor′fēn) codeine.

**3-meth·yl-2-oxo·bu·ta·no·ate de·hy·dro·gen·ase (lip·o·am·ide)** (meth′əl ok″so-bu″tə-no′āt de-hi′dro-jən-ās lip″o-am′īd) [EC 1.2.4.4] an enzyme of the oxidoreductase class that is a component of the multienzyme branched-chain α-keto acid dehydrogenase complex (q.v.). The enzyme catalyzes the oxidative decarboxylation of the branched chain amino acids leucine, isoleucine, and valine, transferring the products formed to the lipoic acid moiety of dihydrolipoamide acyltransferase via a thiamine pyrophosphate cofactor. See also *maple sugar urine disease,* under *disease.* Called also *α-ketoisovalerate dehydrogenase.*

**meth·yl·par·a·ben** (meth″əl-par′ə-bən) [NF] an antifungal compound, closely related to butylparaben and ethylparaben, used as a preservative in pharmaceutic preparations.

**meth·yl·par·a·fy·nol** (meth″əl-par″ə-fi′nol) meparfynol.

**meth·yl·pen·tose** (meth″əl-pen′tōs) a hexose derivative in which carbon 6 exists in reduced form, as a methyl group; e.g., *fucose.* See also *deoxyhexose.*

**meth·yl·pen·ty·nol** (meth″əl-pen′tĭ-nol) meparfynol.

**meth·yl·phen·i·date hy·dro·chlo·ride** (meth″əl-fen′ĭ-dāt) [USP] a central stimulant used in the treatment of attention-deficit/hyperactivity disorder, various types of depression, and narcolepsy; administered orally.

**meth·yl·pred·nis·o·lone** (meth″əl-pred-nis′ə-lōn) [USP] [MeSH: Methylprednisolone] a synthetic glucocorticoid derived from progesterone, used in replacement therapy for adrenal insufficiency and as an anti-inflammatory and immunosuppressant in a wide variety of disorders; administered orally.
**m. acetate** [USP], the 21-acetate ester of methylprednisolone, used topically as an anti-inflammatory and administered by enema or by intramuscular, intra-articular, intrasynovial, or soft-tissue injection in replacement therapy for adrenal insufficiency and as an anti-inflammatory and immunosuppressant in a wide variety of disorders.
**m. hemisuccinate** [USP], the hemisuccinate salt of methylprednisolone, having actions and uses similar to those of the base.
**m. sodium phosphate,** the 21-phosphate disodium salt of methylprednisolone, having actions similar to those of the base.
**m. sodium succinate** [USP], the 21-succinate sodium salt of methylprednisolone having actions and uses similar to those of the base; it is highly soluble in water and is chiefly used for the rapid achievement of high blood levels of methylprednisolone in short-term emergency treatment; administered by intramuscular or intravenous injection.

**meth·yl·pu·rine** (meth″əl-pu′rēn) see under *purine.*

**meth·yl·py·ra·pone** (meth″əl-pi′rə-pōn) metyrapone.

**4-meth·yl-1H-py·ra·zole** (meth″əl-pi′rə-zōl) fomepizole.

**meth·yl·py·ri·dine** (meth″əl-pi′rĭ-dēn) a basic substance oxidized in the body to pyridine-carboxylic acid.

**meth·yl·ro·san·i·line chlo·ride** (meth″əl-ro-zan′ĭ-lēn) gentian violet; see under *gentian.*

**meth·yl·tes·tos·ter·one** (meth″əl-təs-tos′tər-ōn) [USP] [MeSH: Methyltestosterone] a synthetic androgen derived from cholesterol, having actions similar to those of testosterone (q.v.); used as replacement therapy for androgen deficiency in males, in the palliation of certain inoperable mammary cancers, and to prevent postpartum breast pain and engorgement in the non-nursing mother; administered orally or sublingually.

**5-meth·yl·tet·ra·hy·dro·fo·late** (meth″əl-tet″rə-hi″dro-fo′lāt) a substituted, reduced derivative of folic acid, occurring as a source of methyl groups for the regeneration of methionine; it is formed by reduction of 5,10-methylenetetrahydrofolate and is the principal form of folic acid during transport and storage in the body.

**5-meth·yl·te·tra·hy·dro·fo·late–ho·mo·cys·te·ine *S*-meth·yl·trans·fer·ase** (meth″əl-tet″rə-hi″dro-fo′lāt-ho″mo-sis′te-ēn meth″əl-trans′fər-ās) [EC 2.1.1.13] an enzyme of the oxidoreductase class that catalyzes the remethylation of homocysteine to form methionine, using methyltetrahydrofolate as a methyl donor and requiring methylcobalamin as a coenzyme; the reaction also regenerates tetrahydrofolate. Deficiency of enzyme activity can result from any of several defects, including deficiency of the apoenzyme, inability to convert cobalamin specifically to methylcobalamin or, more generally, to either of the cobalamin-containing coenzymes, deficiency of 5,10-methylenetetrahydrofolate reductase ($FADH_2$) activity (q.v.), familial megaloblastic anemia or other defect in absorption or transport of vitamin $B_{12}$, or nutritional deficiency of vitamin $B_{12}$ or folate; it results in homocystinuria, with developmental delay and neurologic abnormalities, and hypomethioninemia. Defects in cobalamin metabolism are characterized additionally by hematologic abnormalities and some also by methylmalonicacidemia (q.v.).

**meth·yl·the·o·bro·mine** (meth″əl-the″o-bro′mēn) caffeine.

**meth·yl·thi·o·nine chlo·ride** (meth″əl-thi′o-nēn) methylene blue.

**meth·yl·trans·fer·ase** (meth″əl-trans′fər-ās) [EC 2.1.1] any member of the sub-subclass of enzymes of the transferase class that catalyzes the transfer of a methyl group from one compound to another. Called also *transmethylase.*

**5-meth·yl·ura·cil** (meth″əl-ūr′ə-sil) thymine.

**meth·yl·xan·thine** (meth″əl-zan′thēn) any of the methylated derivatives of xanthine, including caffeine, theobromine, and theophylline and their derivatives. Methylxanthines relax smooth muscle, stimulate the central nervous system and cardiac muscle, and produce diuresis; they are used clinically as bronchodilators.

**meth·y·ser·gide** (meth″ĭ-ser′jīd) [MeSH: Methysergide] a potent serotonin antagonist having direct vasoconstrictor effects.
**m. maleate** [USP], the maleate salt of methysergide, having the same actions as the base; used as an analgesic in the treatment of vascular (migraine) headache in certain patients, administered orally.

**me·ti·amide** (mə-ti′ə-mīd) [MeSH: Metiamide] an antagonist to histamine, competing for the $H_2$ receptor site on cells.

**me·ti·a·pine** (mə-ti′ə-pēn) a tranquilizer which has been used in the treatment of schizophrenia.

**Met·i·cor·ten** (met″ĭ-kor′tən) trademark for a preparation of prednisone.

**met·myo·glo·bin** (mət-mi″o-glo′bin) [MeSH: Metmyoglobin] a compound formed from myoglobin by oxidation of the ferrous to the ferric state.

**met·o·clo·pra·mide hy·dro·chlo·ride** (met″o-klo′prə-mīd) [USP] a dopamine receptor antagonist that stimulates gastric motility, used as an antiemetic, as an adjunct in gastrointestinal radiology and intestinal intubation, and in the treatment of gastroparesis and gastroesophageal reflux; administered orally, intramuscularly, and intravenously.

**met·o·cu·rine io·dide** (met″o-ku′rēn) a nondepolarizing neuromuscular blocking agent, used as an anesthesia adjunct to induce skeletal muscle relaxation and to reduce the intensity of muscle contractions in convulsive therapy; administered intravenously. Called also *dimethyl tubocurarine iodide.*

**me·to·la·zone** (mə-to′lə-zōn) [USP] [MeSH: Metolazone] a sulfonamide derivative that has a different chemical structure from but the same pharmacological actions as the thiazide diuretics, used in the treatment of hypertension and edema; administered orally.

**me·ton·y·my** (mə-ton′ĭ-me) [*meta-* + Gr. *onyma* name] a disturbance of language seen in schizophrenic disorders in which an inappropriate but related term is used instead of the correct one.

**me·top·a·gus** (mə-top′ə-gəs) metopopagus.

**me·top·ic** (me-top′ik) pertaining to the forehead; frontal.

**me·to·pi·on** (mə-to′pe-on) glabella.

**Met·o·pi·rone** (met″o-pi′rōn) trademark for preparations of metyrapone.

**met·o·pism** (met′o-piz″əm) the persistence of the frontal suture.

**metop(o)-** [Gr. *metōpon* forehead] a combining form denoting relationship to the forehead.

**me·to·pon** (mə-to′pon) a morphine derivative, methyldihydromorphinone hydrochloride, used to relieve pain.

**met·o·pop·a·gus** (met″o-pop′ə-gəs) [*metopo-* + *-pagus*] a craniopagus in which the fusion is in the region of the forehead.

**met·o·pro·lol** (met″o-pro′lol) a cardioselective $\beta_1$-adrenergic blocking agent.
**m. succinate,** the succinate salt of metoprolol, used for the treatment of angina pectoris and hypertension; administered orally.
**m. tartrate** [USP], the tartrate salt of metoprolol, used in the treatment of hypertension, angina pectoris, and myocardial infarction; administered orally and intravenously.

**Met·or·chis** (met-or′kis) [*meta-* + Gr. *orchis* testicle] a genus of trematodes of the family Opisthorchiidae. *M. al′bidus* and *M. conjunc′tus* parasitize cats, dogs, and other mammals.

**met·o·ser·pate hy·dro·chlo·ride** (met″o-ser′pāt) a veterinary sedative used in chickens.

**me·tox·e·nous** (mə-tok′sə-nəs) [*meta-* + Gr. *xenos* host] requiring two hosts for the full cycle of existence; said of certain parasites.

**me·tox·e·ny** (mə-tok′sə-ne) the condition of being metoxenous.

**me·tra** (me′trə) [Gr. *metra* womb] uterus.

**me·tral·gia** (mə-tral′jə) [*metr-* + *-algia*] hysteralgia.

**me·tra·term** (me′trə-tərm) [*metr-* + L. *terminus* boundary] the external opening of the uterus in some tapeworms (Diphyllobothriidae).

**me·tra·to·nia** (me″trə-to′ne-ə) [*metr-* + *atonia*] uterine atony.

**me·tra·tro·phia** (me″trə-tro′fe-ə) [*metr-* + *atrophia*] uterine atrophy.

**Met·ra·zol** (met′rə-zol) trademark for preparations of pentylenetetrazol.

**me·tre** (me′tər) meter.

**met·re·chos·co·py** (met″rə-kos′kə-pe) [Gr. *metron* measure + *ēchō* sound + *-scopy*] combined mensuration, auscultation, and inspection.

**me·trec·to·my** (me-trek′tə-me) [*metr-* + *-ectomy*] hysterectomy.

**me·trec·to·pia** (me″trek-to′pe-ə) [*metr-* + *ectopia*] uterine displacement.

**Met·re·ton** (met′rə-ton) trademark for a preparation of prednisolone sodium phosphate.

**me·treu·ryn·ter** (me″troo-rin′tər) [*metr-* + Gr. *eurynein* to stretch] an inflatable bag for dilating the cervical canal of the uterus.

**me·tria** (me′tre-ə) any inflammatory condition of the uterus during the puerperium.

**met·ric** (met′rik) [Gr. *metron* measure] 1. pertaining to measures based on the meter; see Appendix 5. 2. having the meter as a basis.

**met·ri·fo·nate** (met″rĭ-fo′nāt) trichlorfon.

**met·rio·ce·phal·ic** (met″re-o-sə-fal′ik) [Gr. *metrios* moderate + *cephal-* + *-ic*] having a skull with a vertical index between 72 and 77.

**met·ri·pho·nate** (met″rĭ-fo′nāt) trichlorfon.

**me·tri·tis** (mə-tri′tis) [*metr-* + *-itis*] inflammation of the uterus. Several varieties are named, according to the part of the organ affected—cervical, corporeal, interstitial, and parenchymatous.
**contagious equine m.,** CEM; a highly contagious venereal disease of horses caused by infection with *Haemophilus equigenitalis;* symptoms may include endometritis and salpingitis with a profuse purulent discharge, but sometimes infection is subclinical with only a lowered conception rate.
**m. dis′secans, dissecting m.,** metritis characterized by the passage of fragments or large masses of the necrotic uterine wall.
**puerperal m.,** infection of the uterus of the puerperal woman.

**me·triz·a·mide** (mə-triz′ə-mīd) [MeSH: Metrizamide] a water-soluble, non-ionic, iodinated derivative of benzoic acid used as a radiopaque medium in radiography and computed tomography.

**met·ri·zo·ate so·di·um** (met″rĭ-zo′āt) chemical name: 3-(acetylamino)-5-(acetylmethylamino)-2,4,6-triiodobenzoic acid monosodium salt; a diagnostic radiopaque medium, $C_{12}H_{10}I_3N_2NaO_4$.

**metr(o)-** [Gr. *mētra* uterus] a combining form denoting relationship to the uterus; see also *hyster(o)-.*

**me·tro·cele** (me′tro-sēl) [*metro-* + *-cele*[1]] hernia of the uterus; hysterocele.

**me·tro·col·po·cele** (me″tro-kol′po-sēl) [*metro-* + *colpo-* + *-cele*[1]] hernia of the uterus and the vagina.

**me·tro·cys·to·sis** (me″tro-sis-to′sis) formation of cysts in the uterus.

**me·tro·cyte** (me′tro-sīt) [Gr. *mētēr* mother + *-cyte*] a mother cell.

**Me·tro·din** (me′tro-dēn) trademark for a preparation of urofollitropin.

**me·tro·dyn·ia** (me″tro-din′e-ə) [*metro-* + *-odynia*] hysteralgia.

**me·tro·en·do·me·tri·tis** (me″tro-en″do-me-tri′tis) combined inflammation of the uterus and its mucous membranes.

**me·tro·fi·bro·ma** (me″tro-fi-bro′mə) [*metro-* + *fibroma*] uterine leiomyoma.

**me·trog·e·nous** (mə-troj′ə-nəs) derived from the uterus.

**me·trog·ra·phy** (mə-trog′rə-fe) hysterography.

**me·tro·leu·kor·rhea** (me″tro-loo″ko-re′ə) leukorrhea of uterine origin.

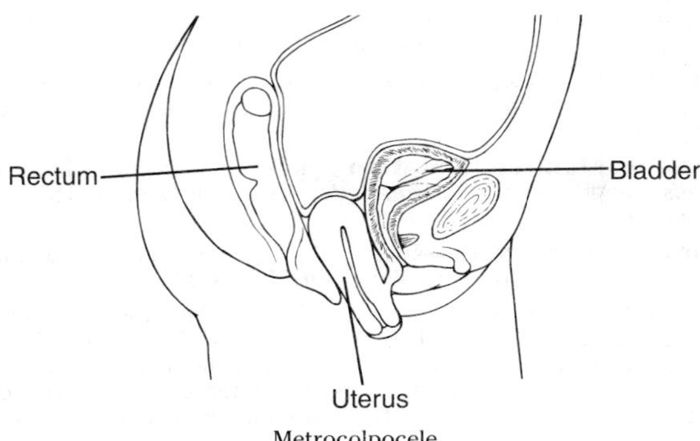


Metrocolpocele.

**me·trol·o·gy** (mə-trol′ə-je) [Gr. *metron* measure + *-logy*] the science which deals with measurement.

**me·tro·lym·phan·gi·tis** (me″tro-lim″fan-ji′tis) inflammation of the uterine lymphatic vessels.

**me·tro·ma·la·cia** (me″tro-mə-la′shə) [*metro-* + *-malacia*] abnormal softening of the uterus.

**me·tro·mal·a·co·ma** (me″tro-mal″ə-ko′mə) metromalacia.

**me·tro·men·or·rha·gia** (me″tro-men″o-ra′je-ə) metrorrhagia combined with menorrhagia.

**met·ro·ni·da·zole** (met″ro-ni′də-zōl) [USP] [MeSH: Metronidazole] an antiprotozoal and antibacterial effective against obligate anaerobes; administered orally and intravaginally in *Trichomonas vaginalis* infection in females and orally in *T. vaginalis* infection in males, in giardiasis, and in intestinal amebiasis. It is also used orally or intravenously in extraintestinal amebiasis and infection by obligate anaerobic bacteria and intravenously for the prophylaxis of colonic perioperative infection.
**m. hydrochloride,** the hydrochloride salt of metronidazole, administered intravenously for the same indications for which the base is used intravenously.

**me·trono·scope** (mə-tron′ə-skōp) an instrument for giving exercises in rhythmic reading to correct poorly coordinated ocular movements.

**me·tro·pa·ral·y·sis** (me″tro-pə-ral′ə-sis) paralysis of the uterus.

**me·tro·path·ic** (me″tro-path′ik) pertaining to or characterized by uterine disorder.

**me·trop·a·thy** (mə-trop′ə-the) [*metro-* + *-pathy*] any uterine disease or disorder.

**me·tro·peri·to·ne·al** (me″tro-per″ĭ-to-ne′əl) pertaining to the uterus and peritoneum, or communicating with the uterine and peritoneal cavities, as a metroperitoneal fistula.

**me·tro·peri·to·ni·tis** (me″tro-per″ĭ-to-ni′tis) [*metro-* + *peritonitis*] inflammation of the peritoneum about the uterus, or peritonitis resulting from infection after metritis.

**me·tro·phle·bi·tis** (me″tro-flə-bi′tis) [*metro-* + *phlebo-* + *-itis*] inflammation of the veins of the uterus.

**Me·tro·pine** (met′ro-pin) trademark for preparations of methylatropine nitrate.

**me·tro·plas·ty** (me″tro-plas′te) reconstructive surgery on the uterus.

**me·trop·o·lis** (mə-trop′ə-lis) [Gr. *mētropolis* mother-state, as opposed to her colonies] the area in which a particular species of organisms commonly occurs.

**me·tro·pto·sis** (me″tro-to′sis) [*metro-* + *-ptosis*] uterine prolapse.

**me·tror·rha·gia** (me″tro-ra′je-ə) [*metro-* + *-rrhagia*] [MeSH: Metrorrhagia] uterine bleeding, usually of variable amount, occurring at completely irregular but frequent intervals, the period of flow sometimes being prolonged.
**m. myopa′thica,** uterine hemorrhage due to insufficient contraction of uterine muscles after parturition.

**me·tror·rhea** (me″tro-re′ə) [*metro-* + *-rrhea*] a free or abnormal uterine discharge.

**me·tror·rhex·is** (me″tro-rek′sis) [*metro-* + *-rrhexis*] rupture of the uterus.

**me·tro·sal·pin·gi·tis** (me″tro-sal″pin-ji′tis) [*metro-* + *salping-* + *-itis*] inflammation of the uterus and oviducts.

**me·tro·sal·pin·gog·ra·phy** (me″tro-sal″ping-gog′rə-fe) hysterosalpingography.

**me·tro·scope** (me′tro-skōp) hysteroscope.

**me·tros·ta·sis** (mə-tros′tə-sis) [Gr. *metron* measure + *-stasis*] a state in which the length of a muscle fiber is relatively fixed, and at which length it contracts and relaxes.

**me·tro·stax·is** (me″tro-stak′sis) [*metro-* + *staxis*] a slight but persistent escape of blood from the uterus.

**me·tro·ste·no·sis** (me″tro-stə-no′sis) [*metro-* + *stenosis*] contraction or stenosis of the cavity of the uterus, as in Asherman's syndrome.

**me·trot·o·my** (mə-trot′ə-me) hysterotomy.

**me·tro·tu·bog·ra·phy** (me″tro-too-bog′rə-fe) hysterosalpingography.

**-metry** [Gr. *metrein* to measure] a word termination denoting the measurement of, or the science of measuring, an object specified by the word stem to which the termination is affixed.

**M. et sig.** abbreviation for L. *mi′sce et sig′na,* mix and write a label.

**Mett's (Mette's) test tubes** (mets) [Emil Ludwig Paul *Mett* (or *Mette*), German physician, born 1867] see under *test* and *tube.*

**Me·tu·bine** (mə-tu′bin) trademark for a preparation of metocurine iodide.

**met·u·la** (met′u-lə) [L., dim. of *meta* cone] a flask-shaped branch of the conidiophore of certain fungi, which has phialides; seen in *Aspergillus, Penicillium,* and other genera. Called also *sterigma.* See Plate 29.

**me·tyr·a·pone** (mə-tēr′ə-pōn) [USP] [MeSH: Metyrapone] an inhibitor of the enzyme steroid 11$\beta$-hydroxylase; used in a test of hypothalamic-pituitary function. See *metyrapone test,* under *tests.*
**m. tartrate,** the tartrate salt of metyrapone, used for the same purpose as the base; administered by intravenous infusion.

**me·ty·ro·sine** (mə-ti′ro-sēn) [USP] an inhibitor of tyrosine 3-monooxygenase, which catalyzes the first step in catecholamine synthesis, used to control hypertensive attacks in pheochromocytoma; administered orally.

**MeV, Mev** megaelectron volt.

**Mev·a·cor** (mev′ə-kor) trademark for a preparation of lovastatin.

**me·val·o·nate** (mə-val′o-nāt) a salt, ester, or anionic form of mevalonic acid.

**me·val·o·nate ki·nase** (mə-val′o-nāt ki′nās) [EC 2.7.1.36] an enzyme of the transferase class that catalyzes the ATP-dependent phosphorylation of mevalonate as a step in the biosynthesis of cholesterol and other isoprenoids. Deficiency of the enzyme causes mevalonicaciduria.

**mev·a·lon·ic ac·id** (mev-ə-lon′ik) [MeSH: Mevalonic Acid] a carboxylic acid precursor of sterols and other isoprenoids; it accumulates abnormally in mevalonicaciduria.

**me·va·lon·ic·ac·id·uria** (mev-ə-lon″ik-as″ĭ-du′re-ə) an inherited aminoacidopathy due to deficiency of mevalonate kinase and characterized by excessive excretion in the urine of mevalonic acid, with variable clinical symptoms including developmental delay, hypotonia, hepatosplenomegaly, and failure to thrive.

**Mex·ate** (mek′sāt) trademark for preparations of methotrexate sodium.

**mex·il·e·tine hy·dro·chlo·ride** (mek′sĭ-lə-tēn) an oral antiarrhythmic agent, similar to lidocaine in structure and action, used in the treatment of ventricular arrhythmias.

**Mex·i·til** (mek′sĭ-til) trademark for a preparation of mexiletine hydrochloride.

**Mey·er's disease** (mi′erz) [Hans Wilhelm *Meyer,* Danish physician, 1824–1895] see under *disease.*

**Mey·er's line, organ, sinus** (mi′erz) [Georg Hermann von *Meyer,* German anatomist, 1815–1892] see under *line, organ,* and *sinus.*

**Mey·er's loop** (mi′ərz) [Adolf B. *Meyer,* American psychiatrist, 1866–1950] see under *loop.*

**Mey·er-Ar·cham·bault loop** (mi′er-ahr-shahm-bo′) [A. *Meyer;* La Salle *Archambault,* American neurologist, 1879–1940] Meyer's loop.

**Mey·er-Betz disease** (mi′ər betz) [Friedrich *Meyer-Betz,* German physician, early 20th century] see under *disease.*

**Mey·er-Schwick·er·ath and Wey·ers syndrome** (mi′er-shvik′ə-raht and vi′erz) [Gerhard Rudolph Edmund *Meyer-Schickerath,* German ophthalmologist, born 1920; Helmut *Weyers,* German pediatrician, 20th century] oculodentodigital dysplasia; see under *dysplasia.*

**Mey·er·hof** (mi′er-hof) Otto Fritz. German physiologist, 1884–1951; co-winner, with Archibald Vivian Hill, of the Nobel prize for medicine or physiology in 1922 for his studies in cellular oxidation and his discovery of the metabolism of lactic acid in muscles.

**Mey·nert's cells, commissure,** etc. (mi'nerts) [Theodor Herman *Meynert,* German neurologist and psychiatrist in Vienna, 1833–1892] see under *cell* and *commissure,* and see *nucleus basalis telencephali* and *tractus habenulointerpeduncularis.*

**me·ze·re·in** (mə-ze're-in) a toxic glycoside found in *Daphne mezereum,* causing severe or even fatal irritation of the alimentary tract in humans and other animals.

**me·ze·re·um** (me-ze're-əm) [L.] the dried bark of *Daphne mezereum,* formerly used as a diaphoretic, diuretic, and stimulant; it is highly irritating to the gastrointestinal tract and produces vesication when rubbed on the skin.

**Mez·lin** (mez'lin) trademark for a preparation of mezlocillin sodium.

**mez·lo·cil·lin so·di·um** (mez″lo-sil'in) [USP] a semisynthetic, broad-spectrum penicillin antibiotic effective against a wide range of gram-positive and gram-negative aerobic and anaerobic bacteria; especially useful in treating mixed infections.

**μF** symbol for *microfarad.*

**M. flac.** abbreviation for L. *membrana flaccida* (pars flaccida membranae tympanicae [TA]).

**M. ft.** abbreviation for L. *mistu'ra fi'at,* let a mixture be made.

**Mg** symbol for *magnesium.*

**mg** symbol for *milligram.*

**mγ** symbol for *milligamma* (millimicrogram, micromilligram, or nanogram).

**μg** symbol for *microgram.*

**μγ** symbol for *microgamma* (micromicrogram, or picogram).

**mgm** former symbol for *milligram.*

**3MH** 3-methylhistidine.

**MHA-TP** microhemagglutination assay–*Treponema pallidum.*

**MHC** major histocompatibility complex.

**MHD** minimum hemolytic dose.

**mho** (mo) [*ohm* spelled backwards, because it is a reciprocal ohm] former name for *siemens.*

**MHz** symbol for megahertz.

**MI** myocardial infarction.

**Mi·a·cal·cin** (me-ə-kal'sin) trademark for a preparation of calcitonin-salmon.

**Mi·an·eh bug** (me'ə-na) [the city of *Mianeh,* Iran] see under *bug.*

**mi·an·ser·in hy·dro·chlo·ride** (me-an'sər-in) a tetracyclic antidepressant with antihistaminic effects; it has also been used in the treatment of chronic tension headache; administered orally.

**mi·as·ma** (mi-az'mə) [Gr. "defilement, pollution"] a supposed noxious emanation from the soil or earth, alleged to be the cause of diseases endemic in certain areas, such as malaria, before the true cause became known. See *tellurism.*

**mi·as·mat·ic** (mi″az-mat'ik) pertaining to or caused by miasma.

**mi·be·fra·dil di·hy·dro·chlo·ride** (mi-bə-fra'dil) a calcium channel blocker used in the treatment of angina and hypertension; administered orally.

**Mi·bel·li's porokeratosis** (me-bel'ēz) [Vittorio *Mibelli,* Italian dermatologist, 1860–1910] porokeratosis.

**MIBG** metaiodobenzylguanidine; see *iobenguane.*

**MIBI** sestamibi.

**mIBG** iobenguane (*m*-iodobenzylguanidine).

**mi·ca** (mi'kə) [L.] any of a group of complex aluminum silicate compounds; see also *mica pneumoconiosis,* under *pneumoconiosis.*

**mi·ca·ceous** (mi-ka'shəs) 1. pertaining to mica. 2. resembling mica, or occurring in silvery gray flakes.

**Mi·ca·nol** (mi'kənol) trademark for a preparation of anthralin.

**Mi·ca·tin** (mi'kə-tin) trademark for preparations of miconazole nitrate.

**mi·ca·tion** (mi-ka'shən) any quick motion, such as winking.

**mi·ca·to·sis** (mi″kə-to'sis) pneumoconiosis due to inhalation of and tissue reaction to mica particles.

**mi·cel·la** (mi-sel'ə) see *micelle.*

**mi·celle** (mi-sel') [MeSH: Micelles] a colloid particle formed by an aggregation of small molecules.

**Mi·chae·lis' constant, stain** (mĭ-ka'lis) [Leonor *Michaelis,* German-born American biochemist, 1875–1949] see under *constant* and *stain.*

**Mi·chae·lis' rhomboid** (mĭ-ka'lis) [Gustav Adolf *Michaelis,* German obstetrician, 1798–1848] see under *rhomboid.*

**Mi·chae·lis-Gut·mann bodies** (mĭ-ka'lis-goot'mahn) [Leonor *Michaelis;* C. *Gutmann,* German physician, 20th century] see under *body.*

**Mi·chae·lis-Men·ten equation** (mĭ-ka'lis-men'tən) [Leonor *Michaelis;* Maude Lenore *Menten,* American physician, 1879–1960] see under *equation.*

**Mi·chel's deafness** (me-shelz') [E.M. *Michel,* French physician, 19th century] see under *aplasia* and *deafness.*

**mi·con·a·zole** (mi-kon'ə-zōl) [USP] [MeSH: Miconazole] an imidazole derivative used as a broad-spectrum antifungal agent; administered by intravenous infusion in the treatment of systemic fungal infections, topically in the treatment of tinea and cutaneous candidiasis, and intravaginally in the treatment of vulvovaginal candidiasis.

**m. nitrate** [USP], a synthetic antifungal agent, used topically in the treatment of tinea pedis, tinea cruris, and tinea corpora due to *Trichophyton rubrum, T. mentagrophytes,* and *Epidermophyton floccosum;* of cutaneous candidiasis, and of tinea versicolor; and intravaginally in the treatment of vulvovaginal candidiasis.

**mi·cra** (mi'krə) plural of *micron.*

**mi·cran·at·o·my** (mi″krən-at'ə-me) [*micr-* + *anatomy*] microscopical anatomy; histology.

**mi·cren·ce·pha·lia** (mi″krən-sə-fa'le-ə) micrencephaly.

**mi·cren·ceph·a·lon** (mi″krən-sef'ə-lon) [*micr-* + *encephalon*] a small brain.

**mi·cren·ceph·a·lous** (mi″krən-sef'ə-ləs) having a small brain.

**mi·cren·ceph·a·ly** (mi″krən-sef'ə-le) [*micr-* + Gr. *enkephalos* brain] abnormal smallness of the brain.

**micr(o)-** [Gr. *mikros* small] combining form denoting small size; used in naming units of measurement to indicate one-millionth ($10^{-6}$) of the unit designated by the root with which it is combined. Symbol $\mu$.

**mi·cro·abra·sion** (mi'kro-ə-bra″zhən) the removal of minute amounts of dental enamel using an abrasive compound in order to correct enamel defects.

**mi·cro·ab·scess** (mi″kro-ab'ses) a very small, localized collection of pus.

**Munro m.,** a small focal collection of pyknotic polymorphonuclear leukocytes within the parakeratotic portion of the stratum corneum, which is one of the cardinal histologic features of active psoriasis, and also found in other dermatoses such as seborrheic dermatitis and Reiter's disease. Called also *Munro's abscess.* Cf. *spongiform pustule.*

**Pautrier's m.,** one of the well-defined collections of mycosis cells located within nonspongiotic intraepidermal vesicles in T-cell lymphoma and mycosis fungoides. Called also *Pautrier's abscess.*

**mi·cro·ad·e·nec·to·my** (mi″kro-ad″ə-nek'tə-me) [*microadenoma* + *-ectomy*] surgical removal of a microadenoma.

**mi·cro·ad·e·no·ma** (mi″kro-ad″ə-no'mə) a pituitary adenoma less than 10 mm in diameter, so that it is too small to be easily visualized by usual radiographic techniques; most endocrine-active adenomas are this size and are detected because of their hormone activities. Cf. *macroadenoma.*

**mi·cro·aero·bic** (mi-kro-ār-o'bik) microaerophilic.

**mi·cro·aero·phile** (mi″kro-ār'o-fīl) a microaerophilic microorganism.

**mi·cro·aero·phil·ic** (mi″kro-ār'o-fil″ik) [*micro-* + *aero-* + *-philic*] requiring oxygen for growth but at lower concentration than is present in the atmosphere; said of bacteria.

**mi·cro·aer·oph·i·lous** (mi″kro-ār-of'ĭ-ləs) microaerophilic.

**mi·cro·aero·to·nom·e·ter** (mi″kro-ār″o-to-nom'ə-tər) an instrument for measuring the volume of gases in the blood.

**mi·cro·ag·gre·gate** (mi″kro-ag'rə-gət) a collection of microscopic particles, such as that of platelets, leukocytes, and fibrin in stored blood.

**mi·cro·al·bu·min·uria** (mi″kro-al-bu-min-u're-ə) an increase in urinary albumin excretion too subtle to be measured by conventional means, often seen with the hyperfiltration of insulin-dependent diabetes mellitus.

**mi·cro·aleu·rio·spore** (mi″kro-ə-loo're-o-spor) a small aleuriospore; the term is sometimes used interchangeably with *microconidium.*

**mi·cro·am·me·ter** (mi″kro-am'me-tər) an instrument for measuring currents in the microampere range.

**mi·cro·am·pere** (mi″kro-am'pēr) one-millionth ($10^{-6}$) ampere. Symbol, $\mu$A.

**mi•cro•anal•y•sis** (mi″kro-ə-nal′ə-sis) [*micro-* + *analysis*] the chemical analysis of minute quantities of material.

**mi•cro•an•as•to•mo•sis** (mi″kro-ən-as″tə-mo′sis) anastomosis between very small tubular structures.

**mi•cro•anat•o•my** (mi″kro-ə-nat′ə-me) histology, especially organology.

**mi•cro•an•eu•rysm** (mi″kro-an′u-riz″əm) a microscopic aneurysm, a characteristic feature of diabetes mellitus.

**mi•cro•an•gio•path•ic** (mi″kro-an″je-o-path′ik) pertaining to or characterized by microangiopathy.

**mi•cro•an•gi•op•a•thy** (mi″kro-an″je-op′ə-the) [*micro-* + *angiopathy*] disease of the small blood vessels.
**diabetic m.**, the presence of generalized basement membrane thickening of capillaries throughout many vascular beds, occurring in diabetics.
**thrombotic m.**, the formation of thrombi in the arterioles and capillaries, as occurs in thrombotic thrombocytopenic purpura and hemolytic uremic syndrome.

**mi•cro•an•gi•os•co•py** (mi″kro-an″je-os′kə-pe) capillaroscopy.

**Mi•cro•as•ca•ceae** (mi″kro-as-ka′se-e) a family of fungi of the order Microascales, subdivision Ascomycotina, which are mostly saprobes; pathogenic genera include *Microascus* and *Pseudallescheria*.

**Mi•cro•as•ca•les** (mi″kro-as-ka′lēz) [*micro-* + *ascus*] an order of perfect fungi of the subphylum Ascomycotina, consisting mainly of saprobes from soil and dung and characterized by prototunicate asci; it includes the family Microascaceae.

**Mi•cro•as•cus** (mi″kro-as′kəs) a genus of fungi of the family Microascaceae. *M. cine′reus* has been isolated from onychomycosis and other human infections.

**mi•cro•bac•te•ria** (mi″kro-bak-tēr′e-ə) [L.] plural of *microbacterium*.

**Mi•cro•bac•te•ri•um** (mi″kro-bak-tēr′e-əm) a genus of coryneform bacteria of uncertain status, consisting of small diphtheroid, gram-positive, rod-shaped organisms, found in dairy products, and characterized by resistance to heat.
**M. fla′vum,** an aerobic species occurring predominantly in dairy products and producing lactic acid without gas in carbohydrate fermentation.
**M. lac′ticum,** an aerobic species occurring in the intestinal tract and producing lactic acid without gas in carbohydrate fermentation.

**mi•cro•bac•te•ri•um** (mi″kro-bak-tēr′e-əm) pl. *microbacte′ria* [L.] 1. an organism belonging to the genus Microbacterium. 2. a microorganism.

**mi•cro•bal•ance** (mi′kro-bal″əns) a balance for measuring minute quantities.

**mi•cro•bar** (mi′kro-bahr) a unit of pressure, being one-millionth ($10^{-6}$) bar.

**mi•crobe** (mi′krōb) [*micro-* + Gr. *bios* life] a minute living organism, a microphyte or microzoon; applied especially to those minute forms of life which are capable of causing disease in animals, including bacteria, protozoa, and fungi.

**mi•cro•bi•al** (mi-kro′be-əl) of or pertaining to or caused by microbes.

**mi•cro•bi•an** (mi-kro′be-ən) 1. pertaining to or of the nature of a microbe. 2. a microbe.

**mi•cro•bic** (mi-kro′bik) microbial.

**mi•cro•bi•ci•dal** (mi-kro″bĭ-si′dəl) [*microbe* + *-cide* + *-al*] destructive to microbes.

**mi•cro•bi•cide** (mi-kro′bĭ-sīd) [*microbe* + *-cide*] an agent that destroys microbes.

**mi•cro•bio•as•say** (mi″kro-bi″o-as′a) the determination of minute quantities of an active substance or nutrient factor by a biologic method.

**mi•cro•bi•o•log•i•cal** (mi″kro-bi″o-loj′ĭ-kəl) pertaining to microbiology.

**mi•cro•bi•ol•o•gist** (mi″kro-bi-ol′ə-jist) one specializing in microbiology.

**mi•cro•bi•ol•o•gy** (mi″kro-bi-ol′ə-je) [*micro-* + *biology*] [MeSH: Microbiology] the science that deals with the study of microorganisms, including algae, bacteria, fungi, protozoa, and viruses.

**mi•cro•bio•pho•tom•e•ter** (mi″kro-bi″o-fo-tom′ə-tər) an instrument for measuring the growth of bacterial cultures by the turbidity of the medium.

**mi•cro•bi•o•ta** (mi″kro-bi-o′tə) the microscopic living organisms of a region; the combined microflora and microfauna of a region.

**mi•cro•bi•ot•ic** (mi″kro-bi-ot′ik) pertaining to the microbiota, or to microscopic living organisms.

**mi•cro•blast** (mi′kro-blast) [*micro-* + *-blast*] an abnormally small erythroblast.

**mi•cro•ble•pha•ria** (mi″kro-blə-fa′re-ə) [*micro-* + *blephar-* + *-ia*] a developmental anomaly characterized by abnormal shortness of the vertical dimensions of the eyelids.

**mi•cro•bleph•a•rism** (mi″kro-blef′ə-riz″əm) microblepharia.

**mi•cro•bleph•a•ry** (mi″kro-blef′ə-re) microblepharia.

**mi•cro•body** (mi″kro-bod′e) [MeSH: Microbodies] 1. any of the membrane-bound, ovoid or spherical, granular cytoplasmic particles containing enzymes and other substances, which originate in the endoplasmic reticulum of vertebrate liver and kidney cells and other cells, and in protozoa, yeast, and many cell types of higher plants. Two types of microbodies are *peroxisomes* (found in vertebrates) and *glyoxysomes* (found in plants and microorganisms). 2. peroxisome.

**mi•cro•bra•chia** (mi″kro-bra′ke-ə) [*micro-* + *brachia*] abnormal smallness of the arms.

**mi•cro•bra•chi•us** (mi″kro-bra′ke-əs) [*micro-* + Gr. *brachiōn* arm] a fetus with abnormally small arms.

**mi•cro•bren•ner** (mi″kro-bren′ər) [*micro-* + Ger. *Brenner* burner] a needle-pointed electric cautery.

**mi•cro•bub•ble** (mi′kro-bub″əl) a very small bubble.

**mi•cro•bu•ret** (mi″kro-bu-ret′) a buret with a capacity of the order of 0.1 to 10 mL, with graduated intervals of 0.001 to 0.02 mL.

**mi•cro•cal•ci•fi•ca•tion** (mi″kro-kal″sĭ-fĭ-ka′shən) a minute area of calcification in the tissues.

**mi•cro•cal•ci•fi•cec•to•my** (mi″kro-kal″sĭ-fĭ-sek′to-me) surgical excision of calcifications.

**mi•cro•ca•lix** (mi″kro-ka′liks) a very small renal calix arising by caliceal branching, usually at the side of a calix of normal size. Written also *microcalyx*.

**mi•cro•ca•lyx** (mi″kro-ka′liks) microcalix.

**mi•cro•car•dia** (mi″kro-kahr′de-ə) [*micro-* + *cardia*] smallness of the heart.

**mi•cro•cen•trum** (mi″kro-sen′trəm) [*micro-* + *centrum*] centrosphere, def. 1.

**mi•cro•ce•pha•lia** (mi″kro-sə-fa′le-ə) microcephaly.

**mi•cro•ce•phal•ic** (mi″kro-sə-fal′ik) pertaining to or exhibiting microcephaly.

**mi•cro•ceph•a•lism** (mi″kro-sef′ə-liz″əm) microcephaly.

**mi•cro•ceph•a•lous** (mi″kro-sef′ə-ləs) microcephalic.

**mi•cro•ceph•a•lus** (mi″kro-sef′ə-ləs) an individual with a very small head.

**mi•cro•ceph•a•ly** (mi″kro-sef′ə-le) [*micro-* + *cephaly*] [MeSH: Microcephaly] abnormal smallness of the head, usually associated with mental retardation.

**mi•cro•chei•lia** (mi″kro-ki′le-ə) [*micro-* + *cheil-* + *-ia*] abnormal smallness of the lips.

**mi•cro•chei•ria** (mi″kro-ki′re-ə) [*micro-* + *cheir-* + *-ia*] abnormal smallness of the hands, as a result of hypoplasia of all the skeletal elements.

**mi•cro•chem•i•cal** (mi″kro-kem′ĭ-kəl) pertaining to microchemistry.

**mi•cro•chem•is•try** (mi″kro-kem′is-tre) [*micro-* + *chemistry*] [MeSH: Microchemistry] the study of chemical reactions using quantities invisible to the naked eye; chemistry which deals with minute quantities (a few milligrams) of substances, using apparatus of small size. Cf. *macrochemistry*.

**mi•cro•cin•e•ma•tog•ra•phy** (mi″kro-sin″ə-mə-tog′rə-fe) [*micro-* + Gr. *kinēma* movement + *graphein* to write] the making of moving picture photographs of microscopic subjects. Called also *microkinematography*. See also *cinemicrography*.

**mi•cro•cir•cu•la•tion** (mi″kro-sir″ku-la′shən) [MeSH: Microcirculation] the flow of blood in the microvasculature of the body.

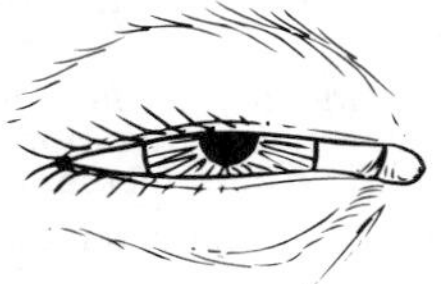
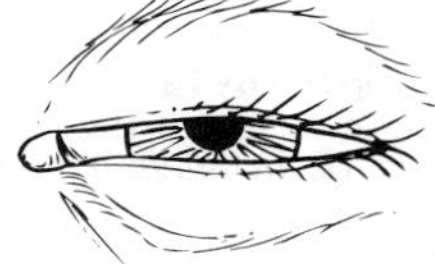

Microblepharia.

**mi·cro·cir·cu·la·to·ry** (mi″kro-sər′ku-lə-tor″e) pertaining to or affecting the microcirculation.

**mi·cro·cli·mate** (mi″kro-kli′mət) [MeSH: Microclimate] the immediate climatic environment, as that of a vector insect.

**mi·cro·cne·mia** (mi″kro-ne′me-ə) [*micro-* + Gr. *knēmē* tibia] abnormal shortness of the leg.

**Mi·cro·coc·ca·ceae** (mi″kro-kŏ-ka′se-e) [*micro-* + Gr. *kokkos* berry] [MeSH: Micrococcaceae] a family of gram-positive, aerobic or facultatively anaerobic bacteria made up of spherical cells that divide primarily in two or three planes, which sometimes remain in contact after division to form clusters or packets. Genera include *Micrococcus, Sarcina,* and *Staphylococcus.*

**mi·cro·coc·ci** (mi″kro-kok′si) plural of *micrococcus.*

**Mi·cro·coc·cus** (mi″kro-kok′əs) [MeSH: Micrococcus] a genus of bacteria of the family Micrococcaceae, consisting of spherical, gram-positive, aerobic cells, usually occurring in irregular masses. Saprophytic and nonpathogenic forms are found in soil, water, dust, and dairy products.

**mi·cro·coc·cus** (mi″kro-kok′əs) pl. *micrococ′ci* [MeSH: Micrococcus] 1. an organism of the genus *Micrococcus.* 2. a spherical microorganism of extremely small size.

**mi·cro·co·lon** (mi″kro-ko′lon) an abnormally small colon.

**mi·cro·col·o·ny** (mi′kro-kol″ə-ne) a microscopic colony of bacteria.

**mi·cro·con·cen·tra·tion** (mi″kro-kon″sən-tra′shən) a minute amount of solute, less than 0.05 per cent of the solution.

**mi·cro·co·nid·i·um** (mi″kro-ko-nid′e-əm) pl. *microconid′ia.* A small, usually single-celled conidium or exospore in a fungus that also produces macroconidia; the term is sometimes used interchangeably with *microaleuriospore.*

**mi·cro·co·ria** (mi″kro-ko′re-ə) [*micro-* + *coro-* + *-ia*] congenital usually hereditary smallness of the pupil.

**mi·cro·cor·nea** (mi″kro-kor′ne-ə) [*micro-* + *cornea*] a usually bilateral developmental anomaly, in which the cornea is unusually small (less than 11 mm after one year of age), due to arrest of development. It may be associated with other ocular abnormalities, such as microphthalmia, hydrophthalmia, multiple defects of the anterior chamber, cataract, and glaucoma, and may be inherited as an X-linked recessive or as an autosomal dominant trait.

**mi·cro·cou·lomb** (mi″kro-koo′lom) a unit of quantity of current electricity, being one one-millionth ($10^{-6}$) of a coulomb. Symbol, $\mu$C.

**mi·cro·cra·nia** (mi″kro-kra′ne-ə) abnormal smallness of the skull, the cranial cavity being reduced in all diameters, and the facial area being disproportionately large in comparison.

**mi·cro·crys·tal** (mi′kro-kris″təl) an extremely minute crystal.

**mi·cro·crys·tal·line** (mi″kro-kris″tə-lin) made up of minute crystals.

**mi·cro·cu·rie** (mi′kro-ku″re) a unit of radioactivity, being one one-millionth ($10^{-6}$) curie, or the quantity of radioactive material in which the number of nuclear disintegrations is $3.7 \times 10^4$ per second. Abbreviated $\mu$C.

**mi·cro·cu·rie-hour** (mi′kro-ku″re-our″) a unit of exposure equivalent to that obtained by exposure for one hour to radioactive material disintegrating at the rate of $3.7 \times 10^4$ atoms per second. Abbreviated $\mu$C-hr.

**mi·cro·cyst** (mi′kro-sist) [*micro-* + *cyst*] 1. a very small cyst. 2. in bacteriology, a type of resting cell developed from the vegetative cells of certain species of Myxobacterales and Nocardiaceae. 3. in mycology, a resting cell produced by certain slime molds. Cf. *macrocyst.*

**Mi·cro·cys·tis** (mi″kro-sis′tis) a genus of cyanobacteria that sometimes contaminates water and can cause cyanobacteria poisoning. Called also *Anacystis.*

**mi·cro·cys·tom·e·ter** (mi″kro-sis-tom′ə-tər) a small portable cystometer.

**mi·cro·cyte** (mi′kro-sīt) [*micro-* + *-cyte*] 1. an abnormally small erythrocyte, i.e., one 5 $\mu$m or less in diameter. Called also *microerythrocyte.* 2. microglial cell.
**hypochromic m.,** a small erythrocyte with less than the usual coloring, as seen in iron deficiency anemia.

**mi·cro·cy·the·mia** (mi″kro-si-the′me-ə) [*microcyte* + *hem-* + *-ia*] a condition in which the erythrocytes are smaller than normal; see also *microcytic anemia,* under *anemia.* Called alse *microcytosis.*

**mi·cro·cyt·ic** (mi″kro-sit′ik) pertaining to or characterized by microcytes.

**mi·cro·cy·to·sis** (mi″kro-si-to′sis) microcythemia.

**mi·cro·cy·to·tox·ic·i·ty** (mi″kro-si″to-tok-sis′ĭ-te) [*micro-* + *cytotoxicity*] the capability of lysing or damaging cells by procedures that use extremely minute amounts of material such as target cells, antibody, and complement (e.g., lymphotoxicity procedures).

**mi·cro·dac·tyl·ia** (mi″kro-dak-til′e-ə) microdactyly.

**mi·cro·dac·ty·ly** (mi″kro-dak′tə-le) [*micro-* + Gr. *daktylos* finger] abnormal smallness of the digits.

**mi·cro·dens·i·tom·e·ter** (mi″kro-dens″ĭ-tom′ə-tər) an instrument used in spectroscopy to measure lines in a spectrum by light transmission measurement.

**mi·cro·der·ma·tome** (mi″kro-dər′mə-tōm) an instrument for cutting very thin skin sections.

**mi·cro·de·ter·mi·na·tion** (mi″kro-de-tər″mĭ-na′shən) a chemical examination in which minute quantities of the substance to be examined are used.

**mi·cro·dis·kec·to·my** (mi″kro-dis-kek′tə-me) debulking of a herniated nucleus pulposus using an operating microscope or loupe for magnification.
**arthroscopic m.,** microdiskectomy performed with instruments introduced into the area of herniation through an arthroscope.

**mi·cro·dis·sec·tion** (mi″kro-di-sek′shən) dissection of tissue or cells under the microscope.

**mi·cro·dont** (mi′kro-dont) [*micro-* + Gr. *odous* tooth] having an abnormally small tooth or teeth.

**mi·cro·don·tia** (mi″kro-don′shə) [*micro-* + *odont-* + *-ia*] a developmental disorder characterized by abnormal smallness of the teeth; it may affect a single tooth or all of the teeth, or teeth of normal size may appear abnormally small in proportion to abnormally large jaws. Called also *microdontism.*

**mi·cro·don·tic** (mi″kro-don′tik) pertaining to or characterized by microdontia.

**mi·cro·don·tism** (mi″kro-don′tiz-əm) microdontia.

**mi·cro·do·sage** (mi′kro-do″səj) dosage in small quantities.

**mi·cro·dose** (mi′kro-dōs) a very small dose.

**mi·cro·drep·a·no·cyt·ic** (mi″kro-drep″ə-no-sit′ik) containing microcytic and drepanocytic elements, as in sickle cell–thalassemia disease.

**mi·cro·drep·a·no·cy·to·sis** (mi″kro-drep″ə-no-si-to′sis) sickle cell–thalassemia disease.

**mi·cro·dys·ge·ne·sia** (mi″kro-dis-jə-ne′zhə) subtle abnormalities of neurons in the area surrounding the hippocampus and cerebellum, seen in cases of epilepsy.

**mi·cro·ecol·o·gy** (mi″kro-ĕ-kol′ə-je) the branch of ecology of parasites concerned with the relationships of the organisms and the environment provided by the hosts.

**mi·cro·eco·sys·tem** (mi″kro-ĕ″ko-sis′təm) a miniature ecological system, occurring naturally or produced in the laboratory for experimental purposes.

**mi·cro·elec·trode** (mi″kro-ə-lek′trōd) [MeSH: Microelectrodes] an electrode with an extremely small tip, used in a voltage clamp or other apparatus to stimulate or record bioelectric potentials of single cells intracellularly or extracellularly.

**mi·cro·elec·tro·pho·re·sis** (mi″kro-e-lek″tro-fə-re′sis) electrophoresis in which migrating particles are observed by light microscopy.

**mi·cro·elec·tro·pho·ret·ic** (mi″kro-e-lek″tro-fə-ret′ik) pertaining to microelectrophoresis.

**mi·cro·em·bo·lus** (mi″kro-em′bo-ləs) pl. *microem′boli.* An embolus of microscopic size.

**mi·cro·en·ceph·a·ly** (mi″kro-ən-sef′ə-le) micrencephaly.

**mi·cro·en·vi·ron·ment** (mi″kro-ən-vi′ron-mənt) the environment at the microscopic or cellular level.

**mi·cro·eryth·ro·cyte** (mi″kro-ə-rith′ro-sīt) microcyte (def. 1).

**mi·cro·es·ti·ma·tion** (mi″kro-es″tĭ-ma′shən) microdetermination.

**mi·cro·far·ad** (mi″kro-far′əd) a unit of electrical capacity, being one one-millionth of a farad ($10^{-6}$ F). Symbol $\mu$F.

**mi·cro·fau·na** (mi″kro-faw′nə) the animal life, visible only under the microscope, which is present in or characteristic of a special location.

**mi·cro·fi·bril** (mi″kro-fi′bril) an extremely small fibril.

**mi·cro·fil·a·ment** (mi″kro-fil′ə-mənt) [MeSH: Microfilaments] any of the submicroscopic filaments composed chiefly of actin, found in the cytoplasmic matrix of almost all cells, often in close association with the microtubules; they are believed by some to have a supportive and cytoskeletal function and/or to mediate movement of the cell and of the organelles within it.

**mi·cro·fil·a·re·mia** (mi″kro-fil″ə-re′me-ə) the presence of microfilariae in the circulating blood.

**mi·cro·fi·la·ria** (mi″kro-fĭ-lar′e-ə) [MeSH: Microfilaria] the prelarval stage of Filarioidea in the blood of man and in the tissues of the vector. This term is sometimes incorrectly used as a genus and is then spelled with a capital M.

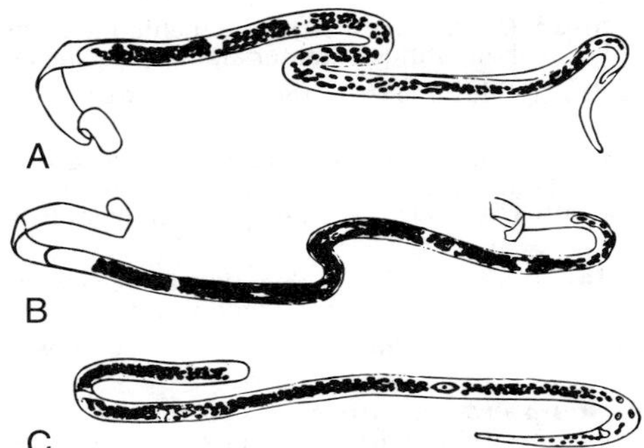


Microfilariae of *(A), Wuchereria bancrofti,* 270 μm × 8.5 μm; *(B), Loa loa,* 275 μm × 7.0 μm; *(C), Onchocerca volvulus,* 320 μm × 7.5 μm. *A* and *B* have sheaths covering the body.

**m. bancrof′ti,** the microfilaria of *Wuchereria bancrofti.*
**m. diur′na,** the microfilaria of *Loa loa.*
**m. lo′a,** the microfilaria of *Loa loa.*
**m. streptocer′ca,** the microfilaria of *Dipetalonema streptocerca,* found in the subcutaneous tissues.
**m. vol′vulus,** the prelarval form of *Onchocerca volvulus,* found in skin snips taken from infected persons.

**mi·cro·film** (mi′kro-film) 1. a trade term for 16- or 35-millimeter film to be used in high-speed automatic machines for the photographic reproduction, in greatly reduced size, of books, documents, forms, or other record files. 2. to photographically reproduce, in greatly reduced size, on film specially designed for the purpose.

**mi·cro·fil·ter** (mi′kro-fil″tər) a filter that removes particles with diameters of 0.1–10.0 μm; used, for example, to remove microbubbles and microaggregates from the blood in cardiopulmonary bypass.

**mi·cro·flo·ra** (mi″kro-flor′ə) the entire population of microorganisms present in or characteristic of a special location.

**mi·cro·flu·or·om·e·try** (mi″kro-flo͞o-rom′ə-tre) cytophotometry.

**mi·cro·frac·ture** (mi″kro-frak′chər) a minute, incomplete break or area of discontinuity in a bone.

**mi·cro·gam·ete** (mi″kro-gam′ēt) [*micro-* + *gamete*] the smaller, often flagellated, actively motile male anisogamete.

**mi·cro·ga·me·to·cyte** (mi″kro-gə-me′to-sīt) [*micro-* + *gametocyte*] microgamont.

**mi·cro·ga·me·to·phyte** (mi″kro-gə-me′to-fīt) [*micro-* + *gameto-* + *-phyte*] the male gametophyte in heterosporous plants, developed from the microspore.

**mi·cro·gam·ma** (mi″kro-gam′ə) picogram.

**mi·cro·gam·ont** (mi″kro-gam′ont) [*micro-* + *gamont*] a gamont that produces microgametes by fission. Called also *microgametocyte.*

**mi·crog·a·my** (mi-krog′ə-me) conjugation or fusion when the gametes are smaller than the somatic cells.

**mi·cro·gas·tria** (mi″kro-gas′tre-ə) [*micro-* + *gastr-* + *-ia*] congenital smallness of the stomach.

**mi·cro·gen·e·sis** (mi″kro-jen′ə-sis) [*micro-* + *-genesis*] abnormally small development of a part.

**mi·cro·gen·ia** (mi″kro-jen′e-ə) [*micro-* + *geni-* + *-ia*] an extremely small chin, caused by underdevelopment of the mandibular symphysis or malocclusion with excessive prominence of alveolar structures. See also *micrognathia.*

**mi·cro·gen·i·tal·ism** (mi″kro-jen′ĭ-təl-iz-əm) [*micro-* + *genitalism*] abnormal smallness of the external genitals.

**mi·crog·lia** (mi-krog′le-ə) [*micro-* + *-glia*] [MeSH: Microglia] the small, non-neural, interstitial cells of mesodermal origin that form part of the supporting structure of the central nervous system. They are of various forms and may have slender branched processes. They are migratory and act as phagocytes to waste products of nerve tissue. See also *microglial cell* and *gitter cell.*

**mi·crog·lia·cyte** (mi-krog′le-ə-sīt) microglial cell.

**mi·crog·li·al** (mi-krog′le-əl) of or pertaining to the microglia.

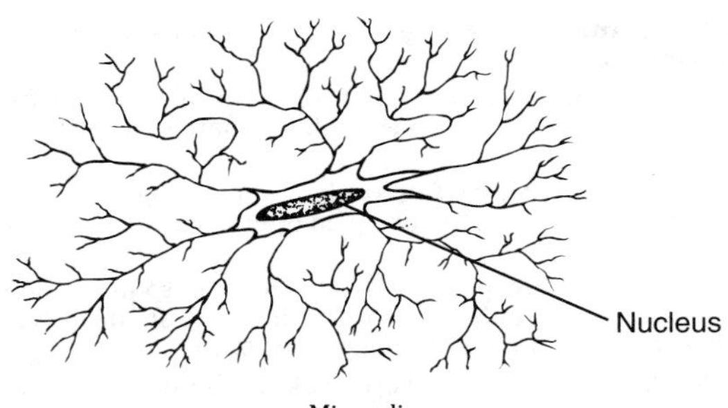


Microglia.

**mi·crog·lio·cyte** (mi-krog′le-o-sīt) microglial cell.

**mi·cro·gli·o·ma** (mi″kro-gli-o′mə) former name for *primary central nervous system lymphoma.*

**mi·cro·gli·o·ma·to·sis** (mi″kro-gli″o-mə-to′sis) former name for *primary central nervous system lymphoma.*

**mi·cro·glob·u·lin** (mi″kro-glob′u-lin) any globulin, or any fragment of a globulin, of low molecular weight.

**$\beta_2$-mi·cro·glob·u·lin** (mi″kro-glob′u-lin) see *beta$_2$-microglobulin.*

**mi·cro·glos·sia** (mi″kro-glos′e-ə) [*micro-* + *gloss-* + *-ia*] undersize of the tongue.

**mi·cro·gna·thia** (mi″kro-na′the-ə) [*micro-* + *gnath-* + *-ia*] 1. abnormal smallness of the mandible; see also *vertical overlap* (def. 1). Called also *bird-beak jaw, parrot jaw, micromandible,* and *brachygnathia.* 2. micromaxilla.

**mi·cro·go·nio·scope** (mi″kro-go′ne-o-skōp) [*micro-* + *gonioscope*] a magnifying gonioscope.

**mi·cro·gram** (mi′kro-gram) a unit of mass (weight) of the metric system, being one one-millionth of a gram ($10^{-6}$ gm), or one one-thousandth of a milligram ($10^{-3}$ mg). Symbol μg (formerly γ). Abbreviated mcg.

**mi·cro·graph** (mi′kro-graf) 1. an instrument for recording extremely minute movements. It acts by making a greatly magnified record on a photographic film of the minute motions of a diaphragm. 2. the photograph of a minute object or specimen (tissue, etc.) as seen through a microscope.
**electron m.,** the photograph of an object through an electron microscope.

**mi·cro·graph·ia** (mi″kro-graf′e-ə) [*micro-* + *graph-* + *-ia*] a dysgraphia in which handwriting is tiny or decreases in size from normal to minute, seen in parkinsonism.

**mi·crog·ra·phy** (mi-krog′rə-fe) [*micro-* + *-graphy*] 1. an account of microscopic objects. 2. microscopy.

**mi·cro·grav·i·ty** (mi′kro-grav″ĭ-te) the minute amount of gravitational force existing in outer space; it results in a weightless condition and enhances the likelihood of certain diseases.

**mi·cro·gyr·ia** (mi″kro-ji′re-ə) [*micro-* + *gyr-* + *-ia*] polymicrogyria.

**mi·cro·gy·rus** (mi″kro-ji′rəs) pl. *microgy′ri* [*micro-* + *gyrus*] an abnormally small, malformed convolution of the brain, as seen in polymicrogyria.

**mi·cro·he·mat·o·crit** (mi″kro-he-mat′ə-krit) a hematocrit determination done on an extremely small quantity of blood, by use of a capillary tube and a high speed centrifuge.

**mi·cro·he·pat·ia** (mi″kro-hə-pat′e-ə) [*micro-* + *hepat-* + *-ia*] smallness of the liver.

**mi·cro·his·tol·o·gy** (mi″kro-his-tol′ə-je) histology.

**mi·cro·in·cin·er·a·tion** (mi″kro-in-sin″ər-a′shən) the incineration of minute specimens of tissue or other substance, for identification from the ash of the elements composing it.

**mi·cro·in·farct** (mi″kro-in′fahrkt) a very small infarct due to obstruction of circulation in capillaries, arterioles, or small arteries.

**mi·cro·in·jec·tor** (mi″kro-in-jek′tər) an instrument for infusion of very small amounts of fluids or drugs into animals or humans.

**mi·cro·in·ter·lock** (mi″kro-in′tər-lok″) the growth of mineralized bone into the porous surface of a specially constructed prosthesis, anchoring the prosthesis into place.

**mi·cro·in·va·sion** (mi″kro-in-va′zhən) microscopic extension of malignant cells into adjacent tissue in carcinoma *in situ.*

**mi·cro·in·va·sive** (mi″kro-in-va′siv) exhibiting or pertaining to microinvasion.

**Mi·cro-K** (mi″kro-ka′) trademark for a preparation of potassium chloride.

**mi·cro·kin·e·ma·tog·ra·phy** (mi″kro-kin″ə-mə-tog′rə-fe) microcinematography.

**mi·cro·ker·a·tome** (mi″kro-kər′ə-tōm) an instrument for removing a thin slice, or creating a thin hinged flap, on the surface of the cornea.

**mi·cro·lam·i·nec·to·my** (mi″kro-lam″ĭ-nek′to-me) excision of the posterior arch of a vertebra using an operative microscope or loupe for magnification.

**mi·cro·lar·yn·gos·co·py** (mi″kro-lar″ing-gos′kə-pe) [*micro-* + *laryngo-* + *scopy*] examination of the interior of the larynx with a laryngoscope with binocular magnification.

**mi·cro·leak·age** (mi″kro-le′kəj) leakage of minute amounts of fluids, debris, and microorganisms through the microscopic space between a dental restoration or its cement and the adjacent surface of the cavity preparation; it may progress through the dentin into the pulp.

**mi·cro·lec·i·thal** (mi″kro-les′ĭ-thəl) [*micro-* + *-lecithal*] containing little yolk; see *microlecithal ovum,* under *ovum.*

**mi·cro·le·sion** (mi″kro-le′zhən) a minute lesion.

**mi·cro·leu·ko·blast** (mi″kro-loo′ko-blast) myeloblast.

**Mi·cro·lite** (mi′kro-līt) trademark for a kit for the preparation of technetium Tc 99m albumin colloid.

**mi·cro·li·ter** (mi′kro-le″tər) [Fr. *microlitre; micro-* + *liter*] a thousandth part of a milliliter or a millionth part of a liter. Usually abbreviated $\mu$L or $\mu$l. Former symbol $\lambda$.

**mi·cro·lith** (mi′kro-lith) [*micro-* + *-lith*] a minute concretion or calculus.

**mi·cro·li·thi·a·sis** (mi″kro-lĭ-thi′ə-sis) [*micro-* + *lithiasis*] the formation of minute concretions in an organ.
**m. alveola′ris pulmo′num, pulmonary alveolar m.,** a condition caused by deposition in the alveoli of the lungs of minute calculi, which appear radiographically as fine, sandlike mottling.

**mi·crol·o·gy** (mi-krol′ə-je) [*micro-* + *-logy*] the science dealing with the handling and preparation of materials for microscopic study.

**mi·cro·man·di·ble** (mi″kro-man′dĭ-bəl) micrognathia, def. 1.

**mi·cro·ma·nip·u·la·tion** (mi″kro-mə-nip″u-la′shən) [MeSH: Micromanipulation] 1. the performance of surgery, injections, dissections, etc., by means of micromanipulators. 2. in the treatment of male infertility, the processing of gametes, as by partial removal of the zona pellucida or direct injection of sperm into the egg, in order to increase the possibility of fertilization.

**mi·cro·ma·nip·u·la·tor** (mi″kro-mə-nip′u-la″tor) an attachment to a microscope for manipulating tiny instruments used in examination and dissection of minute objects under the microscope.

**mi·cro·ma·nom·e·ter** (mi″kro-mə-nom′ə-tər) an apparatus for indicating gas or vapor pressure from a very small sample, as of blood or other fluid.

**mi·cro·mano·met·ric** (mi″kro-man″o-met′rik) relating to gas or vapor pressure from very small samples, as of blood or other fluid.

**mi·cro·mas·tia** (mi″kro-mas′te-ə) abnormal smallness of the mamma.

**mi·cro·max·il·la** (mi″kro-mək-sil′ə) abnormal smallness of the maxilla; called also *micrognathia.*

**mi·cro·ma·zia** (mi″kro-ma′ze-ə) [*micro-* + *maz-* + *-ia*] micromastia.

**mi·cro·meg·a·lop·sia** (mi″kro-meg″ə-lop′se-ə) [*micro-* + *megal-* + *-opsia*] the condition in which objects appear too small or too large, or too small and too large by turns.

**mi·cro·me·lia** (mi″kro-me′le-ə) [*micro-* + *-melia*] a developmental anomaly characterized by abnormal smallness or shortness of the limbs.

**mi·crom·e·lus** (mi-krom′ə-ləs) an individual exhibiting micromelia.

**mi·cro·mere** (mi′kro-mēr) [*micro-* + *-mere*] one of the small blastomeres formed by unequal cleavage of a fertilized oocyte, located in the animal hemisphere and dividing more rapidly than the macromeres of the vegetal hemisphere.

**mi·cro·me·tab·o·lism** (mi″kro-mə-tab′ə-liz-əm) metabolism as studied by micromethods.

**mi·cro·me·tas·ta·sis** (mi″kro-mə-tas′tə-sis) the spread of cancer cells from the primary tumor to distant sites, where they form microscopic secondary tumors.

**mi·cro·meta·stat·ic** (mi″kro-met″ə-stat′ik) 1. pertaining to or caused by micrometastasis. 2. clinically undetectable; said of a metastatic tumor.

**mi·crom·e·ter**[1] (mi-krom′ə-tər) [*micro-* + *-meter*] an instrument for measuring objects seen through the microscope.
**eyepiece m.,** a micrometer that is used in connection with the eyepiece of a microscope.
**filar m.,** an eyepiece micrometer in which the micrometer screw acts upon a slide carrying a movable wire: one revolution of the screw moves the wire 1 mm across the field.
**ocular m.,** eyepiece m.
**stage m.,** a micrometer fastened to the stage of a microscope.

**mi·cro·me·ter**[2] (mi′kro-me″tər) one-millionth ($10^{-6}$) of a meter; symbol $\mu$m. Formerly called *micron* (symbol $\mu$).

**mi·cro·meth·od** (mi″kro-meth′əd) any technique involving use of exceedingly small quantities of material. Cf. *macromethod.*

**mi·crom·e·try** (mi-krom′ə-tre) the measurement of microscopic objects.

**micromicro-** a prefix used in naming units of measurement to indicate one-millionth of one-millionth ($10^{-12}$) of the unit designated by the root with which it is combined. Now supplanted by the prefix *pico-.*

**mi·cro·mo·lar** (mi″kro-mo′lər) denoting a concentration of one millionth ($10^{-6}$) of a mole per liter. Symbol $\mu$M.

**mi·cro·mo·lec·u·lar** (mi″kro-mo-lek′u-lər) composed of small molecules.

**Mi·cro·mo·nos·po·ra** (mi″kro-mə-nos′pə-rə) [*micro-* + Gr. *monos* single + *sporos* seed] [MeSH: Micromonospora] a genus of bacteria of the family Micromonosporaceae, made up of gram-positive, spore-forming, generally aerobic organisms that form a branched mycelium; they occur as saprophytic forms in soil and water. Various species are sources of aminoglycoside antibiotics.
**M. inyoen′sis,** a species that produces sisomicin.
**M. keratoly′ticum,** a species that causes cracked heel disease. See also *keratolysis plantare sulcatum.*
**M. purpu′rea,** a species that produces gentamycin.

**Mi·cro·mo·nos·po·ra·ceae** (mi″kro-mə-nos″pə-ra′se-e) [MeSH: Micromonosporaceae] a family of bacteria of the order Actinomycetales, made up of gram-positive, spore-forming soil organisms that form a true mycelium. It contains the genera *Actinobifida, Microbispora, Micromonospora, Micropolyspora, Thermoactinomyces,* and *Thermomonospora.*

**Mi·crom·y·ces** (mi-krom′ĭ-sēz) [*micro-* + Gr. *mykēs* fungus] in former systems of classification, a genus of bacteria made up of organisms now included in the genus *Mycoplasma.*

**mi·cro·my·e·lia** (mi″kro-mi-e′le-ə) [*micro-* + *myel-* + *-ia*] abnormal smallness of the spinal cord.

**mi·cro·my·elo·blast** (mi″kro-mi′ə-lo-blast) a small, immature myelocyte, observed in micromyeloblastic leukemia.

**mi·cron** (mi′kron) pl. *mi′crons, mi′cra* [Gr. *mikros* small] one-millionth ($10^{-6}$) of a meter; now replaced by the SI unit *micrometer* ($\mu$m). Symbol $\mu$.

**Mi·cro·nase** (mi′kro-nās) trademark for a preparation of glyburide.

**mi·cro·nee·dle** (mi″kro-ne′dəl) a fine glass needle for use in micrurgy.

**Mi·cro·ne·ma** (mi″kro-ne′mə) *Halicephalobus.*

**mi·cro·nem·a·tous** (mi″kro-nem′ə-təs) [*micro-* + Gr. *nēma* thread] said of a conidiophore that is similar morphologically to its hypha.

**mi·cro·neme** (mi″kro-nēm) [*micro-* + Gr. *nēma* thread] any of the electron-dense, convoluted tubular organelles forming part of the apical complex in apicocomplexan protozoa, which are often associated with or give rise to the rhoptries. Called also *sarconeme.*

**mi·cro·neu·rog·ra·phy** (mi″kro-noo͝-rog′rə-fe) the study of conduction in individual nerve fibers or bundles of fibers using a microelectrode.

**mi·cro·neu·ro·sur·gery** (mi″kro-noo͝″ro-sər′jər-e) surgery conducted under high magnification with miniaturized instruments on microscopic vessels and structures of the nervous system.

**mi·cro·nize** (mi′kro-nīz) [Gr. *micron* a small thing] to reduce to a fine powder; to reduce to particles a micron in diameter.

**mi·cro·nod·u·lar** (mi″kro-nod′u-lər) marked by the presence of small nodules.

**mi·cro·nor·mo·blast** (mi″kro-nor′mo-blast) an abnormal red cell precursor in which there has been defective hemoglobin synthesis, characterized by a narrow rim of cytoplasm and an overdeveloped pyknotic nucleus.

**mi·cro·nu·cle·us** (mi″kro-noo′kle-əs) [*micro-* + *nucleus*] [MeSH: Micronuclei] 1. the smaller of two types of nuclei when more than one is present in a cell. 2. in ciliate protozoa, the transcriptively inert, diploid nucleus, much smaller than the macronucleus, that is involved in reproduction.

**mi·cro·nu·tri·ent** (mi″kro-noo′tre-ənt) [MeSH: Micronutrients] any essential dietary element required only in small quantities, e.g., trace minerals.

**mi·cro·nych·ia** (mi″kro-nik′e-ə) [*micr-* + *onych-* + *-ia*] abnormal smallness of the nails of fingers or toes.

**mi·cro·or·chid·ia** (mi″kro-or-kid′e-ə) micro-orchidism.

**mi·cro·or·chi·dism** (mi″kro-or′kĭ-diz-əm) [*micro-* + *orchid-* + *-ism*] abnormal smallness of the testis.

**mi·cro·or·gan·ic** (mi″kro-or-gan′ik) pertaining to a microorganism.

**mi·cro·or·gan·ism** (mi″kro-or′gən-iz-əm) [*micro-* + *organism*] a microscopic organism; those of medical interest include bacteria, viruses, fungi, and protozoa.

**mi·cro·or·gan·is·mal** (mi″kro-or″gən-iz′məl) pertaining to microorganisms.

**mi·cro·par·a·site** (mi″kro-par′ə-sīt) a parasitic microorganism.

**mi·cro·pa·thol·o·gy** (mi″kro-pə-thol′ə-je) [*micro-* + *pathology*] 1. the sum of what is known regarding minute pathologic changes. 2. the pathology of diseases caused by microorganisms.

**mi·cro·pe·nis** (mi″kro-pe′nis) microphallus.

**mi·cro·per·fu·sion** (mi″kro-pər-fu′zhən) perfusion of a minute amount of a substance.

**mi·cro·phage** (mi′kro-fāj) [*micro-* + *-phage*] a small phagocyte, such as a type of actively motile neutrophil. Called also *microphagocyte.*

**mi·cro·phago·cyte** (mi″kro-fag′o-sīt) [*micro-* + *phagocyte*] microphage.

**mi·cro·pha·kia** (mi″kro-fa′ke-ə) [*micro-* + *phak-* + *-ia*] abnormal smallness of the crystalline lens.

**mi·cro·phal·lus** (mi″kro-fal′əs) [*micro-* + *phallus*] abnormal smallness of the penis.

**mi·cro·phone** (mi′kro-fōn) a device for converting an acoustic signal into an electric signal for purposes of amplification or transmission.
**cardiac catheter-m.**, phonocatheter.

**mi·cro·pho·nia** (mi″kro-fo′ne-ə) [*micro-* + *-phonia*] hypophonia.

**mi·cro·phon·ic** (mi″kro-fon′ik) 1. serving to amplify sound. 2. (in the plural) cochlear microphonics.
**cochlear m.**, the electrical potential generated in the hair cells of the organ of Corti in response to acoustic stimulation; called also *cochlear potentials* and *Wever-Bray phenomenon.*

**mi·cro·pho·to·graph** (mi″kro-fo′tə-graf) [*micro-* + *photograph*] a photograph of small size. Cf. *photomicrograph.*

**mi·croph·thal·mia** (mi″krof-thal′me-ə) [*micro-* + *ophthalm-* + *-ia*] microphthalmos.

**mi·croph·thal·mos** (mi″krof-thal′mos) [*micro-* + Gr. *ophthalmos* eye] [MeSH: Microphthalmos] a developmental defect causing moderate or severe reduction in size of the eye. Opacities of the cornea and lens, scarring of the retina and choroid, and other abnormalities may also be present. Cf. *nanophthalmos.*

**mi·croph·thal·mo·scope** (mi″krof-thal′mə-skōp) [*micro-* + *ophthalmoscope*] an instrument for performing fundus microscopy.

**mi·cro·phyte** (mi′kro-fīt) [*micro-* + *-phyte*] a microscopic vegetable organism. Cf. *microzoon.*

**mi·cro·pi·no·cy·to·sis** (mi″kro-pi″no-si-to′sis) the taking up into a cell of specific macromolecules by invagination of the plasma membrane which is then pinched off, resulting in small vesicles in the cytoplasm.

**mi·cro·pi·pet** (mi″kro-pi-pet′) a pipet for handling small quantities of liquids (up to 1 mL).

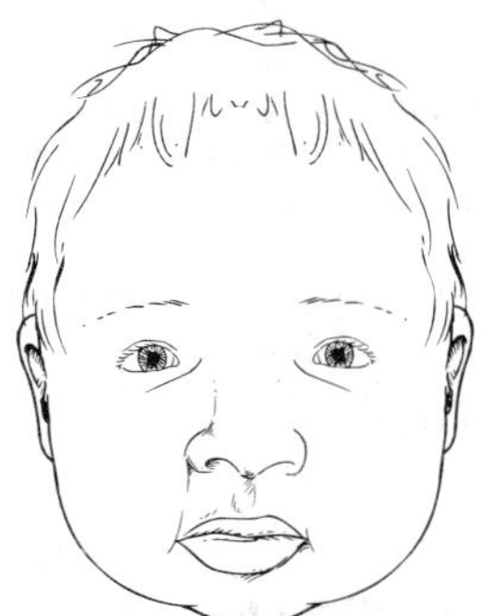

Microphthalmos.

**mi·cro·pi·tu·i·cyte** (mi″kro-pĭ-too′ĭ-sīt) see *pituicyte.*

**mi·cro·pla·sia** (mi″kro-pla′zhə) [*micro-* + *-plasia*] dwarfism.

**mi·cro·pleth·ys·mog·ra·phy** (mi″kro-pleth″is-mog′rə-fe) [*micro-* + *plethysmography*] the recording of minute changes in the size of a part as produced by the circulation of blood in it.

**mi·cro·po·dia** (mi″kro-po′de-ə) [*micro-* + *pod-* + *-ia*] abnormal smallness of the feet.

**mi·cro·po·lar·i·scope** (mi″kro-po-lar′ĭ-skōp) a microscope with a polariscope attached.

**mi·cro·poly·gy·ria** (mi″kro-pol″e-ji′re-ə) polymicrogyria.

**Mi·cro·po·lys·po·ra** (mi″kro-pə-lis′pə-rə) [*micro-* + Gr. *poly* many + *sporos* seed] a genus of bacteria of the family Micromonosporaceae, consisting of gram-positive organisms occurring in branching filaments and forming a spore-producing mycelium.
**M. fae′ni**, a thermophilic species isolated from compost, hay, and grain that is the principal cause of farmer's lung.

**mi·cro·pore** (mi′kro-por) [*micro-* + *pore*] an ultrastructural organelle in the side of the body of apicocomplexan protozoa, consisting of a cytoplasmic ring or cylinder formed by invagination of the outer membrane of the pellicle at the site of a disruption of the inner membrane. Formerly called *micropyle.*

**mi·cro·pre·cip·i·ta·tion** (mi″kro-pre-sip″ĭ-ta′shən) precipitation with a minute amount ($\frac{1}{2}$ to 1 drop or less) of reagent observed under the microscope.

**mi·cro·pre·da·tion** (mi″kro-prə-da′shən) the derivation by an organism of elements essential for its existence from larger organisms of other species which it does not destroy.

**mi·cro·pred·a·tor** (mi″kro-pred′ə-tor) [*micro-* + *predator*] an organism, e.g., the mosquito, that derives elements essential for its existence from other species of organisms, larger than itself, without causing their destruction.

**mi·cro·probe** (mi′kro-prōb) a minute probe, as one used in microsurgery.
**laser m.**, a laser beam utilized to vaporize a minute area of tissue, as in a biopsy specimen, which is then subjected to emission spectrography.

**mi·cro·pro·jec·tion** (mi″kro-pro-jek′shən) [*micro-* + *projection*] the throwing of the image of a microscopic object on a screen.

**mi·cro·pro·jec·tor** (mi″kro-pro-jek′tor) a projector that fits the viewing stage of a microscope and enlarges the image on an illuminated viewing screen.

**mi·cro·pro·lac·ti·no·ma** (mi″kro-pro-lak″tĭ-no′mə) a prolactinoma less than 10 mm in diameter, usually associated with serum prolactin levels of 100 to 500 ng per milliliter.

**mi·cro·pro·so·pus** (mi″kro-pro-so′pəs) [*micro-* + Gr. *prosōpon* face] a fetus with a small or undeveloped face.

**mi·crop·sia** (mi-krop′se-ə) [*micr-* + *-opsia*] a visual disorder in which objects appear smaller than their actual size.

**mi·crop·tic** (mi-krop′tik) pertaining to or affected with micropsia.

**mi·cro·punc·ture** (mi′kro-punk″chər) [MeSH: Punctures] 1. the creation of minute openings by piercing. 2. in renal physiology, the process by which nephron segments are pierced.

**mi·cro·pus** (mi-kro′pəs) [*micro-* + Gr. *pous* foot] a person with micropodia.

**mi·cro·pyle** (mi′kro-pīl) [*micro-* + Gr. *pylē* gate] 1. a minute opening in: (1) the ovum of certain invertebrates, such as arthropods, that permits entrance of a sperm; (2) the apex of the ovule of a seed plant that admits the pollen tube; (3) the covering of a sponge through which geminating cells emerge. 2. former name for *micropore.*

**mi·cro·ra·dio·gram** (mi″kro-ra′de-o-gram) a picture produced by microradiography.

**mi·cro·ra·di·og·ra·phy** (mi″kro-ra″de-og′rə-fe) [*micro-* + *radiography*] [MeSH: Microradiography] a process by which a radiograph of a small or very thin object is produced on fine-grained photographic film under conditions which permit subsequent microscopic examination or enlargement of the radiograph at linear magnifications of up to several hundred and with a resolution approaching the resolving power of the photographic emulsion (about 1000 lines per millimeter).

**mi·cror·chid·ia** (mi″kror-kid′e-ə) [*micro-* + *orchid-* + *-ia*] microorchidism.

**mi·cro·re·frac·tom·e·ter** (mi″kro-re″frak-tom′ə-tər) a refractometer for the discovery of variations in minute structures, such as of blood corpuscles.

**mi·cro·res·pi·rom·e·ter** (mi″kro-res″pĭ-rom′ə-tər) an apparatus for investigating the oxygen utilization of isolated tissues.

**mi·cro·rhin·ia** (mi″kro-rin′e-ə) [*micro-* + *rhin-* + *-ia*] abnormal smallness of the nose.

**mi·cro·roent·gen** (mi″kro-rent′gen) one millionth ($10^{-6}$) roentgen; abbreviated $\mu$R.

**mi·cros·ce·lous** (mi-kros′kə-ləs) [*micro-* + Gr. *skelos* leg] short-legged.

**mi·cro·scler** (mi′kro-sklēr) dolichomorphic.

**mi·cro·scope** (mi′kro-skōp) [*micro-* + *-scope*] an instrument used to obtain an enlarged image of small objects and reveal details of structure not otherwise distinguishable.
**acoustic m.**, one in which very high frequency sound waves (close to one billion cycles per second [one gigahertz]) are focused on the object and the reflected beam is processed electronically and stored for display on a television screen.
**beta ray m.**, one which reveals emission of beta particles from a microscopic specimen by means of a scintillator.
**binocular m.**, a microscope which has two eyepieces, making possible simultaneous viewing with both eyes.
**capillary m.**, an instrument for giving an enlarged image of capillaries, often used for viewing the capillaries of the nail bed.
**centrifuge m.**, a microscope built into a high-speed centrifuge, by which a magnified image of a specimen undergoing centrifugal force may be produced.
**color-contrast m.**, Rheinberg m.
**comparison m.**, an instrument which permits simultaneous viewing of parts of images of two separate specimens, involving two microscopes bridged together with a comparison eyepiece, or one microscope with two body tubes and lens systems.
**compound m.**, one that consists of two lens systems, one above the other, in which the image formed by the system nearer the object (objective) is further magnified by the system nearer the eye (eyepiece).
**corneal m.**, a specially designed instrument with lenses of high magnifying power, for observing minute changes in the cornea and iris.
**darkfield m.**, one with a central stop in the condenser, permitting diversion of the light rays and illumination of the object from the side, so that the details appear light against a dark background. See also *ultramicroscope.*
**electron m.**, one in which an electron beam, instead of light, forms an image for viewing, allowing much greater magnification and resolution. The image may be viewed on a fluorescent screen or may be photographed. Types include the *scanning* and the *transmission electron microscope.*
**fluorescence m.**, one used for the examination of specimens stained with fluorochromes or fluorochrome complexes, e.g., a fluorescein-labeled antibody, which fluoresces in ultraviolet light.
**hypodermic m.**, a combination of a fiberoptic probe (housed in a hypodermic needle) and a microscope for examining cell structure in tissue and muscle without a cutaneous incision.
**infrared m.**, one in which radiation of 800 m$\mu$ or longer wavelength is used as the image-forming energy.
**integrating m.**, one in which a special mechanical stage permits recording of the sizes of the components of the specimen.
**interference m.**, a microscope for observing the same kind of refractile detail as that observed with the phase microscope, but utilizing two separate beams of light which are sent through the specimen and combined with each other in the image plane.
**ion m.**, an electron microscope modified to use ions (e.g., of lithium), instead of electrons.
**laser m.**, see *laser microprobe.*
**light m.**, one in which the specimen is viewed under visible light.
**opaque m.**, one with vertical illumination or with the condenser built around the objective (epimicroscope) for viewing opaque specimens.
**operating m.**, a specially designed magnifying instrument employed in the performance of delicate microsurgical procedures, as in operations on the middle ear, on small blood vessels, or on a vocal cord.
**phase m., phase-contrast m.**, a microscope that converts variations of the refracting index in the object into variations of intensity in the image. Altering the phase relationship of light passing through and that passing around the object allows details of living cells to be seen without the fixation and staining that is normally necessary.
**polarizing m.**, one equipped with a polarizer, analyzer, and means for measurement of the alteration of the polarized light by the specimen.
**polarizing m., rectified,** a polarizing microscope corrected for depolarization from curved lens surfaces so that full apertures can be used.
**projection x-ray m.**, a microscope using soft x-radiation for high resolution; the images may be photographed or observed directly on a fluorescent viewing screen.
**reflecting m.**, one which utilizes mirrors instead of lenses to form the image.
**Rheinberg m.**, a darkfield microscope in which the condenser is modified by having a colored instead of an opaque stop, with the annulus in a complementary color. Called also *color-contrast m.*
**scanning m., scanning electron m.**, an electron microscope in which a beam of electrons scans over a specimen point by point, causing the emission of a secondary beam that makes an image on the fluorescent screen of a cathode ray tube; differences in depth over the surface may be imaged in three dimensions.
**schlieren m.**, one in which light is deviated by the insertion of one or two diaphragms in the optical system, to reveal differences in refractive index in a specimen.
**simple m.**, one which consists of a single lens; a magnifying glass.
**slit lamp m.**, see *slit lamp,* under *lamp.*
**stereoscopic m.**, a binocular biobjective microscope, or a binocular monobjective microscope modified to give a three-dimensional view of the specimen.
**stroboscopic m.**, one which utilizes flashing illumination, permitting analysis of motion in the specimen.
**transmission electron m. (TEM),** an electron microscope that transmits a beam of electrons through the object, forming an image on a screen behind it.
**trinocular m.**, a binocular microscope with a third eyepiece tube for photomicrography or other use.
**ultra-m.**, see *ultramicroscope.*
**ultrasonic m.**, one which utilizes the reflection of ultrasonic or mechanical vibration to reveal the detail of the specimen.
**ultraviolet m.**, a microscope which utilizes reflecting optics or quartz and other ultraviolet-transmitting lenses, with radiation of less than 400 m$\mu$ wavelength as the image-forming energy.
**x-ray m.**, one in which a beam of x-rays is used instead of light, the image usually being reproduced on film.

**mi·cro·scop·ic, mi·cro·scop·i·cal** (mi″kro-skop′ik) 1. of extremely small size; visible only by the aid of the microscope. 2. pertaining or relating to a microscope or to microscopy.

**mi·cro·scop·i·cal** (mi″kro-skop′ĭ-kəl) microscopic.

**mi·cros·co·pist** (mi-kros′kə-pist) a person skilled in using the microscope.

**mi·cros·co·py** (mi-kros′kə-pe) [*micro-* + *-scopy*] [MeSH: Microscopy] examination under or observation by means of the microscope.
**clinical m.**, employment of the microscope in making clinical diagnoses.
**electron m.**, examination by means of the electron microscope.
**epiluminescent m.**, a technique for the examination of pigmented skin lesions in which the lesion is covered with immersion oil and a glass slide to make the epidermis translucent; then it is examined with a binocular surface microscope.
**fluorescence m.**, microscopy of natural fluorescent materials or of specimens stained with fluorochromes, which emit light when exposed to blue or ultraviolet light.
**fundus m.**, examination of the fundus of the eye with an instrument which combines a corneal microscope with an ophthalmoscope.
**immunofluorescence m.**, fluorescence microscopy using immunofluorescence (q.v.) staining methods.
**television m.**, projection on a television screen of the image obtained by use of a flying spot, or scanning, microscope, or by use of a television camera over a microscope.

**mi·cro·sec·ond** (mi′kro-sek″ənd) one-millionth of a second; symbol $\mu$s.

**mi·cro·sec·tion** (mi″kro-sek′shən) an extremely thin section for examination with the microscope.

**mi·cro·seme** (mi′kro-sēm) [*micro-* + Gr. *sēma* sign] having an orbital index of 83 or less.

**mi·cro·shock** (mi′kro-shok″) a term used in cardiology to denote a low level of electric current applied directly to myocardial tissue; as little as 0.1 mA causes ventricular fibrillation. Cf. *macroshock.*

**mi·cro·slide** (mi′kro-slīd) the slide on which objects for microscopic examination are mounted.

**mi·cros·mat·ic** (mi″kros-mat′ik) [*micro-* + *osmatic*] having the sense of smell, but of relatively feeble development, as in man.

**mi·cro·so·ma** (mi″kro-so′mə) [*micro-* + *soma*] a very short but not dwarfish stature.

**mi·cro·so·mal** (mi″kro-so′məl) of or pertaining to microsomes.

**mi·cro·some** (mi′kro-sōm) [*micro-* + *-some*] [MeSH: Microsomes] any of the vesicular fragments of endoplasmic reticulum formed after disruption and centrifugation of cells.

**mi·cro·so·mia** (mi″kro-so′me-ə) [*micro-* + *-somia*] small body size; see also *dwarfism.*
**m. feta′lis,** abnormally small size of the fetus.

**mi·cro·spec·tro·pho·tom·e·ter** (mi″kro-spek″tro-fo-tom′ə-tər) a system combining a microscope with a spectrophotometer.

**mi·cro·spec·tro·scope** (mi″kro-spek′trə-skōp) [*micro-* + *spectro-*

*scope*] a spectroscope to be used in connection with a microscope for the examination of the spectra of microscopic objects.

**mi·cro·sphere** (mi-kro-sfēr′) [MeSH: Microspheres] centrosome.

**mi·cro·sphe·ro·cyte** (mi″kro-sfe′ro-sīt) spherocyte.

**mi·cro·sphero·cy·to·sis** (mi″kro-sfe″ro-si-to′sis) spherocytosis.

**mi·cro·sphero·lith** (mi″kro-sfēr′o-lith) a particle resembling a miniature gallstone in the bile.

**mi·cro·sphyg·mia** (mi″kro-sfig′me-ə) [*micro-* + *sphygm-* + *-ia*] a pulse that is difficult to perceive by the finger.

**mi·cro·sphyg·my** (mi″kro-sfig′me) microsphygmia.

**Mi·cro·spi·ra** (mi″kro-spi′rə) [*micro-* + Gr. *speira* coil] in former systems of classification, a genus of bacteria made up of organisms now assigned to the genus *Vibrio.*

**Mi·cro·spi·ro·ne·ma** (mi″kro-spi″ro-ne′mə) [*micro-* + Gr. *speira* coil + *nema* thread] a genus name once proposed for organisms now included in the genus *Treponema.*

**mi·cro·sple·nia** (mi″kro-sple′ne-ə) [*micro-* + *splen-* + *-ia*] smallness of the spleen.

**mi·cro·sple·nic** (mi″kro-sple′nik) marked by smallness of the spleen.

**Mi·cros·po·ra** (mi-kros′pə-rə) [*micro-* + *spore*] [MeSH: Microspora] a phylum of protozoa found as obligatory intracellular parasites in nearly all major animal groups, being especially common in insects, sometimes causing economically important disease. The spore phase is characterized by the presence of minute unicellular spores, each with an imperforate wall containing one nucleus or a dinucleate sporoplasm and a simple or complex extrusion apparatus with a polar tube or polar cap always present; mitochondria are absent. It comprises two classes: Rudimicrosporea and Microsporea. Called also *Cnidospora.*

**mi·cro·spo·ran·gi·um** (mi″kro-spə-ran′je-əm) pl. *microsporan′gia* [*micro-* + *sporangium*] the sporangium in which microspores develop.

**mi·cro·spore** (mi′kro-spor) [*micro-* + *spore*] 1. the smaller spore form when spores of two sizes are present, as in certain fungi and protozoa. 2. in heterogenous plants, one of four haploid spores, usually smaller than the megaspore, formed in the microsporangium from a microspore mother cell, and from which the microgametophyte, or male gametophyte, develops. See also *pollen.*

**Mi·cro·spor·ea** (mi″kro-spor′e-ə) [MeSH: Microsporea] a class of parasitic protozoa (phylum Microspora), the spores of which have a complex extrusion apparatus of Golgi origin, often including a polaroplast and posterior vacuole and a typically filamentous polar tube extending backward from the polar cap and coiling around inside of the three-layered spore wall; a sporocyst may or may not be present. It comprises two orders: Minisporida and Microsporida.

**Mi·cro·spor·i·da** (mi″kro-spor′ĭ-də) [*micro-* + *spore*] [MeSH: Microsporida] an order of parasitic protozoa (class Microsporea, phylum Microspora) found in invertebrates, especially arthropods, in lower vertebrates, and rarely in higher vertebrates, which have a tendency toward maximum development and varied specialization of accessory spore organelles accompanied by a reduction of sporocysts. It comprises two suborders: Pansporoblastina and Apansporoblastina. Called also *Cnidosporidia* and *Microsporidia.*

**mi·cro·spor·i·dan** (mi″kro-spor′ĭ-dən) 1. any protozoan of the phylum Microspora. 2. pertaining to protozoa of the phylum Microspora. 3. microsporidian.

**Mi·cro·spo·rid·ia** (mi″kro-spə-rid′e-ə) Microsporida.

**mi·cro·spo·rid·ia** (mi″kro-spə-rid′e-ə) a nontaxonomic group comprising organisms of the order Microsporida.

**mi·cro·spo·rid·i·al** (mi″kro-spə-rid′e-əl) pertaining to or caused by microsporidia.

**mi·cro·spo·rid·i·an** (mi″kro-spo-rid′e-ən) 1. any protozoan of the order Microsporida. 2. pertaining to protozoa of the order Microsporida. 3. microsporidan.

**mi·cro·spo·rid·i·o·sis** (mi″kro-spo-rid″e-o′sis) infection with protozoa of the order Microsporida, usually seen in immunocompromised patients; the usual symptoms are diarrhea and wasting. See also *encephalitozoonosis* and *nosematosis.*

**Mi·cros·po·ron** (mi-kros′pə-ron) *Microsporum.*

**mi·cro·spo·ro·sis** (mi″kro-spə-ro′sis) infection with a fungus of genus *Microsporum.*
**m. ni′gra,** tinea nigra.

**mi·cro·ste·a·to·sis** (mi″kro-ste″ə-to′sis) [*micro-* + *steatosis*] fatty change in which numerous small lipid droplets are present in the cytoplasm. Cf *macrosteatosis.*

**Mi·cros·po·rum** (mi-kros′pə-rəm) [*micro* + Gr. *sporos* seed] [MeSH: Microsporum] a genus of Fungi Imperfecti, family Moniliaceae, mostly small-spored ectothrix ringworm fungi (dermatophytes); numerous species are causes of diseases of the skin and hair. As the perfect (sexual) stages are identified, they are classified in the genus *Arthroderma.* Called also *Microsporon.*
**M. audoui′nii,** a small-spored ectothrix that is the most common cause of prepuberal tinea capitis in Europe and of about half the cases in the United States.
**M. ca′nis,** a small-spored ectothrix that commonly causes ringworm in cats and dogs and can be transmitted to children, in whom it causes tinea capitis and tinea corporis. It is also probably the cause of a dermatomycosis in horses. It has perfect (sexual) stages in genus *Arthroderma.* Called also *M. felineum* and *M. lanosum.*
**M. coo′kei,** a common geophilic species that sometimes causes dermatophytosis in rodents, dogs, and humans. Its perfect (sexual) stage is *Arthroderma cajetani.*
**M. feli′neum,** *M. canis.*
**M. ferrugi′neum,** a small-spored ectothrix that is anthropophilic and causes tinea capitis, mainly in children. Called also *Trichophyton ferrugineum.*
**M. ful′vum,** a geophilic species that can be a large-spored ectothrix and cause tinea corporis or tinea capitis.
**M. galli′nae,** *Trichophyton gallinae.*
**M. gyp′seum,** a common geophilic species that can be a large-spored ectothrix and cause tinea capitis and tinea corporis. Its perfect (sexual) stage is *Arthroderma gypsea.*
**M. lano′sum,** *M. canis.*
**M. na′num,** a geophilic species that can be a large-spored ectothrix and cause ringworm in pigs and occasionally in humans. It has perfect (sexual) stages in genus *Arthroderma.*
**M. persi′color,** a geophilic species that usually infects small rodents but occasionally causes tinea capitis or tinea corporis in humans. Its perfect (sexual) stage is *Arthroderma persicolor.*
**M. vanbreuseghe′mii,** a large-spored ectothrix causing dermatophytosis in dogs, cats, humans, and some other mammals. It has perfect (sexual) stages in genus *Arthroderma.*

**Mi·cro·stix-3** (mi′kro-stiks) trademark for a reagent strip with a chemical test area for recognition of nitrite in urine, which turns pink on contact with nitrite, and two culture areas for semiquantification of bacterial growth after 18–24 hours of incubation; one culture area supports both gram-negative and gram-positive organisms, the other, only gram-negative organisms.

**mi·cro·sto·mia** (mi″kro-sto′me-ə) [*micro-* + *stom-* + *-ia*] [MeSH: Microstomia] a congenital anomaly in which the mouth is unusually small.

**mi·cro·stra·bis·mus** (mi″kro-strə-biz′məs) [*micro-* + *strabismus*] strabismus of such slight degree that the deviation is undetectable by the usual methods.

**mi·cro·sur·gery** (mi′kro-sər″jər-e) [MeSH: Microsurgery] dissection of minute structures under the microscope by means of instruments held in the hand, as in microsurgery of the ear and larynx.

**mi·cro·syr·inge** (mi″kro-sə-rinj′) a syringe fitted with a screw-thread micrometer head for the accurate control of minute measurements.

**mi·cro·tech·nic** (mi″kro-tek′nik) micrology.

**mi·cro·the·lia** (mi″kro-the′le-ə) [*micro-* + *thel-* + *-ia*] unusual smallness of the nipples.

**mi·cro·throm·bo·sis** (mi″kro-throm-bo′sis) presence of many small thrombi in the capillaries and other small blood vessels.

**mi·cro·throm·bus** (mi″kro-throm′bəs) pl. *microthrom′bi.* a small thrombus located in a capillary or other small blood vessel.

**mi·cro·tia** (mi-kro′shə) [*micro-* + *ot-* + *-ia*] gross hypoplasia or aplasia of the auricle (pinna) of the ear, with a blind or absent external acoustic meatus.

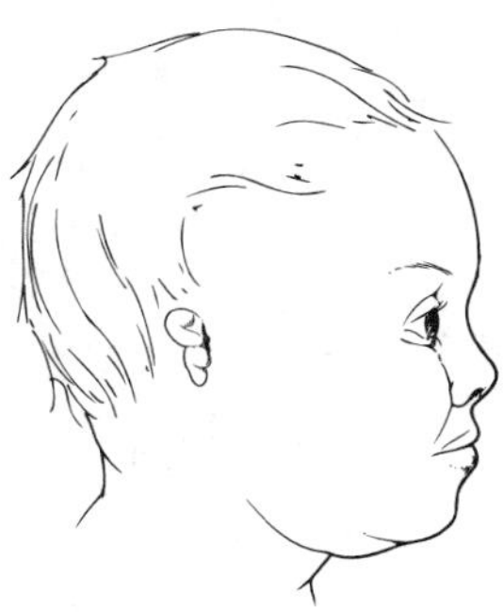

Microtia.

**mi·cro·ti·ter** (mi″kro-ti′tər) a titer of minute quantity.

**mi·cro·tome** (mi′kro-tōm) [*micro-* + *-tome*] an instrument for cutting thin slices of tissue for microscopical study.
**freezing m.**, a microtome for cutting frozen sections.
**rocking m.**, a microtome in which the specimen is held in the end of a lever which passes up and down over a stationary knife.
**rotary m.**, one in which a wheel action is translated into a back-and-forth movement of the specimen being sectioned.
**sliding m.**, one in which the specimen being sectioned is made to slide on a tract.

**mi·crot·o·my** (mi-krot′ə-me) [*micro-* + *-tomy*] [MeSH: Microtomy] the cutting of thin sections; called also *histotomy.*

**mi·cro·to·nom·e·ter** (mi″kro-to-nom′ə-tər) a small tonometer for measuring the oxygen and carbon dioxide tension in arterial blood.

**mi·cro·trans·fu·sion** (mi″kro-trans-fu′zhən) introduction into the circulation of a small quantity of blood of another individual, as sometimes occurs with transplacental passage of a small amount of fetal blood into the maternal circulation.

**mi·cro·trau·ma** (mi″kro-traw′mə) a slight trauma or lesion; a microscopic lesion.

**Mi·cro·trom·bid·i·um aka·mu·shi** (mi″kro-trom-bid′e-əm ah″kah-moo′she) *Trombicula akamushi.*

**mi·cro·tro·pia** (mi″kro-tro′pe-ə) microstrabismus.

**mi·cro·tu·bule** (mi″kro-too′būl) [MeSH: Microtubules] any of the slender, tubular structures composed chiefly of tubulin, found in the cytoplasmic ground substance of nearly all cells; they are involved in maintenance of cell shape and in the movements of organelles and inclusions, and form the spindle fibers of mitosis. In cilia and flagella, they are constantly arranged with two single microtubules in the center and nine pairs of doublets arrayed around the central two.
**subpellicular m.**, any of the microtubules (24 to 26) radiating posteriorly from the polar rings, directly beneath the pellicle, forming part of the apical complex in apicocomplexan protozoa.

**Mi·cro·tus** (mi-kro′təs) [*micro-* + Gr. *ous, ōtos,* ear] a genus of rodents of the family Muridae, including voles found in the Arctic. Various species are reservoirs of *Leptospira interrogans* serovar *hebdomadis.*

**mi·cro·tus** (mi-kro′təs) an individual with microtia.

**mi·cro·unit** (mi′kro-u″nit) one-millionth ($10^{-6}$) of a standard unit; abbreviated $\mu$U.

**mi·cro·vas·cu·lar** (mi″kro-vas′ku-lər) pertaining to the microvasculature.

**mi·cro·vas·cu·la·ture** (mi″kro-vas′ku-lə-chər) the portion of the vasculature of the body comprising the finer vessels, sometimes described as those with an internal diameter of 100 microns or less.

**mi·cro·vas·cu·lop·a·thy** (mi″kro-vas″ku-lop′ə-the) any disorder affecting the microvasculature.
**retinal m.**, HIV-associated retinopathy.

**mi·cro·ves·sel** (mi′kro-ves″əl) any of the finer vessels of the body; cf. *microvasculature.*

**mi·cro·vil·li** (mi″kro-vil′i) [pl. of L. *microvillus* a tuft of hair] [MeSH: Microvilli] minute cylindrical processes on the free surface of a cell, especially cells of the proximal convolution in a renal tubule and of the intestinal epithelium, which increase the surface size of the cell; see also *brush border,* under *border.*

**mi·cro·vil·lus** (mi″kro-vil′əs) [MeSH: Microvilli] a minute process or protrusion from the free surface of a cell; see *microvilli.*

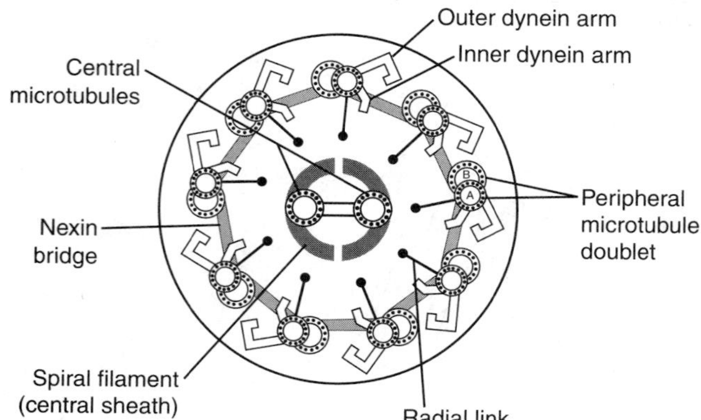


Microtubules in a 9 + 2 array in a cross-section of the axoneme of a cilium.

**mi·cro·vis·co·sim·e·ter** (mi″kro-vis″ko-sim′ə-tər) a viscosimeter for measuring the viscosity of blood plasma, using a small quantity of blood.

**mi·cro·viv·i·sec·tion** (mi″kro-viv″i-sek′shən) microdissection.

**mi·cro·volt** (mi′kro-volt) [*micro-* + *volt*] one-millionth of a volt. Symbol, $\mu$V.

**mi·cro·vol·tom·e·ter** (mi″kro-vol-tom′ə-tər) an instrument for detecting minute changes of electric potential in the body.

**mi·cro·watt** (mi′kro-waht) [*micro-* + *watt*] one-millionth of a watt. Symbol, $\mu$W.

**mi·cro·wave** (mi′kro-wāv) [MeSH: Microwaves] a wave typical of electromagnetic radiation between far infrared and radio waves, generally regarded as extending from 300,000 to 100 megacycles (wavelength of 1 mm to 30 cm).

**Mi·crox** (mi′kroks) former name for Mykrox.

**mi·croxy·cyte** (mi-krok′sĭ-sīt) [*micr-* + *oxy-* + *-cyte*] any finely granular oxyphil cell.

**mi·croxy·phil** (mi-krok′sĭ-fil) microxycyte.

**mi·cro·zoa** (mi″kro-zo′ə) plural of *microzoon.*

**mi·cro·zo·on** (mi″kro-zo′on) pl. *microzo′a* [*micro-* + Gr. *zōon* animal] a microscopic animal organism. Cf. *microphyte.*

**mi·crur·gic** (mi-krur′jik) pertaining to micrurgy.

**mi·crur·gy** (mi′krər-je) [*micro-* + Gr. *ergon* work] micromanipulative technique in the field of a microscope. See *micromanipulator.*

**Mi·cru·roi·des** (mi″kroo-roi′dēz) a genus of venomous snakes of the family Elapidae. *M. euryxan′thus* is the Arizona or Sonoran coral snake of Mexico and the Southwestern United States.

**Mi·cru·rus** (mi-kroo′rəs) a genus of venomous snakes of the family Elapidae. *M. ful′vius* is the Eastern or Texas coral snake, a species found in the southern United States and tropical America whose body is marked with bright red, yellow, and black bands. Called also *Elaps.* See table at *snake.*

**mic·tion** (mik′shən) urination.

**mic·tu·rate** (mik′tu-rāt) urinate.

**mic·tu·ri·tion** (mik″tu-rĭ′shən) [L. *micturire* to urinate] urination.

**MID** minimum infective dose.

**Mi·da·mor** (mi′də-mor) trademark for preparations of amiloride hydrochloride.

**mid·ax·il·la** (mid″ak-sil′ə) the center of the axilla.

**mid·azo·lam** (mid′a-zo-lam″) [MeSH: Midazolam] a benzodiazepine tranquilizer, stronger than diazepam but otherwise similar to diazepam in actions and properties; administered intravenously or intramuscularly.
**m. maleate**, a tranquilizer used in the induction of anesthesia, administered intravenously.

**mid·body** (mid′bod″e) 1. a body or a mass of granules developed in the equatorial region of the spindle during the anaphase of mitosis. 2. the middle region of the trunk.

**mid·brain** (mid′brān″) mesencephalon.

**mid·car·pal** (mid-kahr′pəl) between the two rows of bones of the carpus.

**mid·di·as·tol·ic** (mid″di-ə-stol′ik) occurring in the middle third of diastole.

**mid·dle·piece** (mid′əl-pēs) middle piece; see under *piece.*

**mid·face** (mid′-fās″) the middle of the face, including the nose, nasion, and glabella.

**mid·foot** (mid′foot″) the middle portion of the foot, comprising the region of the navicular, cuboid, and cuneiform bones.

**mid·fron·tal** (mid-fron′təl) pertaining to the middle of the forehead.

**midge** (mij) 1. a small dipterous insect of the family Chironomidae; many species give painful bites, and some are vectors of *Mansonella ozzardi* and *Dipetalonema perstans.* 2. any of several small biting insects resembling the Chironomidae, such as various members of Ceratopogonidae and Culicoides.
**owl m.**, *Phlebotomus.*

**midg·et** (mij′ət) normal dwarf.

**mid·gut** (mid′gut″) 1. the region of the embryonic digestive tube into which the yolk sac opens; it gives rise to most of the intestines. Ahead of it is the foregut and caudal to it is the hindgut. 2. the middle endodermal portion of the alimentary tract of invertebrates, such as arthropods, comprising a stomach and sometimes a midintestine. Defs. 1 and 2 called also *mesenteron.*

**Mid·i·cel** (mid′ĭ-səl) trademark for a preparation of sulfamethoxypyridazine.

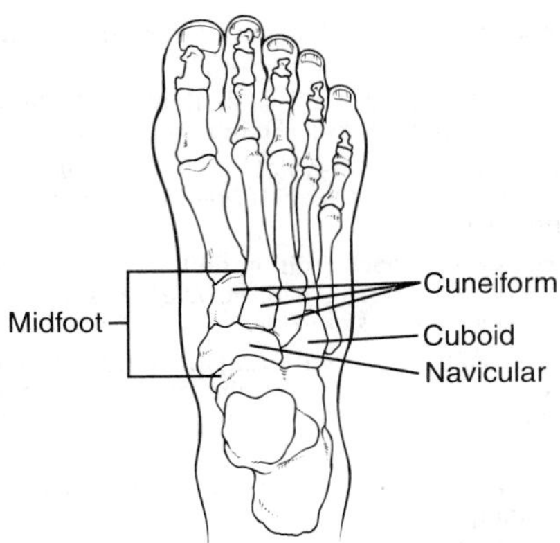


**mid·oc·cip·i·tal** (mid″ok-sip′ĭ-təl) pertaining to or located in the middle of the occiput.

**mid·pain** (mid′pān″) intermenstrual pain.

**mid·pe·riph·e·ry** (mid″pə-rif′ə-re) the middle zone of the fundus.

**mid·plane** (mid′plān″) the median plane of a bilateral structure.

**mid·riff** (mid′rif) 1. diaphragma (def. 1). 2. the middle region of the torso; the region between the inferior border of the breast and the waistline.

**mid·sec·tion** (mid-sek′shən) a cut through the middle of any organ or part.

**mid·ster·num** (mid-stər′nəm) corpus sterni.

**mid·tar·sal** (mid-tahr′səl) between the two rows of bones of the tarsus.

**mid·teg·men·tum** (mid″təg-men′təm) the median or central part of the tegmentum.

**mid·wife** (mid′wīf) an individual who practices midwifery; see *nurse-midwife.*

**mid·wi·fery** (mid′wif-re, mid′wi-fər-e) [MeSH: Midwifery] the practice of assisting in childbirth. See *nurse-midwife* and *obstetrics.*

**Mier·ze·jew·ski effect** (myer″zhə-yef′ske) [Jan Lucian *Mierzejewski,* Polish neurologist and psychiatrist, 1839–1908] see under *effect.*

**Mie·scher's granuloma, granulomatous cheilitis** (me′sherz) [Guido *Miescher,* Swiss dermatologist, 1877–1961] see *granulomatous cheilitis,* under *cheilitis,* and *actinic granulom,* under *granuloma.*

**Mie·scher's tube, tubule** (me′sherz) [Johann Friedrich *Miescher,* Swiss pathologist, 1811–1887] sarcocyst.

**MIF** migration inhibition factor. See under *factor.*

**mi·fe·pris·tone** (mi″fə-pris′tōn) an antiprogestin used to induce abortion in the first trimester; administered orally. Called also *RU-486.*

**mi·graine** (mi′grān) [Fr., from Gr. *hemikrania* an affection of half of the head] [MeSH: Migraine] an often familial symptom complex of periodic attacks of vascular headache, usually temporal and unilateral in onset, commonly associated with irritability, nausea, vomiting, constipation or diarrhea, and often photophobia. Attacks are preceded by constriction of the cranial arteries, often with resultant prodromal sensory (especially ocular) symptoms and the spreading depression of Leão; the migraines themselves commence with the vasodilation that follows. Two primary types are distinguished, *m. with aura* and *m. without aura;* the variety without an aura is more common.
**abdominal m.,** migraine in which abdominal symptoms (nausea and vomiting) are prominent.
**acute confusional m.,** a rare variant of classic migraine occurring in children, marked by attacks of confusion and disorientation, with agitation manifested as a mixture of apprehension and combativeness; headache may not appear at first but always develops eventually.
**m. with aura,** migraine that is preceded by a prodrome of neurologic symptoms, often visual ones such as teichopsia; called also *classic m.*
**m. without aura,** migraine of sudden onset, without a prodrome; called also *common m.*
**basilar m., basilar artery m.,** a type of ophthalmic migraine whose aura fills both visual fields and which may be accompanied by dysarthria and problems of equilibrium such as vertigo and incoordination; the symptoms are in the area supplied by the basilar and posterior cerebral arteries. Called also *Bickerstaff's m.*
**Bickerstaff's m.,** basilar m.
**classic m.,** m. with aura.
**common m.,** m. without aura.
**complicated m.,** migrainous infarction.
**familial hemiplegic m.,** a rare type of hemiplegic migraine that is passed on as an autosomal dominant trait.
**hemiplegic m.,** migraine associated with varying degrees of transient hemiplegia or hemiparesis.
**neurologic m.,** classic m.
**ocular m.,** ophthalmic m.
**ophthalmic m.,** migraine accompanied by amblyopia, teichopsia, or other visual disturbance; see also *basilar m., ophthalmoplegic m.,* and *retinal m.* Called also *ocular m.*
**ophthalmoplegic m.,** periodic migraine accompanied by ophthalmoplegia; called also *Möbius' disease.*
**retinal m.,** a type of ophthalmic migraine with retinal symptoms such as monocular visual loss or blurring, probably because of constriction of one or more retinal arteries.

**mi·grain·eur** (me″gran-oor′) [Fr.] a person who suffers from migraine.

**mi·grain·oid** (mi′grən-oid) [*migraine* + *-oid*] resembling migraine.

**mi·grain·ous** (mi′grən-əs) resembling, or of the nature of migraine.

**mi·gra·tion** (mi-gra′shən) [L. *migratio*] 1. an apparently spontaneous change of place, as of symptoms. 2. diapedesis.
**anodic m.,** the migration of a negatively charged particle toward the positive pole in an electrical field.
**cathodic m.,** the migration of a positively charged particle toward the negative pole in an electrical field.
**external m.,** the passage of an ovum from the ovary to the oviduct of the opposite side without passing through the uterus.
**internal m.,** the passing of an ovum from an ovary into the uterus in the normal way, followed by its entry into the opposite oviduct or, in animals with separate uterine horns, into the opposite horn.
**m. of leukocytes,** leukopedesis.
**m. of ovum,** 1. the passage of the ovum into the uterine tube after its discharge from the ovary. 2. the passage of the ovum through the reproductive tract and through the uterine epithelium into the stroma.
**retrograde m.,** the passage into the upper urinary tract of foreign bodies introduced through the urethra.
**tooth m., pathologic,** drifting of the teeth due to destruction of tooth-supporting structures by periodontal disease or to failure to replace missing teeth. Called also *pathologic tooth wandering.*
**tooth m., physiologic,** change of position of the teeth during their growth and development. Called also *physiologic drift.*
**transperitoneal m.,** external m.

**Mi·gu·la's classification** (me′goo-lahz) [Walter *Migula,* German naturalist, 1863–1938] see under *classification.*

**Mi·ka·nia** (mĭ-ka′ne-ə) [J. G. *Mikan,* Czech botanist, 19th century] a genus of tropical American vines of the family Compositae. *M. gua′co* Humb. & Bonpl. is the medicinal plant guaco.

**mikr(o)-** for words beginning thus, see those beginning *micr(o)-.*

**Mi·ku·licz's angle, cells,** etc. (me′koo-lich″əz) [Johann von *Mikulicz*-Radecki, Polish surgeon, 1850–1905] see under *angle, cell, clamp, disease, drain, operation, pack,* and *syndrome,* and see *periadenitis mucosa necrotica recurrens.*

**mil·am·me·ter** (mil-am′ə-tər) milliammeter.

**Milch's method** (milch′əz) see under *method.*

**mil·dew** (mil′doo) 1. any of various fungi that grow on vegetable or other material, divided into *downy* and *powdery* types. 2. the condition caused by such a fungus.
**downy m., false m.,** a mildew of the family Peronosporaceae.
**powdery m.,** a mildew of the order Erysiphales.

**Miles' operation** (mīlz) [William Ernest *Miles,* British surgeon, 1869–1947] see under *operation.*

**mil·ia** (mil′e-ə) [L.] plural of *milium.*

**mi·li·a·ria** (mil″e-ar′e-ə) [L. *milium* millet] [MeSH: Miliaria] a syndrome of cutaneous changes associated with sweat retention and extravasation of sweat occurring at different levels in the skin; when used alone, it refers to *m. rubra.*
**m. al′ba,** m. crystallina.
**apocrine m.,** Fox-Fordyce disease.
**m. crystalli′na,** miliaria in which the sweat escapes in or just beneath the stratum corneum, producing noninflammatory vesicles which, because of the thinness of the layer covering them, have the appearance of clear droplets. Called also *m. alba* and *sudamina.*
**m. profun′da,** miliaria seen in hot humid climates in which the occlusion of the sweat ducts is in the upper cutis; it almost always occurs following a severe episode of miliaria rubra and may lead to heat intolerance as in tropical anhidrotic asthenia.
**m. ru′bra,** a condition resulting from obstruction to the ducts of the sweat glands, probably caused in part by prolonged maceration of the skin surface; the sweat escapes into the epidermis, producing

pruritic erythematous papulovesicles. The severity of the symptoms fluctuates with the heat load of the individual. Called also *heat rash, lichen tropicus,* and *prickly heat.*

**mil·i·ary** (mil'e-ar-e) [L. *miliaris* like a millet seed] 1. resembling a millet seed. 2. characterized by the formation of minute lesions resembling millet seeds, as in miliary tuberculosis.

**Mil·i·bis** (mil'ĭ-bis) trademark for preparations of glycobiarsol.

**mi·lieu** (mēl-yoo') [Fr.] surroundings: environment.
**m. extérieur** (eks-ta"re-oor'), the external environment.
**m. intérieur,** (ă-ta"re-oor') [Fr. "interior environment"], Claude Bernard's term for the blood and lymph which bathe the cells of the body.

**mil·i·um** (mil'e-əm) pl. *mil'ia* [L. "millet seed"] a tiny epidermal cyst presenting as a firm, white to yellow, smooth, globoid, keratin-containing papule lying superficially within the skin, occurring multiply and usually located on the eyelids, cheeks, and forehead, and found in the pilosebaceous follicles in all age groups, including neonates. Milia may arise de novo or in association with various dermatoses and skin traumas. Called also *whitehead.* See also *Epstein's pearls,* under *pearl.*
**colloid m.,** a small, discrete, translucent, ivory to yellow, firm papule containing an amorphous colloid material, occurring in profuse eruptions, usually located on the face and dorsum of the hands, during middle age. *Multiple eruptive milia* is a similar condition that presents during childhood, and is transmitted as an autosomal dominant condition.

**milk** (milk) [L. *lac*] [MeSH: Milk] 1. the fluid secretion of the mammary gland forming the natural food of young mammals. 2. any whitish milklike substance, e.g., coconut milk or plant latex. 3. a liquid (emulsion or suspension) resembling the secretion of the mammary gland.
**acidophilus m.,** milk fermented with cultures of *Lactobacillus acidophilus;* used in gastrointestinal disorders in attempts to modify the bacterial flora of the intestinal tract.
**m. of bismuth** [USP], a suspension of bismuth hydroxide and bismuth subcarbonate in water, yielding 5.2–5.8 per cent bismuth trioxide; used as an astringent and antacid. Called also *bismuth magma.*
**certified m.,** unpasteurized milk certified to meet specified guidelines for microbial content, processing, and storage and handling temperatures.
**condensed m.,** milk which has been partly evaporated and sweetened with sugar.
**evaporated m.,** milk prepared by evaporation of half its water content.
**fortified vitamin D m.,** vitamin D m.
**homogenized m.,** milk so treated that the fats become intimately combined with the general body of the milk, the emulsified particles of fat being made so minute that the cream does not separate.
**litmus m.,** see *litmus medium* under *culture medium.*
**lowfat m.,** milk having 1 to 2 per cent fat content.
**m. of magnesia** [USP], a suspension of 7.0–8.5 per cent of magnesium hydroxide used as an antacid and cathartic; called also *magnesia magma.*
**modified m.,** milk in which the constituents have been made to correspond in amount to the composition of human milk.
**nonfat m.,** milk having no greater than 0.5 per cent fat content.
**pasteurized m.,** milk that has been specially heat treated to kill bacteria; see *pasteurization.*
**skim m.,** milk from which some or all of the cream has been removed; see *lowfat m.* and *nonfat m.*
**soy m.,** a liquid made from soybeans, used as a milk substitute and a source of calcium for those unable or unwilling to ingest dairy products.
**m. of sulfur,** precipitated sulfur.
**uterine m.,** a white milky substance in the gravid uterus of some species, presumably for nourishment of the embryo.
**vegetable m.,** synthetic milk made out of vegetables.
**vitamin D m.,** cow's milk supplemented with 400 IU of vitamin D per quart.
**witch's m.,** milk secreted in the breast of the newborn child; hexenmilch.

**milk·ing** (milk'ing) the pressing out of the contents of a tubular part, such as the urethra, by running the finger along it.

**Milk·man's syndrome** (milk'manz) [Louis Arthur *Milkman,* American radiologist, 1895–1951] see under *syndrome.*

**milk·pox** (milk'poks) variola minor.

**milk·weed** (milk'wēd) any plant of the genus *Asclepias.*

**milk·wort** (milk'wōrt) any plant of the genus *Polygala.*

**Mil·lard-Gub·ler syndrome (paralysis)** (me-yahr' goo-blār') [Auguste L. J. *Millard,* French physician, 1830–1915; Adolphe Marie *Gubler,* French physician, 1821–1879] see under *syndrome.*

**Mil·ler syndrome** (mil'ər) [Marvin *Miller,* American pediatrician, 20th century] see under *syndrome.*

**Mil·ler Fish·er syndrome** (mil'ər fish'ər) [C. *Miller Fisher,* American neurologist, 20th century] Fisher syndrome.

**Mil·ler-Ab·bott tube** (mil'ər-ab'ət) [T. Grier *Miller,* American physician, 1886–1981; William Osler *Abbott,* American physician, 1902–1943] see under *tube.*

**Mil·ler-Diek·er syndrome** (mil'ər de'kər) [James Quinter *Miller,* American neurologist, born 1926; H. *Dieker,* American physician, 20th century] see under *syndrome.*

**milli-** [L. *mille* thousand] a combining form indicating one thousand (e.g., millipede); used in naming units of measurement to indicate one one-thousandth ($10^{-3}$) of the unit designated by the root with which it is combined. Symbol, m.

**mil·li·am·me·ter** (mil"e-am'me-tər) an ammeter which registers a current in milliamperes.

**mil·li·am·pere** (mil"e-am'pēr) [Fr.] one-thousandth of an ampere. Symbol mA.

**mil·li·bar** (mil'ĭ-bahr) one-thousandth part of a bar.

**mil·li·cou·lomb** (mil"ĭ-koo'lom) a unit of quantity of current electricity, being one one-thousandth ($10^{-3}$) of a coulomb. Symbol mC.

**mil·li·cu·rie** (mil"ĭ-ku're) a unit of radioactivity, being one one-thousandth ($10^{-3}$) curie, or the quantity of radioactive material in which the number of nuclear disintegrations is $3.7 \times 10^7$ per second. Symbol mCi.

**mil·li·cu·rie-hour** (mil"ĭ-ku're-our") a unit of cumulated radioactivity equal to the presence of 1 millicurie for 1 hour. Symbol mCi-hr.

**mil·li·equiv·a·lent** (mil"e-e-kwiv'ə-lənt) the number of grams of a solute contained in one milliliter of a normal solution; symbol mEq.

**mil·li·gram** (mil'ĭ-gram) [*milli-* + *gram*] one-thousandth of a gram. Symbol mg.

**Mil·li·kan-Sie·kert syndrome** (mil'ə-kən-se'kərt) [Clark Harold *Millikan,* American neurologist, born 1915; Robert George *Siekert,* American neurologist, born 1924] vertebrobasilar insufficiency.

**mil·li·lam·bert** (mil"i-lam'bərt) one-thousandth of a lambert.

**mil·li·li·ter** (mil'ĭ-le"tər) [*milli-* + *liter*] a unit of volume in the metric system, being one one-thousandth ($10^{-3}$) liter. Symbol mL or ml.

**mil·li·me·ter** (mil'ĭ-me"tər) a unit of linear measure of the metric system, being one one-thousandth ($10^{-3}$) meter. Symbol mm.

**millimicr(o)-** a prefix used in naming units of measurement to indicate one-thousandth of one-millionth ($10^{-9}$) of the unit designated by the root with which it is combined; now supplanted by the prefix *nan(o)-.*

**mil·li·mi·cro·cu·rie** (mil"ĭ-mi"kro-ku're) nanocurie.

**mil·li·mo·lar** (mil"ĭ-mo'lər) denoting a concentration of 1 millimole per liter. Symbol mM.

**mil·li·mole** (mil'ĭ-mōl) one-thousandth part of a mole (see *mole¹*); symbol mmol.

**mill·ing-in** (mil'ing-in) correction of occlusal disharmonies of natural or artificial teeth by the use of abrasives between their occluding surfaces while they are rubbed together in the mouth or on the articulator. See also *grinding-in, occlusal adjustment,* under *adjustment,* and *selective grinding,* under *grinding.*

**mil·lions** (mil'yənz) a name applied to various small fish that devour mosquito larvae; see *Lebistes reticulatus.*

**mil·li·os·mole** (mil"e-os'mōl) one-thousandth of an osmole. Symbol mOsm.

**mil·li·pede** (mil'ĭ-pēd) any arthropod of the class Diplopoda.

**mil·li·rad** (mil'ĭ-rad) one-thousandth ($10^{-3}$) rad; symbol mrad.

**mil·li·rem** (mil'ĭ-rem) one-thousandth ($10^{-3}$) of a rem; symbol mrem.

**mil·li·roent·gen** (mil'ĭ-rent"gən) one-thousandth ($10^{-3}$) roentgen; symbol mr.

**mil·li·sec·ond** (mil"ĭ-sek'ond) one-thousandth of a second; abbreviated msec; symbol ms.

**mil·li·unit** (mil'ĭ-u"nit) one-thousandth ($10^{-3}$) of a standard unit; symbol mU.

**mil·li·volt** (mil'ĭ-vōlt) one-thousandth of a volt. Symbol mV.

**Mil·lon's test (reaction, reagent)** (me-yawz') [Auguste Nicolas Eugène *Millon,* French chemist, 1812–1867] see under *test.*

**Mills' disease** (milz) [Charles Karsner *Mills,* American neurologist, 1845–1931] ascending hemiplegia.

**Mills-Rein·cke phenomenon** (milz-rīn'kĕ) [Hiram F. *Mills,* American engineer, 1836–1921; Johann Julius *Reincke,* German physician, 19th century] see under *phenomenon.*

**Mil·path** (mil'path) trademark for a preparation of meprobamate and tridihexethyl chloride.

**mil·pho·sis** (mil-fo'sis) [Gr. *milphōsis*] the falling out of the eyelashes. Cf. *madarosis.*

**mil·ri·none** (mil'rĭ-nōn) a cardiotonic.

**Mil·roy's disease (edema)** (mil'roiz) [William Forsyth *Milroy,* American physician, 1855–1942] see under *disease.*

**Milstein** (mil'stīn) Cesar. Argentine-born immunologist in Great Britain, born 1927. Co-winner with Niels Kaj Jerne and Georges J. F. Köhler of the Nobel prize for medicine or physiology in 1984 for his and Köhler's production of monoclonal antibodies.

**Mil·ton's disease, edema** (mil'tonz) [John Laws *Milton,* British dermatologist, 1820–1898] angioedema.

**Mil·town** (mil'toun) trademark for a preparation of meprobamate.

**milz·brand** (milts'brahnt) old name for *anthrax.*

**Mi·ma poly·mor·pha** (me'mə pol″e-mor'fə) *Acinetobacter calcoaceticus.*

**mi·me·sis** (mi-me'sis) [Gr. *mimēsis* imitation] the simulation of one disease or bodily process by another.

**mi·met·ic** (mi-met'ik) [Gr. *mimētikos*] marked by simulation of another bodily process or disease.

**-mimetic** Also used as a word termination indicating simulation of a function, process, etc., designated by the root to which it is affixed, as *sympathomimetic.*

**mim·ic** (mim'ik) mimetic.

**mim·ic·ry** (mim'ik-re″) [Gr. *mimos* to imitate] 1. imitation or simulation. 2. an adaptation for survival in which an organism takes on a resemblance to some other organism or a nonliving object.

**mim·ma·tion** (mĭ-ma'shən) mytacism.

**mi·mo·sis** (mi-mo'sis) mimesis.

**min.** abbreviation for L. *min'imum,* a minim.

**Mi·na·ma·ta disease** (me″nah-mah'tah) [*Minamata* Bay, Japan, source of poisoned seafood that caused the disease in the 1950's] see under *disease.*

**Min·card** (min'kahrd) trademark for a preparation of aminometradine.

**mind** (mīnd) [from A.S. *gemynd;* L. *mens;* Gr. *psychē*] 1. the organ or seat of consciousness; the faculty, or function of the brain, by which an individual becomes aware of his surroundings and of their distribution in space and time, and by which he experiences feelings, emotions, and desires, and is able to attend, to remember, to learn, to reason, and to decide. 2. the organized totality of an organism's mental and psychological processes, conscious and unconscious. 3. the characteristic thought process of a person or group.

**min·er·al** (min'ər-əl) [L. *minerale*] a nonorganic homogeneous solid substance, usually a constituent of the earth's crust.
**trace m.,** a mineral trace element.

**min·er·alo·cor·ti·coid** (min″ər-əl-o-kor'tĭ-koid) any of the group of C21 corticosteroids, principally aldosterone in humans, involved in the regulation of electrolyte and water balance through their effects on ion transport in epithelial cells. They promote retention of sodium, loss of potassium, and the secondary retention of water; some also have varying degrees of glucocorticoid activity. The primary stimulant to aldosterone secretion is angiotensin II.

**Mi·ner·va jac·ket** (mĭ-nər'və) [*Minerva,* Roman goddess of wisdom, because of its resemblance to her armor] see under *jacket.*

**mini-** [*mini*ature] a combining form denoting something smaller than is usual for objects in a given class.

**min·i·fy** (min'ĭ-fi) [L. *minus* less] to render less or diminish; the opposite of magnify.

**mini·lap·a·rot·o·my** (min″e-lap″ə-rot'ə-me) [*mini-* + *laparotomy*] a very short laparotomy incision.

**min·im** (min'im) [L. *minimum* least] a unit of capacity (liquid measure), being one-sixtieth part of a fluid dram, or the equivalent of 0.0616 milliliter. Symbol m.

**min·i·ma** (min'ĭ-mə) [L.] plural of *minimum.*

**min·i·mal** (min'ĭ-məl) [L. *minimus* least] smallest or least; the smallest possible.

**min·i·mum** (min'ĭ-məm) pl. *min'ima* [L. "smallest"] the smallest amount or lowest limit.
**m. audi'bile, m. audible,** auditory threshold.
**m. cognosci'bile,** the threshold of visual recognition of complicated shapes or contours.
**m. legi'bile,** the threshold of visible recognition of form, as of test letters or numbers.
**light m.,** the minimum intensity of light which is visually perceptible in completely darkened surroundings.
**m. sensi'bile,** threshold of consciousness.
**m. separa'bile,** resolution threshold.
**m. visi'bile,** light m.

**mini·plate** (min'e-plāt) a small bone plate.

**Mini·press** (min'ĭ-pres) trademark for a preparation of prazosin hydrochloride.

**Mini·spor·i·da** (min″ĭ-spor'ĭ-də) [*mini-* + *spore*] an order of parasitic protozoa (class Microsporea, phylum Microspora) having a general tendency toward minimum development of accessory spore organelles accompanied by maximum development of sporocysts, and characterized by spores without a well-developed polaroplast, usually with a relatively short polar tube, with little or no endospore.

**Mini·tran** (min'e-tran) trademark for a preparation of nitroglycerin.

**Mini·zide** (min'ĭ-zīd) trademark for preparations of prazosin hydrochloride with polythiazide.

**Min·kow·ski's figure** (min-kof'skēz) [Oskar *Minkowski,* Lithuanian physician in Germany, 1858–1931] see under *figure.*

**Min·kow·ski-Chauf·fard syndrome** (min-kof'ske-sho-fahr') [Oskar *Minkowski;* Anatole-Marie-Emile *Chauffard,* French physician, 1855–1932] hereditary spherocytosis.

**Mi·no·cin** (mĭ-no'sin) trademark for preparations of minocycline hydrochloride.

**mi·no·cy·cline** (mĭ-no-si'klēn) [MeSH: Minocycline] a semisynthetic broad-spectrum antibiotic of the tetracycline group.
**m. hydrochloride** [USP], the monohydrochloride salt of minocycline, used in the treatment of a wide variety of infections due to tetracycline-susceptible bacteria and to some tetracycline-resistant organisms, especially staphylococci, administered orally and intravenously.

**Mi·nor's disease, sign** (me'norz) [Lazar Salomonovich *Minor,* Russian neurologist, 1855–1942] see under *disease* and *sign.*

**Mi·not** (mi'not) George Richards. American physician and pathologist, 1885–1950; co-winner, with William Parry Murphy and George Hoyt Whipple, of the Nobel prize for medicine or physiology in 1934 for their research into the use of liver therapy in pernicious anemia.

**Mi·not-von Wil·le·brand syndrome** (mi'not-fon vil'e-brahnt) [Francis *Minot,* American physician, 1821–1899; Erick Adolf *von Willebrand,* Finnish physician, 1870–1949] see *von Willebrand's disease,* under *disease..*

**mi·nox·i·dil** (mĭ-nok'sĭ-dil) [USP] [MeSH: Minoxidil] a potent, long-acting orally effective vasodilator, acting primarily on arterioles, used as an antihypertensive; also applied topically in the treatment of male pattern baldness of the vertex.

**mint** (mint) 1. any plant of the genus *Mentha.* 2. any of certain other plants resembling those of genus *Mentha.*
**mountain m.,** a plant of the genus *Pycnanthemum.*
**wild m.,** *Mentha canadensis,* a fragrant North American plant that is the source of an essential oil with a lemonlike odor that is used in perfumery. Called also *pennyroyal.*

**Min·te·zol** (min'tə-zol) trademark for a preparation of thiabendazole.

**mi·nute** (mi-nōōt') [L. *minuere* to diminish] extremely small.
**double m's,** acentric chromosomal fragments created by gene amplification and newly integrated into the chromosome; they are tumor markers indicative of solid neoplasms with poor prognosis.

**MIO** minimal identifiable odor.

**mio-** [Gr. *meiōn* smaller] a combining form meaning less, or denoting relationship to contraction.

**Mio·chol** (mi'o-kol) trademark for a preparation of acetylcholine chloride.

**mio·did·y·mus** (mi″o-did'ĭ-məs) [*mio-* + *-didymus*] asymmetrical conjoined twins in which a smaller head is joined to the larger one at the occiput.

**mio·lec·i·thal** (mi″o-les'ĭ-thəl) [*mio-* + *-lecithal*] containing little yolk; see under *ovum.*

**mio·pra·gia** (mi″o-pra'je-ə) [*mio-* + Gr. *prassein* to perform] decreased functional activity.

**mi·o·pus** (mi'o-pəs) [*mio-* + Gr. *ōps* face] a fetus with two fused heads, one face being rudimentary.

**mi·o·sis** (mi-o'sis) [Gr. *meiōsis* diminution] [MeSH: Miosis] 1. contraction of the pupil. 2. meiosis.
**irritative m.,** spastic m.
**paralytic m.,** miosis due to paralysis of the dilator of the iris.

**spastic m.,** miosis due to spasm of the sphincter pupillae.
**spinal m.,** miosis occurring in spinal diseases.

**mi·ot·ic** (mi-ot'ik) 1. pertaining to, characterized by, or producing miosis (def. 1). 2. an agent that causes the pupil to contract. 3. meiotic.

**MIP** maximum inspiratory pressure.

**mi·ra·cid·ia** (mi-rə-sid'e-ə) plural of *miracidium.*

**mi·ra·cid·i·um** (mi-rə-sid'e-əm) pl. *miraci'dia* [Gr. *meirakidion* a boy, lad, stripling] the first stage larva of a trematode which undergoes further development in the body of a snail.

**mir·ac·u·lin** (mir-ak'u-lin) a glycoprotein from the fruit of the tropical plant *Synsepalum dulcificum* which, after it is tasted, is able to change the perception of the taste of acids from sour to sweet.

**Mir·a·don** (mir'ə-don) trademark for a preparation of anisindione.

**mire** (mēr) [Fr., from L. *mirari* to look at] one of the figures on the arm of an ophthalmometer whose images are reflected on the cornea. The measurement of their variations determines the amount of corneal astigmatism.

**mir·in·ca·my·cin hy·dro·chlo·ride** (mir-in'kə-mi"sin) an antibacterial and antimalarial, $C_{19}H_{35}ClN_2O_5S \cdot HCl$.

**MIRL** membrane inhibitor of reactive lysis; see *protectin.*

**mir·ror** (mir'ər) [Fr. *miroir*] a polished surface that reflects sufficient light to yield images of objects in front of it.
**concave m.,** one with a concave reflecting surface.
**convex m.,** one with a convex reflecting surface.
**dental m.,** mouth m.
**frontal m.,** head m.
**Glatzel m.,** a mirror held below the nose for receiving moist breath to assess nasal patency; see also *pneumatype.*
**head m.,** a circular mirror strapped to the head of the examiner to reflect light into a cavity, especially the nose, pharynx, or larynx. Called also *frontal m.*
**mouth m.,** a small mirror, magnifying or nonmagnifying, used to reflect the operating field in the oral cavity, to retract the tissues and tongue, and to protect the tissues from injury during operation. Called also *dental m.* See also *dental reflector,* under *reflector.*
**nasographic m.,** Glatzel m.
**plane m.,** one with a flat reflecting surface.

**mir·taz·a·pine** (mir"taz-ə-pēn) an antidepressant compound unrelated to any of the classes of antidepressants; administered orally.

**mir·ya·chit** (mir-yah'chit) myriachit.

**mis·an·thro·py** (mis-an'thrə-pe) [*miso-* + *anthrop-* + *-ia*] hatred of mankind.

**mis·car·riage** (mis'kar-əj) loss of the products of conception from the uterus before the fetus is viable; spontaneous abortion.

**mis·ce** (mis'e) [L.] mix. Symbol M.

**mis·ceg·e·na·tion** (mĭ-sej"ə-na'shən) [L. *miscere* to mix + *genus* race] the intermarriage or cohabitation of persons of different races, or the interbreeding of races.

**mis·ci·ble** (mis'ĭ-bəl) susceptible of being mixed.

**mis·clas·si·fi·ca·tion** (mis"klas-ĭ-fĭ-ka'shən) assignment of subjects, values, or attributes to inappropriate groups or categories. In *nondifferential m.* the probability or direction of misclassification error is constant across all study groups while in *differential m.* it varies across the groups.

**mis·i·den·ti·fi·ca·tion** (mis"i-den"tĭ-fi"ka'shən) failure to identify correctly persons or objects known to the subject, caused by confusion or memory loss.
**delusional m.,** that due to the mistaken belief that a person or object has been transformed physically or mentally. See also *Capgras' syndrome,* under *syndrome,* and *Frégoli's phenomenon,* under *phenomenon.*

**mis(o)-** [Gr. *misos* hatred] a combining form meaning hatred of.

**mi·sog·a·my** (mĭ-sog'ə-me) [*miso-* + Gr. *gamos* marriage] hatred of or aversion to marriage.

**mi·sog·y·ny** (mĭ-soj'ĭ-ne) [*miso-* + Gr. *gynē* woman] hatred of women.

**mi·so·nid·a·zole** (mi"so-nid'ə-zōl) [MeSH: Misonidazole] a compound structurally related to metronidazole, formerly used as an antitrichomonal and antiprotozoal but now primarily used as a radiosensitizer. Administered orally.

**mi·so·pro·stol** (mi-so-pros'tol) [USP] [MeSH: Misoprostol] a synthetic prostaglandin $E_1$ analog administered orally to treat gastric irritation that is the result of long-term therapy with nonsteroidal anti-inflammatory drugs.

**mist.** abbreviation for L. *mistu'ra,* a mixture.

**mis·tle·toe** (mis'əl-to) any of several parasitic shrubs of the family Loranthaceae. European mistletoe is *Viscum album* and American mistletoe is *Phorandendron flavescens.* Both contain small amounts of toxins such as pressor amines, beta-phenylethylamine, and tyramine.

**mis·tu·ra** (mis-tu'rə) [L.] mixture. Symbol M.
**m. cre'tae,** chalk mixture.

**MIT** monoiodotyrosine.

**Mit.** abbreviation for L. *mit'te,* send.

**mit·ap·sis** (mit-ap'sis) [*mito-* + Gr. *hapsis* joining] the fusion of the chromatin granules in the final stage of cell conjugation.

**Mitch·ell's disease** (mich'əlz) [Silas Weir *Mitchell,* American neurologist, 1829–1914] erythromelalgia.

**Mitch·ell operation** (mich'əl) [Charles L. *Mitchell,* American orthopedic surgeon, born 1901] see under *operation.*

**Mit·chel·la** (mĭ-chel'ə) [John *Mitchell,* American botanist, 18th century] a genus of creeping perennial evergreen herbs of the family Rubiaceae. *M. re'pens* L. is the partridge berry or deerberry, a North American species that when dried is the medicinal herb called *mitchella.*

**mitch·el·la** (mĭ-chel'ə) 1. any plant of the genus *Mitchella.* 2. the dried plant *Mitchella repens,* used as a diuretic, astringent, and antidiarrheal, and formerly as a uterine tonic.

**mite** (mīt) [MeSH: Mites] any arthropod of the order Acarina except the ticks. Most mites are minute and have transparent or semitransparent bodies; they may be parasitic on humans and domestic animals, producing various irritations of the skin (acariasis). Families include Acaridae, Dermanyssidae, and Trombiculidae. Mite genera important to human and veterinary medicine include *Acarapis, Acarus, Allodermanyssus, Bryobia, Cheyletiella, Chorioptes, Demodex, Dermanyssus, Dermatophagoides, Echinolaelaps, Eutrombicula, Glycyphagus, Knemidokoptes, Lynxacarus, Myobia, Neoschoengastia, Notoedres, Ornithonyssus, Otodectes, Pneumonyssus, Psorergates, Psoroptes, Pyemotes, Rhizoglyphus, Sarcoptes, Tetranychus, Trombicula,* and *Tyrophagus.*
**auricular m.,** see *Otodectes.*
**bird m.,** *Dermanyssus gallinae.*
**burrowing m.,** see *Sarcoptes.*
**cheese m.,** *Tyrophagus longior.*
**chicken m.,** *Dermanyssus gallinae.*
**chigger m.,** trombiculid.
**clover m.,** *Bryobia praetiosa.*
**coolie-itch m.,** *Rhizoglyphus parasiticus.*
**copra m.,** *Tyrophagus castellani.*
**depluming m.,** *Knemidokoptes gallinae.*
**face m.,** *Demodex folliculorum.*
**flour m.,** *Tyrophagus farinae.*
**follicle m.,** *Demodex folliculorum.*
**food m.,** *Glycyphagus domesticus.*
**fowl m.,** *Dermanyssus gallinae.*
**hair follicle m.,** *Demodex folliculorum.*
**harvest m.,** chigger.
**house dust m.,** either *Dermatophagoides pteronyssinus* or *D. farinae.*
**itch m.,** see *Notoedres* and *Sarcoptes.*
**kedani m.,** *Trombicula akamushi.*
**louse m.,** *Pyemotes.*
**mange m.,** any of various mites that cause mange; see, e.g., *Chorioptes, Demodex, Knemidokoptes, Notoedres, Otodectes, Psoroptes,* and *Sarcoptes.*
**meal m.,** *Tyrophagus.*
**mouse m.,** *Allodermanyssus sanguineus.*
**mower's m.,** chigger.
**nasal m.,** *Pneumonyssus caninum.*
**northern fowl m.,** *Ornithonyssus sylviarum.*
**onion m.,** *Acarus rhyzoglypticus hyacinthi.*
**poultry m.,** *Dermanyssus gallinae.*
**rat m.,** see *Ornithonyssus.*
**red m.,** chigger.
**scab m.,** see *Psoroptes.*
**spinning m.,** *Bryobia praetiosa.*
**straw m.,** *Pyemotes.*
**tropical fowl m.,** *Ornithonyssus bursa.*
**tropical rat m.,** *Ornithonyssus bacoti.*

**mi·tel·la** (mi-tel'ə) [L.] an arm sling.

**Mith·ra·cin** (mith'rə-sin) trademark for a preparation of mithramycin.

**mith·ra·my·cin** (mith"rə-mi'sin) [USP] plicamycin.

**mith·ri·da·tism** (mith'rĭ-da"tiz-əm) [after *Mithridates,* died 63 B.C., king of Pontus, who reportedly took poisons so as to become immunized against them] the acquisition of immunity to the effects of a poison by ingestion of gradually increasing amounts of it.

**mi·ti·ci·dal** (mi"tĭ-si'dəl) destructive to mites.

**mi·ti·cide** (mi'tĭ-sīd) an agent that is destructive to mites.

**mit·i·gate** (mit'ĭ-gāt) [L. *mitigara* to soften] to moderate; to render milder.

**mi·tis** (mi'tis) [L.] mild.

**mit(o)-** [Gr. *mitos* thread] a combining form meaning threadlike, or denoting relationship to a thread, or to mitosis.

**mi·to·car·cin** (mi"to-kahr'sin) an antineoplastic antibiotic derived from *Streptomyces* species.

**mi·to·chon·dria** (mi"to-kon'dre-ə, mit"o-kon'dre-ə) pl. of *mitochondrion* [*mito-* + *chondri-* + *-ia*] [MeSH: Mitochondria] small spherical to rod-shaped components (organelles) found in the cytoplasm of cells, enclosed in a double membrane, with an internal membrane space between the two units, the inner one infolded into the interior of the organelle as a series of projections (cristae). They are the principal sites of the generation of energy (in the form of ion gradients and adenosine triphosphate [ATP] synthesis) resulting from the oxidation of foodstuffs, and they contain the enzymes of the Krebs and fatty acid cycles and the respiratory pathway. Mitochondria also contain RNA and DNA, by means of which they can independently replicate and code for the synthesis of some of their proteins. Called also *chondriosomes.* See Plates 13 and 14.

**mi·to·chon·dri·al** (mi"to-kon'dre-əl) of or pertaining to mitochondria.

**mi·to·chon·dri·al ATP·ase** (mi-tə-kon'dre-əl a-te-pe'ase) $H^+$-transporting ATP synthase.

**mi·to·chon·dri·on** (mi"to-kon'dre-on) singular of *mitochondria.*

**mi·to·cro·min** (mi"to-kro'min) an antineoplastic antibiotic produced by *Streptomyces viridochromogenes.*

**mi·to·gen** (mi'to-jən) a substance that induces blast transformation; DNA, RNA, and protein synthesis; and proliferation of lymphocytes, e.g., concanavalin A, phytohemagglutinin, pokeweed mitogen, or lipopolysaccharide.
**pokeweed m.,** a lectin isolated from pokeweed *(Phytolacca americana)*; it is a mitogen that stimulates both B and T lymphocytes. Abbreviated PWM.

**mi·to·ge·ne·sia** (mi"to-jə-ne"zhə) mitogenesis.

**mi·to·gen·e·sis** (mi"to-jen'ə-sis) [*mito-* + *-genesis*] the production, or causation, of mitosis in or transformation of a cell.

**mi·to·ge·net·ic** (mi"to-jə-net'ik) pertaining to, inducing, or characterized by mitogenesis.

**mi·to·gen·ic** (mi"to-jen'ik) causing or inducing mitosis or cell transformation.

**mi·to·ki·net·ic** (mit"o-kĭ-net'ik) [*mito-* + *kinetic*] a term applied to the force existing in the kinoplasm of a cell which produces the achromatic spindle in karyokinesis.

**mi·to·lac·tol** (mi"to-lak'tol) [MeSH: Mitolactol] an alkylating agent that has been used as an antineoplastic in the treatment of invasive ovarian carcinoma; administered orally.

**mi·to·mal·cin** (mi"to-mal'sin) an antineoplastic antibiotic produced by *Streptomyces malayensis.*

**mi·tome** (mi'tōm) a thready network of the protoplasm of a cell; the more solid portion of cell protoplasm.

**mi·to·my·cin** (mi"to-mi'sin) an antineoplastic antibiotic produced by *Streptomyces caespitosus* that acts as a bifunctional or trifunctional alkylating agent causing cross-linking of DNA and inhibition of DNA synthesis and is relatively phase-specific for the late $G_1$ and early S phases of the cell cycle. It has activity against many types of carcinoma as well as chronic myelogenous leukemia, but because of its severe toxicity and myelosuppression it is usually used only for palliation in patients who have not responded to other treatment.

**mi·to·plasm** (mi'to-plaz"əm) [*mito-* + *-plasm*] the chromatic substance of a cell nucleus.

**mi·tos·chi·sis** (mĭ-tos'kĭ-sis) [*mito-* + *-schisis*] karyokinesis.

**mi·to·ses** (mi-to'sēz) [MeSH: Mitosis] plural of *mitosis.*

**mi·to·sis** (mi-to'sis) pl. *mito'ses* [*mito-* + *-osis*] [MeSH: Mitosis] a method of indirect division of a cell, consisting of a complex of various processes, by means of which the two daughter nuclei normally receive identical complements of the number of chromosomes characteristic of the somatic cells of the species. It is the process by which the body grows and replaces cells and is divided into four phases: *Prophase:* Formation of paired chromosomes; disappearance of nuclear membrane; appearance of the achromatic spindle; formation of polar bodies. *Metaphase:* Arrangement of chromosomes in the equatorial plane of the central spindle to form the monaster. Chromosomes separate into exactly similar halves. *Anaphase:* The two groups of daughter chromosomes separate and move along the fibers of the central spindle, each toward one of the asters, forming the diaster. *Telophase:* The daughter chromosomes resolve themselves into a reticulum and the daughter nuclei are formed; the cytoplasm divides, forming two complete daughter cells. NOTE: The term *mitosis* is used interchangeably with cell division, but strictly speaking it refers to nuclear division, whereas *cytokinesis* refers to division of the cytoplasm. In some cells, as in many fungi and the fertilized eggs of many insects, nuclear division occurs within the cell unaccompanied by division of the cytoplasm and formation of daughter cells. Cf. *meiosis.*
**heterotypic m.,** mitosis in which the halves of bivalent chromosomes move away from each other toward the poles, as occurs in the first, or reductional, division of meiosis.
**homeotypic m.,** the ordinary type of cell division in mitosis, as occurs also in the second, or equational, division of meiosis.
**multicentric m.,** pluripolar m.
**pathologic m.,** atypical, asymmetrical mitosis indicative of malignancy.
**pluripolar m.,** cell division that results in the formation of more than two daughter cells.

**mi·to·some** (mi'to-sōm) [*mito-* + *-some*] a body formed from the spindle fibers of the preceding mitosis; a spindle remnant.

**mi·to·sper** (mi'to-spər) an antineoplastic substance derived from *Aspergillus glaucus.*

**mi·to·spore** (mi'to-spor) an asexual spore, so called because it is produced by mitosis; when motile it is called a *zoospore.*

**mi·to·tane** (mi'to-tān) [USP] [MeSH: Mitotane] a cytotoxic compound related to the insecticides DDT and TDE (DDD) that causes severe damage to the adrenal cortex, causing a rapid decrease in adrenocorticosteroid production; used for palliation in inoperable adrenocortical carcinoma of both functional and nonfunctional types, administered orally.

**mi·tot·ic** (mi-tot'ik) pertaining to mitosis.

**mi·to·xan·trone hy·dro·chlo·ride** (mi"to-zan'trōn) [USP] an antineoplastic agent of the anthracenedione family, administered intravenously for the treatment of acute nonlymphocytic leukemia.

**mi·tral** (mi'trəl) 1. shaped somewhat like a miter. 2. pertaining to the mitral or bicuspid valve.

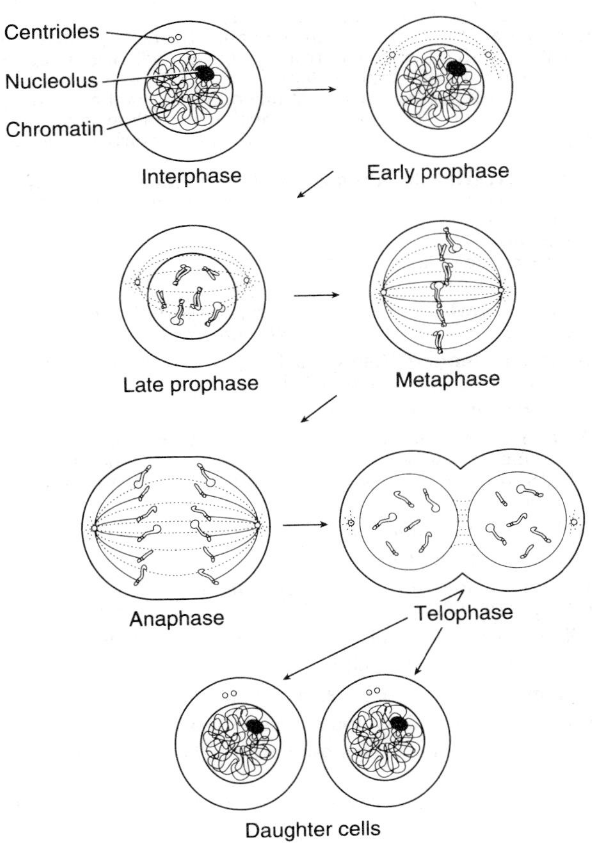


Mitosis shown as occurring in a cell of a hypothetical animal with a diploid chromosome number of six (haploid number three); one pair of chromosomes is short, one pair is long and hooked, and one pair is long and knobbed.

**mi·tral·iza·tion** (mi″trəl-ĭ-za′shən) straightening of the left border and prominence of the pulmonary salient of the cardiac shadow, a configuration commonly seen radiographically in mitral stenosis.

**Mit·su·da antigen, reaction, test** (mit′soo-dah″) [Kensuke *Mitsuda,* Japanese physician, born 1876] see *lepromin,* see under *reaction,* and see *lepromin test,* under *test.*

**mit·tel·schmerz** (mit′əl-shmertz) [Ger. *mittel* mid, middle, + *schmerz* pain, suffering] pain associated with ovulation, usually occurring in the middle of the menstrual cycle.

**mi·va·cu·rium chlo·ride** (mi″və-ku′re-əm) a nondepolarizing neuromuscular blocking agent of short duration administered intravenously as an adjunct to general anesthesia, to facilitate tracheal intubation, and to induce skeletal muscle relaxation during mechanical ventilation.

**Mi·va·cron** (mi′və-kron″) trademark for a preparation of mivacurium chloride.

**mixed** (mikst) affecting various parts at once; showing two or more different characteristics.

**mixo·sco·pia** (mik″so-sko′pe-ə) [Gr. *mixis* intercourse + *skopein* to examine] a paraphilia in which gratification is obtained by the sight of the object of one's desire engaged in sexual intercourse with another.

**mixo·troph** (mik′so-trof) in bacterial physiology, the ability to use alternative sources for metabolism and energy, as being capable of growth in either the absence or presence of light, or with either organic or inorganic compounds for nutrition.

**mixo·troph·ic** (mik″so-trof′ik) having the nutritional characters of both animals and plants.

**Mix·tard** (miks′tərd) trademark for a mixture of 30 per cent insulin injection (regular insulin) and 70 per cent isophane insulin suspension.

**mix·ture** (miks′chər) [L. *mixtura, mistura*] a combination of different drugs or ingredients, as a fluid resulting from mixing a fluid with other fluids, or with solids, or a suspension of a solid in a liquid. See also under *mistura.*
**Chabaud's m.,** a fixative mixture containing alcohol, phenol, formalin, and acetic acid.
**chalk m.,** prepared chalk, with bentonite magma, cinnamon water, and saccharin sodium; used as an antacid.
**Gunning's m.,** a mixture used in estimating the nitrogen in the urine, consisting of 15 mL of concentrated sulfuric acid, 10 g of potassium sulfate, and 0.5 g of copper sulfate.
**kaolin m. with pectin,** a preparation containing kaolin, pectin, powdered tragacanth, benzoic acid, saccharin sodium, glycerin, and peppermint oil in purified water; used as an adsorbent and demulcent.
**Mayer's glycerin-albumin m.,** a mixture of equal parts of white of egg and glycerin, with a little camphor or phenol, for affixing paraffin sections to slides.
**racemic m.,** racemate.
**Ringer's m.,** see under *irrigation.*
**Tellyesniczky's m.,** see under *fluid.*

**Mi·ya·ga·wa·nel·la** (me″yah-gah″wah-nel′ah) [Yoneji *Miyagawa,* Japanese bacteriologist, 1885–1959] *Chlamydia.*

**Mi·ya·sa·to disease** (me-yah-sah′to) [*Miyasato,* surname of the propositus] $\alpha_2$-antiplasmin deficiency.

**MK** monkey lung (cell culture).

**MKS** abbreviation for *meter-kilogram-second* system, a system of measurements in which the units are based on the meter as the unit of length, the kilogram as the unit of mass, and the second as the unit of time.

**mL, ml** symbol for *milliliter.*

**μl** symbol for *microliter.*

**MLA** abbreviation for L. *mento-laeva anterior* (left mentoanterior, a position of the fetus), and for *Medical Library Association.*

**MLBW** moderately low birth weight; see under *infant.*

**MLC** mixed lymphocyte culture.

**MLD** 1. median lethal dose. 2. minimum lethal dose.

**MLNS** mucocutaneous lymph node syndrome.

**MLP** abbreviation for L. *mento-laeva posterior* (left mentoposterior, a position of the fetus).

**MLR** mixed lymphocyte reaction; see *mixed lymphocyte culture,* under *culture.*

**MLT** abbreviation for L. *mento-laeva transversa* (left mentotransverse, a position of the fetus).

**MM** mucous membranes.

**mM** symbol for *millimolar.*

**mm** symbol for *millimeter.*

**mμ** symbol for *millimicron.*

**μM** symbol for *micromolar.*

**μm** symbol for *micrometer.*

**mμCi** symbol for *millimicrocurie.* See *nanocurie.*

**μμCi** symbol for *micromicrocurie.* See *picocurie.*

**mm Hg** millimeter of mercury, a unit of pressure equal to that exerted by a column of mercury at 0°C one millimeter high at mean sea level. It equals $\frac{1}{760}$ atmosphere or 1 torr to within one part in 7 million.

**MMIHS** megacystis-microcolon–intestinal hypoperistalsis syndrome.

**MMPI** [MeSH: MMPI] Minnesota Multiphasic Personality Inventory.

**MMR** measles-mumps-rubella (vaccine); see *measles, mumps, and rubella vaccine live,* under *vaccine.*

**Mn** symbol for *manganese.*

**M'Nagh·ten (Mc·Naugh·ten) rule** (mik-naw′tən) [Daniel *M'Naghten,* died 1865; acquitted of murder in 1843 by a British court on the grounds of insanity] see under *rule.*

**mne·mic** (ne′mik) mnemonic.

**mne·mon·ic** (ne-mon′ik) [Gr. *mnēmonikos* pertaining to memory] pertaining to, characterized by, or promoting recollection, or memory.

**mne·mon·ics** (ne-mon′iks) the cultivation or improvement of memory by special methods or techniques.

**MO** Medical Officer.

**Mo** symbol for *molybdenum.*

**Mo·ban** (mo′bən) trademark for a preparation of molindone hydrochloride.

**Mo·bi·li·na** (mo″bĭ-li′nə) [L. *mobilis* mobile] a suborder of ciliate protozoa of the order Peritrichida, subclass Peritrichia, which are mobile; usually conical, cylindrical, or discoidal; and orally and aborally flattened. They characteristically have a ciliary girdle and a complex thigmotactic apparatus at the aboral end, often with a highly distinctive denticulate ring of "teeth." All species are ectoparasites or endoparasites of fresh water or marine vertebrates and invertebrates, and those found on the gills of fish are pathogenic.

**mo·bil·i·ty** (mo-bil′ĭ-te) [L. *mobilis* mobile] 1. capability of movement, of being moved, or of flowing freely. 2. rate of movement of a charged particle in an applied electric field.
**electrophoretic m.,** 1. the rate of migration (usually in cm/s) per unit electric field strength (usually V/cm) of a charged particle in electrophoresis. Symbol $\mu$. 2. any measure of the rate of migration of an ionic species in electrophoresis, e.g., $\beta$ electrophoretic mobility, designating the electrophoretic mobility of a beta globulin.

**mo·bi·li·za·tion** (mo″bĭ-lĭ-za′shən) the process of making a fixed part or stored substance mobile, as by separating a part from surrounding structures to make it accessible for an operative procedure or by causing release into the circulation for body use of a substance stored in the body.
**stapes m.,** surgical correction of immobility of the stapes, in treatment of deafness resulting from otosclerosis.

**mo·bil·om·e·ter** (mo″bil-om′ə-tər) an instrument for measuring the consistency of liquids such as oil, cream, liquid foods, etc.

**Mo·bi·lun·cus** (mo″bĭ-lung′kəs) [L. *mobilis* motile + *uncus* hook] [MeSH: Mobiluncus] a genus of gram-negative, anaerobic, small, curved, rod-shaped bacteria, frequently isolated from women with bacterial vaginosis.

**Mö·bi·us' disease, sign, syndrome** (mer′be-əs) [Paul Julius *Möbius,* German neurologist, 1853–1907] see under *sign* and *syndrome* and see *ophthalmoplegic migraine,* under *migraine.*

**moc·ca·sin** (mok′ə-sin) any of several species of snakes of the genus *Agkistrodon.*
**highland m.,** copperhead, def. 1.
**water m.,** *Agkistrodon piscivorus,* a venomous semiaquatic crotalid snake with an olive or brown back, found in the southern United States. Called also *cottonmouth.*

**mo·dal·i·ty** (mo-dal′ĭ-te) 1. a method of application of, or the employment of, any therapeutic agent, especially a physical agent. Cf. *mode* (def. 2). 2. a homeopathic term signifying a condition which modifies drug action; a condition under which symptoms develop, becoming better or worse. 3. a specific sensory entity, such as taste.

**mode** (mōd) [L. *modus* measure, manner] 1. the most frequently occurring value or item in a distribution; when data are grouped, it is the midpoint of the grouping with the highest frequency. A distribution with two peaks is bimodal. 2. the manner of interaction

between a ventilator and the person being ventilated, usually defined in terms of what the stimulus is that starts the ventilation. Cf. *modality* (def. 1).
**assist m.,** a mode of positive pressure ventilation in which the patient initiates and terminates all or most breaths and the ventilator gives some amount of support. Cf. *control m.* and *assist-control m.* Called also *assisted m.*
**assist-control m.,** a mode of positive pressure ventilation in which the ventilator is in assist mode unless the patient's respiration rate falls below a certain amount, in which case the ventilator switches to a control mode. When the strength or rate of respiration increases again, the ventilator goes back into assist mode.
**assisted m.,** assist m.
**control m., controlled m.,** a mode of positive pressure ventilation in which the ventilator controls the initiation and volume of breaths. Cf. *assist m.* and *assist-control m.*
**pressure control m.,** a mode of positive pressure ventilation in which each breath is augmented by air at a fixed rate and amount of pressure, with tidal volume not being fixed. See also under *ventilation.*
**pressure support m.,** a mode of positive pressure ventilation similar to the assist mode; the patient breathes spontaneously and breathing is augmented by air at a preset amount of pressure. See also under *ventilation.*

**mod·el** (mod′əl) 1. something that represents or simulates something else; a replica. 2. a reasonable facsimile of the body or any of its parts; used for demonstration and teaching purposes. 3. cast, def. 5. 4. to imitate another's behavior; see *modeling.* 5. a hypothesis or theory.
**animal m.,** any condition found in an animal that is of value in studying a biological phenomenon, e.g., a pathological mechanism of an animal disorder useful in studying human disease.
**Cox proportional hazards m.,** a method of analysis of multiple factors (variables) that influence an actuarial curve of the risk of a given negative outcome such as disease occurrence or death. A hazard rate is computed for each separate variable (e.g., among those patients with that factor who had not previously suffered a negative outcome, how many subsequently suffered the negative outcome during a short interval) and cumulative hazard rates are computed for the combinations of variables that exist in actual situations.
**figure-of-eight m.,** in cardiology, a variation of the leading circle model of reentry in which the interface of refractory tissue is a curved barrier, with the result that the wavefronts split, proceed around each edge of the arc, and return centrally to describe a figure eight configuration.
**fluid mosaic m.,** the generally accepted theory that cell membranes are composed of bilayers made up of external phospholipids and a central hydrophobic region, with membrane proteins floating in the phospholipids and held in position by various chemical and physical bonding mechanisms.
**leading circle m.,** in cardiology, a multidimensional model of reentry that describes the cycle of alternating tissue activation and refractoriness in terms of a functional, rather than anatomical, intertissue interface acting as a barrier around which the wavefronts circle. In the model, their pathway is the smallest circuit in which the head of each wavefront is just within the tail of that preceding and thus is able to excite tissue still in its relative refractory period.
**proportional hazards m.,** Cox proportional hazards m.
**ring m.,** in cardiology, a model describing the mechanism of anatomical reentry, based on a circuit that is formed around an impenetrable barrier to propagation and contains a locus of slow conduction. The locus blocks the initial normal impulse but is traversed by later impulses from the opposite direction that reexcite normal cardiac fibers, which can occur repetitively. There must exist either a segment of slow conduction or overall slow conduction with a locus of unidirectional block, and total conduction time in the circuit must exceed the refractory period of the fibers so that an excitable gap exists between a wavefront head and the tail of that preceding. See also *reentrant mechanism,* under *mechanism.*

**mod·el·ing** (mod′əl-ing) 1. learning vicariously by observation and imitation, which can be used as a form of behavior therapy. 2. developing or using a hypothesis or theory.
**urea kinetic m.,** the tracing of urea kinetics during hemodialysis, considering urea as a representative medium-sized molecule whose clearance is similar to that of other more toxic substances. A series of mathematical equations are used, taking measured serum urea concentrations and using them to develop other parameters such as dialyzer clearance, urea generation rate of the body, protein catabolic rate, and urea distribution volume.

**Mod·er·il** (mod′ər-il) trademark for a preparation of rescinnamine.

**mod·i·fi·ca·tion** (mod″ĭ-fĭ-ka′shən) the process or result of changing the form or characteristics of an object or substance.
**behavior m.,** see under *therapy.*
**effect m.,** the alteration of the association between two variables under study as a function of a third variable.
**racemic m.,** racemate.

**mod·i·fi·er** (mod′ĭ-fi″ər) an agent that changes the form or characteristics of an object or substance.
**biologic response m. (BRM),** a method or agent, such as a cytokine, monoclonal antibody, or vaccine, that alters host-tumor interaction, usually by amplifying the antitumor mechanisms of the immune system, but also by various mechanisms directly or indirectly affecting host or tumor cell characteristics. Called also *biomodulator.*

**mo·di·o·li·form** (mo″de-o′lĭ-form) shaped like the hub of a wheel.

**mo·di·o·lus** (mo-di′o-ləs) [L. "nave," "hub"] [TA] the central pillar or columella of the cochlea; called also *columella cochleae.*

**Mod. praesc.** abbreviation for L. *mo′do praescrip′to,* in the way directed.

**mod·u·la·tion** (mod″u-la′shən) [L. *modulare* to measure] 1. the act of tempering or toning down. 2. in cytology, the normal capacity of cell adaptability to its environment. 3. embryologic induction in a specific region.
**antigenic m.,** alteration or loss of reactivity of cell surface antigens resulting from redistribution of antigenic sites due to the presence of bound antibody.
**biochemical m.,** in combination chemotherapy, the use of one substance to modulate negative side effects of the primary agent, increasing the effectiveness or allowing a higher dose of the primary agent.

**mod·u·la·tor** (mod′u-la″tər) a specific inductor that brings out characteristics peculiar to a definite region.
**selective estrogen receptor m. (SERM),** an agent that activates some estrogen receptors but not others, thereby having estrogen-like effects on target tissues without affecting other tissues that have estrogen receptors.

**mod·u·lus** (mod′u-ləs) pl. *mo′duli* [L., dim. of *modus* quantity] a coefficient that indicates by a numerical value the extent to which a substance has a given property.
**elastic m., m. of elasticity,** a coefficient indicating the ratio between deforming stress to a unit of area of a substance and the extent of resulting deformation.

**Mod·uret·ic** (mod″u-ret′ik) trademark for preparations of amiloride hydrochloride with hydrochlorothiazide.

**MODY** maturity-onset diabetes of youth.

**Moe plate** (mo) [John H. *Moe,* American surgeon, born 1905] see under *plate.*

**Moe·bi·us** see *Möbius.*

**Moel·ler's glossitis** (mer′lerz) [Julius Otto Ludwig *Moeller,* German surgeon, 1819–1887] see under *glossitis.*

**Moel·ler-Bar·low disease** (mer′ler-bahr′lo) [J. O. L. *Moeller;* Sir Thomas *Barlow,* London physician, 1845–1945] see under *disease.*

**Moen·cke·berg** (mern′kĕ-berg) see *Mönckeberg.*

**mo·e·no·my·cins** (mo″ə-no-mi′sinz) bambermycins.

**mo·ex·i·pril hy·dro·chlo·ride** (mo-ek′sĭpril″) an angiotensin-converting enzyme inhibitor used as an antihypertensive; administered orally.

**mo·fe·til** USAN contraction for 2-(4-morpholinyl)ethyl.

**mogi-** [Gr. *mogis* with difficulty] a combining form meaning difficult, or with difficulty.

**mogi·ar·thria** (moj-e-ahr′thre-ə) [*mogi-* + *arthr-*[2] + *-ia*] dysarthria due to defective muscular coordination.

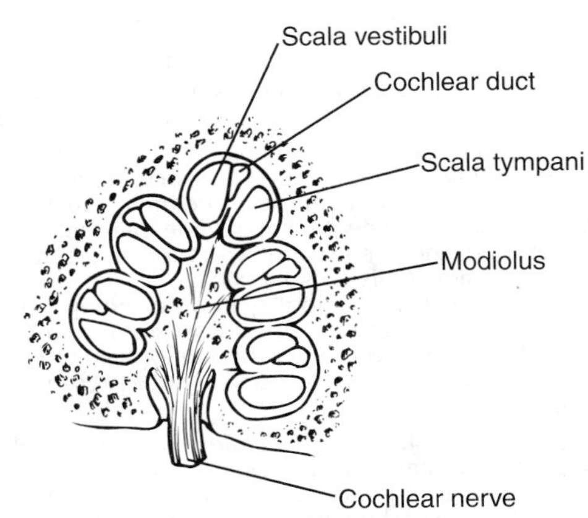

Modiolus in a cross-section through the axis of the cochlea.

**mogi·la·lia** (moj-ĭ-la'le-ə) 1. paralalia. 2. difficulty speaking during psychotherapy, due to resistance.

**mogi·pho·nia** (moj-ĭ-fo'ne-ə) [*mogi-* + *phon-* + *-ia*] dysphonia.

**Mohr syndrome** (mor) [Otto Lous *Mohr,* Norwegian geneticist, 1886–1967] see under *syndrome.*

**Mohr's test** (morz) [Francis *Mohr,* American pharmaceutical chemist, 19th century] see under *test.*

**Moh·ren·heim's fossa (triangle), space** (mo'ren-hīmz) [Baron Joseph Jacob Freiherr von *Mohrenheim,* Austrian surgeon, 1759–1799] see *fossa infraclavicularis* and see under *space.*

**Mohs' chemosurgery, surgery, technique** (mōz) [Frederic Edward *Mohs,* American surgeon, born 1910] see under *technique.*

**moi·e·ty** (moi'ə-te) [Fr. *moitié,* from L. *medietas, medius,* middle] any equal part; a half; also any part or portion.
**carbohydrate m.,** a carbohydrate-derived portion of the structure of a molecule.

**mol** (mol) mole[1].

**mo·lal** (mo'ləl) containing one mole of solute per kilogram of solvent. NOTE: *molal* refers to the weight of the solvent, *molar* to the volume of the solution. Symbol *m.*

**mo·lal·i·ty** (mo-lal'ĭ-te) the number of moles of a solute per kilogram of pure solvent. NOTE: *molality* refers to the weight of the solvent, *molarity* to the volume of the solution.

**mo·lar**[1] (mo'lahr) [MeSH: Molar] 1. pertaining to a mole of a substance, such as molar mass or molar absorptivity, i.e., the quantity of some property associated with a mole of the substance. 2. a measure of the concentration of a solute, expressed as the number of moles of solute per liter of solution (symbol M or *M*) e.g., 0.25M = 0.25 mole per liter (mol/l). The latter notation is used in the SI system.

**mo·lar**[2] (mo'lər) [L. *molaris* belonging to a mill, from *mola* millstone] [MeSH: Molar] 1. molar tooth. 2. pertaining to a molar tooth.
**Moon's m's,** see under *tooth.*
**mulberry m.,** a malformed first molar characterized by dwarfing of the cusps and hypertrophy of the enamel surrounding the cusp with agglomeration of masses of globules, giving it the appearance of a mulberry; seen in congenital syphilis and certain other diseases. Called also *mulberry tooth.*
**sixth-year m.,** the permanent first molar tooth, so called because it usually erupts at the age of 6 years just posterior to the last molar of the deciduous dentition.
**supernumerary m.,** paramolar.
**third m.,** see under *tooth.*
**twelfth-year m.,** the permanent second molar tooth, so called because it usually erupts at the age of 12 years.

**mo·lar·i·form** (mo-lar'ĭ-form) shaped like a molar tooth; showing molarlike characteristics.

**mo·la·ris** (mo-la'ris) [L. "millstone, grinder, molar tooth"] 1. adapted for grinding. 2. one of the molar teeth (dentes molares [TA]).
**m. ter'tius,** wisdom tooth (dens serotinus [TA]).

**mo·lar·i·ty** (mo-lar'ĭ-te) the number of moles of a solute per liter of solution. Cf. *molality.*

**mold** (mōld) [Middle English *moulde*] 1. an imprecise term used to refer to any member of one of the two largest groupings of fungi (the other being the *yeasts*); molds are parasitic and saprobic, and most exist as multicellular filamentous colonies. Common molds are *Mucor, Penicillium, Rhizopus,* and *Aspergillus.* See Plate 29. 2. the deposit or growth produced by such a fungus. 3. a form in which an object is given shape; see also *cast.* 4. an object so shaped. 5. the act of so forming or shaping.
**slime m.,** any member of the fungal class Myxomycetes.
**white m.,** white or slightly gray patches that form on the surface of meat in cold storage and other products due to the growth of fungi.

**mold·ing** (mōld'ing) [L. *modulus* mold, form] 1. the creation of shape, or fashioning of an object. 2. the shaping of the fetal head in adjustment to the size and shape of the birth canal.
**border m.,** the shaping of dental impression material by the manipulation or action of the tissues and structures adjacent to the borders of an impression. Called also *tissue m.*
**compression m.,** a method of molding in which compression is used to pack the material in and to express its excess from the mold.
**injection m.,** the act or process of forcing a plastic material, such as a softened resin, into the mold space under pressure.
**tissue m.,** border m.

**mole**[1] (mōl) [Ger. *Mol,* short for *Molekulargewicht* molecular weight] [MeSH: Moles] that amount of substance (in a system) that contains as many elementary entities (e.g., atoms, ions, molecules, or radicals) as there are carbon atoms in 12 grams of carbon 12 ($^{12}$C); thus one mole equals 6.023 × $10^{23}$ (Avogadro's number) elementary entities. Formerly, the connotation of mole was gram molecular weight (q.v.) and the two terms were sometimes used synonymously. Abbreviated mol.

**mole**[2] (mōl) [A.S. *māl* spot] [MeSH: Moles] a nevocytic nevus; the term is also used to designate a pigmented fleshy growth, and is applied loosely to any blemish of the skin.
**pigmented m.,** see under *nevus.*

**mole**[3] (mōl) [L. *mola* millstone, mole] [MeSH: Moles] a fleshy mass or tumor formed in the uterus by the degeneration or abnormal development of a fertilized ovum.
**blood m.,** a mass in the uterus made up of blood clots, the placenta, and fetal membranes retained after fetal death.
**Breus' m.,** a pathologic change in the placenta found in abortion consisting of accumulation of masses of intervillous hematomas that project into the chorionic space.
**cystic m.,** hydatidiform m.
**false m.,** an intrauterine mass formed from a polyp or neoplasm.
**fleshy m.,** 1. a blood mole which has assumed a fleshlike appearance. 2. one formed by a dead ovum in the uterus.
**hydatid m., hydatidiform m.,** an abnormal pregnancy resulting from a pathologic ovum, with proliferation of the epithelial covering of the chorionic villi and dissolution and cystic cavitation of the avascular stroma of the villi. It results in a mass of cysts resembling a bunch of grapes. Called also *cystic* or *vesicular m.*

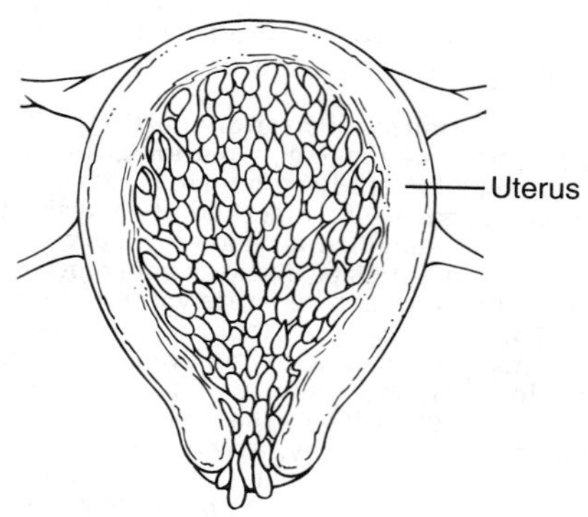

Hydatidiform mole.

**invasive m., malignant m.,** chorioadenoma destruens.
**stone m.,** a mole which has undergone a calcareous degeneration.
**true m.,** a mole which represents the degenerated ovum itself.
**tubal m.,** the mass of blood clot and chorionic villi found after death of the conceptus in a tubal pregnancy.
**vesicular m.,** hydatidiform m.

**mo·lec·u·lar** (mo-lek'u-lər) of, pertaining to, or composed of molecules.

**mol·e·cule** (mol'ə-kūl) [L. *molecula* little mass] a very small mass of matter; the smallest amount of a substance which can exist alone; an aggregation of atoms; specifically, a chemical combination of two or more atoms which form a specific chemical substance. To break up the molecule into its constituent atoms is to change its character. The number and kind of atoms in a molecule vary with the compound.
**adhesion m's, cell adhesion m's (CAM),** cell surface glycoproteins that mediate intercell adhesion in vertebrates.
**cell interaction (CI) m's,** products of cell interaction genes (q.v.).
**CI m's,** cell interaction m's.
**diatomic m.,** one containing two atoms.
**hexatomic m.,** one containing six atoms.
**intercellular adhesion m. 1 (ICAM-1),** a cell membrane glycoprotein containing five immunoglobulin-like domains and expressed on a variety of cells, including B and T lymphocytes, fibroblasts, keratinocytes, and endothelial cells. It functions as a ligand for leukocyte function–associated antigen 1 (LFA-1) and glycoprotein Mac-1 and as a specific receptor for rhinoviruses and *Plasmodium.*
**intercellular adhesion m. 2 (ICAM-2),** a cell membrane glycoprotein containing two immunoglobulin-like domains and having a tissue distribution similar to that of ICAM-1; it serves as a ligand for leukocyte function–associated antigen 1 (LFA-1).
**monatomic m.,** one which consists of a single atom.
**nonpolar m.,** a molecule in which the electrical potential is symmetrically distributed over the molecule.
**polar m.,** a molecule in which the electrical potential is not symmetrically distributed.
**tetratomic m.,** a molecule made up of four atoms.
**triatomic m.,** one composed of three atoms.

**moli·la·lia** (mol″ĭ-la'le-ə) mogilalia.

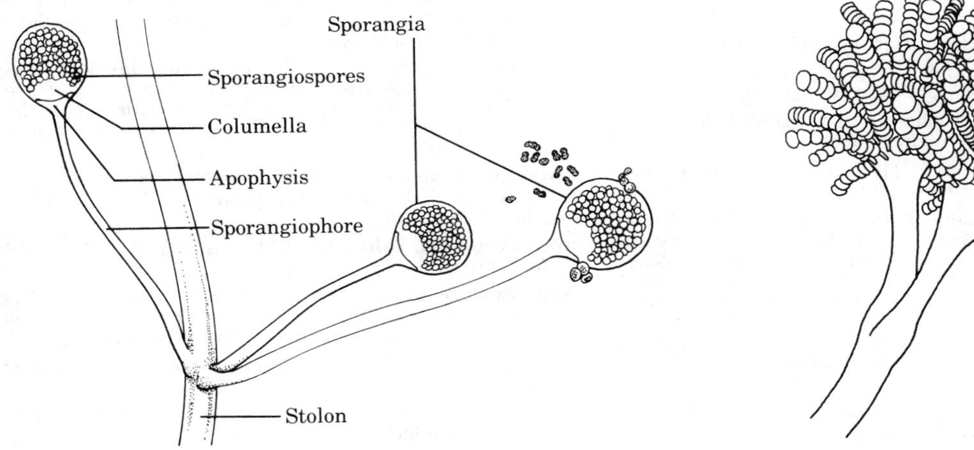


Sporangia of *Absidia* arising from a stolon.

Conidiophores and conidia of *Aspergillus*.

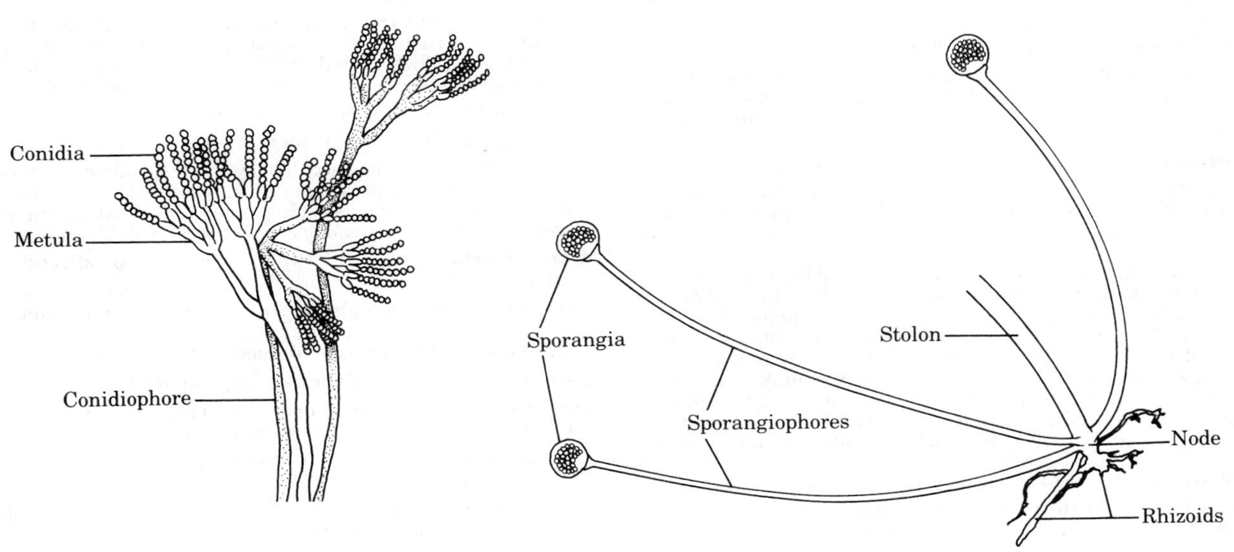


Brushlike conidiophores and parallel chains of conidia of *Penicillium*.

Sporangiophores of *Rhizopus* arising from a node above the rhizoids.

**PLATE 29**—CHARACTERISTIC STRUCTURES OF COMMON MOLDS

**mo·li·men** (mo-li'mən) pl. *moli'mina* [L. "effort"] a laborious effort made for the performance of any normal body function, especially that manifested by a variety of mild but unpleasant symptoms preceding or accompanying the menstrual period.

**mo·lim·i·na** (mo-lim'ĭ-nə) plural of *molimen.*

**mo·lin·done hy·dro·chlo·ride** (mo-lin'dōn) [USP] a dihydroindolone antipsychotic agent, used especially in the treatment of schizophrenia, brief reactive psychosis, and schizophreniform disorders; administered orally.

**Mol-Iron** (mōl-i'ərn) trademark for preparations of ferrous sulfate.

**Mo·lisch's test (reaction)** (mo'lish-əz) [Hans *Molisch,* Czechoslovakian botanist in Vienna, 1856–1937] see under *test.*

**Moll's glands** (molz) [Jacob Antonius *Moll,* Dutch ophthalmologist, 1832–1914] glandulae ciliaris conjunctivales.

**Mol·la·ret's meningitis** (mo-lah-rāz') [Pierre *Mollaret,* French neurologist, born 1898] see under *meningitis.*

**Mol·li·cu·tes** (mol″ĭ-ku'tēz) [L. *mollis* soft + *cutis* skin] [MeSH: Mollicutes] a class of bacteria of the division Tenericutes, made up of cells bounded by a triple-layered membrane; they differ from other bacteria in lacking a true cell wall. The class comprises the smallest microorganisms capable of growth in a cell-free medium, occurring as pleomorphic, coccoid, or filamentous cells with a tendency to produce myeloid structures. It contains a single order, Mycoplasmatales, and the additional genera *Anaeroplasma* and *Thermoplasma.*

**mol·lin** (mol'in) a glycerinated soft soap with excess of fats, used as a vehicle for medicines to be applied externally.

**mol·li·ti·es** (mo-lish'e-ēz) [L.] softness; abnormal softening.
**m. os'sium,** osteomalacia.

**Mol·lus·ca** (mo-lus'kə) [L. *molluscus* soft] [MeSH: Mollusca] a large phylum of invertebrates that have a soft unsegmented body often protected by a calcareous shell; it includes snails, slugs, mussels, oysters, clams, octopuses, nautiluses, squids, cuttlefish, and others.

**mol·lusc·a·ci·dal** (mo-lusk″ə-si'dəl) destructive to snails and other mollusks.

**mol·lusc·a·cide** (mo-lusk'ə-sīd) an agent that kills snails and other mollusks.

**mol·lusc·i·cide** (mo-lus'ĭ-sīd) molluscacide.

**Mol·lus·ci·pox·vi·rus** (mə-lus'kĭ-poks-vi″rəs) [*molluscum contagiosum* + *poxvirus*] [MeSH: Molluscipoxvirus] a proposed genus of the subfamily Chordopoxvirinae (family Poxviridae) containing the molluscum contagiosum virus.

**mol·lus·cous** (mo-lus'kəs) pertaining to molluscum.

**mol·lus·cum** (mo-lus'kəm) [L. *molluscus* soft] the name given to various skin diseases characterized by the formation of soft rounded cutaneous tumors; when used alone it refers to *m. contagiosum.*
**m. contagio'sum,** a common, benign, usually self-limited viral infection of the skin and occasionally the conjunctivae by a poxvirus, transmitted by autoinoculation, close contact, or fomites; it primarily affects children but may also be seen in adolescents and adults, in whom it is often sexually transmitted. The characteristic lesion, occurring singly or in groups, is a flesh-colored or gray umbilicated papule that becomes pearly white and has a caseous core that can be expressed and in which pathognomonic intracytoplasmic inclusions *(molluscum bodies)* containing replicating virions can be found.

**mol·lusk** (mol'əsk) any member of the phylum Mollusca.

**Mo·lo·ney test (reaction)** (mə-lo'ne) [Peter J. *Moloney,* Canadian immunochemist, born 1891] see under *test.*

**molt·ing** (mōlt'ing) [MeSH: Molting] ecdysis.

**Mol wt, mol wt** molecular weight.

**mo·lyb·date** (mo-lib'dāt) any salt of molybdic acid; some are used in tests, especially for the detection of heavy metal ions.

**mo·lyb·de·no·sis** (mo-lib″də-no'sis) molybdenum poisoning.

**mo·lyb·den·um** (mo-lib'də-nəm) [Gr. *molybdos* lead] [MeSH: Molybdenum] a hard, silvery-white, metallic element; symbol, Mo; atomic number, 42; atomic weight, 95.94; specific gravity, 10.2. It is an essential trace element, being a component of the enzymes xanthine oxidase, aldehyde oxidase, and nitrate reductase. Livestock grazing in certain types of pasture may suffer from molybdenum poisoning.

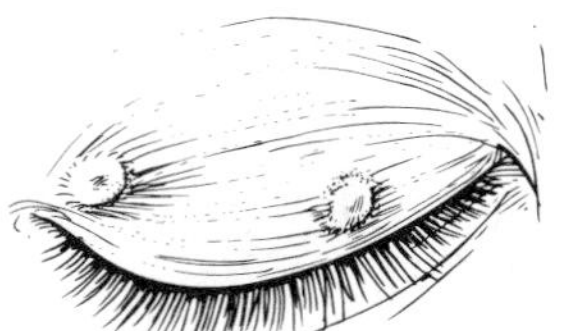
Papules of molluscum contagiosum on the eyelid.

**mo·lyb·dic** (mo-lib'dik) containing molybdenum as a hexavalent element.

**mo·lyb·dic ac·id** (mo-lib'dik) an inorganic acid existing only in solution; commercial molybdic acid is either ammonium molybdate or molybdenum trioxide.

**mo·lyb·do·en·zyme** (mo-lib″do-en'zīm) any enzyme containing a molybdenum cofactor; in humans, those known are aldehyde oxidase, sulfite oxidase, and xanthine dehydrogenase. Molybdenum is part of the redox system for electron transport in all such enzymes so far discovered.

**mo·lyb·do·fla·vo·pro·tein** (mo-lib″do-fla'vo-pro″tēn) a molybdoenzyme that is also a flavoprotein, such as aldehyde oxidase or xanthine oxidase.

**mo·lyb·do·pro·tein** (mo-lib″do-pro'tēn) a protein containing molybdenum.

**mo·lyb·dop·ter·in** (mo″lib-dop'tər-in) the nonmetal portion of a molybdenum cofactor; it is a pterin derivative with an aliphatic side chain that can attach to molybdenum by its two sulfhydryl groups.

**mo·lyb·dous** (mo-lib'dəs) containing molybdenum as a tetravalent element.

**mo·men·tum** (mo-men'təm) [L. "a movement"] the quantity of motion; the product of mass by velocity. Symbol *P.* Called also *linear morphea*

**mo·met·a·sone fu·ro·ate** (mo-met'ə-sōn″) [USP] a synthetic corticosteroid used topically for the relief of inflammation and pruritus in corticosteroid-responsive dermatoses.

**mon·ac·id** (mon-as'id) containing one atom of hydrogen that is replaceable by a base; said of a salt or of an alcohol.

**mon·ad** (mon'əd) [Gr. *monas* a unit, from *monos* single] 1. a single-celled protozoon or a single-celled coccus. 2. a univalent radical or element. 3. in meiosis, one member of a tetrad.

**Mo·na·kow's nucleus, syndrome, tract (bundle, fasciculus, fibers)** (mo-nah'kofz) [Constantin von *Monakow,* Russian-born neurologist in Switzerland, 1853–1930] see *nucleus cuneatus accessorius,* see under *syndrome,* and see *tractus rubrospinalis.*

**mon·am·ide** (mon-am'id) monoamide.

**mon·am·ine** (mon-am'in) monoamine.

**mon·an·gle** (mon'ang-gəl) having only one angle; a dental instrument having only one angulation in the shank connecting the handle, or shaft, with the working portion of the instrument, known as the blade, or nib. Cf. *binangle, quadrangle* (def. 2), and *triple-angle.*

**mon·ar·thric** (mon-ahr'thrik) pertaining to or affecting a single joint.

**mon·ar·thri·tis** (mon″ahr-thri'tis) [*mono-* + *arthritis*] inflammation of a single joint.
**m. defor'mans,** arthritis deformans of a single joint.

**mon·ar·tic·u·lar** (mon″ahr-tik'u-lər) monarthric.

**mon·as·ter** (mon-as'tər) [*mon-* + *aster*] the single star-shaped figure at the end of the prophase in mitosis.

**mon·ath·e·to·sis** (mon″ath-ə-to'sis) [*mon-* + *athetosis*] athetosis of one limb.

**mon·atom·ic** (mon″ə-tom'ik) [*mon-* + *atomic*] 1. monovalent (def. 1). 2. monobasic. 3. consisting of monatomic molecules.

**mon·auch·e·nos** (mon-awk'ə-nəs) a dicephalic fetus with one neck.

**mon·au·ral** (mon-aw'rəl) [*mon-* + *aural*[1]] pertaining to one ear. Called also *monotic* and *uniaural.*

**mon·avi·ta·min·o·sis** (mon″ə-vi″tə-min-o'sis) a deficiency disease in which only one vitamin is lacking in the diet.

**Mön·cke·berg's arteriosclerosis (calcification, degeneration, mesarteritis, sclerosis)** (merng'kĕ-bergz) [Johann Georg *Mönckeberg,* German pathologist, 1877–1925] see under *arteriosclerosis.*

**Monde·ville** (mōnd-vēl') Henri de (1260–1320). a French physician, surgeon to Philip the Fair and Louis X; in his *Chirurgie,* one of the first French surgical texts, Mondeville urged the use of sutures and the avoidance of suppuration in primary healing.

**Mon·di·ni's deafness** (mon-de'nēz) [C. *Mondini,* Italian physician, 1729–1803] see under *cochlea, deafness,* and *deformity.*

**Mon·dor's disease** (mon'dorz) [Henri *Mondor,* French surgeon, 1885–1962] see under *disease.*

**mo•ne•cious** (mo-ne'shəs) monoecious.

**mo•nen•sin** (mo-nen'sin) [USP] [MeSH: Monensin] a veterinary antibiotic, antifungal, and coccidiostat produced by *Streptomyces cinnamonensis;* used as a coccidiostat in poultry, cattle, and sheep.
**m. sodium** [USP], the sodium salt of monensin, having the same uses as the base.

**Mo•ne•ra** (mo-ne'rə) [Gr. *monērēs* single] in some systems of classification, a kingdom comprising unicellular organisms without true nuclei, i.e., the prokaryotes, including bacteria, blue-green algae (now blue-green bacteria), and actinomycetes and viruses. Cf. *Protista.*

**mo•ner•u•la** (mo-ner'u-lə) pl. *moner'ulae* [Gr. *monērēs* single] an impregnated oocyte before it has a cleavage nucleus.

**mon•es•thet•ic** (mon″əs-thet'ik) [*mon-* + *esthetic*] pertaining to or affecting a single sense or sensation.

**mon•es•trous** (mon-es'trəs) completing only one estrous cycle in each sexual season.

**Mon•ge's disease** (mōn'hāz) [Carlos *Monge,* Peruvian pathologist, 1884–1970] chronic mountain sickness.

**mon•go•li•an** (mong-go'le-ən) 1. pertaining to, resembling, or belonging to the Mongols, one of the chief ethnological divisions of Asiatic peoples. 2. a term formerly applied to defects of Down syndrome because of the typical facial characteristics.

**mon•go•lism** (mong'go-liz-əm) term formerly used for *Down syndrome,* because of facial characteristics typical of this condition.
**translocation m.,** translocation Down syndrome; see under *syndrome.*

**mon•go•loid** (mong'go-loid) [see *mongolism*] an individual with Down syndrome.

**Mon•i•e•zia** (mon″ĭ-e'zhə) a genus of cestodes of the family Anoplocephalidae. *M. benedi'ni* and *M. expan'sa* are found in the small intestines of young cattle, goats, and sheep; heavy infestations may cause diarrhea and wasting.

**mon•il•at•ed** (mon'il-āt″əd) moniliform.

**mo•nil•e•thrix** (mo-nil'ə-thriks) [L. *monile* necklace + *-thrix*] an autosomal dominant condition in which the hairs exhibit multiple constrictions, with a beading effect, and are brittle, rarely reaching an inch in length before breaking.

**Mo•nil•ia** (mo-nil'e-ə) [L. *monile* necklace] 1. former name for *Candida.* 2. a genus of imperfect fungi of the family Moniliaceae; its perfect (sexual) stage is *Sclerotinia.*

**Mo•nil•i•a•ceae** (mo-nil″e-a'se-e) in some systems of classification, a form-family of colorless or light-colored Fungi Imperfecti of the form-order Moniliales; genera of medical importance include *Acremonium, Aspergillus, Beauveria, Blastomyces, Botrytis, Coccidioides, Epidermophyton, Fusarium, Histoplasma, Paecilomyces, Paracoccidioides, Penicillium, Scedosporium, Sporothrix, Trichoderma, Trichophyton, Trichothecium,* and *Verticillium.*

**mo•nil•i•al** (mo-nil'e-əl) 1. candidal. 2. pertaining to or caused by *Monilia.*

**Mo•nil•i•a•les** (mo-nil″e-a'lēz) in some systems of classification, a form-order of Fungi Imperfecti of the form-class Hyphomycetes, consisting of fungi whose conidiophores are not organized on conidiomata. It includes the form-families Dematiaceae, Moniliaceae, and Tuberculariaceae. Some authorities call this form-order *Hyphomycetales.*

**mon•i•li•a•sis** (mon-ĭ-li'ə-sis) candidiasis.

**mo•nil•i•form** (mo-nil'ĭ-form) [L. *monile* necklace + *form*] shaped like a necklace or string of beads; called also *monilated.*

**Mo•nil•i•for•mis** (mo-nil″ĭ-for'mis) [MeSH: Moniliformis] a genus of acanthocephalans. *M. monilifor'mis* (formerly *Echinorhynchus moniliformis*) is a parasite of rats, mice, and dogs, and a facultative parasite in humans.

**mo•nil•i•id** (mo-nil'e-id) candidid.

**mo•nil•i•o•sis** (mo-nil″e-o'sis) candidiasis.

**Mon•i•stat** (mon'ĭ-stat) trademark for preparations of miconazole.

**mon•i•tor** (mon'ĭ-tər) [L. "one who reminds," from *monere* to remind, admonish] 1. to check constantly on a state or condition, as on the vital signs of a patient under anesthesia and undergoing surgery, or to determine the amount of exposure to radiation. 2. an apparatus used to observe or record such physiological signs as respiration, pulse, and blood pressure in a patient.
**ambulatory ECG m.,** a portable continuous electrocardiographic recorder, typically monitoring two channels for 24 hours; it is used to detect the frequency and duration of cardiac rhythm disturbances and to assess pacemaker programming. The term is sometimes used synonymously with Holter monitor.
**Holter m.,** a type of ambulatory ECG monitor.

**mon•i•to•ry** (mon'ĭ-tor″e) warning or preliminary; said of early signs of underlying disease.

**Mo•niz** (mo'nēsh) Antonio Caetano de Abreu Friere Egas. Portuguese neurosurgeon and diplomat 1874–1955; co-winner, with Walter Rudolf Hess, of the Nobel prize for medicine or physiology in 1949 for his development of cerebral angiography and the introduction of prefrontal lobotomy as a therapy for certain psychoses.

**mon•key** (mung'ke) [MeSH: Haplorhini] any member of several families of nonhuman primates, usually distinguished as *New World monkeys* (see superfamily Platyrrhina) or *Old World monkeys* (see superfamily Cercopithecoidea).
**cynomolgus m.,** *Macaca fascicularis,* a macaque native to South America, much used in laboratory research. Called also *crab-eating macaque.*
**rhesus m.,** *Macaca mulatta,* a light brown macaque native to India, much used in physiological research. See also *Rh factor,* under *factor.* Called also *rhesus macaque* and *rhesus.*

**mon•key•pox** (mung'ke-poks) a mild, epidemic, exanthematous disease occurring in captive monkeys, which can be transmitted to humans, in whom it causes a disease clinically similar to smallpox.

**monks•hood** (mungks'hood) 1. aconite. 2. Aconitum.

**mon(o)-** [Gr. *monos* single] 1. a combining form meaning one or single, or limited to one part. 2. in chemistry, combined with one atom, group, or radical.

**mono•ac•yl•glyc•er•ol** (mon″o-a″səl-glis'ər-ol) monoglyceride.

**mono•ac•yl•glyc•er•ol lip•ase** (mon″o-a″səl-glis'ə-rol li'pās) acylglycerol lipase.

**mono•am•ide** (mon″o-am'īd) an amide containing one amide group.

**mono•amine** (mon″o-ə-mēn') an amine molecule containing one amino group; biogenic amines in this group include serotonin, dopamine, epinephrine, and norepinephrine.

**mono•amine ox•i•dase** (mon″o-ə-mēn' ok'sĭ-dās) [MeSH: Monoamine Oxidase] amine oxidase (flavin-containing); abbreviated MAO.

**mono•am•in•er•gic** (mon″o-am″in-er'jik) of or pertaining to neurons that secrete monoamine neurotransmitters.

**mono•am•ni•on•ic** (mon″o-am″ne-on'ik) having or developing within a single amniotic cavity, such as monoamnionic twins.

**mono•am•ni•ot•ic** (mon″o-am″ne-ot'ik) monoamnionic.

**mono•ar•tic•u•lar** (mon″o-ahr-tik'u-lər) monarthric.

**mon•o•bac•tam** (mon″o-bak'tam) a class of synthetic antibiotics having a monocyclic beta-lactam nucleus.

**mono•ba•sic** (mon″o-ba'sik) [*mono-* + *basic*] having but one base; a term applied to an acid having only one replaceable atom of hydrogen and therefore yielding only one series of salts, as HCl.

**mono•ben•zone** (mon″o-ben'zōn) a melanin-inhibiting agent used as a depigmenting agent, applied topically to the skin.

**mono•blast** (mon'o-blast) [*mono-* + *-blast*] the earliest precursor in the monocytic series, which matures to develop into the promonocyte; it has a fine chromatin structure and nucleoli are usually visible. Monoblasts are not normally seen in the bone marrow or peripheral blood, but may be seen in myelogenous leukemia.

**mono•blas•to•ma** (mon″o-blas-to'mə) a neoplasm containing monoblasts and monocytes; see *acute monocytic leukemia,* under *leukemia.*.

**mono•blep•sia** (mon″o-blep'se-ə) [*mono-* + Gr. *blepsis* sight + *-ia*] 1. a condition of the vision in which it is more distinct when only one eye is used. 2. a variety of color blindness in which only one color is perceived. See also *monochromatism.*

**mono•bra•chia** (mon″o-bra'ke-ə) [*mono-* + *brachi-* + *-ia*] a developmental anomaly characterized by the presence of a single arm.

**mono•bra•chi•us** (mon″o-bra'ke-əs) an individual exhibiting monobrachia.

**mono•bro•mat•ed** (mon″o-bro'māt-əd) [L. *monobromatus*] having a single atom of bromine in each molecule.

**mono•cal•cic** (mon″o-kal'sik) containing one atom of calcium in the molecule.

**mono•car•box•yl•ic ac•id** (mon″o-kahr″bok-sil'ik) a carboxylic acid containing a single carboxyl group.

**mono•car•di•an** (mon″o-kahr'de-ən) [*mono-* + Gr. *kardia* heart] possessing a heart with a single atrium and ventricle, as that of a shark.

**mono•celled** (mon'o-səld) [*mono-* + *cell*] unicellular.

**mono•cel•lu•lar** (mon″o-sel'u-lər) unicellular.

**mono·ceph·a·lus** (mon″o-sef′ə-ləs) [*mono-* + *-cephalus*] a fetus with one head but with some duplication of its parts.
**m. tet′rapus dibra′chius,** conjoined twins with one head, two arms, and partial or complete duplication of the pelvis, with four legs, the pair belonging to one member often being fused in a single limb.
**m. tri′pus dibra′chius,** conjoined twins with one head, two arms, and partial duplication of the pelvis, with a median third leg or leg rudiment.

**mono·chlo·ro·thy·mol** (mon″o-klor″o-thi′mol) chlorothymol.

**mono·cho·rea** (mon″o-kə-re′-ə) [*mono-* + *chorea*] chorea affecting but one limb.

**mono·cho·ri·al** (mon″o-kor′e-əl) monochorionic.

**mono·cho·ri·on·ic** (mon″o-kor″e-on′ik) [*mono-* + *chorionic*] having or developing in a common chorionic sac; said of monozygotic twins.

**mono·chro·ic** (mon″o-kro′ik) [*mono-* + Gr. *chroa* color] having only one color; monochromatic.

**mono·chro·ma·sy** (mon″o-kro′mə-se) monochromatism.

**mono·chro·mat** (mon″o-kro′mat) a person affected by monochromatism; called also *achromat.*

**mono·chro·mat·ic** (mon″o-kro-mat′ik) 1. existing in or having only one color. 2. pertaining to or affected by monochromatism. 3. staining with only one dye at a time. Cf. *polychromatic.*

**mono·chro·ma·tism** (mon″o-kro′mə-tiz-əm) complete color blindness; inability to discriminate hues, all colors of the spectrum appearing as neutral grays with varying shades of light and dark. Called also *achromatism* and *achromatopsia.*
**cone m.,** that in which there is some cone function and normal visual acuity and which is not associated with nystagmus and photophobia.
**rod m.,** that in which there is complete absence of cone function and which is accompanied by poor vision, photophobia, and nystagmus.

**mono·chro·mato·phil** (mon″o-kro-mat′ə-fil) [*mono-* + *chromato-* + *-phil*] 1. stainable with only one kind of stain. 2. any cell or other element that will take only one stain.

**mono·chro·mo·phil·ic** (mon″o-kro″mo-fil′ik) stainable with only one kind of stain.

**Mono·cid** (mon′o-sid) trademark for a preparation of cefonicid sodium.

**mono·clin·ic** (mon″o-klin′ik) [*mono-* + Gr. *klinein* to incline] a term applied to crystals in which the vertical axis is inclined to one lateral axis, but is at right angles to the other.

**mono·clo·nal** (mon″o-klōn′əl) 1. derived from a single cell. 2. pertaining to a single clone.

**mono·con·tam·i·nat·ed** (mon″o-kən-tam′ĭ-nāt″əd) infected by a single species of microorganism, or by a single type of contaminating agent; see *monoxenic.*

**mono·con·tam·i·na·tion** (mon″o-kən-tam″ĭ-na′shən) experimental infection of a previously germ-free animal by a single infectious agent. See *monoxenic.*

**mono·cor·di·tis** (mon″o-kor-di′tis) inflammation of one vocal cord.

**mono·cra·ni·us** (mon″o-kra′ne-əs) [*mono-* + Gr. *kranion* cranium] monocephalus.

**mono·cro·ta·line** (mon″o-kro′tə-lēn) [MeSH: Monocrotaline] a poisonous pyrrolizidine alkaloid found in various species of *Crotalaria,* the cause of crotalism.

**mono·crot·ic** (mon″o-krot′ik) characterized by monocrotism.

**mo·noc·ro·tism** (mə-nok′rə-tiz-əm) [*mono-* + Gr. *krotos* beat] presence of a monocrotic pulse, with neither an anacrotic nor a dicrotic notch.

**mon·oc·u·lar** (mon-ok′u-lər) [*mono-* + *ocular*] 1. pertaining to or having but one eye. 2. having but one eyepiece, as in a microscope.

**mon·oc·u·lus** (mon-ok′u-ləs) [*mono-* + *oculus*] 1. a bandage for covering one eye. 2. cyclops.

**mono·cy·clic** (mon″o-si′klik) pertaining to one cycle. In chemistry, having a molecular structure containing only one ring.

**mono·cy·e·sis** (mon″o-si-e′sis) [*mono-* + *cyesis*] pregnancy with a single fetus.

**mono·cyte** (mon′o-sīt) [*mono-* + *-cyte*] [MeSH: Monocytes] a mononuclear phagocytic leukocyte, 13 to 25 μm in diameter, with an ovoid or kidney-shaped nucleus, containing lacy, linear chromatin and abundant gray-blue cytoplasm filled with fine reddish and azurophilic granules. Formed in the bone marrow from promonocytes, monocytes are transported to tissues such as the lung and liver, where they develop into macrophages. See also *monocytic series,* under *series.*

**mono·cyt·ic** (mon″o-sit′ik) 1. pertaining to, characterized by, or of the nature of monocytes. 2. pertaining to the monocytic series; see under *series.*

**mono·cy·toid** (mon″o-si′toid) resembling a monocyte.

**mono·cy·to·pe·nia** (mon″o-si″to-pe′ne-ə) [*monocyte* + *-penia*] abnormal decrease in the proportion of monocytes in the blood.

**mono·cy·to·poi·e·sis** (mon″o-si″to-poi-e′sis) [*monocyte* + *-poiesis*] the formation of monocytes.

**mono·cy·to·sis** (mon″o-si-to′sis) increase in the proportion of monocytes in the blood; see also *mononucleosis.*

**Mo·nod** (mŏ-no′) Jacques Lucien. French biochemist, 1910–1976; co-winner with François Jacob and André Michael Lwoff, of the Nobel prize in medicine or physiology for 1965, for discoveries concerning the genetic control of enzymes and virus synthesis.

**mono·dac·tyl·ia** (mon″o-dak-til′e-ə) monodactyly.

**mono·dac·tyl·ism** (mon″o-dak′təl-iz-əm) monodactyly.

**mono·dac·ty·ly** (mon″o-dak′tə-le) [*mono-* + Gr. *daktylos* finger] a developmental anomaly characterized by the presence of only one digit on a hand or foot.

**mono·dal** (mon-o′dəl) [*mono-* + Gr. *hodos* road] having connection with one terminal of a resonator or of a grounded solenoid, so that the patient is a capacitor for entrance and exit of high frequency currents.

**mono·der·mal** (mon″o-der′məl) pertaining to or possessing just one germ cell layer; said of tumors.

**mono·der·mo·ma** (mon″o-dər-mo′mə) a tumor that has developed from one germ layer.

**mono·di·plo·pia** (mon″o-dĭ-plo′pe-ə) [*mono-* + *diplopia*] double vision in one eye only.

**Mono·don·tus** (mon″o-don′təs) *Bunostomum.*

**Mono·dral bro·mide** (mon′o-drəl) trademark for preparations of penthienate bromide.

**mo·noe·cious** (mo-ne′shəs) [*mono-* + Gr. *oikos* house] having reproductive organs typical of both sexes in a single individual.

**mono·es·ter** (mon″o-es′tər) an ester containing a single ester group.

**mon·o·es·trous** (mon″o-es′trus) having just one estrous cycle per annual breeding season. Cf. *polyestrous.*

**mono·eth·a·nol·amine** (mon″o-eth″ə-nōl′ə-mēn) 1. 2-aminoethanol; an amino alcohol found in cephalins and phospholipids, and derived metabolically by decarboxylation of serine. The oleate salt, a sclerosing agent, is called *ethanolamine oleate.* Called also *colamine* and *ethanolamine.* 2. [NF] a purified preparation of monoethanolamine, used as a surfactant in pharmaceuticals.

**mono·eth·yl·gly·cine·xy·li·dide** (mon″o-eth″il-gli″sēn-zi′lĭ-dīd) MEGX; the principal active metabolite of lidocaine, produced in the liver; measurement of the conversion of lidocaine to MEGX is used to assess hepatic function.

**mono·film** (mon′o-film) a monomolecular layer transferred to a prepared plate.

**mo·nog·a·mous** (mə-nog′ə-məs) pertaining to monogamy.

**mo·nog·a·my** (mə-nog′ə-me) [*mono-* + Gr. *gamos* marriage] 1. marriage to a single spouse. 2. the animal mating system in which each individual mates with just one partner for the entire breeding season. Cf. *polygamy.*

**mono·gan·gli·al** (mon″o-gang′gle-əl) affecting a single ganglion.

**mono·gas·tric** (mon″o-gas′trik) [*mono-* + *gastr-* + *-ic*] having but one belly or stomach.

**mono·gen** (mon′o-jən) 1. a monovalent chemical element which combines in only one proportion. 2. an antiserum produced by the use of one antigen (i.e., immunogen).

**mono·gen·e·sis** (mon″o-jen′ə-sis) [*mono-* + *-genesis*] 1. the production of only male or female offspring. 2. the theory that all living things develop from a single cell.

**mono·gen·ic** (mon-o-jen′ik) pertaining to or influenced by a single gene.

**mono·ger·mi·nal** (mon″o-jer′mĭ-nəl) monozygotic.

**mono·glyc·er·ide** (mon″o-glis′ər-īd) a compound consisting of one molecule of fatty acid esterified to glycerol, usually occurring as an intermediate in triglyceride metabolism. Called also *monoacylglycerol.*

**mono·glyc·er·ide ac·yl·trans·fer·ase** (mon″o-glis′ər-īd a″səl-trans′fər-ās) 2-acylglycerol *O*-acyltransferase.

**mono·graph** (mon′o-graf) [*mono-* + *-graph*] an essay or treatise on one subject.

**mono·hor·mo·nal** (mon″o-hor-mo′nəl) secreting a single hormone.

**mono·hy·brid** (mon″o-hi′brid) [*mono-* + *hybrid*] the offspring of parents differing from each other in that each is homozygous for a different allele at a single locus; thus their offspring will be heterozygous at that locus.

**mono·hy·drat·ed** (mon″o-hi′drāt-əd) united with a single molecule of water or a single hydroxyl group.

**mono·hy·dric** (mon″o-hi′drik) containing one atom of replaceable hydrogen.

**mono·in·fec·tion** (mon″o-in-fek′shən) infection with a single kind of organism.

**mono·io·do·ty·ro·sine** (mon″o-i-o″do-ti′ro-sēn) an iodinated amino acid that is an intermediate in the thyroidal biosynthesis of thyroxine and triiodothyronine. Abbreviated MIT.

**mono·kary·on** (mon″o-kar′e-on) [*mono-* + *karyon*] a growth stage in the mycelium of fungi, especially Basidiomycetes, in which each cell has one haploid nucleus.

**mono·kary·ote** (mon″o-kar′e-ōt) a cell having one haploid nucleus.

**mono·kary·ot·ic** (mon″o-kar″e-ot′ik) pertaining to the monokaryon or to a monokaryote.

**mono·kine** (mon′o-kīn) a soluble cytokine that mediates immune responses; it is not an antibody or a complement component and is produced by mononuclear phagocytes (monocytes or macrophages). Cf. *lymphokine.*

**mono·lay·er** (mon″o-la′ər) pertaining to or consisting of a single layer, such as a monolayer sheet of cells in cultures used in studies of viruses.

**mono·lep·sis** (mon″o-lep′sis) [*mono-* + Gr. *lēpsis* a taking] the transmission to the offspring of the characters of one parent, to the exclusion of those of the other.

**mono·loc·u·lar** (mon″o-lok′u-lər) [*mono-* + *loculus*] having but one cavity or compartment, as a cyst.

**mono·ma·nia** (mon″o-ma′ne-ə) [*mono-* + *-mania*] a form of mental disorder characterized by preoccupation with one subject or idea.

**mono·max·il·lary** (mon″o-mak′sĭ-lar″e) pertaining to or affecting one maxilla.

**mono·mel·ic** (mon″o-mel′ik) [*mono-* + *mel-* + *-ic*] affecting one limb.

**mono·mer** (mon′o-mər) [*mono-* + Gr. *meros* part] 1. a simple molecule of a compound of relatively low molecular weight, consisting of simple unrepeated structural units, which can react to form a dimer, trimer, polymer, etc. 2. some basic unit of a molecule, either the molecule itself or some structural or functional subunit of it, e.g., an individual polypeptide chain in a multi-subunit protein.
**fibrin m.,** the material resulting from the highly specific and orderly cleavage of fibrinogen by thrombin; through polymerization, these monomers form macromolecular fibrin.

**mono·mer·ic** (mon″o-mer′ik) 1. pertaining to, made up of, or affecting a single segment, as distinguished from dimeric, polymeric, etc. 2. in genetics, determined by a gene or genes at a single locus either in the heterozygous or homozygous state.

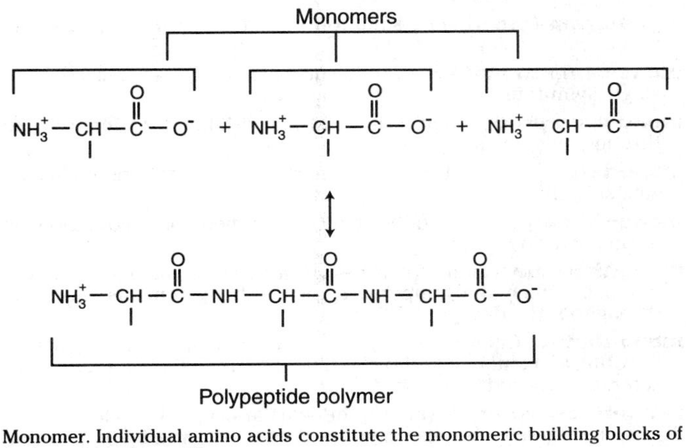

Monomers

$NH_3^+{-}CH{-}C(=O){-}O^- + NH_3^+{-}CH{-}C(=O){-}O^- + NH_3^+{-}CH{-}C(=O){-}O^-$

↕

$NH_3^+{-}CH{-}C(=O){-}NH{-}CH{-}C(=O){-}NH{-}CH{-}C(=O){-}O^-$

Polypeptide polymer

Monomer. Individual amino acids constitute the monomeric building blocks of (polymeric) polypeptides.

**mono·me·tal·lic** (mon″o-mə-tal′ik) having one atom of a metal in the molecule.

**mono·meth·yl·hy·dra·zine** (mon″o-meth″əl-hi′drə-zēn) [MeSH: Monomethylhydrazine] a toxin found in many species of *Gyromitra* mushrooms, acting as an antagonist to pyridoxine; six or more hours after ingestion, patients develop headache, dizziness, malaise, and vomiting, occasionally progressing to delirium, coma, and convulsions.

**mono·mo·lec·u·lar** (mon″o-mo-lek′u-lər) pertaining to or involving one molecule.

**mono·mor·phic** (mon″o-mor′fik) [*mono-* + *morph-* + *-ic*] existing in only one form; maintaining the same form throughout all stages of development.

**mono·mor·phism** (mon″o-mor′fiz-əm) the quality or condition of being monomorphic.

**mono·mor·phous** (mon″o-mor′fəs) composed of lesions all of the same age, form, and shape.

**mon·om·pha·lus** (mon-om′fə-ləs) [*mono-* + *omphalus*] omphalopagus.

**mono·myo·ple·gia** (mon″o-mi′o-ple′jə) [*mono-* + *myo-* + *-plegia*] paralysis restricted to a single muscle.

**mono·myo·si·tis** (mon″o-mi″o-si′tis) [*mono-* + *myositis*] a myositis of the biceps muscle occurring periodically.

**Mo·non·chus** (mo-nong′kəs) a genus of nematodes living in fresh water or moist soil, reportedly found in human urine, probably representing a case of spurious parasitosis.

**mono·neph·rous** (mon″o-nef′rəs) [*mono-* + *nephr-* + *-ous*] affecting one kidney only.

**mono·neu·ral** (mon″o-no͞o′ral) [*mono-* + *neural*] 1. pertaining to or receiving branches from a single nerve. 2. having only one neuron.

**mono·neur·ic** (mon″o-noor′ik) mononeural.

**mono·neu·ri·tis** (mon″o-no͞o-ri′tis) [*mono-* + *neur-* + *-itis*] disease of a single nerve.
**m. mul′tiplex,** see under *mononeuropathy.*

**mono·neu·rop·a·thy** (mon″o-no͞o-rop′ə-the) disease affecting a single nerve.
**cranial m.,** disease of one of the cranial nerves, as the seventh cranial nerve in Bell's palsy.
**multifocal m., multiple m., m. mul′tiplex,** mononeuropathy of several different nerves simultaneously. Called also *mononeuritis multiplex* and *multiple neuropathy.*



**mono·nu·cle·ar** (mon″o-noo′kle-ər) [*mono-* + *nuclear*] 1. having but one nucleus; mononucleate; uninucleated. 2. a cell having a single nucleus, especially a monocyte of the blood or tissues.

**mono·nu·cle·ate** (mon″o-noo′kle-āt) having a single nucleus; mononuclear.

**mono·nu·cle·o·sis** (mon″o-noo″kle-o′sis) 1. excessive numbers of circulating monocytes (see *monocytosis*), usually referring to abnormal types. 2. infectious m.
**chronic m.,** chronic fatigue syndrome.
**cytomegalovirus m.,** a type of acquired cytomegalic inclusion disease; in many respects it resembles infectious mononucleosis, with fever, splenomegaly, hepatic involvement, and atypical lymphocytes with a negative heterophile test, but it does not include pharyngitis or cervical adenopathy. It may occur sporadically or following multiple blood transfusions. See also *postperfusion syndrome,* under *syndrome.*
**infectious m.,** a common, acute, usually self-limited infectious disease caused by the Epstein-Barr virus, characterized by fever, membranous pharyngitis, lymph node and splenic enlargement, lymphocyte proliferation, and the presence of atypical lymphocytes, and giving rise to various immune reactions, including the development of a transient heterophile and a persistent Epstein-Barr virus antibody response. Potential complications include hepatitis and encephalomeningitis. It affects primarily adolescents and young adults, being spread by saliva transfer and possibly other modes; in children the infection is largely subclinical. Called also *glandular fever, Filatov's disease, kissing disease,* and *Pfeiffer's disease.*
**post-transfusion m.,** postperfusion syndrome.

**mono·nu·cle·o·tide** (mon″o-noo′kle-o-tīd) a product obtained by the digestion or hydrolytic decomposition of nucleic acid. It is a compound of phosphoric acid and a pentoside. The latter is a combination of a pentose (ribose or 2-deoxyribose) with one of the following bases: guanine, adenine, cytosine, uracil, or thymine.

**mono·oc·ta·no·in** (mon″o-ok″tə-no′in) a semisynthetic glycerol derivative used to dissolve cholesterol stones in the common and intrahepatic bile ducts; administered as a continuous perfusion via catheter.

**mono·os·te·it·ic** (mon″o-os″te-it′ik) denoting a type of osteitis which affects a single bone.

**mono·ov·u·lar** (mon″o-ov′u-lər) monovular.

**mono·oxy·gen·ase** (mon″o-ok′sĭ-jə-nās″) a term used in the recommended names of some enzymes of the oxidoreductase class; it denotes any enzyme catalyzing the incorporation of one atom from molecular oxygen into a compound while reducing the other atom of oxygen to water; this includes those in which the oxygen acceptor acts also as the hydrogen donor [EC 1.13.12] as well as those in which a second compound acts as the hydrogen donor in a coupled reaction [EC 1.14.13 to 1.14.18 and 1.14.99]. Called also *mixed function oxidase.*

**mono·par·e·sis** (mon″o-pə-re′sis) [*mono-* + *paresis*] paresis of a single limb.

**mono·par·es·the·sia** (mon″o-par″əs-the′zhə) [*mono-* + *paresthesia*] paresthesia of a single limb.

**mo·nop·a·thy** (mo-nop′ə-the) [*mono-* + *-pathy*] a disease affecting a single part.

**mono·pe·nia** (mon″o-pe′ne-ə) monocytopenia.

**mono·pha·gia** (mon″o-fa′je-ə) [*mono-* + *-phagia*] 1. desire for one kind of food only. 2. the eating of only one meal a day.

**mo·noph·a·gism** (mə-nof′ə-jiz-əm) monophagia.

**mono·pha·sia** (mon″o-fa′zhə) [*mono-* + *-phasia*] aphasia with ability to utter but one word or phrase.

**mono·pha·sic** (mon″o-fa′zik) exhibiting only one phase or variation. Cf. *diphasic* and *triphasic.*

**mono·phe·nol mono·oxy·gen·ase** (mon″o-fe′nol mon″o-ok′sĭ-jən-ās″) [EC 1.14.18.1] [MeSH: Monophenol Monooxygenase] any of a group of enzymes of the oxidoreductase class that catalyze the hydroxylation of tyrosine to dopa and the oxidation of dopa to dopaquinone. They are copper proteins that also act on catechols and substituted catechols (i.e., act as catechol oxidases). The reaction is a step in the formation of melanin pigments from tyrosine. Cf. *catechol oxidase.*

**mono·phos·phate** (mon″o-fos′fāt) a salt containing a single phosphate radical.

**mon·oph·thal·mus** (mon″of-thal′məs) [*mono-* + Gr. *ophthalmos* eye] cyclops.

**mono·phy·let·ic** (mon″o-fi-let′ik) [*mono-* + Gr. *phylē* tribe] arising or descended from a single cell type; see *monophyletic theory,* under *theory.*

**mono·phy·le·tism** (mon″o-fi′lə-tiz-əm) monophyletic theory; see under *theory.*

**mono·phy·le·tist** (mon″o-fi′lə-tist) an adherent of the monophyletic theory; see under *theory.*

**mono·phy·odont** (mon″o-fi′o-dont) [*mono-* + Gr. *phyein* to grow + *odous* tooth] having only one set of teeth, and those permanent. Cf. *diphyodont* and *polyphyodont.*

**mon·o·pia** (mon-o′pe-ə) [*mono-* + Gr. *ops* eye + *-ia*] cyclopia.

**mono·plas·mat·ic** (mon″o-plaz-mat′ik) [*mono-* + *plasmatic*] made up of a single substance.

**mono·plast** (mon′o-plast) [*mono-* + *-plast*] a single constituent cell.

**mono·ple·gia** (mon″o-ple′jə) [*mono-* + *-plegia*] paralysis of a limb.

**mono·ple·gic** (mon″o-ple′jik) pertaining to or characterized by monoplegia.

**mono·po·dia** (mon″o-po′de-ə) [*mono-* + *pod-* + *-ia*] monopodial symmelia.

**mono·po·di·al** (mon″o-po′de-əl) having a single median foot; see *symmelia.*

**mono·poi·e·sis** (mon″o-poi-e′sis) monocytopoiesis.

**mono·po·lar** (mon′o-po″lər) said of an electrical apparatus having a single pole, with the ground acting as the second pole. Called also *uniterminal.*

**Mono·pril** (mon′o-pril) trademark for a preparation of fosinopril sodium.

**mon·ops** (mon′ops) [*mono-* + Gr. *ōps* eye] cyclops.

**Mono·psyl·lus** (mon″o-sil′əs) [*mono-* + Gr. *psylla* flea] a genus of fleas. *M. ani′sus* is the common rat flea of Japan and northern China.

**mono·pty·chi·al** (mon″o-ti′ke-əl) [*mono-* + Gr. *ptychē* fold] arranged in a single layer; said of glands whose cells are arranged on the basement membrane in a single layer. Cf. *polyptychial.*

**mono·pus** (mon′o-pəs) [*mono-* + Gr. *pous* foot] sympus monopus.

**mon·or·chia** (mon-or′ke-ə) monorchism.

**mon·or·chid** (mon-or′kid) an individual exhibiting monorchism.

**mon·or·chid·ic** (mon″or-kid′ik) [*mono-* + *orchid-* + *-ic*] pertaining to or characterized by monorchism; having but one descended testicle.

**mon·or·chid·ism** (mon-or′kid-iz-əm) monorchism.

**mon·or·chis** (mon-or′kis) monorchid.

**mon·or·chism** (mon′or-kiz-əm) the condition of having only one testis in the scrotum.

**Mon·or·cho·tre·ma** (mon-or″ko-tre′mə) [*mono-* + Gr. *orchis* testicle + *trēma* aperture] a genus of flukes of the family Heterophyidae, found in birds and mammals in the Middle East and Taiwan, and characterized by having only a single testis. They have as invertebrate host an operculate snail, and as first vertebrate host an edible fish.

**mono·rhin·ic** (mon″o-rin′ik) pertaining to or possessing one nasal cavity.

**mono·sac·cha·ride** (mon″o-sak′ə-rīd) a simple sugar; a carbohydrate that cannot be decomposed by hydrolysis. The monosaccharides are colorless crystalline substances with a sweet taste and all have the general formula $C_nH_{2n}O_n$. They are classified according to the number of carbon atoms in the chain into dioses ($C_2H_4O_2$), trioses ($C_3H_6O_3$), etc., and are further classified as aldoses or ketoses.

**mon·ose** (mon′ōs) a monosaccharide.

**mono·sex·u·al** (mon″o-sek′shoo-əl) showing the traits of one sex only.

**mono·so·di·um glu·ta·mate** (mon″o-so′de-əm) sodium glutamate.

**mono·some** (mon′o-sōm) [*mono-* + *-some*] 1. the unpaired sex chromosome; called also *unpaired allosome.* 2. the single chromosome present in monosomy.

**mono·so·mic** (mon″o-so′mik) pertaining to or characterized by monosomy.

**mono·so·my** (mon′o-so″me) [MeSH: Monosomy] the absence of one chromosome of a homologous pair in the complement of an otherwise diploid cell (2n−1), as seen in Turner's syndrome and various other conditions.

**mono·spasm** (mon′o-spaz-əm) [*mono-* + *spasm*] spasm of a single limb or part. Different varieties are distinguished according to the part affected or to the site of the causal lesion; as, brachial, facial, lateral, peripheral, etc.

**mono·spe·cif·ic** (mon″o-spə-sif′ik) having an effect only on a particular kind of cell or tissue, or reacting with a single antigen, as a monospecific antiserum.

**mono·sper·my** (mon′o-spər″me) [*mono-* + Gr. *sperma* seed] fertilization in which only one spermatozoon enters the ovum.

**Mono·spo·ri·um** (mon″o-spor′e-əm) former name for *Scedosporium.*

**Mono·sto·ma** (mon″o-sto′mə) [Gr. *monos* single + *stoma* mouth] *Paramphistomum.*

**Mono·sto·mum** (mon″o-sto′məm) *Paramphistomum.*

**mon·os·tot·ic** (mon″os-tot′ik) [*mono-* + Gr. *osteon* bone] pertaining to or affecting a single bone.

**mono·stra·tal** (mon″o-stra′təl) pertaining to a single layer or stratum.

**mono·strat·i·fied** (mon″o-strat′ĭ-fīd) disposed in a single layer or stratum.

**mono·sub·sti·tut·ed** (mon″o-sub′stĭ-to͞ot″əd) having only one atom in the molecule replaced.

**mono·symp·tom** (mon″o-simp′tom) [*mono-* + *symptom*] a symptom occurring singly.

**mono·symp·to·mat·ic** (mon″o-simp″tə-mat′ik) expressed by a single symptom.

**mono·syn·ap·tic** (mon″o-sĭ-nap′tik) pertaining to or relayed through only one synapse.

**Mono·tard** (mon′o-tahrd) trademark for preparations of insulin zinc suspension.

**mono·ther·a·py** (mon″o-ther′ə-pe) treatment of a condition by means of a single drug.

**mono·ther·mia** (mon″o-thər′me-ə) [*mono-* + *therm-* + *-ia*] a condition in which the temperature of the body remains the same throughout the day.

**mono·thet·ic** (mon″o-thet′ik) [*mono-* + Gr. *thetikos* fit for placing] denoting a taxonomic group classified on the basis of a single character, as opposed to polythetic.

**mono·thio·glyc·er·ol** (mon″o-thi″o-glis′ər-ol) [NF] a clear, colorless, moderately viscous liquid used as a preservative in pharmaceutical preparations.

**mon·o·tic** (mon-o'tik) [*mono-* + *ot-* + *-ic*] 1. monaural. 2. possessing a single ear.

**mo·not·o·cous** (mo-not'ə-kəs) [*mono-* + *toc-* + *-ous*] giving birth to but one offspring at a time.

**Mono·tre·ma·ta** (mon″o-tre'mə-tə) [MeSH: Monotremata] the lowest order of mammals, including animals which lay eggs similar to those of reptiles, and nourish their young by a mammary gland which has no nipple, in a shallow pouch developed only during lactation. The only living representatives are the spiny anteater and duck-billed platypus. In some systems of classification, considered to be an order of subclass Prototheria, class Mammalia.

**mono·treme** (mon'o-trēm) a member of the order Monotremata.

**mono·trich·ic** (mon″o-trik'ik) monotrichous.

**mon·ot·ri·chous** (mon-ot'rĭ-kəs) [*mono-* + *trich-* + *-ous*] having a single polar flagellum; said of a bacterial cell. See *flagellum.*

**mon·o·trop·ic** (mon″o-trop'ik) [*mono-* + *-tropic*] affecting only one particular kind of bacterium, virus, or tissue. Cf. *polytropic.*

**mono·un·sat·u·rat·ed** (mon″o-ən-sach'ər-āt″əd) of a chemical compound, containing one double or triple bond; used particularly of fatty acids, such as oleic acid.

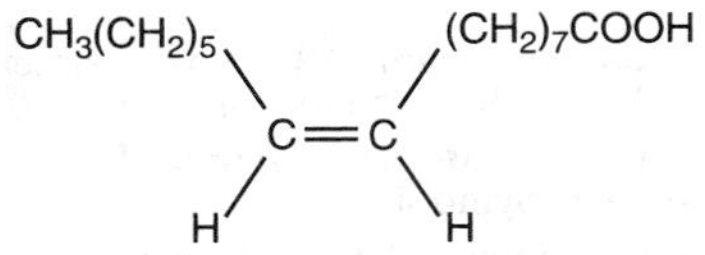

$CH_3(CH_2)_5$ $(CH_2)_7COOH$
C=C
H H

A monounsaturated fatty acid, palmitoleic acid (*cis*-9-hexadecenoic acid).

**mono·ure·ide** (mon″o-u're-id) see *ureide.*

**mono·va·lent** (mon″o-va'lənt) 1. having a valence of one. Called also *univalent.* 2. denoting an antiserum, vaccine, or antitoxin specific for a single antigen or organism.

**mon·ov·u·lar** (mon-ov'u-lər) pertaining to or derived from a single oocyte; said of monozygotic twins.

**mon·ov·u·la·to·ry** (mon-ov'u-lə-tor″e) ordinarily discharging only one ovum in one ovarian cycle.

**mono·xen·ic** (mon″o-zen'ik) [*mono-* + *xen-* + *-ic*] associated with a single species of microorganisms; said of otherwise germ-free animals contaminated by a single type of organism.

**mo·nox·e·nous** (mo-nok'sə-nəs) [*mono-* + *xen-* + *-ous*] homoxenous; requiring only one host in the life cycle; said of certain parasites.

**mon·ox·ide** (mon-ok'sīd) an oxide containing but one atom of oxygen; vernacularly applied to carbon monoxide.

**mono·zy·gos·i·ty** (mon″o-zi-gos'ĭ-te) the state of being monozygotic.

**mono·zy·got·ic** (mon″o-zi-got'ik) pertaining to or derived from one zygote; see under *twins.*

**mono·zy·gous** (mon″o-zi'gəs) monozygotic.

**Mon·ro's bursa, foramen, line, sulcus (fissure)** (mən-rōz') [Alexander *Monro* (Secundus), Scottish anatomist and surgeon, 1733–1817] see *bursa intratendinea, foramen interventriculare,* and *sulcus hypothalamicus,* and see under *line.*

**Mon·ro-Kel·lie doctrine** (mən-ro' kel'e) [Alexander *Monro;* George *Kellie,* Scottish anatomist, late 18th century] see under *doctrine.*

**Mon·ro-Rich·ter line** (mən-ro' rik'ter) [Alexander *Monro;* August Gottlieb *Richter,* German surgeon, 1742–1812] see under *line.*

**mons** (monz) pl. *mon'tes* [L. "mountain"] [TA] a general term for an elevation, or eminence.
**m. pu'bis** [TA], the rounded fleshy prominence over the symphysis pubis.
**m. ure'teris,** a papilla-like elevation of the mucosa of the bladder at its junction with the ureter.
**m. ve'neris,** m. pubis.

**Mon·so·nia** (mon-so'ne-ə) a genus of African and Asian plants of the family Geraniaceae; certain species are used in medicine as astringents or in treatment of dysentery.

**mon·ster** (mon'stər) [L. *monstrum*] [MeSH: Monsters] 1. an animal whose appearance is considered strange or frightening. 2. a term formerly used to denote a fetus or infant with such pronounced developmental anomalies as to be grotesque and usually nonviable. Called also *monstrosity* and *monstrum.*
**acardiac m.,** acardius.
**acraniate m.,** acranius.
**autositic m.,** autosite.
**celosomian m.,** celosomus.
**compound m.,** asymmetrical conjoined twins.
**cyclopic m.,** cyclops.
**diaxial m.,** a fetus that shows duplication of the body axis.
**double m.,** asymmetrical conjoined twins.
**emmenic m.,** an infant that menstruates.
**endocymic m.,** a fetus retained in the uterus, forming the basis of a dermoid tumor.
**Gila m.,** *Heloderma suspectum,* a venomous lizard found especially in Arizona and New Mexico.
**hair m.,** a fetus with a heavy covering of hair.
**monoaxial m.,** a malformed fetus with a single body axis.
**parasitic m.,** 1. in asymmetrical conjoined twins, the smaller, imperfect twin, which is unable to exist alone and is attached to or derives its nutrition from the circulation of the larger, more perfectly developed twin. 2. parasite (def. 2).
**polysomatous m.,** a fetus consisting of multiple components, each of which shows some of the characteristics of a separate individual.
**single m.,** an imprecise term for a fetus with congenital anomalies or duplications but a single body.
**sirenoform m.,** sirenomelus.
**triplet m.,** a fetus with triplication of body parts.
**twin m.,** asymmetrical conjoined twins.

**mon·stros·i·ty** (mon-stros'ĭ-te) [L. *monstrositas*] monster (def. 2).

**mon·strum** (mon'strəm) pl. *mon'stra* [L.] monster (def. 2).
**m. abun'dans,** m. per excessum.
**m. defi'ciens,** m. per defectum.
**m. per defec'tum,** a single fetus in which all or part of an organ is missing.
**m. per exces'sum,** a single fetus in which an organ is enlarged or duplicated.
**m. per fab'ricam alie'nam,** a single fetus in which an organ is wrongly formed or displaced.
**m. sirenofor'me,** sirenomelus.

**mon·tage** (mon-tahzh') an arrangement of electrodes on the scalp for several simultaneous electroencephalographic recordings at multiple sites over a given area or over the entire brain.

**Mon·teg·gia's dislocation, fracture** (mon-tej'əz) [Giovanni Battista *Monteggia,* Italian surgeon, 1762–1815] see under *dislocation* and *fracture.*

**mon·te·lu·kast so·di·um** (mon″təloo'kast) a leukotriene antagonist used as an antiasthmatic in the prophylaxis and chronic treatment of asthma; administered orally.

**mon·tes** (mon'tēz) [L.] plural of *mons.*

**Mont·gom·ery's follicles, glands, tubercles** (mont-gum'ər-ēz) [William Fetherstone *Montgomery,* Irish obstetrician, 1797–1859] see under *tubercle,* and see *Naboth's follicle,* under *follicle,* and *glandulae areolares.*

**mon·tic·u·lus** (mon-tik'u-ləs) gen. and pl. *monti'culi* [L., dim. of *mons*] a small eminence.
**m. cerebel'li,** the projecting or central part of the superior vermis.

**mood** (mo͞od) [A.S. *mōd* disposition] a pervasive and sustained emotion that, when extreme, can color one's whole view of life and markedly affect behavior. Mood is generally used to refer to either elation or depression. See also *mood disorders,* under *disorder.*
**dysphoric m.,** one that is unpleasant.
**elevated m.,** one characterized by an exaggerated sense of well-being, cheerfulness, or elation.
**euthymic m.,** one in the range of normal, being neither elevated nor depressed.
**expansive m.,** one characterized by a lack of restraint in expressing one's feelings, often with an overestimation of self-importance or significance.
**irritable m.,** one that is easily annoyed or provoked to anger.

**mood-con·gru·ent** (mo͞od kong'groo-ənt) consistent with one's mood. The term is used particularly in the classification of mood disorders: in those disorders with psychotic features, *mood-congruent psychotic features* are grandiose delusions or related hallucinations occurring in a manic episode or depressive delusions or related hallucinations in a major depressive episode, while *mood-incongruent psychotic features* are delusions or hallucinations that either contradict or are inconsistent with the prevailing emotions, such as delusions of persecution or of thought insertion in either a manic or a depressive episode.

**mood-in·con·gru·ent** (mo͞od in″kong'groo-ənt) not mood-congruent (q.v.).

**Moon's teeth (molars)** (mo͞onz) [Henry *Moon,* English surgeon, 1845–1892] see under *tooth.*

**Moore's fracture** (mo͞orz) [Edward Mott *Moore,* American surgeon, 1814–1902] see under *fracture.*

**Moore's lightning streaks** (mo͞orz) [Robert Foster *Moore,* British ophthalmologist, 1878–1963] see under *streak.*

**Moore's syndrome** (mōōrz) [Matthew T. *Moore,* American neuropsychiatrist, born 1901] abdominal epilepsy.

**Moor·en's ulcer** (mo'rənz) [Albert *Mooren,* German ophthalmologist, 1828–1899] see under *ulcer.*

**Moor·head foreign body locator** (mōōr'hed) [John J. *Moorhead,* New York surgeon, born 1874] Berman-Moorhead locator.

**MOPP** a regimen of mechlorethamine, Oncovin (vincristine), procarbazine, and prednisone, used in cancer chemotherapy.

**Mor·and's foot, spur** (mor-ahnz') [Sauveur François *Morand,* French surgeon, 1697–1773] see under *foot* and see *calcar avis.*

**mo·ran·tel tar·trate** (mo-ran'təl) an anthelmintic used in sheep and cattle.

**Mor·ax-Ax·en·feld bacillus, conjunctivitis, diplococcus** (mor'ahks-ahk'sen-felt") [Victor *Morax,* Swiss ophthalmologist in Paris, 1866–1935; Theodor *Axenfeld,* German ophthalmologist, 1867–1930] see under *conjunctivitis,* and see *Moraxella (Moraxella) lacunata.*

**Mo·rax·el·la** (mo"rak-sel'ə) [Victor *Morax*] [MeSH: Moraxella] a genus of bacteria of the family Neisseriaceae, made up of gram-negative, short, aerobic, oxidase-positive, nonpigmented organisms found as parasites and pathogens on the mucous membranes of mammals. The genus includes two subgenera: *M. (Moraxella)* occurring as rods, and *M. (Branhamella)* occurring as cocci.
**M. anatipes'tifer,** a species of uncertain status isolated from septicemic disease in ducks, geese, turkeys, and waterfowl; called also *Pasteurella anatipestifer.*
**M. bo'vis,** *M. (M.) bovis.*
**M. (Branhamel'la) catarrha'lis,** a normal inhabitant of the human nasal cavity and nasopharynx, occasionally causing otitis media or respiratory disease (see Moraxella catarrhalis pneumonia, under *pneumonia*). Called also *Branhamella catarrhalis* and *Neisseria catarrhalis.*
**M. lacuna'ta,** *M. (M.) lacunata.*
**M. liquefa'ciens,** *M. (M.) lacunata.*
**M. lwof'fi,** *Acinetobacter calcoaceticus.*
**M. (Moraxel'la) bo'vis,** the etiologic agent of infectious bovine keratoconjunctivitis.
**M. (Moraxel'la) lacuna'ta,** the etiologic agent of conjunctivitis and corneal infections in humans; called also *diplococcus of Morax-Axenfeld, Haemophilus duplex,* and *M. liquefaciens.*

**mor·bid** (mor'bid) [L. *morbidus* sick] 1. pertaining to, affected with, or inducing disease; diseased. 2. unhealthy or unwholesome. 3. characterized by preoccupation with gloomy or unwholesome feelings or thoughts.

**mor·bid·i·ty** (mor-bid'ĭ-te) [MeSH: Morbidity] 1. a diseased condition or state. 2. the incidence or prevalence of a disease or of all diseases in a population. See *morbidity rate,* under *rate.*

**mor·bif·ic** (mor-bif'ik) [L. *morbificus; morbus* sickness + *facere* to make] causing disease.

**mor·big·e·nous** (mor-bij'ə-nəs) producing disease.

**mor·bil·li** (mor-bil'i) [L.] measles.

**mor·bil·li·form** (mor-bil'ĭ-form) [*morbilli* + *form*] like measles; resembling the eruption of measles.

**Mor·bil·li·vi·rus** (mor-bil'ĭ-vi"rəs) [L. *morbilli* measles + *virus*] [MeSH: Morbillivirus] measles-like viruses; a genus of viruses of the subfamily Paramyxovirinae (family Paramyxoviridae) comprising the agents of measles, canine distemper, rinderpest, and peste des petits ruminants.

**mor·bil·lous** (mor-bil'əs) pertaining to measles.

**mor·bus** (mor'bəs) [L.] disease.
**m. cox'ae seni'lis,** hip-joint disease of aged people.
**m. monilifor'mis,** lichen ruber moniliformis.

**MORC** Medical Officers Reserve Corps.

**mor·cel·la·tion** (mor"səl-a'shən) [Fr. *morcellement*] the division of solid tissue (as a tumor) into pieces, followed by its removal piecemeal.

**mor·celle·ment** (mor"səl-maw') morcellation.

**mor·dant** (mor'dənt) [L. *mordere* to bite] 1. a substance capable of intensifying or deepening the reaction of a specimen to a stain; the chief mordants are alum, aniline, oil, and phenol. 2. to subject to the action of a mordant preliminary to staining.

**Mor. dict.** abbreviation for L. *mo're dic'to,* in the manner directed.

**Mo·rel ear, syndrome** (mo-rel') [Augustin Benoit *Morel,* French psychiatrist, 1809–1873] see under *ear,* and see *hyperostosis frontalis interna.*

**Mo·rel·li's test** (mo-rel'ēz) [F. *Morelli,* Italian physician, early 20th century] see under *test.*

**mo·res** (mo'rēz) [L., pl. of *mos* custom] the traditions and habits which are generally regarded as conducive to social welfare.

**Mor·ga·gni's caruncle, foramen,** etc. (mor-gah'nyēz) [Giovanni Battista *Morgagni,* Italian anatomist and pathologist, 1682–1771; professor at Padua, and the founder of pathological anatomy, whose clinicopathological reports were published in 1761 under the title *De sedibus et causis morborum* ("The Seats and Causes of Disease")] see under *caruncle, foramen, fossa, globule, hernia, lacuna, prolapse,* and *tubercle* and see *appendix testis, columnae anales, fossa navicularis urethrae, frenulum valvae ileocaecalis, glandulae urethrales urethrae masculinae, sinus anales,* and *ventriculus laryngis.*

**Mor·ga·gni-Ad·ams-Stokes syndrome** (mor-gah'nye-ad'əmz-stōks) [Giovanni Battista *Morgagni;* Robert *Adams,* Irish physician, 1791–1875; William *Stokes,* Irish physician, 1804–1878] Adams-Stokes syndrome; see under *syndrome.*

**mor·ga·gni·an** (mor-gah'nye-ən) referring to or named after Giovanni Battista Morgagni; see under *cataract* and see *appendix testis* and *appendices vesiculosae epoophori* under *appendix.*

**Mor·gan** (mor'gən) Thomas Hunt. American zoologist, 1866–1945; winner of the Nobel prize for medicine or physiology in 1933 for his research on the pomace fly *Drosophila* in linkage and crossing over, which he used to map the linear arrangement of genes along the chromosome.

**Mor·gan's bacillus** (mor'gənz) [Harry de Reimer *Morgan,* British physician, 1863–1931] *Morganella morganii.*

**mor·gan** (mor'gən) [T.H. *Morgan*] a unit of distance on a linkage map; see *centimorgan.* Symbol M.

**Mor·ga·nel·la** (mor"gə-nel'ə) [H. de R. *Morgan*] a genus of gram-negative, facultatively anaerobic, rod-shaped bacteria of the family Enterobacteriaceae, made up of motile, pleomorphic organisms found in fecal material of humans and other mammals. The organisms resemble *Proteus,* except that they do not produce hydrogen sulfide or liquefy gelatin.
**M. morga'nii,** the single species of the genus. It is a primary cause of urinary tract infections and is an opportunistic pathogen, causing secondary infections of blood, respiratory tract, and wounds. Called also *Proteus morganii* and *Salmonella morganii.*

**morgue** (morg) [Fr.] a place where dead bodies may be temporarily kept, for identification or until claimed for burial.

**mo·ria** (mo're-ə) [Gr. *mōria* folly] an abnormal tendency to joke, particularly inappropriately.

**mor·i·bund** (mor'ĭ-bənd) [L. *moribundus*] in a dying state.

**mor·i·ci·zine hy·dro·chlo·ride** (mor-ĭ'sĭ-zēn) [USP] a phenothiazine derivative used as an antiarrhythmic in the treatment of ventricular arrhythmias; administered orally.

**Mo·rin·ga** (mo-ring'gə) a genus of trees of the family Moringaceae, native to southern Asia and tropical Africa. *M. oli'fera* is the horseradish tree, whose root tastes like horseradish and whose nuts yield an oil that was formerly used in the treatment of rheumatism and dyspepsia.

**Mor·i·son's pouch** (mor'ĭ-sənz) [James Rutherford *Morison,* British surgeon, 1853–1939] see under *pouch.*

**Mo·ri·ta therapy** (mo-re'tah) [Shomei *Morita,* Japanese physician, 20th century] see under *therapy.*

**Mör·ner's reagent, test** (mer'nerz) [Carl Axel Hampus *Mörner,* Swedish chemist, 1854–1917] see under *reagent* and *test.*

**mor·ning glo·ry** (mor'ning glo're) 1. any of various species of *Ipomoea,* which are toxic to humans and can be fatal to ruminants. 2. any of various other plants of the family Convolvulaceae that resemble those of genus *Ipomoea.*

**Mo·ro's reflex** (mo'rōz) [Ernst *Moro,* Austrian pediatrician, 1874–1951] see under *reflex.*

**mo·ron** (mo'ron) [Gr. *mōros* stupid] obsolete, offensive term for a person with mild mental retardation; see *mental retardation,* under *retardation.*

**-morph** [Gr. *morphē* form] a word termination denoting relationship to form or shape, especially an individual or substance possessing a certain form, indicated by the preceding root, as *mesomorph.*

**mor·phal·lac·tic** (mor"fə-lak'tik) pertaining to or characterized by morphallaxis.

**mor·phal·lax·is** (mor"fə-lak'sis) [Gr. *morphē* form + *allaxis* exchange] the renewal of lost tissue or a part by reorganization of the remaining part of the body of an animal.

**mor·phea** (mor-fe'ə) [Gr. *morphē* form] a localized form of scleroderma characterized by the presence of one or more supple, nonindurated, rose and violaceous macules followed by the development of yellowish or ivory-colored discrete patches or plaques in

which the skin is hard, dry, and smooth. The lesions may remain localized or may become generalized. Called also *circumscribed* or *localized scleroderma.* Cf. *systemic scleroderma.*
**generalized m.,** a severe form that may become so extensive as to involve the entire skin, which may lead to progressive disability, contractures of the limbs, and progressive atrophy.
**guttate m.,** a form characterized by multiple small, rounded, atrophic macules, sometimes surrounded by a violaceous zone, and arranged in clusters or lines; it is difficult to distinguish from and believed by some authorities to be the same as lichen sclerosus. Called also *white spot disease.*
**linear m., m. linea'ris,** see under *scleroderma.*

**mor·pheme** (mor'fēm) a meaningful unit of sound.

**mor·phia** (mor'fe-ə) morphine.

**mor·phi·na** (mor-fi'nə) gen. and pl. *morphi'nae* [L.] morphine.

**mor·phine** (mor'fēn) [L. *morphina, morphinum*] [MeSH: Morphine] the principal and most active narcotic alkaloid of opium (q.v.), having powerful analgesic action and some central stimulant action. In the United States, it is usually used in the form of the sulfate salt, while in Germany and Great Britain, the hydrochloride salt is usually preferred. Abuse of morphine and its salts leads to dependence.
**dimethyl m.,** thebaine.
**m. hydrochloride,** the trihydrate hydrochloride salt of morphine, having the same actions as the base; used as a narcotic analgesic, usually administered orally. It is the form usually preferred in Germany and Great Britain.
**m. sulfate** [USP], the pentahydrate sulfate salt of morphine, having the same actions as the base; used as a narcotic analgesic, administered parenterally. It is the form usually preferred in the United States.

**mor·phin·ic** (mor-fin'ik) pertaining to morphine.

**mor·phin·ism** (mor'fin-iz"əm) 1. a pathologic state due to the habitual misuse of morphine. 2. morphine addiction.

**mor·phin·iza·tion** (mor"fin-ĭ-za'shən) subjection to the influence of morphine.

**mor·phi·um** (mor'fe-əm) morphine.

**morph(o)-** [Gr. *morphē* form] a combining form denoting relationship to form or structure.

**mor·pho·dif·fer·en·ti·a·tion** (mor"fo-dif"ər-en"she-a'shən) the arrangement of formative cells in the development of tissues or organs, which leads to production of the ultimate shape of the structure.

**mor·pho·gen** (mor'fo-jən) a diffusible substance in embryonic tissue postulated to form a concentration gradient that influences morphogenesis.

**mor·pho·ge·ne·sia** (mor"fo-jə-ne'se-ə) morphogenesis.

**mor·pho·gen·e·sis** (mor"fo-jen'ə-sis) [*morpho-* + *-genesis*] [MeSH: Morphogenesis] the evolution and development of form, as the development of the shape of a particular organ or part of the body, or the development undergone by individuals who attain the type to which the majority of the individuals of the species approximate.

**mor·pho·ge·net·ic** (mor"fo-jə-net'ik) producing growth; producing form or shape.

**mor·phog·e·ny** (mor-foj'ə-ne) morphogenesis.

**mor·pho·log·i·cal** (mor"fo-loj'ĭ-kəl) pertaining to morphology.

**mor·phol·o·gy** (mor-fol'ə-je) [*morpho-* + *-logy*] 1. the science of the forms and structure of organisms. 2. the form and structure of a particular organism, organ, or part.

**mor·phol·y·sis** (mor-fol'ĭ-sis) [*morpho-* + *-lysis*] destruction of form.

**mor·phom·e·try** (mor-fom'ə-tre) [*morpho-* + *-metry*] the measurement of the forms or structures of organisms.

**mor·phon** (mor'fon) [Gr. *morphōn* forming] an individual organism or structural unit.

**mor·phoph·y·ly** (mor-fof'ə-le) [*morpho-* + Gr. *phylon* tribe] the branch of phylogenesis dealing with the evolutionary development of form.

**mor·pho·phys·ics** (mor"fo-fiz'iks) the study of the physical and chemical causes of development.

**mor·pho·plasm** (mor'fo-plaz"əm) [*morpho-* + *-plasm*] the substance of the cellular reticulum.

**mor·pho·sis** (mor-fo'sis) [Gr. *morphōsis* a shaping, bringing into shape] the process of formation of a part or organ.

**mor·phot·ic** (mor-fot'ik) pertaining to morphosis or formation; concerned in a formative process.

**mor·pio** (mor'pe-o) pl. *morpio'nes* [L.] *Phthirus pubis.*

**mor·pi·on** (mor'pe-on) *Phthirus pubis.*

**Mor·quio's sign, syndrome (disease)** (mor'kyōz) [Luis *Morquio,* Uruguayan pediatrician, 1867–1935] see under *sign* and *syndrome.*

**Mor·quio-Ull·rich disease** (mor'kyo-ool'rik) [Luis *Morquio;* Otto *Ullrich,* German physician, 1894–1957] Morquio's syndrome; see under *syndrome.*

**mor·rhua** (mor'u-ə) [L.] *Gadus morrhua.*

**mor·rhu·ate** (mor'u-āt) a salt, ester, or anionic form of morrhuic acid.
**m. sodium** [USP], the sodium salts of the fatty acids of cod liver oil; used as a sclerosing agent, especially for the treatment of varicose veins and hemorrhoids, injected in solution into varicosities.

**mor·rhu·ic ac·id** (mor'u-ik) a mixture of fatty acids occurring in cod liver oil.

**Mor·ris syndrome** (mor'is) [John McLean *Morris,* American surgeon, born 1914] complete androgen resistance; see under *resistance.*

**mors** (morz) [L.] death.
**m. thy'mica,** a type of sudden infant death syndrome or death of a child formerly thought to occur in thymic asthma and status lymphaticus.

**mor·sal** (mor'səl) [L. *morsus* bite] taking part in mastication; a term applied to the masticating surface of a bicuspid or molar.

**Mor. sol.** abbreviation for L. *mo're so'lito,* in the usual way.

**mor·su·lus** (mor'su-ləs) [L., dim. of *morsus* bite] a troche.

**mor·sus** (mor'səs) [L.] bite; sting.
**m. dia'boli,** the fimbriae at the ovarian extremity of an oviduct.
**m. huma'nus,** a bite by a human being.

**mor·tal** (mor'təl) [L. *mortalis*] 1. subject to death, or destined to die. 2. fatal.

**mor·tal·i·ty** (mor-tal'ĭ-te) [MeSH: Mortality] 1. the quality of being mortal. 2. the mortality rate; see *death rate,* under *rate.* 3. in life insurance, the ratio of actual deaths to expected deaths.

**mor·tar** (mor'tər) [L. *mortarium*] a bell-shaped or urn-shaped vessel of glass, iron, porcelain, or other material, in which drugs are beaten, crushed, or ground with a pestle.

**mor·ti·cian** (mor-tish'ən) [L. *mors* death] an undertaker; a person trained to care for the dead.

**Mor·ti·e·rel·la** (mor"te-ə-rel'ə) a genus of fungi of the family Mortierellaceae, characterized by the lack of a columella and branched, tapering sporangiophores. It occasionally causes indolent human mucormycosis.
**M. wol'fii,** a species, first isolated from soil in India, that causes pneumonia and mycotic abortion in cattle in Australia, New Zealand, England, and the United States.

**Mor·ti·e·rel·la·ceae** (mor"te-ə-rel-a'se-e) a family of fungi of the order Mucorales, having a rudimentary or absent columella and occurring mainly as a soil saprophyte; it includes one pathogenic genus, *Mortierella.*

**mor·ti·fi·ca·tion** (mor"tĭ-fĭ-ka'shən) gangrene.

**Mor·ton's neuralgia (disease, foot, metatarsalgia, toe), neuroma, test** (mor'tənz) [Thomas George *Morton,* American surgeon, 1835–1903] see under *neuralgia* and *test.*

**mor·tu·ary** (mor'choo-ar"e) [L. *mortuarium* tomb] 1. pertaining to death. 2. a place where dead bodies are kept until burial or cremation.

**mor·u·la** (mor'u-lə) [L. *morus* mulberry] [MeSH: Morula] 1. the solid mass of blastomeres formed by cleavage of a zygote. 2. an inclusion body seen in circulating leukocytes in ehrlichiosis, consisting of a membrane-bound cluster of organisms that is formed by binary fission.

**mor·u·lar** (mor'u-lər) 1. pertaining to a morula. 2. resembling a mulberry.

**mor·u·la·tion** (mor"u-la'shən) the process of formation of the morula.

**mor·u·loid** (mor'u-loid) [*morula* + *-oid*] 1. shaped like a mulberry. 2. a bacterial colony in the form of a mulberry-like mass.

**Mor·van's disease, syndrome** (mor-vahz') [Augustin Marie *Morvan,* French physician, 1819–1897] see under *syndrome* and see *syringomyelia.*

**mo·sa·ic** (mo-za'ik) [L. *mosaicus;* Gr. *mouseion*] 1. a pattern made of numerous small pieces fitted together. 2. in genetics, an individual or cell cultures having two or more cell lines that are karyotypically or genotypically distinct but are derived from a single zygote. Cf. *chimera.* 3. in embryology, the condition in the fertilized eggs of some species, such as the sea urchin, whereby the cells of early stages have developed cytoplasm which determines the parts that are to develop. 4. in plant pathology, a viral disease characterized by mottling of the foliage.

**mo·sa·i·cism** (mo-za'ĭ-siz-əm) [MeSH: Mosaicism] in genetics, the presence in an individual of two or more cell lines that are karyotypically or genotypically distinct and are derived from a single zygote. Cf. *chimerism.*
**erythrocyte m.**, the mixture of two blood types in each of nonidentical twins as a result of anastomosis of placental blood vessels.
**confined placental m.**, mosaicism in which a chromosomal abnormality (usually trisomy) is restricted to the placenta; it occurs in about 2 per cent of viable pregnancies and is a possible cause of intrauterine growth restriction.
**gonadal m.**, mosaicism that results from mosaicism within the gonad so that some of the germ cells are mutants. More than one offspring of a gonadal mosaic for a dominant trait may show the trait although it is not manifested in the parent.

**Mosch·co·witz's disease, test (sign)** (mosh'ko-witz) [Eli *Moschcowitz,* American physician, 1879–1964] see *thrombotic thrombocytic purpura,* under *purpura,* and see under *test.*

**Mosch·co·witz's operation** (mosh'ko-witz) [Alexis Victor *Moschcowitz,* American surgeon, 1865–1933] see under *operation.*

**Mos·ler's sign** (mōz'lərz) [Karl Friedrich *Mosler,* German physician, 1831–1911] see under *sign.*

**mOsm** symbol for *milliosmole.*

**mos·qui·to** (məs-ke'to) pl. *mosquitoes* [Sp. "little fly"] any of the gnatlike insects of the family Culicidae; many are bloodsucking and are vectors of human and animal diseases; others are venomous.
**anautogenous m.**, a mosquito that requires a blood meal in the adult stage for the production of viable eggs.
**arygamous m.**, a mosquito that requires large or outdoor spaces for breeding.
**autogenous m.**, a mosquito that can produce viable eggs without a blood meal.
**house m.**, either *Culex pipiens* or *C. quinquefasciatus.*
**steyogamous m.**, a mosquito that can breed in captivity in limited spaces.
**tiger m.**, *Aedes aegypti.*

**mos·qui·to·ci·dal** (məs-ke"to-si'dəl) destructive to mosquitoes.

**mos·qui·to·cide** (mos-ke'to-sīd) [*mosquito* + *-cide*] an agent that is destructive to mosquitoes.

**moss** (mos) 1. any plant of the class Musci. 2. material composed of or derived from a plant of the class Musci.
**Ceylon m.**, *Gracilaria lichenoides.*
**club m.**, 1. any moss of the genus *Lycopodium;* some species have their spores inside small club-shaped structures. 2. any of various other mosses of genera related to *Lycopodium.*
**Irish m.**, 1. *Polytrichum juniperinum.* 2. *Chondrus crispus.* 3. chondrus (def. 2).
**juniper m.**, *Polytrichum juniperinum.*
**pearl m., salt rock m.**, 1. *Chondrus crispus.* 2. chondrus (def. 2).

**Mosse's syndrome** (maws'əz) [Max *Mosse,* German physician, 20th century] see under *syndrome.*

**Mos·so's ergograph, sphygmomanometer** (mos'ōz) [Angelo *Mosso,* Italian physiologist, 1846–1910] see under *ergograph*

**Mo·tais' operation** (mo-tāz') [Ernest *Motais,* French ophthalmologist, 1845–1913] see under *operation.*

**moth** (mawth) [MeSH: Moths] any of numerous flying insects of the order Lepidoptera. See also *insect dermatitis,* under *dermatitis.*
**brown-tail m.**, *Euproctis chrysorrhoea.*
**flannel m.**, *Megalopyge opercularis.*
**io m.**, *Automeris io.*
**meal m.**, a moth that infests grain and meal, such as *Asopia farinalis* or *Pyralis farinalis.*
**peppered m.**, *Biston betularia.*
**silkworm m.**, *Bombyx mori.*
**tussock m.**, *Hemerocampa leukostigma.*

**moth·er** (muth'ər) [L. *mater*] [MeSH: Mothers] 1. the female parent. 2. something from which another thing is derived, as a *mother cell.*

**mo·tile** (mo'təl, mo'tīl) having spontaneous but not conscious or volitional movement.

**mo·til·in** (mo-til'in) [MeSH: Motilin] a polypeptide hormone (2698 daltons, 22 amino acids) secreted by the enterochromaffin cells of the intestine; it increases motility of several portions of the gastrointestinal tract and stimulates pepsin secretion. In humans, its release is stimulated by the presence of acid or fat in the duodenum; its physiologic role in gastrointestinal function is not yet known.

**mo·til·i·ty** (mo-til'ĭ-te) the ability to move spontaneously.

**motion** (mo'shən) [MeSH: Motion] movement.
**brownian m.**, see under *movement.*
**continuous passive m. (CPM)**, promotes healing of articular cartilage.
**range of m.**, see under *exercise.*

**mo·ti·va·tion** (mo"tĭ-va'shən) [MeSH: Motivation] in psychology, any of the forces that activate behavior toward satisfying needs or achieving goals.

**mo·tive** (mo'tiv) in psychology, any state that affects an individual's goal-directed behavior.
**achievement m.**, the desire to achieve for the sake of achievement per se.
**aroused m.**, one that is actively influencing behavior, or that can be inferred from actual behavior.

**mo·to·cep·tor** (mo'to-sep"tor) any muscle sense receptor.

**mo·to·fa·cient** (mo"to-fa'shənt) producing motion; a term applied to that phase of muscular activity by which the muscle produces actual motion, in contradistinction to the *nonmotofacient* phase in which the muscle is contracting without producing motion.

**mo·to·neu·ron** (mo"to-noo͡'ron) a neuron with a motor function; an efferent neuron conveying motor impulses. Called also *motor neuron.*

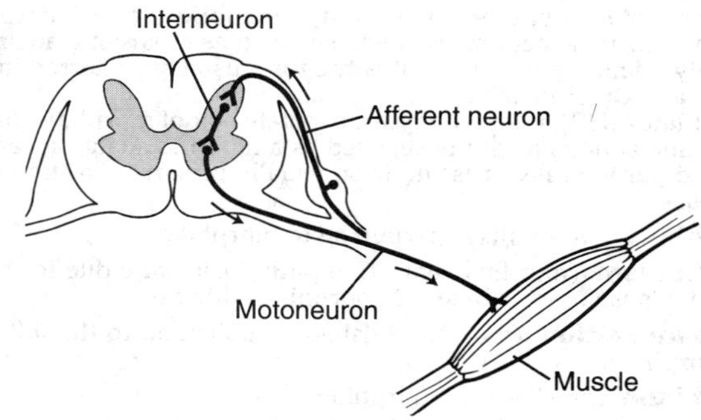


Motoneuron shown as the efferent neuron in a three-neuron reflex arc.

**alpha m's**, neurons of the anterior spinal cord that give rise to the alpha fibers which innervate the skeletal muscle fibers. Cf. *anterior horn cell.*
**beta m's**, neurons of the anterior spinal cord that give rise to the beta fibers that innervate extrafusal and intrafusal muscle fibers.
**gamma m's**, neurons of the anterior spinal cord that give rise to the gamma (fusimotor) fibers which innervate intrafusal fibers of the muscle spindle. Cf. *anterior horn cell* and *gamma loop.*
**heteronymous m's**, those supplying muscles other than the one from which the afferent impulses originate.
**homonymous m's**, those supplying the muscle from which the afferent impulses originate.
**lower m's**, peripheral neurons whose cell bodies lie in the ventral gray columns of the spinal cord and whose terminations are in skeletal muscles.
**peripheral m.**, in a reflex arc, a motoneuron that receives impulses from interneurons. Cf. *peripheral sensory neuron.*
**upper m's**, neurons in the cerebral cortex that conduct impulses from the motor cortex to motor nuclei of the cerebral nerves or to the ventral gray columns of the spinal cord.

**mo·tor** (mo'tər) [L.] 1. a muscle, nerve, or center that effects or produces movement. 2. producing or subserving motion.
**plastic m.**, the tissues of an amputation stump used to secure motion in an artificial limb.

**mo·tor·ic·i·ty** (mo"tər-is'ĭ-te) the faculty of performing movement; power of movement.

**mo·toro·ger·mi·na·tive** (mo"tər-o-jər'mĭ-nə-tiv) developing into the muscles; said of portions of the mesoderm.

**Mo·trin** (mo'trin) trademark for a preparation of ibuprofen.

**MOTT** mycobacteria other than tubercle bacilli. See *nontuberculous mycobacteria,* under *mycobacterium.*

**mot·tling** (mot'ling) a condition of spotting with patches of color.

**mou·lage** (moo-lahzh') [Fr. "molding"] [MeSH: Models, Anatomic] the making of molds or models in wax or plaster, as of a structure or a lesion; also such a mold or model.

**mould** (mōld) mold.

**mould·ing** (mōld'ing) molding.

**mound·ing** (mound'ing) myoedema, def. 1.

**Mou·ni·er-Kuhn's syndrome** (moo-ne-a'kūn) [Pierre *Mounier-Kuhn,* French physician, 20th century] tracheobronchomegaly.

**Mount's syndrome** (mounts) [Lester Adrian *Mount,* American physician, born 1910] Mount-Reback syndrome.

**Mount-Re·back syndrome** (mount-re'bak) [L. A. *Mount;* S. *Reback,* American physician, 20th century] see under *syndrome.*

**mount** (mount) 1. to fix on or in a support. 2. a support, backing, setting, or the like, on which something may be fixed. 3. to prepare specimens and slides for study. 4. a specimen on slide prepared for study.
**wet m.,** a temporary preparation in which a fluid specimen or suspension of a specimen is placed on a slide for microscopic examination and covered with a coverslip to keep it moist instead of being dehydrated and imbedded in a permanent mounting medium.

**mount·ant** (mount'ənt) a medium, such as natural resins, polymers, or glycerol, in which objects are embedded for study, especially with the microscope; called also *mounting medium.*

**mount·ing** (mount'ing) the preparation of specimens and slides for study. The chief media used in mounting large specimens are alcohol and glycerin jelly; for microscopic objects on a slide, Canada balsam and glycerin.
**split cast m.,** 1. a dental cast with key grooves on its base, mounted on an articulator for the purpose of easy removal and accurate replacement. Split remounting metal plates may be used instead of grooves in casts. 2. see under *method.*

**mourn·ing** (mor'ning) 1. the normal psychological processes that follow the loss of a loved one; grief is the accompanying emotional state. Four phases have been described: a short phase of numbness and denial, followed by a phase of yearning and protest marked by intense pining for the dead, followed by a phase of disorganization marked by pain and despair, ending in a phase of detachment and reorganization of love relationships that completes the work of mourning. 2. social expressions of grief, such as funeral and burial services, prayers, the wearing of black or other specific garments, or other rituals.

**mouse** (mous) 1. any of numerous small rodents of the family Muridae, particularly those of the genus *Mus;* some are household pests around the world and others are used as experimental animals. 2. a small weight, or movable structure.
**C.F.W. m.,** (cancer-*f*ree *w*hite mouse), one of a strain of mice bred for use in cancer research laboratories.
**deer m.,** *Peromyscus maniculatus.*
**house m.,** 1. any of several species that live in dwellings of humans. 2. *Mus musculus,* a small usually gray mouse, the most common mouse found around the world in human dwellings, an importation source of destruction of food and a carrier of disease.
**joint m.,** one of the portions of the fringes in the synovial membrane of joints in osteoarthritis which are changed into cartilage and become free in the joints. Cf. *arthrolith* and *arthrophyte.*
**meadow m.,** vole.
**multimammate m.,** *Mastomys natalensis,* a species that lives in close proximity to humans in Africa and is the natural host of Lassa virus. An inbred strain is used in cancer research. Called also *multimammate rat.*
**New Zealand black m.,** NZB m.
**nude m., *nu/nu* m.,** a mouse homozygous for the *nu* gene; these mice are hairless and congenitally athymic and thus lack T lymphocytes.
**NZB m.,** a mouse of an inbred strain that develops an autoimmune disease closely resembling human systemic lupus erythematosus.
**peritoneal m.,** a free body in the peritoneal cavity, probably representing a small mass of omentum or epiploic appendage which has twisted off and become coated with fibrin; it may appear as a soft density on the radiograph.
**pleural m.,** a fibrinous body sometimes seen in the pleural space on a radiograph.
**red-backed m.,** any of several vole species of the genus *Clethrionomys,* which have been implicated as reservoirs of epidemic hemorrhagic fever. Called also *wood m.*
**white-footed m.,** *Peromyscus leucopus.*
**wood m.,** 1. *Apodemus sylvaticus,* a European species that serves as a reservoir of *Leptospira interrogans* serovar *grippotyphosa.* 2. red-backed m.

**mouse·pox** (mous'poks) infectious ectromelia.

**mouth** (mouth) [L. *os, oris*] [MeSH: Mouth] 1. the anterior or proximal opening of the alimentary canal, which is bounded anteriorly by the lips and which contains the tongue and teeth. Called also *os* [TA]. 2. any aperture or opening.
**broken m.,** a condition in aging sheep in which teeth are broken or missing, especially incisors, so that the animals have trouble grazing.
**Ceylon sore m.,** tropical sprue.
**denture sore m.,** denture stomatitis.
**dry m.,** xerostomia.
**glass-blowers' m.,** swelling of the parotid gland in glass-blowers; see also *parotid pneumatocele,* under *pneumatocele.*
**parrot m.,** brachygnathia in a horse.
**purse-string m.,** fissures or scarring caused by syphilitic lesions around the mouth in neonates with congenital syphilis.
**sore m.,** contagious ecthyma.
**tapir m.,** a condition in which the mouth resembles that of a tapir, with the orbicularis oris muscle atrophied and the lips thickened and separated; seen in facioscapulohumeral muscular dystrophy.
**trench m.,** acute necrotizing ulcerative gingivitis; so called because it occurred in the troops in the trenches in World War I.
**watery m.,** a disease of newborn lambs in the British Isles in which they cannot nurse, have excessive abdominal fluid and fluid dripping from the mouth, and soon become comatose and die; the cause is thought to be infection with a strain of *Escherichia coli.*
**white m.,** thrush, def. 1.

**mouth·wash** (mouth'wahsh) a solution for rinsing the mouth, e.g., the official [NF] preparation of potassium bicarbonate, sodium borate, thymol, eucalyptol, methyl salicylate, amaranth solution, alcohol, glycerin, and purified water.

**move·ment** (mo͞ov'mənt) [MeSH: Movement] 1. an act of moving; motion. 2. an act of defecation.
**active m.,** voluntary movement produced by the person's own muscles, as opposed to passive m.
**ameboid m.,** the movement of an ameba or leukocyte by virtue of the flow of cytoplasm, resulting in the protrusion of a pseudopodium, or a movement similar to it.
**angular m.,** a movement which changes the angle between two bones.
**associated m.,** 1. a movement of parts which act together, as of the eyes. 2. contralateral association m. 3. synkinesis.
**automatic m.,** any involuntary movement, such as a reflex, a synkinesia, or a spasm.
**ballistic m's,** a rapid series of related movements, such as saccadic movements of the eyes, set into motion by one complex command from the brain, with no feedback on individual segments before the entire series is finished.
**Bennett m.,** the lateral shift of the mandibular condyles and articular disks in the direction of the working bite as the lower jaw swings in preparation for mastication.
**border m.,** any extreme compass of mandibular movement limited by bone, ligaments, or soft tissues; usually applied to horizontal mandibular movements.
**border tissue m's,** movements produced by action of the muscles and other tissues adjoining the borders of a denture.
**brownian m.,** the random zigzag or dancing motion of minute solute particles suspended in a solvent, due to bombardment by rapidly moving solvent molecules.
**choreic m's, choreiform m's,** irregular, jerky movements of muscles or groups of muscles.
**ciliary m.,** the lashing motion of cilia occurring in certain of the tissues.
**circus m.,** 1. a peculiar circular gait; an involuntary rolling or tumbling movement, the result of lesions of the brain and basal nerve centers. 2. continuous cycling of an excitatory wavefront in a ring or circuit around muscle, such as around a region of cardiac tissue in reentry (q.v.).
**contralateral associated m.,** a movement on the paralyzed side in hemiplegia associated with active movement of the corresponding part on the unaffected side. Called also *associated m.* and *spasmodic synkinesis.*
**dystonic m.,** a large slow, amplified athetoid movement.
**euglenoid m.,** a wormlike writhing movement, usually nonprogressive, resulting from local expansion and contraction of the body, seen in flagellates with thin pellicles and very plastic bodies, as in certain species of the order Euglenida and certain other protozoa.
**excursive m's,** excursion.
**fetal m.,** that of a fetus in the uterus usually observable at about 18 to 20 weeks in a primigravida and at about 16 to 18 weeks in a multipara.
**forced m.,** 1. passive m. 2. involuntary m.
**Frenkel's m's,** see under *exercise.*
**gliding m.,** a translatory movement in which one surface glides over another, without any angular or rotary movements, being the simplest kind of motion of a joint.
**hinge m.,** movement occurring in a single plane, as that occurring in opening or closing of the mouth.
**intermediary m's, intermediate m's,** mandibular movements between the extremes of mandibular excursions.
**involuntary m.,** movement of a limb or other body part caused by involuntary contraction of muscles; common types are athetosis, ballismus, chorea, myoclonus, seizure, tic, and tremor. Called also *forced m.*
**jaw m.,** mandibular m.
**Magnan's m.,** forward and backward movement of the tongue when it is drawn out; observed in general paresis.
**mandibular m.,** any movement of which the mandible is capable. Called also *jaw m.*

**mandibular m., free,** any unhampered movement of the mandible.
**mandibular m's, functional,** those movements of the mandible which occur in the performance of some function, as mastication, swallowing, articulation of vocal sounds, and yawning.
**masticatory m's,** those movements of the mandible occurring in the mastication of food.
**molecular m.,** brownian m.
**morphogenetic m.,** a flowing of cell groups concerned with the formation of germ layers or of organ primordia.
**nucleopetal m.,** the movement of a male pronucleus toward the female pronucleus in the zygote.
**opening m.,** a mandibular movement during jaw separation.
**opening m., posterior,** the opening movement of the mandible about the terminal hinge axis.
**passive m.,** any movement of the body effected by a force entirely outside of the organism; see *passive exercise,* under *exercise.*
**pendular m.,** one of the movements of the small intestine in digestion, consisting of a gentle swinging to and fro of the different loops; these movements are ascribed to rhythmical contractions of the longitudinal muscles. See also *segmentation m.*
**rapid eye m.,** REM; the rapid conjugate movement of the eyes that occurs during REM sleep.
**reflex m.,** reflex (def. 2).
**saccadic m.,** the quick movement of the eye in going from one fixation point to another; see also *saccade.*
**scissors m.,** a movement of the pupillary reflex seen with a retinoscope, resembling the opening and shutting of scissors; it is indicative of irregular astigmatism.
**segmentation m.,** one of the movements of the small intestine in digestion, consisting of small, irregular or rhythmic, circular contractions that segment a portion of the intestine into evenly spaced parts somewhat resembling a string of sausages; see also *pendular m.*
**spontaneous m.,** automatic m.
**Swedish m.,** see under *gymnastics.*
**synkinetic m.,** synkinesis.
**vermicular m's,** the wormlike movements of the intestines in peristalsis.

**mov·er** (mo͞ov′ər) one that moves.
**prime m.,** a muscle that acts directly to bring about a desired movement.

**moxa** (mok′sah) [Japanese] a tuft of soft, combustible substance to be burned upon the skin, popularly used in the Orient as a cautery and counterirritant.

**mox·a·lac·tam** (mok″sə-lak′tam) [MeSH: Moxalactam] a semisynthetic antibiotic chemically related to the third-generation cephalosporins, having a broad spectrum of antibacterial activity and reported to be effective against some β-lactamase producing organisms.
**m. disodium,** the disodium salt of moxalactam, used to treat a wide variety of infections caused by susceptible organisms; administered intramuscularly and intravenously.
**m. disodium for injection,** a sterile mixture of moxalactam disodium and mannitol.

**mox·a·zo·cine** (mok-sa′zo-sēn) an analgesic and antitussive, $C_{18}H_{25}NO_2$.

**mox·i·bus·tion** (mok″sĭ-bus′chən) [MeSH: Moxibustion] counterirritation produced by igniting a cone or cylinder of moxa placed on the skin.

**mox·nid·a·zole** (moks-nid′ə-zōl) an antiprotozoal effective against *Trichomonas.*

**Moy·na·han's syndrome** (moi′nə-hanz) [E. J. *Moynahan,* British physician, 20th century] see under *syndrome.*

**Moy·ni·han's cream, test** (moin′yənz) [Berkeley George Andrew *Moynihan* (Lord Moynihan), British surgeon, 1865–1936] see under *cream* and *test.*

**Mo·zart ear** (mōt′sahrt) [Wolfgang Amadeus *Mozart,* Austrian composer, 1756–1791, who was reported to have this ear deformity] see under *ear.*

**6-MP** 6-mercaptopurine.

**mp** melting point.

**MPD** maximum permissible dose; see under *dose.*

**MPH** Master of Public Health.

**MPI DMSA Kid·ney Re·a·gent** trademark for a kit for the preparation of technetium Tc 99m succimer.

**MPI MDP** trademark for a kit for the preparation of technetium Tc 99m medronate.

**MPI Py·ro·phos·phate** trademark for a preparation of technetium Tc 99m pyrophosphate.

**MPI Tc 99m DTPA** trademark for a kit for the preparation of technetium Tc 99m pentetate.

**MPO** myeloperoxidase.

**MPS** mononuclear phagocyte system; mucopolysaccharidosis.

**MR** mitral regurgitation.

**mR** symbol for *milliroentgen.*

**μR** symbol for *microroentgen.*

**MRA** Medical Record Administrator; magnetic resonance angiography.

**MRACP** Member of Royal Australasian College of Physicians.

**mrad** symbol for *millirad.*

**MRC** Medical Reserve Corps.

**MRCP** Member of the Royal College of Physicians.

**MRCPE** Member of the Royal College of Physicians of Edinburgh.

**MRCP (G'asg)** Member of the Royal College of Physicians and Surgeons of Glasgow *qua* Physician.

**MRCPI** Member of the Royal College of Physicians of Ireland.

**MRCS** Member of the Royal College of Surgeons.

**MRCSE** Member of the Royal College of Surgeons of Edinburgh.

**MRCSI** Member of the Royal College of Surgeons of Ireland.

**MRCVS** Member of the Royal College of Veterinary Surgeons.

**MRD** minimum reacting dose.

**MRDM** malnutrition-related diabetes mellitus.

**mrem** millirem.

**MRI** magnetic resonance imaging.

**MRL** Medical Record Librarian; now called Medical Record Administrator.

**mRNA** messenger RNA; see under *RNA.*

**MS** Master of Surgery; mitral stenosis; multiple sclerosis.

**ms** symbol for *millisecond.*

**μs** symbol for *microsecond.*

**MS Con·tin** (kon′tin) trademark for a preparation of morphine sulfate.

**MSE** Mental Status Examination.

**msec** symbol for *millisecond.*

**MSG** monosodium glutamate.

**MSH** [MeSH: MSH] melanocyte-stimulating hormone (see under *hormone*); it occurs in two forms, α-MSH and β-MSH.

**MSIR** trademark for a preparation of morphine sulfate.

**MSL** midsternal line.

**MSUD** maple syrup urine disease.

**MSLT** multiple sleep latency test.

**MT** Medical Technologist; membrana tympani.

**MTD** maximum tolerated dose.

**mtDNA** mitochondrial DNA; see under *DNA.*

**MTX** methotrexate.

**Mu** Mache unit.

**mU** symbol for *milliunit.*

**mu** (mu) [M, μ] the twelfth letter of the Greek alphabet.

**m.u.** mouse unit.

**μU** symbol for *microunit.*

**MUAP** motor unit action potential.

**Muc.** abbreviation for L. *mucila′go,* mucilage.

**Much's granules** (mooks) [Hans Christian R. *Much,* German physician, 1880–1932] see under *granule.*

**Mu·cha's disease** (moo′kahz) [Viktor *Mucha,* Austrian dermatologist, 1877–1919] acute lichenoid pityriasis.

**Mu·cha-Ha·ber·mann disease** (moo′kah-hah′ber-mahn) [Viktor *Mucha;* Rudolf *Habermann,* German dermatologist, 1884–1941] acute lichenoid pityriasis.

**muci-** [L. *mucus*] a combining form denoting relationship to mucus, or to mucin.

**mu·ci·car·mine** (mu″sĭ-kahr′min) a specific stain for mucin containing carmine and aluminum chloride; used to detect mucin-secreting tissues or tumors and to identify certain fungi.

**mu·ci·car·mi·no·phil·ic** (mu″sĭ-kahr″mĭ-no-fil′ik) pertaining to a cell or other element that stains readily with mucicarmine.

**mu·cif·er·ous** (mu-sif′ər-əs) [*muci-* + *-ferous*] muciparous.

**mu·ci·fi·ca·tion** (mu″sĭ-fĭ-ka′shən) the mucus-producing changes in the vaginal epithelium of laboratory animals during the progestational stage of the ovarian cycle.

**mu·ci·form** (mu'sĭ-form) [*muci-* + *form*] mucoid, def. 1.

**mu·ci·gen** (mu'sĭ-jən) [*muci-* + *-gen*] the substance from which mucin is derived.

**mu·cig·e·nous** (mu-sij'ə-nəs) muciparous.

**mu·ci·gogue** (mu'sĭ-gog) [*muci-* + *-agogue*] 1. stimulating the secretion of mucus. 2. an agent that stimulates the secretion of mucus.

**mu·ci·he·ma·tein** (mu"sĭ-he'mə-tēn) a hematein-based staining fluid for mucins.
**Mayer's m.**, see under *stain.*

**mu·ci·lage** (mu'sĭ-ləj) [L. *mucilago*] [MeSH: Adhesives] 1. an artificial viscid paste of gum or dextrin used in pharmacy as a vehicle or excipient, or in therapy as a demulcent. 2. a naturally formed viscid principle in a plant, consisting of a gum dissolved in the juices of the plant.
**acacia m.**, a preparation of acacia and benzoic acid in purified water, used as a suspending agent for drugs.
**tragacanth m.** [NF], a preparation of tragacanth, benzoic acid, and glycerin in distilled water, used as a protective.

**mu·ci·lag·i·nous** (mu"sĭ-laj'ĭ-nəs) of the nature of mucilage; slimy and adhesive.

**mu·ci·la·go** (mu"sĭ-lah'go) [L.] mucilage.
**m. aca'ciae,** acacia mucilage.
**m. tragacan'thae,** tragacanth mucilage.

**mu·cil·loid** (mu'sĭ-loid) a preparation of a mucilaginous substance.
**psyllium hydrophilic m.**, a powdered preparation of the mucilaginous portion of the seeds of blond psyllium *(Plantago ovata),* used in treatment of simple constipation resulting from lack of bulk.

**mu·cin** (mu'sin) 1. any of a group of protein-containing glycoconjugates with high sialic acid or sulfated polysaccharide content that compose the chief constituent of mucus. 2. more generally, any of a wide variety of glycoconjugates such as mucoproteins, glycoproteins, glycosaminoglycans, and glycolipids.

**mu·ci·no·blast** (mu-sin'o-blast) [*mucin* + *-blast*] the progenitor of a mucous cell.

**mu·ci·noid** (mu'sĭ-noid) [*mucin* + *-oid*] resembling or pertaining to mucin. Called also *mucoid.*

**mu·ci·no·lyt·ic** (mu"sĭ-no-lit'ik) [*mucin* + *-lytic*] dissolving or splitting up mucin.

**mu·ci·no·sis** (mu"sĭ-no'sis) a condition characterized by abnormal deposits of mucopolysaccharides (mucins) in the skin. The mucinoses have been classified as metabolic (myxedema, diffuse or pretibial; lichen myxedematosus; and gargoylism), secondary or catabolic (degeneration in a variety of neoplasms), and localized (follicular, papular, plaquelike, focal, and the myxoid [synovial] cyst).
**follicular m.**, a disease of the pilosebaceous unit, presenting clinically as grouped follicular papules or plaques with associated hair loss, caused by mucinous infiltration of tissues, and usually involving the scalp, face, and neck. Called also *alopecia mucinosis.*
**papular m.**, lichen myxedematosus.

**mu·ci·nous** (mu'sĭ-nəs) resembling or marked by the formation of mucin.

**mu·cin·uria** (mu"sin-u're-ə) [*mucin* + *-uria*] the occurrence of mucin in the urine; it may suggest vaginal contamination.

**mu·cip·a·rous** (mu-sip'ə-rəs) [*mucus* + L. *parere* to produce] producing or secreting mucus. Called also *blennogenic, blennogenous, muciferous,* and *mucigenous.*

**mu·ci·tis** (mu-si'tis) inflammation of the mucous membrane.

**Muck·le-Wells syndrome** (muk'əl-welz) [Thomas James *Muckle,* Canadian pediatrician, 20th century; Michael Vernon *Wells,* English physician, 20th century] see under *syndrome.*

**muc(o)-** [L. *mucus*] a combining form denoting relationship to mucus, or to a mucous membrane.

**mu·co·car·ti·lage** (mu"ko-kahr'tĭ-ləj) a soft cartilage the cells of which are in a mucuslike matrix.

**mu·co·cele** (mu'ko-sēl) [*muco-* + *-cele*[1]] [MeSH: Mucocele] 1. dilatation of a cavity with accumulated mucous secretion. 2. mucus retention cyst. 3. mucus extravasation phenomenon.
**suppurating m.**, a mucocele whose contents are purulent.

**mu·co·cil·i·ary** (mu"ko-sil'e-ar-e) [*muco-* + *ciliary*] pertaining to mucus and to the cilia of the epithelial cells in the respiratory system.

**mu·co·cla·sis** (mu-kok'lə-sis) [*muco-* + Gr. *klasis* a breaking] surgical destruction of the mucous lining of any organ.

**mu·co·co·li·tis** (mu"ko-ko-li'tis) former term for irritable bowel syndrome.

**mu·co·col·pos** (mu"ko-kol'pos) [*muco-s* + *colpo-* + *-ous*] accumulation of mucus in the vaginal canal.

**mu·co·cu·ta·ne·ous** (mu"ko-ku-ta'ne-əs) [*muco-* + *cutaneous*] pertaining to or affecting the mucous membrane and the skin.

**mu·co·cyst** (mu'ko-sist) [*muco-* + *cyst*] any of the paracrystalline, saccular or rod-shaped, subpellicular cystic organelles seen in certain ciliate protozoa, which contain a mucoid material that is expelled through a pore in the pellicle; its function is uncertain but it may be involved in the formation of cysts or protective coverings. Called also *mucigenic body.*

**mu·co·en·ter·itis** (mu"ko-en-tər-i'tis) former term for irritable bowel syndrome.

**mu·co·ep·i·der·moid** (mu"ko-ep"ĭ-dər'moid) composed of mucus-producing and epithelial cells; see under *carcinoma.*

**mu·co·fi·brous** (mu"ko-fi'brəs) composed of mucus and fibrous tissue.

**mu·co·floc·cu·lent** (mu"ko-flok'u-lənt) containing threads of mucus.

**mu·co·gin·gi·val** (mu"ko-jin'jĭ-vəl) pertaining to the oral mucosa and gingiva, or to the line of demarcation between them (mucogingival junction).

**mu·co·gin·gi·vi·tis** (mu"ko-jin"jĭ-vi'tis) inflammation of the gingiva, particularly at the mucogingival junction.

**mu·coid** (mu'koid) [*muc-* + *-oid*] 1. pertaining or relating to, or resembling mucus. Called also *blennoid, muciform,* and *mucous.* 2. mucinoid.

**mu·co·lem·ma** (mu"ko-lem'ə) mucin coat, a noncellular envelope secreted around the rabbit egg and its oolemma by the oviduct.

**mu·co·lip·i·do·sis** (mu"ko-lip"ĭ-do'sis) pl. *mucolipido'ses* [MeSH: Mucolipidosis] any of a group of lysosomal storage diseases in which both glycosaminoglycans (mucopolysaccharides) and lipids accumulate in tissues but without excess of glycosaminoglycans in the urine.
**m. I,** sialidosis, type I.
**m. II,** a rapidly progressing disease of young children, characterized histologically by abnormal fibroblasts containing a large number of dark inclusions which fill the central part of the cytoplasm except for the juxtanuclear zone (I-cells), and clinically by severe growth impairment, minimal hepatomegaly, extreme mental and motor retardation, and clear corneas; inherited as an autosomal recessive trait, it is caused by failure of lysosomal enzymes to be incorporated into lysosomes, due to deficiency of the enzyme UDP-*N*-acetylglucosamine–lysosomal-enzyme *N*-acetylglucosamine-phosphotransferase. Called also *I-cell disease.*
**m. III,** a disorder similar to but milder than mucolipidosis II and thought to be due to the same enzyme deficiency but to a lesser extent. Called also *pseudo-Hurler polydystrophy.*
**m. IV,** an autosomal recessive disorder characterized by psychomotor retardation and severe visual impairment, initially manifest in infancy or childhood as corneal clouding. Sialic acid–containing gangliosides are accumulated due to deficient ganglioside sialidase activity; however the deficiency is not believed to be the primary defect.

**mu·co·lyt·ic** (mu"ko-lit'ik) destroying or dissolving mucin; an agent that so acts.

**mu·co·mem·bra·nous** (mu"ko-mem'brə-nəs) pertaining to or composed of mucous membrane.

**Mu·co·myst** (mu'ko-mist) trademark for a preparation of acetylcysteine.

**mu·co·peri·chon·dri·al** (mu"ko-per"e-kon'dre-əl) pertaining to the mucoperichondrium.

**mu·co·peri·chon·dri·um** (mu"ko-per"e-kon'dre-əm) perichondrium having a mucosal surface, as that of the nasal septum.

**mu·co·peri·os·te·al** (mu"ko-per"e-os'te-əl) consisting of mucous membrane and periosteum.

**mu·co·peri·os·te·um** (mu"ko-per"e-os'te-əm) periosteum having a mucous surface, as in parts of the auditory apparatus.

**mu·co·poly·sac·cha·ride** (mu"ko-pol"e-sak'ə-rīd) 1. glycosaminoglycan. 2. less frequently, any polysaccharide with a high hexosamine content, including the glycosaminoglycans, which are acidic, as well as neutral polysaccharides such as chitin.

**mu·co·pol·y·sac·cha·ri·do·sis** (mu"ko-pol"e-sak"ə-ri-do'sis) pl. *mucopolysaccharido'ses.* Any of a group of lysosomal storage diseases resulting from defects in degradation of the glycosaminoglycans dermatan sulfate, heparan sulfate, keratan sulfate, chondroitin sulfate or a combination of them, which are then excreted in the urine and accumulate in tissues, affecting the bony skeleton, joints,

liver, spleen, eye, ear, skin, teeth, and the cardiovascular, respiratory, and central nervous systems. The prototype for mucopolysaccharidosis is Hurler's syndrome (q.v.).
**m. I (MPS I),** originally, Hurler's syndrome; it now encompasses any of the forms characterized by deficiency of L-iduronidase and by excretion in the urine of dermatan sulfate and heparan sulfate.
**m. IH (MPS I H),** Hurler's syndrome.
**m. IH/S (MPS I H/S),** Hurler-Scheie syndrome.
**m. IS (MPS I S),** Scheie's syndrome.
**m. II (MPS II),** Hunter's syndrome.
**m. III (MPS III),** Sanfilippo's syndrome.
**m. IV (MPS IV),** Morquio's syndrome.
**m. V,** former name for Scheie's syndrome, now classified as *m. IS.*
**m. VI (MPS VI),** Maroteaux-Lamy syndrome.
**m. VII (MPS VII),** Sly's syndrome.

**mu·co·poly·sac·cha·ri·du·ria** (mu″ko-pol″e-sak″ə-rĭ-du′re-ə) an excess of mucopolysaccharides in the urine.

**mu·co·pro·tein** (mu″ko-pro′tēn) a covalently linked conjugate of protein and polysaccharide, the latter containing many hexosamine residues and constituting approximately 4 to 30 per cent of the weight of the compound; mucoproteins occur mainly in mucous secretions. Cf. *glycoprotein.*
**Tamm-Horsfall m.,** a substance produced by cells of the ascending limb of the loop of Henle; it is a normal constituent of urine and is the major protein constituent of urinary casts. Called also *Tamm-Horsfall protein* and *uromodulin.*

**mu·co·pu·ru·lent** (mu″ko-pu′roo-lənt) containing both mucus and pus.

**mu·co·pus** (mu′ko-pəs″) [*muco-* + *pus*] mucus which has the appearance of pus on account of the presence of leukocytes.

**Mu·cor** (mu′kor) [L., "bread mold"] [MeSH: Mucor] a genus of fungi of the family Mucoraceae, order Mucorales, which form delicate, white tubular filaments and spherical, black sporangia; it produces no stolons or rhizoids, and sporangiophores arise at all parts of the thallus. A number of species cause mucormycosis in humans and other animals.
**M. circinelloi′des,** a species found as normal flora in various warm-blooded animals, and sometimes causing opportunistic mucormycosis in humans.
**M. corym′bifer,** *Absidia corymbifera.*
**M. muce′do,** a species of common soil saprobes causing rotting of fruit, baked goods, and insects; it is sometimes isolated from human feet and skin but has not been found to be pathogenic.
**M. pusil′lus,** *Rhizomucor pusillus.*
**M. racemosis′simus,** a species that grows on decaying vegetation and bread, and sometimes causes otomycosis and mucormycosis.
**M. ramo′sus,** *Absidia corymbifera.*
**M. rhizopodifor′mis,** *Rhizopus rhizopodiformis.*

**Mu·co·ra·ceae** (mu″kə-ra′se-e) a family of fungi of the order Mucorales, characterized by having the thallus not segmented or ramified; pathogenic genera include *Absidia, Apophysomyces, Mucor, Rhizomucor,* and *Rhizopus.*

**mu·co·ra·ceous** (mu″kə-ra′shəs) pertaining to fungi of the order Mucorales.

**Mu·co·ra·les** (mu″kə-ra′lēz) [MeSH: Mucorales] an order of perfect fungi of the class Zygomycetes made up of bread molds and related fungi, the majority of which are saprobes; pathogenic species are included in the families Cunninghamellaceae, Mortierellaceae, Mucoraceae, and Saksenaeaceae and cause mainly opportunistic infections such as mucormycosis.

**mu·cor·my·co·sis** (mu″kor-mi-ko′sis) [*Mucor* + *-mycosis*] [MeSH: Mucormycosis] a mycosis due to fungi of the order Mucorales, such as species of *Rhizopus* and less often *Mucor* or *Absidia.* In humans it is usually an opportunistic infection in immunocompromised patients or those with a chronic debilitating disease such as uncontrolled diabetes mellitus. Organisms enter through the respiratory tract, digestive tract, or a skin lesion, and then invade blood vessel walls and are disseminated in the blood; spread along nerve trunks also occurs. The disease may affect the head and neck, the respiratory tract, the digestive tract, or more rarely the skin. Clinical manifestations range from chronic to fulminant. In domestic animals it is a cause of abortion or placentitis in cows and of secondary infections of lesions of rumenitis in ruminants. Related fungi in the class Entomophthorales cause a similar condition called *entomophthoromycosis.* Called also *phycomycosis* and *zygomycosis.*
**cerebral m.,** a fulminant, usually fatal infection of the brain by fungi of the order Mucorales, most often occurring in patients with acidotic diabetes or leukemia or who are receiving immunosuppressive agents; it may be caused by dissemination of fungi from a distant site or by direct extension from the nasopharynx (rhinocerebral mucormycosis).
**cutaneous m.,** mucormycosis of the skin, usually seen in weak, diabetic, or immunocompromised patients; it may result from contamination of a wound or from spread outwards of rhinocerebral mucormycosis. The infecting agent is usually a species of *Rhizopus* and occasionally *Saksenaea vasiformis.*
**pulmonary m.,** lung infection by a fungus of the order Mucorales, usually seen primarily in diabetic or immunocompromised patients; symptoms include bronchitis, cavitation, and hemoptysis and death within a month is common.
**rhinocerebral m.,** cerebral mucormycosis in which the original site of infection is in the ethmoid, sphenoid, or maxillary sinuses, or, in some cases, the palate or pharynx.

**mu·co·sa** (mu-ko′sə) [L. "mucus"] tunica mucosa.
**redundant supraglottic m.,** see under *syndrome.*

**mu·co·sal** (mu-ko′səl) pertaining to the tunica mucosa.

**mu·co·san·guin·e·ous** (mu″ko-sang-gwin′e-əs) composed of mucus and blood.

**mu·co·sec·to·me** (mu-ko-sek′tə-me) [*mucosa* + *-ectomy*] excision of the tunica mucosa, such as in the colon in the treatment of inflammatory bowel disease.

**mu·co·sed·a·tive** (mu″ko-sed′ə-tiv) soothing to the mucous surfaces.

**mu·co·se·rous** (mu″ko-se′rəs) pertaining to or producing both mucus and serum.

**mu·co·sin** (mu-ko′sin) a form of mucin peculiar to the more tenacious varieties of mucus, as that of the nasal and uterine cavities.

**mu·co·si·tis** (mu″ko-si′tis) inflammation of a mucous membrane.

**mu·co·so·cu·ta·ne·ous** (mu-ko″so-ku-ta′ne-əs) mucocutaneous.

**mu·co·stat·ic** (mu″ko-stat′ik) 1. arresting the secretion of mucus. Called also *blennostatic.* 2. denoting the normal relaxed condition of the tissues of the mucosa of the jaws.

**mu·co·sul·fa·ti·do·sis** (mu″ko-sul″fə-tĭ-do′sis) multiple sulfatase deficiency.

**mu·co·tome** (mu′ko-tōm) a dermatome for removing mucous membrane for transplantation; see *Castroviejo dermatome,* under *dermatome.*

**mu·cous** (mu′kəs) [L. *mucosus*] 1. pertaining or relating to, or resembling mucus; mucoid. 2. covered with mucus. 3. secreting, producing, or containing mucus.

**mu·co·vis·ci·do·sis** (mu″ko-vis″ĭ-do′sis) cystic fibrosis of the pancreas (q.v. under *fibrosis*); so called because of the abnormally viscous mucoid secretions observed in the disease.

**mu·cro** (mu′kro) pl. *mucro′nes* [L. "a sharp point"] the pointed end of a part or organ.
**m. ster′ni,** processus xiphoideus.

**mu·cro·nate** (mu′kro-nāt) [*mucro* + *-ate*] 1. having a spinelike tip. 2. sword-shaped; xiphoid.

**mu·cron·i·form** (mu-kron′ĭ-form) spinelike.

**Mu·cu·na** (mu-ku′nə) [L., from Portuguese] a genus of plants of the family Leguminosae. *M. pru′riens* is cowage, an herb native to the East Indies whose seeds contain L-dopa; its pods bear the medicinal but allergenic hairs also called cowage (q.v.).

**mu·cus** (mu′kəs) [L.] [MeSH: Mucus] the free slime of the mucous membranes, composed of secretion of the glands, along with various inorganic salts, desquamated cells, and leukocytes.

**Muel·ler** (me′ler) see *Müller.*

**Muel·le·ri·us** (me-ler′e-əs) a genus of nematodes of the family Protostrongylidae. *M. capilla′ris* is a lungworm that causes hoose in sheep and goats.

**muf·fle** (muf′əl) a part of a furnace, usually removable or replaceable, in which material may be placed for processing, without exposing it to the direct action of the heat source.

**MUGA** multiple gated acquisition; see under *scanning.*

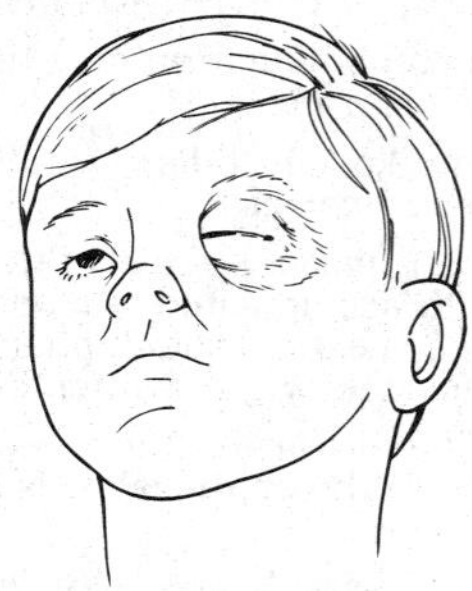
Unilateral facial swelling and exophthalmos in rhinocerebral mucomycosis.

**Muir-Tor·re syndrome** (mūr-tor'e) [E.G. *Muir,* British physician; Douglas P. *Torre,* American dermatologist, b. 1919] Torre's syndrome; see under *syndrome.*

**Mul·der's angle** (mool'derz) [Johannes *Mulder,* Dutch anatomist, 1769–1810] see under *angle.*

**Mules' operation** (mūlz) [Philip Henry *Mules,* English ophthalmologist, 1843–1905] see under *operation.*

**mu·li·e·bria** (mu"le-e'bre-ə) [L.] the female genitalia.

**Mul·ler** (mul'ər) Hermann Joseph. American biologist and geneticist, 1890–1967; winner of the Nobel prize for medicine or physiology in 1946 for his research into spontaneous genetic mutation, which led to a technique to induce mutations artificially by x-rays.

**Mül·ler** (mēl'er) Paul Herrmann. Swiss chemist, 1899–1965; winner of the Nobel prize for medicine or physiology in 1948 for synthesizing DDT and discovering its insecticidal qualities.

**Mül·ler's capsule, duct (canal)** (mūl'erz) [Johannes Peter *Müller,* German physiologist, 1801–1858, the founder of scientific medicine in Germany] see *capsula glomeruli, ductus paramesonephricus,* and *ganglion superius nervi glossopharyngei,* and see under *maneuver* and *tubercle.*

**Mül·ler's fibers (cells, radial cells), muscle** (mūl'erz) [Heinrich *Müller,* German anatomist, 1820–1864] see under *fiber* and *muscle.*

**Mül·ler's fluid (liquid)** (mūl'erz) [Hermann Franz *Müller,* German histologist, 1866–1898] see under *fluid.*

**Mül·ler's sign** (mūl'erz) [Friedrich von *Müller,* German physician, 1858–1941] see under *sign.*

**Mül·ler-Haeck·el law** (mūl'er-hāk'el) [Fritz *Müller,* German naturalist, 1821–1897; Ernst Heinrich *Haeckel,* German biologist, 1834–1919] biogenetic law; see under *law.*

**mull·er** (mul'er) a kind of pestle, flat at the bottom, used for grinding drugs upon a slab of similar material.

**mül·le·ri·an** (mu-ler'e-ən) named for Johannes Peter *Müller,* as müllerian duct and müllerian capsule.

**Mül·le·ri·us** (me-ler'e-əs) Muellerius.

**mul·tan·gu·lar** (məl-tang'gu-lər) having many angles or corners.

**multi-** [L. *multus* many, much] a combining form meaning many or much; see also words beginning *poly-.*

**mul·ti·al·lel·ic** (mul"te-ə-lel'ik) pertaining to or occupied by many alleles at a single gene locus.

**mul·ti·ar·tic·u·lar** (mul"te-ahr-tik'u-lər) pertaining to or affecting many joints.

**mul·ti·bac·il·lary** (mul"tĭ-bas'ĭ-lar"e) pertaining to or made up of a number of bacilli.

**mul·ti·cap·su·lar** (mul"tĭ-cap'su-lər) having many capsules, as a lamellar (pacinian) corpuscle.

**mul·ti·cell** (mul'tĭ-sel) any organ made up of many cells; any group of functionally active cells.

**mul·ti·cel·lu·lar** (mul"tĭ-sel'u-lər) [*multi-* + *cellular*] 1. composed of many cells. 2. containing many hollow spaces.

**mul·ti·cel·lu·lar·i·ty** (mul"tĭ-sel"u-lar'ĭ-te) the state of being composed of many cells; the state of being multicellular.

**mul·ti·cen·tric** (mul"tĭ-sen'trik) [*multi-* + *center*] polycentric.

**mul·ti·cen·tric·i·ty** (mul"tĭ-sən-tris'ĭ-te) polycentricity.

**Mul·ti·ceps** (mul'tĭ-seps) a former genus of cestodes, now classified as part of the genus *Taenia.*
**M. mul'ticeps,** *Taenia multiceps.*
**M. seria'lis,** *Taenia serialis.*

**mul·ti·con·tam·i·nat·ed** (mul"tĭ-kən-tam'ĭ-nat"əd) infected by several different species of microorganisms, or by several different contaminating agents.

**mul·ti·cus·pid** (mul"tĭ-kus'pid) [*multi-* + *cuspid*] having many cusps, such as a tooth with many cusps. Called also *multicuspidate.*

**mul·ti·cus·pi·date** (mul"tĭ-kus'pĭ-dāt) multicuspid.

**mul·ti·cys·tic** (mul"tĭ-sis'tik) polycystic.

**mul·ti·den·tate** (mul"tĭ-den'tāt) [*multi-* + *dentate*] having many teeth or toothlike processes.

**mul·ti·elec·trode** (mul-te-e-lek'trōd) multilead electrode.

**mul·ti·fac·to·ri·al** (mul"tĭ-fak-tor'e-əl) 1. of or pertaining to, or arising through the action of many factors. 2. in genetics, arising as the result of the interaction of several genes and usually, to some extent, of nongenetic factors. Cf. *polygenic.*

**mul·ti·fid** (mul'tĭ-fid) cleft into many parts.

**mul·tif·i·dus** (məl-tif'ĭ-dəs) [L., from *multus* many + *findere* to split] cleft into many parts, as the musculus multifidus.

**mul·ti·fo·cal** (mul"tĭ-fo'kəl) arising from or pertaining to many foci.

**mul·ti·form** (mul'tĭ-form) occurring in several forms; polymorphic.

**mul·ti·gan·gli·on·ic** (mul"tĭ-gang"gle-on'ik) pertaining to, affecting, or possessing many ganglia.

**mul·ti·ges·ta** (mul"tĭ-jes'tə) multigravida.

**mul·ti·glan·du·lar** (mul"tĭ-glan'du-lər) pluriglandular.

**mul·ti·grav·i·da** (mul"tĭ-grav'ĭ-də) [*multi-* + *gravida*] a woman who has been pregnant several times. Also written gravida II, III, etc., according to the number of pregnancies.
**grand m.,** a woman who has had five or more previous pregnancies.

**mul·ti·hal·lu·cal·ism** (mul"te-hal'u-kəl-iz-əm) [*multi-* + *hallucal* + *-ism*] a developmental anomaly characterized by the presence of more than one great toe on one foot.

**mul·ti·hal·lu·cism** (mul"te-hal'u-siz-əm) multihallucalism.

**mul·ti·in·fec·tion** (mul"te-in-fek'shən) infection with several varieties of organisms.

**mul·ti·lo·bar** (mul"tĭ-lo'bər) having numerous lobes.

**mul·ti·lob·u·lar** (mul"tĭ-lob'u-lər) [*multi-* + *lobular*] having many lobules.

**mul·ti·loc·u·lar** (mul"tĭ-lok'u-lər) [*multi-* + *locular*] having many cells or compartments, as a multilocular cyst.

**mul·ti·mam·mae** (mul"tĭ-mam'e) [*multi-* + *mammae*] the condition of having more than two breasts.

**mul·ti·mo·dal** (mul"tĭ-mo'dəl) 1. having more than one mode. 2. of a graph, having several maxima (peaks). 3. multisensory.

**mul·ti·nod·u·lar** (mul"tĭ-nod'u-lər) composed of many nodules.

**mul·ti·nu·cle·ate** (mul"tĭ-noo'kle-āt) polynuclear.

**mul·tip·a·ra** (məl-tip'ə-rə) [*multi-* + *para*] a woman who has had two or more pregnancies which resulted in viable fetuses, whether or not the offspring were alive at birth. Also written para II, III, IV, etc., according to the number of offspring.
**grand m.,** a woman who has had five or more pregnancies which resulted in viable fetuses.

**mul·ti·par·i·ty** (mul"tĭ-par'ĭ-te) 1. the condition of being a multipara. 2. the production of several offspring in one gestation.

**mul·tip·a·rous** (məl-tip'ə-rəs) 1. having had two or more pregnancies which resulted in viable fetuses. 2. producing several ova or offspring at one time.

**mul·ti·ple** (mul'tĭ-pəl) [L. *multiplex*] manifold; occurring in or affecting various parts of the body at once.

**mul·tip·let** (mul'tĭ-plet) multiple discharge.

**mul·ti·plic·i·tas** (mul"tĭ-plis'ĭ-təs) a multiplication; a developmental anomaly characterized by the presence of an abnormal multiplicity of organs, or of a specific organ.
**m. cor'dis,** a developmental anomaly characterized by the presence of a number of separate hearts.

**mul·ti·po·lar** (mul"tĭ-po'lər) [*multi-* + *polar*] having more than two poles or processes.

**mul·ti·pol·li·cal·ism** (mul"tĭ-pol'ĭ-kəl-iz-əm) [*multi-* + *pollical* + *-ism*] a developmental anomaly characterized by the presence of more than one thumb on one hand.

**mul·ti·root·ed** (mul"tĭ-ro͞ot'əd) having many roots; said of molar teeth.

**mul·ti·sen·si·tiv·i·ty** (mul"tĭ-sen"sĭ-tiv'ĭ-te) the condition of being sensitive (allergic) to more than one antigen (allergen).

**mul·ti·sen·so·ry** (mul"te-sen'sə-re) said of certain neurons in the central nervous system that can respond to more than one kind of sensory input.

**mul·ti·syn·ap·tic** (mul"te-sĭ-nap'tik) polysynaptic.

**mul·ti·ter·mi·nal** (mul"tĭ-ter'mĭ-nəl) having several sets of terminals so that several electrodes may be used.

**mul·ti·tu·ber·cu·late** (mul"tĭ-too-ber'ku-lət) having many tubercles.

**mul·ti·va·lent** (mul"tĭ-va'lənt) [*multi-* + L. *valere* to have value] 1. having a valence of two or more. 2. denoting an antiserum, vaccine, or antitoxin specific for more than one antigen or an organism. Called also *polyvalent.*

**mul·ti·va·ri·ate** (mul"tĭ-var'e-āt) involving more than one variable.

**mum·mi·fi·ca·tion** (mum"ĭ-fĭ-ka'shən) conversion into a state resembling that of a mummy, such as occurs in dry gangrene, or the shriveling and drying up of a dead fetus.

**mumps** (mumps) [MeSH: Mumps] an acute infectious disease caused by a paramyxovirus, spread by direct contact, airborne droplet nuclei, fomites contaminated by infectious saliva, and perhaps urine, and usually seen in children under the age of 15, although adults may also be affected. Many cases of mumps are subclinical, but in those that are clinically apparent the principal manifestation is parotitis, usually associated with painful swelling of one or both parotid glands; other salivary glands may also be involved. Infection of other organs may cause complications, chiefly epididymo-orchitis in males, oophoritis in females, meningoencephalitis, and pancreatitis. Called also *epidemic parotitis.*

**iodine m.**, swelling of the salivary and lacrimal glands as a toxic reaction to iodine therapy.

**m. meningoencephalitis,** see under *meningoencephalitis.*

**mu·mu** (mu'mu) a condition characterized by swelling and edema of the spermatic cord, and sometimes swelling of the scrotum, epididymis, and testicle, and by the appearance of a hydrocele; probably an allergic manifestation developing after inoculation by filaria.

**Mun·chau·sen syndrome** (moon'chou-zenz) [Baron Karl Friedrich Hieronymus *Münchhausen,* German soldier and traveler, 1720–1797, a reputed teller of exaggerated tales] [MeSH: Munchausen Syndrome] see under *syndrome.*

**Münch·mey·er's disease** (mĕnch'mi-ərz) [Ernst *Münchmeyer,* German physician, 1846–1880] see under *disease.*

**Mun·ro's microabscess (abscess)** (mən-rōz') [William John *Munro,* English dermatologist, 19th century] see under *microabscess.*

**Mun·ro's point** (mən-rōz') [John Cummings *Munro,* American surgeon, 1858–1910] see under *point.*

**Mun·ro Kerr cesarean section, incision** (mən-ro'kər) [John Martin *Munro Kerr,* Scottish gynecologist and obstetrician, 1868–1955] see under *incision,* and *section.*

**Mun·son's sign** (mun'sənz) [Edward Sterling *Munson,* American ophthalmologist, born 1933] see under *sign.*

**MUP** motor unit potential.

**mu·pir·o·cin** (mu-pir'o-sin) [USP] [MeSH: Mupirocin] an inhibitor of bacterial protein synthesis, produced by fermentation of *Pseudomonas fluorescens* and effective against staphylococci and nonenteric streptococci; applied topically in the treatment of impetigo.

**m. calcium,** the calcium salt of mupirocin, applied intranasally for the treatment of nasal colonization with methicillin-resistant *Staphylococcus aureus.*

**mu·ral** (mu'rəl) [L. *muralis,* from *murus* wall] pertaining to or occurring in the wall of a cavity.

**mu·ram·ic ac·id** (mu-ram'ik) a compound consisting of glucosamine and lactic acid joined by an ether linkage; it occurs naturally as the *N*-acetyl derivative (MurNAc) in peptidoglycan, the characteristic polysaccharide composing bacterial cell walls.

**mu·ram·i·dase** (mu-ram'ĭ-dās) [MeSH: Muramidase] lysozyme.

**Mur·chi·son-Pel-Eb·stein fever** (mur'chĭ-sən-pel-eb'shtīn) [Charles *Murchison,* British physician, 1830–1879; Pieter Klaases *Pel,* Dutch physician, 1852–1919; Wilhelm *Ebstein,* German physician, 1836–1912] Pel-Ebstein fever.

**Mu·rel** (mu'rel) trademark for preparations of valethamate bromide.

**Mu·rex** (mu'reks) a genus of whelks of the family Muricidae. *M. purpu'rea* is a Mediterranean species from which murexine (or purpurine) is obtained.

**mu·rex·ide** (mu-rek'sīd) [L. *murex* purple sea snail] [MeSH: Murexide] ammonium purpurate, a substance formed in Weidel's test for uric acid; a purple color is produced when uric acid is present. See also *Weidel's test* (1), under *tests.*

**mu·rex·ine** (mu-rek'sin) [*Murex* + *-ine,*] a neurotoxic substance derived from the median zone of the hypobranchial gland of gastropods of the genus *Murex* and related species; the substance is called *purpurine* when derived from snails of the genus *Purpura.*

**Mu·ric·i·dae** (mu-ris'ĭ-de) a family of marine snails of the order Neogastropoda, including the genera *Murex* and *Purpura.*

**Mu·ri·dae** (mu'rĭ-de) [MeSH: Muridae] a large family of rodents including many types of mice and rats, as well as gerbils, hamsters, and voles. Some are used as laboratory animals or pets and others are household pests and reservoirs of disease. Genera of medical and laboratory interest include *Clethrionomys, Cricetulus, Cricetus, Gerbillus, Mesocricetus, Microtus, Mus, Neotoma,* and *Rattus.*

**mu·ri·form** (mu'rĭ-form) [L. *murus* wall + *form*] wall-like, used in mycology and bacteriology to describe a spore having both transverse and longitudinal septa.

**Mu·ri·my·ces** (mu"rĭ-mi'sēz) in former systems of classification, a genus of bacteria species of which have been assigned to the genus *Mycoplasma.*

**mu·rine** (mu'rin) [L. *mus, muris* mouse] pertaining to or affecting mice or rats.

**mur·mur** (mur'mər) [L. *murmer*] an auscultatory sound, benign or pathologic, particularly a periodic sound of short duration of cardiac or vascular origin.

**amphoric m.**, see under *resonance.*

**anemic m.**, a cardiac murmur heard in anemic patients.

**aneurysmal m.**, a vascular murmur heard over an aneurysm.

**aortic m.**, a sound generated by blood flowing through a diseased aorta or aortic valve.

**apex m., apical m.**, one heard at the apex of the heart.

**apical diastolic m's,** diastolic murmurs heard at the apex of the heart, indicative of mitral stenosis or other condition causing altered flow through the mitral valve; they consist essentially of low-frequency vibrations, which account for their rumble quality.

**arterial m.**, a murmur (bruit) over an artery, sometimes aneurysmal and sometimes constricted.

**attrition m.**, pericardial friction rub.

**Austin Flint m.**, a presystolic or mid-diastolic murmur heard at the cardiac apex in aortic regurgitation, originating at the mitral valve when blood enters simultaneously from both the aorta and the left atrium.

**basal diastolic m's,** diastolic murmurs at the base of the heart, due to aortic or pulmonic regurgitation.

**bellows m.**, to-and-fro m.

**brain m.**, one produced over a vascular abnormality in the brain.

**cardiac m.**, a sound of finite length generated by turbulence of blood flow through the heart; often classified as systolic, diastolic, or continuous, and further divided on the basis of its timing within systole or diastole. Murmurs are graded from 1 to 6 on the basis of increasing loudness.

**cardiopulmonary m., cardiorespiratory m.**, a sound generated within lung tissue and related to movement of the heart.

**Carey Coombs m.**, a rumbling apical mid-diastolic cardiac murmur occurring in the acute phase of rheumatic fever and disappearing afterward.

**continuous m.**, a humming cardiac murmur extending throughout systole into late diastole or to the end of diastole; it is due to conditions characterized by connections between the aorta and the pulmonary artery or its branches (such as patent ductus arteriosus), by arteriovenous fistulas, or by altered blood flow in arteries or veins. Cf. *systolic m.* and *diastolic m.*

**cooing m.**, a type of musical murmur, resembling the cooing of a bird.

**crescendo m.**, a murmur marked by progressively increasing loudness and abrupt cessation, e.g., the presystolic murmur in mitral stenosis with sinus rhythm.

**Cruveilhier-Baumgarten m.**, a venous murmur heard at the abdominal wall over veins connecting the portal and caval systems.

**deglutition m.**, one heard over the esophagus during the act of swallowing.

**diamond-shaped m.**, a cardiac murmur with a characteristic crescendo-decrescendo pattern of intensity on the phonocardiogram; it is almost always a systolic ejection murmur caused by aortic stenosis.

**diastolic m's,** cardiac murmurs occurring during diastole and usually due to semilunar valve regurgitation or to altered blood flow through atrioventricular valves; they are frequently divided into early and mid-diastolic murmurs.

**Duroziez's m.**, a double murmur over the femoral or other large peripheral artery, due to aortic insufficiency.

**early diastolic m.**, a high frequency murmur beginning immediately after the second heart sound and progressively diminishing in intensity; it results from semilunar valve regurgitation.

**early systolic m.**, a regurgitant cardiac murmur beginning at the first heart sound and diminishing and ending well before the second heart sound; it results from abbreviation of pansystolic murmurs due to special circumstances such as acute mitral regurgitation or ventricular septal defect that is associated with pulmonary hypertension.

**ejection m.**, a type of systolic murmur occurring predominantly in midsystole, at the time of maximal ejection volume and blood flow velocity, such as that heard in aortic or pulmonary stenosis; it is due to ejection of blood into the root of the aorta or pulmonary artery, is diamond-shaped, and ends before the second heart sound. Cf. *regurgitant m.*

**extracardiac m.**, a murmur heard over the heart originating from another structure, such as a cardiopulmonary murmur.

**Flint's m.**, Austin Flint m.

**friction m.**, see under *rub.*

**functional m.**, a cardiac murmur generated in the absence of organic cardiac disease. Called also *innocent m., inorganic m.,* and *physiologic m.*

**Gibson m.**, a long rumbling sound occupying most of systole and diastole, usually localized in the second left interspace near the sternum, and usually indicative of patent ductus arteriosus.

**Graham Steell's m.**, a high-pitched diastolic murmur caused by pulmonary regurgitation secondary to severe pulmonary hypertension;

it is heard at the left sternal edge, level with the second or third costal cartilage.
**Hamman's m.,** see under *sign.*
**heart m.,** cardiac m.
**hemic m.,** one due to an abnormal, usually anemic, condition of the blood.
**holosystolic m.,** pansystolic m.
**hourglass m.,** a cardiac murmur characterized by two periods of maximum loudness joined by a period of decreasing, then increasing, loudness, with the point of lowest intensity midway between the two peaks.
**humming-top m.,** venous hum.
**innocent m., inorganic m.,** functional m.
**late systolic m.,** a regurgitant murmur beginning in the middle or last third of systole and continuing until the second heart sound; it is often associated with a midsystolic click and mitral valve prolapse.
**machinery m.,** a loud, rumbling, continuous murmur named for its sound, such as occurs in patent ductus arteriosus.
**mid-diastolic m.,** a mainly low-frequency murmur beginning a short time after the second heart sound; it is associated with early ventricular filling and is caused by turbulence in the ventricle due to altered flow of blood through one or both atrioventricular valves, such as occurs in mitral or tricuspid stenosis.
**midsystolic m.,** a cardiac murmur, usually an ejection murmur, beginning a short time after the first heart sound and ending before the second heart sound; it is almost always a functional murmur or the result of obstruction to ventricular outflow, such as occurs in aortic or pulmonary stenosis.
**mitral m.,** cardiac murmur due to disease of the mitral valve.
**musical m.,** a cardiac murmur, usually systolic, resulting when the responsible vibrations have a periodic harmonic pattern.
**organic m.,** one due to a lesion in the organ or organ system being examined, e.g., in the heart, in a blood vessel, or in lung tissue.
**pansystolic m.,** a regurgitant cardiac murmur that extends throughout systole and is due to blood flow between two chambers normally of very different pressures in systole; the most common causes are mitral or tricuspid regurgitation and ventricular septal defects. Called also *holosystolic m.*
**pericardial m.,** see under *rub.*
**physiologic m.,** functional m.
**pleuropericardial m.,** a pleural friction sound heard in the pericardial region and resembling a pericardial rub.
**prediastolic m.,** early diastolic m.
**presystolic m.,** a cardiac murmur occurring immediately prior to ventricular ejection, usually associated with atrial contraction and the acceleration of blood flow through a narrowed atrioventricular valve.
**pulmonic m.,** one due to disease of the pulmonary valve or artery.
**regurgitant m.,** a murmur due to regurgitation of blood through an abnormal valvular orifice, usually occurring throughout systole. Cf. *ejection m.*
**Roger's m.,** bruit de Roger.
**seagull m.,** a raucous murmur with musical qualities resembling the call of a seagull, such as that heard occasionally in aortic insufficiency, and attributed specifically to eversion or retroversion of the right anterior aortic cusp.
**seesaw m.,** to-and-fro m.
**Steell's m.,** Graham Steell's m.
**stenosal m.,** a sound produced in an artery by artificial pressure or by a stenosis.
**Still's m.,** a functional low-frequency, vibratory or buzzing, cardiac murmur of childhood, occurring in midsystole and usually of maximal intensity at the lower left sternal border.
**systolic m's,** cardiac murmurs occurring during systole; usually due to mitral or tricuspid regurgitation or to aortic or pulmonary obstruction. They are often subdivided into ejection and regurgitant murmurs and, on the basis of cardiac cycle timing, classified as early, mid-, late, or pansystolic murmurs.
**to-and-fro m.,** a friction sound or murmur heard with both systole and diastole.
**tricuspid m.,** a murmur caused by disease of the tricuspid valve.
**vascular m.,** one heard over a blood vessel; see *arterial m.* and *venous m.*
**venous m.,** a murmur heard over a vein.
**vesicular m.,** vesicular breath sounds; see under *sound.*

**mu·ro·mo·nab-CD3** (mu″ro-mo′nab) [MeSH: Muromonab-CD3] a murine monoclonal antibody to the CD3 antigen of human T cells, which functions as an immunosuppressant in the treatment of acute allograft rejection of renal transplants; administered intravenously.

**Mur·phy** (mər′fe) William Parry. American physician, born in 1892, co-winner with George Richards Minot and George Hoyt Whipple, of the Nobel prize for medicine or physiology in 1934, for their work on anemia.

**Mur·phy button,** etc. (mər′fe) [John Benjamin *Murphy,* American surgeon, 1857–1916] see under *button, percussion, sign,* and *test.*

**Mur·ray** (mər′e) Joseph Edward. American plastic surgeon, born 1919. Co-winner with Edward Donnall Thomas of the Nobel prize for his pioneering work with organ transplantation. He was the first to successfully transplant a kidney.

**Mur·ray Val·ley encephalitis (disease), virus** (mər′e val′e) [*Murray Valley,* Australia, where the disease occurred in epidemics in 1950 and 1951] see under *encephalitis* and *virus.*

**mur·ri·na** (moo-re′nə) [Sp. *morriña*] surra in horses in Central and South America.

**Mus** (mus) [L. "mouse"] a genus of rodents of the family Muridae, including several species of mice. *M. mus′culus* is the house mouse. *M. decuma′nus* and *M. norve′gicus* are former names for *Rattus norvegicus.*
**M. decuma′nus,** former name for *Rattus norvegicus.*
**M. mus′culus,** the common house mouse.
**M. norve′gicus,** former name for *Rattus norvegicus.*
**M. rat′tus rat′tus,** former name for *Rattus rattus.*

**Mus·ca** (mus′kə) [L. "fly"] a genus of flies of the family Muscidae which have their mouth parts adapted for suction only.
**M. autumna′lis,** the face fly, a species commonly found in Europe, the Americas, and parts of Asia and Africa, often crawling on the faces of large mammals such as cattle and horses.
**M. domes′tica,** the common house fly. It may act as a mechanical carrier of the microorganisms of typhoid fever, cholera, dysentery, plague, anthrax, tetanus, trachoma, leprosy, and encephalitis, and of pyogenic bacteria, cysts of some protozoa, and helminth ova. The larvae may cause myiasis.
**M. domes′tica ne′bulo,** a subspecies of *M. domestica* found in India.
**M. domes′tica vici′na,** a subspecies of *M. domestica* common in Egypt and India.
**M. lute′ola,** see *Auchmeromyia.*
**M. sor′bens,** a species of bush flies found in Ethiopia, East Asia, Indonesia, and Australia, believed to transmit conjunctivitis, trachoma, and other infections to humans and livestock.
**M. vomito′ria,** *Calliphora vomitoria.*

**mus·ca** (mus′kə) pl. *mus′cae* [L.] a fly.
**mus′cae hispa′nicae,** cantharides.
**mus′cae volitan′tes,** [L. "flitting flies"], specks seen floating before the eyes; see *floaters.*

**mus·ca·cide** (mus′kə-sīd) [*musca* + *-cide*] 1. destructive to flies. 2. any agent that destroys flies.

**mus·cae** (mus′e) [L.] plural of *musca.*

**mus·car·dine** (mus′kər-din) a fungal infection of silkworms caused by *Beauveria bassiana.*

**mus·ca·rine** (mus′kə-rēn) [MeSH: Muscarine] a cholinomimetic alkaloid occurring in the mushrooms *Amanita muscaria* and various species of the genera *Inocybe* and *Clitocybe;* ingestion causes *muscarinism,* a type of mushroom poisoning characterized by parasympathetic effects such as decrease in heart rate and contractility; bronchoconstriction; dilation of arterioles; increase in motility, tone, and secretion of the stomach and intestines; stimulation of the urinary bladder; and stimulation of the salivary, lacrimal, and sweat glands. See also *muscarinic receptors,* under *receptor.*

**mus·ca·rin·ic** (mus″kə-rin′ik) denoting the effects of muscarine or acetylcholine at muscarinic receptors (q.v.).

**mus·ca·rin·ism** (mus′kə-rin-iz-əm) a type of mushroom poisoning caused by the ingestion of mushrooms containing muscarine.

**mus·ce·ge·net·ic** (mus″e-jə-net′ik) giving rise to muscae volitantes.

**Mus·ci** (mus′ke) [L.] the mosses, a class of lower plants that are cryptogams.

**mus·ci·cide** (mus′ĭ-sīd) muscacide.

**Mus·ci·dae** (mus′ĭ-de) [MeSH: Muscidae] a family of flies of the order Diptera. It includes the genera *Fannia, Haematobia, Glossina, Musca, Muscina,* and *Stomoxys.*

**mus·ci·mol** [mus′kĭ-mol] [MeSH: Muscimol] a neurotoxin similar in chemical structure and activity to ibotenic acid, found in species of *Amanita* mushrooms.

**Mus·ci·na** (mə-si′nə) the nonbiting stable flies, a genus of the family Muscidae which breeds in dung. It is closely related to the housefly and it also frequents dwellings.

**mus·cle** (mus′əl) [MeSH: Muscles] an organ which by contraction produces the movements of an animal organism; there are two varieties: *striated,* including all the muscles in which contraction is voluntary and the heart muscle; and *nonstriated* or *smooth,* including all the involuntary muscles except the heart. Striated muscles are covered with a thin layer of connective tissue *(epimysium)* from which septa *(perimysium)* pass, dividing the muscle into *fasciculi* containing parallel fibers separated by connective tissue septa *(endomysium).* Each fiber consists of sarcoplasm composed of alternate light and dark portions (whence the name *striated muscle*); each contains embedded in it the *myofibrils* and is surrounded by *sarcolemma.* Smooth muscles are composed of elongated, spindle-shaped, nucleated cells arranged parallel to one another and to the long axis of the muscle, and these cells are often grouped into bundles of varying size. The muscles, bundles, and cells are enclosed in an indifferent connective tissue material much as is found in striated muscles. Called also *musculus* [TA].

## Muscle

Muscles are often referred to by their Latin names with the omission of the word *musculus,* e.g., *rectus abdominis* for *musculus rectus abdominis.* For muscles so called, see under *musculus.*

**abductor m. of great toe,** musculus abductor hallucis.
**abductor m. of little finger,** musculus abductor digiti minimi manus.
**abductor m. of little toe,** musculus abductor digiti minimi pedis.
**abductor m. of thumb, long,** musculus abductor pollicis longus.
**abductor m. of thumb, short,** musculus abductor pollicis brevis.
**adductor m., great,** musculus adductor magnus.
**adductor m., long,** musculus adductor longus.
**adductor m., short,** musculus adductor brevis.
**adductor m., smallest,** musculus adductor minimus.
**adductor m. of great toe,** musculus adductor hallucis.
**adductor m. of thumb,** musculus adductor pollicis.
**Aeby's m.,** musculus depressor labii inferioris.
**agonistic m.,** a muscle opposed in action by another muscle, called the antagonist.
**Albinus' m.,** 1. musculus risorius. 2. musculus scalenus medius.
**anconeus m.,** musculus anconeus.
**anconeus m., lateral,** caput laterale musculi tricipitis brachii.
**anconeus m., medial,** caput mediale musculi tricipitis brachii.
**anconeus m., short,** caput laterale musculi tricipitis brachii.
**antagonistic m.,** a muscle that counteracts the action of another muscle, called the agonist.
**antigravity m's,** those muscles, mainly extensors of the knees, hips, and back, that by their tone resist the constant pull of gravity in the maintenance of normal posture.
**antitragicus m., m. of antitragus,** musculus antitragicus.
**appendicular m's,** the muscles of a limb.
**arrector m. of hair,** musculus arrector pili.
**articular m.,** a muscle that has one end attached to the capsule of a joint; called also *musculus articularis.*
**articular m. of elbow,** musculus articularis cubiti.
**articular m. of knee,** musculus articularis genus.
**aryepiglottic m.,** pars ary-epiglottica musculi arytenoidei obliqui.
**arytenoid m., oblique,** musculus arytenoideus obliquus.
**arytenoid m., transverse,** musculus arytenoideus transversus.
**m's of auditory ossicles,** musculi ossiculorum auditoriorum.
**auricular m's,** 1. the extrinsic auricular muscles; see *musculus auricularis anterior, posterior,* and *superior.* 2. musculi auriculares.
**auricular m., anterior,** musculus auricularis anterior.
**auricular m., posterior,** musculus auricularis posterior.
**auricular m., superior,** musculus auricularis superior.
**Bell's m.,** the muscular strands between the ureteric orifices and the uvula vesicae, bounding the trigone of the urinary bladder. Called also *ureteric bridge.*
**biceps m. of arm,** musculus biceps brachii.
**biceps m. of thigh,** musculus biceps femoris.
**bipennate m.,** musculus pennatus.
**Bowman's m.,** musculus ciliaris.
**brachial m.,** musculus brachialis.
**brachioradial m.,** musculus brachioradialis.
**Braune's m.,** musculus puborectalis.
**bronchoesophageal m.,** musculus bronchooesophageus.
**Brücke's m.,** the longitudinal fibers of the ciliary muscle.
**buccinator m.,** musculus buccinator.
**buccopharyngeal m.,** pars buccopharyngea musculi constrictoris pharyngis superioris.
**bulbocavernous m.,** musculus bulbospongiosus.
**canine m.,** musculus levator anguli oris.
**cardiac m.,** the muscle of the heart, comprising the chief component of the myocardium and lining the walls of the large vessels joined to the heart; it is composed of fibers of striated but involuntary muscle. The composition and organization of its fibers resemble those of skeletal muscle, but instead of forming a syncytium, its branched, mononucleate cells are linked end to end by intercalated disks that provide both mechanical and ionic coupling for coordination of the entire muscle.
**Casser's m., casserian m.,** ligamentum mallei anterius.
**ceratocricoid m.,** musculus ceratocricoideus.
**ceratopharyngeal m.,** pars ceratopharyngea musculi constrictoris pharyngis medii.
**cervical m's,** musculi colli.
**Chassaignac's axillary m.,** an occasional muscle bundle extending from the lower edge of the latissimus dorsi across the hollow of the axilla to the brachial fascia or to the lower border of the pectoralis minor.
**chondroglossus m.,** musculus chondroglossus.
**chondropharyngeal m.,** pars chondropharyngea musculi constrictoris pharyngis medii.
**ciliary m.,** musculus ciliaris.
**cleidohyoid m.,** a slip of muscle sometimes seen augmenting the sternohyoid muscle, extending from the hyoid bone to the clavicle.
**coccygeal m.,** musculus coccygeus.
**coccygeal m's,** those connected with the coccyx, including the musculus coccygeus, musculus sacrococcygeus dorsalis, and musculus sacrococcygeus ventralis; called also *musculi coccygei* [TA].
**compressor naris m., compressor m. of naris,** pars transversa musculi nasalis.
**compressor m. of urethra,** musculus compressor urethrae.
**congenerous m's,** muscles having a common action or function.
**constrictor m. of pharynx, inferior,** musculus constrictor pharyngis inferior.
**constrictor m. of pharynx, middle,** musculus constrictor pharyngis medius.
**constrictor m. of pharynx, superior,** musculus constrictor pharyngis superior.
**coracobrachial m.,** musculus coracobrachialis.
**Crampton's m.,** the anterior portion of the ciliary muscle in birds.
**cremaster m.,** musculus cremaster.
**cricoarytenoid m., lateral,** musculus crico-arytenoideus lateralis.
**cricoarytenoid m., posterior,** musculus crico-arytenoideus posterior.
**cricopharyngeal m.,** pars cricopharyngea musculi constrictoris pharyngis inferioris.
**cricothyroid m.,** musculus cricothyroideus.
**cruciate m.,** a muscle in which the fiber bundles are arranged in the shape of an X. Called also musculus cruciatus.
**cutaneous m.,** musculus cutaneus.
**dartos m.,** 1. musculus dartos, def. 1. 2. tunica dartos, def. 1.
**dartos m. of scrotum,** tunica dartos.
**deltoid m.,** musculus deltoideus.
**depressor m., superciliary,** musculus depressor supercilii.
**depressor m. of angle of mouth,** musculus depressor anguli oris.
**depressor m. of lower lip,** musculus depressor labii inferioris.
**depressor m. of septum of nose,** musculus depressor septi nasi.
**detrusor m. of bladder, detrusor urinae m.,** musculus detrusor vesicae.
**diaphragmatic m.,** diaphragma (def. 1).
**digastric m.,** musculus digastricus.
**dilator m.,** musculus dilatator.
**dilator naris m., dilator m. of naris,** pars alaris musculi nasalis.
**dilator pupillae m.,** musculus dilatator pupillae.
**dorsal m's,** musculi dorsi.
**double m.,** myofiber hyperplasia.
**emergency m's,** muscles which ordinarily are not required in the performance of an act but which assist the prime movers when an act is performed with great force.
**epicranial m.,** musculus epicranius.
**epimeric m.,** a muscle derived from an epimere and innervated by a posterior ramus of a spinal nerve.
**epitrochleoanconeus m.,** musculus epitrochleoanconaeus.
**erector m. of penis,** musculus ischiocavernosus.
**erector m. of spine,** musculus erector spinae.
**eustachian m.,** musculus tensor tympani.
**m's of expression,** musculi faciei.
**extensor m. of digits, common, extensor m. of fingers,** musculus extensor digitorum.
**extensor m. of fifth digit, proper,** musculus extensor digiti minimi.
**extensor m. of great toe, long,** musculus extensor hallucis longus.
**extensor m. of great toe, short,** musculus extensor hallucis brevis.
**extensor m. of index finger,** musculus extensor indicis.
**extensor m. of little finger,** musculus extensor digiti minimi.

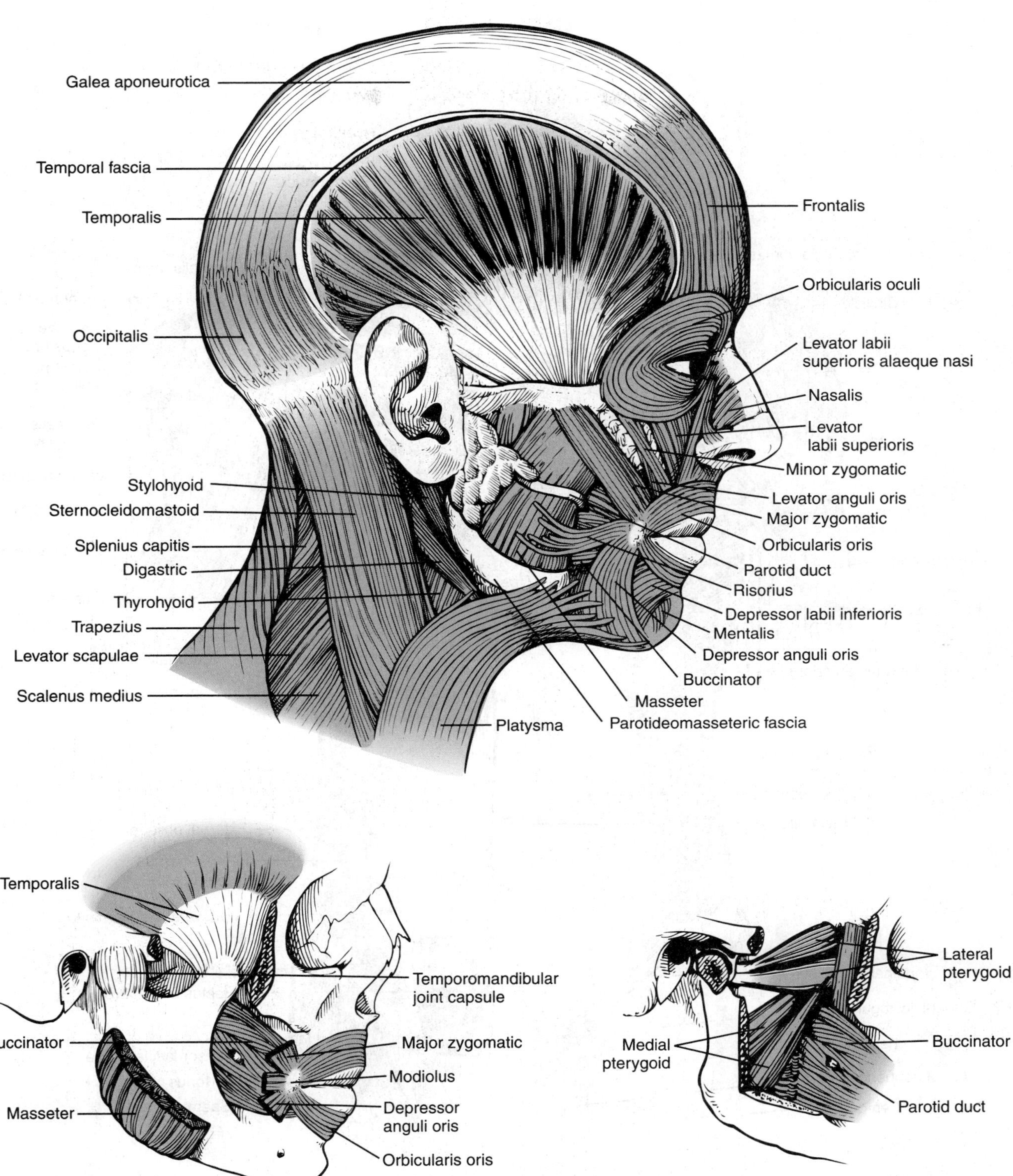


**PLATE 30**—MUSCLES OF THE HEAD AND NECK

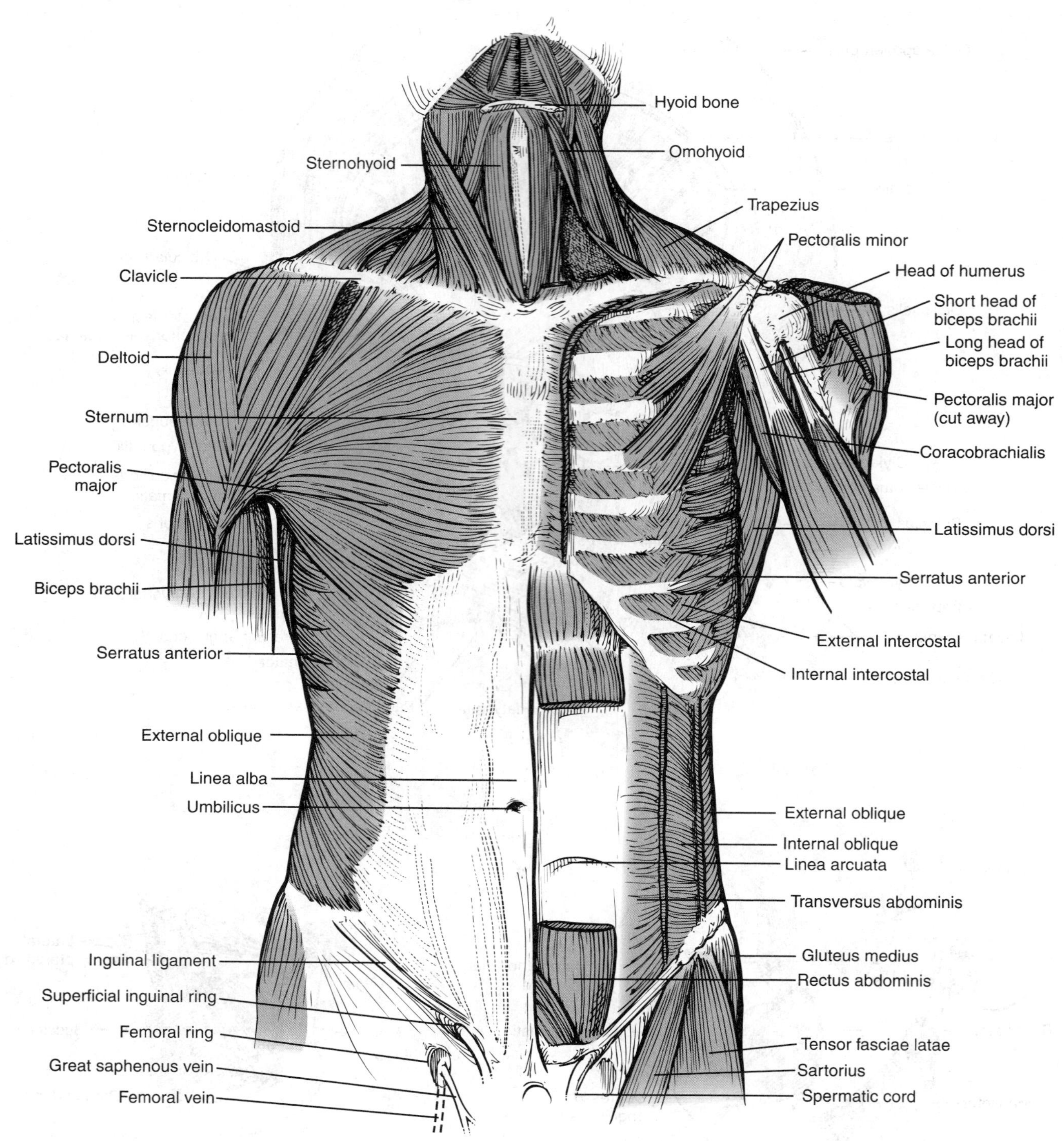


**PLATE 31**—MUSCLES OF THE TRUNK, ANTERIOR VIEW

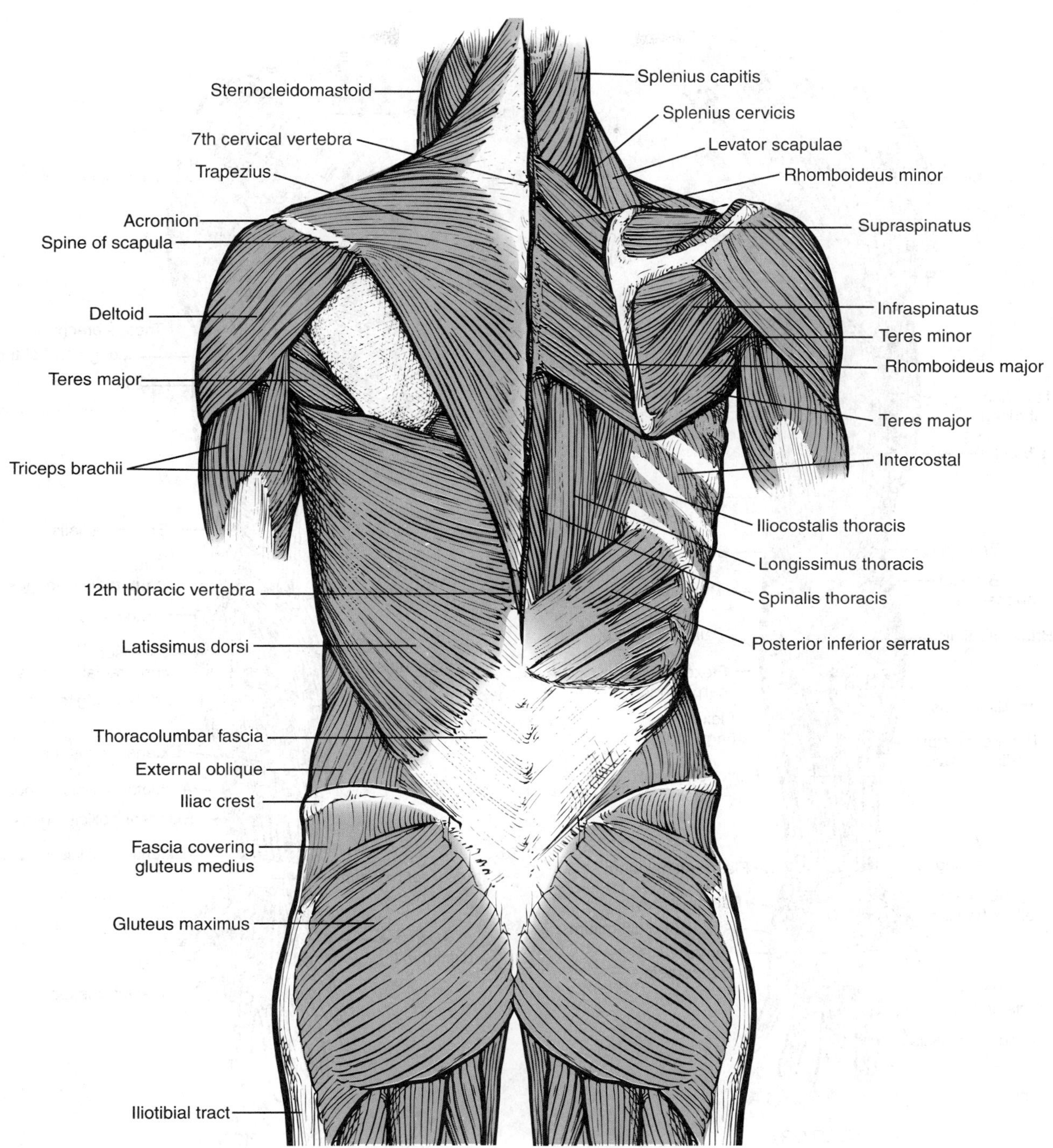


**PLATE 32**—MUSCLES OF THE TRUNK, POSTERIOR VIEW

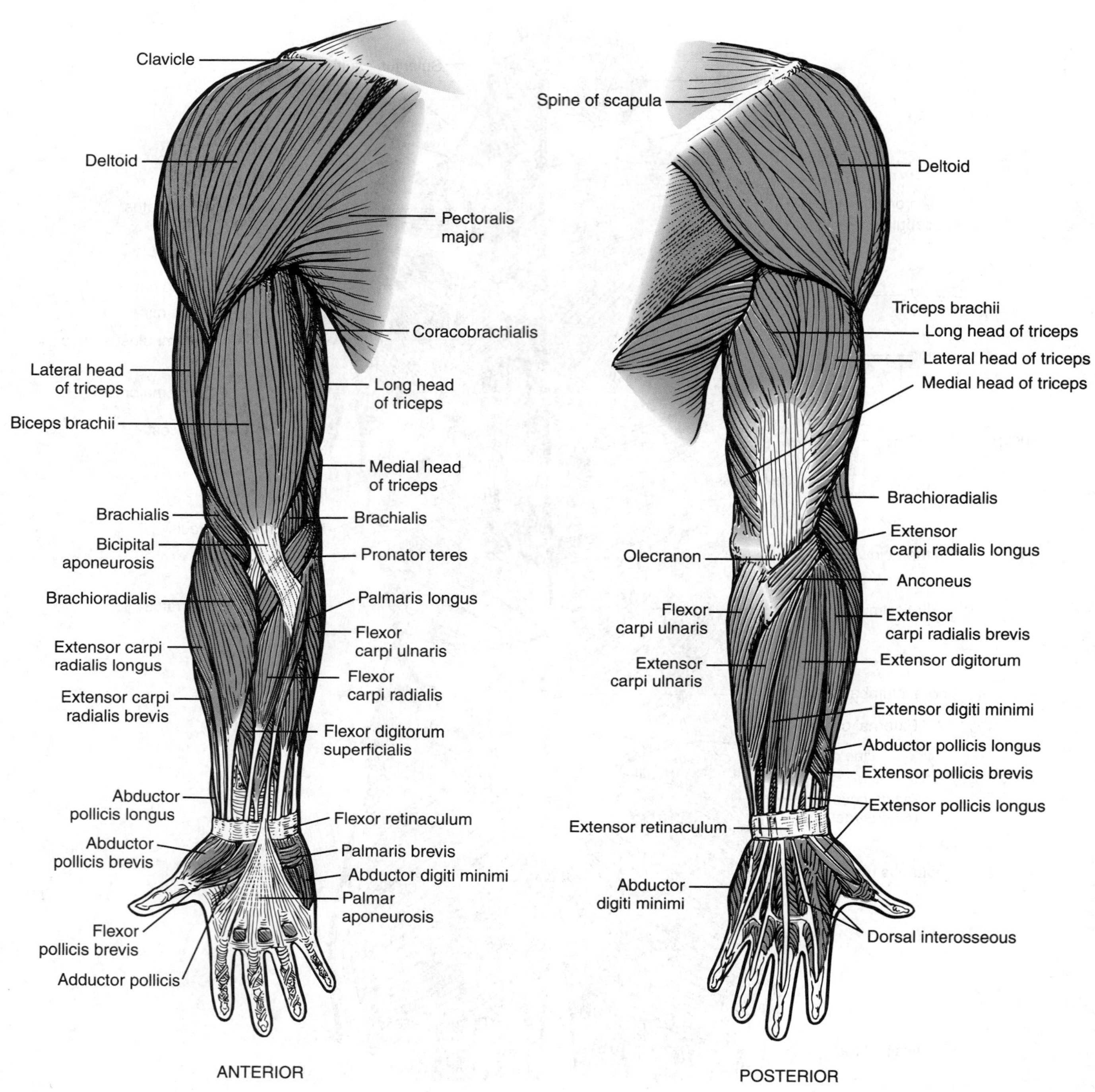


**PLATE 33**—SUPERFICIAL MUSCLES OF THE UPPER LIMB

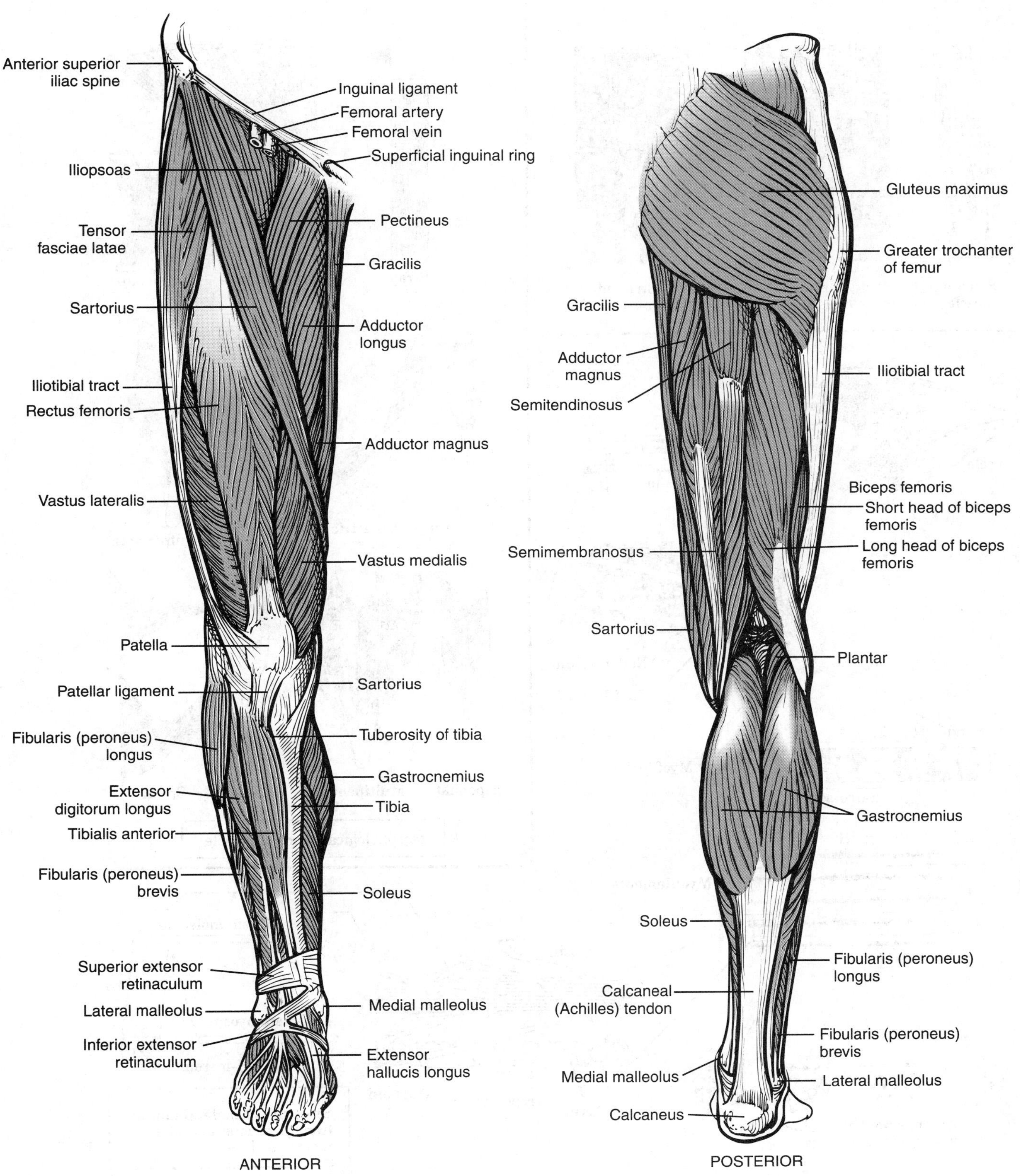


**PLATE 34—**SUPERFICIAL MUSCLES OF THE LOWER LIMB

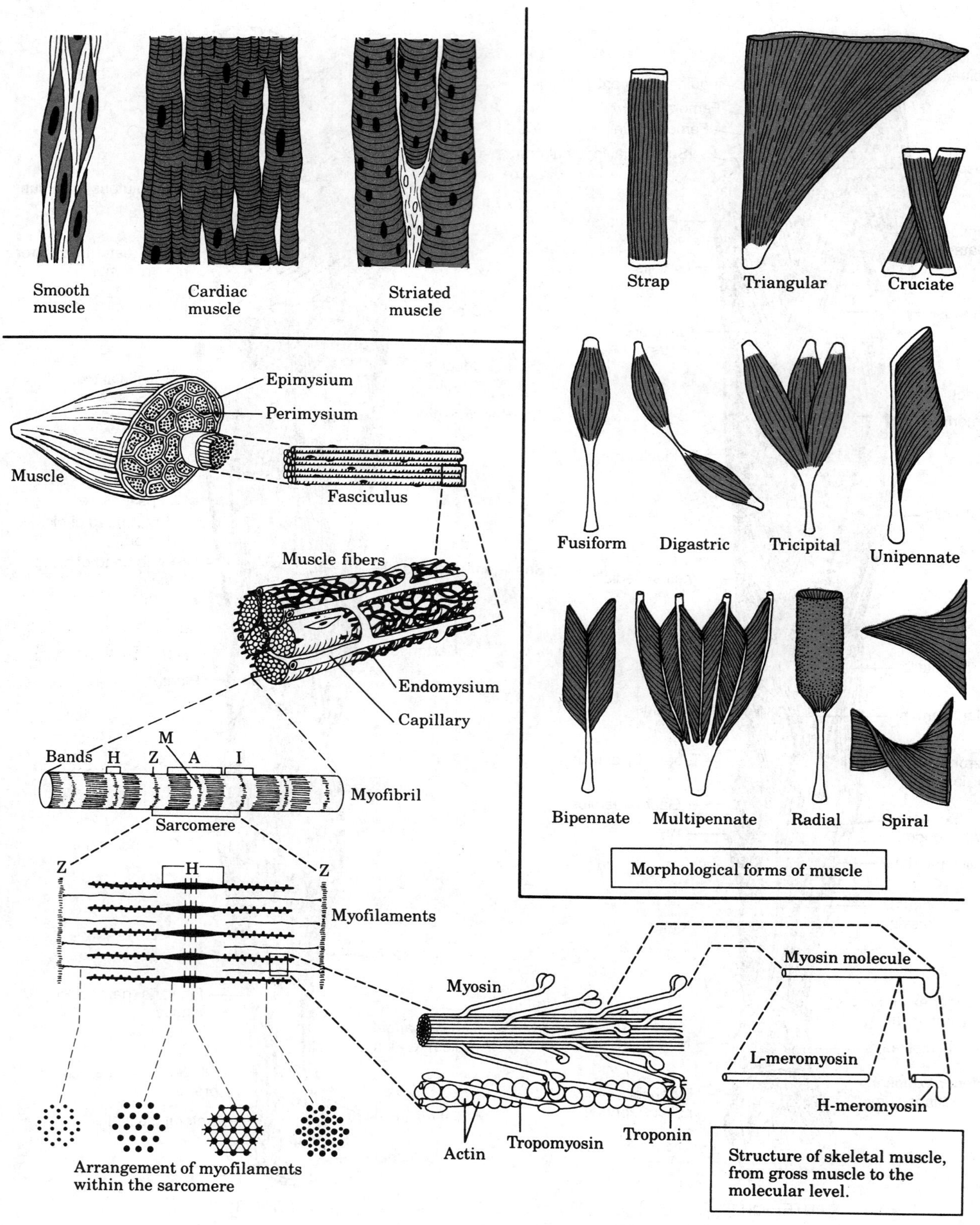


**PLATE 35—**TYPES AND STRUCTURE OF MUSCLE

**extensor m. of thumb, long,** musculus extensor pollicis longus.
**extensor m. of thumb, short,** musculus extensor pollicis brevis.
**extensor m. of toes, long,** musculus extensor digitorum longus.
**extensor m. of toes, short,** musculus extensor digitorum brevis.
**extraocular m's,** musculi externi bulbi oculi.
**extrinsic m.,** a muscle that does not originate in the same limb or part in which it is inserted.
**m's of eye,** musculi externi bulbi oculi.
**facial m's, m's of facial expression,** musculi faciei.
**facial and masticatory m's,** musculi faciales et masticatores.
**fast m.,** white m.
**m's of fauces,** see *musculi palati mollis et faucium.*
**femoral m.,** musculus vastus intermedius.
**fibular m., long,** musculus fibularis longus.
**fibular m., short,** musculus fibularis brevis.
**fibular m., third,** musculus fibularis tertius.
**fixation m's, fixator m's,** accessory muscles that serve to steady a part.
**flexor m., accessory,** musculus quadratus plantae.
**flexor m. of fingers, deep,** musculus flexor digitorum profundus.
**flexor m. of fingers, superficial,** musculus flexor digitorum superficialis.
**flexor m. of great toe, long,** musculus flexor hallucis longus.
**flexor m. of great toe, short,** musculus flexor hallucis brevis.
**flexor m. of little finger, short,** musculus flexor digiti minimi brevis manus.
**flexor m. of little toe, short,** musculus flexor digiti minimi brevis pedis.
**flexor m. of thumb, long,** musculus flexor pollicis longus.
**flexor m. of thumb, short,** musculus flexor pollicis brevis.
**flexor m. of toes, long,** musculus flexor digitorum longus.
**flexor m. of toes, short,** musculus flexor digitorum brevis.
**flexor m. of wrist, radial,** musculus flexor carpi radialis.
**flexor m. of wrist, ulnar,** musculus flexor carpi ulnaris.
**Folius' m.,** ligamentum mallei laterale.
**frontal m.,** venter frontalis musculi occipitofrontalis.
**fusiform m.,** a spindle-shaped muscle; see *musculus fusiformis.*
**gastrocnemius m.,** musculus gastrocnemius.
**gastrocnemius m., lateral,** caput laterale musculi gastrocnemii.
**gastrocnemius m., medial,** caput mediale musculi gastrocnemii.
**Gavard's m.,** the oblique muscular elements of the stomach wall.
**gemellus m., inferior,** musculus gemellus inferior.
**gemellus m., superior,** musculus gemellus superior.
**genioglossus m.,** musculus genioglossus.
**geniohyoid m.,** musculus geniohyoideus.
**glossopalatine m.,** musculus palatoglossus.
**glossopharyngeal m.,** pars glossopharyngea musculi constrictoris pharyngis superioris.
**gluteal m., least,** musculus gluteus minimus.
**gracilis m.,** musculus gracilis.
**Guthrie's m.,** musculus sphincter urethrae.
**hamstring m's,** the muscles of the back of the thigh, including the biceps femoris, the semitendinosus, and the semimembranosus.
**Hilton's m.,** musculus aryepiglotticus.
**Horner's m.,** pars lacrimalis musculi orbicularis oculi.
**Houston's m.,** fibers of the bulbocavernosus muscle compressing the dorsal vein of the penis.
**hyoglossal m., hyoglossus m.,** musculus hyoglossus.
**m's of hyoid bone,** see *musculi infrahyoidei* and *musculi suprahyoidei.*
**hypaxial m's,** musculus longus capitis, musculus longus colli, the vertebral portion of the diaphragm, and musculus sacrococcygeus anterior; called also *subvertebral m's.*
**hypomeric m.,** a muscle derived from a hypomere and innervated by an anterior ramus of a spinal nerve.
**hypothenar m's,** the intrinsic muscles of the little finger; flexing, abducting, and opposing it, and comprising the palmaris brevis, abductor digiti minimi, flexor digiti minimi brevis, and opponens digiti minimi.
**iliac m.,** musculus iliacus.
**iliococcygeal m.,** musculus iliococcygeus.
**iliocostal m.,** musculus iliocostalis.
**iliopsoas m.,** musculus iliopsoas.
**incisive m's of inferior lip,** musculi incisivi labii inferioris.
**incisive m's of lower lip,** musculi incisivi labii inferioris.
**incisive m's of superior lip,** musculi incisivi labii superioris.
**incisive m's of upper lip,** musculi incisivi labii superioris.
**infrahyoid m's,** musculi infrahyoidei.
**infraspinous m.,** musculus infraspinatus.
**inspiratory m's,** the muscles that act during inspiration, such as the diaphragm, and the intercostal and pectoral muscles.
**intercostal m's, external,** musculi intercostales externi.
**intercostal m's, innermost,** musculi intercostales intimi.
**intercostal m's, internal,** musculi intercostales interni.
**interfoveolar m.,** ligamentum interfoveolare.
**interosseous m's, palmar,** musculi interossei palmares.
**interosseous m's, plantar,** musculi interossei plantares.
**interosseous m's, volar,** musculi interossei palmares.
**interosseous m's of foot, dorsal,** musculi interossei dorsales pedis.
**interosseous m's of hand, dorsal,** musculi interossei dorsales manus.
**interspinal m's,** musculi interspinales.
**interspinal m's of loins,** musculi interspinales lumborum.
**interspinal m's of neck,** musculi interspinales cervicis.
**interspinal m's of thorax,** musculi interspinales thoracis.
**intertransverse m's,** musculi intertransversarii.
**intertransverse m's, anterior,** musculi intertransversarii thoracis.
**intertransverse m's, lateral lumbar,** musculi intertransversarii laterales lumborum.
**intertransverse m's, medial lumbar,** musculi intertransversarii mediales lumborum.
**intertransverse m's of neck, anterior,** musculi intertransversarii anteriores cervicis.
**intertransverse m's of neck, posterior,** musculi intertransversarii posteriores laterales cervicis.
**intertransverse m's of thorax,** musculi intertransversarii thoracis.
**intraauricular m's,** the stapedius and tensor tympani muscles.
**intraocular m's,** the intrinsic muscles of the eyeball.
**intrinsic m.,** a muscle that is contained (origin, belly, and insertion) in the same limb or part.
**involuntary m.,** a muscle that is not under the control of the will; such muscles are, for the most part, composed of nonstriated fibers.
**iridic m's,** the muscles controlling the iris.
**ischiocavernous m.,** musculus ischiocavernosus.
**Jarjavay's m.,** a muscle arising from the ramus of the ischium and inserting in the constrictor muscle of the vagina, which acts to depress the urethra.
**Jung's m.,** musculus pyramidalis auriculae.
**Koyter's m.,** musculus corrugator supercilii.
**Landström's m.,** minute muscle fibers in the fascia around and behind the eyeball, attached in front to the anterior orbital fascia and eyelids.
**Langer's m.,** muscular fibers from the insertion of the pectoralis major muscle over the bicipital groove to the insertion of the latissimus dorsi.
**latissimus dorsi m.,** musculus latissimus dorsi.

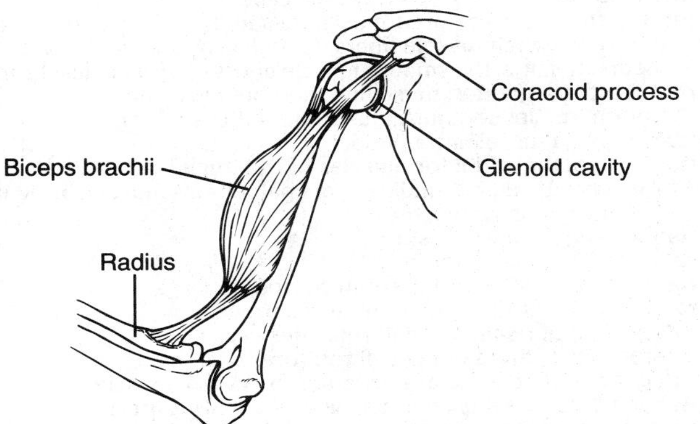

Extrinsic muscle exemplified by the biceps brachii, which originates at the glenoid cavity and the coracoid process and inserts into the tuberosity of the radius.

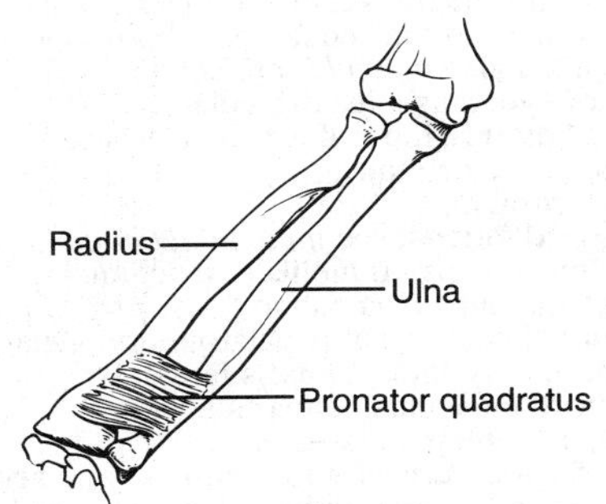

Intrinsic muscle exemplified by the pronator quadratus, which originates at the ulna and inserts into the radius.

**levator m. of angle of mouth,** musculus levator anguli oris.
**levator ani m.,** musculus levator ani.
**levator m. of prostate,** musculus levator prostatae.
**levator m's of ribs,** musculi levatores costarum.
**levator m's of ribs, long,** musculi levatores costarum longi.
**levator m's of ribs, short,** musculi levatores costarum breves.
**levator m. of scapula,** musculus levator scapulae.
**levator m. of thyroid gland,** musculus levator glandulae thyroideae.
**levator m. of upper eyelid,** musculus levator palpebrae superioris.
**levator m. of upper lip,** musculus levator labii superioris.
**levator m. of upper lip and ala of nose,** musculus levator labii superioris alaeque nasi.
**levator m. of velum palatinum,** musculus levator veli palatini.
**lingual m's,** musculi linguae.
**long m. of head,** musculus longus capitis.
**long m. of neck,** musculus longus colli.
**longissimus m.,** musculus longissimus.
**longissimus m. of back,** musculus longissimus thoracis.
**longissimus m. of head,** musculus longissimus capitis.
**longissimus m. of neck,** musculus longissimus cervicis.
**longissimus m. of thorax,** musculus longissimus thoracis.
**longitudinal m. of tongue, inferior,** musculus longitudinalis inferior linguae.
**longitudinal m. of tongue, superior,** musculus longitudinalis superior linguae.
**m's of lower limb,** musculi membri inferioris.
**lumbrical m's of foot,** musculi lumbricales pedis.
**lumbrical m's of hand,** musculi lumbricales manus.
**masseter m.,** musculus masseter.
**m's of mastication, masticatory m's,** musculi masticatorii.
**Merkel's m.,** musculus ceratocricoideus.
**mesothenar m.,** musculus adductor pollicis.
**Müller's m.,** 1. fibrae circulares musculi ciliaris. 2. musculus orbitalis.
**multifidus m's,** musculi multifidi.
**multipennate m.,** musculus multipennatus.
**mylohyoid m.,** musculus mylohyoideus.
**mylopharyngeal m.,** pars mylopharyngea musculi constrictoris pharyngis superioris.
**nasal m.,** musculus nasalis.
**m's of neck,** musculi colli.
**nonstriated m.,** a type of muscle without transverse striations in its constituent fibers; such muscles are almost always involuntary. Called also *smooth m.*
**oblique m. of abdomen, external,** musculus obliquus externus abdominis.
**oblique m. of abdomen, internal,** musculus obliquus internus abdominis.
**oblique m. of auricle,** musculus obliquus auriculae.
**oblique m. of eyeball, inferior,** musculus obliquus inferior bulbi.
**oblique m. of eyeball, superior,** musculus obliquus superior bulbi.
**oblique m. of head, inferior,** musculus obliquus capitis inferior.
**oblique m. of head, superior,** musculus obliquus capitis superior.
**obturator m., external,** musculus obturatorius externus.
**obturator m., internal,** musculus obturatorius internus.
**occipital m.,** venter occipitalis musculi occipitofrontalis.
**occipitofrontal m.,** musculus occipitofrontalis.
**Ochsner's m.,** an inconstant muscular thickening of the duodenal muscle just distal to the opening of the common bile duct.
**ocular m's, oculorotatory m's,** musculi externi bulbi oculi.
**Oddi's m.,** 1. sphincter of Oddi (def. 1). 2. musculus sphincter ampullae hepatopancreaticae.
**Oehl's m.,** muscle fibers in the chordae tendineae of the left atrioventricular valve.
**omohyoid m.,** musculus omohyoideus.
**opposing m. of little finger,** musculus opponens digiti minimi.
**opposing m. of thumb,** musculus opponens pollicis.
**orbicular m.,** a muscle that encircles a body opening, such as the eye or mouth; called also *musculus orbicularis* [TA].
**orbicular m. of eye,** musculus orbicularis oculi.
**orbicular m. of mouth,** musculus orbicularis oris.
**orbital m.,** musculus orbitalis.
**organic m.,** visceral m.
**m's of palate and fauces,** see *musculi palati mollis et faucium.*
**palatine m's,** musculi palati mollis et faucium.
**palatoglossus m.,** musculus palatoglossus.
**palatopharyngeal m.,** musculus palatopharyngeus.
**palmar m., long,** musculus palmaris longus.
**palmar m., short,** musculus palmaris brevis.
**papillary m's,** musculi papillares.
**papillary m. of conus arteriosus,** a septal papillary muscle arising near the septal end of the supraventricular crest and attached to the anterior and septal cusps of the tricuspid valve.
**papillary m. of left ventricle, anterior,** musculus papillaris anterior ventriculi sinistri.
**papillary m. of left ventricle, posterior,** musculus papillaris posterior ventriculi sinistri.
**papillary m. of right ventricle, anterior,** musculus papillaris anterior ventriculi dextri.
**papillary m. of right ventricle, posterior,** musculus papillaris posterior ventriculi dextri.
**papillary m's of right ventricle, septal,** several small papillary muscles in the right ventricle of the heart, arising from the interventricular septum and attaching to adjacent cusps of the tricuspid valve via chordae tendineae.
**pectinate m's of left atrium,** musculi pectinati atrii sinistri.
**pectinate m's of right atrium,** musculi pectinati atrii dextri.
**pectineal m.,** musculus pectineus.
**pectoral m., greater,** musculus pectoralis major.
**pectoral m., smaller,** musculus pectoralis minor.
**m's of pelvic diaphragm,** musculi diaphragmatis pelvis.
**pennate m., penniform m.,** musculus pennatus.
**perineal m's, m's of perineum,** musculi perinei.
**peroneal m., long,** musculus fibularis longus.
**peroneal m., short,** musculus fibularis brevis.
**peroneal m., third,** musculus fibularis tertius.
**pharyngopalatine m.,** musculus palatopharyngeus.
**Phillips' m.,** a muscular slip from the radial collateral ligament of the wrist and the styloid process of the radius to the phalanges.
**piriform m.,** musculus piriformis.
**plantar m.,** musculus plantaris.
**platysma m.,** see *platysma.*
**pleuroesophageal m.,** musculus pleurooesophageus.
**popliteal m.,** musculus popliteus.
**postaxial m.,** a muscle on the dorsal side of a limb.
**preaxial m.,** a muscle on the ventral side of a limb.
**procerus m.,** musculus procerus.
**pronator m., quadrate,** musculus pronator quadratus.
**pronator m., round,** musculus pronator teres.
**psoas m., greater,** musculus psoas major.
**psoas m., smaller,** musculus psoas minor.
**pterygoid m., external,** musculus pterygoideus lateralis.
**pterygoid m., internal,** musculus pterygoideus medialis.
**pterygoid m., lateral,** musculus pterygoideus lateralis.
**pterygoid m., medial,** musculus pterygoideus medialis.
**pterygopharyngeal m.,** pars pterygopharyngea musculi constrictoris pharyngis superioris.
**pubicoperitoneal m.,** ligamentum interfoveolare.
**pubococcygeal m.,** musculus pubococcygeus.
**puboprostatic m.,** musculus puboprostaticus.
**puborectal m.,** musculus puborectalis.
**pubovaginal m.,** musculus pubovaginalis.
**pubovesical m.,** musculus pubovesicalis.
**pyloric sphincter m.,** musculus sphincter pyloricus.
**pyramidal m.,** musculus pyramidalis.
**pyramidal m. of auricle,** musculus pyramidalis auricularis.
**quadrate m.,** musculus quadratus.
**quadrate m. of lower lip,** musculus depressor labii inferioris.
**quadrate m. of sole,** musculus quadratus plantae.
**quadrate m. of thigh,** musculus quadratus femoris.
**quadrate m. of upper lip,** musculus levator labii superioris.
**quadriceps m. of thigh,** musculus quadriceps femoris.
**rectococcygeal m.,** musculus rectococcygeus.
**rectourethral m.,** musculus recto-urethralis.
**rectouterine m.,** musculus recto-uterinus.
**rectovesical m.,** musculus rectovesicalis.
**red m.,** the darker-colored muscle tissue of some mammals, composed of slow twitch muscle fibers. Called also *slow m.* Cf. *white m.*
**Reisseisen's m's,** the smooth muscle fibers of the smallest bronchi.
**rhomboid m., greater,** musculus rhomboideus major.
**rhomboid m., lesser,** musculus rhomboideus minor.
**ribbon m's,** musculi infrahyoidei.
**rider's m's,** the adductor muscles of the thigh.
**Riolan's m.,** 1. ciliary bundle of pars palpebralis musculi orbicularis oculi. 2. musculus cremaster.
**risorius m.,** musculus risorius.
**rotator m's,** musculi rotatores.
**rotator m's, long,** musculi rotatores longi.
**rotator m's, short,** musculi rotatores breves.
**rotator m's of neck,** musculi rotatores cervicis.
**rotator m's of thorax,** musculi rotatores thoracis.
**Rouget's m.,** the circular portion of the ciliary muscle.
**Ruysch's m.,** the muscular tissue of the fundus uteri.
**sacrococcygeal m., anterior,** musculus sacrococcygeus ventralis.
**sacrococcygeal m., dorsal,** musculus sacrococcygeus dorsalis.
**sacrococcygeal m., posterior,** musculus sacrococcygeus dorsalis.

## **Muscle** *Continued*

**sacrococcygeal m., ventral,** musculus sacrococcygeus ventralis.
**sacrospinal m.,** musculus erector spinae.
**salpingopharyngeal m.,** musculus salpingopharyngeus.
**Santorini's m.,** musculus risorius.
**Santorini's m's, circular,** the nonstriated fibers that encircle the urethra beneath the sphincter urethrae.
**sartorius m.,** musculus sartorius.
**scalene m., anterior,** musculus scalenus anterior.
**scalene m., middle,** musculus scalenus medius.
**scalene m., posterior,** musculus scalenus posterior.
**scalene m., smallest,** musculus scalenus minimus.
**Sebileau's m.,** the deeper fibers of the musculus dartos.
**semimembranous m.,** musculus semimembranosus.
**semipennate m.,** musculus semipennatus.
**semispinal m.,** musculus semispinalis.
**semispinal m. of head,** musculus semispinalis capitis.
**semispinal m. of neck,** musculus semispinalis cervicis.
**semispinal m. of thorax,** musculus semispinalis thoracis.
**semitendinous m.,** musculus semitendinosus.
**serratus m., anterior,** musculus serratus anterior.
**serratus m., inferior posterior,** musculus serratus posterior inferior.
**serratus m., superior posterior,** musculus serratus posterior superior.
**Sibson's m.,** musculus scalenus minimus.
**skeletal m's,** striated muscles that are attached to bones and typically cross at least one joint; called also *musculi skeleti.*
**slow m.,** red m.
**smooth m.,** nonstriated m.
**soleus m.,** musculus soleus.
**somatic m's,** musculi skeleti.
**sphincter m.,** musculus sphincter.
**sphincter m. of anus, external,** musculus sphincter ani externus.
**sphincter m. of anus, internal,** musculus sphincter ani internus.
**sphincter m. of bile duct,** musculus sphincter ductus choledochi.
**sphincter m. of hepatopancreatic ampulla,** musculus sphincter ampullae hepatopancreaticae.
**sphincter m. of membranous urethra,** musculus sphincter urethrae.
**sphincter m. of pupil,** musculus sphincter pupillae.
**sphincter m. of pylorus,** musculus sphincter pyloricus.
**sphincter m. of urethra, sphincter urethrae m.,** musculus sphincter urethrae.
**sphincter m. of urinary bladder,** musculus sphincter vesicae urinariae.
**spinal m.,** musculus spinalis.
**splenius m. of head,** musculus splenius capitis.
**splenius m. of neck,** musculus splenius cervicis.
**stapedius m.,** musculus stapedius.
**sternal m.,** musculus sternalis.
**sternocleidomastoid m.,** musculus sternocleidomastoideus.
**sternohyoid m.,** musculus sternohyoideus.
**sternomastoid m.,** musculus sternocleidomastoideus.
**sternothyroid m.,** musculus sternothyroideus.
**strap m's,** muscles of the neck, particularly those of the thyroid cartilage and hyoid bone.
**striated m., striped m.,** any muscle whose fibers are divided by transverse bands into striations, including cardiac and voluntary muscle; often used as a synonym for voluntary muscle. See *muscle.*
**styloglossus m.,** musculus styloglossus.
**stylohyoid m.,** musculus stylohyoideus.
**stylopharyngeus m.,** musculus stylopharyngeus.
**subclavius m.,** musculus subclavius.
**subcostal m's,** musculi subcostales.
**suboccipital m's,** musculi suboccipitales.
**subscapular m.,** musculus subscapularis.
**subvertebral m's,** hypaxial m's.
**supinator m.,** musculus supinator.
**suprahyoid m's,** musculi suprahyoidei.
**supraspinous m.,** musculus supraspinatus.
**suspensory m. of duodenum,** musculus suspensorius duodeni.
**synergic m's, synergistic m's,** muscles that assist one another in action.
**tarsal m., inferior,** musculus tarsalis inferior.
**tarsal m., superior,** musculus tarsalis superior.
**temporal m., temporalis m.,** musculus temporalis.
**temporoparietal m.,** musculus temporoparietalis.
**tensor m. of fascia lata,** musculus tensor fasciae latae.
**tensor m. of tympanic membrane, tensor m. of tympanum,** musculus tensor tympani.
**tensor m. of velum palatinum,** musculus tensor veli palatini.
**teres major m.,** musculus teres major.
**teres minor m.,** musculus teres minor.
**Theile's m.,** musculus transversus perinei superficialis.
**thenar m's,** the abductor and flexor muscles of the thumb.
**thyroarytenoid m.,** musculus thyro-arytenoideus.
**thyroepiglottic m.,** pars thyro-epiglottica musculi thyro-arytenoidei.
**thyrohyoid m.,** musculus thyrohyoideus.
**thyropharyngeal m.,** pars thyropharyngea musculi constrictoris pharyngis inferioris.
**tibial m., anterior,** musculus tibialis anterior.
**tibial m., posterior,** musculus tibialis posterior.
**m's of tongue,** musculi linguae.
**tracheal m.,** musculus trachealis.
**trachelomastoid m.,** musculus longissimus capitis.
**m. of tragus,** musculus tragicus.
**transverse abdominal m.,** musculus transversus abdominis.
**transverse m. of auricle,** musculus transversus auricularis.
**transverse m. of chin,** musculus transversus menti.
**transverse m. of neck,** musculus transversus nuchae.
**transverse perineal m., deep,** musculus transversus perinei profundus.
**transverse perineal m., superficial,** musculus transversus perinei superficialis.
**transverse m. of thorax,** musculus transversus thoracis.
**transverse m. of tongue,** musculus transversus linguae.
**transversospinal m's,** musculi transversospinales.
**trapezius m.,** musculus trapezius.
**m. of Treitz,** musculus suspensorius duodeni.
**triangular m.,** musculus triangularis.
**triceps m. of arm,** musculus triceps brachii.
**triceps m. of calf,** musculus triceps surae.
**trigonal m.,** a submucous muscular sheet of the trigone of the bladder, continuous with muscles of the ureteral wall above and extending to the proximal urethra.
**unipennate m.,** musculus semipennatus.
**unstriated m.,** nonstriated m.
**m's of upper limb,** musculi membri superioris.
**urethrovaginal sphincter m.,** musculus sphincter urethrovaginalis.
**m's of urogenital diaphragm,** musculi diaphragmatis urogenitalis.
**m. of uvula,** musculus uvulae.
**vertical m. of tongue,** musculus verticalis linguae.
**vestigial m.,** a muscle that was once well developed but through evolution has become rudimentary.
**visceral m.,** muscle fibers associated chiefly with the hollow viscera and largely of splanchnic mesodermal origin; except for the striated fibers in the wall of the heart, they are smooth muscle fibers bound together by reticular fibers.
**vocal m.,** musculus vocalis.
**voluntary m.,** any muscle that normally is under the control of the will; such muscles are nearly always composed of striated fibers.
**white m.,** the paler-colored muscle tissue of some mammals, composed of fast twitch muscle fibers. Called also *fast m.* Cf. *red m.*
**Wilson's m.,** musculus sphincter urethrae.
**yoked m's,** muscles that normally act simultaneously and equally, as in moving the eyes.
**zygomatic m., zygomatic m., greater,** musculus zygomaticus major.
**zygomatic m., lesser,** musculus zygomaticus minor.

---

**mus·cle phos·pho·fruc·to·ki·nase** (mus′əl fos″fo-frook″to-ki′nās) the muscle isozyme of 6-phosphofructokinase.

**mus·cle phos·pho·fruc·to·ki·nase de·fi·cien·cy** glycogen storage disease, type VII.

**mus·cle phos·phor·y·lase** (mus′əl fos-for′ə-lās) the muscle isozyme of glycogen phosphorylase.

**mus·cle phos·phor·y·lase de·fi·cien·cy** glycogen storage disease, type V.

**mus·cu·lam·ine** (mus″ku-lam′in) a base isolated from hydrolyzed calf's muscle; it is the same as spermine.

**mus·cu·lar** (mus′ku-lər) [L. *muscularis*] 1. pertaining to or composing muscle. 2. having a well-developed musculature.

**mus·cu·la·ris** (mus″ku-la′ris) [L.] 1. muscular. 2. pertaining to a muscular layer or coat; see *tunica muscularis* and *lamina muscularis mucosae*.
**m. muco′sae,** lamina muscularis mucosae.

**mus·cu·lar·i·ty** (mus″ku-lar′ĭ-te) the condition or quality of being muscular.

**mus·cu·lar·ize** (mus′ku-lər-īz) to change into muscle tissue.

**mus·cu·la·ture** (mus′ku-lə-chər) the muscular apparatus of the body, or of any part of it.

**mus·cu·li** (mus′ku-li) [L.] genitive and plural of *musculus.*

**mus·cu·lo·apo·neu·rot·ic** (mus″ku-lo-ap′o-noo͞-rot′ik) pertaining to a muscle and its aponeurosis.

**mus·cu·lo·cu·ta·ne·ous** (mus″ku-lo-ku-ta′ne-əs) pertaining to or supplying both muscles and skin. Called also *musculodermic.*

**mus·cu·lo·der·mic** (mus″ku-lo-der′mik) musculocutaneous.

**mus·cu·lo·elas·tic** (mus″ku-lo-e-las′tik) composed of muscular and elastic tissue.

**mus·cu·lo·in·tes·ti·nal** (mus″ku-lo-in-tes′tĭ-nəl) pertaining to the muscles and the intestines.

**mus·cu·lo·mem·bra·nous** (mus″ku-lo-mem′brə-nəs) [*musculus* + *membranous*] both muscular and membranous.

**Mus·cu·lo·my·ces** (mus″ku-lo-mi′sēz) in former systems of classification, a genus of bacteria made up of organisms now classified as *Mycoplasma.*

**mus·cu·lo·phren·ic** (mus″ku-lo-fren′ik) [*muscular* + *phrenic*] pertaining to or supplying both the diaphragm and the adjoining muscles.

**mus·cu·lo·skel·e·tal** (mus″ku-lo-skel′ə-təl) pertaining to or comprising the skeleton and the muscles, as musculoskeletal system.

**mus·cu·lo·spi·ral** (mus″ku-lo-spi′rəl) [*musculus* + *spiral*] pertaining to muscles and having a spiral direction, as the nervus radialis.

**mus·cu·lo·ten·di·nous** (mus″ku-lo-ten′dĭ-nəs) pertaining to or composed of muscle and tendon.

**mus·cu·lus** (mus′ku-ləs) gen. and pl. *mus′culi* [L., dim. of *mus* mouse, because of a fancied resemblance to a mouse moving under the skin] [TA] 1. muscle. 2. in plural, TA alternative for *systema musculare.*

## Musculus

The names occurring here are often used without the word *musculus,* e.g. *rectus abdominis* for *musculus rectus abdominis.*

**mus′culi abdo′minis** [TA], the muscles of the abdomen.

**m. abduc′tor dig′iti min′imi ma′nus** [TA], abductor muscle of little finger: *origin,* pisiform bone, flexor carpi ulnaris tendon; *insertion,* medial surface of base of proximal phalanx of little finger; *innervation,* ulnar; *action,* abducts little finger.

**m. abduc′tor dig′iti min′imi pe′dis** [TA], abductor muscle of little toe: *origin,* medial and lateral tubercles of calcaneus, plantar fascia; *insertion,* lateral surface of base of proximal phalanx of little toe; *innervation,* superficial branch of lateral plantar; *action,* abducts little toe.

**m. abduc′tor dig′iti quin′ti ma′nus,** m. abductor digiti minimi manus.

**m. abduc′tor dig′iti quin′ti pe′dis,** m. abductor digiti minimi pedis.

**m. abduc′tor hal′lucis** [TA], abductor muscle of great toe: *origin,* medial tubercle of calcaneus, plantar fascia; *insertion,* medial surface of base of proximal phalanx of great toe; *innervation,* medial plantar; *action,* abducts, flexes great toe.

**m. abduc′tor pol′licis bre′vis** [TA], short abductor muscle of thumb: *origin,* scaphoid, ridge of trapezium, transverse carpal ligament; *insertion,* lateral surface of base of proximal phalanx of thumb; *innervation,* median; *action,* abducts thumb.

**m. abduc′tor pol′licis lon′gus** [TA], long abductor muscle of thumb: *origin,* posterior surfaces of radius and ulna; *insertion,* radial side of base of first metacarpal bone; *innervation,* posterior interosseous; *action,* abducts, extends thumb.

**m. adduc′tor bre′vis** [TA], short adductor muscle: *origin,* outer surface of inferior ramus of pubis; *insertion,* upper part of linea aspera of femur; *innervation,* obturator; *action,* adducts, rotates, flexes thigh.

**m. adduc′tor hal′lucis** [TA], adductor muscle of great toe (2 heads): *origin,* CAPUT OBLIQUUM—bases of second, third, and fourth metatarsals, and sheath of peroneus longus, CAPUT TRANSVERSUM—capsules of metatarsophalangeal joints of three lateral toes; *insertion,* lateral side of base of proximal phalanx of great toe; *innervation,* lateral plantar; *action,* adducts great toe.

**m. adduc′tor lon′gus** [TA], long adductor muscle: *origin,* crest and symphysis of pubis; *insertion,* linea aspera of femur; *innervation,* obturator; *action,* adducts, rotates, flexes thigh.

**m. adduc′tor mag′nus** [TA], great adductor muscle (2 parts): *origin,* DEEP PART—inferior ramus of pubis, ramus of ischium, SUPERFICIAL PART—ischial tuberosity; *insertion,* DEEP PART—linea aspera of femur, SUPERFICIAL PART—adductor tubercle of femur; *innervation,* DEEP PART—obturator, SUPERFICIAL PART—sciatic; *action,* DEEP PART—adducts thigh, SUPERFICIAL PART—extends thigh.

**m. adduc′tor mi′nimus** [TA], smallest adductor muscle: a name given the anterior portion of the adductor magnus muscle; *insertion,* ischium, body and ramus of pubis; *innervation,* obturator and sciatic; *action,* adducts thigh.

**m. adduc′tor pol′licis** [TA], adductor muscle of thumb (2 heads): *origin,* CAPUT OBLIQUUM—sheath of flexor carpi radialis, anterior carpal ligament, capitate bone, and bases of second and third metacarpals, CAPUT TRANSVERSUM—lower two-thirds of anterior surface of third metacarpal; *insertion,* medial surface of base of proximal phalanx of thumb; *innervation,* ulnar; *action,* adducts, opposes thumb.

**m. ancone′us** [TA], anconeus muscle: *origin,* back of lateral epicondyle of humerus; *insertion,* olecranon and posterior surface of ulna; *innervation,* radial; *action,* extends forearm.

**m. antitra′gicus** [TA], antitragicus muscle: *origin,* outer part of antitragus; *insertion,* caudate process of helix and anthelix; *innervation,* temporal and posterior auricular.

**m. arrec′tor pi′li** [TA], arrector muscle of hair: *origin,* papillary layer of skin; *insertion,* a hair follicle; *innervation,* sympathetic; *action,* elevate a hair of skin.

**m. articula′ris,** articular muscle: a muscle that is attached at one end to the synovial capsule of a joint.

**m. articula′ris cu′biti** [TA], articular muscle of elbow: a few fibers of the deep surface of the triceps brachii that insert into the posterior ligament and synovial membrane of the elbow joint.

**m. articula′ris ge′nu,** m. articularis genus.

**m. articula′ris ge′nus** [TA], articular muscle of knee: *origin,* distal fourth of anterior surface of shaft of femur; *insertion,* synovial membrane of knee joint; *innervation,* femoral; *action,* lifts capsule of knee joint.

**m. aryepiglot′ticus,** pars ary-epiglottica musculi arytenoidei obliqui.

**m. arytenoi′deus obli′quus** [TA], oblique arytenoid muscle: one of the intrinsic muscles of the larynx; *origin,* dorsal aspect of muscular process of arytenoid cartilage; *insertion,* apex of opposite arytenoid cartilage; *innervation,* recurrent laryngeal; *action,* closes inlet of larynx.

**m. arytenoi′deus transver′sus** [TA], transverse arytenoid muscle: one of the intrinsic muscles of the larynx; *origin,* dorsal aspect of muscular process of arytenoid cartilage; *insertion,* continuous with thyroarytenoid, apex of opposite cartilage; *innervation,* recurrent laryngeal; *action,* approximates arytenoid cartilages.

**mus′culi auricula′res,** auricular muscles: the intrinsic auricular muscles that extend from one part of the auricle to another, including the helicis major and minor, tragicus, antitragicus, transversus auricularis, and obliquus auricularis.

**m. auricula′ris ante′rior** [TA], anterior auricular muscle: *origin,* superficial temporal fascia; *insertion,* cartilage of ear; *innervation,* facial; *action,* draws the auricle forward.

**m. auricula′ris poste′rior** [TA], posterior auricular muscle: *origin,* mastoid process; *insertion,* cartilage of ear; *innervation,* facial; *action,* draws auricle backward.

**m. auricula′ris supe′rior** [TA], superior auricular muscle: *origin,* galea aponeurotica; *insertion,* cartilage of ear; *innervation,* facial; *action,* raises auricle.

**m. bi′ceps bra′chii** [TA], biceps muscle of arm (2 heads): *origin,* CAPUT LONGUM—upper border of glenoid cavity, CAPUT BREVE—apex of coracoid process; *insertion,* radial tuberosity and fascia of forearm;

*innervation,* musculocutaneous; *action,* flexes forearm, supinates hand.

**m. bi'ceps fe'moris** [TA], biceps muscle of thigh (2 heads): *origin,* CAPUT LONGUM—ischial tuberosity, CAPUT BREVE—linea aspera of femur; *insertion,* head of fibula, lateral condyle of tibia; *innervation,* CAPUT LONGUM—tibial, CAPUT BREVE—peroneal, popliteal; *action,* flexes leg, extends thigh.

**m. bipenna'tus,** TA alternative for *musculus pennatus.*

**m. brachia'lis** [TA], brachial muscle: *origin,* anterior surface of humerus; *insertion,* coronoid process of ulna; *innervation,* radial, musculocutaneous; *action,* flexes forearm.

**m. brachioradia'lis** [TA], brachioradial muscle: *origin,* lateral supracondylar ridge of humerus; *insertion,* lower end of radius; *innervation,* radial; *action,* flexes forearm.

**m. bronchooesopha'geus** [TA], bronchoesophageal muscle: a name given muscular fasciculi arising from the wall of the left bronchus, reinforcing muscles of the esophagus.

**m. buccina'tor** [TA], buccinator muscle: *origin,* buccinator ridge of mandible, alveolar process of maxilla, pterygomandibular ligament; *insertion,* orbicularis oris at angle of mouth; *innervation,* buccal branch of facial; *action,* compresses cheek and retracts angle of the mouth.

**m. buccopharyn'geus,** pars buccopharyngea musculi constrictoris pharyngis superioris.

**mus'culi bul'bi,** musculi externi bulbi oculi.

**m. bulbocaverno'sus,** m. bulbospongiosus.

**m. bulbospongio'sus** [TA], bulbocavernous muscle: *origin,* central point of perineum, median raphe of bulb; *insertion,* fascia of penis (clitoris); *innervation,* pudendal; *action,* constricts bulbous urethra (urethra).

**m. cani'nus,** m. levator anguli oris.

**mus'culi ca'pitis** [TA], the muscles of the head.

**m. ceratocricoi'deus** [TA], ceratocricoid muscle: a name given a muscular fasciculus arising from the cricoid cartilage and inserted on the inferior cornu of the thyroid cartilage, considered one of the intrinsic muscles of the larynx.

**m. ceratopharyn'geus,** pars ceratopharyngea musculi constrictoris pharyngis medii.

**mus'culi cer'vicis,** TA alternative for *musculi colli.*

**m. chondroglos'sus** [TA], chondroglossus muscle: *origin,* medial side and base of lesser cornu of hyoid bone; *insertion,* substance of tongue; *innervation,* hypoglossal; *action,* depresses, retracts tongue.

**m. chondropharyn'geus,** pars chondropharyngea musculi constrictoris pharyngis medii.

**m. cilia'ris** [TA], ciliary muscle: *origin,* scleral spur; *insertion,* outer layers of choroid and ciliary processes; *innervation,* oculomotor, parasympathetic; *action,* affects shape of lens in visual accommodation.

**mus'culi coccy'gei,** coccygeal muscles: the muscles acting upon the coccyx, including the coccygeal and the dorsal and ventral sacrococcygeal muscles.

**m. coccy'geus** [TA], coccygeal muscle: *origin,* ischial spine; *insertion,* lateral border of lower part of sacrum, upper coccyx; *innervation,* third and fourth sacral; *action,* supports and raises coccyx.

**mus'culi col'li** [TA], the muscles of the neck, including the sternocleidomastoid and the longus colli, and the suprahyoid, infrahyoid, and scalene muscles. Called also *cervical muscles* and *musculi cervicis* [TA alternative].

**m. compres'sor na'ris,** pars transversa musculi nasalis.

**m. constric'tor pharyn'gis infe'rior** [TA], inferior constrictor muscle of pharynx: *origin,* under surfaces of cricoid and thyroid cartilages; *insertion,* median raphe of posterior wall of pharynx; *innervation,* glossopharyngeal, pharyngeal plexus, and external and recurrent laryngeal; *action,* constricts pharynx. It is divided into a cricopharyngeal part and a thyropharyngeal part *(pars cricopharyngea* and *pars thyropharyngea).*

**m. constric'tor pharyn'gis me'dius** [TA], middle constrictor muscle of pharynx: *origin,* cornua of hyoid and stylohyoid ligament; *insertion,* median raphe of posterior wall of pharynx; *innervation,* pharyngeal plexus of vagus and glossopharyngeal; *action,* constricts pharynx. It is divided into a ceratopharyngeal part and an chondropharyngeal part *(pars ceratopharyngea* and *pars chondropharyngea).*

**m. constric'tor pharyn'gis supe'rior** [TA], superior constrictor muscle of pharynx: *origin,* medial pterygoid plate, pterygomandibular raphe, mylohyoid ridge of mandible, and mucous membrane of floor of mouth; *insertion,* median raphe of posterior wall of pharynx; *innervation,* pharyngeal plexus of vagus; *action,* constricts pharynx. It is divided into buccopharyngeal, glossopharyngeal, mylopharyngeal, and pterygopharyngeal parts *(pars buccopharyngea, pars glossopharyngea, pars mylopharyngea,* and *pars pterygopharyngea).*

**m. coracobrachia'lis** [TA], coracobrachial muscle: *origin,* coracoid process of scapula; *insertion,* medial surface of shaft of humerus; *innervation,* musculocutaneous; *action,* flexes, adducts arm.

**m. corruga'tor superci'lii** [TA], *origin,* medial end of superciliary arch; *insertion,* skin of eyebrow; *innervation,* facial; *action,* draws eyebrow downward and medially. Called also *Koyter's muscle.*

**m. cremas'ter** [TA], cremaster muscle: *origin,* inferior margin of internal oblique muscle of abdomen; *insertion,* pubic tubercle; *innervation,* genital branch of genitofemoral; *action,* elevates testis.

**m. cricoarytenoi'deus latera'lis** [TA], lateral cricoarytenoid muscle: one of the intrinsic muscles of the larynx; *origin,* lateral surface of cricoid cartilage; *insertion,* muscular process of arytenoid cartilage; *innervation,* recurrent laryngeal; *action,* approximates vocal folds.

**m. cricoarytenoi'deus poste'rior** [TA], posterior cricoarytenoid muscle: one of the intrinsic muscles of the larynx; *origin,* back of cricoid cartilage; *insertion,* muscular process of arytenoid cartilage; *innervation,* recurrent laryngeal; *action,* separates vocal folds.

**m. cricopharyn'geus,** TA alternative for *pars cricopharyngea musculi constrictoris pharyngis inferioris.*

**m. cricothyroi'deus** [TA], cricothyroid muscle: one of the intrinsic muscles of the larynx; *origin,* front and side of cricoid cartilage; *insertion,* lamina of thyroid cartilage; *innervation,* superior laryngeal; *action,* tenses vocal folds.

**m. crucia'tus,** cruciate muscle.

**m. cuta'neus** [TA], cutaneous muscle: striated muscle that inserts into the skin, such as the platysma.

**m. dar'tos,** 1. [TA] dartos muscle: the nonstriated muscle fibers of the tunica dartos, the deeper layers of which help to form the septum of the scrotum. Called also *dartos.* 2. tunica dartos.

**m. deltoi'deus** [TA], deltoid muscle: *origin,* clavicle, acromion, spine of scapula; *insertion,* deltoid tuberosity of humerus; *innervation,* axillary; *action,* abducts, flexes, extends arm.

**m. depres'sor an'guli o'ris** [TA], depressor muscle of angle of mouth: *origin,* lower border of mandible; *insertion,* angle of mouth; *innervation,* facial; *action,* pulls down angle of mouth.

**m. depres'sor la'bii inferio'ris** [TA], depressor muscle of lower lip: *origin,* anterior portion of lower border of mandible; *insertion,* orbicularis oris and skin of lower lip; *innervation,* facial; *action,* depresses lower lip.

**m. depres'sor sep'ti na'si** [TA], depressor muscle of nasal septum: *origin,* incisor fossa of maxilla; *insertion,* ala and septum of nose; *innervation,* facial; *action,* contracts nostril and depresses ala.

**m. depres'sor superci'lii** [TA], superciliary depressor muscle: a name given a few fibers of the orbital part of the orbicularis oculi muscle that are inserted in the eyebrow, which they depress.

**m. detru'sor ve'sicae** [TA], detrusor muscle of bladder: the bundles of smooth muscle fibers forming the muscular coat of the urinary bladder, which are arranged in a longitudinal and a circular layer and, on contraction, serve to expel urine; called also *detrusor urinae* and *detrusor urinae muscle.*

**mus'culi diaphrag'matis pel'vis,** the muscles of the pelvic diaphragm.

**mus'culi diaphrag'matis urogenita'lis,** the muscles of the urogenital diaphragm.

**m. digas'tricus** [TA], digastric muscle: *origin,* VENTER ANTERIOR—digastric fossa on deep surface of inferior border of mandible near symphysis, VENTER POSTERIOR—mastoid notch of temporal bone; *insertion,* intermediate tendon on hyoid bone; *innervation,* VENTER ANTERIOR—mylohyoid, VENTER POSTERIOR—digastric branch of facial; *action,* elevates hyoid bone, lowers jaw.

**m. dilata'tor** [TA], dilator muscle: a general term for a muscle that dilates; called also *dilator.*

**m. dilata'tor pupil'lae** [TA], dilator pupillae muscle: a name given fibers extending radially from the sphincter pupillae to the ciliary margin; *innervation,* sympathetic; *action,* dilates iris.

**m. dila'tor na'ris,** pars alaris musculi nasalis.

**mus'culi dor'si** [TA], dorsal muscles: the muscles of the back.

**m. epicra'nius** [TA], epicranial muscle: a name given the muscular covering of the scalp, including the occipitofrontalis and temporoparietalis muscles, and the galea aponeurotica.

**m. epitrochleoanconae'us,** epitrochleoanconeus muscle: an occasional band of fibers originating at the back of the medial condyle of the humerus and inserting on the medial side of the olecranon process, innervated by a branch of the ulnar nerve.

**m. erec'tor spi'nae** [TA], erector muscle of spine: a name given the fibers of the more superficial of the deep muscles of the back, originating from the sacrum, spines of the lumbar and the eleventh and twelfth thoracic vertebrae, and the iliac crest, which split and insert as the iliocostalis, longissimus, and spinalis muscles (q.v.).

**m. exten'sor car'pi radia'lis bre'vis** [TA], short radial extensor muscle of wrist: *origin,* lateral epicondyle of humerus, *insertion,* base of third metacarpal bone; *innervation,* radial; *action,* extends and abducts wrist joint.

**m. exten'sor car'pi radia'lis lon'gus** [TA], long radial extensor muscle of wrist: *origin,* lateral supracondylar ridge of humerus; *insertion,* base of second metacarpal bone; *innervation,* radial; *action,* extends and abducts wrist joint.

**m. exten'sor car'pi ulna'ris** [TA], ulnar extensor muscle of wrist (2 heads): *origin,* CAPUT HUMERALE—lateral epicondyle of humerus, CA-

PUT ULNARE—dorsal border of ulna; *insertion,* base of fifth metacarpal bone; *innervation,* deep radial; *action,* extends and adducts wrist joint.

**m. exten'sor di'giti mi'nimi** [TA], extensor muscle of little finger: *origin,* common extensor tendon; *insertion,* tendon of extensor digitorum to little finger; *innervation,* deep radial; *action,* extends little finger.

**m. exten'sor di'giti quin'ti pro'prius,** m. extensor digiti minimi.

**m. exten'sor digito'rum** [TA], extensor muscle of fingers: *origin,* lateral epicondyle of humerus; *insertion,* common extensor tendon of each finger; *innervation,* posterior interosseus; *action,* extends wrist joint and phalanges.

**m. exten'sor digito'rum bre'vis** [TA], short extensor muscle of toes: *origin,* dorsal surface of calcaneus; *insertion,* extensor tendons of first, second, third, fourth toes; *innervation,* deep peroneal; *action,* extends toes.

**m. exten'sor digito'rum commu'nis,** m. extensor digitorum.

**m. exten'sor digito'rum lon'gus** [TA], long extensor muscle of toes: *origin,* anterior surface of fibula, lateral condyle of tibia, interosseous membrane; *insertion,* common extensor tendon of four lateral toes: *innervation,* deep peroneal; *action,* extends toes.

**m. exten'sor hal'lucis bre'vis** [TA], short extensor muscle of great toe: a name given the portion of the extensor digitorum brevis muscle that goes to the great toe.

**m. exten'sor hal'lucis lon'gus** [TA], long extensor muscle of great toe: *origin,* front of fibula and interosseous membrane; *insertion,* dorsal surface of base of distal phalanx of great toe; *innervation,* deep peroneal; *action,* dorsiflexes ankle joint, extends great toe.

**m. exten'sor in'dicis** [TA], extensor muscle of index finger: *origin,* dorsal surface of body of ulna, interosseous membrane; *insertion,* common extensor tendon of index finger; *innervation,* posterior interosseous; *action,* extends index finger.

**m. exten'sor in'dicis pro'prius,** m. extensor indicis.

**m. exten'sor pol'licis bre'vis** [TA], short extensor muscle of thumb: *origin,* dorsal surface of radius and interosseous membrane; *insertion,* dorsal surface of proximal phalanx of thumb; *innervation,* posterior interosseous; *action,* extends thumb.

**m. exten'sor pol'licis lon'gus** [TA], long extensor muscle of thumb: *origin,* dorsal surface of ulna and interosseous membrane; *insertion,* dorsal surface of distal phalanx of thumb; *innervation,* posterior interosseous; *action,* extends, abducts thumb.

**mus'culi exter'ni bul'bi o'culi** [TA], extraocular muscles: the six voluntary muscles that move the eyeball, including the superior, inferior, middle, and lateral recti, and the superior and inferior oblique muscles. Called also *musculi bulbi, muscles of eye,* and *ocular muscles.*

**mus'culi extremita'tis inferio'ris,** musculi membri inferioris.

**mus'culi extremita'tis superio'ris,** musculi membri superioris.

**mus'culi facia'les, mus'culi facie'i** [TA], facial muscles: a group of cutaneous muscles of the facial structures, which includes the muscles of the scalp, ear, eyelids, nose, and mouth, and the platysma; called also *muscles of expression* and *muscles of facial expression.*

**m. fibula'ris bre'vis** [TA], short fibular muscle: *origin,* lateral surface of fibula; *insertion,* base of fifth metatarsal bone; *innervation,* superficial peroneal; *action,* abducts, plantar flexes foot. Called also *m. peroneus brevis* [TA alternative] and *short peroneal muscle.*

**m. fibula'ris lon'gus** [TA], long peroneal muscle: *origin,* lateral condyle of tibia, head and lateral surface of fibula; *insertion,* medial cuneiform, first metatarsal; *innervation,* superficial peroneal; *action,* abducts, everts, plantar flexes foot. Called also *m. peroneus longus* [TA alternative] and *long peroneal muscle.*

**m. fibula'ris ter'tius** [TA], third fibular muscle: *origin,* anterior surface of fibula, interosseous membrane; *insertion,* fifth metatarsal; *innervation,* deep peroneal; *action,* everts, dorsiflexes foot. Called also *m. peroneus tertius* [TA alternative] and *third peroneal muscle.*

**m. flex'or accesso'rius,** TA alternative for *m. quadratus plantae.*

**m. flex'or car'pi radia'lis** [TA], radial flexor muscle of wrist: *origin,* medial epicondyle of humerus; *insertion,* base of second metacarpal; *innervation,* median; *action,* flexes and abducts wrist joint.

**m. flex'or car'pi ulna'ris** [TA], ulnar flexor muscle of wrist (2 heads): *origin,* CAPUT HUMERALE—medial epicondyle of humerus, CAPUT ULNARE—olecranon, ulna, intermuscular septum; *insertion,* pisiform, hook of hamate, proximal end of fifth metacarpal; *innervation,* ulnar; *action,* flexes and adducts wrist joint.

**m. flex'or di'giti mi'nimi bre'vis ma'nus** [TA], short flexor muscle of little finger: *origin,* hook of hamate bone, transverse carpal ligament; *insertion,* medial side of proximal phalanx of little finger; *innervation,* ulnar; *action,* flexes little finger.

**m. flex'or di'giti mi'nimi bre'vis pe'dis** [TA], short flexor muscle of little toe: *origin,* base of fifth metatarsal, sheath of long peroneal muscle; *insertion,* lateral surface of base of proximal phalanx of little toe; *innervation,* lateral plantar; *action,* flexes little toe.

**m. flex'or di'giti quin'ti bre'vis ma'nus,** m. flexor digiti minimi brevis manus.

**m. flex'or di'giti quin'ti bre'vis pe'dis,** m. flexor digiti minimi brevis pedis.

**m. flex'or digito'rum bre'vis** [TA], short flexor muscle of toes: *origin,* medial tuberosity of calcaneus, plantar fascia; *insertion,* middle phalanges of four lateral toes; *innervation,* medial plantar; *action,* flexes toes.

**m. flex'or digito'rum lon'gus** [TA], long flexor muscle of toes: *origin,* posterior surface of shaft of tibia; *insertion,* distal phalanges of four lateral toes; *innervation,* posterior tibial; *action,* flexes toes and extends foot.

**m. flex'or digito'rum profun'dus** [TA], deep flexor muscle of fingers: *origin,* shaft of ulna, coronoid process; *insertion,* distal phalanges of fingers; *innervation,* ulnar and anterior interosseous; *action,* flexes distal phalanges.

**m. flex'or digito'rum subli'mis,** m. flexor digitorum superficialis.

**m. flex'or digito'rum superficia'lis** [TA], superficial flexor muscle of fingers (2 heads): *origin,* CAPUT HUMEROULNARE—medial epicondyle of humerus, coronoid process of ulna, CAPUT RADIALE—oblique line of radius, anterior border; *insertion,* middle phalanges of fingers; *innervation,* median; *action,* flexes middle phalanges.

**m. flex'or hal'lucis bre'vis** [TA], short flexor muscle of great toe: *origin,* under surface of cuboid, lateral cuneiform; *insertion,* base of proximal phalanx of great toe; *innervation,* medial plantar; *action,* flexes great toe.

**m. flex'or hal'lucis lon'gus** [TA], long flexor muscle of great toe: *origin,* posterior surface of fibula; *insertion,* base of distal phalanx of great toe; *innervation,* tibial; *action,* flexes great toe.

**m. flex'or pol'licis bre'vis** [TA], short flexor muscle of thumb: *origin,* flexor retinaculum, ridge of trapezium; *insertion,* base of proximal phalanx of thumb; *innervation,* median, ulnar; *action,* flexes and adducts thumb.

**m. flex'or pol'licis lon'gus** [TA], long flexor muscle of thumb: *origin,* anterior surface of radius and coronoid process of ulna; *insertion,* base of distal phalanx of thumb; *innervation,* anterior interosseous; *action,* flexes thumb.

**m. fronta'lis,** venter frontalis musculi occipitofrontalis.

**m. fusifor'mis** [TA], fusiform muscle: a spindle-shaped muscle in which the fibers are approximately parallel to the long axis of the muscle but converge upon a tendon at either end.

**m. gastrocne'mius** [TA], gastrocnemius muscle (2 heads): *origin,* CAPUT MEDIALE—popliteal surface of femur, upper part of medial condyle, and capsule of knee, CAPUT LATERALE—lateral condyle and capsule of knee; *insertion,* aponeurosis unites with tendon of soleus to form calcaneal tendon (Achilles tendon); *innervation,* tibial; *action,* plantar flexes ankle joint, flexes knee joint.

**m. gemel'lus infe'rior** [TA], inferior gemellus muscle: *origin,* tuberosity of ischium; *insertion,* greater trochanter of femur; *innervation,* nerve to quadrate muscle of thigh; *action,* rotates thigh laterally.

**m. gemel'lus supe'rior** [TA], superior gemellus muscle: *origin,* spine of ischium; *insertion,* greater trochanter of femur; *innervation,* nerve to internal obturator; *action,* rotates thigh laterally.

**m. genioglos'sus** [TA], genioglossus muscle: *origin,* mental spine of mandible; *insertion,* hyoid bone and inferior surface of tongue; *innervation,* hypoglossal; *action,* protrudes and depresses tongue.

**m. geniohyoi'deus** [TA], geniohyoid muscle: *origin,* mental spine of mandible; *insertion,* body of hyoid bone; *innervation,* a branch of first cervical nerve through hypoglossal; *action,* elevates, draws hyoid forward.

**m. glossopalati'nus,** m. palatoglossus.

**m. glossopharyn'geus,** pars glossopharyngea musculi constrictoris pharyngis superioris.

**m. glu'teus max'imus** [TA], greatest gluteal muscle: *origin,* lateral surface of ilium, dorsal surface of sacrum and coccyx, sacrotuberous ligament; *insertion,* iliotibial tract of fascia lata, gluteal tuberosity of femur; *innervation,* inferior gluteal; *action,* extends, abducts, and rotates thigh laterally.

**m. glu'teus me'dius** [TA], middle gluteal muscle: *origin,* lateral surface of ilium between anterior and posterior gluteal lines; *insertion,* greater trochanter of femur; *innervation,* superior gluteal; *action,* abducts and rotates thigh medially.

**m. glu'teus mi'nimus** [TA], least gluteal muscle: *origin,* lateral surface of ilium between anterior and inferior gluteal lines; *insertion,* greater trochanter of femur; *innervation,* superior gluteal; *action,* abducts, rotates thigh medially.

**m. gra'cilis** [TA], gracilis muscle: *origin,* lower half of body and entire inferior ramus of pubis; *insertion,* medial surface of shaft of tibia; *innervation,* obturator; *action,* adducts thigh, flexes knee joint.

**m. he'licis ma'jor** [TA], helicis major muscle: *origin,* spine of helix; *insertion,* anterior border of helix; *innervation,* auriculotemporal and posterior auricular (branches of facial); *action,* tenses skin of auditory canal.

**m. he'licis mi'nor** [TA], helicis minor muscle: *origin,* anterior rim of helix; *insertion,* concha; *innervation,* temporal, posterior auricular.

**m. hyoglos'sus** [TA], hyoglossal muscle: *origin,* body and greater cornu of hyoid bone; *insertion,* side of tongue; *innervation,* hypoglossal; *action,* depresses and retracts tongue.

**m. ili'acus** [TA], iliac muscle: *origin,* iliac fossa and base of sacrum; *insertion,* greater psoas tendon and lesser trochanter of femur; *innervation,* femoral; *action,* flexes thigh, trunk on limb.

**m. iliococcy'geus** [TA], iliococcygeal muscle: the posterior portion of the levator ani which originates as far anteriorly as the obturator canal and inserts on the side of the coccyx and the anococcygeal body; *innervation,* third and fourth sacral; *action,* helps to support pelvic viscera and resist increases in intra-abdominal pressure.

**m. iliocosta'lis** [TA], iliocostal muscle: the lateral division of m. erector spinae, which includes the *m. iliocostalis cervicis, m. iliocostalis thoracis,* and *m. iliocostalis lumborum.*

**m. iliocosta'lis cer'vicis** [TA], iliocostal muscle of neck: *origin,* angles of third, fourth, fifth, and sixth ribs; *insertion,* transverse processes of fourth, fifth, and sixth cervical vertebrae; *innervation,* branches of cervical; *action,* extends cervical spine. Called also *m. iliocostalis colli* [TA alternative].

**m. iliocosta'lis col'li,** TA alternative for *m. iliocostalis cervicis.*

**m. iliocosta'lis dor'si,** m. iliocostalis thoracis.

**m. iliocosta'lis lumbo'rum** [TA], iliocostal muscle of loins: *origin,* iliac crest; *insertion,* angles of lower six or seven ribs; *innervation,* branches of thoracic and lumbar; *action,* extends lumbar spine.

**m. iliocosta'lis thora'cis,** iliocostal muscle of thorax: *origin,* upper borders of angles of six lower ribs; *insertion,* angles of six upper ribs and transverse process of seventh cervical vertebra; *innervation,* branches of thoracic; *action,* keeps thoracic spine erect.

**m. iliopso'as** [TA], iliopsoas muscle: a compound muscle consisting of iliacus and psoas major.

**mus'culi incisi'vi la'bii inferio'ris,** incisive muscles of inferior lip: small bundles of muscle fibers, one arising from the incisive fossa of the mandible on each side and passing laterally to the angle of the mouth.

**mus'culi incisi'vi la'bii superio'ris,** incisive muscles of superior lip: small bundles of muscle fibers, one arising from the incisive fossa of the maxilla on each side and passing laterally to the angle of the mouth.

**m. incisu'rae termina'lis** [TA], an inconstant muscular slip continuing forward from the m. tragicus to bridge the incisure of the cartilaginous meatus.

**m. incisu'rae termina'lis [Santori'ni],** m. incisurae helicis.

**mus'culi infrahyoi'dei** [TA], infrahyoid muscles: the muscles that anchor the hyoid bone to the sternum, clavicle, and scapula, including the sternohyoid, omohyoid, sternothyroid, and thyrohyoid muscles.

**m. infraspina'tus** [TA], infraspinous muscle: *origin,* infraspinous fossa of scapula; *insertion,* greater tubercle of humerus; *innervation,* suprascapular; *action,* rotates humerus laterally.

**mus'culi intercosta'les exter'ni** [TA], external intercostal muscles (11 on each side): *origin,* inferior border of rib; *insertion,* superior border of rib below; *innervation,* intercostal; *action,* draw ribs together in respiration and expulsive movements.

**mus'culi intercosta'les inter'ni** [TA], internal intercostal muscles (11 on each side): *origin,* inferior border of rib and costal cartilage; *insertion,* superior border of rib and costal cartilage below; *innervation,* intercostal; *action,* draw ribs together in respiration and expulsive movements.

**mus'culi intercosta'les in'timi** [TA], innermost intercostal muscles: the layer of muscle fibers separated from the internal intercostal muscles by the intercostal nerves.

**mus'culi interos'sei dorsa'les ma'nus** [TA], dorsal interosseous muscles of hand (4): *origin,* by two heads from adjacent sides of metacarpal bones; *insertion,* extensor tendons of second, third, and fourth fingers; *innervation,* ulnar; *action,* abduct, flex proximal phalanges.

**mus'culi interos'sei dorsa'les pe'dis** [TA], dorsal interosseous muscles of foot (4): *origin,* adjacent surfaces of metatarsal bones; *insertion,* base of proximal phalanges of second, third, and fourth toes; *innervation,* lateral plantar; *action,* abduct, flex toes.

**mus'culi interos'sei palma'res** [TA], palmar interosseous muscles (3): *origin,* sides of second, fourth, and fifth metacarpal bones; *insertion,* extensor tendons of second, fourth, and fifth fingers; *innervation,* ulnar; *action,* adduct, flex proximal phalanges, extend middle and distal phalanges.

**mus'culi interos'sei planta'res** [TA], plantar interosseous muscles (3): *origin,* medial surface of third, fourth, and fifth metatarsal bones; *insertion,* medial side of base of proximal phalanges of third, fourth, and fifth toes; *innervation,* lateral plantar; *action,* adduct, flex toes.

**mus'culi interos'sei vola'res,** musculi interossei palmares.

**mus'culi interspina'les** [TA], interspinal muscles: short bands of muscle fibers between spinous processes of contiguous vertebrae, including the *musculi interspinales cervicis, musculi interspinales thoracis,* and *musculi interspinales lumborum.*

**mus'culi interspina'les cer'vicis** [TA], interspinal muscles of neck: paired bands of muscle fibers extending between spinous processes of contiguous cervical vertebrae, innervated by spinal nerves, and acting to extend the vertebral column. Called also *musculi interspinales colli* [TA alternative].

**mus'culi interspina'les col'li,** TA alternative for *musculi interspinales cervicis.*

**mus'culi interspina'les lumbo'rum** [TA], interspinal muscles of loins: paired bands of muscle fibers extending between spinous processes of contiguous lumbar vertebrae, innervated by spinal nerves, and acting to extend the vertebral column.

**mus'culi interspina'les thora'cis** [TA], interspinal muscles of thorax: paired bands of muscle fibers extending between spinous processes of contiguous thoracic vertebrae, innervated by spinal nerves, and acting to extend the vertebral column.

**mus'culi intertransversa'rii** [TA], intertransverse muscles: small muscles passing between the transverse processes of contiguous vertebrae, including the lateral and medial intertransverse muscles of the loins, the intertransverse muscles of the thorax, and the anterior and posterior intertransverse muscles of the neck.

**mus'culi intertransversa'rii anterio'res,** musculi intertransversarii thoracis.

**mus'culi intertransversa'rii anterio'res cer'vicis** [TA], anterior intertransverse muscles of neck: small muscles passing between the anterior tubercles of adjacent cervical vertebrae, innervated by spinal nerves, and acting to bend the vertebral column laterally. Called also *musculi intertransversarii anteriores colli* [TA alternative].

**mus'culi intertransversa'rii anterio'res col'li,** TA alternative for *musculi intertransversarii anteriores cervicis.*

**mus'culi intertransversa'rii latera'les,** musculi intertransversarii laterales lumborum.

**mus'culi intertransversa'rii latera'les lumbo'rum** [TA], lateral lumbar intertransverse muscles: small muscles passing between the transverse processes of adjacent lumbar vertebrae, innervated by spinal nerves, and acting to bend the vertebral column laterally.

**mus'culi intertransversa'rii media'les,** musculi intertransversarii mediales lumborum.

**mus'culi intertransversa'rii media'les lumbo'rum** [TA], medial lumbar intertransverse muscles: small muscles passing from the accessory process of one lumbar vertebra to the mammillary process of the contiguous lumbar vertebra, innervated by spinal nerves, and acting to bend the vertebral column laterally.

**mus'culi intertransversa'rii posterio'res,** musculi intertransversarii posteriores laterales cervicis.

**mus'culi intertransversa'rii posterio'res latera'les cer'vicis** [TA], posterior lateral intertransverse muscles of neck: small muscles passing between the posterior tubercles of adjacent cervical vertebrae, innervated by spinal nerves, and acting to bend the vertebral column laterally. Called also *musculi intertransversarii posteriores laterales colli* [TA alternative].

**mus'culi intertransversa'rii posterio'res latera'les col'li,** TA alternative for *musculi intertransversarii posteriores laterales cervicis.*

**mus'culi intertransversa'rii thora'cis** [TA], intertransverse muscles of thorax: poorly developed muscle bundles extending between the anterior tubercles of adjacent thoracic vertebrae, innervated by spinal nerves, and acting to bend the vertebral column laterally.

**m. ischiocaverno'sus** [TA], ischiocavernous muscle: *origin,* ramus of ischium; *insertion,* crus penis (crus clitoridis); *innervation,* perineal; *action,* maintains erection of penis (clitoris).

**mus'culi laryn'gis** [TA], muscles of larynx: the intrinsic and extrinsic muscles of the larynx, including the oblique and transverse arytenoid, ceratocricoid, lateral and posterior crico-arytenoid, cricothyroid, thyroarytenoid, and vocal muscles.

**m. latis'simus dor'si** [TA], *origin,* spines of lower thoracic vertebrae, lumbar and sacral vertebrae through thoracolumbar fascia, iliac crest, lower ribs, inferior angle of scapula; *insertion,* floor of intertubercular sulcus of humerus; *innervation,* thoracodorsal; *action,* adducts, extends, and rotates humerus medially.

**m. leva'tor an'guli o'ris** [TA], levator muscle of angle of mouth: *origin,* canine fossa of maxilla; *insertion,* orbicularis oris and skin at angle of mouth; *innervation,* facial; *action,* raises angle of mouth.

**m. leva'tor a'ni** [TA], levator ani muscle: a name applied collectively to important muscular components of the pelvic diaphragm, including the pubococcygeus (levator prostatae and pubovaginalis), the puborectalis, and the iliococcygeus muscles.

**mus'culi levato'res costa'rum** [TA], levator muscles of ribs (12 on each side): originating from the transverse processes of the seventh cervical and first to eleventh thoracic vertebrae and inserting medial to the angle of a lower rib (see *musculi levatores costarum breves* and *musculi levatores costarum longi*); innervated by intercostal nerves and aiding in elevation of the ribs in respiration.

**mus'culi levato'res costa'rum bre'ves** [TA], short levator muscles of ribs: the levatores costarum of each side that insert medial to the angle of the rib next below the vertebra of origin.

**mus'culi levato'res costa'rum lon'gi** [TA], long levator muscles of ribs: the lower levatores costarum muscles of each side, which have fascicles extending down to the second rib below the vertebra of origin.

**m. leva'tor glan'dulae thyroi'deae** [TA], levator muscle of thyroid gland: an inconstant muscle originating on the isthmus or pyramid of the thyroid gland and inserting on the body of the hyoid bone.

**m. leva'tor la'bii superio'ris** [TA], levator muscle of upper lip: *origin,* lower orbital margin; *insertion,* muscle of upper lip; *innervation,* facial nerve; *action,* raises upper lip.

**m. leva'tor la'bii superio'ris alae'que na'si** [TA], levator muscle of upper lip and ala of nose: *origin,* nasal process of maxilla; *insertion,* cartilage and skin of ala nasi, and upper lip; *innervation,* infraorbital branch of facial; *action,* raises upper lip and dilates nostril.

**m. leva'tor pal'pebrae superio'ris** [TA], levator muscle of upper eyelid: *origin,* upper border of optic foramen; *insertion,* tarsal plate and skin of upper eyelid; *innervation,* oculomotor; *action,* raises upper lid.

**m. leva'tor prosta'tae** [TA], levator muscle of prostate: a part of the anterior portion of the pubococcygeus muscle, inserted in the prostate and the tendinous center of the perineum; innervated by sacral and pudendal nerves, it supports and compresses the prostate and is involved in control of micturition.

**m. leva'tor sca'pulae** [TA], levator muscle of scapula: *origin,* transverse processes of four upper cervical vertebrae; *insertion,* medial border of scapula; *innervation,* third and fourth cervical; *action,* raises scapula.

**m. leva'tor ve'li palati'ni** [TA], *origin,* apex of petrous portion of temporal bone and cartilaginous part of auditory tube; *insertion,* aponeurosis of soft palate; *innervation,* pharyngeal plexus of vagus; *action,* raises soft palate.

**mus'culi lin'guae** [TA], **mus'culi lingua'les,** muscles of tongue: the extrinsic and intrinsic muscles that move the tongue; called also *lingual muscles.*

**m. longis'simus** [TA], longissimus muscle: the largest element of the m. erector spinae, which includes the *m. longissimus capitis, m. longissimus cervicis,* and *m. longissimus thoracis.*

**m. longis'simus ca'pitis** [TA], longissimus muscle of head: *origin,* transverse processes of four or five upper thoracic vertebrae, articular processes of three or four lower cervical vertebrae; *insertion,* mastoid process of temporal bone; *innervation,* branches of cervical; *action,* draws head backward, rotates head.

**m. longis'simus cer'vicis** [TA], longissimus muscle of neck: *origin,* transverse processes of four or five upper thoracic vertebrae; *insertion,* transverse processes of second to sixth cervical vertebrae; *innervation,* lower cervical and upper thoracic; *action,* extends cervical vertebrae. Called also *m. longissimus colli* [TA alternative].

**m. longis'simus col'li,** TA alternative for *m. longissimus cervicis.*

**m. longis'simus dor'si,** m. longissimus thoracis.

**m. longis'simus thora'cis** [TA], longissimus muscle of thorax: *origin,* transverse and articular processes of lumbar vertebrae and thoracolumbar fascia; *insertion,* transverse processes of all thoracic vertebrae, nine or ten lower ribs; *innervation,* lumbar and thoracic; *action,* extends thoracic vertebrae.

**m. longitudina'lis infe'rior lin'guae** [TA], inferior longitudinal muscle of tongue: *origin,* inferior surface of tongue at base; *insertion,* tip of tongue; *innervation,* hypoglossal; *action,* changes shape of tongue in mastication and deglutition.

**m. longitudina'lis supe'rior lin'guae** [TA], superior longitudinal muscle of tongue: *origin,* submucosa and septum of tongue; *insertion,* margins of tongue; *innervation,* hypoglossal; *action,* changes shape of tongue in mastication and deglutition.

**m. lon'gus ca'pitis** [TA], long muscle of head: *origin,* transverse processes of third to sixth cervical vertebrae; *insertion,* basal portion of occipital bone; *innervation,* branches from first, second, and third cervical; *action,* flexes head.

**m. lon'gus cer'vicis,** TA alternative for *m. longus colli.*

**m. lon'gus col'li** [TA], long muscle of neck: *origin,* SUPERIOR OBLIQUE PORTION—transverse processes of third to fifth cervical vertebrae; INFERIOR OBLIQUE PORTION—bodies of first to third thoracic vertebrae; VERTICAL PORTION—bodies of three upper thoracic and three lower cervical vertebrae; *insertion,* SUPERIOR OBLIQUE PORTION—tubercle of anterior arch of atlas; INFERIOR OBLIQUE PORTION—transverse processes of fifth and sixth cervical vertebrae; VERTICAL PORTION—bodies of second to fourth cervical vertebrae; *innervation,* anterior cervical. *action,* flexes and supports cervical vertebrae. Called also *m. longus cervicis* [TA alternative].

**mus'culi lumbrica'les ma'nus** [TA], lumbrical muscles of hand: *origin,* tendons of flexor digitorum profundus; *insertion,* extensor tendons of four lateral fingers; *innervation,* median and ulnar; *action,* flex metacarpophalangeal joint and extend middle and distal phalanges.

**mus'culi lumbrica'les pe'dis** [TA], lumbrical muscles of foot: *origin,* tendons of flexor digitorum longus; *insertion,* extensor tendons of four lateral toes; *innervation,* medial and lateral plantar; *action,* flex metatarsophalangeal joints, extend distal phalanges.

**m. masse'ter** [TA], masseter muscle: *origin,* PARS SUPERFICIALIS—zygomatic process of maxilla and inferior border of zygomatic arch, PARS PROFUNDA—inferior border and medial surface of zygomatic arch; *insertion,* PARS SUPERFICIALIS—angle and ramus of mandible, PARS PROFUNDA—superior half of ramus and lateral surface of coronoid process of mandible; *innervation,* mandibular division of trigeminal; *action,* raises mandible, closes jaws.

**mus'culi masticato'rii** [TA], masticatory muscles: a group of muscles responsible for the movement of the jaws during mastication, including the masseter, temporal, and medial and lateral pterygoid muscles; called also *muscles of mastication.*

**mus'culi mem'bri inferio'ris** [TA], muscles of inferior limb: the muscles acting on the thigh, leg, and foot.

**mus'culi mem'bri superio'ris** [TA], muscles of superior limb: the muscles acting on the arm, forearm, and hand.

**m. menta'lis** [TA], *origin,* incisive fossa of mandible; *insertion,* skin of chin; *innervation,* facial; *action,* wrinkles skin of chin.

**mus'culi multi'fidi,** multifidus muscles: *origin,* sacrum, sacroiliac ligament, mammillary processes of lumbar, transverse processes of thoracic, and articular processes of cervical vertebrae; *insertion,* spines of contiguous vertebrae above; *innervation,* dorsal branches of spinal nerves; *action,* extend, rotate vertebral column.

**m. multipenna'tus** [TA], multipennate muscle: a muscle in which the fiber bundles converge to several tendons.

**m. mylohyoi'deus** [TA], mylohyoid muscle: *origin,* mylohyoid line of mandible; *insertion,* body of hyoid bone and median raphe; *innervation,* mylohyoid branch of inferior alveolar; *action,* elevates hyoid bone, supports floor of mouth.

**m. mylopharyn'geus,** pars mylopharyngea musculi constrictoris pharyngis superioris.

**m. nasa'lis** [TA], nasal muscle: *origin,* maxilla; *insertion,* PARS ALARIS—ala of nose, PARS TRANSVERSA—by aponeurotic expansion with fellow of opposite side; *innervation,* facial; *action,* PARS ALARIS—aids in widening nostril, PARS TRANSVERSA—depresses cartilage of nose.

**m. obli'quus auri'culae** [TA], **m. obli'quus auricula'ris,** oblique muscle of auricle: *origin,* cranial surface of concha; *insertion,* cranial surface of auricle above concha; *innervation,* temporal and posterior auricular (branches of facial).

**m. obli'quus ca'pitis infe'rior** [TA], inferior oblique muscle of head: *origin,* spinous process of axis; *insertion,* transverse process of atlas; *innervation,* dorsal branches of spinal nerves; *action,* rotates atlas and head.

**m. obli'quus ca'pitis supe'rior** [TA], superior oblique muscle of head: *origin,* transverse process of atlas; *insertion,* occipital bone; *innervation,* dorsal branches of spinal nerves; *action,* extends and moves head laterally.

**m. obli'quus exter'nus abdo'minis** [TA], external oblique muscle of abdomen; *origin,* lower eight ribs at costal cartilages; *insertion,* crest of ilium, linea alba through rectus sheath; *innervation,* lower intercostal; *action,* flexes and rotates vertebral column, compresses abdominal viscera.

**m. obli'quus infe'rior bul'bi** [TA], inferior oblique muscle of eyeball: *origin,* orbital plate of maxilla; *insertion,* sclera; *innervation,* oculomotor; *action,* rotates eyeball upward and outward.

**m. obli'quus infe'rior o'culi,** m. obliquus inferior bulbi.

**m. obli'quus inter'nus abdo'minis** [TA], internal oblique muscle of abdomen: *origin,* inguinal ligament, iliac crest, thoracolumbar fascia; *insertion,* inferior three or four costal cartilages, linea alba, conjoined tendon to pubis; *innervation,* lower intercostal; *action,* flexes and rotates vertebral column, compresses abdominal viscera.

**m. obli'quus supe'rior bul'bi** [TA], superior oblique muscle of eyeball: *origin,* lesser wing of sphenoid above optic foramen; *insertion,* sclera; *innervation,* trochlear; *action,* rotates eyeball downward and outward.

**m. obli'quus supe'rior o'culi,** m. obliquus superior bulbi.

**m. obtura'tor exter'nus,** m. obturatorius externus.

**m. obtura'tor inter'nus,** m. obturatorius internus.

**m. obturato'rius exter'nus** [TA], external obturator muscle: *origin,* pubis, ischium, and superficial surface of obturator membrane; *insertion,* trochanteric fossa of femur; *innervation,* obturator; *action,* rotates thigh laterally.

**m. obturato'rius inter'nus** [TA], internal obturator muscle: *origin,* pelvic surface of hip bone, margin of obturator foramen, ramus of ischium, inferior ramus of pubis, internal surface of obturator membrane; *insertion,* greater trochanter of femur; *innervation,* fifth lumbar, first and second sacral; *action,* rotates thigh laterally.

**m. occipita'lis,** venter occipitalis musculi occipitofrontalis.

**m. occipitofronta'lis** [TA], occipitofrontal muscle: *origin,* VENTER FRONTALIS—galea aponeurotica, VENTER OCCIPITALIS—highest nuchal line of occipital bone; *insertion,* VENTER FRONTALIS—skin of eyebrows and root of nose, VENTER OCCIPITALIS—galea aponeurotica; *innervation,* VENTER FRONTALIS—temporal branch of facial, VENTER OCCIPITALIS—posterior auricular branch of facial; *action,* VENTER FRONTALIS—raises eyebrows, VENTER OCCIPITALIS—draws scalp posteriorly.

**mus'culi o'culi,** musculi externi bulbi oculi.

**m. omohyoi'deus** [TA], omohyoid muscle, comprising two bellies (superior and inferior) connected by a central tendon that is bound to the clavicle by a fibrous expansion of the cervical fascia; *origin,* superior border of scapula; *insertion,* lateral border of hyoid bone; *innervation,* upper cervical through ansa cervicalis; *action,* depresses hyoid bone.

**m. oppo'nens di'giti mi'nimi** [TA], opposing muscle of little finger: *origin,* hook of hamate bone, transverse carpal ligament; *insertion,* medial aspect of fifth metacarpal; *innervation,* eighth cervical through ulnar; *action,* rotates, abducts, and flexes fifth metacarpal.

**m. oppo'nens di'giti quin'ti ma'nus,** m. opponens digiti minimi.

**m. oppo'nens pol'licis** [TA], opposing muscle of thumb: *origin,* ridge of trapezium, flexor retinaculum; *insertion,* radial side of first metacarpal; *innervation,* sixth and seventh cervical through median; *action,* flexes and opposes thumb.

**m. orbicula'ris** [TA], orbicular muscle: a muscle that encircles a body opening, such as the eye or mouth.

**m. orbicula'ris o'culi** [TA], orbicular muscle of eye: the oval sphincter muscle surrounding the eyelids, consisting of three parts: *origin,* PARS ORBITALIS—medial margin of orbit, including frontal process of maxilla, PARS PALPEBRALIS—medial canthus, medial palpebral ligament, PARS LACRIMALIS—posterior lacrimal crest; *insertion,* PARS ORBITALIS—near origin after encircling orbit, PARS PALPEBRALIS—fibers intertwine to form lateral palpebral raphe, PARS LACRIMALIS—lateral palpebral raphe, upper and lower tarsi; *innervation,* facial; *action,* closes eyelids, wrinkles forehead, compresses lacrimal sac.

**m. orbicula'ris o'ris** [TA], orbicular muscle of mouth, comprising a *pars labialis,* fibers restricted to the lips, and a *pars marginalis,* fibers blending with those of adjacent muscles; *innervation,* facial; *action,* closes and protrudes lips.

**m. orbita'lis** [TA], orbital muscle: a thin layer of nonstriated muscle that bridges the inferior orbital fissure; *innervation,* sympathetic branches.

**mus'culi ossiculo'rum auditorio'rum** [TA], muscles of auditory ossicles: the two muscles of the middle ear, the tensor tympani and the stapedius.

**mus'culi os'sis hyoi'dei,** muscles of the hyoid bone; see *musculi infrahyoidei* and *musculi suprahyoidei.*

**mus'culi pala'ti,** see *musculi palati mollis et faucium.*

**mus'culi pala'ti mol'lis et fau'cium** [TA], muscles of soft palate and fauces: the intrinsic and extrinsic muscles that act upon the soft palate *(musculi palati)* and the adjacent pharyngeal wall.

**m. palatoglos'sus** [TA], palatoglossus muscle: *origin,* under surface of soft palate; *insertion,* side of tongue; *innervation,* pharyngeal plexus of vagus; *action,* elevates tongue, constricts fauces.

**m. palatopharyn'geus** [TA], palatopharyngeal muscle: one of the intrinsic muscles of the larynx; *origin,* soft palate; *insertion,* aponeurosis of pharynx, dorsal border of thyroid cartilage; *innervation,* pharyngeal plexus of vagus; *action,* aids in deglutition.

**m. palma'ris bre'vis** [TA], short palmar muscle: *origin,* palmar aponeurosis; *insertion,* skin of medial border of hand; *innervation,* ulnar; *action,* assists in deepening hollow of palm.

**m. palma'ris lon'gus** [TA], long palmar muscle: *origin,* medial epicondyle of humerus; *insertion,* flexor retinaculum, palmar aponeurosis; *innervation,* median; *action,* flexes wrist joint.

**mus'culi papilla'res** [TA], papillary muscles: conical muscular projections from the walls of the cardiac ventricles, attached to the cusps of the atrioventricular valves by the chordae tendineae. There is an anterior and a posterior papillary muscle in each ventricle, as well as a group of small papillary muscles on the septum in the right ventricle.

**m. papilla'ris ante'rior ventri'culi dex'tri** [TA], anterior papillary muscle of right ventricle: the papillary muscle arising from the sternocostal wall of the right ventricle.

**m. papilla'ris ante'rior ventri'culi sinis'tri** [TA], anterior papillary muscle of left ventricle: the papillary muscle arising from the anterior wall of the left ventricle.

**m. papilla'ris poste'rior ventri'culi dex'tri** [TA], posterior papillary muscle of right ventricle: the papillary muscle arising from the diaphragmatic wall of the right ventricle.

**m. papilla'ris poste'rior ventri'culi sinis'tri** [TA], posterior papillary muscle of left ventricle: the papillary muscle arising from the posterior wall of the left ventricle.

**mus'culi pectina'ti a'trii dex'tri** [TA], pectinate muscles of right atrium: small ridges of muscle fibers projecting from the inner walls of the right auricle of the heart and extending in the right atrium to the crista terminalis.

**mus'culi pectina'ti a'trii sinis'tri** [TA], pectinate muscles of left atrium: small ridges of muscle fibers projecting from the inner walls of the left auricle of the heart.

**m. pectin'eus** [TA], pectineal muscle: *origin,* pectineal line of pubis; *insertion,* femur distal to lesser trochanter; *innervation,* obturator and femoral; *action,* flexes, adducts thigh.

**m. pectora'lis ma'jor** [TA], greater pectoral muscle: *origin,* clavicle, sternum, six upper ribs, aponeurosis of obliquus externus abdominis. These origins are reflected in the subdivision of the muscle into clavicular, sternocostal, and abdominal parts; *insertion,* crest of intertubercular groove of humerus; *innervation,* medial and lateral pectoral; *action,* adducts, flexes, rotates arm medially.

**m. pectora'lis mi'nor** [TA], smaller pectoral muscle: *origin,* third, fourth, and fifth ribs; *insertion,* coracoid process of scapula; *innervation,* lateral and medial pectoral; *action,* draws shoulder forward and downward, raises third, fourth, and fifth ribs in forced inspiration.

**m. penna'tus** [TA], pennate muscle: a muscle in which the fibers approach the tendon of insertion from a wide area and are inserted through a large segment of its circumference. Called also *m. bipennatus* [TA alternative] and *bipennate* or *penniform muscle.*

**mus'culi perinea'les, mus'culi perine'i** [TA], muscles of perineum: the muscles participating in formation of the perineum.

**m. perone'us bre'vis,** TA alternative for *m. fibularis brevis.*

**m. perone'us lon'gus** [TA], TA alternative for *m. fibularis longus.*

**m. perone'us ter'tius,** TA alternative for *m. fibularis tertius.*

**mus'culi pharyn'gis** [TA], pharyngeal muscles: the muscular coat of the pharynx, consisting of the three constrictor muscles and the stylopharyngeal, salpingopharyngeal, and palatopharyngeal muscles.

**m. pharyngopalati'nus,** m. palatopharyngeus.

**m. pirifor'mis** [TA], piriform muscle: *origin,* ilium, second to fourth sacral vertebrae; *insertion,* upper border of greater trochanter; *innervation,* first and second sacral; *action,* rotates thigh laterally.

**m. planta'ris** [TA], plantar muscle: *origin,* oblique popliteal ligament, lateral supracondylar line of femur; *insertion,* posterior part of calcaneus; *innervation,* tibial; *action,* plantar flexes foot.

**m. pleurooesopha'geus** [TA], pleuroesophageal muscle: a bundle of smooth muscle usually connecting the esophagus with the left mediastinal pleura.

**m. popli'teus** [TA], popliteal muscle: *origin,* lateral condyle of femur, lateral meniscus; *insertion,* posterior surface of tibia; *innervation,* tibial; *action,* flexes leg, rotates leg medially.

**m. proce'rus** [TA], procerus muscle: *origin,* fascia over nasal bone; *insertion,* skin of forehead; *innervation,* facial; *action,* draws medial angle of eyebrows down.

**m. prona'tor quadra'tus** [TA], *origin,* anterior surface and border of distal third or fourth of ulna; *insertion,* anterior surface and border of distal fourth of shaft of radius; *innervation,* anterior interosseous; *action,* pronates hand.

**m. prona'tor te'res** [TA], (2 heads): *origin,* CAPUT HUMERALE—medial epicondyle of humerus, CAPUT ULNARE—coronoid process of ulna; *insertion,* lateral surface of radius; *innervation,* median; *action,* pronates hand and flexes elbow.

**m. prosta'ticus,** substantia muscularis prostatae.

**m. pso'as ma'jor** [TA], greater psoas muscle: *origin,* lumbar vertebrae; *insertion,* lesser trochanter of femur; *innervation,* second and third lumbar; *action,* flexes thigh or trunk.

**m. pso'as mi'nor** [TA], smaller psoas muscle: *origin,* last thoracic and first lumbar vertebrae; *insertion,* arcuate line, iliopectineal eminence, iliac fascia; *innervation,* first lumbar; *action,* flexes trunk.

**m. pterygoi'deus latera'lis** [TA], lateral pterygoid muscle (2 heads): *origin,* SUPERIOR HEAD—lateral surface of greater wing of sphenoid and infratemporal crest; INFERIOR HEAD—lateral surface of lateral pterygoid plate; *insertion,* neck of condyle of mandible, temporomandibular joint capsule; *innervation,* mandibular division of trigeminal; *action,* protrudes mandible, opens jaws, moves mandible from side to side.

**m. pterygoi'deus media'lis** [TA], medial pterygoid muscle: *origin,* lateral pterygoid plate, tuberosity of maxilla; *insertion,* medial surface of ramus and angle of mandible; *innervation,* mandibular division of trigeminal; *action,* closes jaws.

**m. pterygopharyn'geus,** pars pterygopharyngea musculi constrictoris pharyngis superioris.

**m. pubococcy'geus** [TA], pubococcygeal muscle: the anterior portion of the levator ani, originating anterior to the obturator canal; *insertion,* anococcygeal ligament and side of coccyx; *innervation,* third and fourth sacral; *action,* helps support pelvic viscera and resist increases in intra-abdominal pressure.

**m. puboprosta'ticus** [TA], puboprostatic muscle: smooth muscle fibers contained within the medial puboprostatic ligament, which pass from the prostate anteriorly to the pubis.

**m. puborecta'lis** [TA], puborectal muscle: a portion of the levator ani having a more lateral origin from the pubic bone, and continuous posteriorly with the corresponding muscle of the opposite side; *innervation,* third and fourth sacral; *action,* helps support pelvic viscera and resist increases in intra-abdominal pressure. Called also *Braune's muscle.*

**m. pubovagina'lis** [TA], pubovaginal muscle: a part of the anterior portion of the pubococcygeus muscle, which is inserted into the urethra and vagina; innervated by the sacral and pudendal nerves, it is involved in control of micturition.

**m. pubovesica'lis** [TA], pubovesical muscle: smooth muscle fibers extending from the neck of the urinary bladder to the pubis.

**m. pyramida'lis** [TA], pyramidal muscle: *origin,* anterior aspect of pubis, anterior pubic ligament; *insertion,* linea alba; *innervation,* last thoracic; *action,* tenses abdominal wall.

**m. pyramida'lis auri'culae** [TA], **m. pyramida'lis auricula'ris,** pyramidal muscle of auricle: a prolongation of the fibers of the tragicus to the spina helicis.

**m. quadra'tus** [TA], quadrate muscle: a square-shaped muscle.

**m. quadra'tus fe'moris** [TA], quadrate muscle of thigh: *origin,* upper part of lateral border of tuberosity of ischium; *insertion,* quadrate tubercle of femur, intertrochanteric crest; *innervation,* fourth and fifth lumbar and first sacral; *action,* adducts, rotates thigh laterally.

**m. quadra'tus la'bii inferio'ris,** m. depressor labii inferioris.

**m. quadra'tus la'bii superio'ris,** m. levator labii superioris.

**m. quadra'tus lumbo'rum** [TA], *origin,* crest of ilium, thoracolumbar fascia, lumbar vertebrae; *insertion,* twelfth rib, transverse processes of four upper lumbar vertebrae; *innervation,* first and second lumbar and twelfth thoracic; *action,* flexes lumbar vertebrae laterally.

**m. quadra'tus plan'tae** [TA], quadrate muscle of sole: *origin,* calcaneus and plantar fascia; *insertion,* tendons of flexor digitorum longus; *innervation,* lateral plantar; *action,* aids in flexing toes. Called also *m. flexor accessorius* [TA alternative] or *accessory flexor muscle.*

**m. quad'riceps fe'moris** [TA], quadriceps muscle of thigh: a name applied collectively to the rectus femoris, vastus intermedius, vastus lateralis, and vastus medialis, inserting by a common tendon that surrounds the patella and ends on the tuberosity of the tibia, and acting to extend the leg upon the thigh. See individual components.

**m. rectococcy'geus** [TA], rectococcygeal muscle: smooth muscle fibers originating on the anterior surface of the second and third coccygeal vertebrae and inserting on the posterior surface of the rectum, innervated by autonomic nerves, and acting to retract and elevate the rectum.

**m. rectourethra'lis** [TA], rectourethral muscle: a band of smooth muscle fibers extending from the perineal flexure of the rectum to the membranous urethra in the male.

**m. rectouteri'nus** [TA], rectouterine muscle: a band of fibers running between the cervix of the uterus and the rectum, in the rectouterine fold.

**m. rectovesica'lis** [TA], rectovesical muscle: a band of fibers in the male, connecting the longitudinal musculature of the rectum with the external muscular coat of the bladder.

**m. rec'tus abdom'inis** [TA], *origin,* pubis; *insertion,* xiphoid process, cartilages of fifth, sixth, and seventh ribs; *innervation,* branches of lower thoracic; *action,* flexes lumbar vertebrae, supports abdomen.

**m. rec'tus ca'pitis ante'rior** [TA], *origin,* lateral mass of atlas; *insertion,* basilar process of occipital bone; *innervation,* first and second cervical; *action,* flexes, supports head.

**m. rec'tus ca'pitis latera'lis** [TA], *origin,* upper surface of transverse process of atlas; *insertion,* jugular process of occipital bone; *innervation,* first and second cervical; *action,* flexes, supports head.

**m. rec'tus ca'pitis poste'rior ma'jor** [TA], *origin,* spinous process of axis; *insertion,* occipital bone; *innervation,* suboccipital and greater occipital; *action,* extends head.

**m. rec'tus ca'pitis poste'rior mi'nor** [TA], *origin,* tubercle on dorsal arch of atlas; *insertion,* occipital bone; *innervation,* suboccipital and greater occipital; *action,* extends head.

**m. rec'tus fe'moris** [TA], *origin,* anterior inferior iliac spine, rim of acetabulum; *insertion,* patella, tubercle of tibia; *innervation,* femoral; *action,* extends leg, flexes thigh.

**m. rec'tus infe'rior bul'bi** [TA], inferior rectus muscle: *origin,* anulus tendineus communis; *insertion,* under side of sclera; *innervation,* oculomotor; *action,* adducts, rotates eyeball downward and medially.

**m. rec'tus infe'rior o'culi,** m. rectus inferior bulbi.

**m. rec'tus latera'lis bul'bi** [TA], lateral rectus muscle: *origin,* anulus tendineus communis; *insertion,* lateral side of sclera; *innervation,* abducens; *action,* abducts eyeball.

**m. rec'tus latera'lis o'culi,** m. rectus lateralis bulbi.

**m. rec'tus media'lis bul'bi** [TA], medial rectus muscle: *origin,* anulus tendineus communis; *insertion,* medial side of sclera; *innervation,* oculomotor; *action,* adducts eyeball.

**m. rec'tus media'lis o'culi,** m. rectus medialis bulbi.

**m. rec'tus supe'rior bul'bi** [TA], superior rectus muscle: *origin,* anulus tendineus communis; *insertion,* upper aspect of sclera; *innervation,* oculomotor; *action,* adducts, rotates eyeball upward and medially.

**m. rec'tus supe'rior o'culi,** m. rectus superior bulbi.

**m. rhomboi'deus ma'jor** [TA], greater rhomboid muscle: *origin,* spinous processes of second, third, fourth, and fifth thoracic vertebrae; *insertion,* medial margin of scapula; *innervation,* dorsal scapular; *action,* retracts, elevates scapula.

**m. rhomboi'deus mi'nor** [TA], lesser rhomboid muscle: *origin,* spinous processes of seventh cervical to first thoracic vertebrae, lower part of ligamentum nuchae; *insertion,* medial margin of scapula at root of the spine; *innervation,* dorsal scapular; *action,* adducts, elevates scapula.

**m. riso'rius** [TA], risorius muscle: *origin,* fascia over masseter; *insertion,* skin at angle of mouth; *innervation,* buccal branch of facial; *action,* draws angle of mouth laterally.

**mus'culi rotato'res** [TA], rotator muscles: a series of small muscles deep in the groove between the spinous and transverse processes of the vertebrae, including the *musculi rotatores cervicis, musculi rotatores thoracis,* and *musculi rotatores lumborum.*

**mus'culi rotato'res bre'ves,** short rotator muscles: a name given the musculi rotatores that insert on the lamina of the vertebra next above the vertebra of origin.

**mus'culi rotato'res cer'vicis** [TA], rotator muscles of neck: *origin,* transverse processes of cervical vertebrae; *insertion,* base of spinous process of superjacent vertebrae; *innervation,* spinal nerves; *action,* extend vertebral column and rotate it toward the opposite side.

**mus'culi rotato'res lon'gi,** long rotator muscles: a name given the musculi rotatores that cross one or two segments of the vertebral column and insert into the spine of the vertebra next above.

**mus'culi rotato'res lumbo'rum** [TA], *origin,* transverse processes of lumbar vertebrae; *insertion,* base of spinous process of superjacent vertebrae; *innervation,* spinal nerves; *action,* extend vertebral column and rotate it toward the opposite side.

**mus'culi rotato'res thora'cis** [TA], rotator muscles of thorax: *origin,* transverse processes of thoracic vertebrae; *insertion,* base of spinous process of superjacent vertebrae; *innervation,* spinal nerves; *action,* extend vertebral column and rotate it toward the opposite side.

**m. sacrococcy'geus ante'rior,** m. sacrococcygeus ventralis.

**m. sacrococcy'geus dorsa'lis,** dorsal sacrococcygeal muscle: a muscular slip passing from the dorsal aspect of the sacrum to the coccyx.

**m. sacrococcy'geus poste'rior,** m. sacrococcygeus dorsalis.

**m. sacrococcy'geus ventra'lis,** ventral sacrococcygeal muscle: a musculotendinous slip passing from the lower sacral vertebrae to the coccyx.

**m. sacrospina'lis,** m. erector spinae.

**m. salpingopharyn'geus** [TA], salpingopharyngeal muscle: *origin,* auditory tube near its orifice; *insertion,* posterior part of palatopharyngeus; *innervation,* pharyngeal plexus of vagus; *action,* raises nasopharynx.

**m. sarto'rius** [TA], sartorius muscle: *origin,* anterior superior iliac spine; *insertion,* medial side of proximal end of tibia; *innervation,* femoral; *action,* flexes thigh and leg.

**m. scale'nus ante'rior** [TA], anterior scalene muscle: *origin,* transverse processes of third to sixth cervical vertebrae; *insertion,* scalene tubercle of first rib; *innervation,* second to seventh cervical; *action,* raises first rib, flexes cervical vertebrae forward and laterally, rotates cervical vertebrae to opposite side.

**m. scale'nus me'dius** [TA], middle scalene muscle: *origin,* transverse processes of second to sixth cervical vertebrae; *insertion,* upper surface of first rib; *innervation,* second to seventh cervical; *action,* raises first rib, flexes cervical vertebrae laterally.

**m. scale'nus mi'nimus** [TA], smallest scalene muscle: a band occasionally found between the m. scalenus anterior and the m. scalenus medius. Called also *Sibson's muscle.*

**m. scale'nus poste'rior** [TA], posterior scalene muscle: *origin,* posterior tubercles of transverse processes of fourth to sixth cervical vertebrae; *insertion,* second rib; *innervation,* second to seventh cervical; *action,* raises first and second ribs, flexes cervical vertebrae laterally.

**m. semimembrano'sus** [TA], semimembranous muscle: *origin,* tuberosity of ischium; *insertion,* medial condyle and border of tibia, lateral condyle of femur; *innervation,* tibial; *action,* flexes and rotates leg medially, extends thigh.

**m. semipenna'tus** [TA], semipennate muscle: a muscle in which the fiber bundles approach the tendon of insertion from only one direction and are inserted through only a small segment of its circumference. Called also *m. unipennatus* [TA alternative] and *unipennate muscle.*

**m. semispina'lis** [TA], semispinal muscle: a muscle composed of fibers extending obliquely from the transverse processes of the vertebrae to the spine, except for the semispinalis capitis; it includes the *m. semispinalis capitis, m. semispinalis cervicis,* and *m. semispinalis thoracis.*

**m. semispina'lis ca'pitis** [TA], semispinal muscles of head: *origin,* transverse processes of five or six upper thoracic and four lower cervical vertebrae; *insertion,* occipital bone; *innervation,* suboccipital, greater occipital, and branches of cervical; *action,* extends head.

**m. semispina'lis cer'vicis** [TA], semispinal muscles of neck: *origin,* transverse processes of five or six upper thoracic vertebrae; *insertion,* spinous processes of second to fifth cervical vertebrae; *innervation,* branches of cervical; *action,* extends, rotates vertebral column.

**m. semispina'lis dor'si,** m. semispinalis thoracis.

**m. semispina'lis thora'cis** [TA], semispinal muscles of thorax: *origin,* transverse processes of sixth to tenth thoracic vertebrae; *insertion,* spinous processes of two lower cervical and four upper thoracic vertebrae; *innervation,* spinal nerves; *action,* extends, rotates vertebral column.

**m. semitendino'sus** [TA], semitendinous muscle: *origin,* tuberosity of ischium; *insertion,* upper part of medial surface of tibia; *innervation,* tibial; *action,* flexes and rotates leg medially, extends thigh.

**m. serra'tus ante'rior** [TA], anterior serratus muscle: *origin,* eight or nine upper ribs; *insertion,* medial border of scapula; *innervation,* long thoracic; *action,* draws scapula forward; rotates scapula to raise shoulder in abduction of arm.

**m. serra'tus poste'rior infe'rior** [TA], inferior posterior serratus muscle: *origin,* spines of two lower thoracic and two or three upper lumbar vertebrae; *insertion,* inferior border of four lower ribs; *innervation,* ninth to twelfth thoracic; *action,* lowers ribs in expiration.

**m. serra'tus poste'rior supe'rior** [TA], superior posterior serratus muscle: *origin,* ligamentum nuchae, spinous processes of upper thoracic vertebrae; *insertion,* second, third, fourth, and fifth ribs; *innervation,* first four thoracic; *action,* raises ribs in inspiration.

**mus'culi ske'leti** [TA], skeletal muscles: striated muscles that are attached to bones and typically cross at least one joint.

**m. so'leus** [TA], soleus muscle: *origin,* fibula, popliteal fascia, tibia; *insertion,* calcaneus by tendo calcaneus; *innervation,* tibial; *action,* plantar flexes foot.

**m. sphinc'ter** [TA], sphincter muscle: a ringlike muscle that closes a natural orifice; called also *sphincter.*

**m. sphinc'ter ampul'lae hepatopancrea'ticae** [TA], sphincter muscle of hepatopancreatic ampulla: muscle fibers investing the hepatopancreatic ampulla in the wall of the duodenum; called also *Oddi's muscle, sphincter of Oddi,* and *Glisson's sphincter.*

**m. sphinc'ter a'ni exter'nus** [TA], external sphincter muscle of anus: *origin,* tip of coccyx, anococcygeal ligament; *insertion,* tendinous center of perineum; *innervation,* inferior rectal and fourth sacral; *action,* closes anus. Called also *external anal sphincter.*

**m. sphinc'ter a'ni inter'nus** [TA], internal sphincter muscle of anus: a thickening of the circular lamina of the tunica muscularis at the caudal end of the rectum. Called also *internal anal sphincter.*

**m. sphinc'ter duc'tus bilia'ris,** TA alternative for *m. sphincter ductus choledochi.*

**m. sphinc'ter duc'tus chole'dochi** [TA], an annular sheath of muscle that invests the bile duct within the wall of the duodenum.

**m. sphinc'ter pupil'lae** [TA], sphincter muscle of pupil: circular fibers of the iris, innervated by the ciliary nerves (parasympathetic), and acting to contract the pupil.

**m. sphinc'ter pylo'ri,** m. sphincter pyloricus.

**m. sphinc'ter pylo'ricus** [TA], pyloric sphincter muscle: a thickening of the circular muscle of the stomach around its opening into the duodenum; called also *m. sphincter pylori, pyloric sphincter,* and *sphincter muscle of pylorus.*

**m. sphinc'ter ure'thrae,** sphincter muscle of urethra: *origin,* ramus of pubis; *insertion,* median raphe behind and in front of urethra; *innervation,* perineal; *action,* compresses the membranous part of the urethra. Called also *m. sphincter urethrae membranaceae.*

**m. sphinc'ter ure'thrae membrana'ceae,** m. sphincter urethrae.

**m. sphinc'ter vesi'cae urina'riae,** sphincter muscle of urinary bladder: a circular layer of fibers surrounding the internal urethral orifice, innervated by the vesical nerve, and acting to close the internal orifice of the urethra.

**m. spina'lis** [TA], spinal muscle: the medial division of the erector spinae, including the *m. spinalis capitis, m. spinalis cervicis,* and *m. spinalis thoracis.*

**m. spina'lis ca'pitis** [TA], spinal muscle of head: *origin,* spines of upper thoracic and lower cervical vertebrae; *insertion,* occipital bone; *innervation,* spinal nerves; *action,* extends head.

**m. spina'lis cer'vicis** [TA], spinal muscle of neck: *origin,* spinous processes of seventh cervical and sometimes two upper thoracic vertebrae; *insertion,* spinous processes of axis and sometimes of second to fourth cervical vertebrae; *innervation,* branches of cervical; *action,* extends vertebral column.

**m. spina'lis dor'si,** m. spinalis thoracis.

**m. spina'lis thora'cis** [TA], spinal muscle of thorax: *origin,* spinous processes of two upper lumbar and two lower thoracic; *insertion,* spines of upper thoracic vertebrae; *innervation,* branches of spinal nerves; *action,* extends vertebral column.

**m. sple'nius ca'pitis** [TA], splenius muscle of head: *origin,* lower half of ligamentum nuchae, spines of seventh cervical and three upper thoracic vertebrae; *insertion,* mastoid process of temporal bone, occipital bone; *innervation,* middle and lower cervical; *action,* extends, rotates head.

**m. sple'nius cer'vicis** [TA], splenius muscle of neck: *origin,* spinous processes of third to sixth thoracic vertebrae; *insertion,* transverse processes of two or three upper cervical vertebrae; *innervation,* dorsal branches of lower cervical; *action,* extends, rotates head and neck.

**m. stape'dius** [TA], stapedius muscle: *origin,* interior of pyramid of tympanic cavity; *insertion,* posterior surface of neck of stapes; *innervation,* stapedial branch of facial; *action,* dampens stapedial movement.

**m. sterna'lis** [TA], sternal muscle: a band occasionally found parallel to the sternum on the sternocostal origin of the pectoralis major.

**m. sternocleidomastoi'deus** [TA], sternocleidomastoid muscle (2 heads): *origin,* STERNAL HEAD—manubrium sterni, CLAVICULAR HEAD—clavicle; *insertion,* mastoid process and superior nuchal line of occipital bone; *innervation,* accessory nerve and cervical plexus; *action,* flexes vertebral column, rotates head.

**m. sternohyoi'deus** [TA], sternohyoid muscle: *origin,* manubrium sterni and clavicle; *insertion,* body of hyoid bone; *innervation,* upper ansa cervicalis; *action,* depresses hyoid bone and larynx.

**m. sternothyroi'deus** [TA], sternothyroid muscle: *origin,* manubrium sterni; *insertion,* lamina of thyroid cartilage; *innervation,* ansa cervicalis; *action,* depresses thyroid cartilage.

**m. styloglos'sus** [TA], styloglossus muscle: *origin,* styloid process; *insertion,* margin of tongue; *innervation,* hypoglossal; *action,* raises and retracts tongue.

**m. stylohyoi'deus** [TA], stylohyoid muscle: *origin,* styloid process; *insertion,* body of hyoid bone; *innervation,* facial; *action,* draws hyoid and tongue superiorly and posteriorly.

**m. stylopharyn'geus** [TA], stylopharyngeal muscle: one of the intrinsic muscles of the larynx; *origin,* styloid process; *insertion,* thyroid cartilage and pharyngeal constrictors; *innervation,* pharyngeal plexus, glossopharyngeal; *action,* raises and dilates pharynx.

**m. subcla'vius** [TA], subclavius muscle: *origin,* first rib and its cartilage; *insertion,* lower surface of clavicle; *innervation,* fifth and sixth cervical; *action,* depresses lateral end of clavicle.

**mus'culi subcosta'les** [TA], subcostal muscles: *origin,* inner surface of ribs: *insertion,* inner surface of first, second, third rib below; *innervation,* intercostal; *action,* draw adjacent ribs together, depress ribs.

**mus'culi suboccipita'les** [TA], suboccipital muscles: the muscles situated just below the occipital bone, including the recti capitis posteriores major and minor, the oblique capitis inferior and superior, the recti capitis anterior and lateral, the splenius capitis, and the longus capitis muscles.

**m. subscapula'ris** [TA], subscapular muscle: *origin,* subscapular fossa of scapula; *insertion,* lesser tubercle of humerus; *innervation,* subscapular; *action,* rotates humerus medially.

**m. supina'tor** [TA], supinator muscle: *origin,* lateral epicondyle of humerus, ulna, elbow joint fascia; *insertion,* radius; *innervation,* deep radial; *action,* supinates hand.

**mus'culi suprahyoi'dei** [TA], suprahyoid muscles: the muscles that attach the hyoid bone to the skull, including the digastric, stylohyoid, mylohyoid, and geniohyoid muscles.

**m. supraspina'tus** [TA], supraspinous muscle: *origin,* supraspinous fossa of scapula; *insertion,* greater tubercle of humerus; *innervation,* suprascapular; *action,* abducts humerus.

**m. suspenso'rius duode'ni** [TA], suspensory muscle of duodenum: a flat band of smooth muscle originating from the left crus of the diaphragm, and continuous with the muscular coat of the duodenum at its junction with the jejunum.

**m. tarsa'lis infe'rior** [TA], inferior tarsal muscle: *origin,* inferior rectus muscle; *insertion,* tarsal plate of lower eyelid; *innervation,* sympathetic; *action,* widens palpebral fissure.

**m. tarsa'lis supe'rior** [TA], superior tarsal muscle: *origin,* m. levator palpebrae superioris; *insertion,* tarsal plate of upper eyelid; *innervation,* sympathetic; *action,* widens palpebral fissure.

**m. tempora'lis** [TA], temporal muscle: *origin,* temporal fossa and fascia; *insertion,* coronoid process of mandible; *innervation,* mandibular; *action,* closes jaws.

**m. temporoparieta'lis** [TA], temporoparietal muscle: *origin,* temporal fascia above ear; *insertion,* galea aponeurotica; *innervation,* temporal branches of facial; *action,* tightens scalp.

**m. ten'sor fas'ciae la'tae** [TA], tensor muscle of fascia lata: *origin,* iliac crest; *insertion,* iliotibial band of fascia lata; *innervation,* superior gluteal; *action,* flexes, rotates thigh medially.

**m. ten'sor tym'pani** [TA], tensor muscle of tympanic membrane: *origin,* cartilaginous portion of auditory tube; *insertion,* manubrium of malleus; *innervation,* mandibular; *action,* tenses tympanic membrane.

**m. ten'sor ve'li palati'ni** [TA], *origin,* scaphoid fossa of pterygoid process, wall of auditory tube, spine of sphenoid; *insertion,* aponeurosis of soft palate, horizontal part of palatine bone; *innervation,* mandibular; *action,* tenses soft palate, opens auditory tube.

**m. te'res ma'jor** [TA], teres major muscle: *origin,* inferior angle of scapula; *insertion,* crest of intertubercular sulcus of humerus; *innervation,* lower subscapular; *action,* adducts, extends, rotates arm medially.

**m. te'res mi'nor** [TA], teres minor muscle: *origin,* lateral margin of scapula; *insertion,* greater tuberosity of humerus; *innervation,* axillary; *action,* rotates arm laterally.

**mus'culi thora'cis** [TA], the muscles of the thorax.

**m. thyroarytenoi'deus** [TA], thyroarytenoid muscle: one of the intrinsic muscles of the larynx; *origin,* lamina of thyroid cartilage; *insertion,* muscular process of arytenoid cartilage; *innervation,* recurrent laryngeal; *action,* relaxes, shortens vocal folds.

**m. thyroepiglot'ticus,** pars thyroepiglottica musculi thyroarytenoidei.

**m. thyrohyoi'deus** [TA], thyrohyoid muscle: *origin,* lamina of thyroid cartilage; *insertion,* greater cornu of hyoid bone; *innervation,* first cervical; *action,* raises and changes form of larynx.

**m. thyropharyn'geus,** TA alternative for *pars thyropharyngea musculi constrictoris pharyngis inferioris.*

**m. tibia'lis ante'rior** [TA], anterior tibial muscle: *origin,* lateral condyle and lateral surface of tibia, interosseous membrane; *insertion,* medial cuneiform and base of first metatarsal; *innervation,* deep peroneal; *action,* dorsiflexes and inverts foot.

**m. tibia'lis poste'rior** [TA], posterior tibial muscle: *origin,* tibia, fibula, interosseous membrane; *insertion,* bases of second to fourth metatarsals and tarsals, except talus; *innervation,* tibial; *action,* plantar flexes and inverts foot.

**m. trachea'lis** [TA], tracheal muscle: a transverse layer of smooth fibers in the dorsal portion of the trachea; *insertion,* tracheal cartilages; *innervation,* autonomic fibers; *action,* lessens caliber of trachea.

**m. tra'gicus** [TA], muscle of tragus: a short, flattened vertical band on the lateral surface of the tragus, innervated by the auriculotemporal and posterior auricular nerves.

**mus'culi transversospina'les** [TA], a general term including the semispinalis and multifidus muscles and the rotatores.

**m. transver'sus abdo'minis** [TA], transverse abdominal muscle: *origin,* cartilages of six lower ribs, thoracolumbar fascia, iliac crest, inguinal ligament; *insertion,* linea alba through rectus sheath, conjoined tendon to pubis; *innervation,* lower intercostals, iliohypogastric, ilioinguinal; *action,* compresses abdominal viscera.

**m. transver'sus auri'culae** [TA], **m. transver'sus auricula'ris,** transverse muscle of auricle: *origin,* cranial surface of auricle; *insertion,* circumference of auricle; *innervation,* posterior auricular; *action,* retracts helix.

**m. transver'sus lin'guae** [TA], transverse muscle of tongue: *origin,* median septum of tongue; *insertion,* dorsum and margins of tongue; *innervation,* hypoglossal; *action,* changes shape of tongue in mastication and deglutition.

**m. transver'sus men'ti** [TA], transverse muscle of chin: superficial fibers of the depressor anguli oris which turn back and cross to the opposite side.

**m. transver'sus nu'chae** [TA], transverse muscle of neck: a small muscle often present, passing from the occipital protuberance to the posterior auricular muscle; it may be either superficial or deep to the trapezius.

**m. transver'sus perine'i profun'dus** [TA], deep transverse perineal muscle: *origin,* ramus of ischium; *insertion,* tendinous center of perineum; *innervation,* perineal; *action,* fixes tendinous center of perineum.

**m. transver'sus perine'i superficia'lis** [TA], superficial transverse perineal muscle: *origin,* ramus of ischium; *insertion,* tendinous center of perineum; *innervation,* perineal; *action,* fixes tendinous center of perineum. Called also *Theile's muscle.*

**m. transver'sus thora'cis** [TA], transverse muscle of thorax: *origin,* mediastinal surface of sternum and of xiphoid process; *insertion,* cartilages of second to sixth ribs; *innervation,* intercostal; *action,* draws ribs downward.

**m. trape'zius** [TA], trapezius muscle: *origin,* occipital bone, ligamentum nuchae, spinous processes of seventh cervical and all thoracic vertebrae; *insertion,* clavicle, acromion, spine of scapula; *innervation,* accessory nerve and cervical plexus; *action,* rotates scapula to raise shoulder in abduction of arm, draws scapula backward.

**m. triangula'ris** [TA], triangular muscle: a muscle that is triangular in shape.

**m. tri'ceps bra'chii** [TA], triceps muscle of arm (3 heads): *origin,* CAPUT LONGUM—infraglenoid tubercle of scapula, CAPUT LATERALE—posterior surface of humerus, lateral border of humerus, lateral intermuscular septum, CAPUT MEDIALE—posterior surface of humerus below radial groove, medial border of humerus, medial intermuscular septa; *insertion,* olecranon of ulna; *innervation,* radial; *action,* extends forearm, long head adducts and extends arm.

**m. tri'ceps su'rae** [TA], the gastrocnemius and soleus considered together.

**m. unipenna'tus,** TA alternative for *m. semipennatus.*

**m. u'vulae** [TA], muscle of uvula: *origin,* posterior nasal spine of palatine bone and aponeurosis of soft palate; *insertion,* uvula; *innervation,* pharyngeal plexus of vagus; *action,* raises uvula.

**m. vas'tus interme'dius** [TA], *origin,* anterior and lateral surfaces of femur; *insertion,* patella, common tendon of quadriceps femoris; *innervation,* femoral; *action,* extends leg.

**m. vas'tus latera'lis** [TA], *origin,* capsule of hip joint, lateral aspect of femur; *insertion,* patella, common tendon of quadriceps femoris; *innervation,* femoral; *action,* extends leg.

**m. vas'tus media'lis** [TA], *origin,* medial aspect of femur; *insertion,* patella, common tendon of quadriceps femoris; *innervation,* femoral; *action,* extends leg.

**m. ventricula'ris,** a name applied to fibers of the thyroarytenoid muscle running into the vestibular folds.

**m. vertica'lis lin'guae** [TA], vertical muscle of tongue: *origin,* dorsal fascia of tongue; *insertion,* sides and base of tongue; *innervation,* hypoglossal; *action,* changes shape of tongue in mastication and deglutition.

**m. voca'lis** [TA], vocal muscle: one of the intrinsic muscles of the larynx; *origin,* angle between laminae of thyroid cartilage; *insertion,* vocal process of arytenoid cartilage; *innervation,* recurrent laryngeal; *action,* shortens and relaxes vocal folds.

**m. zygoma'ticus,** m. zygomaticus major.

**m. zygoma'ticus ma'jor** [TA], greater zygomatic muscle: *origin,* zygomatic bone in front of temporal process; *insertion,* angle of mouth; *innervation,* facial; *action,* draws angle of mouth backward and upward.

**m. zygoma'ticus mi'nor** [TA], lesser zygomatic muscle: *origin,* zygomatic bone near maxillary suture; *insertion,* orbicularis oris and levator labii superioris; *innervation,* facial; *action,* draws upper lip upward and laterally.

---

**mush·room** (mush'ro͞om) the fruiting body (basidiocarp) of any of a variety of basidiomycetous fleshy fungi of the order Agaricales, especially one that is edible. Poisonous species are popularly called *toadstools.* See also *agaric.*

**mu·si·co·gen·ic** (mu″zĭ-ko-jen'ik) caused by or in reaction to musical sounds.

**Mus·set's sign** (mu-sāz') [Louis Charles Alfred de *Musset,* French poet, 1810–1857, who died of aortic insufficiency] see under *sign.*

**mus·si·ta·tion** (mus″ĭ-ta'shən) [L. *mussitare* to mutter] the moving of the lips with no utterance of articulate sounds.

**Mus·tard operation** (mus'tərd) [William Thornton *Mustard,* Canadian surgeon, born 1914] see under *operation.*

**mus·tard** (mus'tərd) [L. *sinapis*] [MeSH: Mustard] 1. any of several plants of the genus *Brassica* (formerly classified as genus *Sinapis*); see *black m.* and *white m.* 2. the ripe seeds of black mustard or white mustard; when they are crushed and moistened, volatile oils are liberated that are responsible for the counterirritant, stimulant, and emetic properties of mustard.

**black m., brown m.,** *Brassica nigra* (L.) Koch, a source of oil of mustard and allyl isothiocyanate; used internally as an emetic and externally as a counterirritant (see *mustard plaster,* under *plaster*). Since the plant contains sinigrin, animals consuming large quantities of it may develop fatal gastroenteritis.

**nitrogen m.,** 1. mechlorethamine hydrochloride. 2. *(pl.)* general term for a group of cytotoxic alkylating agents (q.v.) having the general formula $R—N(CH_2CH_2Cl)_2$; they are homologous with the vesicant war gas dichloroethyl sulfide (mustard gas). Those used as antineoplastic and immunosuppressive agents include chlorambucil, cyclophosphamide, ifosfamide, mechlorethamine (nitrogen mustard), melphalan, and uracil mustard.

**L-phenylalanine m.,** melphalan.

**uracil m.,** a cytotoxic alkylating agent that is the uracil derivative of nitrogen mustard, used as an antineoplastic in the treatment of chronic lymphocytic and chronic granulocytic leukemia, non-Hodgkin's lymphoma, mycosis fungoides, and polycythemia vera; now generally replaced by more effective agents.

**white m., yellow m.,** *Brassica alba* (L.) Rabenh.; it is a source of oil of mustard and is used the same as black mustard (q.v.). Since the plant contains sinigrin, animals consuming large quantities of it may develop fatal gastroenteritis.

**Mus·tar·gen** (mus'tər-jən) trademark for a preparation of mechlorethamine hydrochloride.

**mu·ta·cism** (mu'tə-siz-əm) mytacism.

**mu·ta·gen** (mu'tə-jən) [*muta*tion + *gen*esis] a chemical or physical agent that induces or increases genetic mutations by causing changes in DNA.

**mu·ta·gen·e·sis** (mu″tə-jen'ə-sis) [*muta*tion + *-genesis*] [MeSH: Mutagenesis] 1. the production of change. 2. the induction of genetic mutation.
**site-directed m.**, a method for producing a defined DNA mutation; a sequence alteration is made in vitro at a specific nucleotide or region and the altered DNA is reintroduced into cells.

**mu·ta·gen·ic** (mu″tə-jen'ik) 1. causing change. 2. inducing genetic mutation.

**mu·ta·ge·nic·i·ty** (mu″tə-jə-nis'ĭ-te) the property of being able to induce genetic mutation.

**Mu·ta·my·cin** (mu″tə-mi'sin) trademark for a preparation of mitomycin.

**mu·tant** (mu'tənt) [L. *mutare* to change] 1. a gene or organism that has undergone genetic mutation. 2. produced by mutation.

**mu·ta·ro·tase** (mu″tə-ro'tās) aldose 1-epimerase.

**mu·ta·ro·ta·tion** (mu″tə-ro-ta'shən) a change in the optical activity of a freshly prepared solution of a pure compound that occurs because of the formation of diastereoisomers of the original compound having different optical activity, e.g., the equilibration of the $\alpha$ and $\beta$ anomers of glucose.

**mu·tase** (mu'tās) [EC 5.4] any member of a subclass of enzymes of the isomerase class that act as intramolecular transferases, catalyzing the intramolecular shift of an acyl, amino, phosphate, or other chemical group.

**mu·ta·tion** (mu-ta'shən) [L. *mutatio,* from *mutare* to change] [MeSH: Mutation] 1. a change in form, quality, or some other characteristic. 2. in genetics, a permanent transmissible change in the genetic material, usually in a single gene. Also, an individual exhibiting such a change.
**allelic m's**, see *multiple alleles,* under *allele.*
**amber m.**, see *nonsense m.*
**auxotrophic m.**, a mutation resulting in the inability of bacteria to grow on minimal media.
**biochemical m.**, nutritional m.
**chromosomal m.**, a mutation affecting large regions of a chromosome and caused by breakage, e.g., by *deletion,* by *inversion,* in which a section of chromosome is inserted in reverse order, and by *translocation,* in which a piece of one chromosome attaches to another. See also *genomic m.* and *point m.*
**clear plaque m.**, a mutation resulting in clear plaque formation by a temperate phage that usually makes turbid plaques on bacterial lawns.
**cold-sensitive m.**, a conditional mutation producing a gene functional at high temperatures and nonfunctional at low.
**conditional m.**, a mutation affecting an organism's phenotype under restrictive growth conditions but not under permissive growth conditions; the wild type is expressed equivalently under both growth conditions. See also *temperature-sensitive m.*
**conditional lethal m.**, a mutation lethal only under certain environmental or genetic conditions; see also *lethal m.*
**constitutive m.**, a mutation resulting in the formation of a product in the absence of the inducer, either by modifying an operator so that the repressor cannot combine with it or by modifying the regulator so that no repressor is formed.
**forward m.**, a point mutation causing a change from the normal wild type to the mutant; cf. *reverse m.*
**frameshift m.**, a mutation resulting from an addition or subtraction that is not an exact multiple of 3 base pairs in a coding sequence. From the point of mutation onwards, base triplets (codons) are read out of phase; the reading frame of the gene is changed, and a completely different set of amino acids is made into protein. Called also *reading frameshift m.*
**genomic m.**, a mutation affecting the number of chromosomes present, e.g., aneuploidy, in which the genome gains or loses one or more chromosomes, and polyploidy, in which the overall chromosome number is doubled or tripled. See also *chromosomal m.* and *point m.*
**germinal m.**, a mutation in a germ cell; it generally does not affect the phenotype of the individual in which it first occurs but can be transmitted to offspring. See also *somatic m.*
**homoeotic m.**, a mutation interfering with the correct interpretation of positional information.
**induced m.**, a genetic mutation caused by external factors which are experimentally or accidentally produced; see also *spontaneous movement*
**lethal m.**, a mutation that destroys a gene's ability to produce an active form of an indispensable protein or that destroys an organism's ability to reproduce and transmit the mutation to subsequent generations; see also *conditional lethal m.*
**missense m.**, one that changes a codon so that it codes for a different amino acid; cf. *nonsense m.*
**natural m.**, spontaneous movement
**nonsense m.**, a mutation in which one of the three terminator codons in the mRNA (UAG, *amber;* UAA, *ochre;* UGA, *umber* or *opal*), used to signal the end of a polypeptide, appears in the middle of a genetic message, causes premature termination of transcription, and releases incomplete, generally nonfunctional polypeptides from the ribosome. See also *missense m.*
**nutritional m.**, a mutation affecting an organism's ability to produce a molecule, e.g., an amino acid, essential for growth; called also *biochemical m.*
**ochre m.**, see *nonsense m.*
**opal m.**, see *nonsense m.*
**point m.**, a mutation resulting from a change in a single base pair in the DNA molecule, caused by the substitution of one nucleotide for another. See also *chromosomal m.* and *genomic m.*
**reading frameshift m.**, frameshift m.
**reverse m.**, a point mutation causing reversion from the mutant to the normal wild type; cf. *forward m.*
**silent m.**, a mutation that has no detectable phenotypic effect.
**somatic m.**, a mutation in a somatic cell, not in a germ cell; it may affect the phenotype in which it occurs since it provides the basis for mosaicism, but generally the mutation will not be transmitted to offspring. Somatic mutations have been proposed as causes of aging and cancer. See also *germinal m.*
**spontaneous m's**, mutations occurring at a low but measurable rate in all organisms, presumably because of the inherent rates of error in the replication and transmission of a genome. Called also *natural m.* See also *induced m.*
**suppressor m.**, a mutation that partially or completely masks phenotype expression of a mutation but occurs at a different site from the primary mutation (i.e., causes suppression); it may be intragenic or intergenic. The term is used particularly to describe a secondary mutation that restores the ability of a transfer RNA to recognize a nonsense codon that was created by the primary mutation.
**temperature-sensitive (t-s) m.**, a conditional mutation resulting in an abnormality at one temperature, but not at others; see also *cold-sensitive m.*
**umber m.**, see *nonsense m.*
**visible m.**, a mutation affecting a morphological trait and for which screening is done by inspection.

**mu·ta·tion·al** (mu-ta'shən-əl) pertaining to mutation.

**mute** (mūt) [L. *mutus*] 1. unable to speak. 2. one who cannot or will not speak.
**deaf m.**, see *deaf-mute.*

**mu·te·in** (mu'tēn) [from *mu*tant-pro*tein*] a name suggested for a protein arising as a result of a mutation; it is analogous to the wild-type protein but does not necessarily have the same enzymological, immunological, or physicochemical properties.

**mu·ti·la·tion** (mu″tĭ-la'shən) [L. *mutilatio*] the act of depriving an individual of a limb, member, or other important part; deprival of an organ; severe disfigurement.

**Mu·tis·ia** (mu-tiz'e-ə) a genus of shrubs of the family Compositae, native to South America. *M. viciaefo'lia* is a species used as a sedative and in treatment of cardiac, respiratory, and nervous disorders.

**mu·tism** (mu'tiz-əm) [MeSH: Mutism] the condition of being mute.
**akinetic m.**, a state in which the individual can make no spontaneous movement or sound; often caused by a tumor or other lesion in the third ventricle. Cf. *locked-in syndrome.*
**deaf m.**, see *deaf-mutism.*
**elective m.**, selective m.
**selective m.** [DSM-IV], a mental disorder of childhood characterized by continuous refusal to speak in social situations by a child who is able and willing to speak to selected persons.

**mu·tu·al·ism** (mu'choo-əl-iz-əm) symbiosis in which both populations (or individuals) gain from the association and are unable to survive without it.

**mu·tu·al·ist** (mu'tu-əl-ist) any organism or species associated with another in a relationship which is beneficial to both.

**muz·zle** (muz'əl) the most anterior region of the face of various animals, consisting of the nose, jaws, and surrounding structures.

**MV** abbreviation for L. *Med'icus Veterina'rius,* veterinary physician.

**mV** symbol for *millivolt.*

**μV** symbol for *microvolt.*

**M-VAC** a regimen of methotrexate, vinblastine, doxorubicin, and cisplatin used in the treatment of transitional cell carcinoma.

**MVP** mitral valve prolapse.

**MW** molecular weight.

**μW** symbol for *microwatt.*

**Mx** Medex.

**My** myopia.

**my** mayer.

**my·al·gia** (mi-al'jə) [*my-* + *algia*] pain in a muscle or muscles. Called also *myodynia.*
**m. abdo'minis,** pain in the abdominal wall.
**m. ca'pitis,** pain in the scalp muscles, formerly thought to be a cause of tension headache.
**m. cervica'lis,** torticollis.
**epidemic m.,** see under *pleurodynia.*

**My·am·bu·tol** (mi-am'bu-tol) trademark for a preparation of ethambutol hydrochloride.

**My·an·e·sin** (mi-an'ə-sin) trademark for a preparation of mephenesin.

**my·a·sis** (mi-a'sis) myiasis.

**my·as·the·nia** (mi"əs-the'ne-ə) [*my-* + *asthenia*] muscular debility; any constitutional anomaly of muscle.
**m. gas'trica,** weakness and loss of tone in the muscular coats of the stomach; atony of the stomach.
**m. gra'vis,** a disorder of neuromuscular function due to the presence of antibodies to acetylcholine receptors at the neuromuscular junction; characteristics include muscular fatigue and exhaustion tending to fluctuate in severity, without sensory disturbance or atrophy. It may be restricted to one muscle group or become generalized with severe weakness and sometimes ventilatory insufficiency. It may affect any muscle of the body, but especially those of the eye, face, lips, tongue, throat, and neck. Called also *Erb-Goldflam, Goldflam's,* or *Goldflam-Erb disease.*
**m. gra'vis pseudoparaly'tica,** m. gravis.
**m. gravis, familial infantile,** an autosomal recessive disorder seen in infants and characterized by feeding difficulties, episodes of apnea, varying degrees of ophthalmoparesis, and weakness or fatigability after exercise; symptoms often improve with age.
**m. laryn'gis,** phonasthenia.
**neonatal m.,** a transient (a week to a month) myasthenia affecting offspring of myasthenic women, characteristically marked by difficulty in sucking and swallowing.

**my·as·then·ic** (mi"əs-then'ik) pertaining to or characterized by muscular weakness.

**my·a·to·nia** (mi"ə-to'ne-ə) [*my-* + *atonia*] amyotonia.

**my·at·o·ny** (mi-at'ə-ne) amyotonia.

**my·at·ro·phy** (mi-at'rə-fe) [*my-* + *atrophy*] atrophy of a muscle; muscular atrophy.

**My·ce·lex** (mi'sə-leks) trademark for a preparation of clotrimazole.

**my·ce·li·al** (mi-se'le-əl) pertaining to a mycelium.

**my·ce·li·an** (mi-se'le-ən) mycelial.

**my·ce·li·oid** (mi-se'le-oid) resembling a mycelium.

**my·ce·li·um** (mi-se'le-əm) pl. *myce'lia* [*myc-* + Gr. *hēlos* nail] the mass of threadlike processes (hyphae) constituting the fungal thallus.

**my·cete** (mi'sēt) [Gr. *mykēs* fungus] fungus.

**my·ce·the·mia** (mi"sə-the'me-ə) [*myceto-* + *-emia*] fungemia.

**my·ce·tism** (mi'sə-tiz-əm) mycotoxicosis (def. 2).

**my·ce·tis·mus** (mi"sə-tiz'məs) mycotoxicosis (def. 2).
**m. ce'rebris,** a type of mushroom poisoning with hallucinogenic symptoms, caused by ingestion of any of several different species.
**m. cholerifor'mis,** a serious and often fatal type of mushroom poisoning caused by ingestion of *Amanita phalloides, A. verna,* and probably other *Amanita* species that produce phalloidin; it is characterized by abdominal pain, vomiting, diarrhea, bloody stools, protein and casts in the urine, malaise, and cyanosis.
**m. gastrointestina'lis,** a mild form of mushroom poisoning marked by nausea, vomiting, and diarrhea, caused by ingestion of the orange jack-o-lantern mushroom *(Clitocybe illudens)* or any of numerous other species.
**m. nervo'sus,** mushroom poisoning caused by ingestion of *Amanita pantherina* or *A. muscaria,* which elaborate muscarine. It is marked by such symptoms as tearing, sweating, salivation, persistent peristalsis, retching and vomiting, contraction of the pupil and ciliary muscles, acute excitement, delirium, and coma.
**m. sanguina'rius,** a type of mushroom poisoning caused by ingestion of *Helvella esculenta* or other species of *Helvella;* symptoms include hemoglobinuria, abdominal pain, and jaundice.

**mycet(o)-** [Gr. *mykēs,* gen. *mykētos* fungus] a combining form denoting relationship to fungus. See also *myc(o)-.*

**my·ce·to·gen·ic** (mi"səto-jen'ik) mycetogenous.

**my·ce·tog·e·nous** (mi"sə-toj'ə-nəs) [*myceto-* + *-genous*] caused by fungous growths; called also *mycetogenic.*

**my·ce·to·ma** (mi"sə-to'mə) [*myceto-* + *-oma*] a slowly progressive, destructive infection of the cutaneous and subcutaneous tissues, fascia, and bone caused by certain actinomycetes *(actinomycotic m.)* or fungi *(eumycotic m.),* acquired by traumatic implantation of the fungus or bacterium. It usually involves the foot *(Madura foot)* or leg, although the hand or any other site may be inoculated. The primary lesion is a tumefaction, with granulomas, suppurating abscesses, and sinuses discharging grains or granules representing microcolonies of the pathogen. Called also *maduromycosis.* See also illustration and table.
**actinomycotic m.,** that caused by infection with actinomycetes; see table. Called also *actinomycetoma.*
**eumycotic m.,** that caused by infection with true fungi; see table. Called also *eumycetoma.*

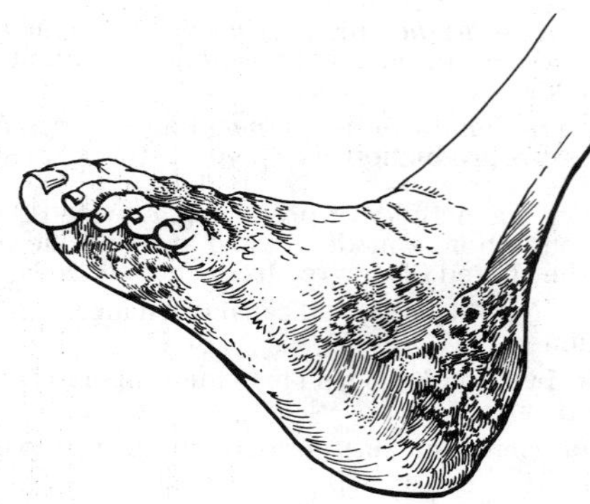

Mycetoma affecting the foot (Madura foot).

**My·ce·to·zoa** (mi-se"to-zo'ə) former name for Myxomycetes when it was considered a group of protozoa.

**My·ce·to·zoi·da** (mi"se-to-zoi'də) former name for Myxomycetes when it was considered a group of protozoa.

**my·cid** (mi'sid) dermatophytid.

**My·cif·ra·din** (mi-sif'rə-din) trademark for preparations of neomycin sulfate.

**Selected Etiologic Agents of Mycetoma**

| Agent | Grain Color |
|---|---|
| Actinomycotic | |
| *Actinomadura madurae* | White to yellow or pink |
| *Actinomadura pellitieri* | Red |
| *Actinomyces israelii* | White to yellow |
| *Nocardia asteroides* | White (when present) |
| *Nocardia brasiliensis* | White |
| *Nocardia otitidis-caviarum* | White to yellow |
| *Nocardiopsis dassonvillei* | Cream color |
| *Streptomyces somaliensis* | Yellow to brown |
| Eumycotic | |
| *Acremonium falciforme* | White to yellow |
| *Acremonium kiliense* | White |
| *Acremonium recifei* | White |
| *Aspergillus nidulans* | White |
| *Corynespora cassicola* | Black |
| *Curvularia geniculata* | Black |
| *Curvularia lunata* | Black |
| *Exophiala jeanselmei* | Black |
| *Fusarium moniliforme* | White |
| *Fusarium oxysporum* | White |
| *Fusarium solani* | White |
| *Leptosphaeria senegalensis* | Black |
| *Leptosphaeria tompkinsii* | Black |
| *Madurella grisea** | Black |
| *Madurella mycetomatis* | Black |
| *Neotestudina rosatii* | White |
| *Phialophora cyanescens* | White |
| *Plenodomus avramii* | Black |
| *Pseudallescheria boydii* | White |
| *Pseudochaetosphaeronema larense* | Black |
| *Pyrenochaeta mackinnonii* | Black |
| *Pyrenochaeta romeroi** | Black |

* Believed to be related if not identical.

**My·ci·guent** (mi′sĭ-gwent″) trademark for preparations of neomycin sulfate.

**myc(o)-** [Gr. *mykēs,* fungus] a combining form denoting relationship to fungus. Also, *mycet(o)-.*

**my·co·bac·te·ria** (mi″ko-bak-tēr-eə) plural of *mycobacterium.*

**My·co·bac·te·ri·a·ceae** (mi″ko-bak-tēr″e-a′se-e) [MeSH: Mycobacteriaceae] a family of bacteria, order Actinomycetales, made up of slightly curved or straight, rod-shaped, gram-positive, aerobic, mesophilic cells, sometimes branching. The organisms are found in soil, water, and dairy products and as parasites in humans and lower animals. The family contains the genus *Mycobacterium.*

**my·co·bac·te·ri·o·sis** (mi″ko-bak-tēr-eo′sis) a disease caused by a mycobacterium, usually excluding *Mycobacterium tuberculosis* (see *nontuberculous mycobacteria* under *mycobacterium*). The incidence of these infections is sharply increased among immunocompromised patients. Called also *atypical tuberculosis.*

**My·co·bac·te·ri·um** (mi″ko-bak-tēr-eəm) [*myco-* + Gr. *baktērion* little rod] [MeSH: Mycobacterium] a genus of bacteria of the family Mycobacteriaceae, order Actinomycetales, occurring as gram-positive, aerobic, mostly slow-growing, slightly curved or straight rods, sometimes branching and filamentous, and distinguished by acid-fast staining. It contains many species, including the highly pathogenic organisms that cause tuberculosis *(M. tuberculosis)* and leprosy *(M. leprae).*
**M. absces′sus,** *M. chelonae.*
**M. africa′num,** a species resembling *M. bovis* and *M. tuberculosis* that is the cause of human disease in tropical Africa.
**M. a′quae,** *M. gordonae.*
**M. a′vium-intracellula′re,** a complex of slow-growing, nonphotochromogenic organisms that cause tuberculosis in birds and swine and are associated with human pulmonary disease, lymphadenitis in children, and serious systemic disease in immunocompromised patients. See also *mycobacteriosis.*
**M. bal′nei,** *M. marinum.*
**M. borstelen′se,** *M. chelonae.*
**M. bo′vis,** a virulent species, isolated originally from tuberculous tubercles in cattle, that causes tuberculosis in humans and lower animals. In humans, the disease is usually acquired by children from infected milk. An attenuated strain of *M. bovis* is used to prepare BCG vaccine.
**M. brunen′se,** *M. avium-intracellulare.*
**M. bu′ruli,** *M. ulcerans.*
**M. chelo′nae,** a rapid-growing, nonphotochromogenic species that is an opportunist pathogen, found in soil and recovered from sputum and soft tissue abscesses throughout the body. It produces synovial lesions, gluteal abscesses, and gross lesions in various organs. Called also *M. abscessus* and *M. borstelense.*
**M. flaves′cens,** a scotochromogenic species isolated from drug-treated tuberculous guinea pigs but considered nonpathogenic for humans.
**M. fortu′itum,** a rapid-growing, nonphotochromogenic species that is potentially pathogenic, producing lesions of lung, bone, or soft tissue following trauma. It has been found in soil and in injection sites of humans, cattle, and cold-blooded animals. Called also *M. ranae.*
**M. gas′tri,** a nonpathogenic species found in soil and gastric and sputum specimens obtained from humans.
**M. gi′ae,** *M. fortuitum.*
**M. gordo′nae,** a scotochromogenic species found in tap water and soil and in human sputum and gastric lavage; it is usually nonpathogenic, but sometimes causes systemic disease in immunocompromised patients.
**M. haba′na,** *M. simiae.*
**M. haemo′philum,** a nonphotochromogenic, pathogenic species that requires hemin for growth; it is a rare cause of ulcerative skin lesions and pulmonary and joint disease in immunocompromised patients.
**M. intracellula′re,** see *M. avium-intracellulare.*
**M. kansa′sii,** a slow-growing, photochromogenic species that is the etiologic agent of a tuberculosis-like disease in humans and is frequently isolated from human pulmonary secretions or tubercles. The incidence of infection is sharply increased among immunocompromised individuals. Called also *M. luciflavum.* See also *photochromogen.*
**M. lep′rae,** the causative agent of human leprosy, not yet cultivated in vitro, isolated from suspect lesions as acid-fast bacilli. They typically occur in intracellular clumps or rounded masses or in groups of bacilli side by side.
**M. lepraemu′rium,** a noncultivable species resembling *M. leprae* in size and shape, which causes a chronic epizootic disease in wild rats; see also *rat leprosy,* under *leprosy.*
**M. littora′le,** *M. xenopi.*
**M. lucifla′vum,** *M. kansasii.*
**M. malmoen′se,** a slow-growing, nonphotochromogenic species associated with pulmonary disease in humans.
**M. maria′num,** *M. scrofulaceum.*
**M. mari′num,** a moderate-growing, photochromogenic species found in aquariums, diseased fish, and swimming pools. It is the cause of cutaneous lesions and granulomas (swimming pool granuloma) in humans. Called also *M. balnei* and *M. platypoecilus.*
**M. micro′ti,** a species producing generalized tuberculosis in field mice and also infecting guinea pigs, rabbits, and calves. It is not virulent for humans and has been used for the preparation of experimental vaccines. Called also *vole bacillus* and *M. tuberculosis* var. *muris.*
**M. minet′ti,** *M. fortuitum.*
**M. moel′leri,** *M. phlei.*
**M. nonchromoge′nicum,** a slow-growing, nonphotochromogenic, nonpathogenic species found in soil.
**M. paraffi′nicum,** *M. scrofulaceum.*
**M. paratuberculo′sis,** the causative agent of Johne's disease, a chronic enteritis of cattle, sheep, and goats; nonpathogenic for man. Called also *Johne's bacillus.*
**M. phle′i,** a rapid-growing, photochromogenic, nonpathogenic species found in grasses and soil. Called also *M. moelleri* and *timothy bacillus.*
**M. platypoe′cilus,** *M. marinum.*
**M. ra′nae,** *M. fortuitum.*
**M. scrofula′ceum,** a slow-growing, scotochromogenic species found in human secretions, particularly pus from suppurating cervical lymphadenitis in children. It also occurs in human sputum and gastric lavage, sometimes in association with pulmonary disease. Called also *M. marianum* and *M. paraffinicum.*
**M. si′miae,** a slow-growing, photochromogenic species that is sometimes pathogenic.
**M. smeg′matis,** a rapid-growing, nonpathogenic, nonphotochromogenic species originally isolated from human smegma and found also in soil and water. Called also *smegma bacillus.*
**M. szul′gai,** a slow-growing, pathogenic species that behaves as a scotochromogen at 37°C. and as a photochromogen at 25°C. It is associated with pulmonary infections but may be found in nonpulmonary sites.
**M. ter′rae,** a slow-growing, nonpathogenic, nonpigmented species found in soil, water, and human sputum and gastric lavage specimens.
**M. trivia′le,** a slow-growing, nonpathogenic, nonpigmented species isolated from sputum and gastric washings.
**M. tuberculo′sis,** a slow-growing, nonphotochromogenic, pathogenic species that is the causative agent of tuberculosis in man, other primates, dogs, guinea pigs, and hamsters. Infection in man is commonly pulmonary; rates of both pulmonary and nonpulmonary disease are sharply increased among immunocompromised individuals. Strains of low virulence have also been isolated from cases of lupus erythematosus, scrofuloderma, and urogenital tuberculosis. Called also *tubercle bacillus* and *M. tuberculosis* var. *hominis.*
**M. tuberculo′sis** var. **a′vium,** *M. avium-intracellulare.*
**M. tuberculo′sis** var. **bo′vis,** *M. bovis.*
**M. tuberculo′sis** var. **ho′minis,** *M. tuberculosis.*
**M. tuberculo′sis** var. **mu′ris,** *M. microti.*
**M. ul′cerans,** a slow-growing, nonphotochromogenic species that causes chronic skin lesions in humans (Buruli ulcer).
**M. vac′cae,** a rapid-growing, scotochromogenic, nonpathogenic species, widely distributed in nature and found in cattle.
**M. xeno′pi,** a slow-growing, scotochromogenic species occurring usually harmlessly in human secretions but occasionally associated with chronic pulmonary disease. Called also *M. littorale.*

**my·co·bac·te·ri·um** (mi″ko-bak-tēr-eəm) pl. *mycobacte′ria* [MeSH: Mycobacterium] an organism of the genus *Mycobacterium.*
**anonymous mycobacteria, atypical mycobacteria,** nontuberculous mycobacteria.
**Group I–IV mycobacteria,** nontuberculous mycobacteria.
**nontuberculous mycobacteria,** mycobacteria other than *M. tuberculosis* or *M. bovis.* They are divided into four groups (Runyon groups) based on pigmentation and rate of growth, each containing several species. Group I includes slow-growing photochromogens; group II slow-growing scotochromogens; group III slow-growing nonphotochromogens; and group IV rapidly growing mycobacteria. Called also *anonymous* or *atypical mycobacteria.*

**my·co·bac·tin** (mi″ko-bak′tin) a complex lipophilic compound found in the cell envelope of certain species of *Mycobacterium;* it is also required for growth by at least one species. Mycobactin chelates iron and facilitates iron transport into the cell.

**My·co·bu·tin** (mi″kə-bu′tin) trademark for a preparation of rifabutin.

**My·co·cen·tros·po·ra** (mi″ko-sen-tros′pə-rə) a genus of Fungi Imperfecti of the form-class Hyphomycetes. *M. aceri′na* has been identified as the cause of verrucose skin lesions.

**My·co·der·ma** (mi″ko-der′mə) a former genus of imperfect fungi whose species are now included in *Candida, Blastomyces, Coccidioi-*

*des,* and *Paracoccidioides. M. ace'ti* is a misnomer for a combination of yeasts that produce acetic acid from fermentation of alcohol.

**my·co·der·ma** (mi″ko-der′mə) tunica mucosa.

**my·co·der·ma·ti·tis** (mi″ko-der″mə-ti′tis) dermatomycosis.

**my·co·flo·ra** (mi″ko-flor′ə) the number and varieties of fungi present in or characteristic of a specific location.

**my·co·he·mia** (mi″ko-he′me-ə) [*myco-* + *-emia*] fungemia.

**my·co·lic ac·ids** (mi-ko′lik) [MeSH: Mycolic Acids] α-alkyl, β-hydroxy substituted long chain fatty acids found in the cell walls of bacteria in the genera *Mycobacterium, Nocardia,* and *Corynebacterium;* they may be responsible for the acid-fast staining properties of these organisms.

**my·col·o·gist** (mi-kol′ə-jist) a person specializing in mycology.

**my·col·o·gy** (mi-kol′ə-je) [*myco-* + *-logy*] [MeSH: Mycology] the science and study of fungi.

**my·co·myr·in·gi·tis** (mi″ko-mir″in-ji′tis) [*myco-* + *myringitis*] myringomycosis.

**my·co·pa·thol·o·gy** (mi″ko-pə-thol′ə-je) the scientific study of the pathologic changes caused by fungi.

**my·co·phage** (mi′ko-fāj) [*myco-* + *-phage*] a virus that infects fungi and may cause their lysis.

**my·coph·a·gy** (mi-kof′ə-je) ingestion of mushrooms and other fungi.

**my·co·pheno·late mo·fe·til** (mi″ko-fen′o-lāt) an immunosuppressive agent used in conjunction with cyclosporine and corticosteroids to prevent rejection of allogeneic renal transplants; administered orally.

**My·co·plas·ma** (mi″ko-plaz′mə) [*myco-* + Gr. *plasma* anything formed or molded] [MeSH: Mycoplasma] a genus of bacteria of the family Mycoplasmataceae, made up of round, highly pleomorphic, gram-negative cells that are bounded by a single triple-layered membrane and lack a true cell wall. Cholesterol or another sterol is required for growth. *M. mycoi′des* causes pleuropneumonia in cattle, and other species comprise the pleuropneumonia-like organisms (see under *organism*). The organisms are parasites and pathogens widely distributed on the mucous membranes of humans, animals, and birds, and are common contaminants of animal cell cultures. Formerly called *Asterococcus.*
**M. agalac′tiae,** a species that causes contagious agalactia in sheep and goats.
**M. bucca′le,** a common inhabitant of the oropharynx of nonhuman primates. Called also *M. orale type 2.*
**M. ca′nis,** a nonpathogenic species commonly found in the throat and respiratory and genital tracts of dogs.
**M. conjunc′tivae,** a species that causes keratoconjunctivitis in sheep and goats.
**M. fau′cium,** a species found occasionally in the oropharynx of humans and frequently in the oropharynx of nonhuman primates. Called also *M. orale type 3.*
**M. fermen′tans,** a species occasionally isolated from the mucosa of the genital tract and oropharynx of humans.
**M. gallisep′ticum,** a pathogen for poultry, causing respiratory disease, encephalitis, and infectious arthritis in chickens and turkeys.
**M. granula′rum,** *Acholeplasma granularum.*
**M. ho′minis,** a common parasitic inhabitant of the vagina and cervix and a potential human pathogen, causing infections of the male and female reproductive tracts. It has also been associated with respiratory disease and pharyngitis.
**M. hyoarthrino′sa,** a species of uncertain status, probably identical to *M. hyosynoviae.*
**M. hyorhi′nis,** a common inhabitant of the nasal cavity in swine; it can cause mycoplasmal polyarthritis or mycoplasmal polyserositis when the animals are under stress.
**M. hyosyno′viae,** a common inhabitant of the nasopharynx of swine; it can cause mycoplasmal polyarthritis when the animals are under stress.
**M. laidla′wii,** *Acholeplasma laidlawii.*
**M. mycoi′des,** the type species of *Mycoplasma,* which is the etiologic agent of pleuropneumonia in cattle and goats. Called also *Bovimyces pleuropneumoniae.*
**M. neuroly′ticum,** a species some strains of which elaborate a neurolytic exotoxin that causes rolling disease in mice.
**M. ora′le,** a species found in the upper respiratory tract of humans and primates. Called also *M. orale type 1* and *M. pharyngis.*
**M. ora′le type 1,** *M. orale.*
**M. ora′le type 2,** *M. buccale.*
**M. ora′le type 3,** *M. faucium.*
**M. pharyn′gis,** *M. orale.*
**M. pneumo′niae,** a species that often causes inapparent infections or mild respiratory tract disease but can also cause a type of primary atypical pneumonia; see also *mycoplasmal pneumonia,* under *pneumonia.* Called also *Eaton agent.*
**M. saliva′rium,** a nonpathogenic species found as part of the normal flora of the human oral cavity and upper respiratory tract.
**M. syno′viae,** a species that causes infectious synovitis in birds.

**my·co·plas·ma** (mi″ko-plaz′mə) pl. *mycoplasmas, mycoplas′mata* [MeSH: Mycoplasma] a bacterium of the class Mollicutes.
**T-strain m.,** *Ureaplasma.*

**my·co·plas·mal** (mi″ko-plaz′məl) of, pertaining to, or caused by *Mycoplasma.*

**My·co·plas·mas** (mi″ko-plaz′məs) Mycoplasmatales.

**My·co·plas·ma·ta·ceae** (mi″ko-plaz″mə-ta′se-e) [MeSH: Mycoplasmataceae] a family of bacteria of the order Mycoplasmatales, class Mollicutes, made up of organisms that require a sterol for growth. It contains the genera *Mycoplasma* and *Ureaplasma.*

**My·co·plas·ma·ta·les** (mi″ko-plaz″mə-ta′ləs) [MeSH: Mycoplasmatales] an order of bacteria of the class Mollicutes, the members of which are bounded by a triple-layered membrane but lack a rigid cell wall. The order is made up of the families Acholeplasmataceae, Mycoplasmataceae, and Spiroplasmataceae, and two genera of uncertain status, *Anaeroplasma* and *Thermoplasma.* Called also *Mycoplasmas.*

**my·co·plas·mo·sis** (mi″ko-plaz-mo′sis) infection with *Mycoplasma*: see also *mycoplasmal pneumonia, polyarthritis,* and *polyserositis.*

**my·co·pre·cip·i·tin** (mi″ko-pre-sip′ĭ-tin) [*myco-* + *precipitin*] a precipitin that will precipitate extracts of yeast and fungi.

**my·co·pus** (mi′ko-pəs) mucus containing pus.

**my·cose** (mi′kōs) trehalose.

**my·co·side** (mi′ko-sīd) a glycolipid that contains mycolic acid and a polysaccharide moiety. A distinctive mycoside found in the cell walls confers immunologic cross-reactivity on cells of *Corynebacterium, Mycobacteria,* and *Nocardia.*

**my·co·sis** (mi-ko′sis) [*myc-* + *-osis*] 1. any disease caused by a fungus. 2. any of various other diseases that were originally thought to be caused by fungi.
**m. fungoi′des,** a chronic or rapidly progressive form of cutaneous T-cell lymphoma (the name is a misnomer because it was formerly thought to be of fungal origin). In some cases it evolves into generalized lymphoma with a tendency for nodal, hematogenous, and visceral involvement. It may be divided generally into three successive stages: the *premycotic stage,* associated with intensely pruritic erythematous, eczematous, or psoriasiform eruptions; the *mycotic stage,* or *stage of infiltrated plaques,* characterized by the presence of abnormal mononuclear cells *(Sézary cells)*; and the *tumor stage,* characterized by mushroomlike tumors that often ulcerate. In a variant type of tumor stage *(d′emblée type)*, tumors may develop without preceding lesions or prodromal symptoms. Called also *granuloma fungoides.*
**m. fungoides d′emblée,** see *m. fungoides.*
**Gilchrist's m.,** blastomycosis (def. 1).
**m. lepto′thrica,** a benign condition of the tonsils and pharynx produced by the bacterium *Leptotrichia buccalis.*
**Posadas' m.,** coccidioidomycosis.
**splenic m.,** siderotic splenomegaly.

**-mycosis** word termination denoting a fungal disease or infection.

**my·cos·ta·sis** (mi-kos′tə-sis) [*myco-* + *stasis*] fungistasis.

**my·co·stat** (mi′ko-stat) fungistat.

**My·co·stat·in** (mi′ko-stat″in) trademark for a preparation of nystatin.

**my·cos·ter·ol** (mi-kos′tə-rol) any of the sterols isolated from fungi.

**my·cot·ic** (mi-kot′ik) 1. pertaining to mycosis. 2. caused by a fungus.

**My·co·tor·u·loi·des** (mi″ko-tor″u-loi′dēz) *Candida.*

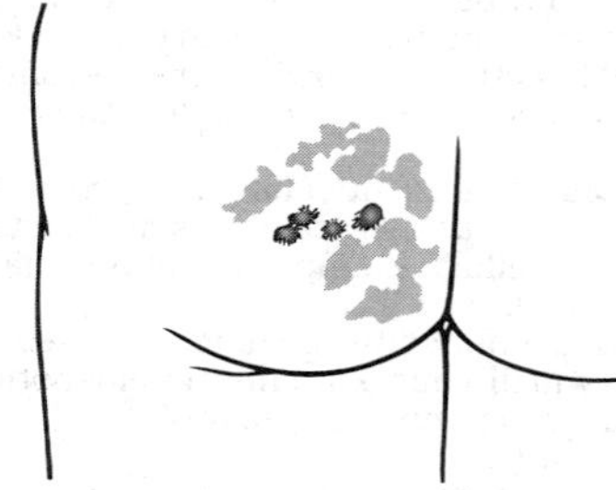

Diffuse patches and sharply demarcated plaques on the buttock in mycosis fungoides.

**my·co·tox·i·co·sis** (mi″ko-tok″sĭ-ko′sis) [MeSH: Mycotoxicosis] 1. poisoning caused by a fungal or bacterial toxin. 2. poisoning resulting from ingestion of fungi. See table, and see also *mushroom poisoning.* Called also *mycetism* and *mycetismus.*

**my·co·tox·in** (mi″ko-tok′sin) a fungal toxin.

**my·co·tox·in·iza·tion** (mi″ko-tok″sin-ĭ-za′shən) inoculation with a mycotoxin.

**myc·tero·xe·ro·sis** (mik″tər-o-ze-ro′sis) [Gr. *myktēr* nostril + *xerosis*] dryness of the nostrils.

**My·dri·a·cyl** (mĭ-dri′ə-səl) trademark for a preparation of tropicamide.

**my·dri·a·sis** (mĭ-dri′ə-sis) [Gr.] [MeSH: Mydriasis] 1. physiologic dilatation of the pupil. 2. morbid dilatation of the pupil. 3. dilatation of the pupil effected by a drug.
**alternating m.**, varying inequality of the pupils, mydriasis occurring first on one side, then on the other; called also *bounding* or *springing m.*
**bounding m.**, alternating m.
**paralytic m.**, that caused by paralysis of the oculomotor nerve.
**spasmodic m., spastic m.**, that due to spasm of the dilator of the iris or to overaction of the sympathetic.
**spinal m.**, that due to lesion of the ciliospinal center of the spinal cord.
**springing m.**, alternating m.

**myd·ri·at·ic** (mid″re-at′ik) 1. dilating the pupil. 2. any drug that dilates the pupil.

**my·ec·to·my** (mi-ek′tə-me) [*my-* + *-ectomy*] excision of a portion of muscle.

**my·ec·to·pia** (mi-ek-to′pe-ə) [*myo-* + *ectopia*] displacement of a muscle.

**my·ec·to·py** (mi-ek′tə-pe) myectopia.

**my·el·al·gia** (mi″ə-lal′jə) [*myel-* + *-algia*] pain in the spinal cord.

**my·el·ap·o·plexy** (mi″əl-ap′o-plek-se) [*myel-* + *apoplexy*] hematomyelia.

**my·el·ate·lia** (mi″el-ə-te′le-ə) [*myel-* + *atelia*] myelodysplasia.

**my·el·at·ro·phy** (mi″əl-at′rə-fe) [*myel-* + *atrophy*] atrophy of the spinal cord.

**my·el·auxe** (mi″əl-awk′se) [*myel-* + Gr. *auxē* increase] morbid increase in size of the spinal cord.

**my·el·emia** (mi″ə-le′me-ə) [*myel-* + *-emia*] myelocytosis.

**my·el·en·ceph·a·li·tis** (mi″əl-en-sef″ə-li′tis) encephalomyelitis.

**my·el·en·ceph·a·lon** (mi″əl-en-sef′ə-lon) [*myel-* + *encephalon*] [MeSH: Medulla Oblongata] 1. [TA] official nomenclature for *medulla oblongata* (q.v.). 2. the posterior of the two brain vesicles formed by specialization of the rhombencephalon in the developing embryo.

**my·el·en·ceph·a·lo·spi·nal** (mi″əl-en-sef″ə-lo-spi′nəl) pertaining to the myelencephalon and spinal cord.

**my·elin** (mi′ə-lin) [Gr. *myelos* marrow] the substance of the cell membrane of Schwann's cells that coils to form the myelin sheath (see under *sheath*); it has a high proportion of lipid to protein and serves as an electrical insulator.

**my·eli·nat·ed** (mi′ə-lĭ-nāt″əd) having a myelin sheath.

**my·eli·na·tion** (mi″ə-lĭ-na′shən) myelinization.

**my·elin·ic** (mi″ə-lin′ik) pertaining to or of the nature of myelin.

**my·eli·ni·za·tion** (mi″ə-lĭ-nĭ-za′shən) the act of furnishing with or taking on myelin; formation of a myelin sheath. Called also *medullation, myelination,* and *myelinogenesis.*

**my·eli·noc·la·sis** (mi″ə-lĭ-nok′lə-sis) [*myelin* + Gr. *klasis* a breaking] myelinolysis.
**acute perivascular m.**, acute disseminated encephalomyelitis.
**postinfection perivenous m.**, postinfection encephalomyelopathy.

**my·elino·gen·e·sis** (mi″ə-lin″o-jen′ə-sis) myelinization.

**my·elino·ge·net·ic** (mi″ə-lin″o-jə-net′ik) producing myelin; producing myelinization.

**my·eli·nog·e·ny** (mi″əl-ĭ-noj′ə-ne) [*myelin* + *-geny*] myelogeny.

**my·eli·nol·y·sis** (mi″ə-lin-ol′ə-sis) demyelination.
**central pontine m.**, a form of widespread demyelination of the pons occurring in alcoholics.

**my·eli·nop·a·thy** (mi″ə-lĭ-nop′ə the) any disease of the myelin; degeneration of the white matter of the brain.

**my·eli·no·sis** (mi″ə-lĭ-no′sis) fat decomposition in which myelin is formed.

**my·elino·tox·ic** (mi″ə-lin-o-tok′sik) having a deleterious effect on myelin; causing demyelination.

**my·elino·tox·ic·i·ty** (mi″ə-lin-o-tok-sis′ĭ-te) the property of being myelinotoxic.

**my·elit·ic** (mi″ə-lit′ik) pertaining to myelitis.

**my·eli·tis** (mi″ə-li′tis) [*myel-* + *-itis*] [MeSH: Myelitis] 1. inflammation of the spinal cord, often part of a more specifically defined disease process. One group of diseases is named according to whether primarily white matter or gray matter is affected (see *leukomyelitis* and *poliomyelitis*); another group is defined by whether there is coexistent disease of the meninges *(meningomyelitis)* or the brain *(encephalomyelitis).* In practice, the term is also used to denote noninflammatory lesions of the spinal cord; see *myelopathy.* 2. inflammation of the bone marrow; see *osteomyelitis.*
**acute m.**, any rapidly developing inflammatory disease of the spinal cord.
**ascending m.**, see under *myelopathy.*
**bulbar m.**, that which involves the medulla oblongata.
**cavitary m.**, syringomyelia.
**central m.**, inflammation affecting chiefly the gray substance of the spinal cord; see *poliomyelitis* and *syringomyelia.*
**chronic m.**, a slowly progressing inflammation of the spinal cord; taking between six weeks and two years after onset to full manifestation of the disease.

**Types of Mycotoxicosis**

| Fungus | Condition(s) Caused | Toxin |
|---|---|---|
| *Acremonium coenophialum* | Fescue foot | Unknown |
| *Acremonium lolii* | Rye grass staggers | Unknown |
| *Alternaria* species | Alternariatoxicosis | Unknown |
| *Aspergillus* (any species) | Aspergillustoxicosis | Various |
| (1) *A. clavatus, A. giganteus, A. terreus* | (Neurotoxicity) | Patulin |
| (2) *A. flavus* et al. | Aflatoxicosis | Aflatoxin |
| (3) *A. ochraceus* | Ochratoxicosis | Ochratoxin |
| *Claviceps paspali* | Paspalum staggers | Unknown |
| *Claviceps purpurea* | Ergotism | Ergot alkaloids |
| *Dendrodochium toxicum* | Dendrodochiotoxicosis | Unknown |
| *Diplodia* species | Diplodiosis | Unknown |
| *Endoconidium temulentum* | Darnel poisoning (endoconidiotoxicosis) | Unknown |
| *Fusarium culmorum, F. roseum* | (Vulvovaginitis) | Zearalenone |
| *Fusarium culmorum, F. roseum, F. moniliforme, F. sporotrichioides* | Forage poisoning (fusariotoxicosis) | T-2 toxin, deoxynivalenol, diacetoxyscirpenol |
| *Myrothecium roridum, M. verrucaria* | Myrotheciotoxicosis | Roridin, verrucarin |
| *Penicillium citrinum* | (Nephrotoxicity) | Citrinin |
| *Penicillium claviforme, P. expansum, P. patulum,* et al. | (Neurotoxicity) | Patulin |
| *Phomopsis leptostromiformis, P. rossiana* | Mycotoxic lupinosis | Phomopsin |
| *Pithomyces chartarum* | Facial eczema of ruminants (pithomycotoxicosis) | Sporidesmin |
| *Rhizoctonia leguminicola* | Slobbers | Slaframine |
| *Stachybotrys atra* | Stachybotryotoxicosis | Roridin, satratoxin, verrucarin |

**compression m.**, see under *myelopathy.*
**concussion m.**, see under *myelopathy.*
**cornual m.**, that which affects the horns of gray matter of the spinal cord; see also *poliomyelitis.*
**diffuse m.**, disseminated m.
**disseminated m.**, a form with several distinct foci in the spinal cord.
**hemorrhagic m.**, hematomyelitis.
**neuro-optic m.**, neuromyelitis optica.
**periependymal m.**, myelitis surrounding the central canal of the spinal cord.
**postinfectious m.**, myelitis occurring after a viral infection; see also *acute disseminated encephalomyelitis.*
**postvaccinal m.**, myelitis occurring after vaccination; see also *acute disseminated encephalomyelitis.* Called also *m. vaccinia.*
**subacute m.**, myelitis that develops over a period of a few weeks; cf. *acute m.* and *chronic m.*
**subacute necrotic m.**, Foix-Alajouanine syndrome.
**syphilitic m.**, myelitis occurring as part of meningovascular neurosyphilis.
**transverse m.**, myelitis in which the functional effect of the lesions spans the width of the entire cord at a given level.
**m. vacci'nia**, postvaccinal m.
**viral m.**, myelitis due to infection of the spinal cord by a virus, such as poliovirus, herpesvirus, or human immunodeficiency virus.

**myel(o)-** [Gr. *myelos* marrow] a combining form denoting relationship to marrow, to the spinal cord, or to myelin.

**my·elo·ab·la·tion** (mi″ə-lo-ab-la′shən) [*myelo-* + *ablation*] severe myelosuppression.

**my·e·lo·ab·la·tive** (mi″ə-lo-ab′lə-tiv) pertaining to or causing myeloablation.

**my·elo·ar·chi·tec·ture** (mi″ə-lo-ahr′kĭ-tek″chər) 1. the arrangement of nerve fibers in the cerebral and cerebellar cortices. 2. the organization of the nerve tracts in the spinal cord and brain stem.

**my·elo·blast** (mi′ə-lo-blast) [*myelo-* + *-blast*] an immature cell found in the bone marrow and not normally in the peripheral blood, the most primitive precursor in the granulocytic series, which develops into the promyelocyte. Myeloblasts have fine, evenly distributed chromatin, several nucleoli, and a nongranular basophilic cytoplasm. Called also *granuloblast.*

**my·elo·blas·te·mia** (mi″ə-lo-blas-te′me-ə) [*myeloblast* + *-emia*] the presence of myeloblasts in the blood, as in acute myeloblastic leukemia.

**my·elo·blas·to·ma** (mi″ə-lo-blas-to′mə) [*myeloblast* + *-oma*] a focal malignant tumor, observed in acute myelogenous leukemia, composed of myeloblasts or early myeloid precursors occurring outside of the bone marrow.

**my·elo·blas·to·ma·to·sis** (mi″ə-lo-blas″to-mə-to′sis) the presence of multiple myeloblastomas.

**my·elo·blas·to·sis** (mi″ə-lo-blas-to′sis) 1. the presence of an excess of myeloblasts in the blood, as in acute myeloblastic leukemia. 2. avian m.
**avian m.**, a neoplastic viral disease of chickens, one of the avian leukosis complex, with proliferation of malignant myeloblasts in the bone marrow, liver, spleen, and kidneys, as well as spontaneous hemorrhages. Called also *myeloblastic leukosis.*

**my·elo·cele** (mi′ə-lo-sēl) [*myelo-* + *-cele*[1]] protrusion of the substance of the spinal cord through a defect in the vertebral arch, with varying degrees of protective covering; cf. *myelomeningocele.*

**my·elo·clast** (mi′ə-lo-klast) [*myelo-* + *-clast*] a cell which splits up myelin sheaths.

**my·elo·cyst** (mi′ə-lo-sist) [*myelo-* + *cyst*] a benign cyst developed from rudimentary medullary canals.

**my·elo·cys·tic** (mi″ə-lo-sis′tik) both myeloid and cystic in structure.

**my·elo·cys·to·cele** (mi″ə-lo-sis′to-sēl) [*myelo-* + *cysto-* + *-cele*[1]] myelomeningocele.

**my·elo·cys·to·me·nin·go·cele** (mi″ə-lo-sis″to-mə-ning′go-sēl) myelomeningocele.

**my·elo·cyte** (mi′ə-lo-sīt) [*myelo-* + *-cyte*] a precursor in the granulocytic series, being a cell intermediate in development between a promyelocyte and a metamyelocyte; in this stage, differentiation of cytoplasmic granules has begun, so that they are specifically basophilic, eosinophilic, or neutrophilic.

**my·elo·cy·the·mia** (mi″ə-lo-si-the′me-ə) myelocytosis.

**my·elo·cyt·ic** (mi″ə-lo-sit′ik) pertaining to myelocytes.

**my·elo·cy·to·ma** (mi″ə-lo-si-to′mə) 1. chronic granulocytic leukemia. 2. myeloma.

**my·elo·cy·to·ma·to·sis** (mi″ə-lo-si″to-mə-to′sis) a neoplastic viral disease of fowl, one of the avian leukosis complex, marked by bone tumors composed of myeloid cells, and sometimes increased numbers of myeloid cells in the circulating blood.

**my·elo·cy·to·sis** (mi″ə-lo-si-to′sis) the presence of an excessive number of myelocytes in the blood; see also *myelodysplasia* (def. 1). Called also *myelocythemia* and *myelosis.*

**my·elo·dys·pla·sia** (mi″ə-lo-dis-pla′zhə) [*myelo-* + *dysplasia*] 1. a neural tube defect (q.v.) causing defective development of any part of the spinal cord, especially the lower segments. Called also *myelatelia.* 2. dysplasia of myelocytes and other elements in bone marrow, which may take the form of myelosuppression or of abnormal proliferation; in the latter case it may precede myelogenous leukemia. See also *myelodysplastic syndrome,* under *syndrome.*

**my·elo·dys·plas·tic** (mi″ə-lo-dis-plas′tik) pertaining to myelodysplasia.

**my·elo·en·ce·phal·ic** (mi″ə-lo-en″sə-fal′ik) cerebrospinal.

**my·elo·en·ceph·a·li·tis** (mi″ə-lo-en-sef″ə-li′tis) [*myelo-* + *encephal-* + *-itis*] inflammation of the spinal cord and brain; called also *encephalomyelitis.*
**eosinophilic m.**, a complex of neurologic symptoms produced by invasion of the central nervous system by *Gnathostoma spinigerum,* including severe nerve root pain, followed by paralysis of extremities and sudden sensorial impairment, accompanied by eosinophilic pleocytosis and bloody or xanthochromic spinal fluid.
**equine protozoal m.**, a condition in horses consisting of myelitis and encephalitis from central nervous system infection with an unknown protozoan, possibly a species of *Sarcocystis*; symptoms include lameness and ataxia, usually asymmetric, progressing to paresis and sometimes blindness, facial paralysis, and dysphagia.

**my·e·lo·en·ceph·a·lop·a·thy** (mi″ə-lo-en-sef″ə-lop′ə-the) encephalomyelopathy.
**equine degenerative m.**, a disease of young horses with degeneration of axons and myelin in the spinal cord and medulla oblongata; spasticity, defective proprioception, and ataxia develop progressively, sometimes ending as paraplegia or paralysis. It may be either hereditary or due to a vitamin E deficiency.

**my·elo·fi·bro·sis** (mi″ə-lo-fi-bro′sis) [MeSH: Myelofibrosis] replacement of the bone marrow by fibrous tissue, occurring in association with a myeloproliferative disorder such as agnogenic myeloid metaplasia or secondary to another unrelated condition. Called also *myelosclerosis.*
**osteosclerosis m.**, myelosclerosis, def. 2.

**my·elof·u·gal** (mi″ə-lof′u-gəl) [*myelo-* + *-fugal*] spinifugal.

**my·elo·gen·e·sis** (mi″ə-lo-jen′ə-sis) 1. myelinization. 2. myelopoiesis.

**my·elo·gen·ic** (mi″ə-lo-jen′ik) 1. myelogenous. 2. myelopoietic.

**my·elog·e·nous** (mi″ə-loj′ə-nəs) [*myelo-* + *-genous*] 1. produced in the bone marrow; called also *myelogenic.* 2. myelinogenetic.

**my·elog·e·ny** (mi″ə-loj′ə-ne) the maturation of the myelin sheaths of nerve fibers in the development of the central nervous system. Cf. *myelinization.*

**my·elo·gone** (mi′ə-lo-gōn″) a white blood cell of the myeloid series having a reticulate violaceous nucleus, well-stained nucleolus, and a deep-blue rim of cytoplasm.

**my·elo·gram** (mi′ə-lo-gram) 1. a radiograph of the spinal cord. 2. a graphic representation of the differential count of cells found in a stained preparation of bone marrow.

**my·elog·ra·phy** (mi″ə-log′rə-fe) [*myelo-* + *-graphy*] [MeSH: Myelography] radiography of the spinal cord after injection of a contrast medium into the subarachnoid space.
**oxygen m.**, myelography in which oxygen is used as the contrast medium.

**my·eloid** (mi′ə-loid) [*myelo-* + *-oid*] 1. resembling bone marrow. 2. having the appearance of myelocytes, but not derived from bone marrow. 3. medullary (def. 2). 4. medullary (def. 3).

**my·eloi·din** (mi″ə-loi′din) [*myelin* + Gr. *eidos* form] a substance resembling myelin, occurring in the pigmented cells of the retina.

**my·eloi·do·sis** (mi″ə-loi-do′sis) the development of myeloid tissue, especially hyperplastic development of such tissue.

**my·elo·ken·tric** (mi″ə-lo-ken′trik) [*myeloid* + Gr. *kentron* stimulus] stimulating myelopoiesis.

**my·elo·li·po·ma** (mi″ə-lo-lĭ-po′mə) [MeSH: Myelolipoma] a rare benign tumor of the adrenal gland, several centimeters in diameter, composed in varying proportions of adipose tissue, lymphocytes, and primitive myeloid cells, probably a developmental abnormality.

**my·elol·y·sis** (mi″ə-lol′ĭ-sis) demyelination.

**my·elo·lyt·ic** (mi″ə-lo-lit′ik) myelinolytic.

**my·elo·ma** (mi″ə-lo′mə) [*myelo-* + *-oma*] a tumor composed of cells of the type normally found in the bone marrow; see *multiple m.*
**giant cell m.**, giant cell tumor of bone.
**indolent m.**, a variant of multiple myeloma in which the tumor cells are hypoproliferative; an M component and bone marrow plasmacytosis are present, but significant bone marrow destruction, hypercalcemia, and Bence Jones proteinuria are absent.
**localized m.**, solitary m.
**multiple m.**, a disseminated type of plasma cell dyscrasia characterized by multiple bone marrow tumor foci and secretion of an M component, associated with widespread osteolytic lesions resulting in bone pain, pathologic fractures, hypercalcemia, and normochromic normocytic anemia; spread to extraosseous sites occurs frequently in advanced disease. Depression of immunoglobulin levels results in increased susceptibility to infection. Bence Jones proteinuria is present in many cases and may result in systemic amyloidosis. Renal failure from calcium nephropathy or extensive cast formation may also occur. Called also *plasma cell m.* See also *myeloma cell*, under *cell*.
**plasma cell m.**, multiple m.
**sclerosing m.**, myeloma associated with osteosclerosis, most often manifested by peripheral neuropathy; the myeloma involved may be localized or a part of multiple myeloma. POEMS syndrome (q.v.) may be present.
**solitary m.**, a variant of multiple myeloma in which there is a single localized tumor focus. Called also *localized m.*

**my·elo·ma·la·cia** (mi″ə-lo-mə la′shə) [*myelo-* + *-malacia*] morbid softening of the spinal cord.

**my·elo·ma·toid** (mi″ə-lo′mə-toid) resembling myeloma.

**my·elo·ma·to·sis** (mi″ə-lo-mə-to′sis) multiple myeloma.

**my·elo·me·nia** (mi″ə-lo-me′ne-ə) [*myelo-* + *men-* + *-ia*] menstrual hemorrhage into the spinal cord, associated with plaques of endometriosis in the spinal canal.

**my·elo·men·in·gi·tis** (mi″ə-lo-men″in-ji′tis) meningomyelitis.

**my·elo·me·nin·go·cele** (mi″ə-lo-mə-ning′go-sēl″) [*myelo-* + *meningocele*] hernial protrusion of the spinal cord and its meninges through a defect in the vertebral arch (spina bifida); cf. *spinal meningocele.* Called also *meningomyelocele* and *myelocystocele.*

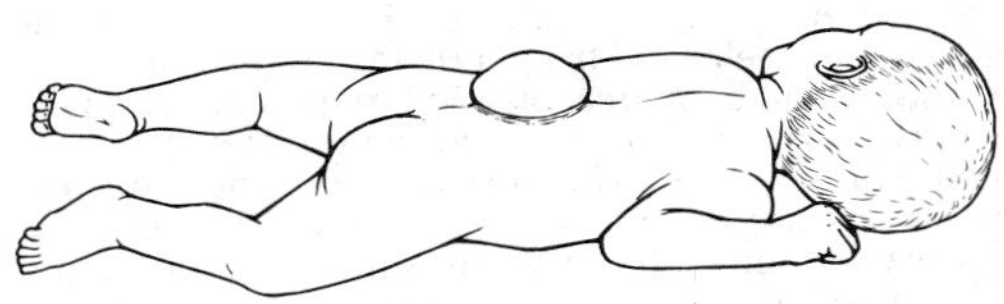

Myelomeningocele.

**my·elo·mere** (mi′ə-lo-mēr) [*myelo-* + *-mere*] one of the segments of the developing brain and spinal cord.

**my·elo·mono·cyt·ic** (mi″ə-lo-mon″o-sit′ik) characterized by both myelocytes and monocytes; said of leukemia.

**my·elo·neu·ri·tis** (mi″ə-lo-noo-ri′tis) neuromyelitis.

**my·elo·op·ti·co·neu·rop·a·thy** (mi″ə-lo-op″tĭ-ko-noo-rop′ə-the) a disorder affecting the spinal cord and optic nerve.
**subacute m.-o.**, a clinical syndrome reported from Japan affecting the spinal cord, optic nerve, and peripheral nerves, preceded by diarrhea. Symptoms include paresthesia in both lower limbs, gait disturbances, visual disturbances, abnormalities of deep tendon reflexes, and psychic disorders. The hydroxyquinolones (especially clioquinol), taken for gastrointestinal disorders, have been implicated as an etiologic factor. Abbreviated SMON.

**my·elo·path·ic** (mi″ə-lo-path′ik) pertaining to or characterized by myelopathy.

**my·elop·a·thy** (mi″ə-lop′ə-the) [*myelo-* + *-pathy*] 1. any of various functional disturbances or pathological changes in the spinal cord, often referring to nonspecific lesions in contrast to the inflammatory lesions of myelitis. 2. a pathological condition of the bone marrow; see also *myelodysplasia* (def. 2).
**anterior m.**, anterior spinal artery syndrome.
**ascending m.**, myelopathy that progresses cephalad along the spinal cord.
**carcinomatous m.**, a rapidly progressive, paraneoplastic myelopathy, most often associated with carcinoma of the lung, but also seen with other carcinomas. It is characterized by a rapidly developing myelopathic syndrome due to necrosis of both the gray and white matter of the spinal cord. Called also *paraneoplastic m.* and *paracarcinomatous m.*
**cervical m.**, compression myelopathy of the cervical spinal cord, a complication that occasionally arises from rheumatoid arthritis or osteoarthritis.
**cervical spondylotic m.**, spondylotic cervical m.
**cervical stenotic m., cervical vertebral stenotic m.**, wobbler syndrome (def. 2).
**chronic progressive m.**, gradually progressive spastic paraparesis associated with infection by human T-lymphotropic virus 1, characterized by progressive difficulty in walking and weakness of the lower extremity, sensory disturbances, and urinary incontinence, with no evidence of spinal compression or motor neuron involvement. Called also *HTLV-1–associated m.* and *tropical spastic paraparesis.*
**compression m.**, myelopathy due to pressure on the spinal cord, as from a tumor.
**concussion m.**, myelopathy due to concussion of the spinal cord (q.v.).
**cystic m.**, syringomyelia.
**descending m.**, myelopathy that progresses caudad along the spinal cord.
**focal m.**, myelopathy affecting a small area only, or several small areas.
**funicular m.**, leukomyelopathy.
**hemorrhagic m.**, myelopathy associated with hemorrhage; see also *hematomyelia.*
**hereditary m.**, an autosomal recessive disease seen in young Afghan hounds, characterized by cavitation and necrosis of the white matter of the spinal cord, with pelvic limb paralysis before the age of one year.
**HTLV-1–associated m.**, chronic progressive m.
**necrotizing m.**, myelopathy marked by necrosis of the spinal cord.
**paracarcinomatous m., paraneoplastic m.**, carcinomatous m.
**radiation m.**, a slowly progressive myelopathy occurring six months or longer after excessive exposure of the spinal cord to radiation, usually in the form of radiation therapy.
**spondylotic cervical m.**, myelopathy secondary to encroachment by cervical spondylosis on the spinal cord within the spinal canal, often in those with a congenitally small spinal canal; called also *cervical spondylotic m.*
**systemic m.**, myelopathy which affects distinct tracts in the spinal cord.
**transverse m.**, myelopathy which extends across the spinal cord.
**traumatic m.**, myelopathy which follows injury to the spinal cord.
**vacuolar m.**, loss of myelin and spongy degeneration of the spinal cord with microscopic vacuolization, similar to that of subacute combined degeneration of the spinal cord, caused by infection with human immunodeficiency virus. Symptoms include spastic paraparesis, sensory ataxia in the lower limbs, and unsteadiness of gait.

**my·elo·per·ox·i·dase** (mi″ə-lo-pər-ok′sĭ-dās) an oxidoreductase that catalyzes the reaction of hydrogen peroxide and halide ions to produce cytotoxic acids (such as hypochlorous acid) and other intermediates; these play a role in oxygen-dependent killing of microorganisms and tumor cells. The enzyme is a hemoprotein found in the azurophil granules of neutrophils and the primary lysosomes of monocytes and it has the green color seen in pus. Deficiency of the enzyme, an autosomal recessive or acquired trait, is usually asymptomatic but may predispose affected individuals to severe fungal infections. Abbreviated MPO.

**my·elo·per·ox·i·dase (MPO) de·fi·cien·cy** an autosomal recessive trait characterized by the complete absence of MPO in azurophil granules of neutrophils and monocytes; the deficiency is usually clinically insignificant.

**my·elop·e·tal** (mi″ə-lop′ə-təl) [*myelo-* + *-petal*] spinipetal.

**my·elo·phage** (mi′ə-lo-fāj″) [*myelo-* + *-phage*] a macrophage which digests or breaks down myelin.

**my·elo·phthis·ic** (mi″ə-lo-tiz′ik) 1. myelosuppressive. 2. causing wasting of the spinal cord.

**my·e·loph·thi·sis** (mi″ə-lof′thĭ-sis) [*myelo-* + *phthisis*] 1. wasting of the spinal cord. 2. bone marrow suppression.

**my·elo·plast** (mi′ə-lo-plast″) [*myelo-* + *-plast*] any leukocyte of the bone marrow.

**my·elo·ple·gia** (mi″ə-lo-ple′jə) [*myelo-* + *-plegia*] spinal paralysis.

**my·elo·poi·e·sis** (mi″ə-lo-poi-e′sis) [*myelo-* + *-poiesis*] the formation of bone marrow or the cells that arise from it. See also *hematopoiesis.* Called also *medullation* and *myelogenesis.*
**ectopic m., extramedullary m.**, the formation of myeloid tissue outside the bone marrow.

**my·elo·poi·et·ic** (mi″ə-lo-poi-et′ik) pertaining to myelopoiesis; called also *myelogenic.*

**my·elo·pore** (mi′ə-lo-por) [*myelo-* + *pore*] a canal or opening in the spinal cord.

**my·elo·pro·lif·er·a·tive** (mi″ə-lo-pro-lif′ər-ə-tiv) pertaining to or characterized by medullary and extramedullary proliferation of bone marrow constituents, including erythroblasts, granulocytes, megakaryocytes, and fibroblasts. See under *disorder* and see also *lymphoproliferative.*

**my·elo·ra·dic·u·li·tis** (mi″ə-lo-rə-dik″u-li′tis) [*myelo-* + *radiculitis*] inflammation of the spinal cord and the posterior nerve roots.

**my·elo·ra·dic·u·lo·dys·pla·sia** (mi″ə-lo-rə-dik″u-lo-dis-pla′zhə) developmental abnormality of the spinal cord and spinal nerve roots.

**my·elo·ra·dic·u·lop·a·thy** (mi″ə-lo-rə-dik″u-lop′ə-the) disease of the spinal cord and spinal nerve roots; called also *radiculomyelopathy.*

**my·elor·rha·gia** (mi″ə-lo-ra′jə) [*myelo-* + *-rrhagia*] hematomyelia.

**my·elo·sar·co·ma** (mi″ə-lo-sahr-ko′mə) a sarcomatous growth made up of myeloid tissue or bone marrow cells; see also *myeloma.*

**my·elo·sar·co·ma·to·sis** (mi″ə-lo-sahr-ko″mə-to′sis) multiple myeloma.

**my·elos·chi·sis** (mi″ə-los′kĭ-sis) [*myelo-* + *-schisis*] a developmental anomaly characterized by a cleft spinal cord, owing to failure of the neural plate to form a complete neural tube or to rupture of the neural tube after closure. Cf. *diastematomyelia* and *spina bifida.*

**my·elo·scle·ro·sis** (mi″ə-lo-sklə-ro′sis) 1. sclerosis of the spinal cord, such as in multiple sclerosis. 2. obliteration of the normal marrow cavity by small spicules of bone; the pathogenesis may be similar to that of myelofibrosis. Called also *osteosclerosis myelofibrosis.* 3. myelofibrosis.

**my·el·o·sis** (mi″ə-lo′sis) 1. myelocytosis. 2. the formation of a tumor of the spinal cord.
**aleukemic m., chronic nonleukemic m.,** agnogenic myeloid metaplasia.
**erythremic m.,** erythroleukemia.
**nonleukemic m.,** agnogenic myeloid metaplasia.

**my·elo·spon·gi·um** (mi″ə-lo-spon′ge-əm) [*myelo-* + Gr. *spongos* sponge] the network from which the neuroglial tissue is developed: it pervades the embryonic neural tube, and is composed of the spongioblasts and their branching processes.

**my·elo·sup·pres·sion** (mi″ə-lo-sə-presh′ən) bone marrow suppression.

**my·elo·sup·pres·sive** (mi″ə-lo-sə-pres′iv) 1. causing bone marrow suppression. 2. an agent causing bone marrow suppression.

**my·elo·syph·i·lis** (mi″ə-lo-sif′ĭ-lis) spinal syphilis.

**my·elo·ther·a·py** (mi″ə-lo-ther′ə-pe) [*myelo-* + *therapy*] the therapeutic use of bone marrow. Cf. *bone marrow transplantation.*

**my·elo·tome** (mi′ə-lo-tōm) [*myelo-* + *-tome*] 1. an instrument for making sections of the spinal cord. 2. an instrument used for cutting the spinal cord squarely across in removing the brain in postmortem examinations.

**my·elot·o·my** (mi″ə-lot′-o-me) the operation of severing tracts in the spinal cord.
**Bischof's m.,** surgical division of the spinal cord longitudinally through the lumbar region to relieve spasticity.
**commissural m.,** longitudinal division of the spinal cord, to sever crossing sensory fibers and produce localized analgesia.

**my·elo·tox·ic** (mi″ə-lo-tok′sik) [*myelo-* + *toxic*] 1. destructive to bone marrow. 2. myelosuppressive. 3. arising from diseased bone marrow.

**my·elo·tox·ic·i·ty** (mi″ə-lo-tok-sis′ĭ-te) the quality of being myelotoxic.

**my·en·ter·ic** (mi″ən-ter′ik) pertaining to the myenteron; see also under *plexus* and *reflex.*

**my·en·ter·on** (mi-en′tər-on) [*my-* + *enteron*] the muscular coat of the intestine.

**My·er·son's sign** (mi′ər-sənz) [Abraham *Myerson,* American neurologist, 1881–1948] see under *sign.*

**my·es·the·sia** (mi″es-the′zhə) [*my-* + *esthesia*] muscle sense (def. 1).

**my·i·a·sis** (mi-i′ə-sis) [Gr. *myia* fly + *-iasis*] [MeSH: Myiasis] a condition caused by infestation of the body by fly maggots.
**creeping m.,** larva migrans caused by fly larvae.
**cutaneous m.,** 1. infestation of an animal by maggots in areas of thick hair or wool and on nearby skin, usually when the area is chronically wet or fouled by feces or urine; sheep are particularly susceptible, and serious cases may result in skin breakdown and death. The maggots are usually larvae of *Phaenicia, Phormia, Chrysomyia,* or *Calliphora* species. Several different types are distinguished according to the part of the body infested; see under *strike.* 2. m. linearis.
**cutaneous blowfly m.,** cutaneous myiasis (def. 1) by blowflies. Called also *blowfly strike* and *fly strike.*
**dermal m.,** 1. cutaneous m. (def. 1). 2. m. linearis. 3. larva migrans.
**intestinal m.,** the presence of living fly larvae in the intestines.
**m. linea′ris,** cutaneous larva migrans (def. 2) caused by fly larvae. Called also *cutaneous* or *dermal m., dermamyiasis,* and *dermatomyiasis.*
**nasal m.,** myiasis in the nasal passages.
**traumatic m., wound m.,** cutaneous myiasis at the site of a wound or ulcer. Called also *wound strike.*

**my·io·ceph·a·lon** (mi-i″o-sef′ə-lon) iridocele.

**my·io·ceph·a·lum** (mi-i″o-sef′ə-ləm) iridocele.

**my·io·des·op·sia** (mi-i″o-dəs-op′se-ə) [Gr. *myiōdes* flylike + *-opsia*] the appearance of muscae volitantes.

**my·io·sis** (mi″i-o′sis) myiasis.

**my·itis** (mi-i′tis) [*my-* + *-itis*] myositis.

**myk(o)-** for words beginning thus, see those beginning *myc(o)-.*

**My·krox** (mi′kroks) trademark for a preparation of metolazone.

**My·ler·an** (mi′lər-an) trademark for a preparation of busulfan.

**My·li·con** (mi′lĭ-kon) trademark for preparations of simethicone.

**my·lo·hy·oid** (mi″lo-hi′oid) [Gr. *myloi* molar teeth + *hyoid*] pertaining to molar teeth and the hyoid bone.

**my·lo·pha·ryn·ge·al** (mi″lo-fə-rin′je-əl) [Gr. *mylai* molar teeth + *pharyngeal*] pertaining to molar teeth and the pharynx.

**My·meth·a·sone** (mi-meth′ə-sōn″) trademark for a preparation of dexamethasone.

**my(o)-** [Gr. *mys,* gen. *myos* muscle] a combining form denoting relationship to muscle.

**myo·ad·en·yl·ate de·am·i·nase** (mi″o-ad′ən-əl-āt de-am′ĭ-nās) the muscle isozyme of AMP deaminase. See *isoenzyme A* under *AMP deaminase.*

**myo·ad·en·yl·ate de·am·i·nase de·fi·cien·cy** a mild autosomal recessive disorder, due to defective AMP deaminase in the purine nucleotide cycle, and characterized clinically by fatigue, cramps, and myalgia after exercise.

**myo·al·bu·min** (mi″o-al-bu′min) an albumin constituting about one per cent of the protein of muscle.

**myo·ar·chi·tec·ton·ic** (mi″o-ahr″kĭ-tek-ton′ik) [*myo-* + *architectonic*] pertaining to the structure of muscle.

**myo·at·ro·phy** (mi″o-at′ro-fe) myatrophy.

**Myo·bia** (mi-o′be-ə) a genus of mites of the family Myobiidae; *M. mus′culi* causes dermatitis in laboratory mice.

**Myo·bi·i·dae** (mi″o-be′ĭ-de) a family of parasitic mites, including the genera *Myobia* and *Radfordia.*

**myo·blast** (mi′o-blast) [*myo-* + *-blast*] an embryonic cell that becomes a cell of muscle fiber; called also *sarcoblast.*

**myo·blas·tic** (mi″o-blas′tik) pertaining to a myoblast.

**myo·blas·to·ma** (mi″o-blas-to′mə) a benign circumscribed tumor-like lesion of soft tissue, possibly consisting of myoblasts.
**granular cell m.,** see under *tumor.*

**myo·blas·to·my·o·ma** (mi″o-blas″to-mi-o′mə) myoblastoma.

**myo·bra·dia** (mi″o-bra′de-ə) [*myo-* + *brady-* + *-ia*] a slow, sluggish reaction of muscle to electric stimulation.

**myo·car·di·al** (mi″o-kahr′de-əl) pertaining to the muscular tissue of the heart; see also under *infarction.*

**myo·car·di·op·a·thy** (mi″o-kahr″de-op′ə-the) [MeSH: Myocardial Diseases] cardiomyopathy.

**myo·car·di·or·rha·phy** (mi″o-kahr″de-or′ə-fe) [*myocardium* + *-rrhaphy*] suture of the myocardium.

**myo·car·dit·ic** (mi″o-kahr-dit′ik) pertaining to myocarditis.

**myo·car·di·tis** (mi″o-kahr-di′tis) [*myo-* + *carditis*] [MeSH: Myocarditis] inflammation of the muscular walls of the heart.
**acute isolated m.,** acute interstitial myocarditis of unknown etiology, marked by sudden onset, absence of endocarditis or pericarditis, and frequently by a fatal outcome; called also *Fiedler's m.* and *idiopathic m.*
**bacterial m.,** myocarditis associated with bacterial infection; it may be caused either by the presence of the organisms in the myocardium or by toxins released from a distant infection.
**chronic m.,** chronic myocardial inflammatory disease; formerly used loosely to indicate any myocardial deficiency.
**diphtheritic m.,** that due to bacterial toxin production in diphtheria; primary lesions are degenerative and necrotic, with a secondary inflammatory response. It is usually subclinical but can cause permanent cardiac damage.
**fibrous m.,** a term formerly used frequently to describe focal or diffuse fibrosis of the myocardium caused by chronic inflammation.

**Fiedler's m.**, acute isolated m.
**giant cell m.**, a subtype of acute isolated myocarditis characterized by the presence of multinucleate giant cells and other inflammatory cells including lymphocytes, plasma cells, and macrophages, and by ventricular dilatation, mural thrombi, and widespread areas of necrosis. The term is sometimes used synonymously with *granulomatous m.* or may be distinguished from it as not including granuloma formation.
**granulomatous m.**, see *giant cell m.*
**hypersensitivity m.**, that due to allergic reactions caused by hypersensitivity to various agents, particularly sulfonamides, penicillins, and methyldopa. It is characterized by interstitial infiltration, principally perivascular, by lymphocytes, plasma cells, macrophages, and eosinophils.
**idiopathic m.**, acute isolated m.
**infectious m.**, that due to infectious agents, including bacteria, viruses, rickettsiae, protozoa, spirochetes, and fungi; they may damage the myocardium by direct invasion, production of toxins, or mediation of an immunological response.
**interstitial m.**, myocarditis affecting chiefly the interstitial fibrous tissue.
**parenchymatous m.**, myocarditis affecting chiefly the muscle substance itself.
**protozoal m.**, myocarditis due to protozoal infection, occurring particularly in Chagas' disease and toxoplasmosis.
**rheumatic m.**, a common sequela of rheumatic fever characterized histologically by perivascular granulomata known as Aschoff bodies or nodules.
**rickettsial m.**, myocarditis associated with infection by rickettsiae; it is frequently subclinical and occurs particularly in Q fever and scrub typhus.
**toxic m.**, degeneration and focal necrosis of myocardial fibers caused by drugs, chemicals, physical agents such as radiation, animal or insect toxins, or other agents or situations causing trauma to the myocardium.
**tuberculous m.**, granulomatous inflammation of the myocardium in tuberculosis, usually resulting from infection elsewhere in the body.
**viral m.**, myocarditis due to viral infection, particularly by enteroviruses; it most often occurs in infants, pregnant women, and immunosuppressed patients.

**myo·car·di·um** (mi″o-kahr′de-əm) [*myo-* + Gr. *kardia* heart] [TA] [MeSH: Myocardium] the middle and thickest layer of the heart wall, composed of cardiac muscle.
**hibernating m.**, see *myocardial hibernation,* under *hibernation.*
**stunned m.**, see *myocardial stunning,* under *stunning.*

**myo·cele** (mi′o-sēl) [*myo-* + *-cele*[1]] hernia of muscle; protrusion of a muscle through its ruptured sheath.

**myo·ce·li·al·gia** (mi″o-se″le-al′jə) [*myo-* + *celi-* + *-algia*] pain in the abdominal muscles.

**myo·ce·li·tis** (mi″o-se-li′tis) [*myo-* + *celi-* + *-itis*] inflammation of the muscles of the abdomen.

**myo·cel·lu·li·tis** (mi″o-sel″u-li′tis) myositis conjoined with cellulitis.

**myo·cho·sis** (mi″o-ko′sis) [*myo-* + Gr. *chōsis* a piling up] shortening of the circular muscle and taeniae of the colon, resulting in a corrugated appearance and a narrowing of the lumen, caused by the deposition of elastin in contracted form; seen in diverticulosis and in prediverticular disease.

**myo·chrome** (mi′o-krōm) [*myo-* + *-chrome*] any member of a group of muscle pigments; see *cytochrome* and *myohematin.*

**Myo·chry·sine** (mi″o-kri′sin) trademark for a preparation of gold sodium thiomalate.

**myo·clo·nia** (mi″o-klo′ne-ə) any disorder characterized by myoclonus.
**m. conge′nita**, congenital tremor syndrome.
**m. epilep′tica**, myoclonus epilepsy.
**m. fibrilla′ris mul′tiplex**, myokymia.
**fibrillary m.**, the twitching of the fibrils of a muscle; see *fibrillation,* def. 2.
**pseudoglottic m.**, hiccup.

**myo·clon·ic** (mi″o-klon′ik) relating to or marked by myoclonus.

**my·oc·lo·nus** (mi-ok′lo-nəs) [*myo-* + *clonus*] [MeSH: Myoclonus] shocklike contractions of a portion of a muscle, an entire muscle, or a group of muscles, restricted to one area of the body or appearing synchronously or asynchronously in several areas. It may be part of a disease process (e.g., epileptic or post-anoxic myoclonus) or be a normal physiological response (e.g., nocturnal myoclonus).
**action m.**, intention m.
**Baltic m.**, myoclonus occurring as part of Baltic myoclonic epilepsy; it is often photosensitive.
**cortical m.**, myoclonus caused by an electrical discharge in the cerebral cortex; it may be a precursor of epilepsia partialis continua.
**cortical reflex m.**, cortical myoclonus caused by an external stimulus.
**epileptic m.**, myoclonus occurring as part of an epileptic aura or seizure; see *myoclonic epilepsy* under *epilepsy.*
**essential m.**, myoclonus of unknown etiology; it may involve single or multiple muscles and may be initiated by excitement or an attempt at voluntary movement. A few cases have been found to be autosomal dominant.
**intention m.**, myoclonus that occurs when voluntary muscle activity is initiated; called also *action m.*
**m. mul′tiplex**, paramyoclonus multiplex.
**nocturnal m.**, nonpathological myoclonic jerks of the limbs occurring as a person is falling asleep or is asleep; in the latter case they may disrupt sleep.
**opsoclonus-m.**, see under *syndrome.*
**palatal m.**, rapid, rhythmic, up-and-down movements of one side or both sides of the palate, often with ipsilateral synchronous clonic movements of muscles of the face, tongue, pharynx, and diaphragm. Called also *palatal nystagmus.*
**reflex m.**, myoclonus in response to an external stimulus; see also *cortical reflex m.* and *reflex epilepsy.*

**myo·coele** (mi′o-sēl) [*myo-* + *-coele*] the cavity within a myotome (def. 2).

**myo·col·pi·tis** (mi″o-kol-pi′tis) [*myo-* + *colp-* + *-itis*] inflammation of the muscular layers of the vaginal wall.

**myo·com·ma** (mi″o-kom′ə) [*myo-* + Gr. *komma* cut] 1. a myotome or muscle segment, as in a fish. 2. the septum between two adjacent myotomes.

**Myo·cop·tes** (mi″o-kop′tēz) a genus of mites of the family Listrophoridae. *M. musculi′nus* is found clinging to the hair of guinea pigs and mice and may cause dermatitis and hair loss.

**my·oc·to·nine** (mi-ok′to-nin) [*myo-* + Gr. *kteinein* to kill] a poisonous alkaloid from *Aconitum lycoctonum.*

**my·oc·u·la·tor** (mi-ok′u-la″tor) [*myo-* + L. *oculus* eye] an ocular instrument, on the principle of the orthoptoscope, which allows fusion and movement laterally, vertically, and in rotation. Cf. *myoscope.*

**myo·cyte** (mi′o-sīt) [*myo-* + *-cyte*] a cell of the muscular tissue.
**Anichkov's m., Anitschkow's m.**, see under *cell.*

**myo·cy·tol·y·sis** (mi″o-si-tol′ĭ-sis) [*myo-* + *cytolysis*] disintegration of muscle fibers.
**coagulative m.**, contraction-band necrosis.
**focal m. of heart**, a miliary lesion characterized by loss of muscular syncytium, preservation of stroma, absence of inflammatory reaction, and eventual necrosis.

**myo·cy·to·ma** (mi″o-si-to′mə) [*myocyte* + *-oma*] a tumor made up of myocytes.

**myo·de·gen·er·a·tion** (mi″o-de-jen″ər-a′shən) [*myo-* + *degeneration*] degeneration of muscle.

**myo·des·op·sia** (mi″o-dəs-op′se-ə) myiodesopsia.

**myo·di·as·ta·sis** (mi″o-di-as′tə-sis) [*myo-* + *diastasis*] separation of a muscle.

**myo·di·op·ter** (mi″o-di-op′tər) the force of ciliary muscle contraction necessary to raise the refraction of the emmetropic eye by 1 diopter from a state of rest.

**myo·dy·nam·ic** (mi″o-di-nam′ik) relating to muscular force.

**myo·dy·nam·ics** (mi″o-di-nam′iks) the physiology of muscular action.

**myo·dy·na·mom·e·ter** (mi″o-di″nə-mom′ə-tər) dynamometer.

**my·odyn·ia** (mi″o-din′e-ə) [*myo-* + *-odynia*] myalgia.

**myo·dys·to·nia** (mi″o-dis-to′ne-ə) [*myo-* + *dys-* + *ton-* + *-ia*] disorder of muscular tone.

**myo·dys·to·ny** (mi″o-dis′tə-ne) myodystonia.

**my·o·dys·tro·phia** (mi″o-dis-tro′fe-ə) 1. muscular dystrophy. 2. myotonic dystrophy.
**m. feta′lis**, amyoplasia congenita.

**myo·dys·tro·phy** (mi″o-dis′trə-fe) 1. muscular dystrophy. 2. myotonic dystrophy.

**myo·ede·ma** (mi″o-ə-de′mə) [*myo-* + *edema*] 1. the rising in a lump by a wasting muscle when struck; called also *mounding.* 2. edema of a muscle.

**myo·elas·tic** (mi″o-e-las′tik) composed of elastic fibers associated with smooth muscle cells.

**myo·elec·tric, myo·elec·tri·cal** (mi″o-e-lek′trik, mi″o-e-lek′trĭ-kəl) pertaining to the electric or electromotive properties of muscle.

**myo·en·do·car·di·tis** (mi″o-en″do-kahr-di′tis) [*myo-* + *endocarditis*] combined myocarditis and endocarditis.

**myo·epi·the·li·al** (mi″o-ep″ĭ-the′le-əl) pertaining to or composed of myoepithelium.

**myo·epi·the·li·o·ma** (mi″o-ep″ĭ-the″le-o′mə) [*myoepithelium* + *-oma*] [MeSH: Myoepithelioma] a benign tumor predominantly composed of myoepithelial cells; a pure myoepithelial neoplasm is rare.

**myo·epi·the·li·um** (mi″o-ep″ĭ-the′le-əm) [*myo-* + *epithelium*] a specialized type of epithelium that has contractile qualities; see *myoepithelial cells,* under *cell.*

**myo·fas·ci·al** (mi″o-fash′e-əl) pertaining to or involving the fascia surrounding and associated with muscle tissue.

**myo·fas·ci·tis** (mi″o-fə-si′tis) [*myo-* + *fascitis*] inflammation of a muscle and its fascia, particularly of the fascial insertion of muscle to bone.

**myo·fi·ber** (mi′o-fi″bər) muscle fiber.

**myo·fi·bril** (mi″o-fi′bril) [MeSH: Myofibrils] a muscle fibril, one of the slender threads which can be rendered visible in a muscle fiber by maceration in certain acids. They run parallel with the long axis of the fiber, and are composed of numerous myofilaments (q.v.). See Plate 35.

**myo·fi·bril·la** (mi″o-fi-bril′ə) pl. *myofibril′lae.* A myofibril.

**myo·fi·bril·lar** (mi″o-fi′brĭ-lər) relating to a myofibril.

**myo·fi·bro·blast** (mi″o-fi′bro-blast) an atypical fibroblast combining the ultrastructural features of a fibroblast and a smooth muscle cell; it has a highly irregular nucleus, a large amount of rough endoplasmic reticulum, and a dense collection of myofilaments.

**myo·fi·bro·ma** (mi″o-fi-bro′mə) [*myo-* + *fibroma*] leiomyoma.
**infantile m.,** congenital generalized fibromatosis.

**myo·fi·bro·ma·to·sis** (mi″o-fi″bro-mə-to′sis) [MeSH: Myofibromatosis] fibromatosis in which there is proliferation of muscle tissue, presenting as solitary or multiple nodules that may involve any organ and almost always occurring in children; it is usually benign, but multifocal lesions involving vital organs may be lethal.
**juvenile m.,** congenital generalized fibromatosis.

**myo·fi·bro·sis** (mi″o-fi-bro′sis) [*myo-* + *fibrosis*] replacement of muscle tissue by fibrous tissue.
**m. cor′dis,** myofibrosis of the heart.

**myo·fi·bro·si·tis** (mi″o-fi″bro-si′tis) inflammation of the perimysium; perimysiitis.

**myo·fila·ment** (mi″o-fil′ə-mənt) [*myo-* + *filament*] [MeSH: Microfilaments] any of the numerous ultramicroscopic threadlike structures occurring in bundles in the myofibrils of striated muscle fibers. The thick *myosin filaments* and the thin *actin filaments* are together responsible for the contractile properties of muscle. Also present are *intermediate filaments,* of uncertain function, composed of desmin and vimentin. See Plate 35.

**myo·func·tion·al** (mi″o-funk′shən-əl) 1. pertaining to muscular function. 2. pertaining to the use of muscles as an adjunct in orthodontic therapy.

**myo·ge·lo·sis** (mi″o-jə-lo′sis) [*myo-* + L. *gelare* to freeze] an area of hardening in a muscle, especially in the gluteus muscle.

**my·o·gen** (mi′o-jən) [*myo-* + *-gen*] an albumin-like protein, constituting 10 per cent of the protein of muscle; it is spontaneously coagulable, passing first into soluble myogen fibrin, and then into myosin fibrin. Cf. *myosin.*

**myo·gen·e·sis** (mi″o-jen′ə-sis) the development of muscle tissue, especially its embryonic development.

**myo·ge·net·ic** (mi″o-jə-net′ik) pertaining to myogenesis.

**my·o·gen·ic** (mi″o-jen′ik) 1. myogenetic. 2. originating in myocytes or muscle tissue.

**my·og·e·nous** (mi-oj′ə-nəs) originating in muscle tissue.

**my·og·lia** (mi-og′le-ə) [*myo-* + *-glia*] a fibrillar substance formed by muscle cells, and present only during early embryogenesis of muscle fibers; called also *border fibrils.*

**myo·glo·bin** (mi′o-glo″bin) [MeSH: Myoglobin] the oxygen-transporting pigment of muscle, a type of hemoprotein resembling a single subunit of hemoglobin, composed of one globin polypeptide chain and one heme group (containing one iron atom); it combines with oxygen released by erythrocytes, stores it, and transports it to the mitochondria of muscle cells, where it generates energy by combustion of glucose to carbon dioxide and water.

**myo·glo·bin·uria** (mi″o-glo″bĭ-nu′re-ə) [MeSH: Myoglobinuria] the presence of myoglobin in the urine, as in deficiency of muscle phosphorylase, in crush injuries, and after vigorous and prolonged exercise in susceptible persons.
**paralytic m.,** azoturia, def. 2.
**familial m., idiopathic m., spontaneous m.,** Meyer-Betz disease.

**myo·glob·u·lin** (mi″o-glob′u-lin) [*myo-* + *globulin*] a globulin found in muscle serum.

**myo·glob·u·lin·uria** (mi″o-glob″u-lĭ-nu′re-ə) the presence of myoglobulin in the urine.

**my·og·na·thus** (mi-og′nə-thəs) [*myo-* + Gr. *gnathos* jaw] a fetus with a supernumerary lower jaw attached to the normally placed lower jaw. See also *dignathus.*

**myo·gram** (mi′o-gram) [*myo-* + *-gram*] the record or tracing made by a myograph.

**myo·graph** (mi′o-graf) [*myo-* + *-graph*] an apparatus for recording the effects of a muscular contraction.

**myo·graph·ic** (mi″o-graf′ik) pertaining to a myograph or to myography.

**my·og·ra·phy** (mi-og′rə-fe) [*myo-* + *-graphy*] [MeSH: Myography] 1. the use of the myograph. 2. a description of the muscles. 3. radiography of muscle tissue after injection of an opaque medium.

**myo·he·ma·tin** (mi″o-he′mə-tin) [*myo-* + *hematin*] MacMunn's name for the cytochrome of muscle tissue, an iron-containing catalyst of tissue oxidation; see *cytochrome.*

**myo·he·mo·glo·bin** (mi″o-he″mo-glo′bin) myoglobin.

**myo·hy·per·tro·phia** (mi″o-hi″pər-tro′fe-ə) muscular hypertrophy.
**m. kymoparaly′tica,** a muscular dystrophy, with paralysis, described by Oppenheim (1914).

**my·oid** (mi′oid) [*my-* + *-oid*] 1. resembling or like a muscle. 2. a substance resembling muscle.
**visual cell m.,** the basophilic inner region of the inner segment of the dendritic process of a retinal rod or cone, lying between the ellipsoid and the soma, and containing agranular endoplasmic reticulum and free ribosomes.

**my·oi·dem** (mi-oi′dəm) myoedema.

**my·oi·de·ma** (mi″oi-de′mə) myoedema.

**my·oi·de·um** (mi-oi′de-əm) myoid tissue.

**my·oid·ism** (mi-o-id′iz-əm) [*myo-* + *idi-* *-ism*] idiomuscular contraction.

***myo*-ino·si·tol** (mi″o-in-o′sĭ-tol) see under *inositol.*

***myo*-ino·si·tol-1 (or 4)-monophos·pha·tase** (mi″o-in-o′sĭ-tol mon″o-fos′fə-tās) [EC 3.1.3.25] an enzyme of the hydrolase class that catalyzes the dephosphorylation of *myo*-inositol 1-phosphate or 4-phosphate enantiomers to form *myo*-inositol. Inhibition of this reaction by lithium breaks the hormonally dependent cycle of degradation and regeneration of phosphoinositides.

**myo·is·che·mia** (mi″o-is-ke′me-ə) [*myo-* + *ischemia*] local deficiency of blood supply in muscle.

**myo·ki·nase** (mi″o-ki′nās) adenylate kinase.

**myo·ki·ne·sis** (mi″o-kĭ-ne′sis) [*myo-* + *-kinesis*] movement of muscles, especially displacement of muscle fibers in operation.

**myo·ki·net·ic** (mi″o-kĭ-net′ik) pertaining to or characterized by myokinesis.

**myo·kym·ia** (mi″o-ki′me-ə) [*myo-* + Gr. *kyma* wave] a benign condition marked by brief spontaneous tetanic contractions of motor units or groups of muscle fibers, usually adjacent groups of fibers contracting alternately. Called also *myoclonia fibrillaris multiplex.*

**myo·lem·ma** (mi″o-lem′ə) [*myo-* + *-lemma*] the sarcolemma.

**myo·li·po·ma** (mi″o-lĭ-po′mə) [*myo-* + *lip-* + *-oma*] a benign mesenchymoma containing fatty or lipomatous elements.

**my·ol·o·gy** (mi-ol′ə-je) [*myo-* + *-logy*] the scientific study of muscles, and the body of knowledge relating thereto.

**my·ol·y·sis** (mi-ol′ĭ-sis) [*myo-* + *-lysis*] disintegration or degeneration of muscle tissue.
**m. cardiotox′ica,** degeneration of the heart muscle occurring in systemic infection.

**my·o·ma** (mi-o′mə) pl. *myomas, myo′mata* [*my-* + *-oma*] [MeSH: Myoma] a benign tumor made up of muscular elements. See also *leiomyoma.*
**m. pre′vium,** leiomyoma uteri.
**m. striocellula′re,** rhabdomyoma.
**uterine m.,** see under *leiomyoma.*

**my·o·ma·gen·e·sis** (mi″o-mə-jen′ə-sis) the production or causation of myoma.

**my·o·ma·la·cia** (mi″o-mə-la′shə) [*myo-* + *-malacia*] morbid softening of a muscle.

**my·o·ma·ta** (mi-o′mə-tə) plural of *myoma.*

**my·o·ma·tec·to·my** (mi″o-mə-tek′tə-me) myomectomy, def. 1.

**my·o·ma·to·sis** (mi″o-mə-to′sis) the formation of multiple myomas.

**my·o·ma·tous** (mi-o′mə-təs) pertaining to or of the nature of a myoma.

**my·o·mec·to·my** (mi″o-mek′tə-me) [*myoma* + *-ectomy*] 1. surgical removal of a myoma (leiomyoma). 2. myectomy.
**abdominal m.**, uterine myomectomy using an abdominal approach. Called also *celiomyomectomy* and *laparomyomectomy*.
**uterine m.**, surgical excision of a uterine myoma (leiomyoma); called also *fibroidectomy* and *fibromectomy*.
**vaginal m.**, uterine myomectomy using a vaginal approach; called also *colpomyomectomy*.

**myo·mel·a·no·sis** (mi″o-mel″ə-no′sis) [*myo-* + *melanosis*] melanosis, or black pigmentation of a portion of the muscular substance.

**myo·mere** (mi′o-mēr) [*myo-* + *-mere*] myotome (def. 2).

**my·om·e·ter** (mi-om′ə-tər) [*myo-* + *-meter*] an apparatus for measuring muscle contraction.

**myo·me·tri·tis** (mi″o-mə-tri′tis) [*myo-* + *metritis*] inflammation of the muscular substance, or myometrium, of the uterus.

**myo·me·tri·um** (mi-o-me′tre-əm) [*myo-* + Gr. *mētra* uterus] [MeSH: Myometrium] TA alternative for *tunica muscularis uteri*.

**myo·mo·hys·ter·ec·to·my** (mi″o-mo-his″tər-ek′tə-me) [*myoma* + *hyster-* + *-ectomy*] surgical removal of a myomatous uterus.

**myo·mot·o·my** (mi″o-mot′ə-me) incision into a myoma.

**my·on** (mi′on) [*myo-* + *-on* neuter ending] a muscular unit.

**myo·ne·cro·sis** (mi″o-nə-kro′sis) necrosis, or death of, individual muscle fibers.
**clostridial m.**, gas gangrene.

**myo·neme** (mi′o-nēm) [*myo-* + Gr. *nēma* thread] any of various fibrillar organelles, known or believed to have contractile properties, commonly seen in the cytoplasm of stalked ciliate protozoa, but also occurring in certain nonciliates and certain nonprotozoans.

**myo·neu·ral** (mi″o-no͞o′rəl) [*myo-* + *neural*] pertaining to both muscle and nerve; said of the nerve terminations in muscles.

**my·on·o·sus** (mi-on′ə-səs) [*myo-* + Gr. *nosos* disease] myopathy.

**my·on·y·my** (mi-on′ĭ-me) [*myo-* + Gr. *onoma* name] nomenclature of the muscles.

**myo·pa·chyn·sis** (mi″o-pə-kin′sis) [*myo-* + *pachynsis*] hypertrophy of muscle.

**myo·pal·mus** (mi″o-pal′məs) muscle twitching.

**myo·pa·ral·y·sis** (mi″o-pə-ral′ĭ-sis) [*myo-* + *paralysis*] paralysis of a muscle.

**myo·par·e·sis** (mi″o-pə-re′sis) muscle weakness.

**myo·path·ia** (mi″o-path′e-ə) myopathy.
**m. infraspina′ta**, a condition marked by the sudden development of pain in the shoulder with tenderness in the infraspinatus muscle.

**myo·path·ic** (mi″o-path′ik) of the nature of a myopathy.

**my·op·a·thy** (mi-op′ə-the) [*myo-* + *-pathy*] any disease of a muscle.
**alcoholic m.**, myopathy affecting alcoholics, commonly characterized by acute myoglobinuria and sometimes by proximal limb weakness.
**capture m.**, a form of exertional rhabdomyolysis seen in wild animals that are captured and put under restraint.
**central core m.**, see under *disease*.
**centronuclear m.**, myotubular m.
**deep pectoral m., degenerative m.**, degeneration and necrosis of areas of the pectoral muscles in turkeys owing to increased pressure on blood vessels and resultant ischemia; in some breeds it is hereditary. Muscles become greenish, resulting in loss of value of the meat. Called also *green muscle disease*.
**distal m.**, an autosomal dominant form of muscular dystrophy, appearing in two types. The first has *onset in infancy,* does not progress past adolescence, and is not incapacitating. The second, *late distal hereditary m.,* sets in usually after age 40, does not affect life span and first affects the small muscles of the hands and feet and then spreads proximally. Called also *distal muscular dystrophy* and *Gowers type muscular dystrophy*.
**fibrotic m.**, fibrosis with adhesions in the thigh muscles of working horses; the muscles eventually become hard and ossified. Called also *ossifying m.*
**glycolytic m.**, any metabolic myopathy resulting from a defect of glycolytic enzyme activity, marked by exercise intolerance and cramping, the accumulation of glycogen in muscle, and recurrent myoglobinuria.
**late distal hereditary m.**, distal myopathy of late onset; called also *distal* or *Gowers' muscular dystrophy, Gowers' syndrome, Welander's distal m.,* and *Welander's m.* or *syndrome*.
**lipid m.**, any metabolic myopathy caused by a defect in fatty acid oxidation, with the accumulation of triglycerides in muscle; manifestations depend on the specific enzyme deficiency and include limb and respiratory weakness, cardiomyopathy, encephalopathy, and myoglobinuria.
**metabolic m.**, myopathy due to disordered metabolism, usually caused by genetic defects or hormonal dysfunction.
**mitochondrial m.**, any of a group of myopathies associated with an increased number of enlarged, often abnormal, mitochondria in muscle fibers and manifested by exercise intolerance, generalized weakness, lactic acidosis, infantile quadriparesis, ophthalmoplegia, and cardiac abnormalities. Underlying metabolic defects include defects in substrate utilization, defects in the coupling of mitochondrial respiration to phosphorylation, and deficiencies in mitochondrial respiratory chain components.
**myotubular m.**, an often fatal X-linked myopathy characterized by myofibers resembling those of early fetal muscle, i.e., with the nucleus located centrally and surrounded by a halo of apparently empty space; called also *centronuclear m.*
**nemaline m.**, a nonprogressive myopathy of uncertain inheritance, characterized histologically by abnormal threadlike structures in muscle cells and clinically by hypotonia with diffuse weakness of the limbs and trunk, usually beginning in infancy.
**nutritional m.**, myopathy due to dietary deficiencies, usually seen in young animals. Two common types are enzootic muscular dystrophy and vitamin E–selenium deficiency syndrome.
**ocular m.**, progressive external ophthalmoplegia.
**ossifying m.**, fibrotic m.
**rod m.**, nemaline m.
**thyrotoxic m.**, weakness and wasting of skeletal muscles, especially in the pelvic and shoulder girdles, accompanying hyperthyroidism.
**Welander's m., Welander's distal m.**, late distal hereditary m.

**my·ope** (mi′ōp) [Gr. *myein* to shut + *ōps* eye] a nearsighted person; one affected with myopia.

**myo·peri·car·di·tis** (mi″o-per″ĭ-kahr-di′tis) [*myo-* + *pericarditis*] myocarditis combined with pericarditis.

**myo·phage** (mi′o-fāj) a phagocyte which destroys the contractile substance of muscle.

**my·oph·a·gism** (mi-of′ə-jiz-əm) [*myo-* + *phag-* + *-ism*] the atrophy, or wasting away, of muscular tissue.

**myo·phone** (mi′o-fōn) [*myo-* + Gr. *phōnē* voice] a device which renders audible the sound of a muscular contraction.

**myo·phos·phor·y·lase** (mi″o-fos-for′ə-lās) the muscle isozyme of glycogen phosphorylase.

**myo·phos·phor·y·lase de·fi·cien·cy** glycogen storage disease, type V.

**my·o·pia** (mi-o′pe-ə) [Gr. *myein* to shut + *-opia*] [MeSH: Myopia] that error of refraction in which rays of light entering the eye parallel to the optic axis are brought to a focus in front of the retina, as a result of the eyeball being too long from front to back *(axial m.)* or of an increased strength in refractive power of the media of the eye *(index m.)* Called also *nearsightedness,* because the near point is less distant than it is in emmetropia with an equal amplitude of accommodation. Symbol M.
**curvature m.**, a form due to changes or increases in the curvature of the refracting surfaces of the eye, especially of the cornea.
**index m.**, a form due to variations in the index of refraction of the media of the eye.
**malignant m., pernicious m.**, progressive myopia, associated with grave disease of the choroid and leading to retinal detachment and blindness.
**primary m.**, simple m.
**prodromal m.**, a condition marked by the return of the ability to do close work without eyeglasses; sometimes seen in incipient cataract.
**progressive m.**, myopia that continues to increase abnormally rapidly in adult life.
**simple m.**, 1. that myopia due to normal growth of the healthy eyeball. It stops increasing at maturity and may be corrected to normal visual acuity. 2. myopia without astigmatism.

**my·op·ic** (mi-op′ik) pertaining to or affected with myopia; nearsighted.

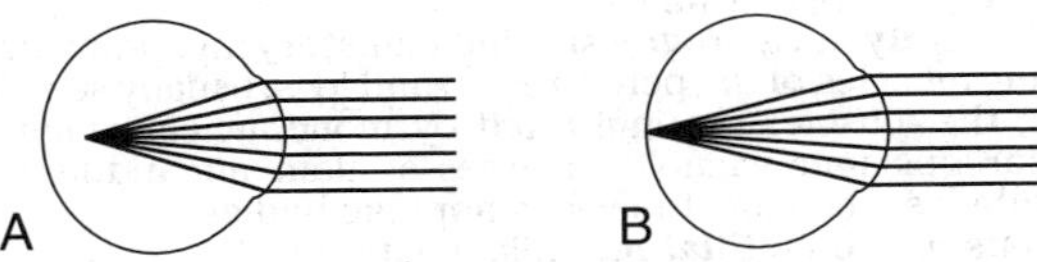

Myopia: error of refraction in a myopic eye *(A),* contrasted with normal refraction in an emmetropic eye *(B).*

**myo·plasm** (mi′o-plaz-əm) [*myo-* + *-plasm*] the contractile part of the muscle cell, or myofibril.

**myo·plas·tic** (mi″o-plas′tik) [*myo-* + *plastic*] performed by the plastic use of muscle; said of operations.

**myo·plas·ty** (mi′o-plas″te) plastic surgery on muscle; an operation in which portions of partly detached muscle are utilized, especially in the field of defects or deformities.

**Myo·po·rum** (mi″o-po′rəm) a genus of shrubs and trees of Australia and New Zealand, many species of which are poisonous to livestock. *M. lae′tum,* the ngaio, causes photosensitization and sometimes fatal hemorrhaging.

**myo·pro·tein** (mi″o-pro′tēn) a protein obtained from muscle tissue.

**my·op·sis** (mi-op′sis) myiodesopsia.

**my·or·rha·phy** (mi-or′ə-fe) [*myo-* + *-rrhaphy*] suture of divided muscle; myosuture.

**my·or·rhex·is** (mi″o-rek′sis) [*myo-* + *-rrhexis*] the rupture of a muscle.

**myo·sal·gia** (mi″o-sal′jə) myalgia.

**myo·sal·pin·gi·tis** (mi″o-sal″pin-ji′tis) [*myo-* + *salpingitis*] inflammation of the muscular tissue of the oviduct.

**myo·sal·pinx** (mi″o-sal′pinks) the muscular tissue of the oviduct.

**my·o·san** (mi′o-sən) a denatured and insoluble form of myosin.

**myo·sar·co·ma** (mi″o-sahr-ko′mə) [*myo-* + *sarcoma*] [MeSH: Myosarcoma] a malignant tumor derived from muscle tissue; see also *leiomyosarcoma* and *rhabdomyosarcoma.*

**myo·schwan·no·ma** (mi″o-shwah-no′mə) schwannoma.

**myo·scle·ro·sis** (mi″o-sklə-ro′sis) [*myo-* + *sclero-* + *-sis*] hardening, or sclerosis, of muscle tissue.

**myo·scope** (mi′o-skōp) [*myo-* + *-scope*] an ocular instrument, on the principle of the orthoptoscope, which allows fusion and movement laterally, vertically, and in rotation. Cf. *myoculator.*

**myo·sep·tum** (mi″o-sep′təm) myocomma.

**my·o·sin** (mi′o-sin) [MeSH: Myosin] a globin which is the most abundant protein (68 per cent) in muscle, occurring chiefly in the A band. Along with actin (q.v.), it is responsible for the contraction and relaxation of muscle. Myosin has enzymatic properties, acting as an ATPase. It is the main constituent of the thick filaments of muscle fibers. Cf. *myogen* and *actomyosin.* See Plate 35.

**my·o·sin ATP·ase** (mi′o-sin a-te-pe′ās) [EC 3.6.1.32] [MeSH: Myosin ATPase] an enzyme activity of muscle that uses the energy derived from the hydrolysis of ATP to drive a cycle of muscular contraction and relaxation. The ATP-hydrolyzing activity occurs in the myosin molecules, but an actomyosin complex is necessary for full activity, in which muscular contraction and relaxation occur by successive making and breaking of cross-bridges between actin and myosin filaments.

**my·o·sin·o·gen** (mi″o-sin′ə-jən) [*myosin* + Gr. *gennan* to produce] myogen.

**my·o·sin·uria** (mi″o-sĭ-nu′re-ə) the presence of myosin in the urine.

**my·o·sis** (mi-o′sis) miosis, def. 1.

**myo·sit·ic** (mi″o-sit′ik) pertaining to myositis.

**myo·si·tis** (mi″o-si′tis) [*myo-* + *-itis*] [MeSH: Myositis] inflammation of a voluntary muscle; called also *myitis* and *initis.*
**acute disseminated m.,** primary multiple m.
**acute progressive m.,** a rare disease in which the inflammation gradually involves the whole muscular system and ends in death by asphyxia and pneumonia.
**m. a frigo′re,** fibrositis resulting from cold or chilling.
**eosinophilic m.,** 1. inflammation of the muscles of mastication in dogs, especially large breeds such as German shepherds; it may be an autoimmune disorder. As the muscles swell, the animal has increased difficulty swallowing. Facial edema may also cause exophthalmos. 2. facial myositis in cattle, usually subclinical and found as a greenish discolored lesion of the meat after the animal is slaughtered.
**m. fibro′sa,** a type in which there is a formation of connective tissue within the muscle substance.
**inclusion body m.,** a progressive inflammatory myopathy primarily involving muscles of the pelvic region and legs, usually seen in older people; the muscles are infiltrated by mononuclear inflammatory cells, sarcoplasmic vacuoles, masses of filaments and filamentous microtubules, and sometimes eosinophilic bodies.
**infectious m., interstitial m.,** inflammation of the connective and septal elements of muscular tissue.
**multiple m.,** polymyositis.
**orbital m.,** see under *pseudotumor.*
**m. ossi′ficans,** myositis which is characterized by bony deposits or by ossification of muscles.
**m. ossi′ficans circumscrip′ta,** a form marked by the formation of a muscular osteoma, such as rider's bone.
**m. ossi′ficans progressi′va,** a progressive disease, beginning in early life, in which the muscles are gradually converted into bony tissue; called also *progressive ossifying m.* and *fibrodysplasia ossificans progressiva.*
**m. ossi′ficans trauma′tica,** myositis ossificans due to injury.
**parenchymatous m.,** that which affects the essential substance of a muscle.
**primary multiple m.,** an acute febrile disease characterized by edema and inflammation of the skin and muscles in various parts of the body; called also *acute disseminated m.*
**progressive ossifying m.,** m. ossificans progressiva.
**proliferative m.,** a benign, rapidly growing, reactive, nodular lesion similar to nodular fasciitis but characterized by fibroblast proliferation within skeletal muscle; histologically it resembles sarcoma.
**m. purulen′ta,** myositis due to bacteremia and associated with suppuration and gangrene. Cf. *pyomyositis.*
**rheumatoid m.,** fibrositis.
**m. sero′sa,** muscle inflammation characterized by a serous exudation.
**spontaneous bacterial m.,** pyomyositis.
**trichinous m.,** myositis in humans or other animals due to the presence of trichinae; see also *trichinosis.*

**myo·spasm** (mi′o-spaz-əm) [*myo-* + *spasm*] spasm (def. 1).

**myo·spas·mia** (mi″o-spaz′me-ə) disease characterized by uncontrollable muscular spasm.

**myo·spher·u·lo·sis** (mi″o-sfĕr″u-lo′sis) an inflammatory giant cell reaction linked to topical use of tetracycline in oil-based ointment on wounds.

**my·os·te·o·ma** (mi-os″te-o′mə) [*my-* + *osteoma*] a muscle tumor containing bony deposits or areas.

**my·os·then·ic** (mi″os-then′ik) [*myo-* + *sthen-* + *-ic*] pertaining to strength of muscle.

**my·os·then·om·e·ter** (mi″os-thən-om′ə-tər) [*myo-* + *stheno-* + *-meter*] dynamometer.

**myo·stro·ma** (mi″o-stro′mə) [*myo-* + *stroma*] the stroma or framework of muscle tissue.

**myo·stro·min** (mi″o-stro′min) a protein occurring in muscle stroma.

**myo·su·ria** (mi″o-su′re-ə) [*myo-* + *-uria*] myosinuria.

**myo·su·ture** (mi″o-soo′chər) [*myo-* + *suture*] the suture of a muscle; myorrhaphy.

**myo·syn·i·ze·sis** (mi″o-sin″ĭ-ze′sis) [*myo-* + Gr. *synizēsis* a sinking down] adhesion of muscles.

**myo·tac·tic** (mi″o-tak′tik) [*myo-* + L. *tactus* touch] pertaining to the proprioceptive sense of muscles.

**my·ot·a·sis** (mi-ot′ə-sis) [*myo-* + Gr. *tasis* stretching] stretching of muscle.

**myo·tat·ic** (mi″o-tat′ik) [*myo-* + Gr. *teinein* to stretch] performed or induced by stretching or extending a muscle.

**myo·ten·on·to·plas·ty** (mi″o-tən-on′to-plas″te) tenomyoplasty.

**myo·teno·si·tis** (mi″o-ten″o-si′tis) [*myo-* + *teno-* + *-itis*] inflammation of a muscle and its tendon.

**myo·te·not·o·my** (mi″o-tə-not′ə-me) [*myo-* + *tenotomy*] surgical division of the tendon of a muscle.

**myo·ther·mic** (mi″o-ther′mik) [*myo-* + *therm-* + *-ic*] pertaining to temperature changes in muscle produced by its activity.

**my·ot·ic** (mi-ot′ik) miotic (def. 2).

**myo·tome** (mi′o-tōm) [*myo-* + *-tome*] 1. an instrument for performing myotomy. 2. the muscle plate or portion of a somite that develops into striated (skeletal) muscle; called also *myomere.* 3. a group of muscles innervated from a single spinal segment.

**myo·tom·ic** (mi″o-tom′ik) pertaining to or derived from a myotome.

**my·ot·o·my** (mi-ot′ə-me) [*myo-* + *-tomy*] the cutting or dissection of a muscle or of muscular tissue.
**Heller's m.,** esophagocardiomyotomy.
**Livaditis' circular m.,** in anastomosis of the upper and lower pouches for esophageal atresia, the lengthening of the upper pouch by circumferential esophagomyotomy.

**Myo·ton·a·chol** (mi″o-tōn′ə-kol) trademark for preparations of bethanechol chloride.

**myo·to·nia** (mi″o-to′ne-ə) [*myo-* + *ton-* + *-ia*] [MeSH: Myotonia] dystonia involving increased muscular irritability and contractility with decreased power of relaxation; cf. *tetanus* (def. 2).

**m. atro'phica,** *myotonic dystrophy;* see under *dystrophy.*
**chondrodystrophic m.,** Schwartz-Jampel syndrome.
**m. conge'nita,** tonic spasm and rigidity of certain muscles when an attempt is made to move them after a period of rest or when mechanically stimulated; the stiffness disappears as the muscles are used. There are autosomal dominant and autosomal recessive forms of the condition. Called also *m. hereditaria.*
**m. dystro'phica,** myotonic dystrophy.
**m. heredita'ria,** m. congenita.
**m. tar'da,** a rare form of myotonia, possibly autosomal recessive myotonia congenita, presenting later in life than the more common forms of myotonia congenita.

**myo·ton·ic** (mi″o-ton'ik) pertaining to or characterized by myotonia.

**my·ot·o·noid** (mi-ot'ə-noid) [*myo-* + *ton-* + *-oid*] resembling myotonia; said of reactions in muscle which are marked by slow contraction or relaxation.

**my·ot·o·nus** (mi-ot'ə-nəs) tonic spasm of a muscle or of a group of muscles.

**myo·troph·ic** (mi″o-trof'ik) 1. increasing the weight of muscle. 2. pertaining to myotrophy.

**my·ot·ro·phy** (mi-ot'rə-fe) [*myo-* + *-trophy*] nutrition of muscle.

**my·o·trop·ic** (mi″o-trop'ik) [*myo-* + *-tropic*] having an affinity for muscle, as myotropic organisms.

**myo·tube** (mi'o-to͞ob″) myotubule.

**myo·tu·bu·lar** (mi″o-too'bu-lər) relating to a myotubule.

**myo·tu·bule** (mi″o-too'būl) a developing muscle fiber with a centrally, rather than peripherally, located nucleus.

**myo·vas·cu·lar** (mi″o-vas'ku-lər) [*myo-* + *vascular*] pertaining to a muscle and its blood vessels.

**Myo·view** (mi'o-vu″) trademark for a kit for the preparation of technetium Tc 99m tetrofosmin.

**myr·cene** (mer'sēn) an essential oil from myrcia oil; it is an olefinic terpene, used in perfumery and pharmaceuticals as an odorant.

**myria-** [Gr. *myrios* numberless] a combining form meaning a great number.

**myr·ia·chit** (mir-yah'chit) [Russ.] a variety of jumping disease seen in Siberia, possibly identical to latah. Called also *miryachit.*

**Myr·i·an·gi·a·les** (mir″e-an″je-a'lēz) former name for Dothideales.

**myr·ia·pod** (mir'e-ə-pod) a member of the Myriapoda; a centipede or millipede.

**Myr·i·ap·o·da** (mir″e-ap'ə-də) [*myria-* + Gr. *pous* foot] a superclass of arthropods, including the classes Chilopoda (centipedes) and Diplopoda (millipedes).

**myr·i·cyl** (mir'ĭ-səl) the radical occurring in beeswax and other waxes.

**my·rin·ga** (mĭ-ring'gə) [L. "membrane," from Gr. *mēninx*] the membrana tympani.

**my·rin·gec·to·my** (mir″in-jek'tə-me) [*myring-* + *-ectomy*] tympanectomy.

**my·rin·gi·tis** (mir″in-ji'tis) [*myringa* + *-itis*] inflammation of the membrana tympani.
**m. bullo'sa, bullous m.,** a form of viral otitis media in which serous or hemorrhagic blebs appear on the membrana tympani and often on the adjacent wall of the auditory meatus.

**myring(o)-** [L. *myringa,* q.v.] a combining form denoting relationship to the membrana tympani.

**my·rin·go·der·ma·ti·tis** (mĭ-ring″go-der″mə-ti'tis) [*myringo-* + *dermatitis*] inflammation of the outer layer of the membrana tympani, with the formation of blebs.

**my·rin·go·my·co·sis** (mĭ-ring″go-mi-ko'sis) [*myringo-* + *-mycosis*] otomycosis of the membrana tympani.

**my·rin·go·plas·ty** (mĭ-ring'go-plas″te) [*myringo-* + *-plasty*] [MeSH: Myringoplasty] surgical restoration of a perforated tympanic membrane by grafting. See also *tympanoplasty.*

**my·rin·go·sta·pe·dio·pexy** (mĭ-ring″go-stə-pe'de-o-pek″se) fixation of the pars tensa of the membrana tympani to the head of the stapes.

**my·rin·go·tome** (mĭ-ring'go-tōm) a knife for use in operating upon the membrana tympani.

**my·rin·got·o·my** (mir″ing-got'o-me) [*myringo-* + *-tomy*] the creation of a hole in the tympanic membrane, as for tympanocentesis. Called also *tympanostomy* and *tympanotomy.*

**my·rinx** (mi'rinks) membrana tympani.

**myr·is·tate** (mir'is-tāt) a salt, ester, or anionic form of myristic acid.

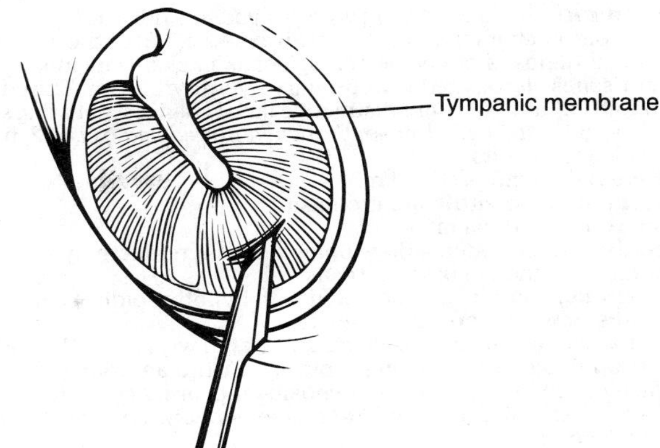

Myringotomy.

**isopropyl m.,** see under *isopropyl.*

**my·ris·tic ac·id** (mĭ-ris'tik) a saturated 14-carbon fatty acid occurring in most animal and vegetable fats, particularly butterfat and coconut, palm, and nutmeg oils. See also table accompanying *fatty acid.*

**My·ris·ti·ca** (mə-ris'tĭ-kə) [Gr. *myrizein* to anoint] a genus of tropical trees of the family Myristicaceae. *M. fra'grans* is the nutmeg, source of nutmeg oil. See also *nutmeg poisoning,* under *poisoning.*

**my·ro·the·cio·tox·i·co·sis** (mi″ro-the″se-o-tok″sĭ-ko'sis) mycotoxicosis in ruminants caused by eating grass or feed contaminated with fungi of the species *Myrothecium,* which contain roridins and verrucarins. In its chronic form animals have intestinal ulcerations and weight loss. In the acute form, characteristics include diarrhea, hepatitis, and pulmonary congestion and edema that can be fatal.

**My·ro·the·ci·um** (mi″ro-the'se-um) a genus of Fungi Imperfecti of the form-class Hyphomycetes that contaminate grasses and contain roridins and verrucarins, causing myrotheciotoxicosis. Certain species contain trichothecenes and can cause alimentary toxic aleukia. Species include *M. ro'ridum* and *M. verruca'ria.*

**myrrh** (mər) [Gr. *murrha*] the oleo-gum-resin obtained from species of *Commiphora;* it has been used as a carminative and a topical oral stimulant.

**myrrh·o·lin** (mir'-o-lin) a mixture of myrrh and fat in equal parts, used as a vehicle for the administration of creosote.

**myr·te·nol** (mər'tə-nol) a terpene alcohol from the volatile oil distilled from the leaves of *Myrtus communis.*

**Myr·tus** (mər'təs) [L.; Gr. *myrtos*] a genus of shrubs of the family Myrtaceae that have white or pink flowers. *M. commu'nis* L. is a European species of myrtle whose leaves are antiseptic and astringent.

**My·so·line** (mi'so-lēn) trademark for preparations of primidone.

**my·so·phil·ia** (mi″so-fil'e-ə) [Gr. *mysos* uncleanness of body or mind + *-philia*] abnormal interest in dirt or filth, with a desire for contact with it that may encompass a paraphilia.

**my·so·pho·bia** (mi″so-fo'be-ə) [Gr. *mysos* uncleanness of body or mind + *-phobia*] irrational fear of dirt and contamination.

**my·so·pho·bic** (mi″so-fo'bik) pertaining to or characterized by mysophobia.

**my·ta·cism** (mi'tə-siz-əm) [Gr. *mytakismos*] a speech disorder consisting of too free use of *m* sounds; called also *mimmation* and *mutacism.*

**My·te·lase** (mi'tə-lās) trademark for a preparation of ambenonium chloride.

**mytho·pho·bia** (mith″o-fo'be-ə) [Gr. *mythos* myth + *-phobia*] irrational fear of myths or of stating an untruth.

**myx·ad·e·ni·tis** (miks″ad-ə-ni'tis) [*myx-* + *aden-* + *-itis*] inflammation of a mucous gland.
**m. labia'lis,** see *cheilitis glandularis.*

**myx·ame·ba** (mik″sə-me'bə) [*myx-* + *ameba*] a uninucleate, naked, free-living ameboid cell without either cilia or flagella produced from a spore, which aggregates and fuses with other myxamebas to form a plasmodium or aggregates without fusion to form a pseudoplasmodium.

**myx·an·gi·tis** (miks″ən-ji'tis) [*myx-* + *angitis*] inflammation of the ducts of mucous glands.

**myx·as·the·nia** (miks″əs-the'ne-ə) [*myxo-* + *asthen-* + *-ia*] deficiency in the secretion of mucus.

**myx·ede·ma** (mik″sə-de′mə) [*myxo-* + *edema*] [MeSH: Myxedema] 1. a condition characterized by dry, waxy swelling of the skin, with abnormal deposits of glycosaminoglycans in skin (mucinosis) and other tissues, associated with primary hypothyroidism. The edema is nonpitting, and there are distinctive facial changes including swollen lips and a thickened nose. Cf. *lichen myxedematosus.* 2. hypothyroidism in adults.
**circumscribed m.**, pretibial m.
**congenital m., infantile m.**, cretinism.
**nodular m.**, pretibial m.
**operative m.**, myxedema developing after thyroidectomy.
**papular m.**, lichen myxedematosus.
**pituitary m.**, myxedema associated with hypothyroidism caused by thyroid stimulating hormone deficiency.
**pretibial m.**, localized myxedema associated with hyperthyroidism and exophthalmos, occurring typically on the anterior (pretibial) surface of the legs, the mucin deposits appearing as both plaques and papules; called also *infiltrative dermopathy, circumscribed m.,* and *nodular m.*
**primary m.**, atrophic thyroiditis.
**secondary m.**, pituitary m.

**myx·edem·a·toid** (mik″sə-dem′ə-toid) [*myxedema* + *-oid*] resembling myxedema.

**myx·edem·a·tous** (mik″sə-dem′ə-təs) pertaining to or characterized by myxedema.

**myx·i·o·sis** (mik″se-o′sis) a discharge of mucus.

**myx(o)-** [Gr. *myxa* mucus] combining form denoting relationship to mucus, or to slime.

**myxo·blas·to·ma** (mik″so-blas-to′mə) myxoma.

**myxo·chon·dro·fi·bro·sar·co·ma** (mik″so-kon″dro-fi″bro-sahr-ko′mə) [*myxo-* + *chondro-* + *fibro-* + *sarcoma*] a malignant mesenchymoma containing myxoid, chondroid, and fibrous elements.

**myxo·chon·dro·ma** (mik″so-kon-dro′mə) [*myxo-* + *chondroma*] chondroma with a stroma resembling primitive mesenchymal tissue.

**myxo·chon·dro·sar·co·ma** (mik″so-kon″dro-sahr-ko′mə) [*myxo-* + *chondro-* + *sarcoma*] chondromyxosarcoma.

**myxo·cys·ti·tis** (mik″so-sis-ti′tis) [*myxo-* + *cystitis*] inflammation of the mucosa of the bladder.

**myxo·cys·to·ma** (mik″so-sis-to′mə) [*myxo-* + *cyst-* + *-oma*] myxoma with cystic degeneration.

**myxo·cyte** (mik′so-sīt) [*myxo-* + *cyte*] one of the characteristic cells of mucous tissue.

**myxo·en·chon·dro·ma** (mik″so-en″kon-dro′mə) [*myxo-* + *enchondroma*] a chondroma in which some of the elements have undergone mucous degeneration.

**myxo·en·do·the·li·o·ma** (mik″so-en″do-the″le-o′mə) hemangioendothelioma with myxomatous degeneration.

**myxo·fi·bro·ma** (mik″so-fi-bro′mə) [*myxoma* + *fibroma*] a fibroma containing myxomatous tissue.
**odontogenic m.**, odontogenic myxoma, particularly one containing large amounts of collagen.

**myxo·fi·bro·sar·co·ma** (mik″so-fi″bro-sahr-ko′mə) [*myxo-* + *fibro-* + *sarcoma*] older term for the myxoid subtype of malignant fibrous histiocytoma.

**myxo·gli·o·ma** (mik″so-gli-o′mə) a glioma which has undergone myxomatous degeneration.

**myxo·glob·u·lo·sis** (mik″so-glob″u-lo′sis) [*myxo-* + *globule* + *-osis*] a cystic condition of the appendix marked by the presence in the cysts of globoid bodies of mucinous character.

**myx·oid** (mik′soid) [*myxo-* + *-oid*] resembling mucus.

**myxo·li·po·ma** (mik″so-lĭ-po′mə) [*myxo-* + *lipoma*] lipoma with foci of myxomatous degeneration.

**myx·o·ma** (mik-so′mə) pl. *myxomas, myxo′mata* [*myx-* + *-oma*] [MeSH: Myxoma] a benign tumor composed of primitive connective tissue cells and stroma resembling mesenchyme. Called also *colloid tumor, gelatinous tumor,* and *mucous tumor.*
**atrial m.**, a benign gelatinous growth usually pedunculated and usually arising from the interatrial septum of the heart in the region of the fossa ovalis; symptoms may include effort dyspnea, loss of weight, fatigue, low-grade fever, polyneuritis, nausea, and palpitations, and sometimes sudden syncopal attacks related to obstruction.
**cystic m.**, myxocystoma.
**enchondromatous m.**, one containing cartilage in the intercellular substance.
**m. fibro′sum**, myxofibroma.
**infectious m.**, myxomatosis cuniculi.
**lipomatous m.**, myxolipoma.
**odontogenic m.**, an uncommon tumor of the jaw, apparently arising from the mesenchymal portion of the tooth germ, and possibly produced by myxomatous degeneration of an odontogenic fibroma.
**m. sarcomato′sum**, myxosarcoma.
**vascular m.**, a myxoma containing many blood vessels.

**myx·o·ma·to·sis** (mik″so-mə-to′sis) 1. a condition marked by the development of multiple myxomas. 2. myxomatous degeneration.
**m. cuni′culi, infectious m.**, an infectious, highly fatal, febrile disease of rabbits caused by the myxoma virus, and characterized by edematous swelling of the mucous membranes and myxomalike tumors of the skin.

**myx·o·ma·tous** (mik-so′mə-təs) of the nature of a myxoma.

**Myxo·my·ce·tes** (mik″so-mi-se′tēz) [*myxo-* + Gr. *mykēs* fungus] the slime molds, a class of perfect fungi found on damp or rotting plant material; they are not pathogenic to humans. They were formerly thought to be groups of protozoa and were called *Mycetozoa* or *Mycetozoida.*

**myxo·my·o·ma** (mik″so-mi-o′mə) [*myxo-* + *myoma*] a myoma with myxomatous degeneration.

**myxo·pap·il·lo·ma** (mik″so-pap″ĭ-lo′mə) myxoma combined with papilloma.

**myxo·poi·e·sis** (mik″so-poi-e′sis) [*myxo-* + *-poiesis*] the formation of mucus.

**myx·or·rhea** (mik″so-re′ə) [*myxo-* + *-rrhea*] blennorrhea.
**m. intestina′lis**, a flow of mucus from the bowel occurring in nervous individuals under mental strain.

**myxo·sar·co·ma** (mik″so-sahr-ko′mə) [*myxo-* + *sarcoma*] [MeSH: Myxosarcoma] a sarcoma containing myxomatous tissue.
**odontogenic m.**, a rare form of odontogenic myxoma characterized by hypercellularity, atypical cytological features, and locally aggressive behavior.

**myxo·sar·co·ma·tous** (mik″so-sahr-ko′mə-təs) relating to or affected with myxosarcoma.

**Myxo·so·ma** (mik″so-so′mə) [*myxo-* + Gr. *soma* body] a genus of parasitic protozoa (suborder Platysporina, order Bivalvulida), characterized by the presence of a mucoid envelope around the spore. *M. cerebra′lis* infects salmonid fishes, causing whirling disease.

**myxo·spor·an** (mik″so-spor′ən) any protozoan of the class Myxosporea.

**Myxo·spor·ea** (mik″so-spor′e-ə) [*myxo-* + *spore*] a class of histozoic or celozoic parasitic protozoa (phylum Myxozoa) found in cold-blooded vertebrates, having spores with one or two sporoplasms and one to six (typically two) polar capsules, each capsule with a coiled polar tube, the probable function of which is anchorage to the host's tissues. The spore membrane usually has two, sometimes up to six, valves. It comprises two orders: Bivalvulida and Multivalvulida.

**myxo·vi·rus** (mik′so-vi″rəs) [*myxo-* + *virus*] [MeSH: Orthomyxoviridae] a group of RNA viruses characterized by special affinities for mucopolysaccharides and glycoproteins, similarities in virion structure, neuraminidase activity, and hemagglutination. Myxoviruses are divided into the families Orthomyxoviridae and Paramyxoviridae.

**Myxo·zoa** (mik″so-zo′ə) [*myxo-* + Gr. *zōon* animal] a phylum of chiefly histozoic or celozoic parasitic protozoa having spores of multicellular origin, with one or more polar capsules and one, two, or three, rarely more, valves, and usually found in fishes but also in amphibians and reptiles. It comprises two classes: Myxosporea and Actinosporea.

**myxo·zo·an** (mik″so-zo′ən) 1. any protozoan of the phylum Myxozoa. 2. pertaining to protozoa of the phylum Myxozoa.

**My·zo·my·ia** (mi″zo-mi′ə) [Gr. *myzan* to suck + *myia* fly] a series of mosquitoes, part of the subgenus *Cellia* of the genus *Anopheles.*

**My·zo·rhyn·chus** (mi″zo-ring′kəs) [Gr. *myzan* to suck + *rhynchos* snout] a series of mosquitoes, part of the subgenus *Anopheles* of the genus *Anopheles.* Several species are carriers of malarial parasites in Asia and Africa.

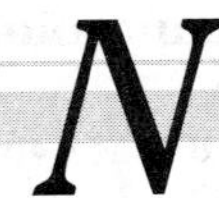

**N** symbol for *newton, nitrogen,* and for *normal* (solution), used with a number designating the strength of the solution relative to the normal, e.g., N/2 or 0.5 N for half-normal.

***N*** symbol for *normal* (see N), *number, Avogadro's number, neutron number,* and (in statistics) *population size.*

**N-** in chemical nomenclature, a prefix indicating that the group or groups named immediately after the symbol are joined to the molecule via its nitrogen atoms.

$N_A$ symbol for *Avogadro's number.*

**n** symbol for *nano-, refractive index,* and *neutron.*

**n.** symbol for L. *ner'vus,* nerve.

***n*** symbol for (haploid) *chromosome number, refractive index,* and (in statistics) *sample size.*

***n-*** symbol for *normal* (def. 2b).

$n_D$ symbol for *refractive index.*

$\nu$ nu, the thirteenth letter of the Greek alphabet; symbol for *degrees of freedom, frequency* (def. 1), *neutrino,* and *kinematic viscosity.*

**NA** Nomina Anatomica; numerical aperture.

**Na** symbol for *sodium* (L. *natrium*).

**nab·i·lone** (nab'ĭ-lōn) a synthetic cannabinoid which acts as a minor tranquilizer and antiemetic.

**Na·both's follicles (cysts, glands)** (nah'bots) [Martin *Naboth,* German anatomist, 1675–1721] see under *follicle.*

**na·bo·thi·an** (nə-bo'the-ən) described by or named in honor of Martin *Naboth.* See under *follicle.*

**na·bu·me·tone** (nə-bu'mə-tōn") a nonsteroidal anti-inflammatory drug used in the treatment of osteoarthritis and rheumatoid arthritis; administered orally.

**na·cre·ous** (na'kre-əs) [Fr. *nacre* mother of pearl] having a grayish-white, translucent color, with a pearl-like luster; said of bacterial colonies.

**Nac·ton** (nak'ton) trademark for a preparation of poldine methylsulfate.

**NAD** [MeSH: NAD] nicotinamide adenine dinucleotide; no appreciable disease.

$NAD^+$ the oxidized form of nicotinamide adenine dinucleotide.

**NADH** the reduced form of nicotinamide adenine dinucleotide.

**NADH cy·to·chrome $b_5$ re·duc·tase** (si'to-krōm re-duk'tās) cytochrome-$b_5$ reductase.

**NADH de·hy·dro·ge·nase (ubi·quin·one)** (de-hi'dro-jən-ās u-bik'win-ōn) [EC 1.6.5.3] an enzyme complex of the inner mitochondrial membrane that catalyzes the transfer of electrons from NADH to ubiquinone, oxidizing the former and reducing the latter in a reaction of the electron transport chain (q.v.). The enzyme complex contains flavoprotein (FMN) and iron-sulfur prosthetic groups and is associated with proton translocation and the resultant synthesis of ATP.

**NADH met·he·mo·glo·bin re·duc·tase** (met-he'mo-glo-bin re-duk'tās) cytochrome-$b_5$ reductase.

**NADH ox·i·dase** (ok'sĭ-dās) NADH peroxidase.

**NADH per·ox·i·dase** (pər-ok'sĭ-dās) [EC 1.11.1.1] an enzyme of the oxidoreductase class that catalyzes the transfer of electrons from NADH to hydrogen peroxide, reducing the latter to water. The enzyme contains FAD.

**NADH-Q re·duc·tase** (re-duk'tās) NADH dehydrogenase (ubiquinone).

**na·dide** (na'dīd) an alcohol and narcotic antagonist; it is the naturally occurring coenzyme nicotinamide adenine dinucleotide.

**$NAD^+$ ki·nase** (ki'nās) [EC 2.7.1.23] an enzyme of the transferase class that catalyzes the phosphorylation of $NAD^+$ to form $NADP^+$.

**na·do·lol** (na-do'lol) [MeSH: Nadolol] a nonselective $\beta$-adrenergic receptor blocker, used in the treatment of angina pectoris and hypertension.

**NADP** [MeSH: NADP] nicotinamide adenine dinucleotide phosphate.

$NADP^+$ the oxidized form of NADP.

**NADPH** the reduced form of NADP.

**NADPH–cy·to·chrome P-450 re·duc·tase** (si'to-krōm re-duk'tās) NADPH–ferrihemoprotein reductase.

**NADPH-fer·ri·he·mo·pro·tein re·duc·tase** (fer"e-he"mo-pro'tēn re-duk'tās) [EC 1.6.2.4] [MeSH: NADPH-Ferrihemoprotein Reductase] an enzyme of the oxidoreductase class that catalyzes the transfer of electrons to cytochromes via oxidation of NADPH. It is a flavoprotein (FMN, FAD) occurring in the endoplasmic reticulum and serving as the initial electron donor in reactions catalyzed by cytochrome P-450 monooxygenases (e.g., unspecific monooxygenase). It can also transfer electrons to cytochromes *b* and *c.* Called also *NADPH–cytochrome P-450 reductase.*

**NADPH met·he·mo·glo·bin re·duc·tase** (met-he'mo-glo"bin re-duk'tās) an enzyme of the erythrocytes that catalyzes the reduction of methemoglobin to hemoglobin via oxidation of NADH. The physiological significance of the enzyme is uncertain; no endogenous intermediate electron carrier has been found, although the enzyme can be activated if methylene blue or other artificial electron acceptor is introduced. Called also *methemoglobin reductase (NADPH).*

**NADPH ox·i·dase** (ok'sĭ-dās) [MeSH: NADPH Oxidase] a plasma membrane–associated enzyme complex that catalyzes the univalent reduction of oxygen using NADPH as an electron donor; the superoxide anion formed acts as an oxidant in the phagocyte microbicidal system, proceeding through a series of electron transfer reactions that form the respirator burst. Various genetic defects in the system result in chronic granulomatous disease.

**$NAD(P)^+$ trans·hy·dro·gen·ase (AB spe·ci·fic)** (trans-hi'dro-jən-ās spə-sif'ik) [EC 1.6.1.2] an enzyme of the inner mitochondrial membrane that uses the energy generated by proton translocation to catalyze the reaction NADH + $NADP^+$ = $NAD^+$ + NADPH. The enzyme is regulated by the relative concentrations of NAD and NADP and by the energy state of the membrane, becoming activated in the presence of excess ATP and electrons from the electron transport chain. The enzyme from heart is A specific with respect to $NAD^+$ and B specific with respect to $NADP^+$.

**$NAD^+$ syn·thase (glu·ta·mine-hy·dro·lys·ing)** (sin'thās gloo'tə-mēn hi'dro-līz"ing) [EC 6.3.5.1] an enzyme of the transferase class that catalyzes the transfer of an amino group from glutamine to desamido-$NAD^+$ to form $NAD^+$.

**Nae·ge·li's leukemia** (na'gĕ-lēz) [Otto *Naegeli,* Swiss hematologist, 1871–1938] acute myelomonocytic leukemia.

**Nae·ge·li's syndrome** (na'gĕ-lēz) [Oskar *Naegeli,* Swiss dermatologist, 1885–1959] Franceschetti-Jadassohn syndrome.

**Nae·gle·ria** (na-glēr'e-ə) [F.P.O. *Nägler,* Austrian bacteriologist, 20th century] [MeSH: Naegleria] a genus of free-living protozoa (order Schizopyrenida, subclass Gymnamoebia) found in fresh water, soil, and sewage, which have both an ameboid and a flagellate stage in their life cycle; in the latter stage, two flagella are present. Certain species, especially *N. fowleri,* are capable of facultative parasitism, and some strains are highly pathogenic and may cause a highly fatal primary amebic meningoencephalitis. Infection is usually acquired by swimming in water contaminated with the organisms.

**nae·gle·ri·a·sis** (na"glə-ri'ə-sis) infection with *Naegleria.*

**naev(o)-** for words beginning thus, see those beginning *nev(o)-.*

**na·fam·o·stat mes·y·late** (nə-fam'o-stat mes'ə-lāt) a proteinase inhibitor used in treatment of acute pancreatitis and as an anticoagulant in hemofiltration.

**naf·a·rel·in ace·tate** (naf'ə-rel"in) a synthetic preparation of gonadotropin-releasing hormone, used in the treatment of central precocious puberty; administered by nasal spray.

**naf·cil·lin so·di·um** (naf-sil'in) [MeSH: Nafcillin] a semisynthetic, acid- and penicillinase-resistant penicillin, used as an antibacterial in severe staphylococcal infections caused by penicillinase-positive organisms; administered orally, intramuscularly, and intravenously.

**Naff·zig·er's operation, syndrome** (naf'zig-ərz) [Howard Christian *Naffziger,* American surgeon, 1884–1961] see under *operation,* and see *scalenus syndrome,* under *syndrome.*

**naf·ro·nyl ox·a·late** (naf'ro-nəl) a vasodilator which has been used in the treatment of peripheral and cerebral vascular disorders.

**naf·ta·lo·fos** (naf'tə-lo-fos) a veterinary anthelmintic.

**naf·ti·fine hy·dro·chlo·ride** (naf'tĭ-fēn) [USP] a broad-spectrum antifungal agent, chemically related to allylamines, applied topically to the skin.

**Naf·tin** (naf'tin) trademark for preparations of naftifine hydrochloride.

**na·ga·na** (nah-gah'nah) [Zulu, from *ngana* feeble, weak] any of various tsetse fly–transmitted types of trypanosomiasis in domestic animals in Africa, including cattle, horses, sheep, goats, dogs, pigs, and camels. It may be acute or chronic and its pathogenicity and symptoms are determined by many factors, such as the trypanosome involved and the species infected. Anemia, fever, and emaciation occur in many species, corneal opacities in horses and dogs, and abortion in cows.

**Na·gel's test** (nah'gelz) [Willibald A. *Nagel,* German physiologist, 1870–1911] see under *test.*

**Na·geotte bracelets, cell** (nah-zhot') [Jean *Nageotte,* Paris histologist, 1866–1948] see under *bracelet* and *cell.*

**Na·ger's acrofacial dysostosis (syndrome)** (nah-zherz') [Félix Robert *Nager,* Swiss otorhinolaryngologist, 1877–1959] see under *dysostosis.*

**Na·ger-De Rey·nier syndrome** (nah-zher'də-ra-ne-a') [F.R. *Nager;* Jean Pierre *de Reynier,* Swiss otologist, born 1914] see *Nager's acrofacial dysostosis,* under *dysostosis.*

**Na·gler effect** (nah'glər) [Joseph *Nagler,* Austrian radiologist, born 1910] see under *effect.*

**Na·gler's reaction (test)** (na'glərz) [F. P. O. *Nagler,* Australian bacteriologist, 20th century] see under *reaction.*

**nai·ad** (ni'ad) [Gr. *nan* to flow] an aquatic, gill-breathing nymph (q.v.) of certain arthropods.

**nail** (nāl) [MeSH: Nails] 1. unguis. 2. a rod of metal, bone, or other material used for fixation of the ends or the fragments of fractured bones.
**eggshell n.,** a fingernail which has become thin and curved upward at its anterior edge.
**hippocratic n.,** see *hippocratic fingers,* under *finger.*
**ingrown n.,** aberrant growth of a toenail, with one or, less often, both lateral margins pushing deeply into the adjacent soft tissues. Called also *ingrowing toenail, onychocryptosis, onyxis,* and *unguis incarnatus.*
**Jewett n.,** a nail for internal fixation of a trochanteric fracture; the nail is fastened to a plate for fixing the head and neck of the bone to the shaft.
**Küntscher n.,** a tubular metal nail for the intramedullary fixation of fractures.
**Neufeld n.,** a device for internal fixation of intertrochanteric fracture of the femur, the V nail section being set at an angle of about 130 degrees to the plate portion.
**parrot beak n.,** a curvation of the fingernail like that of a parrot's beak.
**pitted n's,** nails with surface pits, usually under 1 mm in diameter, seen most often in psoriasis, frequently in alopecia areata, and sometimes unexplained.
**racket n.,** thumbnails that are much shorter than they are wide; rarely, other fingers may be affected. In the commonest form, the distal phalanges of affected digits are shortened as well. It is believed to be an autosomal dominant disorder.
**reedy n.,** a fingernail marked by longitudinal furrows.
**Smith-Petersen n.,** a flanged nail for fixing the head of the femur in fracture of the femoral neck.
**spoon n.,** depression of the central portion of the fingernail, with raising of the edges at the sides.
**turtle-back n.,** a fingernail which is greatly distorted, being more convex than normal.
**watch-crystal n.,** a nail convex lengthwise as well as crosswise, and often as broad as it is long, seen in pulmonary osteoarthropathy and pachydermoperiostosis.

**nail·ing** (nāl'ing) the operation of fixing or fastening of a fractured bone with a nail.
**intramedullary n., marrow n., medullary n.,** the fixation of a fractured long bone by insertion of a steel rod into the marrow cavity of the bone.

**Nai·ro·bi sheep disease** (ni-ro'be) [*Nairobi,* Kenya, where it is particularly prevalent] [MeSH: Nairobi Sheep Disease] see under *disease.*

**Nai·ro·vi·rus** (ni″ro-vi'rəs) [*Nairobi* sheep disease + *virus*] [MeSH: Nairovirus] a genus of viruses of the family Bunyaviridae, containing at least 33 species in seven serogroups; it includes Crimean-Congo hemorrhagic fever virus and Nairobi sheep disease virus. The chief vectors are ticks of the genera *Amblyomma* and *Hyalomma.*

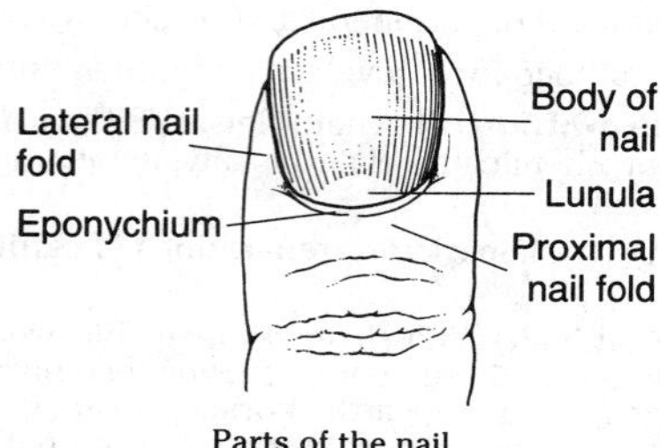

Parts of the nail.

**na·ïve** (nah-ēv') [Fr. "ingenuous, unaffected"] not previously exposed to therapy or treatment.

**Na·ja** (na'jə) a genus of venomous snakes of the family Elapidae found in Asia and Africa, including most of the cobras. *N. ha'je* is the Egyptian cobra; *N. mossambi'ca* is the Mozambique cobra; *N. na'ja* is the Asian cobra; *N. nigricol'lis* is the black-necked cobra; and *N. ni'vea* is the Cape cobra. See table at *snake.*

**na·ja** (nah'jə) [Arabic] 1. Asian cobra. 2. a homeopathic preparation made from the venom of *Naja naja.*

**Na$^+$,K$^+$-ATP·ase** (a-te-pe'ās) an enzyme that spans the plasma membrane and hydrolyzes ATP to provide the energy necessary to drive the cellular sodium pump (q.v.). See also *adenosinetriphosphatase.* In EC nomenclature, called *Na$^+$/K$^+$-exchanging ATPase.*

**Na$^+$/K$^+$-ex·chang·ing ATP·ase** (eks-chānj'ing a-te-pe'ās) [EC 3.6.1.37] EC nomenclature for *Na$^+$,K$^+$-ATPase.*

**Na$^+$/K$^+$-trans·port·ing ATP·ase** (trans-port'ing a-te-pe'ās) Na$^+$,K$^+$-ATPase.

**nal·bu·phine hy·dro·chlo·ride** (nal'bu-fēn) an opioid analgesic, used in the treatment of moderate to severe pain and as an anesthesia adjunct; administered intravenously, intramuscularly, and subcutaneously.

**Nal·fon** (nal'fon) trademark for a preparation of fenoprofen calcium.

**nal·i·dix·ic ac·id** (nal-i-dik'sik) [USP] [MeSH: Nalidixic Acid] a quinolone antibacterial used orally in the treatment of urinary infections caused by gram-negative organisms, especially those caused by *Proteus* species.

**nal·me·fene hy·dro·chlo·ride** (nal'mə-fēn″) a derivative of naltrexone that acts as an opioid antagonist, used in the treatment of opioid toxicity and overdose; administered parenterally.

**Nal·line** (nal'ēn) trademark for a preparation of nalorphine.

**nal·or·phine** (nal'or-fēn, nal-or'fēn) [MeSH: Nalorphine] a drug structurally related to morphine which acts as an antagonist to morphine and related narcotics. Called also *allorphine* and *antorphine.* **n. hydrochloride,** the hydrochloride salt of nalorphine, $C_{19}H_{21}NO_3 \cdot HCl$, occurring as a white or practically white, crystalline powder; used as a narcotic antagonist, chiefly to counteract respiratory depression due to narcotic overdosage, administered intravenously. It is also used to diagnose narcotic addiction; withdrawal symptoms occur following its subcutaneous administration to addicts.

**nal·ox·one hy·dro·chlo·ride** (nal-ok'sōn) a narcotic antagonist structurally related to oxymorphone, used as an antidote to narcotic overdosage, and as an antagonist for pentazocine overdose; administered parenterally.

**nal·trex·one hy·dro·chlo·ride** (nal-trek'sōn) [USP] a synthetic congener of oxymorphone, chemically related to naloxone, that acts as an opioid antagonist; administered orally in the treatment of opioid abuse.

**name** (nām) [MeSH: Names] a word or words used to designate a unique entity and distinguish it from others.
**British Approved N.,** see *BAN.*
**generic n.,** 1. in chemistry, a name applied to a class of compounds, e.g., alkane or halide. 2. nonproprietary n. 3. in biology, the name applied to a genus.
**International Nonproprietary N.,** see INN.
**nonproprietary n.,** a short name coined for a drug or chemical not subject to proprietary (trademark) rights and recommended or recognized by an official body, e.g., a USAN, INN, or BAN.
**pharmacy equivalent n. (PEN),** a shortened name used by pharmacists for a combination of generic drugs when all the names are too long to fit on a prescription label; the new term consists of the prefix *co-* plus an abbreviation for each drug in the combination.
**proprietary n.,** a brand name or trademark under which a proprietary product is marketed. See *proprietary.*
**systematic n.,** in chemical nomenclature, a name of a substance based on the chemical structure of a compound.
**trivial n.,** in chemical nomenclature, a name of a substance that does not reflect its chemical structure; many trivial names are semisystematic, e.g., the *-ol* in glycerol indicates that it is an alcohol.
**United States Adopted N.,** see *USAN.*

**NAMI** National Alliance for the Mentally Ill.

**NAN** *N*-acetylneuraminic acid.

**NANBH** non-A, non-B hepatitis.

**nan·dro·lone** (nan'dro-lōn) [MeSH: Nandrolone] an anabolic steroid that differs from testosterone in not having a methyl group at-

tached to carbon 10 of the steroid nucleus; it has anabolic effects that are more pronounced than its androgenic effects.
**n. decanoate** [USP], an ester of nandrolone having a long duration of action, used in the treatment of severe growth retardation in children and as an adjunct in the treatment of chronic wasting diseases and anemia associated with renal insufficiency; administered intramuscularly.
**n. phenpropionate** [USP], an ester of nandrolone having a moderate duration of action, used in the treatment of metastatic breast cancer and of severe growth retardation in children, and as an adjunct in the treatment of chronic wasting diseases; administered intramuscularly.

**na·nism** (na'niz-əm) [L. *nanus* dwarf] dwarfism.
**mulibrey n.,** a rare autosomal recessive disorder marked by dwarfism and constrictive pericarditis; called mulibrey to denote defects of *mu*scle, *li*ver, *br*ain, and *ey*es. Affected infants have a triangular face often with hypocephaloid skull, muscular hypotonia, squeaky voice, and yellowish dots and pigment dispersion in the ocular fundus.
**pituitary n.,** hypophysial infantilism.
**senile n.,** progeria.

**Nan·niz·zia** (nə-niz'e-ə) a genus of fungi, classified in the family Gymnoascaceae but later found to be the same as *Arthroderma.*

**nann(o)-** see *nano-.*

**Nan·no·mo·nas** (nan″o-mo'nəs) [*nanno-* + Gr. *monas* unit] in some systems of classification, a subgenus of salivarian trypanosomes, including *Trypanosoma congolense, T. dimorphon,* and *T. simiae.*

**nan(o)-** [Gr. *nanos* dwarf] a combining form designating small size; used in naming units of measurement to indicate one-billionth ($10^{-9}$) of the unit designated by the root with which it is combined. Symbol n.

**nano·ce·pha·lia** (nan″o-sə-fa'le-ə) microcephaly.

**nano·ceph·a·lous** (nan″o-sef'ə-ləs) [*nano-* + *cephal-* + *-ous*] microcephalic.

**nano·ceph·a·ly** (nan″o-sef'ə-le) microcephaly.

**nano·cor·mia** (nan″o-kor'me-ə) [*nano-* + Gr. *kormos* trunk + *-ia*] a developmental anomaly characterized by abnormal smallness of the body, or trunk.

**nano·cu·rie** (nan'o-ku're) a unit of radioactivity, being $10^{-9}$ curie, or the quantity of radioactive material in which the number of nuclear disintegrations is $3.7 \times 10$, or 37, per second. Abbreviated nCi. Called also *millimicrocurie.*

**nano·gram** (nan'o-gram) a unit of mass (weight) of the metric system, being one one-billionth ($10^{-9}$) gram; abbreviated ng. Called also *millimicrogram.*

**nan·oid** (nan'oid) [*nano-* + *-oid*] dwarfish.

**nano·li·ter** (nan'o-le″tər) a unit of capacity equal to one-billionth ($10^{-9}$) of a liter; abbreviated nL or nl. Called also *millimicroliter.*

**nano·me·lia** (nan″o-me'le-ə) micromelia.

**nan·om·e·lus** (nan-om'ə-ləs) micromelus.

**nano·me·ter** (nan'o-me″tər) a unit of linear measure equal to one-billionth of a meter, $10^{-9}$ meter; abbreviated nm.

**nan·oph·thal·mia** (nan″of-thal'me-ə) nanophthalmos.

**nan·oph·thal·mos** (nan″of-thal'məs) [*nan-* + Gr. *ophthalmos* eye] microphthalmos in an eye that is otherwise normal. A nanophthalmic eye is very hyperopic and prone to angle-closure glaucoma.

**Nano·phy·e·tus** (nan″o-fi'ə-təs) a genus of trematodes of the family Troglotrematidae; called also *Troglotrema. N. salmin'cola* is found in the kidney and under the skin of various fish, especially salmon and trout, and serves as a vector of *Neorickettsia helminthoeca,* the etiologic agent of salmon poisoning (q.v.). It is transmitted to humans, dogs, cats, foxes, bears, hogs, and other animals by the ingestion of infected raw fish.

**nano·plank·ton** (na″no-plank'ton) plankton of extremely minute size.

**nano·sec·ond** (nan'o-sek″ond) one-billionth ($10^{-9}$) of a second; abbreviated ns. or nsec.

**nano·so·ma** (nan″o-so'mə) dwarfism.

**nano·so·mia** (nan″o-so'me-ə) [*nano-* + *-somia*] dwarfism.

**nano·unit** (nan'o-u″nit) one-billionth ($10^{-9}$) of a standard unit; abbreviated nU.

**nan·ous** (nan'əs) dwarfish.

**na·nu·ka·ya·mi** (nah″noo-kah-yah'me) a leptospirosis marked by fever and jaundice, first reported in Japan and caused by *Leptospira interrogans* (formerly believed to be caused specifically by the serovar *L. hebdomadis);* the animal host is the field vole, *Microtus montebelli.* Called also *nanukayami disease* or *fever, akiyami, seven-day fever, autumn fever,* and *gikiyami.*

**na·nus** (nă'nəs) [L., from Gr. *nanos*] a dwarf.

**NAP** nasion, point A, pogonion; see *angle of convexity.*

**nape** (nāp) the back of the neck (nucha [TA]).

**na·pex** (na'peks) the region of the scalp just inferior to the occipital protuberance.

**naph·az·o·line hy·dro·chlo·ride** (naf-az'o-lēn) [USP] an adrenergic used as a vasoconstrictor, applied topically to the nasal or ocular mucous membranes.

**naph·tha** (naf'thə) [L., from Arabic] any of various volatile, often flammable, liquid hydrocarbon mixtures from petroleum, natural gas, or coal tar, sometimes specifically petroleum benzoin or ligroin; specific fractions are used as solvents, dry cleaning fluids, in synthesis, in varnishes and paints, and as fuels.

**naph·tha·lene** (naf'thə-lēn) a silvery, crystalline hydrocarbon from coal tar oil, used as an intermediate, moth repellent, fungicide, and preservative and formerly used as an antiseptic in diarrhea of typhoid fever; it is toxic by ingestion, inhalation, and skin absorption.
**chlorinated n.,** any of a group of compounds resulting from chlorination of naphthalene; their uses include wood preservatives, varnishes, and machine lubricating oils. Excessive exposure can cause halogen acne in humans, and contamination of cattle feed with them during harvesting or processing can cause hyperkeratosis in the animals. Called also *chloronaphthalene.*

**naph·tha·mine** (naf'thə-mēn) methenamine.

**naph·thol** (naf'thol) a crystalline, antiseptic substance from coal tar occurring in two forms, α- or 1-naphthol and β- or 2-naphthol, used in dyes, organic synthesis, perfumes, insecticides, and pharmaceutical compounds; it is toxic by ingestion and skin absorption. See also under *poisoning.*
**β-n., beta-n.,** see *betanaphthol.*

**naph·tho·late** (naf'tho-lāt″) a naphthol compound in which a base takes the place of hydrogen in the hydroxyl.

**naph·thol·ism** (naf'thol-iz-əm) naphthol poisoning.

**naph·tho·re·sor·cine** (naf″tho-re-sor'sin) a principle in transparent crystals derived from naphthol and resorcinol.

**naph·thyl** (naf'thəl) the radical, $C_{10}H_7$.

**naph·thyl·amine** (naf-thil'ə-mēn) a nitrogen-substituted arylamine, existing as two different isomers, α- or *1-naphthylamine* and β- or *2-naphthylamine.* Both isomers are used in dyes and are carcinogenic.

**na·pi·form** (na'pĭ-form) [L. *napus* turnip + *forma* shape] having the shape or form of a turnip.

**NAPNES** National Association for Practical Nurse Education and Services.

**nap·ra·path** (nap'rə-path) a practitioner of naprapathy.

**na·prap·a·thy** (nə-prap'ə-the) [Czech *napravit* to correct + *-pathy*] a system of therapy employing manipulation of connective tissue (ligaments, muscles, and joints) and dietary measures; said to facilitate the recuperative and regenerative processes of the body.

**Nap·re·lan** (nap'rə-lan) trademark for a preparation of naproxen sodium.

**Na·pro·syn** (nə-pro'sin) trademark for a preparation of naproxen.

**na·prox·en** (nə-prok'sən) [USP] [MeSH: Naproxen] a nonsteroidal anti-inflammatory agent that is a propionic acid derivative, used for treatment of osteoarthritis and rheumatoid arthritis; administered orally or in suppository form. Also available as *naproxen sodium.*

**na·prox·ol** (nə-prok'sōl) an anti-inflammatory, antipyretic, and analgesic used in the treatment of rheumatoid arthritis, administered orally.

**nap·sy·late** (nap'sə-lāt) USAN contraction for 2-naphthalenesulfonate.

**Na·qua** (na'kwə) trademark for a preparation of trichlormethiazide.

**Na·qui·val** (na'kwi-val″) trademark for a preparation of trichlormethiazide with reserpine.

**nar·a·sin** (nar'ə-sin) [USP] a veterinary coccidiostat and growth stimulant.

**Nar·can** (nahr'kan) trademark for a preparation of naloxone hydrochloride.

**nar·cis·sine** (nahr-sis'ēn) lycorine.

**nar·cis·sism** (nahr'sĭ-siz-əm) [from *Narcissus,* a character in Greek mythology who fell in love with his own image reflected in water] [MeSH: Narcissism] dominant interest in oneself; self-love; the state in which the ego is invested in oneself, rather than in another person.
**primary n.**, that occurring in the early infantile phase of object relationship development, when the child has not differentiated himself from the outside world and regards all sources of pleasure as originating within himself.
**secondary n.**, that in which the libido, once attached to external love objects, is redirected back to the self.

**Nar·cis·sus** (nahr-sis'əs) a genus of flowering plants of the family Amaryllidaceae, whose bulbs contain the toxin lycorine. *N. pseudonarcis'sus* L. is the daffodil. *N. tazet'ta* contains the alkaloid tazettine.

**nar·cis·sus** (nahr-sis'əs) any plant of the genus *Narcissus.*

**nar·cis·sis·tic** (nahr"sĭ-sis'tik) pertaining to or characterized by narcissism.

**narco-** [Gr. *narkē* numbness] a combining form denoting relationship to stupor, to a stuporous state, or to narcosis.

**nar·co·anal·y·sis** (nahr"ko-ə-nal'ĭ-sis) a form of psychotherapy that utilizes the slow intravenous administration of barbiturates in order to release suppressed or repressed thoughts, i.e., to disinhibit communication of affect-laden and unacceptable ideas.

**nar·co·hyp·no·sis** (nahr"ko-hip-no'sis) hypnotic suggestions made while the patient is under the influence of a narcotic drug.

**nar·co·lep·sy** (nahr'ko-lep"se) [*narco-* + Gr. *lepsis* a taking hold, a seizure] [MeSH: Narcolepsy] [DSM-IV] recurrent, uncontrollable, brief episodes of sleep, often associated with hypnagogic or hypnopompic hallucinations, cataplexy, and sleep paralysis; called also *Gélineau's syndrome* and *paroxysmal sleep.*

**nar·co·lep·tic** (nahr"ko-lep'tik) pertaining to, characterized by, or producing narcolepsy. By extension, sometimes used to denote an individual who exhibits narcolepsy.

**nar·co·ma** (nahr-ko'mə) a stuporous state produced by narcotics.

**nar·cose** (nahr'kōs) stuporous.

**nar·co·sine** (nahr'ko-sēn) noscapine.

**nar·co·sis** (nahr-ko'sis) [Gr. *narkōsis* a benumbing] a nonspecific and reversible depression of function of the central nervous system marked by stupor or insensibility, produced by opioid drugs and certain other substances.
**basal n.**, narcosis marked by complete unconsciousness, amnesia, and analgesia; see *preanesthesia.*
**nitrogen n.**, a state resembling drunkenness, with euphoria and disorientation, seen in divers below about 30 meters (100 feet) who are breathing compressed air, because of the high nitrogen content of air; some of the nitrogen enters the bloodstream and acts as a narcotic. Sometimes popularly called *rapture of the deep.*

**nar·co·stim·u·lant** (nahr"ko-stim'u-lənt) having both narcotic and stimulant properties.

**nar·cot·ic** (nahr-kot'ik) [Gr. *narkōtikos* benumbing, deadening] 1. pertaining to or producing narcosis. 2. an agent that produces insensibility or stupor, applied especially to the opioids, i.e., to any natural or synthetic drug that has morphine-like actions.

**nar·cot·i·co·ac·rid** (nahr-kot"ĭ-ko-ak'rid) both narcotic and acrid.

**nar·cot·i·co·ir·ri·tant** (nahr-kot"ĭ-ko-ir'ĭ-tənt) both narcotic and irritant.

**nar·co·tine** (nahr'ko-tēn) noscapine.

**nar·co·tize** (nahr'ko-tīz) to put under the influence of a narcotic.

**nar·cous** (nar'kəs) stuporous.

**Nar·dil** (nahr'dil) trademark for a preparation of phenelzine sulfate.

**na·res** (na'rēz) [L., pl. of *na'ris,* q.v.] [TA] the external orifices of the nose; called also *nostrils.*
**anterior n., external n.**, nares.
**posterior n.**, choanae.

**na·ris** (na'ris) [L.] singular of *nares.*

**Nar·one** (nar'ōn) trademark for a preparation of dipyrone.

**Nar·the·ci·um** (nahr-the'se-əm) a genus of herbs of the family Liliaceae, which have yellow flowers. *N. ossifra'gum* is the bog asphodel, a species that can cause yellows, a form of hepatogenous photosensitization, in ruminants that eat it.

**na·sal** (na'zəl) [L. *nasalis*] 1. pertaining to the nose; called also *rhinal.* 2. a speech sound produced by having air flow through the nose, such as *n, ng,* or *m.*

**Na·sal·ide** (na'zəl-īd") trademark for a preparation of flunisolide.

**na·sa·lis** (na-za'lis) [L., from *nasus* nose] nasal.

**Na·sa·rel** (na'zə-rel) trademark for a preparation of flunisolide.

**nas·cent** (nas'ənt, na'sənt) [L. *nascens*] 1. just born; just coming into existence. 2. just liberated from a chemical combination, and hence more reactive because uncombined.

**NASH** nonalcoholic steatohepatitis.

**na·sio·in·i·ac** (na"ze-o-in'e-ak) pertaining to the nasion and the inion.

**na·si·on** (na'ze-on) [L. *nasus* nose] [TA] a cephalometric landmark located where the internasal and nasofrontal sutures meet; it corresponds roughly to the depression at the root of the nose just inferior to the level of the eyebrows.

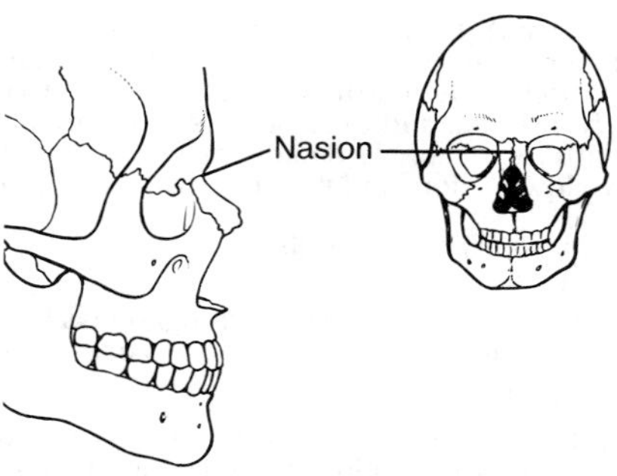


**Nas·myth's membrane** (nas'miths) [Alexander *Nasmyth,* Scottish dental surgeon in London, died 1847] primary (enamel) cuticle.

**NAS-NRC** National Academy of Sciences–National Research Council.

**nas(o)-** [L. *nasus* nose] a combining form denoting relationship to the nose.

**na·so·an·tral** (na"zo-an'trəl) pertaining to the nose and the maxillary antrum (sinus).

**na·so·an·tri·tis** (na"zo-an-tri'tis) rhinoantritis.

**na·so·an·tros·to·my** (na"zo-an-tros'tə-me) surgical formation of a nasoantral window for drainage of an obstructed maxillary sinus.

**na·so·bron·chi·al** (na"zo-brong'ke-əl) pertaining to the nasal cavities and the bronchi.

**na·so·cil·i·ary** (na"zo-sil'e-ar"e) pertaining to or affecting the eyes, brow, and root of the nose, as the nasociliary nerve.

**na·so·eth·moi·dal** (na"zo-eth-moi'dəl) ethmonasal.

**na·so·fron·tal** (na"zo-fron'təl) pertaining to the nose or other nasal structures and the forehead or the frontal bone; called also *frontonasal.*

**na·so·gas·tric** (na"zo-gas'trik) pertaining to the nose and stomach, as in (nasogastric) aspiration of the stomach's contents.

**na·so·la·bi·al** (na"zo-la'be-əl) [*naso-* + *labial*] pertaining to the nose and lip.

**na·so·lac·ri·mal** (na"zo-lak'rĭ-məl) pertaining to the nose and lacrimal apparatus.

**na·so·ma·nom·e·ter** (na"zo-mə-nom'ə-tər) rhinomanometer.

**na·so·oral** (na"zo-or'əl) oronasal.

**na·so·pal·a·tine** (na"zo-pal'ə-tīn) [*naso-* + *palatine*] pertaining to the nose and palate.

**na·so·pha·ryn·ge·al** (na"zo-fə-rin'je-əl) 1. pertaining to the nose and the pharynx. 2. pertaining to the nasopharynx.

**na·so·phar·yn·gi·tis** (na"zo-far"in-ji'tis) [MeSH: Nasopharyngitis] inflammation of the nasopharynx. Called also *epipharyngitis* and *rhinopharyngitis.*

**na·so·pha·ryn·go·la·ryn·go·scope** (na"zo-fə-ring"go-lə-ring'go-skōp) a flexible fiberscope for examining the nasopharynx and larynx.

**na·so·phar·ynx** (na"zo-far'inks) [*naso-* + *pharynx*] [MeSH: Nasopharynx] pars nasalis pharyngis.

**na·so·ros·tral** (na"zo-ros'trəl) pertaining to the nose and the rostrum of the sphenoid bone.

**na·so·scope** (na'zo-skōp) [*naso-* + *-scope*] rhinoscope.

**na·so·sep·tal** (na"zo-sep'təl) pertaining to the nasal septum.

**na·so·sep·ti·tis** (na"zo-sep-ti'tis) inflammation of the nasal septum.

**na·so·si·nu·si·tis** (na"zo-si"nə-si'tis) rhinosinusitis.

**na·so·spi·na·le** (na"zo-spi-na'le) the point at which a horizontal line tangential to the inferior margins of the nasal aperture is intersected by the median plane.

**na·so·tur·bi·nal** (na″zo-tur′bĭ-nəl) pertaining to the nose and a turbinate bone.

**na·sus** (na′səs) [L.] [TA] nose: the specialized structure of the face that serves as the organ of the sense of smell and as part of the respiratory system. See also *n. externus* and *cavitas nasi*.
**n. exter′nus,** the external nose: the part of the nose that protrudes on the face; made up of an osteocartilaginous framework, covered externally by muscles and skin and lined internally by mucous membrane; it has two apertures that open into the nasal cavity and is separated into two halves by the nasal septum.

**na·tal** (na′təl) 1. [L. *natus* birth] pertaining to birth. 2. [L. *nates* buttocks] gluteal.

**na·tal·i·ty** (na-tal′ĭ-te) [L. *natalis* pertaining to birth] birth rate.

**nat·a·my·cin** (nat″ə-mi′sin) [MeSH: Natamycin] a polyene antibiotic used in topical treatment of fungal keratitis, blepharitis, and conjunctivitis.

**na·tes** (na′tēz) sing., *na′tis* [L.] [TA] buttocks: the prominences formed by the gluteal muscles on the lower part of the back; called also *breech* and *clunes* [TA alternative].

**Na·thans** (na′thənz) Daniel. American microbiologist, born 1928; co-winner, with Werner Arber and Hamilton Othanel Smith, of the Nobel prize for medicine or physiology in 1978 for his application of restriction enzymes to molecular genetics.

**na·ti·mor·tal·i·ty** (na″tĭ-mor-tal′ĭ-te) [L. *natus* birth + *mortality*] fetal death rate.

**Na·tion·al For·mu·lary** a book of standards for certain pharmaceuticals and preparations that are not included in the USP. It is revised every five years, and recognized as a book of official standards by the Pure Food and Drugs Act of 1906. Abbreviated NF.

**na·tis** (na′tis) [L. "rump"] singular of *nates*.

**na·tive** (na′tiv) [L. *nativus*] normal to a location; unaltered from its natural state.

**Nat·o·lone** (nat′o-lōn) trademark for a preparation of pregnenolone.

**na·tre·mia** (nə-tre′me-ə) [*natrium* + *-emia*] hypernatremia.

**na·tri·um** (na′tre-əm) gen. *na′trii* [L., from Gr. *nitron* sodium carbonate] sodium.

**na·tri·ure·sis** (na″tre-u-re′sis) [*natrium* + *-uresis*] [MeSH: Natriuresis] the excretion of sodium in the urine; see also *salt-losing syndrome*, under *syndrome*.

**na·tri·uret·ic** (na″tre-u-ret′ik) 1. pertaining to, characterized by, or promoting natriuresis. 2. an agent that promotes natriuresis.

**nat·ru·re·sis** (nat″roo-re′sis) natriuresis.

**nat·ru·ret·ic** (nat″roo-ret′ik) natriuretic.

**nat·u·ral** (nach′ə-rəl) [L. *naturalis*, from *natura* nature] neither artificial nor pathologic.

**Nat·ure·tin** (nat″u-re′tin) trademark for preparations of bendroflumethiazide.

**na·turo·path** (na′chər-o-path″) a practitioner of naturopathy.

**na·turo·path·ic** (na″chər-o-path′ik) pertaining to naturopathy.

**na·tur·op·a·thy** (na″chər-op′ə-the) [MeSH: Naturopathy] a drugless system of therapy, making use of physical forces such as air, light, water, heat, massage, etc.

**nau·sea** (naw′ze-ə) [L.; Gr. *nausia* seasickness] [MeSH: Nausea] an unpleasant sensation, vaguely referred to the epigastrium and abdomen, and often culminating in vomiting.
**n. epide′mica,** an epidemic disease, probably viral gastroenteritis, marked by nausea, vomiting, giddiness, and diarrhea.
**n. gravida′rum,** the morning sickness of pregnancy.

**nau·se·ant** (naw′se-ənt) 1. inducing nausea. 2. an agent that causes nausea.

**nau·se·ate** (naw′se-āt) to affect with nausea.

**nau·seous** (naw′shəs) pertaining to or producing nausea.

**Nav·ane** (Nav′ān) trademark for preparations of thiothixene.

**na·vel** (na′vəl) umbilicus.
**blue n.,** Cullen's sign.
**enamel n.,** either of two depressions between the lateral dental lamina and the developing tooth germ, one pointing distally *(distal enamel n.)* and the other mesially *(mesial enamel n.)*.

**Na·vel·bine** (na-vel′bēn) trademark for a preparation of vinorelbine tartrate.

**na·vi·cu·la** (nə-vĭ′ku-lə) [L. "boat"] frenulum labiorum pudendi.

**na·vic·u·lar** (nə-vik′u-lər) [L. *navicula* boat] boat-shaped, as the navicular bone.

**Nb** symbol for *niobium*.

**NBS** National Bureau of Standards.

**NBT** nitroblue tetrazolium; see under *tests*.

**NBTE** nonbacterial thrombotic endocarditis.

**NCF** neutrophil chemotactic factor.

**NCHS** National Center for Health Statistics.

**NCI** National Cancer Institute.

**nCi** nanocurie.

**NCMH** National Committee for Mental Hygiene.

**NCN** National Council of Nurses.

**NCRP** National Committee on Radiation Protection and Measurements.

**NCV** nerve conduction velocity.

**Nd** symbol for *neodymium*.

**NDA** National Dental Association.

**nDNA** nuclear DNA; see under *DNA*.

**NDV** Newcastle disease virus.

**Nd:YAG** neodymium:yttrium-aluminum-garnet; see under *laser*.

**Ne** symbol for *neon*.

**ne·al·o·gy** (ne-al′ə-je) [Gr. *nealēs* young + *-logy*] the study of the early infant stages of animals.

**near·sight** (nēr′sīt) myopia.

**near·sight·ed** (nēr′sīt-əd) myopic.

**near·sight·ed·ness** (nēr-sīt′əd-nəs) myopia.

**ne·ar·thro·sis** (ne″ahr-thro′sis) [*ne-* + *arthrosis* (def. 1)] 1. a false joint; pseudarthrosis. 2. an artificial joint inserted in total joint replacement.

**Neb·cin** (neb′sin) trademark for preparations of tobramycin sulfate.

**ne·ben·kern** (na-ben′kərn) [Ger. *neben* near, beside + *kern* kernel, nucleus] 1. a name given to several structures of the cell, but especially to the paranucleus. 2. a large mitochondrial mass around the axial filament in the flagellum of the spermatozoon; it is formed by coalescence of smaller mitochondria during spermatogenesis.

**neb·ra·my·cin** (neb″rə-mi′sin) [MeSH: Nebramycin] an aminoglycoside antibacterial complex produced by *Streptomyces tenebrarius*, consisting of eight components; factor 6 (tobramycin) is used clinically as an antibiotic and factor 2 (apramycin) is used as an antibiotic in veterinary medicine.

**neb·u·la** (neb′u-lə) gen. and pl. *ne′bulae* [L. "mist"] 1. a slight corneal opacity or scar that can be seen only by oblique illumination; it seldom interferes with vision. 2. cloudiness in urine. 3. an oily preparation for use in an atomizer.

**neb·u·lar·ine** (neb-u-lar′in) an antibiotic substance isolated from the juice of the fungus *Clitocybe nebularis*, which has tuberculostatic and antimitotic activity, and in high dilutions preferentially inhibits growth of some cancer cells.

**neb·u·li·za·tion** (neb″u-lĭ-za′shən) [L. *nebula* mist] 1. conversion into an aerosol or spray. 2. treatment by an aerosol. Called also *atomization*.

**neb·u·liz·er** (neb′u-līz-ər) [MeSH: Nebulizers and Vaporizers] a device for creating and throwing an aerosol spray. Called also *atomizer*.

**Neb·u·pent** (neb′u-pent) trademark for a preparation of pentamidine isethionate.

**Ne·ca·tor** (ne-ka′tor) [L. "murderer"] [MeSH: Necator] a genus of nematode parasites of the family Ancylostomatidae.
**N. america′nus,** the American or New World hookworm; infection with this parasite causes hookworm disease in humans and occasionally in pigs. It resembles *Ancylostoma duodenale* but is shorter and more slender. Its buccal cavity contains four plates, four pharyngeal lancets, and a dorsal conic tooth. Called also *Ancylostoma americanum* and *Uncinaria americana*.

**ne·ca·to·ri·a·sis** (ne-ka″to-ri′ə-sis) [MeSH: Necatoriasis] hookworm disease in humans or pigs caused by infection with worms of the genus *Necator*.

**ne·ces·si·ty** (nə-ses′ĭ-te) something necessary or indispensable.
**pharmaceutic n., pharmaceutical n.,** a substance having slight or no value therapeutically, but used in the preparation of various pharmaceuticals, including preservatives, solvents, ointment bases, and flavoring, coloring, diluting, emulsifying, and suspending agents; called also *pharmaceutic* or *pharmaceutical aid*.

**neck** (nek) [MeSH: Neck] 1. cervix (def. 1). 2. a constricted part; see also *collum*.
**anatomical n. of humerus,** collum anatomicum humeri.

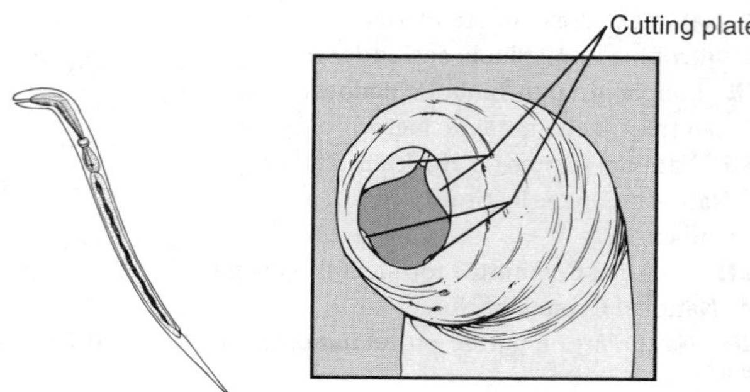


*Necator americanus,* with inset showing dorsal and ventral pairs of cutting plates in a frontal view of the head.

**n. of ankle bone,** collum tali.
**bladder n.,** cervix vesicae.
**bull n.,** marked edema of the anterior neck and submandibular region associated with massive cervical lymphadenopathy.
**n. of condyloid process of mandible,** collum mandibulae.
**dental n.,** cervix dentis.
**n. of dorsal horn of spinal cord,** cervix cornus posterioris medullae spinalis.
**false n. of humerus,** collum chirurgicum humeri.
**n. of femur,** collum femoris.
**n. of fibula,** collum fibulae.
**n. of gallbladder,** collum vesicae biliaris.
**n. of glans penis,** collum glandis penis.
**n. of hair follicle,** collum folliculi pili.
**n. of head of posterior horn of spinal cord,** cervix cornus posterioris medullae spinalis.
**n. of humerus,** collum anatomicum humeri.
**lateral n. of vertebra,** pediculus arcus vertebrae.
**Madelung's n.,** diffuse symmetrical lipomas of the neck.
**n. of malleus,** collum mallei.
**n. of mandible,** collum mandibulae.
**n. of pancreas,** a constricted portion marking the junction of the head and body of the pancreas.
**n. of posterior horn of spinal cord,** cervix cornus posterioris medullae spinalis.
**n. of radius,** collum radii.
**n. of rib,** collum costae.
**n. of scapula,** collum scapulae.
**n. of spermatozoon,** the portion of the tail of a spermatozoon beginning immediately distal to the head and extending to the anterior centriole. See illustration under *spermatozoon.*
**surgical n. of humerus,** collum chirurgicum humeri.
**n. of talus,** collum tali.
**n. of tooth,** cervix dentis.
**true n. of humerus,** collum anatomicum humeri.
**turkey gobbler n.,** submental vertical skin folds due to aging.
**n. of urinary bladder,** cervix vesicae.
**uterine n., n. of uterus,** cervix uteri.
**n. of vertebra, n. of vertebral arch,** pediculus arcus vertebrae.
**webbed n.,** pterygium colli.
**wry n.,** torticollis.

**neck·lace** (nek'ləs) an encircling band around the neck.
**Casal's n.,** an area of erythema and pigmentation around the neck in pellagra; called also *Casal's collar.*

**nec·rec·to·my** (nek-rek'tə-me) [*necro-* + *-ectomy*] excision of necrotic tissue.

**nec·ren·ceph·a·lus** (nek"ren-sef'ə-ləs) [*necro-* + Gr. *enkephalos* brain] encephalomalacia.

**necr(o)-** [Gr. *nekros* dead] a combining form denoting relationship to death or to a dead body, cells, or tissue.

**nec·ro·bac·il·lo·sis** (nek"ro-bas"ĭ-lo'sis) any of various infections with *Fusobacterium necrophorum,* such as foot rot and calf diphtheria in cattle, gangrenous dermatitis in horses, and Schmorl's disease in hogs, cattle, and rabbits. Called also *bacillary necrosis.*
**interdigital n.,** foot rot of cattle.

**nec·ro·bi·o·sis** (nek"ro-bi-o'sis) [*necro-* + *biosis*] swelling, basophilia, and distortion of collagen bundles in the dermis, sometimes with obliteration of normal structure, but without actual necrosis, seen especially in granuloma annulare and necrobiosis lipoidica diabeticorum. Cf. *gangrene* and *necrosis.*
**equine nodular n.,** the existence of numerous firm cutaneous nodules on the sides of the neck and trunk of a horse, filled with degenerated collagen and eosinophils. Called also *collagenolytic granuloma.*
**n. lipoi'dica,** a degenerative disease of dermal connective tissue characterized by development of erythematous papules or nodules in the pretibial area and sometimes elsewhere, extending to form shiny yellow to red plaques that are covered with telangiectatic vessels and have a scaly, atrophic, depressed center. More than half of affected patients have diabetes; the clinical appearance, genetic background for diabetes, and histopathologic findings are similar in both diabetic and nondiabetic patients. See also *diabetic dermopathy,* under *dermopathy,* and *granulomatosis disciformis progressiva et chronica.*
**n. lipoi'dica diabetico'rum,** necrobiosis lipoidica in diabetics.

**nec·ro·bi·ot·ic** (nek"ro-bi-ot'ik) pertaining to or characterized by necrobiosis.

**nec·ro·cy·to·sis** (nek"ro-si-to'sis) [*necro-* + *cyt-* + *-osis*] death and decay of cells.

**nec·ro·cy·to·tox·in** (nek"ro-si"to-tok'sin) a toxin that produces death of cells.

**nec·ro·gen·ic** (nek"ro-jen'ik) [*necro-* + *-genic*] productive of necrosis or death.

**ne·crog·e·nous** (nə-kroj'ə-nəs) originating or arising from dead matter.

**nec·ro·log·ic** (nek"ro-loj'ik) pertaining to necrology.

**ne·crol·o·gist** (nə-krol'ə-jist) an expert in necrology.

**ne·crol·o·gy** (nə-krol'ə-je) [*necro-* + *-logy*] the statistics or records of deaths.

**ne·crol·y·sis** (nə-krol'ĭ-sis) [*necro-* + *-lysis*] separation or exfoliation of tissue due to necrosis.
**toxic epidermal n.,** an exfoliative skin disease seen primarily in adults as a severe cutaneous reaction to various factors, usually drugs but sometimes infections (viral, bacterial, or fungal), neoplastic disease, graft-versus-host reaction, or chemical exposure. It is characterized by full-thickness epidermal necrosis, resulting in subepidermal separation, bulla formation, and dermal inflammatory changes; there is widespread loss of skin, leaving raw areas where the skin surface looks scalded. Called also *Lyell's disease* or *syndrome, nonstaphylococcal scalded skin syndrome,* and *toxic bullous epidermolysis.* Cf. *staphylococcal scalded skin syndrome.*

**nec·ro·ma·nia** (nek"ro-ma'ne-ə) [*necro-* + *-mania*] pathological preoccupation with dead bodies.

**nec·ro·mi·me·sis** (nek"ro-mi-me'sis) [*necro-* + *mimesis*] a delusion in which individuals act as if dead because they believe themselves to be so.

**nec·ro·nec·to·my** (nek"ro-nek'tə-me) [*necro-* + *-ectomy*] necrectomy.

**ne·croph·a·gous** (nə-krof'ə-gəs) [*necro-* + *phag-* + *-ous*] devouring or subsisting on dead bodies.

**nec·ro·phil·ia** (nek"ro-fil'e-ə) [*necro-* + *-philia*] fascination or obsession with death, usually specifically sexual attraction to or sexual contact with dead bodies. Called also *necrophilism.*

**nec·ro·phil·ic** (nek"ro-fil'ik) 1. pertaining to or characterized by necrophilia. 2. showing preference for dead tissue, as necrophilic bacteria.

**ne·croph·i·lism** (nə-krof'ĭ-liz-əm) necrophilia.

**ne·croph·i·lous** (nə-krof'ĭ-ləs) necrophilic.

**ne·croph·i·ly** (nə-krof'ĭ-le) necrophilia.

**nec·ro·pho·bia** (nek"ro-fo'be-ə) [*necro-* + *-phobia*] irrational fear of death or of dead bodies.

**nec·rop·sy** (nek'rop-se) [Gr. *nekros* dead + *opsis* view] examination of a body after death; see *autopsy.*

**nec·ro·sa·dism** (nec"ro-sa'diz-əm) [*necro-* + *sadism*] mutilation of a corpse for the purpose of exciting or gratifying sexual feelings.

**ne·cros·co·py** (nə-kros'kə-pe) [*necro-* + *-scopy*] to examine at necropsy.

**nec·rose** (nek'rōs) to become necrotic or to undergo necrosis.

**nec·ro·ses** (nə-kro'sēz) [Gr.] [MeSH: Necrosis] plural of *necrosis.*

**ne·cro·sis** (nə-kro'sis) pl. *necro'ses* [Gr. *nekrōsis* deadness] [MeSH: Necrosis] the sum of the morphological changes indicative of cell death and caused by the progressive degradative action of enzymes; it may affect groups of cells or part of a structure or an organ.
**acute pancreatic n.,** acute necrotizing pancreatitis.
**acute tubular n.,** acute renal failure with mild to severe damage or necrosis of tubule cells, usually occurring secondary to ischemia or the effects of a nephrotoxin. See also *lower nephron nephrosis.* Called also *vasomotor nephropathy.*
**arteriolar n.,** arteriolonecrosis.
**aseptic n.,** increasing sclerosis and cystic changes in the head of the femur which sometimes follow traumatic dislocation of the hip.

A similar condition sometimes develops in the head of the humerus after shoulder dislocation.
**avascular n.,** coagulation n.
**avascular n. of bone,** osteonecrosis.
**bacillary n.,** necrobacillosis.
**Balser's fatty n.,** gangrenous pancreatitis with omental bursitis and disseminated patches of necrosis of the fatty tissues; pancreatitis with fat necrosis.
**bridging n.,** septa of confluent necrosis bridging adjacent central veins and portal triads of hepatic lobules characteristic of subacute hepatic necrosis.
**caseation n., caseous n.,** caseation (def. 2).
**central n.,** that which affects the central portion of a cell or of a bone or a lobule of the liver.
**cerebrocortical n.,** polioencephalomalacia.
**cheesy n.,** caseation (def. 2).
**coagulation n., coagulative n.,** necrosis in which tissue becomes a dry, opaque, eosinophilic mass containing the outlines of anucleated cells, resulting from the denaturation of proteins following hypoxic injury, such as that caused by ischemia in infarction. Called also *avascular n.* and *ischemic n.*
**colliquative n.,** necrosis in which the necrotic material becomes softened and liquefied.
**contraction band n.,** a cardiac lesion seen in patients with neurologically induced cardiographic changes, in myocardial biopsy specimens, and in cocaine or epinephrine toxicity, characterized by hypercontracted myofibrils with contraction bands and mitochondrial damage; it is caused by calcium ion influx into dying cells, which results in the arrest of cells in the contracted state, following severe ischemia and subsequent reperfusion. Called also *coagulative myocytolysis.*
**cystic medial n.,** changes in the medial layer of the aorta, consisting of degeneration and necrosis of elastic and muscle fibers, mucoid infiltration, and cyst formation, often resulting in dissecting aneurysm; called also *Erdheim's disease* and *medionecrosis of aorta.*
**dietary hepatic n.,** hepatosis dietetica.
**dry n.,** that in which the necrotic tissue becomes dry.
**enzymatic fat n.,** fat n.
**epiphyseal ischemic n.,** degeneration and eventual replacement of the osseous nucleus of an epiphysis, which collapses under pressure and causes distortion of the surrounding healthy tissue; attributed to interference with the blood supply of the epiphysis. It may affect the femur, tibia, tarsal navicular head, humerus, etc. Called also *osteochondrosis* (q.v.).
**Erdheim's cystic medial n.,** changes in the medial layer of the aorta, consisting of degeneration and necrosis of elastic and muscle fibers, mucoid infiltration, and cyst formation, often resulting in dissecting aneurysm; called also *medionecrosis of aorta.*
**exanthematous n.,** an acute necrotizing process involving the gingivae, jaw bones, and contiguous soft tissues, which primarily affects children; it resembles gangrenous stomatitis, except that there is slight odor, a tendency to be self-limited, a low mortality rate, and a normal leukocyte count.
**fat n.,** a condition in which the neutral fats in the cells of adipose tissue are split by enzymatic action into fatty acids and glycerol, producing minute, chalky white areas where the released fatty acids react with calcium, magnesium, and sodium ions to form soaps; it usually affects the pancreas and peripancreatic fat in acute hemorrhagic pancreatitis. Called also *steatonecrosis.*
**fibrinoid n.,** deposition of fibrin and other plasma proteins in the walls of afferent renal arterioles in malignant hypertension, often accompanied by an inflammatory infiltrate within the walls and thrombosis of the vessel lumen. Called also *necrotizing arteriolitis.*
**focal n.,** the presence of small foci of necrosis often seen in the liver in the course of an infection.
**gangrenous n.,** cell death caused by a combination of ischemia and superimposed bacterial infection, combining the features of coagulation and colliquative necrosis.
**gangrenous pulp n.,** necrosis of the pulp tissue due to ischemia with superimposed bacterial infection, representing an advanced stage of untreated pulpitis. Called also *pulp gangrene.* See also *necrotic pulp,* under *pulp.*
**hyaline n.,** Zenker's degeneration.
**infectious bulbar n.,** heel abscess.
**infectious pancreatic n.,** an acute disease affecting fry and young fish, originally seen in salmonids, but also affecting non-salmonids and shellfish, caused by the infectious pancreatic necrosis virus. It is characterized by darkened pigmentation, whirling about the long axis, and massive necrosis of the pancreas, pylorus, and anterior intestine, with the formation of a white exudate.
**ischemic n.,** coagulation n.
**ischemic n. of bone,** osteonecrosis.
**labial n. of rabbits,** a fatal necrobacillosis of rabbits that begins in the lower lip and extends down to the thorax.
**liquefaction n.,** colliquative n.
**massive hepatic n.,** massive necrosis of the liver, a rare complication of viral hepatitis (fulminant hepatitis) that may also result from exposure to hepatotoxins or from drug hypersensitivity. A lobe or the entire liver shrinks, becoming a soft, flabby, yellow-brown to green mass with a wrinkled capsule; there is confluent necrosis of hepatocytes, often with fatty change. Mortality is 60 to 90 per cent. Formerly called *acute parenchymatous hepatitis* and *acute yellow atrophy.*
**medial n.,** medionecrosis.
**mercurial n.,** necrosis due to mercury poisoning.
**mummification n.,** dry gangrene.
**Paget's quiet n.,** a process of local necrosis and sequestrum formation in the superficial layers of the shaft of a long bone with a minimal amount of suppuration around the sequestrum and without sinus formation.
**peripheral n.,** necrosis of the peripheral portions of a liver lobule as in puerperal eclampsia.
**phosphorus n.,** necrosis of the jaw, sometimes associated with deposition of new subperiosteal bone, occurring in workers exposed to yellow phosphorus fumes. Called also *phosphonecrosis* and *phossy jaw.*
**piecemeal n.,** destruction of hepatocytes at the interface between liver parenchyma and portal triads associated with lymphocytic infiltration, characteristic of severe (active) chronic hepatitis and primary biliary cirrhosis.
**postpartum pituitary n.,** necrosis of the pituitary during the postpartum period, often associated with shock and excessive uterine bleeding during delivery, and leading to variable patterns of hypopituitarism; called also *Sheehan's syndrome.*
**pressure n.,** necrosis due to insufficient local blood supply as in decubitus ulcers.
**n. progre'diens,** progressive sloughing.
**progressive emphysematous n.,** gas gangrene.
**radiation n.,** radionecrosis.
**radium n.,** necrosis of bones due to exposure to radium, formerly common in workers in radium plants.
**n. of renal papillae, renal papillary n.,** an accompaniment of acute pyelonephritis, most often seen in diabetics, characterized by necrosis of the renal papillae of one or both kidneys, with sharp demarcation between necrotic and living tissue; called also *necrotizing papillitis* and *necrotizing renal papillitis.*
**septic n.,** necrosis resulting from bacterial infection.
**subacute hepatic n.,** a clinical entity comprising a small group of viral hepatitis cases characterized by bridging necrosis and having an increased incidence of progression to liver failure, chronic active hepatitis, or cirrhosis. Called also *subacute* or *subchronic atrophy of liver* and *submassive hepatic n.*
**subcutaneous fat n.,** adiponecrosis subcutanea neonatorum.
**submassive hepatic n.,** subacute hepatic n.
**superficial n.,** that which affects only the outer layers of a bone.
**syphilitic n.,** necrosis caused by syphilis.
**total n.,** that which affects all parts of a bone.
**n. ustilagi'nea,** dry gangrene from ergotism.
**Zenker's n.,** see under *degeneration.*

**nec·ro·sper·mia** (nek″ro-sper′me-ə) [*necro-* + *sperm-* + *-ia*] a condition in which the spermatozoa of the semen are dead or motionless.

**nec·ro·sper·mic** (nek″ro-sper′mik) pertaining to or characterized by necrospermia.

**ne·crot·ic** (nə-krot′ik) pertaining to or characterized by necrosis.

**nec·ro·tiz·ing** (nek′ro-tīz″ing) causing necrosis.

**ne·crot·o·my** (nə-krot′ə-me) [*necro-* + *-tomy*] 1. dissection of a dead body. 2. the excision of a sequestrum.
**osteoplastic n.,** removal of a sequestrum from a bone after first lifting a flap of the bone, which is replaced after the operation.

**nec·ro·tox·in** (nek″ro-tok′sin) a toxin that kills tissue cells, e.g., the exotoxins secreted by species of *Clostridium* and by *Staphylococcus aureus.*

**nec·ro·zoo·sper·mia** (nek″ro-zo″o-sper′me-ə) necrospermia.

**Nec·tria** (nek′tre-ə) a genus of fungi of the family Hypocreaceae, usually found on wood or various fruits. It contains the perfect (sexual) stage of several species of *Acremonium* and *Fusarium.*

**Nec·tu·rus** (nek-tu′rəs) [MeSH: Necturus] a genus of salamanders having large external gills; employed in physiologic research.

**NED** no evidence of disease.

**nee·dle** (ne′dəl) [L. *acus*] [MeSH: Needles] 1. a sharp instrument for suturing or puncturing. 2. to puncture with a needle, as in discission of the lens for treatment of cataract.
**Abrams' n.,** a biopsy needle designed to reduce the danger of introducing air into tissues, as in pleural biopsy.
**aneurysm n.,** one with a handle, used in ligating blood vessels.
**aspirating n.,** a long, hollow needle for removing fluid from a cavity.
**Brockenbrough n.,** a curved steel transseptal needle within a Brockenbrough transseptal catheter; used to puncture the interatrial septum.

**cataract n.**, one used in removing a cataract.
**Chiba n.**, fine n.
**Cope's n.**, a blunt-ended hooklike needle with a concealed cutting edge and snare, used in biopsy of the pleura, pericardium, peritoneum, and synovium.
**Deschamps' n.**, one with the eye near the point, and a long handle attached; used in ligating deep-seated arteries.
**discission n.**, a special form of cataract needle.
**fine n.**, a very thin, highly flexible steel needle with a narrow inner core used to cannulate very small bile ducts to perform percutaneous (or fine needle) transhepatic cholangiography (see under *cholangiography*). Called also *Chiba n.* and *skinny n.*
**Hagedorn's n's,** surgical needles which are flat from side to side, and have a straight cutting edge near the point and a large eye.
**hypodermic n.**, a short, slender, hollow needle used in injecting drugs beneath the skin.
**knife n.**, a slender knife with a needlelike point, used in discission of a cataract and other ophthalmic operations, as in goniotomy and goniopuncture.
**ligature n.**, a slender steel needle with a long handle and an eye in its curved end, used for passing a ligature underneath an artery.
**Menghini n.**, a needle that does not require rotation to cut loose the tissue specimen in a biopsy of the liver.
**Reverdin's n.**, a surgical needle having an eye which can be opened and closed by means of a slide.
**Seldinger n.**, a needle with a blunt, tapered external cannula with a sharp obturator; used for the initial percutaneous insertion characteristic of the Seldinger technique for arterial or venous access.
**Silverman n.**, an instrument for taking tissue specimens, consisting of an outer cannula, an obturator, and an inner split needle with longitudinal grooves in which the tissue is retained when the needle and cannula are withdrawn.
**skinny n.**, fine n.
**stop n.**, a needle with a shoulder that prevents it from being inserted beyond a certain distance.
**swaged n.**, one permanently attached to the suture material.
**transseptal n.**, a needle used to puncture the interatrial septum in transseptal catheterization.
**Tuohy n.**, one in which the opening at the end is angled 45 degrees so that a catheter or endoscope through its lumen exits at an angle; used for examination or treatment of the epidermal space or subarachnoid space.
**Veress n.**, a hollow needle consisting of a sharp trocar with a slanted end surrounding an inner cylinder with a blunt end; after the trocar is introduced into a body cavity the blunt cylinder is advanced outward so that internal organs are not injured by the sharp edge; used for insufflation of a body cavity, such as for pneumoperitoneum in minimally invasive surgery.
**Vim-Silverman n.**, a needle used in needle biopsy.

**NEFA** nonesterified fatty acids.

**ne·fa·zo·done hy·dro·chlo·ride** (nə-fa'zo-dōn) a compound structurally related to trazodone, used as an antidepressant; administered orally.

**ne·flu·o·ro·pho·tom·e·ter** (nə-floor"o-fo-tom'ə-tər) fluoronephelometer.

**nef·o·pam hy·dro·chlo·ride** (nef'o-pam) a non-opioid analgesic, used for the relief of mild to moderate pain; administered intramuscularly and orally.

**Neg·a·tan** (neg'ə-tan) trademark for a preparation of negatol.

**neg·a·tiv·ism** (neg'ə-tiv-iz"əm) [MeSH: Negativism] resistance or opposition to advice, suggestions, or commands; e.g., in catatonic schizophrenia the patient may lower his arms if asked to raise them or may resist efforts to move them.

**neg·a·tol** (neg'ə-tol) a colloidal product obtained by reacting metacresol sulfonic acid with formaldehyde; used as a parasiticide, germicide, and bacteriostatic, for topical application to the cervix.

**neg·a·tron** (neg'ə-tron) [MeSH: Electrons] the negative electron; see *positron* and *electron.*

**Neg·Gram** (neg'ram) trademark for preparations of nalidixic acid.

**ne·glect** (nə-glekt') [L. *neglegere* to disregard] disregard of or failure to perform some task or function.
**hemispatial n.**, failure to respond to stimuli on one side, usually opposite the side of a lesion in a cerebral hemisphere. Cf. *unilateral n.*
**sensory n.**, unilateral n.
**unilateral n.**, hemiapraxia with failure to pay attention to bodily grooming and stimuli on one side but not on the other, usually due to a lesion in the central nervous system, as after a stroke. Called also *selective inattention.* Cf. *dressing apraxia.*

**Ne·gri bodies** (na'gre) [Adelchi *Negri,* Italian physician, 1876–1912] see under *body.*

**Ne·gri-Ja·cod syndrome** (na'gre-zhah-ko') [Silvio *Negri,* Italian physician, 20th century; Maurice *Jacod,* French physician, 20th century] Jacod's syndrome.

**Ne·gro's phenomenon (sign)** (na'grōz) [Camillo *Negro,* Italian neurologist, 1861–1927] see *cogwheel rigidity,* under *rigidity.*

**Ne·her** (na'her) Erwin. German biophysicist, born 1944. Co-winner with Bert Sakmann of the Nobel prize for medicine or physiology in 1991 for their work on cellular communications involving electrical signals, particularly their study of ion channels.

**NEI** National Eye Institute.

**neigh·bor·wise** (na'bor-wīz) descriptive of the plastic behavior of transplanted embryonic cells or tissue in a manner appropriate to its new and strange location. Cf. *selfwise.*

**Neill-Moo·ser bodies, reaction** (nēl-mo'zer) [Mather Humphrey *Neill,* American physician, 1882–1930; Hermann *Mooser,* Swiss pathologist, 1891–1971] see under *body* and *reaction.*

**Neis·ser's diplococcus** (ni'serz) [Albert Ludwig Siegmund *Neisser,* German physician, 1855–1916] see *Neisseria gonorrhoeae.*

**Neis·ser-Wechs·berg phenomenon** (ni'ser-veks'berg) [Max *Neisser,* German physician, 1869–1938; Friedrich *Wechsberg,* German physician, 1873–1929] see *complement deviation,* under *deviation.*

**Neis·se·ria** (ni-se're-ə) [A.L.S. *Neisser*] [MeSH: Neisseria] a genus of bacteria of the family Neisseriaceae, consisting of gram-negative, oxidase-positive cocci characteristically coffee bean–shaped and paired. The organisms are aerobic or facultatively anaerobic and are part of the normal flora of the oropharynx, nasopharynx, and genitourinary tract. The genus includes the gonococcus, the several meningococcus types, pigmented forms occasionally associated with meningitis, and a number of saprophytic or parasitic but nonpathogenic species.
**N. catarrha'lis,** *Moraxella (Branhamella) catarrhalis.*
**N. flaves'cens,** a species characterized by the production of yellow pigmented colonies. It is sometimes found in the body fluids of patients with meningitis and septicemia.
**N. gonorrhoe'ae,** the specific etiologic agent of gonorrhea, occurring typically as pairs of flattened cells, found primarily in purulent venereal discharges. Called also *diplococcus of Neisser.*
**N. lacta'mica,** a species that ferments lactose, found frequently in throat and nasopharyngeal cultures of infants and young children; it occasionally causes endocarditis and meningitis in humans.
**N. meningi'tidis,** a prominent cause of meningitis and the specific etiologic agent of meningococcal meningitis; it can also cause bacterial pneumonia (see *meningococcal pneumonia,* under *pneumonia*). The species is differentiated serologically into four main groups (A, B, C, D) and several provisional groups; group C is the most important pathogen.
**N. muco'sa,** a species that produces mucoid colonies that are often adherent; it is found in the human nasopharynx and is occasionally pathogenic, causing pneumonia. Called also *Diplococcus mucosus.*
**N. sic'ca,** a species characterized by dry grayish or slimy white or yellow colonies, which is part of the normal flora of the human nasopharynx, saliva, and sputum.
**N. subfla'va,** a species that produces smooth, yellow-pigmented colonies, found in the human nasopharynx and occasionally in cerebrospinal fluid in cases of meningitis.

**Neis·se·ri·a·ceae** (ni-se"re-a'se-e) [MeSH: Neisseriaceae] a family of gram-negative, aerobic cocci and rod-shaped bacteria occurring singly or in pairs, short chains, or masses. The organisms are parasitic or saprophytic, and some produce pigment. The family includes four genera: *Acinetobacter, Kingella, Moraxella,* and *Neisseria.*

**neis·se·ri·al** (ni-se're-əl) of, relating to, or caused by *Neisseria.*

**nekr(o)-** for words beginning thus, see those beginning *necr(o)-.*

**nek·ton** (nek'ton) [Gr. *nēktos* swimming] collective term for marine organisms that swim actively, as contrasted with plankton.

**Né·la·ton's catheter, line, sphincter, syndrome** (na-lah-tawz') [Auguste *Nélaton,* French surgeon, 1807–1873] see under *catheter, line,* and *sphincter,* and see *hereditary sensory radicular neuropathy,* under *neuropathy.*

**nel·fin·a·vir mesy·late** (nel-fin'ə-veer) a protease inhibitor active against the human immunodeficiency virus, causing the formation of immature, noninfectious viral particles, used in the treatment of human immunodeficiency virus infection and acquired immunodeficiency syndrome; administered orally.

**Nel·son's syndrome** (nel'sənz) [Don H. *Nelson,* American internist, born 1925] see under *syndrome.*

**ne·ma** (ne'mə) [Gr. *nēma* thread] a nematode.

**nem·a·line** (nem'ə-lēn) [Gr. *nēma* thread] threadlike or rod-shaped.

**nem·a·thel·minth** (nem"ə-thel'minth) [*nemat-* + *helminth*] a worm of the phylum Nemathelminthes.

**Nem·a·thel·min·thes** (nem″ə-thəl-min′thēz) in some systems of classification, a phylum including the Acanthocephala and Nematoda.

**nem·a·thel·min·thi·a·sis** (nem″ə-thel″min-thi′ə-sis) nematodiasis.

**ne·mat·i·cide** (nə-mat′ĭ-sīd) nematocide.

**nem·a·ti·za·tion** (nem″ə-tĭ-za′shən) nematodiasis.

**nemat(o)-** [Gr. *nēma* thread, gen. *nēmatos*] a combining form denoting relationship to a nematode, or to a threadlike structure.

**nem·a·to·blast** (nem′ə-to-blast) [*nemato-* + *-blast*] spermatid.

**Nem·a·toc·era** (nem″ə-tos′ər-ə) [Gr. *nēma* thread + *keras* horn] a suborder of Diptera characterized by having antennae of many segments; it includes the gnats, mosquitoes, midges, black flies, craneflies, gallflies, and others.

**nem·a·to·cide** (nem′ə-to-sīd″) [*nemato-* + *-cide*] 1. destructive to nematode worms. 2. an agent that destroys nematodes.

**nem·a·to·cyst** (nem′ə-to-sist″) a minute stinging structure, found in the cnidoblasts of jellyfish and other coelenterates, used for anchorage, for defense, and for the capture of prey.

**Nem·a·to·da** (nem″ə-to′də) [Gr. *nēma* thread + *eidos* form] [MeSH: Nematoda] a class of tapered cylindrical helminths, the roundworms, of the phylum Aschelminthes, many species of which are parasites. They are characterized by longitudinally oriented muscles and by a triradiate esophagus. In some systems of classification, they are considered to be a separate phylum. Sometimes called *Nemathelminthes,* or a class under that phylum.

**nem·a·tode** (nem′ə-tōd) any member of the class Nematoda; called also *roundworm* or *round worm* and *eelworm* or *eel worm.*

**nem·a·to·des·ma** (nem″ə-to-dez′mə) pl. *nematodesma′ta* [*nemato-* + Gr. *desmos* band, ligament] a bundle of parallel microtubules serving to support the cytostome and cytopharyngeal apparatus and associated organelles of certain ciliate protozoa; also seen in certain flagellate groups. Called also *trichite.*

**nem·a·to·di·a·sis** (nem″ə-to-di′ə-sis) infection by nematode parasites; called also *nemathelminthiasis, nematization,* and *nematosis.*

**Nem·a·to·di·rus** (nem″ə-to′dĭ-rəs) a genus of nematode parasites belonging to the family Trichostrongylidae, found in the duodenum of ruminants.

**nem·a·toid** (nem′ə-toid) resembling a thread; pertaining to a nematode parasite.

**nem·a·tol·o·gist** (nem″ə-tol′ə-jist) a specialist in nematology.

**nem·a·tol·o·gy** (nem″ə-tol′ə-je) the branch of zoology which deals with nematode worms.

**Nem·a·to·mor·pha** (nem″ə-to-mor′fə) [Gr. *nēma* thread + *morphē* form] a class of the phylum Aschelminthes, consisting of long, slender, cylindrical worms; commonly called *hairworms, horse hairs,* or *hair eels.* They are parasitic as juveniles. In some systems of classification, they are considered to be a separate phylum. Called also *Gordiacea.*

**nem·a·to·sis** (nem″ə-to′sis) nematodiasis.

**nem·a·to·sper·mia** (nem″ə-to-sper′me-ə) [*nemato-* + *sperm-* + *-ia*] spermatozoa having elongated tails.

**Nem·bu·tal** (nem′bu-tal) trademark for preparations of sodium pentobarbital.

**nem·ic** (nem′ik) pertaining to nematodes, or roundworms.

**Nen·cki's test** (nents′kēz) [Marcellus von *Nencki,* Polish physician, 1847–1901] see under *test.*

**ne(o)-** [Gr. *neos* new] 1. a combining form meaning new or recent, or denoting an immature form. 2. in chemistry, a prefix denoting a new chemical compound related in some way to an older one, to whose name it is added.

**neo·ad·ju·vant** (ne″o-aj′oo-vənt) said of preliminary cancer therapy that precedes a necessary second modality of treatment. See under *therapy.*

**Neo-An·ter·gan** (ne″o-an′tər-gən) trademark for a preparation of pyrilamine maleate.

**neo·an·ti·gen** (ne″o-an′tĭ-jən) tumor-associated antigen.

**neo·ar·thro·sis** (ne″o-ahr-thro′sis) nearthrosis.

**neo·bio·gen·e·sis** (ne″o-bi″o-jen′ə-sis) [*neo-* + *biogenesis*] biopoiesis.

**neo·blad·der** (ne″o-blad′ər) a continent urinary reservoir constructed from a detubularized bowel segment or from a segment of the stomach, with implantation of the ureters and urethra; used to replace the bladder following cystectomy.

**neo·blas·tic** (ne″o-blas′tik) [*neo-* + *blast-* + *-ic*] originating in or of the nature of new tissue.

**Neo-Cal·glu·con** (ne″o-kal′gloo-kon) trademark for a preparation of calcium glubionate.

**neo·cer·e·bel·lum** (ne″o-ser″ə-bel′əm) [*neo-* + *cerebellum*] [TA] the phylogenetically newest part of the cerebellum, described as corresponding to the lateral parts of the cerebellum, including the cerebellar hemispheres and the middle portion of the vermis. Because the hemispheres are the primary site of termination of the projections from the pons, the corticopontocerebellar fibers, the term is sometimes equated with *pontocerebellum.* Cf. *archicerebellum* and *paleocerebellum.*

**neo·ci·net·ic** (ne″o-si-net′ik) neokinetic.

**Neo-Cob·e·frin** (ne″o-kob′ə-frin) trademark for a preparation of levonordefrin.

**neo·cor·tex** (ne″o-kor′teks) [*neo-* + *cortex*] [TA] the newer, six-layered portion of the cerebral cortex, showing stratification and organization characteristic of the most highly evolved type of cerebral tissue. Called also *homotypical cortex, isocortex, neopallium,* and *nonolfactory cortex.* See also *archicortex* and *paleocortex,* and see *layers of cerebral cortex,* under *layer.*

**neo·cy·to·sis** (ne″o-si-to′sis) the presence of immature erythrocytes in the blood; see also *erythroblastosis* and *reticulocytosis.*

**neo·dar·win·ism** (ne″o-dahr′win-iz-əm) the concept that species evolve by natural selection only, thus ruling out the inheritance of acquired traits; see *darwinism.*

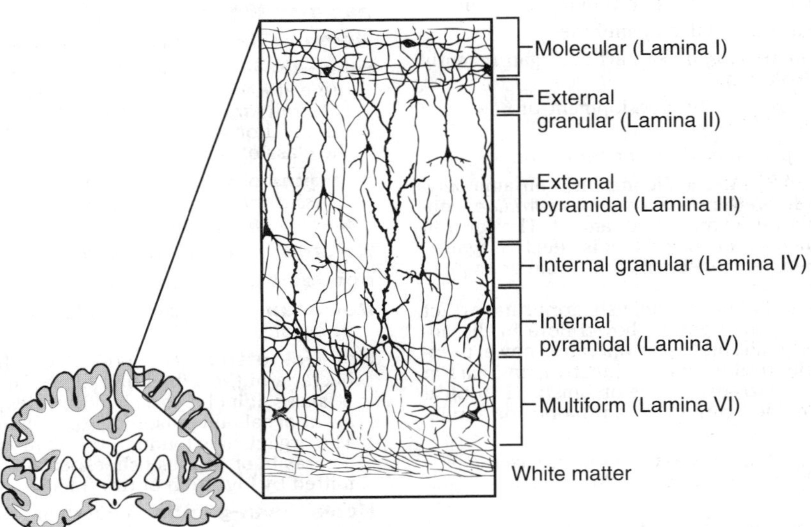


Coronal section through the neocortex, showing the six layers.

**Neo·dec·a·dron** (ne″o-dek′ə-dron) trademark for preparations of dexamethasone sodium phosphate.

**neo·dym·i·um** (ne″o-dim′e-əm) [MeSH: Neodymium] a rare element of atomic number, 60; atomic weight, 144.24; symbol, Nd.

**neo·en·dor·phin** (ne″o-en-dor′fin; -en′dor-fin) either of a pair of opioid peptides, designated $\alpha$ and $\beta$, closely related to and derived from the same precursor as the dynorphins.

**neo·fe·tal** (ne″o-fe′təl) pertaining to the transitional period between the embryonic and fetal stages of the developing human young.

**neo·fe·tus** (ne″o-fe′təs) the embryo at about the eighth week of intrauterine life.

**neo·for·ma·tion** (ne″o-for-ma′shən) a new growth or neoplasm.

**neo·for·ma·tive** (ne″o-for′mə-tiv) concerned with the formation of new tissue.

**ne·og·a·la** (ne-og′ə-lə) [*neo-* + Gr. *gala* milk] the first milk developed after childbirth; see also *colostrum.*

**Neo·gas·trop·o·da** (ne″o-gas-trop′ə-də) an order of marine-dwelling gastropods of the subclass Streptoneura; it includes the family Conidae, which contains some poisonous species, and the genus *Murex.*

**neo·gen·e·sis** (ne″o-jen′ə-sis) [*neo-* + *-genesis*] regeneration.

**neo·ge·net·ic** (ne″o-jə-net′ik) pertaining to neogenesis.

**neo·ger·mi·trine** (ne″o-jer′mĭ-trēn) an alkaloid having antihypertensive properties, isolated from green hellebore *(Veratrum viride).*

**neo·glot·tic** (ne″o-glot′ik) pertaining to a neoglottis.

**neo·glot·tis** (ne″o-glot′is) a surgically constructed glottis created by suturing the pharyngeal mucosa over the superior end of the transected trachea above the primary tracheostoma and making a permanent stoma in the mucosa; it is created to permit phonation after laryngectomy. Called also *pseudoglottis.*

**neo·hip·poc·ra·tism** (ne″o-hĭ-pok′rə-tiz-əm) a school of medicine which tends toward a humanistic view of disease focused on the individual patient and scientific observation by the physician, representing a return to the hippocratic theory and practice, with emphasis on observational and bedside medicine.

**Neo-Hom·bre·ol** (ne″o-hom′bre-ol) trademark for preparations of testosterone propionate.

**neo·in·ti·ma** (ne″o-in′tĭ-mə) in a blood vessel graft or vascular prosthesis, a new layer of endothelial cells on the intimal surface. Cf. *pseudointima.*

**neo·ki·net·ic** (ne″o-kĭ-net′ik) [*neo-* + *kinet-* + *-ic*] to the nervous motor mechanism regulating voluntary muscular control. It is associated with the motor area of cerebral cortex; it is one of the most recently developed functions of the nervous system. Cf. *archeokinetic* and *paleokinetic.*

**neo·lal·ia** (ne″o-lal′e-ə) [*neo-* + *lal-* + *-ia*] speech into which many neologisms are incorporated, as in schizophrenia.

**neo·lal·ism** (ne″o-lal′iz-əm) neolalia.

**ne·ol·o·gism** (ne-ol′ə-jiz-əm) [*neo-* + *log-* + *-ism*] a newly coined word; in psychiatry, a new word whose meaning may be known only to the person using it and may be related to his conflicts.

**Ne·o·loid** (ne′o-loid) trademark for a preparation of castor oil.

**neo·mem·brane** (ne″o-mem′brān) false membrane.

**neo·morph** (ne′o-morf) [*neo-* + *-morph*] a part or organ recently acquired in the course of evolution.

**neo·mor·phism** (ne″o-mor′fiz-əm) the development of new form in the course of evolution.

**neo·mort** (ne′o-mort) a corpse, immediately after death.

**neo·my·cin** (ne″o-mi′sin) [USP] [MeSH: Neomycin] an aminoglycoside antibiotic complex derived from *Streptomyces fradiae,* consisting of three components designated A, B, and C. The form in clinical use is a mixture of neomycins B and C; it is effective against a wide range of aerobic gram-negative bacilli and some gram-positive bacteria.
**n. sulfate** [USP], the sulfate salt of neomycin, used for urinary tract irrigation, administered orally to suppress bowel flora in the adjunctive treatment of hepatic coma and in preoperative bowel preparation, and applied topically to the skin, conjunctiva, and ears in the treatment of infections due to susceptible organisms; in topical preparations it is often combined with other antibiotics or anti-inflammatory steroids.

**ne·on** (ne′on) [Gr. *neos* new] [MeSH: Neon] an inert gaseous element discovered in the air in 1898; symbol, Ne; atomic weight, 20.183; atomic number, 10.

**neo·na·tal** (ne″o-na′təl) [*neo-* + *natal* (def. 1)] pertaining to the first four weeks after birth.

**neo·nate** (ne′o-nāt) 1. newly born. 2. a newborn infant.

**neo·na·tol·o·gist** (ne″o-na-tol′ə-jist) a physician whose primary concern is in the specialty of neonatology.

**neo·na·tol·o·gy** (ne″o-na-tol′ə-je) [MeSH: Neonatology] the art and science of diagnosis and treatment of disorders of the newborn infant.

**neo·pal·li·um** (ne″o-pal′e-əm) [*neo-* + *pallium*] neocortex.

**neo·pla·sia** (ne″o-pla′zhə) the formation of a neoplasm, i.e., the progressive multiplication of cells under conditions that would not elicit, or would cause cessation of, multiplication of normal cells.
**cervical intraepithelial n. (CIN),** dysplasia of the cervical epithelium, often premalignant, characterized by various degrees of hyperplasia, abnormal keratinization, and presence of condylomata.
**gestational trophoblastic n. (GTN),** a group of neoplastic disorders that originate in the placenta, including the benign *hydatidiform mole* and the malignant *chorioadenoma destruens* and *choriocarcinoma.* Called also *gestational trophoblastic disease* and *trophoblastic disease.*
**lobular n.,** lobular carcinoma in situ.
**multiple endocrine n. (MEN),** a group of rare diseases caused by genetic defects that lead to hyperplasia and hyperfunction of two or more components of the endocrine system; three separate types have been distinguished, named *multiple endocrine n., type I, type II,* and *type III* (qq.v.). All forms are transmitted as autosomal dominant traits with varying penetrance. Called also *multiple endocrine adenomatosis, pluriglandular* or *polyendocrine adenomatosis,* and *polyendocrinoma.*
**multiple endocrine n., type I,** a variety that includes tumors of the anterior pituitary, parathyroid glands, and pancreatic islet cells in association with a high incidence of peptic ulcers and sometimes the Zollinger-Ellison syndrome; it is caused by a genetic abnormality on the long arm of chromosome 11. Called also *Wermer's syndrome.*
**multiple endocrine n., type II,** a variety characterized by medullary carcinoma of the thyroid, pheochromocytoma (often bilateral and multiple), and parathyroid hyperplasia. Called also *Sipple's syndrome* and *multiple endocrine n., type IIA.*
**multiple endocrine n., type IIA,** multiple endocrine n., type II.
**multiple endocrine n., type IIB,** multiple endocrine n., type III.
**multiple endocrine n., type III,** a variety resembling type II except that parathyroid hyperplasia is rare, mean survival time is shorter, a marfanoid body habitus may occur, and there may be disfiguring neuromas of the lips, buccal mucosa, and tongue, neurofibromas of the skin, ganglioneuromas of the gastrointestinal tract, thickened corneal nerves, and cafe-au-lait spots. Called also *mucosal neuroma syndrome* and *multiple endocrine n., type IIB.*
**prostatic intraepithelial n.,** neoplastic changes in epithelial cells of prostatic ducts and acini showing some morphologic features of cancer but not involving stromal invasion; these are sometimes precursors of carcinoma or adenocarcinoma.

**neo·plasm** (ne′o-plaz-əm) [*neo-* + *-plasm*] [MeSH: Neoplasms] any new and abnormal growth; specifically a new growth of tissue in which the growth is uncontrolled and progressive (see *neoplasia*). Malignant neoplasms are distinguished from benign in that the former show a greater degree of anaplasia and have the properties of invasion and metastasis. Called also *tumor.*

**neo·plas·tic** (ne″o-plas′tik) 1. pertaining to or like a neoplasm. 2. pertaining to neoplasia.

**neo·plas·ti·gen·ic** (ne″o-plas″tĭ-jen′ik) tumorigenic.

**Ne·op·syl·la** (ne-op′səl-ə) a genus of fleas.

**ne·op·ter·in** (ne-op′tər-in) a pteridine derivative excreted in the urine at low levels; urinary excretion is elevated in some disorders of tetrahydrobiopterin biosynthesis, certain malignant diseases, viral infection, and graft rejection. The term is also used to denote the class of related compounds.

**neo·quas·sin** (ne″o-kwas′in) a crystalline principle, $C_{24}H_{30}O_6$, from *Quassia amara;* it is a phenanthropyran derivative which forms quassin on oxidation.

**Ne·or·al** (ne-or′əl) trademark for preparations of cyclosporine.

**neo·rec·tum** (ne″o-rek′təm) ileoanal reservoir.

**Neo·scan** (ne′o-skan″) trademark for a preparation of gallium Ga 67 citrate.

**Neo·rick·ett·sia** (ne″o-rĭ-ket′se-ə) [*neo-* + *rickettsia*] a genus of bacteria of the tribe Ehrlichieae, family Rickettsiaceae, order Rickettsiales. It includes a single species, *N. helminthoe′ca,* the etiologic agent of salmon poisoning (q.v.) in dogs, wolves, jackals, and foxes. The organism is found in the salmon fluke, *Troglotrema salmincola,* a parasite of various fish, especially salmon and trout, and is transmitted by ingestion of raw infected fish.

**Neo·schoen·gas·tia** (ne″o-shān-gas′te-ə) a genus of mites of the family Trombiculidae. *N. america′na* infests chickens in the southern United States.

**Ne·os·po·ra** (ne-os′pə-rə) [MeSH: Neospora] a genus of protozoa of the phylum Apicomplexa, morphologically similar to *Toxoplasma*. *N. cani′num* is parasitic in dogs and other mammals, causing neosporosis.

**neo·spo·ro·sis** (ne″o-spə-ro′sis) infection of dogs and other animals by *Neospora caninum*; characteristics are similar to those of toxoplasmosis, with neurologic and ophthalmic symptoms predominating.

**neo·sti·bo·san** (ne″o-sti′bo-san) a pentavalent antimony compound, used as an antileishmanial. Called also *ethylstibamine*.

**neo·stig·mine** (ne″o-stig′mēn) [MeSH: Neostigmine] an anticholinesterase used for the symptomatic treatment of myasthenia gravis, for prevention and treatment of postoperative stasis and atony of the gastrointestinal tract or urinary bladder, and for reversal of the effects of nondepolarizing neuromuscular blocking agents (e.g., tubocurarine) after surgery.
**n. bromide** [USP], the bromide salt of neostigmine, used as a cholinergic in the symptomatic control of myasthenia gravis, and to produce miosis in certain forms of glaucoma in patients who have developed tolerance to other miotics; administered orally and applied to the conjunctiva.
**n. methylsulfate** [USP], the methylsulfate salt of neostigmine, used as a cholinergic in the prevention and treatment of postoperative distention and urinary retention, in the symptomatic treatment of myasthenia gravis, as a diagnostic test for myasthenia gravis, and as an antidote for curare principles; administered intravenously and subcutaneously.

**ne·os·to·my** (ne-os′tə-me) [*neo-* + *-stomy*] surgical creation of an artificial opening into an organ or between two organs.

**neo·stri·a·tum** (ne″o-stri-a′təm) [*neo-* + *striatum*] [MeSH: Neostriatum] the later developed portion of the corpus striatum represented by the caudate nucleus and the putamen; called also *striatum*. Cf. *paleostriatum*.

**Neo·stron·gy·lus** (ne″o-stron′jĭ-ləs) a genus of parasitic nematodes of the family Protostrongylidae, some species of which are lungworms of sheep and goats.

**Neo·Syn·a·lar** (ne″o-sin′ə-lahr) trademark for a combination preparation of neomycin sulfate and fluocinolone acetonide.

**Neo·Sy·neph·rine** (ne″o-sĭ-nef′rin) trademark for preparations of phenylephrine hydrochloride.

**ne·ot·e·ny** (ne-ot′ə-ne) [*neo-* + Gr. *teinein* to extend] 1. the tendency to remain in the larval state, although gaining sexual maturity. 2. the retention in an adult organism of some of its ancestor's larval characteristics.

**Neo·tes·tu·di·na** (ne″o-tes″too-di′nə) a genus of bitunicate fungi of the order Dothideales. *N. rosa′tii* is an etiologic agent of eumycotic mycetoma in tropical Africa and Australia.

**neo·thal·a·mus** (ne″o-thal′ə-məs) [*neo-* new + *thalamus*] new thalamus; the phylogenetically new part of the thalamus, i.e., the part connected to the neocortex. Cf. *paleothalamus*.

**Neo·thyl·line** (ne″o-thi′lēn) trademark for preparations of dyphylline.

**Ne·ot·o·ma** (ne-ot′ə-mə) a genus of rodents of western North America, the wood or pack rats.

**Neo·tri·zine** (ne″o-tri′zēn) trademark for preparations of trisulfapyrimidenes.

**Neo·trom·bic·u·la** (ne″o-trom-bik′u-lə) a genus of mites of the family Trombiculidae. *N. autumna′lis* (also called *Trombicula autumnalis*) is a European species whose larva, the *autumn chigger*, causes trombiculiasis of the skin in humans and other animals.

**neo·type** (ne′o-tīp) a strain of bacteria that replaces a type culture which no longer exists, and that agrees with the original description of the taxon and is accepted by international agreement.

**neo·va·gi·na** (ne″o-və-ji′nə) [*neo-* + *vagina*] a surgically created vagina, as after vaginectomy or in male-to-female transsexual surgery.

**neo·vas·cu·lar·iza·tion** (ne″o-vas″ku-lər-ĭ-za′shən) 1. new blood vessel formation in abnormal tissue or in abnormal positions. 2. revascularization. Cf. *angiogenesis* (def. 2).

**ne·pen·thic** (ne-pen′thik) [Gr. *nēpenthēs* free from sorrow] pertaining to or inducing peace and forgetfulness, such as with a psychotropic drug.

**Nep·e·ta** (nep′ə-tə) a genus of Eurasian mints of the family Labiatae. *N. cata′ria* L. is catnip, a plant that contains the volatile aromatic oil nepetalactone, an attractant to cats; its leaves and tops, called *cataria*, are carminative and stimulant for humans.

**nep·e·ta·lac·tone** (nep″ə-tə-lak′tōn) the chief constituent of the aromatic volatile oil from the leaves and tops of *Nepeta cataria*, an attractant to cats.

**nephel(o)-** [Gr. *nephelē* cloud or mist] a combining form denoting relationship to clouds or cloudiness.

**neph·e·lom·e·ter** (nef″ə-lom′ə-tər) an instrument that measures the turbidity of a solution by measuring the amount of light that is scattered at an angle from a beam of light passing through the solution. Cf. *turbidimeter*.

**neph·e·lom·e·try** (nef″ə-lom′ə-tre) [*nephelo-* + *-metry*] measurement of the concentration of a suspension by means of a nephelometer.

**neph·rad·e·no·ma** (nef″rad-ə-no′mə) [*nephr-* + *adenoma*] adenoma of the kidney.

**ne·phral·gia** (nə-fral′jə) [*nephr-* + *-algia*] pain in a kidney.

**ne·phral·gic** (nə-fral′jik) pertaining to or characterized by nephralgia.

**neph·ra·pos·ta·sis** (nef″rə-pos′tə-sis) pyonephrosis.

**neph·rauxe** (nef-rawk′se) [*nephr-* + Gr. *auxē* increase] nephromegaly.

**neph·rec·ta·sia** (nef″rek-ta′zhə) [*nephr-* + *ectasia*] distention of the kidney; sacciform kidney.

**ne·phrec·ta·sis** (nə-frek′tə-sis) nephrectasia.

**ne·phrec·ta·sy** (nə-frek′tə-se) nephrectasia.

**ne·phrec·to·mize** (nə-frek′tə-mīz) to deprive of one or both kidneys by surgical removal.

**ne·phrec·to·my** (nə-frek′tə-me) [*nephr-* + *-ectomy*] [MeSH: Nephrectomy] excision of a kidney.
**abdominal n., anterior n.,** nephrectomy through an incision in the abdominal wall.
**lumbar n.,** nephrectomy through an incision in the loin.
**paraperitoneal n.,** the surgical removal of a kidney by a cut through the side along the twelfth rib.
**posterior n.,** lumbar n.
**radical n.,** removal of a kidney with its fascia after prior ligation of the renal artery and vein, as well as removal of the adjacent adrenal gland and all lymph nodes in the region; done for treatment of renal cell carcinoma.

**neph·re·de·ma** (nef″rə-de′mə) renal congestion; called also *nephremia*.

**neph·rel·co·sis** (nef″rəl-ko′sis) [*nephr-* + *elcosis*] ulceration of the kidney.

**ne·phre·mia** (nə-fre′me-ə) [*nephr-* + *-emia*] nephredema.

**neph·ric** (nef′rik) renal.

**ne·phrid·i·um** (nə-frid′e-əm) former term for *mesonephros*.

**ne·phrit·ic** (nə-frit′ik) 1. pertaining to or affected with nephritis. 2. renal.

**ne·phrit·i·des** (nə-frit′ĭ-dēz) [MeSH: Nephritis] plural of *nephritis*, used as a collective term, to include all types of nephritis.

**ne·phri·tis** (nə-fri′tis) pl. *nephrit′ides* [*nephr-* + *-itis*] [MeSH: Nephritis] inflammation of the kidney; a focal or diffuse proliferative or destructive process which may involve the glomerulus, tubule, or interstitial renal tissue. See also *glomerulonephritis*. Cf. *nephrosis*.
**acute n.,** a type of nephritis that is acute and active, usually characterized by edema, weight gain, proteinuria, microhematuria, and cylindruria. When involvement is primarily glomerular, gross hematuria is common.
**arteriosclerotic n.,** nephrosclerotic nephritis which may result primarily from the aging process, with hyaline changes of the large and small arterioles, or from hypertension, with hyaline and/or muscular changes of the small arterioles in the glomerular hilum. Renal damage occurs primarily through ischemic atrophy of the tubules with resultant focal or diffuse interstitial fibrosis.
**azotemic n.,** nephritis which has resulted in anatomic and functional impairment leading to nitrogen retention.
**bacterial n.,** nephritis caused by microorganisms.
**Balkan n.,** Balkan nephropathy.
**capsular n.,** a form said to affect especially Bowman's capsules.
**n. caseo′sa, caseous n.,** cheesy n.
**cheesy n.,** a chronic suppurative form with caseous deposits.
**chloro-azotemic n.,** nonedematous renal failure with acidosis.
**chronic n.,** active and slowly progressive parenchymal renal disease, usually with a predominantly glomerular lesion.
**congenital n.,** nephritis existing at birth, as in congenital syphilis.
**degenerative n.,** nephrosis.
**n. doloro′sa,** nonspecific involvement of the kidney characterized by painful thickening of the renal capsule due to inflammation of indeterminate etiology, as in some forms of perinephritis.
**dropsical n.,** old name for *nephrotic syndrome*.
**exudative n.,** nephritis with exudation of the blood serum.
**fibrolipomatous n.,** perinephritis in which the perirenal fat has become enmeshed in fibrous tissue proliferation with scarring.

**fibrous n.**, interstitial n.
**glomerular n.**, that which principally affects the glomeruli; see *glomerulonephritis.*
**glomerulocapsular n.**, a term sometimes used to describe glomerulopathy involving primarily the epithelial cells of Bowman's capsules.
**n. gravida'rum**, nephritis or other glomerulopathies complicating pregnancy.
**hemorrhagic n.**, glomerulopathy associated with gross hematuria.
**Heymann's n.**, an experimental model of membranous glomerulonephritis, induced in rats by injection of an antigen preparation derived from tubule brush borders, which causes an autoimmune reaction by the native tubules.
**indurative n.**, a condition marked by atrophy and gross scarring of the kidney due to glomerular, tubular, or interstitial renal disease.
**interstitial n.**, primary or secondary disease of the renal interstitial tissue; it may result from arterial, arteriolar, glomerular, or tubular disease which destroys individual nephrons, or from toxic involvement of interstitial cells and tubules due to systemic diseases such as gout, to drug exposure (as in phenacetin abuse), or to mercury poisoning. Clinically, it may be manifested primarily by loss of concentrating capacity, hyponatremia, hyperkalemia, acidosis, non-nephrotic proteinuria, and abnormal urine sediment. It usually has a chronic course with progressive renal atrophy and loss of function; an acute form (see *acute interstitial n.*) occurs particularly after bacterial infection.
**interstitial n., acute,** nephritis in which inflammatory changes are usually confined to interstitial tissue, usually occurring as a complication of a systemic infection, especially by beta-hemolytic streptococci, although it may have an allergic etiology. The kidneys may be normal in size and appearance, or enlarged, soft, and pale or mottled red or gray. Other signs include a thickened cortex, focal or diffuse interstitial infiltration of leukocytes, and tubular degeneration.
**Lancereaux's n.**, interstitial nephritis allegedly resulting from rheumatic disease.
**lupus n.**, glomerulonephritis (diffuse, focal, or membranous) associated with systemic lupus erythematosus, marked by deposition of antigen-antibody complexes in the mesangium and basement membrane. The morphological findings have been classified into 5 subgroups by the World Health Organization. The clinical course is highly variable and depends in part on the morphological findings.
**Masugi n.**, nephrotoxic serum n.
**nephrotoxic serum n.**, an animal model of antibody-mediated glomerulonephritis produced by injection of heterologous antibody against renal antigens. It occurs in two phases. The *heterologous phase,* occurring within a few hours, consists of the inflammatory response triggered by the nephrotoxic antibody binding to antigens in the glomerular basement membrane (GBM) and resembles anti-GBM antibody disease. The *autologous phase,* occurring 4–6 days later, consists of the host response to the foreign antibody and does not correspond to a human disease.
**parenchymatous n.**, renal parenchymal disease of specific or unknown etiology.
**parenchymatous n., chronic,** chronic disease of the renal parenchyma of specific or nonspecific etiology, usually manifested as a diffuse glomerular, tubular, or interstitial fibrosis.
**pneumococcus n.**, nephritis from infection with pneumococci, occurring usually as a complication of pneumonia or empyema.
**potassium-losing n.**, persistent urinary potassium losses in the presence of hypokalemia. It may be seen in metabolic alkalosis, adrenocortical hormone excess, or in intrinsic renal disease (e.g., renal tubular acidosis or juxtaglomerular cell hyperplasia). Called also *potassium-losing nephropathy.*
**n. of pregnancy**, n. gravidarum.
**productive n.**, nephritis with the development of serous exudate and hypertrophy of the connective tissue stroma.
**n. re'pens**, a condition in which the patient has advanced renal insufficiency and raised blood pressure but without an antecedent history of acute nephritis.
**salt-losing n.**, any intrinsic renal disease causing salt wasting; it usually affects the renal medulla (e.g., medullary cystic disease, polycystic kidney disease, pyelonephritis), resulting in volume depletion and hypotension. See also *salt-losing syndrome,* under *syndrome.* Called also *Thorn's syndrome.*
**saturnine n.**, a form due to chronic lead poisoning.
**scarlatinal n.**, acute nephritis due to scarlet fever.
**subacute n.**, parenchymatous n., chronic.
**suppurative n.**, a form accompanied by abscess of the kidney.
**suppurative n., acute,** a form due to septic infection, generally from operations on the genitourinary tract (then called *surgical kidney*), and marked by the development of multiple abscesses.
**suppurative n., chronic,** is caused by infection with the tubercle bacillus; in this disease cavities are found in the kidney, filled with puslike, cheesy masses and tubercle bacilli.
**syphilitic n.**, a form of nephritis occurring in tertiary syphilis.
**transfusion n.**, a nephropathy following blood transfusion from a donor whose blood is incompatible with that of the recipient.
**tubal n., tubular n.**, a variety that affects principally the tubules.
**tuberculous n.**, see *interstitial n.*
**tubulointerstitial n.**, nephritis of the tubules and interstitial tissues of the kidney, usually seen secondary to a drug sensitization, systemic infection, graft rejection, or autoimmune disease; characteristics include lymphocytes in interstitial infiltrate and within tubules, with mild hematuria and pyuria.
**tubulointerstitial n., hereditary,** familial juvenile nephronophthisis (def. 1).
**vascular n.**, nephrosclerosis.

**ne·phrit·o·gen·ic** (nə-frit″o-jen′ik) giving rise to nephritis.

**nephr(o)-** [Gr. *nephros* kidney] combining form denoting relationship to the kidney.

**neph·ro·ab·dom·i·nal** (nef″ro-ab-dom′ĭ-nəl) pertaining to the kidney and the abdominal wall.

**neph·ro·an·gio·scle·ro·sis** (nef″ro-an″je-o-sklə-ro′sis) hypertension with renal lesions of arterial origin.

**neph·ro·blas·to·ma** (nef″ro-blas-to′mə) [MeSH: Nephroblastoma] Wilms' tumor.

**neph·ro·blas·to·ma·to·sis** (nef″ro-blas-to″mə-to′sis) clusters of microscopic blastema cells, tubules, and stromal cells at the periphery of renal lobes of infants, thought to be a precursor of Wilms' tumor.

**neph·ro·cal·ci·no·sis** (nef″ro-kal″si-no′sis) [*nephro-* + *calcinosis*] [MeSH: Nephrocalcinosis] a condition characterized by precipitation of calcium phosphate in the tubules of the kidney, with resultant renal insufficiency.

**neph·ro·cap·sec·to·my** (nef″ro-kap-sek′to-me) [*nephro-* + *capsule* + *-ectomy*] renal decapsulation.

**neph·ro·car·di·ac** (nef″ro-kahr′de-ak) cardiorenal.

**neph·ro·cele** (nef′ro-sēl) [*nephro-* + *-cele*[1]] hernial protrusion of a kidney.

**neph·ro·col·ic** (nef″ro-kol′ik) [*nephro-* + *colic*] 1. pertaining to the kidney and the colon. 2. renal colic.

**neph·ro·co·lop·to·sis** (nef″ro-ko″lop-to′sis) [*nephro-* + *colo-* + *-ptosis*] downward displacement of the kidney and colon.

**neph·ro·cys·ta·nas·to·mo·sis** (nef″ro-sis″tə-nas″to-mo′sis) [*nephro-* + *cyst-* + *anastomosis*] the surgical formation of a communication between the kidney and the urinary bladder.

**neph·ro·cys·ti·tis** (nef″ro-sis-ti′tis) [*nephro-* + *cyst-* + *-itis*] inflammation of the kidney and bladder.

**neph·ro·cys·to·sis** (nef″ro-sis-to′sis) [*nephro-* + *cyst-* + *-osis*] development of cysts in the kidney.

**neph·ro·er·y·sip·e·las** (nef″ro-er″ĭ-sip′ə-ləs) erysipelas complicated with acute nephritis.

**neph·ro·gas·tric** (nef″ro-gas′trik) pertaining to the kidney and the stomach; renogastric.

**neph·ro·gen·ic** (nef″ro-jen′ik) [*nephro-* + *-genic*] forming kidney tissue.

**ne·phrog·e·nous** (nə-froj′ə-nəs) originating or arising in the kidney.

**neph·ro·gram** (nef′ro-gram) a radiograph of the kidney.

**ne·phrog·ra·phy** (nə-frog′rə-fe) [*nephro-* + *-graphy*] radiography of the kidney.

**neph·ro·he·mia** (nef″ro-he′me-ə) nephredema.

**neph·ro·hy·dro·sis** (nef″ro-hi-dro′sis) hydronephrosis.

**neph·ro·hy·per·tro·phy** (nef″ro-hi-per′tro-fe) [*nephro-* + *hypertrophy*] hypertrophy of the kidney.

**neph·roid** (nef′roid) [*nephro-* + *-oid*] kidney-shaped, or resembling a kidney.

**neph·ro·lith** (nef′ro-lith) [*nephro-* + *-lith*] renal calculus.

**neph·ro·li·thi·a·sis** (nef″ro-lĭ-thi′ə-sis) a condition marked by the presence of renal calculi.

**neph·ro·li·thot·o·my** (nef″ro-lĭ-thot′ə-me) [*nephrolith* + *-tomy*] the removal of renal calculi by incision through the kidney.
**percutaneous n.**, removal of renal calculi using an endoscope that penetrates the skin.

**ne·phrol·o·gist** (nə-frol′ə-jist) an expert in nephrology.

**ne·phrol·o·gy** (nə-frol′ə-je) [*nephro-* + *-logy*] [MeSH: Nephrology] scientific study of the kidney, its anatomy, physiology, pathology, and pathophysiology.

**ne·phrol·y·sis** (nə-frol′ə-sis) [*nephro-* + *-lysis*] 1. solution of kidney substance. 2. the operation of separating the kidney from paranephric adhesions.

**neph·ro·lyt·ic** (nef″ro-lit′ik) pertaining to, characterized by, or producing nephrolysis.

**ne·phro·ma** (nə-fro′mə) [*nephr-* + *-oma*] a tumor of the kidney or of kidney tissue.
**congenital mesoblastic n.,** a renal tumor similar to Wilms' tumor but appearing earlier in infancy and with more infiltration of surrounding tissue than in classic Wilms' tumor.
**embryonal n.,** Wilms' tumor.

**neph·ro·ma·la·cia** (nef″ro-mə-la′shə) [*nephro-* + *-malacia*] softening of the kidney.

**neph·ro·meg·a·ly** (nef″ro-meg′ə-le) [*nephro-* + *-megaly*] enlargement of the kidney.

**neph·ro·mere** (nef′ro-mēr) [*nephro-* + *-mere*] nephrotome.

**neph·ron** (nef′ron) [Gr. *nephros* kidney + *-on* neuter ending] [MeSH: Nephrons] the anatomical and functional unit of the kidney, consisting of the renal corpuscle, the proximal convoluted tubule, the descending and ascending limbs of Henle's loop, the distal convoluted tubule, and the collecting tubule. See illustration accompanying *kidney.*

**neph·ron·oph·thi·sis** (nef″ron-of′thĭ-sis) [*nephron* + *phthisis*] wasting disease of the kidney substance.
**familial juvenile n.,** 1. a progressive hereditary disease of the kidneys characterized clinically by anemia, polyuria, and renal loss of sodium, progressing to chronic renal failure; pathologically, there is tubular atrophy, interstitial fibrosis, glomerular sclerosis, and medullary cysts. Called also *medullary cystic disease, medullary cystic kidney disease,* and *juvenile nephronophthisis–medullary cystic disease complex.* 2. according to some authorities, a variant of the juvenile nephronophthisis–medullary cystic disease complex, of autosomal inheritance and having onset in childhood.

**neph·ro·path·ia** (nef″ro-path′e-ə) nephropathy.
**n. epide′mica ,** a mild, usually asymptomatic form of epidemic hemorrhagic fever, caused by Puumala virus. Proteinuria, elevated creatine levels, and leukocytosis may occur; it is rarely hemorrhagic and seldom fatal.

**neph·ro·path·ic** (nef″ro-path′ik) pertaining to, characterized by, or producing nephropathy.

**ne·phrop·a·thy** (nə-frop′ə-the) [*nephro-* + *-pathy*] disease of the kidneys.
**analgesic n.,** interstitial nephritis with renal papillary necrosis, seen in patients with a history of abuse of analgesics, especially phenacetin.
**Balkan n.,** a slowly progressive type of interstitial nephritis seen in well-defined areas of the former Yugoslavia, as well as Romania, Bulgaria, and Greece. The cause is unknown and has been attributed to chronic lead poisoning, poisoning by grains containing the mycotoxins citrinin and ochratoxin A, or other factors. Called also *Balkan nephritis.*
**diabetic n.,** the nephropathy that commonly accompanies later stages of diabetes mellitus; it begins with hyperfiltration, renal hypertrophy, microalbuminuria, and hypertension; in time proteinuria develops, with other signs of decreasing function leading to end stage renal disease.
**gouty n.,** any of a group of chronic kidney diseases associated with the abnormal production and excretion of uric acid.
**HIV-associated n., human immunodeficiency virus–associated n.,** renal pathology in patients infected with the human immunodeficiency virus, similar to focal glomerular sclerosis, with proteinuria, enlarged kidneys, and dilated tubules containing proteinaceous casts; it may progress to end stage renal disease within weeks.
**hypazoturic n.,** kidney disease with retention of nitrogen.
**IgA n.,** a chronic form of glomerulonephritis marked by hematuria and proteinuria and by deposits of immunoglobulin A in the mesangial areas of the renal glomeruli, with subsequent reactive hyperplasia of mesangial cells. Called also *Berger's disease* and *IgA glomerulonephritis.*
**IgM n.,** mesangial proliferative glomerulonephritis.
**ischemic n.,** nephropathy resulting from partial or complete obstruction of a renal artery with ischemia, accompanied by a significant reduction in the glomerular filtration rate.
**light chain n.,** nephropathy caused by deposition of abnormal light chains (usually kappa chains but sometimes lambda chains) in renal basement membranes, often with nodular glomerulosclerosis; it may be associated with multiple myeloma or some other plasma cell dyscrasia.
**membranous n.,** see under *glomerulonephritis.*
**minimal change n.,** see under *disease.*
**mycotoxic n.,** kidney damage in livestock, usually pigs, due to ochratoxins or citrinin contaminating their food, usually produced by *Penicillium.* Symptoms include edema around the kidneys with degeneration of proximal tubules, fibrosis, polyuria, and enlarged kidneys. Called also *mycotic* or *mold nephrosis.*
**potassium-losing n.,** potassium-losing nephritis.
**reflux n.,** childhood pyelonephritis in which the renal scarring results from vesicoureteric reflux, with radiological appearance of intrarenal reflux.
**sickle cell n.,** chronic kidney pathology seen with sickle cell disease, including microangiopathy with capillary obstruction, dilated or obliterated vasa recta, enlarged glomeruli, interstitial fibrosis, and an increased glomerular filtration rate.
**thin basement membrane n.,** a rare, usually benign disorder characterized by abnormally thin basement membranes of the glomerular capillaries and persistent hematuria; autosomal dominant inheritance is suspected. Called also *benign familial hematuria.*
**urate n.,** any of a group of kidney diseases occurring in patients with hyperuricemia, including an acute form, a chronic form (gouty nephropathy), and nephrolithiasis with the formation of uric acid calculi. Called also *uric acid nephropathy.*
**urate n., acute,** rapidly progressive nephropathy caused by the precipitation of uric acid crystals in the renal tubules, leading to obstruction and acute renal failure, seen especially in patients with lymphoproliferative or myeloproliferative disease, usually after the induction of chemotherapy. Called also *acute uric acid n.*
**urate n., chronic,** gouty n.
**uric acid n.,** urate n.
**uric acid n., acute,** urate n.
**uric acid n., chronic,** gouty n.
**vasomotor n.,** acute tubular necrosis.

**neph·ro·pexy** (nef′ro-pek″se) [*nephro-* + *-pexy*] the fixation or suspension of a floating kidney.

**neph·ro·pha·gi·a·sis** (nef″ro-fə-ji′ə-sis) [*nephro-* + *phag-* + *-iasis*] the devouring of the kidney by certain parasites.

**ne·phroph·thi·sis** (nə-frof′thĭ-sis) [*nephro-* + *phthisis*] 1. nephrotuberculosis. 2. nephronophthisis.

**neph·ro·poi·et·ic** (nef″ro-poi-et′ik) [*nephro-* + Gr. *poiein* to make] nephrogenic.

**neph·rop·to·sia** (nef″rop-to′se-ə) nephroptosis.

**neph·rop·to·sis** (nef″rop-to′sis) [*nephro-* + *-ptosis*] downward displacement of the kidney.

**neph·ro·py·eli·tis** (nef″ro-pi″ə-li′tis) [*nephro-* + *pyelitis*] pyelonephritis.

**neph·ro·py·elog·ra·phy** (nef″ro-pi″ə-log′rə-fe) radiography of the kidney and renal pelvis.

**neph·ro·py·elo·li·thot·o·my** (nef″ro-pi″ə-lo-lĭ-thot′ə-me) [*nephro-* + *pyelo-* + *lithotomy*] removal of a calculus from the renal pelvis by an incision through the kidney substance.

**neph·ro·py·elo·plas·ty** (nef″ro-pi′ə-lo-plas″te) [*nephro-* + *pyelo-* + *-plasty*] plastic operation on the pelvis of the kidney.

**neph·ro·py·o·sis** (nef″ro-pi-o′sis) [*nephro-* + *py-* + *-osis*] pyonephrosis.

**neph·ror·rha·gia** (nef″ro-ra′je-ə) [*nephro-* + *-rrhagia*] hemorrhage from the kidney.

**neph·ror·rha·phy** (nef-ror′ə-fe) [*nephro-* + *-rrhaphy*] the operation of suturing the kidney.

**neph·ro·scle·ria** (nef″ro-skler′e-ə) nephrosclerosis.

**neph·ro·scle·ro·sis** (nef″ro-sklə-ro′sis) [*nephro-* + *sclerosis*] [MeSH: Nephrosclerosis] sclerosis or hardening of the kidney, usually due to renovascular disease.
**arteriolar n.,** nephrosclerosis of arterioles; it is often associated with hypertension, with insidious onset, cylindruria, edema, hypertrophy of the heart, degeneration of the renal tubules, and glomerulonephritis, resulting in renal insufficiency, congestive heart failure, and cerebral hemorrhage. Two types are distinguished: *benign* and *malignant* (q.v.). Called also *intercapillary n.* and *glomerulosclerosis.*
**benign n., benign arteriolar n.,** a type of arteriolar nephrosclerosis usually seen in patients 60 years of age or older, frequently associated with benign hypertension and hyaline arteriolosclerosis; in younger persons, it may occur in diabetics with a predisposition to arteriosclerosis and in those with hypertension resulting from an apparent underlying disease such as pheochromocytoma. Called also *hyaline arteriolar n.*
**hyaline arteriolar n.,** benign n.
**hyperplastic arteriolar n.,** malignant n.
**hypertensive n.,** the most common kind of arteriolar nephrosclerosis, due to hypertension of the renal arterioles.
**intercapillary n.,** arteriolar n.
**malignant n., malignant arteriolar n.,** a rare form of arteriolar nephrosclerosis affecting all the vessels of the body, especially small renal arteries and arterioles, often associated with malignant hy-

pertension and hyperplastic arteriolosclerosis. It may occur without previous hypertension or superimposed on benign hypertension or primary renal disease, especially glomerulonephritis, benign nephrosclerosis, or pyelonephritis. Called also *hyperplastic arteriolar n.* and *Fahr-Volhard disease.*
**senile n.,** nephrosclerosis that is simply a part of the arteriosclerosis common in old age.

**neph·ro·scope** (nef'ro-skōp) an instrument inserted into an incision in the renal pelvis for viewing the inside of the kidney, equipped with three channels for telescope, fiberoptic light input, and irrigation.

**neph·ros·co·py** (nə-fros'kə-pe) visualization of the kidney by means of the nephroscope.

**ne·phro·ses** (nə-fro'sēz) [MeSH: Nephrosis] plural of *nephrosis.*

**ne·phro·sis** (nĕ-fro'sis) pl. *nephro'ses* [*nephr-* + *-osis*] [MeSH: Nephrosis] any disease of the kidneys that includes purely degenerative lesions of the renal tubules, characterized by hypoalbuminemia, hypercholesterolemia, and edema. See also *nephritis* and *nephrotic syndrome.*
**acute n.,** nephrosis marked by scanty urine but with little edema or albuminuria.
**amyloid n.,** renal amyloidosis.
**cholemic n.,** renal disease associated with various types of hepatic or biliary dysfunction, especially those in which there is obstructive jaundice.
**chronic n.,** renal disease characterized by chronic degeneration of the renal epithelium.
**Epstein's n.,** a type of chronic tubular nephritis resulting from systemic metabolic disorder, occurring usually in young persons and in women, and frequently associated with hypothyroidism or other endocrine disturbance.
**glycogen n.,** nephrosis associated with glycogen vacuolation within the proximal convoluted tubules and the loops of Henle.
**hydropic n.,** vacuolar n.
**hypokalemic n.,** vacuolar n.
**infectious avian n.,** infectious bursal disease.
**larval n., lipid n., lipoid n.,** minimal change disease.
**lower nephron n.,** acute tubular necrosis in the lower nephron, seen after severe injuries, especially crushing injury to muscles *(crush syndrome).*
**mold n., mycotic n.,** mycotoxic nephropathy.
**necrotizing n.,** renal disease characterized by necrosis of tubular epithelium of the kidney.
**osmotic n.,** vacuolar n.
**toxic n.,** nephrosis caused by some toxic agent, most frequently and typically by mercury bichloride.
**vacuolar n.,** renal disease in which injury of the renal tubules is associated with vacuolization of the proximal convoluted tubules and sometimes of the loops of Henle and collecting tubules. It is presumed to be caused by disturbances in the normal osmotic relationships within the cells and is seen in various clinical situations, such as after administration of hypertonic solutions, in conditions involving marked alterations in fluid balance, and in severe hypokalemia. Called also *hydropic n., hypokalemic n.,* and *osmotic n.*

**neph·ro·so·ne·phri·tis** (nə-fro"so-nə-fri'tis) [*nephrosis* + *nephritis*] renal disease with nephrotic and nephritic components.
**hemorrhagic n., Korean hemorrhagic n.,** epidemic hemorrhagic fever.

**neph·ro·so·nog·ra·phy** (nef"ro-so-nog'rə-fe) ultrasonic scanning of the kidney.

**neph·ro·spas·is** (nef"ro-spas'is) [*nephro-* + Gr. *span* to draw] movable kidney in which the natural supports of the organ are so weakened that the organ hangs by its pedicle.

**ne·phros·to·li·thot·o·my** (nə-fros'tə-lĭ-thot'ə-me) [*nephrostomy* + *lithotomy*] removal of renal calculi through a nephrostomy tube inserted through the abdominal wall into the renal pelvis.

**ne·phros·to·ma** (nə-fros'tə-mə) [*nephro-* + *stoma*] one of the funnel-shaped and ciliated orifices of excretory tubules that open into the coelom in the embryo, best seen in lower vertebrates.

**neph·ro·stome** (nef'ro-stōm) nephrostoma.

**ne·phros·to·my** (nə-fros'tə-me) [*nephro-* + *-stomy*] the creation of a fistula leading directly into the pelvis of the kidney.
**percutaneous n.,** insertion of a catheter through the skin and into the renal pelvis under the guidance of fluorography or ultrasonography; performed for relief of supravesical obstruction and to gain access to the upper urinary tract for a variety of procedures, such as dilation of strictures or removal of calculi.

**ne·phrot·ic** (nə-frot'ik) pertaining to, resembling, or caused by nephrosis.

**neph·ro·tome** (nef'ro-tōm) one of the segmented divisions of the mesoderm connecting the somite with the lateral plates of unsegmented mesoderm; it is the source of much of the urogenital system. Called also *intermediate cell mass* and *middle plate.*

**neph·ro·to·mo·gram** (nef"ro-to'mo-gram) the sectional radiograph of the kidney obtained by nephrotomography.

**neph·ro·to·mog·ra·phy** (nef"ro-to-mog'rə-fe) radiologic visualization of the kidney by tomography after intravenous introduction of contrast medium as a bolus or by infusion.

**ne·phrot·o·my** (nə-frot'ə-me) [*nephro-* + *-tomy*] a surgical incision into the kidney.
**abdominal n.,** nephrotomy performed through an incision into the abdomen.
**anatrophic n.,** incision into the kidney between its vascular segments, to minimize bleeding and parenchymal injury and to prevent atrophy
**lumbar n.,** nephrotomy performed through an incision into the loin.

**neph·ro·tox·ic** (nef"ro-tok'sik) toxic or destructive to kidney cells.

**neph·ro·tox·ic·i·ty** (nef"ro-tok-sis'ĭ-te) the quality of being toxic or destructive to kidney cells.

**neph·ro·tox·in** (nef"ro-tok'sin) [*nephro-* + *toxin*] a toxin which has a specific destructive effect on kidney cells.

**neph·ro·trop·ic** (nef"ro-trop'ik) having a special affinity for or exerting its principal effect upon kidney tissue.

**neph·ro·tu·ber·cu·lo·sis** (nef"ro-too-ber"ku-lo'sis) [*nephro-* + *tuberculosis*] disease of the kidney due to *Mycobacterium tuberculosis.*

**neph·ro·ure·ter·ec·to·my** (nef"ro-u"re-tər-ek'tə-me) [*nephro-* + *ureterectomy*] excision of a kidney and a whole or part of the ureter.

**neph·ro·ure·tero·cys·tec·to·my** (nef"ro-u-re"tər-o-sis-tek'tə-me) [*nephro-* + *uretero-* + *cystectomy*] excision of the kidney, ureter, and a portion of the bladder wall.

**neph·ry·dro·sis** (nef"rĭ-dro'sis) hydronephrosis.

**neph·ry·drot·ic** (nef"rĭ-drot'ik) pertaining to nephrydrosis.

**Nep·ta·zane** (nep'tə-zān) trademark for a preparation of methazolamide.

**nep·tu·ni·um** (nep-too'ne-əm) [from planet Neptune] [MeSH: Neptunium] a radioactive element of atomic number 93 and atomic weight 237, occurring in certain earths and obtained by splitting the uranium atom with neutrons. It is unstable and changes into plutonium. Symbol Np.

**ne·quin·ate** (nə-kwin'āt) a coccidiostat for poultry.

**Ne·ri's sign** (na'rēz) [Vincenzo *Neri,* Italian neurologist, born 1882] see under *sign.*

**Ne·ri·um** (ne're-əm) a genus of evergreen shrubs of the family Apocynaceae, native to the Mediterranean region and Asia, including the oleanders; most species contain toxic glycosides (see *oleandrism*). Common species include *N. olean'der* and *N. in'dicum.*
**N. olean'der,** L., the common oleander, a popular ornamental flowering garden plant; its roots, flowers, seeds, and bark contain cardiac glycosides and are toxic to humans and livestock. See *oleandrism.*

**Nernst equation, potential** (nernst) [Walther Hermann *Nernst,* German physical chemist, 1864–1941] see under *equation* and *potential.*

**ne·rol** (ne'rol) an essential oil that is a constituent of orange flower oil.

**ner·o·li** (ner'o-le) [It] orange flower oil.

**nerve** (nərv) [L. *nervus*] a cordlike structure made up of a collection of fibers that convey impulses between a part of the central nervous system and some other region of the body. A nerve consists of a connective tissue sheath (epineurium) enclosing bundles of fibers (funiculi or fasciculi); each bundle is in turn surrounded by its own sheath of connective tissue (perineurium), the inner surface of which is formed by a membrane of flattened mesothelial cells. Very small nerves may consist of only one funiculus derived from the parent nerve. Within each such bundle, the individual nerve fibers, which are microscopic in size, are surrounded by interstitial connective tissue (endoneurium). An individual nerve fiber (an axon with its covering sheath) consists of formed elements in a matrix of protoplasm (axoplasm), the entire structure being enclosed in a thin membrane (axolemma). Each nerve fiber is enclosed by a cellular sheath (neurilemma), from which it may or may not be separated by a lipid layer (myelin sheath) derived from neurilemmal cells. Called also *nervus* [TA].

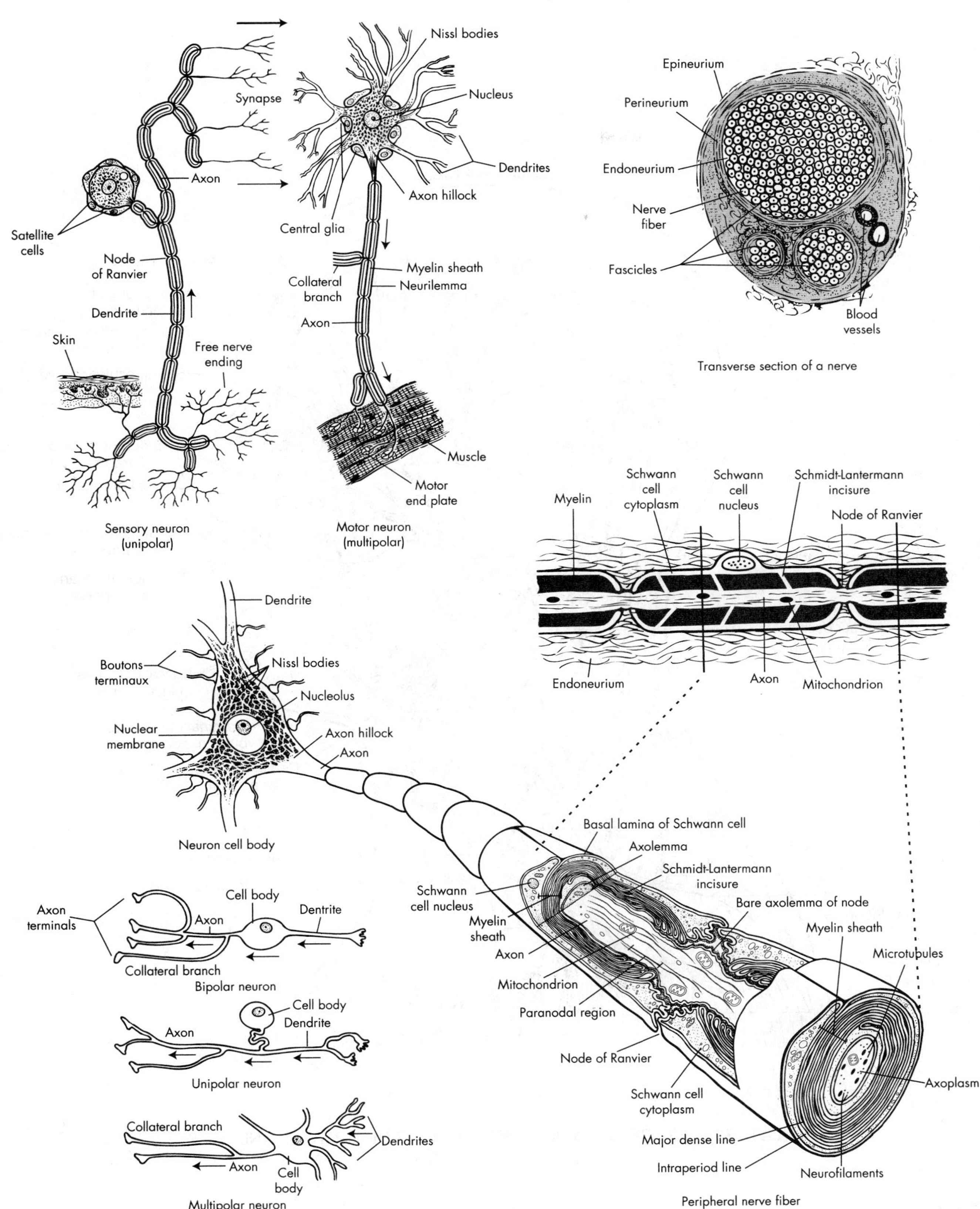


**PLATE 36**—STRUCTURE OF NERVE TISSUE

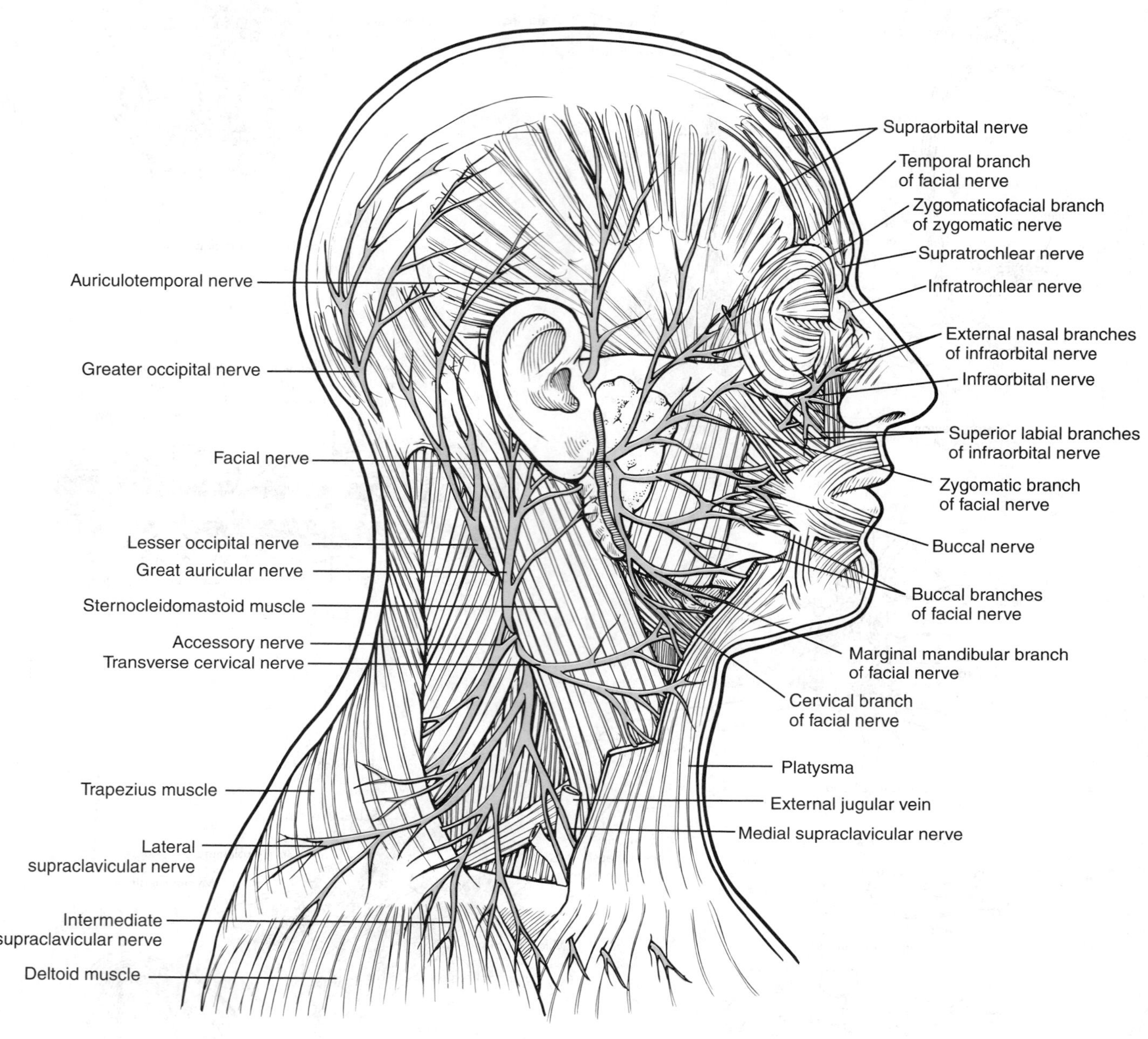


**PLATE 37**—SUPERFICIAL NERVES AND MUSCLES OF THE HEAD AND NECK

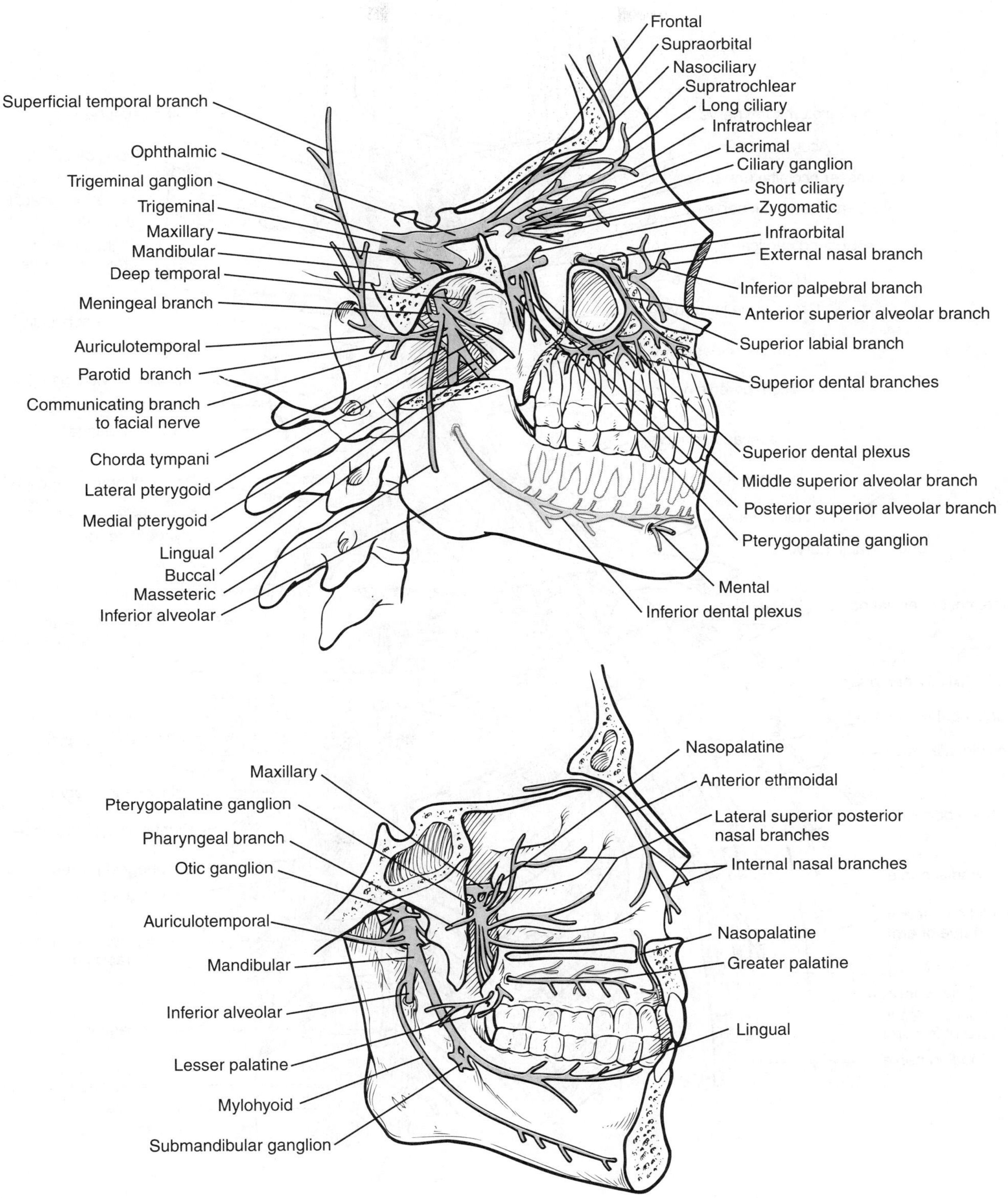


**PLATE 38**—DEEP NERVES SHOWN IN RELATION TO THE BONES OF THE FACE

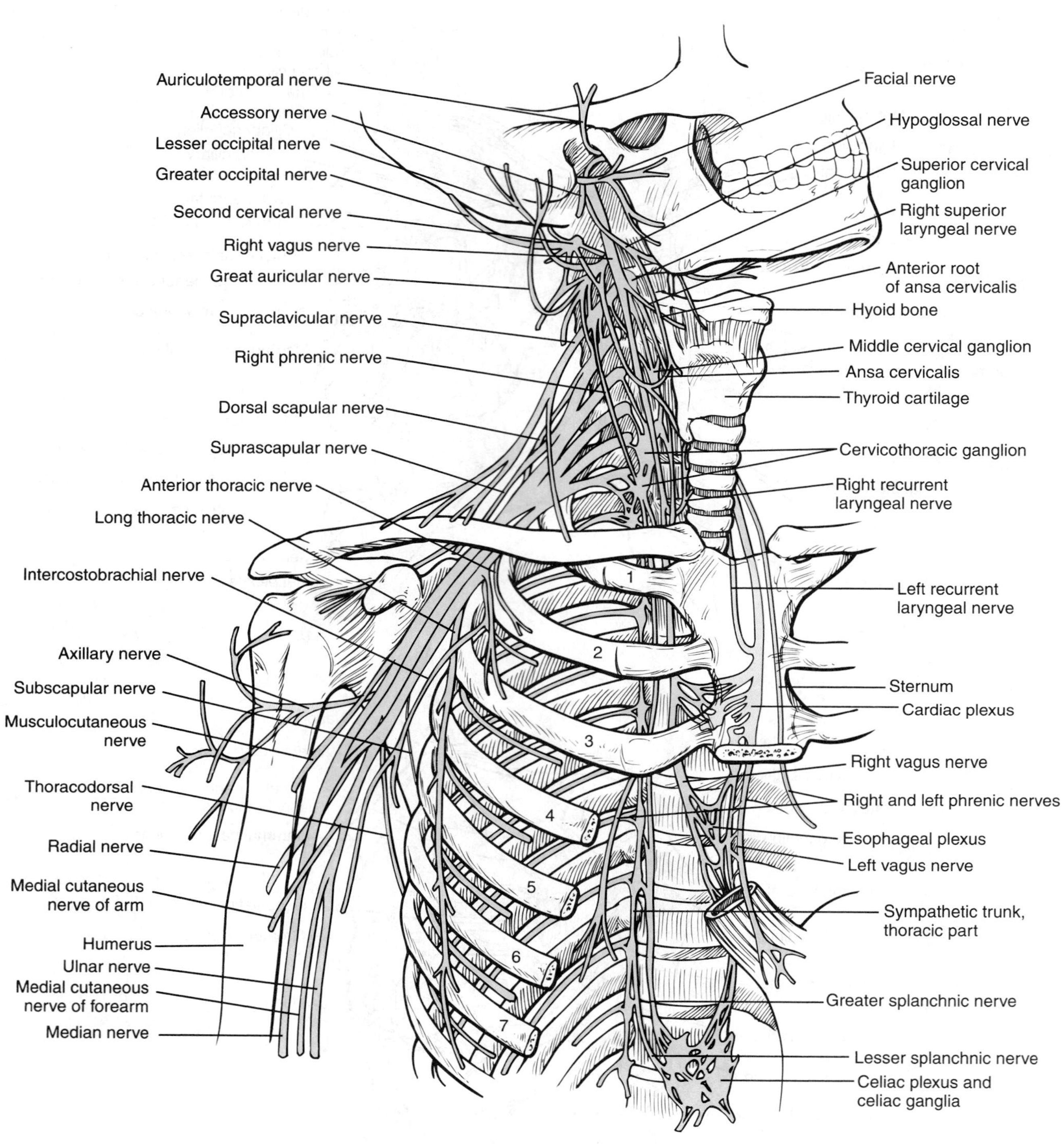


**PLATE 39**—DEEP NERVES OF THE NECK, AXILLA, AND UPPER THORAX

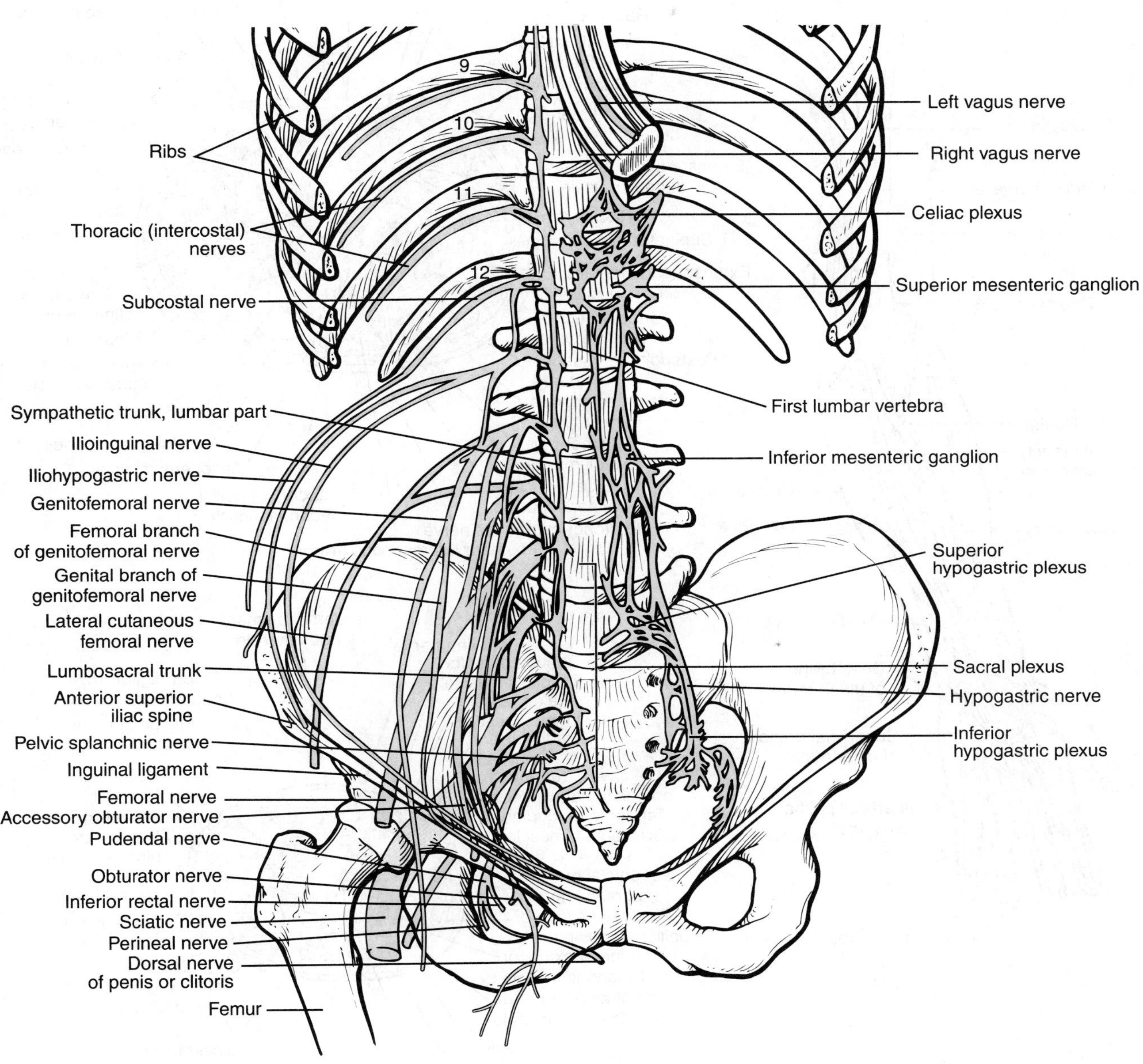


**PLATE 40**—DEEP NERVES OF THE LOWER TRUNK

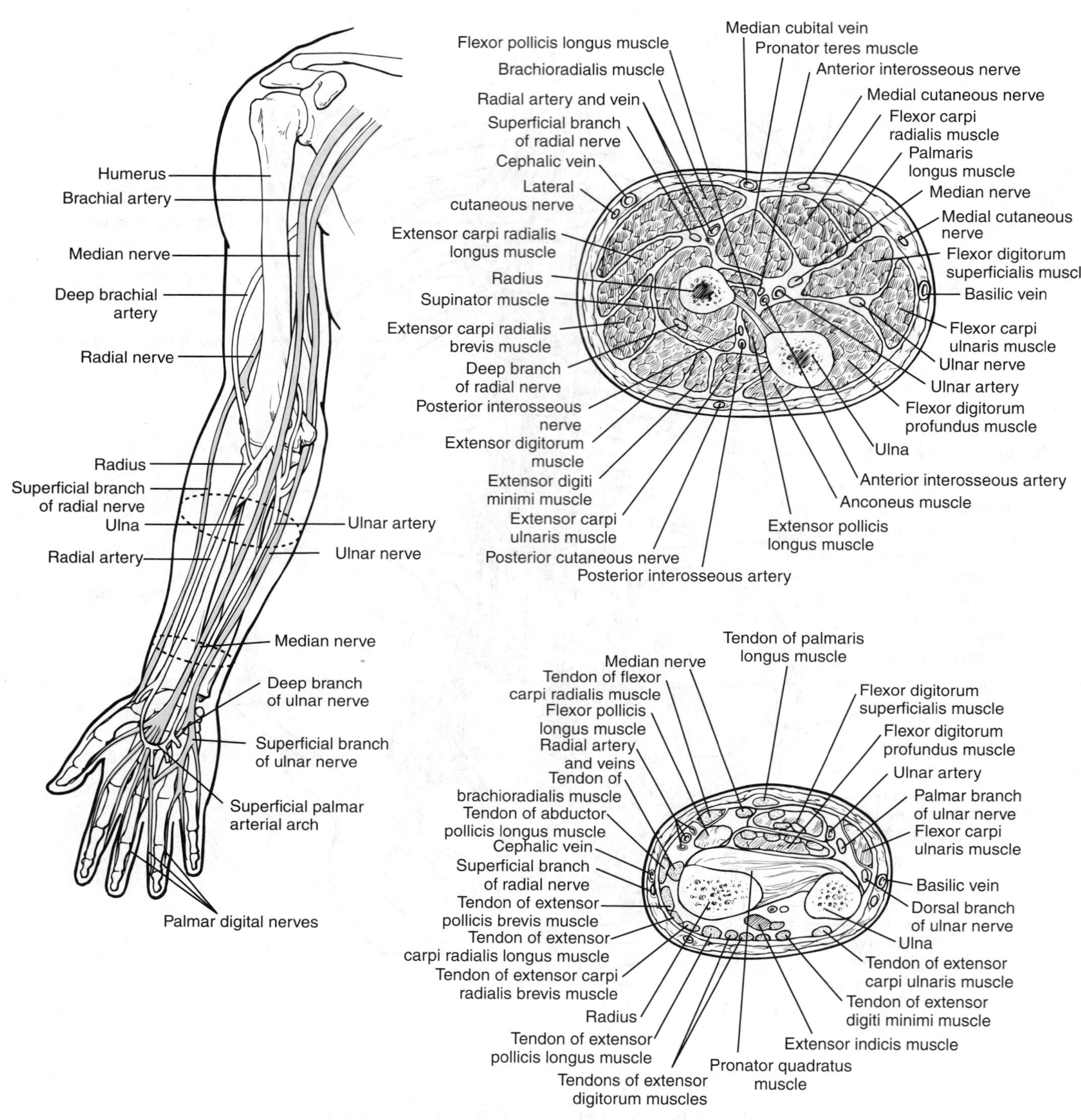


**PLATE 41**—NERVES OF THE UPPER LIMB

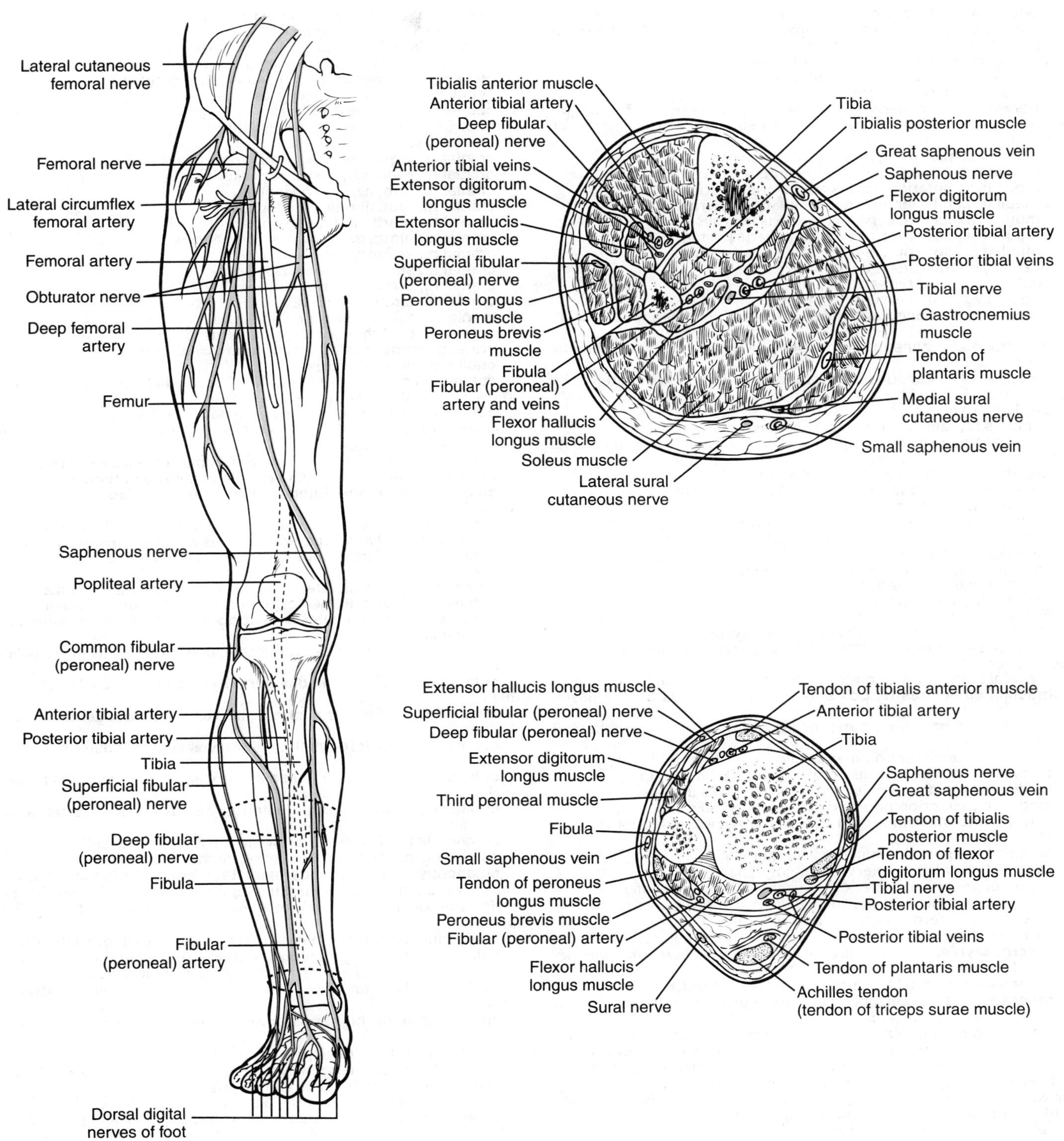


**PLATE 42**—NERVES OF THE LOWER LIMB

## Nerve

For names and descriptions of specific nerves, see under *nervus*.

**abducens n., abducent n.**, nervus abducens.

**accelerator n's**, the cardiac sympathetic nerves, which, when stimulated, accelerate the action of the heart.

**accessory n., accessory n., spinal**, nervus accessorius.

**accessory n., vagal**, ramus internus nervi accessorii.

**acoustic n.**, nervus vestibulocochlearis.

**afferent n.**, any nerve that transmits impulses from the periphery toward the central nervous system, as a sensory nerve; cf. *efferent n.*

**alveolar n., inferior**, nervus alveolaris inferior.

**alveolar n's, superior**, nervi alveolares superiores.

**ampullar n., anterior**, nervus ampullaris anterior.

**ampullar n., inferior**, nervus ampullaris posterior.

**ampullar n., lateral**, nervus ampullaris lateralis.

**ampullar n., posterior**, nervus ampullaris posterior.

**ampullar n., superior**, nervus ampullaris anterior.

**anal n's, inferior**, nervi anales inferiores.

**Andersch's n.**, nervus tympanicus.

**anococcygeal n.**, nervus anococcygeus.

**antebrachial cutaneous n., lateral**, nervus cutaneus antebrachii lateralis.

**antebrachial cutaneous n., medial**, nervus cutaneus antebrachii medialis.

**antebrachial cutaneous n., posterior**, nervus cutaneus antebrachii posterior.

**aortic n.**, Cyon's n.

**Arnold's n.**, ramus auricularis nervi vagi.

**articular n.**, any mixed peripheral nerve that supplies a joint and its associated structures. See also *rami articulares*, under *ramus*.

**auditory n.**, nervus vestibulocochlearis.

**auricular n's, anterior**, nervi auriculares anteriores.

**auricular n., great**, nervus auricularis magnus.

**auricular n., internal**, ramus posterior nervi auricularis magni.

**auricular n., posterior**, nervus auricularis posterior.

**auricular n. of vagus n.**, ramus auricularis nervi vagi.

**auriculotemporal n.**, nervus auriculotemporalis.

**autonomic n.**, nervus autonomicus.

**axillary n.**, nervus axillaris.

**Bell's n.**, nervus thoracicus longus.

**Bock's n.**, ramus pharyngeus ganglii pterygopalatini.

**brachial cutaneous n., inferior lateral**, nervus cutaneus brachii lateralis inferior.

**brachial cutaneous n., medial**, nervus cutaneus brachii medialis.

**brachial cutaneous n., posterior**, nervus cutaneus brachii posterior.

**brachial cutaneous n., superior lateral**, nervus cutaneus brachii lateralis superior.

**buccal n., buccinator n.**, nervus buccalis.

**cardiac n., inferior**, nervus cardiacus cervicalis inferior.

**cardiac n., middle**, nervus cardiacus cervicalis medius.

**cardiac n., superior**, nervus cardiacus cervicalis superior.

**cardiac n's, supreme**, rami cardiaci cervicales superiores nervi vagi.

**cardiac n's, thoracic**, rami cardiaci thoracici.

**caroticotympanic n's**, nervi caroticotympanici.

**caroticotympanic n., inferior**, see *nervi caroticotympanici.*

**caroticotympanic n., superior**, see *nervi caroticotympanici.*

**carotid n's, external**, nervi carotici externi.

**carotid n., internal**, nervus caroticus internus.

**cavernosal n's**, see *nervi cavernosi clitoridis* and *nervi cavernosi penis*, under *nervus.*

**cavernous n's of clitoris**, nervi cavernosi clitoridis.

**cavernous n's of penis**, nervi cavernosi penis; see also *greater* and *lesser cavernous n's of penis.*

**cavernous n. of penis, greater**, a cavernous nerve on the dorsum penis running forward from the plexus prostaticus to supply erectile tissue of the corpus cavernosum penis and the corpus spongiosum.

**cavernous n's of penis, lesser**, cavernous nerves that pierce the proximal tunic of the corpus spongiosum penis and supply the urethra and erectile tissue in the corpus spongiosum.

**celiac n's**, rami coeliaci nervi vagi.

**centrifugal n.**, efferent n.

**centripetal n.**, afferent n.

**cerebral n's**, nervi craniales.

**cervical n's**, nervi cervicales.

**cervical n., descending**, radix inferior ansae cervicalis.

**cervical n., transverse**, nervus transversus colli.

**cervical cardiac n., inferior**, nervus cardiacus cervicalis inferior.

**cervical cardiac n., middle**, nervus cardiacus cervicalis medius.

**cervical cardiac n., superior**, nervus cardiacus cervicalis superior.

**chorda tympani n.**, see *chorda tympani.*

**ciliary n's, long**, nervi ciliares longi.

**ciliary n's, short**, nervi ciliares breves.

**circumflex n.**, nervus axillaris.

**cluneal n's, inferior**, nervi clunium inferiores.

**cluneal n's, middle**, nervi clunium medii.

**cluneal n's, superior**, nervi clunium superiores.

**coccygeal n.**, nervus coccygeus.

**cochlear n.**, nervus cochlearis.

**n. of Cotunnius**, nervus nasopalatinus.

**cranial n's**, nervi craniales.

**cranial n., eighth**, nervus vestibulocochlearis.

**cranial n., eleventh**, nervus accessorius.

**cranial n., fifth**, nervus trigeminus.

**cranial n., first**, nervus olfactorius.

**cranial n., fourth**, nervus trochlearis.

**cranial n., ninth**, nervus glossopharyngeus.

**cranial n., second**, nervus opticus.

**cranial n., seventh**, nervus facialis.

**cranial n., sixth**, nervus abducens.

**cranial n., tenth**, nervus vagus.

**cranial n., third**, nervus oculomotorius.

**cranial n., twelfth**, nervus hypoglossus.

**crural interosseous n.**, nervus interosseus cruris.

**cubital n.**, nervus ulnaris.

**cutaneous n.**, any mixed peripheral nerve that supplies a region of the skin. See also *rami cutanei*, under *ramus.*

**cutaneous n's, femoral**, see *cutaneous n. of thigh, intermediate; cutaneous n. of thigh, medial; nervus cutaneus femoris lateralis;* and *nervus cutaneus femoris posterior.*

**cutaneous n. of abdomen, anterior**, ramus cutaneus anterior [pectoralis/abdominalis] ramorum ventralium nervorum thoracicorum.

**cutaneous n. of arm, inferior lateral**, nervus cutaneus brachii lateralis inferior.

**cutaneous n. of arm, medial**, nervus cutaneus brachii medialis.

**cutaneous n. of arm, posterior**, nervus cutaneus brachii posterior.

**cutaneous n. of arm, superior lateral**, nervus cutaneus brachii lateralis superior.

**cutaneous n. of calf, lateral**, nervus cutaneus surae lateralis.

**cutaneous n. of calf, medial**, nervus cutaneus surae medialis.

**cutaneous n. of foot, intermediate dorsal**, nervus cutaneus dorsalis intermedius.

**cutaneous n. of foot, lateral dorsal**, nervus cutaneus dorsalis lateralis.

**cutaneous n. of foot, medial dorsal**, nervus cutaneus dorsalis medialis.

**cutaneous n. of forearm, dorsal**, nervus cutaneus antebrachii posterior.

**cutaneous n. of forearm, lateral**, nervus cutaneus antebrachii lateralis.

**cutaneous n. of forearm, medial**, nervus cutaneus antebrachii medialis.

**cutaneous n. of forearm, posterior**, nervus cutaneus antebrachii posterior.

**cutaneous n. of neck, anterior**, nervus transversus colli.

**cutaneous n. of neck, transverse**, nervus transversus colli.

**cutaneous n. of thigh, intermediate**, a branch of the anterior cutaneous branch of the femoral nerve; it supplies the skin on the anterior side of the thigh and knee and ends as part of the patellar plexus.

**cutaneous n. of thigh, lateral**, nervus cutaneus femoris lateralis.

**cutaneous n. of thigh, medial**, a branch of the anterior cutaneous branch of the femoral nerve; it supplies the skin on the medial side of the thigh and knee and has a branch that forms part of the patellar plexus.

**cutaneous n. of thigh, posterior**, nervus cutaneus femoris posterior.

**Cyon's n.**, a type of depressor nerve found in rabbits, being a branch of the vagus nerve which when stimulated lowers the blood pressure. Called also *aortic n.* and *Ludwig's n.*

**dental n., inferior**, nervus alveolaris inferior.

**depressor n.**, 1. a nerve that lessens the activity of an organ. 2. an afferent nerve whose stimulation causes a fall in blood pressure.

**diaphragmatic n.**, nervus phrenicus.

**digastric n.**, ramus digastricus nervi facialis.

**digital n's, radial dorsal**, nervi digitales dorsales nervi radialis.

**digital n's, ulnar dorsal**, nervi digitales dorsales nervi ulnaris.

**digital n's of foot, dorsal**, nervi digitales dorsales pedis.

**digital n's of lateral plantar n., common plantar**, nervi digitales plantares communes nervi plantaris lateralis.

**digital n's of lateral plantar n., proper plantar**, nervi digitales plantares proprii nervi plantaris lateralis.

**digital n's of lateral surface of great toe and of medial surface of second toe, dorsal**, nervi digitales dorsales pedis (def. 2).

**digital n's of medial plantar n., common plantar,** nervi digitales plantares communes nervi plantaris medialis.
**digital n's of medial plantar n., proper plantar,** nervi digitales plantares proprii nervi plantaris medialis.
**digital n's of median n., common palmar,** nervi digitales palmares communes nervi mediani.
**digital n's of median n., proper palmar,** nervi digitales palmares proprii nervi mediani.
**digital n's of radial n., dorsal,** nervi digitales dorsales nervi radialis.
**digital n's of ulnar n., collateral palmar,** nervi digitales palmares proprii nervi ulnaris.
**digital n's of ulnar n., common palmar,** nervi digitales palmares communes nervi ulnaris.
**digital n's of ulnar n., dorsal,** nervi digitales dorsales nervi ulnaris.
**digital n's of ulnar n., proper palmar,** nervi digitales palmares proprii nervi ulnaris.
**dorsal n. of clitoris,** nervus dorsalis clitoridis.
**dorsal n. of penis,** nervus dorsalis penis.
**dorsal n. of scapula, dorsal scapular n.,** nervus dorsalis scapulae.
**efferent n.,** any nerve that carries impulses from the central nervous system toward the periphery, as a motor nerve; cf. *afferent n.*
**eighth n.,** nervus vestibulocochlearis.
**eleventh n.,** nervus accessorius.
**encephalic n's,** nervi craniales.
**ethmoidal n., anterior,** nervus ethmoidalis anterior.
**ethmoidal n., posterior,** nervus ethmoidalis posterior.
**exciter n., excitor n.,** a nerve that transmits impulses resulting in an increase in functional activity.
**excitoreflex n.,** a visceral nerve that produces reflex action.
**n. of external acoustic meatus,** nervus meatus acustici externi.
**facial n.,** nervus facialis.
**facial n., temporal,** see *rami temporales nervi facialis.*
**femoral n.,** nervus femoralis.
**femoral cutaneous n., intermediate,** intermediate cutaneous n. of thigh.
**femoral cutaneous n., lateral,** nervus cutaneus femoris lateralis.
**femoral cutaneous n., medial,** medial cutaneous n. of thigh.
**femoral cutaneous n., posterior,** nervus cutaneus femoris posterior.
**fibular n., common,** nervus fibularis communis.
**fibular n., deep,** nervus fibularis profundus.
**fibular n., superficial,** nervus fibularis superficialis.
**fifth n.,** nervus trigeminus.
**first n.,** nervus olfactorius.
**fourth n.,** nervus trochlearis.
**frontal n.,** nervus frontalis.
**furcal n.,** the fourth lumbar nerve, so called because its fibers pass to the lumbar and sacral plexuses.
**fusimotor n's,** those with a special type of nerve ending that innervates intrafusal fibers of the muscle spindle.
**Galen's n.,** ramus communicans nervi laryngei superioris cum nervo laryngeo inferiore.
**gangliated n.,** any nerve of the sympathetic nervous system.
**gastric n's,** truncus vagalis anterior and truncus vagalis posterior.
**genitofemoral n.,** nervus genitofemoralis.
**glossopharyngeal n.,** nervus glossopharyngeus.
**gluteal n's,** 1. the superior and inferior gluteal nerves; see *nervus gluteus superior* and *nervus gluteus inferior.* 2. the cluneal nerves in the lumbar and sacral regions; see *nervi clunium inferiores, nervi clunium medii,* and *nervi clunium superiores.*
**gluteal n., inferior,** 1. nervus gluteus inferior. 2. (in plural) nervi clunium inferiores.
**gluteal n's, middle,** nervi clunium medii.
**gluteal n., superior,** 1. nervus gluteus superior. 2. (in plural) nervi clunium superiores.
**gustatory n's,** sensory nerve fibers innervating the taste buds and associated with taste; they include branches from the lingual and glossopharyngeal nerves. See *rami linguales nervi glossopharyngei* and *rami linguales nervi lingualis,* under *ramus.*
**hemorrhoidal n's, inferior,** nervi anales inferiores.
**Hering's n.,** ramus sinus carotici nervi glossopharyngei.
**hypogastric n.,** nervus hypogastricus.
**hypoglossal n.,** nervus hypoglossus.
**hypoglossal n., descending,** radix superior ansae cervicalis.
**iliohypogastric n.,** nervus iliohypogastricus.
**ilioinguinal n.,** nervus ilioinguinalis.
**iliopubic n.,** nervus iliohypogastricus.
**infraoccipital n.,** nervus suboccipitalis.
**infraorbital n.,** nervus infraorbitalis.
**infratrochlear n.,** nervus infratrochlearis.
**inhibitory n.,** a nerve that transmits impulses resulting in a decrease in functional activity.
**intercostal n's,** nervi intercostales.
**intercostobrachial n's,** nervi intercostobrachiales.
**intermediary n., intermediate n.,** nervus intermedius.
**interosseous n. of forearm, anterior,** nervus interosseus antebrachii anterior.
**interosseous n. of forearm, posterior,** nervus interosseus antebrachii posterior.
**interosseous n. of leg,** nervus interosseus cruris.
**ischiadic n.,** nervus ischiadicus.
**Jacobson's n.,** nervus tympanicus.
**jugular n.,** nervus jugularis.
**labial n's, anterior,** nervi labiales anteriores.
**labial n's, posterior,** nervi labiales posteriores.
**lacrimal n.,** nervus lacrimalis.
**n's of Lancisi,** stria longitudinalis lateralis corporis callosi and stria longitudinalis medialis corporis callosi.
**Langley's n's,** pilomotor n's.
**laryngeal n., external,** ramus externus nervi laryngei superioris.
**laryngeal n., inferior,** nervus laryngeus inferior.
**laryngeal n., internal,** ramus internus nervi laryngei superioris.
**laryngeal n., internal superior,** ramus internus nervi laryngei superioris.
**laryngeal n., recurrent,** nervus laryngeus recurrens.
**laryngeal n., superior,** nervus laryngeus superior.
**Latarjet's n.,** the distal part of the anterior vagal trunk (truncus vagalis anterior), which runs along the lesser curvature of the stomach.
**n. to lateral pterygoid,** nervus pterygoideus lateralis.
**n. to levator ani,** a branch of the sacral plexus that innervates the levator ani muscle.
**lingual n.,** nervus lingualis.
**longitudinal n's of Lancisi,** stria longitudinalis lateralis corporis callosi and stria longitudinalis medialis corporis callosi.
**Ludwig's n.,** Cyon's n.
**lumbar n's,** nervi lumbales.
**lumboinguinal n.,** ramus femoralis nervi genitofemoralis.
**n. of Luschka,** 1. ramus meningeus nervorum spinalium. 2. nervus ethmoidalis posterior.
**mandibular n.,** nervus mandibularis.
**masseteric n.,** nervus massetericus.
**maxillary n.,** nervus maxillaris.
**n. to medial pterygoid,** nervus pterygoideus medialis.
**median n.,** nervus medianus.
**meningeal n.,** ramus meningeus nervi maxillaris.
**mental n.,** nervus mentalis.
**mixed n., n. of mixed fibers,** nervus mixtus.
**motor n.,** nervus motorius.
**motor n. of tongue,** nervus hypoglossus.
**musculocutaneous n.,** nervus musculocutaneus.
**musculocutaneous n. of foot,** nervus fibularis superficialis.
**musculocutaneous n. of leg,** nervus fibularis profundus.
**musculospiral n.,** nervus radialis.
**myelinated n.,** a nerve, especially a peripheral nerve, whose fibers (axons) are encased in a myelin sheath, which in turn is enclosed by a neurilemma. Cf. *unmyelinated n.*
**mylohyoid n., n. to mylohyoid,** nervus mylohyoideus.
**nasociliary n.,** nervus nasociliaris.
**nasopalatine n.,** nervus nasopalatinus.
**ninth n.,** nervus glossopharyngeus.
**obturator n.,** nervus obturatorius.
**obturator n., accessory,** nervus obturatorius accessorius.
**obturator n., internal,** nervus musculi obturatorii interni.
**n. to obturator internus, n. to obturator internus and gemellus superior,** nervus musculi obturatorii interni.
**occipital n., greater,** nervus occipitalis major.
**occipital n., least,** nervus occipitalis tertius.
**occipital n., lesser, occipital n., smaller,** nervus occipitalis minor.
**occipital n., third,** nervus occipitalis tertius.
**oculomotor n.,** nervus oculomotorius.
**olfactory n.,** 1. nervus olfactorius (def. 1). 2. (in the plural) fila olfactoria.
**ophthalmic n.,** nervus ophthalmicus.
**optic n.,** nervus opticus.
**pain n.,** a sensory nerve whose function is the conduction of stimuli which produce the sensation of pain.
**palatine n., anterior,** nervus palatinus major.
**palatine n., greater,** nervus palatinus major.
**palatine n's, lesser,** nervi palatini minores.
**palatine n., medial, palatine n., middle,** see *nervi palatini minores.*
**palatine n., posterior,** see *nervi palatini minores.*
**parasympathetic n.,** any of the nerves of the parasympathetic nervous system; see *parasympathetic system,* under *system.*
**parotid n's,** rami parotidei nervi auriculotemporalis.
**n. to pectineus,** a branch of the femoral nerve that begins just below the inguinal ligament and innervates the pectineus muscle.

**pectoral n., lateral,** nervus pectoralis lateralis.
**pectoral n., medial,** nervus pectoralis medialis.
**perforating cutaneous n.,** nervus cutaneus perforans.
**perineal n's,** nervi perineales.
**peripheral n.,** any nerve outside the central nervous system (outside the brain and spinal cord).
**peroneal n., accessory deep,** nervus peroneus profundus accessorius.
**peroneal n., common,** nervus fibularis communis.
**peroneal n., deep,** nervus fibularis profundus.
**peroneal n., superficial,** nervus fibularis superficialis.
**petrosal n., deep,** nervus petrosus profundus.
**petrosal n., greater, petrosal n., greater superficial,** nervus petrosus major.
**petrosal n., lesser, petrosal n., lesser superficial,** nervus petrosus minor.
**pharyngeal n.,** nervus pharyngeus.
**phrenic n.,** nervus phrenicus.
**phrenic n's, accessory,** nervi phrenici accessorii.
**phrenicoabdominal n's,** rami phrenicoabdominales nervi phrenici.
**pilomotor n's,** the nerves that supply the arrectores pilorum muscles.
**piriform n., n. to piriformis,** nervus musculi piriformis.
**plantar n., lateral,** nervus plantaris lateralis.
**plantar n., medial,** nervus plantaris medialis.
**pneumogastric n.,** nervus vagus.
**popliteal n., external,** nervus fibularis communis.
**popliteal n., internal,** nervus tibialis.
**popliteal n., lateral,** nervus fibularis communis.
**popliteal n., medial,** nervus tibialis.
**presacral n.,** plexus hypogastricus superior.
**pressor n.,** any afferent nerve whose irritation stimulates a vasomotor center and increases intravascular tension.
**pterygoid n., external,** nervus pterygoideus lateralis.
**pterygoid n., internal,** nervus pterygoideus medialis.
**pterygoid n., lateral,** nervus pterygoideus lateralis.
**pterygoid n., medial,** nervus pterygoideus medialis.
**n. of pterygoid canal,** nervus canalis pterygoidei.
**pterygopalatine n's,** nervi pterygopalatini.
**pudendal n.,** nervus pudendus.
**n. to quadratus femoris, n. to quadratus femoris and gemellus inferior,** nervus musculi quadrati femoris.
**radial n.,** nervus radialis.
**radial n., deep,** ramus profundus nervi radialis.
**radial n., superficial,** ramus superficialis nervi radialis.
**rectal n's, inferior,** nervi anales inferiores.
**recurrent n.,** nervus laryngeus recurrens.
**recurrent n., ophthalmic,** ramus meningeus recurrens nervi ophthalmici.
**saccular n.,** nervus saccularis.
**sacral n's,** nervi sacrales.
**saphenous n.,** nervus saphenus.
**n. to sartorius,** a branch of the femoral nerve that arises in common with the intermediate cutaneous nerve and innervates the sartorius muscle.
**scapular n., dorsal,** nervus dorsalis scapulae.
**Scarpa's n.,** nervus nasopalatinus.
**sciatic n.,** nervus ischiadicus.
**sciatic n., small,** nervus cutaneus femoris posterior.
**scrotal n's, anterior,** nervi scrotales anteriores.
**scrotal n's, posterior,** nervi scrotales posteriores.
**second n.,** nervus opticus.
**secretomotor n.,** secretory n.
**secretory n.,** any efferent nerve whose stimulation increases glandular activity.
**sensory n.,** nervus sensorius.
**seventh n.,** nervus facialis.
**sinus n.,** ramus sinus carotici nervi glossopharyngei.
**sinu-vertebral n.,** ramus meningeus nervorum spinalium.
**sixth n.,** nervus abducens.
**somatic n's,** the motor and sensory nerves that supply skeletal muscle and somatic tissues.
**spermatic n., external,** ramus genitalis nervi genitofemoralis.
**sphenopalatine n's,** nervi pterygopalatini.
**n. to sphincter ani,** a branch of the sacral plexus that innervates the sphincter ani muscle.
**spinal n's,** the thirty-one pairs of nerves arising from the spinal cord; see *nervi spinales.*
**splanchnic n's,** the nerves of the blood vessels and viscera, especially the visceral branches of the thoracic, abdominal (lumbar), and pelvic parts of the sympathetic trunks.
**splanchnic n., greater,** nervus splanchnicus major.
**splanchnic n., inferior, splanchnic n., lesser,** nervus splanchnicus minor.
**splanchnic n., least, splanchnic n., lowest,** nervus splanchnicus imus.
**splanchnic n's, lumbar,** nervi splanchnici lumbales.
**splanchnic n's, pelvic,** radix parasympathica gangliorum pelvicorum.
**splanchnic n's, sacral,** nervi splanchnici sacrales.
**stapedial n., stapedius n., n. to stapedius,** nervus stapedius.
**stylohyoid n.,** ramus stylohyoideus nervi facialis.
**stylopharyngeal n.,** ramus musculi stylopharyngei nervi glossopharyngei.
**subclavian n., n. to subclavius,** nervus subclavius.
**subcostal n.,** nervus subcostalis.
**sublingual n.,** nervus sublingualis.
**submaxillary n's,** rami glandulares ganglii submandibularis.
**suboccipital n.,** nervus suboccipitalis.
**subscapular n's,** nervi subscapulares.
**sudomotor n's,** the nerves that innervate the sweat glands.
**supraclavicular n's,** nervi supraclaviculares.
**supraclavicular n's, anterior,** nervi supraclaviculares mediales.
**supraclavicular n's, intermediate,** nervi supraclaviculares intermedii.
**supraclavicular n's, lateral,** nervi supraclaviculares laterales.
**supraclavicular n's, medial,** nervi supraclaviculares mediales.
**supraclavicular n's, middle,** nervi supraclaviculares intermedii.
**supraclavicular n's, posterior,** nervi supraclaviculares laterales [posteriores].
**supraorbital n.,** nervus supraorbitalis.
**suprascapular n.,** nervus suprascapularis.
**supratrochlear n.,** nervus supratrochlearis.
**sural n.,** nervus suralis.
**sural cutaneous n., lateral,** nervus cutaneus surae lateralis.
**sural cutaneous n., medial,** nervus cutaneus surae medialis.
**sympathetic n.,** 1. truncus sympathicus. 2. one of the nerves of the sympathetic nervous system; see *sympathetic system,* under *system.*
**temporal n., anterior deep,** see *nervi temporales profundi.*
**temporal n's, deep,** nervi temporales profundi.
**temporal n., middle deep,** see *nervi temporales profundi.*
**temporal n., posterior deep,** see *nervi temporales profundi.*
**temporal n's, subcutaneous,** rami temporales superficiales nervi auriculotemporalis.
**n. to tensor tympani,** nervus musculi tensoris tympani.
**n. to tensor veli palatini,** nervus musculi tensoris veli palatini.
**tenth n.,** nervus vagus.
**tentorial n.,** ramus meningeus recurrens nervi ophthalmici.
**terminal n.,** nervus terminalis.
**third n.,** nervus oculomotorius.
**thoracic n's,** nervi thoracici.
**thoracic n., long,** nervus thoracicus longus.
**thoracic splanchnic n., greater,** nervus splanchnicus major.
**thoracic splanchnic n., lesser,** nervus splanchnicus minor.
**thoracic splanchnic n., lowest,** nervus splanchnicus imus.
**thoracodorsal n.,** nervus thoracodorsalis.
**tibial n.,** nervus tibialis.
**Tiedemann's n.,** a name given to a plexus of sympathetic nerve fibrils surrounding the central artery of the retina.
**tonsillar n's,** rami tonsillares nervi glossopharyngei.
**transverse n. of neck,** nervus transversus colli.
**trigeminal n.,** nervus trigeminus.
**trochlear n.,** nervus trochlearis.
**twelfth n.,** nervus hypoglossus.
**tympanic n.,** nervus tympanicus.
**ulnar n.,** nervus ulnaris.
**unmyelinated n.,** a nerve whose fibers (axons) are not encased in a myelin sheath, and which may or may not be enclosed by a neurilemma. Cf. *myelinated n.*
**utricular n.,** nervus utricularis.
**utriculoampullary n.,** nervus utriculoampullaris.
**vaginal n's,** nervi vaginales.
**vagus n.,** nervus vagus.
**Valentin's n.,** a nerve sometimes observed connecting the pterygopalatine ganglion and the abducent nerve.
**vascular n's,** nervi vasorum.
**vasoconstrictor n.,** a nerve whose stimulation causes contraction of the blood vessels.
**vasodilator n.,** a nerve whose stimulation causes dilation of the blood vessels.
**vasomotor n.,** any nerve concerned in controlling the caliber of vessels, whether as a vasodilator or a vasoconstrictor.
**vasosensory n.,** any nerve supplying sensory fibers to the vessels.
**vertebral n.,** nervus vertebralis.

## **Nerve** *Continued*

**vestibular n.,** nervus vestibularis.
**vestibulocochlear n.,** nervus vestibulocochlearis.
**vidian n.,** nervus canalis pterygoidei.
**vidian n., deep,** nervus petrosus profundus.
**visceral n.,** nervus autonomicus.
**n. of Willis,** nervus accessorius.
**Wrisberg's n.,** 1. nervus intermedius. 2. nervus cutaneus brachii medialis.
**zygomatic n.,** nervus zygomaticus.
**zygomaticofacial n.,** ramus zygomaticofacialis nervi zygomatici.
**zygomaticotemporal n.,** ramus zygomaticotemporalis nervi zygomatici.

**ner·vi** (ner'vi) [L.] genitive and plural of *nervus.*

**ner·vi·mo·til·i·ty** (ner″vĭ-mo-til'ĭ-te) susceptibility to nervimotion.

**ner·vi·mo·tion** (ner″vĭ-mo'shən) motion effected through the agency of a nerve.

**ner·vi·mo·tor** (ner″vĭ-mo'tor) pertaining to a motor nerve.

**ner·vi·mus·cu·lar** (ner″vĭ-mus'ku-lər) pertaining to the nerve supply of muscles.

**ner·vo·mus·cu·lar** (ner″vo-mus'ku-lər) nervimuscular.

**ner·von·ate** (nər-von'āt) a salt, ester, or anionic form of nervonic acid.

**ner·vone** (ner'vōn) a cerebroside isolated from nerve tissue.

**ner·von·ic ac·id** (nər-von'ik) a polyunsaturated 24-carbon fatty acid occurring in cerebrosides and sphingomyelin. See also table accompanying *fatty acid.*

**ner·vous** (ner'vəs) [L. *nervosus,* from *nervus*] 1. neural (def. 1). 2. unduly excitable or easily agitated.

**ner·vous·ness** (ner'vəs-nəs) excessive excitability and irritability, with mental and physical unrest.

**ner·vus** (ner'vəs) gen. and pl. *ner'vi* [L.] [TA] nerve.

## **Nervus**

Descriptions are given on TA terms, and include anglicized names of specific nerves.

**n. abdu'cens** [TA], abducens nerve (6th cranial): *origin,* a nucleus in the pons, beneath the floor of the fourth ventricle, emerging from the brain stem anteriorly between the pons and medulla oblongata; *distribution,* lateral rectus muscle of eye; *modality,* motor.

**n. accesso'rius** [TA], accessory nerve (11th cranial); *origin,* by cranial roots from the side of the medulla oblongata, and by spinal roots from the side of the spinal cord (from the upper three or more cervical segments); the roots unite to form the trunk of the accessory nerve, which divides into an internal branch (cranial portion) and an external branch (spinal portion); *distribution,* the internal branch to the vagus and thereby to the palate, pharynx, larynx, and thoracic viscera; the external branch branches to the sternocleidomastoid and trapezius muscles; *modality,* parasympathetic and motor.

**n. acus'ticus,** n. vestibulocochlearis.

**n. alveola'ris infe'rior** [TA], inferior alveolar nerve: *origin,* mandibular nerve; *branches,* mylohyoid, inferior dental, mental, and inferior gingival nerves; *distribution*—see individual branches, in this table; *modality,* motor and general sensory.

**ner'vi alveola'res superio'res** [TA], superior alveolar nerves: a term denoting collectively the dental branches arising from the maxillary and infraorbital nerves, viz., *rami alveolares superiores anteriores nervi infraorbitalis, ramus alveolaris superior medius nervi infraorbitalis,* and *rami alveolares superiores posteriores nervi maxillaris.*

**n. ampulla'ris ante'rior** [TA], anterior ampullar nerve: the branch of the vestibular nerve that innervates the ampulla of the anterior semicircular duct, ending around the hair cells of the ampullary crest.

**n. ampulla'ris latera'lis** [TA], lateral ampullar nerve: the branch of the vestibular nerve that innervates the ampulla of the lateral semicircular duct, ending around the hair cells of the ampullary crest.

**n. ampulla'ris poste'rior** [TA], posterior ampullar nerve: the branch of the vestibular nerve that innervates the ampulla of the posterior semicircular duct, ending around the hair cells of the ampullary crest.

**ner'vi ana'les inferio'res** [TA], inferior anal nerves: *origin,* pudendal nerve, or independently from sacral plexus; *distribution,* sphincter ani externus muscle, skin around anus, and lining of anal canal up to pectinate line; *modality,* general sensory and motor. Called also *inferior rectal nerves* and *nervi rectales inferiores* [TA alternative].

**n. anococcy'geus** [TA], anococcygeal nerve: *origin,* coccygeal plexus; *distribution,* sacrococcygeal joint, coccyx, skin over the coccyx; *modality,* general sensory.

**n. articula'ris,** articular nerve.

**ner'vi auricula'res anterio'res** [TA], anterior auricular nerves: *origin,* auriculotemporal nerve; *distribution,* skin of anterosuperior part of external ear; *modality,* general sensory.

**n. auricula'ris mag'nus** [TA], great auricular nerve: *origin,* cervical plexus—C2–C3; *branches,* anterior and posterior rami; *distribution,* skin over parotid gland and mastoid process, and both surfaces of auricle; see individual branches under *ramus; modality,* general sensory.

**n. auricula'ris poste'rior** [TA], posterior auricular nerve: *origin,* facial nerve; *branches,* occipital ramus; *distribution,* auricularis posterior and occipitofrontalis muscles and skin of external acoustic meatus; *modality,* motor and general sensory.

**n. auriculotempora'lis** [TA], auriculotemporal nerve: *origin,* by two roots from the mandibular nerve; *branches,* anterior auricular nerve, nerve of external acoustic meatus, parotid branches, branch to tympanic membrane, and branches communicating with facial nerve; its terminal branches are superficial temporal to the scalp; *distribution*—see individual branches, in this table and under *ramus; modality,* general sensory.

**n. autono'micus** [TA], autonomic nerve: any of the parasympathetic or sympathetic nerves of the autonomic nervous system; called also *n. visceralis* and *visceral nerve.*

**n. axilla'ris** [TA], axillary nerve: *origin,* posterior cord of brachial plexus (C5–C6); *branches,* lateral superior brachial cutaneous nerve and muscular rami; *distribution,* deltoid and teres minor muscles, skin on back of arm; *modality,* motor and general sensory.

**n. bucca'lis** [TA], buccal nerve: *origin,* mandibular nerve; *distribution,* skin and mucous membrane of cheeks, gums, and perhaps the first two molars and the premolars; *modality,* general sensory.

**n. cana'lis pterygoi'dei** [TA], nerve of pterygoid canal: *origin,* union of deep and greater petrosal nerves; *distribution,* pterygopalatine ganglion and branches; *modality,* parasympathetic and sympathetic. Called also *radix facialis.*

**n. cardi'acus cervica'lis infe'rior** [TA], inferior cervical cardiac nerve: *origin,* cervicothoracic ganglion; *distribution,* heart via cardiac plexus; *modality,* sympathetic (accelerator) and visceral afferent (chiefly pain).

**n. cardi'acus cervica'lis me'dius** [TA], middle cervical cardiac nerve: *origin,* middle cervical ganglion; *distribution,* heart; *modality,* sympathetic (accelerator) and visceral afferent (chiefly pain).

**n. cardi'acus cervica'lis supe'rior** [TA], superior cervical cardiac nerve: *origin,* superior cervical ganglion; *distribution,* heart; *modality,* sympathetic (accelerator).

**ner'vi cardi'aci thora'cici,** rami cardiaci thoracici.

**ner'vi caroticotympa'nici** [TA], caroticotympanic nerves: *origin,* internal carotid plexus; inferior and superior nerves can be distinguished; together with tympanic nerve, they form the tympanic plexus; *distribution,* tympanic region and parotid gland; *modality,* sympathetic.

**ner'vi caro'tici exter'ni** [TA], external carotid nerves: *origin,* superior cervical ganglion; *distribution,* cranial blood vessels and glands via the external carotid plexus; *modality,* sympathetic.

**n. caro'ticus inter'nus** [TA], internal carotid nerve: *origin,* superior cervical ganglion; *distribution,* cranial blood vessels and glands via internal carotid plexus; *modality,* sympathetic.

**ner'vi caverno'si clito'ridis** [TA], cavernous nerves of clitoris: *origin,* uterovaginal plexus; *distribution,* erectile tissue of clitoris; *modality,* parasympathetic, sympathetic, and visceral afferent.

**ner'vi caverno'si pe'nis** [TA], cavernous nerves of penis: *origin,* prostatic plexus; *distribution,* erectile tissue of penis; *modality,* sympathetic, parasympathetic, and visceral afferent. See also *greater* and *lesser cavernous nerves of penis,* under *nerve.*

**ner'vi cervica'les** [TA], cervical nerves: the eight pairs of nerves (C1–C8) that arise from the cervical segments of the spinal cord and, except for the last pair, leave the vertebral column above the correspondingly numbered vertebra. The ventral branches of the upper four, on either side, unite to form the cervical plexus, and those of the lower four, together with the ventral branch of the first thoracic nerve, form most of the brachial plexus.

**ner'vi cilia'res bre'ves** [TA], short ciliary nerves: *origin,* ciliary ganglion; *distribution,* smooth muscle and tunics of eye; *modality,* parasympathetic, sympathetic, and general sensory.

**ner'vi cilia'res lon'gi** [TA], long ciliary nerves: *origin,* nasociliary nerve, from ophthalmic nerve; *distribution,* dilator pupillae, uvea, cornea; *modality,* sympathetic and general sensory.

**ner'vi clu'nium inferio'res** [TA], inferior cluneal nerves: general sensory nerve branches of the posterior femoral cutaneous nerve, innervating the skin of the lower part of the buttocks; called also *rami gluteales inferiores, rami clunium inferiores,* and *inferior gluteal nerves.*

**ner'vi clu'nium me'dii** [TA], middle cluneal nerves: general sensory nerve branches of the plexus formed by the lateral branches of dorsal rami of the first four sacral nerves, innervating ligaments of the sacrum and the skin over the posterior buttocks; called also *rami gluteales mediales, rami clunium mediales,* and *middle gluteal nerves.*

**ner'vi clu'nium superio'res** [TA], superior cluneal nerves: general sensory nerve branches of the dorsal rami of the upper lumbar nerves, innervating the skin of the upper part of the buttocks; called also *rami gluteales superiores, rami clunium superiores,* and *superior gluteal nerves.*

**n. coccy'geus** [TA], coccygeal nerve: either of the thirty-first pair of spinal nerves (Co), arising from the coccygeal segment of the spinal cord.

**n. cochlea'ris** [TA], cochlear nerve: the part of the vestibulocochlear nerve concerned with hearing, consisting of fibers that arise from the bipolar cells in the spiral ganglion and have their receptors in the spiral organ of the cochlea. Called also *pars cochlearis nervi octavi,* and *pars cochlearis nervi vestibulocochlearis.*

**ner'vi crania'les** [TA], cranial nerves: the twelve pairs of nerves that are connected with the brain, including the nervi olfactorii (I), and the opticus (II), oculomotorius (III), trochlearis (IV), trigeminus (V), abducens (VI), facialis (VII), vestibulocochlearis (VIII), glossopharyngeus (IX), vagus (X), accessorius (XI), and hypoglossus (XII). Called also *cerebral nerves, encephalic nerves,* and *nervi encephalici.*

**n. cuta'neus,** cutaneous nerve.

**n. cuta'neus antebra'chii latera'lis** [TA], lateral cutaneous nerve of forearm: *origin,* continuation of musculocutaneous nerve; *distribution,* skin over radial side of forearm and sometimes an area of skin of dorsum of hand; *modality,* general sensory. Called also *lateral antebrachial cutaneous nerve.*

**n. cuta'neus antebra'chii media'lis** [TA], medial cutaneous nerve of forearm: *origin,* medial cord of brachial plexus (C8, T1); *branches,* anterior and ulnar; *distribution,* skin of front, medial, and posteromedial aspects of forearm; *modality,* general sensory. Called also *medial antebrachial cutaneous nerve.*

**n. cuta'neus antebra'chii poste'rior** [TA], posterior cutaneous nerve of forearm: *origin,* radial nerve; *distribution,* skin of dorsal aspect of forearm; *modality,* general sensory. Called also *posterior antebrachial cutaneous nerve.*

**n. cuta'neus bra'chii latera'lis infe'rior** [TA], inferior lateral cutaneous nerve of arm: *origin,* radial nerve; *distribution,* skin of lateral surface of lower part of arm; *modality,* general sensory. Called also *inferior lateral brachial cutaneous nerve.*

**n. cuta'neus bra'chii latera'lis supe'rior** [TA], superior lateral cutaneous nerve of arm: *origin,* axillary nerve; *distribution,* skin of back of arm; *modality,* general sensory. Called also *superior lateral brachial cutaneous nerve.*

**n. cuta'neus bra'chii media'lis** [TA], medial cutaneous nerve of arm: *origin,* medial cord of brachial plexus (T1); *distribution,* skin on medial and posterior aspects of arm; *modality,* general sensory. Called also *medial brachial cutaneous nerve.*

**n. cuta'neus bra'chii poste'rior** [TA], posterior cutaneous nerve of arm: *origin,* radial nerve in the axilla; *distribution,* skin on back of arm; *modality,* general sensory. Called also *posterior brachial cutaneous nerve.*

**n. cuta'neus dorsa'lis interme'dius** [TA], intermediate dorsal cutaneous nerve: *origin,* superficial peroneal nerve; *branches,* dorsal digital nerves of foot; *distribution,* skin of front of lower third of leg and dorsum of foot, and skin and joints of adjacent sides of third and fourth, and of fourth and fifth toes; *modality,* general sensory.

**n. cuta'neus dorsa'lis latera'lis** [TA], lateral dorsal cutaneous nerve: *origin,* continuation of sural nerve; *distribution,* skin and joints of lateral side of foot and fifth toe; *modality,* general sensory.

**n. cuta'neus dorsa'lis media'lis** [TA], medial dorsal cutaneous nerve: *origin,* superficial peroneal nerve; *distribution,* skin and joints of medial side of foot and big toe, and adjacent sides of second and third toes; *modality,* general sensory.

**n. cuta'neus femora'lis latera'lis,** n. cutaneus femoris lateralis.

**n. cuta'neus femora'lis poste'rior,** n. cutaneus femoris posterior.

**n. cuta'neus fe'moris latera'lis** [TA], lateral femoral cutaneous nerve: *origin,* lumbar plexus—L2–L3; *distribution,* skin of lateral and front aspects of thigh; *modality,* general sensory. Called also *lateral cutaneous nerve of thigh.*

**n. cuta'neus fe'moris poste'rior** [TA], posterior femoral cutaneous nerve: *origin,* sacral plexus—S1–S3; *branches,* rami clunium inferiores and perineal rami; *distribution,* skin of buttock, external genitalia, and back of thigh and calf; *modality,* general sensory. Called also *posterior cutaneous nerve of thigh.*

**n. cuta'neus per'forans** [TA], perforating cutaneous nerve: one of the inferior clunial nerves which pierces the sacrotuberous ligament and supplies the skin over the inferomedial gluteus maximus; it is absent in one third of the population.

**n. cuta'neus su'rae latera'lis** [TA], lateral sural cutaneous nerve: *origin,* common fibular nerve; *distribution,* skin of lateral side of back of leg, rarely may continue as the sural nerve; *modality,* general sensory. Called also *lateral cutaneous nerve of calf.*

**n. cuta'neus su'rae media'lis** [TA], medial sural cutaneous nerve: *origin,* tibial nerve; usually joins peroneal communicating branch of common peroneal nerve to form the sural nerve; *distribution,* may continue as the sural nerve; *modality,* general sensory. Called also *medial cutaneous nerve of calf.*

**ner'vi digita'les dorsa'les hal'lucis latera'lis et dig'iti secun'di media'lis,** nervi digitales dorsales pedis (def. 2).

**ner'vi digita'les dorsa'les ner'vi radia'lis** [TA], dorsal digital nerves of radial nerve: *origin,* superficial branch of radial nerve; *distribution,* skin and joints of back of thumb, index finger, and part of middle finger, as far distally as the distal phalanx; *modality,* general sensory.

**ner'vi digita'les dorsa'les ner'vi ulna'ris** [TA], dorsal digital nerves of ulnar nerve: *origin,* dorsal branch of ulnar nerve; *distribution,* skin and joints of medial side of little finger, dorsal aspects of adjacent sides of little and ring fingers and of ring and middle fingers; *modality,* general sensory.

**ner'vi digita'les dorsa'les pe'dis,** dorsal digital nerves of foot: 1. [TA] nerves supplying the third, fourth, and fifth toes; *origin,* intermediate dorsal cutaneous nerve; *distribution,* skin and joints of adjacent sides of third and fourth, and of fourth and fifth toes; *modality,* general sensory. 2. [TA] nerves supplying the first and second toes; *origin,* medial terminal division of deep peroneal nerve; *distribution,* skin and joints of adjacent sides of great and second toes; *modality,* general sensory.

**ner'vi digita'les palma'res commu'nes ner'vi media'ni** [TA], common palmar digital nerves of median nerve: *number,* four; *origin,* lateral and medial divisions of median nerve; *branches,* proper palmar digital nerves; *distribution,* thumb, index, middle, and ring fingers, and first two lumbrical muscles—see individual branches, in this table; *modality,* motor and general sensory.

**ner'vi digita'les palma'res commu'nes ner'vi ulna'ris** [TA], common palmar digital nerves of ulnar nerve: *number,* two; *origin,* superficial branch of ulnar nerve; *branches,* proper palmar digital nerves; *distribution,* little and ring fingers—see individual branches, in this table; *modality,* general sensory.

**ner'vi digita'les palma'res pro'prii ner'vi media'ni** [TA], proper palmar digital nerves of median nerve: *origin,* common palmar digital nerves; *distribution,* first two lumbrical muscles, skin and joints of both sides and palmar aspect of thumb, index, and middle fingers, radial side of ring finger, and back of distal aspect of these digits; *modality,* general sensory and motor.

**ner'vi digita'les palma'res pro'prii ner'vi ulna'ris** [TA], proper palmar digital nerves of ulnar nerve: *origin,* the lateral of the two common palmar digital nerves from the superficial branch of the ulnar nerve; *distribution,* skin and joints of adjacent sides of fourth and fifth fingers; *modality,* general sensory.

**ner'vi digita'les planta'res commu'nes ner'vi planta'ris latera'lis** [TA], common plantar digital nerves of lateral plantar nerve: *number,* two; *origin,* superficial branch of lateral plantar nerve; *branches,* the medial nerve gives rise to two proper plantar digital nerves; *distribution,* the lateral one to the musculus flexor digiti minimi brevis pedis and to skin and joints of lateral side of sole and little toe; the medial one to adjacent sides of fourth and fifth toes—see individual branches, in this table; *modality,* motor and general sensory.

**ner'vi digita'les planta'res commu'nes ner'vi planta'ris media'lis** [TA], common plantar digital nerves of medial plantar nerve: *number,* four; *origin,* medial plantar nerve; *branches,* muscular and proper plantar digital nerves; *distribution,* flexor hallucis brevis muscle and first lumbrical muscles, skin and joints of medial side of foot and big toe, and adjacent sides of first and second, second and third, and third and fourth toes—see individual branches, in this table; *modality,* motor and general sensory.

**ner'vi digita'les planta'res pro'prii ner'vi planta'ris latera'lis** [TA], proper plantar digital nerves of lateral plantar nerve: *origin,* common plantar digital nerves; *distribution,* flexor digiti minimi brevis muscle, skin and joints of lateral side of sole and little toe, and adjacent sides of fourth and fifth toes; *modality,* motor and general sensory.

**ner'vi digita'les planta'res pro'prii ner'vi planta'ris media'lis** [TA], proper plantar digital nerves of medial plantar nerve: *origin,* common plantar digital nerves; *distribution,* skin and joints of medial side of first toe, and adjacent sides of first and second, second and third, and third and fourth toes; the nerves extend to the dorsum to supply nail beds and tips of toes; *modality,* general sensory.

**n. dorsa'lis clito'ridis** [TA], dorsal nerve of clitoris: *origin,* pudendal nerve; *distribution,* transversus perinei profundus and sphincter urethrae muscles; corpus cavernosum clitoridis; and skin, prepuce, and glans of clitoris; *modality,* general sensory and motor.

**n. dorsa'lis pe'nis** [TA], dorsal nerve of penis: *origin,* pudendal nerve; *distribution,* transversus perinei profundus and sphincter urethrae muscles; corpus cavernosum penis; and skin, prepuce, and glans of penis; *modality,* general sensory and motor.

**n. dorsa'lis sca'pulae** [TA], dorsal scapular nerve: *origin,* brachial plexus—ventral ramus of C5; *distribution,* rhomboid muscles and occasionally the levator scapulae muscle; *modality,* motor.

**ner'vi encepha'lici,** nervi craniales.

**ner'vi erigen'tes,** radix parasympathica gangliorum pelvicorum.

**n. ethmoida'lis ante'rior** [TA], anterior ethmoidal nerve: *origin,* continuation of nasociliary nerve, from ophthalmic nerve; *branches,* internal, external, lateral, and medial rami; *distribution,* mucosa of upper and anterior nasal septum, lateral wall of nasal cavity, skin of lower bridge and tip of nose; *modality,* general sensory.

**n. ethmoida'lis poste'rior** [TA], posterior ethmoidal nerve: *origin,* nasociliary nerve, from ophthalmic nerve; *distribution,* mucosa of posterior ethmoid cells and of sphenoidal sinus; *modality,* general sensory.

**n. facia'lis** [TA], facial nerve (7th cranial), consisting of two roots: a large motor root, which supplies the muscles of facial expression, and a smaller root, the nervus intermedius (q.v.). *Origin,* inferior border of pons, between olive and inferior cerebellar peduncle; *branches* (of motor root), stapedius and posterior auricular nerves, parotid plexus, digastric, temporal, zygomatic, buccal, lingual, marginal mandibular, and cervical rami, and a communicating ramus with the tympanic plexus; *distribution*—see individual branches, in this table and under *ramus; modality,* motor, parasympathetic, general sensory, special sensory. See also *n. intermediofacialis.*

**n. femora'lis** [TA], femoral nerve: *origin,* lumbar plexus—L2–L4; descending behind the inguinal ligament to the femoral triangle; *branches,* saphenous nerve, muscular and anterior cutaneous rami; *distribution,* the skin of the thigh and leg, the muscles of the front of the thigh, and the hip and knee joints—see individual branches, in this table and under *ramus; modality,* general sensory and motor.

**n. fibula'ris commu'nis** [TA], common fibular nerve: *origin,* sciatic nerve in lower part of thigh; *branches and distribution,* supplies short head of biceps femoris muscle (while still incorporated in sciatic nerve), gives off lateral sural cutaneous nerve and fibular communicating branch as it descends in popliteal fossa, supplies knee and superior tibiofibular joints and tibialis anterior muscle, and divides into superficial and deep fibular nerves; *modality,* general sensory and motor. Called also *n. peroneus communis* [TA alternative] and *common peroneal nerve.*

**n. fibula'ris profun'dus** [TA], deep fibular nerve: *origin,* a terminal branch of common fibular nerve; *branches and distribution,* winds around the neck of the fibula and descends on the interosseous membrane to the front of the ankle; gives off muscular branches, an articular branch, and lateral and medial terminal branches (see under *branch*); *modality,* general sensory and motor. Called also *n. peroneus profundus* [TA alternative] and *deep peroneal nerve.*

**n. fibula'ris superficia'lis** [TA], superficial fibular nerve: *origin,* a terminal branch of common fibular nerve; *branches and distribution,* descends in front of the fibula, supplies peroneus longus and brevis muscles and, in the lower part of the leg, divides into the muscular rami, medial and intermediate dorsal cutaneous nerves—see also individual branches, in this table and under *ramus; modality,* general sensory and motor. Called also *n. peroneus superficialis* [TA alternative] and *superficial peroneal nerve.*

**n. fronta'lis** [TA], frontal nerve: *origin,* ophthalmic division of trigeminal nerve; enters the orbit through the superior orbital fissure; *branches,* supraorbital and supratrochlear nerves; *distribution,* chiefly to the forehead and scalp—see individual branches, in this table; *modality,* general sensory.

**n. genitofemora'lis** [TA], genitofemoral nerve: *origin,* lumbar plexus—L1–L2; *branches,* genital and femoral rami; *distribution*—see individual branches, under *ramus; modality,* general sensory and motor.

**n. glossopharyn'geus** [TA], glossopharyngeal nerve (9th cranial): *origin,* several rootlets from lateral side of upper part of medulla oblongata, between the olive and the inferior cerebellar peduncle; *branches,* tympanic nerve, pharyngeal, stylopharyngeal, tonsillar, and lingual rami, ramus to the carotid sinus, and a ramus communicating with the auricular ramus of the vagus nerve; *distribution,* it has two enlargements (superior and inferior ganglia) and supplies the tongue, pharynx, and parotid gland—see individual branches, in this table and under *ramus; modality,* motor, parasympathetic, and general, special, and visceral sensory.

**n. glu'teus infe'rior** [TA], inferior gluteal nerve: *origin,* sacral plexus—L5–S2; *distribution,* gluteus maximus muscle; *modality,* motor.

**n. glu'teus supe'rior** [TA], superior gluteal nerve: *origin,* sacral plexus—L4–S1; *distribution,* gluteus medius and minimus muscles, tensor fasciae latae, and hip joint; *modality,* motor and general sensory.

**n. hypogas'tricus** [TA], hypogastric nerve: a nerve trunk situated on either side (right and left), interconnecting the superior and inferior hypogastric plexuses.

**n. hypoglos'sus** [TA], hypoglossal nerve (12th cranial): *origin,* several rootlets in the anterolateral sulcus between the olive and the pyramid of the medulla oblongata; it passes through the hypoglossal canal to the tongue; *branches,* lingual rami; *distribution,* styloglossus, hypoglossus, and genioglossus muscles and intrinsic muscles of the tongue; *modality,* motor.

**n. iliohypogas'tricus** [TA], iliohypogastric nerve: *origin,* lumbar plexus—L1 (sometimes T12); *branches,* lateral and anterior cutaneous rami; *distribution,* the skin above the pubis and over the lateral side of the buttock, and occasionally the pyramidalis; *modality,* motor and general sensory. Called also *n. iliopubicus* [TA alternative] and *iliopubic nerve.*

**n. ilioinguina'lis** [TA], ilioinguinal nerve: *origin,* lumbar plexus—L1 (sometimes T12); accompanies the spermatic cord through the inguinal canal; *branches,* anterior scrotal or labial rami; *distribution,* skin of scrotum or labia majora, and adjacent part of thigh; *modality,* general sensory.

**n. iliopu'bicus,** TA alternative for *n. iliohypogastricus.*

**n. infraorbita'lis** [TA], infraorbital nerve: *origin,* continuation of the maxillary nerve, entering the orbit through the inferior orbital fissure, and occupying in succession the infraorbital groove, canal, and foramen; *branches,* middle and anterior superior alveolar, inferior palpebral, internal and external nasal, and superior labial rami; *distribution*—see individual branches, under *ramus; modality,* general sensory.

**n. infratrochlea'ris** [TA], infratrochlear nerve: *origin,* nasociliary nerve from ophthalmic nerve; *branches,* palpebral rami; *distribution,* skin of root and upper bridge of nose and lower eyelid, conjunctiva, lacrimal duct; *modality,* general sensory.

**ner'vi intercosta'les** [TA], intercostal nerves: branches of the first eleven thoracic spinal nerves, situated between the ribs. The first three send branches to the brachial plexus as well as to the thoracic wall; the fourth, fifth, and sixth supply only the thoracic wall; and the seventh through eleventh are thoracoabdominal in distribution. Called also *anterior branches of thoracic nerves, rami anteriores nervorum thoracicum* [TA alternative], *ventral branches of thoracic nerves,* and *rami ventrales nervorum thoracicorum* [TA alternative]. The primary anterior division of the twelfth thoracic nerve is subcostal rather than intercostal in position and is known as the subcostal nerve (see *nervus subcostalis*). It differs in course and relationship from the other anterior branches and so is classified separately.

**ner'vi intercostobrachia'les** [TA], intercostobrachial nerves: two nerves arising from the intercostal nerves and supplying the skin of the arm. The first is constant: *origin,* second intercostal nerve; *distribution,* skin on back and medial aspect of arm; *modality,* general sensory. A second intercostobrachial nerve is often present;*origin,* third intercostal nerve; *distribution,* skin of axilla and medial aspect of arm; *modality,* general sensory.

**n. intermediofacia'lis,** the nervus facialis and the nervus intermedius considered together; so called because they are two radices of the same cranial nerve and, even though they usually occur as separate trunks, they form a common trunk.

**n. interme'dius** [TA], intermediate nerve: the smaller root of the facial nerve, lying between the main root and the vestibulocochlear nerve; it joins the main root at, or merges with, the geniculate ganglion at the geniculum of the facial nerve; *branches,* chorda tympani and greater petrosal nerve; *distribution,* lacrimal, nasal, palatine, submandibular, and sublingual glands, and anterior two-thirds of tongue; *modality,* parasympathetic and special sensory. Called also *Wrisberg's nerve.* See also *n. intermediofacialis.*

**n. interos'seus antebra'chii ante'rior** [TA], anterior interosseous nerve of forearm: *origin,* median nerve; *distribution,* flexor pollicis longus, flexor digitorum profundus, and pronator quadratus muscles, wrist and intercarpal joints; *modality,* motor and general sensory.

**n. interos'seus antebra'chii poste'rior** [TA], posterior interosseous nerve of forearm: *origin,* continuation of deep branch of radial nerve; *distribution,* abductor pollicis longus, extensors of the thumb and second finger, and wrist and intercarpal joints; *modality,* motor and general sensory.

**n. interos'seus cru'ris** [TA], interosseous nerve of leg: *origin,* tibial nerve; *distribution,* interosseous membrane and tibiofibular syndesmosis; *modality,* general sensory. Called also *crural interosseous nerve.*

**n. ischia'dicus** [TA], sciatic nerve, the largest nerve of the body: *origin,* sacral plexus—L4–S3; it leaves the pelvis through the greater sciatic foramen; *branches,* divides into the tibial and common peroneal nerves, usually in lower third of thigh; *distribution*—see individual branches, in this table; *modality,* general sensory and motor. Called also *n. sciaticus.*

**n. jugula'ris** [TA], jugular nerve: a branch of the superior cervical ganglion which communicates with the vagus and glossopharyngeal nerves.

**ner'vi labia'les anterio'res** [TA], anterior labial nerves: *origin,* ilioinguinal nerve; *distribution,* skin of anterior labial region of labia majora, and adjacent part of thigh; *modality,* general sensory.

**ner'vi labia'les posterio'res** [TA], posterior labial nerves: *origin,* pudendal nerve; *distribution,* labium majus; *modality,* general sensory.

**n. lacrima'lis** [TA], lacrimal nerve: *origin,* ophthalmic division of trigeminal nerve, entering the orbit through the superior orbital fissure; *distribution,* lacrimal gland, conjunctiva, lateral commissure of eye, and skin of upper eyelid; *modality,* general sensory.

**n. laryngea'lis infe'rior,** n. laryngeus inferior.

**n. laryngea'lis recur'rens,** n. laryngeus recurrens.

**n. laryngea'lis supe'rior,** n. laryngeus superior.

**n. laryn'geus infe'rior,** inferior laryngeal nerve: *origin,* recurrent laryngeal nerve, especially the terminal portion of this nerve; *distribution,* intrinsic muscles of larynx, except cricothyroid; communicates with the internal laryngeal nerve; *modality,* motor. Called also *n. laryngealis inferior.*

**n. laryn'geus recur'rens** [TA], recurrent laryngeal nerve: *origin,* vagus nerve (chiefly the cranial part of the accessory nerve): *branches,* inferior laryngeal nerve and tracheal, esophageal, and inferior cardiac rami; *distribution*—see individual branches, in this table and under *ramus; modality,* parasympathetic, visceral afferent, and motor. Called also *n. laryngealis recurrens.*

**n. laryn'geus supe'rior** [TA], superior laryngeal nerve: *origin,* inferior ganglion of vagus nerve; *branches,* external, internal, and communicating rami; *distribution,* inferior constrictor of the pharynx, cricothyroid muscle, and mucous membrane of back of tongue and larynx—see individual branches, under *ramus; modality,* motor, general sensory, visceral afferent, and parasympathetic. Called also *n. laryngealis superior.*

**n. lingua'lis** [TA], lingual nerve: *origin,* mandibular nerve, descending to the tongue, first medial to the mandible and then under cover of the mucous membrane of the mouth; *branches,* sublingual nerve, lingual ramus, ramus to the isthmus of the fauces, and rami communicating with the hypoglossal nerve and chorda tympani; *distribution*—see individual branches, in this table and under *ramus; modality,* general sensory.

**ner'vi lumba'les** [TA], **ner'vi lumba'res,** lumbar nerves: the five pairs of nerves (L1–L5) that arise from the lumbar segments of the spinal cord, each pair leaving the vertebral column below the correspondingly numbered vertebra. The ventral branches of these nerves participate in the formation of the lumbosacral plexus.

**n. lumboinguina'lis,** ramus femoralis nervi genitofemoralis.

**n. mandibula'ris** [TA], mandibular nerve, one of three terminal divisions of the trigeminal nerve, passing through the foramen ovale to the infratemporal fossa. *Origin,* trigeminal ganglion; *branches,* meningeal ramus, masseteric, deep temporal, lateral and medial pterygoid, buccal, auriculotemporal, lingual, and inferior alveolar nerves; *distribution,* extensive distribution to muscles of mastication, skin of face, mucous membrane of mouth, and teeth— see individual branches, in this table and under *ramus; modality,* general sensory and motor.

**n. massete'ricus** [TA], masseteric nerve: *origin,* mandibular division of trigeminal nerve; *distribution,* masseter muscle and temporomandibular joint; *modality,* motor and general sensory.

**n. maxilla'ris** [TA], maxillary nerve, one of the three terminal divisions of the trigeminal nerve, passing through the foramen rotundum, and entering the pterygopalatine fossa. *Origin,* trigeminal ganglion; *branches,* meningeal ramus, zygomatic nerve, posterior superior alveolar rami, infraorbital nerve, pterygopalatine nerves, and, indirectly, the branches of the pterygopalatine ganglion; *distribution,* extensive distribution to skin of face and scalp, mucous membrane of maxillary sinus and nasal cavity, and teeth—see individual branches, in this table and under *ramus; modality,* general sensory.

**n. mea'tus acus'tici exter'ni** [TA], nerve of external acoustic meatus: *origin,* auriculotemporal nerve; *distribution,* skin lining external acoustic meatus, and tympanic membrane; *modality,* general sensory.

**n. media'nus** [TA], median nerve: *origin,* lateral and medial cords of brachial plexus—C6–T1; *branches,* anterior interosseous nerve of forearm, common palmar digital nerves, and muscular and palmar rami, and a communicating branch with the ulnar nerve; *distribution,* ultimately, skin on front of lateral part of hand, most of flexor muscles of front of forearm, most of short muscles of thumb and elbow joint, and many joints of hand—see individual branches, in this table and under *ramus; modality,* general sensory.

**n. menin'geus me'dius,** ramus meningeus nervi maxillaris.

**n. menta'lis** [TA], mental nerve: *origin,* inferior alveolar nerve; *branches,* mental, gingival, and inferior labial rami; *distribution,* skin of chin, and lower lip; *modality,* general sensory.

**n. mix'tus** [TA], mixed nerve: a nerve composed of both sensory (afferent) and motor (efferent) fibers.

**n. moto'rius** [TA], motor nerve: a peripheral efferent nerve that conducts impulses from the spinal cord or brain to motor end plates or other terminals, resulting in stimulation of muscle contractions.

**n. mus'culi obturato'rii inter'ni** [TA], nerve to obturator internus: *origin,* ventral branches of ventral rami of L5, S1–S2; *distribution,* posterior gemellus superior muscle and obturator internus muscle; *modality,* general sensory and motor. Called also *n. obturatorius internus* and *obturator nerve.*

**n. mus'culi pirifor'mis** [TA], nerve to piriformis: *origin,* dorsal branches of ventral rami of S1–S2; *distribution,* anterior piriform muscle; *modality,* general sensory and motor. Called also *n. piriformis* and *piriform nerve.*

**n. musculi quadra'ti fe'moris** [TA], nerve to quadratus femoris: *origin,* ventral branches of ventral rami of L4–L5; *distribution,* gemellus inferior, anterior quadratus femoris muscle, hip joint; *modality,* general sensory and motor. Called also *n. quadratus femoris.*

**n. mus'culi tenso'ris tym'pani** [TA], nerve to tensor tympani: *origin,* mandibular nerve via nerve to medial pterygoid muscle and otic ganglion; *distribution,* tensor tympani muscle; *modality,* motor.

**n. mus'culi tenso'ris ve'li palati'ni** [TA], nerve to tensor veli palatini: *origin,* mandibular nerve via nerve to medial pterygoid muscle and otic ganglion; *distribution,* tensor veli palatini muscle; *modality,* motor. Called also *n. tensoris veli palatini.*

**n. musculocuta'neus** [TA], musculocutaneous nerve: *origin,* lateral cord of brachial plexus—C5–C7; *branches,* lateral cutaneous nerve of forearm, and muscular rami; *distribution,* coracobrachialis, biceps brachialis muscles, the elbow joint, and skin of radial side of forearm; *modality,* general sensory and motor.

**n. mylohyoi'deus** [TA], mylohyoid nerve: *origin,* inferior alveolar nerve; *distribution,* mylohyoid muscle, anterior belly of digastric muscle; *modality,* motor. Called also *nerve to mylohyoid.*

**n. nasocilia'ris** [TA], nasociliary nerve: *origin,* ophthalmic division of trigeminal nerve; *branches,* long ciliary, posterior ethmoidal, anterior ethmoidal, and infratrochlear nerves, and a communicating branch to the ciliary ganglion; *distribution*—see individual branches, in this table; *modality,* general sensory.

**n. nasopalati'nus** [TA], nasopalatine nerves: *origin,* pterygopalatine ganglion; *distribution,* mucosa and glands of most of nasal septum and anterior part of hard palate; *modality,* parasympathetic and general sensory.

**n. nervo'rum,** a small nerve supplying the epineurium of a larger nerve.

**n. obturato'rius** [TA], obturator nerve: *origin,* lumbar plexus—L3–L4; *branches,* anterior, posterior, and muscular rami; *distribution,* adductor muscles and gracilis muscle, skin of medial part of thigh, and hip and knee joints—see individual branches, under *ramus; modality,* general sensory and motor.

**n. obturato'rius accesso'rius** [TA], accessory obturator nerve: *origin,* ventral branches of ventral rami of L3–L4; *distribution,* pectineus muscle, hip joint, obturator nerve; *modality,* general sensory and motor.

**n. obturato'rius inter'nus,** n. musculi obturatorii interni.

**n. occipita'lis ma'jor** [TA], greater occipital nerve: *origin,* medial branch of dorsal ramus of C2; *distribution,* semispinalis capitis muscle and skin of scalp as far forward as the vertex; *modality,* general sensory and motor.

**n. occipita'lis mi'nor** [TA], lesser occipital nerve: *origin,* superficial cervical plexus—C2–C3; *distribution,* ascends behind the auricle and supplies some of the skin on the side of the head and on the cranial surface of the auricle; *modality,* general sensory.

**n. occipita'lis ter'tius** [TA], third occipital nerve: *origin,* medial branch of dorsal ramus of C3; *distribution,* skin of upper part of back of neck and head; *modality,* general sensory.

**n. octa'vus** [L. "eighth nerve"], n. vestibulocochlearis.

**n. oculomoto'rius** [TA], oculomotor nerve (3rd cranial): *origin,* brain stem, emerging medial to cerebral peduncles and running forward in the cavernous sinus; *branches,* superior and inferior rami; *distribution,* entering the orbit through the superior orbital fissure, the branches supply the levator palpebrae superioris, all extrinsic eye muscles except the lateral rectus and superior oblique, and carry parasympathetic fibers for the ciliary muscle and sphincter pupillae; *modality,* motor and parasympathetic.

**n. olfacto'rius,** 1. [TA] olfactory nerve (1st cranial): the central processes of the olfactory receptor cells, or fila olfactoria, considered collectively. 2. (in the plural) fila olfactoria.

**n. ophthal'micus** [TA], ophthalmic nerve, one of the three terminal divisions of the trigeminal nerve. *Origin,* trigeminal ganglion; *branches,* tentorial rami, frontal, lacrimal, and nasociliary nerves; *distribution,* eyeball and conjunctiva, lacrimal gland and sac, nasal mucosa and frontal sinus, external nose, upper eyelid, forehead, and scalp—see individual branches, in this table and under *ramus; modality,* general sensory.

**n. op'ticus** [TA], optic nerve (2nd cranial): the so-called nerve of sight, actually part of the central nervous system throughout its course, misnamed as a nerve because of its cordlike appearance; it consists chiefly of axons and central processes of cells of the ganglionic layer of the retina, which leave the orbit through the optic canal, and joins with its opposite number to form the optic chiasm (the medial fibers of each nerve crossing over to the opposite side), then continues as the optic tract to end in the lateral geniculate body.

**ner'vi palati'ni,** see *n. palatinus major* and *nervi palatini minores.*

**n. palati'nus ma'jor** [TA], greater palatine nerve: *origin,* pterygopalatine ganglion; *branches,* posterior inferior (lateral) nasal branches; *distribution,* emerges through the greater palatine foramen and supplies the palate; *modality,* parasympathetic, sympathetic, and general sensory.

**ner'vi palati'ni mino'res** [TA], lesser palatine nerves: *origin,* pterygopalatine ganglion; *distribution,* emerge through the lesser palatine foramen and supply the soft palate and tonsil; *modality,* parasympathetic, sympathetic, and general sensory.

**n. pectora'lis latera'lis** [TA], lateral pectoral nerve: *origin,* lateral cord of brachial plexus or anterior divisions of upper and middle trunks (C5–C7); *distribution,* usually several nerves supplying the musculus pectoralis minor and acromioclavicular and shoulder joints; *modality,* motor and general sensory.

**n. pectora'lis media'lis** [TA], medial pectoral nerve: *origin,* medial cord or lower trunk of brachial plexus (C8, T1); *distribution,* usually several nerves supplying the musculus pectoralis major and musculus pectoralis minor; *modality,* motor.

**ner'vi perinea'les** [TA], perineal nerves: *origin,* pudendal nerve in the pudendal canal; *branches,* muscular branches and posterior scrotal or labial nerves; *distribution,* muscular branches supply the bulbospongiosus, ischiocavernosus, superficial transversus perinei muscles and bulb of the penis and, in part, the sphincter ani externus and levator ani; the scrotal (labial) nerves supply the scrotum or labium majus; *modality,* general sensory and motor.

**n. perone'us commu'nis,** TA alternative for *n. fibularis communis.*

**n. perone'us profun'dus,** TA alternative for *n. fibularis profundus.*

**n. perone'us profun'dus accesso'rius,** accessory deep peroneal nerve: a branch of the superficial fibular nerve that sometimes occurs supplying the musculus peroneus brevis, often extending to the lateral malleolus, and ending in twigs to the musculus extensor digitorum brevis and adjacent joints.

**n. perone'us superficia'lis,** TA alternative for *n. fibularis superficialis.*

**n. petro'sus ma'jor** [TA], greater petrosal nerve: *origin,* intermediate nerve via geniculate ganglion; *distribution,* running forward from the geniculate ganglion, it joins the deep petrosal nerve of the pterygoid canal, and reaches lacrimal, nasal, and palatine glands and nasopharynx, via pterygopalatine ganglion and its branches; *modality,* parasympathetic and general sensory. Called also *radix parasympathica ganglii pterygopalatini* [TA alternative] (which is the term preferred in the official nomenclature when the ganglia of the pars parasympathica are being considered), *radix intermedia ganglii pterygopalatini* [TA alternative], and *parasympathetic root of pterygopalatine ganglion.*

**n. petro'sus mi'nor** [TA], lesser petrosal nerve: *origin,* tympanic plexus; *distribution,* parotid gland via otic ganglion and auriculotemporal nerve; *modality,* parasympathetic. Called also *radix parasympathica ganglii otici* [TA alternative]. NOTE: radix is the term preferred in the official nomenclature when considering the ganglia of the pars parasympathica.

**n. petro'sus profun'dus** [TA], deep petrosal nerve: *origin,* internal carotid plexus; *distribution,* joins greater petrosal nerve to form nerve of pterygoid canal, and supplies lacrimal, nasal, and palatine glands via pterygopalatine ganglion and its branches; *modality,* sympathetic.Called also *radix sympathica ganglii pterygopalatini* [TA alternative]. NOTE: radix is the term preferred in the official nomenclature when considering the ganglia of the pars parasympathica.

**n. pharyn'geus** [TA], pharyngeal nerve: a nerve running from the posterior part of the pterygopalatine ganglion, through the pharyngeal canal with the pharyngeal branch of the maxillary artery, to the mucous membrane of the nasal part of the pharynx posterior to the auditory tube.

**n. phre'nicus** [TA], phrenic nerve: *origin,* cervical plexus—C4–C5; *branches,* pericardiac and phrenicoabdominal rami; *distribution,* pleura, pericardium, diaphragm, peritoneum, and sympathetic plexuses; *modality,* general sensory and motor.

**ner'vi phre'nici accesso'rii** [TA], accessory phrenic nerves: an inconstant contribution of the fifth cervical nerve to the phrenic nerve; when present, they run a separate course to the root of the neck or into the thorax before joining the phrenic nerve.

**n. pirifor'mis,** n. musculi piriformis.

**n. planta'ris latera'lis** [TA], lateral plantar nerve: *origin,* the smaller of terminal branches of tibial nerve; *branches,* muscular, superficial, and deep rami; *distribution,* lying between first and second layers of muscles of sole, it supplies the quadratus plantae, abductor digiti minimi, flexor digiti minimi brevis, adductor hallucis, interossei, and second, third, and fourth lumbrical muscles, and gives off cutaneous and articular twigs to lateral side of sole and fourth and fifth toes—see individual branches, under *ramus; modality,* general sensory and motor.

**n. planta'ris media'lis** [TA], medial plantar nerve: *origin,* the larger of the terminal branches of tibial nerve; *branches,* common plantar digital nerves and muscular rami; *distribution,* abductor hallucis, flexor digitorum brevis, flexor hallucis brevis, and first lumbrical muscles, and cutaneous and articular twigs to the medial side of the sole, and to the first to fourth toes—see individual branches, in this table and under *ramus; modality,* general sensory and motor.

**n. presacra'lis,** TA alternative for *plexus hypogastricus superior.*

**n. pterygoi'deus latera'lis** [TA], lateral pterygoid nerve: *origin,* mandibular nerve; *distribution,* lateral pterygoid muscle; *modality,* motor.

**n. pterygoi'deus media'lis** [TA], medial pterygoid nerve: *origin,* mandibular nerve; *distribution,* medial pterygoid, tensor tympani, and tensor veli palatini muscles; *modality,* motor.

**ner'vi pterygopalati'ni,** pterygopalatine nerves: the two nerves which connect the maxillary nerve to the pterygopalatine ganglion; they are the sensory roots of the ganglion.

**n. puden'dus** [TA], pudendal nerve: *origin,* sacral plexus— S2–S4; *branches,* enters the pudendal canal, gives off the inferior rectal nerve, and then divides into the perineal nerve and dorsal nerve of the penis (clitoris); *distribution,* muscles, skin, and erectile tissue of perineum—see individual branches; *modality,* general sensory, motor, and parasympathetic.

**n. quadra'tus fe'moris,** n. musculi quadrati femoris.

**n. radia'lis** [TA], radial nerve: *origin,* posterior cord of brachial plexus—C6–C8, and sometimes C5 and T1; *branches,* posterior cutaneous and inferior lateral cutaneous nerves of arm, posterior cutaneous nerve of forearm, muscular, deep, and superficial rami; *distribution,* descending in the back of arm and forearm, it is ultimately distributed to skin on back of arm, forearm, and hand, extensor muscles on back of arm and forearm, and elbow joint and many joints of hand—see individual branches, in this table and under *ramus; modality,* general sensory and motor.

**ner'vi recta'les inferio'res,** TA alternative for *nervi anales inferiores.*

**n. saccula'ris** [TA], saccular nerve: the branch of the vestibular nerve that innervates the macula of the saccule.

**ner'vi sacra'les** [TA], sacral nerves: the five pairs of nerves (S1–S5) that arise from the sacral segments of the spinal cord; the ventral branches of the first four pairs participate in the formation of the sacral plexus.

**ner'vi sacra'les et n. coccy'geus** [TA], see *nervi sacrales* and *n. coccygeus.*

**n. saphe'nus** [TA], saphenous nerve: *origin,* termination of femoral nerve, descending first with femoral vessels and then on medial side of leg and foot; *branches,* infrapatellar and medial crural cutaneous rami; *distribution,* knee joint, subsartorial and patellar plexuses, skin on medial side of leg and foot—see individual branches, under *ramus; modality,* general sensory.

**n. scia'ticus,** n. ischiadicus.

**ner'vi scrota'les anterio'res** [TA], anterior scrotal nerves: *origin,* ilioinguinal nerve; *distribution,* skin of anterior scrotal region; *modality,* general sensory.

**ner'vi scrota'les posterio'res** [TA], posterior scrotal nerves: *origin,* perineal nerves; *distribution,* skin of scrotum; *modality,* general sensory.

**n. senso'rius** [TA], sensory nerve: a peripheral afferent nerve that conducts impulses from receptors on a sense organ to the termination of its axon in the spinal cord or brain.

**n. sperma'ticus exter'nus,** ramus genitalis nervi genitofemoralis.

**ner'vi spina'les** [TA], spinal nerves: the thirty-one pairs of nerves that arise from the spinal cord and pass out between the vertebrae, including the eight pairs of cervical, 12 of thoracic, five of lumbar, five of sacral, and one pair of coccygeal nerves.

**n. spino'sus,** TA alternative for *ramus meningeus nervi mandibularis.*

**n. splanch'nicus i'mus** [TA], lowest splanchnic nerve: *origin,* last ganglion of sympathetic trunk or lesser splanchnic nerve; *distribution,* aorticorenal ganglion and adjacent plexus; *modality,* sympathetic and visceral afferent. Called also *lowest thoracic splanchnic nerve* and *n. splanchnicus thoracicus imus.*

**ner'vi splanch'nici lumba'les** [TA], lumbar splanchnic nerves: *origin,* lumbar ganglia or sympathetic trunk; *distribution,* upper nerves join celiac and adjacent plexuses, middle ones go to intermesenteric and adjacent plexuses, and lower ones descend to superior hypogastric plexus; *modality,* preganglionic sympathetic and visceral afferent. Called also *nervi splanchnici lumbares* [TA alternative].

**ner'vi splanch'nici lumba'res,** nervi splanchnici lumbales.

**n. splanch'nicus ma'jor** [TA], greater splanchnic nerve: *origin,* thoracic sympathetic trunk and fifth through tenth thoracic ganglia; *distribution,* descending through the diaphragm or its aortic openings, ends in celiac ganglia and plexuses, with a splanchnic ganglion commonly occurring near the diaphragm; *modality,* preganglionic sympathetic and visceral afferent. Called also *greater thoracic splanchnic nerve* and *n. splanchnicus thoracicus major.*

**n. splanch'nicus mi'nor** [TA], lesser splanchnic nerve: *origin,* ninth and tenth thoracic ganglia of sympathetic trunk; *branches,* renal ramus; *distribution,* pierces the diaphragm, joins the aorticorenal ganglion and celiac plexus, and communicates with the renal and superior mesenteric plexuses; *modality,* preganglionic sympathetic and visceral afferent. Called also *lesser thoracic splanchnic nerve* and *n. splanchnicus thoracicus minor.*

**ner'vi splanch'nici pelvi'ci,** TA alternative for *radix parasympathica gangliorum pelvicorum.*

**ner'vi splanch'nici sacra'les** [TA], sacral splanchnic nerves: *origin,* sacral part of sympathetic trunk; *distribution,* pelvic organs and blood vessels via inferior hypogastric plexus; *modality,* preganglionic sympathetic and visceral afferent.

**n. splanch'nicus thora'cicus i'mus,** n. splanchnicus imus.

**n. splanch'nicus thora'cicus ma'jor,** n. splanchnicus major.

**n. splanch'nicus thora'cicus mi'nor,** n. splanchnicus minor.

**n. stape'dius** [TA], stapedius nerve: *origin,* facial nerve; *distribution,* stapedius muscle; *modality,* motor.

**n. statoacus'ticus,** n. vestibulocochlearis.

**n. subcla'vius** [TA], subclavian nerve: *origin,* upper trunk of brachial plexus—C5; *distribution,* subclavius muscle and sternoclavicular joint; *modality,* motor and general sensory.

**n. subcosta'lis** [TA], subcostal nerve: *origin,* anterior ramus of twelfth thoracic nerve; *distribution,* skin of lower abdomen and lateral side of gluteal region, parts of transversus, oblique, and rectus muscles, and usually the pyramidalis muscle, and adjacent peritoneum; *modality,* general sensory and motor.

**n. sublingua'lis** [TA], sublingual nerve: *origin,* lingual nerve; *distribution,* sublingual gland and overlying mucous membrane; *modality,* parasympathetic and general sensory.

**n. suboccipita'lis** [TA], suboccipital nerve: *origin,* dorsal ramus of first cervical nerve; *distribution,* emerges above posterior arch of atlas and supplies muscles of suboccipital triangle and semispinalis capitis muscle; *modality,* motor.

**ner'vi subscapula'res** [TA], subscapular nerves: *origin,* posterior cord of brachial plexus—C5; *distribution,* usually two or more nerves, upper and lower, supplying subscapularis and teres major muscles; *modality,* motor.

**ner'vi supraclavicula'res** [TA], supraclavicular nerves: a term denoting collectively the common trunk, which is a branch of the cervical plexus (C3–C4) and which emerges under cover of the posterior border of the sternocleidomastoid muscle and divides into the nervi supraclaviculares intermedii, nervi supraclaviculares laterales, and nervi supraclaviculares mediales.

**ner'vi supraclavicula'res interme'dii** [TA], intermediate supraclavicular nerves: *origin,* cervical plexus—C3–C4; *distribution,* descend in the posterior triangle, cross the clavicle, and supply the skin over pectoral and deltoid region; *modality,* general sensory.

**ner'vi supraclavicula'res latera'les** [TA], lateral supraclavicular nerves: *origin,* cervical plexus—C3–C4; *distribution,* descend in the posterior triangle, cross the clavicle, and supply the skin of superior and posterior parts of shoulder; *modality,* general sensory. Called also *nervi supraclaviculares posteriores.*

**ner'vi supraclavicula'res media'les** [TA], medial supraclavicular nerves: *origin,* cervical plexus—C3–C4; *distribution,* descend in posterior triangle, cross the clavicle, and supply the skin of medial infraclavicular region; *modality,* general sensory.

**ner'vi supraclavicula'res posterio'res,** nervi supraclaviculares laterales.

**n. supraorbita'lis** [TA], supraorbital nerve: *origin,* continuation of frontal nerve, from ophthalmic nerve; *branches,* lateral and medial rami; *distribution,* leaves orbit through supraorbital notch or foramen, and supplies the skin of upper eyelid, forehead, anterior scalp (to vertex), mucosa of frontal sinus; *modality,* general sensory.

**n. suprascapula'ris** [TA], suprascapular nerve: *origin,* brachial plexus—C5–C6; *distribution,* descends through suprascapular and spinoglenoid notches and supplies acromioclavicular and shoulder joints, and supraspinatus and infraspinatus muscles; *modality,* motor and general sensory.

**n. supratrochlea'ris** [TA], supratrochlear nerve: *origin,* frontal nerve, from ophthalmic nerve; *distribution,* leaves orbit at medial end of supraorbital margin and supplies the forehead and upper eyelid; *modality,* general sensory.

**n. sura'lis** [TA], sural nerve: *origin,* medial sural cutaneous nerve and peroneal communicating branch of common peroneal nerve; *branches,* lateral dorsal cutaneous nerve and lateral calcaneal rami; *distribution,* skin on back of leg, and skin and joints on lateral side of heel and foot—see individual branches, in this table and under *ramus; modality,* general sensory.

**ner'vi tempora'les profun'di** [TA], deep temporal nerves, usually two in number, anterior and posterior, with a third middle one often seen: *origin,* mandibular nerve; *distribution,* temporal muscles; *modality,* motor.

**n. tenso'ris ve'li palati'ni,** n. musculi tensoris veli palatini.

**n. termina'lis** [TA], terminal nerve: the collection of nerve filaments found in the pia mater between the olfactory bulb and the crista galli, and passing through the cribriform plate to the nasal mucosa; ganglion cells occur along their course.

**ner'vi thora'cici** [TA], thoracic nerves: the twelve pairs of spinal nerves (T1–T12) that arise from the thoracic segments of the spinal cord, each pair leaving the vertebral column below the correspondingly numbered vertebra. They innervate the body wall of the thorax and upper abdomen.

**n. thora'cicus lon'gus** [TA], long thoracic nerve: *origin,* brachial plexus—ventral rami of C5–C7; *distribution,* descends behind brachial plexus to serratus anterior muscle; *modality,* motor.

**n. thoracodorsa'lis** [TA], thoracodorsal nerve: *origin,* posterior cord of brachial plexus—C7–C8; *distribution,* latissimus dorsi muscle; *modality,* motor.

**n. tibia'lis** [TA], tibial nerve: *origin,* sciatic nerve in lower part of thigh; *branches,* interosseous nerve of leg, medial cutaneous nerve of calf, sural nerve, and medial and lateral plantar nerves, and muscular and medial calcaneal rami; *distribution,* while still incorporated in the sciatic nerve, it supplies the semimembranosus and semitendinosus muscles, long head of biceps, and adductor magnus muscle; it supplies the knee joint as it descends in the popliteal fossa and, continuing into the leg, supplies the muscles and skin of the calf and sole of the foot, and the toes—see individual branches, in this table and under *ramus; modality,* general sensory and motor.

**n. transver'sus cervica'lis,** TA alternative for *n. transversus colli.*

**n. transver'sus col'li** [TA], transverse cervical nerve: *origin,* cervical plexus—C2–C3; *branches,* superior and inferior rami; *distribution,* skin on side and front of neck; *modality,* general sensory. Called also *cutaneous* or *transverse nerve of neck* and *n. transversus cervicalis* [TA alternative].

**n. trigemina'lis,** n. trigeminus.

**n. trige'minus** [TA], trigeminal nerve (5th cranial), which emerges from the lateral surface of the pons as a motor and a sensory root, together with some intermediate fibers. The sensory root expands into the trigeminal ganglion, which contains the cells of origin of most of the sensory fibers, and from which the three divisions of the nerve arise. See *n. mandibularis, n. maxillaris,* and *n. ophthalmicus.* The trigeminal nerve is sensory in supplying the face, teeth, mouth, and nasal cavity, and motor in supplying the muscles of mastication.

**n. trochlea'ris** [TA], trochlear nerve (4th cranial): *origin,* the fibers of each trochlear nerve (one on either side) decussate across the median plane and emerge from the back of the brain stem below the corresponding inferior colliculus; *distribution,* runs forward in lateral wall of cavernous sinus, traverses the superior orbital fissure, and supplies superior oblique muscle of eyeball; *modality,* motor.

**n. tympa'nicus** [TA], tympanic nerve: *origin,* inferior ganglion of glossopharyngeal nerve; *branches,* helps form tympanic plexus; *distribution,* mucous membrane of tympanic cavity, mastoid air cells, auditory tube, and, via lesser petrosal nerve and otic ganglion, the parotid gland; *modality,* general sensory and parasympathetic.

**n. ulna'ris** [TA], ulnar nerve: *origin,* medial and lateral cords of brachial plexus—C7–T1; *branches,* muscular, dorsal, palmar, superficial, and deep rami; *distribution,* ultimately to skin on front and back of medial part of hand, some flexor muscles on front of forearm, many short muscles of hand, elbow joint, many joints of hand—see individual branches, under *ramus; modality,* general sensory and motor.

**n. utricula'ris** [TA], utricular nerve: the branch of the vestibular nerve that innervates the macula of the utricle.

**n. utriculoampulla'ris** [TA], utriculoampullary nerve: a nerve that arises by peripheral division of the vestibular nerve, and supplies the utricle and ampullae of the semicircular ducts.

**ner'vi vagina'les** [TA], vaginal nerves: *origin,* uterovaginal plexus; *distribution,* vagina; *modality,* sympathetic and parasympathetic.

**n. va'gus** [TA], vagus nerve (10th cranial): *origin,* by numerous rootlets from lateral side of medulla oblongata in the groove between the olive and the inferior cerebellar peduncle; *branches,* superior and re-

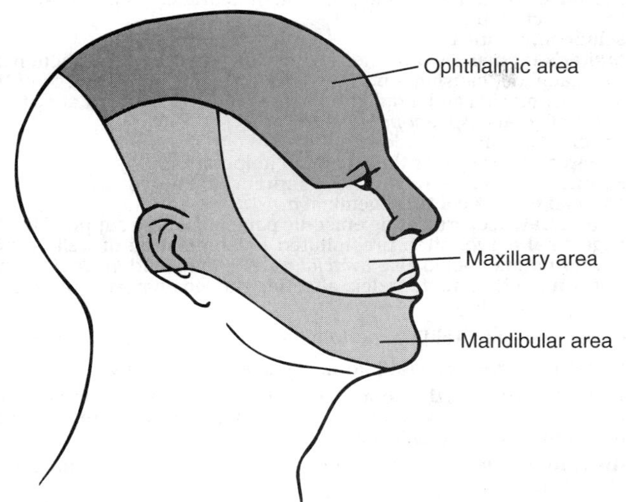


Diagram of the general distribution of the nervus trigeminus (trigeminal nerve). Shown are the three areas, ophthalmic, maxillary, and mandibular, supplied by its three main divisions, the nervi ophthalmicus, maxillaris, and mandibularis, respectively.

current laryngeal nerves, meningeal, auricular, pharyngeal, cardiac, bronchial, gastric, hepatic, celiac, and renal rami, pharyngeal, pulmonary, and esophageal plexuses, and anterior and posterior trunks; *distribution,* descending through the jugular foramen, it presents as a superior and an inferior ganglion, and continues through the neck and thorax into the abdomen. It supplies sensory fibers to the ear, tongue, pharynx, and larynx, motor fibers to the pharynx, larynx, and esophagus, and parasympathetic and visceral afferent fibers to thoracic and abdominal viscera—see individual branches, in this table and under *ramus; modality,* parasympathetic, visceral afferent, motor, general sensory.

**ner'vi vaso'rum** [TA], vascular nerves: the nerve branches that supply the adventitia of the blood vessels.

**n. vertebra'lis** [TA], vertebral nerve: *origin,* cervicothoracic and vertebral ganglia; *distribution,* ascends with vertebral artery and gives fibers to spinal meninges, cervical nerves, and posterior cranial fossa; *modality,* sympathetic.

**n. vestibula'ris** [TA], vestibular nerve: the posterior part of the vestibulocochlear nerve, which is concerned with equilibration. It consists of fibers arising from bipolar cells in the vestibular ganglion, and divides peripherally into a rostral and a caudal part, with receptors in the ampullae of the semicircular canals, the utricle, and the saccule. Called also *pars vestibularis nervi octavi* and *pars vestibularis nervi vestibulocochlearis.*

**n. vestibulocochlea'ris** [TA], vestibulocochlear nerve (8th cranial), which emerges from the brain between the pons and the medulla oblongata, at the cerebellopontine angle and behind the facial nerve. It divides near the lateral end of the internal acoustic meatus into two functionally distinct and incompletely united components, the vestibular nerve and the cochlear nerve, and is connected with the brain by corresponding roots, the vestibular and the cochlear roots. Called also *n. acusticus, n. octavus,* and *acoustic nerve.*

**n. viscera'lis,** n. autonomicus.

**n. zygoma'ticus** [TA], zygomatic nerve: *origin,* maxillary nerve, entering the orbit through the inferior orbital fissure; *branches,* zygomaticofacial and zygomaticotemporal rami; *distribution,* communicates with the lacrimal nerve and supplies the skin of the temple and adjacent part of the face (see individual branches, under *ramus*); *modality,* general sensory.

**Nes·a·caine** (nes'ə-kān) trademark for preparations of chloroprocaine hydrochloride.

**ne·sid·i·ec·to·my** (ne-sid″e-ek'tə-me) [Gr. *nēsidion* islet + *-ectomy*] excision of the pancreatic islets.

**ne·sid·io·blast** (ne-sid'e-o-blast″) [Gr. *nēsidion* islet + *-blast*] [MeSH: Islets of Langerhans] any one of the cells that mature to become the cells of the pancreatic islets.

**ne·sid·io·blas·to·ma** (ne-sid″e-o-blas-to'mə) islet cell tumor.

**ne·sid·io·blas·to·sis** (ne-sid″e-o-blas-to'sis) diffuse proliferation of the pancreatic islet cells.

**Ne·so·kia** (nə-so'ke-ə) a genus of burrowing rodents found in India. *N. bengalen'sis* is the bandicoot.

**Ness·ler's reagent (solution, test)** (nes'lerz) [Julius *Nessler,* German chemist, 1827–1905] see under *reagent.*

**ness·ler·iza·tion** (nes″lər-ĭ-za'shən) treatment with Nessler's reagent.

**nest** (nest) a small mass of cells foreign to the area in which it is found.

**birds' n's,** endocardial pockets.

**Brunn's epithelial n's,** solid or branched glandlike clusters of transitional epithelium occurring in the lamina propria mucosae of the lower urinary tract.

**cell n.,** a mass of closely packed epithelial cells surrounded by a stroma of connective tissue.

**junctional n.,** a nest of dysplastic cells seen at the dermoepidermal junction as part of a junctional nevus.

**Walthard cell n's,** Walthard's islets.

**net** (net) a meshlike structure of interlocking fibers or strands; see also *network, plexus,* and *rete.*

**achromatic n.,** the network within the cell which does not stain with dyes.

**chromidial n.,** a network of chromatin staining material in the cytoplasm of certain cells; it has the properties of active nuclear material.

**neth·a·lide** (neth'ə-līd) pronethalol.

**Neth·er·ton's syndrome** (neth'ər-tənz) [Earl Weldon *Netherton,* American dermatologist, 20th century] see under *syndrome.*

**net·il·mi·cin** (net″il-mi'sin) [MeSH: Netilmicin] a semisynthetic aminoglycoside antibiotic derived from sisomicin, having a range of antibacterial activity similar to that of gentamicin and tobramycin.

**n. sulfate** [USP], the sulfate salt of netilmicin, administered intramuscularly and intravenously in the treatment of a wide variety of infections caused by susceptible gram-negative organisms.

**Net·ro·my·cin** (net″ro-mi'sin) trademark for a preparation of netilmicin sulfate.

**net·tle** (net'əl) any plant of the genus *Urtica.*

**Net·tle·ship-Falls type ocular albinism** (net'əl-ship-fawlz) [Edward *Nettleship,* English ophthalmologist and dermatologist, 1845–1913; Harold Francis *Falls,* American ophthalmologist and geneticist, born 1909] see *X-linked (Nettleship) ocular albinism.*

**net·work** (net'wərk) a meshlike structure of interlocking fibers, strands, or tubules; see also *net, plexus,* and *rete.*

**acromial n.,** rete acromiale.

**arterial n.,** rete arteriosum.

**arterial n., cutaneous,** rete arteriosum dermidis.

**arterial n., subpapillary,** rete arteriosum subpapillare.

**arterial n. of dermis,** rete arteriosum dermidis.

**articular n. of elbow,** rete articulare cubiti.

**articular n. of knee,** rete articulare genus.

**calcaneal n.,** rete calcaneum.

**carpal n., dorsal,** rete carpale dorsale.

**cell n.,** mitome.

**Chiari's n.,** a network of fine fibers which sometimes extend across the interior of the right atrium of the heart from the valve of coronary sinus and the valve of inferior vena cava to the crista terminalis; it is believed to represent incomplete resorption of the septum spurium. It may act as a nucleus for thrombus formation.

**idiotype–anti-idiotype n.,** a regulatory mechanism mounted in response to the unique or idiotypic determinants of lymphocytes or antibodies upon antigenic stimulation. Activation of a B cell results in a clone of plasma cells producing immunoglobulin of a single idiotype, which, because it was previously present in very small quantities, can be recognized as "nonself" and results in the production of anti-idiotypic antibodies directed against its idiotypic determinants. There can also be anti–anti-idiotypic antibodies directed against the second antibodies, antibodies directed against them, and so forth. These antibodies react with antigen receptors

on B cells and T helper and suppressor cells, as well as with circulating antibodies, to enhance or suppress production of the initial antibody by various mechanisms.
**lymphocapillary n.,** rete lymphocapillare.
**malleolar n., lateral,** rete malleolare laterale.
**malleolar n., medial,** rete malleolare mediale.
**neurofibrillar n.,** the network formed by the neurofibrils of a nerve cell.
**patellar n.,** rete patellare.
**peritarsal n.,** a set of lymphatics in the eyelid.
**Purkinje n., subendocardial terminal n.,** rami subendocardiales.
**subpapillary n.,** rete arteriosum subpapillare.
**vascular n., articular,** rete vasculosum articulare.
**venous n.,** rete venosum.
**venous n., plantar, venous n., plantar cutaneous,** rete venosum plantare.
**venous n. of foot, dorsal,** rete venosum dorsale pedis.
**venous n. of hand, dorsal,** rete venosum dorsale manus.

**Neu·bau·er's artery** (noi'bou-erz) [Johann Ernst *Neubauer,* German anatomist, 1742–1777] arteria thyroidea.

**Neu·bau·er-Fisch·er test** (noi'bou-er-fish'er) [Otto *Neubauer,* German physician, 1874–1957; Hans *Fischer,* German physician, 1881–1945] glycyltryptophan test; see under *test.*

**Neu·berg ester** (noi'berg) [Carl *Neuberg,* German biochemist, 1877–1956] see *fructose-6-phosphate.*

**Neu·feld nail** (noo'fēld) [Alonzo John *Neufeld,* American orthopedic surgeon, born 1906] see under *nail.*

**Neu·feld's reaction (test)** (noi'felts) [Fred *Neufeld,* German bacteriologist, 1861–1945] see under *reaction.*

**Neu·mann's law** (noi'mahnz) [Franz Ernst *Neumann,* German physicist, 1798–1895] see under *law.*

**Neu·mann's sheath** (noi'mahnz) [Ernst *Neumann,* German pathologist, 1834–1918] see under *sheath.*

**Neu·po·gen** (noo'po-jən) trademark for a preparation of filgrastim.

**neu·rag·mia** (noo͡-rag'me-ə) [*neur-* + Gr. *agmos* break] the tearing of a nerve trunk.

**neu·ral** (noor'əl) [L. *neuralis*] 1. pertaining to a nerve or to the nerves. 2. situated in the region of the spinal axis, as the neural arch; cf. *hemal.*

**neu·ral·gia** (noo͡-ral'jə) [*neur-* + *-algia*] [MeSH: Neuralgia] pain extending along the course of one or more nerves. Many varieties of neuralgia are distinguished according to the part affected, as brachial, facial, occipital, or supraorbital, or to the cause, as anemic, diabetic, gouty, malarial, or syphilitic.
**cervicobrachial n.,** cervicobrachialgia.
**cervico-occipital n.,** neuralgia in the upper cervical nerves, especially the posterior division of the second cervical nerve.
**cranial n.,** neuralgia along the course of a cranial nerve. Cf. *glossopharyngeal n., trigeminal n.,* and *Ramsay Hunt syndrome,* def. 1.
**n. facia'lis ve'ra,** Ramsay Hunt syndrome, def. 1.
**geniculate n.,** Ramsay Hunt syndrome (def. 1).
**glossopharyngeal n.,** neuralgia affecting the petrosal and jugular ganglia of the glossopharyngeal nerve, marked by severe paroxysmal pain originating on the side of the throat and occasionally extending to the ear. Rarely, attacks may be associated with cardiac slowing or arrest, and syncope.
**hallucinatory n.,** a mental impression of pain without any actual peripheral stimulus.
**Hunt's n.,** Ramsay Hunt syndrome, def. 1.
**idiopathic n.,** neuralgia of unknown etiology, unaccompanied by any structural change.
**intercostal n.,** neuralgia of the intercostal nerves.
**mammary n.,** neuralgic pain in the breast.
**mandibular joint n.,** vertex and occipital pain, otalgia, glossodynia, and pain about the nose and eyes, associated with disturbed function of the temporomandibular joint.
**migrainous n.,** cluster headache.
**Morton's n.,** a form of foot pain, metatarsalgia caused by compression of a branch of the plantar nerve by the metatarsal heads; chronic compression may lead to formation of a neuroma. Called also *Morton's disease, foot, metatarsalgia,* and *toe.*
**nasociliary n.,** Charlin's syndrome.
**occipital n.,** pain in the distribution of the occipital nerves, due to pressure or trauma to the nerve.
**otic n.,** Ramsay Hunt syndrome (def. 1).
**peripheral n.,** pain along the course of a peripheral sensory nerve.
**postherpetic n.,** persistent burning pain and hyperesthesia along the distribution of a cutaneous nerve following an attack of herpes zoster; it may last for a few weeks or many months. It occurs in two forms, *Ramsay Hunt syndrome* (or *herpes zoster auricularis*) and *herpes zoster ophthalmicus.*
**red n.,** erythromelalgia.
**reminiscent n.,** a mental impression of neuralgic pain persisting after the actual pain has ceased.
**sciatic n.,** sciatica.
**Sluder's n.,** neuralgia of the territory supplied by the sphenopalatine ganglion, causing a burning and boring pain in the area of the superior maxilla and a radiation of the pain into the neck and shoulder. Called also *sphenopalatine n.*
**sphenopalatine n.,** Sluder's n.
**stump n.,** neuralgia at the site of an amputation.
**supraorbital n.,** neuralgia of the supraorbital nerve.
**trifacial n., trifocal n.,** trigeminal n.
**trigeminal n.,** excruciating episodic pain in the area supplied by the trigeminal nerve, often precipitated by stimulation of well-defined trigger points. Called also *trifacial n., trifocal n.,* and *tic douloureux.*
**Vail's n., vidian n.,** neuralgia affecting the vidian nerve (nervus canalis pterygoidei).

**neu·ral·gic** (noo͡-ral'jik) pertaining to or of the nature of neuralgia.

**neu·ral·gi·form** (noo͡-ral'ji-form) resembling neuralgia.

**neu·ra·min·ic ac·id** (noor"ə-min'ik) a nine carbon amino sugar formed from mannosamine and pyruvate, mostly important as its *N*-acyl derivatives (sialic acids).

**neu·ra·min·i·dase** (noor"ə-min'ĭ-dās) [MeSH: Neuraminidase] sialidase.

**neu·rana·gen·e·sis** (noor"an-ə-jen'ə-sis) [*neur-* + Gr. *anagennan* to regenerate] regeneration or renewal of nerve tissue.

**neu·ra·poph·y·sis** (noor"ə-pof'ə-sis) [*neur-* + *apophysis*] the structure forming either side of the neural arch.

**neu·ra·prax·ia** (noor"ə-prak'se-ə) [*neur-* + *apraxia*] failure of conduction in a nerve in the absence of structural changes, due to blunt injury, compression, or ischemia; return of function normally ensues. Called also *axonapraxia.* Cf. *axonotmesis* and *neurotmesis.*

**neu·rar·chy** (noor'ahr-ke) [*neur-* + Gr. *archē* rule] the control of the cerebrospinal system over the body.

**neu·rar·throp·a·thy** (noor"ahr-throp'ə-the) neuroarthropathy.

**neu·ras·the·nia** (noor"əs-the'ne-ə) [*neur-* + *asthenia*] [MeSH: Neurasthenia] a term introduced by Beard in 1869, and now virtually obsolete, to refer to a syndrome of chronic mental and physical weakness and fatigue, which was supposed to be caused by exhaustion of the nervous system.

**neu·rax·i·al** (noo͡-rak'se-əl) pertaining to the neuraxis.

**neu·rax·is** (noo͡-rak'sis) [*neur-* + *axis*] the central nervous system.

**neure** (nūr) neuron.

**neu·rec·ta·sia** (noor"ək-ta'zhə) [*neur-* + *ectasia*] neurotony.

**neu·rec·to·my** (noo͡-rek'to-me) [*neur-* + *-ectomy*] the excision of a part of a nerve.

**neu·rec·to·pia** (noor"ək-to'pe-ə) [*neur-* + *ectopia*] displacement of a nerve or abnormal situation of a nerve.

**neu·rec·to·py** (noo͡-rek'tə-pe) neurectopia.

**neu·ren·ter·ic** (noor"ən-ter'ik) [*neur-* + *enteric*] pertaining to the neural tube and archenteron of the embryo, applied especially to the canal interconnecting them.

**neur·epi·the·li·al** (noor"ep-ĭ-the'le-əl) neuroepithelial.

**neur·epi·the·li·um** (noor"ep-i-the'le-əm) neuroepithelium.

**neu·rer·gic** (noo͡-rər'jik) [*neur-* + *erg-* + *-ic*] pertaining to or dependent on nerve action.

**neur·ex·er·e·sis** (noor"ek-ser'ə-sis) [*neur-* + *exeresis*] nerve avulsion.

**neu·ri·a·try** (noo͡-ri'ə-tre) [*neur-* + *-iatry*] clinical neurology.

**neu·ri·dine** (noor'ĭ-dēn) a base isolated from fresh human brain, identical with spermine.

**neu·ri·lem·ma** (noor"ĭ-lem'ə) [*neur-* + *-lemma*] [MeSH: Neurilemma] the thin membrane spirally enwrapping the myelin layers of certain fibers, especially of peripheral nerves, or the axons of certain unmyelinated nerve fibers. Called also *neurolemma, Schwann's membrane, sheath of Schwann,* and *endoneural membrane.* See figure at *nerve.*

**neu·ri·lem·mal** (noor"ĭ-lem'əl) pertaining to a neurilemma.

**neu·ri·lem·mi·tis** (noor"ĭ-lem-i'tis) inflammation of the neurilemma.

**neu·ri·lem·mo·ma** (noor"ĭ-lem-o'mə) [MeSH: Neurilemmoma] neurilemoma.

**neu·ri·lem·o·ma** (noor"ĭ-lem-o'mə) a tumor of a neurilemma, the most common type of neurogenic tumor, usually isolated and en-

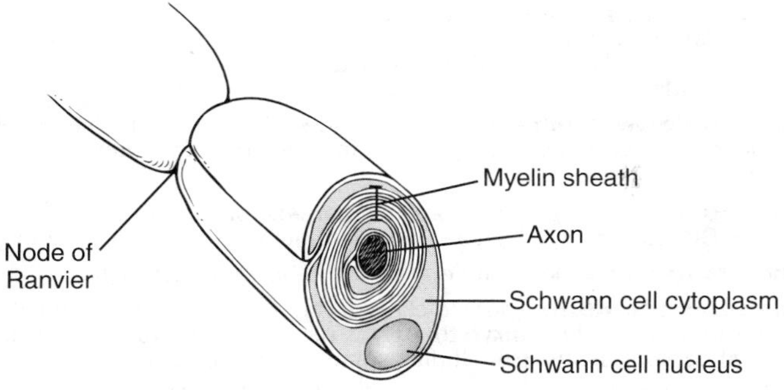


Neurilemma enclosing axon in a peripheral nerve fiber.

capsulated. Most are benign but occasionally they become malignant. Cf. *neurofibroma.* Called also *schwannoma.*
**acoustic n.,** acoustic neuroma.

**neu·ril·i·ty** (n̄oo-ril′ĭ-te) the sum of the attributes and functions of nerve tissue.

**neu·ri·mo·til·i·ty** (noor″ĭ-mo-til′ĭ-te) nervimotility.

**neu·ri·mo·tor** (noor″ĭ-mo′tər) nervimotor.

**neu·rine** (noor′ēn) a poisonous ptomaine with a fishy odor, formed by dehydration of choline during putrefaction and found in decaying fish, fungi, and also in the brain and in many other normal tissues; used in biochemical research.

**neu·ri·no·ma** (noor″ĭ-no′mə) schwannoma.
**acoustic n.,** acoustic neuroma.
**acoustic n., bilateral,** neurofibromatosis 2.

**neu·rit·ic** (n̄oo-rit′ik) pertaining to or affected with neuritis.

**neu·ri·tis** (n̄oo-ri′tis) [*neur-* + *-itis*] [MeSH: Neuritis] inflammation of a nerve, with pain and tenderness, anesthesia and paresthesias, paralysis, wasting, and disappearance of the reflexes. See also *neuropathy.*
**alcoholic n.,** see under *neuropathy.*
**brachial n.,** neuralgic amyotrophy.
**cauda equina n.,** inflammation of the nerve roots of the cauda equina of a horse or dog, usually seen in adults; symptoms include paralysis of the tail and certain abdominal muscles, with incoordination of the hind limbs and often fecal and urinary incontinence. Called also *cauda equina syndrome.*
**dietetic n.,** beriberi.
**fallopian n.,** neuritis of the facial nerve in the fallopian canal.
**Gombault's n.,** progressive hypertrophic neuropathy.
**hypertrophic n., interstitial,** progressive hypertrophic interstitial neuropathy.
**intraocular n.,** papillitis (def. 2).
**lead n.,** see under *neuropathy.*
**leprous n.,** see under *polyneuritis.*
**n. mi′grans, migrating n.,** neuritis affecting first one nerve and then another.
**multiple n.,** polyneuritis.
**n. mul′tiplex ende′mica,** beriberi.
**optic n.,** inflammation of the optic nerve; it is classified as either *intraocular,* affecting the part of the nerve within the eyeball (see *papillitis*) or *retrobulbar,* affecting the portion behind the eyeball (see *retrobulbar optic n.*).
**optic n., hereditary,** Leber's hereditary optic neuropathy.
**optic n., orbital,** retrobulbar optic n.
**optic n., postocular,** retrobulbar optic n.
**optic n., retrobulbar,** inflammation in the portion of the optic nerve that is posterior to the eyeball.
**periaxial n.,** segmental (demyelination) neuropathy.
**peripheral n.,** neuritis of one or more peripheral nerves; cf. *polyneuritis.*
**postfebrile n.,** neuritis following fever; see *acute idiopathic polyneuritis.*
**n. puerpera′lis trauma′tica,** neuritis occurring in parturient women as a result of injury at childbirth.
**radiation n.,** radioneuritis.
**radicular n.,** radiculitis.
**retrobulbar n.,** retrobulbar optic n.
**n. saturni′na,** lead neuropathy.
**sciatic n.,** sciatica.
**segmental n.,** segmental (demyelination) neuropathy.
**serum n.,** see under *neuropathy.*
**shoulder-girdle n.,** neuralgic amyotrophy.
**syphilitic n.,** neuritis due to neurosyphilis.
**toxic n.,** see under *neuropathy.*
**vestibular n.,** see under *neuronitis.*

**neur(o)-** [Gr. *neuron* nerve] combining form denoting relationship to a nerve or nerves, or to the nervous system.

**neu·ro·acan·tho·cy·to·sis** (noor″o-ə-kan″tho-si-to′sis) choreoacanthocytosis.

**neu·ro·al·ler·gy** (noor″o-al′ər-je) allergy in nervous tissue.

**neu·ro·am·e·bi·a·sis** (noor″o-am″e-bi′ə-sis) neuritis due to amebiasis.

**neu·ro·anas·to·mo·sis** (noor″o-ə-nas″tə-mo′sis) surgical formation of an anastomosis between nerves.

**neu·ro·anat·o·my** (noor″o-ə-nat′ə-me) [*neuro-* + *anatomy*] [MeSH: Neuroanatomy] that branch of neurology which is concerned with the anatomy of the nervous system.

**neu·ro·ar·throp·a·thy** (noor″o-ahr-throp′ə-the) [*neuro-* + *arthropathy*] any disease of joint structures associated with disease of the central or peripheral nervous system.

**neu·ro·as·tro·cy·to·ma** (noor″o-as″tro-si-to′mə) [*neuro-* + *astrocytoma*] a glioma composed mainly of astrocytes, closely resembling an astrocytoma and most commonly found in the floor of the third ventricle and the temporal lobes, although it may arise in almost any part of the central nervous system.

**neu·ro·be·hav·ior·al** (noor″o-be-hāv′u-rəl) relating to neurologic status as assessed by observation of behavior.

**neu·ro·bi·ol·o·gist** (noor″o-bi-ol′ə-jist) a specialist in neurobiology.

**neu·ro·bi·ol·o·gy** (noor″o-bi-ol′ə-je) [MeSH: Neurobiology] the biology of the nervous system, including its anatomy, physiology, biochemistry, and so on.

**neu·ro·bio·tax·is** (noor″o-bi″o-tak′sis) [*neuro-* + *biotaxis*] the theory that nerve cell bodies have a tendency during development to migrate in the direction from which they habitually receive their stimuli.

**neu·ro·blast** (noor′o-blast) [*neuro-* + *-blast*] any embryonic cell which develops into a nerve cell or neuron; an immature nerve cell.
**sympathetic n.,** sympathoblast.

**neu·ro·blas·to·ma** (noor″o-blas-to′mə) [MeSH: Neuroblastoma] sarcoma consisting of malignant neuroblasts, usually arising in the autonomic nervous system (sympathicoblastoma) or in the adrenal medulla; it is considered a type of neuroepithelial tumor and affects mostly infants and children up to 10 years of age.
**olfactory n.,** a rare, slow-growing, malignant tumor of neuroectodermal origin that begins in neuroepithelial cells of the olfactory membrane. The tumor appears primarily in the nasal cavity and nasopharynx of adults as a painful swelling and eventually may spread to the sinuses, palate, orbit, and brain. Called also *esthesioneuroblastoma.*

**neu·ro·bor·rel·i·o·sis** (noor″o-bə-rel″e-o′sis) borreliosis affecting the nervous system, most commonly manifested by meningitis, cranial neuritis, or radiculopathy, or a combination of these; severity ranges from mild neuritis to severe meningopolyneuritis (Bannwarth's syndrome).

**neu·ro·ca·nal** (noor″o-kə-nal′) [*neuro-* + *canal*] the vertebral canal (canalis vertebralis).

**neu·ro·car·di·ac** (noor″o-kahr′de-ak) [*neuro-* + *cardiac*] pertaining to the nervous system and the heart.

**neu·ro·cen·tral** (noor″o-sen′trəl) pertaining to the centrum and the two lateral masses of a developing vertebra.

**neu·ro·cen·trum** (noor″o-sen′trəm) one of the embryonic vertebral elements from which the spinous processes of the vertebrae develop.

**neu·ro·cep·tor** (noor′o-sep″tər) [*neuro-* + *-ceptor*] the postsynaptic area of a dendrite or effector organ; see also *postsynaptic membrane,* under *membrane.*

**neu·ro·chem·is·try** (noor″o-kem′is-tre) [MeSH: Neurochemistry] that branch of neurology which is concerned with the chemistry of the nervous system.

**neu·ro·chon·drite** (noor″o-kon′drīt) [*neuro-* + *chondr-* + *-ite*[1]] one of the embryonic cartilaginous elements that develop into the vertebral arch of a vertebra.

**neu·ro·cho·rio·ret·i·ni·tis** (noor″o-kor″e-o-ret″ĭ-ni′tis) [*neuro-* + *chorioretinitis*] inflammation of the optic nerve, choroid, and retina.

**neu·ro·cho·roi·di·tis** (noor″o-kor″oi-di′tis) inflammation of the choroid coat and optic nerves.

**neu·ro·cir·cu·la·to·ry** (noor″o-sər′ku-lə-tor″e) pertaining to the nervous and circulatory systems.

**neu·roc·la·dism** (noo͝-rok′lə-diz-əm) [*neuro-* + Gr. *klados* branch] the formation of new branches by the process of a neuron; especially the force by which, in regeneration of divided nerves, the newly formed axons of the proximal stump become attracted by the peripheral stump so as to form a bridge between the two ends. Called also *odogenesis.*

**neu·ro·com·mu·ni·ca·tions** (noor″o-kə-mu″nĭ-ka′shənz) the branch of neurology dealing with the transfer and integration of information within the nervous system.

**neu·ro·cra·ni·al** (noor″o-kra′ne-əl) pertaining to the neurocranium.

**neu·ro·cra·ni·um** (noor″o-kra′ne-əm) [TA] brain box; the portion of the cranium which encloses the brain; cf. *viscerocranium.*
**cartilaginous n.**, chondrocranium.
**membranous n.**, that part of the neurocranium formed by intramembranous ossification and comprising the bones of the calvaria.

**neu·ro·cris·top·a·thy** (noor″o-kris-top′ə-the) [*neuro-* + *crista* + *-pathy*] any disease arising from maldevelopment of the neural crest.

**neu·ro·cu·ta·ne·ous** (noor″o-ku-ta′ne-əs) pertaining to the nerves and the skin; pertaining to the cutaneous nerves. See also *phakomatosis.*

**neu·ro·cys·ti·cer·co·sis** (noor″o-sis″tĭ-sər-ko′sis) [*neuro-* + *cysticercosis*] infection of the central nervous system with the larval forms (cysticerci) of *Taenia solium;* manifestations are highly variable, depending on the location and number of cysts, and include seizures, hydrocephalus, and a variety of other neurologic dysfunctions, often accompanied by distinctive lesions visible by computed tomography or magnetic resonance imaging.

**neu·ro·cy·tol·o·gy** (noor″o-si-tol′ə-je) that branch of neurology which is concerned with the cellular components of the nervous system.

**neu·ro·cy·tol·y·sin** (noor″o-si-tol′ĭ-sin) a constituent of the venom of certain snakes (rattlesnake, coral snake, cobra), which lyses nerve cells.

**neu·ro·cy·to·ma** (noor″o-si-to′mə) [MeSH: Neurocytoma] 1. medulloepithelioma. 2. ganglioneuroma.

**neu·ro·de·al·gia** (noor″o-de-al′jə) [Gr. *neurōdēs* nervelike + *-algia*] pain in the retina.

**neu·ro·de·atro·phia** (noor″o-de-ə-tro′fe-ə) [Gr. *neurōdēs* nervelike + *atrophia*] retinal atrophy.

**neu·ro·de·gen·er·a·tive** (noor″o-de-jen′ər-ə-tiv) relating to or marked by nervous degeneration.

**neu·ro·den·drite** (noor″o-den′drīt) dendrite.

**neu·ro·den·dron** (noor″o-den′dron) dendrite.

**neu·ro·derm** (noor′o-dərm) that portion of the ectoderm which develops into the neural tube; called also *neural ectoderm.*

**neu·ro·der·ma·ti·tis** (noor″o-dər″mə-ti′tis) [*neuro-* + *dermatitis*] [MeSH: Neurodermatitis] name given to various types of eczematous dermatosis, varying widely between individuals, presumed to be cutaneous responses to prolonged scratching, rubbing, or pinching to relieve pruritus; it may produce polymorphic lesions at the same or different times. Some authorities consider it a psychogenic disorder.
**circumscribed n.**, lichen simplex chronicus.

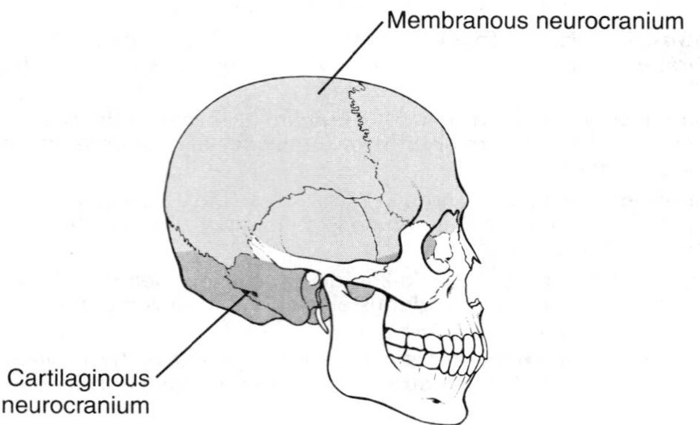


Neurocranium, comprising membranous and cartilaginous portions; the former, the calvaria, includes the frontal and parietal and portions of the temporal, occipital, and sphenoid bones; the latter, the chondrocranium, includes the ethmoid and portions of the occipital, temporal, and sphenoid bones.

**disseminated n.**, atopic dermatitis.
**exudative n.**, nummular eczema.
**localized n.**, lichen simplex chronicus.
**nummular n.**, see under *eczema.*

**neu·ro·de·vel·op·men·tal** (noor″o-de-vel″op-men′təl) [*neuro-* + *developmental*] pertaining to the development of the nervous system.

**neu·ro·din** (noo͝-ro′din) acetyl para-oxyphenylurethane, $C_6H_4(OCOCH_3)NH{\cdot}COOC_2H_5$, used as an antineuralgic and antipyretic.

**neu·ro·dyn·ia** (noor″o-din′e-ə) [*neur-* + *-odynia*] neuralgia.

**neu·ro·ec·to·derm** (noor″o-ek′to-dərm) the portion of the ectoderm of the early embryo that gives rise to the central and peripheral nervous systems, including some glial cells. Cf. *neuroderm.*

**neu·ro·ec·to·der·mal** (noor″o-ek″to-der′məl) pertaining or relating to the neuroectoderm.

**neu·ro·ef·fec·tor** (noor″o-ə-fek′tər) of or relating to the junction between a neuron and the effector organ it innervates.

**neu·ro·elec·tric·i·ty** (noor″o-e″lek-tris′ĭ-te) the electrical signals, currents, or voltages generated by the nervous system.

**neu·ro·en·ceph·a·lo·my·elop·a·thy** (noor″o-en-sef″ə-lo-mi″ə-lop′ə-the) [*neuro-* + *encephalo-* + *myelopathy*] disease involving the brain, spinal cord, and nerves.
**optic n.**, neuromyelitis optica.

**neu·ro·en·do·crine** (noor″o-en′do-krin) pertaining to the interactions between the nervous and endocrine systems and to hormones such as vasopressin and gastrin (neurohormones) that are elaborated in the neurons or neuronlike cells (neuroendocrine cells).

**neu·ro·en·do·cri·nol·o·gy** (noor″o-en″do-krĭ-nol′ə-je) [MeSH: Neuroendocrinology] the study of the interactions among nervous system and endocrine system components.

**neu·ro·en·ter·ic** (noor″o-en-ter′ik) neurenteric.

**neu·ro·epi·der·mal** (noor″o-ep″ĭ-der′məl) [*neuro-* + *epidermal*] pertaining to or giving origin to the nervous and epidermal tissues.

**neu·ro·epi·the·li·al** (noor″o-ep″ĭ-the′le-əl) pertaining to or composed of neuroepithelium.

**neu·ro·epi·the·li·o·ma** (noor″o-ep″ĭ-the″le-o′mə) [MeSH: Neuroepithelioma] medulloepithelioma.

**neu·ro·epi·the·li·um** (noor″o-ep″ĭ-the′le-əm) [*neuro-* + *epithelium*] 1. simple columnar epithelium made up of cells specialized to serve as sensory cells for the reception of external stimuli, as the sensory cells of the cochlea, vestibule, nasal mucosa, and tongue. Called also *neurepithelium* and *sensory epithelium.* 2. the epithelium of the ectoderm, from which the central nervous system is developed.
**n. cris′tae ampulla′ris,** neuroepithelium of ampullary crest: the specialized epithelium of the ampullary crest of the labyrinth, containing receptor cells from some of which cilia (sensory hairs) project into the cupula.
**n. macula′rum,** neuroepithelium of maculae: the specialized epithelium of the maculae of the labyrinth, containing receptor cells from some of which cilia (sensory hairs) project into the statoconic membrane.

**neu·ro·fi·ber** (noor″o-fi′bər) [MeSH: Nerve Fibers] neurofibra.
**afferent n's,** neurofibrae afferentes.
**association n.,** fibra associationis.
**autonomic n's,** neurofibrae autonomicae.
**commissural n.,** fibra commissuralis.
**efferent n's,** neurofibrae efferentes.
**postganglionic n's,** neurofibrae postganglionicae.
**preganglionic n's,** neurofibrae preganglionicae.
**projection n.,** fibra projectionis.
**somatic n's,** neurofibrae somaticae.
**tangential n's,** neurofibrae tangentiales.
**visceral n's,** neurofibrae autonomicae.

**neu·ro·fi·bra** (noor″o-fi′brə) pl. *neurofi′brae* [L.] [TA] [MeSH: Nerve Fibers] nerve fiber: a slender process of a neuron; the term is often synonymous with axon. Nerve fibers are classified on the basis of the presence or absence of a myelin sheath as myelinated or unmyelinated. In the terminology for types of nerve fibers, the word *nerve* is frequently dropped; e.g., *myelinated f's, unmyelinated f's,* etc. Called also *fiber, fibra, and neurofiber.*
**neurofi′brae afferen′tes** [TA], afferent nerve fibers: nerve fibers that convey sensory impulses from the periphery to the central nervous system; classified according to function as somatic afferent and visceral afferent fibers. Called also *afferent neurofibers.*
**n. associatio′nis,** fibra associationis.
**neurofi′brae autono′micae** [TA], autonomic nerve fibers: nerve fibers that innervate smooth muscle and glandular tissues. They ei-

ther stimulate and activate the muscle or tissue *(autonomic efferent fibers)* or receive sensory impulses from them *(autonomic afferent fibers)*. Called also *autonomic neurofibers, neurofibrae viscerales,* and *visceral nerve fibers* or *neurofibers.*
**n. commissura'lis,** fibra commissuralis.
**neurofi'brae efferen'tes** [TA], efferent nerve fibers: nerve fibers that convey motor impulses away from the central nervous system toward the periphery; classified according to function as somatic efferent and visceral efferent fibers. Called also *efferent neurofibers.*
**neurofi'brae postgangliona'res, neurofi'brae postganglio'nicae** [TA], postganglionic nerve fibers: the axons of postganglionic neurons; called also *postganglionic neurofibers.*
**neurofi'brae pregangliona'res, neurofi'brae preganglio'nicae** [TA], preganglionic nerve fibers: the axons of preganglionic neurons; called also *preganglionic neurofibers.*
**n. projectio'nis,** fibra projectionis.
**neurofi'brae soma'ticae** [TA], somatic nerve fibers: nerve fibers that innervate skeletal muscles and somatic tissues. They either stimulate and activate the muscle or tissue *(somatic efferent fibers)* or receive sensory impulses from them *(somatic afferent fibers)*. Called also *somatic fibers* or *neurofibers.*
**neurofi'brae tangentia'les** [TA], tangential fibers: tangentially oriented nerve fibers arranged in striae in the superficial layers of the hippocampus and cerebral cortex; called also *tangential neurofibers.*
**neurofi'brae viscera'les,** neurofibrae autonomicae.

**neu•ro•fi•bril** (noor″o-fi'bril) [MeSH: Neurofibrils] any of the fibrils visible in the perikaryon, dendrites, and axon of a neuron in light microscopy after staining with silver; the fibrils are believed to be neurofilament bundles, and perhaps also neurotubules, that have become coated with silver particles.

**neu•ro•fi•bril•la** (noor″o-fi-bril'ə) pl. *neurofibril'lae.* Neurofibril.

**neu•ro•fi•bril•lar** (noor″o-fi-bril'ər) pertaining to neurofibrils.

**neu•ro•fi•bro•ma** (noor″o-fi-bro'mə) [*neuro-* + *fibroma*] [MeSH: Neurofibroma] a usually benign tumor of peripheral nerves caused by abnormal proliferation of Schwann cells; called also *fibroneuroma.* Cf. *neurilemoma.*
**cutaneous n., dermal n.,** a neurofibroma arising within the skin, occurring as a small, fleshy nodule that may become pedunculated, overlying a palpable subcutaneous lesion.
**plexiform n.,** a fusiform, ropelike enlargement of a nerve, consisting of Schwann cells, fibroblasts, and inflammatory cells in a loose myxoid ground, usually occurring as multiple lesions in neurofibromatosis 1, although occasionally arising as a solitary, spontaneous lesion. Called also *plexiform neuroma* and *Verneuil's neuroma.*
**solitary n.,** a neurofibroma arising along a nerve trunk, occurring as spontaneous lesion without internal manifestations.

**neu•ro•fi•bro•ma•to•sis** (noor″o-fi-bro″mə-to'sis) [MeSH: Neurofibromatosis] a familial condition characterized by developmental changes in the nervous system, muscles, bones, and skin and marked superficially by the formation of multiple pedunculated soft tumors (neurofibromas) distributed over the entire body associated with areas of pigmentation. Called also *multiple neuroma* and *neuromatosis.*
**n. 1 (NF1),** a disorder of autosomal dominant inheritance, marked by developmental changes in the nervous system, muscles, bones, and skin with café au lait spots, intertriginous freckling, Lisch nodules, and multiple pedunculated soft tumors (neurofibromas) distributed over the entire body. Its cause is the absence of the tumor suppressor neurofibromin, which is coded by a gene on chromosome 17q. Called also *von Recklinghausen's disease* and *peripheral n.*
**n. 2 (NF2),** a disorder of autosomal dominant inheritance, characterized by usually bilateral acoustic neuromas (q.v.), sometimes with skin changes like those seen in neurofibromatosis 1, central and peripheral nerve tumors, and presenile lens opacities. It is caused by a defective gene on chromosome 22q that codes for the cytoskeletal protein merlin, which acts as a tumor suppressor. Called also *bilateral acoustic neurinoma, neuroma,* or *neurofibromatosis* and *central n.*
**bilateral acoustic n.,** n. 2.
**central n.,** n. 2.
**peripheral n.,** n. 1.

**neu•ro•fi•bro•min** (noor″ro-fi'bro-min) a GTPase-activating protein that functions as a tumor suppressor; a defect in the gene that codes for this protein is the cause of neurofibromatosis 1.

**neu•ro•fi•bro•sar•co•ma** (noor″o-fi″bro-sahr-ko'mə) [MeSH: Neurofibrosarcoma] a malignant type of schwannoma whose appearance is superficially similar to that of a fibrosarcoma; it may occur in association with neurofibromatosis that is undergoing malignant transformation.

**neu•ro•fil•a•ment** (noor″o-fil'ə-ment) an intermediate filament (q.v.) occurring with neurotubules in the neurons; it has a cytoskeletal function and may be involved in the intracellular transport of metabolites.

**neu•ro•gan•gli•itis** (noor″o-gang″gle-i'tis) ganglionitis.

**neu•ro•gan•gli•on** (noor″o-gang'gle-on) ganglion (def. 2).

**neu•ro•gas•tric** (noor″o-gas'trik) involving the innervation of the stomach.

**neu•ro•gen** (noor'o-jən) the chemical substance by means of which the primary organizer causes the development of the neural plate.

**neu•ro•gen•e•sis** (noor″o-jen'ə-sis) [*neuro-* + *-genesis*] the development of nervous tissue.

**neu•ro•ge•net•ic** (noor″o-jə-net'ik) 1. pertaining to neurogenesis. 2. neurogenic.

**neu•ro•ge•net•ics** (noor″o-jə-net'iks) [*neuro-* + *genetics*] the study of genetic influences on the nervous system, including embryonic development of the nervous system and neurological disorders that have genetic bases.

**neu•ro•gen•ic** (noor″o-jen'ik) [*neuro-* + *-genic*] 1. forming nervous tissue. 2. originating in the nervous system or from a lesion in the nervous system.

**neu•rog•e•nous** (no͞o-roj'ə-nəs) neurogenic.

**neu•rog•lia** (no͞o-rog'le-ə) [*neuro-* + *-glia*] [TA] [MeSH: Neuroglia] the supporting structure of nervous tissue. It consists of a fine web of tissue made up of modified ectodermal elements, in which are enclosed peculiar branched cells known as *neuroglial cells* or *glial cells.* The neuroglial cells are of three types: astrocytes and oligodendrocytes (astroglia and oligodendroglia), which appear to play a role in myelin formation, transport of material to neurons, and maintenance of the ionic environment of neurons; and microcytes (microglia), which phagocytize waste products of nerve tissue. Called also *glia.* See plate accompanying *nerve.*
**interfascicular n.,** oligodendroglia of white matter along the myelin sheaths.
**peripheral n.,** the neurilemma, Schwann cells, and satellite cells of the peripheral nervous system.

**neu•rog•li•al** (no͞o-rog'le-əl) pertaining to the neuroglia.

**neu•rog•lio•cyte** (no͞o-rog'le-o-sīt″) [*neuroglia* + *-cyte*] a cell of the neuroglia.

**neu•rog•lio•cy•to•ma** (no͞o-rog″le-o-si-to'mə) glioma.

**neu•rog•li•o•ma** (no͞o-rog″le-o'mə) glioma.
**n. gangliona're,** ganglioglioma.

**neu•rog•li•o•ma•to•sis** (no͞o-rog″le-o-mə-to'sis) gliomatosis.

**neu•rog•li•o•sis** (no͞o-rog″le-o'sis) gliomatosis.

**neu•ro•gly•co•pe•nia** (noor″o-gli″ko-pe'ne-ə) [*neuro-* + *glycopenia*] chronic hypoglycemia of a degree sufficient to impair brain function, resulting in personality changes and intellectual deterioration that may progress to convulsions, coma, and occasionally even death.

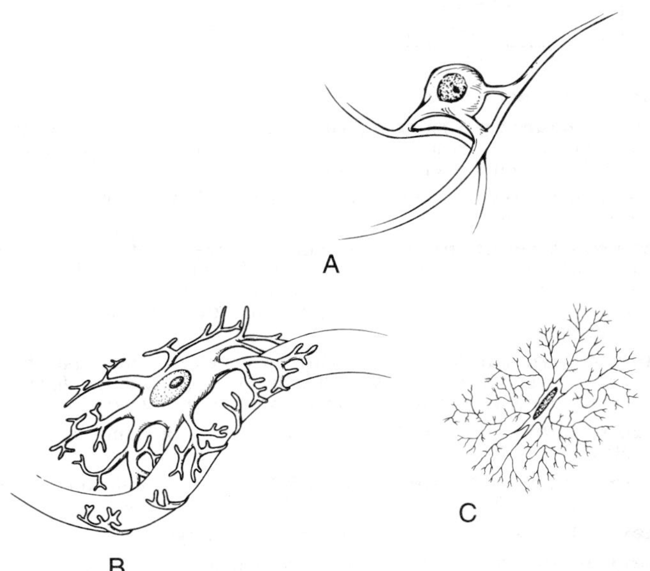

Neuroglia. *(A),* Oligodendrocyte; *(B),* astrocyte; *(C),* microglial cell.

**neu·ro·gram** (noor'o-gram") [*neuro-* + *-gram*] residua of past cerebral activities which make up the brain disposition and thus take part in the formation of personality.

**neu·ro·his·tol·o·gy** (noor"o-his-tol'ə-je) the histology of the nervous system.

**neu·ro·hor·mo·nal** (noor"o-hor-mo'nəl) pertaining to a neurohormone.

**neu·ro·hor·mone** (noor'o-hor"mōn) a hormone secreted by a specialized neuron into the bloodstream, the cerebrospinal fluid, or the intercellular spaces of the nervous system; examples are neuropeptides and other types of neuromodulators. Cf. *neuroendocrine.*

**neu·ro·hu·mor** (noor"o-hu'mər) neurohormone.

**neu·ro·hu·mor·al·ism** (noor"o-hu'mor-əl-iz-əm) the theory that the action of the autonomic nerves on peripheral organs is produced through the medium of chemicals (neurohumors or neurotransmitters) that are liberated at the endings of activated nerves.

**neu·ro·hy·po·phys·e·al** (noor"o-hi"po-fiz'e-əl) neurohypophysial.

**neu·ro·hy·po·phys·ec·to·my** (noor"o-hi"po-fiz-ek'tə-me) [*neuro-* + *hypophysectomy*] surgical removal of the neural lobe of the pituitary gland.

**neu·ro·hy·po·phys·i·al** (noor"o-hi"po-fiz'e-əl) pertaining to the neurohypophysis.

**neu·ro·hy·poph·y·sis** (noor"o-hi-pof'ə-sis) [*neuro-* + *hypophysis*] [TA] the posterior lobe of the hypophysis (pituitary gland), the neural portion of the gland. It consists of the *infundibulum* or *neural stalk,* which is continuous with the hypothalamus, and the *neural lobe,* which is the main body of the neurohypophysis. The median eminence is sometimes classified as part of the neurohypophysis. It serves as a reservoir for the hypothalamic neurohormones vasopressin, oxytocin, and the neurophysins, releasing them as needed. It originates in the embryo as an evagination from the floor of the diencephalon. See also *circumventricular organs.* Called also *posterior pituitary, posterior lobe of hypophysis* or *of pituitary gland,* and *lobus posterior hypophysis* [TA alternative].

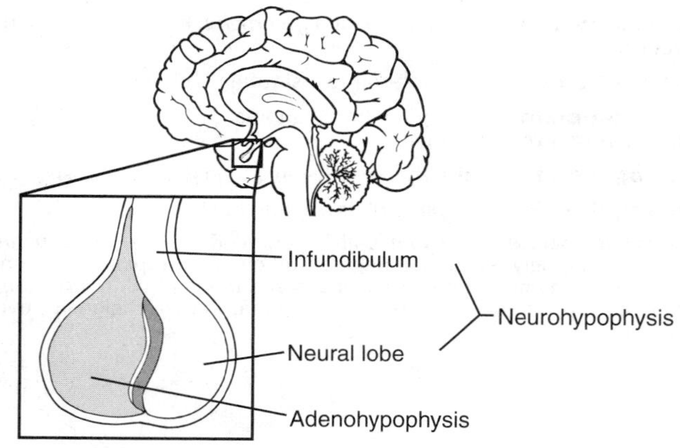


**neu·roid** (noor'oid) resembling a nerve.

**neu·ro·imag·ing** (noor'o-im"ə-jing) the use of radiographic studies and magnetic resonance imaging to detect structural abnormalities in the central nervous system.

**neu·ro·im·mu·no·log·ic** (noor"o-im"u-no-loj'ik) pertaining to neuroimmunology.

**neu·ro·im·mu·nol·o·gy** (noor"o-im"u-nol'ə-je) that branch of science which deals with the interaction of the nervous and immune systems in health and disease, as in the effects of autonomic nervous activity on the immune response and the role of antibodies in myasthenia gravis.

**neu·ro·ker·a·tin** (noor"o-ker'ə-tin) proteinaceous material left after the myelin of a myelin sheath is dissolved away during fixation; it forms a network that probably does not exist *in vivo.*

**neu·ro·ki·nin** (noor"o-ki'nin) [*neuro-* + *kinin*] a kinin that stimulates nerve receptors.

**neu·ro·lab·y·rin·thi·tis** (noor"o-lab"ĭ-rin-thi'tis) inflammation of the neural structures of the labyrinth.

**neu·ro·lath·y·rism** (noor"o-lath'ĭ-riz-əm) lathyrism.

**neu·ro·lem·ma** (noor"o-lem'ə) neurilemma.

**neu·ro·lep·tan·al·ge·sia** (noor"o-lep"tən-əl-je'ze-ə) [*neuroleptic* + *analgesia*] [MeSH: Neuroleptanalgesia] a state of quiescence, altered awareness, and analgesia produced by the administration of a combination of a narcotic analgesic and a neuroleptic agent.

**neu·ro·lep·tan·al·ge·sic** (noor"o-lep"tən-əl-je'zik) 1. pertaining to or producing neuroleptanalgesia. 2. an agent that produces neuroleptanalgesia.

**neu·ro·lep·tan·es·the·sia** (noor"o-lep"tən-əs-the'zhə) [*neuroleptic* + *anesthesia*] a state of neuroleptanalgesia and unconsciousness, produced by the combined administration of a narcotic analgesic and a neuroleptic agent, together with the inhalation of nitrous oxide and oxygen.

**neu·ro·lep·tan·es·thet·ic** (noor"o-lep"tən-əs-thet'ik) 1. pertaining to or producing neuroleptanesthesia. 2. an agent that produces neuroleptanesthesia.

**neu·ro·lep·tic** (noor"o-lep'tik) [*neuro-* + Gr. *lēpsis* a taking hold] a term coined to refer to the effects on cognition and behavior of the original antipsychotic agents, which produced a state of apathy, lack of initiative, and limited range of emotion and in psychotic patients caused a reduction in confusion and agitation and normalization of psychomotor activity. The term is outdated as a synonym for antipsychotic agents because newer agents do not necessarily have such effects. See *antipsychotic.*

**neu·ro·lin·guis·tics** (noor"o-ling-gwis'tiks) the study of language acquisition, processing, and production at the neurological level.

**neu·ro·li·po·ma·to·sis** (noor"o-lĭ-po"mə-to'sis) a condition characterized by the formation of subcutaneous multiple fat deposits, with pressure on the nerves resulting in tenderness, pain, and paresthesias.
**n. doloro'sa,** adiposis dolorosa.

**Neu·ro·lite** (noor'o-līt") trademark for a kit for the preparation of technetium Tc 99m bicisate.

**neu·ro·lo·gia** (noor"o-lo'jə) neurology.

**neu·ro·log·ic** (noor"o-loj'ik) pertaining to neurology or to the nervous system.

**neu·rol·o·gist** (no͞o-rol'ə-jist) a physician whose practice focuses on neurology.

**neu·rol·o·gy** (no͞o-rol'ə-je) [*neuro-* + *-logy*] [MeSH: Neurology] that branch of medical science which deals with the nervous system, both normal and in disease.
**clinical n.,** that specialty concerned with the diagnosis and treatment of disorders of the nervous system.

**neu·ro·lu·es** (noor"o-loo'ēz) neurosyphilis.

**neu·ro·lym·pho·ma·to·sis** (noor"o-lim"fo-mə-to'sis) lymphoblastic infiltration of a nerve.
**n. gallina'rum,** Marek's disease in which neurological symptoms are dominant.

**neu·rol·y·sin** (no͞o-rol'ĭ-sin) a cytolysin which has a specific destructive action upon nerve cells.

**neu·rol·y·sis** (no͞o-rol'ĭ-sis) [*neuro-* + *lysis*] 1. release of a nerve sheath by cutting it longitudinally. 2. the operative breaking up of perineural adhesions. 3. the relief of tension upon a nerve obtained by stretching. 4. destruction or dissolution of nerve tissue; sometimes done as a temporary or permanent measure for the relief of pain or spasticity. See also *rhizotomy.* Called also *nerve block.*
**alcohol n.,** intrathecal neurolysis in which dehydrated alcohol is injected at the point where the dorsal root emerges from the spinal cord.
**chemical n.,** neurolysis (def. 4) by injection of a neurolytic chemical such as glycerol, phenol, or alcohol adjacent to a nerve; see also *chemical rhizotomy.*
**intramuscular n.,** motor point block.
**intrathecal n.,** chemical neurolysis in which a substance is injected under the dura mater of the spinal cord.
**phenol n.,** intrathecal neurolysis in which a solution of 5 to 7.5 per cent phenol in glycerol is injected into a dorsal root ganglion.
**trigeminal n.,** see under *rhizotomy.*

**neu·ro·lyt·ic** (noor"o-lit'ik) pertaining to neurolysis.

**neu·ro·ma** (no͞o-ro'mə) [*neur-* + *-oma*] [MeSH: Neuroma] a tumor growing from a nerve or made up largely of nerve cells and nerve fibers. Many lesions formerly called neuromas are now given more specific names such as *ganglioneuroma, neurilemoma,* or *neurofibroma.*
**acoustic n.,** a progressively enlarging, benign tumor, usually within the internal auditory canal arising from Schwann cells of the vestibular division of the eighth cranial nerve; the symptoms, which vary with the size and location of the tumor, may include hearing loss, headache, disturbances of balance and gait, facial numbness or pain, and tinnitus. It may be unilateral or bilateral (neurofibromatosis 2). Called also *acoustic neurilemoma, neurinoma,* or *schwannoma,* and *acoustic nerve tumor.*

**amputation n.,** traumatic n.
**amyelinic n.,** one containing only nonmedullated nerve fibers.
**n. cu'tis,** neuroma seated in the skin.
**false n.,** 1. a neuroma that does not contain nerve cells. 2. traumatic n.
**ganglionar n., ganglionated n., ganglionic n.,** ganglioneuroma.
**medullated n.,** myelinic n.
**Morton's n.,** the neuroma that results from Morton's neuralgia.
**multiple n.,** 1. neurofibromatosis. 2. neuromatosis.
**myelinic n.,** one that contains myelinated nerve fibers; called also *medullated n.*
**nevoid n.,** n. telangiectodes.
**plexiform n.,** see under *neurofibroma.*
**stump n.,** amputation n.
**n. telangiecto'des,** one which contains an excess of blood vessels; called also *nevoid n.*
**traumatic n.,** a non-neoplastic unorganized bulbous or nodular mass of nerve fibers and Schwann cells produced by hyperplasia of nerve fibers and their supporting tissues after accidental or purposeful sectioning of the nerve. Called also *amputation n., false n.,* and *pseudoneuroma.*
**true n.,** a neuroma made up of nerve tissue; see also *ganglioneuroma.*
**Verneuil's n.,** plexiform neurofibroma.

**neu·ro·ma·la·cia** (noor″o-mə-la′shə) [*neuro-* + *malacia*] necrosis and softening of the nerves.

**neu·ro·ma·la·kia** (noor″o-mə-la′ke-ə) neuromalacia.

**neu·ro·ma·to·sis** (no͞o-ro′mə-to′sis) 1. any disease characterized by multiple neuromas. 2. neurofibromatosis.

**neu·rom·a·tous** (no͞o-rom′ə-təs) affected with or of the nature of neuroma.

**neu·ro·mech·a·nism** (noor″o-mek′ə-niz-əm) the structure and arrangement of the nervous system in relation to function.

**neu·ro·me·di·a·tor** (noor″o-me′de-a-tər) a mediator in the nervous system; see *mediator.*

**neu·ro·me·nin·ge·al** (noor″o-mə-nin′je-əl) pertaining to or affecting nervous tissue and the meninges.

**neu·ro·mere** (noor′o-mēr) [*neuro-* + *-mere*] 1. any of the series of transitory segmental elevations in the wall of the neural tube of the developing embryo; also commonly used to refer to such elevations in the wall of the mature rhombencephalon. 2. a part of the spinal cord to which a pair of dorsal roots and a pair of ventral roots are attached. Called also *neural segment.*

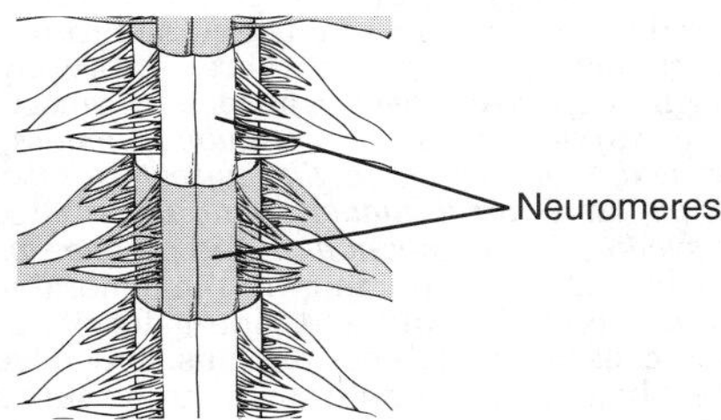


**neu·ro·met·rics** (noor″o-met′riks) a computer-assisted method for evaluating brain functions by quantitative analysis of the results of tests such as the electroencephalogram or measurements of evoked potentials. Data from patients with similar signs or symptoms are compared with a normative data base to identify links between patterns of electrical activity and of behavioral or other symptomatic abnormalities.

**neu·ro·mi·met·ic** (noor″o-mi-met′ik) 1. eliciting a response in effector organs that simulates that elicited by nervous impulses. 2. an agent that elicits such a response.

**neu·ro·mod·u·la·tion** (noor″o-mod″u-la′shən) 1. electrical stimulation of a peripheral nerve, the spinal cord, or the brain for relief of pain; it may be done transcutaneously or with an implanted stimulator. 2. the effect of a neuromodulator on another neuron.

**neu·ro·mod·u·la·tor** (noor″o-mod′u-la″tər) a substance other than a neurotransmitter, released by a neuron and conveying information to adjacent or distant neurons, either enhancing or damping their activities. Neuropeptides are often neuromodulators.

**neu·ro·mo·tor** (noor″o-mo′tər) 1. involving both nerves and muscles. 2. pertaining to nervous impulses to muscles.

**neu·ro·mus·cu·lar** (noor″o-mus′ku-lər) pertaining to muscles and nerves, or to the relationship between them.

**neu·ro·my·al** (noor″o-mi′əl) neuromuscular.

**neu·ro·my·as·the·nia** (noor″o-mi″es-the′ne-ə) [*neuro-* + *myasthenia*] muscular weakness associated with emotional lability.
**epidemic n.,** chronic fatigue syndrome.

**neu·ro·my·eli·tis** (noor″o-mi″ə-li′tis) [*neuro-* + *myelitis*] inflammation of nervous and medullary substance; myelitis attended with neuritis.
**n. op'tica,** combined, but not usually clinically simultaneous, demyelination of the optic nerve and the spinal cord; it is marked by diminution of vision and possibly blindness, flaccid paralysis of the extremities, and sensory and genitourinary disturbances. Called also *Devic's disease, optic neuroencephalomyelopathy, neuro-optic myelitis,* and *ophthalmoneuromyelitis.*

**neu·ro·my·ic** (noor″o-mi′ik) neuromuscular.

**neu·ro·myo·path·ic** (noor″o-mi″o-path′ik) pertaining to neuromyopathy.

**neu·ro·my·op·a·thy** (noor″o-mi-op′ə-the) any disease of both muscles and nerves, especially a muscular disease of nervous origin.
**carcinomatous n.,** a paraneoplastic syndrome of neuromyopathy in patients having carcinoma, usually of the lung. Cf. *carcinomatous polyneuropathy.*

**neu·ro·myo·si·tis** (noor″o-mi″o-si′tis) [*neuro-* + *myositis*] neuritis complicated with myositis.

**neu·ro·myo·to·nia** (noor″o-mi″o-to′ne-ə) [*neuro-* + *myotonia*] myotonia caused by electric activity of a peripheral nerve; characterized by stiffness, delayed relaxation, fasciculations, and myokymia.

**neu·ron** (noor′on) [Gr. "nerve"] [TA] [MeSH: Neurons] any of the conducting cells of the nervous system. A typical neuron consists of a cell body, containing the nucleus and the surrounding cytoplasm (perikaryon); several short radiating processes (dendrites); and one long process (the axon), which terminates in twiglike branches (telodendrons) and may have branches (collaterals) projecting along its course. The axon together with its covering or sheath forms the nerve fiber. See illustration accompanying *nerve.* Called also *nerve cell.*
**afferent n.,** any neuron conducting a nerve impulse that originated at a receptor and is proceeding towards the center. See also *sensory n.,* and see *afferent fiber,* under *fiber.*
**bipolar n.,** a neuron having two processes, one projecting from each end of the cell body; these may be either one axon and one dendrite or two dendrites.
**central n.,** a neuron which belongs entirely to the central nervous system.
**connector n.,** interneuron.
**efferent n.,** any neuron conducting a nerve impulse that originated at the center and is proceeding towards the periphery. See also *efferent fiber,* under *fiber.*
**fusimotor n's,** gamma motoneurons.
**Golgi type I n's,** pyramidal neurons with very long axons, that leave the gray matter of the central nervous system, traverse the white matter, and terminate in the periphery; called also *Golgi type I cells.*
**Golgi type II n's,** stellate neurons with short axons that do not pass out of the gray matter in which the cell body lies, and are especially numerous in the cerebral and cerebellar cortices and in the retina. Called also *Golgi type II cells.*
**intercalary n., intercalated n., internuncial n.,** interneuron.
**local circuit n.,** Golgi type II n.
**motor n.,** motoneuron.
**multiform n.,** multipolar n.
**multimodal n.,** multisensory n.
**multipolar n.,** a neuron with several to many processes; such neurons vary in shape, depending on the arrangement of the processes, with pyramidal and stellate (star) shapes being common. Called also *polymorphic n.*
**multisensory n.,** a neuron in the cerebral cortex or subcortical regions that can receive input from more than one sensory modality; the inputs may be simultaneous, reinforcing each other.
**peripheral sensory n.,** in a reflex arc, a sensory neuron whose fibers end at synapses with interneurons. Cf. *peripheral motoneuron.*
**piriform n's,** Purkinje cells.
**polymorphic n.,** multipolar n.
**postganglionic n's,** neurons in the autonomic nervous system whose cell bodies are situated in the autonomic ganglia and whose purpose is to relay impulses beyond the ganglia. See also *pars parasympathetica* and *pars sympathetica systematis nervosi autonomici,* under *pars.*
**preganglionic n's,** neurons in the autonomic nervous system whose cell bodies lie in the central nervous system and whose efferent fibers terminate in the autonomic ganglia. See also *pars parasympathetica* and *pars sympathetica systematis nervosi autonomici,* under *pars.*
**premotor n.,** upper motoneuron.
**primary sensory n.,** a sensory neuron that is the first in an afferent

pathway, beginning at the receptor and ending at a synapse with a secondary sensory neuron, often within a nucleus of the central nervous system. One common type is the pseudounipolar neuron. **projection n.,** one which serves for the transmission of nervous impulses, whether motor or sensory, between the cerebral cortex and other parts of the nervous system. See also *projection fibers,* under *fiber.*
**pseudounipolar n.,** a unipolar neuron, almost always a primary sensory neuron, that was originally bipolar but whose two processes fused during development to form a single process that bifurcates at a distance from the cell body. One branch is structurally an axon with a myelin sheath but functions as a dendrite, with afferent conduction originating in a nerve ending.
**Purkinje n's,** see under *cell.*
**pyramidal n.,** see under *cell.*
**secondary sensory n.,** a sensory neuron that is the second in an afferent pathway, being stimulated at a synapse by a primary sensory neuron and often extending some distance into the central nervous system.
**sensory n.,** any neuron with a sensory function; an afferent neuron conveying sensory impulses. Cf. *primary sensory n.* and *secondary sensory n.* See illustration accompanying *nerve.*
**spiny n.,** a neuron whose dendrites have many spines (gemmules), such as a Golgi type I neuron.
**unipolar n.,** a neuron with one process only; see also *pseudounipolar n.*

**neu·ro·nal** (noor′o-nəl) pertaining to a neuron or neurons.

**neu·rone** (noor′ōn) neuron.

**neu·ro·neph·ric** (noor″o-nef′rik) pertaining to the innervation of the kidneys.

**neu·ro·ne·vus** (noor″o-ne′vəs) [*neuro-* + *nevus*] an intradermal nevus in which the nevus cells differentiate into neural-like structures, and may clinically resemble neurofibroma or may have the clinical aspect of a giant hairy pigmented nevus. Called also *neural* or *neuroid nevus.*

**neu·ro·ni·tis** (noor″o-ni′tis) 1. inflammation of one or more neurons. 2. former name for acute idiopathic polyneuritis.
**vestibular n.,** a disturbance of vestibular function consisting of a single attack of severe vertigo, usually accompanied by nausea and vomiting but without auditory symptoms; it attacks mainly young to middle-aged adults and usually improves within a few days. Called also *endemic paralytic vertigo, epidemic vertigo, paralytic vertigo,* and *vestibular neuritis.*

**neu·ro·nop·a·thy** (noor″on-op′ə-the) polyneuropathy involving destruction of the cell bodies of neurons.

**neu·rono·phage** (no͝o-ron′o-fāj) [*neuron* + *-phage*] a phagocyte which destroys nerve cells.

**neu·rono·pha·gia** (noor″on-o-fa′jə) the destruction of nerve cells by phagocytic action.

**neu·rono·trop·ic** (noor″on-o-trop′ik) [*neuron* + *-tropic*] having a special affinity for neurons.

**Neu·ron·tin** (no͝o-ron′tin) trademark for a preparation of gabapentin.

**neu·ro·on·col·o·gy** (noor″o-on-kol′ə-je) the field of specialization dealing with tumors of the nervous system.

**neu·ro·oph·thal·mol·o·gy** (noor″o-of″thəl-mol′ə-je) [*neuro-* + *ophthalmology*] the field of specialization dealing with portions of the nervous system related to the eye.

**neu·ro·otol·o·gy** (noor″o-o-tol′ə-je) that part of otology dealing especially with portions of the nervous system related to the ear.

**neu·ro·pace·mak·er** (noor″o-pās′māk-ər) an implant device that relieves pain due to nerve injury.

**neu·ro·pap·il·li·tis** (noor″o-pap″ĭ-li′tis) papillitis, def. 2.

**neu·ro·path·ic** (noor″o-path′ik) pertaining to or characterized by neuropathy.

**neu·ro·patho·gen·e·sis** (noor″o-path″o-jen′ə-sis) development of disease of the nervous system.

**neu·ro·patho·ge·nic·i·ty** (noor″o-path″o-jə-nis′ĭ-te) the quality of producing or the ability to produce pathologic changes in nerve tissue.

**neu·ro·pa·thol·o·gy** (noor″o-pə-thol′ə-je) the branch of medicine dealing with morphological and other aspects of disease of the nervous system.

**neu·rop·a·thy** (no͝o-rop′ə-the) [*neuro-* + *-pathy*] a functional disturbance or pathological change in the peripheral nervous system, sometimes limited to noninflammatory lesions as opposed to those of neuritis; the etiology may be known or unknown. Known etiologies include complications of other diseases (e.g., *diabetic n., amyloid n., porphyric n.*) or of toxic states (e.g., *arsenic n., isoniazid n., lead n., nitrofurantoin n.*). Neuropathies affecting a specific nerve may be named for the nerve (e.g., *femoral n.*). The terms *mononeuropathy* and *polyneuropathy* may be used to denote whether one nerve or several are involved. *Encephalopathy* and *myelopathy* are corresponding terms referring to the brain and spinal cord, respectively.
**acrodystrophic n.,** hereditary sensory radicular n.
**alcoholic n.,** neuropathy due to thiamine deficiency in chronic alcoholism.
**amyloid n.,** see under *polyneuropathy.*
**angiopathic n.,** neuropathy caused by arteritis of the blood vessels supplying the nerves. It is usually a systemic complication of diseases such as Wegener's granulomatosis, temporal arteritis, systemic lupus erythematosus, rheumatoid arthritis, systemic scleroderma, and polyarteritis nodosa; occasional nonsystemic cases occur in the form of a mononeuropathy that is more indolent than the systemic forms.
**arsenic n., arsenical n.,** see under *polyneuropathy.*
**ascending n.,** that which progresses from the feet upwards to affect the thigh, hip, trunk, etc.
**autonomic n.,** any neuropathy of the autonomic nervous system, causing symptoms such as orthostatic hypotension, disordered bowel, bladder, or sexual functions, or abnormal pupillary reflexes; it is a complication of many diseases including Adie's syndrome, chronic alcoholism, diabetes mellitus, dysautonomia, and Shy-Drager syndrome.
**axonal n.,** axonopathy.
**brachial plexus n.,** brachial plexopathy.
**compression n.,** entrapment n.
**Dejerine-Sottas n.,** progressive hypertrophic n.
**Denny-Brown's sensory n., Denny-Brown's sensory radicular n.,** hereditary sensory radicular n.
**descending n.,** that which starts proximally (shoulder, hip) and spreads distally toward the limb extremities (hands, feet).
**diabetic n.,** any of several clinical types of peripheral neuropathy occurring with diabetes mellitus; there are sensory, motor, autonomic, and mixed varieties. The most common kind is a chronic, symmetrical sensory polyneuropathy affecting first the nerves of the lower limbs and often affecting autonomic nerves; pathologically, there is a segmental demyelination of the peripheral nerves. An uncommon acute form is the ischemic variety, accompanied by severe pain, weakness, and wasting of proximal and distal muscles, peripheral sensory impairment, and loss of tendon reflexes. With autonomic involvement there may be orthostatic hypotension, nocturnal diarrhea, retention of urine, impotence, and small diameter of the pupils with sluggish reaction to light.
**entrapment n.,** any of a group of neuropathies in which a peripheral nerve is injured by compression in its course through a fibrous or osseofibrous tunnel or at a point where it abruptly changes its course through deep fascia over a fibrous or muscular band. Examples include *carpal tunnel syndrome, cubital tunnel syndrome, meralgia paresthetica, Morton's neuralgia, musculospiral paralysis, pronator syndrome,* and *tarsal tunnel syndrome.* Called also *nerve compression syndrome, compression n.,* and *pressure n.*
**femoral n.,** neuropathy due to injury to the femoral nerve, characterized by a variety of sensory and motor deficits in the leg; the most common causes are diabetes mellitus, anticoagulant-induced retroperitoneal hemorrhage, and trauma during surgery.
**giant axonal n.,** an autosomal recessive neuropathy of childhood characterized by enlarged axons made up of masses of tightly woven neurofilaments.
**hepatic n.,** neuropathy caused by liver disease, particularly one of three varieties: an asymptomatic or mild demyelinating polyneuropathy, often seen with chronic liver failure; a polyneuritis similar to acute idiopathic polyneuritis, sometimes seen with viral hepatitis; and a painful sensory neuropathy, sometimes seen with biliary cirrhosis.
**hypertrophic n., hereditary,** progressive hypertrophic n.
**hypertrophic n., progressive,** a condition characterized by hyperplasia of the interstitial connective tissue, causing thickening of peripheral nerve trunks and posterior roots, and by sclerosis of the posterior columns of the spinal cord. It is a slowly progressive familial disease beginning in early life, marked by atrophy of distal parts of the legs, and by diminution of tendon reflexes and of sensation. Called also *Dejerine's disease, Dejerine-Sottas atrophy, disease,* or *n., Gombault's degeneration* or *neuritis, interstitial hypertrophic neuritis, hereditary hypertrophic n.,* and *hypertrophic interstitial n.* See also *hereditary motor and sensory n.*
**hypertrophic interstitial n.,** progressive hypertrophic n.
**ischemic n.,** an injury to a peripheral nerve caused by a reduction in blood supply, such as that seen with diabetes mellitus.
**isoniazid n.,** polyneuropathy seen in some patients on isoniazid therapy, consisting of symmetrical numbness and paresthesias of the lower extremities.
**lead n.,** a form of segmental (demyelination) neuropathy seen with chronic lead poisoning; see under *poisoning.*
**Leber's hereditary optic n., Leber's optic n.,** a rare hereditary dis-

order, resulting from a deficit of ATP caused by mutation of a mitochondrial gene involved in ATP manufacture and occurring most commonly in males, with onset usually at about age twenty; it is characterized by degeneration of the optic nerve and papillomacular bundle, resulting in a progressive loss of central vision that may remit spontaneously. Called also *hereditary optic n.* or *atrophy, Leber's optic atrophy,* and *Leber's disease.*
**lumbar plexus n.,** lumbar plexopathy.
**lumbosacral plexus n.,** lumbosacral plexopathy.
**motor n.,** neuropathy or polyneuropathy involving only motor nerves.
**motor and sensory n., hereditary (HMSN),** any of a group of hereditary polyneuropathies involving muscle weakness, atrophy, sensory deficits, and vasomotor changes in the lower limbs. Some diseases in this group have been numbered: types I and II are varieties of Charcot-Marie-Tooth disease and type III is progressive hypertrophic neuropathy. Called also *hereditary sensory and motor n.*
**multiple n.,** 1. polyneuropathy. 2. mononeuropathy multiplex.
**nitrofurantoin n.,** neuropathy seen in some patients being treated with nitrofurantoin; it consists of symmetrical pain and paresthesias in the feet, which may in time spread to the hands.
**nutritional n.,** see under *polyneuropathy.*
**optic n., hereditary,** Leber's hereditary optic n.
**paraneoplastic n.,** see under *polyneuropathy.*
**periaxial n.,** segmental (demyelination) n.
**peripheral n.,** polyneuropathy.
**porphyric n.,** see under *polyneuropathy.*
**pressure n.,** entrapment n.
**sacral plexus n.,** sacral plexopathy.
**sarcoid n.,** a polyneuropathy sometimes occurring in sarcoidosis, characterized by either cranial polyneuritis or spinal nerve deficits; there may be large areas of sensory loss on the trunk.
**segmental (demyelination) n.,** neuropathy in which there is loss of myelin segments; called also *periaxial* or *segmental neuritis* and *periaxial n.*
**senile n.,** mild neuropathy occurring in the elderly, affecting chiefly the nerves of the extremities.
**sensorimotor n.,** neuropathy or polyneuropathy involving both sensory and motor nerves.
**sensory n.,** neuropathy or polyneuropathy of sensory nerves.
**sensory n., hereditary,** hereditary sensory radicular n.
**sensory and autonomic n., hereditary (HSAN),** any of several inherited neuropathies that involve slow ascendance of lesions of the sensory nerves, resulting in pain, distal trophic ulcers, and a variety of autonomic disturbances. Some diseases in this group have been numbered: type I is the autosomal dominant form of hereditary sensory radicular neuropathy; type II is the autosomal recessive form of hereditary sensory radicular neuropathy; and type III is familial dysautonomia.
**sensory and motor n., hereditary,** hereditary motor and sensory n.
**sensory radicular n., hereditary,** a hereditary polyneuropathy characterized by signs of radicular sensory loss in both the upper and lower extremities; shooting pains; chronic, indolent, trophic ulceration of the feet; and sometimes deafness. The pathologic findings are primary degeneration of the dorsal root ganglia together with evidence of degeneration of the olivary nuclei, optic nerves, and cerebellum. Most cases are autosomal dominant but a few autosomal recessive examples have been reported. The dominant form is also called *hereditary sensory and autonomic n. (type I)* and the recessive form is also called *hereditary sensory and autonomic n. (type II).* Called also *acrodystrophic n., hereditary sensory n., Denny-Brown's sensory n.* or *syndrome,* and *ulcerative mutilating acropathy.*
**serum n., serum sickness n.,** a neurologic disorder, usually involving the cervical nerves or brachial plexus, occurring two to eight days after the injection of foreign protein, e.g., an antiserum or antitoxin of animal origin, and characterized by local pain followed by sensory disturbances and paralysis. Called also *serum neuritis.*
**suprascapular n.,** a type of entrapment neuropathy caused by a lesion of the suprascapular nerve at the scapular notch, characterized by pain and weakness at the shoulder joint upon external rotation of the upper arm.
**tomaculous n.,** an autosomal dominant form of neuropathy characterized by pain, weakness, and pressure palsy in the arms and hands; myelin sheaths become swollen and sausage-shaped but there is neither demyelination nor damage to axons.
**toxic n.,** neuropathy caused by ingestion of a toxin; substances commonly implicated are *n*-hexane solvents, organophosphorus insecticides, acrylamide, heavy metals, and a variety of drugs.
**traumatic n.,** neuropathy resulting from trauma.
**vasculitic n.,** angiopathic n.

**neu·ro·pep·tide** (noor″o-pep′tīd) any of several types of molecules found in brain tissue, composed of short chains of amino acids; they include endorphins, enkephalins, vasopressin, and others. They are often localized in axon terminals at synapses and are classified as putative neurotransmitters, although some are also hormones.
**n. Y,** a 36–amino acid peptide found in neurons supplying blood vessels, as well as in the basal ganglia, thalamus, hypothalamus, and dorsal horn of the spinal cord; it is a vasoconstrictor and is believed to play a role in regulation of feeding behavior.

**neu·ro·phar·ma·co·log·i·cal** (noor″o-fahr″mə-ko-loj′ĭ-kəl) pertaining to neuropharmacology.

**neu·ro·phar·ma·col·o·gy** (noor″o-fahr″mə-kol′ə-je) [MeSH: Neuropharmacology] that branch of pharmacology dealing especially with the action of drugs upon various parts and elements of the nervous system.

**neu·ro·phil·ic** (noor″o-fil′ik) neurotropic.

**neu·roph·thal·mol·o·gy** (noor″of-thəl-mol′ə-je) neuro-ophthalmology.

**neu·ro·phy·sin** (noor″o-fi′sin) any of a group of soluble proteins (molecular weights 9500–10,500) derived from the precursors of vasopressin, oxytocin, and related hormones, secreted in the hypothalamus. They serve as binding proteins (carrier proteins) for vasopressin and oxytocin and may contribute to hormone storage and transport.

**neu·ro·phys·i·ol·o·gy** (noor″o-fiz″e-ol′ə-je) [*neuro-* + *physiology*] [MeSH: Neurophysiology] the physiology of the nervous system.

**neu·ro·pil** (noor′o-pil) [*neuro-* + Gr. *pilos* felt] a dense feltwork of interwoven cytoplasmic processes of nerve cells (dendrites and axons) and of neuroglial cells in the gray matter of the central nervous system.

**neu·ro·pile** (noor′o-pīl) neuropil.

**neu·ro·plasm** (noor′o-plaz-əm) [*neuro-* + *-plasm*] the undifferentiated basophilic protoplasm of a nerve cell.

**neu·ro·plas·mic** (noor″o-plaz′mik) of or relating to neuroplasm.

**neu·ro·plas·ty** (noor′o-plas″te) [*neuro-* + *-plasty*] plastic surgery of a nerve.

**neu·ro·plex·us** (noor″o-plek′səs) a plexus of nerves.

**neu·ro·po·di·on** (noor″o-po′de-on) bouton terminal.

**neu·ro·po·di·um** (noor″o-po′de-əm) pl. *neuropo′dia* [*neuro-* + *podium*] bouton terminal.

**neu·ro·pore** (noor′o-por) [*neuro-* + *pore*] the open anterior end (foramen anterius) or the open posterior end (foramen posterius) of the neural tube of the early embryo. These openings gradually close during the fourth week as the primordial spinal cord develops.
**anterior n.,** the embryonic opening in the anterior (or rostral) portion of the forebrain, which closes at the 20-somite stage (about 25 days).
**caudal n.,** posterior n.
**posterior n.,** the embryonic opening at the posterior (or caudal) end of the neural tube, which closes by about the 25-somite stage (about 27 days).
**rostral n.,** anterior n.

**neu·ro·pro·ba·sia** (noor″o-pro-ba′zhə) [*neuro-* + Gr. *pro* forward + *basis* walking] advance along the nerves; said of the action of certain viruses.

**neu·ro·pro·tec·tion** (noor″o-prə-tek′shən) protection against neurotoxicity.

**neu·ro·pro·tec·tive** (noor″o-prə-tek′tiv) guarding or protecting against neurotoxicity.

**neu·ro·psy·chi·a·trist** (noor″o-si-ki′ə-trist) a physician who specializes in neuropsychiatry.

**neu·ro·psy·chi·a·try** (noor″o-si-ki′ə-tre) [*neuro-* + *psychiatry*] the branch of medicine which includes both neurology and psychiatry.

**neu·ro·psy·cho·log·i·cal** (noor″o-si″ko-loj′ĭ-kəl) pertaining to neuropsychology.

**neu·ro·psy·chol·o·gy** (noor″o-si-kol′ə-je) [*neuro-* + *psychology*] [MeSH: Neuropsychology] a discipline combining neurology and psychology to study the relationship between the functioning of the brain and cognitive processes or behavior, using psychological testing and assessment to assay central nervous system function and diagnose specific behavioral or cognitive deficits or disorders.

**neu·ro·psy·cho·met·ric** (noor″o-si″ko-met′rik) pertaining to the quantitative testing of neurological processes underlying cognitive processes and behaviors.

**neu·ro·psy·cho·phar·ma·col·o·gy** (noor″o-si″ko-fahr″mə-kol′ə-je) psychopharmacology.

**neu·ro·ra·di·ol·o·gy** (noor″o-ra″de-ol′ə-je) radiology of the nervous system.

**neu·ro·ret·i·ni·tis** (noor″o-ret″ĭ-ni′tis) inflammation of the optic nerve and retina.

**neu·ro·ret·i·nop·a·thy** (noor″o-ret″ĭ-nop′ə-the) [*neuro-* + *retina* + *-pathy*] a disease of the optic disk and retina.

**hypertensive n.,** swelling of the optic disk and formation of serous and fibrinous precipitates in the retina, occurring in severe hypertension.

**neu·ro·roent·gen·og·ra·phy** (noor″o-rent″gən-og′rə-fe) neuroradiology.

**neu·ror·rha·phy** (noo͝-ror′ə-fe) [*neuro-* + *-rrhaphy*] the suturing of a cut nerve.

**neu·ro·sar·co·clei·sis** (noor″o-sahr″ko-kli′sis) [*neuro-* + *sarco-* + Gr. *kleisis* closure] an operation performed for neuralgia, done by relieving pressure on the affected nerve by partial resection of the bony canal through which it passes, and transplanting the nerve into soft tissues.

**neu·ro·sar·co·ma** (noor″o-sahr-ko′mə) a sarcoma with neural elements.

**neu·ro·schis·to·so·mi·a·sis** (noor″o-skis″to-so-mi′ə-sis) schistosomiasis affecting the central nervous system, most often caused by *Schistosoma japonicum.*

**neu·ro·sci·ence** (noor′o-si″əns) [MeSH: Neurosciences] any of the branches of science dealing with the embryology, anatomy, physiology, biochemistry, pharmacology, etc., of the nervous system.

**neu·ro·sci·en·tist** (noor″o-si′ən-tist) an expert in any of the branches of the neurosciences.

**neu·ro·se·cre·tion** (noor″o-sə-kre′shən) [*neuro-* + *secretion*] [MeSH: Neurosecretion] 1. the secretory activities of nerve cells, as the secretion of releasing hormones, vasopressin, neurotransmitters, etc. 2. the product of such activities; a neurosecretory substance.

**neu·ro·se·cre·to·ry** (noor″o-sə-kre′tə-re) pertaining to neurosecretion.

**neu·ro·seg·men·tal** (noor″o-seg-men′təl) [*neuro-* + *segmental*] of or pertaining to a pair of spinal dorsal and ventral roots or to the area which they supply.

**neu·ro·sen·so·ry** (noor″o-sen′sə-re) pertaining to a sensory nerve.

**neu·ro·ses** (noo͝-ro′sēz) plural of *neurosis.*

**neu·ro·sis** (noo͝-ro′sis) pl. *neuro′ses* [*neur-* + *-osis*] 1. former name for a category of mental disorders characterized by anxiety and avoidance behavior. In general, the term refers to disorders in which the symptoms are distressing to the person, reality testing is intact, behavior does not violate gross social norms, and there is no apparent organic etiology. Classified in DSM-IV under *anxiety disorders, dissociative disorders, mood disorders, sexual disorders,* and *somatoform disorders.* 2. in psychoanalytic theory, the specific etiological process that gives rise not only to neuroses as defined above but also to personality disorders (formerly called character neuroses to emphasize this) and some psychotic disorders. Unconscious conflicts involving opposing wishes or forbidden infantile wishes give rise to an unconscious anticipation of danger (experienced as anxiety) in situations that activate a conflict, and anxiety serves as a signal to trigger unconscious defense mechanisms, the operation of which is visible to the conscious mind and to observers in the form of neurotic symptoms or pathological personality traits.
**actual n.,** *(obs.),* Freud's term for a neurosis caused by sexual excitement without adequate gratification (in which he included neurasthenia and anxiety neurosis), as opposed to psychoneurosis (hysteria, obsessions, phobias) originating in childhood experiences.
**anxiety n.,** *(obs.)* Freud's term for conditions now reclassified as *panic disorder* and *generalized anxiety disorder.*
**cardiac n.,** neurocirculatory asthenia.
**character n.,** a type of character or personality disorder with some neurotic characteristics, particularly one of a predominantly obsessive-compulsive or hysterical nature; see also *neurosis.*
**combat n.,** an older term used for forms of post-traumatic stress disorder in which the traumatic event is combat-related.
**compensation n.,** an obsolete term for a factitious disorder following injury and motivated in part by prospects of financial compensation.
**compulsion n.,** obsessive-compulsive disorder.
**conversion n.,** see under *disorder.*
**depersonalization n.,** see under *disorder.*
**depressive n.,** dysthymic disorder.
**experimental n.,** a state produced in an experimental animal, usually by exposure to frustration or conflict, that resembles human neuroses.
**hypochondriacal n.,** hypochondriasis.
**hysterical n.,** former name for a group of conditions now divided between *conversion disorder* and *dissociative disorders.* See also *hysteria.*
**obsessional n.,** obsessive-compulsive disorder.
**obsessive-compulsive n.,** see under *disorder.*
**pension n.,** compensation n.
**phobic n.,** older term for *phobic disorder;* see *phobia.*
**prison n.,** chronophobia occurring in prisoners having trouble adjusting to a long prison sentence, characterized by feelings of restlessness, panic, anxiety, and claustrophobia.
**transference n.,** a phenomenon occurring during psychoanalysis, in which transference causes the patient to undergo, with the analyst as the object, an intense repetition of childhood conflicts and traumas, reexperiencing impulses, feelings, and fantasies that originally developed in relation to the parents.
**traumatic n.,** older term for *post-traumatic stress disorder.*
**vegetative n.,** acrodynia.
**war n.,** older term for a form of post-traumatic stress disorder in which the traumatic event is war-related.

**neu·ro·skel·e·tal** (noor″o-skel′ə-təl) pertaining to the nervous tissues and the skeletal muscular tissue.

**neu·ro·skel·e·ton** (noor″o-skel′ə-ton) endoskeleton.

**neu·ro·some** (noor′o-sōm) [*neuro-* + *-some*] 1. the body of a nerve cell. 2. any of the minute particles found in the protoplasm of a neuron.

**neu·ro·spasm** (noor′o-spaz-əm) [*neuro-* + *spasm*] a spasm caused by a disorder in the motor nerve supplying the muscle.

**neu·ro·splanch·nic** (noor″o-splangk′nik) pertaining to the cerebrospinal and sympathetic nervous systems; neurovisceral.

**neu·ro·spon·gi·o·ma** (noor″o-spon″je-o′mə) glioma.

**Neu·ros·po·ra** (noo͝-ros′pə-rə) [MeSH: Neurospora] a genus of usually saprobic fungi of the family Sordariaceae, comprising the bread molds; they are capable of converting tryptophan to nicotinic acid and are extensively used in genetic and enzyme research.

**neu·ro·sta·tus** (noor″o-sta′təs) the state or condition of neural symptoms in a case history.

**neu·ro·sur·geon** (noor″o-sur′jən) a physician who specializes in neurosurgery.

**neu·ro·sur·gery** (noor′o-sər″jər-e) [MeSH: Neurosurgery] surgery of the nervous system.
**functional n.,** 1. neurosurgery designed to restore physiological activity of nerves, such as by enhancing conductivity of nerve fibers or improving blood flow to nerve tissue. 2. psychosurgery.
**stereotactic n.,** see under *surgery.*

**neu·ro·su·ture** (noor″o-soo′chər) neurorrhaphy.

**neu·ro·syph·i·lis** (noor″o-sif′ĭ-lis) [*neuro-* + *syphilis*] [MeSH: Neurosyphilis] the central nervous system manifestations of syphilis, which may be divided into two groups: asymptomatic and symptomatic; the latter includes meningovascular and parenchymatous neurosyphilis (see *general paresis,* under *paresis,* and *tabes dorsalis*).
**asymptomatic n.,** neurosyphilis diagnosed when there is a positive VDRL test in the cerebrospinal fluid in the absence of the signs and symptoms of neurologic disease.
**meningovascular n.,** neurosyphilis at the stage of extensive meningeal involvement, secondarily investing and then occluding vessels in their course through the subarachnoid space, resulting in focal or widespread cerebrovascular disease. Called also *meningovascular syphilis.*
**parenchymatous n.,** a form in which there is widespread parenchymal damage; called also *parenchymatous syphilis.* See *general paresis,* under *paresis,* and *tabes dorsalis.*
**paretic n.,** general paresis.
**tabetic n.,** tabes dorsalis.

**neu·ro·ten·di·nous** (noor″o-ten′dĭ-nəs) pertaining to both nerve and tendon.

**neu·ro·ten·sin** (noor″o-ten′sin) [MeSH: Neurotensin] a tridecapeptide found in the small intestine and brain; it induces vasodilatation and hypotension and in the brain it is a neurotransmitter.

**neu·ro·ter·mi·nal** (noor″o-tər′mĭ-nəl) end-organ.

**neu·ro·thele** (noor″o-the′le) [*neuro-* + Gr. *thele* nipple] a sensory papilla located in the papillary layer of the dermis; called also *nerve papilla* and *nervous papilla.*

**neu·rot·ic** (noo͝-rot′ik) 1. pertaining to or characterized by neurosis. 2. a person affected with a neurosis.

**neu·rot·iza·tion** (noo͝″rot-ĭ-za′shən) the regeneration of a nerve after its division.

**neu·rot·me·sis** (noor″ot-me′sis) [*neuro-* + Gr. *tmēsis* cutting apart] partial or complete severance of a nerve, with disruption of the axon and its myelin sheath and the connective tissue elements; regeneration does not occur. Cf. *axonotmesis* and *neurapraxia.*

**neu·ro·tome** (noor′o-tōm) [*neuro-* + *-tome*] 1. a needle-like knife for dissecting the nerves. 2. neuromere (def. 1).

**neu·ro·to·mog·ra·phy** (noor″o-to-mog′rə-fe) tomography of the central nervous system.

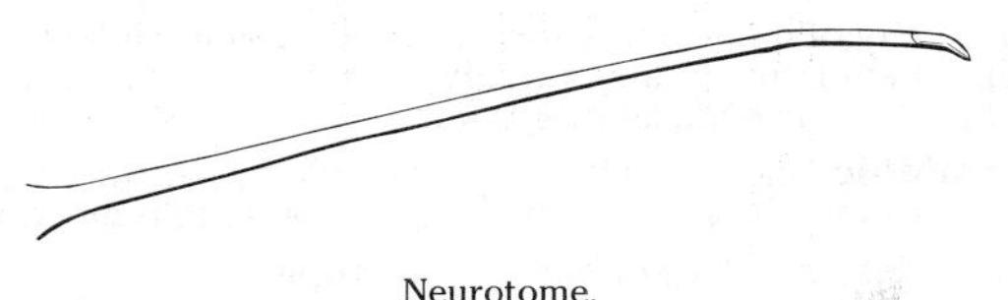
Neurotome.

**neu·rot·o·my** (noo͝-rot′ə-me) [*neuro-* + *-tomy*] interruption of a nerve through surgical cutting or production of artificial lesions.
**radiofrequency n.,** percutaneous radiofrequency rhizotomy.
**retrogasserian n.,** trigeminal rhizotomy.

**neu·rot·o·ny** (noo͝-rot′ə-ne) [*neuro-* + Gr. *teinein* to stretch] the stretching of a nerve; called also *neurectasia.*

**neu·ro·tox·ic** (noor″o-tok′sik) poisonous or destructive to nerve tissue.

**neu·ro·tox·ic·i·ty** (noor″o-tok-sis′ĭ-te) the quality of exerting a destructive or poisonous effect upon nerve tissue.

**neu·ro·tox·in** (noor″o-tok′sin) a toxin that is poisonous to or destroys nerve tissue, especially the exotoxins secreted by *Clostridium botulinum, C. tetani, Corynebacterium diphtheriae,* and *Shigella dysenteriae.*

**neu·ro·trans·duc·er** (noor″o-trans-do͞o s′ər) a neuron that synthesizes and releases hormones which serve as the functional link between the nervous system and the pituitary gland.

**neu·ro·trans·mis·sion** (noor″o-trans-mish′ən) the process by which a neurotransmitter is released, crosses the synapse, and affects the action of the target cell.

**neu·ro·trans·mit·ter** (noor″o-trans′mit-ər) any of a group of substances that are released on excitation from the axon terminal of a presynaptic neuron of the central or peripheral nervous system and travel across the synaptic cleft to either excite or inhibit the target cell. Among the many substances that have the properties of a neurotransmitter are acetylcholine, norepinephrine, epinephrine, dopamine, glycine, γ-aminobutyrate, glutamic acid, substance P, enkephalins, endorphins, and serotonin.
**false n.,** an amine, e.g., octopamine, that can be stored in and released from presynaptic vesicles but that has little effect on postsynaptic receptors.

**neu·ro·trau·ma** (noor″o-traw′mə) [*neuro-* + *trauma*] mechanical injury of a nerve.

**neu·ro·troph·ic** (noor″o-trof′ik) pertaining to neurotrophy.

**neu·ro·tro·phin** (noor′o-tro″fin) any of a family of growth factors that block apoptosis in neurons and thus promote nerve growth; the best-known example is nerve growth factor.

**neu·rot·ro·phy** (noo͝-rot′rə-fe) [*neuro-* + *-trophy*] 1. the nutrition and maintenance of tissues as regulated by nervous influence. 2. the nutrition and maintenance of nervous tissue.

**neu·ro·trop·ic** (noor″o-trop′ik) having a selective affinity for nervous tissue, or exerting its principal effect on the nervous system.

**neu·rot·ro·pism** (noo͝-rot′ro-piz-əm) [*neuro-* + *tropism*] 1. the quality of having a special affinity for nervous tissue. 2. the alleged tendency of regenerating nerve fibers to grow toward specific portions of the periphery.

**neu·rot·ro·py** (noo͝-rot′rə-pe) neurotropism.

**neu·ro·tro·sis** (noor″o-tro′sis) neurotrauma.

**neu·ro·tu·bule** (noor″o-too′būl) a microtubule occurring in a neuron.

**neu·ro·vac·cine** (noor″o-vak-sēn′) vaccinia virus prepared by growing the virus in the brain of a rabbit.

**neu·ro·var·i·co·sis** (noor″o-var″ĭ-ko′sis) a varicose state of the fibers of a nerve.

**neu·ro·va·ri·o·la** (noor″o-və-ri′ə-lə) neurovaccine.

**neu·ro·vas·cu·lar** (noor″o-vas′ku-lər) pertaining to both nervous and vascular elements; pertaining to the nerves that control the caliber of blood vessels.

**neu·ro·veg·e·ta·tive** (noor″o-vej′ə-ta″tiv) pertaining to the vegetative (autonomic) nervous system.

**neu·ro·vir·u·lence** (noor″o-vir′u-ləns) the competence of an infectious agent to produce pathologic effects on the nervous system.

**neu·ro·vir·u·lent** (noor″o-vir′u-lənt) capable of producing pathologic effects on the nervous system.

**neu·ro·vi·rus** (noor′o-vi″rəs) a vaccine virus which has been modified by passing into nervous tissue.

**neu·ro·vis·cer·al** (noor″o-vis′ər-əl) neurosplanchnic.

**neu·ru·la** (noor′u-lə) [*neuro-* + dim. *-ula*] the early embryo during the development of the neural tube from the neural plate, marking the first appearance of the nervous system; the next stage after the gastrula, and occurring 19 to 26 days after fertilization.

**neu·ru·la·tion** (noor″u-la′shən) formation, in the early embryo, of the neural plate, followed by its closure with development of the neural tube.

**neu·rur·gic** (noo͝-rər′jik) neurergic.

**neu·ter** (noo′tər) to castrate an animal; see *spay* and *geld.*

**neu·tral** (noo′trəl) [L. *neutralis; neuter,* neither] in chemistry, neither acid nor basic.

**neu·tral·ism** (noo′trəl-iz-əm) the absence of interaction between coexisting organisms of different species.

**neu·tral·i·ty** (noo-tral′ĭ-te) the state of being neutral.

**neu·tral·iza·tion** (noo″trəl-ĭ-za′shən) the act or process of rendering neutral.
**viral n.,** the process by which antibody alone or antibody plus complement neutralizes the infectivity of a virus. The antibody may coat the virus forming a stable complex or may cause conformational changes in viral structural proteins on binding; either process may interfere with binding of the virion to cellular receptor sites and entry into the cell. Enveloped viruses may be lysed by complement.

**neu·tral·ize** (noo′trəl-īz) to render neutral.

**neu·tra·my·cin** (noo″trə-mi′sin) an antibacterial substance produced by *Streptomyces rimosus.*

**Neu·tra·pen** (noo′trə-pən) trademark for a lyophilized preparation of penicillinase.

**Neu·tra-Phos-K** (noo″trə-fos′ka) trademark for a preparation of potassium phosphate.

**neu·tri·no** (noo-tre′no) [It. "little neutron"] an elementary particle that has no electric charge and no mass, and that very rarely reacts with matter; it is a product of beta decay. Symbol *ν*.

**neu·tro·clu·sion** (noo″trō-kloo′zhən) malocclusion characterized by irregularities of individual teeth, but with normal mesiodistal or normal anteroposterior relation of the mandibular to the maxillary dental arch. Generally regarded as identical with class I in Angle's classification of malocclusion.

**neu·tro·cyte** (noo′tro-sīt) neutrophil (def. 1).

**neu·tro·fla·vine** (noo″tro-fla′vin) acriflavine.

**neu·tron** (noo′tron) [MeSH: Neutrons] an electrically neutral or uncharged particle of matter existing along with protons in the atoms of all elements except the mass 1 isotope of hydrogen. Symbol n.
**epithermal n.,** a neutron having an energy level of a few hundredths of an electron volt to 100 electron volts.
**fast n.,** a neutron having an energy level exceeding $10^5$ electron volts.
**intermediate n.,** a neutron having an energy level of 100 to 100,000 electron volts.
**slow n.,** 1. thermal n. 2. any neutron having an energy level up to 100 electron volts.
**thermal n.,** a neutron having an energy level of about 0.025 electron volt; called also *slow n.*

**neu·tro·pe·nia** (noo″tro-pe′ne-ə) [*neutrophil* + *-penia*] [MeSH: Neutropenia] a decrease in the number of neutrophils in the blood; see also *agranulocytosis.*
**autoimmune n.,** that caused by autoantibodies against the neutrophils; it may occur in isolation, in association with other autoimmune conditions, or secondary to malignancy, infection, or a drug complication. The most common type is alloimmune neonatal neutropenia.
**chronic benign n., chronic familial n.,** a rare familial type of peripheral neutropenia, probably transmitted as an autosomal dominant trait, related to but less severe than agranulocytosis. It is usually seen in children and is characterized by recurrent infections with eventual spontaneous remission, but in a few cases it has persisted into adulthood. Called also *familial benign chronic n.*
**chronic hypoplastic n., congenital n.,** former names for *infantile genetic agranulocytosis.*
**cyclic n.,** 1. a chronic type of neutropenia that abates and recurs, accompanied by malaise, fever, stomatitis, and various types of infections. Called also *periodic n.* 2. a rare autosomal recessive disorder of gray collie dogs in which there is a bone marrow stem cell defect with periodic fluctuations in numbers of circulating neutrophils, platelets, and reticulocytes; during the episodes animals have lethargy, fever, arthralgias, and bacterial infections that can be fatal. Called also *cyclic hematopoiesis* and *gray collie syndrome.*
**drug-induced n.,** that caused by medications; the most common mechanisms are immunological (formation of antibodies destructive to neutrophils or of immune complexes that bind to neutrophils), followed by inhibition of granulopoiesis and direct damage to bone marrow or precursor cells of the granulocytic series.

**familial benign chronic n.**, chronic benign n.
**hypersplenic n.**, primary splenic n.
**idiopathic n.**, agranulocytosis.
**Kostmann's n.**, infantile genetic agranulocytosis.
**malignant n.**, agranulocytosis.
**neonatal n., alloimmune, neonatal n., isoimmune,** neutropenia in the newborn due to *in utero* incompatibility between its immunoglobulin G antigens and those of the mother's blood; the mother's blood produces IgG antineutrophil antibodies that cross the placenta and sensitize fetal neutrophils. Affected infants may have fever, pneumonia, septicemia, and other infections that can be fatal. The condition eventually resolves itself as the infant's immunoglobulin replaces that from the mother.
**periodic n.**, cyclic n.
**peripheral n.**, decrease in the number of neutrophils in the circulating blood.
**primary splenic n.**, a syndrome characterized by splenomegaly, hypercellular bone marrow, profound leukopenia and neutropenia, and susceptibility to infection, occasionally with anemia and thrombocytopenia. Called also *hypersplenic n.*
**severe congenital n.**, infantile genetic agranulocytosis.

**neu·tro·phil** (noo'tro-fil) [*neutro-* + *-phil*] [MeSH: Neutrophils] 1. a mature granular leukocyte that is polymorphonuclear (its nucleus having three to five lobes connected by slender threads of chromatin, and cytoplasm containing fine granules); neutrophils have the properties of chemotaxis, adherence to immune complexes, and phagocytosis. The counterpart in nonhuman mammals is the heterophil. Called also *neutrocyte* and *neutrophilic leukocyte.* 2. any cell, structure, or histologic element readily stainable by neutral dyes.
**band n.**, see under *cell.*
**giant n.**, macropolycyte.
**juvenile n.**, metamyelocyte.
**polymorphonuclear n.**, the usual type of mature neutrophil, which has a multilobar nucleus; see also *polymorphonuclear leukocyte,* under *leukocyte.*
**rod n., stab n.**, band cell.

**neu·tro·phil elas·tase** (noo'tro-fil e-las'tās) leukocyte elastase.

**neu·tro·phil·ia** (noo″tro-fil'e-ə) increase in the number of neutrophils in the blood; it is the most common form of leukocytosis and can have any of numerous causes, including acute infections, intoxications, hemorrhage, and rapidly growing malignant neoplasms. Called also *neutrophilic leukocytosis.*

**neu·tro·phil·ic** (noo″tro-fil'ik) 1. stainable by neutral dyes. 2. neither anthropophilic nor zoophilous; said of certain mosquitoes.

**neu·tro·pism** (noo'tro-piz-əm) neurotropism.

**neu·tro·tax·is** (noo″tro-tak'sis) [*neutrophil* + *-taxis*] the attractive or repellent influence exerted by neutrophils.

**ne·vi** (ne'vi) [L.] plural of *nevus.*

**ne·vir·a·pine** (nə-vir'ə-pēn) an inhibitor of reverse transcriptase, used in combination with nucleoside analogue antiviral agents in the treatment of human immunodeficiency virus infection and acquired immunodeficiency syndrome; administered orally.

**nev(o)-** [L. *naevus* mole] a combining form denoting relationship to a nevus, or mole.

**ne·vo·blast** (ne″vo-blast) [*nevo-* + *-blast*] a neural crest–derived cell postulated to be the precursor of the nevus cell.

**ne·vo·cel·lu·lar** (ne″vo-sel'u-lər) nevocytic.

**ne·vo·cyte** (ne″vo-sīt) [*nevo-* + *-cyte*] nevus cell.

**ne·vo·cyt·ic** (ne-vo-sit'ik) pertaining to or composed of nevus cells.

**ne·void** (ne'void) resembling a nevus.

**ne·vo·li·po·ma** (ne″vo-lĭ-po'mə) [*nevo-* + *lipoma*] a nevus containing a large amount of fibrofatty tissue. Called also *fatty nevus* and *nevus lipomatosus.*

**ne·vo·xan·tho·en·do·the·li·o·ma** (ne″vo-zan″tho-en″do-the″le-o'mə) [*nevo-* + *xantho-* + *endothelioma*] juvenile xanthogranuloma.

**ne·vus** (ne'vəs) pl. *ne'vi* [L. *naevus*] [MeSH: Nevus] 1. any congenital lesion of the skin; a birthmark. 2. a type of hamartoma representing a circumscribed stable malformation of the skin and occasionally of the oral mucosa, which is not due to external causes and therefore presumed to be of hereditary origin. The excess (or deficiency) of tissue may involve epidermal, connective tissue, adnexal, nervous, or vascular elements.

## Nevus

**achromic n.**, n. depigmentosus.
**acquired n.**, a nevus that is not present at birth but appears later in life.
**amelanotic n.**, a nevocytic nevus that contains no pigment. Cf. *n. depigmentosus.*
**n. ane'micus**, a congenital disorder typically characterized by the presence of pale, round, well-defined macules with irregular borders that may have a normal amount of melanin or may lack melanin but are not totally amelanotic. Studies suggest that the disorder is due to a functional incapacity of the blood vessels to dilate as a result of increased sensitivity to catecholamines.
**n. ara'neus**, vascular spider.
**balloon cell n.**, an intradermal nevus, often a brown mole with a subtle yellow halo surrounding it, consisting of balloon cells with pale cytoplasm that contains large vacuoles formed of altered melanosomes; it may be confused with melanoma.
**bathing trunk n.**, see *giant congenital pigmented n.*
**Becker's n.**, a nevus occurring mostly in males in the second to third decade of life consisting of epidermal melanosis, presenting as segmental, uniform, light hyperpigmentation, followed several years later by the growth of long dark hairs from the lesions; the lesions usually have the same pattern of distribution as those of nevus unius lateris (q.v.). Called also *n. spilus tardus* and *pigmented hairy epidermal n.*
**blue n.**, a benign nevus, usually solitary, representing a localized proliferation of dermal melanocytes, which is manifested by a dark blue to black, moderately firm, rounded, sharply defined nodular tumor composed of spindle-shaped melanocytes with slender cytoplasmic processes, occurring often in association with melanin-laden macrophages in a sclerotic dermis. Called also *dermal melanocytoma* and *Jadassohn-Tièche n.* Cf. *cellular blue n.*
**blue rubber bleb n.**, a type of congenital nevus, transmitted as an autosomal dominant trait, characterized by bluish hemangiomas with soft elevated nipple-like centers on the skin surface, in the gastrointestinal tract, and sometimes on mucous membranes; it is sometimes associated with pain, regional hyperhidrosis, and gastrointestinal bleeding.
**cellular n.**, nevocytic n.
**cellular blue n.**, a large blue or blue-black, multilobulated, well-circumscribed nodular tumor, usually congenital, having a tendency to occur on the buttocks and sacrococcygeal region. It is characterized histologically by deeply pigmented, dendritic, spindle-shaped melanocytes alternating with cellular islands of spindle cells with ovoid nuclei and abundant pale cytoplasm in the dermis and subcutaneous tissue. These nevi have a low incidence of malignant transformation to melanoma, in which case they show cellular pleomorphism, mitotic figures, and evidence of invasion into the deep dermis. Called also *dermal melanocytoma.* Cf. *blue n.*
**choroidal n.**, a flat or slightly raised uveal nevus of the choroid, usually brown to gray in color.
**chromatophore n. of Naegeli**, Franceschetti-Jadassohn syndrome.
**n. comedo'nicus**, a rare epidermal nevus thought to represent a developmental abnormality of the pilosebaceous apparatus, characterized by the presence of aggregations of dilated keratin-filled hair follicles, producing large cutaneous patches studded with comedo-like lesions that are usually unilateral and generally localized to areas such as the trunk, an upper extremity, or the neck, sometimes in a linear or zosteriform pattern. The condition is occasionally associated with other lesions such as ichthyosis, nevoid cell carcinoma, vascular nevi, and cataracts.
**compound n.**, a nevocytic nevus composed of fully formed nests of nevus cells in the epidermis as well as newly forming ones in the dermis. Cf. *intradermal n.* and *junction n.*
**congenital n.**, a nevus present at birth, generally larger than acquired nevi; larger lesions are associated with an increased risk of melanoma.
**connective tissue n.**, any of a group of variable-appearing hamartomas involving various components of the connective tissue, usually present at birth or soon thereafter, which may be inherited or acquired, and may be associated with other diseases. They may present clinically as single or multiple nodules, papules, or plaques, or in various combinations of these lesions, but individual lesions usually appear as a plaque composed of firm, flat, closely set, white to ivory or yellow-brown papules, often having a cobblestonelike surface. Called also *juvenile elastoma, n. elasticus,* and *n. elasticus of Lewandowsky.*

**n. depigmento'sus,** a developmental anomaly of melanization producing long bands or streaks of hypopigmentation on the skin, especially on the trunk and extremities, usually unilaterally. Called also *achromic n.* Cf. *amelanotic n.*

**dermal n.,** intradermal n.

**dysplastic n.,** an acquired atypical nevus with an irregular border, indistinct margin, and mixed coloration, often occurring in large numbers, that is characterized by intraepidermal melanocytic dysplasia and often is a precursor of malignant melanoma.

**n. elas'ticus,** 1. pseudoxanthoma elasticum. 2. connective tissue n.

**n. elasticus of Lewandowsky,** connective tissue n.

**epidermal n., epithelial n.,** a circumscribed congenital developmental anomaly resulting in faulty production of mature or nearly mature cutaneous structures, occurring as a result of overproduction of surface or adnexal epithelium. Such nevi vary widely in presentation and are commonly hyperkeratotic.

**fatty n.,** nevolipoma.

**n. flam'meus,** a common congenital vascular malformation involving mature capillaries, presenting as a sharply demarcated, flat, irregularly shaped patch, ranging in color from faint pink to orange *(salmon patch)* to dark red–purple *(port-wine stain),* and usually found on the face and neck. The paler varieties tend to involute during childhood, while the darker ones usually are persistent. See also *capillary hemangioma* (def. 1), under *hemangioma,* and *vascular n.*

**n. fuscoceru'leus acromiodeltoi'deus,** n. of Ito.

**n. fuscoceru'leus ophthalmomaxilla'ris,** n. of Ota.

**giant congenital pigmented n., giant hairy n., giant pigmented n.,** any of a group of large darkly pigmented hairy nevi, present at birth, usually bilaterally symmetric, and having a predilection for the chest, upper back, and shoulders; the area usually covered by bathing trunks; and distal upper and lower extremities. These nevi have been shown to be associated with other cutaneous and subcutaneous lesions, neurofibromatosis and other developmental anomalies, and leptomeningeal melanocytosis, and they also exhibit a predisposition to the development of malignant melanoma.

**hair follicle n.,** trichofolliculoma.

**halo n.,** a pigmented lesion (usually a compound or intradermal nevocytic nevus but sometimes a neuronevus, blue nevus, or malignant melanoma) surrounded by an annular depigmented area. Called also *leukoderma acquisitum centrifugum, Sutton's disease,* and *Sutton's n.*

**hepatic n.,** hemorrhagic infarct of the liver.

**intradermal n.,** a nevocytic nevus, clinically indistinguishable from compound nevus, in which the nests of nevus cells lie exclusively within the dermis. Called also *dermal n.* Cf. *compound n.* and *junction n.*

**n. of Ito,** a mongolian spot–like lesion having the same features as nevus of Ota except for localization to the areas of distribution of the posterior supraclavicular and lateral cutaneous brachial nerves, to involve the shoulder, side of the neck, supraclavicular areas, and upper arm. Called also *n. fuscoceruleus acromiodeltoideus.*

**Jadassohn's sebaceous n.,** n. sebaceus of Jadassohn.

**Jadassohn-Tièche n.,** blue n.

**junction n., junctional n.,** a nevocytic nevus in which the nests of nevus cells are confined to the dermoepidermal junction, which usually presents clinically as a small, discrete, flat or slightly raised macule. Cf. *compound n.* and *intradermal n.*

**n. lipomato'sus,** nevolipoma.

**n. lipomato'sus cuta'neus superficia'lis,** a connective tissue nevus, usually congenital, characterized histologically by the presence of ectopic, mature adipocytes in the dermis, and clinically by multiple or single soft, skin-colored to yellowish papules, nodules, and plaques, usually located on the lower trunk, gluteal region, or thigh.

**melanocytic n.,** a usually pigmented nevus, acquired or hereditary, caused by a disorder of melanocytes.

**neural n., neuroid n.,** neuronevus.

Nevus flammeus.

**nevocellular n.,** nevocytic n.

**nevocytic n., nevus cell n.,** an acquired or inherited tumor composed of nests *(theques)* of nevus cells, usually presenting as tan to deep brown small macules or papules with well-defined, rounded borders, although the clinical appearance is quite variable. Based on the histologic pattern and location of the nevus cells, these nevi are classified as compound, intradermal, and junction. Called also *cellular n.* and *nevocellular n.*

**nuchal n.,** nevus flammeus situated on either side of the posterior midline between the occipital protuberance and the tip of the spine of the fifth cervical vertebra, with the long axis up and down. Called also *Unna's n.*

**organoid n.,** n. sebaceus.

**n. of Ota, Ota's n.,** a persistent mongolian spot–like lesion, usually present at birth, involving the conjunctiva and skin about the eye supplied by the first and second branches of the trigeminal nerve as well as the sclera, ocular muscles, retrobulbar fat, periosteum, and buccal mucosa, usually unilaterally. The skin lesions are manifested as macular bluish or gray-brown patchy areas of pigmentation that grow slowly and become deeper in color. Called also *oculodermal melanocytosis* and *n. fuscoceruleus ophthalmomaxillaris.*

**pigmented n., n. pigmento'sus,** a nevus containing melanin; the term is usually restricted to nevocytic nevi, or moles, but may be applied to other pigmented nevi, e.g., nevus spilus and Becker's nevus.

**pigmented hairy epidermal n.,** Becker's n.

**port-wine n.,** see under *stain.*

**sebaceous n., n. seba'ceus, n. sebaceus of Jadassohn,** a syndrome characterized by single or linear hamartomas of the scalp, face, or neck that change progressively throughout life; many patients have neurologic symptoms (retardation or seizures) or ophthalmologic abnormalities. In children there are yellow or tan waxy patches with hypoplastic sebaceous glands and hair follicles or with scalp alopecia. After puberty the patches become thickened and verrucous, often with papillomatous projections and hyperplastic sebaceous glands, papillary epidermal hyperplasia, and ectopic apocrine glands of the deep dermis. Later some lesions become nodular and may develop benign or malignant adnexal tumors or basal cell carcinoma. Called also *Feuerstein-Mims syndrome* and *linear sebaceous nevus syndrome.*

**spider n.,** vascular spider.

**n. spi'lus,** a smooth-surfaced, tan to brown, macular, epidermal, melanocytic nevus, which is speckled with smaller, darker macules.

**n. spi'lus tar'dus,** Becker's n.

**spindle and epithelioid cell n.,** a benign compound nevus usually seen in children before puberty, composed of spindle and epithelioid cells located mainly in the dermis, sometimes associated with large atypical cells and multinucleate cells, and having a close resemblance to malignant melanoma. It presents as a smooth to slightly scaly pink to red papule or nodule, often with surface telangiectasia. Called also *benign juvenile melanoma, compound melanocytoma, juvenile melanoma,* and *Spitz n.*

**Spitz n.,** spindle and epithelioid cell n.

**n. spongio'sus al'bus muco'sae,** white sponge n.

**stellar n.,** vascular spider.

**strawberry n.,** 1. see under *hemangioma.* 2. vascular n. 3. cavernous hemangioma.

**Sutton's n.,** halo n.

**n. uni'us la'teris,** a verrucous epidermal nevus, ranging from flesh-colored to yellowish brown, but sometimes more deeply pigmented, and occurring in a linear, unilaterally distributed pattern; on the extremities, the lesions usually follow the long axis and may be arranged in continuous or broken spiral streaks, bands, or patches, and on the trunk, they usually have a transverse orientation, as if along the distribution of the intercostal nerves.

**Unna's n.,** nuchal n.

**uveal n.,** a nevus of the uvea, often bilateral and sometimes premalignant; it may be present at birth but more often becomes clinically evident at puberty due to increased pigmentation.

**vascular n., n. vascula'ris, n. vasculo'sus,** a localized overgrowth of blood vessels that are dilated and have thin walls but are otherwise normal; characterized by areas of flat or elevated erythema of various sizes. According to one classification, nonacquired vascular spider, nevus flammeus, strawberry hemangioma, cavernous hemangioma, and lymphangioma circumscriptum are all types of vascular nevi. Called also *strawberry hemangioma, mark,* or *nevus.* Cf. *capillary hemangioma,* def. 1.

**white sponge n.,** a benign autosomal dominant disorder characterized by exuberant and spongy whiteness of the mucous membranes, especially of the oral mucosa, with gray-white, soft, and sometimes friable lesions with fissures and folds; it reaches maximal severity at adolescence or early adulthood without further progression. Called also *familial white folded mucosal dysplasia* and *n. spongiosus albus mucosae.*

**new·born** (noo'born) [MeSH: Infant, Newborn] 1. recently born. 2. newborn infant; see under *infant.*

**New·cas·tle disease** (noo'kas-əl) [*Newcastle,* England, near which it was first observed in 1926] [MeSH: Newcastle Disease] see under *disease.*

**New·ton's law** (noo'tənz) [Sir Isaac *Newton,* English mathematician, physicist, and astronomer, 1643–1727] see under *law.*

**new·ton** (noo'tən) [Sir Isaac *Newton*] the SI unit of force which, when applied in a vacuum to a body having a mass of one kilogram, accelerates it at the rate of one meter per second squared. Symbol, N.

**nex·in** (nek'sin) a substance which serves as a connecting link between the outer pairs of microtubules in cilia and flagella.

**nex·us** (nek'səs) pl. *nex'us* [L. "bond"] 1. a bond, especially one between members of a series or group. 2. gap junction.

**Ne·ze·lof's syndrome** (nĕ-zĕ-lofs') [Christian *Nezelof,* French pediatrician, born 1922] see under *syndrome.*

**NF** National Formulary.

**NF1** neurofibromatosis 1.

**NF2** neurofibromatosis 2.

**NFLPN** National Federation for Licensed Practical Nurses.

**ng** nanogram.

**NGF** nerve growth factor.

**NHC** National Health Council.

**NHLBI** National Heart, Lung, and Blood Institute.

**NHMRC** National Health and Medical Research Council.

**NHS** National Health Service (British).

**$NH_2$-ter·mi·nal** (ter'mĭ-nəl) N-terminal.

**Ni** symbol for *nickel.*

**NIA** National Institute on Aging.

**NIAAA** National Institute on Alcohol Abuse and Alcoholism.

**ni·a·cin** (ni'ə-sin) [USP] [MeSH: Niacin] nicotinic acid, a B complex vitamin that is a constituent of the redox coenzymes nicotinamide adenine dinucleotide (NAD) and nicotinamide adenine dinucleotide phosphate (NADP). Niacin and niacinamide are used for the prophylaxis and treatment of pellagra. Niacin, but not niacinamide, also acts as a vasodilator and to reduce plasma cholesterol and has been used for these effects.

**ni·a·cin·amide** (ni"ə-sin'ə-mīd) [USP] [MeSH: Niacinamide] nicotinamide, a B complex vitamin used in the prophylaxis and treatment of pellagra.

**NIAID** National Institute of Allergy and Infectious Diseases.

**ni·al·amide** (ni-al'ə-mīd) [MeSH: Nialamide] a monoamine oxidase inhibitor that has been used orally as an antidepressant.

**Ni·a·mid** (ni'ə-mid) trademark for a preparation of nialamide.

**NIAMSD** National Institute of Arthritis and Musculoskeletal and Skin Diseases.

**nib** (nib) the working part of a dental condenser, which corresponds to the blade in an excavating or cutting instrument. Called also *condenser point.*

**Nic·a·lex** (nik'ə-leks) trademark for a preparation of aluminum nicotinate.

**ni·car·ba·zin** (ni-kahr'bə-zin) [MeSH: Nicarbazin] a coccidiostat used in poultry.

**ni·car·di·pine hy·dro·chlo·ride** (ni-kahr'dĭ-pēn) a calcium channel blocker structurally related to nifedipine that acts as a vasodilator; administered orally in the treatment of angina and hypertension.

**nic·co·lum** (nik'o-ləm) gen. *nic'coli* [L.] nickel.

**niche** (nich) [Fr. "recess"] a defect in an otherwise even surface, especially a depression or recess in the wall of an organ as seen on a radiograph or by the unaided eye.
**Barclay's n.,** a deformity of the duodenal cap in a duodenal ulcer, seen as a projection on the radiograph.
**ecologic n.,** the place of an organism within its community or ecosystem.
**Haudek's n.,** see under *sign.*
**n. of round window,** fossula fenestrae cochleae.

**nick** (nik) a break in just one strand of a double-stranded nucleic acid.

**NICHHD** National Institute of Child Health and Human Development.

**nick·el** (nik'əl) [L. *niccolum*] [MeSH: Nickel] a silver-white metallic element: symbol, Ni; specific gravity, 8.9; atomic number, 28; atomic weight, 58.71. Long-term excessive exposure to metallic nickel, such as on jewelry, can cause contact dermatitis *(nickel dermatitis);* excessive exposure to nickel fumes can cause nasal cancer and lung cancer.
**n. carbonyl,** a combination of nickel and carbonyl ions, produced in the refining of nickel; it is extremely toxic, causing pulmonary edema and dyspnea, and carcinogenic, causing lung and nasal cancers.

**nick·ing** (nik'ing) localized constrictions in the retinal blood vessels seen in arterial hypertension.

**ni·clo·sa·mide** (nĭ-klo'sə-mīd) [MeSH: Niclosamide] a salicylanilide anthelmintic effective against the tapeworms *Diphyllobothrium latum, Hymenolepis nana, Taenia saginata,* and the adults of *Taenia solium;* administered orally to humans, cats, and dogs.

**Nic·ol prism** (nik'ol) [William *Nicol,* Scottish physicist, 1768–1851] see under *prism.*

**Ni·co·la·do·ni's sign** (nik-o-lə-do'nēz) [Carl *Nicoladoni,* German surgeon, 1847–1902] Branham's sign; see under *sign.*

**Ni·co·las-Fa·vre disease** (ne-ko-lah'fahv'rə) [Joseph *Nicolas,* French physician, 1868–1960; Maurice Jules *Favre,* French physician, 1876–1954] lymphogranuloma venereum.

**Ni·colle** (ne-kol') Charles Jules Henri. French physician and microbiologist, 1866–1936; winner of the Nobel prize for medicine or physiology in 1928 for his demonstration of the transmission of typhus by the body louse.

**Ni·co·nyl** (ni'ko-nəl) trademark for a preparation of isoniazid.

**Nic·o·rette** (nik'o-ret") trademark for a chewing gum containing nicotine polacrilex.

**Nic·o·ti·a·na** (nik"o-she-a'nə) [Jean *Nicot* de Villemain, 1530–1600, who introduced tobacco chewing to the queen of France] a genus of annual plants of the family Solanaceae, native to tropical America. *N. taba'cum* L. and certain other species are sources of tobacco.

**nic·o·tin·a·mide** (nik"o-tin'ə-mīd) niacinamide.
**n. adenine dinucleotide (NAD),** a coenzyme composed of nicotinamide mononucleotide (NMN) coupled to adenosine monophosphate (AMP) by pyrophosphate linkage. It is found widely in nature and is involved in numerous enzymatic reactions in which it serves as an electron carrier by being alternately oxidized ($NAD^+$) and reduced (NADH). Formerly called also *diphosphopyridine nucleotide (DPN).*
**n. adenine dinucleotide phosphate (NADP),** a coenzyme composed of nicotinamide mononucleotide (NMN) coupled by pyrophosphate linkage to the 5′-phosphate of adenosine 2′,5′-bisphosphate. It serves as an electron carrier in numerous reactions, being alternately oxidized ($NADP^+$) and reduced (NADPH). Formerly called also *triphosphopyridine nucleotide (TPN).*
**n. mononucleotide (NMN),** a nucleotide containing covalently linked nicotinamide and ribose 5-phosphate. It is a constituent of NAD and NADP.

**nic·o·tin·ate** (nik"o-tin'āt) the dissociated form of nicotinic acid.
**n. ribonucleotide,** nicotinic acid coupled to ribose 5′-phosphate via an amino linkage; it is an intermediate in the synthesis of NAD.

**nic·o·tine** (nik'o-tēn, nik'o-tin) [L. *nicotiana* tobacco] [USP] [MeSH: Nicotine] a very poisonous, colorless, soluble fluid alkaloid with a pyridine-like odor and a burning taste, obtained from tobacco or produced synthetically. It is used as an agricultural insecticide, in veterinary medicine as an external parasiticide, and in pharmacological and physiological studies for its neurological effects. See also *nicotinic.*
**n. polacrilex** [USP], nicotine bound to an ion exchange resin; used in nicotine chewing gum as an aid to smoking cessation.
**n. sulfate,** the sulfate salt of nicotine, formerly a component of veterinary vermifuges; it can cause poisoning in lambs and calves. See *nicotine sulfate poisoning,* under *poisoning.*

**nic·o·tin·ic** (nik"o-tin'ik) denoting the effect of nicotine and other drugs in initially stimulating and subsequently, in high doses, inhibiting neural impulses at autonomic ganglia and the neuromuscular junction. See also *nicotinic receptors,* under *receptor.*

**nic·o·tin·ic ac·id** (nik"o-tin'ik) niacin.

**nic·o·tin·ism** (nik'o-tin-iz"əm) nicotine poisoning.

**nic·o·tino·lyt·ic** (nik"o-tin-o-lit'ik) [*nicotine* + *-lytic*] destroying or suppressing the toxic action of nicotine.

**β-nic·o·ty·rine** (nik"o-ti'rēn) an alkaloid from tobacco, which occurs as an oily liquid with a characteristic odor, and has insecticidal properties.

**ni·cou·ma·lone** (ni-koo'mə-lōn) acenocoumarol.

**Nic·o·zide** (nik'o-zīd) trademark for preparations of isoniazid.

**nic·ta·tion** (nik-ta′shən) nictitation.

**nic·ti·ta·tion** (nik″tĭ-ta′shən) [L. *nictitare* to wink] the act of winking.

**NIDA** National Institute on Drug Abuse.

**ni·dal** (ni′dəl) pertaining to a nidus.

**ni·da·tion** (ni-da′shən) [L. *nidus* nest] implantation (def. 1).

**NIDD** non–insulin-dependent diabetes mellitus; see *type 2 diabetes mellitus,* under *diabetes.*

**NIDDK** National Institute of Diabetes and Digestive and Kidney Diseases.

**NIDDM** non–insulin-dependent diabetes mellitus; see *type 2 diabetes mellitus,* under *diabetes.*

**ni·di** (ni′di) [L.] plural of *nidus.*

**NIDCR** National Institute of Dental and Craniofacial Research.

**ni·dus** (ni′dəs) pl. *ni′di* [L. "nest"] 1. the point of origin or focus of a morbid process. 2. nucleus, def. 2.
**n. a′vis,** a depression in the cerebellum between the posterior velum and the uvula, the location of the tonsil of the cerebellum.

**NIEHS** National Institute of Environmental Health Sciences.

**Niel·sen method** (nēl′sen) [Holger *Nielsen,* Danish army officer, 1866–1955] see *artificial respiration,* under *respiration.*

**Nie·mann's disease** (ne′mahnz) [Albert *Niemann,* German pediatrician, 1880–1921] Niemann-Pick disease.

**Niemann-Pick cells, disease** (ne′mahn-pik) [A. *Niemann;* Ludwig *Pick,* German physician, 1868–1944] see under *cell* and *disease.*

**ni·fed·i·pine** (ni-fed′ĭ-pēn) [MeSH: Nifedipine] a calcium channel blocker used as a coronary vasodilator in the treatment of coronary insufficiency and angina of effort; also used as an antihypertensive. Administered orally.

**ni·fun·gin** (ni-fun′jin) an antifungal polypeptide derived from *Aspergillus giganteus.*

**ni·fur·ox·ime** (ni″fūr-ok′sēm) a fungicide used in combination with furazolidone (an antibacterial and antiprotozoal agent) in the treatment of bacterial, candidal, and trichomonal vaginitis due to susceptible organisms, administered intravaginally.

**ni·fur·sem·i·zone** (ni″fūr-sem′ĭ-zōn) an antiprotozoal effective against *Histomonas;* used in poultry.

**ni·fur·sol** (ni′fūr-sol) an antiprotozoal effective against *Histomonas;* used in poultry.

**ni·fur·ti·mox** (ni-fūr′tĭ-moks) [MeSH: Nifurtimox] an antitrypanosomal used in the treatment of acute and chronic Chagas' disease.

**night·mare** (nīt′mār) [MeSH: Dreams] a terrifying dream; an anxiety attack during dreaming, accompanied by mild autonomic reactions and usually awakening the dreamer, who recalls the dream but is oriented.

**night·shade** (nīt′shād) 1. any of several flowering plants of the genus *Solanum.* 2. deadly n.; see *belladonna.*
**deadly n.,** belladonna (def. 1).

**NIGMS** National Institute of General Medical Sciences.

**ni·gra** (ni′grə) [L. "black"] the substantia nigra.

**ni·gral** (ni′grəl) pertaining to the substantia nigra.

**ni·gri·cans** (ni′grĭ-kəns) [L.] blackish.

**ni·gri·ti·es** (ni-grish′e-ēz) [L.] blackness.
**n. lin′guae,** black tongue.

**ni·gro·pal·li·dal** (ni″gro-pal′ĭ-dəl) pertaining to the substantia nigra and the globus pallidus.

**ni·gro·sin** (ni′gro-sin) an aniline dye having a special affinity for ganglion cells, used to stain tissues from the central nervous system for study under the microscope.

**ni·gro·stri·a·tal** (ni″gro-stri-a′təl) projecting from the substantia nigra to the corpus striatum; said of a bundle of nerve fibers.

**NIH** National Institutes of Health.

**ni·hil·ism** (ni′il-iz-əm) [L. *nihil* nothing + *-ism*] 1. an attitude of skepticism regarding traditional values and beliefs or their frank rejection. 2. a delusion of nonexistence of part or all of the self or the world.
**therapeutic n.,** skepticism regarding the therapeutic value of drugs or treatment procedures.

**ni·keth·a·mide** (nĭ-keth′ə-mīd) [MeSH: Nikethamide] a central and respiratory stimulant used to counteract respiratory and central nervous system depression and circulatory failure, administered intramuscularly and intravenously.

**Ni·ki·fo·roff's method** (ne-ke′fə-rofs) [Mikhail *Nikiforoff,* Russian dermatologist, 1858–1915] see under *method.*

**Ni·kol·sky's sign** (nĭ-kol′skēz) [Petr Vasilyevich *Nikolsky,* Russian dermatologist, 1858–1940] see under *sign.*

**Ni·lan·dron** (nĭ-lan′drən) trademark for a preparation of nilutamide.

**Ni·le·var** (ni′lə-vahr) trademark for preparations of norethandrolone.

**ni·lu·ta·mide** (nĭ-loo′tə-mīd) a nonsteroidal anti-androgen used as an antineoplastic in treatment of prostatic carcinoma; administered orally.

**Nim·bex** (nim′beks) trademark for a preparation of cisatracurium besylate.

**NIMH** National Institute of Mental Health.

**nim·i·dane** (nim′ĭ-dān) a veterinary acaricide.

**ni·mo·di·pine** (ni-mo′dĭ-pēn) [MeSH: Nimodipine] a calcium channel blocker structurally related to nifedipine, used as a vasodilator in the treatment of cerebral arterial spasm following subarachnoid hemorrhage from a ruptured intracranial aneurysm; administered orally.

**Ni·mo·top** (ni′mo-top) trademark for a preparation of nimodipine.

**NINDS** National Institute of Neurological Disorders and Stroke.

**Nin·hy·drin** (nin-hi′drin) [MeSH: Ninhydrin] trademark for a preparation of triketohydrindene hydrate.

**NINR** National Institute for Nursing Research.

**ni·o·bi·um** (ni-o′be-əm) [named for *Niobe,* of Greek mythology, who was turned into stone] [MeSH: Niobium] chemical element, atomic number, 41; atomic weight, 92.906; symbol, Nb.

**Ni·o·nate** (ni′o-nāt) trademark for a preparation of ferrous gluconate.

**NIOSH** National Institute for Occupational Safety and Health.

**Ni·pent** (ni′pent) trademark for a preparation of pentostatin.

**ni·per·yt** (ni′pər-it) pentaerythritol tetranitrate.

**nip·pers** (nip′ərz) pincers, def. 2.

**nip·ple** (nip′əl) [MeSH: Nipples] 1. papilla mammae. 2. any structure shaped like the papilla mammae.

**Nip·po·stron·gy·lus** (nip″o-stron′jə-ləs) [MeSH: Nippostrongylus]

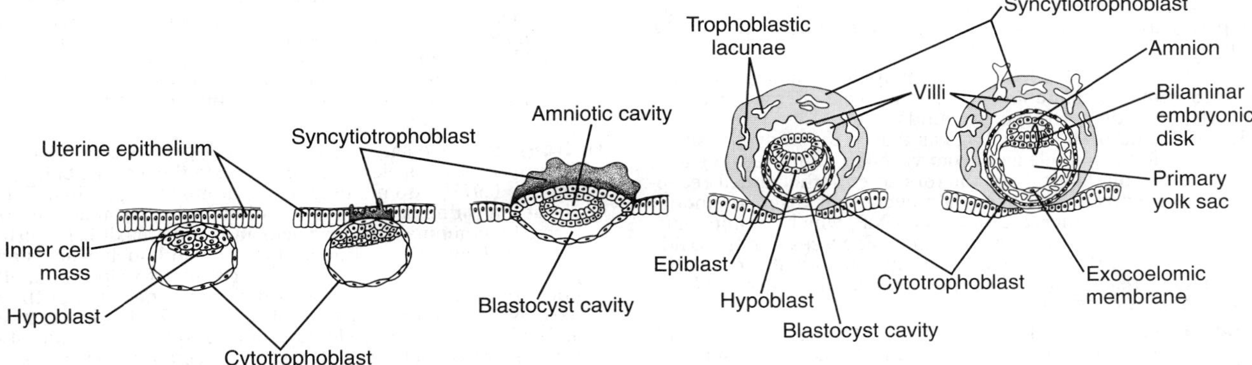


Nidation, occurring over the period between 7 to 10 days after fertilization.

a genus of hookworms of the family Trichostrongylidae. *N. mu'ris* parasitizes rats.

**Nip·ride** (nip'rid) trademark for a preparation of sodium nitroprusside.

**Nir·en·berg** (nir'ən-bərg) Marshall Warren. American biochemist, born 1927; co-winner, with Robert William Holley and Har Gobind Khorana, of the Nobel prize for medicine or physiology in 1968 for their interpretation of the genetic code and its function in protein synthesis.

**ni·rid·a·zole** (nĭ-rid'ə-zōl) [MeSH: Niridazole] an antischistosomal also used in the treatment of intestinal and extraintestinal amebiasis and in dracunculiasis, administered orally.

**ni·sin** (ni'sin) [MeSH: Nisin] a polypeptide antibiotic produced by *Streptococcus lactis* and occurring naturally in certain cheeses. Nisin is active against certain streptococci, *Mycobacterium tuberculosis,* and several other bacteria.

**ni·sol·di·pine** (ni-sol'dĭ-pēn) a calcium channel blocker used in the treatment of hypertension; administered orally.

**Nis·sen operation** (nis'en) [Rudolf *Nissen,* Swiss surgeon, born 1896] see under *fundoplication.*

**Nis·sl bodies (granules, substance), degeneration, method of staining** (nis'əl) [Franz *Nissl,* German neurologist, 1860–1919] see under *body, degeneration,* and *stain.*

**ni·sus** (ni'səs) [L., from *niti* to strive] an effort, strong tendency, or molimen.

**nit** (nit) the egg of a louse.

**Ni·ta·buch's layer (stria, zone)** (ne'tah-books) [Raissa *Nitabuch,* German physician, 19th century] see under *layer.*

**ni·tar·sone** (nĭ-tahr'sōn) an antiprotozoal effective against *Histomonas;* used in poultry.

**ni·ta·zox·a·nide** (ni″tə-zok'sə-nīd) an antimicrobial used in the treatment of cryptosporidiosis in patients with HIV infection and acquired immunodeficiency syndrome.

**ni·ter** (ni'tər) potassium nitrate.

**ni·ti·nol** (ni'tĭ-nol) any of several alloys of nickel and titanium that are resistant to fatigue, have low moduli of elasticity, and return to their original shape after deformation if they are heated; used in orthodontic materials.

**ni·tram·ine** (ni-tram'in) a nitro derivative of an amine, having the group $—NNO_2$.

**ni·trate** (ni'trāt) any salt or ester of nitric acid or the $NO_3^-$ anion; organic nitrates, e.g., nitroglycerin, are used as coronary vasodilators in the treatment of angina pectoris.

**ni·trate re·duc·tase** (ni'trāt re-duk'tās) any of several enzymes occurring in plants and some bacteria and catalyzing the reduction of nitrate to nitrite. The reaction allows plants to use the nitrogen from nitrate for protein synthesis and allows some bacteria, under certain conditions, to use nitrate as a terminal electron acceptor in respiration. A test for nitrate reduction in a bacterial culture is useful in identification of Enterobacteriaceae, mycobacteria, and certain anaerobic bacteria.

**ni·tra·ze·pam** (ni-traz'ə-pam) [MeSH: Nitrazepam] a benzodiazepine tranquilizer used as a sedative and anticonvulsant; administered orally.

**ni·tre** (ni'tər) [L. *nitrum;* Gr. *nitron*] potassium nitrate.
**cubic n.,** sodium nitrate.

**ni·tre·mia** (ni-tre'me-ə) azotemia.

**ni·tren·di·pine** (ni-tren'dĭ-pēn) [MeSH: Nitrendipine] a calcium channel blocker chemically related to nifedipine, used as an antihypertensive and administered orally; its predominant effects are in the peripheral circulation, reducing both systolic and diastolic pressures.

**ni·tric** (ni'trik) pertaining to or containing nitrogen, applied especially to compounds containing nitrogen with a higher valence than that contained in the nitrous compounds.
**n. oxide,** NO; a naturally-occurring gas that in the body is a short-lived dilator substance released from vascular endothelial cells in response to the binding of vasodilators to endothelial cell receptors; it causes activation of guanylate cyclase in vascular smooth muscle, leading to an increase in cyclic GMP, which inhibits muscular contraction and produces relaxation. Excesses of nitric oxide are toxic to cells of the central nervous system and also cause the drop in blood pressure seen in septic shock. Called also *endothelium-derived relaxing factor.*

**ni·tric ac·id** (ni'trik) [MeSH: Nitric Acid] a strong mineral acid, $HNO_3$, an extremely corrosive liquid with a characteristic suffocating odor; it is a strong oxidizing agent that is highly toxic by inhalation and corrosive to skin and mucous membranes.
**fuming n. a.,** nitric acid containing dissolved oxides of nitrogen; it is a very strong oxidizing agent.

**ni·tri·da·tion** (ni″trĭ-da'shən) combination with nitrogen to form a nitride.

**ni·tride** (ni'trīd) a binary compound of nitrogen with a metal.

**ni·tri·fi·ca·tion** (ni″trĭ-fĭ-ka'shən) [*nitric acid* + L. *facere* to make] oxidation of the nitrogen in ammonia and organic compounds to nitrites and to nitrates, carried out by soil bacteria of the family Nitrobacteraceae.

**ni·tri·fi·er** (ni'trĭ-fi″ər) a nitrifying microorganism.

**ni·tri·fy·ing** (ni'trĭ-fi″ing) oxidizing ammonia to nitrite (nitrosification) and then to nitrate.

**ni·trile** (ni'tril) an organic compound containing trivalent nitrogen attached to one carbon atom, —C≡N.

**ni·trilo·tri·ace·tic ac·id** (ni″tril-o-tri-ə-se'tik) [MeSH: Nitrilotriacetic Acid] a chelating agent found in synthetic detergents; in excessive amounts it is an epigenetic carcinogen for kidney and bladder cancer.

**ni·trite** (ni'trīt) any salt or ester of nitrous acid or the $NO_2^-$ anion; organic nitrites, e.g., amyl nitrite, are used as coronary vasodilators in the treatment of angina pectoris.

**ni·tri·toid** (ni'trĭ-toid) resembling a nitrite or the reaction caused by a nitrite.

**ni·tri·tu·ria** (ni″trĭ-tu're-ə) the presence of nitrites in the urine.

**nitro-** a prefix indicating presence of the group $—NO_2$.

**ni·tro·amine** (ni'tro-ə-mēn″) nitramine.

**ni·tro·an·i·line** (ni″tro-an'ĭ-līn) a dye used in paints, paint removers, inks, and solvents; excessive exposure can cause nitroaniline poisoning.

**Ni·tro·bac·te·ra·ceae** (ni″tro-bak″te-ra'se-e) [MeSH: Nitrobacteraceae] a family of soil bacteria, consisting of gram-negative chemolithotrophic organisms that oxidize ammonia or nitrites, commonly known as the nitrifying bacteria.

**ni·tro·bac·te·ria** (ni″tro-bak-te're-ə) plural of *nitrobacterium.*

**ni·tro·bac·te·ri·um** (ni″tro-bak-tēr'e–əm) pl. *nitrobacte'ria* [*nitro-* + *bacterium*] a bacterium that oxidizes nitrites to nitrates.

**ni·tro·ben·zene** (ni″tro-ben'zēn) a poisonous benzene derivative used in the manufacture of aniline. Called also *nitrobenzol* and *oil of mirbane.*

**ni·tro·ben·zol** (ni″tro-ben'zol) nitrobenzene.

**ni·tro·blue te·tra·zo·li·um** (ni'tro-bloo tet″rə-zo'le-əm) [MeSH: Nitroblue Tetrazolium] a yellow water-soluble dye that on reduction is converted to a dark blue water-insoluble formazan; see also under *tests.*

**ni·tro·cel·lu·lose** (ni″tro-sel'u-lōs) pyroxylin.

**Ni·tro-Dur** (ni'tro-dər) trademark for a preparation of nitroglycerin.

**ni·tro·fu·ran** (ni″tro-fu'ran) any of a group of antibacterials, including furazolidone, nitrofurazone, nitrofurantoin, and related compounds, which are effective against a wide range of bacteria.

**ni·tro·fu·ran·to·in** (ni″tro-fu-ran'to-in) [USP] [MeSH: Nitrofurantoin] a synthetic antibacterial effective against many gram-negative and gram-positive organisms, including *Escherichia coli, Staphylococcus pyogenes, Streptococcus pyogenes, Aerobacter aerogenes,* and *Paracolobactrum* species; used in the treatment of urinary tract infections due to susceptible bacteria, administered orally.

**ni·tro·fu·ra·zone** (ni″tro-fu'rə-zōn) [MeSH: Nitrofurazone] an antibacterial effective against a wide variety of gram-negative and gram-positive organisms. It is used topically as a local anti-infective in skin lesions including wounds, burns, skin infections, and ulcers; to aid healing and prevent infection of skin grafts; and in the treatment of otitis media and externa, urethritis, and eye infections. It has also been used orally in the treatment of African trypanosomiasis.

**ni·tro·gen** (ni'tro-jən) [Gr. *nitron* niter + *-gen*] [MeSH: Nitrogen] 1. a colorless, gaseous element found free in the air; symbol, N; specific gravity, 0.9713; atomic number, 7; atomic weight, 14.007. It forms about four fifths of common air. Chemically it is almost inert, but it forms by combination nitric acid and ammonia. It is important biologically, being a constituent of protein and nucleic acids and thus present in all living cells. It will not support respiration; although not a poison, it is fatal if breathed alone, because of the lack of oxygen. It is soluble in the blood and body fluids and when released as bubbles of gas by reduction of atmospheric pressure it causes serious or even fatal symptoms (see *decompression sickness,* under *sickness*). 2. [NF] the official preparation, not less than 99 per cent $N_2$ by volume; used to replace air in pharmaceutical preparations.

**n. 13,** a radioactive isotope of nitrogen, atomic mass 13, having a half-life of 9.97 minutes; it decays by positron emission (1.190 MeV) and is used as a tracer in positron emission tomography.
**amide n.,** that portion of the nitrogen in protein that exists in the form of acid amides.
**n. dioxide,** a brownish, irritant gas, $NO_2$, generated by the decomposition of nitrogen tetroxide or the reaction of metals with concentrated nitric acid. Exposure to heavy concentrations causes lung damage with coughing, dyspnea, and acute bronchiolitis. See also *silo filler's lung,* under *lung.*
**n. mustards,** see under *mustard.*
**nomadic n.,** free nitrogen from the air which enters into plant and animal growth.
**nonprotein n.,** the nitrogenous constituents of the blood exclusive of the protein bodies. It consists of the nitrogen of urea, uric acid, creatine, creatinine, amino acids, polypeptides, and an undetermined part known as *rest nitrogen.*
**n. pentoxide,** a crystalline compound, $N_2O_5$, or nitric anhydride, which combines with water to form nitric acid.
**n. peroxide,** n. tetroxide.
**rest n.,** see *nonprotein n.*
**n. tetroxide,** a poisonous volatile liquid, $N_2O_4$; at room temperature it decomposes to nitrogen dioxide (q.v.). Called also *n. peroxide.*
**urea n.,** see under *urea.*

**ni·tro·gen·ase** (ni'tro-jən-ās) [MeSH: Nitrogenase] an enzyme system of nitrogen-fixing bacteria and blue-green algae that catalyzes the reduction of molecular nitrogen ($N_2$) to ammonia ($NH_3$).

**ni·tro·gen-fix·ing** (ni'tro-jən-fik'sing) accomplishing nitrogen fixation (see under *fixation* ); said of certain bacteria.

**ni·trog·e·nous** (ni-troj'ə-nəs) containing nitrogen.

**ni·tro·glyc·er·in** (ni″tro-glis'ər-in) [MeSH: Nitroglycerin] 1. a colorless to yellow liquid formed by the action of nitric and sulfuric acids on glycerine. It explodes on concussion, but is rendered safe when compounded in tablets with mannitol. 2. [USP] the official preparation of nitroglycerine, having antianginal, antihypertensive, and vasodilator properties; used in medicine chiefly in the prophylaxis and treatment of angina pectoris, administered sublingually.

**Ni·tro·glyn** (ni'tro-glin) trademark for a preparation of nitroglycerin.

**ni·tro·hy·dro·chlo·ric ac·id** (ni″tro-hi″dro-klor'ik) aqua regia.

**Ni·trol** (ni'trol) trademark for preparations of nitroglycerin.

**ni·tro·man·nite** (ni″tro-man'īt) mannitol hexanitrate.

**ni·tro·mer·sol** (ni″tro-mer'sol) [USP] a mercurial compound used as a local anti-infective; applied in solution topically to the skin and mucous membranes. It is also used to disinfect surgical and dental instruments.

**ni·trom·e·ter** (ni-trom'ə-tər) [*nitrogen* + *-meter*] an apparatus for measuring the quantity of nitrogen given off in a reaction.

**ni·tro·naph·tha·lene** (ni″tro-naf'thə-lēn) a compound, used in the alpha form to mask fluorescence in mineral oils and in dye manufacture; its vapors may cause vesication and opacity of the cornea. The beta form is highly toxic by ingestion.

**ni·tro·naph·tha·lin** (ni″tro-naf'thə-lin) nitronaphthalene.

**ni·tro·phe·nol** (ni″tro-fe'nol) an indicator with a pH range of 5 to 7, being colorless at 5 and yellow at 7.

**2-ni·tro·pro·pane** (ni″tro-pro'pān) a flammable yellow liquid prepared by the reaction of propane with nitric acid under pressure; used as a solvent, rocket propellant, and gasoline additive. It is carcinogenic.

**ni·tro·pro·tein** (ni″tro-pro'tēn) a nitrated protein made by treating serum protein with nitric acid.

**ni·tro·prus·side** (ni″tro-prus'īd) [MeSH: Nitroprusside] the anion $[Fe(CN_5)NO]^{2-}$; see *sodium nitroprusside,* under *sodium.*

**ni·tro·sac·cha·rose** (ni″tro-sak'ə-rōs) nitrated sucrose, an explosive and vasodilator used like nitroglycerin.

**ni·tros·amine** (ni-trōs'ə-mēn) any of a group of *N*-nitroso derivatives of secondary amines ($R_2N$—NO), formed by the combining of nitrates with amines; some nitrosamines show carcinogenic activity. Under certain conditions, nitrite-containing foods can form nitrosamines in the mammalian stomach, causing hepatotoxicity and other symptoms.

**ni·tro·sate** (ni'tro-sāt) to convert into a nitroso compound.

**ni·tro·sa·tion** (ni″tro-sa'shən) [MeSH: Nitrosation] conversion into a nitroso compound.

**ni·tro·scan·ate** (ni″tro-skan'āt) an anthelmintic used in dogs.

**ni·trose** (ni'trōs) a term used to include nitric and nitrous acids.

**ni·tro·si·fi·ca·tion** (ni-tro″sĭ-fĭ-ka'shən) the oxidation of ammonia into nitrites.

**ni·tro·si·fy·ing** (ni-tro'sĭ-fi″ing) oxidizing ammonia into nitrites; said of certain bacteria of the family Nitrobacteraceae.

**nitroso-** a prefix indicating presence of the group —NO.

**ni·tro·so·bac·te·ria** (ni-tro″so-bak-te're-ə) plural of *nitrosobacterium.*

**ni·tro·so·bac·te·ri·um** (ni-tro″so-bak-te're-əm) pl. *nitrosobacte'ria.* a bacterium that oxidizes ammonia to nitrites.

***N*-ni·tro·so·di·meth·yl·amine** (ni-tro″so-di-meth'əl-ə-mēn″) a yellow liquid nitrosamine formerly used in rocket fuels, as an antioxidant, and for other purposes; it is sometimes found as a contaminant in fish meal, causing hepatotoxicity and carcinogenesis in humans or animals that eat the meal. Called also *dimethylnitrosamine.*

***N*-ni·tro·so·di·phen·yl·amine** (ni-tro″so-di-fen'əl-ə-mēn″) a bicyclic nitrosamine used as an accelerator in the vulcanization of rubber; it is carcinogenic. Called also *diphenylnitrosamine.*

**ni·tro·so·sub·sti·tu·tion** (ni-tro″so-sub″stĭ-too'shən) the substitution of the radical nitryl for some other radical or atom in a compound.

**ni·tro·so·urea** (ni-tro″so-u're-ə) any of several chemically related antineoplastic agents including carmustine, lomustine, semustine, and the antibiotic streptozocin. Carmustine, lomustine, and semustine are closely related chemically, are highly lipid-soluble, cross the blood-brain barrier, and are used against brain tumors; they act by alkylation, carbamoylation, and inhibition of DNA repair; they are not cross resistant with other alkylating agents and are highly effective against resting ($G_0$) cells; the major side effect is dose-limiting bone marrow suppression. Streptozocin differs from the others in that it is not cross resistant with them, is not myelosuppressive, and does not act by carbamoylation.

**Ni·tro·stat** (ni'tro-stat) trademark for a preparation of nitroglycerin.

**ni·tro·sug·ars** (ni″tro-shoog'ərz) a class of substances which have been used in the treatment of angina pectoris.

**ni·tro·syl** (ni'tro-səl) the univalent radical NO.

**ni·trous** (ni'trəs) pertaining to nitrogen in its lowest valency.

**ni·trous ac·id** (ni'trəs) [MeSH: Nitrous Acid] a weak acid, $HNO_2$, existing only in aqueous solution.

**Ni·tro·vas** (ni'tro-vas) trademark for a preparation of nitroglycerin.

**ni·tro·xan·thic ac·id** (ni″tro-zan'thik) trinitrophenol.

**ni·trox·yl** (ni-trok'səl) nitryl.

**ni·tryl** (ni'trəl) the radical $NO_2$.

**Nitzs·chia** (nich'e-ə) a genus of marine diatoms; *N. pun'gens* is a source of the neurotoxin domoic acid.

**Nix** (niks) trademark for a preparation of permethrin.

**ni·za·ti·dine** (nĭ-za'tĭ-dēn) [USP] [MeSH: Nizatidine] an antagonist to histamine $H_2$ receptors, used to inhibit gastric acid secretion in the treatment of gastric and duodenal ulcer, gastroesophageal reflux, and conditions that cause gastric hypersecretion; administered orally.

**Ni·zo·ral** (ni'zor-al) trademark for preparations of ketoconazole.

**nl** nanoliter.

**NLN** National League for Nursing.

**Nm.** abbreviation for L. *nux moscha'ta,* nutmeg.

**nm** nanometer.

**NMA** National Medical Association.

**NMDA** *N*-methyl-D-aspartate.

**NMN** nicotinamide mononucleotide.

**NMR** nuclear magnetic resonance.

**NMRI** Naval Medical Research Institute, part of the National Naval Medical Center.

**NMS** neuroleptic malignant syndrome.

**N-Mul·ti·stix** (mul'te-stiks) trademark for a reagent strip for testing urine specimens for protein, glucose, ketones, bilirubin, occult blood, urobilinogen, nitrite, and to indicate urinary pH.

**nn.** abbreviation for L. *nervi* (nerves).

**NND** *New and Nonofficial Drugs,* former annual publication of the American Medical Association containing descriptions of agents proposed for use in or on the human body in the prevention, diagnosis, or treatment of disease, which have been evaluated by the Council on Drugs of the AMA.

**No** symbol for *nobelium.*

**No.** abbreviation of L. *nu'mero,* "to the number of."

**No·ack's syndrome** (no'ahks) [Margot *Noack,* German physician, born 1909] acrocephalopolysyndactyly (type I).

**NOAEL** no observed adverse effect level.

**No·bel prize** (no-bel') [MeSH: Nobel Prize] an award usually given annually for outstanding achievement in chemistry, physics, medicine or physiology, literature, and in the interest of world peace. It was established under the terms of the will of the Swedish chemist and engineer Alfred Bernhard Nobel (1833–1896), and was first presented in 1901. An award for achievement in economics has since been added.

**no·bel·i·um** (no-bel'e-əm) [Alfred Bernhard *Nobel*] [MeSH: Nobelium] the chemical element of atomic number 102, atomic weight 253, symbol No, obtained in 1958 by bombardment of $^{246}$Cm with $^{12}$C ions in a heavy ion linear accelerator.

**No·ble's position** (no'bəlz) [Charles Percy *Noble,* American gynecologist, 1863–1935] see under *position.*

**No·car·dia** (no-kahr'de-ə) [Edmond Isidore Etienne *Nocard,* French veterinarian, 1850–1903] [MeSH: Nocardia] a genus of bacteria of the family Nocardiaceae, order Actinomycetales, separable into 30 or more species of which a few are pathogenic and the remainder saprophytic forms. They are gram-positive aerobes, found in the soil, with branching filaments that break into bacillary or coccal forms, and produce chains of spores by simple fragmentation of hyphal branches.
**N. asteroi'des,** an acid-fast filamentous actinomycete, the most common cause of nocardiosis, including pulmonary nocardiosis, in humans; it may also cause actinomycotic mycetoma in humans and nocardial mastitis in cattle.
**N. brasilien'sis,** an acid-fast pathogenic species that produces yellow to brown mycelium with branching filaments, found most commonly in the tropics. They are found in soil and cause nocardiosis and actinomycotic mycetoma in man. Called also *Actinomyces brasiliensis.*
**N. ca'viae,** *N. otitidis-caviarum.*
**N. coeli'aca,** a species that produces the antibiotic substance nocardin.
**N. farci'nica,** a species of acid-fast filamentous actinomycetes of uncertain classification, which may be identical to *N. asteroides;* it is the etiologic agent of bovine farcy and nocardial mastitis, as well as a cause of actinomycotic mycetoma. Called also *Streptothrix farcini* and *S. nocardii.*
**N. lu'tea,** a partially acid-fast species isolated from the lacrimal gland in actinomycosis. Called also *Actinomyces luteus.*
**N. madu'rae,** *Actinomadura madurae.*
**N. oti'tidis-cavia'rum,** a species of widespread distribution that sometimes causes nocardiosis and actinomycotic mycetoma in which the granules secreted in the pus are white. Called also *N. caviae.*

**No·car·di·a·ceae** (no-kahr"de-a'se-e) [MeSH: Nocardiaceae] a family of bacteria of the order Actinomycetales, consisting of the genera *Actinomadura, Nocardia,* and *Nocardiopsis.*

**no·car·di·al** (no-kahr'de-əl) pertaining to or caused by *Nocardia.*

**no·car·di·a·sis** (no"kahr-di'ə-sis) nocardiosis.

**no·car·din** (no-kahr'din) an antibiotic substance from *Nocardia coeliaca,* active against tubercle bacilli.

**no·car·dio·form** (no-kahr'de-o-form") characterized by a fugacious mycelium that breaks into bacillary or coccal forms.

**No·car·di·op·sis** (no-kahr"de-op'sis) a genus of soil bacteria of the family Nocardiaceae, order Actinomycetales, consisting of gram-positive, aerobic, non–acid-fast organisms that form filaments. The organisms resemble *Nocardia* but differ in cell wall type and are not resistant to lysozymes. They are potential pathogens, causing abscesses and pulmonary lesions. *N. dassonvil'lei* can sometimes cause actinomycotic mycetoma.

**no·car·di·o·sis** (no-kahr"de-o'sis) infection with a species of *Nocardia,* usually *N. asteroides,* but occasionally *N. brasiliensis* or *N. otitidis-caviarum;* it takes the form of an acute or chronic suppurative infection with abscess formation, usually of the lungs (see *pulmonary n.*), but with a marked tendency to spread to any organ of the body, especially the brain, skin, or subcutaneous tissues, and sometimes with a fatal outcome. Called also *nocardiasis.*
**bovine n.,** infection of cattle with species of *Nocardia;* see *bovine farcy* and *nocardial mastitis.*
**pulmonary n.,** lung infection with a species of *Nocardia;* it ranges from subclinical to a type of pneumonia with necrosis, cavitation, and abscess formation; it is most common in debilitated or immunocompromised patients. See also Nocardia *pneumonia.*

**Noch·tia** (nok'te-ə) a genus of small nematode worms. *N. noch'ti* infests the stomach of an Indonesian monkey, causing tumors.

**noci-** [L. *nocēre* to injure] a combining form denoting relationship to injury or to a noxious or deleterious agent or influence.

**no·ci·as·so·ci·a·tion** (no"se-ə-so"se-a'shən) the unconscious discharge of nervous energy under the stimulus of trauma, as in surgical shock.

**no·ci·cep·tion** (no"sĭ-sep'shən) pain sense.

**no·ci·cep·tive** (no"sĭ-sep'tiv) pertaining to a nociceptor.

**no·ci·cep·tor** (no"sĭ-sep'tər) [*noci-* + *-ceptor*] [MeSH: Nociceptors] a receptor for pain caused by injury to body tissues; the injury may be from physical stimuli such as mechanical, thermal, or electrical stimuli, or from chemical stimuli such as the presence of a toxin or an excess of a nontoxic substance. Most nociceptors are in either the skin *(cutaneous n's)* or the walls of viscera *(visceral n's).*
**C-fiber n.,** polymodal n.
**cutaneous n's,** nociceptors in the skin, responding to stimuli such as heat, chemicals, and mechanical displacement; the two most common kinds are *polymodal nociceptors* and *mechanical nociceptors.*
**mechanical n.,** a nociceptor of myelinated nerve fibers, activated primarily by strong mechanical displacement of the skin; called also *high-threshold mechanoreceptor.*
**polymodal n.,** a nociceptor of unmyelinated nerve fibers, activated by several different types of stimuli such as heat, mechanical pressure, or chemical mediators of inflammation as a result of tissue injury. Called also *C-fiber n.*

**no·ci·fen·sor** (no"se-fen'sor) [*noci-* + L. *fendere* to defend] protecting against injury; said of a system of nerves in the skin and mucous membranes which are concerned with local defense against injury.

**no·ci·in·flu·ence** (no"se-in'floo-əns) injurious or traumatic influence.

**no·ci·per·cep·tion** (no"sĭ-pər-sep'shən) pain sense.

**Noct.** abbreviation for L. *noc'te,* at night.

**noc·tal·bu·min·uria** (nok"təl-bu"mĭ-nu're-ə) [L. *nox* night + *albuminuria*] the presence of excessive amounts of albumin in the urine secreted during the night.

**noc·tam·bu·la·tion** (nok"tam-bu-la'shən) [L. *noctambulatio; nox* night + *ambulare* to walk] somnambulism.

**noc·tam·bu·lic** (nok"tam-bu'lik) pertaining to or marked by somnambulism.

**Noc·tec** (nok'tek) trademark for preparations of chloral hydrate.

**noc·ti·pho·bia** (nok"tĭ-fo'be-ə) [L. *nox* night + *-phobia*] irrational fear of night and darkness.

**Noct. maneq.** abbreviation for L. *noc'te mane'que,* at night and in the morning.

**noc·tu·ria** (nok-tu're-ə) [L. *nox* night + *-uria*] excessive urination at night; called also *nycturia.*

**noc·tur·nal** (nok-tur'nəl) [L. *nocturnus*] pertaining to, occurring at, or active at night.

**no·dal** (no'dəl) pertaining to a node, particularly the atrioventricular node.

**node** (nōd) [L. *nodus* knot] 1. a small mass of tissue in the form of a swelling, knot, or protuberance, either normal or pathological. 2. in fungi, a swelling on a stolon where the rhizomes arise. See Plate 29.

## Node

For descriptions of specific anatomic structures not found here, see under *nodus.*

**abdominal lymph n's, parietal,** nodi lymphoidei abdominis parietales.
**abdominal lymph n's, visceral,** nodi lymphoidei abdominis viscerales.
**accessory lymph n's,** nodi lymphoidei accessorii.
**anorectal lymph n's,** nodi lymphoidei pararectales.
**n. of anterior border of epiploic foramen,** nodus lymphoideus foraminalis.

**aortic lymph n's,** lumbar lymph n's.
**aortic lymph n's, lateral,** nodi lymphoidei aortici laterales.
**apical lymph n's,** nodi lymphoidei axillares apicales.
**appendicular lymph n's,** nodi lymphoidei appendiculares.
**Aschoff's n., n. of Aschoff and Tawara,** nodus atrioventricularis.
**atrioventricular n., AV n. (AVN),** nodus atrioventricularis.
**axillary lymph n's,** nodi lymphoidei axillares.
**axillary lymph n's, anterior,** nodi lymphoidei axillares pectorales.
**axillary lymph n's, apical,** nodi lymphoidei axillares apicales.
**axillary lymph n's, central,** nodi lymphoidei axillares centrales.
**axillary lymph n's, lateral,** nodi lymphoidei brachiales.
**axillary lymph n's, pectoral,** nodi lymphoidei axillares pectorales.
**axillary lymph n's, posterior, axillary lymph n's, subscapular,** nodi lymphoidei axillares subscapulares.
**Babès' n's,** see under *nodule.*
**Bouchard's n's,** cartilaginous and bony enlargements of the proximal interphalangeal joints of the fingers in degenerative joint disease. Such nodules in the distal interphalangeal joints are called *Heberden's n's.*

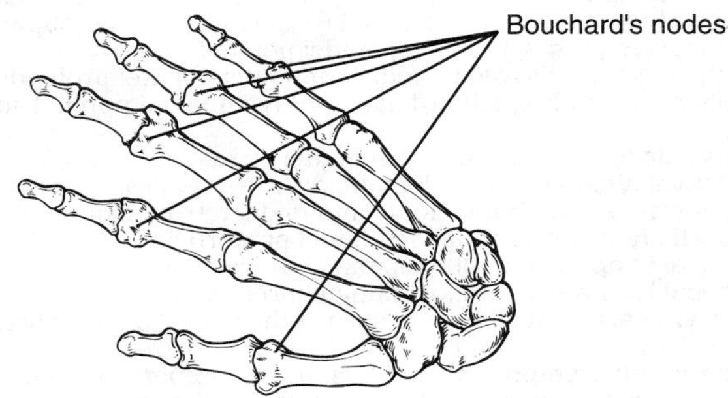


**brachial lymph n's,** nodi lymphoidei brachiales.
**bronchopulmonary lymph n's,** nodi lymphoidei bronchopulmonales.
**buccal lymph n., buccinator lymph n.,** nodus lymphoideus buccinatorius.
**caval lymph n's, lateral,** nodi lymphoidei cavales laterales.
**celiac lymph n's,** nodi lymphoidei coeliaci.
**central lymph n's,** nodi lymphoidei axillares centrales.
**cervical lymph n's, anterior,** nodi lymphoidei cervicales anteriores.
**cervical lymph n's, anterior superficial,** nodi lymphoidei cervicales anteriores superficiales.
**cervical lymph n's, deep anterior,** nodi lymphoidei cervicales anteriores profundi.
**cervical lymph n's, deep lateral,** nodi lymphoidei cervicales laterales profundi.
**cervical lymph n's, inferior deep,** nodi lymphoidei cervicales laterales profundi inferiores.
**cervical lymph n's, prelaryngeal,** nodi lymphoidei prelaryngeales.
**cervical lymph n's, superficial lateral,** nodi lymphoidei cervicales laterales superficiales.
**cervical lymph n's, superior deep,** nodi lymphoidei cervicales laterales profundi superiores.
**Cloquet's n., n. of Cloquet,** the highest of the deep inguinal lymph nodes; called also *Cloquet's gland.*
**colic lymph n's, right/middle/left,** nodi lymphoidei colici dextri/medii/sinistri.
**colic lymph n's, terminal,** lymph nodes associated with the main trunks of the superior and inferior mesenteric arteries, being continuous with the corresponding preaortic lymph nodes.
**cubital lymph n's,** nodi lymphoidei cubitales.
**cystic lymph n.,** nodus lymphoideus cysticus.
**Delphian n.,** a lymph node encased in the fascia in the midline, just anterior to the thyroid isthmus, so called because it is exposed first at surgery and, if diseased, is indicative of disease in the thyroid gland, but not of a specific disease process.
**deltoideopectoral lymph n's, deltopectoral lymph n's,** nodi lymphoidei deltopectorales.
**diaphragmatic lymph n's,** nodi lymphoidei phrenici superiores.
**Dürck's n's,** granulomatous perivascular infiltrations in the cerebral cortex in trypanosomiasis.
**epicolic lymph n's,** minute lymph nodes situated on the wall of the bowel and sometimes in the epiploic appendices.
**epigastric lymph n's, inferior,** nodi lymphoidei epigastrici inferiores.
**n. of epiploic foramen,** nodus lymphoideus foraminalis.
**epitrochlear lymph n's,** nodi lymphoidei cubitales.
**Ewald's n.,** signal n.
**facial lymph n's,** nodi lymphoidei faciales.
**fibular lymph n.,** nodus lymphoideus fibularis.
**Flack's n.,** nodus sinuatrialis.
**foraminal lymph n.,** nodus lymphoideus foraminalis.
**gastric lymph n's, right/left,** nodi lymphoidei gastrici dextri/sinistri.
**gastroepiploic lymph n's, right/left,** nodi lymphoidei gastroomentales dextri/sinistri.
**gastro-omental lymph n's, right/left,** nodi lymphoidei gastroomentales dextri/sinistri.
**gluteal lymph n's, inferior,** nodi lymphoidei gluteales inferiores.
**gluteal lymph n's, superior,** nodi lymphoidei gluteales superiores.
**gouty n.,** a nodule produced by gouty inflammation.
**Heberden's n's,** small hard nodules, formed usually at the distal interphalangeal articulations of the fingers, produced by calcific spurs of the articular cartilage and associated with interphalangeal osteoarthritis. Heredity is an important etiologic factor. Called also *Heberden's sign.* Cf. *Bouchard's n's.*

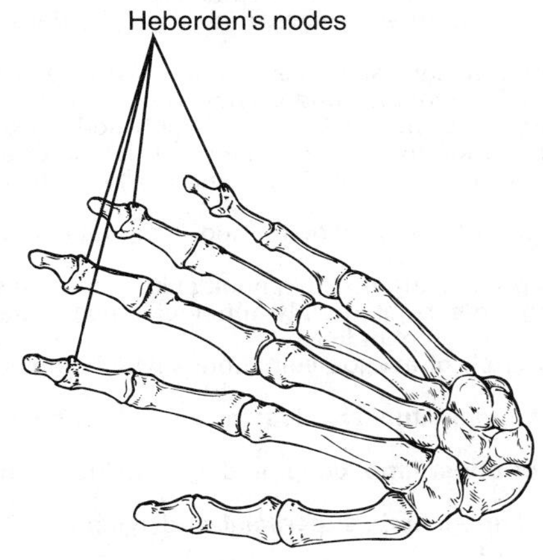


**hemal n's,** nodes found in certain mammals, especially ruminants, having a rich content of erythrocytes within sinuses and an organization much like a lymph node but with no lymphatic supply. They are located near the spleen, the kidney, and large blood vessels along the ventral side of the vertebrae, and their functions are probably like those of the spleen. A special type *(hemolymph nodes)* are found in the pig. The presence of hemal nodes in humans is doubtful. Called also *hemal glands, hemolymph n's,* and *vascular glands.*
**hemolymph n's,** 1. hemal n's. 2. special types of hemal nodes found in the pig, having characteristics midway between those of ordinary lymph nodes and typical hemal nodes, containing both blood and lymphatic vessels, the contents of both of which mix in the sinuses; called also *hemolymph glands.*
**Hensen's n.,** primitive knot.
**hepatic lymph n's,** nodi lymphoidei hepatici.
**hilar lymph n's,** nodi lymphoidei bronchopulmonales.
**ileocolic lymph n's,** nodi lymphoidei ileocolici.
**iliac lymph n's, circumflex,** lymph nodes situated along the deep iliac circumflex vessels.
**iliac lymph n's, common,** nodi lymphoidei iliaci communes.
**iliac lymph n's, external,** nodi lymphoidei iliaci externi.
**iliac lymph n's, intermediate common,** nodi lymphoidei iliaci communes intermedii.
**iliac lymph n's, intermediate external,** nodi lymphoidei iliaci externi intermedii.
**iliac lymph n's, internal,** nodi lymphoidei iliaci interni.
**iliac lymph n's, lateral common,** nodi lymphoidei iliaci communes laterales.
**iliac lymph n's, lateral external,** nodi lymphoidei iliaci externi laterales.
**iliac lymph n's, medial common,** nodi lymphoidei iliaci communes mediales.
**iliac lymph n's, medial external,** nodi lymphoidei iliaci externi mediales.
**iliac lymph n's, promontory common,** nodi lymphoidei iliaci communes promontorii.
**iliac lymph n's, subaortic common,** nodi lymphoidei iliaci communes subaortici.
**infraclavicular lymph n's,** nodi lymphoidei deltopectorales.
**infrahyoid lymph n's,** nodi lymphoidei infrahyoidei.
**inguinal lymph n's, deep,** nodi lymphoidei inguinales profundi.
**inguinal lymph n's, inferior superficial,** nodi lymphoidei inguinales superficiales inferiores.
**inguinal lymph n's, superficial,** nodi lymphoidei inguinales superficiales.

**inguinal lymph n's, superolateral superficial,** nodi lymphoidei inguinales superficiales superolaterales.

**inguinal lymph n's, superomedial superficial,** nodi lymphoidei inguinales superficiales superomediales.

**intercostal lymph n's,** nodi lymphoidei intercostales.

**interiliac lymph n's,** nodi lymphoidei interiliaci.

**interpectoral lymph n's,** nodi lymphoidei interpectorales.

**intrapulmonary lymph n's,** nodi lymphoidei intrapulmonales.

**jugular lymph n's, anterior,** nodi lymphoidei cervicales anteriores superficiales.

**jugular lymph n's, lateral,** nodi lymphatici jugulares laterales.

**jugulodigastric lymph n.,** nodus lymphoideus jugulodigastricus.

**jugulo-omohyoid lymph n.,** nodus lymphoideus juguloomohyoideus.

**juxtaintestinal lymph n's,** nodi lymphoidei mesenterici juxtaintestinales.

**Keith's n., Keith-Flack n.,** nodus sinuatrialis.

**lacunar lymph n., intermediate,** nodus lymphoideus lacunaris intermedius.

**lacunar lymph n., lateral,** nodus lymphoideus lacunaris lateralis.

**lacunar lymph n., medial,** nodus lymphoideus lacunaris medialis.

**lumbar lymph n's,** numerous large lymph nodes extending from the aortic bifurcation to the aortic hiatus of the diaphragm, as three parallel chains: left, intermediate, and right. Called also *aortic lymph n's.*

**lumbar lymph n's, intermediate,** nodi lymphoidei lumbales intermedii.

**lumbar lymph n's, left,** nodi lymphoidei lumbales sinistri.

**lumbar lymph n's, right,** nodi lymphoidei lumbales dextri.

**lymph n.,** nodus lymphoideus.

**lymph n. of arch of azygos vein,** nodus lymphoideus arcus venae azygos.

**lymph n. of ligamentum arteriosum,** nodus lymphoideus ligamenti arteriosi.

**lymph n's of upper limb, deep,** nodi lymphoidei profundi membri superioris.

**lymph n's of upper limb, superficial,** nodi lymphoidei superficiales membri superioris.

**malar lymph n.,** nodus lymphoideus malaris.

**mandibular lymph n.,** nodus lymphoideus mandibularis.

**mastoid lymph n's,** nodi lymphoidei mastoidei.

**mediastinal lymph n's, anterior,** nodi lymphatici mediastinales anteriores.

**mediastinal lymph n's, posterior,** nodi lymphatici mediastinales posteriores.

**mesenteric lymph n's,** nodi lymphoidei mesenterici.

**mesenteric lymph n's, central superior,** nodi lymphoidei mesenterici superiores centrales.

**mesenteric lymph n's, inferior,** nodi lymphoidei mesenterici inferiores.

**mesenteric lymph n's, juxtaintestinal,** nodi lymphoidei mesenterici juxtaintestinales.

**mesenteric lymph n's, superior,** nodi lymphoidei mesenterici superiores.

**mesocolic lymph n's,** nodi lymphoidei mesocolici.

**milker's n's,** 1. milker's nodules, def. 1. 2. paravaccinia, def. 1.

**nasolabial lymph n.,** nodus lymphoideus nasolabialis.

**n. of neck of gallbladder,** nodus lymphoideus cysticus.

**obturator lymph n's,** nodi lymphoidei obturatorii.

**occipital lymph n's,** nodi lymphoidei occipitales.

**Osler's n's,** small, raised, swollen tender areas, about the size of a pea, characteristically bluish but sometimes pink or red, and sometimes having a blanched center, occurring most commonly in the pads of the fingers or toes, in the thenar or hypothenar eminences, or the soles of the feet; they are practically pathognomonic of subacute bacterial endocarditis.

**pancreatic lymph n's,** nodi lymphoidei pancreatici.

**pancreatic lymph n's, inferior,** nodi lymphoidei pancreatici inferiores.

**pancreatic lymph n's, superior,** nodi lymphoidei pancreatici superiores.

**pancreaticoduodenal lymph n's, inferior,** nodi lymphoidei pancreaticoduodenales inferiores.

**pancreaticoduodenal lymph n's, superior,** nodi lymphoidei pancreaticoduodenales superiores.

**paracardial lymph n's,** a group of small lymph nodes forming a chain or ring (annulus lymphaticus cardiae [TA]), around the cardiac opening of the stomach.

**paracolic lymph n's,** nodi lymphoidei paracolici.

**paramammary lymph n's,** nodi lymphoidei paramammarii.

**pararectal lymph n's,** nodi lymphoidei pararectales.

**parasternal lymph n's,** nodi lymphoidei parasternales.

**paratracheal lymph n's,** nodi lymphoidei paratracheales.

**parauterine lymph n's,** nodi lymphoidei parauterini.

**paravaginal lymph n's,** nodi lymphoidei paravaginales.

**paravesicular lymph n's,** nodi lymphoidei paravesicales.

**parietal lymph n's,** nodi lymphoidei parietales.

**parotid lymph n's, deep,** nodi lymphoidei parotidei profundi.

**parotid lymph n's, infra-auricular deep,** nodi lymphoidei parotidei profundi infra-auriculares.

**parotid lymph n's, intraglandular deep,** nodi lymphoidei parotidei profundi intraglandulares.

**parotid lymph n's, preauricular deep,** nodi lymphoidei parotidei profundi preauriculares.

**parotid lymph n's, superficial,** nodi lymphoidei parotidei superficiales.

**Parrot's n's,** Parrot's sign (def. 2).

**pectoral lymph n's,** nodi lymphoidei pectorales.

**pelvic lymph n's, parietal,** nodi lymphoidei pelvis parietales.

**pelvic lymph n's, visceral,** nodi lymphoidei pelvis viscerales.

**pericardial lymph n's, lateral,** nodi lymphoidei pericardiaci laterales.

**peroneal lymph n.,** nodus lymphoideus fibularis.

**phrenic lymph n's, inferior,** nodi lymphoidei phrenici inferiores.

**phrenic lymph n's, superior,** nodi lymphoidei phrenici superiores.

**popliteal lymph n's,** nodi lymphoidei poplitei.

**popliteal lymph n's, deep,** nodi lymphoidei poplitei profundi.

**popliteal lymph n's, superficial,** nodi lymphoidei poplitei superficiales.

**postaortic lymph n's,** nodi lymphoidei retroaortici.

**postcaval lymph n's,** nodi lymphoidei retrocavales.

**postvesicular lymph n's,** nodi lymphoidei retrovesicales.

**preaortic lymph n's,** nodi lymphoidei preaortici.

**precaval lymph n's,** nodi lymphoidei precavales.

**prececal lymph n's,** nodi lymphoidei precaecales.

**prelaryngeal n.,** a lymph node deep in the neck that helps drain the thyroid gland.

**prepericardial lymph n's,** nodi lymphoidei prepericardiaci.

**pretracheal n.,** a lymph node deep in the neck that helps drain the thyroid gland.

**pretracheal lymph n's,** nodi lymphoidei pretracheales.

**prevertebral lymph n's,** nodi lymphoidei prevertebrales.

**prevesicular lymph n's,** nodi lymphoidei prevesicales.

**primitive n.,** primitive knot.

**pulmonary juxtaesophageal lymph n's,** nodi lymphoidei juxtaoesophageales pulmonales.

**pulmonary lymph n's,** nodi lymphoidei intrapulmonales.

**pyloric lymph n's,** nodi lymphoidei pylorici.

**n's of Ranvier,** constrictions occurring on myelinated nerve fibers at regular intervals of about 1 mm; at these sites the myelin sheath is absent and the axon is enclosed only by Schwann cell processes. See illustration at *nerve.*

**rectal lymph n's, superior,** nodi lymphoidei rectales superiores.

**retroaortic lymph n's,** nodi lymphoidei retroaortici.

**retroauricular lymph n's,** nodi lymphoidei mastoidei.

**retrocaval lymph n's,** nodi lymphoidei retrocavales.

**retrocecal lymph n's,** nodi lymphoidei retrocaecales.

**retropharyngeal lymph n's,** nodi lymphoidei retropharyngeales.

**retropyloric n's,** nodi lymphoidei retropylorici.

**retrovesicular lymph n's,** nodi lymphoidei retrovesicales.

**Rosenmüller's n.,** 1. pars palpebralis glandulae lacrimalis. 2. [pl.] nodi lymphoidei inguinales profundi.

**Rotter's n's,** lymph nodes occasionally found between the pectoralis major and minor muscles which often contain metastases from mammary cancer.

**n. of Rouvière,** the most superior of the lateral group of the retropharyngeal lymph nodes, located at the base of the skull.

**SA n.,** nodus sinuatrialis.

**sacral lymph n's,** nodi lymphoidei sacrales.

**Schmorl's n.,** an irregular or hemispherical bone defect in the upper or lower margin of the body of the vertebra.

**sentinel n.,** 1. the first lymph node to receive drainage from a tumor; used to determine whether there is lymphatic metastasis in certain types of cancer. 2. signal n.

**sigmoid lymph n's,** nodi lymphoidei sigmoidei.

**signal n.,** an enlarged supraclavicular lymph node that is often the first sign of an abdominal tumor; called also *sentinel n., Troisier's n., ganglion,* or *sign,* and *Virchow's n.* or *gland.*

**singer's n's,** vocal cord nodules.

**sinoatrial n., sinuatrial n., sinus n.,** nodus sinuatrialis.

**splenic lymph n's,** nodi lymphoidei splenici.

**submandibular lymph n's,** nodi lymphoidei submandibulares.

**submental lymph n's,** nodi lymphoidei submentales.

**subpyloric n's,** nodi lymphoidei subpylorici.

**subscapular lymph n's,** the five to seven lymph nodes extending along the subscapular veins at the lower border of the axilla, which drain the skin and muscles of the dorsal posterior shoulder region and lower part of the back of the neck.

**supraclavicular lymph n's,** nodi lymphoidei supraclaviculares.
**suprapyloric lymph n.,** nodus lymphoideus suprapyloricus.
**supratrochlear lymph n's,** nodi lymphoidei supratrochleares.
**syphilitic n.,** a swelling on a bone due to syphilitic periostitis.
**n. of Tawara,** nodus atrioventricularis.
**teacher's n's,** vocal cord nodules.
**thyroid lymph n's,** nodi lymphoidei thyroidei.
**tibial n., anterior,** nodus lymphoideus tibialis anterior.
**tibial n., posterior,** nodus lymphoideus tibialis posterior.
**tracheal lymph n's,** nodi lymphoidei paratracheales.
**tracheobronchial lymph n's, inferior,** nodi lymphoidei tracheobronchiales inferiores.
**tracheobronchial lymph n's, superior,** nodi lymphoidei tracheobronchiales superiores.
**triticeous n.,** cartilago triticea.
**Troisier's n.,** signal n.
**vesicular lymph n's, lateral,** nodi lymphoidei vesicales laterales.
**Virchow's n.,** signal n.
**visceral lymph n's,** nodi lymphoidei viscerales.

**no·di** (no'di) [L.] genitive and plural of *nodus.*

**no·dose** (no'dōs) [L. *nodosus*] having nodes or projections.

**no·dos·i·ty** (no-dos'ĭ-te) [L. *nodositas*] 1. the quality or condition of being nodose. 2. node.

**no·do·ven·tric·u·lar** (no″do-ven-trik'u-lər) connecting the atrioventricular node to the ventricle.

**nod·u·lar** (nod'u-lər) 1. like a nodule or node. 2. marked with nodules.

**Nod·u·la·ria** (nod″u-lar'e-ə) a genus of cyanobacteria; certain species, such as *N.* spumi'gena, sometimes contaminate water and can cause cyanobacteria poisoning.

**nod·u·lat·ed** (nod'u-lāt″əd) marked with nodules.

**nod·u·la·tion** (nod″u-la'shən) the presence of nodules.

**nod·ule** (nod'ūl) [L. *nodulus* little knot] nodulus.
**accessory thymic n's,** noduli thymici accessorii.
**aggregate n's,** noduli lymphoidei aggregati intestini tenuis.
**Albini's n's,** gray nodules of the size of small grains, sometimes seen on the free edges of the atrioventricular valves of infants; they are remains of fetal structures.
**n's of aortic valve,** noduli valvularum semilunarium valvae aortae.
**apple jelly n's,** minute translucent nodules of a distinctive yellowish or reddish brown color, visible on diascopic examination of the lesions of lupus vulgaris.
**n's of Arantius,** noduli valvularum semilunarium valvae aortae.
**Aschoff's n's,** Aschoff bodies.
**Babès' n's,** collections of microglial cells around neurons in the central nervous system, seen in rabies and other types of viral encephalitis; called also *Babès' nodes* or *tubercles.*
**Bianchi's n's,** noduli valvularum semilunarium valvae aortae.
**Bohn's n's,** inclusion cysts along the buccal and lingual aspects of the dental ridges and on the palate away from the raphe, found in newborn infants; considered to be remnants of mucous-gland tissue trapped during fetal development. Called also *Bohn's pearls.*
**Brenner n's,** nodular masses of tumor in the cyst wall in cases of Brenner tumor.
**Busacca n's,** an accumulation of epithelioid cells and lymphocytes occurring in chronic inflammation of the iris, usually on the anterior surface about the region of the ciliary zone.
**n. of cerebellum,** nodulus vermis.
**cirrhotic n.,** a regenerative nodule surrounded by fibrous septa.
**coal n.,** a palpable lesion of the lung seen in coal workers' pneumoconiosis, containing coal dust, dust-filled macrophages, and collagen fibers; it is larger than and develops from a coal macule.
**cold n.,** a thyroid nodule that is less detectable than surrounding tissues on a radionuclide scan because of low uptake of the tracer; up to one in four may be malignant.
**cortical n's,** nodules of closely packed lymphocytes in the cortical portion of a lymph gland.
**Dalen-Fuchs n's,** small hemispherical mounds principally composed of epithelioid cells and cells of the retinal epithelium, seen in sympathetic ophthalmia and certain other disorders.
**dysplastic n.,** a cluster, at least 1 mm in diameter, of dysplastic hepatocytes, occurring as a precancerous lesion of the liver; called also *adenomatous hyperplasia.*
**Fraenkel's n's,** typhus nodules of the cutaneous blood vessels.
**Gamna n's,** brown or yellow pigmented nodules seen in the spleen in certain cases of enlargement, such as Banti's disease and siderotic splenomegaly; called also *n's tabac.*
**Gandy-Gamna n's,** Gamna n's.
**Hoboken's n's,** dilatations of the outer surface of the umbilical arteries.
**hot n.,** a thyroid nodule that is more detectable than surrounding tissues on a radionuclide scan because of high uptake of the tracer; most are nonmalignant causes of hyperthyroidism, but a small number may be malignant.
**Jeanselme's n's,** gummata of tertiary syphilis and of nonvenereal treponemal diseases, located on joint capsules, bursae, or tendon sheaths; called also *juxta-articular n's.*
**juxta-articular n's,** Jeanselme's n's.
**n's of Kerckring,** noduli valvularum semilunarium valvae aortae.
**Kimmelstiel-Wilson n.,** see under *lesion.*
**Koeppe n's,** white to gray nodules observed at the pupillary border in chronic inflammation of the iris, and consisting of accumulations of epithelioid cells and lymphocytes.
**Lisch n's,** hamartomas of the iris, occurring in neurofibromatosis.
**Lutz-Jeanselme n's,** Jeanselme's n's.
**lymphatic n.,** 1. nodulus lymphoideus. 2. a small dense accumulation of lymphocytes found within the cortex of a lymph node, expressing the cytogenic and defense functions of the tissue.
**lymphatic n's of large intestine, solitary,** see *noduli lymphoidei solitarii,* under *nodulus.*
**lymphatic n's of small intestine, solitary,** see *noduli lymphoidei solitarii,* under *nodulus.*
**lymphatic n's of stomach,** folliculi lymphatici gastrici.
**lymphoid n's of large intestine, solitary,** see *noduli lymphoidei solitarii,* under *nodulus.*
**lymphoid n's of small intestine, aggregated,** noduli lymphoidei aggregati intestini tenuis.
**lymphoid n's of small intestine, solitary,** see *noduli lymphoidei solitarii,* under *nodulus.*
**lymphoid n's of vermiform appendix, aggregated,** noduli lymphoidei aggregati appendicis vermiformis.
**macroregenerative n.,** 1. dysplastic n. 2. a multiacinar regenerative nodule over 5 mm in diameter.
**microglial n's,** typhus nodules occurring in the central nervous system.
**milker's n's,** 1. paravaccinia infection in humans, contracted during milking of infected cows; it consists of purple nodules on the fingers and adjacent areas, which later break down, crust, and heal without scarring. Called also *milker's nodes.* 2. paravaccinia, def. 1.
**Morgagni's n's,** noduli valvularum semilunarium valvae aortae.
**pearly n.,** one of the nodules of bovine tuberculosis.
**primary n.,** a lymph nodule without a germinal center, or apart from a center.
**n's of valves of pulmonary trunk, n's of pulmonary valve,** noduli valvularum semilunarium valvae trunci pulmonalis.
**pulp n.,** denticle, def. 2.
**regenerative n.,** a region of localized proliferation of hepatocytes and underlying stroma arising in response to liver injury.
**regenerative n., large,** a multiacinar regenerative nodule over 5 mm in diameter.
**regenerative n., monoacinar,** a regenerative nodule having a single portal tract.
**regenerative n., multiacinar,** a regenerative nodule having multiple portal tracts; when over 5 mm in diameter, called also *large regenerative* or *macroregenerative n.*
**rheumatic n's,** small, round or oval, mostly subcutaneous nodules resembling Aschoff bodies, seen in cases of rheumatic fever.
**rheumatoid n's,** subcutaneous nodules consisting of central foci of necrosis surrounded by palisade-like coronas of fibroblasts, often seen in patients with rheumatoid arthritis.
**Schmorl's n.,** a nodule seen in radiographs of the spine, due to prolapse of a nucleus pulposus into an adjoining vertebra.
**secondary n.,** germinal center.
**n's of semilunar valves,** noduli valvularum semilunarium.
**siderotic n's,** focal fibrotic lesions characterized by the presence of crystals of iron on the degenerated elastic tissue fibers, seen in the spleen in Banti's disease.
**singer's n's,** vocal cord n's.
**Sister Mary Joseph's n.,** a nodule deep in the subcutis in the um-

bilical area associated with metastasizing intra-abdominal cancer, usually of gastric, ovarian, colorectal, or pancreatic origin.
**surfers' n's,** hyperplastic, fibrosing, rarely ulcerated granulomas 1 to 3 cm in diameter, occurring over bony prominences of the feet and legs of surfers, occurring as a result of repeated trauma from kneeling on surfboards; called also *Malibu disease* and *surfers' knobs* or *knots.*
**n's tabac,** Gamna n's.
**teacher's n's,** vocal cord n's.
**thyroid n's,** pathological nodules in the thyroid gland, often filled with colloid; some are indicative of adenoma or carcinoma. See *cold n., hot n.,* and *warm n.*
**triticeous n.,** cartilago triticea.
**typhoid n.,** a mass of macrophages and other necrotic cells observed in the liver in typhoid fever.
**typhus n's,** minute nodules, originally described in typhus, produced by perivascular infiltration of polymorphonuclear leukocytes and mononuclear cells in rickettsial disease.
**n. of vermis,** nodulus vermis.
**vestigial n.,** tuberculum auriculare.
**vocal n's, vocal cord n's,** small white nodules appearing on the vocal cords in chorditis tuberosa. Called also *singer's n's* or *nodes* and *teacher's n's* or *nodes.*
**warm n.,** a nodule in the thyroid gland that can concentrate radioiodine; usually not carcinomatous.
**Wohlbach's n's,** typhus n's.

**nod·u·li** (no'du-li) [L.] genitive and plural of *nodulus.*

**nod·u·lous** (nod'u-ləs) nodose.

**nod·u·lus** (nod'u-ləs) gen. and pl. *no'duli* [L., dim. of *nodus*] 1. nodule: a small knot or node; used in anatomical nomenclature as a general term to designate a comparatively minute collection of tissue. Cf. *granuloma.* 2. n. vermis.
**n. cerebel'li,** n. vermis.
**n. lympha'ticus,** n. lymphoideus.
**no'duli lympha'tici aggrega'ti intesti'ni te'nuis,** noduli lymphoidei aggregati intestini tenuis.
**no'duli lympha'tici aggrega'ti [Peye'ri],** noduli lymphoidei aggregati intestini tenuis.
**no'duli lympha'tici aggrega'ti proces'sus vermifor'mis,** noduli lymphoidei aggregati appendicis vermiformis.
**no'duli lympha'tici bronchia'les,** lymph nodules situated in the lining of the bronchi.
**no'duli lympha'tici conjunctiva'les,** lymph nodules situated in the conjunctiva.
**no'duli lympha'tici gas'trici,** folliculi lymphatici gastrici.
**no'duli lympha'tici laryn'gei,** folliculi lymphatici laryngei.
**no'duli lympha'tici rec'ti,** folliculi lymphatici recti.
**no'duli lympha'tici solita'rii,** noduli lymphoidei solitarii.
**no'duli lympha'tici solita'rii intesti'ni cras'si,** see *noduli lymphoidei solitarii.*
**no'duli lympha'tici solita'rii intesti'ni te'nuis,** see *noduli lymphoidei solitarii.*
**no'duli lympha'tici vagina'les,** small collections of lymphatic tissue deep to the epithelial surface of the vagina.
**no'duli lympha'tici vesica'les,** collections of lymphatic tissue in the lining of the urinary bladder.
**n. lymphoi'deus,** lymphoid or lymphatic nodule: a small collection of lymphoid tissue found in such organs as the intestines; called also *folliculus lymphaticus, n. lymphaticus,* and *lymph* or *lymphatic follicle.*
**no'duli lymphoi'dei aggrega'ti appen'dicis vermifor'mis** [TA], aggregated lymphoid nodules of vermiform appendix: oval elevated areas of lymphoid tissue occupying the greater part of the submucosa of the vermiform appendix; called also *folliculi lymphatici aggregati processus vermiformis.*
**no'duli lymphoi'dei aggrega'ti intesti'ni te'nuis** [TA], aggregated lymphoid nodules of small intestine: oval elevated areas of lymphoid tissue on the mucosa of the small intestine, composed of many lymphoid follicles closely packed together; called also *noduli lymphatici aggregati [peyeri]* and *Peyer's glands, patches,* or *plaques.*
**no'duli lymphoi'dei liena'les,** TA alternative for *noduli lymphoidei splenici.*
**no'duli lymphoi'dei solita'rii** [TA], solitary lymphatic or lymphoid nodules: small concentrations of lymphoid tissue scattered throughout the mucosa and submucosa of the small and large intestines; called also *noduli lymphatici solitarii, folliculi lymphatici solitarii,* and *solitary lymphatic* or *lymphoid follicles.*
**no'duli lymphoi'dei sple'nici** [TA], splenic lymphoid nodules: aggregations of lymphatic tissue that ensheath the arteries in the spleen. Called also *noduli lymphoidei lienales* [TA alternative], *folliculi lymphatici splenici, folliculi lymphatici lienales, malpighian bodies of spleen, malpighian corpuscles of spleen,* and *white pulp.*
**no'duli lymphoi'dei tonsil'lae lingua'lis** [TA], lymphoid nodules of lingual tonsil: lymphoid nodules on the root of the tongue, associated with the lingual tonsil. Called also *folliculi linguales* and *lingual follicles.*
**no'duli lymphoi'dei tonsil'lae pharyngea'lis** [TA], lymphoid nodules of pharyngeal tonsils: small collections of lymphoid tissue associated with the laryngeal tonsils.
**no'duli thy'mici accesso'rii,** accessory thymic nodules: portions of thymus tissue that have been detached from the stalk and left behind in the caudal migration of the gland in embryonic development.
**no'duli valvula'rum semiluna'rium val'vae aor'tae** [TA], nodules of semilunar cusps of aortic valve: small fibrous tubercles, one at the center of the free margin of each semilunar cusp of the valve. Called also *nodules of aortic valve.*
**no'duli valvula'rum semiluna'rium val'vae trun'ci pulmona'lis** [TA], nodules of semilunar cusps of pulmonary valve: small fibrous tubercles, one at the center of the free margin of each semilunar cusp. Called also *nodules of pulmonary valve.*
**n. ver'mis** [TA], nodule of vermis: the most ventral part of the caudal surface of the vermis, connected on each side to the caudal medullary velum, and forming the central part of the flocculonodular lobe; called also *nodulus, nodule of cerebellum* and *n. cerebelli.*

**no·dus** (no'dəs) gen. and pl. *no'di* [L.] a node or knot; used in anatomical nomenclature as a general term to designate a small mass of tissue.

## Nodus

Descriptions of anatomic structures are given on TA terms, and include anglicized names of specific nodes.

**n. atrioventricula'ris** [TA], atrioventricular node: a small area of specialized cardiac muscle cells and fibers that receives the cardiac impulses from the sinoatrial node and passes them on toward the ventricles, introducing a delay in impulse conduction. It is located in the right atrium between the tricuspid valve and the orifice of the coronary sinus, is composed of a meshwork of (Purkinje) fibers continuous with the atrial muscle fibers and the bundle of His, and is supplied by a branch of the right coronary artery. The node is sometimes subdivided on the basis of electrophysiology into atrionodal (AN), nodal (N), and nodal-His (NH) regions.
**n. lympha'ticus,** TA alternative for *n. lymphoideus.*
**n. lympha'ticus bucca'lis,** n. lymphoideus buccinatorius.
**no'di lympha'tici gastroepiplo'ici dex'tri/sinis'tri,** nodi lymphoidei gastroomentales dextri/sinistri.
**no'di lympha'tici hila'res,** nodi lymphoidei bronchopulmonales.
**no'di lympha'tici jugula'res latera'les,** lateral jugular lymph nodes: deep lateral cervical lymph nodes situated lateral to the internal jugular vein that empty into the jugular trunk.
**no'di lympha'tici lumba'res dex'tri,** nodi lymphoidei lumbales dextri.
**no'di lympha'tici lumba'res interme'dii,** nodi lymphoidei lumbales intermedii.
**no'di lympha'tici lumba'res sinis'tri,** nodi lymphoidei lumbales sinistri.
**no'di lympha'tici paravesicula'res,** nodi lymphoidei paravesicales.
**no'di lympha'tici postvesicula'res,** nodi lymphoidei retrovesicales.
**no'di lympha'tici prevesicula'res,** nodi lymphoidei prevesicales.
**no'di lympha'tici retroauricula'res,** nodi lymphoidei mastoidei.
**no'di lympha'tici retroceca'les,** nodi lymphoidei retrocaecales.
**no'di lympha'tici trachea'les,** nodi lymphoidei paratracheales.
**no'di lympha'tici vesicula'res latera'les,** nodi lymphoidei vesicales laterales.
**n. lymphoi'deus** [TA], lymph node: any of the accumulations of lymphoid tissue organized as definite lymphoid organs, varying from 1 to 25 mm in diameter, situated along the course of lymphatic vessels, and consisting of an outer cortical and an inner medullary part. The lymph nodes are the main source of lymphocytes of the peripheral blood and, as part of the reticuloendothelial system, serve as a defense mechanism by removing noxious agents, such as bacteria and

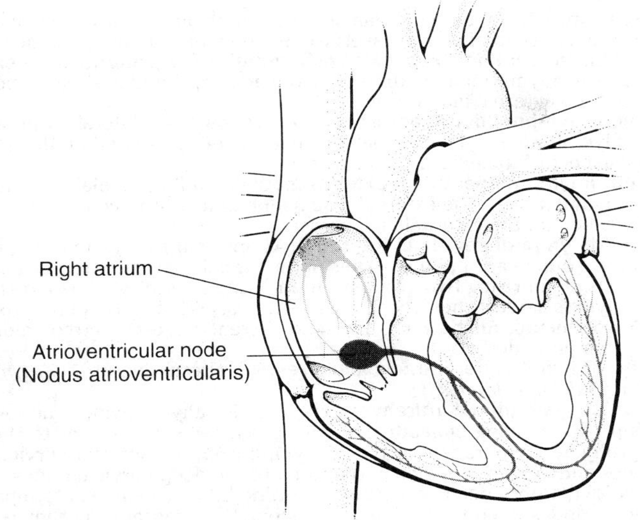


toxins, and probably play a role in antibody production. See also Plate 28. Called also *lymphoglandula* and *lymphonodus* or *n. lymphaticus* [TA alternatives].

**no'di lymphoi'dei abdo'minis parieta'les** [TA], parietal abdominal lymph nodes: the lymph nodes that drain the abdominal walls, comprising the left, intermediate, and lumbar lymph nodes, inferior phrenic lymph nodes, and inferior epigastric lymph nodes.

**no'di lymphoi'dei abdo'minis viscera'les** [TA], visceral abdominal lymph nodes: the numerous lymph nodes that drain the abdominal viscera.

**no'di lymphoi'dei acces'sorii** [TA], accessory nodes: a chain of lymph nodes of the inferior deep lateral cervical group that follow the spinal accessory nerve and receive lymph from the occipital, postauricular, and suprascapular nodes and from the scalp, neck, and shoulder.

**no'di lymphoi'dei anorecta'les,** TA alternative for *nodi lymphoidei pararectales.*

**no'di lymphoi'dei aor'tici latera'les** [TA], lateral aortic lymph nodes: two chains (right and left) of the left lumbar group that are on the left side of the aorta and drain the suprarenal glands, kidneys, ureters, testes, ovaries, pelvic viscera (except the intestines), and posterior abdominal wall.

**no'di lymphoi'dei appendicula'res** [TA], appendicular lymph nodes: lymph nodes situated along the appendicular artery and in the mesoappendix that drain into the ileocolic lymph nodes.

**n. lymphoi'deus ar'cus ve'nae a'zygos** [TA], lymph node of arch of azygos vein: a lymph node sometimes present on the azygos vein at the point where it arches over the root of the lung.

**no'di lymphoi'dei axilla'res** [TA], axillary lymph nodes: the 20 to 30 lymph nodes of the axilla, which receive lymph from all the lymph vessels of the upper limb, most of those of the breast, and the cutaneous vessels from the trunk above the level of the umbilicus. They are divided into groups: apical, central, brachial or lateral, pectoral or anterior, and subscapular or posterior.

**no'di lymphoi'dei axilla'res anterio'res,** TA alternative for *nodi lymphoidei axillares pectorales.*

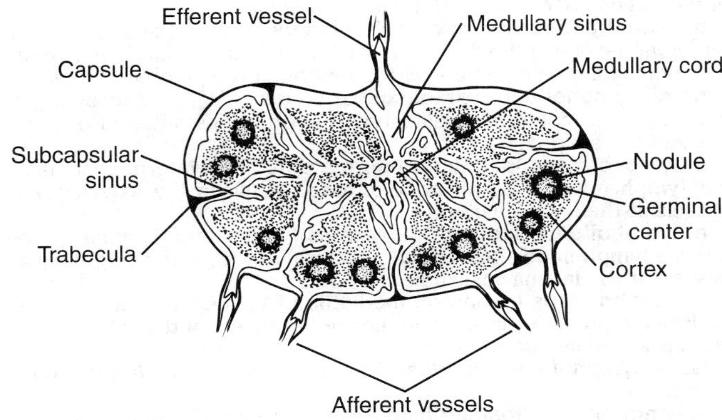


Lymph node (nodus lymphoideus).

**no'di lymphoi'dei axilla'res apica'les** [TA], apical lymph nodes: six to twelve axillary lymph nodes partly posterior to the superior part of the pectoralis minor muscle and partly in the apex of the axilla, receiving afferent vessels that accompany the cephalic vein and draining all other axillary nodes; their efferent vessels unite to form the subclavian trunk.

**no'di lymphoi'dei axilla'res centra'les** [TA], central lymph nodes: three or four axillary lymph nodes embedded in adipose tissue near the base of the axilla; they receive lymph from the lateral, pectoral, and subscapular nodes and drain into the apical nodes.

**no'di lymphoi'dei axilla'res latera'les,** nodi lymphoidei brachiales.

**no'di lymphoi'dei axilla'res pectora'les** [TA], pectoral axillary lymph nodes: four or five axillary lymph nodes along the inferior border of the pectoralis minor muscle near the lateral thoracic artery; they receive lymph from the skin and muscles of the anterior and lateral thoracic walls and mammary gland and drain into the central and apical nodes. Called also *nodi lymphoidei axillares anteriores* [TA alternative] and *anterior axillary lymph nodes.*

**no'di lymphoi'dei axilla'res posterio'res,** TA alternative for *nodi lymphoidei axillares subscapulares.*

**no'di lymphoi'dei axilla'res subscapula'res** [TA], subscapular axillary lymph nodes: six or seven axillary lymph nodes along the inferior margins of the posterior axillary wall along the course of the subscapular artery; they receive lymph from the skin and superficial muscles of the posterior part of the neck and the posterior thoracic wall and drain into the apical and central nodes. Called also *nodi lymphoidei axillares posteriores* [TA alternative] and *posterior axillary lymph nodes.*

**no'di lymphoi'dei brachia'les** [TA], brachial lymph nodes: four to six axillary lymph nodes lying medial to, and behind, the axillary vein, which drain most of the upper limb; called also *lateral axillary lymph nodes.*

**no'di lymphoi'dei bronchopulmona'les** [TA], bronchopulmonary lymph nodes: lymph nodes embedded in the root of the lung, mainly at the hilum that drain into the tracheobronchial lymph nodes; called also *hilar lymph nodes* and *nodi lymphatici hilares.*

**n. lymphoi'deus buccinato'rius** [TA], buccinator lymph node: one of a variable number of facial lymph nodes lying on a line between the angle of the mandible and the mouth, receiving the afferent vessels draining the temporal and infratemporal fossae and nasopharynx; their efferent vessels drain into the superior deep cervical nodes. Called also *buccal lymph node* and *n. lymphaticus buccalis.*

**no'di lymphoi'dei cava'les latera'les** [TA], lateral caval lymph nodes: a group of lymph nodes of the right lumbar group that are on the right side of the inferior vena cava.

**no'di lymphoi'dei cervica'les anterio'res** [TA], anterior cervical lymph nodes: a group of lymph nodes ventral to the larynx and trachea, consisting of superficial vessels on the anterior jugular vein *(nodi lymphoidei cervicales anteriores superficiales)* and deep vessels *(nodi lymphoidei cervicales anteriores profundi)* on the middle cricothyroid ligament as well as ventral to the trachea.

**no'di lymphoi'dei cervica'les anterio'res profun'di** [TA], deep anterior cervical lymph nodes: a group of numerous large lymph nodes that form a chain along the internal jugular vein, extending from the base of the skull to the root of the neck, situated near the pharynx, esophagus, and trachea; they receive lymph from both superficial and deep structures.

**no'di lymphoi'dei cervica'les anterio'res superficia'les** [TA], superficial anterior cervical lymph nodes: lymph nodes along the external jugular vein as it emerges from the parotid gland, being superficial to the sternocleidomastoid muscle; they receive afferent vessels from the auricle and parotid region.

**no'di lymphoi'dei cervica'les latera'les profun'di,** deep lateral cervical lymph nodes: a chain of lymph nodes situated in the posterior cervical triangle; the chain is subdivided into smaller chains of lymph nodes, including a superior group (lateral, anterior, and jugulodigastric nodes) and an inferior group (lateral, anterior, and jugulo-omohyoid nodes).

**no'di lymphoi'dei cervica'les latera'les superficia'les** [TA], superficial lateral cervical lymph nodes: lymph nodes situated along the external jugular vein that send efferent vessels to the deep lateral cervical lymph nodes.

**no'di lymphoi'dei cervica'les latera'les profun'di inferio'res** [TA], inferior deep cervical lymph nodes: a group of lymph nodes adjacent to the carotid sheath, partly deep to the sternocleidomastoid muscle and extending into the subclavian triangle. They receive lymph from the back of the scalp and neck, the tongue, the superficial pectoral region, and part of the arm and drain into the jugular trunk.

**no'di lymphoi'dei cervica'les latera'les profun'di superio'res** [TA], superior deep cervical lymph nodes: a group of lymph nodes adjacent to the carotid sheath deep to the sternocleidomastoid muscle; they receive lymph from a number of structures of the head and neck and drain into the inferior deep cervical nodes or the jugular trunk.

**no′di lymphoi′dei coeli′aci** [TA], celiac lymph nodes: a few nodes along the celiac trunk, which receive lymph from the stomach, spleen, duodenum, liver, and pancreas.

**no′di lymphoi′dei co′lici dex′tri/me′dii/sinis′tri** [TA], colic lymph nodes: a subgroup of the mesocolic lymph nodes, situated along the right, middle, and left colic arteries.

**no′di lymphoi′dei cubita′les** [TA], cubital lymph nodes: one or two superficially placed lymph nodes situated above the medial epicondyle, medial to the basilic vein, the efferent vessels of which accompany the basilic vein and join the deep lymph vessels; called also *epitrochlear lymph nodes.*

**n. lymphoi′deus cys′ticus** [TA], cystic lymph node: a hepatic lymph node situated in the curve of the neck of the gallbladder at the junction of the cystic and common hepatic ducts; called *node of neck of gallbladder.*

**no′di lymphoi′dei deltopectora′les** [TA], deltopectoral lymph nodes: one or two lymph nodes in the groove between the pectoralis major and deltoid muscles, just inferior to the clavicle, which drain into the apical lymph nodes. Called also *nodi lymphoidei infraclaviculares* [TA alternative] and *infraclavicular nodes.*

**no′di lymphoi′dei epigas′trici infe′riores** [TA], inferior epigastric lymph nodes: lymph nodes along the deep epigastric vessels, receiving lymph from the lower abdominal wall.

**no′di lymphoi′dei facia′les** [TA], facial lymph nodes: lymph nodes situated along the course of the facial artery and vein, which receive afferent vessels draining the eyelids, conjunctiva, nose, cheeks, lips, and gums, and send efferent vessels to the submandibular nodes.

**n. lymphoi′deus fibula′ris** [TA], fibular lymph node: a lymph node situated along the peroneal artery; called also *peroneal lymph node.*

**n. lymphoi′deus foramina′lis** [TA], foraminal lymph node: a hepatic lymph node situated along the upper part of the common bile duct; called also *node of anterior border of epiploic foramen* and *node of epiploic foramen.*

**no′di lymphoi′dei gas′trici dex′tri/sinis′tri** [TA], right/left gastric lymph nodes: a few nodes along the right and left gastric arteries that receive lymph from the stomach, spleen, duodenum, liver, and pancreas.

**no′di lymphoi′dei gastroomenta′les dex′tri/sinis′tri** [TA], right/left gastroomental lymph nodes: lymph nodes situated in the greater omentum along the pyloric half of the greater curvature of the stomach in association with the right and left gastroepiploic arteries; called also *nodi lymphatici gastroepiploici dextri/sinistri* and *right/left gastroepiploic lymph nodes.*

**no′di lymphoi′dei glutea′les inferio′res** [TA], inferior gluteal lymph nodes: the internal iliac lymph nodes situated along the inferior gluteal artery.

**no′di lymphoi′dei glutea′les superio′res** [TA], superior gluteal lymph nodes: the internal iliac lymph nodes situated along the superior gluteal artery.

**no′di lymphoi′dei hepa′tici** [TA], hepatic lymph nodes: a variable number of lymph nodes situated along the proper and common hepatic arteries and the bile ducts that receive lymph from the stomach, spleen, duodenum, liver, and pancreas; two are fairly common: the cystic node and the foraminal node.

**no′di lymphoi′dei ileoco′lici** [TA], ileocolic lymph nodes: nodes in the region of the ileocolic junction, draining adjacent structures and draining into the superior mesenteric lymph node.

**no′di lymphoi′dei ili′aci commu′nes** [TA], common iliac lymph nodes: the four to six lymph nodes grouped at the sides and dorsal to the common iliac vessels, comprising five groups: medial, intermediate, lateral, subaortic, and promontory; they receive afferent vessels from the lateral and internal iliac lymph nodes and send efferent vessels to the lateral aortic lymph nodes.

**no′di lymphoi′dei ili′aci commu′nes interme′dii** [TA], intermediate common iliac lymph nodes: the common iliac lymph nodes situated between the common iliac vessels.

**no′di lymphoi′dei ili′aci commu′nes latera′les** [TA], lateral common iliac lymph nodes: the common iliac lymph nodes situated on the lateral aspect of the common iliac vessels.

**no′di lymphoi′dei ili′aci commu′nes media′les** [TA], medial common iliac lymph nodes: the common iliac lymph nodes situated on the medial aspect of the common iliac vessels.

**no′di lymphoi′dei ili′aci commu′nes promonto′rii** [TA], promontory common iliac lymph nodes: the common iliac lymph nodes situated in front of the sacral promontory.

**no′di lymphoi′dei ili′aci commu′nes subaor′tici** [TA], subaortic common iliac lymph nodes: the common iliac lymph nodes situated below the bifurcation of the aorta.

**no′di lymphoi′dei ili′aci exter′ni** [TA], external iliac lymph nodes: the eight to ten nodes along the external iliac vessels, comprising five groups: medial, intermediate, lateral, interiliac, and obturator lymph nodes; they receive afferent vessels from the inguinal lymph nodes, deep part of the abdominal wall below the umbilicus, and some pelvic viscera and send efferent vessels to the common iliac lymph nodes.

**no′di lymphoi′dei ili′aci exter′ni interme′dii** [TA], intermediate external iliac lymph nodes: the external iliac lymph nodes situated between the external iliac vessels.

**no′di lymphoi′dei ili′aci exter′ni latera′les** [TA], lateral external iliac lymph nodes: the external iliac lymph nodes situated on the lateral aspect of the external iliac vessels.

**no′di lymphoi′dei ili′aci exter′ni media′les** [TA], medial external iliac lymph nodes: the external iliac lymph nodes situated on the medial aspect of the external iliac vessels.

**no′di lymphoi′dei ili′aci inter′ni** [TA], internal iliac lymph nodes: nodes grouped around the origins of the branches of the internal iliac vessels, comprising two groups: superior and inferior gluteal and sacral lymph nodes; they receive afferent vessels from the pelvic viscera, perineum, and buttocks and send efferent vessels to the common iliac lymph nodes.

**no′di lymphoi′dei infraclavicula′res,** TA alternative for *nodi lymphoidei deltopectorales.*

**no′di lymphoi′dei infrahyoi′dei** [TA], infrahyoid lymph nodes: lymph nodes lying beneath the deep cervical fascia anterior to the thyrohyoid membrane that receive lymph from the anterior cervical nodes and epiglottic region and drain into the deep cervical nodes.

**no′di lymphoi′dei inguina′les profun′di** [TA], deep inguinal lymph nodes: nodes deep to the fascia lata along the femoral vein; they receive lymph from the deep structures of the lower limb and from the penis or clitoris, and superficial inguinal lymph nodes and drain into the external iliac lymph nodes.

**no′di lymphoi′dei inguina′les superficia′les** [TA], superficial inguinal lymph nodes: lymph nodes situated in the subcutaneous tissue inferior to the inguinal ligament on either side of the proximal part of the greater saphenous vein, comprising two upper (supermedial and superolateral) groups and one lower (inferior) group; they drain the skin of the lower abdominal wall, penis, scrotum or labia majora, perineum, and buttocks.

**no′di lymphoi′dei inguina′les superficia′les inferio′res** [TA], inferior superficial inguinal lymph nodes: the lower superficial inguinal lymph nodes situated below the opening of the saphenous vein.

**no′di lymphoi′dei inguina′les superficia′les superolatera′les** [TA], superolateral superficial inguinal lymph nodes: the upper superficial inguinal nodes situated on the lateral side of the opening of the saphenous vein.

**no′di lymphoi′dei inguina′les superficia′les superomedia′les** [TA], superomedial superficial inguinal lymph nodes: the upper superficial inguinal lymph nodes situated on the medial side of the opening of the saphenous vein.

**no′di lymphoi′dei intercosta′les** [TA], intercostal lymph nodes: lymph nodes in the back of the thorax, along the intercostal vessels.

**no′di lymphoi′dei interili′aci** [TA], interiliac lymph nodes: the external iliac lymph nodes situated between the external and internal iliac vessels and the obturator artery.

**no′di lymphoi′dei interpectora′les** [TA], interpectoral lymph nodes: small inconstant lymph nodes that may occur between the mammary gland and apical lymph nodes.

**no′di lymphoi′dei intrapulmona′les** [TA], intrapulmonary lymph nodes: nodes located along the larger bronchi within the lung substance, through which lymph from the lung drains. Called also *nodi lymphoidei pulmonales* and *pulmonary lymph nodes.*

**no′di lymphoi′dei jugula′res anterio′res,** TA alternative for *nodi lymphoidei cervicales anteriores superficiales.*

**n. lymphoi′deus jugulodigas′tricus** [TA], jugulodigastric lymph node: one of the deep lateral cervical lymph nodes lying on the internal jugular vein at the level of the greater cornu of the hyoid bone, i.e., just below the posterior belly of the digastric muscle; called also *hauptganglion of Küttner* and *Küttner's ganglion.*

**n. lymphoi′deus juguloomohyoi′deus** [TA], jugulo-omohyoid lymph node: one of the deep lateral cervical lymph nodes lying on the internal jugular vein just above the tendon of the omohyoid muscle.

**no′di lymphoi′dei juxtaoesophagea′les** [TA], juxtaesophageal lymph nodes: posterior mediastinal lymph nodes situated on both sides of the esophagus.

**n. lymphoi′deus lacuna′ris interme′dius** [TA], intermediate lacunar lymph node: a lymph node situated between the external iliac vessels at the lacuna vasorum.

**n. lymphoi′deus lacuna′ris latera′lis** [TA], lateral lacunar lymph node: a lymph node situated on the lateral aspect of the external iliac vessels at the lacuna vasorum.

**n. lymphoi′deus lacuna′ris media′lis** [TA], medial lacunar lymph node: a lymph node situated on the medial aspect of the external iliac vessels at the lacuna vasorum.

**no′di lymphoi′dei liena′les,** TA alternative for *nodi lymphoidei splenici.*

**n. lymphoi′deus ligamen′ti arterio′si** [TA], lymph node of ligamentum arteriosum: the lowest anterior mediastinal lymph node situated anterior to the ligamentum arteriosum.

**no'di lymphoi'dei lingua'les** [TA], deep cervical lymph nodes receiving afferent vessels from the tongue.

**no'di lymphoi'dei lumba'les dex'tri** [TA], right lumbar lymph nodes: the chain of lumbar lymph nodes situated partly in front of the vena cava and partly behind it on the psoas major muscle, comprising three groups: lateral caval, precaval, and retrocaval (postcaval) lymph nodes. Called also *nodi lymphatici lumbares dextri.*

**no'di lymphoi'dei lumba'les interme'dii** [TA], intermediate lumbar lymph nodes: the chain of lumbar lymph nodes that lie in the median plane, between the left and right lumbar lymph nodes. Called also *nodi lymphatici lumbares intermedii.*

**no'di lymphoi'dei lumba'les sinis'tri** [TA], left lumbar lymph nodes: the chain of lumbar lymph nodes situated at the side of the abdominal aorta on the psoas major muscle, comprising three groups: right and left lateral aortic, preaortic, and retroaortic (postaortic) lymph nodes. Called also *nodi lymphatici lumbares sinistri.*

**n. lymphoi'deus mala'ris** [TA], malar lymph node: one of a variable number of facial lymph nodes situated in the region of the zygomatic minor muscle.

**n. lymphoi'deus mandibula'ris** [TA], mandibular lymph node: one of a variable number of facial lymph nodes situated near the angle of the mandible, into which lymph from some of the superficial tissues of the head and neck is drained.

**no'di lymphoi'dei mastoi'dei** [TA], mastoid lymph nodes: lymph nodes, two or three on each side, that are superficial to the mastoid attachment of the sternocleidomastoid muscle and deep to the posterior auricular muscle; they drain the nasal fossae and paranasal sinuses, hard and soft palate, middle ear, and nasopharynx and oropharynx. Called also *nodi lymphatici retroauriculares* and *retroauricular lymph nodes.*

**no'di lymphoi'dei mem'bri superio'ris profun'di,** nodi lymphoidei profundi membri superioris.

**no'di lymphoi'dei mem'bri superio'ris superficia'les,** nodi lymphoidei superficiales membri superioris.

**no'di lymphoi'dei mesente'rici,** mesenteric lymph nodes: nodes that lie at the root of the mesentery, receiving lymph from parts of the small intestine, cecum, appendix, and large intestine; they comprise three groups: the juxtaintestinal, central superior, and inferior mesenteric lymph nodes.

**no'di lymphoi'dei mesente'rici inferio'res** [TA], inferior mesenteric lymph nodes: nodes situated along the inferior mesenteric vessels and receiving lymph from the adjacent region; they comprise two groups: the sigmoid and superior rectal lymph nodes.

**no'di lymphoi'dei mesente'rici juxtaintestina'les** [TA], juxtaintestinal mesenteric lymph nodes: the mesenteric lymph nodes situated close to the wall of the intestine between the branches of the jejunal and ileal arteries; they drain into the superior mesenteric lymph node.

**no'di lymphoi'dei mesente'rici superio'res** [TA], superior mesenteric lymph nodes: mesenteric lymph nodes situated along the superior mesenteric artery and draining various other groups of nodes in the region.

**no'di lymphoi'dei mesente'rici superio'res centra'les** [TA], central superior mesenteric lymph nodes: the middle group of superior mesenteric nodes, situated along the ileal and jejunal branches of the superior mesenteric artery.

**no'di lymphoi'dei mesocol'ici** [TA], mesocolic lymph nodes: lymph nodes situated in the mesocolon, comprising two groups: paracolic and colic (right, middle, and left colic); they drain through the superior mesenteric lymph node.

**n. lymphoi'deus nasolabia'lis** [TA], nasolabial lymph node: one of a variable number of facial lymph nodes situated near the junction of the superior labial and facial arteries, which drains the upper lip and external nose into the submandibular node.

**no'di lymphoi'dei obturato'rii** [TA], obturator lymph nodes: the external iliac lymph nodes situated in the obturator canal.

**no'di lymphoi'dei occipita'les** [TA], occipital lymph nodes: several small nodes near the occipital insertion of the semispinalis capitis muscle.

**no'di lymphoi'dei pancrea'tici** [TA], pancreatic lymph nodes: nodes found along the pancreatic arteries that drain lymph from the pancreas to the pancreaticosplenic lymph nodes.

**no'di lymphoi'dei pancrea'tici inferio'res** [TA], inferior pancreatic lymph nodes: lymph nodes associated with the inferior pancreatic artery.

**no'di lymphoi'dei pancrea'tici superio'res** [TA], superior pancreatic lymph nodes: lymph nodes associated with the superior pancreatic artery.

**no'di lymphoi'dei pancreaticoduodena'les inferio'res** [TA], inferior pancreaticoduodenal lymph nodes: lymph nodes situated along the inferior pancreaticoduodenal artery.

**no'di lymphoi'dei pancreaticoduodena'les superio'res** [TA], superior pancreaticoduodenal lymph nodes: lymph nodes situated along the superior pancreaticoduodenal artery.

**no'di lymphoi'dei paracol'ici** [TA], paracolic lymph nodes: a subgroup of the mesocolic lymph nodes, situated along the medial borders of the ascending and descending colon and along the mesenteric borders of the transverse and sigmoid colon.

**no'di lymphoi'dei paramamma'rii** [TA], paramammary lymph nodes: lymph nodes on the lateral mammary gland that drain into the axillary lymph nodes.

**no'di lymphoi'dei pararecta'les** [TA], pararectal lymph nodes: lymph nodes situated around the rectum, embedded in its muscular coat; they drain into the inferior mesenteric, sacral, internal iliac, common iliac, and superficial inguinal nodes. Called also *anorectal lymph nodes* and *nodi lymphoidei anorectales* [TA alternative].

**no'di lymphoi'dei parasterna'les** [TA], parasternal lymph nodes: nodes located along the course of the internal thoracic artery, which drain the mammary gland, abdominal wall, and diaphragm.

**no'di lymphoi'dei paratrachea'les** [TA], paratracheal lymph nodes: lymph nodes on either side of the esophagus, extending upward into the neck, which receive lymph from the esophagus, trachea, and tracheobronchial lymph nodes.

**no'di lymphoi'dei parauteri'ni** [TA], parauterine lymph nodes: lymph nodes situated around the uterus, consisting of superficial (beneath the peritoneum) and deep (in the substance of the uterine wall) nodes: they drain into the lumbar, external and internal iliac, sacral, and superficial inguinal lymph nodes.

**no'di lymphoi'dei paravagina'les** [TA], paravaginal lymph nodes: lymph nodes situated around the vagina; they drain into the external and internal iliac, common iliac, and superficial inguinal lymph nodes.

**no'di lymphoi'dei paravesica'les** [TA], paravesicular lymph nodes: lymph nodes situated around the urinary bladder, comprising three groups: perivesicular, postvesicular, and lateral vesicular lymph nodes; they drain into the external and internal iliac lymph nodes and, in association with some lymph nodes from the prostate, into the sacral and common iliac lymph nodes.

**no'di lymphoi'dei parieta'les** [TA], parietal lymph nodes: lymph nodes that receive lymph from the walls of a body cavity; cf. *nodi lymphoidei viscerales.*

**no'di lymphoi'dei paroti'dei profun'di** [TA], deep parotid lymph nodes: lymph nodes on the lateral wall of the pharynx lying deep to or embedded in the deep substance of the parotid gland, through which lymph drains from the external acoustic meatus, auditory tube, tympanum, soft palate, and posterior nasal cavity.

**no'di lymphoi'dei paroti'dei profun'di infraauricula'res** [TA], infra-auricular deep parotid lymph nodes: deep parotid lymph nodes situated below the ear.

**no'di lymphoi'dei paroti'dei profun'di intraglandula'res** [TA], intraglandular deep parotid lymph nodes: deep parotid lymph nodes situated within the substance of the parotid gland.

**no'di lymphoi'dei paroti'dei profun'di preauricula'res** [TA], preauricular deep parotid lymph nodes: deep parotid lymph nodes situated in front of the ear.

**no'di lymphoi'dei paroti'dei superficia'les** [TA], superficial parotid lymph nodes: lymph nodes lying in the subcutaneous tissue of the parotid gland directly in front of the tragus.

**no'di lymphoi'dei pel'vis parieta'les** [TA], parietal pelvic lymph nodes: the lymph nodes that drain the wall of the pelvis, including the common iliac, external iliac, and internal iliac lymph nodes.

**no'di lymphoi'dei pel'vis viscera'les** [TA], visceral pelvic lymph nodes: the lymph nodes that drain the pelvic viscera, including the paravesicular, parauterine, paravaginal, and pararectal lymph nodes.

**no'di lymphoi'dei pericardi'aci latera'les** [TA], **no'di lymphoi'dei pericardia'les latera'les,** lateral pericardial lymph nodes: lymph nodes accompanying the pericardiacophrenic artery.

**no'di lymphoi'dei phre'nici inferio'res** [TA], inferior phrenic lymph nodes: parietal lymph nodes accompanying the inferior vessels of the diaphragm.

**no'di lymphoi'dei phre'nici superio'res** [TA], superior phrenic lymph nodes: several nodes on the thoracic surface of the diaphragm, receiving lymph from the intercostal spaces, pericardium, diaphragm, and liver; called also *diaphragmatic lymph nodes.*

**no'di lymphoi'dei poplitea'les,** nodi lymphoidei poplitei.

**no'di lymphoi'dei poplitea'les profun'di,** nodi lymphoidei poplitei profundi.

**no'di lymphoi'dei poplitea'les superficia'les,** nodi lymphoidei poplitei superficiales.

**no'di lymphoi'dei popli'tei** [TA], popliteal lymph nodes: lymph nodes embedded in the fat of the popliteal fossa, comprising superficial and deep groups; their efferent vessels accompany the femoral vessels to the deep inguinal lymph nodes.

**no'di lymphoi'dei popli'tei profun'di** [TA], deep popliteal lymph nodes: the popliteal lymph nodes situated at the sides of the popliteal vessels.

**no′di lymphoi′dei popli′tei superficia′les** [TA], superficial popliteal lymph nodes: the popliteal lymph nodes situated at the termination of the small saphenous vein.

**no′di lymphoi′dei postaor′tici,** TA alternative for *nodi lymphoidei retroaortici.*

**no′di lymphoi′dei postcava′les,** TA alternative for *nodi lymphoidei retrocavales.*

**no′di lymphoi′dei postvesica′les,** TA alternative for *nodi lymphoidei retrovesicales.*

**no′di lymphoi′dei preaor′tici** [TA], preaortic lymph nodes: a group of lymph nodes of the left lumbar group that is in front of the aorta and drains the abdominal part of the alimentary canal and its derivatives.

**no′di lymphoi′dei precaeca′les** [TA], prececal lymph nodes: lymph nodes situated in front of the cecum that drain into the anterior ileocolic lymph nodes.

**no′di lymphoi′dei precava′les** [TA], precaval lymph nodes: a group of lymph nodes of the right lumbar group that is in front of the inferior vena cava.

**no′di lymphoi′dei prececa′les,** nodi lymphoidei precaecales.

**no′di lymphoi′dei prelaryngea′les, no′di lymphoi′dei prelaryn′gei** [TA], prelaryngeal lymph nodes: deep anterior cervical lymph nodes situated in front of the larynx that help drain the thyroid gland.

**no′di lymphoi′dei prepericardi′aci** [TA], **no′di lymphoi′dei prepericardia′les,** prepericardial lymph nodes: lymph nodes situated between the pericardium and sternum.

**no′di lymphoi′dei pretrachea′les** [TA], pretracheal lymph nodes: deep anterior cervical lymph nodes situated in front of the trachea near the inferior thyroid veins.

**no′di lymphoi′dei prevertebra′les** [TA], prevertebral lymph nodes: lymph nodes situated in back of the thoracic aorta.

**no′di lymphoi′dei prevesica′les** [TA], prevesicular lymph nodes: the paravesicular lymph nodes situated in front of the urinary bladder.

**no′di lymphoi′dei profun′di mem′bri superio′ris** [TA], deep lymph nodes of upper limb: the lymph nodes situated internal to the deep fascia of the upper limb, most of which are grouped in the axilla; they accompany the radial, ulnar, interosseous, and brachial arteries and end in the brachial axillary lymph nodes.

**no′di lymphoi′dei pulmona′les,** nodi lymphoidei intrapulmonales.

**no′di lymphoi′dei pylo′rici** [TA], pyloric lymph nodes: lymph nodes found anterior to the head of the pancreas, receiving lymph from the pyloric part of the stomach. They are subdivided into three groups: suprapyloric, subpyloric, and retropyloric nodes.

**no′di lymphoi′dei recta′les superio′res** [TA], superior rectal lymph nodes: a group of lymph nodes of the inferior mesenteric group, situated along the superior rectal artery.

**no′di lymphoi′dei retroaor′tici** [TA], retroaortic lymph nodes: a group of lymph nodes of the left lumbar group, situated behind the aorta and formed by peripheral nodes of the right and left lateral aortic lymph nodes. Called also *postaortic lymph nodes* and *nodi lymphoidei postaortici* [TA alternative].

**no′di lymphoi′dei retrocaeca′les** [TA], retrocecal lymph nodes: lymph nodes situated in back of the cecum that drain into the posterior ileocecal lymph nodes.

**no′di lymphoi′dei retrocava′les** [TA], retrocaval lymph nodes: a group of lymph nodes of the right lumbar group situated behind the inferior vena cava. Called also *postcaval lymph nodes* and *nodi lymphoidei postcavales* [TA alternative].

**no′di lymphoi′dei retropharyngea′les** [TA], retropharyngeal lymph nodes: deep lateral cervical lymph nodes, one median and two lateral groups, situated behind the upper part of the pharynx, especially concerned with drainage of the nasal fossae, paranasal sinuses, hard and soft palates, middle ear, nasopharynx, and oropharynx.

**no′di lymphoi′dei retropylo′rici** [TA], retropyloric lymph nodes: pyloric lymph nodes situated posterior to the pylorus.

**no′di lymphoi′dei retrovesica′les** [TA], retrovesicular lymph nodes: the paravesicular lymph nodes situated in back of the urinary bladder. Called also *postvesicular lymph nodes* and *nodi lymphoidei postvesicales* [TA alternative].

**no′di lymphoi′dei sacra′les** [TA], sacral lymph nodes: the internal iliac lymph nodes situated along the lateral and median sacral vessels; they receive lymph from the rectum and posterior pelvic wall.

**no′di lymphoi′dei sigmoi′dei** [TA], sigmoid lymph nodes: a group of lymph nodes of the inferior mesenteric group, situated along the sigmoid arteries.

**no′di lymphoi′dei sple′nici** [TA], splenic lymph nodes: lymph nodes in the capsule and larger trabeculae of the spleen that drain into adjacent lymph nodes; called also *nodi lymphoidei lienales* [TA alternative].

**no′di lymphoi′dei submandibula′res** [TA], submandibular lymph nodes: the three to six nodes alongside the submandibular gland, through which lymph drains from the adjacent skin and mucous membrane.

**no′di lymphoi′dei submenta′les** [TA], submental lymph nodes: nodes under the chin into which the lymph from some of the superficial tissues of the head and neck is drained.

**no′di lymphoi′dei subpylo′rici** [TA], subpyloric lymph nodes: pyloric lymph nodes located inferior to the pylorus.

**no′di lymphoi′dei superficia′les mem′bri superio′ris** [TA], superficial lymph nodes of upper limb: the lymph nodes of the upper limb that are superficially placed, such as the cubital lymph nodes; all except those in the hand and on the back of the forearm converge toward and accompany the superficial veins.

**no′di lymphoi′dei superio′res centra′les,** nodi lymphoidei mesenterici superiores centrales.

**no′di lymphoi′dei supraclavicula′res** [TA], supraclavicular lymph nodes: the deep lateral cervical lymph nodes situated inferior to the omohyoid muscle, extending into the omoclavicular portion of the posterior triangle of the neck.

**n. lymphoi′deus suprapylo′ricus** [TA], suprapyloric lymph node: a pyloric lymph node located superior to the duodenum on the right gastric artery.

**no′di lymphoi′dei supratrochlea′res** [TA], supratrochlear lymph nodes: one or two lymph nodes superficial to the deep fascia proximal to the medial epicondyle and medial to the basilic vein and draining into the deep lymph vessels.

**no′di lymphoi′dei thyroi′dei** [TA], thyroid lymph nodes: deep anterior cervical lymph nodes situated around the thyroid gland.

**n. lymphoi′deus tibia′lis ante′rior** [TA], anterior tibial lymph node: a lymph node situated along the anterior tibial artery.

**n. lymphoi′deus tibia′lis poste′rior** [TA], posterior tibial lymph node: a lymph node situated along the posterior tibial artery.

**no′di lymphoi′dei tracheobronchia′les inferio′res** [TA], inferior tracheobronchial lymph nodes: nodes in the angle of the bifurcation of the trachea, receiving lymph from adjacent structures.

**no′di lymphoi′dei tracheobronchia′les superio′res** [TA], superior tracheobronchial lymph nodes: nodes between the trachea and the bronchus on either side, receiving lymph from adjacent structures.

**no′di lymphoi′dei vesica′les latera′les** [TA], lateral vesicular lymph nodes: the paravesicular lymph nodes situated in relation to the lateral umbilical ligament.

**no′di lymphoi′dei viscera′les** [TA], visceral lymph nodes: lymph nodes that receive lymph from the viscera in a body cavity; cf. *nodi lymphoidei parietales.*

**n. sinuatria′lis** [TA], sinoatrial node: a microscopic collection of atypical cardiac muscle fibers (Purkinje fibers) at the superior end of the sulcus terminalis, at the junction of the superior vena cava and the right atrium. The cardiac rhythm normally takes its origin in this node, which thus is known also as the *cardiac pacemaker.* Called also *sinuatrial* or *sinus node.*

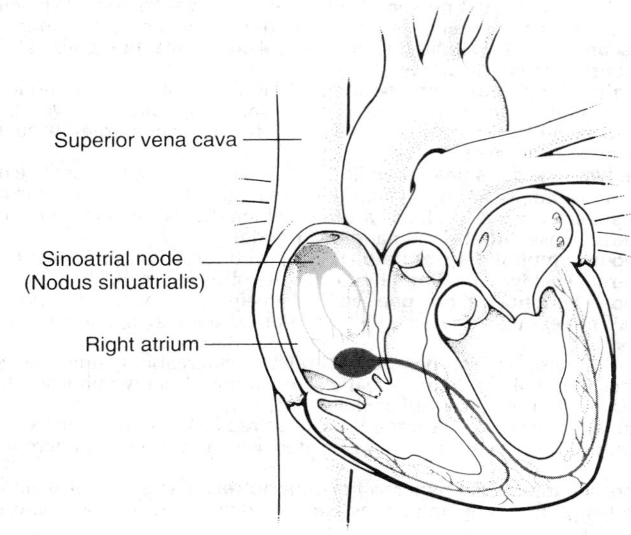

**NOEL** no observed effect level.

**no·e·ma·tacho·graph** (no-e″mə-tak′o-graf) [Gr. *noēma* thought + *tacho-* + *-graph*] a device for registering the time required in a mental operation.

**no·e·ma·ta·chom·e·ter** (no-e″mə-tə-kom′ə-tər) [Gr. *noēma* thought + *tacho-* + *-meter*] a device for measuring the time required in a mental operation.

**no·e·mat·ic** (no″e-mat′ik) pertaining to thought or the operation of the mind.

**no·e·sis** (no-e′sis) [Gr. *noēsis* thought] the operation of the intellect; cognition.

**no·et·ic** (no-et′ik) pertaining to the intellect or to cognition.

**no·gal·a·my·cin** (no-gal″ə-mi′sin) [MeSH: Nogalamycin] an antineoplastic antibiotic produced by a variant of *Streptomyces nogalater.*

**noise** (noiz) [MeSH: Noise] unwanted variations in a signal that result from imperfections in the transmission of the signal, e.g., electrical signals in electrodiagnosis other than those being studied (most often originating within the electrical apparatus). See also *signal-to-noise ratio,* under *ratio.*
**end-plate n.,** the monophasic type of end-plate activity.

**Nol·va·dex** (nol′və-deks″) trademark for a preparation of tamoxifen citrate.

**no·ma** (no′mə) [Gr. *nomai* eating sores] [MeSH: Noma] 1. a severe gangrenous process usually seen in debilitated and malnourished children, beginning as a small vesicle or ulcer on the gingiva that rapidly becomes necrotic and spreads to destroy large areas of the buccal and labial mucosa and tissues of the face, resulting in severe disfigurement or even death. Bacteria implicated in the etiology include fusiform bacilli, *Treponema vincentii,* and *Bacteroides melaninogenicus.* Called also *cancrum oris* and *gangrenous stomatitis.* 2. gangrenous erosions similar to those of the face but involving the genitalia; see *erosive balanitis,* under *balanitis,* and *erosive vulvitis,* under *vulvitis.*
**n. vul′vae,** erosive vulvitis.

**no·mad·ic** (no-mad′ik) wandering; unsettled; free.

**no·men** (no′mən) pl. *no′mina* [L.] a name.
**no′mina genera′lia** [TA], general terminology: terms that denote a general structure type to which a number of specific structures belong.

**no·men·cla·ture** (no′mən-kla′chər) [*nomen* + *calare* to call] [MeSH: Nomenclature] a classified system of names, as of anatomical structures, organisms, etc. See *Terminologia Anatomica.*
**binomial n.,** the nomenclature used in scientific classification of living organisms in which each organism is designated by two latinized names (genus and species), both of which must always be used because species names are not necessarily unique. NOTE: The genus name is always capitalized, the species name is not, and both are italicized, e.g., *Escherichia coli.* When a name is repeated the genus name may be abbreviated by its initial, e.g., *E. coli.*

**no·mi·fen·sine mal·e·ate** (no″mĭ-fen′sēn) a central nervous system stimulant used as an antidepressant.

**No·mi·na Ana·to·mi·ca** (no′mĭ-nə an″ə-tom′ĭ-kə) [L. "anatomical names"] the official body of anatomical nomenclature, applied specifically to that revised by the International Anatomical Nomenclature Committee appointed by the Fifth International Congress of Anatomists held at Oxford in 1950, and approved by the Sixth International Congress of Anatomists (Paris, 1955) with revisions approved by the Seventh (New York, 1960), Eighth (Wiesbaden, 1965), Tenth (Tokyo, 1975), Eleventh (Mexico City, 1980), and Twelfth (London, 1985) International Congresses of Anatomists. It has been superseded by *Terminologia Anatomica* [TA] (1998).

**nom(o)-** [Gr. *nomos* custom, law] a combining form denoting relationship to usage or law.

**no·mo·gen·e·sis** (no″mo-jen′ə-sis) [*nomo-* + *-genesis*] the theory of evolution according to which the course of evolution is fixed and predetermined by law, no place being left for chance.

**no·mo·gram** (nom′o-gram) [*nomo-* + *-gram*] a figure consisting of three or more straight or curved lines, each graduated for a different variable and aligned in such a way that a straightedge crossing all of the scales cuts the scales at values of the variable that have a specified mathematical or empirical relationship. Called also *nomograph.*

**no·mo·graph** (nom′o-graf) nomogram.

**no·mo·top·ic** (no″mo-top′ik) [*nomo-* + *top-* + *-ic*] occurring at a normal place; occurring normally.

**non·ad·her·ent** (non″ad-hēr′ənt) not adherent to or connected with adjacent structures.

**no·nan** (no′nən) [L. *nonus* ninth] recurring every ninth day, or at intervals of eight days.

**non·an·ti·gen·ic** (non″an-tĭ-jen′ik) not antigenic; not eliciting an immune response in a particular animal.

**non·a·pep·tide** (non″ə-pep′tīd) [L. *nonus* ninth + *peptide*] a peptide containing nine amino acids.

**non com·pos men·tis** (non kom′pos men′tis) [L.] not of sound mind, and so not legally responsible.

**non·con·duc·tor** (non″kən-duk′tər) any substance that does not readily transmit electricity, light, or heat.

**non·de·po·lar·iz·er** (non″de-po′lər-īz-ər) a muscle relaxant that produces striate muscle paralysis by competitive interference with the transmission of nerve impulses from nerve ending to muscle receptor.

**non·dis·junc·tion** (non″dis-junk′shən) failure *(a)* of two homologous chromosomes to pass to separate cells during the first division of meiosis, or *(b)* of the two chromatids of a chromosome to pass to separate cells during mitosis or during the second meiotic division. As a result, one daughter cell has an extra chromosome and the other has one too few. If this happens in meiosis, after fertilization an *aneuploid* individual may develop, e.g., a child with trisomy 21 (Down syndrome).

**non·elec·tro·lyte** (non″e-lek′tro-līt) a substance that does not dissociate into ions; in solution it is a nonconductor of electricity.

**non·heme** (non′hēm) not bound within a porphyrin ring; said of iron so contained within a protein.

**non·ho·mo·ge·ne·i·ty** (non-ho″mo-jə-ne′ĭ-te) the lack of homogeneity; the state of not being homogeneous.

**no·ni·grav·i·da** (no″ne-grav′ĭ-də) [L. *nonus* ninth + *gravida*] a woman pregnant for the ninth time. Written gravida IX.

**non·in·fec·tious** (non″in-fek′shəs) not infectious; not spread by contact, inhalation, etc.; not able to spread disease.

**non·in·vo·lu·tion** (non″in-vo-loo′shən) failure of a part to return to normal size and condition after enlargement from functional activity, as noninvolution of the uterus after pregnancy.

**no·nip·a·ra** (no-nip′ə-rə) [L. *nonus* ninth + *para*] a woman who has had nine pregnancies which resulted in viable offspring. Written para IX.

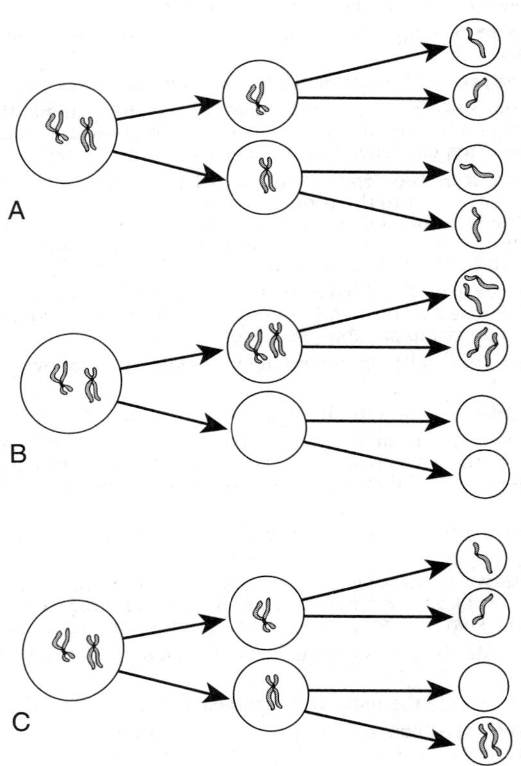


Nondisjunction. Normal meiosis *(A)* is contrasted with failure of homologous chromosomes to separate in meiosis I *(B)* or of sister chromatids to separate in meiosis II *(C).*

**non·med·ul·lat·ed** (non-med'u-lāt"əd) unmyelinated.

**non·met·al** (non-met'əl) any chemical element that is not a metal or a metalloid.

**non·my·eli·nat·ed** (non-mi'ə-lĭ-nāt"əd) unmyelinated.

**Non·ne-Mil·roy disease** (non'ə-mil'roi) [Max *Nonne,* German neurologist, 1861–1939; William Forsyth *Milroy,* American physician, 1855–1942] see *Milroy's disease,* under *disease.*

**Non·ne-Mil·roy-Meige syndrome** (non'ə-mil'roi-mezh) [M. *Nonne;* W. F. *Milroy;* Henri *Meige,* French physician, 1866–1940] see *Milroy's disease,* under *disease.*

**non-neu·ro·nal** (non"no͞o-ro'nəl) pertaining to or composed of nonconducting cells of the nervous system, e.g., neuroglial cells.

**non·nu·cle·at·ed** (non-noo'kle-āt"əd) without a nucleus; cf. *anuclear.*

**non·oc·clu·sion** (non"o-cloo'zhən) open bite malocclusion.

**non·ol·i·gu·ric** (non-ol"ĭ-gu'rik) not pertaining to, characterized by, or conducive to oliguria.

**non·on·co·gen·ic** (non"on-ko-jen'ik) not giving rise to tumors or causing tumor formation.

**non·opaque** (non"o-pāk') not opaque to x-rays; radiolucent.

**non·ose** (non'ōs) [L. *nonus* ninth] a monosaccharide containing nine atoms of carbon in the molecule.

**no·nox·y·nol** (no-nok'sĭ-nōl) [MeSH: Nonoxynol] nonylphenoxypolyethoxyethanol. A group of compounds of the general composition $C_{15}H_{24}O(C_2H_4O)_n$, which are assigned numbers according to the approximate value of *n*: *nonoxynol 4* is $C_{15}H_{24}O(C_2H_4O)_4$, or $C_{23}H_{40}O_5$; *nonoxynol 9* is $C_{33}H_{60}O_{10}$; *nonoxynol 15* is $C_{45}H_{84}O_{16}$; *nonoxynol 30* is $C_{75}H_{144}O_{31}$. Nonoxynol 4, 15, and 30 are nonionic surfactants, and nonoxynol 9 is used as a spermaticide. Nonoxynol 10, in which *n* varies from 6 to 16, is used as a pharmaceutical surfactant.

**non·para·met·ric** (non"par-ə-met'rik) denoting statistical methods or tests requiring neither parameters nor distributional assumptions.

**non·par·ous** (non-par'əs) nulliparous.

**non·pho·to·chro·mo·gen** (non"fo-to-kro'mə-jən) a microorganism that does not produce pigment in the presence of light. The term is specifically applied to mycobacteria that do not produce carotenoid pigmentation; included in this group is the common pathogen *Mycobacterium avium–intracellulare.*

**non·po·lar** (non-po'lər) not having poles; not exhibiting dipole characteristics.

**non repetat.** abbreviation for L. *non repeta'tur,* do not repeat.

**non·re·spond·er** (non-re-spon'dər) a person or animal that after vaccination against a given virus does not show any immune response when challenged with the virus.

**non·ro·ta·tion** (non"ro-ta'shən) [*non-* + L. *rotare* to turn] failure of rotation of a part to the proper position.
**n. of the intestine,** failure of rotation of the intestine during embryonic development, so that the small intestine lies on the right side of the abdomen and the large intestine on the left.

**non·se·cre·tor** (non"se-kre'tor) an individual with A or B type blood whose saliva and other body secretions do not contain the A or B blood group antigens; see also *secretor.*

**non·self** (non'self) in immunology, pertaining to foreign antigens. Cf. *self.*

**non·sep·tate** (non-sep'tāt) without a septum or septa.

**non·spe·cif·ic** (non"spə-sif'ik) 1. not due to any single known cause, as to a particular pathogen. 2. not directed against a particular agent, but rather having a general effect, as nonspecific therapy.

**non·union** (non-ūn'yən) failure of the ends of a fractured bone to unite.

**non·va·lent** (non-va'lənt) [L. *non* not + *valere* to be able] having no chemical valency: not capable of entering into chemical composition; said of argon, helium, and the other inert gases.

**non·vi·a·ble** (non-vi'ə-bəl) [L. *non* not + *viable*] not capable of living.

**no·nyl** (no'nəl) the monovalent radical $C_9H_{19}$.

**Noo·nan's syndrome** (noo'nənz) [Jacqueline Anne *Noonan,* American pediatrician, born 1928] see under *syndrome.*

**noo·trop·ic** (no"o-trop'ik) [Gr. *noos, nous* mind + *-tropic*] having positive effects on organically impaired cognition or nervous system function; said of certain drugs.

**no·pal·in G** (no'pal-in) bluish eosin; see under *eosin.*

**NOPHN** National Organization for Public Health Nursing.

**nor-** chemical prefix denoting *(a)* a compound (e.g., norleucine) of normal structure (having an unbranched chain of carbon atoms) that is isomeric with one (e.g., leucine) having a branched chain, or *(b)* a compound (e.g., norepinephrine) whose chain or ring contains one less methylene ($CH_2$) group than does that of its homologue (e.g., epinephrine).

**nor·adren·a·line** (nor"ə-dren'ə-lin) norepinephrine.

**nor·ad·ren·er·gic** (nor"ə-drən-er'jik) activated by or secreting norepinephrine.

**nor·an·dro·sten·o·lone** (nor-an"dro-sten'ə-lōn) nandrolone.

**Nor·cu·ron** (nor-kūr'on) trademark for a preparation of vecuronium bromide.

**nor·def·rin hy·dro·chlo·ride** (nor-def'rin) an adrenergic agent isomeric with epinephrine, having significant central stimulant action and almost no vasoconstrictor action; the levo-isomer, *levonordefrin* (q.v.), is usually used when vasoconstriction is desired. Called also *homoarterenol hydrochloride.*

**no·re·flow** (no-re'flo) see under *phenomenon.*

**nor·epi·neph·rine** (nor"ep-ĭ-nef'rin) [MeSH: Norepinephrine] 1. one of the naturally occurring catecholamines, a neurohormone released by the postganglionic adrenergic nerves and some brain neurons; it is a major neurotransmitter that acts on $\alpha$- and $\beta_1$-adrenergic receptors. It is also secreted by the adrenal medulla in response to splanchnic stimulation and is stored in the chromaffin granules. It is a powerful vasopressor and is released in the body usually in response to hypotension or stress. Called also *noradrenaline.* 2. a pharmaceutical preparation of the same substance, usually seen in the form of the bitartrate salt.
**n. bitartrate** [USP], the bitartrate salt of the levorotatory isomer of norepinephrine, having the vasoconstrictor actions of the parent compound; used to restore the blood pressure in certain cases of acute hypotension, and as an adjunct in the treatment of cardiac arrest and profound hypotension, administered by intravenous infusion. Called also *levarterenol bitartrate.*
**n. hydrochloride,** the hydrochloride salt of norepinephrine, having actions similar to those of the parent compound; called also *arterenol.*

**nor·eth·an·dro·lone** (nor"əth-an'drə-lōn) [MeSH: Norethandrolone] a synthetic androgen equal to testosterone in anabolic activity, but having less androgenic activity.

**nor·eth·in·drone** (nor-eth'in-drōn) [USP] [MeSH: Norethindrone] a progestin having some anabolic, estrogenic, and androgenic properties; used in the treatment of amenorrhea, abnormal uterine bleeding due to hormonal imbalance, and endometriosis, administered orally. Also used, alone or in combination with an estrogen component, as an oral contraceptive.
**n. acetate** [USP], the acetate salt of norethindrone, having the same appearance, actions, uses, and route of administration as the base.

**nor·eth·is·ter·one** (nor"əth-is'tər-ōn) norethindrone.

**nor·ethy·no·drel** (nor"ə-thi'no-drəl) [USP] [MeSH: Norethynodrel] a progestin used in combination with an estrogen component as an oral contraceptive, to control endometriosis, for the treatment of hypermenorrhea, and to produce cyclic withdrawal bleeding.

**Nor·flex** (nor'fleks) trademark for a preparation of orphenadrine citrate.

**nor·flox·a·cin** (nor-flok'sə-sin) [MeSH: Norfloxacin] a fluorinated 4-quinolone antibacterial effective against penicillin-resistant *Neisseria gonorrhoeae;* administered orally.

**Nor·ge·sic** (nor-je'zik) trademark for a preparation of orphenadrine citrate.

**nor·ges·ti·mate** (nor-jes'tĭ-māt) a synthetic progestin used in combination with an estrogen component as an oral contraceptive.

**nor·ges·trel** (nor-jes'trəl) [USP] [MeSH: Norgestrel] a potent progestin used in combination with an estrogen component as an oral contraceptive.

**nor·hyo·scy·amine** (nor-hi"o-si'ə-mēn) an alkaloid from plants of the family Solanaceae, having properties like those of hyoscyamine. Called also *pseudohyoscyamine* and *solandrine.*

**Nor·iso·drine** (nor-i'so-drin) trademark for preparations of isoproterenol.

**nor·leu·cine** (nor-loo'sēn) [MeSH: Norleucine] chemical name: 2-aminohexanoic acid. A nonessential amino acid extracted from the leucine fraction of the decomposition of the proteins of nervous tissue. It has been synthesized.

**Nor·lu·tate** (nor-loo'tāt) trademark for a preparation of norethindrone acetate.

**Nor·lu·tin** (nor-loo'tin) trademark for a preparation of norethindrone.

**norm** (norm) [L. *norma* rule] a fixed or ideal standard.

**nor·ma** (nor'mə) [L.] 1. an outline established to define the aspects of the cranium 2. a norm or typical standard.
**n. ante'rior,** n. facialis.
**n. basa'lis,** TA alternative for *n. inferior.*
**n. basila'ris,** n. inferior.
**n. facia'lis** [TA], the outline of the skull as viewed from the front; called also *anterior, facial,* or *frontal aspect of cranium, n. anterior,* and *n. frontalis* [TA alternative].
**n. fronta'lis,** TA alternative for *n. facialis.*
**n. infe'rior** [TA], the outline of the inferior aspect of the skull, viewed from above; called also *n. basalis* [TA alternative] and *n. basilaris.*
**n. latera'lis** [TA], the outline of the skull as viewed from either side; called also *temporal aspect of cranium* and *n. temporalis.*
**n. occipita'lis** [TA], **n. poste'rior,** the outline of the skull as viewed from behind; called also *occipital aspect of cranium.*
**n. sagitta'lis,** the outline of a sagittal section through the skull.
**n. supe'rior** [TA], the outline of the superior surface of the skull; called also *superior* or *vertical aspect of cranium* and *n. verticalis* [TA alternative].
**n. tempora'lis,** n. lateralis.
**n. ventra'lis,** basis cranii externa.
**n. vertica'lis,** TA alternative for *n. superior.*

**nor·mal** (nor'məl) [L. *norma* rule] 1. agreeing with the regular and established type. 2. in chemistry, *(a)* denoting a solution containing in each 1000 mL 1 g equivalent weight of the active substance, symbol N or *N*; *(b)* denoting aliphatic hydrocarbons in which no carbon atom is combined with more than 2 other carbon atoms, symbol *n-*; *(c)* denoting salts formed from acids and bases in such a way that no acidic hydrogen of the acid remains nor any of the basic hydroxyl of the base.

**nor·mal·i·ty** (nor-mal'ĭ-te) 1. the state of being normal. 2. the number of gram-equivalent weights of solute per liter of solution.

**nor·mal·iza·tion** (nor″məl-ĭ-za'shən) 1. the process of bringing or restoring to the normal standard. 2. in statistics, the process of transforming data so that it has no units but is expressed in terms of standard deviations from the mean.

**nor·meta·neph·rine** (nor-met″ə-nef'rin) [MeSH: Normetanephrine] a methylated metabolite of norepinephrine excreted in the urine and found in certain tissues.

**norm(o)-** [L. *norma* rule] a combining form meaning conforming to the rule; normal or usual.

**nor·mo·blast** (nor'mo-blast) [*normo-* + *-blast*] [MeSH: Erythroblasts] 1. a term often used as a synonym of erythroblast, but sometimes specifically denoting nucleated cells in a normal course of erythrocyte maturation, as distinguished from megaloblasts (q.v.); when the term is used with this meaning, the developmental stages of the nucleated cells of the erythrocytic series (q.v.) are generally named pronormoblasts *(proerythroblasts)* and basophilic, polychromatophilic, and orthochromatic normoblasts (see under *erythroblast*). 2. orthochromatic erythroblast.
**acidophilic n.,** orthochromatic erythroblast.
**basophilic n.,** a nucleated immature erythrocyte, having cytoplasm generally similar to that of the earlier proerythroblast but sometimes even more basophilic, and usually regular in outline. The nucleus is still relatively large, but the chromatin strands are thicker and more deeply staining, giving a coarser appearance; the nucleoli have disappeared. Called also *prorubricyte, early n.,* and *basophilic* or *early erythroblast.*
**early n.,** basophilic erythroblast.
**eosinophilic n.,** orthochromatic erythroblast.
**intermediate n.,** polychromatophilic erythroblast.
**late n., orthochromatic n., oxyphilic n.,** see under *erythroblast.*
**polychromatic n., polychromatophilic n.,** see under *erythroblast.*

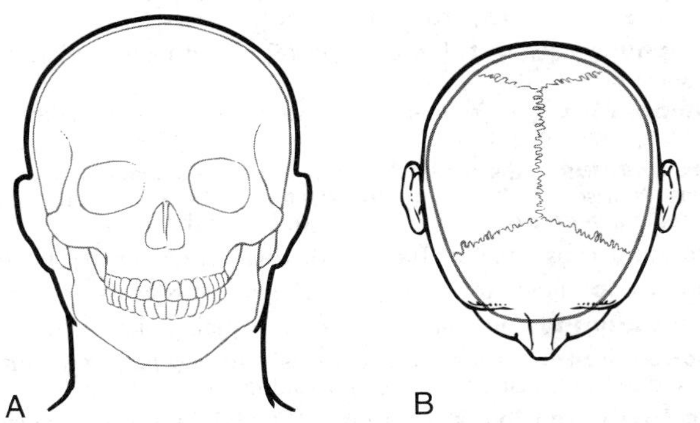

*(A),* Norma facialis; *(B),* norma verticalis.

**nor·mo·blas·tic** (nor″mo-blas'tik) relating to or having the character of a normoblast.

**nor·mo·blas·to·sis** (nor″mo-blas-to'sis) excessive production of normoblasts by the bone marrow.

**nor·mo·cal·ce·mia** (nor″mo-kal-se'me-ə) a normal level of calcium in the blood.

**nor·mo·cal·ce·mic** (nor″mo-kal-se'mik) pertaining to or characterized by normocalcemia.

**nor·mo·cap·nia** (nor″mo-kap'ne-ə) eucapnia.

**nor·mo·cap·nic** (nor″mo-kap'nik) eucapnic.

**nor·mo·cho·les·ter·ol·emia** (nor″mo-kə-les″tər-ol-e'me-ə) a normal level of cholesterol in the blood.

**nor·mo·cho·les·ter·ol·emic** (nor″mo-kə-les″tər-ol-e'mik) pertaining to, characterized by, or tending to produce a normal level of cholesterol in the blood.

**nor·mo·chro·ma·sia** (nor″mo-kro-ma'zhə) [*normo-* + Gr. *chrōma* color] 1. a normal staining reaction in a cell or tissue. 2. normochromia.

**nor·mo·chro·mia** (nor″mo-kro'me-ə) normal color (hemoglobin content) of the red blood cells; see also *normochromic anemia,* under *anemia.* Called also *normochromasia* and *orthochromia.*

**nor·mo·chro·mic** (nor″mo-kro'mik) 1. having a normal color. 2. having a normal hemoglobin content; called also *orthochromic.*

**nor·mo·crin·ic** (nor″mo-krin'ik) pertaining to normal secretion or to normal endocrine action.

**nor·mo·cyte** (nor'mo-sīt) [*normo-* + *-cyte*] an erythrocyte that is normal in size, shape, and color. Called also *normoerythrocyte.*

**nor·mo·cyt·ic** (nor″mo-sit'ik) relating to or having the character of a normocyte.

**Nor·mo·cy·tin** (nor″mo-si'tin) trademark for preparations of concentrated crystalline vitamin $B_{12}$. See *cyanocobalamin.*

**nor·mo·cy·to·sis** (nor″mo-si-to'sis) a normal state of the blood in respect to the erythrocytes.

**Nor·mo·dyne** (nor'mo-dīn) trademark for a preparation of labetalol hydrochloride.

**nor·mo·eryth·ro·cyte** (nor″mo-ə-rith'ro-sīt) normocyte.

**nor·mo·gly·ce·mia** (nor″mo-gli-se'me-ə) euglycemia.

**nor·mo·gly·ce·mic** (nor″mo-gli-se'mik) euglycemic.

**nor·mo·ka·le·mia** (nor″mo-kə-le'me-ə) a normal level of potassium in the blood.

**nor·mo·ka·le·mic** (nor″mo-kə-le'mik) pertaining to, characterized by, or conducive to normokalemia.

**nor·mo·lip·i·de·mic** (nor″mo-lip″ĭ-de'mik) pertaining to or characterized by normal levels of lipids in the blood.

**nor·mo·or·tho·cy·to·sis** (nor″mo-or″tho-si-to'sis) [*normo-* + *orthocytosis*] an increase in total numbers of leukocytes in the blood but with a normal proportion between the different varieties; see also *absolute leukocytosis.*

**nor·mo·skeo·cy·to·sis** (nor″mo-ske″o-si-to'sis) [*normo-* + Gr. *skaios* left + *-cyte* + *-osis*] a condition of the leukocytes of the blood in which the number is normal, but many immature forms (deviation to the left) are present.

**nor·mo·sper·mic** (nor″mo-sper'mik) producing spermatozoa normal in number and motility.

**nor·mo·sthen·uria** (nor″mo-sthən-u're-ə) [*normo-* + *stheno-* + *-uria*] 1. the secretion of urine of varying specific gravity within the normal range. 2. normally active urination.

**nor·mo·ten·sion** (nor″mo-ten'shən) normal tone, tension, or pressure.

**nor·mo·ten·sive** (nor″mo-ten'siv) 1. characterized by normal tone, tension, or pressure, as by normal blood pressure. 2. a person with normal blood pressure.

**nor·mo·ther·mia** (nor″mo-ther'me-ə) [*normo-* + *therm-* + *-ia*] a normal state of temperature, especially normal body temperature (37°C or 98.6°F).

**nor·mo·ther·mic** (nor″mo-ther'mik) pertaining to or characterized by normal temperature; neither hyperthermic nor hypothermic.

**nor·mo·to·nia** (nor″mo-to'ne-ə) normal tone or tension.

**nor·mo·ton·ic** (nor″mo-ton'ik) pertaining to or characterized by normotonia.

**nor·mo·troph·ic** (nor″mo-trof'ik) of normal development; exhibiting neither hypertrophy nor hypotrophy.

**nor·mo·uri·ce·mia** (nor″mo-u″rĭ-se′me-ə) a normal value of uric acid in the blood.

**nor·mo·uri·ce·mic** (nor″mo-u″rĭ-se′mik) pertaining to or characterized by normouricemia.

**nor·mo·uri·cu·ria** (nor″mo-u″rĭ-ku′re-ə) a normal amount of uric acid in the urine.

**nor·mo·uri·cu·ric** (nor″mo-u″rĭ-ku′rik) pertaining to or characterized by normouricuria.

**nor·mo·vo·le·mia** (nor″mo-vo-le′me-ə) [*normo-* + *volume* + *-emia*] normal blood volume.

**nor·mo·vo·le·mic** (nor″mo-vo-le′mik) pertaining to or characterized by normovolemia; having a normal volume of circulating fluid (plasma) in the body.

**Nor·ox·in** (nor-ok′sin) trademark for a preparation of norfloxacin.

**Nor·pace** (nor′pās) trademark for a preparation of disopyramide phosphate.

**Nor·pram·in** (nor′prəm-in) trademark for a preparation of desipramine hydrochloride.

**nor·pseu·do·ephed·rine** (nor-soo″do-ə-fed′rēn) a nervous system stimulant from the leaves of the shrub *Catha edulis.*

**Nor·rie's disease** (nor′ēz) [Gordon *Norrie,* Danish ophthalmologist, 1855–1941] see under *disease.*

**Nor·ris' corpuscles** (nor′is-əz) [Richard *Norris,* English physiologist, 1831–1916] see under *corpuscle.*

**North·ern blot technique (blot analysis, blot hybridization, blot test)** (nor′thərn) [facetious coinage by analogy with *Southern blot technique*] see under *technique.*

**North·rop** (north′rop) John Howard. American chemist, born 1891; co-winner, with James Batcheller Sumner and Wendell Meredith Stanley, of the Nobel prize for chemistry in 1946 for isolation and crystallization of enzymes and for isolating virus proteins in pure form.

**nor·trip·ty·line hy·dro·chlo·ride** (nor-trip′tə-lēn) [USP] a tricyclic antidepressant of the dibenzocycloheptadiene class, used to treat symptoms of depression and to relieve chronic, severe pain; administered orally.

**Nor·vasc** (nor′vask) trademark for a preparation of amlodipine besylate.

**Nor·vir** (nor′vir) trademark for a preparation of ritonavir.

**Nor·walk gastroenteritis, virus** (nor′wawk) [*Norwalk,* Ohio, location of the outbreak from which the virus was isolated] see under *gastroenteritis* and *virus.*

**nos·az·on·tol·o·gy** (nos-az″on-tol′ə-je) nosetiology.

**nos·ca·pine** (nos′kə-pēn) [MeSH: Noscapine] an alkaloid of opium used as an antitussive, administered orally.
**n. hydrochloride,** the hydrochloride salt of noscapine, having the same actions, uses, and route of administration as the base.

**nose** (nōz) [L. *nasus;* Gr. *rhis*] [MeSH: Nose] 1. nasus. 2. nasus externus.
**cleft n.,** a developmental anomaly resulting from incomplete union of the paired nasal primordia.
**collie n.,** nasal solar dermatitis.
**external n.,** nasus externus.
**saddle n., saddle-back n., swayback n.,** concavity of the contour of the bridge of the nose due to collapse of cartilaginous or bony support, or both; it was once most often due to congenital syphilis, but is now more commonly the result of trauma, surgery, a congenital epidermal defect, or leprosy.

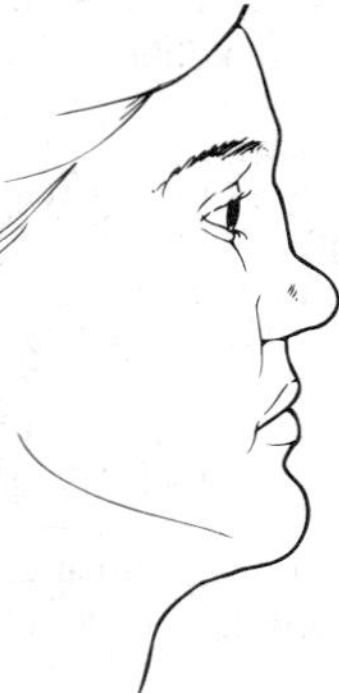

Saddle nose.

**nose·bleed** (nōz′blēd) epistaxis.

**nose·gay** (nōz′ga) a name applied to an anatomical structure resembling a small bunch of flowers.
**Riolan's n.,** the group of muscles that take their origin from the styloid process of the temporal bone.

**No·se·ma** (no-se′mə) [Gr. *nosēma* sickness] [MeSH: Nosema] a genus of intracellular protozoa (suborder Apansporoblastina, order Microsporida), formerly thought to be identical to *Encephalitozoon;* they are parasitic in invertebrates, and especially pathogenic in insects.
**N. a′pis,** the etiologic agent of nosema disease of bees.
**N. bomby′cis,** the etiologic agent of the disease pébrine in silkworms.
**N. cuni′culi,** *Encephalitozoon cuniculi.*
**N. ocula′rum,** a species that causes corneal infections in humans.

**no·se·ma·to·sis** (no-se″mə-to′sis) 1. infection with protozoa of the genus *Nosema.* 2. former name for *encephalitozoonosis.*

**nos·en·ceph·a·lus** (nos″ən-sef′ə-ləs) [*noso-* + Gr. *enkephalos* brain] a fetus with cranium bifidum.

**nose·piece** (nōz′pēs) the portion of a microscope nearest to the stage, which bears the objective or objectives, constructed so as to permit change of the objective without disturbing the focus of the instrument.
**quick-change n.,** one bearing a single objective, which may be quickly attached to or removed from a microscope.
**rotating n.,** one bearing more than one objective, designed to permit the one selected to be rotated into place, with its axis coincident with the optical axis of the microscope.

**nos·eti·ol·o·gy** (nos″e-te-ol′ə-je) [*nos-* + *etiology*] the study of the causation of disease.

**no·si·hep·tide** (no″sĭ-hep′tīd) a veterinary growth stimulant.

**nos(o)-** [Gr. *nosos* disease] a combining form denoting relationship to disease.

**nos·och·tho·nog·ra·phy** (nos″ok-tho-nog′rə-fe) [*noso-* + Gr. *chthōn* land + *-graphy*] geomedicine.

**noso·co·mi·al** (nos″o-ko′me-əl) [*noso-* + Gr. *komeion* to take care of] pertaining to or originating in the hospital; said of an infection not present or incubating prior to admittance to the hospital, but generally occurring 72 hours after admittance; the term is usually used to refer to patient disease, but hospital personnel may also acquire nosocomial infection. Cf. *iatrogenic.*

**noso·gen·e·sis** (nos″o-jen′ə-sis) pathogenesis.

**noso·gen·ic** (nos″o-jen′ik) pathogenic.

**no·sog·e·ny** (no-soj′ə-ne) [*noso-* + *-geny*] pathogenesis.

**noso·ge·og·ra·phy** (nos″o-je-og′rə-fe) [*noso-* + *geo-* + *-graphy*] geomedicine.

**no·sog·ra·phy** (no-sog′rə-fe) [*noso-* + *-graphy*] a written account or description of diseases.

**noso·log·ic** (nos″o-loj′ik) pertaining to the classification of disease.

**no·sol·o·gy** (no-sol′ə-je) [*noso-* + *-logy*] the science of the classification of diseases. Called also *nosonomy* and *nosotaxy.*

**no·som·e·try** (no-som′ə-tre) [*noso-* + *-metry*] the measurement of the morbidity rate.

**noso·my·co·sis** (nos″o-mi-ko′sis) mycosis.

**no·son·o·my** (no-son′ə-me) [*noso-* + Gr. *nomos* law] nosology.

**noso·para·site** (nos″o-par′ə-sīt) [*noso-* + *parasite*] an organism found in conjunction with a disease which it is able to modify, but not to produce.

**noso·pho·bia** (nos″o-fo′be-ə) [*noso-* + *-phobia*] irrational dread of sickness or of some particular disease.

**noso·phyte** (nos′o-fīt) [*noso-* + *-phyte*] a pathogenic plant microorganism.

**noso·poi·et·ic** (nos″o-poi-et′ik) [*noso-* + Gr. *poiein* to make] causing or producing disease.

**Noso·psyl·lus** (nos″o-sil′əs) [*noso-* + Gr. *psylla* flea] a genus of fleas. *N. fascia′tus,* the common rat flea of North America and Europe, is a vector of murine typhus and probably of plague.

**noso·taxy** (nos′o-tak″se) [*noso-* + Gr. *taxis* arrangement] nosology.

**noso·tox·ic** (nos″o-tok′sik) producing nosotoxicosis.

**noso·tox·ic·i·ty** (nos″o-tok-sis′ĭ-te) the quality of being nosotoxic.

**noso·tox·i·co·sis** (nos″o-tok″sĭ-ko′sis) [*noso-* + *toxicosis*] any disease due to or associated with poisoning.

**noso·tox·in** (nos″o-tok′sin) [*noso-* + *toxin*] any toxin causing or associated with disease.

**no·sot·ro·phy** (no-sot′rə-fe) [*noso-* + *-trophy*] the care and nursing of the sick.

**noso·trop·ic** (nos″o-trop′ik) [*noso-* + *-tropic*] directed against or opposed to a disease.

**nos·tril** (nos′tril) naris; see *nares.*

**nos·trum** (nos′trəm) [L.] a quack, patent, or secret remedy.

**no·tal·gia** (no-tal′jə) [*not-* + *-algia*] dorsalgia.

**no·tan·ce·pha·lia** (no″tən-sə-fa′le-ə) [*not-* + *an-* + *cephal-* + *-ia*] congenital absence of the posterior aspect of the skull.

**no·tan·en·ce·pha·lia** (no″tən-ən-sə-fa′le-ə) [*not-* + *anencephalia*] absence of the cerebellum.

**notch** (noch) an indentation or depression, especially one on the edge of a bone or other organ. See also *incisura.*
**acetabular n.,** incisura acetabuli.
**angular n. of stomach,** incisura angularis gastris.
**antegonial n.,** a notch on the mandible at the border between the body and ramus.
**anterior n. of auricle,** incisura anterior auriculae
**aortic n.,** dicrotic n.
**auricular n.,** incisura anterior auriculae.
**n. of cardiac apex,** incisura apicis cordis.
**cardiac n. of left lung,** incisura cardiaca pulmonis sinistri.
**cardiac n. of stomach, cardial n.,** incisura cardialis.
**n. in cartilage of acoustic meatus,** incisura cartilaginis meatus acustici.
**cerebellar n., anterior,** incisura cerebelli anterior.
**cerebellar n., posterior,** incisura cerebelli posterior.
**clavicular n. of sternum,** incisura clavicularis sterni.
**coracoid n.,** incisura scapulae.
**costal n's of sternum,** incisurae costales sterni.
**cotyloid n.,** incisura acetabuli.
**dicrotic n.,** a small downward deflection in the arterial pulse or pressure contour immediately following closure of the aortic valve and preceding the dicrotic wave; sometimes used as a marker for the end of systole or the ejection period.
**ethmoidal n. of frontal bone,** incisura ethmoidalis ossis frontalis.
**fibular n., fibular n. of tibia,** incisura fibularis tibiae.
**frontal n.,** incisura frontalis.
**n. of gallbladder,** fossa vesicae biliaris.
**gastric n.,** incisura angularis gastris.
**greater n. of ischium,** incisura ischiadica major.
**interarytenoid n.,** incisura interarytenoidea.
**interclavicular n.,** incisura jugularis sterni.
**intercondylar n. of femur,** fossa intercondylaris femoris.
**interlobar n.,** incisura ligamenti teretis.
**intertragic n.,** incisura intertragica.
**intervertebral n.,** see *incisura vertebralis inferior* and *incisura vertebralis superior.*
**ischiadic n., greater,** incisura ischiadica major.
**ischiadic n., lesser,** incisura ischiadica minor.
**ischial n., greater,** incisura ischiadica major.
**ischial n., lesser,** incisura ischiadica minor.
**jugular n. of manubrium of sternum,** incisura jugularis sterni.
**jugular n. of occipital bone,** incisura jugularis ossis occipitalis.
**jugular n. of sternum,** incisura jugularis sterni.
**jugular n. of temporal bone,** incisura jugularis ossis temporalis.
**Kernohan's n.,** a groove in the cerebral peduncle caused by displacement of the brain stem against the tentorium in some cases of transtentorial herniation.
**lacrimal n. of maxilla,** incisura lacrimalis maxillae.
**lesser n. of ischium,** incisura ischiadica minor.
**n. for ligamentum teres,** incisura ligamenti teretis.
**mandibular n.,** incisura mandibulae.
**mastoid n.,** incisura mastoidea ossis temporalis.
**nasal n. of frontal bone,** margo nasalis ossis frontalis.
**nasal n. of maxilla,** incisura nasalis maxillae.
**palatine n.,** 1. incisura pterygoidea. 2. incisura sphenopalatina ossis palatini.
**pancreatic n.,** incisura pancreatis.
**parietal n. of temporal bone,** incisura parietalis ossis temporalis.
**parotid n.,** the notch between the ramus of the mandible and the mastoid process of the temporal bone.
**popliteal n.,** fossa intercondylaris femoris.
**preoccipital n.,** incisura preoccipitalis.
**presternal n.,** incisura jugularis sterni.
**pterygoid n.,** incisura pterygoidea.
**radial n., radial n. of ulna,** incisura radialis ulnae.
**rivinian n., Rivinus' n.,** incisura tympanica.
**sacrosciatic n., greater,** incisura ischiadica major.
**sacrosciatic n., lesser,** incisura ischiadica minor.
**scapular n.,** incisura scapulae.
**sciatic n., greater,** incisura ischiadica major.
**sciatic n., lesser,** incisura ischiadica minor.
**semilunar n. of mandible,** incisura mandibulae.
**semilunar n. of scapula,** incisura scapulae.
**Sibson's n.,** an inward bend of the left upward limit of precordial dullness in acute pericardial effusion.
**sigmoid n.,** incisura mandibulae.
**sphenopalatine n. of palatine bone,** incisura sphenopalatina ossis palatini.
**sternal n.,** incisura jugularis sterni.
**supraorbital n.,** incisura supraorbitalis.
**suprascapular n.,** incisura scapulae.
**suprasternal n.,** incisura jugularis sterni.
**tentorial n.,** incisura tentorii cerebelli.
**terminal n. of auricle,** incisura terminalis auricularis.
**thyroid n., inferior,** incisura thyroidea inferior.
**thyroid n., superior,** incisura thyroidea superior.
**trigeminal n.,** a notch in the superior border of the petrosal portion of the temporal bone, near the apex, for transmission of the trigeminal nerve.
**trochlear n. of ulna,** incisura trochlearis ulnae.
**tympanic n.,** incisura tympanica.
**ulnar n., ulnar n. of radius,** incisura ulnaris radii.
**umbilical n.,** incisura ligamenti teretis.
**vertebral n., inferior,** incisura vertebralis inferior.
**vertebral n., superior,** incisura vertebralis superior.

**No·tech·is** (no-tek′is) a genus of extremely venomous Australian snakes of the family Elapidae. *N. scuta′tus* is the tiger snake. See table at *snake.*

**no·ten·ceph·a·lo·cele** (no″ten-sef′ə-lo-sēl″) [*not-* + *encephalocele*] occipital encephalocele.

**no·ten·ceph·a·lus** (no″ten-sef′ə-ləs) [*noto-* + Gr. *enkephalos* brain] a fetus affected with notencephalocele.

**Noth·na·gel's bodies, syndrome** (not′nah-gelz) [Carl Wilhelm Hermann *Nothnagel,* Austrian physician, 1841–1905] see under *body* and *syndrome.*

**not(o)-** [Gr. *nōton* back] a combining form denoting relationship to the back.

**no·to·chord** (no′to-kord) [*noto-* + *chord*] [MeSH: Notochord] the rod-shaped body, composed of cells derived from the mesoblast of the primitive node of the embryo, defining the primitive axis of the body; it is the common factor of all species of the phylum Chordata. It is the center of development of the axial skeleton. Called also *chorda dorsalis.*

**no·to·chor·do·ma** (no″to-kor-do′mə) chordoma.

**No·to·ed·res** (no″to-ed′rēz) a genus of mange mites of the family Sarcoptidae. *N. ca′ti* is the itch mite, which causes a persistent, sometimes fatal, mange in cats and may also infest rabbits and humans.

**no·to·ed·ric** (no″to-ed′rik) pertaining to or caused by *Notoedres.*

**no·to·gen·e·sis** (no″to-jen′ə-sis) [*noto-* + *-genesis*] the development of the notochord.

**no·tom·e·lus** (no-tom′ə-ləs) [*noto-* + Gr. *melos* limb] a fetus with accessory limbs on the back.

**not-self** (not′self) nonself.

**no·tum** (no′təm) [Gr. *nōton* back] 1. the dorsal part of the body. 2. the dorsal element of each segment of an arthropod.

**nou·me·nal** (noo′mə-nəl) [Gr. *noumenon* a thing thought] pertaining to rational intuition independent of sensory perception.

**No·val·din** (no-val′din) trademark for preparations of dipyrone.

**No·van·trone** (no-van′trōn) trademark for a preparation of mitoxantrone hydrochloride.

**no·vo·bio·cin** (no″vo-bi′o-sin) [MeSH: Novobiocin] an antibiotic obtained from *Streptomyces niveus* and other *Streptomyces* species, effective chiefly against staphylococci and other gram-positive organisms.
**n. calcium,** the calcium salt of novobiocin, having the same actions as the base; used in the treatment of infections in children due to susceptible bacteria resistant to other antibiotics, administered orally.
**n. sodium,** the sodium salt of novobiocin, having the same appearance, actions, uses, and mode of administration as the calcium salt; usually used in adults.

**No·vo·cain** (no′və-kān) trademark for preparations of procaine hydrochloride.

**No·vo-Met·for·min** (no″vo-met-for′min) trademark for a preparation of metformin.

**no·vo·scope** (no′və-skōp) [L. *novus* new + *scope*] Fornai's instrument for auscultatory percussion.

**Nov·rad** (nov′rad) trademark for preparations of levopropoxyphene napsylate.

**No·vy's rat disease** (no'vēz) [Frederick George *Novy,* American bacteriologist, 1864–1957] see under *disease.*

**noxa** (nok'sə) pl. *nox'ae* [L. "harm"] an injurious agent, act, or influence.

**nox·ious** (nok'shəs) [L. *noxius*] hurtful; not wholesome; pernicious; damaging to tissue.

**NP-59** iodomethylnorcholesterol.

**Np** symbol for *neptunium.*

**NPA** National Perinatal Association.

**NPN** nonprotein nitrogen.

**NPO** abbreviation for L. *nil per os,* nothing by mouth.

**NRC** normal retinal correspondence.

**NREM** non–rapid eye movement (see under *sleep*).

**ns** symbol for *nanosecond.*

**NSAIA** nonsteroidal antiinflammatory analgesic; see under *drug.*

**NSAID** nonsteroidal antiinflammatory drug.

**NSCLC** non–small cell lung carcinoma (or cancer).

**nsec** symbol for *nanosecond.*

**NSNA** National Student Nurse Association.

**NSR** normal sinus rhythm.

**NST** nonstress test.

**N-ter·min·al** (ter'min-əl) the amino ($NH_2$) end of a polypeptide chain, conventionally written to the left; called also *$NH_2$-terminal.*

**NTP** normal temperature and pressure; National Toxicology Program.

**nU** symbol for *nanounit.*

**nu** (noo) [N, ν] the thirteenth letter of the Greek alphabet.

**Nu·bain** (nu'bān) trademark for a preparation of nalbuphine hydrochloride.

**nu·bec·u·la** (noo-bek'u-lə) [L., dim. of *nubes* cloud] nebula.

**nu·bil·i·ty** (noo-bil'ĭ-te) [L. *nubilitas;* from *nubere* to marry] marriageableness; fitness to marry; said of the female.

**nu·cha** (noo'kə) [L.] the nape, or posterior aspect of the neck.

**nu·chal** (noo'kəl) pertaining to the nucha, or posterior aspect of the neck.

**Nuck's canal, diverticulum** (nooks) [Anton *Nuck,* Dutch anatomist, 1650–1692] see *processus vaginalis peritonei.*

**nu·cle·ar** (noo'kle-ər) pertaining to a nucleus.

**nu·cle·ase** (noo'kle-ās) a general term for enzymes of the hydrolase class that catalyze the cleavage of phosphodiester linkages in nucleic acids to form nucleotides or oligonucleotides [EC 3.1.11–31]. The nucleases are classified in subgroups on the basis of their substrate specificity; they may be endonucleases or exonucleases, each of which may be specific for the ribonucleic acids (ribonucleases) or deoxyribonucleic acids (deoxyribonucleases).

**nu·cle·at·ed** (noo'kle-āt"əd) [L. *nucleatus*] having a nucleus or nuclei.

**nu·clei** (noo'kle-i) [L.] genitive and plural of *nucleus.*

**nu·cle·ic ac·id** (noo-kle'ik) a high-molecular-weight nucleotide polymer. There are two types: *deoxyribonucleic acid* (DNA) and *ribonucleic acid* (RNA) (q.v.).
**infectious n. a.,** viral nucleic acid capable of infecting a cell and inducing the production of viruses.

**nu·cle·ide** (noo'kle-īd) any compound of nucleic acid with a metallic element.

**nu·cle·i·form** (noo'kle-ĭ-form) shaped like a nucleus.

**nu·cle·in** (noo'kle-in) a decomposition product of nucleoprotein intermediate between native nucleoprotein and nucleic acid. It is a colorless, amorphous compound, soluble in dilute alkalis, but insoluble in dilute acids. The nucleins consist of nucleic acid and bases which vary in the different nucleins.

**nu·cle·in·ic ac·id** (noo-kle-in'ik) nucleic acid.

**nucle(o)-** [L. *nucleus,* q.v.] a combining form denoting relationship to a nucleus.

**nu·cleo·cap·sid** (noo"kle-o-kap'sid) [MeSH: Nucleocapsid] a unit of viral structure, consisting of a capsid (protein coat) with the enclosed nucleic acid; some simple viruses are naked nucleocapsids, while in others the nucleocapsids form part of a more complex structure.

**nu·cleo·chy·le·ma** (noo"kle-o-ki-le'mə) [*nucleo-* + Gr. *chylos* juice] the ground substance of the nucleus of a cell as distinguished from that of the cytoplasm.

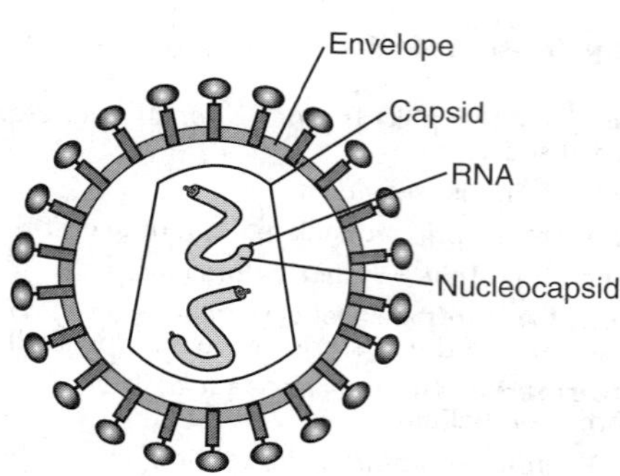


Nucleocapsid in a schematic diagram of HIV-1; molecules of protease, integrase, and reverse transcriptase, which also occur within the capsid, are omitted for simplicity.

**nu·cleo·chyme** (noo'kle-o-kīm) [*nucleo-* + *chyme*] karyolymph.

**nu·cleo·cy·to·plas·mic** (noo"kle-o-si"to-plaz'mik) pertaining to the nucleus and the cytoplasm of cells.

**nu·cle·of·u·gal** (noo"kle-of'u-gəl) [*nucleo-* + *-fugal*] moving away from a nucleus.

**nu·cleo·glu·co·pro·tein** (noo"kle-o-gloo"ko-pro'tēn) a combination of a nucleoprotein with a carbohydrate.

**nu·cleo·his·tone** (noo"kle-o-his'tōn) a complex nucleoprotein made up of deoxyribonucleic acid (DNA) and a histone, the principal constituent of chromatin.

**nu·cleo·hy·a·lo·plasm** (noo"kle-o-hi'ə-lo-plaz"əm) linin.

**nu·cle·oid** (noo'kle-oid) 1. resembling a nucleus. 2. the nuclear region of a bacterium, consisting of a dense, centrally located, irregularly shaped region containing DNA material without a surrounding nuclear membrane. 3. the genetic material (nucleic acid) of a virus, situated in the center of the virion.

**nu·cle·o·lar** (noo-kle'o-lər) pertaining to a nucleolus.

**nu·cle·o·li** (noo-kle'o-li) [L.] plural of *nucleolus.*

**nu·cle·o·li·form** (noo"kle-o'lĭ-form) resembling a nucleolus.

**nu·cle·o·lin** (noo-kle'o-lin) the substance composing the nucleolus of a cell.

**nu·cle·o·li·nus** (noo"kle-o-li'nəs) a deeply staining granule in the nucleolus.

**nu·cle·o·loid** (noo'kle-o-loid) resembling a nucleolus.

**nu·cle·ol·o·lus** (noo"kle-ol'o-ləs) a minute spot within the nucleolus.

**nu·cleo·lo·ne·ma** (noo"kle-o"lo-ne'mə) [*nucleolus* + Gr. *nēma* thread] a network of strands formed by organization of a finely granular substance, perhaps containing ribonucleic acid, in the nucleolus of a cell.

**nu·cleo·lo·neme** (noo"kle-o'lo-nēm) nucleolonema.

**nu·cleo·lo·nu·cle·us** (noo"kle-o-lo-noo'kle-əs) a nucleololus.

**nu·cle·o·lus** (noo-kle'ə-ləs) gen. and pl. *nucle'oli* [L., dim. of *nucleus*] a rounded refractile body present in the nucleus of most cells, which is the site of synthesis of ribosomal RNA, becoming enlarged during periods of synthesis and atrophied during quiescent periods; it consists of a mixed granular (pars granulosa) and a fibrillar (pars fibrosa) portion. Multiple nucleoli occur in some cells. Called also *micronucleus.*
**chromatin n., false n., nucleinic n.,** karyosome.
**secondary n.,** a mass sometimes seen near a nucleolus, and looking like a separated portion of the latter.

**nu·cleo·lymph** (noo'kle-o-limf") karyolymph.

**nu·cleo·mi·cro·some** (noo"kle-o-mi'kro-sōm) [*nucleo-* + *micro-* + *-some*] any of the minute segments of a chromatin fiber.

**nu·cle·on** (noo'kle-on) a particle of the atomic nucleus, a proton or a neutron.

**nu·cle·on·ic** (noo"kle-on'ik) pertaining to a nucleus.

**nu·cle·on·ics** (noo"kle-on'iks) the study of atomic nuclei and their reactions; nuclear physics.

**nu·cle·op·e·tal** (noo"kle-op'ə-təl) [*nucleo-* + *-petal*] moving toward a nucleus.

**nu·cleo·phago·cy·to·sis** (noo"kle-o-fag"o-si-to'sis) the engulfing of the nuclei of other cells by phagocytes; see *tart cell,* under *cell.*

**nu·cleo·phile** (noo'kle-o-fil") an electron donor in chemical reactions involving covalent catalysis in which the donated electrons bond other chemical groups (electrophiles).

**nu·cleo·phil·ic** (noo″kle-o-fil′ik) 1. having an affinity for nuclei. 2. being or serving as a nucleophile.

**nu·cleo·plasm** (noo′kle-o-plaz″əm) [*nucleo-* + *-plasm*] the protoplasm composing the nucleus of a cell; karyoplasm. Cf. *cytoplasm.*

**nu·cleo·plas·min** (noo′kle-o-plaz″min) any of a family of acidic nuclear proteins that act as molecular chaperones, mediating the assembly of nucleosomes; nucleoplasmin transiently reduces the positive charges on histone proteins to prevent incorrect nonspecific aggregation of histones and DNA.

**nu·cleo·pro·tein** (noo″kle-o-pro′tēn) a substance composed of a simple basic protein, usually a histone or protamine, combined with a nucleic acid.
**deoxyribose n.,** a deoxyribonucleic acid–protein complex.
**ribose n.,** a ribonucleic acid–protein complex.

**nu·cleo·re·tic·u·lum** (noo″kle-o-rə-tik′u-ləm) [*nucleo-* + *reticulum*] any intranuclear network.

**nu·cleo·si·dase** (noo″kle-o-si′dās) a term used in the recommended names of some glycosidases hydrolyzing *N*-glycosyl linkages [EC 3.2.2] to denote those catalyzing the cleavage of a nucleoside to form a purine or pyrimidine base and a sugar.

**nu·cleo·side** (noo′kle-o-sīd″) a heterocyclic nitrogenous base, particularly a purine or pyrimidine, in *N*-glycosidic linkage with a sugar, particularly a pentose; it is often used specifically to denote a compound obtained by hydrolysis of nucleic acids, a purine or pyrimidine linked to ribose or deoxyribose, e.g., adenosine or cytidine.

**nu·cleo·side-di·phos·phate ki·nase** (noo′kle-o-sīd di′fos-fāt ki′nās) [EC 2.7.4.6] [MeSH: Nucleoside-Diphosphate Kinase] an enzyme of the transferase class with broad specificity that catalyzes the reversible transfer of a phosphate from ATP to a nucleoside diphosphate to form a nucleoside triphosphate. The reaction is part of the mechanism that regenerates high-energy nucleotides for metabolic processes and conserves the purine-pyrimidine pool.

**nu·cleo·side-phos·phate ki·nase** (noo′kle-o-sīd fos′fat ki′nās) [EC 2.7.4.4] [MeSH: Nucleoside-Phosphate Kinase] any enzyme of the transferase class that catalyzes the transfer of a phosphate from ATP to a nucleoside phosphate to form a nucleoside diphosphate. The reaction is part of the mechanism that regenerates high energy nucleotides for metabolic processes and conserves the purine-pyrimidine pool. Specific enzymes exist for individual nucleosides (e.g., adenylate kinase).

**nu·cleo·side phos·phor·y·lase** (noo′kle-o-sīd″ fos-for′ə-lās) any of the enzymes of the sub-subclass pentosyltransferases [EC 2.4.2] that catalyze the phosphorolysis of a nucleoside to form the free base and a ribose (or deoxyribose) 1-phosphate as a step in the degradation of nucleic acids and nucleotides. See also *purine-nucleoside phosphorylase* and *pyrimidine-nucleoside phosphorylase.*

**nu·cle·o·sis** (noo″kle-o′sis) nuclear proliferation; abnormal increase in the production of nuclei, such as occurs in the subsarcolemmal nuclei of muscle following injury.

**nu·cleo·some** (noo′kle-o-sōm) [*nucleo-* + *-some*] [MeSH: Nucleosomes] a specific complex of histone and DNA in eukaryotic cells, seen under the electron microscope as beadlike bodies on a string of DNA.

**nu·cleo·spin·dle** (noo″kle-o-spin′dəl) the spindle-shaped body in mitosis.

**nu·cleo·ti·dase** (noo″kle-o-ti′dās) [EC 3.1.3.31] 1. an enzyme of the hydrolase class that catalyzes the cleavage of a nucleotide to a nucleoside and orthophosphate. 2. any of several enzymes catalyzing this reaction, individual enzymes being named for their specificities (e.g., 5′-nucleotidase, polynucleotide 3′-phosphatase).

**5′-nu·cleo·ti·dase** (noo″kle-o-ti′dās) [EC 3.1.3.5] a membrane-bound, cytoplasmic nucleotidase specifically cleaving phosphate from the 5′ position of nucleotides to yield nucleosides. The enzyme acts on a wide range of 5′-nucleotides and the reaction is part of the main nucleotide degradation pathway.

**nu·cleo·tide** (noo′kle-o-tīd) a phosphate ester of a nucleoside, particularly the 5′-phosphate of a pyrimidine or purine in *N*-glycosidic linkage with ribose or deoxyribose, as occurs in nucleic acid.
**cyclic n's,** nucleotides in which the phosphate group forms a ring, as in AMP and GMP.

**nu·cleo·tid·yl** (noo″kle-o-tid′əl) a nucleotide residue.

**nu·cleo·tid·yl·trans·fer·ase** (noo″kle-o-tid′əl-trans′fər-ās) [EC 2.7.7] any member of a sub-subclass of enzymes of the transferase class that catalyze the transfer of a nucleotidyl group from a nucleoside di- or triphosphate donor group to an acceptor group.

**nu·cleo·tox·in** (noo″kle-o-tok′sin) 1. a toxin from cell nuclei. 2. any toxin exerting a deleterious effect on cell nuclei.

**nu·cle·us** (noo′kle-əs) gen. and pl. *nu′clei* [L., dim. of *nux* nut] 1. the central core of a body or object. 2. a cell nucleus: a spheroid body within a cell, consisting of a number of characteristic organelles visible with the light microscope, a thin nuclear membrane, a nucleolus or nucleoli, irregular granules of chromatin and linin, and a diffuse nucleoplasm. 3. [TA] a group of nerve cells ordinarily located within the central nervous system and bearing a direct relationship to the fibers of a particular nerve. 4. in organic chemistry, the combination of atoms forming the central element or basic framework of the molecule of a specific compound or class of compounds. 5. see *atomic n.*

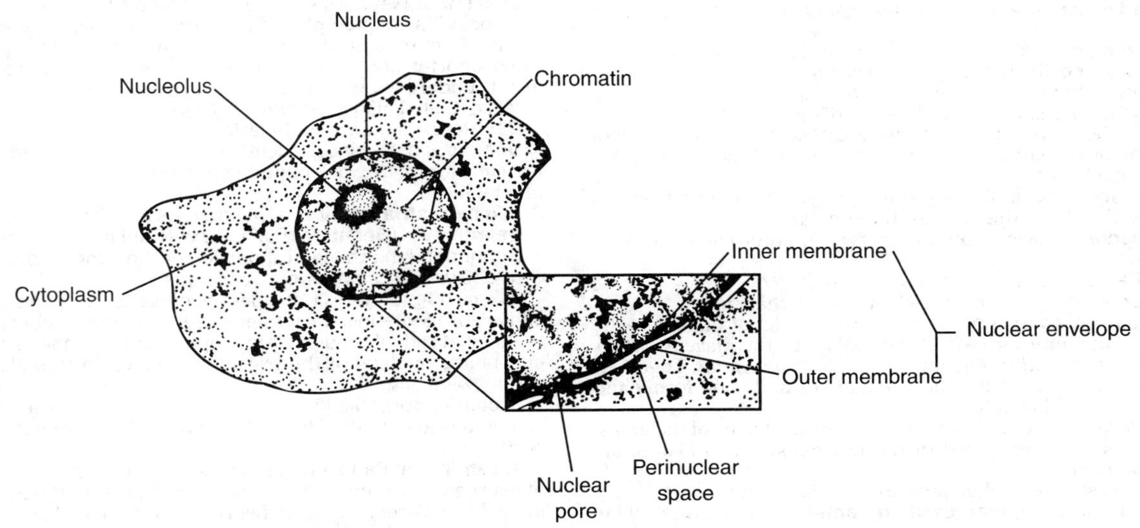


Diagram of a cell, showing the chromatin-rich nucleus bounded by the double-membraned nuclear envelope.

## Nucleus

Descriptions of anatomic structures are given on TA terms, and include anglicized names of specific nuclei.

**abducens n., n. abdu'cens,** n. nervi abducentis.

**n. of abducens nerve, n. abducen'tis,** n. nervi abducentis.

**n. accesso'rius colum'nae anterio'ris medul'lae spina'lis,** n. nervi accessorii.

**nu'clei accesso'rii ner'vi oculomoto'rii** [TA], accessory nuclei of oculomotor nerve: a collection of small cells located dorsal to the upper part of the somatic groups of the oculomotor nuclear complex, comprising the parasympathetic outflow via the ciliary ganglion to the ciliary muscle and sphincter pupillae of the eye; called also *Edinger's* or *Edinger-Westphal nuclei, nuclei oculomotorii accessorii* and *nuclei oculomotorii autonomici.*

**accessory n. of anterior column of spinal cord,** n. nervi accessorii.

**accessory basal amygdaloid n.,** a nucleus in the basolateral part of the amygdaloid body.

**n. of accessory nerve,** n. nervi accessorii.

**accessory oculomotor nuclei, accessory nuclei of oculomotor nerve,** nuclei accessorii nervi oculomotorii.

**accessory olivary n., dorsal,** n. olivaris accessorius posterior.

**accessory olivary n., medial,** n. olivaris accessorius medialis.

**accessory olivary n., posterior,** n. olivaris accessorius posterior.

**accessory n. of ventral column of spinal cord,** n. nervi accessorii.

**n. accum'bens** [TA], **n. accum'bens sep'ti,** a collection of pleomorphic cells in the caudal part of the anterior horn of the lateral ventricle of the olfactory tubercle, lying between the head of the caudate nucleus and the anterior perforated substance.

**acoustic nuclei, nuclei of acoustic nerve,** vestibulocochlear nuclei.

**n. a'lae cine'reae,** n. posterior nervi vagi.

**n. ambi'guus** [TA], ambiguous nucleus: the nucleus of origin of motor fibers of the vagus, glossopharyngeal, and accessory nerves that supply the striated muscles of the larynx and pharynx. It consists of an intermittent cell column in the middle of the lateral funiculus of the medulla oblongata, between the caudal end of the medulla and the level of exit of the glossopharyngeal nerve.

**n. amyg'dalae,** corpus amygdaloideum.

**n. amyg'dalae centra'lis** [TA], central amygdaloid nucleus: a nucleus in the corticomedial part of the amygdaloid body, providing the major relay for projections from the amygdala to the brainstem and also receiving numerous return projections.

**n. amyg'dalae cortica'lis** [TA], cortical amygdaloid nucleus: a nucleus in the corticomedial part of the amygdaloid body.

**n. amyg'dalae latera'lis** [TA], lateral amygdaloid nucleus: a nucleus in the basolateral part of the amygdaloid body.

**n. amyg'dalae media'lis** [TA], medial amygdaloid nucleus: a nucleus in the corticomedial part of the amygdaloid body.

**amygdaloid n.,** corpus amygdaloideum.

**amygdaloid n., basal,** a nucleus in the basolateral part of the amygdaloid body.

**amygdaloid n., central,** n. amygdalae centralis.

**amygdaloid n., cortical,** n. amygdalae corticalis.

**amygdaloid n., lateral,** n. amygdalae lateralis.

**amygdaloid n., medial,** n. amygdalae medialis.

**n. an'sae lenticula'ris** [TA], **n. of ansa lenticularis,** a collection of neurons in the ansa lenticularis as it curves around the medial edge of the globus pallidus.

**n. ante'rior hypotha'lami** [TA], anterior hypothalamic nucleus: a nucleus of nerve cells in the anterior hypothalamic region.

**anterior medial n. of oculomotor nerve,** n. anteromedialis nervi oculomotorii.

**anterior olfactory n.,** n. olfactorius anterior.

**anterior nuclei of thalamus,** nuclei anteriores thalami.

**nu'clei anterio'res tha'lami** [TA], anterior nuclei of thalamus: the three nuclei in the anterior part of the thalamus: the *nucleus anteroventralis, nucleus anterodorsalis,* and *nucleus anteromedialis.* Together, they receive connections from the mammillary body and fornix and project fibers to the cingulate body.

**n. anterodorsa'lis tha'lami** [TA], anterodorsal nucleus of thalamus: one of the three anterior nuclei of the thalamus; called also *n. anterosuperior thalami.*

**n. anteroinfe'rior tha'lami,** n. anteroventralis thalami.

**anterolateral n. of spinal cord, n. anterolatera'lis medul'lae spina'lis** [TA], a group of nerve cells in the gray substance of the anterolateral region of the anterior column of the spinal cord; called also *ventrolateral n. of spinal cord* and *n. ventrolateralis medullae spinalis.*

**anteromedial n. of spinal cord,** n. anteromedialis medullae spinalis.

**anteromedial n. of thalamus,** n. anteromedialis thalami.

**n. anteromedia'lis medul'lae spina'lis** [TA], anteromedial nucleus of spinal cord: a group of nerve cells in the gray matter of the anteromedial region of the anterior column of the spinal cord; called also *ventromedial n. of spinal cord* and *n. ventromedialis medullae spinalis.*

**n. anteromedia'lis ner'vi oculomoto'rii** [TA], anterior medial nucleus of oculomotor nerve: ventrally placed cells in the lateral part of the oculomotor nuclear complex *(nucleus nervi oculomotorii);* they are distinct from the dorsally placed cells in the middle third of the complex and have a somatic motor function. Called also *ventral medial n. of oculomotor nerve* and *ventromedial n. of oculomotor nuclear complex.*

**n. anteromedia'lis tha'lami** [TA], anteromedial nucleus of thalamus: one of the three anterior nuclei of the thalamus.

**n. anterosupe'rior tha'lami,** n. anterodorsalis thalami.

**n. anteroventra'lis tha'lami** [TA], anteroventral nucleus of thalamus: one of the three anterior nuclei of the thalamus; called also *n. anteroinferior thalami.*

**arcuate n. of hypothalamus,** n. arcuatus hypothalami.

**arcuate n. of medulla oblongata,** n. arcuatus medullae oblongatae.

**n. arcua'tus hypotha'lami** [TA], arcuate nucleus of hypothalamus: a nucleus of nerve cells in the posterior hypothalamic region, extending into the median eminence and almost entirely surrounding the base of the infundibulum. Called also *infundibular n., n. infundibularis* [TA alternative] and *n. semilunaris* [TA alternative].

**n. arcua'tus medul'lae oblonga'tae** [TA], arcuate nucleus of medulla oblongata: one of the group of small, irregular areas of gray substance found on the ventromedial aspect of the pyramid of the medulla oblongata.

**nu'clei a'reae H, $H_1$, $H_2$,** nuclei campi perizonalis.

**n. of atom, atomic n.,** the central core of an atom, constituting almost all of its mass but only a small part of its volume, and composed of protons and neutrons, the protons being positively charged and their number (atomic number) being fixed for all the atoms of each element and equal to the number of the orbiting electrons. The neutrons, which bear no charge, may vary in number, accounting for the isotopes of an element.

**auditory nuclei,** vestibulocochlear nuclei.

**nuclei of auditory nerve,** vestibulocochlear nuclei.

**autonomic oculomotor nuclei,** nuclei accessorii nervi oculomotorii.

**Balbiani's n.,** yolk n.

**basal nuclei,** nuclei basales.

**basal n. of telencephalon,** n. basalis telencephali.

**nu'clei basa'les** [TA], basal nuclei: specific interconnected groups of masses of gray substance deep in the cerebral hemispheres and in the upper brain stem. Although various subcortical nuclei have been considered to be part of the basal nuclei, in official anatomical terminology the term includes the nucleus caudatus, nucleus lentiformis, corpus striatum, capsula interna, and corona radiata (including the capsula externa and capsula extrema). Called also *basal ganglia.*

**basal n. of Meynert, n. basalis of Meynert,** n. basalis telencephali.

**n. basa'lis telence'phali** [TA], basal nucleus of telencephalon: a group of neurons in the basal forebrain that has wide projections to the neocortex and is rich in acetylcholine and choline acetyltransferase. It undergoes degeneration in paralysis agitans and Alzheimer's disease. Called also *n. basalis of Meynert* and *Meynert's n.*

**Bechterew's n.,** n. vestibularis superior.

**Béclard's n.,** a vascular lentil-shaped center of ossification seen in the cartilage of the lower epiphysis of the femur during the latter part of fetal life.

**bed n. of stria terminalis,** n. striae terminalis.

**Bekhterev's (Bechterew's) n.,** n. vestibularis superior.

**Blumenau's n.,** the lateral portion of the cuneate nucleus.

**n. of Burdach's column,** n. cuneatus.

**n. caeru'leus** [TA], a compact aggregation of pigmented neurons subjacent to the locus caeruleus; it is sometimes considered one of the medial reticular nuclei. At its upper end it connects with the mesencephalic nucleus of the trigeminal nerve. Written also *n. ceruleus* and *n. coeruleus.*

**n. cam'pi dorsa'lis** [TA], nucleus of dorsal field: the group of nerve cell bodies among the fibers of field $H_1$ of Forel. See also *nuclei campi perizonalis.*

**n. cam'pi media'lis** [TA], nucleus of medial field: any of the groups of neurons scattered along the caudomedial border of the zona incerta in field H of Forel (prerubral field). Called also *n. of prerubral field* and *n. of tegmental field.* See also *nuclei campi perizonalis.*

**nu'clei cam'pi perizona'lis** [TA], nuclei of perizonal field: the group of nuclei in the ventral thalamus comprising the nucleus of the prerubral field (field H of Forel) and neurons scattered along the thalamic and lenticular fasciculi in fields $H_1$ and $H_2$ of Forel.

**n. cam'pi ventra'lis** [TA], nucleus of ventral field: the group of nerve cell bodies among the fibers of field $H_2$ of Forel. See also *nuclei campi perizonalis.*

**caudal n., central,** n. caudalis centralis.

**nuclei of caudal colliculus,** nuclei colliculi inferioris.

**n. cauda'lis centra'lis,** central caudal nucleus: an unpaired collection of cells in the caudal third of the oculomotor nuclear complex

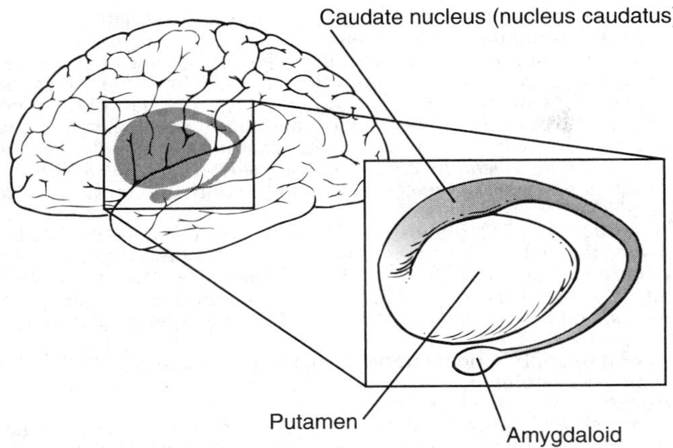


Nucleus caudatus (caudate nucleus) in a lateral view of the left side of the brain.

(nucleus nervi oculomotorii [TA]), located in the median raphe somewhat dorsal to the lateral nuclei. Called also *central caudate n.*

**n. cauda'tus** [TA], caudate nucleus: an elongated, arched gray mass closely related to the lateral ventricle throughout its entire extent and consisting of a head, body, and tail. The caudate nucleus and putamen form a functional unit (the neostriatum) of the corpus striatum.

**cell n., cellular n.,** nucleus (def. 2).

**central n. of spinal cord,** n. centralis medullae spinalis.

**central caudate n.,** n. caudalis centralis.

**central lateral n. of thalamus,** n. centralis lateralis thalami.

**central medial n. of thalamus,** n. centralis medialis thalami.

**n. centra'lis latera'lis tha'lami** [TA], central lateral nucleus of thalamus: one of the smaller intralaminar nuclei of the dorsal thalamus, situated in the dorsal part of the internal medullary lamina.

**n. centra'lis media'lis tha'lami** [TA], medial central nucleus of thalamus: one of the smaller intralaminar nuclei, situated medially in the internal medullary lamina.

**n. centra'lis medul'lae spina'lis** [TA], **n. centra'lis medul'lae spina'lis,** central nucleus of spinal cord: a group of nerve cells in the gray substance in the central region of the anterior column of the spinal cord.

**n. centra'lis supe'rior ra'phes,** n. raphes medianus.

**n. centromedia'nus tha'lami** [TA], centromedian nucleus of thalamus: the largest and most caudal of the intralaminar nuclei of the dorsal thalamus; its main connections are with the corpus striatum.

**cerebellar n., lateral,** n. lateralis cerebelli.

**cerebellar n., medial,** n. medialis cerebelli.

**nu'clei cerebella'res, nu'clei cerebel'li** [TA], cerebellar nuclei: four accumulations of gray substance embedded in the white substance of the cerebellum, comprising the nucleus dentatus, nucleus emboliformis, nucleus globosus, and nucleus fastigii; called also *intracerebellar nuclei* and *roof nuclei* (q.v.).

**n. ceru'leus,** n. caeruleus.

**cervical n., lateral,** n. cervicalis lateralis.

**n. cervica'lis latera'lis** [TA], lateral cervical nucleus: a small group of cells in the lateral funiculus of the first and second cervical segments of the spinal cord, comprising a relay station in a spinocervicothalamic path.

**cholane n.,** a cyclopentenophenanthrene structure forming the basis of the specific compounds, found in the bile acids; the sterols; toad poisons; digitalis, strophanthus, ouabain, and other heart aglycones; the sex hormones; and some carcinogenic hydrocarbons.

**Clarke's n.,** n. thoracicus posterior.

**cleavage n.,** segmentation n.

**cochlear nuclei,** nuclei cochleares.

**cochlear n., anterior,** n. cochlearis anterior.

**cochlear n., dorsal, cochlear n., posterior,** n. cochlearis posterior.

**cochlear n., ventral,** n. cochlearis anterior.

**nuclei of cochlear nerve,** nuclei cochleares.

**nu'clei cochlea'res** [TA], cochlear nuclei: the two nuclei, *anterior* and *posterior,* partly encircling the inferior cerebellar peduncle (lentiform body) at the junction of the medulla oblongata and the pons, in which the fibers of the cochlear part of the vestibulocochlear nerve terminate; called also *nuclei of cochlear nerve* and *nuclei nervi cochlearis.*

**n. cochlea'ris ante'rior** [TA], anterior cochlear nucleus: the anterior of the two cochlear nuclei; located on the anterolateral aspect of the inferior cerebellar peduncle; it receives the larger, ascending branches of the cochlear nerve. Called also *ventral cochlear n.* and *n. cochlearis ventralis.*

**n. cochlea'ris dorsa'lis, n. cochlea'ris poste'rior** [TA], posterior cochlear nucleus: the posterior of the two cochlear nuclei, located on the dorsal aspect of the inferior cerebellar peduncle; it forms an eminence (the *auditory tubercle*) on the lateral part of the vestibular area of the floor of the fourth ventricle. Called also *dorsal cochlear n.*

**n. cochlea'ris ventra'lis,** n. cochlearis anterior.

**n. coeru'leus,** n. caeruleus.

**nu'clei colli'culi cauda'lis, nu'clei colli'culi inferio'ris** [TA], nuclei of inferior colliculus: the large oval-shaped group of nerve cells that make up most of the substance of the inferior colliculus. Called also *nuclei of caudal colliculus* and *nuclei colliculi caudalis.*

**n. commis'surae posterio'ris** [TA], nucleus of posterior commissure: a nucleus of the rostral midbrain tegmentum, located adjacent to the posterior commissure and near the oculomotor nucleus.

**n. commissura'lis ner'vi va'gi** [TA], commissural nucleus of vagus nerve: a group of noradrenergic neurons that encloses the dorsolateral aspect of the nucleus of the hypoglossal nerve and approaches the ependymal floor of the fourth ventricle.

**n. commissura'lis rhomboida'lis** [TA], rhomboid nucleus: one of the median nuclei of the thalamus, bordering the third ventricle and ventral to the central medial nucleus; see *nuclei mediani thalami.* Called also *n. rhomboidalis.*

**compact n.,** a cellular nucleus with an inconspicuous nuclear membrane and minute chromatin granules throughout its substance.

**conjugation n.,** fertilization n.

**n. cor'poris genicula'ti latera'lis,** lateral geniculate nucleus.

**nu'clei cor'poris genicula'ti media'lis** [TA], medial geniculate nuclei: nuclei within the medial geniculate body, composed of ventral *(n. ventralis corporis geniculati medialis),* medial *(n. medialis magnocellularis corporis geniculati medialis),* and dorsal *(n. dorsalis corporis geniculati medialis)* nuclei that receive ascending auditory and some nonauditory fibers and project to the auditory cortex. Called also *nuclei of medial geniculate body.*

**n. cor'poris mammilla'ris media'lis/latera'lis,** see *n. mammillaris lateralis* and *n. mammillaris medialis.*

**n. of of cranial nerve,** n. nervi cranialis.

**cuneate n.,** n. cuneatus.

**cuneate n., accessory, cuneate n., lateral,** n. cuneatus accessorius.

**n. cunea'tus** [TA], cuneate nucleus: a nucleus in the medulla oblongata at the rostral end of the fasciculus cuneatus, in which the fibers of this fasciculus synapse; the cells project to the thalamus via the medial lemniscus.

**n. cunea'tus accesso'rius** [TA], accessory cuneate nucleus: a group of nerve cells lying lateral to the nucleus cuneatus that relay impulses from upper limb fibers in the fasciculus cuneatus to the cerebellum (rostral spinocerebellar tract) via external arcuate fibers and the inferior cerebellar peduncle; called also *lateral cuneate n.*

**n. cuneifor'mis** [TA], **n. cuneifor'mis mesencepha'licus,** cuneiform nucleus: a large nucleus in the mesencephalon representing a widening and continuation of the tracts from the medial column reticular nuclei.

**Darkshevich's n.,** a small nucleus dorsal to the medial longitudinal fasciculus in the central gray matter at the rostral end of the cerebral aqueduct; it is believed to receive fibers from the fasciculus and from the superior colliculus.

**daughter n.,** a new cell nucleus formed in mitosis by the diaster.

**Deiters' n.,** n. vestibularis lateralis.

**dental n.,** pulpa dentis.

**dentate n., dentate n. of cerebellum,** n. dentatus.

**n. denta'tus** [TA], dentate nucleus: the largest of the cerebellar nuclei, lying in the white matter of the cerebellum just lateral to the emboliform nucleus, and receiving Purkinje cell fibers from the neocerebellum; its axons form most of the superior cerebellar peduncle and project chiefly to the contralateral red nucleus and thalamus. It is the term preferred in official terminology when considering humans, and is frequently also used to describe nonhuman primates. Cf. *n. lateralis cerebelli.*

**diploid n.,** a cell nucleus containing the number of chromosomes typical of the somatic cells of the particular species.

**dorsal n. of Clarke,** n. thoracicus posterior.

**dorsal column nuclei,** the nucleus cuneatus and nucleus gracilis, which are at the upper end of the dorsal column of the spinal cord.

**n. of dorsal field,** n. campi dorsalis.

**dorsal lateral n. of thalamus,** n. dorsalis lateralis thalami.

**dorsal n. of medial geniculate body,** n.dorsalis corporis geniculati medialis.

**dorsal medial n. of thalamus,** n. mediodorsalis thalami.

**dorsal n. of oculomotor nerve,** n. dorsalis nervi oculomotorii.

**dorsal raphe n.,** n. raphes posterior.

**dorsal nuclei of thalamus,** nuclei dorsales thalami.

**dorsal n. of vagus nerve,** n. posterior nervi vagi.

**n. dorsa'lis cor'poris genicula'ti latera'lis** [TA], dorsal lateral geniculate nucleus: the large dorsal part of the lateral geniculate nucleus, consisting of six concentrically arranged cell layers in a dome-shaped mound, which receive crossed and uncrossed fibers of the optic tract that are connected with the visual cortex. See also *n. ventralis corporis geniculati lateralis.*

**n. dorsa'lis cor'poris genicula'ti media'lis** [TA], dorsal nucleus of medial geniculate body: the larger, dorsal part of the medial geniculate nucleus, receiving ascending auditory fibers from the inferior colliculus as well as afferent projections from some nonauditory areas of the brain stem, and projecting to the auditory cortex.

**n. dorsa'lis hypotha'lami** [TA], dorsal hypothalamic nucleus: a nerve cell nucleus situated in the dorsal portion of the intermediate hypothalamic region.

**n. dorsa'lis latera'lis tha'lami** [TA], lateral dorsal nucleus of thalamus: a nucleus in the dorsal lateral part of the thalamus having extensive connections with the cerebral cortex.

**n. dorsa'lis ner'vi oculomoto'rii** [TA], dorsal nucleus of oculomotor nerve: a group of dorsally placed cells in the lateral part of the oculomotor nuclear complex (nucleus nervi oculomotorii); they are distinct from the ventrally placed cells in the middle third of the complex and have a somatic motor function. Called also *posterior n. of oculomotor nerve.*

**n. dorsa'lis ner'vi va'gi,** TA alternative for *n. posterior nervi vagi.*

**n. dorsa'lis ra'phes,** n. raphes posterior.

**nu'clei dorsa'les tha'lami** [TA], dorsal nuclei of thalamus: the nuclei forming the posterior end of the dorsal thalamus, including the nuclei pulvinares, nucleus dorsalis lateralis, and nucleus lateralis posterior.

**dorsolateral n. of oculomotor nuclear complex,** n. dorsalis nervi oculomotorii.

**dorsolateral n. of spinal cord, n. dorsolatera'lis medul'lae spina'lis,** n. posterolateralis medullae spinalis.

**dorsomedial n. of intermediate hypothalamus,** n. dorsomedialis hypothalamicae intermediae.

**dorsomedial n. of thalamus,** n. mediodorsalis thalami.

**dorsomedial n. of spinal cord, n. dorsomedia'lis medul'lae spina'lis,** n. posteromedialis medullae spinalis.

**n. dorsomedia'lis hypothalami'cae interme'diae** [TA], dorsomedial nucleus of intermediate hypothalamus: a group of nerve cell bodies found in the dorsal part of the intermediate hypothalamic region.

**droplet nuclei,** small pathogen-containing particles of respiratory secretions expelled into the air by coughing, which are reduced by evaporation to small, dry particles that can remain airborne for long periods; this is one possible mechanism for transmission of infection from one individual to another *(droplet infection).*

**drumstick n.,** a leukocyte nucleus that has a drumstick.

**Edinger's nuclei, Edinger-Westphal nuclei,** nuclei accessorii nervi oculomotorii.

**n. embolifor'mis** [TA], emboliform nucleus: a small cerebellar nucleus that lies between the dentate nucleus and globose nucleus and contributes to the superior cerebellar peduncles. It is the term preferred in official terminology when considering humans, and is frequently also used to describe nonhuman primates. Cf. *n. interpositus inferior.*

**enamel n.,** in the cap stage of odontogenesis, a slight indentation in the outer dental epithelium of a developing tooth, in the end of the enamel cord; a temporary structure that disappears before enamel formation begins.

**n. endopeduncula'ris** [TA], endopeduncular nucleus: a small nucleus in the internal capsule of the hypothalamus adjacent to the medial edge of the globus pallidus.

**entopeduncular n., n. entopeduncula'ris,** n. endopeduncularis.

**n. of facial nerve, n. facia'lis,** n. nervi facialis.

**fastigial n., n. fastigia'tus,** n. fastigii.

**n. fasti'gii** [TA], fastigial nucleus: the most medial of the cerebellar nuclei, near the midline in the roof of the fourth ventricle; it projects to the pons and medulla oblongata, chiefly to the vestibular nuclei. It is the term preferred in official terminology when considering humans, and is frequently also used to describe nonhuman primates. Cf. *n. medialis cerebelli.*

**fertilization n.,** the nucleus produced by fusion of the male and female pronuclei in the fertilized oocyte; called also *conjugation n., zygote n.,* and *synkaryon.*

**nu'clei formatio'nis reticula'ris trun'co encepha'lico,** nuclei reticulares.

**free n.,** a cell nucleus from which the other elements of the cell have disappeared.

**n. gelatino'sus,** n. pulposus disci intervertebralis.

**geniculate n., dorsal lateral,** n. dorsalis corporis geniculati lateralis.

**geniculate n., lateral,** a nucleus within the lateral geniculate body, composed of a small ventral part (n. ventralis corporis geniculati lateralis) and large dorsal part (n. dorsalis corporis geniculati lateralis).

**geniculate nuclei, medial,** nuclei corporis geniculati medialis.

**geniculate n., ventral lateral,** n. ventralis corporis geniculati lateralis.

**n. genicula'tus latera'lis,** lateral geniculate nucleus.

**nu'clei genicula'ti media'les,** nuclei corporis geniculati medialis.

**germ n., germinal n.,** pronucleus.

**gigantocellular n., n. gigantocellula'ris** [TA], either of a symmetrical pair of large medial column reticular nuclei located in the superior part of the medulla oblongata and the posterior part of the pons, lateral to the nucleus raphes magnus and inferior to the caudal pontine reticular nucleus; its neurons are serotoninergic. Called also *gigantocellular intermediate reticular n.* and *gigantocellular reticular n.*

**gingival n.,** a part of the cerebellum in the third and fourth months of fetal life.

**n. globo'sus** [TA], globose nucleus: a cerebellar nucleus that lies between the emboliform nucleus and the nucleus fastigii and projects its fibers via the superior cerebellar peduncle (brachium conjunctivum). It is the term preferred in official terminology when considering humans, and is frequently also used to describe nonhuman primates. Cf. *n. interpositus posterior.*

**n. of glossopharyngeal nerve,** n. nervi glossopharyngei.

**n. of Goll's column,** n. gracilis.

**gonad n.,** micronucleus ( def. 1).

**n. gra'cilis** [TA], gracile nucleus: a nucleus in the medulla oblongata at the rostral end of the fasciculus gracilis of the cord, in which the fibers of the fasciculus gracilis synapse; the cells project to the thalamus via the medial lemniscus. Called also *n. of Goll's column.*

**nuclei of habenula, nu'clei habe'nulae,** see *n. habenularis lateralis* and *n. habenularis medialis.*

**habenular n., lateral,** n. habenularis lateralis.

**habenular n., medial,** n. habenularis medialis.

**n. habenula'ris latera'lis** [TA], lateral habenular nucleus: the more dispersed of the two nerve cell groups situated deep to the habenular trigone; it receives fibers from the stris medullaris thalami and projects to the raphe nuclei, reticular formation of mesencephalon, pars compacta of substantia nigra, and hypothalamus and basal forebrain.

**n. habenula'ris media'lis** [TA], medial habenular nucleus: the more densely packed of the two nerve cell groups situated deep to the habenular trigone; it receives fibers from the stria medullaris thalami and projects to the interpeduncular nucleus of the midbrain.

**haploid n.,** a cell nucleus containing half of the number of chromosomes typical of the somatic cells of a particular species.

**hypoglossal n., n. of hypoglossal nerve, n. hypoglossa'lis,** n. nervi hypoglossi.

**hypothalamic n., anterior,** n. anterior hypothalami.

**hypothalamic n., dorsal,** n. dorsalis hypothalami.

**hypothalamic n., dorsomedial,** n. dorsomedialis hypothalamicae intermediae.

**hypothalamic n., posterior,** n. posterior hypothalami.

**hypothalamic n., ventrolateral, hypothalamic n., ventromedial,** n. ventromedialis hypothalami.

**n. hypothala'micus ante'rior,** n. anterior hypothalami.

**n. hypothala'micus dorsa'lis,** n. dorsalis hypothalami.

**n. hypothala'micus dorsomedia'lis,** n. dorsomedialis hypothalamicae intermediae.

**n. hypothala'micus poste'rior,** n. posterior hypothalami.

**n. hypothala'micus ventrolatera'lis, n. hypothala'micus ventromedia'lis,** n. ventromedialis hypothalami.

**nuclei of inferior colliculus,** nuclei colliculi inferioris.

**n. infe'rior ner'vi trigemina'lis, inferior n. of trigeminal nerve,** n. spinalis nervi trigemini.

**infundibular n.,** nucleus arcuatus hypothalami.

**n. infundibula'ris,** TA alternative for *n. arcuatus hypothalami.*

**n. intercala'tus** [TA], intercalated nucleus: a group of nerve cells between the dorsal nucleus of the vagus nerve and the nucleus of the hypoglossal nerve, forming part of the perihypoglossal nuclear complex; called also *Staderini's n.*

**n. intermediolatera'lis medul'lae spina'lis** [TA], intermediolateral nucleus of spinal cord: a nucleus situated in the substantia intermedia lateralis of thoracic and upper lumbar levels of the spinal cord, which forms the lateral horn, and whose cells give rise to the preganglionic sympathetic outflow.

**n. intermediomedia'lis medul'lae spina'lis** [TA], intermediomedial nucleus of spinal cord: a nucleus composed of scattered cells in the substantia intermedia centralis, medial to the nucleus intermediolateralis; it is most prominent in the cervical spinal cord and is thought to be propriospinal in its connections.

**n. interpeduncula'ris** [TA], interpeduncular nucleus: a nucleus situated between the cerebral peduncles immediately dorsal to the interpeduncular fossa, which receives the fasciculus retroflexus.

**interposed n., anterior,** n. interpositus anterior.

**interposed n., posterior,** n. interpositus posterior.

**n. interpo'situs ante'rior** [TA], n. emboliformis; the term is preferred in official terminology when considering nonprimate mammals, and is occasionally used to refer to primates.

**n. interpo'situs poste'rior** [TA], n. globosus; the term is preferred in official terminology when considering nonprimate mammals, and is occasionally used to refer to primates.

**interstitial n. of Cajal,** nucleus interstitialis.

**n. interstitia'lis** [TA], interstitial nucleus: a nucleus at the rostral end of the medial longitudinal fasciculus in the mesencephalic tegmentum; its chief connections are reciprocal with vestibular nuclei and it also projects to the spinal cord.

**intracerebellar nuclei,** nuclei cerebelli.

**intralaminar nuclei of thalamus, nu'clei intralamina'res tha'lami** [TA], the nuclei within the internal medullary lamina of the thalamus, lying between the medial dorsal nucleus above and the lateral posterior nucleus below; included are the centromedian, paracentral, parafascicular, central lateral, and central medial nuclei. Formerly called also *reticular nuclei of thalamus* and *nuclei reticulares thalami.*

**Kölliker-Fuse n.,** n. subparabrachialis.

**large cell auditory n.,** n. vestibularis lateralis.

**lateral dorsal n. of thalamus,** n. dorsalis lateralis thalami.

**n. of lateral geniculate body,** lateral geniculate nucleus.

**nuclei of lateral lemniscus,** nuclei lemnisci lateralis.

**lateral n. of mammillary body,** n. mammillaris lateralis.

**n. of lateral olfactory stria,** a nucleus in the corticomedial part of the amygdaloid body.

**lateral posterior n. of thalamus,** n. lateralis posterior thalami.

**lateral ventral nuclei of thalamus,** nuclei ventrales laterales thalami.

**n. latera'lis cerebel'li** [TA], n. dentatus; the term is preferred in official terminology when considering nonprimate mammals, and is occasionally used to refer to primates.

**n. latera'lis dorsa'lis tha'lami,** n. dorsalis lateralis thalami.

**n. latera'lis poste'rior tha'lami** [TA], lateral posterior nucleus of thalamus: a nucleus in the ventral lateral part of the thalamus having major connections with the cingulate gyrus.

**nu'clei lemnis'ci latera'lis** [TA], nuclei of lateral lemniscus: several diffuse cell groups interposed in the course of the lateral lemniscus through the pons.

**n. of lens,** n. lentis.

**lenticular n., n. lenticula'ris,** n. lentiformis.

**n. lentifor'mis** [TA], lentiform nucleus: the part of the corpus striatum somewhat resembling a biconvex lens, divided into an external, larger, lateral part (putamen) and an internal, smaller, lighter colored medial part (globus pallidus), which is in turn subdivided into a smaller, medial, and a larger, lateral part by the medial medullary lamina; called also *lenticular n.* and *n. lenticularis.*

**n. len'tis** [TA], nucleus of lens: the harder internal part of the lens of the eye.

**linear n., inferior,** n. linearis inferioris.

**linear n., intermediate,** n. linearis intermedius.

**linear n., superior,** n. linearis superior.

**n. linea'ris inferio'ris** [TA], inferior linear nucleus: a raphe nucleus located in the mesencephalon.

**n. linea'ris interme'dius** [TA], intermediate linear nucleus: a raphe nucleus located in the mesencephalon.

**n. linea'ris supe'rior** [TA], superior linear nucleus: a raphe nucleus located in the mesencephalon.

**n. of Luys,** nucleus subthalamicus.

**magnus raphe n.,** n. raphes magnus.

**n. mammilla'ris latera'lis** [TA], lateral nucleus of mammillary body: the smaller of the two main nuclei of the mammillary body, which receive fibers from the basal olfactory areas and the fornix, and project to the thalamus and midbrain via mammillothalamic and mammillotegmental fasciculi.

**n. mammilla'ris media'lis** [TA], medial nucleus of mammillary body: the larger, predominant mass of cells, forming the medial of the two main nuclei of the mammillary body, which receive fibers from the basal olfactory areas and the fornix, and project to the thalamus and midbrain via mammillothalamic and mammillotegmental fasciculi.

**masticatory n.,** n. motorius nervi trigemini.

**medial central n. of thalamus,** former name for *n. centromedianus thalami.*

A

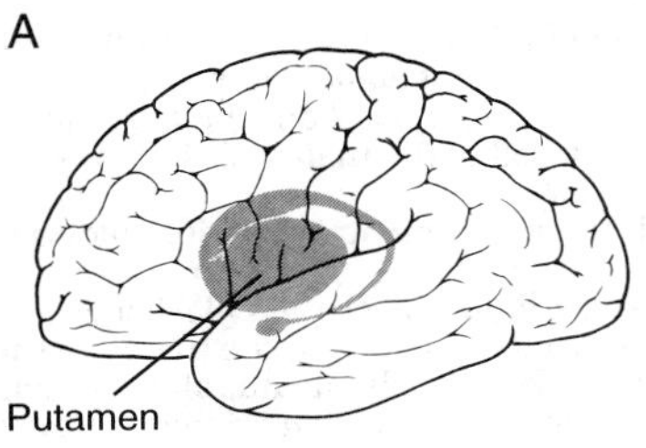


B

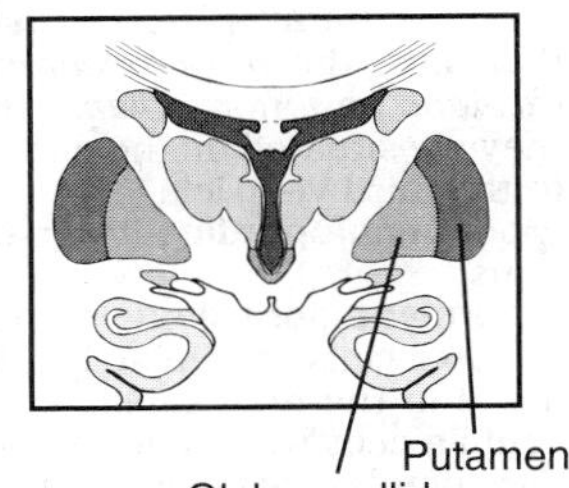


Nucleus lentiformis (lentiform nucleus), comprising the putamen and globus pallidus. *(A),* Lateral view of left hemisphere; *(B),* frontal section.

**medial dorsal n. of thalamus,** n. mediodorsalis thalami.

**n. of medial field,** nucleus campi medialis.

**nuclei of medial geniculate body,** nuclei corporis geniculati medialis.

**medial magnocellular n. of medial geniculate body,** nucleus medialis magnocellularis corporis geniculati medialis.

**medial n. of mammillary body,** n. mammillaris medialis.

**medial nuclei of thalamus,** nuclei mediales thalami.

**n. media'lis cerebel'li** [TA], n. fastigii; the term is preferred in official terminology when considering nonprimate mammals, and is occasionally used to refer to primates.

**n. media'lis dorsa'lis tha'lami,** n. mediodorsalis thalami.

**n. media'lis magnocellula'ris cor'poris genicula'ti media'lis** [TA], the medial of the medial geniculate nuclei; it receives afferent projections from both auditory and nonauditory neurons of the brainstem, from the fibers of the inferior colliculus and deep layers of the superior colliculus, and projects to the auditory cortex and adjacent insular and opercular fields.

**nu'clei media'les tha'lami** [TA], medial nuclei of thalamus: groups of nerve cells lying between the internal medullary lamina laterally and projecting toward the ependymal lining of the third ventricle medially; included are the large nucleus mediodorsalis and a series of smaller nuclei of uncertain significance and connections.

**median raphe n.,** n. raphes medianus.

**median nuclei of thalamus,** nuclei mediani thalami.

**nu'clei media'ni tha'lami** [TA], median nuclei of thalamus: small groups of nonspecific nerve cells scattered in the periventricular gray substance, separating the medial part of the thalamus from the ependyma of the third ventricle, and partly forming the interthalamic adhesion; included in the group are the anterior and posterior paraventricular nuclei, nucleus parataenialis, nucleus commissuralis rhomboidalis, and nucleus reuniens.

**n. mediodorsa'lis tha'lami** [TA], medial dorsal nucleus of thalamus: the largest of the medial nuclei of the thalamus, having a rostral magnocellular part and a caudolateral parvocellular part, both of which make extensive intrathalamic connections with most of the other thalamic nuclei. Called also *dorsomedial n. of thalamus.*

**n. of mesencephalic tract of trigeminal nerve, mesencephalic trigeminal n., mesencephalic n. of trigeminal nerve,** n. mesencephalicus nervi trigemini.

**n. mesencepha'licus ner'vi trige'mini** [TA], **n. mesencepha'licus trigemina'lis,** mesencephalic n. of trigeminal nerve: one of the nuclei of the trigeminal nerve, consisting of a slender column of cells in the lateral central gray matter of the superior part of the fourth ventral and cerebral aqueduct. It is the only central nervous system site of primary sensory neurons; its cells resemble posterior root ganglion cells. The peripheral processes of the cells, which form the mesencephalic tract, carry proprioceptive impulses; the central processes have widespread cerebellar and brain stem connections, including the motor nucleus of the trigeminal nerve. Called also *n. tractus mesencephalici nervi trigeminalis.*

**Meynert's n.,** n. basalis telencephali.

**midline nuclei of thalamus,** nuclei mediani thalami.

**Monakow's n.,** n. cuneatus accessorius.

**motor n.,** any collection of cells of the central nervous system giving origin to motor fibers of a nerve.

**motor n. of facial nerve,** n. nervi facialis.

**n. moto'rius ner'vi trige'mini** [TA], motor nucleus of trigeminal nerve: the nucleus of origin of the motor fibers of the trigeminal nerve, located in the dorsolateral part of the pons, just medial to the main sensory nucleus and the entering sensory root.

**n. moto'rius trigemina'lis,** n. motorius nervi trigemini.

**n. ner'vi abducen'tis** [TA], nucleus of abducens nerve: the nucleus of origin of the abducens nerve; it lies in the lower part of the pons and forms the lateral part of the facial colliculus in the floor of the fourth ventricle; fibers of the facial nerve form a complicated loop about the nucleus. Called also *abducens n., n. abducens,* and *n. abducentis.*

**n. ner'vi accesso'rii** [TA], nucleus of accessory nerve: an irregularly shaped group of nerve cells formed by the axons of nerve cells entering the spinal part of the accessory nerve; found at the anterior border of the anterior column of the spinal cord in an intermediate or central position. Called also *n. accessorius columnae anterioris medullae spinalis* and *accessory n. of anterior column of spinal cord.*

**nu'clei ner'vi cochlea'ris,** nuclei cochleares.

**n. ner'vi crania'lis** [TA], nucleus of cranial nerve: any of the nerve cells in the central nervous system that give rise to, or transmit or receive impulses from, the motor and sensory components of the cranial nerves.

**n. ner'vi facia'lis,** 1. [TA] nucleus of facial nerve: the nucleus of origin of the motor fibers of the facial nerve, which innervate the muscles of facial expression; the nucleus lies in the ventrolateral part of the lower pons, and its emerging fibers form a complicated loop about the nucleus of the abducens nerve. Called also *n. facialis* and *motor n.*

*of facial nerve.* 2. a collective name for the superior salivatory nucleus, the nucleus solitarius, and an adjacent motor nucleus.

**n. ner'vi glossopharyn'gei,** nucleus of glossopharyngeal nerve: the nucleus of origin and termination of the glossopharyngeal nerve, located in the medulla oblongata, comprising the inferior salivatory nucleus, the rostral part of the nucleus ambiguus, and the nucleus solitarius.

**n. ner'vi hypoglos'si** [TA], nucleus of hypoglossal nerve: the nucleus of origin of the hypoglossal nerve, forming a column in the central gray matter of the medial eminence from below the level of the inferior olive to the upper part of the medulla oblongata. Called also *hypoglossal n.* and *n. hypoglossalis.*

**n. ner'vi oculomoto'rii** [TA], nucleus of oculomotor nerve: a nuclear complex that is the origin of the fibers of the oculomotor nerve, situated in the tegmentum of the mesencephalon immediately ventral to the central gray matter, between the medial longitudinal fasciculi. The complex comprises larger paired dorsolateral and ventromedial somatic groups (see *n. dorsalis nervi oculomotorii* and *n. anteromedialis nervi oculomotorii*) as well as scattered small nuclei that have a parasympathetic function. Innervation of the superior rectus of one eye originates in the contralateral oculomotor nerve nucleus; the other elements of the nucleus supply ipsilateral eye muscles via the oculomotor nerve.

**n. ner'vi phre'nici** [TA], nucleus of phrenic nerve: a centrally positioned group of nerve cells in the gray substance of the anterior column of the spinal cord, extending from the third to the seventh cervical segments, which innervate the diaphragm; called also *phrenic n., phrenic n. of anterior column of spinal cord* and *n. phrenicus columnae anterioris medullae spinalis.*

**n. ner'vi puden'di** [TA], nucleus of pudendal nerve: a group of somatomotor neurons in the ventral horns of the spinal cord at the S1 and S2 levels, innervating the musculature of the pelvic floor and the external urethral and external anal sphincters. Called also *Onuf's n.*

**nu'clei ner'vi trigemina'lis, nu'clei ner'vi trige'mini,** nuclei of trigeminal nerve.

**n. ner'vi trochlea'ris** [TA], nucleus of trochlear nerve: the nucleus of origin of the motor fibers of the trochlear nerve; it lies in the central gray matter on the dorsal surface of the medial longitudinal fasciculus in the lower part of the mesencephalon. Called also *n. trochlearis* and *trochlear nucleus.*

**nu'clei ner'vi va'gi,** nuclei of vagus nerve: the nuclei of origin and termination of the vagus nerve, situated in the medulla oblongata, comprising the dorsal nucleus of the vagus nerve, the nucleus ambiguus, and the nuclei tractus solitarii.

**nu'clei ner'vi vestibulocochlea'ris,** vestibulocochlear nuclei.

**obscurus raphe n., n. obscu'rus ra'phes,** n. raphes obscurus.

**oculomotor n., n. of oculomotor nerve, n. oculomoto'rius,** n. nervi oculomotorii.

**nu'clei oculomoto'rii accesso'rii, nu'clei oculomoto'rii autono'mici,** nuclei accessorii nervi oculomotorii.

**n. olfacto'rius ante'rior** [TA], anterior olfactory nucleus: scattered groups of neurons intermingled with the olfactory tract that run caudally from the end of the olfactory bulb; some of them receive synaptic stimuli from the fibers of the olfactory tract.

**n. oliva'ris accesso'rius dorsa'lis,** n. olivaris accessorius posterior.

**n. oliva'ris accesso'rius media'lis** [TA], medial accessory olivary nucleus: the band of gray substance that lies medial to the inferior olivary nucleus and projects fibers to the opposite side of the cerebellum, especially to the vermis.

**n. oliva'ris accesso'rius poste'rior** [TA], posterior accessory olivary nucleus: the band of cells that lies posterior to the inferior olivary nucleus and projects fibers to the opposite side of the cerebellum, especially to the vermis. Called also *n. olivaris accessorius dorsalis* and *dorsal accessory olivary n.*

**nu'clei oliva'res cauda'les,** complexus olivaris inferior.

**n. oliva'ris crania'lis,** n. olivaris superior.

**nu'clei oliva'res inferio'res,** TA alternative for *complexus olivaris inferior.*

**n. oliva'ris rostra'lis, n. oliva'ris supe'rior** [TA], superior olivary nucleus: a band of gray substance located laterally at the level of the pontomedullary junction superior to the inferior olivary nucleus; its fibers form the olivocochlear tract. Called also *superior olivary complex, n. olivaris cranialis,* and *cranial* or *rostral olivary n.*

**olivary n.,** 1. complexus olivaris inferior. 2. oliva.

**olivary nuclei, caudal,** complexus olivaris inferior.

**olivary n., cranial,** n. oliva'ris supe'rior.

**olivary n., dorsal accessory,** n. olivaris accessorius posterior.

**olivary nuclei, inferior,** complexus olivaris inferior.

**olivary n., posterior accessory,** n. olivaris accessorius posterior.

**olivary n., rostral, olivary n., superior,** n. olivaris superior.

**Onuf's n., n. of Onufrowicz,** n. nervi pudendi.

**n. ori'ginis** [TA], nucleus of origin: any of the groups of nerve cells in the central nervous system from which arise the motor, or efferent, fibers of the cranial nerves.

**pallidal raphe n., n. pal'lidus ra'phes,** n. raphes pallidus.

**parabrachial nuclei,** nuclei parabrachiales.

**parabrachial n., lateral,** n. parabrachialis lateralis.

**parabrachial n., medial,** n. parabrachialis medialis.

**nu'clei parabrachia'les** [TA], the nucleus parabrachialis lateralis, nucleus parabrachialis medialis, and nucleus subparabrachialis considered collectively.

**n. parabrachia'lis latera'lis** [TA], lateral parabrachial nucleus: either of a pair of lateral column reticular nuclei located symmetrically on the border between the pons and the mesencephalon, adjacent to the brachium of the caudal colliculus and lateral to the cuneiform and subcuneiform nuclei.

**n. parabrachia'lis media'lis** [TA], medial parabrachial nucleus: either of a pair of lateral column reticular nuclei located symmetrically in the pons, near the caudal border of the mesencephalon, lateral to the nucleus reticularis pontis rostralis and nucleus reticularis pontis caudalis.

**n. paracentra'lis tha'lami** [TA], paracentral nucleus of thalamus: one of the smaller reticular nuclei of the dorsal thalamus, situated ventrolateral to the dorsal medial nucleus and medial to the central lateral nucleus.

**n. parafascicula'ris tha'lami** [TA], parafascicular nucleus of thalamus: one of the smaller reticular nuclei of the dorsal thalamus, situated medial to the centromedian nucleus and ventral to the dorsal medial nucleus.

**paragigantocellular n., lateral, n. paragigantocellula'ris latera'lis** [TA], either of a pair of lateral column reticular nuclei located symmetrically at the level of the facial nucleus, rostral to the nucleus retroambiguus.

**paramedian n., dorsal, paramedian n., posterior,** n. paramedianus posterior.

**n. paramedia'nus dorsa'lis, n. paramedia'nus poste'rior** [TA], posterior paramedian nucleus: a group of nerve cells near the posterior surface of the medulla oblongata, forming part of the perihypoglossal nuclear complex; called also *dorsal paramedian n.*

**n. parasolita'rius** [TA], parasolitary nucleus: an aggregation of nerve cells situated ventrolateral to the solitary nucleus.

**nu'clei parasympa'thici sacra'les** [TA], sacral parasympathetic nuclei: a group of nerve cells in the second through the fourth sacral segments of the spinal cord, located lateral to the central canal and central gelatinous substance, between the bases of the anterior and posterior gray columns; the cells are the source of the pelvic or sacral outflow of parasympathetic preganglionic fibers.

**n. parataenia'lis tha'lami** [TA], **paratenial n. of thalamus,** one of the median nuclei of the thalamus, situated ventral and medial to the stria medullaris; see *nuclei mediani thalami.*

**paraventricular n. of hypothalamus,** n. paraventricularis hypothalami.

**paraventricular nuclei of thalamus,** nuclei paraventriculares thalami.

**paraventricular n. of thalamus, anterior,** n. paraventricularis anterior thalami.

**paraventricular n. of thalamus, posterior,** n. paraventricularis posterior thalami.

**n. paraventricula'ris ante'rior tha'lami** [TA], anterior paraventricular nucleus of thalamus: the anterior of the two nuclei paraventriculares thalami (q.v.).

**n. paraventricula'ris hypotha'lami** [TA], paraventricular nucleus of hypothalamus: a sharply defined band of cells in the wall of the third ventricle in the anterior hypothalamic region; many of its cells are neurosecretory in function, secreting oxytocin, which is carried to the posterior lobe of the pituitary gland by the fibers of the paraventriculohypophysial tract.

**n. paraventricula'ris poste'rior tha'lami** [TA], posterior paraventricular nucleus of thalamus: the posterior of the two nuclei paraventriculares thalami (q.v.).

**nu'clei paraventricula'res tha'lami** [TA], paraventricular nuclei of thalamus: the *n. paraventricularis anterior thalami* and *n. paraventricularis posterior thalami,* two of the nuclei mediani thalami (q.v.); they are situated on the dorsomedial wall of the thalamus, juxtaposed to the third ventricle.

**pedunculopontine tegmental n.,** n. tegmentalis pedunculopontinus.

**perihypoglossal nuclei, nu'clei perihypoglossa'les** [TA], a group of nerve cells immediately adjacent to the nucleus of the hypoglossal nerve in the gray substance of the medulla oblongata, all of which contain cells with characteristics suggestive of reticular connections; the complex includes the nucleus intercalatus, the nucleus paramedianus dorsalis, the nucleus prepositus, and the sublingual nucleus. Called also *perihypoglossal nuclear complex.*

**n. periventricula'ris poste'rior** [TA], posterior periventricular nucleus: a nucleus of nerve cells in the intermediate hypothalamic area, lying in the posterior part of the third ventricle.

**nuclei of perizonal field,** nuclei campi perizonalis.

**Perlia's n.,** a group of cells in the midline of the oculomotor nuclear complex, thought to be associated with ocular convergence.

**phenanthrene n.,** cholane n.

**phrenic n., phrenic n. of anterior column of spinal cord, n. of phrenic nerve,** n. nervi phrenici.

**n. phre'nicus colum'nae anterio'ris medul'lae spina'lis,** n. nervi phrenici.

**polymorphic n.,** a cell nucleus that assumes an irregular form or splits up into more or less completely separated lobes, such as the nuclei in the polymorphonuclear leukocytes (neutrophils).

**nuclei of pons, pontine nuclei,** nuclei pontis.

**pontine raphe n., pontine n. of raphe,** n. raphes pontis.

**pontine reticular n., caudal, pontine reticular n., inferior intermediate,** n. reticularis pontis caudalis.

**pontine reticular nuclei, intermediate,** see *n. reticularis pontis caudalis* and *n. reticularis pontis rostralis.*

**pontine reticular n., oral, pontine reticular n., superior intermediate,** n. reticularis pontis rostralis.

**pontine reticular n., tegmental,** n. reticularis tegmenti pontis.

**pontine n. of trigeminal nerve, n. ponti'nus ner'vi trigemina'lis,** n. principalis nervi trigemini.

**nu'clei pon'tis** [TA], nuclei of pons: masses of nerve cells scattered throughout the ventral part of the pons, in which the longitudinal fibers of the pons terminate, and whose axons in turn cross to the opposite side and form the middle cerebellar peduncle, which projects fibers to the neocerebellum.

**n. pon'tis ra'phes,** n. raphes pontis.

**n. of posterior commissure,** n. commissurae posterioris.

**n. poste'rior hypotha'lami** [TA], **posterior n. of hypothalamus,** posterior hypothalamic nucleus: a nucleus of nerve cells in the posterior hypothalamic region, above the lateral and medial nuclei of the mammillary body; it has major brain stem connections via periventricular fibers and the dorsal longitudinal fasciculus.

**n. poste'rior ner'vi va'gi** [TA], posterior nucleus of vagus nerve: the nucleus of origin of the parasympathetic fibers of the vagus nerve, situated in the trigone of the vagus nerve in the floor of the fourth ventricle, lateral to the nucleus of the hypoglossal nerve; called also *dorsal vagal n., dorsal n. of vagus nerve, n. alae cinereae, n. vagalis dorsalis* and *n. dorsalis nervi vagi* [TA alternative].

**posterior n. of oculomotor nerve,** n. dorsalis nervi oculomotorii.

**posterior periventricular n.,** n. periventricularis posterior.

**posterior raphe n., n. poste'rior ra'phes,** n. raphes posterior.

**posterior nuclei of thalamus,** nuclei posteriores thalami.

**posterior n. of vagus nerve,** n. posterior nervi vagi.

**nu'clei posterio'res tha'lami** [TA], posterior nuclear complex of thalamus: groups of nerve cells anterior to the pulvinar, forming an ill-defined complex that receives afferents from the spinothalamic tract and superior and inferior colliculi.

**n. posterolatera'lis medul'lae spina'lis** [TA], posterolateral nucleus of spinal cord: a group of nerve cells in the posterolateral gray substance of the anterior column of the spinal cord; called also *dorsolateral n. of spinal cord.*

**n. posteromedia'lis medul'lae spina'lis** [TA], posteromedial nucleus of spinal cord: a group of nerve cells in the posteromedial gray substance of the anterior column of the spinal cord; called also *dorsomedial n. of spinal cord.*

**pregeniculate n.,** n. ventralis corporis geniculati lateralis.

**n. pregenicula'tus,** TA alternative for *n. ventralis corporis geniculati lateralis.*

**preoptic n., lateral,** n. preopticus lateralis.

**preoptic n., medial,** n. preopticus medialis.

**preoptic n., median,** n. preopticus medianus.

**preoptic n., periventricular,** n. preopticus periventricularis.

**n. preop'ticus latera'lis** [TA], lateral preoptic nucleus: a nucleus of nerve cells in the preoptic area of the basal forebrain.

**n. preop'ticus media'lis** [TA], medial preoptic nucleus: a nucleus of nerve cells in the preoptic area of the basal forebrain, ventral to the anterior commissure.

**n. preop'ticus media'nus** [TA], median preoptic nucleus: a nucleus of nerve cells in the preoptic area of the basal forebrain.

**n. preop'ticus periventricula'ris** [TA], periventricular preoptic nucleus: a nucleus of nerve cells in the preoptic area of the basal forebrain; the nucleus is situated adjacent to the wall of the preoptic recess of the third ventricle.

**n. prepo'situs** [TA], prepositus nucleus: a group of nerve cells rostral to the hypoglossal nucleus and nucleus intercalatus and caudal to the abducent nucleus; it forms part of the perihypoglossal nuclei.

**n. of prerubral field,** n. campi medialis.

**nu'clei pretecta'les** [TA], pretectal nuclei: various groups of nerve cells in the pretectal area which receive impulses chiefly from the optic tract; they project to the nucleus accessorius of the oculomotor nerve and constitute the midbrain center for the pupillary light reflex.

**principal sensory n. of trigeminal nerve, n. principa'lis ner'vi trige'mini** [TA], the nucleus of termination of afferent fibers of the trigeminal nerve, carrying impulses for sensations of touch and pressure, located in the dorsolateral part of the middle of the pons, just lateral to the entering trigeminal root fibers. Called also *pontine n. of trigeminal nerve, n. pontinus nervi trigeminalis,* and *n. sensorius principalis nervi trigeminalis.*

**n. pro'prius** [TA], a column of large neurons that extends throughout the posterior column of the spinal cord, ventral to the gelatinous substance; it corresponds to some of the cell constituents of Rexed's laminae III and IV.

**n. of pudendal nerve,** n. nervi pudendi.

**n. pulpo'sus,** n. pulposus disci intervertebralis.

**n. pulposus, herniated,** herniation of intervertebral disk.

**n. pulpo'sus dis'ci intervertebra'lis** [TA], **pulpy n. of intervertebral disk,** a semifluid mass of fine white and elastic fibers that forms the central portion of an intervertebral disk; it has been regarded as the persistent remains of the embryonic notochord.

**nu'clei pulvina'res tha'lami** [TA], pulvinar nuclei: a subgroup of the dorsal thalamic nuclei consisting of those that form the prominent, cushion-like medial portion of the posterior extremity of the thalamus (the pulvinar).

**raphe nuclei, nuclei of raphe,** nuclei raphes.

**nu'clei ra'phes** [TA], raphe nuclei: the median column reticular nuclei, a subgroup of the reticular nuclei of the brain stem, found in narrow longitudinal sheets along the raphae of the medulla oblongata, pons, and mesencephalon; they include many neurons that synthesize serotonin. Their ascending fibers project to parts of the limbic system and their descending fibers project to other brain stem nuclei, the medulla oblongata, and the pons. In the group are the *nucleus raphes magnus, nucleus raphes obscurus, nucleus raphes pallidus, nucleus raphes pontis, nucleus raphes posterior, nucleus raphes medianus, nucleus linearis inferioris, nucleus linearis intermedius,* and *nucleus linearis superior.*

**n. ra'phes dorsa'lis,** n. raphes posterior.

**n. ra'phes mag'nus** [TA], magnus raphe nucleus: a raphe nucleus partially overlapping the nucleus pallidus and nucleus obscurus in the medulla oblongata and projecting upward into the posterior part of the pons; its neurons are serotoninergic.

**n. ra'phes media'nus** [TA], median raphe nucleus: a raphe nucleus in the anterior part of the pons; its neurons are serotoninergic. Called also *superior central n.*

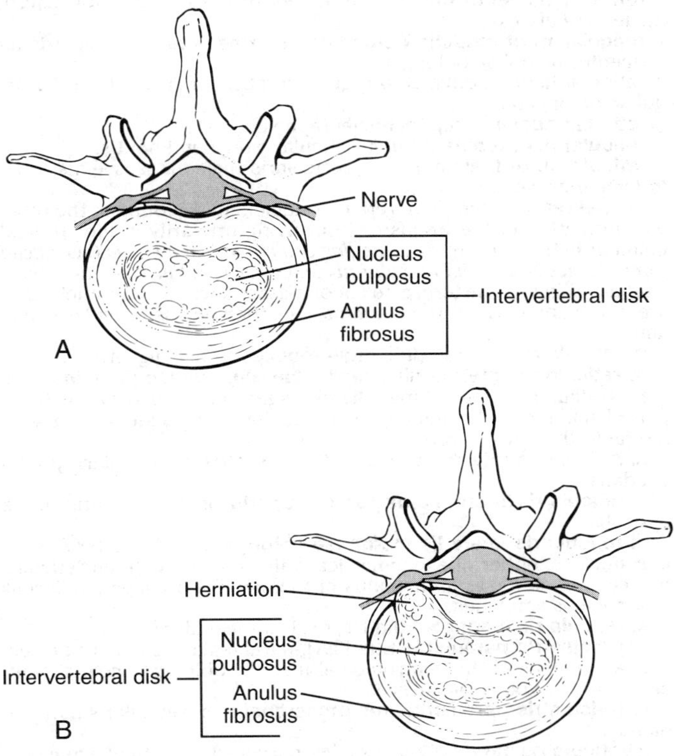


Intervertebral disk in transverse section, showing the nucleus pulposus and the anulus fibrosus. *(A),* Normal disk; *(B),* herniation of the nucleus pulposus.

**n. ra'phes obscu'rus** [TA], obscurus raphe nucleus: a raphe nucleus of the medulla oblongata closely associated with the nucleus pallidus raphes; its neurons are serotoninergic.

**n. ra'phes pal'lidus** [TA], pallidal raphe nucleus: a raphe nucleus of the medulla oblongata closely associated with the nucleus raphes obscurus; its neurons are serotoninergic.

**n. ra'phes pon'tis** [TA], pontine raphe nucleus: a raphe nucleus in the central part of the pons; its neurons are serotoninergic.

**n. ra'phes poste'rior** [TA], posterior raphe nucleus: a large raphe nucleus extending from the anterior part of the pons through the mesencephalon; its neurons are serotoninergic. Called also *dorsal raphe n.* and *n. raphes dorsalis.*

**red n.,** n. ruber.

**reproductive n.,** micronucleus (def. 1).

**reticular nuclei,** nuclei reticulares.

**reticular n., caudal pontine,** n. reticularis pontis caudalis.

**reticular n., gigantocellular, reticular n., gigantocellular intermediate,** n. gigantocellularis.

**reticular n., lateral,** 1. n. reticularis lateralis medullae oblongatae. 2. see *lateral column reticular nuclei.*

**reticular nuclei, lateral column,** a pair of symmetrical groups of scattered small reticular nuclei of the brain stem, each arranged in a column lateral to the medial column reticular nuclei; most of their neurons are associative in nature. Included are the nucleus reticularis lateralis medullae oblongatae, nucleus tegmenti pedunculopontinus, nucleus reticularis parvocellularis, nucleus paragigantocellularis lateralis, nucleus parabrachialis lateralis, nucleus parabrachialis medialis and nucleus subparabrachialis.

**reticular n., magnocellular,** n. gigantocellularis.

**reticular nuclei, medial column,** two groups of reticular nuclei of the brainstem, located symmetrically in the central parts of the two halves of the tegmentum; their neurons are often large, with long axons, and have dendrites and preterminal axons at right angles to the long axis of the brainstem. Included are the nucleus gigantocellularis, nucleus reticularis tegmenti pontis, nucleus reticularis pontis caudalis, nucleus reticularis pontis rostralis, nucleus cuneiformis, and nucleus subcuneiformis.

**reticular nuclei, median column,** nuclei raphes.

**reticular n., oral pontine,** n. reticularis pontis rostralis.

**reticular n., paramedian,** n. reticularis paramedianus.

**reticular n., parvocellular,** nucleus reticularis parvocellularis.

**reticular nuclei, pontine,** 1. any of the reticular nuclei located in the pons. 2. see *n. reticularis pontis caudalis, n. reticularis pontis rostralis,* and *n. reticularis tegmenti pontis.*

**reticular n., tegmental pontine,** n. reticularis tegmenti pontis.

**reticular nuclei of brain stem, nuclei of the reticular formation,** nuclei reticulares.

**reticular n. of medulla oblongata, intermediate,** n. reticularis intermedius medullae oblongatae.

**reticular n. of medulla oblongata, lateral,** n. reticularis lateralis medullae oblongatae.

**reticular nuclei of raphe,** nuclei raphes.

**reticular n. of tegmentum,** n. reticularis tegmenti pontis.

**reticular n. of thalamus,** 1. n. reticularis thalami. 2. see *nuclei intralaminares thalami.*

**nu'clei reticula'res** [TA], reticular nuclei: nuclei found in the reticular formation of the brainstem, occurring primarily in longitudinal columns in three groups: the *median column reticular nuclei* (see *nuclei raphes*), *medial column reticular nuclei* (q.v.), and *lateral column reticular nuclei* (q.v.). The term also encompasses several other nuclei that are not in any of the three columns, e.g., the nucleus reticularis thalami.

**n. reticula'ris interme'dius gigantocellula'ris,** n. gigantocellularis.

**n. reticula'ris interme'dius medul'lae oblonga'tae** [TA], intermediate reticular nucleus of medulla oblongata: either of a symmetrical pair of small medial column reticular nuclei in the medulla oblongata lateral to the nucleus raphes obscurus.

**n. reticula'ris interme'dius pon'tis inferio'ris,** n. reticularis pontis caudalis.

**n. reticula'ris interme'dius pon'tis superio'ris,** n. reticularis pontis rostralis.

**n. reticula'ris latera'lis medul'lae oblonga'tae** [TA], lateral reticular nucleus: either of a symmetrical pair of lateral column reticular nuclei, each in a lateral funiculus of the medulla oblongata adjacent to a nucleus ambiguus.

**n. reticula'ris magnocellula'ris,** n. gigantocellularis.

**n. reticula'ris paramedia'nus** [TA], paramedian reticular nucleus: a small nucleus in the ventromedial medulla oblongata near the nucleus of the hypoglossal nerve.

**n. reticula'ris paramedia'nus precerebel'li,** n. reticularis paramedianus.

**n. reticula'ris parvocellula'ris** [TA], parvocellular reticular nucleus: either of a pair of principal lateral column reticular nuclei, lying lateral to the nucleus gigantocellularis and adjacent to the nucleus ambiguus.

**n. reticula'ris pon'tis cauda'lis** [TA], caudal pontine reticular nucleus: a medial column reticular nucleus in the pons, located next to the nucleus reticularis tegmenti pontis and superior to the gigantocellular nucleus. Called also *n. reticularis intermedius pontis inferioris* and *inferior intermediate pontine reticular n.*

**n. reticula'ris pon'tis ora'lis, n. reticula'ris pon'tis rostra'lis** [TA], oral pontine reticular nucleus: either of a symmetrical pair of medial column reticular nuclei in the central part of the pons, one on either side of the superior central nucleus. Called also *n. reticularis intermedius pontis superioris* and *superior intermediate pontine reticular n.*

**nu'clei reticula'res ra'phes,** nuclei raphes.

**n. reticula'ris tegmenta'lis pedunculoponti'nus,** n. tegmentalis pedunculopontinus.

**n. reticula'ris tegmenta'lis ponti'nus, n. reticula'ris tegmen'ti pon'tis** [TA] tegmental pontine reticular nucleus: either of a pair of medial column reticular nuclei located symmetrically in the posterior part of the pons between the nucleus raphes pontis and the nucleus reticularis pontis caudalis. Called also *reticulotegmental n.*

**n. reticula'ris tha'lami** [TA], 1. [TA] reticular nucleus of thalamus: a thin layer of cells on the lateral surface of the thalamus, within and lateral to the external medullary lamina. 2. see *nuclei intralaminares thalami.*

**reticulate n. of thalamus, n. reticula'tus tha'lami,** n. reticularis thalami.

**reticulotegmental n.,** n. reticularis tegmenti pontis.

**n. retroambi'guus** [TA], retroambiguus nucleus: a nucleus near the nucleus ambiguus, with motor fibers that control both inspiratory and expiratory muscles.

**retrodorsal n. of spinal cord, n. retrodorsolatera'lis medul'lae spina'lis,** n. retroposterolateralis medullae spinalis.

**retrofacial n., n. retrofacia'lis** [TA], a small nucleus between the nucleus ambiguus and the facial nucleus, believed to be a source of vagal efferent visceral fibers.

**retroposterolateral n. of spinal cord, n. retroposterolatera'lis medul'lae spina'lis** [TA], a group of nerve cells in the gray substance of the retroposterolateral region of the anterior column of the spinal cord, which innervates the digital muscles.

**n. reu'niens** [TA], one of the median nuclei of the thalamus; it is situated near the interthalamic adhesion, bordering the third ventricle, ventral to the central medial nucleus; see *nuclei mediani thalami.*

**rhomboid n., n. rhomboida'lis,** n. commissuralis rhomboidalis.

**Roller's n.,** 1. sublingual n. 2. cells near the hilum of the inferior olivary nucleus.

**roof nuclei,** a term sometimes used to refer to the nuclei cerebelli because some of them are situated in close proximity to the roof of the fourth ventricle of the brain.

**n. ru'ber** [TA], red nucleus: a distinctive oval nucleus (pink in fresh specimens because of an iron-containing pigment in many of the cells) centrally placed in the upper mesencephalic reticular formation; it receives fibers from the deep cerebellar nuclei and cerebral cortex and projects fibers to the cerebellum, brain stem, spinal cord, and probably to the thalamus. See also: *pars magnocellularis nuclei rubri* and *pars parvocellularis nuclei rubri.*

**sacral parasympathetic nuclei,** nuclei parasympathici sacrales.

**n. saliva'rius infe'rior,** n. salivatorius inferior.

**n. saliva'rius supe'rior,** n. salivatorius superior.

**salivary n., inferior,** n. salivatorius inferior.

**salivary n., superior,** n. salivatorius superior.

**n. salivato'rius infe'rior** [TA], inferior salivatory nucleus: the inferior part of the column of scattered cells in the posterolateral part of the reticular formation in the lower pons and upper medulla oblongata; they comprise the parasympathetic outflow of the glossopharyngeal nerve for the supply of the parotid gland. Called also *inferior salivary n.,* and *n. salivarius inferior.*

**n. salivato'rius supe'rior** [TA], superior salivatory nucleus: an ill-defined column of scattered cells in the posterolateral part of the reticular formation of the posterior pons, continuous with the inferior salivatory nucleus; its cells comprise the parasympathetic outflow of the facial nerve for the supply of the lacrimal, nasal, palatine, submandibular, and sublingual glands. Called also *superior salivary n.* and *n. salivarius superior.*

**salivatory n., caudal,** n. salivatorius inferior.

**salivatory n., inferior,** n. salivatorius inferior.

**salivatory n., rostral, salivatory n., superior,** n. salivatorius superior.

**sanded n.,** a hepatocyte nucleus seen in chronic hepatitis B, having a characteristic appearance caused by the presence of large amounts of hepatitis B surface antigen; a similar phenomenon is seen in hepatitis D.

**Schwalbe's n.,** n. vestibularis medialis.

**Schwann's n.,** the nucleus of a Schwann cell.

**segmentation n.,** the fertilization nucleus after cleavage has begun. Called also *cleavage n.*

**n. semiluna'ris,** TA alternative for *n. arcuatus hypothalami.*

**n. senso'rius infe'rior ner'vi trigemina'lis,** n. spinalis nervi trigemini.

**n. senso'rius principa'lis ner'vi trigemina'lis,** n. principalis nervi trigemini.

**sensory n.,** the nucleus of termination of the afferent (sensory) fibers of a peripheral nerve.

**sensory n. of trigeminal nerve, inferior, sensory n. of trigeminal nerve, lower,** n. spinalis nervi trigemini.

**sensory n. of trigeminal nerve, principal,** n. principalis nervi trigemini.

**septal n., lateral,** n. septalis lateralis.

**septal n., medial,** n. septalis medialis.

**n. septa'lis latera'lis** [TA], lateral septal nucleus: a nucleus in the septal area, continuous with the gray lamina of the septum pellucidum; it has afferent and cholinergic efferent connections with a variety of forebrain and brain stem areas including the hippocampus, the lateral hypothalamus, the tegmentum, and the amygdaloid bodies.

**n. septa'lis media'lis** [TA], medial septal nucleus: a nucleus in the septal area, coextensive with the diagonal band of Broca; it has afferent and cholinergic efferent connections with a variety of forebrain and brain stem areas including the hippocampus, the lateral hypothalamus, the tegmentum, and the amygdaloid bodies.

**shadow n.,** a cell nucleus that does not stain and appears as a faint shadow under the microscope.

**Siemerling's n.,** one of the subdivisions of the nucleus nervi oculomotorius.

**nu'clei solita'rii, solitary nuclei, nuclei of solitary tract,** nuclei tractus solitarii.

**somatic n.,** macronucleus.

**sperm n.,** the male pronucleus.

**spherical n.,** n. globosus.

**spinal n. of accessory nerve,** n. spinalis nervi accessorii.

**n. of spinal tract of trigeminal nerve, spinal n. of trigeminal nerve,** n. spinalis nervi trigemini.

**n. spina'lis ner'vi accesso'rii,** spinal nucleus of accessory nerve: the group of cells in the anterior horn of the upper five or six levels of the cervical spinal cord that form the spinal roots of the accessory nerve; continuous rostrally with the nucleus ambiguus.

**n. spina'lis ner'vi trige'mini** [TA], spinal nucleus of trigeminal nerve: a column of cells that lies along the medial aspect of the spinal tract, extending from the level of entry of the trigeminal nerve in the pons to the second cervical segment of the spinal cord, where it is continuous with the dorsal gray column. The nucleus has several cytoarchitectonic subdivisions and the fibers of the spinal tract end in it. Called also *inferior n. of trigeminal nerve, n. inferior nervi trigeminalis, inferior* or *lower sensory n. of trigeminal nerve,* and *n. of spinal tract of trigeminal nerve.*

**Spitzka's n.,** Perlia's n.

**Staderini's n.,** n. intercalatus.

**Stilling's n.,** n. thoracicus posterior.

**n. stri'ae termina'lis** [TA], bed nucleus of stria terminalis: the collection of scattered groups of neurons between the fibers near the anterior end of the stria terminalis; they serve a relay function.

**striate n.,** a term loosely applied to the neostriatum, to a nucleus of the corpus striatum, or to the corpus striatum itself.

**n. subcaeru'leus** [TA], **n. subceru'leus,** a group of neurons subjacent to the nucleus caeruleus in the anterior part of the pons; sometimes considered part of the medial column reticular nuclei.

**n. subcuneifor'mis** [TA], subcuneiform nucleus: a nucleus in the mesencephalon adjacent to and closely associated with the cuneiform nucleus.

**sublingual n.,** a sharply defined nucleus immediately ventral to the nucleus of the hypoglossal nerve, forming part of the perihypoglossal nuclear complex; called also *Roller's n.*

**subparabrachial n., n. subparabrachia'lis** [TA], either of a pair of parabrachial nuclei that constitute part of the lateral column reticular nuclei; it is a pneumotaxic center lying ventral to the medial and lateral parabrachial nuclei in the pons. Called also *Kölliker-Fuse n.*

**n. subthala'micus** [TA], subthalamic nucleus: a biconvex mass of gray matter on the medial side of the junction of the internal capsule and the crus cerebri; its chief connections are with the globus pallidus. Called also *n. of Luys* and *Luys' body.*

**superior central n., superior central raphe n.,** n. raphes medianus.

**n. of superior olive,** n. olivaris superior.

**suprachiasmatic n., n. suprachiasma'ticus** [TA], a small nucleus in the supraoptic region of the hypothalamus, just above the optic chiasm; it influences rhythmical aspects of hypothalamic functions in many vertebrate species, including humans.

**n. supraop'ticus** [TA], supraoptic nucleus: a sharply defined nucleus of nerve cells in the anterior hypothalamic region, immediately above the lateral part of the optic chiasm; many of its cells are neurosecretory in function, secreting antidiuretic hormone, which is carried to the posterior lobe of the pituitary gland by the fibers of the supraopticohypophysial tract; other cells are osmoreceptors which respond to increased osmotic pressure to signal the release of antidiuretic hormone by the posterior lobe of the pituitary gland.

**n. tec'ti,** n. fastigii.

**tegmental nuclei, anterior,** nuclei tegmentales anteriores.

**tegmental n., laterodorsal, tegmental n., lateroposterior,** n. tegmentalis posterolateralis.

**tegmental nuclei, ventral,** nuclei tegmentales anteriores.

**n. of tegmental field,** n. campi medialis.

**tegmental pedunculopontine reticular n.,** n. tegmentalis pedunculopontinus.

**nu'clei tegmenta'les anterio'res** [TA], anterior tegmental nuclei: several masses of neurons of the mesencephalic tegmentum, situated ventral to the medial longitudinal fasciculus. Called also *ventral tegmental nuclei.*

**n. tegmenta'lis pedunculoponti'nus** [TA], tegmental pedunculopontine nucleus: a nucleus at the posterior end of the mesencephalon, sometimes considered one of the lateral column reticular nuclei. It merges anteriorly into the cuneiform and subcuneiform nuclei.

**n. tegmenta'lis posterolatera'lis** [TA], lateroposterior tegmental nucleus: a nucleus of nerve cells in the mesencephalic tegmentum, situated dorsal to the nucleus of the trochlear nerve. Called also *laterodorsal tegmental n.*

**nu'clei tegmen'ti, nuclei of tegmentum,** see *nuclei tegmentales anteriores* and *n. tegmentalis posterolateralis.*

**terminal n., n. terminatio'nis** [TA], terminator nucleus: any of the groups of nerve cells within the central nervous system upon which the axons of primary afferent neurons of various cranial nerves synapse.

**thalamic nuclei,** nuclei of thalamus.

**thalamic nuclei, anterior,** nuclei anteriores thalami.

**thalamic nuclei, medial,** nuclei mediales thalami.

**thalamic nuclei, median,** nuclei mediani thalami.

**thalamic nuclei, posterior,** nuclei posteriores thalami.

**thalamic n., reticular,** 1. n. reticularis thalami. 2. see *nuclei intralaminares thalami.*

**thalamic nuclei, ventral,** nuclei ventrales thalami.

**nuclei of thalamus,** the nuclei and nuclear groups in the thalamus. Groups are the *nuclei anteriores thalami, nuclei dorsales thalami, nuclei mediales thalami, nuclei mediani thalami, nuclei intralaminares thalami, nuclei posteriores thalami,* and *nuclei ventrales thalami.* The *nucleus reticularis thalami* and *nucleus subthalamicus* are also thalamic nuclei.

**thoracic n., thoracic n., dorsal, thoracic n., posterior,** n. thoracicus posterior.

**n. thora'cicus,** n. thoracicus posterior.

**n. thora'cicus dorsa'lis,** TA alternative for *n. thoracicus posterior.*

**n. thora'cicus poste'rior** [TA], posterior thoracic nucleus: a well-defined column of cells in the medial part of the posterior column of the spinal cord, immediately posterior to the intermediate column, usually extending from the eighth cervical segment caudally to the third or fourth lumbar segment; it gives rise to the ipsilateral posterior spinocerebellar tract. Called also *columna thoracica, thoracic column, Clarke's column* or *nucleus, dorsal nucleus of Clarke, dorsal thoracic nucleus, nucleus thoracicus dorsalis* [TA alternative], and *Stilling's column* or *nucleus.*

**n. trac'tus mesencepha'lici ner'vi trigemina'lis,** n. mesencephalicus nervi trigemini.

**nu'clei trac'tus solita'rii** [TA], nuclei of solitary tract: any of various nuclei of termination of the visceral afferent fibers of the facial, glossopharyngeal, and vagus nerves, which enter the tractus solitarius. The nuclei surround the tractus solitarius and their caudal ends join with the caudal ends of the corresponding nuclei of the opposite side. Called also *solitary nuclei* and *nuclei solitarii.*

**nuclei of trapezoid body,** a group of nerve cell bodies of the superior olivary complex, lying within the fibers of the trapezoid body.

**triangular n.,** 1. n. vestibularis medialis. 2. n. triangularis septi.

**triangular septal n.,** n. triangularis septi.

**n. triangula'ris,** n. vestibularis medialis.

**n. triangula'ris sep'ti** [TA], triangular septal nucleus: a nucleus of nerve cells of the caudal region of the septum pellucidum.

**trigeminal nuclei,** nuclei of trigeminal nerve.

**trigeminal mesencephalic n.,** n. mesencephalicus nervi trigeminalis.

**trigeminal motor n.,** n. motorius nervi trigemini.

**nuclei of trigeminal nerve,** four nuclei located along the trigeminal nerve, chiefly in the pons and medulla oblongata but also extending as far down as the upper cervical spinal cord. See *n. mesencephalicus nervi trigemini, n. motorius nervi trigemini, n. principalis nervi trigemini,* and *n. spinalis nervi trigemini.*

**trochlear n., n. of trochlear nerve,** n. nervi trochlearis.

**n. trochlea'ris,** n. nervi trochlearis.

**trophic n.,** macronucleus.

**nu'clei tubera'les latera'les** [TA], lateral tuberal nuclei: nerve cell nuclei situated ventrally in the intermediate hypothalamic region, mainly in the lateral hypothalamic area.

**vagal n., dorsal, n. vaga'lis dorsa'lis,** n. posterior nervi vagi.

**nuclei of vagus nerve,** nuclei nervi vagi.

**ventral anterior n. of thalamus,** n. ventralis anterior thalami.

**n. of ventral field,** n. campi ventralis.

**ventral intermediate n. of thalamus,** n. ventralis intermedius thalami.

**ventral lateral nuclei of thalamus,** nuclei ventrales laterales thalami.

**ventral medial nuclei of thalamus,** nuclei ventrales mediales thalami.

**ventral medial n. of oculomotor nerve,** n. anteromedialis nervi oculomotorii.

**ventral posterior nuclei of thalamus,** nuclei ventrobasales thalami.

**ventral principal n. of medial geniculate body,** n. ventralis corporis geniculati medialis.

**ventral nuclei of thalamus,** nuclei ventrales thalami.

**n. ventra'lis ante'rior tha'lami** [TA], ventral anterior nucleus of thalamus: a nucleus anteriorly located within the ventral nuclei of the thalamus, posterior to the reticular nucleus, anterior to the ventral lateral nucleus, and lateral and medial to the internal and external medullary laminae, respectively; it is subdivided into magnocellular and principal divisions.

**n. ventra'lis cor'poris genicula'ti latera'lis** [TA], ventral lateral geniculate nucleus: the smaller, ventral part of the lateral geniculate nucleus, projecting toward the zona incerta of the ventral thalamus. Called also *pregeniculate n.* and *n. pregeniculatus* [TA alternative].

**n. ventra'lis cor'poris genicula'ti media'lis** [TA], ventral principal nucleus of medial geniculate body: the principal relay nucleus of the medial geniculate nuclei, receiving ascending auditory fibers from the inferior colliculus and relaying information on sound intensity and frequency and its binaural properties to the auditory cortex.

**n. ventra'lis interme'dius tha'lami** [TA], ventral intermediate nucleus of thalamus: a nucleus medially located within the ventral nuclei of the thalamus.

**nu'clei ventra'les latera'les tha'lami** [TA], ventral lateral nuclei of thalamus: nuclei ventrolaterally located within the ventral thalamic nuclei, subdivided into anterior and posterior nuclei; called also *ventral lateral complex of thalamus.*

**nu'clei ventra'les media'les tha'lami,** 1. [TA] ventral medial complex of thalamus: a group of nuclei located in the medial portion of the ventral thalamic nuclei. 2. in the singular, a former name for *n. ventralis intermedius thalami.*

**nu'clei ventra'les posterio'res tha'lami,** nuclei ventrobasales thalami.

**n. ventra'lis posterolatera'lis tha'lami** [TA], the more lateral of the two posterior ventral nuclei of the thalamus; it is the terminus of the spinothalamic tract and the medial lemniscus and it projects to the postcentral gyrus.

**n. ventra'lis posteromedia'lis tha'lami** [TA], the more medial of the two posterior ventral nuclei of the thalamus; it is the secondary trigeminal tract and sends axons to the somesthetic area of the postcentral gyrus for the face.

**nu'clei ventra'les tha'lami** [TA], ventral nuclei of thalamus: a large group of nuclei lying between the internal medullary lamina and the internal capsule; it includes ventral anterior, ventral intermediate, ventral lateral, ventral medial, ventrobasal and other nuclei, which relay impulses to various specific areas of the cerebral cortex.

**nu'clei ventrobasa'les tha'lami** [TA], ventrobasal complex of thalamus: the nuclei that form the posterior ventral part of the ventral nuclei of the thalamus, comprising a posterolateral nucleus and a posteromedial nucleus; see *n. ventralis posterolateralis thalami* and *n. ventralis posteromedialis thalami.* Called also *ventral posterior nuclei of thalamus* and *nuclei ventrales posteriores thalami.*

**ventrolateral n. of hypothalamus,** n. ventromedialis hypothalami.

**ventrolateral nuclei of thalamus,** nuclei ventrales thalami.

**ventrolateral n. of spinal cord,** n. anterolateralis medullae spinalis.

**n. ventrolatera'lis hypotha'lami,** n. ventromedialis hypothalami.

**n. ventrolatera'lis medul'lae spina'lis,** n. anterolateralis medullae spinalis.

**nu'clei ventrolatera'les tha'lami,** nuclei ventrales thalami.

**ventromedial n. of hypothalamus,** n. ventromedialis hypothalami.

**ventromedial n. of oculomotor nuclear complex,** n. anteromedialis nervi oculomotorii.

**ventromedial n. of spinal cord, n. ventromedia'lis medul'lae spina'lis,** n. anteromedialis medullae spinalis.

**n. ventromedia'lis hypotha'lami** [TA], ventromedial hypothalamic nucleus: a group of nerve cell bodies found in the ventral portion of the intermediate hypothalamic region; it is involved in diverse functions, e.g., food intake and sexual behavior. Called also *ventrolateral hypothalamic n.* and *ventromedial* or *ventrolateral n. of hypothalamus.*

**vesicular n.,** a form of cell nucleus, the membrane of which stains deeply, while the central part is rather pale.

**vestibular n., caudal,** n. vestibularis inferior.

**vestibular n., cranial,** n. vestibularis superior.

**vestibular n., inferior,** n. vestibularis inferior.

**vestibular n., lateral,** n. vestibularis lateralis.

**vestibular n., medial, vestibular n., middle,** n. vestibularis medialis.

**vestibular n., rostral, vestibular n., superior,** n. vestibularis superior.

**nu'clei vestibula'res** [TA], vestibular nuclei: the four cellular masses in the lateral floor of the fourth ventricle: the *superior, lateral, medial,* and *inferior vestibular nuclei,* in which the short ascending and longer descending branches of the pars vestibularis nervi octavi terminate and in which cerebellar projections are received. The nuclei give rise to a widely dispersed special sensory system through projections to motor nuclei in the brain stem and cervical cord via the medial longitudinal fasciculi from all the vestibular nuclei to the cerebellum (chiefly from the inferior and medial nuclei), and to motor cells throughout the spinal cord (from the lateral nucleus). Additional connections of the nuclei provide for conscious perception of, and autonomic reactions to, labyrinthine stimulation. Called also *acoustic nuclei, nuclei of acoustic nerve,* and *nuclei nervi vestibularis.*

**n. vestibula'ris cauda'lis,** n. vestibularis inferior.

**n. vestibula'ris infe'rior** [TA], inferior vestibular nucleus: a vestibular nucleus that lies lateral to the middle nucleus and medial to the inferior cerebellar peduncle.

**n. vestibula'ris latera'lis** [TA], lateral vestibular nucleus: a vestibular nucleus composed of large multipolar nerve cells that lies immediately superior to the inferior vestibular nucleus; its upper end becomes continuous with the superior vestibular nucleus. Called also *Deiters' n.* and *large cell auditory n.*

**n. vestibula'ris media'lis** [TA], medial vestibular nucleus: a vestibular nucleus that lies in the floor of the fourth ventricle and extends upward from the medulla oblongata and pons; called also *triangular n., n. triangularis,* and *Schwalbe's n.*

**n. vestibula'ris rostra'lis, n. vestibula'ris supe'rior** [TA], superior vestibular nucleus: a small vestibular nucleus that lies above the lateral vestibular nucleus. Called also *Bekhterev's n.* and *cranial* or *rostral vestibular n.*

**vestibulocochlear nuclei, nuclei of vestibulocochlear nerve,** the vestibular and cochlear nuclei considered together; see *nuclei vestibulares* and *nuclei cochleares.*

**Voit's n.,** a cerebellar nucleus accessory to the dentate nucleus.

**Westphal's nuclei,** nuclei accessorii nervi oculomotorii.

**yolk n.,** a special area of the cytoplasm of an ovum in which the synthetic activities leading to the accumulation of food supplies in the oocyte are apparently initiated; called also *vitelline body* and *Balbiani's n.* or *body.*

**zygote n.,** fertilization n.

**nu·clide** (noo'klīd) a species of atom characterized by the atomic number, mass number, and quantum state of its nucleus, and capable of existing for a measurable lifetime (generally greater than $10^{-10}$ sec). Thus nuclear isomers are separate nuclides, but promptly decaying excited nuclear states and unstable intermediates in nuclear reactions are not so considered.

**radioactive n.,** radionuclide.

**nu·do·pho·bia** (noo″do-fo'be-ə) [L. *nudus* unclothed, bare + *-phobia*] an abnormal aversion to being unclothed.

**Nu·el's spaces** (ne-elz') [Jean Pierre *Nuel,* Belgian oculist, 1847–1920] see under *space.*

**NUG** necrotizing ulcerative gingivitis; see *acute necrotizing ulcerative gingivitis.*

**Nuhn's glands** (noonz) [Anton *Nuhn,* German anatomist, 1814–1889] glandulae linguales anteriores.

**nul·lip·a·ra** (nə-lip'ə-rə) [L. *nullus* none + *para*] a woman who has never borne a viable child. Also written para 0.

**nul·li·par·i·ty** (nul″ĭ-par'ĭ-te) the condition or fact of being nulliparous.

**nul·lip·a·rous** (nə-lip'ə-rəs) having never given birth to a viable infant.

**nul·li·som·ic** (nul″ĭ-som′ik) lacking one pair of chromosomes.

**numb** (num) [A.S. *niman*] anesthetic (def. 1).

**num·ber** (num′bər) [Fr. *nombre,* from L. *numerus*] a symbol, as a figure or word, expressive of a certain value or of a specified quantity determined by count.
**acetyl n.,** the number of milligrams of potassium hydroxide necessary to neutralize the acetic acid saponified from 1 gram of acetylated fat; it represents the extent to which hydroxyl groups are present.
**acid n.,** the number of milligrams of potassium hydroxide necessary to neutralize the free fatty acids in 1 gram of fat; it represents a measure of the amount of free fatty acids in the fat.
**atomic n.,** the number of protons in the nucleus of a nuclide; all the atoms of a chemical element have the same atomic number; sometimes indicated by a subscript preceding the symbol of a chemical element (e.g., $_1H$). Symbol *Z.*
**Avogadro's n.,** the number of molecules in one mole of a substance: $6.023 \times 10^{23}$. Symbol $N$ or $N_A$.
**Brinell hardness n.,** a number indicative of the degree of relative hardness of a material, calculated after measuring the diameter of the impression made by a steel ball pressed under a known load into the surface of the material being tested; equal to the load in kilograms divided by the surface area of the indentation in square millimeters.
**chromosome n.,** the number of chromosomes present in the somatic cells of an organism; the normal individual receives, at conception, one set of chromosomes (the haploid number, symbol *n*) from each of the gametes forming the zygote, thus acquiring the diploid number *(2n).* In humans, *n* equals 23.
**copy n.,** 1. the number of times a given gene is physically represented in the genome. 2. the average number of times a specific plasmid occurs in a bacterial cell.
**CT n's,** attenuation values determined for each pixel in a CT scan on a scale in which water is 0, compact bone +1000, and air −1000. See *Hounsfield unit* under *unit.*
**dibucaine n.,** an expression of the percentage of inhibition of the enzyme cholinesterase in a serum sample by dibucaine; used to differentiate between normal and abnormal serum cholinesterase phenotypes. Normal or usual is about 80; intermediate is about 60; abnormal or atypical is about 20. Abbreviated DN.
**hardness n.,** a number indicative of the degree of relative hardness of materials. See *Brinell, Knoop, Rockwell,* and *Vickers hardness n.*
**Hehner n.,** the percentage of water insoluble fatty acids obtainable from a fat or oil.
**Hittorf n.,** the fraction of the total electric current passing through an electrolytic solution that is carried by a given ion species; called also *transference n.* and *transport n.*
**hydrogen n.,** the amount of hydrogen that one gram of a fat can absorb; it represents the quantity of unsaturated fatty acids in the fat.
**iodine n.,** the amount of iodine in grams which 100 grams of a fat or oil can absorb; it is inversely related to the amount of unsaturated fatty acids present in the fat or oil.
**isotopic n.,** the number which when added to twice the atomic number gives the atomic weight.
**Knoop hardness n.,** a number indicative of the degree of relative hardness of a material, calculated from the load employed and the length of the long axis of the impression made by the rhomboidal pyramid of a diamond pressed into the surface of the material being tested. It is the test most commonly used in dental practice to test the hardness of teeth.
**linking n.,** in topology (def. 3), the total number of times one strand of the DNA double helix winds around the other in a right hand direction, given a DNA molecule with constrained ends. Two molecules differing only in linking number are topoisomers.
**Loschmidt's n.,** the number of molecules per unit volume of an ideal gas at standard temperature and pressure; Avogadro's number divided by 22.4 liters per mole.
**mass n.,** the number of nucleons (protons plus neutrons) in the atom of a nuclide; generally indicated by a superscript preceding the symbol of a chemical element (e.g., $^{131}I$) to denote a specific isotope. Symbol *A.*
**neutron n.,** the number of neutrons in a nucleus, representing the difference between the mass number and the atomic number. Symbol *N.*
**oxidation n.,** a number assigned to each atom in a molecule or ion that represents the number of electrons theoretically gained (positive oxidation numbers) or lost (negative numbers) in converting the atom to the elemental form. Oxidation numbers are assigned according to the following rules. The oxidation number of atoms in an elemental form is zero, and the oxidation number of a monatomic ion equals the ionic charge. Group I and Group II metals always have oxidation numbers of +1 and +2, respectively. Fluorine always has an oxidation number of −1; oxygen always of −2, except in peroxides and superoxides (where it is −1) and in compounds containing O—F bonds. Hydrogen always has an oxidation number of +1, except in metal hydrides (where it is −1). Oxidation numbers are assigned to other atoms so that the sum for all atoms in a neutral compound equals zero and the sum for all atoms in a polyatomic ion equals the ionic charge. Called also *oxidation state.*
**polar n.,** the number of valences (positive or negative) possessed by an atom in any particular compound.
**Polenske n.,** the number of milliliters of tenth normal potassium hydroxide required to neutralize the insoluble, volatile fatty acids from 5 g of the fat.
**Reichert-Meissl n.,** the number of milliliters of tenth normal potassium hydroxide (KOH) required to neutralize the soluble volatile fatty acids distilled from 5 g of fat after it has been saponified with KOH and then made acid with orthophosphoric acid or sulfuric acid.
**Reynolds' n.,** the velocity of flow of a fluid multiplied by the diameter of the vessel and divided by the kinematic viscosity of the circulating fluid. It is lower for turbulent flow and higher for laminar flow, and is used for characterizing the conditions for the onset of turbulence. Symbol $R_e$.
**Rockwell hardness n.,** a number indicative of the degree of relative hardness of materials, determined by measuring the depth of the impression made by a steel or diamond penetrator pressed into the surface of the material being tested. There are a number of Rockwell hardness tests and scales, using various combinations of loads and penetrators; the load and penetrator combination must always be specified when stating a Rockwell hardness number.
**saponification n.,** the number of milligrams of potassium hydroxide required to saponify the fatty acids in 1 gram of a fat or oil; it is inversely related to the average molecular weight of the fatty acid molecules.
**tooth n.,** a number assigned to each of the permanent teeth in consecutive order, with 1 for the upper right third molar, proceeding across to 16 for the upper left third molar, and 17 for the lower left third molar, proceeding across to 32 for the lower right third molar.
**transference n., transport n.,** Hittorf n.
**triangulation n. (T),** a number expressing the multiple of 60 subunits that a viral capsid with icosahedral symmetry contains, so called because it expresses the number of subtriangles into which each face of the capsid is divided.
**turnover n.,** the number of molecules of substrate acted upon by one molecule of enzyme per minute.
**twisting n.,** in topology (def. 3), the number of ordinary (Watson-Crick) helical turns in a DNA molecule with constrained ends. Abbreviated *T.*
**Vickers hardness n.,** a number indicative of the degree of relative hardness of materials, determined by measuring the long diagonals of indentation made by pressing the pyramidal point of a diamond into the surface of the material being tested; equal to the load in kilograms divided by the area, in square millimeters, of the recovered indentation; called also *diamond pyramid hardness.*
**wave n.,** in light waves, the reciprocal of the wavelength expressed as a fraction of a centimeter.
**writhing n.,** in topology (def. 3), the number of superhelical turns in a DNA molecule with constrained ends. Abbreviated *W.*

**numb·ness** (num′nəs) anesthesia (def. 1).

**num·mu·lar** (num′u-lər) [L. *nummularis*] 1. coin-sized and coin-shaped. 2. made up of round, flat disks. 3. piled, like coins, in a rouleau.

**Nu·mor·phan** (noo-mor′fən) trademark for preparations of oxymorphone hydrochloride.

**nun·na·tion** (nən-a′shən) [Heb. *nun* letter N] 1. a speech disorder consisting of too frequent use of *n* sounds. 2. hypernasality.

**Nu·per·cain·al** (noo″pər-kān′əl) trademark for a preparation of dibucaine.

**Nu·per·caine** (noo′pər-kān) trademark for preparations of dibucaine.

**Nu·prin** (noo′prin) trademark for a preparation of ibuprofen.

**N-Uri·stix** (u′rĭ-stiks) trademark for a reagent strip designed for testing for nitrite, glucose, and protein in urine.

**Nu·ro·max** (noor′o-maks″) trademark for a preparation of doxacurium chloride.

**nurse** (ners) [MeSH: Nurses] 1. a person who is especially prepared in the scientific basis of nursing and who meets certain prescribed standards of education and clinical competence. 2. to provide services that are essential to or helpful in the promotion, maintenance, and restoration of health and well-being. 3. to breast-feed an infant. See also *nursing.*
**clinical n. specialist,** a registered nurse with a high degree of knowledge, skill, and competence in a specialized area of nursing. These skills are made directly available through the provision of nursing care to clients and are indirectly available through guidance and planning of care with other nursing personnel. Clinical nurse specialists hold a master's degree in nursing, preferably with an emphasis in clinical nursing. Called also *n. specialist.*

**n. clinician,** a registered nurse, referred to as a *nurse clinician* or as a *n. practitioner,* who has well-developed competencies in utilizing a broad range of cues. These cues are used for prescribing and implementing both direct and indirect nursing care and for articulating nursing therapies with other planned therapies. Nurse clinicians demonstrate expertise in nursing practice and ensure ongoing development of expertise through clinical experience and continuing education. Generally, minimal preparation for this role is the baccalaureate degree.
**community n.,** the name given in Great Britain to a public health nurse, from the fact that such a nurse was placed in charge of each one of the districts into which the city or community was divided. See also *public health n.*
**community health n.,** public health n.
**district n.,** community n.
**general duty n.,** a registered nurse, usually one who has not undergone training beyond the basic nursing program, who sees to the general nursing care of patients in a hospital or other health agency.
**graduate n.,** a graduate of a school of nursing; often used to designate one who has not been registered or licensed to practice. Called also *trained n.*
**hospital n.,** one employed by a hospital.
**licensed practical n.,** a graduate of a school of practical nursing whose qualifications have been examined by a state board of nursing and who has been legally authorized to practice as a licensed practical or vocational nurse (L.P.N. or L.V.N.), under the supervision of a physician or registered nurse.
**licensed vocational n.,** see *licensed practical n.*
**monthly n.,** a nurse who attends confinement cases.
**occupational health n.,** an especially prepared registered nurse employed by an institution to apply nursing principles and procedures for the promotion, restoration, and maintenance of optimal health of its employees as compared to a nurse who performs normal nursing functions in an occupational setting.
**office n.,** a registered nurse employed by a physician in his office to perform or to assist him in the performance of certain procedures.
**practical n.,** a person who has had practical experience in nursing care but who is not a graduate of any kind of nursing school; not to be confused with a licensed practical nurse.
**n. practitioner,** see *n. clinician.*
**private n., private duty n.,** one who attends an individual patient, usually on a fee-for-service basis, and who may specialize in a specific class of diseases; called also *special n.*
**probationer n.,** a person who has entered a school of nursing and is under observation to determine her fitness for the nursing profession; applied principally to nursing students enrolled in hospital schools of nursing.
**public health n.,** an especially prepared registered nurse employed in a community agency to safeguard the health of persons in the community, giving care to the sick in their homes, promoting health and well-being by teaching families how to keep well, and assisting in programs for the prevention of disease. Called also *community health n.* and *visiting n.*
**Queen's n.,** in Great Britain, a district nurse who has been trained at or in accordance with the regulations of the Queen Victoria Jubilee Institute for Nurses.
**registered n.,** a graduate nurse who has been legally authorized (registered) to practice after examination by a state board of nurse examiners or similar regulatory authority, and who is legally entitled to use the designation RN.
**school n.,** an especially prepared registered nurse employed in a school system or public health agency to assist in safeguarding the health of students and to teach health practices.
**scrub n.,** one who directly assists the surgeon in the operating room.
**special n.,** 1. a private nurse. 2. a nurse who specializes in a particular class of cases.
**n. specialist,** clinical n. specialist.
**student n.,** a person enrolled in a basic program of nursing education.
**trained n.,** graduate n.
**visiting n.,** see *public health n.*
**wet n.,** a woman who breast-feeds the infant of another.

**nurse-mid·wife** (ners-mid'wīf) an individual educated in the two disciplines of nursing and midwifery, who possesses evidence of certification according to the requirements of the American College of Nurse-Midwives. Abbreviated CNM (Certified Nurse-Midwife).

**nurse-mid·wi·fery** (ners-mid'wi-fər-e) the independent management of care of essentially normal newborns and women, antepartally, intrapartally, postpartally, and/or gynecologically, occurring within a health care system which provides for medical consultation, collaborative management, or referral, and is in accord with the functions, standards, and qualifications as defined by the American College of Nurse-Midwives.

**nur·se·ry** (ner'sə-re) [MeSH: Nurseries] the department in a hospital where newborn infants are cared for.
**day n., day care n.,** an institution devoted to the care of young children during the day.

**nurs·ing** (ners'ing) [MeSH: Nursing] the provision, at various levels of preparation, of services that are essential to or helpful in the promotion, maintenance, and restoration of health and well-being or in the prevention of illness, as of infants, of the sick and injured, or of others for any reason unable to provide such services for themselves. Sometimes designated according to the age of the patients being cared for (e.g., pediatric or geriatric nursing), or their particular health problems (e.g., gynecologic, medical, obstetrical, orthopedic, psychiatric, surgical, urological nursing, or the like), or the setting in which the services are provided (e.g., office, school, or occupational health nursing). See also *nurse.*

**Nuss·baum's experiment** (noos'boumz) [Moritz *Nussbaum,* German histologist, 1850–1915] see under *experiment.*

**nut** (nut) [L. *nux;* Gr. *karyon*] [MeSH: Nuts] a seed element, as of various trees, usually enclosed in a coating of variable hardness.
**areca n., betel n.,** areca (def 2).
**ground n.,** peanut.
**physic n., purging n.,** 1. *Jatropha curcas.* 2. *J. multifida.* 3. the seed of either of these trees, which contains a purgative oil and a phytotoxin that can be fatal to humans or other animals.

**nu·ta·tion** (noo-ta'shən) [L. *nutatio*] the act of nodding, especially involuntary nodding.

**nu·ta·to·ry** (noo'tə-tor"e) [L. *nutare* to keep nodding, to sway] pertaining to nodding.

**nut·gall** (nut'gawl) [L. *galla*] an excrescence growing on oak trees (genus *Quercus*), especially *Q. alba* (the white oak), produced by insect eggs and larvae embedded in the plant tissues; it is a source of gallic and tannic acids, which are used in various pharmaceuticals for their astringent properties. Called also *gall, Aleppo gall, Smyrna gall,* and *gallnut.*

**nut·meg** (nut'meg) 1. *Myristica fragrans.* 2. the seed of *M. fragrans;* see also under *oil* and *poisoning.*

**Nu·tra·cort** (noo'trə-kort") trademark for preparations of hydrocortisone.

**neu·tra·ceu·ti·cals** (noo"trə-soo'tĭ-kəlz) functional foods.

**nu·tri·ent** (noo'tre-ənt) [L. *nutriens*] 1. nourishing; providing nutrition. 2. a food or other substance that provides energy or building material for the survival and growth of a living organism; called also *nutriment.*
**essential n's,** those nutrients (proteins, minerals, carbohydrates, fats, vitamins) necessary for growth, normal functioning, and maintaining life; they must be supplied by food, since they cannot be synthesized by the body.
**secondary n.,** a substance that stimulates the intestinal microflora to synthesize other nutrients.

**nu·tri·lite** (noo'trĭ-līt) a substance essential in minute amounts in the nutrition of a microorganism.

**nu·tri·ment** (noo'trĭ-mənt) [L. *nutrimentum*] nutrient (def. 2).

**nu·tri·ol·o·gy** (noo"tre-ol'ə-je) the science of nutrition; the study of foods and their use in diet and therapy.

**nu·tri·tion** (noo-trĭ'shən) [L. *nutritio*] [MeSH: Nutrition] the taking in and metabolism of nutrients (food and other nourishing material) by an organism so that life is maintained and growth can take place.
**adequate n.,** see under *diet.*
**enteral n.,** the delivery of nutrients in liquid form directly into the stomach, duodenum, jejunum; used when the patient's condition precludes oral intake.
**total parenteral n. (TPN),** total parenteral alimentation.

**nu·tri·tion·al** (noo-trĭ'shən-əl) relating to or affecting nutrition.

**nu·tri·tion·ist** (noo-trĭ'shən-ist) a specialist in food and nutrition.

**nu·tri·tious** (noo-trĭ'shəs) [L. *nutritius*] affording nourishment or nutrition.

**nu·tri·tive** (noo'trĭ-tiv) nutritional.

**nu·tri·ture** (noo'trĭ-chur") the status of the body in relation to nutrition, generally or in regard to a specific nutrient, such as protein.

**Nu·tro·pin** (noo'trə-pin) trademark for a preparation of growth hormone of rDNA origin.

**nux** (nuks) gen. *nu'cis* [L.] nut.
**n. vo'mica,** the dried ripe seed of *Strychnos nux-vomica* L. (Loganiaceae), containing several alkaloids, principally strychnine and brucine. It has been used as a bitter tonic and central nervous system stimulant, and in veterinary medicine it is used as a bitter tonic and in the treatment of inappetence, atony of the rumen, and chronic indigestion.

**nvCJD** new variant Creutzfeldt-Jakob disease.

**nyc·tal·gia** (nik-tal'jə) [*nyct-* + *-algia*] pain that occurs in sleep only.

**nyc·ta·lope** (nik'tə-lōp) a person affected with nyctalopia.

**nyc·ta·lo·pia** (nik"tə-lo'pe-ə) [*nyct-* + Gr. *alaos* blind + *-opia*] night blindness; failure or imperfection of vision at night or in a dim light, with good vision only on bright days.

**nyc·ta·pho·nia** (nik"tə-fo'ne-ə) [*nyct-* + *aphonia*] elective mutism with loss of voice during the night.

**nyc·tero·hem·er·al** (nik"tər-o-hem'ər-əl) nyctohemeral.

**nyct(o)-** [Gr. *nyx*, gen. *nyctos* night] a combining form denoting relationship to night or to darkness.

**nyc·to·hem·er·al** (nik"to-hem'ər-əl) [*nycto-* + Gr. *hēmera* day] pertaining to both night and day.

**nyc·to·phil·ia** (nik"to-fil'e-ə) [*nycto-* + *-philia*] a preference for darkness or for night.

**nyc·to·pho·bia** (nik"to-fo'be-ə) [*nycto-* + *phobia*] irrational fear of darkness.

**nyc·to·pho·nia** (nik"to-fo'ne-ə) [*nycto-* + *phon-* + *-ia*] elective mutism with loss of voice during the day but not at night.

**nyc·tu·ria** (nik-tu're-ə) [*nyct-* + *-uria*] 1. frequent urination during the night, especially the passage of more urine at night than during the day. 2. nocturia.

**NYD** not yet diagnosed.

**Ny·dra·zid** (ni'drə-zid) trademark for preparations of isoniazid.

**nyl·i·drin hy·dro·chlo·ride** (nil'ĭ-drin) a synthetic adrenergic used as a peripheral vasodilator; administered orally, intramuscularly, and subcutaneously.

**ny·lon** (ni'lon) a synthetic polymerized plastic which in fiber form is used as a nonabsorbable suture material.

**nymph** (nimf) [Gr. *nymphē* a bride] [MeSH: Nymph] a stage in the life cycle of certain arthropods, such as ticks, between the larva and the adult; it somewhat resembles the adult but is small, sexually immature, and wingless. Cf. *naiad.*

**nym·pha** (nim'fə) gen. and pl. *nym'phae* [L., from Gr. *nymphē*] labium minus pudendi.
**n. of Krause,** clitoris.

**nym·phec·to·my** (nim-fek'tə-me) [*nymph-* + *-ectomy*] excision of the labia minora.

**nym·phi·tis** (nim-fi'tis) inflammation of the labia minora.

**nymph(o)-** [L. *nympha*] a combining form denoting relationship to the nymphae, or labia minora.

**nym·pho·ca·run·cu·lar** (nim"fo-kə-rung'ku-lər) pertaining to the labia minora and the caruncula hymenalis.

**nym·pho·hy·me·ne·al** (nim"fo-hi"mə-ne'əl) pertaining to the labia minora and the hymen.

**nym·pho·ma·nia** (nim"fo-ma'ne-ə) [*nympho-* + *-mania*] abnormal, excessive, insatiable sexual desire in the female. Cf. *satyriasis.*

**nym·pho·ma·ni·ac** (nim"fo-ma'ne-ak) 1. affected with nymphomania. 2. one who is affected with nymphomania.

**nym·phon·cus** (nim-fong'kəs) [*nympho-* + Gr. *onkos* mass, bulk] swelling of the labia minora.

**nym·phot·o·my** (nim-fot'o-me) [*nympho-* + *-tomy*] surgical incision of the labia minora or clitoris.

**Nys·sen-van Bo·gaert syndrome** (ni'sen-vahn-bo'gārt) [René *Nyssen,* Belgian neurologist, 1891–1972; Ludo *van Bogaert,* Belgian neurologist, born 1897] metachromatic leukodystrophy (adult form); see under *leukodystrophy.*

**Nyss·o·rhyn·chus** (nis"o-ring'kəs) [Gr. *nyssa* prick + *rhynchos* snout] a subgenus of mosquitoes of the genus *Anopheles;* several species act as carriers of the malarial parasite in tropical America.

**nys·tag·mic** (nis-tag'mik) pertaining to or characterized by nystagmus.

**nys·tag·mi·form** (nis-tag'mĭ-form) nystagmoid.

**nys·tag·mo·graph** (nis-tag'mo-graf) [*nystagmus* + *-graph*] an instrument for recording the movements of the eyeball in nystagmus.

**nys·tag·moid** (nis-tag'moid) resembling nystagmus.

**nys·tag·mus** (nis-tag'məs) [Gr. *nystagmos* drowsiness, from *nystazein* to nod] [MeSH: Nystagmus] an involuntary, rapid, rhythmic movement of the eyeball, which may be horizontal, vertical, rotatory, or mixed, i.e., of two varieties.
**amaurotic n.,** nystagmus in the blind or in those with defects of central vision; called also *ocular n.*
**amblyopic n.,** nystagmus due to any lesion interfering with central vision.
**ataxic n.,** a unilateral nystagmus occurring in multiple sclerosis and marked by impaired lateral conjugate gaze.
**aural n.,** vestibular n.
**caloric n.,** rotatory nystagmus induced by irrigating the ears with warm or cold water or air; see *caloric test,* under *test.*
**central n.,** a jerk nystagmus due to a lesion somewhere in the neurologic pathways regulating gaze.
**Cheyne's n., Cheyne-Stokes n.,** a peculiar rhythmic eye movement resembling Cheyne-Stokes respiration in its rhythm.
**congenital n., congenital hereditary n.,** nystagmus usually present at birth, usually horizontal and pendular, but occasionally jerky and pendular; the nystagmus may be caused by or associated with optic atrophy, coloboma, albinism, bilateral macular lesions, congenital cataract, severe astigmatism, and glaucoma.
**convergence n.,** a rhythmic oscillation of the eyes, in which they have a rapid adduction movement relative to each other alternating with a slow abduction movement; usually caused by a tumor of the aqueduct of Sylvius, third ventricle, or midbrain. It is often accompanied by retraction nystagmus.
**disjunctive n.,** nystagmus in which the eyes swing toward and away from each other.
**dissociated n.,** nystagmus in which the movements in the two eyes are dissimilar.
**downbeat n.,** a vertical nystagmus with the fast phase downward, occurring in lesions at the cervicomedullary junction.
**electrical n.,** galvanic n.
**end-position n.,** nystagmus occurring in normal individuals at extremes of gaze; called also *pseudonystagmus.*
**fixation n.,** nystagmus which appears only on gazing fixedly at an object.
**galvanic n.,** a vestibular nystagmus caused by electrical stimulation of the labyrinth of the inner ear; called also *electrical n.*
**gaze n.,** nystagmus made apparent by looking to the right or to the left.
**gaze paretic n.,** a form of gaze nystagmus seen in patients recovering from central nervous system lesions; the eyes fail to stay fixed to the affected side with a cerebral or pontine lesion. If the defect is in vertical gaze it usually signifies a lesion in the pretectal area.
**jerk n., jerky n.,** nystagmus which consists of a slow movement in one direction, followed by a rapid return movement in the opposite direction; called also *resilient n.* and *rhythmical n.*
**labyrinthine n.,** vestibular n.
**latent n.,** nystagmus which occurs only when one eye is covered.
**lateral n.,** nystagmus in which the movement of the eyes is from side to side.
**miner's n.,** an occupational disease of coal miners consisting of abnormal eye movements associated with other signs and symptoms; it is considered by some to be related to poor lighting and by others as a functional disorder.
**ocular n.,** amaurotic n.
**opticokinetic n., optokinetic n.,** the normal nystagmus occurring when looking at objects passing across the field of vision, as in viewing from a moving railroad car or automobile. It can be induced for testing purposes to check ocular and vestibular functioning.
**oscillating n.,** pendular n.
**palatal n.,** see under *myoclonus.*
**paretic n.,** a false nystagmus occurring when there is a weakness of the ocular muscles.
**pendular n.,** nystagmus in which the oscillations of the eyes have an equal rate, amplitude, direction, and type of movement; called also *oscillating n., undulatory n.,* and *vibratory n.*
**periodic alternating n.,** a rare form of jerk nystagmus with rhythmic changes in amplitude and direction and with intervals of quiet between periods.
**positional n.,** that which occurs, or is altered in form or intensity, on assumption of certain positions of the head.
**railroad n.,** optokinetic n.
**resilient n.,** jerk n.
**retraction n., n. retracto'rius,** 1. a spasmodic retraction of the eyeball backward into the orbit, occurring on attempted movement of the eye; it is a sign of disease of the midbrain. 2. sylvian syndrome; see under *syndrome.*
**rhythmical n.,** jerk n.
**rotatory n.,** nystagmus in which the movement is about the visual axis.
**secondary n.,** nystagmus occurring after the abrupt cessation of rotation of the head, caused by the labyrinthine fluid continuing to move.
**see-saw n.,** that in which one eye moves up as the other moves down.
**spontaneous n.,** that occurring without specific stimulation of the vestibular system.

**undulatory n.**, pendular n.
**unilateral n.**, nystagmus manifest in only one eye.
**upbeat n.**, a vertical nystagmus with the fast phase upward, occurring in lesions of the vermis cerebelli.
**vertical n.**, an up-and-down movement of the eyes.
**vestibular n.**, nystagmus due to disturbance of the vestibular system; eye movements are rhythmic, with a slow and a fast component. Called also *aural n.* and *labyrinthine n.* Cf. *vestibular vertigo.*
**vibratory n.**, pendular n.
**voluntary n.**, rapid rhythmic eye movements, up to 80 a second, that can be produced at will by some normal individuals.

**nys·tag·mus-my·oc·lo·nus** (nis-tag′məs-mi-ok′lə-nəs) a rare congenital condition in which there is nystagmus together with abnormal involuntary movements of the extremities and trunk.

**nys·ta·tin** (nis′tə-tin) [USP] [MeSH: Nystatin] a polyene antifungal produced by the growth of *Streptomyces noursei,* specifically effective against *Candida albicans;* used in the treatment of vaginal, intestinal, oral, or cutaneous candidal infections, administered orally and topically. Called also *fungicidin.*

**nys·tax·is** (nis-tak′sis) [Gr.] nystagmus.

**Ny·sten's law** (ne-stawz′) [Pierre Hubert *Nysten,* Belgian pediatrician in France, 1771–1818] see under *law.*

**nyx·is** (nik′sis) [Gr. "pricking"] puncture, or paracentesis.

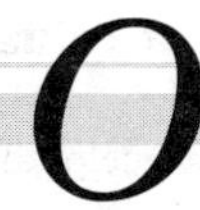

**O** symbol for *oxygen* and *ohne Hauch.*

**O.** symbol for *L. octa'rius* (pint) and *o'culus* (eye).

**o-** chemical symbol for *ortho-.*

**Ω** the Greek capital letter omega; symbol for *ohm.*

**ω** omega, the twenty-fourth letter of the Greek alphabet.

**ω-** a prefix designating (1) the carbon atom farthest from the principal functional group, as in *ω*-oxidation; and (2) the last in a series of related entities or terms.

**OA** ocular albinism.
**OA1,** ocular albinism, type 1; see *X-linked (Nettleship) ocular albinism,* under *albinism.*
**OA2,** ocular albinism, type 2; see *Forsius-Eriksson syndrome,* under *syndrome.*

**OAE** otoacoustic emissions.

**OAF** osteoclast activating factor.

**oak** (ōk) 1. any tree of the genus *Quercus.* 2. any of certain trees that resemble those of *Quercus.*
**poison o.,** 1. *Rhus diversiloba.* 2. *Rhus quercifolia.*
**white o.,** *Quercus alba,* source of white oak bark (see under *bark*).

**OAP** a regimen of Oncovin (vincristine), ara-C (cytarabine), and prednisone, used in cancer chemotherapy.

**oari(o)-** [Gr. *ōarion,* dim. of *ōon* egg] for words beginning thus, see those beginning *oophor (o)-* and *ovari (o)-.*

**oa·sis** (o-a'sis) pl. *oa'ses* [Gr. "a fertile islet in a desert"] an island or spot of healthy tissue in a diseased area.

**OAT** ornithine aminotransferase.

**oath** (ōth) a solemn declaration or affirmation.
**o. of Hippocrates, hippocratic o.,** see under *H.*

**oat·meal** (ōt'mēl) meal made from oats *(Avena sativa),* used in the preparation of a bland, nutritious food.
**colloidal o.** [USP], a colloidal extract from oatmeal, used as an emollient in dermatologic preparations.

**OB** obstetrics.

**ob·ce·ca·tion** (ob"se-ka'shən) incomplete blindness.

**ob·du·cent** (ob-doo'sənt) [L. *obducere* to draw over, to cover] serving as a cover; covering.

**ob·duc·tion** (ob-duk'shən) [L. *obductio*] a medicolegal autopsy.

**O'Beirne's sphincter** (o-birnz') [James *O'Beirne,* Irish surgeon, 1786–1862] see under *sphincter.*

**obe·li·ac** (o-be'le-ak) pertaining to the obelion.

**obe·li·ad** (o-be'le-ad) toward the obelion.

**obe·li·on** (o-be'le-on) [Gr., dim. of *obelos* a spit] a point on the sagittal suture where it is crossed by a line which connects the parietal foramina.

**Ober's operation, test (sign)** (o'bərz) [Frank Roberts *Ober,* American orthopedic surgeon, 1881–1960] see under *operation* and *test.*

**obese** (o-bēs') [L. *obesus*] excessively fat.

**obes·i·ty** (o-bēs'ĭ-te) [L. *obesus* fat] [MeSH: Obesity] an increase in body weight beyond the limitation of skeletal and physical requirement, as the result of an excessive accumulation of fat in the body. Called also *adiposity, adiposis, corpulency,* and *pimelosis.*
**adult-onset o.,** obesity beginning in adulthood and characterized by increase in size (hypertrophy) of adipose cells with no increase in number; called also *hypertrophic o.*
**alimentary o.,** exogenous o.
**endogenous o.,** obesity due to metabolic (endocrine) abnormalities or genetic defects that affect the synthesis of enzymes involved in intermediate metabolism.
**exogenous o.,** obesity due to overeating; called also *alimentary o.* and *simple o.*
**hyperinsulinar o.,** obesity due to excessive insulin secretion, associated with hypoglycemia and increased appetite.
**hyperplastic-hypertrophic o.,** lifelong o.
**hypertrophic o.,** adult-onset o.
**hypogonadal o.,** obesity associated with hypogonadism.
**hypothyroid o.,** obesity associated with hypothyroidism.
**lifelong o.,** obesity beginning in childhood and characterized by an increase both in number (hyperplasia) and in size (hypertrophy) of adipose cells; called also *hyperplastic-hypertrophic o.*
**morbid o.,** the condition of weighing two or three, or more, times the ideal weight; so called because it is associated with many serious and life threatening disorders (diabetes mellitus, atherosclerosis, hypertension, pickwickian syndrome, etc.).
**simple o.,** exogenous o.

**obes·og·e·nous** (o"bēs-oj'ə-nəs) producing or causing obesity.

**Obe·sum·bac·te·ri·um** (o-be"səm-bak-tēr'e-əm) [L. *obesum* fat + *bacterium*] a genus of gram-negative, facultatively anaerobic, rod-shaped bacteria of the family Enterobacteriaceae, occurring as a brewery contaminant. The type species is *O. pro'teus.*

**obex** (o'beks) [L. "barrier"] [TA] the ependyma-lined junction of the taeniae of the fourth ventricle of the brain at the inferior angle.

**obi·dox·ime chlo·ride** (ŏ-bĭ-dok'sēm) [MeSH: Obidoxime Chloride] a cholinesterase reactivator which has been used to counter organophosphorus poisoning.

**ob·jec·tive** (ob-jek'tiv) [L. *objectivus*] 1. perceptible to the external senses. 2. a result for whose achievement an effort is made. 3. the lens or system of lenses in a microscope (or telescope) that is nearest to the object under examination.
**achromatic o.,** a microscope objective in which the chromatic aberration is corrected for two colors and the spherical aberration is corrected for one color.
**apochromatic o.,** a microscope objective in which the chromatic aberration is corrected for three colors and the spherical aberration is corrected for two colors.
**dry o.,** a microscope objective designed to be used without a liquid between its tip and the cover glass over the specimen.
**flat field o.,** a microscope objective that provides an image in which all parts of the field are simultaneously in focus.
**fluorite o.,** a microscope objective in which some of the lenses are made from fluorite instead of glass.
**immersion o.,** a microscope objective designed to have its tip and the cover glass over the specimen connected by a liquid instead of by air. The liquid may be water (water immersion) or a specially prepared oil (oil immersion).
**semiapochromatic o.,** a type of microscope objective in which spherical aberration and chromatic aberration are both corrected for two colors.

**ob·li·gate** (ob'lĭ-gāt) [L. *obligatus*] not facultative; necessary; compulsory; capable of survival only under particular conditions, as an obligate aerobe.

**oblique** (o-blēk') [L. *obliquus*] slanting; inclined; between a horizontal and a perpendicular direction.
**external o.,** musculus obliquus externus abdominis.
**internal o.,** musculus obliquus internus abdominis.

**obliq·ui·ty** (o-blik'wĭ-te) the state of being oblique, or slanting.
**Litzmann's o.,** inclination of the fetal head so that the posterior parietal bone presents to the parturient canal; called also *posterior asynclitism.*
**Nägele's o.,** the position of the fetal head in which the anterior parietal bone presents to the parturient canal, the biparietal diameter being oblique in relation to the brim of the pelvis; called also *anterior asynclitism.*
**o. of pelvis,** inclination of the pelvis.

**obli·quus** (o-bli'kwəs) [L.] oblique.

**oblit·er·a·tion** (ob-lit"ər-a'shən) [L. *obliteratio*] complete removal, whether by disease, degeneration, surgical procedure, irradiation, or otherwise.
**cortical o.,** cortical achromia; a condition in which the cerebral cortex is marked by areas in which the ganglion cells have disappeared.

**ob·lon·ga·ta** (ob"long-gah'tə) [L.] oblong, sometimes used informally to refer to the medulla oblongata.

**ob·lon·ga·tal** (ob"long-ga'təl) pertaining to the medulla oblongata.

**ob·nu·bi·la·tion** (ob-noo"bĭ-la'shən) clouding of consciousness.

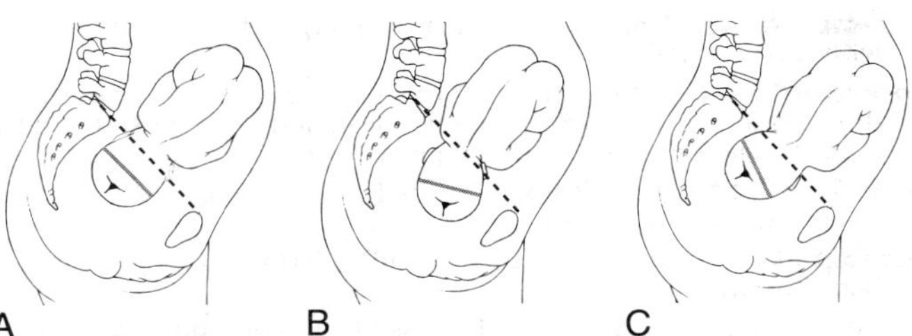


Obliquity. *(A)* Concordance of the fetal and pelvic planes, synclitism; *(B)* Litzmann's obliquity (posterior asynclitism); *(C)* Nägele's obliquity (anterior asynclitism).

**O'Bri·en akinesia** (o-bri'ən) [Cecil Starling *O'Brien,* American ophthalmologist, 1889–1977] see under *akinesia.*

**ob·serv·er** (ob-sər'vər) one who takes note of or watches.
**participant o.,** in certain psychoanalytic theory, the role of the therapist; not merely examining the overt and covert behavior of the patient but also participating by analyzing his or her own reactions as well as their relevance to the therapy.

**ob·ses·sion** (ob-sesh'ən) [L. *obsessio*] a recurrent, persistent thought, image, or impulse that is unwanted and distressing (ego-dystonic) and comes involuntarily to mind despite attempts to ignore or suppress it. Common obsessions involve thoughts of violence, contamination, and self-doubt.

**ob·ses·sive** (ob-ses'iv) pertaining to or characterized by obsession.

**ob·ses·sive-com·pul·sive** (əb-ses'iv-kəm-pul'siv) pertaining to obsessions and compulsions, to obsessive-compulsive disorder, or to obsessive-compulsive personality disorder.

**ob·so·les·cence** (ob″so-les'əns) [L. *obsolescere* to grow old] the cessation or the beginning of the cessation of any physiologic process.

**ob·stet·ric, ob·stet·ri·cal** (ob-stet'rik, ob-stet'rĭ-kəl) [L. *obstetricius*] pertaining to obstetrics.

**ob·ste·tri·cian** (ob″stə-trĭ'shən) [L. *obstetrix* midwife] one who practices obstetrics.

**ob·stet·rics** (ob-stet'riks) [L. *obstetricia*] [MeSH: Obstetrics] that branch of surgery which deals with the management of pregnancy, labor, and the puerperium.

**ob·sti·pa·tion** (ob″stĭ-pa'shən) [L. *obstipatio*] intractable constipation.

**ob·struc·tion** (ob-struk'shən) [L. *obstructio*] 1. the act of blocking or clogging. 2. the state or condition of being clogged. Cf. *atresia.* Called also *blockage, closure,* and *occlusion.*
**chronic airflow o., chronic airway o.,** name given to a group of disorders in which the upper or lower airways are chronically obstructed; it includes chronic bronchitis, emphysema, and other types of chronic obstructive pulmonary disease.
**closed-loop o.,** intestinal obstruction caused by the closing off of both ends of a bowel segment, as by volvulus.
**false colonic o.,** Ogilvie's syndrome; see under *syndrome.*
**intestinal o.,** any hindrance to the passage of the intestinal contents. See also *ileus.*

**ob·stru·ent** (ob'stroo-ənt) [L. *obstruens*] 1. causing obstruction or blocking. 2. any agent or agency that causes obstruction.

**ob·tund** (ob-tund') [L. *obtundere* to blunt] 1. to render dull or blunt. 2. to render a sensation less acute. 3. to reduce the level of alertness.

**ob·tun·da·tion** (ob″tən-da'shən) clouding of consciousness.

**ob·tun·dent** (ob-tun'dənt) [L. *obtundens*] 1. having the power to soothe pain. 2. causing obtundation. 3. a soothing or partially anesthetic medicine.

**ob·tu·ra·tion** (ob″tə-ra'shən) obstruction.
**canal o., root canal o.,** in root canal therapy, filling of the canal completely and densely with a nonirritating hermetic sealing agent. Called also *root canal filling.*

**ob·tu·ra·tor** (ob'tə-ra'tor) [L.] 1. any structure, natural or artificial, that closes an opening. 2. speech-aid prosthesis.

**ob·tu·sion** (ob-too'zhən) [L. *obtusio*] blunting of sensation and perception.

**OCA** oculocutaneous albinism.

**oc·cip·i·tal** (ok-sip'ĭ-təl) [L. *occipitalis*] pertaining to the occiput; located near the occipital bone, as the occipital lobe of the brain.

**oc·cip·i·ta·lis** (ok-sip″ĭ-ta'lis) [L., from *occiput,* q.v.] 1. [TA] pertaining to the occiput or to the occipital bone; occipital. 2. the posterior part of the occipitofrontalis muscle.

**oc·cip·i·tal·iza·tion** (ok-sip″ĭ-təl-ĭ-za'shən) synostosis of the atlas with the occipital bone.

**oc·cip·i·to·an·te·ri·or** (ok-sip″ĭ-to-an-te're-or) having the occiput directed forward toward the pubis (designating the position of the fetus in relation to the maternal pelvis).

**oc·cip·i·to·at·loid** (ok-sip″ĭ-to-at'loid) pertaining to the occipital bone and the atlas.

**oc·cip·i·to·ax·oid** (ok-sip″ĭ-to-ak'soid) pertaining to the occipital bone and the axis.

**oc·cip·i·to·bas·i·lar** (ok-sip″ĭ-to-bas'ĭ-lər) pertaining to the occiput and the base of the skull.

**oc·cip·i·to·breg·mat·ic** (ok-sip″ĭ-to-breg-mat'ik) pertaining to the occiput and the bregma.

**oc·cip·i·to·cal·car·ine** (ok-sip″ĭ-to-kal'kar-īn) both occipital and calcarine.

**oc·cip·i·to·cer·vi·cal** (ok-sip″ĭ-to-ser'vĭ-kəl) pertaining to the occiput and the neck.

**oc·cip·i·to·fa·cial** (ok-sip″ĭ-to-fa'shəl) pertaining to the occiput and the face.

**oc·cip·i·to·fron·tal** (ok-sip″ĭ-to-fron'təl) pertaining to the occiput and the forehead.

**oc·cip·i·to·fron·ta·lis** (ok-sip″ĭ-to-fron-ta'lis) occipitofrontal; see under *musculus.*

**oc·cip·i·to·mas·toid** (ok-sip″ĭ-to-mas'toid) pertaining to the occipital bone and the mastoid process of the temporal bone.

**oc·cip·i·to·men·tal** (ok-sip″ĭ-to-men'təl) pertaining to the occiput and the chin.

**oc·cip·i·to·pa·ri·e·tal** (ok-sip″ĭ-to-pə-ri'ə-təl) pertaining to the occipital and parietal bones or lobes of the brain.

**oc·cip·i·to·pos·te·ri·or** (ok-sip″ĭ-to-pos-te're-or) having the occiput directed toward the back, or turned toward the sacrum (designating the position of the fetus in relation to the maternal pelvis).

**oc·cip·i·to·tem·po·ral** (ok-sip″ĭ-to-tem'pə-rəl) pertaining to the occipital and the temporal bones.

**oc·cip·i·to·tha·lam·ic** (ok-sip″ĭ-to-thə-lam'ik) pertaining to the occipital lobe and the thalamus.

**oc·ci·put** (ok'sĭ-pət) [L.] [TA] the posterior part of the head; called also *o. cra'nii* and *o. of cranium.*

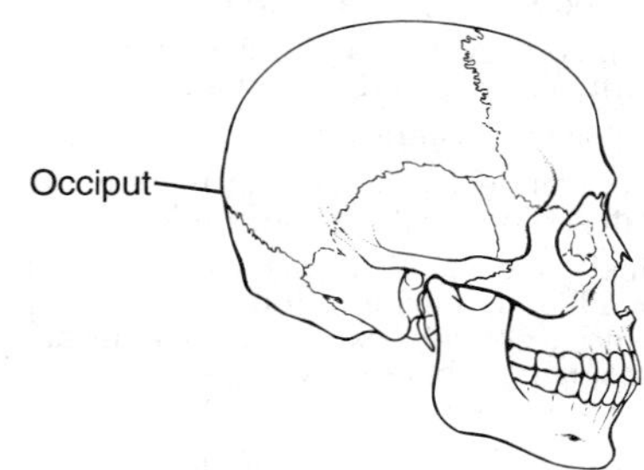


**oc·clude** (ŏ-klōōd') 1. to fit close together. 2. to close tight, as to bring the mandibular teeth into contact with the teeth in the maxilla. 3. obstruct.

**oc·clud·er** (ŏ-klōōd'ər) a form of dental articulator.

**oc·clu·sal** (ŏ-kloo'zəl) 1. pertaining to occlusion. 2. pertaining to the contacting surfaces of opposing teeth or of opposing occlusion rims, or to the masticating surfaces of the premolar and molar teeth.

**oc·clu·sion** (o-kloo'zhən) [L. *occlusio*] 1. obstruction. 2. the trapping of a liquid or gas within cavities in a solid or on its surface. 3. the relationship between all of the components of the masticatory system in normal function, dysfunction, and parafunction. See also *bite* and *malocclusion.* 4. momentary closure of part of the vocal tract, which produces a plosive.
**abnormal o.,** malocclusion.
**acentric o.,** a condition in which the habitual voluntary closure pattern of the mandible does not coincide with centric relation, producing primary premature tooth contacts in the centric path of closure.
**anatomic o.,** that in which the arrangement of natural teeth in the same arch and in opposing arches is defined by dental or skeletal landmarks rather than functional criteria.
**anterior o.,** mesioclusion.
**balanced o.,** that in which the occlusal contact of the teeth on the working side of the jaw is accompanied by the harmonious contact of the teeth of the opposite (balancing) side. The occlusion of artificial teeth may be *mechanically balanced,* as on an articulator, without reference to physiologic considerations, or *physiologically balanced,* functioning in harmony with the temporomandibular joint and the neuromuscular system.
**buccal o.,** the position of a posterior tooth when it is outside (buccal to) the line of occlusion.
**centric o.,** that in the vertical and horizontal position of the mandible in which the cusps of the mandibular and maxillary teeth interdigitate maximally. Ideally, the lingual cusps of the maxillary bicuspids make contact with the marginal ridges of the mandibular bicuspids and the marginal ridges of the second bicuspid and first molar. The mesial lingual cusps of the maxillary molar occlude in the central fossae of the mandibular molars, while the distal cusps of the maxillary molars occlude on the marginal ridges of the mandibular molars. Similarly, the supporting cusps of the mandibular

teeth occlude on the marginal ridges and fossae of the maxillary molars and bicuspids.
**coronary o.,** complete obstruction of an artery of the heart, usually from progressive atherosclerosis (sometimes complicated by thrombosis), rarely from embolism, arteritis, or dissecting aneurysm.
**distal o.,** the position of a lower tooth when it is distal to its opposite number in the maxilla. Called also *postnormal o.*
**eccentric o.,** acentric o.
**edge-to-edge o., end-to-end o.,** that in which the anterior maxillary and mandibular teeth meet along their incisal edges when the mandible is in centric position. Called also *edge-to-edge bite* and *end-to-end bite.*
**enteromesenteric o.,** obstruction of blood vessels in both the mesentery and the wall of the intestine.
**functional o.,** such contact of the maxillary and mandibular teeth as will provide the highest efficiency in the centric position and during all excursive movements of the jaw that are essential to mastication, without producing trauma.
**habitual o.,** the consistent relationship of the teeth in the maxilla to those of the mandible when the teeth in both jaws are brought into maximum contact, such relationship varying from individual to individual; the ideal habitual occlusion is centric occlusion, but it is seldom attained without corrective dental treatment.
**hyperfunctional o.,** traumatic o.
**ideal o.,** perfect interdigitation of the upper and lower teeth.
**labial o.,** the position of an anterior tooth when it is outside (labial to) the line of occlusion.
**lateral o.,** the occlusion of the teeth when the lower jaw is moved to the right or left of centric position.
**lingual o.,** malocclusion in which the tooth is lingual to the line of the normal dental arch. Called also *linguoclusion.*
**mechanically balanced o.,** see *balanced o.*
**mesial o.,** the position of a lower tooth when it is mesial to its opposite number in the maxilla. Called also *prenormal o.*
**neutral o.,** normal o.
**normal o.,** the contact of the upper and lower teeth in the centric relationship.
**pathogenic o.,** an occlusal relationship that is capable of producing pathologic changes in the supporting tissues. See also *traumatic o.*
**physiologically balanced o.,** see *balanced o.*
**posterior o.,** distoclusion.
**postnormal o.,** distal o.
**prenormal o.,** mesial o.
**protrusive o.,** mesioclusion.
**retrusive o.,** distoclusion.
**spherical form of o.,** an arrangement of teeth that places their occlusal surfaces on the surface of an imaginary sphere, about 8 inches in diameter, with its center above the level of the teeth; see also *Monson curve,* under *curve.*
**terminal o.,** the relationship of opposing occlusal surfaces that provides the maximum natural or planned contact and/or intercuspation.
**traumatic o.,** progressive injury to the supporting structure of the teeth as a result of occlusal dysfunction. Called also *hypofunctional o.* See also *traumatogenic o.*
**traumatogenic o.,** abnormal occlusion capable of producing injury to the teeth, residual ridges, and periodontal structures. See *traumatic o.*
**working o.,** the contact made between the teeth on the side toward which the mandible is moved.

**oc·clu·sive** (ŏ-kloo'siv) pertaining to or effecting occlusion.

**oc·clu·so·cer·vi·cal** (ŏ-kloo"so-ser'vĭ-kəl) pertaining to the occlusal surface and the neck of a tooth.

**oc·clu·som·e·ter** (ok"loo-som'ə-tər) gnathodynamometer.

**oc·clu·so·re·ha·bil·i·ta·tion** (o-kloo"zo-re"hə-bil"ĭ-ta'shən) occlusal rehabilitation.

**oc·cult** (ŏ-kult') [L. *occultus*] obscure; concealed from observation; difficult to understand.

**oc·cu·pan·cy** (ok'u-pən-se) the period of time during which a unit quantity of a substance, administered in a specified way, is present in, or occupies, a part of the body before it is excreted or broken down.

**OCD** obsessive-compulsive disorder.

**ocel·lus** (o-sel'əs) [L., dim. of *oculus* eye] 1. a rudimentary eye with photosensitive pigmented cells, such as a small simple eye or eyespot of some insects and other invertebrates. 2. a roundish, eyelike patch of color.

**och·le·sis** (ok-le'sis) [Gr. *ochlēsis* crowding] any disease due to overcrowding.

**Ochoa** (o-cho'ah) Severo. Spanish-born American physician and biochemist, 1905–1993; co-winner, with Arthur Kornberg, of the Nobel prize for medicine or physiology in 1959 for discovering the mechanisms in the biological synthesis of deoxyribonucleic acid and ribonucleic acid.

**ochra·tox·i·co·sis** (o"krə-tok"sĭ-ko'sis) a type of mycotoxicosis usually seen in pigs and sometimes poultry or dogs after they eat grain or flour products contaminated by ochratoxin-producing molds such as *Aspergillus ochraceus* or *Penicillium viridicatum.* Characteristics include kidney damage with anorexia, prostration, and sometimes death. Balkan nephritis is closely related and may be a rare form of ochratoxicosis in humans. See also *mycotoxic nephropathy.*

**ochra·tox·in** (o"krə-tok'sin) any of a group of mycotoxins produced by *Aspergillus ochraceus* and certain species of *Penicillium,* sometimes found contaminating grains, peanuts, and green coffee beans. It has been implicated in cases of hepatic carcinoma and Balkan nephritis. The most common and the most toxic is ochratoxin A, which causes ochratoxicosis in pigs, fowl, dogs, and other animals that eat contaminated grain or flour products.

**ochrom·e·ter** (o-krom'ə-tər) [Gr. *ōchros* paleness + *-meter*] an instrument for measuring the capillary blood pressure by registering the force necessary to compress a finger by a rubber balloon until blanching of the skin occurs.

**Ochro·my·ia** (o"kro-mi'ə) *Cordylobia.*

**ochro·no·sis** (o"krə-no'sis) [Gr. *ōchros* yellow + *nos-* + *-sis*] [MeSH: Ochronosis] generalized deposition of dark pigment in the connective tissues, usually secondary to alkaptonuria (q.v.). It is characterized by urine that darkens on standing and visible dusky discoloration of the sclerae and ears. The pigment is believed to be composed of homogentisic acid and related polymers.
**exogenous o.,** ochronosis induced by exposure to chemicals such as phenolic compounds or hydroquinone.

**ochro·no·sus** (o"krə-no'səs) ochronosis.

**ochro·not·ic** (o"krə-not'ik) pertaining to, characterized by, or caused by ochronosis.

**Ochs·ner's muscle, ring** (oks'nərz) [Albert John *Ochsner,* American surgeon, 1858–1925] see under *muscle* and *ring.*

**oc·ry·late** (ok'rə-lāt) a type of cyanoacrylate adhesive used in surgery.

**OCT** ornithine carbamoyltransferase; oxytocin challenge test.

**octa-** [Gr. *oktō,* L. *octo* eight] a combining form meaning eight.

**oc·ta·dec·a·no·ate** (ok"tə-dek"ə-no'āt) stearate.

**oc·ta·de·ca·no·ic ac·id** (ok"tə-dek"ə-no'ik) systematic name for *stearic acid;* see also table at *fatty acid.*

**oc·ta·meth·yl pyro·phos·phor·amide** (ok"tə-meth'əl pir"o-fos-for'ə-mīd") an organophosphorus compound used as a systemic insecticide for plants. Called also *schradan.* Abbreviated OMPA.

**oc·tan** (ok'tan) [L. *octo* eight] recurring every eighth day, or after intervals of seven days.

**oc·tane** (ok'tān) an oily hydrocarbon occurring in petroleum.

**oc·ta·no·ic ac·id** (ok"tə-no'ik) systematic name for *caprylic acid.* See also table accompanying *fatty acid.*

**oc·ta·pep·tide** (ok"tə-pep'tīd) a peptide which on hydrolysis yields eight amino acids.

**oc·ta·ri·us** (ok-tar'e-us) [L.; from *octo* eight] a pint; the eighth part of a gallon. Symbol O.

**oc·ta·va·lent** (ok"tə-va'lənt) [*octa-* + *valens* able] having a valence of eight.

**oc·tet** (ok-tet') a group of eight identical or similar objects or entities, as the group of eight electrons (four pairs) in the outer, or valence, shell of an atom, which pairs may or may not be shared with another atom.

**oc·ti·ci·zer** (ok"tĭ-si'zər) a plasticizer for pharmaceuticals.

**oc·ti·grav·i·da** (ok"tĭ-grav'ĭ-də) [*octa-* + *gravida*] a woman pregnant for the eighth time; also written gravida VIII.

**Oc·tin** (ok'tin) trademark for preparations of isometheptene mucate.

**oc·tip·a·ra** (ok-tip'ə-rə) [*octa-* + *para*] a woman who has had eight pregnancies which resulted in viable offspring; also written para VIII.

**oc·to·cryl·ene** (ok'to-kril"ēn) [USP] a sunscreen that absorbs ultraviolet light in the UVB range.

**Oc·to·my·ces** (ok"to-mi'sēz) former name for *Saccharomyces.*

**oc·to·pam·ine** (ok"to-pam'ēn) [MeSH: Octopamine] a sympathomimetic amine thought to result from inability of the diseased liver to metabolize tyrosine; it is called a false neurotransmitter, since it can be stored in presynaptic vesicles, replacing norepinephrine, but has little effect on postsynaptic receptors. It is used as the hydrochloride salt in treatment of hypotension.

**oc·to·pus** (ok'tə-pəs) any of numerous carnivorous marine mollusks having eight tentacles.
**blue-ringed o.,** *Hapalochlaena maculosa,* a venomous species found along the coast of Australia that when excited bites its enemy and secretes tetrodotoxin. See *tetrodotoxism.*

**oc·tose** (ok'tōs) a monosaccharide containing eight carbon atoms in the molecule.

**oc·tox·y·nol 9** (ok-toks'ĭ-nol) [NF] [MeSH: Octoxynol] a clear, pale yellow, viscous liquid used as a surfactant in pharmaceutical preparations. Called also *octylphenoxy polyethoxyethanol.*

**Oc·treo·scan** (ok-tre'o-skan″) trademark for a preparation of indium In 111 pentetreotide.

**oc·tre·o·tide** (ok-tre'o-tīd) [MeSH: Octreotide] a synthetic analogue of somatostatin, having actions similar to those of somatostatin but having a prolonged duration of effect; used as the acetate salt as a treatment adjunct for the palliative treatment of diarrhea associated with gastrointestinal endocrine tumors and for the palliative treatment of the symptoms of hyperinsulinemia in pancreatic tumors, and to decrease the secretion of growth hormone in acromegaly.
**o. acetate,** the acetate salt of octreotide, having the same actions and uses as the base; administered subcutaneously.

**oc·tyl·phe·noxy poly·eth·oxy·eth·a·nol** (ok″təl-fə-nok'se pol″e-əth-ok″se-eth'ə-nol) octoxynol 9.

**oc·tyl sal·i·cyl·ate** (ok'til sal″ĭ-sil'āt) [USP] a substituted salicylate that absorbs ultraviolet light in the UVB range, used as a sunscreen.

**oc·u·fil·con** (ok″u-fil'kon) any of three hydrophilic contact lens materials, designated A, B, or C.

**oc·u·lar** (ok'u-lər) [L. *ocularis, from oculus* eye] 1. of, pertaining to, or affecting the eye. 2. eyepiece.

**oc·u·len·tum** (ok″u-len'təm) pl. *oculen'ta.* An eye ointment.

**oc·u·li** (ok'u-li) [L.] genitive and plural of *oculus.*

**oc·u·list** (ok'u-list) ophthalmologist.

**oc·u·lis·tics** (ok″u-lis'tiks) the treatment of diseases of the eye.

**ocul(o)-** [L. *oculus* eye] a combining form denoting relationship to the eye.

**oc·u·lo·ceph·a·lo·gyr·ic** (ok″u-lo-sef″ə-lo-gi'rik) [*oculo-* + *cephalo-* + *gyr-* + *-ic*] pertaining to the movements of the head in connection with vision.

**oc·u·lo·cu·ta·ne·ous** (ok″u-lo-ku-ta'ne-əs) pertaining to or affecting both the eyes and the skin.

**oc·u·lo·fa·cial** (ok″u-lo-fa'shəl) pertaining to the eyes and the face.

**oc·u·lo·gy·ra·tion** (ok″u-lo-ji-ra'shən) movement of the eye about the anteroposterior axis.

**oc·u·lo·gy·ric** (ok″u-lo-ji'rik) pertaining to, characterized by, or causing oculogyration; see also under *crisis.*

**oc·u·lo·man·dib·u·lo·dys·ceph·a·ly** (ok″u-lo-man-dib″u-lo-dis-sef'ə-le) [*oculo-* + *mandibulo-* + *dyscephaly*] malformation of the cranium and facial bones with optic abnormalities; see *oculomandibulofacial syndrome,* under *syndrome.*

**oc·u·lo·met·ro·scope** (ok″u-lo-met'rə-skōp) [*oculo-* + *metro-* + *-scope*] an instrument for performing retinoscopy in which the trial lenses are rotated before the eyes without effort on the part of the examiner.

**oc·u·lo·mo·tor** (ok″u-lo-mo'tor) [*oculo-* + *motor*] pertaining to or effecting movements of the eye.

**oc·u·lo·my·co·sis** (ok″u-lo-mi-ko'sis) [*oculo-* + *mycosis*] ophthalmomycosis.

**oc·u·lo·na·sal** (ok″u-lo-na'səl) pertaining to the eye and the nose.

**oc·u·lop·a·thy** (ok″u-lop'ə-the) ophthalmopathy.

**oc·u·lo·pu·pil·lary** (ok″u-lo-pu'pĭ-lar-e) pertaining to the pupil of the eye.

**oc·u·lo·spi·nal** (ok″u-lo-spi'nəl) pertaining to the eye and the spinal cord.

**oc·u·lo·zy·go·mat·ic** (ok″u-lo-zi″go-mat'ik) pertaining to the eye and the zygomatic arch (zygoma).

**oc·u·lus** (ok'u-ləs) gen. and pl. *o'culi* [L.] [TA] the organ of vision; see *eye.* Symbol O.

**Oc·u·sert** (ok'u-sərt) trademark for a drug delivery system placed in the cul-de-sac of the eyes and providing a sustained release of pilocarpine.

**OD** optical density; Doctor of Optometry; outside diameter; popular term for *overdose;* [L.] *o'culus dex'ter,* right eye.

**ODA** abbreviation for L. *occipito-dextra anterior* (right occipito-anterior, a position of the fetus).

**odax·es·mus** (o″dak-sez'məs) [Gr. *odaxēsmos* an itching] the biting of the tongue or cheek in an epileptic seizure.

**odax·et·ic** (o″dak-set'ik) [Gr. *odaxētikos*] causing a biting or itching sensation.

**ODC** orotidine 5′-phosphate decarboxylase.

**Od·di's sphincter (muscle)** (od'ēz) [Ruggero *Oddi,* Italian physician, 1864–1913] see under *sphincter.*

**od·di·tis** (od-i'tis) inflammation of Oddi's muscle.

**odds** (odz) the ratio of a part to the remainder; it is a means of expressing the chance that a particular event will occur. See also under *ratio.*

**odo·gen·e·sis** (od″o-jen'ə-sis) [Gr. *hodos* pathway + *-genesis*] neurocladism.

**odon·tal·gia** (o-don-tal'jə) [*odont-* + *-algia*] toothache.

**odon·tal·gic** (o-don-tal'jik) pertaining to or characterized by toothache.

**odon·tec·to·my** (o″don-tek'tə-me) [*odont-* + *-ectomy*] excision or removal of a tooth; tooth extraction.

**odon·ti·at·ro·gen·ic** (o-don″te-at″ro-jen'ik) [*odont-* + *iatro-* + *-genic*] occurring as a result of treatment by a dentist.

**odon·tic** (o-don'tik) [*odont-* + *-ic*] pertaining to the teeth; dental.

**odont(o)-** [Gr. *odous,* gen. *odontos* tooth] a combining form denoting relationship to a tooth or to the teeth.

**odon·to·am·e·lo·blas·to·ma** (o-don″to-am″ə-lo-blas-to'mə) ameloblastic odontoma.

**odon·to·blast** (o-don'to-blast) [*odonto-* + *-blast*] [MeSH: Odontoblasts] one of the columnar connective tissue cells which deposit dentin and form the outer surface of the dental pulp adjacent to the dentin.

**odon·to·blas·to·ma** (o-don″to-blas-to'mə) a tumor made up of odontoblasts.

**odon·to·both·ri·on** (o-don″to-both're-on) [*odonto-* + Gr. *bothrion* a small trench] one of the dental alveoli.

**odon·to·both·ri·tis** (o-don″to-both-ri'tis) alveolitis.

**odon·to·cla·mis** (o-don″to-kla'mis) [*odonto-* + Gr. *klamys* cloak] dental operculum.

**odon·to·clast** (o-don'to-klast) [*odonto-* + *-clast*] [MeSH: Osteoclasts] cementoclast.

**odon·to·gen** (o-don'to-jen) [*odonto-* + *-gen*] the substance which develops into the dentin of the teeth.

**odon·to·gen·e·sis** (o-don″to-jen'ə-sis) [*odonto-* + *genesis*] [MeSH: Odontogenesis] the development and formation of the teeth; it has been divided into three stages: the *lamina-bud stage, cap stage,* and *bell stage.*
**o. imperfec'ta,** dentinogenesis imperfecta.

**odon·to·ge·net·ic** (o-don″to-jə-net'ik) pertaining to odontogenesis.

**odon·to·gen·ic** (o-don″to-jen'ik) 1. forming teeth. 2. arising in tissues which give origin to the teeth.

**odon·tog·e·nous** (o″don-toj'ə-nəs) 1. arising or originating in the teeth. 2. originating in a dental condition.

**odon·to·gram** (o-don'to-gram) [*odonto-* + *-gram*] the tracing made by an odontograph.

**odon·to·graph** (o-don'to-graf) [*odonto-* + *-graph*] an instrument for recording the unevenness of surface of tooth enamel.

**odon·tog·ra·phy** (o″don-tog'rə-fe) [*odonto-* + *-graphy*] 1. a description of the teeth. 2. the use of the odontograph. Called also *dentography.*

**odon·to·iat·ria** (o-don″to-i-at're-ə) [*odonto-* + Gr. *iatreia* cure] dental therapeutics.

**odon·toid** (o-don'toid) [*odont-* + *-oid*] toothlike; resembling a tooth.

**odon·to·lith** (o-don'to-lith) [*odonto-* + *-lith*] dental calculus.

**odon·to·li·thi·a·sis** (o-don″to-lĭ-thi'ə-sis) [*odonto-* + *lith-* + *-iasis*] a condition marked by the presence of dental calculus.

**odon·tol·o·gist** (o″don-tol'ə-jist) a dentist.

**odon·tol·o·gy** (o″don-tol'ə-je) [*odonto-* + *-logy*] 1. the sum of knowledge regarding the teeth. 2. dentistry.

**odon·tol·y·sis** (o-don-tol'ĭ-sis) [*odonto-* + *-lysis*] tooth resorption.

**odon·to·ma** (o-don-to'mə) [*odont-* + *-oma*] [MeSH: Odontoma]

1. any tumor of odontogenic origin. 2. a mixed tumor of odontogenic origin, in which both the epithelial and mesenchymal cells exhibit complete differentiation, resulting in the formation of tooth structures.
**o. adamanti'num,** ameloblastic o.
**ameloblastic o.,** a rare, slow-growing, mixed tumor of odontogenic origin that combines the characteristics of composite odontoma and ameloblastoma, and occurs more commonly on the mandible than on the maxilla.
**composite o.,** an odontogenic tumor of the jaws, most commonly of the molar region, composed of both the ectodermal and mesodermal components of the tooth apparatus. A type that consists of calcified dental tissue exhibiting complete differentiation, resulting in the formation of enamel and dentin that bear resemblance to normal tooth structures, is known as *compound composite odontoma;* a type in which calcified dental tissue presents a disorganized mass bearing no similarity to normal tooth structure is known as *complex composite odontoma.*
**composite o., complex,** a composite odontoma in which the calcified dental tissues occur in an irregular mass, and there is no morphologic similarity to even rudimentary teeth.
**composite o., compound,** a composite odontoma in which the enamel and dentin are laid down so that the structure bears a superficial anatomic resemblance to normal teeth.
**coronal o., coronary o.,** odontoma associated with the crown of a tooth, or one formed at the time when the crown of the tooth was developing.
**dilated o.,** d. in dente.
**embryoplastic o.,** a soft odontoma formed in the period that precedes the formation of the dental tissues.
**fibrous o.,** an odontoma containing fibrous elements.
**mixed o.,** an odontogenic neoplasm containing different elements of the tooth structure.
**radicular o.,** one associated with the root of a tooth, or one formed at the time when the root of the tooth was developing.

**odon·ton·o·my** (o″don-ton'ə-me) [*odonto-* + Gr. *onoma* name] the nomenclature of dentistry; a system of terminologies in all branches of dentistry and related fields. Called also *dentonomy.*

**odon·to·path·ic** (o-don″to-path'ik) relating to disease of the teeth.

**odon·top·a·thy** (o″don-top'ə-the) [*odonto-* + *-pathy*] any disease of the teeth.

**odon·to·peri·os·te·um** (o-don″to-per″e-os'te-əm) periodontium, def. 1.

**odon·to·pho·bia** (o-don″to-fo'be-ə) [*odonto-* + *-phobia*] an irrational fear associated with teeth, as that aroused by the sight of teeth, or abnormal dread of dental operations.

**odon·to·plas·ty** (o-don'to-plas″te) recontouring of a tooth surface, such as to enhance calculus and plaque control and morphology of the gingiva.

**odon·to·pri·sis** (o-don″to-pri'sis) [*odonto-* + Gr. *prisis* sawing] bruxism.

**odon·to·ra·dio·graph** (o-don″to-ra'de-o-graf) a radiograph of a tooth or of the teeth.

**odon·to·schism** (o-don'to-skiz-əm) [*odonto-* + Gr. *schisma* cleft] fissure of a tooth.

**odon·tos·co·py** (o″don-tos'kə-pe) [*odonto-* + *-scopy*] the taking of dental impressions.

**odon·to·sei·sis** (o-don″to-si'sis) [*odonto-* + Gr. *seisis* a shaking] looseness of the teeth.

**odon·to·sis** (o″don-to'sis) [*odont-* + *-osis*] the formation or eruption of the teeth.

**odon·to·the·ca** (o-don″to-the'kə) [*odonto-* + *theca*] the dental sac.

**odon·tot·o·my** (o″don-tot'ə-me) [*odonto-* + *-tomy*] the operation of cutting into a tooth, especially incision into an occlusal groove.

**odon·to·trip·sis** (o-don″to-trip'sis) [*odonto-* + *tripsis*] wearing away of the teeth.

**odor** (o'dər) [L.] [MeSH: Odors] a volatile emanation that is perceived by the sense of smell.
**minimal identifiable o.,** minimum perceptible o., the lowest concentration of a substance in air, or in another medium, which still permits its identification by the sense of smell, see also *olfact.*

**odor·ant** (o'dər-ənt) any substance capable of eliciting olfactory excitation, i.e., of stimulating the sense of smell.

**odor·a·tism** (o″dər-a'tiz-əm) osteolathyrism.

**odor·if·er·ous** (o″dər-if'ər-əs) [*odor* + *-ferous*] fragrant; emitting an odor.

**odor·im·e·ter** (o″dər-im'ə-tər) an instrument for performing odorimetry.

**odor·im·e·try** (o″dər-im'ə-tre) measurement of the strength of olfactory stimuli.

**odor·i·phore** (o-dor'ĭ-for) osmophore.

**odor·i·vec·tor** (o″dər-ĭ-vek'tər) a substance which gives off an odor.

**odor·og·ra·phy** (o″dər-og'rə-fe) [*odor* + *-graphy*] a description of odors.

**ODP** abbreviation for L. *occipito-dextra posterior* (right occipitoposterior, a position of the fetus).

**ODT** abbreviation for L. *occipito-dextra transversa* (right occipitotransverse, a position of the fetus).

**odyn·acu·sis** (o″din-ə-ku'sis) [*odyno-* + *acou-* + *-sis*] painful hearing.

**-odynia** [Gr. *odynē* pain] a word ending denoting a painful condition.

**odyn(o)-** [Gr. *odynē* pain] a combining form meaning pain.

**odyn·om·e·ter** (o″din-om'ə-tər) [*odyno-* + *-meter*] algesimeter.

**od·y·no·pha·gia** (od″ĭ-no-fa'jə) [*odyno-* + *-phagia*] a dysphagia in which swallowing causes pain.

**oe-** for words beginning thus, see also those beginning with *e-.*

**Oeci·a·cus** (e-si'ə-kəs) a genus of insects related to bedbugs but having hairy bodies covered by long silklike coats; they are found on birds and in their nests. *O. hiru'dinis* is found on barn swallows in Europe and sometimes invades homes and attacks humans, causing severe irritation. *O. vica'rius* is found on swallows in North America.

**oed·i·pism** (ed'ĭ-piz-əm) [from *Oedipus,* King of Thebes, who blinded himself after unknowingly killing his father and marrying his mother.] intentional injury of one's own eyes.

**Oed·i·pus complex** (e'dĭ-pəs) [*Oedipus,* character in Greek legend who was raised by a foster parent and later unwittingly killed his father and married his mother] [MeSH: Oedipus Complex] see under *complex.*

**Oehl's muscle** (ərlz) [Eusebio *Oehl,* Italian anatomist, 1827–1903] see under *muscle.*

**Oeh·ler's symptom** (er'lerz) [Johannes *Oehler,* German physician, born 1879] see under *symptom.*

**Oenan·the** (e-nan'the) the dropworts, a genus of umbelliferous plants that grow in wet places in the Birtish Isles. The roots of several species contain poisonous alcohols that can cause fatal convulsions and opisthotonos in ruminants.

**oenan·thol** (e-nan'thol) heptanal.

**oer·sted** (ər'sted) [Hans Christian *Oersted,* Danish physicist, 1777–1851] an older unit of magnetic field strength, largely replaced by the SI unit amperes per meter.

**oesophag(o)-** for words beginning thus, see those beginning *esophag(o)-.*

**Oesoph·a·go·don·tus** (e-sof″ə-go-don'təs) a genus of nematodes of the family Strongylidae. *O. robus'tus* is a blood-sucking parasite in the colon of the horse.

**oesoph·a·go·sto·mi·a·sis** (e-sof″ə-go-sto-mi'ə-sis) [MeSH: Oesophagostomiasis] infection with nematodes of the genus *Oesophagostomum.* See *nodular worm disease,* under *disease.*

**Oesoph·a·gos·to·mum** (e-sof″ə-gos'to-məm) [*Oesophagus* + Gr. *stoma* mouth] [MeSH: Oesophagostomum] the nodular worms, a genus of nematodes of the family Strongylidae, parasitic in the intestines of various animals; the larvae often encyst in the intestinal wall, while the adults are mostly free in the lumen. See *nodular worm disease,* under *disease.*
**O. bifur'cum,** a parasite that forms tumors in the large intestine of monkeys and occasionally of man in Africa and the Philippines.
**O. brevicau'dum,** a species that causes nodular worm disease in pigs.
**O. columbia'num,** a species that causes nodular worm disease in sheep and goats in the southern United States.
**O. denta'tum,** a species that causes nodular worm disease in pigs.
**O. radia'tum,** a species that causes nodular worm disease in cattle.
**O. stephanos'tomum,** a species, normally parasitic in gorillas; a single human case has been recorded from Brazil.
**O. venulo'sum,** a species that causes nodular worm disease in ruminants.

**oesoph·a·gus** (ə-sof'ə-gəs) [Gr. *oisophagos,* gullet, related to *phagein* to eat] [TA] the esophagus.

**oestr-** for words beginning thus, see also those beginning *estr-.*

**oes·tri·a·sis** (es-tri'ə-sis) infestation with larvae of flies of the genus *Oestrus.*

**Oes·tri·dae** (es'trĭ-de) a family of flies, including the bot, heel, and warble flies. They are very hairy diptera with rudimentary mouth parts and with the antennae inserted into round pits. Genera include *Cuterebra, Dermatobia, Gasterophilus, Hypoderma, Oestrus,* and *Rhinoestrus.*

**Oes·trus** (es'trəs) [Gr. *oistros* gadfly] a genus of botflies of the family Oestridae, which may cause ophthalmomyiasis; called also *Cephalomyia.*
**O. ho'minis,** *O. ovis.*
**O. o'vis,** a species of botfly whose larvae infest nasal cavities and sinuses of sheep; they may cause ocular myiasis in man.

**OFD** oral-facial-digital; see under *syndrome.*

**of·fi·cial** (o-fĭ'shəl) [L. *officialis; officum* duty] recognized by the current U. S. Pharmacopeia or National Formulary, and meeting the standards established by the respective authority.

**of·fic·i·nal** (o-fis'ĭ-nəl) [L. *officinalis; officina* shop] denoting pharmaceutical preparations that are regularly kept at pharmacies. Cf. *magistral.*

**oflox·a·cin** (o-flok'sə-sin) [USP] [MeSH: Ofloxacin] a broad-spectrum fluorinated 4-quinolone antibacterial with actions similar to those of norfloxacin, effective against a wide variety of gram-negative organisms; administered orally in the treatment of prostatitis, sexually transmitted diseases, and infections of the lower respiratory tract, urinary tract, and skin, and applied topically in the treatment of bacterial corneal ulcers.

**Ogen** (o'jən) trademark for preparations of estropipate.

**Og·il·vie's syndrome** (o'gil-vēz) [Sir William Heneage *Ogilvie,* English surgeon, 1887–1971] see under *syndrome.*

**OGTT** oral glucose tolerance test.

**Ogu·chi's disease** (o-goo'chēz) [Chuta *Oguchi,* Japanese ophthalmologist, 1875–1945] see under *disease.*

**Oha·ra's disease** (o-hah'rahz) [Shoichiro *Ohara,* Japanese physician, 20th century] see under *disease.*

**OH-Cbl** hydroxocobalamin.

**17-OHCS** 17-hydroxycorticosteroid.

**Ohm's law** (ōmz) [George Simon *Ohm,* German physicist, 1787–1854] see under *law.*

**ohm** (ōm) [George S. *Ohm*] the SI unit of electrical resistance, being equivalent to that of a column of mercury one square millimeter in cross-section and 106 centimeters long. Symbol Ω.

**ohm·am·me·ter** (ōm"am'me"tər) an ohmmeter and ammeter combined.

**ohm·me·ter** (ōm'me-tər) an instrument for measuring electric resistance in ohms.

**ohne Hauch** (o'nə houkh) [Ger. "without breath" cf. *Hauch*] see *O antigen,* under *antigen* and *O colony* under *colony.* Symbol O.

**OI** osteogenesis imperfecta.

**OIC** osteogenesis imperfecta congenita; see *osteogenesis imperfecta,* under *osteogenesis.*

**-oid** [Gr. *-oeidēs,* from *eidos* form] a word termination denoting resemblance to the thing specified by the stem to which it is affixed, as ovoid.

**Oid·i·um** (o-id'e-əm) [dim. of Gr. *ōon* egg] 1. the imperfect (asexual) stage of powdery mildews (order Erysiphales), which cause many plant diseases. 2. a former genus of fungi which is now included in the genera *Candida, Geotrichum,* and *Olpitrichum.*

**oid·i·um** (o-id'e-əm) a short cylindrical asexual spore formed by the fragmentation of a hypha.

**OIH** orthoiodohippurate; see *iodohippurate sodium.*

**oil** (oil) [L. *oleum*] [MeSH: Oils] 1. an unctuous, combustible substance which is liquid, or easily liquefiable, on warming, and is soluble in ether but insoluble in water. Such substances, depending on their origin, are classified as animal, mineral, or vegetable oils. Depending on their behavior on heating, they are classified as volatile or fixed. 2. a fat that is liquid at room temperature.

## Oil

**almond o.** [NF], a preparation of the fixed oil obtained from the seed of *Prunus amygdalus,* the almond; used as an emollient, perfume, and oleaginous vehicle and as an ingredient of rose water ointment. Called also *expressed* or *sweet almond o.*

**almond o., bitter,** the volatile oil obtained from the bitter almond or from other kernels containing amygdalin; used in perfumery and liqueurs and formerly as a topical antipruritic.

**almond o., expressed, almond o., sweet,** almond o.

**American wormseed o.,** chenopodium o.

**anise o.,** a volatile oil distilled from the dried, ripe fruit of *Pimpinella anisum* or of *Illicium verum;* used as a flavoring agent for drugs, and has been used as a carminative and expectorant.

**apricot kernel o.,** persic o.

**arachis o.,** peanut o.

**argemone o.,** an oil from the seeds of *Argemone mexicana*; it contains the toxic alkaloid sanguinarine. In certain countries it may be found as a contaminant of cooking oil and may cause epidemic dropsy.

**bergamot o.,** a volatile oil obtained by expression from the rind of the fresh fruit of bergamot *(Citrus bergamia),* used as a perfuming agent and insecticide.

**betula o.,** methyl salicylate.

**bhilawanol o.,** the oil of a nut grown in India, used for marking laundry; it is the cause, through induction of eczematous contact sensitization, of dhobie itch.

**birch o., sweet,** methyl salicylate.

**birch tar o., rectified,** a pyroligneous oil obtained by dry distillation of the bark and wood of various birches (genus *Betula*), especially *B. alba,* rectified by steam distillation; used topically in the treatment of eczema and other dermatitides.

**cade o.,** juniper tar.

**cajeput o., o. of cajeput,** a volatile oil from the fresh leaves and twigs of *Melaleuca leucadendron* and other species of *Melaleuca;* used as a stimulant, expectorant, counterirritant, and external parasiticide, and in veterinary medicine as a rubefacient and parasiticide in the treatment of ringworm. Spelled also *cajuput o.*

**camphorated o.,** camphor liniment.

**canola o.,** rapeseed oil, specifically that prepared from plants bred to contain lowered amounts of erucic acid.

**caraway o.,** a volatile oil distilled from the dried ripe fruit of *Carum carvi,* yielding at least 50 per cent by volume of carvone; used as a flavoring agent for drugs and as a carminative.

**cardamom o.,** a volatile oil distilled from the seed of the cardamom plant *(Elettaria cardamomum),* used as a flavoring agent in pharmaceutical preparations.

**cassia o.,** cinnamon o.

**castor o.** [USP], a fixed oil obtained from the seed of *Ricinus communis;* used as a cathartic and as a plasticizer for pharmaceutical preparations, and has been used as a bland emollient to the skin in certain dermatoses.

**castor o., aromatic** [USP], a mixture of cinnamon, clove, and castor oils, with saccharin, vanillin, and alcohol, used as a cathartic.

**cedar o., cedarwood o., o. of cedar wood,** a volatile oil from the wood of the red cedar, *Juniperus virginiana,* used as a clearing agent in microscopical techniques; the thicker fraction is used as the immersion medium with oil-immersion objectives.

**chenopodium o.,** a volatile oil obtained from species of *Chenopodium;* formerly used as an anthelmintic. Called also *American wormseed o.*

**chloriodized o.,** an iodine monochloride addition product of vegetable oil; formerly used as a radiopaque medium in radiography of the uterus and uterine tubes, and of the bronchi.

**cinnamon o.,** a volatile oil distilled with steam from the leaves and twigs of *Cinnamomum cassia;* used as a flavoring agent for pharmaceuticals and formerly used as a carminative.

**citronella o.,** a fragrant oil extracted from *Cymbopogon nardus,* used as an insect repellent.

**clove o.,** a volatile oil, consisting chiefly of eugenol, distilled from the clove (q.v.); used as a flavor in pharmaceutical preparations, and as a topical germicide and analgesic in dentistry.

**coconut o.,** the fixed oil obtained by expression or extraction from the kernels of seeds of *Cocos nucifera;* used as an ointment base and edible oil and in soap, chocolate, and candle formulations.

**cod liver o.** [USP], the partially destearinated fixed oil obtained from fresh livers of *Gadus morrhua* and other species of the family Gadidae; used as a source of vitamin A and vitamin D. In veterinary medicine, it is also used topically to promote wound healing and in abscesses, burns, and dermatoses.

**cod liver o., nondestearinated** [NF], the entire fixed oil obtained from fresh livers of *Gadus morrhua* and other species of the family Gadidae; used as a source of vitamins A and D.

**coriander o.**, a volatile oil distilled with steam from the dried ripe fruit of *Coriandrum sativum;* used as a flavoring agent.

**corn o.** [NF], a refined fixed oil obtained from the embryo of *Zea mays;* used as a solvent and vehicle for various medicinal agents and as a vehicle for injections. It has also been promoted as a source of polyunsaturated fatty acids in special diets.

**cottonseed o.** [NF], the fixed oil obtained by expression from the seeds of cultivated varieties of cotton (genus *Gossypium*). It is widely used in soaps, oleomargarine, lubricants, cosmetics, and salad and cooking oils. In veterinary medicine, used as delousing agent, usually combined with two parts of pine tar for ear ticks of horses, and as a mild emollient and laxative for small animals.

**croton o.**, the thick, fixed oil of the seeds of *Croton tiglium;* it is a drastic purgative and counterirritant, unsafe for human use, and is used as a standard irritant in pharmacological research.

**o. of dill**, an oil distilled from the dried ripe fruits of *Anethum graveolens,* used as an aromatic carminative and as a source of carvone.

**distilled o.**, volatile o.

**drying o.**, a type of fixed oil which thickens and hardens on exposure to the air, especially when spread out in a thin layer, being converted to a solid by absorption and reaction with oxygen.

**empyreumatic o.**, a volatile oil formed by the destructive distillation of organic material.

**essential o., ethereal o.**, volatile o.

**ethiodized o.** [USP], an iodine addition product of the ethyl ester of the fatty acids of poppyseed oil, used as a radiopaque medium in hysterosalpingography and lymphography.

**eucalyptus o.**, a volatile oil distilled with steam from the fresh leaf of *Eucalyptus globulus* and other species of *Eucalyptus;* used as a pharmaceutical flavoring agent, and as a veterinary and human expectorant and local antiseptic. See also *eucalyptol.*

**expressed o., fatty o.**, fixed o.

**fennel o.**, a volatile oil distilled from fennel (the seeds of *Foeniculum vulgare*), used as a flavoring agent for pharmaceuticals and formerly as a carminative.

**fixed o.**, an oil that does not evaporate on warming. Such oils, consisting of a mixture of fatty acids and their esters, are classified as *solid* (chiefly stearin), *semisolid* (chiefly palmitin), and *liquid* (chiefly olein). They are also classified as *drying, semidrying,* and *nondrying,* depending on their tendency to solidify when exposed, in a thin film, to air. Called also *expressed o.* and *fatty o.*

**flaxseed o.**, linseed o.

**gaultheria o.**, methyl salicylate.

**groundnut o.**, peanut o.

**Haarlem o.**, juniper tar.

**halibut liver o.**, a fixed oil obtained from the liver of the halibut (genus *Hippoglossus*); used as a source of vitamins A and D.

**iodized o.**, an iodine addition product of vegetable oil; used as radiopaque medium in radiography of the uterus and uterine tubes.

**juniper o.**, a volatile oil distilled with steam from the dried ripe fruit of *Juniperus communis;* used to preserve surgical gut sutures and has been used as a diuretic.

**lavender o., lavender flowers o.**, a volatile oil distilled with steam from the fresh flowering tops of *Lavandula angustifolia* subsp. *angustifolia* or prepared synthetically; used as a perfume in pharmaceutical preparations.

**lemon o.** [NF], the volatile oil obtained by expression from the fresh peel of the fruit of *Citrus limon;* used as a flavoring agent.

**linseed o.**, the fixed oil obtained from the dried ripe seed of *Linum usitatissimum;* used as an emollient in liniments, pastes, and medicinal soaps, and in veterinary medicine as a laxative. Called also *flaxseed o.* and *raw linseed o.*

**o. of male fern**, a dark green oleoresin from the root of the male fern, *Dryopteris filix-mas;* it contains about 24 per cent of crude filicin and is used as an anthelmintic.

**mineral o.** [USP], a mixture of liquid hydrocarbons obtained from petroleum, with a specific gravity of 0.845–0.905; used as a cathartic and as a solvent and oleaginous vehicle in pharmaceutical preparations. Called also *heavy liquid petrolatum, liquid petrolatum, liquid paraffin, petrolatum liquidum,* and *white mineral o.*

**mineral o., light** [NF], **mineral o., light white,** a mixture of liquid hydrocarbons obtained from petrolatum, with a specific gravity of 0.818–0.880; used as a vehicle for drugs and also as a laxative. Called also *light liquid paraffin* and *light liquid petrolatum.*

**mineral o., white,** mineral o.

**o. of mirbane,** nitrobenzene.

**o. of mustard,** an oil derived from the seeds of mustard (q.v.); *volatile o. of mustard* is another name for *allyl isothiocyanate.*

**myristica o.,** nutmeg o.

**neroli o.,** orange flower o.

**nondrying o.,** a type of fixed oil that does not harden but rather remains sticky to the touch indefinitely when exposed in a thin film to air.

**nutmeg o.,** the volatile oil distilled with steam from the dried kernels of the ripe seeds of *Myristica fragrans;* used as a flavoring agent in pharmaceutical preparations. Called also *myristica o.*

**olive o.** [NF], the fixed oil obtained from the ripe fruit of *Olea europaea;* used as a setting retardant for dental cements and as a topical emollient, and has been used as a laxative. Called also *sweet o.*

**orange o.,** the volatile oil obtained by expression from the fresh peel of the ripe fruit of *Citrus sinensis;* used as a flavoring agent in pharmaceuticals. Called also *sweet orange o.*

**orange o., bitter,** a volatile oil obtained from the fresh peel of the fruit of *Citrus aurantium;* used as a flavoring agent.

**orange o., sweet,** orange o.

**orange flower o.,** a volatile oil distilled from the fresh flowers of *Citrus aurantium,* used as a flavoring agent and perfume. Called also *neroli o.*

**peach kernel o.,** persic o.

**peanut o.** [NF], the refined fixed oil obtained from peanuts *(Arachis hypogaea)*; used as a solvent and oleaginous vehicle for drugs, and as a laxative in veterinary medicine. Called also *arachis o.* and *groundnut o.*

**peppermint o.** [NF], the volatile oil distilled from the fresh aboveground parts of the flowering plant of *Mentha piperita,* used as a flavor in pharmaceutical preparations, and as a gastric stimulant and carminative.

**persic o.,** an oil expressed from the kernels of varieties of *Prunus armeniaca,* the apricot, or from *P. persica,* the peach; used as a vehicle for drugs.

**pine o.,** the volatile oil obtained by steam distillation of the wood of *Pinus palustris* and other species of *P.;* used as a deodorant and disinfectant.

**pine needle o., pine needle o., dwarf,** the volatile oil distilled with steam from the fresh leaf of the Swiss mountain pine, *Pinus mugo,* and its variety *P. mugo,* var. *pumilio;* used as a perfume and flavoring agent.

**rapeseed o.,** the oil expressed from seeds of *Brassica napus,* used in the manufacture of soaps, margarines, and lubricants. An edible variety, called canola oil (q.v.), has been developed.

**ricinus o.,** castor o.

**rose o.** [NF], the volatile oil distilled with steam from the fresh flowers of *Rosa alba, R. centifolia, R. damascena,* or *R. gallica,* used as a perfuming agent and flavoring agent. Called also *attar of roses.*

**rosemary o.,** the volatile oil distilled with steam from the fresh flowering tops of *Rosmarinus officinalis,* used as a flavoring or perfuming agent.

**safflower o.,** an oily liquid extracted from the seeds of the safflower, *Carthamus tinctorius;* used as a dietary supplement in the management of hypercholesterolemia.

**sandalwood o., santal o.,** a viscid oily liquid with a characteristic odor and taste, distilled with steam from the dried heartwood of *Santalum album* (sandalwood); formerly used as a urinary antiseptic.

**sassafras o.,** the volatile oil distilled from the root of *Sassafras albidum;* it is the source of the beverage root beer and is used as a pharmaceutical flavoring agent. It is also applied to insect bites and stings and has been used as a topical antiseptic, pediculicide, and carminative. It contains safrene and safrole.

**savin o.,** an acrid oil from the fresh tops of *Juniperus sabina,* the chief constituent of which is sabinol; it has been used in folk medicine as an emmenagogue, anthelmintic, and antirheumatic, and is used in perfumery. It may cause hematuria and violent gastrointestinal irritation when administered internally; fatal poisoning has resulted from its use as an abortifacient.

**semidrying o.,** a fixed oil that dries incompletely or slowly when exposed in a thin film to air.

**sesame o.** [NF], the refined fixed oil obtained from the seed of *Sesamum indicum;* it is used as a solvent and oleaginous vehicle for drugs, and has been used internally as a laxative and externally as a skin softener.

**shark liver o.,** the oil extracted from the liver of the soupfin shark *(Galeorhinus zyopterus* and *Hypoprion brevirostris)*; used as a protectant and emollient in topical preparations.

**silicone o.,** a long-chain silicone polymer with a viscosity of 5000 to 5400 centistokes, injected into the vitreous to maintain retinal tamponade in the management of complicated retinal detachment; called also *polydimethylsiloxane.*

**spearmint o.,** the volatile oil distilled with steam from the fresh overground parts of *Mentha spicata* or *M. cardiaca,* yielding at least 55 per cent by volume of carvone; used as a flavor for pharmaceutical preparations.

**o. of spike,** a volatile oil obtained from a broad-leaved variety of lavender, *Lavandula latifolia;* used in perfumery, and formerly in home remedies as an emmenagogue and abortive.

**sweet o.,** olive o.

**tar o., rectified,** the volatile oil from *Pinus palustris* Mill. (Pinaceae) and pine tar rectified by steam distillation; in veterinary medicine, administered internally as a stimulant expectorant and externally as an antipruritic, antiseptic, and stimulant for skin diseases. Also used as a disinfectant and deodorizer.

**theobroma o.,** cocoa butter.

**thyme o.,** the volatile oil distilled from the flowering plant of *Thymus vulgaris;* used as a flavoring agent for drugs, and has been used as a rubefacient, expectorant, counterirritant, antiseptic, and carminative.

**turpentine o.,** the volatile oil distilled from turpentine; its chief constituent is pinene, which is used in the synthetic production of camphor. It is used as a counterirritant and rubefacient.

**turpentine o., rectified,** turpentine oil rectified by use of sodium hydroxide; used as an inhalation expectorant.

**volatile o.,** an oil that evaporates readily; such oils are usually found in aromatic plants, to which they give odor and other characteristics. Most consist of a mixture of two or more terpenes. Called also *distilled, essential,* or *ethereal o.*

**wintergreen o.,** methyl salicylate.

**oint·ment** (oint'mənt) [L. *unguentum*] a semisolid preparation for external application to the body, and usually containing a medicinal substance. Called also *unguent, unction,* and *salve.*

**belladonna o.,** a preparation of pilular belladonna extract and diluted alcohol in yellow ointment; used locally as an analgesic.

**benzoic and salicylic acids o.** [USP], a preparation of benzoic acid and salicylic acid in a ratio of about 2:1 in a water-soluble base, used topically as an antifungal and keratolytic agent in the treatment of tinea pedis; called also *Whitfield's o.*

**bland lubricating ophthalmic o.** [USP], an ointment composed of white petrolatum and mineral oil; it may also contain lanolin, modified lanolin, or lanolin alcohols.

**calamine o.,** a preparation containing calamine, yellow wax, anhydrous lanolin, and petrolatum; used as an astringent protective application.

**carbolic acid o.,** phenol o.

**coal tar o.** [USP], a preparation of coal tar, polysorbate 80, and zinc oxide paste, used as a topical antieczematic and antipsoriatic.

**erythromycin ophthalmic o.** [USP], a preparation of erythromycin in a suitable ointment base; used as a topical antibacterial in the treatment of superficial infections of the conjunctiva and cornea by susceptible organisms.

**hydrophilic o.** [USP], a water-in-oil emulsion consisting of methylparaben, propylparaben, sodium lauryl sulfate, propylene glycol, stearyl alcohol, white petrolatum, and purified water; used as an ointment base.

**iodochlorhydroxyquin and hydrocortisone o.,** an ointment containing 90 to 110 per cent of the labeled amounts of iodochlorhydroxyquin and of hydrocortisone; used for its local anti-infective effect and the anti-inflammatory and antipruritic activity of glucocorticoids in a wide range of dermatoses, applied topically.

**penicillin o.,** a preparation of calcium penicillin, crystalline penicillin, or procaine penicillin in a suitable ointment base, with or without incorporation of a suitable anesthetic.

**phenol o.,** a preparation of phenol, glycerin, and white ointment, containing 1.8–2.2 per cent of phenol; used as an antipruritic. Called also *carbolic acid o.*

**pine tar o.,** a preparation of pine tar, yellow wax, and yellow ointment, used as a local antieczematic and rubefacient.

**polyethylene glycol o.** [NF], a mixture of polyethylene glycol 4000 and polyethylene glycol 400, used as a water-soluble ointment base.

**resorcinol o., compound** [USP], preparation of resorcinol, zinc oxide, bismuth subnitrate, juniper tar, yellow wax, petrolatum, anhydrous lanolin, and glycerin, used as a topical antifungal and keratolytic; applied topically.

**rose water o.** [USP], a preparation of spermaceti, white wax, almond oil, sodium borate, stronger rose water, purified water, and rose oil, used as an emollient and ointment base.

**rose water o., petrolatum,** an ointment prepared with spermaceti, white wax, mineral oil, sodium borate, rose water, purified water, and rose oil.

**scarlet red o.,** a preparation of scarlet red, olive oil, anhydrous lanolin, and petrolatum, applied locally as a protective agent.

**simple o.,** white o.

**tar o., compound,** a preparation of rectified tar oil, benzoin tincture, zinc oxide, yellow wax, lard, and cottonseed oil, used locally as an antibacterial and irritant.

**white o.** [USP], an oleaginous ointment base prepared from white wax and white petrolatum.

**Whitfield's o.,** benzoic and salicylic acids o.

**yellow o.** [USP], a mixture of yellow wax and petrolatum, used as an ointment base for drugs.

**Oken's body (corpus), canal** (o'kenz) [Lorenz *Oken,* German physiologist, 1779–1851] see *mesonephros* and *ductus mesonephricus.*

**OKT3** trademark for a preparation of muromonab-CD3.

**OL** [L.] *o'culus lae'vus,* left eye.

**Ol.** abbreviation for L. *o'leum,* oil.

**-ol** suffix indicating that the substance is an alcohol or a phenol, i.e., a hydroxyl derivative of a hydrocarbon.

**OLA** abbreviation for L. *occipito-laeva anterior* (left occipito-anterior, a position of the fetus).

**ol·amine** (ol'ə-mēn) USAN contraction for ethanolamine.

**Old·field's syndrome** (ōld'fēldz) [Michael C. *Oldfield,* British physician, 20th century] see under *syndrome.*

**Olea** (o'le-ə) a genus of small trees or shrubs of the family Oleaceae, which have drupaceous fruit. *O. europae'a* L. is the commonly cultivated olive tree, source of olive oil. *O. oleas'ter* is the wild olive or oleaster.

**olea**[1] (o'le-ə) [L.] olive (def. 1).

**olea**[2] (o'le-ə) [L.] plural of *oleum.*

**ole·ag·i·nous** (o″le-aj'ĭ-nəs) [L. *oleaginus*] oily; greasy; unctuous.

**ole·an·der** (o″le-an'dər) *Nerium oleander.*

**ole·an·drin** (o″le-an'drin) a cardiac glycoside from oleander *(Nerium oleander)* that has been used in cardiac insufficiency.

**ole·an·drism** (o″le-an'driz-əm) poisoning of humans or other animals by oleander, which contains cardiac glycosides. Characteristics include gastroenteritis with vomiting and diarrhea, increased pulse rate, and increased respiration, sometimes ending fatally.

**ole·ate** (o'le-āt) 1. a salt, anion, or ester of oleic acid. 2. a solution of an alkaloid or other basic drug in oleic acid, used as an ointment.

**olec·ra·nal** (o-lek'rə-nəl) pertaining to the olecranon.

**olec·ran·ar·thri·tis** (o-lek″rən-ahr-thri'tis) [*olecranon* + *arthritis*] anconitis.

**olec·ran·ar·throp·a·thy** (o-lek″rən-ahr-throp'ah-the) [*olecranon* + *arthro-* + *-pathy*] disease of the elbow joint.

**olec·ra·noid** (o-lek'rə-noid) resembling the olecranon.

**olec·ra·non** (o-lek'rə-non) pl. *olec'rana* [Gr. *ōlekranon*] [TA] the proximal bony projection of the ulna at the elbow, its anterior surface forming part of the trochlear notch.

**ole·fin** (o'lə-fin) [*oleo-* + L. *facere* to make] any of a class of unsaturated aliphatic hydrocarbons having one or more double bonds; those with one double bond are called alkenes.

**ole·ic ac·id** (o-le'ik) [MeSH: Oleic Acid] 1. a monounsaturated 18-carbon fatty acid, liquid at room temperature and occurring in most

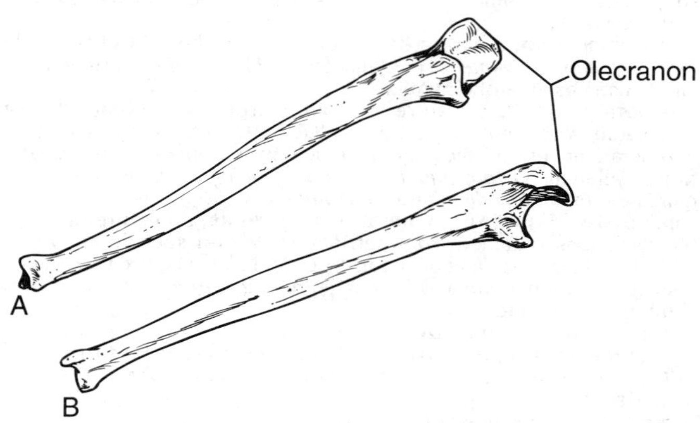


Olecranon in anterior *(A)* and lateral *(B)* views of the ulna.

animal fats and vegetable oils. See also table accompanying *fatty acid.* 2. [NF] a preparation consisting mainly of oleic acid with some palmitic and stearic acids, manufactured from fats and oils that are derived from edible sources unless the mixture is for external use only; used as an emulsifying agent and to assist absorption of some drugs by the skin.

**ole·in** (o'le-in) the triglyceride formed from oleic acid, occurring in most fats and oils.

**olen·itis** (o-lən-i'tis) anconitis.

**ole(o)-** [L. *oleum* oil] a combining form denoting relationship to oil.

**oleo·chryso·ther·a·py** (o″le-o-kris″o-ther'ə-pe) [*oleo-* + *chrysotherapy*] therapeutic administration of gold salts in oily suspensions.

**oleo·cre·o·sote** (o″le-o-kre'ə-sōt) the oleic acid ester of creosote.

**oleo·gran·u·lo·ma** (o″le-o-gran″u-lo'mə) paraffinoma.

**oleo·in·fu·sion** (o″le-o-in-fu'zhən) a preparation made by infusing a drug in oil.

**ole·o·ma** (o″le-o'mə) [*oleo-* + *-oma*] paraffinoma.

**ole·om·e·ter** (o″le-om'ə-tər) [*oleo-* + *-meter*] an instrument for testing the purity of oil.

**oleo·pal·mi·tate** (o″le-o-pal'mĭ-tāt) an oleate and a palmitate of the same base.

**oleo·peri·to·ne·og·ra·phy** (o″le-o-per″ĭ-to-ne-og'rə-fe) radiography of the peritoneum following the injection of iodized oil.

**oleo·res·in** (o″le-o-rez'in) [*oleo-* + *resin*] 1. any natural combination of a resin and a volatile oil such as exudes from pines and other plants. 2. a compound prepared by exhausting a drug by percolation with a volatile solvent, such as acetone, alcohol, or ether, and evaporating the solvent.
**aspidium o.**, oil of male fern.
**capsicum o.** [USP], the extract from capsicum obtained by percolation, with either acetone or ether as the menstruum; used as an irritant and carminative.

**oleo·sac·cha·rum** (o″le-o-sak'ə-rəm) eleosaccharum.

**oleo·ste·ar·ate** (o″le-o-ste'ər-āt) an oleate and a stearate of the same base.

**oleo·sus** (o″le-o'səs) [L.] oily; greasy.

**oleo·ther·a·py** (o″le-o-ther'ə-pe) [*oleo-* + *therapy*] treatment with oil, particularly treatment by the injection of oil.

**oleo·tho·rax** (o″le-o-tho'raks) a method of collapse therapy in which oil or paraffin was inserted into part of the thoracic cavity.

**oleo·vi·ta·min** (o″le-o-vi'tə-min) a preparation of fish liver oil or edible vegetable oil containing one or more fat-soluble vitamins or their derivatives.
**o. A and D** [USP], an oily preparation containing vitamin A and natural or synthetic vitamin D; used as a dietary supplement.

**oleo·yl** (o-le'o-əl) the acyl radical of oleic acid.

**ole·um** (o'le-əm) gen. *o'lei,* pl. *o'lea* [L.] oil.

**ol·fact** (ol'fakt) a unit of odor, the minimum perceptible odor, being the minimum concentration of a substance in solution which can be perceived by a large number of normal individuals, expressed in terms of grams per liter.

**ol·fac·tant** (ol-fak'tənt) odorant.

**ol·fac·tion** (ol-fak'shən) [L. *olfacere* to smell] 1. the sense of smell; the ability to perceive and distinguish odors. 2. the act of perceiving and distinguishing odors.

**ol·fac·tism** (ol-fak'tiz-əm) a sensation of smell produced by other than olfactory stimuli.

**ol·fac·tol·o·gy** (ol″fak-tol'ə-je) the science of the sense of smell. Called also *osmics.*

**ol·fac·tom·e·ter** (ol″fak-tom'ə-tər) [*olfactus* + *-meter*] an apparatus for testing the sensitiveness of perception of odors.

**ol·fac·tom·e·try** (ol″fak-tom'ə-tre) the measurement of the sense of smell.

**ol·fac·to·ry** (ol-fak'tə-re) [L. *olfacere* to smell] pertaining to olfaction, or the sense of smell.

**ol·fac·tus** (ol-fak'təs) gen. *olfac'tus.* Olfaction (def. 1); see also *organum olfactus.*

**ol·i·gak·i·su·ria** (ol″ĭ-gak″ĭ-su're-ə) [Gr. *oligakis* few times + *-uria*] a condition in which urination occurs at long intervals.

**ol·i·ge·mia** (ol″ĭ-je'me-ə) hypovolemia.

**olig(o)-** [Gr. *oligos* little, few] a combining form meaning *(a)* few, little, or scanty, *(b)* less than normal, or *(c)* deficient. Cf. *pauci-.*

**ol·i·go·am·ni·os** (ol″ĭ-go-am'ne-os) [*oligo-* + *amnios*] oligohydramnios.

**ol·i·go·an·al·ge·sia** (ol″ĭ-go-an″əl-je'zhə) the use of analgesics too infrequently or at doses insufficient to relieve pain.

**ol·i·go·an·u·ria** (ol″ĭ-go-an-u're-ə) oliguria in which there is a temporary complete cessation of urinary flow.

**ol·i·go·arth·ri·tis** (ol″ĭ-go-ahr-thri'tis) arthritis of a small number of joints.

**ol·i·go·as·tro·cy·to·ma** (ol″ĭgo-as″tro-si-to'mə) a mixed glioma consisting of elements derived from astrocytes and elements derived from oligodendrogliocytes.

**ol·i·go·blast** (ol'ĭ-go-blast″) a primitive oligodendrocyte.

**ol·i·go·chro·ma·sia** (ol″ĭ-go-kro-ma'se-ə) hypochromia (def. 1).

**ol·i·go·cys·tic** (ol″ĭ-go-sis'tik) [*oligo-* + *cystic*] containing only a few cysts.

**ol·i·go·dac·ty·ly** (ol″ĭ-go-dak'tə-le) [*oligo-* + Gr. *daktylos* finger] hypodactyly.

**ol·i·go·den·dria** (ol″i-go-den'dre-ə) oligodendroglia.

**ol·i·go·den·dro·blas·to·ma** (ol″ĭ-go-den″dro-blas-to'mə) oligodendroglioma.

**ol·i·go·den·dro·cyte** (ol″ĭ-go-den'dro-sīt) [*oligodendro*glia + *-cyte*] [MeSH: Oligodendroglia] a cell of the oligodendroglia.

**ol·i·go·den·drog·lia** (ol″ĭ-go-dən-drog'le-ə) [*oligo-* + *dendro-* + *neuroglia*] [MeSH: Oligodendroglia] 1. the non-neural cells of ectodermal origin forming part of the adventitial structure (neuroglia) of the central nervous system; projections of the surface membrane of each of these cells (oligodendrocytes) fan out and coil around the axon of many neurons to form myelin sheaths in the white matter. With microglia, they form the perineuronal satellites in the gray matter. 2. the tissue composed of such cells.

**ol·i·go·den·dro·gli·o·ma** (ol″ĭ-go-den″dro-gli-o'mə) [MeSH: Oligodendroglioma] a usually benign neoplasm derived from and composed of oligodendrocytes in varying stages of differentiation; the majority are seen in adults in the white matter of the brain. Called also *oligodendroblastoma.*

**ol·i·go·dip·sia** (ol″ĭ-go-dip'se-ə) [*oligo-* + *dipsia*] hypodipsia.

**ol·i·go·don·tia** (ol″ĭ-go-don'she-ə) [*olig-* + *odont-* + *-ia*] absence of many teeth, usually associated with small size of the existing teeth and other anomalies.

**ol·i·go·dy·nam·ic** (ol″ĭ-go-di-nam'ik) [*oligo-* + *dynamic*] active in very minute quantities; said especially of heavy metal ions ($Hg^{2+}$, $Ag^{+}$) to describe toxic effect on cells and organisms.

**ol·i·go·en·ceph·a·lon** (ol″ĭ-go-ən-sef'ə-lon) [*oligo-* + *encephalon*] micrencephalon.

**ol·i·go·ga·lac·tia** (ol″ĭ-go-gə-lak'she-ə) [*oligo-* + *galact-* + *-ia*] hypogalactia.

**ol·i·go·gen·ic** (ol″ĭ-go-jen'ik) [*oligo-* + *genic*] produced by a few genes at most; used in reference to certain hereditary characters.

**ol·i·gog·lia** (ol″ĭ-gog'le-ə) oligodendroglia.

**ol·i·go-1,4-1,4-glu·can·trans·fer·ase** (ol″ĭ-go-gloo″kan-trans'fər-ās) an enzyme activity catalyzing the transfer of short $\alpha$-1,4 linked glucose chains from side chains of limit dextrins to new $\alpha$-1,4 linkages on main chains or glucose, thereby exposing $\alpha$-1,6 branch points for debranching and further degradation. The enzyme activity is the transferase activity of amylo-1,6-glucosidase (q.v.).

**ol·i·go-1,6-glu·co·si·dase** (ol'ĭ-go-gloo-ko'sĭ-dās) [EC 3.2.1.10] [MeSH: Oligo-1,6-Glucosidase] EC nomenclature for *α-dextrinase.*

**ol·i·go·glu·co·side** (ol″ĭ-go-gloo'ko-sīd) an oligosaccharide composed of glucose residues. Cf. *polyglucoside.*

**ol·i·go·hy·dram·ni·os** (ol″ĭ-go-hi-dram'ne-os) [*oligo-* + *hydro-* + *amnion*] [MeSH: Oligohydramnios] the presence of less than the normal amount of amniotic fluid; defined as 500 mL or less at term and smaller amounts at earlier gestational ages.

**ol·i·go·hy·dru·ria** (ol″ĭ-go-hi-droo're-ə) [*oligo-* + *hydruria*] abnormally high concentration of the urine.

**Ol·i·go·hy·me·no·phor·ea** (ol″ĭ-go-hi″mə-no-for'e-ə) [*oligo-* + *hymen* + Gr. *phoros* bearing] [MeSH: Oligohymenophorea] a class of ciliate protozoa (phylum Ciliophora), characterized by the presence of an oral apparatus that is usually well developed and situated at least partially in a buccal cavity and by oral ciliature that is clearly distinct from the somatic ciliature, consisting of a paraoral membrane on the right side and a few compound organelles on the left. Some species are loricate, and colony formation is common in some groups. It comprises two subclasses: Hymenostomatia and Peritrichia.

**ol·i·go·hy·per·men·or·rhea** (ol″ĭ-go-hi″pər-men″o-re'ə) infrequent menstruation with excessive menstrual flow.

**ol·i·go·hy·po·men·or·rhea** (ol″ĭ-go-hi″po-men″o-re'ə) infrequent menstruation with diminished menstrual flow.

**ol·i·go·lec·i·thal** (ol″ĭ-go-les′ĭ-thəl) [*oligo-* + *-lecithal*] possessing only a little yolk.

**ol·i·go·meg·a·ne·phro·nia** (ol″ĭ-go-meg″ə-nə-fro′ne-ə) [*oligo-* + *mega-* + *nephron* + *-ia*] congenital renal hypoplasia in which there is a reduction in the number of lobes and of total number of nephrons, and hypertrophy of the nephrons.

**ol·i·go·meg·a·neph·ron·ic** (ol″ĭ-go-meg″ə-nəf-ron′ik) 1. characterized by a reduced number of and hypertrophy of the nephrons. 2. pertaining to oligomeganephronia.

**ol·i·go·men·or·rhea** (ol″ĭ-go-men″o-re′ə) [*oligo-* + *meno-* + *-rrhea*] [MeSH: Oligomenorrhea] infrequent menstrual flow, occurring at intervals of 35 days to 6 months.

**ol·i·go·mer** (ol′ĭ-go-mər) [*oligo-* + Gr. *meros* part] a polymer formed by the combination of relatively few monomers.

**ol·i·go·me·tal·lic** (ol″ĭ-go-mə-tal′ik) containing only small quantities of metals.

**ol·i·go·mor·phic** (ol″ĭ-go-mor′fik) [*oligo-* + *morph-* + *-ic*] passing through only a few forms of growth; said of microorganisms.

**ol·i·go·nec·ro·sper·mia** (ol″ĭ-go-nek″ro-sper′me-ə) [*oligo-* + *necro-* + *sperm-* + *-ia*] a condition of the spermatic fluid in which there is diminution of the number of spermatozoa, some of which are dead.

**ol·i·go·ni·tro·phil·ic** (ol″ĭ-go-ni″tro-fil′ik) [*oligo-* + *nitrogen* + *-philic*] absorbing nitrogen from the air and from media containing combined nitrogen; said of microorganisms.

**ol·i·go·nu·cle·o·tide** (ol″ĭ-go-noo′kle-o-tīd) [*oligo-* + *nucleotide*] a polymer made up of a few (2–20) nucleotides. In molecular genetics, a short sequence synthesized to match a region where a mutation is known to occur, and then used as a probe (oligonucleotide probe).

**ol·i·go·ov·u·la·tion** (ol″ĭ-go-ov″u-la′shən) maturation and discharge of fewer than the normal number of ova from the ovaries.

**ol·i·go·pep·tide** (ol″ĭ-go-pep′tīd) the structure formed by the linkage of a few amino acids.

**ol·i·go·phos·pha·tu·ria** (ol″ĭ-go-fos″fə-tu′re-ə) deficiency in the excretion of phosphates in the urine.

**ol·i·gop·nea** (ol″ĭ-gop-ne′ə) [*oligo-* + *-pnea*] hypopnea.

**ol·i·go·py·rene, ol·i·go·py·rous** (ol″ĭ-go-pi′rēn, ol″ĭ-go-pi′rəs) [*oligo-* + Gr. *pyrēn* stone of fruit] deficient in nuclear or chromatin material.

**ol·i·go·sac·cha·ride** (ol″ĭ-go-sak′ə-rīd) a carbohydrate that on hydrolysis yields a small number of monosaccharides (from two to four, or according to some definitions up to ten). Cf. *polysaccharide.*

**ol·i·go·sper·ma·tism** (ol″ĭ-go-sper′mə-tiz-əm) oligospermia.

**ol·i·go·sper·mia** (ol″ĭ-go-sper′me-ə) [*oligo-* + *sperm-* + *-ia*] [MeSH: Oligospermia] deficiency in the number of spermatozoa in the semen.

**ol·i·go·syn·ap·tic** (ol″ĭ-go-sin-ap′tik) [*oligo-* + *synaptic*] involving a few synapses in series and therefore a sequence of only a few neurons; called also *paucisynaptic.* Cf. *polysynaptic.*

**ol·i·go·tro·phia** (ol″ĭ-go-tro′fe-ə) [*oligo-* + *troph-* + *-ia*] malnutrition.

**ol·i·go·troph·ic** (ol″ĭ-go-trof′ik) pertaining to or characterized by malnutrition.

**ol·i·got·ro·phy** (ol″ĭ-got′rə-fe) malnutrition.

**ol·i·go·zo·o·sper·ma·tism** (ol″ĭ-go-zo″o-sper′mə-tiz-əm) oligospermia.

**ol·i·go·zo·o·sper·mia** (ol″ĭ-go-zo″o-sper′me-ə) oligospermia.

**ol·i·gu·re·sis** (ol″ĭ-gu-re′sis) oliguria.

**ol·i·gu·ria** (ol″ĭ-gu′re-ə) [*oligo-* + *-uria*] [MeSH: Oliguria] excretion of a diminished amount of urine in relation to the fluid intake, usually defined as less than 400 mL per 24 hours. Called also *hypouresis* and *oliguresis.*

**ol·i·gu·ric** (ol″ĭ-gu′rik) pertaining to or characterized by oliguria.

**olis·the** (o-lis′the) olisthy.

**olis·thet·ic** (o-lis-thet′ik) exhibiting or affected by olisthy.

**olis·thy** (o-lis′the) [Gr. *olisthanein* to slip] a slipping, as the slipping of the bones of a joint from their normal relation in the joint.

**oli·va** (o-li′və) gen. and pl. *oli′vae* [L.] [TA] olive: a rounded elevation, lateral to the upper part of each pyramid of the medulla oblongata, between the ventrolateral and dorsolateral sulci; it is formed by an irregular mass of gray substance *(nucleus olivaris caudalis)* located just beneath its surface and is linked by fiber systems to the pons and cerebellum. Called also *inferior olive, olivary body,* and *olivary nucleus.*

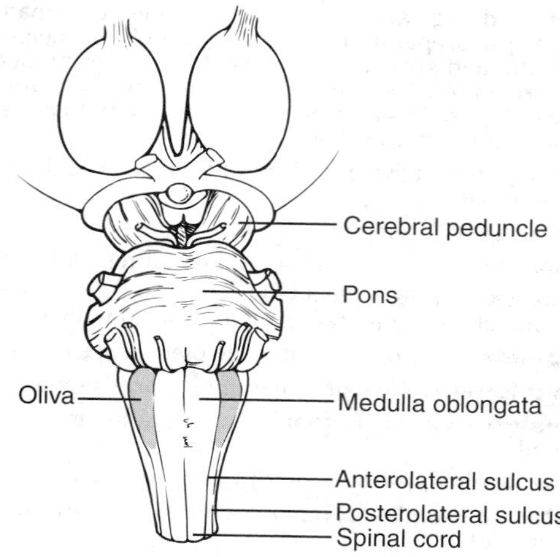


Oliva (olive) shown in an anterior (inferior) view of the brain.

**ol·i·vary** (ol′ĭ-var″e) [L. *olivarius*] 1. shaped like an olive. 2. pertaining to the oliva.

**ol·ive** (ol′iv) [L. *oliva*] 1. any tree of the genus *Olea.* 2. the fruit of one of these trees, especially *O. europaea,* which yields olive oil (see under *oil*). 3. oliva.

**accessory o's,** the nucleus olivaris accessorius posterior and the nucleus olivaris accessorius medialis; see under *nucleus.*

**inferior o.,** oliva.

**pyloric o.,** the enlarged pylorus of infantile hypertrophic pyloric stenosis as identified by palpation.

**spurge o.,** mezereum.

**superior o.,** nucleus dorsalis corporis trapezoidei.

**Ol·i·ver's sign** (ol′ĭ-vərz) [William Silver *Oliver,* English physician, 1836–1908] tracheal tugging.

**ol·i·vif·u·gal** (ol″ĭ-vif′u-gəl) [*oliva* + *-fugal*[2]] moving or conducting away from the oliva.

**ol·i·vip·e·tal** (ol″ĭ-vip′ə-təl) [*oliva* + *-petal*] passing or conducting toward the oliva.

**ol·i·vo·pon·to·cer·e·bel·lar** (ol″ĭ-vo-pon″to-ser″ə-bel′ər) pertaining to the olivae, the middle peduncles, and the cortex of the cerebellum.

**Ol·lier's disease, law, layer** (o-le-āz′) [Léopold Louis Xavier Edouard *Ollier,* French surgeon, 1830–1900] see *enchondromatosis,* and see under *law* and *layer.*

**Ol·lier-Thiersch graft** (o-le-a′ tērsh) [L.L.X.E. *Ollier;* Karl *Thiersch,* German surgeon, 1822–1895] see under *graft.*

**Ol·lu·la·nus** (ol″u-lan′us) a genus of nematodes. *O. tricus′pis* is a small worm found in the stomachs of pigs and cats that causes gastritis.

**Ol. oliv.** abbreviation for L. *o′leum oli′vae,* olive oil.

**OLP** abbreviation for L. *occipito-laeva posterior* (left occipitoposterior, a position of the fetus).

**Ol·pi·trich·um** (ol-pĭ-trik′əm) a genus of Fungi Imperfecti of the form-family Moniliaceae, which contains species of the former genera *Oidium* and *Acladium;* they are found in soil, and are sometimes isolated from infected wounds.

**ol·sal·a·zine so·di·um** (ol-sal′ə-zēn) a compound consisting of two molecules of mesalamine linked by an azo bond, used in the treatment of ulcerative colitis; administered orally.

**Ols·hau·sen's operation** (olz′hou-zenz) [Robert von *Olshausen,* German obstetrician, 1835–1915] see under *operation.*

**Ol·shev·sky tube** (ol-shev′ske) [Dimitry E. *Olshevsky,* American physician, born 1900] see under *tube.*

**OLT** abbreviation for L. *occipito-laeva transversa* (left occipitotransverse, a position of the fetus).

**o.m.** abbreviation for L. *om′ni ma′ne,* every morning.

**-oma** [Gr. *ōma,* noun-forming suffix] a word termination meaning tumor or neoplasm of the part indicated by the stem to which it is attached.

**oma·ceph·a·lus** (o″mə-sef′ə-ləs) [*om-* + *a-*[1] + *-cephalus*] omocephalus.

**oma·gra** (o-ma′grə) [*om-* + *-agra*] gout in the shoulder.

**omal·gia** (o-mal′jə) [*om-* + *-algia*] pain in the shoulder.

**omar·thri·tis** (o″mahr-thri′tis) [*om-* + *arthr-* + *-itis*] inflammation of the shoulder joint.

**oma·sal** (o-ma′səl) pertaining to the omasum.

**oma·si·tis** (o″mə-si′tis) inflammation of the omasum.

**oma·sum** (o-ma′səm) [L.] [MeSH: Omasum] the third stomach of a ruminant; its walls are lined with many folia that have rough surfaces, serving to grind up food. Called also *manyplies* and *psalterium.*

**Om·bré·danne's operation** (om-bra-dahnz′) [Louis *Ombrédanne,* Paris surgeon, 1871–1956] see under *operation.*

**omega** (o-ma′gə) [Ω, ω] the twenty-fourth, and final, letter of the Greek alphabet. See also *ω-*.

**ome·ga pep·ti·dase** (o-ma′gə pep′tĭ-dās) [EC 3.4.19] any of a group of exopeptidases that catalyze the cleavage of a substituted N- or C-terminal amino acid residue from a peptide chain.

**Omenn's syndrome** (o′menz) [Gilbert Stanley *Omenn,* American internist, born 1941] histiocytic medullary reticulosis; see under *reticulosis.*

**omen·ta** (o-men′tə) [L.] plural of *omentum.*

**omen·tal** (o-men′təl) pertaining to the omentum.

**omen·tec·to·my** (o″mən-tek′tə-me) [*omentum* + *-ectomy*] excision of all or a portion of the omentum.

**omen·ti·tis** (o″mən-ti′tis) inflammation of the omentum.

**omen·to·fix·a·tion** (o-men″to-fik-sa′shən) omentopexy.

**omen·to·pexy** (o-men′to-pek″se) [*omentum* + *-pexy*] in general, an operation in which omentum is fastened to some other tissue, especially one in which omentum is used as a circulatory bridge to reduce congestion or provide vascular nutrition.

**omen·to·plas·ty** (o-men′to-plas″te) [*omentum* + *-plasty*] the use of omental grafts to cover raw surfaces in abdominal surgery.

**omen·to·por·tog·ra·phy** (o-men″to-por-tog′rə-fe) radiography of the hepatic portal veins after injection of a contrast medium into the gastroepiploic vein in the base of the omentum.

**omen·tor·rha·phy** (o″mən-tor′ə-fe) [*omentum* + *-rrhaphy*] suture or repair of the omentum.

**omen·tot·o·my** (o″mən-tot′ə-me) [*omentum* + Gr. *temnein* to cut] incision of the omentum.

**omen·to·vol·vu·lus** (o-men″to-vol′vu-ləs) volvulus of the omentum.

**omen·tum** (o-men′təm) pl. *omen′ta* [L. "fat skin"] [MeSH: Omentum] a fold of peritoneum extending from the stomach to adjacent organs in the abdominal cavity; see *o. majus* and *o. minus.*

- **colic o., gastrocolic o.,** o. majus.
- **gastrohepatic o.,** o. minus.
- **gastrosplenic o.,** ligamentum gastrosplenicum.
- **greater o.,** o. majus.
- **lesser o.,** 1. ligamentum hepatogastricum. 2. o. minus.
- **o. ma′jus** [TA], greater omentum: a prominent peritoneal fold suspended from the greater curvature of the stomach and passing inferiorly a variable distance in front of the intestines; it is attached to the anterior surface of the transverse colon.
- **o. mi′nus** [TA], lesser omentum: a peritoneal fold joining the lesser curvature of the stomach and the first part of the duodenum to the porta hepatis.
- **pancreaticosplenic o.,** a fold of peritoneum connecting the tail of the pancreas and the visceral surface of the spleen.
- **splenogastric o.,** ligamentum gastrosplenicum.

**omen·tum·ec·to·my** (o-men″təm-ek′tə-me) [*omentum* + *-ectomy*] omentectomy.

**omep·ra·zole** (o-mep′rə-zōl) [USP] [MeSH: Omeprazole] a substituted benzimidazole used as a gastric acid secretion inhibitor in the treatment of symptomatic gastroesophageal reflux disease and in conjunction with clarithromycin in the treatment of duodenal ulcer associated with *Helicobacter pylori* infection; administered orally.

**om·i·cron** (om′ĭ-kron) [O, *o*] the fifteenth letter of the Greek alphabet.

**omi·tis** (o-mi′tis) [*omo-* + *-itis*] inflammation of the shoulder.

**om·ma·tid·i·um** (om″ə-tid′e-əm) pl. *ommatid′ia* [Gr. dim. of *omma* eye] one of the units of the compound eye of arthropods, itself complete with all the functional and structural elements of the eye (including lens, retina, photoreceptor cells).

**Om·ma·ya reservoir** (o-mi′yə) [Ayub Khan *Ommaya,* Pakistani neurosurgeon in the United States, born 1930] see under *reservoir.*

**Omn. bih.** abbreviation for L. *om′ni biho′ra,* every two hours.

**Omn. hor.** abbreviation for L. *om′ni ho′ra,* every hour.

**Om·ni·paque** (om′nĭ-pāk) trademark for preparations of iohexol.

**Om·ni·pen** (om′nĭ-pən) trademark for preparations of ampicillin.

**om·nip·o·tence** (om-nip′ə-tens) fantasies of special abilities and power and superiority to others; occurring in infancy and sometimes later in life as a defense mechanism or as an expression of delusional thinking.

**Om·ni·scint** (om′nĭ-sint″) trademark for a preparation of indium In III satumonab pendetide.

**om·niv·o·rous** (om-niv′ə-rəs) [L. *omnis* all + *vorare* to eat] subsisting upon both plants and animals.

**Omn. noct.** abbreviation for L. *om′ni noc′te,* every night.

**om(o)-** [Gr. *ōmos* shoulder] a combining form denoting relationship to the shoulder.

**omo·ceph·a·lus** (o″mo-sef′ə-ləs) [*omo-* + *-cephalus*] a fetus with no upper limbs and an incomplete head.

**omo·cla·vic·u·lar** (o″mo-klə-vik′u-lər) pertaining to the shoulder and the clavicle.

**omo·dyn·ia** (o″mo-din′e-ə) [*omo-* + *-odynia*] omalgia.

**omo·hy·oid** (o″mo-hi′oid) pertaining to the shoulder and the hyoid bone.

**omo·pha·gia** (o″mo-fa′je-ə) [Gr. *ōmos* raw + *-phagia*] the eating of raw food.

**omo·ster·num** (o″mo-ster′nəm) the interarticular cartilage at the joint between the sternum and clavicle.

**OMPA** octamethyl pyrophosphoramide.

**om·pha·lec·to·my** (om″fə-lek′tə-me) [*omphalo-* + *-ectomy*] excision of the umbilicus.

**om·phal·el·co·sis** (om″fəl-əl-ko′sis) [*omphalo-* + *helcosis*] ulceration of the umbilicus.

**Om·pha·lia** (om-fa′le-ə) a genus of mushrooms of the family Agaricaceae. *O. lapides′cens* is dried and used as an anthelmintic called *raigan* in Chinese medicine.

**om·phal·ic** (om-fal′ik) [Gr. *omphalikos*] umbilical.

**om·pha·li·tis** (om″fə-li′tis) [*omphalo-* + *-itis*] inflammation of the umbilicus.

- **o. of birds,** infection of the yolk sac with bacteria normally found in the alimentary tract and on the skin of the hen, leading to death of the embryo or of the chick up to ten days after hatching; called also *mushy chick disease.*

**omphal(o)-** [Gr. *omphalos* navel] a combining form denoting relationship to the umbilicus.

**om·pha·lo·an·gi·op·a·gous** (om″fə-lo-an″je-op′ə-gəs) [*omphalo-* + *angio-* + *-pagus*] allantoidoangiopagous.

**om·pha·lo·an·gi·op·a·gus** (om″fə-lo-an″je-op′ə-gəs) allantoidoangiopagus.

**om·pha·lo·cele** (om′fə-lo-sēl″) [*omphalo-* + *-cele*[1]] protrusion at birth of part of the intestine through a large defect in the abdominal wall at the umbilicus, the protruding bowel being covered only by a thin transparent membrane composed of amnion and peritoneum. Cf. *umbilical hernia.* Called also *umbilical eventration.*

**om·pha·lo·cho·ri·on** (om″fə-lo-kor′e-on) the structure formed by fusion of the yolk sac with the chorion; a choriovitelline placenta.

**om·pha·lo·did·y·mus** (om″fə-lo-did′ĭ-məs) [*omphalo-* + *-didymus*] gastrodidymus.

**om·pha·lo·gen·e·sis** (om″fə-lo-jen′ə-sis) [*omphalo-* + *-genesis*] development of the umbilicus or yolk sac in the embryo.

**om·pha·lo·is·chi·op·a·gus** (om″fə-lo-is-ke-op′ə-gəs) [*omphalo-* + *ischio-* + *-pagus*] conjoined twins united at the umbilicus and the ischia.

**om·pha·lo·ma** (om″fə-lo′mə) [*omphalo-* + *-oma*] a tumor of the umbilicus.

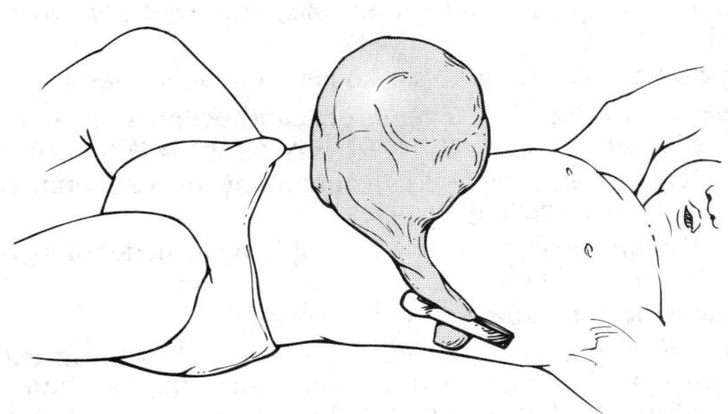

Omphalocele.

**om·pha·lo·mes·a·ra·ic** (om″fə-lo-mes″ə-ra′ik) omphalomesenteric.

**om·pha·lo·mes·en·ter·ic** (om″fə-lo-mes″ən-ter′ik) pertaining to the umbilicus and mesentery.

**om·pha·lon·cus** (om″fə-long′kəs) [*omphalo-* + Gr. *onkos* mass, bulk] omphaloma.

**om·pha·lop·a·gus** (om″fə-lop′ə-gəs) [*omphalo-* + *-pagus*] conjoined twins united in the region of the umbilicus.

**om·pha·lo·phle·bi·tis** (om″fə-lo-flə-bi′tis) [*omphalo-* + *phlebitis*] 1. inflammation of the umbilical veins. 2. infection with suppurative lesions of the umbilicus in young animals; see also *navel ill,* under *ill.*

**om·pha·lor·rha·gia** (om″fə-lo-ra′jə) [*omphalo-* + *-rrhagia*] hemorrhage from the umbilicus.

**om·pha·lor·rhea** (om″fə-lo-re′ə) [*omphalo-* + *-rrhea*] an effusion of lymph at the navel.

**om·pha·lor·rhex·is** (om″fə-lo-rek′sis) [*omphalo-* + *-rrhexis*] rupture of the umbilicus.

**om·pha·lo·site** (om′fə-lo-sīt″) [*omphalo-* + Gr. *sitos* food] an underdeveloped member of allantoidoangiopagous twins, which is joined to the more developed member (autosite) by the vessels of the umbilical cord.

**om·pha·lot·o·my** (om″fə-lot′ə-me) [*omphalo-* + *-tomy*] the cutting of the umbilical cord.

**om·pha·lus** (om′fə-ləs) [Gr. *omphalos*] umbilicus.

**Om. quar. hor.** abbreviation for L. *om′ni quadran′te ho′ra,* every quarter of an hour.

**o.n.** abbreviation for L. *om′ni noc′te,* every night.

**onan·ism** (o′nə-niz-əm) [*Onan,* son of Judah] 1. coitus interruptus. 2. masturbation.

**ona·ye** (o-nah′ye) an extremely strong poison from the seeds of *Strophanthus hispidus.*

**onch(o)-** see *onco-*[2].

**On·cho·cer·ca** (ong″ko-ser′kə) [Gr. *onkos* tumor + *kerkos* tail] [MeSH: Onchocerca] a genus of nematode parasites of the superfamily Filarioidea that infect humans and ruminants. The adults live and breed in subcutaneous fibroid nodules; the young (the microfilariae) are carried by the lymph and are found chiefly in the skin, subcutaneous connective tissues, and eyes.
**O. caecu′tiens,** *O. volvulus.*
**O. cervica′lis,** a species found in the cervical ligament of horses and mules.
**O. gibso′ni,** a species that produces subcutaneous nodular swellings on the legs of cattle and zebras.
**O. vol′vulus,** a common parasite of humans breeding in fast-flowing rivers and streams in tropical regions of the Americas and Africa, particularly West Africa. It is the etiologic agent of human onchocerciasis and is transmitted by the bites of buffalo gnats of the genus *Simulium,* in which the parasite passes part of its life cycle. Formerly called *Filaria volvulus* and *O. caecutiens.*

**on·cho·cer·ci·a·sis** (ong″ko-sər-ki′ə-sis) [*Onchocerca* + *-iasis*] [MeSH: Onchocerciasis] infection with worms of the genus *Onchocerca.* Human infection is caused by *O. volvulus,* with heavy infestations usually characterized by the firm subcutaneous nodules called *onchocercomas;* a persistent dermatitis with a pruritic papular rash, sometimes associated with edema, lichenification, thickening, wrinkling, and atrophy of the skin, with areas of leukoderma; lymphadenitis; and ocular lesions, related to invasion and local death of the microfilariae *(eye worms),* which may progress to optic neuritis, optic atrophy, and blindness. Called also *onchocercosis* and *volvulosis.* There are many local and regional names such as *craw-craw, river blindness,* and *sowdah.*

**on·cho·cer·co·ma** (ong″ko-sər-ko′mə) [*Onchocerca* + *-oma*] a firm, usually freely movable and nontender subcutaneous nodule containing a tangled mass of adult *Onchocerca volvulus* worms; seen in onchocerciasis.

**on·cho·cer·co·sis** (ong″ko-sər-ko′sis) onchocerciasis.

**On·ci·co·la** (on-sik′ə-lə) a genus of acanthocephalous parasites. *O. ca′nis* is found in the intestines of dogs in Texas and Nebraska.

**onc(o)-**[1] [Gr. *onkos* mass, bulk] a combining form denoting relationship to a tumor, swelling, or mass.

**onc(o)-**[2] [Gr. *onkos* barb, hook] a combining form denoting relationship to a barb or hook.

**On·co·cer·ca** (ong″ko-ser′kə) *Onchocerca.*

**on·co·cyte** (ong′ko-sīt) a large epithelial cell with an extremely acidophilic and granular cytoplasm, containing vast numbers of mitochondria; such cells undergo neoplastic transformation.

**on·co·cyt·ic** (ong″ko-sit′ik) composed of or containing oncocytes.

**on·co·cy·to·ma** (ong″ko-si-to′mə) [*oncocyte* + *-oma*] 1. a usually benign adenoma composed of oncocytes with granular, eosinophilic cytoplasm; often used specifically for a tumor of the salivary glands. Called also *oncocytic adenoma, oxyphilic adenoma,* and *oxyphil cell tumor.* 2. Hürthle cell adenoma.
**renal o.,** a benign neoplasm of the kidney that resembles a renal cell carcinoma but is encapsulated and not invasive; most patients are middle-aged and have few overt symptoms from the tumor.

**on·co·cy·to·sis** (on″ko-si-to′sis) metaplasia of oncocytes.

**on·co·fe·tal** (ong″ko-fe′təl) [*onco-*[1] + *fetal*] occurring both in tumor tissue and during fetal development; see under *antigen.*

**on·co·gene** (ong′ko-jēn) a gene capable under certain conditions of causing the initial and continuing conversion of normal cells into cancer cells. The term may be used to denote such a gene occurring in a viral genome (v-*onc*) or a cellular gene derived from alteration of a proto-oncogene (c-*onc*). See table for selected oncogenes associated with human neoplasms.
**viral o.,** an oncogene carried by a virus into a cell, where it becomes incorporated into the DNA of the cell.

**on·co·gen·e·sis** (ong″ko-jen′ə-sis) [*onco-*[1] + *-genesis*] the production or causation of tumors. Called also *tumorigenesis.*

**on·co·ge·net·ic** (ong″ko-jə-net′ik) pertaining to or characterized by oncogenesis.

**on·co·gen·ic** (ong″ko-jen′ik) giving rise to tumors (either benign or malignant) or causing tumor formation; said especially of tumor-inducing viruses. Cf. *tumorigenic.*

**on·co·ge·nic·i·ty** (ong″ko-jə-nis′ĭ-te) the quality or property of being able to cause tumor formation.

**on·cog·e·nous** (ong-koj′ə-nəs) arising in or originating from a tumor.

**on·coi·des** (ong-koi′dēz) [*onco-*[1] + Gr. *eidos* form] turgid swelling; intumescence.

**on·co·lip·id** (ong″ko-lip′id) [*onco-*[1] + *lipid*] a structurally altered lipid moiety of a lipoprotein molecule found in the plasma of cancer patients.

**on·col·o·gy** (ong-kol′ə-je) [*onco-*[1] + *-logy*] the sum of knowledge concerning tumors; the study of tumors.

**on·col·y·sate** (ong-kol′ĭ-sāt) any agent that lyses or destroys tumor cells. Cf. *cytotoxicity.*

**on·col·y·sis** (ong-kol′ĭ-sis) [*onco-*[1] + *-lysis*] the lysis or destruction of tumor cells.

**on·co·lyt·ic** (ong″ko-lit′ik) pertaining to, characterized by, or causing oncolysis; see also *cytotoxicity.* Called also *tumoricidal.*

**on·co·ma** (ong-ko′mə) [Gr. *onkōma*] tumor.

**On·co·me·la·nia** (ong″ko-mə-la′ne-ə) a genus of fresh water snails of the family Bulimidae, found in eastern Asia and nearby Pacific islands; some species transmit schistosomiasis japonica. Formerly called *Katayama.*

**on·com·e·ter** (ong-kom′ə-tər) an instrument for measuring oncotic pressure.

**On·co·Scint CR/OV** (on′ko-sint″) trademark for a preparation of indium In 111 satumomab pendetide.

**on·co·sis** (ong-ko′sis) [*onco-*[1] + *-osis*] a morbid condition characterized by the development of tumors.

**on·co·sphere** (ong′ko-sfēr) [*onco-*[2] + *sphere*] the larva of the tapeworm contained within the external embryonic envelope and armed with six hooks; it may be found in the feces.

**on·co·ther·a·py** (ong″ko-ther′ə-pe) [*onco-*[1] + *therapy*] the treatment of tumors.

**on·co·thlip·sis** (ong″ko-thlip′sis) [*onco-*[1] + Gr. *thlipsis* pressure] pressure caused by a tumor.

**on·cot·ic** (ong-kot′ik) 1. pertaining to, caused by, or marked by swelling. 2. see under *pressure.*

**on·cot·o·my** (ong-kot′ə-me) [*onco-*[1] + *-tomy*] the incision of a tumor or swelling.

**on·co·trop·ic** (ong″ko-trop′ik) [*onco-*[1] + *-tropic*] having a special affinity or attraction for tumor cells; called also *tumoraffin.*

**On·co·vin** (on′ko-vin) trademark for a preparation of vincristine sulfate.

**On·co·vi·ri·nae** (on″ko-vir-i′ne) the RNA tumor viruses: a former subfamily of the Retroviridae, containing the type B, C, and D retroviruses.

**on·co·vi·rus** (ong′ko-vi″rəs) [*onco-*[1] + *virus*] [MeSH: Retroviridae] any of the tumor-producing RNA viruses of the family Oncovirinae, classified in four groups (A, B, C, and D) on the basis of morphology, and also grouped by host range (feline, avian, human, etc.). Type A viral particles comprise intracytoplasmic and intracisternal inclusion bodies; types B, C, and D are genera.

**on·dan·se·tron hy·dro·chlo·ride** (on-dan'sə-tron) [USP] an antiemetic used in conjunction with cancer chemotherapy; administered intravenously.

**On·dine's curse** (on-dēnz') [*Ondine,* sea nymph in German mythology who cursed an unfaithful human lover by abolishing the automaticity of his bodily functions] primary alveolar hypoventilation.

**-one** a suffix used in chemistry to indicate *(a)* quintivalent nitrogen, and *(b)* a compound having two hydrocarbon radicals attached to the carbonyl group; a ketone.

**onei·ric** (o-ni'rik) pertaining to or characterized by dreaming or oneirism.

**onei·rism** (o-ni'riz-əm) an abnormal dreamlike state of consciousness.

**oneir(o)-** [Gr. *oneiros* dream] a combining form denoting relationship to a dream.

**onei·ro·gen·ic** (o″ni-ro-jen'ik) producing a dreamlike state; capable of causing dreams.

**onei·rog·mus** (o″ni-rog'məs) [Gr. *oneirōgmos* an effusion during sleep] emission of semen accompanying dreams.

**onei·roid** (o'ni-roid) resembling a dream.

**onei·rol·o·gy** (o″ni-rol'ə-je) [*oneiro-* + *-logy*] the science of dreams and their interpretation.

**onei·ro·phre·nia** (o-ni″ro-fre'ne-ə) [*oneiro-* + *phren-* + *-ia*] a form of schizophrenia characterized by clouding of consciousness.

**onei·ros·co·py** (o″ni-ros'kə-pe) [Gr. *oneiroskopilkos* of the interpretation of dreams] analysis of dreams for the purpose of diagnosing the patient's mental state.

**oni·um** (o'ne-əm) a term applied to a cation in which nitrogen has its maximum covalency, as in the ammonium ion $NH_4^+$. The compounds include betaines, cholines, and amine oxides.

**on·kino·cele** (ong-kin'o-sēl) [Gr. *onkos* swelling + *is* fiber + *-cele*[1]] a swollen condition of a tendon sheath.

**on·lay** (on'la) [MeSH: Inlays] 1. a graft applied or laid on the surface of an organ or structure. 2. a cast metal restoration that overlays cusps, thus lending strength to the restored tooth.
**epithelial o.,** an epithelial graft, the edges of which are not completely approximated to the edges of the wound, thus permitting new epithelium to grow out around the margin; see also under *inlay.*

**on·o·mato·ma·nia** (on″ə-mat″ə-ma'ne-ə) [Gr. *onoma* name + *-mania*] irresistible preoccupation with specific words or names.

**on·o·mato·pho·bia** (on″ə-mat″ə-fo'be-ə) [Gr. *onoma* name + *-phobia*] irrational fear of hearing a particular word or name.

**on·o·mat·o·poe·ia** (on″ə-mat″ə-pe'ə) [Gr. *onoma* name + *poiein* to make] the formation of meaningless words that imitate sounds, such as may occur to excess in some cases of schizophrenia.

**on·o·mato·poi·e·sis** (on″ə-mat″ə-poi-e'sis) onomatopoeia.

**on·to·gen·e·sis** (on″to-jen'ə-sis) ontogeny.

**on·to·ge·net·ic** (on″to-jə-net'ik) ontogenic.

**on·to·gen·ic** (on″to-jen'ik) pertaining to ontogeny.

**on·tog·e·ny** (on-toj'ə-ne) [Gr. *ōn* existing + *-geny*] the development of the individual organism. Cf. *phylogeny.*

**Onu·fro·wicz's nucleus** (o-noo'fro-wich-ez) [B. *Onufrowicz,* early 20th century] see under *nucleus.*

**ony·al·ai, ony·al·ia** (o″ne-al'a-e) a nutritional disorder seen in Central Africa, marked by the formation on the palatal and buccal mucous membranes of blebs containing semicoagulated blood; there are no signs of constitutional disorder. It is a form of thrombocytopenic purpura.

**on·y·cha·tro·phia** (on″ĭ-kə-tro'fe-ə) [*onych-* + *atrophia*] atrophy of the nail(s).

**on·y·chat·ro·phy** (on″ĭ-kat'rə-fe) onychatrophia.

**on·y·chaux·is** (on″ĭ-kawk'sis) [*onych-* + Gr. *auxein* to increase] simple hypertrophy of the nail(s) without deformity. Called also *hyperonychia.* Cf. *onychogryphosis.*

**on·y·chec·to·my** (on″ĭ-kek'tə-me) [*onych-* + *-ectomy*] 1. excision of a nail or nail bed. 2. removal of the claws of an animal; called also *declawing.*

**onych·ia** (o-nik'e-ə) [*onych-* + *-ia*] inflammation of the matrix of the nail resulting in shedding of the nail. Called also *onychitis.* See also *paronychia.*

**on·y·chi·tis** (on″ĭ-ki'tis) [*onych-* + *-itis*] onychia.

**onych(o)-** [Gr. *onyx,* gen. *onychos* nail] a combining form denoting relationship to the nails.

**on·y·choc·la·sis** (on″ĭ-kok'lə-sis) [*onycho-* + Gr. *klasis* breaking] breaking of the nail.

**on·y·cho·cryp·to·sis** (on″ĭ-ko-krip-to'sis) [*onycho-* + *crypto-* + *-sis*] ingrown nail.

**on·y·cho·dys·tro·phy** (on″ĭ-ko-dis'trə-fe) [*onycho-* + *dystrophy*] dystrophia unguium.

**on·y·cho·gen·ic** (on″ĭ-ko-jen'ik) [*onycho-* + *-genic*] producing or forming nail substance.

**on·y·cho·gram** (o-nik'o-gram) a tracing made by the onychograph.

**on·y·cho·graph** (o-nik'o-graf) [*onycho-* + *-graph*] an instrument for observing and recording the nail pulse and capillary circulation.

**on·y·cho·gry·pho·sis** (on″ĭ-ko-grĭ-fo'sis) [*onycho-* + *gryposis*] hypertrophy of the nail(s), producing a hooked or incurved clawlike deformity. Called also *onychogryposis.* Cf. *onychauxis.*

**on·y·cho·gry·po·sis** (on″ĭ-ko-grĭ-po'sis) onychogryphosis.

**on·y·cho·het·ero·to·pia** (on″ĭ-ko-het″ər-o-to'pe-ə) [*onycho-* + *heterotopia*] a condition in which the nails are abnormally situated.

**on·y·chol·y·sis** (on″ĭ-kol'ĭ-sis) [*onycho-* + *-lysis*] separation of the nail plate from the nail bed, usually beginning at the free margin and progressing proximally.

**on·y·cho·ma·de·sis** (on″ĭ-ko-mə-de'sis) [*onycho-* + Gr. *madēsis* loss of hair] periodic separation of the proximal portions of the nail plate from the matrix and bed with subsequent shedding of the nails. Called also *defluvium unguium* and *onychoptosis.*

**on·y·cho·ma·la·cia** (on″ĭ-ko-mə-la'shə) [*onycho-* + *malacia*] softening of the nail(s).

**on·y·cho·my·co·sis** (on″ĭ-ko-mi-ko'sis) [*onycho-* + *mycosis*] [MeSH: Onychomycosis] tinea unguium.
**dermatophytic o.,** tinea unguium.

**on·y·cho·os·teo·dys·pla·sia** (on″ĭ-ko-os″te-o-dis-pla'zhə) [*onycho-* + *osteo-* + *dysplasia*] 1. osteo-onychodysplasia (def. 1). 2. nail-patella syndrome.

**on·y·cho·path·ic** (on″ĭ-ko-path'ik) pertaining to onychopathy or any disease of the nails.

**on·y·cho·pa·thol·o·gy** (on″ĭ-ko-pə-thol'ə-je) [*onycho-* + *pathology*] the study of diseases of the nails.

**on·y·chop·a·thy** (on″ĭ-kop'ə-the) [*onycho-* + *-pathy*] disease or deformity of the nail(s). Called also *onychosis.*

**on·y·cho·pha·gia** (on″ĭ-ko-fa'jə) [*onycho-* + *-phagia*] the habit of biting the nails.

**on·y·choph·a·gy** (on″ĭ-kof'ə-je) [*onycho-* + *-phagy*] onychophagia.

**on·y·chop·to·sis** (on″ĭ-kop-to'sis) [*onycho-* + *-ptosis*] onychomadesis.

**on·y·chor·rhex·is** (on″ĭ-ko-rek'sis) [*onycho-* + *-rrhexis*] longitudinal striation of the nail plate with brittleness and breakage.

**on·y·cho·schi·zia** (on″ĭ-ko-skiz'e-ə) [*onycho-* + *schiz-* + *-ia*] splitting or lamination of the nail plate, usually in the horizontal plane at the free edge.

**on·y·cho·sis** (on″ĭ-ko'sis) [*onycho-* + *-osis*] onychopathy.

**on·y·cho·til·lo·ma·nia** (on″ĭ-ko-til″o-ma'ne-ə) compulsive picking or tearing at the nails.

**on·y·chot·o·my** (on″ĭ-kot'ə-me) [*onycho-* + *-tomy*] incision of a nail.

**Ony·ge·na·les** (on″ĭ-jə-na'lēz) an order of keratinophilic perfect fungi of the subphylum Ascomycotina, series Prototunicatae; medically important genera include *Ajellomyces* and *Arthroderma.*

**o'nyong-nyong** (o-nyong'nyong) ["severe joint pain" in the language of the Acholi people of East Africa] an acute, nonfatal febrile disease due to an alphavirus, transmitted by anopheline mosquitoes, occurring in Uganda, Kenya, Tanzania, Malawi, and Senegal, and clinically resembling dengue and chikungunya; it is characterized by lymphadenitis, joint pains, and an extremely pruritic morbilliform skin rash. Called also *o'nyong-nyong fever.*

**on·yx** (on'iks) [Gr. "nail"] 1. a fingernail or toenail; see *unguis* [TA]. 2. a variety of hypopyon.

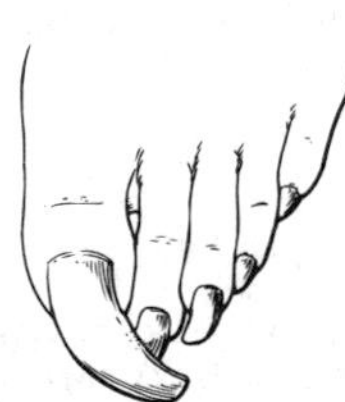

Onychogryphosis.

**on·yx·is** (ə-nik′sis) ingrown nail.

**oo-** [Gr. *ōon* egg] a combining form denoting relationship to an egg or ovum; see also words beginning *ov(o)-*.

**oo·blast** (o′o-blast) [*oo-* + *-blast*] a primordial cell from which an oocyte (ovum) ultimately is developed.

**oo·ceph·a·lus** (o″o-sef′ə-ləs) [*oo-* + *-cephalus*] an individual characterized by an egg-shaped head.

**Oo·cho·ris·ti·ca** (o″o-ko-ris′tĭ-kə) a large genus of tapeworms, family Linstowiidae, which are parasitic in birds, reptiles, and mammals.

**oo·ci·ne·sia** (o″o-sĭ-ne′zhə) ookinesis.

**oo·cy·e·sis** (o″o-si-e′sis) [*oo-* + *cyesis*] ovarian pregnancy.

**oo·cyst** (o′o-sist) [*oo-* + *cyst*] the encysted or encapsulated zygote in the life cycle of sporozoan protozoa, which by the process of sporogony develops into a sporozoite or a sporocyst containing sporozoites.

**oo·cyte** (o′o-sīt) [*oo-* + *-cyte*] [MeSH: Oocytes] a developing egg cell in one of two stages: The *primary oocyte* (one that has begun but not completed the first maturation division) is derived from an oogonium by differentiation near the time of birth. The *secondary oocyte* (one in the period between the first and second maturation division) is derived from a primary oocyte shortly before ovulation by a division that splits off the first polar body. Ovulation follows. If fertilized, the secondary oocyte divides into an ootid and the second polar body; otherwise it perishes.

**oog·a·mous** (o-og′ə-məs) heterogamous.

**oog·a·my** (o-og′ə-me) 1. the fertilization of a large nonmotile oocyte by a small, motile male gamete or sperm, as seen in certain algae. 2. heterogamy.

**oo·gen·e·sis** (o″o-jen′ə-sis) [*oo-* + *-genesis*] [MeSH: Oogenesis] the process of formation of female gametes (oocytes).

**oo·ge·net·ic** (o″o-jə-net′ik) 1. pertaining to oogenesis. 2. producing oocytes. Called also *oogenic, ovogenetic,* and *ovogenic.*

**oo·gen·ic** (o″o-jen′ik) oogenetic.

**oo·go·ni·um** (o″o-go′ne-əm) pl. *oogo′nia* [*oo-* + Gr. *gonē* generation] 1. a primordial oocyte during fetal development; it is derived from a primordial germ cell, multiplies rapidly, then becomes encapsulated in primordial follicle cells and, near time of birth, becomes a primary oocyte by entering into prophase of first maturation division. 2. in certain fungi and algae, the female gametangium containing one or more eggs (oospheres).

**oo·ki·ne·sis** (o″o-kĭ-ne′sis) [*oo-* + *-kinesis*] the mitotic movements of the oocyte during maturation and fertilization.

**oo·ki·nete** (o″o-ki′nēt, o″o-kĭ-net′) [*oo-* + Gr. *kinetos* movable] the motile, worm-shaped zygote of certain protozoa, such as *Plasmodium,* which is found in the insect vector.

**oo·lem·ma** (o″o-lem′ə) [*oo-* + *-lemma*] zona pellucida, def. 1.

**Oo·my·ce·tes** (o″o-mi-se′tēz) [*oo-* + Gr. *mykēs* fungus] [MeSH: Oomycetes] a class of funguslike organisms of the subphylum Mastigomycotina, having sporangia of different kinds and cell walls made up of cellulose, in which reproduction takes place sexually by biflagellate spores. Some authorities classify them with Fungi and others with Protista. The orders Peronosporales and Saprolegniales include animal pathogens.

**oo·my·co·sis** (o-o-mi-ko′sis) infection by fungi of the class Oomycetes, such as *Pythium* species in horses or *Saprolegnia* species in fish.

**oo·pha·gia** (o″o-fa′je-ə) oophagy.

**ooph·a·gy** (o-of′ə-je) [Gr. *ōophagein* to eat eggs] the eating of eggs; said of insects whose diet consists largely of eggs.

**ooph·or·al·gia** (o″of-ər-al′jə) [*oophor-* + *-algia*] pain in an ovary.

**ooph·o·rec·to·mize** (o″of-ə-rek′tə-mīz) to surgically remove one or both of the ovaries; See also *castrate* and *spay.*

**ooph·o·rec·to·my** (o″of-ə-rek′tə-me) [*oophor-* + *-ectomy*] the removal of an ovary or ovaries; if done bilaterally, the individual is incapable of reproduction (see *castration*). Called also *ovariectomy.*

**ooph·o·ri·tis** (o″of-ə-ri′tis) [*oophor-* + *-itis*] [MeSH: Oophoritis] inflammation of an ovary.
 **o. paroti′dea,** oophoritis occurring in association with infection by the virus causing mumps.

**oophor(o)-** [Gr. *ōophoros* bearing eggs] a combining form denoting relationship to the ovary.

**ooph·o·ro·cys·tec·to·my** (o-of″ə-ro-sis-tek′tə-me) [*oophoro-* + *cyst-* + *-ectomy*] excision of an ovarian cyst.

**ooph·o·ro·cys·to·sis** (o-of″ə-ro-sis-to′sis) [*oophoro-* + *cyst* + *-osis*] the formation of ovarian cysts.

**ooph·o·rog·e·nous** (o-of″ə-roj′ə-nəs) derived from the ovary.

**ooph·o·ro·hys·ter·ec·to·my** (o-of″ə-ro-his″tər-ek′tə-me) [*oophoro-* + *hysterectomy*] surgical removal of the uterus and ovaries.

**ooph·o·ro·ma** (o-of″ə-ro′mə) a term formerly used for an ovarian tumor; of historic interest.
 **o. follicula′re,** Brenner's name for Brenner tumor.

**ooph·o·ron** (o-of′ə-ron) [Gr. *ōon* egg + *pherein* to bear] ovarium.

**ooph·o·rop·a·thy** (o-of″ə-rop′ə-the) [*oophoro-* + *-pathy*] any disease of the ovaries. Called also *ovariopathy.*

**ooph·o·ro·pexy** (o-of′ə-ro-pek″se) ovariopexy.

**ooph·o·ro·plas·ty** (o-of′ə-ro-plas″te) plastic surgery of the ovary.

**ooph·o·ro·sal·pin·gec·to·my** (o-of″ə-ro-sal″pin-jek′tə-me) [*oophoro-* + *salpingectomy*] salpingo-oophorectomy.

**ooph·o·ro·sal·pin·gi·tis** (o-of″ə-ro-sal″pin-ji′tis) salpingo-oophoritis.

**ooph·o·ros·to·my** (o-of″ə-ros′tə-me) [*oophoro-* + *-stomy*] the making of an opening into an ovarian cyst.

**ooph·o·rot·o·my** (o-of″ə-rot′o-me) incision of an ovary.

**ooph·or·rha·gia** (o-of″ə-ra′jə) [*oophoro-* + *-rrhagia*] severe hemorrhage from an ovary.

**oo·phyte** (o′o-fīt) [*oo-* + *-phyte*] any member of the generation in the life history of mosses, ferns, etc., in which the sexual organs are produced.

**oo·plasm** (o′o-plaz-əm) the cytoplasm of an oocyte.

**oo·sperm** (o′o-spərm) [*oo-* + *sperm*] a recently fertilized oocyte.

**oo·sphere** (o″o-sfēr) 1. an unfertilized female gamete of certain fungi; when fertilized by an antheridium it becomes an oospore. 2. the large, nonmotile, fertile gamete of certain algae and fungi.

**Oos·po·ra** (o-os′pə-rə) [*oo-* + Gr. *sporos* seed] a genus of Fungi Imperfecti of the form-family Moniliaceae that is associated with disease of citrus trees and potatoes. *O. lac′tis* is now called *Geotrichum candidum* and *O. tozeu′ri* is now called *Madurella mycetomi.*

**oo·spo·ran·gi·um** (o″o-spə-ran′je-əm) oosphere, def. 1.

**oo·spore** (o′o-spor) [*oo-* + *spore*] 1. in certain fungi that have sexual spores, the final developmental stage after fusion of sexually differentiated gametes. 2. the thick-walled, resting zygote formed from a fertilized oosphere.

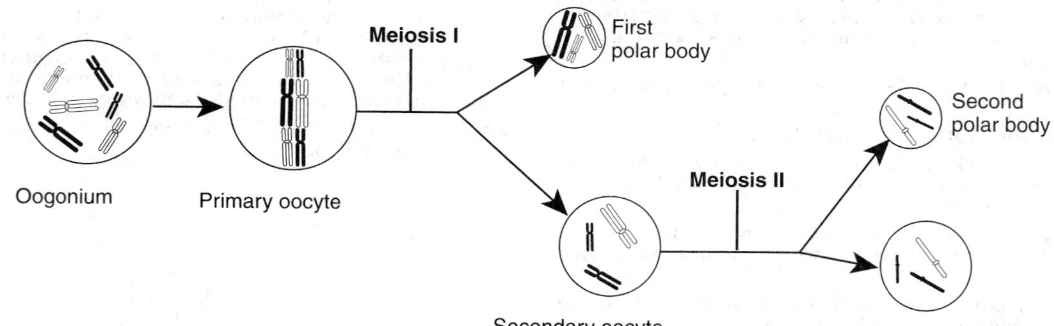


Oogenesis, depicting only six of the 46 double-stranded chromosomes (oogonium, primary oocyte), three of the 23 double-stranded chromosomes (secondary oocyte, first polar body) and three of the 23 single-stranded chromosomes (ovum, second polar body) occurring in human oogensis, and showing random assortment of homologous chromosome pairs. Progression through meiosis II is only completed if fertilization occurs, although fertilization and the male chromosomal contribution to the ovum are omitted here. Crossing over, which may occur in meiosis I, has also been omitted.

**oo•the•ca** (o″o-the′kə) [*oo-* + *theca*] 1. an egg case, such as is found in some lower animals. 2. an ovary.

**oothec(o)-** [Gr. *ōon* egg + *thēkē* case] for words beginning thus, see those beginning *oophor(o)-* and *ovari(o)-*.

**oo•tid** (o′o-tid) a mature oocyte (ovum); one of four cells derived from the two consecutive divisions of the primary oocyte, and corresponding to the spermatids derived from division of the primary spermatocyte. In mammals, the second maturation division is not completed unless fertilization occurs; hence the ootid has male as well as female pronuclear (haploid) elements.

**oo•type** (o′o-tīp) [*oo-* + Gr. *typos* impression] in some trematodes, a dilated portion of the uterus into which the oviduct opens and where the ovum is fertilized, provided with the yolk, and invested with a shell.

**oo•zo•oid** (o″o-zo′oid) [*oo-* + *zo-* + *-oid*] an individual developed from an ovum, that is, as a result of sexual reproduction. Cf. *blastozooid.*

**opac•i•fi•ca•tion** (o-pas″ĭ-fĭ-ka′shən) 1. the development of opacity, as of the cornea or lens. 2. the rendering of a tissue or organ opaque to radiation by introduction of a contrast medium.

**opac•i•ty** (o-pas′ĭ-te) [L. *opacitas*] 1. the condition of being opaque. 2. an opaque spot or area. See also *cataract.*

**opal•es•cent** (o″pəl-es′ənt) showing a milky iridescence, like an opal.

**opal•gia** (o-pal′jə) [Gr. *ōps* face + *-algia*] facial neuralgia.

**Opa•li•na** (o″pə-li′nə) [L. *opalus* opal] a genus of ciliate parasitic protozoa (order Opalinida, class Opalinatea) found as endocommensals in the colon of frogs and toads. The life cycle of *O. ranarum* involves asexual reproduction in adult frogs and sexual reproduction in tadpoles.

**Opa•li•na•ta** (o″pə-lĭ-na′tə) a subphylum of parasitic, flat, leaf-like, multinucleate protozoa (phylum Sarcomastigophora) found as endocommensals in anurans and less often in fish, salamanders, and reptiles. They have cilia arranged in multiple oblique longitudinal rows over the entire body surface, but differ from the Ciliophora in that they possess only one type of nucleus (i.e., no differentiated micronuclei and macronuclei) and they reproduce sexually. It comprises one class: Opalinatea.

**Opa•li•na•tea** (o″pə-lĭ-na′te-ə) a class of parasitic ciliated protozoa (subphylum Opalinata, phylum Mastigophora) with characters of the subphylum. It comprises one order: Opalinida.

**opa•line** (o′pə-lēn) [L. *opalus* opal] having the appearance of an opal.

**opa•lin•id** (o″pə-lin′id) 1. pertaining or referring to protozoa of the subphylum Opalinata. 2. any protozoan of the subphylum Opalinata.

**Opa•lin•i•da** (o″pə-lin′ĭ-də) an order of ciliated parasitic protozoa (class Opalinatea, subphylum Opalinata) with characters of the class. *Opalina* is a representative genus.

**opaque** (o-pāk′) [L. *opacus* dark] impervious to light rays, or by extension to x-rays or other electromagnetic radiations; neither transparent nor translucent.

**open** (o′pən) 1. exposed to the air; not covered by unbroken skin. 2. interrupted (as a circuit) so that an electric current cannot pass. 3. not obstructed or closed. 4. pertaining to a clinical trial or other experiment in which both the subjects and the persons administering the test are aware of which treatment is administered to which subject. Cf. *single blind, double blind,* and *triple blind.*

**open•ing** (o′pən-ing) an aperture, orifice, or open space; see also *inlet* and *outlet.* Anatomic nomenclature for various types of openings includes *aditus, apertura, foramen, fossa, hiatus,* and *ostium.*
**o. in adductor magnus muscle,** hiatus tendineus.
**anterior o. of stomach,** ostium pyloricum.
**aortic o.,** ostium aortae.
**aortic o. in diaphragm,** hiatus aorticus.
**atrioventricular o., left,** ostium atrioventriculare sinistrum.
**atrioventricular o., right,** ostium atrioventriculare dextrum.
**o. of bladder,** ostium urethrae internum.
**o. of coronary artery,** see under *ostium.*
**cardiac o.,** ostium cardiacum.
**caval o.,** foramen venae cavae.
**o. of coronary sinus,** ostium sinus coronarii.
**cutaneous o. of male urethra,** ostium urethrae externum masculinae.
**duodenal o. of stomach,** ostium pyloricum.
**esophageal o. in diaphragm,** hiatus oesophageus.
**external o. of aqueduct of vestibule,** apertura externa aqueductus vestibuli.
**external o. of canaliculus of cochlea,** apertura externa canaliculi cochleae.
**o. of frontal sinus,** apertura sinus frontalis.
**o. of Hunter's canal, inferior,** hiatus tendineus.
**ileocecal o.,** ostium ileale.
**inferior o. of pelvis,** apertura pelvis inferior.
**inferior o. of sacral canal,** hiatus sacralis.
**inferior o. of thorax,** apertura thoracis inferior.
**inferior o. of tympanic canaliculus,** apertura inferior canaliculi tympanici.
**o. of inferior vena cava,** ostium venae cavae inferioris.
**o. to lesser sac of peritoneum,** foramen omentale.
**nasal o. of facial skeleton,** apertura piriformis.
**orbital o., o. of orbital cavity, anterior,** aditus orbitalis.
**ovarian o. of uterine tube,** ostium abdominale tubae uterinae.
**pharyngeal o. of auditory tube,** ostium pharyngeum tubae auditivae.
**piriform o.,** apertura piriformis.
**o. of pulmonary trunk,** ostium trunci pulmonalis.
**o's of pulmonary veins,** ostia venarum pulmonalium.
**pyloric o.,** ostium pyloricum.
**saphenous o.,** hiatus saphenus.
**semilunar o. of ethmoid bone,** hiatus semilunaris.
**o. of sphenoidal sinus,** apertura sinus sphenoidalis.
**superior o. of pelvis,** apertura pelvis superior.
**superior o. of thorax,** apertura thoracis superior.
**superior o. of tympanic canaliculus,** apertura superior canaliculi tympanici.
**o. of superior vena cava,** ostium venae cavae superioris.
**tendinous o.,** hiatus tendineus.
**thoracic o., inferior, thoracic o., lower,** apertura thoracis inferior.
**thoracic o., superior, thoracic o., upper,** apertura thoracis superior.
**tympanic o. of auditory tube,** ostium tympanicum tubae auditivae.
**o. for tympanic branch of glossopharyngeal nerve,** apertura inferior canaliculi tympanici.
**tympanic o. of canaliculus of chorda tympani,** apertura tympanica canaliculi chordae tympani.
**uterine o. of uterine tube,** ostium uterinum tubae uterinae.
**o. of vermiform appendix,** ostium appendicis vermiformis.
**vesicourethral o.,** ostium urethrae internum.

**op•er•a•ble** (op′ər-ə-bəl) subject to being operated upon with a reasonable degree of safety; appropriate for surgical removal.

**op•er•ant** (op′ər-ənt) in psychology, any response that is not elicited by specific external stimuli but that recurs at a given rate in a particular set of circumstances. See also *conditioning.*

**op•er•ate** (op′ər-āt) 1. to perform an operation. 2. an individual that has undergone a specific experimental surgical procedure, in contrast to the normal control.

**operating room technician** [MeSH: Operating Room Technicians] the job title formerly used for SURGICAL TECHNOLOGIST.

**op•er•a•tion** (op″ər-a′shən) [L. *operatio*] 1. any act performed with instruments or by the hands of a surgeon; a surgical procedure. 2. the process or act of functioning, doing, or performing.

## Operation

For terms not found here, see also *method, procedure, surgery,* and *technique.*

**Abbe o.,** attachment of a triangular, full-thickness flap from the median portion of the lower lip to fill a defect in the upper lip.

**Adams' o.,** 1. subcutaneous intracapsular division of the neck of the femur for ankylosis of the hip. 2. subcutaneous division of the palmar fascia at various points for Dupuytren's contracture. 3. excision of a wedge-shaped piece from the eyelid for relief of ectropion.

**Akin o.,** resection of the medial prominence of the first metatarsal head and cuneiform osteotomy of the proximal phalanx of the great toe, done for hallux valgus.

**Albee's o.,** operation for ankylosis of the hip, consisting of cutting off the upper surface of the head of the femur and freshening a corresponding point on the acetabulum, and permitting the two freshened surfaces to rest in contact.

**Albee-Delbet o.,** an operation for fracture of the neck of the femur, done by drilling a hole through the trochanter and the neck and head of the femur and inserting a bone peg in this hole.

**Albert's o.,** excision of the knee to secure ankylosis for the cure of flail joint.

**Alexander's o., Alexander-Adams o.,** shortening of the round ligaments to repair displacement of the uterus.

**Alouette's o.,** see under *amputation.*

**Ammon's o.,** 1. blepharoplasty by a flap from the cheek. 2. dacryocystotomy. 3. for epicanthus: resection of a spindle-shaped piece of skin over the bridge of the nose, undermining the flaps of the epicanthal fold and closing with sutures.

**Amussat's o.,** a long transverse incision for exposure of the colon.

**Anagnostakis' o.,** 1. an operation for entropion. 2. an operation for trichiasis.

**Aries-Pitanguy o.,** see under *mammaplasty.*

**Asch o.,** an operation for deflection of the nasal septum by reinserting resected pieces of cartilage and holding them in place with a splint; of historical interest.

**Babcock's o.,** a former method of treating varicose veins, consisting of excision using a long probe with an acorn tip.

**Baldy's o., Baldy-Webster o.,** Webster's o.

**Barkan's o.,** goniotomy.

**Barker's o.,** 1. an excision of the hip joint by an anterior cut. 2. a special method of excising the astragalus by an incision extending from just above the external malleolus forward and inward to the dorsum of the foot.

**Barraquer's o.,** phacoerysis.

**Barsky's o.,** an operation for repair of a cleft hand with a missing central ray and a deep central V-shaped cleft, consisting in closing the cleft, bringing the ring and index fingers closer together, and correcting the associated syndactyly, if present.

**Barton's o.,** an operation for ankylosis consisting of sawing through the bone and removing a V-shaped piece.

**Basset's o.,** a method of dissecting the inguinal glands in radical operations for cancer of the vulva.

**Bassini's o.,** repair of inguinal hernia, with high ligation of the sac, reinforcement of the floor of the canal, and placement of the spermatic cord under the external oblique anastomosis.

**Battle's o.,** an operation for appendicitis in which the rectus muscle is temporarily retracted.

**Beer's o.,** a flap method for cataract.

**Belsey Mark IV o.,** fundoplication for gastroesophageal reflux with the fundus being wrapped 270 degrees around the circumference of the esophagus, leaving its posterior wall free; done through a thoracic incision. Called also *Belsey Mark IV fundoplication.*

**Berger's o.,** interscapulothoracic amputation.

**Berke o.,** an operation for ptosis of the upper eyelid, consisting of (1) a modification of the Blaskovics operation, with resection of the levator muscle through a skin incision and excision of excess muscle, or (2) a modification of the Motais operation, with suspension of the ptotic lid from the superior rectus muscle.

**Bevan's o.,** an operation for an undescended testicle, by which the testicle is brought down permanently into the scrotum.

**Bier's o.,** see under *amputation.*

**Biesenberger's o.,** see under *mammaplasty.*

**Bigelow's o.,** lithotripsy.

**Billroth's o.,** 1. partial resection of the stomach with anastomosis of the severed end of the duodenum to the end of the resected stomach (Billroth I), or with anastomosis of the resected stomach to the jejunum (Billroth II). Called also *Billroth gastrectomy.* 2. excision of the tongue by making a transverse incision below the symphysis of the jaw and joining it by two incisions, one on each side, parallel to the body of the mandible, with preliminary ligation of the lingual arteries.

**Blair-Brown o.,** repair of a cleft lip by the use of a lateral flap one-half the length of the lip.

**Blalock-Hanlon o.,** a palliative operation for transposition of the great vessels, consisting of the creation of an interatrial septal defect.

**Blalock-Taussig o.,** the side-to-side anastomosis of the left subclavian artery to the left pulmonary artery (sometimes the right subclavian to the right pulmonary artery) in order to shunt some of the systemic circulation into the pulmonary circulation; performed as palliative treatment of tetralogy of Fallot or other congenital anomalies associated with insufficient pulmonary arterial flow.

**Blaskovics o.,** an operation for ptosis of the upper eyelid, consisting of excision of the levator muscle and the tarsus through a conjunctival approach.

**Bozeman's o.,** hysterocystocleisis.

**Bricker's o.,** the surgical creation of an ileal conduit with a flat stoma for the collection of urine; the flat contour is achieved by suturing the ileal mucosa to the skin.

**Brock's o.,** transventricular closed valvotomy.

**Browne o.,** a urethroplasty for hypospadias repair, in which an intact strip of epithelium is left on the ventral surface of the penis to form the roof of the urethra, and the floor of the urethra is formed by epithelialization from the lateral wound margins.

**Brunschwig's o.,** a technique of pancreatoduodenectomy.

**Buck's o.,** cuneiform excision of the patella and the ends of tibia and fibula.

**Burow's o.,** a method of excising triangles of skin at the base of the pedicle of a skin flap to facilitate advancement.

**Caldwell-Luc o.,** 1. antrostomy in which an opening is made into the maxillary sinus by way of an incision into the supradental fossa opposite the premolar teeth, usually done to remove tooth roots or abnormal tissue from the sinus. 2. in compound zygomaticomaxillary fractures, the packing of the maxillary sinus by approaching the antrum through the canine fossa of the maxilla above the tooth apices, thus allowing reduction of displaced fragments of the zygoma by upward and outward pressure. Called also *Luc's o.*

**Carpue's o.,** Indian rhinoplasty.

**Cecil's o.,** 1. a two-stage urethroplasty for hypospadias repair, with construction of a new urethral segment buried in the scrotum, followed by separation of the new urethra from the scrotum. 2. a three-stage urethroplasty for repair of urethral stricture, with excision of the strictured area through an incision on the ventral surface of the penis, followed by the steps of the operation used for hypospadias repair.

**Charles' o.,** treatment of elephantiasis and other types of massive lymphedema of the lower limb by excision of subcutaneous tissue followed by skin grafting.

**Chopart's o.,** see under *amputation.*

**Colonna's o.,** 1. a reconstruction operation for intracapsular fracture of the femoral neck. 2. a common type of capsular arthroplasty of the hip.

**Commando's o.,** an operation for management of oral cancer, consisting in resection of the primary lesion and the regional lymphatic nodes.

**concrete o's,** a stage in reasoning or functioning usually seen in children between the ages of approximately 7 and 11, following the stage of preoperational thinking and preceding that of formal operations; it is characterized by comprehension of relational terms, decrease in egocentricity and increase in the ability to appreciate the perspective of others, understanding of the reversibility of events and ideas as well as of conservation of volume and quantity, and the beginning of logical thought, although it is initially restricted to objects immediately present.

**Conway o.,** see under *mammaplasty.*

**cosmetic o.,** one intended to remove or correct a deformity in an esthetically acceptable manner.

**Cotte's o.,** removal of the presacral nerve.

**Cotting's o.,** operation for ingrowing toenail, consisting in cutting off the side of the toe down to and including the ingrowing edge of the nail.

**Dandy's o.,** trigeminal rhizotomy using an approach through the posterior cranial fossa.

**Daviel's o.,** extraction of cataract through a corneal incision without cutting the iris.

**Denis Browne o.,** Browne o.

**Denonvilliers' o.,** plastic correction of a defective ala nasi by transferring a triangular flap from the adjacent side of the nose.

**Dieffenbach's o.,** plastic closure of triangular defects by displacing a quadrangular flap toward one side of the triangle.

**Dittel's o.,** enucleation of an enlarged prostate through an external incision; of historical interest.

**Duhamel o.,** the treatment of congenital megacolon by a modification of the pull-through operation and establishment of a longitudinal anastomosis between the proximal ganglionated segment of colon and the rectum, leaving the rectum in situ.

**Dührssen's o.,** vaginofixation of the uterus.

**Duplay's o.,** a method of urethroplasty for repair of hypospadias, employing a buried skin strip.

**Dupuy-Dutemps o.,** blepharoplasty of the lower lid with tissue from the opposing lid.

**Dupuytren's o.,** shoulder disarticulation.

**Elliot's o.,** a method of trephining the sclerocornea for the relief of increased tension in glaucoma.

**Emmet's o.,** 1. a method of repairing a lacerated perineum. 2. trachelorrhaphy, or suture of the edges of a lacerated cervix uteri. 3. surgical creation of a vesicovaginal fistula to secure drainage of the bladder in cystitis.

**equilibrating o.,** tenotomy of the direct antagonist of a paralyzed eye muscle.

**Esser's o.,** epithelial inlay.

**Estes' o.,** implantation of an ovary into a uterine cornu; performed for sterility when the tubes are absent.

**Estlander's o.,** 1. resection of one or more ribs in empyema so as to allow the chest wall to collapse and close the abnormal cavity; of historical interest. 2. rotation of a triangular flap from the side of the lower lip to fill a defect in the lateral upper lip.

**Eversbusch's o.,** an operation for ptosis of the upper eyelid, consisting of resection of the levator muscle through a skin incision.

**exploratory o.,** surgical incision into an area of the body followed by inspection and palpation of organs and tissues to determine the cause of unexplained symptoms.

**Fergusson's o.,** removal of the maxilla through an incision running along the junction of the nose with the cheek, around the ala of the nose to the median line, and then down to bisect the upper lip. Called also *Fergusson's incision.*

**Finney's o.,** see under *pyloroplasty.*

**flap o.,** 1. any operation involving the raising of a flap of tissue. 2. in periodontics, an operation to secure greater access to granulation tissue and osseous defects, consisting of detachment of the gingivae, the alveolar mucosa, and/or a portion of the palatal mucosa. 3. see under *amputation.*

**formal o's,** a form of thinking following the stage of concrete operations and representing the final, most mature state of thinking; usually occurring after the age of 11 and characterized by the emergence of true logical thought, with the capability for deductive reasoning, abstract thinking, formulation and testing of hypotheses, appreciation for multiple perspectives on an issue, and the manipulation of ideas and concepts.

**Fothergill o.,** Manchester o.

**Franco's o.,** suprapubic cystotomy.

**Frank's o.,** Ssabanejew-Frank o.

**Frazier-Spiller o.,** trigeminal rhizotomy using an approach through the middle cranial fossa.

**Fredet-Ramstedt o.,** pyloromyotomy.

**Freund's o.,** resection of cartilages of the chest wall to restore elasticity and improve respiratory mechanics; of historical interest.

**Freyer's o.,** a method of performing suprapubic enucleation of the hypertrophied prostate; of historical interest.

**Frost-Lang o.,** insertion of a gold ball to take the place of an enucleated eyeball.

**Fukala's o.,** removal of the lens of the eye for the treatment of marked myopia.

**Fuller's o.,** perineal incision and drainage of the seminal vesicles; of historical interest.

**Gifford's o.,** delimiting keratotomy.

**Gigli's o.,** lateral section of the os pubis by means of Gigli's wire saw; done to permit delivery of the fetus in difficult labor.

**Gilliam's o.,** an operation for retroversion of the uterus by drawing a loop of each round ligament through the abdominal wall and fixing the loops to the abdominal fascia.

**Gillies o.,** 1. operation for correction of ectropion utilizing a split-thickness skin graft and a mold. 2. a technique for reducing fractures of the zygoma and zygomatic arch through an incision in the temporal region above the hairline.

**Girdlestone o.,** Girdlestone resection.

**Glenn o.,** an operation for congenital cyanotic heart disease, consisting of anastomosis of the superior vena cava to the right pulmonary artery.

**Gonin's o.,** treatment of retinal detachment by thermocautery of the fissure in the retina performed through an opening in the sclera.

**Graefe's o.,** removal of the cataractous lens by a scleral cut, with laceration of the capsule and iridectomy.

**Gritti's o.,** see under *amputation.*

**Grondahl-Finney o.,** esophagogastroplasty in which the orifice between the esophagus and stomach is enlarged.

**Guyon's o.,** see under *amputation.*

**Halsted's o.,** 1. an operation for inguinal hernia with transposition of the spermatic cord above the external oblique aponeurosis. 2. radical mastectomy.

**Hancock's o.,** see under *amputation.*

**Hartley-Krause o.,** excision of the gasserian ganglion and its roots to relieve trigeminal neuralgia; of historical interest.

**Hartmann's o.,** see under *procedure.*

**Haultain's o.,** a modification of the Huntington operation (q.v.) for replacement of a chronically inverted uterus, involving a posterior incision in the uterus through the cervical ring.

**Heath's o.,** division of the ascending rami of the lower jaw with a saw for ankylosis, performed within the oral cavity; rarely done.

**Heine's o.,** cyclodialysis in glaucoma.

**Heineke-Mikulicz o.,** see under *pyloroplasty.*

**Heller's o.,** esophagocardiomyotomy.

**Herbert's o.,** displacement of a wedge-shaped flap of sclera in order to form a filtering cicatrix in glaucoma.

**Hey's o.,** see under *amputation.*

**Hibbs' o.,** a spinal fusion operation done by fracturing the spinous processes of the vertebrae and pressing the tip of each downward to rest in the denuded area caused by the fracture of its elbow below.

**Hochenegg's o.,** total excision of the rectum with preservation of the anal sphincter; of historical interest.

**Hoffa's o., Hoffa-Lorenz o.,** Lorenz's o.

**Holth's o.,** excision of the sclera by punch operation.

**Homans' o.,** a formerly common treatment for elephantiasis and other types of massive edema of the lower limb, consisting of excision of subcutaneous tissue and redundant skin on the lateral and medial aspects.

**Horsley's o.,** excision of an area of motor cortex for relief of athetoid and convulsive movements of an upper extremity; of historical interest.

**Huggins' o.,** orchiectomy performed for cancer of the prostate.

**Hunter's o.,** a former method of treating aneurysm, consisting of ligation of the artery on the proximal side of the aneurysm above the first collateral.

**Huntington's o.,** transabdominal repair of a chronically inverted uterus. It is done by grasping the invaginated portion of the uterus with forceps; as the uterus is pulled up, additional forceps are placed sequentially lower down, and upward traction is applied. After the uterus is in place, the position is maintained by packing through the vagina.

**Indian o.,** see under *rhinoplasty.*

**interposition o.,** Watkins' o.

**interval o.,** an operation performed during the interval between two acute attacks of a disease, as in appendicitis.

**Irving's sterilization o.,** a method of tubal ligation in which the uterine tubes are ligated and severed and the proximal ends are sewn into the myometrium.

**Italian o.,** tagliacotian rhinoplasty.

**Jaboulay's o.,** hemipelvectomy.

**Jantene o.,** a type of arterial switch procedure (q.v.).

**Kader's o.,** gastrostomy by which the feeding tube is introduced through a valvelike flap which closes on withdrawal of the tube.

**Kasai o.,** portoenterostomy.

**Kazanjian's o.,** 1. a technique of surgical extension of the buccal vestibular sulcus of edentulous ridges to increase their height and to improve denture retention. 2. the use of extraskeletal fixation for support in compound zygomaticomaxillary fractures: a small hole is drilled through the infraorbital rim, and a stainless steel wire is inserted with both ends brought out through the wound, where they are twisted together into a loop or hook. Rubber band traction between the suspension wire and an outrigger on a head cap provides support for the zygomatic fragments.

**Keller o.,** sagittal resection of the medial prominence of the first metatarsal head and excision of the base of the proximal phalanx of the great toe; done for hallux valgus.

**Kelly's o.,** an operation for correction of stress incontinence in women; the site of the internal urinary sphincter is identified with a balloon catheter and the connective tissue between the vagina and the urethra and the floor of the bladder are sutured to form a wide shelf of firm tissue supporting the urethra and bladder.

**Killian's o.,** excision of the anterior wall of the frontal sinus, removal of the diseased tissue, and formation of a permanent communication with the nose.

**Killian-Freer o.,** submucous resection of the nasal septum, including the septal cartilage, vomer, and perpendicular plate of the ethmoid.

**King's o.,** arytenoidopexy.

**Knapp's o.,** (for cataract), the formation of a peripheral opening in the capsule behind the iris, without iridectomy.

**Kocher's o.,** 1. a method of excising the ankle joint by a cut below the outer malleolus, division of the peroneal tendons, removal of the diseased tissues, and suture of the divided tendons. 2. a method of reducing a subcoracoid dislocation of the humerus. 3. excision of the tongue through an incision extending from the symphysis of the jaw to the hyoid bone and thence to the mastoid process. 4. see under *maneuver.* 5. a method of pylorectomy.

**Kondoleon's o.,** a formerly common treatment for elephantiasis and other types of lymphedema by the removal of strips of subcutaneous tissue; it was later modified as Homans' operation.

**Körte-Ballance o.,** anastomosis of the facial and hypoglossal nerves.

**Kraske's o.,** removal of the coccyx and part of the sacrum for access to a carcinoma of the rectum.

**Krause's o.,** extradural excision of the gasserian ganglion for trigeminal neuralgia; of historical interest.

**Krönlein's o.,** resection of the outer wall of the orbit for the removal of an orbital tumor without excising the eye.

**Küstner o.,** replacement of an inverted uterus through an incision made in the cervix and uterus along the posterior surface.

**Lagrange's o.,** sclerectoiridectomy.

**Landolt's o.,** the formation of a lower eyelid with a double pedicle or bridge flap of eyelid skin taken from the upper lid.

**Lane's o.,** the operation of dividing the ileum near the cecum, closing the distal portion and anastomosing the proximal end with the upper part of the rectum or lower part of the sigmoid, thus eliminating the colon from the fecal current.

**Lapidus o.,** a procedure for correction of hallux valgus, involving wedge resection and fusion of the innermost cuneometatarsal joint and establishment of a bridge between the bases of the first and second metatarsals.

**Larrey's o.,** see under *amputation.*

**Latzko's o.,** 1. Latzko's cesarean section. 2. a method of repairing a vesicovaginal fistula by using mucosa denuded from the posterior wall of the vagina as a flap to cover the fistula.

**Le Fort's o., Le Fort-Neugebauer o.,** the operation of uniting the anterior and posterior vaginal walls along the middle line for the repair or prevention of prolapse of the uterus.

**Lempert's fenestration o.,** an operation for otosclerosis, consisting of drilling a small window into the lateral semicircular canal and then placing a flap of skin over the fistula.

**Lisfranc's o.,** 1. see under *amputation.* 2. shoulder disarticulation.

**Lorenz's o.,** an operation for congenital dislocation of the hip, consisting in reduction of the dislocation, and keeping the head of the femur fixed against the rudimentary acetabulum until a socket is formed.

**Lowsley's o.,** an operation for repair of simple epispadias, consisting in closing the glandular cleft urethra, splitting the glans, and burying the repaired urethra deep in the soft tissue so that the orifice will be positioned at the normal site.

**Luc's o.,** Caldwell-Luc o.

**Lynch's o.,** incision of the frontal sinus and removal of its floor and contents; done in cases of expanding mucoceles, pyoceles, and tumors of the sinus.

**McBride o.,** resection of the medial prominence of the first metatarsal head, medial capsulorrhaphy, resection of the fibular sesamoid, and transfer of the adductor tendon to the neck of the first metatarsal; done for hallux valgus.

**McBurney's o.,** an operation for inguinal hernia: the sac is exposed, ligated, and cut off at the internal ring; the skin is turned in and stitched to the underlying tendinous and ligamentous structures.

**McDonald o.,** an operation for incompetent cervix, in which the cervical os is closed with a purse-string suture.

**Macewen's o.,** an operation for the radical cure of hernia by closing the internal ring with a pad made of the hernial sac.

**McGill's o.,** suprapubic transvesical prostatectomy.

**magnet o.,** removal of a fragment of steel or iron from the eyeball by means of a powerful magnet.

**major o.,** an operation of major surgery (q.v.).

**Manchester o.,** an operation for uterine prolapse comprising dilation and curettage, anterior repair, amputation of the vaginal portion of the cervix, shortening of the cardinal ligaments, and posterior colpoperineorrhaphy.

**Marshall-Marchetti-Krantz o.,** an operation for the correction of stress incontinence, the anterior portion of the urethra, vesical neck, and bladder being sutured to the posterior surface of the pubic bone.

**Matas' o.,** endoaneurysmorrhaphy.

**Maydl's o.,** 1. colostomy in which the colon is drawn out through the wound and maintained in position by placing a glass rod beneath it until adhesions have formed; of historical interest. 2. insertion of the ureters into the rectum for exstrophy of the bladder; of historical interest.

**Mayo's o.,** 1. excision of the pyloric end of the stomach, followed by closure of both duodenum and stomach and the construction of an independent posterior gastrojejunostomy. 2. a former method of treating umbilical hernia, consisting of excision followed by transverse overlapping of the abdominal aponeuroses. 3. a former method of treating varicose veins, consisting of removal with a long-handled stripper.

**Meller's o.,** an operation for excision of the tear sac.

**Mikulicz's o.,** 1. removal of the sternocleidomastoid muscle for torticollis. 2. Heineke-Mikulicz pyloroplasty. 3. tarsectomy in which the heel, os calcis, and astragalus are removed, the articular surfaces of the tibia, fibula, cuboid, and scaphoid are excised, and the foot brought into line with the leg; called also *Vladimiroff o.* 4. enterectomy in stages, including exteriorization of the section of intestine to be resected, usually the colon; resection of the exteriorized loop; elimination of the fecal fistula by crushing the spur between the two barrels of the anastomosis; and closure of the fecal fistula.

**Miles' o.,** surgical treatment for cancer of the lower sigmoid and rectum, with removal of the pelvic colon, mesocolon, and adjacent lymph nodes, and wide perineal excision of the rectum and anus, and a permanent colostomy.

**Millin-Read o.,** an operation for the correction of stress incontinence employing the suprapubic approach.

**minor o.,** an operation of minor surgery (q.v.).

**Mitchell o.,** a procedure for correction of hallux valgus, involving distal osteotomy of the first metatarsal.

**Moschcowitz's o.,** an operation for the repair of a femoral hernia by the inguinal approach.

**Motais' o.,** an operation for ptosis, consisting of transplanting the middle portion of the tendon of the superior rectus muscle of the eyeball into the upper lid.

**Mules' o.,** evisceration of the eyeball, with insertion of an artificial vitreous.

**Mustard o.,** correction of transposition of great vessels by construction of an intra-atrial baffle, composed of pericardial tissue or synthetic material, to direct the systemic and pulmonary venous blood into the left and right ventricles, respectively.

**Naffziger's o.,** excision of the superior and lateral walls of the orbit for exophthalmos.

**Nissen o.,** see under *fundoplication.*

**Ober's o.,** medial subtalar syndesmotomy for clubfoot.

**Olshausen's o.,** the operation of fixing or suturing the uterus to the abdominal wall for the cure of retroversion.

**Ombrédanne's o.,** transscrotal orchiopexy.

**open o.,** an operation in which the tissues and organs are exposed to view through a surgical incision.

**Partsch's o.,** a technique for marsupialization of dental cyst.

**Patey's o.,** modified radical mastectomy.

**Péan's o.,** hip joint amputation in which the vessels are ligated as the operation goes on.

**Pereyra o.,** a surgical technique for the correction of stress incontinence: a loop of suture or other material is inserted through the paraurethral tissue near the bladder neck and attached to the abdominal fascia in order to elevate the bladder.

**Phelps' o.,** an open and direct incision through the sole and inner side of the foot, done for talipes.

**Phemister o.,** use of an onlay graft of cancellous bone without internal fixation, for treatment of a stable but ununited fracture.

**plastic o.,** one in which the shape of a part or the character of its covering is altered by transplantation of tissue, etc.

**Polya's o.,** anastomosis of the transected end of the stomach to the side of the jejunum following subtotal gastrectomy.

**Pomeroy's o.,** a method of sterilization in the female, in which the fallopian tube is picked up about two inches from the uterine cornua, a chromic gut ligature tied around the loop without crushing it, and the tied loop is then resected.

**Potts o.,** anastomosis between the descending aorta and left pulmonary artery as palliative treatment of congenital pulmonary stenosis. Called also *Potts anastomosis* or *shunt.*

**pull-through o.,** surgery on the intestine in which a diseased segment is removed and a proximal segment is pulled down and through the part just beyond the removed part. See *ileoanal pull-through anastomosis, Duhamel o., Soave o.,* and *Swenson's o.*

**radical o.,** see under *surgery.*

**Ramstedt's o.,** pyloromyotomy.

**Rastelli o.,** an operation for correction of large ventricular septal defects with pulmonary infundibular and valvular stenosis; an intraventricular patch is placed so that blood flows through the septal defect and out the aorta, and a prosthesis is placed to establish continuity between the right ventricle and the pulmonary artery.

**Regnoli's o.,** excision of the tongue through a median opening below the lower jaw, reaching from the chin to the hyoid bone.

**Ridell o.,** obliteration of the frontal sinus by removal of the anterior wall and floor and sometimes posterior walls of the sinus; for treatment of malignant tumors.

**Roux-en-Y o.,** see under *anastomosis.*

**Saemisch's o.,** transfixion of the cornea and of the base of the ulcer for the cure of hypopyon.

**Scanzoni's o.,** see under *maneuver.*

**Schauta's o.,** radical hysterectomy by the vaginal route.

**Schede's o.,** 1. resection of the thorax for chronic empyema. 2. in cases of necrotic bone, excision of dead bone and diseased tissue, after which the cavity is permitted to fill with a blood clot that is kept moist and aseptic and eventually becomes organized.

**Scheie's o.,** 1. scleral cauterization with peripheral iridectomy for treatment of glaucoma. 2. a technique for needling and aspiration of cataract.

**Sédillot's o.,** a flap operation for restoring the upper lip.

**Senning o.,** surgical creation of two interatrial channels for crossing the systemic and pulmonary venous circulations in transposition of the great vessels.

**Serre's o.,** an operation for correction of skin contractures that distort the angle of the mouth, involving switching of a skin and subcutaneous tissue flap from one lip to another.

**Shirodkar's o.,** an operation for incompetent cervix in which the cervical os is closed with a surrounding purse-string suture.

**Silver o.,** resection of the medial prominence of the first metatarsal head, medial capsulorrhaphy of the first metatarsophalangeal joint, and sectioning of the adductor tendon; done for hallux valgus.

**Sistrunk o.,** a surgical procedure for removal of thyroglossal cysts and sinuses.

**Smith's o.,** extraction of an immature cataract with an intact capsule.

**Soave o.,** treatment of congenital megacolon by an endorectal pull-through operation, with normal colon connected to the anus through a rectum denuded of mucosa.

**Spinelli's o.,** the operation of splitting the anterior wall of the prolapsed inverted uterus, reversing the organ, and restoring it to the correct position.

**Ssabanejew-Frank o.,** a method of performing gastrostomy by pulling a cone of the stomach through an incision in the left rectus muscle and suturing it to the skin.

**State o.,** the treatment of congenital megacolon (Hirschsprung's disease) by end-to-end anastomosis of the colon from above the aganglionic segment to the upper part of the rectum.

**Stein o.**, an operation for reconstruction of the lower lip with flaps taken from the upper lip.

**Steindler o.**, surgical correction of pes cavus by stripping muscle and fascia from the plantar calcaneal surface.

**Stokes' o.**, Gritti-Stokes amputation.

**Strömbeck o.**, see under *mammaplasty*.

**Sturmdorf's o.**, conical excision of the diseased endocervix.

**Swenson's o.**, an operation for congenital megacolon, consisting of removal of the rectum and the aganglionic segment of the intestine and an ileoanal pull-through procedure with preservation of the anal sphincters.

**Syme's o.**, see under *amputation*.

**tagliacotian o.**, see under *rhinoplasty*.

**Talma's o.**, omentopexy in treatment of ascites; of historical interest.

**Tanner's o.**, an operation for bleeding esophageal varices in which the terminal end of the esophagus, the cardia, and the proximal portion of the stomach are freed of all external vascular and ligamentous connections, and the stomach is transected below the cardia.

**Teale's o.**, see under *amputation*.

**Thiersch's o.**, removal of thin split-thickness skin grafts by means of a razor, skin-graft cutting knife, or a dermatome.

**Thompson's o.**, a formerly common treatment for elephantiasis and other types of massive lymphedema of the lower limb, consisting of excision of some subcutaneous tissue and burying of a dermal flap among the underlying muscles.

**Torek o.**, 1. an operation for an undescended testicle. 2. an operation for the excision of the thoracic part of the esophagus; of historical interest.

**Torkildsen's o.**, ventriculocisternal shunt.

**Toti's o.**, dacryocystorhinostomy.

**Toupet's o.**, see under *fundoplication*.

**Trendelenburg's o.**, 1. an early method for treating varicose veins, consisting of ligation of the great saphenous vein. 2. synchondroseotomy. 3. transthoracic pulmonary embolectomy.

**van Hook's o.**, ureteroureterostomy.

**Vineberg o.**, implantation of the internal mammary artery into the myocardium to enhance the growth of collateral circulation.

**Vladimiroff o.**, Mikulicz's o., def. 3.

**von Burow's o.**, Burow's o.

**Waters' o.**, a form of extraperitoneal cesarean section.

**Waterston o.**, anastomosis between the ascending aorta and right pulmonary artery as palliative treatment of congenital pulmonary stenosis. Called also *Waterston anastomosis* or *shunt*.

**Watkins' o.**, an operation for prolapse and procidentia uteri in which the bladder is separated from the anterior wall of the uterus so that the uterus is left in a position to support the entire bladder. Called also *interposition o.*

**Webster's o.**, for retrodisplacement of the uterus: the round ligaments are passed through the perforated broad ligaments and fixed to the back of the uterus.

**Wertheim's o.**, radical hysterectomy; removal of the uterus, tubes, parametrium, tissues surrounding the upper vagina, and pelvic lymphatics.

**Whipple's o.**, see under *procedure*.

**White's o.**, castration for hypertrophy of the prostate.

**Whitehead's o.**, treatment of hemorrhoids by excision.

**Whitman's o.**, 1. an operation for arthroplasty of the hip joint. 2. a method of astragalectomy.

**Witzel's o.**, see under *gastrostomy*.

**Wölfler's o.**, anterior gastrojejunostomy for pyloric obstruction; of historical interest.

**Young's o.**, 1. an operation for penile epispadias, with formation of a new urethral tube. 2. perineal prostatectomy.

**Ziegler's o.**, V-shaped iridectomy for forming an artificial pupil.

---

**op·er·a·tive** (op′ər-ə-tiv) [L. *operativus*] 1. pertaining to an operation. 2. effective; not inert.

**op·er·a·tor** (op′ər-a-tor) [L. "worker"] 1. one who performs an operation, or operates a mechanical device. 2. operator gene.

**op·er·a·tory** (op′ər-ə-tor″e) the working area of a dental office, in which treatment is provided to patients.

**oper·cu·la** (o-per′ku-lə) [L.] plural of *operculum*.

**oper·cu·lar** (o-per′ku-lər) pertaining to an operculum.

**oper·cu·late** (o-pər′ku-lāt) having an operculum; said of an ascus.

**oper·cu·lec·to·my** (o-per″ku-lek′tə-me) the surgical removal of a mucosal flap partially or completely covering an unerupted tooth.

**oper·cu·li·tis** (o-per″ku-li′tis) pericoronitis.

**oper·cu·lum** (o-per′ku-ləm) pl. *oper′cula* [L.] 1. a lid or covering structure, such as the mucous plug obstructing the cervix of the gravid uterus in various animals. 2. one of the opercula of the insula; see *pars opercularis gyri frontalis inferioris, o. frontoparietale,* and *o. temporale*. 3. in fungi, a small cap on an ascus that pops open when the mature organism is ready to eject its spores.

**cartilaginous o.**, discus articularis articulationis temporomandibularis.

**dental o.**, the hood of gingival tissue overlying the crown of an erupting tooth; called also *odontoclamis* and *tooth hood*.

**frontal o., o. fronta′le** 1. [TA] the portion of the insular opercula within the frontal lobe; it corresponds to the pars orbitalis, pars triangularis, and pars opercularis of the inferior frontal gyrus together with the lower end of the precentral gyrus. 2. the portion of the insular opercula lying between the anterior and ascending rami of the lateral sulcus, corresponding to the pars opercularis gyri frontalis inferioris; when used this way, the term is contrasted with the operculum frontoparietale. It may also be expanded to include the pars orbitalis gyri frontalis inferioris, in which case the frontal operculum is said to have two parts: frontal and orbital. 3. the anterior portion of the operculum frontoparietale, corresponding to the pars opercularis gyri frontalis inferior.

**frontoparietal o., o. frontoparieta′le,** the part of the cerebrum that covers the upper portion of the insula; from anterior to posterior, it consists of the part of the inferior frontal gyrus behind the ascending branch of the lateral sulcus (corresponding to the pars opercularis gyri frontalis inferior), the lower ends of the precentral and postcentral gyri, and the anterior and lower part of the inferior parietal lobule. The term is used in contrast with operculum frontale (def. 2) (q.v.), although its frontal, as opposed to parietal, portion may itself be called *operculum frontale* (see *o. frontale,* def. 3).

**opercula of insula,** the areas of the cerebral cortex overlapping above and below the insular lobe (insula) of the cerebral hemisphere forming part of the lips of the lateral sulcus, and separated by the rami of the lateral sulcus; see *o. frontale, o. frontoparietale,* and *o. temporale*.

**occipital o.**, a part of the occipital lobe of the brain demarcated by the sulcus lunatus, when the latter structure is present.

**parietal o., o. parieta′le** [TA], the portion of the insular opercula within the parietal lobe, corresponding to the lower end of the postcentral gyrus and the anterior and lower part of the inferior parietal lobule. It has often been considered as a portion of the operculum frontoparietale (q.v.).

**temporal o., o. tempora′le** [TA], the parts of the superior temporal gyrus and transverse temporal gyri that cover the lower portion of the insula.

**trophoblastic o.**, the plug of trophoblast that helps close the gap in the endometrium made by the implanting blastocyst.

**op·er·on** (op′ər-on) [L. *opera* work + Gr. *-on* neuter ending] [MeSH: Operon] in prokaryotes, a chromosomal segment constituting a functional unit of transcription and so of genetic regulation. It comprises one or more structural genes, their promoter, and an operator region that through interaction with a regulator protein controls the structural genes.

**ophi·a·sis** (o-fi′ə-sis) [Gr. *ophis* snake] a form of alopecia areata of long duration, involving the temporal and occipital margins of the scalp in a continuous band.

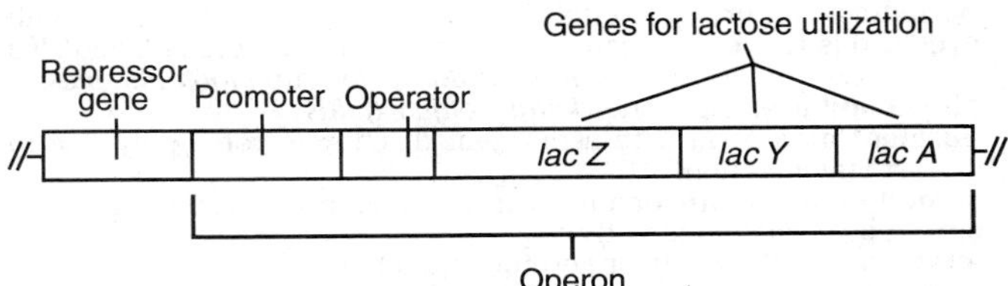


*Escherichia coli lac* operon. In the absence of lactose, the product of the repressor gene binds the operator region and prevents transcription of genes involved in lactose utilization by blocking movement of the RNA polymerase from promoter to structural gene region; the operon is repressed. If lactose is added, an inducer binds the repressor protein, lessening its affinity for the operator. The RNA polymerase can then proceed from promoter to structural genes, so that operon is derepressed, or expressed.

**Ophid·ia** (o-fid′e-ə) [Gr. *ophidion* serpent] a suborder of Reptilia, the snakes. See table at *snake.*

**ophi·di·a·sis** (o″fĭ-di′ə-sis) ophidism.

**ophid·ic** (o-fid′ik) pertaining to, caused by, or derived from snakes.

**ophi·dism** (o′fĭ-diz-əm) poisoning by snake venom.

**Oph·i·oph·a·gus** (of″e-of′ə-gəs) [Gr. *ophis* snake + *phagein* to eat] a genus of venomous snakes of the family Elapidae. *O. han′nah* is the king cobra. See also table at *snake.*

**ophi·o·tox·emia** (o″fe-o-tok-se′me-ə) [Gr. *ophis* snake + *toxemia*] poisoning by snake venom.

**ophi·tox·emia** (o″fe-tok-se′me-ə) ophiotoxemia.

**Oph·ry·o·gle·ni·na** (of″re-o-glə-ni′nə) [Gr. *ophrys* eyebrow + *glēnē* socket] a suborder of large, chiefly freshwater, histophagous ciliate protozoa of the order Hymenostomatida, characterized by a polymorphous life cycle and an oral apparatus including three ciliary organelles on the left and an associated watchglass organelle on the right. Several species cause disease in marine and freshwater fish, resulting in great economic loss. *Ichthyophthirius* is a representative genus.

**oph·ry·on** (of′re-on) [Gr. *ophrys* eyebrow + *-on* neuter ending] the middle point of the transverse supraorbital line.

**oph·ry·o·sis** (of″re-o′sis) [Gr. *ophrys* eyebrow] spasm of the eyebrow.

**Oph·thaine** (of′thān) trademark for a preparation of proparacaine hydrochloride.

**oph·thal·mag·ra** (of″thəl-mag′rə) [*ophthalm-* + *-agra*] sudden pain in the eye.

**oph·thal·mal·gia** (of″thəl-mal′jə) [*ophthalm-* + *-algia*] pain in the eye.

**oph·thal·ma·tro·phia** (of″thəl-mə-tro′fe-ə) [*ophthalm-* + *atrophia*] atrophy of the eye.

**oph·thal·mec·to·my** (of″thəl-mek′tə-me) [*ophthalm-* + *-ectomy*] the surgical removal of an eye; enucleation of the eyeball.

**oph·thal·men·ceph·a·lon** (of″thəl-mən-sef′ə-lon) [*ophthalm-* + *encephalon*] the retina, optic nerve, and visual apparatus of the brain.

**oph·thal·mia** (of-thal′me-ə) [Gr., from *ophthalmos* eye] severe inflammation of the eye or of the conjunctiva or deeper structures of the eye.
**actinic ray o.,** actinic conjunctivitis.
**Brazilian o.,** keratomalacia.
**catarrhal o.,** a severe form of simple conjunctivitis.
**caterpillar o.,** o. nodosa.
**contagious o.,** infectious keratoconjunctivitis.
**o. eczemato′sa,** phlyctenulosis.
**Egyptian o.,** trachoma.
**electric o., flash o.,** actinic conjunctivitis.
**gonorrheal o.,** acute and severe purulent ophthalmia due to gonorrheal infection.
**granular o.,** trachoma.
**hepatic o.,** retinochoroidal degeneration with nyctalopia due to liver disease.
**infectious o.,** infectious keratoconjunctivitis.
**metastatic o.,** choroiditis due to metastasis or to pyemia.
**migratory o.,** sympathetic o.
**mucous o.,** catarrhal o.
**o. neonato′rum,** any hyperacute purulent conjunctivitis occurring during the first ten days of life, usually contracted during birth from infected vaginal discharge of the mother; it formerly referred only to gonorrheal infections. An iatrogenic form sometimes occurs after administration of silver nitrate. Called also *neonatal conjunctivitis.*
**neuroparalytic o.,** keratitis due to lesion of branches of the fifth nerve or of the gasserian ganglion.
**o. nivia′lis,** snow blindness.
**o. nodo′sa,** inflammation of the conjunctiva produced by caterpillar hairs, and marked by the formation of a round, gray swelling where each hair is embedded. Called also *nodular conjunctivitis.*
**periodic o.,** recurrent uveitis in horses; it may occur in one or both eyes and is the leading cause of blindness in the horse. Called also *equine recurrent uveitis, recurrent iridocyclitis,* and *moon blindness.*
**phlyctenular o.,** see under *keratoconjunctivitis.*
**purulent o.,** a form with a purulent discharge, commonly due to gonorrheal infection.
**scrofulous o.,** keratoconjunctivitis associated with tuberculosis.
**spring o.,** vernal conjunctivitis.
**strumous o.,** phlyctenular keratoconjunctivitis.
**sympathetic o., transferred o.,** granulomatous inflammation of the uveal tract of the uninjured eye (the sympathizing eye) following some weeks after a wound involving the uveal tract of the other eye (the exciting eye). The end result is bilateral granulomatous inflammation of the entire uveal tract. Called also *sympathetic uveitis.*
**ultraviolet ray o.,** actinic conjunctivitis.
**varicose o.,** a variety associated with varicosity of the veins of the conjunctiva.

**oph·thal·mi·ac** (of-thal′me-ak) a person affected with ophthalmia.

**oph·thal·mi·at·rics** (of″thəl-me-at′riks) [*ophthalm-* + *-iatrics*] the treatment of eye diseases.

**oph·thal·mic** (of-thal′mik) pertaining to the eye.

**oph·thal·mit·ic** (of″thəl-mit′ik) pertaining to ophthalmitis.

**oph·thal·mi·tis** (of″thəl-mi′tis) [*ophthalm-* + *-itis*] inflammation of the eye.

**ophthalm(o)-** [Gr. *ophthalmos* eye] a combining form denoting relationship to the eye.

**oph·thal·mo·blen·nor·rhea** (of-thal″mo-blen″o-re′ə) [*ophthalmo-* + *blennorhea*] gonorrheal or purulent ophthalmia.

**oph·thal·mo·cele** (of-thal′mo-sēl) exophthalmos.

**oph·thal·mo·co·pia** (of-thal″mo-ko′pe-ə) [*ophthalmo-* + Gr. *kopos* weariness] asthenopia, or eyestrain; fatigue of the eyes.

**oph·thal·mo·des·mi·tis** (of-thal″mo-dez-mi′tis) [*ophthalmo-* + *desmitis*] inflammation of the ocular tendons.

**oph·thal·mo·di·a·phan·o·scope** (of-thal″mo-di-ə-fan′o-skōp) [*ophthalmo-* + *diaphanoscope*] an instrument to examine the interior or the retina of the eye by transillumination.

**oph·thal·mo·di·as·tim·e·ter** (of-thal″mo-di″əs-tim′ə-tər) [*ophthalmo-* + *diastema* + *-meter*] an instrument for determining the proper distance at which to place lenses for the two eyes.

**oph·thal·mo·do·ne·sis** (of-thal″mo-də-ne′sis) [*ophthalmo-* + Gr. *donēsis* trembling] a trembling motion of the eyes.

**oph·thal·mo·dy·na·mom·e·ter** (of-thal″mo-di″nə-mom′ə-tər) [*ophthalmo-* + *dynamo-* + *-meter*] 1. an instrument for measuring the retinal arterial pressure. 2. an instrument for determining the near point of convergence.

**oph·thal·mo·dy·na·mom·e·try** (of-thal″mo-di″nə-mom′ə-tre) [MeSH: Ophthalmodynamometry] 1. determination of retinal arterial pressure by ophthalmodynamometer. 2. determination of the near point of convergence by an ophthalmodynamometer.

**oph·thal·mo·dyn·ia** (of-thal″mo-din′e-ə) ophthalmalgia.

**oph·thal·mo·ei·ko·nom·e·ter** (of-thal″mo-i″ko-nom′ə-tər) [*ophthalmo-* + Gr. *eikōn* image + *-meter*] an instrument used to determine both the refraction of the eye and the relative size and shape of the ocular images.

**oph·thal·mo·graph** (of-thal′mo-graf) [*ophthalmo-* + *-graph*] an instrument for photographing the movements of the eye during reading.

**oph·thal·mog·ra·phy** (of″thəl-mog′rə-fe) [*ophthalmo-* + *-graphy*] description or photography of the eyes.

**oph·thal·mo·gy·ric** (of-thal″mo-ji′rik) oculogyric.

**oph·thal·mo·leu·ko·scope** (of-thal″mo-loo′ko-skōp) [*ophthalmo-* + *leukoscope*] an apparatus for testing color perception by means of colors produced by polarized light.

**oph·thal·mo·lith** (of-thal′mo-lith) [*ophthalmo-* + *-lith*] a lacrimal calculus.

**oph·thal·mo·log·ic** (of″thəl-mə-loj′ik) pertaining to ophthalmology.

**oph·thal·mol·o·gist** (of″thəl-mol′ə-jist) a physician who specializes in the diagnosis and medical and surgical treatment of diseases and defects of the eye and related structures.

**oph·thal·mol·o·gy** (of″thəl-mol′ə-je) [*ophthalmo-* + *-logy*] [MeSH: Ophthalmology] that branch of medicine dealing with the eye, its anatomy, physiology, pathology, etc.

**oph·thal·mo·ma·la·cia** (of-thal″mo-mə-la′shə) [*ophthalmo-* + *malacia*] abnormal softness of the eye.

**oph·thal·mom·e·ter** (of″thəl-mom′ə-tər) keratometer.

**oph·thal·mo·met·ro·scope** (of-thal″mo-met′rə-skōp) [*ophthalmo-* + *metro-* + *-scope*] an ophthalmoscope with an attachment for measuring the refraction of the eye.

**oph·thal·mom·e·try** (of″thəl-mom′ə-tre) keratometry.

**oph·thal·mo·my·co·sis** (of-thal″mo-mi-ko′sis) [*ophthalmo-* + *mycosis*] any disease of the eye caused by a fungus; called also *oculomycosis.*

**oph·thal·mo·my·ia·sis** (of-thal″mo-mi-i′ə-sis) [*ophthalmo-* + *myiasis*] infection of the eye by the larvae of the fly *Oestrus ovis.*

**oph·thal·mo·my·itis** (of-thal″mo-mi-i′tis) [*ophthalmo-* + *myitis*] inflammation of the muscles that move the eyeball.

**oph·thal·mo·myo·si·tis** (of-thal″mo-mi″o-si′tis) [*ophthalmo-* + *myositis*] inflammation of the eye muscles.

**oph·thal·mo·my·ot·o·my** (of-thal″mo-mi-ot′ə-me) [*ophthalmo-* + *myotomy*] surgical division of the muscles of the eye.

**oph·thal·mo·neu·ri·tis** (of-thal″mo-no͞o-ri′tis) optic neuritis.

**oph·thal·mo·neu·ro·my·eli·tis** (of-thal″mo-noo͝″ro-mi″ə-li′tis) neuromyelitis optica.

**oph·thal·mop·a·thy** (of″thəl-mop′ə-the) [*ophthalmo-* + *-pathy*] any disease of the eye.
**dysthyroid o.**, see under *orbitopathy.*
**external o.**, any disease of the eyelids, cornea, conjunctiva, or eye muscles.
**Graves' o.**, see under *orbitopathy.*
**infiltrative o.**, ocular changes, most often seen in thyroid disorders, caused by increased water content of the orbital contents, including discomfort, lacrimation, exophthalmos, edema, chemosis, and conjunctival infection; if the changes are severe, malignant exophthalmos results.
**internal o.**, any disease of the deep or more essential parts of the eye.

**oph·thal·mo·pha·com·e·ter** (of-thal″mo-fa-kom′ə-tər) [*ophthalmo-* + *phacometer*] an ophthalmometer used to determine the refractive power of the lens.

**oph·thal·mo·phan·tom** (of-thal″mo-fan′tom) a model of the eye used in demonstration.

**oph·thal·mo·phle·bot·o·my** (of-thal″mo-flə-bot′ə-me) [*ophthalmo-* + *phlebotomy*] phlebotomy to relieve congestion of the conjunctival veins.

**oph·thal·moph·thi·sis** (of″thəl-mof′thĭ-sis) [*ophthalmo-* + *phthisis*] ophthalmomalacia.

**oph·thal·mo·plas·ty** (of-thal′mo-plas″te) [*ophthalmo-* + *-plasty*] plastic surgery of the eye or of its appendages.

**oph·thal·mo·ple·gia** (of-thal″mo-ple′jə) [*ophthalmo-* + *-plegia*] [MeSH: Ophthalmoplegia] paralysis of the eye muscles.
**basal o.**, ophthalmoplegia due to a lesion at the base of the brain.
**exophthalmic o.**, external ocular paresis and exophthalmos of Graves' disease.
**external o.**, paralysis of the external ocular muscles.
**fascicular o.**, ophthalmoplegia due to lesion in the pons varolii.
**internal o.**, paralysis of the iris and ciliary apparatus.
**internuclear o.**, a horizontal ocular motor disturbance due to a lesion of the medial longitudinal fasciculus.
**nuclear o.**, that which is due to some lesion of the nuclei of the motor nerves of the eye.
**orbital o.**, ophthalmoplegia due to lesion in the orbit.
**Parinaud's o.**, Parinaud syndrome.
**partial o.**, paralysis of either one or two of the eye muscles.
**o. plus**, Kearns-Sayre syndrome.
**progressive external o.**, a slowly progressing, bilateral myopathy often affecting only the extraocular muscles, but sometimes also the orbicularis oculi. The levators of the upper lids are usually affected first, with ptosis resulting, followed by progressive, total ocular paresis. Called also *ocular myopathy.*
**total o., o. tota′lis**, that affecting both the extrinsic and intrinsic muscular apparatus of the eye.

**oph·thal·mo·ple·gic** (of-thal″mo-ple′jik) pertaining to ophthalmoplegia.

**oph·thal·mop·to·sis** (of-thal″mop-to′sis) [*ophthalmo-* + *ptosis*] exophthalmos.

**oph·thal·mor·rha·gia** (of-thal″mo-ra′je-ə) [*ophthalmo-* + *-rrhagia*] hemorrhage from the eye.

**oph·thal·mor·rhea** (of-thal″mo-re′ə) [*ophthalmo-* + *-rrhea*] oozing of blood from the eye.

**oph·thal·mor·rhex·is** (of-thal″mo-rek′sis) [*ophthalmo-* + *rhexis*] rupture of the eyeball.

**oph·thal·mo·scope** (of-thal′mə-skōp) [*ophthalmo-* + *-scope*] an instrument containing a perforated mirror and lenses used to examine the interior of the eye; called also *funduscope.*
**binocular o.**, an ophthalmoscope by which the fundus of the eye is viewed with both eyes through two eyepieces; called also *stereo-ophthalmoscope.*
**direct o.**, one that produces an upright, or unreversed, image of approximately 15 times magnification.
**indirect o.**, one that produces an inverted, or reversed, direct image of 2 to 5 times magnification, depending on the dioptic power to the examining lens.

**oph·thal·mos·co·py** (of″thəl-mos′kə-pe) [MeSH: Ophthalmoscopy] the examination of the interior of the eye with the ophthalmoscope. Called also *funduscopy.*
**direct o.**, direct, close-range ophthalmoscopic observation of the fundus; the image is virtual, erect, and magnified.
**indirect o.**, ophthalmoscopic examination of the fundus with the interposition of a strong convex lens between the observer and the patient; the image is real and inverted.
**medical o.**, ophthalmoscopy performed to diagnose local or systemic diseases such as diabetes mellitus, hypertension, and cerebral tumor.
**metric o.**, that performed for the measurement of refraction.

**oph·thal·mo·spec·tro·scope** (of-thal″mo-spek′tro-skōp) an instrument used in ophthalmospectroscopy.

**oph·thal·mo·spec·tros·co·py** (of-thal″mo-spek-tros′kə-pe) [*ophthalmo-* + *spectroscopy*] ophthalmoscopic and spectroscopic examination of the ocular fundus.

**oph·thal·mos·ta·sis** (of″thəl-mos′tə-sis) [*ophthalmo-* + *stasis*] fixation of the eye with the ophthalmostat.

**oph·thal·mo·stat** (of-thal′mo-stat) [*ophthalmo-* + Gr. *histanai* to halt] an instrument for holding the eye steady during operation.

**oph·thal·mo·sta·tom·e·ter** (of-thal″mo-stə-tom′ə-tər) exophthalmometer.

**oph·thal·mo·ste·re·sis** (of-thal″mo-stə-re′sis) [*ophthalmo-* + Gr. *steresis* privation, loss] loss of an eye.

**oph·thal·mo·syn·chy·sis** (of-thal″mo-sin′kĭ-sis) [*ophthalmo-* + *synchysis*] effusion into the eye.

**oph·thal·mo·ther·mom·e·ter** (of-thal″mo-thər-mom′ə-tər) [*ophthalmo-* + *thermometer*] an apparatus for recording the temperature of the eye.

**oph·thal·mot·o·my** (of″thəl-mot′ə-me) [*ophthalmo-* + *-tomy*] the operation of incising the eyeball.

**oph·thal·mo·to·nom·e·ter** (of-thal″mo-tə-nom′ə-tər) tonometer.

**oph·thal·mo·to·nom·e·try** (of-thal″mo-tə-nom′ə-tre) [*ophthalmo-* + *tono-* + *-metry*] the indirect estimation of intraocular pressure by determining the resistance of the eyeball to indentation by an applied force; called also *tonometry.*

**oph·thal·mo·tox·in** (of-thal″mo-tok′sin) [*ophthalmo-* + *toxin*] a toxin acting on the eye.

**oph·thal·mo·trope** (of-thal′mo-trōp) [*ophthalmo-* + Gr. *trepein* to turn] a mechanical eye that moves like a real eye, used for demonstrating the action of the ocular muscles.

**oph·thal·mo·tro·pom·e·ter** (of-thal″mo-tro-pom′ə-tər) strabismometer.

**oph·thal·mo·tro·pom·e·try** (of-thal″mo-tro-pom′ə-tre) strabismometry.

**oph·thal·mo·vas·cu·lar** (of-thal″mo-vas′ku-lər) pertaining to the blood vessels of the eye.

**oph·thal·mo·xe·ro·sis** (of-thal″mo-ze-ro′sis) xerophthalmia.

**oph·thal·mox·ys·ter** (of-thal″moks-is′ter) [*ophthalmo-* + *xyster*] an instrument for scraping the conjunctiva.

**Oph·thet·ic** (of-thet′ik) trademark for a preparation of proparacaine hydrochloride.

**Oph·tho·chlor** (of′tho-klor) trademark for a preparation of chloramphenicol.

**-opia** [Gr. *ōps* eye] a combining form denoting condition or a defect of the eye, or of vision.

**opi·an** (o′pe-ən) noscapine.

**opi·a·nine** (o-pi′ə-nin) noscapine.

**opi·ate** (o′pe-ət) a remedy containing or derived from opium; also any drug that induces sleep.

**Opie paradox** (o′pe) [Eugene Lindsay *Opie,* American pathologist, 1873–1971] see under *paradox.*

**opi·oid** (o′pe-oid) 1. any synthetic narcotic that has opiate-like activities but is not derived from opium. 2. any of a group of naturally occurring peptides that bind at or otherwise influence opiate receptors of cell membranes; they may have either opiate-like or opiate antagonist effects. They include the dynorphins, endorphins, and enkephalins.

**opip·ra·mol hy·dro·chlo·ride** (o-pip′rə-mol) a tricyclic antidepressant with mild tranquilizing properties.

**Opi·so·cros·tis** (o″pĭ-so-kros′tis) a genus of fleas. *O. bru′neri* is a squirrel flea that may be a vector of sylvatic plague.

**opis·the** (o-pis′the) [Gr. *opisthen* behind] the posterior daughter organism after transverse division of a ciliate protozoan; cf. *proter.*

**opis·the·nar** (o-pis′the-nər) [*opistho-* + *thenar*] the dorsum of the hand.

**opis·thi·o·ba·si·al** (o-pis″the-o-ba′se-əl) pertaining to or connecting the opisthion and basion.

**opis·thi·on** (o-pis′the-on) [Gr. *opisthion* rear, posterior] [TA] a craniometric landmark located at the midpoint of the posterior border of the foramen magnum.

**opis·thio·na·si·al** (o-pis″the-o-na′ze-əl) connecting the opisthion and nasion.

**opisth(o)-** [Gr. *opisthen* behind, at the back] a combining form meaning backward or denoting relationship to the back.

**opis·tho·cra·ni·on** (o-pis″tho-kra′ne-on) [*opistho-* + Gr. *kranion* the upper part of the head] a craniometric landmark determined instrumentally to indicate the posterior end of the maximum cranial length measured along the midline of the glabella.

**opis·tho·ge·nia** (o-pis″tho-je′ne-ə) defective development of the jaws following ankylosis of the jaw. Cf. *retrognathia.*

**opis·thog·na·thism** (o″pis-thog′nə-thiz-əm) retrognathism.

**opis·tho·mas·ti·gote** (o″pis-tho-mas′tĭ-gōt) [*opistho-* + *mastigote*] any of the bodies representing the morphologic stage in the life cycle of trypanosomatid protozoa of the genus *Herpetomonas,* in which the kinetoplast and basal body are posterior to the nucleus and the flagellum runs through the body of the cell to emerge anteriorly as a free-flowing structure. Cf. *amastigote, choanomastigote, epimastigote, promastigote,* and *trypomastigote.*

**opis·tho·po·reia** (o-pis″tho-po-ri′ə) [*opistho-* + Gr. *poreia* walk] retropulsion (def. 2).

**opis·thor·chi·a·sis** (o″pis-thor-ki′ə-sis) [MeSH: Opisthorchiasis] infection of the biliary tract by liver flukes of the genus *Opisthorchis.* In heavy infections there is local injury to the distal bile capillaries and surrounding liver tissue; this may ultimately develop into cirrhosis of the liver with areas of necrosis and fatty degeneration. See also *clonorchiasis.* Called also *opisthorchosis.*

**Opis·thor·chi·i·dae** (o″pis-thor-ki′ĭ-de) a family of trematodes; it includes the genera *Metorchis, Opisthorchis, Parametorchis,* and *Pseudamphistomum.*

**Opis·thor·chis** (o″pis-thor′kis) [*opistho-* + *orchis*] [MeSH: Opisthorchis] a genus of trematodes of the family Opisthorchiidae, characterized by having the testes near the posterior end of the body.
**O. feli′neus,** the Siberian liver fluke found in the liver of cats, dogs, pigs, and humans; infection (see *opisthorchiasis* ) results from ingestion of infected fish, such as *Leuciscus rutilis, Idus melanotus,* and related species.
**O. nover′ca,** *Amphimerus noverca.*
**O. sinen′sis,** the common liver fluke of China, Japan, Korea, Taiwan, and Indochina, found in the bile ducts of humans, cats, dogs, and other species that consume fresh water fish containing larvae. Larval development requires two intermediate hosts, the first a snail of the genus *Parafossarulus* or *Bithynia,* the second a fresh water fish of the carp family. Called also *Clonorchis sinensis* and *Distoma sinensis.*
**O. tenuicol′lis,** a species found in the bile ducts and sometimes the intestines of cats, dogs, pigs, and sometimes other mammals including humans.
**O. viver′rini,** a species that causes opisthorchiasis in the civet cat and sometimes humans in Thailand.

**opis·thor·cho·sis** (o″pis-thor-ko′sis) opisthorchiasis.

**opis·thot·ic** (o″pis-thot′ik) [*opistho-* + *otic*] situated behind the ear.

**opis·thot·o·noid** (o″pis-thot′ə-noid) resembling opisthotonos.
**o. feta′lis,** an exaggerated deflection attitude of the fetus during labor, which may persist during the neonatal period, but which gradually changes to a more normal posture.

**opis·thot·o·nos** (o″pis-thot′ə-nəs) [*opistho-* + Gr. *tonos* tension] a form of spasm consisting of extreme hyperextension of the body; the head and the heels are bent backward and the body bowed forward.

**opis·thot·o·nus** (o″pis-thot′ə-nəs) opisthotonos.

**Opitz's disease** (o′pit-səz) [Hans *Opitz,* German pediatrician, 20th century] see under *disease.*

**Opitz's syndrome** (o′pit-səz) [John Marius *Opitz,* German-born pediatrician in United States, born 1935] see under *syndrome.*

**Opitz-Fri·as syndrome** (o′pits-fre′ahs) [J. M. *Opitz;* Jaime L. *Frías,* Chilean pediatrician, 20th century] see under *syndrome.*

**opi·um** (o′pe-əm) [L., from Gr. *opion*] [USP] [MeSH: Opium] the air-dried milky exudate obtained from the unripe capsules of *Papaver somniferum* or *P. album.* Various principles and derivatives of opium, including some 20 alkaloids, notably morphine, codeine, papaverine, and thebaine, are used for their narcotic and analgesic effects. Because it is highly addictive, the production of opium is restricted, and the cultivation of the plants from which it is obtained is prohibited by most nations under an international agreement. Called also *crude o.* and *gum o.*
**crude o.,** see *opium.*
**denarcotized o., deodorized o.,** powdered opium freed from certain nauseating constituents by extraction with purified petroleum benzin.
**granulated o., o. granula′tum,** opium reduced to a coarse powder.
**gum o.,** see *opium.*
**powdered o.** [USP], **o. pulvera′tum,** opium dried and reduced to a very fine powder; it may contain any of the diluents, except starch, permitted in powdered extracts. See also *paregoric.*

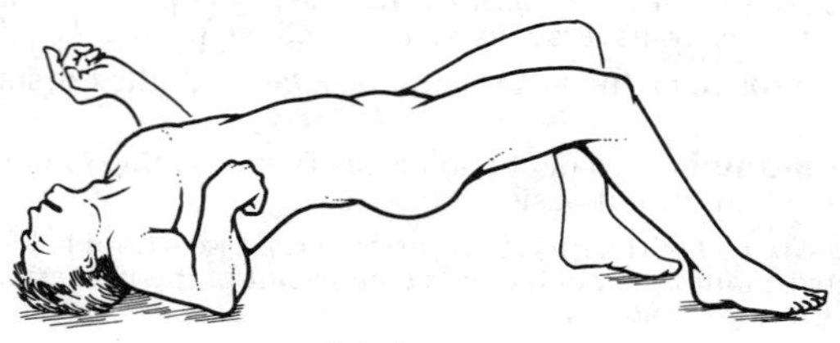

Opisthotonos.

**opo·ceph·a·lus** (o″po-sef′ə-ləs) [Gr. *ōps* face + *-cephalus*] a fetus with the ears fused to the head, one orbit, no mouth, and no nose.

**opo·did·y·mus** (o″po-did′ĭ-məs) [Gr. *ōps* face + *-didymus*] a fetus with two fused heads and with the sense organs partially fused.

**opod·y·mus** (o-pod′ĭ-məs) opodidymus.

**opos·sum** (o-pos′əm) [Algonquian] [MeSH: Opossums] a member of any of several genera of marsupial mammals; see *Didelphis.*

**Op·pen·heim's, reflex (sign)** (op′en-hīmz) [Hermann *Oppenheim,* German neurologist, 1858–1919] see under *reflex.*

**op·po·nens** (o-po′nənz) [L.] opposing; said of an opposing structure, as musculus opponens.

**op·por·tu·nis·tic** (op″ər-too-nis′tik) 1. denoting a microorganism that does not ordinarily cause disease but that, under certain circumstances (e.g., impaired immune responses resulting from other disease or drug treatment), becomes pathogenic. 2. denoting a disease or infection caused by such an organism.

**op·pos·i·ti·po·lar** (o-poz″ĭ-tĭ-po′lər) having two poles on opposite sides of a cell.

**OPRT** orotate phosphoribosyltransferase.

**-opsia** [Gr. *opsis* sight] a combining form denoting a condition or a defect of vision.

**op·si·al·gia** (op″se-al′jə) [Gr. *ōps* face + *-algia*] Ramsay Hunt syndrome, def. 1.

**op·sin** (op′sin) [MeSH: Opsin] a protein of the retinal rods (scotopsin) and cones (photopsin) that combines with 11-*cis*-retinal to form visual pigments; see *retinal* (def. 2). The opsins are also named according to the color of pigment: iodopsin (violet), rhodopsin (purple), etc. See illustration at *visual cycle,* under *cycle.*

**op·si·om·e·ter** (op″se-om′ə-tər) optometer.

**op·si·uria** (op″se-u′re-ə) [Gr. *opse* late + *-uria*] the condition in which more urine is excreted during fasting than during digestion.

**op·so·clo·nia** (op″so-klo′ne-ə) opsoclonus.

**op·so·clo·nia, op·so·clo·nus** (op″so-klo′ne-ə, op″so-klo′nəs) a condition characterized by nonrhythmic horizontal and vertical oscillations of the eyes, observed in various disorders of the brain stem or cerebellum.
**o.-myoclonus,** see under *syndrome.*

**op·son·ic** (op-son′ik) pertaining to opsonins.

**op·so·nin** (op′sə-nin) [Gr. *opsōnein* to buy victuals] any substance that binds to particulate antigens and induces their phagocytosis by macrophages and neutrophils. In current usage the term is used to refer to substances of two types, opsonizing antibodies (IgM, IgG1, and IgG3 immunoglobulins specific for the antigen) and certain complement fragments (C3b, C3d, and C4b, which become bound to the antigen during complement activation), both of which trigger phagocytosis by binding to specific cell-surface receptors, Fc receptors, and C3b receptors on neutrophils and macrophages and C3d receptors on macrophages.
**immune o.,** opsonizing antibody; see *opsonin.*

**op·so·ni·za·tion** (op″sə-nĭ-za′shən) the rendering of bacteria and other cells subject to phagocytosis by the action of an opsonin.

**op·so·nize** (op′sə-nīz) to function as an opsonin.

**op·so·no·cy·to·phag·ic** (op″sə-no-si″to-faj′ik) denoting the phagocytic activity of blood in the presence of serum opsonins and homologous leukocytes.

**op·so·no·pha·go·cy·to·sis** (op″so-no-fa″go-si-to′sis) phagocytosis by macrophages and monocytes in the presence of specific serum opsonins.

**op·so·no·phil·ia** (op″sə-no-fil′e-ə) [*opsonin* + *-philia*] affinity for opsonins.

**op·so·no·phil·ic** (op″sə-no-fil′ik) having an affinity for opsonins.

**op·tes·the·sia** (op″təs-the′zhə) [*opt-* + *esthesia*] visual sensibility; ability to perceive visual stimuli.

**op·tic** (op′tik) [Gr. *optikos* of or for sight] [MeSH: Optics] of or pertaining to the eye.

**Op·ti·caine** (op′tĭ-kān″) trademark for a preparation of tetracaine hydrochloride.

**op·ti·cal** (op′tĭ-kəl) [L. *opticus;* Gr. *optikos*] pertaining to or subserving vision.

**op·ti·cian** (op-tish′ən) an expert in opticianry.

**op·ti·cian·ry** (op-tish′ən-re) the science of optics as applied to filling and adapting of ophthalmic prescriptions and products.

**op·ti·co·chi·as·mat·ic** (op″tĭ-ko-ki″az-mat′ik) pertaining to the optic nerves and chiasma.

**op·ti·co·cil·i·ary** (op″tĭ-ko-sil′e-ar-e) pertaining to the optic and ciliary nerves.

**op·ti·co·ki·net·ic** (op″tĭ-ko-kĭ-net′ik) optokinetic.

**op·ti·co·na·si·on** (op″tĭ-ko-na′se-on) the distance from the posterior edge of the optic foramen to the nasion.

**op·ti·co·pu·pil·lary** (op″tĭ-ko-pu′pĭ-lar-e) pertaining to the optic nerve and the pupil.

**op·tics** (op′tiks) [Gr. *optikos* of or for sight] [MeSH: Optics] the science which treats of light and of vision.
**fiber o.**, see *fiberoptics.*

**op·ti·mal** (op′ti-məl) the best; the most favorable.

**op·tim·e·ter** (op-tim′ə-tər) optometer.

**Op·ti·mine** (op′tĭ-mēn″) trademark for a preparation of azatadine maleate.

**op·ti·mum** (op′tĭ-məm) [L. "best"] that condition of surroundings which is conducive to the most favorable activity or function.

**opt(o)-** [Gr. *optos* seen] a combining form denoting relationship to vision or sight.

**op·to·chi·as·mic** (op″to-ki-az′mik) opticochiasmatic.

**op·to·gram** (op′to-gram) [*opto-* + *-gram*] the retinal image formed by the bleaching of the visual purple under the influence of light.

**op·to·ki·net·ic** (op″to-kĭ-net′ik) [*opto-* + *kinetic*] pertaining to movement of the eyes and of objects in the visual field, as in nystagmus.

**op·to·me·ninx** (op″to-me′ningks) [*opto-* + Gr. *mēninx* membrane] the retina.

**op·tom·e·ter** (op-tom′ə-tər) [*opto-* + *-meter*] an instrument formerly used to measure ocular refraction; called also *opsiometer, optimeter,* and *refractometer.*

**op·tom·e·trist** (op-tom′ə-trist) a person trained and licensed in accordance with state law to diagnose, manage, and treat conditions of the human eye and visual system. See *optometry.*

**op·tom·e·try** (op-tom′ə-tre) [*opto-* + *-metry*] [MeSH: Optometry] the professional practice consisting of examination of the eyes to evaluate health and visual abilities, diagnosis of eye diseases and conditions of the eye and visual system, and provision of treatment by such means as the prescription of eyeglasses and contact lenses and the use of vision therapy, low vision aids, drugs (in most states), and certain surgical procedures.

**op·to·my·om·e·ter** (op″to-mi-om′ə-tər) [*opto-* + *myometer*] a device used in measuring the power of the extrinsic ocular muscles.

**op·to·phone** (op′tə-fōn) [*opto-* + Gr. *phōnē* voice] an instrument by means of which light and darkness are made discernible to the blind through their sense of hearing, the light waves being transformed into sound waves.

**op·to·type** (op′to-tīp) test type.

**Opun·tia** (o-pun′she-ə) the prickly pears, a large genus of cacti. *O. vulga′ris* is used as a remedy in homeopathic practice.

**OPV** poliovirus vaccine live oral.

**OR** operating room.

**ora**[1] (o′rə) gen. and pl. *o′rae* [L.] an edge or margin.
**o. serra′ta re′tinae** [TA], the irregular anterior margin of the pars optica of the retina, lying internal to the junction of the choroid and the ciliary body.

**ora**[2] (o′rə) [L.] plural of *os*[1].

**orad** (o′rad) [*ora-* + *-ad*[1]] toward the mouth.

**orae** (o′re) [L.] genitive and plural of *ora*[1].

**Or·a·graf·in** (or″ə-graf′in) trademark for a preparation of the calcium or the sodium salt of ipodate.

**oral** (or′əl) [L. *oralis*] 1. pertaining to the mouth, taken through or applied in the mouth, as an oral medication or an oral thermometer. 2. see *facies lingualis dentis.*

**ora·le** (o-ra′le) a craniometric landmark, being the point in the midline of the maxillary suture just lingual to the central incisors in the alveolar process.

**oral·i·ty** (o-ral′ĭ-te) in psychoanalytic theory, the psychic organization of all the sensations, impulses, and personality traits derived from the oral stage of psychosexual development.

**oral·o·gy** (o-ral′ə-je) [*oral* + *-logy*] stomatology.

**Ora·morph** (or′ə-morf″) trademark for a preparation of morphine sulfate.

**or·ange** (or′ənj) [L. *aurantium*] 1. *Citrus aurantium.* 2. the yellow, edible fruit of *C. aurantium;* there are two varieties, *bitter orange* and *sweet orange;* the peels of both are used in making various pharmaceutical preparations. See also under *oil* and *syrup.* 3. a color between red and yellow. 4. a dye or stain that produces an orange color.
**o. III,** methyl o.
**acid o. 10,** o. G.
**acridine o.**, see under *acridine.*
**ethyl o.**, an indicator with a pH range of 2 to 4.
**o. G,** an acid azo dye used as a counterstain in histology and cytology and as a component of Mallory's acid fuchsin, orange G, and aniline blue stains.
**gold o.**, methyl o.
**methyl o.** [USP], an orange-yellow powder, the sodium salt of dimethylaminoazobenzene sulfonic acid, used as an indicator with a pH range of 3.2 to 4.4 and a color change from pink to yellow. Called also *gold o., helianthin, o. III,* and *Poirrier's o.*
**Poirrier's o.**, methyl o.
**victoria o.**, a salt of dinitrocresol used in histology as a stain.
**wool o.**, o. G.

**or·an·ge·o·phil** (or-an′je-o-fĭl) [*orange* + *-phil*] 1. staining readily with orange dyes. 2. a cell or other histologic element that stains readily with orange dyes. 3. somatotroph.

**orang·u·tan** (ə-rang′ə-tan″) [Malayan "wild man"] *Pongo pygmaeus,* an anthropoid ape native to Indonesia, used for laboratory studies because it is susceptible to some human diseases.

**Ora·sone** (or′ə-sōn″) trademark for preparations of prednisone.

**Ora-Tes·tryl** (or″ə-tes′trəl) trademark for a preparation of fluoxymesterone.

**Or·be·li phenomenon (effect)** (or-ba′le) [Leon Algarovich *Orbeli,* Russian physiologist, 1882–1958] see under *phenomenon.*

**or·bic·u·lar** (or-bik′u-lər) [L. *orbicularis*] circular, or rounded.

**or·bic·u·la·re** (or-bik″u-la′re) [L.] processus lenticularis incudis.

**or·bic·u·li** (or-bik′u-li) genitive and plural of *orbiculus.*

**or·bic·u·lus** (or-bik′u-ləs) gen. and pl. *orbic′uli* [L., dim. of *orbis* orb, circle] [TA] a general term denoting a structure shaped like a small circle, or disk.
**o. cilia′ris** [TA], ciliary disk: the thin part of the ciliary body extending between its crown and the ora serrata retinae; called also *pars plana corporis ciliaris.*

**or·bit** (or′bit) [MeSH: Orbit] the bony cavity that contains the eyeball; see *orbita* [TA].

**or·bi·ta** (or′bĭ-tə) gen. and pl. *or′bitae* [L. "mark of a wheel, circuit"] [TA] orbit: the bony cavity that contains the eyeball and its associated muscles, vessels, and nerves; the ethmoid, frontal, lacrimal, nasal, palatine, sphenoid, and zygomatic bones, and the maxilla contribute to its formation.

**or·bi·tae** (or′bĭ-te) [L.] genitive and plural of *orbita.*

**or·bi·tal** (or′bĭ-təl) 1. pertaining to the orbit. 2. in an atom, the wave function describing the probability of occurrence of an electron of a particular energy level of an atom or molecule; each orbital can hold two electrons of opposing spin.

**or·bi·ta·le** (or″bĭ-ta′le) an anthropometric landmark, the lowest point on the inferior margin of the orbit.

**or·bi·ta·lis** (or″bĭ-ta′lis) [L.] pertaining to the orbit.

**or·bi·tog·ra·phy** (or″bĭ-tog′rə-fe) [*orbit* + *-graphy*] visualization of the orbit and its contents using radiography or computed tomography.

**or·bi·to·na·sal** (or″bĭ-to-na′zəl) pertaining to the orbit and the nose.

**or·bi·to·nom·e·ter** (or″bĭ-to-nom′ə-tər) [*orbit* + *tonometer*] an instrument for measurement of the backward displacement of the eyeball produced by a given pressure exerted against its anterior aspect; called also *piezometer.*

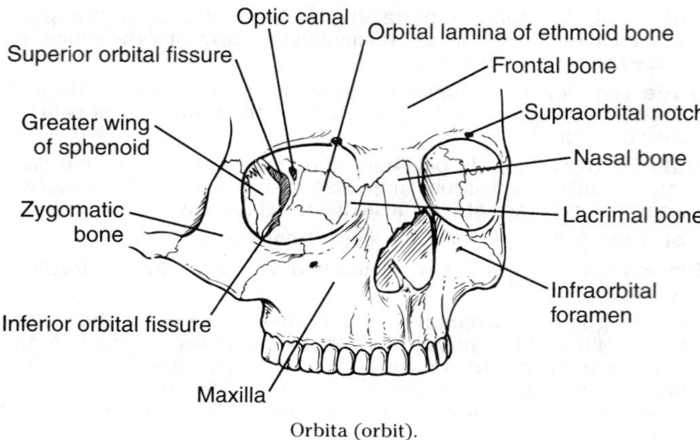

Orbita (orbit).

**or·bi·to·nom·e·try** (or″bĭ-to-nom′ə-tre) the measurement of the backward displacement of the eyeball under varying pressures.

**or·bi·top·a·gus** (or″bĭ-top′ə-gəs) [*orbit* + *-pagus*] conjoined twins in which the smaller parasitic fetus is attached to the orbit of the larger twin.

**or·bi·top·a·thy** (or″bĭ-top′ə-the) [*orbit* + *-pathy*] disease affecting the orbit and its contents.
**dysthyroid o.,** the ocular changes associated with thyroid dysfunction, most often Graves' disease, including endocrine exophthalmos, malignant exophthalmos, and infiltrative ophthalmopathy; called also *dysthyroid ophthalmopathy.*
**Graves' o.,** dysthyroid orbitopathy occurring in Graves' disease. Called also *Graves' ophthalmopathy.*

**or·bi·to·stat** (or′bĭ-to-stat) [*orbit* + Gr. *statos* placed] an instrument for measuring the axis of the orbit.

**or·bi·to·tem·po·ral** (or″bĭ-to-tem′pə-rəl) pertaining to the orbital and temporal regions.

**or·bi·tot·o·my** (or″bĭ-tot′ə-me) [*orbit* + *-tomy*] the operation of incising or opening into the orbit through the orbital margin.

**Or·bi·vi·rus** (or′bĭ-vi″rəs) [L. *orbis* circle + *virus*] [MeSH: Orbivirus] orbiviruses; a genus of viruses of the family Reoviridae, separable into at least 14 antigenically distinct groups, and infecting a variety of vertebrates, including humans. It includes the human pathogens Orungo virus and Kemerovo virus and the agents of bluetongue and African horse sickness. Mosquitoes, sandflies, and ticks are vectors.

**or·bi·vi·rus** (or′bĭ-vi″rəs) [MeSH: Orbivirus] any virus of the genus *Orbivirus.*

**or·ce·in** (or-se′in) a brown coloring matter, derived from orcinol and soluble in alcohol; used as a specific stain for elastic tissue.

**or·chec·to·my** (or-kek′tə-me) orchiectomy.

**or·chel·la** (or-shel′ə) a histologic stain composed of 5 mL of acetic acid and 40 mL each of alcohol and water, colored to a dark red with archil from which excess of ammonia has been driven off.

**or·chi·al·gia** (or″ke-al′jə) [*orchi-* + *-algia*] pain in a testis. Called also *orchidalgia, orchiodynia,* and *testalgia.*

**or·chic** (or′kik) testicular.

**or·chi·cho·rea** (or″kĭ-kə-re′ə) [*orchi-* + *chorea*] a twitching or jerking movement of a testis.

**or·chi·dal·gia** (or″kĭ-dal′jə) orchialgia.

**or·chi·dec·to·my** (or″kĭ-dek′tə-me) orchiectomy.

**or·chid·ic** (or-kid′ik) testicular.

**or·chi·di·tis** (or″kĭ-di′tis) orchitis.

**orchid(o)-** [Gr. *orchidion,* dim. of *orchis* testis] a combining form denoting relationship to the testes.

**or·chi·do·epi·did·y·mec·to·my** (or″kĭ-do-ep″ĭ-did″ĭ-mek′tə-me) [*orchido-* + *epididymis* + *-ectomy*] the operation of excising the testis and epididymis.

**or·chi·dom·e·ter** (or″kĭ-dom′ə-tər) an instrument for measuring the testis.
**Prader o.,** a string of plastic models of testicular shape, marked according to their volume in cubic centimeters; used for measuring the size of the testes in genital development.

**or·chi·don·cus** (or″kĭ-dong′kəs) [*orchido-* + Gr. *onkos* tumor] testicular tumor.

**or·chi·dop·a·thy** (or″kĭ-dop′ə-the) orchiopathy.

**or·chi·do·pexy** (or′kĭ-do-pek″se) orchiopexy.

**or·chi·do·plas·ty** (or′kĭ-do-plas″te) orchioplasty.

**or·chi·dop·to·sis** (or″kĭ-dop-to′sis) [*orchido-* + *-ptosis*] downward displacement of the testis, a condition due to varicocele or relaxation of the scrotum.

**or·chi·dor·rha·phy** (or″kĭ-dor′ə-fe) orchiopexy.

**or·chi·dot·o·my** (or″kĭ-dot′ə-me) orchiotomy.

**or·chi·ec·to·my** (or″ke-ek′tə-me) [*orchio-* + Gr. *-ectomy*] [MeSH: Orchiectomy] excision of one or both testes; if it is bilateral, the individual is incapable of reproduction (see *castration*).
**radical inguinal o.,** surgical removal of a testis and of the spermatic cord up to the internal inguinal ring.

**or·chi·epi·did·y·mi·tis** (or″ke-ep″ĭ-did″ĭ-mi′tis) [*orchio-* + *epididymis* + *-itis*] inflammation of a testis and an epididymis.

**or·chi·lyt·ic** (or″kĭ-lit′ik) [*orchio-* + *-lytic*] destroying testicular tissue.

**orchi(o)-** [Gr. *orchis,* gen. *orchios* testis] a combining form denoting relationship to the testes.

**or·chio·blas·to·ma** (or″ke-o-blas-to′mə) yolk sac tumor.

**or·chio·ca·tab·a·sis** (or″ke-o-kə-tab′ə-sis) [*orchio-* + Gr. *katabasis* descent] the descent of the testes.

**or·chio·cele** (or′ke-o-sēl″) [*orchio-* + *-cele*[1]] 1. hernial protrusion of a testis. 2. scrotal hernia. 3. testicular tumor.

**or·chio·dyn·ia** (or″ke-o-din′e-ə) orchialgia.

**or·chi·on·cus** (or″ke-ong′kəs) [*orchio-* + Gr. *onkos* tumor] testicular tumor.

**or·chio·neu·ral·gia** (or″ke-o-noo͞-ral′jə) [*orchio-* + *neuralgia*] orchialgia.

**or·chi·op·a·thy** (or″ke-op′ə-the) [*orchio-* + *-pathy*] any disease of the testis. Called also *orchidopathy* and *testopathy.*

**or·chio·pexy** (or′ke-o-pek″se) [*orchio-* + *-pexy*] surgical fixation in the scrotum of an undescended testis.

**or·chio·plas·ty** (or′ke-o-plas″te) [*orchio-* + *-plasty*] plastic surgery of the testis.

**or·chi·or·rha·phy** (or″ke-or′ə-fe) [*orchio-* + *-rrhaphy*] orchiopexy.

**or·chi·os·cheo·cele** (or″ke-os′ke-o-sēl″) [*orchio-* + *oscheo-* + *-cele*[1]] scrotal tumor with scrotal hernia.

**or·chio·scir·rhus** (or″ke-o-skir′əs) [*orchio-* + Gr. *skirrhos* hard] hardening of the testis.

**or·chi·ot·o·my** (or″ke-ot′ə-me) [*orchio-* + *-tomy*] incision and drainage of a testis.

**Or·chis** (or′kis) [Gr. *orchis* testicle, so called because the roots or rhizomes of certain species resemble testicles] a genus of orchids, flowering plants of the family Orchidaceae; some species are medicinal.

**or·chis** (or′kis) [Gr.] TA alternative for *testis.*

**or·chit·ic** (or-kit′ik) pertaining to, causing, or affected with orchitis.

**or·chi·tis** (or-ki′tis) [*orchio-* + *-itis*] [MeSH: Orchitis] inflammation of a testis. The disease is marked by pain, swelling, and a feeling of weight. It may occur idiopathically, or it may be associated with conditions such as mumps, gonorrhea, filarial disease, syphilis, or tuberculosis.
**metastatic o.,** an infection brought to the testis by the blood stream, as in mumps.
**spermatogenic granulomatous o.,** orchitis in which the normal structure of the testis has been replaced by gray-white granulomatous tissue without evident necrosis; it is thought to be in some way a reaction to spermatozoa.
**traumatic o.,** orchitis following trauma, vas ligation, or surgical manipulation, without evidence of previous disease, believed to be due to an infectious process resulting from lowered resistance of the injured tissues to bacteria.
**o. variolo′sa,** orchitis occurring in smallpox.

**or·chi·to·lyt·ic** (or″kĭ-to-lit′ik) orchilytic.

**or·chot·o·my** (or-kot′ə-me) orchiotomy.

**or·cin** (or′sin) orcinol.

**or·ci·nol** (or′sĭ-nol) an antiseptic principle derived mainly from lichens, used as a reagent in various tests; called also *orcin.*

**or·der** (or′dər) [L. *ordo* a line, row, or series] a taxonomic category subordinate to a class and superior to a family; see *taxon.*

**or·der·ly** (or′dər-le) an attendant in a hospital who works under the direction of a nurse.

**or·di·nal** (or'dĭ-nəl) being of a specified position in a ranked, often numbered, series (e.g., first, second, third, etc.).

**or·di·nate** (or'dĭ-nət) [L. *ordinare* to arrange in order] in a two-dimensional coordinate system, the distance of a point from the horizontal *(x)* axis, measured along a line parallel to the *y*-axis. Denoted by *y*. Cf. *abscissa*.

**orel·la·nine** (o-rel'ə-nēn) a toxic chemical found in certain species of *Cortinarius* mushrooms in Europe and Japan; ingestion causes gastritis, chills, headaches, myalgias, and occasionally renal tubular necrosis progressing to renal failure.

**orel·line** (or'ə-lēn) a toxic chemical found in certain species of *Cortinarius* mushrooms in Europe and Japan; ingestion causes gastritis, chills, headaches, myalgias, and occasionally renal tubular necrosis progressing to renal failure.

**ore·o·se·li·num** (o″re-o-se-li'num) [L.] *Peucedanum oreoselinum,* a plant used in homeopathic practice as a diuretic.

**Oret·ic** (o-ret'ik) trademark for a preparation of hydrochlorothiazide.

**Oret·i·cyl** (o-ret'ĭ-səl) trademark for preparations of hydrochlorothiazide with deserpidine.

**orex·i·gen·ic** (o-rek″sĭ-jen'ik) [Gr. *orexis* appetite + *-genic*] increasing or stimulating the appetite.

**orf** (orf) contagious ecthyma.

**or·gan** (or'gən) [L. *organum;* Gr. *organnon*] a somewhat independent part of the body that performs a special function or functions; see *organum* [TA].
**accessory o's of eye,** organa oculi accessoria.
**acoustic o.,** organum spirale.
**Bidder's o.,** an anterior portion, ovarian in character, of the gonad of male toads.
**cell o.,** a structural part of a cell having some definite function in its life or reproduction, as a nucleus or a centrosome.
**cement o.,** the embryonic tissue that develops into the cement layer of the tooth.
**Chievitz's o.,** an embryonic outgrowth behind the parotid gland which may merge into the latter or may disappear.
**circumventricular o's,** several small structures located around the edges of the third and fourth ventricles, lacking the regular blood-brain barrier and thus serving as significant sites for neural-endocrine interaction. They include the area postrema, the median eminence, the subcommissural organ, the subfornical organ, and the organum vasculosum of the lamina terminalis. Sometimes also included are the funiculus separans, the neurohypophysis, and the pineal body.
**o. of Corti,** organum spirale.
**critical o.,** the organ or organ system in which a specific radioactive material tends to concentrate, and thus the organ receiving the highest level of exposure to the radioactivity.
**digestive o's,** those concerned with the ingestion, digestion, and assimilation of food (*systema digestorium* [TA]).
**effector o.,** effector (def. 2).
**enamel o.,** a circumscribed knoblike mass of ectodermal cells arising from the dental lamina; it produces the enamel cap from which the dental enamel develops.
**end o.,** end-organ; see under *E*.
**extraperitoneal o.,** organum extraperitoneale.
**genital o's,** organa genitalia.
**genital o's, external,** see *organa genitalia feminina externa* and *organa genitalia masculina externa,* under *organum*.
**genital o's, female,** see *organa genitalia feminina externa* and *organa genitalia feminina interna,* under *organum*.
**genital o's, internal,** see *organa genitalia feminina interna* and *organa genitalia masculina interna,* under *organum*.
**genital o's, male,** see *organa genitalia masculina externa* and *organa genitalia masculina interna,* under *organum*.
**o. of Giraldés,** paradidymis.
**Golgi tendon o.,** an encapsulated nerve ending found in tendons of mammalian muscles and acting as a mechanoreceptor; arranged in series with the muscle, it is sensitive to mechanical distortion induced by either passive stretch of the tendon or isometric contraction of the muscle and thus signals muscle tension, being the receptor responsible for the lengthening reaction, or clasp-knife reflex. Called also *Golgi's corpuscle, tendon o.* or *spindle,* and *neurotendinous o.* or *spindle*.
**gustatory o.,** organum gustatorium.
**holdfast o.,** holdfast.
**intromittent o.,** any male copulatory organ, e.g., the human penis or the claspers seen especially in male insects and cartilaginous fishes, used to transfer sperm to the female reproductive tract.
**Jacobson's o.,** organum vomeronasale.
**lateral line o's,** a system of sense organs arranged in longitudinal canals in the skin of fishes and amphibians; they contain mechanoreceptors that are sensitive to changes in pressure and current and to vibrations of low frequency and thus aid in localizing objects.
**Marchand's o.,** see under *adrenal*.
**o's of mastication,** masticatory apparatus.
**Meyer's o.,** an area of circumvallate papillae on either side of the posterior part of the tongue.
**neurotendinous o.,** Golgi tendon o.
**olfactory o.,** organum olfactorium.
**parapineal o.,** a median dorsal outgrowth of the pineal body in certain lower vertebrates such as tailless amphibians, primitive fishes, and lizards; its principal cell type is an apparent photoreceptor. In some species it may specialize to form an extracranial epiphyseal eye. Called also *parietal o.*
**parenchymal o., parenchymatous o.,** organon parenchymatosum.
**parietal o.,** parapineal o.
**primitive fat o.,** brown adipose tissue.
**reproductive o's,** organa genitalia.
**reproductive o's, female,** see *organa genitalia feminina externa* and *organa genitalia feminina interna,* under *organum*.
**reproductive o's, male,** see *organa genitalia masculina externa* and *organa genitalia masculina interna,* under *organum*.
**retroperitoneal o.,** organum extraperitoneale.
**Rosenmüller's o.,** epoöphoron.
**rudimentary o.,** 1. a primordium. 2. an imperfectly or incompletely developed organ.
**Ruffini's o.,** see under *corpuscle*.
**segmental o.,** the pronephros, mesonephros, and metanephros together.
**sense o's, sensory o's,** organa sensuum. See under *organum*.
**o. of shock, shock o.,** the organ which reacts in anaphylactic shock; those organs whose responses determine the nature and, to a large extent, the outcome of a given anaphylactic reaction.
**o's of special sense,** organa sensuum; see under *organum*.
**spiral o.,** organum spirale.
**subcommissural o.,** organum subcommissurale.
**subfornical o.,** organum subfornicale.
**target o.,** an organ that is affected by a specific hormone, as the adrenal cortex by corticotropin.
**tendon o.,** Golgi tendon o.
**terminal o.,** the organ situated at either end of a reflex neural arc.
**urinary o's,** organa urinaria.
**vascular o. of lamina terminalis,** organum vasculosum of lamina terminalis.
**vestibulocochlear o.,** organum vestibulocochleare.
**vestigial o.,** an undeveloped organ that, in the embryo or in some more or less remote ancestor, was well developed and functional.
**vomeronasal o.,** organum vomeronasale.
**Weber's o.,** utriculus prostaticus.
**o's of Zuckerkandl,** corpora para-aortica.

**or·ga·na** (or'gə-nə) plural of *organum* [L.] and *organon* [Gr.].

**or·ga·nel·la** (or″gə-nel'ə) pl. *organel'lae* [L., dim. of *organum*] organelle.

**or·ga·nel·lae** (or″gə-nel'e) [L.] plural of *organella*.

**or·ga·nelle** (or″gə-nel') [L. *organella,* dim. of *organum* organ] [MeSH: Organelles] any of the membrane-bound organized cytoplasmic structures of distinctive morphology and function present in all eukaryotic cells. Organelles include such structures as nucleus, mitochondria, lysosomes, peroxisomes, Golgi apparatus, and endoplasmic reticulum, as well as chloroplasts in plants, and cilia, flagella, and the cytopharynx in protozoa. See Plates 13 and 14.
**holdfast o.,** holdfast.

**or·gan·ic** (or-gan'ik) 1. pertaining to or arising from an organ or the organs; cf. *functional,* def. 2. 2. having an organized structure. 3. arising from an organism. 4. pertaining to substances derived from living organisms. 5. denoting chemical substances containing covalently bound carbon atoms. 6. pertaining to or cultivated by the use of animal or vegetable fertilizers, rather than synthetic chemicals.

**or·gan·i·cist** (or-gan'ĭ-sist) one who believes in organicism.

**Or·gan·i·din** (or-gan'ĭ-din) trademark for a preparation of iodinated glycerol.

**or·gan·ism** (or'gə-niz-əm) any individual living thing, whether animal or plant.
**consumer o's,** the organisms of an ecosystem, plants or animals, that eat other plants or animals.
**nitrifying o's,** those nitrogen bacteria which are capable of oxidizing ammonia to nitrites and nitrates.
**nitrosifying o's,** those nitrogen bacteria which are capable of oxidizing ammonia to nitrites.
**pleuropneumonia-like o's,** PPLO; originally, a group of filtrable microorganisms similar to *Mycoplasma mycoides,* the causative agent of pleuropneumonia in cattle, which have been isolated from man and other animals (e.g., sheep, goats, dogs, rats, mice). They are

now classified as bacteria and have been assigned to various species of the genus *Mycoplasma.*

**or·ga·ni·za·tion** (or″gə-nĭ-za′shən) 1. the process of organizing or of becoming organized. 2. the replacement of blood clots by fibrous tissue. 3. [MeSH: Organizations] an organized body, group, or structure.

**or·ga·nize** (or′gə-nīz) 1. to provide with an organic structure. 2. to form into organs.

**or·ga·niz·er** (or′gə-nīz″ər) a part of an embryo which so influences some other part as to bring about and direct its histological and morphological differentiation. Parts developing as a result of induction, and inducing in their turn are classified as organizers of the second grade, third grade, and so on. Cf. *activator* (def. 2) and *inductor.*
**nucleolar o., nucleolus o.,** material responsible for organization of the nucleolus of a cell; it is thought to comprise slender strands of heterochromatin by which satellites are attached to the rest of the chromosome.
**primary o.,** the dorsal lip region of the blastopore.
**procentriole o.,** deuterosome.
**secondary o.,** one of second grade, such as the optic cup, which exerts influence on the developing lens.
**tertiary o.,** one of third grade, such as the tympanic ring, which exerts influence on the tympanic membrane.

**organ(o)-** [Gr. *organon* organ] a combining form meaning organic, or denoting relationship to an organ.

**or·ga·no·chlo·rine** (or″gə-no-klor′ēn) any compound of chlorine and organic elements, such as the chlorinated hydrocarbons.

**or·ga·no·fac·tion** (or″gə-no-fak′shən) organogenesis.

**or·ga·no·fer·ric** (or″gə-no-fer′ik) containing iron and some organic compound.

**or·ga·no·gel** (or-gan′o-jəl) a gel in which an organic liquid takes the place of water.

**or·ga·no·gen·e·sis** (or″gə-no-jen′ə-sis) [*organo-* + *-genesis*] the origin and development of organs.

**or·ga·no·ge·net·ic** (or″gə-no-jə-net′ik) pertaining to organogenesis.

**or·ga·no·gen·ic** (or″gə-no-jen′ik) originating in an organ.

**or·ga·nog·e·ny** (or″gə-noj′ə-ne) organogenesis.

**or·ga·nog·ra·phy** (or″gə-nog′rə-fe) [*organo-* + *-graphy*] the radiographic visualization of the organs of the body.

**or·ga·noid** (or′gə-noid) [*organ* + *-oid*] [MeSH: Organoids] 1. resembling an organ. 2. a structure which resembles an organ.

**or·ga·no·lep·tic** (or″gə-no-lep′tik) [*organo-* + Gr. *lambanein* to seize] 1. making an impression on an organ of special sense. 2. capable of receiving a sense impression.

**or·ga·nol·o·gy** (or″gə-nol′ə-je) [*organo-* + *-logy*] the sum of what is known regarding the organs of the body.

**or·ga·no·meg·a·ly** (or″gə-no-meg′ə-le) [*organo-* + *-megaly*] visceromegaly.

**or·ga·no·mer·cu·ri·al** (or″gə-no-mər-ku′re-əl) any mercury-containing organic compound, e.g., the diuretic mercaptomerin.

**or·ga·no·me·tal·lic** (or″gə-no-mə-tal′ik) consisting of a metal in combination with an organic radical; used particularly for a compound in which the metal is linked directly to a carbon atom.

**or·ga·non** (or′gə-non) pl. *or′gana* [Gr. "tool, instrument"] organum.
**o. parenchymato′sum,** a parenchymatous organ.

**or·ga·nop·a·thy** (or″gə-nop′ə-the) [*organo-* + *-pathy*] organic disease.

**or·ga·no·pexy** (or″gə-no-pek′se) [*organo-* + *-pexy*] the surgical fixation of an organ, especially of the uterus.

**or·ga·no·phil·ic** (or″gə-no-fil′ik) [*organo-* + *-philic*] organotropic.

**or·ga·noph·i·lism** (or-gə-nof′ĭ-liz-əm) organotropism.

**or·ga·no·phos·phate** (or″gə-no-fos′fāt) phosphate esterified to organic compounds such as glucose or sorbitol; see *organophosphorus.*

**Organochlorine Insecticides (Chlorinated Hydrocarbons)**

| | |
|---|---|
| Aldrin | Endrin |
| Chlordane | Heptachlor |
| Chlordecone | Lindane |
| DDT (dichlorodiphenyltrichloroethane) | Methoxychlor |
| Dieldrin | TDE (tetradichlorodiphenylethane; DDD) |
| Endosulfan | Toxophene (camphochlor) |

**Organophosphorus Insecticides**

| | |
|---|---|
| Acephate | Malathion |
| Azinphos-methyl | Methyl demeton |
| Chlorfenvinphos | Methyl parathion |
| Chlorothion | Mevinphos |
| Chlorpyrifos | Naled |
| Coumaphos | Parathion |
| Demeton | Phorate |
| Diazinon | Ronnel |
| Dichlorvos | Octamethyl pyrophosphoramide |
| Dicrotophos | Temephos |
| Dimethoate | Tetraethyl pyrophosphate (TEPP) |
| Dioxathion | Trichlorfon |
| Disulfoton | |
| Ethyl *p*-nitrophenyl benzenethiophosphonate (EPN) | |

**or·ga·no·phos·pho·rus** (or″gə-no-fos′for-əs) a compound containing phosphorus bound to an organic molecule; several organophosphorus compounds are used as insecticides, and they are highly toxic cholinesterase inhibitors. See *organophosphorus compound poisoning,* under *poisoning.*

**or·ga·no·tax·is** (or″gə-no-tak′sis) [*organo-* + *-taxis*] a tendency to selective migration to some particular organ.

**or·ga·no·ther·a·py** (or″gə-no-ther′ə-pe) [*organo-* + *therapy*] [MeSH: Organotherapy] the treatment of disease by the administration of animal endocrine organs or their extracts; called also *Brown-Séquard's treatment.*

**or·ga·no·trope** (or′gə-no-trōp″) an organotropic element or agent.

**or·ga·no·troph·ic** (or″gə-no-trof′ik) [*organo-* + *-trophic*] heterotrophic.

**or·ga·no·trop·ic** (or″gə-no-trop′ik) pertaining to or characterized by organotropism.

**or·ga·not·ro·pism** (or″gə-not′rə-piz-əm) [*organo-* + *tropism*] the special affinity of chemical compounds or of pathogenic agents for particular tissues or organs of the body.

**or·ga·not·ro·py** (or″gə-not′rə-pe) organotropism.

**or·ga·num** (or′gə-nəm) pl. *or′gana* [L., from Gr. *organon* tool, instrument] [TA] an organ: a somewhat independent part of the body that is arranged according to a characteristic structural plan, and performs a special function or functions; it is composed of various tissues, one of which is primary in function. Called also *organon.*
**o. extraperitonea′le,** extraperitoneal organ: any of the abdominal viscera, e.g., the kidneys, lying on the posterior abdominal wall and invested by peritoneum only on the anterior surface; called also *o. retroperitoneale* and *retroperitoneal organ.*
**or′gana genita′lia,** genital organs: the various internal and external organs that are concerned with reproduction; see *organa genitalia feminina externa, organa genitalia feminina interna, organa genitalia masculina externa,* and *organa genitalia masculina interna.* See Plate 50.
**or′gana genita′lia femini′na exter′na** [TA], external female genital organs: the external genitalia of the female, comprising the pudendum femininum, clitoris, and urethra feminina.
**or′gana genita′lia femini′na inter′na** [TA], internal female genital organs: the various organs in the female that are concerned with reproduction, including the ovary, uterine tube, uterus, and vagina. See Plate 50.
**or′gana genita′lia masculi′na exter′na** [TA], external male genital organs: the external genitalia in the male, comprising the penis, scrotum, and urethra masculina.
**or′gana genita′lia masculi′na inter′na** [TA], internal male genital organs: the various organs in the male that are concerned with reproduction, including the testis, epididymis, ductus deferens, seminal vesicle, ejaculatory duct, prostate, and bulbourethral gland. See Plate 50.
**o. gustato′rium** [TA], gustatory organ: the organ of taste, comprising the taste buds, most of which are found within the epithelial covering of the tongue; called also *o. gustus* [TA alternative].
**o. gus′tus,** TA alternative for *o. gustatorium.*
**or′gana o′culi accesso′ria,** the accessory organs of the eye, including the ocular muscles and fascia, and the eyebrows, eyelids, conjunctiva, and lacrimal apparatus. Called also *adnexa oculi.* See Plate 17.
**o. olfacto′rium** [TA], olfactory organ: the specialized structures subserving the function of the sense of smell, including the olfactory region of the nasal mucosa containing the bipolar cells of origin of the olfactory nerves, together with the olfactory glands; called also *o. olfactus* [TA alternative].

**o. olfac'tus,** TA alternative for *o. olfactorium.*
**o. retroperitonea'le,** o. extraperitoneale.
**or'gana senso'ria,** organa sensuum.
**or'gana sen'suum** [TA], sense organs: organs that receive stimuli that give rise to sensations, i.e., organs that translate certain forms of energy into nerve impulses that are perceived as special sensations; they are characterized by highly specialized neuroreceptors and relationships, and include the visual, vestibulocochlear, olfactory, and gustatory organs. Called also *organa sensoria* and *organs of special sense.*
**o. spira'le** [TA], spiral organ: the organ, resting on the basilar membrane in the cochlear duct, that contains the special sensory receptors for hearing; it consists of neuroepithelial hair cells and several types of supporting cells, including the inner and outer pillar cells, inner and outer phalangeal cells, border cells, and Hensen's cells. Called also *organ of Corti.*
**o. subcommissura'le** [TA], subcommissural organ: a group of tall columnar ciliated ependymal cells lining the dorsal aspect of the cerebral aqueduct, situated dorsoventral to the commissure of the epithalamus; it is one of the circumventricular organs and may have neuroendocrine and neurosecretory functions.
**o. subfornica'le** [TA], subfornical organ: a group of specialized ependymal cells, similar to those of the subcommissural organ, projecting toward the cavity of the third ventricle from its anterior wall between the columns of the fornix; it is one of the circumventricular organs. Called also *intercolumnar tubercle.*
**or'gana urina'ria, or'gana uropoë'tica,** urinary organs: the organs concerned with the production and excretion of urine, including the kidneys, ureters, bladder, and urethra. See Plate 50.
**o. vasculosum of lamina terminalis,** an area of the lamina terminalis hypothalami where many neurons pass through a double-layered capillary bed and the blood-brain barrier is modified; it has a superficial capillary layer that receives blood from nearby arteries and drains into a deeper layer, from which blood passes to the cerebral veins. It is one of the *circumventricular organs.*
**o. vestibulocochlea're** [TA], vestibulocochlear organ: a collective term in official anatomical nomenclature applied to those structures outside the central nervous system that are concerned with balance and hearing, and comprising the internal, middle, and external ear. See Plate 16.
**o. vomeronasa'le** [TA], vomeronasal organ: a short rudimentary canal just above the vomeronasal cartilage, opening in the side of the nasal septum and passing from there blindly upward and backward; called also *Jacobson's organ.*

**or·gasm** (or'gaz-əm) [Gr. *orgasmos* swelling, or *organ* to swell, to be lustful] [MeSH: Orgasm] the apex and culmination of sexual excitement.

**or·go·tein** (or'go-tēn) any of a group of water-soluble congeners derived from red blood cells, liver, and other tissues, of molecular weight about 33,000 with compact conformation maintained by about 4 gram-atoms of divalent metal; produced from beef liver as a copper-zinc mixed chelate having superoxide dismutase activity. Orgotein has anti-inflammatory properties and has been used as an antirheumatic.

**Or·i·ba·si·us** (or"ĭ-ba'se-əs) [325–403 A.D.] Roman physician and medical writer, physician to the Emperor Julian. His *magnum opus* was an encyclopedia of medicine in seventy volumes, of which only one third survive; these are invaluable for they contain extracts from the works of many important physicians of antiquity (e.g., Dioscorides, Galen, Antyllus).

**ori·en·ta·tion** (or"e-ən-ta'shən) [MeSH: Orientation] 1. awareness of one's environment, with reference to place, time, and people. 2. the relative positions of atoms or groups in chemical compounds.

**or·i·fice** (or'ĭ-fis) [L. *orificium*] 1. the entrance or outlet of any cavity in the body. 2. any foramen, meatus, or opening. Called also *ostium* [TA] and *orificium.*
**abdominal o. of uterine tube,** ostium abdominale tubae uterinae.
**aortic o.,** ostium aortae.
**o. of aqueduct of vestibule, external,** apertura externa aqueductus vestibuli.
**atrioventricular o., left,** ostium atrioventriculare sinistrum.
**atrioventricular o., right,** ostium atrioventriculare dextrum.
**cardiac o.,** ostium cardiacum.
**o. of coronary sinus,** ostium sinus coronarii.
**duodenal o. of stomach,** ostium pyloricum.
**epiploic o.,** foramen omentale.
**external o. of urethra, external urethral o.,** see *ostium urethrae externum femininae* and *ostium urethrae externum masculinae.*
**external o. of uterus,** ostium uteri.
**hymenal o.,** o. vaginae.
**ileal o., o. of ileal papilla,** ostium ileale.
**o. of inferior vena cava,** ostium venae cavae inferioris.
**internal o. of urethra, internal urethral o.,** ostium urethrae internum.
**o. of maxillary sinus,** hiatus maxillaris.
**mitral o.,** ostium atrioventriculare sinistrum.
**pharyngeal o. of auditory tube,** ostium pharyngeum tubae auditivae.
**pilosebaceous o's,** the openings of the hair follicles, giving egress to the secretion of the sebaceous glands whose ducts open into the follicles, and to the hairs.
**pulmonary o., o. of pulmonary trunk,** ostium trunci pulmonalis.
**o. of pulp canal,** foramen apicis dentis.
**reticulo-omasal o.,** a sphincter between the reticulum and the omasum of a ruminant.
**o. of superior vena cava,** ostium venae cavae superioris.
**tricuspid o.,** ostium atrioventriculare dextrum.
**tympanic o. of auditory tube,** ostium tympanicum tubae auditivae.
**o. of ureter, ureteral o.,** ostium ureteris.
**uterine o. of uterine tube,** ostium uterinum tubae uterinae.
**vaginal o.,** o. vaginae.
**vesicourethral o.,** ostium urethrae internum.

**or·i·fi·cia** (or"ĭ-fish'e-ə) [L.] plural of *orificium.*

**or·i·fi·cial** (or"ĭ-fish'əl) pertaining to an orifice.

**or·i·fi·ci·um** (or"ĭ-fish'e-əm) pl. *orifi'cia* [L.] an opening or orifice, especially the entrance or outlet of any cavity or tube. Called also *ostium* [TA].
**o. exter'num isth'mi, o. exter'num u'teri,** ostium uteri.
**o. hy'menis,** o. vaginae.
**o. inter'num isth'mi, o. inter'num u'teri,** the internal orifice of the cervix uteri, opening into the cavity of the uterus.

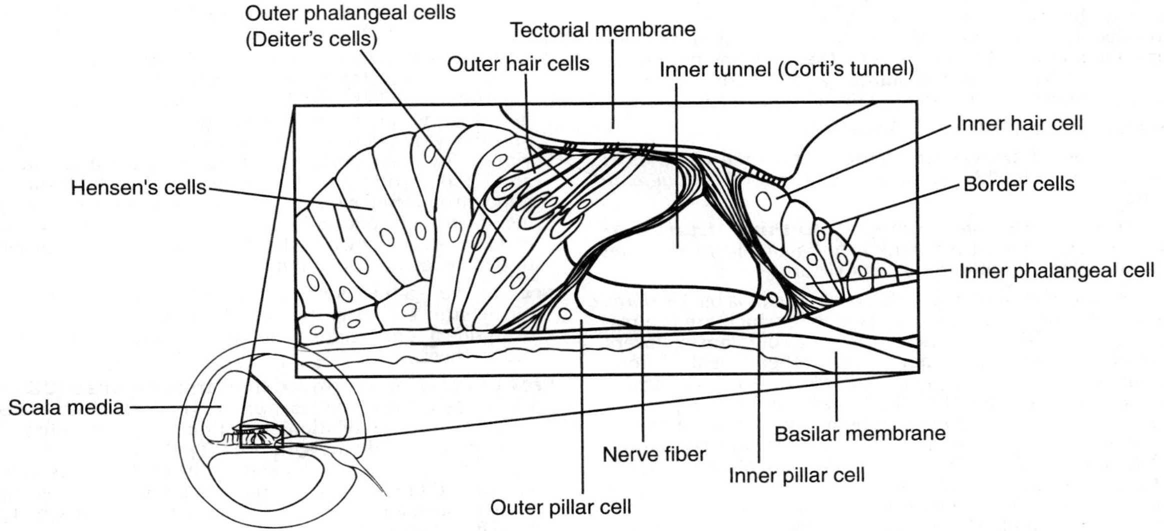


Detail of the organum spirale (spiral organ) in the cochlear duct in the inner ear.

**o. ure′teris,** ostium ureteris.
**o. ure′thrae exter′num mulie′bris,** ostium urethrae externum femininae.
**o. ure′thrae exter′num viri′lis,** ostium urethrae externum masculinae.
**o. ure′thrae inter′num,** ostium urethrae internum.
**o. vagi′nae,** o. vaginae.

**or·i·gin** (or′ĭ-jin) [L. *origo* beginning] the source or beginning of anything, especially the more proximal, fixed end or attachment of a muscle (as distinguished from its insertion), or the site of emergence of a peripheral nerve from the central nervous system.

**Or·i·mune** (or′ĭ-mūn) trademark for a preparation of live oral poliovirus vaccine.

**Or·i·nase** (or′ĭ-nās) trademark for a preparation of tolbutamide.

**ori·no·ther·a·py** (o-ri″no-ther′ə-pe) [Gr. *oreinos* pertaining to mountains + *therapy*] treatment by living in high, mountainous regions.

**or·li·stat** (or′lĭ-stat) a pancreatic lipase inhibitor that prevents the digestion, and therefore absorption, of dietary fat, used in the treatment of obesity; administered orally.

**Or·mond's disease** (or′məndz) [John Kelso *Ormond,* American physician, born 1886] retroperitoneal fibrosis; see under *fibrosis.*

**Orn** ornithine.

**Or·ni·dyl** (or′nĭ-dil″) trademark for a preparation of eflornithine hydrochloride.

**or·ni·thine** (or′nĭ-thēn) [MeSH: Ornithine] an amino acid produced in the urea cycle by the splitting off of urea from arginine and is itself converted into citrulline. On decomposition, it gives rise to putrescine.

**or·ni·thine ami·no·trans·fer·ase** (or′nĭ-thēn ə-mē″no-trans′fər-ās) [MeSH: Ornithine Aminotransferase] an enzyme of the transferase class that catalyzes the conversion of ornithine to $\Delta^1$-pyrroline 5-carboxylate via transfer of the ornithine amino group to an α-keto acid (e.g., α-ketoglutarate). The reaction is important in the degradation of ornithine from excess dietary tissue arginine, in the biosynthesis of proline, and in the de novo synthesis of ornithine. The enzyme is a mitochondrial matrix protein occurring in most cells; deficiency of it, an autosomal recessive trait, causes gyrate atrophy of choroid and retina. Abbreviated OAT. In EC nomenclature called *ornithine–oxo-acid transaminase.*

**or·ni·thine car·ba·mo·yl·trans·fer·ase** (or′nĭ-thēn kahr″bə-mo″əl-trans′fər-ās) [EC 2.1.3.3] [MeSH: Ornithine Carbamoyltransferase] an enzyme of the transferase class that catalyzes the carbamoylation of ornithine by carbamoyl phosphate to form citrulline. The reaction occurs in liver mitochondria as part of the urea cycle (see illustration at *urea cycle*). Called also *ornithine transcarbamoylase (OTC).* Abbreviated OCT.

**or·ni·thine car·ba·mo·yl·trans·fer·ase (OCT) de·fi·cien·cy** an X-linked aminoacidopathy involving the biosynthesis of urea; most hemizygous males show complete deficiency and do not survive the neonatal period; heterozygous females show varying degrees of deficiency and age of onset. Characteristic signs include hyperammonemia, neurologic abnormalities, and oroticaciduria. Called also *ornithine transcarbamoylase (OTC) deficiency.*

**or·ni·thine de·car·box·y·lase** (or′nĭ-thēn de″kahr-bok′sə-lās) [EC 4.1.1.17] [MeSH: Ornithine Decarboxylase] a cytosolic enzyme of the lyase class that catalyzes the decarboxylation of ornithine to form putrescine; the reaction occurs in the conversion of arginine to spermine and spermidine and in the synthesis of γ-aminobutyric acid via putrescine. The enzyme requires pyridoxal phosphate as a cofactor and is concentrated in rapidly proliferating cells.

**or·ni·thin·emia** (or″nĭ-thĭ-ne′me-ə) hyperornithinemia.

**or·ni·thine–oxo-ac·id trans·am·i·nase** (or′nĭ-thēn ok′so as′id trans-am′ĭ-nās″) [EC 2.6.1.13] EC nomenclature for *ornithine aminotransferase.*

**or·ni·thine trans·car·ba·mo·yl·ase, or·ni·thine trans·car·bam·y·lase (OTC)** (or′nĭ-thēn trans″kahr-bə-mo′əl-ās, or′nĭ-thēn trans″kahr-bam′ə-lās) ornithine carbamoyltransferase.

**Or·ni·thod·o·ros** (or″nĭ-thod′ə-ros) [Gr. *ornis, ornithos* bird + *doros* bag] a genus of argasid ticks, many species of which are the reservoirs and vectors of the spirochetes *(Borrelia)* of relapsing fevers and of other infectious agents for humans and other animals. Among the important vectors are: *O. as′perus, O. tartakov′skyi, O. tholoza′ni,* and *O. verruco′sus* in Russia, the Middle East, and other parts of Asia; *O. erra′ticus* and *O. norman′di* in Spain and North Africa; *O. duge′si, O. herm′sii, O. par′keri,* and *O. turica′ta* in Mexico and the western United States; *O. ru′dis* and *O. tala′je* in Central and South America; *O. savi′gnyi* in Africa, Arabia, and India; *O. mouba′ta* (the tampan tick) in South Africa; and *O. gur′neyi* in Australia.
**O. coria′ceus,** a tick found in California that attacks cattle, deer, and humans; its bite is painful and irritating because of the presence of a toxin, and may transmit *Chlamydia* and cause enzootic bovine abortion. Called also *pajaroello* and *pajaroello tick.*

**Or·ni·tho·nys·sus** (or″nĭ-tho-nis′əs) a genus of mites of the family Dermanyssidae; formerly called *Liponyssus.*
**O. baco′ti,** the rat mite or tropical rat mite; a species whose bite may cause a painful dermatitis (rat-mite dermatitis), and which experimentally transmits murine typhus; formerly called *Leiognathus bacoti* and *Liponyssus bacoti.*
**O. bur′sa,** the tropical fowl mite, commonly found on chickens and wild birds or in their nests.
**O. sylvia′rum,** the northern fowl mite, commonly a parasite of many domestic and wild fowl.

**or·ni·tho·sis** (or″nĭ-tho′sis) [Gr. *ornis, ornithos* bird + *-osis*] [MeSH: Ornithosis] 1. psittacosis in nonpsittacine birds or humans. 2. any kind of psittacosis.

**oro-**[1] [L. *os,* gen. *oris* mouth] a combining form denoting relationship to the mouth.

**oro-**[2] [Gr. *oros* whey, serum] see *orrho-.*

**oro·lin·gual** (or″o-ling′gwəl) [*oro-*[1] + *lingual*] pertaining to the mouth and tongue.

**oro·man·dib·u·lar** (o″ro-man-dib′u-lər) [*oro-*[1] + *mandibular*] pertaining to the mouth and mandible.

**oro·max·il·lary** (or″o-mak′sĭ-lar″e) pertaining to the mouth and the maxillary region.

**oro·men·in·gi·tis** (or″o-men″in-ji′tis) orrhomeningitis.

**oro·na·sal** (or″o-na′səl) [*oro-*[1] + *nasal*] pertaining to the mouth and nose.

**oro·pha·ryn·ge·al** (or″o-fə-rin′je-əl) 1. pertaining to the mouth and the pharynx; called also *pharyngo-oral.* 2. pertaining to the oropharynx (pars oralis pharyngis).

**oro·phar·ynx** (or″o-far′inks) [*oro-*[1] + *pharynx*] [MeSH: Oropharynx] pars oralis pharyngis.

**Orop·syl·la** (o″rop-sil′ə) a genus of fleas.
**O. idahoen′sis,** a rodent flea of the western United States, implicated in the transmission of sylvatic plague.
**O. monta′na,** former name for *Diamanus montanus.*
**O. silantie′wi,** a flea of the Manchuria marmot or tarbagan, capable of transmitting plague.

**or·o·so·mu·coid** (or″o-so-mu′koid) [MeSH: Orosomucoid] α1-acid glycoprotein; see under *glycoprotein.*

**or·o·tate** (or′o-tāt) a dissociated form of orotic acid.

**or·o·tate phos·pho·ri·bo·syl·trans·fer·ase (OPRT)** (or′o-tāt fos″fo-ri″bo-səl-trans′fər-ās) [EC 2.4.2.10] [MeSH: Orotate Phosphoribosyltransferase] an enzyme activity of the transferase class that catalyzes the transfer to orotate of a ribosyl group from phosphoribosylpyrophosphate (PRPP) to form orotidine 5′-phosphate as a step in the synthesis of pyrimidine nucleotides. The catalytic sites for this activity and for orotidine 5′-phosphate decarboxylase (ODC) activity occur on a single protein, called *UMP synthase;* deficiency of both activities, an autosomal recessive trait, causes hereditary oroticaciduria, type I.

**orot·ic ac·id** (ə-rot′ik) [MeSH: Orotic Acid] uracil-6-carboxylic acid, an intermediate in the biosynthesis of the pyrimidine nucleotides.

**orot·ic·ac·i·du·ria** (ə-rot″ik-as″ĭ-du′re-ə) 1. excess of orotic acid in the urine, occurring in several metabolic disorders and also resulting from administration of some drugs. 2. an autosomal recessive defect of pyrimidine metabolism due to deficiency of orotate phosphoribosyltransferase (OPRT) or orotidine-5′-phosphate decarboxylase (ODC). Manifestations include crystalluria and excessive excretion of orotic acid in the urine, megaloblastic anemia with hypochromic, microcytic circulating erythrocytes, and physical and mental growth retardation. There are two biochemical types: *type I* is due to deficiency of both OPRT and ODC activities; *type II* is due to deficiency of ODC activity only.

**orot·i·dine** (ə-rot′ĭ-dēn) a nucleoside, orotic acid linked by its N1 nitrogen to the C1 carbon of ribose; a phosphorylated derivative, orotidine 5′-phosphate, is an intermediate in pyrimidine nucleotide biosynthesis.

**orot·i·dine-5′-phos·phate de·car·box·y·lase (ODC)** (ə-rot′ĭ-dēn fos′fāt de″kahr-bok′sə-lās) an enzyme of the lyase class that catalyzes the decarboxylation of orotidine 5′-phosphate to form uridine monophosphate in the synthesis of pyrimidine nucleotides. The catalytic sites for this activity and for the orotate phosphoribosyltransferase (OPRT) activity are on a single protein. Deficiency of ODC activity only, an autosomal recessive trait, results in oroticaciduria, type II.

**orot·i·dyl·ate** (ə-rot″ĭ-dil′āt) a dissociated form of orotidylic acid.

**orot·i·dyl·ate de·car·box·y·lase** (ə-rot″ĭ-dil′āt de″kahr-bok′sə-lās) orotidine-5′-phosphate decarboxylase.

**orot·i·dyl·ic ac·id** (ə-rot″ĭ-dil′ik) phosphorylated orotidine, usually referring to orotidine 5′-phosphate (see *orotidine*).

**Oroya fever** (o-roi′ə) [*Oroya,* Peru, where the earliest cases were reported in 1885] see under *fever.*

**or·phen·a·drine** (or-fen′ə-drēn) [MeSH: Orphenadrine] the *ortho*-methyl analogue of diphenhydramine, having anticholinergic, antihistaminic, antispasmodic, and euphoric actions. Called also *mephenamine.*
**o. citrate** [USP], the citrate salt of orphenadrine, used as a skeletal muscle relaxant in acute spasm of voluntary muscles, regardless of location, especially post-traumatic, discogenic, and tension spasms, administered orally, intramuscularly, and intravenously.
**o. hydrochloride,** the hydrochloride salt of orphenadrine, used in the treatment of parkinsonian and drug-induced extrapyramidal reactions, administered orally.

**Orr treatment (method, technique)** (or) [Hiram Winnett *Orr,* American orthopedic surgeon, 1877–1956] see under *treatment.*

**orrho-** [Gr. *orrhos* whey, serum] a combining form denoting relationship to serum.

**or·rho·men·in·gi·tis** (or″o-men″in-ji′tis) [*orrho-* + *meningitis*] inflammation of a serous membrane.

**or·ris** (or′is) 1. any of several species of herbs of the genus *Iris,* especially *I. florentina.* 2. the peeled, dried, and powdered, fragrant root of *Iris florentina* and other species of *I.;* used in dentifrices, toilet and dusting powders, and perfumery. Called also *orris root.*

**ORS** oral rehydration salts.

**Or·si-Groc·co method** (or″se-grok′o) [Francesco *Orsi,* Italian physician, 1828–1890; Pietro *Grocco,* Italian physician, 1857–1916] see under *method.*

**ORT** oral rehydration therapy.

**or·the·sis** (or-the′sis) pl. *orthe′ses.* Orthosis.

**or·thet·ic** (or-thet′ik) orthotic.

**or·thet·ics** (or-thet′iks) orthotics.

**or·the·tist** (or′thə-tist) orthotist.

**ortho-** [Gr. *orthos* straight] 1. a combining form meaning straight, normal, or correct. 2. symbol *o-*; in organic chemistry, a prefix indicating a 1,2-substituted benzene ring, e.g., *o*-xylene (1,2-dimethylbenzene) or *o*-nitrophenol (2-nitrophenol). 3. in inorganic chemistry, a prefix indicating the common form of an acid as opposed to dimeric or polymeric anhydrides indicated by the prefixes *pyro-* and *meta-,* respectively.

Two examples of disubstituted benzene derivatives with substituents in the *ortho-* position. *(A), o*-xylene (1,2-dimethylbenzene); *(B), o*-nitrophenol.

**or·tho·ac·id** (or″tho-as′id) an acid containing as many hydroxyl groups as the valence of the acidulous element.

**or·tho·ar·te·ri·ot·o·ny** (or″tho-ahr-tēr-e-ot′ə-ne) [*ortho-* + *arterio-* + *tonos* tension] normal arterial pressure.

**or·tho·bi·o·sis** (or″tho-bi-o′sis) [*ortho-* + *biosis*] proper living; living in accordance with all the laws of health.

**or·tho·ce·phal·ic** (or″tho-sə-fal′ik) [*ortho-* + *cephalic*] having a head with a vertical index of 70.1 to 75.

**or·tho·ceph·a·lous** (or″tho-sef′ə-ləs) orthocephalic.

**or·tho·cho·rea** (or″tho-kə-re′ə) [*ortho-* + *chorea*] choreic movements in the erect posture.

**or·tho·chro·mat·ic** (or″tho-kro-mat′ik) 1. normochromic. 2. denoting a photographic emulsion sensitive to all colors except red.

**or·tho·chro·mia** (or″tho-kro′me-ə) [*ortho-* + *chrom-* + *-ia*] normochromia.

**or·tho·chro·mic** (or″tho-kro′mik) normochromic (def. 1).

**or·tho·chro·mo·phil** (or″tho-kro′mo-fil) [*ortho-* + *chromo-* + *-phil*] staining normally with neutral stains.

**Or·tho·clone OKT3** (or′tho-klōn) trademark for a preparation of muromonab-CD3.

**or·tho·cre·sol** (or″tho-kre′sol) one of the three isomeric forms of cresol.

**or·tho·cy·to·sis** (or″tho-si-to′sis) [*ortho-* + *-cyte* + *-osis*] the presence of mature cells only in the blood.

**or·tho·dac·ty·lous** (or″tho-dak′tə-ləs) [*ortho-* + *dactyl-* + *-ous*] having straight digits.

**or·tho·den·tin** (or″tho-den′tin) [*ortho-* + *dentin*] straight-tubed dentin, as seen in the teeth of mammals.

**or·tho·de·ox·ia** (or″tho-de-ok′se-ə) accentuation of arterial hypoxemia in the erect position, improved by assumption of a recumbent position.

**or·tho·di·chlo·ro·ben·zene** (or″tho-di-klor″o-ben′zēn) *o*-dichlorobenzene.

**or·tho·dig·i·ta** (or″tho-dij′ĭ-tə) [*ortho-* + *digitus*] the art of correcting deformities of the toes and fingers.

**or·tho·don·tia** (or″tho-don′shə) orthodontics.

**or·tho·don·tic** (or″tho-don′tik) pertaining to orthodontics.

**or·tho·don·tics** (or″tho-don′tiks) [*ortho-* + *odont-* + *-ic*] [MeSH: Orthodontics] that branch of dentistry concerned with the supervision, guidance, and correction of the growing or mature dentofacial structures. Called also *dentofacial orthopedics* and *orthodontology.*
**corrective o.,** that phase of orthodontics concerned with the reduction or elimination of an existing malocclusion and its attendant sequelae.
**interceptive o.,** that phase of orthodontics concerned with elimination of a condition that might lead to the development of malocclusion.
**preventive o., prophylactic o.,** that phase of orthodontics concerned with preservation of the integrity of proper occlusion through the use of orthodontic procedures and devices.
**surgical o.,** orthodontic therapy involving surgical procedures or orthognathic surgery, including resections and ostectomies, cosmetic surgery, the surgical uncovering of impacted teeth, and positioning and transpositioning of teeth.

**or·tho·don·tist** (or″tho-don′tist) a dentist who specializes in orthodontics.

**or·tho·don·tol·o·gy** (or″tho-don-tol′ə-je) orthodontics.

**or·tho·drom·ic** (or″tho-drom′ik) [Gr. *orthodromein* to run straight forward] conducting impulses in the normal direction; said of nerve fibers. Cf. *antidromic.*

**or·tho·gen·e·sis** (or″tho-jen′ə-sis) [*ortho-* + *genesis*] 1. progressive evolution in a given direction, in contrast with variations in several directions. 2. the theory that the course of evolution is fixed and predetermined; monogenesis.

**or·tho·gen·ics** (or″tho-jen′iks) eugenics.

**or·tho·gly·ce·mic** (or″tho-gli-se′mik) [*ortho-* + *glyc-* + *hemic*] having the normal amount of sugar in the blood.

**Or·thog·na·tha** (or-thog′nə-thə) a suborder of spiders (order Araneae) of temperate and tropical areas of the world; Theraphosidae and Dipluridae are families of medical importance.

**or·thog·nath·ia** (or″thog-nath′e-ə) [*ortho-* + *gnath-* + *-ia*] the branch of oral medicine dealing with the cause and treatment of malposition of the bones of the jaw.

**or·thog·na·thic** (or″thog-na′thik) 1. pertaining to orthognathia. 2. orthognathous.

**or·thog·na·thous** (or-thog′nə-thəs) [*ortho-* + *gnath-* + *-ous*] pertaining to or characterized by minimal protrusion of the mandible or minimal prognathism, with a gnathic index of 98 or less. Called also *orthognathic.*

**or·tho·grade** (or′tho-grād) [*ortho-* + L. *gradi* to walk] characterized by walking with the body upright, such as the bipeds. Cf. *pronograde.*

**Or·tho·hep·ad·na·vi·rus** (or″tho-hep-ad′nə-vi″rəs) [*ortho-* + hepadnavirus] hepatitis B viruses that infect mammals; a genus of the family Hepadnaviridae that includes hepatitis B virus and species infecting ground squirrels and woodchucks.

**or·tho·hy·droxy·ben·zo·ic ac·id** (or″tho-hi-drok″se-ben-zo′ik) salicylic acid.

**or·tho·io·do·hip·pu·rate** (or″tho-i″o-do-hip′ūr-āt) see *iodohippurate sodium.*

**or·thol·i·dine** (or-thol′ĭ-dēn) ortho-tolidine.

**or·tho·me·lic** (or″tho-me′lik) [*ortho-* + *mel-* + *-ic*] correcting deformities of the limbs.

**or·thom·e·ter** (or-thom′ə-tər) exophthalmometer.

**or·tho·mo·lec·u·lar** (or″tho-mo-lek′u-lər) [*ortho-* + *molecular*] relating to or aimed at restoring the optimal concentrations and functions at the molecular level of the substances (e.g., vitamins) normally present in the body. See also under *psychiatry.*

**or·tho·mor·phia** (or″tho-mor′fe-ə) [*ortho-* + *morph-* + *-ia*] the surgical and mechanical correction of deformities.

**Or·tho·myxo·vi·ri·dae** (or″tho-mik″so-vir′ĭ-de) [*ortho-* + *myxo-* + *virus* + *-idae*] [MeSH: Orthomyxoviridae] the influenzaviruses: a family of RNA viruses having a pleomorphic virion, which may be roughly spherical and 80–120 nm in diameter or filamentous and up to several micrometers long, consisting of a lipid bilayer envelope with large peplomers, surrounding a helical nucleocapsid. The genome consists of seven (influenza C virus) or eight (influenza A virus and influenza B virus) molecules of linear negative-sense single-stranded RNA (total MW approximately $5 \times 10^6$, total size 10.0–13.6 kb). Viruses contain seven to nine major polypeptides, including a transcriptase and a neuramidase, and are sensitive to lipid solvents, radiation, and disinfectants. Replication occurs in the nucleus and cytoplasm, and assembly is by budding on the plasma membrane. There are three genera: *Influenzavirus A, B, Influenzavirus C,* and the Thogoto-like viruses.

**or·tho·myxo·vi·rus** (or″tho-mik′so-vi″rəs) [MeSH: Orthomyxoviridae] any virus belonging to the family Orthomyxoviridae.

**or·tho·neu·tro·phil** (or″tho-noo′tro-fil) orthochromophil.

**or·tho·pae·dic** (or″tho-pe′dik) orthopedic.

**or·tho·pae·dics** (or″tho-pe′diks) orthopedics.

**or·tho·pan·to·graph** (or″tho-pan′to-graf″) panoramic radiograph.

**Or·tho·pan·to·mo·graph** (or″tho-pan′to-mo-graf) trademark for the equipment used in pantomography.

**or·tho·pe·dic** (or″tho-pe′dik) [*ortho-* + *ped-* + *-ic*] [MeSH: Orthopedics] pertaining to the correction of deformities of the musculoskeletal system; pertaining to orthopedics.

**or·tho·pe·dics** (or″tho-pe′diks) [*ortho-* + *ped-* + *-ic*] [MeSH: Orthopedics] that branch of surgery which is specially concerned with the preservation and restoration of the function of the skeletal system, its articulations, and associated structures.
**dentofacial o.,** orthodontics.
**functional jaw o.,** the use of muscle force to effect changes in jaw position and tooth alignment with a removable orthodontic appliance.

**or·tho·pe·dist** (or″tho-pe′dist) an orthopedic surgeon.

**or·tho·per·cus·sion** (or″tho-pər-kush′ən) [*ortho-* + *percussion*]

**or·thoph·o·ny** (or-thof′ə-ne) [*ortho-* + Gr. *phōnē* voice] the direct and correct production of sound.

**or·tho·pho·ria** (or″tho-fo′re-ə) [*ortho-* + *phoria*] the absence of heterophoria; the normal condition in which the visual axes remain parallel after the visual fusional stimuli have been partially or entirely eliminated.

**or·tho·phor·ic** (or″tho-for′ik) pertaining to or marked by orthophoria.

**or·tho·phos·phate** (or″tho-fos′fāt) an anion or salt of orthophosphoric acid or of any of its esters; it is the major intracellular anion. Abbreviated $P_i$. Called also *inorganic phosphate.*

**or·tho·phos·phor·ic ac·id** (or″tho-fos-for′ik) a strong mineral acid, $H_3PO_4$, the monomeric form of phosphoric acid (q.v.).

**or·tho·phre·nia** (or″tho-fre′ne-ə) [*ortho-* + *phren-* + *-ia*] soundness of mind.

**or·tho·pia** (or-tho′pe-ə) [*orth-* + *-opia*] the prevention or correction of strabismus.

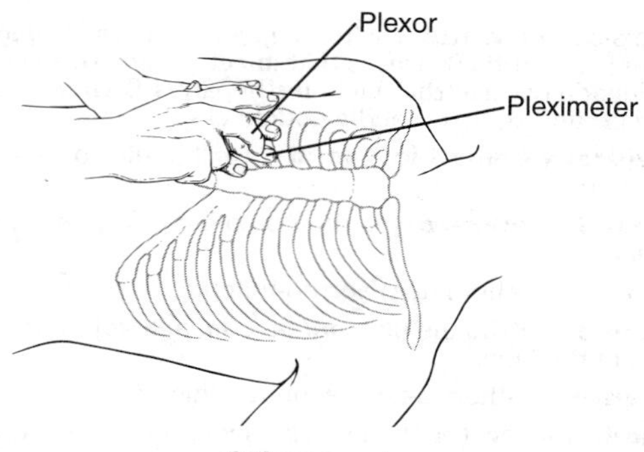


Orthopercussion.

**or·tho·ples·sim·e·ter** (or″tho-plə-sim′ə-tər) an instrument used to take the place of the pleximeter finger in orthopercussion.

**or·thop·nea** (or″thop-ne′ə) [*ortho-* + *-pnea*] dyspnea that is relieved by assuming an upright position. Cf. *platypnea.*
**two-pillow o.,** orthopnea that is relieved by elevating the head and chest from the recumbent position by the use of two pillows; see also *orthopneic position,* under *position.*

**or·thop·ne·ic** (or″thop-ne′ik) pertaining to or marked by orthopnea.

**or·tho·pod** (or′tho-pod) orthopedist.

**Or·tho·pox·vi·rus** (or′tho-poks-vi″rəs) [*ortho-* + *poxvirus*] [MeSH: Orthopoxvirus] a genus of viruses of the subfamily Chordopoxvirinae (family Poxviridae) with nucleic acid homology and serologic cross-reactivity that cause generalized infections with a rash in mammals, including camelpox, cowpox, ectromelia, monkeypox, and vaccinia viruses. The virtually extinct agent of smallpox, variola virus, belongs to this genus.

**or·tho·pox·vi·rus** (or′tho-poks-vi″rəs) [MeSH: Orthopoxvirus] a virus of the genus *Orthopoxvirus.*

**or·tho·prax·is** (or″tho-prak′sis) orthopraxy.

**or·tho·praxy** (or′tho-prak-se) [*ortho-* + Gr. *prassein* to make] the mechanical correction of deformities.

**or·tho·psy·chi·a·try** (or″tho-si-ki′ə-tre) [*ortho-* + *psychiatry*] [MeSH: Orthopsychiatry] an interdisciplinary field that combines psychiatry with principles of psychology, sociology, social work, and other fields in the study and practice of maintaining or restoring mental health, emphasizing a prophylactic approach to mental disease.

**Or·thop·tera** (or-thop′tər-ə) [*ortho-* + Gr. *pteron* wing] [MeSH: Orthoptera] an order of biting insects that do not undergo metamorphosis; they include the grasshoppers, locusts, crickets, and cockroaches.

**or·thop·tic** (or-thop′tik) [MeSH: Orthoptics] correcting obliquity of one or both visual axes.

**or·thop·tics** (or-thop′tiks) [MeSH: Orthoptics] a technique of eye exercises designed to correct the visual axes of eyes not properly coordinated for binocular vision.

**or·thop·tist** (or-thop′tist) an expert in orthoptics.

**or·thop·to·scope** (or-thop′to-skōp) [*ortho-* + *opto-* + *-scope*] an instrument for orthoptic or exercise treatment in anomalies of the ocular muscles, strabismus, or amblyopia.

**Or·tho·reo·vi·rus** (or″tho-re′o-vi″rəs) [*ortho-* + *r*espiratory *e*nteric *o*rphan + *virus*] a genus of viruses of the family Reoviridae, formerly classed as echoviruses, separable into three serotypes. No causative relationship to any disease has been proved in humans, although reoviruses have been isolated from both healthy individuals and patients with a variety of diseases. In other mammals reoviruses are associated with respiratory and enteric disease, and in chickens and turkeys, with arthritis.

**or·tho·rhom·bic** (or″tho-rom′bik) having three unequal axes intersected at right angles.

**or·thor·rhach·ic** (or″tho-rak′ik) [*ortho-* + *rhachi-* + *-ic*] having a vertebral column with practically no curvature in the lumbar region; cf. *koilorrhachic* and *kyrtorrhachic.*

**or·tho·scope** (or′tho-skōp) [*ortho-* + *-scope*] an apparatus that neutralizes the corneal refraction by means of a layer of water; it is used in examining the eye.

**or·tho·scop·ic** (or″tho-skop′ik) 1. pertaining to orthoscopy or an orthoscope. 2. having normal, undistorted vision. 3. pertaining to an optical system that produces undistorted images.

**or·thos·co·py** (or-thos′kə-pe) examination of the eye by means of the orthoscope.

**or·tho·sis** (or-tho′sis) pl. *ortho′ses* [Gr. *orthōsis* making straight] an orthopedic appliance or apparatus used to support, align, prevent, or correct deformities or to improve the function of movable parts of the body. See also *brace* and *splint.*
**ankle-foot o. (AFO),** any orthotic device for the lower limb that encloses the ankle and foot and does not extend above the knee; often there is a cuff or other device in the region of the knee or upper calf to take weight off the limb.
**balanced forearm o.,** a forearm orthosis consisting of a trough to support the forearm attached by a mechanism to the back of a wheelchair so that small movements of the shoulder girdle or the trunk produce motion at the elbow; for patients with severe weakness or paralysis of the shoulder or elbow.
**cervical o.,** a rigid plastic orthosis that encircles the neck and supports the chin and the back of the head; used in the treatment of injuries to the cervical spine.
**dynamic o.,** a support or protective apparatus for the hand or any

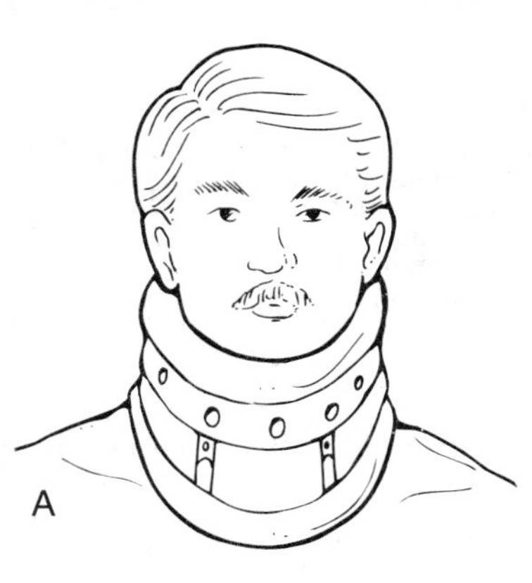

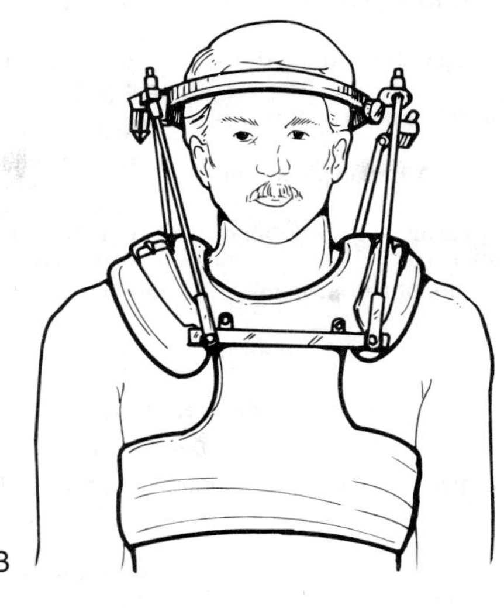

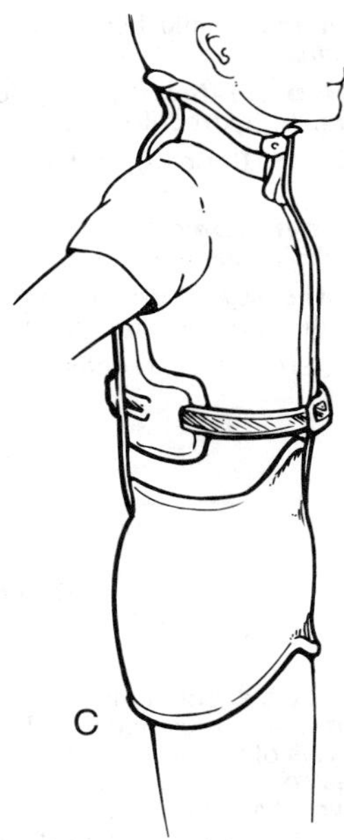


*(A),* cervical orthosis; *(B),* halo orthosis; *(C),* lumbosacral orthosis.

other part of the body that also aids in initiating and performing motion of that part or adjacent parts and assists in dealing with the forces resulting from the action, thus assisting in those motions necessary to perform the activities of daily living.
**Engen extension o.,** an orthosis for extension contracture of the knee or elbow that provides three points of pressure: one over the apex of the deformity and two on the opposite side of the limb at a distance.
**flexor hinge o.,** a dynamic orthosis for a weak or paralyzed hand, activated by movements of the wrist; metacarpophalangeal flexion is accomplished via a spring and hinge mechanism when the wrist extends.
**functional o.,** dynamic o.
**halo o.,** a cervical orthosis that provides maximal rigidity of the cervical spine, consisting of a metal or plastic halo attached to the upper skull by tongs or pins and linked by upright bars to a rigid jacket on the chest.
**hip-knee-ankle-foot o. (HKAFO),** any orthotic device for the lower limb that encloses the knee, ankle, and foot and extends to the hip, often being attached by means of a strap in the pelvic region; used for patients with paralysis of the lower limbs for whom walking is unlikely. Called also *long leg brace.*
**hyperextension o.,** a thoracolumbosacral orthosis that maintains hyperextension of the spine following compression fractures in the lower thoracic or upper lumbar regions.
**ischial weight-bearing o.,** a hip-knee-ankle-foot orthosis that transmits weight from the ischium to the ground; there is usually a large cuff in the ischial region to absorb weight and provide attachment for the upright bars; the knee and ankle may be either allowed movement with hinges or kept rigid.
**knee-ankle-foot o. (KAFO),** any orthotic device for the lower limb that extends from above the knee to the ankle and foot; called also *leg brace.*
**lumbosacral o. (LSO),** a spinal orthosis that encircles the body in the lumbosacral region; different types vary in width, from belts to corsets, as well as in rigidity.
**opponens o.,** one that holds the thumb metacarpal in maximal abduction and the thumb phalanges in extension to treat adduction contracture of the thumb.
**patellar tendon-bearing o.,** an ankle-foot orthosis designed to take weight off the heel and ankle by means of a cuff in the lower knee region and metal uprights to the shoe sole.
**pneumatic o.,** a plastic garment with inflatable tubes that surround the trunk or limbs; inflation of a tube provides stabilization and rigidity for the enclosed body part.
**poster o.,** a cervical orthosis with rigid upright posts, sometimes adjustable in length, extending from flat plates in the chin and occipital regions down to plates or a jacket on the chest and back.
**resting o.,** static o.
**serial stretch o's,** a series of static orthoses to keep a body part with a flexion contracture on gentle passive stretch; at each therapy session the joint is extended as far as it will comfortably go and a splint is shaped to hold it at that angle; eventually an optimal position of extension is reached.
**SOMI o.,** sternal-occipital-mandibular immobilizer.
**spinal o.,** a corset or other orthosis that surrounds part or all of the trunk to support or align the vertebral column or to prevent movement following trauma; see *lumbosacral o.* and *thoracolumbosacral o.*
**standing o.,** a device to maintain the patient in a standing position for improvement in posture and prevention of leg contractures and other deformities; used in lower limb paralysis.
**static o.,** an orthosis that does not allow motion of the part, primarily serving for support only.
**therapeutic o.,** dynamic o.
**thoracolumbosacral o. (TLSO),** a spinal orthosis that goes over the lumbar, sacral, and thoracic regions and thus limits movement of the thorax; different types vary in rigidity and in the kind of support given to the thorax.
**Toronto Legg-Perthes o.,** a knee-ankle-foot orthosis that treats or prevents deformities resulting from conditions such as Legg-Calvé-Perthes disease by holding the hips abducted at 45° while permitting hip flexion, knee flexion, and ambulation.

**or·tho·stat·ic** (or″tho-stat′ik) [*ortho-* + *-static*] pertaining to or caused by standing erect.

**or·tho·stat·ism** (or′tho-stat″iz-əm) an erect standing position of the body.

**or·tho·ster·eo·scope** (or″tho-ster′e-o-skōp) an apparatus for stereoradiography.

**or·tho·ther·a·py** (or″tho-ther′ə-pe) [*ortho-* + *therapy*] treatment of disorders by correction of posture.

**or·thot·ic** (or-thot′ik) serving to protect or to restore or improve function; pertaining to the use or application of orthoses.

**or·thot·ics** (or-thot′iks) the field of knowledge relating to orthoses and their use.

**or·thot·ist** (or-thot′ist) [Gr. *orthōtēr* a restorer or preserver] a person skilled in orthotics and practicing its application in individual cases.

**or·tho-tol·u·eno-azo-be·ta-naph·thol** (or″tho-tol″u-ēn″o-az″o-ba″tə-naf′thol) a poisonous dye used in processing citrus fruits.

**or·thot·o·nos** (or-thot′ə-nəs) [*ortho-* + Gr. *tonos* tension] tetanic fixation of the head, body, and limbs in a rigid straight line.

**or·thot·o·nus** (or-thot′ə-nəs) orthotonos.

**or·tho·top·ic** (or″tho-top′ik) [*ortho-* + *top-* + *-ic*] occurring at the normal place or upon the proper part of the body; pertaining to a tissue transplant grafted into its normal anatomical position.

**or·tho·tro·pia** (or″tho-tro′pe-ə) 1. absence of strabismus. 2. a condition of the eye in which there is no deviation of the visual axis with respect to a given meridian of the eye, e.g., hypotropia without lateral deviation.

**or·tho·trop·ic** (or″tho-trop′ik) pertaining to or characterized by orthotropia.

**or·tho·vol·tage** (or′tho-vōl″təj) in radiotherapy, voltage in the range of 140 to 400 kilovolts, as contrasted to *supervoltage* and *megavoltage.*

**Or·thox·ine** (or-thok'sēn) trademark for preparations of methoxyphenamine hydrochloride.

**or·thu·ria** (or-thu're-ə) [*ortho-* + *-uria*] normal frequency of urination.

**Ort·ner's syndrome** (ort'nerz) [Norbert *Ortner,* Austrian physician, 1865–1935] see under *syndrome.*

**Or·to·la·ni's sign (click)** (or-to-lah'nēz) [Marius *Ortolani,* Italian orthopedic surgeon, 20th century] see under *sign.*

**Oru·dis** (o-roo'dis) trademark for a preparation of ketoprofen.

**Or·u·vail** (or'oo-vāl) trademark for a preparation of ketoprofen.

**Ory·za** (o-ri'zə) [L., from Gr. *oryza* rice] a genus of cereal plants of the grass family (Gramineae). *O. sati'va* is rice.

**OS** [L.] *o'culus sinis'ter,* left eye.

**Os** symbol for *osmium.*

**os**[1] (os) gen. *o'ris,* pl. *o'ra* [L. "an opening, or mouth"] 1. any orifice of the body. 2. [TA] the mouth; the anterior or proximal opening of the digestive apparatus. See *mouth.*
**o. exter'num u'teri,** ostium uteri.
**o. of uterus, external,** ostium uteri.

**os**[2] (os) gen. *os'sis,* pl. *os'sa* [L.] [TA] bone (q.v.).

## Os

Descriptions are given on TA terms, and include anglicized names of specific bones.

**o. aceta'buli,** acetabulum.
**o. acromia'le,** a movable joint between the spine of the scapula and the epiphysis of the acromion.
**o. basila're,** basioccipital bone.
**o. bre've** [TA], short bone: one whose main dimensions are approximately equal, e.g., one of the bones of the carpus or tarsus.
**o. cal'cis,** calcaneus.
**o. capita'tum** [TA], capitate bone: the bone in the distal row of carpal bones lying between the trapezoid and hamate bones.
**o. carpa'le dista'le pri'mum,** o. trapezium.
**o. carpa'le dista'le quar'tum,** o. hamatum.
**o. carpa'le dista'le secun'dum,** o. trapezoideum.
**o. carpa'le dista'le ter'tium,** o. capitatum.
**o.'sa carpa'lia,** TA alternative for *ossa carpi.*
**o.'sa car'pi** [TA], carpal bones: the eight bones of the wrist (carpus), including the *o. capitatum, o. hamatum, o. lunatum, o. pisiforme, o. scaphoideum, o. trapezium, o. trapezoideum,* and *o. triquetrum.* Called also *ossa carpalia* [TA alternative].
**o. centra'le** [TA], central bone: an accessory bone sometimes found on the back of the carpus.
**o. centra'le tar'si,** o. naviculare.
**o. coc'cygis** [TA], coccygeal bone: the small bone caudad to the sacrum in humans, formed by union of four (sometimes five or three) rudimentary vertebrae, and forming the caudal extremity of the vertebral column; called also *coccyx* [TA alternative], *vertebrae coccygeae* [TA alternative], and *tail bone.*
**o. coro'nae,** small pastern bone; see *pastern bone,* under *bone.*
**o. cos'tae, o. costa'le,** costa (def. 2).
**o. cox'ae** [TA], the hip bone, which comprises the ilium, ischium, and pubis. Called also *o. pelvicum* and *pelvic bone.*
**o.'sa crania'lia,** ossa cranii.
**o.'sa cra'nii** [TA], cranial bones: the bones of the cranium, including the occipital, temporal, parietal, frontal, ethmoid, sphenoid, lacrimal, and nasal bones; the concha nasalis; and the vomer. Some authorities also include the maxilla, the palatine bone, and the zygomatic bone. Called also *ossa cranialia.*
**o. cuboi'deum** [TA], cuboid bone: a bone on the lateral side of the tarsus between the calcaneus and the fourth and fifth metatarsal bones.
**o. cuneifor'me interme'dium** [TA], intermediate cuneiform bone: the intermediate and smallest of the three wedge-shaped tarsal bones located medial to the cuboid and between the navicular and the first three metatarsal bones; called also *o. cuneiforme secundum.*
**o. cuneifor'me latera'le** [TA], lateral cuneiform bone: the most lateral of the three wedge-shaped tarsal bones located medial to the cuboid and between the navicular and the first three metatarsal bones; called also *o. cuneiforme tertium.*
**o. cuneifor'me media'le** [TA], medial cuneiform bone: the medial and largest of the three wedge-shaped tarsal bones located medial to the cuboid and between the navicular and the first three metatarsal bones; called also *o. cuneiforme primum.*
**o. cuneifor'me pri'mum,** o. cuneiforme mediale.
**o. cuneifor'me secun'dum,** o. cuneiforme intermedium.
**o. cuneifor'me ter'tium,** o. cuneiforme laterale.
**o.'sa digito'rum ma'nus** [TA], bones of digits of hand: the 14 bones that compose the skeleton of the fingers—two for the thumb and three for each finger. Called also *phalanges digitorum manus* [TA alternative] and *phalanges of fingers.*
**o.'sa digito'rum pe'dis** [TA], bones of digits of foot: the bones that compose the skeleton of the toes—two for the great toe and often the fifth toe and three for each of the other toes. Called also *phalanges digitorum pedis* [TA alternative] and *phalanges of toes.*
**o. epitympa'nicum,** a bone of very early fetal life that becomes the posterior portion of the squama that aids in forming the mastoid cells.
**o. ethmoida'le** [TA], ethmoid bone: the cubical bone located between the orbits and consisting of the lamina cribrosa, the lamina perpendicularis, and the paired lateral masses.
**o.'sa facia'lia, o.'sa facie'i,** facial bones.
**o. femora'le,** femur (def. 1).
**o. fe'moris,** TA alternative for *femur* (def. 1).
**o.'sa fonticulo'rum,** sutural bones (ossa suturalia [TA]) often present at the fontanelles.
**o. fronta'le** [TA], frontal bone: a single bone that closes the anterior part of the cranial cavity and forms the skeleton of the forehead; it is developed from two halves, the line of separation (the frontal or metopic suture) sometimes persisting in adult life.
**o. hama'tum** [TA], hamate bone: the medial bone in the distal row of carpal bones.

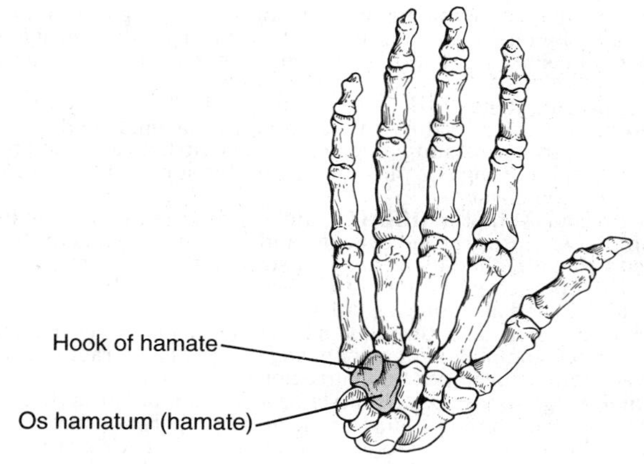


**o. hyoi'deum** [TA], hyoid bone: a horseshoe-shaped bone situated at the base of the tongue, just superior to the thyroid cartilage.
**o. ilia'cum,** o. ilium.
**o. i'lii, o. i'lium** [TA], iliac bone: the expansive superior portion of the os coxae (hip bone); it is a separate bone in early life. Called also *ilium* and *o. iliacum* [TA alternatives]. See Plate 45.
**o. in'cae,** o. interparietale.
**o. incisi'vum** [TA], incisive bone: the portion of the maxilla that bears the incisor teeth. In humans, the embryonic bone called the premaxilla fuses with the maxilla proper to form the adult bone. In most other vertebrates it persists as an independent bone. Called also *premaxilla* [TA alternative].
**o. innomina'tum,** o. coxae.
**o. intercuneifor'me,** an occasionally occurring bone situated between the medial and intermediate cuneiform bones.
**o. interme'dium,** o. lunatum.
**o. intermetatar'seum,** an occasionally occurring accessory bone situated between the proximal ends of the first and second metatarsal bones.
**o. interparieta'le** [TA], interparietal bone: the portion of the squamous part of the occipital bone that lies superior to the highest nuchal line when this portion remains separate throughout life.
**o. irregula're** [TA], irregular bone: a bone that is not readily classified as long, short, or flat; e.g., skull and hip bones and vertebrae.

**o. is'chii** [TA], the ischial bone: the inferior dorsal portion of the hip bone (os coxae); it is a separate bone in early life. Called also *ischium* [TA alternative]. See illustration accompanying *skeleton.*

**o. lacrima'le** [TA], lacrimal bone: a thin scalelike bone at the anterior part of the medial wall of the orbit, articulating with the frontal and ethmoid bones and the maxilla and inferior nasal concha. Called also *o. unguis.*

**o. lon'gum** [TA], long bone: a bone that has a longitudinal axis of considerable length, consisting of a body or shaft (the diaphysis) and an expanded portion (the epiphysis) at each end that is usually articular; typically found in the limbs.

**o. luna'tum** [TA], lunate bone: the bone in the proximal row of carpal bones lying between the scaphoid and triquetral bones.

**o. mag'num,** o. capitatum.

**o.'sa ma'nus** [TA], the bones of the hand: the carpals, metacarpals, and phalanges.

**o.'sa mem'bri inferio'ris** [TA], bones of inferior limb: the os coxae, pelvis, patella, tibia, fibula, tarsus, metatarsus, and digits of the foot.

**o.'sa mem'bri superio'ris** [TA], bones of superior limb: the humerus, radius, ulna, carpus, metacarpus, and digits of the hand.

**o.'sa metacarpa'lia,** TA alternative for *ossa metacarpi.*

**o. metacarpa'le ter'tium,** TA alternative for *o. metacarpi tertium.*

**o.'sa metacar'pi** [TA], metacarpal bones: the five cylindrical bones of the hand (metacarpals), which articulate proximally with the bones of the carpus and distally with the proximal phalanges of the fingers; numbered from that articulating with the proximal phalanx of the thumb to the most lateral one articulating with the proximal phalanx of the little finger. Called also *metacarpals* and *ossa metacarpalia* [TA alternative]. See also *o. metacarpi tertium.*

**o. metacar'pi ter'tium** [TA], third metacarpal bone: the middle metacarpal bone, which presents the styloid process on the dorsal surface of the radial side of its base. Called also *o. metacarpale tertium* [TA alternative].

**o.'sa metatarsa'lia,** TA alternative for *ossa metatarsi.*

**o.'sa metatar'si** [TA], metatarsal bones: the five bones (metatarsals) extending from the tarsus to the phalanges of the toes, being numbered in the same sequence from the most medial to the most lateral. Called also *ossa metatarsalia* [TA alternative].

**o. multan'gulum ma'jus,** o. trapezium.

**o. multan'gulum mi'nus,** o. trapezoideum.

**o. nasa'le** [TA], nasal bone: either of the two small, oblong bones that together form the bridge of the nose.

**o. navicula're** [TA], navicular bone: the ovoid-shaped tarsal bone that is situated between the talus and the three cuneiform bones; called also *o. naviculare pedis.*

**o. navicula're ma'nus,** o. scaphoideum.

**o. navicula're pe'dis,** o. naviculare.

**o. navicula're pe'dis retarda'tum,** Köhler's bone disease (def. 1).

**o. occipita'le** [TA], occipital bone: a single trapezoid-shaped bone situated at the posterior and inferior part of the cranium, articulating with the two parietal and two temporal bones, the sphenoid bone, and the atlas; it contains a large opening, the foramen magnum.

**o. odontoi'deum,** an anomalous bone that replaces all or part of the dens axis and is not attached to the atlas.

**o. orbicula're,** processus lenticularis incudis.

**o. in o.,** a radiation-induced injury appearing on radiographs as a vertebra within a vertebra.

**o. palati'num** [TA], palatine bone: the irregularly shaped bone forming the posterior part of the hard palate, the lateral wall of the nasal fossa between the medial pterygoid plate and the maxilla, and the posterior part of the floor of the orbit.

**o. parieta'le** [TA], parietal bone: either of the two quadrilateral bones forming part of the superior and lateral surfaces of the skull, and joining each other in the midline at the sagittal suture.

**o. pe'dis,** coffin bone.

**o.'sa pe'dis** [TA], the bones of the foot: the bones making up the skeleton of the foot, including the tarsal and metatarsal bones and the phalanges.

**o. pel'vicum,** o. coxae.

**o. pe'nis,** baculum.

**o. perone'um,** a sesamoid bone sometimes formed in the tendon of the peroneus longus muscle.

**o. pisifor'me** [TA], pisiform bone: the medial bone of the proximal row of carpal bones.

**o. pla'num,** 1. [TA] flat bone: any bone whose thickness is slight, sometimes consisting of only a thin layer of compact bone, or two layers with intervening spongy bone and marrow; usually bent or curved, rather than flat. 2. lamina orbitalis ossis ethmoidalis.

**o. pneuma'ticum** [TA], pneumatic bone: a bone that contains air-filled cavities or sinuses.

**o. pri'api,** baculum.

**o. pu'bis** [TA], pubic bone: the anterior inferior part of the hip bone (os coxae) on either side, articulating with its fellow in the anterior midline at the pubic symphysis; it is a separate bone in early life; called also *pubis* [TA alternative].

**o. radia'le,** o. scaphoideum.

**o. sacra'le,** o. sacrum.

**o. sa'crum** [TA], the sacrum: the wedge-shaped bone formed usually by five fused vertebrae that are lodged dorsally between the two hip bones (ossa coxae); called also *o. sacrale* and *vertebrae sacrales* [TA] alternative.

**o. scaphoi'deum** [TA], scaphoid bone: the most lateral bone of the proximal row of carpal bones; called also *o. naviculare manus.*

**o. sedenta'rium,** tuber ischiadicum.

**o.'sa sesamoi'dea ma'nus** [TA], sesamoid bones of hand, usually located in the palmar region in the tendons of the flexor pollicis brevis and adductor pollicis muscles. See *sesamoid bones,* under *bone.*

**o.'sa sesamoi'dea pe'dis** [TA], sesamoid bones of foot, usually located in the metatarsal region, particularly in the tendon of the flexor hallucis brevis muscle. See *sesamoid bones,* under *bone.*

**o. sphenoida'le** [TA], sphenoid bone: a single irregular, wedge-shaped bone at the base of the skull, forming a part of the floor of the anterior, middle, and posterior cranial fossae.

**o. subtibia'le,** an occasionally occurring bone found over the tip of the medial malleolus.

**o.'sa suprasterna'lia** [TA], suprasternal bones: ossicles occasionally occurring in the ligaments of the sternoclavicular articulation.

**o. suturale** [TA], sutural bone: any of the small irregular bones in the sutures between the bones of the skull, most frequently in the course of the lambdoid suture and often at the fontanelles *(ossa fonticulorum);* called also *epactal bone* and *wormian bone.*

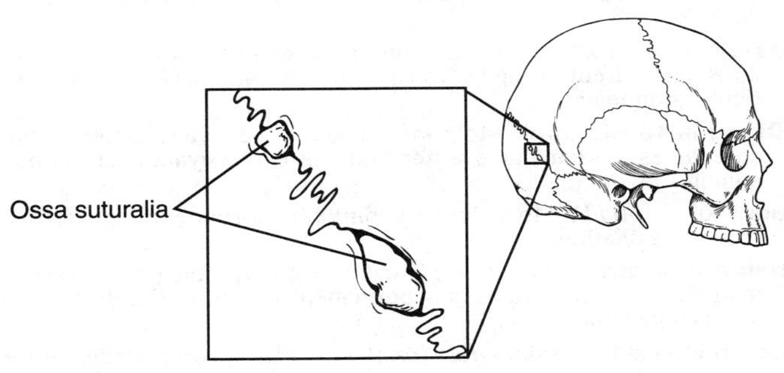


**o.'sa tarsa'lia,** TA alternative for *ossa tarsi.*

**o. tarsa'le dista'le pri'mum,** o. cuneiforme mediale.

**o. tarsa'le dista'le quar'tum,** o. cuboideum.

**o. tarsa'le dista'le secun'dum,** o. cuneiforme intermedium.

**o. tarsa'le dista'le ter'tium,** o. cuneiforme laterale.

**o.'sa tar'si** [TA], bones of tarsus: the seven bones of the ankle (tarsus), including the calcaneus, o. cuboideum, ossa cuneiforme intermedium, laterale, and mediale, o. naviculare, and talus. Called also *ossa tarsalia* [TA alternative].

**o. tar'si fibula're,** calcaneus.

**o. tar'si tibia'le,** talus.

**o. tempora'le** [TA], temporal bone: one of the two irregular bones forming part of the lateral surfaces and base of the skull, and containing the organs of hearing. It is divided anatomically into four parts: the *mastoid, petrous, squamous,* and *tympanic parts (pars mastoidea, pars petrosa, pars squamosa,* and *pars tympanica).*

**o.'sa tho'racis,** the bones of the thorax; see *skeleton thoracis.*

**o. tibia'le exter'num,** a small anomalous bone situated in the angle between the navicular bone and the head of the talus.

**o. trape'zium** [TA], trapezium bone: the most lateral bone of the distal row of carpal bones; called also *o. multangulum majus.*

**o. trapezoi'deum** [TA], trapezoid bone: the bone in the distal row of carpal bones lying between the trapezium and capitate bones; called also *o. multangulum minus.*

**o. trigo'num** [TA], an external tubercle at the back of the talus, sometimes occurring as a separate bone.

**o. trique'trum** [TA], triquetral bone: the bone in the proximal row of carpal bones lying between the lunate and pisiform bones; called also *triangular bone.*

**o. un'guis,** o. lacrimale.

**o. vesalia'num pe'dis,** vesalian bone: the proximal and external part of the tuberosity of the fifth metatarsal bone.

**o.'sa Wor'mi,** see *os suturale.*

**o. zygoma'ticum** [TA], zygomatic bone: the quadrangular bone of the cheek, articulating with the frontal bone, the maxilla, the zygomatic process of the temporal bone, and the greater wing of the sphenoid bone.

**OSAS** obstructive sleep apnea syndrome; see *sleep apnea*.

**osa·zone** (o'sə-zōn) any of a series of compounds obtained by heating a sugar with phenylhydrazine and an acid; the resulting crystals are characteristic of specific sugars and have been used to identify them. See also individual compounds; e.g., *glucosazone*.

**Os·bil** (os'bil) trademark for a preparation of iobenzamic acid.

**os·che·al** (os'ke-əl) [Gr. *oscheon* scrotum] scrotal.

**os·che·itis** (os″ke-i'tis) [*oscheo-* + *-itis*] inflammation of the scrotum.

**osche(o)-** [Gr. *oschē* scrotum] a combining form denoting relationship to the scrotum.

**os·cheo·cele** (os'ke-o-sēl″) [*oscheo-* + *-cele*[1]] tumor or swelling of the scrotum.

**os·cheo·hy·dro·cele** (os″ke-o-hi'dro-sēl) [*oscheo-* + *hydrocele*] hydrocele in the sac of a scrotal hernia.

**os·cheo·lith** (os'ke-o-lith) [*oscheo-* + *-lith*] a concretion in the sebaceous glands of the scrotum.

**os·che·o·ma** (os″ke-o'mə) [*oscheo-* + *-oma*] a tumor of the scrotum.

**os·che·on·cus** (os″ke-ong'kəs) [*oscheo-* + Gr. *onkos* mass, bulk] oscheoma.

**os·cheo·plas·ty** (os'ke-o-plas″te) [*oscheo-* + *-plasty*] plastic surgery of the scrotum.

**os·chi·tis** (os-ki'tis) oscheitis.

**os·cil·la·tion** (os″ĭ-la'shən) [L. *oscillare* to swing] a backward and forward motion, like a pendulum; see also *vibration, fluctuation,* and *variation.*

**os·cil·la·tor** (os'ĭ-la″tor) an apparatus for producing oscillations; an electric circuit designed to generate alternating current at a particular frequency.

**Os·cil·la·to·ria** (ə-sil″ə-to're-ə) a genus of cyanobacteria that sometimes contaminates water and can cause cyanobacteria poisoning.

**oscillo-** [L. *oscillare* to swing] a combining form denoting relationship to oscillation.

**os·cil·lo·gram** (ŏ-sil'o-gram) [*oscillo-* + *-gram*] the graphic record made by an oscillograph or a permanent record of the display on the oscilloscope.

**os·cil·lo·graph** (ŏ-sil'o-graf) [*oscillo-* + *-graph*] an instrument for producing a permanent record of variations in electrical voltage over time.

**os·cil·lom·e·ter** (os″ĭ-lom'ə-tər) [*oscillo-* + *-meter*] an instrument for measuring oscillations of any kind, such as changes in the volume of the arteries accompanying the heart beat. See also *sphygmo-oscillometer.*

**os·cil·lo·met·ric** (os″ĭ-lo-met'rik) pertaining to the oscillometer.

**os·cil·lop·sia** (os″ĭ-lop'se-ə) [*oscillo-* + *-opsia*] oscillating vision, a condition in which objects seem to move back and forth, to jerk, or to wiggle; it sometimes accompanies downbeat nystagmus.

**os·cil·lo·scope** (ŏ-sil'o-skōp) [*oscillo-* + *-scope*] an instrument that displays a visual representation of electrical variations on the fluorescent screen of a cathode-ray tube.

**Os·cil·lo·spi·ra** (ə-sil″o-spi'rə) [*oscillo-* + Gr. *speira* spiral] a genus of endospore-forming, rod-shaped bacteria of uncertain affiliation, formerly classified in the family Oscillospiraceae, found in the alimentary tract of herbivorous animals, and made up of anaerobic, motile cells. It contains a single species, *O. guilliermon'di.*

**Os·cil·lo·spi·ra·ceae** (ə-sil″o-spi-ra'se-e) in former systems of classification, a family of bacteria of the order Caryophanales, including the single genus *Oscillospira.*

**Os·ci·nis pal·li·pes** (os'ĭ-nis pal'ĭ-pēz) *Hippelates pallipes.*

**os·ci·tate** (os'ĭ-tāt) to yawn.

**os·ci·ta·tion** (os″ĭ-ta'shən) [L. *oscitatio*] yawning.

**os·cu·lum** (os'ku-ləm) pl. *os'cula* [L.] a minute opening.

**-ose** a suffix indicating that the substance is a carbohydrate.

**Os·good-Schlat·ter disease** (oz'good-shlaht'er) [Robert Bayley *Osgood,* American orthopedist, 1873–1956; Carl *Schlatter,* Swiss surgeon, 1864–1934] see under *disease.*

**OSHA** Occupational Safety and Health Administration.

**-osis** [Gr.] a word termination denoting a process, especially a disease or morbid process, and sometimes conveying the meaning of abnormal increase. See also *-sis.*

**Os·ler's disease, maneuver, nodes,** etc. (ōs'lərz) [Sir William *Osler,* Canadian-born physician, 1849–1919; successively professor of medicine in McGill University, the University of Pennsylvania, Johns Hopkins University, and the University of Oxford] see *hereditary hemorrhagic telangiectasia,* under *telangiectasia;* see *polycythemia vera,* and see under *maneuver, node, sign,* and *triad.*

**Os·ler-Va·quez disease** (ōs'lər-vah-kāz') [Sir William *Osler;* Louis Henri *Vaquez,* French physician, 1860–1936] polycythemia vera.

**Os·ler-We·ber-Ren·du disease** (ōs'lər va'bər ron-du') [Sir William *Osler;* Frederick Parkes *Weber,* British physician, 1863–1962; Henri Jules Louis Marie *Rendu,* French physician, 1844–1902] hereditary hemorrhagic telangiectasia.

**os·mate** (oz'māt) a salt containing the $OsO_4^{2-}$ anion, e.g., potassium osmate $K_2OsO_4$.

**os·mat·ic** (oz-mat'ik) [Gr. *osmasthai* to smell] 1. pertaining to the sense of smell. 2. having a sense of smell; applied to a category of animals subdivided further into macrosmatic and microsmatic. Cf. *anosmatic.*

**os·ma·tion** (oz-ma'shən) olfaction.

**os·me·sis** (oz-me'sis) [Gr. *osmēsis* smelling] olfaction (def. 2).

**os·mes·the·sia** (oz″mes-the'zhə) [*osm-* + *esthesia*] olfaction (def. 1).

**os·mic** (oz'mik) containing osmium.

**os·mic ac·id** (oz'mik) 1. osmium tetroxide. 2. the hypothetical acid, $H_2OsO_4$, which forms osmate salts.

**os·mi·cate** (oz'mĭ-kāt) to stain or impregnate with osmium tetroxide (osmic acid).

**os·mics** (oz'miks) [Gr. *osmē* odor] olfactology.

**os·mi·dro·sis** (oz″mĭ-dro'sis) [*osmo-*[1] + *hidro-* + *-sis*] bromhidrosis.

**os·mi·fi·ca·tion** (oz″mĭ-fĭ-ka'shən) treatment with osmium or osmic acid, as in histologic technique.

**os·mi·oph·i·lic** (oz″me-o-fil'ik) [*osmic* acid + *-philic*] staining easily with osmium or osmium tetroxide.

**os·mio·pho·bic** (oz″me-o-fo'bik) [*osmic* acid + *phobia*] resistant to staining with osmium or osmium tetroxide.

**os·mi·um** (oz'me-əm) [Gr. *osmē* odor; so named because of the odor of the vapor, $OsO_4$, produced by oxidation of the element] [MeSH: Osmium] 1. a very hard, gray, toxic, and nearly infusible metal; atomic number, 76; atomic weight, 190.2; symbol, Os. 2. a homeopathic trituration of metallic osmium.
**o. tetroxide,** $OsO_4$, a colorless or light yellow crystalline compound with a pungent odor, used as a fixative in preparing histologic specimens; if splashed in the eyes it can cause conjunctivitis, corneal damage, and in severe cases blindness. Called also *osmic acid.*

**osm(o)-**[1] [Gr. *osmē* odor] a combining form denoting relationship to odors.

**osm(o)-**[2] [Gr. *ōsmos* impulse] a combining form denoting relationship to osmosis.

**os·mo·cep·tor** (oz'mo-sep″tor) osmoreceptor.

**os·mol** (oz'mōl) osmole.

**os·mo·lal·i·ty** (oz″mo-lal'ĭ-te) the concentration of osmotically active particles in solution expressed in terms of osmoles of solute per kilogram of solvent. The osmolality is directly proportional to the colligative properties of solutions: osmotic pressure, boiling point elevation, freezing point depression, and vapor pressure lowering.

**os·mo·lar** (oz-mo'lər) pertaining to the concentration of osmotically active particles in solution.

**os·mo·lar·i·ty** (oz″mo-lar'ĭ-te) the concentration of osmotically active particles in solution expressed in terms of osmoles of solute per liter of solution.

**os·mole** (oz'mōl) the amount of substance that dissociates in solution to form one mole of osmotically active particles, e.g., 1 mole of glucose, which is not ionizable, forms 1 osmole of solute, but 1 mole of sodium chloride forms 2 osmoles of solute. Symbol Osm. Abbreviated *osmol.*

**os·mol·o·gy**[1] (oz-mol'ə-je) [*osmo-*[1] + *-logy*] osphresiology.

**os·mol·o·gy**[2] (oz-mol'ə-je) [*osmo-*[2] + *-logy*] that branch of physical chemistry that treats of osmosis.

**os·mo·lute** (oz'mo-lo͞ot″) an osmotically active solute.

**os·mom·e·ter** (oz-mom'ə-tər) [*osmo-*[2] + *-meter*] a device for measuring osmotic concentration or pressure.
**freezing-point o.,** an osmometer using freezing-point depression measurement for analysis of osmotic pressure (number of particles, molecules, or ions) of solutions.
**Hepp o.,** an osmometer in which very small quantities of material

can be used and a direct reading of the osmotic pressure may be made.

**membrane o.,** an osmometer in which diffusion through a semipermeable membrane indicates the osmotic pressure of macromolecules (number of molecules or ions) in a solution.

**os·mo·phil·ic** (oz″mo-fil′ik) [*osmo-*$^2$ + *-philic*] having an affinity for solutions with a high osmotic pressure.

**os·mo·pho·bia** (oz″mo-fo′be-ə) [*osmo-*$^1$ + *-phobia*] irrational fear of odors.

**os·mo·phore** (oz′mo-for) [*osmo-*$^1$ + *-phore*] the group of atoms in a molecule of a compound that is responsible for its characteristic odor.

**os·mo·re·cep·tor** (oz″mo-re-sep′tor) 1. [*osmo-*$^2$ + *receptor*] any of a group of specialized neurons in the supraoptic nuclei of the hypothalamus that are stimulated by increased osmolality (chiefly, increased sodium concentration) of the extracellular fluid; their excitation promotes the release of antidiuretic hormone by the posterior pituitary. 2. [*osmo-*$^1$ + *receptor*] olfactory receptor.

**os·mo·reg·u·la·tion** (oz″mo-reg″u-la′shən) maintenance of osmolarity by a simple organism or body cell with respect to the surrounding medium.

**os·mo·reg·u·la·to·ry** (oz″mo-reg′u-lə-tor″e) pertaining to osmoregulation.

**os·mose** (os′mōs) to pass through a membrane by osmosis.

**os·mo·sis** (oz-mo′sis, os-mo′sis) [Gr. *ōsmos* impulsion] [MeSH: Osmosis] the diffusion of pure solvent across a membrane in response to a concentration gradient, usually from a solution of lesser to one of greater solute concentration.

**reverse o.,** the passage of solvent across a semipermeable membrane going from a solution of greater to one of lesser solute concentration, i.e., in the opposite direction from the usual; it is caused by application of hydrostatic pressure to the solution with greater concentration.

**os·mo·sol·o·gy** (oz″mo-sol′ə-je) the science of osmosis.

**os·mo·stat** (oz′mo-stat″) the regulatory centers that control the osmolality of the extracellular fluid.

**os·mo·tax·is** (oz″mo-tak′sis) [*osmo-*$^2$ + *-taxis*] the movement of cells as affected by the density of the liquid containing them.

**os·mo·ther·a·py** (oz″mo-ther′ə-pe) [*osmo-*$^2$ + *therapy*] treatment by the intravenous injection of hypertonic solutions to produce dehydration.

**os·mot·ic** (oz-mot′ik) pertaining to or of the nature of osmosis.

**osphresi(o)-** [Gr. *osphrēsis* smell] a combining form denoting relationship to odors.

**os·phre·si·ol·o·gy** (os″fre-ze-ol′ə-je) [*osphresio-* + *-logy*] the sum of knowledge regarding odors and the sense of smell.

**os·phre·sis** (os-fre′sis) [Gr. *osphrēsis* smell] olfaction (def. 1).

**os·phret·ic** (os-fret′ik) olfactory.

**os·sa** (os′ə) [L.] plural of *os*$^2$.

**os·sa·ture** (os′ə-chər) the arrangement of bones in the body or in a part.

**os·se·in** (os′e-in) the collagen of bone.

**os·se·let** (os′ə-let) an exostosis on the inner aspect of a horse's knee or on the lateral aspect of the fetlock.

**osse(o)-** [L. *osseus* bony, from *os* bone] pertaining to bone or containing a bony element.

**os·seo·al·bu·moid** (os″e-o-al′bu-moid) a protein derived from bone after hydration of the collagen.

**os·seo·apo·neu·rot·ic** (os″e-o-ap″o-no͞o-rot′ik) pertaining to bone and the aponeurosis of a muscle.

**os·seo·car·ti·lag·i·nous** (os″e-o-kahr″tĭ-laj′ĭ-nəs) osteochondral.

**os·seo·fi·brous** (os″e-o-fi′brəs) made up of fibrous tissue and bone.

**os·seo·in·te·gra·tion** (os″e-o-in″tə-gra′shən) [*osseo-* + *integration*] [MeSH: Osseointegration] direct anchorage of an implant by the formation of bony tissue around it without growth of fibrous tissue at the bone-implant interface. See also *osseointegrated implant,* under *implant.*

**os·seo·mu·cin** (os″e-o-mu′sin) the homogeneous ground substance that binds together the collagen and elastic fibrils of bony tissue.

**os·seo·mu·coid** (os″e-o-mu′koid) a mucin existing in bone.

**os·se·ous** (os′e-əs) [L. *osseus*] of the nature or quality of bone; bony.

**os·si·cle** (os′ĭ-kəl) [L. *ossiculum*] a small bone.

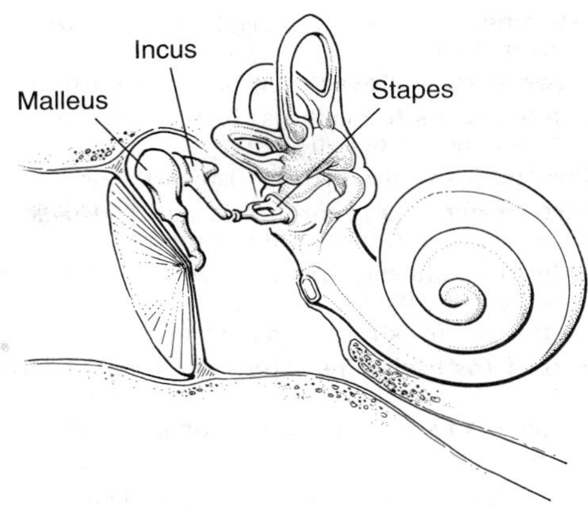


Auditory ossicles.

**Andernach's o's,** see *os suturale.*

**auditory o's,** ossicula auditus; see under *ossiculum.*

**o. of Bertin,** concha sphenoidalis.

**epactal o's,** see *os suturale.*

**episternal o's,** ossa suprasternalia.

**intercalcar o's,** see *os suturale.*

**Kerckring's (Kerkring's) o.,** see under *center.*

**Riolan's o's,** small bones occasionally seen in the suture between the mastoid portion of the temporal bone and the occipital bone.

**sphenoturbinal o.,** concha sphenoidalis.

**wormian o's,** see *os suturale.*

**os·sic·u·la** (o-sik′u-lə) [L.] plural of *ossiculum.*

**os·sic·u·lar** (ə-sik′u-lər) pertaining to an ossicle.

**os·sic·u·lec·to·my** (os″ĭ-ku-lek′tə-me) [*ossiculum* + *-ectomy*] surgical removal of an ossicle, or of the ossicles, of the ear.

**os·si·cu·lot·o·my** (os″ĭ-ku-lot′ə-me) [*ossiculum* + *-tomy*] surgical incision of the ossicles of the ear.

**os·sic·u·lum** (ə-sik′u-ləm) pl. *ossi′cula* [L.] [TA] ossicle.

**ossi′cula audito′ria,** TA alternative for *ossicula auditus.*

**ossi′cula audi′tus** [TA], auditory ossicles: the malleus, incus, and stapes, the small bones of the middle ear, which transmit vibrations from the tympanic membrane to the oval window. Called also *ossicula auditoria* [TA alternative] and *ossicular chain.*

**os·si·des·mo·sis** (os″ĭ-dəs-mo′sis) osteodesmosis.

**os·sif·er·ous** (ə-sif′ər-əs) [*os*$^2$ + *-ferous*] producing bone.

**os·sif·ic** (ə-sif′ik) [L. *os* bone + *facere* to make] forming or becoming bone.

**os·si·fi·ca·tion** (os″ĭ-fĭ-ka′shən) [L. *ossificatio*] the formation of bone or of a bony substance; the conversion of fibrous tissue or of cartilage into bone or a bony substance.

**cartilaginous o.,** ossification that occurs in and replaces cartilage.

**ectopic o.,** a pathological condition in which bone arises in tissues not in the osseous system and in connective tissues usually not manifesting osteogenic properties.

**endochondral o.,** cartilaginous o.

**heterotopic o.,** the formation of bone in abnormal locations, secondary to pathology either at the local site or elsewhere.

**intramembranous o.,** ossification that occurs in and replaces connective tissue, as occurs in the calvaria and in periosteal bone formation.

**metaplastic o.,** the development of bony substance in normally soft structures.

**perichondral o.,** that which occurs in a layered manner beneath the perichondrium or, later, the periosteum.

**periosteal o.,** a type of intramembranous bone formation.

**os·sif·lu·ence** (ə-sif′loo-əns) softening of bony tissue.

**os·si·form** (os′ĭ-form) resembling bone.

**os·si·fy·ing** (os′ĭ-fi″ing) changing or developing into bone.

**os·si·phone** (os′ĭ-fōn) [L. *os,* pl. *ossa* bone + Gr. *phōnē* voice] an early type of hearing aid that used bone conduction.

**os·tal·gia** (os-tal′jə) ostealgia.

**os·tar·thri·tis** (os″tahr-thri′tis) osteoarthritis.

**os·te·al** (os′te-əl) bony; osseous.

**os·te·al·bu·moid** (os″te-al′bu-moid) osseoalbumoid.

**os·te·al·gia** (os″te-al′jə) [*oste-* + *-algia*] pain in a bone or in the bones.

**os·te·ana·bro·sis** (os″te-an″ə-bro′sis) [*osteo-* + Gr. *anabrōsis* eating up] atrophy of bone.

**os·te·ana·gen·e·sis** (os″te-an″ə-jen′ə-sis) osteoanagenesis.

**os·te·anaph·y·sis** (os″te-ə-naf′ĭ-sis) [*osteo-* + Gr. *anaphyein* to reproduce] reproduction of bone.

**os·te·ar·thri·tis** (os″te-ahr-thri′tis) osteoarthritis.

**os·te·ar·throt·o·my** (os″te-ahr-throt′ə-me) [*osteo-* + *arthro-* + *-tomy*] excision of an articular end of a bone.

**os·tec·to·my** (os-tek′tə-me) [*osteo-* + *-ectomy*] the excision of a bone or a portion of a bone.

**os·te·ec·to·my** (os″te-ek′tə-me) ostectomy.

**os·te·ec·to·pia** (os″te-ek-to′pe-ə) [*osteo-* + *-ectopia*] displacement of a bone.

**os·te·ec·to·py** (os″te-ek′tə-pe) osteectopia.

**os·te·in** (os′te-in) ossein.

**os·te·ite** (os′te-īt) an independent bony element or center of ossification.

**os·te·itis** (os″te-i′tis) [*osteo-* + *-itis*] [MeSH: Osteitis] inflammation of a bone, involving the haversian spaces, canals, and their branches, and generally the medullary cavity, and marked by enlargement of the bone, tenderness, and a dull, aching pain. See also *osteomyelitis.*
**acute o.**, osteomyelitis, usually of septic origin.
**o. albumino′sa,** osteitis with accumulation of a sticky, albuminous liquid.
**alveolar o.**, dry socket.
**carious o.**, osteomyelitis.
**o. carno′sa,** o. fungosa.
**caseous o.**, tuberculous caries of bone.
**central o.**, endosteitis.
**chronic o.**, central caries or bone abscess; often due to tuberculosis, sometimes syphilitic.
**chronic nonsuppurative o.**, sclerosing nonsuppurative osteomyelitis.
**o. conden′sans,** condensing o.
**o. conden′sans generalisa′ta,** osteopoikilosis.
**o. conden′sans i′lii,** a condition marked by an area of dense sclerosis on the iliac side of the sacroiliac joint.
**condensing o.**, osteitis with hard deposits of earthy salts in the affected bone; called also *formative o.* and *sclerosing o.*
**cortical o.**, periostitis.
**o. defor′mans,** a disease of bone marked by repeated episodes of increased bone resorption followed by excessive attempts at repair, resulting in weakened deformed bones of increased mass. There may be bowing of long bones and deformation of flat bones; pain and pathological fractures are associated. When it affects the bones of the skull, deafness may result. Called also *Paget's disease of bone.*
**o. fibro′sa cys′tica, o. fibro′sa cys′tica generalisa′ta,** rarefying osteitis with fibrous degeneration and formation of cysts, and with the presence of fibrous nodules on the affected bones; it is due to marked osteoclastic activity secondary to hyperfunction of the parathyroid gland. Called also *Recklinghausen's* or *von Recklinghausen's disease.*
**o. fibro′sa dissemina′ta,** polyostotic fibrous dysplasia.
**o. fibro′sa localisa′ta,** monostotic fibrous dysplasia.
**o. fibro′sa osteoplas′tica,** o. fibrosa cystica.
**formative o.**, condensing o.
**o. fragi′litans,** osteogenesis imperfecta.
**o. fungo′sa,** chronic osteitis in which the haversian canals are dilated and filled with granulation tissue.
**Garré's o.**, sclerosing nonsuppurative osteomyelitis.
**o. granulo′sa,** o. fungosa.
**gummatous o.**, a chronic form associated with syphilis.
**necrotic o.**, osteomyelitis.
**o. ossi′ficans,** condensing o.
**parathyroid o.**, o. fibrosa cystica.
**pedal o.**, inflammation of the pedal (coffin) bone of the forefoot of a horse, due to overwork, corns, or repeated trauma such as that due to an irregular conformation of the hoof surface. Called also *peditis.*
**productive o.**, condensing o.
**o. pu′bis,** 1. sclerosis of the pubic bones, in the region of the symphysis, usually observed as an incidental finding in radiography of the pelvis. 2. a symptom-producing inflammatory condition of the pubic bones in the region of the symphysis, which may be associated with surgical procedures on pelvic structures or with pregnancy, infection of the urinary tract, degenerative changes, rheumatic disease, or other conditions.
**rarefying o.**, a bone disease in which the inorganic matter is lessened and the hard bone becomes cancellated.
**sclerosing o.**, 1. sclerosing nonsuppurative osteomyelitis. 2. condensing o.
**secondary hyperplastic o.**, hypertrophic pulmonary osteoarthropathy.
**vascular o.**, rarefying osteitis in which the spaces formed become occupied by blood vessels.

**os·tem·bry·on** (os-tem′bre-on) [*osteo-* + Gr. *embryon* fetus] lithopedion.

**os·tem·py·e·sis** (os″təm-pi-e′sis) [*osteo-* + *empyesis*] suppuration within a bone.

**Os·ten·sin** (os-ten′sin) trademark for a preparation of trimethidinium methosulfate.

**oste(o)-** [Gr. *osteon* bone] a combining form denoting relationship to a bone or to the bones.

**os·teo·acu·sis** (os″te-o-ə-ku′sis) [*osteo-* + Gr. *akousis* hearing] bone conduction.

**os·teo·ana·gen·e·sis** (os″te-o-an′ə-jen′ə-sis) [*osteo-* + Gr. *anagenesis*] regeneration of bone.

**os·teo·an·es·the·sia** (os″te-o-an″əs-the′zhə) the insensitiveness of bone.

**os·teo·an·eu·rysm** (os″te-o-an′u-riz-əm) aneurysm in a bone.

**os·teo·ar·thrit·ic** (os″te-o-ahr-thrit′ik) pertaining to or affected with osteoarthritis.

**os·teo·ar·thri·tis** (os″te-o-ahr-thri′tis) [*osteo-* + *arthr-* + *-itis*] [MeSH: Osteoarthritis] a noninflammatory degenerative joint disease seen mainly in older persons, characterized by degeneration of the articular cartilage, hypertrophy of bone at the margins, and changes in the synovial membrane. It is accompanied by pain, usually after prolonged activity, and stiffness, particularly in the morning or with inactivity. Called also *degenerative arthritis, hypertrophic arthritis,* and *degenerative joint disease.*
**o. defor′mans, o. defor′mans ende′mica, endemic o.**, Kashin-Bek disease.
**hyperplastic o.**, hypertrophic pulmonary osteoarthropathy.
**interphalangeal o.**, a localized form of arthritis involving the finger joints, characterized by the formation of nodosities (Bouchard's nodes and Heberden's nodes) and degenerative changes with intermittent inflammatory episodes, and leading eventually to deformities and ankyloses.

**os·teo·ar·throp·a·thy** (os″te-o-ahr-throp′ə-the) [*osteo-* + *arthropathy*] any disease of the joints and bones.
**familial o. of fingers,** Thiemann's disease.
**hypertrophic o., idiopathic, hypertrophic o., primary,** pachydermoperiostosis.
**hypertrophic pulmonary o.**, symmetrical osteitis of the four limbs, chiefly localized to the phalanges and the terminal epiphyses of the long bones of the forearm and leg, sometimes extending to the proximal ends of the limbs and the flat bones, and accompanied by a dorsal kyphosis and some affection of the joints. It is often secondary to chronic conditions of the lungs and heart. Called also *hyperplastic osteoarthritis, Marie-Bamberger disease* or *syndrome, pulmonary o.,* and *secondary hypertrophic o.*
**pulmonary o., secondary hypertrophic o.**, hypertrophic pulmonary o.

**os·teo·ar·thro·sis** (os″te-o-ahr-thro′sis) osteoarthritis.
**o. juveni′lis,** Köhler's bone disease (def. 1).

**os·teo·ar·throt·o·my** (os″te-o-ahr-throt′ə-me) ostearthrotomy.

**os·teo·ar·tic·u·lar** (os″te-o-ahr-tik′u-lər) pertaining to or affecting bones and joints.

**os·teo·blast** (os′te-o-blast″) [*osteo-* + *-blast*] [MeSH: Osteoblasts] a cell that arises from a fibroblast and that, as it matures, is associated with the production of bone.

**os·teo·blas·tic** (os″te-o-blas′tik) pertaining to or composed of osteoblasts.

**os·teo·blas·to·ma** (os″te-o-blas-to′mə) [*osteoblast* + *-oma*] [MeSH: Osteoblastoma] a benign, painful, rather vascular tumor of bone characterized by the formation of osteoid tissue and primitive bone; called also *giant osteoid osteoma.*

**os·teo·ca·chec·tic** (os″te-o-kə-kek′tik) pertaining to or characterized by osteocachexia.

**os·teo·ca·chex·ia** (os″te-o-kə-kek′se-ə) cachexia due to chronic bone disease; also chronic disease of bone.

**os·teo·cal·cin** (os″te-o-kal′sin) [MeSH: Osteocalcin] a vitamin K–dependent, calcium-binding bone protein, the most abundant noncollagen protein in bone; increased serum concentrations are a marker of increased bone turnover in disease states. Called also *bone Gla protein.*

**os·teo·camp·sia** (os″te-o-kamp′se-ə) [*osteo-* + Gr. *kamptein* to bend] curvature or bending of a bone, as in rickets.

**os·teo·camp·sis** (os″te-o-kamp′sis) osteocampsia.

**os·teo·car·ti·lag·i·nous** (os″te-o-kahr″tĭ-laj′ĭ-nəs) pertaining to or composed of bone and cartilage.

**os·teo·cele** (os′te-o-sēl) [*osteo-* + *-cele*[1]] 1. bony tumor of the testis or scrotum. 2. a hernia containing bone.

**os·teo·ce·men·tum** (os″te-o-se-men′təm) [*osteo-* + *cementum*] a hard bonelike secondary cementum, typically arranged in concentric layers around the root and frequently showing numerous resting lines, such as that occurring in hypercementosis.

**os·teo·chon·dral** (os″te-o-kon′drəl) pertaining to or composed of bone and cartilage; pertaining to a bone and its articular cartilage. Called also *osseocartilaginous.*

**os·teo·chon·dri·tis** (os″te-o-kon-dri′tis) [*osteo-* + *chondr-* + *-itis*] [MeSH: Osteochondritis] inflammation of both bone and cartilage.
**calcaneal o.,** Haglund's disease.
**o. defor′mans juveni′lis,** osteochondrosis of the capitular epiphysis of the femur; see *osteochondrosis.*
**o. defor′mans juveni′lis dor′si,** osteochondrosis of vertebrae; see *osteochondrosis.*
**o. dis′secans,** osteochondritis resulting in the splitting of pieces of cartilage into the joint, particularly the knee joint or shoulder joint.
**o. ischiopu′bica,** a condition observed in the radiograph, consisting of granular-looking bodies at the junction of the ischium and os pubis in children.
**juvenile deforming metatarsophalangeal o.,** Köhler's bone disease (def. 2).
**o. necro′ticans,** a condition marked by necrosis and destruction in the cartilage of the sesamoid bone of the great toe.
**o. os′sis metacar′pi et metatar′si,** Thiemann's disease (q.v.) affecting both the fingers and toes.

**os·teo·chon·dro·dys·pla·sia** (os″te-o-kon″dro-dis-pla′zhə) [*osteo-* + *chondro-* + *dys-* + *-plasia*] [MeSH: Osteochondrodysplasias] Morquio's syndrome.

**os·teo·chon·dro·dys·tro·phia** (os″te-o-kon″dro-dis-tro′fe-ə) Morquio's syndrome.
**o. defor′mans,** Morquio's syndrome.

**os·te·o·chon·dro·dys·tro·phy** (os″te-o-kon″dro-dis′trə-fe) Morquio's syndrome.
**familial o.,** Morquio's syndrome.

**os·teo·chon·dro·fi·bro·ma** (os″te-o-kon″dro-fi-bro′mə) fibrosing osteochondroma.

**os·teo·chon·drol·y·sis** (os″te-o-kon-drol′ĭ-sis) osteochondritis dissecans.

**os·teo·chon·dro·ma** (os″te-o-kon-dro′mə) [*osteo-* + *chondroma*] [MeSH: Osteochondroma] a benign tumor consisting of projecting adult bone capped by cartilage projecting from the lateral contours of endochondral bones. Called also *chondrosteoma, osteocartilaginous exostosis,* and *osteoenchondroma.*
**fibrosing o.,** a tumor containing the elements of osteoma, chondroma, and fibroma.

**os·teo·chon·dro·ma·to·sis** (os″te-o-kon″dro-mə-to′sis) [MeSH: Osteochondromatosis] a condition marked by the presence of multiple osteochondromas, such as occurs in multiple cartilaginous exostoses or enchondromatosis; the term is sometimes used to denote one of the two conditions specifically, usually the former.
**multiple o.,** osteochondromatosis.
**synovial o.,** a rare condition in which cartilage bodies are formed in the synovial membrane of the joints, tendon sheaths, or bursae, later undergoing secondary calcification and ossification; some of the bodies may become detached and remain as viable, growing structures in the synovial spaces.

**os·teo·chon·dro·myx·o·ma** (os″te-o-kon″dro-mik-so′mə) [*osteochondroma* + *myxoma*] osteochondroma containing myxoid elements.

**os·teo·chon·drop·a·thy** (os″te-o-kon-drop′ə-the) [*osteo-* + *chondro-* + *-pathy*] any morbid condition affecting both bone and cartilage, or marked by abnormal enchondral ossification.
**polyglucose (dextran) sulfate–induced o.,** an experimentally produced disorder of enchondral ossification characterized by a deficient formation of bone matrix in the metaphyses of long bones.

**os·teo·chon·dro·sar·co·ma** (os″te-o-kon″dro-sahr-ko′mə) [*osteo-* + *chondrosarcoma*] chondrosarcoma occurring in bone; used for those tumors including cartilaginous foci but not neoplastic foci of bone.

**os·teo·chon·dro·sis** (os″te-o-kon-dro′sis) a disease of the growth or ossification centers in children that begins as a degeneration or necrosis followed by regeneration or recalcification. Called also *epiphyseal ischemic necrosis* (q.v.). It may affect (1) the calcaneus (os calcis), a condition sometimes called *apophysitis;* (2) the capitular epiphysis (head) of the femur, a condition known as *Legg-Calvé-Perthes disease, Perthes disease, Waldenström's disease, coxa plana,* and *pseudocoxalgia;* (3) the ilium; (4) the lunate (semilunar) bone, known as *Kienböck's disease;* (5) head of the second metatarsal bone, known as *Freiberg's infraction;* (6) the navicular (tarsal scaphoid); (7) the tuberosity of the tibia, called *Osgood-Schlatter disease* and *Schlatter's disease;* (8) the vertebrae, called *Scheuermann's disease* or *kyphosis, juvenile kyphosis, vertebral epiphysitis,* and *kyphosis dorsalis juvenilis;* (9) the capitellum of the humerus, called *Panner's disease.*
**o. defor′mans ti′biae,** aseptic necrosis of the medial condyle of the tibia, producing lateral bowing of the leg; called also *Blount's disease, nonrachitic bowleg,* and *tibia vara.*

**os·teo·chon·drous** (os″te-o-kon′drəs) [*osteo-* + *chondr-* + *-ous*] composed of bone and cartilage.

**os·teo·cla·sia** (os″te-o-kla′zhə) [*osteo-* + Gr. *klasis* a breaking + *-ia*] the absorption and destruction of bone tissue.

**os·te·oc·la·sis** (os″te-ok′lə-sis) [*osteo-* + Gr. *klasis* a breaking] the surgical fracture or refracture of bones.

**os·teo·clast** (os′te-o-klast″) [*osteo-* + *-clast*] [MeSH: Osteoclasts] 1. a large multinuclear cell associated with the absorption and removal of bone; osteoclasts become highly active in the presence of parathyroid hormone, causing increased bone resorption and release of bone salts (phosphorus and, especially, calcium) into the extracellular fluid. 2. an instrument for use in the surgical fracture or refracture of bones.

**os·teo·clas·tic** (os″te-o-klas′tik) pertaining to or of the nature of an osteoclast; destructive to bone.

**os·teo·clas·to·ma** (os″te-o-klas-to′mə) [*osteoclast* + *-oma*] giant cell tumor of bone.

**os·teo·clas·ty** (os′te-o-klas″te) osteoclasis.

**os·teo·com·ma** (os″te-o-kom′ə) [*osteo-* + Gr. *komma* fragment] any of the pieces or members of a series of bony structures, as a vertebra.

**os·teo·cope** (os′te-o-kōp″) [*osteo-* + Gr. *kopos* pain] a severe pain in a bone or in the bones, generally a symptom of syphilitic bone disease.

**os·teo·cop·ic** (os″te-o-kop′ik) pertaining to or characterized by osteocope.

**os·teo·cra·ni·um** (os″te-o-kra′ne-əm) [*osteo-* + *cranium*] the fetal cranium during its stage of ossification.

**os·teo·cys·to·ma** (os″te-o-sis-to′mə) [*osteo-* + *cystoma*] a bone cyst.

**os·teo·cyte** (os″te-o-sīt″) [MeSH: Osteocytes] an osteoblast that has become embedded within the bone matrix, occupying a flat oval cavity (bone lacuna [q.v.]) and sending, through the canaliculi, slender cytoplasmic processes that make contact with processes of other osteocytes.

**os·teo·den·tin** (os″te-o-den′tin) [*osteo-* + *dentin*] dentin that resembles bone: seen in the teeth of certain fish and pathologically in other lower species, and in man, being produced by rapid formation of secondary dentin, with entrapment of cells.

**os·teo·den·ti·no·ma** (os″te-o-den″tĭ-no′mə) an odontoma composed of bone and dentin.

**os·teo·der·mia** (os″te-o-der′me-ə) [*osteo-* + *derm-* + *-ia*] osteoma cutis.

**os·teo·des·mo·sis** (os″te-o-des-mo′sis) [*osteo-* + *desmo-* + *-sis*] 1. the formation of bone and tendon. 2. ossification of tendon.

**os·teo·di·as·ta·sis** (os″te-o-di-as′tə-sis) [*osteo-* + *diastasis*] the separation of two adjacent bones.

**os·te·odyn·ia** (os″te-o-din′e-ə) [*osteo-* + *-odynia*] pain in a bone.

**os·teo·dys·plas·ty** (os″te-o-dis-plas′te) [*osteo-* + *dys-* + *-plasty*] abnormal development of bone.
**o. of Melnick and Needles,** a hereditary disorder, transmitted as an autosomal dominant trait, in which there are severe congenital bone abnormalities manifested by striking facies (exophthalmos, full cheeks, micrognathia, and malalignment of the teeth), flaring of the metaphyses of long bones, S-like curvature of the leg bones, irregular constrictions in the ribs, and sclerosis of the base of the skull.

**os·teo·dys·tro·phia** (os″te-o-dis-tro′fe-ə) osteodystrophy.
**o. cys′tica,** osteitis fibrosa cystica.
**o. fibro′sa,** osteitis fibrosa cystica.

**os·teo·dys·tro·phy** (os″te-o-dis′trə-fe) defective bone formation.
**Albright's hereditary o.,** pseudohypoparathyroidism.
**renal o.,** a condition resulting from chronic kidney disease, characterized by impaired renal function, elevated serum phosphorus with low or normal serum calcium levels, and stimulation of parathyroid function. Bone disease includes a variable mixture of oste-

itis fibrosa cystica, osteomalacia, osteoporosis, and sometimes osteosclerosis. Onset is usually in childhood, resulting in renal dwarfism.

**os·teo·ec·ta·sia** (os″te-o-ek-ta′zhə) [*osteo-* + *ectasia*] bowing of the bones.
**familial o.,** hyperostosis corticalis deformans juvenilis.

**os·teo·ec·to·my** (os″te-o-ek′tə-me) ostectomy.

**os·teo·en·chon·dro·ma** (os″te-o-en″do-kon-dro′mə) osteochondroma.

**os·teo·epiph·y·sis** (os″te-o-ə-pif′ĭ-sis) [*osteo-* + *epiphysis*] any bony epiphysis.

**os·teo·fi·bro·ma** (os″te-o-fi-bro′mə) [*osteo-* + *fibroma*] a benign tumor containing both osseous and fibrous elements.

**os·teo·fi·bro·ma·to·sis** (os″te-o-fi″bro-mə-to′sis) polyostotic form of fibrous dysplasia of bone.
**cystic o.,** Jaffe-Lichtenstein disease.

**os·teo·flu·o·ro·sis** (os″te-o-flo͞o-ro′sis) skeletal changes, usually consisting of osteomalacia and osteosclerosis, caused by the chronic intake of excessive quantities of fluorides. See also *fluorosis,* def. 2.

**os·teo·gen** (os′te-o-jen″) [*osteo-* + *-gen*] the substance composing the inner layer of the periosteum, from which bone is formed.

**os·teo·gen·e·sis** (os″te-o-jen′ə-sis) [*osteo-* + *-genesis*] [MeSH: Osteogenesis] formation of bone; the development of the bones.
**o. imperfec′ta (OI),** a collagen disorder due to defective biosynthesis of type I collagen and generally characterized by brittle, osteoporotic, easily fractured bones. Other defects that may appear include blue sclerae, wormian bones, lax joints, and dentinogenesis imperfecta. OI is variable in manifestation and severity and has great molecular, genetic, and clinical heterogeneity. There are four major types (I–IV) plus variants of OI. *Type I,* the classic, most common, mildest type, is autosomal dominant; called also *o. imperfecta with blue sclerae* and *o. imperfecta tarda.* Its eponymic synonyms include *Adair Dighton's, Eddowes', Ekman's, Lobstein's, Spurway's,* and *van der Hoeve's syndrome. Type II,* the perinatal lethal type, has at least three clinical and genetic subtypes and may be an autosomal dominant trait, an autosomal recessive trait, or an autosomal dominant new mutation. The dominant type is also called *o. imperfecta congenita, neonatal lethal form,* and *lethal perinatal OI.* The recessive form is also called *o. imperfecta congenita, Vrolik type of osteogenesis imperfecta, Vrolik's disease,* and *lethal perinatal OI. Type III,* the progressive deforming type, may be autosomal recessive or a new mutation; called also *o. imperfecta, progressively deforming, with normal sclerae. Type IV* is an autosomal dominant form, called also *o. imperfecta with normal sclerae.*
**o. imperfec′ta conge′nita (OIC),** o. imperfecta (type II), recessive form.
**o. imperfec′ta cys′tica,** a disorder in which the marrow spaces contain myxomatous fibroid tissue, the x-ray showing cystic changes.
**o. imperfec′ta tar′da (OIT),** o. imperfecta (type I).

**os·teo·ge·net·ic** (os″te-o-jə-net′ik) forming bone; concerned in bone formation.

**os·te·o·gen·ic** (os″te-o-jen′ik) [*osteo-* + *-genic*] derived from or composed of any tissue that is concerned in the growth or repair of bone.

**os·te·og·e·nous** (os″te-oj′ə-nəs) osteogenic.

**os·te·og·e·ny** (os″te-oj′ə-ne) osteogenesis.

**os·te·og·ra·phy** (os″te-og′rə-fe) [*osteo-* + *-graphy*] a description of the bones.

**os·teo·ha·lis·ter·e·sis** (os″te-o-hə-lis″tər-e′sis) [*osteo-* + *hal-* + *sterein* to deprive] loss or deficiency of the mineral elements of bones.

**os·teo·hema·chro·ma·to·sis** (os″te-o-hem″ə-kro″mə-to′sis) [*osteo-* + *hema-* + *chromato-* + *-sis*] discoloration of the bone by blood pigment, such as occurs in congenital erythropoietic porphyria in cattle.

**os·teo·hy·da·tid·o·sis** (os″te-o-hi″də-tid-o′sis) hydatid disease of bone.

**os·te·oid** (os′te-oid) [*osteo-* + *-oid*] 1. resembling bone. 2. the organic matrix of bone; young bone that has not undergone calcification.

**os·teo·in·duc·tion** (os″te-o-in-duk′shən) the act or process of stimulating osteogenesis.

**os·teo·lath·y·rism** (os″te-o-lath′ĭ-riz-əm) a skeletal disorder produced in laboratory animals by diets containing the sweet pea *(Lathyrus odoratus)* or its active principle, β-aminopropionitrile, or other aminonitriles. Characterized, in rats, by hernias, dissecting aortic aneurysms, lameness of the hind legs, exostoses, and kyphoscoliosis and other skeletal deformities, apparently as the result of defective aging of collagen tissue.

**os·teo·lipo·chon·dro·ma** (os″te-o-lip″o-kon-dro′mə) [*osteo-* + *lipo-* + *chondroma*] a benign cartilaginous tumor containing osseous and fatty elements.

**os·teo·li·po·ma** (os″te-o-lĭ-po′mə) [*osteo-* + *lipoma*] lipoma with osseous metaplasia.

**Os·teo·lite** (os′te-o-līt″) trademark for a kit for the preparation of technetium Tc 99m medronate.

**os·teo·lo·gia** (os″te-o-lo′jə) osteology; the nomenclature relating to the bones.

**os·te·ol·o·gist** (os″te-ol′ə-jist) a specialist in osteology.

**os·te·ol·o·gy** (os″te-ol′ə-je) [*osteo-* + *-logy*] the scientific study of the bones; applied also to the body of knowledge relating to the bones.

**os·te·ol·y·sis** (os″te-ol′ĭ-sis) [*osteo-* + *-lysis*] [MeSH: Osteolysis] dissolution of bone; applied especially to the removal or loss of the calcium of bone.

**os·teo·lyt·ic** (os″te-o-lit′ik) relating to, characterized by, or promoting osteolysis.

**os·te·o·ma** (os″te-o′mə) [*oste-* + *-oma*] [MeSH: Osteoma] a benign, slow-growing tumor composed of well-differentiated, densely sclerotic, compact bone, usually arising in membrane bones, particularly the skull and facial bones.
**cavalryman's o.,** osteoma at the insertion of the adductor femoris longus muscle.
**compact o.,** a small, dense, compact tumor of mature lamellar bone with little medullary space, usually occurring in the craniofacial or nasal bones.
**o. cu′tis,** a cutaneous ossification manifested by the development of one or more hard, round to irregular, sharply defined tumors of varying size within the dermis or subcutis. Called also *osteodermia* and *osteosis cutis.*
**o. du′rum, o. ebur′neum,** compact o.
**giant osteoid o.,** osteoblastoma.
**ivory o.,** compact o.
**o. medulla′re,** an osteoma containing marrow spaces.
**osteoid o.,** a small, benign but painful, circumscribed tumor of spongy bone occurring especially in the bones of the extremities and vertebrae, most often in young persons.
**o. spongio′sum, spongy o.,** osteoma containing cancellated bone.
**trabecular o.,** o. spongiosum.

**os·teo·ma·la·cia** (os″te-o-mə-la′shə) [*osteo-* + *-malacia*] [MeSH: Osteomalacia] inadequate or delayed mineralization of osteoid in mature cortical and spongy bone; it is the adult equivalent of rickets and accompanies that disorder in children. The etiology of osteomalacia and its clinical and biochemical manifestations are as described for rickets (q.v.).
**antacid-induced o.,** osteomalacia in which low dietary phosphorus intake coupled to excessive, chronic consumption of aluminum hydroxide–containing antacids leads to phosphate depletion, characterized by hypophosphatemia, nephrolithiasis, anorexia, muscle weakness, and bone loss.
**anticonvulsant o.,** osteomalacia occurring in anticonvulsant rickets of children or anticonvulsant rickets occurring in adults.
**familial hypophosphatemic o.,** osteomalacia occurring in familial hypophosphatemic rickets.
**hepatic o.,** osteomalacia as a complication of cholestatic liver disease, which may lead to severe bone pain and multiple fractures.
**oncogenic o., oncogenous o.,** osteomalacia occurring in association with usually benign mesenchymal neoplasms. The tumors appear to produce a substance that impairs renal tubular functions such as phosphate transport and hydroxylation of 25-hydroxyvitamin D; hypophosphatemia secondary to reduced renal resorption of phosphate is a major cause of the bone disease.
**puerperal o.,** osteomalacia occurring as a consequence of exhaustion of skeletal stores of calcium and phosphorus by repeated pregnancies and lactation.
**renal tubular o.,** osteomalacia occurring as a consequence of acidosis and hypercalciuria, resulting from inability to produce an acid urine or ammonia because of deficient activity of the renal tubules.
**senile o.,** softening of bones in old age due to vitamin D deficiency.

**os·teo·ma·la·cic** (os″te-o-mə-la′sik) pertaining to or characterized by osteomalacia.

**os·teo·mal·a·co·sis** (os″te-o-mal″ə-ko′sis) osteomalacia.

**os·teo·ma·toid** (os″te-o′mə-toid) resembling an osteoma.

**os·teo·ma·to·sis** (os″te-o-mə-to′sis) the formation of multiple osteomas.

**os·teo·me·at·al** (os″te-o-me-at′əl) pertaining to a nasal meatus and one of the bones of the face.

**os•teo•mere** (os′te-o-mēr″) [*osteo-* + *-mere*] one of a series of similar bony structures, such as the vertebrae.

**os•te•om•e•try** (os″te-om′ə-tre) [*osteo-* + *-metry*] the measurement of bones.

**os•teo•mi•o•sis** (os″te-o-mi-o′sis) [*osteo-* + *mio-* + *-sis*] disintegration of bone.

**os•teo•my•elit•ic** (os″te-o-mi″ə-lit′ik) marked by or characteristic of osteomyelitis.

**os•teo•my•eli•tis** (os″te-o-mi″ə-li′tis) [*osteo-* + *myelitis*] [MeSH: Osteomyelitis] inflammation of bone caused by infection, usually by a pyogenic organism, although any infectious agent may be involved. It may remain localized or may spread through the bone to involve the marrow, cortex, cancellous tissue, and periosteum.
**acute hematogenous o.,** osteomyelitis resulting from localization of blood-borne bacteria in bone, usually seen in the long bones of children following blunt trauma or adjacent infection; the most common infecting organism is *Staphylococcus aureus.* When it spreads to the joints it is known as *septic* or *bacterial arthritis.*
**conchiolin o.,** a condition seen in workers in mother-of-pearl, probably due to the inhaled dust being deposited in the bone marrow. Cf. *coniosis.*
**diffuse sclerosing o.,** chronic diffuse inflammatory response of bone to low-grade infection, with inflammatory cell infiltrate, fibrous replacement of marrow, and dense sclerotic masses of trabecular bone. Polymorphonuclear leukocytes, plasma cells, and focal osteoblasts may be present. Oral lesions occur predominantly in the mandible of older persons and are often sequelae of chronic periodontal disease.
**focal sclerosing o.,** chronic confined inflammatory response of bone to low-grade infection, with formation of dense trabecular bony masses with little interstitial marrow tissue. It occurs particularly in the mandible of children and young adults, adjacent to the apex of a tooth with long-term pulpitis. Called also *condensing osteitis.*
**Garré's o.,** sclerosing nonsuppurative o.
**salmonella o.,** osteomyelitis due to salmonella organisms; it occurs more frequently than normal in sickle cell disease.
**sclerosing nonsuppurative o.,** chronic idiopathic osteomyelitis involving the long bones, particularly the tibia and femur, and characterized by a diffuse inflammatory reaction, increased density and spindle-shaped sclerotic thickening of the cortex, and an absence of suppuration; called also *Garré's o., osteitis,* or *disease,* and *chronic nonsuppurative osteitis.*
**typhoid o.,** a type of osteomyelitis that usually occurs in the late convalescent stage of typhoid fever.
**o. variolo′sa,** osteomyelitis due to, or occurring as a complication of, smallpox.

**os•teo•my•elo•dys•pla•sia** (os″te-o-mi″ə-lo-dis-pla′zhə) [*osteo-* + *myelo-* + *dys-* + *-plasia*] a condition characterized by thinning of the osseous tissue of bones and increase in size of the marrow cavities, accompanied by leukopenia and fever.

**os•teo•my•elog•ra•phy** (os″te-o-mi″ə-log′rə-fe) radiographic visualization of bone marrow.

**os•teo•myxo•chon•dro•ma** (os″te-o-mik″so-kon-dro′mə) osteochondromyxoma.

**os•te•on** (os′te-on) [Gr. *"bone"*] the basic unit of structure of compact bone, comprising a haversian canal and its concentrically arranged lamellae, of which there may be 4 to 20, each 3 to 7 microns thick, in a single (haversian) system; such units are directed mainly in the long axis of the bone.

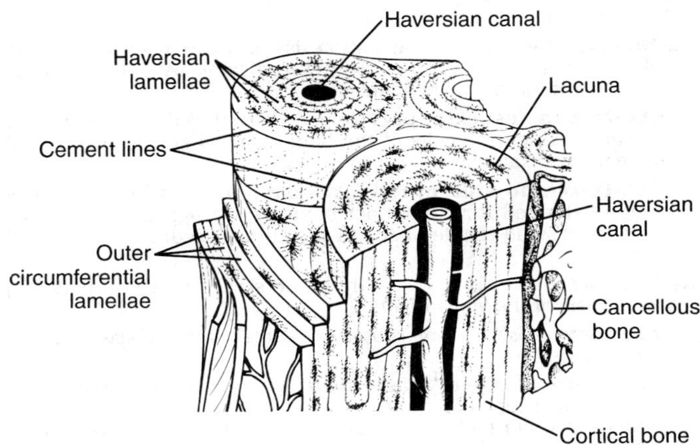

Osteons in the shaft of a long bone.

**os•te•one** (os′te-ōn) osteon.

**os•teo•ne•cro•sis** (os″te-o-nə-kro′sis) [*osteo-* + *necrosis*] [MeSH: Osteonecrosis] necrosis of bone due to obstruction of its blood supply. Called also *avascular* or *ischemic necrosis of bone.*

**os•teo•nec•tin** (os″te-o-nek′tin) [*osteo-* + L. *nectere* to fasten] [MeSH: Osteonectin] a phosphoprotein that binds both collagen and calcium and serves as a regulator of mineralization, found in bone and blood platelets.

**os•teo•neu•ral•gia** (os″te-o-nōō-ral′jə) [*osteo-* + *neuralgia*] neuralgia of a bone.

**os•te•on•o•sus** (os″te-on′ə-səs) osteopathy, def. 1.

**os•teo-odon•to•ma** (os″te-o-o″don-to′mə) ameloblastic odontoma.

**os•teo•on•y•cho•dys•pla•sia** (os″te-o-on″ĭ-ko-dis-pla′zhə) [*osteo-* + *onycho-* + *dysplasia*] 1. abnormal development of nails and bones; called also *onycho-osteodysplasia.* 2. nail-patella syndrome.
**hereditary o.-o.,** nail-patella syndrome.

**os•teo•path** (os′te-o-path) a practitioner of osteopathy.

**os•teo•path•ia** (os″te-o-path′e-ə) osteopathy, def. 1.
**o. conden′sans,** myelosclerosis, def. 2.
**o. conden′sans dissemina′ta, o. conden′sans generalisa′ta,** osteopoikilosis.
**o. hemorrha′gica infan′tum,** Moeller-Barlow disease.
**o. hyperosto′tica conge′nita,** melorheostosis.
**o. hyperosto′tica mul′tiplex infan′tilis,** diaphyseal dysplasia.
**o. stria′ta,** multiple condensations of cancellous bone beginning at the epiphyseal line and extending into the diaphysis, an abnormality seen only on radiographic examination.

**os•teo•path•ic** (os″te-o-path′ik) pertaining to osteopathy.

**os•teo•pa•thol•o•gy** (os″te-o-pə-thol′ə-je) any disease of bone.

**os•te•op•a•thy** (os″te-op′ə-the) [*osteo-* + *-pathy*] 1. any disease of a bone. 2. a system of therapy founded by Andrew Taylor Still (1828–1917), based on the theory that the body can make its own remedies against disease and other toxic conditions when it is in normal structural relationship and has favorable environmental conditions and adequate nutrition. It uses generally accepted physical, medicinal, and surgical methods of diagnosis and therapy, while placing chief emphasis on maintenance of normal body mechanics and on manipulative methods of detecting and correcting faulty structure.
**alimentary o.,** hunger o.
**disseminated condensing o.,** osteopoikilosis.
**hunger o.,** disturbances of the skeletal system observed in famine areas, characterized by a reduction in the amount of normally calcified bone, and attributed to dietary deficiencies and associated hormonal dysfunction.
**hypertrophic o.,** a condition in dogs similar to the hypertrophic pulmonary osteoarthropathy of humans; characteristics include hyperostosis of the limbs and later other skeletal regions, sometimes associated with tumors, tuberculosis, or other pulmonary conditions. Called also *acropachia.*
**myelogenic o.,** any bone disease due to the impaired relation between the medullary and osseous tissues.

**os•teo•pe•cil•ia** (os″te-o-pə-sil′e-ə) [*osteo-* + *pecil-* + *-ia*] osteopoikilosis.

**os•teo•pe•di•on** (os″te-o-pe′de-on) [*osteo-* + Gr. *paidion* child] lithopedion.

**os•teo•pe•nia** (os″te-o-pe′ne-ə) [*osteo-* + *-penia*] reduced bone mass due to a decrease in the rate of osteoid synthesis to a level insufficient to compensate normal bone lysis. The term is also used to refer to any decrease in bone mass below the normal.

**os•teo•pen•ic** (os″te-o-pen′ik) pertaining to osteopenia.

**os•teo•peri•os•te•al** (os″te-o-per″e-os′te-əl) pertaining to bone and its periosteum.

**os•teo•peri•os•ti•tis** (os″te-o-per″e-os-ti′tis) [*osteo-* + *periostitis*] inflammation of a bone and its periosteum. Called also *periosteitis.*
**alveolodental o.,** periodontitis.

**os•teo•pe•tro•sis** (os″te-o-pe-tro′sis) [*osteo-* + Gr. *petra* stone + *-osis*] [MeSH: Osteopetrosis] a rare genetic disease characterized by abnormally dense bone, due to defective resorption of immature bone. It occurs in two forms: a severe autosomal recessive form occurring in utero, infancy, or childhood, and a benign autosomal dominant form occurring in adolescence or adulthood. In the recessive form, the proliferation of bone obliterates the marrow cavity, causing anemia and hepatosplenomegaly, and narrowing the foramina of the skull, causing compression of cranial nerves, which may result in deafness and blindness. Fractures are common in both forms. Called also *Albers-Schönberg* or *marble bones disease, ivory bones,* and *marble bones.*

**o. gallina'rum**, a neoplastic viral disease of chickens, one of the avian leukosis complex, marked by thickening of the diaphyses of long bones.

**os·teo·phage** (os'te-o-fāj) [*osteo-* + *-phage*] osteoclast, def. 1.

**os·teo·pha·gia** (os"te-o-fa'je-ə) [*osteo-* + *-phagia*] the eating of bone due to a craving for phosphorus.

**os·teo·phle·bi·tis** (os"te-o-flə-bi'tis) [*osteo-* + *phleb-* + *-itis*] inflammation of the veins of a bone.

**os·te·oph·o·ny** (os"te-of'ə-ne) [*osteo-* + Gr. *phōnē* voice] bone conduction.

**os·teo·phy·ma** (os"te-o-fi'mə) [*osteo-* + *phyma*] osteophyte.

**os·teo·phyte** (os'te-o-fīt") [*osteo-* + *-phyte*] a bony excrescence or osseous outgrowth. Called also *osteophyma.*

**os·teo·phy·to·sis** (os"te-o-fi-to'sis) a condition characterized by the formation of osteophytes.

**os·teo·plaque** (os'te-o-plak) a layer of bone.

**os·teo·plast** (os'te-o-plast) [*osteo-* + *-plast*] osteoblast.

**os·teo·plas·tic** (os"te-o-plas'tik) 1. osteogenic. 2. pertaining to osteoplasty.

**os·teo·plas·ti·ca** (os"te-o-plas'tĭ-kə) osteitis fibrosa cystica.

**os·teo·plas·ty** (os'te-o-plas"te) [*osteo-* + *-plasty*] plastic surgery of the bones.

**os·teo·poi·ki·lo·sis** (os"te-o-poi"kĭ-lo'sis) [*osteo-* + *poikil-* + *-osis*] [MeSH: Osteopoikilosis] an autosomal dominant trait in which there are multiple sclerotic foci in the ends of long bones and scattered stippling in round and flat bones, usually without symptoms and diagnosed fortuitously by x-ray examination.

**os·teo·poi·ki·lot·ic** (os"te-o-poi"kĭ-lot'ik) pertaining to or characterized by osteopoikilosis.

**os·teo·pon·tin** (os"te-o-pon'tin) an acidic calcium-binding phosphoprotein with a high affinity for hydroxyapatite, involved in bone mineralization and in dystrophic calcification.

**os·teo·po·ro·sis** (os"te-o-pə-ro'sis) [*osteo-* + *por-*[1] + *-osis*] [MeSH: Osteoporosis] reduction in the amount of bone mass, leading to fractures after minimal trauma.
**o. circumscrip'ta cra'nii**, demineralization of the bones of the skull, characteristic of the destructive or osteolytic phase of Paget's disease; called also *Schüller's disease.*
**o. of disuse**, decrease in bone substance as a result of lack of reformation of laminae in the absence of functional stress that ordinarily leads to their replacement in new stress lines.
**postmenopausal o.**, that occurring in women within 3 to 20 years after menopause, affecting trabecular bone more than cortical bone, and manifested mainly by vertebral fractures of the painful crush type, hip fracture, Colles' fracture, and increased tooth loss.
**post-traumatic o.**, loss of bone substance following an injury in which there is damage to a nerve, sometimes due to an increased blood supply caused by the neurogenic insult, or to disuse secondary to pain. It is one component of reflex sympathetic dystrophy. Called also *Sudeck's atrophy.*
**senile o.**, that occurring in men and women over 70, manifested mainly by hip and vertebral fractures of the painless multiple wedge type leading to dorsal kyphosis.

**os·teo·po·rot·ic** (os"te-o-pə-rot'ik) pertaining to or characterized by osteoporosis.

**os·te·op·sath·y·ro·sis** (os"te-op-sath"ĭ-ro'sis) [*osteo-* + Gr. *psathyros* friable] osteogenesis imperfecta.

**os·teo·ra·dio·ne·cro·sis** (os"te-o-ra"de-o-nĕ-kro'sis) [MeSH: Osteoradionecrosis] necrosis of bone following irradiation.

**os·te·or·rha·gia** (os"te-o-ra'jə) [*osteo-* + *-rrhagia*] hemorrhage from bone.

**os·te·or·rha·phy** (os"te-or'ə-fe) [*osteo-* + *-rrhaphy*] the suturing or wiring of bones.

**os·teo·sar·co·ma** (os"te-o-sahr-ko'mə) [*osteo-* + *sarcoma*] [MeSH: Osteosarcoma] a malignant primary neoplasm of bone composed of a malignant connective tissue stroma with evidence of malignant, osteoid, bone, or cartilage formation. Classical osteosarcoma is a poorly differentiated tumor affecting mainly young adults, most often involving the long bones, and is classified as *osteoblastic, chondroblastic,* or *fibroblastic* according to which histologic component predominates. Called also *osteogenic sarcoma.*
**chondroblastic o.**, see *osteosarcoma.*
**classical o.**, see *osteosarcoma.*
**extraosseous o.**, a rare neoplasm occurring in the soft tissues of the body, generally in the thighs, composed of sarcomatous tissue that produces malignant osteoid and bone; it is histologically identical to osteosarcoma occurring in bone.
**fibroblastic o.**, see *osteosarcoma.*
**gnathic o.**, o. of jaw.
**high-grade surface o.**, a highly malignant osteosarcoma histologically identical to classical osteosarcoma but located on the surface of a bone.
**intracortical o.**, a rare form of osteosarcoma affecting mainly young adults, consisting of an osteolytic lesion confined within the cortex of a bone with a surrounding area of cortical sclerosis.
**intraosseous low-grade o.**, a well-differentiated osteosarcoma of low malignancy arising within a bone, composed of spindle cells arranged in interlacing bundles separated by collagen fibers, with invasion of fatty marrow or extraosseous soft tissue.
**o. of jaw**, a variant of osteosarcoma occurring in the mandible or maxilla, having a slightly older age of onset than classical osteosarcoma, with less tendency to metastasize than other osteosarcomas.
**juxtacortical o.**, parosteal o.
**multicentric o.**, the occurrence of osteosarcomas in more than one bone or in different sites on the same bone; lesions may be synchronous or metachronous.
**osteoblastic o.**, see *osteosarcoma.*
**parosteal o.**, a variant of osteosarcoma consisting of a slowly growing tumor that arises from the cortex of a bone and grows outward, eventually surrounding the bone; it resembles cancellous bone and is characterized histologically by a fibrous stroma containing bony spicules and trabeculae. It affects adults in the second through fifth decades of life and is less malignant than classical osteosarcoma. Called also *juxtacortical o.* and *parosteal sarcoma.*
**periosteal o.**, a variant of osteochondroma consisting of a soft, lobulated tumor arising from the periosteum of a long bone and growing outward from the bone; histologically it is a chondroblastic osteosarcoma.
**small-cell o.**, a variant of osteosarcoma resembling Ewing's sarcoma, composed of small round to spindle-shaped cells arranged in sheets or separated into lobules by fibrous septa, and having areas of osteoid and sometimes chondroid formation; called also *polyhistiocytoma* and *multipotential primary sarcoma of bone.*
**telangiectatic o.**, an aggressive, lytic form occurring as a soft, cystic tumor containing aneurysmally dilated blood-filled spaces lined by pleomorphic cells producing osteoid foci.

**os·teo·sar·co·ma·to·sis** (os"te-o-sahr-ko"mə-to'sis) the simultaneous occurrence of multiple osteosarcomas; synchronous multicentric osteosarcoma.

**os·teo·sar·co·ma·tous** (os"te-o-sahr-ko'mə-təs) of the nature of osteosarcoma.

**os·teo·scle·ro·sis** (os"te-o-sklə-ro'sis) [*osteo-* + *sclerosis*] [MeSH: Osteosclerosis] the hardening or abnormal density of bone, as in eburnation and condensing osteitis.
**o. conge'nita**, achondroplasia.
**o. fra'gilis**, osteopetrosis.
**o. fra'gilis generalisa'ta**, osteopoikilosis.
**o. myelofibrosis**, myelosclerosis, def. 2.

**os·teo·scle·rot·ic** (os"te-o-sklə-rot'ik) pertaining to or characterized by osteosclerosis.

**os·teo·sep·tum** (os"te-o-sep'təm) [*osteo-* + *septum*] pars ossea septi nasi.

**os·te·o·sis** (os"te-o'sis) the formation of bony tissue, especially the infiltration of connective tissue with bone.
**o. cu'tis**, osteoma cutis.
**o. ebur'nisans monome'lica**, melorheostosis.
**parathyroid o.**, osteitis fibrosa cystica.

**os·teo·su·ture** (os'te-o-soo"chər) [*osteo-* + *suture*] osteorrhaphy.

**os·teo·syn·o·vi·tis** (os"te-o-sin"o-vi'tis) synovitis together with osteitis of the neighboring bones.

**os·teo·syn·the·sis** (os"te-o-sin'thə-sis) [*osteo-* + *synthesis*] surgical fastening of the ends of a fractured bone by sutures, rings, plates, or other mechanical means.

**os·teo·ta·bes** (os"te-o-ta'bēz) [*osteo-* + *tabes*] a disease, chiefly of infants, in which the cells of the bone marrow are destroyed and the marrow disappears.

**os·teo·throm·bo·phle·bi·tis** (os"te-o-throm"bo-flə-bi'tis) inflammation extended through intact bone by a progressive thrombophlebitis of small venules, such as sometimes occurs in the mastoid bone.

**os·teo·throm·bo·sis** (os"te-o-throm-bo'sis) [*osteo-* + *thrombosis*] thrombosis of the veins of a bone.

**os·teo·tome** (os'te-o-tōm") [*osteo-* + *-tome*] a chisel-like knife for cutting bone.

**os·te·ot·o·my** (os"te-ot'ə-me) [*osteo-* + *-tomy*] [MeSH: Osteotomy] the surgical cutting of a bone.
**angulation o.**, in midhumeral amputation, the bending of a small terminal of the humerus at a right angle to the bone shaft so as to provide a projection that locks the prosthesis to the bone.
**block o.**, osteotomy in which a section of bone is removed.

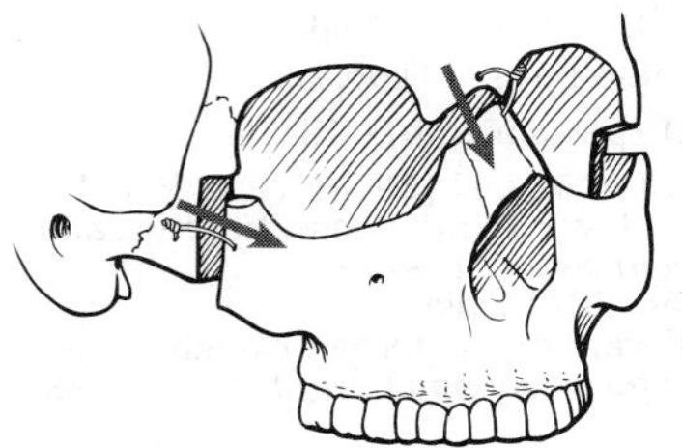
Le Fort III osteotomy.

**cuneiform o.,** the removal of a wedge of bone.
**cup-and-ball o.,** osteotomy in which the distal fragment is pointed and the proximal fragment is recessed.
**displacement o.,** surgical division of a bone and shifting of the divided ends to change the alignment of the bone or to alter weight-bearing stresses.
**innominate o.,** pelvic osteotomy to deepen the acetabulum in congenital dislocation of the hip.
**inverted L o.,** a type of osteotomy performed on the mandible to correct prognathism, the cut being an inverted L shape made in the ramus just below the condyle.
**Le Fort o.,** transverse sectioning and repositioning of the maxilla; the incision for each of the three types *(Le Fort I, II,* and *III o's)* is placed along the line defined by the corresponding Le Fort fracture (q.v.).
**linear o.,** the sawing or linear cutting of a bone.
**Lorenz's o.,** osteotomy of the neck of the femur by a V-shaped cutting of the femur so as to prevent displacement of the shaft.
**pelvic o.,** pubiotomy.
**sagittal ramus o.,** sagittal split o.
**sagittal split o.,** sagittal splitting of mandible; see under *splitting.*
**sandwich o.,** a surgical technique for augmenting an atrophic mandible; it is similar to a visor osteotomy (q.v.) but the split is a horizontal one confined between the mental foramina so that only the anterior portion of the cranial fragment is lifted upward.
**total maxillary o.,** Le Fort I o.; see *Le Fort o.*
**vertical ramus o.,** a type of osteotomy performed to correct prognathism; the ramus is resected in a vertical line proceeding from the sigmoid notch to the angle area of the lower border of the mandible.
**visor o.,** a surgical technique for augmenting an atrophic mandible, performed by splitting the mandible sagittally and sliding the cranial fragment upward, then supporting the structure with interposed grafts. Cf. *sandwich o.*
**visor/sandwich o.,** a combination of the visor and sandwich osteotomies in which the cut is in the vertical plane posterior to the mental foramina and at a 45° angle in the anterior region.

**os·teo·tribe, os·teo·trite** (os′te-o-trīb″, os′te-o-trīt″) [*osteo-* + Gr. *tribein* to rub] an instrument for rasping carious bone.

**os·te·ot·ro·phy** (os″te-ot′rə-fe) [*osteo-* + *-trophy*] nutrition of bone.

**os·te·ot·y·lus** (os″te-ot′ə-ləs) [*osteo-* + Gr. *tylos* callus] the callus enclosing the end of a broken bone.

**Os·ter·ta·gia** (os″tər-ta′jə) [Robert von *Ostertag,* German veterinarian, 1864–1940] [MeSH: Ostertagia] a genus of attenuated nematode stomach worms of the family Trichostrongylidae, found mostly in cysts on the wall of the abomasum of cattle and other ruminants. It closely resembles *Teladorsagia.*

**os·ter·ta·gi·a·sis** (os″tər-tə-ji′ə-sis) [MeSH: Ostertagiasis] infection of the abomasum of a ruminant by nematodes of the genus *Ostertagia.* In lambs and calves, if there are large numbers of adult worms the host may suffer from anorexia and diarrhea. In older animals, when the resident worm population yields large numbers of larvae, the result is edema and thickening of the abomasal mucosa, with chronic diarrhea and emaciation that can be fatal.

**os·ter·tag·i·o·sis** (os″tər-taj″e-o′sis) ostertagiasis.

**os·thex·ia, os·thexy** (os-thek′se-ə, os′thək-se) [*osteo-* + Gr. *hexis* condition] abnormal ossification.

**os·tia** (os′te-ə) [L.] plural of *ostium.*

**os·ti·al** (os′te-əl) pertaining to an ostium.

**os·ti·ole** (os′te-ōl) a pore, such as in a perithecium or pycnidium.

**os·tio·me·a·tal** (os″te-o-me-a′təl) [*ostium* + *meatal*] pertaining to the opening of the urinary, nasal, or acoustic meatus.

**os·ti·tis** (os-ti′tis) osteitis.

**os·ti·um** (os′te-əm) pl. *os′tia* [L.] [TA] an opening, aperture, or orifice.
**o. abdomina′le tu′bae uteri′nae** [TA], abdominal orifice of uterine tube: the funnel-shaped opening by which the uterine tube communicates with the pelvic cavity.
**o. aor′tae** [TA], aortic opening: the opening between the left ventricle and the ascending aorta; guarded by the aortic valve. Called also *aortic orifice.*
**o. appen′dicis vermifor′mis** [TA], opening of vermiform appendix: the orifice between the vermiform appendix and the cecum.
**o. atrioventricula′re dex′trum** [TA], right atrioventricular opening: the opening between the right atrium and the right ventricle of the heart, guarded by the right atrioventricular valve; called also *tricuspid orifice* and *right atrioventricular orifice.*
**o. atrioventricula′re sinis′trum** [TA], left atrioventricular opening; the opening between the left atrium and the left ventricle of the heart, guarded by the left atrioventricular valve; called also *mitral orifice* and *left atrioventricular orifice.*
**o. cardi′acum** [TA], cardiac opening: the orifice between the esophagus and the cardiac part of the stomach (cardia)

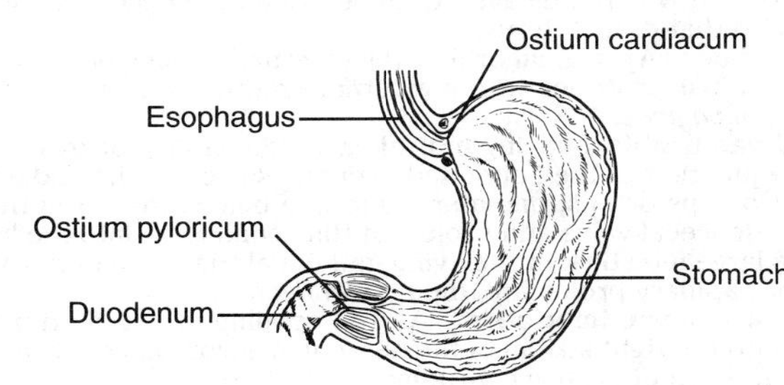


**coronary o., o. of coronary artery,** either of the two openings in the aortic sinus that mark the origins of the left and right coronary arteries.
**ethmoid o., ethmoidal o., o. of ethmoidal sinus, o. of ethmoid sinus,** any of various small openings connecting an ethmoidal sinus or air cell to the nasal cavity.
**frontal o., frontal sinus o., o. of frontal sinus,** apertura sinus frontalis.
**o. ilea′le** [TA], opening of ileal papilla: the orifice at the junction of the ileum and cecum, which is rounded at the left (anterior) end and pointed at the right (posterior) end. It has two lips, one above and one below, that form the so-called ileocecal valve; in the living individual the ileum forms a conical projection, the *papilla ilealis.* Called also *o. ileocaecale* and *o. ileocecale.*
**o. ileocaeca′le, o. ileoceca′le,** o. ileale.
**o. inter′num u′teri,** o. uterinum tubae uterinae.
**maxillary o., maxillary sinus o., o. of maxillary sinus,** hiatus maxillaris.
**o. pharyn′geum tu′bae auditi′vae** [TA], pharyngeal opening of auditory tube: the opening at the inferior end of either auditory tube, located on each of the lateral walls of the pharynx, posterior and inferior to the posterior end of the inferior nasal concha. Called also *o. pharyngeum tubae auditoriae* [TA alternative] and *pharyngeal orifice of auditory tube.*
**o. pharyn′geum tu′bae audito′riae,** TA alternative for *o. pharyngeum tubae auditivae.*
**o. pri′mum,** an opening in the lowest aspect of the septum primum of the embryonic heart, posteriorly in the neighborhood of the primordial atrioventricular valves. Called also *interatrial foramen primum.*
**o. primum, persistent,** an endocardial cushion defect characterized by a cleft in the basal portion of the atrial septum, usually associated with cleft mitral valve.
**o. pylo′ricum** [TA], pyloric opening: the orifice between the stomach and the duodenum.
**o. secun′dum,** an opening high in the septum primum of the embryonic heart, approximately where the foramen ovale will develop. Called also *interatrial foramen secundum.*
**o. si′nus corona′rii** [TA], opening of coronary sinus: an opening in the wall of the right atrium, situated between the opening of the inferior vena cava and the atrioventricular opening, the lower part of which is covered by the valve of the coronary sinus. Called also *orifice of coronary sinus.*
**sinusoidal o.,** any of the openings of the anterior cardiac veins into the right atrium of the heart.
**sphenoid o., sphenoid sinus o., o. of sphenoid sinus,** apertura sinus sphenoidalis.
**o. trun′ci pulmona′lis** [TA], opening of pulmonary trunk, guarded by the pulmonary valve.
**o. tympa′nicum tu′bae auditi′vae** [TA], tympanic opening of auditory tube: the opening of the auditory tube on the carotid wall of the tympanic cavity. Called also *o. tympanicum tubae auditoriae* [TA alternative] and *tympanic orifice of auditory tube.*
**o. tympa′nicum tu′bae audito′riae,** TA alternative for *o. tympanicum tubae auditivae.*

**o. ure'teris** [TA], orifice of ureter: the opening of the ureter in the bladder; called also *orificium ureteris* and *ureteral orifice.*
**o. ure'thrae exter'num femini'nae** [TA], external orifice of female urethra: the opening of the urethra into the vestibule; it is surrounded by a sphincter of striated muscle derived from the bulbocavernosus muscle. Called also *orificium urethrae externum muliebris.*
**o. ure'thrae exter'num masculi'nae** [TA], external orifice of male urethra: the slitlike opening of the urethra on the tip of the glans penis; called also *orificium urethrae externum virilis.*
**o. ure'thrae inter'num** [TA], internal orifice of urethra: the opening between the bladder and the urethra; called also *orificium urethrae internum.*
**o. u'teri** [TA], ostium of uterus: the external opening of the cervix of the uterus into the vagina; called also *orificium externum uteri* and *external orifice of uterus.*
**o. uteri'num tu'bae uteri'nae** [TA], uterine orifice of uterine tube: the point at which the cavity of the uterine tube becomes continuous with that of the uterus.
**o. vagi'nae** [TA], vaginal orifice: the external opening of the vagina, situated just posterior to the external urethral orifice; called also *orificium vaginae.*
**o. val'vae ilea'lis,** opening of ileal valve: the slitlike or oval orifice at the junction of the ileum and cecum, as seen in the cadaver. It has two flaps or lips, one above and one below, that form the so-called ileocecal valve and project at thickened folds into the lumen of the large intestine; in the living individual the ileum forms a conical or papillary projection, the *papilla ilealis.*
**o. ve'nae ca'vae inferio'ris** [TA], the opening of the inferior vena cava into the right atrium of the heart; it is accompanied by a valve that, in the adult, is usually rudimentary.
**o. ve'nae ca'vae superio'ris** [TA], the opening of the superior vena cava into the right atrium of the heart; it is unaccompanied by a valve.
**os'tia vena'rum pulmona'lium** [TA], the openings of the pulmonary veins (in the human, usually four) into the left atrium of the heart; they are unaccompanied by valves.

**os·to·mate** (os'tə-māt) one who has undergone enterostomy or ureterostomy.

**os·to·my** (os'tə-me) [MeSH: Ostomy] a general term referring to any operation in which an artificial opening is formed between two hollow organs or between one or more such viscera and the abdominal wall for discharge of intestinal contents or of urine.

**-ostomy** [Gr. *stoma* mouth] a word termination denoting an operation in which an artificial opening is formed, with the organ into which the opening is made denoted by the combining form to which the word termination is attached.

**os·to·sis** (os-to'sis) osteogenesis.

**os·tra·ceous** (os-tra'shəs) [Gr. *ostrakon* shell] shaped like or resembling an oyster shell.

**os·tra·co·sis** (os"trə-ko'sis) [Gr. *ostrakon,* shell] bone change that takes on the consistency of oyster shell.

**os·treo·tox·ism** (os"tre-o-tok'siz-əm) [Gr. *ostreon* oyster + *toxikon* poisoning] poisoning caused by the eating of contaminated oysters.

**Os·trum-Furst syndrome** (os'trəm-fərst) [Herman William *Ostrum,* American physician, born 1893; William *Furst,* American physician, 20th century] see under *syndrome.*

**Os·wal·do·cru·zia** (oz-wahl"do-kroo'ze-ə) [G. *Oswaldo Cruz,* Brazilian physician, 1872–1917] a genus of nematodes of the family Trichostrongylus, inhabiting the lungs and intestines of reptiles and amphibians.

**OT** 1. abbreviation for *old term* in anatomy. 2. Old tuberculin.

**Ota's nevus** (o'tahz) [Masao T. *Ota,* Japanese dermatologist, 1885–1945] see under *nevus.*

**otal·gia** (o-tal'je-ə) [Gr. *ōtalgia*] pain in the ear; called also *earache* and *otodynia.*
**o. denta'lis,** reflex pain in the ear due to dental disease.
**geniculate o.,** Ramsay-Hunt syndrome, def. 1.
**o. intermit'tens,** otalgia of an intermittent type.
**reflex o.,** referred pain (q.v.) in the ear, usually from a lesion of the buccal cavity or nasopharynx.
**secondary o.,** otalgia due to inflammation of the geniculate ganglion.
**tabetic o.,** otalgia in tabes dorsalis due to degeneration of the nerve of Wrisberg.

**otal·gic** (o-tal'jik) 1. pertaining to earache. 2. an earache remedy.

**OTC** 1. over the counter; applied to drugs not required by law to be sold on prescription only. 2. ornithine transcarbamoylase; see *ornithine carbamoyltransferase.*

**OTD** organ tolerance dose; see under *dose.*

**otic** (o'tik) [Gr. *ōtikos*] pertaining to the ear; called also *aural.*

**otio·bio·sis** (o"te-o-bi-o'sis) otobiosis.

**Oti·o·bi·us** (o"te-o'be-əs) *Otobius.*

**otit·ic** (o-tit'ik) pertaining to otitis.

**oti·tis** (o-ti'tis) [*ot-* + *-itis*] [MeSH: Otitis] inflammation of the ear, often with pain, fever, hearing loss, tinnitus, and vertigo. See also *o. externa, o. media,* and *o. interna.*
**aviation o.,** barotitis media.
**o. desquamati'va,** otitis externa or media in which there are overdevelopment and desquamation of the cutaneous or mucous epithelium.
**o. exter'na,** inflammation of the external auditory canal.
**o. externa, acute,** acute infection of the cartilaginous external auditory meatus, caused by either a fungus *(otomycosis)* or a bacteria *(acute bacterial otitis externa).* It is common in swimmers and in hot, humid weather. Symptoms include pain and swelling, sometimes with formation of a circumscribed furuncle *(circumscribed otitis externa).* Called also *swimmer's ear* and *tank ear.*
**o. externa, acute bacterial,** acute otitis externa caused by a bacterial infection, usually with a species of *Pseudomonas* and less often with *Staphylococcus* and formation of a furuncle. See also *circumscribed o. externa.*
**o. externa, acute fungal,** otomycosis.
**o. externa, circumscribed,** acute bacterial o. externa in a limited area with formation of a furuncle, which may obstruct the canal; usually due to a staphylococcal infection. Cf. *diffuse o. externa.* Called also *furuncular o. externa* and *furuncular o.*
**o. externa, diffuse,** otitis externa involving a relatively wide area, without formation of a furuncle. Cf. *circumscribed o. externa.*
**o. externa, fungal,** otomycosis.
**o. externa, furuncular,** circumscribed o. externa.
**o. externa, malignant,** a progressive, necrotizing, frequently fatal infection of the external auditory canal and base of the skull, caused by *Pseudomonas aeruginosa;* it affects chiefly elderly diabetic and immunocompromised patients. Called also *necrotizing o. externa.*
**o. externa, necrotizing,** malignant o. externa.
**external o.,** o. externa.
**furuncular o.,** circumscribed o. externa.
**o. inter'na,** labyrinthitis.
**o. me'dia,** inflammation of the middle ear; subtypes are distinguished by length of time from onset *(acute* versus *chronic)* and by type of discharge *(serous* versus *suppurative).*
**o. media, adhesive,** tympanic membrane atelectasis.
**o. media, atelectatic,** tympanic membrane atelectasis.
**o. media, catarrhal,** serous o. media.
**o. media, mucoid,** serous otitis media in which the secretion is particularly viscous.
**o. media, purulent,** suppurative o. media.
**o. media, secretory,** serous o. media.
**o. media, serous,** chronic otitis media marked by serous effusion into the middle ear. Called also *secretory* or *catarrhal o. media.*
**o. media, suppurative,** otitis media with a discharge of pus (otorrhea); infecting bacteria are usually *Streptococcus* species, *Haemophilus influenzae,* or *Staphylococcus pyogenes.* It may be either acute or chronic. See also *Gradenigo's syndrome.* Called also *purulent otitis media.*
**parasitic o.,** otoacariasis.

**ot(o)-** [Gr. *ous,* gen. *ōtos* ear] a combining form denoting relationship to the ear.

**oto·ac·a·ri·a·sis** (o"to-ak"ə-ri'ə-sis) [*oto-* + *acariasis*] infection of the ears of cats, dogs, and domestic rabbits with the mite *Otodectes;* see also *otodectic mange.* Called also *otocariasis* and *parasitic otitis.*

**oto·bi·o·sis** (o"to-bi-o'sis) infestation by *Otobius.*

**Oto·bi·us** (o-to'be-əs) [*oto-* + Gr. *bios* manner of living] a genus of argasid ticks, the spinous ear ticks. The nymphs of *O. lago'philus* of rabbits and *O. megni'ni* of cattle and other domestic animals may attack the ears of humans.

**oto·ca·ri·a·sis** (o"to-kə-ri'ə-sis) otoacariasis.

**Oto·cen·tor** (o"to-sen'tor) *Anocentor.*

**oto·ceph·a·lus** (o"to-sef'ə-ləs) [*oto-* + *-cephalus*] an individual exhibiting otocephaly.

**oto·ceph·a·ly** (o"to-sef'ə-le) [*oto-* + *-cephaly*] a congenital anomaly characterized by lack of a lower jaw and by ears that are united inferior to the face.

**oto·cer·e·bri·tis** (o"to-ser"ə-bri'tis) [*oto-* + *cerebritis*] otoencephalitis.

**oto·co·nia** (o"to-ko'ne-ə) [*oto-* + *coni-* + *-ia*] plural of otoconium.

**otoc·o·nite** (o-tok'o-nīt) statoconium.

**oto·co·ni·um** (o"to-ko'ne-əm) [L.] statoconium.

**oto·cra·ni·al** (o"to-kra'ne-əl) pertaining to the otocranium.

**oto·cra·ni·um** (o"to-kra'ne-əm) [*oto-* + *cranium*] the area of the petrous part of the temporal bone surrounding the osseous labyrinth.

**oto·cyst** (o'to-sist) [*oto-* + *cyst*] 1. the auditory vesicle of the embryo, the primordium of the internal ear. 2. the auditory sac of certain animals.

**Oto·dec·tes** (o″to-dek'tēz) [*oto-* + Gr. *dēktēs* a biter] a genus of mange mites of the family Psoroptidae. *O. cyno'tis* infests the external ear canal of cats, dogs, foxes, and ferrets, causing otodectic mange and otoacariasis.

**oto·dec·tic** (o″to-dek'tik) pertaining to or caused by *Otodectes.*

**oto·dyn·ia** (o″to-din'e-ə) [*oto-* + *-odynia*] otalgia.

**oto·en·ceph·a·li·tis** (o″to-ən-sef″ə-li'tis) [*oto-* + *encephalitis*] inflammation of the brain due to an extension from an inflamed middle ear. See also *otitis media.*

**oto·gen·ic** (o″to-jen'ik) otogenous.

**otog·e·nous** (o-toj'ə-nəs) [*oto-* + *-genous*] originating within the ear.

**otog·ra·phy** (o-tog'rə-fe) [*oto-* + *-graphy*] a description of the ear.

**oto·lar·yn·gol·o·gy** (o″to-lar″ing-gol'ə-je) [*oto-* + *laryngo-* + *-logy*] [MeSH: Otolaryngology] that branch of medicine concerned with medical and surgical treatment of the head and neck, including the ears, nose, and throat. Called also *otorhinolaryngology.*

**oto·lite** (o'to-līt) 1. statoconium. 2. otolith (def. 2).

**oto·lith** (o'to-lith) [*oto-* + *-lith*] [MeSH: Otolithic Membrane] 1. statoconium. 2. a calcareous mass in the inner ear of vertebrates or in the otocyst of invertebrates.

**oto·log·ic** (o″to-loj'ik) pertaining to otology.

**otol·o·gist** (o-tol'ə-jist) a physician who specializes in otology.

**otol·o·gy** (o-tol'ə-je) [*oto-* + *-logy*] that branch of medicine that deals with the medical treatment and surgery of the ear, and its anatomy, physiology, and pathology.

**oto·mas·toid·itis** (o″to-mas″toid-i'tis) mastoiditis combined with otitis media, usually of the suppurative type.

**oto·mu·cor·my·co·sis** (o″to-mu″kor-mi-ko'sis) mucormycosis affecting the ear.

**Oto·my·ces** (o″to-mi'sēz) [*oto-* + Gr. *mykēs* fungus] former name for *Aspergillus.*

**oto·my·co·sis** (o″to-mi-ko'sis) [*oto-* + *-mycosis*] fungal infection of the external auditory meatus, usually by a species of *Aspergillus,* marked by pruritus and exudative inflammation; there may be secondary bacterial infection. It is more common in hot weather and tropical climates. Called also *Hong Kong, hot weather, Singapore,* or *tropical ear* and *fungal* or *acute fungal otitis externa.*
**o. aspergilli'na, Aspergillus o.,** that caused by a species of *Aspergillus,* usually *A. niger.* Called also *aural aspergillosis.*

**oto·my·ia·sis** (o″to-mi-i'ə-sis) infestation of the ear by larvae.

**oto·neu·ral·gia** (o″to-nōō-ral'jə) [*oto-* + *neuralgia*] neuralgic pain in the ear.

**oto·neu·ro·log·ic** (o″to-noo″ro-loj'ik) pertaining to those portions of the nervous system relating to the ear.

**oto·neu·rol·o·gy** (o″to-nōō-rol'o-je) neuro-otology.

**oto·pha·ryn·ge·al** (o″to-fə-rin'je-əl) pertaining to the ear and pharynx.

**oto·plas·ty** (o'to-plas″te) [*oto-* + *-plasty*] plastic surgery of the ear, done to correct deformities and defects.

**oto·py·or·rhea** (o″to-pi″o-re'ə) [*oto-* + *pyorrhea*] otorrhea that is purulent.

**oto·rhi·no·lar·yn·gol·o·gy** (o″to-ri″no-lar″in-gol'ə-je) [*oto-* + *rhino-* + *laryngo-* + *-logy*] otolaryngology.

**oto·rhi·nol·o·gy** (o″to-ri-nol'ə-je) [*oto-* + *rhino-* + *-logy*] that branch of medicine which treats of the nose and ear and their diseases.

**otor·rhea** (o″to-re'ə) [*oto-* + *-rrhea*] a discharge from the ear, especially a purulent one.
**cerebrospinal fluid o.,** escape of cerebrospinal fluid through the external auditory meatus due to fracture or other pathology of the temporal bone; cf. *cerebrospinal fluid fistula.*

**oto·sal·pinx** (o″to-sal'pinks) [*oto-* + *salpinx*] tuba auditiva.

**oto·scle·ro·sis** (o″to-sklə-ro'sis) [*oto-* + *sclerosis*] [MeSH: Otosclerosis] otospongiosis of the bony labyrinth, especially adjacent to the footplate of the stapes; it may cause bony ankylosis of the stapes, resulting in conductive hearing loss. Cochlear otosclerosis may also develop, resulting in sensorineural hearing loss.

**oto·scle·rot·ic** (o″to-sklə-rot'ik) characterized by otosclerosis.

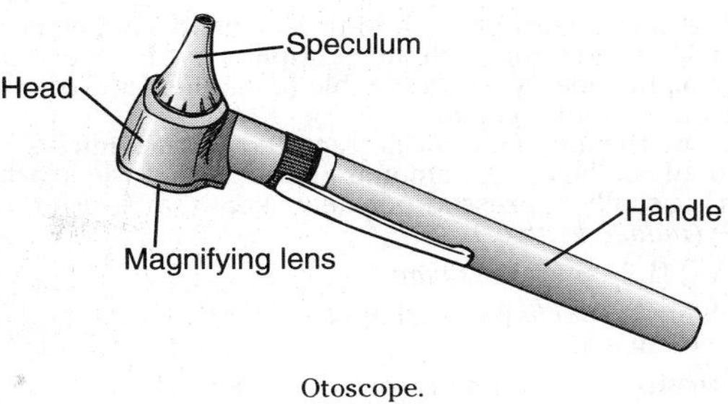


Otoscope.

**oto·scope** (o'to-skōp) [*oto-* + *-scope*] an instrument for inspecting or auscultating the ear; called also *auriscope.*
**Siegle's o.,** an otoscope that gives a view of the drum membrane when subjected to condensed or rarefied air.

**otos·co·py** (o-tos'kə-pe) examination of the ear by means of the otoscope.

**oto·sis** (o-to'sis) a false impression of sounds uttered by others.

**oto·spon·gi·o·sis** (o″to-spon″je-o'sis) the formation of spongy bone in the bony labyrinth of the ear; see *otosclerosis.*

**oto·tox·ic** (o″to-tok'sik) causing damage to the vestibulocochlear nerve or the organs of hearing and balance. See also *ototoxicity.*

**oto·tox·ic·i·ty** (o″to-tok-sis'ĭ-te) the quality of causing damage to the vestibulocochlear nerve or the organs of hearing and balance. See also *ototoxic hearing loss,* under *hearing loss.*

**Otri·vin** (o'trĭ-vin) trademark for preparations of xylometazoline hydrochloride.

**Ot·to's disease, pelvis** (ot'o) [Adolph Wilhelm *Otto,* German surgeon, 1786–1845] see under *disease* and *pelvis.*

**OU** [L.] *o'culus uter'que,* each eye.

**oua·ba·in** (wah-ba'in) [MeSH: Ouabain] a cardiac glycoside consisting of a molecule of rhamnose linked to a steroid nucleus, obtained principally from the seeds of *Strophanthus gratus* (Wall & Hock.) Baill. (Apocynaceae), having the same actions as digitalis but producing digitalization more rapidly; used in the emergency treatment of acute congestive heart failure, administered intravenously. Called also *G-strophanthin* or *strophanthin-G.*

**Ouch·ter·lo·ny technique** (ok'tər-lo″ne) [Orjan Thomas Gunnarson *Ouchterlony,* Swedish bacteriologist, born 1914] see *immunodiffusion.*

**oulec·to·my** (oo-lek'tə-me) 1. ulectomy, def. 1. 2. gingivectomy.

**ouli·tis** (oo-li'tis) gingivitis.

**ounce** (ouns) [L. *uncia*] a measure of weight in both the avoirdupois and the apothecaries' system; abbreviation oz. The ounce *avoirdupois* is one sixteenth of a pound, or 437.5 grains (28.3495 g). The *apothecaries'* ounce is one twelfth of a pound, or 480 grains (31.103 gm); symbol ℥.
**fluid o.,** a unit of capacity (liquid measure) of the apothecaries' system, being 8 fluid drams, or the equivalent of 29.57 mL. Abbreviated fl oz.

**-ous** 1. a suffix meaning possessing, having, or full of, e.g., cancerous. 2. in chemistry, a suffix used to indicate an ion or acid exhibiting the lower of two oxidation states, the other being indicated by the suffix *-ic.*

**out·breed·ing** (out'brēd-ing) the mating of totally unrelated individuals, which frequently results in the production of offspring that show more vigor, as measured in terms of growth, survival, and fertility, than the parents (heterosis); called also *crossbreeding.*

**out·let** (out'lət) a means by which something escapes.
**pelvic o.,** apertura pelvis inferior.
**thoracic o.,** apertura thoracis inferior.

**out·li·er** (out'li-ər) in statistics, an observation so distant from the central mass of the data that it noticeably influences results; it is often considered an error and removed from the data, although not necessarily appropriately so.

**out·pa·tient** (out'pa-shənt) [MeSH: Outpatients] a patient who comes to the hospital, clinic, or dispensary for diagnosis and/or treatment but does not occupy a bed.

**out·pock·et·ing** (out-pok'ət-ing) evagination.

**out·pouch·ing** (out'pouch-ing) the obtrusion of a layer or part to form a pouch; evagination.

**out·put** (out'poot) the yield; the total of anything produced by any functional system of the body.
**cardiac o. (CO),** the effective volume of blood expelled by either

ventricle of the heart per unit of time (usually volume per minute); it is equal to the stroke volume multiplied by the heart rate.
**energy o.,** the energy a body is able to manifest in work or activity.
**stroke o.,** see under *volume.*
**urinary o.,** the amount of urine excreted by the kidneys.
**work o. of the heart,** the amount of energy that the heart converts to work; usually expressed per heart beat *(stroke work o.)* or per minute *(minute work o.).*

**ova** (o'və) [L.] plural of *ovum.*

**oval** (o'vəl) [L. *ovalis*] egg-shaped; having the outline of the long section of an egg.

**ov·al·bu·min** (ōv"al-bu'min) [*ovum* + *albumin*] [MeSH: Ovalbumin] an albumin obtainable from the whites of eggs.

**ova·lo·cy·tary** (o"və-lo-si'tar-e) elliptocytary.

**ovalo·cyte** (o'və-lo-sīt) elliptocyte.

**ovalo·cy·to·sis** (o-val"o-si-to'sis) elliptocytosis.

**ovar·i·al·gia** (o-var"e-al'jə) oophoralgia.

**ovar·i·an** (o-var'e-ən) pertaining to an ovary or ovaries.

**ovar·i·ec·to·my** (o-var"e-ek'tə-me) [MeSH: Ovariectomy] oophorectomy.

**ovari(o)-** [L. *ovarium* ovary] a combining form denoting relationship to the ovary.

**ovar·io·cele** (o-var'e-o-sēl) [*ovario-* + *-cele*[1]] hernial protrusion of an ovary.

**ovar·io·cen·te·sis** (o-var"e-o-sən-te'sis) [*ovario-* + *-centesis*] surgical puncture of an ovary.

**ovar·io·cy·e·sis** (o-var"e-o-si-e'sis) [*ovario-* + *cyesis*] ovarian pregnancy.

**ovar·io·dys·neu·ria** (o-var"e-o-dis-noor'e-ə) [*ovario-* + *dys-* + *neur-* + *-ia*] neuralgic pain in the ovary.

**ovar·io·gen·ic** (o-var"e-o-jen'ik) arising in the ovary.

**ovar·io·hys·ter·ec·to·my** (o-var"e-o-his"tər-ek'tə-me) oophorohysterectomy.

**ovar·i·op·a·thy** (o-var"e-op'ə-the) [*ovario-* + *-pathy*] oophoropathy.

**ovar·io·pexy** (o-var"e-o-pek'se) [*ovario-* + *-pexy*] the operation of elevating and fixing an ovary to the abdominal wall.

**ovar·i·or·rhex·is** (o-var"re-o-rek'sis) [*ovario-* + *-rrhexis*] rupture of an ovary.

**ovar·io·sal·pin·gec·to·my** (o-var"e-o-sal"pin-jek'tə-me) salpingo-oophorectomy.

**ovar·i·os·to·my** (o-var"e-os'tə-me) oophorostomy.

**ovar·io·tes·tis** (o-var"e-o-tes'tis) ovotestis.

**ovar·i·ot·o·my** (o-var"e-ot'ə-me) [*ovario-* + *-tomy*] 1. oophorectomy. 2. removal of an ovarian tumor.
**abdominal o.,** ovariotomy performed through the abdominal wall.
**vaginal o.,** ovariotomy performed through the vagina.

**ovar·io·tu·bal** (o-var"e-o-too'bəl) tubo-ovarian.

**ova·ri·tis** (o"və-ri'tis) oophoritis.

**ova·ri·um** (o-var'e-əm) pl. *ova'ria* [L.] [TA] ovary: the female gonad, one of the two sexual glands in which the ova are formed. It is a flat oval body along the lateral wall of the pelvic cavity, attached to the posterior surface of the broad ligament. It consists of stroma and ovarian follicles in various stages of maturation, and is covered by a modified peritoneum.
**o. masculi'num,** appendix testis.

**ova·ry** (o'və-re) [MeSH: Ovary] ovarium.
**oyster o's,** hypertrophied, edematous ovaries usually seen in hydatidiform mole.
**polycystic o's,** 1. ovaries containing multiple, small follicular cysts filled with yellow or blood-stained, thin serous fluid, characteristic of polycystic ovary syndrome. 2. polycystic ovary syndrome.

**OVD** occlusal vertical dimension; see *vertical dimension,* under *dimension.*

**over·bite** (o'vər-bīt) vertical overlap (def. 1).
**deep o.,** closed bite.
**horizontal o.,** see under *overlap.*
**vertical o.,** see under *overlap.*

**over·clo·sure** (o"vər-klo'zhər) the loss of occlusal vertical dimension.
**reduced interarch distance o.,** the loss of occlusal or contact vertical dimension.

**over·com·pen·sa·tion** (o"vər-kom"pən-sa'shən) conscious or unconscious exaggerated correction for a real or imagined physical or psychological deficiency.

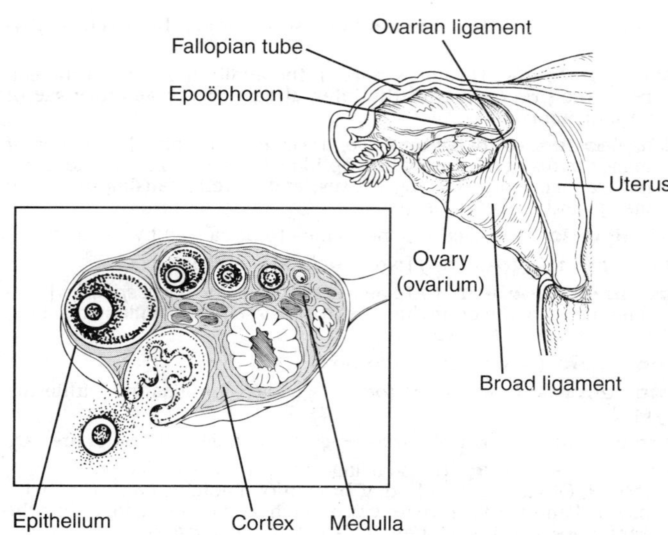


Ovarium (ovary). Inset shows the ovarian microstructure, with the stages of ovarian follicle development depicted counterclockwise from the top right, showing follicles progressively more mature: from primordial to primary, secondary, then tertiary, followed by ovulation, and finally corpora lutea from maturation to degeneration.

**over·cor·rec·tion** (o"vər-kə-rek'shən) the use of too powerful lenses in correcting defect of vision.

**over·den·ture** (o"vər-den'chər) overlay denture.

**over·de·ter·mi·na·tion** (o"vər-de-ter"mĭ-na'shən) in psychoanalytic theory, the concept that every dream, disorder, aspect of behavior, or other emotional reaction or symptom has multiple causative factors.

**over·do·sage** (o"vər-do'səj) 1. the administration of an excessive dose. 2. the condition resulting from an excessive dose.

**over·dose** (o'vər-dōs) [MeSH: Overdose] 1. to administer an excessive dose. 2. an excessive dose.

**over·drive** (o'vər-drīv) in cardiology, a more rapid heart rate produced in the correction of an underlying pathologic rhythm; see also under *pacing.*

**over·erup·tion** (o"vər-e-rup'shən) supraclusion.

**over·ex·ten·sion** (o"vər-ek-sten'shən) extension, as of a limb, beyond the normal limit.

**over·flow** (o'vər-flo) the continuous escape of a fluid, as of the tears or the urine.
**motor o.,** contralateral associated movement.

**over·graft·ing** (o"vər-graft'ing) the application of a second skin graft over a previously healed graft from which the epithelium has been removed, as a means of reinforcing split-thickness grafts.

**over·growth** (o'vər-grōth) excessive growth of a part, due either to increase in size of the constituent cells (hypertrophy) or to an increase in their number (hyperplasia).

**over·hang** (o'vər-hang) the extension, over the margins of a tooth cavity, of an excessive amount of filling material.

**over·hy·dra·tion** (o"vər-hi-dra'shən) a state of excess fluids in the body.

**over·in·fla·tion** (o"vər-in-fla'shən) hyperinflation.
**congenital lobar o.,** see under *emphysema.*
**nonobstructive pulmonary o.,** compensatory emphysema.
**obstructive pulmonary o.,** localized obstructive emphysema.

**over·jet** (o'vər-jet) horizontal overlap.

**over·jut** (o'vər-jət) horizontal overlap.

**over·lap** (o'vər-lap) 1. to cover and extend beyond a certain point. 2. anything that lies or extends over and partially covers something.
**horizontal o.,** extension of the incisal or buccal cusp ridges of the maxillary teeth labially or buccally to the incisal margins and ridges of the mandibular teeth when the jaws are in habitual occlusion. Called also *horizontal overbite, overjet,* and *overjut.*
**vertical o.,** 1. extension of the incisal ridges of the maxillary anterior teeth below the incisal ridges of the mandibular anterior teeth when the jaws are in centric occlusion. Cf. *micrognathia.* Called also *overbite* or *over bite* and *vertical overbite.* 2. the distance that the teeth lap over their antagonists. 3. the relationship of the maxillary in-

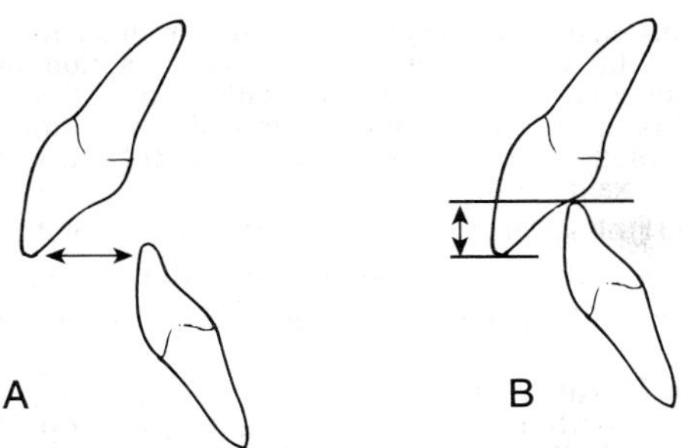

*(A),* Horizontal overlap (overjet); *(B),* vertical overlap (overbite).

cisors to the mandibular incisors when the incisal edges pass each other in centric occlusion.

**over·lay** (o′vər-la) an increment; a later addition superimposed upon an already existing mass, state, or condition.
**emotional o.,** psychogenic o.
**psychogenic o.,** the emotionally determined increment to an existing organic symptom or disability.

**over·load** (o′vər-lōd) excess.
**iron o.,** an excess of iron in the body; see *hemochromatosis, hemosiderosis,* and *siderosis.*

**over·match·ing** (o′vər-mach′ing) in statistics, matching of too many variables or matching variables too closely when selecting cases and controls for study, so that true causal relationships between variables may be obscured, irrelevant variables may be included, or the study may become too complex and specific for appropriate controls to be reasonably obtained.

**over·reach·ing** (o″vər-rēch′ing) an error of gait in the horse, in which the toe of the hind hoof strikes the heel of the forefoot.

**over·re·sponse** (o″vər-re-spons′) abnormally intense response or reaction to a stimulus.

**over·rid·ing** (o″vər-rīd′ing) 1. the slipping of either part of a fractured bone past the other. 2. extending beyond the usual position.

**over·sens·ing** (o′vər-sens″ing) inappropriate sensing of electrical signals by an artificial cardiac pacemaker, either extracardiac signals or cardiac signals other than those it is set to detect; in demand pacemakers the result is slowed or irregular pacemaker output.

**over·stain** (o′vər-stān) to stain a tissue excessively, so that certain elements may be properly stained when the excess of stain is washed out.

**over·strain** (o′vər-strān) an abnormal degree of fatigue brought about by activity; it is intermediate between fatigue and actual exhaustion.

**over·stress** (o′vər-stres) excessive activity resulting in overstrain.

**over·toe** (o′vər-to) hallux valgus in which the great toe overlies its fellows.

**over·tone** (o′vər-tōn) any whole number multiple of a fundamental tone.
**psychic o.,** the consciousness of a fringe or halo of associated relations that surrounds every image presented to the mind.

**over·trans·fu·sion** (o″vər-trans-fu′zhən) overloading of the circulation by excessive transfusion of blood or other fluid; see *hypervolemia.*

**over·ven·ti·la·tion** (o″vər-ven″tĭ-la′shən) hyperventilation.

**over·weight** (o′vər-wāt) excessive increase in adipose tissue (obese overweight) or in muscle and skeletal tissue (muscular overweight).

**ovi-** see *ov(o)-.*

**ovi·cide** (o′vĭ-sīd) an agent destructive to the ova of certain organisms.

**ovi·du·cal** (o′vĭ-doo-kəl) pertaining to the oviducts.

**ovi·duct** (o′vĭ-dəkt) [*ovi-* + *duct*] [MeSH: Oviducts] 1. a passage through which ova leave the maternal organism or pass to an organ that communicates with the exterior of the body. 2. a uterine tube (tuba uterina [TA]).

**ovi·duc·tal** (o″vĭ-duk′təl) pertaining to an oviduct.

**ovif·er·ous** (o-vif′ər-əs) [*ovi-* + *-ferous*] producing ova.

**ovi·form** (o′vĭ-form) [*ovi-* + *form*] egg-shaped; ovoid.

**ovi·gen·e·sis** (o″vĭ-jen′ə-sis) [*ovi-* + *-genesis*] oogenesis.

**ovi·ge·net·ic** (o″vĭ-jə-net′ik) oogenetic.

**ovi·gen·ic** (o″vĭ-jen′ik) oogenetic.

**ovig·e·nous** (o-vij′ə-nəs) oogenetic.

**ovi·germ** (o′vĭ-jərm) [*ovi-* + *germ*] ooblast.

**ovig·er·ous** (o-vij′ər-əs) [*ovi-* + L. *gerere* to bear] producing or containing ova.

**ovine** (o′vīn) [L. *ovinus* of a sheep] pertaining to, characteristic of, or derived from sheep.

**ovi·par·i·ty** (o″vĭ-par′ĭ-te) the quality of being oviparous.

**ovip·a·rous** (o-vip′ə-rəs) [*ovi-* + L. *parere* to bring forth, produce] producing eggs from which the young are hatched outside the body of the maternal organism. Cf. *ovoviviparous* and *viviparous.*

**ovi·po·si·tion** (o″vĭ-po-zi′shən) [*ovi-* + L. *ponere* to place] [MeSH: Oviposition] the act of laying or depositing eggs.

**ovi·pos·i·tor** (o″vĭ-pos′ĭ-tor) a specialized organ by means of which many female insects deposit their eggs in various plant structures or in the soil.

**ovi·sac** (o′vĭ-sak) [*ovi-* + *sac*] a graafian follicle (see *folliculi ovarici vesiculosi* under *folliculus*).

**ovist** (o′vist) one who believes that the undeveloped embryo exists preformed in the ovum. Cf. *animalculist.*

**ovi·um** (o′ve-əm) ootid.

**ov(o)-** [L. *ovum* egg] a combining form denoting relationship to an egg, or to ova. Also, *ovi-.* See also words beginning *oo-.*

**ovo·cyte** (o′vo-sīt) [MeSH: Oocytes] oocyte.

**ovo·gen·e·sis** (o″vo-jen′ə-sis) oogenesis.

**ovo·glob·u·lin** (o″vo-glob′u-lin) the globulin of white of egg.

**ovo·go·ni·um** (o″vo-go′ne-əm) oogonium.

**ovoid** (o′void) [*ovo-* + *-oid*] 1. egg-shaped. 2. an egg-shaped structure.
**myelin o's,** small oval compartments containing myelin that are formed by the breaking up of the myelin sheath in wallerian degeneration.

**ovo·lac·to·veg·e·tar·i·an** (o″vo-lak″to-vej″ə-tar′e-ən) one who practices ovolactovegetarianism.

**ovo·lac·to·veg·e·tar·i·an·ism** (o″vo-lak″to-vej″ə-tar′e-ə-niz″əm) restriction of the diet to vegetables, dairy products, and eggs, eschewing other foods of animal origin.

**ovo·lyt·ic** (o″vo-lit′ik) splitting up egg albumin.

**ovo·mu·cin** (o″vo-mu′sin) [MeSH: Ovomucin] a glycoprotein from the white of egg.

**ovo·mu·coid** (o″vo-mu′koid) [*ovo-* + *mucoid*] a glycoprotein derivable from egg white.

**ovo·plasm** (o′vo-plaz-əm) [*ovo-* + *-plasm*] ooplasm.

**ovo·tes·tis** (o″vo-tes′tis) an abnormal gonad containing both testicular and ovarian tissue, seen in hermaphroditism. Called also *ovariotestis.*

**ovo·trans·fer·rin** (o″vo-trans-fer′in) an iron-binding protein in egg white having the same properties as transferrin.

**ovo·veg·e·tar·i·an** (o″vo-vej″ə-tar′e-ən) one who practices ovovegetarianism.

**ovo·veg·e·tar·i·an·ism** (o″vo-vej″ə-tar′e-ə-niz″əm) restriction of the diet to vegetables and eggs, eschewing other foods of animal origin.

**ovo·vi·tel·lin** (o″vo-vi-tel′in) vitellin.

**ovo·vivi·par·i·ty** (o″vo-viv″ĭ-par′ĭ-te) the quality of being ovoviviparous.

**ovo·vi·vip·a·rous** (o″vo-vi-vip′ə-rəs) [*ovo-* + *vivi-* + *-parous*] bearing living young that hatch from large, yolk-filled eggs inside the body of the maternal organism, the embryo being nourished by food stored in the egg; said of lizards, etc. Cf. *oviparous* and *viviparous.*

**Ov·rette** (ōv-ret′) trademark for a preparation of norgestrel.

**ovu·lar** (ov′u-lər) 1. pertaining to an ovule. 2. pertaining to an oocyte (ovum).

**ovu·la·tion** (ov″u-la′shən) [MeSH: Ovulation] the discharge of a secondary oocyte from a vesicular follicle of the ovary.
**amenstrual o.,** that which occurs in the absence of menstrual bleeding.
**anestrous o.,** that which occurs in animals unaccompanied by other events of estrus.
**paracyclic o.,** supplementary o.
**supplementary o.,** an extra ovulation in a particular estrous cycle; called also *paracyclic o.*

**ov·u·la·to·ry** (ov′u-lə-tor″e) pertaining to ovulation.

**ovule** (o′vūl) [L. *ovulum*] 1. the ovum within the ovarian (graafian) follicle. 2. any small, egglike structure. 3. the megasporangium en-

closed within one or more integuments that, after fertilization, becomes a plant seed.
**graafian o's,** folliculi ovarici vesiculosi.
**primitive o., primordial o.,** a rudimentary ovum within the ovary.

**ovu·log·e·nous** (ov″u-loj′ə-nəs) producing or developing from an ovule or ovum.

**ovum** (o′vəm) pl. *o′va,* gen. *o′vi* [L.] [MeSH: Ovum] 1. the female reproductive cell which, after fertilization, becomes a zygote that develops into a new member of the same species. Called also *egg.* 2. [TA] the human mature oocyte: a round cell about 0.1 mm in diameter, produced in the ovary, where there is deposited around it a noncellular covering *(oolemma; zona pellucida; zona radiata).* It consists of protoplasm that contains some yolk, enclosed by a thin cell wall *(vitelline membrane).* There is a large nucleus *(germinal vesicle),* within which is a nucleolus *(germinal spot).* 3. the term was formerly extended to include any early stage of the conceptus.
**alecithal o.,** one with only a small amount of yolk, or almost no yolk, as in the ova of mammals and many of the invertebrates; called also *oligolecithal o.*
**blighted o.,** a zygote in which development has become arrested, and abnormality or degeneration is evident.
**Bryce-Teacher o.,** a human embryo that was thought to be the youngest known ovum at the time of its study in 1908; now known to be a pathological specimen.
**centrolecithal o.,** one in which the yolk is centrally located, and surrounded by a peripheral layer of cytoplasm, as the ova of arthropods.
**cleidoic o.,** one that possesses within itself sufficient nutritive material for the production of a complete embryo and so needs to absorb nothing from its environment except oxygen, as a bird's egg.
**ectolecithal o.,** one in which the yolk is situated peripherally.
**Hertig-Rock ova,** 34 fertilized ova, ranging from 1 to 17 days of age, 21 of which were normal, and 13 abnormal to one degree or another; discovered between 1938 and 1953, they constitute the only series of such early human conceptuses in existence.
**holoblastic o.,** one that undergoes total cleavage.
**isolecithal o.,** one with yolk evenly distributed throughout the cytoplasm.
**macrolecithal o.,** one with much yolk.
**Mateer-Streeter o.,** an embryo about 18 days old, first described in 1920.
**medialecithal o.,** one with a medium amount of yolk.
**megalecithal o.,** macrolecithal o.
**meroblastic o.,** one that undergoes partial cleavage.
**microlecithal o.,** miolecithal o.
**Miller o.,** an embryo 10 or 11 days old, first described in 1913.
**miolecithal o.,** one containing little yolk.
**oligolecithal o.,** alecithal o.
**permanent o.,** an ovum ready for fertilization.
**Peters' o.,** an embryo about 13 or 14 days old, first described in 1899.
**primitive o., primordial o.,** an oocyte very early in its development.
**telolecithal o.,** one in which the yolk is increasingly concentrated toward one pole.

**Owen's lines** (o′ənz) [Sir Richard *Owen,* English anatomist and paleontologist, 1804–1892] see under *line.*

**Ow·ren's disease** (o′renz) [Paul Arnor *Owren,* Norwegian hematologist, born 1905] parahemophilia.

**ox-** see *oxy-.*

**ox·ac·id** (oks-as′id) oxyacid.

**ox·a·cil·lin so·di·um** (oks″ə-sil′in) [USP] a semisynthetic penicillinase-resistant penicillin, used primarily in the treatment of infections due to penicillin-resistant staphylococci, administered orally, intramuscularly, or intravenously.

**ox·al·al·de·hyde** (ok″səl-al′də-hīd) glyoxal.

**ox·a·late** (ok′sə-lāt) a salt of oxalic acid; see also *oxalate poisoning,* under *poisoning..*

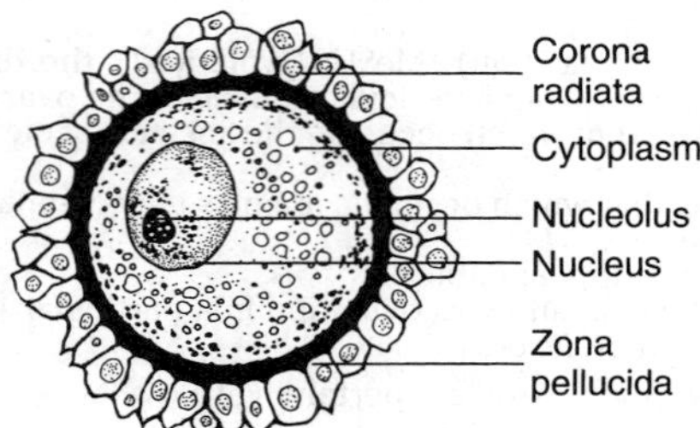

Human ovum.

**ammonium o.,** odorless crystals or white granules formed by evaporation of the product obtained by the reaction of equivalent amounts of ammonia solution and oxalic acid.
**balanced o.,** a mixture of ammonium and potassium oxalates in a 3:2 ratio, used as an anticoagulant in the collection of blood for laboratory examination.

**ox·a·lat·ed** (ok′sə-lāt″əd) treated with oxalate solution.

**ox·a·la·tion** (ok″sə-la′shən) treatment with oxalate solution.

**ox·a·le·mia** (ok″sə-le′me-ə) [*oxalate* + *-emia*] an excess of oxalates in the blood.

**ox·al·ic ac·id** (ok-sal′ik) a strong dicarboxylic acid, HOOC-COOH, occurring in foods such as spinach and rhubarb or produced in the body by metabolism of glyoxylic acid or ascorbic acid; it is not metabolized but excreted in the urine. Ingestion of a diet rich in oxalates or a genetic disorder of glycine metabolism (primary hyperoxaluria) may lead to the formation of calcium oxalate renal calculi. See also *oxalate poisoning,* under *poisoning.*

**Ox·a·lid** (ok′sə-lid) trademark for a preparation of oxyphenbutazone.

**ox·al·ism** (ok′səl-iz-əm) oxalate poisoning.

**ox·a·lo·ac·e·tate** (ok″sə-lo-as′ə-tāt) an anionic form of oxaloacetic acid.

**ox·a·lo·ace·tic ac·id** (ok″sə-lo-ə-se′tik) an intermediate in the tricarboxylic acid cycle (q.v.); it is convertible to aspartic acid by a transamination reaction.

**ox·a·lo·sis** (ok″sə-lo′sis) generalized deposition of calcium oxalate in renal and extrarenal tissues, as may occur in primary hyperoxaluria.

**ox·al·uria** (ok″səl-u′re-ə) hyperoxaluria.

**ox·al·ur·ic ac·id** (ok″səl-ūr′ik) the amide of oxalic acid and urea, which occurs in urine.

**ox·a·lyl** (ok′sə-ləl) the divalent group, $(C{:}O)_2$, formed from oxalic acid by the loss of two hydroxyl groups.

**ox·a·lyl·urea** (ok″sə-ləl-u′re-ə) 1. oxaluric acid. 2. parabanic acid.

**ox·am·ide** (ok-sam′id) the diamide of oxalic acid; it will give the biuret reaction.

**ox·am·ni·quine** (oks-am′nĭ-kwin) [MeSH: Oxamniquine] an antischistosomal especially effective against *Schistosoma mansoni.*

**Ox·an·drin** (ok-san′drin) trademark for a preparation of oxandrolone.

**ox·an·dro·lone** (ok-san′dro-lōn) [USP] [MeSH: Oxandrolone] an androgenic steroidal lactone that promotes retention of nitrogen, potassium, and phosphorus, and is used to accelerate anabolism and/or to arrest excessive catabolism.

**ox·an·tel pam·o·ate** (oks′ən-təl) an anthelmintic effective against *Trichuris.*

**ox·a·pro·zin** (ok″sə-pro′zin) a nonsteroidal antiinflammatory drug, administered orally.

**ox·az·e·pam** (ok-saz′ə-pam) [USP] [MeSH: Oxazepam] a benzodiazepine used as an anxiolytic in the treatment of anxiety disorders and anxiety associated with depression, for short-term relief of anxiety symptoms, especially in the elderly, and for the treatment of the symptoms of acute alcohol withdrawal; administered orally.

**ox·et·o·rone fu·mar·ate** (ok-set′o-rōn fu′mə-rāt) an analgesic specific in migraine.

**ox·fen·da·zole** (oks-fen′də-zōl) [USP] a benzimidazole anthelmintic used to treat ruminant infestatations by either roundworms or tapeworms.

**ox·gall** (oks′gawl) see *ox bile extract,* under *extract.*

**ox·i·ben·da·zole** (ok″sĭ-ben′də-zōl) a benzimidazole anthelmintic used to treat roundworm and lungworm infestations in horses and other ruminants.

**ox·i·dant** (ok′sĭ-dənt) the electron acceptor in an oxidation-reduction (redox) reaction.

**ox·i·dase** (ok′sĭ-dās) a term used in the recommended names of some oxidoreductases to denote those in which molecular oxygen is the hydrogen acceptor.
**mixed function o.,** monooxygenase.

**ox·i·da·tion** (ok″sĭ-da′shən) the act of oxidizing or state of being oxidized. Chemically it consists in the increase of positive charges on an atom or the loss of negative charges. Most biological oxidations are accomplished by the removal of a pair of hydrogen atoms (dehydrogenation) from a molecule. Such oxidations must be accompanied by reduction of an acceptor molecule. *Univalent o.* indicates loss of one electron; *divalent o.,* the loss of two electrons.
**alpha o.,** oxidation of a fatty acid at the alpha carbon, that adjacent

to the carboxyl group, as occurs in the metabolism of phytanic acid. Written also *α-oxidation.*

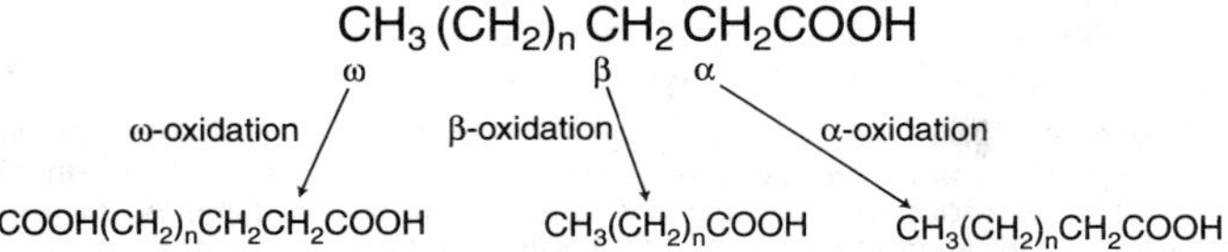


Oxidation of a saturated fatty acid having $(n + 4)$ carbon atoms; α-oxidation yields a saturated fatty acid of one fewer carbons, β-oxidation a saturated fatty acid of two fewer carbon atoms, and ω-oxidation a dicarboxylic acid with no loss of carbon atoms.

**beta o.,** oxidation of a fatty acid at the beta carbon atom, the second carbon from the carboxyl group, with the result that the two end carbons are split off as acetic acid (acetylcoenzyme A) and with the formation of a fatty acid containing two fewer carbon atoms. Written also *β-oxidation.*
**biological o.,** the enzymatic process by which food is metabolized, resulting in the release of energy. See also *oxidation.*
**coupled o.,** the enzymatic oxidation of two donor molecules, with the incorporation of oxygen into one of the donors.
**omega o.,** a minor pathway of fatty acid oxidation in which the ω-carbon is oxidized, forming an α,ω-dicarboxylic acid. Written also *ω-oxidation.*

**ox·i·da·tion-re·duc·tion** (ok″sĭ-da′shən-re-duk′shən) [MeSH: Oxidation-Reduction] the chemical reaction whereby electrons are removed (oxidation) from atoms of the substance being oxidized and transferred to atoms being reduced (reduction). Called also *redox.*

**ox·i·da·tive** (ok′sĭ-da-tiv) referring to the process of oxidation; being capable of an oxidizing reaction.

**ox·ide** (ok′sīd) [L. *oxidum*] any compound of oxygen with an element or radical.
**arsenous o.,** arsenic trioxide.
**diethyl o.,** ether.
**ferric o., red,** a red pigment used as a coloring agent in preparations for application to the skin.
**ferric o., yellow,** a yellow pigment used as a coloring agent in preparations for application to the skin.
**nitric o.,** NO, a naturally occurring gas that in the body is a short-lived dilator substance released from vascular endothelial cells in response to the binding of vasodilators to endothelial cell receptors; it causes activation of guanylate cyclase in vascular smooth muscle, leading to an increase in cyclic GMP, which inhibits muscular contraction and produces relaxation. Excess nitric oxide is toxic to cells of the central nervous system and causes the hypotension seen in septic shock. Called also *endothelial-derived relaxant factor* and *endothelium-derived relaxing factor.*
**nitrous o.** [USP], dinitrogen monoxide, $N_2O$, a colorless, odorless gas that is a weak inhalational anesthetic; it is nonflammable but supports combustion; primarily used in combination with a potent halogenated inhalational anesthetic (halothane, isoflurane, or enflurane) to produce general anesthesia; use as a sole agent requires high concentrations that may cause hypoxia. Called also *laughing gas.*

**ox·i·dize** (ok′sĭ-dīz) to combine or cause to combine with oxygen, or to lose electrons. See *oxidation.*

**ox·i·do·re·duc·tase** (ok″sĭ-do-re-duk′tās) [EC 1] any member of a class of enzymes that catalyze the reversible transfer of electrons from a substrate that becomes oxidized (hydrogen or electron donor) to a substrate that becomes reduced (hydrogen or electron acceptor). The class includes dehydrogenases, hydroxylases, oxidases, oxygenases, peroxidases, and reductases.

**ox·i·do·sis** (ok″sĭ-do′sis) acidosis.

**ox·i·dro·nate** (ok″sĭ-dro′nāt) HDP, HMDP; a hydroxymethylene-substituted diphosphonate compound having an affinity for sites of osteoid mineralization; complexed with technetium 99m it is used in bone imaging. See table at *technetium.*

**ox·il·or·phan** (ok″sil-or′fən) a narcotic antagonist, $C_{20}H_{27}NO_2$.

**ox·im** (ok′sim) oxime.

**ox·ime** (ok′sēm) any of a series of compounds containing the CH(=NOH) group, formed by the action of hydroxylamine on an aldehyde or a ketone.

**ox·im·e·ter** (ok-sim′ə-tər) a photoelectric device for determining the oxygen saturation of the blood.
**CO-o.,** a device that uses spectrophotometry to measure relative blood concentrations of oxyhemoglobin, carboxyhemoglobin, methemoglobin, and reduced hemoglobin.
**ear o.,** a pulse oximeter for attachment to the ear, by which oxygen saturation of the blood flowing through the ear can be determined.
**finger o.,** a pulse oximeter whose sensor is attached to a finger, so that the oxygenation of blood flowing through the finger can be determined.
**intracardiac o.,** an instrument for measuring the concentration of oxygen or dye in blood within the heart; see also *oxygen gas analyzer,* under *analyzer.*
**pulse o.,** an oximeter that measures the oxygen saturation of arterial blood by passing a beam of red and infrared light through a pulsating capillary bed, the ratio of red to infrared transmission varying with the oxygen saturation of the blood; because it responds only to pulsatile objects, it does not detect nonpulsating objects like skin and venous blood.
**whole blood o.,** an oximeter for determination of oxygen saturation of removed specimens of blood.

**ox·im·e·try** (ok-sim′ə-tre) [MeSH: Oximetry] determination of the oxygen saturation of arterial blood using an oximeter.

**ox·ine** (ok-sēn′) oxyquinoline.

**ox·i·per·o·mide** (ok″se-per′o-mīd) a dopamine-receptor antagonist used as a tranquilizer.

**ox·ir·ane** (ok′sĭ-rān) ethylene oxide.

**ox·met·i·dine mes·y·late** (oks-met′ĭ-dēn mes′ə-lāt) a histamine $H_2$ receptor antagonist.

**oxo-** the approved prefix in formal nomenclature for *keto-,* as in *oxoglutarate* for *ketoglutarate.* Terms prefixed with *keto-* are the common forms in the United States.

**3-oxo·ac·id CoA-trans·fer·ase** (ok″so-as′id ko-a′ trans′fər-ās) [EC 2.8.3.5] an enzyme of the transferase class that catalyzes the shift of coenzyme A (CoA) from succinyl CoA to acetoacetic acid to form acetoacetyl CoA; the reaction is part of a mechanism by which free β-hydroxybutyrate can be converted to acetyl CoA and used as fuel. The enzyme is present in muscle and nerve tissue but absent from liver, and it can also act on some related keto acids. Called also *3-ketoacid CoA transferase.*

**oxo·ac·id-ly·ase** (ok″so-as″id-li′ās) [EC 4.1.3] any member of a sub-subclass of enzymes of the lyase class that catalyze the cleavage of a C—C bond of a 3-hydroxy acid.

**oxo·glu·ta·rate de·hy·dro·gen·ase (lip·o·am·ide)** (ok″so-gloo′tə-rāt de-hi′dro-jən-ās lip″o-am′īd) [EC 1.2.4.2] EC nomenclature for *α-ketoglutarate dehydrogenase.*

**2-oxo·glu·tar·ic ac·id** (ok″so-gloo-tar′ik) α-ketoglutaric acid.

**2-oxo·iso·val·er·ate de·hy·dro·gen·ase (lip·o·am·ide)** (ok″so-i″so-val′er-āt de-hi′dro-jən-ās lip″o-am′īd) 3-methyl-2-oxobutanoate dehydrogenase (lipoamide).

**oxo·lin·ic ac·id** (ok-so-lin′ik) [MeSH: Oxolinic Acid] a synthetic antibacterial used orally for urinary tract infections caused by gram-negative organisms, including *Escherichia coli, Proteus* species, and *Klebsiella* species.

**oxo·ni·um** (ok-so′ne-əm) containing tetravalent basic oxygen.

**oxo·phen·ar·sine hy·dro·chlo·ride** (ok″so-fən-ahr′sēn) an arsenical with antispirochetal and antitrypanosomal properties; rarely used in the treatment of syphilis and trypanosomiasis.

**oxo·ste·roid** (ok″so-ster′oid) ketosteroid.

**5-oxo·pro·li·nase (ATP-hy·dro·lyz·ing)** (ok″so-pro′lĭ-nās hi′dro-li-zing) [EC 3.5.2.9] an enzyme of the hydrolase class that catalyzes the ATP-dependent linearization of 5-oxoproline to form glutamate; the reaction is a part of the mechanism of transport of amino acids into tissue cells by the γ-glutamyl cycle.

**5-oxo·pro·line** (ok″so-pro′lēn) a ninhydrin-negative, acidic lactam of glutamic acid occurring at the N-terminus of several peptides and proteins. Called also *pyroglutamic acid* or *pyroglutamate.*

**5-oxo·pro·lin·u·ria** (ok″so-pro″lin-u′re-ə) 1. excess of 5-oxoproline in the urine. 2. generalized deficiency of glutathione synthetase.

**ox·pen·tif·yl·line** (oks″pən-tif′ə-lēn) pentoxifylline.

**ox·pren·o·lol hy·dro·chlo·ride** (oks-pren′ə-lol) [USP] a beta-adrenergic blocking agent having the same actions as propranolol (q.v.).

**Ox·sor·a·len** (ok-sor′ə-lən) trademark for preparations of methoxsalen.

**ox·triph·yl·line** (oks-trif′ə-lēn) [USP] the choline salt of theophylline, used as a bronchodilator in the prevention and treatment of symptoms of asthma and of reversible bronchospasm associated with chronic bronchitis or emphysema; administered orally.

**oxy-** [Gr. *oxys* keen] a combining form *(a)* meaning sharp, quick, or sour, *(b)* denoting relationship to acid, or *(c)* denoting the presence of oxygen in a compound. Also, *ox-.*

**oxy·ac·id** (ok″se-as′id) an acid containing both oxygen and hydrogen atoms. When there are two common oxyacids of the same element, that with the higher oxidation state is designated by the suffix

*-ic,* that with the lower by *-ous.* When additional oxidation states occur, the prefix *hypo-* may be used to indicate a lower state and *per-* to indicate a higher state; e.g., hypochlorous acid ($HClO$), chlorous acid ($HClO_2$), chloric acid ($HClO_3$), and perchloric acid ($HClO_4$). Called also *oxo acid* and *oxacid.*

**oxy·acoia** (ok″se-ə-koi′ə) hyperacusis.

**oxy·ben·zene** (ok″se-ben′zēn) phenol (def. 1).

**oxy·ben·zone** (ok″se-ben′zōn) [USP] a sunscreening agent applied topically to the skin.

**oxy·blep·sia** (ok″se-blep′se-ə) [*oxy-* + Gr. *blepsis* vision + *-ia*] oxyopia.

**oxy·bu·ty·nin chlo·ride** (ok″se-bu′tĭ-nin) an anticholinergic that has a direct antispasmodic effect on smooth muscle; used in the treatment of uninhibited neurogenic bladder and reflex neurogenic bladder, administered orally.

**oxy·bu·tyr·ia** (ok″se-bu-tir′e-ə) the presence of hydroxybutyric acid in urine.

**oxy·bu·tyr·ic ac·id** (ok″se-bu-tir′ik) hydroxybutyric acid.

**oxy·bu·tyr·ic·ac·i·de·mia** (ok″se-bu-tir″ik-as″ĭ-de′me-ə) oxybutyria.

**oxy·cal·o·rim·e·ter** (ok″se-kal″o-rim′ə-tər) Benedict's apparatus for determining the caloric value of food by burning a sample in a combustion chamber and measuring the volume of oxygen consumed.

**Oxy·cel** (ok′sĭ-sel) trademark for preparations of oxidized cellulose.

**oxy·ce·pha·lia** (ok″se-sə-fa′le-ə) oxycephaly.

**oxy·ce·phal·ic** (ok″se-sə-fal′ik) pertaining to or characterized by oxycephaly.

**oxy·ceph·a·lous** (ok″se-sef′ə-ləs) oxycephalic.

**oxy·ceph·a·ly** (ok″se-sef′ə-le) [*oxy-* + *-cephaly*] a condition in which the top of the head is pointed or conical owing to premature closure of the coronal and lambdoid sutures. Called also *acrocephaly, hypsicephaly, turricephaly, steeple head* or *skull,* and *tower head* or *skull.*

**oxy·chlo·ride** (ok″se-klor′īd) an element or radical combined with oxygen and chlorine.

**oxy·chlo·ro·sene** (ok″se-klor′o-sēn) the hypochlorous acid complex of a mixture of the phenyl sulfonate derivatives of aliphatic hydrocarbons, having actions similar to those of chlorine; used as a topical anti-infective.
**o. sodium,** the sodium salt of oxychlorosene, used like the base.

**oxy·cho·line** (ok″se-ko′lin) muscarine.

**oxy·chro·mat·ic** (ok″se-kro-mat′ik) [*oxy-* + *chromat-* + *-ic*] staining with acid dyes; acidophilic.

**oxy·chro·ma·tin** (ok″se-kro′mə-tin) [*oxy-* + *chromatin*] that part of the chromatin that stains with acid aniline dyes; called also *lanthanin.*

**oxy·ci·ne·sia** (ok″se-sĭ-ne′zhə) [*oxy-* + *cinesi-* + *-ia*] kinesialgia.

**oxy·clo·za·nide** (ok″se-klo′zə-nīd) [MeSH: Oxyclozanide] a salicylanilide anthelmintic used against adult liver flukes in cattle and sheep.

**oxy·co·done** (ok″se-ko′dōn) [MeSH: Oxycodone] an opioid agonist analgesic derived from morphine derivative.
**o. hydrochloride** [USP], the hydrochloride salt of oxycodone, used as an analgesic; administered orally or rectally.
**o. terephthalate** [USP], a salt of oxycodone used as an analgesic, administered orally.

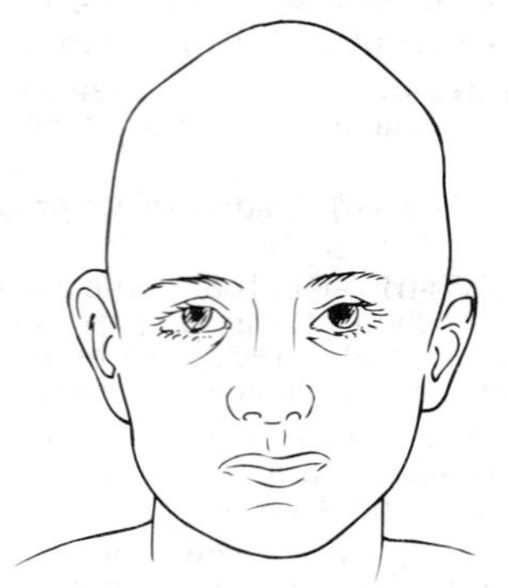

Oxycephaly.

**Oxy·Con·tin** (ok″se-kon′tin) trademark for a preparation of oxycodone hydrochloride.

**oxy·cy·a·nide** (ok″se-si′ə-nīd) the oxide of any binary compound of cyanogen.

**oxy·ecoia** (ok″se-e-koi′ə) hyperacusis.

**ox·y·gen** (ok′sĭ-jən) [Gr. *oxys* sour + *gennan* to produce] [MeSH: Oxygen] a gaseous element existing free in the air and in combination in most nonelementary solids, liquids, and gases; atomic number, 8; atomic weight, 15.999; symbol, O. There are three naturally occurring isotopes, with atomic weights of 16, 17, and 18 (heavy oxygen). Oxygen constitutes 20 per cent by weight of the atmospheric air; it is the essential agent in the respiration of plants and animals and, although noninflammable, is necessary to support combustion. It forms the characteristic constituent of ternary acids. It is administered by inhalation in some pulmonary and cardiac disorders.
**o. 15,** an artificial radioactive isotope of oxygen, atomic mass 15, having a half-life of 2.04 minutes; it decays by positron emission (1.70 MeV) and is used as a tracer in the measurement of regional blood volume and flow and oxygen metabolism by positron emission tomography.
**heavy o.,** an isotope of oxygen of atomic weight 18.
**high pressure o.,** hyperbaric o.
**hyperbaric o.,** oxygen under greater than atmospheric pressure. Called also *high-pressure o.*
**molecular o.,** dioxygen, $O_2$.
**singlet o.,** a highly reactive, dimagnetic excited state ($^1O_2$) of dioxygen that rapidly decays with the emission of visible light to the paramagnetic (triplet) ground state. Singlet oxygen is highly reactive and is thought to be involved in the oxidative killing of ingested microorganisms by neutrophils; it is produced spontaneously during the respiratory burst by spontaneous reactions of hydrogen peroxide with superoxide and hypochlorite ions.

**ox·y·gen·ase** (ok′sĭ-jən-ās) [EC 1.13] any member of a subclass of enzymes of the oxidoreductase class that catalyze the oxidation of a single substrate (hydrogen donor) with incorporation of one or both atoms of oxygen from molecular oxygen into the substance oxidized.

**ox·y·gen·ate** (ok′sĭ-jə-nāt) to add oxygen to.

**ox·y·gen·a·tion** (ok″sĭ-jə-na′shən) the act, process, or result of oxygenating.
**extracorporeal membrane o. (ECMO),** a technique for providing respiratory support by circulating the blood through an artificial lung consisting of two compartments separated by a gas-permeable membrane, with the blood on one side and the ventilating gas on the other; used in newborns and occasionally in adults with acute respiratory distress syndrome.

**ox·y·gen·a·tor** (ok′sĭ-jə-na″tor) [MeSH: Oxygenators] a device that mechanically oxygenates venous blood extracorporeally. It is used in combination with one or more pumps for maintaining circulation during open heart surgery and for assisting the circulation in patients seriously ill with some cardiac and pulmonary disorders. Called also *artificial lung.*
**bubble o.,** a device in which a stream of pure oxygen is broken up into small bubbles that diffuse through a column of blood, with gas exchange occurring on the bubbles' surface; the oxygenated blood is defoamed and collected in a reservoir for return to the patient's circulatory system.
**disk o.,** rotating disk o.
**film o.,** a device, encased in a container of oxygen, that makes possible the production of a thin film of blood to facilitate the exchange of gases; see *rotating disk o.* and *screen o.*
**intravascular o.,** a device consisting of hundreds of hollow fibers through which oxygen is drawn by a vacuum pump; it is implanted in the vena cava, where gas exchange occurs as blood flows over the fibers. Used to provide part of the gas exchange needs of patients with acute respiratory failure, allowing mechanical ventilation to be performed at reduced pressures, thus reducing or preventing oxygen toxicity and barotrauma.
**membrane o.,** a device in which blood and oxygen are separated by a semipermeable membrane, generally of Teflon or polypropylene, across which gas exchange occurs. The membrane may be arranged as a series of parallel plates or as a number of hollow fibers; in the latter arrangement, the blood may flow inside the fibers, which are surrounded by gas, or the blood may flow outside the fibers and the gas inside the fibers.
**pump-o.,** see *pump-oxygenator.*
**rotating disk o.,** a formerly used type of film oxygenator in which parallel disks in series rotate through an extracorporeal pool of venous blood in a container of oxygen; gaseous exchange occurs between the thin film of blood on the exposed surfaces of the disks and the oxygen in the container.
**screen o.,** a formerly used type of film oxygenator in which the venous blood is passed over a series of screens in a container of oxy-

gen, gaseous exchange taking place in the thin film of blood produced on the screens.

**ox·y·gen·ic** (ok″sĭ-jen′ik) containing oxygen.

**oxy·hem·a·to·por·phy·rin** (ok″se-hem″ə-to-por′fĭ-rin) a pigment sometimes found in the urine, closely allied to hematoporphyrin.

**oxy·heme** (ok′se-hēm) heme.

**oxy·he·mo·chro·mo·gen** (ok″se-he″mo-kro′mo-jən) heme.

**oxy·he·mo·cy·a·nine** (ok″se-he″mo-si′ə-nēn) hemocyanin charged with oxygen.

**oxy·he·mo·glo·bin** (ok″se-he′mo-glo″bin) hemoglobin that contains bound $O_2$, a compound formed from hemoglobin on exposure to alveolar gas in the lungs, with formation of a covalent bond with oxygen and without change of the charge of the ferrous state.

**oxy·hy·dro·ceph·a·lus** (ok″se-hi″dro-sef′ə-ləs) hydrocephalus in which the top of the head assumes a pointed shape.

**oxy·hy·per·gly·ce·mia** (ok″se-hi″pər-gli-se′me-ə) a condition in which there is slight glycosuria and an oral glucose tolerance curve that rises about 180–200 mg per 100 mL but returns to fasting values $2\frac{1}{2}$ hours after ingestion of the glucose.

**oxy·io·dide** (ok″se-i′o-dīd) an element or radical combined with oxygen and iodine.

**Oxy·lo·bi·um** (ok″se-lo′be-um) a genus of leguminous plants, many of which contain fluoroacetates and can cause fatal fluoroacetate poisoning in livestock.

**oxy·met·az·o·line hy·dro·chlo·ride** (ok″se-mət-az′o-lēn) [USP] an adrenergic, used topically as a vasoconstrictor to reduce swelling and congestion of the nasal mucosa.

**oxy·meth·o·lone** (ok″se-meth′ə-lōn) [USP] [MeSH: Oxymetholone] an anabolic-androgenic steroid, administered orally.

**ox·ym·e·try** (ok-sim′ə-tre) oximetry.

**oxy·mor·phone hy·dro·chlo·ride** (ok″se-mor′fōn) [USP] a semisynthetic compound, used as a narcotic analgesic.

**oxy·myo·glo·bin** (ok″se-mi″o-glo′bin) a compound formed from myoglobin on exposure to atmospheric conditions, with formation of a covalent bond with oxygen and without change of the charge of the ferrous state.

**oxy·myo·he·ma·tin** (ok″se-mi″o-he′mə-tin) oxidized myohematin from muscle.

**oxy·ner·von** (ok″se-ner′von) a cerebroside isolated from the brain.

**oxy·neu·rine** (ok″se-noor′in) betaine.

**ox·yn·tic** (ok-sin′tik) [Gr. *oxynō* to make acid] secreting acid, as the parietal (oxyntic) cells.

**ox·yn·to·mod·u·lin** (ok-sin″to-mod′u-lin) a major form of enteroglucagon.

**oxy·opia** (ok″se-o′pe-ə) [*oxy-* + *-opia*] acuteness of vision; called also *oxyblepsia.*

**oxy·op·ter** (ok″se-op′tər) [*oxy-* + Gr. *optēr* observer] a unit of measurement of visual acuity, being the reciprocal value of the visual angle expressed in degrees. An oxyopter (1 degree) is equivalent to 60 Snellen units (60′) and corresponds to the counting of fingers at 1 meter.

**oxy·o·sis** (ok″se-o′sis) [*oxy-* + *-osis*] acidosis.

**oxy·para·plas·tin** (ok″se-par″ə-plas′tin) the oxyphilic part of paraplastin.

**oxy·phen·bu·ta·zone** (ok″se-fən-bu′tə-zōn) [MeSH: Oxyphenbutazone] a derivative of phenylbutazone, having similar toxicity and anti-inflammatory, analgesic, and antipyretic actions; administered orally in the treatment of arthritis, gout, and similar conditions.

**oxy·phen·cy·cli·mine hy·dro·chlo·ride** (ok″se-fən-si′klĭ-mēn) an anticholinergic, having antispasmodic, antisecretory, and antimotility activities; used especially in the treatment of peptic ulcer and spasm of the gastrointestinal tract, administered orally.

**oxy·phe·ni·sa·tin** (ok″se-fə-ni′sə-tin) a cathartic, administered as an enema to cleanse the bowel before surgery or colon examination.
**o. acetate,** the diacetyl derivative of oxyphenisatin, used as a cathartic, administered orally.

**oxy·phe·no·ni·um bro·mide** (ok″se-fə-no′ne-əm) a quaternary ammonium anticholinergic having antisecretory, antispasmodic, and antimotility activities; used in the treatment of peptic ulcer and other gastrointestinal disorders in which hypermotility and spasm are a feature, administered orally.

**oxy·phen·yl·eth·yl·amine** (ok″se-fen″əl-eth″əl-am′ēn) tyramine.

**oxy·phil** (ok′se-fil) 1. (in pl.) oxyphil cells. 2. (in pl.) Askanazy cells. 3. acidophilic.

**oxy·phil·ic** (ok″se-fil′ik) [*oxy-* + *-philic*] acidophilic.

**ox·yph·i·lous** (ok-sif′ĭ-ləs) acidophilic.

**oxy·pho·nia** (ok″se-fo′ne-ə) [Gr. *oxyphōnia*] an abnormally sharp quality or pitch of the voice.

**Oxy·pho·to·bac·te·ria** (ok″se-fo″to-bak-tēr′e-ə) [*oxy-* + *photo-* + *bacteria*] a class of bacteria of the division Gracilicutes, kingdom Procaryotae, made up of gram-negative aerobic organisms that derive energy from light (phototrophic metabolism), using water as an electron donor and producing oxygen. The class includes the blue-green bacteria (Cyanobacteria) and the green prokaryotic algae (Prochlorophyta).

**oxy·plasm** (ok′se-plaz-əm) the oxyphil part of the cytoplasm.

**oxy·pu·rine** (ok″se-pu′rin) a purine containing oxygen. The oxypurines include hypoxanthine or monoxypurine, xanthine or dioxypurine, and uric acid or trioxypurine.

**oxy·pur·i·nol** (ok″se-pūr′ĭ-nol) [MeSH: Oxypurinol] the active metabolite of allopurinol, a xanthine oxidase inhibitor responsible for much of the activity of allopurinol against gout.

**oxy·quin·o·line** (ok″sĭ-kwin′o-lēn) [MeSH: Oxyquinoline] a dicyclic aromatic compound used as a bacteriostatic and fungistatic in the preparation of fungicides and as a disinfectant; it is also used as a chelating agent.
**o. sulfate** [NF], the sulfate salt of oxyquinoline, used as a complexing agent for pharmaceuticals; it is also used as a topical antiseptic and disinfectant.

**oxy·rhine** (ok′se-rīn) [*oxy-* + Gr. *rhis* nose] having a sharp-pointed nose.

**oxy·salt** (ok′se-sawlt) any salt of an oxoacid.

**oxy·san·to·nin** (ok″se-san′to-nin) a compound formed in the body from ingested santonin.

**Oxy·spi·ru·ra** (ok″se-spi-roo′rə) a genus of nematodes of the family Thelaziidae. *O. manso′ni* is found under the nictitating membrane of chickens and other fowl.

**ox·yt·a·lan** (ok-sit′ə-lən) a connective tissue fiber resistant to acid hydrolysis, found in humans and certain other animals such as monkeys, in structures subjected to mechanical stress including tendons, ligaments, adventitia, connective tissue sheaths surrounding skin appendages, and the periodontal membranes. It stains with aldehyde fuchsin after appropriate oxidation. On electron microscopic examination, fibrillar and amorphous components are revealed. Called also *oxytalan fiber.*

**ox·yt·a·lan·ol·y·sis** (ok-sit″ə-lən-ol′ĭ-sis) destruction of oxytalan fibers.

**oxy·tet·ra·cy·cline** (ok″sĭ-tet″rə-si′klēn) [USP] [MeSH: Oxytetracycline] a broad-spectrum antibiotic of the tetracycline group produced by *Streptomyces rimosus,* effective against a wide range of both gram-positive and gram-negative organisms, used as an antibacterial and as an adjunct in the treatment of amebiasis; administered intramuscularly.
**o. calcium** [USP], the calcium salt of oxytetracycline, used as an antibacterial; administered orally.
**o. hydrochloride** [USP], the monohydrochloride salt of oxytetracycline, used as an antibacterial and antirickettsial; administered orally and by intravenous infusion.

**oxy·to·cia** (ok-sĭ-to′se-ə) [*oxy-* + *toc-* + *-ia*] rapid labor.

**oxy·to·cic** (ok-sĭ-to′sik) 1. pertaining to, characterized by, or promoting oxytocia. 2. an agent that hastens evacuation of the uterus by stimulating contractions of the myometrium.

**oxy·to·cin** (ok″sĭ-to′sin) [USP] [MeSH: Oxytocin] 1. a nonapeptide secreted by the magnocellular neurons of the hypothalamus and stored in the neurohypophysis along with vasopressin. It promotes uterine contractions and milk ejection and contributes to the second stage of labor. 2. [USP] a preparation of this substance obtained from the neurohypophyses of domestic food animals or produced synthetically; it is administered intramuscularly or by intravenous infusion to induce labor, increase the force of uterine contractions, contract uterine muscle after delivery of the placenta, control postpartum hemorrhage, or stimulate milk ejection. In veterinary medicine it is used to stimulate letdown of milk in cows with agalactia.
**o. citrate,** the citrate salt of oxytocin, used to initiate or stimulate labor in selected patients, administered buccally.

**Oxy·tro·pis** (ok″se-tro′pis) a genus of leguminous plants, related botanically to *Astragalus;* like *A.,* it is one of the groups called *locoweed* that causes locoism in grazing animals.

**ox·yt·ro·pism** (ok-sit′ro-piz-əm) [*oxygen* + *tropism*] response of living cells to the stimulus of oxygen.

**Oxy·u·ra·nus** (ok″se-u-ra′nəs) a genus of venomous snakes of the family Elapidae. *O. scutella′tus* is the taipan of Australia and New Guinea.

**oxy·uria** (ok″se-u′re-ə) oxyuriasis.

**oxy·uri·a·sis** (ok″se-u-ri′ə-sis) [MeSH: Oxyuriasis] 1. infection of a human or other animal with oxyurids. 2. enterobiasis.

**oxy·uri·cide** (ok″se-u′rĭ-sīd) [*oxyuris* + *-cide*] an agent that destroys oxyurids.

**oxy·urid** (ok-se-u′rid) any member of the superfamily Oxyuroidea. Called also *pinworm* and *seatworm.*

**Oxy·uri·dae** (ok″se-u′rĭ-de) a family of nematodes, many of which are intestinal parasites. Genera of medical or veterinary interest are *Enterobius, Oxyuris,* and *Syphacia.*

**oxy·uri·fuge** (ok″se-u′rĭ-fūj) [*oxyuris* + *-fuge*] an agent that promotes the expulsion of oxyurids.

**oxy·uri·o·sis** (ok″se-u″re-o′sis) oxyuriasis.

**Oxy·uris** (ok″se-u′ris) [Gr. *oxys* sharp + *oura* tail] a genus of intestinal nematodes of the family Oxyuridae. *O. e′qui,* the largest known pinworm, is found in the cecum, colon, and rectum of the horse. *O. vermicula′ris* has been renamed *Enterobius vermicularis.*

**oxy·uroid** (ok-se-u′roid) oxyurid.

**Oxy·uroi·dea** (ok″se-u″roi-de′ə) [MeSH: Oxyuroidea] the oxyurids, a superfamily of small nematode phasmids with a bulbous esophagus, usually found as parasites in the cecum and colon of vertebrates, but sometimes found in insects and other invertebrates. The single family of medical or veterinary interest is *Oxyuridae.* In some systems of classification, Oxyuroidea is considered to be an order.

**Oz** an antigenic marker distinguishing immunoglobulin human λ light chain subtypes.

**oz** ounce.

**oze·na** (o-ze′nə) [Gr. *ozaina* a fetid polypus in the nose] a late stage of atrophic rhinitis with a thick mucopurulent discharge, mucosal crusting, and fetor, often associated with the presence of *Klebsiella pneumoniae* subsp. *ozaenae.*

**oze·nous** (o′zə-nəs) pertaining to or of the nature of ozena.

**ozone** (o′zōn) [Gr. *ozē* stench] [MeSH: Ozone] a bluish explosive gas or blue liquid, an allotropic and more active form of oxygen, $O_3$ that is formed when oxygen is exposed to the silent discharge of electricity. It is an antiseptic and disinfectant. Ozone is a major air pollutant and is irritating and toxic to the respiratory system.

**ozo·nom·e·ter** (o″zo-nom′ə-tər) [*ozone* + *-meter*] an instrument for estimating the ozone in the air.

**ozo·no·phore** (o-zo′nə-for) [*ozone* + *-phore*] 1. one of the granular elements of cell cytoplasm. 2. old term for erythrocyte.

**ozo·sto·mia** (o″zo-sto′me-ə) [Gr. *ozē* stench + *stom-* + *-ia*] halitosis.

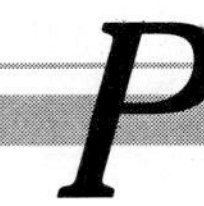

**P** symbol for *phosphorus, phosphate group* (in biochemistry), *para, peta-, poise, posterior, premolar,* and *pupil.*

***P*** symbol for *power, pressure,* and *probability.*

**$P_1$** symbol for *parental generation.*

**$P_2$** symbol for *pulmonic second sound.*

**$P_{CO_2}$** symbol for *carbon dioxide partial pressure* or *tension.*

**$P_i$** symbol for *orthophosphate.*

**$P_{O_2}$** symbol for *oxygen partial pressure* or *tension.*

**p** symbol for *pico-, proton,* and for the short arm of a chromosome.

**p150,95** glycoprotein p150,95; see *complement receptor 3 (CR3),* under *receptor.*

***p*** symbol for *momentum* and (in statistics) for the probability that a specific event will occur. Cf. *q.*

***p*-** symbol for *para-*[2].

**Π** the Greek capital letter pi, used in mathematics to indicate a product;

$$\Pi^n_{i=1} x_i = x_1 \times x_2 \times \ldots \times x_n .$$

***π*** pi, the sixteenth letter of the Greek alphabet; mathematical symbol for the ratio of the diameter and circumference of a circle: approximately 3.1415926536; symbol for *osmotic pressure.*

**Φ** the Greek capital letter phi, used as the symbol for magnetic flux.

***φ*** phi, the twenty-first letter of the Greek alphabet.

***ψ*** psi, the twenty-third letter of the Greek alphabet; symbol in molecular biology for *pseudouridine.*

**PA** posteroanterior; physician assistant; pulmonary artery.

**Pa** symbol for *protactinium* and *pascal.*

**Paas' disease** (pahz) [Hermann R. *Paas,* German physician, born 1900] see under *disease.*

**PAB** para-aminobenzoic acid; see *p-aminobenzoic acid.*

**PABA** para-aminobenzoic acid; see *p-aminobenzoic acid.*

**Pab·a·late** (pab′ə-lāt) trademark for a combination preparation of sodium salicylate and aminobenzoate sodium. **P.-SF,** trademark for a combination preparation of potassium salicylate and aminobenzoate potassium.

**Pab·a·nol** (pab′ə-nol) trademark for a preparation of aminobenzoic acid.

**PAC** premature atrial complex; see *atrial premature complex,* under *complex.*

**pa·ca** (pă′kə) [Sp., from Tupi] *Cuniculus paca,* a large nocturnal burrowing rodent of Central and South America; it is sometimes a reservoir for parasites such as *Echinococcus vogelii.*

**pac·chi·o·ni·an depressions, foramen, granulations (bodies)** (pahk″e-o′ne-ən) [Antonio *Pacchioni,* Italian anatomist, 1665–1726] see *foveolae granulares, foramen diaphragmatis [sellae],* and *granulationes arachnoideales.*

**pace·mak·er** (pās′ma-kər) 1. an object or substance that influences the rate at which a certain phenomenon occurs. 2. the natural cardiac pacemaker or an artificial cardiac pacemaker. 3. in biochemistry, a substance whose rate of reaction sets the pace for a series of interrelated reactions.

## Pacemaker

**AAI p.,** atrial demand inhibited p.

**AAIR p.,** an atrial demand inhibited pacemaker that is responsive to the patient's respiratory rate and thus to exercise and metabolic needs.

**AAT p.,** atrial demand triggered p.

**antitachycardia p.,** an implanted pacemaker that terminates tachycardia by delivering one or more pacing stimuli; it may require arrhythmia detection and device activation by the patient or may detect arrhythmias and deliver stimuli automatically.

**AOO p.,** atrial asynchronous p.

**artificial p., artificial cardiac p.,** a device that uses electrical impulses to reproduce or regulate the rhythms of the heart. Battery-driven and connected to the heart by leads and electrodes, it may be temporary or permanent and is inserted transvenously, transcutaneously, epicardially, or via the esophagus or coronary artery. Most pacemakers are either triggered or inhibited to modify output by sensing the intracardiac potential of one or more cardiac chambers; they have some degree of programmability and may also have antitachycardia functions. A five-letter code is used to categorize pacemakers by their combinations of these features; see table. Popularly called *pacemaker.*

**asynchronous p.,** an artificial cardiac pacemaker that delivers stimuli at a fixed rate, independent of any atrial or ventricular activity.

**asynchronous atrial p.,** atrial asynchronous p.

**asynchronous ventricular p.,** ventricular asynchronous p.

**atrial asynchronous p.,** an artificial cardiac pacemaker that stimulates the atrium at a constant rate, without sensing atrial or ventricular activity; rarely used except to initiate or terminate some tachycardias. Called also *AOO p.*

**atrial demand inhibited p.,** an artificial cardiac pacemaker that delivers stimuli to the atrium at a fixed rate in the absence of sensed atrial activity; spontaneous cardiac activity causes inhibition of pacemaker output, termination of the current stimulation cycle, and initiation of a new cycle. Called also *AAI p.*

**atrial demand triggered p.,** an artificial cardiac pacemaker that delivers stimuli to the atrium at a fixed rate in the absence of sensed atrial activity; spontaneous cardiac activity triggers pacemaker output, which falls ineffectively in the myocardial refractory period and initiates a new pacemaker stimulation cycle. Called also *AAT p.*

**atrial synchronous ventricular p.,** a dual chamber cardiac pacemaker that senses atrial activity and delivers a ventricular stimulus after a preset interval; used in patients with impaired atrioventricular conduction but normal sinus node function. Called also *VAT p.* See also *atrial synchronous ventricular inhibited p.*

**atrial synchronous ventricular inhibited p.,** a dual chamber cardiac pacemaker similar to an atrial synchronous ventricular pacemaker but able to sense ventricular as well as atrial activity. Called also *VDD p.*

**atrioventricular junctional p.,** an ectopic pacemaker occurring in the atrioventricular junction.

**atrioventricular (AV) sequential p.,** an artificial cardiac pacemaker used in patients with abnormal sinus node function and impaired AV conduction; it senses ventricular, and sometimes atrial, activity and in addition to stimulating the atrium also stimulates the ventricle after an appropriate delay. Committed versions invariably deliver the ventricular stimulus while noncommitted versions deliver it only in the absence of interim ventricular activity. See also *DVI p., DDD p.,* and *DDI p.*

**automatic p.,** universal p.

**bipolar p.,** an implanted cardiac pacemaker in which the lead contains both electrodes, anode and cathode, and is thus a complete circuit.

**cardiac p.,** the group of cells rhythmically initiating the heart beat, characterized physiologically by a slow loss of membrane potential during diastole. Usually the pacemaker site is the sinoatrial node. See also *artificial cardiac p.*

**cilium p.,** the biological regulator which controls the frequency of the beat of the cilia of cells by determining the rate of contraction and excitation.

**DDD p.,** an artificial cardiac pacemaker that can sense and pace both the atria and ventricles; it is capable of operating in both triggered and inhibited modes as necessary.

**DDDR p.,** a universal pacemaker that is responsive to the patient's respiratory rate and thus to exercise and metabolic needs.

**DDI p.,** a type of atrioventricular sequential pacemaker that delivers impulses to the atrium and ventricles on the basis of sensed ventricular and atrial activity, although the latter can only inhibit atrial impulses and cannot trigger ventricular stimulation. Cf. *DVI p.* and *DDD p.*

**demand p.,** an implanted cardiac pacemaker in which the generator stimulus is inhibited for a set interval (refractory period) by a signal derived from depolarization (normal or ectopic), thus minimizing the risk of pacemaker-induced ventricular fibrillation.

**NASPE/BPEG* Generic (NBG) Pacemaker Code**

| Position† | I | II | III | IV | V |
|---|---|---|---|---|---|
| Category | Chamber(s) Paced | Chamber(s) Sensed | Response to Sensing | Programmability, Rate Modulation | Antitachyarrhythmia Function(s) |
| | O = None<br>A = Atrium<br>V = Ventricle<br>D = Dual (A + V) | O = None<br>A = Atrium<br>V = Ventricle<br>D = Dual (A + V) | O = None<br>T = Triggers pacing<br>I = Inhibits pacing<br>D = Dual (T + I) | O = None<br>P = Simple programmable<br>M = Multiprogrammable<br>C = Communicating<br>R = Rate modulation | O = None<br>P = Pacing (antitachyarrhythmia)<br>S = Shock<br>D = Dual (P + S) |
| Manufacturers' Designation Only | S = Single (either A or V) | S = Single (either A or V) | | | |

* NASPE, North American Society of Pacing and Electrophysiology; BPEG, British Pacing and Electrophysiology Group.
† Positions I through III describe only antibradyarrhythmia functions of the pacemaker.

**dual chamber p.**, a pacemaker having two leads, one in the atrium and one in the ventricle, so that electromechanical synchrony between the chambers can be approximated.
**DVI p.**, a type of atrioventricular sequential pacemaker that delivers impulses to the atrium and ventricle on the basis of sensed ventricular activity only. Cf. *DDI p.* and *DDD p.*
**ectopic p.**, any biological cardiac pacemaker other than the sinus node; under normal conditions it is not active.
**escape p.**, an ectopic pacemaker that assumes control of cardiac impulse propagation because of failure of the sinoatrial node to generate one or more normal impulses.
**external p.**, an artificial cardiac pacemaker located outside the body with output wires connected to circular chest electrodes, with a wire sewn directly into the heart, or with an electrode inserted through an intravenous catheter.
**fixed-rate p.**, an artificial cardiac pacemaker set to pace at only a single rate.
**fully automatic p.**, universal p.
**gastric p.**, a saddle-shaped area of the greater curvature of the stomach at the junction of its proximal and middle thirds, where originate electric potentials which regulate the frequency of gastric contractions.
**p. of heart**, cardiac p.
**implanted p., internal p.**, an artificial cardiac pacemaker completely implanted into the subcutaneous tissue.
**junctional p.**, atrioventricular junctional p.
**latent p.**, ectopic p.
**radiofrequency p.**, a cardiac pacemaker consisting of an antenna coil on the skin and a subcutaneously implanted receiving coil with an electrode inserted into the ventricular myocardium. Pulses from a lightweight radio transmitter carried by the patient are transmitted to the pacemaker.
**rate responsive p.**, an artificial cardiac pacemaker that can deliver stimuli at a rate adjustable to some parameter independent of atrial activity, such as respiratory rate, physical activity level, blood temperature, or mixed venous oxygen saturation level.
**runaway p.**, a malfunctioning artificial cardiac pacemaker that abruptly accelerates its pacing rate, resulting in pacemaker-induced ventricular tachycardia.
**secondary p.**, ectopic p.
**single chamber p.**, an implanted cardiac pacemaker having only one lead, which is placed in either the atrium or the ventricle.
**synchronous p.**, an implanted cardiac pacemaker that synchronizes the electromechanical events in the atrium with those of the ventricle by delivering stimuli in response to sensed activity in the atrium, ventricle, or both.
**transthoracic p.**, an external cardiac pacemaker delivering stimuli through the chest wall, such as one connected to the heart by percutaneous pacing wires introduced through a transthoracic needle or one in which large electrodes are placed on the skin over the heart.
**transvenous p.**, an artificial cardiac pacemaker, either external or implantable, that is connected to the heart by pacing leads passed through the venous circulation.
**unipolar p.**, an implanted cardiac pacemaker in which the lead has a single stimulating electrode, the cathode, with the anode connected to an indifferent electrode, usually the outer surface of the pulse generator.
**universal p.**, a term sometimes used to describe a DDD pacemaker, emphasizing that because it can be programmed to operate in one of numerous possible pacemaker modes under specific circumstances, it can be made to most closely approximate normal electrophysiologic functioning under a variety of conditions.
**VAT p.**, atrial synchronous ventricular p.
**VDD p.**, atrial synchronous ventricular inhibited p.
**ventricular p.**, an ectopic pacemaker occurring in a ventricle.
**ventricular asynchronous p.**, an artificial cardiac pacemaker that stimulates the ventricle at a constant rate, without sensing atrial or ventricular activity; rarely used except to initiate or terminate some tachycardias. Called also *VOO p.*
**ventricular demand inhibited p.**, an artificial cardiac pacemaker that delivers stimuli to the ventricle at a fixed rate in the absence of sensed ventricular activity; spontaneous cardiac activity causes inhibition of pacemaker output, termination of the current stimulation cycle, and initiation of a new cycle. Called also *VVI p.*
**ventricular demand triggered p.**, an artificial cardiac pacemaker that delivers stimuli to the ventricle at a fixed rate in the absence of sensed ventricular activity; spontaneous cardiac activity triggers pacemaker output, which falls ineffectively in the myocardial refractory period and initiates a new cycle of pacemaker stimulation. Called also *VVT p.*
**VOO p.**, ventricular asynchronous p.
**VVI p.**, ventricular demand inhibited p.
**VVIR p.**, a ventricular demand inhibited pacemaker that is responsive to the patient's respiratory rate and thus to exercise and metabolic needs.
**VVT p.**, ventricular demand triggered p.
**wandering atrial p.**, a condition in which the site of origin of the impulses controlling the heart rate shifts from one point to another within the atria, including the sinus node, changing with almost every beat. P waves and PR intervals vary, and the rate of impulse formation is somewhat irregular. It occurs when the rate of sinus impulses falls below a critical level or fails.

**pachy-** [Gr. *pachys* thick] a combining form meaning thick.

**pachy·bleph·a·ron** (pak″e-blef′ə-ron) [*pachy-* + Gr. *blepharon* eyelid] a thickening of the eyelid, chiefly near the border.

**pachy·bleph·a·ro·sis** (pak″e-blef″ə-ro′sis) pachyblepharon.

**pachy·ce·pha·lia** (pak″e-sə-fa′le-ə) pachycephaly.

**pachy·ce·phal·ic** (pak″e-sə-fal′ik) pertaining to or characterized by pachycephaly.

**pachy·ceph·a·lous** (pak″e-sef′ə-ləs) pachycephalic.

**pachy·ceph·a·ly** (pak″e-sef′ə-le) [*pachy-* + *-cephaly*] abnormal thickness of the bones of the skull, as in acromegaly.

**pachy·chei·lia** (pak″e-ki′le-ə) [*pachy-* + *cheil-* + *-ia*] thickening of the lips.

**pachy·chro·mat·ic** (pak″e-kro-mat′ik) [*pachy-* + *chromat-* + *-ic*] having thick chromatin threads.

**pachy·dac·tyl·ia** (pak″e-dak-til′e-ə) pachydactyly.

**pachy·dac·ty·ly** (pak″e-dak′tə-le) [*pachy-* + Gr. *daktylos* finger] abnormal enlargement of the fingers and toes.

**pachy·der·ma** (pak″e-der′mə) [*pachy-* + *derma*] abnormal thickening of the skin. See also *elephantiasis.*

**pachy·der·ma·to·cele** (pak″e-dər-mat′o-sēl) [*pachy-* + *dermato-* + *-cele*[1]] plexiform neuroma which attains large dimensions and produces a condition resembling elephantiasis.

**pachy·der·ma·tous** (pak″e-der′mə-təs) thick-skinned; pertaining or relating to pachyderma. Called also *pachydermic.*

**pachy·der·mic** (pak″e-der′mik) pachydermatous.

**pachy·der·mo·peri·os·to·sis** (pak″e-der″mo-per″e-os-to′sis) [*pachy-* + *dermo-* + *periostosis*] a condition believed to be inherited as an autosomal dominant trait, chiefly characterized by thickening of the skin of the head and distal extremities, deep folds and furrows of the skin of the forehead, cheeks, and scalp *(cutis verticis gyrata),* seborrhea, hyperhidrosis, periostosis of the long bones, digital clubbing, and spadelike enlargement of the hands and feet. It is more prevalent in the male and is usually first evident during adolescence. Called also *acropachyderma with pachyperiostitis, idiopathic* or *primary hypertrophic osteoarthropathy,* and *Touraine-Solente-Golé syndrome.*

**pachy·glos·sia** (pak″e-glos′e-ə) [*pachy-* + *gloss-* + *-ia*] abnormal thickness of the tongue.

**pa·chyg·na·thous** (pə-kig′nə-thəs) [*pachy-* + *gnath-* + *-ous*] having a large jaw. See also *macrognathia* and *prognathism.*

**pachy·gy·ria** (pak″e-ji′re-ə) [*pachy-* + *gyr-* + *-ia*] macrogyria.

**pachy·lep·to·men·in·gi·tis** (pak″e-lep″to-men″in-ji′tis) [*pachy-* + *lepto-* + *mening-* + *-itis*] inflammation of the dura and pia together.

**pachy·men·in·ges** (pak″e-mə-nin′jēz) plural of *pachymeninx.*

**pachy·men·in·gi·tis** (pak″e-men″in-ji′tis) [*pachy-* + *mening-* + *-itis*] inflammation of the dura mater; the symptoms of the disease resemble those of meningitis. Cf. *leptomeningitis.*
**cerebral p.,** inflammation of the dura of the brain.
**circumscribed p.,** pachymeningitis limited to a definite area of the dura.
**external p.,** inflammation of the outer layers of the dura.
**hypertrophic cervical p.,** hypertrophic spinal pachymeningitis in the cervical region.
**hypertrophic spinal p.,** a diffuse fibrosing form of pachymeningitis in the spinal canal; it may be due to tuberculosis, syphilis, or an unknown cause.
**internal p.,** that which affects the inner layer of the dura.
**p. intralamella′ris,** intradural abscess.
**purulent p.,** abscess on the dura mater; see *extradural, intradural,* and *subdural abscess,* under *abscess.*
**spinal p.,** inflammation of the dura of the spinal column.
**syphilitic p.,** that which is caused by syphilis; see also *hypertrophic spinal p.*

**pachy·men·in·gop·a·thy** (pak″e-men″in-gop′ə-the) [*pachymeninx* + *-pathy*] any noninflammatory disease of the dura mater.

**pachy·me·ninx** (pak″e-me′ninks) pl. *pachymenin′ges* [*pachy-* + *meninx*] [TA] the dura mater. NOTE: In official nomenclature, this term is used as the preferred term when contrasting this structure with the leptomeninx, which comprises the arachnoidea mater and the pia mater (arachnoidea mater et pia mater).

**pachy·me·ter** (pə-kim′ə-tər) [*pachy-* + *meter*] an instrument used to determine thickness.

**pachy·ne·ma** (pak″e-ne′mə) [*pachy-* + Gr. *nēma* thread] a postsynaptic stage of mitosis in which the chromatin is in the form of thick spireme threads.

**pa·chyn·sis** (pə-kin′sis) [Gr.] a thickening, especially an abnormal thickening.

**pa·chyn·tic** (pə-kin′tik) pertaining to or characterized by abnormal thickening.

**pachy·onych·ia** (pak″e-o-nik′e-ə) [*pachy-* + *onych-* + *-ia*] thickening of the nails.
**p. conge′nita,** an autosomal dominant syndrome characterized by increased thickness of the nails that progresses to onychogryphosis; hyperkeratosis of the palms, soles, knees, and elbows; widespread tiny cutaneous horns; leukoplakia of the mucous membranes; and usually hyperhidrosis of the hands and feet. Bullae may develop on the palms and soles following trauma. Called also *Jadassohn-Lewandowsky syndrome.*

**pachy·peri·os·ti·tis** (pak″e-per″e-os-ti′tis) periostitis of long bones resulting in abnormal thickness of the bones.

**pachy·peri·to·ni·tis** (pak″e-per″ĭ-to-ni′tis) [*pachy-* + *peritonitis*] peritonitis with thickening of the affected membrane.

**pachy·pleu·ri·tis** (pak″e-ploo͞-ri′tis) [*pachy-* + *pleuritis*] 1. fibrothorax. 2. pleural fibrosis.

**pachy·sal·pin·gi·tis** (pak″e-sal″pin-ji′tis) [*pachy-* + *salping-* + *-itis*] chronic interstitial inflammation of the muscular coat of the oviduct, producing thickening; called also *mural salpingitis* and *parenchymatous salpingitis.*

**pachy·sal·pin·go·ova·ri·tis** (pak″e-sal-ping″go-o″var-i′tis) chronic parenchymatous inflammation of the ovary and oviduct.

**pachy·tene** (pak′e-tēn) [Gr. *pachytēs* thickness] in meiosis (q.v.), the stage following synapsis (zygotene) in which the homologous chromosome threads (synaptonemal complex) shorten, thicken, and continue to intertwine, and each of the conjoined (bivalent) chromosomes separate into two sister chromatids, which are held together by a centromere, to form a tetrad. During this phase the chromatids break up and corresponding regions of the nonsister chromatids of the paired chromosomes are exchanged in a process known as crossing over. See also *diplotene, leptotene,* and *zygotene.*

**pachy·vag·i·nal·itis** (pak″e-vaj″ĭ-nəl-i′tis) [*pachy-* + *vaginalitis*] inflammatory thickening of the tunica vaginalis of the testis.

**pach·y·vag·i·ni·tis** (pak″e-vaj″ĭ-ni′tis) [*pachy-* + *vaginitis*] chronic vaginitis with thickening of the vaginal walls.
**cystic p.,** emphysematous vaginitis.

**pac·ing** (pās′ing) setting of the pace, or regulation of the rate of.
**antitachycardia p.,** delivery of cardiac pacing stimuli timed to terminate a tachyarrhythmia.
**asynchronous p.,** cardiac pacing in which impulse generation by the pacemaker occurs at a fixed rate, independent of underlying cardiac activity.
**atrial p.,** regulation of the rate of the heartbeat by means of an intracardiac electrode inserted in the atrium or by temporary placement of an esophageal electrode.
**bipolar p.,** a form of cardiac pacing in which both electrodes contact the cardiac tissue; inappropriate sensing of electromagnetic interference and extracardiac stimulation are less frequent than in unipolar pacing.
**burst p.,** overdrive p.
**cardiac p.,** regulation of the rate of contraction of the heart muscle by an artificial cardiac pacemaker.
**competitive p.,** underdrive p.
**continuous p.,** continuous delivery of cardiac pacing stimuli, either at a normal or overdrive rate, to prevent tachycardias.
**coupled p.,** a variation of paired pacing in which the patient's natural depolarization serves as the first of the two stimuli, with the second induced by an artificial cardiac pacemaker.
**diaphragm p., diaphragmatic p.,** electrophrenic respiration.
**dual chamber p.,** control of the heart rate by means of an artificial cardiac pacemaker that paces, senses, or does both in the atria and in the ventricles.
**epicardial p.,** a method for temporary pacing or sensing of the atria or ventricles by attaching the pacing leads to the epicardial surface; usually used in the diagnosis and treatment of postoperative dysrhythmias.
**esophageal p.,** transesophageal p.
**overdrive p.,** the process of increasing the heart rate by means of an artificial cardiac pacemaker in order to suppress certain arrhythmias.
**paired p.,** cardiac pacing in which two impulses are delivered to the heart in close succession, the second generally just at the end of the refractory period induced by the first; used to slow tachyarrhythmias and to improve cardiac performance.
**phrenic p.,** electrophrenic respiration.
**physiologic p.,** cardiac pacing in which the pacemaker stimulates cardiac activity such that it duplicates as closely as possible the normally conducted sinus rhythm.
**ramp p.,** cardiac pacing in which stimuli are delivered at a rapid but continually altering rate, either from faster to slower *(rate decremental* or *tune down),* from fast to faster *(cycle length decremental* or *ramp up),* or in some cyclic combination of increasing and decreasing rates; it is used to terminate tachyarrhythmias.
**single chamber p.,** control of the heart rate by an artificial cardiac pacemaker that paces and senses in either atria or ventricles, usually in the latter.
**synchronous p.,** cardiac pacing in which information about sensed activity in one or more cardiac chambers is used to determine the timing of impulse generation by the pacemaker.
**transcutaneous p.,** a temporary method for cardiac pacing, in which large surface, high impedance electrodes are applied to the anterior and posterior chest walls to deliver high current stimuli of long duration for pacing of the ventricles.
**transesophageal p.,** a temporary method for cardiac pacing using leads placed within the esophagus to effect temporary atrial pacing in the diagnosis and treatment of dysrhythmias.
**transthoracic p.,** a method for temporary cardiac pacing in which a hooked pacing lead is attached to the ventricular endocardium by insertion through the chest wall or epigastric area and then the ventricular wall; it is used in emergency situations, usually cardiac arrest, as an alternative to transcutaneous pacing.
**transvenous p.,** a permanent or temporary method for cardiac pacing in which the pacing leads, inserted by means of a catheter, are

connected to the endocardium via the venous circulation; the pulse generator may be implanted or external.
**ultrafast train p., ultrarapid p.,** a form of overdrive pacing in which a short series of pacing stimuli are delivered at a rate equivalent to 3000 to 6000 beats per minute to terminate a tachyarrhythmia.
**underdrive p.,** a method for terminating certain slow ventricular or supraventricular tachycardias by means of slow asynchronous pacing, with stimuli delivered at a rate not an even fraction of the tachycardia rate, in order to capture the heart rate.
**unipolar p.,** a form of cardiac pacing using only a single electrode in contact with the cardiac tissue, with the indifferent electrode generally part of the pulse generator metal housing.
**ventricular p.,** cardiac pacing in which the stimulus from the pacemaker is delivered to the ventricle.

**Pa·ci·ni's corpuscles** (pah-che'nēz) [Filippo *Pacini,* Italian anatomist, 1812–1883] see under *corpuscle.*

**pa·cin·i·an** (pə-sin'e-ən) named for Filippo Pacini; see *corpusculum lamellosum.*

**pack** (pak) 1. treatment by wrapping a patient in blankets or sheets or a limb in towels, wet or dry and either hot or cold; also the blankets, sheets, or towels used for this purpose. 2. a tampon.
**cold p.,** blankets, sheets, or towels that have been dipped in cold water, for wrapping the body or an extremity.
**dry p.,** dry, hot blankets or towels for wrapping the body or an extremity.
**full p.,** one which encloses the entire body.
**half p.,** a pack applied from the axillae to below the knees.
**hot p.,** hot blankets or towels, wet or dry, for wrapping the body or an extremity.
**Hydrocollator p.,** trademark for a hot pack containing silicate gel in a porous bag that is soaked in hot water and laid over cloth over a body part.
**ice p.,** a folded towel filled with crushed ice, often used in place of an icebag.
**Mikulicz p.,** layers of mesh or gutta-percha sewn together at the edges, packed with strips of gauze, often placed in a denuded pelvic area to wall off the unperitonealized surfaces but also used for packing off abdominal viscera to improve operative exposure.
**one sheet p.,** a wet pack consisting of only one large sheet.
**partial p.,** a wet pack covering only a portion of the body.
**periodontal p.,** a surgical dressing applied over the surgical wound following periodontal operations to provide a matrix for the regeneration of tissue and enhance healing processes.
**salt p.,** a wet pack utilizing sheets or blankets wrung out after immersion in salt water.
**three-quarters p.,** a wet pack extending upward from the toes as far as the axillae.
**throat p.,** a moistened gauze pack used as a posterior pharyngeal seal around a noncuffed endotracheal tube.
**wet p., wet-sheet p.,** wet blankets or sheets, hot or cold, for wrapping an extremity or the entire body.

**pack·er** (pak'ər) an instrument for introducing dressing into the uterus or vagina, or into another body cavity or wound.

**pack·ing** (pak'ing) 1. the act of filling a wound or cavity with gauze, sponges, pads, or other material. 2. the material used for filling a cavity.

**pac·li·tax·el** (pak″lĭ-tak'səl) [MeSH: Paclitaxel] an antineoplastic agent that acts by promoting and stabilizing the polymerization of microtubules, isolated from the Pacific yew tree *(Taxus brevifolia);* used investigationally in the treatment of ovarian carcinoma and melanoma, breast cancer, and lung cancer. Administered intravenously.

**pad** (pad) a cushion-like mass of soft material.
**abdominal p.,** a pad for the absorption of discharges from abdominal wounds; also for packing off abdominal viscera to improve exposure during surgical procedures.
**buccal fat p.,** corpus adiposum buccae.
**dinner p.,** a pad placed over the abdomen before a plaster jacket is applied. The pad is then removed, leaving space under the jacket to provide for expansion of the abdomen after eating.
**infrapatellar fat p.,** corpus adiposum infrapatellare.
**gum p's,** edentulous segments of the maxilla and the mandible that correspond to the underlying primary teeth.
**heating p.,** a hollow pad with an electric mechanism inside that can be adjusted to a variety of temperatures; used for superficial warming of body parts.
**knuckle p's,** nodules about the size of a split pea on the dorsal surface of the interphalangeal joints, consisting of new growths of fibrous tissue, with thickening of the dermis and epidermis, and frequently associated with camptodactyly and Dupuytren's contracture; they are probably of genetic origin.
**occlusal p.,** a pad which covers the occlusal surface of a tooth.
**Passavant's p.,** see under *bar.*
**retromolar p.,** a mass of tissue, often pear-shaped, located at the distal termination of the mandibular residual ridge, and made up of the retromolar papilla and the retromolar glandular prominence.
**retropatellar fat p.,** corpus adiposum infrapatellare.
**sucking p., suctorial p.,** corpus adiposum buccae.

**Pad·gett's dermatome** (paj'əts) [Earl Calvin *Padgett,* American surgeon, 1893–1946] see under *dermatome.*

**pad·i·mate A** (pad'ĭ-māt) a substituted aminobenzoate having properties similar to those of *p*-aminobenzoic acid, used as a sunscreen.

**pad·i·mate O** (pad'ĭ-māt) a substituted aminobenzoate having properties similar to those of *p*-aminobenzoic acid, used as a sunscreen.

**pae-** for words beginning thus, see also those beginning *pe-.*

**Pae·cil·o·my·ces** (pe-sil″o-mi'sēz) [MeSH: Paecilomyces] a genus of soil-inhabiting Fungi Imperfecti of the form-class Hyphomycetes, form-family Moniliaceae, which morphologically resembles *Penicillium.* Species have caused mycotic keratitis, endocarditis, endophthalmitis, and opportunistic infections. See also *paecilomycosis.*

**pae·ci·lo·my·co·sis** (pe″sĭ-lo-mi-ko'sis) a fungal infection with species of *Paecilomyces. P. lilacinus* infection is most often oculomycosis; both *P. lilacinus* and *P. varioti* cause mycotic endocarditis that can be fatal. Various species cause systemic infections in cats and dogs.

**Pae·der·us** (pe'dər-əs) a genus of blister beetles (family Meloidae), native to South America, Asia, and Africa, from which pederin has been isolated.

**paed(o)-** see *ped(o)-¹.*

**PAF** platelet activating factor.

**PAF-ac·e·ther** (əs-e'thər) see *platelet activating factor,* under *factor.*

**PAGE** polyacrylamide gel electrophoresis.

**Pa·get's cell, disease, necrosis, test** (pă'jəts) [Sir James *Paget,* English surgeon, 1814–1899] see under *cell, disease, necrosis,* and *test.*

**Pag·et-Schroet·ter syndrome** (paj'ət-shrər'tər) [Sir James *Paget;* Kristelli Leopold von *Schroetter,* Austrian physician, 1837–1908] see under *syndrome.*

**pa·get·ic** (pə-jet'ik) affected with or relating to Paget's disease.

**pag·et·oid** (paj'ə-toid) resembling or characteristic of Paget's disease.

**Pag·i·tane** (paj'ĭ-tān) trademark for a preparation of cycrimine hydrochloride.

**pa·go·pha·gia** (pa″go-fa'je-ə) [Gr. *pagos* frost + *-phagia*] the ingestion of extraordinary amounts of ice, often related to iron lack.

**pa·go·plex·ia** (pa″go-plek'se-ə) [Gr. *pagos* frost + *plēgē* stroke] frostbite.

**-pagus** [Gr. *pagos* that which is fixed] a word termination denoting a symmetrical pair of twins conjoined at the site indicated by the stem to which it is affixed, as *craniopagus, pygopagus, thoracopagus.*

**PAH, PAHA** *p*-aminohippuric acid.

**Pah·vant Val·ley fever, plague** (pah'vant) [*Pahvant Valley,* Utah, where some of the first cases were reported] tularemia.

**PAI** plasminogen activator inhibitor.

**pain** (pān) [L. *poena, dolor;* Gr. *algos, odynē*] [MeSH: Pain] a more or less localized sensation of discomfort, distress, or agony, resulting from the stimulation of specialized nerve endings. It serves as a protective mechanism insofar as it induces the sufferer to remove or withdraw from the source.
**bearing-down p.,** pain accompanying uterine contractions during the second stage of labor.
**boring p.,** a sensation as of being pierced with a long, slender, twisting object; called also *terebrant p.*
**central p.,** pain due to a lesion in the central nervous system.
**chest p.,** see *pectoralgia, pleuralgia,* and *thoracalgia.*
**dilating p's,** those of the first stage of labor.
**expulsive p's,** those of the second stage of labor.
**false p's,** ineffective pains which resemble labor pains, but which are not accompanied by effacement and dilatation of the cervix.
**fulgurant p's,** lightning p's.
**gas p's,** pains caused by distention of the stomach or intestines by accumulations of air or other gases, occurring as a result of ingestion of gas-forming foods.
**girdle p.,** a painful sensation as of a cord about the waist.
**griping p.,** colic, def. 2.
**growing p's,** recurrent quasirheumatic limb pains peculiar to early youth.
**heterotopic p.,** referred p.
**homotopic p.,** pain that is felt at the point of injury.

**hunger p.,** pain coming on at the time for feeling hunger for the next meal; it is a symptom of gastric disorder.
**intermenstrual p.,** pain occurring during the period between the menses, usually about halfway, accompanying extrusion of the ovum.
**jumping p.,** a peculiar pain in joint diseases when the bone is laid bare by ulceration of the cartilage.
**labor p's,** the rhythmic pains of increasing severity and frequency, caused by contractions of the uterus during childbirth.
**lancinating p.,** a sharp, darting pain.
**lightning p's,** the cutting and intense darting pains of tabes dorsalis; called also *fulgurant p's* and *shooting p's.*
**middle p.,** intermenstrual p.
**osteocopic p.,** osteocope.
**phantom limb p.,** pain felt as though arising in an absent (amputated) limb; see under *limb.*
**postprandial p.,** abdominal pain occurring after eating a meal.
**premonitory p's,** mild uterine contractions before the beginning of true labor.
**psychic p.,** psychalgia (def. 1).
**psychogenic p.,** symptoms of physical pain having psychological origin.
**referred p.,** pain felt in a part other than that in which the cause that produced it is situated.
**rest p.,** a continuous burning pain of the lower leg and foot, beginning or worsening after reclining and being relieved by sitting or standing; it is due to ischemia.
**root p.,** pain caused by disease of the sensory nerve roots and felt in the cutaneous areas supplied by the affected roots.
**shooting p's,** lightning p's.
**starting p's,** pain and muscular spasm in the early stages of sleep.
**terebrant p., terebrating p.,** boring p.
**wandering p.,** a pain which repeatedly changes its location.

**paint** (pānt) [MeSH: Paint] 1. a liquid designed for application to the surface, as of the body or a tooth. 2. to apply a liquid to a specific area as a remedial or protective measure.
**antiseptic p.,** a term used to describe immunoglobulin A secreted onto the surfaces of mucous membranes and affording local protection against agents possessing homologous antigens.
**Castellani's p.,** carbol-fuchsin solution.

**pair** (par) 1. a combination of two related, similar, or identical entities or objects. 2. in cardiology, two successive premature beats, particularly two ventricular premature complexes. Called also *couplet.*
**base p.,** either of the two pairs—guanine and cytosine, adenine and thymine—of purine-pyrimidine bases joined by hydrogen bonds that make up DNA. In RNA, uracil replaces thymine.
**buffer p.,** a buffer system consisting of an acid and its conjugate base.
**ion p.,** the free electron and the positively charged residual atom that result from the ejection of an orbital electron by ionizing radiation.

**pair·ing** (par'ing) the act or process of joining into pairs.
**base p.,** the bonding of purines and pyrimidines in DNA; see under *pair.*
**somatic p.,** the close association of homologous pairs of polytene chromosomes, as in meiotic prophase; such chromosomes are considered to be in a permanent prophase.

**pa·ja·ro·e·llo** (pah-hah-ro-a'yo) *Ornithodoros coriaceus.*

**Pa·jot's law, maneuver** (pah-zhōz') [Charles *Pajot,* French obstetrician, 1816–1896] see under *law* and *maneuver.*

**pak·u·rin** (pak'u-rin) an arrow poison derived from the sap of a tree in Colombia; it has a digitalis-like action on the heart.

**Pal's stain** (pahlz) [Jacob *Pal,* Austrian physician, 1863–1936] see under *stain.*

**Pal·ade** (pəl-ād') George Emil. Romanian-born American cytologist, born 1912; co-winner, with Albert Claude and Christian René de Duve, of the Nobel prize for medicine or physiology for 1974 for his work on mitochondria, ribosomes, and microsomes in the structural and functional organization of the cell.

**palae(o)-** for words beginning thus, see those beginning *pale(o)-.*

**pa·la·ta** (pə-la'tə) [L.] plural of *palatum.*

**pal·a·tal** (pal'ə-təl) 1. pertaining to the palate. 2. pertaining to the lingual surface of a maxillary tooth. 3. a consonantal speech sound produced with part of the tongue near the hard palate, such as *y, ch,* or *j.*

**pal·ate** (pal'ət) [MeSH: Palate] palatum.
**artificial p.,** speech-aid prosthesis.
**bony p., bony hard p.,** palatum osseum.
**cleft p.,** congenital fissure of the soft palate or both the soft and hard palates, due to faulty fusion of the palatine processes; it typically opens through the roof of the mouth into the nasal cavity and extends anteriorly to the premaxilla, where it deviates to the right or left, following the line of fusion. Called also *palatoschisis, uranoschisis,* and *uranostaphyloschisis* (cleft of both the hard and the soft palate).
**hard p.,** palatum durum.
**pendulous p.,** uvula.
**premaxillary p., primary p., primitive p.,** primordial p.
**primordial p.,** that portion of the palate in embryonic development that forms first, being contributed by the median nasal process. Called also *premaxillary* or *primary p.*
**secondary p.,** in embryonic development, the part of the palate that forms later than the primordial palate, by fusion of the lateral palatine processes.
**smokers' p.,** stomatitis nicotina.
**soft p.,** palatum molle.

**pal·a·tine** (pal'ə-tīn) [L. *palatinus*] pertaining to the palate.

**pal·a·ti·tis** (pal"ə-ti'tis) 1. inflammation of the palate. 2. lampas.

**palat(o)-** [L. *palatum* palate] a combining form denoting relationship to the palate; sometimes used instead of lingu(o)- in terms referring to the lingual surface of maxillary teeth.

**pal·a·to·glos·sal** (pal"ə-to-glos'əl) pertaining to the palate and tongue.

**pal·a·tog·na·thous** (pal"ə-tog'nə-thəs) [*palato-* + *gnath-* + *-ous*] having a cleft palate.

**pal·a·to·graph** (pal'ə-to-graf) [*palato-* + *-graph*] an instrument used in palatography.

**pal·a·tog·ra·phy** (pal"ə-tog'rə-fe) the recording of the movements of the palate in speech. See also *palatomyography.*

**pal·a·to·max·il·lary** (pal"ə-to-mak'sĭ-lar"e) pertaining to the palate and the maxilla.

**pal·a·to·my·og·ra·phy** (pal"ə-to-mi-og'rə-fe) [*palato-* + *myo-* + *-graphy*] the recording of muscular movements of the palate.

**pal·a·to·na·sal** (pal"ə-to-na'zəl) [*palato-* + *nasal*] nasopalatine.

**pal·a·top·a·gus** (pal"ə-top'ə-gəs) [*palato-* + *-pagus*] symmetrical twins conjoined at the palate.

**pal·a·to·pha·ryn·ge·al** (pal"ə-to-fə-rin'je-əl) pertaining to the palate and pharynx.

**pal·a·to·pha·ryn·go·plas·ty** (pal"ə-to-fə-ring'go-plas"te) a trimming back of excess palatal and pharyngeal tissue, done in order to widen the airway and relieve obstructive sleep apnea or severe snoring. Called also *uvulopalatoplasty* and *uvulopalatopharyngoplasty.*

**pal·a·to·plas·ty** (pal'ə-to-plas"te) [*palato-* + *-plasty*] plastic reconstruction of the palate, including cleft palate operations; cf. *staphyloplasty* and *palatorrhaphy.* Called also *uraniscoplasty* and *uranoplasty.*

**pal·a·to·ple·gia** (pal"ə-to-ple'jə) [*palato-* + *-plegia*] paralysis of the palate.

**pal·a·to·prox·i·mal** (pal"ə-to-prok'sĭ-məl) pertaining to the palatal (lingual) and proximal surface of a maxillary tooth.

**pal·a·tor·rha·phy** (pal"ə-tor'ə-fe) surgical correction of a cleft palate, the cleft involving the soft palate and the soft tissues over the hard palate; cf. *palatoplasty.* Called also *staphylorrhaphy, uraniscorrhaphy,* and *uranorrhaphy.*

**pal·a·tos·chi·sis** (pal"ə-tos'kĭ-sis) [*palato-* + *-schisis*] cleft palate.

**pa·la·tum** (pə-la'təm) gen. *pala'ti,* pl. *pala'ta* [L.] [TA] the palate: the partition separating the nasal and oral cavities, consisting anteriorly of a hard bony part and posteriorly of a soft fleshy part.
**p. du'rum** [TA], hard palate: the anterior part of the palate, char-

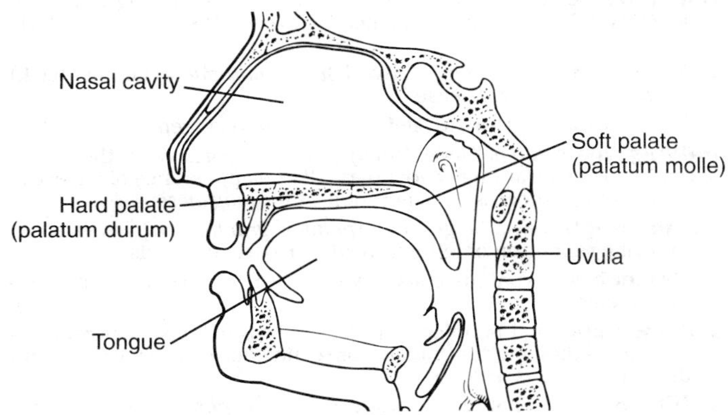

acterized by an osseous framework, covered superiorly by mucous membrane of the nasal cavity and, on its oral surface, by mucoperiosteum.
**p. fis'sum,** cleft palate.
**p. mol'le** [TA], soft palate: the fleshy part of the roof of the mouth, extending from the posterior edge of the hard palate; from its free inferior border is a projection of variable length, the uvula. Called also *velum palatinum* [TA alternative].
**p. os'seum** [TA], bony palate: the bony part of the anterior two-thirds of the roof of the mouth, formed by the palatine processes of the maxillae and the horizontal plates of the palatine bones. Called also *bony hard palate.*

**pale(o)-** [Gr. *palaios* old] a combining form meaning old. Also, *palae(o)-.*

**pa·leo·cer·e·bel·lar** (pa″le-o-ser″ə-bel′ər) pertaining to or affecting the paleocerebellum.

**pa·leo·cer·e·bel·lum** (pa″le-o-ser″ə-bel′əm) [*paleo-* + *cerebellum*] [TA] the phylogenetically second oldest part of the cerebellum, namely the vermis of the anterior lobe and the pyramis, uvula, and paraflocculus of the posterior lobe. Because this corresponds roughly to the primary site of termination of the major spinocerebellar afferents, the term is sometimes equated with *spinocerebellum.* Cf. *archicerebellum* and *neocerebellum.*

**pa·leo·cor·tex** (pa″le-o-kor′teks) [*paleo-* + *cortex*] [TA] that portion of the cerebral cortex that, with the archicortex, develops in association with the olfactory system, and which is phylogenetically older and less stratified than the neocortex. It is composed chiefly of the piriform cortex and the parahippocampal gyrus. Spelled also *palaeocortex.*

**pa·leo·gen·e·sis** (pa″le-o-jen′ə-sis) palingenesis, def. 2.

**pa·leo·ge·net·ic** (pa″le-o-jə-net′ik) [*paleo-* + *genetic*] originated in the past; not newly acquired. Said of traits, structures, etc., of species.

**pa·leo·pa·thol·o·gy** (pa″le-o-pə-thol′ə-je) [*paleo-* + *pathology*] [MeSH: Paleopathology] the study of disease in bodies preserved from ancient times, such as mummies.

**pa·leo·sen·sa·tion** (pa″le-o-sən-sa′shən) [*paleo-* + *sensation*] the sensation of severe pain and marked variations of temperature, as compared with phylogenetically newer sensations such as those of light touch and moderate variations of temperature and the epicritic sensations.

**pa·leo·stri·a·tal** (pa″le-o-stri-a′təl) pertaining to the paleostriatum.

**pa·leo·stri·a·tum** (pa″le-o-stri-a′təm) [*paleo-* + *striatum*] the phylogenetically older part of the corpus striatum represented by the globus pallidus. Cf. *neostriatum.*

**pa·leo·thal·a·mus** (pa″le-o-thal′ə-məs) [*paleo-* + *thalamus*] old thalamus; a term applied occasionally to the phylogenetically older part of the thalamus, i.e., the medial portion which lacks reciprocal connections with the neopallium.

**pali-** [Gr. *palin* backward, or again] a combining form meaning again, often denoting pathologic repetition. Also, *palin-.*

**pali·ci·ne·sia** (pal″ĭ-sĭ-ne′zhə) palikinesia.

**Pali·co·u·rea** (pal″ĭ-ko-u′re-ə) a genus of Brazilian plants, some species of which contain fluoroacetates and can cause fatal fluoroacetate poisoning in livestock.

**pali·ki·ne·sia** (pal″ĭ-kĭ-ne′zhə) [*pali-* + *kinesi-* + *-ia*] a dyskinesia involving pathologic repetition of movements; called also *palicinesia.*

**pali·la·lia** (pal″ĭ-la′le-ə) [*pali-* + *lal-* + *-ia*] palinphrasia.

**palin-** see *pali-.*

**pal·in·drome** (pal′in-drōm) [Gr. *palindromos* a running back] in genetics, a DNA or RNA sequence that reads the same in both directions.

**pal·in·dro·mia** (pal″in-dro′me-ə) [Gr. *palindromia* a running back] the recurrence of a disease.

**pal·in·dro·mic** (pal″in-dro′mik) returning; recurrent.

**pal·in·gen·e·sis** (pal″in-jen′ə-sis) [*palin-* + *genesis*] 1. the regeneration or restoration of a lost part. 2. the appearance of ancestral characters in successive generations. Cf. *cenogenesis.*

**pal·in·gra·phia** (pal″in-gra′fe-ə) [*palin-* + *graph-* + *-ia*] dysgraphia involving repetition of letters, words, or parts of words.

**pa·lin·mne·sis** (pal″in-ne′sis) [*palin-* + Gr. *-mnēsis* memory] remote memory.

**pal·i·nop·sia** (pal″ĭ-nop′se-ə) [*palin-* + *-opsia*] visual perseveration; the pathologic continuance or recurrence of a visual sensation after the stimulus is gone.

**pal·in·phra·sia** (pal″in-fra′zhə) [*palin-* + Gr. *phrasis* speech + *-ia*] a dysphasia involving repetition of words or phrases; see *stuttering.* Called also *palilalia* and *paliphrasia.*

**pali·phra·sia** (pal″ĭ-fra′ze-ə) palinphrasia.

**pal·i·sade** (pal″ĭ-sād′) [Fr. *palissade,* from L. *palus* stake] the arrangement of cells or cellular structures side by side in rows, like pickets in a fence; it is characteristic of some fungi and bacterial cell smears and of cells seen in tissue sections in certain normal and disease states.

**pal·la·di·um** (pə-la′de-əm) [L.] [MeSH: Palladium] 1. a rare, hard, noble metal resembling platinum; symbol, Pd; specific gravity, 12.16; atomic number, 46; atomic weight, 106.4. It is lighter in weight than platinum and of a neutral color, and is used in alloys for dental and orthodontic appliances. 2. a homeopathic preparation of the same metal.

**pall·an·es·the·sia** (pal″ən-əs-the′zhə) [Gr. *pallein* to shake + *anesthesia*] loss or lack of pallesthesia (vibration sense). Called also *apallesthesia.*

**pall·es·the·sia** (pal″es-the′zhə) [Gr. *pallein* to shake + *esthesia*] the ability to feel mechanical vibrations on or near the body, such as when a vibrating tuning fork is placed over a bony prominence. Called also *vibration sense.*

**pall·es·thet·ic** (pal″əs-thet′ik) pertaining to pallesthesia, or vibration sense.

**pal·li·al** (pal′e-əl) pertaining to the pallium.

**pal·li·ate** (pal′e-āt) to reduce the severity of; to relieve.

**pal·li·a·tive** (pal′e-ə-tiv) [L. *palliatus* cloaked] 1. affording relief but not cure. 2. an alleviating medicine.

**pal·li·dal** (pal′ĭ-dəl) pertaining to the globus pallidum.

**pal·li·dec·to·my** (pal″ĭ-dek′tə-me) surgical excision of the globus pallidus or extirpation of it by other means (chemopallidectomy).

**pal·li·do·an·sec·tion** (pal″ĭ-do-ən-sek′shən) surgical section of the globus pallidus and ansa lenticularis.

**pal·li·do·an·sot·o·my** (pal″ĭ-do-ən-sot′ə-me) production of lesions in the globus pallidus and ansa lenticularis.

**pal·li·dof·u·gal** (pal″ĭ-dof′u-gəl) [*pallidum* + *-fugal*] conducting impulses away from the globus pallidus.

**pal·li·dot·o·my** (pal″ĭ-dot′ə-me) [*pallidum* + *-tomy*] a stereotaxic surgical technique for producing lesions in the globus pallidus for treatment of extrapyramidal disorders.

**pal·li·dum** (pal′ĭ-dəm) [L. "pale"] globus pallidus.
**p. I,** globus pallidus medialis.
**p. II,** globus pallidus lateralis.

**pal·li·um** (pal′e-əm) [L. "cloak"] 1. [TA] cortex cerebri. 2. the cortex cerebri during its period of development.

**pal·lor** (pal′or) [L.] [MeSH: Pallor] paleness; decrease or absence of the skin coloration.

**palm** (pahm, pahlm) [L. *palma*] 1. palma. 2. any of a large family of mostly tropical trees. Genera of medical interest include *Areca* and *Cocos.*
**betel p.,** *Areca catechu.*
**coconut p.,** *Cocos nucifera.*
**handball p.,** contusion of the palm of the hand occurring in handball players.
**tripe p.,** a paraneoplastic syndrome in which the palm of the hand is thickened, velvety, and rugose, similar to tripe; often a sign of new or recurrent pulmonary or gastric malignancy.

**pal·ma** (pahl′mə) gen. and pl. *pal′mae* [L.] [TA] palm: the flexor surface of the hand. Called also *vola* [TA alternative] and *regio palmaris* [TA alternative].
**pal′mae plica′tae,** the branching folds of the mucosa of the vagina.

**Pal·ma·ceae** (pahl-ma′se-e) Palmae.

**Pal·mae** (pahl′me) the palms, a family of evergreen trees, shrubs, and woody vines, generally found in tropical regions. Genera of medical interest include *Areca, Cocos, Copernicia,* and *Cycas.* Called also *Palmaceae.*

**pal·mae** (pahl′me) [L.] genitive and plural of *palma.*

**pal·mar** (pahl′mər) [L. *palmaris; palma* palm] pertaining to the palm.

**pal·mar·is** (pahl-mar′is) [TA] palmar; a general term designating relationship to the palm of the hand. Called also *volaris* [TA alternative].

**pal·ma·ture** (pahl′mə-chər) [L. *palma* palm] a webbed state of the fingers.

**Pal·maz stent** (pahl-maz′) [J. C. *Palmaz,* American vascular surgeon, 20th century] see under *stent.*

**pal·mi·tal** (pal′mĭ-təl) an aldehyde lipid, the aldehyde form of palmitate; see *plasmalogen.*

**pal·mi·tate** (pal'mĭ-tāt) the anionic form of palmitic acid.

**pal·mit·ic ac·id** (pal-mit'ik) [MeSH: Palmitic Acid] a 16-carbon saturated fatty acid found in most fats and oils, particularly associated with stearic acid. It is one of the most prevalent saturated fatty acids in body lipids. See also table accompanying *fatty acid.*

**pal·mi·tin** (pal'mĭ-tin) a crystallizable and saponifiable fat from various fats and oils; glyceryl tripalmitate.

**pal·mi·to·le·ate** (pal"mĭ-to'le-āt) a salt (soap), ester, or anionic form of palmitoleic acid.

**pal·mi·to·le·ic ac·id** (pal"mĭ-to-le'ik) a monounsaturated 16-carbon fatty acid occurring in many oils, particularly those derived from marine animals. See also table accompanying *fatty acid.*

**pal·mi·to·yl** (pal"mĭ-to'əl) the acyl radical of palmitic acid. As palmitoyl CoA, a thioester formed with coenzyme A, it can act as a donor of fatty acyl groups in lipid biosynthesis.

**palp** (palp) a sensory or feeding appendage, especially one of the jointed sensory appendages attached to the mouth of arthropods.

**palp·a·ble** (pal'pə-bəl) perceptible by touch.

**pal·pate** (pal'pāt) [L. *palpare* to touch] to examine by the hand; to feel.

**pal·pa·tion** (pal-pa'shən) [L. *palpatio*] [MeSH: Palpation] the act of feeling with the hand; the application of the fingers with light pressure to the surface of the body for the purpose of determining the consistency of the parts beneath in physical diagnosis.
**bimanual p.,** examination with both hands.
**light touch p.,** light palpation of the surface of the abdomen and thorax with the fingertips for the purpose of finding the outlines of the organs.

**pal·pa·tom·e·try** (pal"pə-tom'ə-tre) [*palpation* + *-metry*] measurement of the amount of pressure that can be borne without causing pain.

**pal·pa·to·per·cus·sion** (pal"pə-to-pər-kŭ'shən) palpation combined with percussion.

**pal·pe·bra** (pal'pə-brə) gen. and pl. *pal'pebrae* [L.] [TA] eyelid; either of the two movable folds that protect the anterior surface of the eyeball.
**p. infe'rior** [TA], lower eyelid: the inferior of the paired movable folds that protect the surface of the eyeball.
**p. supe'rior** [TA], upper eyelid: the superior of the paired movable folds that protect the surface of the eyeball.
**p. ter'tia,** nictitating membrane.

**pal·pe·brae** (pal'pə-bre) [L.] genitive and plural of *palpebra.*

**pal·pe·bral** (pal'pə-brəl) pertaining to an eyelid.

**pal·pe·bral·is** (pal"pə-bra'lis) [L.] pertaining to an eyelid.

**pal·pe·brate** (pal'pə-brāt) [L. *palpebrare* to wink] 1. to wink. 2. having eyelids.

**pal·pe·bra·tion** (pal"pə-bra'shən) 1. the act of winking. 2. abnormally frequent winking, as from a tic.

**pal·pe·bri·tis** (pal"pə-bri'tis) blepharitis.

**pal·pi·ta·tion** (pal"pĭ-ta'shən) [L. *palpitare* to move frequently and rapidly] a subjective sensation of an unduly rapid or irregular heart beat.

**pal·pus** (pal'pəs) pl. *pal'pi* [L. *palpare* to touch softly] one of the articulated sensory structures attached to the mouthparts of arthropods.

**PALS** periarterial lymphoid sheath.

**pal·sy** (pawl'ze) paralysis.
**Bell's p.,** unilateral facial paralysis of sudden onset, due to lesion of the facial nerve and resulting in characteristic distortion of the face.
**birth p.,** see under *paralysis.*
**brachial p.,** see under *paralysis.*
**cerebral p.,** any of a group of persisting, nonprogressive motor disorders appearing in young children and resulting from brain damage caused by birth trauma or intrauterine pathology. The disorders are characterized by delayed or abnormal motor development, such as spastic paraplegia, hemiplegia, or tetraplegia, which is often accompanied by mental retardation, seizures, or ataxia. See also *spastic paraplegia* and *Little's disease.*
**crossed leg p.,** palsy of the peroneal nerve caused by sitting with one leg crossed over the other.
**divers' p.,** weakness of an area of the body owing to decompression sickness.
**Erb's p., Erb-Duchenne p.,** see under *paralysis.*
**facial p.,** Bell's p.
**ischemic p.,** see under *paralysis.*
**Klumpke's p.,** see under *paralysis.*
**maternal obstetric p.,** paralysis affecting some portion of the mother's lower limb due to compression of a nerve during delivery, usually when the fetus is large and the mother is small and has difficult labor. The most common cause is compression of the lumbosacral plexus or its nerves by the fetal head or forceps, resulting in unilateral footdrop.
**printer's p.,** a condition observed in printers due to chronic antimony poisoning, and marked by neuritis with paralysis, pain in the pelvic region, and papular eruption.
**progressive bulbar p.,** progressive paralysis and atrophy of the muscles of the lips, tongue, mouth, pharynx, and larynx due to lesions of the motor nuclei of the lower brain stem. It is a chronic, generally fatal disease with onset usually in late adulthood but also earlier in patients with amyotrophic lateral sclerosis, syringobulbia, or multiple sclerosis. See also *progressive bulbar p. of childhood* and *Brown-Vialetto-van Laere syndrome.* Called also *bulbar, glossolabial, glossopharyngolabial, labial, labioglossolaryngeal, labioglossopharyngeal,* or *progressive bulbar paralysis;* and *Duchenne's paralysis* or *syndrome.*
**progressive bulbar p. of childhood, progressive infantile bulbar p.,** a rare type of progressive bulbar palsy that occurs in young children. Called also *Fazio-Londe atrophy* or *disease.*
**progressive supranuclear p.,** Steele-Richardson-Olszewski syndrome.
**pseudobulbar p.,** see under *paralysis.*
**Saturday night p.,** musculospiral paralysis.
**scriveners' p.,** writers' cramp.
**shaking p.,** paralysis agitans.
**spastic bulbar p.,** pseudobulbar paralysis.
**tardy median p.,** carpal tunnel syndrome.
**tardy ulnar p.,** cubital tunnel syndrome that occurs months to years after injury to the elbow.
**wasting p.,** spinal muscular atrophy.

**Pal·u·drine** (pal'u-drin) trademark for a preparation of proguanil hydrochloride.

**2-PAM** pralidoxime.

**L-PAM** melphalan.

**pam·a·brom** (pam'ə-brom) [USP] a mild diuretic used in preparations for the relief of premenstrual syndrome.

**pam·a·to·lol sul·fate** (pam"ə-to'lol) an antiadrenergic (β-receptor), $(C_{16}H_{26}N_2O_4)_2 \cdot H_2SO_4$.

**Pam·e·lor** (pam'ə-lor) trademark for preparations of nortriptyline hydrochloride.

**pam·id·ro·nate** (pam"ĭ-dro'nāt) ADP; an aminohydroxypropylidene-substituted diphosphonate compound with an affinity for sites of osteoid mineralization; used as the disodium salt to treat moderate to severe hypercalcemia associated with malignancy; administered by intravenous infusion. Complexed with technetium 99m, it is used in bone imaging; see table at *technetium.*

**Pam·ine** (pam'ēn) trademark for preparations of methscopolamine bromide.

**Pam·i·syl** (pam'ĭ-səl) trademark for preparations of aminosalicylic acid.

**pam·o·ate** (pam'o-āt) USAN contraction for 4,4′-methylenebis [3-hydroxy-2-naphthoate].

**pam·pin·i·form** (pam-pin'ĭ-form) [L. *pampinus* tendril + *form*] shaped like a tendril.

**pam·pin·ocele** (pam-pin'o-sēl) [L. *pampinus* tendril + *-cele*[1]] varicocele.

**PAN** polyarteritis nodosa.

**Pan** (pan) a genus of primates of the family Pongidae. *P. troglody'tes* is the chimpanzee.

**pan-** [Gr. *pan* all] prefix signifying all.

**Pan·a·cea** (pan"ə-se'ə) [Gr. *Panakeia*] one of two sisters, the other being Hygeia, who were the daughters of Aesculapius.

**pan·a·cea** (pan"ə-se'ə) [Gr. *panakeia*] 1. a universal remedy. 2. an ancient name for a healing herb or its juice.

**pan·ac·i·nar** (pan-as'ĭ-nər) affecting many acini uniformly, including respiratory bronchioles, alveolar ducts, and alveolar sacs.

**Pan·a·fil** (pan'ə-fil) trademark for a preparation of chlorophyllin copper complex, papain, and urea.

**pan·ag·glu·tin·a·ble** (pan"ə-gloo'tĭ-nə-bəl) agglutinable with every type of blood serum from the same species, e.g., red blood cells agglutinable with sera of all human blood groups.

**pan·ag·glu·ti·na·tion** (pan"ə-gloo"tĭ-na'shən) agglutination (e.g., of red blood cells) by the serum of all blood groups of the same species.

**pan·ag·glu·ti·nin** (pan"ə-gloo'tĭ-nin) [*pan-* + *agglutinin*] an agglutinin which agglutinates the red blood cells of all blood groups in the same species.

**pan·an·gi·itis** (pan″an-je-i′tis) [*pan-* + *angiitis*] inflammation involving all the coats of the vessel.
**diffuse necrotizing p.,** panangiitis with extensive involvement of the blood vessels.

**pan·ar·te·ri·tis** (pan″ahr-tə-ri′tis) polyarteritis (def. 1).
**p. nodo′sa,** polyarteritis nodosa.

**pan·ar·thri·tis** (pan″ahr-thri′tis) [*pan-* + *arthr-* + *-itis*] inflammation of all the joints or of all the structures of a joint.

**pan·at·ro·phy** (pan-at′rə-fe) [*pan-* + *atrophy*] atrophy affecting several parts; general atrophy.

**pan·au·to·no·mic** (pan-aw″tə-no′mik) pertaining to or affecting the entire autonomic (sympathetic and parasympathetic) nervous system.

**Pan·ax** (pan′aks) the ginsengs, a genus of perennial herbs of the family Araliaceae, native to parts of Asia and eastern North America. *P. gin′seng* is Chinese ginseng and *P. quinquefo′lius* is American ginseng; both yield the root used in Chinese medicine. See *ginseng* (def. 2).

**pan·blas·tic** (pan-blas′tik) [*pan-* + *blast-* + *-ic*] pertaining to each of the layers of the blastoderm.

**pan·bron·chi·o·li·tis** (pan-brong″ke-o-li′tis) a chronic type of infectious inflammation of the airways limited to the bronchioles, seen mainly in East Asia and nearby island countries.

**pan·car·di·tis** (pan″kahr-di′tis) [*pan-* + *carditis*] diffuse inflammation of the heart, involving the pericardium, myocardium, and endocardium.

**pan·chro·mat·ic** (pan″kro-mat′ik) [*pan-* + *chromatic*] sensitive to all colors; applied to photographic emulsions.

**pan·chro·mia** (pan-kro′me-ə) the condition of staining with various dyes.

**Pan·coast's suture** (pan′kōsts) [Joseph *Pancoast,* American surgeon, 1805–1882] see under *suture.*

**Pan·coast's syndrome, tumor** (pan′kōsts) [Henry Khunrath *Pancoast,* American radiologist, 1875–1939] see under *syndrome,* and see *pulmonary sulcus tumor,* under *tumor.*

**pan·co·lec·to·my** (pan″ko-lek′tə-me) excision of the entire colon with creation of an ileostomy.

**pan·co·li·tis** (pan″ko-li′tis) inflammation of the entire colon.
**necrotizing amebic p.,** a rare but highly fatal complication of amebic dysentery, clinically resembling fulminant ulcerative colitis.

**pan·cre·al·gia** (pan″kre-al′jə) pancreatalgia.

**pan·cre·as** (pan′kre-əs) gen. *pancre′atis,* pl. *pancre′ata* [L., from Gr. *pankreas,* from *pan* all + *kreas* flesh] [TA] [MeSH: Pancreas] a large, elongated, racemose gland situated transversely behind the stomach, between the spleen and the duodenum. Its right extremity, the *head,* is larger and directed downward; the left extremity, or *tail,* is transverse and terminates close to the spleen. It is subdivided into lobules by septa that extend into the gland from the thin, areolar tissue that forms an indefinite capsule. The endocrine part *(endocrine pancreas)* consists of the islets of Langerhans, which contain beta cells that produce insulin, alpha cells that produce glucagon, and delta cells that produce somatostatin; all three of these hormones are secreted directly into the bloodstream. Some islets contain PP cells that secrete pancreatic polypeptide. The exocrine part *(exocrine pancreas)* consists of pancreatic acini, secretory units that produce and secrete into the duodenum pancreatic juice, which contains enzymes essential to protein digestion.
**aberrant p.,** an exclave of pancreatic tissue occurring most commonly as a firm yellow nodule in the stomach, duodenum, or jejunum, but encountered also in other sites.

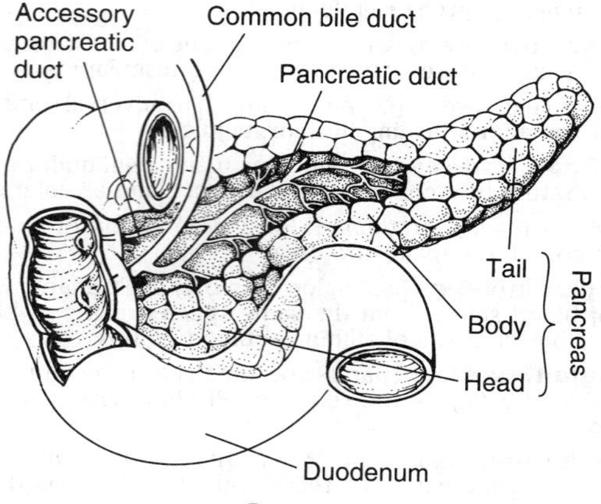

Pancreas.

**p. accesso′rium** [TA], **accessory p.,** an inconstant separate part of the head of the pancreas, usually an unattached uncinate process.
**annular p.,** a developmental anomaly in which the pancreas forms a ring entirely surrounding the duodenum.
**Aselli's p.,** the mesenteric lymph nodes of certain carnivores. Called also *Aselli's glands.*
**p. divi′sum,** a developmental anomaly in which the pancreas is present as two separate structures, each with its own duct.
**dorsal p.,** an embryonic outpocketing or bud from the endodermal lining of the gut on the dorsal wall cephalad to the level of the hepatic diverticulum, which forms most of the pancreas and its main duct.
**endocrine p.,** that part of the pancreas that acts as an endocrine gland, consisting of the islets of Langerhans, which secrete insulin, glucagon, somatostatin, and sometimes pancreatic polypeptide directly into the bloodstream. See *pancreas.* Called also *endocrine part of pancreas.*
**exocrine p.,** that part of the pancreas that acts as an exocrine gland, consisting of the pancreatic acini, which produce pancreatic juice and secrete it into the duodenum to aid in protein digestion. See *pancreas.* Called also *exocrine part of pancreas.*
**lesser p.,** processus uncinatus pancreatis.
**ventral p.,** an embryonic outpocketing or bud from the endodermal lining of the gut on the ventral wall, in the caudal angle between the gut and the hepatic diverticulum, which forms the head of the pancreas and the stem of its main duct.
**Willis' p., Winslow's p.,** processus uncinatus pancreatis.

**Pan·cre·ase** (pan′kre-ās) trademark for a preparation of pancrelipase.

**pan·cre·a·ta** (pan-kre′ə-tə) [L.] plural of *pancreas.*

**pan·cre·a·tal·gia** (pan″kre-ə-tal′jə) [*pancreas* + *-algia*] pain in the pancreas.

**pan·cre·a·tec·to·my** (pan″kre-ə-tek′tə-me) [*pancreat-* + *-ectomy*] [MeSH: Pancreatectomy] surgical removal of the pancreas.

**pan·cre·at·ic** (pan″kre-at′ik) [L. *pancreaticus*] pertaining to the pancreas.

**pan·cre·at·ic elas·tase II** (pan″kre-at′ik e-las′tās) [EC 3.4.21.71] a serine endopeptidase that catalyzes the cleavage of peptide bonds, preferentially clearing on the carboxyl side of leucine, methionine, and phenylalanine residues. Secreted by the pancreas as the proenzyme proelastase and activated in the duodenum via cleavage by trypsin, it is involved in protein digestion. In a given species, usually either pancreatic elastase or pancreatic elastase II is expressed; in humans it is the latter.

**pan·cre·at·ic lip·ase** (pan″kre-at′ik li′pās) see under *lipase.*

**pancreatic(o)-** [*pancreatic,* q.v.] a combining form denoting relationship to the pancreas, or to the pancreatic duct.

**pan·cre·at·i·co·du·o·de·nal** (pan″kre-at″ĭ-ko-doo″o-de′nəl) pertaining to the pancreas and duodenum.

**pan·cre·at·i·co·du·o·de·nos·to·my** (pan″kre-at″ĭ-ko-doo″o-də-nos′tə-me) surgical anastomosis of the pancreatic duct, or the divided end of the transected pancreas, with the duodenum.

**pan·cre·at·i·co·en·ter·os·to·my** (pan″kre-at″ĭ-ko-en″tər-os′tə-me) surgical anastomosis of the pancreatic duct, or the divided end of the transected pancreas, with the intestine.

**pan·cre·at·i·co·gas·tros·to·my** (pan″kre-at″ĭ-ko-gas-tros′tə-me) surgical anastomosis of the pancreatic duct, or the divided end of the transected pancreas, with the stomach.

**pan·cre·at·i·co·je·ju·nos·to·my** (pan″kre-at″ĭ-ko-jə-joo-nos′tə-me) [MeSH: Pancreaticojejunostomy] surgical anastomosis of the pancreatic duct, or the divided end of the transected pancreas, with the jejunum.

**pan·cre·at·i·co·splen·ic** (pan″kre-at″ĭ-ko-splen′ik) pertaining to the pancreas and spleen.

**pan·cre·a·tin** (pan′kre-ə-tin) [USP] [MeSH: Pancreatin] a substance from the pancreas of the hog or the ox that contains enzymes such as amylase, trypsin, and lipase; used as a digestive aid in pancreatic insufficiency and to peptonize milk and other foods.

**pan·cre·a·ti·tis** (pan″kre-ə-ti′tis) [MeSH: Pancreatitis] acute or chronic inflammation of the pancreas, which may be asymptomatic or symptomatic, and which is due to autodigestion of a pancreatic tissue by its own enzymes. It is caused most often by alcoholism or biliary tract disease; less commonly it may be associated with hyperlipemia, hyperparathyroidism, abdominal trauma (accidental or operative injury), vasculitis, or uremia.
**acute p.,** a form characterized by sudden onset of abdominal pain, nausea, and vomiting.
**acute hemorrhagic p.,** 1. a condition due to autolysis of pancreatic tissue caused by the escape of enzymes into its substance, resulting

in hemorrhage into the parenchyma and surrounding tissues. Blood staining of the lateral abdominal wall (Grey Turner's sign) or periumbilical area (Cullen's sign) may result. 2. acute necrotizing p.
**acute necrotic p., acute necrotizing p.,** a condition usually seen in middle-aged obese dogs that eat a high-fat diet; characteristics include necrosis of the pancreas with abdominal pain and vomiting. Clinical signs include hyperlipidemia and elevated serum amylase or lipase. If untreated, it may progress to hyperglycemia, shock, coma, and death. Called also *acute pancreatic necrosis* and *acute hemorrhagic p.*
**calcareous p.,** pancreatitis accompanied by the formation of calculi; pancreatic calcification is usually associated with exocrine insufficiency and diabetes mellitus.
**centrilobar p.,** pancreatitis located around the branches of the pancreatic duct.
**chronic p.,** a form marked usually by chronic abdominal pain and by progressive fibrosis and loss of exocrine (steatorrhea) and endocrine (diabetes mellitus) function; recurrent attacks of acute pancreatitis *(chronic relapsing p.)* are often superimposed.
**chronic relapsing p.,** see *chronic p.*
**interstitial p.,** pancreatitis in which there is overgrowth of the inter- and intra-acinar connective tissue and frequently a corresponding atrophy of the glandular tissue.
**perilobar p.,** fibrosis of the pancreas surrounding collections of atrophic acini.
**purulent p.,** purulent inflammation of the pancreas.

**pancreat(o)-** [L. *pancreas,* q.v.] a combining form denoting relationship to the pancreas.

**pan·cre·a·to·blas·to·ma** (pan″kre-ə-to-blas-to′mə) a rare type of malignant pancreatic tumor, having an uncertain origin and usually affecting children.

**pan·cre·a·to·du·o·de·nec·to·my** (pan″kre-ə-to-doo″o-də-nek′tə-me) excision of the head of the pancreas along with the encircling loop of the duodenum.

**pan·cre·a·to·du·o·de·nos·to·my** (pan″kre-ə-to-doo″o-də-nos′tə-me) pancreaticoduodenostomy.

**pan·cre·a·to·en·ter·os·to·my** (pan″kre-ə-to-en″tər-os′tə-me) pancreaticoenterostomy.

**pan·cre·a·to·gen·ic** (pan″kre-ə-to-jen′ik) pancreatogenous.

**pan·cre·a·tog·e·nous** (pan″kre-ə-toj′ə-nəs) arising in or from the pancreas.

**pan·cre·a·to·gram** (pan″kre-at′o-gram) the x-ray film produced by pancreatography.

**pan·cre·a·tog·ra·phy** (pan″kre-ə-tog′rə-fe) radiography of the pancreas performed during surgical exploration, a water-soluble contrast medium being injected into the pancreatic duct and the film being made while the abdomen is open.
**endoscopic retrograde p.,** that in which the radiopaque medium is injected into the pancreatic duct at the ampulla of Vater via a cannula introduced through a fiberoptic endoscope. See also *endoscopic retrograde cholangiopancreatography,* under *cholangiopancreatography.*

**pan·cre·ato·lith** (pan″kre-at′o-lith) [*pancreato-* + *-lith*] pancreatic calculus.

**pan·cre·a·to·li·thec·to·my** (pan″kre-ə-to-lĭ-thek′tə-me) [*pancreatolith* + *-ectomy*] removal of a calculus from the pancreas.

**pan·cre·a·to·li·thi·a·sis** (pan″kre-ə-to-lĭ-thi′ə-sis) the presence of calculi in the pancreas or its ductal system, usually associated with pancreatic exocrine (digestive enzymes) and endocrine (insulin) insufficiency, accompanied by steatorrhea, weight loss, and diabetes mellitus. Called also *pancreatic lithiasis.*

**pan·cre·a·to·li·thot·o·my** (pan″kre-ə-to-lĭ-thot′ə-me) [*pancreatolith* + *-tomy*] incision of the pancreas for the removal of a calculus.

**pan·cre·a·tol·y·sis** (pan″kre-ə-tol′ĭ-sis) pancreolysis.

**pan·cre·a·to·lyt·ic** (pan″kre-ə-to-lit′ik) pancreolytic.

**pan·cre·at·o·my** (pan-kre-at′ə-me) pancreatotomy.

**pan·cre·a·top·a·thy** (pan″kre-ə-top′ə-the) [*pancreato-* + *-pathy*] pancreopathy.

**pan·cre·a·tot·o·my** (pan″kre-ə-tot′ə-me) [*pancreato-* + *-tomy*] incision of the pancreas.

**pan·cre·a·to·trop·ic** (pan″kre-ə-to-trop′ik) [*pancreato-* + *-tropy*] having an affinity for or an influence on the pancreas.

**pan·cre·a·trop·ic** (pan″kre-ə-trop′ik) pancreatotropic.

**pan·cre·ec·to·my** (pan″kre-ek′tə-me) pancreatectomy.

**pan·cre·li·pase** (pan″kre-li′pās) [USP] a standardized preparation of hog pancreas, containing enzymes, principally lipase, with amylase and protease, and having the same actions as those of the pancreatic juice; used as a digestive aid in conditions of pancreatic insufficiency.

**pan·creo·li·thot·o·my** (pan″kre-o-lĭ-thot′ə-me) pancreatolithotomy.

**pan·cre·ol·y·sis** (pan″kre-ol′ĭ-sis) [*pancreas* + *-lysis*] destruction of pancreatic tissue by pancreatic enzymes.

**pan·creo·lyt·ic** (pan″kre-o-lit′ik) pertaining to or producing pancreolysis.

**pan·cre·op·a·thy** (pan″kre-op′ə-the) [*pancreas* + *-pathy*] any disease of the pancreas. Called also *pancreatopathy.*

**pan·creo·priv·ic** (pan″kre-o-priv′ik) lacking a pancreas.

**pan·creo·ther·a·py** (pan″kre-o-ther′ə-pe) therapeutic use of pancreas tissue or of extracts of the pancreas containing digestive enzymes; pancreatic replacement therapy, used in pancreatic insufficiency with malabsorption.

**pan·cre·o·trop·ic** (pan″kre-o-trop′ik) pancreatotropic.

**pan·creo·zy·min** (pan′kre-o-zi″min) cholecystokinin.

**pan·cu·ro·ni·um bro·mide** (pan″ku-ro′ne-əm) a nondepolarizing skeletal muscle relaxant, with curariform action; used as an adjunct to anesthesia and may be used to facilitate mechanical ventilation; administered intravenously.

**pan·cys·ti·tis** (pan″sis-ti′tis) cystitis involving the entire thickness of the wall of the urinary bladder, as occurs in interstitial cystitis.

**pan·cy·to·pe·nia** (pan″si-to-pe′ne-ə) [*pan-* + *cytopenia*] [MeSH: Pancytopenia] deficiency of all cellular elements of the blood. See also *erythropenia, leukopenia,* and *thrombocytopenia.*
**congenital p., Fanconi's p.,** Fanconi's syndrome (def. 1).
**tropical canine p.,** canine ehrlichiosis.

**pan·dem·ic** (pan-dem′ik) [*pan-* + Gr. *dēmos* people] 1. a widespread epidemic of a disease. 2. widely epidemic; distributed or occurring widely throughout a region, country, or continent or globally.

**pan·dem·ic·i·ty** (pan″dəm-is′ĭ-te) the state of being pandemic.

**Pan·der's islands, layer** (pahn′derz) [Heinrich Christian *Pander,* German anatomist, 1794–1865] see under *island* and *layer.*

**pan·dic·u·la·tion** (pan″dik-u-la′shən) [L. *pandiculari* to stretch one's self] the act of stretching and yawning.

**pan·el** (pan′əl) 1. a list of names. 2. a group of individuals participating in a specific discussion or activity. 3. a list of names of the medical professionals who are willing to care for insured persons for a stipulated yearly fee under the system of medical insurance carried on by insurance groups under the supervision of the government in Great Britain. 4. the list of the insured persons assigned as clients to a physician under the British National Health Insurance Act. 5. a series of chemical substances, such as drugs or antigens, to which a given animal, tissue, or substance is exposed to test for reactions. 6. a group of related laboratory measurements that reflect the state of function of an organ or system.

**pan·en·ceph·a·li·tis** (pan″ən-sef″ə-li′tis) encephalitis, probably of viral origin, which produces intranuclear or intracytoplasmic inclusion bodies of type A (Cowdry's classification), which result in parenchymatous lesions affecting the gray and white matter of the brain simultaneously.
**Pette-Döring p.,** a form of subacute encephalitis characterized by involvement of both the gray and white matter of the brain, and with a predilection for the basal ganglia.
**subacute sclerosing p. (SSPE),** a rare and devastating form of leukoencephalitis usually affecting children and adolescents. Insidious in onset, it characteristically produces progressive cerebral dysfunction over a course of several weeks or months and death within a year. Pathologically, in addition to the lesions of the white matter, there are demyelination and intranuclear inclusion bodies in nerve cells and oligodendroglia. High titers of measles virus in the serum and cerebrospinal fluid have indicated a linkage between this condition and earlier measles infection. Called also *Dawson's encephalitis, subacute inclusion body encephalitis, subacute sclerosing leukoencephalopathy, van Bogaert's encephalitis,* and *van Bogaert's sclerosing leukoencephalitis.*

**pan·en·dog·ra·phy** (pan″ən-dog′rə-fe) the recording of events observed through a panendoscope.

**pan·en·do·scope** (pan-en′do-skōp) 1. an endoscope for wide-angle viewing. 2. a cystoscope that permits wide-angle viewing of the urinary bladder and urethra.
**oral p.,** an illuminated tubular device that permits visual observation and audiovisual recording of the larynx and vocal cords during production of speech sounds.

**pan·en·dos·co·py** (pan″ən-dos′kə-pe) observation by means of a panendoscope.

**pan·epi·zo·ot·ic** (pan-ep″ĭ-zo-ot′ik) panzootic.

**pan·es·the·sia** (pan″əs-the′zhə) [*pan-* + *esthesia*] the sum of the sensations experienced.

**pan·es·thet·ic** (pan″əs-thet′ik) relating to panesthesia.

**Pa·neth's cells** (pah′nets) [Josef *Paneth,* Austrian physician, 1857–1890] see under *cell.*

**pang** (pang) a sudden, piercing pain.
**breast p.,** angina pectoris.
**brow p.,** 1. supraorbital neuralgia. 2. hemicrania (def. 1).

**pan·gen·e·sis** (pan-jen′ə-sis) [pan- + *genesis*] Darwin's hypothesis of the inheritance of acquired characteristics. According to the hypothesis, true reproductive power lies not in the germ cells but in the totality of the somatic cells (hence "pangenesis"). The somatic cells generate pangenes that circulate freely in the blood, reproduced by division, and collect in the germ cells, where they combine with and alter earlier pangenes in correspondence to recent changes in the peripheral organs.

**pan·glos·sia** (pan-glos′e-ə) [*pan-* + Gr. *glōssa* tongue] abnormal or pathologic garrulity.

**Pan·go·nia** (pan-go′ne-ə) the zimbs, a genus of tabanid flies found in Ethiopia that feed on the blood of humans and other mammals.

**Pan·he·ma·tin** (pan-he′mə-tin) trademark for a preparation of hemin.

**pan·he·ma·to·pe·nia** (pan-he″mə-to-pe′ne-ə) [*pan-* + *hemato-* + *-penia*] pancytopenia.

**Pan·hep·rin** (pan-hep′rin) trademark for a preparation of heparin sodium.

**pan·hy·drom·e·ter** (pan″hi-drom′ə-tər) [*pan-* + *hydrometer*] an instrument for ascertaining the specific gravity of any liquid.

**pan·hy·per·emia** (pan″hi-pər-e′me-ə) [*pan-* + *hyperemia*] a generalized hyperemia or plethora.

**pan·hy·po·gam·ma·glob·u·lin·emia** (pan-hi″po-gam′ə-glob″u-lin-e′me-ə) [*pan-* + *hypogammaglobulinemia*] hypogammaglobulinemia; deficiency of all immunoglobulin classes.

**pan·hy·po·go·nad·ism** (pan-hi″po-go′nad-iz-əm) underdevelopment of all the genital tissues with decreased functional activities of the gonads.

**pan·hy·po·pi·tu·i·ta·rism** (pan-hi″po-pĭ-too′ĭ-tə-riz-əm) generalized or particularly severe hypopituitarism, which in its complete form leads to absence of gonadal function and insufficiency of thyroid and adrenal cortical function. Dwarfism, regression of secondary sex characters, loss of libido, weight loss, fatigability, bradycardia, hypotension, pallor, depression, and many other manifestations may occur. When cachexia is a prominent feature, it is called *hypophysial* or *pituitary cachexia.* Called also *Simmonds' disease.*
**prepubertal p.,** inadequate production of all adenohypophysial hormones that begins before puberty and is associated with subnormal growth. See also *hypophysial infantilism,* under *infantilism.*

**pan·hys·ter·ec·to·my** (pan″his-tər-ek′tə-me) [*pan-* + *hysterectomy*] complete removal of the uterus and cervix; total hysterectomy.

**pan·hys·tero-ooph·o·rec·to·my** (pan-his″tər-o-o″of-ə-rek′tə-me) excision of the body of the uterus, cervix, and ovary.

**pan·hys·tero·sal·pin·gec·to·my** (pan-his″tər-o-sal″pin-jek′tə-me) excision of the body of the uterus, cervix, and uterine tube.

**pan·hys·ter·o·sal·pin·go-ooph·o·rec·to·my** (pan-his″tər-o-sal″ping-go-o″of-ə-rek′tə-me) excision of the uterus, cervix, uterine tube, and ovary.

**pan·ic** (pan′ik) [from Gr. *Pan* woodland deity who was considered to be the cause of sudden or groundless fear] [MeSH: Panic] acute, extreme anxiety with disorganization of personality and function.
**homosexual p.,** an acute, extreme anxiety reaction brought on by circumstances that induce the unconscious fear of being homosexual or of succumbing to homosexual impulses.

**Pan·i·cum** (pan′ĭ-kum) a genus of grasses used for hay and cereal, including panic grass and millet. Certain species may cause oxalate poisoning and others may cause hepatogenous photosensitization in ruminants.

**pan·im·mu·ni·ty** (pan″ĭ-mu′nĭ-te) [*pan-* + *immunity*] immunity to several infections caused by bacteria and viruses.

**Pan·iz·za's plexus** (pah-nēt′səz) [Bartolomeo *Panizza,* Italian anatomist, 1785–1867] see under *plexus.*

**pan·leu·ko·pe·nia** (pan″loo-ko-pe′ne-ə) a highly contagious and often fatal disease of cats, caused by a parvovirus; characteristics include leukopenia, inactivity, anorexia, diarrhea, and vomiting. Called also *feline* or *infectious feline agranulocytosis, cat* or *feline enteritis, cat* or *feline distemper,* and *cat plague.*

**pan·mix·ia** (pan-mik′se-ə) panmixis.

**pan·mix·is** (pan-mik′sis) [*pan-* + Gr. *mixis* mixture] random mating, i.e., choice of mate uninfluenced by the genotypes of the mates.

**pan·mu·ral** (pan-mu′rəl) [*pan-* + *mural*] pertaining to or affecting the entire wall.

**Pan·my·cin** (pan-mi′sin) trademark for preparations of tetracycline.

**pan·my·eloid** (pan-mi′ə-loid) pertaining to all the elements of the bone marrow.

**pan·my·elo·pa·thia** (pan-mi″ə-lo-path′e-ə) panmyelopathy.

**pan·my·elop·a·thy** (pan″mi-ə-lop′ə-the) [*pan-* + *myelopathy*] myelopathy involving all the elements of the bone marrow.
**constitutional infantile p., Fanconi's p.,** Fanconi's syndrome (def. 1).

**pan·my·e·loph·thi·sis** (pan-mi″ə-lof′thĭ-sis) aplastic anemia.

**Pan·ner's disease** (pahn′ərz) [Hans Jessen *Panner,* Danish radiologist, 1871–1930] see under *disease.*

**pan·nic·u·lal·gia** (pə-nik″u-lal′jə) adiposalgia.

**pan·nic·u·lec·to·my** (pə-nik″u-lek′tə-me) surgical excision of the abdominal apron of superficial fat in an obese patient.

**pan·nic·u·li** (pə-nik′u-li) [L.] genitive and plural of *panniculus.*

**pan·nic·u·li·tis** (pə-nik″u-li′tis) [*panniculus* + *-itis*] [MeSH: Panniculitis] an inflammatory reaction of the subcutaneous fat, which may involve the connective tissue septa between the fat lobes, the septa lobules and vessels, or the fat lobules, characterized by the development of single or multiple cutaneous nodules. Cf. *steatitis.* Called also *adipositis.*
**cytophagic histiocytic p.,** a severe variant of relapsing febrile nodular nonsuppurative panniculitis characterized by lobules infiltrated by histiocytes that have phagocytized erythrocytes, leukocytes, and platelets; it is sometimes accompanied by systemic conditions that can be fatal, such as multiorgan failure, coagulopathies with hemorrhaging, and overwhelming infection.
**LE p.,** lupus erythematosus profundus.
**lobular p.,** relapsing febrile nodular nonsuppurative p.
**lupus p.,** lupus erythematosus profundus.
**nodular nonsuppurative p.,** relapsing febrile nodular nonsuppurative p.
**relapsing febrile nodular nonsuppurative p.,** a form of panniculitis characterized by recurrent episodes of fever accompanied by crops of single or multiple, erythematous, tender or painless subcutaneous nodules on the lower extremities and trunk, which resolve and usually leave a depression in the skin. The condition is most often seen in women, and it may occur alone or it may be associated with numerous other disorders. Called also *Christian-Weber disease, nodular nonsuppurative p.,* and *Weber-Christian p., disease,* or *syndrome.*
**subacute nodular migratory p.,** a condition considered by some to be the same as *erythema nodosum migrans,* characterized by the development on the anterior and lateral aspects of the lower extremities, particularly in women, of discrete nodules that spread centrifugally with erythematous borders and central clearing (giving the appearance of migration) and coalesce to form plaques that eventually involute, usually with residual pigmentation.
**Weber-Christian p.,** relapsing febrile nodular nonsuppurative p.

**pan·nic·u·lus** (pə-nik′u-ləs) gen. and pl. *panni′culi* [L., dim. of *pannus* cloth] a layer of membrane.
**p. adipo′sus** [TA], the subcutaneous fat: a layer of fat underlying the dermis. Called also *pannus.*
**p. carno′sus,** a thin muscular layer within the superficial fascia of animals with a hairy coat; in humans it is represented mainly by the platysma myoides.

**pan·nus** (pan′əs) [L. "a piece of cloth"] 1. superficial vascularization of the cornea with infiltration of granulation tissue. 2. an inflammatory exudate overlying the lining layer of synovial cells on the inside of a joint, usually occurring in patients with rheumatoid or other inflammatory arthritis and sometimes resulting in fibrous ankylosis of the joint. 3. panniculus adiposus.
**degenerative p., p. degenerati′vus,** 1. a connective-tissue growth between the epithelium of the cornea and Bowman's membrane. 2. chronic superficial keratitis.
**glaucomatous p.,** degeneration and desquamation of corneal epithelium due to edema in advanced glaucoma.
**phlyctenular p.,** pannus associated with phlyctenular keratitis, the vascularization running all the way around the periphery of the limbus and extending toward the center.
**p. sic′cus,** pannus of the cornea associated with dryness of the cornea and conjunctiva.
**p. trachomato′sus,** pannus occurring secondarily to trachoma, the small fine branching vessels always appearing at the upper limbus and running down under the epithelium into the cornea.

**pa·nod·ic** (pə-nod′ik) panthodic.

**pano·pho·bia** (pan″o-fo′be-ə) panphobia.

**pan·oph·thal·mia** (pan″of-thal′me-ə) panophthalmitis.

**pan·oph·thal·mi·tis** (pan″of-thəl-mi′tis) [*pan-* + *ophthalmitis*] [MeSH: Panophthalmitis] inflammation of all the structures or tissues of the eye.

**pan·op·tic** (pan-op′tik) [*pan-* + *opt-* + *-ic*] rendering everything visible; said of a stain which differentiates all the tissues of a specimen. See *Giemsa stain,* under *stain.*

**pan·os·te·itis** (pan″os-te-i′tis) [*pan-* + *oste-* + *-itis*] inflammation of every part of a bone.

**pan·os·ti·tis** (pan″os-ti′tis) panosteitis.

**pan·oti·tis** (pan″o-ti′tis) [*pan-* + *ot-* + *-itis*] an inflammation of all the parts or structures of the ear.

**pan·pho·bia** (pan-fo′be-ə) [*pan-* + *-phobia*] fear of everything; a vague and persistent dread of some unknown evil.

**pan·proc·to·co·lec·to·my** (pan-prok″to-ko-lek′tə-me) excision of the entire rectum and colon, with creation of an ileal stoma.

**pan·ret·i·nal** (pan-ret′ĭ-nəl) pertaining to or encompassing the entire retina.

**Pansch's fissure** (pahn′shəz) [Adolf *Pansch,* German anatomist, 1841–1887] see under *fissure.*

**pan·scle·ro·sis** (pan″sklə-ro′sis) [*pan-* + *sclerosis*] complete induration of a part or organ.

**pan·si·nu·itis** (pan″si-nu-i′tis) pansinusitis.

**pan·si·nus·ec·to·my** (pan″si-nəs-ek′tə-me) excision of the diseased membrane of all of the paranasal sinuses on one side.

**pan·si·nus·itis** (pan″si-nəs-i′tis) [*pan-* + *sinus* + *-itis*] inflammation involving all of the paranasal sinuses on one side.

**pan·sper·mia** (pan-sper′me-ə) [*pan-* + *sperm-* + *-ia*] 1. the doctrine of Anaxagoras and Democritus that the elements were a mixture of all the seeds of things. 2. panspermy.

**pan·sper·mic** (pan-sper′mik) pertaining to panspermy.

**pan·sper·my** (pan-sper′me) [*pan-* + Gr. *sperma* seed] the 19th-century hypothesis, opposed to spontaneous generation, that the atmosphere is full of invisible germs or reproductive bodies of plants and animals and that these germs penetrate the minutest crevices and develop upon finding a suitable soil or environment. See also *biogenesis* (def. 1). Called also *panspermia.*

**pan·sphyg·mo·graph** (pan-sfig′mo-graf) [*pan-* + *sphygmo-* + *-graph*] a device for recording cardiac, pulse, and chest movements at the same time.

**pan·sporo·blast** (pan-spor′o-blast) [*pan-* + *sporo-* + *-blast*] a disporoblastic sporont, i.e., a sporoblast that develops into two or more spores, with or without an enclosing membrane; characteristic of certain protozoa. See *Apansporoblastina* and *Pansporoblastina.*

**Pan·sporo·blas·ti·na** (pan″spor-o-blas-ti′nə) a suborder of parasitic protozoa (order Microsporida, class Microsporea) in which the sporulation sequence occurs in the host cell within a more or less persistent intracellular sporocyst (with a pansporoblastic membrane); organisms are often dimorphic, with another sporulation sequence not involving such a membrane. The sporoblasts and spores are usually uninucleate when the membrane is present and dinucleate when it is absent. Representative genera include *Amblyospora, Pleistophora,* and *Thelohania.*

**Pan·stron·gy·lus** (pan-stron′jə-ləs) [MeSH: Panstrongylus] a genus of cone-nosed bugs of the family Reduviidae, species of which are vectors of *Trypanosoma.*
**P. genicula′tus,** a vector of *Trypanosoma cruzi* in Panama and Brazil.
**P. infes′tans,** *Triatoma infestans.*
**P. megis′tus,** an important vector of *Trypanosoma cruzi* in Brazil; its local name is *barbeiro* because it frequently bites the face. Formerly called *Triatoma megista.*

**pan·ta·chro·mat·ic** (pan″tə-kro-mat′ik) [*pant-* + *achromatic*] entirely achromatic.

**pan·tal·gia** (pan-tal′jə) [*pant-* + *-algis*] pain over the whole body.

**pan·ta·mor·phia** (pan″tə-mor′fe-ə) [*pant-* + *amorphia*] complete or general deformity.

**pan·ta·mor·phic** (pan″tə-mor′fik) formless.

**pan·tan·en·ceph·a·ly** (pan″tan-ən-sef′ə-le) [*pant-* + *anencephaly*] complete anencephaly.

**pan·tan·ky·lo·bleph·a·ron** (pan-tang″kə-lo-blef′ə-ron) [*pant-* + *ankyloblepharon*] general adhesion of the eyelids to the eyeball and to each other.

**pan·ta·tro·phia** (pan″tə-tro′fe-ə) panatrophy.

**pan·tat·ro·phy** (pan-tat′rə-fe) panatrophy.

**Pan·ter·ic** (pan-ter′ik) trademark for a preparation of pancreatin.

**pan·te·the·ine** (pan-tə-the′in) [MeSH: Pantetheine] a naturally occurring amide of pantothenic acid and β-mercaptoethanolamine; it is an intermediate in the biosynthesis of coenzyme A, a growth factor for *Lactobacillus bulgaricus* and certain other bacteria, and a cofactor in certain enzyme complexes (e.g., in fatty acid or polypeptide synthesis).

**pan·the·nol** (pan′thə-nol) [USP] the alcohol derivative of pantothenic acid; is converted in the body to pantothenic acid, a member of the B-complex vitamins. Called also *pantothenyl alcohol* and *pantothenol.* The term is sometimes used to refer to the D(+) form of panthenol; see *dexpanthenol.*

**pan·thod·ic** (pan-thod′ik) [*pan-* + Gr. *hodos* way] radiating in every direction; said of nerve impulses.

**Pan·tho·lin** (pan′tho-lin) trademark for a preparation of calcium pantothenate.

**pant·ing** (pant′ing) rapid shallow breathing with a small tidal volume; cf. *tachypnea.*

**pant(o)-** [Gr. *pas,* gen. *pantos* all] a combining form meaning all, the whole.

**pan·to·chro·mism** (pan″to-kro′miz-əm) [*panto-* + *chrom-* + *-ism*] the phenomenon of existing in two or more differently colored forms, as a salt.

**pan·to·graph** (pan′to-graf) [*panto-* + *-graph*] an instrument for copying a plane figure to any desired scale.

**pan·to·ic ac·id** (pan-to′ik) a constituent of pantothenic acid remaining after cleavage of β-alanine.

**pan·to·mo·gra·phic** (pan-to″mo-graf′ik) pertaining to pantomography.

**pan·to·mog·ra·phy** (pan″to-mog′rə-fe) a method of tomography for visualization of body curved surfaces at any depth. In dentistry, it may be used for radiography of the maxillary and mandibular dental arches and their associated structures. Called also *panoramic radiography.*

**pan·to·mor·phia** (pan″to-mor′fe-ə) [*panto-* + *morph-* + *-ia*] 1. general or perfect symmetry. 2. ability to assume various shapes, as an ameba.

**pan·to·mor·phic** (pan″to-mor′fik) able to assume any shape.

**Pan·to·paque** (pan-to-pāk′) trademark for a preparation of iophendylate.

**pan·to·pho·bia** (pan″to-fo′be-ə) [*panto-* + *-phobia*] panphobia.

**pan·to·scop·ic** (pan″to-skop′ik) [*panto-* + Gr. *skopein* to examine] adapted to view both near and distant objects; a term applied to bifocal lenses.

**pan·to·then·ate** (pan-to′thən-āt) a salt of pantothenic acid.

**pan·to·the·nic ac·id** (pan″to-then′ik) [MeSH: Pantothenic Acid] the amide of β-alanine and pantoic acid, a B complex vitamin that is a constituent of coenzyme A; it is distributed ubiquitously in foods, and a deficiency syndrome has not been demonstrated in humans except by experimental administration of the pantothenic acid antagonist ω-methylpantothenic acid.

**pan·to·the·nol** (pan″to-the′nol) 1. panthenol. 2. dexpanthenol.

**pan·to·trop·ic** (pan″to-trop′ik) pantropic.

**pan·to·yl·tau·rine** (pan″to-əl-taw′rēn) a competitive inhibitor of pantothenic acid derived by replacement of the carboxyl group by a sulfonyl group; it is the amide of pantoic acid and taurine. Called also *thiopanic acid.*

**pan·trop·ic** (pan-trop′ik) [*pan-* + *-tropic*] having an affinity for many tissues; capable of attacking derivatives of any of the three embryonic layers.

**pan·tur·bi·nate** (pan-tur′bĭ-nāt) the entire structure of a nasal concha, including bone and soft tissue.

**Pa·num's area** (pah′noomz) [Peter Ludwig *Panum,* Danish physiologist, 1820–1885] see under *area.*

**pa·nus** (pa′nəs) [L. "swelling"] a lymphatic gland inflamed but not suppurating.

**pan·uve·itis** (pan″u-ve-i′tis) [MeSH: Panuveitis] inflammation of the entire uveal tract.

**Pan·war·fin** (pan-wawr′fin) trademark for a preparation of warfarin sodium.

**pan·zo·ot·ic** (pan″zo-ot′ik) [*pan-* + *zootic*] 1. occurring pandemically among animals. 2. a disease that is pandemic among animals. Called also *panepizootic.*

**PAP** 1. peroxidase-antiperoxidase; see under *technique.* 2. placental alkaline phosphatase.

**pa·pa·in** (pə-pa′in, pə-pi′in) [EC 3.4.22.2] [MeSH: Papain] 1. an enzyme of the hydrolase class that catalyzes the hydrolysis of proteins and peptides with preferential cleavage at bonds containing arginine, lysine, and glycine residues. It is obtained from the latex of the papaya tree, *Carica papaya.* 2. [USP] a purified preparation of papain used as a protein digestant and as a topical application for enzymatic débridement and promotion of normal healing of surface lesions.

**Pa·pa·ni·co·laou's stain, test (smear)** (pă″pə-nĭ″ko-la′o͞oz) [George Nicolas *Papanicolaou,* Greek physician and anatomist in the United States, 1883–1962] see under *stain* and *test.*

**Pa·pav·er** (pə-pav′ər) [MeSH: Papaver] a genus of flowering herbs of the family Papaveraceae. *P. somni′ferum,* a pink to purple species, and *P. al′bum,* a silvery white species, are the source of opium (q.v.) and of the poppy seeds (devoid of narcotic alkaloids) that are used as a condiment.

**Pa·pav·er·a·ceae** (pap″ə-vər-a′se-e) the poppies, a family of plants with often brightly colored flowers. It includes the genera *Argemone, Eschscholtzia,* and *Papaver.*

**pa·pav·er·ine hy·dro·chlo·ride** (pə-pav′ər-in) [USP] the hydrochloride salt of an opium alkaloid, which also may be synthesized; used as a smooth muscle relaxant, especially in the treatment of cerebral and peripheral ischemia associated with arterial spasm and myocardial ischemia complicated by arrhythmias, administered orally and intramuscularly.

**pa·paw** (paw′paw) 1. *Carica papaya.* 2. papaya (def. 2). 3. *Asimina triloba.* 4. the fruit of *A. triloba,* which is edible, although ingestion may cause severe skin irritation in sensitive persons; called also *pawpaw.*

**pa·pa·ya** (pah-pah′yah) [Sp.] 1. *Carica papaya.* 2. the fruit of *Carica papaya,* which contains the enzyme papain. Called also *papaw.*

**pa·per** (pa′pər) [MeSH: Paper] a substance manufactured in thin sheets, prepared from wood, rags, or other fibrous substance which has first been reduced to a pulp.
**alkannin p.,** filter paper dipped in an alcoholic solution of alkannin; alkalis turn it blue, acids red.
**aniline acetate p.,** filter paper dipped into a mixture of aniline, water, and glacial acetic acid and then dried.
**articulating p.,** paper strips coated with ink- or dye-containing wax, used for the marking or locating of occlusal interferences or deflective or interceptive occlusal contacts.
**azolitmin p.,** filter paper saturated with a solution of azolitmin; acids turn it purple to bright red, alkalis turn it blue.
**biuret p.,** filter paper previously dipped in Gies' biuret reagent, dried, and cut into strips.
**blue litmus p.,** see *litmus p.*
**Congo red p.,** wet filter paper with a 0.2 per cent solution of Congo red in water, dried, and cut in strips.
**filter p.,** a porous, unsized paper used as a filter.
**litmus p.,** bibulous paper impregnated with a solution of litmus, dried, and cut into strips. If slightly alkaline, the paper is blue and is used as a test for acids, which turn it red; if slightly acid, it is red and alkalis turn it blue.
**niter p.,** paper impregnated with potassium nitrate, ignited, and used as a moxa or by inhalation in asthma; called also *saltpeter p.*
**potassium nitrate p.,** niter p.
**red litmus p.,** see *litmus p.*
**saltpeter p.,** niter p.
**test p.,** paper that is impregnated with litmus or other indicator.
**turmeric p.,** paper dyed yellow with turmeric; alkalis turn it brown.

**Pa·pez circuit** (pah-pez′) [James Wenceslas *Papez,* American anatomist, 1883–1958] see under *circuit.*

**pa·pil·la** (pə-pil′ə) gen. and pl. *papil′lae* [L.] a small nipple-shaped projection, elevation, or structure.
**acoustic p.,** organum spirale.
**Bergmeister's p.,** 1. a small mass of neuroglial cells in the center of the embryonic optic disk, surrounding the bulb of the hyaloid artery. 2. a congenital anomaly consisting of a glial veil attached to the anterior aspect of the optic disk, resulting from glial proliferation around the remnants of the posterior part of the hyaloid vessel system.
**bile p.,** p. duodeni major.
**circumvallate papillae,** papillae vallatae.
**papil′lae co′nicae,** conical papillae: sparsely scattered large elevations on the tongue surface, often considered a modified type of filiform papillae.
**conoid papillae of tongue,** papillae conicae.
**p. co′rii,** TA alternative for *p. dermis.*
**p. of corium,** p. dermis.
**dental p., dentinal p., p. den′tis** [TA], a small mass of condensed mesenchymal tissue in the enamel organ, which differentiates into the dentin and dental pulp.
**p. der′matis, p. der′mis** [TA], dermal papilla: any of the conical extensions of the collagen fibers, the capillary blood vessels, and sometimes the nerves of the dermis into corresponding spaces among the downward- or inward-projecting rete ridges on the under surface of the epidermis. On the forehead and ear these are less prominent; on the face, neck, and pubes the relations are reversed and "rete pegs" extend inward or downward into spaces among a network of dermal ridges. Called also *p. corii* [TA alternative], *p. of corium,* and *skin p.*
**p. duc′tus paroti′dei** [TA], papilla of parotid duct: the small papilla marking the orifice of the parotid duct in the mucous membrane of the cheek.
**p. duode′ni ma′jor** [TA], major duodenal papilla: a small elevation at the site of the opening of the conjoined common bile duct and pancreatic duct into the lumen of the duodenum. Called also *p. duodeni [Santorini].* See also *p. duodeni minor.*
**p. duode′ni mi′nor** [TA], minor duodenal papilla: a small elevation at the site of the opening of the accessory pancreatic duct into the lumen of the duodenum. See also *p. duodeni major.*
**p. duode′ni [Santori′ni],** p. duodeni major.
**papil′lae filifor′mes** [TA], filiform papillae: threadlike elevations that cover most of the tongue surface.
**papil′lae folia′tae** [TA], foliate papillae: parallel mucosal folds on the margins of the tongue at the junction of its body and root.
**papil′lae fungifor′mes** [TA], fungiform papillae: knoblike projections on the tongue, scattered singly among the filiform papillae.
**p. gingiva′lis** [TA], gingival papilla: a cone-shaped pad of the interdental gingiva filling the space between two contiguous teeth up to the contact area, as viewed from the labial, buccal, or lingual aspect; called also *interdental p., p. interdentalis* [TA alternative], and *interproximal p.* See also *interdental gingiva,* under *gingiva.*
**hair p.,** p. pili.
**ileal p., p. ilea′lis** [TA], the conical projection formed by the terminal ileum at the junction of the cecum and the ileum and extending into the large intestine, as seen in the living individual; called also *ileocecal p., p. ileocaecalis,* and *valva ilealis.* See also *ostium papillae ilealis.*

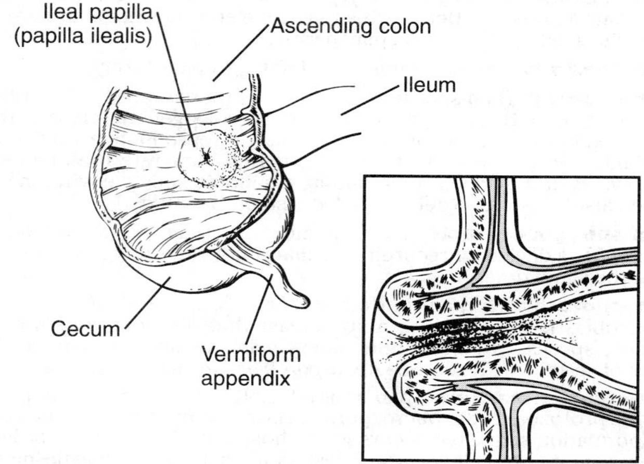


**p. ileocaeca′lis, ileocecal p.,** p. ilealis.
**p. incisi′va** [TA], incisive papilla: a rounded projection at the anterior end of the raphe of the palate.
**interdental p.,** p. gingivalis.
**p. interdenta′lis,** TA alternative for *p. gingivalis.*
**interproximal p.,** p. gingivalis.
**p. lacrima′lis** [TA], lacrimal papilla: a papilla in the conjunctiva near the medial angle of the eye.
**papil′lae lenticula′res,** lenticular papillae: a series of papillae of the tongue resembling, but less elevated than, the fungiform papillae.
**papil′lae lingua′les** [TA], lingual papillae: the filiform, fungiform, vallate, foliate, and conical papillae of the tongue.
**major duodenal p.,** p. duodeni major.
**p. mam′mae, p. mamma′ria** [TA], **mammary p.,** nipple of the breast: the pigmented projection on the anterior surface of the mammary gland, surrounded by the areola; the lactiferous ducts open onto it. Called also *mammilla, nipple, teat,* and *thelium.*
**minor duodenal p.,** p. duodeni minor.
**nerve p., nervous p.,** neurothele.
**p. ner′vi op′tici,** discus nervi optici.
**optic p.,** discus nervi optici.
**palatine p.,** p. incisiva.
**parotid p., p. paroti′dea,** p. ductus parotidei.
**p. pi′li,** hair papilla: the fibrovascular mesodermal papilla enclosed within the hair bulb.
**p. rena′lis** [TA], renal papilla: one of the blunted apices of the renal pyramids, which project into the renal sinus.
**retromolar p.,** a small papilla of gingival tissue located at the foot of the ramus of the mandible and attached to the most inferior part of the anterior border of the ramus.
**p. of Santorini,** p. duodeni major.
**simple papillae of tongue,** papillae filiformes.
**skin p.,** p. dermis.
**p. spira′lis,** organum spirale.
**sublingual p.,** caruncula sublingualis.
**tactile p.,** corpusculum tactus.

**urethral p.,** a slight elevation in the vestibule of the vagina on which is situated the external orifice of the urethra.
**papil'lae valla'tae** [TA], vallate papillae: the largest papillae of the tongue, 8 to 12 in number, arranged in the form of a V anterior to the sulcus terminalis of the tongue.
**p. of Vater,** p. duodeni major.

**pa·pil·lae** (pə-pil'e) [L.] genitive and plural of *papilla.*

**pap·il·lary** (pap'ĭ-lar″e) pertaining to or resembling a papilla, or nipple.

**pap·il·late** (pap'ĭ-lāt) marked by nipplelike elevations.

**pap·il·lec·to·my** (pap″ĭ-lek'tə-me) [*papilla* + *-ectomy*] excision of a papilla.

**pa·pil·le·de·ma** (pap″il-ə-de'mə) [MeSH: Papilledema] choked disk; edema of the optic disk (papilla), most commonly due to increased intracranial pressure, malignant hypertension, or thrombosis of the central retinal vein.

**pap·il·lif·er·ous** (pap″ĭ-lif'ər-əs) [*papilla* + *-ferous*] bearing papillae.

**pa·pil·li·form** (pə-pil'ĭ-form) [*papilla* + *form*] shaped like a papilla.

**pa·pil·li·tis** (pap″ĭ-li'tis) [*papilla* + *-itis*] 1. inflammation of a papilla. 2. a form of optic neuritis involving the optic papilla (disk).
**necrotizing p., necrotizing renal p.,** renal papillary necrosis.

**pa·pil·lo·ad·e·no·cys·to·ma** (pə-pil″o-ad″ə-no-sis-to'mə) papillary cystadenoma (def. 1).

**pa·pil·lo·car·ci·no·ma** (pə-pil″o-kahr″sĭ-no'mə) papillary carcinoma.

**pap·il·lo·ma** (pap″ĭ-lo'mə) [*papilla* + *-oma*] [MeSH: Papilloma] a benign epithelial neoplasm producing finger-like or verrucous projections from the epithelial surface. Called also *papillary tumor, villoma,* and *villous p.* or *tumor.*
**choroid plexus p.,** a slow-growing benign tumor of the choroid plexus that often invades the leptomeninges. In children it is usually in a lateral ventricle but in adults it is more often in the fourth ventricle. Hydrocephalus is common, either from obstruction or from tumor secretion of cerebrospinal fluid. If it undergoes malignant transformation it is called a *choroid plexus carcinoma.*
**cockscomb p.,** papilloma of the uterine cervix that occurs during pregnancy and regresses following delivery; it is a small, red lesion that projects above the surrounding mucosa and resembles a cockscomb.
**cutaneous p.,** acrochordon.
**fibroepithelial p.,** a type of papilloma containing extensive fibrous tissue; called also *fibropapilloma.*
**hirsutoid p's of penis,** pearly penile papules.
**intracanalicular p.,** an arborizing, nonmalignant growth within the ducts of certain glands, especially of the breast.
**intracystic p.,** a papilloma formed within a cyst of a cystadenoma.
**intraductal p.,** a tumor in a lactiferous duct, usually attached to the wall by a stalk; a distinction is often made between the solitary type (tumors found in just one duct and often benign) and the multiple type (tumors found in several or many ducts, often bilaterally, and often premalignant). The solitary type often has a serous or bloody discharge from the nipple, whereas the multiple type does not.
**inverted p.,** papilloma in which the proliferating epithelial cells invaginate into the underlying stroma; it usually occurs in the nasal cavity, urinary bladder, or oral soft tissues *(inverted ductal p.)* of middle-aged males.
**inverted ductal p.,** an intraductal papilloma of the salivary glands, presenting as a nodular submucosal mass in the oral cavity of adults.
**inverted schneiderian p.,** a neoplasm of the nasal wall, having destructive capacity, a tendency to recur, and a potential for malignancy.
**rabbit p.,** a viral disease of rabbits marked by the formation of horny warts. These papillomas were the first mammalian tumors shown to be induced by a virus (by Shope in 1933) and the first to be transmitted by purified viral DNA. Called also *Shope p.*
**Shope p.,** rabbit p.
**squamous p.,** a papilloma composed of squamous epithelium, such as commonly occurs in the oral cavity.
**villous p.,** papilloma.

**pap·il·lo·ma·to·sis** (pap″ĭ-lo-mə-to'sis) the development of multiple papillomas.
**bovine p.,** an infectious disease of cattle, caused by a papillomavirus and characterized by the development of multiple warts with connective tissue proliferation, occurring mainly on the teats and udder in dairy cattle and the head and neck in beef cattle; calves are affected more often than adults.
**canine oral p., canine viral p.,** a benign viral disease of young dogs, characterized by papillomas on the oral mucous membranes that usually resolve spontaneously in a few weeks; the cause is a papillomavirus.
**confluent and reticulate p.,** a progressive, pruritic papillomatosis, probably a genodermatosis, seen chiefly in girls, especially those at or near puberty, beginning in the intramammary and midback areas as slightly keratotic pigmented papules that increase in size and spread over the trunk and other body areas; centrally located lesions tend to become confluent and peripherally located ones to become reticulate. Called also *Gougerot-Carteaud syndrome.*
**equine p.,** an infectious disease of horses, caused by a papillomavirus and characterized by the development of warts, usually around the face but occasionally around the genitals; it primarily affects animals younger than two years old.
**florid p. of nipple,** nipple adenoma.
**juvenile laryngeal p., juvenile laryngotracheobronchial p., recurrent respiratory p.,** the recurrent growth of benign squamous cell papillomas in the larynx and trachea, caused by the human papillomavirus, and leading to severe narrowing of the airway that may require frequent treatments; onset is in childhood or early adulthood.
**subareolar duct p.,** nipple adenoma.

**pap·il·lom·a·tous** (pap″ĭ-lo'mə-təs) of the nature of a papilloma.

**Pa·pil·lo·ma·vi·rus** (pap″ĭ-lo'mə-vi″rəs) [*papilloma* + *virus*] [MeSH: Papillomavirus] papillomaviruses; a genus of viruses family Papovaviridae that induce papillomas in humans and in many animal species. Papillomaviruses are highly species-specific and have a tropism for squamous epithelium; some have been associated with malignancy.

**pap·il·lo·ma·vi·rus** (pap″ĭ-lo'mə-vi″rəs) [MeSH: Papillomavirus] any virus of the genus *Papillomavirus.*
**bovine p.,** species (BPV-1, -2, and -4) that cause bovine papillomatosis; there are at least six types with no immunological cross-reactivity, each type producing a characteristic lesion. Called also *bovine papillomatosis virus.*
**cottontail rabbit p.,** a species that causes rabbit papilloma.
**equine p.,** a species that causes equine papillomatosis.
**human p. (HPV),** any of a number of species, comprising at least 70 types, that cause warts, particularly plantar warts and genital warts, on the skin and mucous membranes in humans, transmitted by either direct or indirect contact; some are associated with malignancies of the genital tract.
**rabbit p.,** cottontail rabbit p.

**Pa·pil·lon-Le·fèvre syndrome** (pah″pe-yaw' lə-fev'rə) [M.M. *Papillon,* French dermatologist, 20th century; Paul *Lefèvre,* French dermatologist, 20th century] see under *syndrome.*

**pap·il·lo·ret·i·ni·tis** (pap″ĭ-lo-ret″ĭ-ni'tis) inflammation of the optic papilla extending to the retina.

**pap·il·lo·sphinc·ter·ot·o·my** (pap″ĭ-lo-sfingk″tər-ot'ə-me) surgical division of the sphincter of the major duodenal papilla (Oddi's sphincter).

**pap·il·lo·tome** (pap'ĭ-lo-tōm″) a cutting instrument for incising the major duodenal papilla.

**pap·il·lot·o·my** (pap″ĭ-lot'ə-me) incision of a papilla, as of the duodenal papilla.

**Pa·po·va·vi·ri·dae** (pə-po″və-vir'ĭ-de) [MeSH: Papovaviridae] the papovaviruses: a family of DNA viruses having a nonenveloped icosahedral virion 40 nm (polyomaviruses) or 55 nm (papillomaviruses) in diameter with 72 capsomers in skew arrangement. The genome consists of a single circular molecule of double-stranded DNA (MW $3–5 \times 10^6$, size 5 kbp for polyomaviruses and 8 kbp for papillomaviruses). Viruses contain five to seven structural proteins and are resistant to ether, acids, and heat. Replication and assembly occur in the nucleus; virions are released by cell destruction. Host range is generally narrow; transmission is by contact or by airborne particles, and many species are oncogenic. There are two genera, *Papovavirus* and *Polyomavirus.*

**pa·po·va·vi·rus** (pə-po'və-vi″rəs) [from *pa*pilloma *po*lyoma *va*cuolating agent (SV40) + *virus*] [MeSH: Papovaviridae] any virus of the family Papovaviridae.
**lymphotropic p. (LPV),** a polyomavirus originally isolated from a B-lymphoblastic cell line of an African green monkey; antigenically related viruses are widespread in primates and may infect humans.

**Pap·pen·heim's stain** (pahp'ən-hīmz) [Artur *Pappenheim,* German physician, 1870–1916] see under *stain.*

**pap·pose** (pap'ōs) having a downy surface.

**pap·u·lar** (pap'u-lər) [L. *papularis*] consisting of, characterized by, or pertaining to a papule.

**pap·u·la·tion** (pap″u-la'shən) the production of papules.

**pap·ule** (pap'ūl) [L. *papula*] a small circumscribed, superficial, solid elevation of the skin less than 1 cm (0.5 cm according to some authorities) in diameter.
**Gottron's p's,** a cutaneous manifestation pathognomonic of dermatomyositis, consisting of flat-topped violaceous papules on the

dorsal aspect of the interphalangeal joints of the hand, which develop central atrophy with hypopigmentation and telangiectasia; see also *Gottron's sign* (def. 1).. Called also *Gottron's sign.*
**moist p., mucous p.,** condyloma latum.
**painful piezogenic pedal p's,** piezogenic p's.
**pearly penile p's,** numerous tiny white, dome-shaped asymptomatic angiofibromas occurring circumferentially around the penile coronal sulcus. Called also *hirsutoid papillomas of penis.*
**piezogenic p's,** transitory, noninflammatory, soft, sometimes painful, large papules appearing above the heel on the side of one or both feet, elicited by weight bearing associated with prolonged standing or running, and presumed to result from temporary herniation of fat tissue together with its blood vessels and nerves through connective tissue defects. They disappear when the pressure is removed. Called also *painful fat herniation* and *painful piezogenic pedal p's.*
**prurigo p.,** see *prurigo.*
**split p's,** fissured papular syphilides sometimes seen at the corners of the mouth.

**pap·u·lo·er·y·the·ma·tous** (pap″u-lo-er″ə-them′ə-təs) marked by papules on an erythematous surface.

**pap·u·loid** (pap′u-loid) resembling a papule; papular.

**pap·u·lo·pus·tu·lar** (pap″u-lo-pus′tu-lər) characterized by the presence of papules and pustules.

**pap·u·lo·sis** (pap-u-lo′sis) a state marked by the presence of multiple papules.
**bowenoid p.,** benign reddish brown papules occurring primarily on the genitalia, particularly the penis, in young adults; a viral etiology is suspected and the histologic features are those of squamous cell carcinoma in situ, identical to Bowen's disease.
**lymphomatoid p.,** a usually benign, self-healing, recurrent eruption of hemorrhagic papules, similar to acute lichenoid pityriasis (of which it may be a variant); lesions occur asynchronously primarily on the trunk and extremities and, after healing, either leave macular scars or form crusted scales or a central necrotic mass. Histologic features may suggest malignancy and include clusters of large mononuclear cells with dark-staining nuclei and large pale-staining histoid cells.
**malignant atrophic p.,** an often fatal disease occurring most often in men, characterized by endovasculitis of the skin, gastrointestinal tract, and sometimes other organs, resulting in ischemic infarction of involved tissues. Cutaneous lesions occur in crops of erythematous papules that become umbilicated with characteristic porcelain-white centers with telangiectatic borders, many of which atrophy and leave white scars. Called also *Degos' disease* or *syndrome.*

**pap·u·lo·squa·mous** (pap″u-lo-squa′məs) both papular and scaly; used to denote a group of dermatoses so characterized, including psoriasis, pityriasis rosea, lichen planus, seborrheic dermatitis, and parapsoriasis.

**pap·u·lo·ve·sic·u·lar** (pap″u-lo-və-sik′u-lər) characterized by the presence of papules and vesicles.

**pap·y·ra·ceous** (pap″ĭ-ra′shəs) [L. *papyraceus*] like paper; chartaceous.

**par-** see *para-.*

**para** (par′ə) [L. *parere* to bring forth, to bear] a woman who has produced viable young regardless of whether the child was living at birth. Used with Roman numerals to designate the number of pregnancies that have resulted in the birth of viable offspring, as *para 0* (none—nullipara), *para I* (one—primipara), *para II* (two—secundipara), *para III* (three—tripara), *para IV* (four—quadripara), etc. Since the number indicates how many pregnancies, a multiple birth counts as just one in the calculation. Symbol P. Cf. *gravida.*

**para-** [Gr. *para* to, at, or from the side of] 1. a prefix meaning *(a)* beside, near, *(b)* resembling, *(c)* accessory to, *(d)* beyond, *(e)* apart from, *(f)* abnormal. 2. symbol *p-*; in organic chemistry, a prefix indicating a 1,4-substituted benzene ring, e.g., *p*-xylene (1,4-dimethylbenzene) or *p*-nitrophenol (4-nitrophenol).

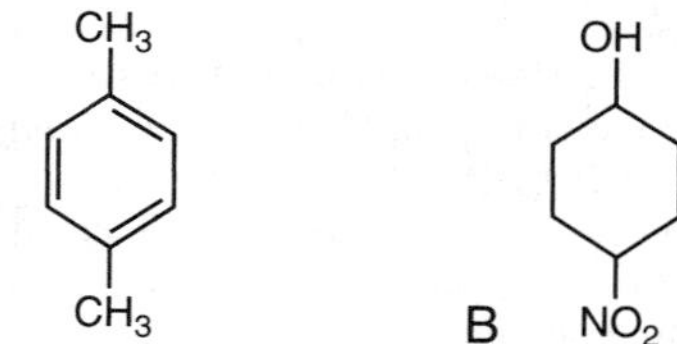


Two examples of disubstituted benzene derivatives with substituents in the *para-* position. *(A), p*-xylene (1,4-dimethylbenzene); *(B), p*-nitrophenol.

**para·ad·ven·ti·tial** (par″ə-ad″vən-tĭ′shəl) near the tunica adventitia.

**para·am·i·no·ben·zo·ic ac·id** (par″ə-ə-me″no-bən-zo′ik) *p*-aminobenzoic acid.

**para·ami·no·hip·pu·ric ac·id** (par″ə-ə-me″-no-hĭ-pūr′ik) *p*-aminohippuric acid.

**para·ami·no·sal·i·cyl·ic ac·id** (par″ə-ə-me″no-sal-ĭ-sil′ik) *p*-aminosalicylic acid.

**para·an·al·ge·sia** (par″ə-an″əl-je′ze-ə) analgesia of the lower part of the body, including the lower limbs. Called also *paranalgesia.*

**para·an·es·the·sia** (par″ə-an″əs-the′zhə) anesthesia of the lower part of the body and of the legs. Called also *paranesthesia.*

**para·aor·tic** (par″ə-a-or′tik) situated near or next to the aorta.

**para·ap·pen·di·ci·tis** (par″ə-ə-pen″dĭ-si′tis) inflammation of tissues adjacent to the vermiform appendix.

**para·ban·ic ac·id** (par″ə-ban′ik) the cyclic anhydride of oxaluric acid, an oxidation product of urea.

**par·ab·i·on** (par-ab′e-on) parabiont.

**par·ab·i·ont** (par-ab′e-ont) [*para-* + Gr. *bioun* to live] one of two or more organisms living in a condition of parabiosis.

**para·bio·sis** (par″ə-bi-o′sis) [*para-* + *biosis*] [MeSH: Parabiosis] the union of two individuals, as of conjoined twins or of experimental animals by surgical operation.
**dialytic p.,** the circulation of the blood of two individuals through a dialyzer, separated by a membrane which permits the removal of harmful material from the recipient's blood and the contribution of essential factors from the donor's blood.
**vascular p.,** the crossing of the circulation between two individuals by anastomosis of blood vessels.

**para·bi·ot·ic** (par″ə-bi-ot′ik) pertaining to or characterized by parabiosis.

**para·blast** (par′ə-blast) [*para-* + *-blast*] that part of the mesoblast from which the blood vessels, lymphatics, etc., are developed.

**para·blas·tic** (par″ə-blas′tik) pertaining to the parablast.

**para·bu·lia** (par″ə-bu′le-ə) [*para-* + Gr. *boulē* will + *-ia*] perversion of the will, as when an individual intends to perform a particular action but halts and substitutes either an opposite action or an unrelated alternative; usually seen in schizophrenics.

**para·car·di·ac** (par″ə-kahr′de-ak) beside the heart.

**para·car·mine** (par″ə-kahr′mēn) a staining medium consisting of carminic acid, calcium chloride, and alcohol.

**para·ca·sein** (par″ə-ka′sēn) the chemical product of the action of rennin on casein; see *casein.*

**par·a·cel·si·an** (par″ə-sel′se-ən) pertaining to or named for Paracelsus.

**Par·a·cel·sus** (par″ə-sel′səs) (pseudonym of Philipus Aureolus Theophrastus Bombastus von Hohenheim, Swiss physician and alchemist [1493–1541]) the "Luther of Medicine," he defied the authority of Galen and Avicenna and condemned all medical teaching not based on experience. His alchemical researches led to the introduction of such substances as lead, sulfur, iron, and arsenic into pharmaceutical chemistry. Although he was far ahead of his time in many of his observations (e.g., on metabolic and on occupational diseases), much of his thinking was made obscure by his mysticism.

**para·cen·es·the·sia** (par″ə-se″nəs-the′zhə) [*para-* + *cenesthesia*] any abnormality of the general sense of well-being.

**para·cen·te·sis** (par″ə-sən-te′sis) [*para-* + *-centesis*] [MeSH: Paracentesis] surgical puncture of a cavity with a needle or other hollow instrument for diagnostic or therapeutic aspiration of fluid.

**para·cen·tet·ic** (par″ə-sən-tet′ik) pertaining to or accomplished by paracentesis.

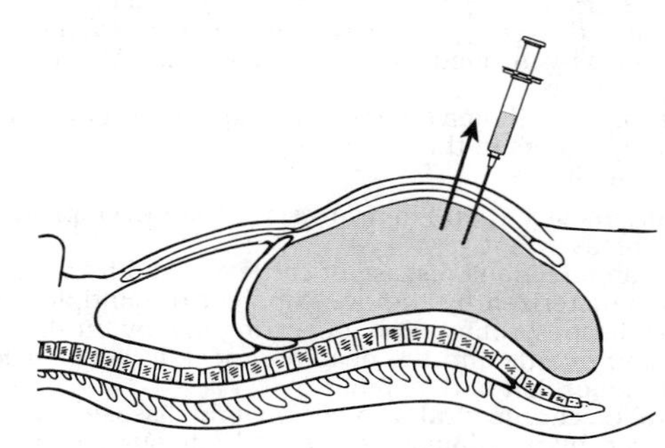

Paracentesis of the abdominal cavity.

**para·cen·tral** (par″ə-sen′trəl) near a center.

**para·ceph·a·lus** (par″ə-sef′ə-ləs) [*para-* + *-cephalus*] a fetus with a rudimentary or misshapen head, imperfect sense organs, and defective trunk or limbs.

**para·cer·e·bel·lar** (par″ə-ser″ə-bel′ər) pertaining to the lateral part of the cerebellum.

**para·cer·vix** (par″ə-ser′viks) [*para-* + *cervix*] [TA] the inferior part of the parametrium.

**par·ac·et·al·de·hyde** (par-as″ət-al′də-hīd) paraldehyde.

**par·ac·et·am·ol** (par-as″ət-am′ol) acetaminophen.

**pa·ra·chlo·ro·met·a·xy·le·nol** (par″ə-klor″o-met″ə-zi′lə-nol) chloroxylenol.

**para·chlo·ro·phe·nol** (par″ə-klor″o-fe′nol) [USP] an antibacterial effective against most gram-negative organisms; used as a topical anti-infective.
**camphorated p.** [USP], a preparation of 33–37 per cent parachlorophenol and 63–67 per cent camphor, used as a dental anti-infective; applied topically to the root canals and the periapical region.

**para·chol·era** (par″ə-kol′ər-ə) a disease resembling Asiatic cholera, but caused by an organism other than *Vibrio cholerae.*

**para·chor·dal** (par″ə-kor′dəl) [*para-* + *chordal*] situated beside the notochord; see *parachordal cartilages,* under *cartilage.*

**Par·a·chor·do·des** (par″ə-kor-do′dēz) a genus of the class Nematomorpha. A few cases of human infection with the species *P. pustilo′sus, P. tolosa′nus,* and *P. viola′ceus* have been reported from France and Italy.

**para·chro·ma·tin** (par″ə-kro′mə-tin) a chromatophil substance contained in the finer part of the nuclear substance, as in the nucleoplasm of the spindle in karyokinesis.

**para·chro·ma·tism** (par″ə-kro′mə-tiz-əm) dichromasy.

**para·chro·ma·top·sia** (par″ə-kro″mə-top′se-ə) dichromasy.

**para·ci·ne·sia** (par″ə-si-ne′zhə) parakinesia.

**para·ci·ne·sis** (par″ə-si-ne′sis) parakinesia.

**para·clin·i·cal** (par″ə-klin′ĭ-kəl) pertaining to abnormalities (e.g., morphological or biochemical) underlying clinical manifestations (e.g., chest pain or fever).

**Para·coc·cid·i·oi·des** (par″ə-kok-sid″e-oi′dēz) [MeSH: Paracoccidioides] a genus of Fungi Imperfecti of the form-family Moniliaceae. *P. brasilien′sis* (called also *Blastomyces brasiliensis*) is the species that causes paracoccidioidomycosis; organisms proliferate by multiple budding yeast cells in the tissues, and produce white aerial mycelia and single or double conidia in media at 25°C. or in soil.

**para·coc·cid·i·oi·do·my·co·sis** (par″ə-kok-sid″e-oi″do-mi-ko′sis) [MeSH: Paracoccidioidomycosis] an often fatal infection caused by *Paracoccidioides brasiliensis.* The primary infection begins in the lungs and spreads to the mucocutaneous areas, particularly the buccal mucosa, and may extend to the adjacent skin, tonsils, gastrointestinal lymphatics, liver, and spleen. Called also *Almeida's* or *Lutz-Splendore-Almeida disease, Brazilian* or *South American blastomycosis,* and *paracoccidioidal granuloma.*

**para·co·li·tis** (par″ə-ko-li′tis) inflammation of the outer coat of the colon.

**Para·col·o·bac·trum** (par″ə-kol″o-bak′trəm) in former systems of classification, a genus of bacteria made up of nonlactose-fermenting coliform organisms that are now assigned to various other genera.

**para·col·pi·tis** (par″ə-kol-pi′tis) [*para-* + *colp-* + *-itis*] inflammation of the tissues around the vagina.

**para·col·pi·um** (par″ə-kol′pe-əm) [*para-* + Gr. *kolpos* vagina] the connective and other tissues that surround the vagina.

**para·cone** (par′ə-kōn) [*para-* + Gr. *kōnos* cone] the mesiobuccal cusp of a maxillary tooth of mammals, which normally occludes between the paraconid and hypoconid of the corresponding lower molar.

**para·co·nid** (par″ə-ko′nid) the mesiobuccal cusp of a mandibular molar tooth.

**para·cor·tex** (par″ə-kor′teks) [*para-* + *cortex*] thymus-dependent area.

**par·acou·sis** (par″ə-koo′sis) paracusia.

**para·cox·al·gia** (par″ə-kok-sal′jə) a condition marked by pain simulating that of coxitis.

**para·crine** (par′ə-krin) [*para-* + Gr. *krinein* to separate] denoting a type of hormone function in which hormone synthesized in and released from endocrine cells binds to its receptor in nearby cells of a different type and affects their function.

**par·acu·sia** (par″ə-ku′se-ə) 1. any deficiency in the sense of hearing; see also *deafness.* Called also *paracusis* and *paracousis.* 2. auditory hallucination.
**p. lo′ci,** inability to locate correctly the origin of sounds.
**p. willisia′na,** paradoxic hearing loss.

**par·acu·sis** (par″ə-ku′sis) paracusia.
**p. of Willis,** paradoxic hearing loss.

**para·cys·tic** (par″ə-sis′tik) [*para-* + *cyst-* + *-ic*] situated near the bladder.

**para·cys·ti·tis** (par″ə-sis-ti′tis) [*para-* + *cyst-* + *-itis*] inflammation of the tissues around the bladder.

**para·cys·ti·um** (par″ə-sis′te-əm) [*para-* + Gr. *kystis* bladder] the connective and other tissues around the bladder.

**para·cyt·ic** (par″ə-sit′ik) [*para-* + *cyt-* + *-ic*] denoting cell elements present in the blood or other part of the organism, but enthetic or not normal to it.

**para·den·tal** (par″ə-den′təl) 1. having some connection with or relation to the science or practice of dentistry. 2. periodontal.

**para·den·ti·tis** (par″ə-dən-ti′tis) periodontitis.

**para·den·ti·um** (par″ə-den′she-əm) periodontium, def. 2.

**para·den·to·sis** (par″ə-dən-to′sis) juvenile periodontitis.

**para·derm** (par′ə-dərm) [*para-* + *-derm*] the part of the vitellus of the ovum that furnishes cells which contribute to the body of the embryo.

**para·des·mose** (par″ə-des′mōs) [*para-* + *desmose*] the connection between extranuclear centrioles during mitosis in certain protozoa; see *desmose.*

**para·did·y·mal** (par″ə-did′ĭ-məl) 1. pertaining to the paradidymis. 2. beside the testis.

**para·did·y·mis** (par″ə-did′ĭ-mis) [*para-* + Gr. *didymos* testis] [TA] a body made up of a few convoluted tubules in the anterior part of the spermatic cord, considered to be a remnant of the mesonephros; called also *organ of Giraldés, parepididymis,* and *massa innominata.*

**para·di·meth·yl·ami·no·benz·al·de·hyde** (par″ə-di-meth″əl-ə-me″no-ben-zal′də-hīd) white or pale yellow crystals or crystalline powder, used in the preparation of Ehrlich's aldehyde reagent and in the determination of urobilinogen and porphobilinogen.

**Para·di·one** (par″ə-di′ōn) trademark for preparations of paramethadione.

**para·dip·sia** (par″ə-dip′se-ə) [*para-* + *dipsia*] an abnormally increased appetite for fluids, which are ingested without relation to bodily need.

**para·dox** (par′ə-doks) [Gr. *paradoxos* incredible] a statement which seems to be, though it may not be, absurd or self-contradictory.
**Opie p.,** necrotizing local anaphylaxis sometimes acts as a specific protective mechanism.
**Simpson's p.,** a form of extreme confounding (q.v.) such that an association between two variables is actually reversed after adjusting for a third.
**Weber's p.,** the elongation of a muscle which has been so stretched that it cannot contract.

**para·dox·i·cal** (par″ə-dok′sĭ-kəl) occurring at variance with the normal rule.

**para·dys·en·tery** (par″ə-dis′ən-ter′e) a diarrhea resembling mild dysentery, caused by *Shigella flexneri.*

**para·ec·cri·sis** (par″ə-ek′rĭ-sis) [*para-* + *-eccrisis*] disordered secretion or excretion.

**para·epi·lep·sy** (par″ə-ep′ĭ-lep-se) minor focal epilepsy.

**para·esoph·a·ge·al** (par″ə-e-sof″ə-je′əl) alongside, near, or about the esophagus.

**para·falx** (par″ə-falks′) situated near the falx cerebri or falx cerebelli.

**Par. aff.** abbreviation for L. *pars affec′ta,* the part affected.

**par·af·fin** (par′ə-fin) [L. *parum* little + *affinis* akin] [MeSH: Paraffin] 1. [NF] a purified mixture of solid hydrocarbons obtained from petroleum, occurring as an odorless, tasteless, colorless or white, more or less translucent mass; used as a stiffening agent in pharmaceutical preparations. 2. alkane.
**hard p.,** paraffin, def. 1.
**liquid p.,** mineral oil.
**liquid p., light,** light mineral oil.
**soft p., white,** white petrolatum.
**soft p., yellow,** petrolatum.
**synthetic p.** [NF], paraffin synthesized by catalytic conversion of carbon monoxide and hydrogen to a mixture of paraffin hydrocarbons; used as a stiffening agent in pharmaceutical preparations.

**par·af·fin·o·ma** (par″ə-fin-o′mə) a chronic granuloma produced by prolonged continuous exposure to the irritation of paraffin.

**Par·a·fi·la·ria** (par″ə-fĭ-lar′e-ə) a genus of nematodes of the superfamily Filarioides that infect ruminants. *P. bovi′cola* causes dermatorrhagia parasitica (summer bleeding) in cattle. *P. multipapillo′sa* causes the same condition in horses.

**Par·a·flex** (par′ə-fleks) trademark for a preparation of chlorzoxazone.

**para·floc·cu·lus** (par″ə-flok′u-ləs) [*para-* + *flocculus*] a small lobe of the cerebellar hemisphere, located immediately cranial to the flocculus and sometimes forming a prominent part of the cerebellum. Called also *accessory flocculus.*
**p. ventra′lis,** TA alternative for *tonsilla cerebelli.*
**ventral p.**, tonsilla cerebelli.

**Para·fon for·te** (par′ə-fon for′tā) trademark for a preparation of chlorzoxazone.

**para·for·mal·de·hyde** (par″ə-for-mal′də-hīd) a white, crystalline polymer of formaldehyde.

**Para·fos·sar·u·lus** (par″ə-fŏ-sar′u-ləs) a genus of fresh water snails of the family Bulimidae.
**P. manchou′ricus,** a species found in eastern Asia and nearby islands. It is the foremost intermediate host of the liver fluke *Opisthorchis sinensis* in Japan and the second most important in China, as well as a carrier of the flukes *O. felineus* and *Echinochasmus perfoliatus.*

**para·func·tion** (par′ə-funk″shən) disordered or abnormal function.

**para·func·tion·al** (par″ə-funk′shən-əl) characterized by disordered or abnormal function.

**para·gam·ma·cism** (par″ə-gam′ə-siz-əm) [*para-* + Gr. *gamma,* the Greek letter G] gammacism.

**para·gan·glia** (par″ə-gang′gle-ə) plural of *paraganglion.*

**para·gan·gli·o·ma** (par″ə-gang″gle-o′mə) [MeSH: Paraganglioma] a tumor of the tissue composing the paraganglia.
**medullary p.**, pheochromocytoma.
**nonchromaffin p.**, chemodectoma.

**para·gan·gli·on** (par″ə-gang′gle-on) pl. *paragan′glia.* A collection of chromaffin cells, derived from neural ectoderm, occurring elsewhere than in the adrenal medulla, usually near the sympathetic ganglia and in relation to the aorta and its branches. Most, if not all, paraganglia secrete epinephrine or norepinephrine. Called also *chromaffin body* and *pheochrome body.*

**para·gen·i·ta·lis** (par″ə-gen″ĭ-ta′lis) [*para-* + L. *genitalis* genital] 1. in lower vertebrates, the urinary part of the mesonephros, caudal to the genital part. 2. in higher animals, the paradidymis or paroöphoron.

**para·geu·sia** (par″ə-goo′zhə) [*para-* + Gr. *geusis* taste + *-ia*] 1. perversion of the sense of taste. 2. a bad taste in the mouth. Called also *dysgeusia.*

**para·geu·sic** (par″ə-goo′zik) pertaining to or characterized by parageusia.

**par·ag·na·thus** (pə-rag′nə-thəs) [*para-* + Gr. *gnathos* jaw] 1. a fetus with a supernumerary jaw. 2. in asymmetrical conjoined twins, a parasitic fetus attached laterally to the jaw of the more developed fetus.

**par·ag·no·sis** (par″əg-no′sis) [*para-* + Gr. *gnōsis* knowledge] diagnosis, after death, based on contemporaneous accounts of the diseases which affected historical characters.

**par·a·gon·i·mi·a·sis** (par″ə-gon″ĭ-mi′ə-sis) [MeSH: Paragonimiasis] infection with flukes of the genus *Paragonimus;* characterized by bronchitis, bronchiectasis, and tuberculoid symptoms. Called also *lung fluke disease, paragonimosis,* and *pulmonary distomiasis.*

**par·a·gon·i·mo·sis** (par″ə-gon″ĭ-mo′sis) paragonimiasis.

**Par·a·gon·i·mus** (par″ə-gon′ĭ-məs) [*para-* + Gr. *gonimos* productive; having generative power] [MeSH: Paragonimus] a genus of trematodes of the family Troglotrematidae; they have two invertebrate hosts, the first a snail such as *Semisulcospira,* and the second a crab or crayfish such as *Potamon* or *Eriocheir.*
**P. africa′nus,** a species of the Congo and Cameroon that parasitizes humans and carnivores.
**P. heterotre′ma,** a species infecting humans in Thailand and China.
**P. kellicot′ti,** a species closely allied to *P. westermani,* found in cats, dogs, and hogs in the United States.
**P. rin′geri,** *P. westermani.*
**P. westerma′ni,** the lung fluke; it is oval or pear-shaped, pink to reddish brown in color, and found in cysts in the lungs and sometimes in the pleura, liver, abdominal cavity, and elsewhere. It causes parasitic hemoptysis in humans and other animals, especially in Asia. Infection is acquired through ingestion of infected freshwater crabs or crayfish. Called also *Distoma westermani, D. ringeri,* and *D. pulmonale.*

**Par·a·gor·di·us** (par″ə-gor′de-əs) a genus of sometimes parasitic worms of the class Nematomorpha. Human infections with *P. cinc′tus, P. tricuspida′tus,* and *P. va′rius* have been reported.

**para·gram·ma·tism** (par″ə-gram′ə-tizm) 1. paraphasia. 2. agrammatism.

**para·gran·u·lo·ma** (par″ə-gran″u-lo′mə) Hodgkin's disease, lymphocyte predominance type.

**para·gra·phia** (par″ə-gra′fe-ə) [*para-* + *graph-* + *-ia*] dysgraphia in which the patient makes mistakes in spelling or writes one word in place of another.

**para·he·mo·phil·ia** (par″ə-he″mo-fil′e-ə) deficiency of coagulation factor V, an autosomal recessive trait causing a hemorrhagic tendency that is highly variable in intensity.

**para·he·pat·ic** (par″ə-hə-pat′ik) [*para-* + *hepat-* + *-ic*] beside the liver.

**para·hep·a·ti·tis** (par″ə-hep″ə-ti′tis) perihepatitis.

**para·hip·po·cam·pal** (par″ə-hip″o-kam′pəl) situated near the hippocampus.

**para·hor·mone** (par″ə-hor′mōn) [*para-* + *hormone*] a substance not conventionally accepted as a true hormone but that exerts hormonelike actions.

**para·hyp·no·sis** (par″ə-hip-no′sis) [*para-* + *hypnosis*] abnormal sleep, as under hypnosis or during general anesthesia; sometimes characterized by a suggestible state, somnambulism, or an unusual partial awareness of the surroundings.

**para·hy·poph·y·sis** (par″ə-hi-pof′ĭ-sis) an accessory mass of pituitary tissue.

**para·in·fec·tious** (par″ə-in-fek′shəs) pertaining to manifestations of infectious disease that are caused by the immune response to the infectious agent.

**para·ker·a·tin·ized** (par″ə-ker′ə-tin-īzd″) pertaining to epithelium in which parakeratosis has occurred.

**para·ker·a·to·sis** (par″ə-ker″ə-to′sis) [MeSH: Parakeratosis] persistence of the nuclei of the keratinocytes into the stratum corneum (horny layer) of the skin. Parakeratosis is normal in the epithelium of true mucous membranes of the mouth and vagina.
**inherited p.**, an autosomal recessive disease of cattle in Europe and North America in which calves around one month of age develop exanthems and parakeratosis on the legs, head, and neck; growth is stunted and they may die within three months. The cause is deficient uptake of zinc by the intestine, and zinc supplements may be curative. Called also *Adema disease.*
**p. ostra′cea,** p. scutularis.
**ruminal p.**, rumenitis with acidosis and hardening and enlargement of the ruminal papillae, most commonly seen in animals fed concentrated, pelleted feed.
**p. scutula′ris,** a rare disease of the legs and scalp marked by the formation of hard crusts that envelop the hairs with incrustations. Called also *p. ostracea.*
**p. variega′ta,** retiform parapsoriasis.

**para·ki·ne·sia** (par″ə-kĭ-ne′zhə) [*para-* + *kinesi-* + *-ia*] 1. abnormality of motor function resulting in distortion of movements; cf. *dyskinesia.* Called also *paracinesia* and *paracinesis.* 2. in ophthalmology, irregular action of an individual ocular muscle.

**para·ki·net·ic** (par″ə-kĭ-net′ik) pertaining to or characterized by parakinesia.

**Pa·ral** (pə-ral′) trademark for preparations of paraldehyde.

**para·la·lia** (par″ə-la′le-ə) [*para-* + *lal-* + *-ia*] any disturbance of speech, especially the utterance of a vocal sound other than the one desired. Called also *dyslalia* and *mogilalia.*
**p. litera′lis,** incorrect utterance of certain consonant sounds, often as part of stuttering. Called also *literal paraphasia.*

**para·lamb·da·cism** (par″ə-lam′də-siz-əm) [*para-* + *lambdacism*] lambdacism.

**par·al·de·hyde** (par-al′də-hīd) [USP] [MeSH: Paraldehyde] a polymerization product of acetaldehyde, having rapid-acting sedative and hypnotic properties; used to control insomnia, excitement, agitation, delirium, and convulsions; administered rectally and intramuscularly and by intravenous infusion.

**par·al·de·hyd·ism** (par-al′də-hīd″iz-əm) a condition produced by excessive use of paraldehyde; called also *paraldehyde poisoning.*

**para·lex·ia** (par″ə-lek′se-ə) [*para-* + *alexia*] dyslexia.

**para·lex·ic** (par″ə-lek′sik) pertaining to or affected with paralexia.

**par·al·ge·sia** (par″əl-je′ze-ə) [*para-* + *algesi-* + *-ia*] any condition marked by abnormal and painful sensations; a painful paresthesia.

**par·al·ges·ic** (par″əl-je′sik) pertaining to or affected with paralgesia.

**par·al·gia** (par-al′jə) paralgesia.

**para·li·nin** (par″ə-li′nin) [*para-* + *linin*] karyolymph.

**par·al·lac·tic** (par″ə-lak′tik) pertaining to parallax.

**par·al·lag·ma** (par″ə-lag′mə) [Gr.] displacement of a bone or of the fragments of a broken bone.

**par·al·lax** (par′ə-laks) [Gr. "change of position"] an apparent displacement of an object due to a change in the observer's position. **binocular p.,** the seeming difference in position of an object as seen separately by one eye and then by the other, the head remaining stationary. Types include *crossed, direct,* and *vertical p.* **crossed p.,** binocular parallax occurring in exophoria; when one eye is covered, the object viewed seems to move away from the open eye and toward the covered eye. **direct p.,** binocular parallax occurring in esophoria; when one eye is covered, the object viewed seems to move toward the open eye and away from the covered eye. **heteronymous p.,** crossed p. **homonymous p.,** direct p. **stereoscopic p.,** binocular p. **uncrossed p.,** direct p. **vertical p.,** binocular parallax occurring in vertical diplopia or heterophoria; the object seen seems to move vertically when each eye is closed in turn.

**par·al·lel** (par′ə-lel) [L. *parallelus*] 1. pertaining to straight lines or planes that do not intersect. 2. pertaining to electric circuit components connected "in parallel" so that the current flow divides, each branch passing through one component, and rejoins; applied by extension to any similar parallel circuit, e.g., the systemic circulation to the various organs. Cf. *series.*

**par·al·lel·om·e·ter** (par″ə-ləl-om′ə-tər) [*parallel* + *-meter*] an instrument for determining the exact parallel relationships of lines, surfaces, and structures in dental prostheses and casts.

**par·al·ler·gic** (par″ə-ler′jik) pertaining to or marked by parallergy.

**par·al·ler·gy** (par-al′ər-je) a condition in which an allergic state, produced by specific sensitization, predisposes the body to react to other allergens with clinical manifestations that differ from the original reaction.

**para·lo·gia** (par″ə-lo′jə) [*para-* + *log-* + *-ia*] disturbance of the reasoning faculty; marked by delusional or illogical speech. **thematic p.,** that limited to one subject, on which the mind dwells insistently. Cf. *monomania.*

**pa·ral·o·gism** (pə-ral′o-jiz-əm) the use of fallacious, meaningless, or illogical thought or language, primarily characteristic of schizophrenia.

**pa·ral·o·gy** (pə-ral′ə-je) anatomical similarity that has no phylogenetic or functional implication.

**pa·ral·y·ses** (pə-ral′ĭ-sēz) [MeSH: Paralysis] plural of *paralysis.*

**pa·ral·y·sis** (pə-ral′ĭ-sis) pl. *paral′yses* [*para-* + *-lysis*] [MeSH: Paralysis] loss or impairment of motor function in a part due to lesion of the neural or muscular mechanism; also, by analogy, impairment of sensory function (sensory paralysis). See also subentries under *hemiplegia, palsy,* and *paraplegia.*

## Paralysis

**abducens p.,** paralysis of the external rectus muscle of the eye due to lesion of the abducens nerve, with internal strabismus and diplopia.

**p. of accommodation,** paralysis of the ciliary muscles so as to prevent accommodation of the eye.

**acute ascending spinal p.,** acute idiopathic polyneuritis.

**p. a′gitans,** parkinsonism of unknown etiology, usually occurring in late life, although a juvenile form has been described. It is a slowly progressive disease characterized by masklike facies, resting tremor, slowing of voluntary movements, festinating gait, peculiar posture, and muscle weakness, sometimes with excessive sweating and feelings of heat. Pathologically, there is degeneration within the nuclear masses of the extrapyramidal system and loss of melanin-containing cells from the substantia nigra and a corresponding reduction in dopamine levels in the corpus striatum. Called also *Parkinson's disease* and *shaking palsy.*

**alternate p., alternating p.,** alternate hemiplegia.

**ambiguo-accessorius p.,** Schmidt's syndrome (def. 1).

**ambiguo-accessorius-hypoglossal p.,** Jackson's syndrome.

**ambiguohypoglossal p.,** Tapia's syndrome.

**ambiguospinothalamic p.,** Avellis' syndrome.

**arsenical p.,** paralysis due to arsenic poisoning.

**ascending p.,** spinal paralysis that progresses cephalad.

**Avellis' p.,** see under *syndrome.*

**Bell's p.,** see under *palsy.*

**bilateral p.,** diplegia; paralysis on both sides.

**birth p.,** paralysis due to injury received at birth.

**brachial p., brachial plexus p.,** paralysis of an arm from lesion of the brachial plexus; subdivided into *lower* and *upper brachial plexus paralysis* depending on which trunk of the plexus is affected.

**brachial plexus p., lower,** atrophic paralysis of the muscles of the arm and hand due to lesions of the eighth cervical or first dorsal nerve (lower trunk of the brachial plexus). When due to birth trauma it is called *Klumpke-Dejerine p.*

**brachial plexus p., upper,** paralysis of arm muscles due to destruction of the fifth and sixth cervical roots (upper trunk of the brachial plexus); small hand muscles are unaffected. When due to birth trauma it is called *Erb-Duchenne p.*

**brachiofacial p.,** paralysis affecting the face and an arm.

**Brown-Séquard's p.,** 1. see under *syndrome.* 2. a flaccid paralysis seen in disorders of the urinary tract.

**bulbar p.,** progressive bulbar palsy.

**cage p.,** a complex nutritional deficiency resembling osteomalacia, sometimes seen in captive primates.

**centrocapsular p.,** that which is due to lesions of the internal capsule.

**cerebral p.,** any paralysis due to an intracranial lesion; see *cerebral palsy,* under *palsy.*

**Chastek p.,** progressive ataxia and paralysis in silver foxes due to thiamine deficiency following a dietary change from meat to raw fish that contains a thiamine-destroying enzyme.

**compression p.,** paralysis such as crutch paralysis or decubitus paralysis that is caused by pressure on a nerve. Called also *pressure p.*

**congenital abducens-facial p., congenital oculofacial p.,** Möbius syndrome.

**conjugate p.,** loss of ability to perform some of the parallel ocular movements.

**coonhound p.,** acute polyradiculoneuritis.

**crossed p., cruciate p.,** paralysis affecting one side of the face and the opposite side of the body. See also *alternate hemiplegia.*

**crural p.,** that which chiefly affects the thigh or thighs.

**crutch p.,** compression paralysis of one or both arms, due to pressure of the crutch in the axilla.

**Cruveilhier's p.,** spinal muscular atrophy.

**curled toe p.,** a sign of riboflavin deficiency in young chickens; the toes show varying degrees of flexing so that the chick has difficulty walking. Severe deficiency is lethal.

**decubitus p.,** paralysis due to pressure on a nerve from lying for a long time in one position.

**Dejerine-Klumpke p.,** Klumpke's p.

**diaphragmatic p.,** paralysis of the diaphragm, usually unilaterally; called also *phrenoplegia.*

**diphtheric p., diphtheritic p.,** a partial paralysis that often follows diphtheria, chiefly affecting the soft palate and throat muscles. Called also *postdiphtheritic p.*

**divers' p.,** decompression sickness.

**Duchenne's p.,** 1. progressive bulbar palsy. 2. Erb-Duchenne p.

**Duchenne-Erb p.,** Erb-Duchenne p.

**Erb's p.,** 1. Erb-Duchenne p. 2. Erb's spastic paraplegia.

**Erb-Duchenne p.,** upper brachial paralysis, caused by birth injury; called also *Erb's* or *Erb-Duchenne palsy; Duchenne's, Duchenne-Erb,* or *Erb's p.;* and *Duchenne-Erb syndrome.*

**facial p.,** weakening or paralysis of the facial nerve, as in Bell's palsy or Millard-Gubler syndrome.

**false p.,** pseudoparalysis.

**Felton's p.,** see under *phenomenon.*

**flaccid p.,** any paralysis accompanied by loss of muscle tone and absence of tendon reflexes in the paralyzed part. Cf. *spastic p.*

**fowl p.**, see *Marek's disease*, under *disease*.
**functional p.**, a temporary paralysis which is apparently not caused by a nerve lesion; some forms may be psychogenic.
**p. of gaze**, paralysis due to pathological processes which implicate the supranuclear oculomotor centers or pathways and result in either lateral or vertical gaze paralysis.
**general p.**, see under *paresis*.
**glossolabial p., glossopharyngolabial p.**, progressive bulbar palsy.
**Gubler's p.**, Millard-Gubler syndrome.
**hereditary cerebrospinal p.**, hereditary spastic paraplegia.
**hyperkalemic periodic p.**, see *familial periodic p.*
**hypoglossal p.**, paralysis due to a lesion of the hypoglossal nucleus or the hypoglossal nerve at any point.
**hypokalemic periodic p.**, see *familial periodic p.*
**hysterical p.**, apparent loss of power of movement in a part, in the absence of an organic neurological cause.
**immune p., immunologic p.**, immunologic unresponsiveness induced by administration of large doses of antigen; now called *immunologic tolerance*.
**infantile p.**, the major illness of poliomyelitis; see *poliomyelitis*.
**infantile cerebral ataxic p.**, cerebral palsy with ataxia.
**infantile cerebrocerebellar diplegic p.**, cerebral palsy with spastic paraplegia and ataxia.
**infantile spinal p.**, spinal paralytic poliomyelitis.
**infectious bulbar p.**, pseudorabies.
**ischemic p.**, local paralysis due to an impairment of the circulation, as by embolism, thrombosis, or trauma; see also *Volkmann's contracture*, under *contracture*.
**Jamaica ginger p.**, a form of paralysis of the extremities, especially the legs, that was seen in the 1930s after a type of Jamaican ginger extract ("jake") was accidentally contaminated with the organophosphorus compound tri-*o*-tolyl phosphate and then consumed. Called also *Jamaica ginger polyneuritis*.
**juvenile p.**, general paralysis in young persons.
**juvenile p. a'gitans, juvenile p. agitans (of Hunt),** a condition developing in early life, usually familial but occasionally occurring sporadically, marked by increased muscle tonus with the characteristic attitude and facies of paralysis agitans, due to progressive degeneration of the globus pallidus; involvement of the substantia nigra and pyramidal tracts may occur. Called also *paleostriatal syndrome, pallidal atrophy, pallidal syndrome*, and *Ramsay Hunt syndrome*.
**Klumpke's p., Klumpke-Dejerine p.**, lower brachial plexus paralysis caused by birth injury, particularly during breech deliveries; called also *Klumpke's palsy* and *Dejerine-Klumpke* or *Klumpke-Dejerine syndrome*.
**Kussmaul's p., Kussmaul-Landry p.**, acute idiopathic polyneuritis.
**labial p., labioglossolaryngeal p., labioglossopharyngeal p.**, progressive bulbar palsy.
**lambing p.**, pregnancy toxemia in ewes.
**Landry's p.**, acute idiopathic polyneuritis.
**laryngeal p.**, paralysis of one of the laryngeal muscles, usually because of a lesion of the vagus nerve or the recurrent laryngeal nerve; seen in disorders such as Avellis' syndrome, Jackson's syndrome, and Vernet's syndrome. Called also *laryngoparalysis* and *laryngoplegia*.
**lead p.**, paralysis caused by lead poisoning, due to a peripheral neuritis, and marked by wristdrop.
**lingual p.**, paralysis of the tongue.
**Lissauer's p.**, an apoplectiform type of general paresis.
**local p.**, paralysis of one muscle or group of muscles.
**masticatory p.**, paralysis of the muscles of mastication; see also *trismus* and *trigeminal p.*
**maternal obstetric p.**, see under *palsy*.
**medullary tegmental p's**, paralyses due to lesions of the medullary tegmentum: they include alternate hemiplegia, Tapia's syndrome, syndrome of Babinski-Nageotte, and Cestan's syndrome.
**Millard-Gubler p.**, see under *syndrome*.
**mimetic p.**, paralysis of the facial muscles.
**mixed p.**, combined motor and sensory paralysis.
**motor p.**, paralysis of voluntary muscles.
**musculospiral p.**, paralysis of the extensor muscles of the wrist and fingers, most often due to compression of the musculospiral (radial) nerve and, depending upon the site of the nerve injury, sometimes accompanied by weakness of extension of the elbow; called also *radial p.* and *Saturday night palsy*.
**myopathic p.**, paralysis due to disease of the muscle itself.
**normokalemic periodic p.**, see *familial periodic p.*
**p. notario'rum**, writers' cramp.
**nuclear p.**, any paralysis due to a lesion in a nucleus of origin.
**obstetric p.**, birth p.
**ocular p.**, see *amaurosis, cycloplegia*, and *ophthalmoplegia*.
**oculomotor p.**, paralysis of the oculomotor nerve; seen in disorders such as Benedikt's syndrome, Claude's syndrome, Nothnagel's syndrome, and Weber's syndrome.
**parotitic p.**, paralysis accompanying mumps.
**parturient p.**, see under *paresis*.
**periodic p.**, 1. any of various diseases characterized by episodic flaccid paralysis or muscular weakness. 2. familial periodic p.
**periodic p., familial**, an autosomal dominant condition marked by recurring attacks of rapidly progressive flaccid paralysis; there are three types: *I*, associated with a fall in serum potassium *(hypokalemic periodic p.)*; *II*, associated with a rise in serum potassium *(hyperkalemic periodic p.*; called also *Gamstorp's disease)*; and *III*, with normal potassium levels *(normokalemic periodic p.)*.
**periodic p., thyrotoxic**, recurrent episodes of generalized or local paralysis accompanied by hypokalemia, occurring in association with Graves' disease and most often affecting males in the third decade of life; attacks occur especially after exercise or a high-carbohydrate or high-sodium meal and generally last 3 to 12 hours.
**peripheral p.**, loss of power due to some lesion of the nervous mechanism between the nucleus of origin and the muscle.
**peroneal p.**, crossed leg palsy.
**phonetic p.**, vocal fold p.
**postdiphtheritic p.**, diphtheritic p.
**postdormital p.**, sleep paralysis occurring upon waking.
**postepileptic p.**, Todd's p.
**posthemiplegic p.**, residual weakness after a stroke.
**posticus p.**, paralysis of the posterior cricothyroid muscle. See also *laryngeal p.*
**Pott's p.**, see under *paraplegia*.
**predormital p.**, sleep paralysis occurring prior to falling asleep.
**pressure p.**, compression p.
**progressive bulbar p.**, see under *palsy*.
**pseudobulbar p.**, spastic weakness of the muscles innervated by the cranial nerves, i.e., the muscles of the face, pharynx, and tongue, due to bilateral lesions of the corticospinal tract; symptoms include dysphagia, dysarthria, and spastic facial jerks, sometimes accompanied by uncontrolled weeping or laughing and Cheyne-Stokes respiration. Called also *supranuclear p.* and *spastic bulbar palsy*.
**pseudohypertrophic muscular p.**, see under *dystrophy*.
**radial p.**, 1. musculospiral p. 2. in quadrupeds such as horses and dogs, paralysis of elbow and knee muscles owing to injury to the radial nerve. Called also *dropped elbow*.
**Ramsay Hunt p.**, juvenile p. agitans (of Hunt).
**range p.**, Marek's disease.
**reflex p.**, paralysis ascribable to peripheral irritation; in some cases secondary changes occur in the spinal cord, and the paralysis ceases to be truly reflex.
**Remak's p.**, paralysis of the extensor muscles of the fingers and wrist; called also *Remak's type*.
**rucksack p.**, a disorder of motor and sensory function of the upper extremities as a result of damage to the brachial plexus caused by the wearing of a backpack.
**sensory p.**, loss of sensation resulting from a morbid process.
**serum p.**, peripheral nerve paralysis following administration of serum.
**sleep p.**, paralysis occurring at awakening or sleep onset; it represents extension of the atonia of REM sleep into the waking state and is often seen in those suffering from narcolepsy or sleep apnea. Called also *waking p.* See also *postdormital p.* and *predormital p.*
**spastic p.**, paralysis marked by spasticity of the muscles of the paralyzed part and increased tendon reflexes, due to upper motor neuron lesions. See also *spastic paraplegia*. Cf. *flaccid p.*
**spinal p.**, paralysis due to a lesion of the spinal cord; called also *myeloplegia*.
**spinomuscular p.**, paralysis due to lesion of the gray matter of the spinal cord; see also *spinal muscular atrophy*, under *atrophy*.
**supranuclear p.**, pseudobulbar p.
**suprascapular p.**, paralysis of the suprascapular muscle in a horse due to damage to its nerve. Called also *slipped shoulder, shoulder slip*, and *sweeney* or *sweeny*.
**tegmental mesencephalic p.**, Benedikt's syndrome.
**tick p.**, a progressive ascending flaccid motor paralysis seen in children and domestic animals following the bite of certain ticks. In the northwestern United States and western Canada it is usually caused by *Dermacentor andersoni*, and in other parts of the world numerous other ticks have been implicated, including species of *Haemaphysalis*, and *Rhipicephalus*. It is usually the result of toxins from a tick's saliva that enter the central nervous system of the host.
**Todd's p.**, hemiparesis or monoparesis lasting for a few minutes or hours, or occasionally for several days, after an epileptic seizure; called also *postepileptic p.*
**trigeminal p.**, paralysis due to a lesion of the trigeminal (fifth) nerve, marked by sensory loss in the face and weakness of the muscles of mastication.
**vasomotor p.**, paralysis of vasomotor muscles; see also *vasoparesis*. Called also *angioparalysis*.

**vocal cord p., vocal fold p.,** paralysis of one or both or the vocal cords; the voice is weakened but not lost. See also *laryngeal p.* Called also *phonetic p.*

**Volkmann's ischemic p.,** see under *contracture.*

**waking p.,** sleep p.

**wasting p.,** spinal muscular atrophy.

**Weber's p.,** see under *syndrome.*

**writers' p.,** writers' cramp.

**par·a·lys·or** (par'ə-līz"or) paralyzer.

**par·a·lyt·ic** (par"ə-lit'ik) [Gr. *paralytikos*] 1. affected with or pertaining to paralysis. 2. a person affected with paralysis.

**par·a·lyt·o·gen·ic** (par"ə-lit"o-jen'ik) causing paralysis.

**par·a·lyz·ant** (par'ə-līz"ənt) 1. causing paralysis. 2. an agent that paralyzes.

**par·a·lyze** (par'ə-līz) to put into a state of paralysis.

**par·a·lyz·er** (par'ə-līz"ər) a substance which hinders or prevents a chemical reaction; an inhibitor.

**para·mag·net·ic** (par"ə-mag-net'ik) characterized by or exhibiting paramagnetism.

**para·mag·ne·tism** (par"ə-mag'nə-tiz-əm) [*para-* + *magnetism*] the property of being attracted by a magnet, and of assuming a position parallel to that of a magnetic force, but not of becoming permanently magnetized.

**para·mas·ti·gote** (par"ə-mas'tĭ-gōt) [*para-* + *mastigote*] having an accessory flagellum by the side of a larger one.

**para·mas·ti·tis** (par"ə-mas-ti'tis) [*para-* + *mastitis*] inflammation of the tissues around the mammary gland.

**para·mas·toid** (par"ə-mas'toid) near the mastoid process.

**para·me·a·tal** (par"ə-me-a'təl) situated near or around a meatus.

**par·a·me·cia** (par"ə-me'she-ə) plural of *paramecium.*

**Par·a·me·ci·um** (par"ə-me'she-əm) [Gr. *paramēkēs* oblong] [MeSH: Paramecium] a genus of ovoid or elongated freshwater protozoa (suborder Peniculina, order Hymenostomatida), some species of which are visible to the naked eye. Certain species have been used as test organisms in cytological, genetic, and other research.

**par·a·me·ci·um** (par"ə-me'she-əm) pl. *parame'cia* [MeSH: Paramecium] an organism belonging to the genus *Paramecium.*

**para·me·di·an** (par"ə-me'de-ən) [*para-* + *median*] situated near the midline or median plane.

**para·med·i·cal** (par"ə-med'i-kəl) having some connection with or relation to the science or practice of medicine; adjunctive to the practice of medicine in the maintenance or restoration of health and normal functioning. Paramedical workers include physical, occupational, and speech therapists, medical social workers, pharmacists, technicians, and so on.

**para·me·nia** (par"ə-me'ne-ə) [*para-* + *men-* + *-ia*] disordered or difficult menstruation.

**para·me·ni·sci·tis** (par"ə-me-nĭ-si'tis) inflammation of the parameniscus.

**para·me·nis·cus** (par"ə-mə-nis'kəs) the structure or area around the menisci (semilunar fibrocartilages) of the knee.

**para·me·si·al** (par"ə-me'se-əl) [*para-* + Gr. *mesos* middle] paramedian.

**pa·ram·e·ter** (pə-ram'ə-tər) [*para-* + *-meter*] 1. a constant in a mathematical expression that distinguishes specific cases, having a definite, fixed value in one case but different values in other cases. For example, in the equation of a straight line, $y = mx + b$, $m$ and $b$ are parameters that specify a particular straight line; changing $m$ changes the slope of the line, while changing $b$ changes the point at which the line crosses the $y$-axis. 2. in statistics, a value that specifies one of the various members of a family of probability distributions, e.g., the mean or variance of a normal distribution. A parameter is often thought of as the "true value" or "population value" as opposed to the observed value or sample value. 3. a variable whose measure is indicative of a quantity or function that cannot itself be precisely determined by direct methods; e.g., blood pressure and pulse rate are parameters of cardiovascular function, and the level of glucose in blood and urine is a parameter of carbohydrate metabolism.

**para·meth·a·di·one** (par"ə-meth"ə-di'ōn) an anticonvulsant, occurring as a clear, colorless liquid, used especially in the treatment of petit mal epilepsy, administered orally.

**para·meth·a·sone ac·e·tate** (par"ə-meth'ə-sōn) [USP] a glucocorticoid, used chiefly for its anti-inflammatory and antiallergic actions, administered orally.

**Para·me·tor·chis** (par"ə-mə-tor'kis) a genus of trematodes of the family Opisthorchiidae. *P. complex'us* is found in the bile ducts of cats and dogs, sometimes causing jaundice or gastrointestinal disorders.

**para·me·tri·al** (par"ə-me'tre-əl) 1. pertaining to the parametrium. 2. parametric[1].

**para·met·ric**[1] (par"ə-me'trik) [*para-* + *metr-* + *-ic*] situated near the uterus; parametrial.

**para·met·ric**[2] (par"ə-met'rik) [*para-* + *metric*] pertaining to or defined in terms of a parameter.

**para·me·trit·ic** (par"ə-mə-trit'ik) pertaining to parametritis.

**para·me·tri·tis** (par"ə-mə-tri'tis) [MeSH: Parametritis] inflammation of the parametrium.

**posterior p.,** inflammation of the cellular tissue around the uterosacral ligaments.

**para·me·tri·um** (par"ə-me'tre-əm) pl. *parame'tria* [*para-* + Gr. *mētra* uterus] [TA] the extension of the subserous coat of the supracervical portion of the uterus laterally between the layers of the broad ligament.

**par·am·i·do·ac·e·to·phe·none** (par-am"ĭ-do-as"ə-to-fe'nōn) $NH_2 \cdot C_6H_4 \cdot CO \cdot CH_3$; used in Ehrlich's diazo reaction.

**para·mi·tome** (par"ə-mi'tōm) [*para-* + *mitome*] hyaloplasm, def. 1.

**par·am·ne·sia** (par"am-ne'zhə) [*para-* + *amnesia*] a disturbance of memory in which reality and fantasy are confused; cf. *dysmnesia.*

**Par·amoe·ba** (par"ə-me'bə) [*para-* + *ameba*] a genus of parasitic or free-living ameboid protozoa (suborder Conopodina, order Amoebida), characterized by the presence of both a nucleus and a nucleus-like body; some authorities consider the latter to be a protistan hyperparasite and not a secondary nucleus. Formerly called *Craigia.*

**para·mo·lar** (par"ə-mo'lər) [*para-* + *molar*] a supernumerary tooth, usually small and rudimentary, sometimes found in the maxilla buccally or lingually to a molar or interproximally between two of the first three molars. Called also *supernumerary molar.*

**Par·a·mo·nos·to·mum** (par"ə-mo-nos'to-məm) a genus of trematodes. *P. par'vum* infects ducks and chickens in North America.

**Par·am·phis·to·ma·ti·dae** (par"am-fis"to-mat'ĭ-de) [MeSH: Paramphistomatidae] the paramphistomes, a family of parasitic trematodes. Most (such as genera *Calicophoron, Cotylophoron,* and *Paramphistomum*) infest primarily ruminants, but genera *Gastrodiscoides* and *Watsonius* also cause paramphistomiasis in humans.

**Par·am·phis·to·ma·toi·dea** (par"am-fis-to"mə-toi'de-ə) a superfamily of trematodes that includes the family Paramphistomatidae.

**pa·ram·phi·stome** (pə-ram'fĭ-stōm) any member of the family Paramphistomatidae, pear-shaped trematodes that have the sucker near the posterior end and infest the intestines of ruminants and occasionally humans or other mammals, causing paramphistomiasis. See also *ruminal fluke.* Called also *amphistome* and *conical fluke.*

**par·am·phis·to·mi·a·sis** (par"am-fis-to-mi'ə-sis) infestation by intestinal flukes of the family Paramphistomatidae. Most genera are usually found in the stomachs or small intestines of ruminants; genera *Gastrodiscoides* in Asia and *Watsonius* in Africa are sometimes found in the duodenum of humans and other animals. Adult worms may be present without any clinical signs, but immature worms cause more severe manifestations such as enteritis, severe diarrhea, anorexia, and hemorrhaging. In flocks of cattle or sheep with heavy infestations, the mortality may be over 90 per cent. Called also *amphistomiasis.*

**Par·am·phis·to·mum** (par"am-fis'to-məm) a genus of trematodes of the family Paramphistomatidae. *P. cer'vi* is found in the rumen and reticulum of ruminants, causing paramphistomiasis.

**para·mu·cin** (par″ə-mu′sin) a colloid substance found in ovarian cysts, which differs from mucin and pseudomucin in the fact that it reduces Fehling's solution before boiling with acid.

**para·mu·sia** (par″ə-mu′ze-ə) [*para-* + Gr. *mousa* music + *-ia*] partial or complete loss of the power of correct musical expression; cf. *amusia.*

**par·am·y·loi·do·sis** (par-am″ə-loi-do′sis) accumulation of an atypical form of amyloid in tissues.

**para·my·oc·lo·nus** (par″ə-mi-ok′lə-nəs) [*para-* + *myoclonus*] myoclonus in several unrelated muscles.
**p. mul′tiplex,** a term coined by Friedreich to describe a form of myoclonus of unknown etiology starting in the muscles of the upper arms and shoulders and spreading to other parts of the upper body. Called also *Friedreich's disease* and *myoclonus multiplex.*

**para·myo·sin** (par″ə-mi′o-sin) a muscle protein found in the catch muscle fibers of mollusks and annelids; it has a molecular weight of about 137,000 and shows pronounced symmetry; called also *tropomyosin A.*

**par·a·my·o·sin·o·gen** (par″ə-mi″o-sin′o-jən) a protein resembling myosinogen (myogen) derived from muscle plasma.

**para·myo·to·nia** (par″ə-mi″o-to′ne-ə) [*para-* + *myo-* + *ton-* + *-ia*] tonic spasms caused by a disorder of muscular tonicity; cf. *myotonia.*
**p. conge′nita,** an autosomal dominant disorder clinically similar to myotonia congenita, except that the precipitating factor is exposure to cold, the myotonia is aggravated by activity, and only the proximal muscles of the limbs, eyelids, and tongue are affected. Called also *Eulenburg disease.*

**Par·a·myxa** (par″ə-mik′sə) [*para-* + Gr. *myxa* mucus] a genus of parasitic protozoa (order Paramyxida, class Paramyxea) having characters of the class.

**Par·a·myx·ea** (par″ə-mik′se-ə) a class of parasitic protozoa (phylum Ascetospora) having bicellular spores, each consisting of a parietal cell and one sporoplasm, an uninterrupted spore wall, and no polar tube. It comprises one order: Paramyxida.

**Par·a·myx·i·da** (par″ə-mik′sĭ-də) an order of parasitic protozoa (class Paramyxea, phylum Ascetospora) having characters of the class. *Paramyxa* is a representative genus.

**Para·myxo·vi·ri·dae** (par″ə-mik″so-vir′ĭ-de) [MeSH: Paramyxoviridae] the paramyxoviruses: a family of RNA viruses having a pleomorphic, usually roughly spherical but occasionally filamentous virion 150–300 nm in diameter, consisting of a lipid bilayer membrane with large peplomers surrounding a helical nucleocapsid. The genome consists of a single molecule of negative-sense single-stranded RNA (MW 5–7 × $10^6$, size 16 kb). Viruses contain six to ten major polypeptides, including a transcriptase, and are sensitive to lipid solvents, detergents, disinfectants, and extremes of pH; thermostability varies according to genus. Replication occurs in the cytoplasm and assembly is by budding through the plasma membrane. Host range is generally narrow in nature but broad in cultured cells, and transmission is horizontal, chiefly airborne. There are two subfamilies, Paramyxovirinae and Pneumovirinae.

**Para·myxo·vi·ri·nae** (par″ə-mik″so-vir-i′ne) a subfamily of the family Paramyxoviridae, containing three genera: *Morbillivirus, Paramyxovirus,* and *Rubulavirus.*

**Para·myxo·vi·rus** (par″ə-mik′so-vi″rəs) [*para-* + *myxovirus*] [MeSH: Paramyxovirus] a genus of viruses of the subfamily Paramyxovirinae (family Paramyxoviridae) that cause chiefly respiratory infections in a variety of vertebrate hosts.

**para·myxo·vi·rus** (par″ə-mik′so-vi″rəs) [MeSH: Paramyxovirus] any virus belonging to the family Paramyxoviridae.
**avian p. 1,** Newcastle disease virus.

**par·an·al·ge·sia** (par″an-al-je′ze-ə) para-analgesia.

**Par·an·a·plas·ma** (par-an″ə-plaz′mə) [*para-* + *an-* neg. + *plasma*] in former systems of classification, a genus of bacteria the organisms of which have been assigned to the genus *Anaplasma.*

**para·neo·plas·tic** (par″ə-ne″o-plas′tik) [*para-* + *neoplastic*] pertaining to changes produced in tissue remote from a tumor or its metastases; see also *paraneoplastic syndrome,* under *syndrome.*

**para·neph·ric** (par″ə-nef′rik) 1. near the kidney; called also *pararenal* and *adrenal.* 2. adrenal (def. 1).

**para·ne·phri·tis** (par″ə-nə-fri′tis) [*para-* + *nephritis*] 1. inflammation of the connective tissue around and near the kidney. 2. adrenalitis.

**para·ne·phro·ma** (par″ə-nə-fro′mə) a tumor of the adrenal gland.

**par·an·es·the·sia** (par″an-əs-the′zhə) para-anesthesia.

**para·neu·ral** (par″ə-noor′əl) [*para-* + *neural*] beside or alongside a nerve.

**para·ni·tro·sul·fa·thi·a·zole** (par″ə-ni″tro-sul″fə-thi′ə-zōl) a sulfonamide, used as an antibacterial in the treatment of nonspecific ulcerative colitis and of proctitis, administered by rectal injection.

**par·a·noia** (par″ə-noi′ah) 1. a term used to describe behavior characterized by well-systematized delusions of persecution, delusions of grandeur, or a combination of the two. There are several disorders in which paranoia may occur: see *delusional disorder, shared psychotic disorder, paranoid personality,* and *paranoid schizophrenia.* 2. former name for the condition now called *delusional disorder.*

**par·a·noi·ac** (par″ə-noi′ak) 1. a person afflicted with paranoia. 2. pertaining to or characterized by paranoia.

**par·a·noid** (par′ə-noid) 1. resembling paranoia. 2. paranoiac.

**par·a·no·mia** (par″ə-no′me-ə) [*para-* + Gr. *onoma* name + *-ia*] anomic aphasia.

**Para·no·plo·ceph·a·la** (par″ə-no″plo-sef′ə-lə) a genus of tapeworms of the family Anoplocephalidae. *P. mamilla′na* infests the stomach and intestines of horses.

**para·nor·mal** (par″ə-nor′məl) beyond the normal or natural; said of phenomena such as extrasensory perception.

**para·nu·cle·ar** (par″ə-noo′kle-ər) 1. beside a nucleus. 2. pertaining to a paranucleus.

**para·nu·cle·o·lus** (par″ə-noo-kle′ə-ləs) a small basophil body in the enclosing sac of the cell nucleus.

**para·nu·cle·us** (par″ə-noo′kle-əs) [*para-* + *nucleus*] a body resembling the nucleus, sometimes seen in the cell cytoplasm near the nucleus.

**para·om·phal·ic** (par″ə-om-fal′ik) [*para-* + *omphalic*] alongside the umbilicus.

**para·op·er·a·tive** (par″ə-op′ər-ə-tiv) pertaining to the accessories essential to operative surgery, such as care of instruments and gloves, sterilization, etc.

**para·oral** (par″ə-or′əl) administered by some route other than by the mouth; said of medication.

**par·aor·tic** (par″a-or′tik) para-aortic.

**para·os·mia** (par″ə-os′me-ə) parosmia.

**para·pan·cre·at·ic** (par″ə-pan″kre-at′ik) situated near the pancreas.

**para·pa·re·sis** (par″ə-pə-re′sis) [*para-* + *paresis*] a partial paralysis of the lower extremities.
**tropical spastic p.,** chronic progressive myelopathy.

**para·pe·de·sis** (par″ə-pə-de′sis) [*para-* + Gr. *pēdēsis* a leaping] passage of body substances into channels not normally conveying them, as of bile pigments into the blood capillaries.

**para·peri·to·ne·al** (par″ə-per″ĭ-to-ne′əl) near the peritoneum.

**para·per·tus·sis** (par″ə-pər-tus′is) [*para-* + *pertussis*] an acute respiratory disease clinically indistinguishable from mild or moderate pertussis, caused by *Bordetella parapertussis.* See also *pertussis-like syndrome,* under *syndrome.*

**para·pes·tis** (par″ə-pes′tis) ambulatory plague.

**para·pha·ryn·ge·al** (par″ə-fə-rin′je-əl) situated near the pharynx.

**para·pha·sia** (par″ə-fa′zhə) [*para-* + *-phasia*] a type of dysphasia in which the patient employs wrong words or uses words in wrong and senseless combinations; called also *paragrammatism, paraphemia,* and *paraphrasia.*
**central p.,** that due to a brain lesion.
**literal p.,** paralalia literalis.
**thematic p.,** incoherent speech characterized by wandering from the subject.

**para·pha·sic** (par″ə-fa′sik) characterized by paraphasia.

**para·phe·mia** (par″ə-fe′me-ə) [*para-* + *-phemia*] paraphasia.

**para·phen·yl·ene·di·amine** (par″ə-fen″əl-ēn-di′ə-mēn) *p*-phenylenediamine.

**pa·ra·phia** (pə-ra′fe-ə) [*para-* + Gr. *haphē* touch + *-ia*] a disorder of the sense of touch; called also *dysaphia, parapsia, parapsis,* and *pseudapsia.*

**para·phil·ia** (par″ə-fil′e-ə) [*para-* + *-philia*] [MeSH: Paraphilias] [DSM-IV] a psychosexual disorder characterized by recurrent intense sexual urges, by sexually arousing fantasies, or by behavior involving use of a nonhuman object, the suffering or humiliation of oneself or one's partner, or children or other nonconsenting partners; included are exhibitionism, fetishism, frotteurism, pedophilia, sexual masochism, sexual sadism, transvestic fetishism, and voyeurism.

**para·phil·i·ac** (par″ə-fil′e-ak) 1. pertaining to paraphilia. 2. an individual exhibiting paraphilia.

**para·phi·mo·sis** (par″ə-fi-mo′sis) [*para-* + *phimosis*] [MeSH: Paraphimosis] retraction of phimotic foreskin, causing a painful swelling of the glans that, if severe, may cause dry gangrene unless corrected. See also *phimosis*.

**para·pho·nia** (par″ə-fo′ne-ə) [*para-* + *phon-* + *-ia*] dysphonia.

**para·phra·sia** (par″ə-fra′zhə) paraphasia.

**para·phre·nia** (par″ə-fre′ne-ə) [*para-* + *phren-* + *-ia*] 1. older term for a condition theoretically lying midway between paranoia and schizophrenia, in which there are fantastic, absurd, well-systematized delusions without severe personality deterioration; use of this term is discouraged. 2. periphrenitis.

**para·phren·ic** (par″ə-fren′ik) 1. pertaining to or characterized by paraphrenia. 2. an individual exhibiting paraphrenia.

**para·phre·ni·tis** (par″ə-frə-ni′tis) [*para-* + *phrenitis*] periphrenitis.

**para·phys·e·al** (par″ə-fiz′e-əl) pertaining to the paraphysis.

**pa·raph·y·sis** (pə-raf′ĭ-sis) [Gr. "offshoot"] 1. a thin-walled derivative of the roof plate of the telencephalon, present only temporarily in the human embryo and fetus; called also *paraphyseal body*. 2. a sterile thread alongside the spore sac or sexual organs in the hymenial layer of some fungi, especially ascomycetes; also found in mosses and ferns.

**para·pin·e·al** (par″ə-pin′e-əl) pertaining to the parapineal organ of certain lower vertebrates.

**para·plasm** (par′ə-plaz-əm) [*para-* + *-plasm*] 1. hyaloplasm (def. 1). 2. an abnormal growth.

**para·plas·mic** (par″ə-plaz′mik) pertaining to paraplasm.

**para·plas·tic** (par″ə-plas′tik) [*para-* + *plastic*] exhibiting an abnormal formative power; of the nature of a paraplasm.

**para·plas·tin** (par″ə-plas′tin) a substance resembling parachromatin in the cytoplasm and nucleus of a cell.

**Para·plat·in** (par″ə-plat′in) trademark for a preparation of carboplatin.

**para·plec·tic** (par″ə-plek′tik) [Gr. *paraplēktikos*] paraplegic.

**para·ple·gia** (par″ə-ple′jə) [*para-* + *-plegia*] [MeSH: Paraplegia] paralysis of the legs and lower part of the body.
**alcoholic p.**, paraplegia due to chronic alcoholism and probably dependent upon peripheral neuritis.
**ataxic p.**, subacute combined degeneration of spinal cord; see under *degeneration*.
**cerebral p.**, paraplegia caused by bilateral cerebral lesions.
**flaccid p.**, flaccid paralysis in the lower limbs. Cf. *spastic p.*
**peripheral p.**, that which is due to a lower motor neuron lesion.
**Pott's p.**, that which is due to vertebral caries or spinal tuberculosis; called also *Pott's paralysis*.
**senile p.**, spastic paraplegia in the elderly, usually caused by transverse lesions of the spinal cord or by anterolateral sclerosis. Called also *tetanoid p.*
**spastic p.**, any of a group of diseases marked by spasticity of the muscles of the paralyzed part and increased tendon reflexes, due to damage to the corticospinal tract. Most varieties are hereditary (see *hereditary spastic p.*), but one variety *(Little's disease)* is caused by birth injury or intrauterine conditions. See also *cerebral palsy*, under *palsy*. Called also *spastic diplegia*.
**spastic p., congenital,** Little's disease.
**spastic p., Erb's, spastic p., Erb's syphilitic,** an uncommon form of meningovascular syphilis marked by progressive spasticity and weakness of the legs, paraplegia, muscular atrophy, paresthesia, increased knee and ankle reflexes, and incontinence. Called also *cerebrospinal syphilis, Erb's paralysis, Erb-Charcot disease,* and *syphilitic p.*
**spastic p., hereditary,** any of a group of hereditary disorders consisting of gradually developing paralysis in one, two, or all four limbs, with spasticity. There is degeneration of corticospinal tracts but sensory abnormalities are not present. Called also *hereditary cerebrospinal paralysis*.
**spastic p., infantile,** Little's disease.
**spastic p., tropical,** chronic progressive myelopathy.
**p. supe′rior,** paralysis of both arms.
**syphilitic p.,** Erb's spastic p.
**tetanoid p.,** senile p.
**toxic p.,** paraplegia due to the effects of neurotoxins.

**para·ple·gic** (par″ə-ple′jik) 1. pertaining to or of the nature of paraplegia. 2. an individual affected with paraplegia.

**para·ple·gi·form** (par″ə-ple′jĭ-form) resembling paraplegia.

**para·po·di·um** (pa-rə-po′de-əm) pl. *parapo′dia* [*para-* + Gr. *pous* foot] 1. a standing orthosis for paralyzed children, consisting of a footplate with shoes, bars parallel to the legs, and a padded frame that supports the abdomen and thorax. 2. one of the paired segmented appendages of marine annelids.

**par·apoph·y·sis** (par″ə-pof′ĭ-sis) [*para-* + *apophysis*] the lower transverse process of a vertebra (processus transversus vertebrae [TA]), or its homologue.

**Para·pox·vi·rus** (par″ə-poks′vi-rəs) [*para-* + *poxvirus*] [MeSH: Parapoxvirus] a genus of viruses of the subfamily Chordopoxvirinae (family Poxviridae) with serologic cross reactivity, comprising viruses of ungulates, including orf virus, pseudocowpox virus, and bovine papular stomatitis virus.

**para·pox·vi·rus** (par″ə-poks′vi-rəs) [MeSH: Parapoxvirus] any member of the genus *Parapoxvirus*.

**para·prax·ia** (par″ə-prak′se-ə) parapraxis.

**para·prax·is** (par″ə-prak′sis) pl. *paraprax′es* [*para-* + *praxis*] a faulty action, as a slip of the tongue or misplacement of an object; attributed by Freud to unconscious motives.

**para·proc·ti·tis** (par″ə-prok-ti′tis) [*paraproctium* + *-itis*] inflammation of the paraproctium; perirectal inflammation.

**para·proc·ti·um** (par″ə-prok′she-əm) [*para-* + Gr. *prōktos* anus] the tissues that surround the rectum and the anus.

**para·pro·fes·sion·al** (par″ə-pro-fesh′ən-əl) 1. a person who is specially trained in a particular field or occupation to assist a professional such as a physician. 2. allied health professional. 3. pertaining to a paraprofessional.

**para·pros·ta·ti·tis** (par″ə-pros″tə-ti′tis) inflammation of the tissues near the prostate gland.

**para·pro·tein** (par″ə-pro′tēn) M component.

**para·pro·tein·emia** (par″ə-pro″tēn-e′me-ə) [MeSH: Paraproteinemias] plasma cell dyscrasia.

**par·ap·sia** (par-ap′se-ə) paraphia.

**par·ap·sis** (par-ap′sis) [*para-* + Gr. *hapsis* touch] paraphia.

**para·pso·ri·a·sis** (par″ə-so-ri′ə-sis) pl. *parapsori′ases* [*para-* + *psoriasis*] [MeSH: Parapsoriasis] any of a group of slowly evolving erythrodermas having common characteristics of scaling, resistance to treatment, and chronicity. The group includes acute and chronic lichenoid pityriasis and large and small plaque parapsoriasis.
**acute p.,** acute lichenoid pityriasis.
**atrophic p.,** large plaque p.
**chronic p.,** chronic lichenoid pityriasis.
**p. gutta′ta, guttate p.,** 1. chronic lichenoid pityriasis. 2. small plaque p.
**large plaque p.,** a chronic, asymptomatic or mildly symptomatic eruption consisting of red-blue, oval, poorly defined, flat, sometimes indurated large plaques with superficial scaling, which preferentially involves the trunk, especially the hips and buttocks, proximal extremities, and breasts in women. It may progress to cutaneous T-cell lymphoma, particularly if atrophy and poikiloderma are prominent features. See also *retiform p.*
**p. lichenoi′des,** retiform p.
**p. en plaques,** see *large plaque p.* and *small plaque p.*
**poikilodermatous p., poikilodermic p.,** 1. large plaque p. 2. retiform p.
**retiform p.,** a chronic eruption consisting of red to brown, scaly lesions with a netlike distribution, intermixed with which are deep red plaques, some exhibiting lichenoid papules, which is histologically similar to large-plaque parapsoriasis (considered by some authorities to be a variant) except that atrophy and poikiloderma are prominent features. It is the form of parapsoriasis from which cutaneous T-cell lymphoma is most likely to arise. Called also *p. lichenoides, p. variegata,* and *parakeratosis variegata*.
**small plaque p.,** a benign, asymptomatic, chronic eruption consisting of small to moderate sized, red-blue to yellow plaques, occurring chiefly on the trunk and proximal extremities, which have distinct, thin borders and fine, adherent scales, giving the surface a cigarette paper–like appearance. Called also *p. guttata* and *xanthoerythrodermia perstans*.
**p. variega′ta,** retiform p.
**p. variolifor′mis acu′ta,** acute lichenoid pityriasis.
**p. variolifor′mis chro′nica,** chronic lichenoid pityriasis.

**para·psy·chol·o·gy** (par″ə-si-kol′ə-je) [*para-* + *psychology*] [MeSH: Parapsychology] the study of psychical effects and experiences which appear to fall outside the scope of physical law, e.g., telepathy and clairvoyance.

**para·pyk·no·mor·phous** (par″ə-pik″no-mor′fəs) [*para-* + *pyknomorphous*] neither pyknomorphous nor apyknomorphous, but between the two; staining moderately well. Said of certain nerve cells.

**para·pyle** (par′ə-pīl) [*para-* + Gr. *pylē* gate] an opening other than the astropyle in the capsular membrane of certain marine planktonic protozoa.

**para·py·ram·i·dal** (par″ə-pĭ-ram′i-dəl) beside or near a pyramid.

**para·quat** (par′ə-kwaht) [MeSH: Paraquat] a poisonous dipyridilium compound whose dichloride and dimethylsulfate salts are used as contact herbicides. See *paraquat poisoning*, under *poisoning*.

**para·rec·tal** (par″ə-rek′təl) beside the rectum.

**para·re·du·cine** (par″ə-re-doo′sin) [*para-* + *reducin*] a leukomaine found in the urine.

**para·re·flex·ia** (par″ə-re-flek′se-ə) dysreflexia.

**para·re·nal** (par″ə-re′nəl) paranephric (def. 1).

**para·rhi·zo·cla·sia** (par″ə-ri″zo-kla′zhə) [*para-* + *rhizo-* + Gr. *klasis* destruction + *-ia*] inflammatory destruction of the deep layers of the alveolar process and the periodontal ligament around the roots of a tooth. Cf. *perirhizoclasia.*

**para·rho·ta·cism** (par″ə-ro′tə-siz-əm) [*para-* + *rhotacism*] rhotacism.

**para·ro·san·i·line** (par″ə-ro-zan′ĭ-lēn) a basic dye occurring as colorless to red crystals, the chief constituent of basic fuchsin (q.v.).
**p. pamoate**, an antischistosomal, $[(C_{19}H_{18}N_3)_2 \cdot C_{23}H_{14}O_6] \cdot 2H_2O$.

**par·ar·rhyth·mia** (par″ə-rith′me-ə) parasystole.

**Par·a·sac·cha·ro·my·ces** (par″ə-sak″ə-ro-mi′sēz) *Candida.*

**para·sa·cral** (par″ə-sa′krəl) situated near the sacrum.

**Par·a·sal** (par′ə-sal) trademark for preparations of aminosalicylic acid.

**para·sal·pin·ge·al** (par″ə-sal-pin′je-əl) situated beside or in the wall of the fallopian or uterine tube.

**para·sal·pin·gi·tis** (par″ə-sal″pin-ji′tis) [*para-* + *salping-* + *-itis*] inflammation of the tissues around a fallopian or uterine tube.

**para·scap·u·lar** (par″ə-skap′u-lər) near the scapula.

**Par·as·car·is** (pər-as′kər-is) a genus of nematodes of the family Ascarididae. *P. equo′rum* is a large parasite that hatches in a horse's intestine and migrates around the body, causing coughing, diarrhea, and other symptoms similar to those of ascariasis.

**para·scar·la·ti·na** (par″ə-skahr″lə-te′nə) Duke's disease.

**para·scar·let** (par″ə-skahr′lət) Duke's disease.

**para·sel·lar** (par″ə-sel′ər) near or around the sella turcica.

**para·sex·u·al** (par″ə-sek′shoo-əl) accomplished by other than sexual means, as by genetic study of *in vitro* somatic cell hybrids rather than by pedigree studies.

**para·sex·u·al·i·ty** (par″ə-sek″shoo-al′ĭ-te) abnormal sexuality; usually a paraphilia.

**para·sig·ma·tism** (par″ə-sig′mə-tiz-əm) [*para-* + *sigmatism*] sigmatism.

**para·si·noi·dal** (par″ə-si-noi′dəl) [*para-* + *sino-* + *-oid* + *-al*[1]] situated along the course of a sinus.

**para·si·nu·soi·dal** (par″ə-si″nə-soi′dəl) [*para-* + *sinusoid* + *-al*[1]] sinusoidal.

**par·a·site** (par′ə-sīt) [Gr. *parasitos*] [MeSH: Parasites] 1. a plant or animal which lives upon or within another living organism at whose expense it obtains some advantage. See *symbiosis.* 2. the smaller, less complete component of asymmetrical conjoined twins, which is attached to and dependent on the autosite.
**accidental p.**, an organism parasitizing an animal other than the usual host, as *Dirofilaria* in humans.
**allantoic p.**, with twins in utero, a weaker twin that takes its blood supply from the stronger through its umbilical circulation.
**animal p.**, any parasite that is a member of the animal kingdom, such as a protozoan, helminth, annelid, or arthropod. Called also *zooparasite.*
**celozoic p.**, a parasite which lives in a body cavity.
**cytozoic p.**, a parasite which lives in body cells, as a plasmodium.
**diheteroxenic p.**, a parasite which requires two intermediate hosts.
**ectophytic p.**, a plant ectoparasite.
**ectozoic p.**, an animal ectoparasite.
**endophytic p.**, a plant endoparasite.
**entozoic p.**, a parasite which lives in the lumen of the intestine.
**eurytrophic p.**, an ectoparasite which can feed on various hosts.
**facultative p.**, an organism which may be parasitic upon another but which is capable of independent existence.
**hematozoic p.**, a parasite which lives in the blood.
**incidental p.**, accidental p.
**intermittent p.**, a parasite which lives in its host only at times, being free living during the interval; called also *occasional p.*
**karyozoic p.**, a parasite which lives in cell nuclei.
**malarial p.**, *Plasmodium.*
**obligatory p.**, a parasite which cannot live apart from its host.
**occasional p.**, intermittent p.
**periodic p.**, a parasite that resides in its host for short periods.
**permanent p.**, a parasite which lives in its host from early life until maturity or death of the parasite.
**plant p.**, vegetable p.
**specific p.**, one normal to its current host.
**spurious p.**, an organism which is parasitic on hosts other than humans, but which may pass through the human body without causing harm.
**stenotrophic p.**, an ectoparasite which can feed on one host only.
**temporary p.**, a parasite which lives free of its host during part of its life cycle.
**teratoid p.**, in asymmetrical conjoined twins, a parasite that appears as a tumorlike mass.
**vegetable p.**, any parasite of the vegetable kingdom, such as a fungus.

**par·a·si·te·mia** (par″ə-si-te′me-ə) [MeSH: Parasitemia] the presence of parasites (especially malarial parasites) in the blood.

**par·a·sit·ic** (par″ə-sit′ik) [Gr. *parasitikos*] pertaining to, of the nature of, or caused by a parasite.

**par·a·sit·i·ci·dal** (par″ə-sit″ĭ-si′dəl) destructive to parasites.

**par·a·sit·i·cide** (par″ə-sit′ĭ-sīd) [*parasite* + *-cide*] 1. destructive to parasites. 2. an agent that is destructive to parasites.

**par·a·sit·i·fer** (par″ə-sit′ĭ-fər) [*parasite* + L. *ferre* to bear] an organism which serves as the host of a parasite.

**par·a·sit·ism** (par″ə-si′tiz-əm) 1. symbiosis in which one population (or individual) adversely affects the other but cannot live without it. 2. infection or infestation with parasites.

**para·sit·iza·tion** (par″ə-sit″ĭ-za′shən) infection or infestation with a parasite.

**par·a·sito·gen·ic** (par″ə-sit″o-jen′ik) [*parasite* + *-genic*] caused by parasites.

**par·a·si·toid** (par′ə-si″toid) resembling a parasite.

**par·a·si·tol·o·gist** (par″ə-si-tol′ə-jist) an expert in parasitology.

**par·a·si·tol·o·gy** (par″ə-si-tol′ə-je) [*parasite* + *-logy*] [MeSH: Parasitology] the science or study of parasites and parasitism.

**par·a·si·to·sis** (par″ə-si-to′sis) infection or infestation with parasites.

**par·a·si·to·trope** (par″ə-si′to-trōp) parasitotropic.

**par·a·si·to·trop·ic** (par″ə-si″to-trop′ik) [*parasite* + *-tropic*] having special affinity for parasites.

**par·a·si·tot·ro·pism** (par″ə-si-tot′rə-piz-əm) parasitotropy.

**par·a·si·tot·ro·py** (par″ə-si-tot′rə-pe) the affinity of a drug for infective parasites.

**para·so·ma** (par″ə-so′mə) paranucleus.

**para·som·nia** (par″ə-som′ne-ə) [*para-* + *somn-* + *-ia*] [DSM-IV] a category of sleep disorders in which abnormal physiological or behavioral events occur during sleep, due to inappropriately timed activation of physiological systems; it includes nightmare disorder, sleep terror disorder, and sleepwalking disorder. Cf. *dyssomnia.*

**para·spa·di·as** (par″ə-spa′de-əs) [*para-* + Gr. *spadon* a rent] a developmental anomaly in which the urethra opens upon one side of the penis.

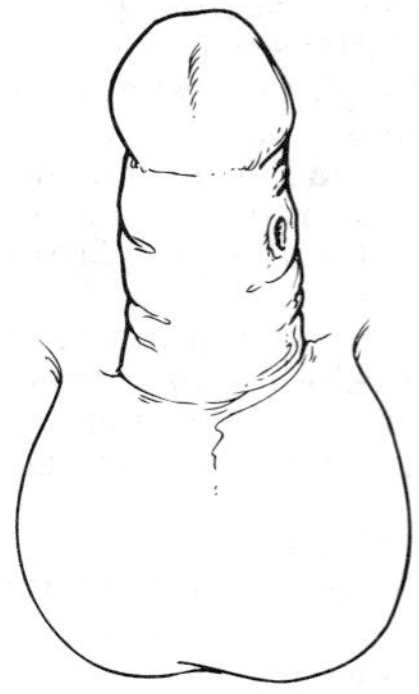

Paraspadias.

**para·spe·cif·ic** (par″ə-spə-sif′ik) having curative properties in addition to the specific one.

**para·sple·nic** (par″ə-sple′nik) beside the spleen.

**para·ster·nal** (par″ə-ster′nəl) [*para-* + *sternal*] situated beside the sternum.

**para·stru·ma** (par″ə-stroo′mə) a goiterlike enlargement of a parathyroid gland.

**para·sui·cide** (par″ə-soo′ĭ-sīd) attempted suicide, emphasizing that in most such attempts death is not the desired outcome.

**para·sym·pa·thet·ic** (par″ə-sim″pə-thet′ik) of or pertaining to that division of the autonomic nervous system made up of the ocular, bulbar, and sacral divisions; see under *system.*

**para·sym·path·i·co·to·nia** (par″ə-sim-path″ĭ-ko-to′ne-ə) vagotonia.

**para·sym·pa·tho·lyt·ic** (par″ə-sim″pə-tho-lit′ik) [*parasympathetic* + *-lytic*] 1. producing effects resembling those of interruption of the parasympathetic nerve supply to a part. 2. an agent that opposes the effects of impulses conveyed by the parasympathetic nerves. Called also *anticholinergic.*

**para·sym·pa·tho·mi·met·ic** (par″ə-sim″pə-tho-mĭ-met′ik) [*parasympathetic* + *-mimetic*] 1. producing effects resembling those of stimulation of the parasympathetic nerve supply to a part. 2. an agent that produces effects similar to those produced by stimulation of the parasympathetic nerves. Called also *cholinergic.*

**para·syn·ap·sis** (par″ə-sin-ap′sis) [*para-* + *synapsis*] the union of chromosomes side by side during meiosis. Cf. *telosynapsis.*

**para·syn·de·sis** (par″ə-sin-de′sis) parasynapsis.

**para·syno·vi·tis** (par″ə-sin″o-vi′tis) [*para-* + *synovitis*] inflammation of the tissues about a synovial sac.

**para·sys·to·le** (par″ə-sis′tə-le) [*para-* + *systole*] [MeSH: Parasystole] a cardiac irregularity attributed to the interaction of two foci that independently initiate cardiac impulses at different rates; as a rule, one of these foci is the sinoatrial node (the normal pacemaker), and the ectopic focus is usually in the ventricle. Each focus, and thus each rhythm, is protected from the influence of the other. **ventricular p.,** parasystole in which the ectopic focus is in the ventricle.

**para·tar·si·um** (par″ə-tahr′se-əm) [*para-* + *tarsus*] the side of the tarsus of the foot.

**para·ten·ic** (par″ə-ten′ik) denoting an intermediate host, sometimes called transfer host, of a parasite that is not essential to (neither hindering nor hastening) the completion of the parasite's life cycle.

**para·ten·on** ((par″ə-ten′on) [*para-* + Gr. *tenōn* tendon] the fatty areolar tissue filling the interstices of the fascial compartment in which a tendon is situated.

**para·thi·on** (par″ə-thi′on) [MeSH: Parathion] an organophosphorus agricultural insecticide that is highly toxic to humans and other animals. See *organophosphorus compound poisoning,* under *poisoning.*

**para·thor·mone** (par″ə-thor′mōn) parathyroid hormone.

**para·thy·mia** (par″ə-thi′me-ə) [*para-* + *-thymia*] a perverted, contrary, or inappropriate mood; characteristic of schizophrenia.

**para·thy·rin** (par″ə-thi′rin) parathyroid hormone.

**par·a·thy·roid** (par″ə-thi′roid) [*para-* + *thyroid*] 1. situated beside the thyroid gland. 2. in the plural, parathyroid glands.

**para·thy·roid·al** (par″ə-thi-roi′dəl) pertaining to the parathyroid glands.

**para·thy·roid·ec·to·mize** (par″ə-thi″roid-ek′tə-mīz) to excise the parathyroid gland(s).

**para·thy·roid·ec·to·my** (par″ə-thi″roid-ek′tə-me) [*parathyroid* + *-ectomy*] [MeSH: Parathyroidectomy] excision of the parathyroid gland(s).

**para·thy·roid·in** (par″ə-thi′roid-in) an extract of the parathyroid glands that exerts the skeletal, renal, and gastrointestinal actions of parathyroid hormone.

**para·thy·roid·o·ma** (par″ə-thi″roid-o′mə) parathyroid adenoma or carcinoma.

**para·thy·ro·pri·val** (par″ə-thi″ro-pri′vəl) hypoparathyroid.

**para·thy·ro·pri·via** (par″ə-thi″ro-pri′ve-ə) hypoparathyroidism.

**para·thy·ro·priv·ic** (par″ə-thi″ro-priv′ik) hypoparathyroid.

**para·thy·rop·ri·vous** (par″ə-thi-rop′rĭ-vəs) hypoparathyroid.

**para·thy·ro·troph·ic** (par″ə-thi″ro-trof′ik) parathyrotropic.

**para·thy·ro·trop·ic** (par″ə-thi″ro-trop′ik) having an affinity for or stimulating the growth or hormonal secretion of the parathyroid glands.

**para·to·nia** (par″ə-to′ne-ə) [*para-* + *ton-* + *-ia*] any disorder of muscle tone, such as gegenhalten; cf. *myotonia* and *dystonia.*

**para·tope** (par′ə-tōp) [*para-* + *-tope*] [MeSH: Binding Sites, Antibody] an antigen-binding site of an antibody molecule. Cf. *epitope.*

**para·tose** (par′ə-tōs) an unusual sugar found to be a polysaccharide somatic antigen of *Salmonella* species.

**para·tra·cho·ma** (par″ə-trə-ko′mə) inclusion conjunctivitis.

**para·troph·ic** (par″ə-trof′ik) [*para-* + *-trophic*] requiring living material or complex protein matter for food. Cf. *metatrophic.*

**pa·rat·ro·phy** (pə-rat′rə-fe) [*para-* + *-trophy*] dystrophy.

**para·tu·ber·cu·lo·sis** (par″ə-tə-ber″ku-lo′sis) [MeSH: Paratuberculosis] 1. a disease resembling tuberculosis but not due to *Mycobacterium tuberculosis.* 2. Johne's disease.

**para·tu·ber·cu·lous** (par″ə-tə-ber′ku-ləs) 1. having an indirect relation to tuberculosis. 2. due to conditions produced by tuberculosis. 3. pertaining to paratuberculosis.

**para·type** (par′ə-tīp) any strain of bacteria, other than the holotype, that is specifically stated to be the one on which the original description of the taxon was based.

**para·typh·li·tis** (par″ə-tif-li′tis) [*para-* + *typhl-* + *-itis*] inflammation of the postperitoneal tissue of the cecum.

**para·ty·phoid** (par″ə-ti′foid) [*para-* + *typhoid*] 1. see under *fever.* 2. any infection due to any of the *Salmonella* serotypes except *S. typhi;* see *enteric fever,* under *fever,* and *salmonellosis.*

**para·typ·ic** (par″ə-tip′ik) paratypical.

**para·typ·i·cal** (par″ə-tip′ĭ-kəl) differing from the type.

**para·um·bil·i·cal** (par″ə-əm-bil′ĭ-kəl) alongside the umbilicus.

**para·un·gual** (par″ə-ung′gwəl) [*para-* + *ungual*] near or beside a nail.

**para·ure·thra** (par″ə-u-re′thrə) an accessory urethral canal.

**para·ure·thral** (par″ə-u-re′thrəl) near the urethra.

**para·ure·thri·tis** (par″ə-u″rə-thri′tis) inflammation of the tissues near the urethra.

**para·uter·ine** (par″ə-u′tər-in) alongside the uterus.

**para·vac·cin·ia** (par″ə-vak-sin′e-ə) [*para-* + *vaccinia*] 1. a viral infection of cattle caused by a parapoxvirus, producing lesions similar to those of cowpox and infectious ecthyma on the udders and teats of cows and on the oral mucosa of suckling calves; it begins as small red papules that evolve to vesicles, pustules, and scabbing. It may be transmitted to humans during milking, producing milker's nodules (q.v.); there may then be retransmission to uninfected cows. Called also *pseudocowpox.* 2. milker's nodules.

**para·vag·i·nal** (par″ə-vaj′ĭ-nəl) beside or alongside of the vagina.

**para·vag·i·ni·tis** (par″ə-vaj″ĭ-ni′tis) inflammation of the tissue about the vagina.

**para·ve·nous** (par″ə-ve′nəs) beside a vein.

**para·ver·te·bral** (par″ə-ver′tə-brəl) beside the vertebral column.

**para·vis·cer·al** (par″ə-vis′er-əl) beside a viscus or the visceral branches of the aorta.

**par·ax·i·al** (par-ak′se-əl) [*para-* + *axial*] situated alongside an axis.

**par·ax·on** (par-ak′son) [*para-* + *axon*] a collateral branch of an axon.

**para·zone** (par′ə-zōn) one of the white bands alternating with the dark bands (diazones) in the layers of enamel prisms and seen in cross-section of a tooth.

**par·ben·da·zole** (par-ben′də-zōl) a veterinary benzimidazole anthelmintic with nematocidal action.

**par·co·na·zole hy·dro·chlo·ride** (par-ko′nə-zōl) an antifungal, $C_{17}H_{16}Cl_2N_2O_3 \cdot HCl$.

**Pa·ré** (pah-ra′) Ambroise (1510–1590) chief surgeon to three French kings and the greatest surgeon of the 16th century. Paré reformed the treatment of gunshot wounds by abolishing cauterization with boiling oil. He also practiced ligation of arteries after amputation and reintroduced podalic version into obstetrics. His famous aphorism, *Je le pansay, et Dieu le guarit* ("I dressed him and God healed him"), first appeared in 1585, in the fourth edition of his collected works, which he wrote in French to make more accessible.

**par·ec·ta·sia** (par″ek-ta′zhə) parectasis.

**par·ec·ta·sis** (par-ek′tə-sis) [*para-* + *ectasis*] excessive stretching or distention of a part or organ.

**Par·e·drine** (par′ə-drēn) trademark for preparations of hydroxyamphetamine hydrobromide.

**par·e·gor·ic** (par″ə-gor′ik) [Gr. *parēgorikos* consoling] [USP] a preparation of powdered opium, anise oil, benzoic acid, camphor, diluted alcohol, and glycerin; used as an antiperistaltic, especially in the treatment of diarrhea, administered orally.

**Pa·rel·a·pho·stron·gy·lus** (pə-rel″ə-fo-stron′jĭ-lus) a genus of nematodes of the family Protostrongylidae. *P. te′nuis* is normally a harmless parasite of the white-tailed deer, but sometimes it invades the central nervous system of other ruminant species, including sheep and goats, causing fatal neurological disease.

**par·el·e·i·din** (par″əl-e′ĭ-din) the keratin precursor of epidermal cells derived from eleidin of the stratum lucidum.

**par·en·ce·pha·lia** (par″ən-sə-fa′le-ə) [*para-* + *encephal-* + *-ia*] congenital defect of the brain.

**par·en·ceph·a·lo·cele** (par″ən-sef′ə-lo-sēl) [*parencephalon* + *-cele*[1]] encephalocele with hernial protrusion of the cerebellum.

**par·en·ceph·a·lous** (par″ən-sef′ə-ləs) [*para-* + *encephal-* + *-ous*] having a congenital deformity of the brain.

**pa·ren·chy·ma** (pə-reng′kĭ-mə) [Gr. "anything poured in beside"] the essential elements of an organ; used in anatomical nomenclature as a general term to designate the functional elements of an organ, as distinguished from its framework, or stroma.
**p. glandula′re prosta′tae,** p. prostatae.
**p. prosta′tae** [TA], parenchyma of prostate: the aggregation of 30 to 50 small compound tubulosaccular or tubuloalveolar glands that make up the bulk of the prostate; called also *p. glandulare prostatae.*
**p. tes′tis** [TA], **p. of testis,** the seminiferous tubules, which are located within the lobules of the testis.

**pa·ren·chy·mal** (pə-reng′kĭ-məl) pertaining to or of the nature of parenchyma.

**par·en·chym·a·ti·tis** (par″əng-kim″ə-ti′tis) inflammation of a parenchyma.

**par·en·chym·a·tous** (par″əng-kim′ə-təs) pertaining to or of the nature of parenchyma.

**par·en·chym·u·la** (par″əng-kim′u-lə) the embryonic stage succeeding that called the closed blastula.

**Par·en·do·my·ces** (par″en-do-mi′sēz) a former genus of fungi, now included in the genus *Candida.*

**pa·ren·tal** (pə-ren′təl) of, pertaining to, or derived from the parents.

**pa·ren·ter·al** (pə-ren′tər-əl) [*para-* + *enteral*] not through the alimentary canal but rather by injection through some other route, such as subcutaneous, intramuscular, intraorbital, intracapsular, intraspinal, intrasternal, or intravenous.

**par·epi·did·y·mis** (par″ep-ĭ-did′ĭ-mis) paradidymis.

**par·epi·gas·tric** (par″ep-ĭ-gas′trik) near the epigastrium.

**pa·re·sis** (pə-re′sis) [Gr. "relaxation"] [MeSH: Paresis] slight or incomplete paralysis.
**benign enzootic p.,** a mild variety of infectious porcine encephalomyelitis.
**general p.,** parenchymatous neurosyphilis in which chronic meningoencephalitis causes gradual loss of cortical function, resulting in progressive dementia and generalized paralysis, which generally occurs 10 to 20 years after the initial infection of syphilis. Called also *Bayle's disease, dementia paralytica, paralytic dementia, paretic neurosyphilis,* and *syphilitic meningoencephalitis.*
**inherited spastic p.,** a hereditary condition seen in calves during the first year of life, characterized by excessive tonic contractions of the gastrocnemius muscle of first one and later both of the hind legs, with rigidity of the hocks so that the animal is lame and because of lack of exercise fails to gain weight. Called also *Elso heel.*
**parturient p.,** paralysis in a cow near the time of delivery, usually accompanied by hypocalcemia and due to a metabolic disorder. See also *downer cow syndrome,* under *syndrome.* Called also *milk fever* and *parturient fever* or *paralysis.*

**par·es·the·sia** (par″əs-the′zhə) [*para-* + *-esthesia*] [MeSH: Paresthesia] an abnormal touch sensation, such as burning, prickling, or formication, often in the absence of an external stimulus.
**Bernhardt's p.,** meralgia paresthetica.
**postoperative p.,** prolonged paresthesia after surgery done with a local anesthetic, especially around the mouth due to injury of the mental nerve or mandibular nerve.

**par·es·thet·ic** (par″əs-thet′ik) pertaining to or marked by paresthesia.

**pa·ret·ic** (pə-ret′ik) pertaining to or affected with paresis.

**par·fo·cal** (pahr-fo′kəl) [L. *par* equal + *focal*] retaining correct focus on changing powers in microscopy.

**par·gy·line hy·dro·chlo·ride** (par′gə-lēn) a monoamine oxidase inhibitor used in the treatment of moderate to severe hypertension; administered orally.

**Par·ham band** (pahr′əm) [Frederick William *Parham,* American surgeon, 1856–1927] see under *band.*

**par·i·ca** (par′ĭ-kə) [Port.] a narcotic snuff prepared from seeds of species of *Piptadenia,* Brazilian trees; the seeds contain dimethyltryptamine and related psychotomimetic indole alkaloids. Called also *cohoba.*

**pa·ric·ine** (pə-ris′in) a quinoline alkaloid from the bark of *Cinchona succirubra,* the red cinchona.

**par·i·es** (par′e-ēz) pl. *pari′etes* [L.] [TA] wall: a general term for the wall of an organ or body cavity.
**p. ante′rior gas′tris** [TA], anterior wall of stomach: the wall of the stomach directed toward the anterior surface of the body. Called also *anterior gastric wall.*
**p. ante′rior vagi′nae** [TA], anterior wall of vagina: the wall of the vagina that is intimately associated with the posterior wall of the bladder and urethra.
**p. ante′rior ventri′culi,** p. anterior gastris.
**p. caro′ticus cavita′tis tympa′nicae, p. caro′ticus cavita′tis tym′pani** [TA], carotid wall of tympanic cavity: the anterior wall of the cavity, related to the carotid canal, in which is lodged the internal carotid artery.
**p. exter′nus duc′tus cochlea′ris** [TA], external wall of cochlear duct: the part of the ductal wall adjacent to the outer wall of the cochlea.
**p. infe′rior or′bitae** [TA], inferior wall of orbit: an inner orbital surface formed by surfaces of the maxilla, the zygomatic bone, and the palatine bone; called also *floor of orbit.*
**p. jugula′ris cavita′tis tympa′nicae, p. jugula′ris cavita′tis tym′pani** [TA], jugular wall of tympanic cavity: the floor of the tympanic cavity, which is in intimate relation with the jugular fossa, which lodges the bulb of the internal jugular vein.
**p. labyrin′thicus cavita′tis tympa′nicae, p. labyrin′thicus cavita′tis tym′pani** [TA], labyrinthic wall of tympanic cavity: the wall of the cavity facing medially toward the inner ear; it contains the fenestra vestibuli, the fenestra cochleae, and the promontory. Called also *medial wall of tympanic cavity.*
**p. latera′lis or′bitae** [TA], lateral wall of orbit: an inner orbital surface formed by the orbital surfaces of the great wing of the sphenoid bone, the zygomatic bone, and the zygomatic process of the frontal bone.
**p. mastoi′deus cavita′tis tympa′nicae, p. mastoi′deus cavita′tis tym′pani** [TA], mastoid wall of tympanic cavity: the posterior wall of the cavity, related to the mastoid portion of the temporal bone.
**p. media′lis or′bitae** [TA], medial wall of orbit: an inner orbital surface formed by parts of the maxillary, lacrimal, ethmoid, and sphenoid bones.
**p. membrana′ceus cavita′tis tympa′nicae, p. membrana′ceus cavita′tis tym′pani** [TA], membranous wall of tympanic cavity: the outer wall of the tympanic cavity, formed mainly by the tympanic membrane.
**p. membrana′ceus tra′cheae** [TA], membranous wall of trachea: the posterior part of the wall of the trachea where the cartilaginous rings are deficient.
**p. poste′rior gas′tris** [TA], posterior wall of stomach: the wall of the stomach directed toward the posterior surface of the body. Called also *posterior gastric wall.*
**p. poste′rior vagi′nae** [TA], posterior wall of vagina: the vaginal wall intimately associated with the anterior wall of the rectum.
**p. poste′rior ventri′culi,** p. posterior gastris.
**p. supe′rior or′bitae** [TA], superior wall of orbit: an inner orbital surface formed chiefly by the orbital plate of the frontal bone and the orbital surface of the lesser wing of the sphenoid bone; called also *roof of orbit.*
**p. tegmenta′lis cavita′tis tympa′nicae, p. tegmenta′lis cavita′tis tym′pani** [TA], tegmental wall of tympanic cavity: the upper surface of the cavity, formed by part of the petrous portion of the temporal bone. Called also *roof of tympanic cavity* and *roof of tympanum.* See also *tegmen tympani.*
**p. tympa′nicus duc′tus cochlea′ris** [TA], tympanic wall of cochlear duct: the wall of the cochlear duct that separates it from the scala tympani, composed of the osseous spiral laminae and the basilar membrane. Called also *membrana spiralis ductus cochlearis* [TA alternative] and *spiral membrane of cochlear duct.*
**p. vestibula′ris duc′tus cochlea′ris** [TA], vestibular wall of cochlear duct: the thin anterior wall of the cochlear duct, which separates it from the scala vestibuli; called also *membrana vestibularis ductus cochlearis* [TA alternative] and *vestibular membrane of cochlear duct.*

**pa·ri·e·tal** (pə-ri′ə-təl) [L. *parietalis*] 1. of or pertaining to the walls of a cavity. 2. pertaining to or located near the parietal bone, as the parietal lobe.

**pa·ri·e·tes** (pə-ri′ə-tēz) [L.] plural of *paries.*

**pa·ri·e·ti·tis** (pə-ri″ə-ti′tis) inflammation of the wall of an organ.

**parieto-** [L. *paries,* gen. *parietis* wall] combining form denoting a relation to the parietal bone, the parietal lobe, or a wall of a cavity or organ.

**pa·ri·e·to·fron·tal** (pə-ri″ə-to-frun′təl) pertaining to the parietal and frontal bones, gyri, or fissures.

**pa·ri·e·tog·ra·phy** (pə-ri″ə-tog′rə-fe) radiographic visualization of the walls of an organ.
**gastric p.,** radiographic visualization of the stomach wall by special technique, as a means of detecting early gastric neoplasm.

**pa·ri·e·to·oc·cip·i·tal** (pə-ri″ə-to-ok-sip′ĭ-təl) pertaining to the parietal and occipital bones or lobes.

**pa·ri·e·to·sphe·noid** (pə-ri″ə-to-sfe′noid) pertaining to the parietal and sphenoid bones.

**pa·ri·e·to·splanch·nic** (pə-ri″ə-to-splank′nik) parietovisceral.

**pa·ri·e·to·squa·mo·sal** (pə-ri″ə-to-skwah-mo′səl) pertaining to the parietal bone and the squamous portion of the temporal bone.

**pa·ri·e·to·tem·po·ral** (pə-ri″ə-to-tem′por-əl) pertaining to the parietal and temporal bones or lobes.

**pa·ri·e·to·vis·ce·ral** (pə-ri″ə-to-vis′ə-rəl) both parietal and visceral; pertaining to the walls of a cavity and the viscera within it.

**Pa·ri·naud's syndrome, oculoglandular syndrome** (pah-rĭ-nōz′) [Henri *Parinaud,* French ophthalmologist, 1844–1905] see under *syndrome.*

**pa·ri pas·su** (par′e pas′oo) [L., "at equal pace"] coincidentally with; to the same proportion or degree.

**par·i·ty**[1] (par′ĭ-te) [L. *parere* to bring forth, produce] [MeSH: Parity] para; the condition of a woman with respect to her having borne viable offspring. Cf. *gravidity.*

**par·i·ty**[2] (par′ĭ-te) [L. *par* equal] equality; close correspondence or similarity.

**Park's aneurysm** (pahrks) [Henry *Park,* English surgeon, 1744–1831] see under *aneurysm.*

**Par·ker's fluid** (pahr′kərz) [George Howard *Parker,* American zoologist, 1864–1955] see under *fluid.*

**Parkes Web·er syndrome** (pahrks va′bər) [Frederick *Parkes Weber,* English physician, 1863–1962] Sturge-Weber syndrome.

**Par·kin·son's disease, facies (sign)** (pahr′kin-sənz) [James *Parkinson,* English physician, 1755–1824] see *paralysis agitans,* and under *facies.* See also *parkinsonism.*

**par·kin·so·ni·an** (pahr″kin-sōn′e-ən) named for James Parkinson or pertaining to parkinsonism; see under *crisis, facies,* and *syndrome.*

**par·kin·son·ism** (pahr′kin-sən-iz″əm) a group of neurological disorders characterized by hypokinesia, tremor, and muscular rigidity. See *parkinsonian syndrome,* under *syndrome,* and see *paralysis agitans (Parkinson's disease).*
**postencephalitic p.,** parkinsonian syndrome.

**Par·lo·del** (par′lo-del″) trademark for a preparation of bromocriptine mesylate.

**Par·nate** (par′nāt) trademark for a preparation of tranylcypromine sulfate.

**par·oc·cip·i·tal** (par″ok-sip′ĭ-təl) [*para-* + *occipital*] near the occipital bone.

**par·ol·i·vary** (par-ol′ĭ-var″e) [*para-* + *olivary*] situated near the olive or olivary nucleus.

**par·o·mo·my·cin** (par′o-mo-mi″sin) [MeSH: Paromomycin] an aminoglycoside antibiotic derived from *Streptomyces rimosus* var. *paromomycinus,* which is effective against a wide variety of gram-negative, gram-positive, and acid-fast bacteria.
**p. sulfate** [USP], the sulfate salt of paromomycin, used orally as an antiamebic.

**Pa·ro·na's space** (pah-ro′nahz) [Francesco *Parona,* Italian orthopedic surgeon, 1861–1910] see under *space.*

**par·onych·ia** (par″o-nik′e-ə) [*para-* + *onych-* + *-ia*] [MeSH: Paronychia] inflammation involving the folds of tissue surrounding the nail. Called also *perionychia.* See also *onychia.*
**herpetic p.,** see under *whitlow.*
**p. tendino′sa,** septic inflammation of the sheath of the tendon of a finger.

**par·o·nych·i·al** (par″o-nik′e-əl) 1. pertaining to paronychia. 2. pertaining to the nail folds.

**par·ooph·o·ric** (par″o-o-fo′rik) pertaining to the paroöphoron.

**par·ooph·o·ri·tis** (par″o-of-o-ri′tis) 1. inflammation of the paroöphoron. 2. inflammation of the tissues about the ovary.

**par·oöph·o·ron** (par″o-of′ə-ron) [*para-* + Gr. *ōon* egg + *pherein* to bear] [TA] an inconstantly present small group of coiled tubules between the layers of the mesosalpinx, being a remnant of the excretory part of the mesonephros.

**par·oph·thal·mia** (par″of-thal′me-ə) [*para-* + *ophthalmia*] inflammation of the connective tissue around the eye.

**par·oph·thal·mon·cus** (par″of-thəl-mong′kəs) [*para-* + *ophthalm-* + *onkos* mass] a tumor situated near the eye.

**par·op·sis** (pər-op′sis) parablepsia.

**par·or·chid·i·um** (par″or-kid′e-əm) [*para-* + Gr. *orchis* testicle] misplacement of a testis or testes.

**par·or·chis** (par-or′kis) the epididymis.

**par·orex·ia** (par″o-rek′se-ə) [*para-* + Gr. *orexis* appetite] disordered appetite, with craving for unusual foods; sometimes used synonymously with pica.

**par·os·mia** (par-oz′me-ə) [*para-* + *osm-*[1] + *-ia*] any disease or perversion of olfaction. Called also *dysosmia* and *paraosmia.* See also *anosmia.*

**par·os·te·al** (par-os′te-əl) pertaining to the outer surface of the periosteum.

**par·os·te·itis** (par″os-te-i′tis) [*para-* + *osteitis*] inflammation of the tissues around a bone.

**par·os·te·o·sis** (par″os-te-o′sis) [*para-* + *osteo-* + *-osis*] ossification of the tissues outside of the periosteum.

**par·os·ti·tis** (par″os-ti′tis) parosteitis.

**par·os·to·sis** (par″os-to′sis) parosteosis.

**pa·rot·ic** (pə-rot′ik) [*para-* + *otic*] situated or occurring near the ear.

**pa·rot·id** (pə-rot′id) [*para-* + Gr. *ous* ear] situated or occurring near the ear, as the parotid gland.

**pa·rot·i·de·an** (pə-rot″ĭ-de′ən) pertaining to the parotid gland.

**pa·rot·i·dec·to·my** (pə-rot″ĭ-dek′tə-me) [*parotid* + *-ectomy*] excision of the parotid gland.

**pa·rot·i·di·tis** (pə-rot″ĭ-di′tis) parotitis.

**pa·rot·i·do·scir·rhus** (pə-rot″ĭ-do-skir′əs) [*parotid* + *scirrh-* + *-ous*] hardening of the parotid gland.

**par·o·tin** (par′o-tin) [MeSH: Parotin] an acidic globulin extractable from human parotid gland, which may have some hormonal properties; in rabbits, it promotes mesenchymal growth and calcification of teeth, lowers serum calcium levels, and affects the leukocyte count.

**par·oti·tis** (par″o-ti′tis) [MeSH: Parotitis] inflammation of the parotid gland. Called also *parotiditis.*
**epidemic p.,** mumps.
**p. phlegmono′sa,** that associated with suppuration.
**postoperative p.,** an acute parotitis due to infection (usually with staphylococci) of the parotid gland following a surgical procedure; it is marked by rapid onset, frequently with severe pain and rapid swelling of the glands, and by trismus, low-grade fever, headache, malaise, and leukocytosis. It affects generally debilitated patients, usually middle-aged or older, suffering from dehydration, suppression of salivary secretion, vomiting, or mouth-breathing.
**staphylococcal p.,** postoperative parotitis caused by staphylococci.

**par·ous** (par′əs) [L. *parere* to bring forth, produce] having borne one or more viable offspring.

**par·ovar·i·an** (par″o-var′e-ən) 1. situated beside the ovary. 2. pertaining to the parovarium (epoöphoron).

**par·ovar·i·ot·o·my** (par″o-var″e-ot′ə-me) [*parovarium* + *-tomy*] incision into the parovarium.

**par·ova·ri·tis** (par″o-və-ri′tis) inflammation of the parovarium (epoöphoron).

**par·ova·ri·um** (par″o-var′e-əm) [*para-* + *ovarium*] epoöphoron.

**par·ox·e·tine hy·dro·chlo·ride** (pə-rok′sə-tēn) a selective serotonin reuptake inhibitor used in the treatment of depression, obsessive-compulsive disorder, and panic disorder; administered orally.

**par·ox·ysm** (par′ok-siz-əm) [Gr. *paroxysmos*] 1. a sudden recurrence or intensification of symptoms. 2. a spasm or seizure.

**par·ox·ys·mal** (par″ok-siz′məl) recurring in paroxysms.

**Par·pan·it** (par-pan′it) trademark for a preparation of caramiphen hydrochloride.

**Par·rot's atrophy of newborn, pseudoparalysis,** etc. (pah-rōz′) [Joseph Marie Jules *Parrot,* French physician, 1829–1883] see under *pseudoparalysis* and *sign,* see *marasmus,* and see *ciliospinal reflex,* under *reflex.*

**Par·ry's disease** (par′ēz) [Caleb Hillier *Parry,* English physician, 1755–1822] toxic nodular goiter.

**Par·ry-Rom·berg syndrome** (par′e-rom′berg) [C.H. *Parry;* Moritz Heinrich *Romberg,* German physician, 1795–1873] facial hemiatrophy.

**pars** (pahrz) pl. *par′tes* [L.] 1. a division or part. 2. [TA] a general term for a particular portion of a larger area, organ, or structure.

## Pars

Descriptions are given on TA terms, and include anglicized names of specific parts.

**p. abdomina'lis aor'tae** [TA], abdominal part of aorta: the distal part of the descending aorta, which is the continuation of the thoracic part and gives rise to the inferior phrenic, lumbar, median sacral, superior and inferior mesenteric, middle suprarenal, renal, and testicular or ovarian arteries, and celiac trunk. Called also *abdominal aorta* and *aorta abdominalis* [TA alternative].

**p. abdomina'lis autono'mica,** abdominal autonomic part: the portion of the autonomic nervous system contained within the abdomen; part of its parasympathetic components (the vagus nerves) arise from the medulla oblongata and the sacral spinal cord, and its sympathetic components arise from the thoracic and upper lumbar cord. Called also *abdominal* or *lumbar part of autonomic nervous system* and *p. abdominalis systematis autonomici.*

**p. abdomina'lis duc'tus thora'cici** [TA], the abdominal part of the thoracic duct; see *ductus thoracicus.*

**p. abdomina'lis eso'phagi,** p. abdominalis oesophagi.

**p. abdomina'lis mus'culi pectora'lis majo'ris** [TA], abdominal part of pectoralis major muscle: the portion of the muscle that originates from the aponeurosis of the obliquus externus abdominis.

**p. abdomina'lis oeso'phagi** [TA], abdominal part of esophagus: the part of the esophagus below the diaphragm, joining the stomach. Written also *p. abdominalis esophagi.* Called also *abdominal esophagus.*

**p. abdomina'lis syste'matis autono'mici,** p. abdominalis autonomica.

**p. abdomina'lis ure'teris** [TA], abdominal part of ureter: that portion of the ureter extending from the kidney to the terminal line of the pelvis.

**p. ala'ris mus'culi nasa'lis** [TA], alar part of nasalis muscle: the part of the nasalis muscle arising from the maxilla on either side above the lateral incisor tooth and attaching to the alar cartilage of the nose; it assists in opening the nasal aperture. Called also *dilator muscle of naris* and *dilator naris.*

**p. alveola'ris mandi'bulae** [TA], alveolar part of mandible: the superior portion of the body of the mandible, which contains sockets for the teeth.

**p. amor'pha,** the spherical, finely granular body surrounded by the nucleolonema of the nucleolus.

**p. ana'lis rec'ti,** canalis analis.

**p. ante'rior commissu'rae anterio'ris** [TA], **p. ante'rior commissu'rae rostra'lis,** anterior part of anterior commissure: the smaller anterior part of the commissure, whose fibers interconnect the two olfactory bulbs.

**p. ante'rior dor'si lin'guae** [TA], anterior part of dorsum of tongue: the part of the dorsum of the tongue anterior to the terminal sulcus. Called also *p. presulcalis dorsi linguae* [TA alternative].

**p. ante'rior facie'i diaphragma'ticae he'patis** [TA], anterior part of diaphragmatic surface of liver: the part directed toward the ventral surface of the body.

**p. ante'rior for'nicis vagi'nae** [TA], the anterior part of the fornix of the vagina; called also *anterior fornix.*

**p. ante'rior lo'buli quadrangula'ris anterio'ris** [TA], anterior part of anterior quadrangular lobule: the anterior division of the lobulus quadrangularis anterior cerebelli. Called also *p. ventralis lobuli quadrangularis anterioris* [TA alternative].

**p. ante'rior pedun'culi ce'rebri,** crus cerebri (def. 1).

**p. ante'rior pon'tis,** p. basilaris pontis.

**p. anula'ris vagi'nae fibro'sae digito'rum ma'nus** [TA], annular part of fibrous sheaths of fingers: strong transverse bands of fibrous tissue, one in the vagina fibrosa of each finger, crossing the flexor tendons at the level of the upper half of the proximal phalanx; called also *annular ligaments of fingers.*

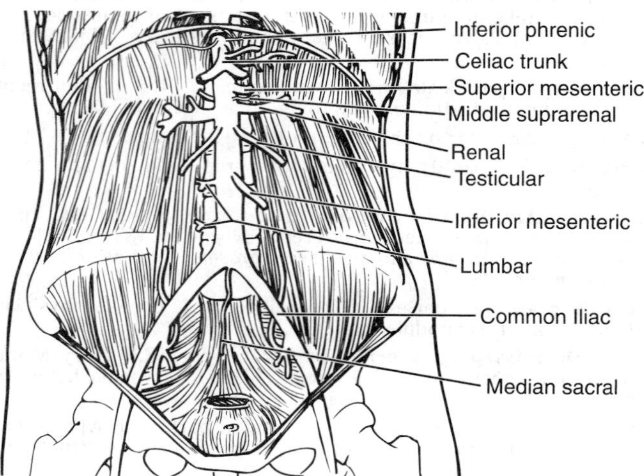


Pars abdominalis aortae (abdominal aorta) and its branches.

**p. anula'ris vagi'nae fibro'sae digito'rum pe'dis** [TA], annular part of fibrous sheaths of toes: fibrous bands in the toes resembling those of similar name in the fingers; called also *annular ligaments of toes.*

**p. aryepiglot'tica mus'culi arytenoi'dei obliq'ui** [TA], aryepiglottic part of oblique arytenoid muscle: an inconstant fascicle of the oblique arytenoid muscle, originating from the apex of the arytenoid cartilage and inserting on the lateral margin of the epiglottis. Called also *aryepiglottic muscle* and *musculus aryepiglotticus.*

**p. ascen'dens aor'tae** [TA], ascending part of aorta: the proximal portion of the aorta, arising from the left ventricle, and giving origin to the right and left coronary arteries before continuing as the arch of the aorta. Called also *aorta ascendens* [TA alternative] and *ascending aorta.*

**p. ascen'dens duode'ni** [TA], ascending part of duodenum: the terminal part of the duodenum, ending at the duodenojejunal flexure.

**p. atlan'tica arte'riae vertebra'lis** [TA], **p. atlan'tis arte'riae vertebra'lis,** atlantal part of vertebral artery: the part of the vertebral artery winding behind the lateral mass of the atlas to lie in a groove on the upper surface of the posterior arch of the atlas. Called also *second part of vertebral artery.*

**p. autono'mica syste'matis nervo'si periphe'rici,** TA alternative for *divisio autonomica systematis nervosi peripherici.*

**p. basa'lis arte'riae pulmona'lis dex'trae** [TA], basal part of right pulmonary artery: the part of the pulmonary artery supplying the basal segments of the inferior lobe of the right lung, comprising the anterior, lateral, medial, and basal segmental arteries.

**p. basa'lis arte'riae pulmona'lis sinis'trae** [TA], basal part of left pulmonary artery: the part of the pulmonary artery supplying the basal segments of the inferior lobe of the left lung, comprising the anterior, lateral, medial, and basal segmental arteries.

**p. basila'ris os'sis occipita'lis** [TA], basilar part of occipital bone: a quadrilateral plate of the occipital bone that projects superiorly and anteriorly from the foramen magnum.

**p. basila'ris pon'tis** [TA], basilar part of pons: the part of the pons connecting the cerebrum, cerebellum, and medulla oblongata. It is a broad transverse band that arches across the anterior surface of the superior end of the rhombencephalon; on each side it narrows to enter the cerebellum as the middle cerebellar peduncle. It comprises longitudinal fibers originating at the cerebral cortex, transverse fibers, and the pontine nuclei. Called also *p. anterior pontis* and *p. ventralis pontis.*

**p. basolatera'lis cor'poris amygdaloi'dei,** basolateral part of amygdaloid body: a part comprising lateral, basal, and accessory basal amygdaloid nuclei.

**p. buccopharyn'gea mus'culi constricto'ris pharyn'gis supe'rio'ris** [TA], buccopharyngeal part of superior constrictor muscle of pharynx: the part of the superior constrictor muscle arising from the pterygomandibular raphe; called also *buccopharyngeal muscle* and *musculus buccopharyngeus.*

**p. calcaneocuboi'dea ligamen'ti bifurca'ti,** ligamentum calcaneocuboideum.

**p. calcaneonavicula'ris ligamen'ti bifurca'ti,** ligamentum calcaneonaviculare.

**p. cana'lis ner'vi op'tici** [TA], intracanalicular part of optic nerve: the part of the nerve that runs through the optic canal. Called also *p. intracanalicularis nervi optici.*

**p. cardi'aca gas'tris,** TA alternative for *cardia.*

**p. cardi'aca ventri'culi,** cardia.

**p. cartilagi'nea sep'ti na'si** [TA], cartilaginous part of nasal septum: the plate of cartilage forming the anterior part of the nasal septum.

**p. cartilagi'nea syste'matis skeleta'lis** [TA], the cartilaginous part of the skeletal system; the cartilages of the body.

**p. cartilagi'nea tu'bae auditi'vae** [TA], cartilaginous part of auditory tube: the part of the tube that is chiefly supported by the tubal cartilage, extending from the pars ossea to the pharyngeal orifice of the auditory tube. Called also *p. cartilaginea tubae auditoriae* [TA alternative].

**p. cartilagi'nea tu'bae audito'riae,** TA alternative for *p. cartilaginea tubae auditivae.*

**p. cauda'lis ner'vi vestibula'ris,** p. inferior nervi vestibularis.

**p. caverno'sa arte'riae caro'tidis inter'nae** [TA], cavernous part of internal carotid artery: the part located in the cavernous sinus; it has numerous branches.

**p. centra'lis syste'matis nervo'si** [TA], the central nervous system, consisting of the brain and spinal cord. Called also *systema nervosum centrale* [TA alternative].

**p. centra'lis ventri'culi latera'lis** [TA], central part of lateral ventricle: the part of the lateral ventricle found within the parietal lobe;

it communicates with the frontal, occipital, and temporal horns. Called also *body of lateral ventricle.*

**p. ceratopharyn'gea mus'culi constricto'ris pharyn'gis me'dii** [TA], ceratopharyngeal part of middle constrictor muscle of pharynx: the part of the middle constrictor muscle arising from the greater cornu of the hyoid bone; called also *musculus ceratopharyngeus* and *ceratopharyngeal muscle.*

**p. cerebra'lis arte'riae caro'tidis inter'nae** [TA], cerebral part of internal carotid artery: the terminal part of the artery, which divides into the anterior and middle cerebral arteries in the middle cranial fossa.

**p. cervica'lis arte'riae caro'tidis inter'nae** [TA], cervical part of internal carotid artery: an unbranched part located in the carotid triangle of the neck.

**p. cervica'lis arte'riae vertebra'lis,** TA alternative for *p. transversaria arteriae vertebralis.*

**p. cervica'lis duc'tus thora'cici** [TA], the cervical part of the thoracic duct; see *ductus thoracicus.*

**p. cervica'lis eso'phagi,** p. cervicalis oesophagi.

**p. cervica'lis medul'lae spina'lis** [TA], cervical part of spinal cord: the part of the cord that is within the cervical part of the vertebral canal and gives rise to the eight pairs of cervical spinal nerves *(segmenta cervicalia medullae spinalis [1–8]).*

**p. cervica'lis oeso'phagi** [TA], cervical part of esophagus: the part of the esophagus located in the cervical region, posterior to the trachea and the recurrent laryngeal nerves, anterior to the longus colli muscle and vertebral column, and medial to the lobes of the thyroid gland and the common carotid arteries. Written also *p. cervicalis esophagi.* Called also *cervical esophagus.*

**p. cervica'lis tra'cheae** [TA], the part of the trachea located in the cervical region, related anteriorly to the jugular venous arch, sternohyoid and sternothyroid muscles, isthmus of thyroid gland, inferior thyroid veins, thymus, arteria thyroidea ima, posteriorly to the esophagus and recurrent laryngeal nerves, and laterally to the lobes of the thyroid gland and common carotid arteries.

**p. chondropharyn'gea mus'culi constricto'ris pharyn'gis me'dii** [TA], chondropharyngeal part of middle constrictor muscle of pharynx: the part of the middle constrictor muscle arising from the lesser cornu of the hyoid bone; called also *chondropharyngeal muscle musculus chondropharyngeus.*

**p. cilia'ris re'tinae** [TA], ciliary part of retina: the two layers of epithelium lining the basal lamina of the ciliary body.

**p. clavicula'ris mus'culi pectora'lis majo'ris** [TA], clavicular part of pectoralis major muscle: the portion of the muscle that originates from the clavicle.

**p. coccy'gea medul'lae spina'lis** [TA], coccygeal part of spinal cord: the part of the cord that is within the coccygeal part of the vertebral canal and gives rise to the coccygeal spinal nerves *(segmenta coccygea medullae spinalis [1–3]).*

**p. cochlea'ris ner'vi octa'vi, p. cochlea'ris ner'vi vestibulocochlea'ris,** nervus cochlearis.

**p. col'lis oeso'phagi,** TA alternative for *p. cervicalis oesophagi.*

**p. compac'ta substan'tiae ni'grae** [TA], compact part of substantia nigra: the posterior part of the substantia nigra, medium-sized cells, many of which are pigmented.

**p. convolu'ta lo'buli cortica'lis re'nis,** convoluted part of cortical lobule of kidney: the part of the renal cortex that surrounds the intracortical prolongations of the pyramids and is composed of convoluted tubules.

**p. corneosclera'lis reti'culi trabecula'ris** [TA], corneoscleral part of trabecular reticulum: the anterior part of the trabecular reticulum, situated between the venous sinus of the sclera, the scleral spur, and the posterior limiting lamina of the cornea.

**par'tes corpo'ris huma'ni** [TA], the parts of the human body; a category in official anatomical terminology.

**p. cortica'lis arte'riae ce'rebri me'diae,** p. terminalis arteriae cerebri mediae.

**p. cortica'lis arte'riae ce'rebri posterior'is,** p. terminalis arteriae cerebri posterioris.

**p. corticomedia'lis cor'poris amygdaloi'dei,** corticomedial part of amygdaloid body: the part comprising central, medial, and cortical amygdaloid nuclei, the nucleus of the lateral olfactory stria, and the transitional anterior amygdaloid area; called also *p. olfactoria corporis amygdaloidei.*

**p. costa'lis diaphrag'matis** [TA], costal part of diaphragm: the part of the thoracic diaphragm arising from the inner surfaces of the ribs and their cartilages.

**p. crania'lis par'tis parasympa'thici divisio'nis autono'mici syste'matis nervo'si** [TA], cranial part of parasympathetic part of autonomic division of nervous system: the part of the parasympathetic nervous system that includes cranial nerves III, VII, IX, and X and the ciliary, pterygopalatine, otic, and submandibular ganglia.

**p. cricopharyn'gea mus'culi constricto'ris pharyn'gis inferio'ris** [TA], cricopharyngeal part of inferior constrictor muscle of pharynx: the part of the inferior constrictor muscle arising from the cricoid cartilage; called also *cricopharyngeal muscle* or *sphincter* and *musculus cricopharyngeus* [TA alternative].

**p. crucifor'mis vagi'nae fibro'sae digito'rum ma'nus** [TA], cruciate part of fibrous sheaths of fingers: one of the diagonal bundles of the fascia of the fingers that cross each other on the dorsal surface of each digit at the level of the distal end of the proximal phalanx; called also *ligamenta cruciata digitorum manus* and *cruciate ligaments of fingers.*

**p. crucifor'mis vagi'nae fibro'sae digito'rum pe'dis** [TA], cruciate part of fibrous sheaths of toes: one of the bundles of fascial fibers in the toes resembling those of similar name in the fingers; called also *ligamenta cruciata digitorum pedis* and *cruciate ligaments of toes.*

**p. cupula'ris reces'sus epitympa'nici** [TA], cupular space: the part of the epitympanic recess above the head of the malleus.

**p. descen'dens aor'tae** [TA], the continuation of the aorta from the arch of the aorta, in the thorax, to the point of its division into the common iliac arteries, in the abdomen; divided anatomically into a thoracic part *(pars thoracica aortae)* and an abdominal part *(pars abdominalis aortae).* Called also *aorta descendens* [TA alternative] and *descending aorta.*

**p. descen'dens duode'ni** [TA], descending part of duodenum: the part between the superior and inferior parts, into which the bile and pancreatic ducts open.

**p. dex'tra facie'i diaphragma'ticae he'patis** [TA], right part of diaphragmatic surface of liver: the portion that is directed toward the right side of the body.

**p. dista'lis adenohypophy'seos** [TA], distal part of adenohypophysis: the part that makes up the main body of the gland. Called also *p. distalis lobi anterioris hypophyseos* [TA alternative].

**p. dista'lis lo'bi anterio'ris hypophy'seos,** TA alternative for *p. distalis adenohypophyseos.*

**p. dorsa'lis cor'poris genicula'ti latera'lis,** nucleus dorsalis corporis geniculati lateralis.

**p. dorsa'lis cor'poris genicula'ti media'lis,** nucleus dorsalis corporis geniculati medialis.

**p. dorsa'lis dience'phali,** the dorsal part of the diencephalon, above the hypothalamic sulcus, comprising the epithalamus, dorsal thalamus, and metathalamus.

**p. dorsa'lis lo'buli quadrangula'ris anterio'ris,** TA alternative for *pars posterior lobuli quadrangularis anterioris.*

**p. dorsa'lis pedun'culi ce'rebri,** p. posterior pedunculi cerebri.

**p. dorsa'lis pon'tis,** tegmentum pontis.

**p. dura'lis fi'li termina'lis** [TA], dural part of filum terminale: the downward prolongation of the spinal dura mater from the lower border of the second sacral vertebra to the first coccygeal vertebral segment. Called also *dural terminal filament, external terminal filament, f. durae matris spinale, f. terminale durale, f. terminale externum* and *terminal filament of spinal dura mater.*

**p. endocri'na pancre'atis,** endocrine pancreas.

**p. exocri'na pancre'atis,** exocrine pancreas.

**p. feta'lis placen'tae,** fetal placenta: the nonmaternal part of the placenta, derived not from the fetus but from the trophoblast that envelops the fetus; from within outward, it consists of amnion, chorionic plate, and chorionic villi. Called also *placenta foetalis.*

**p. fibro'sa,** the portion of the nucleolus containing chiefly filaments.

**p. flac'cida membra'nae tympa'nicae** [TA], the small portion of the tympanic membrane, between the anterior and posterior mallear folds; it is lax and thin. Called also *membrana flaccida, Rivinus' membrane,* and *Shrapnell's membrane.*

**p. functiona'lis,** stratum functionale.

**p. glossopharyn'gea mus'culi constricto'ris pharyn'gis superio'ris** [TA], glossopharyngeal part of superior constrictor muscle of pharynx: the part of the superior constrictor muscle arising from the side of the root of the tongue. Called also *glossopharyngeal muscle* and *musculus glossopharyngeus.*

**p. granulo'sa,** the portion of the nucleolus containing chiefly granules.

**p. horizonta'lis arte'riae ce'rebri me'diae,** TA alternative for *p. sphenoidalis arteriae cerebri mediae.*

**p. horizonta'lis duode'ni** [TA], horizontal part of duodenum: the part of the duodenum between the descending and ascending parts, crossing from right to left ventral to the third lumbar vertebra; called also *p. inferior duodeni* [TA alternative] and *inferior part of duodenum.*

**p. ili'aca li'neae termina'lis,** linea arcuata ossis ilii.

**p. infe'rior duode'ni,** TA alternative for *p. horizontalis duodeni.*

**p. infe'rior ner'vi vestibula'ris** [TA], inferior part of vestibular nerve: the inferior branch of the nerve, which has filaments that end in the ampullary crest of the posterior semicircular ducts and the macula of the saccule. Called also *p. caudalis nervi vestibularis.*

**p. infe'rior ve'nae lingula'ris** [TA], inferior part of lingular vein: a venous branch that drains the inferior lingular segment of the left lung and drains into the lingular vein. Called also *inferior lingular segmental vein.*

**p. inferoposte'rior lo'buli quadrangula'ris,** lobulus simplex cerebelli.

**p. inflex'a,** bar, def. 5.

**p. infraclavicula'ris plex'us brachia'lis** [TA], infraclavicular part of brachial plexus: the part of the brachial plexus that lies in the axilla, below the level of the clavicle. In it arise the medial and lateral pectoral, musculocutaneous, medial brachial cutaneous, medial antebrachial cutaneous, median, ulnar, radial, subscapular, thoracodorsal, and axillary nerves.

**p. infraloba'ris ra'mi poste'rior** [TA], infralobar part of posterior branch: a tributary to the posterior branch of the right superior pulmonary vein; called also *infralobar vein.*

**p. infrasegmenta'lis,** p. intersegmentalis.

**p. infundibula'ris adenohypophy'seos,** p. tuberalis adenohypophyseos.

**p. insula'ris arte'riae ce'rebri me'diae** [TA], insular part of middle cerebral artery: collectively, the branches of the middle cerebral artery supplying the insula and adjacent areas, comprising the arteriae insulares, arteria frontobasilaris lateralis, and arteriae temporales anterior, media, and posterior.

**p. interarticula'ris,** the part of the lamina between the superior and inferior articular processes of a lumbar vertebra.

**p. intercartilagi'nea ri'mae glot'tidis** [TA], the part of the rima glottidis between the arytenoid cartilages; called also *intercartilaginous glottis, respiratory glottis,* and *interarytenoid space.*

**p. interme'dia adenohypophy'seos** [TA], intermediate part of adenohypophysis: an ill-defined region between the two lobes of the hypophysis; some systems of nomenclature consider it part of the neurohypophysis. In humans a defined structure develops during embryogenesis, but only scattered cells are retained when the gland matures. Called also *p. intermedia lobi anterior hypophyseos* [TA alternative].

**p. interme'dia bulbo'rum vesti'buli,** commissura bulborum vestibuli.

**p. interme'dia lo'bi anterio'ris hypophy'seos,** TA alternative for *p. intermedia adenohypophyseos.*

**p. interme'dia ure'thrae masculi'nae** [TA], intermediate part of male urethra: the portion of the urethra between the pars prostatica and pars spongiosa, and traversing the urogenital diaphragm and the deep perineal space. Called also *membranous part of male urethra* and *p. membranacea urethrae masculinae* [TA alternative].

**p. intermembrana'cea ri'mae glot'tidis** [TA], the part of the rima glottidis between the vocal folds. Called also *glottis vocalis.*

**p. intersegmenta'lis** [TA], intersegmental part: any of the veins lying between and draining adjacent bronchopulmonary segments and supplying a main branch of a right or left pulmonary vein; called also *infrasegmental vein, intersegmental vein,* and *p. infrasegmentalis.*

**p. intersegmenta'lis ra'mi poste'rior,** TA alternative for *p. intralobaris rami posterior.*

**p. interstitia'lis tu'bae uteri'nae,** p. uterina tubae uterinae.

**p. intracanalicula'ris ner'vi op'tici,** p. canalis nervi optici.

**p. intracrania'lis arte'riae vertebra'lis** [TA], intracranial part of vertebral artery: the part of the vertebral artery that ascends medially in front of the medulla oblongata where, at about the lower border of the pons, it joins the opposite artery to form the basilar artery. Called also *fourth part of vertebral artery.*

**p. intracrania'lis ner'vi op'tici** [TA], intracranial part of optic nerve: the part of the nerve that lies between the optic canal and the optic chiasm.

**p. intralamina'ris ner'vi op'tici intraocula'ris** [TA], intralaminar part of intraocular optic nerve: the portion of the intraocular part of the optic nerve that runs through the lamina cribrosa of the sclera.

**p. intraloba'ris ra'mi poste'rior** [TA], intralobar part of posterior branch: a tributary of the posterior branch of the right superior pulmonary vein; called also *intersegmental vein* and *p. intersegmentalis rami posterior* [TA alternative].

**p. intraocula'ris ner'vi op'tici** [TA], intraocular part of optic nerve: the part of the nerve that is within the eyeball, separated into postlaminar, intralaminar, and prelaminar parts (see *p. postlaminaris nervi optici, p. intralaminaris nervi optici,* and *p. prelaminaris nervi optici*).

**p. intrasegmenta'lis** [TA], intrasegmental part: any of the small veins lying within a bronchopulmonary segment and draining into one of the main branches of a right or left pulmonary vein.

**p. iri'dica re'tinae** [TA], iridial part of retina: the two layers of pigmented epithelium lining the posterior part of the iris.

**p. labia'lis mus'culi orbicula'ris o'ris** [TA], labial part of orbicularis oris muscle: the part of the muscle whose fibers are restricted to the lips.

**p. lacrima'lis mus'culi orbicula'ris oc'uli** [TA], the part of the orbicularis oculi muscle that arises from the posterior lacrimal ridge of the lacrimal bone, to become continuous with the palpebral portion.

**p. laryn'gea pharyn'gis** [TA], laryngopharynx: the portion of the pharynx that lies below the upper edge of the epiglottis and opens into the larynx and esophagus.

**p. latera'lis ar'cus pe'dis longitudina'lis** [TA], lateral part of longitudinal arch of foot: the part of the arch formed by the calcaneus, the cuboid bone, and the lateral two metatarsal bones. Called also *lateral arch* and *lateral longitudinal arch.*

**p. latera'lis for'nicis vagi'nae** [TA], the lateral part of the fornix of the vagina; called also *lateral fornix.*

**p. latera'lis musculo'rum intertransversario'rum posterio'rum cer'vicis** [TA], the lateral part of the posterior intertransverse muscles of the neck.

**p. latera'lis os'sis occipita'lis** [TA], lateral part of occipital bone: one of the paired parts of the occipital bone that form the lateral boundaries of the foramen magnum, each being prominently characterized by the presence of one of the occipital condyles.

**p. latera'lis os'sis sa'cri** [TA], lateral part of sacrum: the part or mass of the sacrum on either side lateral to the dorsal and pelvic sacral foramina; called also *lateral mass of sacrum.*

**p. latera'lis ve'nae lo'bi me'dii** [TA], lateral part of middle lobar vein: a venous branch draining the lateral segment of the middle lobe of the right lung, emptying into the middle lobar vein. Called also *lateral segmental vein of right lung.*

**p. lenticulothala'micus cap'sulae inter'nae,** p. thalamolenticularis capsulae internae.

**p. li'bera mem'bri inferio'ris** [TA], the bones of the thigh, leg, and foot. Called also *skeleton membri inferioris liberi.*

**p. li'bera mem'bri superio'ris** [TA], the bones of the arm, forearm, and hand. Called also *skeleton membri superioris liberi.*

**p. lumba'lis diaphrag'matis** [TA], lumbar part of diaphragm: the portion of the thoracic diaphragm that arises from the lumbar vertebrae, comprising the right and left diaphragmatic crura, the right crus arising from the superior three or four vertebrae, and the left from the superior two or three.

**p. lumba'lis medul'lae spina'lis** [TA], **p. lumba'ris medul'lae spina'lis,** lumbar part of spinal cord: the part of the cord that is within the lower thoracic part of the vertebral canal (in adults) and gives rise to the five pairs of lumbar spinal nerves *(segmenta lumbalia medullae spinalis [1–5]).*

**p. magnocellula'ris nu'clei ru'bri** [TA], magnocellular part of red nucleus: in humans, the posterior part of the red nucleus, containing a complement of large multipolar cells; the number of these cells is relatively decreased in comparison to the small cells scattered throughout the nucleus; cf. *p. parvocellularis nuclei rubri.*

**p. margina'lis mus'culi orbicula'ris o'ris** [TA], marginal part of orbicularis oris muscle: the part of the muscle whose fibers blend with those of adjacent muscles.

**p. mastoi'dea os'sis tempora'lis,** mastoid part of temporal bone.

**p. media'lis ar'cus pe'dis longitudina'lis** [TA], the part of the longitudinal arch that is foot formed by the calcaneus, talus, navicular, cuneiform, and the first three metatarsal bones. Called also *medial arch* and *medial longitudinal arch.*

**p. media'lis musculo'rum intertransversario'rum posterio'rum cer'vicis,** the medial part of the posterior intertransverse muscles of the neck.

**p. media'lis ve'nae lo'bi me'dii** [TA], medial part of middle lobar vein: a venous branch draining the medial segment of the middle lobe of the right lung, emptying into the middle lobar vein. Called also *medial segmental vein of right lung.*

**p. membrana'cea sep'ti atrio'rum, p. membrana'cea sep'ti interventricula'ris** [TA], membranous part of interventricular septum: the very small, completely membranous area of the interventricular septum of the heart; situated near the root of the aorta, it can be viewed between the opposed margins of the right and posterior semilunar valves of the aorta.

**p. membrana'cea sep'ti na'si** [TA], membranous septum of nose: the anterior inferior part of the nasal septum, beneath the cartilaginous part; it is composed of skin and subcutaneous tissues. Called also *membranous nasal septum* and *membranous septum of nose.*

**p. membrana'cea ure'thrae masculi'nae,** TA alternative for *p. intermedia urethrae masculinae.*

**p. mo'bilis sep'ti na'si** [TA], mobile part of nasal septum: the part of the nasal septum at the apex of the nose, formed by skin, subcutaneous tissue, the greater alar cartilages, the membranous septum, and the columella; called also *septum mobile nasi.*

**p. muscula'ris sep'ti interventricula'ris** [TA], muscular part of interventricular septum of heart: the thick muscular partition forming the greater part of the septum between the ventricles of the heart.

**p. mylopharyn'gea mus'culi constricto'ris pharyn'gis superio'ris** [TA], mylopharyngeal part of superior constrictor muscle of pharynx: the part of the superior constrictor muscle arising from the mylohyoid ridge of the mandible; called also *mylopharyngeal muscle* and *musculus mylopharyngeus.*

**p. nasa'lis os'sis fronta'lis** [TA], nasal part of frontal bone: the small, irregularly shaped process that projects inferiorly from the medial part of the squama of the frontal bone to articulate with the nasal bones and the frontal processes of the maxillae. Called also *prefrontal bone* and *nasal process of frontal bone.*

**p. nasa'lis pharyn'gis** [TA], nasopharynx: the part of the pharynx that lies above the level of the soft palate.

**p. nervo'sa neurohypophy'seos,** TA alternative for *lobus nervosus neurohypophyseos.*

**p. nervo'sa re'tinae,** neural part of retina: the internal, transparent, light-sensitive portion of the optic nerve part of the retina (cf. *p. pigmentosa retinae*), comprising nine layers seen by light microscopy, named from within outward: internal limiting membrane, nerve fiber layer, ganglion cell layer, inner plexiform layer, inner nuclear layer, outer plexiform layer, outer nuclear layer, outer limiting membrane, and layer of rods and cones; the various layers are connected transversely by fibers of connective tissue *(Müller's fibers).* See illustration at *retina.* Called also *cerebral* or *nervous layer of retina,* and *cerebral stratum of retina.*

**p. obli'qua mus'culi cricothyroi'dei** [TA], the fibers of the cricothyroid muscle that are inserted into the inferior horn, caudal margin, and inner surface of the thyroid cartilage.

**p. occlu'sa arte'riae umbilica'lis** [TA], the portion of an umbilical artery that atrophies at birth when the placental circulation ceases to become the medial umbilical ligament. Cf. *p. patens arteriae umbilicalis.*

**p. olfacto'ria cavita'tis na'si** [TA], olfactory region: the superior part of the nasal cavity, the mucosa of which contains most of the receptors for the sense of smell.

**p. olfacto'ria cor'poris amygdaloi'dei,** p. corticomedialis corporis amygdaloidei.

**p. opercula'ris gy'ri fronta'lis inferio'ris** [TA], opercular part of inferior frontal gyrus: the part of the inferior frontal gyrus lying posterior to the ascending ramus of the lateral sulcus and pars triangularis and overlapping the insular lobe (insula). In the hemisphere dominant for speech, it is Broca's motor speech area. See also *operculum frontale* and *operculum frontoparietale.*

**p. op'tica re'tinae** [TA], optic part of retina: the part of the retina that contains receptors sensitive to light, extending posteriorly from the ora serrata on the inner surface of the choroid and continuous at the optic disk with the optic nerve; it consists of an outer pigmented layer (*p. pigmentosa*) and an inner, multilayered nervous layer (*purpura nervosa*). See also *retina.*

**p. ora'lis pharyn'gis** [TA], oropharynx: the division of the pharynx lying between the soft palate and the upper edge of the epiglottis.

**p. orbita'lis glan'dulae lacrima'lis** [TA], orbital part of lacrimal gland: the main part of the lacrimal gland, limited in front by the orbicularis muscle and the orbital septum; called also *glandula lacrimalis superior.*

**p. orbita'lis gy'ri fronta'lis inferio'ris** [TA], orbital part of inferior frontal gyrus: the part of the inferior frontal gyrus lying below the anterior ramus of the lateral sulcus, which curves around the superciliary border to the orbital surface of the frontal lobe of the cerebral hemisphere anterior to the pars triangularis. See also *operculum frontale* (defs. 1,2).

**p. orbita'lis mus'culi orbicula'ris oc'uli** [TA], orbital part of orbicularis oculi muscle: the part of the orbicularis oculi muscle that arises from the medial margin of the orbit and surrounds it and the palpebral part of the muscle, inserting near the site of origin.

**p. orbita'lis ner'vi op'tici** [TA], orbital part of optic nerve: the part of the nerve located between the optic canal and the eyeball.

**p. orbita'lis os'sis fronta'lis** [TA], orbital part of frontal bone: the horizontal part of the bone; it forms the greater part of the roof of the orbit and of the floor of the anterior cranial fossa and is separated from its fellow of the other side by the ethmoid incisure. Called also *orbital plate of frontal bone.*

**p. os'sea sep'ti na'si** [TA], the bony part of the nasal septum, composed posterosuperiorly of the perpendicular plate of the ethmoid bone and posteroinferiorly of the vomer. Called also *bony* or *osseous nasal septum* and *septum nasi osseum* [TA].

**p. os'sea syste'matis skeleta'lis** [TA], the osseous part of the skeletal system; the bones of the body.

**p. os'sea tu'bae auditi'vae** [TA], osseous part of auditory tube: the part of the tube that lies within the temporal bone, extending from the tympanic orifice to the pars cartilaginea of the auditory tube. Called also *p. ossea tubae auditoriae* [TA alternative].

**p. os'sea tu'bae audito'riae,** TA alternative for *p. ossea tubae auditivae.*

**p. palpebra'lis glan'dulae lacrima'lis** [TA], palpebral part of lacrimal gland: the part of the gland that projects laterally into the upper eyelid; called also *glandula lacrimalis inferior,* and *Rosenmüller's gland* or *node.*

**p. palpebra'lis mus'culi orbicula'ris o'culi** [TA], palpebral part of orbicularis oculi muscle: the part of the orbicularis oculi muscle that is contained in the eyelids, originating from the medial palpebral ligament and inserting in the lateral canthus.

**p. parasympa'thica divisio'nis autono'mici syste'matis nervo'si** [TA], official terminology for *parasympathetic nervous system*; see under *system.*

**p. parvocellula'ris nu'clei ru'bri** [TA], parvocellular part of red nucleus: the complement of small multipolar cells scattered throughout the red nucleus; in humans, these cells predominate over the large cells in the caudal part of the nucleus; cf. *p. magnocellularis nuclei rubri.*

**p. pa'tens arte'riae umbilica'lis** [TA], patent part of umbilical artery: the proximal section of the fetal umbilical cord, which remains patent in the adult, although reduced in size. Cf. *p. occlusa arteriae umbilicalis.*

**p. pel'vica autono'mica,** pelvic autonomic part: the portion of the autonomic nervous system contained within the pelvis; it comprises four or five sacral ganglia and is continuous superiorly with the abdominal part. Called also *p. pelvica systematis autonomici.*

**p. pel'vica par'tis parasympathe'ticae syste'matis nervo'si autono'mici** [TA], pelvic part of parasympathetic part of autonomic division of nervous system: the part of the parasympathetic nervous system that includes the second to fourth anterior sacral roots and the sacral splanchnic nerves.

**p. pel'vica syste'matis autonom'ici,** p. pelvica autonomica.

**p. pel'vica ure'teris** [TA], pelvic part of ureter: the portion of the ureter that extends from the terminal line of the pelvis to the urinary bladder.

**p. periphe'rica syste'matis nervo'si** [TA], the peripheral part of the nervous system, consisting of the nerves and ganglia outside the brain and spinal cord; called also *peripheral nervous system* and *systema nervosum periphericum* [TA alternative].

**p. petro'sa arte'riae caro'tidis inter'nae** [TA], petrous part of internal carotid artery: the portion of the artery located in the carotid canal.

**p. petro'sa os'sis tempora'lis** [TA], petrous part of temporal bone: a pyramid of dense bone located at the base of the cranium; one of the three parts of the temporal bone, it houses the organ of hearing. Some anatomists divide it into petrous and mastoid subparts and call it the *petromastoid part of temporal bone.* Called also *pyramid of temporal bone.*

**p. pharyn'gea lo'bi anterio'ris hypophy'seos,** pharyngeal hypophysis.

**p. pia'lis fi'li termina'lis** [TA], pial part of filum terminale: the prolongation of the spinal pia mater, surrounded by extensions of the dural and arachnoid meninges, from the conus medullaris to the lower border of the second sacral vertebra. Called also *f. terminale internum, f. terminale piale,* and *internal* or *pial terminal filament.*

**p. pigmento'sa re'tinae,** pigmented part of retina: a layer of pigmented epithelium, the outer of the two parts of the optic part of the retina (cf. *p. nervosa retinae*), extending from the entrance of the optic nerve to the pupillary margin of the iris; see also *retina.* Called also *pigmented layer* or *stratum of retina, stratum pigmenti bulbi oculi,* and *stratum pigmenti retinae.*

**p. pla'na cor'poris cilia'ris,** orbiculus ciliaris.

**p. plica'ta cor'poris cilia'ris,** corona ciliaris.

**p. postcommunica'lis arte'riae ce'rebri anterio'ris** [TA], postcommunical part of anterior cerebral artery: collectively, the branches of the anterior cerebral artery that supply the cortex of the medial parts of the frontal and parietal lobes, comprising arteriae frontobasalis medialis, callosomarginalis (and its rami), paracentralis, precunealis, and parieto-occipitalis. Called also *arteria pericallosa* and *pericallosal artery.*

**p. postcommunica'lis arte'riae ce'rebri posterio'ris** [TA], postcommunical part of posterior cerebral artery: collectively, the branches of the posterior cerebral artery that supply cerebral peduncles, posterior thalamus, colliculi, and pineal and medial geniculate bodies, and choroid plexuses of lateral and third ventricles, comprising the arteriae posterolaterales and rami thalamici, choroidei posteriores mediales and laterales, and pedunculares.

**p. poste'rior commissu'rae anterio'ris** [TA], **p. poste'rior commissu'rae rostra'lis,** posterior part of anterior commissure: the larger posterior portion of the commissure, whose fibers interconnect the middle and inferior temporal gyri, the parahippocampal gyri, and the amygdaloid bodies of the two sides.

**p. poste'rior dor'si lin'guae** [TA], posterior part of dorsum of tongue: the part of the dorsum of the tongue posterior to the terminal sulcus. Called also *p. postsulcalis dorsi linguae* [TA alternative].

**p. poste'rior facie'i diaphragma'ticae he'patis** [TA], posterior part of diaphragmatic surface of liver: the part directed toward the dorsal surface of the body; called also *facies posterior hepatis.*

**p. poste'rior for'nicis vagi'nae** [TA], the posterior part of the fornix of the vagina; called also *posterior fornix.*

**p. poste'rior lo'buli quadrangula'ris anterio'ris** [TA], posterior part of anterior quadrangular lobule: the posterior division of the lobulus quadrangularis anterior cerebelli. Called also *p. dorsalis lobuli quadrangularis anterioris* [TA alternative].

**p. poste'rior pedun'culi ce'rebri,** posterior part of cerebral peduncle: the part of the peduncle that is posterior to the substantia nigra, continuous across the median plane and forming the tegmentum of the mesencephalon. Called also *p. dorsalis pedunculi cerebri.*

**p. poste'rior pon'tis,** tegmentum pontis.

**p. postlamina'ris ner'vi op'tici intraocula'ris** [TA], postlaminar part of intraocular optic nerve: that portion of the intraocular part of the optic nerve that is posterior to the lamina cribrosa of the sclera.

**p. postsulca'lis dor'si lin'guae,** TA alternative for *p. posterior dorsi linguae.*

**p. precommunica'lis arte'riae ce'rebri anterio'ris** [TA], precommunical part of anterior cerebral artery: collectively, the branches of the anterior cerebral artery that supply the thalamus and corpus striatum, comprising arteriae centrales anteromediales, centralis brevis and longa, and communicans anterior, and rami centrales anteromediales.

**p. precommunica'lis arte'riae ce'rebri posterio'ris** [TA], precommunical part of posterior cerebral artery: collectively, the branches of the posterior cerebral artery anterior to its point of junction with the posterior communicating branch of the internal carotid artery, comprising the arteriae centrales posterolaterales.

**p. prelamina'ris ner'vi op'tici intraocula'ris** [TA], prelaminar part of intraocular optic nerve: that portion of the intraocular part of the optic nerve that is anterior to the lamina cribrosa of the sclera.

**p. presulca'lis dor'si lin'guae,** TA alternative for *p. anterior dorsi linguae.*

**p. prevertebra'lis arte'riae vertebra'lis** [TA], prevertebral part of vertebral artery: the part of the artery before it ascends through the transverse processes of the upper six cervical vertebrae. Called also *first part of vertebral artery.*

**p. profun'da glan'dulae paroti'deae** [TA], deep part of parotid gland: that part of the gland located deep to the facial nerve.

**p. profun'da mus'culi masse'teris** [TA], deep part of masseter muscle: the part whose fibers arise from the medial surface of the zygomatic arch and the fascia over the temporal muscle, and are directed in a vertical inferior direction.

**p. profun'da mus'culi sphinc'teris a'ni exter'nus** [TA], deep part of sphincter ani externus muscle: the part of the muscle that surrounds the upper part of the anal canal.

**p. prosta'tica ure'thrae masculi'nae** [TA], prostatic part of male urethra: the part of the urethra that passes through the prostate.

**p. pterygopharyn'gea mus'culi constricto'ris pharyn'gis superio'ris** [TA], pterygopharyngeal part of superior constrictor muscle of pharynx: the part of the superior constrictor muscle arising from the caudal part and hamulus of the medial pterygoid plate; called also *pterygopharyngeal muscle* and *musculus pterygopharyngeus.*

**p. pylo'rica gas'tris** [TA], pyloric part of stomach: the caudal third of the stomach, consisting of the pyloric antrum and canal, and distinguished by the presence of the pyloric glands and by the absence of parietal cells; called also *p. pylorica ventriculi* [TA alternative].

**p. pylo'rica ventri'culi,** TA alternative for *p. pylorica gastris.*

**p. quadra'ta,** quadrate part: the quadrilateral portion of the medial segment of the left hepatic lobe.

**p. radia'ta lo'buli cortica'lis re'nis,** radiate part of cortical lobule of kidney: any of the intracortical prolongations of the renal pyramids; called also *processus Ferreini lobuli corticalis renis* and *pyramid of Ferrein.*

**p. rec'ta mus'culi cricothyroi'dei** [TA], the fibers of the cricothyroid muscle that are inserted into the caudal margin of the thyroid cartilage.

**p. rec'ta tu'buli rena'lis,** tubulus rectus proximalis.

**p. respirato'ria cavita'tis na'si** [TA], respiratory region: the part of the nasal cavity inferior to the olfactory region.

**p. reticula'ris substan'tiae ni'grae** [TA], reticular part of substantia nigra: the anterior part of the substantia nigra, which contains fewer cells than the pars compacta, only some of which contain a small amount of pigment.

**p. retrolentifor'mis cap'sulae inter'nae** [TA], retrolentiform part of internal capsule: that part of the internal capsule resting on the lateral surface of the thalamus behind the lentiform nucleus, and containing the posterior thalamic radiation. Called also *retrolenticular* or *retrolentiform limb of internal capsule.*

**p. rostra'lis ner'vi vestibula'ris,** p. superior nervi vestibularis.

**p. sacra'lis li'neae termina'lis,** the sacral part of the terminal line of the pelvis.

**p. sacra'lis medul'lae spina'lis** [TA], sacral part of spinal cord: the part of the cord that is within the lumbar part of the vertebral canal and gives rise to the five pairs of sacral spinal nerves *(segmenta sacralia medullae spinalis [1–5]).*

**p. sphenoida'lis arte'riae ce'rebri me'diae** [TA], sphenoidal part of middle cerebral artery: collectively, the branches of the middle cerebral artery that supply the internal capsule, thalamus, and corpus striatum, comprising the arteriae anterolaterales and rami mediales and laterales. Called also *p. horizontalis arteriae cerebri mediae* [TA alternative].

**p. spina'lis ner'vi accesso'rii,** TA alternative for *radix spinalis nervi accessorii.*

**p. spongio'sa ure'thrae masculi'nae** [TA], spongiose part of male urethra: the portion of the urethra within the corpus spongiosum of the penis.

**p. squamo'sa os'sis tempora'lis** [TA], squamous part of temporal bone: the flat, scalelike, anterior and superior portion of the temporal bone; called also *squama temporalis.*

**p. sterna'lis diaphrag'matis** [TA], sternal part of diaphragm: the portion of the thoracic diaphragm that arises from the inner aspect of the xiphoid process of the sternum.

**p. sternocosta'lis mus'culi pectora'lis majo'ris** [TA], sternocostal part of pectoralis major muscle: the portion of the muscle that originates from the sternum and the ribs.

**p. subcuta'nea mus'culi sphinc'teris a'ni exter'nus** [TA], subcutaneous part of sphincter ani externus muscle: the part of the muscle that surrounds the lowermost portion of the anal canal.

**p. sublentifor'mis cap'sulae inter'nae** [TA], sublentiform part of internal capsule: the part of the internal capsule lying anterior to the posterior part of the lentiform nucleus, and containing the temporopontine, geniculocalcarine, and auditory radiation fibers. Called also *sublenticular limb of internal capsule* and *sublentiform limb of internal capsule.*

**p. superficia'lis glan'dulae paroti'deae** [TA], superficial part of parotid gland: that part of the parotid gland located superficial to the facial nerve.

**p. superficia'lis mus'culi masse'teris** [TA], superficial part of masseter muscle: the part of the muscle whose fibers arise from the anterior part of the zygomatic arch and are directed inferiorly and posteriorly.

**p. superficia'lis mus'culi sphinc'teris a'ni exter'nus** [TA], superficial part of sphincter ani externus muscle: the part of the muscle that lies just deep to the pars subcutanea, extending farther toward the rectum.

**p. supe'rior duode'ni** [TA], superior part of duodenum: the part of the duodenum adjacent to the pylorus, forming the superior flexure.

**p. supe'rior facie'i diaphragma'ticae he'patis** [TA], superior part of diaphragmatic surface of liver: the part that is directed cranially.

**p. supe'rior ner'vi vestibula'ris** [TA], superior part of vestibular nerve: the superior branch of the nerve, which has filaments that end in the ampullary crests of the anterior and lateral semicircular ducts and the macula of the utricle. Called also *p. rostralis nervi vestibularis.*

**p. supe'rior ve'nae lingula'ris** [TA], superior part of lingular vein: a venous branch that drains the superior lingular segment of the left lung and drains into the lingular vein. Called also *superior lingular segmental vein.*

**p. supraclavicula'ris plex'us brachia'lis** [TA], supraclavicular part of brachial plexus: the part of the brachial plexus lying in the cervical region above the level of the clavicle, in which arise the dorsal scapular, long thoracic, and suprascapular nerves, and the nerve to the subclavius muscle.

**p. sympa'thica divisio'nis autono'mici syste'matis nervo'si** [TA], official terminology for *sympathetic nervous system*; see under *system.*

**p. ten'sa membra'nae tympa'nicae** [TA], the larger portion of the tympanic membrane; it is tense and firm. Called also *membrana tensa* and *membrana vibrans.*

**p. termina'lis arte'riae ce'rebri me'diae,** terminal part of middle cerebral artery: collectively, the branches of the middle cerebral artery that supply the lateral surface of the hemisphere, comprising the arteriae sulci centralis, precentralis, and postcentralis, arteriae parietales anterior et posterior, and arteria gyri angularis. Called also *p. corticalis arteriae cerebri mediae.*

**p. termina'lis arte'riae ce'rebri posterio'ris,** terminal part of posterior cerebral artery: collectively, the branches of the posterior cerebral artery that supply the cortex of the temporal and parietal lobes, comprising arteriae occipitalis lateralis and medialis and their rami. Called also *p. corticalis arteriae cerebri posterioris.*

**p. thalamolenticula'ris cap'sulae inter'nae,** thalamolenticular part of internal capsule: the part of the posterior limb of the internal capsule adjacent to the thalamus and lentiform nucleus, consisting of fibers of the thalamic radiations and corticospinal, corticorubral, corticoreticular, and corticothalamic fibers; sometimes the thalamoparietal fibers and the central thalamic radiations are also included. Called also *p. lenticulothalamicus capsulae internae.*

**p. thora'cica aor'tae** [TA], thoracic part of aorta: the proximal portion of the descending aorta, which proceeds from the arch of the aorta and gives rise to the bronchial, esophageal, pericardiac, and mediastinal branches, and the superior phrenic, posterior intercostal III to XI, and subcostal arteries; it is continuous through the diaphragm with the abdominal aorta. Called also *aorta thoracalis, thoracic aorta,* and *aorta thoracica* [TA alternative].

**p. thora'cica autono'mica** [TA], thoracic autonomic part: the portion of the autonomic nervous system contained within the thorax; its sympathetic components are derived from the upper thoracic spinal cord and its parasympathetic components from the vagus nerves. It also contains preganglionic sympathetic fibers that reach abdominal

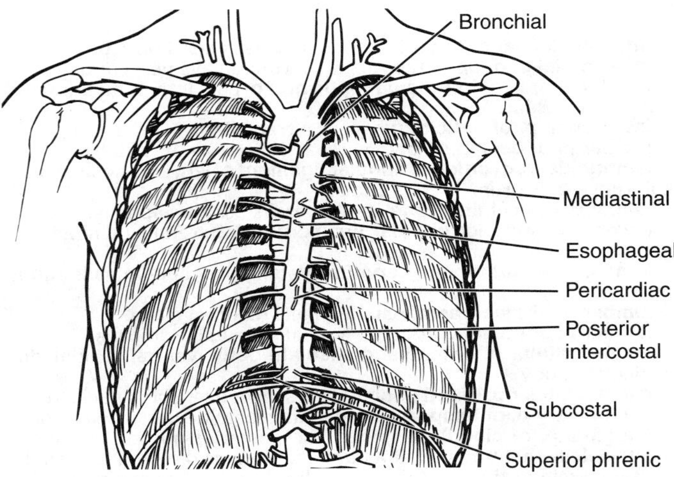


Pars thoracica aortae (thoracic aorta) and the arteries and branches to which it gives rise.

viscera by way of thoracic splanchnic nerves. Called also *p. thoracica systematis autonomici.*

**p. thora′cica duc′tus thora′cici** [TA], the thoracic part of the thoracic duct; see *ductus thoracicus.*

**p. thora′cica eso′phagi,** p. thoracica oesophagi.

**p. thora′cica medul′lae spina′lis** [TA], thoracic part of spinal cord: the part of the cord that is within the upper three fourths of the thoracic part of the vertebral canal (in the adult) and gives rise to the twelve pairs of thoracic spinal nerves *(segmenta thoracica medullae spinalis [1–12]).*

**p. thora′cica oeso′phagi** [TA], thoracic part of esophagus: the part of the esophagus located in the thoracic region, posterior to the trachea and pericardium and anterior to the vertebral column. Written also *p. thoracica esophagi.* Called also *thoracic esophagus.*

**p. thora′cica syste′matis autono′mici,** p. thoracica autonomica.

**p. thora′cica tra′cheae** [TA], the part of the trachea that lies posteriorly in the superior mediastinum, separated from the upper four thoracic vertebrae by the esophagus.

**p. thyroepiglot′tica mus′culi thyroarytenoi′dei** [TA], thyro-epiglottic part of cricoarytenoid muscle: fibers of the thyroarytenoid muscle that continue to the margin of the epiglottis; it closes the inlet to the larynx. Called also *thyroepiglottic muscle* and *musculus thyro-epiglotticus.*

**p. thyropharyn′gea mus′culi constricto′ris pharyn′gis inferio′ris** [TA], thyropharyngeal part of inferior constrictor muscle of pharynx: the part of the inferior constrictor muscle arising from the thyroid cartilage; called also *thyropharyngeal muscle* and *musculus thyropharyngeus* [TA alternative].

**p. tibiocalca′nea ligamen′ti collatera′lis media′lis** [TA], tibiocalcaneal part of medial collateral ligament: the middle portion of the superficial fibers of the medial collateral ligament of the ankle joint, attached superiorly to the medial malleolus of the tibia and inferiorly into nearly the entire length of the sustentaculum tali of the calcaneus. Called also *calcaneotibial ligament, ligamentum calcaneotibiale,* and *tibiocalcaneal* or *tibiocalcanean ligament.*

**p. tibionavicula′ris ligamen′ti collatera′lis media′lis** [TA], tibionavicular part of medial collateral ligament: the anterior portion of the superficial fibers of the medial collateral ligament of the ankle joint, attached superiorly to the anterior surface of the medial malleolus of the tibia and inferiorly to the navicular bone and the margin of the calcaneonavicular ligament. Called also *ligamentum tibionaviculare* and *tibionavicular ligament.*

**p. tibiotala′ris ante′rior ligamen′ti collatera′lis media′lis** [TA], anterior tibiotalar part of medial collateral ligament: the deeper portion of the medial collateral ligament of the ankle joint, attached superiorly to the medial malleolus of the tibia and inferiorly to the medial surface of the talus. Called also *ligamentum talotibiale anterius* and *anterior talotibial ligament.*

**p. tibiotala′ris poste′rior ligamen′ti collatera′lis media′lis** [TA], posterior tibiotalar part of medial collateral ligament: the posterior portion of the superficial fibers of the medial collateral ligament of the ankle joint, attached superiorly to the posterior part of the medial malleolus of the tibia and inferiorly to the medial surface of the talus. Called also *ligamentum talotibiale posterius* and *posterior talotibial ligament.*

**p. transver′sa mus′culi nasa′lis** [TA], transverse part of nasalis muscle: the part of the nasalis muscle arising from the maxilla on either side just lateral to the nasal notch and inserting on the bridge of the nose; it compresses the nasal opening. Called also *compressor muscle of naris* and *compressor naris.*

**p. transver′sa ra′mi sinis′tri ve′nae por′tae he′patis** [TA], the transverse part of the left branch of the hepatic portal vein.

**p. transversa′ria arte′riae vertebra′lis** [TA], transverse part of vertebral artery: the part of the vertebral artery in the transverse processes of the upper six cervical vertebrae, which provides spinal and muscular branches; called also *p. cervicalis arteriae vertebralis* [TA alternative] and *third* or *cervical part of vertebral artery.*

**p. triangula′ris gy′ri fronta′lis inferio′ris** [TA], triangular part of inferior frontal gyrus: the wedge-shaped part of the inferior frontal lobe that lies between the anterior and ascending branches of the lateral sulcus of the cerebral hemisphere bordered by the pars orbitalis anteriorly and the pars opercularis posteriorly. See also *operculum frontale* (defs. 1,2).

**p. tubera′lis adenohypophy′seos** [TA], tubular part of adenohypophysis: a part consisting of a thin cloak of cells on the anterior and lateral surfaces of the infundibulum. It provides a vascular communication between the hypothalamus and the pituitary gland and secretes some hormones. Called also *p. infundibularis adenohypophyseos* and *p. tuberalis lobi anterioris hypophyseos* [TA alternative].

**p. tubera′lis lo′bi anterio′ris hypophy′seos,** TA alternative for *p. tuberalis adenohypophyseos.*

**p. tympa′nica os′sis tempora′lis** [TA], tympanic part of temporal bone: the curved bony plate, developed from the annulus tympanicus of the fetus, forming the anterior and inferior walls and part of the posterior wall of the external auditory meatus in the adult; called also *tympanic plate.*

**p. umbilica′lis ra′mi sinis′tri ve′nae por′tae he′patis** [TA], umbilical part of left branch: the part of the left branch of the hepatic portal vein that passes from the hilum of the liver to the umbilicus.

**p. uteri′na placen′tae,** uterine placenta: the maternally contributed part of the placenta, derived from the decidua basalis; called also *maternal placenta* and *placenta uterina.*

**p. uteri′na tu′bae uteri′nae** [TA], uterine part of uterine tube: the proximal part of the uterine tube, located within the wall of the uterus.

**p. uvea′lis reti′culi trabecula′ris** [TA], uveal part of trabecular reticulum: the posterior part of the trabecular reticulum, situated between the scleral spur, the ciliary body, and the anterior iris.

**p. vaga′lis ner′vi accesso′rii,** TA alternative for *radix cranialis nervi accessorii.*

**p. ventra′lis cor′poris genicula′ti latera′lis,** nucleus ventralis corporis geniculati lateralis.

**p. ventra′lis cor′poris genicula′ti media′lis,** nucleus ventralis corporis geniculati medialis.

**p. ventra′lis dience′phali,** the ventral part of the diencephalon, below the hypothalamic sulcus, comprising the ventral thalamus (subthalamus) and the hypothalamus.

**p. ventra′lis lo′buli quadrangula′ris anterio′ris,** TA alternative for *pars anterior lobuli quadrangularis anterioris.*

**p. ventra′lis pedun′culi ce′rebri,** crus cerebri (def. 1).

**p. ventra′lis pon′tis,** p. basilaris pontis.

**p. vertebra′lis facie′i costa′lis pulmo′nis** [TA], vertebral part of costal surface of lung: the part of the costal surface of each lung related behind to the sides of the vertebral bodies.

**p. vestibula′ris ner′vi octa′vi, p. vestibula′ris ner′vi vestibulocochlea′ris,** nervus vestibularis.

**Par•si•dol** (pahr′sĭ-dol) trademark for a preparation of ethopropazine hydrochloride.

**pars pla•ni•tis** (pahrz pla-ni′tis) [MeSH: Pars Planitis] a granulomatous uveitis of the pars plana of the ciliary body.

**part** (pahrt) [L. *pars* a portion, piece, share] a division or portion.

## Part

For names of parts of various anatomical structures not found here, see under *pars*.

**abdominal autonomic p., abdominal p. of autonomic nervous system,** pars abdominalis autonomica.
**abdominal p. of esophagus,** pars abdominalis oesophagi.
**alar p. of nasal muscle,** pars alaris musculi nasalis.
**annular p. of fibrous sheaths of fingers,** pars anularis vaginae fibrosae digitorum manus.
**annular p. of fibrous sheaths of toes,** pars anularis vaginae fibrosae digitorum pedis.
**anterior p. of anterior commissure,** pars anterior commissurae anterioris cerebri.
**anterior p. of anterior quadrangular lobule,** pars anterior lobuli quadrangularis anterioris.
**anterior p. of cerebral peduncle,** crus cerebri (def. 1).
**anterior p. of dorsum of tongue,** pars anterior dorsi linguae.
**anterior p. of pons,** pars basilaris pontis.
**autonomic p. of peripheral nervous system,** divisio autonomica systematis nervosi peripherici.
**basal p. of left pulmonary artery,** pars basalis arteriae pulmonis sinistri.
**basal p. of right pulmonary artery,** pars basalis arteriae pulmonis dextri.
**basilar p. of occipital bone,** pars basilaris ossis occipitalis.
**basilar p. of pons,** pars basilaris pontis.
**basolateral p. of amygdaloid body,** pars basolateralis corporis amygdaloidei.
**broad p. of anterior annular ligament of leg,** retinaculum musculorum extensorum superius pedis.
**cardiac p. of stomach, cardial p. of stomach,** cardia.
**central p. of lateral ventricle,** pars centralis ventriculi lateralis.
**cervical p. of esophagus,** pars cervicalis oesophagi.
**cervical p. of spinal cord,** pars cervicalis medullae spinalis.
**cervical p. of vertebral artery,** pars transversaria arteriae vertebralis.
**coccygeal p. of spinal cord,** pars coccygea medullae spinalis.
**colic p. of omentum,** omentum majus.
**compact p. of substantia nigra,** pars compacta substantiae nigrae.
**condylar p. of occipital bone,** pars lateralis ossis occipitalis.
**corticomedial p. of amygdaloid body,** pars corticomedialis corporis amygdaloidei.
**costal p. of diaphragm,** pars costalis diaphragmatis.
**cranial p. of parasympathetic p. of autonomic division of nervous system,** pars cranialis partis parasympathici divisionis autonomici systematis nervosi.
**craniosacral p. of autonomic nervous system,** parasympathetic nervous system; see under *system* (*pars parasympathica divisionis autonomici systematis nervosi* [TA]).
**cruciate p. of fibrous sheaths of fingers,** pars cruciformis vaginae fibrosae digitorum manus.
**cruciate p. of fibrous sheaths of toes,** pars cruciformis vaginae fibrosae digitorum pedis.
**dorsal p. of anterior quadrangular lobule,** pars posterior lobuli quadrangularis anterioris.
**dorsal p. of lateral geniculate body,** the part of the lateral geniculate body overlying the dorsal part of the lateral geniculate nucleus.
**dorsal p. of lateral geniculate nucleus,** nucleus dorsalis corporis geniculati lateralis.
**dorsal p. of medial geniculate body,** the part of the medial geniculate body overlying the dorsal part of the medial geniculate nucleus. Called also *parvocellular p. of medial geniculate body*.
**dorsal p. of medial geniculate nucleus,** nucleus dorsalis corporis geniculati medialis.
**dural p. of filum terminale,** pars duralis fili terminalis.
**endocrine p. of pancreas,** endocrine pancreas.
**exoccipital p. of occipital bone,** pars lateralis ossis occipitalis.
**exocrine p. of pancreas,** exocrine pancreas.
**first p. of vertebral artery,** pars transversaria arteriae vertebralis.
**fourth p. of vertebral artery,** pars intracranialis arteriae vertebralis.
**horizontal p. of middle cerebral artery,** pars sphenoidalis arteriae cerebri mediae.
**inferior p. of duodenum,** pars horizontalis duodeni.
**inferior p. of rhomboid fossa,** the triangular caudal portion of the rhomboid fossa, extending downward from the rostral part of the taeniae with its apex (the calamus scriptorius) being continuous with the wall of the central canal of the medulla oblongata.
**inferior p. of vestibular nerve,** pars inferior nervi vestibularis.
**infraclavicular p. of brachial plexus,** pars infraclavicularis plexus brachialis.
**intermediate p. of male urethra,** pars intermedia urethrae masculinae.
**intermediate p. of rhomboid fossa,** the wide central portion of the rhomboid fossa, between the superior foveae rostrally and the beginning of the taeniae caudally.
**interstitial p. of uterine tube, intramural p. of uterine tube,** pars uterina tubae uterinae.
**intracanalicular p. of optic nerve,** p. canalis nervi optici.
**intracranial p. of optic nerve,** pars intracranialis nervi optici.
**intralaminar p. of intraocular optic nerve,** pars intralaminaris nervi optici intraocularis.
**intraocular p. of optic nerve,** pars intraocularis nervi optici.
**jugular p. of occipital bone,** pars lateralis ossis occipitalis.
**lambdoidal p. of anterior annular ligament of leg,** retinaculum musculorum extensorum inferius pedis.
**lateral p. of occipital bone,** pars lateralis ossis occipitalis.
**lower p. of anterior annular ligament of leg,** retinaculum musculorum extensorum inferius pedis.
**lumbar p. of autonomic nervous system,** pars abdominalis autonomica.
**lumbar p. of diaphragm,** pars lumbalis diaphragmatis.
**lumbar p. of spinal cord,** pars lumbalis medullae spinalis.
**magnocellular p. of medial geniculate body,** ventral p. of medial geniculate body.
**magnocellular p. of red nucleus,** pars magnocellularis nuclei rubri.
**mammillary p. of temporal bone,** pars mastoidea ossis temporalis.
**marginal p. of cingulate sulcus,** the posterior portion of the cingulate sulcus that turns off at a right angle and is directed toward the dorsal margin of the cerebral hemisphere, separating the precuneus and the paracentral lobule.
**mastoid p. of temporal bone,** the posterior portion of the pars petrosa ossis temporalis, bounded anteriorly by the external acoustic meatus and articulating superiorly with the parietal bone and posteriorly with the occipital bone. Called also *mastoid bone*.
**membranous p. of male urethra,** pars intermedia urethrae masculinae.
**nasal p. of frontal bone,** pars nasalis ossis frontalis.
**occipital p. of occipital bone,** squama occipitalis.
**orbital p. of optic nerve,** pars orbitalis nervi optici.
**parasympathetic p. of autonomic division of nervous system,** pars parasympathica divisionis autonomici systematis nervosi; see *parasympathetic nervous system,* under *system*.
**parietal p. of pelvic fascia,** fascia superior diaphragmatis pelvis.
**parvocellular p. of medial geniculate body,** dorsal p. of medial geniculate body.
**parvocellular p. of red nucleus,** pars parvocellularis nuclei rubri.
**pectineal p. of inguinal ligament,** ligamentum lacunare.
**pelvic autonomic p., pelvic p. of autonomic nervous system,** pars pelvica autonomica.
**pelvic p. of parasympathetic p. of autonomic division of nervous system,** pars pelvica partis parasympathici divisionis autonomici systematis nervosi.
**petromastoid p. of temporal bone, petrous p. of temporal bone,** 1. a name given to the pars petrosa ossis temporalis when the petrous and mastoid parts are considered separate entities. 2. the anterior portion of the pars petrosa ossis temporalis, excluding the mastoid part.
**pial p. of filum terminale,** pars pialis fili terminalis.
**posterior p. of anterior commissure,** pars posterior commissurae anterioris.
**posterior p. of anterior quadrangular lobule,** pars posterior lobuli quadrangularis anterioris.
**posterior p. of cerebral peduncle,** pars dorsalis pedunculi cerebri.
**posterior p. of dorsum of tongue,** pars posterior dorsi linguae.
**posterior p. of pons,** tegmentum pontis.
**postlaminar p. of intraocular optic nerve,** pars postlaminaris nervi optici intraocularis.
**postsphenoid p., postsphenoidal p., postsphenoidal p. of sphenoid bone,** the posterior portion of the sphenoid bone; in the fetus it consists of separate basisphenoid, pterygoid, and alisphenoid parts, first cartilaginous and later bony, which fuse to each other and to the presphenoid part before birth. Called also *postsphenoid bone*.
**postsulcal p. of dorsum of tongue,** pars posterior dorsi linguae.
**prelaminar p. of intraocular optic nerve,** pars prelaminaris nervi optici intraocularis.
**presenting p.,** 1. that portion of the fetus that is touched by the examining finger through the uterine cervix and, during labor, is bounded by the girdle of resistance. 2. that portion of the body of the fetus that is farthest forward in the birth canal or is closest to it.
**presphenoid p., presphenoidal p., presphenoidal p. of sphenoid bone,** the anterior portion of the sphenoid bone; it develops separately in the fetus and unites with the postsphenoidal part between the seventh and eighth months of intrauterine life. Called also *presphenoid bone*.
**presulcal p. of dorsum of tongue,** pars anterior dorsi linguae.
**reticular p. of substantia nigra,** pars reticularis substantiae nigrae.
**retrolentiform p. of internal capsule,** pars retrolentiformis capsulae internae.
**sacral p. of spinal cord,** pars sacralis medullae spinalis.
**second p. of vertebral artery,** pars atlantica arteriae vertebralis.

**sphenoid p. of middle cerebral artery,** pars sphenoidalis arteriae cerebri mediae.
**spinal p. of accessory nerve,** radix spinalis nervi accessorii.
**squamous p. of frontal bone,** squama frontalis.
**squamous p. of occipital bone,** squama occipitalis.
**squamous p. of temporal bone,** pars squamosa ossis temporalis.
**sternal p. of diaphragm,** pars sternalis diaphragmatis.
**sternocostal p. of diaphragm,** pars costalis diaphragmatis.
**sublentiform p. of internal capsule,** pars sublentiformis capsulae internae.
**subphrenic p. of esophagus,** pars abdominalis esophagi.
**superior p. of anterior annular ligament of leg,** retinaculum musculorum extensorum superius pedis.
**superior p. of rhomboid fossa,** the triangular rostral portion of the rhomboid fossa, continuous at its apex with the wall of the cerebral aqueduct and terminating at an imaginary line drawn between the superior foveae.
**superior p. of vestibular nerve,** pars superior nervi vestibularis.
**supraclavicular p. of brachial plexus,** pars supraclavicularis plexus brachialis.
**sympathetic p. of autonomic division of nervous system,** pars sympathica divisionis autonomici systematis nervosi; see *sympathetic nervous system,* under *system.*
**tabular p. of occipital bone,** squama occipitalis.
**tendinous p. of epicranius muscle,** galea aponeurotica.
**thalamolenticular p. of internal capsule,** pars thalamolenticularis capsulae internae.
**third p. of quadriceps femoris muscle,** musculus adductor minimus.
**third p. of vertebral artery,** pars transversaria arteriae vertebralis.
**thoracic autonomic p., thoracic p. of autonomic nervous system,** pars thoracica autonomica.
**thoracic p. of esophagus,** p. thoracica oesophagi.
**thoracic p. of spinal cord,** pars thoracica medullae spinalis.
**thoracolumbar p. of autonomic nervous system,** sympathetic nervous system; see under *system (pars sympathica divisionis autonomici systematis nervosi* [TA]).
**transverse p. of anterior annular ligament of leg,** retinaculum musculorum extensorum superius pedis.
**transverse p. of nasal muscle,** pars transversa musculi nasalis.
**tympanic p. of temporal bone,** pars tympanica ossis temporalis.
**vagal p. of accessory nerve,** radix cranialis nervi accessorii.
**vaginal p. of cervix,** portio vaginalis cervicis.
**ventral p. of anterior quadrangular lobule,** pars anterior lobuli quadrangularis anterioris.
**ventral p. of cerebral peduncle,** crus cerebri (def. 1).
**ventral p. of lateral geniculate body,** the part of the lateral geniculate body overlying the ventral part of the lateral geniculate nucleus.
**ventral p. of lateral geniculate nucleus,** nucleus ventralis corporis geniculati lateralis.
**ventral p. of medial geniculate body,** the part of the medial geniculate body overlying the ventral part of the medial geniculate nucleus; called also *magnocellular p. of medial geniculate body.*
**ventral p. of medial geniculate nucleus,** nucleus ventralis corporis geniculati medialis.
**ventral p. of pons,** p. basilaris pontis.
**vertebral p. of diaphragm,** pars lumbalis diaphragmatis.
**visceral p. of pelvic fascia,** fascia pelvis visceralis.

**Part. aeq.** abbreviation for L. *par'tes aequa'les,* equal parts.

**par·tal** (pahr'təl) pertaining to parturition.

**par·tes** (pahr'tēz) [L.] plural of *pars.*

**Par·the·ne·um** (pahr-the'ne-əm) a genus of flowering herbs of the family Compositae. *P. hystero'phorus* is wild feverfew, a common cause of airborne contact dermatitis.

**par·the·no·gen·e·sis** (pahr"thə-no-jen'ə-sis) [Gr. *parthenos* virgin + *-genesis*] [MeSH: Parthenogenesis] a modified form of sexual reproduction by the development of a gamete without fertilization, as occurs in some plants and invertebrates, especially arthropods, e.g., honey bees and wasps, and in certain lizards. It may occur as a natural phenomenon or be induced by chemical, thermal, or mechanical stimulation *(artificial p.).*

**par·the·no·pho·bia** (pahr"thə-no-fo'be-ə) [Gr. *parthenos* virgin + *-phobia*] irrational fear of girls.

**par·tho·gen·e·sis** (pahr"tho-jen'ə-sis) parthenogenesis.

**par·tial·ism** (pahr'shəl-iz-əm) a paraphilia characterized by exclusive focus on a body part of the sexual partner.

**par·ti·cle** (pahr'tĭ-kəl) [L. *particula,* dim. of *pars* part] a tiny mass of material.
**alpha p.,** a positively charged particle ejected from the nucleus of a radioactive atom, being a high-speed ionized atom of helium. A stream of these particles constitutes alpha rays.
**attraction p.,** a small particle in the center of the centrosome.
**beta p.,** an electron emitted from an atomic nucleus during beta decay.
**colloid p's,** the particles making up the disperse phase of a colloid. See *colloid,* def. 2.
**Dane p.,** an intact hepatitis B virion.
**disperse p's,** colloid p's.
**elementary p.,** any of the subatomic particles, including electrons, protons, neutrons, positrons, neutrinos, muons, etc.
**elementary p's of mitochondria,** numerous minute, club-shaped granules with spherical heads attached to the inner membrane of a mitochondrion.
**high-velocity p's,** subatomic particles, such as electrons, protons, and deuterons, given high speeds in an accelerator.
**nuclear p's,** Howell-Jolly bodies.
**viral p., virus p.,** virion.
**Zimmermann's elementary p.,** old term for *platelet.*

**par·tic·u·late** (pahr-tik'u-lət) composed of separate particles.

**par·ti·tion** (pahr-tĭ'shən) something that separates or divides into parts.
**oropharyngeal p.,** a protective barrier between the oral cavity and the pharynx made of moistened gauze sponges, useful during general anesthesia when a nasal mask is used.

**par·ti·tion·ing** (pahr-tĭ'shən-ing) dividing into parts.
**gastric p.,** a form of gastroplasty in which a small stomach pouch is formed whose filling signals satiety; used in treatment of morbid obesity. Called also *gastric stapling.*

**par·tri·cin** (pahr-tri'sin) an antifungal and antiprotozoal produced by *Streptomyces aureofaciens,* consisting of a mixture in a constant ratio (about 1:1) of two polyene substances having very similar structures and biological properties. See also *mepartricin.*

**par·tu·ri·ent** (pahr-tu're-ənt) [L. *parturiens*] 1. giving birth, or pertaining to childbirth. 2. by extension, a woman in labor.

**par·tu·ri·fa·cient** (pahr"tu-re-fa'shənt) [L. *parturire* to have the pains of labor + *-facient*] 1. inducing or facilitating childbirth. 2. an agent that induces or facilitates childbirth.

**par·tu·ri·om·e·ter** (pahr"tu-re-om'ə-tər) [L. *parturitio* childbirth + *-meter*] a device used in measuring the expulsive power of the uterus.

**par·tu·ri·tion** (pahr"tu-rĭ'shən) [L. *parturitio*] childbirth.

**par·tus** (pahr'təs) [L.] 1. labor. 2. childbirth.

**Part. vic.** abbreviation for L. *parti'tis vi'cibus,* in divided doses.

**pa·ru·lis** (pə-roo'lis) [*para-* + Gr. *oulon* gum] an elevated nodule at

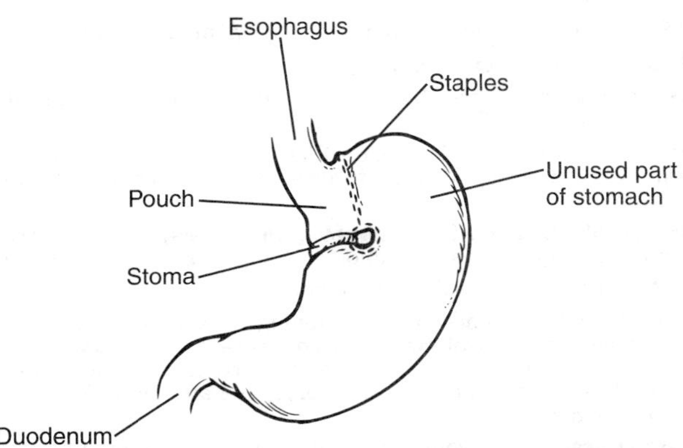

Gastric partitioning using a vertical banded gastroplasty.

the site of a fistula draining a chronic periapical abscess. Called also *gumboil* (or *gum boil*).

**par·um·bil·i·cal** (par″əm-bil′ĭ-kəl) alongside the umbilicus.

**par·u·ria** (par-u′re-ə) [*para-* + *-uria*] any disorder of the urine or abnormal state of the urine or its discharge.

**par·vi·cel·lu·lar** (pahr″vĭ-sel′u-lər) [L. *parvus* small + *cellular*] composed of small cells.

**par·vo·cel·lu·lar** (pahr″vo-sel′u-lər) parvicellular.

**par·vo·line** (par′vo-lin) an amber-colored liquid poison from decaying fish or horse flesh.

**par·vo·vi·ral** (pahr′vo-vi″vəl) pertaining to or caused by parvoviruses.

**Par·vo·vi·ri·dae** (pahr″vo-vir′ĭ-de) [MeSH: Parvoviridae] the parvoviruses: a family of DNA viruses having a nonenveloped virion 18–26 nm in diameter composed of 60 copies of the capsid protein with icosahedral symmetry. The genome consists of a single molecule of linear single-stranded DNA (MW 1.5–2.2 × $10^6$, size 4–6 kb). Viruses contain 2–4 major polypeptides, depending on the species, and are resistant to heat, lipid solvents, deoxycholate, and nucleases but sensitive to formalin, β-propiolactone, hydroxylamine, oxidizing agents, and ultraviolet radiation. Replication and assembly occur in the nucleus and require S-phase cellular function in the host cell or the presence of helper virus. Host range is narrow and transmission may be vertical or by mechanical vectors. There are two subclasses: Densovirinae, comprising genera that infect invertebrates, and Parvovirinae, comprising genera that infect vertebrates.

**Par·vo·vi·ri·nae** (pahr″vo-vir-i′ne) a subfamily of the family Parvoviridae, containing parvoviruses that infect vertebrates; it comprises three genera: *Dependovirus, Erythrovirus,* and *Parvovirus.*

**Par·vo·vi·rus** (pahr′vo-vi″rəs) [*parvo-* + *virus*] [MeSH: Parvovirus] parvoviruses; a genus of viruses of the subfamily Parvovirinae (family Parvoviridae) that infect mammals and birds. Viruses multiply in the nucleus and require S-phase cellular functions for replication. Transmission is transplacental or by mechanical vector. Human parvoviruses cause transient aplastic crisis, acute arthritis, erythema infectiosum, hydrops fetalis, spontaneous abortion, and fetal death. Animal pathogens include bovine, canine, feline, and goose parvoviruses, feline panleukopenia virus, mink enteritis virus, Aleutian mink disease virus, and various murine parvoviruses.

**par·vo·vi·rus** (pahr′vo-vi″rəs) [L. *parvus* small + *virus*] [MeSH: Parvovirus] any virus belonging to the family Parvoviridae.
**bovine p.**, a virus of the genus *Parvovirus* infecting cattle that causes diarrhea in calves; infection during the first or second trimesters of gestation may result in abortion. Infection is widespread and antibody to the virus can be found in a high proportion of adult cattle.
**canine p.**, a virus of the genus *Parvovirus* that causes myocarditis in dogs and a type of enteritis called canine parvovirus disease; it is sometimes considered to be a species-specific variant of feline parvovirus.
**feline p.**, a virus of the genus *Parvovirus* that primarily affects cats. Canine parvovirus, feline panleukopenia virus, and mink enteritis virus are sometimes considered to be host-specific variant strains.
**goose p.**, a virus of the genus *Parvovirus* that causes a highly fatal disease of young geese affecting the liver, thyroid, and pancreas.
**human p. B19**, B19 virus.
**human p. RA-1**, a species belonging to the genus *Parvovirus* that has been associated with rheumatoid arthritis.

**par·vule** (pahr′vūl) [L. *parvulus* very small] a very small pill, pellet, or granule.

**Par·y·phos·to·mum** (par″e-fos′to-məm) a genus of flukes related to *Echinostoma.*

**PAS** *p*-aminosalicylic acid; periodic acid–Schiff (see under *reaction*).

**PASA** *p*-aminosalicylic acid.

**Pas·cal's law** (pahs-kahlz′) [Blaise *Pascal,* French mathematician and physicist, 1623–1662] see under *law.*

**pas·cal** (pas-kal′, pas′kal) [after Blaise *Pascal*] the SI unit of pressure, which corresponds to a force of one newton per square meter; symbol Pa.

**Pa·schen's bodies (corpuscles, granules)** (pah′shenz) [Enrique *Paschen,* German pathologist, 1860–1936] see under *body.*

**PASG** pneumatic antishock garment.

**pas·pal·ism** (pas′pəl-iz-əm) poisoning of livestock by ingestion of excessive amounts of *Paspalum commersonii* or *P. scrobiculatum,* grasses containing neurotoxic hydrocarbons; characteristics include tremor, convulsions, and coma. See also *paspalum staggers,* under *staggers.*

**Pas·pa·lum** (pas′pə-ləm) a genus of grasses commonly eaten by livestock in Asia and Africa. Some species contain a toxic hydrocarbon that can cause paspalism; other species are sometimes contaminated with an ergot and cause paspalum staggers.

**pas·pa·lum** (pas′pə-ləm) any grass of the genus *Paspalum.*

**pas·sage** (pas′əj) 1. a channel. 2. an evacuation of the bowels. 3. introduction of infectious material into an experimental animal or culture medium, followed by recovery of the infectious agent. 4. the act of moving from one place to another. 5. the introduction of a catheter, probe, sound, or bougie through a natural channel such as the urethra.
**blind p.**, successive transfer of infection through experimental animals, chick embryo, or tissue culture, when overt lesions of disease are not apparent, at least in the earlier members of the series.
**false p.**, fistula.
**serial p.**, the successive transfer of a virus or other infectious agent through a series of experimental animals, tissue culture, or synthetic media, with growth occurring in each medium. The process is usually used to attenuate a pathogenic agent.

**Pas·sa·vant's bar (cushion, pad, ridge)** (pahs′ə-vahnts) [Philip Gustav *Passavant,* German surgeon, 1815–1893] see under *bar.*

**pas·sen·ger** (pas′ən-jər) the fetus or any of the fetal membranes during labor.

**pas·ser** (pas′ər) one who or that which conveys something from one place to another.
**foil p.**, a pointed or forked instrument used to carry pellets of gold foil through an annealing flame or from the annealing tray to the prepared cavity for compaction. Called also *foil carrier.*

**Pas·si·flo·ra** (pas″ĭ-flo′rə) [L. *passio* passion + *flora*] the passion flowers, a genus of twining vines of the family Passifloraceae, having brightly colored flowers and found in tropical parts of the Americas. Many of the plants, such as *P. incarna′ta* L., were formerly used medicinally for their sedative and anodyne properties; they also contain cyanogenetic glycosides and have caused cyanide poisoning in livestock.

**pas·si·vate** (pas′ĭ-vāt) to make the surface of a chemically reactive metal (base metal) less reactive by forming a stable surface reaction compound, usually a metallic oxide.

**pas·si·va·tion** (pas″ĭ-va′shən) 1. reduction of reactivity of the surface of a chemically reactive metal *(base metal).* 2. the process of making such a surface less reactive.

**pas·sive** (pas′iv) [L. *passivus*] neither spontaneous nor active; not produced by active efforts.

**pas·siv·ism** (pas′iv-iz-əm) a submissive attitude or behavior, particularly submission to the will of a sexual partner.

**pas·siv·i·ty** (pə-siv′ĭ-te) 1. in psychology, an unwillingness, inability, or other failure to take initiative or personal responsibility for routine life events. 2. in dentistry, the condition of rest assumed by the teeth, surrounding tissue, and denture when a removable partial denture is in place but not under masticatory pressure.

**Past.** abbreviation for *Pasteurella.*

**paste** (pāst) [L. *pasta*] a semisolid preparation, generally for external use, of a fatty base, a viscous or mucilaginous base, or a mixture of starch and petrolatum.
**dextrinated p.**, a preparation of dextrin, glycerin, and distilled water, used as a vehicle.
**Ihle's p.**, an ointment containing resorcin, starch, and zinc oxide in soft paraffin.
**Lassar's p.**, zinc oxide and salicylic acid p.
**Lassar's betanaphthol p.**, a paste containing betanaphthol, precipitated sulfur, soft soap, and petrolatum.
**Lassar's plain zinc p.**, zinc oxide p.
**triamcinolone acetonide dental p.** [USP], a preparation of triamcinolone acetonide in an emollient paste; used in the treatment of steroid-responsive oral inflammatory lesions and ulcerative lesions due to trauma, applied topically.
**zinc oxide p.** [USP], a preparation of zinc oxide and starch in white petrolatum, used topically as an astringent and protectant; called also *Lassar's plain zinc p.*
**zinc oxide and salicylic acid p.** [USP], **zinc oxide p. with salicylic acid** a mixture of zinc oxide paste and salicylic acid, used topically as an astringent and local protective. Called also *Lassar's p.*

**pas·ter** (pās′tər) the portion of a bifocal lens ground for near vision.

**pas·tern** (pas′tərn) the portion of a horse's foot just proximal to the hoof. See also under *bone* and *joint.*

**Pas·teur** (pahs-toor′) Louis (1822–1895). French chemist, author of the germ theory of disease, and founder of microbiology, virology, and immunology. Pasteur is famous for disproving spontaneous generation and for his work in stereochemistry, lactic and alcoholic fermentation, microbiology and diseases of wine and beer, diseases of silkworms, anaerobiosis, virulent diseases (anthrax, chicken cholera), and preventive inoculation with attenuated microbes (especially against rabies). Pasteur's work enabled Joseph Lister to develop antiseptic surgery.

**Pas·teur's effect (reaction), theory** (pahs-toorz') [Louis *Pasteur*] see under *effect* and *theory.*

**Pas·teur·el·la** (pas″tər-el'ə) [Louis *Pasteur*] [MeSH: Pasteurella] a genus of gram-negative, facultatively anaerobic, ovoid to rod-shaped bacteria of the family Pasteurellaceae, made up of nonmotile fermentative organisms. Bipolar staining is common. They are parasitic on humans, wild and domestic animals, and birds, and are potential pathogens, causing abscesses and septicemias in humans and respiratory and septic infections in sheep, cattle, and fowl.
**P. aero'genes,** a species occurring in swine that is a possible cause of abortion in swine and of human wound infections following swine bites.
**P. anapes'tifer,** *P. anatipestifer.*
**P. anatipes'tifer,** a species of uncertain affiliation that causes infectious avian serositis. Called also *Moraxella anatipestifer* and *Pfeifferella anatipestifer.*
**P. haemoly'tica,** a species that is part of the normal flora of cattle and sheep and is the etiologic agent of hemorrhagic septicemia in sheep and goats, shipping fever in cattle, and a cholera-like disease in fowl; it occasionally is found in human infections.
**P. multoci'da,** a species that is part of the normal flora of the mouth and respiratory tract of many species of mammals and birds; several different biotypes and serotypes are recognized. In animals it causes hemorrhagic septicemias, pneumonia, local abscesses, and intestinal disease. Human disease is usually from infection of a cat or dog bite or scratch, with localized swelling, abscesses, bronchiectasis, pneumonia, meningitis, and septicemia. See also *P. multocida pneumonia,* under *pneumonia.* Formerly called *P. septica.*
**P. novi'cida,** *Francisella novicida.*
**P. pes'tis,** *Yersinia pestis.*
**P. pfaf'fii,** a species of uncertain status that is the etiologic agent of an epidemic septicemia in canaries.
**P. pneumotro'pica,** a species occurring normally and as an occasional pathogen in rodents; it is of importance as a human pathogen.
**P. pseudotuberculo'sis,** former name for *Yersinia pseudotuberculosis.*
**P. sep'tica,** *P. multocida.*
**P. septicae'miae,** a species of uncertain status that causes septicemia in young geese.
**P. tularen'sis,** *Francisella tularensis.*
**P. ure'ae,** a species with no known animal host. It has been isolated from human infections of the upper respiratory tract and occasionally from the nasal passages of healthy humans.

**Pas·teur·el·la·ceae** (pas″tər-el-a'se-e) [MeSH: Pasteurellaceae] a family of facultatively anaerobic, nonmotile, gram-negative, coccoid to rod-shaped bacteria, occurring as parasites in mammals and birds. It contains the genera *Actinobacillus, Haemophilus,* and *Pasteurella.*

**Pas·teur·el·leae** (pas″tər-el'e-e) in former systems of classification, a tribe of bacteria that included the genus *Pasteurella.*

**pas·teur·el·lo·sis** (pas″tər-ə-lo'sis) infection of humans or animals by species of *Pasteurella;* several different species cause disease.
**pneumonic p.,** infection of the lungs of animals with *Pasteurella* species, usually *P. haemolytica* or *P. multocida.* Cattle infected with *P. haemolytica* may develop fulminating, fatal lobar pneumonia; infected sheep, goats, and pigs may develop various types of pneumonia, some fatal.
**septicemic p.,** hemorrhagic septicemia.

**pas·teur·iza·tion** (pas″chər-ĭ-za'shən) [Louis *Pasteur*] the process of heating milk or other liquids, e.g., wine or beer, to destroy microorganisms that would cause spoilage. Milk is either held at 62°C for 30 minutes *(holding method* or *low temperature holding method)* or heated rapidly to 80°C and held for 15 to 30 seconds *(flash method* or *high temperature short time).* The procedure kills most pathogenic bacteria while retaining the flavor of the liquid.

**pas·teur·iz·er** (pas'chər-īz″ər) an instrument used in pasteurization.

**Pas·tia's lines (sign)** (pahs'te-ahz) [Chessec *Pastia,* Romanian physician, born 1878] see under *line.*

**pas·til** (pas'til) pastille.

**pas·tille** (pas-tēl') [Fr.] 1. a troche in which the active ingredient is incorporated in a mass of sweetened gum, glycerin, and gelatin base. 2. an aromatic mass to be burnt as a fumigant. 3. A small disk of paper coated with platinocyanide of barium or other substance. The green color changes to brown when exposed to x-rays. Formerly used to estimate the amount of x-ray administered and also to test the intensity of ultraviolet radiation.

**PAT** paroxysmal atrial tachycardia; see *paroxysmal tachycardia,* under *tachycardia.*

**Pa·tau's syndrome** (pah-touz') [Klaus *Patau,* German-born American geneticist, 20th century] trisomy 13 syndrome.

**patch** (pach) [L. *pittacium;* Gr. *pittakion*] 1. an area differing from the rest of a surface, in either color or texture, or both, but not elevated above it. 2. a macule 1 cm or more in diameter.
**ash-leaf p.,** ash-leaf m.
**Bitot's p's,** see under *spot.*
**cotton-wool p's,** see under *spot.*
**herald p.,** the solitary lesion that precedes the general eruption in pityriasis rosea.
**Hutchinson's p.,** salmon p. (def. 1).
**lance-ovate p.,** ash-leaf m.
**MacCallum's p.,** a sheet of granulation tissue in the deeper layers of the endocardium formed by extensive confluence of Aschoff nodules in the myocardium in rheumatic fever.
**mucous p.,** a flat, rounded, grayish white erosion covered by a soggy membrane with an erythematous zone, occurring most often on the oral mucosa, and sometimes on the anogenital mucosa, in early active secondary syphilis. It contains vast numbers of treponemata and is therefore highly contagious.
**Peyer's p's,** noduli lymphoidei aggregati intestini tenuis.
**salmon p.,** 1. a salmon-colored spot in the cornea in syphilis of that structure; called also *Hutchinson's p.* 2. a salmon-colored nevus flammeus, usually found over the eyelids, between the eyes, or on the mid forehead; it usually fades completely in time.
**shagreen p.,** see under *skin.*
**smokers' p's,** stomatitis nicotina.
**soldiers' p's,** milk spots, def. 1.

**pat·e·fac·tion** (pat″ə-fak'shən) [L. *patefacere* to lay open] the act of laying open.

**Pa·tel·la's disease** (pah-tel'ahz) [Vincenzo *Patella,* Italian physician, 1856–1928] see under *disease.*

**pa·tel·la** (pə-tel'ə) [L., dim of *patera* a shallow dish] [TA] [MeSH: Patella] a triangular sesamoid bone, about 5 cm in diameter, situated at the front of the knee in the tendon of insertion of the quadriceps extensor femoris muscle. Called also *knee cap.*
**p. al'ta,** an abnormally high patella, the Insall-Salvati ratio being greater than 1.2; called also *high-riding p.*
**p. ba'ja** (bah'hah), an abnormally low patella, having an Insall-Salvati ratio of less than 1.0; called also *low-riding p.* and *p. infra.*
**p. biparti'ta, bipartite p.,** a patella that is divided into two parts.
**p. cu'biti,** an anomalous sesamoid bone sometimes occurring over the extensor surface of the elbow joint.
**floating p.,** a patella that is separated from the condyles by a large effusion in the knee.
**high-riding p.,** p. alta.
**p. in'fra,** p. baja.
**low-riding p.,** p. baja.
**p. parti'ta,** a patella that is divided into two or more parts.
**slipping p.,** a patella that is easily movable and readily dislocated.
**p. triparti'ta, tripartite p.,** a patella that is divided into three parts.

**pa·tel·lar** (pə-tel'ər) [L. *patellarius*] of or pertaining to the patella.

**pat·el·lec·to·my** (pat″ə-lek'tə-me) [*patella* + *-ectomy*] excision or removal of the patella.

**pat·el·li·form** (pə-tel'ĭ-form) shaped like the patella.

**pa·tel·lo·fem·o·ral** (pə-tel″o-fem'ə-rəl) pertaining to the patella and the femur.

**pat·en·cy** (pa'tən-se) [L. *patens* open] the condition of being widely open.
**probe p. of foramen ovale,** incomplete physical closure of the foramen ovale postnatally, although functional closure occurs, so that

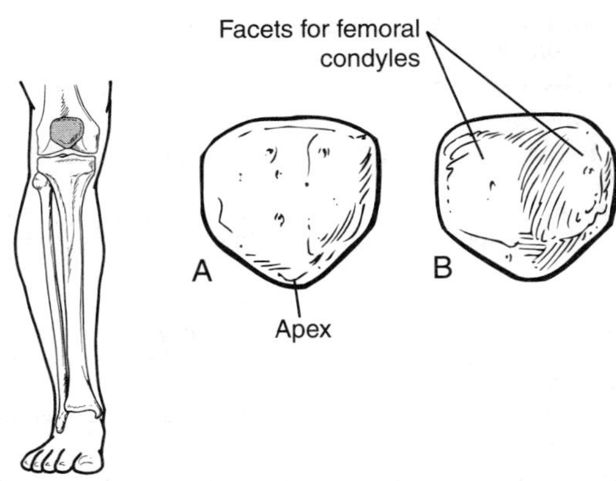

Patella. The right patella is shown in anterior *(A)* and posterior *(B)* aspects.

a probe may be passed between the atria in the adult. It occurs in 20 to 25 per cent of all hearts.

**pat·ent** (pa'tənt) [L. *patens*] [MeSH: Patents] 1. open, unobstructed, or not closed. 2. apparent, evident.

**Pat·er·son's syndrome** (pat'ər-sənz) [Donald Ross *Paterson,* Welsh laryngologist, 1863–1939] Plummer-Vinson syndrome.

**Pat·er·son–Brown Kel·ly syndrome** (pat'ər-sən-broun-kel'e) [D. R. *Paterson;* A. *Brown Kelly,* Scottish laryngologist, 1865–1941] Plummer-Vinson syndrome.

**Pat·er·son-Kel·ly syndrome** (pat'ər-sən-kel'e) [D. R. *Paterson;* A. *Brown Kelly*] Plummer-Vinson syndrome.

**Pa·tey's operation** (pa'tēz) [David Howard *Patey,* English surgeon, 1899–1977] see *modified radical mastectomy,* under *mastectomy.*

**path** (path) 1. a particular course that is followed, or a route that is ordinarily traversed. 2. pathway (def. 2).
**alvear p.,** see under *fasciculus.*
**condyle p.,** the course followed by the mandibular condyle in the temporomandibular joint during the various movements of the mandible.
**copulation p.,** the course taken by the male and female pronuclei as they approach each other in a fertilized ovum.
**incisor p.,** the course followed by the incisal edges of the lower anterior teeth in movement of the mandible from the position of normal occlusion to that of edge-to-edge contact with opposing incisors.
**p. of insertion,** that direction or path of a removable partial denture that permits the proper relation of the prosthesis to the hard and soft tissues on insertion, on removal, in function, and at rest. Called also *p. of removal.*
**ionization p.,** the trail of ion pairs produced by ionizing radiation in its passage through matter; called also *ionization track.*
**lateral condyle p.,** the path of the condyle in the glenoid fossa when a lateral mandibular movement is made.
**milled-in p's,** 1. the contours carved by various mandibular movements into the occluding surface of an occlusion rim by teeth or studs placed in the opposing occlusion rim. The curves or contours may be carved into wax, modeling plastic, or plaster of Paris. 2. gliding movements of occlusion rims, which are composed of materials, including abrasives.
**occlusal p.,** the course followed by the occlusal surfaces of the lower teeth in movements of the mandible.
**occlusal p., generated,** a registration of the paths of movement of the occlusal surfaces of mandibular teeth on a plastic or abrasive surface attached to the maxillary arch.
**p. of removal,** p. of insertion.

**pa·the·ma** (pə-the'mə) pl. *pathemas* or *pathem'ata* [Gr. *pathēma* disease] any disease state or morbid condition.

**path·er·gia** (path-er'je-ə) pathergy.

**path·er·gic** (path'ər-jik) characterized by pathergy.

**path·er·gy** (path'ər-je) [*path-* + Gr. *ergon* work] 1. an abnormal reaction to an allergen, either a subnormal reaction or an excessive reaction. 2. the condition of being allergic to numerous antigens; polyvalent allergy.

**pa·thet·ic** (pə-thet'ik) [L. *patheticus;* Gr. *pathētikos*] pertaining to the trochlear nerve.

**path·find·er** (path'fīnd-ər) 1. an instrument for locating strictures of the urethra. 2. root canal probe.

**Pa·thi·lon** (pă'thĭ-lon) trademark for a preparation of tridihexethyl chloride.

**path(o)-** [Gr. *pathos* disease] a combining form denoting relationship to disease.

**patho·an·a·tom·i·cal** (path″o-an″ə-tom'ĭ-kəl) pertaining to anatomic pathology.

**patho·anat·o·my** (path″o-ə-nat'ə-me) anatomic pathology.

**patho·bi·ol·o·gy** (path″o-bi-ol'ə-je) pathology.

**Path·o·cil** (path'o-sil) trademark for a preparation of dicloxacillin sodium.

**patho·cli·sis** (path″o-klis'is) a specific elemental sensitivity to specific toxins, or a specific affinity of certain toxins for certain systems of organs.

**path·odon·tia** (path″o-don'shə) dental pathology.

**patho·for·mic** (path″o-for'mik) [*patho-* + *form* + *-ic*] pertaining to the beginning of disease; said particularly of symptoms at the beginning of mental disorder.

**patho·gen** (path'o-jən) [*patho-* + *-gen*] any disease-producing microorganism.

**patho·gen·e·sis** (path″o-jen'ə-sis) [*patho-* + *genesis*] the development of morbid conditions or of disease; more specifically the cellular events and reactions and other pathologic mechanisms occurring in the development of disease.
**drug p.,** the production of symptoms of disease by the use of drugs.

**patho·ge·net·ic** (path″o-jə-net'ik) pertaining to pathogenesis.

**path·o·gen·ic** (path-o-jen'ik) giving origin to disease or to morbid symptoms.

**patho·ge·nic·i·ty** (path″o-jə-nis'ĭ-te) the quality of producing or the ability to produce pathologic changes or disease.

**path·og·e·ny** (path-oj'ə-ne) pathogenesis.

**pa·thog·no·mon·ic** (path″og-no-mon'ik) [*patho-* + Gr. *gnōmonikos* fit to give judgment] specifically distinctive or characteristic of a disease or pathologic condition; a sign or symptom on which a diagnosis can be made.

**path·og·no·my** (pə-thog'nə-me) [*patho-* + Gr. *gnōmē* a means of knowing] the science of the signs and symptoms of disease.

**path·og·nos·tic** (path″og-nos'tik) pathognomonic.

**pa·thog·ra·phy** (pə-thog'rə-fe) [*patho-* + *-graphy*] a history or description of disease.

**patho·log·ic** (path″o-loj'ik) 1. indicative of or caused by a morbid condition. 2. pertaining to pathology.

**patho·log·i·cal** (path″o-loj'ĭ-kəl) pertaining to pathology; pathologic.

**pa·thol·o·gist** (pə-thol'ə-jist) an expert in pathology.
**speech p.,** a person skilled and certified in speech pathology. Cf. *speech therapist.*

**pa·thol·o·gy** (pə-thol'ə-je) [*patho-* + *-logy*] [MeSH: Pathology] 1. that branch of medicine which treats of the essential nature of disease, especially of the structural and functional changes in tissues and organs of the body that cause or are caused by disease. 2. the structural and functional manifestations of disease.
**anatomic p.,** the anatomical study of changes in the function, structure, or appearance of organs or tissues, including postmortem examinations and the study of biopsy specimens. Called also *morbid* or *pathological anatomy* and *pathoanatomy.*
**cellular p.,** that which regards the cells as starting points of the phenomena of disease as first proposed by Virchow.
**clinical p.,** pathology applied to the solution of clinical problems, especially the use of laboratory methods in clinical diagnosis.
**comparative p.,** that which institutes comparisons between various diseases of the human body and those of the lower animals.
**dental p.,** the branch of pathology that treats dental changes in disease. Called also *pathodontia.* See also *oral p.*
**experimental p.,** the study of artificially induced disease processes.
**functional p.,** the study of the changes of function due to morbid tissue changes.
**general p.,** that which takes cognizance of pathologic conditions that may occur in various diseases and in different organs.
**geographical p.,** the study and comparison of variations in morbidity and mortality in different geographic regions to determine the relationship between these variations and environmental conditions found in each region. Called also *geopathology.*
**internal p.,** medical p.
**medical p.,** that which relates to morbid processes that are not accessible to operative intervention. Cf. *surgical p.*
**oral p.,** the branch of pathology that treats the structural and functional changes in cells, tissues, and organs of the oral cavity that cause or are caused by disease. See also *dental p.*
**special p.,** the study of the pathology of particular diseases or organs.
**speech p.,** a field of the health sciences dealing with the evaluation of speech, language, and voice disorders and the rehabilitation of patients with such disorders not amenable to medical or surgical treatment.
**surgical p.,** the pathology of disease processes that are surgically accessible for diagnosis or treatment.

**patho·mi·me·sis** (path″o-mi-me'sis) [*patho-* + *mimesis*] mimicry of a disease or disorder, particularly malingering.

**patho·mim·ic·ry** (path″o-mim'ĭ-kre) mimicry of a disease or disorder, particularly malingering.

**patho·mor·phism** (path″o-mor'fiz-əm) abnormal morphology.

**patho·neu·ro·sis** (path″o-noo͞-ro'sis) hysterical symptoms due to a chronic disease process.

**patho·no·mia** (path-o-no'me-ə) [*patho-* + *nom-* + *-ia*] the sum of knowledge regarding the laws of disease.

**pa·thon·o·my** (pə-thon'ə-me) pathonomia.

**patho·pho·bia** (path″o-fo'be-ə) [*patho-* + *-phobia*] nosophobia.

**patho·phys·i·ol·o·gy** (path″o-fiz″e-ol'ə-je) the physiology of disordered function.

**patho·poi·e·sis** (path″o-poi-e'sis) [*patho-* + *-poiesis*] 1. the causation of disease. 2. the tendency of an individual to become diseased.

**patho·psy·chol·o·gy** (path″o-si-kol′ə-je) [*patho-* + *psychology*] the psychology of mental disease.

**patho·psy·cho·sis** (path″o-si-ko′sis) a psychosis arising from organic disease, such as brain tumor, encephalitis, etc.

**pa·tho·sis** (pə-tho′sis) [*patho-* + *-osis*] a condition of disease; a morbid condition.

**pa·thot·ro·pism** (pə-thot′rə-piz″əm) [*patho-* + *tropism*] the tendency of drugs to pass to diseased areas.

**path·way** (path′wa) 1. a path or course, especially a course followed in the attainment of a specific end. 2. the nerve structures through which an impulse passes between groups of nerve cells or between the central nervous system and an organ or muscle; see also *tract.* 3. metabolic p.

**accessory conducting p.,** myocardial fibers that propagate the atrial contraction impulse to the ventricles but are not a part of the normal atrioventricular conducting system; impulses conducted over such a pathway can cause preexcitation (q.v.). See also *Kent's bundle,* under *bundle; Mahaim fibers,* under *fiber;* and *atriohisian tracts,* under *tract.*

**afferent p.,** the nerve structures through which an impulse, especially a sensory impression, is conducted to the cerebral cortex; see also terms under *tract.*

**alternative complement p.,** a pathway of complement activation initiated by a variety of factors other than those initiating the classical pathway, including IgA immune complexes, bacterial endotoxins, microbial polysaccharides, and cell walls. It does not include factors C1, C2, and C4 of the classical complement pathway but does include factors B and D and properdin. See illustration at *complement.* The term is sometimes used to denote specifically those steps occurring prior to initiation of formation of the membrane attack complex (C5–C9).

**amphibolic p.,** a group of metabolic reactions with a dual function, providing small metabolites for further catabolism to end products or for use as precursors in synthetic, anabolic reactions. The tricarboxylic cycle system is an example. See also *anabolism* and *catabolism.*

**atrioventricular p.,** Kent's bundle.

**auditory p.,** any of the various sensory pathways for hearing, conducting impulses between the organ of Corti and the cerebral cortex.

**auditory p. central,** the auditory pathway in the central nervous system that runs through the central tract of the auditory nerve.

**circus p.,** the ring or circuit traversed by an excitatory wavefront exhibiting circus movement; see also *reentry.*

**classical complement p.,** the enzymatic cascade containing all the components of complement, C1 through C9, primarily activated by the binding of C1 to antigen-antibody complexes containing IgM, IgG1, IgG2, or IgG3. See illustration at *complement.* The term is sometimes used to denote specifically those steps occurring prior to initiation of formation of the membrane attack complex (C5–C9).

**common p. of coagulation,** the steps in the mechanism of coagulation from the activation of factor X through the conversion of fibrinogen to fibrin. See also *intrinsic p. of coagulation* and *extrinsic p. of coagulation.*

**concealed accessory p.,** an accessory pathway that conducts impulses unidirectionally from the ventricles to the atria; thus it is not associated with preexcitation but can participate in supraventricular tachycardia.

**efferent p.,** the nerve structures through which an impulse passes away from the brain, especially for the innervation of muscles, effector organs, or glands; see also terms under *tract.*

**Embden-Meyerhof p.** (of glucose metabolism), the series of enzymatic reactions in the anaerobic conversion of glucose to lactic acid, resulting in energy in the form of adenosine triphosphate (ATP).

**Embden-Meyerhof-Parnas p.,** Embden-Meyerhof p.

**Entner-Doudoroff p.,** a series of enzymatic reactions in bacteria that convert glucose to pyruvate by way of the intermediate 2-keto-3-deoxy-6-phosphogluconate, forming ATP. It is the major pathway of glucose metabolism in certain strains of *Pseudomonas* and *Zymomonas.*

**extrinsic p. of coagulation,** the mechanism that produces fibrin following tissue injury, beginning with formation of an activated complex between tissue factor and activated factor VII and leading to activation of factor X, which induces the reactions of the common pathway of coagulation. Cf. *intrinsic p. of coagulation.*

**final common p.,** a motor pathway consisting of the motor neurons by which nerve impulses from many central sources pass to a muscle or gland in the periphery.

**gustatory p.,** any of the sensory pathways for taste, conducting impulses from the taste buds through the thalamus to the cerebral cortex.

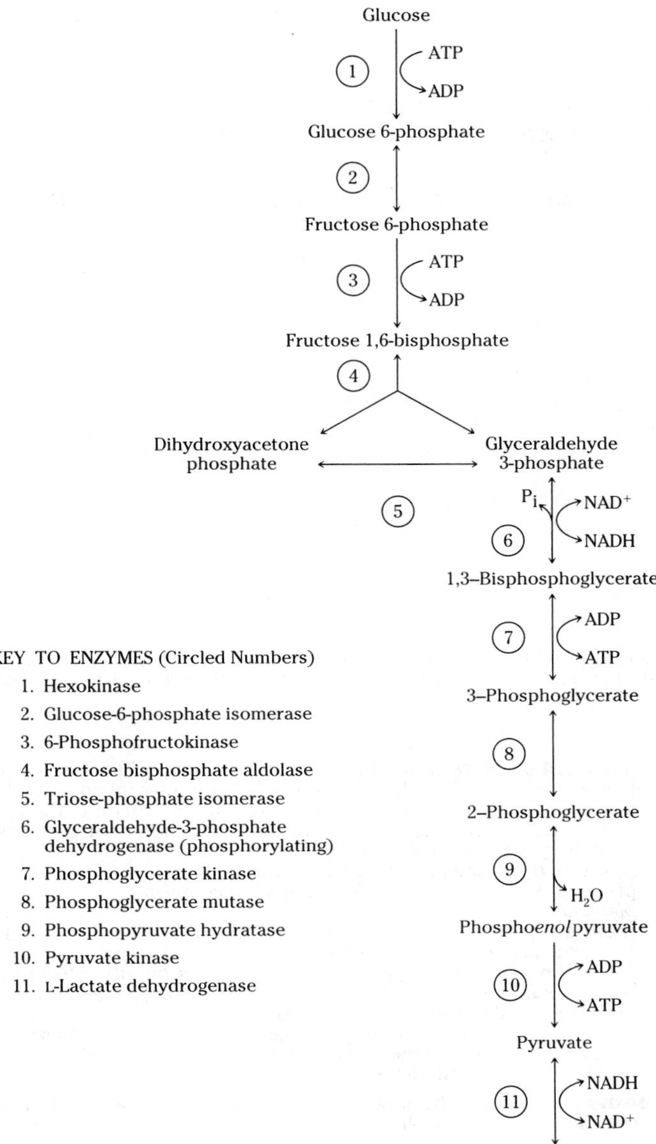


Embden-Meyerhof pathway of glucose metabolism, showing also the conversion of pyruvate to lactate.

**internuncial p.,** a correlation tract connecting different centers or neurons within the central nervous system.

**intrinsic p. of coagulation,** a sequence of reactions leading to fibrin formation, beginning with the contact activation of factor XII, followed by the sequential activation of factors XI and IX and resulting in the activation of factor X, which in activated form initiates the common pathway of coagulation. Cf. *extrinsic p. of coagulation.*

**lipoxygenase p.,** a pathway for the formation of leukotrienes and hydroxyeicosatetraenoic acids from arachidonic acid. It is initiated by oxidation of arachidonic acid by arachidonate lipoxygenases and the reactions occur in the cytosol of leukocytes, mast cells, platelets, and lung tissue cells. See illustration.

**metabolic p.,** a series of enzymatic reactions that converts one biological material to another.

**motor p.,** an efferent pathway conducting impulses from the central nervous system to a muscle; see also under *tract.*

**olfactory p.,** the sensory pathway for smell, conducting impulses from the osmoreceptors to the cerebral cortex by way of the olfactory nerves and olfactory tract.

**pentose phosphate p.,** a major branching of the Embden-Meyerhof pathway of carbohydrate metabolism: a pathway of hexose oxidation in which glucose-6-phosphate undergoes two successive oxidations by NADP, the final one being an oxidative decarboxylation to form a pentose phosphate. Called also *phosphogluconate p., hexose monophosphate shunt,* and *pentose shunt.*

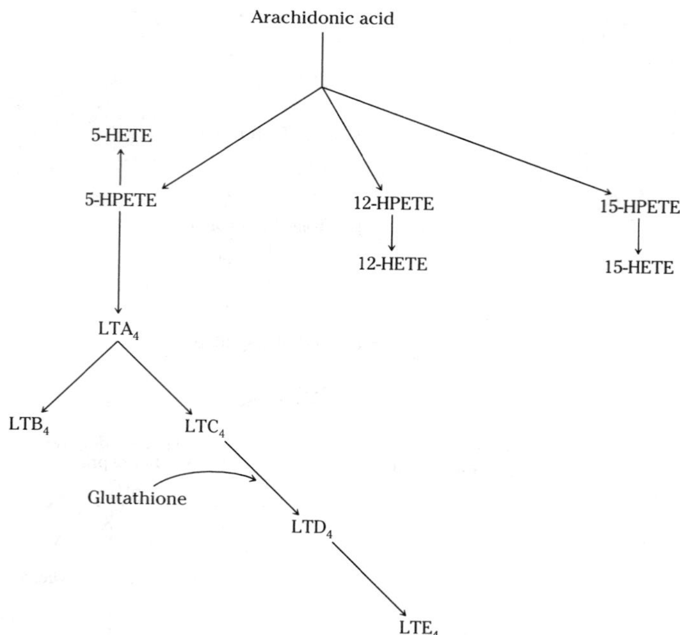


Lipoxygenase pathway of leukotriene and hydroxyeicosatetraenoic acid synthesis. *HPETE,* hydroperoxyeicosatetraenoic acid; *HETE,* hydroxyeicosatetraenoic acid; *LT,* leukotriene.

**perforant p., perforating p.,** a pathway of fibers originating in the lateral part of the entorhinal area, perforating the subiculum of the hippocampus, and running into the stratum moleculare of the hippocampus, where these fibers synapse with others that go to the dentate gyrus. Called also *perforating fasciculus.*
**phosphogluconate p.,** pentose phosphate p.
**properdin p.,** former name for *alternative complement p.;* see *complement.*
**reentrant p.,** that over which the impulse is conducted in reentry (q.v); see also *reentrant mechanism,* under *mechanism.*
**sensory p.,** an afferent pathway that conducts impulses from the receptors in the sense organs to one of the primary receiving areas of the cerebral cortex; see also under *tract.*
**visual p.,** the sensory pathway for sight, conducting impulses from the photoreceptors to the cerebral cortex by way of the optic nerve, optic tract, and optic radiation.

**-pathy** [Gr. *-patheia,* from *pathos* feeling, disease] a word termination denoting *(a)* a feeling, *(b)* a disease, *(c)* a system of treating disease.

**pa·tient** (pa'shənt) [L. *patiens*] [MeSH: Patients] a person who is ill or who is undergoing treatment for disease.

**Pat·rick's test (sign)** (pat'riks) [Hugh Talbot *Patrick,* American neurologist, 1860–1938] see under *test.*

**pa·tri·lin·e·al** (pat″rĭ-lin'e-əl) [L. *pater* father + *linea* line] descended through the male line.

**pat·ro·cli·nous** (pat″ro-kli'nəs) [Gr. *patēr* father + *klinein* to incline] inheriting or inherited from the father; having characters inherited from the father. Cf. *matroclinous.*

**pa·tro·gen·e·sis** (pat″ro-jen'ə-sis) [Gr. *patēr* father + *genesis*] androgenesis.

**pat·ten** (pat'ən) a metallic framework fitted to the base of a shoe to equalize leg length.

**pat·tern** (pat'ərn) 1. a design to be followed or a device to be used in the construction or fabrication of something. 2. the particular design or arrangement of figures. 3. a characteristic set of traits or actions, as behavior patterns.
**action p., fixed action p.,** a genetically determined sequence of stereotyped acts elicited by specific stimuli and peculiar to a species, such as a courting dance.
**full interference p.,** an interference pattern in which all the motor unit action potentials overlap with others so that none can be measured individually.
**interference p.,** electrical activity in a muscle recorded during maximal voluntary contraction; since a large number of activated motor units are firing asynchronously, some or all of their action potentials overlap (interfere with each other on the recording) and cannot be measured separately. Cf. *full interference p., reduced interference p.,* and *discrete activity.*
**occlusal p.,** the form or design of the occluding surfaces of a tooth or teeth; these forms may be based upon natural or modified anatomic or nonanatomic concepts of teeth.
**recruitment p.,** a description of the sequence of recruitment in a muscle; see also *recruitment frequency* and *recruitment rate.*
**reduced interference p.,** an interference pattern in which only some of the motor unit action potentials overlap each other.
**wax p.,** a reproduction of missing tooth structure or a dental appliance made from casting wax, from which the outline of the mold is made for the casting of a restoration or an appliance.

**pat·u·lin** (pat'u-lin) [MeSH: Patulin] a toxic and carcinogenic antibiotic derived from cultures of various fungi, especially *Aspergillus* and *Penicillium;* it causes tremor, paralysis, and death in animals that eat contaminated grain products. Called also *clavacin, claviformin,* and *penicidin.*

**pat·u·lous** (pat'u-ləs) [L. *patulus*] spreading widely apart; open; distended.

**pauci-** [L. *paucus* few] a combining form denoting few. Cf. *olig(o)-.*

**pau·ci·ar·tic·u·lar** (paw″se-ahr-tik'u-lər) [*pauci-* + *articular*] pertaining to or involving only a few joints.

**pau·ci·syn·ap·tic** (paw″se-sin-ap'tik) [*pauci-* + *synaptic*] oligosynaptic.

**Paul-Bun·nell test** (pawl-bə-nel') [John Rodman *Paul,* American physician, 1893–1971; Walls Willard *Bunnell,* American physician, 1902–1966] see under *test.*

**Paul-Bun·nell-Da·vid·sohn test** (pawl-bə-nel'-da'vid-son) [J. R. *Paul;* W. W. *Bunnell;* Israel *Davidsohn,* American pathologist, 1895–1979] see under *test.*

**Paul-Mix·ter tube** (pawl-mik'stər) [Frank Thomas *Paul,* English surgeon, 1851–1941; Samuel Jason *Mixter,* American surgeon, 1855–1926] see under *tube.*

**paunch** (pawnch) rumen.

**pause** (pawz) an interruption, or rest.
**compensatory p.,** the pause in impulse generation occurring after an extrasystole, designated as *full* if the sinus node is not reset and the total length of the aberrant plus the following cycle is equivalent to that of two normal cycles, or *incomplete, less than full,* or *noncompensatory* if the sinus node is reset and the normal cycle length disrupted.
**noncompensatory p.,** see *compensatory p.*
**sinus p.,** a transient interruption in the sinus rhythm, of a duration that is not an exact multiple of the normal cardiac cycle. See also *sinus arrest,* under *arrest.*
**ventricular p.,** a momentary delay in rhythmicity in ventricular tachycardia.

**Pau·tri·er's microabscess (abscess)** (po-tre-āz') [Lucien Marius Adolphe *Pautrier,* French dermatologist, 1876–1959] see under *microabscess.*

**pa·vé** (pah-va') [Fr. "paved," "cobbled"] pseudomembranelle, def. 1.

**pave·ment·ing** (pāv'mənt-ing) adhesion of leukocytes to the lining endothelium of the vessels of an injured part, which occurs as the circulation slows down within the vessels in response to the inflammatory process.

**Pa·vet·ta** (pə-vet'ə) a genus of shrubs found in southern Africa; various species are poisonous to sheep and cattle, causing gousiekte.

**pa·vil·ion** (pə-vil'yən) [L. *papilio* butterfly, tent] a dilated or flaring expansion at the end of a passage.
**p. of the oviduct,** ostium uterinum tubae uterinae.
**p. of the pelvis,** the upper, flaring portion of the pelvis.

**Pav·lov** (pahv'lof) Ivan Petrovich. Russian physiologist and experimental psychologist, 1849–1936; winner of the Nobel prize for medicine or physiology in 1904 for his work on the physiology of digestion, in which he established fistulas from various parts of dogs' digestive tracts and obtained secretions of the salivary glands, pancreas, and liver without upsetting the nerves and blood supply.

**Pav·lov's pouch, stomach** (pahv'lofs) [I. P. *Pavlov*] see under *pouch* and *stomach.*

**pav·lov·i·an con·di·tion·ing** (pav-lov'e-ən) [I.P. *Pavlov*] see *conditioning.*

**pa·vor** (pa'vor) [L.] terror.
**p. diur'nus** [L. "day terrors"], attacks of anxiety in children occurring during the afternoon nap.
**p. noctur'nus** [L. "night terrors"], a sleep disturbance usually occurring in children and characterized by extreme anxiety occurring shortly after sleep onset, with fear and signs of autonomic arousal,

inability to be comforted, poor recall of any dream, and later amnesia for the event. Repeated occurrences are called *sleep terror disorder.*

**Pav·u·lon** (pav′u-lon) trademark for a preparation of pancuronium bromide.

**paw** (paw) the foot of an animal that is equipped with claws or nails, especially that of a digitigrade or carnivorous animal.
**monkey p.,** see under *hand.*

**Paw·lik's triangle (trigone)** (pahv′liks) [Karel J. *Pawlik,* Czech gynecologist, 1849–1914] see under *triangle.*

**PAWP** pulmonary artery wedge pressure.

**paw·paw** (paw′paw) 1. papaw (def. 3). 2. papaw (def. 4).

**Pax·il** (pak′sil) trademark for a preparation of paroxetine hydrochloride.

**Pax·il·lus** (pak-sil′əs) a genus of mushrooms of the family Agaricaceae. *P. involu′tus* is considered edible but can cause gastroenteritis and in some individuals causes systemic reactions including syncope, hemoglobinuria, and decreased haptoglobins in the blood.

**Pax·i·pam** (pak′sĭ-pam″) trademark for a preparation of halazepam.

**Payr's clamp, disease** (pīrz) [Erwin *Payr,* German surgeon, 1871–1946] see under *clamp* and *disease.*

**PB** abbreviation for *Pharmacopoeia Britannica,* British Pharmacopoeia.

**Pb** symbol for *lead* [L. *plumbum*].

**PBG** porphobilinogen.

**PBI** protein-bound iodine.

**PBPC** peripheral blood progenitor cells.

**PBZ** trademark for preparations of tripelennamine citrate and tripelennamine hydrochloride.

**PC** phosphocreatine; sometimes used to designate phosphatidylcholine.

**P.C.** abbreviation for L. *pon′dus civi′le,* avoirdupois weight.

**p.c.** abbreviation for L. *post ci′bum,* after meals.

**PCA** passive cutaneous anaphylaxis.

**PCB** polychlorinated biphenyl; see under *biphenyl.*

**PcB** abbreviation for *near point of convergence to the intercentral base line.*

**PCE** pseudocholinesterase; see *cholinesterase.*

**PCEC** purified chick embryo cell vaccine.

**PCG** phonocardiogram.

**pCi** picocurie.

**$Pco_2$** symbol for *carbon dioxide partial pressure* or *tension;* also written $PCO_2$, $pco_2$, and $pCO_2$.

**PCOS** polycystic ovary syndrome.

**PCP** phencyclidine hydrochloride; *Pneumocystis carinii* pneumonia.

**PCR** polymerase chain reaction.

**PCT** porphyria cutanea tarda.

**PCV** packed cell volume.

**PCWP** pulmonary capillary wedge pressure.

**PD** prism diopter; interpupillary distance; peritoneal dialysis.

**Pd** symbol for *palladium.*

**PDA** 1. patent ductus arteriosus. 2. posterior descending (coronary) artery; see *ramus interventricularis posterior arteriae coronariae dextrae.*

**PE** phosphatidylethanolamine.

**pea** (pe) [Gr. *pisos*] [MeSH: Peas] 1. the leguminous vine *Pisum sativum.* 2. the edible seed of *P. sativum.* 3. any of numerous other leguminous vines resembling *P. sativum.* 4. the edible seed of one of these other leguminous vines.
**rosary p.,** 1. *Abrus precatorius.* 2. jequirity bean, so called because it is sometimes used to make rosary beads.

**peak** (pēk) the top or upper limit of a graphic tracing or of any variable.
**Bragg p.,** a peak in the Bragg curve reflecting a sharp increase in the intensity of ionization produced by an ionizing particle just before its velocity falls to zero.
**kilovolts p.,** the highest kilovoltage used in producing a radiograph; abbreviated kVp.

**Pé·an's forceps** (pa-ahz′) [Jules Émile *Péan,* French surgeon, 1830–1898] see under *forceps.*

**pea·nut** (pe′nut) [MeSH: Peanuts] 1. *Arachis hypogaea.* 2. the edible tuber of *A. hypogaea;* see also under *oil.*

**pearl** (pərl) 1. a small medicated granule, or a glass globule with a single dose of volatile medicine, as amyl nitrite. 2. a rounded mass of tough sputum as seen in the early stages of an attack of bronchial asthma.
**Bohn's p's,** see under *nodule.*
**Elschnig's p's,** see under *body.*
**enamel p.,** enameloma.
**epidermic p's, epithelial p's,** rounded concentric masses of epithelial cells and keratin found in certain squamous cell carcinomas.
**Epstein's p's,** small whitish-yellow cysts *(milia)* on each side of the raphe of the hard palate of the newborn.
**gouty p.,** a sodium urate concretion on the cartilage of the ear in gouty persons.
**Laënnec's p's,** soft casts of the smaller bronchial tubes expectorated in bronchial asthma. Cf. *Curschmann's spirals.*

**PEARS** porcine epidemic abortion and respiratory syndrome.

**Pear·son's correlation coefficient** (pēr′sənz) [Karl *Pearson,* British statistician, 1857–1936] see under *coefficient.*

**Pear·son's syndrome** (pēr′sənz) [H. A. *Pearson,* American physician, 20th century] see under *syndrome.*

**peau** (po) [Fr.] skin.
**p. de chagrin** (də shah-gră′) [Fr.], shagreen skin.
**p. d'orange** (do-rahj′) [Fr. "orange skin"], a dimpled condition of the skin, resembling that of an orange.

**peb·ble** (peb′əl) a kind of rock crystal from which lenses are sometimes cut.

**pé·brine** (pa-brēn′) [Fr.] an infectious protozoal disease of silkworms caused by *Nosema bombycis.* Cf. *nosema disease.*

**pe·ca·zine** (pe′kə-zēn) mepazine.

**pec·cant** (pek′ənt) [L. *peccans* sinning] unhealthy; causing illness or disease.

**pec·ca·ti·pho·bia** (pek″ə-tĭ-fo′be-ə) [L. *peccata* sins + *-phobia*] irrational fear of sinning.

**pechy·agra** (pek″e-ag′rə) [Gr. *pēchys* forearm + *-agra*] gout of the elbow.

**pecil(o)-** for words beginning thus, see those beginning *poikil(o)-.*

**Pec·quet's cistern (reservoir), duct** (pĕ-kāz′) [Jean *Pecquet,* French anatomist, 1622–1674] see *cisterna chyli* and *ductus thoracicus.*

**pec·ten** (pek′tən) pl. *pec′tines* [L.] 1. a comb; applied to certain anatomical structures because of a fancied resemblance to a comb. 2. p. analis. 3. a pleated projection of choroid into the vitreous in the eye of birds, extending forward from the optic disk.
**p. of anal canal, p. ana′lis** [TA], the zone in the lower half of the anal canal between the anocutaneous line and the anal verge; called also *pecten.*
**p. os′sis pu′bis** [TA], the anterior border of the superior ramus of the pubis, beginning at the pubic tubercle and continuing to the iliopubic eminence; called also *pectineal line.*

**pec·te·nine** (pek′tə-nin) a poisonous alkaloidal compound from a Mexican cactus, *Cereus pecten.*

**pec·te·ni·tis** (pek″tə-ni′tis) inflammation of the pecten of the anus.

**pec·te·no·sis** (pek″tə-no′sis) stenosis of the anal canal caused by a rigid, inelastic ring of tissue of variable width and thickness, between the anal groove and anal crypts, producing pain on defecation, bleeding, and anal irritation.

**pec·te·not·o·my** (pek″tə-not′ə-me) [*pecten* + *-tomy*] surgical correction of pectenosis by incision of the ring of tissue causing it.

**pec·tic** (pek′tik) relating to pectin.

**pec·tic ac·id** (pek′tik) a complex acid occurring in fruits, containing partially demethylated polymeric galacturonic acids.

**pec·tin** (pek′tin) [Gr. *pēktos* congealed] a homosaccharidic polymer of sugar acids of fruit that forms gels with sugar at the proper pH. A purified form [USP] obtained from the acid extract of the inner portion of the rind of citrus fruits or from apple pomace is used as the protective component of various formulations employed in the treatment of diarrhea and as a suspending agent in pharmaceutical preparations. It is also used in the preparation of certain foods, such as jams and jellies.

**pec·ti·nate** (pek′tĭ-nāt) [*pecten* + *-ate*] shaped like a comb.

**Pec·ti·na·tus** (pek″tĭ-na′təs) [L. *pectinatus* combed] a genus of gram-negative, anaerobic, slightly curved, rod-shaped bacteria of the family Bacteroidaceae, made up of motile cells with lateral flagella. They are found in spoiled packaged beer. The type species is *P. cerevisii′philus.*

**pec·tin·e·al** (pek-tin'e-əl) [L. *pecten,* comb, pubes] pertaining to the os pubis.

**pec·tin·i·form** (pek-tin'ĭ-form) [*pecten* + *form*] comb-shaped.

**pec·ti·za·tion** (pek″tĭ-za'shən) [Gr. *pēktikos* curdling] the process of changing to a gel or coagulate.

**Pec·to·bac·te·ri·um** (pek″to-bak-tēr-e-əm) a genus of gram-negative, facultatively anaerobic, rod-shaped organisms of the family Enterobacteriaceae, made up of plant pathogens. The organisms are not human pathogens but have been occasionally isolated from clinical specimens. Formerly called *Erwinia.*

**pec·to·lyt·ic** (pek″to-lit'ik) [*pectin* + *-lytic*] capable of effecting the digestion of pectin.

**pec·to·ra** (pek'tə-rə) [L.] plural of *pectus.*

**pec·to·ral** (pek'tə-rəl) [L. *pectoralis*] thoracic.

**pec·to·ral·gia** (pek″tə-ral'jə) [*pectoral* + *-algia*] 1. pain in the pectoral muscles; called also *stethalgia, thoracalgia,* and *thoracodynia.* 2. thoracalgia (def. 1).

**pec·to·ra·lis** (pek″tə-ra'lis) [L., from *pectus,* q.v.] thoracic.

**pec·to·ril·o·quy** (pek″tə-ril'ə-kwe) [*pectus* + L. *loqui* to speak] voice sounds of increased resonance heard through the chest wall; cf. *egophony* and *bronchophony.* Called also *pectorophony.*
**aphonic p.,** the sound of the whispered voice transmitted through a serous, but not through a purulent, exudate within the pleura. Called also *Baccelli's sign.*
**whispered p., whispering p.,** the transmission of the sound of whispered words through the walls of the chest, heard upon auscultation and indicating an area of consolidation. Called also *whispered bronchophony* or *voice.*

**pec·to·roph·o·ny** (pek″tə-rof'ə-ne) [L. *pectus* breast + Gr. *phōnē* voice] pectoriloquy.

**pec·tose** (pek'tōs) protopectin.

**pec·tous** (pek'təs) pertaining to, composed of, or resembling pectin; having a firm, jelly-like consistence.

**pec·tun·cu·lus** (pek-tung'ku-ləs) [L., dim of *pecten* comb] any one of the series of small longitudinal ridges on the aqueduct of Sylvius.

**pec·tus** (pek'təs) gen. *pec'toris,* pl. *pec'tora* [L.] [TA] the front of the chest.
**p. carina'tum** [L. "keeled breast"], a condition of the chest in which the sternum is prominent, due to obstruction of infantile respiration or to rickets; called also *chicken breast, pigeon breast, keeled chest,* and *pigeon chest.*
**p. excava'tum** [L. "hollowed breast"], a chest in which there is a funnel-shaped depression in the middle of the anterior thoracic wall, with the deepest part in the sternum. Called also *foveated* or *funnel chest, funnel breast, p. recurvatum,* and *koilosternia.*
**p. gallina'tum,** p. carinatum.
**p. recurva'tum,** p. excavatum.

**ped·al** (ped'əl) [L. *pedalis; pes* foot] pertaining to the foot or feet.

**pe·dar·throc·a·ce** (pe″dahr-throk'ə-se) [*ped-*[1] + *arthrocace*] caries of the joints in children.

**pe·da·tro·phia** (pe″də-tro'fe-ə) [*ped-*[1] + *atrophia*] marasmus.

**ped·er·ast** (ped'ər-ast) one who practices pederasty.

**ped·er·as·ty** (ped'ər-as″te) [*ped-*[1] + Gr. *erastēs* lover] anal intercourse between a man and a boy.

**ped·er·in** (ped'ər-in) a crystalline toxin isolated from blister beetles of the genus *Paederus.*

**pe·des** (pe'dēz) [L.] plural of *pes.*

**pedi-** see *ped(o)-*[2].

**Pe·di·a·flor** (pe'de-ə-flor) trademark for a preparation of sodium fluoride.

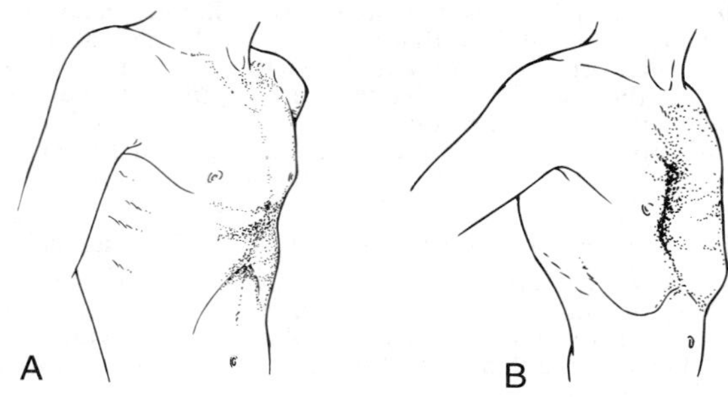

*(A),* Pectus carinatum; *(B),* pectus excavatum.

**pedi·al·gia** (ped″e-al'jə) [*pedi-* + *-algia*] podalgia.

**Pe·di·a·my·cin** (pe″de-ə-mi'sin) trademark for preparations of erythromycin ethylsuccinate.

**pe·di·at·ric** (pe″de-at'rik) pertaining to pediatrics.

**pe·di·a·tri·cian** (pe″de-ə-trĭ'shən) a physician who specializes in pediatrics.

**pe·di·at·rics** (pe″de-at'riks) [*ped-*[1] + *-iatrics*] [MeSH: Pediatrics] that branch of medicine which treats of the child and its development and care and of the diseases of children and their treatment.

**pe·di·at·rist** (pe″de-at'rist) pediatrician.

**pe·di·at·ry** (pe'de-at″re) pediatrics.

**ped·i·cel** (ped'ĭ-sel) a footlike part, especially any of the secondary processes of a podocyte which interdigitate with those of other podocytes in a renal corpuscle; called also *foot process.*

**ped·i·cel·la·ria** (ped″ĭ-sə-lar'e-ə) pl. *pedicella'riae.* a modified spine with a flexible head, seen in sea urchins and related animals, used in grooming, food getting, and self-defense and the principal site of venom glands.

**ped·i·cel·late, ped·i·cel·lat·ed** (pĕ-dis'ĭ-lāt; ped'ĭ-sel-āt″ed) pediculate; pedunculated.

**ped·i·cel·la·tion** (ped″ĭ-səl-a'shən) the development or possession of a pedicle.

**ped·i·cle** (ped'ĭ-kəl) [L. *pediculus* little foot] a footlike, stemlike, or narrow basal part or structure, as the stalk by which a nonsessile tumor is attached to normal tissue, or the narrow strip of flap tissue through which it receives its blood supply. Called also *pediculus.*
**cone p.,** the thick triangular or club-shaped ending of a retinal cone cell, which synapses with the bipolar and horizontal cells in the outer plexiform layer.
**p. of lung,** radix pulmonis.
**p. of vertebral arch,** pediculus arcus vertebrae.

**ped·i·cled** (ped'ĭ-kəld) having a pedicle.

**pe·dic·u·lar** (pə-dik'u-lər) [L. *pedicularis*] pertaining to or caused by lice.

**pe·dic·u·late** (pə-dik'u-lāt) [L. *pediculatus*] provided with a pedicle; pedunculated.

**pe·dic·u·la·tion** (pə-dik″u-la'shən) [L. *pediculatio*] 1. infestation with lice. 2. the formation of a pedicle.

**pe·dic·u·li** (pə-dik'u-li) plural of *pediculus.*

**pe·dic·u·li·cide** (pə-dik'u-lĭ-sīd) [*pediculus* + *-cide*] 1. destroying lice. 2. an agent that destroys lice.

**Ped·i·cu·li·dae** (ped″ĭ-ku'lĭ-de) a family of lice (order Anoplura) that includes the genera Pediculus and Phthirus, which feed on human blood.

**Pe·dic·u·loi·des** (pə-dik″u-loi'dēz) former name for *Pyemotes.*

**pe·dic·u·lo·sis** (pə-dik″u-lo'sis) [*pediculus* + *-osis*] [MeSH: Pediculosis] infestation with lice of the family Pediculidae, especially infestation with *Pediculus humanus.*
**p. capilli'tii, p. cap'itis,** infestation of the hair of the head by lice.
**p. cor'poris,** infestation of the body by lice.
**p. inguina'lis,** phthiriasis inguinalis.
**p. palpebra'rum,** infestation of the eyelashes by lice.
**p. pu'bis,** phthiriasis inguinalis.
**p. vestimen'ti, p. vestimento'rum,** infestation of the clothing by lice.

**pe·dic·u·lous** (pə-dik'u-ləs) infested with lice.

**Pe·dic·u·lus** (pə-dik'u-ləs) [MeSH: Pediculus] a genus of sucking lice (order Anoplura), of the family Pediculidae. *Pediculus humanus.*
**P. huma'nus,** a species that feeds on human blood, is a major vector of epidemic typhus, trench fever, and relapsing fever, and causes skin reactions, especially in sensitized persons. It includes two subspecies, *P. humanus capitis* and *P. humanus corporis.*
**P. huma'nus cap'itis,** the head louse, found on the scalp hair.
**P. huma'nus cor'poris,** the body or clothes louse, which lives on the clothing when feeding is not taking place; called also *P. humanus humanus, P. humanus vestimento'rum,* and *P. vestimenti.*
**P. huma'nus huma'nus,** *P. humanus corporis.*
**P. huma'nus vestimento'rum,** *P. humanus corporis.*
**P. inguina'lis, P. pu'bis,** *Phthirus pubis.*
**P. vestimen'ti,** *P. humanus corporis.*

**pe·dic·u·lus** (pə-dik'u-ləs) pl. *pedic'uli* [L.] [MeSH: Pediculus] 1. louse. 2. pedicle: a footlike or stemlike part.
**p. ar'cus ver'tebrae** [TA], pedicle of vertebral arch: one of the paired parts of the vertebral arch that connect a lamina to the vertebral body; called also *radix arcus vertebrae.*
**p. pulmo'nis,** radix pulmonis.

**ped·i·cure** (ped'ĭ-kūr) [*pedi-* + *cure*] professional care and treatment of the feet.

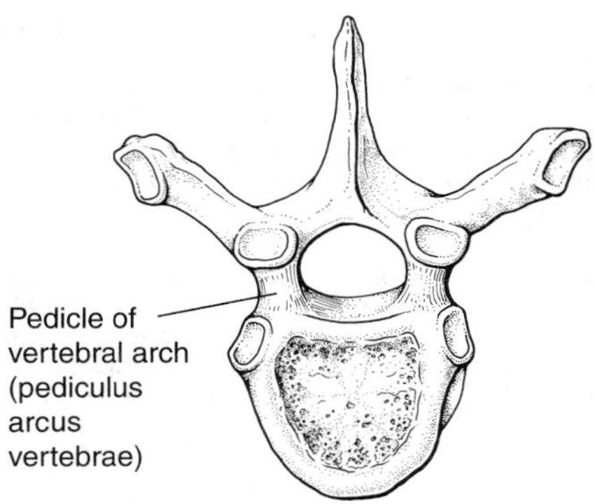


**ped·i·gree** (ped'ĭ-gre) [Fr. *pied de grue,* "crane's foot" (from the shape of the stemma)] [MeSH: Pedigree] a table, chart, diagram, or list of an individual's ancestors, used in human genetics in the analysis of inheritance.

**Pe·di·o·coc·cus** (pe″de-o-kok'əs) [Gr. *pedion* a plane surface + *kokkos* berry] [MeSH: Pediococcus] a genus of microaerophilic saprophytic, gram-positive, nonmotile cocci of the family Streptococcaceae. They usually occur in pairs or tetrads, and are found most commonly in fermenting plant products.
**P. acidilacti'ci,** a species found in sauerkraut and fermenting mashes.
**P. cerevi'siae,** a species found in spoiled beer and brewer's yeast.
**P. halophi'lus,** a species found in anchovies and soy mash.
**P. pentosa'ceus,** a species occurring commonly in fermenting products, such as pickles, sauerkraut, etc.
**P. uri'nae-e'qui,** a species originally isolated from horse urine, also often found in brewer's yeast.

**pe·dio·don·tia** (pe″de-o-don'shə) pediatric dentistry.

**pe·dio·nal·gia** (pe″de-o-nal'jə) [Gr. *pedion* metatarsus + *-algia*] pain in the sole of the foot. Cf. *podalgia.*

**Ped·i·pal·pa** (ped″ĭ-pal'pə) the whip scorpions, an order of arachnids (not true scorpions) that are nonvenomous but sometimes have irritating secretions; it includes the genus *Mastigoproctus.*

**pedi·pha·lanx** (ped″ĭ-fa'lanks) [*pedi-* + *phalanx*] a phalanx of a digit of the foot.

**pe·di·tis** (pə-di'tis) [*ped-*[2] + *-itis*] pedal osteitis.

**ped(o)-**[1] [Gr. *pais,* gen. *paidos* child] a combining form denoting relationship to a child. Also, *paed(o)-.*

**ped(o)-**[2] [L. *pes,* gen. *pedis* foot] a combining form denoting relationship to the foot. Also, *pedi-.*

**pe·do·baro·graph** (pe″do-bar'o-graf) [*pedo-* + *baro-* + *graph*] an apparatus for recording dynamic variations in downward pressure by different areas of the sole of a foot as a person stands upright or walks. A common type places the subject above a sheet of deformable white film over a glass plate; light reflects differently at different areas on the under side of the plate according to variations in pressure on the plastic sheet, and the differences are recorded.

**pe·do·bar·og·ra·phy** (pe″do-bə-rog'rə-fe) [*pedo-* + *baro-* + *-graphy*] measurement of dynamic variations in downward pressure by different areas of the sole of a foot, using a pedobarograph.

**pe·do·don·tia** (pe″do-don'shə) pediatric dentistry.

**pe·do·don·tics** (pe-do-don'tiks) [*pedo-*[1] + *odont-* + *-ic*] pediatric dentistry.

**pe·do·don·tist** (pe-do-don'tist) pediatric dentist.

**pe·do·dy·na·mom·e·ter** (pe″do-di-nə-mom'ə-tər) [*pedo-*[2] + *dynamometer*] a dynamometer used for leg muscles.

**pe·dog·a·my** (pe-dog'ə-me) [*pedo-*[1] + Gr. *gamos* marriage] endogamy, def. 1.

**pe·do·gen·e·sis** (pe″do-jen'ə-sis) [*pedo-*[1] + *-genesis*] the production of offspring by young or larval forms.

**pe·do·graph** (pe'do-graf) [*pedo-*[2] + *-graph*] an imprint on paper of the weight-bearing surface of the foot, surrounded by a pencil-marked contour of the upper foot.

**pe·dol·o·gist** (pe-dol'ə-gist) a specialist in pedology.

**pe·dol·o·gy** (pe-dol'ə-je) [*pedo-*[1] + *-logy*] the systematical study of the life and development of children.

**pe·dom·e·ter** (pə-dom'ə-tər) [*pedo-*[2] + *-meter*] an instrument for recording the number of steps taken in walking.

**pe·do·mor·phic** (pe″do-mor'fik) pertaining to or characterized by pedomorphism.

**pe·do·mor·phism** (pe″do-mor'fiz-əm) [*pedo-*[1] + *morph-* + *-ism*] the retention in the adult organism of highly progressive species of bodily characters which at an earlier stage of evolutionary history were actually only infantile.

**pe·dop·a·thy** (pə-dop'ə-the) [*pedo-*[2] + *-pathy*] any disease of the foot.

**pe·do·phil·ia** (pe″do-fil'e-ə) [*pedo-*[1] + *-philia*] [MeSH: Pedophilia] [DSM-IV] a paraphilia in which an adult has recurrent, intense sexual urges or sexually arousing fantasies of engaging in or repeatedly engages in sexual activity with a prepubertal child.

**pe·do·phil·ic** (pe″do-fil'ik) pertaining to or characterized by pedophilia.

**pe·do·pho·bia** (pe″de-o-fo'be-ə) [*pedo-*[1] + *-phobia*] irrational fear or dread of children.

**pe·dor·thic** (pə-dor'thik) pertaining to pedorthics.

**pe·dor·thics** (pə-dor'thiks) [*pedo-*[2] + *ortho-* + *-ic*] the design, manufacture, fit, and modification of shoes and related foot appliances as prescribed for amelioration of painful and/or disabling conditions of the foot and limb.

**pe·dor·thist** (pə-dor'thist) a person skilled in pedorthics and practicing its application in individual cases.

**pe·dun·cle** (pə-dung'kəl) 1. pedunculus. 2. the stalk by which a nonsessile tumor is attached to normal tissue.
**anterior p. of thalamus,** radiatio thalami anterior.
**caudal p. of thalamus,** radiatio thalami inferior.
**central p. of thalamus,** radiatio thalami centralis.
**cerebellar p's,** pedunculi cerebellares
**cerebellar p., caudal,** pedunculus cerebellaris inferior.
**cerebellar p., cranial,** pedunculus cerebellaris superior.
**cerebellar p., inferior,** pedunculus cerebellaris inferior.
**cerebellar p., middle,** pedunculus cerebellaris medius.
**cerebellar p., pontine,** pedunculus cerebellaris medius.
**cerebellar p., rostral,** pedunculus cerebellaris superior.
**cerebellar p., superior,** pedunculus cerebellaris superior.
**p's of cerebellum,** pedunculi cerebellares.
**cerebral p., p. of cerebrum,** pedunculus cerebri.
**p. of flocculus,** pedunculus flocculi.
**inferior p. of thalamus,** radiatio thalami inferior.
**p. of mammillary body,** a bundle formed by a convergence of afferent fibers in the midbrain tegmentum; it ends in the mammillary body.
**olfactory p.,** in comparative neuroanatomy, the olfactory stalk, especially the region of its attachment to the cerebral hemisphere.
**pineal p., p. of pineal body,** habenula, def. 2.
**posterior p. of thalamus,** radiatio thalami posterior.
**superior p. of thalamus,** radiatio thalami centralis.
**thalamic p's,** p's of thalamus.
**p's of thalamus,** thalamic radiations.

**pe·dun·cu·lar** (pə-dung'ku-lər) pertaining to a peduncle.

**pe·dun·cu·lat·ed** (pə-dung'ku-lāt-əd) provided with a peduncle; opposed to sessile.

**pe·dun·cu·lus** (pə-dung'ku-ləs) pl. *pedun'culi* [L.] [TA] peduncle: a stemlike part; a general term for collections of nerve fibers coursing between different areas in the central nervous system.
**pedun'culi cerebella'res** [TA], cerebellar peduncles: three large bundles of projection fibers on each side of the cerebellum that connect it with other parts of the brain and spinal cord; see *p. cerebellaris inferior, p. cerebellaris medius,* and *p. cerebellaris superior.* Called also *pedunculi cerebelli.*
**p. cerebella'ris cauda'lis,** p. cerebellaris inferior.
**p. cerebella'ris infe'rior** [TA], inferior cerebellar peduncle: a large bundle of nerve fibers connecting the medulla oblongata and spinal cord with the cerebellum (especially the archeocerebellum and paleocerebellum). It courses along the lateral border of the fourth ventricle and turns posteriorly into the cerebellum. Called also *p. cerebellaris caudalis, caudal cerebellar peduncle,* and *restiform body.*
**p. cerebella'ris me'dius** [TA], **p. cerebella'ris ponti'nus,** middle cerebellar peduncle: a large bundle of projection fibers originating in the contralateral pontine nuclei and entering the cerebellum, conveying impulses from the cerebral cortex to the neocerebellum; it is continuous with the pons at the line of attachment of the trigeminal nerve. Called also *brachium pontis* and *pontine cerebellar peduncle.*
**p. cerebella'ris rostra'lis,** p. cerebellaris superior.
**p. cerebella'ris supe'rior** [TA], superior cerebellar peduncle: a large bundle of projection fibers arising chiefly in the dentate nucleus of each cerebellar hemisphere (the neocerebellum) and ascending to decussate in the mesencephalon; its fibers end mostly in the red nucleus and thalamus. Spinocerebellar fibers to the palaeocerebellum lie adjacent to each peduncle. Called also *p. cerebellaris rostralis, cranial cerebellar peduncle, rostral cerebellar peduncle,* and *brachium conjunctivum.*
**pedun'culi cerebel'li,** pedunculi cerebellares.

**p. cerebra'lis, p. ce'rebri** [TA], peduncle of cerebrum: either of the two large masses of substance that descend from each cerebral hemisphere, being separated by the interpeduncular fossa until they converge where they enter the pons; they form the ventral part of the mesencephalon. Each peduncle is divided into an anterior part, consisting of a bundle of nerve fiber tracts (basis pedunculi cerebri), and a posterior part, which is continuous across the median plane, forming the tegmentum of the mesencephalon; the parts are separated by the substantia nigra. The term also has been used to denote the right or left half of the midbrain, each consisting of an anterior part, the crus cerebri, and a posterior or tegmental part, the tegmentum. Called also *cerebral peduncle.*
**p. cor'poris pinea'lis,** habenula, def. 2.
**p. floc'culi** [TA], peduncle of flocculus: a narrow band of afferent and efferent nerve fibers that connects the nodulus of the cerebellum to the flocculus; its dorsal part is continuous with the anterolateral part of the caudal medullary velum, from which most of its fibers are derived.
**p. thala'micus infe'rior,** radiatio thalami inferior.

**peel** (pēl) [L. *pilare* to deprive of hair] 1. the outer covering of something. 2. to remove such an outer covering.
**bitter orange p.,** the dried rind of unripe but fully grown fruit of *Citrus aurantium* Linné, used as a pharmaceutical flavoring agent.
**chemical p.,** chemabrasion.
**lemon p.,** the outer, yellow rind of the fresh ripe fruit of *Citrus limon,* used as a source of lemon oil.

**PEEP** positive end-expiratory pressure; see under *pressure.*

**PEF** peak expiratory flow.

**PEFR** peak expiratory flow rate.

**PEG** pneumoencephalography; polyethylene glycol.
**PEG-ADA, PEG-adenosine deaminase,** pegademase.

**peg** (peg) a projecting structure.
**rete p's,** rete ridges.

**peg·ad·e·mase** (peg-ad'ə-mās) adenosine deaminase derived from bovine intestine and attached covalently to polyethylene glycol, used in replacement therapy for adenosine deaminase deficiency in patients with severe combined immunodeficiency; administered intramuscularly.

**Peg·a·none** (peg'ə-nōn) trademark for a preparation of ethotoin.

**Peg·a·num** (peg'ə-nəm) a genus of herbs of the family Zygophyllaceae. *P. harma'la* L. is African rue, a species whose seeds contain the hallucinogens harmine and harmaline.

**pe·gli·col 5 ole·ate** (pə-gli'kol) a product obtained by alcoholysis of natural vegetable oils in the presence of polyethylene glycols of molecular weights between 200 and 400, consisting of a mixture of partially mixed esters of glycerin and these polyethylene glycols; the average number of ethylene glycol units is 5. It is used as an emulsifying agent in pharmaceutical preparations. Called also *polyoxyl 5 oleate.*

**peg·o·ter·ate** (peg'o-ter'āt) a condensation polymer used as a suspending agent in pharmaceutical preparations.

**peg·ox·ol 7 ste·a·rate** (peg-ok'sōl) a mixture of mono- and distearic esters of ethylene glycol and of polyoxyethylene glycol, the latter having an average molecular weight of 450; the average number of ethylene glycol units is 7. It is used as an emulsifying agent in pharmaceutical preparations.

**Pel-Eb·stein fever (disease, pyrexia)** (pel-eb'shtīn) [Pieter Klaases *Pel,* Dutch physician, 1852–1919; Wilhelm *Ebstein,* German physician, 1836–1912] see under *fever.*

**pe·lade** (pə-lahd') [Fr.] alopecia areata.

**pel·age** (pel'əj) [Fr.] 1. the hairy coat of mammals. 2. the hairs of the body, limbs, and head collectively.

**Pel·a·mis** (pel'ə-mis) a genus of sea snakes (family Hydrophiidae). *P. bico'lor* is a venomous species found in the Indian Ocean. *P. platu'rus* is the yellow-bellied sea snake, a venomous species found in many parts of the Indian and Pacific Oceans.

**Pel·e·cyp·o·da** (pel"e-sip'o-də) [Gr. *pelekys* hatchet + *podos* foot] the bivalves: a class of mollusks which are laterally compressed and have a pair of dorsally hinged lateral shells (valves) and a hatchet-shaped foot for digging; it includes the clams, oysters, and scallops. Called also *Bivalvia.*

**Pel·ger's nuclear anomaly** (pel'gərz) [Karel *Pelger,* Dutch physician, 1885–1931] see under *anomaly.*

**Pel·ger-Hu·ët nuclear anomaly** (pel'gər-hu'ət) [Karel *Pelger;* G. J. *Huët,* Dutch physician, 1879–1970] see under *anomaly.*

**pel·i·o·sis** (pel"e-o'sis) [Gr. *peliōsis* extravasation of blood] purpura.
**bacillary p.,** the presence in the liver or spleen of disseminated vasoproliferative lesions containing colonies of *Bartonella henselae* or *B. quintana.*
**p. he'patis, p. of liver,** the presence of blood-filled lacunae in the parenchyma of the liver, giving it a mottled blue appearance.

**Pe·li·zae·us-Merz·ba·cher disease** (pa"le-tsa'oos-merts'bahkər) [Friedrich *Pelizaeus,* German physician, 1850–1917; Ludwig *Merzbacher,* German physician, 1875–1942] familial centrolobar sclerosis.

**pel·lag·ra** (pə-lag'rə) [It. *pelle* skin + *agra* rough] [MeSH: Pellagra] a clinical deficiency syndrome due to deficiency of niacin (or failure to convert tryptophan to niacin) and characterized by dermatitis, inflammation of mucous membranes, diarrhea, and psychic disturbances. The dermatitis occurs on the portions of the body exposed to light or trauma. Mental symptoms include depression, irritability, anxiety, confusion, disorientation, delusions, and hallucinations.
**monkey p.,** pellagra in caged monkeys, manifested by anorexia, diarrhea, vomiting, emaciation, and finally death.
**p. si'ne pella'gra,** pellagra in which the characteristic dermatitis is not present.
**typhoid p.,** pellagra characterized by continued high temperature.

**pel·lag·ra·gen·ic** (pə-lag"rə-jen'ik) causing pellagra.

**pel·lag·ral** (pə-lag'rəl) pertaining to or caused by pellagra.

**pel·lag·rin** (pə-lag'rin) a person affected with pellagra.

**pel·la·groid** (pə-lag'roid) a condition resembling pellagra.

**pel·lag·rose** (pə-lag'rōs) pellagrous.

**pel·la·gro·sis** (pel"ə-gro'sis) the dermal syndrome of pellagra characterized by skin pigmentation, erythema, and hyperkeratosis.

**pel·lag·rous** (pə-lag'rəs) affected with or of the nature of pellagra.

**pel·lant** (pel'ənt) [L. *pellere* to drive] depurative.

**pel·late** (pel'āt) to repel or tend to separate.

**Pel·le·gri·ni's disease** (pel"ə-gre'nēz) [Augusto *Pellegrini,* Italian surgeon, born 1877] see under *disease.*

**Pel·le·gri·ni-Stie·da disease** (pel"ə-gre'ne-shte'də) [A. *Pellegrini;* Alfred *Stieda,* German surgeon, 1869–1945] see *Pellegrini's disease* under *disease.*

**pel·let** (pel'ət) 1. a small pill or granule, such as a small rod- or ovoid-shaped, sterile mass composed of essentially pure steroid hormones, to be implanted under the skin to provide for their slow absorption. 2. a small pill made from sucrose and impregnated with a medicine, used in homeopathic practice.

**pel·li·cle** (pel'ĭ-kəl) [L. *pellicula*] 1. a thin skin or film, such as a thin film on the surface of a liquid. 2. in protozoology, a living outer layer of denser cytoplasm containing the peripheral and surface organelles of ciliate protozoa.
**brown p.,** a brownish gray to black film formed over a period of time on the surfaces of the teeth, resulting from poor oral hygiene and brushing habits. See also *dental plaque,* under *plaque.*

**pel·lic·u·lar, pel·lic·u·lous** (pə-lik'u-lər, pə-lik'u-ləs) pertaining to or characterized by a pellicle.

**Pel·liz·zi's syndrome** (pə-le'tsēz) [G. B. *Pellizzi,* Italian physician, early 20th century] epiphyseal syndrome.

**pel·lu·cid** (pə-loo'sid) [L. *pellucidus,* from *per* through + *lucere* to shine] translucent.

**pel(o)-** [Gr. *pēlos* mud] a combining form denoting relationship to mud.

**Pe·lo·bi·on·ti·da** (pe"lo-bi-on'tĭ-də) [*pelo-* + Gr. *bioun* a living being] an order of large, free-living cylindrical, monopodial, multinucleate ameboid protozoa (subclass Gymnamoebia, class Lobosea) found in soil and water, and characterized by the presence of bacterial and other inclusions and numerous nonmotile cilia. *Pelomyxa* is a representative genus.

**Pel·o·de·ra** (pel"o-der'ə) *Rhabditis.*

**Pe·lo·myxa** (pe"lo-mik'sə) [*pelo-* + Gr. *myxa* mucus] a genus of protozoa (order Pelobiontida, subclass Gymnamoebida), including *P. carolinensis (Chaos chaos),* the giant ameba, which may attain a diameter of 5 mm.

**pe·lo·ther·a·py** (pe"lo-ther'ə-pe) [*pelo-* + *therapy*] the therapeutic use of earth or mud.

**pel·ta** (pel'tə) [L. "a shield"] a crescent-shaped membranous structure arising from or covering the axostyle of certain parasitic flagellate protozoa, especially trichomonads.

**pel·tate** (pel'tāt) [L. *pelta;* Gr. *peltē* shield] shield-shaped.

**pel·ves** (pel'vēs) [L.] plural of *pelvis.*

**pel·vic** (pel'vik) pertaining to the pelvis.

**pel·vi·cal·i·ce·al, pel·vi·cal·y·ce·al** (pel"vĭ-kal"ĭ-se'əl) pertaining to the renal pelves and calices.

**pel•vi•cel•lu•li•tis** (pel″vĭ-sel″u-li′tis) parametritis.

**pel•vi•ceph•a•log•ra•phy** (pel″vĭ-sef″ə-log′rə-fe) [*pelvis* + *cephalo-* + *-graphy*] radiographic measurement of the fetal head and of the birth canal.

**pel•vi•ceph•a•lom•e•try** (pel″vĭ-sef″ə-lom′ə-tre) [*pelvis* + *cephalo-* + *-metry*] measurement of the diameters of the head of the fetus in relation to those of the mother's pelvis.

**pel•vi•fem•o•ral** (pel″vĭ-fem′ə-rəl) pertaining to or affecting the pelvis and femur.

**pel•vi•fix•a•tion** (pel″vĭ-fik-sa′shən) surgical fixation of an organ to the pelvic cavity.

**pel•vi•li•thot•o•my** (pel″vĭ-lĭ-thot′ə-me) pyelolithotomy.

**pel•vim•e•ter** (pel-vim′ə-tər) [*pelvis* + *-meter*] an instrument for measuring the diameters and capacity of the pelvis.

**pel•vim•e•try** (pel-vim′ə-tre) [MeSH: Pelvimetry] the measurement of the dimensions and capacity of the pelvis.
**combined p.,** pelvimetry in which measurements are made both within and outside the body.
**instrumental p.,** measurement of the pelvis with the pelvimeter.
**manual p.,** that which is performed with the hands.
**x-ray p.,** the measurement of the maternal pelvis and the fetal head using radiographic techniques.

**pel•vi•og•ra•phy** (pel″ve-og′rə-fe) pelvioradiography.

**pel•vio•il•eo•neo•cys•tos•to•my** (pel″ve-o-il″e-o-ne″o-sis-tos′tə-me) anastomosis of renal pelvis to an isolated segment of the ileum, which is then anastomosed to the urinary bladder.

**pel•vio•li•thot•o•my** (pel″ve-o-lĭ-thot′ə-me) pyelolithotomy.

**pel•vio•ne•os•to•my** (pel″ve-o-ne-os′tə-me) ureteropyeloneostomy.

**pel•vio•peri•to•ni•tis** (pel″ve-o-per″ĭ-to-ni′tis) pelvic peritonitis.

**pel•vio•plas•ty** (pel′ve-o-plas″te) pyeloplasty.

**pel•vio•ra•di•og•ra•phy** (pel″ve-o-ra″de-og′rə-fe) radiography of the organs of the pelvis.

**pel•vi•os•co•py** (pel″ve-os′kə-pe) [*pelvis* + *-scopy*] 1. the inspection or visual examination of the pelvis or pelvic viscera, as with a laparoscope or pelviscope. 2. pyeloscopy.

**pel•vi•os•to•my** (pel″ve-os′tə-me) pyelostomy.

**pel•vi•ot•o•my** (pel″ve-ot′ə-me) [*pelvis* + *-tomy*] 1. the cutting of the pelvic bones. 2. pyelotomy.

**pel•vi•peri•to•ni•tis** (pel″ve-per″ĭ-to-ni′tis) pelvic peritonitis.

**pel•vi•ra•di•og•ra•phy** (pel″vĭ-ra″de-og′rə-fe) pelvioradiography.

**pel•vi•rec•tal** (pel″vĭ-rek′təl) pertaining to the pelvis and the rectum.

**pel•vis** (pel′vis) pl. *pel′ves* [L. "basin"] [MeSH: Pelvis] 1. [TA] the inferior portion of the trunk of the body, bounded anteriorly and laterally by the two hip bones and posteriorly by the sacrum and coccyx. The pelvis is divided by a plane passing through the terminal lines into the *p. major* superiorly and the *p. minor* inferiorly. The superior boundary of the pelvic cavity is the *inlet* (*apertura pelvis superior* [TA]), and the inferior boundary of the pelvis minor is the *outlet* (*apertura pelvis inferior* [TA]), which is bounded by the coccyx, the symphysis pubis, and the ischium of either side. The outlet is closed by the coccygeus and levator ani muscles and the perineal fascia, which form the *floor of the pelvis.* The inlet and outlet each have three important diameters: an anteroposterior (conjugate), an oblique, and a transverse, the relations of which determine types variously classified by different authors (see illustration under *diameter*). 2. any basinlike structure.
**android p.,** a pelvis characterized by a wedge-shaped inlet and narrowness of the anterior segment; used as a general designation of a female pelvis showing characters typical of the pelvis in the male.
**anthropoid p.,** a female pelvis characterized by a long anteroposterior diameter of the inlet, which equals or exceeds the transverse diameter.
**assimilation p.,** a pelvis in which the transverse processes of the last lumbar vertebra are fused with the sacrum (*high-assimilation p.*—including six vertebral segments), or the last sacral vertebra may fuse with the first coccygeal body (*low-assimilation p.*—including only four vertebral segments).
**beaked p.,** one with the pelvic bones laterally compressed and their anterior junction pushed forward, as in osteomalacia.
**bony p.,** p. ossea.
**brachypellic p.,** an oval type of pelvis, the transverse diameter of the inlet exceeding the anteroposterior diameter by 1 to 3 cm.
**contracted p.,** a pelvis in which there is a diminution of 1.5 to 2 cm in any important diameter; when all dimensions are proportionately diminished it is a generally contracted pelvis *(p. justo minor).*
**cordate p., cordiform p.,** one that is somewhat heart shaped.
**coxalgic p.,** one deformed in consequence of hip-joint disease.
**dolichopellic p.,** an elongated pelvis, the anteroposterior diameter of the inlet being greater than the transverse diameter.
**dwarf p.,** a small pelvis seen in several types of dwarfism.
**extrarenal p.,** see under *p. rena′lis.*
**false p.,** p. major.
**flat p.,** one in which the anteroposterior dimension is abnormally reduced.
**frozen p.,** a condition, due to infection or carcinoma, in which the adnexa and uterus are fixed in the pelvis.
**funnel-shaped p.,** a female pelvis with a normal inlet, but a greatly narrowed outlet.
**giant p.,** p. justo major.
**greater p.,** p. major.
**gynecoid p.,** a pelvis having a rounded oval shape with a well rounded anterior and posterior segment; it represents the normal female pelvis.
**high-assimilation p.,** see *assimilation p.*
**infantile p.,** a generally contracted pelvis characterized by an oval shape, a high sacrum, and marked inclination of the walls.
**p. jus′to ma′jor,** a pelvis that is unusually large, with all its dimensions equally increased.
**p. jus′to mi′nor,** a pelvis that is unusually small, with all its dimensions equally reduced; see also *contracted p.*
**juvenile p.,** infantile p.
**kyphoscoliotic p.,** an irregularly contracted pelvis due to rachitic kyphoscoliosis.
**kyphotic p.,** one characterized by increase of the conjugate diameter at the brim, with decrease of the transverse diameter at the outlet, due to close proximity of the ischial spines and tuberosities.
**large p.,** p. major.
**lesser p.,** p. minor.
**lordotic p.,** one associated with an anterior curvature in the lumbar region of the vertebral column.

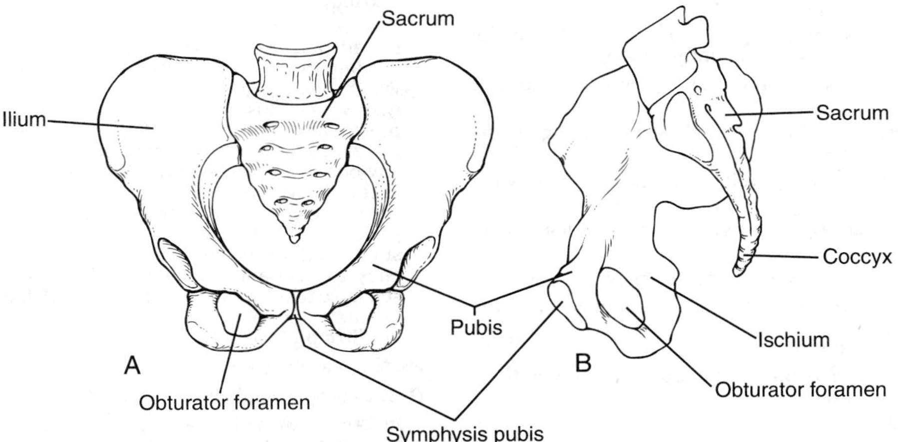


Pelvis. Anterior *(A)* and internal *(B)* aspects.

**low-assimilation p.,** see *assimilation p.*
**p. ma'jor** [TA], greater pelvis: the part of the pelvis superior to a plane passing through the iliopectineal lines.
**mesatipellic p.,** a round type of pelvis, the transverse diameter of the inlet being equal to the anteroposterior diameter or being greater by 1 cm. or less.
**p. mi'nor** [TA], lesser pelvis: the part of the pelvis inferior to a plane passing through the iliopectineal lines; see *pelvis.*
**p. na'na,** dwarf p.
**p. obtec'ta,** a kyphotic pelvis in which the vertebral column extends horizontally across the pelvic inlet.
**p. os'sea,** bony pelvis: the ring of bone forming the skeleton of the pelvis, supporting the vertebral column and resting upon the inferior members, and composed of the two hip bones anteriorly and laterally, and the sacrum and coccyx posteriorly.
**osteomalacic p.,** deformity of the pelvis due to absorption by the bones of their calcium salts, as a result of which the bones become soft and so flexible that they may be stretched or pushed together and cause narrowing of the pelvic inlet.
**Otto p.,** a pelvis in which the acetabulum is depressed, permitting the head of the femur to protrude intrapelvically; see *arthrokatadysis.*
**p. pla'na,** flat p.
**platypellic p., platypelloid p.,** a pelvis characterized by flattening of the pelvic inlet, with a short anteroposterior and a wide transverse diameter.
**Prague p.,** spondylolisthetic p.
**pseudo-osteomalacic p.,** a deformed pelvis simulating one affected with osteomalacia, but resulting from other causes.
**pseudospider p.,** a congenitally small, long, thin renal pelvis with calices that may simulate renal tumor urographically.
**rachitic p.,** one distorted as a result of rickets.
**p. rena'lis** [TA], renal pelvis: the expansion from the upper end of the ureter into which the calices of the kidney open; ordinarily lodged within the renal sinus, under certain conditions, as in a long kidney or obstruction of the ureteropelvic junction, a large part of it may be outside the kidney *(extrarenal p.).*
**Rokitansky's p.,** spondylolisthetic p.
**round p.,** one with an inlet of nearly circular outline.
**scoliotic p.,** one deformed as a result of scoliosis.
**simple flat p.,** one with a shortened anteroposterior diameter.
**small p.,** p. minor.
**spider p.,** a renal pelvis which in the pyelogram shows the calices as narrow, string-like extensions, resembling the legs of a spider.
**p. spino'sa,** a rachitic pelvis with the crest of the pubis very sharp.
**split p.,** one with a congenital separation at the symphysis pubis, often associated with exstrophy of the bladder.
**spondylolisthetic p.,** one in which the last, or rarely the fourth or third, lumbar vertebra is dislocated in front of the sacrum, more or less occluding the pelvic brim. Called also *Prague p.* and *Rokitansky's p.*
**p. spu'ria,** p. major.
**triangular p.,** one with a triangular inlet.
**true p.,** p. minor.
**p. of ureter,** p. renalis.

**pel·vi·sa·cral** (pel″vĭ-sa'krəl) pertaining to the pelvis and the sacrum.

**pel·vi·sa·crum** (pel″vĭ-sa'krəm) the pelvis and the sacrum together.

**pel·vi·scope** (pel'vĭ-skōp) an apparatus for viewing the pelvis or its contents; cf. *laparoscope* and *pelvioscopy.*

**pel·vis·co·py** (pel-vis'kə-pe) pelvioscopy.

**pel·vi·sec·tion** (pel″vĭ-sek'shən) [*pelvis* + *section*] a cutting of the pelvis bones, such as pubiotomy and symphysiotomy.

**pel·vi·ster·num** (pel″vĭ-ster'nəm) the cartilage of the symphysis pubis.

**pel·vi·tro·chan·te·ri·an** (pel″vĭ-tro-kan-tĕr'e-ən) relating to the pelvis and the great trochanter of the femur.

**pel·vi·ure·ter·al** (pel″ve-u-re'tər-əl) relating to the renal pelvis and the ureter.

**pel·vi·ure·tero·ra·di·og·ra·phy** (pel″ve-u-re″tər-o-ra″de-og'rə-fe) ureteropyelography.

**pel·vos·co·py** (pel-vos'kə-pe) [*pelvis* + *-scopy*] pelvioscopy.

**pel·vo·spon·dy·li·tis** (pel″vo-spon″də-li'tis) inflammation of the pelvic portion of the spine.
**p. ossi'ficans,** ankylosing spondylitis.

**pelyc(o)-** [Gr. *pelyx,* gen. *pelykos* bowl] for words beginning thus, see those beginning *pelvi-* and *pyel(o)-.*

**PEM** protein-energy malnutrition.

**pem·o·line** (pem'o-lēn) [MeSH: Pemoline] a central nervous system stimulant used in the treatment of attention-deficit/hyperactivity disorder; administered orally.

**pem·phi·goid** (pem'fĭ-goid) [*pemphigus* + *-oid*] 1. like or resembling pemphigus. 2. any of a group of dermatological syndromes similar to but clearly distinguishable from those of the pemphigus group. The term is often used alone to designate *bullous p.*
**benign mucosal p., benign mucous membrane p.,** cicatricial p.
**bullous p.,** a usually mild, relatively benign, self-limited subepidermal blistering skin disease, sometimes with oral involvement, predominantly affecting the elderly, and characterized clinically by the presence of large, tense bullae that rupture and leave denuded areas, which have a tendency to heal spontaneously. It is characterized histologically by a cleft formation at the dermoepidermal junction, and immunofluorescent studies reveal deposition of complement, usually with immunoglobulin G at the dermoepidermal junction at the level of the lamina lucida of the basement membrane.
**bullous p., localized,** a variant of bullous pemphigoid beginning at a localized site, such as on the scalp, trunk, or extremity, especially a lower extremity, and remaining confined to that site throughout the course of the disease. A localized chronic form has been reported.
**cicatricial p.,** a benign, chronic, usually bilateral, subepidermal blistering disease chiefly involving the mucous membranes, especially those of the mouth and eye *(ocular pemphigus),* which heals by scarring and may lead to a slowly progressive shrinkage of the affected mucous membranes and connective tissues, and eventually to blindness if untreated. Called also *benign mucosal p.* and *benign mucous membrane p.*
**p. gestationis,** herpes gestationis.
**localized chronic p.,** see *localized bullous p.*

**pem·phi·gus** (pem'fĭ-gəs) [Gr. *pemphix* blister] [MeSH: Pemphigus] any in a group of chronic, relapsing, sometimes fatal skin diseases characterized clinically by the development of successive crops of vesicles and bullae, histologically by acantholysis, and immunologically by serum autoantibodies directed against antigens in the intracellular zones of the epidermis. The specific disease is usually indicated by a modifying term, but the term *pemphigus* is often used alone to designate *p. vulgaris.* Cf. *pemphigoid.*
**benign familial p.,** a benign, persistently recurrent bullous and vesicular autosomal dominant dermatitis involving chiefly the sides of the neck, axillae, groin, and flexural and apposing surfaces of the body, and characterized by crops of lesions, which may remain localized or become generalized, that rupture, undergo erosion, and become thickly crusted. The histopathologic features are suggestive of keratosis follicularis as well as pemphigus. Called also *Hailey-Hailey disease.*
**Brazilian p.,** fogo selvagem.
**p. erythemato'sus,** a variant of pemphigus foliaceus, with which it is histologically identical, characterized clinically by a lupus erythematosus–like rash on the nose, cheeks, and ears and seborrhea-like lesions elsewhere on the body; and immunologically by granular deposition of immunoglobulin and complement along the dermoepidermal junction. These findings suggest the coexistence of lupus erythematosus and pemphigus in the same individual. Called also *Senear-Usher syndrome.*
**p. folia'ceus,** a superficial, relatively mild and chronic form of pemphigus, usually occurring in the fourth and fifth decades of life, and characterized by the development of small flaccid bullae that rupture and crust and localized or generalized exfoliation. The lesions may be found on the scalp, face, and trunk, or they may spread to become generalized.
**ocular p.,** cicatricial pemphigoid involving the conjunctivae.
**South American p.,** fogo selvagem.
**p. ve'getans,** a variant of pemphigus vulgaris characterized by the development of proliferating verrucous granulations, sometimes with pustules at their periphery, which seemingly arise from denuded bullae, and have a tendency to coalesce into patches. According to some authorities, there are two types: a *Hallopeau type,* which has a more benign course and prognosis; and a *Neumann type,* which closely resembles pemphigus vulgaris in all respects.
**p. vegetans, benign,** the Hallopeau type of pemphigus vegetans.
**p. vulga'ris,** the most common and severe form of pemphigus, usually occurring between the ages of 40 and 60, characterized by the chronic development of flaccid, easily ruptured bullae upon apparently normal skin and mucous membranes, beginning focally but progressing to become generalized, leaving large, weeping, denuded surfaces that become partially crusted over with little or no tendency to heal and that enlarge by confluence. In untreated cases, sepsis, cachexia, and electrolyte imbalance may occur and lead to death.
**wildfire p.,** fogo selvagem.

**PEN** pharmacy equivalent name.

**Pen·brit·in** (pen-brit'in) trademark for preparations of ampicillin.

**pen·bu·to·lol sul·fate** (pen-bu'tə-lol) [USP] a beta-adrenergic blocking agent with intrinsic sympathomimetic activity; used in the treatment of hypertension.

**pen·ci·clo·vir** (pen-si'klo-vir) an antiviral compound that inhibits viral DNA synthesis and replication in human herpesviruses 1 and 2, used in the treatment of recurrent herpes labialis; applied topically.

**Pen·de's sign** (pen'dāz) [Nicola *Pende,* Italian physician, 1880–1970] André-Thomas sign.

**pen·del·luft** (pen'də-looft″) [Ger. "pendulum breath"] the movement of air back and forth between the lungs, resulting in increased dead space ventilation.

**Pen·dred's syndrome** (pen'dredz) [Vaughan *Pendred,* English physician, 1869–1946] see under *syndrome.*

**pen·du·lar** (pen'du-lər) having a pendulum-like movement.

**pen·du·lous** (pen'du-ləs) [L. *pendere* to hang] hanging loosely; dependent.

**Pen·e·cort** (pen'ə-kort″) trademark for preparations of hydrocortisone.

**pe·nec·to·my** (pe-nek'tə-me) [*penis* + *-ectomy*] surgical removal of the penis.

**pen·e·tra·bil·i·ty** (pen″ə-trə-bil'ĭ-te) the ability of x-rays to penetrate matter.

**pen·e·trance** (pen'ə-trəns) [L. *penetrare* to enter into] in genetics, the frequency of expression of a genotype. If it is less than 100 per cent, the trait is said to exhibit *reduced penetrance* or *lack of penetrance.* In an individual who has a genotype that characteristically produces an abnormal phenotype but is phenotypically normal, the trait is said to be *nonpenetrant.*

**pen·e·trat·ing** (pen'ə-trāt-ing) [L. *penetrans*] piercing; entering deeply.

**pen·e·tra·tion** (pen″ə-tra'shən) [L. *penetratio*] 1. the act of piercing or entering deeply, as by a sharp object, radiation, or a chemical or drug. 2. focal depth.

**pen·e·trom·e·ter** (pen″ə-trom'ə-tər) 1. step wedge; a device for measuring the penetrability of x-rays. 2. an apparatus for registering the resistance of semisolid material to penetration.

**-penia** [Gr. *penia* poverty, need] a word termination indicating an abnormal reduction in number of the element denoted by the root to which it is affixed, as leukopenia.

**pe·ni·al** (pe'ne-əl) penile.

**pen·i·ci·din** (pen″ĭ-si'din) patulin.

**pen·i·cil·la·mine** (pen″ĭ-sil'ə-mēn) [USP] [MeSH: Penicillamine] a degradation product of penicillin which chelates certain heavy metals; used orally to reduce the blood copper level in the treatment of hepatolenticular degeneration and to promote excretion of cystine by forming a more soluble penicillamine-cystine disulfide. It is also used in the treatment of refractory rheumatoid arthritis.

**pen·i·cil·li** (pen″ĭ-sil'i) [L.] genitive and plural of *penicillus.*

**pen·i·cil·li·ary** (pen″ĭ-sil'e-ar″e) [L. *penicillum* brush] resembling a brush or broom.

**pen·i·cil·lic ac·id** (pen″ĭ-sil'ik) [MeSH: Penicillic Acid] an antibiotic substance produced by several species of *Penicillium* and *Aspergillus;* it has antibacterial activity but is also toxic to animal tissues, causing nephrotoxicity and other damage.

**pen·i·cil·lin** (pen″ĭ-sil'in) any of a large group of natural or semisynthetic antibacterial antibiotics derived directly or indirectly from strains of fungi of the genus *Penicillium* and other soil-inhabiting fungi grown on special culture media, which exert a bacteriocidal as well as a bacteriostatic effect on susceptible bacteria by interfering with the final stages of the synthesis of peptidoglycan, a substance in the bacterial cell wall. The penicillins, despite their relatively low toxicity for the host, are active against many bacteria, especially gram-positive pathogens (streptococci, staphylococci, pneumococci); clostridia; some gram-negative forms (gonococci, meningococci); some spirochetes (*Treponema pallidum* and *T. pertenue*); and some fungi. Certain strains of some target species, e.g., staphylococci, secrete the enzyme penicillinase, which inactivates penicillin and confers resistance to the antibiotic.
**aluminum p.,** the aluminum salt of penicillin prepared from extracts of cultures of *Penicillium notatum* or *P. chrysogenum.*
**benzathine p.,** p. G benzathine.
**benzyl p. potassium,** p. G. potassium.
**benzyl p. sodium,** p. G sodium.
**clemizole p.,** the clemizole salt of penicillin G, the combination of which produces a repository form of penicillin G with antihistaminic properties.
**dimethoxyphenyl p. sodium,** methicillin sodium.
**p. G,** the most widely used form and the first of the penicillins developed for medicinal use. It is used in the form of the benzathine, potassium, procaine, and sodium salts, principally in the treatment of infections due to penicillin-susceptible gram-positive bacteria, gram-negative cocci, *Treponema pallidum,* and *Actinomyces israelii.* Called also *benzylpenicillin.*
**p. G benzathine** [USP], a salt having a long-sustained action, obtained by combining penicillin G with *N,N′*-bis(phenylmethyl)-1,2-ethanediamine (2:1); administered orally and intramuscularly.
**p. G potassium,** a salt of penicillin G, administered orally and by intravenous injection or infusion.
**p. G procaine,** a salt having a long-sustained action, obtained by combining penicillin G with procaine (1:1); administered intramuscularly.
**p. G sodium** [USP], a salt having a potency of 1500–1750 U per mg; administered intramuscularly and intravenously.
**isoxazolyl p.,** a group of semisynthetic penicillins, including oxacillin, cloxacillin, and dicloxacillin, which combine resistance to penicillinase with acid stability and activity against gram- positive bacteria.
**p. N,** adicillin.
**p. O,** a penicillin produced biosynthetically by adding a precursor to the culture medium; penicillin O and its potassium and sodium salts have actions similar to those of penicillin G and are said to be hypoallergenic.
**p. O potassium,** see *p. O.*
**p. O sodium,** see *p. O.*
**phenoxymethyl p.,** p. V.
**potassium phenoxymethyl p.,** p. V potassium.
**p. V** [USP], a semisynthetic oral penicillin prepared from cultures of the mold *Penicillium* in the presence of 2-phenoxyethanol with an autolysate of yeast as the source of nitrogen. It is a broad-spectrum antibiotic having pharmacologic and toxic properties similar to those of other penicillins, and is less potent than penicillin G. Called also *phenoxymethyl p.*
**p. V benzathine** [USP], the benzathine salt of penicillin V, administered orally.
**p. V potassium** [USP], the potassium salt of penicillin V, administered orally.

**pen·i·cil·lin·ase** (pen″ĭ-sil'ĭ-nās) [MeSH: Penicillinase] a *β*-lactamase (q.v.) preferentially cleaving penicillins.

**pen·i·cil·lin-fast** (pen″ĭ-sĭl'in-fast) resistant to the action of penicillin; said of certain strains of bacteria.

**pen·i·cil·li·o·sis** (pen'ĭ-sil″e-o'sis) infection of humans or other animals with species of *Penicillium.* In humans it is rare and usually manifested as a pulmonary infection with fever, coughing, and leukocytosis; in other animals it may cause necrotic rhinitis, mycotoxic nephropathy, or neurological symptoms.

**Pen·i·cil·li·um** (pen″ĭ-sil'e-əm) [L. *penicillum* brush] [MeSH: Penicillium] a genus of Fungi Imperfecti of the form-class Hyphomycetes, form-family Moniliaceae; they develop fruiting organs resembling a broom or phalanges. Many species are commonly found in the human environment and are thought to occasionally cause penicilliosis. When identified, the perfect (sexual) stage is classified in the family Eurotiaceae.
**P. chryso'genum,** a species from which various penicillins are obtained.
**P. citreovi'ride,** a species that sometimes contaminates rice and contains the toxin citreoviridin, which can cause cardiac damage or neurotoxicity.
**P. citri'num,** a species that sometimes contaminates corn and contains the mycotoxin citrinin, which has caused nephropathy and hepatic necrosis in rats and chickens and possibly Balkan nephritis in humans.
**P. clavifor'me,** a toxic species that contains patulin.
**P. crusta'ceum,** *P. glaucum.*
**P. cyclo'pium,** a species that contains mycotoxins such as patulin and penicillic acid.
**P. expan'sum,** a toxic species that contains patulin.
**P. glau'cum,** a common bluegreen mold; called also *P. crustaceum.*
**P. griseoful'vum,** a species that yields the antibiotic griseofulvin.
**P. leu'copus,** a toxic species that contains patulin.
**P. meli'nii,** a toxic species that contains patulin.
**P. nota'tum,** a species from which various penicillins and the enzyme glucose oxidase are obtained.
**P. pa'tulum,** *P. uticale.*
**P. purpuroge'num,** a species that sometimes contaminates corn and contains the toxin rubratoxin, which causes hepatotoxicity in livestock.
**P. ru'brum,** a species that sometimes contaminates corn and contains the toxin rubratoxin, which causes hepatotoxicity in livestock.
**P. utica'le,** a toxic species that produces patulin; called also *P. patulum.*
**P. viridica'tum,** a species that sometimes contaminates grain and contains the mycotoxins citrinin and ochratoxins; it has caused nephropathy in rats and possibly Balkan nephritis in humans.

**pen·i·cil·lo·yl pol·y·ly·sine** (pen″ĭ-sil'o-əl pol″e-li'sēn) benzylpenicilloyl polylysine.

**pen·i·cil·lus** (pen″ĭ-sil'əs) gen. and pl. *penicil'li* [L. "brush"] a structure resembling a brush in appearance.

**penicil'li arte'riae liena'lis, penicil'li arte'riae sple'nicae** [TA], brushlike groups of arterial branches of the lobules of the spleen.

**Pe•nic•u•li•na** (pə-nik'u-li'nə) [MeSH: Peniculina] a suborder of large, free-living, monomorphic, mainly freshwater protozoa (order Hymenostomatida, subclass Hymenostomatia), characterized by the presence of explosive fusiform trichocysts and three peniculi, often located deep in the buccal cavity; nematodesmata and preoral and postoral sutures and an oral groove occur often. Many species have algal and gram-negative endosymbionts. *Paramecium* is a representative species.

**pe•nic•u•lus** (pə-nik'u-ləs) pl. *penic'uli* ["little brush"] a modified membrane manifested as a band of fused cilia in the left wall in the buccal cavity of certain ciliate protozoa.

**pe•nile** (pe'nīl) pertaining to or affecting the penis.

**pen•il•lam•ine** (pen"il-am'in) an amine derived from penillic acid by the removal of a molecule of carbon dioxide.

**pen•il•lo•al•de•hyde** (pen"ĭ-lo-al'də-hīd) an aldehyde derived from penicillin.

**pe•nis** (pe'nis) [L.] [TA] [MeSH: Penis] the male organ of copulation and of urinary excretion, comprising a root, body, and extremity, or glans penis. The root is attached to the descending portions of the pubic bone by the *crura,* the latter being the extremities of the corpora cavernosa. The body consists of two parallel cylindrical bodies, the *corpora cavernosa,* and beneath them the *corpus spongiosum,* through which the urethra passes. The glans is covered with mucous membrane and ensheathed by the prepuce, or foreskin. The penis is homologous with the clitoris in the female.
**clubbed p.**, a condition in which the penis is curved when erect.
**concealed p.**, a rudimentary penis concealed beneath the skin of the scrotum, perineum, abdomen, or thigh.
**corkscrew p.**, a defect seen in bulls in which some parts of the penile tunica albuginea stretch more than others during erection, so that a spiral deviation prevents insertion and copulation. Called also *spiral deviation of the penis.*
**double p.**, an anomaly resulting when the urethral groove completely divides the penile shaft during development of the embryo.
**p. palma'tus,** webbed p.
**p. plas'tica,** Peyronie's d..
**webbed p.**, a penis that is enclosed by the skin of the scrotum; called also *p. palmatus.*

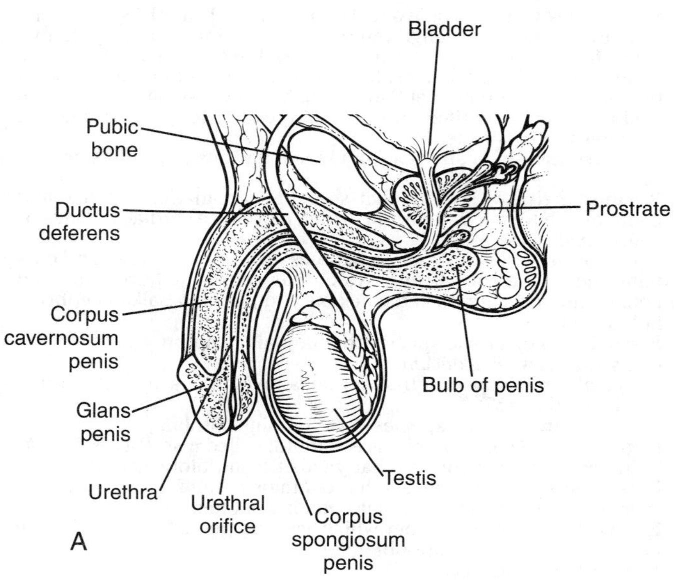


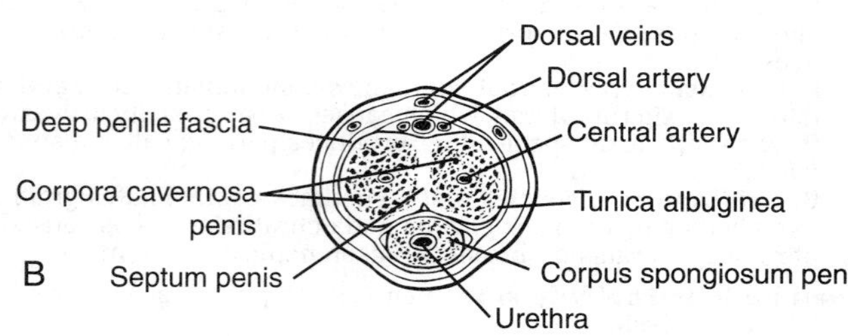


Penis. *(A),* Median sagittal section; *(B),* transverse section.

**pe•nis•chi•sis** (pe-nis'kĭ-sis) [*penis* + *-schisis*] a fissured state of the penis, as epispadias, hypospadias, or paraspadias.

**pe•ni•tis** (pe-ni'tis) inflammation of the penis.

**pen•nate** (pen'āt) penniform.

**pen•ni•form** (pen'ĭ-form) [L. *penna* feather + *form*] shaped like a feather; looking like a feather.

**pen•ny•ro•yal** (pen"e-roi'əl) 1. any of various mint plants, especially *Mentha pulegium,* whose oil was formerly used as a diaphoretic, aromatic, and emmenagogue. 2. wild mint.

**pe•no•scro•tal** (pe"no-skro'təl) relating to the penis and the scrotum.

**Pen•rose drain** (pen'rōz) [Charles Bingham *Penrose,* American gynecologist, 1862–1925] see under *drain.*

**pen•ta** (pen'tə) pentachlorophenol.

**pen•ta•ba•sic** (pen"tə-ba'sik) having five replaceable atoms of hydrogen in the molecule.

**pen•ta•chlo•ro•phe•nol** (pen"tə-klo"ro-fen'ol) [MeSH: Pentachlorophenol] a compound used as an insecticide for termite control, an herbicide, and a fungicidal wood preservative; its use has been restricted because it can cause severe toxic reactions in humans and other animals, such as convulsions, contact dermatitis, and lung, liver, and kidney damage. Called also *penta.*

**pen•ta•chro•mic** (pen"tə-kro'mik) [*penta-* + *chrom-* + *-ic*] 1. pertaining to or exhibiting five colors. 2. able to distinguish only five of the seven colors of the spectrum.

**pen•ta•cyc•lic** (pen"tə-sīk'lik) containing five fused rings or closed chains in the molecular structure.

**pen•tad** (pen'tad) 1. any group of five. 2. a pentavalent element or radical.

**pen•ta•dac•tyl** (pen"tə-dak'təl) [*penta-* + *dactyl*] having five fingers or toes on the hand or foot.

**pen•ta•ene** (pen'tə-ēn) a suffix denoting a chemical compound in which there are five conjugated double bonds.

**pen•ta•eryth•ri•tol** (pen"tə-ə-rith'rĭ-tol) an alcohol prepared by treating acetaldehyde with formaldehyde in an aqueous solution of calcium hydroxide; used in synthetic resins and in paints and varnishes.
**p. chloral,** petrichloral.
**p. tetranitrate,** the nitric acid ester of pentaerythritol, having vasodilator action similar to nitroglycerin, occurring as a white, crystalline powder that may explode on percussion. Called also *niperyt, pentaerythrityl tetranitrate, penthrit, pentrinitrol,* and *PTEN.*

**pen•ta•eryth•ri•tyl** (pen"tə-ə-rith'rĭ-təl) pentaerythritol.
**p. tetranitrate,** pentaerythritol tetranitrate.

**pen•ta•gas•trin** (pen"tə-gas'trin) [MeSH: Pentagastrin] a synthetic pentapeptide consisting of *β*-alanine and the C-terminal tetrapeptide of gastrin; used as a test of gastric secretory function.

**pen•tal•o•gy** (pən-tal'ə-je) a combination of five elements or factors, as five concurrent defects or symptoms.
**Cantrell's p., p. of Cantrell,** a cleft in the inferior part of the sternum associated with midline abdominal defects such as omphalocele, defective pericardium and diaphragm with communication between the pericardial and peritoneal cavities, and cardiac anomalies such as ventricular septal defect or less often atrial septal defect, tetralogy of Fallot, or left ventricular diverticulum.
**p. of Fallot,** the four defects of the tetralogy of Fallot accompanied by patent foramen ovale or atrial septal defect.

**pen•ta•mer** (pen'tə-mər) 1. a polymer consisting of five monomers. 2. a viral capsomer having five structural units.

**pen•ta•meth•a•zene** (pen"tə-meth'ə-zēn) azamethonium.

**pen•ta•meth•yl•ene•di•amine** (pen"tə-meth"əl-ēn-di'ə-mēn) cadaverine.

**pen•ta•meth•yl•ene•tet•ra•zol** (pen"tə-meth"əl-ēn-tet'rə-zol) pentylenetetrazol.

**pen•ta•meth•yl•mel•amine** (pen"tə-meth"əl-mel'ə-mēn) PMM; an active metabolite of hexamethylmelamine (q.v.), also under investigation as an antineoplastic agent.

**pen•tam•i•dine** (pən-tam'ĭ-dēn) [MeSH: Pentamidine] an anti-infective used as the isethionate salt and effective against *Pneumocystis carinii.*

**pen•tane** (pen'tān) *n*-pentane; an aliphatic hydrocarbon of the methane series, $C_5H_{12}$, obtained by distillation of petroleum and occurring as a clear, colorless, flammable liquid. It produces anesthesia when inhaled, ingested, or injected.

**pen•ta•pep•tide** (pen"tə-pep'tīd) a polypeptide containing five amino acids.

**pen•ta•pi•per•ide meth•yl•sul•fate** (pen″tə-pi′pər-īd) a synthetic quaternary ammonium anticholinergic used in the treatment of peptic ulcer and other disorders in which gastrointestinal hypermotility and hypersecretion are features; administered orally. Called also *pentapiperium methylsulfate.*

**pen•ta•pi•per•i•um meth•yl•sul•fate** (pen″tə-pi-per′e-əm) pentapiperide methylsulfate.

**pen•ta•pyr•ro•li•din•i•um bi•tar•trate** (pen″tə-pĭ-ro″lĭ-din′e-əm) pentolinium tartrate.

**pen•ta•so•my** (pen″tə-so′me) [*penta-* + Gr. *sōma* body] the presence of three additional chromosomes of one type (e.g., 5 X chromosomes) in an otherwise diploid cell (2n + 3).

**Pen•ta•span** (pen′tə-span″) trademark for a preparation of pentastarch.

**pen•ta•starch** (pen′tə-stahrch″) an artificial colloid derived from a waxy starch composed of more than 90 per cent amylopectin that has been etherified so that an average of 4 to 5 of the OH groups in every 10 D-glucopyranose units of the starch polymer have been converted to $OCH_2CH_2OH$ groups; used as an adjunct in leukapheresis to increase the erythrocyte sedimentation rate.

**Pen•tas•to•ma** (pən-tas′to-mə) [*penta-* + Gr. *stoma* mouth] former name of *Linguatula.*
**P. denticula′tum,** old name for *Linguatula serrata.*

**pen•ta•stome** (pen′tə-stōm) an individual of the class Pentastomida; called also *pentastomid* and *tongue worm.*

**pen•ta•sto•mi•a•sis** (pen″tə-sto-mi′ə-sis) infection with pentastomids.

**pen•ta•sto•mid** (pen″tə-sto′mid) pentastome.

**Pen•ta•sto•mida** (pen″tə-sto′mid-ə) a class of Arthropoda, the tongue worms, consisting of degenerate wormlike parasites, without circulatory or respiratory systems. The adults, otherwise without appendages, possess two pairs of hooks near the mouth. The larvae bear two or three pairs of rudimentary legs. Adults live in the respiratory passages and body cavities of reptiles, birds, and mammals. Families of importance in human and veterinary medicine include Porocephalidae and Linguatulidae.

**pen•ta•tom•ic** (pen″tə-tom′ik) [*pent-* + *atom*] 1. containing five atoms. 2. containing five replaceable hydrogen atoms.

**Pen•ta•tricho•mo•nas** (pen″tə-trik″o-mo′nəs) [*penta-* + *tricho-* + Gr. *monas* unit, from *monos* single] in some systems of classification, a genus of parasitic flagellated protozoa established to include the species of *Trichomonas* having five anterior flagella, i.e., *T. hominis.*

**pen•ta•va•lent** (pen″tə-va′lənt) having a chemical valence of five; capable of combining with five atoms of hydrogen.

**pen•taz•o•cine** (pən-taz′o-sēn) [MeSH: Pentazocine] a synthetic analgesic used in the form of the hydrochloride and lactate salts.
**p. hydrochloride** [USP], the hydrochloride salt of pentazocine, administered orally.
**p. lactate** [USP], the lactate salt of pentazocine, administered parenterally.

**pent•dyo•pent** (pent-di′o-pent) [*pent-* + Gr. *dyo* two + *pente* five (i.e., 525), referring to the spectroscopic line of the substance] a substance derived from blood pigment, occurring in the urine in certain diseases.

**pen•te•tate** (pen′tə-tāt) a salt, anion, ester, or complex of pentetic acid.
**p. calcium trisodium,** the calcium trisodium salt of pentetic acid, used as a chelating agent, especially in the treatment of plutonium poisoning. Called also *calcium trisodium pentetate.*

**pen•te•tic ac•id** (pen-tet′ik) [USP] diethylenetriamine pentaacetic acid, DTPA; a chelating agent (iron) with the general properties of the edetates. Complexed with radioisotopes it is used as an imaging agent; its uses as a technetium complex (Tc 99m) include renal and brain imaging, renal perfusion studies, assessment of glomerular filtration rate, radionuclide cisternography, and lung imaging; as a complex with indium (In 111) it is used in radionuclide cisternography.

**pen•te•tre•o•tide** (pen″tə-tre′o-īd) a conjugate of pentetic acid and the somatostatin analogue octreotide; it binds to somatostatin receptors and is used as the $^{111}$In chelate in the imaging of tumors having somatostatin receptors.

**pen•thi•e•nate bro•mide** (pen-thi′ə-nāt) a quaternary ammonium anticholinergic, used orally, mainly in the treatment of gastric ulcer.

**Pen•thrane** (pen′thrān) trademark for a preparation of methoxyflurane.

**pen•thrit** (pen′thrit) pentaerythritol tetranitrate.

**Pen•tids** (pen′tidz) trademark for preparations of penicillin G potassium.

**pen•to•bar•bi•tal** (pen″to-bahr′bĭ-təl) [USP] [MeSH: Pentobarbital] a short- to intermediate-acting barbiturate used as a sedative and hypnotic, administered orally. Called also *pentobarbitone.*
**p. sodium** [USP], the sodium salt of pentobarbital, used as a sedative, anticonvulsant, preanesthetic in surgery, an adjunct to anesthesia, and an amnesic in obstetrics.

**pen•to•bar•bi•tone** (pen″to-bahr′bĭ-tōn) pentobarbital.

**pen•to•lin•i•um tar•trate** (pen″to-lin′e-əm) [MeSH: Pentolinium Tartrate] a ganglionic blocking agent used as an antihypertensive, administered orally, intramuscularly, and subcutaneously.

**pen•to•san** (pen′to-san) any member of the class of polysaccharides composed of pentose residues, e.g., arabans or xylans. They occur widely in plants, serving structural and storage functions.

**pen•to•sa•zone** (pen″tōs′ə-zōn) any osazone formed from a pentose.

**pen•tose** (pen′tōs) a monosaccharide containing five carbon atoms in a molecule.

**pen•tos•emia** (pen″to-se′me-ə) the presence of pentose in the blood.

**pen•to•side** (pen′to-sīd) any glycoside in which the sugar component is a pentose, the most important being the nucleosides.

**pen•to•stat•in** (pen″to-stat′in) [MeSH: Pentostatin] a drug used experimentally in the treatment of hairy cell leukemia refractory to interferon alfa. Called also *deoxycoformycin.*

**pen•tos•uria** (pen″to-su′re-ə) excretion of pentoses in the urine.
**alimentary p.,** urinary excretion of pentoses, probably xylose and arabinose, as a normal consequence of excessive ingestion of some fruits such as cherries, plums, and grapes, or their juices.
**essential p.,** a benign autosomal recessive deficiency of L-xylulose reductase resulting in urinary excretion of high levels of the pentose L-xylulose. Called also L-xylulosuria.

**pen•tos•uric** (pen″to-su′rik) affected with pentosuria.

**pen•to•syl** (pen′tə-səl) a radical of pentose.

**pen•to•syl•trans•fer•ase** (pen″tə-səl-trans′fər-ās) [EC 2.4.2] any member of a sub-subclass of enzymes of the transferase class that catalyze the transfer of a pentose group from one compound to another.

**Pen•to•thal** (pen′to-thol) trademark for preparations of thiopental sodium.

**pen•tox•ide** (pən-tok′sīd) an oxide containing five atoms of oxygen in a molecule.

**pen•tox•i•fyl•line** (pen″tok-sif′ə-lin) [MeSH: Pentoxifylline] a xanthine derivative that reduces blood viscosity and increases erythrocyte flexibility, microcirculatory flow, and tissue oxygenation; used for the symptomatic treatment of intermittent claudication, administered orally.

**pen•tri•ni•trol** (pen″trĭ-ni′trol) pentaerythritol trinitrate.

**Pen•tri•tol** (pen′trĭ-tol) trademark for a preparation of pentaerythritol tetranitrate.

**Pen•try•ate** (pen-tri′āt) trademark for preparations of pentaerythritol trinitrate.

**pen•tu•lose** (pen′tu-lōs) ketopentose.

**pent•yl•ene•tet•ra•zol** (pen″tə-lēn-tet′rə-zol) a synthetic camphor-like compound used to induce convulsions in the electroencephalographic evaluation of epilepsy and, formerly, in the treatment of mental disorders (see *convulsive therapy,* under *therapy*).

**pen•um•bra** (pə-num′brə) [L. *pēne* almost + *umbra*] 1. the area of a shadow where there is partial illumination; it surrounds the umbra. 2. in radiography, an area of blurring around the edges of a structure.
**ischemic p.,** an area of moderately ischemic brain tissue surrounding an area of more severe ischemia; blood flow to this area may be enhanced in order to prevent the spread of a cerebral infarction.

**Pen-Vee** (pen′ve) trademark for preparations of penicillin V.

**pe•ot•o•my** (pe-ot′ə-me) [Gr. *peos* penis + *-tomy*] penectomy.

**PEP** phospho*enol*pyruvate; preejection period.

**Pep•cid** (pep′sid) trademark for preparations of famotidine.

**pep•lo•mer** (pep′lo-mər) [*peplos* + Gr. *meros* part] one of the knob-like projections, generally composed of glycoproteins, on the surface of the lipoprotein envelope of many enveloped viruses.

**pep•los** (pep′lōs) [Gr. "robe"] envelope (def. 2).

**pep•per** (pep′ər) [L. *piper*] 1. black p. 2. any of the various plants

of the genus *Piper,* or their fruits. 3. any of various plants of the genus *Capsicum,* or their fruits.
**black p.,** 1. *Piper nigrum.* 2. the dried unripe fruit of *P. nigrum* and other plants of the same genus. It contains piperine, minor alkaloids, fat, protein, and resins; used chiefly as a spice, it also has diaphoretic, carminative, and gastric secretagogue properties.
**cayenne p.,** capsicum.
**Java p.,** *Piper cubeba.*
**red p.,** capsicum.
**tailed p.,** *Piper cubeba.*
**white p.,** the decorticated ripe fruit of the same plants as black pepper; having milder flavor than the black variety.

**pep·per·mint** (pep'ər-mint) 1. *Mentha piperita.* 2. [NF] the dried leaves and flowering tops of *M. piperita,* which have carminative, gastric stimulant, and counterirritant properties; used as an oil, spirit, or water extract as a flavored vehicle for drugs.

**pep·sic** (pep'sik) peptic.

**pep·sin** (pep'sin) any of several enzymes of the gastric juice that catalyze the hydrolysis of proteins to form polypeptides.
**p. A** [EC 3.4.23.1], an enzyme of the hydrolase class that catalyzes the hydrolysis of proteins with preferential cleavage at phenylalanine, tryptophan, tyrosine, and leucine residues. It is secreted by the gastric mucosa in the form of pepsinogen and has an optimum pH of 1.5 to 2.0.
**p. B** [EC 3.4.23.2], pepsin similar to pepsin A, formed from pig pepsinogen B. A related enzyme is found in human beings.
**p. C,** pepsin similar to pepsin A but highly active with hemoglobin as substrate. In EC nomenclature called *gastricsin.*

**pep·sin·ate** (pep'sin-āt) to treat or charge with pepsin.

**pep·sin·ia** (pep-sin'e-ə) the secretion of pepsin; it may be normal, excessive (hyperpepsinia), or deficient (hypopepsinia).

**pep·sin·if·er·ous** (pep″sin-if'ər-əs) [*pepsin* + *-ferous*] producing or secreting pepsin.

**pep·sin·o·gen** (pep-sin'ə-jən) [MeSH: Pepsinogen] a proenzyme secreted by chief cells, mucous neck cells, and pyloric gland cells, which is converted into pepsin in the presence of gastric acid or of pepsin itself.

**pep·sin·uria** (pep″sĭ-nu're-ə) the presence of pepsin in the urine; it may be associated with duodenal ulcer because of the increased volume of gastric secretion.

**pep·stat·in** (pep-stat'in) any of the pentapeptide pepsin inhibitors obtained from several species of *Streptomyces,* identified as pepstatin A, B, and C. The A component has been used in the treatment of gastric ulcer.

**Pep·tav·lon** (pep-tav'lon) trademark for a preparation of pentagastrin.

**pep·tic** (pep'tik) [Gr. *peptikos*] pertaining to pepsin or to digestion; related to the action of gastric juices.

**pep·ti·dase** (pep'tĭ-dās) [EC 3.4] any member of a subclass of enzymes of the hydrolase class that catalyze the hydrolysis of peptide bonds; it comprises the exopeptidases and endopeptidases. Called also *peptide hydrolase.*

**pep·tide** (pep'tīd) any member of a class of compounds of low molecular weight that yield two or more amino acids on hydrolysis. They are the constituent parts of proteins and are formed by loss of water from the $NH_2$ and COOH groups of adjacent amino acids. Peptides are known as di-, tri-, tetra- (etc.) peptides depending on the number of amino acids in the molecule. See also *polypeptide.*
**atrial natriuretic p. (ANP),** a hormone involved in natriuresis and the regulation of renal and cardiovascular homeostasis. It is generally 28 amino acids in length but varies somewhat; it is synthesized as a prohormone in the granules of the myocytes of the atrium and is released into the circulation in response to atrial dilatation or increased intravascular fluid volume. It causes natriuresis, diuresis, and renal vasodilation; reduces circulating concentrations of renin, aldosterone, and antidiuretic hormone; and thereby normalizes circulating blood pressure and volume. Called also *atriopeptin* and *atrial natriuretic factor.*
**C p.,** the connecting peptide chain that is removed when proinsulin is cleaved to form insulin.
**calcitonin gene–related p.,** a 37–amino acid polypeptide encoded by the calcitonin gene, widely distributed in the central and peripheral nervous systems and also occurring in the adrenal medulla and gastrointestinal tract; it is a potent vasodilator and a neurotransmitter.
**corticotropin-like intermediate lobe p. (CLIP),** a peptide with a sequence identical to the C-terminal 22 residues of adrenocorticotropic hormone, found in the intermediate lobe of the pituitary gland in lower animals; the function, if any, is unknown. It is also produced by human fetuses and may be a regulator of the fetal adrenal glands.
***N*-formylmethionyl p's,** di- and tripeptides in which the *N*-terminal amino acid residue is *N*-formylmethionine (fMet), which are produced by bacteria in protein synthesis (fMet initiates each polypeptide chain in prokaryotes but is often removed after translation) and which are chemotactic for granulocytes and macrophages but not lymphocytes.
**gastrin-releasing p.,** a 27–amino acid linear neuropeptide structurally and functionally related to bombesin; it mediates neural release of antral gastrin, causes bronchoconstriction and respiratory tract vasodilation, stimulates growth and mitogenesis of cells in culture, and may act as an excitatory neurotransmitter of enteric interneurons.
**opioid p.,** opioid (def. 2).
**parathyroid hormone–like p., parathyroid hormone–related p.,** a peptide somewhat homologous to parathyroid hormone at its amino terminus; it is secreted by certain types of cancer cells and causes hypercalcemia, apparently by acting on the parathyroid receptor, stimulating adenylate cyclase, increasing bone resorption, and inhibiting bone formation. Called also *parathyroid hormone–like protein.*
**signal p.,** signal sequence.
**vasoactive intestinal p. (VIP),** vasoactive intestinal polypeptide.

**pep·tide hy·dro·lase** (pep'tīd hi'dro-lās) peptidase.

**pep·ti·der·gic** (pep″tĭ-der'jik) 1. having an action resembling that of a peptide hormone. 2. activated by, characteristic of, or secreting a peptide hormone or a neuropeptide.

**pep·ti·do·gly·can** (pep″tĭ-do-gli'kən) [MeSH: Peptidoglycan] a high-molecular-weight polymer that forms the tough, rigid structure of bacterial cell walls. It is made up of three parts: (1) a backbone, composed of alternating *N*-acetylglucosamine and *N*-acetylmuramic acid; (2) a set of identical tetrapeptide side-chains attached to *N*-acetylmuramic acid; and (3) a set of identical peptide cross-bridges. The backbone is the same in all bacterial species; however, the tetrapeptide side-chains and the peptide cross-bridges vary from species to species.

**pep·ti·dyl-di·pep·ti·dase** (pep″tĭ-dəl″ di-pep'tĭ-dās) [EC 3.4.15] any member of a sub-subclass of enzymes of the hydrolase class that catalyze the cleavage of a dipeptide residue from a free C-terminal end of a peptide or polypeptide.

**pep·ti·dyl-di·pep·ti·dase A** (pep'tĭ-dəl di-pep'tĭ-dās) [EC 3.4.15.1] [MeSH: Peptidyl-Dipeptidase A] an enzyme of the hydrolase class that catalyzes the cleavage of a dipeptide from the C-terminal end of an oligopeptide; it is a zinc protein found on the luminal surface of vascular endothelial cells in the lungs and other tissues. When catalyzing the cleavage of angiotensin I to form the activated angiotensin II, it is also called *angiotensin-converting enzyme;* when catalyzing the cleavage and inactivation of kinins, it is also called *kininase II.* Called also *dipeptidyl carboxypeptidase I.*

**pep·ti·za·tion** (pep″tĭ-za'shən) increase in the degree of dispersion of a colloid solution; the liquefaction of a colloid gel to form a sol.

**Pep·to·coc·ca·ceae** (pep″to-kok-a'se-e) [Gr. *pepton* digestion + *kokkus* berry] [MeSH: Peptococcaceae] a family of anaerobic, nonmotile, usually gram-positive bacteria, made up of spherical cells occurring singly or in pairs, tetrads, chains, or irregular masses. They are found in the mouth and intestinal and respiratory tracts of man and other animals, in the human female urogenital tract, and in soil. The family includes the genera *Peptococcus, Peptostreptococcus,* and *Ruminococcus.*

**Pep·to·coc·cus** (pep″to-kok'əs) [Gr. *pepton* digestion + *kokkus* berry] [MeSH: Peptococcus] a genus of gram-positive, anaerobic, coccoid bacteria of the family Peptococcaceae, occurring singly or in pairs, tetrads, or irregular masses, which are chemo-organotrophic and capable of fermenting protein decomposition products. It is part of the normal flora of the human mouth, upper respiratory tract, and large intestine, sometimes causes human infections of soft tissues and bacteremias, and is also found in other animals and soil.
**P. anaero'bius,** a microaerophilic or obligate anaerobe found in the appendix and the female genital tract, and in cystitis and draining sinus. Called also *Diplococcus magnus.*
**P. asaccharoly'ticus,** a species that does not ferment sugars and is found in the human large intestine, oral cavity, pleura, uterus, and vagina and in cows with mastitis.
**P. constella'tus,** a microaerophilic or obligate anaerobe found in purulent pleurisy and in the tonsils, appendix, nose, throat, gums, and infrequently the skin and vagina. Called also *Diplococcus constellatus.*
**P. mag'nus,** a species with large (1–2 $\mu$m in diameter) cells that is recovered most frequently from clinical specimens. It is a cause of septic arthritis and soft tissue infections.

**pep·to·gen·ic** (pep″to-jen'ik) [Gr. *peptein* to digest + *-genic*] 1. producing pepsin or peptones. 2. promoting digestion.

**pep·tog·e·nous** (pep-toj′ə-nəs) peptogenic.

**pep·tol·y·sis** (pep-tol′ĭ-sis) [*peptone* + *-lysis*] the hydrolysis of peptones.

**pep·to·lyt·ic** (pep″to-lit′ik) denoting an agent or process that hydrolyzes peptones.

**pep·tone** (pep′tōn) [Gr. *pepton* digesting] a derived protein, or a mixture of cleavage products produced by the partial hydrolysis of a native protein either by an acid or by an enzyme. Peptones are readily soluble in water, and are not precipitatable by heat, by alkalis, or by saturation with ammonium sulfate.

**pep·ton·ic** (pep-ton′ik) pertaining to or containing peptone.

**pep·to·nize** (pep′to-nīz) to convert a protein into peptone by the action of an acid or enzyme.

**pep·ton·uria** (pep″to-nu′re-ə) the presence of peptones in the urine.
**enterogenous p.,** that which is due to disease of the intestine.
**hepatogenous p.,** that which is due to disease of the liver.
**nephrogenic p.,** that which is due to disease of the kidney.
**puerperal p.,** that which occurs during the puerperium.
**pyogenic p.,** that which is associated with a suppurative process.

**Pep·to·strep·to·coc·cus** (pep″to-strep″to-kok′əs) [Gr. *pepton* digestion + *streptos* twisted + *kokkos* berry] [MeSH: Peptostreptococcus] a genus of gram-positive, coccoid bacteria of the family Peptococcaceae, made up of obligately anaerobic, chemo-organotrophic cells. Part of the normal human flora of the mouth, upper respiratory tract, and large intestine, they are also opportunistic pathogens causing soft tissue infections and bacteremias.
**P. anaero′bius,** a species that ferments glucose only, isolated in humans from cases of gangrene, infected wounds, puerperal fever, appendicitis, pleurisy, paranasal sinusitis, and osteomyelitis, and from the intestinal tract, oral cavity, and genital secretions. Called also *Streptococcus foetidus.*
**P. lanceola′tus,** a species having large ovoid cells with pointed ends, occurring in short chains and in pairs, which has been isolated from humans in cases of diarrhea, dental infection, vulvovaginitis, and abscesses. Called also *Streptococcus lanceolatus.*
**P. mi′cros,** a nonfermentative species having small spheroid cells, isolated from cases of purulent pleurisy, puerperal sepsis, appendicitis, brain and dental abscesses, and actinomycosis. Called also *Streptococcus micros.*
**P. par′vulus,** a species with small spherical cells occurring in pairs and short chains, isolated from the human respiratory tract and oral cavity.
**P. produc′tus,** a species with spherical cells, occurring in chains, isolated from cases of gangrene and pelvic abscesses and from blood and urine.

**pep·to·tox·in** (pep″to-tok′sin) any toxin or poisonous base developed from a peptone; also a poisonous alkaloid or ptomaine occurring in certain peptones and putrefying proteins.

**per-** [L. *per* through] 1. a prefix meaning throughout in space or time, or completely or extremely. 2. a prefix used in chemical terms to denote a large amount or to designate combination of an element in its highest valence.

**per·a·ceph·a·lus** (per″ə-sef′ə-ləs) [*per-* + *acephalus*] a fetus with neither head nor upper limbs, and with a defective thorax.

**per·ac·e·tate** (per-as′ə-tāt) a salt or derivative of peracetic acid.

**per·ace·tic ac·id** (per″ə-se′tik) [MeSH: Peracetic Acid] peroxyacetic acid, $CH_3COOOH$, a strong oxidizing agent.

**per·ac·id** (per-as′id) an acid containing more than the usual quantity of oxygen.

**per·acid·i·ty** (per″ə-sid′ĭ-te) excessive acidity.

**per·acute** (per″ə-kūt′) [L. *peracutus*] excessively acute or sharp.

**Per·an·dren** (pər-an′drən) trademark for a preparation of testosterone.

**per anum** (pər a′nəm) [L.] through the anus.

**per·ar·tic·u·la·tion** (per″ahr-tik″u-la′shən) [*per-* + *articulation*] diarthrosis.

**Per·a·zil** (per′ə-zil) trademark for preparations of chlorcyclizine hydrochloride.

**per·cen·tile** (pər-sen′tīl) [*per cent* + *-ile* (by analogy with *quartile, quintile,* etc.)] any one of the 99 values that divide the range of a probability distribution or sample into 100 intervals of equal probability or frequency, e.g., 45 per cent of a population scores below the 45th percentile.

**per·cept** (per′sept) 1. something perceived. 2. the mental image of an object in space perceived by the senses.

**per·cep·tion** (pər-sep′shən) [L. *percipere* to take in completely] [MeSH: Perception] the conscious mental registration of a sensory stimulus.
**depth p.,** the proper recognition of depth or the relative distances to different objects in space.
**extrasensory p. (ESP),** knowledge of, or response to, an external thought or objective event by means other than the senses.
**stereognostic p.,** stereognosis.

**per·cep·tive** (pər-sep′tiv) 1. pertaining to perception. 2. having keen perception.

**per·cep·tiv·i·ty** (per″sep-tiv′ĭ-te) ability to receive sense impressions.

**per·cep·to·ri·um** (per″sep-tor′e-əm) sensorium.

**per·chlo·rate** (pər-klo′rāt) a salt or ester of perchloric acid.

**per·chlor·ic ac·id** (pər-klor′ik) [MeSH: Perchloric Acid] a strong mineral acid and oxidizing agent, $HClO_4$.

**per·chlo·ride** (pər-klor′īd) a chloride that contains more chlorine than the ordinary chloride; an organic compound in which all the hydrogen atoms are substituted by chlorine, as in perchloroethylene (tetrachloroethylene), $C_2Cl_4$.

**per·chlor·meth·ane** (per″klor-meth′ān) carbon tetrachloride.

**per·chlor·meth·yl·for·mate** (per″klor-meth″əl-for′māt) diphosgene.

**per·chlor·o·eth·y·lene** (pər-klor″o-eth′ə-lēn) tetrachloroethylene.

**per·cip·i·ent** (pər-sip′e-ənt) 1. pertaining to perception. 2. an individual who perceives or is capable of perception.

**Per·co·cet** (pər′ko-set) trademark for a preparation of oxycodone hydrochloride and acetaminophen.

**Per·co·dan** (pər′ko-dan) trademark for a preparation of oxycodone hydrochloride and aspirin.

**per·co·late** (per′ko-lāt) [L. *percolare*] 1. to strain; to submit to percolation. 2. to trickle slowly through a substance. 3. a liquid that has been submitted to percolation.

**per·co·la·tion** (per″kə-la′shən) [L. *percolatio*] the extraction of the soluble parts of a drug by causing a liquid solvent to flow slowly through it.

**per·co·la·tor** (per′kə-la″tər) a vessel used in percolating drugs.

**Per·coll** (per′col) trademark for a colloidal suspension of silica used in density gradient centrifugation.

**per con·tig·u·um** (pər kon-tig′u-əm) [L.] in contiguity: arranged in such a way that the edges touch.

**per con·tin·u·um** (pər kon-tin′u-əm) [L.] in continuity: without separation or break.

**Per·cor·ten** (pər-kor′tən) trademark for preparations of desoxycorticosterone.

**per·cuss** (pər-kus′) [L. *percutere*] to subject to percussion.

**per·cus·si·ble** (pər-kus′ĭ-bəl) discoverable on percussion.

**per·cus·sion** (pər-kŭ′shən) [L. *percussio*] [MeSH: Percussion] 1. the act of striking a part with short, sharp blows as an aid in diagnosing the condition of the underlying parts by the sound obtained. 2. a method of massage; see *tapotement.*
**auscultatory p.,** auscultation, usually by stethoscope, of the sound produced by percussion.
**bimanual p.,** the usual manner of percussion in which the middle finger of the left hand is placed against the body wall and is struck a quick blow with the end of the bent right middle finger.
**comparative p.,** percussion of two or more areas in order to compare the sounds obtained.
**deep p.,** percussion in which a firm blow is struck in order to obtain a note from a deep-seated tissue.

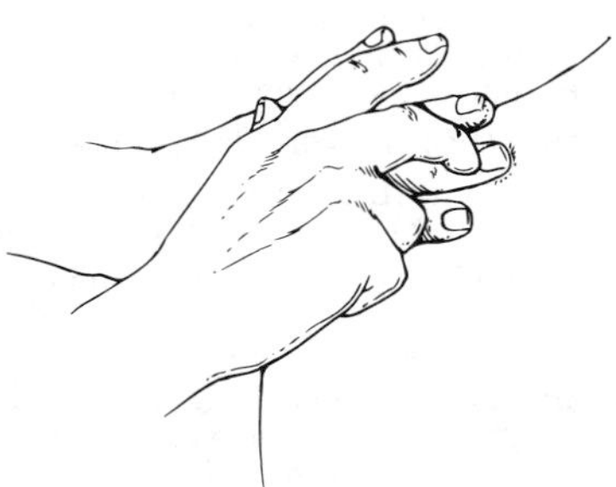

Bimanual percussion.

**direct p.,** immediate p.
**drop p., drop stroke p.,** instrumental percussion in which the plexor is allowed to fall by its own weight on to the pleximeter, the elements considered in the examination being the sound heard, the vibrations felt in the handle of the plexor, and the rebound of the plexor seen. Called also *Lerch's p.*
**finger p.,** that in which the fingers of one hand are used as a plexor, and those of the other as a pleximeter.
**fist p.,** percussion in which the fist is brought down with a moderate thump over the area to be tested.
**Goldscheider's p.,** 1. threshold p. 2. orthopercussion.
**immediate p.,** that in which no pleximeter is used.
**instrumental p.,** that in which a plexor or hammer is used.
**Korányi's p.,** see under *auscultation.*
**Lerch's p.,** drop p.
**mediate p.,** that in which a pleximeter is employed.
**Murphy's p.,** piano p.
**palpatory p.,** a combination of palpation and percussion, affording tactile rather than auditory impressions.
**paradoxical p.,** resonance of the chest combined with abundant rales as in acute edema of the lungs.
**pencil p.,** Plesch's p.
**piano p.,** percussion by striking the body by the four fingers one after the other, beginning with the little finger; called also *Murphy's p.*
**Plesch's p.,** percussion within the intercostal spaces to avoid setting the ribs into vibration, the pleximeter finger with the first interphalangeal joint flexed at a right angle.
**pleximetric p.,** mediate p.
**respiratory p.,** percussion during respiration so as to bring out the difference in the percussion notes of inspiration and expiration.
**slapping p.,** percussion made by a slapping blow: used in comparing the resonance.
**strip p.,** percussion which starts from above and progresses downward, thus covering a "strip" of the chest wall.
**tangential p.,** percussion with the pleximeter placed vertically on the body, the strokes being applied to the pleximeter in a direction parallel with the surface of the skin.
**threshold p.,** percussion performed by tapping lightly with the finger upon a glass rod pleximeter, one end of which, fitted with a rubber cap, rests upon an intercostal space, the rod being held at an angle to the surface of the thorax and parallel to the borders of the organ to be delimited. This method confines the percussion vibrations to a very restricted area. Called also *Goldscheider's p.*
**topographic p.,** the demarcation and outlining of a dull area by percussion to determine the boundaries of organs or parts of organs.

**per·cus·sor** (pər-kus'ər) a vibrator that produces relatively coarse movements.

**per·cu·ta·ne·ous** (per″ku-ta'ne-əs) [*per-* + *cutaneous*] performed through the skin, as injection of radiopaque material in radiological examination, or the removal of tissue for biopsy accomplished by a needle. Cf. *transdermal.*

**per cu·tem** (pər ku'təm) [L.] through the skin; see *percutaneous* and *transdermal.*

**per·cu·teur** (per″ku-tər') [Fr.] an instrument for therapeutic or diagnostic percussion.

**per·en·ceph·a·ly** (per″ən-sef'ə-le) [Gr. *pēra* pouch + *enkephalos* brain] porencephalia.

**per·en·ni·al** (pə-ren'e-əl) [L. *perennis,* from *per* through + *annus* year] lasting through the year or for several years.

**Pe·rey·ra procedure** (pə-ra'rah) [Armand Joseph *Pereyra,* American obstetrician and gynecologist, born 1904] see under *procedure.*

**Pé·rez's sign** (pa'-rāths) [Jorjen (George) Victor *Pérez,* Spanish physician, 1851–1920] see under *sign.*

**per·fect** (pər'fəkt) said of a fungus that can reproduce sexually (with sexual spores). Cf. *imperfect.*

**per·fec·tion·ism** (pər-fek'shən-iz-əm) the setting for oneself or others of a standard of flawless work or performance, or at least of one that is higher than the situation requires.

**per·fil·con A** (pər-fil'kon) a hydrophilic contact lens material.

**per·fla·tion** (pər-fla'shən) [L. *perflatio*] the act of blowing air into a space in order to force out secretions or other substances.

**per·flu·bron** (pər-floo'bron) [USP] a brominated fluorocarbon used as a contrast agent in magnetic resonance imaging of the gastrointestinal tract; administered orally.

**per·flu·o·ro·chem·i·cal** (pər-floor″o-kem'ĭ-kəl) an inert chemical substance with a high oxygen-carrying capacity; some can be emulsified with surfactants and transfused for temporary transport of oxygen in the blood. See also *Fluosol-DC.*

**per·fo·rans** (per'fə-ranz) pl. *perforan'tes* [L.] penetrating, perforating; a term applied to various muscles, nerves, arteries, and veins that perforate other structures.
**p. ma'nus,** musculus flexor digitorum profundus.

**per·fo·rat·ed** (per'fə-rāt″əd) [L. *perforatus*] pierced with holes.

**per·fo·ra·tion** (per″fə-ra'shən) [L. *perforare* to pierce through] 1. the act of boring or piercing through a part. 2. a hole made through a part or substance.
**Bezold's p.,** perforation of the inner surface of the mastoid bone; see also *Bezold's abscess.*
**mechanical p.,** an artificial opening or hole made by boring, piercing, or cutting through a structure or surface, such as the root of a tooth.
**pathologic p.,** an opening or hole produced in a tissue surface or structure by a pathologic process, such as internal resorption of a tooth.
**root p.,** perforation of the root of a tooth, occurring either iatrogenically during treatment or pathologically from internal resorption.

**per·fo·ra·tor** (per'fə-ra″tor) an instrument for piercing the bones, and especially for perforating the fetal head.

**per·fo·ra·to·ri·um** (per″fə-rə-to're-əm) acrosome.

**per·for·in** (pər'fə-rin) a protein expressed by cytotoxic lymphocytes and forming a transmembrane pore at the site of target cell lysis.

**per·for·mance** (pər-for'məns) 1. the execution of an action. 2. the act or process of functioning, sometimes measured by a performance scale or a performance test.
**ventricular p.,** the execution of the pumping function of the ventricles, depending on preload, afterload, cardiac contractility, and heart rate; it is measured by cardiac output or work and expressed on a per stroke or per minute basis.

**per·fri·ca·tion** (per″frĭ-ka'shən) [L. *perfricare* to rub] rubbing with an ointment or embrocation.

**per·frig·er·a·tion** (pər-frij″ər-a'shən) [*per-* + L. *frigere* to be cold] frostbite.

**per·fu·sate** (pər-fu'zāt) a liquid that has been passed over or through the vessels of an organ or tissue.

**per·fuse** (pər-fūz') to pour over or through.

**per·fu·sion** (pər-fu'zhən) [MeSH: Perfusion] 1. the act of pouring over or through, especially the passage of a fluid through the vessels of a specific organ. 2. a liquid poured over or through an organ or tissue.
**isolation-p.,** see under *technique.*
**luxury p.,** abnormally increased flow of blood to an area of the brain, leading to swelling; causes include trauma, nearby cerebral infarction, and epileptogenic focus.
**regional p.,** administration of a therapeutic agent directly to the region of the body that contains disease, commonly done by injecting the agent into a large artery supplying the region.

**per·fu·sion·ist** (pər-fu'zhən-ist) a technologist who operates the heart-lung machine during cardiopulmonary bypass.

**per·go·lide mes·y·late** (per'go-līd mes'ĭ-lāt) a long-acting ergot derivative with dopaminergic properties.

**per·hex·i·line mal·e·ate** (pər-hek'sĭ-lēn) a coronary vasodilator used in the prophylaxis of angina of effort and has been used to control certain cardiac arrhythmias.

**peri-** [Gr. *peri* around] a prefix meaning near or around.

**peri·ac·i·nal** (per″e-as'ĭ-nəl) [*peri-* + *acinus*] situated around an acinus.

**peri·ac·i·nous** (per″e-as'ĭ-nəs) around an acinus.

**Per·i·ac·tin** (per″e-ak'tin) trademark for preparations of cyproheptadine hydrochloride.

**peri·ad·e·ni·tis** (per″e-ad″ə-ni'tis) [*peri-* + *aden-* + *-itis*] inflammation of the tissues around a gland.
**p. muco'sa necro'tica recur'rens,** a recurrent disease of the mucous membranes of unknown etiology, generally considered to be a severe form of recurrent aphthous stomatitis, characterized by deep crateriform ulcers with inflamed borders that leave scars after healing. It usually involves the mucosa of the lips, cheeks, tongue, palate, and anterior tonsillar pillars, but the pharynx, larynx, and genitalia may also be affected. Called also *Mikulicz's aphthae, recurring scarring aphthae,* and *Sutton's disease.*

**peri·ad·ven·ti·tial** (per″e-ad″vən-tĭ'shəl) outside the adventitia.

**peri·am·pul·lary** (per″e-am'pu-lar″e) situated around an ampulla, as around the hepatopancreatic ampulla.

**peri·anal** (per″e-a'nəl) [*peri-* + *anal*] near or around the anus; cf. *circumanal.*

**peri·an·gi·itis** (per″e-an″je-i'tis) [*peri-* + *angiitis*] inflammation of the tissue surrounding a blood or lymph vessel. Called also *perivasculitis.*

**peri·an·gio·cho·li·tis** (per″e-an″je-o-ko-li′tis) pericholangitis.

**peri·an·gi·o·ma** (per″e-an-je-o′mə) [*peri-* + *angi-* + *-oma*] a tumor that surrounds a blood vessel.

**peri·anth** (per′e-anth) [*peri-* + Gr. *anthos* flower] the floral envelope, including the calyx and corolla.

**peri·aor·tic** (per″e-a-or′tik) around the aorta.

**peri·aor·ti·tis** (per″e-a″or-ti′tis) inflammation of the tissues around the aorta.

**peri·apex** (per″e-a′peks) the tissue that surrounds the root apex of a tooth (the periodontal ligament and alveolar bone).

**peri·ap·i·cal** (per″e-ap′ĭ-kəl) [*peri-* + *apic-* + *-al*[1]] situated at or surrounding the apex of a tooth.

**peri·ap·pen·di·ci·tis** (per″e-ə-pen″dĭ-si′tis) [*peri-* + *appendic-* + *-itis*] inflammation of the tissues around the vermiform appendix.
**p. decidua′lis,** a condition in tubal pregnancy in which, on account of adhesions between the appendix and the fallopian tube, decidual cells are present on the peritoneum of the appendix.

**peri·ap·pen·dic·u·lar** (per″e-ap″ən-dik′u-lər) around the vermiform appendix.

**peri·apt** (per′e-apt) [Gr. *periapton* amulet] a substance worn in the belief that it wards off disease.

**peri·aq·ue·duc·tal** (per″e-ak″wĭ-duk′təl) around an aqueduct.

**peri·ar·te·ri·al** (per″e-ahr-tēr′e-əl) around an artery.

**peri·ar·te·ri·tis** (per″e-ahr″tə-ri′tis) [*peri-* + *arteritis*] inflammation of the external coats of an artery and of the tissues around the artery.
**p. gummo′sa,** accumulation of gummas on the blood vessels in syphilis.
**p. nodo′sa,** 1. polyarteritis nodosa. 2. a group comprising classic polyarteritis nodosa, allergic granulomatous angiitis, and many systemic necrotizing vasculitides with clinicopathologic characteristics overlapping the two former disorders.
**syphilitic p.,** p. gummosa.

**peri·ar·thric** (per″e-ahr′thrik) [*peri-* + Gr. *arthron* joint] around a joint.

**peri·ar·thri·tis** (per″e-ahr-thri′tis) [MeSH: Periarthritis] inflammation of the tissues around a joint.
**p. of shoulder,** that occurring in the structures around the shoulder joint, including tendinitis, adhesive capsulitis, and various types of bursitis.

**peri·ar·tic·u·lar** (per″e-ahr-tik′u-lər) [*peri-* + *articular*] situated around a joint.

**peri·atri·al** (per″e-a′tre-əl) around the atrium of the heart.

**peri·au·ric·u·lar** (per″e-aw-rik′u-lər) around the concha of the ear.

**peri·ax·i·al** (per″e-ak′se-əl) [*peri-* + *axial*] situated around an axis.

**peri·ax·il·lary** (per″e-ak′sĭ-lar″e) situated or occurring around the axilla.

**peri·ax·o·nal** (per″e-ak′sə-nəl) [*peri-* + *axonal*] occurring around an axon.

**peri·blast** (per′ĭ-blast) [*peri-* + *-blast*] the portion of the blastoderm of telolecithal eggs the cells of which lack complete cell membranes.

**peri·bron·chi·al** (per″ĭ-brong′ke-əl) situated around a bronchus.

**peri·bron·chi·o·lar** (per″ĭ-brong-ki′o-lər) situated around the bronchioles.

**peri·bron·chio·li·tis** (per″ĭ-brong″ke-o-li′tis) inflammation of the tissues around the bronchioles.

**peri·bron·chi·tis** (per″ĭ-brong-ki′tis) a form of bronchitis consisting of inflammation and thickening of the peribronchial tissue.

**peri·bul·bar** (per″ĭ-bul′bər) surrounding the bulb of the eye.

**peri·bur·sal** (per″ĭ-bur′səl) surrounding a bursa.

**peri·cal·i·ce·al** (per″ĭ-kal″ĭ-se′əl) situated near to or around a renal calix.

**peri·cal·lo·sal** (per″ĭ-kə-lo′səl) situated around the corpus callosum.

**peri·cal·y·ce·al** (per″ĭ-kal″ĭ-se′əl) pericaliceal.

**peri·can·a·lic·u·lar** (per″ĭ-kan″ə-lik′u-lər) occurring around a canaliculus or canaliculi.

**peri·cap·il·lary** (per″ĭ-kap′ĭ-lar″e) around a capillary.

**peri·cap·su·lar** (per″ĭ-kap′su-lər) surrounding a capsule.

**peri·car·dec·to·my** (per″ĭ-kahr-dek′tə-me) pericardiectomy.

**peri·car·di·al** (per″ĭ-kahr′de-əl) pertaining to the pericardium.

**peri·car·di·cen·te·sis** (per″ĭ-kahr″de-sən-te′sis) pericardiocentesis.

**peri·car·di·ec·to·my** (per″ĭ-kahr″de-ek′tə-me) [*pericardium* + *-ectomy*] [MeSH: Pericardiectomy] excision of the pericardium.

**peri·car·dio·cen·te·sis** (per″ĭ-kahr″de-o-sən-te′sis) [*pericardium* + *-centesis*] surgical puncture of the pericardial cavity for the aspiration of fluid.

**peri·car·di·ol·y·sis** (per″ĭ-kahr″de-ol′ĭ-sis) [*pericardium* + *-lysis*] the operation of freeing adhesions between the visceral and parietal pericardium or between the pericardium and surrounding tissues or organs.

**peri·car·dio·me·di·as·ti·ni·tis** (per″ĭ-kahr″de-o-me″de-as-tĭ-ni′tis) [*pericardium* + *mediastinitis*] pericarditis with mediastinitis; inflammation of the pericardium and mediastinum.

**peri·car·dio·phren·ic** (per″ĭ-kahr″de-o-fren′ik) pertaining to the pericardium and the diaphragm.

**peri·car·dio·pleu·ral** (per″ĭ-kahr″de-o-ploor′əl) pertaining to the pericardium and the pleura.

**peri·car·di·or·rha·phy** (per″ĭ-kahr″de-or′ə-fe) [*pericardium* + *-rrhaphy*] the operation of suturing a wound in the pericardium.

**peri·car·di·os·co·py** (per″ĭ-kahr″de-os′ko-pe) [*pericardium* + *-scopy*] visualization of the parietal pericardium and epicardium using a flexible fiberoptic bronchoscope or endoscope.

**peri·car·di·os·to·my** (per″ĭ-kahr″de-os′tə-me) [*pericardium* + *-ostomy*] the creation of an opening into the pericardium, usually for the drainage of effusions.

**peri·car·di·ot·o·my** (per″ĭ-kahr″de-ot′ə-me) [*pericardium* + *-tomy*] surgical incision of the pericardium.

**peri·car·dit·ic** (per″ĭ-kahr-dit′ik) pertaining to pericarditis.

**peri·car·di·tis** (per″ĭ-kahr-di′tis) [*pericardium* + *-itis*] [MeSH: Pericarditis] inflammation of the pericardium.
**acute benign p.,** idiopathic p.
**acute idiopathic p., acute nonspecific p.,** idiopathic p.
**adhesive p.,** a condition resulting from the presence of dense fibrous tissue between the parietal and visceral layers of the pericardium. There may be complete obliteration of the pericardial cavity, or there may be adhesions extending from the pericardium to the mediastinum (mediastinopericarditis), diaphragm, and chest wall (accretio cordis, accretio pericardii).
**amebic p.,** pericarditis occurring as a result of rupture of an amebic abscess of the liver through the diaphragm.
**bacterial p.,** pericarditis produced by bacterial infection, particularly by staphylococci or gram-negative bacilli. See also *purulent p.*
**bread-and-butter p.,** fibrinous pericarditis in which the fibrinous exudate forms a thick shaggy coat over the pericardium, with adhesions between the layers.
**carcinomatous p.,** that which is associated with malignant disease of the pericardium.
**cholesterol p.,** pericarditis characterized by cholesterol-laden effusion, resulting from deposition of cholesterol crystals and subsequent inflammatory response including infiltration of the pericardium by lymphocytes, plasma cells, macrophages, and giant cells.
**chronic constrictive p., constrictive p.,** a chronic form in which a fibrotic, thickened, adherent pericardium restricts diastolic filling and cardiac output. It is usually a consequence of a series of events beginning with an acute episode in which fibrin and sometimes calcium are deposited on the pericardial surface, followed by fibrotic scarring and thickening of the pericardium and obliteration of the pericardial space.
**dry p.,** pericarditis not associated with effusion.
**p. with effusion,** pericarditis associated with the collection of a serous or purulent exudate in the pericardial cavity.
**effusive constrictive p.,** a form characterized by pericardial effusion in the presence of visceral pericardial constriction, manifest as continued elevation of right atrial pressure after pericardiocentesis; it often leads to chronic constrictive pericarditis.
**external p.,** that which chiefly affects the outer surface of the pericardium.
**fibrinous p., fibrous p.,** pericarditis characterized by a fibrinous exudate, sometimes accompanied by a small amount of serous effusion; it is usually manifest as a pericardial friction rub. It often progresses to adhesive pericarditis. Cf. *serofibrinous p.*
**fungal p.,** that due to fungal infection, usually histoplasmosis or coccidioidomycosis.
**hemorrhagic p.,** that in which the exudate is bloody as well as serous, serofibrinous, or purulent; causes include tuberculosis, uremia, severe acute infections, and neoplasia.
**idiopathic p.,** an acute serofibrinous pericarditis of unknown cause; recurrent attacks are not unusual. Called also *acute benign p.*
**localized p.,** a term usually denoting chronic pericarditis with thickened white or milky epicardial areas.
**neoplastic p.,** pericarditis associated with primary or secondary neoplastic infiltration of the pericardium, often characterized by serous or bloody pericardial effusion, constriction, arrhythmia, or tamponade.

**p. obli'terans, obliterating p.,** an adhesive pericarditis which leads to the obliteration of the pericardial cavity.
**postcardiotomy p.,** a form occurring as a complication following cardiac surgery, characterized by effusion and rarely by constriction.
**postinfarction p.,** an acute form developing within one week after myocardial infarction, manifested as pericardial pain, dyspnea, and a pericardial rub.
**post-irradiation p.,** pericardial inflammation, acute or chronic, resulting from high dose radiotherapy, often beginning as exudative effusion with fibrin deposits and sometimes progressing to chronic pericardial effusion or constrictive pericarditis. It may present decades after radiation exposure.
**purulent p.,** a form characterized by pus formation, usually due to bacterial infection, and less often to fungal or viral infection, which may be spread from neighboring tissues, through the blood or lymphatic systems, or via direct implantation in wounds. It is characterized by fibrinopurulent or purulent exudates and often results in constrictive pericarditis and tamponade.
**radiation p.,** post-irradiation p.
**rheumatic p.,** the form associated with active rheumatic heart disease, characterized by a fibrinous, serofibrinous, or purulent exudate, sparse to densely shaggy fibrin deposits, chest pain, and pericardial friction rub.
**serofibrinous p.,** pericarditis characterized by a fibrinous exudate accompanied by substantial serous effusion, otherwise resembling fibrinous pericarditis.
**serous p.,** pericarditis characterized by serous effusion, usually produced by a nonbacterial inflammation.
**p. sic'ca,** acute fibrinous pericarditis without effusion.
**suppurative p.,** purulent p.
**traumatic p.,** 1. pericarditis caused by penetrating or nonpenetrating injury to the pericardium, such as that due to bullet wounds, improper catheter placement, or radiation; it is characterized by pericardial pain and friction and may lead to hemopericardium or tamponade. 2. injury to the pericardium of a cow that has ingested metallic debris or some other hard foreign object; the object migrates from the reticulum through the diaphragm and lodges against the pericardium, causing inflammation. Exudated fluid collects in the pericardial sac until it finally interferes with the heart's pumping efficiency. Called also *hardware disease* and *traumatic reticulopericarditis.*
**tuberculous p.,** a variety caused by tuberculous disease, characterized by effusion of fluid containing fibrin, blood, and sometimes caseous debris, thick shaggy deposits of fibrin, pericardial friction rub, and adhesion of the pericardial layers; it often results in chronic constrictive pericarditis.
**uremic p.,** pericarditis occurring as a complication of uremia; it is characterized by shaggy, vascular, fibrinous exudate on the visceral and parietal pericardial surfaces.
**viral p.,** pericarditis associated with viral infection, usually by coxsackievirus or echovirus, characterized by pericardial friction rub, substantial effusion, and fibrin deposition; it appears to be the cause of at least some cases of idiopathic pericarditis.

**peri·car·di·um** (per″ĭ-kahr'de-əm) [L.; *peri-* + Gr. *kardia* heart] [MeSH: Pericardium] 1. [TA] the fibroserous sac that surrounds the heart and the roots of the great vessels, comprising an external layer of fibrous tissue *(p. fibrosum)* and an inner serous layer *(p. serosum).* The base of the pericardium is attached to the central tendon of the diaphragm. 2. pericardial sinus.
**adherent p.,** a pericardium that is abnormally connected with the heart by dense fibrous tissue, as in adhesive pericarditis.
**bread-and-butter p.,** a pericardium having a thick fibrinous deposit on its surfaces.
**calcified p.,** a pericardium containing deposits of lime salts.

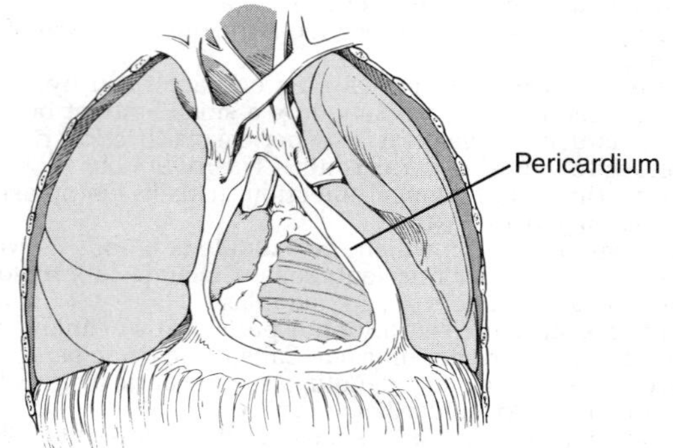

Anterior cutaway view of the pericardium surrounding the heart.

**p. fibro'sum** [TA], **fibrous p.,** the external layer of the pericardium, consisting of fibrous tissue.
**parietal p.,** lamina parietalis pericardii serosi.
**p. sero'sum** [TA], **serous p.,** the inner serous portion of the pericardium consisting of two layers, the *lamina parietalis pericardii serosi,* which is apposed to the fibrous pericardium, and the *lamina visceralis pericardii serosi,* or *epicardium,* which is reflected onto the roots of the great vessels and the heart. The space between the two layers is the *cavitas pericardialis.*
**shaggy p.,** a pericardium coated with a roughened layer of fibrinous exudate.
**visceral p.,** lamina visceralis pericardii serosi.

**peri·car·dot·o·my** (per″ĭ-kahr-dot'ə-me) pericardiotomy.

**peri·carp** (per'ĭ-kahrp″) [*peri-* + *carp*] the seed vessel or ripened ovary of a flower.

**peri·cary·on** (per″ĭ-kar'e-on) perikaryon.

**peri·ce·cal** (per″ĭ-se'kəl) surrounding the cecum.

**peri·ce·ci·tis** (per″ĭ-sə-si'tis) inflammation of the tissues around the cecum.

**peri·cel·lu·lar** (per″ĭ-sel'u-lər) [*peri-* + *cellular*] surrounding a cell.

**peri·ce·men·tal** (per″ĭ-se-men'təl) pertaining to the pericementum (periodontal ligament).

**peri·ce·men·ti·tis** (per″ĭ-se″men-ti'tis) inflammation of the pericementum (periodontal ligament). See *periodontitis.*
**apical p.,** apical abscess.
**chronic suppurative p.,** marginal periodontitis.

**peri·ce·men·tum** (per″ĭ-se-men'təm) [*peri-* + *cementum*] the periodontal ligament.

**peri·cen·tral** (per″ĭ-sen'trəl) surrounding a center.

**peri·cen·tri·o·lar** (per″ĭ-sen″tre-o'lər) situated around a centriole.

**peri·ce·phal·ic** (per″ĭ-sə-fal'ik) surrounding the head.

**peri·cho·lan·gi·tis** (per″ĭ-ko″lan-ji'tis) [*peri-* + *cholangi-* + *-itis*] inflammation of the tissues that surround the bile ducts.

**peri·cho·le·cys·ti·tis** (per″ĭ-ko″le-sis-ti'tis) inflammation of the tissues around the gallbladder.
**gaseous p.,** emphysematous cholecystitis.

**peri·chon·dri·al** (per″ĭ-kon'dre-əl) pertaining to or composed of perichondrium.

**peri·chon·dri·tis** (per″ĭ-kon-dri'tis) inflammation of the perichondrium.

**peri·chon·dri·um** (per″ĭ-kon'dre-əm) [*peri-* + Gr. *chondros* cartilage] [TA] the layer of dense fibrous connective tissue which invests all cartilage except the articular cartilage of synovial joints.

**peri·chon·dro·ma** (per″ĭ-kon-dro'mə) [*perichondrium* + *-oma*] a tumor arising from the perichondrium.

**peri·chord** (per'ĭ-kord) the investing sheath of the notochord.

**peri·chor·dal** (per″ĭ-kor'dəl) [*peri-* + *chordal*] situated around the notochord.

**peri·cho·ri·oi·dal** (per″ĭ-kor″e-oi'dəl) perichoroidal.

**peri·cho·roi·dal** (per″ĭ-kor-oi'dəl) surrounding the choroid coat.

**Per·i·clor** (per'ĭ-klor) trademark for a preparation of petrichloral.

**peri·co·lic** (per″ĭ-ko'lik) around the colon, as pericolic membrane.

**peri·co·li·tis** (per″ĭ-ko-li'tis) [*peri-* + *colo-* + *-itis*] inflammation around the colon, especially of the peritoneal coat of the colon.
**p. dex'tra,** pericolitis affecting the ascending colon.
**membranous p.,** a morbid condition resulting from the presence of Jackson's membrane (q.v.).
**p. sinis'tra,** inflammation of the surrounding connective tissue and peritoneum of the descending colon.

**peri·co·lon·itis** (per″ĭ-ko″lon-i'tis) pericolitis.

**peri·col·pi·tis** (per″ĭ-kol-pi'tis) [*peri-* + *colp-* + *-itis*] inflammation of the tissues around the vagina.

**peri·con·chal** (per″ĭ-kong'kəl) [*peri-* + *concha* + *-al*[1]] situated around a concha; cf. *periauricular.*

**peri·con·chi·tis** (per″ĭ-kong-ki'tis) [*peri-* + *concha* + *-itis*] periorbititis.

**peri·cor·ne·al** (per″ĭ-kor'ne-əl) surrounding the cornea.

**peri·cor·o·nal** (per″ĭ-kə-ro'nəl) around the crown of a tooth.

**peri·cor·o·ni·tis** (per″ĭ-kor″o-ni'tis) [*peri-* + *corona* + *-itis*] [MeSH: Pericoronitis] inflammation of the gingiva surrounding the crown of a tooth. Called also *operculitis.*

**peri·cox·itis** (per″ĭ-kok-si'tis) inflammation of the tissues about the hip joint.

**peri·cra·ni·al** (per″ĭ-kra′ne-əl) pertaining to the pericranium.

**peri·cra·ni·tis** (per″ĭ-kra-ni′tis) inflammation of the external periosteum of the skull.

**peri·cra·ni·um** (per″ĭ-kra′ne-əm) [*peri-* + *cranium*] [TA] the external periosteum of the skull; called also *periosteum externum cranii* [TA alternative].

**peri·cryp·tal** (per″ĭ-krip′təl) located around a crypt.

**peri·cy·cle** (per″ĭ-si′kəl) [*peri-* + Gr. *kyklos* circle] a layer of parenchymal cells capable of being transformed into meristem to give rise to the root cambium and cork cambium and to branch roots.

**peri·cys·tic** (per″ĭ-sis′tik) situated about a cyst.

**peri·cys·ti·tis** (per″ĭ-sis-ti′tis) [*peri-* + *cyst-* + *-itis*] inflammation of the tissues around the bladder.

**peri·cys·ti·um** (per″ĭ-sis′te-əm) the vascular envelope of certain cysts.

**peri·cyte** (per′ĭ-sit) [*peri-* + *-cyte*] one of the peculiar elongated cells with the power of contraction, found wrapped about the outside of precapillary arterioles, postcapillary venules, and capillaries; called also *adventitial, pericapillary, perithelial,* or *perivascular cell.*

**peri·cy·ti·al** (per″ĭ-si′te-əl) situated around a cell.

**peri·cy·to·ma** (per″ĭ-si-to′mə) hemangiopericytoma.

**peri·dec·to·my** (per″ĭ-dek′tə-me) peritectomy.

**peri·def·er·en·ti·tis** (per″ĭ-def″ər-ən-ti′tis) inflammation of the tissues surrounding the ductus deferens.

**peri·den·drit·ic** (per″ĭ-dən-drit′ik) surrounding the dendrites.

**peri·dens** (per″ĭ-dens) a supernumerary tooth appearing elsewhere than in the midline of the dental arch.

**peri·den·tal** (per″ĭ-den′təl) periodontal, def. 1.

**peri·derm** (per′ĭ-dərm) [*peri-* + *-derm*] 1. the large-celled outer layer of the bilaminar fetal epidermis. In the human it is loosened by the hair which grows beneath it, and generally disappears before birth. Called also *epitrichium.* 2. the cuticle (eponychium and hyponychium), the only part of the periderm which persists after birth.

**peri·der·mal** (per″ĭ-der′məl) pertaining to the periderm.

**peri·des·mic** (per″ĭ-dez′mik) around a ligament; pertaining to the peridesmium.

**peri·des·mi·tis** (per″ĭ-dez-mi′tis) inflammation of the peridesmium.

**peri·des·mi·um** (per″ĭ-dez′me-əm) [*peri-* + Gr. *desmion* band] the areolar membrane which covers the ligaments.

**Peri·dex** (per′ĭ-deks) trademark for a preparation of chlorhexidine gluconate.

**pe·rid·ia** (pə-rid′e-ə) plural of *peridium.*

**peri·did·y·mis** (per″ĭ-did′ĭ-mis) [*peri-* + Gr. *didymos* testicle] the tunica vaginalis testis.

**peri·did·y·mi·tis** (per″ĭ-did″ĭ-mi′tis) inflammation of the perididymis; called also *vaginitis testis.*

**pe·rid·i·um** (pə-rid′e-əm) pl. *perid′ia* [Gr. *pēridion* small leather bag or wallet] the outer coat or limiting membrane enveloping the fruiting body of certain fungi and protozoa.

**peri·di·ver·tic·u·lar** (per″ĭ-di″vər-tik′u-lər) around a diverticulum.

**peri·di·ver·tic·u·li·tis** (per″ĭ-di″vər-tik″u-li′tis) inflammation of structures around a diverticulum of the intestine.

**peri·don·ti·um** (per″ĭ-don′she-əm) periodontium, def. 1.

**peri·duc·tal** (per″ĭ-duk′təl) surrounding a duct, particularly a duct of the mammary gland.

**peri·duc·tile** (per″ĭ-duk′tīl) periductal.

**peri·du·o·de·ni·tis** (per″ĭ-doo″o-də-ni′tis) inflammation around the duodenum, a condition marked by a deformed duodenum surrounded and fixed by peritoneal adhesions.

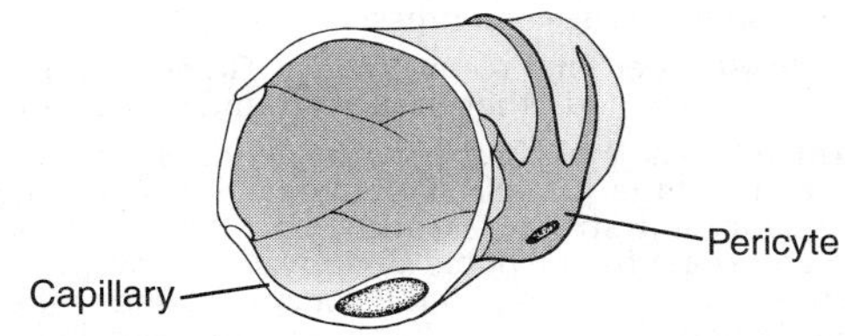


Pericyte, its processes wrapped around the capillary epithelium.

**peri·du·ral** (per″ĭ-doo′rəl) around or external to the dura mater.

**peri·du·ro·gram** (per″ĭ-doo′ro-gram) the film obtained in peridurography.

**peri·du·rog·ra·phy** (per″ĭ-do͞o-rog′rə-fe) [*peri-* + *dura* + Gr. *graphein* to write] radiography of the spinal canal and interspaces after injection of a contrast medium in the peridural space.

**peri·en·ceph·a·li·tis** (per″e-en-sef″ə-li′tis) [*peri-* + *encephalitis*] meningoencephalitis.

**peri·en·ceph·a·log·ra·phy** (per″e-en-sef″ə-log′rə-fe) radiography of the cerebral meninges.

**peri·en·ter·ic** (per″e-en-ter′ik) situated around the intestine.

**peri·en·ter·itis** (per″e-en″tər-i′tis) [*peri-* + *enter-* + *-itis*] inflammation of the peritoneal coat of the intestine; visceral peritonitis.

**peri·en·ter·on** (per″e-en′tər-on) [*peri-* + *enteron*] the primordial embryonic cavity surrounding the viscera.

**peri·ep·en·dy·mal** (per″e-ep-en′də-məl) situated around the ependyma.

**peri·esoph·a·ge·al** (per″e-ə-sof′ə-je-əl) situated around the esophagus.

**peri·esoph·a·gi·tis** (per″e-ə-sof′ə-ji′tis) inflammation of the tissues around the esophagus.

**peri·fas·cic·u·lar** (per″ĭ-fə-sik′u-lər) surrounding a fasciculus of nerve or muscle fibers.

**peri·fis·tu·lar** (per″ĭ-fis′tu-lər) around a fistula.

**peri·fo·cal** (per″ĭ-fo′kəl) around or surrounding a focus, such as a focus of infection.

**peri·fol·lic·u·lar** (per″ĭ-fŏ-lik′u-lər) surrounding a follicle.

**peri·fol·lic·u·li·tis** (per″ĭ-fŏ-lik″u-li′tis) inflammation around the hair follicles.

**p. ca′pitis absce′dens et suffo′diens,** a rare chronic suppurative disease of the scalp, usually seen in young adults, especially men, marked by numerous follicular and perifollicular reactions with the formation of nodules that become fluctuant and rupture to produce intercommunicating draining sinuses, followed by healing with severe scarring and alopecia. Called also *dissecting cellulitis of scalp* and *folliculitis abscedens et suffodiens.*

**superficial pustular p.,** Bockhart's impetigo.

**peri·gan·gli·itis** (per″ĭ-gang″gle-i′tis) inflammation of tissues around a ganglion.

**peri·gan·gli·on·ic** (per″ĭ-gang″gle-on′ik) situated around a ganglion.

**peri·gas·tric** (per″ĭ-gas′trik) situated around the stomach; pertaining to the peritoneal coat of the stomach.

**peri·gas·tri·tis** (per″ĭ-gas-tri′tis) [*peri-* + *gastr-* + *-itis*] inflammation of the peritoneal coat of the stomach.

**peri·gem·mal** (per″ĭ-jem′əl) surrounding a taste bud or other bud.

**peri·glan·du·lar** (per″ĭ-glan′du-lər) surrounding a gland or glands.

**peri·glan·du·li·tis** (per″ĭ-glan″du-li′tis) inflammation of the tissues about a glandule or glandules.

**peri·gli·al** (per″ĭ-gli′əl) surrounding the neuroglial cells.

**peri·glos·si·tis** (per″ĭ-glŏ-si′tis) inflammation of the tissues around the tongue.

**peri·glot·tic** (per″ĭ-glot′ik) situated around the tongue.

**peri·graft** (per′ĭ-graft) situated or occurring around a graft.

**peri·he·pat·ic** (per″e-hə-pat′ik) [*peri-* + *hepatic*] situated or occurring around the liver.

**peri·hep·a·ti·tis** (per″e-hep″ə-ti′tis) [*peri-* + *hepat-* + *-itis*] inflammation of the peritoneal capsule of the liver and of the tissues around the liver.

**p. chro′nica hyperplas′tica,** a disease in which the peritoneal covering of the liver becomes converted into a white mass resembling the icing of a cake; called also *frosted liver, icing liver, sugar-icing liver,* and *zuckergussleber.*

**gonococcal p.,** perihepatitis due to extension of gonorrheal infection; see also *Fitz-Hugh–Curtis syndrome,* under *syndrome.*

**peri·her·ni·al** (per″e-her′ne-əl) situated or occurring around a hernia.

**peri·hi·lar** (per″e-hi′lər) around a hilus, e.g., around the pulmonary hilum.

**peri·im·plan·ti·tis** (per″e-im-plan-ti′tis) inflammation of the tissue around a dental implant, often with tissue breakdown.

**peri·in·su·lar** (per″e-in′su-lər) surrounding an island, particularly the insula.

**peri·is·let** (per″e-i′lət) situated around the islets of Langerhans.

**peri·je·ju·ni·tis** (per″ĭ-je″joo-ni′tis) inflammation around the jejunum.

**peri·kar·ya** (per″ĭ-kar′e-ə) plural of perikaryon.

**peri·kary·on** (per″ĭ-kar′e-on) [*peri-* + *karyon*] the cell body as distinguished from the nucleus and the processes; applied particularly to neurons.

**peri·ker·at·ic** (per″ĭ-kə-rat′ik) surrounding the cornea.

**peri·ky·ma** (per″ĭ-ki′mə) singular of *perikymata.*

**peri·ky·ma·ta** (per″ĭ-ki′mə-tə) [*peri-* + Gr. *kyma* wave] the numerous small transverse ridges on the surface of the enamel of permanent teeth, representing overlapping prism groups; continued abrasion erodes the enamel surface and obliterates them.

**peri·lab·y·rinth** (per″ĭ-lab′ĭ-rinth) the tissue surrounding the labyrinth of the ear.

**peri·lab·y·rin·thi·tis** (per″ĭ-lab″ĭ-rin-thi′tis) circumscribed labyrinthitis.

**peri·la·ryn·ge·al** (per″ĭ-lə-rin′je-əl) situated around the larynx.

**peri·len·tic·u·lar** (per″ĭ-len-tik′u-lər) surrounding the lens of the eye.

**peri·le·sion·al** (per″ĭ-le′zhən-əl) located or occurring around a lesion.

**peri·lig·a·men·tous** (per″ĭ-lig″ə-men′təs) situated around a ligament.

**Pe·ril·la** (pə-ril′ə) a genus of herbs found in North America. *P. frutes′cens,* a type of wild mint, contains a poisonous ketone and can cause fatal emphysema in ruminants.

**peri·lo·bar** (per″ĭ-lo′bər) surrounding a lobe.

**peri·lob·u·li·tis** (per″ĭ-lob-u-li′tis) inflammation of the tissues surrounding the lobules of the lung.

**peri·lymph** (per′ĭ-limf) [MeSH: Perilymph] perilympha.

**peri·lym·pha** (per″ĭ-lim′fə) [*peri-* + *lympha*] [TA] perilymph: the fluid contained within the space separating the membranous labyrinth from the osseous labyrinth; it is entirely separate from the endolymph.

**peri·lym·phad·e·ni·tis** (per″ĭ-lim-fad″ə-ni′tis) inflammation of the tissues around a lymph gland.

**peri·lym·phan·ge·al** (per″ĭ-lim-fan′je-əl) located around a lymphatic vessel.

**peri·lym·phan·gi·tis** (per″ĭ-lim″fan-ji′tis) inflammation of the tissues around a lymphatic vessel.

**peri·lym·phat·ic** (per″ĭ-lim-fat′ik) 1. pertaining to the perilymph. 2. around a lymphatic vessel.

**peri·man·dib·u·lar** (per″ĭ-man-dib′u-lər) situated around or surrounding the mandible.

**peri·mas·ti·tis** (per″ĭ-mas-ti′tis) [*peri-* + *mast-* + *-itis*] inflammation of the connective tissue around the mammary gland.

**peri·med·ul·lary** (per″ĭ-med′u-lar″e) surrounding a medulla, as the medulla oblongata or the marrow of a bone.

**peri·men·in·gi·tis** (per″ĭ-men″in-ji′tis) [*peri-* + *mening-* + *-itis*] pachymeningitis.

**peri·meno·pau·sal** (per″ĭ-men″o-paw′zəl) occurring during or pertaining to perimenopause.

**pe·rim·e·ter** (pə-rim′ə-tər) [*peri-* + *-meter*] 1. a line forming the boundary of a plane figure. 2. an apparatus for determining the extent of the peripheral visual field on a curved surface.
**dental p.,** an instrument for measuring the circumference of a tooth.

**peri·met·ric** (per″ĭ-met′rik) 1. pertaining to a perimeter. 2. around the uterus. 3. pertaining to the perimetrium.

**peri·me·trit·ic** (per″ĭ-mə-trit′ik) pertaining to or characterized by perimetritis.

**peri·me·tri·tis** (per″ĭ-mə-tri′tis) [*peri-* + *metr-* + *-itis*] inflammation of the perimetrium.

**peri·me·tri·um** (per″ĭ-me′tre-əm) [*peri-* + Gr. *mētra* uterus] TA alternative for *tunica serosa uteri.*

**peri·met·ro·sal·pin·gi·tis** (per″ĭ-met″ro-sal″pin-ji′tis) inflammation of the uterus and uterine tubes and of surrounding tissues.
**encapsulating p.,** perimetrosalpingitis with formation of a membrane about the organs involved.

**pe·rim·e·try** (pə-rim′ə-tre) [*peri-* + *-metry*] [MeSH: Perimetry] determination of the extent of the peripheral visual field by use of a perimeter; cf. *perioptometry.*

**peri·mol·y·sis** (per″ĭ-mol′ĭ-sis) [shortened from *perimylolysis,* q.v.] erosion of the lingual surfaces of the anterior teeth and the occlusal surfaces of the posterior teeth by acid decalcification; commonly seen in anorexia nervosa and also in other conditions involving chronic regurgitation.

**peri·my·elis** (per″ĭ-mi′ə-lis) [*peri-* + Gr. *myelos* marrow] endosteum.

**peri·my·eli·tis** (per″ĭ-mi″ə-li′tis) 1. inflammation of the perimyelis (endosteum). 2. spinal meningitis.

**peri·my·elog·ra·phy** (per″ĭ-mi″ə-log′rə-fe) [*peri-* + *myelo-* + *-graphy*] radiologic examination after injecting iodized oil or other contrast fluid into the subarachnoid space of the spinal cord.

**peri·my·lol·y·sis** (per″ĭ-mĭ-lol′ĭ-sis) [*peri-* + Gr. *mylos* molar + *lysis*] perimolysis.

**peri·myo·car·di·tis** (per″ĭ-mi″o-kahr-di′tis) [*peri-* + *myocarditis*] combined pericarditis and myocarditis.

**peri·myo·en·do·car·di·tis** (per″ĭ-mi″o-en″do-kahr-di′tis) pericarditis associated with myocarditis and endocarditis.

**peri·myo·si·tis** (per″ĭ-mi″o-si′tis) inflammation of the connective tissue around muscles.

**peri·mys·ia** (per″ĭ-mis′e-ə) plural of *perimysium.*

**peri·mys·i·al** (per″ĭ-mis′e-əl) pertaining to the perimysium.

**peri·mys·i·itis** (per″ĭ-mis″e-i′tis) inflammation of the perimysium; myofibrositis.

**peri·mys·itis** (per″ĭ-mis-i′tis) perimysiitis.

**peri·mys·i·um** (per″ĭ-mis′e-əm) pl. *perimys′ia* [*peri-* + Gr. *mys* muscle] [TA] the connective tissue demarcating a fascicle of skeletal muscle fibers; called also *internal p.,* or *p. internum.*
**external p., p. exter′num,** epimysium.
**internal p., p. inter′num,** perimysium.

**peri·na·tal** (per″ĭ-na′təl) [*peri-* + *natal*] pertaining to or occurring in the period shortly before and after birth; variously defined as beginning with completion of the twentieth to twenty-eighth week of gestation and ending 7 to 28 days after birth.

**peri·na·tol·o·gist** (per″ĭ-na-tol′ə-jist) a specialist in perinatology.

**peri·na·tol·o·gy** (per″ĭ-na-tol′ə-je) [*perinatal* + *-logy*] [MeSH: Perinatology] the branch of medicine (obstetrics and pediatrics) dealing with the fetus and infant during the perinatal period.

**peri·ne·al** (per″ĭ-ne′əl) pertaining to the perineum.

**peri·neo·cele** (per″ĭ-ne′o-sēl) [*perineum* + *-cele*[1]] a hernia lying between the rectum and the prostate, or between the rectum and vagina; perineal hernia.

**peri·ne·om·e·ter** (per″ĭ-ne-om′ə-tər) an instrument for measuring the strength of contractions of the perivaginal muscles.

**peri·neo·plas·ty** (per″ĭ-ne′o-plas″te) [*perineum* + *-plasty*] plastic surgery of the perineum.

**peri·ne·or·rha·phy** (per″ĭ-ne-or′ə-fe) [*perineum* + *-rrhaphy*] suture of the perineum, performed for the repair of a laceration.

**peri·neo·scro·tal** (per″ĭ-ne″o-skro′təl) pertaining to the perineum and scrotum.

**peri·ne·ot·o·my** (per″ĭ-ne-ot′ə-me) [*perineum* + *-tomy*] surgical incision through the perineum.

**peri·neo·vag·i·nal** (per″ĭ-ne″o-vaj′ĭ-nəl) pertaining to or communicating with the perineum and vagina, as a perineovaginal fistula.

**peri·neo·vag·i·no·rec·tal** (per″ĭ-ne″o-vaj′ĭ-no-rek′təl) pertaining to the perineum, vagina, and rectum.

**peri·neo·vul·var** (per″ĭ-ne″o-vul′vər) pertaining to the perineum and the vulva.

**peri·neph·ri·al** (per″ĭ-nef′re-əl) pertaining to the perinephrium.

**peri·neph·ric** (per″ĭ-nef′rik) surrounding the kidney; called also *perirenal.*

**peri·ne·phrit·ic** (per″ĭ-nə-frit′ik) pertaining to or characterized by perinephritis.

**peri·ne·phri·tis** (per″ĭ-nə-fri′tis) [*peri-* + *nephr-* + *-itis*] [MeSH: Perinephritis] inflammation of the perinephrium; it is marked by fever, local pain, and tenderness on pressure.

**peri·neph·ri·um** (per″ĭ-nef′re-əm) [*peri-* + Gr. *nephros* kidney] the peritoneal envelope and other tissues around the kidney.

**peri·ne·um** (per″ĭ-ne′əm) [Gr. *perinaion, perineos* the space between the anus and scrotum] [MeSH: Perineum] 1. [TA] the pelvic floor and the associated structures occupying the pelvic outlet; it is bounded anteriorly by the pubic symphysis, laterally by the ischial tuberosities, and posteriorly by the coccyx. 2. the region between the thighs, bounded in the male by the scrotum and anus and in the female by the vulva and anus.

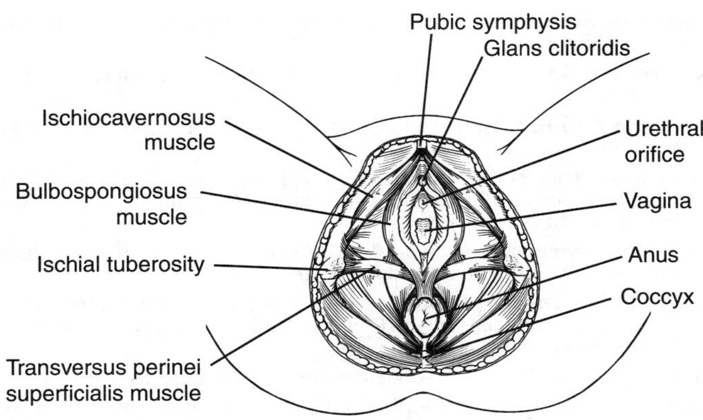


Perineum in a female; the diamond-shaped area between the pubic symphysis and coccyx can be divided into anterior urogenital and posterior anal triangles by drawing a line transversely between the ischial tuberosities.

**peri•neu•ral** (per″ĭ-noor′əl) surrounding a nerve or nerves.

**peri•neu•ri•al** (per″ĭ-noor′e-əl) pertaining to the perineurium.

**peri•neu•rit•ic** (per″ĭ-noo͞-rit′ik) pertaining to or suffering from perineuritis.

**peri•neu•ri•tis** (per″ĭ-noo͞-ri′tis) inflammation of the perineurium.

**peri•neu•ri•um** (per″ĭ-noor′e-um) [*peri-* + Gr. *neuron* nerve] [TA] an intermediate layer of connective tissue in a peripheral nerve, surrounding each bundle (fasciculus) of nerve fibers. See also *epineurium* and *endoneurium.*

**peri•nod•al** (per″ĭ-no′dəl) situated or occurring around a node.

**peri•nu•cle•ar** (per″ĭ-noo′kle-ər) situated or occurring around a nucleus.

**peri•oc•u•lar** (per″e-ok′u-lər) situated or occurring around the eye.

**pe•ri•od** (pe′re-od) [Gr. *periodos* a going around, circuit, period] an interval or division of time; the time for the regular recurrence of a phenomenon.

**absolute refractory p.,** the portion of the refractory period when a nerve or muscle fiber cannot respond to a stimulus, as contrasted with the relative refractory period.

**child-bearing p.,** the duration of the reproductive ability in the human female, roughly from puberty to menopause.

**ejection p.,** the second phase of ventricular systole, being the period intervening between the opening and closing of the semilunar valves, during which the blood is being discharged into the aortic and pulmonary arteries. It can be divided into an initial *period of rapid ejection* followed by a *period of reduced ejection* as aortic and ventricular pressures decline from their peak. Called also *ejection phase* and *sphygmic p.* See illustration at *cardiac cycle,* under *cycle.*

**$G_1$ p.,** the period in the mitotic cycle from the end of the previous division to the start of DNA synthesis (S period).

**$G_2$ p.,** the period of the mitotic cycle from the end of DNA synthesis (S period) to the beginning of mitosis.

**gestational p.,** the duration of pregnancy (from conception to delivery), which in the human female averages about 266 days.

**half-life p.,** see *half-life.*

**incubation p.,** 1. the interval of time required for development. 2. the interval of time between the receipt of infection and the onset of the consequent illness or the first symptoms of the illness *(prodromal stage).* 3. the interval of time between the entrance into a vector of an infectious agent and the time at which the vector is capable of transmitting the infection. See also *generation time* (def. 1), under *time.* Called also *latent p.*

**isoelectric p.,** on an electrocardiogram, the period between the end of the S wave and the beginning of the T wave, when no potential is recorded because the electrical forces are acting in different directions and neutralize each other.

**isometric p.,** isovolumic p.

**isovolumetric p., isovolumic p.,** in the cardiac cycle, an interval during which the cardiac muscle fibers are contracting or relaxing but the valves are all closed, so that ventricular pressure changes rapidly while volume remains constant; see *p. of isovolumic relaxation* and *p. of isovolumic contraction.*

**p. of isovolumic contraction,** the first phase of ventricular systole, being the short period (0.5 second) lasting from atrioventricular valve closing to semilunar valve opening; as the muscle fibers contract, the ventricular pressure rises rapidly but the ventricular blood volume remains constant. See illustration at *cardiac cycle,* under *cycle.*

**p. of isovolumic relaxation,** a short interval (0.05 second) during ventricular diastole, immediately following the ejection period and lasting from semilunar valve closing to atrioventricular valve opening; as the muscle fibers relax, the ventricular pressure drops and the ventricular blood volume remains constant. See illustration at *cardiac cycle,* under *cycle.*

**lag p.,** the time which elapses between the introduction of a microorganism into a nutrient medium and the initiation of exponential growth.

**latency p.,** 1. latent p. 2. see under *stage.*

**latent p.,** a seemingly inactive period, such as that between exposure to an infection and manifestation of symptoms *(incubation p.)* or between the presentation of a stimulus and the response (*latency,* def. 2).

**M p.,** the period of active mitosis.

**menstrual p., monthly p.,** the time of menstruation.

**pacemaker refractory p.,** the interval immediately following either pacemaker sensing or pacing, during which improper inhibition of the pacemaker by inappropriate signals is prevented by temporary inactivation of pacemaker sensing.

**preejection p. (PEP),** the interval between the onset of ventricular depolarization and the onset of ventricular ejection; it is one of the systolic time intervals (q.v.) used in assessing left ventricular performance and is calculated by subtracting the left ventricular ejection time from the electromechanical systole.

**prefunctional p.,** the time span during morphological and histological development before physiological activity begins.

**prodromal p.,** see under *stage.*

**quarantine p.,** the length of time, usually the maximal incubation period of the disease, which must elapse before a person exposed to contagion is regarded as incapable of transmitting or acquiring the disease. See also *quarantine.*

**p. of rapid ventricular filling,** see *p. of ventricular filling.*

**reaction p.,** 1. the stage of rallying from shock after trauma. 2. reaction time, the time that elapses between stimulation and the consequent reaction.

**p. of reduced ventricular filling,** diastasis; see also *p. of ventricular filling.*

**refractory p.,** the period of depolarization of the cell membrane after excitation, during which the nerve or muscle fiber cannot respond to a second stimulus. See also *absolute refractory p.* and *relative refractory p.*

**relative refractory p.,** the brief period following the absolute refractory period, during which there is repolarization of the cell membrane to the extent that the fiber can respond to a strong stimulus, although the normal resting potential has not been reached.

**S p.,** the period of DNA synthesis in the mitotic cycle.

**safe p.,** the period during the menstrual cycle when conception is considered least likely to occur; it is approximately the ten days after menstruation begins, and the ten days preceding menstruation.

**silent p.,** 1. an interval in the course of a disease in which the symptoms become very mild or disappear for a time. 2. a short period of electrical silence in a muscle, such as is seen just after abrupt unloading.

**sphygmic p.,** ejection p.

**p. of ventricular filling,** in the cardiac cycle, the interval in diastole lasting from atrioventricular valve opening to the start of ventricular contraction and valve closure, during which the ventricular blood volume increases and the pressure drops. The interval is frequently divided into an initial rapid phase of filling and a subsequent slowed phase (diastasis). See also illustration at *cardiac cycle,* under *cycle.*

**Wenckebach p.,** the steadily lengthening P–R interval occurring in successive cardiac cycles in Wenckebach block.

**per•io•date** (per-i′o-dāt) a salt of periodic acid.

**pe•ri•od•ic** (pēr′e-od′ik) [Gr. *periodikos*] recurring at regular intervals of time.

**per•iod•ic ac•id** (per″i-o′dik) [MeSH: Periodic Acid] a strong mineral acid and oxidizing agent, $HIO_4$.

**pe•ri•o•dic•i•ty** (pēr″e-o-dis′ĭ-te) [MeSH: Periodicity] recurrence at regular intervals of time.

**filarial p.,** the periodic increase of microfilariae in the peripheral blood: nocturnal periodicity occurs in *Wuchereria bancrofti* infection in most endemic areas and in *Brugia malayi* infection; diurnal periodicity occurs in *Loa loa* infection.

**lunar p.,** recurrence synchronized with phases of the moon, as the reproductive phenomena in some lower animals.

**malarial p.,** the more or less regular recurrence of paroxysms at intervals of one, two, or three days in malaria; see under *malaria.*

**peri•odon•tal** (per″e-o-don′təl) [*peri-* + *odont-* + *-al*[1]] 1. pertaining to or occurring around a tooth; peridental. 2. pertaining to the periodontal ligament or periodontium.

**peri•odon•tia** (per″e-o-don′shə) 1. plural of *periodontium.* 2. periodontics.

**peri·odon·tics** (per″e-o-don′tiks) [*peri-* + *odont-* + *-ic*] [MeSH: Periodontics] that branch of dentistry dealing with the study and treatment of diseases of the periodontium.

**peri·odon·tist** (per″e-o-don′tist) a dentist who specializes in periodontics.

**peri·odon·ti·tis** (per″e-o-don-ti′tis) [*peri-* + *odont-* + *-itis*] [MeSH: Periodontitis] inflammatory reaction of the tissues surrounding a tooth (periodontium), usually resulting from the extension of gingival inflammation (gingivitis) into the periodontium. Periodontitis has been classified in five clinical types: *prepubertal, juvenile, rapidly progressive, and adult p.,* and *necrotizing ulcerative gingivoperiodontitis.* Called also *alveolodental osteoperiostitis, cementoperiostitis,* and *paradentitis.*
**adult p.,** the most common form of periodontitis, usually occurring after the age of 35, and usually manifested by slow progression of tissue destruction, which may ultimately result in loss of the teeth.
**apical p.,** inflammatory reaction of the tissues surrounding the root of a tooth.
**chronic apical p.,** periapical granuloma.
**juvenile p.,** a rare form of periodontitis that has an onset at puberty, is more common in females, and is manifested by deep periodontal pockets, usually involving the first molars and incisors. It may be associated with rapidly progressive periodontitis in later life. Called also *paradentosis* and *periodontosis.*
**marginal p.,** a chronic destructive inflammatory periodontal disease that begins as a simple marginal gingivitis and may migrate along the tooth toward the apex, producing periodontal pockets, usually with pus formation, and destruction of the periodontal and alveolar structures, causing the teeth to become loose. Called also *simple p., chronic suppurative pericementitis, Fauchard's disease, pyorrhea, pyorrhea alveolaris, Riggs' disease,* and *schmutz pyorrhea.*
**prepubertal p.,** a rare form of periodontitis, probably having an onset soon after eruption of the primary teeth. It occurs in a localized form that involves only some teeth, and in a generalized form that causes rapid destruction of alveolar bone and may or may not affect the permanent teeth.
**rapidly progressive p.,** generalized periodontitis occurring after puberty and before the age of 30 to 35 in those who may or may not have had juvenile periodontitis, characterized by severe and rapid bone destruction, which may progress to abscess formation and tooth loss, or may enter a short or prolonged dormant period.
**simple p., p. sim′plex,** marginal p.

**peri·odon·ti·um** (per″e-o-don′she-əm) pl. *periodon′tia* [*peri-* + Gr. *odous* tooth] [TA] [MeSH: Periodontium] 1. the tissues that invest or help to invest and support the teeth, including the periodontal ligament, gingivae, cementum, and alveolar and supporting bone. 2. periodontal ligament. Called also *alveolar periosteum, odontoperiosteum, paradentium,* and *peridontium.*
**p. insertio′nis** [TA], free gingiva: the unattached portion of the gingiva, forming the wall of the gingival crevice. Called also *unattached gingiva* and *free gum.* See also *margo gingivalis.*
**p. protectio′nis** [TA], **p. protecto′ris,** attached gingiva: the part of the gingiva that is firm and resilient and is bound to the underlying cementum and the alveolar bone, thus being immovable.

**peri·odon·tol·o·gy** (per″e-o-don-tol′ə-je) [*peri-* + *odont-* + *-logy*] the branch of dentistry that deals with the scientific study of the structures and function of the periodontium in health and disease; broader in scope than *periodontics,* which is limited to the diagnosis, prevention, and treatment of periodontal disease, although the two terms are sometimes used interchangeably.

**peri·odon·to·sis** (per″e-o-don-to′sis) juvenile periodontitis.

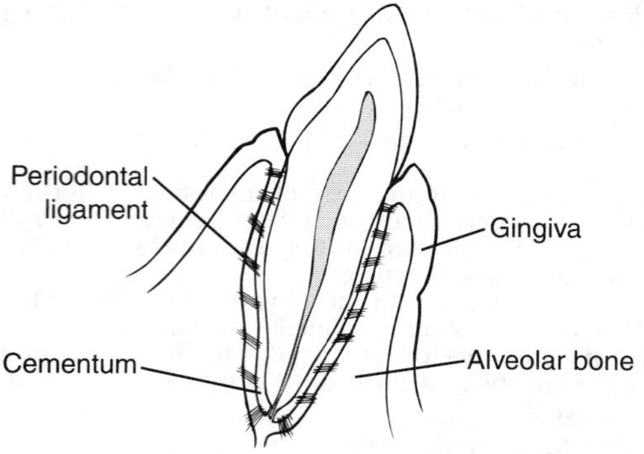


Periodontium, showing the periodontal ligament attaching the cementum of the tooth root to the alveolar bone of the socket; the collagen fibers of the ligament are grouped into bundles.

**peri·om·phal·ic** (per″e-om-fal′ik) [*peri-* + *omphal-* + *-ic*] around the umbilicus.

**peri·onych·ia** (per″e-o-nik′e-ə) 1. paronychia. 2. plural of *perionychium.*

**peri·onych·i·um** (per″e-o-nik′e-əm) [*peri-* + Gr. *onyx* nail] eponychium.

**peri·onyx** (per″e-o′niks) [*peri-* + *onyx*] [TA] a relic of the eponychium persisting as a band across the root of the nail, first seen in the eighth month of fetal life.

**peri·ooph·o·ri·tis** (per″e-o-of″o-ri′tis) [*peri-* + *oophoritis*] inflammation of the tissues around the ovary.

**peri·ooph·o·ro·sal·pin·gi·tis** (per″e-o-of″o-ro-sal″pin-ji′tis) [*peri-* + *oophoro-* + *salping-* + *-itis*] inflammation of the tissues around the ovary and oviducts.

**peri·oo·the·ci·tis** (per-e-o″o-the-si′tis) perioophoritis.

**peri·op·er·a·tive** (per″e-op′ər-ə-tiv) pertaining to the period extending from the time of hospitalization for surgery to the time of discharge.

**peri·oph·thal·mia** (per″e-of-thal′me-ə) periophthalmitis.

**peri·oph·thal·mic** (per″e-of-thal′mik) situated around the eye.

**peri·oph·thal·mi·tis** (per″e-of″thəl-mi′tis) [*peri-* + *ophthalmitis*] inflammation of the tissues around the eye.

**peri·ople** (per′e-o″pəl) [*peri-* + Gr. *hoplē* hoof] the layer of soft, light-colored horn covering the outer aspect of the hoof in ungulates.

**peri·op·tom·e·try** (per″e-op-tom′ə-tre) [*peri-* + *opto-* + *-metry*] the measurement of the peripheral acuity of vision or of the limits of the visual field; cf. perimetry.

**peri·oral** (per″e-or′əl) [*peri-* + *oral*] around or near the mouth; cf. *circumoral.*

**peri·or·bit** (per″e-or′bit) periorbita.

**peri·or·bi·ta** (per″e-or′bĭ-tə) [*peri-* + *orbita*] [TA] the periosteal covering of the bones forming the orbit, or eye socket.

**peri·or·bi·tal** (per″e-or′bĭ-təl) situated around the orbit, or eye socket.

**peri·or·bi·ti·tis** (per″e-or″bĭ-ti′tis) inflammation of the periorbita.

**peri·or·chi·tis** (per″e-or-ki′tis) [*peri-* + *orchi-* + *-itis*] inflammation of the tunica vaginalis testis. Called also *vaginalitis.*
**p. adhaesi′va,** a variety in which the two layers of the tunica vaginalis are more or less adherent.
**p. purulen′ta,** periorchitis which goes on to pus formation.

**peri·or·chi·um** (per″e-or′ke-əm) the parietal layer of the tunica vaginalis testis.

**peri·ost** (per′e-ost) periosteum.

**peri·os·te·al** (per″e-os′te-əl) pertaining to the periosteum.

**peri·os·te·itis** (per″e-os″te-i′tis) periostitis.

**peri·os·teo·de·ma** (per″e-os″te-o-de′mə) periosteoedema.

**peri·os·teo·ede·ma** (per″e-os″te-o-ə-de′mə) edema of the periosteum.

**peri·os·te·o·ma** (per″e-os-te-o′mə) a morbid bony growth surrounding a bone.

**peri·os·teo·med·ul·li·tis** (per″e-os″te-o-med″u-li′tis) inflammation of the periosteum and bone marrow.

**peri·os·teo·my·eli·tis** (per″e-os″te-o-mi″ə-li′tis) [*peri-* + *osteo-* + *myelitis*] inflammation of the entire bone, including periosteum and marrow.

**peri·os·teo·phyte** (per″e-os′te-o-fīt″) [*periosteum* + *-phyte*] a bony outgrowth on the periosteum.

**peri·os·teo·sis** (per″e-os″te-o′sis) periostosis.

**peri·os·teo·tome** (per″e-os′te-o-tōm) an instrument for cutting the periosteum; also an instrument for separating the periosteum from the bone.

**peri·os·te·ot·o·my** (per″e-os″te-ot′ə-me) [*peri-* + *osteo-* + *-tomy*] surgical incision or slitting of the periosteum.

**peri·os·te·ous** (per″e-os′te-əs) pertaining to or of the nature of periosteum.

**peri·os·te·um** (per″e-os′te-əm) [*peri-* + Gr. *osteon* bone] [TA] [MeSH: Periosteum] a specialized connective tissue covering all bones of the body, and possessing bone-forming potentialities; in adults, it consists of two layers that are not sharply defined, the external layer being a network of dense connective tissue containing blood vessels, and the deep layer composed of more loosely arranged collagenous bundles with spindle-shaped connective tissue cells and a network of thin elastic fibers.

**alveolar p., p. alveola're,** periodontium, def. 1.
**p. exter'num cra'nii,** TA alternative for pericranium.

**peri·os·ti·tis** (per″e-os-ti′tis) [MeSH: Periostitis] inflammation of the periosteum. The condition is generally chronic, and is marked by tenderness and swelling of the bone and an aching pain. Acute periostitis is due to infection, is characterized by diffuse suppuration, severe pain, and constitutional symptoms, and usually results in necrosis.
**p. albumino'sa, albuminous p.,** a form accompanied by the exudation of a clear, albuminous liquid into a flattened cavity beneath the periosteum; called also *serous abscess* and *periosteal gangrene.*
**diffuse p.,** a noncircumscribed periostitis of the long bones.
**hemorrhagic p.,** a form in which blood is extravasated beneath the periosteum.
**p. hyperplas'tica,** hypertrophic pulmonary osteoarthropathy.
**p. inter'na cra'nii,** external pachymeningitis.
**precocious p.,** syphilitic osteoperiostitis occurring as an early symptom.

**peri·os·to·ma** (per″e-os-to′mə) periosteoma.

**peri·os·to·med·ul·li·tis** (per″e-os″to-med″u-li′tis) periosteomedullitis.

**peri·os·to·sis** (per″e-os-to′sis) the abnormal deposition of periosteal bone; the condition manifested by development of periosteomas. Called also *periosteosis.*
**hyperplastic p.,** infantile cortical hyperostosis.

**peri·os·tos·te·itis** (per″e-os-tos″te-i′tis) osteoperiostitis.

**peri·os·to·tome** (per″e-os′to-tōm) periosteotome.

**peri·os·tot·o·my** (per″e-os-tot′ə-me) periosteotomy.

**peri·otic** (per″e-o′tik) [*peri-* + *otic*] 1. situated about the ear, especially the internal ear. 2. pars petrosa ossis temporalis.

**peri·ova·ri·tis** (per″e-o″və-ri′tis) perioophoritis.

**peri·ovu·lar** (per″e-o′vu-lər) surrounding an ovum.

**peri·pan·cre·at·ic** (per″ĭ-pan″kre-at′ik) surrounding the pancreas.

**peri·pan·cre·a·ti·tis** (per″ĭ-pan″kre-ə-ti′tis) [*peri-* + Gr. *pancreat-* + *-itis*] inflammation of tissues around the pancreas.

**peri·pap·il·lary** (per″ĭ-pap′ĭ-lar″e) located around the optic papilla.

**peri·par·tum** (per″ĭ-pahr′təm) occurring during the last month of gestation or the first few months after delivery, with reference to the mother.

**peri·pa·tel·lar** (per″ĭ-pə-tel′ər) around the patella, or knee cap.

**peri·pa·tet·ic** (per″ĭ-pə-tet′ik) [Gr. *peripatētikos* given to walking about while teaching or disputing] walking about; used especially in reference to typhoid patients who are ambulatory.

**peri·pe·ni·al** (per″ĭ-pe′ne-əl) around the penis.

**peri·pha·ci·tis** (per″ĭ-fə-si′tis) [*peri-* + *phac-* + *-itis*] inflammation surrounding the capsule of the lens of the eye.

**peri·pha·ki·tis** (per″ĭ-fə-ki′tis) periphacitis.

**peri·pha·ryn·ge·al** (per″ĭ-fə-rin′je-əl) situated around the pharynx.

**pe·riph·er·ad** (pə-rif′ər-əd) toward the periphery.

**pe·riph·er·al** (pə-rif′ər-əl) pertaining to or situated at or near the periphery; situated away from a center or central structure.

**peri·phe·ra·lis** (pə-rĭ″fə-ra′lis) [L., from Gr. *peripherein* to carry around] peripheral; TA alternative for *periphericus.*

**pe·riph·er·aphose** (pə-rif′ər-ə-fōs) [*periphery* + *aphose*] a subjective sensation of a dark spot in the line of vision, originating in the peripheral ocular mechanism; cf. *peripherophose.*

**peri·pher·ic** (per″ĭ-fer′ik) peripheral.

**peri·phe·ri·cus** (per″ĭ-fer′ĭ-kəs) [L., from Gr. *peripherein* to carry around] [TA] peripheral; a general term denoting location away from a center or central structure. Called also *peripheralis* [TA alternative].

**pe·riph·ero·cen·tral** (pə-rif″ər-o-sen′trəl) both peripheral and central.

**pe·riph·ero·phose** (pə-rif′ər-o-fōz) [*periphery* + *phose*] any phose or subjective sensation of light originating in the peripheral ocular mechanism; cf. *peripheraphose.*

**pe·riph·ery** (pə-rif′ər-e) [Gr. *periphereia,* from *peri* around + *pherein* to bear] the outward part or surface or structure; the portion of a system outside the central region.

**peri·phle·bit·ic** (per″ĭ-flə-bit′ik) pertaining to periphlebitis.

**peri·phle·bi·tis** (per″ĭ-flə-bi′tis) [*peri-* + *phlebitis*] inflammation of the tissues around a vein or of its external coat.
**sclerosing p.,** Mondor's disease.

**peri·pho·ria** (per″ĭ-for′e-ə) [*peri-* + *-phoria*] cyclophoria.

**peri·phre·ni·tis** (per″ĭ-frə-ni′tis) [*peri-* + *phrenitis*] inflammation of the diaphragm and structures around it. Called also *paraphrenitis.*

**Per·i·pla·ne·ta** (per″ĭ-plə-ne′tə) [Gr. *periplanasthai* to wander about] [MeSH: Periplaneta] a genus of cockroaches (order Blattaria). *P. america'na* is the American cockroach and *P. australa'siae* is the Australian cockroach.

**peri·plasm** (per′ĭ-plaz-əm) [*peri-* + *-plasm*] periplasmic space.

**peri·plas·mic** (per″ĭ-plas′mik) around the plasma membrane; between the plasma membrane and the cell wall of a bacterium.

**peri·pleu·ral** (per″ĭ-ploor′əl) surrounding the pleura.

**peri·pleu·ri·tis** (per″ĭ-ploo-ri′tis) [*peri-* + *pleur-* + *-itis*] inflammation of the tissues between the pleura and the chest wall.

**peri·plo·cin** (per″ĭ-plo′sin) a crystallizable glycoside from a woody vine, *Periploca graeca* L. (Asclepiadaceae); it acts like digitalin as a heart tonic and slower of the pulse.

**peri·plo·cy·ma·rin** (per″ĭ-plo-si′mə-rin) a cardiac glycoside from the bark and wood of *Periploca graeca* L. (Asclepiadaceae).

**peri·plog·e·nin** (per″ĭ-ploj′ə-nin) an aglycone sterol derivative from periplocin and periplocymarin.

**peri·po·lar** (per″ĭ-po′lər) situated about a pole or poles.

**peri·po·le·sis** (per″ĭ-po-le′sis) [Gr. *peripolēsis* a going about] the movement of one cell around another; used to refer to the clustering of lymphocytes around macrophages in lymphoid tissue.

**peri·po·ri·tis** (per″ĭ-por-i′tis) a staphylococcal infection complicating miliaria, with inflammation around the sweat pores, usually affecting infants; called also *periporitis staphylogenes.*

**peri·por·tal** (per″ĭ-por′təl) situated around the portal vein.

**peri·proc·tic** (per″ĭ-prok′tik) [*peri-* + *proct-* + *-ic*] situated around the anus.

**peri·proc·ti·tis** (per″ĭ-prok-ti′tis) [*peri-* + *proct-* + *-itis*] inflammation of the tissues surrounding the rectum and anus.

**peri·pros·tat·ic** (per″ĭ-pros-tat′ik) situated about the prostate.

**peri·pros·ta·ti·tis** (per″ĭ-pros″tə-ti′tis) inflammation of the tissues and structures around the prostate gland.

**peri·py·le·phle·bi·tis** (per″ĭ-pi″le-flə-bi′tis) [*peri-* + *pylephlebitis*] inflammation of the tissue about the portal vein.

**peri·py·lo·ric** (per″ĭ-pi-lor′ik) around the pylorus or the pyloric part of the stomach (see *pars pylorica gastris*).

**peri·ra·dic·u·lar** (per″ĭ-rə-dik′u-lər) around or surrounding a root, especially the root of a tooth.

**peri·rec·tal** (per″ĭ-rek′təl) around the rectum.

**peri·rec·ti·tis** (per″ĭ-rek-ti′tis) periproctitis.

**peri·re·nal** (per″ĭ-re′nəl) perinephric.

**peri·rhi·nal** (per″ĭ-ri′nəl) [*peri-* + *rhin-* + *-al*[1]] situated about the nose.

**peri·rhi·zo·cla·sia** (per″ĭ-ri″zo-kla′zhə) [*peri-* + Gr. *rhizo-* + *klasis* destruction] inflammatory destruction of tissues immediately around the root of a tooth, i.e., the pericementum, cementum, and superficial layers of the alveolar process. Cf. *pararhizoclasia.*

**peri·sal·pin·gi·tis** (per″ĭ-sal″pin-ji′tis) [*peri-* + *salping-* + *-itis*] inflammation of the tissues and peritoneum around a uterine tube.

**peri·sal·pin·go·ova·ri·tis** (per″ĭ-sal-ping″go-o″və-ri′tis) inflammation involving the ovary and the tissues around the uterine tube.

**peri·sal·pinx** (per″ĭ-sal′pinks) the peritoneal cover of the upper border of the uterine tube.

**peri·scle·ri·um** (per″ĭ-skle′re-əm) [*peri-* + Gr. *sklēros* hard] fibrous tissue surrounding ossifying cartilage.

**peri·scop·ic** (per″ĭ-skop′ik) [*peri-* +Gr. *skopein* to examine] affording a wide range of vision; said of microscopical and meniscus lenses.

**peri·sig·moid·itis** (per″ĭ-sig″moid-i′tĭs) inflammation of the peritoneal covering of the sigmoid flexure.

**peri·sin·u·ous** (per″ĭ-sin′u-əs) situated around a sinus.

**peri·sin·u·si·tis** (per″i-si″nə-si′tis) inflammation of the tissues around a sinus.

**peri·sin·u·soi·dal** (per″ĭ-si″nə-soi′dəl) surrounding a sinusoid.

**peri·sper·ma·ti·tis** (per″ĭ-sper″mə-ti′tis) inflammation of the tissues about the spermatic cord.
**p. sero'sa,** encysted hydrocele of the spermatic cord.

**peri·splanch·nic** (per″ĭ-splank′nik) [*peri-* + *splanchn-* + *-ic*] around a viscus or the viscera.

**peri·splanch·ni·tis** (per″ĭ-splank-ni′tis) inflammation around the viscera; perivisceritis.

**peri·splen·ic** (per″ĭ-splen′ik) occurring around the spleen.

**peri·sple·ni·tis** (per″ĭ-splə-ni′tis) [*peri-* + *splen-* + *-itis*] inflammation of the peritoneal coat of the spleen and of the structures around it.
**p. cartilagi′nea,** inflammatory overgrowth of the capsule of the spleen, causing a thickening of cartilaginous hardness.

**peri·spon·dyl·ic** (per″ĭ-spon-dil′ik) around a vertebra.

**peri·spon·dy·li·tis** (per″ĭ-spon″də-li′tis) [*peri-* + *spondyl-* + *-itis*] inflammation of the parts around a vertebra.
**Gibney's p.,** a painful condition of the spinal muscles.

**Peri·spo·ri·a·ceae** (per″ĭ-spor″e-a′se-e) Moniliaceae.

**Pe·ris·so·dac·ty·la** (pə-ris″o-dak′tə-lə) [Gr. *perissos* odd + *daktylos* finger] [MeSH: Perissodactyla] an order of mammals, the ungulates with an odd number of toes, including the horse, tapir, and rhinoceros. Cf. *Artiodactyla.*

**pe·ris·so·dac·ty·lous** (pə-ris″o-dak′tə-ləs) 1. having an odd number of digits on a hand or foot. 2. pertaining to the Perissodactyla.

**peri·stal·sis** (per″ĭ-stal′sis) [*peri-* + Gr. *stalsis* contraction] [MeSH: Peristalsis] the movement by which the alimentary canal and other tubular organs that have both longitudinal and circular muscle fibers propel their contents; it consists of a wave of contraction passing along the tube for variable distances.
**mass p.,** strong usually brief bursts of peristaltic movements, which propel intestinal contents through long stretches of the intestine or colon, often resulting in defecation.
**retrograde p.,** reversed p.
**reversed p.,** that which impels the contents of the intestine cephalad.

**peri·stal·tic** (per″ĭ-stal′tik) of the nature of peristalsis.

**peri·stal·tin** (per″ĭ-stal′tin) a glycoside of cascara sagrada.

**peri·staph·y·line** (per″ĭ-staf′ə-lin) [*peri-* + *staphyline*] situated around the uvula.

**peri·sto·mal** (per″ĭ-sto′məl) [*peri-* + Gr. *stoma* mouth] around the mouth.

**peri·stome** (per′ĭ-stōm) [*peri-* + Gr. *stoma* mouth] 1. in ciliate protozoa, the buccal area and its encircling adoral zone of membranelles. 2. buccal cavity.

**peri·sto·mi·al** (per″ĭ-sto′me-əl) pertaining or relating to the peristome or to the area around the cytostome of ciliate protozoa.

**peri·stru·mi·tis** (per″ĭ-stroo-mi′tis) inflammation extending from an inflamed goiter to the surrounding structures.

**peri·stru·mous** (per″ĭ-stroo′məs) around or near a goiter.

**peri·syl·vi·an** (per″-ĭ-sil′ve-ən) near the sylvian fissure (sulcus lateralis cerebri).

**peri·sy·no·vi·al** (per″ĭ-sĭ-no-ve′əl) around a synovial structure.

**peri·syr·in·gi·tis** (per″ĭ-sir″in-ji′tis) inflammation of tissues around ducts of the sweat glands.

**peri·tec·to·my** (per″ĭ-tek′tə-me) [*peri-* + *ectomy*] excision of a ring of conjunctiva behind the limbus, followed by cauterization of the trench thus made.

**peri·ten·din·e·um** (per″ĭ-tən-din′e-əm) the connective tissue investing larger tendons and extending as septa between the fibers composing them.

**peri·ten·di·ni·tis** (per″ĭ-ten″dĭ-ni′tis) tenosynovitis.
**p. calca′rea,** a painful condition marked by calcareous deposits in tendons and in peritendinous, capsular, and ligamentous tissues.
**p. cre′pitans,** tenosynovitis crepitans.
**p. sero′sa,** ganglion (def. 3).

**peri·ten·di·nous** (per″ĭ-ten′dĭ-nəs) around a tendon.

**peri·te·non** (per″ĭ-te′non) [*peri-* + Gr. *tenōn* tendon] the connective tissue structures associated with a tendon.

**peri·ten·o·ne·um** (per″ĭ-ten″o-ne′əm) the loose connective tissue covering the surface of tendons and ligaments and penetrating inside to separate the substance into bundles.

**peri·ten·o·ni·tis** (per″ĭ-ten″o-ni′tis) tenosynovitis.

**peri·ten·on·ti·tis** (per″ĭ-ten″on-ti′tis) tenosynovitis.

**peri·the·ci·um** (per″ĭ-the′se-əm) [*peri-* + Gr. *thēkē* case] the flask-shaped fruiting body of certain molds and ascomycetous fungi (see *ascocarp*) having a pore for the escape of spores.

**peri·the·li·al** (per″ĭ-the′le-əl) pertaining to the perithelium.

**peri·the·li·o·ma** (per″ĭ-the″le-o′mə) hemangiopericytoma.

**peri·the·li·um** (per″ĭ-the′le-əm) [*peri-* + *thelium*] the layer of connective tissue that surrounds the capillaries and smaller vessels.
**Eberth's p.,** a partial layer of cells on the external surface of the capillaries.

**peri·tho·rac·ic** (per″ĭ-thə-ras′ik) surrounding the thorax.

**peri·thy·roi·di·tis** (per″ĭ-thi″roi-di′tis) inflammation of the thyroid capsule.

**pe·rit·o·mist** (pə-rit′ə-mist) one who performs peritomy (circumcision).

**pe·rit·o·my** (pə-rit′ə-me) [*peri-* + *-tomy*] 1. surgical incision of the conjunctiva and subconjunctival tissue about the whole circumference of the cornea; usually done as part of enucleation and retinal detachment procedure. 2. circumcision.

**peritone(o)-** [L. *peritoneum,* q.v.] a combining form denoting relationship to the peritoneum.

**peri·to·ne·al** (per″ĭ-to-ne′əl) pertaining to the peritoneum.

**peri·to·ne·al·gia** (per″ĭ-to″ne-al′jə) pain in the peritoneum.

**peri·to·ne·al·ize** (per″ĭ-to-ne′əl-īz) to cover with peritoneum.

**peri·to·neo·cen·te·sis** (per″ĭ-to″ne-o-sən-te′sis) [*peritoneo-* + *-centesis*] puncture of the peritoneal cavity with a needle for the purpose of obtaining fluid.

**peri·to·neo·cly·sis** (per″ĭ-to″ne-o-kli′sis) injection of water or other fluids into the peritoneal cavity.

**peri·to·ne·og·ra·phy** (per″ĭ-to″ne-og′rə-fe) radiography of the peritoneum.

**peri·to·neo·mus·cu·lar** (per″ĭ-to-ne″o-mus′ku-lər) pertaining to or composed of peritoneum and muscle.

**peri·to·ne·op·a·thy** (per″ĭ-to-ne-op′ə-the) [*peritoneo-* + *-pathy*] any disease of the peritoneum.

**peri·to·neo·peri·car·di·al** (per″ĭ-to-ne″o-per″ĭ-kahr′de-əl) pertaining to the peritoneum and pericardium.

**peri·to·neo·pexy** (per″ĭ-to′ne-o-pek″se) [*peritoneo-* + *-pexy*] fixation of the uterus by the vaginal route.

**peri·to·neo·plas·ty** (per″ĭ-to′ne-o-plas″te) [*peritoneo-* + *-plasty*] the operation of covering denuded areas of abdominal viscera or of the abdominal cavity with peritoneum; peritonization.

**peri·to·neo·scope** (per″ĭ-to′ne-o-skōp″) laparoscope.

**peri·to·ne·os·co·py** (per″ĭ-to″ne-os′kə-pe) laparoscopy.

**peri·to·neo·tome** (per″ĭ-to-ne′o-tōm) an area of the peritoneum supplied with afferent nerve fibers by a single posterior root.

**peri·to·ne·ot·o·my** (per″ĭ-to″ne-ot′ə-me) celiotomy.

**peri·to·neo·ve·nous** (per″ĭ-to-ne″o-ve′nəs) communicating with the peritoneal cavity and the venous system; see under *shunt.*

**peri·to·ne·um** (per″ĭ-to-ne′əm) [L., from Gr. *peritonaion,* from *per* around + *teinein* to stretch] [TA] [MeSH: Peritoneum] the serous membrane lining the abdominopelvic walls *(parietal p.)* and investing the viscera *(visceral p.).* A strong, colorless membrane with a smooth surface, it forms a double-layered sac that is closed in the male and is continuous with the mucous membrane of the uterine tubes in the female. The potential space between the parietal and visceral peritoneum is called the *peritoneal cavity* (see *cavitas peritonealis* [TA]).
**abdominal p.,** p. parietale.
**intestinal p.,** p. viscerale.
**p. parieta′le** [TA], parietal peritoneum: the peritoneum that lines the abdominal and pelvic walls and the inferior surface of the thoracic diaphragm.
**p. urogenita′le** [TA], urogenital peritoneum: the peritoneum lining the urogenital structures in the lower pelvis.
**p. viscera′le** [TA], visceral peritoneum: a continuation of the parietal peritoneum reflected at various places over the viscera, forming a complete covering for the stomach, spleen, liver, ascending portion of the duodenum, jejunum, ileum, transverse colon, sigmoid flexure, upper end of rectum, uterus, and ovaries; it also partially covers the descending and transverse portions of the duodenum, the cecum, ascending and descending colon, the middle part of the rectum, the posterior wall of the bladder, and the upper portion of the vagina. It holds the viscera in position by its folds, some of which form the *mesenteries,* connecting portions of the intestine with the posterior abdominal wall; other folds, the *omenta,* are attached to the stomach; and still others form the *ligaments* of the liver, spleen, stomach, kidneys, bladder, and uterus. The potential space between the visceral and the parietal peritoneum is the peritoneal cavity, which consists of the *pelvic peritoneal cavity* below and the *general peritoneal cavity* above. The general cavity communicates by the epiploic foramen with the cavity of the greater omentum, which is also known as the *lesser peritoneal cavity.*

**peri·to·nism** (per′ĭ-to-niz-əm) a condition of shock simulating peritonitis, but without inflammation of the peritoneum.

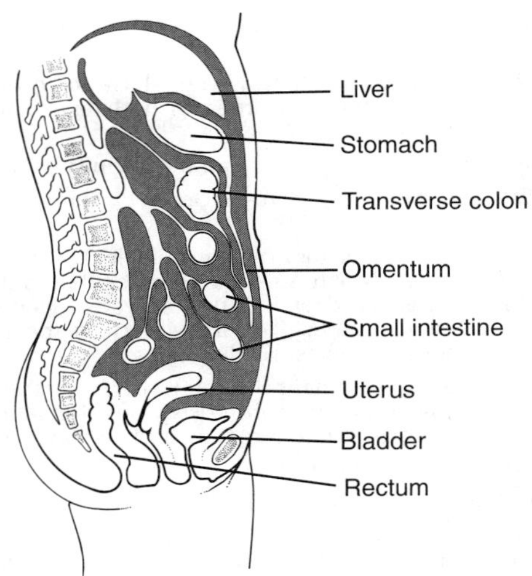


Course of the peritoneum (enclosing shaded area) in a median sagittal section of a female.

**peri·to·ni·tis** (per″ĭ-to-ni′tis) [MeSH: Peritonitis] inflammation of the peritoneum, with exudations of serum, fibrin, cells, and pus, usually accompanied by abdominal pain and tenderness, constipation, vomiting, and moderate fever.
**adhesive p.,** a type characterized by adhesions between adjacent serous surfaces.
**bacterial p.,** peritonitis caused by a bacterial infection, usually with species of *Staphylococcus, Pseudomonas,* or *Mycobacterium.*
**benign paroxysmal p.,** familial Mediterranean fever.
**bile p., biliary p.,** choleperitoneum.
***Candida* p.,** that caused by a species of *Candida,* generally seen as a complication of peritoneal dialysis; symptoms include abdominal pain with or without mild fever, nausea, and vomiting.
**chemical p.,** peritonitis due to chemical irritation.
**p. chro′nica fibro′sa encap′sulans,** a chronic peritonitis marked by the formation on the intestine of a white coating of fibrous tissue undergoing hyaline degeneration; called also *iced intestine* and *zuckergussdarm.*
**circumscribed p.,** a type limited to a portion of the peritoneum. Called also *localized p.*
**p. defor′mans,** a chronic type with shortening of the mesentery so that the intestines are drawn up in loops toward the spine.
**diaphragmatic p.,** a type affecting the peritoneal surface of the diaphragm.
**diffuse p.,** general p.
**p. encap′sulans, encysted p.,** peritoneal abscess.
**feline infectious p.,** a usually fatal contagious viral disease of domestic cats and other felines, caused by a coronavirus; characteristics include slow onset, persistent fever, and varying effects of peritonitis such as pleural or peritoneal effusions and granulomas.
**fibrocaseous p.,** tuberculous peritonitis with fibrous and caseous degeneration.
**fungal p.,** peritonitis caused by a fungus, usually seen as a complication of peritoneal dialysis, although it may be seen following abdominal surgery. The most common type is *Candida* p.
**gas p.,** peritonitis with accumulation of gas in the peritoneum.
**general p.,** inflammation of the greater part of the peritoneum. Called also *diffuse p.*
**hemorrhagic p.,** peritonitis accompanied by hemorrhagic effusion.
**localized p.,** circumscribed p.
**meconium p.,** peritonitis resulting from perforation of the bowel into the peritoneal cavity *in utero* or shortly after birth, resulting in escape of meconium into the peritoneal cavity; it occurs most often as a complication of meconium ileus in fibrocystic disease of the pancreas.
**pelvic p.,** 1. perimetritis. 2. peritonitis situated in the pelvis.
**perforative p.,** a type due to a perforation in the digestive tract.
**periodic p.,** familial Mediterranean fever.
**puerperal p.,** peritonitis following childbirth.
**purulent p.,** peritonitis with the formation of pus.
**sclerosing p.,** any of several rare complications of long-term peritoneal dialysis; the peritoneum becomes either opaque or tan, wrinkled, and dry. Severe forms, which are often fatal, include formation of a fibrous sac around the small intestine *(sclerosing encapsulating peritonitis),* intestinal obstruction, and calcification of the peritoneum. Called also *peritoneal sclerosis.*
**sclerosing encapsulating p.,** sclerosing peritonitis with formation of a fibrous sac around the intestine; it often progresses to fatal necrosis or obstruction.
**septic p.,** that which is due to a pyogenic microorganism.
**serous p.,** a type accompanied by a copious liquid exudation.
**silent p.,** peritonitis that is asymptomatic.
**spontaneous bacterial p.,** bacterial infection of ascitic fluid without evidence of an intra-abdominal source of infection; seen as a complication of cirrhosis.
**terminal p.,** primary peritonitis in the late stages of a wasting disease.
**traumatic p.,** simple acute peritonitis due to trauma.
**tuberculous p.,** a type of bacterial peritonitis caused by *Mycobacterium tuberculosis.*

**peri·to·ni·za·tion** (per″ĭ-to-nĭ-za′shən) the operation of covering a denuded surface of an abdominal organ or the abdominal wall with peritoneum; peritoneoplasty.

**peri·to·nize** (per′ĭ-to-nīz) to cover with peritoneum.

**peri·ton·sil·lar** (per″ĭ-ton′sĭ-lər) situated around a tonsil.

**peri·ton·sil·li·tis** (per″ĭ-ton″sĭ-li′tis) inflammation of the peritonsillar tissues.

**peri·tra·che·al** (per″ĭ-tra′ke-əl) situated around the trachea.

**Per·i·trate** (per′ĭ-trāt) trademark for preparations of pentaerythritol tetranitrate.

**peri·trich** (per′ĭ-trik) 1. any ciliate protozoan of the subclass Peritrichia. 2. peritrichous.

**Peri·trich·ia** (per″ĭ-trik′e-ə) [*peri-* + Gr. *thrix* hair] a subclass of typically cone-shaped, ciliate protozoa (class Oligohymenophorea, phylum Ciliophora), characterized by the presence of a prominent oral ciliary field covering the apical end of the body and spiraling counterclockwise into the infundibulum, a paroral membrane and adoral membranelles that become peniculi, and much reduced somatic ciliature. Many are stalked and sedentary, and others are mobile, all with an aboral scopula. The free-swimming larvae have a locomotory posterior ciliary girdle. It comprises one order: Peritrichida.

**Peri·trich·i·da** (per″ĭ-trik′ĭ-də) an order of ciliate protozoa (subclass Peritrichia, class Oligohymenophorea) having characters of the subclass. It comprises two suborders: Sessilina and Mobilina.

**pe·rit·ri·chous** (pə-rit′rĭ-kəs) [*peri-* + *trich-* + *-ous*] 1. having flagella over the entire surface; said of a bacterial cell; see *flagellum.* 2. of flagella, occurring over the entire surface of a bacterial cell. 3. having cilia around the cytostome only; said of Ciliophora. Called also *peritrich.*

**peri·tro·chan·ter·ic** (per″ĭ-tro″kan-ter′ik) situated about a trochanter.

**peri·typh·lic** (per″ĭ-tif′lik) [*peri-* + *typhl-* + *-ic*] around the cecum; pericecal.

**peri·typh·li·tis** (per″ĭ-tif-li′tis) [*peri-* + *typhl-* + *-itis*] inflammation of the peritoneum surrounding the cecum; appendicitis.
**p. actinomyco′tica,** actinomycosis whose principal seat is pericecal.

**peri·um·bil·i·cal** (per″e-əm-bil′ĭ-kəl) situated around the umbilicus.

**peri·un·gual** (per″e-ung′gwəl) around the nail.

**peri·ure·ter·al** (per″ĭ-u-re′tər-əl) around the ureter.

**peri·ure·ter·ic** (per″ĭ-u″rə-ter′ik) about the ureter.

**peri·ure·ter·itis** (per″ĭ-u-re″tər-i′tis) [*peri-* + *ureter-* + *-itis*] inflammation of the tissues around a ureter.

**peri·ure·thral** (per″ĭ-u-re′thrəl) occurring around the urethra.

**peri·ure·thri·tis** (per″ĭ-u″re-thri′tis) [*peri-* + *urethr-* + *-itis*] inflammation of the tissues around the urethra; spongiitis.

**peri·uter·ine** (per″ĭ-u′tər-in) around the uterus.

**peri·vag·i·nal** (per″ĭ-vaj′ĭ-nəl) around the vagina.

**peri·vag·i·ni·tis** (per″ĭ-vaj″ĭ-ni′tis) pericolpitis.

**peri·vas·cu·lar** (per″ĭ-vas′ku-lər) near a vessel.

**peri·vas·cu·lar·i·ty** (per″ĭ-vas′ku-lar′ĭ-te) an infiltrate of cellular elements of mesodermal origin (polymorphonuclear leukocytes, lymphocytes, etc.) in the perivascular spaces, as in those of the cerebral parenchyma.

**peri·vas·cu·li·tis** (per″ĭ-vas″ku-li′tis) periangiitis.

**peri·ve·nous** (per″ĭ-ve′nəs) around a vein.

**peri·ven·tric·u·lar** (per″ĭ-vən-trik′u-lər) around a ventricle; see also under *system.*

**peri·ver·te·bral** (per″ĭ-ver′tə-brəl) around a vertebra.

**peri·ves·i·cal** (per″ĭ-ves′ĭ-kəl) [*peri-* + *vesic-* + *-al*[1]] occurring around the bladder.

**peri·ve·sic·u·lar** (per″ĭ-və-sik′u-lər) around a seminal vesicle.

**peri·ve·sic·u·li·tis** (per″ĭ-və-sik″u-li′tis) inflammation of tissue around the seminal vesicle.

**peri·vis·cer·al** (per″ĭ-vis′ər-əl) occurring around a viscus or the viscera.

**peri·vis·cer·itis** (per″ĭ-vis″ər-i′tis) inflammation around a viscus or around the viscera.

**peri·vi·tel·line** (per″ĭ-vi-tel′īn) situated around a vitellus or yolk.

**peri·win·kle** (per′ĭ-wing″kəl) 1. any of several woody herbs of the genus *Vinca*. 2. *Vinca rosea*.
**Madagascar p.,** *Vinca rosea*.
**minor p.,** *Vinca minor*.

**per·lèche** (per-lesh′) [Fr.] single or multiple fissures at the corners of the mouth, which may be unilateral or bilateral and may spread to the lips and cheeks. It may be due to a primary or superimposed infection, such as with *Candida albicans,* staphylococci, or streptococci; poor hygiene; drooling of saliva; overclosure of the jaws in edentulous patients or those with ill-fitting dentures; ariboflavinosis; or other causes. Called also *angular cheilitis, cheilosis,* or *stomatitis, migrating cheilitis,* and *intertrigo labialis.*

**Per·lia's nucleus** (per′le-ahz) [Richard *Perlia,* German ophthalmologist, late 19th century] see under *nucleus.*

**Perl·man syndrome** (pərl′mən) [M. *Perlman,* Israeli physician, 20th century] see under *syndrome.*

**Perls' test (stain)** (perlz) [Max *Perls,* German pathologist, 1843–1881] see under *test.*

**per·ma·nence** (pər′mə-nens) the quality or condition of lasting without essential change.
**object p.,** the concept, usually appreciated during the second year of life, that an object continues to exist even when removed from view.

**per·man·ga·nate** (pər-mang′gə-nāt) the $MnO_4^-$ anion, which has a deep purple color in aqueous solution and is a strong oxidizing agent, or a salt containing this ion.

**per·man·gan·ic ac·id** (per″mang-gan′ik) an unstable strong acid and oxidizing agent, $HMnO_4$, existing only in aqueous solution; its salts are permanganates.

**per·me·a·bil·i·ty** (per″me-ə-bil′ĭ-te) [MeSH: Permeability] the property or state of being permeable; see also *osmosis.*

**per·me·a·ble** (per′me-ə-bəl) [L. *per* through + *meare* to pass] not impassable; pervious; permitting passage of a substance.

**per·me·ase** (pər′me-ās) former term for transport protein.

**per·me·ate** (per′me-āt″) 1. to penetrate or pass through, as through a filter. 2. the constituents of a solution or suspension that pass through a filter.

**per·me·a·tion** (per″me-a′shən) the act of spreading through or penetrating a substance, tissue, or organ, as by a disease process, such as cancer.

**per·meth·rin** (pər-meth′rin) a pyrethroid insecticide applied topically in the treatment of infestations by *Pediculus humanus capitis, Sarcoptes scabiei,* and various species of ticks. In veterinary medicine, used in ear tags for cattle to combat biting flies and in flea collars for cats and dogs.

**Per·mi·til** (per′mĭ-til) trademark for a preparation of fluphenazine hydrochloride.

**perm·se·lec·tiv·i·ty** (pərm″-sə-lek-tiv′ĭ-te) restriction of the permeation of macromolecule across a glomerular capillary wall. A major factor is molecule size relative to the size of the pores through the wall; other important factors include the electrical charge of the molecule versus that of the wall or pore and the physical configuration of the molecule.

**per·na** (per′nə) a chlorinated naphthalene, which may cause a serious acne in persons handling it.

**per·na·sal** (pər-na′səl) [*per-* + *nasal*] performed through the nose.

**per·nic·i·o·si·form** (per-nish″e-o′sĭ-form) seemingly pernicious; a term applied to a condition which is apparently, but not actually, pernicious or malignant.

**per·ni·cious** (pər-nish′əs) [L. *perniciosus*] harmful; tending towards a fatal outcome.

**per·nio** (per′ne-o) pl. *pernio′nes* [L.] chilblain.

**pero-** [Gr. *pēros* maimed] a combining form meaning deformed.

**pe·ro·bra·chi·us** (pe″ro-bra′ke-əs) [*pero-* + Gr. *brachiōn* arm] a fetus with deformed arms.

**pe·ro·ceph·a·lus** (pe″ro-sef′ə-ləs) [*pero-* + *-cephalus*] strophocephalus.

**pe·ro·chi·rus** (pe″ro-ki′rəs) [*pero-* + Gr. *cheir* hand] a fetus with malformed hands.

**pe·ro·cor·mus** (pe″ro-kor′məs) [*pero-* + Gr. *kormos* trunk] perosomus.

**pe·ro·dac·ty·lus** (pe″ro-dak′tə-ləs) [*pero-* + Gr. *daktylos* finger] a fetus with deformity of fingers or toes, or both, especially absence of one or more digits.

**pe·ro·me·lia** (per″o-me′le-ə) congenital deformity of the limbs.

**pe·rom·e·lus** (pe-rom′ə-ləs) [*pero-* + Gr. *melos* limb] a fetus with malformed limbs.

**Pe·ro·mys·cus** (pe″ro-mis′kəs) a genus of mice. *P. leu′copus* is the white-footed mouse, a North American species that is the primary reservoir for the eastern deer tick that spreads Lyme disease. *P. manicula′tus* is the deer mouse, a North American species that is a reservoir for various disease-spreading ticks.

**pero·nar·thro·sis** (per″o-nahr-thro′sis) [Gr. *peronē* anything pointed for piercing or pinning + *arthrosis*] an articulation in which the surfaces are convex in one direction and concave in the other.

**per·o·ne** (pər-o′ne) the fibula.

**per·o·ne·al** (per″o-ne′əl) 1. fibular. 2. pertaining to the outer side of the leg.

**pe·ro·ne·a·lis** (pə-ro″ne-a′lis) peroneal; TA alternative for *fibularis.*

**pe·ro·neo·tib·i·al** (per″o-ne″o-tib′e-əl) tibiofibular.

**pe·ro·nia** (pe-ro′ne-ə) [Gr. *pēros* maimed] developmental anomaly.

**Pe·ro·no·spo·ral·es** (per″o-no-spə-ra′lēz) [Gr. *peronē* pin + *spora* seed] an order of funguslike organisms of the class Oomycetes, saprobes and plant parasites that reproduce asexually by zoospores and conidia and sexually by oospores. Animal pathogens are included in the family Pythiaceae.

**Per. op. emet.** abbreviation for L. *perac′ta operatio′ne emet′ici,* when the action of the emetic is over.

**pe·ro·pus** (pe′ro-pəs) [*pero-* + Gr. *pous* foot] a fetus with malformed legs and feet.

**per·oral** (pər-or′əl) [*per-* + *oral*] performed through or administered through the mouth.

**per os** (pər os) [L.] by mouth.

**pe·ro·sis** (pə-ro′sis) a disease of chicks marked by bone deformities, associated with deficiency of dietary factors such as choline and manganese.

**pe·ro·so·mus** (pe″ro-so′məs) [*pero-* + Gr. *sōma* body] a fetus with greatly deformed body or trunk.

**pe·ro·splanch·nia** (pe″ro-splank′ne-ə) [*pero-* + *splanchn-* + *-ia*] a developmental anomaly characterized by malformation of the viscera.

**per·os·se·ous** (pər-os′e-əs) [*per-* + *osseous*] transmitted through bone.

**pe·rot·ic** (pə-rot′ik) pertaining to or characterized by perosis.

**per·ox·i·dase** (pər-ok′sĭ-dās) [MeSH: Peroxidase] a term used in the recommended names of enzymes of the oxidoreductase class that catalyze the oxidation of organic substrates by hydrogen peroxide, which is reduced to water. [EC 1.11] These enzymes are heme proteins, found frequently in plants and occasionally in animal tissues.

**per·ox·ide** (pər-ok′sīd) that oxide of any element which contains more oxygen than any other. More correctly applied to compounds

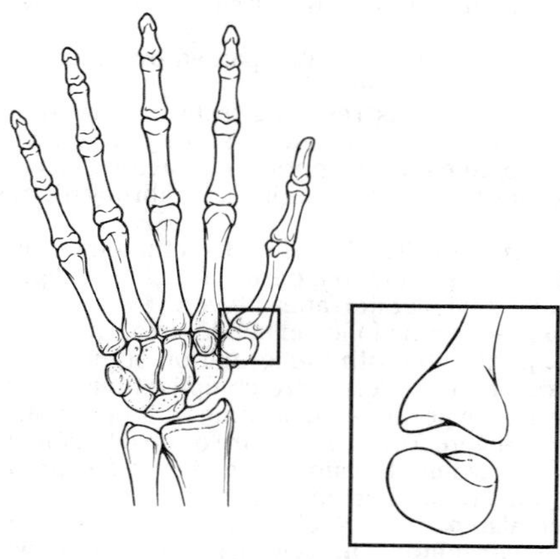
Peronarthrosis.

having such linkage as —O—O—; for instance, hydrogen peroxide, H—O—O—H.

**per·ox·i·some** (pər-ok′sĭ-sōm) [MeSH: Microbodies] 1. any of the microbodies present in vertebrate animal cells, especially liver and kidney cells, which are rich in the enzymes peroxidase, catalase, D-amino acid oxidase, and, to a lesser extent, urate oxidase; their functions are not fully understood, but they participate in metabolic oxidations involving hydrogen peroxide, purine metabolism, cellular lipid metabolism, and gluconeogenesis. Similar structures *(glyoxysomes),)* containing the enzymes of the glyoxylate cycle, are found in certain plants and microorganisms. 2. microbody.

**peroxy-** a prefix indicating the substitution of —O—O— for —O—, as in peroxyacetic acid.

**per·oxy·ace·tic ac·id** (pər-ok″se-ə-se′tik) peracetic acid.

**per·oxy·dol** (pər-ok′sĭ-dol) sodium perborate.

**per·phen·a·zine** (pər-fen′ə-zēn) [USP] [MeSH: Perphenazine] a phenothiazine antipsychotic agent used orally and intramuscularly as an antipsychotic agent and also used as an antiemetic.

**per pri·mam** (pər pri′məm) [L.] see *per primam intentionem.*

**per pri·mam in·ten·ti·o·nem** (pər pri′məm in-ten″she-o′nəm) [L.] by first intention; see under *healing.*

**per rec·tum** (pər rek′təm) [L.] by way of the rectum.

**Per·rin-Fer·ra·ton disease** (pə-ră′-fer″ə-taw′) [Maurice *Perrin,* French surgeon, 1826–1889; Louis *Ferraton,* French surgeon, born 1860] snapping hip.

**Per·ron·ci·to's apparatus (spirals)** (per″on-che′tōz) [Aldo *Perroncito,* Italian histologist, 1882–1929] see under *apparatus.*

**Per·ry bag** (per′e) [Murle *Perry,* American colostomy patient, 20th century] see under *bag.*

**per·salt** (per′sawlt) a salt of a peracid; a salt the acid radical of which has a higher valence than the protosalt.

**per sal·tum** (pər sawl′təm) [L.] by a leap or bound; denoting a sudden evolutionary development without intermediate stages.

**Per·san·tine** (pər-san′tēn) trademark for preparations of dipyridamole.

**per se·cun·dam** (pər se-kun′dəm) [L.] see *per secundam intentionem.*

**per se·cun·dam in·ten·ti·o·nem** (pər se-kun′dəm in-ten″she-o′nəm) [L.] by second intention; see under *healing.*

**per·sev·er·a·tion** (pər-sev″ər-a′shən) the inappropriate persistence or repetition of a thought or act after the causative stimulus has ceased or in response to different stimuli, e.g., answering a question correctly and then inappropriately repeating that answer to succeeding questions; most often associated with brain lesions but also seen in schizophrenia.

**per·sis·tence** (pər-sis′təns) continuation of a behavior or characteristic at a time when it would normally be expected to have disappeared.

**hereditary p. of fetal hemoglobin,** continued production of fetal hemoglobin beyond the point when it is normally replaced by hemoglobin A. Heterozygotes are asymptomatic, while homozygotes have hypochromic microcytic erythrocytes and may have a mild type of thalassemia.

**per·sis·ter** (pər-sis′tər) [L. *persistere* persist, from *per* through + *sistere* to stand still] in bacteriology, a microorganism that resists a generally toxic level of a drug but is not genetically resistant.

**per·so·na** (pər-so′nə) [L. "mask"] in jungian psychology, the personality mask or facade presented by a person to the world, as opposed to the *anima,* the inner being.

**per·so·nal·i·ty** (per″sə-nal′ĭ-te) [MeSH: Personality] the characteristic way that a person thinks, feels, and behaves; the relatively stable and predictable part of a person's thought and behavior; it includes conscious attitudes, values, and styles as well as unconscious conflicts and defense mechanisms. See also under *disorder, trait,* and *type.*

**alternating p.,** dissociative identity disorder.

**anancastic p.,** obsessive-compulsive p. (disorder).

**antisocial p. (disorder)** [DSM-IV], a personality disorder characterized by continuous and chronic antisocial behavior in which the rights of others or generally accepted social norms are violated; associated personality traits include impulsiveness, egocentricity, inability to tolerate boredom or frustration, irritability and aggressiveness, recklessness, disregard for truth, and inability to maintain consistent, responsible functioning at work, at school, or as a parent. The concept of a personality disorder that predisposes an individual toward criminality has a long history. Among the terms that have been applied to this disorder are *moral insanity, psychopathic personality,* and *sociopathic personality.*

**as-if p.,** one resembling normalcy but lacking real, enduring emotion, the person adopting and appearing to express ordinary characteristics but then able to summarily discard them and adopt others as situations change.

**avoidant p. (disorder)** [DSM-IV], a personality disorder characterized by social discomfort, hypersensitivity to criticism, low self-esteem, and an aversion to activities that involve significant interpersonal contact; there is a proclivity to anxiety, an exaggeration of difficulties, a desire for affection and acceptance that is restrained for fear of rejection, and an avoidance of risks or new activities for fear of embarrassment.

**borderline p. (disorder)** [DSM-IV], a personality disorder marked by a pervasive instability of mood, self-image or sense of self, and interpersonal relationships; impulsive and self-damaging acts are common, as are uncontrolled anger, fears of abandonment, chronic feelings of emptiness, recurrent self-mutilating behavior and suicide threats, and transient, stress-induced periods of paranoia and dissociation.

**compulsive p.,** obsessive-compulsive p. (disorder).

**cyclothymic p.,** a temperament characterized by rapid, frequent swings between sad and cheerful moods. See also *cyclothymic disorder,* under *disorder.*

**dependent p. (disorder)** [DSM-IV], a personality disorder marked by an excessive need to be taken care of, with submissiveness and clinging and preoccupation with fears of being abandoned; features include need for advice and reassurance in decision making, yielding of responsibility, initiative, and independence, avoidance of disagreement for fear of loss of support, voluntarily undertaking unpleasant tasks to ensure further care, and discomfort or helpless feelings when alone, with an indiscriminate rush to a new relationship.

**depressive p. (disorder),** a personality disorder characterized by a persistent and pervasive pattern of depressive cognitions and behaviors, such as chronic unhappiness, low self-esteem, pessimism, critical and derogatory attitudes toward oneself and others, feelings of guilt or remorse, and an inability to relax or feel enjoyment.

**double p., dual p.,** dissociative identity disorder.

**histrionic p. (disorder)** [DSM-IV], a personality disorder marked by excessive emotionality and attention-seeking behavior; there is overconcern with physical attractiveness, sexual seductiveness, intolerance of delayed gratification, and rapid shifting and shallow expression of emotions.

**hysterical p.,** former name for *histrionic p.*

**multiple p. (disorder),** dissociative identity disorder.

**narcissistic p. (disorder)** [DSM-IV], a personality disorder characterized by grandiosity (in fantasy or behavior), a lack of social empathy combined with a hypersensitivity to the judgment of others, interpersonal exploitiveness, enviousness, arrogance, a sense of entitlement, and a need for constant signs of admiration.

**negativistic p. (disorder),** passive-aggressive p. (disorder)

**obsessive p.,** obsessive-compulsive p. (disorder).

**obsessive-compulsive p. (disorder)** [DSM IV], a personality disorder characterized by an emotionally constricted manner that is unduly conventional, serious, rigid, stubborn, and stingy, by preoccupation with trivial details, rules, order, organization, schedules, and lists to the extent that the major point of an activity is lost or task completion is delayed, by reluctance to delegate tasks or work cooperatively unless everything is done one's own way, and by excessive devotion to work and productivity to the detriment of interpersonal relationships. This is not the same as *obsessive-compulsive disorder,* which is an anxiety disorder.

**paranoid p. (disorder)** [DSM-IV], a personality disorder marked by a view of other people as hostile, devious, and untrustworthy and a combative response to disappointments or to events experienced as rebuffs or humiliations. Notable are a questioning of the loyalty of friends, the bearing of grudges, a tendency to read threatening meanings into benign remarks, and unfounded suspicions of the fidelity of a partner. Unlike delusional disorder or paranoid schizophrenia, in which delusional or hallucinatory persecution occurs, it is not characterized by psychosis.

**passive-aggressive p. (disorder),** a personality disorder characterized by an indirect resistance to demands for adequate social and occupational performance, such as by obstructionism, procrastination, or forgetfulness, and by negative, defeatist attitudes.

**sadistic p. (disorder),** a pervasive pattern of cruel, demeaning, and aggressive behavior; satisfaction is gained in intimidating, coercing, humiliating, and inflicting pain and suffering on others.

**schizoid p. (disorder)** [DSM-IV], a personality disorder marked by detachment from social relationships and a restricted range of emotional experience and expression. Qualifying characteristics include lack of capacity for, or interest in, social relationships or family life, coldness, aloofness, consistent preference for solitary activities, lack of pleasure in activities, flattened affectivity, and indifference to praise, criticism, or the feelings of others.

**schizotypal p. (disorder)** [DSM-IV], a personality disorder characterized by marked deficits in social and interpersonal competence

and eccentricities in ideation, appearance, and behavior; ideas of reference are common, as are odd beliefs or magical thinking, cognitive or perceptual distortions, little capability or desire for close relationships, excessive social anxiety, suspiciousness, and occasional paranoid ideation. It differs from schizophrenia, to which it is related, in having only transient psychotic episodes, if any.
**seclusive p., shut-in p.,** former name for *schizoid p.*
**self-defeating p. (disorder),** a persistent pattern of behavior detrimental to the self, including being drawn to problematic situations or relationships, failing to accomplish tasks crucial to life objectives, excessive self-sacrifice, inviting criticism and anger, undermining of pleasurable experiences, and inability to enjoy the rewards of success.
**split p.,** an obsolete term formerly used colloquially for either schizophrenia or dissociative identity disorder.

**per·son·o·log·ic** (per″sən-ə-loj′ik) pertaining to personology.

**per·so·nol·o·gy** (per″sə-nol′ə-je) the holistic study of personality, seeking understanding of the aspects of a person through knowledge of the whole.

**per·spi·ra·tio** (per″spĭ-ra′she-o) [L.] perspiration.
**p. insensi′bilis,** insensible perspiration.

**per·spi·ra·tion** (per″spĭ-ra′shən) [L. *perspira′re* to breathe through] 1. sweating; the functional secretion of sweat. 2. sweat.
**insensible p.,** those evaporative losses of water from the moist surfaces of the body (such as the skin and respiratory tree) not due to the secretory activity of glands.
**sensible p.,** perspiration due to secretory activity of sweat glands.

**per·sua·sion** (pər-swa′zhən) in psychiatry, a therapeutic approach based on direct suggestion and guidance intended to influence favorably attitudes, behavior, and goals.

**per·sul·fate** (pər-sul′fāt) a salt of persulfuric acid.

**per·sul·fide** (pər-sul′fīd) a sulfide which contains more sulfur than the ordinary sulfide.

**per·sul·fur·ic acid** (per″səl-fūr′ik) peroxymonosulfuric acid, $H_2SO_5$, a strong oxidizing agent.

**per·tech·ne·tate** (pər-tek′nə-tāt) a salt or ester containing the ion $TcO_4^-$; see under *technetium* and *uptake.*

**Per·thes′ disease, test** (per′təz) [Georg Clemens *Perthes,* German surgeon, 1869–1927] see *osteochondrosis,* and see *tourniquet test,* under *tests.*

**Per·tik′s diverticulum** (per′tiks) [Otto *Pertik,* Hungarian physician, 1852–1913] see under *diverticulum.*

**Per·to·frane** (per′to-frān) trademark for a preparation of desipramine hydrochloride.

**per tu·bam** (pər too′bəm) [L.] through a tube.

**per·tu·ba·tion** (per″too-ba′shən) perflation or insufflation of the uterine tubes to render them patent.

**per·tu·cin** (pər-tu′sin) a bacteriocin produced by *Pseudomonas pertucinogena* that inhibits the growth of *Bordetella pertussis.*

**per·tus·sis** (pər-tus′is) [L. *per* intensive + *tussis*] an acute, highly contagious infection of the respiratory tract, usually affecting young children and caused by *Bordetella pertussis;* similar illnesses are caused by *B. parapertussis* and *B. bronchiseptica.* It is characterized by a *catarrhal stage,* beginning after an incubation period of about two weeks, with slight fever, sneezing, runny nose, and dry cough. After one or two weeks the *paroxysmal stage* begins and lasts three to four weeks; it has the characteristic paroxysmal cough, consisting of a deep inspiration, followed by a series of quick, short coughs that continue until the air is expelled from the lungs and end with a long shrill, whooping inspiration, due to spasmodic closure of the glottis. Finally there is the *convalescent stage,* in which paroxysms diminish and finally cease. See also *parapertussis,* and see *pertussis-like syndrome,* under *syndrome.* Called also *whooping cough.*

**per·tus·soid** (pər-tus′oid) [*pertussis* + *-oid*] resembling pertussis.

**per va·gi·nam** (pər və-ji′nəm) through the vagina.

**per·ver·sion** (pər-ver′zhən) [*per-* + *version*] 1. a turning aside from the normal course; a morbid alteration of function which may occur in emotional, intellectual, or volitional fields. 2. sexual p.; see under *deviation.*

**per·vi·ous** (per′ve-əs) [L. *pervius*] permeable.

**pes** (pes) gen. *pe′dis* pl. *pe′des* [L.] 1. [TA] foot (def. 1). 2. any footlike part.
**p. abduc′tus,** a deformed foot in which the anterior part is displaced so that it lies laterally to the vertical axis of the leg.
**p. adduc′tus,** a deformed foot in which the anterior part is displaced so that it lies medially to the vertical axis of the leg.
**p. anseri′nus** [L. "goose's foot"], 1. plexus intraparotideus. 2. the combined insertion of the tendinous expansions of the sartorius, gracilis, and semitendinosus muscles.

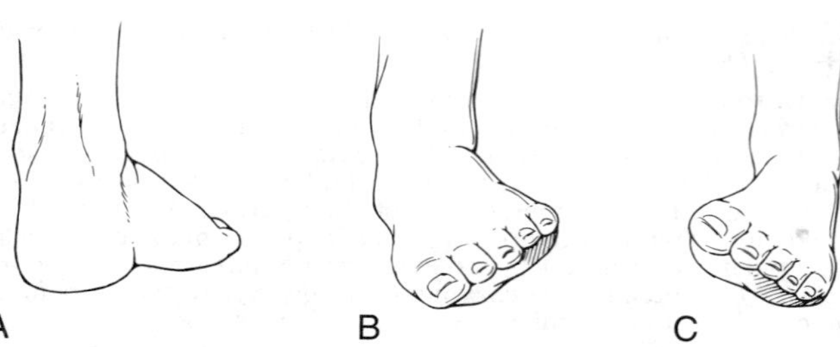

*(A),* Pes abductus; *(B),* pes pronatus; *(C),* pes supinatus.

**p. calcaneoca′vus,** see under *talipes.*
**p. cavova′rus,** see under *talipes.*
**p. ca′vus,** see under *talipes.*
**p. equinoval′gus,** talipes equinovalgus.
**p. equinova′rus,** talipes equinovarus.
**p. gi′gas,** macropodia.
**p. hippocam′pi** [TA], a formation of two or three elevations on the rostral end of the ventricular surface of the hippocampus; called also *digitationes hippocampi.*
**p. pedun′culi,** crus cerebri (def. 1).
**p. planoval′gus, p. pla′nus,** flatfoot.
**p. prona′tus,** a deformed foot in which the outer border of the anterior part is higher than the inner border.
**p. supina′tus,** a deformed foot in which the inner border of the anterior part is higher than the outer border.
**p. val′gus,** flatfoot.
**p. valgus, congenital convex,** rocker-bottom foot (def. 1).
**p. va′rus,** talipes varus.

**pes·sa·ry** (pes′ə-re) [L. *pessarium*] [MeSH: Pessaries] 1. an instrument placed in the vagina to support the uterus or rectum or as a contraceptive device. 2. a medicated vaginal suppository.
**cup p.,** a pessary the top of which has a cuplike shape to fit the ostium uteri.
**diaphragm p.,** a diaphragm for insertion into the vagina as an occlusive contraceptive.
**doughnut p.,** an inflated soft rubber pessary shaped like a doughnut.
**Hodge's p.,** a pessary designed for use in retrodisplacement of the uterus.
**Menge's p.,** a ring pessary with a fixed crossbar holding a detachable stem.
**ring p.,** a round or ring-shaped pessary.
**Smith's p.,** a pessary designed for use in retrodisplacement of the uterus.
**stem p.,** a pessary with a stem for introduction into the canal of the cervix uteri.

**pest** (pest) 1. plague. 2. anything, particularly an animal, that is harmful to humans.
**avian p., chicken p., fowl p.,** 1. Newcastle disease. 2. fowl plague.
**p. of small ruminants,** peste des petits ruminants.

**peste** (pest) [Fr.] plague.
**p. des petits ruminants (PPR)** (da pə-te′ ru-me-nah′) [Fr.], pest of small ruminants; a highly fatal viral disease of sheep and goats, prevalent in central and west Africa and the Middle East, caused by a virus of the genus *Morbillivirus* and characterized by fever, necrotic stomatitis, gastroenteritis, and pneumonia. Called also *kata, pseudorinderpest,* and *stomatitis-pneumoenteritis syndrome* or *complex.*

**pes·ti·ce·mia** (pes″tĭ-se′me-ə) [*pestis* + *-emia*] septicemic plague.

**pes·ti·cide** (pes′tĭ-sīd) a poison used to destroy pests of any sort, such as a fungicide, herbicide, insecticide, rodenticide, anthelmintic, etc.

**pes·tif·er·ous** (pes-tif′ər-əs) [*pestis* + *-ferous*] causing or propagating a pestilence.

**pes·ti·lence** (pes′tĭ-ləns) [L. *pestilentia*] any virulent contagious or infectious epidemic disease; also an epidemic of such a disease.

**pes·ti·len·tial** (pes″tĭ-len′shəl) of the nature of a pestilence; producing an epidemic disease.

**pes·tis** (pes′tis) [L.] plague.
**p. am′bulans,** ambulatory plague.
**p. bubo′nica,** bubonic plague.
**p. equo′rum,** African horse sickness.
**p. ful′minans, p. ma′jor,** the severe form of bubonic plague.
**p. mi′nor,** ambulatory plague.
**p. si′derans,** septicemic plague.

**Pes·ti·vi·rus** (pes′tĭ-vi″rəs) [L. *pestis* plague + *virus*] [MeSH: Pestivirus] mucosal disease viruses; a genus of viruses of the family Flaviviridae comprising bovine diarrhea virus, hog cholera virus, and border disease virus of sheep.

**pes·tle** (pes'əl) [L. *pestillum*] an implement for pounding drugs in a mortar.

**pes·tol·o·gy** (pes-tol'ə-je) the branch of science concerned with pests.

**PET** positron emission tomography.

**peta-** [Gr. *pente* five, because it is fifth in the series of prefixes for multiples] a combining form used in naming units of measurement to indicate a quantity one quadrillion ($10^{15}$) times the unit designated by the root with which it is combined. Symbol, P.

**-petal** [L. *petere* to seek] a word termination meaning directed or moving toward, the point of reference being indicated by the word stem to which it is affixed, as centripetal (toward a center), corticipetal (toward the cortex).

**pet·a·lo·bac·te·ria** (pet″ə-lo-bak-tēr'e-ə) [Gr. *petalon* leaf + *bacteria*] bacteria which become so aggregated as to form thin pellicles.

**pe·te·chia** (pə-te'ke-ə) pl. *pete'chiae* [L.] a pinpoint, nonraised, perfectly round, purplish red spot caused by intradermal or submucous hemorrhage. Cf. *ecchymosis.*
**calcaneal petechiae,** black heel.

**pe·te·chiae** (pə-te'ke-e) plural of *petechia.*

**pe·te·chi·al** (pə-te'ke-əl) characterized by or of the nature of petechiae.

**Pe·ters' anomaly** (pa'tərz) [Albert *Peters,* German ophthalmologist, 1862–1938] see under *anomaly.*

**Pe·ters' ovum** (pa'tərz) [Hubert *Peters,* Austrian gynecologist, 1859–1934] see under *ovum.*

**Pe·ter·sen's bag** (pa'tər-sənz) [Christian Ferdinand *Petersen,* German surgeon, 1845–1908] see under *bag.*

**peth·i·dine hy·dro·chlo·ride** (peth'ĭ-din) meperidine hydrochloride.

**pet·i·o·late, pet·i·o·lat·ed** (pet'e-o-lāt, pet'e-o-lāt-əd) having a stalk or petiole.

**pet·i·ole** (pet'e-ōl) a stem, stalk, or pedicle.
**epiglottic p.,** petiolus epiglottidis.

**pet·i·oled** (pet'e-ōld) petiolate.

**pe·ti·o·lus** (pə-ti'o-ləs) [L., dim. of *pes* foot] a stem, stalk, or pedicle.
**p. epiglot'tidis** [TA], epiglottic petiole: the pointed lower end of the epiglottic cartilage, which is attached to the back of the thyroid cartilage.

**Pe·tit's canal, sinus** (pə-tēz') [François Pourfour du *Petit,* French anatomist and surgeon, 1664–1741] see *spatia zonularia* and *sinus aortae.*

**Pe·tit's hernia, ligament, triangle** (pə-tēz') [Jean Louis *Petit,* French surgeon, 1674–1750] see under *hernia,* see *uterosacral ligament,* under *ligament,* and see *trigonum lumbale inferius.*

**Pe·tit's law** (pə-tēz') [Alexis Therese *Petit,* French physicist, 1791–1820] Dulong and Petit's law; see under *law.*

**pe·tit mal** (pə-te'mahl) [Fr. "little illness"] see under *epilepsy.*

**Pe·tri dish, plate** (pe'tre) [Julius Richard *Petri,* German bacteriologist, 1852–1921] see under *dish* and *plate.*

**pet·ri·chlo·ral** (pet″rĭ-klor'əl) a derivative of chloral with pharmacological properties similar to those of chloral hydrate; used as a hypnotic and sedative.

**Pe·tri·el·lid·i·um** (pe″tre-əl-id'e-əm) former name for *Pseudallescheria.*

**pet·ri·fac·tion** (pet″rĭ-fak'shən) [L. *petra* stone + *facere* to make] conversion into a stonelike substance.

**pé·tris·sage** (pa″trĭ-sahzh') [Fr.] massage in which the muscles are kneaded and pressed.

**pet·roc·cip·i·tal** (pet″rok-sip'ĭ-təl) petro-occipital.

**pet·ro·late** (pet'ro-lāt) petrolatum.

**pet·ro·la·tum** (pet″ro-la'təm) [L.] [USP] [MeSH: Petrolatum] a purified mixture of semisolid hydrocarbons obtained from petroleum; used as an ointment base. It is also used as a protective dressing and soothing application to the skin. Called also *mineral jelly, petroleum jelly, yellow soft paraffin,* and *petrolate.*
**p. al'bum,** white p.
**hydrophilic p.** [USP], a mixture of cholesterol, stearyl alcohol, and white wax, in white petrolatum; used as an absorbent ointment base and topical protectant.
**liquid p.,** mineral oil.
**liquid p., heavy,** mineral oil.
**liquid p., light,** light mineral oil.
**p. li'quidum,** mineral oil.
**p. li'quidum le've,** light mineral oil.
**white p.** [USP], a wholly or nearly decolorized, purified mixture of semisolid hydrocarbons obtained from petroleum; used as an oleaginous ointment base and topical protectant.

**pe·tro·le·um** (pə-tro'le-əm) [L. *petra* stone + *oleum*] [MeSH: Petroleum] a thick natural mixture of solid, liquid, and gaseous hydrocarbons obtained from beneath the surface of the earth. It consists mainly of a mixture of various alkanes, cycloalkanes, and aromatic hydrocarbons as well as small amounts of sulfur, nitrogen, and oxygen compounds.
**p. benzin,** a colorless, volatile, flammable fraction from petroleum distillation, containing largely hydrocarbons of the methane series; it has been variously described as a special grade of ligroin or as a separate but similar fraction with a lower boiling range (35–80°C). It is used chiefly as an extractive solvent.
**p. ether,** a volatile, flammable petroleum distillate, as ligroin or petroleum benzin; sometimes specifically one of these.

**pet·rol·iza·tion** (pet″rol-ĭ-za'shən) the spreading of petroleum on water for the purpose of destroying mosquito larvae therein.

**pet·ro·mas·toid** (pet″ro-mas'toid) 1. pertaining to the petrous portion of the temporal bone and its mastoid process. 2. otocranium.

**pet·ro·oc·cip·i·tal** (pet″ro-ok-sip'ĭ-təl) pertaining to the petrous portion of the temporal bone and to the occipital bone.

**pet·ro·pha·ryn·ge·us** (pet″ro-fə-rin'je-əs) an occasional muscle arising from the lower surface of the petrous portion of the temporal bone and inserted into the pharynx.

**pe·tro·sal** (pə-tro'səl) pertaining to the petrous portion of the temporal bone.

**pet·ro·sec·to·my** (pet″ro-sek'to-me) [*petrous* + *-ectomy*] excision of the air cells of the apex of the petrous portion of the temporal bone.

**pet·ro·si·tis** (pet″ro-si'tis) inflammation of the petrous portion of the temporal bone.

**pe·tro·so·mas·toid** (pĕ-tro″so-mas'toid) petromastoid.

**pet·ro·sphe·noid** (pet″ro-sfe'noid) pertaining to the sphenoid bone and the petrous portion of the temporal bone.

**pet·ro·squa·mo·sal** (pet″tro-skwə-mo'səl) pertaining to the petrous and squamous portions of the temporal bone.

**pet·ro·squa·mous** (pet″ro-skwa'məs) petrosquamosal.

**pet·rous** (pet'rəs) [L. *petrosus*] resembling a rock; hard; stony.

**pet·rous·itis** (pet″rəs-i'tis) petrositis.

**Pet·te-Döring panencephalitis** (pet'ə-der'ing) [Heinrich Wilhelm *Pette,* German neurologist, 1887–1964; Gerhard *Döring,* German neurologist, born 1909] see under *panencephalitis.*

**Peu·ced·a·num** (pu-sed'ə-nəm) a genus of herbs of the family Umbelliferae, native to Europe and Asia. *P. oreoseli'num* (L.) Munch. is oreoselinum, a medicinal plant.

**Peu·ce·tia** (pu-se'te-ə) a genus of spiders. *P. vi'ridans* is the lynx spider.

**Peutz-Jeg·hers syndrome** (pərtz-ja'gerz) [J.L.A. *Peutz,* Dutch physician, 1886–1957; Harold *Jeghers,* American physician, born 1904] [MeSH: Peutz-Jeghers Syndrome] see under *syndrome.*

**pex·ia** (pek'se-ə) pexis.

**pex·ic** (pek'sik) [Gr. *pēxis* fixation] having the power of fixing substances; said of tissues.

**pex·in** (pek'sin) chymosin.

**pex·is** (pek'sis) [Gr. *pēxis*] 1. the fixation of matter by a tissue. 2. surgical fixation, usually by suturing.

**-pexy** [Gr. *pēxis* fixation] a word termination meaning fixation.

**Pey·er's patches (glands, insulae, plaques)** (pi'ərz) [Johann Conrad *Peyer,* Swiss anatomist, 1653–1712] noduli lymphoidei aggregati intestini tenuis.

**pey·o·te** (pa-yo'ta) [Sp., from Nahuatl *peyotl*] 1. any of several Mexican cacti of the genus *Lophophora,* especially *L. williamsii* or mescal. 2. a hallucinogenic substance whose active principle is mescaline, found in the flowering heads of *Lophophora williamsii* and consumed in various North American Indian cultures as part of religious ceremonies. Called also *peyotl.*

**pey·o·tl** (pa-yo'təl) [Nahuatl] peyote.

**Pey·ro·nie's disease** (pa-ro-nēz') [François de la *Peyronie,* French surgeon, 1678–1747] see under *disease.*

**Pey·rot's thorax** (pa-rōz') [Jean Joseph *Peyrot,* French surgeon, 1843–1918] see under *thorax.*

**Pez·i·za·les** (pez″ĭ-za'lēz) an order of perfect fungi of the subphylum Ascomycotina, series Unitunicatae, usually saprobes, characterized by fleshy ascocarps of various shapes that form as a hymenium, as well as operculate asci. Families of medical significance include Ascobolaceae and Helvellaceae; other families include edible species such as truffles and morels.

**Pfan·nen·stiel's incision** (fahn'ən-shtēlz) [Hermann Johann *Pfannenstiel,* German gynecologist, 1862–1909] see under *incision.*

**Pfeif·fer's bacillus, phenomenon (reaction)** (fi'fərz) [Richard Friedrich Johann *Pfeiffer,* German bacteriologist, 1858–1945] see *Haemophilus influenzae,* and see under *phenomenon.*

**Pfeif·fer's disease (glandular fever)** (fi'fərz) [Emil *Pfeiffer,* German physician, 1846–1921] infectious mononucleosis.

**Pfeif·fer·el·la** (fi"fər-el'ə) [R. F. J. *Pfeiffer*] in former systems of classification, a genus of bacteria made up of organisms now classified in various other genera.
**P. anatipes'tifer,** *Moraxella anatipestifer.*

**Pflü·ger's cords, tubes** (fle'gərz) [Edward Friedrich Wilhelm *Pflüger,* German physiologist, 1829–1910] see *ovarian tubes,* under *tube.*

**Pfuhl's sign** (fo͞olz) [Eduard *Pfuhl,* German physician, 1852–1905] see under *sign.*

**PG** prostaglandin; *Pharmacopoeia Germanica.*

**pg** picogram.

**$PGD_2$, $PGE_2$, $PGF_{2\alpha}$, $PGI_2$,** etc. symbols for various prostaglandins; see *prostaglandin.*

**Pgp** P-glycoprotein.

**Ph** symbol for *Pharmacopeia* and *phenyl.*

**pH** the symbol relating the hydrogen ion ($H^+$) concentration or activity of a solution to that of a given standard solution. Numerically the pH is approximately equal to the negative logarithm of $H^+$ concentration expressed in molarity. pH 7 is neutral; above it alkalinity increases and below it acidity increases.

**PHA** phytohemagglutinin (def. 2).

**pha·ci·tis** (fə-si'tis) phakitis.

**phac(o)-** [Gr. *phakos* lentil, or lentil-shaped object] a combining form denoting relationship *(a)* to a lens, as the crystalline lens, or *(b)* a mole, freckle or nevus, as in phacomatosis. See also words beginning *phak(o)-.*

**phaco·ana·phy·lax·is** (fak"o-an"ə-fə-lak'sis) [*phaco-* + *anaphylaxis*] hypersensitivity to the protein of the crystalline lens of the eye, induced by escape of material from the lens capsule.

**phaco·cele** (fak'o-sēl) [*phaco-* + *-cele*] the dislocation of the eye lens from its proper place; hernia of the eye lens.

**phaco·cyst** (fak'o-sist) [*phaco-* + *cyst* (def. 1)] the capsule of the lens (capsula lentis [TA]).

**phaco·cys·tec·to·my** (fak"o-sis-tek'tə-me) [*phacocyst* + *ectomy*] excision of a portion of the capsule of the lens for cataract.

**phaco·cys·ti·tis** (fak"o-sis-ti'tis) [*phacocyst* + *-itis*] inflammation about the capsule of the crystalline lens; called also *phacohymenitis.*

**phaco·emul·si·fi·ca·tion** (fak"o-e-mul"sĭ-fĭ-ka'shən) [*phaco-* + L. *emulgēre* to milk out] [MeSH: Phacoemulsification] a method of cataract extraction in which the lens is fragmented by ultrasonic vibrations and simultaneously irrigated and aspirated.

**phaco·ery·sis** (fak"o-ə-re'sis) [*phaco-* + Gr. *eryein* to drag away] removal of the lens in cataract by means of suction with an instrument known as an erysiphake; called also *Barraquer's method* or *operation.*

**phaco·glau·co·ma** (fak"o-glaw-ko'mə) [*phaco-* + *glaucoma*] the structural changes in the lens produced by glaucoma.

**phaco·hy·men·itis** (fak"o-hi"mən-i'tis) phacocystitis.

**phac·oid** (fak'oid) [*phaco-* + *-oid*] shaped like a lens or a lentil.

**phac·oid·itis** (fak"oi-di'tis) phakitis.

**pha·coido·scope** (fə-koid'ə-skōp) phacoscope.

**pha·col·y·sin** (fə-kol'ĭ-sin) [*phaco-* + *lysin*] an albumin from the lens of the eye; used in the treatment of early cataract.

**pha·col·y·sis** (fə-kol'ĭ-sis) [*phaco-* + *lysis*] discission of the crystalline lens, followed by extraction.

**phaco·lyt·ic** (fak"o-lit'ik) pertaining to or causing dissolution of the crystalline lens.

**pha·co·ma** (fə-ko'mə) phakoma.

**phaco·ma·la·cia** (fak"o-mə-la'shə) [*phaco-* + *malacia*] softening of the lens; a soft cataract.

**phac·o·ma·to·sis** (fak"o-mə-to'sis) phakomatosis.

**phaco·meta·cho·re·sis** (fak"o-met"ə-ko-re'sis) [*phaco-* + Gr. *metachōrēsis* displacement] displacement of the crystalline lens.

**phaco·met·e·ce·sis** (fak"o-met"ə-se'sis) [*phaco-* + Gr. *metoikēsis* migration] phacometachoresis.

**pha·com·e·ter** (fə-kom'ə-tər) lensometer.

**phaco·pal·in·gen·e·sis** (fak"o-pal"in-jen'ə-sis) [*phaco-* + *palingenesis* (def. 1)] re-formation of the crystalline lens.

**phaco·pla·ne·sis** (fak"o-plə-ne'sis) [*phaco-* + Gr. *planēsis* wandering] abnormal mobility of the crystalline lens.

**phaco·scle·ro·sis** (fak"o-sklə-ro'sis) [*phaco-* + *sclerosis*] hardening of the crystalline lens; a hard cataract.

**phaco·scope** (fak'o-skōp) [*phaco-* + *-scope*] an instrument for viewing accommodative changes of the eye lens; called also *phacoidoscope.*

**pha·cos·co·py** (fə-kos'kə-pe) the examination of the eye with a phacoscope.

**phaco·sco·tas·mus** (fak"o-sko-taz'məs) [*phaco-* + Gr. *skotasmos* a clouding] the clouding of the lens of the eye.

**phaco·tox·ic** (fak"o-tok'sik) exerting a deleterious effect upon the crystalline lens.

**Phae·ni·cia** (fe-nish'ə) a genus of greenbottle flies of the family Calliphoridae that are metallic green or blue; some species are important causes of cutaneous myiasis in domestic animals. Called also *Lucilia.*
**P. cupri'na,** a sheep maggot fly of worldwide distribution, causing cutaneous myiasis; its larvae also cause various forms of myiasis in humans. Called also *Lucilia cuprina.*
**P. serica'ta,** a sheep maggot fly of the British Isles that often causes cutaneous myiasis; its larvae (maggots) have also been introduced into infected wounds to facilitate healing. Called also *Lucilia sericata.*

**phae(o)-** [Gr. *phaios* dun, dusky] a combining form meaning brown dusky. See also *pheo-.*

**phaeo·hy·pho·my·co·sis** (fe"o-hi"fo-mi-ko'sis) [*phaeo-* + *hyphomycosis*] a hyphomycosis in which the infecting fungus is dark in color, usually of the form-family Dematiaceae. Most are opportunistic infections.

**phaeo·spo·ro·tri·cho·sis** (fe"o-spor"o-trĭ-ko'sis) phaeohyphomycosis.

**phage** (fāj) [MeSH: Bacteriophages] bacteriophage.

**-phage** [Gr. *phagein* to eat] a word termination denoting one that eats or destroys.

**phag·e·de·na** (faj"ə-de'nə) [Gr. *phagedaina; phagein* to eat] a progressive and rapidly spreading and sloughing ulceration.

**phag·e·den·ic** (faj"ə-den'ik) pertaining to or characterized by phagedena. See under *ulcer.*

**-phagia** [Gr. *phagein* to eat] a word termination denoting relationship to eating or swallowing. Also, *-phagy.*

**phag(o)-** [Gr. *phagein* to eat] a combining form denoting relationship to eating or consumption by ingestion or engulfing.

**phago·cyt·a·ble** (fag'o-sīt"ə-bəl) susceptible to phagocytosis.

**phago·cyte** (fag'o-sīt) [*phago-* + *-cyte*] [MeSH: Phagocytes] any cell capable of ingesting particulate matter, such as a *microphage, macrophage,* or *monocyte.* Such cells ingest microorganisms and other particulate antigens that are opsonized (coated with antibody or complement), a process mediated by specific cell-surface receptors (Fc receptors and complement receptors). Other cell types exhibit phagocytosis, but not specific phagocytosis of opsonized particles.
**alveolar p.,** see under *macrophage.*
**mononuclear p.,** any cell of the monocyte-macrophage lineage, including macrophages, monocytes, and their precursors in the monocytic series.

**phago·cyt·ic** (fag"o-sit'ik) 1. pertaining to or exhibiting phagocytosis. 2. pertaining to phagocytes.

**phago·cy·tin** (fag"o-si'tin) any of several poorly characterized basic proteins with bactericidal activity found in the granules of neutrophils. See *cationic proteins,* under *protein.*

**phago·cyt·ize** (fag'o-sīt"īz) phagocytose.

**phago·cy·tol·y·sis** (fag"o-si-tol'ĭ-sis) [*phagocyte* + *-lysis*] solution or destruction of phagocytes.

**phago·cy·to·lyt·ic** (fag"o-si"to-lit'ik) pertaining to phagocytolysis.

**phago·cy·tose** (fag"o-si'tōs) to ingest particles by the process of phagocytosis.

**phago·cy·to·sis** (fag"o-si-to'sis) [MeSH: Phagocytosis] endocytosis of particulate material, such as microorganisms or cell fragments. The material is taken into the cell in membrane-bound vesicles (phagosomes) that originate as pinched off invaginations of the plasma membrane. Phagosomes fuse with lysosomes, forming phagolysosomes in which the engulfed material is killed and digested. See *phagocyte.*

**induced p.**, phagocytosis aided by subjecting bacteria to the action of opsonins in the blood.
**spontaneous p.**, phagocytosis of bacteria taking place in an indifferent medium, or phagocytosis of nonantigenic particles.
**surface p.**, enhanced phagocytosis by macrophages and neutrophils of microorganisms or other particulate antigens that are trapped against surfaces, e.g., other leukocytes, fibrin clots, or tissue surfaces; it does not require opsonins.

**phago·cy·tot·ic** (fag″o-si-tot′ik) pertaining to or characterized by phagocytosis.

**phago·log·i·cal** (fag″o-loj′ĭ-kəl) pertaining to phage.

**pha·gol·y·sis** (fə-gol′ĭ-sis) phagocytolysis.

**phago·ly·so·some** (fag″o-li′so-sōm) [MeSH: Phagosomes] the digestive vacuole formed when the membranes of pre-existent lysosomes within the cytoplasm merge with the phagosome; the lysosomes then discharge their hydrolytic enzymes, resulting in digestion of the phagocytized material.

**phago·lyt·ic** (fag″o-lit′ik) phagocytolytic.

**phago·ma·nia** (fag″o-ma′ne-ə) [*phago-* + *-mania*] an insatiable craving for food, or an obsessive preoccupation with the subject of eating.

**phago·pho·bia** (fag″o-fo′be-ə) [*phago-* + *-phobia*] irrational fear of eating.

**phago·plasm** (fa′go-plaz-əm) [*phago-* + *plasm*] the digestive enzyme–rich cytoplasm of the cytopharyngeal area in certain ciliate protozoa.

**phago·some** (fag′o-sōm) [*phago-* + *-some*] [MeSH: Phagosomes] the membrane-bounded vesicle in a phagocyte formed by invagination of the cell membrane and the phagocytized material; called also *phagocytotic vesicle.* See also *phagolysosome.*

**phago·troph** (fag′o-trof) a holozoic organism.

**phago·troph·ic** (fag″o-trof′ik) [*phago-* + *-trophic*] holozoic.

**phago·type** (fag′o-tīp) phage type; see under *type.*

**-phagy** see *-phagia.*

**pha·ki·tis** (fa-ki′tis) [*phak-* + *-itis*] inflammation of the crystalline lens.

**phak(o)-** [Gr. *phakos* a lentil, or lentil-shaped object; a spot on the body, a freckle] for words beginning thus, see also those beginning *phac(o)-.*

**pha·ko·ma** (fə-ko′mə) [*phak-* + *-oma*] any of the hamartomas found characteristically in the phakomatoses; one example is the herald lesion of tuberous sclerosis (see *tuber,* def. 2). Written also *phacoma.*

**phak·o·ma·to·sis** (fak″o-mə-to′sis) pl. *phakomato′ses* [*phakoma* + *-osis*] any of a group of congenital and hereditary developmental anomalies having in common selective involvement of the tissues of ectodermal origin (i.e., central nervous system, eye, and skin) and the development of disseminated glial hamartomas (phakomas) in these tissues. The major syndromes in the group are neurofibromatosis, tuberous sclerosis, Sturge-Weber syndrome, von Hippel-Lindau disease, and ataxia-telangiectasia. Called also *neurocutaneous syndrome.* Written also *phacomatosis.*

**pha·lan·ge·al** (fə-lan′je-əl) pertaining to a phalanx.

**phal·an·gec·to·my** (fal″ən-jek′tə-me) excision of a phalanx of a finger or toe.

**pha·lan·ges** (fə-lan′jēz) plural of *phalanx.*

**phal·an·gette** (fal″ən-jet′) [Fr.] the distal phalanx of a digit; see *phalanx distalis digitorum manus* and *phalanx distalis digitorum pedis.*
**drop p.**, dropping of the distal phalanx of a finger and loss of power to extend it when the hand is prone.

**phal·an·gi·tis** (fal″ən-ji′tis) inflammation of one or more phalanges.

**phal·an·gi·za·tion** (fal″ən-jĭ-za′shən) surgical separation of the terminal portion of fused digits, without complete extirpation of the connecting web.

**phalang(o)-** [L. *phalanx,* q.v.] a combining form denoting relationship to a phalanx or to the phalanges.

**pha·lan·go·pha·lan·ge·al** (fə-lang″go-fə-lan′je-əl) pertaining to two adjoining phalanges of a finger or toe.

**phal·an·go·sis** (fal″ən-go′sis) [*phalang-* + *-osis*] a condition in which the eyelashes grow in rows.

**pha·lanx** (fa′lanks) pl. *phalan′ges* [Gr. "a line or array of soldiers"] 1. [TA] any of the bones of the fingers or toes; see *ossa digitorum manus* and *ossa digitorum pedis,* under *os.* 2. any one of a set of plates (made up of supporting cells, q.v.) which are disposed in rows and make up the reticular membrane of the organ of Corti.

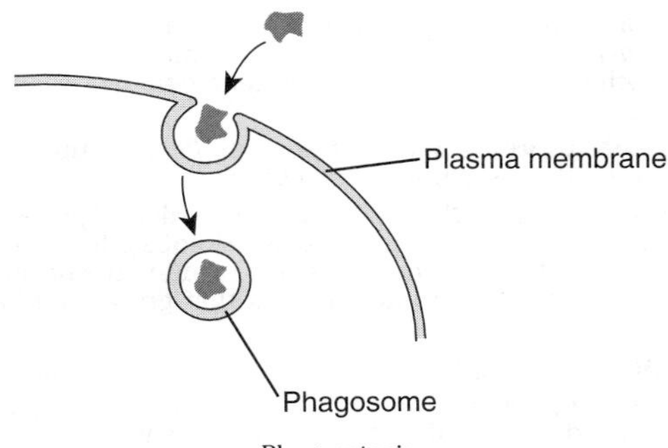

Phagocytosis.

**Deiters' phalanges,** modified cuticular plates forming the ends of sustentacular epithelial cells of the reticular membrane of the organ of Corti.
**phalan′ges digito′rum ma′nus,** TA alternative for *ossa digitorum manus.*
**phalan′ges digito′rum pe′dis,** TA alternative for *ossa digitorum pedis.*
**p. dista′lis digito′rum ma′nus** [TA], distal phalanx of fingers: any one of the five terminal bones of the fingers, articulating, except in the thumb, with the phalanx media; called also *p. tertia digitorum manus.*
**p. dista′lis digito′rum pe′dis** [TA], distal phalanx of toes: any one of the five terminal bones of the toes, articulating, except in the great toe, with the phalanx media; called also *p. tertia digitorum pedis.*
**phalanges of fingers,** ossa digitorum manus.
**p. me′dia digito′rum ma′nus** [TA], middle phalanx of fingers: any one of the four bones of the fingers (excluding the thumb) situated between the proximal and distal phalanges; called also *p. secunda digitorum manus.*
**p. me′dia digito′rum pe′dis** [TA], middle phalanx of toes: any one of the four bones of the toes (excluding the great toe) situated between the proximal and distal phalanges; called also *p. secunda digitorum pedis.*
**p. pri′ma digito′rum ma′nus,** p. proximalis digitorum manus.
**p. pri′ma digito′rum pe′dis,** p. proximalis digitorum pedis.
**p. proxima′lis digito′rum ma′nus** [TA], proximal phalanx of fingers: any one of the five bones of the fingers that articulate with the metacarpal bones and, except in the thumb, with the phalanx media; called also *p. prima digitorum manus.*
**p. proxima′lis digito′rum pe′dis** [TA], proximal phalanx of toes: any one of the five bones of the toes that articulate with the metatarsal bones and, except in the great toe, with the phalanx media; called also *p. prima digitorum pedis.*
**p. secun′da digito′rum ma′nus,** p. media digitorum manus.
**p. secun′da digito′rum pe′dis,** p. media digitorum pedis.
**p. ter′tia digito′rum ma′nus,** p. distalis digitorum manus.
**p. ter′tia digito′rum pe′dis,** p. distalis digitorum pedis.
**phalanges of toes,** ossa digitorum pedis.
**ungual p. of fingers,** p. distalis digitorum manus.
**ungual p. of toes,** p. distalis digitorum pedis.

**Pha·lar·is** (fə-lar′is) a genus of North American and European

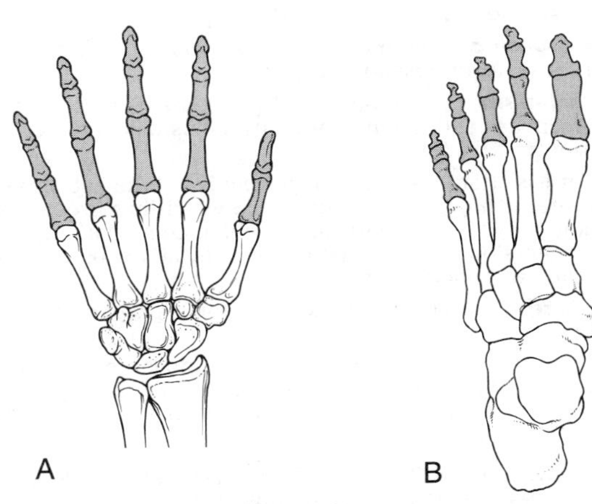

Phalanges of the hand *(A)* and foot *(B).*

grasses commonly found in pastures, certain species of which are called *canary grass.* Various species sometimes cause *Phalaris* staggers and other toxic conditions, including fatal heart failure, in ruminants.

**Pha·len's maneuver** (fa'lənz) [George S. *Phalen,* American orthopedist, born 1911] see under *maneuver.*

**Phal·la·les** (fə-la'lēz) the stinkhorns, an order of perfect fungi of the subphylum Basidiomycotina, class Holobasidiomycetes; most species have a fetid mucinous substance around the basidiospores, which are exposed by an internal stalk that grows and breaks out of the basidiocarp.

**phal·lal·gia** (fə-lal'jə) [*phall-* + *-algia*] pain in the penis.

**phal·lan·as·tro·phe** (fal"ən-as'trə-fe) [*phall-* + Gr. *anastrophē* a turning upward] upward distortion of the penis.

**phal·lan·eu·rysm** (fə-lan'u-riz-əm) [*phall-* + *aneurysm*] aneurysm of the penis.

**phal·lec·to·my** (fə-lek'tə-me) [*phall-* + *-ectomy*] penectomy.

**phal·li** (fal'i) genitive and plural of *phallus.*

**phal·lic** (fal'ik) [Gr. *phallikos*] pertaining to the phallus, or penis.

**phal·li·form** (fal'ĭ-form) [*phallus* + *form*] shaped like the phallus or penis.

**phal·lin** (fal'in) a poisonous hemolytic glycoside from *Amanita phalloides.*

**phal·li·tis** (fə-li'tis) [*phall-* + *-itis*] penitis.

**phall(o)-** [Gr. *phallos* penis] a combining form denoting relationship to the penis.

**phal·lo·camp·sis** (fal"o-kamp'sis) [*phallo-* + Gr. *kampsis* bending] curvature of the penis when erect.

**phal·lo·cryp·sis** (fal"o-krip'sis) [*phallo-* + Gr. *krypsis* hiding] retraction of the penis.

**phal·lo·dyn·ia** (fal"o-din'e-ə) [*phallo-* + *-odynia*] phallalgia.

**phal·loid** (fal'oid) [*phallo-* + *-oid*] resembling a penis.

**phal·loi·din** (fə-loi'din) [MeSH: Phalloidine] a heat-stable, bicyclic hexapeptide poison from the mushroom *Amanita phalloides;* see *mushroom poisoning,* under *poisoning.*

**phal·loi·dine** (fə-loi'dēn) [MeSH: Phalloidine] phalloidin.

**phal·lon·cus** (fə-long'kəs) [*phallo-* + Gr. *onkos* mass] a morbid swelling or tumor of the penis.

**phal·lo·plas·ty** (fal'o-plas"te) [*phallo-* + *-plasty*] plastic surgery of the penis.

**phal·lor·rha·gia** (fal"o-ra'jə) [*phallo-* + *-rrhagia*] hemorrhage from the penis.

**phal·lot·o·my** (fə-lot'ə-me) [*phallo-* + *-tomy*] incision of the penis.

**phal·lo·tox·in** (fal'o-tok"sin) any of a group of potent hepatotoxins found in species of *Amanita* mushrooms; because they are not well absorbed in the human gastrointestinal tract, they usually do not do as much damage as the amatoxins do.

**phal·lus** (fal'əs) pl. *phal'li* [Gr. *phallos*] 1. penis. 2. a representation of the penis. 3. the rudiment of embryonic tissue that develops into the penis or clitoris.

**phaner(o)-** [Gr. *phaneros* visible] a combining form meaning visible or apparent.

**phan·er·o·gam** (fan'ər-o-gam) [*phanero-* + Gr. *gamos* marriage] a true seed-bearing plant.

**phan·ero·ge·net·ic** (fan"ər-o-jə-net'ik) phanerogenic.

**phan·er·o·gen·ic** (fan"ər-o-jen'ik) [*phanero-* + *-genic*] having a known cause, as opposed to *idiopathic.*

**phan·ero·plasm** (fan'ər-o-plaz-əm) [*phanero-* + *-plasm*] membranous organelles and nonmembranous inclusions in the cytoplasm; cf. *cytosol.*

**phan·er·o·sis** (fan"ər-o'sis) [Gr. *phanerōsis*] the act of becoming visible; the setting free of a substance which has previously been undemonstrable owing to its being held in combination.
**fat p.,** conversion in the tissues of invisible fatty substances into fat which can be stained and seen.

**Phan·o·dorn** (fan'o-dorn) trademark for a preparation of cyclobarbital.

**phan·tasm** (fan'taz-əm) [Gr. *phantasma* appearance] an impression or image not evoked by actual stimuli, and usually recognized as false by the observer; called also *phantom.* Cf. *hallucination.*

**phan·ta·sy** (fan'tə-se) fantasy.

**phan·to·geu·sia** (fan"to-goo'zhə) a parageusia consisting of continuous abnormal taste in the mouth, usually metallic or salty, in the absence of any external stimulus.

**phan·tom** (fan'təm) [Gr. *phantasma* an appearance] 1. phantasm. 2. a model of the body or of a specific part thereof. 3. in radiology, a device that simulates the conditions encountered when radiation or radioactive material is deposited *in vivo* and permits a quantitative estimation of its effects.

**phan·tos·mia** (fant-oz'me-ə) [Gr. *phantasia* imagination + *osm-*[1] + *-ia*] a parosmia consisting of a sensation of smell in the absence of any external stimulus.

**phan·u·rane** (fan'u-rān) canrenone.

**phar** pharmacy; pharmaceutical; pharmacopeia. Also, *pharm.*

**Phar B** abbreviation for L. *Pharmaciae Baccalaureus,* Bachelor of Pharmacy.

**Phar C** Pharmaceutical Chemist.

**phar·ci·dous** (fahr'sĭ-dəs) [Gr. *pharkis* wrinkled] wrinkled.

**Phar D** abbreviation for L. *Pharmaciae Doctor,* Doctor of Pharmacy.

**Phar G** Graduate in Pharmacy.

**Phar M** abbreviation for L. *Pharmaciae Magister,* Master of Pharmacy.

**pharm** see *phar.*

**phar·ma·cal** (fahr'mə-kəl) pertaining to pharmacy.

**phar·ma·ceu·tic** (fahr"mə-soo'tik) [Gr. *pharmakeutikos*] pertaining to pharmacy or to drugs.

**phar·ma·ceu·ti·cal** (fahr"mə-soo'tĭ-kəl) 1. pertaining to pharmacy or to drugs. 2. a medicinal drug.

**phar·ma·ceu·tics** (fahr"mə-soo'tiks) 1. pharmacy (def. 1). 2. pharmaceutical preparations.

**phar·ma·ceu·tist** (fahr"mə-soo'tist) a pharmacist.

**phar·ma·cist** (fahr'mə-sist) [MeSH: Pharmacists] one who is licensed to prepare and sell or dispense drugs and compounds, and to make up prescriptions. Called also *apothecary, druggist,* and *chemist* (British).

**pharmaco-** [Gr. *pharmakon* medicine] a combining form denoting relationship to a drug or medicine.

**phar·ma·co·an·gi·og·ra·phy** (fahr"mə-ko-an"je-og'rə-fe) [*pharmaco-* + *angiography*] angiography in which visualization is enhanced by manipulating the flow of blood by the administration of vasodilating and vasoconstricting agents.

**phar·ma·co·chem·is·try** (fahr"mə-ko-kem'is-tre) pharmaceutical chemistry.

**phar·ma·co·di·ag·no·sis** (fahr"mə-ko-di"əg-no'sis) [*pharmaco-* + *diagnosis*] the employment of drugs in the diagnosis of disease.

**phar·ma·co·dy·nam·ic** (fahr"mə-ko-di-nam'ik) [*pharmaco-* + *dynamic*] pertaining to pharmacodynamics.

**phar·ma·co·dy·nam·ics** (fahr"mə-ko-di-nam'iks) [*pharmaco-* + *dynamics*] the study of the biochemical and physiological effects of drugs and the mechanisms of their actions, including the correlation of actions and effects of drugs with their chemical structure; also, such effects on the actions of a particular drug or drugs.

**phar·ma·co·eco·nom·ics** (fahr"mə-ko-ek"ə-nom'iks) the study of economic factors regarding the cost of drug therapy, including their impact on health care systems and society.

**phar·ma·co·en·do·cri·nol·o·gy** (fahr"mə-ko-en"do-krĭ-nol'ə-je) the study of the influence of drugs on the activity of the endocrine glands, and of the effects of very high levels of hormones on organs and tissues.

**phar·ma·co·ge·net·ics** (fahr"mə-ko-jə-net'iks) [MeSH: Pharmacogenetics] the scientific study of the relationship between genetic factors and the nature of responses to drugs.

**phar·ma·cog·nos·tics** (fahr"mə-kog-nos'tiks) pharmacognosy.

**phar·ma·cog·no·sy** (fahr"mə-kog'nə-se) [*pharmaco-* + Gr. *gnōsis* knowledge] [MeSH: Pharmacognosy] that branch of pharmacology which deals with the biological, biochemical, and economic features of natural drugs and their constituents.

**phar·ma·cog·ra·phy** (fahr"mə-kog'rə-fe) [*pharmaco-* + *-graphy*] an account or written description of drugs.

**phar·ma·co·ki·net·ics** (fahr"mə-ko-kĭ-net'iks) [MeSH: Pharmacokinetics] the activity or fate of drugs in the body over a period of time, including the processes of absorption, distribution, localization in tissues, biotransformation, and excretion.

**phar·ma·co·log·ic** (fahr"mə-ko-loj'ik) pertaining to pharmacology or to the properties and reactions of drugs.

**phar·ma·col·o·gist** (fahr"mə-kol'ə-jist) one who makes a study of the actions of drugs.

**phar·ma·col·o·gy** (fahr"mə-kol'ə-je) [*pharmaco-* + *-logy*] [MeSH: Pharmacology] the science that deals with the origin, nature, chemistry, effects, and uses of drugs; it includes pharmacognosy, pharmacokinetics, pharmacodynamics, pharmacotherapeutics, and toxicology.

**phar·ma·co·ma·nia** (fahr″mə-ko-ma′ne-ə) [*pharmaco-* + *-mania*] uncontrollable desire to take or to administer medicines.

**phar·ma·co·met·rics** (fahr″mə-ko-met′riks) [*pharmaco-* + Gr. *metron* measure] the comparative evaluation of drug activity, distinguished from bioassay in that substances with different chemical constitutions are compared.

**phar·ma·co·or·yc·tol·o·gy** (fahr″mə-ko-or″ik-tol′ə-je) [*pharmaco-* + Gr. *oryktos* excavated + *-logy*] the study of mineral drugs.

**phar·ma·co·pe·dia, phar·ma·co·pe·dics** (fahr″mə-ko-pe′de-ə, fahr″mə-ko-pe′diks) [*pharmaco-* + Gr. *paideia* instruction] the science which deals with the properties and preparations of drugs.

**phar·ma·co·pe·ia** (fahr″mə-ko-pe′ə) [*pharmaco-* + Gr. *poiein* to make] an authoritative treatise on drugs and their preparations; a book containing a list of products used in medicine, with descriptions, chemical tests for determining identity and purity, and formulas for certain mixtures of these substances. It also generally contains a statement of average dosage. The first United States pharmacopeia was published on December 15, 1820, printed in both Latin and English, and its 272 pages included 217 drugs which were considered worthy of recognition. See *USP.*

**phar·ma·co·pe·ial** (fahr″mə-ko-pe′əl) pertaining to or recognized by the pharmacopeia.

**phar·ma·co·pho·bia** (fahr″mə-ko-fo′be-ə) [*pharmaco-* + *-phobia*] irrational fear of drugs or medicines.

**phar·ma·co·phore** (fahr′mə-ko-for″) [*pharmaco-* + *-phore*] the group of atoms in a drug molecule which is responsible for the action of the compound.

**phar·ma·co·poe·ia** (fahr″mə-ko-pe′ə) pharmacopeia.

**phar·ma·co·psy·cho·sis** (fahr″mə-ko-si-ko′sis) [*pharmaco-* + *psychosis*] any psychosis due to alcohol, drugs, or poisons.

**phar·ma·co·ra·di·og·ra·phy** (fahr″mə-ko-ra″de-og′rə-fe) radiographic examination of a body organ under the influence of a drug that best facilitates such examination.

**phar·ma·co·ther·a·peu·tics** (fahr″mə-ko-ther″ə-pu′tiks) [*pharmaco-* + *therapeutics*] study of the uses of drugs in the treatment of disease.

**phar·ma·co·ther·a·py** (fahr″mə-ko-ther′ə-pe) [*pharmaco-* + *therapy*] the treatment of disease by drugs. Cf. *chemotherapy.* Called also *drug therapy* or *treatment.*

**phar·ma·cy** (fahr′mə-se) [Gr. *pharmakon* medicine] [MeSH: Pharmacy] 1. the branch of the health sciences dealing with the preparation, dispensing, and proper utilization of drugs. 2. a place where drugs are compounded or dispensed.
**chemical p.,** pharmaceutical chemistry.
**galenic p.,** the pharmacy of vegetable medicines.

**Pharm D** abbreviation for Doctor of Pharmacy.

**phar·yn·gal·gia** (far″in-gal′jə) [*pharyng-* + *-algia*] pharyngodynia.

**pha·ryn·ge·al** (fə-rin′je-əl) [L. *pharyngeus*] pertaining to the pharynx.

**phar·yn·gec·ta·sia** (far″in-jək-ta′zhə) pharyngoesophageal diverticulum.

**phar·yn·gec·to·my** (far″in-jek′tə-me) [*pharyng-* + *-ectomy*] [MeSH: Pharyngectomy] surgical removal of a part of the pharynx.

**phar·yn·ge·us** (far″in-je′əs) [L.] pharyngeal.

**phar·yn·gism** (far′in-jiz-əm) pharyngospasm.

**phar·yn·gis·mus** (far″in-jiz′məs) pharyngospasm.

**phar·yn·git·ic** (far″in-jit′ik) affected with or of the nature of pharyngitis.

**pha·ryn·gi·tid** (fə-rin′jĭ-tid) a cutaneous eruption occurring in pharyngitis.

**phar·yn·gi·tis** (far″in-ji′tis) [*pharyng-* + *-itis*] [MeSH: Pharyngitis] inflammation of the pharynx. See also *faucitis* and *tonsillitis.* Called also *sore throat.*
**acute p.,** inflammation of the throat with dryness and pain, especially on swallowing, followed by moisture of the pharynx, congestion of the mucous membrane, and fever.
**aphthous p.,** herpangina.
**atrophic p.,** a type of chronic pharyngitis involving wasting of the submucous tissue, dryness, and thickened secretions. Called also *p. sicca.*
**chronic p.,** pharyngitis with repeated acute episodes; the most common types are atrophic pharyngitis and hypertrophic pharyngitis.
**diphtheritic p.,** faucial diphtheria.
**gangrenous p.,** a form characterized by gangrenous patches.
**p. herpe′tica,** herpangina.
**hypertrophic p.,** a type of chronic pharyngitis with thickening of the mucous membranes, which contain nodules of lymphoid tissue; it is often due to repeated faulty habits of speaking.
**membranous p.,** a general term for any type in which there is a fibrous exudate and formation of a false membrane; it is seen in Vincent's angina, diphtheria, and other conditions.
**plague p.,** pharyngeal plague.
**p. sic′ca,** atrophic p.
**streptococcal p.,** an acute variety caused by infection with *Streptococcus pyogenes;* it occurs in epidemics and is usually spread by droplets or in air, although it can also be spread by direct contact and in food. Characteristics include intense local hyperemia, sometimes with enlargement of cervical lymph nodes and a yellow exudate. Called also *septic sore throat, streptococcal sore throat,* and *streptococcal tonsillitis.*
**ulcerative p., p. ulcero′sa,** pharyngitis with ulceration of the mucous membrane.
**vesicular p.,** herpangina.

**pharyng(o)-** [Gr. *pharynx* pharynx] a combining form denoting relationship to the pharynx.

**pha·ryn·go·cele** (fə-ring′go-sēl) [*pharyngo-* + *-cele*[2]] pharyngoesophageal diverticulum.

**pha·ryn·go·cer·a·to·sis** (fə-ring″go-ser″ə-to′sis) keratosis pharyngea.

**pha·ryn·go·con·junc·ti·vi·tis** (fə-ring″go-kən-junk″tĭ-vi′tis) inflammation involving the pharynx and conjunctiva, the result of a viral infection.

**pha·ryn·go·dyn·ia** (fə-ring″go-din′e-ə) [*pharyng-* + *-odynia*] pain in the pharynx; called also *pharyngalgia.*

**pha·ryn·go·epi·glot·tic** (fə-ring″go-ep″ĭ-glot′ik) pertaining to the pharynx and epiglottis.

**pha·ryn·go·epi·glot·tid·e·an** (fə-ring″go-ep″ĭ-glŏ-tid′e-ən) pharyngoepiglottic.

**pha·ryn·go·esoph·a·ge·al** (fə-ring″go-ə-sof′ə-je″əl) pertaining to the pharynx and esophagus.

**pha·ryn·go·glos·sal** (fə-ring″go-glos′əl) glossopharyngeal.

**pha·ryn·go·ker·a·to·sis** (fə-ring″go-ker″ə-to′sis) keratosis pharyngea.

**pha·ryn·go·la·ryn·ge·al** (fə-ring″go-lə-ring′je-əl) pertaining to the pharynx and the larynx.

**pha·ryn·go·lar·yn·gi·tis** (fə-ring″go-lar″in-ji′tis) [*pharyngo-* + *laryngitis*] laryngopharyngitis.

**pha·ryn·go·lith** (fə-ring′go-lith) [*pharyngo-* + *-lith*] a concretion in the walls of the pharynx.

**phar·yn·gol·o·gy** (far″ing-gol′ə-je) [*pharyngo-* + *-logy*] the study, diagnosis, and treatment of the pharynx and its diseases.

**phar·yn·gol·y·sis** (far″ing-gol′ĭ-sis) [*pharyngo-* + *-lysis*] pharyngoparalysis.

**pha·ryn·go·max·il·lary** (fə-ring″go-mak′sĭ-lar″e) pertaining to the pharynx and the maxillae.

**pha·ryn·go·my·co·sis** (fə-ring″go-mi-ko′sis) [*pharyngo-* + *mycosis*] any fungal disease of the pharynx.

**pha·ryn·go·na·sal** (fə-ring″go-na′səl) nasopharyngeal, def. 1.

**pha·ryn·go·oral** (fə-ring″go-or′əl) oropharyngeal, def. 1.

**pha·ryn·go·pal·a·tine** (fə-ring″go-pal′ə-tīn) palatopharyngeal.

**pha·ryn·go·pa·ral·y·sis** (fə-ring″go-pə-ral′ĭ-sis) [*pharyngo-* + *paralysis*] paralysis of the pharyngeal muscles. Called also *pharyngolysis* and *pharyngoplegia.*

**pha·ryn·gop·a·thy** (far″ing-gop′ə-the) [*pharyngo-* + *-pathy*] disease of the pharynx.

**pha·ryn·go·plas·ty** (fə-ring″go-plas′te) [*pharyngo-* + *-plasty*] plastic operation on the pharynx.
**Hynes p.,** a technique of pharyngoplasty accomplished by muscle transposition.

**pha·ryn·go·ple·gia** (fə-ring″go-ple′jə) pharyngoparalysis.

**pha·ryn·go·rhi·nos·co·py** (fə-ring″go-ri-nos′kə-pe) examination of the nasopharynx and posterior nares with the rhinoscope.

**pha·ryn·gor·rha·gia** (fə-ring″go-ra′jə) [*pharyngo-* + *-rrhagia*] hemorrhage from the pharynx.

**pha·ryn·go·sal·pin·gi·tis** (fə-ring″go-sal″pin-ji′tis) inflammation of the pharynx and the eustachian tube.

**pha·ryn·go·scle·ro·ma** (fə-ring″go-sklə-ro′mə) scleroma of the pharynx, usually from extension of rhinoscleroma.

**pha·ryn·go·scope** (fə-ring′go-skōp) [*pharyngo-* + *-scope*] an instrument for inspecting the pharynx.

**phar·yn·gos·co·py** (far″ing-gos′kə-pe) direct visual examination of the pharynx.

**pha·ryn·go·spasm** (fə-ring′go-spaz-əm) [*pharyngo-* + *spasm*] spasm of the pharyngeal muscles. Called also *pharyngism* and *pharyngismus.*

**pha·ryn·go·ste·no·sis** (fə-ring″go-stə-no′sis) [*pharyngo-* + *stenosis*] narrowing of the lumen of the pharynx.

**pha·ryn·gos·to·ma** (far″ing-gos′tə-mə) [*pharyngo-* + *stoma*] the opening formed by pharyngostomy.

**pha·ryn·go·stome** (fə-ring′go-stōm″) pharyngostoma.

**phar·yn·gos·to·my** (far″ing-gos′tə-me) [*pharyngo-* + *-stomy*] [MeSH: Pharyngostomy] the surgical creation of an artificial opening into the pharynx.

**pha·ryn·go·tome** (fə-ring′go-tōm) a cutting instrument used in pharyngeal surgery.

**phar·yn·got·o·my** (far″ing-got′ə-me) [*pharyngo-* + *-tomy*] surgical incision of the pharynx.
**external p.,** pharyngotomy done through an incision on the external surface of the neck.
**internal p.,** that which is performed from within the pharynx.
**lateral p.,** the opening of the pharynx from one side.
**subhyoid p.,** external pharyngotomy done through the thyrohyoid membrane.

**pha·ryn·go·ton·sil·li·tis** (fə-ring″go-ton″sĭ-li′tis) inflammation of the pharynx and tonsils.

**pha·ryn·go·ty·phoid** (fə-ring″go-ti′foid) enteric fever with angina and sore patches on the tonsils.

**pha·ryn·go·xe·ro·sis** (fə-ring″go-ze-ro′sis) [*pharyngo-* + *xerosis*] dryness of the pharynx.

**phar·ynx** (far′inks) [Gr. "the throat"] [TA] [MeSH: Pharynx] the musculomembranous passage between the mouth and posterior nares and the larynx and esophagus. The part above the level of the soft palate is the *nasopharynx,* which communicates with the auditory tube. The lower portion consists of two sections—the *oropharynx,* which lies between the soft palate and the upper edge of the epiglottis, and the *hypopharynx,* which lies below the upper edge of the epiglottis and opens into the larynx and esophagus. Called also *throat.*

**phase** (fāz) [Gr. *phasis* an appearance] 1. the view that a thing presents to the eye. 2. any one of the varying aspects or stages through which a disease or process may pass. 3. in physical chemistry, any physically or chemically distinct, homogeneous, and mechanically separable part of a system. 4. on an electrodiagnostic recording, that portion of a wave that is between any two consecutive times it crosses the baseline.
**alpha p.,** the estrous stage of the ovarian cycle.
**alveolar p.,** the fourth period or phase in lung development, beginning after the terminal saccular phase in utero and lasting until a child is about eight years old. The terminal alveolar saccules subdivide several more times and mature alveoli form.
**anal p.,** see under *stage.*
**beta p.,** the progestational stage of the ovarian cycle.
**canalicular p.,** the second period or phase of lung development in utero, lasting in different parts of the lungs from the sixteenth or seventeenth week to the twenty-fourth week or later. Basic structures of the gas-exchanging parts of the lungs form and become vascular, and primitive alveoli called the terminal saccules begin to form, enabling respiration to begin. Fetuses delivered after respiration begins may be viable. This is followed by the *terminal saccular phase*

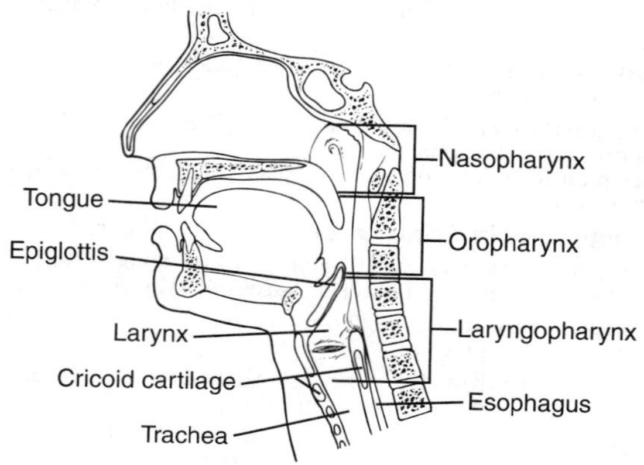


Pharynx, divided into the nasopharynx, oropharynx, and laryngopharynx.

**cholesteric p.,** a liquid crystal phase that exhibits molecular orientation and arrangement both within and between equispaced planes, being arranged in parallel rows within a layer but twisted slightly between layers so as to form a helix through the layers.
**continuous p.,** a phase that is physically uninterrupted; the continuous portion of a colloid system (see *dispersion medium*).
**p. of decline,** the stage in the growth of a bacterial culture in which the number of live organisms gradually decreases.
**disperse p., dispersed p.,** the internal or discontinuous portion of a colloid system; it is analogous to the solute in a solution. Called also *internal p.* Cf. *dispersion medium.*
**ejection p.,** see under *period.*
**embryonic p.,** the earliest phase of lung development in utero, lasting from the third week after conception to the sixth or seventh week. A ventral diverticulum arises from the caudal end of the laryngotracheal groove and grows into lung buds and the primordial trachea. This is followed by the *pseudoglandular phase.*
**erythrocytic p.,** that phase in the life cycle of a malarial plasmodium in which the parasites multiply in the red blood cells.
**estrin p.,** proliferative stage.
**exponential p.,** logarithmic p.
**external p.,** dispersion medium.
**$G_1$ p.,** a part of the cell cycle during interphase, lasting from the end of cell division (the M phase) until the start of DNA synthesis (the S phase).
**$G_2$ p.,** a relatively quiescent part of the cell cycle during interphase, lasting from the end of DNA synthesis (the S phase) until the start of cell division (the M phase).
**genital p.,** see under *stage.*
**growth p.,** one of the stages in the growth of a neoplasm.
**growth p., radial,** an early growth phase of melanoma in which tumor cells are spreading laterally in the epidermis and have not spread into the dermis as in the vertical growth phase.
**growth p., vertical,** a growth phase of melanoma more advanced than the radial growth phase; tumor cells are spreading from the epidermis into deeper layers such as the dermis and run the risk of metastasizing.
**nematic p.,** a liquid crystal phase that exhibits molecular orientation without periodicity, having an irregular threadlike surface with little viscosity.
**internal p.,** disperse p.
**isovolumetric contraction p., isovolumic contraction p.,** period of isovolumic contraction.
**isovolumetric relaxation p., isovolumic relaxation p.,** period of isovolumic relaxation.
**lag p.,** the early period following bacterial inoculation into a new medium, a time of stationary population during which the cells adjust to the new environment and synthesize enzymes and intermediates for the subsequent logarithmic phase.
**latency p.,** see under *stage.*
**logarithmic p.,** the stage in the growth of a bacterial culture when a plot of the logarithm of the number of cells against time gives a straight-upward line. Called also *exponential p.*
**M p.,** the part of the cell cycle during which mitosis occurs; subdivided into prophase, metaphase, anaphase, and telophase.
**m p.,** see *cell cycle,* under *cycle.*
**meiotic p.,** that stage in meiosis in which the reduction of the chromosomes occurs; called also *reduction p.*
**motofacient p.,** see *motofacient.*
**negative p.,** the initial lowering of the antibody titer following the injection of corresponding antigen.
**nonmotofacient p.,** see *motofacient.*
**oral p.,** see under *stage.*
**phallic p.,** see under *stage.*
**positive p.,** the rise in antibody titer that follows the negative phase.
**postmeiotic p.,** the stage following the reduction of the chromosomes in meiosis.
**premeiotic p., prereduction p.,** the stage in meiosis which precedes the reduction of the chromosomes.
**pseudoglandular p.,** the first period or phase of lung development in utero, lasting in different parts of the lung from the sixth or seventh to the sixteenth or seventeenth week. Repeated branching of bronchi and bronchioles takes place to form primitive conductive airways, and the lungs resemble exocrine glands. Fetuses delivered during this phase are not viable because respiration does not begin until the following *canalicular phase.*
**reduction p.,** meiotic p.
**resting p.,** former term for interphase.
**reversal p.,** in the process of bone turnover, the period between resorption and formation, during which the cement substance is deposited.
**S p.,** a part of the cell cycle, near the end of interphase, during which DNA is synthesized; it comes between the $G_1$ and $G_2$ phases.
**s p.,** see *cell cycle,* under *cycle.*

**smectic p.**, a liquid crystal phase that exhibits molecular orientation and arrangement in equispaced planes but no periodicity within the planes, having separate layers with little viscosity.
**stance p.**, that part of the gait cycle in which the foot is in contact with the floor and the leg bears the body weight, comprising heel strike, mid stance, and push-off.
**stationary p.**, the stage in the growth of a bacterial culture when the bacteria undergoing division are in equilibrium with those dying, and the number of bacterial cells remains nearly constant.
**swing p.**, that part of the gait cycle in which the foot does not touch the floor and the opposite leg bears the body weight, comprising acceleration, swing through, and deceleration.
**synaptic p.**, synapsis.
**terminal sac p., terminal saccular p.**, the third phase of lung development in utero, lasting in different parts of the lungs from the twenty-fourth week or later until near term. Walls of the air spaces become thinner and the spaces divide into alveolar saccules with adjacent capillaries; type I and type II alveolar cells begin functioning and surfactant is secreted. This is followed by the *alveolar phase.*
**ventricular filling p.**, see under *period.*

**pha·sein** (fa'sēn) phasin.

**pha·se·o·lam·in** (fə-se″o-lam'in) an alpha-amylase inhibitor purified from the kidney bean *(Phaseolus vulgaris);* it is the basis of starch-blocker tablets.

**pha·se·o·lin** (fa-se'o-lin) a globulin from the kidney bean, *Phaseolus vulgaris,* which has antifungal properties.

**pha·se·o·lu·na·tin** (fa″se-o-loo'nə-tin) linamarin.

**Pha·se·o·lus** (fa″ze-o'ləs) a large genus of plants of the family Leguminosae, including many edible beans. *P. limen'sis* (the lima bean) and other varieties contain the cyanogen linamarin and can cause cyanide poisoning in animals consuming them in large amounts. *P. vulga'ris* is the kidney bean, a source of phaseolamin and phaseolin.

**-phasia** [Gr. *phasis* speech + *-ia*] combining form denoting a manner of speaking, usually one that is disordered.

**phase-spe·cif·ic** (fāz-spə-sif'ik) having maximum activity during a certain phase of the cell growth cycle; see under *agent.*

**pha·sin** (fa'sin) any of a group of nitrogenous substances found in seeds, bark, and other plant tissues, which agglutinate red blood corpuscles.

**phas·mid** (faz'mid) 1. one of a pair of caudal chemoreceptors occurring in certain nematodes. The class Nematoda is sometimes divided into two subclasses, Phasmidia and Aphasmidia, on the basis of the presence or absence of these organs. 2. a nematode belonging to the Phasmidia. Cf. *aphasmid.*

**Phas·mid·ia** (faz-mid'e-ə) a subclass of Nematoda comprising those organisms possessing phasmids. The following superfamilies are of medical or veterinary importance: Rhabditoidea, Strongyloidea, Oxyuroidea, Ascaridoidea, Spiruroidea, Filarioidea, and Dracunculoidea.

**Pha·zyme** (fa'zīm) trademark for a preparation of simethicone.

**PhB** British Pharmacopoeia.

**PhD** Doctor of Philosophy.

**Phe** phenylalanine.

**Phelps' operation** (felps) [Abel Mix *Phelps,* American surgeon, 1851–1902] see under *operation.*

**Phe-Mer-Nite** (fe'mər-nīt) trademark for preparations of phenylmercuric nitrate.

**Phe·mer·ol** (fe'mər-ol) trademark for preparations of benzethonium.

**phem·fil·con A** (fem-fil'kon) a hydrophilic contact lens material.

**-phemia** [Gr. *phēmē* speech + *-ia*] combining form denoting a manner of speaking, usually one that is disordered.

**Phem·is·ter graft, oper·ation** (fem'is-tər) [Dallas Burton *Phemister,* American surgeon, 1882–1951] see under *graft* and *operation.*

**phem·i·tone** (fem'ĭ-tōn) mephobarbital.

**phe·nac·e·mide** (fə-nas'ə-mīd) an oral anticonvulsant used in the treatment of psychomotor, grand mal, and petit mal epilepsy, and in the management of mixed seizures.

**phe·nac·e·tin** (fə-nas'ə-tin) [MeSH: Phenacetin] the ethyl ether of acetaminophen, which is its major active metabolite, an analgesic and antipyretic; now little used because of its toxicity.

**phen·a·cet·o·lin** (fen″ə-set'ə-lin) a red powder used as an indicator: it has a pH range of 5 to 6, being yellow at 5 and red at 6.

**phe·nan·threne** (fĕ-nan'thrēn) a tricyclic aromatic hydrocarbon occurring in coal tar and isomeric with anthracene; used in the synthesis of dyes and pharmaceuticals. It is toxic and carcinogenic.

***o*-phe·nan·thro·line** (fə-nan'thrə-lēn) the *ortho* (1,10) isomeric form of phenanthroline, it is a metal chelator often used as an indicator.

**phen·an·to·in** (fen'ən-to″in) mephenytoin.

**phen·ar·sa·zine chlor·ide** (fen-ahr'sə-zēn) diphenylamine chlorarsine.

**phe·nate** (fe'nāt) phenolate.

**phen·a·zone** (fen'ə-zōn) antipyrine.

**phen·a·zo·pyr·i·dine hy·dro·chlo·ride** (fen″ə-zo-pir'ĭ-dēn) [USP] a urinary analgesic used orally in cystitis, urethritis, pyelonephritis, and prostatitis. Formerly used as a urinary antiseptic.

**phen·cy·cli·dine hy·dro·chlo·ride** (fen-si'klĭ-dēn) a potent veterinary analgesic and anesthetic; it is sometimes used illicitly by humans in cases of drug abuse, leading to serious psychological disturbances. Abbreviated PCP.

**phen·di·met·ra·zine tar·trate** (fen″di-met'rə-zēn) [USP] a sympathomimetic amine with pharmacologic activity similar to that of the amphetamines, used as an appetite suppressant; administered orally.

**phene** (fēn) [gr. *phainein* to show] advanced stages of the developmental sequence determined by gene action, sometimes with environmental factors, resulting in a special phenotype.

**phen·el·zine sul·fate** (fen'əl-zēn) [USP] a monoamine oxidase inhibitor used as an antidepressant, administered orally.

**Phen·er·gan** (fen'ər-gən) trademark for preparations of promethazine hydrochloride.

**phe·neth·i·cil·lin** (fə-neth″ĭ-sil'in) a semisynthetic acid-resistant penicillin which is a methyl analogue of penicillin V.
**p. potassium,** the monopotassium salt of phenethicillin, used as an antibacterial, especially in certain infections due to susceptible organisms, such as streptococcal infections of the upper respiratory tract, pneumococcal infections of the respiratory tract, staphylococcal infections of the skin and soft tissues, and fusospirochetosis. It is administered orally.

**phen·eth·yl·bi·guan·ide** (fen-eth″əl-bi'gwahn-īd) phenformin.

**phen·for·min hy·dro·chlo·ride** (fen-for'min) an oral hypoglycemic agent related to buformin and phenformin, no longer available in the United States because of a high incidence of fatal lactic acidosis associated with its use.

**phen·go·pho·bia** (fen″go-fo'be-ə) irrational fear of daylight.

**phe·nin·da·mine tar·trate** (fə-nin'də-mēn) an antihistaminic used for symptomatic relief in hypersensitivity reactions and as a component of cough preparations; administered orally.

**phen·in·di·one** (fen″in-di'ōn) [MeSH: Phenindione] one of the indanedione anticoagulants, having a rapid onset and short duration of action; administered orally.

**phen·ir·amine mal·e·ate** (fən-ir'ə-mēn) an antihistaminic occurring as a white crystalline powder; administered orally. Called also *prophenpyridamine maleate.*

**phen·met·ra·zine hy·dro·chlo·ride** (fən-met'rə-zēn) [USP] a central nervous system stimulant used as an anorexic. Abuse of this drug may lead to habituation; see *amphetamine.*

**phen(o)-** [Gr. *phainein* to show] 1. a combining form denoting a showing or displaying. 2. in chemistry, a prefix denoting a compound derived from benzene.

**phe·no·bar·bi·tal** (fe″no-bahr'bĭ-təl) [USP] [MeSH: Phenobarbital] a long-acting barbiturate, used as a sedative, hypnotic, and anticonvulsant, administered orally. Called also *phenobarbitone* and *phenylethylbarbituric acid.*
**p. sodium** [USP], the monosodium salt of phenobarbital, having the actions and uses of the base; administered orally, rectally, intravenously, intramuscularly, and subcutaneously.

**phe·no·bar·bi·tone** (fe″no-bahr'bĭ-tōn) phenobarbital.

**phe·no·copy** (fe'no-kop″e) [*pheno-* (def. 1) + *copy*] 1. an environmentally induced phenotype mimicking one usually produced by a specific genotype. 2. an individual exhibiting such a phenotype. 3. the simulated trait in a phenocopy.

**phe·no·de·vi·ant** (fe″no-de've-ənt) [*pheno-* (def. 1) + *deviant*] an individual whose phenotype differs significantly from that of the typical phenotype in the population.

**phe·no·ge·net·ics** (fe″no-jə-net'iks) [*pheno-* (def. 1) + *genetics*] the science which attempts to explain the chain of causality between genotype and phenotype.

**phe·nol** (fe'nol) 1. [USP] an extremely poisonous, colorless to light pink, crystalline compound obtained by the distillation of coal tar, and converted, by the addition of 10 per cent water, into a clear liquid with a peculiar odor and a burning taste. Used as an antimicrobial agent. Called also *carbolic acid, hydroxybenzene,* and *oxybenzene.* See also *phenol poisoning,* under *poisoning.* 2. a generic term for any organic compound containing one or more hydroxyl groups attached to an aromatic or carbon ring.

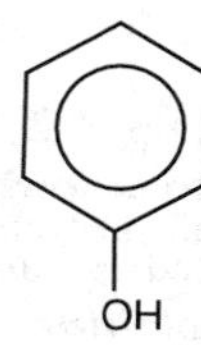

Phenol.

**liquefied p.** [USP], an aqueous solution of phenol, used as a topical antipruritic. Called also *phenylic alcohol.*
**p. red,** phenolsulfonphthalein.

**phe·no·late** (fe'nə-lāt) 1. to treat with phenol for purposes of sterilization. 2. a salt formed by union of a base with phenol, in which a monovalent metal, such as sodium or potassium, replaces the hydrogen of the hydroxyl group.

**phe·no·lat·ed** (fe'nə-lāt″əd) charged with phenol.

**Phe·no·lax** (fe'no-laks) trademark for a preparation of phenolphthalein.

**phe·nol·emia** (fe″nol-e'me-ə) the presence of phenols in the blood.

**phe·nol·ic** (fe-nol'ik) pertaining to or derived from phenol.

**phe·nol·iza·tion** (fe″nol-ĭ-za'shən) treatment by subjection to the action of phenol.

**phe·nol·o·gist** (fe-nol'ə-jist) an expert or specialist in phenology.

**phe·nol·o·gy** (fe-nol'ə-je) [*pheno-* (def. 1) + *-logy*] a study of the effects of climate upon the life and health of living organisms.

**phe·nol·phthal·ein** (fe″nol-thal'ēn) a cathartic and pH indicator, with a range of 8.5 (colorless) to 9.0 (red).

**phe·nol·sul·fon·phthal·ein** (fe″nol-sul″fon-thal'ēn) [MeSH: Phenolsulfonphthalein] a bright to dark red, crystalline powder administered by intramuscular or intravenous injection as a test of renal function and as a qualitative test for residual bladder urine. Called also *phenol red.* Abbreviated PSP. See also under *tests.*

**phe·nol·tet·ra·chlo·ro·phthal·ein** (fe″nol-tet″rə-chlor″o-thal'ēn) a coal tar derivative, used intravenously in tests of liver function.

**phe·nol·uria** (fe″nol-u're-ə) the presence of phenols in the urine.

**phe·nom** (fe'nom) in some systems of classification, a group or "cluster" of strains of phenotypically related organisms. Called also *phenon.* See also *numerical taxonomy,* under *taxonomy.*

**phe·nom·e·nol·o·gy** (fə-nom″ə-nol'ə-je) in psychiatry, the study of phenomena in their own right rather than inferring causes, based on the theory that behavior is determined by the way the person perceives reality rather than by objective external reality.

**phe·nom·e·non** (fə-nom'ə-non) pl. *phenom'ena.* Any sign or objective symptom; any observable occurrence or fact.

## Phenomenon

See also under *sign, symptom,* and *syndrome.*

**Anderson's p.,** clumps of red blood cells in the feces, seen on microscopic examination in amebic dysentery.
**aqueous-influx p.,** entrance into conjunctival or subconjunctival vessels of clear fluid (aqueous humor), deriving from an aqueous vein during compression of its recipient vessel by a glass rod. Called also *Ascher's positive glass-rod p.* Cf. *blood-influx p.*
**arm p.,** Pool's p. (def. 2).
**Arthus p.,** see under *reaction.*
**Ascher's negative glass-rod p.,** blood-influx p.
**Ascher's positive glass-rod p.,** aqueous-influx p.
**Aschner's p.,** oculocardiac reflex.
**Ashman's p.,** aberrant ventricular activation resulting in a short cardiac cycle that follows a normal or long cycle; it is associated with supraventricular premature beats and with atrial fibrillation.
**Aubert's p.,** an optical illusion in which a bright vertical line in a dark room tilts to one side when an observer tilts his head to the opposite side.
**Austin Flint p.,** see under *murmur.*
**autokinetic visible light p.,** the apparent spontaneous movement of a pin-point source of light as seen by certain susceptible persons when they gaze steadily at it in a completely blacked-out room.
**Babinski's p.,** see under *reflex.*
**Becker's p.,** increased pulsation of the retinal arteries, one manifestation of Graves' orbitopathy. Called also *Becker's sign.*
**Bell's p.,** an outward and upward rolling of the eyeball on the attempt to close the eye; it occurs on the affected side in peripheral facial paralysis (Bell's palsy).
**blood-influx p.,** filling of conjunctival or subconjunctival vessels with blood during compression by a glass rod of the recipient vessel of an aqueous vein. This and the aqueous-influx phenomenon, depending on minute pressure differences between blood and aqueous humor, differ in glaucomatous eyes and those with normal intraocular pressure. Called also *Ascher's negative glass-rod p.*
**booster p.,** on a tuberculin test, an initial false negative result due to a diminished amnestic response that becomes positive on subsequent testing.
**Bordet-Gengou p.,** complement fixation.
**Bowditch staircase p.,** treppe.
**brake p.,** the tendency of a muscle to maintain itself in its normal resting position; called also *Rieger's p.*
**break-off p.,** a state of disconnectedness or unreality experienced by high-altitude pilots. Its symptomatic sensations are apparently indescribable in understandable physical terms, but the condition could be the result of a loss of all the physical sense perceptions.
**Chase-Sulzberger p.,** Sulzberger-Chase p.
**cheek p.,** in meningitis if pressure is exerted on both cheeks just under the zygomas there is reflex upward jerking of both arms with simultaneous bending of both elbows.
**clasp-knife p.,** see under *rigidity.*
**cogwheel p.,** see under *rigidity.*
**Collie p.,** when pure neon is enclosed in a glass tube with a globule of mercury and shaken it glows with a bright, orange-red color, and when the globule rolls it appears to be followed by a flame.
**Cushing's p.,** a rise in systemic blood pressure as a result of an increase in intracranial pressure.
**Dale p.,** see under *reaction.*
**Danysz's p.,** decrease of the neutralizing influence of an antitoxin when a toxin is added to it in divided portions instead of all at once.
**dawn p.,** the early-morning increase in plasma glucose concentration and thus insulin requirement in a patient with insulin-dependent diabetes mellitus.
**Debré's p.,** absence of measles rash at the site of injection of convalescent measles serum which has not prevented the appearance of the eruption.
**Dejerine-Lichtheim p.,** Lichtheim's sign.
**Denys-Leclef p.,** phagocytosis taking place in a test tube on mixing therein leukocytes, bacteria, and immune serum specific for the bacteria.
**d'Herelle's p.,** Twort-d'Herelle p.
**doll's head p.,** an abnormal extraocular muscle manifestation of many ophthalmologic syndromes and conditions: the eyes depress as the head is bent backward.
**Doppler p.,** see under *effect.*
**Duckworth's p.,** arrest of breathing before stoppage of the heart's action in certain fatal brain conditions.
**Erben's p.,** see under *reflex.*
**face p., facialis p.,** Chvostek's sign.
**fall-and-rise p.,** the drop in the number of bacteria that occurs at the beginning of drug treatment and the gradual rise that follows, even while treatment continues.
**Felton's p.,** immunologic unresponsiveness or tolerance to pneumococcal polysaccharide induced in mice by administration of large doses of the antigen.
**Fick's p.,** a fogging of vision, with the appearance of halos around light, occurring in individuals wearing contact lenses.
**finger p.** (in hemiplegia), 1. extension of all the fingers or of the thumb and index finger, on pressure against the pisiform bone; called also Gordon's sign. 2. Souques' p.
**first-set p.,** the immunological reaction of the body against a tissue or organ in a host not previously sensitized against the graft antigens. Called also *first-set rejection.* See also *second-set p.*
**flicker p.,** flicker.

**Frégoli's p.,** a form of delusional misidentification in which the subject believes that a stranger, particularly a persecutor, is disguised as various people familiar to the subject. Cf. *Capgras' syndrome.*

**Friedreich's p.,** the tympanic note of skodaic resonance in pleuritis with effusion varies in pitch during inspiration and expiration, being raised on inspiration.

**Galassi's pupillary p.,** orbicularis pupillary reflex.

**Gärtner's p.,** the degree of fullness of the veins of the arm as it is raised above the level of the heart and the point at which the veins collapse indicate the degree of pressure in the right atrium.

**Gengou p.,** complement fixation.

**glass-rod p., negative,** blood-influx p.

**glass-rod p., positive,** aqueous-influx p.

**Goldblatt p.,** see under *hypertension.*

**Gowers' p.,** Gowers' sign (def. 2).

**Grasset's p., Grasset-Gaussel p.,** inability of a patient to raise both legs at the same time, though he can raise either alone; seen in incomplete organic hemiplegia.

**Gunn's p.,** see under *syndrome.*

**Gunn's pupillary p.,** Marcus Gunn's pupillary p.

**halisteresis p.,** selective withdrawal of bone salt from already calcified tissue.

**Hamburger p.,** chloride shift.

**Hammerschlag's p.,** abnormal fatigability toward continuous sounds of gradually decreasing intensity.

**Hata p.,** increase in severity of an infectious disease when a small dose of a chemotherapeutical remedy is given.

**Hecht p.,** Rumpel-Leede p.

**Hektoen p.,** when antigens are introduced into the animal body in allergic states, there may exist an increased range of new antibody production which may include production of antibodies concerned in previous infections and immunizations.

**Herendeen p.,** rarely occurring rapid enlargement of a giant cell tumor of bone for several weeks to months after therapeutic irradiation of the lesion.

**Hering's p.,** a faint murmur heard with the stethoscope over the lower end of the sternum for a short time after death.

**Hertwig-Magendie p.,** skew deviation.

**hip-flexion p.,** in paraplegia, when the patient attempts to rise from a lying position, he flexes the hip of the paralyzed side.

**Hochsinger's p.,** pressure on the inner side of the biceps muscle produces closure of the fist in tetany.

**Hoffmann's p.,** increased excitability to electrical stimulation in the sensory nerves; the ulnar nerve is usually tested. Called also *Hoffmann's sign.*

**Holmes' p., Holmes-Stewart p.,** rebound p.

**Houssay p.,** hypoglycemia and marked increase in sensitiveness to insulin produced in an Houssay animal (an experimental animal deprived of both the pancreas and the pituitary gland).

**Hunt's paradoxical p.,** in dystonia musculorum deformans, if the examiner attempts forcible plantar flexion of the foot that is in dorsal spasm there is produced increase of the dorsal spasm, but if the patient is ordered to extend the foot he will perform plantar flexion.

**iceberg p.,** cases of clinically apparent disease represent only a small fraction of the total cases of disease, inapparent cases, including preclinical, subclinical, chronic, and latent disease, being even more prevalent.

**jaw-winking p.,** Gunn's syndrome.

**Kienböck's p.,** paradoxical diaphragm p.

**Koch's p.,** if a guinea pig that has been previously infected with tuberculosis organisms is reinjected intracutaneously, the skin over the injected area undergoes necrosis and a superficial ulcer develops; the ulcer heals quickly and infection of regional lymph nodes is retarded. The phenomenon demonstrates development of ability to localize tubercle bacilli, which is the principle underlying tuberculin tests (q.v.). Called also *Koch's reaction.*

**Koebner's p.,** a cutaneous response seen in certain dermatoses, e.g., psoriasis, lichen planus, and infectious eczematoid dermatitis, manifested by the appearance on uninvolved skin of lesions typical of the skin disease at the site of trauma, on scars, or at points where articles of clothing (e.g., a belt) produce pressure. Called also *isomorphic effect.*

**Kohnstamm's p.,** aftermovement.

**Kühne's muscular p.,** Porret's p.

**Leede-Rumpel p.,** Rumpel-Leede p.

**Le Grand-Geblewics p.,** a flickering colored light (40–50 per second) observed indirectly is perceived as a constant white light.

**Leichtenstern's p.,** see under *sign.*

**Lewis' p.,** hydrophagocytosis.

**Liacopoulos p.,** nonspecific immunosuppression to an antigen induced by administration of large doses of an unrelated antigen.

**Liesegang's p.,** the peculiar periodic formation of a precipitate in concentric banded rings, waves, or spirals when two electrolytes diffuse into and meet in a colloid gel.

**Lucio's p.,** a local exacerbation reaction occurring in diffuse lepromatous leprosy, characterized histologically by ischemic necrosis of the epidermis as a result of necrotizing vasculitis of small blood vessels of the subpapillary plexus, and clinically by the eruption of crops of small erythematous lesions with central necrosis; the eschar may be shed, revealing ulceration, with eventual scar formation. Cf. *erythema nodosum leprosum.*

**Lust's p.,** abduction with dorsal flexion of the foot on tapping the common peroneal nerve just below the head of the fibula; indicative of spasmophilia. Called also *peroneal nerve p., Lust's sign,* and *peroneal sign.*

**Marcus Gunn's p.,** Gunn's syndrome.

**Marcus Gunn's pupillary p.,** with unilateral optic nerve or retinal disease, a difference between the pupillary reflexes of the two eyes when a light is shone alternately into each one with the other eye covered; on the affected side there is abnormally slight contraction or even dilation of the pupil. See also *swinging flashlight test,* under *test.* Called also *Gunn's pupillary p.* or *sign* and *Marcus Gunn's pupillary sign.*

**Meirowsky p.,** darkening of existing melanin, perhaps by oxidation, beginning within seconds and complete within minutes to a few hours after exposure to long-wave ultraviolet radiation. See also *tan* (def. 2).

**Mills-Reincke p.,** the mortality from all diseases decreases as a result of water purification.

**mucus extravasation p.,** extravasation of mucus into the surrounding connective tissue from a damaged minor salivary gland excretory duct, followed by an inflammatory reaction leading to the formation of a pool of macrophages and mucin surrounded by a wall of granulation tissue; visible as a small nodule or vesicle on the oral mucosa. Called also *mucocele.* Cf. *mucus retention cyst,* under *cyst.*

**Negro's p.,** cogwheel rigidity.

**Neisser-Wechsberg p.,** complement deviation.

**no-reflow p.,** when blood flow is restored to a part following prolonged ischemia, there is initial hyperemia followed by a gradual decline in perfusion until there is almost no blood flow.

**Orbeli p.,** when the response of a nerve-muscle preparation is diminishing because of fatigue, stimulation of the sympathetic nerve increases the height of the contractions.

**orbicularis p.,** orbicularis pupillary reflex.

**paradoxical diaphragm p.,** one hemidiaphragm moves upward on inspiration and downward on expiration, opposite to the movements on the contralateral side; seen in phrenic nerve paralysis and diaphragmatic eventration.

**paradoxical p. of dystonia,** Hunt's paradoxical p.

**paradoxical pupillary p.,** 1. reversed pupillary reflex. 2. see under *reflex* (def. 2).

**peroneal nerve p.,** Lust's p.

**Pfeiffer's p.,** the lysis of *Vibrio cholerae* when injected into the peritoneal cavity of an immunized guinea pig; the term is also used to describe the in vitro lysis of cholera vibrios or other bacteria when incubated with specific antibody and complement.

**phi p.,** the perception of the sequential flashing of a stationary row of lights as a moving light.

**Piltz-Westphal p.,** orbicularis pupillary reflex.

**pivot shift p.,** a sign of anterior cruciate ligament disruption: with the knee held at 20° flexion and in neutral rotation and with the muscles relaxed (which lets the femur drop down if the anterior cruciate ligament is torn), a slight valgus or axial force is applied to the knee; subluxation or reduction of the tibia occurs if the anterior cruciate ligament is torn. Called also *pivot shift sign* or *test.*

**Pool's p.,** 1. Schlesinger's sign. 2. in tetany, the arm muscles contract when the arm is raised above the head with the forearm extended, so as to cause stretching of the brachial plexus.

**Porret's p.,** the passage of a continuous current through a living muscle fiber causes an undulation proceeding from the positive toward the negative pole.

**psi p.** [*psy*che], an experience or effect that appears to be produced without physical agency or intermediation.

**Purkinje p.,** as the intensity of illumination decreases and the eye becomes scotopic, the region of maximum visual acuity shifts from red-yellow to blue-green, the reds becoming less luminous, the blues more luminous. Called also *Purkinje effect* or *shift.*

**Queckenstedt's p.,** see under *sign.*

**radial p.,** the involuntary dorsal flexion of the wrist which occurs on palmar flexion of the fingers.

**Raynaud's p.,** intermittent bilateral ischemia of the fingers, toes, and sometimes ears and nose, with severe pallor and often paresthesias and pain, usually brought on by cold or emotional stimuli and relieved by heat; it is usually due to an underlying disease or anatomical abnormality. When it is idiopathic or primary it is called *Raynaud's disease.*

**rebound p.,** a manifestation of loss of coordination between groups of antagonistic muscles of the extremities in cerebellar dysfunction. It is usually tested by having the patient rest an elbow on a table and try to flex that arm against the resistance of the examiner; when the resistance is suddenly withdrawn, the affected arm rebounds to the patient's chest, whereas the normal arm flexes only slightly, the flexion being arrested by contraction of antagonistic muscles (the triceps). Cf. *André Thomas sign* (def. 1). Called also *Holmes'* or *Holmes-Stewart p., Holmes' sign,* and *Stewart-Holmes sign.*

**reclotting p.,** thixotropy.

**release p.,** the unhampered activity of a lower center when a higher inhibiting control is removed.

**Rieger's p.,** brake p.

**R on T p.,** the occurrence of a premature ventricular complex near the peak of the T wave in electrocardiography; it may lead to ventricular tachycardia or fibrillation.

**Rumpel-Leede p.,** the appearance of minute subcutaneous hemorrhages below the area at which a tourniquet is applied not too tightly for ten minutes upon the upper arm; characteristic of scarlet fever and hemorrhagic diathesis.

**Rust's p.,** in caries or cancer of the upper cervical vertebrae, the patient supports his head with his hands when rising from or assuming a lying position; see also under *syndrome.*

**satellite p.,** the more luxuriant development of a colony of microorganisms when in the neighborhood of a foreign colony, as shown by *Haemophilus influenzae* when contaminated by *Staphylococcus pyogenes* var. *aureus.*

**Schellong-Strisower p.,** fall of systolic blood pressure on assuming an erect posture from the lying down position.

**Schlesinger's p.,** see under *sign.*

**Schramm's p.,** a funnel-like deformity of the posterior urethra, seen in spinal cord disease and tabes dorsalis.

**Schultz-Charlton p.,** see under *reaction.*

**second-set p.,** the accelerated and intensified rejection by the recipient of a second graft of tissue from the same donor as a consequence of the primary immune response (i.e., antibody production and cell-mediated immunity) induced by the first graft. Called also *second-set rejection.*

**Sherrington's p.,** the response of the hind limb musculature on stimulation of a motor nerve which has previously been degenerated.

**shot-silk p.,** see under *retina.*

**Shwartzman p.,** see under *reaction.*

**Somogyi p.,** a rebound phenomenon occurring in diabetes: overtreatment with insulin induces hypoglycemia, which initiates the release of epinephrine, adrenocorticotropic hormone, glucagon, and growth hormone, which stimulate lipolysis, gluconeogenesis, and glycogenolysis, which in turn result in hyperglycemia. Called also *rebound hyperglycemia* and *Somogyi effect.*

**Soret p.,** see under *effect.*

**Souques' p.,** a phenomenon seen in incomplete hemiplegia, consisting of involuntary extension and separation of the fingers when the arm is raised; called also *finger p.*

**springlike p.,** André Thomas sign (def. 1).

**staircase p.,** treppe.

**Staub-Traugott p.,** after a glucose load is administered, subsequent loads, given after a short interval, are disposed of at an accelerated rate. See also *Staub-Traugott effect,* under *effect.*

**Straus' p.,** see under *reaction.*

**Strümpell's p.,** tibialis sign.

**Sulzberger-Chase p.,** abolition of dermal contact hypersensitivity to sensitizing agents, e.g., picryl chloride, produced by prior oral feeding of the agent.

**Theobald Smith's p.,** guinea pigs that have been used for standardizing diphtheria antitoxin and have thus been injected with a small dose of blood serum become highly susceptible to the serum and may die quickly if given a large second dose of the same serum a few weeks later. See *anaphylaxis.*

**toe p.,** Babinski's reflex.

**Trousseau's p.,** spasmodic contractions of muscles provoked by pressure upon the nerves which go to them; seen in tetany.

**Tullio's p.,** vertigo induced by high-intensity sounds.

**Twort-d'Herelle p.,** the phenomenon of transmissible bacterial lysis; bacteriophagia. When to a broth culture of typhoid or dysentery bacilli there is added a drop of filtered broth emulsion of the stool from a convalescent typhoid or dysentery patient, complete lysis of the bacterial culture will occur in a few hours. If a drop of this lysed culture is added to another culture of the bacilli, lysis will take place exactly as in the first. A drop of this culture will then dissolve a third culture, and so on through hundreds of transfers. d'Herelle attributed this phenomenon to the action of an ultramicroscopic parasite of bacteria, which he named the *bacteriophage.* See *bacterial virus,* under *virus.*

**Tyndall p.,** see under *effect.*

**Wedensky's p.,** on applying a series of rapidly repeated stimuli to a nerve, the muscle contracts quickly in response to the first stimulus and then fails to respond further; but if the stimuli are applied to the nerve at a slower rate, the muscle responds to all of them.

**Wenckebach p.,** see under *block.*

**Westphal's p.,** 1. (A.K.O. Westphal) orbicularis pupillary reflex. 2. (C.F.O. Westphal) see under *sign.*

**Westphal-Piltz p.,** orbicularis pupillary reflex.

**Wever-Bray p.,** cochlear microphonic.

**Williams' p.,** the tympanic note of skodaic resonance in pleuritis with effusion varies in pitch with the opening and closing of the patient's mouth.

**phe·non** (fe′non) phenom.

**phe·no·pro·pa·zine hy·dro·chlo·ride** (fe″no-pro′pə-zēn) ethopropazine hydrochloride.

**phe·no·thi·a·zine** (fe″no-thi′ə-zēn) 1. a greenish, tasteless compound prepared by fusing diphenylamine with sulfur; used as a veterinary anthelmintic. Called also *dibenzothiazine* and *thiodiphenylamine.* 2. any of a group of antipsychotic agents (e.g., chlorpromazine) resembling phenothiazine in molecular structure, i.e., all sharing a three-ring structure in which two benzene rings are joined by a sulfur and nitrogen atom. They are potent adrenergic blocking agents, their pharmacologic actions including central nervous system depression, prolongation and potentiation of the effects of narcotic and hypnotic drugs, hypotensive activity, and antispasmodic, antihistaminic, and antiemetic activity. See also *antipsychotic.*

**phe·no·type** (fe′no-tīp) [*pheno-* (def. 1) + *type*] [MeSH: Phenotype] 1. the entire physical, biochemical, and physiological makeup of an individual as determined both genetically and environmentally, as opposed to genotype. 2. the expression of a single gene or gene pair.

**Bombay p.,** a rare blood phenotype produced by the interaction of genes of the ABO blood group and a rare recessive gene at a different locus, resulting in a complete lack of H antigen; cells of individuals with this phenotype lack A, B, and H antigens, and their serum contains anti-A, anti-B, and anti-H antigen.

**McLeod p.,** a rare blood phenotype with X-linked inheritance in which several antigens of the Kell blood group are weakly expressed; affected individuals sometimes have an anemic condition called *McLeod syndrome.*

**phe·no·typ·ic** (fe″no-tip′ik) pertaining to or expressive of the phenotype.

**phen·ox·ide** (fən-ok′sīd) phenolate (def. 2).

**phenoxy-** a prefix indicating the presence of the group $—OC_6H_5$, composed of phenyl and an atom of oxygen.

**phe·noxy·benz·amine hy·dro·chlo·ride** (fə-nok″se-ben′zə-mēn) [USP] an irreversible α-adrenergic blocking agent, chemically related to the nitrogen mustards, with a long duration of action; used to control hypertension and sweating in pheochromocytoma, to treat Raynaud's phenomenon, and to treat micturition disorders resulting from neurogenic bladder dysfunction or prostatic obstruction; administered orally.

**phe·no·zy·gous** (fe″no-zi′gəs) [*pheno-* (def. 1) + *zyg-* + *-ous*] having the cranium much narrower than the face, so that the zygomatic arches are seen when the skull is viewed from above. Cf. *cryptozygous.*

**phen·pro·cou·mon** (fen-pro′koo-mon) [MeSH: Phenprocoumon] one of the synthetic coumarin anticoagulants, having a more rapid onset and longer-acting effects than dicumarol and having a marked cumulative effect; administered orally.

**phen·pro·meth·amine hy·dro·chlo·ride** (fen″pro-meth′ə-mēn) phenylpropylmethylamine hydrochloride.

**phen·pro·pi·o·nate** (fən-pro′pe-ə-nāt″) USAN contraction for 3-phenylpropionate.

**phen·sux·i·mide** (fən-suk′sĭ-mīd) [USP] an anticonvulsant used mainly in the treatment of petit mal epilepsy, administered orally.

**phen·ter·mine** (fen′tər-mēn) [MeSH: Phentermine] an adrenergic

isomeric with amphetamine, used as an anorexic; administered orally as a complex with an ion-exchange resin to produce a sustained action.
**p. hydrochloride,** the water-soluble hydrochloride salt of phentermine, used as an anorexic, administered orally.

**phen·tol·amine** (fən-tol'ə-mēn) [MeSH: Phentolamine] an antiadrenergic which blocks the hypertensive action of epinephrine and norepinephrine and most smooth muscle responses involving alpha-adrenergic cell receptors.
**p. hydrochloride,** the monohydrochloride salt of phentolamine, having the same antiadrenergic actions as the base; used mainly in the treatment of peripheral vascular diseases and to prevent and control hypertension due to pheochromocytoma; administered orally.
**p. mesylate** [USP], the methanesulfonate salt of phentolamine, having the same antiadrenergic actions as the base; used mainly in the diagnosis of pheochromocytoma and in the prevention and treatment of cutaneous necrosis and sloughing when extravasation of norepinephrine occurs after intravenous administration; administered intramuscularly and intravenously.

**Phen·u·rone** (fen'u-rōn) trademark for a preparation of phenacemide.

**phen·yl** (fen'əl, fe'nəl) the monovalent radical $C_6H_5$—, derived from benzene by removal of hydrogen. Symbol Ph.
**p. carbinol,** benzyl alcohol.
**p. hydrate, p. hydroxide,** phenol (def. 1).
**p. mercury acetate,** phenylmercuric acetate.
**p. mercury nitrate,** phenylmercuric nitrate.
**p. salicylate,** a compound formerly used as an analgesic, antipyretic, intestinal antiseptic, and enteric coating for tablets, and in the prevention of sunburn. In veterinary medicine, it is sometimes used internally as an antipyretic and externally as an antiseptic. Called also *salol.*

**phen·yl·a·ce·tic ac·id** (fen"əl-ə-se'tik) a catabolite of phenylalanine excessively formed and excreted, sometimes conjugated with glutamine, in phenylketonuria.

**phen·yl·ac·e·tyl·urea** (fen"əl-as"ə-tēl-u-re'ə) phenacemide.

**phen·yl·al·a·nine** (fen"əl-al'ə-nēn) [MeSH: Phenylalanine] an aromatic essential amino acid, $\alpha$-amino-$\beta$-phenylpropionic acid; most of that ingested is hydroxylated to form tyrosine, which is used for protein synthesis, but small amounts are transaminated to phenylpyruvic acid or decarboxylated. Symbols Phe and F. See also table at *amino acid.*

**phen·yl·al·a·nine hy·drox·y·lase** (fen"əl-al'ə-nēn hi-drok'sə-lās) [MeSH: Phenylalanine Hydroxylase] phenylalanine 4-monooxygenase.

**phen·yl·al·a·nine hy·drox·y·lase de·fi·cien·cy** phenylketonuria.

**phen·yl·al·a·nine mono·ox·y·gen·ase** (fen"əl-al'ə-nēn mon"o-ok'sə-jən-ās) [EC 1.14.16.1] a monooxygenase that activates molecular oxygen to catalyze the oxidation of phenylalanine to tyrosine, activating oxygen via oxidation of the cofactor tetrahydrobiopterin to dihydrobiopterin. Deficiency of the enzyme results in hyperphenylalaninemia.

**phen·yl·al·a·nin·emia** (fen"əl-al"ə-nĭ-ne'me-ə) hyperphenylalaninemia.

**phen·yl·al·a·nyl** (fen"əl-al'ə-nəl) the acyl radical of phenylalanine.

***N*-phen·yl·an·thra·nil·ic ac·id** (fen"əl-an"thrə-nil'ik) 2-(phenylamino)benzoic acid: the parent compound of the fenamate analgesics.

**phen·yl·bu·ta·zone** (fen"əl-bu'tə-zōn) [MeSH: Phenylbutazone] a congener of aminopyrine and antipyrine, having analgesic, antipyretic, anti-inflammatory, and mild uricosuric properties; used especially in the treatment of gout, rheumatoid arthritis, ankylosing spondylitis, and other rheumatoid conditions, administered orally. It is given for periods of less than one week because it can cause aplastic anemia and agranulocytosis. Called also *diphebuzol.*

**phen·yl·car·bi·nol** (fen"əl-kahr'bĭ-nol) benzyl alcohol.

**phen·yl·di·meth·yl·py·ra·zo·lon** (fen"əl-di-meth"əl-pi-ra'zo-lon) antipyrine.

**phe·ny·lene** (fen'ə-lēn) a divalent radical, $=C_6H_4$.

***p*-phen·yl·ene·di·amine** (par"ə-fen"əl-ēn-di'ə-mēn) a diamino derivative of benzene used as a dye for hair, garments, and other textiles, as a photographic developing agent, and in a variety of other industrial processes; it is a strong allergen, causing contact dermatitis and bronchial asthma.

**phen·yl·eph·rine** (fen"əl-ef'rin) [MeSH: Phenylephrine] a direct-acting sympathomimetic amine that stimulates $\alpha$-adrenergic receptors and is a powerful vasoconstrictor.
**p. hydrochloride** [USP], the hydrochloride salt of phenylephrine, used as a vasoconstrictor; used topically to decongest nasal and laryngeal mucous membranes and to produce mydriasis without cycloplegia, and intravenously to maintain blood pressure during spinal and inhalation anesthesia, to treat vascular failure in drug-induced shock, shocklike states, and hypotension, and to prolong spinal anesthesia. It is also administered orally as a component of combination antihistaminic-decongestant preparations.
**p. tannate,** the tannate salt of phenylephrine, used as a decongestant in combination antihistaminic-decongestant preparations; administered orally.

**phen·yl·eth·yl·bar·bi·tu·ric ac·id** (fen"əl-eth"əl-bahr"bĭ-tu'rik) phenobarbital.

**phen·yl·gly·co·lic ac·id** (fen"əl-gli-ko'lik) mandelic acid.

**phen·yl·hy·dra·zine** (fen"əl-hi'drə-zēn) a diazo derivative of aniline, used as a reagent for sugars, ketones, and aldehydes.

**phe·nyl·ic** (fə-nil'ik) pertaining to phenyl.

**phen·yl·in·dane·di·one** (fen"əl-in-dān'de-ōn) phenindione.

**phen·yl·ke·ton·uria** (fen"əl-ke"to-nu're-ə) [MeSH: Phenylketonuria] the most severe manifestation of hyperphenylalaninemia due to phenylalanine 4-monooxygenase deficiency, with accumulation and excretion of phenylalanine, phenylpyruvic acid, and related compounds and inherited as an autosomal recessive trait; it is characterized by severe mental retardation, tumors, seizures, hypopigmentation of hair and skin, eczema, and mousy odor, all preventable by early restriction of dietary phenylalanine. Called also *classic p.* Abbreviated PKU or PKU1. See also *hyperphenylalaninemia.*
**atypical p.,** malignant hyperphenylalaninemia.
**classic p.,** phenylketonuria.
**maternal p.,** abnormal fetal development in pregnant women with PKU, probably due to intrauterine exposure of the fetus to high levels of phenylalanine. Miscarriages are frequent and most surviving offspring are severely mentally retarded, often with microcephaly, low birth weight, and congenital anomalies.
**transient p.,** transient hyperphenylalaninemia.

**phen·yl·lac·tic ac·id** (fen"əl-lak'tik) a product of phenylalanine catabolism produced by reduction of phenylpyruvic acid; it is formed and excreted in excess in phenylketonuria.

**phen·yl·mer·cu·ric** (fen"əl-mər-ku'rik) denoting a compound containing the radical $C_6H_5Hg$—, forming various antiseptic, antibacterial, and fungicidal salts.
**p. acetate** [NF], a compound with properties similar to those of phenylmercuric nitrate; used as a bacteriostatic preservative in pharmaceutical preparation, and in solution as a vaginal douche for adjunctive therapy in trichomonal, candidal, bacterial, and mixed infections and nonspecific leukorrhea. It is also widely used as a herbicide, especially for crabgrass. Called also *phenyl mercury acetate.*
**p. nitrate,** the normal salt, $C_6H_5HgNO_3$, which is converted to the basic compound (basic phenylmercuric nitrate) in aqueous solution or in moist air.
**p. nitrate, basic** [NF], an antibacterial and antifungal compound of phenylmercuric nitrate and its hydroxide; used as a bacteriostatic preservative in pharmaceuticals, and as an antiseptic for various topical uses.

**phen·yl·meth·a·nol** (fen"əl-meth'ə-nol) benzyl alcohol.

**phen·yl·pro·pa·nol·amine** (fen"əl-pro"pə-nol'ə-mēn) an adrenergic structurally and pharmacologically related to amphetamine and ephedrine, used as a vasoconstrictor and bronchodilator.
**p. bitartrate** [USP], the bitartrate salt of phenylpropanolamine, administered orally as a nasal decongestant in combination cold preparations.
**p. hydrochloride** [USP], the hydrochloride salt of phenylpropanolamine, applied topically as a vasoconstrictor to decongest mucous membranes and administered orally to produce bronchodilation in the symptomatic control of allergic manifestations. It has also been used as a central nervous system stimulant and as an anorexic.

**phen·yl·pro·pyl·meth·yl·am·ine hy·dro·chlo·ride** (fen"əl-pro"pəl-meth"əl-am'ēn) an adrenergic with chiefly $\alpha$-receptor activity, used mainly as a vasoconstrictor to decongest mucous membranes, applied topically by inhalation. Called also *phenpromethamine hydrochloride.*

**phen·yl·py·ru·vic ac·id** (fen"əl-pi-roo'vik) a metabolite of phenylalanine, excessively formed and excreted in phenylketonuria because the major pathway of phenylalanine catabolism, via hydroxylation, is blocked.

**phen·yl·thio·car·ba·mide** (fen"əl-thi"o-kahr'bə-mīd) phenylthiourea.

**phen·yl·thio·urea** (fen"əl-thi"o-u-re'ə) [MeSH: Phenylthiourea] a compound used in genetics in dry crystal form or in 5 per cent solution. The ability to taste it is inherited as a dominant trait, the compound being intensely bitter to approximately 70 per cent of the population, and nearly tasteless to the rest. Called also *phenylthiocarbamide (PTC).*

**phen·yl·tol·ox·amine cit·rate** (fen″əl-tol-ok′sə-mēn) an isomer of diphenhydramine, used as an antihistaminic, mainly to decongest the nasal mucosa, administered orally.

**phen·y·to·in** (fen′ĭ-to-in″) [USP] [MeSH: Phenytoin] an anticonvulsant and cardiac depressant used in the treatment of all forms of epilepsy except petit mal and as an antiarrhythmic, administered orally. Called also *diphenylhydantoin.*
**p. sodium** [USP], the monosodium salt of phenytoin, having the same appearance, actions, and uses as the base; administered orally and intravenously.

**phe(o)-** [Gr. *phaios* dun, dusky] a combining form meaning brown or dusky. See also *phae(o)-.*

**pheo·chrome** (fe′o-krōm) [*pheo-* + *-chrome*] chromaffin.

**pheo·chro·mo·blast** (fe″o-kro′mo-blast) any of the embryonic structures which develop into pheochrome (chromaffin) cells.

**pheo·chro·mo·blas·to·ma** (fe″o-kro″mo-blas-to′mə) pheochromocytoma.

**pheo·chro·mo·cyte** (fe″o-kro′mo-sīt) [*pheochrome* + *-cyte*] a chromaffin cell.

**pheo·chro·mo·cy·to·ma** (fe″o-kro″mo-si-to′mə) [*pheochromocyte* + *-oma*] [MeSH: Pheochromocytoma] a usually benign, well-encapsulated, lobular, vascular tumor of chromaffin tissue of the adrenal medulla or sympathetic paraganglia. Because of increased secretion of epinephrine and norepinephrine, hypertension is a cardinal symptom; it may be persistent or intermittent. During severe attacks, there may be headache; sweating; palpitation and tremor; pallor or flushing of the face; nausea and vomiting; pain in the chest and abdomen; and paresthesias of the extremities. Called also *medullary chromaffinoma, medullary paraganglioma, chromaffin cell tumor,* and *pheochromoblastoma.*

**phe·re·sis** (fə-re′sis) [Gr. *aphairesis* removal] apheresis.

**pher·o·mone** (fer′o-mōn) a substance secreted to the outside of the body by an individual and perceived (as by smell) by a second individual of the same species, releasing a specific reaction of behavior in the percipient.

**pheth·ar·bi·tal** (feth-ahr′bĭ-təl) a nonhypnotic barbiturate which has been used as an anticonvulsant and in the treatment of unconjugated hyperbilirubinemia.

**PhG** Graduate in Pharmacy; Pharmacopoeia Germanica (German pharmacopeia).

**phi** (fi) [Φ, φ] the twenty-first letter of the Greek alphabet.

**phi·al** (fi′əl) a vial or small bottle.

**Phi·al·e·mo·ni·um** (fi″əl-ə-mo′ne-əm) a genus of Fungi Imperfecti of the form-class Hyphomycetes, form-family Dematiaceae, closely related to *Acremonium* and *Phialophora. P. obova′tum* has been isolated from hyalohyphomycosis.

**phi·a·lide** (fi′ə-līd) [Gr. *phialis,* dim. of *phialē* a broad flat vessel] 1. a flask-shaped conidiogenous cell formed in blastic conidiogenesis, projecting from the mycelium and not increasing in length with successive conidium formation. 2. the end cell of a phialophore.

**phi·a·lo·co·nid·i·um** (fi″ə-lo-kə-nid′e-əm) phialospore.

**Phi·a·loph·o·ra** (fi″ə-lof′ə-rə) [MeSH: Phialophora] a genus of Fungi Imperfecti of the form-class Hyphomycetes, form-family Dematiaceae. *P. jeansel′mei* and *P. spini′fera* have been reclassified in genus *Exophiala. P. verruco′sa* causes chromoblastomycosis.

**phi·a·lo·phore** (fi′ə-lo-for″) in certain fungi, the branch of the mycelium that bears at its tip the phialospores.

**phi·a·lo·spore** (fi′ə-lə-spor) a spore borne at the end of a phialide or a phialophore.

**-phil** [Gr. *philos* loving, dear] a word termination denoting one having an affinity for something. Also, *-phile.*

**-phile** see *-phil.*

**-philia** [Gr. *philein* to love] a word termination denoting *(a)* an abnormal craving or attraction or *(b)* an affinity for an object denoted by the word stem to which it is affixed.

**phi·li·a·ter** (fĭ-li′ə-tər) [Gr. *philos* fond + *iatreia* healing] a person interested in medical science, particularly a medical student.

**-philic** [Gr. *philos* loving] a word termination meaning having an affinity for.

**Phil·ip's glands** (fil′ips) [Sir Robert William *Philip,* Scottish physician, 1857–1939] see under *gland.*

**Phi·lippe-Gom·bault tract** (fe-lēp′gom-bo′) [Claudien *Philippe,* French pathologist, 1866–1903; François Alexis Albert *Gombault,* French neurologist, 1844–1904] Gombault-Philippe triangle.

**Phil·ly·rea** (fĭ-lir′e-ə) a genus of evergreen shrubs of the family Oleaceae, native to the Mediterranean region. *P. latifo′lia* L. has leaves and bark that contain the medicinal substance phillyrin.

**phil·ly·rin** (fil′ĭ-rin) a crystalline substance that has antimalarial properties, extracted from the leaves and bark of evergreens of the genus *Phillyrea,* especially *P. latifolia* L.

**phil·trum** (fil′trəm) [Gr. *philtron* love potion] [TA] the vertical groove in the median portion of the upper lip, a part of the prolabium.

**phi·mo·sis** (fi-mo′sis) [Gr. *phimōsis* a muzzling or closure] [MeSH: Phimosis] constriction of the preputial orifice so that the prepuce cannot be retracted back over the glans.

**phi·mot·ic** (fi-mot′ik) pertaining to phimosis.

**pHi·so·Hex** (fi′so-heks) trademark for an emulsion containing hexachlorophene.

**phle·bal·gia** (flə-bal′jə) [*phleb-* + *-algia*] pain in a vein or varix.

**phleb·an·gi·o·ma** (fleb″an-je-o′mə) [*phleb-* + *angioma*] venous aneurysm.

**phleb·ar·te·ri·ec·ta·sia** (fleb″ahr-tēr″e-ək-ta′zhə) [*phleb-* + *arteriectasia*] vasodilation.

**phleb·ec·ta·sia** (fleb″ek-ta′zhə) [*phleb-* + *-ectasia*] varicosity (def. 1).
**p. laryn′gis,** permanent dilatation of the veins of the larynx, especially those of the vocal cords.

**phle·bec·ta·sis** (flə-bek′tə-sis) varicosity (def. 1).

**phle·bec·to·my** (flə-bek′to-me) [*phleb-* + *-ectomy*] excision of a vein, or of a part of a vein.

**phleb·ec·to·pia** (fleb″ek-to′pe-ə) [*phleb-* + *-ectopia*] displacement of a vein.

**phle·bec·to·py** (flə-bek′to-pe) phlebectopia.

**phleb·em·phrax·is** (fleb″əm-frak′sis) [*phleb-* + *emphraxis*] obstruction of a vein by a plug or clot.

**phle·bis·mus** (flə-biz′məs) obstruction and consequent dilation of veins.

**phle·bit·ic** (flə-bit′ik) pertaining to phlebitis.

**phle·bi·tis** (flə-bi′tis) [*phleb-* + *-itis*] [MeSH: Phlebitis] inflammation of a vein; when accompanied by thrombus formation it is called *thrombophlebitis.*
**adhesive p.,** phlebitis which tends to the obliteration of the vein; called also *plastic p.* and *proliferative p.*
**blue p.,** phlegmasia cerulea dolens.
**p. mi′grans, migrating p.,** thrombophlebitis migrans.
**obliterating p., obstructive p.,** phlebitis that obstructs a vein.
**plastic p.,** adhesive p.
**productive p.,** phlebosclerosis.
**proliferative p.,** adhesive p.
**puerperal p.,** septic inflammation of uterine or other veins following childbirth.
**septic p.,** that which is related to a septic process, as in erysipelas, peritonitis, or endometritis. In it the thrombus breaks down and septic emboli are carried to distant parts of the body. Called also *suppurative p.*
**sinus p.,** inflammation of a cerebral sinus.
**suppurative p.,** septic p.

**phleb(o)-** [Gr. *phleps,* gen. *phlebos* vein] a combining form denoting relationship to a vein or veins. See also words beginning *ven(o)-.*

**phle·boc·ly·sis** (flə-bok′lĭ-sis) [*phlebo-* + *clysis*] injection of fluid into a vein.
**drip p., slow p.,** phleboclysis in which the solution is instilled slowly, drop by drop.

**phlebo·fi·bro·sis** (fleb″o-fi-bro′sis) phlebosclerosis.

**phle·bog·e·nous** (flə-boj′ə-nəs) originating in a vein.

**phlebo·gram** (fleb′o-gram) [*phlebo-* + *-gram*] 1. radiograph of a vein taken during phlebography. 2. a tracing of the venous pulse (see illustration at *pulse*) made with a phlebograph or sphygmograph. Called also *venogram.*

**phlebo·graph** (fleb′o-graf) [*phlebo-* + *-graph*] an instrument for recording the venous pulse.

**phle·bog·ra·phy** (flə-bog′rə-fe) [*phlebo-* + *-graphy*] [MeSH: Phlebography] 1. angiography of veins. 2. the graphic recording of the venous pulse. Called also *venography.*
**ascending p.,** that in which contrast medium is injected into a vein in the foot and observed as it ascends toward the heart.
**descending p.,** a method for detecting reversed flow of blood: contrast medium is injected into the common femoral vein with the patient in an upright position; since it is heavier than blood the contrast medium may move downward spontaneously or when en-

couraged by a Valsalva maneuver, thus indicating any incompetent valves or other areas of reversed flow.

**phleb·oid** (fleb′oid) [*phlebo-* + *-oid*] 1. resembling a vein. 2. venose.

**phlebo·lith** (fleb′o-lith) [*phlebo-* + *-lith*] a calculus in a vein; called also *vein stone.*

**phlebo·li·thi·a·sis** (fleb″o-lĭ-thi′ə-sis) [*phlebo-* + *lithiasis*] the presence or development of phleboliths.

**phle·bol·o·gy** (flə-bol′ə-je) [*phlebo-* + *-logy*] the study of the veins and their diseases.

**phlebo·ma·nom·e·ter** (fleb″o-mə-nom′ə-tər) a manometer for the direct measurement of venous blood pressure.

**phlebo·me·tri·tis** (fleb″o-mə-tri′tis) [*phlebo-* + *metr-* + *-itis*] inflammation of the veins of the uterus.

**phlebo·phle·bos·to·my** (fleb″o-flə-bos′tə-me) operative anastomosis of vein to vein; called also *venovenostomy.*

**phleb·oph·thal·mot·o·my** (fleb″of-thəl-mot′ə-me) ophthalmophlebotomy.

**phlebo·pi·ezom·e·try** (fleb″o-pi″ə-zom′ə-tre) [*phlebo-* + *piezo-* + *-metry*] measurement of the venous pressure.

**phlebo·plas·ty** (fleb′o-plas″te) [*phlebo-* + *-plasty*] plastic operation for the repair of a vein.

**phlebo·rhe·og·ra·phy** (fleb″o-re-og′rə-fe) [*phlebo-* + *rheography*] a technique for measuring venous volume changes in response to respiration and to compression of the foot or calf, employing a plethysmograph having cuffs applied to the abdomen, thigh, upper, mid, and lower calf, and foot; used in the diagnosis of deep venous thrombosis.

**phle·bor·rha·phy** (flə-bor′ə-fe) [*phlebo-* + *-rrhaphy*] the suturing of a vein; called also *venorrhaphy, venesuture,* and *venisuture.*

**phleb·or·rhex·is** (fleb″o-rek′sis) [*phlebo-* + *-rrhexis*] rupture of a vein.

**phlebo·scle·ro·sis** (fleb″o-sklə-ro′sis) [*phlebo-* + *sclerosis*] fibrous thickening of the walls of the veins; called also *phlebofibrosis, proliferative endophlebitis, venofibrosis, venosclerosis,* and *venous sclerosis.*

**phle·bo·sis** (flə-bo′sis) abnormal noninflammatory changes in the veins.

**phleb·os·ta·sia** (fleb″os-ta′zhə) phlebostasis.

**phle·bos·ta·sis** (flə-bos′tə-sis) [*phlebo-* + *-stasis*] 1. venous stasis. 2. temporary sequestration of a portion of the blood from the general circulation by application of tourniquets on an extremity.

**phlebo·ste·no·sis** (fleb″o-stə-no′sis) [*phlebo-* + *stenosis*] stenosis or constriction of a vein.

**phlebo·throm·bo·sis** (fleb″o-throm-bo′sis) [*phlebo-* + *thrombosis*] presence of a clot in a vein, unassociated with inflammation of the wall of the vein. Cf. *thrombophlebitis.* Called also *venous thrombosis.*

**phle·bot·o·mist** (flə-bot′ə-mist) one who practices phlebotomy.

**phle·bot·o·mize** (flə-bot′ə-mīz) to remove blood by phlebotomy.

**Phle·bot·o·mus** (flə-bot′ə-məs) [*phlebo-* + Gr. *tomos* a cutting] [MeSH: Phlebotomus] a genus of very small, bloodsucking sandflies of the family Psychodidae, many species of which are vectors of disease-causing organisms.
**P. argen′tipes,** the vector of visceral leishmaniasis in India.
**P. chinen′sis,** the vector of visceral leishmaniasis in China.
**P. lon′gipes,** a vector of *Leishmania aethiopica,* the etiologic agent of diffuse cutaneous leishmaniasis in Kenya and Ethiopia.
**P. ma′jor,** a vector of *Leishmania donovani infantum* in the Mediterranean region.
**P. marti′ni,** the major vector of visceral leishmaniasis in East Africa.
**P. nogu′chii,** a species found in Peru which may transmit *Bartonella bacilliformis,* the etiologic agent of Carrión's disease; called also *Lutzomyia noguchi.*
**P. orienta′lis,** the vector of visceral leishmaniasis in the Sudan.
**P. papata′si,** a species that is the vector of the virus of phlebotomus fever, or protozoa of the *Leishmania tropica* complex and of *L. donovani infantum.*
**P. pe′difer,** a vector of *Leishmania aethiopica,* the etiologic agent of diffuse cutaneous leishmaniasis in Kenya and Ethiopia.
**P. pernicio′sus,** a vector of *Leishmania donovani infantum* in the Mediterranean region.
**P. sergen′ti,** a vector of *Leishmania tropica,* the etiologic agent of dry cutaneous leishmaniasis.
**P. verruca′rum,** a vector of *Bartonella bacilliformis,* the etiologic agent of Carrión's disease.

**phle·bot·o·my** (flə-bot′ə-me) [*phlebo-* + *-tomy*] [MeSH: Phlebotomy] 1. incision of a vein, as for the letting of blood. 2. needle puncture of a vein for the drawing of blood. Called also *venepuncture, venesection, venipuncture, venisection,* and *venotomy.*
**bloodless p.,** phlebostasis, def. 2.

**Phlebovirus** (fleb′o-vi″rəs) [*Phlebotomus* + *virus*] [MeSH: Phlebovirus] sandfly fever viruses and uukuviruses; a genus of the family Bunyaviridae. Viruses are classified in two antigenic groups, the sandfly fever group and the Uukuniemi group. The sandfly fever group includes at least 39 species in nine serogroups and ungrouped species; the Uukuniemi group (the uukuviruses), which was previously recognized as a separate genus, contains 12 species in a single serogroup. The sandfly fever group includes the pathogens sandfly fever–Naples, sandfly fever–Sicilian, Toscana, and Rift Valley fever viruses; most sandfly fever viruses are transmitted by sandflies of the genus *Phlebotomus,* but some are mosquito-borne. Uukuviruses are tick-borne and include no known human pathogens.

**phlegm** (flem) [Gr. *phlegma*] 1. abnormally thick mucus secreted by the mucosa of the respiratory passages during certain infectious processes. 2. in humoralism, one of the four humors of the body.

**phleg·ma·sia** (fleg-ma′zhə) [Gr. "heat, inflammation"] old term for inflammation.
**p. al′ba do′lens,** phlebitis of the femoral vein, occasionally following parturition or an acute febrile illness; it is characterized by swelling of the leg, usually without redness. Called also *galactophlebitis, thrombotic p., milk leg,* and *white leg.*
**cellulitic p.,** swelling and inflammation of the leg after childbirth from infection of the connective tissue.
**p. ceru′lea do′lens,** an acute fulminating form of deep venous thrombosis, with reactive arterial spasm and pronounced edema of the extremity and severe cyanosis, purpuric areas, and petechiae; called also *blue phlebitis.*
**thrombotic p.,** p. alba dolens.

**phleg·mat·ic** (fleg-mat′ik) [Gr. *phlegmatikos*] characterized by an excess of the supposed humor called phlegm; hence, heavy, dull, and apathetic.

**phleg·mon** (fleg′mon) [Gr. *phlegmonē*] 1. a spreading, diffuse inflammatory reaction to infection with microaerophilic streptococci, which forms a suppurative or gangrenous and undermining lesion that may extend into deep subcutaneous tissues and muscles, creating multiple small pockets of pus. Called also *phlegmonous cellulitis.* Cf. *cellulitis* and *erysipelas.* 2. a solid, swollen, inflamed mass of pancreatic tissue occurring as a complication of acute pancreatitis, which may subside spontaneously or become secondarily infected and develop into an abscess. Cf. *pseudocyst,* def. 2.
**pancreatic p.,** see *phlegmon,* def. 2.
**periurethral p.,** an extensive fulminating phlegmon originating in and about the urethra and usually accompanied by massive gangrene of the genital and perigenital tissues; called also *periurethral cellulitis.*
**pharyngeal p.,** swelling and necrosis of the wall of the pharynx in cattle, with toxemia and respiratory distress; it may be fatal. Infection with *Fusobacterium necrophorum* is sometimes the cause. Called also *intermandibular cellulitis.*

**phleg·mon·ous** (fleg′mən-əs) pertaining to or attended by phlegmon; see under *cellulitis.*

**Phle·um** (fle′əm) a genus of grasses (family Gramineae). *P. praten′se* is timothy or timothy grass, a North American species used as fodder for cattle and horses; its pollen causes hay fever in susceptible people. When infested with *Claviceps purpurea,* it can cause ergotism in animals.

**phlo·gis·tic** (flo-jis′tik) [Gr. *phlogistos*] inflammatory.

**phlo·gis·ton** (flo-jis′ton) [Gr. *phlogistos* burnt up, inflammable] a term and general chemical theory of fire or inflammability proposed by George Ernst Stahl in 1702, warmly defended by Joseph Priestley, denied and disproved by Antoine Laurent Lavoisier (1775), and defunct after 1800. Phlogiston was a material substance thought to be present in and compounded with all combustible bodies and was released by combustion, the other structures of the substance being left behind. Liberation of phlogiston thus would correspond to oxidation, and combination with phlogiston, to reduction.

**phlog(o)-** [Gr. *phlox,* gen. *phlogos* flame] a combining form denoting relationship to inflammation.

**phlo·go·cyte** (flo′go-sīt) [*phlogo-* + *-cyte*] a cell characteristic of tissue in an inflamed state; a plasma cell.

**phlo·go·cy·to·sis** (flo″go-si-to′sis) presence of phlogocytes (plasma cells) in the blood.

**phlo·go·gen** (flo′go-jən) a body that has the power of causing inflammation.

**phlo·go·gen·ic** (flo″go-jen′ik) [*phlogo-* + *-genic*] causing inflammation.

**phlo·gog·e·nous** (flo-goj′ə-nəs) phlogogenic.

**phlo·got·ic** (flo-got′ik) inflammatory.

**phlo·rhi·zin** (flo-ri′zin) [Gr. *phloios* bark + *rhiza* root] [MeSH: Phlorhizin] a bitter glycoside from the root bark of apple, cherry, plum, and pear trees; it causes glycosuria *(phlorhizin glycosuria)* by blocking the tubular reabsorption of glucose. Spelled also *phlorizin* and *phlorrhizin.*

**phlo·rhi·zin hy·dro·lase** (flo-ri'zin hi'dro-lās) glycosylceramidase.

**phlo·rhi·zi·nize** (flo-ri'zi-nīz) to bring under the influence of phlorhizin.

**phlo·rid·zin** (flo-rid'zin) phlorhizin.

**phlo·rid·zin·ize** (flo-rid'zi-nīz) phlorhizinize.

**phlo·ri·zin** (flo-ri'zin) phlorhizin.

**phlo·ro·glu·cin** (flor"o-gloo'sin) [*phlorhizin* + Gr. *glykys* sweet] the aglycone of many glycosides, obtained from the bark of apple and other trees, and used as a reagent for pentoses, pentosans, glycuronates, hydrochloric acid in gastric juice, etc. It is an excellent decalcifier of bone specimens. See *Günzburg's test,* under *tests.*

**phlo·ro·glu·ci·nol** (flor"o-gloo'sĭ-nol) [MeSH: Phloroglucinol] phloroglucin.

**phlor·rhi·zin** (flo-ri'zin) phlorhizin.

**phlox·ine** (flok'sin) a brick-red acid dye said to have a destructive action on cancer cells.
**p. B,** a red acid dye used as a plasma stain in histology and as a component of Mallory's phloxine–methylene blue stain.

**phlyc·ten** (flik'tən) phlyctena.

**phlyc·te·na** (flik-te'nə) pl. *phlycte'nae* [Gr. *phlyktaina*] 1. a blister made by a burn. 2. a small vesicle containing lymph seen on the conjunctiva in certain conditions. Called also *phlycten.*

**phlyc·te·nar** (flik'tə-nər) pertaining to or marked by phlyctenae.

**phlyc·te·noid** (flik'tə-noid) [*phlycten* + *-oid*] resembling a phlyctena.

**phlyc·ten·u·la** (flik-ten'u-lə) pl. *phlycten'ulae* [L.] phlyctenule.

**phlyc·ten·u·lar** (flik-ten'u-lər) associated with the formation of phlyctenules or vesicles, or of prominences that look like vesicles.

**phlyc·ten·ule** (flik'tən-ūl) [L. *phlyctaenula;* Gr. *phlyktaina* blister] a small vesicle, or an ulcerated nodule of the cornea or of the conjunctiva.

**phlyc·ten·u·lo·sis** (flik"tən-u-lo'sis) an eye condition marked by the formation of phlyctenules, as phlyctenular keratoconjunctivitis, conjunctivitis, or ophthalmia.
**allergic p.,** phlyctenulosis due to allergy.
**tuberculous p.,** phlyctenulosis due to tuberculous allergy.

**pho·bia** (fo'be-ə) [Gr. *phobos* fear + *-ia*] [MeSH: Phobic Disorders] a persistent, irrational, intense fear of a specific object, activity, or situation (the phobic stimulus), fear that is recognized as being excessive or unreasonable by the individual himself. When a phobia is a significant source of distress or interferes with social functioning, it is considered a mental disorder (sometimes called a *phobic disorder*); in DSM-IV phobias are classified with the anxiety disorders and are subclassified as agoraphobia, specific phobias, and social phobias.
**simple p.,** specific p.
**social p.** [DSM-IV], an anxiety disorder characterized by fear and avoidance of social or performance situations in which the individual fears possible embarrassment and humiliation, e.g., fears of speaking, performing, or eating in public. Panic attacks may occur.
**specific p.** [DSM-IV], an anxiety disorder characterized by persistent and excessive or unreasonable fear of a circumscribed, well-defined object or situation, in contrast to fear of being alone or of public places (agoraphobia) or fear of embarrassment in social situations (social phobia). Common specific phobias involve fear of animals, particularly dogs, snakes, insects, and mice; fear of closed spaces (claustrophobia); and fear of heights (acrophobia).

**-phobia** a word termination denoting irrational fear of or an aversion to the subject indicated by the stem to which it is affixed.

**pho·bic** (fo'bik) of the nature of or pertaining to a phobia.

**pho·bo·pho·bia** (fo"bo-fo'be-ə) [Gr. *phobos* fear + *-phobia*] irrational fear of one's own fears or of acquiring a phobia.

**Pho·ca·ne·ma** (fo"kə-ne'mə) a genus of nematodes of the family Anisakidae; different stages of development are found in marine fishes and sea animals and cause anisakiasis in other animals including humans who eat raw or inadequately cooked seafood.

**Pho·cas' disease** (fo-kahz') [B. Gerasime *Phocas,* French surgeon, 1861–1937] see under *disease.*

**pho·co·me·lia** (fo"ko-me'le-ə) [Gr. *phōkē* seal + *-melia*] a type of meromelia characterized by absence of the proximal portion of a limb or limbs, the hands or feet being attached to the trunk of the body by a single small, irregularly shaped bone.

**pho·com·e·lus** (fo-kom'ə-ləs) [Gr. *phōkē* seal + *melos* limb] an individual exhibiting phocomelia.

**Pho·ma** (fo'mə) a genus of Fungi Imperfecti of the form-class Coelomycetes, widely found on plants and in the soil. Several species have been occasionally isolated from cases of phaeohyphomycosis.

**pho·mop·sin** (fo-mop'sin) a mycotoxin found in *Phomopsis leptostromiformis* and *P. rossiana;* it causes mycotoxic lupinosis in grazing animals.

**Pho·mop·sis** (fo-mop'sis) a genus of Fungi Imperfecti of the form-class Coelomycetes. *P. leptostromifor'mis* and *P. rossia'na* infest plants of the genus *Lupinus* and contain phomopsins, mycotoxins that cause mycotoxic lupinosis in grazing livestock.

**phon** (fōn) [Gr. *phōnē* voice] a unit of the subjective loudness of a sound.

**pho·naco·scope** (fo-nak'o-skōp) the apparatus used in phonacoscopy.

**pho·na·cos·co·py** (fo"nə-kos'kə-pe) [*phon-* + *acou-* + *-scopy*] combined auscultation and percussion by means of a bell-shaped resonating chamber containing a percussion hammer, which is held on the anterior thoracic wall while the examiner listens at the back of the thorax.

**pho·nal** (fo'nəl) 1. pertaining to sound. 2. vocal.

**phon·as·the·nia** (fo"nəs-the'ne-ə) [*phon-* + *asthenia*] weakness of voice or difficult phonation from overuse, debilitation, or old age. Called also *myasthenia laryngis* and *vocal fatigue.*

**pho·na·tion** (fo-na'shən) [MeSH: Phonation] the utterance of vocal sounds. See also *speech.*
**subenergetic p.,** hypophonia.
**superenergetic p.,** hyperphonia.

**pho·na·to·ry** (fo'nə-tor"e) pertaining to phonation.

**pho·neme** (fo'nēm) [Gr. *phōnēma* a thing spoken] the smallest speech sound in a language that is distinguishable from others in its class.

**phon·en·do·scope** (fōn-en'do-skōp) [*phon-* + *endoscope*] a stethoscopic device that intensifies auscultatory sounds, consisting of a shallow metal cup closed by a diaphragm.

**pho·net·ic** (fə-net'ik) [Gr. *phonētikos*] pertaining to the articulated sounds of speech; called also *phonic.*

**pho·net·ics** (fə-net'iks) [MeSH: Phonetics] the science of vocal sounds; called also *phonology.*

**pho·ni·at·rics** (fo"ne-at'riks) [*phon-* + *-iatrics*] logopedics.

**phon·ic** (fon'ik, fo'nik) 1. pertaining to sound. 2. vocal. 3. phonetic.

**pho·nism** (fo'niz-əm) a form of synesthesia in which a sensation of hearing is produced by the effect of something seen, felt, tasted, smelled, or thought of.

**phon(o)-** [Gr. *phōnē* voice] a combining form denoting relationship to sound, often specifically the sound of the voice.

**pho·no·an·gi·og·ra·phy** (fo"no-an"je-og'rə-fe) the recording and analysis of arterial bruits to estimate the extent of arterial stenosis.

**pho·no·aus·cul·ta·tion** (fo"no-aws"kəl-ta'shən) auscultation in which a tuning fork is placed over the organ to be examined and its vibrations are listened to through a stethoscope placed over the same organ.

**pho·no·car·di·o·gram** (fo"no-kahr'de-o-gram) [*phono-* + *cardiogram*] the graphic record produced by phonocardiography.

**pho·no·car·dio·graph** (fo"no-kahr'de-o-graf) [*phono-* + *cardiograph*] the instrument used in phonocardiography, generally comprising a microphone, amplifier, filters, and a recording device.
**fetal p.,** an instrument which provides continuous, instantaneous recording of fetal heart sounds.

**pho·no·car·dio·graph·ic** (fo"no-kahr"de-o-graf'ik) pertaining to phonocardiography or to a phonocardiogram.

**pho·no·car·di·og·ra·phy** (fo"no-kahr"de-og'rə-fe) [*phono-* + *cardiography*] [MeSH: Phonocardiography] the graphic representation of heart sounds, murmurs, or any acoustic phenomena emanating from the heart; in clinical use, the term usually includes recording of the pulse tracings (carotid, apex, and jugular venous) for completeness, and is often combined with other noninvasive methods such as echocardiography.
**intracardiac p.,** the graphic registration of sounds produced by action of the heart by means of a phonocatheter passed into one of the heart chambers.

**pho·no·cath·e·ter** (fo"no-kath'ə-tər) a device similar in appearance to a conventional catheter, with a microphone at the tip; used in recording the sounds of the heart and great vessels.

**pho·no·cath·e·ter·i·za·tion** (fo"no-kath"ə-tər-ĭ-za'shən) the use

of a phonocatheter for the detection of sounds produced by the circulatory system.
**intracardiac p.,** the passage of a phonocatheter into a chamber of the heart, for the detection of sounds as an aid in diagnosis of cardiac defects.

**pho·no·gram** (fo'no-gram) [*phono-* + *-gram*] a graphic record of a sound, as of a heart sound.

**pho·nol·o·gy** (fə-nol'ə-je) [*phono-* + *-logy*] phonetics.

**pho·no·my·oc·lo·nus** (fo"no-mi-ok'lə-nəs) myoclonus in which a sound is heard on auscultation of an affected muscle, indicating fibrillar contractions.

**pho·no·myo·gram** (fo"no-mi'o-gram) [*phono-* + *myo-* + *-gram*] a tracing of the sound produced by muscle action.

**pho·no·my·og·ra·phy** (fo"no-mi-og'rə-fe) the recording of muscle sounds by an oscillograph to which the sounds are transmitted by a microphone placed over the muscle.

**pho·no·pho·bia** (fo"no-fo'be-ə) [*phono-* + *-phobia*] irrational fear of sounds or of speaking aloud.

**pho·nop·sia** (fo-nop'se-ə) [*phon-* + *-opsia*] a type of photism consisting of a sensation of seeing colors when sounds are heard.

**pho·no·re·no·gram** (fo"no-re'no-gram) a graphic representation by means of a paper recording of pulsations of the renal artery obtained by use of a phonocatheter passed through a ureter into the pelvis of the kidney.

**pho·no·scope** (fo'no-skōp) [*phono-* + *scope*] an instrument for auscultatory percussion.

**pho·nos·co·py** (fo-nos'kə-pe) 1. the delimiting of solid and hollow organs (liver, heart, lungs, etc.) by listening with a stethoscope while percussion is made in the vicinity. 2. the use of the phonoscope.

**pho·no·se·lec·to·scope** (fo"no-sə-lek'tə-skōp) [*phono-* + *select* + *-scope*] an instrument for auscultation by means of which the lower (normal) range of the pulmonary sounds are eliminated, thus emphasizing the higher-pitched pathologic elements.

**pho·no·stetho·graph** (fo"no-steth'o-graf) an instrument by which the chest sounds are amplified, filtered, and recorded.

**Pho·ran·den·dron** (for"an-den'drən) a genus of North American parasitic plants of the family Loranthaceae. *P. flaves'cens* (Pursh.) Nutt. is American mistletoe, which was formerly used as an oxytocic.

**phor·bol** (for'bol) a polycyclic alcohol occurring naturally in croton oil; it is the parent compound of the phorbol esters.
**p. ester,** any of several esters of phorbol that are potent cocarcinogens; they are structurally similar to diacylglycerol and can activate protein kinase C. They are used frequently in research to enhance the induction of mutagenesis or tumors by carcinogens.

**-phore** [Gr. *phoros* carrying] a word termination denoting a carrier of the object designated by the stem to which it is affixed, as a melanophore.

**-phoresis** [Gr. *phorēsis* a being carried] a word termination indicating transmission, as electrophoresis.

**pho·ria** (for'e-ə) [MeSH: Strabismus] heterophoria.

**pho·ria·scope** (for'e-ə-skōp) [*phoria* + *-scope*] a prism-refracting instrument for use in orthoptic training.

**Phor·mia** (for'me-ə) the blackbottle flies, a genus of blue, black, or green flies of the family Calliphoridae.
**P. regi'na,** a blowfly which causes a cutaneous myiasis of sheep in the United States and Canada. The larvae (maggots) have also been introduced into infected wounds to facilitate healing.

**pho·ro·blast** (for'o-blast) [Gr. *phoros* carrying + *-blast*] fibroblast.

**pho·ro·cyte** (for'o-sīt) a connective tissue cell.

**pho·ro·cy·to·sis** (fo"ro-si-to'sis) proliferation of connective tissue cells.

**pho·rom·e·ter** (fə-rom'ə-tər) [Gr. *phora* movement, range + *-meter*] 1. an instrument to test oculomotor balance. 2. a phoro-optometer.

**pho·rom·e·try** (fə-rom'ə-tre) use of the phorometer.

**pho·ront** (for'ont) [Gr. *phora* producing + *ontos* being] the encysted stage or form in the life cycle of certain ciliate protozoa, produced by a tomite and developing into a trophont.

**pho·ro-op·tom·e·ter** (for"o-op-tom'ə-tər) [Gr. *phora* movement, range + *opto-* + *-meter*] an instrument to test ocular ductions, phorias, refractions, and vergences.

**Pho·rop·tor** (fo-rop'tor) trademark for a phorometer fitted with a battery of cylindrical lenses.

**pho·ro·scope** (for'o-skōp) [Gr. *phora* movement, range + *-scope*] a fixed trial frame for eye testing, with a head rest that may be fastened to the table or the wall.

**pho·ro·tone** (for'o-tōn) [Gr. *phora* movement, range + *tonos* tension] an instrument for exercising the muscles of the eye.

**pho·ro·zo·on** (for"o-zo'on) [Gr. *phoros* fruitful + *zōon* animal] the asexual stage in the life history of an organism.

**phose** (fōz) [Gr. *phōs* light] any subjective visual sensation, as of light or color; see *aphose, centraphose, centrophose, chromophose, peripheraphose, peripherophose,* etc.

**phos·gene** (fos'jēn) [MeSH: Phosgene] carbonic dichloride, $CCl_2O$; a highly toxic, colorless gas that causes rapidly fatal pulmonary edema or pneumonia on inhalation; used in the synthesis of a number of organic compounds and formerly used as a war gas.

**phos·gen·ic** (fos-jen'ik) [*phose* + *-genic*] producing light.

**pho·sis** (fo'sis) the production of a phose.

**Phos·Lo** (foz-lo') trademark for a preparation of calcium acetate.

**phos·pha·gen** (fos'fə-jən) any of a group of high energy compounds that are substituted derivatives of phosphoguanidine; they act as reservoirs of phosphate bond energy, donating phosphoryl groups to phosphorylate ADP when ATP levels are low. Phosphocreatine is the phosphagen of vertebrates.

**phos·pha·gen·ic** (fos"fə-jen'ik) producing or forming phosphate.

**phos·pha·tase** (fos'fə-tās) a term used in the recommended names of some enzymes of the hydrolase class that are phosphoric monoester hydrolases [EC 3.1.3], catalyzing the release of inorganic phosphate from phosphoric esters. See also *acid phosphatase* and *alkaline phosphatase.*

**phos·phate** (fos'fāt) [L. *phosphas*] 1. any salt of phosphoric acid or its anions, particularly referring to orthophosphate (inorganic phosphate). 2. any ester of phosphoric acid or of one of its salts or anions; an organic phosphate (q.v.).
**acid p.,** any phosphate in which only one or two of the three replaceable hydrogen atoms are taken up or replaced.
**alkaline p.,** a phosphate of an alkaline metal, as sodium or potassium.
**ammoniomagnesium p., ammonium magnesium p.,** a double salt of ammonium and magnesium with orthophosphoric acid, closely allied to and often associated with triple phosphate. See *struvite.*
**carbamoyl p.,** an important intermediate compound in the formation of pyrimidine and citrulline, the latter being a step in urea formation.
**chromic p. P 32** [USP], the phosphate salt of chromium, labeled with radiophosphorus ($^{32}P$); a colloidal suspension administered intraperitoneally or intrapleurally in the treatment of intraperitoneal or intrapleural effusions resulting from metastatic disease and intrastitially in the treatment of certain ovarian and prostate carcinomas.
**dicalcium p.,** dibasic calcium phosphate; see under *calcium.*
**earthy p.,** a phosphate of any one of the alkaline earth metals.
**energy rich p.,** high energy p.
**ferric p.,** a yellowish white powder, insoluble in water or acetic acid, used as a feed and food supplement, especially to enrich bread, and as a fertilizer.
**ferric p., soluble,** ferric phosphate rendered soluble by the presence of sodium citrate; used as a hematinic.
**high-energy p.,** an ester, amide, or anhydride of phosphoric acid that contains a high-energy phosphate bond (q.v.), e.g., ATP or phosphocreatine.
**inorganic p.,** a salt of phosphoric acid or of any of its anions, usually orthophosphate.
**normal p.,** any phosphate in which all the replaceable hydrogen atoms in phosphoric acid are replaced.
**organic p.,** any ester of phosphoric acid with an organic alcohol, e.g., phospholipids, phosphoproteins, nucleotides, nucleic acids, sugar phosphates, and many small phosphorylated molecules involved in intermediary metabolism.
**polyestradiol p.,** a polymeric ester of phosphoric acid and estradiol, used as a palliative in prostatic carcinoma.
**stellar p.,** calcium phosphate occurring in star-shaped masses of crystals in urinary sediment.
**tricresyl p.,** tritolyl p.
**trimagnesium p.,** tribasic magnesium phosphate; see *magnesium phosphate,* under *magnesium.*
**tri-*o*-cresyl p., triorthocresyl p.,** tri-*o*-tolyl p.
**tri-*o*-tolyl p., triorthotolyl p.,** the highly toxic ortho isomer of tritolyl phosphate; when ingested, it can cause paralysis. See *Jamaica ginger paralysis,* under *paralysis.* Called also *triorthocresyl p.* and *tri-o-cresyl p.*
**triple p.,** a calcium, ammonium, and magnesium phosphate, sometimes found in the urine. See also *struvite.*
**tritolyl p.,** a mixture of isomers prepared from creosote and other organic compounds; used as a flame retardant, in the manufacture of vinyl plastics, and for other industrial purposes. One of the isomers, tri-*o*-tolyl phosphate, is highly toxic. Called also *tricresyl p.*

**phos·phat·ed** (fos'fāt-əd) containing phosphates.

**phos·pha·te·mia** (fos″fə-te′me-ə) hyperphosphatemia.

**phos·phat·ic** (fos-fat′ik) pertaining to or containing phosphates.

**phos·pha·ti·date** (fos″fə-ti′dāt) 1. the anionic form of phosphatidic acid. 2. any of the group of phospholipids derived from phosphatidic acid.

**phos·pha·ti·date cy·ti·dyl·yl·trans·fer·ase** (fos″fə-ti′dāt si″tĭ-dil″əl-trans′fər-ās) [EC 2.7.7.41] an enzyme of the transferase class that catalyzes the synthesis of CDPdiacylglycerol from CTP and a phosphatidate as a step in the cycle of degradation and resynthesis of phosphoinositides.

**phos·pha·ti·date phos·pha·tase** (fos″fə-ti′dāt fos′fə-tās) [EC 3.1.3.4] [MeSH: Phosphatidate Phosphatase] an enzyme of the hydrolase class that catalyzes the cleavage of a phosphate group from a phosphatidate to form a diglyceride; the reaction is a step in the synthesis of triglycerides.

**phos·pha·tide** (fos′fə-tīd) a phospholipid (q.v.), particularly one derived from phosphatidic acid. The term is sometimes used as a synonym of phosphoglyceride.

**phos·pha·ti·dic ac·id** (fos″fə-ti′dik) glycerol esterified with long-chain fatty acyl groups at C1 and C2 and phosphorylated at C3; it is the simplest phosphoglyceride (q.v.), the parent compound of most important membrane phospholipids, and a key intermediate in the biosynthesis and degradation of many phosphoglycerides.

**phos·pha·ti·do·sis** (fos″fə-tĭ-do′sis) [*phosphatide* + *-osis*] lipidosis in which the fatty accumulations are phosphatides.

**phos·pha·ti·dyl** (fos″fə-ti′dəl) a term denoting a compound containing a phosphatidic acid group; used also as a prefix to denote such a compound.

**phos·pha·ti·dyl·cho·line** (fos″fə-ti″dəl-ko′lēn) a phospholipid in which choline is attached to the phosphate group of phosphatidic acid by an ester linkage; it is a major component of cell membrane and is localized preferentially in the outer surface of the plasma membrane. Abbreviated PC. Also called *lecithin*.

**phos·pha·ti·dyl·cho·line–ster·ol *O*-ac·yl·trans·fer·ase** (fos″fə-ti″dəl-ko′lēn ster′ol a″səl-trans′fər-ās) [EC 2.3.1.43] an enzyme of the transferase class, secreted by the liver, that catalyzes the formation of cholesteryl esters in high-density lipoproteins by transferring long-chain fatty acid residues from phosphatidyl choline to a sterol. The reaction is a step in the synthesis of lipoproteins. Deficiency of the enzyme, an autosomal recessive trait, is called lecithin–cholesterol acyltransferase (LCAT) deficiency. Called also *lecithin–cholesterol acyltransferase*.

**phos·pha·ti·dyl·eth·a·nol·amine** (fos″fə-ti″dəl-eth″ə-nol′ə-mēn) a phospholipid in which ethanolamine is attached to the phosphate group of phosphatidic acid by an ester linkage; it is a major constituent of cell membranes and is localized preferentially in the inner surface of the plasma membrane. Abbreviated PE.

**phos·pha·ti·dyl·ino·si·tol (PI)** (fos″fə-ti″dəl-ĭ-no′sĭ-tol) a phospholipid in which the sugar inositol is attached to the phosphate group of phosphatidic acid by an ester linkage and the fatty acyl groups are usually arachidonate and stearate; additional phosphates can be attached to the sugar. It is a minor constituent of cell membranes found primarily in the plasma membrane. It is converted by specific kinases to mono- and diphosphorylated forms, phosphoinositides involved in hormonally activated calcium mobilization.

**p. 4,5-bisphosphate (PIP$_2$),** a polyphosphoinositide occurring as a minor constituent of the plasma membrane and involved in calcium-mediated responses to hormones; its breakdown to the second messengers diacylglycerol and inositol 1,4,5-triphosphate is a primary event resulting in increases in intracellular calcium.

**p. 4-phosphate (PIP),** a phosphoinositide occurring as a minor constituent of the plasma membrane; an intermediate in the formation of phosphatidylinositol 4,5-bisphosphate from phosphatidylinositol.

**phos·pha·ti·dyl·ino·si·tol de·acyl·ase** (fos″fə-ti′dəl-ĭ-no′sĭ-tol de-a′səl-ās) [EC 3.1.1.52] formal EC nomenclature for a phospholipase A$_2$ specific for phosphatidylinositol. See *phospholipase A$_2$*.

**1-phos·pha·ti·dyl·ino·si·tol phos·pho·di·es·ter·ase** (fos″fə-ti″dəl-ĭ-no′sĭ-tol fos″fo-di-es′tər-ās) [EC 3.1.4.10] a phospholipase C specific for phosphoinositides, occurring in all tissues. It is part of a mechanism for mobilization of calcium in response to hormones; it is activated by hormonal binding via a G protein and begins the cycle of phosphoinositide metabolism. It can also play a role in the liberation of arachidonic acid from phosphatidylinositol.

**phos·pha·ti·dyl·ser·ine** (fos″fə-ti″dəl-ser′ēn) a phospholipid in which serine is attached to the phosphate group of phosphatidic acid by an ester linkage; it is an important constituent of cell membranes and is localized preferentially in the inner surface of the plasma membrane. Abbreviated PS.

**phos·pha·top·to·sis** (fos″fə-top-to′sis) [*phosphate* + *-ptosis*] the spontaneous precipitation of the earthy phosphates from the urine; phosphaturia.

**phos·pha·tu·ria** (fos″fə-tu′re-ə) 1. a high percentage of phosphates in any given specimen of urine. 2. ready precipitation of the earthy phosphates from the urine; phosphatoptosis.

**phos·phene** (fos′fēn) [Gr. *phōs* light + *phainein* to show] [MeSH: Phosphenes] an objective visual sensation that appears with the eyes closed and in the absence of visual light.

**accommodation p.,** the streak of light surrounding the visual field seen in the dark after accommodation.

**phos·phide** (fos′fīd) any binary compound of phosphorus and another element or radical.

**phos·phine** (fos′fēn) 1. hydrogen phosphide, PH$_3$; a toxic malodorous gas and radical. 2. any of a group of organic compounds derived from this; they are similar to amines but are weaker bases. 3. coal tar dye extremely destructive to infusorial life; it is used as a stain. Called also *Philadelphia yellow*.

**phos·phite** (fos′fīt) any salt of phosphorous acid.

**Phos·pho·col P 32** (fos′fo-kol) trademark for a preparation of chromic phosphate P 32.

**phos·pho·cre·a·tine (PC)** (fos″fo-kre′ə-tin) [MeSH: Phosphocreatine] the phosphagen of vertebrates, a substituted derivative of phosphoguanidine. It is an important storage form of high-energy phosphate, the energy source for muscle contraction; as ATP levels diminish with muscular exertion, the phosphoryl group of phosphocreatine can be donated to ADP to replenish ATP.

**phos·pho·di·es·ter** (fos″fo-di-es′tər) a diester of phosphoric acid.

**phos·pho·di·es·ter·ase** (fos″fo-di-es′tər-ās) a term used in the recommended names of some phosphoric diester hydrolases [EC 3.1.4] of the hydrolase class that catalyze the hydrolysis of one of the two ester linkages in a phosphodiester compound.

**phos·pho·*enol*·py·ru·vate** (fos″fo-e″nol-pi′roo-vāt) a high-energy compound that is a phosphorylated ester of the enol form of pyruvate; it is an intermediate in the Embden-Meyerhof pathway of glucose metabolism, in gluconeogenesis, and in the synthesis of some amino acids. Abbreviated PEP.

**phos·pho·*enol*·py·ru·vate car·boxy·ki·nase (GTP)** (fos″fo-e″nol-pi′roo-vāt kahr-bok″se-ki′nās) [EC 4.1.1.32] an enzyme of the lyase class that catalyzes the decarboxylation and phosphorylation of oxaloacetate to form phospho*enol*pyruvate, using GTP as a phosphate donor. The enzyme occurs in both the mitochondria and cytosol of mammalian liver, and the reaction is part of the mechanism of gluconeogenesis. Deficiency of the enzyme in mitochondria or cytosol, an autosomal recessive trait, causes infant hypoglycemia. Called also *phosphopyruvate carboxykinase*.

**phos·pho·eth·a·nol·amine** (fos″fo-eth″ə-nol′ə-mēn) an intermediate in the biosynthesis of phosphatidylethanolamine; elevated levels are excreted in the urine in a number of conditions, including hypophosphatasia, pseudohypophosphatasia, and metabolic bone disease.

**phos·pho·fruct·al·do·lase** (fos″fo-frook-tal′do-lās) fructose-bisphosphate aldolase.

**phos·pho·fruc·to·ki·nase 1** (fos″fo-frook″to-ki′nās) 6-phosphofructokinase.

**phos·pho·fruc·to·ki·nase 2** (fos″fo-frook″to-ki′nās) 6-phosphofructo-2-kinase.

**6-phos·pho·fruc·to·ki·nase** (fos″fo-frook″to-ki′nās) [EC 2.7.1.11] [MeSH: 6-Phosphofructokinase] an enzyme of the transferase class that catalyzes the phosphorylation of fructose 6-phosphate by ATP to form fructose 1,6-bisphosphate. The reaction is essentially irreversible and is a committed step and a key site of regulation in the Embden-Meyerhof pathway of glucose metabolism. Numerous isozymes occur; deficiency of the muscle isoenzyme, an autosomal recessive trait, is the cause of glycogen storage disease, type VII. Called also *phosphofructokinase 1*.

**6-phos·pho·fruc·to-2-ki·nase** (fos″fo-frook″to-ki′nās) [EC 2.7.1.105] an enzyme activity that catalyzes the phosphorylation of fructose 6-phosphate by ATP to form fructose 2,6-bisphosphate; it occurs on the same polypeptide as the enzyme activity fructose-2,6-bisphosphate 2-phosphatase (q.v.). In liver, the two activities form part of a mechanism for regulating carbohydrate metabolism. The liver enzyme activity is inhibited via phosphorylation by cyclic-AMP–dependent protein kinase, thus diminishing the rate of formation of fructose 2,6-bisphosphate and slowing glycolysis. Called also *phosphofructokinase 2*.

**phos·pho·glob·u·lin** (fos″fo-glob′u-lin) a phosphoprotein with globulin as the protein moiety.

**phos·pho·glu·co·ki·nase** (fos″fo-gloo″ko-ki′nās) [EC 2.7.1.10] an enzyme of the transferase class that catalyzes the phosphorylation of glucose 1-phosphate glucose 1,6-bisphosphate. The reaction product is a necessary intermediate in the phosphoglucomutase reaction.

**phos•pho•glu•co•mu•tase** (fos″fo-gloo″ko-mu′tās) [EC 5.4.2.2] [MeSH: Phosphoglucomutase] an enzyme of the isomerase class requiring the presence of the intermediate glucose 1,6-bisphosphate to catalyze the interconversion of glucose 1-phosphate and glucose 6-phosphate, a step in the formation and utilization of glycogen. It also catalyzes the interconversion of the 1-phosphate and 5-phosphate isomers of ribose.

**6-phos•pho•glu•co•nate** (fos″fo-gloo′kə-nāt) gluconate, the hexonic acid derivative of glucose, phosphorylated at the 6 carbon; it is an intermediate in the pentose phosphate pathway.

**phos•pho•glu•co•nate 2-de•hy•dro•gen•ase (de•car•box•y•lat•ing)** (fos″fo-gloo′kə-nāt de-hi′dro-jən-ās de″kahr-bok′sə-lāt-ing) [EC 1.1.1.44] an enzyme of the oxidoreductase class that catalyzes the oxidative decarboxylation of 6-phosphogluconate to form ribulose 5-phosphate, reducing $NADP^+$ to NADPH. The reaction is a step in the pentose phosphate pathway of glucose metabolism.

**6-phos•pho•glu•co•no•lac•ton•ase** (fos″fo-gloo″-kə-no-lak′tə-nās) [EC 3.1.1.31] an enzyme of the hydrolase class that catalyzes the formation of 6-phosphogluconate from the corresponding lactone as a step in the pentose phosphate pathway.

**phos•pho•glu•cose isom•er•ase** (fos″fo-gloo′kōs i-som′ər-ās) glucose-6-phosphate isomerase.

**3-phos•pho•glyc•er•al•de•hyde** (fos″fo-glis″ər-al′də-hīd) a triose phosphate which results from the splitting of fructose 1,6-diphosphate in muscle metabolism.

**phos•pho•glyc•er•ate** (fos″fo-glis′ər-āt) an anionic form of phosphoglyceric acid; the 2- and 3-phosphate forms, 2-phosphoglycerate and 3-phosphoglycerate, are enzymatically interconvertible intermediates in the Embden-Meyerhof pathway (q.v.) of glucose metabolism.

**phos•pho•glyc•er•ate ki•nase** (fos″fo-glis′ər-āt ki′nās) [EC 2.7.2.3] [MeSH: Phosphoglycerate Kinase] an enzyme of the transferase class that catalyzes the ATP-dependent phosphorylation of 3-phosphoglycerate to form 1,3-bisphosphoglycerate. The reaction is an important energy-transducing step in carbohydrate metabolism. As written, the reaction drives gluconeogenesis; the reverse reaction generates ATP in the catabolism of glucose (see illustration at *Embden-Meyerhof pathway,* under *pathway*). Deficiency of the enzyme, an X-linked trait, causes hemolytic anemia, mental retardation, and behavioral and neurologic abnormalities.

**phos•pho•glyc•er•ate mu•tase** (fos″fo-glis′ər-āt mu′tās) [EC 5.4.2.1] [MeSH: Phosphoglycerate Mutase] an enzyme of the isomerase class that catalyzes the interconversion of 3-phosphoglycerate and 2-phosphoglycerate, a step in the Embden-Meyerhof pathway (see illustration at *pathway*). The enzyme requires the presence of a small amount of 2,3-bisphosphoglycerate, which is also an intermediate. Called also *phosphoglyceromutase.*

**phos•pho•gly•cer•ic ac•id** (fos″fo-glĭ-ser′ik) a phosphate ester of glyceric acid.

**phos•pho•glyc•er•ide** (fos″fo-glis′ər-īd) a phospholipid in which the phosphate group of a phosphatidic acid is joined in ester linkage to an alcohol moiety, commonly choline, ethanolamine, glycerol, inositol, or serine, forming the corresponding phosphatidyl compound. The phosphoglycerides are a major component of cell membranes.

**phos•pho•glyc•ero•mu•tase** (fos″fo-glis″ər-o-mu′tās) phosphoglycerate mutase.

**phos•pho•gly•co•pro•tein** (fos″fo-gli″ko-pro′tēn) a phosphorus-containing glycoprotein.

**phos•pho•guan•i•dine** (fos″fo-gwahn′ĭ-dēn) 1. phosphorylated guanidine, a high energy compound. 2. a term sometimes used to denote one of the phosphagens because these compounds are substituted derivatives of phosphoguanidine.

**phos•pho•hex•ose isom•er•ase** (fos″fo-hek″sōs i-som′ər-ās) glucose-6-phosphate isomerase.

**phos•pho•ino•si•tide** (fos″fo-in-o′sĭ-tīd) any of a number of phosphorylated inositol-containing compounds that play roles in cell activation and calcium mobilization in response to hormones.

**phos•pho•lam•ban** (fos″fo-lam′ban) a 22-kilodalton membrane-bound polypeptide of the sarcoplasmic reticulum that stimulates cardiac relaxation; upon phosphorylation by a cyclic AMP–dependent protein kinase, it activates the calcium pump, stimulating the uptake and storage of calcium by the sarcoplasmic reticulum and resulting in relaxation of cardiac muscle.

**Phos•pho•line** (fos′fo-lēn) trademark for a preparation of echothiophate iodide.

**phos•pho•lip•ase** (fos″fo-lip′ās) any of a number of enzymes that catalyze the hydrolysis of specific ester bonds in phospholipids. Individual enzymes are grouped on the basis of the bond they hydrolyze and are further categorized as carboxylic acid esterases (p. $A_1$, p. $A_2$) or phosphodiesterases (p. C, p. D).

**p. $A_1$** [EC 3.1.1.32], any esterase that catalyzes the hydrolysis of the terminal acyl group from a phospholipid, generating a free fatty acid and a lysophospholipid. The enzyme occurs in various forms in all mammalian tissues, particularly the liver and pancreas, and in bee and snake venoms.

**p. $A_2$** [EC 3.1.1.4], any esterase that catalyzes the hydrolysis of the central acyl group from a membrane phospholipid, generating a free fatty acid and a lysophospholipid; this reaction is important in the digestion of dietary phospholipids, and it liberates arachidonic acid for a variety of processes, such as platelet activation. The enzyme occurs in various forms in all mammalian tissues and in snake and bee venoms. EC nomenclature for the enzyme specifically hydrolyzing phosphatidylinositol is *phosphatidylinositol deacylase.*

**p. C** [EC 3.1.4.3], any esterase that catalyzes the hydrolysis of the phosphoric ester bond of a membrane phospholipid, generating a phosphorylated alcohol and diacylglycerol. Important in the digestion of dietary phospholipids and in various processes dependent on hormonally induced calcium mobilization or arachidonic acid production, they occur in all mammalian tissues and as toxic secretion products of pathogenic bacteria. EC nomenclature for the isozyme specifically hydrolyzing phosphatidylinositol-1-phosphate is *1-phosphatidylinositol phosphodiesterase.*

**p. D** [EC 3.1.4.4], any esterase that catalyzes the hydrolysis of the alcohol group from a phospholipid, generating the corresponding phosphatidate. It occurs in various forms, predominantly in plants, but in humans it may be part of a mechanism to generate diacylglycerol for the mobilization of calcium in response to hormones.

**phos•pho•lip•id** (fos″fo-lip′id) any lipid that contains phosphorus, including those with a glycerol backbone (phosphoglycerides and plasmalogens) or a backbone of sphingosine or related substance (sphingomyelins). Phospholipids are the major form of lipid in all cell membranes.

**phos•pho•lip•i•de•mia** (fos″fo-lip″ĭ-de′me-ə) the presence of phospholipid in the blood.

**phos•pho•man•no•mu•tase** (fos″fo-man″o-mu′tās) [EC 5.4.2.8] an enzyme of the isomerase class that catalyzes the interconversion of mannose 6-phosphate and mannose 1-phosphate.

**phos•pho•man•nose isom•er•ase** (fos″fo-man′ōs i-som′ər-ās) mannose-6-phosphate isomerase.

**phos•pho•mo•lyb•dic ac•id** (fos″fo-mo-lib′dik) a strong acid and oxidizing agent used as a protein precipitant and color reagent; alkaloids, xanthine, uric acid, and other substances reduce phosphomolybdic acid to molybdenum blue. It is also used in histology as a mordant.

**phos•pho•mono•es•ter** (fos″fo-mon″o-es′tər) a monoester in which phosphate is the ester group.

**phos•pho•mono•es•ter•ase** (fos″fo-mon″o-es′tər-ās) any of a group of enzymes that act as phosphatases on phosphomonoester substrates; however, the term is usually used to denote acid phosphatase or alkaline phosphatase specifically.

**phos•pho•mu•tase** (fos″fo-mu′tās) any of the phosphotransferases of the isomerase class, which catalyze the intramolecular transfer of a phosphate group.

**phos•pho•nate** (fos′fo-nāt) a salt, anion, or ester of phosphonic acid.

**phos•pho•ne•cro•sis** (fos″fo-nə-kro′sis) phosphorus necrosis.

**phos•phon•ic ac•id** (fos-fon′ik) the compound $HPO(OH)_2$, or substituted derivatives of the form $RPO_3H_2$.

**phos•pho•ni•um** (fos-fo′ne-əm) the univalent radical $PH_4^+$, forming compounds analogous to those of ammonium.

**phos•pho•pe•nia** (fos″fo-pe′ne-ə) [*phosphorus* + *-penia*] deficiency of phosphorus in the body.

**phos•pho•pro•tein** (fos″fo-pro′tēn) a protein to which one or more phosphate groups are attached at serine or threonine (rarely tyrosine) residues.

**phos•pho•pro•tein phos•pha•tase** (fos″fo-pro′tēn fos′fə-tās) [EC 3.1.3.16] [MeSH: Phosphoprotein Phosphatase] an enzyme of the hydrolase class that catalyzes the cleavage of phosphoryl groups from phosphoproteins. Enzymes with this activity are involved in digestion and in the regulation of a variety of enzymes undergoing phosphorylation-dephosphorylation cycles. Called also *protein phosphatase.*

**p. p. 1,** protein phosphatase 1.

**phos•pho•pto•maine** (fos″fo-to′mān) any of a class of toxic compounds found in the blood in phosphorus poisoning.

**phos•pho•py•ru•vate car•boxy•ki•nase** (fos″fo-pi′roo-vāt kahr-bok″se-ki′nās) phospho*enol*pyruvate carboxykinase (GTP).

**phos·pho·py·ru·vate hy·dra·tase** (fos″fo-pi′roo-vāt hi′drə-tās) [EC 4.2.1.11] [MeSH: Phosphopyruvate Hydratase] an enzyme of the lyase class that catalyzes the dehydration of 2-phosphoglycerate to form phospho*enol*pyruvate, a part of the Embden-Meyerhof pathway of glucose catabolism (see illustration at *pathway*). Called also *enolase.*

**phos·pho·rat·ed** (fos′fo-rāt″əd) charged or combined with phosphorus.

**phos·pho·res·cence** (fos″fo-res′əns) the emission of light without appreciable heat; it is characterized by the emission of absorbed light after a delay and at a considerably longer wavelength than that of the absorbed light. Cf. *fluorescence.*

**phos·pho·res·cent** (fos″fo-res′ənt) pertaining to or exhibiting phosphorescence.

**phos·pho·ri·bo·isom·er·ase** (fos″fo-ri″bo-i-som′ər-ās) ribose-5-phosphate isomerase.

**phos·pho·ri·bo·syl·amine** (fos″fo-ri″bo-sil′ə-mēn) an intermediate product in the synthesis of purines formed from phosphoribosylpyrophosphate and glutamine; excessive production is often a factor in primary gout.

**phos·pho·ri·bo·syl·py·ro·phos·phate** (fos″fo-ri″bo-səl-pi″ro-fos′fāt) an intermediate in the formation of purines and of purine and pyrimidine nucleotides; abbreviated PRPP.

**phos·pho·ri·bo·syl·py·ro·phos·phate syn·the·tase** (fos″fo-ri″bo-səl-pi″ro-fos′fāt sin′thə-tās) ribose-phosphate pyrophosphokinase.

**phos·pho·ri·bo·syl·trans·fer·ase** (fos″fo-ri″bo-səl-trans′fər-ās) a term used in the recommended and trivial names of some pentosyltransferases [EC 2.4.2] to denote those that catalyze the transfer of ribose 5-phosphate, usually from phosphoribosylpyrophosphate, to a purine or pyrimidine to form a 5′ nucleotide and inorganic pyrophosphate. These enzymes are important in the biosynthesis of nucleotides.

**phos·phor·ic ac·id** (fos-for′ik) 1. orthophosphoric acid, the monomeric form $H_3PO_4$. 2. a general term encompassing the monomeric (orthophosphoric acid), dimeric (pyrophosphoric acid), and polymeric (metaphosphoric acid) forms of the acid. Phosphoric acid is an important metabolite; see *phosphate* and specific acids and salts.
**p. a., diluted** [NF], a preparation of phosphoric acid in purified water, containing 9.5–10.5 g phosphoric acid per mL; it is used as a solvent in pharmaceutical preparations and orally as a gastric acidifier.
**p. a., glacial,** metaphosphoric acid.

**phos·pho·rism** (fos′fo-riz″əm) chronic phosphorus poisoning; see under *poisoning.*

**phos·pho·rized** (fos′fo-rīzd) containing phosphorus.

**phos·pho·rol·y·sis** (fos″fo-rol′ĭ-sis) cleavage of a chemical bond with simultaneous addition of the elements of phosphoric acid to the residues, as in the splitting of the glycosidic bonds of glycogen catalyzed by the enzyme phosphorylase in carbohydrate metabolism. The reaction is analogous to hydrolysis.

**phos·phoro·scope** (fos′for-ə-skōp) an instrument for measuring phosphorescence.

**phos·pho·rous** (fos′fə-rəs) pertaining to or containing phosphorus.

**phos·pho·rous ac·id** (fos-for′əs) a reducing inorganic acid, $H_3PO_3$, which readily absorbs oxygen to form phosphoric acid.

**phos·phor·pe·nia** (fos″for-pe′ne-ə) phosphopenia.

**phos·phor·uria** (fos″for-u′re-ə) [*phosphorus* + *-uria*] the presence of free phosphorus in the urine.

**phos·pho·rus** (fos′fə-rəs) [Gr. *phōs* light + *phorein* to carry] [MeSH: Phosphorus] a nonmetallic, allotropic element: poisonous and highly inflammable; symbol, P; atomic number, 15; atomic weight, 30.974. It occurs in three forms—*white* (yellow), *red,* and *black.* It is obtainable from bones, urine, and especially minerals, such as apatite. Phosphorus is an essential element in the diet; it is a major component of the mineral phase of bone and is abundant in all tissues, being involved in some form in almost all metabolic processes. Free phosphorus causes a fatty degeneration of the liver and other viscera, and the inhalation of its vapor often leads to necrosis of the lower jaw. Therapeutically, it was once used in rickets, osteomalacia, nervous and cerebral diseases, scrofula, and tuberculosis, as a genital stimulant in sexual exhaustion, and as a tonic in conditions of exhaustion.
**p. 32,** a radioisotope of phosphorus, atomic mass 32, having a half-life of 14.28 days and emitting only beta particles (1.71 MeV); its therapeutic uses include treatment of polycythemia vera, chronic myelocytic leukemia, chronic lymphocytic leukemia, certain ovarian and prostate carcinomas, palliation of metastatic skeletal disease, and treatment of metastatic intrapleural and intraperitoneal effusions.
**amorphous p.,** red p.
**black p.,** black lustrous crystals, resembling coal, insoluble in organic solvents, produced by heating white phosphorus under very high pressure.
**ordinary p.,** white p.
**red p.,** a dark red amorphous powder, which is infusible and insoluble in carbon disulfide, and is not poisonous; called also *amorphous p.*
**white p.,** a usually white, sometimes yellow, waxy solid, very inflammable and exceedingly poisonous, which was formerly used in medicine to treat various disorders. Called also *yellow* or *ordinary p.*
**yellow p.,** white p.

**phos·pho·ryl** (fos′fə-rəl) the trivalent chemical radical ≡P:O.

**phos·phor·y·lase** (fos-for′ə-lās) 1. any of a group of enzymes catalyzing phosphorolysis of glycosides, transferring the cleaved glycosyl group to inorganic phosphate. The term is usually qualified by adding the name of the substrate acted upon; when used alone it usually denotes glycogen phosphorylase (q.v.) in animals or starch phosphorylase in plants. 2. any of a group of transferases that catalyze the transfer of a phosphate group to an organic acceptor.
**hepatic p. deficiency,** glycogen storage disease, type VI.
**muscle p. deficiency,** glycogen storage disease, type V.

**phos·phor·y·lase ki·nase** (fos-for′ə-lās ki′nās) [EC 2.7.1.38] [MeSH: Phosphorylase Kinase] an enzyme of the transferase class that catalyzes the phosphorylation of (inactive) glycogen phosphorylase *b* to form (active) glycogen phosphorylase *a,* a step in the cascade of reactions regulating glycogenolysis. The enzyme is itself activated via phosphorylation by cyclic-AMP–dependent protein kinase, and one of its four subunits is identical to calmodulin. Deficiency of the enzyme in liver, an X-linked trait, causes phosphorylase *b* kinase deficiency.

**phos·phor·y·lase *b* ki·nase** (fos-for′ə-lās ki′nās) phosphorylase kinase.

**phos·phor·y·lase *b* ki·nase de·fi·cien·cy** an X-linked disorder of glycogen storage caused by a deficiency of phosphorylase kinase in liver; it is characterized in affected males by hepatomegaly, occasional fasting hypoglycemia, and some growth retardation, but is mostly benign. Its classification as a particular type of glycogen storage disease has been controversial; it has been included in type VI and called type VIII and (formerly) type IX.

**[phos·phor·y·lase] phos·pha·tase** (fos-for′ə-lās fos′fə-tās″) [EC 3.1.3.17] an enzyme of the hydrolase class that catalyzes the cleavage of a phosphoryl group from (active) glycogen phosphorylase *a* to form (inactive) phosphorylase *b;* the reaction is part of the mechanism of regulation of glycogenolysis. Recently, this enzyme has been considered to be an activity of the more general enzyme *protein phosphatase 1.*

**phos·phor·y·la·tion** (fos-for″ə-la′shən) [MeSH: Phosphorylation] the metabolic process of introducing a phosphate group into an organic molecule.
**oxidative p.,** the formation of high-energy phosphate bonds by phosphorylation of ADP to ATP coupled to the transfer of electrons from reduced coenzymes (NADH or $FADH_2$) to molecular oxygen via the electron transport chain (see illustration at *chain* ). Three molecules of ATP per NADH and two per $FADH_2$ are produced as a result of a proton gradient created across the mitochondrial inner membrane by the electron transport chain.
**substrate-level p.,** the formation of high-energy phosphate bonds by phosphorylation of ADP to ATP (or GDP to GTP) coupled to cleavage of a high-energy metabolic intermediate, e.g., succinyl CoA in the tricarboxylic acid cycle.

**phos·pho·ryl·y·sis** (fos″fə-ril′ĭ-sis) phosphorolysis.

**phos·pho·sug·ar** (fos′fo-shoog″ər) a sugar in which a hydroxyl group has been esterified with a phosphate group.

**Phos·pho·tec** (fos′fo-tek) trademark for a kit for the preparation of technetium Tc 99m pyrophosphate.

**phos·pho·trans·fer·ase** (fos″fo-trans′fər-ās) an enzyme that catalyzes the transfer of a phosphate group, either from one molecule to another [EC 2.7.1–4.2.7.9] or within the same molecule [EC 5.4.2].

**phos·pho·tri·ose** (fos″fo-tri′ōs) triose phosphate.

**phos·pho·tung·state** (fos″fo-tung′stāt) a salt of phosphotungstic acid.

**phos·pho·tung·stic ac·id** (fos″fo-tung′stik) [MeSH: Phosphotungstic Acid] a strong acid and oxidizing agent used as a protein precipitant and color reagent; alkaloids, nitrogenous bases, and other substances reduce phosphotungstic acid to tungsten blue. It is also used in histology as a mordant for hematoxylin and other dyes.

**phos·pho·vi·tel·lin** (fos″fo-vi-tel′in) phosvitin.

**phos·phu·re·sis** (fos″fu-re′sis) the urinary excretion of phosphorus (phosphates).

**phos·phu·ret·ic** (fos″fu-ret′ik) pertaining to, characterized by, or promoting the urinary excretion of phosphorus (phosphates).

**phos·phu·ria** (fos-fu′re-ə) phosphaturia.

**phos·vi·tin** (fos-vi′tin) [MeSH: Phosvitin] a phosphoprotein isolated from vitellin in egg yolk; called also *phosphovitellin.*

**phot** (fōt) [Gr. *phōs* light] the CGS unit of illumination, being one lumen per square centimeter.

**pho·tal·gia** (fo-tal′jə) [*phot-* + *-algia*] ocular pain caused by light.

**pho·tal·lo·chro·my** (fo-tal′ə-kro″me) [*phot-* + *allo-* + *-chrome*] allotropic change with color alteration due to light, as the change of yellow into red phosphorus.

**pho·tau·gia·pho·bia** (fo-taw″je-ə-fo′be-ə) [Gr. *phōtaugeia* glare + *phobia*] abnormal intolerance of glare.

**pho·te·ryth·rous** (fo″tə-rith′rəs) deuteranopic.

**pho·tes·the·sis** (fo″təs-the′sis) [*phot-* + *esthesis*] sensitiveness to light.

**pho·tic** (fo′tik) pertaining to light.

**pho·tism** (fo′tiz-əm) a synesthesia in which a sensation of color or light is associated with a sensation of hearing, taste, smell, or touch.

**phot(o)-** [Gr. *phōs,* gen. *phōtos* light] combining form denoting relationship to light.

**pho·to·abla·tion** (fo″to-ab-la′shən) volatilization of tissue by ultraviolet rays emitted by a laser.

**pho·to·ac·tin·ic** (fo″to-ak-tin′ik) giving off both luminous and actinic rays.

**pho·to·ac·tive** (fo″to-ak′tiv) reacting chemically to sunlight or ultraviolet radiation.

**pho·to·ag·ing** (fo″to-āj′ing) premature aging of the skin due to long-term exposure to ultraviolet irradiation such as in sunlight. See also *actinic elastosis,* under *elastosis.*

**pho·to·al·ler·gen** (fo″to-al′ər-jən) an agent that elicits an allergic response to light.

**pho·to·al·ler·gic** (fo″to-ə-ler′jik) pertaining to, characterized by, or producing photoallergy.

**pho·to·al·ler·gy** (fo″to-al′ər-je) [*photo-* + *allergy*] a delayed immunologic type of photosensitivity involving a chemical substance to which the individual has become previously sensitized and radiant energy. See also *photoallergic contact dermatitis,* under *dermatitis.* Cf. *phototoxicity.*

**pho·to·au·to·troph** (fo″to-aw′to-trōf) a photoautotrophic organism.

**pho·to·au·to·troph·ic** (fo″to-aw″to-trōf′ik) requiring for growth only inorganic compounds with carbon dioxide as the sole source of carbon (autotrophic) and deriving energy from photosynthesis; said of algae and certain photosynthetic bacteria.

**pho·to·bac·te·ria** (fo″to-bak-tēr′e-ə) [*photo-* + *bacteria*] bacteria that derive energy from light by the process of photosynthesis. See also *Oxyphotobacteria.*

**pho·to·bi·o·log·ic, pho·to·bi·o·log·i·cal** (fo″to-bi″ə-loj′ik, fo″to-bi″ə-loj′ĭ-kəl) pertaining to photobiology or to the effect of light on living organisms.

**pho·to·bi·ol·o·gy** (fo″to-bi-ol′ə-je) [*photo-* + *biology*] [MeSH: Photobiology] that department of biology which deals with the effect of light on living organisms, including the study of photosynthesis.

**pho·to·bi·ot·ic** (fo″to-bi-ot′ik) [*photo-* + *biotic*] living or thriving only in the light; said of certain organisms such as green plants.

**pho·to·ca·tal·y·sis** (fo″to-kə-tal′ĭ-sis) the promotion or stimulation of a reaction by light.

**pho·to·cat·a·lyst** (fo″to-kat′ə-list) a substance by means of which sunlight is utilized, as chlorophyll in the photosynthesis of carbohydrates by green plants.

**pho·to·cat·a·lyt·ic** (fo″to-kat″ə-lit′ik) promoted or stimulated by light; pertaining to, characterized by, or causing photocatalysis.

**pho·to·cat·a·lyz·er** (fo″to-kat′ə-līz″ər) photocatalyst.

**pho·to·cep·tor** (fo″to-sep′tor) photoreceptor.

**pho·to·chem·i·cal** (fo″to-kem′ə-kəl) pertaining to the chemical properties of light; chemically reactive in the presence of light or other radiation.

**pho·to·chem·is·try** (fo″to-kem′is-tre) [*photo-* + *chemistry*] [MeSH: Photochemistry] the branch of chemistry which deals with the chemical properties or effects of light rays or other radiation.

**pho·to·che·mo·ther·a·py** (fo″to-ke″mo-ther′ə-pe) [MeSH: Photochemotherapy] 1. treatment by means of drugs (e.g., methoxsalen) that react to ultraviolet radiation or sunlight. 2. photodynamic therapy.

**pho·to·chro·mo·gen** (fo″to-kro′mə-jən) [*photo-* + *chromo-* + *-gen*] a microorganism whose pigmentation develops as a result of exposure to light, e.g., *Mycobacterium kansasii* (pathogenic for man), which is yellow-orange if grown in the light, and almost colorless if grown in the dark. See also *nontuberculous mycobacteria,* under *mycobacterium.*

**pho·to·chro·mo·gen·ic** (fo″to-kro″mə-jen′ik) pertaining to or characterized by photochromogenicity.

**pho·to·chro·mo·ge·nic·i·ty** (fo″to-kro″mə-jə-nis′ĭ-te) the property of microorganisms of forming pigment consequent to light exposure; induction occurs within a few minutes in the shorter wavelengths of visible light, pigmentation then occurring within 24 hours if conditions permit continued growth.

**pho·to·co·ag·u·la·tion** (fo″to-ko-ag″u-la′shən) [*photo-* + *coagulation*] condensation of protein material by the controlled use of an intense beam of light (e.g., xenon arc light or argon laser); used especially in treatment of retinal detachment and destruction of abnormal retinal vessels, or of intraocular tumor masses.

**pho·to·con·vul·sive** (fo″to-kən-vul′siv) photoparoxysmal.

**pho·to·cu·ta·ne·ous** (fo″to-ku-ta′ne-əs) [*photo-* + *cutaneous*] pertaining to a dermatitis in which exposure to light is an important factor.

**pho·to·der·ma·ti·tis** (fo″to-der″mə-ti′tis) an abnormal state of the skin in which light is an important causative factor.

**pho·to·der·ma·to·sis** (fo″to-der″mə-to′sis) a morbid condition produced in the skin by exposure to light.

**pho·to·de·tec·tor** (fo″to-de-tek′tər) a detector responsive to radiant energy.

**pho·to·dis·rup·tion** (fo″to-dis-rup′shən) disruption of tissues by laser-produced rapid ionization of molecules.

**pho·tod·ro·my** (fo-tod′rə-me) [*photo-* + Gr. *dromos* running] the phenomenon of moving toward *(positive p.)* or away from *(negative p.)* light, as in the case of particles in suspension.

**pho·to·dy·nam·ic** (fo″to-di-nam′ik) [*photo-* + *dynamic*] powerful in the light; used particularly for the action exerted by fluorescent substances in the light.

**pho·to·dy·nam·ics** (fo″to-di-nam′iks) the science of the activating effects of light on living organisms.

**pho·to·dyn·ia** (fo″to-din′e-ə) [*photo-* + *-odynia*] photalgia.

**pho·to·dys·pho·ria** (fo″to-dis-for′e-ə) [*photo-* + *dysphoria*] intolerance of light; photophobia.

**pho·to·elec·tric** (fo″to-e-lek′trik) pertaining to the electric effects of light or other radiation.

**pho·to·elec·tron** (fo″to-e-lek′tron) an electron emitted from a metallic surface when the latter is illuminated with light, especially with light of short wavelength.

**pho·to·er·y·the·ma** (fo″to-er″ĭ-the′mə) erythema due to exposure to light.

**pho·to·es·thet·ic** (fo″to-əs-thet′ik) [*photo-* + *esthetic*] pertaining to or having the sensation of light.

**pho·to·flu·o·ro·gram** (fo″to-floor′o-gram) the film produced in photofluorography.

**pho·to·flu·o·rog·ra·phy** (fo″to-floor-og′rə-fe) [MeSH: Photofluorography] the photographic recording of fluoroscopic images on small films, using a fast lens: a procedure used in mass radiography of the chest. Called also *fluororadiography,* and formerly *abreuography.*

**pho·to·flu·o·ro·scope** (fo″to-floor′o-skōp) a form of fluoroscope used in making either observations or photographs by means of x-rays.

**Pho·to·frin** (fo′to-frin) trademark for a preparation of porfimer sodium.

**pho·to·gas·tro·scope** (fo″to-gas′tro-skōp) [*photo-* + *gastro-* + *-scope*] an apparatus for photographing the interior of the stomach.

**pho·to·gen·ic** (fo″to-jen′ik) 1. produced by light, as photogenic epilepsy. 2. producing or emitting light; phosphorescent.

**pho·to·glot·tog·ra·phy** (fo″to-glŏ-tog′rə-fe) glottography using a photoelectric transducer to measure changes in transillumination of the glottis during phonation or respiration.

**pho·to·hal·ide** (fo″to-hal′īd) any halogen salt that is sensitive to light.

**pho·to·he·mo·ta·chom·e·ter** (fo″to-he″mo-tə-kom′ə-tər) [*photo-* + *hemo-* + *tacho-* + *-meter*] a device for making a photographic record of the speed of the blood current.

**pho·to·hen·ric** (fo″to-hen′rik) [*photo-* + *henry*] denoting a change in inductive capacity due to the action of light.

**pho·to·het·ero·troph** (fo″to-het′ər-o-trōf) [*photo-* + *hetero-* + *troph*] a photoheterotrophic organism.

**pho·to·het·ero·troph·ic** (fo″to-het″ər-o-trōf′ik) deriving nourishment from organic compounds and energy from visible light.

**pho·tohm·ic** (fo-to′mik) denoting a change in electric resistance produced by light.

**pho·to·in·ac·ti·va·tion** (fo″to-in-ak″tĭ-va′shən) inactivation, as of complement, by light.

**pho·to·ki·ne·sis** (fo″to-kĭ-ne′sis) [*photo-* + *-kinesis*] a change in the rate of motion in response to light, as an increase or decrease in motility of bacteria with a change in illumination.

**pho·to·ki·net·ic** (fo″to-kĭ-net′ik) [*photo-* + *kinet-* + *-ic*] pertaining to photokinesis.

**pho·to·ky·mo·graph** (fo″to-ki′mo-graf) a camera with a moving film for recording movements, as of the string in a string galvanometer; called also a *recording camera.*

**pho·tol·o·gy** (fo-tol′ə-je) [*photo-* + *-logy*] the branch of physics which treats of light.

**pho·to·lu·min·es·cence** (fo″to-loo″mĭ-nes′əns) the quality of being luminescent after being exposed to light or other electromagnetic radiation.

**pho·tol·y·sis** (fo-tol′ĭ-sis) [MeSH: Photolysis] 1. chemical decomposition or change by the action of light or other form of radiant energy. 2. lysis or solution of cells under the influence of light.

**pho·to·lyte** (fo′to-līt) [*photo-* + Gr. *lyein* to dissolve] any substance decomposable by the action of light.

**pho·to·lyt·ic** (fo″to-lit′ik) decomposed by radiant energy; pertaining to photolysis.

**pho·to·ma** (fo-to′mə) a flash of light sparks or color with no objective basis.

**pho·to·mag·ne·tism** (fo″to-mag′nə-tiz-əm) magnetism induced by the action of light.

**pho·tom·e·ter** (fo-tom′ə-tər) [*photo-* + *-meter*] 1. a device for measuring the intensity of infrared, ultraviolet, or visible light. 2. a device for testing the sensitivity of the eye to light by determining the light minimum.
**flame p.,** an instrument for analyzing the light emitted by a substance in a flame; commonly used for determination of sodium, potassium, lithium, and calcium in biological materials.
**flicker p.,** an instrument in which the frequency of a flickering light can be controlled, for use in performing the flicker test.
**Förster's p.,** photoptometer.

**pho·tom·e·try** (fo-tom′ə-tre) [*photo-* + *-metry*] [MeSH: Photometry] the measurement of light.
**flicker p.,** see *flicker.*

**pho·to·mi·cro·graph** (fo″to-mi′kro-graf) [*photo-* + *micro-* + *-graph*] the photograph of a minute object as seen under the light microscope, produced by ordinary photographic methods. Cf. *microphotograph.*

**pho·to·mi·crog·ra·phy** (fo″to-mi-krog′rə-fe) [MeSH: Photomicrography] the production of photomicrographs.

**pho·to·mi·cro·scope** (fo″to-mi′kro-skōp) a microscope and camera combined for making photomicrographs.

**pho·to·mi·cros·co·py** (fo″to-mi-kros′kə-pe) photography of enlarged pictures of minute objects with the photomicroscope.

**pho·to·mor·pho·gen·e·sis** (fo″to-mor″fo-jen′ə-sis) the regulation of form by light, as in the induction of flowering in plants by a minimal period of daylight.

**pho·to·myo·clon·ic** (fo″to-mi″o-klon′ik) photomyogenic.

**pho·to·my·o·gen·ic** (fo″to-mi″o-jen′ik) photomyoclonic; denoting an electroencephalographic response to photic stimulation (brief flashes of light) marked by myoclonus of the facial muscles.

**pho·ton** (fo′ton) [Gr. *phōs,* gen. *phōtos* light] a particle with no mass and no charge, the quantum electromagnetic radiation.

**pho·ton·cia** (fo-ton′se-ə) [*photo-* + *onc-*[1] + *-ia*] swelling due to the action of light.

**pho·to-onych·ol·y·sis** (fo″to-o″nĭ-kol′ĭ-sis) onycholysis resulting from exposure to sunlight or ultraviolet rays, as after treatment with the tetracyclines, methoxypsoralen, or other photoactive drugs.

**pho·to·par·ox·ys·mal** (fo″to-par″ok-siz′məl) photoconvulsive; denoting an abnormal electroencephalographic response to photic stimulation (brief flashes of light), marked by diffuse paroxysmal discharge recorded as spike-wave complexes; the response may be accompanied by minor seizures.

**pho·top·a·thy** (fo-top′ə-the) [*photo-* + *-pathy*] a pathologic effect produced by light.

**pho·to·per·cep·tive** (fo″to-pər-sep′tiv) [*photo-* + *perceptive*] able to perceive light.

**pho·to·pe·ri·od** (fo′to-pēr″e-əd) [MeSH: Photoperiod] the period of time per day that an organism is exposed to daylight or to artificial light.

**pho·to·pe·ri·od·ic** (fo″to-pēr″e-od′ik) pertaining to the photoperiod or to photoperiodism.

**pho·to·pe·ri·o·dic·i·ty** (fo″to-pe″re-o-dis′ĭ-te) photoperiodism.

**pho·to·pe·ri·od·ism** (fo″to-pe′re-əd-iz-əm) the physiologic and behavioral reactions brought about in organisms by changes in the duration of daylight and darkness in a 24-hour period. Called also *photoperiodicity.*

**pho·to·phar·ma·col·o·gy** (fo″to-fahr″mə-kol′ə-je) [*photo-* + *pharmacology*] the study of the effects of light and other radiations on drugs and on their pharmacological action.

**pho·to·phe·re·sis** (fo″to-fə-re′sis) [*photo-* + *pheresis*] [MeSH: Photopheresis] a technique for treating cutaneous T-cell lymphoma; after administration of a photoactive chemical, such as methoxsalen, blood is circulated out of the patient, through a source of ultraviolet radiation, and returned. The therapeutic effect is believed to involve stimulation of the host immune system.

**pho·to·phil·ic** (fo″to-fil′ik) [*photo-* + *-philic*] thriving in light; said of organisms.

**pho·to·pho·bia** (fo″to-fo′be-ə) [*photo-* + *-phobia*] abnormal visual intolerance of light.

**pho·to·pho·bic** (fo″to-fo′bik) pertaining to or characterized by photophobia.

**pho·to·phos·phor·y·la·tion** (fo″to-fos″for-ə-la′shən) [MeSH: Photophosphorylation] the formation of ATP occurring in chloroplasts during photosynthesis; it is analogous to oxidative phosphorylation.
**cyclic p.,** that in which ATP formation is coupled with liberation of the energy arising from a cyclic flow of electrons from the ferredoxin-reducing system back to the chlorophyll.

**pho·toph·thal·mia** (fo″tof-thal′me-ə) [*phot-* + *ophthalmia*] ophthalmia caused by intense light, such as electric light, rays of welding arc, or reflection from snow (ophthalmia nivialis).
**flash p.,** ophthalmia produced by exposure to a welding arc.

**pho·to·pia** (fo-to′pe-ə) day vision; see also *light adaptation.*

**pho·top·ic** (fo-top′ik) pertaining to vision in the light; said of the eye which has become light-adapted.

**pho·to·pig·ment** (fo″to-pig′mənt) a pigment, such as a retinal pigment, that is unstable in the presence of light.

**pho·to·ple·thys·mo·graph** (fo″to-plə-thiz′mo-graf) the diode and sensor apparatus used in photoplethysmography.

**pho·to·ple·thys·mog·ra·phy** (fo″to-pleth″iz-mog′rə-fe) [MeSH: Photoplethysmography] a technique for assessing blood flow by placing a diode that emits infrared light, along with a sensor, on the surface of the skin over a blood vessel; the amount of light reflected back to the sensor is inversely proportional to the number of red blood cells flowing through the vessel.

**pho·to·prod·uct** (fo′to-prod″əkt) a substance synthesized in the body by the action of light.

**pho·to·pro·tec·tion** (fo″to-pro-tek′shən) the protection of some cells by exposure to light in the near ultraviolet light range prior to exposure to light in the far ultraviolet range.

**pho·top·sia** (fo-top′se-ə) [*photo-* + *-opsia*] an appearance as of sparks or flashes due to retinal irritation.

**pho·top·sin** (fo-top′sin) the opsin of the cones of the retina that combines with 11-*cis* retinal to form photochemical pigments (iodopsins). See illustration at *visual cycle,* under *cycle.*

**pho·top·sy** (fo-top′se) photopsia.

**pho·to·ptar·mo·sis** (fo″to-tahr-mo′sis) [*photo-* + Gr. *ptarmos* sneezing + *-osis*] sneezing caused by the influence of light.

**pho·top·tom·e·ter** (fo″top-tom′ə-tər) [*phot-* + *opto-* + *-meter*] a device for testing the acuity of vision by determining the smallest amount of light that will render an object just visible; called also *Förster's photometer*

**pho·top·tom·e·try** (fo″top-tom′ə-tre) [*photo-* + *opto-* + *-metry*] determination of the flicker fusion threshold. See *flicker.*

**pho·to·ra·di·a·tion** (fo″to-ra″de-a′shən) photodynamic therapy.

**pho·to·ra·di·om·e·ter** (fo″to-ra″de-om′ə-tər) an apparatus for measuring the quantity of x-rays penetrating any given surface.

**pho·to·re·ac·tion** (fo″to-re-ak′shən) a chemical reaction initiated or affected by light; called also *photochemical reaction.*

**pho·to·re·ac·ti·va·tion** (fo″to-re-ak″tĭ-va′shən) the reversal of the biological effects of ultraviolet radiation on cells by subsequent exposure to visible light; called also *photoreversal.*

**pho·to·re·cep·tion** (fo″to-re-sep′shən) [*photo-* + *re-* + *-ceptor*] the process of detecting radiant energy, usually of wavelengths between 370 and 760 nm, being the range of visible light.

**pho·to·re·cep·tive** (fo″to-re-sep′tiv) sensitive to stimulation by light.

**pho·to·re·cep·tor** (fo″to-re-sep′tor) [MeSH: Photoreceptors] a nerve end-organ or receptor sensitive to light; see also *visual cells,* under *cell.*

**pho·to·res·pi·ra·tion** (fo″to-res″pĭ-ra′shən) a process carried out by certain plants, occurring as a result of oxidation of glycolic acid (a product of photosynthesis released by chloroplasts) by glycolic acid oxidase, an enzyme present in the glyoxosomes, ultimately causing an increased output of carbon dioxide.

**pho·to·ret·i·ni·tis** (fo″to-ret″ĭ-ni′tis) inflammation of the retina due to exposure to intense light, which may result in transient central scotoma.

**pho·to·re·ver·sal** (fo″to-re-ver′səl) photoreactivation.

**pho·to·scan** (fo′to-skan) a two-dimensional representation (map) of the gamma rays emitted by a radioisotope, revealing its varying concentration in a body tissue, differing from a scintiscan only in that the printout mechanism is a light source exposing a photographic film.

**pho·to·scan·ner** (fo″to-skan′ər) the system of equipment used in the making of a photoscan.

**pho·to·scope** (fo′to-skōp) [*photo-* + *-scope*] a kind of fluoroscope.

**pho·tos·co·py** (fo-tos′kə-pe) [*photo-* + *-scopy*] fluoroscopy.

**pho·to·sen·si·tive** (fo″to-sen′sĭ-tiv) exhibiting an abnormally heightened reactivity to sunlight.

**pho·to·sen·si·tiv·i·ty** (fo″to-sen″sĭ-tiv′ĭ-te) [*photo-* + *sensitivity*] an abnormal cutaneous response involving the interaction between photosensitizing substances and sunlight or filtered or artificial light at wavelengths of 280–400 nm. There are two main types: *photoallergy* and *phototoxicity.*

**pho·to·sen·si·ti·za·tion** (fo″to-sen″sĭ-tĭ-za′shən) 1. the process of photosensitizing. 2. abnormally heightened reactivity of the skin to sunlight.
**hepatogenous p.,** that caused by accumulation in body tissues of a photosensitizing substance because of inadequate hepatic clearance; it often occurs in ruminants when plants break down in the stomach under anaerobic conditions and form phylloerythrin.

**pho·to·sen·si·tize** (fo″to-sen′sĭ-tīz) [*photo-* + *sensitize*] to sensitize a substance, organism, cell, or tissue to the influence of light. See *photosensitivity,* and see *photodynamic therapy,* under *therapy.*

**pho·to·sta·ble** (fo′to-sta″bəl) unchanged by the influence of light.

**pho·to·stetho·scope** (fo″to-steth′ə-skōp) a lamp which transforms sounds amplified by a microphone into pulsations of light; used for recording the heartbeats of the fetus.

**pho·to·syn·the·sis** (fo″to-sin′thə-sis) [*photo-* + *synthesis*] [MeSH: Photosynthesis] a chemical combination caused by the action of light; specifically the formation of carbohydrates (with release of molecular oxygen) from carbon dioxide and water in the chlorophyll tissue of plants and blue-green algae under the influence of light. In bacteria, photosynthesis employs hydrogen sulfide, molecular hydrogen, and other reduced compounds in place of water, so that molecular oxygen is not released. See also *light reaction* and *dark reaction,* under *reaction.* Cf. *chemosynthesis.*

**pho·to·tac·tic** (fo″to-tak′tik) of, pertaining to, or exhibiting phototaxis.

**pho·to·tax·is** (fo″to-tak′sis) [*photo-* + *taxis*] taxis of an organism elicited in response to the source of light stimulus; called also *heliotaxis.*

**pho·to·ther·a·py** (fo″to-ther′ə-pe) [*photo-* + *therapy*] [MeSH: Phototherapy] 1. the treatment of disease, e.g., herpes simplex, psoriasis, neonatal hyperbilirubinemia, or seasonal affective disorder, by exposure to light, especially by variously concentrated light rays or specific wavelengths. 2. photodynamic therapy.
**ultraviolet p.,** the use of ultraviolet radiation (which may be type A, B, or C, or a combination of types) in the treatment of skin diseases. The radiation is generated by an artificial source such as an arc lamp and may be used in combination with photosensitizing drugs; see also *photochemotherapy.*

**pho·to·ther·mal** (fo″to-ther′məl) pertaining to the heat produced by radiant energy.

**pho·to·ther·my** (fo′to-ther″me) [*photo-* + Gr. *thermē* heat] the heat effects produced by radiant energy.

**pho·to·tim·er** (fo′to-tīm″ər) a device used in radiology and photography to control the exposure interval by terminating the exposure when the amount of incident radiation or light reaches a preset quantity.

**pho·tot·o·nus** (fo-tot′ə-nəs) [*photo-* + *tonus*] the sensitivity of an organism to light.

**pho·to·tox·ic** (fo″to-tok′sik) [*photo-* + *toxic*] pertaining to, characterized by, or producing phototoxicity.

**pho·to·tox·ic·i·ty** (fo″to-tok-sis′ĭ-te) [*photo-* + *toxicity*] a nonimmunologic, chemically induced type of photosensitivity. See also *phototoxic dermatitis,* under *dermatitis.* Cf. *photoallergy.*

**pho·to·trans·duc·tion** (fo″to-trans-duk′shən) [MeSH: Phototransduction] visual transduction.

**pho·to·troph·ic** (fo″to-trof′ik) [*photo-* + *-trophic*] capable of deriving energy from light, as in certain green plants and bacteria. Cf. *chemotrophic.*

**pho·to·trop·ic** (fo″to-trop′ik) exhibiting phototropism.

**pho·tot·ro·pism** (fo-tot′rə-piz-əm) [*photo-* + *trop-* + *-ism*] [MeSH: Phototropism] 1. tropism of an organism in response to the source of light stimulus. 2. change of color produced in a substance by the action of light.

**pho·to·va·por·iza·tion** (fo″to-va″por-ĭ-za′shən) laser-produced vaporization of intracellular and extracellular fluids to provide an incision with cauterization of adjacent vessels.

**pho·tron·re·flec·tom·e·ter** (fo″tron-re″flek-tom′ə-tər) an apparatus for measuring turbidity.

**pho·tu·ria** (fo-tu′re-ə) [*photo-* + *-uria*] the excretion of urine having a luminous appearance.

**PHPPA** *p*-hydroxyphenylpyruvic acid.

**Phrag·mo·ba·sid·io·my·ce·tes** (frag″mo-bə-sid″e-o-mi-se′tēz) [Gr. *phragma* fence + *basidium* + Gr. *mykēs* fungus] a class of perfect fungi of the subphylum Basidiomycotina, characterized by having a septate basidium.

**Phrag·mo·ba·sid·io·my·ce·ti·dae** (frag″mo-bə-sid″e-o-mi-set′ĭ-de) name given to Phragmobasidiomycetes when it is considered a subclass.

**phrag·mo·plast** (frag′mo-plast) [Gr. *phragmos* enclosure + *-plast*] the barrel-shaped spindle formed in the equatorial plane during mitosis of plant cells; it precedes the formation of the cell plate.

**phren** (fren) [Gr. *phrēn*] 1. diaphragma (def. 1). 2. the mind, as seat of the intellect, or the heart, as seat of the passions.

**phre·nal·gia** (fre-nal′jə) [*phren-* + *-algia*] pain in the diaphragm; called also *diaphragmalgia* and *phrenodynia.*

**phre·nec·to·my** (fre-nek′tə-me) [*phren-* + *-ectomy*] the removal of all or a part of the diaphragm.

**phren·em·phrax·is** (fren″em-frak′sis) [*phreni*c nerve + *emphraxis*] phreniclasia.

**phren·ic** (fren′ik) [L. *phrenicus;* Gr. *phrēn* diaphragm, mind] 1. pertaining to the diaphragm of the body; called also *diaphragmatic.* 2. pertaining to the mind.

**phren·i·cec·to·my** (fren″ĭ-sek′tə-me) [*phrenic* nerve + *-ectomy*] resection of the phrenic nerve, causing paralysis of the diaphragm; called also *phreniconeurectomy.*

**phreni·cla·sia, phreni·cla·sis** (fren″ĭ-kla′zhə, fren″ĭ-kla′sis) [*phrenic* nerve + Gr. *klasis* crushing] crushing of the phrenic nerve with a clamp, causing paralysis of the diaphragm. Called also *phrenemphraxis* and *phrenicotripsy.*

**phren·i·co·ex·air·e·sis** (fren″ĭ-ko-ek-sar′ə-sis) phrenicoexeresis.

**phren·i·co·ex·er·e·sis** (fren″ĭ-ko-ek-ser′ə-sis) [*phrenic* nerve + *exeresis*] avulsion of the phrenic nerve; cf. *phrenicectomy* and *phreniclasia.* Called also *phrenicoexairesis.*

**phren·i·co·neu·rec·to·my** (fren″ĭ-ko-no͞o-rek′tə-me) phrenicectomy.

**phren·i·cot·o·my** (fren″ĭ-kot′ə-me) [*phrenic* nerve + *-tomy*] surgical division of the phrenic nerve and its accessory for the purpose of causing one-sided paralysis of the diaphragm.

**phren·i·co·trip·sy** (fren″ĭ-ko-trip′se) [*phrenic* nerve + *-tripsy*] phreniclasia.

**phre·ni·tis** (frə-ni′tis) [*phren-* + *-itis*] inflammation of the diaphragm; called also *diaphragmitis.*

**phren(o)-** [Gr. *phrēn,* gen. *phrenos* diaphragm, mind] a combining form denoting relationship to the diaphragm, the phrenic nerve, or the mind.

**phreno·col·ic** (fren″o-kol′ik) pertaining to or connecting the diaphragm and colon.

**phreno·dyn·ia** (fren″o-din′e-ə) [*phreno-* + *-odynia*] phrenalgia.

**phreno·gas·tric** (fren″o-gas′trik) pertaining to the diaphragm and the stomach.

**phreno·glot·tic** (fren″o-glot′ik) pertaining to the diaphragm and the glottis.

**phreno·graph** (fren′o-graf) [*phreno-* + *-graph*] an apparatus for recording the movements of the diaphragm.

**phreno·he·pat·ic** (fren″o-hə-pat′ik) [*phreno-* + *hepatic*] pertaining to the diaphragm and the liver.

**phre·nol·o·gist** (frə-nol′ə-jist) a person who practices phrenology.

**phre·nol·o·gy** (frə-nol′ə-je) [*phreno-* + *-logy*] [MeSH: Phrenology] the theory, popular in the 18th and 19th centuries, that mental faculties could be determined by the location of bumps and other topographical features on the skull.

**phreno·peri·car·di·tis** (fren″o-per″ĭ-kahr-di′tis) [*phreno-* + *pericarditis*] a condition in which the apex of the heart is attached to the diaphragm by adhesions.

**phreno·ple·gia** (fren″o-ple′jə) [*phreno-* + *-plegia*] diaphragmatic paralysis.

**phren·op·to·sis** (fren″op-to′sis) [*phreno-* + *-ptosis*] downward displacement of the diaphragm.

**phren·o·sin, phren·o·sine** (fren′o-sin; fren′o-sēn) a cerebroside occurring in the brain and other nervous tissue; it is composed of sphingosine linked to galactose and cerebronic acid.

**phreno·spasm** (fren′o-spaz-əm) [*phreno-* + *spasm*] spasm of the diaphragm.

**phreno·splen·ic** (fren″o-splen′ik) pertaining to or connecting the diaphragm and the spleen.

**phren·o·trop·ic** (fren″o-trop′ik) [*phreno-* + *-tropic*] exerting its principal effect upon the mind.

**phric·to·path·ic** (frik″to-path′ik) [Gr. *phriktos* producing a shudder + *pathos* disease] causing a shudder; a term applied to a peculiar sensation caused by irritating a hysterical anesthetic area during recovery.

**phry·nin** (fri′nin) a poisonous substance obtainable from the skin and secretions of various toads; its properties resemble those of digitalin.

**phryno·der·ma** (frin″o-der′mə) [Gr. *phrynē* toad + *derma*] follicular hyperkeratosis.

**phry·nol·y·sin** (fri-nol′ĭ-sin) [Gr. *phrynē* toad + *lysin*] the lysin or toxin from the venom of the fire toad *(Bombinator igneus)*.

**phthal·ate** (thal′āt) a salt, anion, or ester of phthalic acid.

**phthal·ein** (thal′ēn) any one of a series of coloring matters formed by the condensation of phthalic anhydride with the phenols; some of them have a purgative action. See *phenolphthalein*.
**alpha-naphthol p.**, an indicator used in the determination of hydrogen ion concentration; it has a pH range of 9.3–10.5.
**orthocresol p.**, an indicator used in the determination of hydrogen ion concentration; it has a pH range of 8.2–9.8.

**phthal·ein·om·e·ter** (thal″ēn-om′ə-tər) an instrument for use in performing phenolsulfonphthalein tests.

**phthal·ic ac·id** (thal′ik) any of the isomers, but usually the ortho- isomer, of the dicarboxylic acid–substituted benzene ring; the ortho- isomer is used in dye manufacture.

**phthal·in** (thal′in) any one of a series of colorless compounds formed by reduction of phthalein.

**phthal·yl·sul·fa·cet·amide** (thal″əl-sul″fə-set′ə-mīd) a sulfonamide used as an intestinal antibacterial, administered orally. Called also *phthalylsulfonazole*.

**phthal·yl·sul·fa·thi·a·zole** (thal″əl-sul″fə-thi′ə-zōl) a sulfonamide used as an intestinal antibacterial, administered orally.

**phthal·yl·sul·fon·a·zole** (thal″əl-səl-fon′ə-zōl) phthalylsulfacetamide.

**phthi·o·col** (thi′o-kol) an antibiotic substance produced by *Mycobacterium tuberculosis* and having some vitamin K activity.

**phthi·o·ic ac·id** (thi-o′ik) a branched-chain fatty acid occurring in the cell wall of *Mycobacterium tuberculosis*.

**phthir·i·a·sis** (thir-i′ə-sis) [Gr. *phtheiriasis*, from *phtheir* louse] infestation with crab or pubic lice; see also *pediculosis*.
**p. inguina′lis, pubic p.**, infestation with lice of the species *Phthirus pubis;* it is usually limited to the pubic hairs but may occur on other areas, as the eyelashes.

**Phthir·us** (thir′əs) [Gr. *phtheir* louse] a genus of sucking lice (order Anoplura), of the family Pediculidae, which feed on human blood.
**P. pu′bis**, the pubic or crab louse which infests the hair of the pubic region and which is sometimes found in other hairy areas of the body, such as the eyebrows, eyelashes, and axillae.

**phthi·sis** (thi′sis; ti′sis) [Gr. *phthisis*, from *phthiein* to decay] 1. a wasting away of the body or a part of the body. 2. old name for *pulmonary tuberculosis*.
**aneurysmal p.**, the clinical symptoms of chest pain and cough, at first dry and later productive, sometimes with hemoptysis, produced by aneurysm of the ascending aorta and the aortic arch.
**p. bul′bi**, shrinkage and wasting of the eyeball.
**p. cor′neae**, the shriveling and disappearance of the cornea after suppurative keratitis.
**essential p. of the eye**, ophthalmomalacia.
**ocular p.**, ophthalmomalacia.

**phyco-** [Gr. *phykos* seaweed] a combining form denoting relationship to seaweed or algae.

**phy·co·chrome** (fi′ko-krōm) [*phyco-* + *-chrome*] 1. a blue-green pigment from various fresh-water algae of the simplest type. 2. any of the algae that contain both chlorophyll and a blue pigment; the blue-green algae.

**phy·co·chro·mo·pro·tein** (fi″ko-kro″mo-pro′tēn) a colored, conjugated protein, with respiratory function, found in various seaweeds.

**phy·co·eryth·rin** (fi″ko-ə-rith′rin) [MeSH: Phycoerythrin] a red, fluorescent, algal protein that can be coupled to various biological molecules to make them more easily assayed.

**Phy·co·my·ce·tes** (fi″ko-mi-se′tēz) [*phyco-* + Gr. *mykēs* fungus] [MeSH: Phycomycetes] in some systems of classification, a class of fungi comprising the common water, leaf, and bread molds, which includes Oomycetes and Zygomycetes as subclasses.

**phy·co·my·ce·to·sis** (fi″ko-mi-sə-to′sis) mucormycosis.

**phy·co·my·ce·tous** (fi′ko-mi-se′təs) of or pertaining to fungi of the group Phycomycetes.

**phy·co·my·co·sis** (fi″ko-mi-ko′sis) 1. mucormycosis. 2. zygomycosis.
**subcutaneous p.**, entomophthoromycosis basidiobolae.

**phy·go·ga·lac·tic** (fi″go-gə-lak′tik) [Gr. *pheugein* to avoid + *galactic*] checking the secretion of milk; galactophygous.

**phy·la** (fi′lə) plural of *phylum*.

**phy·lac·tic** (fə-lak′tik) [Gr. *phylaktikos* preservative] serving to protect; pertaining to or producing phylaxis.

**phy·lax·is** (fə-lak′sis) [Gr. "a guarding"] protection against infection; the bodily defense against infection.

**phy·let·ic** (fi-let′ik) pertaining to a phylum, or to phylogeny.

**Phyl·lan·thus** (fə-lan′thəs) a genus of herbs, shrubs, and trees of the family Euphorbiaceae, found in tropical and subtropical regions. *P. eng′leri* is a species found in southern Africa whose local name is suicide plant; when the bark or root is smoked it causes death.

**phyl·lid·ea** (fə-lid′e-ə) bothridium.

**phyll(o)-** [Gr. *phyllon* leaf] a combining form denoting relationship to leaves, or to chlorophyll.

**phyl·lode** (fil′ōd) [*phyllo-* + *-oid*] resembling a leaf; a term applied to tumors which on section show a lobulated, leaflike appearance.

**phyl·lo·er·y·thrin** (fil″o-er′ĭ-thrin) a derivative of chlorophyll formed in the intestinal canal of ruminant animals and found also in their bile. In cases of hepatic insufficiency it may accumulate in the tissues and cause photosensitization (see *yellows*).

**phyl·lo·lith** (fil′o-lith) a small concretion 100 to 200 μm in diameter formed of concentric strata, occurring in cavities in renal tuberculosis.

**phyl·lo·quin·one** (fil″o-kwin′ōn) phytonadione.

**phy·lo·gen·e·sis** (fi″lo-jen′ə-sis) phylogeny.

**phy·lo·ge·net·ic** (fi″lo-jə-net′ik) phylogenic.

**phy·lo·gen·ic** (fi-lo-jen′ik) pertaining to phylogeny.

**phy·log·e·ny** (fi-loj′ə-ne) [Gr. *phylon* tribe + *-geny*] [MeSH: Phylogeny] the complete developmental history of a race or group of animals. Cf. *ontogeny*.

**phy·lum** (fi′ləm) pl. *phy′la* [L.; Gr. *phylon* race] a primary or main division of a kingdom, composed of a group of related classes; in the taxonomy of plants, the term *division* is used instead.

**phy·ma** (fi′mə) pl. *phy′mata* [Gr. "a growth"] any skin tumor or cutaneous tubercle, especially a circumscribed swelling on the skin, larger than a tubercle, and produced by exudation into the subcutaneous tissue or the corium.

**phy·ma·ta** (fi'mə-tə) [Gr.] plural of *phyma.*

**phy·ma·to·rhu·sin** (fi"mə-to-roo'sin) [Gr. *phyma,* gen. *phymatos* a growth + *rhysis* flow] a dark pigment from hair and melanotic tumors; it is a form of melanin.

**phy·ma·tor·rhys·in** (fi"mə-to-ris'in) phymatorhusin.

**Phy·sa·lia** (fi-sa'le-ə) a genus of cnidarians of the class Hydrozoa, all called Portuguese man-of-war, characterized by a large, purple air sac that allows them to float on the surface of the water, and from which many long tentacles of stinging polyps hang. The tentacles are equipped with nematocysts that are able to penetrate the skin of man, causing intense pain; paralysis sometimes results from numerous stings.

**phy·sal·i·des** (fi-sal'ĭ-dēz) plural of *physalis.*

**phys·a·lif·er·ous** (fis"ə-lif'ər-əs) [*physalis* + *-ferous*] physaliphorous.

**phy·sal·i·form** (fĭ-sal'ĭ-form) [*physalis* + *form*] resembling bubbles.

**phy·sal·i·phore** (fĭ-sal'ĭ-for) [*physalis* + *-phore*] physaliphorous cell; sometimes used incorrectly for the vacuole within such a cell.

**phys·a·liph·o·rous** (fis"ə-lif'ə-rəs) [*physalis* + Gr. *phoros* bearing] containing bubbles or vacuoles.

**phys·a·lis** (fis'ə-lis) pl. *physal'ides* [Gr. *physallis* bubble] a vacuole cavity found in certain cells, such as the giant cells of sarcoma or chordoma.

**phys·al·li·za·tion** (fis"əl-ĭ-za'shən) [Gr. *physallis* bubble] the formation of a permanent froth when a liquid is shaken together with a gas.

**Phys·a·lop·tera** (fis"ə-lop'tər-ə) [Gr. *physallis* bubble + *pteron* wing] a genus of nematodes of the family Physalopteridae, superfamily Spiruroidea, found in the stomach and intestine of birds and mammals, including humans.
**P. cauca'sica,** a species occurring in the Caucasus and in Africa.
**P. mor'dens,** *P. caucasica.*
**P. ra'ra,** a species found in the stomach of dogs.
**P. trunca'ta,** a species found in the proventriculus of chickens and pheasants.

**phys·a·lop·ter·i·a·sis** (fis"ə-lop-tər-i'ə-sis) infection with *Physaloptera.*

**Phys·a·lop·ter·i·dae** (fis"əl-op-ter'ĭ-de) a family of nematodes of the superfamily Spiruroidea; they infect birds and mammals. The one genus of veterinary interest is *Physaloptera.*

**phys·e·al** (fiz'e-əl) pertaining to growth, or to the segment of tubular bone which is concerned mainly with growth (the physis).

**phys·iat·rics** (fiz"e-at'riks) [*physi-* + *-iatrics*] physiatry.

**phys·iat·rist** (fiz"e-at'rist) a physician who specializes in physiatry.

**phys·iat·ry** (fiz"e-at're) [*physi-* + *-iatry*] the branch of medicine that deals with the prevention, diagnosis, and treatment of disease or injury, and the rehabilitation from resultant impairments and disabilities, using physical agents such as light, heat, cold, water, electricity, therapeutic exercise, and mechanical apparatus, and sometimes pharmaceutical agents. Called also *physiatrics* and *physical medicine.* See also *rehabilitation* (def. 2).

**phys·ic** (fiz'ik) [Gr. *physikos* natural] [MeSH: Physics] 1. the art of medicine and of therapeutics. 2. a medicine, especially a cathartic.

**phys·i·cal** (fiz'ĭ-kəl) [Gr. *physikos*] pertaining to the body, to material things, or to physics.

**phy·si·cian** (fĭ-zish'ən) [MeSH: Physicians] 1. an authorized practitioner of medicine, as one graduated from a college of medicine or osteopathy and licensed by the appropriate board. See also *doctor.* 2. one who practices medicine as distinct from surgery.
**p. assistant,** one who has been trained in an accredited program and certified by an appropriate board to perform certain of a physician's duties, including history taking, physical examination, diagnostic tests, treatment, certain minor surgical procedures, etc., all under the responsible supervision of a licensed physician. Abbreviated P.A. See also *Medex.* Called also *physician's assistant.*
**attending p.,** a physician who attends a hospital at stated times to visit the patients and give directions as to their treatment.
**emergency p.,** a specialist in emergency medicine.
**family p.,** a medical specialist who plans and provides the comprehensive primary health care of all members of a family, regardless of age or sex, on a continuing basis.
**resident p.,** resident.

**Phy·sick's pouches** (fiz'iks) [Philip Syng *Physick,* American surgeon, 1768–1837] see under *pouch.*

**phys·i·co·chem·i·cal** (fiz"ĭ-ko-kem'ĭ-kəl) pertaining to physics and chemistry.

**phys·ics** (fiz'iks) [Gr. *physis* nature] [MeSH: Physics] the science of the laws and phenomena of nature, but especially of the forces and general properties of matter and energy.

**physi(o)-** [Gr. *physis* nature] a combining form meaning physical, or denoting relationship to nature or physiology.

**phys·io·chem·i·cal** (fiz"e-o-kem'ĭ-kəl) pertaining to physiologic chemistry, or clinical chemistry.

**phys·io·chem·is·try** (fiz"e-o-kem'is-tre) physiologic chemistry, or clinical chemistry.

**phys·io·gen·e·sis** (fiz"e-o-jen'ə-sis) embryology.

**phys·i·og·no·my** (fiz"e-og'nə-me) [*physio-* + Gr. *gnōmōn* a judge] [MeSH: Physiognomy] 1. the determination of temperament and character from facial features. 2. physiognosis.

**phys·i·og·no·sis** (fiz"e-og-no'sis) [*physio-* + Gr. *gnōsis* knowledge] diagnosis by means of the facial expression or appearance.

**phys·i·o·log·ic** (fiz"e-o-loj'ik) normal; not pathologic; characteristic of or conforming to the normal functioning or state of the body or a tissue or organ; physiological.

**phys·i·o·log·i·cal** (fiz"e-o-loj'ĭ-kəl) pertaining to physiology; physiologic.

**phys·i·o·log·i·co·an·a·tom·i·cal** (fiz"e-o-loj"ĭ-ko-an"ə-tom'ĭ-kəl) pertaining to physiology and anatomy.

**phys·i·ol·o·gist** (fiz"e-ol'ə-jist) a specialist in the study of physiology.

**phys·i·ol·o·gy** (fiz"e-ol'ə-je) [*physio-* + *-logy*] [MeSH: Physiology] 1. the science which treats of the functions of the living organism and its parts, and of the physical and chemical factors and processes involved. 2. the basic processes underlying the functioning of a species or class of organism, or any of its parts or processes.
**animal p.,** the physiology of animals other than humans; called also *zoophysiology* and *zoodynamics.*
**comparative p.,** a study of organ functions in various types of animals, vertebrate and invertebrate, in an effort to find fundamental relations in the physiology of members of the entire animal kingdom.
**dental p.,** the study of the function and functional form of the teeth and supporting tissues.
**general p.,** the science of the general laws of life and functional activity.
**hominal p.,** human physiology.
**morbid p., pathologic p.,** the study of disordered function or of function in diseased tissues.
**special p.,** the physiology of particular organs.
**vegetable p.,** the physiology of plants.

**phys·i·ol·y·sis** (fiz"e-ol'ĭ-sis) [*physio-* + *-lysis*] natural dissolution and disintegration of tissue.

**phys·io·med·i·cal·ism** (fiz"e-o-med'ĭ-kəl-iz-əm) [*physio-* + *medicalism*] a system of medical treatment in which only plant remedies are used, excluding those which are poisonous.

**phys·i·om·e·try** (fiz"e-om'ə-tre) [*physio-* + *-metry*] measurement of the physiologic functions of the body by serologic and physiologic methods.

**phys·i·on·o·my** (fiz"e-on'ə-me) [*physio-* + Gr. *nomos* law] the science of the laws of nature.

**phys·io·patho·log·ic** (fiz"e-o-path"ə-loj'ik) pertaining to both the physiologic and pathologic conditions.

**phys·io·pa·thol·o·gy** (fiz"e-o-pə-thol'ə-je) [*physio-* + *pathology*] the science of functions in disease, or as modified by disease.

**phys·i·oph·y·ly** (fiz"e-of'ə-le) [*physio-* + Gr. *phylon* tribe] the evolution of bodily functions.

**phys·io·ther·a·pist** (fiz"e-o-ther'ə-pist) physical therapist.

**phys·io·ther·a·py** (fiz"e-o-ther'ə-pe) [*physio-* + *therapy*] physical therapy.

**phy·sique** (fĭ-zēk') bodily structure, organization, and development.

**phy·sis** (fi'sis) [Gr. *phyein* to generate] the segment of tubular bone which is concerned mainly with growth in length of the bone. It consists of four zones: zone of resting cartilage, zone of proliferating cartilage, zone of hypertrophy, and zone of calcification.

**physo-** [Gr. *physa* air] a combining form denoting relationship to air or gas.

**phy·so·cele** (fi'so-sēl) [*physo-* + *-cele*[1]] 1. a tumor filled with gas. 2. a hernial sac filled with gas.

**Phy·so·ceph·a·lus** (fi"so-sef'ə-ləs) a genus of nematodes of the superfamily Spiruroidea. *P. sexala'tus* is found in the stomach of pigs.

**phy·so·hem·a·to·me·tra** (fi"so-hem"ə-to-me'trə) [*physo-* + *hemato-* + *metra*] the presence of gas and blood within the uterus.

**phy·so·hy·dro·me·tra** (fi″so-hi″dro-me′trə) [*physo-* + *hydro-* + *metra*] the presence of gas and fluid within the uterus.

**phy·so·me·tra** (fi″so-me′trə) [*physo-* + *metra*] air or gas in the uterine cavity.

**Phy·sop·sis** (fi-sop′sis) a subgenus of snails (genus *Bulinus*), several species of which are the intermediate hosts of *Schistosoma haematobium* and other animal schistosomes.

**phy·so·pyo·sal·pinx** (fi″so-pi″o-sal′pinks) [*physo-* + *pyo-* + *salpinx*] presence of pus and gas in the uterine tube.

**Phy·so·stig·ma** (fi″so-stig′mə) [*physo-* + Gr. *stigma* stigma] a genus of tropical plants of the family Leguminosae. *P. veneno′sum* Balf. is the Calabar bean.

**phy·so·stig·mine** (fi″zo-stig′mēn) [USP] [MeSH: Physostigmine] a cholinergic alkaloid having anticholinesterase activity and obtained from the dried ripe seed (Calabar bean) of *Physostigma venenosum;* used topically to produce miosis and decrease of intraocular pressure in glaucoma and parenterally to reverse the central nervous system effects produced by overdosage of anticholinergic drugs (anticholinergic syndrome). Called also *eserine.*
**p. salicylate** [USP], the salicylate salt of physostigmine with the same properties as the alkaloid.
**p. sulfate** [USP], the sulfate salt of physostigmine with the same properties as the alkaloid.

**phy·so·stig·min·ism** (fi″so-stig′min-iz-əm) poisoning by physostigmine.

**phy·tag·glu·ti·nin** (fi″tə-gloo′tĭ-nin) a phytotoxin which has the power of agglutinating red blood corpuscles.

**phy·tal·bu·min** (fi″tal-bu′min) [*phyto-* + *albumin*] vegetable albumin.

**phy·tan·ate** (fi′tən-āt) a salt or anionic form of phytanic acid.

**phy·tan·ic ac·id** (fi-tan′ik) [MeSH: Phytanic Acid] an unusual 20-carbon branched-chain fatty acid occurring at high levels in dairy products and ruminant fats and accumulated in tissues of patients with Refsum's disease and several peroxisomal disorders.

**phy·tan·ic ac·id α-hy·droxy·lase** (fi-tan′ik as′id hi-drok′sə-lās) an enzyme that catalyzes the alpha oxidation of phytanic acid, hydroxylating its alpha carbon; the reaction requires molecular oxygen and is stimulated by NADPH and by ferric iron. Deficiency of the enzyme, an autosomal recessive trait, causes Refsum's disease.

**6-phy·tase** (fi′tās) [EC 3.1.3.26] [MeSH: 6-Phytase] an enzyme of the hydrolase class, present at a low level in ileal mucosa, that hydrolyzes excess dietary phytic acid.

**phy·tate** (fi′tāt) an anionic form of phytic acid.

**-phyte** [Gr. *phyton* plant] a combining form denoting a plant or a pathological growth.

**phy·tic ac·id** (fi′tik) [MeSH: Phytic Acid] inositol hexaphosphate, a compound occurring in the leaves of plants.

**phyt(o)-** [Gr. *phyton* plant] a combining form denoting relationship to a plant or plants.

**phy·to·a·lex·in** (fi″to-ə-lek′sin) any of a group of compounds formed in plants in response to fungal infection, physical damage, chemical injury, or a pathogenic process. Phytoalexins inhibit or destroy the invading agent.

**phy·to·an·a·phy·lac·to·gen** (fi″to-an″ə-fə-lak′to-jən) [*phyto-* + *anaphylactogen*] an antigen of plant origin that is capable of inducing anaphylaxis; called also *phytosensitinogen.*

**phy·to·be·zoar** (fi″to-be′zor) [*phyto-* + *bezoar*] a gastric concretion composed of vegetable matter such as skins, seeds, and the fibers of fruit and vegetables.

**phy·to·chem·is·try** (fi″to-kem′is-tre) [*phyto-* + *chemistry*] the study of plant chemistry, including the chemical processes that take place in plants, the nature of plant chemicals, and the various applications of such chemicals to science and industry.

**phy·to·chin·in** (fi″to-kin′in) a substance isolated from the leaves of certain grasses, said to have an effect on carbohydrate metabolism resembling that of insulin.

**phy·to·dem·ic** (fi″to-dem′ik) [*phyto-* + *epidemic*] an epidemic attack of any disease of plants.

**phy·to·de·tri·tus** (fi″to-de-tri′təs) detritus produced by the disintegration and decomposition of vegetable organisms. Cf. *zoodetritus.*

**phy·to·flag·el·late** (fi″to-flaj′ə-lāt) [*phyto-* + *flagellate*] a plantlike flagellate protozoan of the class Phytomastigophorea. Cf. *zooflagellate.*

**phy·to·gen·e·sis** (fi″to-jen′ə-sis) [*phyto-* + *-genesis*] the origin and development of plants.

**phy·to·ge·net·ic, phy·to·gen·ic** (fi″to-jə-net′ik, fi″to-jen′ik) phytogenous.

**phy·tog·e·nous** (fi-toj′ə-nəs) [*phyto-* + *-genous*] derived from a plant, or caused by a vegetable growth.

**phy·to·hem·ag·glu·ti·nin** (fi″to-hēm″ə-gloo′tĭ-nin) a lectin isolated from the red kidney bean *(Phaseolus vulgaris);* it is a hemagglutinin that agglutinates mammalian erythrocytes and a mitogen that stimulates predominantly T lymphocytes. Abbreviated PHA.

**phy·to·hor·mone** (fi″to-hor′mōn) [*phyto-* + *hormone*] any of the hormones produced naturally in plants and which are active in minute amounts in controlling growth and other functions at a site remote from the place of production. There are three principal types: auxins, cytokinins, and gibberellins. Called also *plant hormone.*

**phy·toid** (fi′toid) [*phyto-* + *-oid*] resembling a plant.

**phy·tol** (fi′tol) [MeSH: Phytol] an unsaturated aliphatic alcohol related to xanthophyll, to the carotenoids, and to vitamin A, that exists in chlorophyll as an ester; used in the preparation of vitamin E and phytonadione.

**Phy·to·lac·ca** (fi″to-lak′ə) a genus of perennial herbs. *P. america′na* is the pokeweed (q.v.) of North America, which contains oxalate and saponins and is medicinal but can be toxic to livestock.

**Phy·to·mas·ti·goph·o·ra** (fi″to-mas″tĭ-gof′ə-rə) Phytomastigophorea.

**Phy·to·mas·ti·goph·o·rea** (fi″to-mas″tĭ-go-for′e-ə) [*phyto-* + Gr. *mastix* whip + *phoros* bearing] [MeSH: Phytomastigophorea] a class comprising all of the plantlike, as opposed to animal-like, protozoa (subphylum Mastigophora, phylum Sarcomastigophora), which are collectively known as the phytoflagellates. Phytomastigophoreans are characterized by the presence of chromatophores and usually one or two emergent flagella, with ameboid forms occurring in some groups. They are mostly free-living and are typically autotrophic. These organisms are sometimes classified with the algae. Called also *Phytomastigophora.* Cf. *Zoomastigophorea.*

**phy·to·mas·ti·goph·o·re·an** (fi″to-mas″tĭ-gə-for′e-ən) a protozoan of the class Phytomastigophorea.

**phy·to·men·a·di·one** (fi″to-men″ə-di′ōn) phytonadione.

**phy·to·mi·to·gen** (fi″to-mi′to-jən) a substance of plant origin that induces mitosis in human cells.

**phy·to·na·di·one** (fi″to-nə-di′ōn) [MeSH: Phytonadione] 1. a fat-soluble vitamin of the K group (q.v.) with a phytyl side chain, found in green plants or prepared synthetically and having prothrombinogenic properties. 2. [USP] a preparation of phytonadione used as a prothrombinogenic agent in the treatment of hypoprothrombinemia due to various causes; administered orally and parenterally. Called also *phylloquinone* and *vitamin* $K_1$.

**phy·to·no·sis** (fi″to-no′-sis) [*phyto-* + *nos-* + *-sis*] any morbid condition due to a plant.

**phy·to·par·a·site** (fi″to-par′ə-sīt) [*phyto-* + *parasite*] any parasitic vegetable organism or species.

**phy·to·path·o·gen·ic** (fi″to-path″o-jen′ik) producing disease in plants.

**phy·to·pa·thol·o·gy** (fi″to-pə-thol′ə-je) [*phyto-* + *pathology*] 1. the study of plant diseases and their control. 2. the pathology of morbid conditions caused by schizomycetes and other vegetable parasites.

**phy·top·a·thy** (fi-top′ə-the) [*phyto-* + *-pathy*] any disease of plants.

**phy·toph·a·gous** (fi-tof′ə-gəs) [*phyto-* + *phag-* + *-ous*] eating vegetable food.

**phy·to·pho·to·der·ma·ti·tis** (fi″to-fo″to-der″mə-ti′tis) [*phyto-* + *photo-* + *dermatitis*] phototoxic dermatitis induced by the sequential exposure to certain plants containing psoralen-type photosensitizers and then to sunlight. It is manifested by burning erythema, followed by edema and the development of small vesicles that coalesce into large bullae, and this is followed by intense residual hyperpigmentation in the areas of the skin that come in contact with the psoralen photosensitizer.

**phy·to·plank·ton** (fi″to-plank′ton) [*phyto-* + *plankton*] [MeSH: Phytoplankton] the minute plant (vegetable) organisms which, with those of the animal kingdom, make up the plankton of natural waters.

**phy·to·plasm** (fi′to-plaz-əm) [*phyto-* + *-plasm*] vegetable protoplasm.

**phy·to·pre·cip·i·tin** (fi″to-pre-sip′ĭ-tin) a precipitin produced by immunization with protein substances of plant origin.

**phy·to·sen·si·tin·o·gen** (fi″to-sen″sĭ-tin′ə-jən) [*phyto-* + *sensitinogen*] phytoanaphylactogen.

**phy·to·sis** (fi-to′sis) [*phyto-* + *-osis*] any disease caused by a phytoparasite.

**phy·tos·ter·ol** (fi-tos′tər-ol″) a plant sterol. See also *sitosterol.*

**phy·tos·ter·ol·emia** (fi-tos″tər-ol-e′me-ə) sitosterolemia.

**phy·to·ther·a·py** (fi″to-ther′ə-pe) [*phyto-* + *therapy*] treatment by use of plants.

**phy·to·tox·ic** (fi″to-tok′sik) 1. pertaining to a phytotoxin, or plant poison. 2. inhibiting the growth of plants.

**phy·to·tox·in** (fi″to-tok′sin) 1. any toxic substance of plant origin. 2. any of a group of exotoxins produced by certain species of higher plants; they are resistant to proteolytic digestion, and are effective when taken by mouth. Included are abrin, crotin, ricin, and robin.

**phy·to·tri·cho·be·zoar** (fi″to-tri″ko-be′zor) [*phyto-* + *tricho-* + *bezoar*] a bezoar composed of both plant fibers and hair.

**phy·to·vi·tel·lin** (fi″to-vi-tel′in) vitellin of vegetable origin.

**phy·tox·y·lin** (fi-tok′sə-lin) [*phyto-* + Gr. *xylon* wood] a substance resembling pyroxylin; used in preparing celloidin sections.

**PI** phosphatidylinositol.

**pI** the pH of a solution containing a solute at its isoelectric point.

**pi** (pi) [Π, π] the sixteenth letter of the Greek alphabet.

**pia** (pi′ə, pe′ə) [L.] 1. tender; soft. 2. pia mater.

**pia-ar·ach·ni·tis** (pi″ə-ar″ak-ni′tis) leptomeningitis.

**pia-arach·noid** (pi″ə-ə-rak′noid) [*pia* + *arachnoid*] the pia mater and the arachnoid considered together as one functional unit; the leptomeninges.

**pia-glia** (pi″ə-gli′ə) a membrane formed by the fusion of the pia mater and the membrana limitans; it constitutes one of the layers of the pia-arachnoid.

**pia-in·ti·ma** (pi′ə in′tĭ-mə) [*pia* + *intima*] pia-glia.

**pi·al** (pi′əl, pe′əl) pertaining to the pia mater.

**pia ma·ter** (pi′ə ma′tər, pe′ə mah′tər) [L. "tender mother"] [TA] [MeSH: Pia Mater] the innermost of the three membranes (meninges) covering the brain and spinal cord, investing them closely and extending into the depths of the fissures and sulci; it consists of reticular, elastic, and collagenous fibers.
**p. m. crania′lis** [TA], the pia mater covering the brain, very thin over the cerebral cortex, and thicker over the brain stem; the blood vessels for the brain ramify within it and, as they enter the brain, are accompanied for a short distance by a pial sheath. Called also *p. m. encephali* [TA alternative].
**p. m. ence′phali,** TA alternative for *p. m. cranialis.*
**p. m. spina′lis** [TA], the pia mater covering the spinal cord and consisting of collagenous fibers, which also form the denticulate ligament, and reticular fibers, which closely invest the cord, form the various septa, and form an investment for the rootlets.

**pi·an** (pe-ahn′) [Fr.] yaws.
**p. bois,** a form of New World cutaneous leishmaniasis occurring in the forests of the Guianas and northern Brazil, caused by *Leishmania viannia guyanensis,* transmitted chiefly by *Lutzomyia umbratilis,* and characterized by the presence of multiple, widespread, deep skin ulcers with nodular lymphatic metastases. Called also *forest yaws.*
**hemorrhagic p.,** verruga peruana.

**pi·ar·ach·ni·tis** (pi″ar″ak-ni′tis) leptomeningitis.

**pi·arach·noid** (pi″ə-rak′noid) pia-arachnoid.

**pi·as·tri·ne·mia** (pi-as″trĭ-ne′me-ə) [It. *piastre* coin + *hem-* + *-ia*] thrombocythemia.

**pi·blok·to** (pĭ-blok′to) [Eskimo] a culture-specific syndrome seen chiefly among Eskimo women, marked by sudden, short-lived attacks of screaming, crying, running naked through the snow, and other dangerous or irrational acts, sometimes with suicidal or homicidal tendencies, often followed by convulsive seizures and coma.

**pi·ca** (pi′kə) [L. "magpie" (because this bird eats or carries away odd objects)] [MeSH: Pica] compulsive eating of nonnutritive substances, such as ice (pagophagia), dirt (geophagia), gravel, flaking paint or plaster, clay, hair (trichophagia), or laundry starch (amylophagia). Pica and unusual food cravings (citta) are sometimes seen in pregnant women. Pica also occurs in some patients with iron or zinc deficiencies. In children this syndrome, classified with the eating disorders in DSM-IV, is a rare mental disorder with onset typically in the second year of life; it usually remits in childhood but may persist into adolescence.

**Pichia** (pich′e-ə) [MeSH: Pichia] a genus of fungi of the subphylum Ascomycotina, order Endomycetales. It contains the perfect (sexual) stage of a few species of *Candida.*

**Pick's bodies, disease** (piks) [Arnold *Pick,* Czechoslovakian psychiatrist, 1851–1924] see under *body* and *disease* (def. 1).

**Pick's cells, disease** (piks) [Ludwig *Pick,* German physician, 1868–1935] see under *cell,* and *Niemann-Pick disease,* under *disease.*

**pick** (pik) any pointed or other sharp device for removing objects from areas that are difficult to access.
**apical p.,** see under *elevator.*
**crane p.,** an elevator for the removal of root fragments of mandibular molar teeth fractured during extraction.
**root p.,** apical elevator.

**pick·ling** (pik′ling) the process of cleansing newly cast metallic surfaces and removal of oxides and other impurities from metal objects by immersion in an acid solution.

**pick·wick·i·an syndrome** (pik-wik′e-ən) [from the description of Joe, the fat boy in Dickens' *Pickwick Papers*] [MeSH: Pickwickian Syndrome] see under *syndrome.*

**pico-** [from It. *piccolo* small] a combining form used in naming units of measurement to indicate one-trillionth ($10^{-12}$) of the unit designated by the root with which it is combined. Symbol p.

**pi·co·cu·rie** (pi″ko-ku′re) a unit of radioactivity, being one-trillionth ($10^{-12}$) curie, or the quantity of radioactive material in which the number of nuclear disintegrations is $3.7\times10^{-2}$, or 0.037, per second. Abbreviated pCi. Called also *micromicrocurie.*

**pi·co·gram** (pi′ko-gram) a unit of mass (weight) of the metric system, being $10^{-12}$ gram. Abbreviated pg. Called also *microgamma* and *micromicrogram.*

**pi·co·pi·co·gram** (pi″ko-pi′ko-gram) a unit of mass (weight) of the metric system, being $10^{-12}$ picogram, or $10^{-24}$ gram. Abbreviated ppg.

**Pi·cor·na·vi·ri·dae** (pĭ-kor″nə-vir′ĭ-de) [MeSH: Picornaviridae] the picornaviruses: a family of RNA viruses having a nonenveloped icosahedral virion 22–30 nm in diameter without surface features. The genome consists of a single molecule of positive-sense single-stranded RNA (MW approximately $2.5 \times 10^6$, size 7.2–8.5 kb). Viruses contain four major polypeptides and are resistant to lipid solvents but sensitive to ultraviolet radiation. Replication and assembly occur in the cytoplasm; virions are released by cell destruction. Host range is narrow and transmission is chiefly mechanical. There are five genera: *Aphthovirus, Cardiovirus, Enterovirus, Hepatovirus,* and *Rhinovirus.*

**pi·cor·na·vi·rus** (pi-kor′nə-vi″rəs) [*pico-* + *r*ibo*n*ucleic *a*cid + *virus*] [MeSH: Picornaviridae] any virus belonging to the family Picornaviridae.

**pi·co·unit** (pi″ko-u′nit) one trillionth part of a unit ($10^{-12}$).

**Pi·cras·ma** (pi-kraz′mə) a genus of tropical trees of the family Simaroubaceae. *P. excel′sa* (Sw.) Planch. is the bitterwood or Jamaica quassia, source of the medicine quassia.

**pic·rate** (pik′rāt) any salt of picric acid.

**pic·ric ac·id** (pik′rik) trinitrophenol.

**picr(o)-** [Gr. *pikros* bitter] 1. a combining form meaning bitter. 2. denoting relationship to picric acid.

**pic·ro·car·mine** (pik″ro-kahr′min) a stain prepared from picric acid and carmine and used in microscopy. It consists of a mixture of carmine, ammonia, and distilled water, to which is added an aqueous solution of picric acid.

**pic·ro·geu·sia** (pik″ro-goo′zhə) [*picro-* + Gr. *geusis* taste + *-ia*] a pathologic bitter taste.

**pic·rol** (pik′rol) a colorless and odorless, bitter, antiseptic powder which contains about 53 per cent iodine; used as a substitute for iodoform and corrosive sublimate.

**pic·ro·ni·gro·sin** (pik″ro-ni-gro′sin) a solution of picric acid and nigrosin in alcohol, used as a stain.

**pic·ro·podo·phyl·lin** (pik″ro-pod″o-fil′in) a crystalline isomer of podophyllotoxin from *Podophyllum peltatum* L. (Berberidaceae); it is also obtainable from podophyllotoxin.

**Pic·ror·rhi·za** (pik″ro-ri′zə) [*picro-* + Gr. *rhiza* root] a genus of herbs of the family Scrophulariaceae, native to the Himalayas; the rhizome of *P. kurro′a* Royle is tonic and antiperiodic.

**pic·ro·sac·cha·rom·e·ter** (pik″ro-sak″ə-rom′ə-tər) an instrument used in estimating diabetic sugar.

**pic·ro·scle·ro·tine** (pik″ro-skle′ro-tin) a poisonous alkaloid occurring in ergot of rye.

**pic·ro·tox·in** (pik″ro-tok′sin) [MeSH: Picrotoxin] an active principle obtained from the seed (cocculus indicus) of *Anamirta cocculus;* it stimulates all portions of the central nervous system by blocking presynaptic inhibition of neural impulses and can cause convulsions. It has been used medicinally as an antidote in the treatment of poisoning by central nervous system depressant drugs, especially the barbiturates, administered intravenously.

**pic·ro·tox·in·ism** (pik″ro-tok′zin-iz-əm) poisoning by picrotoxin, with hyperactivity of the central nervous system and convulsions.

**PID** pelvic inflammatory disease.

**PIE** pulmonary interstitial emphysema.

**pie·bald** (pi'bawld) exhibiting piebaldism.

**pie·bald·ism** (pi'bawld-iz-əm) [MeSH: Piebaldism] a congenital autosomal dominant pigmentary disorder of the skin due to absence of functioning melanocytes and melanin, resulting in patchy areas of depigmentation or hypopigmentation, often occurring in association with white forelock. Called also *albinismus circumscriptus* and *localized* or *partial albinism.* Cf. *leukoderma* and *vitiligo.*

**piece** (pēs) a part or portion.
**chief p.,** principal p.
**connecting p.,** 1. middle p. 2. the neck of a spermatozoon.
**end p.,** the terminal portion of the tail, or flagellum, of a spermatozoon; called also *terminal filament.* See illustration under *spermatozoon.*
**middle p.,** the portion of the tail of a spermatozoon limited by the anterior centriole and by the anulus; called also *connecting p.* See also illustration under *spermatozoon.*
**principal p.,** the main portion of the tail of a spermatozoon, beginning at the anulus and gradually tapering toward the end piece; called also *chief p.* See illustration under *spermatozoon.*
**secretory p.,** see under *component.*

**pi·e·dra** (pya'drə) [Sp.] [MeSH: Piedra] a fungal infection of the hair shaft characterized by the presence of dark or pale, firm, irregular nodules composed of fungal elements.
**black p.,** piedra caused by *Piedraia hortae,* characterized by small black or brown gritty nodules on the shafts of the scalp hair; usually seen in tropical regions.
**white p.,** piedra caused by *Trichosporon beigelii,* characterized by white to light brown nodules on the hair of the beard, axilla, or groin, softer than the nodules of the black variety; usually seen in tropical regions. Called also *trichosporosis.*

**Pi·e·draia** (pi"ə-dri'ə) a genus of fungi of the family Piedraiaceae. *P. hor'tae* is parasitic on hair, causing black piedra.

**Pi·e·drai·a·ceae** (pi"ə-dri-a'se-e) a family of fungi of the order Dothideales, including the genus *Piedraia.*

**pier** (pēr) intermediate abutment.

**Pi·erre Ro·bin syndrome** (pyār-ro-bă') [*Pierre Robin,* French dentist, 1867–1950] [MeSH: Pierre Robin Syndrome] see under *syndrome.*

**Pier·sol's point** (pēr'solz) [George Arthur *Piersol,* American anatomist, 1856–1924] see under *point.*

**pi·eses·the·sia** (pi-e"zes-the'zhə) [Gr. *piesis* pressure + *esthesia*] pressure sense.

**pi·esim·e·ter** (pi"ə-sim'ə-tər) [Gr. *piesis* pressure + *-meter*] an instrument for testing the sensitiveness of the skin to pressure.
**Hales' p.,** a glass tube inserted into an artery for the purpose of ascertaining the blood pressure by the height to which the blood rises in the tube.

**-piesis** [Gr. *piesis* a pressing or squeezing] a word termination meaning pressure, as in otopiesis.

**pi·ezal·lo·chro·my** (pi"ə-zal'ə-kro-me) [*piez-* + *allochromy*] change of color of a substance caused by crushing.

**pi·ezes·the·sia** (pi"ə-zes-the'zhə) [*piez-* + *esthesia*] pressure sense.

**piez(o)-** [Gr. *piezein* to press] a combining form denoting relationship to pressure.

**pi·ezo·chem·is·try** (pi-e'zo-kem"is-tre) [*piezo-* + *chemistry*] that branch of chemistry which deals with the effect of pressure on chemical phenomena.

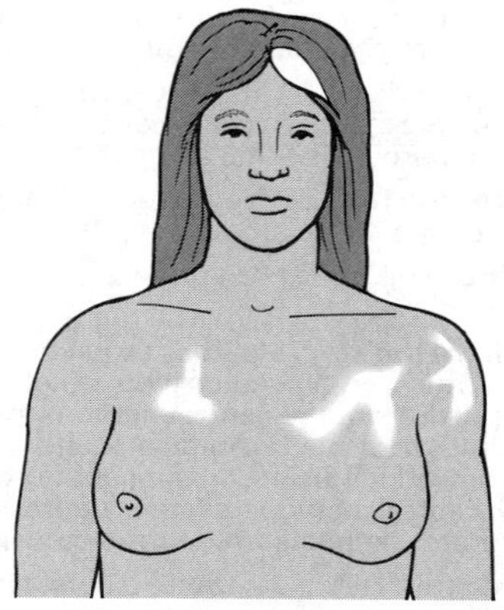

Hypopigmented epidermal patches and white forelock characteristic of piebaldism.

**pi·ezo·elec·tric** (pi-e"zo-e-lek'trik) pertaining to or characterized by piezoelectricity.

**pi·ezo·elec·tri·ci·ty** (pi-e"zo-e-lek-tris'ĭ-te) [*piezo-* + *electricity*] electrical current generated by mechanical stress in quartz and certain other crystals; analogously, the converse property of expansion or contraction of these materials in response to an applied electric field.

**pi·ezom·e·ter** (pi"ə-zom'ə-tər) [*piezo-* + *-meter*] 1. piesimeter. 2. orbitonometer.

**PIF** prolactin-inhibiting factor.

**pig** (pig) [MeSH: Swine] a domesticated form of *Sus scrofa,* a farm animal with cloven hoofs that is raised for its meat.
**dancing p., shaker p.,** a pig suffering from congenital tremor syndrome.

**pig·eon·pox** (pij'ən-poks) a type of fowlpox seen in pigeons, characterized by pox lesions of the oral mucosa and the eyelids, sometimes resulting in blindness.

**pig·ment** (pig'mənt) [L. *pigmentum* paint] 1. any normal or abnormal coloring matter of the body. 2. a paintlike medicinal preparation to be applied to the skin.
**bile p.,** any one of the coloring matters of the bile; they are bilirubin, biliverdin, bilifuscin, biliprasin, choleprasin, bilihumin, and bilicyanin.
**blood p.,** hematogenous p.
**endogenous p.,** a pigment derived from material normally present in the body.
**exogenous p.,** a pigment inhaled or ingested and deposited in the lungs and other tissues.
**fatty p.,** lipid p.
**hematogenous p.,** any of the pigments derived from hemoglobin, such as hematoidin, hematoporphyrin, hemofuscin, hemosiderin, and methemoglobin.
**hepatogenous p.,** bile pigment formed in the liver.
**lipid p.,** any of various pigments having lipid characteristics, some of which also contain protein or iron, the most important one being lipofuscin. Called also *fatty p.*
**lipochrome p.,** lipochrome.
**malarial p.,** a pigment formed by the malarial parasite from the pigment of the blood and deposited largely in the spleen and liver.
**melanotic p.,** melanin.
**respiratory p's,** substances, such as hemoglobin, myoglobin, or the cytochromes, which take part in the oxidation processes of the animal body.
**retinal p's,** the photopigments in retinal rods and cones that respond to certain colors of light and initiate the process of vision; see also *chlorolabe, cyanolabe, erythrolabe,* and *rhodopsin.* Called also *visual p's.*
**visual p's,** retinal p's.
**wear and tear p's,** lipochromes.

**pig·men·tary** (pig'mən-tar"e) pertaining to or of the nature of a pigment.

**pig·men·ta·tion** (pig"mən-ta'shən) [MeSH: Pigmentation] the deposition of coloring matter; the coloration or discoloration of a part by a pigment.

**pig·ment·ed** (pig'mən-təd) colored by deposit of pigment.

**pig·men·to·gen·e·sis** (pig"mən-to-jen'ə-sis) [*pigment* + *genesis*] the production of pigment.

**pig·men·to·gen·ic** (pig"mən-to-jen'ik) inducing the formation or deposit of pigment.

**pig·men·tol·y·sis** (pig"mən-tol'ĭ-sis) [*pigment* + *-lysis*] destruction of pigment.

**pig·men·to·phage** (pig-men'to-fāj) [*pigment* + *-phage*] any pigment-devouring cell, especially such a cell of the hair; called also *chromophage.*

**pig·men·to·phore** (pig-men'to-for") [*pigment* + *-phore*] chromatophore.

**pi·itis** (pi-i'tis) inflammation of the pia mater.

**pik·ro·my·cin** (pik-ro-mi'sin) proactinomycin A.

**Pil.** abbreviation of L. *pilula,* pill, or *pil'ulae,* pills.

**Pi·la** (pi'lə) a genus of freshwater snails of the family Pilidae. *P. co 'nica* is the second intermediate host of the fluke *Echinostoma ilocanum* in the Philippines.

**pi·la** (pi'lə) pl. *pi'lae* [L.] a pillar or pillarlike structure, such as a trabecula of spongy bone.

**pi·lae** (pi'le) [L.] genitive and plural of *pila.*

**pi·lar, pil·a·ry** (pi'lər, pil'ə-re) [L. *pilaris*] pertaining to the hair.

**pi·las·ter** (pi-las′tər) ridge.
**p. of Broca,** linea aspera.

**Pil·cher bag** (pil′chər) [Lewis Stephen *Pilcher,* American surgeon, 1845–1934] see under *bag.*

**pile** (pīl) 1. [L. *pila* pillar] an aggregation of similar elements for generating electricity. 2. [L. *pila* a ball] a hemorrhoid.
**muscular p.,** layers of muscular tissue so arranged as to generate an electric current.
**prostatic p.,** enlarged prostate attended by hemorrhage.
**sentinel p.,** a hemorrhoid-like thickening of the mucous membrane at the lower end of a fissure of the anus.
**thermoelectric p.,** a set of slender metallic bars which, on exposure to heat, generates a current of electricity that moves an index and is made to register delicate changes of temperature.
**voltaic p.,** a battery for current electricity made up of a series of metallic disks.

**piles** (pīlz) hemorrhoids.

**pi·le·us** (pi′le-əs) [L. "a close-fitting felt cap"] caul.

**pi·li** (pi′li) [L.] genitive and plural of *pilus.*

**pi·li·al** (pi′le-əl) pertaining to a pilus or pili.

**pi·li·ate** (pi′le-at) having pili; said of bacteria.

**Pil·i·dae** (pil′ĭ-de) a family of fresh water snails of the order Mesogastropoda; it includes the genus *Pila.*

**pi·li·form** (pi′lĭ-form) shaped like or resembling hair.

**pi·li·mic·tio** (pi″lĭ-mik′she-o) pilimiction.

**pi·li·mic·tion** (pi″lĭ-mik′shən) [*pili* + *miction*] passing of urine containing hair or hairlike threads of mucus.

**pi·lin** (pi′lin) the protein that composes bacterial pili.

**pill** (pil) [L. *pilula*] a small globular or oval medicated mass to be swallowed. Pills contain, in addition to the active drug, a diluent (or filler) and an excipient to give the mass adhesiveness, firmness, and plasticity, so that the pill can be worked by hand or machine to the desired pillular form. Cf. *tablet.*
**chalybeate p's,** ferrous carbonate p's.
**enteric p.,** one coated with a substance, such as salol, which will not dissolve in the stomach.
**ferrous carbonate p's,** pills containing ferrous sulfate, potassium carbonate, sucrose, tragacanth, althea, glycerin, water; used as a hematinic.
**ferruginous p's,** ferrous carbonate p's.
**radio p.,** telemetering capsule.

**pil·lar** (pil′ər) [L. *pila*] a supporting column, usually occurring in pairs.
**anterior p. of fauces,** arcus palatoglossus.
**anterior p. of fornix,** columna fornicis.
**articular p's,** column-like structures formed by the articulation of the superior and inferior articular processes of the vertebrae; see *processus articularis inferior vertebrarum* and *processus articularis superior vertebrarum.*
**p's of Corti's organ,** pillar cells.
**p's of diaphragm,** see *pars lumbalis diaphragmatis.*
**posterior p. of fauces,** arcus palatopharyngeus.
**posterior p. of fornix,** crus fornicis.
**p's of soft palate,** see *arcus palatoglossus* and *arcus palatopharyngeus.*
**Uskow's p's,** two folds of the embryo attached to the dorsolateral portion of the body wall; from these pillars and the septum transversum the diaphragm is formed.

**pil·let** (pil′ət) 1. pilule. 2. pellet.

**pil·lion** (pil′yən) a temporary replacement for an amputated leg.

**pil·low** (pil′o) a case or bag stuffed with soft material.
**Frejka p.,** a therapeutic device consisting of a pillow held wedged

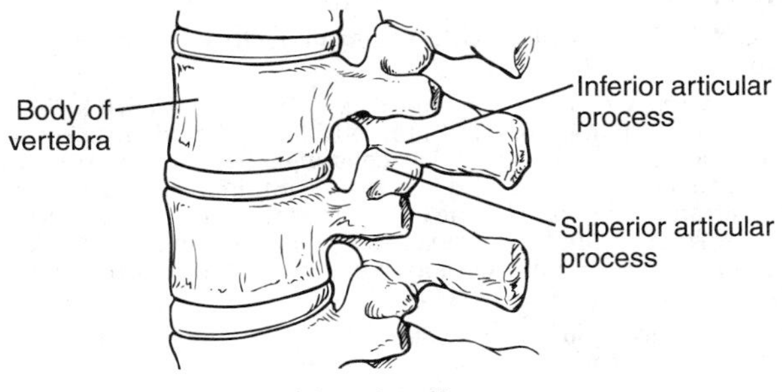

Articular pillar.

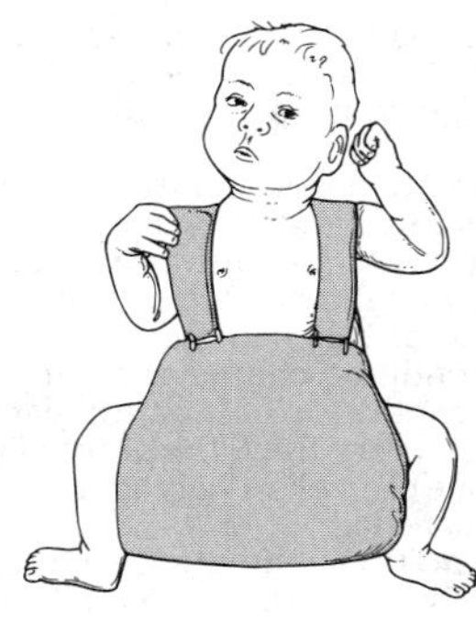
Frejka pillow.

between the thighs of an infant; it corrects congenital hip dislocation by maintaining the femurs in abduction and flexion; called also *Frejka pillow splint.*

**pill-roll·ing** (pil-rōl′ing) see under *tremor.*

**pil(o)-** [L. *pilus* hair] a combining form denoting relationship to hair, or resembling or composed of hair.

**pi·lo·be·zoar** (pi″lo-be′zor) trichobezoar.

**pi·lo·car·pine** (pi″lo-kahr′pēn) [USP] [MeSH: Pilocarpine] a cholinomimetic alkaloid obtained from leaves of plants of the genus *Pilocarpus,* having predominantly muscarinic effects. When applied to the eye, it produces miosis and a transient rise and persistent fall in intraocular pressure. Used in the treatment of glaucoma, and administered by iontophoresis to produce sweating in the sweat chloride test for cystic fibrosis.
**p. hydrochloride** [USP], the monohydrochloride salt of pilocarpine, with the same properties as the alkaloid.
**p. nitrate** [USP], the nitrate salt of pilocarpine, having the same actions and uses as the alkaloid.

**Pi·lo·car·pus** (pi″lo-kahr′pəs) [Gr. *pilos* wool or hair wrought into felt + *karpos* fruit] a genus of shrubs of the family Rutaceae, native to tropical regions of the Americas; *P. jaboran′di* and *P. microphyl′lus* have leaves that yield pilocarpine.

**pi·lo·cys·tic** (pi″lo-sis′tik) [*pilo-* + *cystic*] hollow, or cystlike, and containing hairs; said of certain dermoid tumors.

**pi·lo·cyt·ic** (pi″lo-sit′ik) composed of fiber-shaped cells.

**pi·lo·erec·tion** (pi″lo-e-rek′shən) [*pilo-* + *erection*] [MeSH: Piloerection] erection of the hair.

**pi·lo·leio·myo·ma** (pi″lo-li″o-mi-o′mə) [*pilo-* + *leiomyoma*] cutaneous leiomyoma, single or multiple, arising from the arrectores pilorum muscles.

**pi·lo·ma·tri·co·ma** (pi″lo-ma″trĭ-ko′mə) [*pilo-* + *matrix* + *-oma*] a solitary benign calcifying tumor of hair follicle origin manifested as a sharply circumscribed, firm intracutaneous nodule, usually occurring on the face, neck, or upper extremity, and most often presenting before the age of 20. Histological features include a fibrous stroma surrounding nests of basophilic cells and ghost, or shadow, cells. Called also *benign calcifying* or *calcified epithelioma, calcifying epithelioma of Malherbe,* and *Malherbe's calcifying epithelioma.*

**pi·lo·ma·trix·o·ma** (pi″lo-ma″trik-so′mə) [MeSH: Pilomatrixoma] older name for *pilomatricoma.*

**pi·lo·mo·tor** (pi″lo-mo′tər) [*pilo-* + *motor*] pertaining to the arrector muscles, the contraction of which produces cutis anserina (goose flesh) and the erection of the hairs.

**pi·lo·ni·dal** (pi″lo-ni′dəl) [*pilo-* + L. *nidus* nest] pertaining to, characterized by, or having a nidus or tuft of hairs.

**pi·lose** (pi′lōs) [L. *pilosus*] hairy; covered with hair.

**pi·lo·se·ba·ceous** (pi″lo-sə-ba′shəs) pertaining to the hair follicles and sebaceous glands.

**Piltz's reflex, sign** (pilts′əz) [Jan *Piltz,* Polish neurologist, 1870–1931] see *attention reflex of pupil* and *orbicularis pupillary reflex,* under *reflex.*

**Piltz-West·phal phenomenon** (pilts-vest′fahl) [Jan *Piltz;* Alexander Karl Otto *Westphal,* German neurologist, 1863–1941] orbicularis pupillary reflex.

**pi·lu·la** (pĭ′lu-lə) pl. *pi′lulae* [L.] pill.

**pil·u·lar** (pil′u-lər) resembling or pertaining to a pill.

**pil·ule** (pil′ūl) [L. *pilula*] 1. a small pill. 2. pellet.

**pi·lus** (pi′ləs) gen. and pl. *pi′li* [L.] 1. [TA] hair. 2. [pl.] in micro-

biology, the minute filamentous appendages of certain bacteria; they are considerably smaller and less rigid than flagella and are associated with antigenic properties and sex functions of the cell; called also *fimbria.*
**pi'li annula'ti,** a condition in which the individual hairs appear to be marked by alternating bands of white as a result of some barrier in the hair which prevents passage of light and causes the rays to be reflected back, giving the appearance of white bands.
**pi'li canali'culi,** uncombable hair syndrome.
**pi'li cunicula'ti,** a condition characterized by burrowing hairs.
**F p.,** in bacterial genetics, a hollow tubular pilus possessed by (male) $F^+$ cells, which carry the F (fertility) plasmid. It forms a connection with a (female) $F^-$ cell in bacterial conjugation to allow the transfer of genetic material.
**pi'li incarna'ti,** a condition characterized by ingrown hairs.
**pi'li incarna'ti recur'vi,** a condition characterized by ingrown hairs that have repenetrated the skin after growing from the hair follicles.
**pi'li multige'mini,** multiple hairs growing from the same follicle, as a result of deep division of its base, producing, in effect, a cluster of separate papillae.
**pi'li tor'ti,** a condition characterized by twisted hair.
**pi'li trian'guli et canali'culi,** uncombable hair syndrome.

**Pima** (pim'ə) trademark for a preparation of potassium iodide.

**pim·e·li·tis** (pim″ə-li'tis) [*pimel-* + *-itis*] inflammation of the adipose tissue.

**pimel(o)-** [Gr. *pimelē* lard] a combining form denoting relationship to fat.

**pim·e·lo·ma** (pim″ə-lo'mə) [*pimel-* + *-oma*] lipoma.

**pim·e·lop·ter·yg·i·um** (pim″ə-lo-tər-ij'e-əm) [*pimel-* + *pterygium*] a fatty outgrowth upon the conjunctiva.

**pim·el·or·thop·nea** (pim″əl-or″thop-ne'ə) [*pimel-* + *orthopnea*] dyspnea while lying down, due to obesity. Called also *piorthopnea.*

**pim·e·lo·sis** (pim″ə-lo'sis) [*pimel-* + *-osis*] 1. conversion into fat. 2. obesity.

**pim·el·uria** (pim″ə-lu're-ə) [*pimel-* + *-uria*] lipuria.

**pi·min·o·dine es·y·late** (pĭ-min'o-dēn) a synthetic narcotic analgesic administered orally, intramuscularly, and subcutaneously.

**pi·mo·zide** (pi'mə-zīd) [MeSH: Pimozide] an antipsychotic agent, a diphenylbutylpiperidine, used in the treatment of Gilles de la Tourette's syndrome.

**Pim·pi·nel·la** (pim″pĭ-nel'ə) [L.] a genus of plants of the family Umbelliferae. *P. ani'sum* L. is anise, the source of anise oil. *P. saxifra'ga* L. is the Burnet saxifrage, whose root is tonic, diuretic, emmenagogue, and carminative.

**pim·ple** (pim'pəl) a papule or pustule, usually of the face, neck, or upper trunk, most often due to acne vulgaris.

**pin** (pin) 1. a long slender metal rod for the fixation of the ends of fractured bones. 2. a peg or dowel by means of which an artificial crown is fixed to the root of a tooth.
**friction-locked p., friction-retained p.,** a metal pin slightly larger than a hole drilled into dentin, forced into the hole and retained in place solely by friction.
**Steinmann p.,** a metal rod for the internal fixation of fractures.

**Pi·na·ceae** (pi-na'se-e) a large family of evergreen trees and shrubs that have cones and either needles or leaves. It includes the genera *Abies, Pinus,* and *Tsuga.*

**pin·a·cy·a·nole** (pin″ə-si'ə-nōl) an aniline dye used as a tissue stain and for sensitizing photographic plates for red.

**Pi·nard's maneuver** (pe-nahrz') [Adolphe *Pinard,* French obstetrician, 1844–1934] see under *maneuver.*

**pince-ci·seaux** (pans″se-zo') [Fr. "forceps-scissors"] a cutting forceps used in iridotomy.

**pin·cers** (pin'sərz) 1. forceps (def. 1). 2. the median deciduous incisors of the horse; called also *nippers.*

**pinch** (pinch) 1. to press an object tightly between the thumb and one finger. 2. an act of pinching; used as means of assessing hand dexterity. See also *grip.*
**key p.,** lateral p.
**lateral p.,** the act of pinching an object between the tip of the thumb and the radial side of the forefinger, as when turning a key.
**pulp p.,** the act of pinching an object between the terminal pulp of the thumb and that of one finger.
**tip p., tip to tip p.,** pulp p.

**Pind·borg tumor** (pind'borg) [Jens J. *Pindborg,* Danish oral pathologist, born 1921] see *calcifying epithelial odontogenic tumor,* under *tumor.*

**pin·do·lol** (pin'də-lol) [USP] [MeSH: Pindolol] a beta-adrenergic blocking agent with intrinsic sympathomimetic activity; its uses are similar to those of propranolol.

**pin·done** (pin'dōn) an indanedione anticoagulant used as a rodenticide; it can cause fatal anticoagulant rodenticide poisoning (q.v.) in many mammalian species.

**pine**[1] (pīn) [L. *pinus*] 1. any tree of the genus *Pinus.* 2. any of numerous other coniferous trees.
**longleaf p.,** *Pinus palustris.*
**southern p.,** *Pinus palustris.*
**Swiss mountain p.,** *Pinus mugo.*
**white p.,** 1. *Pinus strobus.* 2. the dried inner bark of *P. strobus,* used as an ingredient in compound white pine syrup.

**pine**[2] (pīn) pining.

**pin·e·al** (pin'e-əl) [L. *pinealis; pinea* pine cone] 1. pertaining to the pineal body. 2. shaped like a pine cone.

**pin·e·al·ec·to·my** (pin″e-əl-ek'tə-me) [*pineal* body + *-ectomy*] excision of the pineal body.

**pin·e·al·ism** (pin'e-əl-iz″əm) any condition due to presumed abnormalities of pineal gland secretion; see also *hyperpinealism* and *hypopinealism.*

**pin·e·a·lo·blas·to·ma** (pin″e-ə-lo-blas-to'mə) a type of neuroepithelial tumor that is a pinealoma in which the pineal cells are not well differentiated. Called also *pineoblastoma.*

**pin·e·a·lo·cyte** (pin'e-ə-lo-sīt″) the principal cell of the pineal body, an epithelioid cell with pale-staining cytoplasm, prominent nucleoli, and large nuclei that may be irregularly infolded or lobulated; cords of these cells make up the body of the pineal body. See also *interstitial cells,* under *cell.* Called also *chief cell* and *pineal cell.*

**pin·e·a·lo·cy·to·ma** (pin″e-ə-lo-si-to'mə) pinealoma.

**pin·e·a·lo·ma** (pin″e-ə-lo'mə) [MeSH: Pinealoma] an uncommon tumor of the pineal body composed of neoplastic nests of large epithelial cells; symptoms include hydrocephalus, conjugate paralysis of upward gaze, disturbances of gait, and precocious puberty, the last possibly due to the suppression of pineal secretion of melatonin. Called also *pinealocytoma* and *pineocytoma.*
**ectopic p.,** pinealoma arising from pineal rests in the midline area, resulting in diabetes insipidus, compression of the optic chiasm, and hypopituitarism.

**pin·e·a·lop·a·thy** (pin″e-ə-lop'ə-the) any disease of the pineal gland.

**pi·nene** (pi'nēn) a terpene found in turpentine and many essential oils; used as a solvent and in the manufacture of camphor, insecticides, and synthetic pine oil.

**pin·eo·blas·to·ma** (pin″e-o-blas-to'mə) pinealoblastoma.

**pin·eo·cy·to·ma** (pin″e-o-si-to'mə) pinealoma.

**pin·gue·cu·la** (ping-gwĕ'ku-lə) gen. and pl. *pingue'culae* [L. "somewhat fatty"] a yellowish spot of proliferation on the bulbar conjunctiva near the sclerocorneal junction, usually on the nasal side; seen in elderly people.

**pin·gui·cu·la** (ping-gwĭ'ku-lə) pinguecula.

**pin·i·form** (pin'ĭ-form) [L. *pinea* pine cone + *form*] conical or cone-shaped.

**pin·ing** (pīn'ing) enzootic marasmus in Scotland due to cobalt deficiency; called also *pine.*

**pink·eye** (pink'i) 1. acute contagious conjunctivitis. 2. infectious keratoconjunctivitis.

**pin·ledge** (pin'lej) a flat floor or shoulder prepared within the tooth structure, into which pin holes are drilled to accommodate pins in a pin-retained cast restoration.

**pin·na** (pin'ə) [L. "wing"] auricula (def. 1).

**pin·nal** (pin'əl) pertaining to the auricle of the ear; see *auricular.*

**pino·cyte** (pin'o-, pi'no-sīt) a cell that exhibits pinocytosis.

**pino·cyt·ic** (pin″o-, pi″no-sit'ik) pertaining to a pinocyte or to pinocytosis.

**pino·cy·to·sis** (pin″o-, pi″no-si-to'sis) [Gr. *pinein* to drink + *cyto-* + *-osis*] [MeSH: Pinocytosis] the imbibition of liquids by cells, especially the mechanism by which cells ingest extracellular fluid and its contents; it involves the formation of minute incuppings or invaginations (caveolae) by the cell membrane, which close and pinch off to form free, fluid-filled vesicles *(pinosomes)* in the cytoplasm. It is thought to be a method of active transport across the cell membrane.

**pino·cy·tot·ic** (pin″o-, pi″no-si-tot'ik) pertaining to or characterized by pinocytosis.

**pino·some** (pin'o-, pi'no-sōm) [Gr. *pinein* to drink + *-some*] any of

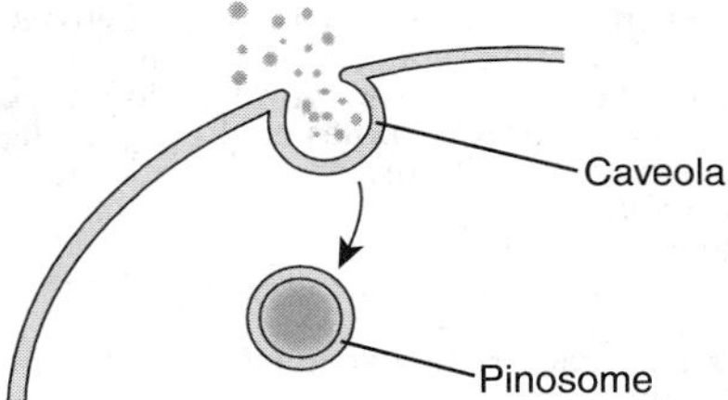


Pinocytosis of small fluid droplets.

the small fluid-filled vesicles found in the cytoplasm during pinocytosis, formed by invaginations of the cell membrane (caveolae) which pinch off and become free. Called also *pinocytotic vesicle.*

**Pi·no·yel·la** (pi″no-yel′ə) former name for *Trichophyton.*

**Pins' sign** (pins) [Emil *Pins,* Austrian physician, 1845–1913] Ewart's sign.

**pint** (pīnt) a measure of capacity (liquid measure), being 16 fluid ounces, or the equivalent of 473.17 milliliters; symbol O (L. *octarius*), or abbreviated pt. The imperial pint is equal to 20 fluid ounces.

**pin·ta** (pēn′tah) [Sp. "painted"] [MeSH: Pinta] a form of treponematosis, being a chronic dyschromic dermatosis endemic in certain parts of tropical America and characterized by the presence on the skin of spots, which may be white, coffee-colored, blue, red, or violet. It is caused by *Treponema carateum* (the Wassermann reaction is usually positive), and is believed to be transmitted usually by direct person-to-person contact.

**pin·tid** (pin′tid) one of the flat erythematous skin lesions constituting the spreading eruption occurring in the second stage of pinta.

**Pi·nus** (pi′nus) the pines, a large genus of coniferous evergreen trees of the family Pinaceae. *P. mu′go* is the Swiss mountain pine; it and its dwarf variant, *P. mu′go* var. *pumi′lio* are sources of pine needle or dwarf pine needle oil (see under *oil*). *P. palus′tris* Mill. is the longleaf or southern pine of the southern United States, a source of pine oil, rosin, turpentine, and other products. *P. stro′bus* L. is the white pine of eastern North America, source of white pine flavoring (see under *syrup*).

**pi·nus** (pi′nəs) [L.] glandula pinealis.

**pin·worm** (pin′werm) oxyurid.

**pi(o)-** [Gr. *piōn* fat] a combining form denoting relationship to fat. See also words beginning *lip(o)-.*

**pio·epi·the·li·um** (pi″o-ep″ĭ-the′le-əm) [*pio-* + *epithelium*] epithelium in which fatty matter is deposited.

**pi·on** (pi′on) [*pi* *meson*] [MeSH: Mesons] a subatomic particle, which may be positive, negative, or neutral, with mass intermediate between that of an electron and that of a proton; it carries the force that binds the atomic nucleus together. It is an example of a meson.

**Pi·oph·i·la** (pi-of′ĭ-lə) a genus of flies. *P. ca′sei* is a fly whose larva is the cheese skipper, a common cause of intestinal myiasis.

**pi·or·thop·nea** (pi″or-thop′ne-ə, pi″or-thop-ne′ə) [*pio-* + *orthopnea*] pimelorthopnea.

**Pi·o·trow·ski's sign (reflex)** (pe″o-trov′skēz) [Alexander *Piotrowski,* German neurologist, born 1878] see under *sign.*

**PIP** phosphatidylinositol 4-phosphate.

**PIP$_2$** phosphatidylinositol 4,5-bisphosphate.

**pi·pam·pe·rone** (pĭ-pam′pə-rōn) a tranquilizer that has been used in the treatment of schizophrenia.

**Pip·a·nol** (pip′ə-nol) trademark for a preparation of trihexyphenidyl hydrochloride.

**pip·az·e·thate hy·dro·chlo·ride** (pĭ-paz′ə-thāt) a nonnarcotic antitussive; administered orally.

**pip·ecol·ic ac·id** (pip″ə-kol′ik) a cyclic amino acid occurring as an intermediate in a minor pathway of lysine degradation and at elevated levels in blood in cerebrohepatorenal syndrome and in hyperlysinemia.

**pi·pen·zo·late bro·mide** (pi-pen′zo-lāt) a synthetic quaternary nitrogen anticholinergic used mainly for adjunctive therapy in the treatment of peptic ulcer, administered orally.

**Pi·per** (pi′pər) [L. "pepper"] a genus of plants of the family Piperaceae, native to southern Asia, Malaysia, and Indonesia. *P. bet′le* is betel, whose leaf is used in the masticatory also called betel. *P. cube′ba* L. f. is the tailed or Java pepper, whose fruit, the cubeb, is medicinal but can cause cubebism. *P. ni′grum* L. is black pepper (see under *pepper*).

**pi·per·a·cet·a·zine** (pi″pər-ə-set′ə-zēn) an antipsychotic used in the treatment of various forms of schizophrenia in adults, administered orally.

**pi·per·a·cil·lin** (pi-per′ə-sil″in) [USP] [MeSH: Piperacillin] a semisynthetic broad-spectrum penicillin effective against gram-negative bacteria.
**p. sodium** [USP], the sodium salt of piperacillin, used in the treatment of infections caused by susceptible organisms and in intraabdominal surgery for the prevention of infection; administered intramuscularly or intravenously.

**pi·per·az·i·dine** (pi″pər-az′ĭ-dēn) piperazine.

**pi·per·a·zine** (pi′pər-ə-zēn″) [USP] an anthelmintic used in humans and domestic and farm animals against *Ascaris lumbricoides* and *Enterobius vermicularis;* it causes a flaccid paralysis of the worm musculature by altering cell membrane permeability and causing hyperpolarization of the membrane. Called also *diethylenediamine* and *piperizadine.*
**p. citrate** [USP], the citrate salt of piperazine, used for humans and domestic and farm animals in the treatment of intestinal roundworm and pinworm infections; administered orally.
**p. edetate calcium,** a compound prepared by the reaction of edetate with calcium carbonate and piperazine; used like the citrate salt.
**p. phosphate,** the phosphate salt of piperazine, used for humans and domestic and farm animals in the treatment of intestinal roundworm and trematode infections.
**p. tartrate,** the tartrate salt of piperazine, used like the citrate salt.

**pi·per·id·o·late hy·dro·chlo·ride** (pi″pər-id′ə-lāt) a synthetic tertiary anticholinergic occurring as a white or cream-colored powder, having the ability to reduce motility of smooth muscle, especially that of the gastrointestinal tract; used as an antispasmodic in functional gastrointestinal disorders, administered orally.

**pi·per·ine** (pi′pər-ēn) [L. *piperinum*] A crystallizable, slightly soluble aromatic pungent alkaloid from *Piper nigrum,* used as an insecticide.

**pi·per·ism** (pi′pər-iz-əm) [L. *piper* pepper] poisoning by pepper.

**pi·per·o·caine hy·dro·chlo·ride** (pi′pər-o-kān″) a local anesthetic used for topical, infiltration, regional, spinal, and caudal anesthesia.

**pi·per·o·nyl bu·tox·ide** (pi-pər′o-nəl) [MeSH: Piperonyl Butoxide] a synergist used mainly in veterinary medicine in combination with pyrethrins in insecticides and pediculicides.

**pi·per·ox·an hy·dro·chlo·ride** (pi″pər-oks′ən) an alpha-adrenergic blocking agent formerly used in diagnostic tests for pheochromocytoma and to counteract the effects of epinephrine release before and during surgery for removal of pheochromocytoma.

**pi·pet** (pi-pet′) pipette.

**pi·pette** (pi-pet′) [Fr.] 1. a glass or transparent plastic tube used in measuring or transferring small quantities of liquid or gas. 2. to dispense fluid or gas by means of a pipette.

**Pi·pi·zan** (pi′pĭ-zən) trademark for a preparation of piperazine.

**pi·po·bro·man** (pĭ″po-bro′mən) [MeSH: Pipobroman] an antineoplastic alkylating agent used in the treatment of polycythemia vera, administered orally.

**Pip·ra·cil** (pip″rə-sil) trademark for a preparation of piperacillin sodium.

**pi·pra·drol hy·dro·chlo·ride** (pĭ′prə-drol) a central nervous system stimulant used mainly as an antidepressant, administered orally.

**Pip·ta·de·nia** (pip″tə-de′ne-ə) a genus of tropical shrubs and trees of the family Leguminosae. Some species from Brazil yield seeds that are made into the narcotic psychotomimetic snuff called *parica.*

**Pip·to·ceph·a·lis** (pip″to-sef′ə-lis) a genus of fungi of the order Zoopagales; some species contain trichothecenes and can cause alimentary toxic aleukia.

**pi·qûre** (pe-kūr′) [Fr.] puncture, especially Bernard's (diabetic) puncture.

**Pi·ra·caps** (pi′rə-kaps) trademark for a preparation of tetracycline hydrochloride.

**pir·ben·i·cil·lin so·di·um** (pir-ben″ĭ-sil′in) an antibacterial, $C_{24}H_{25}N_6NaO_5S$.

**pir·bu·ter·ol ace·tate** (pir-bu′tər-ol) a beta-adrenergic bronchodilating agent administered by aerosol for inhalation.

**pir·bu·ter·ol hy·dro·chlo·ride** (pir-bu′tər-ol) a sympathomimetic agent specific for beta$_2$ receptors, used as bronchodilator in the prevention and treatment of reversible bronchospasm; administered by inhalation.

**Pi·re·nel·la** (pi″rə-nel′ə) a genus of snails of the family Cerithiidae, order Mesogastropoda. *P. co'nica* is a species found in Egypt that is a host of the intestinal fluke *Heterophyes heterophyes.*

**pir·en·ze·pine hy·dro·chlo·ride** (pir″ən-zĕ′pēn) an antagonist of certain muscarinic receptors that has minimal anticholinergic effects and does not cross the blood-brain barrier, used to inhibit gastric secretion in hyperacidity and peptic ulcer.

**pir·i·form** (pir′ĭ-form) [L. *pirum* a pear + *form*] pear-shaped.

**Pir·o·goff's amputation, angle, triangle** (pīr′o-gofs) [Nikolai Ivanovich *Pirogoff,* Russian surgeon, 1810–1881] see under *amputation,* see *venous angle,* under *angle* and see *hypoglossohyoid triangle,* under *triangle.*

**pi·ro·plasm** (pi′ro-plaz-əm) any protozoan of the subclass Piroplasmia. Called also *piroplasmid.*

**Pi·ro·plas·ma** (pi″ro-plaz′mə) former name for *Babesia.*

**Pi·ro·plas·mia** (pi″ro-plaz-me′ə) [L. *pirum* pear + *plasma*] [MeSH: Piroplasmia] a subclass of heteroxenous parasitic protozoa (class Sporozoea, subphylum Apicomplexa), occurring as piriform, round, or rod-shaped cells or ameboid cells without a conoid, oocysts, spores, pseudocysts, and flagella, and usually without subpellicular microtubules but with a polar ring and rhoptries. Locomotion is accomplished by flexion, by gliding, or, in sexual stages of certain species, by large axopodium-like organelles *(strahlen).* They are parasitic in the erythrocytes and other circulating and fixed cells of the host, with merogony occurring in vertebrates and sporogony in invertebrates, and producing sporozoites with a single-membraned wall. Ticks are the vectors of most of the piroplasmids. It comprises a single order: Piroplasmida.

**pi·ro·plas·mid** (pi″ro-plaz′mid) 1. pertaining or relating to protozoa of the subclass Piroplasmia. 2. piroplasm.

**Pi·ro·plas·mi·da** (pi″ro-plaz′mĭ-də) [MeSH: Piroplasmida] an order of protozoa (subclass Piroplasmia, class Sporozoea) having the characters of the subclass. Representative genera include *Babesia, Cytauxzoon, Dactylosoma,* and *Theileria.*

**pi·ro·plas·mo·sis** (pi″ro-plaz-mo′sis) 1. babesiosis. 2. infection by any species of Piroplasmida.
**tropical p.,** see under *theileriasis.*

**pir·o·xan·trone hy·dro·chlo·ride** (pir″o-zan′trōn) a cytotoxic compound that causes DNA strand breaks and cross-linking; used investigationally in the treatment of carcinoma of the breast.

**pir·ox·i·cam** (pir-ok′sĭ-kam) [MeSH: Piroxicam] a nonsteroidal anti-inflammatory agent of the oxicam family having a long plasma half-life; used for once-a-day treatment of rheumatoid arthritis and osteoarthritis.

**Pir·quet's test (reaction)** (pir-kāz′) [Clemens Freiherr von *Pirquet,* Austrian pediatrician, 1874–1929] see under *test.*

**pis·ci·cide** (pis′ĭ-sīd) any substance poisonous to fish.

**Pis·cid·ia** (pĭ-sid′e-ə) [L. *piscis* fish + *caedere* to kill] a genus of trees of the family Leguminosae. *P. pisci'pula* (L.) Sarg. (formerly called *P. erythri'na* L.) is Jamaica dogwood, whose bark is a mild anodyne.

**pis·ci·din** (pĭ-si′din) a neutral principle from *Piscidia piscipula* (L.) Sarg., an anodyne and antispasmodic.

**pi·si·form** (pi′sĭ-form) [L. *pisum* pea + *form*] resembling a pea in shape and size.

**pi·si·for·mis** (pi″sĭ-for′mis) [L.] pisiform.

**Pis·ka·cek's sign** (pis′kə-cheks″) [Ludwig *Piskacek,* Austrian obstetrician, 1854–1933] see under *sign.*

**Pis·ta·cia** (pis-ta′shə) a genus of shrubs and small trees of the family Anacardiaceae, native to various parts of the Northern Hemisphere. *P. lentis'cus* is the mastic tree, source of mastic.

**pis·til** (pis′til) [L. *pistillus* a pestle] gynecium.

**Pi·sum** (pi′səm) a genus of vines of the family Leguminosae. *P. sati'vum* is the pea.

**PIT** plasma iron turnover.

**pit** (pit) 1. a hollow fovea or indentation. 2. a pockmark. 3. a small depression or fault in the dental enamel, considered as belonging to Class I of Black's classification (see table at *caries*). See also *fissure* (def. 3). 4. to indent, or to become and remain for a short period of time indented by pressure. 5. a small depression in the nail plate seen in psoriasis.
**anal p.,** proctodeum.
**arm p.,** the axilla or axillary fossa.
**auditory p.,** a distinct depression appearing in each auditory placode, marking the beginning of embryonic development of the internal ear. Called also *otic p.* or *depression.*
**basilar p.,** a pit in the crown of an incisor tooth above its neck.
**coated p's,** small pits in the plasma membrane of many cells that are involved in the receptor-mediated endocytosis of low-density lipoprotein (LDL), insulin, and other ligands. The pits are coated with a protein, clathrin, on the cytoplasmic surface and may be taken into the cell to form vacuoles enclosing the ligands.
**costal p.,** fovea costalis inferior.
**ear p.,** preauricular p.
**gastric p's,** foveolae gastricae.
**Gaul's p's,** depressions in the corneal epithelium seen in neuroparalytic keratitis.
**Herbert's p's,** a characteristic defect left after the healing of a limbal follicle in trachoma.
**lens p.,** a pitlike depression in the ectoderm of the lens placode where the primordial lens is developing.
**nasal p.,** olfactory p.
**oblong p. of arytenoid cartilage,** fovea oblonga cartilaginis arytenoideae.
**olfactory p.,** the primordium of a nasal cavity.
**otic p.,** auditory p.
**postanal p.,** foveola coccygea.
**preauricular p.,** a slight depression anterior to the helix and superior to the tragus, sometimes leading to a congenital preauricular cyst or fistula. Called also *ear p.*
**primitive p.,** a depression in the primitive node of the primitive streak at the cranial end of the primitive groove; it may open abnormally into a neurenteric canal.
**pterygoid p.,** see under *fovea.*
**p. of the stomach,** the epigastrium or fossa epigastrica.
**suprameatal p.,** foveola suprameatica.
**triangular p. of arytenoid cartilage,** fovea triangularis cartilaginis arytenoideae.

**pitch** (pich) [L. *pix*] 1. a dark, lustrous, more or less viscous residue from the distillation of tar and other substances. Domestic animals and livestock sometimes eat pitch-containing substances and can die from pitch poisoning (see under *poisoning*). 2. any of various bituminous substances such as natural asphalt. 3. a resin from the sap of some coniferous trees. 4. the quality of sound dependent principally on its frequency.
**Burgundy p.,** an aromatic, oily resin from *Abies* (or *Picea*) *excelsa,* the Norway spruce of Europe, much used in plasters.
**Canada p.,** a resin from *Tsuga canadensis,* the hemlock tree, useful in plasters, etc.

**pitch·blende** (pich′blend) a black mineral containing uranium oxide; from it are obtained radium, polonium, and uranium.

**pith** (pith) 1. to pierce the spinal cord or brain; see *pithing.* 2. the soft tissue found in plant stems that often disappears so that the stem becomes hollow. 3. the central core of colorless parenchymatous cells in stems and some roots.

**pith·e·coid** (pith′ə-koid) [Gr. *pithēkos* ape + *-oid*] apelike.

**pith·ing** (pith′ing) destruction of the brain and spinal cord by thrusting a blunt needle into the spinal canal and cranium; done on animals to destroy sensibility preparatory to experimenting on their living tissues.

**Pith·o·my·ces** (pith″o-mi′sez) a genus of Fungi Imperfecti of the form-family Dematiaceae. *P. charta'rum* contains sporidesmin and causes facial eczema of ruminants.

**pith·o·my·co·tox·i·co·sis** (pith″o-mi″ko-tok″sĭ-ko′sis) a form of mycotoxicosis in animals from ingestion of fungi of the genus *Pithomyces,* resulting in liver damage and facial eczema of ruminants (see under *eczema*).

**Pi·to·cin** (pĭ-to′sin) trademark for preparations of oxytocin.

**Pi·tres' rule, sign** (pe′trə) [Jean Albert *Pitres,* French physician, 1848–1927] see under *rule* and *sign.*

**Pi·tres·sin** (pĭ-tres′in) trademark for vasopressin injection.

**pit·ting** (pit′ing) 1. the formation, usually by scarring, of a small depression. 2. the removal from erythrocytes, by the spleen, of certain structures, such as iron granules, without destruction of the cells. 3. remaining indented for a few minutes after removal of firm pressure; see under *edema.*

**pi·tu·i·cyte** (pĭ-too′ĭ-sīt) [*pitui*tary + *-cyte*] any of the dominant and distinctive fusiform cells of the neurohypophysis, which are intermingled with nerve fibers and are regarded as specialized neuroglial cells. According to their morphological appearance on staining with silver, four subtypes are distinguished: adeno-, fibro-, reticulo-, and micropituicytes.

**pi·tu·i·ta** (pĭ-too′ĭ-tə) [L.] a glutinous mucus.

**pi·tu·i·ta·rism** (pĭ-too′ĭ-tə-riz″əm) disorder of pituitary function; see *hyperpituitarism* and *hypopituitarism.*

**pi·tu·i·tary** (pĭ-too′ĭ-tar″e) [L. *pituita* phlegm] 1. hypophysial. 2. hypophysis. 3. a preparation of some part of the pituitary gland of animals (e.g., cattle, pigs, sheep), used therapeutically.

**anterior p.,** 1. adenohypophysis. 2. a preparation of the dried, partially defatted, powdered adenohypophysis of hogs, sheep, or cattle.
**pharyngeal p.,** see under *hypophysis.*
**posterior p.,** 1. neurohypophysis. 2. a powdered preparation of the dried neurohypophysis of certain food animals, having the pharmacological actions of its hormones, *oxytocin* and *vasopressin;* used mainly as an antidiuretic in the treatment of central diabetes insipidus, administered subcutaneously, by nasal inhalation, or by topical application to the nasal mucosa. It may be used to stimulate smooth muscle tissue, especially to produce vasoconstriction in the presence of hemorrhage.
**whole p.,** a preparation of the dried, partially defatted, powdered whole pituitary gland of certain food animals.

**pi·tu·i·tec·to·my** (pĭ-too″ĭ-tek′tə-me) hypophysectomy.

**pi·tu·i·tous** (pĭ too′ĭ-təs) [L. *pituitosus*] pertaining to mucus or characterized by its secretion.

**Pi·tu·i·trin** (pĭ-too′ĭ-trin) trademark for posterior pituitary injection.

**pit·y·ri·a·sis** (pit″ĭ-ri′ə-sis) [Gr. *pityron* bran + *-iasis*] [MeSH: Pityriasis] any of various skin diseases characterized by the formation of fine, branny scales.
**p. al′ba,** a common skin disorder most often seen in young children and adolescents, usually involving the face, especially the cheeks and the area around the mouth, and characterized by the presence of round or oval, slightly scaling, hypopigmented patches; it usually involutes spontaneously. Called also *erythroderma streptogenes, p. maculata,* and *p. simplex.*
**lichenoid p., acute,** an acute or subacute, sometimes relapsing, widespread macular, papular, or vesicular eruption that tends to crusting, necrosis, and hemorrhage, which heals, leaving pigmented depressed scars, followed by the development of a new crop of lesions. Occasionally, progression to the chronic lichenoid form may occur. Called also *acute parapsoriasis; Habermann's, Mucha-Habermann,* or *Mucha's disease; parapsoriasis varioliformis acuta;* and *p. lichenoides et varioliformis acuta.*
**lichenoid p., chronic,** a chronic brown to red-brown scaly macular eruption, distributed chiefly over the trunk, characterized histologically by epidermal alterations and a perivascular lymphocytic infiltrate. It may represent progression of the acute lichenoid form or arise de novo. Called also *chronic* or *guttate parapsoriasis, parapsoriasis guttata,* and *parapsoriasis varioliformis chronica.*
**p. lichenoi′des acu′ta,** acute lichenoid p.
**p. lichenoi′des chro′nica,** chronic lichenoid p.
**p. lichenoi′des et variolifor′mis acu′ta,** acute lichenoid p.
**p. lin′guae,** benign migratory glossitis.
**p. macula′ta,** p. alba.
**p. ni′gra,** tinea nigra.
**p. ro′sea,** a common acute or subacute, self-limited exanthematous disease of unknown etiology, the onset of which is marked by the presence of a solitary erythematous or salmon- or fawn-colored herald plaque, most often seen on the trunk, arms, or thighs, followed by the development of papular or macular lesions, similar to but smaller than the initial lesion, which have vesicular borders subsequently that tend to peel and produce a scaly collarette.
**p. rotun′da,** a form of acquired ichthyosis manifested by circular or oval, brown, scaly, sharply demarcated patches on the trunk and extremities, which become worse during the winter and improve in the summer.
**p. ru′bra (Hebra),** exfoliative dermatitis.
**p. ru′bra pila′ris,** a chronic inflammatory cutaneous disease characterized by tiny acuminate, reddish brown follicular papules topped by central horny plugs in which are embedded hairs, partial or complete; disseminated yellowish pink scaling patches; and often solid confluent hyperkeratosis of the palms and soles with a tendency to fissuring.
**p. sic′ca,** dandruff, def. 2.
**p. sim′plex,** p. alba.
**p. versi′color,** tinea versicolor.

**pit·y·roid** (pit′ĭ-roid) [Gr. *pityron* bran + *-oid*] furfuraceous; branny.

**Pit·y·ros·po·ron** (pit″ĭ-ros′pə-ron) former name for *Malassezia.*

**Pit·y·ros·po·rum** (pit″ĭ-ros′pə-rəm) [Gr. *pityron* bran + *sporos* seed] former name for *Malassezia. P. orbicula′re* is *M. furfur* and *P. ova′le* is *M. ovalis.*

**piv·a·late** (piv′ə-lāt) USAN contraction for trimethylacetate.

**piv·am·pi·cil·lin hy·dro·chlo·ride** (piv-am″pĭ-sil′in) a derivative of ampicillin, having the same broad spectrum of antibacterial activity and uses as ampicillin. Available as *pentazocine hydrochloride, p. pamoate,* and *p. probenate.*

**piv·ot** (piv′ət) 1. that on which something turns, such as a dowel or short post. 2. the point of rotation for a removable partial denture.
**occlusal p.,** an elevation contrived on the occlusal surface, usually in the molar region, designed to act as a fulcrum and to induce sagittal mandibular rotation.

**pix·el** (pik′sel) [contraction of *pix* (short for *pictures*) + *el*ement] a two-dimensional region defining a unit of area on a video display screen.

**pi·zo·ty·line** (pĭ-zo′tĭ-lēn) [MeSH: Pizotyline] an anabolic, antidepressant, and serotonin inhibitor used in treatment of migraine.

**piz·zle** (piz′əl) popular term used in veterinary medicine for the penis of an animal.

**PJRT** permanent junctional reciprocating tachycardia.

**PJT** paroxysmal junctional tachycardia; see *paroxysmal tachycardia,* under *tachycardia.*

**PK** pyruvate kinase.

**p$K_a$** the negative logarithm of the ionization constant of an acid ($K_a$); the buffering power of a buffer system is greatest when its p$K_a$ equals the pH.

**PKU, PKU1** phenylketonuria.

**pla·ce·bo** (plə-se′bo) [L. "I will please"] any dummy medical treatment; originally, a medicinal preparation having no specific pharmacological activity against the patient's illness or complaint given solely for the psychophysiological effects of the treatment; more recently, a dummy treatment administered to the control group in a controlled clinical trial in order that the specific and nonspecific effects of the experimental treatment can be distinguished—i.e., the experimental treatment must produce better results than the placebo in order to be considered effective.
**active p., impure p.,** a substance having pharmacologic properties that are not relevant to the condition being treated.

**place·ment** (plās′mənt) position or arrangement, as of the teeth.
**lingual p.,** displacement of a tooth toward the tongue.

**pla·cen·ta** (plə-sen′tə) pl. *placentas* or *placen′tae* [L. "a flat cake"] [MeSH: Placenta] a fetomaternal organ characteristic of true mammals during pregnancy, joining mother and offspring, providing endocrine secretion and selective exchange of soluble, bloodborne substances through an apposition of uterine and trophoblastic vascularized parts. According to species, the area of vascular apposition may be *diffuse, cotyledonary, zonary,* or *discoid;* the nature of apposition may be *labyrinthine* or *villous;* and the intimacy of apposition may vary according to what layers are lost of those originally interposed between maternal and fetal blood (maternal endothelium, uterine connective tissue, uterine epithelium, chorion, extraembryonic mesoderm, and endothelium of villous capillary). The chorion may be joined by and receive blood vessels from either the yolk sac or the allantois, and the uterine lining may be largely shed with the chorion at birth *(deciduate p.)* or may separate from the chorion and remain *(nondeciduate p.).* The human placenta is *discoid, villous, hemochorial, chorioallantoic,* and *deciduate.* After birth, it weighs about 600 g and is about 16 cm in diameter and 2 cm thick, discounting the decidua basalis and the maternal blood

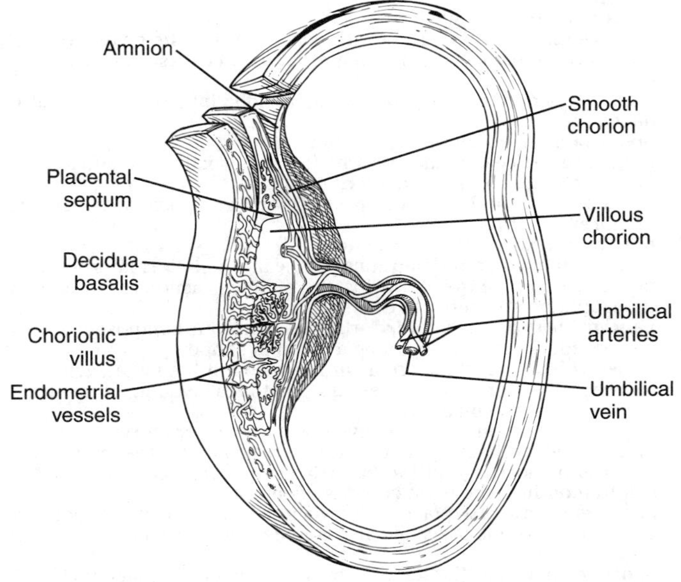

Section through a late-term uterus and placenta.

in the intervillous space (a principal functional part into which the chorionic villi dip and which leaks out at birth). The villi are grouped into adjoining cotyledons making about 20 velvety bumps on the side of the placenta facing the uterus; the side facing the fetus is smooth and covered with amnion, a thin avascular layer that continues past the edges of the placenta to line the entire hollow sphere of chorion except where it is reflected to cover the umbilical cord. The umbilical cord joins fetus and placenta and usually joins the placenta near the center, although it sometimes inserts at the edge, on the nonplacental chorion, or on an accessory placenta.

**accessory p.**, one separate from the main placenta.

**p. accre'ta**, abnormal adherence of part or all of the placenta to the uterine wall, with partial or complete absence of the decidua basalis, especially of the spongiosum layer.

**adherent p.**, one which adheres closely to the uterine wall.

**annular p.**, one which extends around the interior of the uterus like a ring or belt.

**battledore p.**, one with marginal insertion of the cord.

**bidiscoidal p.**, one consisting of two separate discoidal masses, as in the macaques.

**bilobate p.**, **bilobed p.**, a placenta consisting of two lobes.

**p. biparti'ta**, **bipartite p.**, bilobate p.

**chorioallantoic p.**, one in which the allantois joins the chorion or provides its major blood supply.

**choriovitelline p.**, one in which the yolk sac becomes an intermediary in the fetal-maternal relationship.

**p. circumvalla'ta**, **circumvallate p.**, a placenta in which a dense peripheral ring is raised from the surface and the attached membranes are doubled back over the edge of the placenta.

**cirsoid p.**, **p. cirsoi'des**, a placenta the vessels of which appear to be varicose.

**deciduate p.**, **deciduous p.**, a placenta or type of placentation in which the decidua or maternal parts of the placenta separate from the uterus and are cast off together with the fetal (or more precisely, trophoblastic) parts.

**p. diffu'sa**, a placenta in which placental tissue is distributed over the chorionic membrane, as in swine.

**p. dimidia'ta**, **dimidiate p.**, bilobate p.

**discoid p.**, **p. discoi'dea**, a disk-shaped placenta.

**Duncan p.**, one that is expelled with the chorionic surface outward; cf. *Schultze's p.*

**duplex p.**, bilobate p.

**endotheliochorial p.**, one in which syncytial trophoblast embeds maternal vessels bared to their endothelial lining.

**epitheliochorial p.**, one in which the uterine epithelial lining is not eroded but merely lies in apposition to the chorion.

**p. fenestra'ta**, one which has spots where placental tissue is lacking.

**fetal p.**, **p. foeta'lis**, pars fetalis placentae.

**fundal p.**, one attached to the fundus of the uterus in the normal manner.

**furcate p.**, lobed p.

**hemochorial p.**, one in which maternal blood comes in direct contact with the chorion, as in humans.

**hemoendothelial p.**, one in which maternal blood comes in contact with the endothelium of chorionic vessels.

**horseshoe p.**, a crescentic form of placenta sometimes occurring in twin pregnancy.

**incarcerated p.**, retained p.

**p. incre'ta**, placenta accreta with penetration of the myometrium.

**labyrinthine p.**, one in which maternal blood courses in channeled trophoblasts.

**lobed p.**, one that is more or less subdivided into lobes; called also *furcate p.*

**maternal p.**, pars uterina placentae.

**p. membrana'cea**, a placenta which is abnormally thin and spread out over a large area of the uterine wall.

**multilobate p.**, **multilobed p.**, **p. multiparti'ta**, a placenta consisting of more than three lobes.

**p. nappifor'mis**, p. circumvallata.

**nondeciduate p.**, **nondeciduous p.**, one in which the maternal component remains in the uterus instead of being cast off together with the trophoblastic derivatives.

**panduriform p.**, **p. pandurifor'mis**, a placenta composed of two halves side by side, resembling a violin in shape.

**p. percre'ta**, placenta accreta with invasion of the myometrium all the way to its peritoneal covering, sometimes invading other structures such as the bladder.

**p. pre'via**, a placenta which develops in the lower uterine segment, in the zone of dilatation, so that it covers or adjoins the internal os; painless hemorrhage in the last trimester, particularly during the eighth month, is the most common symptom.

**p. pre'via centra'lis**, placenta previa in which the placenta entirely covers the internal os; called also *complete, total,* or *central placenta previa.*

**p. pre'via margina'lis**, placenta previa in which the placenta is just palpable at the margin of the os; called also *lateral* or *marginal placenta previa.*

**p. pre'via partia'lis**, placenta previa in which the internal os is partially covered; called also *incomplete* or *partial placenta previa.*

**p. reflex'a**, one in which the margin is thickened, appearing to turn back on itself.

**p. renifor'mis**, a kidney-shaped placenta.

**retained p.**, one that is either adherent or incarcerated and in consequence fails to be expelled after childbirth.

**Schultze's p.**, a placenta that is delivered with the gestation sac inside out, the amnion providing a smooth, glistening surface. Cf. *Duncan p.*

**p. spu'ria**, an accessory placenta that has no blood vessel attachment to the main placenta.

**p. succenturia'ta**, **succenturiate p.**, an accessory portion attached to the main placenta by an artery and vein.

**syndesmochorial p.**, one in which the lining epithelium of the uterus is the only maternal tissue eroded.

**p. tri'loba**, **trilobate p.**, a placenta having three lobes.

**p. triparti'ta**, **tripartite p.**, trilobate p.

**p. trip'lex**, trilobate p.

**p. uteri'na**, **uterine p.**, maternal p.

**velamentous p.**, one in which the umbilical cord is attached on the adjoining membranes.

**villous p.**, one characterized by the presence of villi which are outgrowths of the chorion.

**yolk-sac p.**, choriovitelline p.

**zonary p.**, **zonular p.**, 1. annular p. 2. a belt-shaped placenta, as occurs in carnivores.

**pla·cen·tal** (plə-sen'təl) 1. pertaining to the placenta. 2. a mammal whose young receive nourishment *in utero* by means of a placenta.

**Pla·cen·ta·lia** (pla″sən-ta'le-ə) a division of mammals whose embryos are nourished through a placenta; it includes all mammals except marsupials and monotremes.

**pla·cen·ta·tion** (pla″sən-ta'shən) [MeSH: Placentation] the process of placenta formation and the result, especially with respect to taxonomically relevant aspects of structure. See *placenta.*

**pla·cen·ti·tis** (pla″sən-ti'tis) inflammation of the placenta.

**pla·cen·to·gen·e·sis** (plə-sen″to-jen'ə-sis) [*placenta* + *genesis*] the origin and development of the placenta.

**pla·cen·to·gram** (plə-sen'to-gram″) a film taken in placentography.

**pla·cen·tog·ra·phy** (pla″sən-tog'rə-fe) radiological visualization of the placenta after the injection of a contrast medium.

**indirect p.**, radiographic measurement of the space between the placenta and the presenting head of the fetus, for the recognition of placenta previa.

**pla·cen·toid** (plə-sen'toid) resembling the placenta.

**pla·cen·tol·o·gist** (pla″sən-tol'ə-jist) a specialist in placentology.

**pla·cen·tol·o·gy** (pla″sən-tol'ə-je) the scientific study of the development, structure, and functioning of the placenta.

**comparative p.**, the scientific study of the development, structure, and functioning of the placenta in different species of animals.

**pla·cen·to·ma** (pla″sən-to'mə) deciduoma.

**pla·cen·top·a·thy** (pla″sən-top'ə-the) any disease of the placenta.

**Pla·ci·do's disk** (plah'se-dōz) [Antonio *Placido* da Costa, Portuguese ophthalmologist, 1848–1916] see under *disk.*

**Plac·i·dyl** (plas'ĭ-dəl) trademark for a preparation of ethchlorvynol.

**plac·ode** (plak'ōd) [Gr. *plax* plate + *eidos* form] a platelike structure, especially a thickened plate of ectoderm in the early embryo, from which a sense organ develops.

**auditory p.**, a thickened ectodermal plate located midway alongside the hindbrain in the early embryo, from which the internal ear ultimately develops. Called also *auditory saucer* and *otic p.*

**dorsolateral p's**, a series of placodes giving rise to the acoustic and lateral line organs.

**epibranchial p's**, a series of placodes located dorsal to the pharyngeal (branchial) grooves; they contribute to adjacent cerebral ganglia.

**lens p.**, a thickened area of ectoderm directly overlying the optic vesicle in the early embryo, from which the lens develops.

**olfactory p.**, an oval area of thickened ectoderm on either ventrolateral surface of the head of the early embryo, constituting the first indication of the olfactory organ.

**otic p.**, auditory p.

**plac·oid** (plak'oid) platelike or plaquelike.

**pla·fond** (plah-fon') [Fr. "ceiling"] the inferior articular surface of the tibia; so called from its vaulted shape.

**pla·gio·ce·phal·ic** (pla″je-o-sə-fal'ik) characterized by plagiocephaly.

**pla·gio·ceph·a·lism** (pla″je-o-sef′ə-liz-əm) plagiocephaly.

**pla·gio·ceph·a·ly** (pla″je-o-sef′ə-le) [Gr. *plagios* oblique + *-cephaly*] an unsymmetrical and twisted condition of the head, resulting from irregular closure of the cranial sutures.

**plague** (plāg) [L. *plaga, pestis;* Gr. *plēgē* stroke] [MeSH: Plague] 1. a severe acute or chronic enzootic or epizootic bacterial infection caused by *Yersinia pestis,* which occurs both endemically and epidemically worldwide; it is primarily a disease of urban and sylvatic rodents and is transmitted to humans by the bite of infected fleas, especially species of *Leptopsylla, Nosopsylla,* and *Xenopsylla,* or by contact with or ingestion of infected animals. Human-to-human infection usually occurs by inhalation of plague bacilli–laden droplet aerosols. The most common forms in humans are bubonic plague, pulmonic plague, and septicemic plague. 2. any of various contagious diseases in animals. Called also *pest* and *pestis.*
**ambulatory p.,** a mild form of bubonic plague, usually occurring only in endemic areas, with lymphadenitis, fever, headache, prostration, and a short course. Called also *parapestis, pestis ambulans,* and *pestis minor.*
**avian p.,** fowl p.
**black p.,** see *bubonic p.*
**bubonic p.,** the most common form of plague, typically characterized by abrupt onset of fever, chills, weakness, and headache, followed by pain, tenderness, and lymphadenopathy (buboes) of the regional lymph nodes, most often the inguinal, femoral, axillary, and cervical nodes, associated with a marked hemorrhagic tendency and the development of disseminated intravascular coagulation and necrotic purpura and extensive symmetrical gangrene (which may have led to the epithet "black death"). Hematogenous dissemination may establish suppurative foci throughout the body. Severe complications include pneumonia (see *pulmonic p.*) and septicemia (see *septicemic p.*). Called also *glandular p., pestis bubonica, pestis fulminans,* and *pestis major.*
**cat p.,** panleukopenia.
**cattle p.,** rinderpest.
**duck p.,** an acute contagious herpesvirus infection of ducks, which may also affect geese and swans. It is characterized by vascular damage, with hemorrhage into the tissues and free blood in the body cavities, exanthematous lesions of the mucosa of the digestive tract, lesions of the lymphoid organs, and retrograde changes in the parenchymatous organs. Called also *duck virus enteritis.*
**equine p.,** African horse sickness.
**fowl p.,** a highly contagious viral disease of domestic fowls caused by an influenza virus of serogroup A; it ranges from a mild to a fulminant, fatal infection. Characteristics include respiratory distress, sinusitis, diarrhea, bloodstained oral and nasal discharges, and edema around the head. Called also *avian influenza, pest,* or *p.* and *fowl pest.*
**glandular p.,** bubonic p.
**hemorrhagic p.,** see *bubonic p.*
**meningeal p.,** plague meningitis.
**Pahvant Valley p.,** tularemia.
**pharyngeal p.,** a rare clinical form of plague that may resemble acute tonsillitis, thought to be due to inhalation or ingestion of plague bacilli. Called also *plague pharyngitis.*
**pneumonic p.,** a rapidly progressive, highly contagious, and often fatal pneumonia in which there is extensive involvement of the lungs and productive cough with mucoid, blood-stained, foamy, plague bacillus–laden sputum. It may occur as a primary infection, due to inhalation of droplet nuclei expelled during coughing, or as a secondary complication of bubonic plague, due to hematogenous spread of infection from buboes to the lungs; in the latter case it may subsequently be associated with human-to-human transmission and cause a primary infection. Called also *plague pneumonia* and *pulmonic p.*
**pulmonic p.,** pneumonic p.
**septicemic p.,** acute fulminating, high-density bacteremia occurring in the acute stage of bubonic plague, or as a so-called primary infection that may present and result in death before the appearance of buboes or of pulmonic manifestations. Called also *pesticemia, pestis siderans, plague septicemia,* and *siderating p.*
**siderating p.,** septicemic p.
**swine p.,** hemorrhagic septicemia of swine.
**sylvatic p.,** plague occurring in the woods, such as that widely spread among ground squirrels and other wild rodents of the western United States.

**pla·kins** (pla′kinz) substances similar to leukins that can be extracted from blood platelets.

**pla·na** (pla′nə) [L.] plural of *planum.*

**pla·nar·i·an** (plə-nar′e-ən) any of the free-living flatworms of the class Turbellaria, which are used extensively in biologic studies of regeneration.

**plan·chet** (plan′chət) a metal disk on which radioactive samples are mounted and prepared for determination of radioactivity.

**Planck's constant, theory** (plahngks) [Max Karl Ernst Ludwig *Planck,* German physicist, 1858–1947] see under *constant,* and see *quantum theory,* under *theory.*

**plane** (plān) [L. *planus*] 1. a surface such that a straight line connecting any two of its points lies wholly in the surface. In craniotomy and cephalometry, the term plane is sometimes used interchangeably with line because when viewed from the side (lateral projection), as in a radiograph, it appears as a line. 2. a specified level, as the plane of anesthesia. 3. to rub away or abrade; see *planing.* 4. a superficial incision in the wall of a cavity or between tissue layers, especially in plastic surgery, made so that the precise point of entry into the cavity or between the layers can be determined.
**Addison's p's,** a series of planes used as landmarks in the topography of the thorax and abdomen.
**Aeby's p.,** one passing through the nasion and basion, perpendicular to the median plane of the cranium.
**auricular p. of sacral bone,** facies auricularis ossis sacri.
**auriculoinfraorbital p.,** Frankfort horizontal p.
**axial p.,** one parallel with the long axis of a structure.
**axiolabiolingual p.,** one parallel with the long axis of an anterior tooth and passing through its labial and lingual surfaces.
**axiomesiodistal p.,** one parallel with the long axis of a tooth and passing through its mesial and distal surfaces.

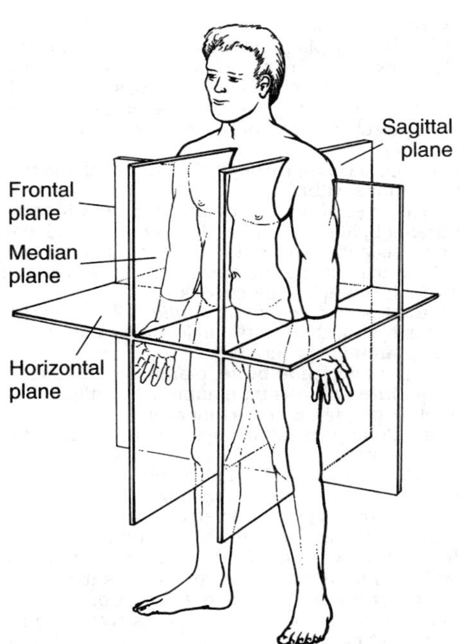

Planes of the body, with subject in the anatomical position.

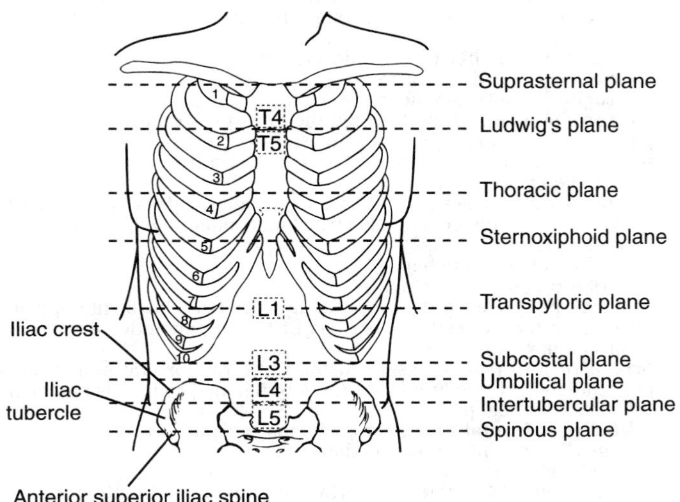

Planes of the trunk.

**Baer's p.**, one passing through the superior borders of the zygomatic arches.
**base p.**, an imaginary plane upon which is estimated the retention of an artificial denture.
**biparietal p.**, the transverse plane that passes through the two parietal eminences.
**bite p.**, 1. biteplane. 2. occlusal p.
**Blumenbach's p.**, a plane determined by the base of a skull from which the mandible has been removed.
**Bolton-nasion p.**, nasion-postcondylare p.
**Broadbent-Bolton p.**, nasion-postcondylare p.
**Broca's p.**, visual p.
**buccolingual p.**, one passing through the buccal and lingual surfaces of a posterior tooth.
**coronal p's**, plana frontalia.
**cusp p.**, the small imaginary plane in which buccal cusp tips and lingual cusp tips are located on posterior teeth.
**Daubenton's p.**, one passing through the opisthion and the inferior edges of the orbits; called also *Daubenton's line*.
**eye-ear p.**, Frankfort horizontal p.
**facial p.**, any of several planes passing through craniometric or cephalometric landmarks of the face.
**Frankfort horizontal p.**, a horizontal plane represented in profile by a line between the lowest point on the margin of the orbit and the highest point on the margin of the external acoustic (auditory) meatus.
**frontal p's**, plana frontalia.
**frontoparallel p.**, any plane parallel to the frontal plane.
**guide p., guiding p.**, 1. any plane that guides movement. 2. an orthodontic appliance used to correct crossbite of anterior teeth. 3. two or more vertically parallel surfaces of abutment teeth, so shaped as to direct the path of placement and removal of a partial denture.
**Hensen's p.**, one passing through the center of a series of sarcous elements of a muscle fibril.
**Hodge's p's**, a series of planes running parallel with the pelvic inlet, the first parallel being in the inlet, the second parallel touching the arch of the pubis and striking the inferior part of the second sacral vertebra, the third cutting the spines of the ischia, and the fourth passing through the tip of the coccyx.
**horizontal p.**, 1. see *plana horizontalia*. 2. in dentistry, a plane passing through a tooth at right angles to its long axis.
**interiliac p.**, planum supracristale.
**interparietal p. of occipital bone**, planum occipitale.
**interspinal p., interspinous p.**, planum interspinale.
**intertubercular p.**, planum intertuberculare.
**labiolingual p.**, one passing through the labial and lingual surfaces of an anterior tooth.
**Listing's p.**, a transverse vertical plane perpendicular to the anteroposterior axis of the eye, and containing the center of motion of the eyes; in it lie the transverse and vertical axes of ocular rotation.
**Ludwig's p.**, a horizontal plane transecting the trunk at about the level of the joint between the fourth and fifth thoracic vertebrae.
**mean foundation p.**, the mean of the various irregularities in form and inclination of the basal seat (denture-supporting tissues). The ideal condition for denture stability exists when the mean foundation plane is most nearly at right angles to the direction of force.
**Meckel's p.**, one passing through the auricular and alveolar points.
**median p.**, planum medianum.
**median-raphe p.**, the median plane of the head.
**median sagittal p.**, planum medianum.
**mesiodistal p.**, one passing through the mesial and distal surfaces of a tooth.
**midclavicular p.**, linea medioclavicularis.
**midpelvic p.**, pelvic p., narrow.
**midsagittal p.**, planum medianum.
**Morton's p.**, one passing through the most projecting points of the parietal and occipital protuberances.
**nasal p.**, the flat area between the nostrils on the muzzle of an animal. Called also *planum nasale*.
**nasion-postcondylare p.**, one passing at right angles to the median plane, and determined in profile by a line connecting the nasion and postcondylare.
**nuchal p.**, planum nuchale.
**occipital p.**, planum occipitale.
**occlusal p., p. of occlusion**, the hypothetical horizontal plane formed by the contacting surfaces of the upper and lower teeth when the jaws are closed.
**orbital p.**, 1. a plane passing through the two orbital points and perpendicular to the Frankfort horizontal plane; called also *planum orbitale*. 2. visual p.
**orbital p. of frontal bone**, pars orbitalis ossis frontalis.
**paramedian p's**, plana paramediana.
**parasagittal p.**, sagittal p's.
**pelvic p.**, one determined by certain landmarks of the hip bone.
**pelvic p., narrow**, an ovoid plane passing through the apex of the pubic arch, the spines of the ischia, and the end of the sacrum.
**pelvic p., wide**, an irregularly ovoid plane passing from the middle of the pubis to the junction of the second and third sacral vertebrae, at about the center of the excavation of the pelvis.
**pelvic p. of outlet**, a plane passing through the arch of the pubis, the rami of the pubis, the ischial tuberosities, and the tip of the coccyx; see *apertura pelvis inferior*.
**popliteal p. of femur**, facies poplitea femoris.
**principal p.**, in radiology, the plane which contains the central ray of a radiation beam.
**p's of reference**, planes which are referred to as a guide to the location of specific anatomical sites, or of other planes.
**p. of regard**, one passing through the center of rotation and the point of fixation in the eye.
**sagittal p's**, plana sagittalia.
**semicircular p. of frontal bone**, facies temporalis ossis frontalis.
**semicircular p. of parietal bone**, planum temporale.
**semicircular p. of squama temporalis**, facies temporalis partis squamosae.
**spinous p.**, a horizontal plane transecting the trunk at the level of the anterior superior iliac spine.
**sternal p.**, planum sternale.
**sternoxiphoid p.**, a horizontal plane transecting the trunk at about the level of the xiphisternal joint.
**subcostal p.**, planum subcostale.
**supracrestal p., supracristal p.**, planum supracristale.
**suprasternal p.**, a horizontal plane transecting the trunk at the level of the jugular notch.
**temporal p.**, planum temporale.
**thoracic p.**, a horizontal plane transecting the trunk at about the level of the fourth intercostal space.
**tooth p.**, any hypothetical plane passing through a tooth.
**transpyloric p.**, planum transpyloricum.
**transtubercular p.**, planum intertuberculare.
**transverse p's**, plana transversalia.
**umbilical p.**, a horizontal plane transecting the trunk at the level of the umbilicus.
**vertical p.**, any plane of the body perpendicular to a horizontal plane and dividing the body into left and right, or front and back portions, as the sagittal and frontal planes.
**visual p.**, one passing through the visual axes of the two eyes; called also *Broca's p.* and *orbital p.*

**pla·ni·gram** (pla'nĭ-gram) tomogram.

**pla·nig·ra·phy** (plə-nig'rə-fe) tomography.

**pla·nim·e·ter** (plə-nim'ə-tər) [L. *planus* plane + *-meter*] an instrument used in measuring the area of surfaces.

**plan·ing** (plān'ing) 1. the plastic surgery procedure of abrading disfigured skin to promote reepithelialization with minimal scarring. It may be done by means of sandpaper, emery paper, low- or high-speed wire brushes, etc. (surgical planing; dermabrasion), or by application of caustic substances such as phenol or trichloroacetic acid (chemical planing; chemabrasion). 2. see *root p.*
**root p.**, smoothing of the root surface of a tooth after subgingival scaling or curettage.

**plani·tho·rax** (plan"ĭ-thor'aks) a diagram of the front and back of the chest.

**plank·ton** (plank'ton) [Gr. *planktos* wandering] [MeSH: Plankton] a collective name for the minute free-floating organisms, vegetable and animal, which live in practically all natural waters.

**pla·no·cel·lu·lar** (pla"no-sel'u-lər) made up of flat cells.

**pla·no·con·cave** (pla"no-kon'kāv) flat on one side and concave on the other; see under *lens*.

**pla·no·con·vex** (pla"no-kon'veks) flat on one side and convex on the other; see under *lens*.

**pla·no·cyte** (pla'no-sīt) [Gr. *planē* wandering + *-cyte*] ameboid cell.

**pla·nor·bid** (plə-nor'bid) 1. a snail of the family Planorbidae. 2. pertaining to snails of the family Planorbidae.

**Pla·nor·bi·dae** (plə-nor'bĭ-de) [L. *planus* flat + *orbis* ring + *-idae*] a large family of pulmonate fresh-water snails (suborder Basommatophora, order Pulmonata), many species of which are intermediate hosts of pathogenic trematodes; it includes the genera *Biomphalaria, Bulinus, Segmentina,* and *Planorbis* (the type genus).

**Pla·nor·bis** (plə-nor'bis) a genus of snails of the family Planorbidae. Several species act as intermediate hosts for trematodes such as *Schistosoma mansoni, Fasciolopsis buski,* and species of *Echinostoma*.

**plan·ta** (plan'tə) [L.] [TA] sole: the undersurface of the foot. Called also *regio plantaris* [TA alternative].
**p. pe'dis**, former name for *planta*.

**plan·tag·i·nis se·men** (plan-taj'ĭ-nis se'mən) [L.] plantago seed.

**Plan·ta·go** (plan-ta'go) [MeSH: Plantago] the psylliums, a genus of herbs of the family Plantaginaceae whose seeds are used medicinally. There are three important species, *P. in'dica* L., *P. ova'ta* Forskal (blond psyllium), and *P. psyl'lium* L. (Spanish psyllium). See *plantago seed,* under *seed* and *psyllium hydrophilic mucilloid,* under *mucilloid.*

**plan·tal·gia** (plan-tal'jə) [L. *planta* sole + *-algia*] a painful condition of the sole of the foot.

**plan·tar** (plan'tər) pertaining to the sole of the foot.

**plan·ta·ris** (plan-ta'ris) [L., from *planta* sole of the foot] [TA] plantar; a term designating relationship to the sole of the foot.

**plan·ta·tion** (plan-ta'shən) [L. *plantare* to plant] the insertion or application of tissue, such as a tooth, or of other material, in or on the human body. Types include *implantation, replantation,* and *transplantation.*

**plan·ti·grade** (plan'tĭ-grād) [L. *planta* sole + *gradi* to walk] characterized by walking on the full sole of the foot; said of animals such as bears and humans. Cf. *digitigrade* and *unguligrade.*

**plan·u·la** (plan'u-lə) 1. a larval coelenterate. 2. something resembling such an animal.

**invaginate p.,** gastrula.

**pla·num** (pla'nəm) pl. *pla'na* [L.] 1. plane. 2. in anatomical nomenclature, a more or less flat surface of a bone or other structure.

**pla'na corona'lia,** TA alternative for plana frontalia

**pla'na fronta'lia** [TA], frontal planes: planes passing longitudinally through the body from side to side, at right angles to the median plane, and dividing the body into front and back parts. So called because such planes roughly parallel the frontal suture of the skull. Called also *plana coronalia* or *coronal planes* because one of these planes passes through the coronal suture.

**pla'na horizonta'lia** [TA], horizontal planes: planes at right angles to the long axis of the body.

**p. interspina'le** [TA], interspinous plane: a horizontal plane transecting the trunk at the level of the anterior superior iliac spines; called also *interspinal line* or *plane.*

**p. intertubercula're** [TA], intertubercular plane: a horizontal plane transecting the trunk at the level of the iliac tubercles; called also *intertubercular line.*

**plana, li'neae et re'giones,** planes, lines, and regions: a section of the *Terminologia Anatomica* that contains terms used to describe the surface anatomy of the body.

**p. media'num** [TA], median plane: the imaginary plane passing longitudinally through the middle of the body from front to back and dividing it into right and left halves. Called also *median sagittal* and *midsagittal plane.*

**p. nasa'le,** nasal plane.

**p. nucha'le,** nuchal plane: the outer surface of the occipital bone between the foramen magnum and the superior nuchal line.

**p. occipita'le** [TA], occipital plane: the outer surface of the occipital bone superior to the superior nuchal line.

**p. orbita'le,** orbital plane (def. 1).

**pla'na paramedia'na** [TA], paramedian planes: sagittal planes other than the median plane.

**p. popli'teum fe'moris,** facies poplitea femoris.

**pla'na sagitta'lia** [TA], sagittal planes: vertical planes that pass through the body parallel to the median plane (or to the sagittal suture) and divide the body into left and right portions. Included here are the *median* and *paramedian planes.*

**p. semiluna'tum,** the rounded end of a crista ampullaris in a semicircular canal.

**p. sterna'le,** sternal plane: the anterior surface of the sternum.

**p. subcosta'le** [TA], subcostal plane: a horizontal plane transecting the trunk at the level of the inferior margins of the tenth costal cartilages; called also *infracostal line.*

**p. supracrista'le** [TA], supracristal plane: a horizontal plane transecting the trunk at the summits of the iliac crests at the level of the fourth lumbar spinous process; called also *supracrestal line* or *plane* and *interiliac plane.*

**p. tempora'le** [TA], temporal plane: the depressed area on the side of the skull inferior to the inferior temporal line.

**p. transpylo'ricum** [TA], transpyloric plane: a horizontal plane half way between the superior margins of the manubrium sterni and the symphysis pubica, which usually does not correspond to the level of the pylorus.

**pla'na trans'versalia** [TA], transverse planes: horizontal planes of the body dividing the body into superior and inferior portions.

**pla·nu·ria** (pla-nu're-ə) [Gr. *planasthai* to wander + *-uria*] the discharge of urine from an abnormal site.

**plaque** (plak) [Fr.] 1. any patch or flat area. 2. a superficial, solid, elevated skin lesion equal to or greater than 1.0 cm (0.5 cm according to some authorities) in diameter. Cf. *papule.*

**argyrophil p's,** senile p's.

**atheromatous p.,** fibrous p.

**attachment p's,** small regions of increased density along the sarcolemma of skeletal muscles to which myofilaments seem to attach; cf. *dense bodies,* under *body.*

**bacterial p.,** dental p.

**bacteriophage p.,** a cleared, usually circular, area on a bacterial lawn plate, occurring as a result of lysis of cells by a bacteriophage.

**dental p.,** a soft, thin film of food debris, mucin, and dead epithelial cells deposited on the teeth, providing the medium for the growth of various bacteria. The main inorganic components are calcium and phosphorus, with small amounts of magnesium, potassium, and sodium; the organic matrix consists of polysaccharides, proteins, carbohydrates, lipids, and other components. Plaque plays an important etiologic role in the development of dental caries and periodontal and gingival diseases and provides the base for the development of materia alba; calcified plaque forms dental calculus. Called also *bacterial p.*

**ear p.,** epidermal hyperplasia of the inner surface of the ear in a horse, with raised white plaques resembling papillomas.

**eosinophilic p.,** an ulcerated, circumscribed, raised skin lesion seen in cats, usually on the abdomen or groin, with eosinophilia of the adjacent dermis; it is part of the eosinophilic granuloma complex.

**fibrofatty p., fibrolipid p.,** fibrous p.

**fibromyelinic p's,** areas of overgrowth of medullated fibers and sheaths in areas of incomplete arteriosclerotic necrosis in the cerebral cortex.

**fibrous p.,** the lesion of atherosclerosis, a white to yellow area within an artery that causes the intimal surface to bulge into the lumen; it is composed of some lipid, cell debris and smooth muscle cells, but mostly collagen, and, in older persons, calcium. Called also *atheromatous p.*

**Hollenhorst p's,** atheromatous emboli containing cholesterol crystals in the retinal arterioles, a warning sign of impending serious cardiovascular disease such as stroke, myocardial infarction, aortic aneurysm, or occlusion of the retinal arterioles.

**Hutchinson's p's,** a persistent cutaneous manifestation of sarcoidosis consisting of flat-surfaced, slightly elevated, large, lobulated, nodular plaques, which show a predilection for the cheeks, nose, arms, and buttocks, usually occurring bilaterally and symmetrically.

**p's jaunes** [Fr. "yellow plaques"], old traumatic injuries on the surface of the brain, appearing as depressed, yellowish-brown patches on the crests of the gyri.

**Lichtheim p's,** areas of degeneration in the cerebral white matter that are seen in pernicious anemia.

**MacCallum's p's,** irregular thickenings induced by subendocardial lesions, usually occurring in the left atrium, in rheumatic heart disease.

**neuritic p's,** senile p's.

**Peyer's p's,** noduli lymphoidei aggregati intestini tenuis.

**pleural p's,** opaque white plaques on the parietal pleura, visible radiographically in cases of asbestosis.

**Randall's p's,** small calcium concretions within the tip of the renal papillae; they may project through the surface and serve as foci for the deposition of urinary salts.

**Redlich-Fisher miliary p's,** thickened, dark colored areas in the neuroglia reticulum of the brain, seen in cases of senile psychoses.

**senile p's,** microscopic argyrophilic masses composed of fragmented axon terminals and dendrites surrounding a core of amyloid; seen in small amounts in the cerebral cortex of normal elderly people and in larger amounts in those with Alzheimer's disease. Called also *argyrophil p's* and *neuritic p's.*

**talc p's,** plaques of opaque material on the pleural surfaces of talc miners and processors suffering from talc pneumoconiosis.

**Pla·que·nil** (pla'kwə-nil) trademark for a preparation of hydroxychloroquine sulfate.

**Plas·bu·min** (plaz-bu'min) trademark for a preparation of albumin human.

**-plasia** [Gr. *plasis* molding, from *plassein* to mold] a combining form denoting development or formation.

**plasm** (plaz'əm) plasma.

**germ p.,** *(obs.),* Weismann's term for the reproductive and hereditary substance of individuals which is passed on from the germ cell in which an individual originates in direct continuity to the germ cells of succeeding generations. By it new individuals are produced and hereditary characters are transmitted. Cf. *somatoplasm.*

**-plasm** [Gr. *plasma* anything formed or molded] a word termination denoting the constituent substance of cells.

**plas·ma** (plaz'mə) [Gr. "anything formed or molded"] [MeSH: Plasma] 1. the fluid portion of the blood in which the particulate components are suspended. *Plasma* is to be distinguished from *serum,* which is the cell-free portion of the blood from which the fibrinogen has been separated in the process of clotting. Called also *blood p.* 2. the lymph deprived of its corpuscles or cells. 3. a glycerite of starch used in preparing ointments. 4. cytoplasm or protoplasm.

**antihemophilic human p.,** normal human plasma that has been processed promptly to preserve the antihemophilic properties of the original blood; used for temporary correction of bleeding tendency in hemophilia.

**blood p.,** plasma (def. 1).
**citrated p.,** blood plasma treated with sodium citrate, which prevents clotting.
**fresh frozen p.,** plasma separated from whole blood and frozen within 8 hours; it contains all coagulation factors including the labile factors V and VIII.
**normal human p.,** sterile plasma obtained by pooling approximately equal amounts of the liquid portion of citrated whole blood from eight or more adult humans, used as a blood volume replenisher.
**oxalate p.,** blood plasma to which ammonium oxalate has been added, formerly used to prevent clotting.
**pooled p.,** a mixture of plasma from several donors.
**salt p.,** blood plasma to which a neutral salt has been added to prevent clotting, such as citrated plasma.
**seminal p.,** the fluid portion of the semen, in which the spermatozoa are suspended.
**true p.,** blood plasma drawn directly from the blood without any change in its gas content.

**plas·ma·blast** (plaz′mə-blast) [*plasma* + *-blast*] the earliest precursor in the plasmacytic series, which matures to form the proplasmacyte and ultimately the mature plasma cell; it may itself be a derivative of the lymphoblast.

**plas·ma·cyte** (plaz′mə-sīt) [*plasma* + *-cyte*] [MeSH: Plasma Cells] plasma cell.

**plas·ma·cyt·ic** (plaz″mə-sit′ik) pertaining to, characterized by, or of the nature of a plasma cell.

**plas·ma·cy·to·ma** (plaz″mə-si-to′mə) [*plasmacyte* + *-oma*] [MeSH: Plasmacytoma] 1. plasma cell dyscrasia. 2. solitary myeloma.
**multiple p. of bone,** multiple myeloma.

**plas·ma·cy·to·sis** (plaz″mə-si-to′sis) the presence of excess plasma cells in the blood.

**plas·ma·gel** (plaz′mə-jel) a relatively rigid peripheral layer of cytoplasm which is devoid of granules.

**plas·ma·gene** (plaz′mə-jēn) [cyto*plasm* + *gene*] in human beings, a gene found on the mitochondrial chromosome (q.v.); called also *cytogene.*

**plas·ma·haut** (plaz′mə-hout) [Ger.] the superficial layer of the protoplasm of a cell.

**plas·mal** (plaz′məl) a long-chain fatty acid aldehyde produced during hydrolysis of plasmalogens.

**plas·ma·lem·ma** (plaz″mə-lem′ə) [*plasma* + *-lemma*] 1. plasma membrane. 2. a thin peripheral layer of the ectoplasm in a fertilized oocyte.

**plas·ma·lo·gen** (plaz-mal′ə-jən) any of various phospholipids in which the group at one C1 of glycerol is an ether-linked alcohol in place of an ester-linked fatty acid, found in myelin sheaths of nerve fibers, cell membranes of muscle, and platelets.

**Plas·ma·nate** (plaz′mə-nāt) trademark for a commercial preparation of human plasma protein fraction.

**plas·ma·phe·re·sis** (plaz″mə-fə-re′sis) [*plasma* + *apheresis*] [MeSH: Plasmapheresis] the removal of plasma from withdrawn blood, with retransfusion of the formed elements into the donor; generally, type-specific fresh frozen plasma or albumin is used to replace the withdrawn plasma. The procedure may be done for purposes of collecting plasma components or for therapeutic purposes.

**plas·mar·rhex·is** (plaz″mə-rek′sis) [*plasma* + *-rrhexis*] dissolution of the cytoplasm.

**plas·mat·ic** (plaz-mat′ik) pertaining to or of the nature of plasma; called also *plasmic.*

**plas·ma·tog·a·my** (plaz″mə-tog′ə-me) plasmogamy.

**plas·ma·tor·rhex·is** (plaz″mə-to-rek′sis) [*plasma* + *-rrhexis*] the bursting of a cell due to the pressure exerted from within.

**plas·mic** (plaz′mik) 1. plasmatic. 2. rich in protoplasm.

**plas·mid** (plaz′mid) [*plasm* + *-id*] an extrachromosomal self-replicating structure found in bacterial cells that carries genes for a variety of functions not essential for cell growth. Plasmids consist of cyclic double-stranded DNA molecules, replicating independently of the chromosomes and transmitting through successive cell divisions genes specifying such functions as antibiotic resistance (R plasmid); conjugation (F plasmid); the production of enzymes, toxins, and antigens; and the metabolism of sugars and other organic compounds. Plasmids can be transferred from one cell to another by conjugation and by transduction. Some plasmids may also become integrated into the bacterial chromosome; these are known as *episomes.*
**conjugative p.,** a plasmid that is transferred from one bacterial cell to another during conjugation.
**F p.,** a conjugative plasmid found in $F^+$ (male) bacterial cells that leads with high frequency to its transfer and much less often to transfer of the bacterial chromosome. A cell possessing the F plasmid ($F^+$, male) can form a conjugation bridge (F pilus) to a cell lacking the F plasmid ($F^-$, female), through which genetic material may pass from one cell to another. Called also *F* or *fertility factor, F element,* and *sex factor.*
**F′ p.,** a hybrid F plasmid that contains also a segment of the host chromosome.
**oligomeric p.,** a plasmid that contains repeating segments of a determinant, formed by recombination between strands during replication and resulting in gene amplification.
**R p., resistance p.,** a conjugative factor in bacterial cells that promotes resistance to agents such as antibiotics, metal ions, ultraviolet radiation, and bacteriophage. R plasmids are large with two functionally distinct parts: a resistance transfer factor (RTF), consisting of genes for autonomous replication and conjugation; and a resistance determinant (R determinant) containing the genes for resistance (R genes); called also *R factor.*

**plas·min** (plaz′min) [EC 3.4.21.7] [MeSH: Plasmin] a serine endopeptidase that catalyzes the hydrolysis of peptide bonds on the carboxyl side of lysine or arginine residues. The enzyme occurs in plasma as plasminogen, which is activated via cleavage by the plasminogen activators prourokinase, u-plasminogen activator (urokinase), and t-plasminogen (tissue plasminogen activator). Plasmin solubilizes fibrin clots and also degrades various proteins including fibrinogen and coagulation factors V and VII. Plasminogen is activated for therapeutic thrombolysis by recombinant forms of physiologic activators and by streptokinase, a streptococcal enzyme. Called also *fibrinolysin.*

**plas·min·o·gen** (plaz-min′ə-jən) [MeSH: Plasminogen] the inactive precursor of plasmin; called also *profibrinolysin.*

**plas·min·o·gen ac·ti·va·tor** see under *activator.*

**plasm(o)-** [Gr. *plasma* anything formed or molded] a combining form denoting relationship to plasma, or to the substance of a cell.

**plas·mo·cyte** (plaz′mo-sīt) [*plasmo-* + *-cyte*] a plasma cell.

**plas·mo·cy·to·ma** (plaz″mo-si-to′mə) [*plasmo-* + *-cyte* + *-oma*] 1. plasma cell dyscrasia. 2. solitary myeloma.

**plas·mo·dia** (plaz-mo′de-ə) plural of *plasmodium.*

**plas·mo·di·al** (plaz-mo′de-əl) pertaining to plasmodia.

**plas·mo·di·blast** (plaz-mo′dĭ-blast) syncytiotrophoblast.

**plas·mo·di·ci·dal** (plaz″mo-dĭ-si′dəl) [*plasmodia* + L. *caedere* to kill] destructive to plasmodia.

**plas·mo·di·cide** (plaz-mo′dĭ-sīd) an agent that is destructive to plasmodia.

**plas·mo·di·tropho·blast** (plaz-mo″di-trof′o-blast) syncytiotrophoblast.

**Plas·mo·di·um** (plaz-mo′de-əm) [Gr. *plasma* anything formed or molded] [MeSH: Plasmodium] the malarial parasite: a genus of coccidian protozoa (suborder Haemosporina, order Eucoccidiida), parasitic in the erythrocytes of mammals, including humans, nonhuman primates, and rodents, birds, and reptiles, mainly lizards; it is transmitted to the bloodstream of mammals by the bite of female anopheline mosquitoes, in whose saliva the sporozoites are concentrated. From the bloodstream, the sporozoites migrate directly to the liver (exoerythrocytic stage), where they develop and multiply within the parenchymal cells as merozoites, which then burst the hepatocytes and invade erythrocytes. Erythrocytic schizogony then occurs and merozoites are free to invade other erythrocytes. Some merozoites develop into gametocytes, which are ingested by mosquitoes and begin the sexual stage, which ends with development of sporozoites. Avian malaria is transmitted by culicine mosquitoes; the vectors of reptilian malaria are unknown.
**P. falci′parum,** the species which causes falciparum malaria in man; it is characterized by thin "signet-ring" forms of trophozoites and the "crescent" form of the gametes.
**P. mala′riae,** the species which causes quartan malaria in man. It is characterized by bandlike trophozoites and schizonts with six to twelve merozoites usually arranged in a rosette-like configuration.
**P. ova′le,** a species found primarily in East and Central Africa that causes ovale malaria, and is characterized by oval or fimbriated infected red blood cells.
**P. vi′vax,** the species causing vivax malaria, characterized by the ameboid activity and irregular form of its trophozoites, and by Schüffner's dots in parasitized red blood cells.

**plas·mo·di·um** (plaz-mo′de-əm) pl. *plasmo′dia* [*plasmo-* + Gr. *eidos* form] [MeSH: Plasmodium] 1. a protozoan of the genus *Plasmodium.* 2. a multinucleate continuous mass of protoplasm formed by aggregation and fusion of myxamebae; also, a protozoan whose body consists of such a mass. Cf. *pseudoplasmodium.*
**exoerythrocytic p.,** a malarial parasite outside a red blood cell; in human malaria this is generally considered to represent the hepatic stage.

**plas·mog·a·my** (plaz-mog′ə-me) [*plasmo-* + Gr. *gamos* marriage] the union of two or more cells with their nuclei remaining separate; in fertilization, karyogamy follows. Called also *plasmatogamy* and *plastogamy.* Cf. *karyogamy.*

**plas·mo·gen** (plaz′mo-jən) [*plasmo-* + *-gen*] the essential part of protoplasm; bioplasm, def. 2.

**plas·moid** (plas′moid) an abnormal protein cellular element; see also under *humor.*

**plas·mol·y·sis** (plaz-mol′ĭ-sis) [*plasmo-* + *-lysis*] contraction or shrinking of the protoplasm of a plant cell due to the loss of water by osmotic action.

**plas·mo·lyt·ic** (plaz″mo-lit′ik) tending toward, pertaining to, or characterized by plasmolysis.

**plas·mo·lyz·a·bil·i·ty** (plaz″mo-līz″ə-bil′ĭ-te) the power of undergoing plasmolysis.

**plas·mo·lyz·a·ble** (plaz″mo-līz′ə-bəl) capable of undergoing plasmolysis.

**plas·mo·lyze** (plaz′mo-līz) to subject to plasmolysis.

**plas·mo·ma** (plaz-mo′mə) 1. plasma cell dyscrasia. 2. solitary myeloma.

**plas·mon** (plaz′mon) [*cytoplasm* + Gr. *-on* neuter ending] the sum total of all non-nuclear extrachromosomal genetic material; in human beings, the mitochondrial chromosome (q.v.). See also *genome.*

**plas·mor·rhex·is** (plaz″mo-rek′sis) [*plasmo-* + *-rhexis*] plasmatorrhexis.

**plas·mos·chi·sis** (plaz-mos′kĭ-sis) [*plasmo-* + *-schisis*] the splitting of protoplasm into fragments.

**plas·mo·sin** (plaz′mo-sin) a protein constituent of cytoplasm.

**plas·mot·o·my** (plaz-mot′ə-me) [*plasmo-* + *-tomy*] reproduction by the separation from the mother cell of smaller masses of protoplasm, each containing several nuclei.

**plas·mo·tropho·blast** (plaz″mo-trof′o-blast) syncytiotrophoblast.

**plas·son** (plas′on) [Gr. *plassōn* forming] the protoplasm of a cytode, or non-nucleated cell.

**-plast** [Gr. *plastos* formed] a word termination denoting any primitive organized unit of living matter, e.g. a granule, an organelle, or a cell.

**plas·tein** (plas′tēn) the protein synthesized by pepsin from the peptic digestion products of protein.

**plas·ter** (plas′tər) [L. *emplastrum*] 1. a gypsum material which hardens when mixed with water, used for immobilizing or making impressions of body parts. 2. a pastelike mixture which can be spread over the skin and which is adhesive at body temperature. Plasters may be protectant, counterirritant, etc.
**impression p.,** a gypsum preparation used for the making of impressions of structures in the mouth.
**mustard p.,** a uniform mixture of powdered black mustard and a solution of suitable adhesive, spread on an appropriate backing material; used as a local irritant.
**p. of Paris,** calcium sulfate hemihydrate reduced to a fine powder; the addition of water produces a porous mass that hardens rapidly. It has been used extensively in making casts and bandages to support or immobilize body parts, and in dentistry for pouring dental impressions.
**salicylic acid p.** [USP], a uniform mixture of salicylic acid in a suitable base, spread on paper, cotton cloth, or other backing material; used as a topical keratolytic.

**plas·ter of Par·is** (par′is) [*Paris,* France, site of gypsum deposits from which it was first made in the early 19th century] see under *plaster.*

**plas·tic** (plas′tik) [L. *plasticus;* Gr. *plastikos*] 1. tending to build up tissues or to restore a lost part. 2. conformable; capable of being molded. 3. a high-molecular-weight polymeric material, usually organic, capable of being molded, extruded, drawn, or otherwise shaped and then hardened into a form. 4. material that can be molded.

**plas·tic·i·ty** (plas-tis′ĭ-te) the capability of being molded.
**synaptic p.,** the ability of synapses to change as circumstances require. They may alter function, such as increasing or decreasing their sensitivity; or they may increase or decrease in actual numbers. This phenomenon is thought to be the main source of the overall plasticity of nervous system pathways.

**plas·ti·ci·zer** (plas′tĭ-si″zər) any of a group of agents, usually organic, added to other organic or synthetic substances to make them soft and flexible.

**plas·tin** (plas′tin) 1. linin. 2. spongioplasm (def. 1).

**plas·to·chon·dria** (plas″to-kon′dre-ə) granular mitochondria.

**plas·to·dy·na·mia** (plas″to-di-na′me-ə) [Gr. *plastos* formed + *dynam-* + *-ia*] power or ability to develop.

**plas·tog·a·my** (plas-tog′ə-me) [Gr. *plastos* formed matter + *gamos* marriage] plasmogamy.

**plas·to·gel** (plas′to-jel) a gel possessing great plasticity.

**plas·to·some** (plas′to-sōm) [Gr. *plastos* formed + *-some*] one of the stainable granules or threads of the cytoplasm.

**plas·tron** (plas′tron) [Fr. "breast-plate"] the sternum and costal cartilages.

**-plasty** [Gr. *plassein* to form] a word termination denoting plastic surgery.

**plate** (plāt) [Gr. *platē*] 1. a flat structure or layer, such as a thin layer of bone; see also *lamina, layer,* etc. 2. a dental plate. Sometimes, by extension, incorrectly used to designate a complete denture. 3. a flat vessel, usually a Petri dish, containing sterile solid medium for the culture of microorganisms. 4. to prepare a culture medium in a Petri dish, or to inoculate such a medium with a bacterial culture.
**alar p.,** lamina alaris.
**anal p.,** the anal part of the cloacal membrane.
**auditory p.,** the bony roof of the external acoustic meatus.
**axial p.,** the primitive streak of the embryo.
**basal p.,** 1. lamina basalis. 2. the fused parachordal cartilages, precursors of the occipital bone. 3. the portion of the decidua basalis that becomes an integral part of the placenta.
**base p.,** see *baseplate.*
**bite p.,** a removable orthodontic appliance, generally made of acrylic resin, that makes use of adhesion to the palate to provide part of the anchorage needed for the desired tooth movement; used to stimulate eruption of the posterior teeth and to decrease the amount of anterior overbite. Written also *biteplate.*
**bone p.,** a metal bar with perforations for the insertion of screws, used to immobilize fractured segments.
**cardiogenic p.,** an area of splanchnic mesoderm, at first cephalad and later in the pharyngeal region of the embryo, from which the heart arises.
**cell p.,** a thickening midway of the mitotic spindle in plants that forms a dividing septum between the future daughter cells.
**chorionic p.,** the part of the inner chorionic wall in the area of its uterine attachment, which gives rise to chorionic villi.
**compression p.,** a type of bone plate in which the screws are arranged so that they compress the defect and actively promote closure.
**cortical p.,** a layer of compact bone overlying the spongiosa of the alveolar process on the vestibular and oral aspects of the mandible and maxilla.
**cough p.,** a plate of culture medium on which a patient with a respiratory infection, especially pertussis, coughs.
**counting p.,** in bacteriology, a plate marked off in square centimeters. A Petri dish culture of microorganisms is placed on the plate and colonies per square centimeter are counted. The number of colonies per plate is calculated by multiplying the average count per square centimeter by the area of the Petri dish.
**p. of cranial bone, inner,** lamina interna ossis cranii.
**p. of cranial bone, outer,** lamina externa ossis cranii.
**cribriform p.,** fascia cribrosa.
**cribriform p. of ethmoid bone,** lamina cribrosa ossis ethmoidalis.
**cuticular p.,** terminal web.
**cutis p.,** dermatome, def. 3.
**deck p.,** roof p.
**dental p.,** a plate of acrylic resin, metal, or other material, which is fitted to the shape of the mouth and serves for the support of artificial teeth.
**dermomyotome p.,** the portion of the embryonic somite remaining after migration of the sclerotomic tissue.

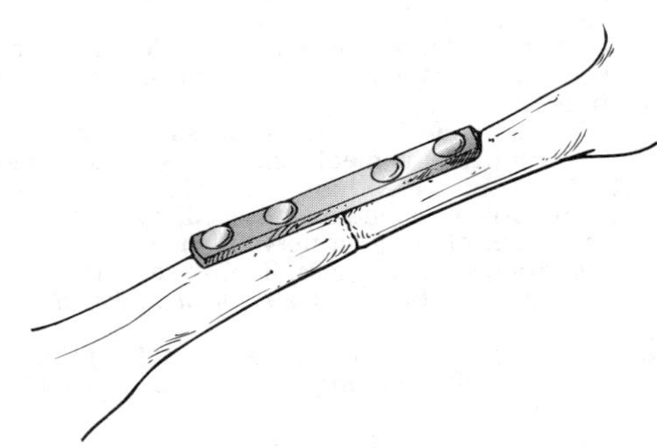

Bone plate.

**die p.,** a plate of metal containing dies for forming the cusps in shell crowns.
**dorsal p.,** roof p.
**dorsolateral p.,** lamina alaris.
**Eggers' p.,** bone plate used for maintaining apposition of bone segments.
**end p.,** see *end plate,* under *E.*
**epiphyseal p.,** cartilago epiphysialis.
**equatorial p.,** the platelike collection of chromosomes at the equator of the spindle in karyokinesis.
**ethmovomerine p.,** the central part of the ethmoid bone in the fetus.
**floor p.,** the unpaired ventral longitudinal zone of the neural tube, forming the floor of that tube; called also *ventral p.* and *bodenplatte.*
**foot p.,** 1. basis stapedis. 2. a flattened expansion at the end of the limb end of the embryo, the precursor of the foot.
**force p.,** force platform.
**frontal p.,** a fetal plate of cartilage between the sides of the ethmoid cartilage and the sphenoid bone.
**frontonasal p.,** a fetal plate from which the external nose is developed.
**growth p.,** cartilago epiphysialis.
**hand p.,** a flattened expansion at the end of the limb bud of the embryo, the precursor of the hand.
**horizontal p. of palatine bone,** lamina horizontalis ossis palatini.
**Ishihara's p.'s,** the pseudoisochromic plates used in Ishihara's test.
**jumping the bite p.,** Kingsley appliance.
**Kingsley p.,** see under *appliance.*
**Kühne's terminal p's,** the motor end-plates of nerves in the muscle spindles.
**Lane p's,** steel plates with holes for screws, used in fixing the fragments of a fractured bone.
**lateral mesoblastic p.,** the thickened portion of either side of the mesoblast.
**lawn p.,** a plate of solid culture medium inoculated by swab or with a liquid inoculum so as to produce a uniform confluent growth of microorganisms, used for assay of bacteriophage.
**lingual p.,** a major partial denture connector formed as a lingual bar extended to cover the cingula of the lower anterior teeth. When used on the maxillary arch it is often referred to as a *palatal p.*
**medullary p.,** neural p.
**mesial p.,** nephrotome.
**metaphase p.,** equatorial p.
**middle p.,** nephrotome.
**Moe p.,** a stainless steel plate for internal fixation of intertrochanteric fractures of the femur.
**motor end p.,** see under *end plate.*
**muscle p.,** myotome (def. 2).
**nail p.,** 1. stratum corneum unguis. 2. stratum germinativum unguis.
**nephrotome p.,** nephrotome.
**neural p.,** the thickened plate of ectoderm in the embryo from which the neural tube develops.
**notochordal p.,** head process.
**oral p.,** oropharyngeal membrane.
**orbital p. of ethmoid bone,** lamina orbitalis ossis ethmoidalis.
**orbital p. of frontal bone,** pars orbitalis ossis frontalis.
**palatal p.,** see *lingual p.*
**paper p.,** lamina orbitalis ossis ethmoidalis.
**parachordal p.,** basal p., def. 2.
**parietal p.,** lamina perpendicularis ossis ethmoidalis.
**perpendicular p. of ethmoid bone,** lamina perpendicularis ossis ethmoidalis.
**perpendicular p. of palatine bone,** lamina perpendicularis ossis palatini.
**Petri p.,** a Petri dish containing a nutrient medium ready for inoculation with the microorganism to be cultured.
**polar p's, pole p's,** platelike bodies at the end of the spindle in certain forms of mitosis.
**pour p.,** a bacterial culture poured into a Petri dish from a test tube in which the medium has been inoculated.
**prechordal p., prochordal p.,** thickened endoderm, cephalad of the notochord, that combines with ectoderm to become the oropharyngeal membrane.
**pterygoid p., lateral,** lamina lateralis processus pterygoidei.
**pterygoid p., medial,** lamina medialis processus pterygoidei.
**quadrigeminal p.,** lamina tecti mesencephali.
**reticular p.,** a form of nerve ending in the ciliary body consisting of very fine reticulations of granular nerve fiber.
**roof p.,** the unpaired dorsal longitudinal zone of the neural tube, forming the roof of that tube; called also *deck p., dorsal p.,* and *deckplatte.*
**segmental p.,** a plate of mesoblast on either side of the notochord at the posterior end of the embryo, from which the mesoblastic segments are formed.
**Sherman p.,** a chrome-cobalt alloy or stainless steel bone plate which can be affixed to a fracture site with screws; often used in open reduction of mandibular fractures.
**spiral p.,** lamina spiralis ossea.
**spring p.,** a dental prosthesis held in place by the elasticity of the base material which abuts against natural teeth.
**Strasburger's cell p.,** midbody, def. 1.
**streak p.,** a plate of solid culture medium in which the infectious material is inoculated in streaks across the surface.
**subgerminal p.,** a sheet of protoplasm forming the floor of the segmentation cavity of the ovum.
**tarsal p's,** see *tarsus superior palpebrae* and *tarsus inferior palpebrae.*
**tectal p.,** lamina tecti mesencephali.
**terminal p.,** lamina terminalis hypothalami.
**tympanic p.,** pars tympanica ossis temporalis.
**urethral p.,** an endodermal plate that gives rise to the terminal portion of the spongy urethra.
**vascular foot p.,** pericapillary end foot.
**ventral p.,** floor p.
**ventrolateral p.,** lamina basalis.
**vertical p. of palatine bone,** lamina perpendicularis ossis palatini.
**wing p.,** lamina alaris.

**pla·teau** (plă-to') [Fr.] an elevated and level area.
**tibial p.,** either of the bony surfaces of the tibia, internal and external, closest to the condyles of the femur.
**ventricular p.,** a nearly level part of the intraventricular curve of blood pressure corresponding to the middle of the ejection period of the ventricle.

**plate·let** (plāt'lət) [MeSH: Blood Platelets] a disk-shaped structure, 2 to 4 $\mu$m in diameter, found in the blood of all mammals and chiefly known for its role in blood coagulation; platelets, which are formed in the megakaryocyte and released from its cytoplasm in clusters, lack a nucleus and DNA but contain active enzymes and mitochondria. See also under *factor,* and see *thrombocytic series,* under *series.* Called also *blood disk, blood p.,* and *thrombocyte.*
**blood p.,** platelet.
**giant p.,** an abnormal large platelet whose membrane lacks glycoprotein Ib so that the platelet cannot bind von Willebrand's factor or adhere to the surface of a blood vessel; seen in the Bernard-Soulier syndrome.
**gray p.,** an abnormal platelet with deficient alpha granules, giving it a gray appearance on a Wright's stain smear; seen in the bleeding disorder called *gray platelet syndrome.*

**plate·let·phe·re·sis** (plāt″lət-fə-re'sis) [*platelet* + *pheresis*] [MeSH: Plateletpheresis] thrombocytapheresis.

**plat·form** (plat'form) a flat horizontal surface higher than the level of the areas around it.
**force p.,** a small platform that measures variations in downward force between different points on its surface, for assessing stability of stance and posture as a person stands on it; see posturography. Called also *force plate.*

**plat·ing** (plāt'ing) 1. the act of preparing a bacterial culture on a plate of solid medium in a Petri dish; the preparation of a plate culture. 2. the application of plates to fractured bones for the purpose of holding the fragments in place.

**pla·tin·ic** (plə-tin'ik) containing platinum in its higher valency.

**Pla·ti·nol** (plat'ĭ-nol) trademark for a preparation of cisplatin.

**plat·i·no·sis** (plat'ĭ-no'sis) [*platinum* + *-osis*] a morbid condition caused by exposure to soluble platinum salts, with involvement of the upper respiratory tract and allergic skin manifestations.

**plat·i·nous** (plat'ĭ-nəs) containing platinum in its lower valency.

**plat·i·num** (plat'ĭ-nəm) [L.] [MeSH: Platinum] a heavy, soft, whitish metal, resembling tin: symbol, Pt; atomic number, 78; atomic weight, 195.09; specific gravity, 21.37. It also occurs as a black powder *(p. black)* and a spongy substance *(spongy p.).* Metallic platinum is insoluble except in nitrohydrochloric acid, and is fusible only at very high temperatures; it is therefore used in the manufacture of chemical apparatus. Platinum black and spongy platinum have a strong affinity for oxygen, and act as powerful oxidizing and catalytic agents.
**p. chloride,** platinic tetrachloride, a poisonous substance used as a chemical reagent and formerly in syphilis.

**platy-** [Gr. *platys* broad] a combining form meaning broad or flat.

**platy·ba·sia** (plat″ĭ-ba'se-ə) [*platy-* + *bas-* + *-ia*] [MeSH: Platybasia] bulging upwards of the floor of the posterior cranial fossa adjacent to the foramen magnum due to softening of skull bones or a developmental anomaly; see also *basilar invagination,* under *invagination.* Called also *basilar impression.*

**platy·ce·lous** (plat″ĭ-se'ləs) [*platy-* + *cel-*$^2$ + *-ous*] having vertebral centra that are flat in front, or cephalad, and concave caudad.

**platy·ce·phal·ic** (plat″ĭ-sə-fal'ik) [*platy-* + *cephal-* + *-ic*] wide headed; having a breadth-height index of less than 70.

**plat·y·ceph·a·ly** (plat″ĭ-sef′ə-le) the state of being platycephalic.

**platy·cne·mia** (plat″ik-ne′me-ə) compression of the tibia from side to side.

**platy·cne·mic** (plat″ik-ne′mik) [*platy-* + Gr. *knēmē* leg] having the tibia compressed from side to side.

**platy·co·ria** (plat″ĭ-kor′e-ə) [*platy-* + *cor-* + *-ia*] a dilated condition of the pupil.

**platy·cra·nia** (plat″ĭ-kra′ne-ə) [*platy-* + *crani-* + *-ia*] artificial flattening of the skull.

**platy·glos·sal** (plat″ĭ-glos′əl) [*platy-* + *gloss-* + *-al*[1]] having a broad, flat tongue.

**platy·hel·minth** (plat″ĭ-hel′minth) any member of the phylum Platyhelminthes; called also *flatworm.*

**Platy·hel·min·thes** (plat″ĭ-həl-min′thēz) [*platy-* + Gr. *helmins* worm] the flatworms, a phylum of acoelomate, dorsoventrally flattened, bilaterally symmetrical invertebrates; classes include Turbellaria, Trematoda, and Cestoidea.

**platy·hi·er·ic** (plat″e-hi-er′ik) [*platy-* + *hier-* + *-ic*] having a wide sacrum; having a sacral index exceeding 100.

**platy·kne·mia** (plat″ik-ne′me-ə) platycnemia.

**platy·kur·tic** (plat″ĭ-kur′tik) [*platy-* + Gr. *kurtos* convex] pertaining to a probability distribution less concentrated about the mean, i.e., having a broader, flatter peak than the normal distribution with the same variance. Cf. *leptokurtic.*

**platy·me·ria** (plat″ĭ-me′re-ə) the condition of being platymeric.

**platy·me·ric** (plat″ĭ-me′rik) [*platy-* + *mer-*[2] + *-ic*] having a femur that is excessively compressed from front to back.

**platy·mor·phia** (plat″ĭ-mor′fe-ə) [*platy-* + *morph-* + *-ia*] having a flat shape; in ophthalmology, a flattened eyeball, resulting in a short anteroposterior axis and hypermetropia.

**platy·mor·phic** (plat″ĭ-mor′fik) pertaining to or characterized by platymorphia.

**platy·my·ar·i·an** (plat″ĭ-mi-ar′e-ən) [*platy-* + Gr. *mys* muscle] having all muscle cells lying next to the hypodermis, their sarcoplasm being uncovered on three sides next to the body cavity; said of the muscle arrangement in certain nematodes.

**platy·my·oid** (plat″ĭ-mi′oid) [*platy-* + *myo-* + *-oid*] having the contractile stratum arranged in an even lamina; said of certain muscle cells.

**Platy·no·so·mum** (plat″ĭ-no-so′mum) a genus of trematodes of the family Dicrocoeliidae. *P. fasto′sum* infests the liver and bile ducts of domestic cats in the southeastern United States and the Caribbean after they eat infested lizards or toads.

**platy·pel·lic** (plat″ĭ-pel′ik) [*platy-* + Gr. *pella* bowl] having a wide, flat pelvis.

**platy·pel·loid** (plat″ĭ-pel′oid) platypellic.

**platy·phyl·line** (plat″ĭ-fil′ēn) an alkaloid from *Senecio platyphyllus* and other species of *Senecio.*

**pla·typ·nea** (plə-tip′ne-ə) [*platy-* + *-pnea*] dyspnea induced by assumption of the upright position and relieved by assumption of a recumbent position; the opposite of *orthopnea.*

**platy·po·dia** (plat″ĭ-po′de-ə) [*platy-* + *pod-* + *-ia*] abnormal flatness of the foot; flatfoot.

**Plat·yr·rhi·na** (plat″ĭ-ri′nə) [*platy-* + Gr. *rhis* nose] the New World monkeys, a superfamily of the order Primates (suborder Anthropoidea), characterized by a broad nasal septum and often a prehensile tail.

**plat·yr·rhine** (plat′ĭ-rīn) [*platy-* + Gr. *rhis* nose] having a broad nose; having a nasal index exceeding 53.

**pla·tys·ma** (plə-tiz′mə) [Gr.] [TA] a platelike muscle that originates from the fascia of the cervical region and inserts in the mandible and the skin around the mouth. It is innervated by the cervical branch of the facial nerve, and acts to wrinkle the skin of the neck and to depress the jaw.

**pla·tys·mal** (plə-tiz′məl) pertaining to the platysma.

**platy·spon·dyl·ia** (plat″ĭ-spon-dil′e-ə) platyspondylisis.

**platy·spon·dyl·i·sis** (plat″ĭ-spon-dil′ĭ-sis) [*platy-* + *spondyl-* + *-sis*] congenital flattening of the vertebral bodies.

**Platy·spo·ri·na** (plat″ĭ-spə-ri′nə) [*platy-* + *spore*] a suborder of parasitic protozoa (order Bivalvulida, class Myxosporea), usually having bilaterally symmetrical spores with two polar capsules at one pole of the spore in a sutural plane. A representative genus is *Myxosoma.*

**platy·staph·y·line** (plat″ĭ-staf′ə-lēn) [*platy-* + *staphyline*] having a broad, flat palate.

**platy·sten·ceph·a·lia** (plat″ĭ-sten″sə-fa′le-ə) platystencephaly.

**platy·sten·ce·phal·ic** (plat″ĭ-sten″sə-fal′ik) exhibiting or pertaining to platystencephaly.

**platy·sten·ceph·a·lism** (plat″ĭ-sten-sef′ə-liz-əm) platystencephaly.

**platy·sten·ceph·a·ly** (plat″ĭ-sten-sef′ə-le) [Gr. *platystatos* widest + *enkephalos* brain + *-ia*] a form of dolichocephalism in which the occiput is very wide and pentagonal, the jaws prognathic; observed among South Africans.

**platy·trope** (plat′ĭ-trōp) [*platy-* + Gr. *trepein* to turn] either of two symmetrical parts on opposite sides of the body; a lateral homologue.

**plau·ra·cin** (plaw′rə-sin) an antibiotic complex produced by *Actinoplanes auranticolor;* used as a veterinary growth stimulant.

**Pla·vix** (pla′viks) trademark for a preparation of clopidogrel bisulfate.

**plec·tron** (plek′tron) [Gr. *plēktron* anything to strike with] the hammer form assumed by certain bacilli during sporulation.

**PLED** periodic lateralized epileptiform discharge.

**pledge** (plej) a solemn statement of intention.
**Nightingale p.**, a statement of principles for the nursing profession, formulated by a committee in 1893 and subscribed to by student nurses at the time of the capping ceremonies.

**pled·get** (plej′ət) a small compress or tuft, as of gauze or cotton.

**pleg·a·pho·nia** (pleg″ə-fo′ne-ə) [Gr. *plēgē* stroke + *aphonia*] auscultation of the chest during percussion over the larynx or trachea in cases in which the patient cannot or is not allowed to speak. The vibrations produced by the percussion take the place of those of the vocal cords.

**-plegia** [Gr. *plēgē* a blow, stroke] a word termination meaning paralysis, or a stroke.

**Pleg·i·sol** (ple′jĭ-sol) trademark for a cardioplegic solution containing sodium, potassium, magnesium, calcium, and chloride.

**plei·a·des** (pli′ə-dēz) [in Greek mythology, seven daughters of Atlas who were placed by Zeus among the stars and form part of the constellation Taurus] a mass of enlarged lymph nodes.

**pleio-** see *pleo-.*

**pleio·chlo·ru·ria** (pli″o-klor-u′re-ə) an excess of chlorides in the urine.

**pleio·tro·pia** (pli″o-tro′pe-ə) pleiotropy.

**plei·o·trop·ic** (pli″o-trop′ik) pertaining to or characterized by pleiotropy; producing many effects in the phenotype.

**plei·ot·ro·pism** (pli-ot′rə-piz-əm) pleiotropy.

**plei·ot·ro·py** (pli-ot′rə-pe) [*pleio-* + *-tropy*] the ability of a gene to manifest itself in more than one way, i.e., to produce more than one phenotypic expression.

**Pleis·toph·o·ra** (plīs-tof′ə-rə) [Gr. *pleistos* most, very many] a genus of parasitic protozoa (suborder Pansporoblastina, order Microsporida) found in the muscles of tropical freshwater fish.

**plek·tron** (plek′tron) [Gr.] plectron.

**Plen·dil** (plen′dil) trademark for a preparation of felodipine.

**pleo-** [Gr. *pleiōn* more] a combining form meaning more, excessive, or multiple. Also, *pleio-.*

**pleo·caryo·cyte** (ple″o-kar′e-o-sīt) pleokaryocyte.

**pleo·chro·ic** (ple″o-kro′ik) pleochromatic.

**pleo·chro·ism** (ple′o-kro″-iz-əm) the condition of being pleochromatic.

**pleo·chro·mat·ic** (ple″o-kro-mat′ik) exhibiting pleochromatism.

**pleo·chro·ma·tism** (ple″o-kro′mə-tiz-əm) [*pleo-* + *chromat-* + *-ism*] the property possessed by some crystals of transmitting one color in one position and the complementary color in a position at right angles to the first.

**pleo·cy·to·sis** (ple″o-si-to′sis) presence of a greater than normal number of cells in the cerebrospinal fluid.

**pleo·karyo·cyte** (ple″o-kar′e-o-sīt) a large nucleated cell found in cachectic disease such as cancer and tuberculosis.

**pleo·mas·tia** (ple″o-mas′te-ə) [*pleo-* + *mast-* + *-ia*] polymastia.

**pleo·mas·tic** (ple″o-mas′tik) polymastic.

**pleo·ma·zia** (ple″o-ma′ze-ə) [*pleo-* + *maz-* + *-ia*] polymastia.

**pleo·mor·phic** (ple″o-mor′fik) [*pleo-* + *morph-* + *-ic*] occurring in various distinct forms; exhibiting pleomorphism.

**pleo·mor·phism** (ple″o-mor′fiz-əm) 1. the assumption of various distinct forms by a single organism or species. 2. in cytomorphology, variation in the size and shape of cells or nuclei. 3. the property of crystallizing in two forms.

**pleo·mor·phous** (ple″o-mor′fəs) pleomorphic.

**pleo·nasm** (ple′o-naz-əm) [Gr. *pleonasmos* exaggeration] polymeria.

**pleo·nex·ia** (ple″o-nek′se-ə) [Gr. "greediness"] a psychiatric disorder characterized by greediness; excessive desire for acquisition of wealth or objects.

**ple·on·os·te·o·sis** (ple″on-os″te-o′sis) [*pleo-* + *oste-* + *-osis*] abnormally increased ossification; premature and excessive ossification.
**Léri's p.,** a hereditary syndrome resulting from premature ossification of epiphyses of the long bones, with broadening and deformity of the digits, flexion contractures of the fingers, broadening and stiffness of the toes and joints, shortening of stature, limitation of movement, and mongolian facies. Inherited as an autosomal dominant trait, the deformities become apparent during the first few years of life.

**pleo·no·tia** (ple″o-no′she-ə) [*pleo-* + *ot-* + *-ia*] a developmental anomaly characterized by the presence of a supernumerary ear located on the neck.

**ple·op·tics** (ple-op′tiks) [*pleo-* + *optics*] a technique of eye exercises designed to develop fuller vision of an amblyopic eye and assure proper binocular cooperation.

**ple·ro·cer·coid** (ple″ro-ser′koid) [Gr. *plēroun* to complete + *cerc-* + *-oid*] the wormlike completed larval stage of certain cestode tapeworms, found in the tissues of vertebrates and invertebrates.

**ple·ro·sis** (ple-ro′sis) the restoration of lost tissue, as after illness.

**Plesch's percussion** (plesh′əz) [Johann *Plesch,* German physician in England, 20th century] see under *percussion.*

**Ple·sio·mo·nas** (ple″se-o-mo′nəs) [Gr. *plēsios* near + *monas* unit, from *monos* single] [MeSH: Plesiomonas] a genus of gram-negative, facultatively anaerobic bacteria of the family Vibrionaceae, consisting of rod-shaped organisms with polar flagella. They are found in the mammalian intestinal tract and in aquatic animals, and may cause diarrhea in humans.
**P. shigelloi′des,** the type species of Plesiomonas, isolated from numerous animal sources and from the human intestinal tract, a cause of infectious diarrhea in humans, especially in tropical and subtropical areas.

**ple·sio·mor·phism** (ple″se-o-mor′fiz-əm) [Gr. *plesios* near + *morph-* + *-ism*] similarity in form.

**ple·sio·mor·phous** (ple″se-o-mor′fəs) pertaining to or characterized by plesiomorphism.

**ples·ses·the·sia** (ples″es-the′zhə) [Gr. *plēssein* to strike + *esthesia*] palpatory percussion; percussion with one hand against a palpating finger of the other hand.

**ples·si·graph** (ples′ĭ-graf) [Gr. *plessein* to strike + *-graph*] a form of pleximeter designed to enable the user to mark out the limits of an area.

**ples·sim·e·ter** (plə-sim′ə-tər) pleximeter.

**ples·si·met·ric** (ples″ĭ-met′rik) pleximetric.

**ples·sor** (ples′or) plexor.

**pleth·o·ra** (pleth′ə-rə) [L.; Gr. *plēthōrē* fullness, satiety] 1. an excess of blood in a part. 2. by extension, a red florid complexion.

**ple·thor·ic** (plə-thor′ik) 1. abundant. 2. containing excessive blood; see *plethora* (def. 1). Called also *sanguine* and *sanguineous.*

**ple·thys·mo·gram** (ple-thiz′mo-gram) a tracing made by the plethysmograph.

**ple·thys·mo·graph** (ple-thiz′mo-graf) [Gr. *plēthysmos* increase + *-graph*] an instrument for determining and registering variations in the volume of an organ, part, or limb and in the amount of blood present or passing through it; also used for recording variations in the size of parts and in the blood supply.
**body p.,** a device for measuring change in body volume, used especially in measuring intrathoracic gas volumes.
**digital p.,** one that registers the change in blood volume taking place in a single finger.
**finger p.,** a digital plethysmograph for a finger.

**ple·thys·mog·ra·phy** (ple″thiz-mog′rə-fe) [MeSH: Plethysmography] the recording of the changes in the size of a part, particularly as modified by the circulation of the blood in it.
**air p., air-cuff p.,** a technique for measuring venous hemodynamics, usually in the legs: with the patient supine with legs elevated, a pneumatic cuff attached to a recording device is applied to the limb; volume changes are recorded during a series of exercises.
**dynamic venous p.,** the measurement of changes in limb circumference in response to exercise or passive compression of the limb.
**impedance p.,** a technique for detecting blood volume changes in a part by measuring changes in electrical resistance; used in the diagnosis of deep venous thrombosis. Electrodes are placed around the calf and a pneumatic cuff around the thigh is inflated just enough to cause venous occlusion and then rapidly deflated. The drop in voltage is recorded; it is smaller in a leg with deep venous thrombosis than in a normal leg.
**strain-gauge p.,** a technique for recording changes in limb circumference employing a rubber tube filled with a conductive fluid; as the tube expands and contracts, the resistance in the fluid changes in proportion to the circumference of the limb; used in the evaluation of deep venous thrombosis and chronic venous insufficiency.
**venous occlusion p.,** the measurement of changes in limb circumference in response to temporary obstruction of venous return.

**pleu·ra** (ploor′ə) gen. and pl. *pleu′rae* [Gr. "rib, side"] [TA] [MeSH: Pleura] the serous membrane investing the lungs and lining the thoracic cavity, completely enclosing a potential space known as the pleural cavity. There are two pleurae, right and left, entirely distinct from each other. The pleura is moistened with a serous secretion which facilitates the movements of the lungs in the chest.
**cervical p.,** cupula pleurae.
**p. costa′lis,** costal pleura: the part of the parietal pleura lining the rib cage.
**p. diaphragma′tica,** diaphragmatic pleura: the part of the parietal pleura covering the diaphragm.
**p. mediastina′lis,** mediastinal pleura: the part of the parietal pleura that covers the lateral face of the mediastinum and the structures within it.
**p. parieta′lis** [TA], parietal pleura: the portion of the pleura lining the walls of the thoracic cavity.
**p. pericardi′aca,** pericardiac pleura: the portion of the mediastinal pleura covering the pericardium and firmly attached to it.
**p. pulmona′lis,** TA alternative for *p. visceralis.*
**pulmonary p.,** p. visceralis.
**p. viscera′lis** [TA], visceral pleura: the portion of the pleura investing the lungs and lining their fissures, completely separating the different lobes; called also *p. pulmonalis* [TA alternative] and *pulmonary p.*

**pleu·ra·cen·te·sis** (ploor″ə-sən-te′sis) thoracentesis.

**pleu·ra·cot·o·my** (ploor″ə-kot′ə-me) thoracotomy.

**pleu·rae** (ploor′e) [L.] genitive and plural of *pleura.*

**pleu·ral** (ploor′əl) pertaining to the pleura.

**pleu·ral·gia** (ploo͝-ral′jə) [*pleur-* + *-algia*] 1. pleurodynia (def. 1). 2. costalgia (def. 2).

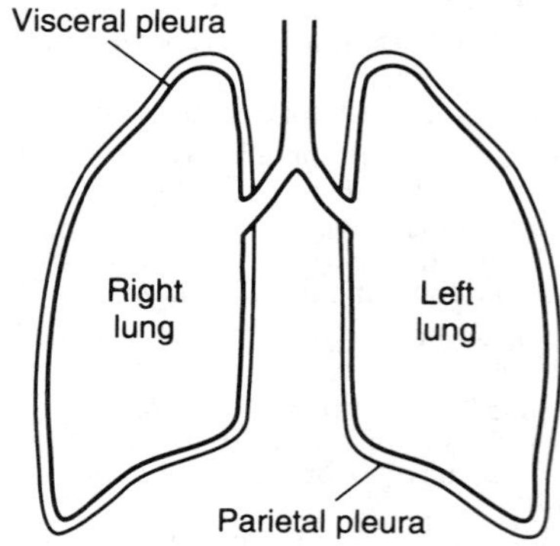


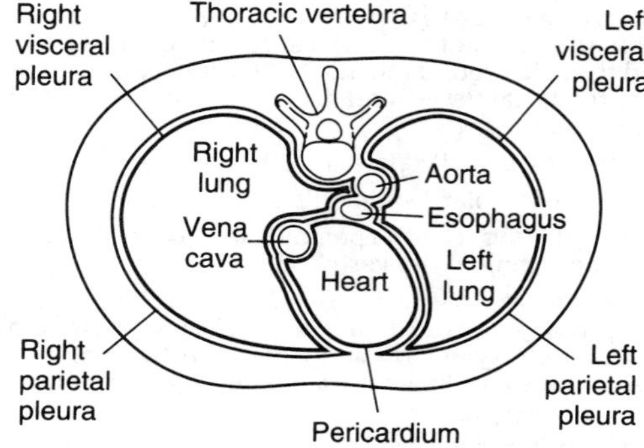


Pleura; for purpose of illustration, the pleural cavity is shown as an actual space.

**pleu·ram·ni·on** (plo͞o-ram′ne-on) an amnion that develops by a process of folding of the somatopleure, a characteristic of many mammals but not man.

**pleu·ra·poph·y·sis** (ploor″ə-pof′ĭ-sis) [*pleur-* + *apophysis*] a rib, or its homologue; a rib considered as part of a vertebra.

**pleu·rec·to·my** (plo͞o-rek′tə-me) [*pleur-* + *-ectomy*] excision of a portion of the pleura.

**pleu·ri·sy** (ploor′ĭ-se) [Gr. *pleuritis*] [MeSH: Pleurisy] inflammation of the pleura, with exudation into its cavity and upon its surface; there are both *dry* and *wet* types (see *dry p.* and *p. with effusion*). The inflamed surfaces of the pleura may become permanently united by adhesions. The symptoms include localized chest pain and dry cough; as effusion occurs there is dyspnea but a diminution of pain. Called also *pleuritis.*
**adhesive p.,** that in which exudate forms dense adhesions between the visceral and parietal pleurae, which partially or totally obliterate the pleural space.
**blocked p.,** encysted p.
**cholesterol p.,** a type resembling pseudochylothorax, with effusion fluid high in cholesterol.
**chylous p.,** chylothorax.
**circumscribed p.,** encysted p.
**costal p.,** inflammation of the parietal pleura.
**diaphragmatic p.,** a variety limited to parts near the diaphragm.
**diffuse p.,** pleurisy in which the inflammation involves the entire surface of the pleura.
**dry p.,** fibrinous p.
**p. with effusion,** pleurisy with a pleural effusion (see under *effusion*); types are named according to the type of exudate, such as *chylous p., hemorrhagic p., purulent p.,* and *serous p.*. Called also *exudative p.* and *wet p.*
**encysted p.,** a form with adhesions that circumscribe the effused material. Called also *blocked p., circumscribed p.,* and *sacculated p.*
**exudative p.,** p. with effusion.
**fibrinous p.,** pleurisy in which exudate forms fibrinous adhesions between the visceral and parietal pleurae, which partially or totally obliterate the pleural space. See also *encysted p.* Called also *adhesive p., dry p.,* and *fibrinous* or *fibrosing pleuritis.*
**hemorrhagic p.,** pleurisy with effusion (q.v.) in which the exudate is bloody. See also *hemothorax.*
**indurative p.,** dry pleurisy marked by thickening and hardening of the pleura.
**interlobular p.,** encysted pleurisy enclosed between the lobes of the lung. Called also *interlobitis.*
**mediastinal p.,** a variety that affects the pleural folds about the mediastinum.
**plastic p., proliferating p.,** dry p.
**pulmonary p.,** inflammation of the pleura that covers the lungs; called also *corticopleuritis* and *visceral p.*
**purulent p.,** empyema (def. 2).
**sacculated p.,** encysted p.
**serofibrinous p.,** pleurisy with effusion (q.v.) with a watery exudate and fibrinous deposits.
**serous p.,** pleurisy with effusion (q.v.) in which the exudate is serous. See also *hydrothorax.*
**suppurative p.,** empyema (def. 2).
**visceral p.,** pulmonary p.
**wet p.,** p. with effusion.

**pleu·rit·ic** (plo͞o-rit′ik) pertaining to or of the nature of pleurisy.

**pleu·ri·tis** (ploo-ri′tis) pleurisy.
**fibrinous p., fibrosing p.,** fibrinous pleurisy.
**lupus p.,** pleurisy, pleural effusion, and fever in patients with systemic lupus erythematosus.
**rheumatoid p.,** pleurisy, pleural effusion, and often empyema in patients with rheumatoid arthritis.
**tuberculous p.,** pleurisy with pleural effusion and multiple tubercles on the pleura in patients with primary tuberculosis.
**uremic p.,** pleurisy, usually of the fibrinous type, with pleural effusion in patients with uremia, often accompanying uremic pericarditis; there are often painful friction rubs and hemothorax.

**pleu·ri·tog·e·nous** (ploor″ĭ-toj′ə-nəs) causing pleurisy.

**pleur(o)-** [Gr. *pleura* rib, side] combining form denoting relationship to the pleura, to the side, or to a rib.

**pleu·ro·bron·chi·tis** (ploor″o-brong-ki′tis) pleurisy and bronchitis combined.

**pleu·ro·cele** (ploor′o-sēl) [*pleuro-* + *-cele*[1]] pneumonocele (def. 1).

**pleu·ro·cen·te·sis** (ploor″o-sen-te′sis) [*pleuro-* + *-centesis*] thoracentesis.

**pleu·ro·cen·trum** (ploor″o-sen′trəm) [*pleuro-* + *centrum*] the lateral element of the vertebral column.

**Pleu·ro·cer·i·dae** (ploor″o-ser′ĭ-de) a family of snails of the order Mesogastropoda that includes the genus *Goniobasis.*

**pleu·ro·cho·le·cys·ti·tis** (ploor″o-ko″le-sis-ti′tis) [*pleuro-* + *cholecystitis*] inflammation of the pleura and the gallbladder.

**pleu·ro·cu·ta·ne·ous** (ploor″o-ku-ta′ne-əs) pertaining to the pleura and the skin.

**pleu·rod·e·sis** (plo͞o-rod′ə-sis) [*pleuro-* + *-desis*] [MeSH: Pleurodesis] the artificial production of adhesions between the parietal and the visceral pleura for treatment of persistent pneumothorax or severe pleural effusion; formerly done by physically irritating the pleural surface, it is now usually done with a chemical sclerosing agent.

**pleur·odont** (ploor′o-dont) [*pleur-* + Gr. *odous* tooth] having teeth attached by one side on the inner surface of the jaw elements, as in certain lizards.

**pleu·ro·dyn·ia** (ploor″o-din′e-ə) [*pleur-* + *-odynia*] 1. pain in the pleural cavity. 2. costalgia (def. 2). Called also *pleuralgia.*
**epidemic p.,** an acute, febrile, infectious disease, generally occurring in epidemics among persons under the age of 20, and characterized by sudden sharp paroxysmal pain in the chest over the ribs or in the upper abdomen; relapses occur frequently after asymptomatic periods. It is caused by infection with group A coxsackieviruses or other enteroviruses. Called also *Bornholm, Daae's,* or *Sylvest's disease, devil's grip,* and *epidemic myalgia.*

**pleu·ro·esoph·a·ge·al** (ploor″o-e-sof″ə-je′əl) pertaining to the pleura and esophagus.

**pleu·ro·eso·pha·ge·us** (ploor″o-e-so-fa′je-əs) [L.] pleuroesophageal; see under *musculus.*

**pleu·ro·gen·ic** (ploor″o-jen′ik) pleurogenous.

**pleu·rog·e·nous** (plo͞o-roj′ə-nəs) [*pleuro-* + *-genous*] originating in the pleura.

**pleu·rog·ra·phy** (plo͞o-rog′rə-fe) [*pleuro-* + *-graphy*] radiographic examination of the pleural cavity.

**pleu·ro·hep·a·ti·tis** (ploor″o-hep″ə-ti′tis) [*pleuro-* + *hepat-* + *-itis*] hepatitis with inflammation of a portion of the pleura near the liver.

**pleu·ro·lith** (ploor′o-lith) [*pleuro-* + *-lith*] a concretion found in the pleura; calcified pleural plaque.

**pleu·rol·y·sis** (plo͞o-rol′ĭ-sis) [*pleuro-* + *-lysis*] surgical separation of pleural adhesions.

**pleu·ro·me·lus** (ploor″o-me′ləs) [*pleuro-* + Gr. *melos* limb] an individual with a supernumerary limb arising laterally from the thorax.

**pleu·ro·pa·ri·e·to·pexy** (ploor″o-pə-ri′ə-to-pek″se) [*pleuro-* + *parieto-* + *-pexy*] fixation of the visceral pleura to the parietal pleura, thus binding the lung to the chest wall. See also *pleurodesis.*

**pleu·ro·peri·car·di·al** (ploor″o-per″ĭ-kahr′de-əl) pertaining to both the pleura and the pericardium.

**pleu·ro·peri·car·di·tis** (ploor″o-per″ĭ-kahr-di′tis) [*pleuro-* + *pericarditis*] inflammation involving both the pleura and the pericardium.

**pleu·ro·peri·to·ne·al** (ploor″o-per″ĭ-to-ne′əl) pertaining to both the pleura and the peritoneum, or communicating with both the pleural and the peritoneal cavity, as a pleuroperitoneal fistula.

**pleu·ro·pneu·mo·nia** (ploor″o-no͞o-mo′ne-ə) [MeSH: Pleuropneumonia] 1. pleurisy complicated with pneumonia; called also *pleuritic pneumonia, pneumonopleuritis,* and *pneumopleuritis.* 2. a contagious disease of cattle and goats caused by infection with *Mycoplasma mycoides;* see *contagious bovine p.* and *contagious caprine p.*
**contagious bovine p.,** pleuropneumonia in cattle, characterized by septicemia, fever, dyspnea, sequestra of infection within the lungs, abnormal lung sounds, and often death.
**contagious caprine p.,** pleuropneumonia in goats, characterized by cough, dyspnea, abnormal lung sounds, and often an early death.

**pleu·ro·pneu·mo·nol·y·sis** (ploor″o-no͞o″mo-nol′ĭ-sis) [*pleuro-* + *pneumono-* + *lysis*] division of adhesions between the lung and the parietal pleura; see also *pleurolysis.*

**pleu·ro·pul·mo·nary** (ploor″o-pul′mə-nar″e) pertaining to the pleura and lungs.

**pleu·ros·co·py** (ploor-os′kə-pe) [*pleuro-* + *-scopy*] thoracoscopy.

**pleu·ro·so·ma** (ploor″o-so′mə) pleurosomus.

**pleu·ro·so·mus** (ploor″o-so′məs) [*pleuro-* + Gr. *sōma* body] a fetus with protrusion of the intestine and imperfect development of one upper limb.

**pleu·ro·thot·o·nos** (ploor″o-thot′ə-nəs) [Gr. *pleurothen* from the side + *tonos* tension] tetanic bending of the body to one side.

**pleu·ro·thot·o·nus** (ploor″o-thot′ə-nəs) pleurothotonos.

**pleu·ro·tin** (plo͞o-ro′tin) a toxic antibiotic obtained from the mushroom *Pleurotus griseus;* it shows activity against staphylococcus (of boils) and tubercle bacillus.

**pleu·ro·tome** (ploor'o-tōm) an area of the lung supplied with afferent nerve fibers by a single posterior spinal root.

**pleu·rot·o·my** (plo͞o-rot'ə-me) thoracotomy.

**pleu·ro·ty·phoid** (ploor"o-ti'foid) acute pleurisy followed by and complicated with typhoid fever.

**pleu·ro·vis·cer·al** (ploor"o-vis'ər-əl) pertaining to the pleura and the viscera.

**plex·al** (plek'səl) pertaining to a plexus.

**plex·ec·to·my** (plek-sek'tə-me) [*plexus* + *-ectomy*] surgical excision of a plexus.

**plex·i·form** (plek'sĭ-form) resembling a plexus or network.

**plex·im·e·ter** (plek-sim'ə-tər) [Gr. *plexis* stroke + *-meter*] 1. a plate to be struck in mediate percussion. 2. a diascope; a glass plate used to show the condition of the skin under pressure.

**plex·i·met·ric** (plek"sĭ-met'rik) pertaining to or performed by a pleximeter.

**plex·im·e·try** (plek-sim'ə-tre) the use of the pleximeter.

**plex·i·tis** (plek-si'tis) inflammation of a nerve plexus.

**plex·o·gen·ic** (plek'so-jen"ik) giving rise to a plexus or plexiform structure.

**plex·om·e·ter** (plek-som'ə-tər) pleximeter.

**plex·op·a·thy** (plek-sop'ə-the) any disorder of a plexus, especially of nerves.
**brachial p.,** any neuropathy of the brachial plexus; see also *brachial paralysis* and *thoracic outlet syndrome.* Called also *brachial plexus neuropathy, brachial syndrome,* and *cervicobrachial syndrome.*
**lumbar p.,** neuropathy of the lumbar plexus.
**lumbosacral p.,** lumbar and sacral plexopathies considered together.
**sacral p.,** neuropathy of the sacral plexus.

**plex·or** (plek'sor) a hammer used in performing percussion.

**plex·us** (plek'səs) pl. *plexus* or *plexuses* [L. "braid"] [TA] a general term for a network of lymphatic vessels, nerves, or veins. See also *net, network,* and *rete.*

## Plexus

Descriptions are given on TA terms, and include anglicized names of specific plexuses.

**annular p.,** a plexus of nerve fibers encircling the corneal margin.
**p. of anterior cerebral artery,** a thin plexus of sympathetic nerve fibers accompanying the anterior cerebral artery.
**aortic p., abdominal,** p. aorticus abdominalis.
**aortic p., thoracic,** p. aorticus thoracicus.
**p. aor'ticus,** a network of lymphatic vessels about the aorta.
**p. aor'ticus abdomina'lis** [TA], abdominal aortic plexus: an unpaired plexus composed of interconnecting bundles of fibers that arise from the celiac and superior mesenteric plexuses and descend along the aorta. Receiving branches from the lumbar splanchnic nerves, it becomes the superior hypogastric plexus below the bifurcation of the aorta. Branches of the plexus are distributed along the adjacent branches of the aorta.
**p. aor'ticus thoraca'lis, p. aor'ticus thora'cicus** [TA], thoracic aortic plexus: a plexus around the thoracic aorta formed by filaments from the sympathetic trunks and vagus nerves, and from which fine twigs accompany branches of the aorta. It is continuous below with the celiac plexus and the abdominal aortic plexus.
**p. arte'riae ova'ricae,** p. ovaricus.
**ascending pharyngeal p.,** a nerve plexus accompanying the ascending pharyngeal artery.
**Auerbach's p.,** p. myentericus.
**auricular p., posterior,** a sympathetic nerve plexus on the posterior auricular artery.
**p. autono'micus** [TA], autonomic plexus: any of the extensive networks of nerve fibers and cell bodies associated with the autonomic nervous system; found particularly in the thorax, abdomen, and pelvis, and containing sympathetic, parasympathetic, and visceral afferent fibers.
**p. basila'ris** [TA], basilar plexus: a venous plexus of the dura mater situated over the basilar part of the occipital bone and the posterior portion of the body of the sphenoid, extending from the cavernous sinus to the foramen magnum, and communicating with other dural sinuses.
**Batson's p.,** the vertebral plexus (def. 1), considered as a whole system.
**biliary p.,** a network of bile ducts said to be sometimes observable in the liver.
**p. brachia'lis** [TA], brachial plexus: a plexus originating from the ventral branches of the last four cervical spinal nerves and most of the ventral branch of the first thoracic spinal nerves. Situated partly in the neck and partly in the axilla, it is composed successively of ventral branches and trunks (supraclavicular part) which are related to the subclavian artery and which give off the dorsal scapular, long thoracic, subclavius, and suprascapular nerves. The infraclavicular part consists of divisions which lie approximately behind the clavicle and cords and branches in the axilla in relation to the axillary artery. Its branches are medial and lateral pectoral, medial brachial cutaneous, medial antebrachial cutaneous, median, ulnar radial, subscapular, thoracodorsal, and axillary nerves.
**cardiac p.,** p. cardiacus.
**cardiac p., anterior,** superficial cardiac p.
**cardiac p., deep, cardiac p., great,** the larger part of the cardiac plexus, situated between the aortic arch and the tracheal bifurcation.

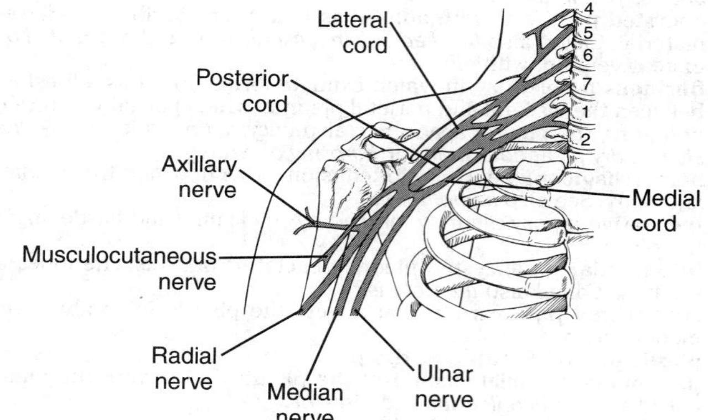


Plexus brachialis (brachial plexus). Anterior view, showing the most major branches.

**cardiac p., superficial,** the part of the cardiac plexus that lies beneath the aortic arch to the right of the ligamentum arteriosum.
**p. cardi'acus** [TA], cardiac plexus: the plexus around the base of the heart, chiefly in the epicardium. It is formed by cardiac branches from the vagus nerves and the sympathetic trunks and ganglia, contains visceral afferent fibers, and shows subdivisions related to the arch of the aorta, right and left atria, and right and left coronary arteries. The cardiac plexus is continuous with the right and left pulmonary plexuses.
**p. caro'ticus commu'nis** [TA], common carotid plexus: a nerve plexus on the common carotid artery, formed by branches of the internal and external carotid plexuses and the cervical sympathetic ganglia.
**p. caro'ticus exter'nus** [TA], external carotid plexus: a nerve plexus located around the external carotid artery, formed by the external carotid nerves from the superior cervical ganglion, and supplying sympathetic fibers which accompany the branches of the external carotid artery.
**p. caro'ticus inter'nus** [TA], internal carotid plexus: a nerve plexus on the internal carotid artery, formed by the internal carotid nerve, which supplies sympathetic fibers to the branches of the internal carotid artery, to the tympanic plexus, to the nerves in the cavernous sinus, and, directly or indirectly, to the cranial parasympathetic ganglia through which they pass.
**carotid p.,** p. caroticus internus.
**carotid p., common,** p. caroticus communis.
**carotid p., external,** p. caroticus externus.
**carotid p., internal,** p. caroticus internus.
**p. caverno'sus** [TA], a plexus of sympathetic nerve fibers related to the cavernous sinus of the dura mater.
**p. caverno'sus con'chae** [TA], cavernous plexus of concha: any of

the numerous venous plexuses in the thick mucous membrane of the nasal conchae.

**cavernous p.,** p. cavernosus.

**cavernous p. of concha,** p. cavernosus conchae.

**celiac p., p. celi'acus,** p. coeliacus.

**cervical p.,** p. cervicalis.

**cervical p., posterior,** a plexus in the posterior cervical region, formed by dorsal rami of the first three or four cervical spinal nerves.

**p. cervica'lis** [TA], cervical plexus: a nerve plexus formed by the ventral branches of the upper four cervical nerves; arranged as an irregular series of loops, it gives off superficial branches (lesser occipital, greater auricular, transverse cervical, and supraclavicular nerves), and deep branches (phrenic, accessory phrenic, ansa cervicalis, and muscular nerves).

**choroid p's,** infoldings of blood vessels of the pia mater covered by a thin coat of ependymal cells that form tufted projections into the third, fourth, and lateral ventricles of the brain; they are supplied by the choroidal arteries, and they secrete the cerebrospinal fluid. See *p. choroideus ventriculi lateralis, p. choroideus ventriculi tertii,* and *p. choroideus ventriculi quarti.*

**choroid p., inferior,** p. choroideus ventriculi quarti.

**p's of choroid artery,** delicate nerve plexuses accompanying the choroid arteries.

**choroid p. of fourth ventricle,** p. choroideus ventriculi quarti.

**choroid p. of lateral ventricle,** p. choroideus ventriculi lateralis.

**choroid p. of third ventricle,** p. choroideus ventriculi tertii.

**p. choroi'deus ventri'culi latera'lis** [TA], choroid plexus of lateral ventricle: vascular, fringelike folds of the pia mater in the floor of the pars centralis and the roof of the temporal horn of the lateral ventricle, concerned with production of the cerebrospinal fluid.

**p. choroi'deus ventri'culi quar'ti** [TA], choroid plexus of fourth ventricle: vascular fringelike folds of the pia mater in the roof of the posterior part of the fourth ventricle and extending into and through the lateral recesses, concerned with production of the cerebrospinal fluid.

**p. choroi'deus ventri'culi ter'tii** [TA], choroid plexus of third ventricle: vascular, fringelike folds of the pia mater in the roof of the third ventricle, concerned with production of the cerebrospinal fluid.

**ciliary ganglionic p.,** an autonomic plexus derived from the long and short ciliary nerves, lying on the ciliary muscle, and supplying the dilator and sphincter muscles of the pupil.

**p. coccy'geus** [TA], coccygeal plexus: a small plexus formed by the ventral branches of the coccygeal and the fifth sacral nerves, and a communication from the fourth sacral nerve, and giving off the anococcygeal nerves.

**p. coeli'acus,** 1. [TA] celiac plexus: a prevertebral plexus that lies on the front and sides of the aorta at the origins of the celiac trunk and superior mesenteric and renal arteries. It contains the paired celiac ganglia, the superior mesenteric ganglion (or ganglia), and small unnamed ganglionic masses. Branches of the plexus extend along all of the adjacent arteries. Called also *solar p.* Also spelled *p. celiacus.* 2. a plexus composed of lymphatic vessels, the superior mesenteric lymph nodes, and the celiac lymph nodes behind the stomach, duodenum, and pancreas. Called also *celiac p.* and *p. celiacus.*

**colic p., left,** the part of the inferior mesenteric plexus that accompanies the left colic artery.

**colic p., middle,** the part of the superior mesenteric plexus that accompanies the middle colic artery.

**colic p., right,** the part of the superior mesenteric plexus that accompanies the right colic artery.

**coronary p's, gastric,** p. gastrici.

**coronary p. of heart, anterior,** a plexus of sympathetic nerve fibers anterior to the heart and related chiefly to the branches of the left coronary artery. Called also *right coronary p. of heart.*

**coronary p. of heart, left,** posterior coronary p. of heart.

**coronary p. of heart, posterior,** a plexus of sympathetic nerve fibers posterior to the heart and related chiefly to the branches of the right coronary artery. Called also *left coronary p. of heart.*

**coronary p. of heart, right,** anterior coronary p. of heart.

**coronary p's of stomach, superior,** p. gastrici.

**crural p.,** p. femoralis.

**Cruveilhier's p.,** posterior cervical p.

**cystic p.,** a nerve plexus near the gallbladder, related to the cystic artery.

**p. deferentia'lis** [TA], deferential plexus: the subdivision of the inferior hypogastric plexus that supplies nerve fibers to the ductus deferens. Called also *p. of ductus deferens.*

**p. denta'lis infe'rior** [TA], inferior dental plexus: a plexus of nerve fibers from the inferior alveolar nerve, situated around the roots of the lower teeth.

**p. denta'lis supe'rior** [TA], superior dental plexus: a plexus of fibers from the superior alveolar nerves, situated around the roots of the upper teeth.

**diaphragmatic p.,** phrenic p.

**p. of ductus deferens,** p. deferentialis.

**p. ente'ricus** [TA], enteric plexus: a plexus of autonomic nerve fibers within the wall of the digestive tube, and made up of the submucosal, myenteric, and subserosal plexuses; it contains visceral afferent fibers, sympathetic postganglionic fibers, parasympathetic preganglionic and postganglionic fibers, and parasympathetic postganglionic cell bodies.

**epigastric p.,** p. coeliacus.

**esophageal p., p. esophagea'lis, p. esopha'geus,** p. oesophageus.

**Exner's p.,** superficial tangential fibers in the molecular layer of the cerebral cortex; called also *molecular p.*

**facial p., p. of facial artery,** a nerve plexus along the facial artery.

**p. femora'lis** [TA], femoral plexus: a plexus accompanying the femoral artery, derived chiefly from the aortic plexus by way of the common and external iliac plexuses.

**gastric p's,** p. gastrici.

**gastric p., inferior,** the inferior portion of the gastric plexuses, located on the greater curvature of the stomach.

**gastric p., left,** superior gastric p.

**gastric p., superior,** the superior portion of the gastric plexuses, accompanying the left gastric artery on the lesser curvature of the stomach; called also *left gastric p.*

**p. gas'trici** [TA], gastric plexuses: subdivisions of the celiac portion of the prevertebral plexuses, accompanying the gastric arteries and branches and supplying nerve fibers to the stomach.

**gastroepiploic p., left,** inferior gastric p.

**Heller's p.,** an arterial network in the submucosa of the intestine.

**hemorrhoidal p.,** p. venosus rectalis.

**hemorrhoidal p., middle,** p. rectalis medius.

**hemorrhoidal p., superior,** p. rectalis superior.

**p. hepa'ticus** [TA], hepatic plexus: a subdivision of the celiac plexus accompanying the hepatic artery to the liver.

**Hovius' p.,** a venous plexus in the ciliary region connected with the sinus venosus sclerae. Called also *Leber's p.*

**p. hypogas'tricus,** 1. hypogastric plexus: the hypogastric portion of the prevertebral plexuses; see *p. hypogastricus inferior* and *p. hypogastricus superior.* 2. a plexus of lymphatic vessels in the hypogastric region.

**p. hypogas'tricus infe'rior** [TA], inferior hypogastric plexus: the plexus formed on each side at the front of the lower part of the sacrum by the junction of the hypogastric and pelvic splanchnic nerves; branches are given off to the pelvic organs. Called also *pelvic p., p. pelvicus* [TA alternative] and *p. pelvina.*

**p. hypogas'tricus supe'rior** [TA], superior hypogastric plexus: the downward continuation of the aortic plexus; it lies in front of the upper part of the sacrum, just below the bifurcation of the aorta, receives fibers from the lower lumbar splanchnic nerves, and divides into the right and left hypogastric nerves. Called also *nervus presacralis* [TA alternative] or *presacral nerve.*

**ileocolic p.,** the part of the superior mesenteric plexus that accompanies the ileocolic artery.

**p. ili'acus** [TA], iliac plexus: any of the plexuses derived chiefly from the aortic plexus and accompanying the common iliac arteries.

**p. ili'acus exter'nus,** a lymphatic plexus situated about the external iliac vessels.

**incisive p.,** a branch of the inferior dental plexus, innervating the canine and incisor teeth of the lower jaw.

**infraorbital p.,** a nerve plexus situated deep to the levator labii superioris muscle, formed by superior labial branches of the infraorbital nerve and branches of the facial nerve.

**p. inguina'lis,** inguinal plexus: a lymphatic plexus situated near the end of the long saphenous vein and along the femoral artery and vein in the iliopectineal fossa.

**intercavernous p.,** a network of venous channels connecting the two cavernous sinuses across both the roof and the floor of the pituitary fossa.

**intermesenteric p., lumboaortic,** p. aorticus abdominalis.

**p. intermesente'ricus** [TA], intermesenteric plexus: the part of the aortic plexus that is located between the origins of the superior and inferior mesenteric arteries.

**interradial p.,** either of the two striae of Baillarger, external or internal; see *stria laminae granularis internae* and *stria laminae pyramidalis internae.*

**intestinal p., submucous,** p. submucosus.

**intramural p.,** a plexus of autonomous intrinsic nerve cells and fibers which are confined entirely to the intestinal and bladder walls, and which take part in or regulate local reflexes and activity.

**p. intraparoti'deus** [TA], parotid plexus: a plexus formed by anastomosis of the terminal branches of the temporal, zygomatic, buccal, marginal mandibular, and cervical rami of the facial nerve, arising in the parotid gland. Called also *p. parotideus.*

**intrascleral p.,** a network of vessels in the sclera, receiving junctional branches from the sinus venosus sclerae.

**ischiadic p.,** p. sacralis.

**Jacobson's p.**, p. tympanicus.

**p. jugula'ris**, jugular plexus: a plexus of lymphatic vessels along the internal jugular vein.

**Leber's p.**, Hovius' p.

**lienal p.**, p. splenicus.

**p. liena'lis**, TA alternative for *p. splenicus.*

**lingual p.**, a nerve plexus accompanying the lingual artery.

**p. lumba'lis**, 1. [TA] lumbar plexus: a plexus formed by the ventral branches of the second to fifth lumbar nerves in the psoas major muscle (the branches of the first lumbar nerve often are included). The lower division of the fourth lumbar nerve joins the fifth, and the lumbosacral trunk thus formed becomes part of the sacral plexus. The branches of the first lumbar nerve are the ilioinguinal and iliohypogastric nerves; branches of the plexus proper are the genitofemoral, lateral femoral cutaneous, obturator, and femoral nerves. 2. a lymphatic plexus in the lumbar region.

**p. lumba'ris**, p. lumbalis (def. 1).

**p. lumbosacra'lis** [TA], lumbosacral plexus: a term applied to the lumbar and sacral nerve plexuses together, because of their continuous nature.

**lymphatic p.**, an interconnecting network of lymph vessels, i.e., the lymphocapillary vessels, collecting vessels, and trunks, which provides drainage of lymph in a one-way flow.

**p. lympha'ticus axilla'ris** [TA], axillary lymphatic plexus: a plexus of lymph vessels and nodes in the fossa axillaris.

**maxillary p.**, a nerve plexus that accompanies the maxillary artery.

**maxillary p., external**, p. of facial artery.

**p. of medial cerebral artery**, a thin plexus of sympathetic nerve fibers accompanying the middle cerebral artery.

**Meissner's p.**, p. submucosus.

**meningeal p.**, a nerve plexus accompanying the middle meningeal artery.

**p. mesente'ricus infe'rior** [TA], inferior mesenteric plexus: a subdivision of the aortic plexus accompanying the inferior mesenteric artery.

**p. mesenter'icus supe'rior** [TA], superior mesenteric plexus: a subdivision of the celiac plexus accompanying the superior mesenteric artery.

**molecular p.**, Exner's p.

**p. myente'ricus** [TA], myenteric plexus: that part of the enteric plexus within the tunica muscularis. Called also *Auerbach's p.*

**nasopalatine p.**, a nerve plexus near the incisor foramen.

**nerve p.**, a plexus made up of intermingled nerve fibers.

**p. nervo'rum spina'lium** [TA], plexus of spinal nerves: a plexus formed by the intermingling of the fibers of two or more spinal nerves, such as the brachial or lumbosacral plexus.

**nervous p.**, nerve p.

**occipital p.**, a nerve plexus accompanying the occipital artery.

**p. oesophagea'lis, p. oesopha'geus** [TA], esophageal plexus: a plexus surrounding the esophagus formed by branches of the left and right vagi and sympathetic trunks and containing also visceral afferent fibers from the esophagus; it is subdivided into anterior and posterior parts.

**ophthalmic p.**, a nerve plexus accompanying the ophthalmic artery.

**p. ova'ricus** [TA], ovarian plexus: a subdivision of the aortic plexus, accompanying the ovarian arteries; called also *p. arteriae ovaricae.*

**p. pampinifor'mis** [TA], 1. pampiniform plexus: in the male, a plexus of veins from the testicle and the epididymis, constituting part of the spermatic cord. 2. in the female, a plexus of ovarian veins in the broad ligament.

**p. pancrea'ticus** [TA], pancreatic plexus: a subdivision of the celiac plexus, accompanying pancreatic arteries.

**Panizza's p's**, two plexuses of the lymph vessels in the lateral fossae of the frenum of the prepuce.

**papillary p.**, superficial vascular p.

**parotid p., p. paroti'deus**, p. intraparotideus.

**patellar p.**, a plexus of nerve fibers in front of the knee, formed by communications between branches of the saphenous nerves and the femoral cutaneous nerves.

**pelvic p.**, p. hypogastricus inferior.

**p. pel'vicus**, TA alternative for *p. hypogastricus inferior.*

**p. pelvi'na**, p. hypogastricus inferior.

**p. periarteria'lis** [TA], periarterial plexus: a network of autonomic and sensory nerve fibers in the adventitia of an artery, some of which follow the course of the artery to reach and innervate other structures and some of which innervate the artery itself.

**pericorneal p.**, anastomosing branches of the anterior conjunctival arteries, arranged in a superficial conjunctival and a deep episcleral layer about the cornea.

**pharyngeal p.**, 1. p. pharyngeus. 2. p. pharyngeus nervi vagi.

**pharyngeal p. of vagus nerve**, p. pharyngeus nervi vagi.

**pharyngeal p., ascending**, a nerve plexus accompanying the ascending pharyngeal artery.

**p. pharyngea'lis**, p. pharyngeus.

**p. pharyngea'lis ner'vi va'gi**, p. pharyngeus nervi vagi.

**p. pharyn'geus** [TA], pharyngeal plexus: a venous plexus posterolateral to the pharynx, formed by the pharyngeal veins, communicating with the pterygoid venous plexus, and draining into the internal jugular vein. Called also *p. pharyngealis.*

**p. pharyn'geus ner'vi va'gi** [TA], pharyngeal plexus of vagus nerve: a plexus formed chiefly by fibers from branches of the vagus nerves, but also containing fibers from the glossopharyngeal nerves and sympathetic trunks, and supplying motor, general sensory, and sympathetic innervation to the muscles and mucosa of the pharynx and soft palate, except for the tensor veli palatini muscle. Called also *p. pharyngealis nervi vagi.*

**phrenic p.**, a nerve plexus accompanying the inferior phrenic artery to the diaphragm and suprarenal glands.

**popliteal p.**, a plexus of nerve fibers accompanying the popliteal artery.

**presacral p.**, p. venosus sacralis.

**prevertebral p's**, autonomic nerve plexuses situated in the thorax, abdomen, and pelvis, anterior to the vertebral column; they consist of visceral afferent fibers, preganglionic parasympathetic fibers, preganglionic and postganglionic sympathetic fibers, and ganglia containing sympathetic ganglion cells, and they give rise to postganglionic fibers. The major plexuses are cardiac, pulmonary, esophageal, celiac, mesenteric, and hypogastric. All are closely related to the aorta; those in the abdomen and pelvis supply adjacent viscera by subdivisions which accompany the branches of the aorta and which are named usually after these branches, but sometimes according to the organ supplied.

**primary p.**, a network of capillaries that arise from the superior

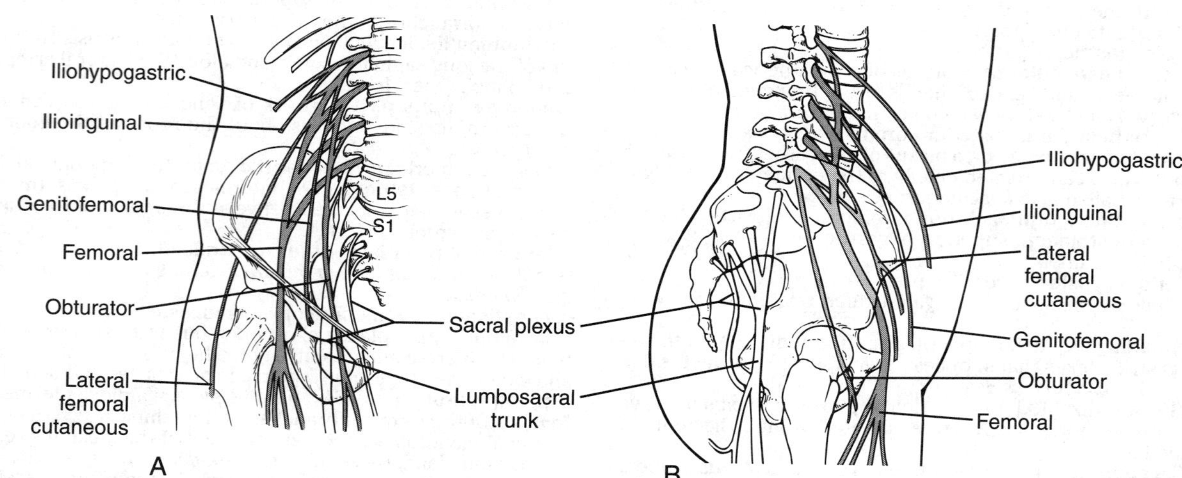


Plexus lumbalis (lumbar plexus) in anterior *(A)* and lateral *(B)* views, with the divisions forming the lumbosacral trunk shown unshaded, as is the sacral plexus.

hypophysial arteries, extend into the median eminence of the hypothalamus, then return to the surface, where they are collected into veins that supply the sinusoids of the adenohypophysis.

**prostatic p.,** 1. p. prostaticus. 2. p. venosus prostaticus.

**prostaticovesical p.,** the plexus venosus vesicalis in the male; called also *vesicoprostatic p.*

**p. prosta'ticus** [TA], prostatic plexus: a subdivision of the inferior hypogastric plexus that supplies nerve fibers to the prostate and adjacent organs. Called also *Santorini's p.*

**p. pterygoi'deus** [TA], pterygoid plexus: a network of veins corresponding to the second and third parts of the maxillary artery; situated on the lateral surface of the medial pterygoid muscle and on both surfaces of the lateral pterygoid muscle, and draining into the facial vein. Called also *p. venosus pterygoideus.*

**pudendal p., p. pudenda'lis,** p. venosus prostaticus.

**p. pulmona'lis** [TA], a nerve plexus formed by several strong trunks of the vagus nerve that are joined at the root of the lung by branches from the sympathetic trunk and cardiac plexus. The plexus is often described as having anterior and posterior parts (see *anterior pulmonary p.* and *posterior pulmonary p.*); filaments from each accompany the blood vessels and bronchi into the lungs.

**pulmonary p., anterior,** the smaller portion of the pulmonary plexus, located in front of the root of the lung and interconnected with the posterior pulmonary plexus.

**pulmonary p., posterior,** the larger portion of the pulmonary plexus, located behind the root of the lung and interconnected with the anterior pulmonary plexus.

**Quénu's hemorrhoidal p.,** a lymphatic plexus found in the perianal skin.

**p. of Raschkow,** a delicate plexus of nerve fibers beneath the odontoblasts in the dental papilla during the formation of dentin.

**p. recta'lis infe'rior** [TA], inferior rectal plexus: a plexus accompanying the inferior rectal artery, derived chiefly from the inferior rectal nerve.

**p. recta'lis me'dius** [TA], middle rectal plexus: a subdivision of the inferior hypogastric plexus, in proximity with and supplying nerve fibers to the rectum; called also middle hemorrhoidal p.

**p. recta'lis supe'rior** [TA], superior rectal plexus: a plexus accompanying the superior rectal artery to the rectum, derived from the inferior mesenteric and hypogastric plexuses. Called also *superior hemorrhoidal p.*

**p. rena'lis** [TA], renal plexus: a subdivision of the celiac plexus, accompanying the renal artery.

**sacral p.,** 1. p. sacralis. 2. p. venosus sacralis.

**sacral p., anterior,** p. venosus sacralis.

**sacral lymphatic p.,** p. sacralis medius.

**p. sacra'lis** [TA], sacral plexus: a plexus that lies in front of the piriform muscle, arising from the ventral branches of the last two lumbar nerves (which form the lumbosacral trunk) and the first four sacral nerves. It has twelve named branches, five supplying pelvic structures (the nerves to the piriformis, to levator ani and coccygeus, and to sphincter ani muscles, the pelvic splanchnic nerves and the pudendal nerve) and seven helping supply the buttocks and lower limbs (superior and inferior gluteal, posterior femoral cutaneous, perforating cutaneous, and sciatic nerves, and nerves to the quadratus femoris and obturator internus muscles).

**p. sacra'lis me'dius,** a fine network of lymphatic vessels in the hollow of the sacrum.

**Santorini's p.,** 1. p. prostaticus. 2. p. venosus prostaticus.

**Sappey's subareolar p.,** a lymphatic plexus situated beneath the areola of the nipple.

**solar p.,** p. coeliacus.

**spermatic p.,** 1. p. testicularis. 2. p. pampiniformis (def. 1).

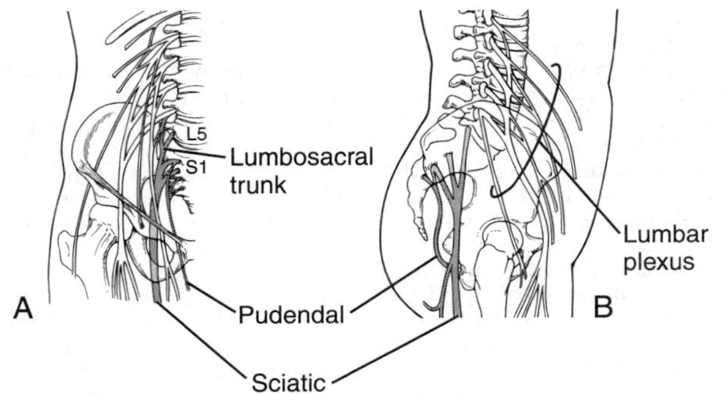


Plexus sacralis (sacral plexus), shaded, in anterior *(A)* and lateral *(B)* views. The lumbar plexus is shown unshaded.

**p. of spinal nerves,** p. nervorum spinalium.

**p. sple'nicus** [TA], splenic plexus: a subdivision of the celiac plexus, which accompanies the splenic artery; called also *lienal p.* and *p. lienalis* [TA alternative].

**Stensen's p.,** the venous network around the parotid duct.

**stroma p.,** superficial and deep nerve fibrils within the substantia propria of the cornea.

**p. subcla'vius** [TA], subclavian plexus: a sympathetic nerve plexus on the subclavian artery, arising from the cervicothoracic ganglion, contributing fibers to the phrenic nerve and to the branches of the subclavian artery, and continuing to the axillary artery.

**subendocardial terminal p.,** rami subendocardiales.

**submucosal p., p. submuco'sus** [TA], submucous plexus: the part of the enteric plexus that is situated in the submucosa.

**subpapillary p.,** superficial vascular p.

**subsartorial p.,** a nerve plexus deep to the sartorius muscle, formed by communications between branches of the medial femoral cutaneous nerve and the saphenous and obturator nerves.

**p. subsero'sus** [TA], subserosal plexus: the part of the enteric plexus situated deep to the serosal surface of the tunica serosa.

**subtrapezius p.,** a term sometimes applied to a small plexus situated deep to the trapezius muscle, formed by communications between branches of the accessory nerve and cervical nerves.

**supraradial p.,** Kaes-Bekhterev layer.

**p. suprarena'lis** [TA], suprarenal plexus: a subdivision of the celiac plexus, in proximity with and supplying nerve fibers to an adrenal (suprarenal) gland.

**temporal p., superficial,** a plexus of nerve fibers accompanying the superficial temporal artery.

**p. testicula'ris** [TA], testicular plexus: a subdivision of the aortic plexus accompanying the testicular arteries; called also *spermatic p.*

**thyroid p., inferior,** a nerve plexus accompanying the inferior thyroid artery to the larynx, pharynx, and thyroid region.

**thyroid p., superior,** a nerve plexus accompanying the superior thyroid artery to the larynx, pharynx, and thyroid region.

**tonsillar p.,** a plexus around the tonsil, formed by communications between the middle and posterior palatine nerves and the tonsillar branches of the glossopharyngeal nerve; fibers are supplied to the tonsil, soft palate, and region of the fauces.

**Trolard's p.,** p. venosus canalis hypoglossi.

**p. tympa'nicus** [TA], **p. tympa'nicus [Jacobso'ni],** tympanic plexus: a nerve plexus on the promontory of the middle ear, formed by the tympanic and caroticotympanic nerves. It gives off the lesser petrosal nerve and a branch of the greater petrosal nerve and sends sensory fibers to the mucous membrane of the tympanic cavity, the auditory tube, and the mastoid air cells.

**p. urete'ricus** [TA], ureteric plexus: a plexus supplying the ureter and derived from the renal and hypogastric plexuses.

**uterine p.,** 1. the part of the uterovaginal plexus that supplies nerve fibers to the cervix and lower part of the uterus. 2. p. venosus uterinus.

**p. uterovagina'lis,** 1. [TA] uterovaginal plexus: the subdivision of the inferior hypogastric plexus that supplies nerve fibers to the uterus, ovary, vagina, urethra, and erectile tissue of the vestibule. 2. see *p. venosus uterinus* and *p. venosus vaginalis.*

**vaginal p.,** 1. the part of the uterovaginal plexus that supplies nerve fibers to the walls of the vagina. 2. p. venosus vaginalis.

**vascular p.,** 1. p. vasculosus. 2. p. vascularis.

**vascular p., deep,** a plexus of arterioles and venules found between the dermis and the tela subcutanea, with many interconnections to the superficial vascular plexus; its arterial part is known as the *cutaneous arterial network* or *arterial network of dermis.*

**vascular p., superficial,** a plexus of arterioles and venules found between the papillary and reticular layers of the dermis, with many interconnections to the deep vascular plexus; its arterial part is known as the *subpapillary network* or *rete.* Called also *papillary* or *subpapillary p.*

**p. vascula'ris** [TA], vascular plexus: a plexus of peripheral nerves through which blood vessels receive innervation.

**p. vasculo'sus** [TA], vascular plexus: a network of intercommunicating blood vessels.

**p. veno'sus** [TA], venous plexus: a network of interconnecting veins.

**p. veno'sus areola'ris** [TA], areolar venous plexus: a venous plexus in the areola around the nipple, formed by branches of the internal thoracic veins and draining into the lateral thoracic vein. Called also *p. venosus mamillae.*

**p. veno'sus cana'lis hypoglos'si** [TA], venous plexus of hypoglossal canal: a venous plexus surrounding the hypoglossal nerve in its canal, and connecting the occipital sinus with the vertebral vein and with the longitudinal vertebral venous sinuses. Called also *rete canalis hypoglossi* and *Trolard's p.*

**p. veno'sus caro'ticus inter'nus** [TA], internal carotid venous plexus: a venous plexus around the petrosal portion of the internal carotid artery, through which the cavernous sinus communicates with the internal jugular vein.

**p. veno'sus fora'minis ova'lis** [TA], venous plexus of foramen ovale: a venous plexus that connects the cavernous sinus through the foramen ovale with the pterygoid plexus and the pharyngeal plexus; called also *rete foraminis ovalis.*

**p. veno'sus mammil'lae,** p. venosus areolaris.

**p. veno'sus prosta'ticus** [TA], prostatic venous plexus: a venous plexus around the prostate gland, receiving the deep dorsal vein of the penis and draining through the vesical plexus and the prostatic veins; called also *p. pudendalis.*

**p. veno'sus pterygoi'deus,** p. pterygoideus.

**p. veno'sus recta'lis** [TA], rectal venous plexus: a venous plexus that surrounds the lower part of the rectum and drains into the rectal veins; called also *hemorrhoidal p.*

**p. veno'sus sacra'lis** [TA], sacral venous plexus: the plexus on the pelvic surface of the sacrum that receives the sacral intervertebral veins, anastomoses with neighboring lumbar and pelvic veins, and drains into the middle and lateral sacral veins.

**p. veno'sus suboccipita'lis** [TA], suboccipital venous plexus: that part of the external vertebral plexus which lies on and in the suboccipital triangle, receives the occipital veins of the scalp, and drains into the vertebral vein.

**p. veno'sus uteri'nus** [TA], uterine venous plexus: the venous plexus around the uterus, draining into the internal iliac veins by way of the uterine veins.

**p. veno'sus vagina'lis** [TA], vaginal venous plexus: a venous plexus in the walls of the vagina, which drains into the internal iliac veins by way of the internal pudendal veins.

**p. veno'sus vertebra'lis exter'nus ante'rior** [TA], anterior external vertebral venous plexus: the venous plexus formed by the anterior external group of veins of the vertebral column that lies on the anterior aspects of the vertebral bodies. See also *venae spinales anteriores.*

**p. veno'sus vertebra'lis exter'nus poste'rior** [TA], posterior external vertebral venous plexus: the venous plexus formed by the posterior external group of veins of the vertebral column that lie on the posterior aspects of the laminae and around the spinous, articular, and transverse processes of the vertebrae. See also *venae spinales posteriores.*

**p. veno'sus vertebra'lis inter'nus ante'rior** [TA], anterior internal vertebral venous plexus: the venous plexus formed by the anterior internal group of veins of the vertebral column that lies on the posterior aspects of the vertebral bodies and intervertebral disks, on either side of the posterior longitudinal ligament. See also *venae spinales anteriores.*

**p. veno'sus vertebra'lis inter'nus poste'rior** [TA], posterior internal vertebral venous plexus: the venous plexus formed by the posterior internal group of veins of the vertebral column that lie on either side of the midline in front of the vertebral arches and ligamenta flava. See also *venae spinales posteriores.*

**p. veno'sus vesica'lis** [TA], vesical venous plexus: a venous plexus surrounding the upper part of the urethra and the neck of the bladder, communicating with the vaginal plexus in the female and with the prostatic plexus in the male.

**venous p.,** p. venosus.

**venous p., areolar,** p. venosus areolaris.

**venous p., hemorrhoidal,** p. venosus rectalis.

**venous p., internal carotid,** p. venosus caroticus internus.

**venous p., prostatic,** p. venosus prostaticus.

**venous p., rectal,** p. venosus rectalis.

**venous p., sacral,** p. venosus sacralis.

**venous p., suboccipital,** p. venosus suboccipitalis.

**venous p., uterine,** p. venosus uterinus.

**venous p., vaginal,** p. venosus vaginalis.

**venous p., vesical,** p. venosus vesicalis.

**venous p. of foot, dorsal,** rete venosum dorsale pedis.

**venous p. of foramen ovale,** p. venosus foraminis ovalis.

**venous p. of hand, dorsal,** rete venosum dorsale manus.

**venous p. of hypoglossal canal,** p. venosus canalis hypoglossi.

**vertebral p.,** 1. a plexus of veins related to the vertebral column; see terms beginning *p. venosus vertebralis.* 2. p. vertebralis.

**vertebral p's, external,** see *p. venosus vertebralis externus anterior* and *p. venosus vertebralis externus posterior.*

**vertebral p's, internal,** see *p. venosus vertebralis internus anterior* and *p. venosus vertebralis internus posterior.*

**p. vertebra'lis** [TA], vertebral plexus: a nerve plexus accompanying the vertebral artery, formed by fibers from the vertebral and cervicothoracic ganglia and carrying sympathetic fibers to the posterior cranial fossa via cranial nerves.

**vesical p.,** 1. p. vesicalis. 2. p. venosus vesicalis.

**p. vesica'le,** p. vesicalis.

**p. vesica'lis,** 1. [TA] vesical plexus: the subdivision of the inferior hypogastric plexus that supplies sympathetic nerve fibers to the urinary bladder and parts of the ureter, ductus deferens, and seminal vesicle; called also *p. vesicale.* 2. p. venosus vesicalis.

**vesicoprostatic p.,** prostaticovesical p.

**vidian p.,** nervus canalis pterygoidei.

**-plexy** [Gr. *plēxis* a stroke] word termination meaning a stroke or seizure.

**pli·ca** (pli'kə) gen. and pl. *pli'cae* [L.] [TA] fold: general anatomical nomenclature for a ridge or fold, as of peritoneum or other membrane.

## Plica

Descriptions are given on TA terms, and include anglicized names of specific folds.

**pli'cae ala'res** [TA], alar folds: a pair of folds of the synovial membrane of the knee joint; attached to the medial and lateral margins of the articular surface of the patella, they pass posteriorly, converge, and become continuous with the infrapatellar synovial fold (see *p. synovialis infrapatellaris*).

**pli'cae ampulla'res tu'bae uteri'nae,** the folds of the mucous coat lining the ampulla of the uterine tube.

**p. aryepiglot'tica** [TA], aryepiglottic fold: a fold of mucous membrane extending on each side between the lateral border of the epiglottis and the summit of the arytenoid cartilage.

**p. axilla'ris ante'rior,** anterior axillary fold.

**p. axilla'ris poste'rior,** posterior axillary fold.

**pli'cae caeca'les** [TA], cecal folds: the folds of peritoneum on either side of the retrocecal recess, which may connect the cecum to the abdominal wall; written also *plicae cecales.*

**p. caeca'lis vascula'ris** [TA], vascular cecal fold: the fold of peritoneum that covers the anterior cecal vessels, forming the superior ileocecal recess; written also *p. cecalis vascularis.*

**pli'cae ceca'les,** plicae caecales.

**p. ceca'lis vascula'ris,** p. caecalis vascularis.

**p. chor'dae tym'pani** [TA], a fold in the mucous membrane of the tympanic cavity overlying the chorda tympani nerve.

**pli'cae cilia'res** [TA], ciliary folds: low ridges in the furrows between the ciliary processes.

**pli'cae circula'res** [TA], **pli'cae circula'res [kerck'ringi], pli'cae conniven'tes,** circular folds: the permanent transverse folds of the luminal surface of the small intestine, involving both the mucosa and submucosa.

**p. cor'dae uteroinguina'lis,** ligamentum teres uteri.

**p. duodena'lis infe'rior** [TA], inferior duodenal fold: a thin fold of peritoneum that bounds the inferior duodenal recess; called also *p. duodenomesocolica* [TA alternative] or *duodenomesocolic fold.*

**p. duodena'lis supe'rior** [TA], superior duodenal fold: a fold of peritoneum covering the inferior mesenteric vein and the ascending branch of the left colic artery; called also *p. duodenojejunalis* [TA alternative] or *duodenojejunal fold.*

**p. duodenojejuna'lis,** TA alternative for *p. duodenalis superior.*
**p. duodenomesoco'lica,** TA alternative for *p. duodenalis inferior.*
**p. epigas'trica,** TA alternative for *p. umbilicalis lateralis.*
**epiglottic p.,** either of the glossoepiglottic folds; see *p. glosso-epiglottica lateralis* and *p. glosso-epiglottica mediana.*
**p. fimbria'ta** [TA], fimbriated fold: the lobulated fold running posteriorly and laterally from the anterior extremity of the frenulum of the tongue.
**pli'cae gas'tricae** [TA], gastric folds: the series of folds in the mucous membrane of the stomach; they are oriented chiefly longitudinally and partially disappear when the stomach is distended.
**p. gastropancrea'tica** [TA], gastropancreatic fold: a crescentic fold of peritoneum formed by the left gastric artery as it runs from the posterior abdominal wall to the lesser curvature of the stomach; called also *left gastropancreatic fold.* Cf. *p. hepatopancreatica.*
**p. glossoepiglot'tica latera'lis** [TA], lateral glossoepiglottic fold: either of two folds of mucous membrane extending, one on either side, between the base of the tongue and the epiglottis.
**p. glossoepiglot'tica media'na** [TA], median glossoepiglottic fold: a single fold of mucous membrane between the two lateral glossoepiglottic folds, connecting the base of the tongue and the epiglottis.
**p. hepatopancrea'tica** [TA], hepatopancreatic fold: a crescentic fold of peritoneum formed by the hepatic artery as it runs forward from the posterior abdominal wall to the lesser omentum; called also *right gastropancreatic fold.* Cf. *p. gastropancreatica.*
**p. hypogas'trica,** p. umbilicalis medialis.
**p. ileocaeca'lis** [TA], **p. ileoceca'lis,** ileocecal fold: a fold of peritoneum at the left border of the cecum, extending from the ileum above to the appendix below.
**p. incudia'lis** [TA], **p. incu'dis,** incudal fold: a variable fold in the tunica mucosa of the tympanic cavity, passing from the roof of the cavity to the body and short crus of the incus.
**infrapatellar p.,** p. synovialis infrapatellaris.
**p. interarytenoi'dea** [TA], interarytenoid fold: a median fold formed by mucous membrane anterior to the transverse arytenoid muscle as it protrudes into the larynx as the muscle approximates the arytenoid cartilages.
**p. interurete'rica** [TA], interureteric fold: a fold of mucous membrane extending across the bladder between the two ureteric orifices, produced by a transverse bundle of muscle fibers; called also *p. ureterica* and *interureteric ridge.*
**pli'cae i'ridis** [TA], iridial folds: the numerous minute folds on the posterior surface of the iris.
**p. lacrima'lis** [TA], **p. lacrima'lis [Has'neri],** lacrimal fold: a fold of mucous membrane at the lower opening of the nasolacrimal duct.
**p. longitudina'lis duode'ni** [TA], longitudinal fold of duodenum: a mucosal ridge running longitudinally on the inner surface of the medial wall of the descending part of the duodenum.
**p. luna'ta,** p. semilunaris conjunctivae.
**p. mallea'ris ante'rior membra'nae tym'panicae** [TA], anterior malleolar fold of tympanic membrane: the line in the tympanic membrane that extends anteriorly from the mallear prominence and demarks the pars tensa from the pars flaccida.
**p. mallea'ris ante'rior tu'nicae muco'sae cavita'tis tympa'nicae** [TA], anterior malleolar fold of mucous coat of tympanic cavity: a fold in the tunica mucosa of the tympanic cavity, reflected from the tympanic membrane over the anterior process and ligament of the malleus and part of the chorda tympani nerve.
**p. mallea'ris poste'rior membra'nae tym'panicae** [TA], posterior malleolar fold of tympanic membrane: the line in the tympanic membrane that extends posteriorly from the mallear prominence and demarks the pars tensa from the pars flaccida.
**p. mallea'ris poste'rior tu'nicae muco'sae cavita'tis tympan'icae** [TA], posterior malleolar fold of mucous coat of tympanic cavity: a fold of the tunica mucosa of the tympanic cavity, extending from the manubrium of the malleus to the posterior wall of the cavity.
**mediopatellar p.,** p. synovialis mediopatellaris.
**p. membra'nae tym'pani exter'na ante'rior,** p. mallearis anterior membranae tympanicae.
**p. membra'nae tym'pani exter'na poste'rior,** p. mallearis posterior membranae tympanicae.
**pli'cae muco'sae vesi'cae bilia'ris** [TA], folds of tunica mucosa of gallbladder: the folds in the mucosa that bound the polygonal spaces, giving the interior a honeycombed appearance; called also *plicae mucosae vesicae felleae* [TA alternative] and *rugae vesicae biliaris* [TA alternative].
**pli'cae muco'sae vesi'cae fel'leae,** TA alternative for *plicae mucosae vesicae biliaris.*
**p. ner'vi laryn'gei supe'rior** [TA], a fold of mucous membrane in the larynx, overlying the superior laryngeal nerve.
**pli'cae palati'nae transver'sae** [TA], transverse palatine folds: four to six transverse ridges on the anterior part of the hard palate. Called also *palatine folds, palatine rugae,* and *rugae palatinae.*
**pli'cae palma'tae** [TA], palmate folds: a system of folds on the anterior and posterior walls of the cervical canal of the uterus, consisting of a median longitudinal ridge and shorter elevations extending laterally and upward. Called also *arbor vitae uteri.*
**p. palpebronasa'lis** [TA], epicanthus.
**p. paraduodena'lis** [TA], paraduodenal fold: an occasionally found peritoneal fold containing a branch of the left colic artery; see also *Treitz's arch,* under *arch.*
**p. pubovesica'lis,** a fold of peritoneum between the pubis and bladder.
**pli'cae rec'ti,** see *plicae transversae recti.*
**p. rectouteri'na** [TA], **p. rectouteri'na [Doug'lasi],** rectouterine fold: a crescentic fold of peritoneum extending from the rectum to the base of the broad ligament on either side, forming the rectouterine pouch.
**p. salpingopalati'na** [TA], salpingopalatine fold: the mucosal fold passing caudally from the auditory tube to the lateral pharyngeal wall.
**p. salpingopharyn'gea** [TA], salpingopharyngeal fold: a mucosal fold passing caudally from the posterior lip of the pharyngeal orifice of the auditory tube to the lateral pharyngeal wall.
**pli'cae semiluna'res co'li** [TA], semilunar folds of colon: crescentic folds in the wall of the large intestine, projecting into the lumen between the haustra.
**p. semiluna'ris conjuncti'vae** [TA], semilunar fold of conjunctiva: a fold of mucous membrane at the medial angle of the eye.
**p. semiluna'ris fau'cium** [TA], semilunar fold of fauces: a curved fold interconnecting the palatoglossal and palatopharyngeal arches and forming the upper boundary of the supratonsillar fossa.
**pli'cae sigmoi'deae co'li,** plicae semilunares coli.
**p. spira'lis** [TA], spiral fold: a spirally arranged elevation in the mucosa of the first part of the cystic duct; called also *valvula spiralis [Heisteri].*
**p. stapedia'lis** [TA], **p. stape'dis,** stapedial fold: a mucosal fold that passes from the posterior wall of the tympanic cavity along the tympanic membrane and surrounds the stapes.
**p. sublingua'lis** [TA], sublingual fold: the elevation on the floor of the mouth under the tongue, covering part of the sublingual gland and containing its excretory ducts.
**suprapatellar p.,** p. synovialis suprapatellaris.
**p. synovia'lis** [TA], synovial fold: an extension of the synovial membrane from its free inner surface into the joint cavity.
**p. synovia'lis infrapatella'ris** [TA], infrapatellar synovial fold: a large process of synovial membrane, containing some fat, which projects into the knee joint; attached to the infrapatellar adipose body, it passes posteriorly and superiorly to the intercondylar fossa of the femur.
**p. synovia'lis mediopatella'ris,** mediopatellar synovial fold: a fold of synovial membrane in the knee joint, extending obliquely along the medial wall of the joint and inserting on the synovial lining of the infrapatellar fat pad.
**p. synovia'lis suprapatella'ris,** suprapatellar synovial fold: a widely variable fold of synovial membrane in the knee joint, most often occurring as a crescent-shaped medial fold extending from the inferior surface of the quadriceps tendon to the medial edge of the knee joint.
**pli'cae transver'sae rec'ti** [TA], **pli'cae transversa'les rec'ti,** transverse folds of rectum: permanent transverse folds in the rectum, usually three in number (two on the left and one on the right), involving the tunica mucosa and tela submucosa, and the circular layer of the tunica muscularis. Called also *Houston's valves.*
**p. triangula'ris** [TA], triangular fold: a fold of mucous membrane extending backward from the palatoglossal arch and covering the anteroinferior part of the palatine tonsil.
**pli'cae tuba'les tu'bae uteri'nae, pli'cae tuba'riae tu'bae uteri'nae** [TA], tubal folds of uterine tube: the folds of the mucous lining of the uterine tube, which are high and complex in the ampulla.
**p. umbilica'lis latera'lis,** 1. [TA] lateral umbilical fold: a laterally placed fold of peritoneum on either side of the inferior part of the anterior abdominal wall, overlying the inferior epigastric vessels; called also *p. epigastrica* or *epigastric fold.* 2. p. umbilicalis medialis.
**p. umbilica'lis me'dia,** p. umbilicalis mediana.
**p. umbilica'lis media'lis** [TA], medial umbilical fold: the fold of peritoneum that covers the obliterated umbilical artery.
**p. umbilica'lis media'na** [TA], median umbilical fold: the fold of peritoneum that covers the median umbilical ligament; called also *p. umbilicalis media.*
**p. ura'chi,** p. umbilicalis mediana.
**p. urete'rica,** p. interureterica.
**pli'cae vagi'nae,** rugae vaginales.
**p. ve'nae ca'vae sinis'trae** [TA], fold of left vena cava: a triangular fold of visceral pericardium occurring between the left superior pulmonary vein and the left pulmonary artery and enclosing the ligament of the left vena cava.
**p. ventricula'ris,** p. vestibularis.

**p. vesica'lis transver'sa** [TA], transverse vesical fold: a transverse fold of the peritoneum extending from the bladder onto the pelvic wall when the bladder is empty.
**p. vestibula'ris** [TA], vestibular fold: a fold of mucous membrane covering muscle in the larynx, separating the ventricle from the vestibule; called also *false vocal cord, false vocal fold,* and *p. ventricularis.*
**pli'cae villo'sae gas'tris** [TA], villous folds of stomach: a fine network of furrows demarcating the gastric areas; called also *plicae villosae ventriculi.*
**pli'cae villo'sae ventri'culi,** plicae villosae gastris.
**p. voca'lis** [TA], vocal fold: a fold of mucous membrane covering the vocalis muscle in the larynx, forming the inferior boundary of the ventricle; called also *chorda vocalis, labium vocale,* and *true vocal cord.*

**pli•cae** (pli'se) genitive and plural of *plica.*

**pli•ca•my•cin** (pli″ka-mi'sin) [USP] [MeSH: Plicamycin] an antineoplastic antibiotic, produced by *Streptomyces plicatus,* that binds to DNA and inhibits RNA synthesis in a manner similar to dactinomycin; it is used for treatment of advanced testicular carcinoma. It also has an inhibiting effect on osteoclasts and is used to treat hypercalcemia and hypercalciuria caused by metastatic malignancy or advanced parathyroid carcinoma. Formerly called *mithramycin.*

**pli•cate** (pli'kāt) [L. *plicatus*] plaited or folded.

**pli•cat•ic acid** (plĭ-kat'ik) a water-soluble organic acid found in the wood of *Thuja plicata,* the western red cedar; it causes asthma in susceptible workers.

**pli•ca•tion** (pli-ka'shən) the taking of tucks in any structure to shorten it, or in the walls of a hollow viscus; a folding.

**pli•cot•o•my** (pli-kot'ə-me) [*plica* + *-tomy*] surgical division of the posterior fold of the tympanic membrane.

**pli courbe** (ple ko͞orb) [Fr.] gyrus angularis.

**pli•ers** (pli'ərz) small tong-jawed pincers for bending metals or holding small objects; various forms are much used in dentistry.

**Plim•mer's bodies** (plim'ərz) [Henry George *Plimmer,* English zoologist, 1857–1918] see under *body.*

**plint** (plint) plinth.

**plinth** (plinth) a padded table for a patient to sit or lie on while performing therapeutic exercises.

**-ploid** [Gr. *-ploos* -fold as in *diploos* twofold + *-oid*] a word termination denoting (in adjectives) the condition in regard to degree of multiplication of chromosome sets in the karyotype, or (in nouns) an individual or cell having chromosome sets of the particular degree of multiplication in the karyotype indicated by the root to which it is added, as aneuploid, polyploid.

**ploi•dy** (ploi'de) [MeSH: Ploidies] the status of the chromosome set in the karyotype; used also as a word termination denoting the condition in regard to the degree of multiplication of chromosome sets, as aneuploidy, diploidy, haploidy.

**plom•bage** (plom-bahzh') [Fr., "sealing, stopping"] a former method of collapse therapy in which part of the thoracic cavity was surgically filled with inert material.

**plop** (plop) a dull, faintly explosive sound made on contact by a falling or dropped object.
**tumor p.,** a sound made in early diastole by movement of a pedunculated atrial tumor but easily confused with an opening snap or a third heart sound.

**plo•sive** (plo'siv) a consonantal speech sound produced by closing off the oral cavity and then releasing with a burst of air, such as an initial *p.* Called also *stop.*

**plot** (plot) 1. to locate points on a graph. 2. to draw a graph. 3. a graph so produced.
**box p.,** a graphic representation of a frequency distribution of a set of data; for each group is drawn a rectangle with upper and lower limits representing the interquartile range, horizontal line within the rectangle representing the median, and vertical tails ("whiskers") extending above and below the rectangle representing the minimum and maximum values.
**bull's-eye p.,** a polar map of the entire myocardium arranged in multiple concentric circles, representing thallium distribution in the myocardium during exercise testing. Called also *polar p.*
**Eadie-Hofstee p.,** graphic representation of a linear transformation of the Michaelis-Menten equation (q.v.) of enzyme kinetics; $v$ is graphed as a function of $v$/[S], resulting in an $x$-intercept of $V_{max}/K_m$, $y$-intercept of $V_{max}$, and slope of $-K_m$.
**Lineweaver-Burk p.,** the double reciprocal plot of an enzyme-catalyzed reaction, obtained from the Lineweaver-Burk equation by graphing $1/v$ as a function of 1/[S]. If the reaction obeys Michaelis-Menten kinetics a straight line is obtained with $x$-intercept of $-1/K_m$, $y$-intercept of $1/V_{max}$, and slope of $K_m/V_{max}$. Although unreliable for large values of $1/v$, the plot is widely used. It is also sometimes used in the classification of enzyme inhibitors, which all cause distinctive alterations in the graph.

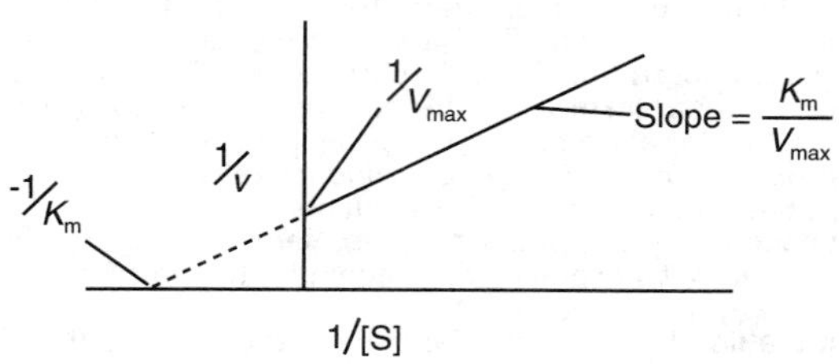

Lineweaver-Burk plot.

**polar p.,** bull's-eye p.
**Scatchard p.,** a graph used in analyzing reversible binding of ligands and receptors, based on the Hill equation where the Hill coefficient is 1.0 (i.e., successive ligands bind independently). The concentration of ligand is varied while that of the receptor is held constant and the ratio of bound to free ligand is plotted as a function of bound ligand.

**plo•to•ly•sin** (plo″to-li'sin) the hemotoxic fraction of plototoxin.

**plo•to•spas•min** (plo″to-spaz'min) the neurotoxic fraction of plototoxin.

**Plo•to•sus** (plo-to'səs) a genus of catfish. *P. linea'tus* is a venomous species found in the Indian and Pacific Oceans; it has plototoxin on its spines and may be deadly to humans or other animals that are cut or scratched by the spines.

**plo•to•tox•in** (plo″to-tok'sin) a toxic substance derived from the catfish *Plotosus lineatus,* said to be composed of a hemotoxic fraction *(plotolysin)* and a neurotoxic fraction *(plotospasmin).*

**PLP** proteolipid protein.

**PLT** 1. primed lymphocyte typing. 2. abbreviation for *p*sittacosis-*l*ymphogranuloma venereum-*t*rachoma (group of organisms); see *Chlamydia.*

**plug** (plug) a lumpy mass that closes or obstructs an opening.
**closing p.,** Schlusskoagulum.
**copulation p.,** vaginal p.
**Dittrich's p's,** yellowish or gray caseous masses of various sizes, consisting of granular debris, fat globules, fatty acid crystals, and bacteria, frequently found in the sputum in cases of bronchiectasis or putrid bronchitis. Called also *Traube's p's.*
**Ecker's p.,** a plug of cells in the primordial mouth of the gastrula.
**epithelial p.,** a mass of ectodermal cells that temporarily closes the external naris of the fetus.
**Imlach's fat p.,** a mass of fatty tissue sometimes found at the mesial angle of the external inguinal ring.
**mucous p.,** 1. a plug formed by secretions of the mucous glands of the cervix uteri and closing the cervical canal during pregnancy. 2. abnormally thick mucus occluding the bronchi and bronchioles, as in asthma or bronchopulmonary aspergillosis.
**Traube's p's,** Dittrich's p's.
**vaginal p.,** a plug that forms in the vaginas of animals, especially rodents, after coitus; it consists of a mass of coagulated sperm and mucus; called also *copulation p.*
**yolk p.,** the mass of yolk cells protruding from the blastopore of amphibians at the end of gastrulation.

**Plugge's test** (plo͞o'gəz) [Pieter Cornelis *Plugge,* Dutch biochemist, 1847–1897] see under *test.*

**plug•ger** (plug'ər) a dental instrument used for packing, condensing, and compacting filling material into a tooth cavity.

**amalgam p.**, one for packing and condensing plastic amalgam in a prepared tooth cavity.

**plum·ba·go** (pləm-ba′go) graphite.

**plum·bic** (plum′bik) [L. *plumbicus* leaden] pertaining to or containing lead.

**plum·bism** (plum′biz-əm) lead poisoning.

**plum·bo·ther·a·py** (plum″bo-ther′ə-pe) [*plumbum* + *therapy*] the therapeutic use of lead, especially its salts.

**plum·bum** (plum′bəm) gen. *plum′bi* [L.] lead[1].

**plu·mer·i·cin** (ploo″mər-i′sin) a principle, isolated from the roots of *Plumeria multiflora* Muell.-Arg., Apocynaceae, which shows *in vitro* activity against fungi and bacteria, including *Mycobacterium tuberculosis*.

**Plum·mer's disease, sign** (plum′ərz) [Henry Stanley *Plummer*, American physician, 1874–1936] see under *disease* and *sign*.

**Plum·mer-Vin·son syndrome** (plum′ər-vin′son) [H.S. *Plummer;* Porter Paisley *Vinson,* American surgeon, 1890–1959] [MeSH: Plummer-Vinson Syndrome] see under *syndrome*.

**plu·mose** (ploo′mōs) [L. *plumosus*, Fr. *pluma* feather] feathery; resembling a feather.

**plum·u·la** (plum′u-lə) a set of delicate cross-furrows occasionally found on the upper wall of the aqueduct of Sylvius.

**pluri-** [L. *plus*, gen. *pluris* more] a combining form meaning several or more.

**plu·ri·glan·du·lar** (ploor″ĭ-glan′du-lər) [*pluri-* + L. *glandula*] pertaining to, derived from, or affecting several glands. Cf. *polyendocrine*. Called also *multiglandular* and *polyglandular*.

**plu·ri·grav·i·da** (ploor″ĭ-grav′ĭ-də) [*pluri-* + *gravida*] multigravida.

**plu·ri·loc·u·lar** (ploor″ĭ-lok′u-lər) multilocular.

**plu·ri·men·or·rhea** (ploor″ĭ-men″o-re′ə) increased frequency of menstrual periods.

**plu·ri·nu·cle·ar** (ploor″ĭ-noo′kle-ər) polynuclear.

**plu·ri·or·i·fi·cial** (ploor″ĭ-or″ĭ-fish′əl) [*pluri-* + *orificial*] pertaining to or affecting several orifices of the body.

**plu·rip·a·ra** (ploo-rip′ə-rə) [*pluri-* + *para*] multipara.

**plu·ri·par·i·ty** (ploor″ĭ-par′ĭ-te) multiparity.

**plu·ri·po·lar** (ploor″ĭ-po′lər) multipolar.

**plu·rip·o·tent** (plo͝o-rip′o-tənt) pluripotential.

**plu·ri·po·ten·tial** (ploor″ĭ-po-ten′shal) pertaining to or characterized by pluripotentiality.

**plu·ri·po·ten·ti·al·i·ty** (ploor″ĭ-po-ten″she-al′ĭ-te) [*pluri-* + L. *potentia* power] 1. possession of the power of developing (as embryonic cells) or acting in any one of several possible ways. 2. affecting more than one organ or tissue.

**plu·ri·re·sis·tant** (ploor″ĭ-re-zis′tənt) resistant to several drugs.

**plu·ri·tis·su·lar** (ploor″ĭ-tis′u-lər) composed of several tissues.

**plu·ri·vis·cer·al** (ploor″ĭ-vis′ər-əl) [*pluri-* + *visceral*] pertaining to or affecting several viscera, or organs.

**plu·to·ni·um** (ploo-to′ne-əm) [named from the planet *Pluto*] [MeSH: Plutonium] a heavy, metallic, radioactive element of atomic number 94, atomic weight 242, obtained by the addition of neutrons to uranium, thereby changing it into neptunium and then into plutonium. Symbol Pu.

**Pm** symbol for *promethium*.

**PMB** polymorphonuclear basophil leukocytes; see *granular leukocytes,* under *leukocyte*.

**PME** polymorphonuclear eosinophil leukocytes; see *granular leukocytes,* under *leukocyte*.

**PMI** point of maximal impulse; see under *point*.

**P mi·trale** (pe mi-tra′le) in electrocardiography, a pattern of abnormally wide, notched P waves, indicative of prolonged depolarization in a large left atrium; it is commonly associated with mitral valve disease.

**PMM** pentamethylmelamine.

**PMMA** polymethyl methacrylate.

**PMN** polymorphonuclear neutrophil leukocytes; see *granular leukocytes,* under *leukocyte*.

**PMR** proportionate mortality ratio.

**PMSG** pregnant mare serum gonadotropin.

**-pnea** [Gr. *pnoia* breath] a word termination denoting relationship to breathing.

**pneo-** [Gr. *pnein* to breathe] a combining form denoting relationship to the breath.

**pneo·gas·ter** (ne′o-gas″tər) [*pneo-* + Gr. *gastēr* the belly] the respiratory tract of the embryo.

**PNET** primitive neuroectodermal tumor.

**pneuma-** see *pneumato-*.

**pneu·mar·thro·gram** (noo-mahr′thro-gram) [*pneumo-* + *arthro-* + *-gram*] a radiograph of a joint after it has been injected with air.

**pneu·mar·throg·ra·phy** (noo″mahr-throg′rə-fe) radiography of a joint after it has been injected with air or gas as a contrast medium; called also *pneumoarthrography*.

**pneu·mar·thro·sis** (noo″mahr-thro′sis) [*pneumo-* + *arthro-* + *-osis*] 1. the presence of gas or air in a joint. 2. the inflation of a joint with air or gas for the purpose of aiding radiographic examination.

**pneu·mat·ic** (noo-mat′ik) [Gr. *pneuma,* gen. *pneumatos,* air, breath] 1. pertaining to air. 2. respiratory.

**pneu·mat·ics** (noo-mat′iks) the science which deals with the physical properties of gases.

**pneu·ma·tin·u·ria** (noo″mə-tĭ-nu′re-ə) pneumaturia.

**pneu·ma·tism** (noo′mə-tiz-əm) [from Gr. *pneuma* air, breath, spirit] a theory, first associated with Empedocles of Acragas, that combines the folk belief of blood's being the seat of innate heat, and the then current philosophical speculation on pneuma, to establish the heart both as center of the vascular system and as the main organ distributing pneuma, life, and heat by the veins, arteries, and nerves. Pneumatism was rejected by the contemporary, growing Coan School (and therefore by Hippocrates of Cos) and by Aristotle, but was accepted by Erasistratus, Diocles, Athenaeus, and ultimately Galen. Pneumatism reigned till William Harvey.

**Pneu·ma·tist** (noo′mə-tist) an eclectic medical school founded by Athenaeus of Attalia on the principle of pneumatism. Agathinus of Sparta, Archigenes of Apamea, Aretaeus of Cappadocia, Erasistratus, and Antyllus were some of its adherents.

**pneu·ma·ti·za·tion** (noo″mə-tĭ-za′shən) the formation of pneumatic cells or cavities in tissue, especially such formation in the temporal bone.

**pneu·ma·tized** (noo′mə-tīzd) 1. filled with air. 2. containing pneumatic cells.

**pneumat(o)-** [Gr. *pneuma,* gen. *pneumatos* breath] combining form denoting relationship to air or gas, or to respiration. Also, *pneuma-*.

**pneu·ma·to·car·dia** (noo″mə-to-kahr′de-ə) [*pneumato-* + *cardia*] the presence of air in the heart.

**pneu·ma·to·cele** (noo-mat′o-sēl) [*pneumato-* + *-cele*[1]] 1. a tumor or cyst formed by air or other gas filling an adventitious pouch, such as a laryngocele, tracheocele, or gaseous swelling of the scrotum. Called also *aerocele* and *pneumocele*. 2. a usually benign, thin-walled, air-containing cyst of the lung, as in staphylococcal pneumonia. Called also *pneumocele* and *pneumonocele*.
**p. cra′nii, extracranial p.,** gaseous tumors beneath the scalp after a fracture of the skull that communicates with the paranasal sinuses.
**intracranial p.,** pneumocephalus.
**parotid p.,** enlargement of the parotid glands as a result of blowing air into the parotid ducts. See also *glass-blowers' mouth,* under *mouth*.

**pneu·ma·to·ceph·a·lus** (noo″mə-to-sef′ə-ləs) pneumocephalus.

**pneu·ma·to·gram** (noo-mat′o-gram) spirogram.

**pneu·ma·to·graph** (noo-mat′o-graf″) spirograph.

**pneu·ma·to·no·me·ter** (noo″mə-tə-nom′ə-tər) [*pneuma-* + *tonometer*] an applanation tonometer in which air pressure applied through a silicone-rubber membrane in direct contact with the cornea is used to flatten the cornea.

**pneu·ma·to·sis** (noo″mə-to′sis) [Gr. *pneumatōsis*] the presence of air or gas in an abnormal situation in the body.
**p. co′li,** p. cystoides intestinalis.
**p. cystoi′des intestina′lis, p. cystoi′des intestino′rum,** the presence of thin-walled, gas-containing cysts in the intestinal wall either subserosally or submucosally. Called also *intestinal emphysema, p. coli,* and *intestinal p.*
**intestinal p., p. intestina′lis,** p. cystoides intestinalis.

**pneu·ma·tu·ria** (noo″mə-tu′re-ə) [*pneumato-* + *-uria*] passage of gas in the urine, usually as a result of a fistula between the bladder and intestine.

**pneu·ma·type** (noo′mə-tīp) [*pneuma-* + Gr. *typos* type] a breath picture; a deposition of moist breath on a glass surface or mirror, used in the diagnosis of nasal obstructions.

**pneu·mec·to·my** (noo-mek′tə-me) [*pneum-* + *-ectomy*] pneumonectomy.

**pneum(o)-** [Gr. *pneuma* breath] a combining form denoting relationship to *(a)* respiration, *(b)* the lungs, *(c)* air, *(d)* pneumonia.

**pneu·mo·al·veo·log·ra·phy** (noo″mo-al″ve-o-log′rə-fe) radiography of the alveoli of the lungs.

**pneu·mo·am·ni·os** (noo″mo-am′ne-os) the presence of gas in the amniotic fluid.

**pneu·mo·an·gi·og·ra·phy** (noo″mo-an″je-og′rə-fe) pulmonary angiography.

**pneu·mo·ar·throg·ra·phy** (noo″mo-ahr-throg′rə-fe) pneumarthrography.

**pneu·mo·ba·cil·lus** (noo″mo-bə-sil′əs) [*pneumo-* + *bacillus*] *Klebsiella pneumoniae.*
**Friedländer's p.,** *Klebsiella pneumoniae.*

**pneu·mo·bil·ia** (noo″mo-bil′e-ə) [*pneumo-* + *bile* + *-ia*] the presence of gas in the biliary system.

**pneu·mo·bul·bar** (noo″mo-bul′bər) pertaining to the lungs and to the respiration center in the medulla oblongata.

**pneu·mo·bul·bous** (noo″mo-bul′bəs) pneumobulbar.

**pneu·mo·car·di·al** (noo″mo-kahr′de-əl) cardiopulmonary.

**pneu·mo·cele** (noo′mo-sēl″) [*pneumo-* + *-cele*[1]] 1. pneumonocele (def. 1). 2. pneumatocele (def. 1). 3. pneumatocele (def. 2).

**pneu·mo·cen·te·sis** (noo″mo-sən-te′sis) [*pneumo-* + *-centesis*] pneumonocentesis.

**pneu·mo·ceph·a·lus** (noo″mo-sef′ə-ləs) [Gr. *pneuma* air + *-cephalus*] [MeSH: Pneumocephalus] the presence of air in the intracranial cavity; called also *intracranial pneumatocele, pneumatocephalus, pneumocrania,* and *pneumoencephalocele.*

**pneu·mo·cho·le·cys·ti·tis** (noo″mo-ko″le-sis-ti′tis) emphysematous cholecystitis.

**pneu·mo·coc·cal** (noo″mo-kok′əl) pertaining to or caused by pneumococci.

**pneu·mo·coc·ce·mia** (noo″mo-kok-se′me-ə) the presence of pneumococci in the blood.

**pneu·mo·coc·ci** (noo″mo-kok′si) plural of *pneumococcus.*

**pneu·mo·coc·cic** (noo″mo-kok′sik) pertaining to or caused by pneumococci.

**pneu·mo·coc·ci·dal** (noo″mo-kok-si′dəl) destroying pneumococci.

**pneu·mo·coc·col·y·sis** (noo″mo-kok-ol′ĭ-sis) [*pneumococcus* + *-lysis*] solubilization of pneumococci.

**pneu·mo·coc·co·sis** (noo″mo-kok-o′sis) infection with pneumococci; see *lobar pneumonia,* under *pneumonia.*

**pneu·mo·coc·co·su·ria** (noo″mo-kok″o-su′re-ə) the presence in the urine of pneumococci or of pneumococcus polysaccharide.

**pneu·mo·coc·cus** (noo″mo-kok′əs) pl. *pneumococ′ci* [*pneumo-* + *coccus*] an individual organism of the species *Streptococcus pneumoniae.*

**pneu·mo·co·lon** (noo″mo-ko′lon) [*pneumo-* + *colon*] the presence of air in the colon, often introduced as an aid to diagnosis.

**pneu·mo·co·ni·o·sis** (noo″mo-ko″ne-o′sis) [*pneumo-* + *coniosis*] [MeSH: Pneumoconiosis] deposition of large amounts of dust or other particulate matter in the lungs, and the subsequent tissue reaction, usually seen in workers in certain occupations and in residents of areas with excessive particulate matter in the air. The definition is usually limited to conditions caused by inorganic dusts, in contrast to those such as byssinosis that are caused by organic dusts. Types range from nearly harmless forms to destructive or fatal conditions and are often named for the implicated substance, such as *aluminosis, anthracosis, asbestosis, graphitosis, siderosis,* or *silicosis.* See table. Called also *pneumokoniosis* and *pneumonoconiosis.*
**antimony p.,** mild pneumoconiosis seen in workers with antimony and its compounds; excessive buildup of antimony in the body may result in antimony poisoning.
**bauxite p.,** a progressive form of pneumoconiosis caused by inhalation of bauxite fumes containing fine particles of alumina and silica. It begins with alveolitis and progresses to emphysema, often with pneumothorax. Called also *bauxite lung, bauxite workers' disease, corundum smelter's lung,* and *Shaver's disease.* Cf. *aluminosis.*
**coal workers' p.,** a form caused by deposition of large amounts of coal dust in the lungs, and typically characterized by centrilobular

**Types of Pneumoconiosis**

| Name | Causative Type of Dust |
|---|---|
| Aluminosis | Aluminum |
| Antimony pneumoconiosis | Antimony |
| Asbestosis | Asbestosis |
| Baritosis | Barium; barite |
| Bauxite pneumoconiosis | Bauxite |
| Cadmiosis | Cadmium |
| Calcicosis | Dusts containing calcium |
| Chalicosis | Miscellaneous stones |
| Coal workers' pneumoconiosis | Coal dust |
| Anthracosis | Anthracite coal |
| Bituminosis | Bituminous coal |
| Cobaltosis | Cobalt |
| Elevator disease | Miscellaneous grains |
| Hard metal disease | Tungsten carbide, titanium carbide, tantalum carbide |
| Kaolin pneumoconiosis (kaolinosis) | Kaolin |
| Mica pneumoconiosis (micatosis) | Mica |
| Polyvinyl chloride pneumoconiosis | Polyvinyl chloride |
| Schistosis | Slate |
| Siderosis | Iron |
| Silicosis | Silica |
| Diatomite fibrosis | Diatomaceous earth |
| Fuller's earth pneumoconiosis | Fuller's earth |
| Graphite pneumoconiosis (graphitosis) | Graphite |
| Hematite pneumoconiosis | Hematite |
| Mixed dust pneumoconioses: | |
| Anthracosilicosis | Anthracite coal, silica |
| Calcicosilicosis | Calcium dusts, silica |
| Labrador lung | Iron, silica, anthophyllite |
| Siderosilicosis | Iron ore, silica |
| Stannosis | Tin oxide |
| Tabacosis | Dried tobacco leaves |
| Talc pneumoconiosis (talcosis) | Talc |
| Titanium dioxide pneumoconiosis | Titanium dioxide |
| Welder's lung | Iron oxide |

emphysema. Different varieties of coal have different risks; those with certain types of contaminants may cause other types of pneumoconiosis. See also *anthracosis* and *bituminosis.* Called also *black, coal miner's,* or *miner's lung.*
**collagenous p.,** that in which permanent scarring results, due to fibrogenic dust, such as asbestos or silica, or to altered tissue response to nonfibrogenic dust.
**fuller's earth p.,** a rare type of silicatosis caused by inhalation of the dust of fuller's earth, seen in workers with long-term heavy exposure.
**graphite p.,** silicosis due to inhalation of graphite dust, which often contains up to 10 per cent silica. Called also *graphitosis* and *graphite fibrosis.*
**hematite p.,** mixed dust pneumoconiosis (silicosiderosis) seen in long-term miners of hematite; some patients show diffuse fibrosis throughout a lung while others show nodules primarily in upper lobes.
**kaolin p.,** silicatosis caused by inhaling particles of kaolin. Called also *kaolinosis.*
**mica p.,** silicatosis due to inhalation of and tissue reaction to mica particles; called also *micatosis.*
**mixed dust p.,** pneumoconiosis that is caused by more than one type of dust, such as anthracosilicosis, calcicosilicosis, or silicosiderosis.
**noncollagenous p.,** that in which the stromal reaction is minimal, consisting chiefly of reticulin fibers.
**polyvinyl chloride p.,** a rare form of pneumoconiosis caused by excessive inhalation of polyvinyl chloride dust.
**rheumatoid p.,** Caplan's syndrome.
**p. sidero'tica,** siderosis, def. 1.
**talc p.,** a type of silicatosis caused by the inhalation of talc; symptoms include shortness of breath, cough, fatigue, weakness, and weight loss. Prolonged exposure may result in pulmonary fibrosis. Called also *talcosis.*
**titanium dioxide p.,** a mild form of pneumoconiosis seen in workers inhaling excessive amounts of titanium dioxide dust.

**pneu·mo·cra·nia** (noo″mo-kra′ne-ə) pneumocephalus.

**pneu·mo·cra·ni·um** (noo″mo-kra′ne-əm) pneumocephalus.

**pneu·mo·cys·ti·a·sis** (noo″mo-sis-ti′ə-sis) interstitial plasma cell pneumonia.

**pneu·mo·cys·tic** (noo″mo-sis′tik) pertaining to or caused by *Pneumocystis.*

**Pneu·mo·cys·tis** (noo″mo-sis′tis) [*pneumo-* + *cyst*] a genus of yeastlike fungi.
**P. cari′nii,** the causative agent of interstitial plasma cell pneumonia, which can also cause extrapulmonary disease in immunocompromised patients.

**pneu·mo·cys·tis** (noo″mo-sis′tis) an individual organism of the genus *Pneumocystis.*

**pneu·mo·cys·tog·ra·phy** (noo″mo-sis-tog′rə-fe) cystography following the injection of air into the bladder.

**pneu·mo·cys·to·sis** (noo″mo-sis-to′sis) interstitial plasma cell pneumonia.

**pneu·mo·cys·to·to·mog·ra·phy** (noo″mo-sis″to-to-mog′rə-fe) tomography after inflation of the bladder with air.

**pneu·mo·cyte** (noo-mo-sīt′) alveolar cell.

**pneu·mo·der·ma** (noo″mo-der′mə) [*pneumo-* + *derma*] subcutaneous emphysema.

**pneu·mo·dy·nam·ics** (noo″mo-di-nam′iks) [*pneumo-* + *dynamics*] 1. the dynamics of the respiratory process. 2. the study of the forces exerted in the process of breathing.

**pneu·mo·em·py·e·ma** (noo″mo-em″pi-e′mə) pyopneumothorax.

**pneu·mo·en·ceph·a·li·tis** (noo″mo-ən-sef″ə-li′tis) Newcastle disease.
**avian p.,** Newcastle disease.

**pneu·mo·en·ceph·a·lo·cele** (noo″mo-en-sef′ə-lo-sēl) [*pneumo-* + *encephalo-* + *-cele*[2]] pneumocephalus.

**pneu·mo·en·ceph·a·lo·gram** (noo″mo-ən-sef′ə-lo-gram) the radiograph obtained by pneumoencephalography.

**pneu·mo·en·ceph·a·log·ra·phy (PEG)** (noo″mo-ən-sef″ə-log′rə-fe) [MeSH: Pneumoencephalography] radiographic visualization of the fluid-containing structures of the brain after cerebrospinal fluid is intermittently withdrawn by lumbar puncture and replaced by air, oxygen, or helium; this procedure is no longer performed, having been replaced by metrizamide cisternography. Abbreviated PEG.

**pneu·mo·en·ceph·a·lo·my·elo·gram** (noo″mo-ən-sef″ə-lo-mi-el′o-gram) the radiograph obtained by pneumoencephalomyelography.

**pneu·mo·en·ceph·a·lo·my·elog·ra·phy** (noo″mo-ən-sef″ə-lo-mi″ə-log′rə-fe) radiographic visualization of the brain and spinal cord after cerebrospinal fluid is removed by lumbar puncture and replaced by gas.

**pneu·mo·en·ceph·a·los** (noo″mo-ən-sef′ə-los) [*pneumo-* + Gr. *enkephalos* brain] pneumocephalus.

**pneu·mo·en·ter·itis** (noo″mo-en″tər-i′tis) [*pneumo-* + *enter-* + *-itis*] inflammation of the lung and intestine.

**pneu·mo·fas·cio·gram** (noo″mo-fas′e-o-gram) a radiograph of tissue after injection of air into the fascial spaces.

**pneu·mo·ga·lac·to·cele** (noo″mo-gə-lak′to-sēl) [*pneumo-* + *galacto-* + *-cele*[1]] a tumor containing gas and milk.

**pneu·mo·gas·tric** (noo″mo-gas′trik) [*pneumo-* + *gastric*] pertaining to the lungs and stomach.

**pneu·mo·gas·trog·ra·phy** (noo″mo-gas-trog′rə-fe) [*pneumo-* + *gastrography*] radiography of the stomach after the injection of air.

**pneu·mo·gram** (noo′mo-gram) 1. a radiogram made after the injection of air into the part. 2. spirogram.

**pneu·mo·graph** (noo′mo-graf) spirograph.

**pneu·mog·ra·phy** (noo-mog′rə-fe) 1. radiography of a part after injection of a gas. 2. spirography.
**cerebral p.,** radiography of the brain by pneumoencephalography or ventriculography.
**retroperitoneal p.,** radiography of the abdominal organs after retroperitoneal injection of air or oxygen.

**pneu·mo·gy·no·gram** (noo″mo-gi′no-gram) a radiograph of the female reproductive organs after injection of air into the uterus.

**pneu·mo·he·mia** (noo″mo-he′me-ə) [*pneumo-* + *hem-* + *-ia*] air embolism.

**pneu·mo·he·mo·peri·car·di·um** (noo″mo-he″mo-per″ĭ-kahr′de-əm) [*pneumo-* + *hemo-* + *pericardium*] the presence of air or gas and blood in the pericardial cavity.

**pneu·mo·he·mo·tho·rax** (noo″mo-he″mo-thor′aks) hemopneumothorax.

**pneu·mo·hy·dro·me·tra** (noo″mo-hi″dro-me′trə) [*pneumo-* + *hydro-* + *metra*] a collection of gas and fluid in the uterine cavity.

**pneu·mo·hy·dro·peri·car·di·um** (noo″mo-hi″dro-per″ĭ-kahr′de-əm) [*pneumo-* + *hydro-* + *pericardium*] the presence of air or gas and fluid in the pericardial cavity.

**pneu·mo·hy·dro·tho·rax** (noo″mo-hi″dro-thor′aks) hydropneumothorax.

**pneu·mo·kid·ney** (noo″mo-kid′ne) [*pneumo-* + *kidney*] the presence of gas in the kidney pelvis.

**pneu·mo·ko·ni·o·sis** (noo″mo-ko″ne-o′sis) pneumoconiosis.

**pneu·mo·lith** (noo′mo-lith) [*pneumo-* + *-lith*] a calculus or concretion in the lung, usually composed of calcium salts. Called also *lung calculus* and *pulmolith.*

**pneu·mo·li·thi·a·sis** (noo″mo-lĭ-thi′ə-sis) the presence of concretions in the lungs.

**pneu·mol·o·gy** (noo-mol′ə-je) [*pneumo-* + *-logy*] the study of disease of the air passages.

**pneu·mol·y·sis** (noo-mol′ĭ-sis) pneumonolysis.

**pneu·mo·ma·la·cia** (noo″mo-mə-la′shə) [*pneumo-* + *-malacia*] morbid softening of lung tissue.

**pneu·mo·mas·sage** (noo″mo-mə-sahzh′) [*pneumo-* + *massage*] air massage of the tympanum by the alternate compression and rarefaction of the air in the external auditory canal. Called also *pneumatic massage.*

**pneu·mo·me·di·as·ti·no·gram** (noo″mo-me″de-əs-ti′no-gram) the film produced by pneumomediastinography.

**pneu·mo·me·di·as·ti·nog·ra·phy** (noo″mo-me″de-as″tĭ-nog′rə-fe) radiography of the mediastinum after injection of nitrous oxide or oxygen through a needle introduced back of the trachea or behind the manubrium.

**pneu·mo·me·di·as·ti·num** (noo″mo-me″de-əs-ti′nəm) [*pneumo-* + *mediastinum*] the presence of air or gas in the mediastinum, which may interfere with respiration and circulation, and may lead to such conditions as pneumothorax or pneumopericardium. It may occur as a result of trauma or a pathologic process, or it may be induced deliberately as a diagnostic procedure. Called also *Hamman's disease* or *syndrome* and *mediastinal emphysema.* See illustration.

**pneu·mo·mel·a·no·sis** (noo″mo-mel″ə-no′sis) [*pneumo-* + *melanosis*] the blackening of the lung tissue by inhaled coal dust, as in coal workers' pneumoconiosis.

**pneu·mo·my·co·sis** (noo″mo-mi-ko′sis) [*pneumo-* + *mycosis*] any fungal disease of the lungs.

**pneu·mo·my·elog·ra·phy** (noo″mo-mi″ə-log′rə-fe) [*pneumo-* +

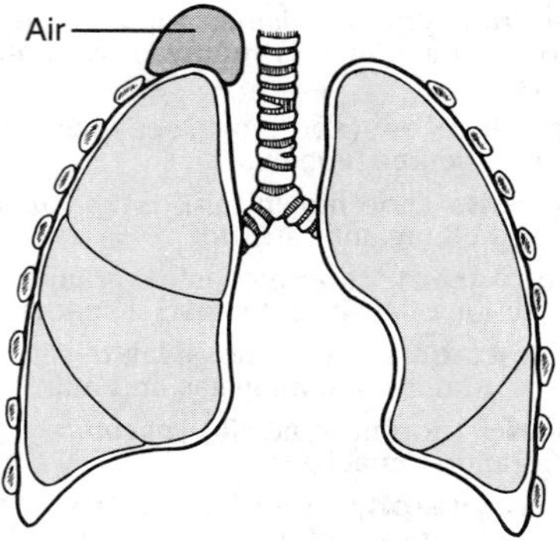

Pneumomediastinum.

*myelo-* + *-graphy*] radiographic examination after withdrawal of cerebrospinal fluid and injection of air or gas into the spinal canal.

**pneu•mo•nec•ta•sia** (noo″mo-nək-ta′zhə) pulmonary emphysema.

**pneu•mo•nec•ta•sis** (noo″mo-nek′tə-sis) [*pneumon-* + *ectasis*] pulmonary emphysema.

**pneu•mo•nec•to•my** (noo″mo-nek′tə-me) [*pneumon-* + *-ectomy*] [MeSH: Pneumonectomy] the excision of lung tissue, especially of an entire lung. Cf. *pneumonoresection.* Called also *pulmonectomy.*

**pneu•mo•nere** (noo′mo-nēr) one of the end-buds that cap the primordial bronchi.

**pneu•mo•nia** (noo-mo′ne-ə) [Gr. *pneumōnia*] [MeSH: Pneumonia] inflammation of the lungs with consolidation. Human pneumonias are most often categorized according to causative organism (such as *amebic p., bacterial p., interstitial plasma cell p., primary atypical p.,* and *viral p.*) or location (such as *apical p., bronchial p.,* and *lobar p.*). See also *pneumonitis.*

## Pneumonia

***Acinetobacter calcoaceticus* p.,** a sometimes fatal type of bacterial pneumonia seen in immunocompromised patients, caused by infection with the normally ubiquitous *Acinetobacter calcoaceticus.* It is usually bronchopneumonia, and characteristics include acute onset of dyspnea with fever, productive cough, chest pain, and abscess formation or empyema.

**acute p.,** severe pneumonia of rapid onset.

**adenovirus p.,** viral pneumonia caused by an adenovirus; it is usually mild, but in neonates and the immunocompromised it can be fatal. Characteristics range from interstitial inflammation without necrosis to a necrotizing bronchitis and bronchiolitis with desquamation that may occlude the lumen, and areas of hemorrhagic consolidation alternating with areas of atelectasis.

**p. al′ba,** a fatal desquamative pneumonia of the newborn resulting from congenital syphilis and characterized by white fatty degeneration of the lungs, which appear pale and virtually airless. Called also *white p.* and *white lung.*

**alcoholic p.,** pneumonia associated with alcoholism.

**amebic p.,** pneumonia resulting from so-called amebic abscesses in the lung caused by *Entamoeba histolytica.*

**anaerobic p.,** any pneumonia caused by anaerobic bacteria, usually due to aspiration of contaminated secretions from the mouth, pharynx, or paranasal sinuses, such as with the increased bacterial load of periodontal disease or some other infection. It usually runs a protracted course, progressing to lung cavitation with abscesses and putrid or bloody expectorations.

**anthrax p.,** inhalational anthrax.

**apex p., apical p.,** lobar pneumonia limited to the apex of the lung.

***Aspergillus* p.,** a type of fungal pneumonia sometimes seen in pulmonary aspergillosis.

**aspiration p.,** pneumonia due to the entrance of foreign matter, such as food particles or oral secretions, into the respiratory passages or lungs. Called also *deglutition p.* and *inhalation p.*

**atypical p.,** primary atypical p.

**atypical interstitial p.,** fog fever.

**bacterial p.,** pneumonia caused by bacteria, such as *Streptococcus pneumoniae, S. hemolytica, Staphylococcus aureus, Klebsiella pneumoniae, Mycoplasma pneumoniae,* and others.

**bronchial p.,** bronchopneumonia.

**bronchial p., atypical,** primary atypical p.

**brooder p.,** a lung disease of chicks and other young birds, acquired from moldy grain or straw; it is a form of aspergillosis, usually caused by *Aspergillus fumigatus.*

***Candida* p.,** pulmonary candidiasis.

**caseous p.,** tuberculous pneumonia in which necrotic lung tissue is of semisolid consistency and the cut surface resembles cheese. Called also *cheesy p.*

**cat p.,** feline pneumonitis.

**central p.,** lobar pneumonia beginning in the hilum of a lobe of the lung. Called also *core p.*

**cheesy p.,** caseous p.

***Chlamydia pneumoniae* p.,** a mild form of primary atypical pneumonia caused by infection with *Chlamydia pneumoniae,* characterized by fever, rales, and infiltration of a middle or lower lobe; the recovery period is usually prolonged.

***Chlamydia trachomatis* p.,** a mild type of bacterial pneumonia, usually seen in infants whose mothers are infected with *Chlamydia trachomatis;* characteristics include coughing, tachypnea, and eosinophilia.

**coccidioidal p.,** pneumonia following primary coccidioidomycosis. It varies from a slowly-developing disease with chronic cough, chest pain, hemoptysis, and fever to a more rapidly spreading acute condition, usually seen in immunocompromised patients, with cavitation, spread to other organ systems, and frequently a fatal outcome.

**cold agglutinin p.,** primary atypical p.

**contusion p.,** pneumonia following an injury to the thorax; called also *traumatic p.*

**core p.,** central p.

**cryptogenic organizing p.,** bronchiolitis obliterans with organizing pneumonia.

**cytomegalovirus p.,** viral pneumonia caused by infection with cytomegalovirus, an often fatal disease seen in immunocompromised patients; symptoms include fever, a nonproductive cough, and dyspnea.

**deglutition p.,** aspiration p.

**dermal p.,** a condition produced by injection of virulent pneumococci into the skin of rabbits.

**desquamative interstitial p.,** chronic pneumonia of unknown etiology, characterized by prominence of intra-alveolar macrophages (which were formerly thought to be desquamated large alveolar cells); it is associated with dyspnea and often a nonproductive and harsh cough, and typically occurs in smokers.

**p. dis′secans,** p. interlobularis purulenta.

**double p.,** that which affects both lungs.

**Eaton agent p.,** mycoplasmal p.

**embolic p.,** 1. pneumonia due to embolism of a blood vessel or vessels of the lungs. 2. in cattle, pneumonia that sometimes follows caudal vena caval thrombosis (q.v.); it often involves abscesses with suppurative pneumonia and aneurysms that may rupture, causing pulmonary hemorrhage that can be either minor or massive and fatal.

***Enterobacter* p.,** a rare type of bacterial pneumonia, usually bronchopneumonia, caused by infection with species of *Enterobacter,* most commonly *E. aerogenes* or *E. cloacae;* it is usually nosocomial and seen in debilitated patients.

**enzootic p.,** any of several types of mild pneumonias that affect young animals, especially lambs, piglets, and calves, usually caused by viruses or species of *Mycoplasma.*

**eosinophilic p.,** 1. see *acute* and *chronic eosinophilic p.* 2. PIE syndrome (def. 2).

**eosinophilic p., acute,** a condition resembling chronic eosinophilic pneumonia but with a more rapid onset and more limited duration, accompanied by acute respiratory failure and diffuse pulmonary infiltrates.

**eosinophilic p., chronic,** a chronic interstitial lung disease characterized by cough, dyspnea, malaise, fever, night sweats, weight loss, eosinophilia, and a chest film revealing nonsegmental, nonmigratory infiltrates in the lung periphery.

***Escherichia coli* p.,** a rare type of bacterial pneumonia caused by infection with *Escherichia coli,* usually in the bronchi or a lower lobe, seen most often in debilitated patients or infants.

**fibrous p.,** a form characterized by an increase in scar tissue during the healing process.

**fibrous p., chronic,** idiopathic pulmonary fibrosis.

**Friedländer's p., Friedländer's bacillus p.,** *Klebsiella* p.

**fungal p.,** pneumonia caused by inhaled fungi, usually *Histoplasma capsulatum, Blastomyces dermatitidis,* or *Coccidioides immitis*; in Central and South America it may be caused by *Paracoccidioides brasiliensis.* Numerous other fungi, such as *Aspergillus* and *Candida,* infect immunocompromised patients. See also *histoplasmosis, North American blastomycosis, coccidioidomycosis,* and *paracoccidioidomycosis.*

**gangrenous p.,** gangrene of the lung.

**giant cell p.,** a rare, often fatal form of interstitial pneumonia caused by the measles virus, affecting children with disease of the reticuloendothelial system (such as leukemia), as well as immunocompromised or otherwise weakened adults; characteristics include multinucleate giant cell inclusion bodies, high fever, tachypnea, hypoxemia, and a harsh dry cough. Called also *Hecht's p.*

**glanders p.,** pneumonia associated with glanders, characterized by caseous or calcified granules and pulmonary consolidation; seen in both humans and horses. Called also *p. malleosa.*

***Haemophilus influenzae* p.,** bacterial pneumonia caused by infection with *Haemophilus influenzae,* seen mainly in young children and debilitated or immunocompromised adults; it sometimes progresses to life-threatening conditions such as meningitis, pericarditis, endocarditis, and epiglottitis that can cause obstruction of the airway.

**Hecht's p.,** giant cell p.

**herpes simplex virus p.,** a type of viral pneumonia seen in neonates or immunocompromised patients, caused by spread of a herpes simplex virus infection into the lungs; characteristics include dyspnea, cough, and hypoxemia in conjunction with other manifestations of the herpesvirus infection.

**hypostatic p.,** pneumonia due to dorsal decubitus in weak or aged persons.

**infectious p. of goats,** contagious caprine pleuropneumonia.

**influenzal p., influenza virus p.,** viral pneumonia caused by an influenza virus, usually the type A virus; some cases are mild, but it can develop into a fulminant condition characterized by high fever, prostration, severe dyspnea, and massive (sometimes rapidly fatal) pulmonary hemorrhagic edema with consolidation. It may be accompanied by a superinfection with bacterial pneumonia.

**inhalation p.,** 1. aspiration p. 2. bronchopneumonia due to the inhalation of irritating substances.

**p. interlobula'ris purulen'ta,** pneumonia with interlobular empyema.

**interstitial p.,** 1. any of various types of pneumonia characterized by thickening of the interstitial tissue. 2. idiopathic pulmonary fibrosis.

**interstitial p., acute,** the acute form of idiopathic pulmonary fibrosis, now thought to represent a sequel to the acute respiratory distress syndrome. Called also *Hamman-Rich syndrome.*

**interstitial p., giant cell,** a type of pneumonia similar to idiopathic pulmonary fibrosis but with interstitial exudate containing large numbers of irregularly shaped multinucleate giant cells; it is thought to represent the pathologic appearance of hard metal disease.

**interstitial p., lymphocytic, interstitial p., lymphoid,** lymphocytic interstitial pneumonitis.

**interstitial p., usual,** idiopathic pulmonary fibrosis.

**interstitial plasma cell p.,** a pulmonary disease caused by *Pneumocystis carinii,* occurring in premature or malnourished infants and immunocompromised persons. It is characterized by dyspnea, tachypnea, fever, cough, and cyanosis, with cellular detritus containing plasma cells appearing in the lungs; if untreated it leads to pulmonary consolidation, hypoxemia, and death. Called also *pneumocystosis, pneumocystiasis,* and Pneumocystis carinii *p.*

**intrauterine p.,** pneumonia contracted by the fetus *in utero;* it may result in the death of the fetus or the birth of an infant with fully developed pneumonia.

***Klebsiella* p.,** an acute type of bacterial pneumonia caused by infection with *Klebsiella pneumoniae,* usually lobar in type and often limited to the right upper lobe; characteristics include large amounts of inflammatory, sometimes bloody, mucoid exudates in the lung. Called also *Friedländer's bacillus p.*

***Legionella* p.,** pneumonia caused by a species of *Legionella;* see *legionnaire's disease* and *Pittsburgh p.*

**lipid p., lipoid p.,** a rare type of aspiration pneumonia caused by aspiration of oil; mineral oils and vegetable oils usually cause lower grade, chronic inflammation while animal fats tend to cause more acute inflammation and sometimes pulmonary hemorrhage. Called also *oil-aspiration p.*.

**lobar p.,** 1. a type of acute bacterial pneumonia with abundant edema, usually limited to just one lobe of a lung; the most common kind is pneumococcal pneumonia. 2. pneumococcal p.

**lobular p.,** bronchopneumonia.

**Löffler's p.,** see under *syndrome.*

**Louisiana p.,** a form of pneumonia seen in Louisiana, caused by a strain of *Chlamydia psittaci.*

**p. malleo'sa,** glanders p.

**measles virus p.,** viral pneumonia caused by the measles virus; it ranges from a mild type occurring during a bout of measles to severe, even fatal, giant cell pneumonia.

**meningococcal p.,** a rare type of bacterial pneumonia caused by the meningococcus *Neisseria meningitidis;* many cases are subclinical, but some infections become overwhelming, with fever, pleural effusion, and even death. Called also Neisseria meningitidis p.

**metastatic p.,** suppurative pneumonia due to bloodborne infection in bacteremia.

**migratory p.,** pneumonia that spreads from one lobe of the lung to others; called also *wandering p.*

***Moraxella* p., *Moraxella catarrhalis* p.,** a usually mild type of bacterial pneumonia caused by infection with *Moraxella (Branhamella) catarrhalis,* generally seen in patients with some other debilitating condition, especially smokers with chronic obstructive pulmonary disease. Symptoms include fever and dyspnea.

***Mycoplasma* p., mycoplasmal p.,** the most common form of primary atypical pneumonia (q.v.), caused by *Mycoplasma pneumoniae* and occurring most frequently in young adults; called also *Eaton agent p.*

**necrotizing p.,** necrosis of lung tissue in bacterial pneumonia, which may range from small abscesses to massive areas.

***Neisseria meningitidis* p.,** meningococcal p.

***Nocardia* p.,** the pneumonia seen with severe pulmonary nocardiosis.

**obstructive p.,** that due to obstruction of the air passages, as by bronchogenic carcinoma.

**oil-aspiration p.,** lipid p.

**organizing p.,** pneumonia characterized by formation of numerous small foci of loose connective tissue called Masson bodies in the bronchioles and alveoli. It may be seen following injury, associated with interstitial lung conditions, or as part of the syndrome called *bronchiolitis obliterans with organizing pneumonia* or *cryptogenic organizing p.*.

**ovine progressive p.,** a chronic viral disease of sheep caused by a retrovirus, characterized by progressive weight loss and dyspnea that can be fatal. A demyelinating meningoencephalitis may occur, with paresis of the hind limbs progressing to total paralysis and death. The respiratory form is also called *maedi* and the meningoencephalitic form *visna; maedi-visna* is used to describe the entire syndrome.

**parainfluenza virus p.,** viral pneumonia caused by the parainfluenza 3 virus, usually seen in children or immunocompromised adults; characteristics include fever, cough, and dyspnea.

***Pasteurella multocida* p.,** a rare type of bacterial pneumonia caused by infection with *Pasteurella multocida,* usually seen in patients with chronic lung disease; characteristics include fever, cough, and dyspnea, sometimes with empyema.

**Pittsburgh p.,** a type of pneumonia resembling legionnaires' disease, caused by *Legionella micdadei,* and occurring as a nosocomial infection especially in immunocompromised patients.

**plague p.,** pneumonic plague.

**plasma cell p.,** interstitial plasma cell p.

**pleuritic p.,** pleuropneumonia (def. 1).

**pneumococcal p.,** a type of acute pneumonia usually caused by *Streptococcus pneumoniae,* with inflammation of one or more lobe(s) of the lung; characteristics include chills followed by sudden fever, dyspnea, tachypnea, pain in the side, and coughing with bloodstained sputum. It usually begins in the lower lobe, which becomes congested *(stage of congestion),* then red and solid *(red hepatization),* and later gray from degeneration of the exudates *(gray hepatization).* In most patients this is followed by the *stage of resolution,* during which the exudates degenerate and are absorbed. Called also *lobar p.*

**pneumocystis p., *Pneumocystis carinii* p.,** interstitial plasma cell p.

**primary atypical p.,** a general term applied to any of numerous acute infectious pulmonary diseases, formerly referring to any type other than bacterial pneumonia; causative organisms include *Mycoplasma pneumoniae* (see *mycoplasmal p.*), species of *Rickettsia* and *Chlamydia,* and various viruses (see *viral p.*). All are marked by extensive but tenuous pulmonary infiltration and by fever, malaise, myalgia, sore throat, and a cough that at first is nonproductive but becomes productive and paroxysmal. Called also *atypical p., atypical bronchial p.,* and *cold agglutinin p.*

***Proteus* p.,** a rare type of bacterial pneumonia caused by infection with species of *Proteus,* usually *P. mirabilis* or *P. vulgaris;* it usually affects debilitated or immunocompromised patients and is characterized by consolidation with abscesses in the upper lobes.

***Pseudomonas aeruginosa* p.,** a form of bacterial pneumonia, usually nosocomial, seen in young children and debilitated or immunocompromised adults, caused by infection with *Pseudomonas aeruginosa;* characteristics include fever and coughing with lung nodules that may be either firm or hemorrhagic and may progress to necrosis of the alveoli with cavitation.

**purulent p.,** suppurative p.

**Q fever p.,** a type of bacterial pneumonia occurring as part of Q fever (infection with *Coxiella burnetii*); it is usually benign and self-limited, with granulomatous infiltrates and linear atelectasis visible radiographically.

**respiratory syncytial virus p.**, viral pneumonia caused by respiratory syncytial virus, seen in infants and young children and occasionally in immunocompromised or otherwise debilitated adults; characteristics include fever, cough, dyspnea, wheezing, and crackles.

**rheumatic p.**, a rare, usually fatal complication of acute rheumatic fever characterized by extensive pulmonary consolidation and rapidly progressive functional deterioration and by alveolar exudate (with the presence of Masson bodies), interstitial infiltrates, and necrotizing arteritis.

***Rhodococcus equi* p.**, a type of bacterial pneumonia seen in immunocompromised persons, caused by infection with *Rhodococcus equi,* often after contact with an infected animal; it is often subacute, with consolidation and cavitation visible radiographically.

**secondary p.**, pneumonia seen as a complication of some other disorder, such as influenza or a fungal infection.

***Serratia* p.**, a rare type of bacterial pneumonia, usually nosocomial, caused by infection with *Serratia marcescens;* it is often fatal to immunocompromised patients.

**staphylococcal p.**, a common type of bacterial pneumonia, usually bronchopneumonia, caused by infection with *Staphylococcus,* particularly *S. aureus.* Since many strains of *Staphylococcus* are antibiotic-resistant, this type is often seen in hospitals in patients on antibiotic therapy after surgery; it also commonly infects debilitated patients such as those suffering from other respiratory infections or viral infections such as influenza. Characteristics include fever, dyspnea, rales, pleural effusion, and empyema.

**streptococcal p.**, pneumonia caused by a streptococcus other than *S. pneumoniae,* usually *Streptococcus pyogenes;* pleural effusion, with or without empyema, is particularly common.

**suppurative p.**, pneumonia with formation of abscesses in the lungs. Called also *purulent p.*

**terminal p.**, pneumonia developing during some other disease and hastening a fatal termination.

**traumatic p.**, contusion p.

**tuberculous p.**, pneumonia occurring as part of the earliest reaction to infection by *Mycobacterium tuberculosis;* see also *caseous p.* and *exudative tuberculosis*

**tularemic p.**, pulmonary tularemia.

**typhoid p.**, pneumonia with typhoid symptoms or accompanying typhoid fever; children may develop bronchopneumonia and adults may develop lobar pneumonia, with suppuration and empyema.

**unresolved p.**, pneumonia in which the lung signs fail to clear up within the usual period.

**varicella p., *Varicella zoster* p.**, viral pneumonia developing as a complication two to six days after the appearance of varicella (chickenpox), seen in adults more often than children. Symptoms may be severe, with violent cough, hemoptysis, and severe chest pains. Radiologically, there are numerous nodular densities, which may coalesce, at the base of each lung, and often enlarged lymph nodes in the hilar region; small nodular calcifications may persist.

**ventilator-associated p.**, the most common type of nosocomial pneumonia, a frequently fatal type seen in patients breathing with a ventilator; it is usually caused by aspiration of contaminated secretions or stomach contents and may be bacterial, viral, or fungal.

**verminous p.**, mild to severe dyspnea and fever in domestic animals due to the presence in the bronchioles or lungs of nematode lungworms, usually of species of *Dictyocaulus, Filaroides, Metastrongylus, Muellerius,* or *Protostrongylus.* Acute episodes may be fatal. In sheep, cattle, goats, and pigs it is called hoose. It also occurs in horses, donkeys, dogs, and cats.

**viral p.**, any of numerous pneumonias caused by a virus, such as an adenovirus, influenza virus, parainfluenza virus, or respiratory syncytial virus.

**wandering p.**, migratory p.

**white p.**, p. alba.

**woolsorter's p.**, inhalational anthrax.

---

**pneu·mon·ic** (noo-mon'ik) [Gr. *pneumonikos*] 1. pertaining to pneumonia. 2. pulmonary (def. 1).

**pneu·mo·ni·tis** (noo"mo-ni'tis) [*pneumon-* + *-itis*] inflammation of the lungs. See also *pneumonia.*

**acute lupus p.**, a type of pneumonitis that accompanies systemic lupus erythematosus; characteristics include rapid onset, fever, dyspnea, and coughing.

***Ascaris* p.**, the most common type of Löffler's syndrome, caused by presence in the lungs of the nematode *Ascaris lumbricoides.* Called also *pulmonary ascariasis.*

**aspiration p.**, see under *pneumonia.*

**chemical p.**, pneumonitis caused by the inhalation of chemical irritants; the extent of the injury reflects the concentration of the irritants and the duration of exposure.

**cholesterol p.**, pneumonitis characterized by chronic inflammatory changes and deposition of excessive amounts of cholesterol in the tissues. It is often lobar or segmental in distribution and may resemble primary or metastatic tumor.

**feline p.**, a fatal pneumonitis with conjunctivitis in cats, caused by a strain of *Chlamydia psittaci.*

**granulomatous p.**, pneumonitis with granulomas, usually resulting from an infection or inhalation of organic dust by a hypersensitive person.

**hypersensitivity p.**, a respiratory hypersensitivity reaction to repeated inspiration of organic particles, usually in an occupational setting, with onset a few hours after exposure to the allergen. Characteristics include fever, fatigue, chills, unproductive cough, tachycardia, and tachypnea; in the chronic form there is interstitial fibrosis with collagenous thickening of the alveolar septa. There are many specific types (see table). Called also *allergic* or *extrinsic allergic alveolitis.*

**interstitial p., lymphocytic,** an insidious, slowly progressive interstitial lung disease of unknown etiology, marked by diffuse peribronchial and interstitial infiltration of the lungs by lymphocytes, plasma cells, and lymphoblasts; usually seen in immunocompromised patients, especially children, or accompanying Sjögren's syndrome. Called also *lymphocytic* or *lymphoid interstitial pneumonia.*

**malarial p.**, pneumonitis caused by *Plasmodium falciparum,* characterized by cough with bloody sputum and coarse rales; in severe cases thromboses may result from the agglutination of parasitized erythrocytes in small blood vessels of the lung.

**manganese p.**, pneumonitis affecting the lower airways and alveoli, caused by inhaling manganese dust or fumes; it may be acute, in which form it is often fatal, or it may be chronic and recurring. See also *manganese poisoning,* under *poisoning.*

**mercury p.**, a sometimes fatal pneumonitis with tracheitis, bronchitis, and bronchiolitis, accompanied by the symptoms of mercury poisoning, caused by the inhalation of mercury fumes.

**mouse p.**, a bronchopneumonia of laboratory mice caused by a strain of *Chlamydia trachomatis.*

**pneumocystis p.**, interstitial plasma cell pneumonia.

**radiation p.**, lung inflammation resulting from radiation exposure, usually radiation therapy, with coughing, dyspnea, and alveolar infiltration, leading to mild to severe or even fatal fibrosis 6 to 9 months after the exposure.

**trimellitic anhydride p.**, hemorrhagic pneumonitis with intra-alveolar hemorrhage and alveolar cell hyperplasia caused by inhalation of trimellitic anhydride fumes.

**uremic p.**, pneumonitis associated with uremia; a butterfly or bat-wing configuration of opacities on the chest radiograph indicates pulmonary edema.

**pneumon(o)-** [Gr. *pneumon* lung] a combining form denoting relationship to the lungs.

**pneu·mo·no·cele** (noo-mon'o-sēl) 1. hernial protrusion of lung tissue, as through a fissure in the chest wall. Called also *pleurocele* and *pneumocele.* 2. pneumatocele (def. 2).

**pneu·mo·no·cen·te·sis** (noo-mo"no-sən-te'sis) [*pneumono-* + *-centesis*] paracentesis of a lung; called also *pneumocentesis.*

**pneu·mo·no·coc·cus** (noo"mo-no-kok'əs) pneumococcus.

**pneu·mo·no·co·ni·o·sis** (noo-mo"no-ko"ne-o'sis) pneumoconiosis.

**pneu·mo·no·cyte** (noo-mon'o-sīt) alveolar cell.

**granular p's,** type II alveolar cells.

**membranous p's,** type I alveolar cells.

**pneu·mo·no·en·ter·itis** (noo-mo"no-en"tər-i'tis) pneumoenteritis.

**pneu·mo·nog·ra·phy** (noo"mo-nog'rə-fe) pneumography.

**pneu·mo·no·ko·ni·o·sis** (noo-mo"no-ko"ne-o'sis) pneumoconiosis.

**Types of Hypersensitivity Pneumonitis**

| Disease | Source of Antigen | Most Likely Antigen |
|---|---|---|
| Bagassosis | Moldy bagasse (pressed sugar cane) | *Thermoactinomyces* spp. and other actinomycetes |
| Cheese handler's (or washer's) disease or lung | Moldy cheese casings | *Penicillium* spp. |
| Duck fever | Duck feathers | Duck proteins |
| Epoxy resin lung | Hot epoxy resin | Phthalic anhydride |
| Farmer's (harvester's, thresher's) lung | Moldy or contaminated hay | *Aspergillus* spp.; *Micropolyspora faeni, Thermoactinomyces vulgaris* and other actinomycetes |
| Grain handler's lung | Moldy grain | Miscellaneous fungi |
| Humidifier lung | Contaminated air conditioners, humidifiers, or dehumidifiers | Amebae, *Cephalosporium* spp., *Penicillium* spp., *Thermoactinomyces* and other actinomycetes |
| Malt worker's lung | Moldy barley | *Aspergillus* spp. |
| Maple bark disease | Moldy maple bark | *Cryptostroma corticale* |
| Meat wrapper's lung | Meat wrappers or labels | Phthalic anhydride |
| Miller's lung | Insect-infested wheat | *Sitophilus granarius* |
| Pigeon breeder's (bird breeder's) lung | Pigeon feces | Pigeon immunoglobulin A |
| Sequoiosis | Moldy sawdust | *Aureobasidium, Graphium* |
| Suberosis | Moldy cork dust | *Penicillium* spp. |
| Turkey handler's disease | Turkey proteins | Turkey products |
| Wood pulp worker's disease | Moldy wood pulp | *Alternaria* spp. |
| Wood trimmer's disease | Moldy wood trimmings | *Mucor, Rhizopus* |

**pneu·mo·no·lip·i·do·sis** (noo-mo″no-lip″ĭ-do′sis) lipid pneumonia.

**pneu·mo·nol·y·sis** (noo″mo-nol′ĭ-sis) [*pneumono-* + *-lysis*] [MeSH: Pneumonolysis] division of the tissues attaching the lung to the wall of the chest cavity so that the lung collapses inward; it was formerly a common method of collapse therapy (q.v.) and is still sometimes done to allow access during thoracic surgery. Called also *pneumolysis.*

**pneu·mo·no·mo·ni·li·a·sis** (noo-mo″no-mo″nĭ-li′ə-sis) pulmonary candidiasis.

**pneu·mo·no·my·co·sis** (noo-mo″no-mi-ko′sis) pneumomycosis.

**pneu·mo·nop·a·thy** (noo″mo-nop′ə-the) [*pneumono-* + *-pathy*] any disease of the lung. Called also *pneumonosis* and *pneumopathy.* **eosinophilic p.,** 1. Löffler's syndrome. 2. any condition associated with eosinophilic infiltration of the lung parenchyma.

**pneu·mo·no·pexy** (noo-mo′no-pek″se) [*pneumono-* + *-pexy*] surgical fixation of the lung to the thoracic wall; see also *pleuroparietopexy* and *pleurodesis.* Called also *pneumopexy.*

**pneu·mo·no·pleu·ri·tis** (noo-mo″no-plo͞o-ri′tis) pleuropneumonia (def. 1).

**pneu·mo·no·re·sec·tion** (noo-mo″no-re-sek′shən) surgical resection of a portion of the lung. Cf. *pneumonectomy.* Called also *pneumoresection.*

**pneu·mo·nor·rha·gia** (noo-mo″no-ra′je-ə) pulmonary hemorrhage.

**pneu·mo·nor·rha·phy** (noo″mo-nor′ə-fe) [*pneumono-* + *-rrhaphy*] suture of the lung.

**pneu·mo·no·sis** (noo″mo-no′sis) pneumonopathy.

**pneu·mo·no·ther·a·py** (noo-mo″no-ther′ə-pe) pneumotherapy.

**pneu·mo·not·o·my** (noo″mo-not′ə-me) [*pneumono-* + *-tomy*] surgical incision of the lung. Called also *pneumotomy.*

**Pneu·mo·nys·soi·des** (noo″mo-nis-oi′dēz) a genus of mites of the family Halarachnidae. Its distinction from the genus *Pneumonyssus* has been questioned.

**Pneu·mo·nys·sus** (noo″mo-nis′əs) a genus of mites of the family Halarachnidae. *P. cani′num* infests the nasal passages of dogs, causing nasal acariasis. *P. simi′cola* is found in the lungs of monkeys.

**pneu·mo·par·oti·tis** (noo″mo-par″o-ti′tis) pneumatic inflation of the parotid gland.

**pneu·mop·a·thy** (noo-mop′ə-the) pneumonopathy.

**pneu·mo·peri·car·di·um** (noo″mo-per″ĭ-kahr′de-əm) [*pneumo-* + *pericardium*] [MeSH: Pneumopericardium] the presence of air or gas in the cavity of the pericardium.

**pneu·mo·peri·to·ne·al** (noo″mo-per″ĭ-to-ne′əl) pertaining to or characterized by pneumoperitoneum.

**pneu·mo·peri·to·ne·um** (noo″mo-per″ĭ-to-ne′əm) [*pneumo-* + *peritoneum*] [MeSH: Pneumoperitoneum] the presence of gas or air in the peritoneal cavity; it may occur spontaneously, as in subphrenic abscess, or be deliberately introduced as an aid to radiologic examination and diagnosis *(diagnostic p.).*

**pneu·mo·peri·to·ni·tis** (noo″mo-per″ĭ-to-ni′tis) [*pneumo-* + *peritonitis*] peritonitis with the accumulation of air or gas in the peritoneal cavity.

**pneu·mo·pexy** (noo′mo-pek″se) pneumonopexy.

**pneu·mo·pha·gia** (noo″mo-fa′jə) [*pneumo-* + *-phagia*] aerophagia.

**pneu·mo·pho·nia** (noo″mo-fo′ne-ə) a form of dysphonia characterized by a breathy voice.

**pneu·mo·plas·ty** (noo′mo-plas″te) plastic surgery to a lung. **reduction p.,** surgical removal of nonfunctional lung tissue in cases of advanced emphysema, such as bullectomy in bullous emphysema where giant bullae are compressing the functional lung tissue.

**pneu·mo·pleu·ri·tis** (noo″mo-plo͞o-ri′tis) pleuropneumonia (def. 1).

**pneu·mo·pre·cor·di·um** (noo″mo-pre-kor′de-əm) [*pneumo-* + *precordium*] the presence of air in the precordial space.

**pneu·mo·pre·peri·to·ne·um** (noo″mo-pre-per″ĭ-to-ne′əm) the presence of air or gas in the preperitoneal space; it may occur spontaneously or be deliberately introduced as an aid to radiologic examination and diagnosis.

**pneu·mo·py·elog·ra·phy** (noo″mo-pi″ə-log′rə-fe) [*pneumo-* + *pyelo-* + *-graphy*] pyelography in which oxygen or air, instead of an opaque solution, is injected into the renal pelvis.

**pneu·mo·pyo·peri·car·di·um** (noo″mo-pi″o-per″ĭ-kahr′de-əm) pyopneumopericardium.

**pneu·mo·pyo·tho·rax** (noo″mo-pi″o-thor′aks) [*pneumo-* + *pyo-* + *thorax*] pyopneumothorax.

**pneu·mo·ra·chi·cen·te·sis** (noo″mo-ra″ke-sen-te′sis) [*pneumo-* + *rachi-* + *-centesis*] pneumorachis (def. 2).

**pneu·mo·ra·chis** (noo″mo-ra′kis) [pneumo- + *rachis*] 1. the presence of a gaseous collection in the spinal canal. 2. the injection of gas into the spinal canal for the facilitation of myelographic examination. See *pneumoencephalomyelography.*

**pneu·mo·ra·di·og·ra·phy** (noo″mo-ra″de-og′rə-fe) [*pneumo-* + *radiography*] [MeSH: Pneumoradiography] radiography of a part following the injection of air or oxygen, as in pneumoperitoneum.

**pneu·mo·re·sec·tion** (noo″mo-re-sek′shən) pneumonoresection.

**pneu·mo·re·tro·peri·to·ne·um** (noo″mo-re″tro-per″ĭ-to-ne′əm) the presence of air or gas in the retroperitoneal space.

**pneu·mor·rha·gia** (noo″mo-ra′jə) [*pneumo-* + *-rrhagia*] pulmonary hemorrhage.

**pneu·mo·se·ro·sa** (noo″mo-se-ro′sə) injection of air into a joint cavity for fluoroscopy.

**pneu·mo·se·ro·tho·rax** (noo″mo-se″ro-thor′aks) hydropneumothorax.

**pneu·mo·sil·i·co·sis** (noo″mo-sil″ĭ-ko′sis) silicosis.

**pneu·mo·si·nus di·la·tans** (noo″mo-si′nəs di-la′təns) abnormal dilatation of the sphenoidal sinuses with remodeling but without erosion or thinning of the sinus bony walls. The sinuses are well aerated and the mucosa is normal.

**pneu·mo·tacho·graph** (noo″mo-tak′o-graf) pneumotachygraph.

**pneu·mo·ta·chom·e·ter** (noo″mo-tə-kom′ə-tər) a transducer used in measuring expired air flow.

**pneu·mo·tach·y·graph** (noo″mo-tak′ĭ-graf) [*pneumo-* + *tachy-* + *-graph*] an instrument for recording the velocity of the respired air.

**pneu·mo·tax·ic** (noo″mo-tak′sik) [*pneumo-* + Gr. *taxis* arrangement] relating to the regulation of the rate of respiration; see under *center.*

**pneu·mo·ther·a·py** (noo″mo-ther′ə-pe) the treatment of diseases of the lungs. Called also *pneumonotherapy.*

**pneu·mo·ther·mo·mas·sage** (noo″mo-ther″mo-mə-sahzh′) [*pneumo-* + *thermo-* + *massage*] the application to the body of hot condensed air to produce an effect resembling massage.

**pneu·mo·tho·rax** (noo″mo-thor′aks) [*pneumo-* + *thorax*] [MeSH: Pneumothorax] an accumulation of air or gas in the pleural space; three types are distinguished: *traumatic p., primary spontaneous p.,* and *secondary spontaneous p.* It was formerly sometimes induced for treatment of pulmonary tuberculosis; see *artificial p.*
**artificial p.,** pneumothorax induced intentionally by artificial means; formerly used as a method of collapse therapy (q.v.) in treatment of pulmonary tuberculosis. Called also *induced p.* and *therapeutic p.*
**catamenial p.,** pneumothorax occurring in conjunction with menstrual periods, believed to represent a consequence of pleural endometriosis.
**clicking p.,** pneumothorax in which there is a clicking sound synchronous with the heart beat.
**closed p.,** pneumothorax in which pulmonary air leaks into the pleural cavity through a wound in a lung.
**diagnostic p.,** temporary artificial pneumothorax employed for the purpose of clearly demonstrating the parietal or visceral pleura on chest films in order to detect and localize tumors of the pleura.
**induced p.,** artificial p.
**open p.,** pneumothorax in which the pleural cavity is exposed to the atmosphere through an open wound in the chest wall. See also *sucking wound.*
**pressure p.,** tension p.
**spontaneous p., primary,** a pneumothorax without an obvious external cause, such as from a ruptured subpleural bleb.
**spontaneous p., secondary,** a pneumothorax resulting from a known pathologic condition.
**tension p.,** pneumothorax in which the pressure within the pleural space is greater than atmospheric pressure; this may occur when air enters under positive pressure, such as when caused by positive pressure ventilation, or when the tissues around the opening into the pleural cavity act as valves, allowing air to enter but not to escape. The resultant positive pressure in the cavity displaces the mediastinum to the opposite side, with consequent interference with respiration. Called also *pressure p.*
**therapeutic p.,** artificial p.
**traumatic p.,** that resulting from chest trauma, such as accompanying a penetrating wound, a fractured rib, or abrupt pressure on a lung.
**valvular p.,** tension p.

**pneu·mo·to·mog·ra·phy** (noo″mo-to-mog′rə-fe) tomography performed after injection of air or other gas into the region or organ being visualized.

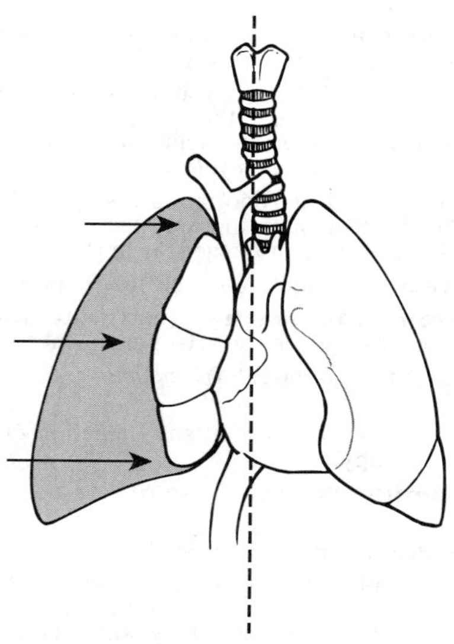
Tension pneumothorax.

**pneu·mot·o·my** (noo-mot′ə-me) pneumonotomy.

**pneu·mo·trop·ic** (noo″mo-trop′ik) 1. having a selective affinity for pulmonary tissue; exerting its principal effect upon the lungs. 2. having a selective affinity for pneumococci.

**pneu·mot·ro·pism** (noo-mot′rə-piz-əm) the predilection of an agent or organism for lung tissue.

**pneu·mo·uria** (noo″mo-u′re-ə) pneumaturia.

**Pneu·mo·vax** (noo′mo-vaks″) trademark for a pneumococcal vaccine containing capsular polysaccharides (antigens) from 14 types of pneumococci.
**P. 23,** trademark for a pneumococcal vaccine containing capsular polysaccharides from 23 types of pneumococci.

**pneu·mo·ven·tri·cle** (noo″mo-ven′trĭ-kəl) [*pneumo-* + *ventricle*] pneumocephalus in one of the cerebral ventricles; called also *pneumoventriculi.*

**pneu·mo·ven·tric·u·li** (noo″mo-ven-trik′u-li) pneumoventricle.

**pneu·mo·ven·tric·u·log·ra·phy** (noo″mo-vən-trik″u-log′rə-fe) ventriculography of the cerebral ventricles after the injection of air or gas.

**Pneu·mo·vi·ri·nae** (noo″mo-vir-i′ne) a subfamily of the Paramyxoviridae containing a single genus, *Pneumovirus.*

**Pneu·mo·vi·rus** (noo′mo-vi″rəs) [*pneumo-* + *virus*] [MeSH: Pneumovirus] respiratory syncytial viruses; a genus of viruses of the subfamily Pneumovirinae (family Paramyxoviridae) that includes human and bovine respiratory syncytial viruses.

**pneu·sis** (noo′sis) [Gr. *pneusis* a blowing] ventilation (def. 2).

**PNH** paroxysmal nocturnal hemoglobinuria.

**-pnoea** see *-pnea.*

**PO** abbreviation for L. *per os,* by mouth, orally.

**$Po_2$** symbol for *oxygen partial pressure* or *tension.*

**Po** symbol for *polonium.*

**$pO_2$, $pO_2$** symbol for *oxygen partial pressure* or *tension.*

**POA** pancreatic oncofetal antigen.

**Poa** (po′ə) a genus of grasses (family Gramineae). *P. praten′sis* is Kentucky bluegrass or June grass, whose pollen causes hay fever.

**Pocill.** abbreviation for L. *pocil′lum,* a small cup.

**pock** (pok) a pustule, especially one of the lesions of smallpox.

**pock·et** (pok′ət) a saclike space. See also *pouch, recess,* and *cavity.*
**complex p.,** a spiral type of periodontal pocket involving more than one surface of the tooth, but communicating with the gingival margin only along the surface at which it originates.
**compound p.,** a periodontal pocket involving more than one tooth surface, and communicating with the marginal gingiva along each of the involved surfaces.
**endocardial p's,** sclerotic thickenings of the mural endocardium, occurring most often on the left ventricular septum below an insufficient aortic valve; called also *regurgitant p's* and *birds' nests.*
**gingival p.,** a gingival sulcus deepened by pathological conditions, caused by gingival enlargement with no destruction of the periodontal tissue. Called also *relative p.*
**infrabony p., intra-alveolar p.,** intrabony p.
**intrabony p.,** intrabony p., a periodontal pocket in which the bottom is apical to the level of the adjacent alveolar bone.
**pacemaker p.,** the subcutaneous area in which the pulse generator and pacing leads of an internal pacemaker are implanted, usually developed in the prepectoralis fascia or the retromammary area.
**periodontal p.,** a gingival sulcus that extends abnormally deep into the periodontal ligament apically to the original level of the resorbed alveolar crest.
**Rathke's p.,** see under *pouch.*
**regurgitant p's,** endocardial p's.
**relative p.,** gingival p.
**retraction p.,** a localized area of atelectasis where the tympanic membrane bulges inward; it may be a precursor of a serious condition such as cholesteatoma or ossicular discontinuity.
**Seessel's p.,** see under *pouch.*
**simple p.,** a periodontal pocket involving only one tooth surface.
**subcrestal p.,** intrabony p.
**suprabony p., supracrestal p.,** a periodontal pocket in which the bottom is coronal to the underlying bone.
**p's of Zahn,** shallow pockets with miniature leaflets, resembling cusps of the semilunar valve, produced in the endocardium of the left ventricle by the regurgitant aortic stream in the presence of insufficiency of the aortic valve.

**pock·mark** (pok′mahrk) a depressed scar left by a pustule, especially one left by a lesion of smallpox.

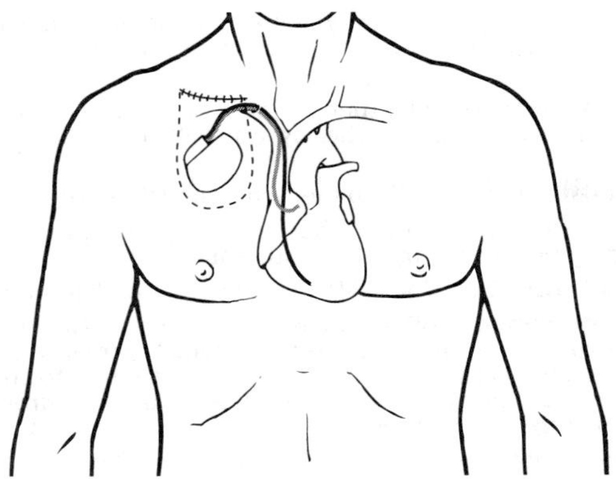

Pacemaker pocket in the prepectoral fascia.

**Pocul.** abbreviation for L. *po'culum,* cup.

**poc·u·lum** (pok'u-ləm) [L.] cup.
**p. Dio'genis,** [L. "Diogenes' cup"], the concave palm of the hand.

**po·dag·ra** (po-dag'rə) [*pod-* + *-agra*] gouty pain in the great toe.

**pod·a·gral** (pod'ə-grəl) pertaining to or characterized by podagra.

**po·dag·ric** (po-dag'rik) podagral.

**pod·a·grous** (pod'ə-grəs) podagral.

**po·dal·gia** (po-dal'jə) [*pod-* + *-algia*] pain in the foot; cf. *podagra* and *tarsalgia.* Called also *pedialgia* and *pododynia.*

**po·dal·ic** (po-dal'ik) [Gr. *pous* foot] pertaining to or accomplished by means of the feet; see under *version.*

**pod·ar·thri·tis** (pod"ahr-thri'tis) [*pod-* + *arthritis*] inflammation of the joints of the feet.

**pod·ede·ma** (pod"ə-de'mə) edema of the feet.

**pod·en·ceph·a·lus** (pod"ən-sef'ə-ləs) [*pod-* + Gr. *enkephalos* brain] a fetus whose brain, without a cranium, hangs by a pedicle.

**po·di·at·ric** (po"de-at'rik) pertaining to podiatry.

**po·di·a·trist** (po-di'ə-trist) a specialist in podiatry; formerly called *chiropodist.*

**po·di·a·try** (po-di'ə-tre) [*pod-* + *-iatry*] [MeSH: Podiatry] the specialized field that deals with the study and care of the foot, including its anatomy, pathology, medical and surgical treatment, etc. Formerly called *chiropody.*

**pod(o)-** [Gr. *pous,* gen. *podos* foot] a combining form denoting relationship to the foot.

**podo·cyte** (pod'o-sīt) [*podo-* + *-cyte*] a modified epithelial cell of the capsular epithelium of the renal glomerulus, having a small perikaryon and a number of primary and secondary footlike radiating processes (pedicels) that interdigitate with those of other podocytes and embrace the basal lamina of glomerular capillaries.

**po·do·dem·o·di·co·sis** (po"do-dem"ə-dĭ-ko'sis) [*podo-* + *demodicosis*] chronic infection of the skin of the feet of dogs or cats by mites of the genus *Demodex,* with pyoderma, alopecia, and scaling.

**podo·derm** (pod'o-dərm) [*podo-* + *-derm*] on hoofed animals, that portion of the skin that continues downward within the horn capsule of the hoof.

**po·do·der·ma·ti·tis** (po"do-der"mə-ti'tis) [*podo-* + *dermatitis*] foot rot of cattle.

**podo·dy·na·mom·e·ter** (pod"o-di"nə-mom'ə-tər) a dynamometer used for leg muscles.

**podo·dyn·ia** (pod"o-din'e-ə) [*pod-* + *-odynia*] podalgia.

**po·dof·i·lox** (po-dof'ĭ-loks) a biologically stable preparation of podophyllotoxin prepared by either chemical synthesis or purification from plant extracts; used especially in topical applications to treat genital warts.

**podo·gram** (pod'o-gram) [*podo-* + *-gram*] a print of, or an outline tracing of, the sole of the foot.

**podo·graph** (pod'o-graf) [*podo-* + *-graph*] the instrument used in the making of a podogram.

**po·dol·o·gy** (po-dol'ə-je) [*podo-* + *-logy*] podiatry.

**podo·phyl·lin** (pod"o-fil'in) [MeSH: Podophyllin] podophyllum resin.

**podo·phyl·lo·tox·in** (pod"o-fil"o-tok'sin) [*Podophyllum* + *toxin*] [MeSH: Podophyllotoxin] a highly toxic compound, the main active component of podophyllum; it has cathartic and antineoplastic properties. Less toxic derivatives such as etoposide and teniposide are used as antineoplastics.

**Podo·phyl·lum** (pod"o-fil'əm) [*podo-* + Gr. *phyllon* leaf] [MeSH: Podophyllum] a genus of perennial North American herbs of the family Berberidaceae. *P. pelta'tum* L. is the source of podophyllotoxin and podophyllum resin.

**podo·phyl·lum** (pod"o-fil'əm) [USP] [MeSH: Podophyllum] the dried rhizome and roots of *Podophyllum peltatum;* see *podophyllum resin,* under *resin.* Called also *Indian apple, mandrake, mandrake root, May apple,* and *vegetable calomel.*

**Po·do·stro·ma** (po"do-stro'mə) a genus of fungi of the family Hypocreaceae, including the perfect (sexual) stage of some species of *Trichoderma.*

**podo·troch·li·tis** (pod"o-trok-li'tis) [*podo-* + *trochlea* + *-itis*] navicular disease.

**po·do·troch·lo·sis** (po"do-trok-lo'sis) [*podo-* + L. *trochlea* pulley + *-osis*] navicular disease.

**poe-** for words beginning thus, see those beginning *pe-.*

**Poe·cil·ia** (pe-sil'e-ə) [Gr. *poikilos* spotted, mottled; varied] [MeSH: Poecilia] a genus of minnows; called also *Girardinus.*
**P. reticula'ta,** a species used, especially in tropical America, to control mosquitoes; they eat the larvae of *Anopheles.* Called also *Girardinus poeciloides.*

**po·go·ni·a·sis** (po"go-ni'ə-sis) [Gr. *pōgōn* beard + *-iasis*] 1. excessive growth of the beard. 2. the growth of a beard on a woman. See also *hirsutism.*

**po·go·ni·on** (po-go'ne-on) [Gr., dim. of *pōgōn* beard] a craniometric landmark, being the most anterior point in the contour of the chin in the sagittal plane.

**pOH** an infrequently used symbol used in expressing the approximate concentration of hydroxide ions in a solution.

**-poiesis** [Gr. *poiein* to make] a word termination meaning formation.

**-poietin** [Gr. *poiein* to make] a word termination used in names of hormones to indicate involvement in regulation of the numbers of various cell types in the peripheral blood.

**poikil(o)-** [Gr. *poikilos* spotted, mottled; varied] a combining form meaning mottled, variable, or irregular.

**poi·ki·lo·blast** (poi'kĭ-lo-blast") [*poikilo-* + *-blast*] an abnormally shaped erythroblast.

**poi·ki·lo·car·y·no·sis** (poi"kĭ-lo-kar"ĭ-no'sis) [*poikilo-* + *cary-* + *-osis*] Darier's term for the formation of various types and arrangements of cells which occurs in Bowen's disease.

**poi·ki·lo·cyte** (poi'kĭ-lo-sīt") [*poikilo-* + *-cyte*] an abnormally shaped erythrocyte, such as a burr cell, sickle cell, target cell, acanthocyte, elliptocyte, schistocyte, spherocyte, or stomatocyte.

**poi·ki·lo·cy·the·mia** (poi"kĭ-lo-si-the'me-ə) poikilocytosis.

**poi·ki·lo·cy·to·sis** (poi"kĭ-lo-si-to'sis) [*poikilocyte* + *-osis*] presence of poikilocytes in the blood; called also *poikilocythemia.*

**poi·ki·lo·der·ma** (poi"kĭ-lo-der'mə) a condition characterized by pigmentary and atrophic changes in the skin, giving it a mottled appearance.

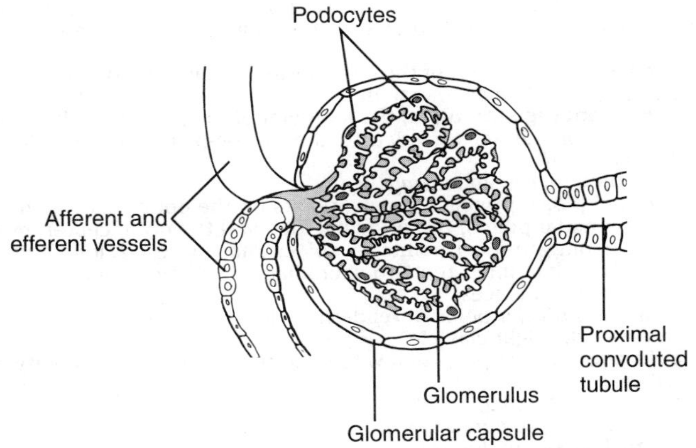


Podocytes in a diagrammatic view of a renal glomerulus within the glomerular capsule, their processes interdigitating along the capillary surfaces.

**p. atro'phicans vascula're,** p. vasculare atrophicans.
**p. of Civatte,** a skin condition seen almost exclusively on sun-exposed areas in middle-aged women, manifested as a reticulated blotchy reddish brown hyperpigmentation and telangiectasia with interspersed atrophic pale puncta localized to the face, neck, and upper chest, and believed to be associated with some type of photosensitivity mechanism.
**p. congenita'le,** Rothmund-Thomson syndrome.
**p. vascula're atro'phicans,** a localized or generalized, chronic, slightly scaling, patchy dermatitis characterized by hyper- and hypopigmentation, atrophy, telangiectases, and sometimes bright red papules, and an erythematous cigarette paper–like appearance of the skin resembling radiodermatitis, which usually occurs symmetrically on the breasts, buttocks, and flexural areas. It may be idiopathic or occur as a manifestation of various other dermatoses. It responds to treatment with systemic antibiotics. Called also *p. atrophicans vasculare.*

**poi·ki·lo·ploid** (poi'kĭ-lo-ploid") [*poikilo-* + *-ploid*] 1. pertaining to or characterized by poikiloploidy. 2. an individual having different cells with varying numbers of chromosomes.

**poi·ki·lo·ploidy** (poi'kĭ-lo-ploi"de) the state of having varying numbers of chromosomes in different cells.

**poi·ki·los·mo·sis** (poi"kil-oz-mo'sis) the processes by which a cell or tissue adjusts the osmolarity of its fluid to that of its immediate environment.

**poi·ki·los·mot·ic** (poi"kil-oz-mot'ik) pertaining to poikilosmosis.

**poi·ki·lo·sta·sis** (poi"kĭ-lo-sta'sis) [*poikilo-* + *-stasis*] the maintenance of stability in the body state (internal environment) by behavioral activities involving movement and selection by the whole organism.

**poi·ki·lo·therm** (poi-kil'o-therm") [*poikilo-* + Gr. *thermē* heat] 1. an animal that exhibits poikilothermy; a so-called cold-blooded animal. 2. ectotherm.

**poi·ki·lo·ther·mal** (poi"kĭ-lo-ther'məl) poikilothermic.

**poi·ki·lo·ther·mic** (poi"kĭ-lo-ther'mik) 1. pertaining to or characterized by poikilothermy. 2. ectothermic.

**poi·ki·lo·ther·mism** (poi"kĭ-lo-ther'miz-əm) poikilothermy.

**poi·ki·lo·ther·my** (poi"kĭ-lo-ther'me) [*poikilo-* + Gr. *thermē* heat] 1. the exhibition of body temperature which varies with the environmental temperature. 2. the ability of organisms to adapt themselves to variations in the temperature of their environment. Cf. *homeothermy.* 3. ectothermy.

**poi·ki·lo·throm·bo·cyte** (poi-kil"o-throm'bo-sīt) [*poikilo-* + *thrombocyte*] a blood platelet of abnormal shape.

**poi·ki·lo·thy·mia** (poi"kĭ-lo-thi'me-ə) [*poikilo-* + *-thymia*] a mental condition characterized by abnormal variations of mood.

**point** (point) [L. *punctum*] 1. a small area or spot; the sharp end of an object. 2. to approach the surface, like the pus of an abscess, at a definite spot or place. 3. a tapered, pointed endodontic instrument used for exploring the depth of the root canal in root canal therapy; called also *root canal p.* 4. an anthropometric landmark from which measurements are made. 5. an elongated silver or gutta-percha cone used in root canal obturation.

## Point

**p. A,** subspinale.
**absorbent p.,** in root canal therapy, a cone of variable width and taper, usually made of paper or a paper product, used to dry or maintain a liquid disinfectant in the canal. Called also *paper p.*
**Addison's p.,** the midpoint of the epigastric region.
**alveolar p.,** the center of the anterior margin of the alveolar arch.
**apophysiary p.,** subnasal p.
**p. Ar,** articulare.
**p. of Arrhigi,** an electrode site in electrocardiography, 2 to 3 cm to the left of the seventh thoracic vertebra.
**p. B,** supramentale.
**p. Ba,** basion.
**Barker's p.,** a point 1.25 inches above and 1.25 inches behind the middle external auditory meatus, the proper spot to apply the trephine in abscess of the temporosphenoid lobe.
**p. Bo,** Bolton p.
**Boas' p.,** a tender area to the left of the twelfth thoracic vertebra in patients with gastric ulcer.
**boiling p.,** the temperature at which a liquid will boil (at sea level water boils at 100°C, or 212°F); specifically, the temperature at which the equilibrium vapor pressure of a liquid phase equals or slightly exceeds the atmospheric pressure.
**boiling p., normal,** the temperature at which a liquid boils at one atmosphere pressure.
**Bolton p.,** a craniometric landmark located at the top of the convex curvature of the retrocondylar fossa, posterior to the condyle and between it and the basal surface of the occipital bone. Called also *p. Bo.*
**Brewer's p.,** the point of the costovertebral angle, tenderness over which points to kidney infection.
**Broadbent registration p.,** the midpoint of the perpendicular from the center of the sella turcica to the nasion-postcondylare plane. Called also *p. R.*
**Cannon's p.,** see under *ring.*
**cardinal p's,** 1. principal points; points on the optic axis which include the nodal points, the principal foci, and the optic center; may include conjugate focal points of object and image. 2. four points within the pelvic inlet: the two sacroiliac articulations and the two iliopectineal eminences.
**Chauffard's p.,** a point of tenderness in gallbladder disease, situated under the right clavicle.
**cold rigor p.,** that point of low temperature at which the activity of a cell ceases.
**condenser p.,** nib.
**conjugate p.,** see under *focus.*
**contact p.,** see under *area.*
**convenience p.,** a small depression at the edge of the floor of the prepared cavity, placed there to retain the first piece of direct filling gold during the process of compaction.
**p. of convergence,** 1. the point at which the lines of sight cross. 2. the point to which rays of light incline.
**corresponding p's,** points upon the two retinae whose impressions unite to produce a single perception. Cf. *disparate p's.*
**Cova's p.,** a point at the apex of the costolumbar angle which is tender on pressure in cases of pyelitis of pregnancy.
**craniometric p.,** any one of a set of points of reference assumed for use in craniometry.
**critical p.,** the point of coincidence of the gas and liquid phases, at which the temperature is the critical temperature and the pressure is the critical pressure, and the substance exists as a single phase.
**deaf p.,** one of certain points near the ear where a vibrating tuning-fork cannot be heard.
**Desjardins' p.,** a point on the abdomen 5 to 7 cm from the umbilicus, on a line joining it to the right axilla; it lies over the head of the pancreas.

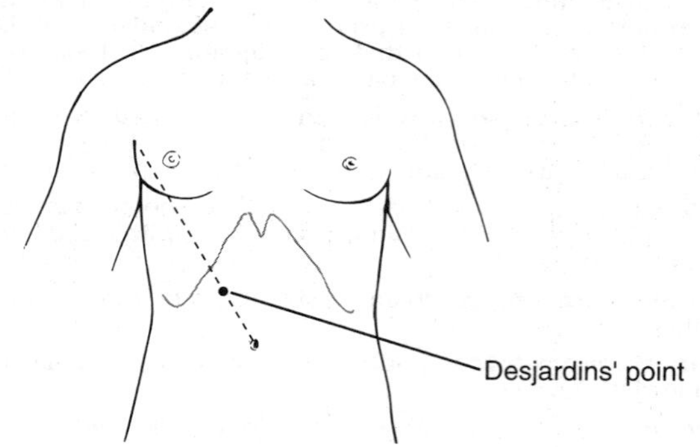


**p. of direction,** see *position* (def. 2).
**disparate p's,** points on the retina which are not paired exactly. Cf. *corresponding p's.*
**p. of dispersion,** in optics, virtual focus.
**p. of divergence,** the conjugate focus from which the light proceeds.
**dorsal p.,** in hepatic colic, a point, tender on pressure, situated between the spinous processes of the vertebrae at the border of the right scapula at the level of the fourth and fifth intercostal spaces at a distance of about 2 or 3 cm from the middle line. Called also *Pauly's p.*
**E p.,** in the apexcardiogram, the peak of the large positive deflection

that represents outward motion of the ventricle during systole; it normally coincides with the onset of ejection.

**p. of election,** that point at which any particular surgical operation is done by preference.

**Erb's p.,** a point two or three centimeters above the clavicle and beyond the posterior border of the sternomastoid, at the level of the transverse process of the sixth cervical vertebra; stimulation here contracts various arm muscles.

**eye p.,** 1. the bright circle seen at the crossing point or nearest the approximation of the rays above the microscopical ocular. 2. See under *spot.*

**far p.,** the remotest point at which an object is clearly seen when the eye is at rest; called also *punctum remotum.*

**p. of fixation,** 1. the point or object on which the eyes are directed and one's sight is fixed; called also *p. of regard.* 2. the point on the retina, usually the fovea, on which are focused the rays coming from an object directly regarded.

**focal p.,** see *focus* (def. 1), and *cardinal p.* (def. 1).

**freezing p.,** the temperature at which a liquid begins to freeze; that of pure water is 0°C, or 32°F. It is often used interchangeably with *melting p.* but should be reserved for substances being cooled while melting point is used for substances being heated.

**fusion p.,** melting p.

**glenoid p.,** the center of the glenoid cavity of the scapula.

**gutta-percha p.,** see under *cone.*

**Hallé's p.,** a point on the surface of the abdomen corresponding to the point where the ureter crosses the pelvic brim. It is the point of intersection between a horizontal line connecting the anterior superior iliac spines and a vertical line projected superiorly from the pubic spine.

**hinge-axis p.,** a reference point on the skin corresponding with the terminal hinge axis of the mandible.

**hysteroepileptogenous p., hysterogenic p.,** a point on which, if pressure such as tickling is exerted, a hysteric or hysteroepileptic attack may be produced.

**ice p.,** the true melting point of ice, being the temperature of equilibrium between ice and air-saturated water under one atmosphere pressure.

**identical p's,** corresponding p's.

**p. of incidence,** see *refraction,* def. 2.

**isobestic p.,** the wavelength at which two substances have the same absorptivity, such that if the sum of the concentrations of the compounds in solution is held constant, the absorbance at this point will be invariant as the ratio of the two compounds is varied; existence of one or more such points is indicative of chemical equilibrium between the two compounds.

**isoelectric p.,** the pH of a solution at which a charged molecule does not migrate in an electric field.

**isoionic p.,** the pH of a solution at which a specific ion (usually a protein) contains as many negative charges as positive charges.

**J p.,** the point of intersection between the end of the QRS complex and the onset of the ST segment in electrocardiography.

**jugal p.,** the point of the angle formed by the masseteric and maxillary edges of the malar bone (os zygomaticum).

**jugomaxillary p.,** the point at the anteroinferior angle of the malar bone (os zygomaticum).

**Keen's p.,** a point for puncture of the lateral ventricles; 3 cm above and 3 cm behind the external auditory meatus.

**Kienböck-Adamson p's,** points and lines to be marked on the scalp to indicate the areas for the application of x-ray therapy in order to produce temporary epilation for the treatment of tinea capitis.

**Kocher's p.,** a point for puncture of the lateral ventricles; 2.5 cm from the midline, 3.5 cm in front of the bregma.

**Krafft p.,** the temperature above which conjugated bile salts form polymolecular aggregates (micelles) of about 3 to 10 nm in diameter.

**lacrimal p.,** punctum lacrimale.

**Lanz's p.,** a point which indicates the position of the vermiform appendix; it is situated on a line connecting the two anterior superior iliac spines one third of the distance from the right spine.

**McBurney's p.,** a point situated about one-third the distance between the right anterior superior iliac spine and the umbilicus. It corresponds with the normal position of the base of the appendix and is a point of special tenderness in acute appendicitis.

**McEwen's p.,** a point above the inner canthus of the eye which is tender in acute frontal sinusitis.

**Mackenzie's p.,** a point of tenderness in gallbladder disease in the upper segment of the rectus muscle.

**malar p.,** a point on the external tubercle of the malar bone (os zygomaticum).

**p. of maximal impulse (PMI),** the point on the chest where the impulse of the left ventricle is felt most strongly, normally in the fifth costal interspace inside the left mammillary line.

**maximum occipital p.,** the point in the occipital bone situated furthest from the glabella.

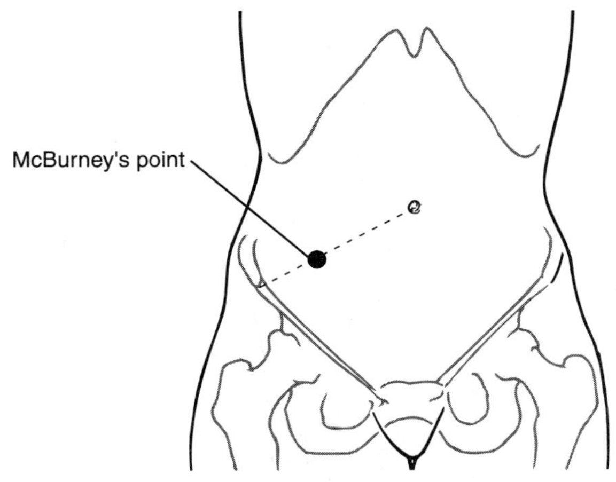


**median mandibular p.,** a craniometric landmark, being the point on the anteroposterior center of the mandibular ridge in the median plane, at the site of former mandibular symphysis.

**Méglin's p.,** a point where the greater palatine nerve emerges from the great palatine foramen.

**melting p.,** the minimum temperature at which a solid begins to liquefy. Abbreviated mp. See also *freezing p.* Cf. *melting temperature* and *fusion temperature.*

**mental p.,** pogonion.

**metopic p.,** glabella.

**motor p.,** 1. the point at which a motor nerve enters a muscle. 2. any point on the skin over a muscle at which the application of galvanic stimulation will cause contraction of a corresponding muscle.

**Munro's p.,** a point midway between the umbilicus and the left anterior iliac spine; used for performing abdominal puncture.

**nasal p.,** nasion.

**near p.,** the nearest point at which the eye can distinctly perceive an object; the nearest point of clear vision; called also *punctum proximum.*

**near p., absolute,** the near point for either eye alone with accommodation relaxed.

**near p., relative,** the near point for both eyes with the employment of accommodation.

**nodal p's,** one of two points on the axis of an optical system so situated that a ray falling on one will produce a parallel ray emerging through the other.

**O p.,** the nadir of the apexcardiogram, occurring in early diastole at the time of mitral valve opening.

**occipital p.,** the posterior point on the occipital bone.

**ossification p.,** centrum ossificationis.

**ossification p., primary,** centrum ossificationis primarium.

**ossification p., secondary,** centrum ossificationis secundarium.

**paper p.,** absorbent p.

**Pauly's p.,** dorsal p.

**phrenic-pressure p.,** a point along the phrenic nerve between the sternocleidomastoid and the scalenus anticus on the right side; pressure on the point suggests gallbladder disease.

**Piersol's p.,** a point indicating the location of the vesical orifice.

**p. Po,** porion.

**pour p.,** the temperature at which a liquid just begins to flow.

**preauricular p.,** a point on the posterior root of the zygomatic arch just anterior to the auricular point.

**pressure p.,** 1. a point that is particularly sensitive to pressure. 2. one of various locations on the body at which digital pressure may be applied for the control of hemorrhage.

**pressure-arresting p.,** a point at which pressure arrests spasm.

**pressure-exciting p.,** a point at which pressure produces spasm.

**principal p's,** cardinal p's (def. 1).

**p. R,** Broadbent registration p.

**Ramond's p.,** a point of tenderness in gallbladder disease between the heads of the sternocleidomastoid muscle.

**reflection p.,** the point from which a ray of light is reflected.

**refraction p.,** the point at which a ray of light is refracted.

**p. of regard,** p. of fixation (def. 1).

**retromandibular tender p.,** a point behind the superior extremity of the inferior maxilla below the lobule of the ear and in front of the mastoid process. Pressure on this point elicits extreme pain in meningitis.

**p. of reversal,** in retinoscopy, the point at which there is neutralization of movement because the reflex motion is changing to the opposite direction.

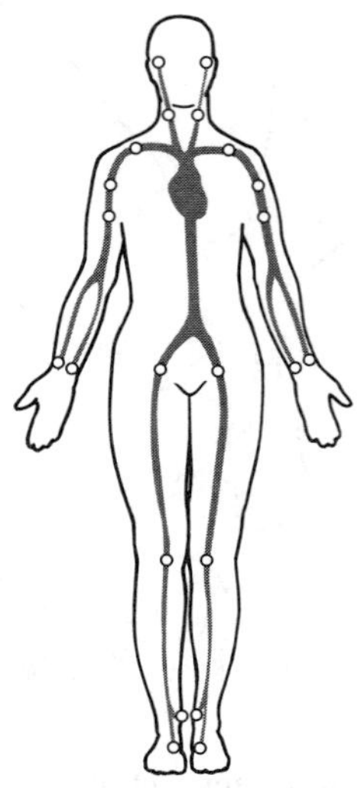

Various pressure points used to control hemorrhage.

**Robson's p.,** the point of greatest tenderness in gallbladder inflammation, situated opposite the junction of the middle and lower third of a line drawn from the right nipple to the umbilicus.
**root canal p.,** point (def. 3).
**p. SE,** sphenoethmoidal suture (def. 2).
**set p.,** see under *S.*
**silver p.,** in root canal therapy, a tapered and elongated silver plug that is cemented into the canal as a filling. Called also *silver cone.*
**p. SO,** spheno-occipital synchondrosis (def. 2).
**spinal p.,** subnasal p.
**stereoidentical p's,** points in space outside of the region within which fusion of double images occurs.
**subnasal p.,** the central point of the root of the anterior nasal spine.
**subtemporal p.,** the point where the sphenotemporal suture and infratemporal crest intersect.
**supra-auricular p.,** a point at the root of the zygomatic process of the temporal bone, directly superior to the auricular point.
**supraclavicular p.,** a point above the clavicle and outside of the sternomastoid where the application of a stimulus causes contraction of the biceps brachii, deltoideus, brachialis, and brachioradialis muscles.
**supranasal p.,** ophryon.
**supraorbital p.,** 1. ophryon. 2. in neuralgia, a tender spot just superior to the supraorbital notch.
**sylvian p.,** a point on the surface of the skull from 29 to 32 mm behind the external angular process of the frontal bone.
**thermal death p.,** the lowest temperature at which a broth culture of microorganisms can be heat-killed in a 10-minute exposure time.
**trigger p.,** a particular spot on the body on which pressure or other stimulus will give rise to specific sensations or symptoms.
**triple p.,** the temperature and pressure at which three different phases of a substance are in equilibrium. The *triple point of water* (ice, liquid, vapor) is 273.15°K.
**vital p.,** a point in the medulla oblongata, at the respiratory center, puncture of which causes immediate death.
**Vogt's p., Vogt-Hueter p.,** a point at the intersection of a horizontal line two fingerbreadths above the zygoma with a vertical line a thumbbreadth behind the ascending sphenofrontal process; here trephination may be performed in traumatic meningeal hemorrhage.
**Voillemier's p.,** a point on the linea alba 6.5 cm below the line which joins the anterior superior iliac spinous processes; here the bladder may be punctured in obese or edematous patients.
**p. Z,** a point formed by a line perpendicular to the nasion-menton line through the anterior nasal spine.
**Ziemssen's motor p.,** motor p.

**point·er** (point'ər) a contusion at a bony eminence.
**hip p.,** contusion of the bone of the iliac crest or avulsion of muscle attachments of the iliac crest.

**Poi·ri·er's glands, line** (pwah-re-āz') [Paul *Poirier,* French surgeon, 1853–1907] see under *gland* and *line.*

**poise** (poiz; Fr. pwahz) [J. M. *Poiseuille*] the unit of viscosity of a liquid, being number of grams per centimeter per second. Symbol P. The commonly used unit is the *centipoise,* or one one-hundredth of a poise.

**Poi·seuille's law, space** (pwah-swēz') [Jean Leonard Marie *Poiseuille,* French physiologist, 1799–1869] see under *law* and *space.*

**poi·son** (poi'zən) [L. *potio* draft] any substance that, when relatively small amounts are ingested, inhaled, or absorbed, or applied to, injected into, or developed within the body, has chemical action that causes damage to structure or disturbance of function, producing symptoms, illness, or death. See also *toxin* and *venom.*
**acrid p.,** one that produces irritation or inflammation, such as the mineral acids, oxalic acid, the caustic alkalis, antimony, arsenic, the salts of copper, some of the compounds of lead, silver nitrate, and the salts of zinc, iodine, cantharides, or phosphorus.
**acronarcotic p., acrosedative p.,** a poison that may produce either irritation, narcotism (or sedation), or both together; most common ones are from plant sources. Stramonium and belladonna are examples of acronarcotics and aconite is an acrosedative.
**arrow p.,** a preparation of plant alkaloids used on arrows in certain primitive societies.
**catalyst p.,** a substance firmly bound to the active areas on the surface of a catalyst, which prevents the adsorption of the reactants for the desired chemical reaction.
**corrosive p.,** any poison which acts by directly destroying tissue.
**fatigue p.,** kenotoxin.
**fugu p.,** tetrodotoxin.
**hemotropic p.,** a poison which has a special affinity for erythrocytes.
**irritant p.,** acrid p.
**mitotic p.,** a toxic principle that interferes with cell division.
**muscle p.,** one that interferes with normal action or functioning of muscle.
**narcotic p's,** poisons causing stupor or delirium, such as opium and hyoscyamus.
**puffer p.,** tetrodotoxin.
**sedative p's,** those which directly depress the vital centers, as hydrocyanic acid, potassium cyanide, hydrogen sulfide, and other of the poisonous gases.
**shellfish p.,** saxitoxin.
**toot p.,** a poison from *Coriaria sarmentosa,* a plant of New Zealand.
**vascular p.,** a poison which acts by affecting the blood vessels.
**whelk p.,** a toxic substance localized in the salivary gland of the whelk; its principal ingredient is tetramethylammonium hydroxide.
See also under *poisoning.*

**poi·son·ing** (poi'zən-ing) [MeSH: Poisoning] the symptoms, illness, or death produced by a poison; see also *intoxication.*

**akee p.**, Jamaican vomiting sickness.
**aluminum p.**, the toxic effects of high levels of aluminum or aluminum compounds in the body. In the gastrointestinal tract aluminum inhibits absorption of calcium, fluorides, iron, and phosphates; inhalation of bauxite fumes may cause pulmonary fibrosis (see *aluminosis*); and aluminum in the bloodstream may lead to neurological symptoms that can be fatal (see *dialysis encephalopathy,* under *encephalopathy*).
**anticholinergic p.**, poisoning caused by overdosage with an anticholinergic agent or by ingestion of plants such as jimsonweed that contain belladonna alkaloids. It is characterized by dry mouth, hot, dry, flushed skin, fixed and dilated pupils, sinus tachycardia, urinary retention, disorientation, agitation, impairment of short-term memory, slurred speech, hallucinations, respiratory depression, seizures, and coma; in rare cases death may occur. Treatment is by induced emesis and administration of activated charcoal; physostigmine may be used in severe cases to reverse the anticholinergic effects.
**anticoagulant rodenticide p.**, accidental poisoning of domestic animals or livestock, with death from hemorrhaging, after consuming an anticoagulant rodenticide such as an indanedione or warfarin derivative. They may eat the poison itself or may eat rodents that died from such rodenticides.
**antimony p.**, poisoning due to ingestion of antimony compounds, such as from industrial exposure; the symptoms are similar to those of acute arsenic poisoning, with vomiting a prominent symptom. Called also *stibialism.*
**arsenic p.**, poisoning due to systemic exposure to inorganic pentavalent arsenic. *Acute arsenic poisoning,* which may result in shock and death, is marked by erythematous skin eruptions, vomiting, diarrhea, abdominal pain, muscular cramps, and swelling of the eyelids, feet, and hands. *Chronic arsenic poisoning* (called also *arsenicalism* and *arsenism*), due to the ingestion of small amounts over a long period of time, is marked by pigmentation of the skin accompanied by scaling, hyperkeratosis of the palms and soles, transverse white lines on the fingernails (Mees' lines), headache, peripheral neuropathy, and confusion.
**barium p.**, poisoning from excessive ingestion of barium or one of its salts, characterized by gastrointestinal symptoms such as stomach pain, nausea, vomiting, and diarrhea, followed by severe, sometimes fatal hypokalemia with paralysis.
**beryllium p.**, berylliosis.
**bismuth p.**, poisoning from excessive or chronic ingestion of bismuth or its salts; symptoms include anuria, stomatitis, dermatitis, and diarrhea. Called also *bismuthism* and *bismuthosis.*
**blister beetle p.**, cantharidin p.
**blood p.**, septicemia.
**blue-green algae p.**, cyanobacteria p.
**bongkrek p.**, poisoning from bongkrek, a Javanese dish prepared by means of molds from copra press cake. When the fermentation process is faulty, severe poisoning occurs, with vomiting, profuse perspiration, muscle cramps, and coma. Called also *tempeh p.*
**boron p.**, poisoning of humans or other animals by boron, boric acid, or a borate salt such as sodium borate (borax). Symptoms include weakness, ataxia, tremors, convulsions, and often death.
**bracken p.**, poisoning of animals after eating *Pteridium aquilinum* (bracken). In monogastric animals it consists of severe intoxication due to enzymatic destruction of thiamine by a thiaminase present in the plant; in ruminants it is apparently due to a dialyzable small molecule that causes bone marrow hypoplasia and eventual death. See also *enzootic bovine hematuria,* under *hematuria.*
**broom p.**, poisoning of humans or other animals by ingestion of *Cytisus scoparius* or other brooms, leguminous shrubs that contain sparteine and cytisine. Characteristics include nausea, vomiting, dizziness, and sometimes clonic convulsions with fatal respiratory paralysis.
**buckthorn p.**, poisoning of humans or other animals that consume the fruit of *Karwinskia humboldtiana* (buckthorn), which contains a neurotoxin. Demyelination and axonal degeneration occur in peripheral nerves, slowly progressing to muscle weakness, paralysis, and death.
**cadmium p.**, poisoning from excessive ingestion of cadmium or breathing in of its fumes; symptoms include nausea, vomiting, salivation, diarrhea, abdominal pain, and occasionally cardiovascular collapse. Long-term exposure may cause renal disease with tubulopathy and proteinuria.
**callistin shellfish p.**, poisoning caused by ingestion of the gastropod shellfish *Callista brevisphonata*; an outbreak occurred in Japan in the 1950s. It was believed to be due to a choline present in the ovaries of the shellfish.
**cantharidin p.**, poisoning of horses or ruminants by hay contaminated with blister beetles whose bodies contain cantharidin; signs include hyperemia or erosions of the oral and esophageal mucosa, frequent urination, and sometimes shock and death. Called also *blister beetle p.* and *cantharidism.*
**carbamate p.**, poisoning of humans or other animals by exposure to excessive amounts of carbamate insecticides; characteristics include salivation, tremors, dyspnea, and occasionally convulsions.
**carbon disulfide p.**, a condition occurring in workers who excessively inhale fumes of carbon disulfide; characteristics include weakness, sleeplessness, and visual impairment, and sometimes gastric ulcers, encephalopathy, and paralysis.
**carbon monoxide p.**, poisoning due to the inhalation of carbon monoxide and the resulting change of oxyhemoglobin to carboxyhemoglobin (see *carboxyhemoglobinemia*); it may result in tissue hypoxia, cellular anoxia, damage to the central nervous system, and death.
**cobalt p.**, poisoning from long-term excessive exposure to cobalt, seen in those who work with cobalt and formerly in beer drinkers because for years cobalt was added to beer as a foam stabilizer. Symptoms include nausea, vomiting, tinnitus, nerve deafness, and cardiomyopathy *(beer-drinkers' cardiomyopathy).*
**copper p.**, poisoning by copper or copper salts. In humans it usually follows excessive intake of medicinal cupric sulfate or results from an enzyme deficiency such as Menkes' syndrome or Wilson's disease. Characteristics include vomiting, which may be bluegreen, hypotension, jaundice, and coma that may end in death. In animals it is most common in ruminants and pigs after excessive intake of medicinal or fungicidal copper; acute poisoning is characterized by vomiting and convulsions, while chronic poisoning is marked by liver and kidney damage. Chronic buildup of liver copper stores resulting in release of copper into the bloodstream may cause symptoms similar to those of acute poisoning and may be fatal.
**corn cockle p.**, githagism.
**cyanide p.**, poisoning of humans or other animals by cyanide compounds, potent rapid-acting substances that cause cellular hypoxia by formation of an inactive complex of cytochrome oxidase and cyanide. Characteristics include nausea without vomiting, dizziness, convulsions, opisthotonos, and death from respiratory paralysis. The usual cause in livestock and other animals is ingestion of plants containing cyanogenetic compounds (see table). In humans it is usually the result of exposure to hydrogen cyanide liquid or gas that is given off by a fungicide, insecticide, or other substance. Cyanide is detoxified by the liver enzyme thiosulfate sulfurtransferase, which catalyzes the reaction of cyanide with thiosulfate to form thiocyanide.
**cyanobacteria p.**, poisoning in humans or other animals by cyanobacteria, usually as a result of drinking contaminated water. The most common genera of such bacteria are Anabaena, Aphanizomenon, Gloeotrichia, Microcystis (Anacystis), Nodularia, and Oscillatoria. In most cases it is a subacute condition characterized by liver damage with jaundice and sometimes bloody diarrhea and photosensitization. Drinking of heavily contaminated water may cause acute symptoms including muscle tremors, ataxia, dyspnea, cyanosis, and hyperesthesia so that a slight touch may cause convulsions and opisthotonos, which can be fatal. Called also *blue-green algae p.*
**darnel p.**, a type of rye grass poisoning of humans or other animals after ingesting the seeds of darnel, *Lolium temulentum,* probably only when they are contaminated with a mold such as *Endoconidium temulentum* (see *endoconidiotoxicosis*); in humans this happens when moldy seeds accidentally contaminate flour. Characteristics include giddiness, staggering, vertigo, vomiting, and visual disturbances.
**djenkol bean p.**, poisoning by the djenkol bean; symptoms vary from lumbar pain, vomiting, and diarrhea to hematuria and proteinuria progressing to anuria and renal failure. Called also *djenkolism.*
**elasmobranch p.**, a form of ichthyosarcotoxism seen in humans or other animals after ingestion of certain toxic sharks and skates. One type results from eating the muscle tissue of the shark *Somniosus microcephalus.* Another type is hypervitaminosis A from eating the liver of any of various species.
**ergot p.**, ergotism.
**esowasure-gai p.**, Japanese name for *callistin shellfish p.*
**fish p.**, ichthyosarcotoxism.
**fluoride p., chronic, fluorine p., chronic,** fluorosis.
**fluoroacetate p.**, poisoning of humans or other animals by fluoroacetate compounds. Carnivores are affected when they eat small animals that have died from fluoroacetate rodenticides, and ruminants are affected when they eat fluoroacetate-containing plants such as *Acacia georginae* or species of *Dichapetalum, Gastrolobium, Oxylobium,* or *Palicourea.* Poisoning in humans is usually caused by ingestion of rodenticides. Fluoroacetate blocks one of the steps in the tricarboxylic acid cycle, causing symptoms that are often fatal such as neurological problems ranging from ataxia and agitation to convulsions, and heart problems such as severe tachycardia and cardiomyopathy.
**food p.**, a group of illnesses varying in severity from mild and self-limited to life threatening, caused by ingestion of contaminated food or food that is inherently poisonous. Various microorganisms may cause it, the most common being pathogenic bacteria or their products (toxins), e.g., *Staphylococcus aureus, Bacillus cereus, Campylobacter, Clostridium botulinum, C. perfringens, Escherichia coli, Vibrio cholerae, V. parahaemolyticus, Shigella* species, *Salmonella* species, and

**Plants That Can Cause Cyanide Poisoning**

| Latin Name | Common Name |
|---|---|
| *Acacia leucophloea; A. sieberana* | Acacias |
| *Adenia digitata* | |
| *Andrachne decaisnei* | Andrachne |
| *Anthemis cotula* | Mayweed |
| *Aquilegia vulgaris* | Columbine |
| *Bahia oppositifolia* | |
| *Brachyachne* spp. | |
| *Bridelia exaltata* | Scrub ironbark tree |
| *Calotis scapigera* | |
| *Canthium vaccinifolium* | |
| *Cercocarpus* spp. | |
| *Chenopodium* (certain species) | |
| *Chloris distichophylla* | Rhodes grass, windmill grass |
| *Cynodon* spp. | Couch grass |
| *Dactyloctenium radulans* | |
| *Digitaria sanguinais* | A type of crab grass |
| *Dimorphotheca ecklonis* | South African daisy |
| *Eleusine indica* | Crab grass, crow's foot grass |
| *Eremophila maculata* | A type of native fuchsia |
| *Eriobotrya japonica* | Loquat |
| *Eschscholtzia* spp. | Eschscholtzia, California poppy |
| *Eucalyptus* spp. | Eucalyptus |
| *Euphorbia* spp. | Spurge |
| *Florestina tripteris* | |
| *Glyceria striata* | Manna grass |
| *Gooida lotifolia* | |
| *Grevillea* spp. | Silky oak |
| *Gyrostemon ramulosus* | |
| *Hakea* spp. | Cushionflower |
| *Haloragis heterophylla* | Raspwort, raspweed |
| *Heterodendron oleifolium* | (Australian) rosewood |
| *Holcus lanatus* | Velvet grass, Yorkshire fog |
| *Hydrangea* spp. | Hydrangea |
| *Indigofera australis* | Indigo plant |
| *Lambertia* spp. | (Australian) honeysuckle |
| *Linum* spp. | Flax |
| *Lotonis laxa* | |
| *Lotus* spp. | Bird's foot trefoil |
| *Loudonia roei* | |
| *Macadamia ternifolia* | Macadamia |
| *Manihot esculenta* | Cassawa, manioc |
| *Nerium oleander* | Oleander |
| *Panicum* spp. | Coolah grass, klein grass, Guinea grass |
| *Passiflora* spp. | Passion flower |
| *Phaseolus limensis* | Lima bean |
| *Phyllanthus gasstroemii* | |
| *Poranthera microphylla* | |
| *Prunus* spp. | Apricot, cherry, peach, plum, sloe |
| *Pyrus* spp. | Pear |
| *Sambucus nigra* | Elder |
| *Sorghum* spp. | Johnson grass, sudan grass |
| *Stillingia treculeana* | Queen's delight |
| *Suckleya suckleyana* | |
| *Trifolium repens* | White clover, Landino clover |
| *Triglochin* spp. | Arrowgrass |
| *Vicia sativa* | Vetch |
| *Xylomelum angustifolium* | Sandplain woody pear |
| *Zea mays* | Corn |
| *Zieria* spp. | |

*Yersinia enterocolitica.* Bacterial food poisoning is usually manifested as acute gastroenteritis but may be associated with such syndromes as botulism, typhoid fever, and cholera. Neurologic symptoms can also be caused by food poisoning as a result of ingestion of chemically toxic foods, such as certain mushrooms and berries, or may involve substances such as heavy metals, mercury, or insecticides.

**forage p.,** a type of mycotoxicosis seen in domestic animals, especially horses, resulting from ingestion of food contaminated with a fungus, usually *Fusarium moniliforme.* It causes neurotoxicity, particularly inflammation or softening of the white matter of the brain, with symptoms such as ataxia, tremor, circling, dimmed vision, drowsiness, and sometimes death. See also *moldy corn p.* Called also *leukoencephalitis, leukoencephalomalacia, mycotoxic leukoencephalomalacia,* and *sleepy staggers.*

**fugu p.,** tetrodotoxism (def. 1).

**gossypol p.,** poisoning from eating cottonseed cake that contains a high proportion of gossypol; most often seen in pigs.

**Gymnothorax p.,** a form of ichthyosarcotoxism produced by ingestion of certain moray eels of the genus *Gymnothorax.*

**heavy metal p.,** poisoning with any of the heavy metals, particularly arsenic, lead, mercury, antimony, cadmium, or thallium.

**iodine p.,** iodism.

**iron p.,** poisoning from ingestion of excessive iron or iron-containing compounds, such as in children who eat iron supplement tablets like candy; symptoms include ulceration of the gastrointestinal tract, vomiting, vasodilation with shock, metabolic acidosis, liver injury, and coagulation disturbances.

**larkspur p.,** poisoning of humans, cattle. or sheep by the fresh leaves and roots of certain species of *Delphinium* (larkspur), which contain delphinine and other alkaloids. Ingestion sometimes results in instantaneous death, probably from paralysis of the heart, and sometimes causes neurological symptoms of less rapid onset that may also terminate in paralysis and asphyxia.

**lead p.,** poisoning due to the absorption or ingestion of lead or one of its salts. The symptoms include loss of appetite, weight loss, colic, constipation, insomnia, headache, dizziness, irritability, moderate hypertension, albuminuria, anemia, a blue line at the edge of the gums *(lead line),* encephalopathy (especially in children), and peripheral neuropathy leading to paralysis. Called also *plumbism.*

**loco p., locoweed p.,** locoism.

**manganese p.,** poisoning by manganese, usually caused by inhalation of manganese dust. Symptoms include neurotoxicity with a syndrome resembling paralysis agitans, and inflammation throughout the respiratory system; see also *manganese pneumonitis,* under *pneumonitis.* Called also *manganism.*

**meat p.,** acute, often severe gastroenteritis, most often caused by meat contaminated with *Bacillus cereus, Clostridium perfringens,* invasive *Escherichia coli, Salmonella, Staphylococcus aureus,* or *Yersinia enterocolitica.*

**mercury p.,** acute or chronic disease caused by mercury and its salts. The *acute* form, due to ingestion, is marked by severe abdominalgia, metallic taste in the mouth, vomiting, bloody diarrhea with watery stools, oliguria or anuria (usually at onset), and corrosion and ulceration of the entire digestive tract. The *chronic* form, due to absorption by the skin and mucous membranes, inhalation of vapors, or ingestion of mercury salts, is marked by stomatitis, metallic taste in the mouth, a blue line along the border of the gum, sore hypertrophied gums that bleed easily, loosening of the teeth, erethism, excessive secretion of saliva, tremors, and incoordination.

**milk p.,** see under *sickness.*

**moldy corn p.,** forage poisoning occurring when animals eat corn contaminated with the fungus *Fusarium moniliforme,* which contains toxic fumonisins. Called also *cornstalk disease.*

**molybdenum p.,** poisoning due to ingestion of large amounts of molybdenum, characterized by weakness, diarrhea, and loss of hair pigmentation; seen primarily in livestock that graze in certain kinds of pastures (see *teart*). Called also *molybdenosis.*

**mushroom p.,** poisoning resulting from ingestion of mushrooms; potentially deadly types result from ingestion of *Amanita phalloides, A. verna, A. virosa,* and species of *Chlorophyllum, Galerina,* and *Lepiota,* which contain neurotoxic amatoxins. The clinical course usually begins with nausea, vomiting, abdominal pain, and diarrhea, followed by a quiescent period of up to 48 hours, and then signs and symptoms of severe hepatic, renal, and central nervous system damage followed by death.

**mussel p.,** see *shellfish p.*

**naphthol p.,** the toxic condition brought on by the ingestion or absorption through the skin of naphthol, characterized by anemia, jaundice, convulsions, and coma. Called also *naphtholism.*

**neurotoxic shellfish p.,** see *shellfish p.*

**nicotine p.,** poisoning by ingestion of excessive amounts of nicotine, usually seen in children who eat cigarettes or in workers who handle wet tobacco leaves; symptoms include stimulation followed by depression of the central and autonomic nervous systems and occasionally death due to respiratory paralysis. See also *green tobacco sickness.* Called also *nicotinism.*

**nicotine sulfate p.,** poisoning of lambs or calves by nicotine sulfate, formerly used as a component of vermifuges. Symptoms include tremors, rapid respiration, recumbency, and convulsions; severe cases may end in death.

**nitrite p.,** poisoning of ruminants grazing on nitrate-rich plants; the nitrates break down into nitrites in the body. Plants naturally rich in nitrates include *Chenopodium album, Salvia reflexa,* and species of *Amaranthus.* Poisoning can also occur in fields heavily dosed with certain fertilizers (see *ammonium nitrate* and *sodium nitrate*). Characteristics include gastroenteritis, diarrhea, potentially fatal methemoglobinemia with anemic anoxia, dyspnea, tremors, and cyanosis.

**nitroaniline p.,** poisoning by nitroaniline, a dye used in paints, inks, and other products, characterized by intense methemoglobinemia.

**nutmeg p.,** severe toxic symptoms produced by ingestion of powdered nutmeg, characterized by narcosis with periods of delirium and excitability.

**organophosphorus compound p.,** poisoning of humans or other animals by excessive exposure to an organophosphorus compound (see table at *organophosphorus*); it often ends fatally. Humans, sheep, and pigs show primarily neurologic signs such as axonopathy and paralysis; cattle, horses, dogs, and cats more often have ataxia or tremors and diarrhea.

**oxalate p.,** poisoning of humans or other animals by oxalic acid or oxalates, usually by ingesting large quantities of oxalate-containing plants (see table). Characteristics include gastroenteritis, hypotension, hypocalcemia, muscle weakness and twitching, nephrosis, and hyperoxaluria. Called also *oxalism.*

**oxygen p.,** see under *toxicity.*

**paraldehyde p.,** paraldehydism.

**paralytic shellfish p.,** see *shellfish p.*

**paraquat p.,** poisoning by paraquat that has been either ingested or absorbed through the skin. Contact with concentrated solutions causes irritation of the skin, cracking and shedding of the nails, and delayed healing of cuts and wounds. After ingestion of large doses, potentially fatal renal and hepatic failure may develop, followed by pulmonary insufficiency.

**parathyroid p.,** the increase in metastatic calcification of organs, particularly the kidneys, when a high calcium diet is given a patient with hyperparathyroidism.

**phenol p.,** poisoning due to ingestion or absorption through the skin of phenol; symptoms include colic, local irritation, corrosion, seizures, cardiac arrhythmias, shock, and respiratory arrest. Called also *carbolism.*

**phosphorus p.,** a condition resulting from ingestion or inhalation of phosphorus, manifested by mandibular necrosis (see *phosphorus necrosis*), toothache, anorexia, weakness, and anemia.

**pitch p.,** an often fatal disorder of domestic animals or livestock, particularly pigs, after they lick or chew on pitch-containing substances such as the tarred walls and floors of pigpens or clay pigeons used in target practice; characteristics include liver damage, inappetence, depression, weakness, jaundice, and anemia.

**puffer p., puffer fish p.,** tetrodotoxism (def. 1).

**ragwort p.,** seneciosis.

**rodenticide p.,** accidental poisoning of domestic animals or livestock by the effects of rodenticides, either when they directly eat the poison or when they eat rodents that died from the poison. See also *fluoroacetate p.* and *anticoagulant rodenticide p.*

**rye grass p.,** poisoning of an animal or occasionally a human by eating rye grass (genus *Lolium*), usually consisting of mycotoxicosis when the grass is moldy. Common types are darnel poisoning and rye grass staggers. See also *endoconidiotoxicosis.*

**salmon p.,** poisoning in canines, other carnivores, or sometimes humans, usually in the Pacific Northwest, from eating raw fish, especially salmon and trout, that are parasitized by the fluke *Troglotrema salmincola,* which serves as a vector of various rickettsiae. When the etiologic agent is *Neorickettsia helminthoeca*, animals or humans suffer from hemorrhagic enteritis. A milder form, caused by an unknown rickettsia, is called *Elokomin fluke fever.*

**salt p.,** poisoning of animals, especially pigs and birds, due to ingestion of too much salt in the absence of available water, marked by excessive thirst, diarrhea, and vomiting, often culminating in death.

**saturnine p.,** lead p.

**sausage p.,** see *allantiasis* and *botulism.*

**scombroid p.,** a form of ichthyosarcotoxism caused by the ingestion of a toxic histamine-like substance produced by the action of bacteria on histidine, a normal component of fish flesh. Scombroid fish (tuna, bonito, mackerel, etc.) are particularly susceptible to bacterial decomposition, and when inadequately preserved contaminated fish are eaten the symptoms of the illness, including epigastric pain, nausea, vomiting, headache, dysphagia, thirst, urticaria, and pruritus, develop and usually last for less than 24 hours.

**selenium p.,** poisoning of livestock from grazing on plants that have absorbed excessive selenium from the soil. Areas of selenium-rich soil have been found in the northern Great Plains of North America, Ireland, Israel, China, Russia, and elsewhere. *Chronic selenium poisoning* (called also *alkali disease*) is characterized by cirrhosis of the liver, anemia, loss of hair, erosions of long bones, and emaciation. *Acute selenium poisoning* (called also *blind staggers*) is characterized by impaired vision, an unsteady gait, and increasing incoordination with respiratory failure and often death within 24 hours. Called also *selenosis.*

***Senecio* p.,** seneciosis.

**shellfish p.,** an acute intoxication caused by ingestion of bivalve mollusks contaminated with saxitoxin, a neurotoxin secreted by certain dinoflagellates, protozoa that are an important component of marine plankton. The *paralytic* form is caused by species of *Gonyaulax,* and is characterized by paresthesias of the mouth, lips, face, and limbs, nausea, vomiting, and diarrhea; in rare severe cases muscle weakness or paralysis and respiratory embarrassment and death may occur. The *neurotoxic* form is milder, self-limited, not associated with paralysis, and caused by species of *Gymnodinium.*

**tempeh p.,** bongkrek p.

**tetrachloroethane p.,** a form of poisoning in munition workers caused by inhalation of fumes of tetrachloroethane, and marked by toxic jaundice, headache, anorexia, and gastrointestinal disturbance.

**tetraodon p.,** tetrodotoxism (def. 1).

**thallium p.,** poisoning, usually of children or domestic animals, due to ingestion of thallium compounds, marked by alopecia, by a variety of neurologic and psychic symptoms, including ataxia, restlessness, delirium, hallucinations, delusions, semicoma, blindness, and by liver and kidney damage. Called also *thallitoxicosis* and *thallotoxicosis.*

**TNT p.,** trinitrotoluene p.

**tobacco p.,** poisoning by tobacco, usually taking the form of nicotine poisoning (q.v.). Called also *tabagism* and *tobaccoism.*

**trinitrotoluene p.,** a form of poisoning in munition workers that work with trinitrotoluene, characterized by dermatitis, gastritis with abdominal pain, vomiting, constipation, flatulence, and blood changes. Called also *TNT p.*

**urea p.,** poisoning of ruminants by excessive consumption of urea, leading to hyperammonemia with tremors, incoordination, dyspnea, convulsions, and sometimes death.

**Plants That Can Cause Oxalate Poisoning**

| Latin Name | Common Name |
|---|---|
| *Amaranthus retroflexus* | Pigweed, prince's feather |
| *Atriplex* spp. | Salt bush |
| *Beta* spp. | Beet |
| *Calandrinia* spp. | Parakeelia |
| *Emex australis* | |
| *Enchylaena tomentosa* | Barrier salt bush |
| *Halogeton glomeratus* | Halogeton |
| *Oxalis* spp. | Oxalis |
| *Panicum antidotale* | Blue panic grass |
| *Portulaca oleracea* | Purslane |
| *Rheum rhaponticum* | Rhubarb |
| *Rumex* spp. | Dock, sorrel |
| *Salsola kali* | Tumbleweed, Russian thistle |
| *Sarcobatus vermiculatus* | Greasewood |
| *Setaria sphacelata* | |
| *Threlkeldia proceriflora* | |
| *Trianthema* spp. | Hogweed, pigweed |

**Selenium Accumulators: Plants That Can Cause Selenium Poisoning**

| Latin Name | Common Name |
|---|---|
| *Acacia cana* | Acacia |
| *Aster* spp. | Aster |
| *Astragalus* (certain species only)* | Andrachne |
| *Atriplex* spp. | Salt bush, orache |
| *Castilleja* spp. | Paintbrush |
| *Comandra pallida* | |
| *Greyia* spp. | |
| *Grindelia* spp. | Gumweed |
| *Gutierrezia* spp. | Broomweed, snakeweed |
| *Machaeranthera* spp. | |
| *Morinda reticulata* | |
| *Neptunia amplexicaulis* | Selenium weed |
| *Oonopsis* spp.* | |
| *Penstemon* spp. | Penstemon |
| *Sideranthus* spp. | |
| *Stanleya* spp. | Prince's plume |
| *Xylorrhiza* spp.* | |

* These plants grow preferentially in selenium-rich soils and are called *selenium indicators.*

**whelk p.**, poisoning caused by ingestion of whelks that contain whelk poison (q.v.); characterized by intense headache, dizziness, nausea, and vomiting.

**zinc p.**, a rare type of poisoning, usually due to inhalation of zinc or zinc oxide fumes, most commonly in metal workers; symptoms include fever, chills, myalgia, diarrhea, vomiting, and pneumonitis. Called also *zincalism.*

---

**poi·son ivy** (poi'zən i've) *Rhus radicans.*

**poi·son oak** (poi'zən ōk) 1. *Rhus diversiloba.* 2. *Rhus quercifolia.*

**poi·son·ous** (poi'zən-əs) toxic (def. 1).

**poi·son su·mac** (poi'zən soo'mak) *Rhus vernix.*

**Pois·son distribution** (pwah-sawn') [Siméon Denis *Poisson,* French mathematician, 1781–1840] [MeSH: Poisson Distribution] see under *distribution.*

**poke·root** (pōk'root) pokeweed.

**poke·weed** (pōk'wēd) *Phytolacca americana,* a tall perennial herb of North America; its root has emetic and purgative properties and has been used as an antirheumatic. See also *pokeweed mitogen,* under *mitogen.* Cattle and pigs that eat excessive amounts of it sometimes suffer fatal gastroenteritis and diarrhea because of its content of oxalates and saponins. Called also *pokeroot.*

**pol·a·cril·in** (pol"ə-kril'in) methacrylic acid ester with divinylbenzene; a synthetic ion-exchange resin, supplied in the hydrogen or free acid form; a pharmaceutic aid.

**p. potassium,** a synthetic ion exchange resin, prepared through polymerization of methacrylic acid and divinylbenzene, and then further neutralized with potassium hydroxide to form the potassium salt of methacrylic acid and divinylbenzene. It is supplied as a pharmaceutical-grade ion-exchange resin in a particle size of 100- to 500-mesh; a tablet disintegrant.

**Po·land's syndrome** (po'ləndz) [Alfred *Poland,* British physician, 1820–1872] see under *syndrome.*

**po·lar** (po'lər) [L. *polaris* pertaining to a pole, from *polus* (q.v.)] 1. of or pertaining to a pole; see also under *compound.* 2. being at opposite ends of a spectrum of manifestations, as polar forms of leprosy.

**Po·lar·amine** (po-lar'ə-mēn) trademark for preparations of dexchlorpheniramine maleate.

**po·la·rim·e·ter** (po"lə-rim'ə-tər) [*polar* + *-meter*] a device for measuring the rotation of plane polarized light; a polariscope.

**po·la·rim·e·try** (po"lə-rim'ə-tre) measurement of the rotation of plane polarized light by a liquid or solid.

**po·lar·i·scope** (po-lar'ĭ-skōp) [*polar* + *-scope*] an instrument for the measurement of polarized light.

**po·lar·i·scop·ic** (po"lər-ĭ-skop'ik) pertaining to the polariscope or to polariscopy.

**po·lar·is·co·py** (po"lər-is'kə-pe) the science of polarized light and the use of the polariscope.

**po·lar·is·tro·bom·e·ter** (po-lar"is-tro-bom'ə-tər) a form of polarimeter used for delicate analyses.

**po·lar·i·ty** (po-lar'ĭ-te) 1. the fact or condition of having poles. 2. the exhibition of opposite effects at the two extremities. 3. the presence of an axial gradient and exhibition by a nerve of both anelectrotonus and catelectrotonus. 4. the orientation of intracellular structures to the tissue as a whole.

**dynamic p.,** the specialization of a nerve cell with reference to the flow of impulses.

**po·lar·iza·tion** (po"lər-i-za'shən) 1. the presence or establishment of polarity. 2. the production of that condition in light by virtue of which its vibrations take place all in one plane or else in circles and ellipses. 3. the accumulation of bubbles of hydrogen gas on the negative plate of a galvanic battery, so that the generation of electricity is impeded. 4. the separation of electric charge so that there is directionality of flow, as between two poles (the anode and the cathode) of an electrolysis cell, or such as that across a biological membrane, which results in a membrane potential. See also *depolarization* and *repolarization.*

**circular p.,** that polarization which causes vibration in circles.

**elliptical p.,** that which causes the vibration in ellipses.

**linear p.,** the production of polarization such that the light vibrations are all in one plane, the electromagnetic wave vector pointing in a fixed direction and having some amplitude of vibration.

**plane p.,** linear p.

**rotatory p.,** circular or elliptical polarization, as distinguished from plane polarization.

**po·lar·ize** (po'lər-īz) 1. to imbue with polarity. 2. to put into a state of polarization.

**po·lar·iz·er** (po'lə-rīz"ər) an appliance for polarizing light.

**po·laro·gram** (po-lar'o-gram) the curve of current versus voltage obtained in polarography.

**po·laro·gra·phic** (po"lər-o-graf'ik) pertaining to polarography.

**po·lar·og·ra·phy** (po"lər-og'rə-fe) [MeSH: Polarography] an electrochemical technique for identifying and estimating the concentration of reducible elements by means of the dual measurement of the current flowing through an electrochemical cell (which contains the test solution) and the electrical potential between the two electrodes as the potential is increased at a constant rate by an external voltage source. As the voltage reaches the standard electrode potential of the test substance, there is a sharp increase in current flow. The indicator electrode is usually a dropping mercury electrode.

**Po·lar·oid** (po'lər-oid) trademark for a sheet (film) polarizer utilizing oriented crystals used as a substitute for Nicol prisms and for reducing glare through lenses and windshields.

**po·laro·plast** (po-lar'o-plast) [*polar* + *plast*] an organelle in microsporidans that imbibes water, swells, and exerts pressure to rupture the polar cap and evert the polar tube through which the sporoplasm escapes to infect the host.

**pol·dine meth·yl·sul·fate** (pol'dēn) a synthetic quaternary nitrogen anticholinergic used as an adjunct in the treatment of peptic ulcer and gastrointestinal disorders associated with hyperacidity, hypermotility, and spasm, administered orally.

**pole** (pōl) [L. *polus;* Gr. *polos*] 1. either extremity of an axis, as of the fetal ellipse, or of an organ of the body; called also *polus* or *extremitas.* 2. either one of two points which have opposite physical qualities (electric or other).

**animal p.,** the site of an ovum to which the nucleus is approximated, and from which the polar bodies pinch off. Also, in nonmammalian species, the pole of an egg less heavily laden with yolk than the vegetal pole and therefore exhibiting faster cell division.

**anterior p. of eyeball,** polus anterior bulbi oculi.

**anterior p. of lens,** polus anterior lentis.

**antigerminal p.,** vegetal p.

**cephalic p.,** the end of the fetal ellipse at which the head of the fetus is situated.

**frontal p. of cerebral hemisphere, frontal p. of hemisphere of cerebrum,** polus frontalis hemispherii cerebri.

**germinal p.,** animal p.

**inferior p. of kidney,** extremitas inferior renis.

**inferior p. of testis,** extremitas inferior testis.

**nutritive p.,** vegetal p.

**occipital p. of cerebral hemisphere, occipital p. of hemisphere of cerebrum,** polus occipitalis hemispherii cerebri.

**pelvic p.,** the end of the fetal ellipse at which the breech of the fetus is situated.

**posterior p. of eyeball,** polus posterior bulbi oculi.

**posterior p. of lens,** polus posterior lentis.

**temporal p. of cerebral hemisphere, temporal p. of hemisphere of cerebrum,** polus temporalis hemispherii cerebri.

**upper p. of kidney,** extremitas superior renis.

**upper p. of testis,** extremitas superior testis.

**vegetal p., vegetative p., vitelline p.,** that pole of an ovum at which the greater amount of food yolk is deposited. Cf. *animal p.*

**po·li** (po'li) [L.] genitive and plural of *polus.*

**pol·i·ca·pram** (pol"ĭ-ka'prəm) microcrystals of colloid dimensions used as a tablet binder for pharmaceutical preparations.

**po·lice·man** (pə-lēs'mən) a glass rod with a piece of rubber tubing on one end, used as a stirring rod and transfer tool in chemical analysis.

**poli·clin·ic** (pol"e-klin'ik) [Gr. *polis* city + *clinic*] a city hospital, infirmary, or clinic. Cf. *polyclinic.*

**pol·i·do·ca·nol** (pol″ĭ-do-ka′nol) laureth 9.

**pol·i·en·ceph·a·li·tis** (pol″e-ən-sef″ə-li′tis) polioencephalitis.

**pol·i·en·ceph·a·lo·my·eli·tis** (pol″e-en-sef″ə-lo-mi″ə-li′tis) cerebral poliomyelitis.

**pol·i·fep·ro·san 20** (pol″e-fep′ro-san) a biodegradable polyanhydride copolymer that binds to carmustine so that it does not degrade as fast as usual, thus controlling local delivery of the medication.

**po·lio** (po′le-o) poliomyelitis.

**poli(o)-** [Gr. *polios* gray] a combining form denoting relationship to the gray matter of the nervous system.

**po·lio·ci·dal** (po″le-o-si′dəl) neutralizing the poliomyelitis virus.

**po·lio·clas·tic** (po″le-o-klas′tik) [*polio-* + Gr. *klastos* breaking] destroying the gray matter of the nervous system; a term applied to the viruses of poliomyelitis, epidemic encephalitis, and rabies.

**po·lio·dys·tro·phia** (po″le-o-dis-tro′fe-ə) poliodystrophy.
**p. ce′rebri, p. ce′rebri progressi′va, p. ce′rebri progressi′va infanti′lis,** Alpers' disease.

**po·lio·dys·tro·phy** (po″le-o-dis′trə-fe) [*polio-* + *dystrophy*] atrophy of the cerebral gray matter.
**progressive cerebral p., progressive infantile p.,** Alpers' disease.

**po·lio·en·ceph·a·li·tis** (po″le-o-ən-sef″ə-li′tis) [*polio-* + *encephalitis*] 1. inflammatory disease of the gray substance of the brain. 2. cerebral poliomyelitis.
**inferior p.,** progressive bulbar palsy.

**po·lio·en·ceph·a·lo·ma·la·cia** (po″le-o-en-sef″ə-lo-mə-la′shə) a highly fatal disease of cattle, sheep, and pigs, caused by a thiamine deficiency; symptoms include edema of the brain with muzzle twitching, opisthotonos, blindness, and inability to stand. Called also *pseudoencephalomalacia* and *cerebrocortical necrosis.*

**po·lio·en·ceph·a·lo·me·nin·go·my·eli·tis** (po″le-o-ən-sef″ə-lo-mə-ning″go-mi″ə-li′tis) inflammation of the gray matter of the brain and spinal cord and of the meninges covering it.

**po·lio·en·ceph·a·lo·my·eli·tis** (po″le-o-en-sef″ə-lo-mi″ə-li′tis) cerebral poliomyelitis.

**po·lio·en·ceph·a·lop·a·thy** (po″le-o-ən-sef″ə-lop′ə-the) [*polio-* + *encephalo-* + *-pathy*] disease of the gray matter of the brain.

**po·lio·en·ceph·a·lo·trop·ic** (po″le-o-ən-sef″ə-lo-trop′ik) having a special affinity for the gray substance of the brain.

**po·lio·my·el·en·ceph·a·li·tis** (po″le-o-mi″əl-en-sef″ə-li′tis) cerebral poliomyelitis.

**po·lio·my·eli·ti·ci·dal** (po″le-o-mi″ə-lĭ′tĭ-si″dəl) having the power of destroying poliomyelitis virus.

**po·lio·my·eli·tis** (po″le-o-mi″ə-li′tis) [*polio-* + *myel-* + *-itis*] [MeSH: Poliomyelitis] an acute infectious disease occurring sporadically or in epidemics and caused by a virus, usually a poliovirus but occasionally a coxsackievirus or echovirus. It is characterized clinically by fever, sore throat, headache, and vomiting, often with stiffness of the neck and back. In the *minor illness (abortive poliomyelitis)* these may be the only symptoms. The *major illness,* which may or may not be preceded by the minor illness, is characterized by involvement of the central nervous system, stiff neck, pleocytosis in the spinal fluid, and perhaps paralysis. (See *nonparalytic p.* and *paralytic p.*) There may be subsequent atrophy of groups of muscles, ending in contraction and permanent deformity. Called also *polio.* The major illness is also called *infantile paralysis, acute anterior p., anterior p., Heine-Medin disease,* and *Medin's disease.*
**abortive p.,** the minor illness of poliomyelitis; see *poliomyelitis.*
**acute anterior p.,** the major illness of poliomyelitis; see *poliomyelitis.*
**acute lateral p.,** spinal paralytic p.
**anterior p.,** the major illness of poliomyelitis; see *poliomyelitis.*
**ascending p.,** poliomyelitis that is first manifested in the legs and rapidly ascends cephalad.
**bulbar p.,** a serious form of poliomyelitis in which the medulla oblongata is affected, and in which there may be dysfunction of the swallowing mechanism, and respiratory and circulatory distress.
**cerebral p.,** poliomyelitis that extends into the brain; called also *polioencephalitis, poliomyeloencephalitis, polioencephalomyelitis,* and *Strümpell's disease.*
**endemic p.,** poliomyelitis occurring sporadically or in a small number of cases, particularly during periods of warm weather, in most countries throughout the world.
**epidemic p.,** poliomyelitis occurring in epidemic form.
**mouse p., murine p.,** Theiler's disease.
**nonparalytic p.,** the major illness of poliomyelitis when it does not involve paralysis.
**paralytic p.,** the major illness of poliomyelitis when it involves paralysis.
**porcine p.,** infectious porcine encephalomyelitis.
**postinoculation p.,** postvaccinal p.
**post-tonsillectomy p.,** acute poliomyelitis appearing within a short time after tonsillectomy.
**postvaccinal p.,** acute poliomyelitis appearing after a person has been vaccinated against poliomyelitis or some other disease. It may occur as a reaction to the vaccine or may be the result of infection by a new virus, usually another enterovirus or a resistant poliovirus.
**spinal paralytic p.,** the classic form of the major illness of poliomyelitis, with the appearance of flaccid paralysis in one or more limbs. Called also *acute lateral p.* and *infantile spinal paralysis.*

**po·lio·my·elo·en·ceph·a·li·tis** (po″le-o-mi″ə-lo-en-sef″ə-li′tis) cerebral poliomyelitis.

**po·lio·my·elop·a·thy** (po″le-o-mi″ə-lop′ə-the) [*polio-* + *myelo-* + *-pathy*] any disease primarily affecting the gray matter of the spinal cord.

**po·lio·neu·ro·mere** (po″le-o-noor′o-mēr) [*polio-* + *neuro-* + *-mere*] one of the primordial segments of the gray matter of the spinal cord.

**po·li·o·sis** (po″le-o′sis) [Gr. *polios* gray] circumscribed depigmentation of the hair, particularly of the scalp, in association with a pathologic condition. Cf. *achromotrichia, canities,* and *leukotrichia.*

**po·lio·vi·ral** (po′le-o-vi″rəl) pertaining to or caused by polioviruses.

**po·lio·vi·rus** (po′le-o-vi″rəs) [*poliomyelitis* + *virus*] [MeSH: Polioviruses] a virus of the genus Enterovirus that is the etiologic agent of poliomyelitis, separable, on the basis of specificity of neutralizing antibody, into three serotypes, designated types 1, 2, and 3. Over the years, type 1 has been responsible for about 85 per cent of all paralytic poliomyelitis and for most epidemics, and type 3 for about 10 per cent of paralytic poliomyelitis and for occasional epidemics. Type 2 has been responsible for about 5 per cent of paralytic poliomyelitis.
**murine p.,** Theiler's virus.

**poli·pro·pene** (pol″e-pro′pēn) a tablet excipient for pharmaceutical preparations.

**pol·ish·ing** (pol′ish-ing) the creation of a smooth and glossy finish on a surface, as of a denture.

**poli·sog·ra·phy** (pol″ĭ-sog′rə-fe) [*poly-* + *iso-* + *-graphy*] radiography in which several exposures are made in the same film.

**Po·lis·tes** (po-lis′tēz) a genus of wasps of the family Vespidae, having painful stings.

**Pol·it·zer's bag, cone, method (test)** (pol′it-zərz) [Adam *Politzer,* Hungarian-born otologist in Austria, 1835–1920] see under *bag* and *method;* see *politzerization;* and see *cone of light,* under *cone.*

**pol·it·zer·iza·tion** (pol″it-zər-ĭ-za′shən) [Adam *Politzer*] inflation of the middle ear by means of a Politzer bag. Called also *Politzer's method.*
**negative p.,** displacement of secretion from a cavity through negative pressure produced by means of a Politzer bag.

**pol·kis·sen** (pōl-kis′ən) [Ger. "pole cushion"] the region of the juxtaglomerular apparatus between the glomerulus and the afferent and efferent arterioles, containing lacelike cells (the lacis cells) and lying in close contact with the mesangium and the macula densa; called also *lacis.*

**poll** (pōl) the back part of the head, especially that of an animal.

**pol·la·ki·dip·sia** (pol″ə-kə-dip′se-ə) [Gr. *pollakis* often + *dipsia*] a condition characterized by abnormally frequent occurrence of the sensation of thirst.

**pol·la·ki·su·ria** (pol″ə-kĭ-su′re-ə) pollakiuria.

**pol·la·ki·uria** (pol″ə-ke-u′re-ə) [Gr. *pollakis* often + *-uria*] unduly frequent passage of the urine.

**polled** (pōld) having no horns; said of cattle that have been bred for this inherited trait.

**pol·len** (pol′ən) [MeSH: Pollen] the mass of microspores (male fertilizing elements) of flowering plants. Many pollens, especially the airborne pollens, are allergens; i.e., they produce proteinaceous antigens capable of sensitizing susceptible persons and producing allergic symptoms.

**pol·le·no·gen·ic** (pol″ə-no-jen′ik) [*pollen* + *-genic*] caused by the pollen of plants.

**pol·le·no·sis** (pol″ə-no′sis) hay fever.

**pol·lex** (pol′əks) pl. *pol′lices* [L.] [TA] thumb: the first digit of the hand; it is the most preaxial of the five fingers, having only the two phalanges and being apposable to the other four fingers. Called also *digitus primus (I) manus* [TA alternative] and *first finger.*
**p. exten′sus,** backward deviation of the thumb.
**p. flex′us,** permanent flexion of the thumb.
**p. val′gus,** deviation of the thumb toward the ulnar side.

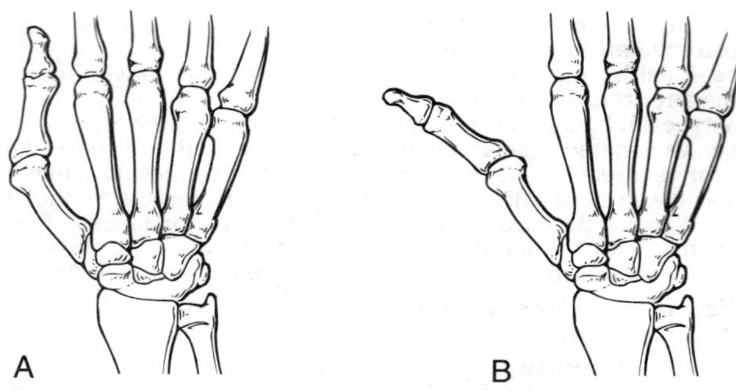

*(A),* Pollex valgus; *(B),* pollex varus.

**p. va'rus,** deviation of the thumb toward the radial side.

**pol·li·cal** (pol'ĭ-kəl) [L. *pollex,* gen. *pollicis* thumb] pertaining to the thumb.

**pol·lic·i·za·tion** (pol″is-ĭ-za'shən) [L. *pollex* thumb] the replacement or rehabilitation of a thumb, especially surgical construction of a thumb from the index finger or great toe.

**pol·li·na·tion** (pol″ĭ-na'shən) the transfer of pollen from anther to stigma of a flowering plant.

**pol·li·ni·um** (po-lin'e-əm) an aggregation of pollen grains held together by a mucilaginous fluid and transported as a whole during pollination.

**pol·li·no·sis** (pol″ĭ-no'sis) hay fever.

**pol·lo·dic** (pə-lod'ik) [Gr. *polloi* many + *hodos* way] panthodic.

**pol·lu·tion** (pə-loo'shən) [L. *pollutio*] the act of defiling or making impure.

**po·lo·cytes** (po'lo-sīts) [Gr. *polos* pole + *-cyte*] polar bodies; see under *body.*

**po·lo·ni·um** (pə-lo'ne-əm) [L. *Polonia* Poland] [MeSH: Polonium] a rare metal resembling bismuth, discovered in 1898 in pitchblende; atomic number, 84; atomic weight, 210; symbol, Po. It is radioactive, but less so than radium.

**pol·ox·a·lene** (pol-ok'sə-lēn) [USP] [MeSH: Poloxalene] a liquid poloxamer, having a molecular weight of approximately 3000; used as a surfactant in pharmaceutical preparations and in the prevention of bloat in ruminants.

**pol·ox·al·kol** (pol-ok'sal-kol) poloxamer 188.

**pol·ox·a·mer** (pol-ok'sə-mər) any of a series of nonionic surfactants of the polyoxypropylene-polyoxyethylene copolymer type, having the general formula $HO(C_2H_4O)_a(C_3H_6O)_b$- $(C_2H_4O)_c$ H, where *a = c;* the molecular weights of the members of the series vary from about 1000 to more than 16,000. The term is used in conjunction with a numerical suffix for individual unique identification of products that may be used as a food, drug, or cosmetic. Poloxamers may be surfactants, emulsifiers, or stabilizers.
**p. 182L,** a liquid poloxamer, having an average molecular weight of 2450; used as a food additive and pharmaceutic aid.
**p. 188,** a waxy poloxamer, having an average molecular weight of 8350; used as a cathartic, administered orally. Called also *poloxalkol.*
**p. 331,** a liquid poloxamer, having an average molecular weight of 3800; used as a food additive.

**pol·ster** (pōl'stər) a small bulge, as on a vessel wall.

**pol·toph·a·gy** (pol-tof'ə-je) [Gr. *poltos* porridge + *-phagy*] thorough chewing of the food.

**po·lus** (po'ləs) gen. and pl. *po'li* [L., from Gr. *polos* axis] [TA] pole: either extremity of an axis, or the extremity of an organ.
**p. ante'rior bul'bi o'culi** [TA], anterior pole of eyeball: the center of the anterior curvature of the eyeball.
**p. ante'rior len'tis** [TA], anterior pole of lens: the central point of the anterior surface of the lens.
**p. fronta'lis hemisphe'rii ce'rebri** [TA], frontal pole of cerebral hemisphere: the most prominent part of the anterior end of each hemisphere.
**p. occipita'lis hemisphe'rii ce'rebri** [TA], occipital pole of cerebral hemisphere: the most posterior prominence of the occipital lobe of the hemisphere.
**p. poste'rior bul'bi o'culi** [TA], posterior pole of eyeball: the center of the posterior curvature of the eyeball.
**p. poste'rior len'tis** [TA], posterior pole of lens: the central point of the posterior surface of the lens.
**p. tempora'lis hemisphe'rii ce'rebri** [TA], temporal pole of cerebral hemisphere: the prominent anterior end of the temporal lobe of a hemisphere.

**poly** (pol'e) colloquial name for *polymorphonuclear leukocyte.*

**poly-** [Gr. *polys* many] a combining form meaning many or much.

**poly A** [MeSH: Poly A] polyadenylate; polyadenylic acid.

**Pol·ya's oper·ation** (pōl'yahz) [Jenö (Eugene) *Polya,* Hungarian surgeon, 1876–1944] see under *operation.*

**poly·ac·id** (pol″e-as'id) capable of neutralizing several molecules of an acid radical; said of a base or basic radical.

**poly·ac·rylo·ni·trile** (pol″e-ə-kril″o-ni'trīl) a polymer of acrylonitrile used as a hemodialyzer membrane; it is more permeable by diffusion than cuprophane for larger molecules, but fluid removal is rapid and not entirely predictable.

**poly·ad·e·ni·tis** (pol″e-ad″ə-ni'tis) [*poly-* + *adenitis*] inflammation (adenitis) of several or many glands.

**poly·ad·e·no·ma** (pol″e-ad″ə-no'mə) adenoma of many glands.

**poly·ad·e·no·ma·to·sis** (pol″e-ad″ə-no-mə-to'sis) multiple adenomas in a part.

**poly·ad·e·nop·a·thy** (pol″e-ad″ə-nop'ə-the) 1. polyadenosis. 2. polyendocrinopathy.

**poly·ad·e·no·sis** (pol″e-ad″ə-no'sis) disorder of several glands, particularly of several endocrine glands. Cf. *polyadenopathy.*

**poly·ad·e·nous** (pol″e-ad'ə-nəs) [*poly-* + *aden-* + *-ous*] 1. polyendocrine. 2. pluriglandular.

**poly·aden·y·late** (pol″e-ə-den'ə-lāt) the salt, ester, or anionic form of polyadenylic acid. Abbreviated poly A.

**poly·aden·y·lat·ed** (pol″e-ə-den'ə-la″təd) having a polyadenylate tail.

**poly·aden·y·la·tion** (pol″e-ə-den″ə-la'shən) the formation of the polyadenylate tail on eukaryotic RNA molecules or at the 3′ end of viral mRNA, catalyzed by polynucleotide adenylyltransferase.

**poly·ad·e·nyl·ic ac·id** (pol″e-ad″ə-nil'ik) a homopolymer composed solely of adenylic acid residues; see also *polyadenylate tail,* under *tail.* Abbreviated poly A.

**poly·ag·glu·ti·na·tion** (pol″e-ə-gloo″tĭ-na'shən) an abnormal condition of erythrocytes in which they agglutinate upon exposure to almost any normal serum due to antigens in their membranes that react to common serum antibodies.

**poly·al·co·hol·ism** (pol″e-al'kə-hol-iz-əm) intoxication or poisoning by a mixture of different alcohols.

**poly·al·ve·o·lar** (pol″e-al-ve'o-lər) having more than the usual number of alveoli, such as a polyalveolar lobe of a lung.

**poly·am·ine** (pol″e-am'ēn) any compound, e.g., spermine and spermidine, containing two or more amine groups; polyamines are low molecular weight cations and are synthesized within cells to provide intermediates for protein synthesis.

**poly·an·dry** (pol″e-an'dre) [*poly-* + Gr. *aner* man] 1. polygamy (q.v.) in which a woman is concurrently married to more than one man. 2. an animal mating system seen in polygamous species, in which the female mates with more than one male. 3. union of two or more male pronuclei with a female pronucleus, resulting in polyploidy of the zygote. Cf. *polygyny.*

**poly·an·gi·itis** (pol″e-an″je-i'tis) inflammation involving multiple blood or lymph vessels.
**microscopic p.,** inflammation of small vessels, usually in the kidneys but sometimes also in the lungs, skin, and nervous system; characteristics are similar to those of polyarteritis nodosa with focal segmental glomerulonephritis and presence of antineutrophil cytoplasmic autoantibodies.

**poly A poly·mer·ase** (pol'e a pə-lim'ər-ās) [MeSH: Poly A Polymerase] polynucleotide adenylyltransferase.

**poly·ar·ter·i·tis** (pol″e-ahr″tə-ri'tis) [*poly-* + *arteritis*] 1. multiple inflammatory and destructive arterial lesions; called also *panarteritis.* 2. p. nodosa.
**p. nodo'sa (PAN),** a form of systemic necrotizing vasculitis involving the small and medium-sized arteries with signs and symptoms resulting from infarction and scarring of the affected organ system. Called also *arteritis nodosa, Kussmaul's* or *Kussmaul-Maier disease, necrotizing arteritis, panarteritis nodosa,* and *periarteritis nodosa.*

**poly·ar·thric** (pol″e-ahr'thrik) [*poly-* + *arthr-* + *-ic*] pertaining to or affecting many joints.

**poly·ar·thri·tis** (pol″e-ahr-thri'tis) [*poly-* + *arthr-* + *-itis*] an inflammation of several joints together.
**chlamydial p.,** an infectious disease of sheep, and occasionally calves and pigs, in the United States, Australia, and New Zealand,

caused by infection with *Chlamydia psittaci*; characteristics include joint enlargement with edema, fever, and anorexia.
**chronic secondary p.,** Jaccoud's syndrome.
**chronic villous p.,** chronic inflammation of the synovial membrane of several joints.
**p. des'truens,** rheumatoid arthritis.
**epidemic p.,** a denguelike disease caused by the Ross River virus, occurring in Australia, New Guinea, and elsewhere in the western Pacific, characterized by polyarthritis, rash, and fever and transmitted by mosquitoes.
**infectious p., infectious porcine p.,** Glasser's disease.
**mycoplasmal p.,** infection in pigs by *Mycoplasma hyorhinis* or *M. hyosynoviae,* often occurring after unusual stresses; characteristics include polyarthritis, swollen joints, and lameness. *M. hyorhinis* infection may be accompanied by polyserositis (see *mycoplasmal polyserositis*).
**nonsuppurative p.,** joint swelling without suppuration in lambs as a result of infection by *Erysipelothrix rhusiopathiae* through a wound. In the acute form, animals have fever and leg pain for two to three weeks; in the chronic form they have permanently swollen joints and are lame.
**peripheral p.,** that limited to peripheral joints; asymmetric involvement is common and the number of joints affected tends to be limited. Often the knees and ankles are more involved than the hands or feet.
**p. rheuma'tica acu'ta,** rheumatic fever.
**tuberculous p.,** pulmonary hypertrophic osteoarthropathy.

**poly·ar·tic·u·lar** (pol″e-ahr-tik′u-lər) [*poly-* + *articular*] affecting many joints.

**poly·atom·ic** (pol″e-ə-tom′ik) [*poly-* + *atomic*] composed of several atoms.

**poly·auxo·troph** (pol″e-awk′so-trōf) [*poly-* + *auxo-* + *-trophic*] an organism, especially a mutant, which requires multiple growth factors.

**poly·auxo·troph·ic** (pol″e-awk″so-trōf′ik) requiring multiple growth factors; used especially with reference to a single mutation that causes a multiple requirement.

**poly·avi·ta·min·o·sis** (pol″e-a-vi″tə-min-o′sis) [*poly-* + *avitaminosis*] a deficiency disease in which more than one vitamin is lacking in the diet.

**poly·ax·on·ic** (pol″e-ak-son′ik) pertaining to or having several axons.

**poly·ba·sic** (pol″e-ba′sik) [*poly-* + *basic*] 1. denoting any acid which has several hydrogen atoms replaceable by a base. 2. denoting any salt of a polybasic acid formed by replacing some or all of its hydrogen atoms by a base.

**poly·blen·nia** (pol″e-blen′e-ə) [*poly-* + *blenn-* + *-ia*] the secretion of an excessive quantity of mucus.

**poly·car·bo·phil** (pol″e-kahr′bo-fil) [USP] a pharmacologically inert polyacrylic acid cross-linked with divinyl glycol, used as a gastrointestinal absorbent in the treatment of diarrhea.

**poly·cel·lu·lar** (pol″e-sel′u-lər) multicellular.

**poly·cen·tric** (pol″e-sen′trik) having many centers.

**poly·cen·tric·i·ty** (pol″e-sən-tris′ĭ-te) the state or quality of being polycentric.

**poly·chei·ria** (pol″e-ki′re-ə) [*poly-* + *cheir-* + *-ia*] the condition of having more than two hands.

**poly·che·mo·ther·a·py** (pol″e-ke″mo-ther′ə-pe) combination chemotherapy.

**poly·chlo·ru·ria** (pol″e-klor-u′re-ə) an increased excretion of chlorine in the urine.

**poly·cho·lia** (pol″e-ko′le-ə) [*poly-* + *chol-* + *-ia*] excessive flow or secretion of bile.

**poly·chon·dri·tis** (pol″e-kon-dri′tis) inflammation involving many cartilages of the body.
**chronic atrophic p., p. chro′nica atro′phicans,** relapsing p.
**relapsing p.,** a disease of unknown etiology with a chronic course and sometimes recurrence, marked by inflammatory and degenerative lesions of cartilage in the joints, ears, nose, trachea, bronchi, and elsewhere, with deformities such as floppy ear and saddle nose; if the tracheal or bronchial wall collapses, respiratory obstruction may occur. The aorta, sclera, and cornea are also affected. Called also *chronic atrophic p., p. chronica atrophicans,* and *polychondropathia.*

**poly·chon·dro·path·ia** (pol″e-kon″dro-path′e-ə) relapsing polychondritis.

**poly·chon·drop·a·thy** (pol″e-kon-drop′ə-the) relapsing polychondritis.

**poly·chrest** (pol′e-krest) [*poly-* + Gr. *chrēstos* useful] 1. useful in many conditions. 2. a remedy useful in many diseases.

**poly·chro·ma·sia** (pol″e-kro-ma′zhə) 1. variation in the hemoglobin content of the erythrocytes of the blood. 2. polychromatophilia.

**poly·chro·ma·tia** (pol″e-kro-ma′shə) polychromatophilia.

**poly·chro·mat·ic** (pol″e-kro-mat′ik) [*poly-* + *chromatic*] exhibiting many colors. Cf. *monochromatic.*

**poly·chro·mato·cyte** (pol″e-kro-mat′o-sīt) polychromatophil.

**poly·chro·ma·to·cy·to·sis** (pol″e-kro″mə-to-si-to′sis) polychromatophilia.

**poly·chro·mato·phil** (pol″e-kro-mat′o-fil) [*poly-* + *chromato-* + *-phil*] a cell or other element that is stainable with various stains or colors; called also *polychromatocyte* and *polychromophil.*

**poly·chro·ma·to·phil·ia** (pol″e-kro″mə-to-fil′e-ə) 1. the quality of being stainable with various different stains or tints. 2. a condition in which the erythrocytes, on staining, show shades of blue tinged with pink; seen in various types of anemia. Called also *polychromasia, polychromatocytosis,* and *polychromophilia.*

**poly·chro·ma·to·phil·ic** (pol″e-kro″mə-to-fil′ik) pertaining to or characterized by polychromatophilia.

**poly·chro·ma·to·sis** (pol″e-kro″mə-to′sis) an excess of abnormally staining erythrocytes in the blood; see *polychromatophilia,* def. 2.

**poly·chro·me·mia** (pol″e-kro-me′me-ə) [*poly-* + *chrom-* + *-emia*] hyperhemoglobinemia.

**poly·chro·mic** (pol″e-kro′mik) pertaining to or exhibiting many colors.

**poly·chro·mo·phil** (pol″e-kro′mo-fil) polychromatophil.

**poly·chro·mo·phil·ia** (pol″e-kro″mo-fil′e-ə) polychromatophilia.

**poly·chy·lia** (pol″e-ki′le-ə) [*poly-* + *chyle* + *-ia*] excessive production of chyle.

**Poly·cil·lin** (pol″e-sil′in) trademark for preparations of ampicillin.

**poly·clin·ic** (pol″e-klin′ik) [*poly-* + *clinic*] a hospital and school where diseases and injuries of many kinds are studied and treated clinically.

**poly·clo·nal** (pol″e-klo′nəl) 1. derived from different cells. 2. of or pertaining to several clones.

**poly·co·ria** (pol″e-kor′e-ə) 1. [*poly-* + Gr. *korē* pupil + *-ia*] the existence of more than one pupil in an eye. 2. [*poly-* + Gr. *koros* surfeit + *-ia*] the deposit of reserve material in an organ or tissue so as to produce enlargement.
**p. spu′ria,** a condition in which the iris contains several openings or holes.
**p. ve′ra,** the existence in the eye of several pupils, each with its own sphincter.

**poly·crot·ic** (pol″e-krot′ik) [*poly-* + Gr. *krotos* beat] said of a pulse tracing that has secondary waves to each beat.

**pol·yc·ro·tism** (pol-ik′rə-tiz-əm) presence of a polycrotic pulse.

**poly·cy·clic** (pol″e-sik′lik, -si′klik) [*poly-* + *cyclic*] containing more than one ring or cycle (frequency).

**Poly·cy·cline** (pol″e-si′klēn) trademark for preparations of tetracycline.

**poly·cy·e·sis** (pol″e-si-e′sis) [*poly-* + *cyesis*] multiple pregnancy.

**poly·cys·tic** (pol″e-sis′tik) [*poly-* + *cystic*] containing or made up of many cysts.

**poly·cyte** (pol′e-sīt) [*poly-* + *-cyte*] an abnormal polymorphonuclear leukocyte of normal size but with more than the usual number of lobes in the nucleus. Cf. *macropolycyte.*

**poly·cy·the·mia** (pol″e-si-the′me-ə) [*poly-* + *cyt-* + *hem-* + *-ia*] [MeSH: Polycythemia] an increase in the total red cell mass of the blood, characterized as either *absolute p.* or *relative p.* Called also *erythrocythemia, hypercythemia,* and *hypererythrocythemia.*
**absolute p.,** an increase in red cell mass caused by a sustained overactivity of the erythroid component of the bone marrow, which may occur as a compensatory physiologic response to tissue hypoxia (see *secondary p.*), or as the principal manifestation of polycythemia vera. Cf. *relative p.*
**appropriate p.,** see *secondary p.*
**benign p.,** stress p.
**compensatory p.,** see *secondary p.*
**hypertonic p., p. hyperto′nica,** stress p.
**inappropriate p.,** see *secondary p.*
**myelopathic p., primary p.,** p. vera.
**relative p.,** a decrease in plasma volume without the change in red blood cell mass of absolute polycythemia, so that the erythrocytes become more concentrated (elevated hematocrit). It occurs in both acute forms (a transient condition due to marked loss of body fluid, lowered fluid intake, or a combination) and chronic forms (see *stress p.*). Called also *spurious p.* and *pseudopolycythemia.*

**relative p., chronic,** stress p.
**p. ru'bra, p. ru'bra ve'ra,** p. vera.
**secondary p.,** any absolute increase in the total red cell mass other than polycythemia vera, occurring as a physiologic response to tissue hypoxia. It may be *compensatory* and *appropriate,* adjusting for general tissue hypoxia, such as that associated with pulmonary disease, alveolar hypoventilation, cardiovascular disease, or prolonged exposure to high altitude, or resulting from defective hemoglobin or drugs, or it may be *inappropriate,* reflecting excessive erythropoietin production due to renal or extrarenal disorders. Called also *erythrocytosis.*
**splenomegalic p.,** p. vera.
**spurious p.,** 1. relative p. 2. stress p.
**stress p.,** a chronic type of relative polycythemia, seen most often in middle-aged, mildly obese males who are active, anxiety-prone, and hypertensive, occurring without the characteristic symptoms associated with polycythemia vera, i.e., without leukocytosis, splenomegaly, and thrombocytosis. Called also *benign erythrocytosis* or *polycytosis, Gaisböck's disease, pseudopolycythemia,* and *chronic relative, hypertonic,* or *spurious p.*
**p. ve'ra,** a myeloproliferative disorder of unknown etiology, characterized by abnormal proliferation of all hematopoietic bone marrow elements and an absolute increase in red cell mass and total blood volume. The skin of the face is often ruddy and swollen, and ecchymoses are common. Most patients have splenomegaly, leukocytosis, and thrombocythemia. Hematopoiesis is also reactive in extramedullary sites (liver and spleen), and in time myelofibrosis occurs. Called also *erythremia, p. rubra* or *p. rubra vera, myelopathic* or *splenomegalic p.,* and *Osler's, Osler-Vaquez, Vaquez',* or *Vaquez-Osler disease.* Cf. *secondary p.*

**poly·dac·tyl·ia** (pol″e-dak-til′e-ə) polydactyly.

**poly·dac·tyl·ism** (pol″e-dak′təl-iz-əm) polydactyly.

**poly·dac·ty·ly** (pol″e-dak′tə-le) [*poly-* + Gr. *daktylos* finger + *-ia*] [MeSH: Polydactyly] a developmental anomaly characterized by the presence of supernumerary digits (fingers or toes) on the hands or feet.

**poly·de·oxy·ri·bo·nu·cleo·tide** (pol″e-de-ok″se-ri″bo-noo′kle-o-tīd) a polymer of deoxyribonucleotides; deoxyribonucleic acid.

**poly·de·oxy·ri·bo·nu·cle·o·tide syn·thase (ATP)** (pol″e-de-ok″se-ri″bo-noo′kle-o-tīd sin′thās) DNA ligase (ATP).

**poly·dip·sia** (pol″e-dip′se-ə) [*poly-* + *dipsia*] chronic excessive thirst and intake of fluid; it may have an organic cause, such as the dehydration of diabetes mellitus, diabetes insipidus, or a reaction to medication, or be of psychological origin.
**psychogenic p.,** polydipsia without an organic basis, occurring as a result of a mental disorder.

**poly·di·meth·yl·si·lox·ane** (pol″ī-di-meth″il-si-lok′sān) silicone oil.

**poly·di·ox·an·one** (pol″e-di-ok′sə-nōn) [MeSH: Polydioxanone] a synthetic polymer used as an absorbable suture material.

**poly·dis·per·soid** (pol″e-dis-per′soid) a colloid in which the disperse phase consists of particles having different degrees of dispersion.

**poly·drug** (pol′e-drug) more than one drug; used particularly for concurrent abuse of multiple drugs.

**poly·dys·pla·sia** (pol″e-dis-pla′zhə) [*poly-* + *dysplasia*] faulty development in several types of tissue or several organs or systems.
**hereditary ectodermal p.,** anhidrotic ectodermal dysplasia.

**poly·dys·spon·dy·lism** (pol″e-dis-pon′də-liz-əm) malformation of several vertebrae, associated with dwarfed stature, low intelligence, and malformation of the sella turcica.

**poly·dys·troph·ic** (pol″e-dis-tro′fik) pertaining to or exhibiting polydystrophy.

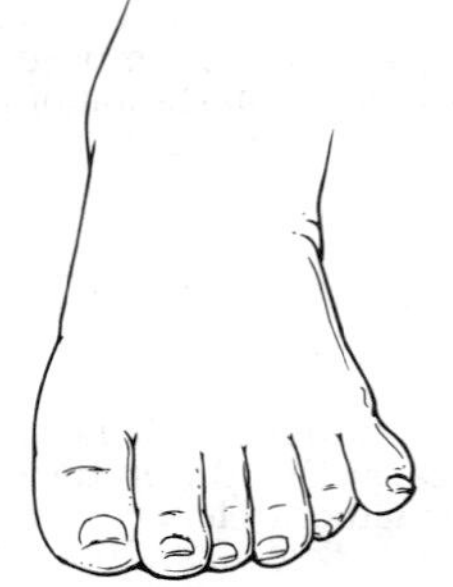

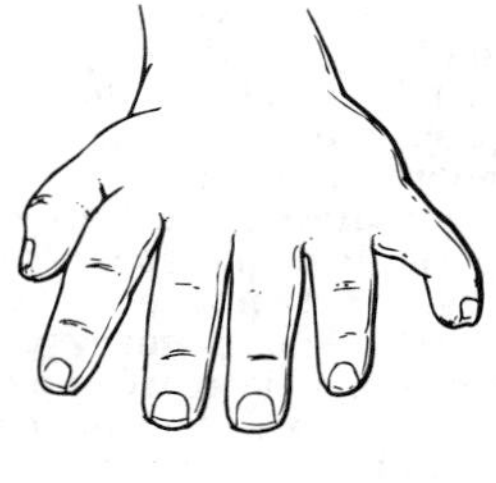

Polydactyly.

**poly·dys·tro·phy** (pol″e-dis′trə-fe) dystrophy of several tissues or structures, as may occur in congenital anomalies.
**pseudo-Hurler p.,** mucolipidosis III.

**poly·elec·tro·lyte** (pol″e-e-lek′tro-līt) a large polymer compound of many monomers, each of which carries one or more ionic groups.

**poly·em·bry·o·ma** (pol″e-em″bre-o′mə) a rare type of germ cell tumor consisting of embryoid bodies and believed to comprise both embryonic and extraembryonic differentiation.

**poly·em·bry·o·ny** (pol″e-em-bri′o-ne) [*poly-* + *embryo*] the production of two or more embryos from the same ovum or seed.

**poly·en·do·crine** (pol″e-en′do-krin) pertaining to or affecting several endocrine glands. Called also *polyadenous.*

**poly·en·do·cri·no·ma** (pol″e-en″do-krĭ-no′mə) multiple endocrine neoplasia.

**poly·en·do·cri·nop·a·thy** (pol″e-en″do-krĭ-nop′ə-the) endocrinopathy involving several glands.

**pol·y·ene** (pol′e-ēn) 1. an aliphatic or alicyclic compound with a carbon chain of four or more atoms and several conjugated double bonds. 2. any of a group of polyene antifungal antibiotics (e.g., amphotericin, candicidin, or nystatin) produced by species of *Streptomyces* that damage cell membranes by forming complexes with sterols.

**poly·er·gic** (pol″e-er′jik) able to act in several different ways.

**poly·es·the·sia** (pol″e-əs-the′zhə) [*poly-* + *esthesia*] a dysesthesia in which a single object seems to be felt in several different places, such as may be seen in tabes dorsalis (see *Remak's symptom*).

**poly·es·tra·di·ol phos·phate** (pol″e-es″trə-di′ol) a polymer of estradiol phosphate having estrogenic activity similar to that of estradiol; used in the palliative therapy of prostatic carcinoma, administered intramuscularly.

**poly·es·trous** (pol″e-es′trəs) completing two or more estrous cycles per annual breeding season. Cf. *monestrous.*

**poly·ether** (pol″e-e′thər) an elastomer made from cyclic ether, used in paste form as an impression material for fixed partial prosthodontic structures, inlays for single quadrants, and dental impressions.

**poly·eth·y·lene** (pol″e-eth′ə-lēn) polymerized ethylene, $(—CH_2—CH_2—)_n$, a synthetic plastic material, forms of which have been used in reparative surgery.
**p. glycol** [NF], PEG; a generic name for mixtures of condensation polymers of ethylene oxide and water, represented by the general formula $H(OCH_2CH_2)_n$ OH, in which *n* is greater than or equal to 4. The term is used in combination with a numeric suffix which indicates the approximate average molecular weight. Those with average molecular weights between 200 and 700 are liquid and those above 1000 are waxlike solids: *p. glycol 3000* (*n* varies from 5 to 5.75) is used as a solvent and dispensing agent in pharmaceutical preparations; *p. glycol 400* (*n* varies from 8.2 to 9.1), *p. glycol 600* (*n* varies from 12.5 to 13.9), and *p. glycol 1500* (*n* varies from 29 to 36) are used as ointment and suppository bases; *p. glycol 1540* (*n* varies from 28 to 36) is used as a vehicle in pharmaceutical preparations; *p. glycol 4000* (*n* varies from 68 to 84) and *p. glycol 6000* (*n* varies from 158 and 204) are used as ointment and suppository bases and as tablet excipients. Called also *macrogol.*
**p. glycol monomethyl ether** [NF], any of a series of addition polymers of ethylene oxide and methanol, represented by the general formula $CH_3(OHC_2CH_2)_nOH$, in which *n* is the average number of oxyethylene groups. Nominal molecular weights range from 350 to 10,000, the viscosity increasing and the solubility in water and in organic solvents decreasing as the molecular weight increases. Used as an excipient in pharmaceutical preparations.
**p. terephthalate,** any of a group of thermoplastic, fiber-forming polyesters used in textile manufacture; see *Dacron.*

**poly·fer·ose** (pol″e-fer′ōs) a chelate complex of iron and a polymerized derivative of sucrose; a hematinic.

**Po·lyg·a·la** (po-lig′ə-lə) [*poly-* + Gr. *gala* milk] the milkworts, a genus of plants of the family Polygalaceae, having many species. *P. se'nega* L. is seneca or senega snakeroot, a North American species that yields senega. *P. klotz'chii* is a Brazilian species that causes fatal gastrointestinal and neurological disorders in cattle.

**poly·ga·lac·tia** (pol″e-gə-lak′she-ə) [*poly-* + *galact-* + *-ia*] excessive secretion of milk.

**po·lyg·a·lin** (pə-lig′ə-lin) senegenin.

**po·lyg·a·mous** (pə-lig′ə-məs) pertaining to polygamy.

**po·lyg·a·my** (pə-lig′ə-me) [*poly-* + Gr. *gamos* marriage] 1. the concurrent marriage of a woman or man to more than one spouse, as opposed to *monogamy.* 2. animal mating in which the individual mates with more than one partner. See also *polyandry* and *polygyny.*

**poly·gan·gli·on·ic** (pol″e-gang″gle-on′ik) [*poly-* + *ganglionic*]

1. having or pertaining to several or many ganglia. 2. affecting several lymphatic glands.

**poly·gel·ine** (pol″e-jel′ēn) [MeSH: Polygeline] a polymer of urea and polypeptides derived from denatured gelatin; used as a plasma expander in hypovolemia.

**poly·gene** (pol′e-jēn) [*poly-* + *gene*] one of a group of nonallelic genes (multiple factors or cumulative genes) that interact to influence the same character in the same way so that the effect is cumulative.

**poly·gen·ic** (pol″e-jēn′ik) pertaining to or determined by the action of several different genes. Called also *quantitative.* Cf. *multifactorial.*

**poly·glac·tin 910** (pol″e-glak′tin) [MeSH: Polyglactin 910] a type of multifilament braided material made of purified lactides and glycolides, used in absorbable sutures.

**poly·glan·du·lar** (pol″e-glan′du-lər) pluriglandular.

**poly·glu·co·side** (pol″e-gloo′ko-sīd) a polysaccharide composed of glucose residues. Cf. *oligoglucoside.*

**poly·gly·col·ic ac·id** (pol″e-gli-kol′ik) [MeSH: Polyglycolic Acid] a polymer of glycolic acid used for absorbable sutures.

**po·lyg·na·thus** (po-lig′nə-thəs, pol″e-nath′əs) [*poly-* + Gr. *gnathos* jaw] asymmetrical conjoined twins with the parasitic twin attached to the jaw of the larger twin. See also *hypognathus.*

**pol·y·gon** (pol′e-gon) a planar figure bounded by three or more line segments.
**frequency p.,** a graphic method for displaying a frequency distribution, obtained from a histogram by placing a dot at the midpoint of the top of each bar, with a line connecting the dots outlining the polygon.

**Poly·go·na·tum** (pol″e-go-na′təm) [*poly-* + Gr. *gony* knee] a genus of plants of the family Liliaceae. *P. biflo′rum* (Walt.) Ell. is Solomon's seal, a perennial herb of eastern North America used as a tonic, diuretic, emetic, and purgative; at high doses it is a cardiac poison.

**poly·gram** (pol′e-gram) a tracing made by a polygraph.

**poly·graph** (pol′e-graf) [*poly-* + *-graph*] an instrument for simultaneously recording various physiological responses as represented by mechanical or electrical impulses, such as respiratory movements, pulse wave, blood pressure, and the psychogalvanic reflex. Such phenomena reflect emotional reactions which are of use in detecting deception. Popularly known as *lie detector.*

**po·lyg·y·ny** (pə-lij′ĭ-ne) [*poly-* + Gr. *gynē* woman] 1. polygamy (q.v.) in which a man is married concurrently to more than one woman. 2. an animal mating system seen in polygamous species, in which the male mates with more than one female. 3. union of two or more female pronuclei with a male pronucleus, resulting in polyploidy of the zygote. Cf. *polyandry.*

**poly·gy·ria** (pol″e-ji′re-ə) polymicrogyria.

**poly·he·dral** (pol″e-he′drəl) [*poly-* + Gr. *hedra* seat, base] having many faces or sides.

**poly·hi·dro·sis** (pol″e-hi-dro′sis) [*poly-* + *hidr-* + *-osis*] hyperhidrosis.

**poly·his·tio·cy·to·ma** (pol″e-his″te-o-si-to′mə) small-cell osteosarcoma.

**poly·hy·brid** (pol″e-hi′brid) [*poly-* + *hybrid*] a hybrid whose parents differ from each other in more than three characters.

**poly·hy·dram·ni·os** (pol″e-hi-dram′ne-os) [*poly-* + *hydr-* + *amnion*] [MeSH: Polyhydramnios] hydramnios.

**poly·hy·dric** (pol″e-hi′drik) containing more than two hydroxyl groups.

**poly·hy·dru·ria** (pol″e-hi-droo′re-ə) [*poly-* + *hydr-* + *-uria*] abnormal dilution of the urine.

**poly·hy·per·men·or·rhea** (pol″e-hi″pər-men″o-re′ə) [*poly-* + *hyper-* + *menorrhea*] frequent menstruation with abnormally profuse discharge.

**poly·hy·po·men·or·rhea** (pol″e-hi″po-men″o-re′ə) [*poly-* + *hypo-* + *menorrhea*] frequent menstruation with deficient amount of discharge.

**poly·id·ro·sis** (pol″e-i-dro′sis) hyperhidrosis.

**poly·in·fec·tion** (pol″e-in-fek′shən) [*poly-* + *infection*] mixed infection.

**poly·ion·ic** (pol″e-i-on′ik) containing several different ions (e.g., potassium, sodium, etc.), as a polyionic solution.

**poly·iso·pre·noid** (pol″e-i′so-pre-noid″) any isoprenoid that contains multiple isoprene units, such as rubber.

**poly·karyo·cyte** (pol″e-kar′e-o-sīt) [*poly-* + *karyo-* + *-cyte*] [MeSH: Giant Cells] a giant cell containing several nuclei.

**poly·ki·ne·ty** (pol″e-ki′ne-te) [*poly-* + *kinety*] a row of closely arranged cilia that descends in a counterclockwise spiral into the infundibulum of peritrichous ciliate protozoa.

**Poly·kol** (pol′ĭ-kol) trademark for preparations of poloxalkol.

**poly·lac·tic ac·id** (pol″e-lak′tik) a hydrophobic hydroxy acid polymer that is formed into granules and used as a surgical dressing material for dental extraction sites, primarily for prevention of postoperative alveolar osteitis.

**poly·lec·i·thal** (pol″e-les′ĭ-thəl) [*poly-* + *-lecithal*] macrolecithal.

**poly·lep·tic** (pol″e-lep′tik) [*poly-* + Gr. *lambanein* to seize] having many remissions and exacerbations.

**poly·lo·gia** (pol″e-lo′jə) [*poly-* + *log-* + *-ia*] logorrhea.

**poly·ly·sine** (pol″e-li′sēn) [MeSH: Polylysine] a polypeptide composed of lysine molecules in peptide linkage; used as a carrier for the benzylpenicilloyl moiety in the detection of penicillin sensitivity; see *penicilloyl polylysine.*

**poly·ma·con** (pol″e-ma′kon) a hydrophilic contact lens material.

**poly·mas·tia** (pol″e-mas′te-ə) [*poly-* + *mast-* + *-ia*] the presence of more than one pair of mammae, or breasts. Called also *pleomastia.*

**poly·mas·tic** (pol″ĭ-mas′tik) pertaining to or characterized by polymastia.

**Poly·mas·ti·gi·da** (pol″e-mas″tĭ-gi′də) an order of protozoa of the class Zoomastigophorea, subphylum Mastigophora, consisting of small organisms possessing three to eight or more flagella and usually one or two nuclei, although some are multinucleate; they are found in the digestive tract of various arthropods and vertebrates. It includes the genera *Callimastix, Enteromonas, Copromastix, Chilomastix, Hexamita, Giardia,* and *Trichomonas.*

**poly·mas·ti·gote** (pol″e-mas′tĭ-gōt) a mastigote having several to many flagella.

**poly·ma·zia** (pol″e-ma′ze-ə) polymastia.

**poly·me·lia** (pol″e-me′le-ə) [*poly-* + *-melia*] a developmental anomaly characterized by the presence of supernumerary limbs.

**po·lym·e·lus** (pə-lim′ə-ləs) an individual exhibiting polymelia.

**poly·me·nia** (pol″e-me′ne-ə) polymenorrhea.

**poly·men·or·rhea** (pol″e-men″o-re′ə) [*poly-* + *menorrhea*] abnormally frequent menstruation, defined as that occurring at regular intervals of less than 21 days.

**poly·mer** (pol′ĭ-mər) [*poly-* + Gr. *meros* part] a compound formed by the joining of smaller molecules, referred to as monomers. The term is generally used to refer either to a macromolecule made up of a large number of monomers linked by covalent bonds, e.g., polypeptides, nucleic acids, polysaccharides, and plastics, or to a protein made up of several subunits linked by covalent or noncovalent bonds, e.g., hemoglobin or IgM immunoglobulin.
**addition p.,** a compound formed by the repeated combination of smaller molecules (monomers) without the formation of any other products (e.g., polyethylene).
**condensation p.,** a compound formed by the repeated reaction of smaller molecules, involving at the same time the elimination of water or other simple compound (e.g., nylon).
**cross-linked p.,** a polymer that has cross-linking; strength and resistance to solvents make many such polymers suitable for use in dental materials.
**polysulfide p.,** see under *rubber.*

**po·lym·er·ase** (pə-lim′ər-ās) any enzyme that catalyzes polymerization, especially of nucleotides to polynucleotides.

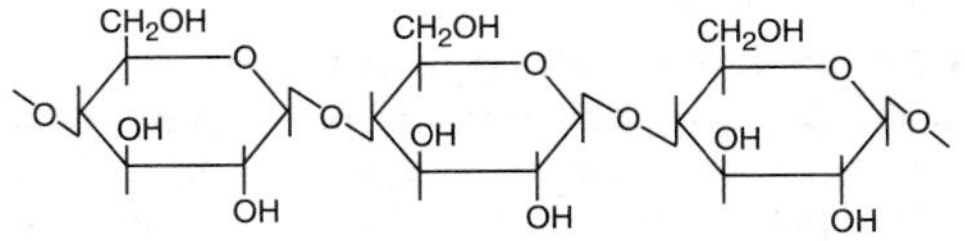

Cellulose

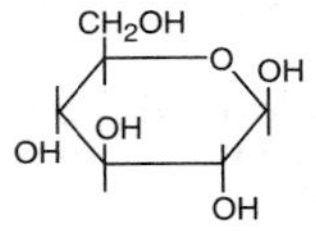

β-D-Glucose

The polymer cellulose consists of linked repeating units of the monomer β-D-glucose.

**poly·me·ria** (pol″e-me′re-ə) [*poly-* + *mer-*[1] + *-ia*] a developmental anomaly characterized by the presence of supernumerary parts or organs of the body.

**poly·mer·ic** (pol″ĭ-mer′ik) exhibiting the characteristics of a polymer.

**po·lym·er·iza·tion** (pə-lim″ər-ĭ-za′shən) the act or process of forming a compound (polymer), usually of high molecular weight, by the combination of simpler molecules (monomers).

**poly·mer·ize** (pə-lim′ər-īz) to subject to or to undergo polymerization.

**poly·meta·car·pia** (pol″e-met″ə-kahr′pe-ə) [*poly-* + *metacarpus* + *-ia*] presence of more than the normal number of metacarpal bones.

**poly·meta·phos·phate** (pol″e-met″ə-fos′fāt) a phosphate polymer that serves as a phosphate reserve in microorganisms, appearing as a metachromatic granule.

**poly·meta·tar·sia** (pol″e-met″ə-tahr′se-ə) [*poly-* + *metatarsus* + *-ia*] presence of more than the normal number of metatarsal bones.

**poly·meth·yl·meth·ac·ryl·ate** (pol″e-meth″əl-meth-ak′rəl-āt) polymethyl methacrylate; see under *methacrylate*.

**poly·mi·cro·bi·al** (pol″e-mi-kro′be-əl) [*poly-* + *microbe*] characterized by the presence of several species of microorganisms.

**poly·mi·cro·bic** (pol″e-mi-kro′bik) polymicrobial.

**poly·mi·cro·gy·ria** (pol″e-mi″kro-ji′re-ə) [*poly-* + *micro-* + *gyr-* + *-ia*] a developmental anomaly of the brain characterized by development of numerous small convolutions (microgyri), causing mental retardation. Called also *microgyria* and *polygyria*.

**poly·mi·cro·lipo·ma·to·sis** (pol″e-mi″kro-lip″o-mə-to′sis) [*poly-* + *micro-* + *lipomatosis*] lipomatosis marked by the presence in the subcutaneous tissues of numerous small lipomas.

**poly·mi·cro·tome** (pol″e-mi′kro-tōm) [*poly-* + *microtome*] a microtome which cuts several sections at once.

**Po·lym·nia** (pə-lim′ne-ə) [Gr.; one of the nine Muses] a genus of plants of the family Compositae, having yellow or white flowers. *P. uveda′lia* L., the leafcup or bearsfoot, is anthelmintic, alterative, antispasmodic, and laxative.

**poly·morph** (pol′e-morf) colloquial term for *polymorphonuclear leukocyte*.

**poly·mor·phic** (pol″e-mor′fik) [*poly-* + *morph-* + *-ic*] occurring in several or many forms; appearing in different forms at different stages of development.

**poly·mor·phism** (pol″e-mor′fiz-əm) [*poly-* + *morph-* + *-ism*] the ability to exist in several different forms.
**balanced p.**, a state of equilibrium in which gene frequencies are maintained by a balance between mutation and selection.
**genetic p.**, the occurrence together in the same population of two or more genetically determined phenotypes in such proportions that the rarest of them cannot be maintained merely by recurrent mutation.
**restriction fragment length p. (RFLP)**, in molecular genetics, a polymorphism in DNA sequence that can be detected on the basis of differences in fragment lengths of DNA produced by digestion with a specific restriction endonuclease.

**poly·mor·pho·cel·lu·lar** (pol″e-mor″fo-sel′u-lər) [*poly-* + *morpho-* + *cellular*] having cells of many forms.

**poly·mor·pho·cyte** (pol″e-mor′fo-sīt) polymorphonuclear leukocyte.

**poly·mor·pho·nu·cle·ar** (pol″e-mor″fo-noo′kle-ər) [*poly-* + *morpho-* + *nuclear*] having a nucleus deeply lobed or so divided that it appears to be multiple.

**poly·mor·phous** (pol″e-mor′fəs) polymorphic.

**Poly·mox** (pol′ĭ-moks) trademark for preparations of amoxicillin.

**poly·my·al·gia** (pol″e-mi-al′jə) myalgia affecting several muscles.
**p. arteri′tica, p. rheuma′tica**, a syndrome in the elderly characterized by proximal joint and muscle pain and a high erythrocyte sedimentation rate; it is sometimes associated with giant cell arteritis.

**poly·my·ar·i·an** (pol″e-mi-ar′e-ən) [*poly-* + Gr. *mys* muscle] having many muscle cells in each quadrant of a cross section, the cells being coelomyarian in type; said of the muscle arrangement in certain nematodes.

**poly·my·oc·lo·nus** (pol″e-mi-ok′lə-nəs) myoclonus in several muscles or groups simultaneously or in rapid succession; it occurs in myoclonic epilepsy and in some types of poisoning.

**poly·my·op·a·thy** (pol″e-mi-op′ə-the) disease affecting several muscles simultaneously.

**poly·myo·si·tis** (pol″e-mi″o-si′tis) [*poly-* + *myositis*] [MeSH: Polymyositis] a chronic, progressive inflammatory disease of skeletal muscle, occurring in both children and adults, and characterized by symmetrical weakness of the limb girdles, neck, and pharynx, usually associated with pain and tenderness, and sometimes preceded or followed by manifestations typical of scleroderma, arthritis, systemic lupus erythematosus, or Sjögren's syndrome. It is also sometimes associated with malignancy, and may be accompanied by characteristic skin lesions (see *dermatomyositis*).
**trichinous p.**, trichinosis.

**poly·myx·in** (pol″e-mik′sin) [MeSH: Polymyxin] the generic name for five polypeptide antibiotics (designated A, B, C, D, and E) derived from strains of the soil bacterium *Bacillus polymyxa*, having specific activity against gram-negative bacteria, including *Pseudomonas aeruginosa, Proteus vulgaris, Escherichia coli, Hemophilus influenzae, Aerobacter aerogenes*, and *Klebsiella pneumoniae*. The least toxic members of the group are polymyxins B, usually used in the form of the sulfate salt, and E (see *colistin*).
**p. B sulfate** [USP], the sulfate salt of the least toxic member of the polymyxin group, occurring as a buff-colored powder; used in the treatment of various systemic, urinary tract, ophthalmic, otic, and cutaneous infections due to susceptible gram-negative bacteria, especially *Pseudomonas aeruginosa*, administered orally, parenterally, and topically.

**poly·ne·sic** (pol″e-ne′sik) [*poly-* + Gr. *nēsos* island] multiple and insular; occurring in many foci.

**poly·neu·ral** (pol″e-noor′əl) [*poly-* + *neural*] pertaining to or supplied by several nerves.

**poly·neu·ral·gia** (pol″e-noo͝-ral′jə) neuralgia of several nerves.

**poly·neu·ric** (pol″e-noor′ik) polyneural.

**poly·neu·rit·ic** (pol″e-noo͝-rit′ik) pertaining to or affected with polyneuritis.

**poly·neu·ri·tis** (pol″e-noo͝-ri′tis) [*poly-* + *neur-* + *-itis*] [MeSH: Polyneuritis] inflammation of several peripheral nerves at once; called also *multiple neuritis*.
**acute febrile p., acute idiopathic p.**, rapidly progressive ascending motor neuron paralysis of unknown etiology, frequently after an enteric or respiratory infection. An autoimmune mechanism following viral infection has been postulated. It begins with paresthesias of the feet, followed by flaccid paralysis of the legs, ascending to the arms, trunk, and face and is attended by slight fever, bulbar palsy, absent or lessened tendon reflexes, and an increase in the protein of the cerebrospinal fluid without corresponding increase in cells. Called also *Barré-Guillain syndrome, Guillain-Barré p.* or *syndrome, acute postinfectious p., postinfectious p., acute ascending spinal paralysis, acute infective p., acute postinfectious polyneuropathy*, and *Landry's paralysis* or *syndrome*.
**acute infective p., acute postinfectious p.**, acute idiopathic p.
**anemic p.**, see under *polyneuropathy*.
**cranial p.**, mononeuritis multiplex involving several cranial nerves, characterized by facial palsy or any of various ocular conditions; sometimes seen as part of sarcoid neuropathy.
**endemic p., p. ende′mica**, beriberi.
**Guillain-Barré p.**, acute idiopathic p.
**Jamaica ginger p.**, see under *paralysis*.
**leprous p.**, sensory or sensorimotor polyneuritis due to inflammation of nerve trunks in association with leprosy.
**postinfectious p.**, acute idiopathic p.

**poly·neu·ro·myo·si·tis** (pol″e-noor″o-mi″o-si′tis) polyneuritis with polymyositis.

**poly·neu·rop·a·thy** (pol″e-noo͝-rop′ə-the) [*poly-* + *neuropathy*] neuropathy of several peripheral nerves simultaneously; called also *multiple* or *peripheral neuropathy*. Some conditions that are actually polyneuropathies are called neuropathies; see under *neuropathy*.
**acute postinfectious p.**, acute idiopathic polyneuritis.
**amyloid p.**, polyneuropathy caused by amyloidosis; symptoms may include dysfunction of the autonomic nervous system, carpal tunnel syndrome, and sensory disturbances in the extremities such as numbness, hyperesthesia, or paresthesia. See also *familial amyloid p.*
**Andrade type familial amyloid p.**, Portuguese type familial amyloid p.
**anemic p.**, polyneuropathy seen in subacute combined degeneration of the spinal cord (q.v.).
**arsenic p., arsenical p.**, polyneuropathy seen in cases of chronic arsenic poisoning, characterized by sensory disturbances of the extremities and sometimes by a syndrome resembling acute febrile polyneuritis.
**carcinomatous p.**, paraneoplastic polyneuropathy seen with carcinoma, especially of the lung; it consists of sensory and sensorimotor disturbances such as dysesthesias, paresthesias, and unsteadiness of gait. Cf. *carcinomatous neuromyopathy*.
**critical illness p.**, an idiopathic sensorimotor type of polyneuropathy seen in critically ill patients such as those who are on ventilators or receiving intensive medication.

**diphtheritic p.,** Dejerine's syndrome (def. 3).
**erythredema p.,** acrodynia.
**familial amyloid p.,** autosomal dominant amyloid polyneuropathy occurring in hereditary amyloidosis; major subtypes are *Portuguese type familial amyloid p., Indiana type familial amyloid p.,* and *Finnish type familial amyloid p.*
**Finnish type familial amyloid p.,** a slowly progressive form of familial amyloid polyneuropathy whose earliest symptom is usually lattice dystrophy of the cornea. Later developments include cranial nerve palsy, paresis along the upper branch of the facial nerve, and renal amyloidosis. Called also *Meretoja type familial amyloid p.* and *Meretoja's syndrome.*
**Indiana type familial amyloid p.,** a slowly progressive form of familial amyloid polyneuropathy with upper limb neuropathy in the distribution of the median nerves, leading to carpal tunnel syndrome and eventually trophic ulcers; ocular symptoms such as vitreous deposits may occur. Called also *Rukavina type familial amyloid p., Maryland type familial amyloid p.,* and *Rukavina's syndrome.*
**inflammatory demyelinating p.,** see under *polyradiculoneuropathy.*
**Iowa type familial amyloid p.,** a slowly progressive type of familial amyloid polyneuropathy affecting both the upper and lower limbs; renal amyloidosis is present and uremia is eventually fatal. It may be an advanced form of Portuguese type familial amyloid polyneuropathy. Called also *Van Allen type familial amyloid p.* and *Van Allen's syndrome.*
**Japanese type familial amyloid p.,** Portuguese type familial amyloid p.
**Maryland type familial amyloid p.,** Indiana type familial amyloid p.
**Meretoja type familial amyloid p.,** Finnish type familial amyloid p.
**nutritional p.,** polyneuropathy due to nutritional deficits, as seen with beriberi, pellagra, alcoholism, malabsorption syndromes, Strachan's syndrome, and other conditions. Cf. *anemic p.*
**paraneoplastic p.,** a paraneoplastic syndrome, sometimes seen with carcinoma, multiple myeloma, or Hodgkin's disease, consisting of polyneuropathy with sensory or sensorimotor symptoms. Cf. *carcinomatous pericarditis* Called also *paraneoplastic neuropathy.*
**porphyric p.,** a severe, often symmetrical type of polyneuropathy that occurs with some varieties of porphyria.
**Portuguese type familial amyloid p.,** familial amyloid polyneuropathy with lower limb neuropathy, autonomic dysfunction, and paresis; death occurs within 7 to 10 years. Called also *Andrade type familial amyloid p., Japanese type familial amyloid p.,* and *Andrade's syndrome.*
**Rukavina type familial amyloid p.,** Indiana type familial amyloid p.
**symmetrical sensory p.,** sensory neuropathy in the limbs, especially their distal parts, seen in diabetes mellitus; it usually develops slowly but occasionally has an acute onset.
**uremic p.,** polyneuropathy caused by the uremia of chronic renal failure, characterized by painless bilateral sensorimotor deficits of the lower limbs and later the upper limbs.
**Van Allen type familial amyloid p.,** Iowa type familial amyloid p.

**poly·neu·ro·ra·dic·u·li·tis** (pol″e-noor″o-rə-dik″u-li′tis) [*poly-* + *neuro-* + *radiculitis*] acute idiopathic polyneuritis.

**poly·nu·cle·ar** (pol″e-noo′kle-ər) pertaining to or having several nuclei; cf. *polymorphonuclear.* Called also *multinucleate* and *polynucleate.*

**poly·nu·cle·ate** (pol″e-noo′kle-āt) polynuclear.

**poly·nu·cle·at·ed** (pol″e-noo′kle-āt″əd) polynuclear.

**poly·nu·cle·o·lar** (pol″e-noo-kle′o-lər) having several nucleoli.

**poly·nu·cleo·tide** (pol″e-noo′kle-o-tīd) any polymer of mononucleotides; nucleic acid.

**poly·nu·cleo·tide aden·yl·yl·trans·fer·ase** (pol″e-noo′kle-o-tīd ə-den″əl-əl-trans′fər-ās) [EC 2.7.7.19] an enzyme of the transferase class that catalyzes the sequential addition of ATP-derived adenylate residues to the 3′ end of a polynucleotide. The enzyme does not require a template. The reaction produces the polyadenylate (poly A) tail characteristic of most eukaryotic messenger RNA molecules. Called also *poly A polymerase.*

**poly·nu·cle·o·tide phos·phor·y·lase** (pol″e-noo′kle-o-tīd fosfor′ə-lās) [MeSH: Polynucleotide Phosphorylase] polyribonucleotide nucleotidyltransferase.

**poly·odon·tia** (pol″e-o-don′shə) [*poly-* + *odont-* + *-ia*] the presence of supernumerary teeth.

**poly·ol** (pol′e-ol) an alcohol containing more than two hydroxyl groups, e.g., sugar alcohols, inositol. Called also *polyhydric alcohol.*

**poly·ol de·hy·dro·gen·ase** (pol′e-ol de-hi′dro-jən-ās) L-iditol 2-dehydrogenase.

**poly·o·ma** (pol″e-o′mə) a tumor caused by an oncogenic virus of broad host range, originally isolated from parotid gland tumors of mice inoculated with Gross leukemia virus; see also *polyomavirus.*

**Poly·o·ma·vi·rus** (pol″e-o′mə-vi″rəs) [*poly-* + *-oma* + *virus*] [MeSH: Polyomavirus] polyomaviruses; a genus of viruses of the Papovaviridae that induce tumors in experimental animals. Two polyomaviruses (BK virus and JC virus) infect humans; others, including simian virus 40 (SV40), infect other mammals.

**poly·o·ma·vi·rus** (pol′e-o-mə-vi″rəs) [MeSH: Polyomavirus] any member of the genus *Polyomavirus.*

**poly·onych·ia** (pol″e-o-nik′e-ə) [*poly-* + *onych-* + *-ia*] the occurrence of supernumerary nails.

**poly·opia** (pol″e-o′pe-ə) [*poly-* + *-opia*] the condition in which one object appears as two or more objects.
**binocular p.,** diplopia.
**p. monophthal′mica,** a condition in which an object looked at by one eye appears double.

**poly·op·sia** (pol″e-op′se-ə) polyopia.

**poly·opy** (pol′e-o″pe) polyopia.

**poly·or·chi·dism** (pol″e-or′kĭ-diz-əm) a developmental anomaly characterized by the presence of more than two testes.

**poly·or·chis** (pol″e-or′kis) [*poly-* + *orchis*] a person with more than two testes.

**poly·or·chism** (pol″e-or′kiz-əm) polyorchidism.

**poly·os·tot·ic** (pol″e-os-tot′ik) [*poly-* + L. *os* bone] pertaining to or affecting many bones.

**poly·otia** (pol″e-o′shə) [*poly-* + *ot-* + *-ia*] the condition of having more than two ears.

**poly·ov·u·lar** (pol″e-ov′u-lər) pertaining to or produced from more than one ovum, as polyovular twins.

**poly·ov·u·la·to·ry** (pol″e-ov′u-lə-tor″e) ordinarily discharging several ova in one ovarian cycle.

**poly·oxy·eth·y·lene 50 ste·a·rate** (pol″e-oks″e-eth′ə-lēn) polyoxyl 50 stearate.

**poly·ox·yl** (pol″e-oks′əl) any of various mixtures of the mono- and distearate esters of mixed polyoxyethylene diols and the corresponding free diols. The term is used in combination with an identifying number which indicates the average polymer length in oxyethylene units: *p. 8 stearate* and *p. 40 stearate* [USP], in which the average polymer lengths in oxyethylene units are equivalent to about 8 and 40, respectively, are used as surfactants in pharmaceutical preparations.
**p. 5 oleate,** peglicol 5 oleate.
**p. 10 oleyl ether,** see under *ether.*
**p. 20 celostearyl ether,** see under *ether.*
**p. 50 stearate,** a mixture of the mono- and distearate esters of mixed polyoxyethylene diols and the corresponding free diols, the average polymer length being equivalent to about 50 oxyethylene units, occurring as a soft, cream-colored, waxy solid; used as a surfactant and emulsifying agent in pharmaceutical preparations. Called also *polyoxyethylene 50 stearate.*

**pol·yp** (pol′ip) [Gr. *polypous* a morbid excrescence] [MeSH: Polyps] a morbid excrescence, or protruding growth, from mucous membrane; classically applied to a growth on the mucous membrane of the nose, the term is now applied to such protrusions from any mucous membrane.
**adenomatous p.,** a benign neoplastic growth representing proliferation of epithelial tissue in the lumen of the sigmoid colon, rectum, or stomach, seen in up to 50 per cent of people over age 60 and widely variable in malignant potential.
**adenomatous p. of the colon,** an adenomatous polyp in the sigmoid colon or rectum, sometimes preneoplastic; both tubular and villous varieties have been described. It may be sessile or pedunculated and solitary or multiple.
**adenomatous p. of the stomach,** a type of adenomatous polyp usually found in the antrum of the stomach, with branching tubules or fingerlike projections and glandular tissue; it may be premalignant or a sign of malignancy nearby. Called also *gastric adenoma.*
**aural p.,** a polyp in the ear; common sites include the external canal, mucosa of middle ear, and eustachian tube.
**cardiac p.,** a ball thrombus or tumor attached by a pedicle to the inside of the heart.
**cervical p.,** a common, relativeiy innocuous tumor of the uterine cervix, usually of the endocervical canal; size varies widely. Such tumors may produce irregular vaginal bleeding.
**choanal p's,** nasal polyps that project posteriorly into the nasopharynx.
**cholesterol p's,** small polypoid excrescences consisting of cholesterol and other lipids, seen projecting into the lumen of the gallbladder in cholesterolosis.
**cystic p.,** a polyp in which the fibrous network is coarse, thus stimulating or producing cysts; called also *hydatid p.*
**endocervical p.,** cervical p.
**endometrial p's,** small, sessile, benign projecting masses on the endometrium, composed of an edematous stroma containing cystically dilated glands.

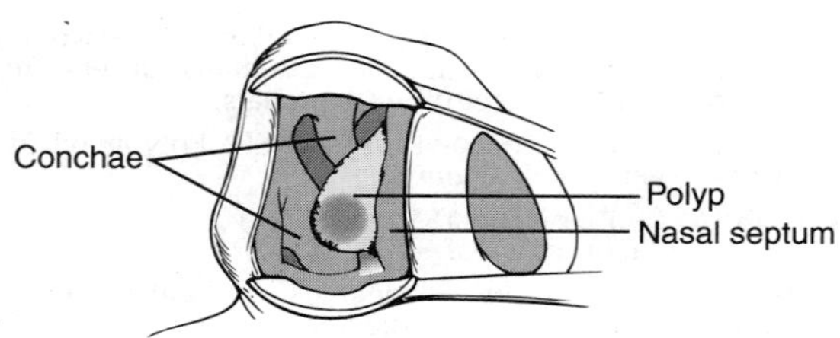


Nasal polyp visible in an inferior view of the nose.

**fibrinous p.,** an intrauterine polyp made up of fibrin from retained blood; it may grow from portions of an ovum or from a thrombus at the placental site.
**fibroepithelial p.,** acrochordon.
**gelatinous p.,** myxoma.
**gum p.,** a small pedunculated growth on the gingiva.
**hydatid p.,** cystic p.
**hyperplastic p.,** pseudopolyp.
**inflammatory p.,** pseudopolyp.
**juvenile p's,** small, benign hemispheric hamartomas of the large intestine occurring sporadically in children; histologically, there is an abundant loose fibrovascular stroma containing widely spaced glands; called also *retention p's*.
**laryngeal p's, p's of larynx,** smooth, rounded, sessile or pedunculated swellings, occurring on the true vocal cords; caused by edema in the lamina propria of the mucous membrane.
**lymphoid p's,** rare, benign tumors of the colon composed of aggregates of lymphoid tissue, usually covered by a fairly regular colonic mucosa.
**nasal p's,** focal accumulations of edema fluid in the mucosa of the nose, with hyperplasia of the associated submucosal connective tissue.
**regenerative p.,** pseudopolyp.
**retention p's,** juvenile p's.

**poly·para·si·tism** (pol″e-par′ə-si-tiz″əm) infection or infestation by more than one variety of parasite.

**poly·path·ia** (pol″e-path′e-ə) [*poly-* + *path-* + *-ia*] the presence of several diseases at once.

**poly·pec·to·my** (pol″ĭ-pek′tə-me) [*polyp* + *-ectomy*] surgical removal of a polyp.

**poly·pep·tide** (pol″e-pep′tīd) [*poly-* + *peptide*] a peptide that on hydrolysis yields more than two amino acids; called tripeptides, tetrapeptides, and so on according to the number of amino acids contained. See also *peptide*.
**gastric inhibitory p. (GIP), glucose-dependent insulinotropic p.,** a polypeptide hormone (molecular weight 5165; 43 amino acids) synthesized by K cells in the midzone of the duodenal and jejunal mucosa and released in response to oral glucose, fat, or amino acids; it is a potent insulin stimulant, increases insulin secretion, and inhibits gastric secretion and motility.
**islet amyloid p. (IAPP),** amylin.
**pancreatic p.,** a hormone (4200 daltons, 36 amino acids) secreted by special endocrine cells in the periphery of some pancreatic islets, the exocrine pancreas, and the intestine; it inhibits pancreatic enzyme secretion and gallbladder contraction, but its physiologic role has not been identified.
**parathyroid-like p.,** a polypeptide with activity like that of parathyroid hormone, causing hypercalcemia; it is produced by tumors of the islet cells and some other organs in type I multiple endocrine neoplasia.
**vasoactive intestinal p. (VIP),** a peptide hormone (3326 daltons, 28 amino acids) widely distributed throughout the body but found in highest concentrations in the nervous system and gut; it is released locally from nerve endings or endocrine cells. Its primary actions are thought to be to serve as a neurotransmitter, to relax smooth muscles of the circulation, gut, and genitourinary system, to increase secretion of water and electrolytes from the pancreas and gut, and to release hormones from the pancreatic islets, gut, and hypothalamus. It is found in excess with VIPomas and the Verner-Morrison syndrome. Called also *vasoactive intestinal peptide*.

**poly·pep·ti·de·mia** (pol″e-pep″tĭ-de′me-ə) [*polypeptide* + *-emia*] the presence of polypeptides in the blood.

**poly·pep·ti·dor·rha·chia** (pol″e-pep″tĭ-do-ra′ke-ə) [*polypeptide* + *rhachi-* + *-ia*] the presence of polypeptides in the spinal fluid.

**poly·peri·os·ti·tis** (pol″e-per″e-os-ti′tis) inflammation of the periosteum of several bones.
**p. hyperesthe′tica,** a chronic disease of the periosteum attended by extreme hyperesthesia of the skin and soft parts.

**poly·pha·gia** (pol″e-fa′jə) [*poly-* + *-phagia*] excessive eating; gluttony. See also *bulimia*. Called also *hyperphagia*.

**poly·pha·lan·gia** (pol″e-fə-lan′jə) side-by-side duplication of one or more of the phalanges of a digit.

**poly·pha·lan·gism** (pol″e-fə-lan′jiz-əm) polyphalangia.

**poly·phar·ma·ceu·tic** (pol″e-fahr″mə-soo′tik) pertaining to several drugs, especially to the administration of several drugs together.

**poly·phar·ma·cy** (pol″e-fahr′mə-se) [*poly-* + Gr. *pharmakon* drug] [MeSH: Polypharmacy] 1. the administration of many drugs together. 2. the administration of excessive medication.

**poly·phase** (pol′e-fāz) [*poly-* + *phase*] having several phases; containing colloids of several types.

**poly·pha·sic** (pol″e-fa′zik) having or existing in many phases; having unlike particles in the disperse phase.

**poly·phen·ic** (pol″e-fen′ik) see *pleiotropism*.

**poly·phe·nol ox·i·dase** (pol″e-fe′nol ok′sĭ-dās) see *catechol oxidase*.

**poly·pho·bia** (pol″e-fo′be-ə) [*poly-* + *-phobia*] irrational fear of many things.

**poly·phos·pho·ino·si·tide** (pol″e-fos″fo-in-o′sĭ-tīd) a multiply phosphorylated phosphoinositide (q.v.), such as phosphatidylinositol 4,5-bisphosphate.

**poly·phra·sia** (pol″e-fra′zhə) logorrhea.

**poly·phy·let·ic** (pol″e-fi-let′ik) [*poly-* + *phyletic*] arising or descending from more than one cell type; see *polyphyletic theory*, under *theory*.

**poly·phy·le·tism** (pol″e-fi′lə-tiz-əm) polyphyletic theory; see under *theory*.

**poly·phy·le·tist** (pol″le-fi′lə-tist) an adherent of the polyphyletic theory; see under *theory*.

**poly·phy·odont** (pol″e-fi′o-dont) [*poly-* + Gr. *phyein* to produce + *odous* tooth] developing several sets of teeth successively throughout life. Cf. *diphyodont* and *monophyodont*.

**poly·pi** (pol′ĭ-pi) [L.] plural of *polypus*.

**po·lyp·i·form** (po-lip′ĭ-form) resembling a polyp; polypoid.

**poly·plas·tic** (pol″e-plas′tik) [*poly-* + *plastic*] 1. containing many structural or constituent elements. 2. undergoing many changes of form.

**Poly·plax** (pol′e-plaks) a genus of sucking lice (order Anoplura), which parasitize rodents. *P. miacan′tha* is found on rats; *P. serra′ta* infests rabbits and transmits tularemia; and *P. spinulo′sa*, the most common louse of rats, transmits murine typhus.

**poly·ploid** (pol′e-ploid) [*poly-* + ha*ploid*] 1. having more than two full sets of homologous chromosomes. There may be three (triploid), four (tetraploid), five (pentaploid), six (hexaploid), seven (heptaploid), eight (octaploid), etc. 2. an individual or cell having more than two full sets of homologous chromosomes. Polyploid organisms, especially plants, are larger than normal and have larger cells. Affected animals are often abnormal in appearance and usually infertile. Cf. *aneuploid*.

**poly·ploi·dy** (pol′e-ploi″de) [MeSH: Polyploidy] the state of having more than two full sets of homologous chromosomes (see *polyploid*).

**pol·yp·nea** (pol″ip-ne′ə) [*poly-* + *-pnea*] hyperpnea.

**pol·yp·ne·ic** (pol″ip-ne′ik) hyperpneic.

**poly·po·dia** (pol″e-po′de-ə) [*poly-* + *pod-* + *-ia*] the presence of supernumerary feet.

**pol·yp·oid** (pol′ĭ-poid) [*polyp* + *-oid*] resembling a polyp.

**poly·poi·do·sis** (pol″e-poi-do′sis) polyposis.

**Po·lyp·o·ra·ceae** (pə-lip″ə-ra′se-e) [MeSH: Polyporaceae] a large family of fungi of the order Aphyllophorales; it includes the genus *Polyporus*.

**Po·lyp·o·ra·les** (pə-lip″ə-ra′lēz) Aphyllophorales.

**pol·yp·o·rous** (pə-lip′ə-rəs) having many pores.

**Pol·yp·o·rus** (pə-lip′ə-rəs) [*poly-* + Gr. *poros* pore] a genus of fungi of the family Polyporaceae. Some species are important pathogens of trees. *P. officina′lis* contains agaricic acid and is the source of larch agaric.

**poly·po·sia** (pol″e-po′zhə) [*poly-* + *-posia*] ingestion of abnormally increased amounts of fluids for long periods of time. Cf. *hyperposia*.

**pol·yp·osis** (pol″ĭ-po′sis) the development of multiple polyps on a part.
**p. co′li,** familial adenomatous p.
**familial p., familial adenomatous p.,** multiple adenomatous polyps with high malignant potential, lining the mucous membrane of the intestine, particularly the colon, beginning at about puberty. It oc-

curs in several autosomal dominant conditions, including Gardner's syndrome, Peutz-Jeghers syndrome, and Turcot's syndrome. Called also *p. coli., familial intestinal p.,* and *multiple familial p.*
**familial intestinal p.,** familial adenomatous p.
**gastric p.,** the presence of multiple polyps on the gastric mucosa.
**intestinal p.,** the presence of multiple polyps in the colon.
**juvenile p., juvenile intestinal p.,** the occurrence of more than ten juvenile polyps (q.v.) in a single patient, occurring both sporadically and as an autosomal dominant trait and appearing in the first or second decade of life.
**multiple familial p.,** familial adenomatous p.

**po·lyp·o·tome** (po-lip'ə-tōm) a cutting instrument for removing polyps.

**po·lyp·o·trite** (po-lip'ə-trīt) [*polyp* + L. *terere* to crush] an instrument for crushing polyps.

**poly·pous** (pol'ĭ-pəs) of the nature of a polyp; polyp-like.

**poly·prag·ma·sy** (pol″e-prag'mə-se) [*poly-* + Gr. *pragma* a doing] polypharmacy.

**poly·pro·py·lene** (pol″e-pro'pə-lēn″) a widely used synthetic crystalline, thermoplastic polymer with a molecular weight of 40,000 or more, having the general formula $(C_3H_5)_n$. Medical uses include the manufacture of nonabsorbable sutures, surgical casts, and semipermeable membranes for membrane oxygenators.
**p. carbonate** [NF], a clear, colorless, mobile liquid, $C_4H_6O_3$, used as solvent in oral and topical pharmaceuticals and as a gelling agent.

**poly·pty·chi·al** (pol″e-ti'ke-əl) [*poly-* + Gr. *ptychē* fold] arranged in several layers; said of glands whose cells are arranged on the basement membrane in several layers. Cf. *monoptychial.*

**poly·pus** (pol'ĭ-pəs) pl. *pol'ypi* [L., from Gr. *polypous,* from *poly-* + *pous* foot] a polyp.
**p. cys'ticus,** cystic polyp.
**p. hydatido'sus,** cystic polyp.

**poly·ra·dic·u·li·tis** (pol″e-rə-dik″u-li'tis) [*poly-* + *radiculitis*] [MeSH: Polyradiculitis] inflammation of the nerve roots.

**poly·ra·dic·u·lo·neu·ri·tis** (pol″e-rə-dik″u-lo-no͝o-ri'tis) [*poly-* + *radiculoneuritis*] [MeSH: Polyradiculoneuritis] 1. acute idiopathic polyneuritis. 2. a disease in dogs similar to human acute idiopathic polyneuritis, usually seen in the form of acute polyradiculoneuritis.
**acute p.,** a common type of ascending paralysis in dogs, clinically similar to human acute idiopathic polyneuritis; ventral roots of spinal nerves, and other peripheral nerves, undergo segmental demyelination. It was first seen in hunting dogs that had had fights with raccoons. The exact etiology is unclear. Called also *coonhound paralysis.*

**poly·ra·dic·u·lo·neu·rop·a·thy** (pol″e-rə-dik″u-lo-no͝o-rop'ə-the) 1. any disease of the peripheral nerves and spinal nerve roots. 2. acute idiopathic polyneuritis.
**acute inflammatory demyelinating p.,** acute idiopathic polyneuritis.
**chronic inflammatory p., chronic inflammatory demyelinating p.,** a rare form of symmetrical motor neuron paralysis similar to acute idiopathic polyneuritis but progressing more slowly or in a fluctuating pattern. The fluctuating variety is sometimes called *chronic relapsing p.*
**chronic relapsing p.,** see *chronic inflammatory demyelinating p.*
**inflammatory demyelinating p.,** see *acute idiopathic polyneuritis* and *chronic inflammatory demyelinating p.*

**poly·ra·dic·u·lop·a·thy** (pol″e-rə-dik″u-lop'ə-the) disease of several spinal nerve roots.

**poly·ri·bo·nu·cleo·tide** (pol″e-ri″bo-noo'kle-o-tīd) a polymer of ribonucleotides; ribonucleic acid.

**poly·ri·bo·nu·cleo·tide nu·cleo·ti·dyl·trans·fer·ase** (pol″e-ri″bo-noo'kle-o-tīd noo″kle-o-ti'dəl trans'fər-ās) [EC 2.7.7.8] an enzyme of the transferase class that catalyzes the reversible phosphorolysis of RNA molecules or other polyribonucleotides to yield nucleoside diphosphate residues. The bacterial enzyme was used in research elucidating the genetic code. Called also *polynucleotide phosphorylase.*

**poly·ri·bo·some** (pol″e-ri'bo-sōm) [MeSH: Polyribosomes] a complex made up of ribosomal subunits assembled among themselves by the filaments of messenger RNA containing the genetic information; they play a role in the synthesis of peptides. Called also *ergosome* and *polysome.*

**pol·yr·rhea** (pol″ĭ-re'ə) [*poly-* + *-rrhea*] a copious fluid discharge.

**poly·sac·cha·ride** (pol″e-sak'ə-rīd) a carbohydrate that on hydrolysis yields a large number of monosaccharides (variously defined as five or more to eleven or more). Cf. *oligosaccharide.*
**bacterial p's,** polysaccharides found in bacteria and especially in bacterial capsules.
**core p.,** the constant part of the heteropolysaccharide chain of lipopolysaccharide.

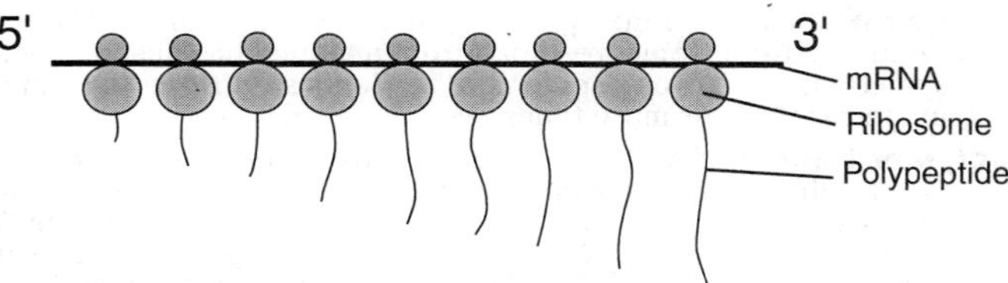


Schematic diagram of polyribosomes synthesizing nascent polypeptide chains from a messenger RNA (mRNA) template, the direction proceeding 5′ to 3′.

**immune p's,** polysaccharides which can function as specific antigens, such as capsular substances.
**O-specific p.,** the variable part of the heteropolysaccharide chain of lipopolysaccharide (q.v.); it is responsible for the antigenic specificity.
**pneumococcus p.,** a polysaccharide derived from the capsule of *Streptococcus pneumoniae.* More than 80 immunologically distinct types have been identified which form the basis of pneumococcal typing. The structure of some is known: Type I is a polymer of trisaccharide units containing galacturonic acids; Type 2 is a polymer of glucose; Type 3 is a high molecular weight polymer of glucose and glucuronic acid units (cellobiuronic acid); and Type 8 consists of glucose and glucuronic acid units alternating with glucosyl-galactose residues.
**specific p's,** soluble polysaccharides obtained from various microorganisms which in high dilution precipitate specifically the antisera to the corresponding organisms.

**poly·sce·lia** (pol″e-se'le-ə) [*poly-* + Gr. *skelos* leg + *-ia*] a developmental anomaly characterized by the presence of more than two legs.

**po·lys·ce·lus** (pə-lis'ə-ləs) [*poly-* + Gr. *skelos* leg] an individual exhibiting polyscelia.

**poly·scope** (pol'e-skōp) [*poly-* + *-scope*] diaphanoscope.

**poly·sen·si·tiv·i·ty** (pol″e-sen″sĭ-tiv'ĭ-te) sensitivity to a number of different stimuli.

**poly·sen·so·ry** (pol″e-sen'sə-re) multisensory.

**poly·se·ro·si·tis** (pol″e-se-ro-si'tis) [*poly-* + *serositis*] general inflammation of serous membranes with serous effusion; see also *Concato's disease.*
**familial recurrent p.,** familial Mediterranean fever.
**mycoplasmal p.,** infection of the serous and synovial membranes of pigs by *Mycoplasma hyorhinis,* with acute lameness, fever, and other signs of mild septicemia. It may be accompanied by mycoplasmal polyarthritis. Called also *porcine p.*
**periodic p.,** familial Mediterranean fever.
**porcine p.,** 1. Glasser's disease. 2. mycoplasmal p.
**recurrent p.,** familial Mediterranean fever.

**poly·si·a·lia** (pol″e-si-a'le-ə) [*poly-* + *sial-* + *-ia*] ptyalism.

**poly·si·a·lic ac·id** large hydrated polysaccharide similar to K1 of *Escherichia coli*

**poly·si·lox·ane** (pol″e-si'lok-sān) a rubberlike addition polymer of siloxane, used in a variety of impression materials.

**poly·sin·u·itis** (pol″e-sin″u-i'tis) polysinusitis.

**poly·si·nu·sec·to·my** (pol″e-si″nə-sek'tə-me) excision of the diseased membrane of several of the paranasal sinuses.

**poly·si·nu·si·tis** (pol″e-si″nəs-i'tis) [*poly-* + *sinusitis*] inflammation of several sinuses at once.

**poly·so·mat·ic** (pol″e-so-mat'ik) characterized by or pertaining to polysomaty.

**poly·so·ma·ty** (pol″e-so'mə-te) [*poly-* + chromo*some*] the state of having reduplicated chromatin in the nucleus. The term is applied both to the condition of increase in chromosome number resulting from a previous endomitotic cycle (endopolyploidy, def. 3) and to increase in the amount of chromatin per chromosome (polyteny).

**poly·some** (pol'e-sōm) [MeSH: Polyribosomes] polyribosome.

**poly·so·mia** (pol″e-so'me-ə) [*poly-* + *-somia*] a doubling or tripling of the body of a fetus. See also *conjoined twins,* under *twin.*

**poly·so·mic** (pol″e-so'mik) 1. pertaining to or exhibiting polysomy. 2. an individual exhibiting polysomy.

**poly·som·nog·ra·phy** (pol″e-som-nog'rə-fe) [*polygraph* + *somni-* + *-graphy*] [MeSH: Polysomnography] the polygraphic recording during sleep of multiple physiologic variables, both directly and indirectly related to the state and stages of sleep, to assess possible biological causes of sleep disorders.

**poly·so·mus** (pol″e-so'məs) [*poly-* + Gr. *sōma* body] conjoined twins exhibiting polysomia.

**poly·so·my** (pol″e-so′me) [*poly-* + chromo*some*] an excess of a particular chromosome, resulting from meiotic chromosomal nondisjunction. The chromosome may be duplicated three (trisomy), four (tetrasomy), or more times.

**poly·sor·bate** (pol″e-sor′bāt) a generic name for esters of sorbitol and its anhydrides condensed with polymers of ethylene oxide, used as surfactant agents: *p. 20,* $C_{58}H_{114}O_{26}$, is polyoxyethylene 20 sorbitan monolaurate; *p. 40,* $C_{62}H_{122}O_{26}$, is polyoxyethylene 20 sorbitan monopalmitate; *p. 60,* $C_{64}H_{126}O_{26}$, is polyethylene 20 sorbitan monostearate; *p. 65,* $C_{100}H_{194}O_{28}$, is polyethylene 20 sorbitan tristearate; *p. 80,* $C_{64}H_{124}O_{26}$, is polyethylene 20 sorbitan monooleate; *p. 85,* $C_{100}H_{188}O_{28}$, is polyethylene 20 sorbitan trioleate. *Polysorbates 20, 40, 60,* and *80* are official in NF.

**poly·sper·mia** (pol″e-sper′me-ə) [*poly-* + *sperm-* + *-ia*] 1. excessive secretion of semen. 2. polyspermy.

**poly·sper·mism** (pol″e-sper′miz-əm) polyspermia.

**poly·sper·my** (pol″e-sper′me) fertilization of an oocyte by more than one spermatozoon. Called also *polyspermia.*
**pathological p.,** entrance of more than one spermatozoon into a mature oocyte when entrance of only one is the rule; usually development is abnormal and the embryo is not viable.
**physiological p.,** entrance of more than one spermatozoon into an oocyte, occurring normally in certain species, but with only one spermatozoon participating fully in the development of the embryo.

**poly·spike** (pol″e-spīk) containing multiple spikes; said of electroencephalographic wave complexes.

**poly·sple·nia** (pol″e-sple′ne-ə) the presence of multiple spleens or splenuli.

**poly·stich·ia** (pol″e-stik′e-ə) [*poly-* + Gr. *stichos* row + *-ia*] the presence of two or more rows of eyelashes upon a lid.

**poly·sty·rene** (pol″e-sti′rēn) a hard, transparent, thermoplastic synthetic resin produced by the polymerization of styrene; used in the construction of denture bases.

**poly·sul·fide** (pol″e-sul′fīd) 1. a sulfide that has two or more atoms of sulfur. 2. containing polysulfides; see under *rubber.*

**polysulfone** (pol″e-sul′fōn) a synthetic thermoplastic polymer used as a hemodialyzer membrane.

**poly·sus·pen·soid** (pol″e-səs-pen′soid) a suspension colloid in which the particles are of different degrees of dispersion.

**poly·sy·nap·tic** (pol″e-sĭ-nap′tik) involving many synapses in series and therefore a sequence of many neurons; called also *multisynaptic.* Cf. *oligosynaptic.*

**poly·syn·dac·ty·ly** (pol″e-sin-dak′tə-le) [*poly-* + *syndactyly*] an association of polydactyly and syndactyly of varying degrees of both the hand and foot.

**poly·syn·o·vi·tis** (pol″e-sin″o-vi′tis) [*poly-* + *synovitis*] general inflammation of the synovial membranes.

**poly·tef** (pol′ĭ-tef) a polymer of tetrafluoroethylene, used as a surgical implant material for prostheses, such as artificial vessels and orbital floor implants and for many applications in skeletal augmentation and skeletal fixation. Also used widely in industry, e.g., as an antistick coating for cooking utensils. See also *polymer fume fever,* under *fever.* Called also *polytetrafluoroethylene (PTFE).*

**poly·ten·di·ni·tis** (pol″e-ten″dĭ-ni′tis) inflammation affecting several tendons.

**poly·ten·di·no·bur·si·tis** (pol″e-ten″dĭ-no-bər-si′tis) associated bursitis and tendinitis in several parts of the body.

**poly·tene** (pol′e-tēn) [*poly-* + Gr. *tainia* (L. *taenia*) band] composed of or containing many strands of chromatin (chromonemata).

**poly·teno·syn·o·vi·tis** (pol″e-ten″o-sin″o-vi′tis) inflammation of several or many tendon sheaths at the same time.

**poly·te·ny** (pol″ĭ-te′ne) reduplication of chromonemata in the chromosome without separation into distinct daughter chromosomes. See also *polysomaty.*

**poly·tet·ra·flu·o·ro·eth·y·lene (PTFE)** (pol″e-tet″rə-floor″o-roeth′ə-lēn) [MeSH: Polytetrafluoroethylene] polytef.

**poly·the·lia** (pol″e-the′le-ə) [*poly-* + *thel-* + *-ia*] the condition of having more than one pair of nipples.

**poly·the·lism** (pol″e-the′liz-əm) polythelia.

**poly·thene** (pol′e-thēn) polyethylene; a formerly used name that is still used in England.

**poly·thet·ic** (pol″e-thet′ik) [*poly-* + Gr. *thetikos* fit for placing] denoting a taxonomic group classified on the basis of several characters, as opposed to a monothetic group.

**poly·thi·a·zide** (pol″ĭ-thi′ə-zīd) [MeSH: Polythiazide] a thiazide diuretic, used in the treatment of hypertension and edema; administered orally.

**po·lyt·o·cous** (po-lit′ə-kəs) [*poly-* + *toc-* + *-ous*] giving birth to several offspring at one time.

**poly·to·mo·gram** (pol″e-to′mo-gram) the record produced by polytomography.

**poly·to·mo·graph·ic** (pol″e-to″mo-graf′ik) pertaining to polytomography.

**poly·to·mog·ra·phy** (pol″e-to-mog′rə-fe) tomography of tissue at several predetermined planes.

**poly·trau·ma** (pol″e-traw′mə) the occurrence of injuries to more than one body system.

**poly·trich·ia** (pol″e-trik′e-ə) [*poly-* + *trich-* + *-ia*] hypertrichosis.

**poly·tri·cho·sis** (pol″e-trĭ-ko′sis) hypertrichosis.

**Po·lyt·ri·chum** (po-lit′rĭ-kəm) [*poly-* + Gr. *thrix* hair] a genus of mosses, *P. juniperi′num* Willd., the haircap or juniper moss, is diuretic.

**poly·tro·phia** (pol″e-tro′fe-ə) [*poly-* + *troph-* + *-ia*] excessive nutrition.

**poly·troph·ic** (pol″e-trof′ik) pertaining to or characterized by polytrophia.

**po·lyt·ro·phy** (po-lit′rə-fe) polytrophia.

**poly·trop·ic** (pol″e-trop′ik) [*poly-* + *trop-* + *-ic*] affecting many kinds of bacteria, viruses, or tissues. Cf. *monotropic.*

**poly·un·guia** (pol″e-ung′gwe-ə) polyonychia.

**poly·un·sat·u·rat·ed** (pol″e-ən-sach′ər-āt″əd) of a chemical compound, containing two or more double or triple bonds; used particularly of fatty acids, such as linoleic acid.

**poly·ure·thane** (pol″e-u′rə-thān) any of a group of thermoplastic polymers, artificial rubbers that occur as fibers, coatings, moldable resins, elastomers, and foams; some are used in dentistry, particularly in maxillofacial prostheses.

**poly·uria** (pol″e-u′re-ə) [*poly-* + *-uria*] [MeSH: Polyuria] the passage of a large volume of urine in a given period, a characteristic of diabetes. Cf. *diuresis.*

**poly·va·lent** (pol″e-va′lənt) having more than one valence.

**poly·vi·nyl** (pol″e-vi′nəl) a polymerization product of a monomeric vinyl compound, as polyvinyl chloride.
**p. acetate,** a light- and heat-stable resin formed by the polymerization of vinyl acetate.
**p. alcohol,** see under *alcohol.*
**p. chloride,** a tasteless, odorless, clear hard resin formed by the polymerization of vinyl chloride; its many uses include packaging, clothing, and insulation of pipes and wires. Workers in its manufacture are at risk primarily because of the toxicity of vinyl chloride. Excessive inhalation of its dust can cause polyvinyl chloride pneumoconiosis.

**poly·vi·nyl·pyr·rol·i·done** (pol″e-vi″nəl-pĭ-rōl′ĭ-dōn) povidone.

**po·made** (po-mād′) pomatum.

**Po·mat·i·op·sis** (po-mat″e-op′sis) a genus of amphibious freshwater snails of the family Bulimidae, native to the United States. *P. cincinnatien′sis* and *P. lapida′ria* are intermediate hosts of the lung fluke *Paragonimus kellicotti.*

**po·ma·tum** (po-ma′təm) [L., from *pomum* apple] a medicated ointment for the hair.

**POMC** pro-opiomelanocortin.

**POMP** a regimen of prednisone, oncovin (vincristine), methotrexate, and 6-mercaptopurine, used in cancer chemotherapy.

**Pom·pe's disease** (pom′pəz) [Johann Cassianius *Pompe,* Dutch physician, 20th century] glycogen storage disease (type II).

**pom·pho·ly·he·mia** (pom″fo-le-he′me-ə) [*pompholyx* + *hem-* + *-ia*] the presence of bubbles of gas in the blood, as in decompression sickness.

**pom·pho·lyx** (pom′fo-liks) [Gr. "bubble"] a recurrent eczematous reaction characterized by the development of a vesicular eruption on the palms and soles, particularly along the sides and between the digits, accompanied by pruritus, and a burning sensation and hyperhidrosis. It is a self-limited condition usually lasting a few weeks. Called also *dyshidrotic eczema,* and formerly *cheiropompholyx* and *dyshidrosis.*

**pon·ceau 3B** (pon-so′) scarlet red; see under *red.*

**Pon·cet's disease, rheumatism** (paw-sāz′) [Antonin *Poncet,* French surgeon, 1849–1913] see under *disease* and *rheumatism.*

**Pond.** abbreviation for L. *pon′dere,* by weight.

**pon·der·a·ble** (pon′dər-ə-bəl) [L. *ponderabilis; pondus* weight] having weight.

**pon·der·al** (pon′dər-əl) [L. *pondus,* weight] pertaining to weight.

**Pon·di·min** (pon'dĭ-mēn) trademark for a preparation of fenfluramine hydrochloride.

**pon·do·stat·u·ral** (pon″do-stat'u-rəl) pertaining to weight and stature.

**po·ne·si·a·trics** (po-ne″ze-at'triks) [Gr. *ponēsis* toil, exertion + *-iatrics*] a system of therapy in which misdirected neurophysiologic reactions are made perceptible (as by the oscilloscope, electromyograph, etc.) and used as a guide in recognizing and correcting such undesirable responses (dysponesis).

**Pon·gi·dae** (pon'jĭ-de) [MeSH: Pongidae] the anthropoid apes, a family of primates that includes gibbons, gorillas, orangutans, and chimpanzees. Some are used in laboratory experiments because of their relationship to humans. See also *Anthropoidea* and *Hominoidea.*

**Pon·go** (pong'go) a genus of primates of the family Pongidae. *P. pyg'maeus* is the orangutan.

**pon(o)-** [Gr. *ponos* toil, suffering, pain] a combining form denoting relationship to hard work or to pain.

**po·no·graph** (po'no-graf) [*pono-* + *-graph*] an instrument for estimating and recording sensitiveness of contracting muscles to pain.

**pons** (ponz) gen. *pon'tis* pl. *pon'tes* [L. "bridge"] [MeSH: Pons] 1. bridge: any slip of tissue connecting two parts of an organ. 2. [TA] the part of the central nervous system lying between the medulla oblongata and the mesencephalon, superior to the cerebellum; it consists of an anterior and a posterior part (see *pars basilaris pontis* and *tegmentum pontis*). Called also *p. cerebelli.* See Plate 11. See also *brainstem.*

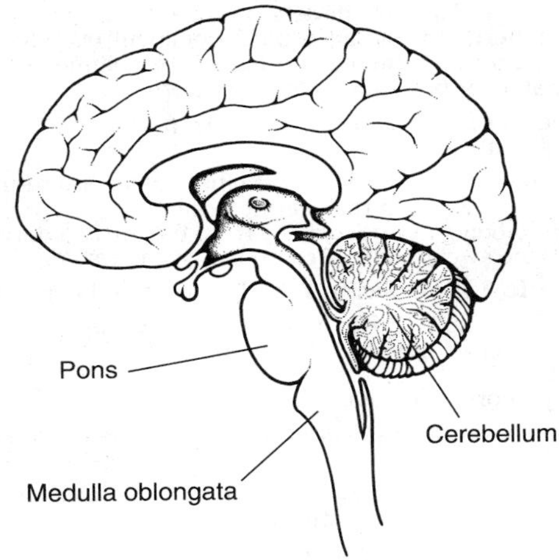


**p. cerebel'li,** pons (def. 2).
**p. et cerebel'lum,** TA alternative for *metencephalon* (def. 1).
**p. he'patis,** an occasional projection of fibers partially bridging the longitudinal fissure of the liver.

**Pon·stel** (pon'stel) trademark for a preparation of mefenamic acid.

**pon·tes** (pon'tēz) [L.] plural of *pons.*

**Pon·ti·ac fever** (pon'te-ak) [*Pontiac,* Michigan, where an outbreak occurred among occupants of a single building in 1968] see under *fever.*

**pon·tic** (pon'tik) [L. *pons,* gen. *pontis* bridge] an artificial tooth on a fixed partial denture, which replaces the lost natural tooth, restores its function, and usually occupies the space previously occupied by the natural crown.

**pon·tic·u·lar** (pon-tik'u-lər) pertaining to a ponticulus.

**pon·tic·u·lus** (pon-tik'u-ləs) pl. *ponti'culi* [L., dim. of *pons* bridge] 1. a small ridge or bridgelike structure. 2. p. auriculae.
**p. auri'culae,** a ridge of bone running posteriorly from the vestibular fenestra, delineating the superior margin of the tympanic sinus and providing the site of attachment of the posterior auricular muscle.

**pon·tile** (pon'tīl, pon'tēl) pertaining to the pons; pontine.

**pon·tine** (pon'tīn, pon'tēn) pertaining to the pons; pontile.

**pont(o)-** [L. *pons,* gen. *pontis* bridge] a prefix denoting relationship to the pons.

**pon·to·bul·bar** (pon″to-bul'bər) pertaining to, affecting, or regulated by the pons and the region of the medulla oblongata situated dorsad to it.

**pon·to·bul·bia** (pon″to-bul'be-ə) syringomyelia extending into the medulla oblongata and pons.

**Pon·to·caine** (pon'to-kān) trademark for preparations of tetracaine.

**pon·to·cer·e·bel·lar** (pon″to-ser″ə-bel'ər) 1. pertaining to the pons and the cerebellum. 2. pertaining to the pontocerebellum (neocerebellum [TA]).

**pon·to·cer·e·bel·lum** (pon″to-ser″ə-bel'um) [*ponto-* + *cerebellum*] [TA] the portion of the cerebellum whose afferent inflow is predominantly supplied by corticopontocerebellar fibers, roughly corresponding to the cerebellar hemispheres; therefore, the term is sometimes equated with neocerebellum, which is the anatomical division of the cerebellum comprising the lateral parts, including most of the hemispheres and the middle portion of the vermis. Cf. *spinocerebellum* and *vestibulocerebellum.*

**pon·to·med·ul·lary** (pon″to-med'u-lar″e) pertaining to the pons and the medulla oblongata.

**pon·to·mes·en·ce·phal·ic** (pon″to-mes″ən-sə-fal'ik) pertaining to or involving the pons and the mesencephalon.

**pon·toon** (pon-tōōn') [Fr. *ponton;* L. *ponto* boat] a loop or knuckle of the small intestine.

**pon·to·pe·dun·cu·lar** (pon″to-pə-dung'ku-lər) pertaining to, affecting, or communicating with the pons and cerebral peduncles.

**Pool's phenomenon** (pōōlz) [Eugene Hillhouse *Pool,* New York surgeon, 1874–1949] 1. see under *phenomenon.* 2. Schlesinger's sign.

**Pool-Schles·in·ger sign** (pōōl-shla'zing-ər) [E. H. *Pool;* Hermann *Schlesinger,* Austrian physician, 1868–1934] Schlesinger's sign.

**pool** (pōōl) 1. a common reservoir on which to draw; a supply available to be used by a group. 2. to create such a reservoir or supply, such as the mixing of plasma from several donors. 3. an accumulation, as of blood in any part of the body due to retardation of the venous circulation.
**gene p.,** the totality of the genes possessed by all of the members of a population.
**metabolic p.,** the entire mass of labile and reactive substances in the body, to which and from which innumerable substances continuously pass; also used in a restricted sense to mean the extracellular pool or the potassium pool.
**storage p.,** the area of a platelet organelle such as a dense body or an alpha granule where specific chemical constituents are stored; see *storage pool disease,* under *disease.*

**pop·les** (pop'lez) [L. "ham"] [TA] the posterior part of the knee; see *regio genus posterior.*

**pop·lit·e·al** (pop-lit'e-əl) [L. *poples* ham] pertaining to the posterior surface of the knee; see *fossa poplitea.*

**pop·py** (pop'e) 1. any plant of the family Papaveraceae. 2. the flower of such a plant.
**California p.,** *Eschscholtzia californica.*
**prickly p.,** *Argemone mexicana.*

**pop·u·la·tion** (pop″u-la'shən) [L. *populatio,* from *populus* people] [MeSH: Population] 1. the individuals collectively constituting a certain category or inhabiting a specified geographic area. 2. in genetics, a stable group of randomly interbreeding individuals. 3. in statistics, a theoretical concept used to describe an entire group or collection of units, finite or infinite; from it a sample can be drawn.
**genetic p.,** deme.

**Pop·u·lus** (pop'u-lus) the poplars, a genus of deciduous flowering trees of the family Salicaceae, found in the Northern Hemisphere. *P. can'dicans* Aiton has buds that contain volatile oils and resins and are used medicinally. See *balm of Gilead* (def. 5).

**POR** problem-oriented record; see under *record.*

**por·ade·nia** (por″ə-de'ne-ə) poradenitis.

**por·ad·e·ni·tis** (por-ad″ə-ni'tis) [*por-*[1] + *adenitis*] a disease of the iliac lymph nodes characterized by the formation of small abscesses. Called also *poradenia.*
**p. nos'tras, subacute inguinal p., p. vene'rea,** lymphogranuloma venereum.

**por·ad·e·no·lym·phi·tis** (por-ad″ə-no-lim-fi'tis) [*por-*[1] + *adeno-* + *lymphitis*] lymphogranuloma venereum.

**Por·ak-Du·ran·te syndrome** (po-rahk'-du-rahnt') [Charles *Porak,* French physician, 1845–1921; Gustave *Durante,* French physician, 1865–1934] osteogenesis imperfecta (type II), recessive form; see under *osteogenesis.*

**por·al** (por'əl) pertaining to or having pores.

**por·ce·lain** (por'sə-lən) 1. a white, translucent, dense ceramic material produced by fusing under high temperature of a mixture of feldspar, kaolin, quartz, whiting, and other substances. 2. dental p.
**dental p.,** a type of porcelain used in dental restorations, either jacket crowns or inlays, artificial teeth, or metal-ceramic crowns. It

is essentially a mixture of particles of feldspar and quartz, the feldspar melting first and providing a glass matrix for the quartz.

**por·ce·la·ne·ous** (por″sə-la′ne-əs) pertaining to or resembling porcelain.

**por·cine** (por′sīn) [L. *porcus* a pig, hog] pertaining to, characteristic of, or derived from domesticated pigs or other members of the family Suidae. Called also *suid.*

**pore** (por) [L. *porus* from Gr. *poros* passage] a small opening; called also *porus* [TA].
**acoustic p., external,** porus acusticus externus.
**acoustic p., internal,** porus acusticus internus.
**alveolar p's,** openings between adjacent pulmonary alveoli that permit passage of air from one to another; called also *pores of Kohn.*
**biliary p.,** ductus choledochus.
**birth p.,** metraterm.
**dilated p. of Winer,** a solitary pore on the face, back, or extremities, filled by a keratinous plug that is surrounded by hyperplastic follicular epithelium.
**Galen's p.,** canalis inguinalis.
**gustatory p.,** porus gustatorius.
**interalveolar p's, p's of Kohn,** alveolar p's.
**nuclear p's,** small octagonal openings in the nuclear envelope at sites where the two nuclear membranes are in contact, which together with the annuli form the pore complex. See also Plate 13.
**slit p's,** small slitlike spaces between the pedicels of the podocytes of the renal glomerulus; called also *filtration slits.*
**sweat p.,** porus sudoriferus.
**taste p.,** porus gustatorius.

**por·en·ce·pha·lia** (por″en-sə-fal′e-ə) porencephaly.

**por·en·ce·phal·ic** (por″en-sə-fal′ik) pertaining to or characterized by porencephaly. Called also *porencephalous.*

**por·en·ceph·a·li·tis** (por″en-sef″ə-li′tis) porencephaly associated with an inflammatory process, such as polioencephalitis.

**por·en·ceph·a·lous** (por″en-sef′ə-ləs) porencephalic.

**por·en·ceph·a·ly** (por″en-sef′ə-le) the presence of one or more cavities in the brain, which may or may not communicate with the arachnoid space, most often occurring in fetal life or early infancy. The two types are *encephaloclastic p.* and *schizencephalic p.* Called also *cerebral porosis, perencephaly,* and *porencephalia.*
**encephaloclastic p.,** a type in which the cavities are residues of destructive lesions after birth.
**schizencephalic p.,** a type in which the cavities are the result of maldevelopment of the brain. Called also *schizencephaly.*

**por·fi·mer so·di·um** (por′fĭ-mər) a hematoporphyrin derivative used as photosensitizer in photodynamic therapy for esophageal carcinoma; administered intravenously.

**por·fi·ro·my·cin** (por″fĭ-ro-mi′sin) [MeSH: Porfiromycin] the methyl derivative of mitomycin C; an antineoplastic antibiotic derived from *Streptomyces aridus.*

**po·ri** (po′ri) [L.] genitive and plural of *porus.*

**Po·rif·e·ra** (pə-rif′ə-rə) [L. *porus* pore + *ferre* to bear] [MeSH: Porifera] the phylum of sponges; the body is perforated with many pores to admit water, from which food is strained.

**po·rin** (por′in) any of a class of transmembrane matrix proteins found in the outer membranes of some gram-negative bacteria; they form trimers that contain channels for a variety of hydrophilic molecules.

**po·rio·ma·nia** (por″e-o-ma′ne-ə) [Gr. *poreia* walking + *-mania*] an irresistible impulse to travel, run away, or wander off.

**po·ri·on** (por′e-on) [*por-*[1] + *-on* neuter ending] a craniometric landmark, being the most lateral point on the roof of the bony external acoustic meatus, vertically over the middle of the meatus. Called also *point Po.*

**por(o)-**[1] [Gr. *poros,* passage] a combining form denoting relationship to a duct, passageway, opening, or pore.

**por(o)-**[2] [Gr. *pōros* callus, stone] a combining form denoting relationship to a callus or calculus.

**po·ro·car·ci·no·ma** (por″o-kahr″sĭ-no′mə) [*poro-*[1] + *carcinoma*] carcinoma arising in or from the intraepidermal portion of the sweat gland.
**eccrine p.,** a porocarcinoma arising from the opening to an eccrine sweat duct, usually occurring as a plaque, ulcer, or pedunculated mast on an extremity.

**po·ro·ceph·a·li·a·sis** (por″o-sef″ə-li′ə-sis) infection with parasites of the order Porocephalida.

**Poro·ce·phal·i·da** (por″o-sə-fal′ĭ-də) an order of the class Pentastomida, wormlike degenerate arthropods, including the families Porocephalidae and Linguatulidae.

**Poro·ce·phal·i·dae** (por″o-sə-fal′ĭ-de) a family of arthropods of the order Porocephalida, class Pentastomida, having cylindrical bodies. Adults are found in the lungs of reptiles, and the larvae are found in various vertebrates, including man. It includes the genera *Armillifer, Porocephalus,* and *Pentastoma.*

**po·ro·ceph·a·lo·sis** (por″o-sef″ə-lo′sis) porocephaliasis.

**Po·ro·ceph·a·lus** (por″o-sef′ə-ləs) [*poro-*[1] + *-cephalus*] a genus of wormlike arthropods of the order Porocephalida, family Porocephalidae. The species which parasitize man, formerly classified in this genus, are now assigned to other genera.
**P. armilla′tus,** *Armillifer armillatus.*
**P. constric′tus,** *Armillifer armillatus.*

**po·ro·fo·con** (por″o-fo′kon) either of two hydrophobic contact lens materials, designated A or B.

**po·ro·ker·a·to·sis** (por″o-ker″ə-to′sis) [*poro-*[2] + *keratosis*] [MeSH: Porokeratosis] a rare, chronic, progressive autosomal dominant skin disorder, seen most often in males, usually first appearing in early childhood, and characterized clinically by the presence of crater-like patches with central atrophy and an elevated thick keratotic border that enlarge to form circinate, serpiginous, or gyrate lesions, and histologically by a cornoid lamella (q.v.). Called also *p. of Mibelli.*
**disseminated superficial actinic p.,** an autosomal dominant skin disorder occurring on sun-exposed skin in individuals over 16 years of age, especially in females, and characterized by the presence of numerous superficial, annular, keratotic, brownish red macules, the centers of which become depressed and the borders form a sharp ridge.
**p. of Mibelli,** porokeratosis.
**p. palma′ris et planta′ris dissemina′ta,** a distinctive form of porokeratosis inherited as an autosomal dominant trait, in which hundreds of gyrate and annular porokeratotic plaques occur on the soles or palms or both, and later elsewhere.

**po·ro·ker·a·tot·ic** (por″o-ker″ə-tot′ik) pertaining to or affected with porokeratosis.

**po·ro·ma** (pə-ro′mə) [Gr. *pōrōma* callus] a general term for a neoplasm arising in or from the eccrine pore.
**eccrine p.,** a benign tumor arising from the intraepidermal portion of the eccrine sweat duct, often on the palm or sole.

**po·ro·plas·tic** (por″o-plas′tik) both porous and plastic.

**po·ro·sis** (pə-ro′sis) 1. [Gr. *pōrōsis* callosity] the formation of the callus in the repair of a fractured bone. 2. [Gr. *poros* passage] cavity formation.
**cerebral p.,** porencephalia.

**po·ros·i·ty** (pə-ros′ĭ-te) [MeSH: Porosity] 1. the condition of being porous. 2. a pore.

**po·rot·ic** (pə-rot′ik) pertaining to or characterized by porosis favoring the growth of connective tissue.

**po·rot·o·my** (pə-rot′o-me) [*poro-*[1] + *-tomy*] meatotomy.

**por·ous** (por′əs) penetrated by pores and open spaces.

**por·phin** (por′fin) a heterocyclic structure composed of four pyrrole rings connected by methylidyne (—CH═) bridges; it is the parent skeleton of the porphyrins.

**por·pho·bi·lin·o·gen** (por″fo-bĭ-lin′ə-jən) [MeSH: Porphobilinogen] the immediate precursor of the porphyrins, a pyrrole ring with acetyl, propionyl, and aminomethyl side chains; four molecules of porphobilinogen are condensed to form one molecule of uroporphyrinogen III, which is then converted successively to coproporphyrinogen III, protoporphyrin IX, and heme. Porphobilinogen is produced in excess and excreted in the urine in acute intermittent porphyria and several other porphyrias. Abbreviated PBG.

**por·pho·bi·lin·o·gen de·am·in·ase** (por″fo-bĭ-lin′ə-jən de-am′in-ās) [MeSH: Porphobilinogen Deaminase] hydroxymethylbilane synthase.

**por·pho·bi·lin·o·gen syn·thase** (por″fo-bĭ-lin′o-jən sin′thās) [EC 4.2.1.24] an enzyme of the lyase class that catalyzes the condensation of two molecules of δ-aminolevulinate to form porphobilinogen in the synthesis of porphyrins. The enzyme is inhibited by minute quantities of lead poisoning. Genetic deficiency of the enzyme causes a porphyria similar to acute intermittent porphyria but with high urinary levels of δ-aminolevulinic acid, coproporphyrinogen III, and protoporphyrin but not porphobilinogen. Called also *aminolevulinate dehydratase.*

**por·pho·bi·lin·o·gen·uria** (por″fo-bĭ-lin′o-jə-nu′re-ə) the excretion of urine containing porphobilinogen.

**por·phy·ria** (por-fēr′e-ə) [Gr. *porphyra* purple] [MeSH: Porphyria] any of a group of disturbances of porphyrin metabolism, characterized biochemically by marked increase in formation and excretion of porphyrins or their precursors and clinically by various neuro-

logic and cutaneous manifestations. Disorders are generally classified as hepatic, erythropoietic, and sometimes erythrohepatic, depending on the location of expression of the biochemical defect.
**acute p.,** acute intermittent p.
**acute intermittent p. (AIP),** a hereditary hepatic porphyria manifested by recurrent attacks of abdominal pain, gastrointestinal dysfunction, and neurologic disturbances and by excessive amounts of δ-aminolevulinic acid and porphobilinogen in the urine; it is caused by an autosomal dominant defect in hydroxymethylbilane synthase. Called also *acute p., intermittent acute p., Swedish p.,* and *pyrroloporphyria.*
**congenital erythropoietic p. (CEP),** 1. an autosomal recessive porphyria in which increased synthesis of uroporphyrinogen I relative to uroporphyrinogen III occurs in bone marrow erythroblasts; it is characterized by cutaneous photosensitivity, leading to mutilating skin lesions, by hemolytic anemia and splenomegaly, and by greatly increased urinary excretion of uroporphyrin I and coproporphyrin I. Erythrodontia and hypertrichosis are invariably present. It appears to be due to deficiency of uroporphyrinogen-III synthase. Called also *congenital photosensitive p., Günther's disease,* and *erythropoietic uroporphyria.* 2. an autosomal recessive disease of cattle, swine, and cats similar to the human disease.
**congenital photosensitive p.,** congenital erythropoietic p.
**p. cuta'nea tar'da (PCT),** the most common form of porphyria, characterized by cutaneous photosensitivity that causes scarring bullae, hyperpigmentation, facial hypertrichosis, and sometimes sclerodermatous thickenings and alopecia; it is frequently associated with alcohol abuse, liver disease, or hepatic siderosis. Urinary levels of uroporphyrin and coproporphyrin are increased and activity of uroporphyrinogen decarboxylase is decreased. The etiology is debated, but two types, which may not be allelic, are generally recognized: an autosomal dominant (or *familial*) form in which enzyme activity is reduced to half normal in liver, erythrocytes, and fibroblasts, and a *sporadic* (but probably also familial) form in which the reduction is confined to the liver. Both types are believed to be heterozygous and clinical expression occurs in adulthood, precipitated by disease or environmental factors; a more severe homozygous form begins in childhood and is called *hepatoerythropoietic p.*
**p. cuta'nea tar'da heredita'ria,** older name for *variegate porphyria.*
**p. cuta'nea tar'da symptoma'tica,** older name for *p. cutanea tarda.*
**cutaneous hepatic p.,** p. cutanea tarda.
**erythrohepatic p.,** porphyria in which abnormal overproduction of porphyrins and precursors occurs in both liver and bone marrow; when this category is used in classifying porphyrias, it usually includes only erythropoietic protoporphyria.
**erythropoietic p.,** porphyria in which excessive formation of porphyrin or its precursors occurs in bone marrow erythroblasts. The most common form is congenital erythropoietic porphyria; a less common type is erythropoietic protoporphyria. It occurs in both humans and cattle.
**hepatic p.,** porphyria in which the excess formation of porphyrin or its precursors is found in the liver; it includes acute intermittent porphyria, variegate porphyria, and hereditary coproporphyria.
**hepatoerythropoietic p. (HEP),** a severe homozygous form of porphyria cutanea tarda believed to result from an autosomal dominant defect in uroporphyrinogen decarboxylase activity; it is clinically identical to porphyria cutanea tarda but onset is in early childhood and enzyme activity in liver, erythrocytes, and fibroblasts is virtually absent.
**mixed p.,** variegate p.
**South African genetic p.,** variegate p.
**Swedish p.,** acute intermittent p.
**symptomatic p.,** p. cutanea tarda.
**p. variega'ta, variegate p. (VP),** an autosomal dominant hepatic porphyria characterized by various combinations of chronic cutaneous photosensitivity with lesions and extreme skin fragility, attacks of abdominal pain, neuropathy, and gastrointestinal dysfunction. Fecal protoporphyrin and coproporphyrin are elevated continually and urinary coproporphyrin, δ-aminolevulinic acid, and porphobilinogen are elevated during acute attacks. It is caused by partial deficiency of protoporphyrinogen oxidase activity. Called also *mixed p., South African genetic p.,* and *protocoproporphyria.*

**por·phy·rin** (por'fə-rin) any of a group of compounds containing the porphin structure, four pyrrole rings connected by methylidyne (—CH=) bridges in a cyclic configuration, to which a variety of side chains may be attached. The nature of the side chains is indicated by a prefix, such as *coproporphyrin, deuteroporphyrin, etioporphyrin, hematoporphyrin, mesoporphyrin, protoporphyrin,* or *uroporphyrin.*. Structural isomers are indicated by roman numerals. Free porphyrins are rarely found in tissues except in disorders of heme biosynthesis *(porphyrias),* but they do occur in the prosthetic groups of hemoglobin, myoglobin, and cytochromes, complexed with metal ions. The term is sometimes used to include porphin or to denote porphin specifically. See also *porphyrinogen* and *chlorophyll.*

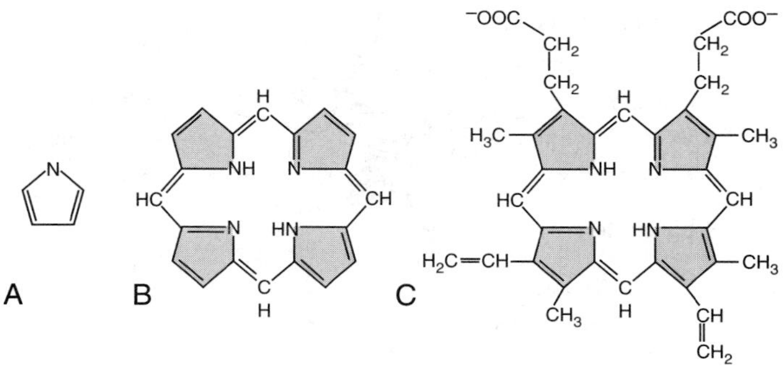

Porphyrin. *(A),* Pyrrole ring; *(B),* porphin ring; *(C),* protoporphyrin IX.

**por·phy·rin·emia** (por"fĭ-rĭ-ne'me-ə) the presence of porphyrin in the plasma or serum.

**por·phy·rin·o·gen** (por"fə-rin'ə-jən) the reduced form of a porphyrin, containing pyrrole rings linked by methylene (—$CH_2$—) instead of methylidyne bridges. The porphyrinogen forms are the functional intermediates in the biosynthesis of heme and if oxidized to their corresponding porphyrins, such as occurs in porphyrias, are irreversibly removed from the biosynthetic pathway and accumulate in tissues. Their nomenclature corresponds to that of the porphyrins.

**por·phy·rin·uria** (por"fə-rĭ-nu're-ə) excessive excretion of one or more porphyrins in the urine.

**por·phy·ris·mus** (por"fĭ-ris'məs) the psychic and emotional disturbances that occur in attacks of acute intermittent porphyria.

**por·phy·ri·za·tion** (por"fĭ-rĭ-za'shən) pulverization; reduction to a powder: so called because it was performed on a porphyry tablet.

**Por·phy·ro·mo·nas** (por"fĭ-ro-mo'nəs) [Gr. *porphyra* purple + *monas* unit, from *monos* single] a genus of gram-negative, obligately anaerobic, nonmotile, non–spore-forming, rod-shaped bacteria that are normal inhabitants of the mucous membranes of the oral cavity; organisms have been isolated from oral infections. Included here are species formerly included in the genus *Bacteroides.*
**P. asaccharoly'tica,** a bile-sensitive, pigmented species that is part of the normal flora of the mucous membranes. Organisms are also important pathogens, causing infections of the head, neck, and other parts of the body. Called also *Bacteroides asaccharolyticus* and *B. melaninogenicus* subsp. *asaccharolyticus.*
**P. endodonta'lis,** a bile-sensitive, pigmented species isolated from the root canal; called also *Bacteroides endodontalis.*
**P. gingiva'lis,** a pigmented, bile-sensitive species isolated from the human gingival crevice; called also *Bacteroides gingivalis.*

**por·phy·rox·ine** (por"fĭ-rok'sin) an opium alkaloid, $C_{19}H_{23}O_4N$.

**por·phyr·uria** (por"fir-u're-ə) porphyrinuria.

**Por·ro's cesarean section** (por'ōz) [Edoardo *Porro,* Italian obstetrician, 1842–1902] see *cesarean section,* under *section.*

**por·ta** (por'tə) pl. *por'tae* [L.] an entrance or portal; used in anatomical nomenclature to designate an opening, especially the site of entrance to an organ of the blood vessels and other structures supplying or draining it.
**p. he'patis** [TA], hepatic portal: the transverse fissure on the visceral surface of the liver where the portal vein and hepatic artery enter the liver and the hepatic ducts leave.
**p. lie'nis,** hilum splenicum.
**p. of lung,** hilum pulmonis.
**p. omen'ti, p. of omentum,** foramen epiploicum.
**p. pulmo'nis,** hilum pulmonis.
**p. re'nis,** hilum renale.
**p. of spleen,** hilum splenicum.

**por·ta·ca·val** (por"tə-ka'vəl) pertaining to or connecting the portal vein and the vena cava.

**por·tal** (por'təl) 1. porta. 2. pertaining to a porta, or entrance, especially to the porta hepatis.
**hepatic p.,** porta hepatis.
**intestinal p., anterior,** the region of opening of the embryonic foregut into the yolk sac or unclosed midgut.
**intestinal p., posterior,** the region of opening of the embryonic hindgut into the yolk sac or unclosed midgut.

**porte-ai·guille** (port"a-gwe') [Fr.] a surgeon's needle holder.

**porte-pol·ish·er, porte-pol·ish·er** (port-pol'ish-ər) a hand instrument constructed to hold a wooden point, to be used in a dental engine for applying polishing paste to and burnishing teeth.

**Por·ter** (por'tər) Rodney Robert. British biochemist, 1917–1985; co-winner, with Gerald Maurice Edelman, of the Nobel prize for

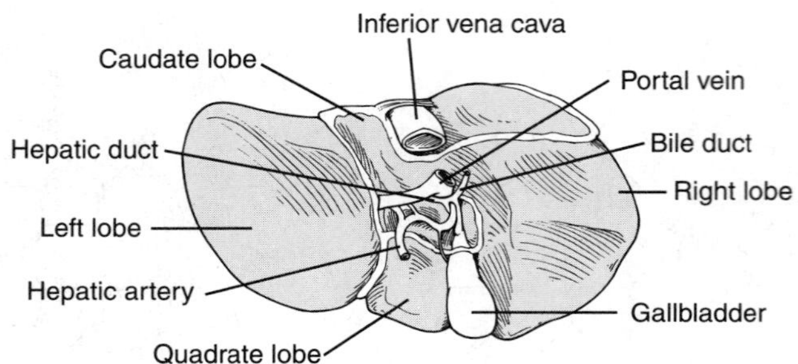

Porta hepatis on the visceral surface of the liver.

physiology or medicine in 1972, for his work on the chemical structure of antibodies, producing the Fc (fragment crystallizable) and the Fab (fragment antigen-binding) portions using pepsin.

**Por·ter's sign** (por'tərz) [William Henry *Porter,* Irish physician, 1790–1861] tracheal tugging; see under *tugging.*

**Por·ter-Sil·ber chromogens, reaction** (por'tər sil'bər) [Curt Culwell *Porter,* American biochemist, born 1914; Robert Howard *Silber,* American biochemist, born 1915] see under *chromogen* and *reaction.*

**Por·te·us maze test** (por'te-əs) [Stanley David *Porteus,* Australian-born psychologist in United States, 1883–1972] see under *test.*

**por·tio** (por'she-o) pl. *portio'nes* [L.] [TA] portion; in anatomical nomenclature, a term used for a division of a larger structure. See also *pars* and *part.*
**p. supravagina'lis cer'vicis** [TA], supravaginal portion of cervix: the part of the cervix uteri that does not protrude into the vagina.
**p. vagina'lis cer'vicis** [TA], vaginal portion of cervix: the part of the cervix uteri that protrudes into the vagina and is lined with stratified squamous epithelium; called also *ectocervix* and *exocervix.*

**por·tion** (por'shən) a part or division of a larger structure; called also *portio* [TA], *part,* and *pars.*

**por·ti·o·nes** (por"she-o'nēz) [L.] plural of *portio.*

**port·lig·a·ture** (port-lig'ə-chər) [Fr. *porte-ligature*] an instrument for applying a ligature in a deep wound.

**por·to·en·ter·os·to·my** (por"to-en"tər-os'tə-me) surgical anastomosis of the jejunum to an intrahepatic biliary radicle; done to establish a conduit from the intrahepatic bile ducts to the intestine in biliary atresia or stenosis or common duct tumor. Called also *hepatic* or *Kasai's p.* and *Kasai operation.*

**por·to·gram** (por'to-gram) a radiograph of the portal vein.

**por·tog·ra·phy** (por-tog'rə-fe) [MeSH: Portography] radiography of the portal vein after injection of opaque material.
**portal p.,** portography after injection of opaque material into the superior mesenteric vein or one of its branches after laparotomy has been performed.
**splenic p.,** portography after percutaneous injection into the substance of the spleen, usually through the ninth intercostal space in the midaxillary line, of opaque material, which passes immediately into the splenic vein, and then into the portal vein, permitting visualization of those two vessels.

**por·to·je·ju·nos·to·my** (por"to-je"joo-nos'tə-me) portoenterostomy.

**por·to·sys·tem·ic** (por"to-sis-tem'ik) connecting the portal and systemic venous circulation.

**por·to·ve·no·gram** (por"to-ve'no-gram) portogram.

**por·to·ve·nog·ra·phy** (por"to-ve-nog'rə-fe) portography.

**Por·tu·guese man-of-war** (por'chə-gēs) any cnidarian of the genus *Physalia.*

**po·rus** (por'əs) gen. and pl. *po'ri* [L., from Gr. *poros* passage] [TA] pore: any of various small openings in the body.
**p. acus'ticus exter'nus** [TA], the outer end of the external acoustic meatus.
**p. acus'ticus inter'nus** [TA], the opening of the internal acoustic meatus.
**p. gale'ni,** canalis inguinalis.
**p. gustato'rius** [TA], gustatory pore: the small opening of a taste bud onto the surface of the tongue. Called also *taste pore.*
**p. op'ticus,** the opening in the sclera for passage of the optic nerve.
**p. sudori'ferus,** sweat pore: the opening of the duct of the sweat gland on the surface of the skin; called also *pore of sweat duct.*

**Po·sa·das' mycosis** (po-sah'dahs) [Alejandro *Posadas,* Argentine pathologist, 1870–1920] coccidioidomycosis.

**Po·sa·das-Wer·ni·cke disease** (po-sah'dahs-ver'nĭ-ke) [A. *Posadas;* Robert *Wernicke,* Argentine pathologist, 1854–1922] coccidioidomycosis.

**-posia** [Gr. *posis* a drink + *-ia*] a word termination denoting relationship to drinking, or to intake of fluids.

**Pos·i·cor** (poz'ĭ-kor) trademark for a preparation of mibefradil dihydrochloride.

**po·si·tion** (pə-zish'ən) [L. *positio*] 1. a bodily posture or attitude assumed by the patient to achieve comfort in certain conditions, or the particular disposition of the body and extremities to facilitate the performance of certain diagnostic or therapeutic procedures. 2. in obstetrics, the situation of the fetus in the pelvis, determined and described by the relation of a given arbitrary point (point of direction) in the presenting part to a given arbitrary point in the coronal plane of the maternal pelvis. For the various possible positions see accompanying table. Cf. *presentation.*

## Position

**Albert's p.,** a semirecumbent position of the patient for radiography as a means of determining the diameters of the superior strait of the pelvis.
**anatomical p.,** the position of the human body, standing erect, with the face directed anteriorly and with the upper limbs at the sides and the palms turned anteriorly (supinated); used as the position of reference in description of site or direction of various structures or parts as established in official anatomical nomenclature.
**batrachian p.,** a lying position of infants in which the lower limbs are flexed, abducted, and resting on the bed on their outer aspects, somewhat resembling the legs of a frog. Called also *froglike p.*
**Bozeman's p.,** one in which the patient is strapped to supports in the knee-elbow position.
**Brickner p.,** a position for treating shoulder disability, secured by tying the patient's wrist to the head of the bed with his arm supported on a pillow and raising the head of the bed; thus traction with abduction and external rotation is obtained.
**Caldwell's p.,** a radiographic position with the forehead and nose against the x-ray plate, used with Caldwell's projection.
**Casselberry's p.,** a prone position employed after intubation so that the patient may swallow without danger of fluid entering the tube.
**centric p.,** the rest position of the mandible, as it is influenced by the muscle tone, while the patient remains standing or is sitting with

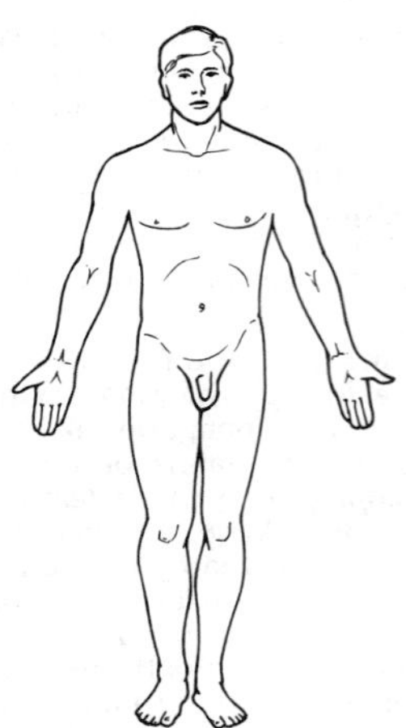
Anatomical position.

**Positions of the Fetus in Various Presentations**

| Presentation | Point of Direction | Position | Abbreviation |
|---|---|---|---|
| *Cephalic Presentation* | | | |
| Vertex | Occiput | Left occipitoanterior | LOA |
| | | Left occipitoposterior | LOP |
| | | Left occipitotransverse | LOT |
| | | Right occipitoanterior | ROA |
| | | Right occipitoposterior | ROP |
| | | Right occipitotransverse | ROT |
| Face | Chin | Left mentoanterior | LMA |
| | | Left mentoposterior | LMP |
| | | Left mentotransverse | LMT |
| | | Right mentoanterior | RMA |
| | | Right mentoposterior | RMP |
| | | Right mentotransverse | RMT |
| Brow | Brow | Left frontoanterior | LFA |
| | | Left frontoposterior | LFP |
| | | Left frontotransverse | LFT |
| | | Right frontoanterior | RFA |
| | | Right frontoposterior | RFP |
| | | Right frontotransverse | RFT |
| *Pelvic Presentation (Breech)* | | | |
| Complete breech (feet crossed and thighs flexed on abdomen) | Sacrum | Left sacroanterior | LSA |
| | | Left sacroposterior | LSP |
| | | Left sacrotransverse | LST |
| | | Right sacroanterior | RSA |
| | | Right sacroposterior | RSP |
| | | Right sacrotransverse | RST |
| Incomplete breech | Sacrum | Same designations as above, adding the qualifications footling, knee, etc. | |
| *Shoulder Presentation (Transverse Lie)* | | | |
| Shoulder | Scapula | Left scapuloanterior | LScA |
| | | Left scapuloposterior | LScP |
| | | Right scapuloanterior | RScA |
| | | Right scapuloposterior | RScP |

jaw open, from which the teeth will come into centric occlusion when the jaw is closed.

***cis* p.**, see under *configuration.*

**coiled p.**, the attitude of a patient on his side with hips and knees flexed and thighs drawn up to the body.

**decubitus p.**, the position of an individual lying on a horizontal surface, designated, according to the portion of the body resting on the surface, *dorsal decubitus* (lying on the back), *left lateral decubitus* (on the left side), *right lateral decubitus* (on the right side), or *ventral decubitus* (on the abdomen).

**Depage's p.**, a prone position with the pelvis raised to form the apex of an inverted V, while the trunk and lower limbs form the branches of the V.

**dorsal p.**, the posture of a person lying on his back; called also *supine p.*

**dorsal elevated p.**, position of the patient lying on the back, with shoulders and head elevated.

**dorsal recumbent p.**, position of patient on back, with lower limbs flexed and rotated outward; used in vaginal examination, application of obstetrical forceps, etc.

**dorsal rigid p.**, position on the back with hips and knees flexed and thighs drawn up to the body.

**dorsosacral p.**, lithotomy p.

**Duncan's p.**, the position of the placenta with its margin presenting at the os for delivery.

**eccentric p.**, see under *relation.*

**Edebohls' p.**, a dorsal position, the knees and thighs drawn up, legs flexed on the thighs, and thighs flexed on the abdomen, the hips raised, and the thighs abducted; called also *Simon's p.*

**Elliot's p.**, position of a patient on the operating table with lower chest elevated by placing a support under the lower costal margin; used in operations on the gallbladder.

**emprosthotonos p.**, emprosthotonos.

**English p.**, the patient on the left side, the right thigh and knee drawn up; called also *lateral recumbent p.*

**figure four p.**, the patient lies with the side of the body upwards and the superior leg flexed with its ankle resting on the knee of the opposite leg so that the legs are in the shape of the number four.

**Fowler's p.**, the position in which the head of the patient's bed is raised 18 or 20 inches above the level; the knees are also elevated.

**froglike p.**, batrachian p.

**frontal anterior p.**, frontoanterior p.

**frontal posterior p.**, frontoposterior p.

**frontal transverse p.**, frontotransverse p.

**frontoanterior p.**, a position of the fetus in cephalic presentation in labor, with its brow directed toward the right (RFA) or left (LFA) anterior quadrant of the maternal pelvis.

**frontoposterior p.**, a position of the fetus in cephalic presentation in labor, with its brow directed toward the right (RFP) or left (LFP) posterior quadrant of the maternal pelvis.

**frontotransverse p.**, a position of the fetus in cephalic presentation in labor, with its brow directed toward the right (RFT) or left (LFT) iliac fossa of the maternal pelvis.

**Fuchs p.**, a radiographic position which gives an oblique view of the zygomatic arch projected free of superimposed structures.

**genucubital p.**, knee-elbow p.

**genufacial p.**, the position of the patient resting on his knees and face.

**genupectoral p.**, knee-chest p.

**hinge p.**, the position of the condyle in the temporomandibular joint from which an opening by hinge movement is possible beyond the amplitude of rest position.

**hinge p., condylar,** the position of the condyles in the glenoid fossa at which hinge axis movement is possible.

**hinge p., mandibular,** a position of the mandible that allows the condyles to move on the hinge axis during the opening or closing of the jaws.

**hinge p., terminal,** centric relation.

**horizontal p.**, the position assumed by a person lying on his back with limbs extended.

**jackknife p.**, Kraske p.

**Jones' p.**, acute flexion of the forearm for the treatment of fracture of the internal condyle of the humerus.

**knee-chest p.**, the position of a patient on his knees with the chest resting on the table. See Plate 43.

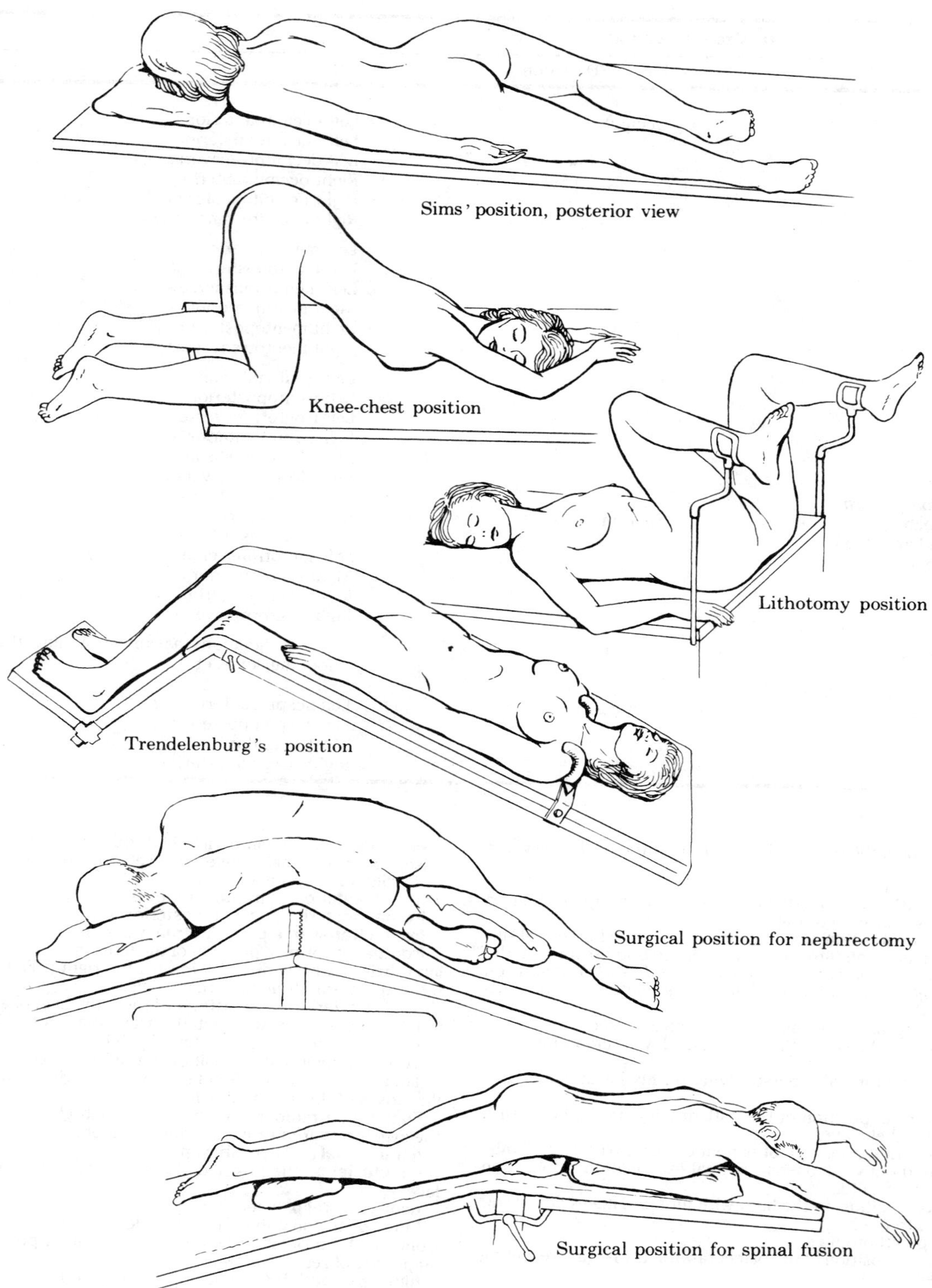


**PLATE 43**—VARIOUS POSITIONS USED IN EXAMINATION OR TREATMENT

**knee-elbow p.,** the position of a patient resting on knees and elbows with the chest elevated from the table.

**kneeling-squatting p.,** squatting position with the knees flexed acutely and pressed against the abdomen while the body is held erect; often effective in digital palpation of high rectal lesions.

**Kraske p.,** a prone position with the buttocks raised.

**lateral recumbent p.,** English p.

**lithotomy p.,** the patient in dorsal decubitus with hips and knees flexed and the thighs abducted and externally rotated; called also *dorsosacral p.* See Plate 43.

**Mayer p.,** a radiographic position that gives a unilateral superoinferior view of the temporomandibular joint, external auditory canal, and mastoid and petrous processes; helpful in demonstrating fractures and malformations of the temporomandibular joint and in the study of bony atresia of the external auditory canal.

**mentoanterior p.,** a position of the fetus in cephalic presentation in labor, with its chin directed toward the right (RMA) or left (LMA) anterior quadrant of the maternal pelvis.

**mentoposterior p.,** a position of the fetus in cephalic presentation in labor, with its chin directed toward the right (RMP) or left (LMP) posterior quadrant of the maternal pelvis.

**mentotransverse p.,** a position of the fetus in cephalic presentation in labor, with its chin directed toward the right (RMT) or left (LMT) iliac fossa of the maternal pelvis.

**mentum anterior p.,** mentoanterior p.

**mentum posterior p.,** mentoposterior p.

**mentum transverse p.,** mentotransverse p.

**Noble's p.,** position of the patient standing up, leaning forward and supporting the upper body on the arms; used in examining the kidney.

**occipitoanterior p.,** a position of the fetus in cephalic presentation in labor, with its occiput directed toward the right (ROA) or left (LOA) anterior quadrant of the maternal pelvis.

**occipitoposterior p.,** a position of the fetus in cephalic presentation in labor, with its occiput directed toward the right (ROP) or left (LOP) posterior quadrant of the maternal pelvis.

**occipitosacral p.,** a position of the fetus in cephalic presentation in labor, with the occiput presenting directly behind, or rotated squarely into the hollow of the sacrum.

**occipitotransverse p.,** a position of the fetus in cephalic presentation in labor, with its occiput directed toward the right (ROT) or left (LOT) iliac fossa of the maternal pelvis.

**occiput anterior p.,** occipitoanterior p.

**occiput posterior p.,** occipitoposterior p.

**occiput sacral p.,** occipitosacral p.

**occiput transverse p.,** occipitotransverse p.

**occlusal p.,** a functional position of the jaws in which contact between some or all of the upper and lower teeth occurs when the mandible is closed, which may or may not coincide with centric occlusion. Called also *occlusal relation.*

**opisthotonos p.,** opisthotonos.

**orthopnea p.,** the patient assumes an upright or a semivertical position by using two or more pillows to support his head and chest from the recumbent position, or he sits upright in a chair. Used when the patient has difficulty in breathing except in the upright position (orthopnea).

**orthotonos p.,** orthotonos.

**physiologic rest p.,** rest p.

**posterior border p.,** the most posterior position of the mandible at any specific vertical relation to the maxillae. Called also *posterior border jaw relation.*

**prone p.,** patient lying face down.

**rest p.,** the position of the mandible when its muscles are at rest, the body is in the upright standing or sitting position, and the eyes are focused toward the horizon; the lips are slightly touching and the distance between the upper and lower teeth has a free-way space of about 2 to 5 mm. Called also *physiologic rest p.* and *rest jaw relation.*

**Robson's p.,** the patient lying supine with a sandbag placed beneath the eleventh and twelfth ribs; used in surgery on the biliary tract.

**Rose's p.,** one intended to prevent aspiration or swallowing of blood, as from an injured lip: the patient is supine with head hanging over the end of the table in full extension so as to enable bleeding to be over the margins of the inverted upper incisors.

**sacroanterior p.,** a position of the fetus in breech presentation in labor, with its sacrum directed toward the right (RSA) or left (LSA) anterior quadrant of the maternal pelvis.

**sacroposterior p.,** a position of the fetus in breech presentation in labor, with its sacrum directed toward the right (RSP) or left (LSP) posterior quadrant of the maternal pelvis.

**sacrotransverse p.,** a position of the fetus in breech presentation in labor, with its sacrum directed toward the right (RST) or left (LST) iliac fossa of the maternal pelvis.

**sacrum anterior p.,** sacroanterior p.

**sacrum posterior p.,** sacroposterior p.

**sacrum transverse p.,** sacrotransverse p.

**scapula anterior p.,** scapuloanterior p.

**scapula posterior p.,** scapuloposterior p.

**scapuloanterior p.,** a position of the fetus in transverse lie in labor, with its head to the right (RScA) or left (LScA) of the maternal pelvis, and its back anterior.

**scapuloposterior p.,** a position of the fetus in transverse lie in labor, with its head to the right (RScP) or left (LScP) of the maternal pelvis, and its back posterior.

**scorbutic p.,** a pseudoparalytic position characteristic of advanced infantile scurvy, in which the infant lies quietly with the legs flexed at the knees and the hips flexed and externally rotated.

**semiaxial p.,** a radiographic position of the head in which the central ray enters at an angle; see *half-axial projection,* under *projection.* Called also *Titterington's p.*

**semi-Fowler p.,** a position similar to Fowler's position but with the head less elevated.

**semiprone p.,** Sims' p.

**semireclining p.,** a partly reclining position seen in heart disease, asthma, and pleural effusion.

**Simon's p.,** Edebohls' p.

**Sims' p.,** the patient lies on the left side with the right knee and thigh flexed and the left arm parallel along the back; for vaginal examination. Called also *semiprone p.* See Plate 43.

**submentovertex p.,** the position of the head for a submentovertex projection.

**supine p.,** dorsal p.

**Titterington's p.,** semiaxial p.

***trans* p.,** see under *configuration.*

**Trendelenburg's p.,** one in which the patient is supine on the table or bed, the head of which is tilted downward 30 to 40 degrees, and the table or bed angulated beneath the knees. See Plate 43.

**tripod p.,** 1. a position assumed by the patient with abdominal weakness or meningeal irritation while sitting in bed, in which he supports himself with his hands in a plane posterior to his pelvis. 2. a sitting position assumed by the patient with respiratory insufficiency, in which his hands are placed anterior to the frontal plane. See also *tripoding.*

**Valentine's p.,** the patient supine and the hips flexed by means of a double inclined plane; used in irrigating the urethra.

**verticosubmental p.,** the position of the head for a verticosubmental projection.

**Waters' p.,** the position of the head in Waters' projection.

**Waters' p., reverse,** a mento-occipital radiographic position used to demonstrate the facial bones when the patient cannot be placed in a prone position; helpful in demonstrating fractures of the orbits, maxillary sinuses, zygomatic bones, and zygomatic arches.

---

**po·si·tion·er** (pə-zish'ən-ər) a resilient elastoplastic removable appliance fitted over the occlusal surfaces of the teeth to obtain limited tooth movement and stabilization, usually at the end of orthodontic treatment.

**tooth p.,** see *positioner.*

**pos·i·tive** (poz'ĭ-tiv) [L. *positivus*] having a value greater than zero; indicating existence or presence of a condition, organism, etc., as chromatin positive or Wassermann positive; characterized by affirmation or cooperation.

**pos·i·tro·ceph·a·lo·gram** (poz″ĭ-tro-sef'ə-lo-gram) [*positron* + *cephalo-* + *-gram*] a record produced by the emission of positrons by isotopes of arsenic administered to facilitate localization of brain tumors.

**pos·i·tron** (poz'ĭ-tron) [*posi*tive elec*tron*] [MeSH: Electrons] the antiparticle of the electron, a positive electron; a particle having the mass of the electron but a positive electric charge. Symbol $e^+$.

**po·so·log·ic** (po″sə-loj'ik) pertaining to doses.

**po·sol·o·gy** (po-sol′ə-je) [Gr. *posos* how much + *-logy*] the science of dosage, or a system of dosage.

**Pos·sum** (pos′əm) [*P*atient-*O*perated *S*elector *M*echanism] trademark for a machine designed for the disabled by which, when breathed into in the correct manner, the individual can operate the telephone, ring bells, turn on the television, switch off a light, type a letter, or perform any of a number of other functions by no movement other than that involved in respiration.

**post** (pōst) 1. a piece of material firmly secured in an upright position, usually to support something. 2. dowel.
**abutment p., implant p.,** implant abutment.

**post-** [L. *post* after] a prefix meaning after or behind.

**post·al·bu·min** (pōst″al-bu′min) a serum protein with an electrophoretic mobility between albumin and alpha-globulin at pH 8.6.

**post·au·ra·le** (pōst″aw-ra′le) a cephalometric landmark, the most posterior point on the helix of the ear.

**post·au·ric·u·lar** (pōst″aw-rik′u-lər) posterior to the auricle of the ear.

**post·ax·i·al** (pōst-ak′se-əl) posterior to an axis. In anatomical usage, this refers to the medial (ulnar) aspect of the upper limb, and the lateral (fibular) aspect of the lower limb.

**post·bra·chi·al** (pōst-bra′ke-əl) on the posterior part of the upper arm.

**post·bul·bar** (pōst-bul′bər) posterior or distal to a bulb, such as the medulla oblongata, or distal to the pileus ventriculi (duodenal bulb).

**post·cap·il·lary** (pōst-kap′ĭ-lar′e) 1. located just to the venous side of a capillary. 2. venous capillary.

**post·car·di·ot·o·my** (pōst″kahr-de-ot′ə-me) occurring after or as a consequence of operating on the heart.

**post·cath·e·ter·iza·tion** (post-kath″ə-tər″i-za′shən) following catheterization.

**post·ca·va** (pōst-ka′və) vena cava inferior.

**post·ca·val** (pōst-ka′vəl) pertaining to the inferior vena cava.

**post·cen·tral** (pōst-sen′trəl) posterior to a center, as the postcentral gyrus.

**post·ci·bal** (pōst-si′bəl) [*post-* + L. *cibum* food] postprandial.

**post ci·bum** (pōst si′bəm) [L.] after meals (after food).

**post·con·dy·la·re** (pōst-kon″də-lar′e) the highest point of the curvature posterior to the occipital condyle.

**post·cra·ni·al** (pōst-kra′ne-əl) posterior or inferior to the cranium.

**post·cu·bi·tal** (pōst-ku′bi-təl) on the dorsal side of the forearm.

**post·di·as·tol·ic** (pōst″di-əs-tol′ik) occurring after diastole.

**post·di·crot·ic** (pōst″di-krot′ik) occurring after the dicrotic notch and wave of the sphygmogram.

**post·diph·ther·it·ic** (pōst-dif-thə-rit′ik) occurring after an attack of diphtheria.

**post·dor·mi·tal** (pōst-dor′mĭ-təl) pertaining to or occurring during the postdormitum.

**post·dor·mi·tum** (pōst-dor′mĭ-təm) the period of increasing consciousness interposed between sound sleep and wakening.

**post·dys·en·ter·ic** (pōst″dis-en-ter′ik) following dysentery.

**post·ec·dy·sis** (pōst-ek′dĭ-sis) [*post-* + *ecdysis*] the concluding phase of ecdysis in certain crustaceans and arthropods, during which the endocuticle is secreted and calcification of the skeleton occurs.

**post·em·bry·on·ic** (pōst″em-bre-on′ik) [*post-* + *embryonic*] occurring after the embryonic stage.

**pos·te·ri·ad** (pos-te′re-ad) toward the posterior surface of the body.

**pos·ter·i·or** (pos-tēr′e-or) [L. "behind"; neut. *posterius*] 1. situated in back of, or in the back part of, a structure. 2. [TA] in humans and other bipeds, towards the back surface of the body; called also *dorsal.* 3. in quadrupeds, a term sometimes used as a synonym for *caudal.*

**postero-** [L. *posterus* behind] a combining form denoting relationship to the posterior part.

**pos·tero·an·te·ri·or** (pos″tər-o-an-tēr′e-or) from back to front, or from the posterior to the anterior surface, such as the direction of a radiographic projection.

**pos·tero·clu·sion** (pos″tər-o-kloo′zhən) distoclusion.

**pos·tero·ex·ter·nal** (pos″tər-o-ek-ster′nəl) situated on the outer side of a posterior aspect.

**pos·tero·in·fe·ri·or** (pos″tər-o-in-fēr′e-or) posterior and inferior.

**pos·tero·in·ter·nal** (pos″tər-o-in-tər′nəl) situated within and toward the posterior surface.

**pos·tero·lat·er·al** (pos″tər-o-lat′ər-əl) situated posteriorly and to one side.

**pos·tero·me·di·al** (pos″tər-o-me′de-əl) situated toward the middle of the posterior surface.

**pos·tero·me·di·an** (pos″tər-o-me′de-ən) situated on the midline of the posterior surface.

**pos·tero·pa·ri·e·tal** (pos″tər-o-pə-ri′ə-təl) situated at the posterior part of the parietal bone.

**pos·tero·su·pe·ri·or** (pos″tər-o-soo-pēr′e-or) situated posteriorly and inferiorly.

**pos·tero·tem·po·ral** (pos″tər-o-tem′po-rəl) situated at the posterior part of the temporal bone.

**post·gan·gli·on·ic** (pōst″gang-gle-on′ik) situated posterior or distal to a ganglion; said especially of autonomic nerve fibers so located.

**post·gle·noid** (pōst-gle′noid) posterior to the glenoid cavity of the scapula.

**post·glo·mer·u·lar** (pōst″glo-mer′u-lər) located or occurring distal to a glomerulus of the kidney.

**pos·thet·o·my** (pos-thet′ə-me) [Gr. *posthē* foreskin + *-tomy*] circumcision.

**pos·thio·plas·ty** (pos′the-o-plas″te) [Gr. *posthē* foreskin + *-plasty*] plastic surgery of the prepuce.

**pos·thi·tis** (pos-thi′tis) [Gr. *posthē* foreskin + *-itis*] inflammation of the prepuce.
**enzootic p.,** see under *balanoposthitis.*

**pos·tho·lith** (pos′tho-lith) [Gr. *posthē* foreskin + *-lith*] a preputial concretion or calculus.

**post·hu·mous** (pos′tu-məs) [L. *postumus* coming after] 1. occurring after death. 2. born after the father's death.

**post·hy·oid** (pōst-hi′oid) posterior to the hyoid bone.

**post·hyp·not·ic** (pōst″hip-not′ik) following the hypnotic state.

**post·ic·tal** (pōst-ik′təl) [*post-* + *-ictal*] occurring after a seizure or sudden attack.

**pos·ti·cus** (pos-ti′kəs) [L.] posterior.

**post·in·farc·tion** (pōst″in-fahrk′shən) following infarction, particularly myocardial infarction.

**post·is·chi·al** (pōst-is′ke-əl) posterior to the ischium.

**post·lin·gual** (pōst-ling′gwəl) 1. occurring after the development of language. 2. posterior to the tongue or to a lingula.

**post·mas·tec·to·my** (pōst″mas-tek′tə-me) following mastectomy.

**post·mas·toid** (pōst-mas′toid) posterior to the mastoid process of the temporal bone.

**post·ma·ture** (pōst″mə-choor′) overly developed, as a postmature infant. Cf. *postterm pregnancy,* under *pregnancy.*

**post·ma·tur·i·ty** (pōst″mə-choor′ĭ-te) overdevelopment; the condition of a postmature infant. See also *dysmaturity syndrome,* under *syndrome.*

**post·me·di·as·ti·nal** (pōst″me-de-əs-ti′nəl) 1. posterior to the mediastinum. 2. pertaining to the posterior mediastinum.

**post·me·di·as·ti·num** (pōst″me-de-əs-ti′nəm) mediastinum posterius.

**post·mei·ot·ic** (pōst″mi-ot′ik) [*post-* + *meiotic*] occurring after or pertaining to the time following meiosis.

**post·meno·pau·sal** (pōst″men-o-paw′zəl) occurring after the menopause.

**post·men·strua** (pōst-men′stroo-ə) the period immediately following cessation of menstrual flow.

**post·mes·en·ter·ic** (pōst″mes-ən-ter′ik) 1. posterior to the mesentery. 2. in the posterior part of the mesentery.

**post·mi·ni·mus** (pōst-mĭ′nĭ-məs) pl. *postmi′nimi* [*post-* + L. *minimus* small] digitus postminimus.

**post·mi·ot·ic** (pōst″mi-ot′ik) postmeiotic.

**post·mi·tot·ic** (pōst″mi-tot′ik) 1. pertaining to the time following or occurring after mitosis in normally dividing cells. 2. pertaining to cells that stop dividing after reaching maturity, as cells of the mammalian heart or central nervous system.

**post·mor·tal** (pōst-mor′təl) occurring after death.

**post mor·tem** (pōst mor′təm) [L.] after death.

**post·mor·tem** (pōst-mor'təm) occurring or performed after death; pertaining to the period after death.

**post·na·ri·al** (pōst-na're-əl) pertaining to the choanae of the nose; called also *choanal.*

**post·nar·is** (pōst-na'ris) choana.

**post·na·sal** (pōst-na'zəl) [*post-* + *nasal*] posterior to the nose.

**post·na·tal** (pōst-na'təl) occurring after birth, with reference to the newborn. Cf. *postpartum.*

**post·op·er·a·tive** (pōst-op'ər-ə-tive) occurring after a surgical operation.

**post·pal·a·tine** (pōst-pal'ə-tīn) posterior to the palate or the palatine bone.

**post·par·tal** (pōst-pahr'təl) postpartum.

**post par·tum** (pōst pahr'təm) [L.] after childbirth, or after delivery.

**post·par·tum** (pōst-pahr'təm) occurring after childbirth, or after delivery, with reference to the mother. Cf. *postnatal.*

**post·pran·di·al** (pōst-pran'de-əl) occurring after a meal; called also *postcibal.*

**post·pu·ber·al** (pōst-pu'bər-əl) postpubertal.

**post·pu·ber·tal** (pōst-pu'bər-təl) occurring in or pertaining to the period following puberty.

**post·pu·ber·ty** (pōst-pu'bər-te) the period following puberty.

**post·pu·bes·cence** (pōst″pu-bes'əns) postpuberty.

**post·pu·bes·cent** (pōst″pu-bes'ənt) postpubertal.

**post·re·nal** (pōst-re'nəl) 1. located behind a kidney. 2. occurring after leaving a kidney, such as renal failure that results from processes impairing normal excretion of urine after it has been formed. Cf. *prerenal.*

**post·ro·lan·dic** (pōst″ro-lan'dik) posterior to the fissure of Rolando (sulcus centralis).

**Post sing. sed. liq.** abbreviation for L. *post sin'gulas se'des liq'uidas,* after every loose stool.

**post·si·nu·soi·dal** (pōst″si-nə-soi'dəl) located beyond a sinusoid or affecting the circulation beyond a sinusoid; used especially to denote the location of vascular resistance in portal hypertension.

**post·sphe·noid** (pōst-sfe'noid) pertaining to the posterior portion of the body of the sphenoid bone.

**post·sphe·noi·dal** (pōst″sfə-noi'dəl) postsphenoid.

**post·splen·ic** (pōst-splen'ik) posterior to the spleen.

**post·ste·not·ic** (pōst″stə-not'ik) distal to a stenosed segment.

**post·syl·vi·an** (pōst-sil've-ən) posterior to the sylvian fissure (sulcus lateralis).

**post·sy·nap·tic** (pōst″sĭ-nap'tik) situated beyond or distal to a synapse, or occurring after the synapse is crossed.

**post-term** (pōst-tərm') extending beyond term; said of pregnancy or of an infant.

**post-trau·mat·ic** (pōst″traw-mat'ik) occurring as a result of or after injury.

**pos·tu·late** (pos'tu-lāt) [L. *postulatum* demanded] anything assumed or taken for granted.
**Koch's p's,** a statement of the kind of experimental evidence required to establish the etiologic relationship of a given microorganism to a given disease. The conditions included are (1) the microorganism must be observed in every case of the disease; (2) it must be isolated and grown in pure culture; (3) the pure culture must, when inoculated into a susceptible animal, reproduce the disease; and (4) the microorganism must be observed in, and recovered from, the experimentally diseased animal.

**pos·tur·al** (pos'chər-əl) pertaining to posture or position.

**pos·ture** (pos'choor) [L. *postura*] [MeSH: Posture] the attitude of the body.
**Drosin's p's,** three postures for eliciting tenderness in appendicitis.

**pos·tu·rog·ra·phy** (pos″chər-og″rə-fe) testing procedures for upright posture, balance, and sense of equilibrium. The patient stands on a force platform and measurements are taken of head position, hip position, and downward force of the feet; further assessments are done under various conditions of changing visual stimuli and platform position.

**post·vac·ci·nal** (pōst-vak'sĭ-nəl) occurring after or as a consequence of vaccination for smallpox.

**post·vac·cin·i·al** (pōst″vak-sin'e-əl) occurring after or as a consequence of vaccinia.

**post·ve·ne·re·al** (pōst″və-nēr'e-əl) following infection with an organism that causes sexually transmitted disease.

**post·vi·tal** (pōst-vi'təl) see *postvital staining,* under *staining.*

**post·zone** (pōst'zōn) see *zone of antigen excess,* under *zone.*

**post·zy·got·ic** (pōst″zi-got'ik) occurring after the completion of fertilization and formation of the zygote.

**Po·ta·ba** (po'tə-bə) trademark for preparations of aminobenzoate potassium.

**pot·a·ble** (po'tə-bəl) [L. *potabilis*] fit to drink; drinkable.

**pot AGT** potential abnormality of glucose tolerance.

**Po·tain's sign** (po-taz') [Pierre Carl Edouard *Potain,* French physician, 1825–1901] see under *sign.*

**Pot·a·mon** (pot'ə-mon) a genus of fresh water crabs (order Decapoda). *P. dentricula'ris, P. dehaa'ni,* and *P. rath'buni* are hosts of the metacercariae of the lung fluke *Paragonimus westermani* in East Asia.

**pot·ash** (pot'ash) impure potassium carbonate.
**caustic p.,** potassium hydroxide.
**sulfurated p.** [USP], a mixture of potassium polysulfides and potassium thiosulfate, used as a source of sulfide in pharmaceutical preparations such as white lotion (q.v.).

**pot·as·se·mia** (pot″ə-se'me-ə) [*potassium* + *-emia*] hyperkalemia.

**po·tas·sic** (po-tas'ik) containing potash.

**po·tas·si·um** (po-tas'e-əm) [L.] [MeSH: Potassium] a metallic element of the alkali group, many of whose salts are used in medicine. It is a soft, silver-white metal, melting at 58° F.; atomic number, 19; atomic weight, 39.102; specific gravity, 0.87; symbol, K (L. *kalium*). Potassium is the chief cation of muscle and most other cells (intracellular fluid); see also *sodium-potassium pump,* under *pump.*
**p. 42,** a radioisotope of potassium, atomic mass 42, having a half-life of 12.36 hours and emitting beta particles (3.52 MeV) and gamma rays (0.187 MeV); as the labeled chloride salt it is used as a tracer in studies of potassium interchange in the body.
**p. acetate** [USP], an electrolyte replenisher and urinary and systemic alkalizer, administered by intravenous infusion and orally. Formerly used as a diuretic and expectorant. Called also *diuretic salt* and *sal diureticum.*
**p. acid phosphate,** monobasic p. phosphate.
**p. acid tartrate,** p. bitartrate.
**p. alum,** see under *alum.*
**p. aspartate and magnesium aspartate,** a mixture of $C_4H_6KNO_4 \cdot \frac{1}{2}H_2O$ and $C_8H_{12}MgN_2O_8 \cdot 4H_2O$; used as a nutrient.
**p. bicarbonate** [USP], pharmaceutic necessity in the preparation of Randall's solution; may be used as an electrolyte replenisher, antacid, and urinary alkalizer.
**p. bitartrate** [USP], a compound formerly administered orally as an osmotic laxative and used in veterinary medicine as a laxative for small animals and as a diuretic for large animals; now administered rectally with sodium bicarbonate to produce carbon dioxide, which promotes defecation by distending the rectal ampulla. It is used for the relief of constipation, for the evacuation of the colon before surgical or diagnostic procedures, and for pre- and postpartum bowel emptying.
**p. bromide,** a sedative used occasionally for grand mal seizures. See also *bromide.*
**p. carbonate** [USP], a compound, $K_2CO_3$, formerly used as a systemic alkalizer and diuretic, but now used chiefly in pharmaceutical and chemical manufacturing procedures.
**p. chloride** [USP], an electrolyte replenisher, administered orally or by intravenous infusion.
**p. citrate** [USP], a systemic alkalizer, electrolyte replenisher, diuretic, and expectorant, usually administered orally. It is sometimes used in veterinary medicine as a nonirritating diuretic.
**p. cyanide,** an extremely poisonous compound, KCN, occurring as a white granular powder or as fused pieces; formerly used medicinally and now used for various industrial processes and to fumigate fruit trees. See also *cyanide poisoning,* under *poisoning.*
**p. dihydrogen phosphate,** p. phosphate, monobasic.
**p. ferricyanide,** deep-red crystals used in a delicate test for ferrous salts.
**p. gluconate** [USP], an electrolyte replenisher used in the prophylaxis and treatment of hypokalemia, administered orally.
**p. glycerophosphate,** a colorless to slightly yellow viscous substance, $K_2C_3H_5(OH)_2PO_4$, formerly used as a tonic.
**p. guaiacolsulfonate,** $C_7H_7KO_5S$, occurring as white crystals or crystalline powder; used as an expectorant.
**p. hydroxide** [NF], an alkalizer used in pharmaceutical preparations.
**p. iodate,** a compound formerly used as a topical antiseptic; now limited to veterinary use, as a feed additive as a source of iodine.
**p. iodide** [USP], an expectorant, used as a source of iodine in thyrotoxic crisis and in the preparation of thyrotoxic patients for thy-

roidectomy, and as an antifungal in the treatment of lymphocutaneous sporotrichosis; administered orally.
**p. mercuric iodide,** a complex containing about 25.5 per cent of mercury; used as a germicide, and as an ingredient of various reagents.
**p. metaphosphate** [NF], a white powder used as a buffering agent in pharmaceutical preparations.
**p. myronate,** sinigrin.
**p. nitrate** [USP], a compound, $KNO_3$, occurring as a white granular or crystalline powder or as colorless transparent prisms; used as a food preservative and formerly used as an oral diuretic. Called also *niter* and *saltpeter.*
**p. oxalate,** colorless, odorless crystals used extensively as a reagent.
**p. penicillin G,** penicillin G potassium.
**p. perchlorate** [USP], a thyroid inhibitor that has been used in the treatment of thyrotoxicosis.
**p. permanganate** [USP], the potassium salt of permanganic acid, having bactericidal, fungicidal, astringent, and oxidizing properties; used in solution as a topical anti-infective. Because of its oxidizing activity, it is also used in solutions as a gastric lavage for certain poisons.
**p. phenoxymethyl penicillin,** penicillin V potassium.
**p. phosphate, p. phosphate, dibasic** [USP], a compound, $K_2HPO_4$, occurring as colorless or white, granules or powder, which has been used as a cathartic. Called also *dipotassium phosphate.*
**p. phosphate, monobasic** [NF], a compound, $KH_2PO_4$, occurring as colorless crystals or as a white, granular or crystalline powder; used as a buffering agent in pharmaceutical preparations and as a urinary acidifier.
**p. salicylate,** the potassium salt of salicylic acid, used as an analgesic, antipyretic, and anti-inflammatory; administered orally.
**p. sodium tartrate** [USP], a compound, $C_4H_4KNaO_6{\cdot}4H_2O$, occurring as colorless crystals or as a white crystalline powder; used as a cathartic. Called also *Preston's salt and Rochelle salt.*
**p. sorbate** [NF], a mold and yeast inhibitor, used as a preservative in pharmaceutical preparations.
**p. sulfate,** $K_2SO_4$, occurring as colorless or white crystals or as a white powder or granules, which has an extremely irritant action on the stomach and intestines; has been used as a cathartic.
**p. tartrate,** a purgative and cathartic.
**p. thiocyanate,** KSCN, occurring as colorless, transparent, prismatic crystals; used as a reagent, and formerly as an antihypertensive agent.

**Po·tas·si·um Tri·plex** (po-tas'e-əm tri'pləks) trademark for Randall's solution.

**po·ten·cy** (po'tən-se) [L. *potentia* power] 1. the ability of the male to perform sexual intercourse. 2. the relationship between the therapeutic effect of a drug and the dose necessary to achieve that effect; a drug with a higher potency will require a smaller dose to produce a given effect. Clinically, potency has little use except as a means to compare the relative activities of pharmaceutic agents. Cf. *efficacy.* 3. the ability of an embryonic part to develop and complete its destiny.
**prospective p.,** the total developmental possibilities of which an embryonic part is capable.
**reactive p.,** see *competence.*

**po·ten·tia** (po-ten'she-ə) [L.] power.

**po·ten·tial** (po-ten'shəl) [L. *potentia* power] 1. existing and ready for action but not yet active. 2. the work per unit charge necessary to move a charged body in an electric field from a reference point (usually infinity) to another point, measured in volts. The difference in potential between two points is measured by the work necessary to move a unit positive charge from one to the other.
**action p. (AP),** the electrical activity developed in a muscle or nerve cell during activity. It may be elicited by electrical, chemical, or mechanical stimulation, by temperature change, and so on; see also *all or none* and *discharge* (def. 4).

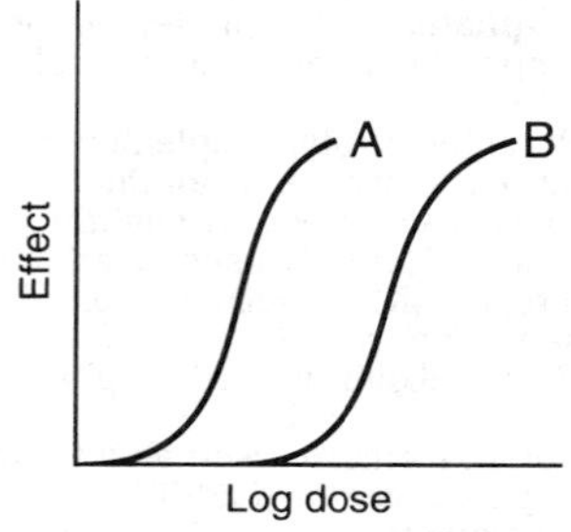


Dose-effect curve for two drugs of different potency: Drug A is more potent than drug B.

**after-p.,** afterpotential.
**auditory evoked p. (AEP),** in electroencephalography, changes in waves in response to sound; see also *brain stem auditory evoked p.*
**bioelectric p.,** the varying electric potential which accompanies all biochemical processes, as those manifested in the electrocardiogram and the electroencephalogram.
**biotic p.,** the maximum rate at which a population can increase when the age ratio is stable and all environmental conditions are ideal. Called also *reproductive p.*
**bizarre high-frequency p.,** complex repetitive discharge.
**brain stem auditory evoked p. (BAEP),** that portion of the auditory evoked potential that comes from the brain stem; abnormalities can be analyzed to evaluate comas, to support diagnosis of multiple sclerosis, and to detect early posterior fossa tumors.
**cochlear p's,** see under *microphonic.*
**compound action p.,** see *compound muscle action p.* and *compound nerve action p.*
**compound muscle action p. (CMAP),** a group of almost simultaneous action potentials from several muscle fibers in the same area; they are usually evoked by stimulation of the supplying motor nerve and are recorded as one multipeaked summated action potential. See also *A wave, F waves, H wave,* and *M wave,* under *wave.*
**compound nerve action p.,** a group of almost synchronous nerve fiber action potentials from the trunk of a motor, sensory, or mixed nerve: they are usually evoked by nerve stimulation and are recorded as a multipeaked summated action potential.
**compound sensory nerve action p.,** sensory nerve action p.
**cortical evoked p.,** an evoked potential recorded from the cerebral cortex. Called also *evoked cortical p.*
**demarcation p.,** injury p.
**electric p., electrical p.,** potential, def. 2.
**electrode p.,** redox p.
**end plate p.,** an action potential that occurs in a stimulated motor end plate, causing initiation of an action potential in the adjacent muscle fiber.
**event-related p.,** a change in waveforms on the electroencephalogram just after a sensory, motor, or cognitive stimulus; cf. *evoked p., readiness p.,* and *contingent negative variation.*
**evoked p. (EP),** the electrical signal recorded from a sensory receptor, nerve, muscle, or area of the central nervous system that has been stimulated, usually by electricity. See also *auditory evoked p., somatosensory evoked p.,* and *visual evoked p.*
**evoked cortical p.,** cortical evoked p.
**excitatory postsynaptic p.,** a transient decrease in membrane polarization induced in a postsynaptic neuron when subjected to a volley of impulses over an excitatory afferent pathway; summation of such potentials may cause discharge by the neuron. Abbreviated EPSP.
**fasciculation p.,** an electrical potential that occurs with a fasciculation, similar in appearance to a motor unit action potential but occurring spontaneously. These may appear singly or in groups; complex or iterative ones occur in motor unit disorders.
**fibrillation p.,** an abnormal spiked electrical potential associated with fibrillation of a muscle fiber; it occurs spontaneously in some myopathic disorders or may be provoked by movement of a needle electrode.
**generator p.,** the depolarization produced in neural receptors in response to specific kinds of physical stimuli; called also *receptor p.*
**inhibitory postsynaptic p.,** a transient hyperpolarization of membrane potential induced in a postsynaptic neuron when subjected to a volley of impulses over an inhibitory afferent pathway, resulting in a diminished responsiveness of the neuron. Abbreviated IPSP.
**injury p.,** the difference in recorded electrical potential between the intact longitudinal surface and the injured end of a muscle or nerve; called also *demarcation p.*
**membrane p.,** the electric potential which exists on the two sides of a membrane or across the wall of a cell.
**morphogenetic p.,** the degree of strength or ability of an embryonic part to develop into a specific structure.
**motor unit p. (MUP), motor unit action p. (MUAP),** the sum of the recorded action potentials of all the muscle fibers in one motor unit.
**muscle action p.,** compound muscle action p.
**muscle fiber action p.,** the action potential recorded on a muscle fiber spreading in both directions away from the plate region to initiate a contraction; see also *single fiber electromyography.*
**myotonic p.,** see under *discharge.*
**negative after-p.,** see under *afterpotential.*
**Nernst p.,** the voltage produced across a membrane by a concentration gradient of an ion that can diffuse through pores in the membrane while oppositely charged ions cannot pass through the membrane; see *Nernst equation* under *equation.*
**nerve p., nerve action p.,** 1. compound nerve action p. 2. nerve fiber action p.
**nerve fiber action p.,** an action potential recorded from a single nerve fiber; see also *compound nerve action p.*
**pacemaker p.,** the slow diastolic depolarization of cell membranes that normally occurs in the sinoatrial node, atrioventricular node,

and His-Purkinje system; under some abnormal conditions it can also occur in atrial and ventricular muscle fibers.
**positive after-p.,** see under *afterpotential.*
**postsynaptic p.,** a change in polarization of a postsynaptic neuron; see *excitatory postsynaptic p.* and *inhibitory postsynaptic p.*
**readiness p.,** a negative potential on the electroencephalogram, which slowly increases and reaches a maximum just before a voluntary movement in a limb; called also *Bereitschaftspotential.*
**receptor p.,** generator p.
**redox p.,** the electrochemical potential of an oxidation-reduction half reaction under prevailing conditions measured with respect to the standard reduction potential of the hydrogen gas/proton redox couple, which is defined as zero. It is related to its own standard reduction potential by the Nernst equation. Symbol $E$ or $E_h$.
**reproductive p.,** biotic p.
**resting p.,** the potential difference across the membrane of a normal cell at rest, i.e., the difference in potential between the outside and inside of a cell at rest; cf. *action p.*
**resting membrane p.,** resting p.
**satellite p.,** a small abnormal action potential separated from the main motor unit action potential and regularly preceding or following each main action potential on the recording.
**sensory p., sensory nerve action p. (SNAP),** a compound nerve action potential recorded from a sensory nerve or from the sensory branch of a mixed nerve. Called also *compound sensory nerve action p.*
**serrated action p.,** an action potential whose waveform has several changes in direction without crossing the baseline.
**somatosensory evoked p. (SEP),** waves recorded from the spinal cord or cerebral hemisphere after electrical stimulation or physiological activation of peripheral sensory fibers; analysis of deviations in latency or amplitude can detect or characterize lesions of the peripheral or sensory conduction pathways.
**spike p.,** the initial very large change in potential of an excitable cell membrane during excitation.
**standard electrode p., standard reduction p.,** the electrochemical potential developed by a half-cell under standard conditions (1 atm pressure; specified temperature, usually 25°C; substances in solution at 1 M concentration) compared to the potential of the hydrogen gas/proton redox couple ($2H^+ + 2e^- \rightleftarrows H_2$) under standard conditions, which by definition has an $E°$ of exactly 0 V. Symbol $E°$.
**transmembrane p.,** membrane p.
**visual evoked p. (VEP), visual evoked cortical p.,** in electroencephalography, changes in the evoked cortical potential when the eye is stimulated by light; variations are diagnostic for abnormalities of the visual system and for other disorders, particularly neurological disorders such as multiple sclerosis, that have visual symptoms.
**zero p.,** in electricity, an arbitrary reference point (usually the potential of the earth) used as a zero value in comparison to other electrical potentials.
**zeta p.,** the electric potential across a solid-liquid interface. The zeta potential at the surface of erythrocytes is the net potential produced by both the negative charges on the cell surface and the positive charges in a cloud of cations attracted by the surface charge and forming a layer over the surface; it is responsible for a repelling force between erythrocytes that resists agglutination or rouleau formation.

**po·ten·tial·iza·tion** (po-ten″shəl-ĭ-za′shən) potentiation (def. 1).

**po·ten·ti·a·tion** (po-ten″she-a′shən) 1. the increasing of potency; particularly, the synergistic action of two drugs, being greater than the sum of the effects of each used alone. 2. posttetanic p.
**long-term p.,** a change in efficacy of synapses at monosynaptic junctions lasting from a few days to several weeks, first observed in the hippocampus, dentate gyrus, and nearby areas but now observed elsewhere in the brain. It is thought to be related to long-term information storage and thus to memory.
**posttetanic p.,** an incrementing response, without change of action potential amplitude, that occurs with repetitive nerve stimulation.

**po·ten·ti·a·tor** (po-ten′she-a-tor) an agent that enhances another agent so that the combined effect is greater than the sum of the effects of each one alone.

**po·ten·ti·om·e·ter** (po-ten″she-om′ə-tər) an instrument for the accurate measuring of voltage.

**po·ti·fi·ca·tion** (po″tĭ-fĭ-ka′shən) the process of making water fit to drink. Applied to sea water, it is the process of removing sufficient salts to render the remaining fluid safe for drinking.

**Pott's aneurysm, disease,** etc. (pots) [Sir Percivall *Pott,* English surgeon, 1714–1788] see *aneurysmal varix,* under *varix;* see *tuberculosis of spine;* and see under *abscess, curvature, fracture, paraplegia,* and *tumor.*

**Pot·ter's facies, syndrome** (pot′ərz) [Edith Louise *Potter,* American physician, born 1901] see under *facies* and see *oligohydramnios sequence,* under *sequence.*

**Pot·ter version** (pot′ər) [Irving W. *Potter,* American obstetrician, 1868–1956] see under *version.*

**Potts operation (anastomosis, shunt)** (pots) [Willis John *Potts,* American surgeon, 1895–1968] see under *operation.*

**pouce** (pōōs) [Fr.] the thumb or great toe.
**p. flottant** (pōōs flah-tahn′) [Fr. "floating thumb (great toe)"], a deformity of the thumb or great toe associated with a number of congenital anomalies and with microvascular and plastic surgery.

**pouch** (pouch) a pocketlike sac or saccule. See also *pocket, cavity,* and *recess.*
**abdominovesical p.,** the pouch formed by reflection of the peritoneum from the anterior abdominal wall to the distended bladder.
**anal p.,** the expanded end of the hindgut in certain insects.
**anterior p. of Tröltsch,** recessus anterior membranae tympanicae.
**Blake's p.,** a blind pocket of arachnoid connected with the fourth ventricle and the subarachnoid space near the medulla oblongata as a result of abnormal development of the membranous lamina of the auditory tube.
**branchial p.,** pharyngeal p.
**craniobuccal p., craniopharyngeal p.,** Rathke's p.
**p. of Douglas,** excavatio recto-uterina.
**enterocoelic p.,** a diverticulum of the enteron of the embryo.
**guttural p's,** large mucous sacs in the horse, which are ventral diverticula of the eustachian tube, situated between the base of the cranium and the atlas dorsally and the pharynx ventrally.
**Hartmann's p.,** an abnormal sacculation of the neck of the gallbladder.
**Heidenhain p.,** a small pocket of the stomach which has been surgically separated from the body of the stomach, and thus vagally denervated, and which drains to the exterior; used in the experimental study of gastric physiology. Cf. *Pavlov p.*
**hypophyseal p.,** Rathke's p.
**ileoanal p.,** see under *reservoir.*
**ileocecal p.,** a peritoneal pouch at the ileocecal junction.
**J p.,** an ileoanal reservoir created by lateral anastomosis of two loops of ileum 15 to 20 cm long.
**Kock p.,** the most common kind of continent ileal reservoir, with a capacity of 500 to 1000 mL and a valve made by intussusception of the terminal ileum.
**laryngeal p.,** sacculus laryngis.
**Morison's p.,** a pouch of peritoneum inferior to the liver and to the right of the right kidney and extending inferiorly to the transverse mesocolon.
**obturator p.,** paravesical p.
**paracystic p.,** the lateral part of the excavatio vesico-uterina.
**pararectal p.,** the lateral part of the excavatio recto-uterina.
**paravesical p.,** the lateral part of the uteroabdominal pouch, beside the bladder and in which the obturator canal opens; called also *obturator p.*
**Pavlov p.,** a pocket of stomach which has been surgically separated from the body of the stomach by a mucosal septum, but which retains vagal innervation and muscular connection, and which drains to the exterior; used in the experimental study of gastric physiology. Cf. *Heidenhain p.*
**perineal p., deep,** saccus profundus perinei.
**perineal p., subcutaneous,** saccus subcutaneus perinei.
**perineal p., superficial,** compartimentum superficiale perinei.
**pharyngeal p.,** a lateral diverticulum of the pharynx that meets a corresponding pharyngeal groove in the embryonic ectoderm, forming a closing membrane that may rupture and complete the gill slit as observed in lower vertebrates. Called also *branchial p.* and *visceral p.*
**Physick's p's,** inflamed sacculations between the rectal valves, with mucous discharge.
**posterior p. of Tröltsch,** recessus posterior membranae tympanicae.
**Prussak's p.,** recessus superior membranae tympanicae.
**Rathke's p.,** a diverticulum from the embryonic buccal cavity, from which the adenohypophysis is developed; its lumen persists in adults as small colloid-filled cysts and clefts at the juncture of the pars distalis and the neurohypophysis. Called also *craniobuccal p., craniopharyngeal p., hypophyseal p.,* and *Rathke's pocket.*
**rectouterine p., rectovaginal p.,** excavatio recto-uterina.
**rectovesical p.,** excavatio rectovesicalis.
**S p.,** an ileoanal reservoir created by lateral anastomosis of three sections of ileum each 10 to 15 cm long in a configuration resembling the letter S.
**Seessel's p.,** a transient outpouching of the embryonic pharynx rostrad of the oropharyngeal membrane and caudal to Rathke's pouch.
**uteroabdominal p.,** the compartment of the pelvic cavity anterior to the uterus and broad ligaments.
**uterovesical p., vesicouterine p.,** excavatio vesico-uterina.
**visceral p.,** pharyngeal p.
**Willis' p.,** omentum minus.
**Zenker's p.,** pulsion diverticulum.

**pouch·itis** (pouch-i'tis) [*pouch* + *-itis*] [MeSH: Pouchitis] inflammation of the mucosa or occasionally of the full thickness of the intestinal wall of an ileal or ileoanal reservoir.

**pou·drage** (poo-drahzh') [Fr.] the application of powder to a surface, as between the visceral and parietal layers of the pericardium or pleura to promote their fusion in pleurodesis.

**poul·tice** (pōl'tis) [L. *puls* pap; Gr. *kataplasma*] a soft, moist mass about the consistency of cooked cereal, spread between layers of muslin, linen, gauze, or towels and applied hot to a given area in order to create moist local heat or counterirritation.

**pound** (pound) [L. *pondus* weight; *libra* pound] a unit of mass (weight) of both the avoirdupois and the apothecaries' system. The avoirdupois pound contains 16 ounces, or 7000 grains, and is the equivalent of 453.592 gm. The apothecaries' pound contains 12 ounces, or 5760 grains, and is the equivalent of 373.242 gm. Abbreviated lb.

**Pou·part's ligament, line** (poo-pahrz') [François *Poupart,* French anatomist, 1661–1708] see *ligamentum inguinale,* and see under *line.*

**Po·van** (po'van) trademark for a preparation of pyrvinium pamoate.

**pov·er·ty** (pov'ər-te) [MeSH: Poverty] the absence or scarcity of requisite substance or elements.
**p. of content,** disordered speech in which quantity is normal but content is altered so that very little or nothing is communicated.
**p. of movement,** the akinesia or bradykinesia seen in subjects with parkinsonism.

**po·vi·done** (po'vĭ-dōn) [USP] [MeSH: Povidone] a synthetic polymer principally consisting of linear 1-vinyl-2-pyrrolidone groups, produced as a series of products having mean molecular weights ranging from about 10,000 to about 700,000; used as a dispersing and suspending agent, and has been used as a tablet binder, coating agent, and viscosity-increasing agent in pharmaceutical preparations. Formerly called *polyvinylpyrrolidone (PVP).* See also *povidone-iodine.*

**po·vi·done-io·dine** (po'vĭ-dōn i'o-dīn) [USP] [MeSH: Povidone-Iodine] a complex produced by reacting iodine with the polymer povidone, which slowly releases iodine; it occurs as a yellowish brown, amorphous powder and is used as a topical anti-infective. Abbreviated PVP-I.

**Pow·as·san encephalitis, virus** (po-wah'sən) [*Powassan,* Ontario, Canada, where the disease was first observed in 1958] see under *encephalitis* and *virus.*

**pow·der** (pou'dər) [L. *pulvis*] a substance made up of an aggregation of small particles, as that obtained by the grinding or trituration of a solid drug. Called also *pulvis.*
**bleaching p.,** chlorinated lime.
**p. of chalk, aromatic,** a preparation of chalk, cinnamon, myristica, clove, cardamom, and sucrose; formerly used as an antacid, stimulant, and astringent.
**p. of chalk, aromatic, with opium,** aromatic powder of chalk containing 2.5 per cent of powdered opium.
**chalk p., compound,** a powder containing prepared chalk, finely powdered acacia, and sucrose; it is an antacid used in treatment of diarrhea.
**clioquinol topical p., compound** [USP], a preparation of clioquinol, boric acid, lactic acid, zinc stearate, and lactose; used as a local anti-infective in the treatment of vaginitis due to *Trichomonas vaginalis, Candida albicans, Trichophyton,* or mixed bacteria, administered by intravaginal insufflation.
**Dalmatian insect p.,** pyrethrum flowers; see under *flower.*
**dusting p.,** a fine powder used as a substitute for talc.
**dusting p., absorbable,** an absorbable powder prepared by processing cornstarch, with not more than 2 per cent of magnesium oxide; used for dusting surgeons' rubber gloves and other purposes for which talc is used in the hospital.
**effervescent p's, compound,** Seidlitz p's.
**furazolidone and nifuroxime p.,** a preparation containing 0.09 to 0.11 per cent furazolidone and 0.45 to 0.55 per cent nifuroxime in a suitable, slightly acidified powder base; used in the treatment of candidal, trichomonal, and bacterial vaginitis, administered intravaginally.
**glycyrrhiza p., compound,** senna p., compound.
**Goa p.,** a bitter, brownish yellow to umber brown powder deposited in irregular interspaces of the wood of *Andira araroba* Aguiar (Leguminosae), a large leguminous tree common in Brazil. It is the source of chrysarobin.
**impalpable p.,** a powder so fine that its particles cannot be felt as distinct bodies.
**iodochlorhydroxyquin p., compound,** compound clioquinol p.
**licorice p., compound, p. of liquorice, compound,** senna p., compound.
**Persian insect p.,** pyrethrum flowers; see under *flower.*
**Seidlitz p's,** a combination of sodium bicarbonate, potassium sodium tartrate, and tartaric acid, used as a cathartic; called also *compound effervescent p's.* See also under *tests.*
**senna p., compound,** a yellow powder prepared from fennel oil; powdered sucrose, senna, and glycyrrhiza; and washed sulfur; used as a laxative.
**sodium bicarbonate and calcium carbonate p.,** a mixture of precipitated calcium carbonate and sodium bicarbonate: antacid; widely used in treatment of peptic ulcer in combination with sodium bicarbonate and magnesium oxide powder.
**sodium bicarbonate and magnesium oxide p.,** a mixture of magnesium oxide and sodium carbonate; used as an antacid and laxative.
**triacetin p.,** a preparation containing 90 to 110 per cent of the labeled amount of triacetin in a suitable powder base; used as an antifungal in superficial skin infections, applied topically.
**zinc sulfate p., compound,** a preparation of salicylic acid, zinc sulfate, phenol, eucalyptol, menthol, thymol, and boric acid; used as an antiseptic.

**pow·er** (pou'ər) [L. *posse* to have power] 1. capability; potency; the ability to act. 2. a measure of magnification, as of a microscope. 3. the rate at which work is done. Symbol *P.* The SI unit of power is the watt. 4. of a statistical test: the probability of correctly rejecting the null hypothesis when a specified alternative holds true; it is equal to 1 minus the probability of a Type II error.
**candle p.,** the numerical expression, in international candles, of the luminous intensity of a light source.
**carbon dioxide-combining p., $CO_2$-combining p.,** ability of the blood plasma to combine with carbon dioxide, defined as the total $CO_2$ bound in plasma as bicarbonate at a $pCO_2$ of 40 mmHg at 25°C. Cf. *alkali reserve.*
**defining p.,** the ability of a lens to make an object clearly visible.
**resolving p.,** the ability of the eye or of a lens to make separately visible small objects that are close together, thus revealing the structure of an object; see also *resolution.*

**pox** (poks) [variant of *pocks,* from A.S. *pocc* pustule, spot] 1. any eruptive or pustular disease, especially one caused by a virus; see specific entries: *chickenpox, cowpox, horsepox, rabbitpox,* etc. 2. former name for syphilis.

**Pox·vi·ri·dae** (poks″vir'ĭ-de) [MeSH: Poxviridae] the poxviruses: a family of DNA viruses having a brick-shaped or ovoid virion 220–450 × 140–260 nm consisting of an envelope containing lipid and tubular or globular protein structures surrounding a DNA-containing core and one or two lateral bodies. The genome consists of a single molecule of double-stranded DNA (size 130–375 kbp). Viruses contain over 100 proteins; some are ether-resistant while others are ether-sensitive. Replication and assembly occur in the cytoplasm; virions are released by cell destruction or budding. Host range is narrow and transmission 7 is by fomites, airborne particles, arthropod vectors, or contact. There are two subfamilies: Chordopoxvirinae (poxviruses of vertebrates) and Entomopoxvirinae (poxviruses of insects).

**pox·vi·rus** (poks'vi-rəs) [MeSH: Poxviridae] any virus belonging to the family Poxviridae.

**PP** abbreviation for L. *punc'tum prox'imum,* near point of accommodation.

**$PP_i$** pyrophosphate.

**PPD** purified protein derivative (tuberculin); see under *tuberculin.*

**ppg** picopicogram.

**PPLO** pleuropneumonia-like organisms; see under *organism.*

**ppm** parts per million.

**PPR** peste des petits ruminants.

**Ppt** precipitate; prepared.

**P pul·mo·nale** (pe pul″mo-na'le) in electrocardiography, a pattern of tall, peaked P waves in leads II, III, and $aV_F$, indicative of enlargement of the right atrium; it is often associated with pulmonary disease.

**PR** prosthion; pulmonic regurgitation.

**P.R.** L. *punc'tum remo'tum,* far point of accommodation.

**Pr** 1. presbyopia; prism. 2. symbol for praseodymium.

**PRA** panel-reactive antibody.

**prac·tice** (prak'tis) [Gr. *praktikē*] the utilization of one's knowledge in a particular profession, the practice of medicine being the exercise of one's knowledge in the practical recognition and treatment of disease.
**contract p.,** the treatment of the members of a specified group for a lump sum, or at so much per member.
**family p.,** the medical specialty concerned with the planning and provision of the comprehensive primary health care of all members of a family, regardless of age or sex, on a continuing basis.

**general p.**, the provision of comprehensive medical care as a continuing responsibility regardless of age of the patient or presence of a condition that may temporarily require the services of a specialist.
**group p.**, see under *medicine.*
**panel p.**, see under *panel.*
**solo p.**, the provision of care by a single, self-employed physician or dentist assisted only by auxiliary personnel. Cf. *group medicine.*

**prac·ti·tion·er** (prak-tish'ən-ər) one who has complied with the requirements of and who is engaged in the practice of medicine, dentistry, or nursing.
**nurse p.**, see *nurse clinician,* under *nurse.*

**prac·to·lol** (prak'to-lol) [MeSH: Practolol] a beta-adrenergic blocking agent having the same actions as propranolol (q.v.). Its use has been found to be associated with an allergic reaction of the eyes, skin, mucous membranes, and ears.

**Pra·der-Wil·li syndrome** (prah'dər-vil'ə) [Andrea *Prader,* Swiss pediatrician, born 1919; Heinrich *Willi,* Swiss pediatrician, 1900–1971] [MeSH: Prader-Willi Syndrome] see under *syndrome.*

**prae-** [L. "before"] a prefix meaning before, in front of; for words beginning thus, see also those beginning *pre-.*

**prae·cox** (pre'koks) [L.] premature, early; see *dementia praecox.*

**prae·pu·ti·um** (pre-pu'she-əm) [L.] preputium.

**prag·mat·ag·no·sia** (prag"mat-ag-no'zhə) [Gr. *pragma* object + *agnosia*] agnosia.

**prag·mat·am·ne·sia** (prag"mat-am-ne'zhə) [Gr. *pragma* object + *amnesia*] visual agnosia.

**pral·i·dox·ime** (pral"ĭ-doks'ēm) a cholinesterase reactivator capable of acting as an antagonist to certain anticholinesterases. Called also *2-PAM.*
**p. chloride** [USP], the chloride salt of pralidoxime, used as an antidote in the treatment of poisoning due to organophosphates having anticholinesterase activity and to counteract the effects of overdosage by anticholinesterases used in the treatment of myasthenia gravis, administered orally and by intravenous infusion.

**pra·mox·ine hy·dro·chlo·ride** (pram-ok'sēn) [USP] a local anesthetic applied topically to the skin and rectal mucous membranes, for temporary relief of pain and pruritus associated with skin and anorectal disorders.

**pran·di·al** (pran'de-əl) [L. *prandium* breakfast] pertaining to a meal, especially dinner.

**Pran·tal** (pran'təl) trademark for preparations of diphemanil methylsulfate.

**pra·seo·dym·i·um** (pra"ze-o-dim'e-əm) [MeSH: Praseodymium] a rare earth element; atomic number, 59; atomic weight, 140.907; symbol, Pr.

**P. rat. aetat.** abbreviation for L. *pro ratio'ne aeta'tis,* in proportion to age.

**pra·tique** (prah-tēk') [Fr.] a certificate which releases an incoming vessel from quarantine. It is given by the quarantine officer to the master, and when presented to the collector of the port admits the boat to entry.

**Praus·nitz-Küst·ner reaction (test)** (prous'nits-kēst'ner) [Otto Carl Willy *Prausnitz,* German hygienist, 1876–1963; Heinz *Küstner,* German gynecologist, 1897–1963] see under *reaction.*

**Prav·a·chol** (prav'ə-kol) trademark for a preparation of pravastatin sodium.

**prav·a·sta·tin so·di·um** (prav'ə-stat"in) an antihyperlipidemic agent that is an inhibitor of hydroxymethylglutaryl-CoA reductase, used to lower blood lipid levels in the treatment of hypercholesterolemia; administered orally.

**Prax·ag·o·ras of Cos** [c. 340 B.C.] a Greek physician who succeeded Diocles as leader of the Dogmatists. He was apparently the first Greek physician to recognize the difference between arteries (carriers of air) and veins (carriers of blood), and to comment on the pulse.

**prax·i·ol·o·gy** (prak"se-ol'ə-je) [*praxis* + *-logy*] the study of conduct, rather than of thought or consciousness.

**prax·is** (prak'sis) [Gr. "action"] the doing or performance of action.

**pra·ze·pam** (praz'ə-pam) [MeSH: Prazepam] a benzodiazepine used as an anxiolytic in the treatment of anxiety disorders and for the short-term relief of anxiety symptoms; administered orally.

**pra·zi·quan·tel** (pra"zĭ-kwahn'təl) [MeSH: Praziquantel] an anthelmintic used in dogs and cats against fluke and tapeworm infestations.

**pra·zo·sin hy·dro·chlo·ride** (pra'zo-sin) a quinazoline derivative with vasodilator properties, used as an oral antihypertensive.

**pre-** [L. *prae-* before] a prefix meaning before, in front of.

**pre·adap·ta·tion** (pre"a-dap-ta'shən) the acquisition in an ancestral group of certain characters that usually are adaptive to the ancestral mode of life yet at the same time enable a shift in mode of life; for example, lungs in fish ancestral to tetrapods.

**pre·ad·i·po·cyte** (pre-ad'ĭ-po-sīt") a precursor to an adipocyte.

**pre·ag·o·nal** (pre-ag'ə-nəl) preceding the death agony.

**pre·al·bu·min** (pre"al-bu'min) [MeSH: Prealbumin] transthyretin.

**pre·an·es·thet·ic** (pre"an-əs-thet'ik) occurring before administration of an anesthetic.

**pre·aor·tic** (pre"a-or'tik) anterior to the aorta.

**pre·atax·ic** (pre"ə-tak'sik) occurring before or preceding ataxia.

**pre·au·ra·le** (pre"aw-ra'le) a cephalometric landmark, the point at which a straight line from the postaurale, perpendicular to the long axis of the auricle, meets the base of the auricle.

**pre·au·ric·u·lar** (pre"aw-rik'u-lər) anterior to the auricle of the ear.

**pre·ax·i·al** (pre-ak'se-əl) anterior to an axis; in anatomical usage, this refers to the lateral (radial) aspect of the upper limb, and the medial (tibial) aspect of the lower limb.

**pre·bac·il·lary** (pre-bas'ĭ-lar"e) occurring before the entrance of bacilli into the system, or before they become discoverable.

**pre·base** (pre'bās) that part of the dorsum of the tongue lying anterior to the base.

**pre·be·ta·lipo·pro·tein·emia** (pre-ba"tə-lip"o-pro"te-ne'me-ə) hyperprebetalipoproteinemia.

**pre·bi·ot·ic** (pre"bi-ot'ik) denoting the period before the existence of life on earth.

**pre·blad·der** (pre-blad'ər) an extensive cavity formed anterior to the orifice of the bladder within the capsule of the prostate.

**pre·can·cer** (pre'kan-sər) a condition which tends eventually to become malignant.

**pre·can·cer·ous** (pre-kan'sər-əs) pertaining to a pathologic process that tends to become malignant.

**pre·cap·il·lary** (pre-kap'ĭ-lar"e) 1. located just to the arterial side of a capillary. 2. arterial capillary.

**pre·car·ci·nom·a·tous** (pre-kahr"sĭ-nom'ə-təs) preceding the development of carcinoma.

**pre·car·di·ac** (pre-kahr'de-ak) anterior to the heart.

**pre·car·di·um** (pre-kahr'de-əm) [*pre-* + Gr. *kardia* heart] precordium.

**pre·car·ti·lage** (pre-kahr'tĭ-ləj) embryonic cartilaginous tissue.

**pre·ca·va** (pre-ka'və) vena cava superior.

**pre·ce·men·tum** (pre"sə-men'təm) cementoid.

**pre·cen·tral** (pre-sen'trəl) anterior to a center, as the precentral gyrus.

**pre·chor·dal** (pre-kor'dəl) situated cranial to the notochord; called also *prochordal.*

**pre·cip·i·ta·ble** (pre-sip'ĭ-tə-bəl) capable of being precipitated.

**pre·cip·i·tant** (pre-sip'ĭ-tənt) a substance which causes a chemical or mechanical precipitation.

**pre·cip·i·tate** (pre-sip'ĭ-tāt) [L. *praecipitare* to cast down] 1. to cause a substance in solution to settle down in solid particles. 2. [L. *praecipitatum*] a deposit made or substance thrown down by precipitation. 3. occurring with undue rapidity, as precipitate labor. 4. in immunology, the product of interaction between soluble macromolecular antigen and the homologous antibody, e.g., the antigen-antibody complex formed as a consequence of the reaction of pneumococcus capsular polysaccharide in solution with specific antiserum.
**immune p.**, see *precipitate.*
**keratic p's**, see under *keratitis punctata.*
**keratic p's, mutton-fat,** coalescent precipitates forming translucent rings with opaque centers in the anterior chamber, and occurring in uveitis.

**pre·cip·i·ta·tion** (pre-sip"ĭ-ta'shən) [L. *praecipitatio*] [MeSH: Precipitation] the act or process of precipitating.
**aluminum p.**, a technique for production of antibody to specific antigen, using precipitation of antigen by aluminum salts *(aluminum adjuvant);* the absorbed antigen forms a depot at the site of inoculation, from which it is slowly released for a prolonged antibody repsonse.
**group p.**, precipitation by a precipitin in a specific antiserum of an antigen common to a group of closely related microorganisms.

**pre·cip·i·tin** (pre-sip'ĭ-tin) an antibody to antigen that specifically aggregates the macromolecular antigen *in vivo* or *in vitro* to give a visible precipitate.

**pre·cip·i·tin·o·gen** (pre-sip″ĭ-tin′o-jən) the soluble antigen which stimulates the formation of precipitins and is capable of reacting with them *in vitro* and *in vivo*.

**pre·cip·i·to·gen** (pre-sip′ĭ-to-jən) precipitinogen.

**pre·ci·sion** (pre-sizh′ən) 1. the quality of being sharply or exactly defined; for example, a measurement with three significant figures is more precise than a measurement with two. Cf. *accuracy*. 2. in statistics, the extent to which a measurement procedure gives the same results when repeated under identical conditions. Under certain conditions, may be called *reliability, repeatability,* or *reproducibility*.

**pre·clin·i·cal** (pre-klin′ĭ-kəl) before a disease becomes clinically recognizable.

**pre·clot·ting** (pre-klot′ing) the forcing of a patient's blood through the interstices of a knitted vascular prosthesis prior to implantation to render the graft temporarily impervious to blood by disposition of fibrin and platelets in the interstices; after implantation fibrous ingrowth from the recipient replaces the fibrin-platelet network.

**pre·co·cious** (pre-ko′shəs) developed more than is usual at a given age.

**pre·coc·i·ty** (pre-kos′ĭ-te) unusually early development of mental or physical traits.
**sexual p.**, precocious puberty.

**pre·cog·ni·tion** (pre″kog-nish′ən) [*pre-* + *cognition*] the extrasensory perception of a future event.

**pre·col·lag·e·nous** (pre″ko-laj′ə-nəs) [*pre-* + *collagenous*] denoting an incomplete stage in the formation of collagen.

**pre·co·ma** (pre-ko′mə) the neuropsychiatric state preceding coma, as in hepatic encephalopathy.

**pre·con·scious** (pre-kon′shəs) the part of the mind that is not in immediate awareness but can be consciously recalled with effort, one of the systems of Freud's topographic model of the mind. Cf. *conscious* and *unconscious*.

**pre·con·di·tion·ing** (pre″kən-dish′ən-ing) the creation of a state in which a stimulus applied later will incur a certain response.
**ischemic p.**, an adaptive response of myocardium injured reversibly by a brief episode of ischemia that increases its resistance to subsequent ischemic episodes.

**pre·cor·dia** (pre-kor′de-ə) pl. of *precordium*.

**pre·cor·di·al** (pre-kor′de-əl) pertaining to the precordium.

**pre·cor·di·al·gia** (pre-kor″de-al′jə) [*precordium* + *-algia*] pain in the precordium.

**pre·cor·di·um** (pre-kor′de-əm) pl. *precor′dia* [L., from *pre-* + *cor*, gen. *cordis*, heart] the region of the anterior surface of the body covering the heart and stomach; it comprises the epigastric region and the inferior part of the thorax.

**Pre·cose** (pre′kōs) trademark for a preparation of acarbose.

**pre·cos·tal** (pre-kos′təl) anterior to the ribs.

**pre·crit·i·cal** (pre-krit′ĭ-kəl) previous to the occurrence of the crisis.

**pre·cu·ne·ate** (pre-ku′ne-āt) pertaining to the precuneus.

**pre·cu·ne·us** (pre-ku′ne-əs) [*pre-* + *cuneus*] [TA] a small wedge-shaped convolution on the medial surface of the parietal lobe of the cerebrum, bounded posteriorly by the medial part of the parietooccipital sulcus and anteriorly by the paracentral lobule.

**pre·cur·sor** (pre′kər-sor) [L. *praecursor* a forerunner] something that precedes. In biological processes, a substance from which another, usually more active or mature substance is formed. In clinical medicine, a sign or symptom that heralds another.

**Pre·date** (pre′dāt) trademark for preparations of prednisolone.

**pre·da·tion** (pre-da′shən) the derivation by an organism of elements essential for its existence from organisms of other species which it consumes and destroys.

**pre·da·tor** (prĕ′də-tor) [L. *praedator* a plunderer, pillager] an organism that derives elements essential for its existence from organisms of other species, which it consumes and destroys.

**pre·den·tin** (pre-den′tin) the soft fibrillar substance composing the primitive dentin and forming the inner layer of the circumpulpar dentin; called also *dentinoid*.

**pre·di·a·be·tes** (pre-di″ə-be′tēz) a state of latent impairment of carbohydrate metabolism, in which the criteria for diabetes mellitus are not all satisfied; sometimes controllable by diet alone.

**pre·di·as·to·le** (pre″di-as′tə-le) the interval immediately preceding diastole in the cardiac cycle.

**pre·di·a·stol·ic** (pre″di-ə-stol′ik) 1. pertaining to the beginning of diastole. 2. occurring just before diastole.

**pre·di·crot·ic** (pre″di-krot′ik) occurring before the dicrotic notch and wave of the sphygmogram.

**pre·di·ges·tion** (pre″di-jes′chən) the partial artificial digestion of food before its ingestion.

**pre·dis·pos·ing** (pre″dis-pōz′ing) conferring a tendency to disease.

**pre·dis·po·si·tion** (pre″dis-pə-zish′ən) [*pre-* + *disposition*] a latent susceptibility to disease which may be activated under certain conditions, as by stress.

**pre·di·ver·tic·u·lar** (pre-di″vər-tik′u-lər) denoting a condition of thickening of the muscular wall of the colon and increased intraluminal pressure but without herniation of the mucosa, i.e., without evidence of diverticulosis.

**Pred·ni·cen-M** (pred′nĭ-sen″) trademark for a preparation of prednisone.

**pred·ni·mus·tine** (pred″nĭ-mus′tēn) [MeSH: Prednimustine] an ester of chlorambucil and prednisone, used as an antineoplastic in the treatment of non-Hodgkin's lymphoma; administered orally.

**pred·nis·o·lone** (pred-nis′ə-lōn″) [USP] [MeSH: Prednisolone] a synthetic glucocorticoid derived from cortisol, administered orally in replacement therapy for adrenocortical insufficiency and as an anti-inflammatory in a wide variety of conditions.
**p. acetate** [USP], the 21-acetate ester of prednisolone, administered by intra-articular, intramuscular, or soft-tissue injection in replacement therapy for adrenal insufficiency and as an anti-inflammatory and immunosuppressant in a wide variety of disorders and applied topically to the conjunctiva in the treatment of allergy and inflammation.
**p. hemisuccinate** [USP], an ester of hydrocortisone, having actions and uses similar to those of the base.
**p. sodium phosphate** [USP], a water-soluble ester of prednisolone, having a rapid onset and short duration of action; administered by intravenous or intramuscular injection when rapid effect is needed, or applied topically to the conjunctiva.
**p. sodium succinate for injection** [NF], sterile prednisolone sodium succinate prepared from the succinate ester of prednisolone with the aid of sodium carbonate; used as a glucocorticoid.
**p. tebutate** [USP], an ester of prednisolone having a slow onset and long duration of action, used as an anti-inflammatory; administered by intra-articular, intralesional, or soft-tissue injection.

**pred·ni·sone** (pred′nĭ-sōn) [USP] [MeSH: Prednisone] a synthetic glucocorticoid derived from cortisone, administered orally as an anti-inflammatory and immunosuppressant in a wide variety of disorders.

**pre·dor·mi·tal** (pre-dor′mĭ-təl) pertaining to or occurring in the predormitum.

**pre·dor·mi·tum** (pre-dor′mĭ-təm) the period of waning consciousness interposed between the waking state and sound slumber.

**pre·eclamp·sia** (pre″e-klamp′se-ə) a complication of pregnancy characterized by hypertension, edema, and/or proteinuria; when convulsions and coma are associated, it is called *eclampsia*.

**pre·ejec·tion** (pre″e-jek′shən) occurring prior to ejection.

**pre·em·bryo** (pre-em′bre-o) denoting the early stages of development of the zygote, occurring during the first three days after fertilization.

**pre·epi·glot·tic** (pre″ep-ĭ-glot′ik) anterior to the epiglottis.

**pre·ex·ci·ta·tion** (pre-ek″si-ta′shən) premature activation of a portion of the ventricles due to transmission of cardiac impulses along an accessory pathway not subject to the physiologic delay of the atrioventricular node. See also *preexcitation syndrome*, under *syndrome*. The term is sometimes used as a synonym for *Wolff-Parkinson-White syndrome*. Called also *ventricular pacemaker*

**pre·for·ma·tion** (pre″for-ma′shən) the theory of early physiologists that the fully formed animal or plant exists in a minute form in the germ cell. Opposed to the theory of *epigenesis*. See *animalculist* and *ovist*.

**pre·for·ma·tion·ist** (pre″for-ma′shən-ist) a believer in the theory of preformation.

**pre·fron·tal** (pre-fron′təl) situated in the anterior part of the frontal lobe or region.

**pre·func·tion·al** (pre-funk′shən-əl) denoting the period in embryological development during which the organ rudiments are formed but are incapable of performing their specific functions.

**pre·gan·gli·on·ic** (pre″gang-gle-on′ik) situated anterior or proximal to a ganglion; said especially of autonomic nerve fibers so located.

**pre·gen·i·tal** (pre-jen′ĭ-təl) pertaining to the early stages of psychosexual development (oral and anal), before the genitals have become the dominant influence on sexual behavior.

**preg·nan·cy** (preg′nən-se) [L. *praegnans* with child] [MeSH: Pregnancy] the condition of having a developing embryo or fetus in the body, after union of an ovum and spermatozoon. In women, duration of pregnancy from conception to delivery is about 266 days. Pregnancy is marked by cessation of the menses; nausea on arising in the morning (morning sickness); enlargement of the breasts and pigmentation of the nipples; progressive enlargement of the abdomen. The absolute signs of pregnancy are fetal movements, sounds of the fetal heart, and demonstration of the fetus by x-ray or ultrasound.
**abdominal p.,** ectopic pregnancy with development of the fetus in the abdominal cavity.
**ampullar p.,** ectopic pregnancy in which the ovum has been arrested in the ampulla of the oviduct.
**bigeminal p.,** twin p.
**broad ligament p.,** ectopic pregnancy with development of the fertilized ovum in the broad ligament.
**cervical p.,** ectopic pregnancy with the development of the ovum within the cervical canal.
**combined p.,** simultaneous existence of intrauterine and ectopic pregnancy.
**compound p.,** superimposition of an intrauterine pregnancy on a previously existing ectopic pregnancy, generally a lithopedion.
**cornual p.,** pregnancy in one of the horns of a bicornate uterus.
**ectopic p.,** development of the fertilized ovum outside of the uterine cavity; called also *extrauterine p.*
**exochorial p.,** graviditas exochorialis.
**extrauterine p.,** ectopic p.
**fallopian p.,** tubal p.
**false p.,** absence of the menses and presence of other signs of pregnancy, without occurrence of conception and development of an embryo. It may be due to psychogenic factors, to a tumor or mole, or to endocrine disorders. Called also *pseudocyesis, pseudopregnancy,* and *spurious p.*
**gemellary p.,** twin p.
**heterotopic p.,** combined p.
**hydatid p.,** that which is accompanied by the formation of a hydatid mole.
**hysteric p.,** false pregnancy due to psychogenic factors.
**interstitial p.,** ectopic pregnancy with gestation in that part of the oviduct which is within the wall of the uterus.
**intraligamentary p., intraligamentous p.,** ectopic pregnancy within the broad ligament.
**intramural p.,** interstitial p.
**intraperitoneal p.,** ectopic pregnancy within the peritoneal cavity.
**membranous p.,** pregnancy in which the fetus has broken through its membranous envelope and lies in contact with the uterine walls.
**mesenteric p.,** tuboligamentary p.
**molar p.,** conversion of the fertilized ovum into a mole.
**multiple p.,** pregnancy in which two or more fetuses exist simultaneously; it may be *monovular* (resulting from the fertilization of a single ovum) or *polyovular* (resulting from the fertilization of more than one ovum). When more than two fetuses coexist, they may come from one ovum or be the result of combined monovular and polyovular twinning. Called also *multiple gestation.*

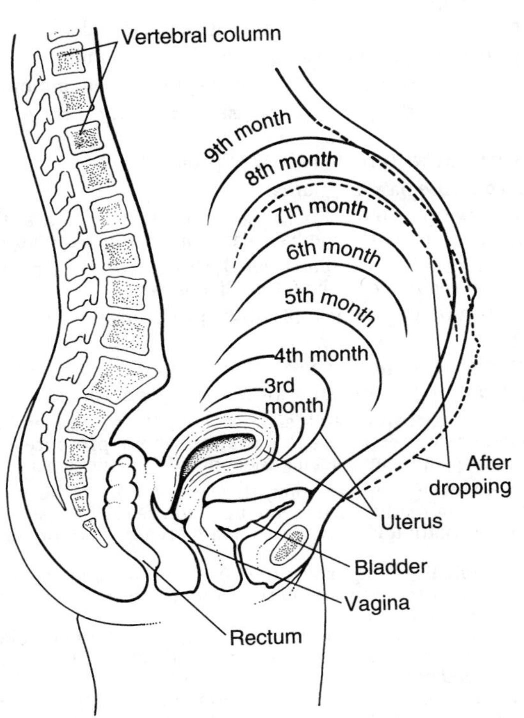

Pregnancy—Uterine levels.

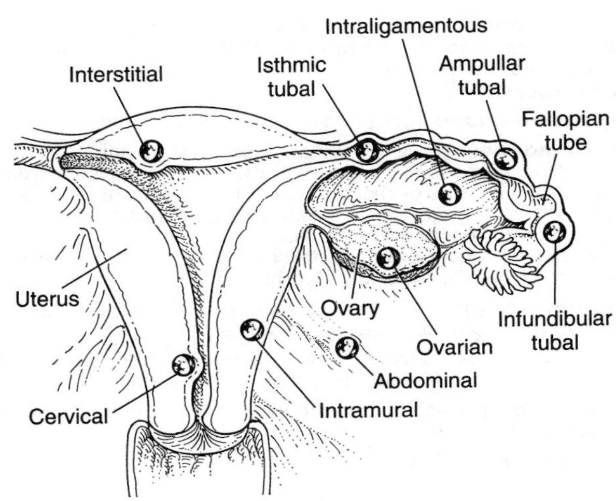

Diagram showing locations of ectopic (extrauterine) pregnancy.

**mural p.,** interstitial p.
**nervous p.,** false pregnancy due to psychogenic factors.
**ovarian p.,** ectopic pregnancy occurring within an ovary.
**ovario-abdominal p.,** ectopic pregnancy that begins ovarian, but afterward becomes abdominal.
**oviductal p.,** tubal p.
**parietal p.,** interstitial p.
**phantom p.,** false pregnancy due to psychogenic factors.
**plural p.,** pregnancy with more than one fetus.
**post-term p.,** pregnancy that has extended beyond 42 completed weeks from the onset of the last menstrual period or 40 completed weeks from conception. Called also *prolonged p.* See also *postmature infant,* under *infant.*
**prolonged p.,** post-term p.
**pseudointraligamentary p.,** an ectopic pregnancy in which a sac has been formed in such a way as to simulate an intraligamentary pregnancy.
**sarcofetal p.,** pregnancy with both a fetus and a mole.
**sarcohysteric p.,** false pregnancy due to a mole.
**spurious p.,** false p.
**stump p.,** pregnancy in the cervical stump remaining after a supracervical hysterectomy.
**tubal p.,** ectopic pregnancy within an oviduct.
**tuboabdominal p.,** ectopic pregnancy occurring partly in the fimbriated end of the oviduct and partly in the abdominal cavity.
**tuboligamentary p.,** ectopic pregnancy partly in the tube and partly in the broad ligament.
**tubo-ovarian p.,** ectopic pregnancy occurring partly in the ovary and partly in the oviduct.
**tubouterine p.,** ectopic pregnancy partly within the uterus and partly in an oviduct.
**twin p.,** gestation with development of two fetuses.
**uteroabdominal p.,** pregnancy with one fetus in the uterus and another in the abdominal cavity.
**uterotubal p.,** tubouterine p.

**preg·nane** (preg′nān) a type of saturated 21-carbon steroid hydrocarbon nucleus that is the parent structure of many steroids; two groups of steroids are distinguished as those stemming from 5$\alpha$-pregnane and those stemming from 5$\beta$-pregnane. In the latter group are progesterones, ketones, and several corticosteroids.

**preg·nane·di·ol** (preg″nān-di′ol) [MeSH: Pregnanediol] any of several biologically inactive dihydroxy derivatives of progesterone; pregnanediols are metabolic degradation products, found especially in urine of women during pregnancy or the luteal phase of the menstrual cycle.

**preg·nane·tri·ol** (preg″nān-tri′ol) [MeSH: Pregnanetriol] a metabolite of 17$\alpha$-hydroxyprogesterone, normally occurring in small amounts in body fluids and urine, but greatly increased in disorders of the adrenal cortex in which 21-hydroxylation of the steroid nucleus is impaired, as in the most common form of congenital adrenocortical hyperplasia with virilism.

**preg·nant** (preg′nənt) [L. *praegnans*] with child; containing developing young. Called also *gravid.*

**preg·nene** (preg′nēn) a term used in steroid hormone nomenclature to refer to an unsaturated 21-carbon structure with one double bond and three methyl groups; the $\delta^4$ and $\delta^5$ pregnene steroid nucleus forms the basis of most of the biologically active progestins and corticosteroids.

**preg·nen·in·o·lone** (preg″nēn-in′o-lōn) ethisterone.

**preg·ne·no·lone** (preg-nēn′ə-lōn) [MeSH: Pregnenolone] 1. an intermediate compound in the synthesis of the steroid hormones, formed by cleavage of the side chain of cholesterol between C-20 and C-22. 2. a synthetic preparation of this hormone, used in the treatment of rheumatoid arthritis.
**p. succinate,** a nonhormonal sterol derivative that has been used in the treatment of rheumatoid arthritis.

**pre·go·ni·um** (pre-go′ne-əm) a recess on the lower edge of the body of the mandible anterior to the angle.

**pre·hal·lux** (pre-hal′əks) a supernumerary bone of the foot sometimes found growing from the medial border of the scaphoid.

**pre·hen·sile** (pre-hen′sil) [L. *prehendere* to lay hold of] adapted for grasping or seizing.

**pre·hen·sion** (pre-hen′shən) [L. *prehensio*] the act of seizing or grasping.

**pre·he·pat·ic** (pre″he-pat′ik) anterior to the liver or (of the portal circulation) before the liver is reached.

**pre·he·pat·i·cus** (pre″hə-pat′ĭ-kəs) [*pre-* + Gr. *hēpar* liver] a mass of vascular and connective tissue in the embryo that develops into the interstitial tissue of the liver.

**Prehn's sign** (prānz) [D.T. *Prehn,* American physician, 20th century] see under *sign.*

**pre·hor·mone** (pre-hor′mōn) a hormone precursor consisting of the hormone with its signal sequence in place. See also *prohormone.*

**pre·hy·oid** (pre-hi′oid) anterior to the hyoid bone.

**pre·hy·po·phys·e·al** (pre″hi-po-fiz′e-əl) adenohypophysial.

**pre·hy·po·phys·i·al** (pre″hi-po-fiz′e-əl) adenohypophysial.

**pre·hy·poph·y·sis** (pre″hi-pof′ĭ-sis) adenohypophysis.

**pre·ic·tal** (pre-ik′təl) [*pre-* + *ictal*] occurring before a stroke or an attack, as before an acute epileptic attack.

**pre·in·va·sive** (pre″in-va′siv) not yet invading other tissues; see *carcinoma in situ.*

**pre·io·ta·tion** (pre″i-o-ta′shən) [*pre-* + *iota*] a speech disorder in which an initial *i* sound is converted to *yi.*

**Prei·ser's disease** (pri′zerz) [Georg Karl Felix *Preiser,* German orthopedic surgeon, 1879–1913] see under *disease.*

**Preisz-No·card bacillus** (prīs-no-kahr′) [Hugo von *Preisz,* Hungarian bacteriologist, 1860–1940; Edmond Isidore Etienne *Nocard,* French veterinarian, 1850–1903] *Corynebacterium pseudotuberculosis.*

**pre·kal·li·kre·in** (pre-kal″ĭ-kre′in) [MeSH: Prekallikrein] a plasma protein that is the proenzyme of plasma kallikrein, being cleaved and activated by activated coagulation factor XII.

**pre·lac·te·al** (pre-lak′te-əl) preceding the establishment of milk flow; a term applied to the feeding of a newborn baby with carbohydrate-electrolyte solutions to reduce initial weight loss until breast feeding is fully established.

**pre·leu·ke·mia** (pre-loo-ke′me-ə) [MeSH: Preleukemia] myelodysplastic syndrome.

**pre·leu·ke·mic** (pre-loo-ke′mik) pertaining to or affected with a myelodysplastic syndrome (preleukemia).

**pre·lim·bic** (pre-lim′bik) situated anterior to a limbus; specifically, anterior to the limbus fossae ovalis.

**pre·lin·gual** (pre-ling′gwəl) occurring before the development of language.

**pre-β-lipo·pro·tein** (pre″ba-tə-lip″o-pro′tēn) see under *lipoprotein.*

**pre·load** (pre′lōd) the mechanical state of the heart at the end of diastole, the magnitude of the maximal (end-diastolic) ventricular volume or the end-diastolic pressure stretching the ventricles, calculated as: in isolated cardiac muscle, the force stretching the resting muscle to a given length prior to contraction; in the intact heart, the stress on the ventricular wall at the end of diastole, determined largely by the venous return, total blood volume and its distribution, and atrial activity. It is usually measured as left ventricular end-diastolic volume.

**pre·lo·cal·iza·tion** (pre″lo-kəl-ĭ-za′shən) the localization in the egg or blastomere of materials that will develop into a particular tissue or organ.

**pre·lo·co·mo·tion** (pre″lo-ko-mo′shən) the movements of a child made with the intention of moving from place to place before motor coordination is sufficiently developed to enable it to walk.

**Prel·one** (pre′lōn) trademark for a preparation of prednisolone.

**pre·ma·lig·nant** (pre″mə-lig′nənt) precancerous.

**Prem·a·rin** (prem′ə-rin) trademark for preparations of conjugated estrogens.

**pre·ma·ture** (pre-mə-choor′) [L. *praematurus* early ripe] 1. occurring before the proper time. 2. a premature infant; see under *infant.*

**pre·ma·tur·i·ty** (pre″mə-choor′ĭ-te) underdevelopment; the condition of a premature infant.

**pre·max·il·la** (pre″mak-sil′ə) 1. TA alternative for *os incisivum.* 2. the embryonic bone derived from the median nasal prominences that later fuses with the maxilla to form the os incisivum.

**pre·max·il·lary** (pre-mak′sĭ-lar′e) 1. anterior to the maxilla proper. 2. os incisivum. 3. pertaining to the premaxilla or to the os incisivum.

**pre·med·i·cal** (pre-med′ĭ-kəl) preceding and preparing for the regular medical course of study, as premedical education.

**pre·med·i·cant** (pre-med′ĭ-kənt) a drug used for premedication.

**pre·med·i·ca·tion** (pre″med-ĭ-ka′shən) [MeSH: Premedication] preliminary medication, particularly to produce narcosis prior to inhalation anesthesia.

**pre·mei·ot·ic** (pre″mi-ot′ik) [*pre-* + *meiotic*] occurring before or pertaining to the time preceding meiosis.

**pre·me·nar·chal** (pre″mə-nahr′kəl) pertaining to the period before menstruation is established; occurring prior to the menarche.

**pre·me·nar·che** (pre″mə-nahr′ke) the period before menstruation is established; preceding the menarche.

**pre·me·nar·che·al** (pre″mə-nahr′ke-əl) premenarchal.

**pre·men·strua** (pre-men′stroo-ə) [L.] plural of *premenstruum.*

**pre·men·stru·al** (pre-men′stroo-əl) occurring before menstruation.

**pre·men·stru·um** (pre-men′stroo-əm) pl. *premenstrua* [L.] the period immediately preceding occurrence of the menstrual flow.

**pre·mi·tot·ic** (pre″mi-tot′ik) occurring before or pertaining to the time preceding mitosis.

**pre·mo·lar** (pre-mo′lər) [*pre-* + *molar*[2]] 1. situated in front of the molar teeth. 2. premolar tooth.

**pre·mon·i·to·ry** (pre-mon′ĭ-tor-e) [L. *praemonitorius*] serving as a warning.

**pre·mono·cyte** (pre-mon′o-sīt) promonocyte.

**pre·mor·bid** (pre-mor′bid) occurring before the development of signs or symptoms of disease.

**pre·mor·tal** (pre-mor′təl) occurring just before death.

**pre·mu·ni·tion** (pre″mu-nish′ən) infection immunity.

**pre·mu·ni·tive** (pre-mu′nĭ-tiv) pertaining to premunition.

**pre·my·elo·blast** (pre-mi′ə-lo-blast″) an early form of a myeloblast.

**pre·my·elo·cyte** (pre-mi′ə-lo-sīt″) promyelocyte.

**pre·na·res** (pre-na′rēz) nares.

**pre·na·sa·le** (pre″na-sa′le) a cephalometric landmark, the most projecting point, in the median plane, at the tip of the nose.

**pre·na·tal** (pre-na′təl) [*pre-* + *natal*] existing or occurring before birth, with reference to the fetus. Cf. *antepartal.*

**pre·neo·plas·tic** (pre″ne-o-plas′tik) preceding the development of a tumor.

**pre·op·er·a·tive** (pre-op′ər-ə-tiv) preceding an operation.

**pre·op·tic** (pre-op′tik) anterior to the optic chiasma.

**pre·oxy·gen·a·tion** (pre-ok″sĭ-jən-a′shən) the prolonged breathing of oxygen before exposure to low atmospheric pressure at high altitudes, as prophylaxis against decompression sickness.

**prep·a·ra·tion** (prep″ə-ra′shən) [L. *praeparatio*] 1. the act or process of making ready. 2. a medicine made ready for use. 3. an anatomic or pathologic specimen made ready and preserved for study.
**biomechanical p.,** the procedures involved in exposing, enlarging, cleansing, and shaping the pulp chamber and root canal of a tooth by mechanical means.
**cavity p.,** a procedure for establishing in a tooth the biochemically acceptable form necessary to receive and retain a restoration. See also *prepared cavity,* under *cavity.*
**corrosion p.,** an anatomic preparation made by injecting the parts to be retained and dissolving the rest of the tissues with some corrosive substance.

**heart-lung p.**, an animal in which only the heart and lungs are kept alive, the blood from the aorta being diverted into an external system of tubes, simulating the systemic circulation, and back via a reservoir to the right atrium; used in studies of heart function.
**impression p.**, a preparation of bacteria on a slide for examination, made by lightly touching a coverglass to a colony.
**touch p.**, impression p.

**pre·par·tal** (pre-pahr′təl) [*pre-* + *partal*] antepartum.

**pre·pa·tent** (pre-pa′tənt) before becoming apparent or manifest; in malariology the term is applied to the period elapsing between infection and detection of parasites in the blood.

**Pre-Pen** (pre′pen) trademark for a preparation of benzylpenicilloyl polylysine.

**pre·per·cep·tion** (pre″pər-sep′shən) in psychology, anticipation of a perception.

**pre·peri·to·ne·al** (pre-per″ĭ-to-ne′əl) situated between the parietal peritoneum and the abdominal wall, or occurring anterior to the peritoneum.

**pre·pon·der·ance** (pre-pon′dər-əns) [*pre-* + L. *pondere* to weigh] the condition of having greater weight, force, or influence.
**ventricular p.**, disproportionate hypertrophy between the ventricles of the heart; diagnosed by the electrocardiograph.

**pre·po·ten·tial** (pre″po-ten′shəl) the slow diastolic depolarization of the cell membranes of the cardiac pacemaker.

**pre·pran·di·al** (pre-pran′de-əl) before meals.

**pre·pro·hor·mone** (pre″pro-hor′mōn) a hormone preproprotein.

**pre·pro·in·su·lin** (pre″pro-in′su-lin) the intraglandular precursor of proinsulin, containing a signal sequence at the N-terminal.

**pre·pro·pro·tein** (pre″pro-pro′tēn) a precursor that is cleaved to form a proprotein.

**pre·pros·thet·ic** (pre″pros-thet′ik) performed or occurring before insertion of a prosthesis.

**pre·pro·tein** (pre-pro′tēn) a protein precursor that contains a signal sequence that must be cleaved off to form the protein or proprotein.

**pre·pu·ber·al** (pre-pu′bər-əl) prepubertal.

**pre·pu·ber·tal** (pre-pu′bər-təl) occurring before puberty; pertaining to the period of accelerated growth preceding gonadal maturity.

**pre·pu·ber·ty** (pre-pu′bər-te) the period preceding puberty.

**pre·pu·bes·cence** (pre″pu-bes′əns) prepuberty.

**pre·pu·bes·cent** (pre″pu-bes′ənt) prepubertal.

**pre·puce** (pre′pūs) 1. preputium. 2. preputium penis.
**p. of clitoris**, preputium clitoridis.
**p. of penis**, preputium penis.
**redundant p.**, a condition in which there is excessive growth of the foreskin, so that it cannot be drawn back over the glans.

**pre·pu·tial** (pre-pu′shəl) pertaining to the prepuce.

**pre·pu·ti·ot·o·my** (pre-pu″she-ot′ə-me) [*preputium* + *-tomy*] incision of the preputium penis on the dorsum or side of the penis, to relieve the constriction in phimosis.

**pre·pu·ti·um** (pre-pu′she-əm) prepuce: a covering fold of skin.
**p. clito′ridis** [TA], prepuce of clitoris: a fold formed by the union of the labia minora anterior over the clitoris and united with the glans clitoris.
**p. pe′nis** [TA], prepuce of penis: the fold of skin covering the glans penis; called also *foreskin*.

**pre·py·lor·ic** (pre″pi-lor′ik) anterior to or just proximal to the pylorus or the pyloric part of the stomach *(pars pylorica gastris)*.

**pre·re·nal** (pre-re′nəl) 1. anterior to a kidney. 2. occurring before the kidney is reached, such as acute renal failure in which the kidney does not receive adequate blood flow. Cf. *postrenal*.

**Pres·a·mine** (pres′ə-mēn) trademark for a preparation of imipramine hydrochloride.

**presby-** [Gr. *presbys* old man] a combining form meaning old or denoting relationship to old age.

**pres·by·acu·sia** (pres″be-ə-ku′se-ə) presbycusis.

**pres·by·at·rics** (pres-be-at′riks) [*presby-* + *-iatrics*] geriatrics.

**pres·by·car·dia** (pres″be-kahr′de-ə) [*presby-* + *cardia*] impaired cardiac function attributed to the aging process, occurring in association with recognizable changes of senescence in the body and in the absence of convincing evidence of other forms of heart disease.

**pres·by·cu·sis** (pres″bĭ-ku′sis) [*presby-* + *acou-* + *-sis*] [MeSH: Presbycusis] a progressive, bilaterally symmetric perceptive hearing loss occurring with age.

**pres·by·esoph·a·gus** (pres″be-ə-sof′ə-gəs) a condition characterized by alteration in motor function of the esophagus as a result of degenerative changes occurring with advancing age.

**pres·by·ope** (pres′be-ōp) one who is presbyopic.

**pres·by·opia** (pres″be-o′pe-ə) [*presby-* + *-opia*] [MeSH: Presbyopia] hyperopia and impairment of vision due to advancing years or to old age; it is dependent on diminution of the power of accommodation from loss of elasticity of the crystalline lens, causing the near point of distinct vision to be removed farther from the eye. Abbreviated Pr.

**pres·by·op·ic** (pres″be-op′ik) pertaining to presbyopia.

**pre·scap·u·la** (pre-skap′u-lə) the suprascapular portion of the scapula.

**pre·scap·u·lar** (pre-skap′u-lər) 1. anterior to the scapula. 2. pertaining to the prescapula.

**pre·scle·rot·ic** (pre″sklə-rot′ik) occurring before sclerosis takes place.

**pre·scribe** (pre-skrīb′) [L. *praescribere* to write before] to designate in writing a remedy for administration.

**pre·scrip·tion** (prĭ-skrip′shən) [L. *praescriptio*] [MeSH: Prescriptions, Drug] a written direction for the preparation and administration of a remedy. A prescription consists of the heading or *superscription*—that is, the symbol ℞ or the word Recipe, meaning "take"; the *inscription*, which contains the names and quantities of the ingredients; the *subscription*, or directions for compounding; and the *signature*, usually introduced by the sign S. for *sig′na*, "mark," which gives the directions for the patient which are to be marked on the receptacle.
**shotgun p.**, an irrational prescription that contains a number of ingredients given with the idea that one or more of them may be effective.

**pre·se·nile** (pre-se′nīl) pertaining to a condition resembling senility but occurring in early or middle life.

**pre·se·nil·i·ty** (pre″sə-nil′ĭ-te) premature old age.

**pre·se·ni·um** (pre-se′ne-əm) the period immediately preceding old age.

**pre·sent** (pre-zent′) [L. *praesentare* to show] to appear or to show, as to appear first at the os uteri (said of a fetus; see *presenting part*, under *part*), or to appear for examination, treatment, etc. (said of a patient).

**pre·sen·ta·tion** (pre″zən-ta′shən) [L. *praesentatio*] in obstetrics, that portion of the fetus which is touched by the examining finger through the cervix or, during labor, is bounded by the girdle of resistance.
**antigen p.**, the activity in which macrophages ingest and partially digest antigens and then present the processed antigen on their surfaces to B and T lymphocytes. The presented antigen is more immunogenic than unprocessed antigen, possibly because it has been broken down into pieces more easily recognized by B and T cells, because it remains on the surface of the presenting cell for a long time, or because it is presented in association with self MHC antigen and thus able to stimulate helper T cells. The principal antigen-presenting cells are dendritic cells in B-dependent areas of lymphoid tissues, interdigitating cells in T-dependent areas, and Langerhans cells in the epidermis.
**breech p.**, presentation of the buttocks or feet of the fetus in labor.
**breech p., complete**, presentation of the buttocks of the fetus in labor, with the feet alongside the buttocks, the thighs flexed upon the fetal abdomen, and the distal legs flexed upon the thighs; the fetus in essence is in the same attitude as in vertex presentation but with polarity reversed.
**breech p., frank**, presentation of the buttocks of the fetus in labor, with the legs extended against the trunk and the feet lying against the face.
**breech p., incomplete**, presentation of the fetus in labor, with one or both feet or one or both knees of the fetus prolapsed into the maternal vagina.
**brow p.**, presentation of the fetal brow in labor.
**cephalic p.**, presentation of any part of the fetal head in labor, including occiput, brow, or face.
**compound p.**, prolapse of an extremity of the fetus (an arm or leg, or both), alongside the head, or of one or both arms alongside a presenting breech, at the beginning of labor.
**face p.**, the presentation of the face of the fetus in labor.
**footling p.**, presentation of the fetus in labor with one (single footling) or both feet (double footling) prolapsed into the maternal vagina.
**funis p.**, presentation of the umbilical cord in labor.
**parietal p.**, presentation of the parietal portion of the fetal head in labor.
**pelvic p.**, breech p.
**placental p.**, placenta previa.

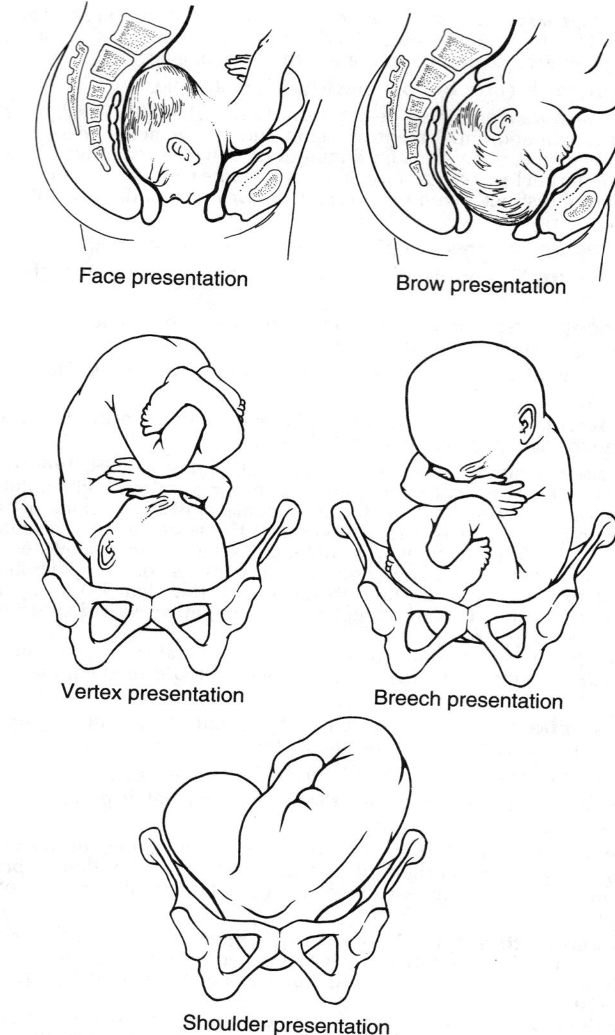


**shoulder p.**, presentation of the fetal shoulder in labor; see also *oblique lie* and *transverse lie*, under *lie*.
**torso p.**, transverse lie.
**transverse p.**, see under *lie*.
**trunk p.**, transverse lie.
**vertex p.**, the presentation of the vertex of the fetal head in labor.

**pre·sep·tal** (pre-sep′təl) anterior to a septum.

**pre·ser·va·tive** (pre-zer′və-tiv) a substance or preparation added to a product for the purpose of destroying or inhibiting the multiplication of microorganisms.

**pre·si·nu·soi·dal** (pre″si-nə-soi′dəl) anterior to a sinusoid or affecting the circulation before the sinusoids are reached; used especially to denote the location of vascular resistance in portal hypertension.

**pre·so·mite** (pre-so′mīt) [*pre-* + *somite*] referring to embryos before the appearance of somites; in the human, before 19 days postfertilization.

**pre·sper·ma·tid** (pre-sper′mə-tid) secondary spermatocyte.

**pre·sphe·noid** (pre-sfe′noid) pertaining to the anterior part of the body of the sphenoid bone.

**pre·sphe·noi·dal** (pre″sfə-noi′dəl) presphenoid.

**pre·spon·dy·lo·lis·the·sis** (pre-spon″də-lo-lis-the′sis) a congenital defect in the last lumbar vertebra consisting of a bilateral defect in the neural arches at the pedicles.

**pres·som·e·ter** (pres-om′ə-tər) manometer.
**Jarcho p.**, an instrument especially designed for measuring pressure during injection of radiopaque material into the uterus in hysterosalpingography.

**pres·sor** (pres′or) tending to increase blood pressure; said of nerves and chemical substances.

**pres·so·re·cep·tive** (pres″o-re-sep′tiv) sensitive to stimuli due to vasomotor activity, such as blood pressure.

**pres·so·re·cep·tor** (pres″o-re-sep′tər) [MeSH: Pressoreceptors] baroreceptor.

**pres·so·sen·si·tive** (pres″o-sen′sĭ-tiv) pressoreceptive.

**pres·sure** (presh′ər) [L. *pressura*] [MeSH: Pressure] force per unit area; symbol *P*. The SI unit for pressure is the Pascal (Pa), which is one newton per square meter of area.
**after p.**, a sense of pressure that lasts for a short period after removal of the actual pressure.
**alveolar p.**, the pressure exerted by the air in the pulmonary alveoli.
**arterial p.**, blood p. (def. 2).
**atmospheric p.**, the pressure exerted by the atmosphere, usually considered as the downward pressure of air onto a unit of area of the earth's surface; the unit of pressure at sea level is one *atmosphere*. Pressure decreases with increasing attitude. See also *atmosphere* (def. 2).
**back p.**, the pressure caused by the damming back of the blood in a heart chamber and its tributaries, due to an obstructive heart valve or failing myocardium.
**barometric p.**, atmospheric p.
**biting p.**, occlusal p.
**blood p.**, 1. the pressure of blood against the walls of any blood vessel. 2. the pressure of the blood on the walls of the arteries, dependent on the energy of the heart action, the elasticity of the walls of the arteries, and the volume and viscosity of the blood. The *maximum* or *systolic blood pressure* occurs near the end of the stroke output of the left ventricle of the heart. The *minimum* or *diastolic blood pressure* occurs late in ventricular diastole. *Mean blood pressure* is the average of the blood pressure levels, and *basic blood pressure* is that during quiet rest or basal conditions. See also *hypertension* and *hypotension*.
**capillary p.**, the blood pressure in the capillaries.
**central venous p. (CVP)**, the venous pressure as measured at the right atrium, obtained by means of a central venous catheter whose distal end is attached to a manometer.
**cerebrospinal p.**, the pressure or tension of the cerebrospinal fluid, normally 100–150 mm as measured by the manometer.
**continuous positive airway p. (CPAP)**, a method of positive pressure ventilation used with patients who are breathing spontaneously, in which pressure in the airway is maintained above the level of atmospheric pressure throughout the respiratory cycle. The purpose is to keep the alveoli open at the end of expiration and thus increase oxygenation and reduce the work of breathing. Cf. *positive end-expiratory p.*
**critical p.**, the smallest amount of pressure necessary to liquefy a gas at the critical temperature.
**diastolic p.**, see *blood p.*
**Donders' p.**, increase of manometric pressure with the instrument placed on the trachea on opening the chest of a dead body; due to collapse of the lung.
**end-diastolic p.**, the pressure in the ventricles at the end of diastole; usually measured in the left ventricle as an approximation of the end-diastolic volume, or preload.
**endocardial p.**, pressure of blood within the heart.
**filling p.**, see *mean circulatory filling p.*
**hydrostatic p.**, the pressure at any level in fluid at rest due solely to the weight of the fluid above it.
**intra-abdominal p.**, the pressure between the viscera within the abdominal cavity.
**intracranial p. (ICP)**, the pressure in the space between the skull and the brain, i.e., the pressure of the subarachnoidal fluid.
**intraocular p.**, the pressure of the fluids of the eye against the tunics. It is produced by continual renewal of the fluids within the interior of the eye, and is altered in certain pathological conditions (e.g., glaucoma). It may be roughly estimated by palpation of the eye or measured, directly or indirectly, with specially devised instruments, the tonometers. Normal intraocular pressure is symbolized Tn. Called also *intraocular tension*.
**intrapleural p.**, pleural p.
**intrathecal p.**, pressure within a sheath, particularly the pressure of the cerebrospinal fluid within the subarachnoid membrane.
**intrathoracic p.**, pleural p.
**intraventricular p.**, the pressure within one ventricle of the heart.
**maximum expiratory p.**, MEP; a measure of the strength of respiratory muscles, obtained by having the patient exhale as strongly as possible against a mouthpiece; the maximum value is near total lung capacity.
**maximum inspiratory p.**, MIP; a measure of the strength of respiratory muscles, obtained by having the patient inhale as strongly as possible with the mouth against a mouthpiece; the maximum value is near the residual volume.
**mean arterial p. (MAP)**, the average pressure within an artery over a complete cycle of one heartbeat; in the brachial artery,

$$\text{MAP} = \text{diastolic pressure} + \frac{\text{systolic pressure} - \text{diastolic pressure}}{3}.$$

**mean circulatory filling p.**, a measure of the average (arterial and venous) pressure necessary to cause filling of the circulation with blood; it varies with blood volume and is directly proportional to the rate of venous return and thus to cardiac output.
**negative p.**, a pressure less than that of the atmosphere.
**occlusal p.**, pressure exerted on the occlusal surfaces of the teeth when the jaws are brought into apposition. Called also *biting p.*
**oncotic p.**, the osmotic pressure due to the presence of colloids in a solution; in the case of plasma–interstitial fluid interaction, it is the force that tends to counterbalance the capillary blood pressure.
**osmotic p.**, the pressure required to stop osmosis through a semipermeable membrane between a solution and pure solvent; it is proportional to the osmolality of the solution and also to other colligative properties of the solution, including freezing point depression, vapor pressure depression, and boiling point elevation. Symbol $\pi$.
**osmotic p., effective**, that part of the total osmotic pressure of a solution which governs the tendency of its solvent to pass through a semipermeable bounding membrane or across another boundary.
**partial p.**, the pressure exerted by each of the components of a gas mixture.
**perfusion p.**, the difference between the arterial and venous pressures through an organ or capillary bed.
**pleural p.**, the pressure between the visceral pleura and the parietal pleura in the pleural cavity. Called also *intrapleural* or *intrathoracic p.*
**positive p.**, pressure greater than that of the atmosphere.
**positive end-expiratory p. (PEEP)**, a method of positive pressure ventilation used in conjunction with mechanical ventilation; pressure is maintained above the level of atmospheric pressure at the end of exhalation. This is achieved by preventing the complete release of gas during exhalation, usually by means of a valve within the circuit. The purpose is to increase the volume of gas remaining in the lungs at the end of expiration, thus reducing the shunting of blood through the lungs and improving gas exchange; done in acute respiratory failure to allow reduction of inspired $O_2$ concentrations. Cf. *continuous positive airway p.*
**pulmonary artery wedge p. (PAWP), pulmonary capillary wedge p. (PCWP)**, intravascular pressure as measured by a catheter wedged into the distal pulmonary artery; it permits indirect measurement of the mean left atrial pressure.
**pulse p.**, the difference between the systolic and diastolic pressures.
**selection p.**, an effect produced by a given gene that determines the frequency of a given allele; it may be advantageous for survival *(positive selection pressure)* or disadvantageous *(negative selection pressure)*.
**solution p.**, the force that tends to bring into solution the molecules of a solid contained in the solvent.
**systolic p.**, see *blood p.*
**transpulmonary p.**, the pressure difference between the inner and outer surfaces of the lung, i.e., the pressure tending to inflate or deflate the lungs; equal to the difference between the alveolar pressure and the pleural pressure.
**urethral p.**, the inward pressure exerted by the walls of the urethra, which must be counteracted in order for urine to flow through; see also under *profile*.
**venous p.**, the blood pressure in a vein, such as central venous pressure or wedged hepatic vein pressure.
**wedge p.**, blood pressure measured by a small catheter wedged into a vessel, occluding it; see *pulmonary capillary wedge p.* and *wedged hepatic vein p.*
**wedged hepatic vein p.**, the venous pressure measured with a catheter wedged into the hepatic vein. The difference between wedged and free hepatic vein pressures is used to locate the site of obstruction in portal hypertension; it is elevated in that due to cirrhosis but low in cardiac ascites or portal vein thrombosis.

**pre·su·bic·u·lum** (pre″soo-bik′u-ləm) [TA] a modified six-layered cortex situated between the subiculum and the main part of the parahippocampal gyrus.

**pre·sump·tive** (pre-zump′tiv) referring to the expected fate of an embryonic part on the basis of established fate mapping.

**pre·syl·vi·an** (pre-sil′ve-ən) pertaining to the anterior or ascending branch of the sylvian fissure (sulcus lateralis).

**pre·symp·tom** (pre-simp′tom) an indication that is a forerunner of the actual symptoms of a condition.

**pre·symp·to·mat·ic** (pre″simp-to-mat′ik) existing before the appearance of symptoms.

**pre·syn·ap·tic** (pre″sĭ-nap′tik) situated before or proximal to a synapse, or occurring before the synapse is crossed.

**pre·sys·to·le** (pre-sis′to-le) the interval immediately preceding systole.

**pre·sys·tol·ic** (pre″sis-tol′ik) 1. pertaining to the beginning of systole. 2. occurring just before systole.

**pre·tar·sal** (pre-tahr′səl) anterior to the tarsus.

**pre·tec·tal** (pre-tek′təl) anterior to the tectum mesencephali.

**pre·tec·tum** (pre-tek′təm) pretectal area.

**pre·throm·bot·ic** (pre-throm-bot′ik) preceding the development of thrombosis.

**pre·thy·roid** (pre-thi′roid) anterior to the thyroid gland or thyroid cartilage.

**pre·thy·roi·de·al** (pre″thi-roi′de-əl) prethyroid.

**pre·thy·roi·de·an** (pre-thi-roi′de-ən) prethyroid.

**pre·tu·ber·cu·lo·sis** (pre″too-ber″ku-lo′sis) tuberculosis in an incipient and occult stage before any symptoms of the disease have appeared.

**pre·ure·thri·tis** (pre″u-re-thri′tis) inflammation of the vestibule of the vagina around the urethral orifice.

**Prev·a·cid** (prev′ə-sid) trademark for a preparation of lansoprazole.

**prev AGT** previous abnormality of glucose tolerance.

**prev·a·lence** (prev′ə-ləns) [L. *praevalēre* to prevail] [MeSH: Prevalence] the number of cases of a disease that are present in a population at a specified time, either at a point in time *(point p.)* or over a period of time *(period p.)*; when the term is unmodified, the former meaning is usually inferred. See *prevalence rate,* under *rate*. Cf. *incidence*.

**pre·ven·tive** (pre-ven′tiv) serving to avert the occurrence of.

**pre·ven·tric·u·lus** (pre″ven-trik′u-ləs) ostium cardiacum.

**pre·ves·i·cal** (pre-ves′ĭ-kəl) [*pre-* + *vesical*] anterior to the bladder.

**pre·vi·a·ble** (pre-vi′ə-bəl) not yet viable; said of a fetus incapable of extrauterine existence.

**pre·vi·ta·min** (pre-vi′tə-min) a precursor of a vitamin.
**p. $D_3$**, the immediate precursor to cholecalciferol, produced as a thermally labile intermediate upon irradiation of 7-dehydrocholesterol in the skin; at body temperature, it spontaneously rearranges to form cholecalciferol in approximately three days.

**Pré·vost's law, sign** (pra-vōz′) [Jean Louis *Prévost,* Swiss physician, 1838–1927] see under *law* and *sign*.

**Pre·vo·tel·la** (pre″vo-tel′ə) [André Romain Prévot, French microbiologist, 20th century] a genus of gram-negative, obligately anaerobic, moderately saccharolytic, bile-sensitive bacteria, consisting of nonmotile, non–spore-forming, pleomorphic rod-shaped organisms. They are normal inhabitants of the mucous membranes and are found especially in the oral cavity, colon, and vagina; some cause human infections. Included here are a number of species formerly included in the genus *Bacteroides*.
**P. bi′via**, a bile-sensitive, nonpigmented species that is moderately fermentative, found in the female genital tract and in the oral cavity, and isolated from infections of the urogenital tract and abdominal region and from breast abscesses. Called also *Bacteroides bivius*.
**P. buc′cae**, a nonpigmented species that is a normal inhabitant of the gingival crevice and has been isolated from chest drainage, blood, sinus aspirates, and peritoneal fluid; called also *Bacteroides buccae*.
**P. cor′poris**, a pigmented species that has been isolated from various clinical specimens; called also *Bacteroides corporis*.
**P. denti′cola**, a pigmented species that is a normal inhabitant of the gingival crevice and has been isolated from various clinical specimens; called also *Bacteroides denticola*.
**P. di′siens**, a nonpigmented, weakly fermentative species found in infections of the oral cavity and the female genital tract, and as part of the normal flora of the vagina and mouth; called also *Bacteroides disiens*.
**P. heparinoly′tica**, a nonpigmented species that has been isolated from infections of the oral cavity and respiratory tract and from the genital tract; called also *Bacteroides heparinolyticus*.
**P. interme′dia**, a weakly fermentative species isolated from the human gingival crevice and various clinical specimens. Called also *Bacteroides intermedius* and *B. melaninogenicus* subsp. *intermedius*.
**P. melaninoge′nica**, a coccoid species that produces a black hematin pigment, part of the normal flora of the mucous membranes. It is also an important pathogen in oral, lung, and brain abscesses and occurs in other mixed infections. Called also *Bacteroides melaninogenicus* and *B. melaninogenicus* subsp. *melaninogenicus*.
**P. ora′lis**, a nonpigmented, strongly fermentative species found principally in the gingival sulcus, which is occasionally associated with infections of the oral cavity and the respiratory and genital tracts; called also *Bacteroides oralis*.

**P. o'ris,** a nonpigmented species that is a normal inhabitant of the gingival crevice and has been isolated from systemic infections; abscesses of the face, neck, and chest; abdominal wound drainage; blood; and peritoneal and spinal fluid. Called also *Bacteroides oris.*
**P. rumini'cola,** a nonpigmented, strongly fermentative species isolated from the rumens of cattle, sheep, and elk, and from human abscesses and feces.

**Prey·er's reflex, test** (pri'ərz) [Thierry Wilhelm *Preyer,* German physiologist, 1841–1897] see *auricle reflex,* under *reflex* and see under *test.*

**pre·zone** (pre'zōn) prozone.

**pre·zy·ga·poph·y·sis** (pre″zi-gə-pof'ĭ-sis) processus articularis superior vertebrarum.

**pre·zy·got·ic** (pre-zi-got'ik) occurring before the completion of fertilization and formation of the zygote.

**PRF** prolactin-releasing factor.

**pri·a·pism** (pri'ə-piz″əm) [L. *priapismus;* Gr. *priapismos*] [MeSH: Priapism] persistent abnormal erection of the penis, usually without sexual desire, and accompanied by pain and tenderness. It is seen in diseases and injuries of the spinal cord, and may be caused by vesical calculus and certain injuries to the penis.
**secondary p.,** priapism caused by obstruction to the outflow of blood through the dorsal vein at the root of the penis.

**pri·a·pi·tis** (pri″ə-pi'tis) penitis.

**pri·a·pus** (pri-a'pəs) penis.

**Price-Jones curve** (prīs-jōnz) [Cecil *Price-Jones,* English physician, 1863–1943] see under *curve.*

**prick** 1. a light puncture. 2. to puncture lightly.
**nail p.,** pricked foot.

**pril·o·caine hy·dro·chlo·ride** (pril'o-kān) [USP] a local anesthetic administered intravenously to produce peripheral nerve block, epidural or caudal block, and infiltration and regional anesthesia.

**Pril·o·sec** (pril'o-sek) trademark for a preparation of omeprazole.

**prim·a·quine phos·phate** (prim'ə-kwēn) [USP] an 8-aminoquinoline compound used as an antimalarial against the extraerythrocytic forms of *Plasmodium vivax* and *P. ovale* and the gametocytes of *P. falciparum,* used especially in the treatment of relapsing vivax malaria; administered orally, sometimes in conjunction with other antimalarials.

**pri·mary** (pri'mar-e) [L. *primarius* principal; *primus* first] first in order or in time of development; principal.

**pri·mate** (pri'māt) [MeSH: Primates] an individual belonging to the order Primates.

**Pri·ma·tes** (pri-ma'tēz) [L. *primus* first] [MeSH: Primates] an order of mammals, including human beings, apes, monkeys, and lemurs. Families include Cercopithecidae, Hominidae, Lemuridae, and Pongidae.

**Pri·max·in** (pri-mak'sin) trademark for a preparation of imipenem and cilastatin sodium.

**primed** (prīmd) immunologically activated by initial exposure to antigen; said of cells of the immune system.

**prim·er** (prīm'ər) 1. a substance that prepares for or facilitates the action of another. 2. in genetics, a short piece of DNA or RNA complementary to a given DNA sequence; it acts as the nucleating point from which replication proceeds via DNA polymerase.
**cavity p.,** a substance that enhances adaptation of resin filling materials to cavity walls by inducing wetting between the resinous material and the treated dentin and enamel surfaces.

**prim·i·done** (prim'ĭ-dōn) [USP] [MeSH: Primidone] an anticonvulsant used in the treatment of grand mal, focal, and psychomotor epileptic seizures, administered orally. Called also *desoxyphenobarbital.*

**pri·mi·grav·id** (pri″mĭ-grav'id) pregnant for the first time.

**pri·mi·grav·i·da** (pri″mĭ-grav'ĭ-də) [L. *prima* first + *gravida*] a woman pregnant for the first time; also written gravida I.

**pri·mip·a·ra** (pri-mip'ə-rə) pl. *primip'arae* [L. *prima* first + *para*] a woman who has had one pregnancy that resulted in a fetus that attained a weight of 500 g or a gestational age of 20 weeks, regardless of whether the infant was living at birth, and regardless of whether it was a single or multiple birth. Also written *para I.*

**pri·mi·par·i·ty** (pri″mĭ-par'ĭ-te) the condition or fact of being a primipara.

**pri·mip·a·rous** (pri-mip'ə-rəs) bearing or having borne but one child.

**pri·mit·iae** (pri-mish'e-e) [L. pl., "first things"] that part of the amniotic fluid discharged before the fetus is extruded.

**prim·i·tive** (prim'ĭ-tiv) [L. *primitivus*] first in point of time; existing in a simple or early form; showing little evolution.

**pri·mor·di·al** (pri-mor'de-əl) [L. *primordialis*] original or primitive; of the simplest and most undeveloped character.

**pri·mor·di·um** (pri-mor'de-əm) pl. *primor'dia* [L. "the beginning"] the earliest discernible indication during embryonic development of an organ or part; called also *anlage* or *rudiment.*

**Pri·mu·la** (pri'mu-lə) a genus of flowering plants of the family Primulaceae. *P. obco'nica* is the cultivated primula plant, a common cause of allergic contact dermatitis.

**prin·ceps** (prin'seps) [L.] principal; chief.

**Prin·ci·pen** (prin'sĭ-pen) trademark for preparations of ampicillin.

**prin·ci·ple** (prin'sĭ-pəl) [L. *principium*] 1. a chemical component. 2. a substance on which certain of the properties of a drug depend. 3. a law of conduct.
**active p.,** any constituent of a drug that helps confer upon it a medicinal property.
**Doppler p.,** see under *effect.*
**Fick p.,** a restatement of the law of conservation of mass used in making indirect measurements: the amount of a substance taken up or released by an organ is the product of the blood flow to the organ and the concentration difference of the substance between the arterial and venous systems. It is usually applied as the Fick method (q.v.) or one of the indicator dilution methods (q.v.) to determine cardiac output.
**immediate p.,** any one of the more or less complex substances of definite chemical constitution into which a heterogeneous substance can be readily resolved.
**Le Chatelier p.,** if a biological system is subjected to stress, it will act in such a way as to reduce the stress.
**organic p.,** immediate p.
**pleasure p., pleasure-pain p.,** in psychoanalytic theory, an inborn tendency to avoid pain and seek pleasure through the immediate reduction of tension by either direct or fantasied gratification; cf. *reality p.*
**proximate p.,** immediate p.
**reality p.,** in psychoanalytic theory, the ego functions that modify the demands of the pleasure principle to meet the demands and requirements of the external world.

**Prin·gle's disease** (pring'gəlz) [John James *Pringle,* British dermatologist, 1855–1922] adenoma sebaceum, def. 1.

**Pri·ni·vil** (prin'ĭ-vil) trademark for a preparation of lisinopril.

**Prin·zide** (prin'zīd) trademark for a combination preparation of lisinopril and hydrochlorothiazide.

**pri·on** (pri'on) [*pro*tein *in*fectious agent] any of several protease-resistant, insoluble, transmissible isoforms of the 27–30 kD core of prion protein that cause a group of progressive neurodegenerative diseases *(prion diseases)* in humans and animals. Prions have a pleated sheet conformation rather than the $\alpha$ helix structure that is normal for prion protein, lack detectable nucleic acid, and do not elicit an immune response.

**Pris·co·line hy·dro·chlor·ide** (pris'ko-lēn) trademark for preparations of tolazoline hydrochloride.

**prism** (priz'əm) [Gr. *prisma*] a solid with a triangular or polygonal cross section. A triangular prism splits up a ray of light into its constituent colors and turns or deflects light rays toward its base. Prisms are used to correct deviations of the eyes, since they alter the apparent situation of objects. Abbreviated Pr.
**adamantine p's, enamel p's,** prismata adamantina; see under *prisma.*
**Maddox p.,** two prisms with their bases together; used in testing for torsion of the eyeball.
**Nicol p.,** two slabs of Iceland spar cemented together and deflecting a ray of light in such a way that it is split in two, one part (the ordinary ray) being totally reflected and the other (polarized ray) passing through.
**Risley's p.,** a prism that rotates in a metal frame marked with a scale; used in testing ocular muscles for imbalance.

**pris·ma** (priz'mə) pl. *pris'mata* [Gr.] prism.
**pris'mata adaman'tina,** adamantine prisms: the structural units of the tooth enamel, consisting of parallel rods or prisms composed mainly of hydroxyapatite crystals and organic substance and held together with a cement substance, each prism being enveloped in a sheath. Called also *enamel prisms* or *rods.*

**pris·ma·ta** (priz'mə-tə) [Gr.] plural of *prisma.*

**pris·mat·ic** (priz-mat'ik) shaped like a prism; produced by a prism.

**pris·moid** (priz'moid) resembling a prism.

**pris·mop·tom·e·ter** (priz″mop-tom'ə-tər) [*prism* + *optometer*] an instrument for testing the eye by means of a revolving prism.

**pris·mo·sphere** (priz'mo-sfēr) [*prism* + *sphere*] a prism combined with a globular lens.

**pris·op·tom·e·ter** (priz"op-tom'ə-tər) prismoptometer.

**Pri·vine hy·dro·chlo·ride** (pri'vēn) trademark for preparations of naphazoline hydrochloride.

**PRL, Prl** prolactin.

**p.r.n.** abbreviation for L. *pro re na'ta,* according as circumstances may require.

**Pro** proline.

**pro-** [L. and Gr. "before"] 1. a prefix signifying before or in front of. 2. a prefix denoting a precursor, as of an enzyme or hormone.

**pro·ac·cel·er·in** (pro"ak-sel'ər-in) [MeSH: Factor V] factor V; see under *coagulation factors,* at factor.

**Pro·ac·ti·no·my·ces** (pro"ak-tĭ-no-mi'sēz) *Nocardia.*

**pro·ac·ti·no·my·cin** (pro-ak"tĭ-no-mi'sin) a group of antibiotic substances, designated A, B, and C, from cultures of *Nocardia gardneri,* which acts against gram-positive bacteria.

**pro·ac·ti·va·tor** (pro-ak'tĭ-va"tor) the inactive precursor form of an activator, or a factor that requires a chemical change, usually by an enzyme, to become an activator.
**C3 p. (C3PA),** former name for *factor B.*

**pro·al** (pro'əl) characterized by forward movement.

**pro·am·ni·on** (pro-am'ne-on) that part of the embryonal area at the ventral and lateral sides of the head which remains without mesoderm for some time.

**pro·ar·rhyth·mia** (pro"ə-rith'me-ə) cardiac arrhythmia that is either drug-induced or drug-aggravated.

**pro·ar·rhyth·mic** (pro"ə-rith'mik) inducing or aggravating arrhythmia.

**pro·at·las** (pro-at'ləs) a rudimentary vertebra that lies in front of the atlas in certain vertebrates; sometimes seen as an anomaly in humans.

**pro·az·amine chlo·ride** (pro-az'ə-mēn) promethazine hydrochloride.

**prob·a·bil·i·ty** (prob"ə-bil'ĭ-te) [*probabilis* probable, from *probare* to test or examine] [MeSH: Probability] the likelihood of occurrence of a specified event; it is often represented as a number between 0 (never) and 1 (always) that corresponds to the long-run trial at which an event occurs in a sequence of random independent trials under identical conditions, as the number of trials approaches infinity. Symbol *P.*
**significance p.,** *P* value.

**pro·bac·te·rio·phage** (pro"bak-te're-o-fāj") prophage.

**pro·band** (pro'band) [Ger.; from L. *probandus* "the one to be tested"] an affected person ascertained independently of his relatives in a genetic study. Called also *propositus.*

**pro·bang** (pro'bang) a flexible rod with a ball, tuft, or sponge at one end; used in applying medications to or removing matter from the esophagus or larynx.

**Pro-Ban·thine** (pro-ban-thīn') trademark for preparations of propantheline bromide.

**pro·bar·bi·tal** (pro-bahr'bĭ-təl) a barbiturate of intermediate duration, used as a sedative in the form of its calcium and sodium salts.

**probe** (prōb) [L. *proba; probare* to test] 1. a slender, flexible instrument designed for introduction into a wound, cavity, or sinus tract for purposes of exploration. 2. a radioactive or chemiluminescent DNA or RNA sequence used to detect the presence of a complementary sequence by molecular hybridization (q.v.). DNA probes are used clinically to detect and identify infectious disease agents.
**Anel's p.,** a delicate probe for the lacrimal puncta and canals.
**blood flow p.,** an implanted cuff that fits around a surgically exposed artery or vein to detect blood flow.
**blunt p.,** a probe with a blunt end.
**Bowman's p.,** one of a set of probes for use on the nasolacrimal ducts.
**Brackett's p's,** delicate and flexible probes of silver wire for exploring dental fistulas.
**bullet p.,** one used for detecting the presence or determining the location of a bullet.
**drum p.,** a probe with an attachment that emits a sound when it comes in contact with a foreign body.
**electric p.,** one that on contact with a foreign body completes an electric circuit, thereby producing a sound.
**eyed p.,** one with a slit near one end through which a ligature or tape may be drawn.
**fiberoptic p.,** a flexible probe made up of a bundle of fine glass fibers optically aligned to transmit an image.
**lacrimal p.,** one designed for use on the lacrimal passages.
**oligonucleotide p.,** see *oligonucleotide.*
**periodontal p., pocket p.,** one graduated in millimeters, used to measure the depth and determine the outline of a periodontal pocket and the condition of the crevicular epithelium.
**root canal p.,** in root canal therapy, a hand-operated instrument consisting of a slender, flexible, smooth or edged wire, used for tracing the course of and exploring root canals. Called also *pathfinder, pathfinder broach,* and *smooth broach.*
**scissors p.,** a long, delicate pair of scissors that can be used as a probe.
**uterine p.,** a probe for uterine exploration.
**vertebrated p.,** a flexible probe made up of joined links.

**pro·ben·e·cid** (pro-ben'ə-sid) [USP] [MeSH: Probenecid] a uricosuric agent that acts by inhibiting the carrier-mediated transport of organic acids in the renal tubule, which increases the excretion of uric acid by blocking its tubular reabsorption and decreases the excretion of penicillins and certain other acidic drugs by blocking their tubular secretion; used in the treatment of hyperuricemia of gout and as an adjunct in penicillin therapy.

**pro·bit** (pro'bit) [contraction of "*prob*ability un*it*"] a normal variate having mean 5 and standard deviation 1. In quantal biologic assays, the observed responses are often converted to probits (the fraction responding is converted to the probit that cuts off the same fraction of the area under the normal frequency curve) in order to fit a linear log dose–response curve, a procedure based on the assumption that the response thresholds are normally distributed.

**pro·bos·cis** (pro-bos'is) [*pro-* + Gr. *boskein* to feed, graze] any tubular process or structure of the head or snout of an animal, usually used in feeding.
**p. latera'lis,** a rare congenital deformity marked by absence of the medial and lateral nasal processes and the globular processes; on the affected side, the nasal cavity, choana, and nasal bones are absent and there is a tubular appendage (proboscis) above the medial canthus.

**pro·bu·col** (pro'bu-kōl) [MeSH: Probucol] an anticholesteremic, used especially as an adjunct to diet for the reduction of elevated serum cholesterol in primary cholesterolemia, administered orally.

**pro·cain·amide hy·dro·chlo·ride** (pro-kān'ə-mīd) [USP] a cardiac depressant used in the treatment of cardiac arrhythmias, administered orally and intramuscularly, and by intravenous infusion. Called also *procaine amide hydrochloride.*

**pro·caine** (pro'kān) [MeSH: Procaine] a benzoic acid derivative with local anesthetic activity.
**p. amide hydrochloride,** procainamide hydrochloride.
**p. hydrochloride** [USP], the monohydrochloride salt of procaine; used to produce infiltration, epidural, and peripheral nerve block, and spinal anesthesia.
**p. penicillin G,** see under *penicillin.*

**pro·cal·lus** (pro-kal'əs) the granulation tissue formed about the site of fracture of a bone that develops into callus.

**Pro·can** (pro'kan) trademark for a preparation of procainamide hydrochloride.

**pro·car·ba·zine hy·dro·chlo·ride** (pro-kahr'bə-zēn) [USP] an alkylating agent specific for the S phase of the cell cycle used as an antineoplastic, primarily in combination with mechlorethamine, vincristine, and prednisone (MOPP) in the treatment of advanced Hodgkin's disease; it is also used in the treatment of non-Hodgkin's lymphoma, primary brain tumors, lung carcinoma, multiple myeloma, malignant melanoma, and polycythemia vera; administered orally.

**pro·car·boxy·pep·ti·dase** (pro"kahr-bok"se-pep'tĭ-dās) a proenzyme of a carboxypeptidase.

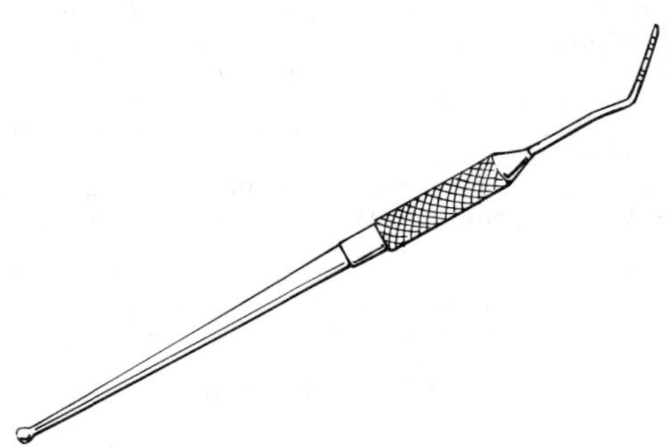

Periodontal probe, its tip marked in millimeter gradations.

**pro·car·cin·o·gen** (pro″kahr-sin′ə-jən) a chemical substance that becomes carcinogenic only after it is altered by metabolic processes.

**Pro·car·dia** (pro-kahr′de-ə) trademark for a preparation of nifedipine.

**pro·cary·on** (pro-kar′e-on) prokaryon.

**pro·caryo·sis** (pro″kar-e-o′sis) prokaryosis.

**Pro·caryo·tae** (pro-kar″e-o′te) [*pro-* + Gr. *karyon* nut, kernel] a kingdom comprising all prokaryotic organisms and consisting of cellular organisms that lack a true nucleus (the bacteria). In one system of classification, it has two subdivisions, Cyanobacteria and Bacteria. In another system, the two subdivisions are Photobacteria and Scotobacteria. More recently the prokaryotes have been arranged in four divisions based on biochemical and phylogenetic analysis and the presence or absence and type of their cell walls: I. Gracilicutes (those with thick, gram-negative–type cell walls); II. Firmicutes (those with thick, strong, gram-positive–type cell walls); III. Tenericutes (those without a cell wall); and IV. Mendosicutes (those with faulty cell walls).

**pro·cary·ote** (pro-kar′e-ōt) prokaryote.

**pro·cary·ot·ic** (pro″kar-e-ot′ik) prokaryotic.

**Pro·ca·via** (pro-ka′ve-ə) a genus of rock hyraxes that live in deserts and hilly regions of Africa and the Middle East; they are common reservoirs for *Leishmania aethiopica,* the cause of Ethiopian cutaneous leishmaniasis.

**pro·ce·dure** (pro-se′jər) [L. *procedere,* from *pro* forward + *cedere* move] [MeSH: Methods] a series of steps by which a desired result is accomplished. See also under *maneuver, method, operation, surgery,* and *technique.*

**abdomino-Peña pull-through p.,** for urinary continence used in treatment of cloacal exstrophy

**Anderson p.,** reconstruction of the hypopharynx and cervical esophagus by the use of bilateral rectangular flaps.

**arterial switch p.,** a one-stage method for anatomical correction of transposition of great arteries, in which both coronary arteries are transposed to the posterior artery, and the aorta and pulmonary arteries are transected, contraposed, and anastomosed.

**endocardial resection p. (ERP),** surgical removal of a portion of left ventricular endocardium and underlying myocardium containing an arrhythmogenic area (as determined by intraoperative cardiac mapping) from the base of an aneurysm or infarction; done to relieve ventricular tachycardia in patients with ischemic heart disease.

**endorectal pull-through p.,** ileoanal pull-through p.

**extended endocardial resection p. (EERP),** surgical removal of all visible endocardial fibrosis around the base of a left ventricular aneurysm; done to relieve ventricular tachycardia in patients with ischemic heart disease in whom intraoperative cardiac mapping is not possible.

**Fick p.,** see under *method.*

**Fontan p.,** functional correction of tricuspid atresia by anastomosis of, or insertion of a nonvalved prosthesis between, the right atrium and the pulmonary artery with closure of the interatrial communication; it is also used in other selected congenital conditions.

**Fulkerson's p.,** a modification of Maquet's procedure in which the tibial tubercle pedicle is shifted medially as well as elevated and held in place with a screw.

**Gomori-Takamatsu p.,** a method for localizing the alkaline phosphatase enzyme: a tissue secretion is incubated in a buffered solution containing the substrate, glycerophosphate, and calcium ions; hydrolysis of the substrate releases phosphoric acid, and it combines with calcium and precipitates as calcium phosphate. This colorless precipitate is converted to brown cobalt sulfide, which is readily visualized with the microscope.

**Hartmann's p.,** resection of a diseased portion of the colon, with the proximal end of the colon brought out as a colostomy and the distal stump or rectum being closed by suture. Bowel continuity can later be restored. Called also *Hartmann's colostomy* or *operation.*

**ileoanal pull-through p.,** see under *anastomosis.*

**Jannetta p.,** microvascular decompression.

**Kock p.,** see under *ileostomy.*

**Ladd's p.,** surgical cutting of Ladd's bands to correct intestinal malrotation and obstruction.

**MAGPI p.,** surgical correction of hypospadias with chordee by meatoplasty and glanuloplasty to advance the meatal orifice distally.

**Maquet's p.,** anterior displacement of the tibial tubercle by creation of a long pedicle of tibial tubercle, which is elevated and held in place by a bone graft taken from the iliac crest; done for relief of severe patellofemoral pain.

**maze p.,** the surgical division of the normal conduction pathways between the sinoatrial node and the atrioventricular node by a series of incisions in the left atrium to create a maze of conduction pathways; its purpose is to allow a normal impulse to activate the atrium while eliminating macroreentrant circuits; done for the relief of atrial fibrillation.

**Mitrofanoff's p.,** for urinary continence, used in treatment of cloacal exstrophy

**push-back p.,** see under *technique.*

**Rovsing's p.,** surgical unroofing of renal cysts followed by aspiration of their fluid.

**Sugiura p.,** esophageal transection with paraesophageal devascularization and devascularization of the abdominal esophagus and proximal stomach; performed for the treatment of bleeding esophageal varices.

**Thal p.,** fundoplication of less than the entire circumference of the lower esophagus; done to correct a benign stricture or gastroesophageal reflux.

**V-Y p.,** a method of repairing a skin defect in which a V-shaped flap is made proximal to the defect; the flap is transferred to the defect, and the secondary defect thus created is closed to produce a Y-shaped scar.

**Whipple p.,** radical pancreatoduodenectomy with removal of the distal third of the stomach, the entire duodenum, and the head of the pancreas, with gastrojejunostomy, choledochojejunostomy, and pancreaticojejunostomy.

**Womack p.,** splenectomy with resection of the superior half of the greater curvature of the stomach, devascularization, and transgastric suturing of the varices; performed for variceal bleeding resulting from portal hypertension.

**Young-Dees-Leadbetter p.,** repositioning of the ureters to a more superior position on the bladder and construction of a new bladder neck sphincter using the trigonal muscle; done for the treatment of urinary incontinence.

**pro·ce·lous** (pro-se′ləs) [*pro-* + *cel-*[2] + *-ous*] concave on the anterior surface; said of the vertebral centra of certain animals.

**pro·cen·tri·ole** (pro-sen′tre-ol) the immediate precursor of centrioles and ciliary basal bodies; it is developed in proximity to either a preexisting centriole or a deuterosome.

**pro·ce·phal·ic** (pro″sə-fal′ik) [*pro-* + *cephal-* + *-ic*] pertaining to the anterior part of the head.

**pro·cer·coid** (pro-ser′koid) one of the larval stages of fish tapeworms.

**pro·ce·rus** (pro-se′rəs) [L.] long; slender.

**proc·ess** (pros′es; pro′ses) [L. *processus*] 1. a prominence or projection, as of bone; for names of specific anatomic structures not found here, see official terms under *processus.* 2. a series of operations, events, or steps leading to the achievement of a specific result; used also as a verb to designate subjection to such a series designed to produce desired changes in the original material, or achieve other result.

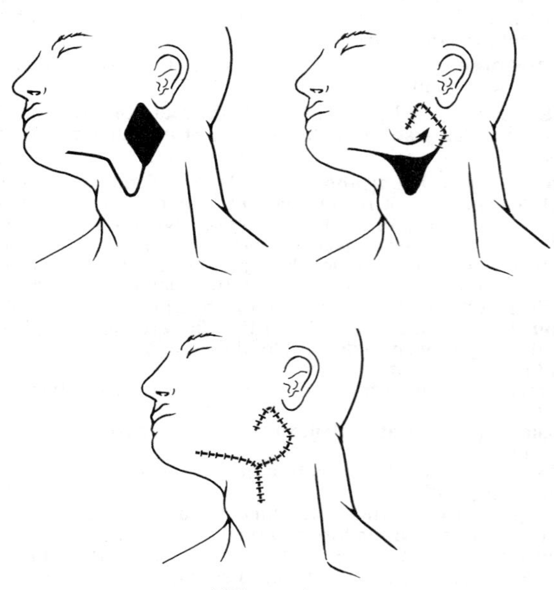

V-Y procedure.

## Process

For descriptions of specific anatomic structures not listed here, see under *processus.*

**A.B.C. p.**, see under *method.*
**accessory p. of sacrum, spurious,** crista sacralis lateralis.
**acromial p., acromion p.,** acromion.
**alar p. of sacrum,** crista sacralis lateralis.
**alveolar p.,** that portion of bone in either the maxilla or the mandible which surrounds and supports the teeth. In the maxilla, it is called *processus alveolaris maxillae* (q.v.); in the mandible, *pars alveolaris mandibulae.*
**anconeal p. of ulna,** olecranon.
**articular p. of axis, anterior,** facies articularis anterior axis.
**articular p. of coccyx, false,** cornu coccygeum.
**articular p. of sacrum, spurious,** crista sacralis medialis.
**ascending p. of vertebra,** see *processus articularis superior vertebra.*
**axillary p. of mammary gland,** processus axillaris glandulae mammariae.
**basilar p.,** pars basilaris ossis occipitalis.
**calcaneal p. of cuboid bone, calcanean p. of cuboid bone,** processus calcaneus ossis cuboidei.
**capitular p.,** the articular process on a vertebra for the head of a rib.
**caudate p.,** processus caudatus hepatis.
**ciliary p's,** processus ciliares.
**Civinini's p. of external pterygoid plate,** processus pterygospinosus.
**clinoid p.,** any of three processes of the sphenoid bone; see *processus clinoideus anterior, medius,* and *posterior.*
**condyloid p. of vertebra, inferior,** processus articularis inferior vertebrae.
**condyloid p. of vertebra, superior,** processus articularis superior vertebrae.
**conoid p.,** tuberculum conoideum.
**coracoid p.,** processus coracoideus scapulae.
**coronoid p.,** see *processus coronoideus mandibulae* and *ulnae.*
**costal p.,** processus costiformis.
**cubital p. of humerus,** see *trochlea humeri* and *capitulum humeri.*
**Deiters' p.,** axon, def. 2.
**dendritic p.,** dendrite.
**dental p.,** processus alveolaris maxillae.
**dentoid p. of axis,** dens axis.
**descending p. of vertebra,** see *processus articularis inferior vertebrae.*
**ensiform p. of sphenoid bone,** ala minor ossis sphenoidalis.
**ensiform p. of sternum,** processus xiphoideus.
**epiphyseal p.,** epiphysis.
**falciform p. of fascia lata,** margo falciformis hiatus saphenus.
**falciform p. of pelvic fascia,** arcus tendineus fasciae pelvis.
**falciform p. of rectus abdominis muscle,** falx inguinalis.
**folian p., p. of Folius,** processus anterior mallei.
**foot p.,** pedicel.
**frontonasal p.,** former name for the frontonasal prominence.
**funicular p.,** the portion of the tunica vaginalis surrounding the spermatic cord.
**hamate p. of ethmoid bone,** processus uncinatus ossis ethmoidalis.
**hamular p. of lacrimal bone,** hamulus lacrimalis.
**hamular p. of sphenoid bone,** hamulus pterygoideus.
**hamular p. of unciform bone,** hamulus ossis hamati.
**head p.,** an axial strand of cells in the embryo extending forward from the primitive knot; called also *notochordal plate.*
**inframalleolar p. of calcaneus,** trochlea fibularis calcanei.
**intercondylar p. of tibia,** eminentia intercondylaris.
**internal p. of humerus,** processus supracondylaris humeri.
**jugular p. of occipital bone, lateral,** processus paramastoideus ossis occipitalis.
**jugular p. of occipital bone, middle,** processus intrajugularis ossis occipitalis.
**lacrimal p., lacrimal p. of inferior nasal concha,** processus lacrimalis conchae nasalis inferioris.
**lateral p. of calcaneus,** sustentaculum tali.
**lateral p. of cartilage of nasal septum,** processus lateralis cartilaginis septi nasi.
**lateral p. of mammary gland,** processus axillaris glandulae mammariae.
**long p. of incus,** crus longum incudis.
**malar p.,** processus zygomaticus maxillae.
**mammillary p. of lumbar vertebra,** processus mammillaris.
**mammillary p's of sacrum, oblique,** see *crista sacralis intermedia.*
**mandibular p.,** former name for the mandibular prominence.
**marginal p. of zygomatic bone,** tuberculum marginale ossis zygomatici.
**mastoid p.,** processus mastoideus ossis temporalis.
**maxillary p.,** former name for the maxillary prominence.
**mental p.,** protuberantia mentalis.
**nasal p., lateral,** former name for the lateral nasal prominence.
**nasal p., medial, nasal p., median,** former name for the medial nasal prominence.
**nasal p. of frontal bone,** pars nasalis ossis frontalis.
**p. of nerve cell, p. of neuron,** a threadlike or cordlike cytoplasmic extension of a nerve cell body; see *axon* (def. 1) and *dendrite.*
**oblique p. of vertebra, inferior,** processus articularis inferior vertebrae.
**oblique p. of vertebra, superior,** processus articularis superior vertebrae.
**occipital p. of occipital bone,** pars basilaris ossis occipitalis.
**p. of odontoblast, odontoblastic p.,** one of the slender protoplasmic processes in a dentinal tubule, which is a cytoplasmic extension of the cell body; odontoblastic processes extend from the dentinoenamel junction and cementodentinal junction to the cell bodies of odontoblasts in the dental pulp. Called also *dentinal fiber* and *Tomes' fiber* or *fibril.*
**odontoid p. of axis,** dens axis.
**olecranon p. of ulna,** olecranon.
**palatine p., lateral,** a shelflike projection developing from the medial aspect of each maxillary prominence of the upper jaw in the embryo, later fusing with each other and with the nasal septum to form the palate.
**palatine p., median,** a shelflike projection developing from each median nasal prominence in the embryo, which participates with its fellow in forming the premaxillary portion of the upper jaw.
**paracondyloid p. of occipital bone, paroccipital p. of occipital bone,** processus paramastoideus ossis occipitalis.
**paramastoid p. of occipital bone,** processus paramastoideus ossis occipitalis.
**posterior p. of cartilage of nasal septum,** processus posterior cartilaginis septi nasi.
**pterygoid p.,** processus pterygoideus ossis sphenoidalis.
**Rau's p., ravian p.,** processus anterior mallei.
**short p. of incus,** crus breve incudis.
**short p. of malleus,** processus lateralis mallei.
**sphenoidal p. of cartilage of nasal septum,** processus posterior cartilaginis septi nasi.
**spinous p.,** a slender, more or less sharp-pointed projection; see *spina.*
**spinous p. of sacrum, spurious,** crista sacralis mediana.
**spinous p. of tibia,** 1. eminentia intercondylaris. 2. tuberculum intercondylare mediale.
**Stieda's p.,** processus posterior tali.
**styloid p. of fibula,** apex capitis fibulae.
**sucker p.,** pericapillary end foot.
**synovial p.,** plica synovialis.
**temporal p. of mandible,** processus coronoideus mandibulae.
**Todd's p.,** see *fibrae intercrurales.*
**Tomes' p.,** 1. [Charles Sissmore Tomes] a finger-like projection of the ameloblast, occurring during the secretory phase of the cell during amelogenesis, which extends from the point of separation of the adjacent cell membrane to the distal free surface. 2. [Sir John Tomes] p. of odontoblast.
**transverse p. of sacrum,** crista sacralis lateralis.
**transverse p. of vertebrae, accessory,** processus accessorius.
**trochlear p. of calcaneus,** trochlea fibularis calcanei.
**unciform p. of scapula,** processus coracoideus scapulae.
**uncinate p. of cervical vertebra,** uncus corporis vertebrae cervicalis.
**uncinate p. of ethmoid bone,** processus uncinatus ossis ethmoidalis.
**uncinate p. of pancreas,** processus uncinatus pancreatis.
**uncinate p. of unciform bone,** hamulus ossis hamati.
**ungual p. of third phalanx of foot,** tuberositas phalangis distalis pedis.
**vermiform p.,** appendix vermiformis.

**pro·ces·sus** (pro-ses′əs) pl. *proces′sus* [L.] [TA] a process: a prominence or projection; in anatomical terminology, a general term for such a mass projecting from a larger structure.

## Processus

Descriptions are given on TA terms, and include anglicized names of specific processes.

**p. accesso'rius** [TA], accessory process: a small nodule that projects backward from the posterior surface of the transverse process and lateral to and below the mammillary process of a lumbar vertebra. Such a process also occurs on the tenth, eleventh, and twelfth thoracic vertebrae.

**p. accesso'rii spu'rii,** crista sacralis lateralis.

**p. alveola'ris maxil'lae** [TA], alveolar process of maxilla: the thick parabolically curved ridge that projects downward and forms the free lower border of the maxilla; it is in front of and lateral to the palatine process and it bears the teeth. Called also *dental process.*

**p. ante'rior mal'lei** [TA], **p. ante'rior mal'lei [Fo'lii],** anterior process of malleus: a slender bony process that arises from the anterior aspect of the neck of the malleus, passes anteriorly and inferiorly to the petrotympanic fissure, and is attached to the petrous portion of the temporal bone by ligamentous fibers. Called also *apophysis of Rau, p. gracilis, process of Folius, long process of malleus,* and *Rau's* or *ravian process.*

**p. articula'ris infe'rior ver'tebrae** [TA], inferior articular process of vertebra: a process on either side of a vertebra, springing from the inferior surface of the arch near the junction of the lamina and pedicle; it bears a surface that faces anteriorly and inferiorly, articulating with the superior articular process of the vertebra below. Called also *zygapophysis inferior* [TA alternative].

**p. articula'ris supe'rior os'sis sa'cri** [TA], superior articular process of sacrum: either of two processes projecting backward and medialward from the first sacral vertebra at the junctions between the body and the alae; they articulate with the inferior articular processes of the fifth lumbar vertebra.

**p. articula'ris supe'rior ver'tebrae** [TA], superior articular process of vertebra: a process on either side of a vertebra, springing from the superior surface of the arch near the junction of the lamina and pedicle; it bears a surface that faces posteriorly and superiorly, articulating with the inferior articular process of the vertebra above. Called also *zygapophysis superior* [TA alternative].

**p. axilla'ris glan'dulae mamma'riae** [TA], axillary process of mammary gland: the superolateral part of the mammary gland that extends toward the axilla; called also *lateral process of mammary gland, axillary tail,* and *p. lateralis glandulae mammariae* [TA alternative].

**p. bre'vis mal'lei,** p. lateralis mallei.

**p. calca'neus os'sis cuboi'dei** [TA], calcaneal process of cuboid bone: a process projecting posteriorly from the inferomedial angle of the cuboid bone that supports the anterior calcaneus; called also *calcanean process of cuboid bone.*

**p. cauda'tus he'patis** [TA], caudate process: the right of the two processes seen on the caudate lobe of the liver.

**p. cilia'res** [TA], ciliary processes: about 70 meridionally arranged ridges or folds projecting from the crown of the ciliary body; they secrete the aqueous humor into the posterior chamber of the eye.

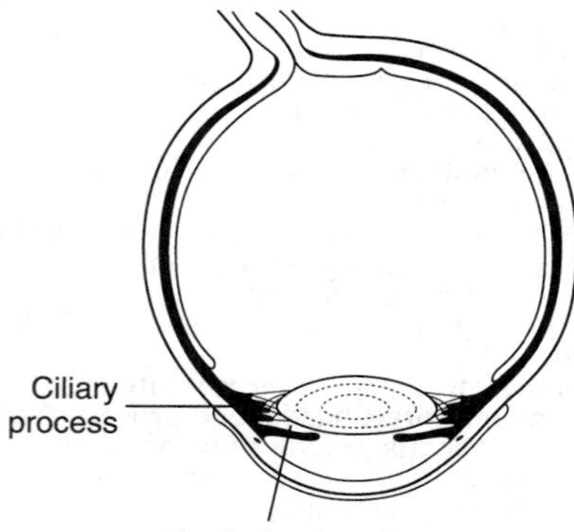


**p. clinoi'deus ante'rior** [TA], anterior clinoid process: the bony process found on the medial extremity of the posterior border of the lesser wing of the sphenoid bone.

**p. clinoi'deus me'dius** [TA], middle clinoid process: either of two small inconstant eminences on the internal surface of the sphenoid bone, one on either side of the anterior part of the hypophyseal fossa.

**p. clinoi'deus poste'rior** [TA], posterior clinoid process: either of two tubercles found on the superior angle of either side of the dorsum sellae of the sphenoid bone, and giving attachment to the tentorium of the cerebellum.

**p. cochlearifor'mis** [TA], cochleariform process: a small hollow cone of bone at the end of the septum canalis musculotubarii, just anterior to the vestibular window, with an opening through which the tendon of the tensor tympani passes.

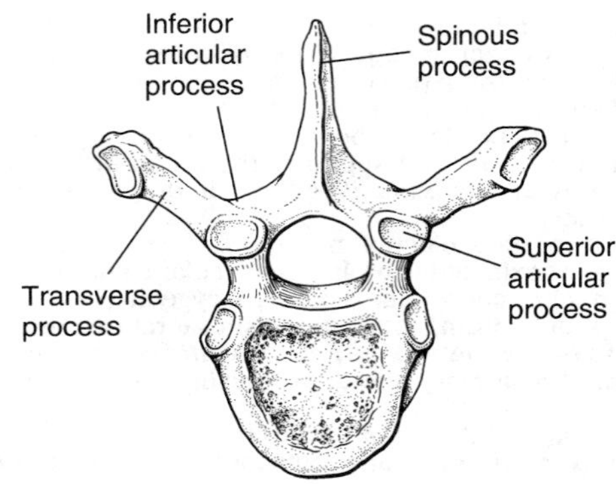


Processes of a thoracic vertebra.

**p. condyla'ris mandi'bulae** [TA], **p. condyloi'deus mandi'bulae,** condylar process of mandible: the posterior process on the ramus of the mandible that articulates with the mandibular fossa of the temporal bone.

**p. coracoi'deus sca'pulae** [TA], coracoid process of scapula: a strong curved process that arises from the upper part of the neck of the scapula and overhangs the shoulder joint.

**p. coronoi'deus mandi'bulae** [TA], coronoid process of mandible: the anterior part of the upper end of the ramus of the mandible, to which the temporal muscle is attached.

**p. coronoi'deus ul'nae** [TA], coronoid process of ulna: a wide eminence at the proximal end of the ulna, forming the anterior and inferior part of the trochlear incisure.

**p. costa'lis ver'tebrae,** TA alternative for *p. costiformis.*

**p. costifor'mis** [TA], costal process: a process that projects laterally from the transverse process of a lumbar vertebra and resembles a rib. Called also *p. costalis* [TA alternative].

**p. ethmoida'lis con'chae nasa'lis inferio'ris** [TA], ethmoidal process of inferior nasal concha: a bony projection above and behind the maxillary process of the inferior nasal concha.

**p. falcifor'mis ligamen'ti sacrotubera'lis** [TA], falciform process of sacrotuberal ligament: a prolongation of the sacrotuberal ligament, continuing forward along the inner border of the ramus of the ischium from the point of attachment of the ligament on the tuber of the ischium.

**p. Ferrei'ni lo'buli cortica'lis re'nis,** pars radiata lobuli corticalis renis.

**p. fronta'lis maxil'lae** [TA], frontal process of maxilla: a large, strong, irregular process of bone that projects upward from the body of the maxilla, its medial surface forming part of the lateral wall of the nasal cavity.

**p. fronta'lis os'sis zygoma'tici** [TA], **p. frontosphenoida'lis os'sis zygoma'tici,** frontal process of zygomatic bone: the strong, superiorly projecting triangular process of the zygomatic bone lying posterior to the malar surface and between the orbital and temporal surfaces; it unites superiorly with the zygomatic process of the frontal bone and posteriorly with the greater wing of the sphenoid bone.

**p. gra'cilis,** p. anterior mallei.

**p. intrajugula'ris os'sis occipita'lis** [TA], intrajugular process of occipital bone: a small process that subdivides the jugular notch of the occipital bone into a lateral and a medial part.

**p. intrajugula'ris os'sis tempora'lis** [TA], intrajugular process of temporal bone: a small ridge on the petrous part of the temporal bone that separates the jugular notch into a medial and a lateral part, corresponding to similar parts of the jugular notch of the facing occipital bone.

**p. jugula'ris os'sis occipita'lis** [TA], jugular process of occipital bone: either of two processes on the occipital bone that project laterally from the occipital condyles and form the posterior boundary of the jugular foramen.

**p. lacrima'lis con'chae nasa'lis inferio'ris** [TA], lacrimal process of inferior nasal concha: a process of the inferior nasal concha that articulates with the lacrimal bone.

**p. latera'lis cartila'ginis sep'ti na'si** [TA], lateral process of cartilage of nasal septum: a lateral expansion of the septal cartilage on either side of the nose, fused with the lateral nasal cartilage.

**p. latera'lis glan'dulae mamma'riae,** TA alternative for *p. axillaris glandulae mammariae.*

**p. latera'lis mal'lei** [TA], lateral process of malleus: a small tapered process that projects laterally from the base of the manubrium mallei and produces the mallear prominence.

**p. latera'lis ta'li** [TA], lateral process of talus: a large low process on the lateral surface of the talus, articulating with the lateral malleolus.

**p. latera'lis tu'beris calca'nei** [TA], lateral process of tuberosity of calcaneus: a rough process projecting downward from the lower lateral portion of the tuber calcanei.

**p. lenticula'ris incu'dis** [TA], lenticular process of incus: a small process on the medial side of the tip of the long limb of the incus, which articulates with the head of the stapes.

**p. mammilla'ris** [TA], mammillary process: a tubercle on each superior articular process of the lumbar vertebrae and on the tenth, eleventh, and twelfth thoracic vertebrae.

**p. mastoi'deus os'sis tempora'lis** [TA], mastoid process of temporal bone: a conical process projecting forward and downward from the external surface of the petrous part of the temporal bone just posterior to the external acoustic meatus.

**p. maxilla'ris con'chae nasa'lis inferio'ris** [TA], maxillary process of inferior nasal concha: a bony process descending from the ethmoid process of the inferior nasal concha.

**p. media'lis tu'beris calca'nei** [TA], medial process of tuberosity of calcaneus: a rough process projecting downward from the lower medial portion of the tuber calcanei.

**p. muscula'ris cartila'ginis arytenoi'deae** [TA], muscular process of arytenoid cartilage: the lateral and posterior lower angular projection of the arytenoid cartilage to which the cricoarytenoid muscles are attached.

**p. orbita'lis os'sis palati'ni** [TA], orbital process of palatine bone: a pyramidal process on the uppermost part of the palatine bone, one surface of it forming the posterior angle of the floor of the orbit.

**p. palati'nus maxil'lae** [TA], palatine process of maxilla: a horizontally arched plate of bone that helps to form the lower part of the maxilla and with its fellow of the opposite side the anterior two thirds of the hard palate.

**p. papilla'ris he'patis** [TA], papillary process of liver: the left of the two processes seen on the caudate lobe of the liver.

**p. paramastoi'deus os'sis occipita'lis** [TA], paramastoid process of occipital bone: a process that in humans is represented by a tubercle on the inferior surface of the jugular process.

**p. poste'rior cartila'ginis sep'ti na'si** [TA], posterior process of cartilage of nasal septum: a narrow flat strip of cartilage that extends backward and upward along the groove on the upper margin of the vomer and below the perpendicular plate of the ethmoid bone, from the septal cartilage nearly to the sphenoid bone. Called also *p. sphenoidalis cartilaginis septi nasi* [TA alternative] and *sphenoidal process of cartilage of nasal septum.*

**p. poste'rior ta'li** [TA], posterior process of talus: a backward projection from the posterior portion of the talus, divided into two unequal parts by the sulcus tendinis musculi flexoris hallucis longi tali.

**p. pterygoi'deus os'sis sphenoida'lis** [TA], pterygoid process of sphenoid bone: either of two processes on the sphenoid bone descending from the points of junction of the greater wings and body of the bone, and each consisting of a lateral and a medial plate (see *lamina lateralis processus pterygoidei* and *lamina medialis processus pterygoidei*).

**p. pterygospino'sus** [TA], **p. pterygospino'sus [Civini'ni],** pterygospinous process: a small spine on the posterior edge of the lateral pterygoid plate of the sphenoid bone, giving attachment to the pterygospinous ligament.

**p. pyramida'lis os'sis palati'ni** [TA], pyramidal process of palatine bone: a strong process projecting downward, backward, and laterally from the lateral part of the posterior margin of the palatine bone and helping to form the pterygoid fossa.

**p. retromandibula'ris glan'dulae paro'tidis,** an irregularly wedge-shaped portion of the parotid gland passing medially behind the ramus of the mandible almost to the wall of the pharynx.

**p. sphenoida'lis cartila'ginis sep'ti na'si,** TA alternative for *p. posterior cartilaginis septi nasi.*

**p. sphenoida'lis os'sis palati'ni** [TA], sphenoid process of palatine bone: an irregular mass of bone that projects superiorly and medially from the posterior portion of the superior margin of the perpendicular portion of the palatine bone, and articulates with the body of the sphenoid bone and with the ala vomeris.

**p. spino'sus ver'tebrae** [TA], spinous process of vertebra: a part of the vertebra projecting backward from the arch, giving attachment to muscles of the back.

**p. styloi'deus fi'bulae,** apex capitis fibulae.

**p. styloi'deus os'sis metacarpa'lis III,** TA alternative for *p. styloideus ossis metacarpi III.*

**p. styloi'deus os'sis metacar'pi III** [TA], styloid process of third metacarpal bone: a prominent process projecting proximally from the base of the third metacarpal bone. Called also *p. styloideus ossis metacarpalis III* [TA alternative].

**p. styloi'deus os'sis tempora'lis** [TA], styloid process of temporal bone: a long spine projecting inferiorly from the inferior surface of the temporal bone just anterior to the stylomastoid foramen, giving attachment to three muscles and two ligaments.

**p. styloi'deus ra'dii** [TA], styloid process of radius: a blunt projection from the lateral surface of the distal end of the radius.

**p. styloi'deus ul'nae** [TA], styloid process of ulna: the medial, nonarticular process on the distal extremity of the ulna.

**p. supracondyla'ris hu'meri** [TA], **p. supracondyloi'deus hu'meri,** supracondylar process of humerus: a small inconstant process just proximal to the medial epicondyle of the humerus, giving rise to the ligament of Struthers.

**p. tempora'lis os'sis zygoma'tici** [TA], temporal process of zygomatic bone: the posterior blunt process of the zygomatic bone that articulates with the zygomatic process of the temporal bone to form the zygomatic arch.

**p. transver'sus ver'tebrae** [TA], transverse process of vertebra: a process on either side of a vertebra, projecting laterally from the junction between the lamina and the pedicle.

**p. trochlea'ris calca'nei,** trochlea fibularis calcanei.

**p. tuba'rius,** an angular process that projects posteriorly from the middle of the posterior edge of the medial pterygoid plate of the sphenoid bone; it provides support for the pharyngeal end of the auditory tube.

**p. uncina'tus os'sis ethmoida'lis** [TA], uncinate process of ethmoid bone: a curved plate of bone that extends inferiorly and posteriorly from the anterior part of the ethmoid labyrinth.

**p. uncina'tus pancre'atis** [TA], uncinate process of pancreas: the left and caudal part of the head of the pancreas, which hooks around behind the pancreatic vessels; called also *lesser pancreas* and *Willis'* or *Winslow's pancreas.*

**p. vagina'lis os'sis sphenoida'lis** [TA], vaginal process of sphenoid bone: a small plate on the inferior surface of the body of the sphenoid bone on either side, running medially from the medial pterygoid plate to articulate with the ala of the vomer and with the sphenoid process of the palatine bone.

**p. vagina'lis peritone'i,** a diverticulum of the peritoneal membrane extending into the inguinal canal, accompanying the round ligament in the female, or the testis in its descent into the scrotum in the male *(processus vaginalis testis);* usually completely obliterated in the female. Called also *canal of Nuck* or *Nuck's diverticulum.*

**p. vermifor'mis,** appendix vermiformis.

**p. voca'lis** [TA], vocal process: the process of the arytenoid cartilage to which the vocal ligament is attached.

**p. xiphoi'deus** [TA], xiphoid process: the pointed process of cartilage, supported by a core of bone, connected with the lower end of the body of the sternum. Called also *ensiform, mucronate,* or *xiphoid cartilage; xiphoid bone;* and *xiphisternum.*

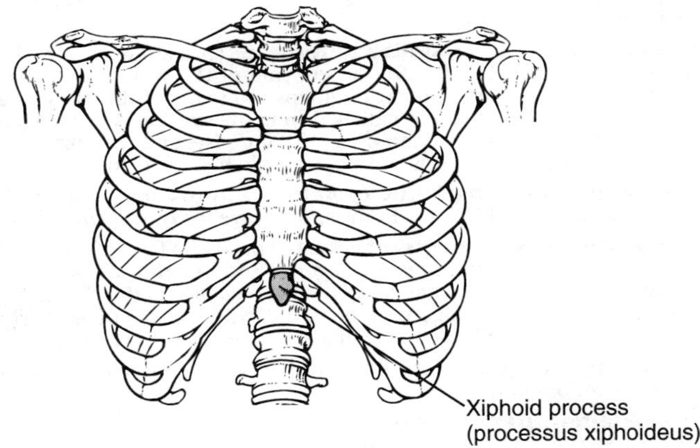


**p. zygoma'ticus maxil'lae** [TA], zygomatic process of maxilla: the rough triangular eminence that articulates with the zygomatic bone and marks the separation of the facies anterior, infratemporalis, and orbitalis.

**p. zygoma'ticus os'sis fronta'lis** [TA], zygomatic process of frontal bone: a thick, strong process of the frontal bone, situated at the lateral end of the supraorbital margin and articulating with the zygomatic bone, and from which the temporal line starts.

**p. zygoma'ticus os'sis tempora'lis** [TA], zygomatic process of temporal bone: a long, strong process arising from the inferior portion of the squamous part of the temporal bone, passing anteriorly from just superior to the entrance of the external acoustic meatus to join the zygomatic bone and thus forming the zygomatic arch. It has an anterior root and a posterior root extending along the temporal bone.

**pro·chei·lon** (pro-ki'lon) [*pro-* + Gr. *cheilon* lip] tuberculum labii superioris.

**Pro·chlo·ro·phy·ta** (pro"klo-ro-fi'tə) [*pro-* + *chloro-* + Gr. *phyton* plant] a subgroup of bacteria of the class Oxyphotobacteria, consisting of prokaryotic, unicellular, green, spheroid to ovoid organisms found associated with sea squirts in tropical coastal waters. They contain chlorophyll and are photosynthetic, using water as an electron donor and producing oxygen, and they fix carbon dioxide.

**pro·chlor·pem·a·zine** (pro"klor-pem'ə-zēn) prochlorperazine.

**pro·chlor·per·a·zine** (pro"klor-per'ə-zēn) [USP] [MeSH: Prochlorperazine] a phenothiazine derivative used chiefly as an antiemetic, administered rectally. Called also *prochlorpemazine*.
**p. edisylate** [USP], the ethanedisulfonate salt of prochlorperazine, used as an antiemetic and tranquilizer, administered orally, intramuscularly, and intravenously.
**p. maleate** [USP], the maleate salt of prochlorperazine, used as an antiemetic and tranquilizer, administered orally.

**pro·chon·dral** (pro-kon'drəl) occurring previous to the formation of cartilage.

**pro·chor·dal** (pro-kor'dəl) prechordal.

**pro·chro·mo·some** (pro-kro'mə-sōm) a chromosome-like body occurring in resting nuclei.

**pro·chy·mo·sin** (pro-ki'mo-sin) the inactive precursor of chymosin (rennin), converted to chymosin by pepsin or autocatalytically.

**pro·ci·den·tia** (pro"sĭ-den'shə) [L.] 1. prolapse. 2. specifically, prolapse of the uterus to such a degree that the cervix protrudes from the vaginal outlet.

**pro·co·ag·u·lant** (pro"ko-ag'u-lənt) 1. tending to favor the occurrence of coagulation. 2. a precursor of a natural substance necessary to coagulation of the blood.

**pro·col·la·gen** (pro-kol'ə-jən) [MeSH: Procollagen] the precursor molecule of collagen, synthesized in the fibroblast, osteoblast, etc., and cleaved to form collagen extracellularly.

**pro·col·la·gen C-en·do·pep·ti·dase** (pro-kol'ə-jən en"do-pep'tĭdās) [EC 3.4.24.19] an extracellular endopeptidase that catalyzes the cleavage of the C-terminal extension from procollagen, a step in the synthesis of collagen fibers. The enzyme does not require the procollagen substrate to be an intact trimer.

**pro·col·la·gen C-pro·tein·ase** (pro-kol'ə-jən pro'tēn-ās) procollagen C-endopeptidase.

**pro·col·la·gen ga·lac·to·syl·trans·fer·ase** (pro-kol'ə-jən gal"aktōs"əl-trans'fər-ās) [EC 2.4.1.50] an enzyme of the transferase class that catalyzes the attachment of galactose to hydroxylysine residues in the synthesis of collagen. The donor of the galactose moiety is UDPgalactose, and the enzyme is specific for collagen that is not yet in triple helical form.

**pro·col·la·gen glu·co·syl·trans·fer·ase** (pro-kol'ə-jən gloo"kosəl-trans'fər-ās) [EC 2.4.1.66] an enzyme of the transferase class that catalyzes the attachment of glucose to some of the galactose-containing hydroxylysine residues during the synthesis of collagen. The donor of the glucose moiety is UDPglucose, and the enzyme is specific for collagen that is not yet in triple helical form.

**pro·col·la·gen-ly·sine 5-di·oxy·gen·ase** (pro-kol'ə-jən li'sēn di-ok'sĭ-jən-ās) [EC 1.14.11.4] EC nomenclature for *lysyl hydroxylase*.

**pro·col·la·gen N-en·do·pep·ti·dase** (pro-kol'ə-jən en"do-pep'tĭdās) [EC 3.4.24.14] [MeSH: Procollagen N-Endopeptidase] an extracellular endopeptidase that catalyzes the cleavage of the N-terminal extension from procollagen, a step in the synthesis of collagen. The enzyme requires an intact procollagen trimer as a substrate.

**pro·col·la·gen N-pro·tein·ase** (pro-kol'ə-jən pro'tēn-ās) procollagen N-endopeptidase.

**pro·col·la·gen pep·ti·dase** (pro-kol'ə-jən pep'tĭ-dās) an endopeptidase that catalyzes the cleavage of specific terminal segments from procollagen chains, specifically used to denote procollagen N-endopeptidase (q.v.) and procollagen C-endopeptidase (q.v.).

**pro·col·la·gen-pro·line di·oxy·gen·ase** (pro-kol'ə-jən pro'lēn di-ok'sə-jən-ās) [EC 1.14.11.2] [MeSH: Procollagen-Proline Dioxygenase] EC nomenclature for *prolyl 4-hydroxylase*.

**pro·col·la·gen-pro·line 3-di·oxy·ge·nase** (pro-kol'ə-jən pro'lēn di-ok'sə-jən-ās) [EC 1.14.11.7] EC nomenclature for *prolyl 3-hydroxylase*.

**pro·con·cep·tive** (pro"kən-sep'tiv) 1. aiding or favoring conception. 2. an agent that facilitates or promotes conception.

**pro·con·ver·tin** (pro"kən-ver'tin) [MeSH: Factor VII] factor VII; see under *coagulation factors*, at *factor*.

**pro·cre·a·tion** (pro"kre-a'shən) [L. *procreatio*] the entire process of bringing a new individual into the world.

**pro·cre·a·tive** (pro'kre-a"tiv) concerned in procreation; able to beget.

**Pro·crit** (pro'krit) trademark for a preparation of epoetin alfa.

**proc·tal·gia** (prok-tal'jə) [*proct-* + *-algia*] neuralgia of the lower rectum.
**p. fu'gax**, episodic severe pain in the rectum, often awakening the individual at night; it is attributed to spasm of the levator ani and coccygeal muscles.

**proc·ta·tre·sia** (prok"tə-tre'zhə) [*proct-* + *atresia* ] imperforate anus.

**proc·tec·ta·sia** (prok"tek-ta'zhə) [*proct-* + *ectasia*] dilatation of the rectum or of the anus.

**proc·tec·to·my** (prok-tek'tə-me) [*proct-* + *ectomy*] surgical removal of the rectum.

**proc·ten·clei·sis** (prok"tən-kli'sis) [*proct-* + Gr. *enkleiein* to shut in] constriction, or stenosis, of the lower rectum; a rectal stricture.

**proc·teu·ryn·ter** (prok'tu-rin"tər) [*proct-* + Gr. *eurynein* to widen] a baglike device used in dilating the rectum.

**proc·teu·ry·sis** (prok-tu'rĭ-sis) dilatation of the rectum by means of a procteurynter.

**proc·ti·tis** (prok-ti'tis) [*proct-* + *-itis*] [MeSH: Proctitis] inflammation of the rectum.
**factitial p.**, radiation p.
**radiation p.**, radiation colitis in the rectum. Called also *factitial p.*
**ulcerative p.**, recurrent ulceration of the mucosa of the rectum, of unknown cause, probably a variant of ulcerative colitis.

**proct(o)-** [Gr. *prōktos* anus] a combining form designating relationship to the rectum.

**proc·to·cele** (prok'to-sēl) [*procto-* + *-cele*[1]] rectocele.

**proc·to·coc·cy·pexy** (prok"to-kok'sĭ-pek"se) [*procto-* + *coccyx* + *-pexy*] fixation of the rectum to the coccyx by sutures.

**proc·to·co·lec·to·my** (prok"to-ko-lek'tə-me) surgical removal of the rectum and colon. Called also *coloproctectomy*.

**proc·to·co·li·tis** (prok"to-ko-li'tis) [MeSH: Proctocolitis] inflammation of the colon and rectum; called also *coloproctitis* and *rectocolitis*.

**proc·to·co·lon·os·co·py** (prok"to-ko"lən-os'kə-pe) the inspection of the interior of the rectum and lower portion of the colon.

**proc·to·col·po·plas·ty** (prok"to-kol'po-plas"te) [*procto-* + *colpo-* + *-plasty*] operative repair of a rectovaginal fistula.

**proc·to·cys·to·plas·ty** (prok"to-sis'to-plas"te) [*procto-* + *cysto-* + *-plasty*] a plastic operation on the rectum and bladder; operative closure of a rectovesical fistula.

**proc·to·cys·tot·o·my** (prok"to-sis-tot'ə-me) [*procto-* + *cysto-* + *-tomy*] incision into the bladder from the rectum.

**proc·to·dae·um** (prok"to-de'əm) proctodeum.

**proc·to·de·um** (prok"to-de'əm) [*proct-* + Gr. *hodaios* pertaining to a way] an invagination of the surface ectoderm of the embryo at the point where later the anus is formed; called also *anal pit*.

**proc·to·dyn·ia** (prok"to-din'e-ə) [*proct-* + *-odynia*] pain in or about the anus.

**Proc·to·foam-HC** (prok'to-fōm) trademark for an aerosol foam containing 1 per cent hydrocortisone acetate and 1 per cent pramoxine hydrochloride; used to relieve anorectal inflammation, pain, swelling, and pruritus.

**proc·to·gen·ic** (prok"to-jen'ik) [*procto-* + *-genic*] derived from the anus or rectum.

**proc·tog·ra·phy** (prok-tog'rə-fe) radiography of the rectum, especially of its movements.

**proc·to·log·ic** (prok"to-loj'ik) pertaining to proctology.

**proc·tol·o·gist** (prok-tol'ə-jist) a physician who specializes in proctology.

**proc·tol·o·gy** (prok-tol'ə-je) [*procto-* + *-logy*] the branch of medicine concerned with disorders of the rectum and anus.

**proc·to·pa·ral·y·sis** (prok"to-pə-ral'ĭ-sis) [*procto-* + *paralysis*] paralysis of the muscles of the anus and rectum.

**proc·to·peri·neo·plas·ty** (prok"to-per"ĭ-ne'o-plas"te) plastic repair of the anus and perineum.

**proc·to·peri·ne·or·rha·phy** (prok"to-per"ĭ-ne-or'ə-fe) proctoperineoplasty.

**proc·to·pexy** (prok'to-pek"se) [*procto-* + *-pexy*] fixation of the rectum to some adjacent tissue or organ by suture.

**proc·to·plas·ty** (prok'to-plas"te) [*procto-* + *-plasty*] plastic surgery of the rectum.

**proc·to·ple·gia** (prok″to-ple′jə) [*procto-* + *-plegia*] proctoparalysis.

**proc·top·to·sis** (prok″top-to′sis) [*procto-* + *-ptosis*] prolapse of the anus.

**proc·tor·rha·gia** (prok″to-ra′jə) bleeding from the rectum.

**proc·tor·rha·phy** (prok-tor′ə-fe) [*procto-* + *-rrhaphy*] surgical repair of the rectum. Called also *rectorrhaphy.*

**proc·tor·rhea** (prok″to-re′ə) [*procto-* + *-rrhea*] a mucous discharge from the anus.

**proc·to·scope** (prok′to-skōp) [*procto-* + *-scope*] a speculum or tubular instrument with appropriate illumination for inspecting the rectum. Called also *rectoscope.*
**Tuttle's p.,** a rectal speculum with an electric light at its extremity and an arrangement for inflating the rectal ampulla.

**proc·tos·co·py** (prok-tos′kə-pe) [*procto-* + *-scopy*] [MeSH: Proctoscopy] inspection of the rectum with a proctoscope. Called also *rectoscopy.*

**proc·to·sig·moid** (prok″to-sig′moid) rectosigmoid.

**proc·to·sig·moi·dec·to·my** (prok″to-sig″moi-dek′tə-me) [*procto-* + *sigmoid* + *ectomy*] excision of the anus, rectum, and sigmoid flexure.

**proc·to·sig·moi·di·tis** (prok″to-sig″moi-di′tis) inflammation of the rectum and sigmoid colon.

**proc·to·sig·moi·do·scope** (prok″to-sig-moid′o-skōp) an instrument for illuminating and viewing the rectum and sigmoid colon. Called also *rectoromanoscope.*

**proc·to·sig·moi·dos·co·py** (prok″to-sig″moi-dos′kə-pe) examination of the rectum and sigmoid with the sigmoidoscope. Called also *rectoromanoscopy.*

**proc·to·spasm** (prok′to-spaz-əm) [*procto-* + *spasm*] spasm of the rectum.

**proc·tos·ta·sis** (prok-tos′tə-sis) [*procto-* + *-stasis*] constipation due to anesthesia of the rectum to the stimulus of defecation.

**proc·to·ste·no·sis** (prok″to-stə-no′sis) [*procto-* + *stenosis*] stricture of the rectum. Called also *rectostenosis.*

**proc·tos·to·my** (prok-tos′tə-me) [*procto-* + *-stomy*] surgical creation of an artificial opening from the body surface into the rectum.

**proc·to·tome** (prok′to-tōm) a knife for proctotomy.

**proc·tot·o·my** (prok-tot′ə-me) [*procto-* + *-tomy*] incision into the rectum, as for relief of rectal stricture.
**external p.,** that done at or below the sphincter.
**internal p.,** that done above the sphincter.

**pro·cum·bent** (pro-kum′bənt) prone.

**pro·cur·sive** (pro-kur′siv) [L. *procursivus*] characterized by a tendency to run forward.

**pro·cur·va·tion** (pro″kər-va′shən) [L. *procurvare* to bend forward] a bending forward, as of the body.

**pro·cu·ti·cle** (pro-ku′tĭ-kəl) [*pro-* + *cuticle*] the layer of the exoskeleton of certain crustaceans and arthropods beneath the epicuticle, which contains chitin as the principal constituent; it is composed of an endocuticle and an exocuticle.

**pro·cy·cli·dine hy·dro·chlo·ride** (pro-si′klĭ-dēn) [USP] a synthetic anticholinergic used as a skeletal muscle relaxant in the treatment of parkinsonism, administered orally.

**pro·do·lic ac·id** (pro-do′lik) an anti-inflammatory.

**pro·dro·ma** (pro-dro′mə) pl. *prodro′mata* [Gr. *prodromē* a running forward] prodrome.

**pro·dro·mal** (pro-dro′məl) premonitory; indicating the onset of a disease or morbid state.

**pro·dro·ma·ta** (pro-dro′mə-tə) [Gr.] plural of *prodroma.*

**pro·drome** (pro′drōm) [L. *prodromus;* Gr. *prodromos* forerunning] a premonitory symptom or precursor; a symptom indicating the onset of a disease.

**pro·dro·mic** (pro-dro′mik) prodromal.

**pro·drug** (pro′drəg) [*pro-* + *drug*] a compound that, on administration, must undergo chemical conversion by metabolic processes before becoming an active pharmacological agent; a precursor of a drug.

**prod·uct** (prod′əkt) something produced.
**advanced glycation end p's,** irreversible products of the glycation of proteins, causing tissue damage; seen when blood glucose concentrations are chronically elevated such as in diabetes mellitus and aging.
**Amadori p.,** a chemically reversible product formed by the combination of Schiff bases.
**cleavage p.,** a substance formed by the splitting of a compound molecule into simpler molecules.
**contact activation p.,** a product of the interaction of blood coagulation factors XII and XI, which functions to activate factor IX.
**decay p.,** a nuclide, which may be stable or radioactive, resulting from the radioactive disintegration of a radionuclide, being formed either directly or as the result of successive transformations in a radioactive series. Called also *daughter.*
**end p.,** the final product resulting from completion of a chain of metabolic reactions.
**fibrin degradation p's, fibrinogen degradation p's, fibrin split p's,** the protein fragments produced upon enzymatic digestion of fibrin and fibrinogen by plasmin. Abbreviated FDP.
**fission p.,** an isotope, usually radioactive, of an element in the middle of the periodic table, produced by fission of a heavy element, such as uranium, under bombardment by high energy particles.
**ion p.,** the product of the concentrations of ions in a chemical reaction, each raised to the power of its coefficient in the balanced reaction. The ion product of water, $K_W$, is a constant equivalent to $10^{-14}$ at 25°C.
**primary gene p.,** 1. a protein or polypeptide, frequently an enzyme, directly produced by transcription and translation of a gene, rather than by metabolic processing. 2. the unprocessed RNA molecule produced by transcription of a gene.
**solubility p.,** see under *constant.*
**spallation p's,** the many different chemical elements produced in small quantities in nuclear fission.
**substitution p.,** a chemical product obtained by substituting for one element in a molecule an atom or a radical of some other substance.

**pro·duc·tive** (pro-duk′tiv) producing or forming; said especially of an inflammation that produces new tissue or of a cough that brings forth sputum or mucus.

**pro·ec·dy·sis** (pro-ek′dĭ-sis) [*pro-* + *ecdysis*] the period of preparation for the process of ecdysis, during which the new cuticle is laid down and the old one ultimately detached from it.

**pro·emi·al** (pro-e′me-əl) [L. *prooemium* a prelude] prodromal.

**pro·en·ceph·a·lon** (pro″ən-sef′ə-lon) prosencephalon.

**pro·en·ceph·a·lus** (pro″ən-sef′ə-ləs) [*pro-* + Gr. *enkephalos* brain] a fetus with a frontal encephalocele.

**pro·en·zyme** (pro-en′zīm) an inactive precursor that can be converted to the active enzyme. Proenzymes, containing extra-long polypeptide chains that block activity, are activated by acid or enzymatic hydrolysis to remove the inhibiting portion.

**pro·eryth·ro·blast** (pro″ə-rith′ro-blast) [MeSH: Erythroblasts] the earliest of the immature forms recognizable as a precursor of the mature erythrocyte. It is round, with a large nucleus occupying most of the cell and surrounded by a small amount of cytoplasm that is a clear deep blue, often stains unevenly, and shows a pale perinuclear halo. The nucleus is round and reddish-purple with several nucleoli and consists of a network of fairly uniformly distributed chromatin strands that give it a finely reticular appearance. This term may be used to refer to cells in either normal or abnormal maturation, but some authorities limit it to those involved in normal maturation, in contrast to *promegaloblasts,* in which case it is a synonym of *pronormoblast.* Called also *rubriblast.*

**pro·eryth·ro·cyte** (pro″ə-rith′ro-sīt) any precursor of an erythrocyte; the term was not adopted by any scheme of red cell morphological development. See *erythrocytic series,* under *series.*

**pro·es·tro·gen** (pro-es′tro-jən) a substance that has no estrogenic activity itself but can be metabolized in the body to active estrogen.

**pro·es·trum** (pro-es′trəm) proestrus.

**pro·es·trus** (pro-es′trəs) [*pro-* + L. *oestrus*] [MeSH: Proestrus] in female mammals that have estrous cycles, the period of heightened follicular activity preceding estrus. Called also *proestrum.*

**Proetz test** (prōt′səz) [Arthur Walter *Proetz,* American otolaryngologist, 1888–1966] see under *test.*

**-profen** a suffix indicating an anti-inflammatory agent of the ibuprofen type (propionic acid derivatives).

**pro·fes·sion·al** (pro-fesh′ə-nəl) 1. pertaining to one's profession or occupation. 2. one who is a specialist in a particular field or occupation.
**allied health p.,** a person with special training and licensed when necessary, who works under the supervision of a health professional with responsibilities bearing on patient care. Called also *paraprofessional.*

**Pro·fes·sion·al Stan·dards Re·view Or·gan·i·za·tion (PSRO)** an organization of physicians, and in some cases allied health professionals, in a designated area, state, or community established to monitor health care services paid for through Medicare, Medicaid, and Maternal and Child Health programs to assure that services provided are medically necessary, meet professional standards, and are provided in the most economic medically appropriate health care agency or institution. The requirement for the establishment of PSRO's was added to the Social Security Amendments of 1972 (Public Law 92-603).

**pro·fi·bri·nol·y·sin** (pro″fi-brĭ-nol′ĭ-sin) plasminogen.

**Pro·fi·chet's syndrome** (pro″fe-shāz′) [Georges Charles *Profichet,* French physician, born 1873] see under *syndrome.*

**pro·file** (pro′fīl) 1. a simple outline of the shape or form of an object, such as the head or face, viewed from the side. 2. a graph, table, or other summary representing quantitatively a set of characteristics subjected to tests.
**antigenic p.,** the total antigenic content and structure of a tissue or cell.
**biophysical p.,** a numeric scoring system used to assess the well-being of the fetus in high-risk pregnancies, based on the nonstress test combined with sonographic evaluation of fetal breathing, fetal movements, fetal tone, amniotic fluid volume, and, sometimes, the echogenicity of the placenta.
**urethral pressure p.,** UPP; a record of the resistance of the urethra to fluid flow, measured as variations in urethral pressure (q.v.). A liquid or gas is pumped into the bladder with a catheter in place and the catheter is slowly withdrawn while measurements are taken of the pressure at various points in the urethra. It is usually done from the internal orifice to the external orifice in females and from the internal orifice to the sphincter urethrae muscle in males.

**pro·fil·in** (pro-fil′in) an actin-binding protein that forms a complex with G-actin and prevents it from polymerizing to form F-actin. It also binds to phosphatidylinositol bisphosphate, providing a link between actin organization and signal transduction. See also *gelsolin.*

**pro·fil·om·e·try** (pro″fīl-om′ə-tre) the recording of a series of measurements to obtain a profile.
**urethral pressure p.,** the measurement of urethral pressures for a urethral pressure profile.

**pro·fla·vine** (pro-fla′vin) [MeSH: Proflavine] an acriflavine derivative which is a disinfectant bacteriostatic against many gram-positive bacteria. It has been used in the form of the dihydrochloride and hemisulfate salts as a topical antiseptic, and was formerly used as a urinary antiseptic. Called also *diaminoacridine.*

**pro·flu·vi·um** (pro-floo′ve-əm) [L.] a flowing forth.
**p. se′minis,** a flowing from the vagina of the semen deposited during coitus.

**pro·fon·dom·e·ter** (pro″fon-dom′ə-tər) an apparatus for locating a foreign body by the fluoroscope by obtaining three lines of sight which intersect at the foreign body.

**pro·fun·da·plas·ty** (pro-fun′də-plas″te) reconstruction of the occluded or stenosed deep femoral artery (arteria profunda femoris); called also *profundoplasty.*

**pro·fun·do·plas·ty** (pro-fun′də-plas″te) profundaplasty.

**pro·fun·dus** (pro-fun′dəs) [L.] [TA] deep; a term denoting a structure situated deeper than another from the surface of the body.

**prog·a·mous** (prog′ə-məs) [*pro-* + *gamo-* + *-ous*] previous to fertilization of the oocyte (ovum).

**pro·gas·ter** (pro′gas-tər) [*pro-* + *gaster*] archenteron.

**pro·gas·trin** (pro-gas′trin) an inactive precursor of gastrin.

**pro·ge·nia** (pro-je′ne-ə) [*pro-* + *geni-* + *-ia*] prognathism.

**pro·gen·i·tal** (pro-jen′ĭ-təl) on the external surface of the genitals.

**pro·gen·i·tor** (pro-jen′ĭ-tor) [L.] 1. a parent or ancestor. 2. stem cell.

**prog·e·ny** (proj′ə-ne) [L. *progignere* to bring forth] offspring, or descendants.

**pro·ge·ria** (pro-je′re-ə) [*pro-* + *ger-* + *-ia*] [MeSH: Progeria] a syndrome of uncertain genetic inheritance, characterized by precocious senility of striking degree, with death from coronary artery disease frequently occurring before 10 years of age. Cf. *infantilism.* Called also *Hutchinson-Gilford syndrome.*

**pro·ges·ta·gen** (pro-jes′tə-jən) progestational agent.

**pro·ges·ta·tion·al** (pro″jəs-ta′shən-əl) 1. a term applied to that phase of the menstrual cycle just before menstruation, when the corpus luteum is active and the endometrium secreting. 2. having effects similar to those of progesterone; see also under *agent.*

**pro·ges·te·rone** (pro-jes′tə-rōn) [MeSH: Progesterone] 1. the principal progestational hormone of the body, liberated by the corpus luteum, placenta, and in minute amounts by the adrenal cortex; it prepares the uterus for the reception and development of the fertilized ovum by transforming the endometrium from the proliferative to the secretory stage and maintains an optimal intrauterine environment for sustaining pregnancy. 2. [USP] the same principle isolated from pregnant sows or prepared synthetically, used, usually in the form of synthetic derivatives, as a progestin in the treatment of functional uterine bleeding, abnormalities of the menstrual cycle, and threatened abortion, administered orally and intramuscularly. Called also *progestational hormone.*

**pro·ges·tin** (pro-jes′tin) 1. progestational agent. 2. former name for the crude hormone of the corpus luteum.

**pro·ges·to·gen** (pro-jes′to-jən) progestational agent.

**pro·glos·sis** (pro-glos′is) [Gr. *proglōssis*] the tip or apex of the tongue.

**pro·glot·tid** (pro-glot′id) [*pro-* + *glottis*] one of the segments making up the body of a tapeworm. See *strobila.*

**pro·glot·tis** (pro-glot′is) pl. *proglot′tides.* proglottid.

**pro·glu·mide** (pro-gloo′mīd) [MeSH: Proglumide] an anticholinergic reported to have a specific inhibitory effect on gastric secretion.

**Pro·gly·cem** (pro-gli′səm) trademark for a preparation of oral diazoxide.

**prog·na·thia** (pro-na′the-ə) prognathism.

**prog·na·thic** (prog-nath′ik, prog-na′thik) prognathous.

**prog·na·thism** (prog′nə-thiz-əm) [*pro-* + *gnath-* + *-ism*] [MeSH: Prognathism] a condition marked by abnormal protrusion of the mandible. Called also *caput progeneum, exognathia, progenia,* and *prognathia.*

**prog·na·thom·e·ter** (prog″nə-thom′ə-tər) [*prognathous* + *-meter*] an instrument or device for measuring the degree of prognathism.

**prog·na·thous** (prog′nə-thəs) [*pro-* + *gnath-* + *-ous*] pertaining to or characterized by protrusion of the lower jaw or prognathism; having projecting jaws; having a gnathic index above 103, the teeth being in mesioclusion. Called also *prognathic.*

**prog·nose** (prog-nōs′) prognosticate.

**prog·no·sis** (prog-no′sis) [Gr. *prognōsis* foreknowledge] [MeSH: Prognosis] a forecast as to the probable outcome of an attack of disease; the prospect as to recovery from a disease as indicated by the nature and symptoms of the case.

**prog·nos·tic** (prog-nos′tik) 1. affording an indication as to prognosis. 2. a symptom or sign on which a prognosis may be based.

**prog·nos·ti·cate** (prog-nos′tĭ-kāt) to forecast the probable outcome of an attack of disease.

**prog·nos·ti·cian** (prog″nos-tish′ən) one who is skilled in prognosis.

**pro·go·no·ma** (pro″go-no′mə) [*pro-* + *gon-* + *-oma*] a tumor due to misplacement of tissue as the result of fetal atavism to a stage which does not occur in the life history of the species, but which does occur in ancestral forms of the species.
**melanotic p.,** melanotic neuroectodermal tumor.

**Pro·graf** (pro′graf) trademark for preparations of tacrolimus.

**pro·gran·u·lo·cyte** (pro-gran′u-lo-sīt″) promyelocyte.

**pro·grav·id** (pro-grav′id) [*pro-* + *gravid*] denoting the phase of the endometrium, under the influence of the corpus luteum, during which it is prepared for pregnancy.

**pro·gres·sion** (prə-gresh′ən) 1. the act of moving or walking forward; see also *gait.* 2. the process of spreading or becoming more severe.
**backward p.,** retropulsion.
**cross-legged p.,** scissors gait.
**saltatory p.,** saltation (def. 5).

**pro·gres·sive** (pro-gres′iv) advancing; going forward; going from bad to worse; increasing in scope or severity.

**pro·guan·il hy·dro·chlo·ride** (pro-gwahn′əl) an antimalarial used

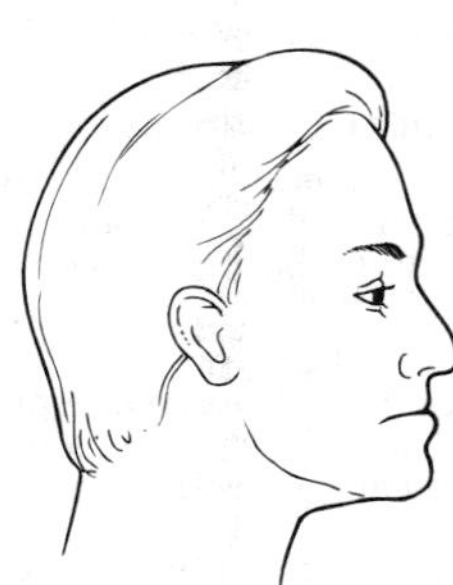

Prognathism.

in the prophylaxis and treatment of malaria, administered orally. Seldom used in the United States because of the development of resistance by the malarial parasite to proguanil. Called also *chloroguanide hydrochloride*.

**Pro·gyn·on** (pro-jin′on) trademark for preparations of estradiol.

**Pro·HIB·iT** (pro-hib′it) trademark for a preparation of *Haemophilus influenzae* b conjugate vaccine.

**pro·hor·mone** (pro-hor′mōn) any substance that can be converted into a hormone; see also *prehormone*. Called also hormonogen.

**pro·in·flam·ma·to·ry** capable of stimulating inflammation.

**pro·in·su·lin** (pro-in′su-lin) [MeSH: Proinsulin] a precursor of insulin, with a molecular weight of 8,000 to 10,000; it has minimal hormonal activity and is converted to insulin by removal of the connecting C peptide, leaving the two (A and B)-chain, active insulin molecule.

**pro·jec·tion** (pro-jek′shən) [*pro-* + L. *jacēre* to throw] [MeSH: Projection] 1. a throwing forward, especially the act of referring impressions made on the sense organs to their proper source, so as to locate correctly the objects producing them. 2. the connection between the cerebral cortex and other parts of the nervous system or organs of special sense. 3. the act of extending or jutting out, or a part that juts out. 4. in psychiatry, an unconscious defense mechanism in which a person attributes to someone else unacknowledged ideas, thoughts, feelings, and impulses that he finds undesirable or unacceptable in himself. 5. the orientation of a radiographic machine in relation to the body or a body part; called also *view*.
**anteroposterior (AP) p.**, a radiographic projection in which the central ray goes from the front to the back of the body or part, with the film at the back.
**axial p.**, a radiographic projection in which the central ray goes from the base to the vertex or from the vertex to the base of a structure.
**axillary p.**, a radiographic projection in which the patient is supine, the arm is abducted, and the central ray enters the axilla at an angle; performed to visualize structures in the shoulder region.
**brow-down p.**, a posteroanterior projection of the head with the patient prone.
**brow-up p.**, an anteroposterior projection of the head with the patient supine.
**Caldwell's p.**, a posteroanterior projection of the head, used for viewing the frontal and anterior ethmoidal sinuses; the central ray enters the back of the head from a slightly superior angle.
**carpal tunnel p.**, a radiographic projection with the wrist hyperextended and the central ray entering the proximal palm at an angle, for visualization of bones and other structures of the proximal palm and wrist.
**cross-table p.**, a radiographic projection of the spine, pelvis, or leg with the patient either prone or supine on a table and the central ray entering laterally.
**Didiée's p.**, a rare type of radiographic projection for evaluation of an unstable or repeatedly dislocating shoulder that may have a subtle condition such as the Hill-Sachs lesion; the patient lies prone and the central ray enters the shoulder from a lateral oblique direction.
**dorsoplantar p.**, a radiographic projection of the foot with the central ray passing from the dorsal surface to the plantar surface.
**eccentric p.**, referred sensation.
**erroneous p.**, a misjudging of the position of an object, due to weakness or palsy of the eye muscles. Called also *false paralysis*.
**frog-leg p.**, an anteroposterior projection of the abducted hips.
**frontal p.**, a radiographic projection in which the central ray is perpendicular to the frontal plane; it may be either anteroposterior or posteroanterior.
**half-axial p.**, a radiographic projection of the head with the central ray at an angle to the frontal and medial planes; it may be either anteroposterior or posteroanterior. Called also *semiaxial p.*
**Heinig's p.**, a radiographic projection for visualization of the sternum and sternoclavicular joint; the arm closer to the tube is abducted over the head and the central ray enters the body from an inferior lateral direction, angling towards the opposite shoulder.
**Hermodsson's p.**, a rare type of radiographic projection for evaluation of an unstable or repeatedly dislocating shoulder that may have a subtle condition such as the Hill-Sachs lesion; the patient stands with the affected arm behind the back and the hand over the lumbar vertebrae, and the central ray enters laterally to the scapula from an inferior posterior direction.
**Hughston's p.**, a radiographic projection of the patellofemoral region, with the patient prone, the legs at 50 to 60 degrees of flexion, and the central ray at 45 degrees from vertical passing tangentially across the knee.
**inferosuperior p.**, any radiographic projection in which the central ray enters the body or a body part from below.
**lateral p.**, a radiographic projection in which the central ray enters the body or part from the side and is perpendicular to the medial or axial plane.
**Laurin's p.**, an axial radiograph of the knees made with the patient seated with the knees flexed at 30 degrees and the legs together; the x-ray tube is placed between the patient's feet and the film is placed against the anterior thighs perpendicular to the beam.
**Merchant's p.**, an axial radiograph of the knees made with the patient supine and the knees flexed at 45 degrees over the table end with the legs together; the tube is angled 30 degrees below the horizontal and the film is held on the tibia perpendicular to the beam.
**mortise p.**, an anteroposterior projection of the ankle with the foot rotated internally 15 to 20 degrees so that the bases of the tibia and fibula are no longer in front of the talus.
**notch p.**, 1. Stryker's notch p. 2. a radiographic projection for visualization of the intercondylar notch of the femur.
**oblique p.**, a radiographic projection in which the central ray enters the body or part at an angle to the frontal and medial or axial planes.
**open-mouth p.**, an anteroposterior projection of the cervical spine, particularly the axis and atlas, done through the open mouth with the patient supine and the central ray pointing vertically downward.
**pillar p.**, a radiographic projection of the articular pillars of the cervical spine, usually with the patient supine and the central ray angled slightly towards the feet from a position above the face; for an unobstructed view, the head may be rotated so that the mandible is not above the spine.
**posteroanterior (PA) p.**, a radiographic projection in which the central ray goes from the back to the front of the body, with the film at the front.
**radiographic p.**, projection (def. 5).
**Schüller's p.**, a lateral projection of the head, with the beam originating 30° above horizontal; it allows a view of the antrum, part of the attic, and the head of the malleus.
**semiaxial p.**, half-axial p.
**Settegast's p.**, a tangential projection of the patellofemoral region, usually with the patient prone, the knee flexed more than 90 degrees, and the central ray directed vertically downward at the knee. Called also *sunrise p.*
**Stenvers p.**, an oblique projection of the head, done with the head rotated 45° so that the petrous part of the temporal bone is perpendicular to the beam; it allows a view of the petrous apex, the labyrinth, and the internal acoustic meatus.
**stress p.**, a radiographic projection of a movable joint, such as the wrist or knee, while it is under significant stress.
**Stryker's notch p.**, a rare type of radiographic projection for evaluation of an unstable or repeatedly dislocating shoulder that may have a subtle condition such as the Hill-Sachs lesion. The patient lies supine with the elbow on the affected side vertical and the hand next to or above the head; the central ray enters anteriorly and angles slightly upwards towards the coracoid process. Called also *notch p.*
**submentovertex p.**, a radiographic projection of the head with the central ray entering under the chin and directed toward the vertex.
**sunrise p.**, Settegast's p.
**swimmer's p.**, a radiographic projection of the cervical or thoracic spine with the patient lying supine on a table, the neck hyperextended, the arm nearer the camera parallel to the body, and the arm nearer the film placed above the head; the central ray enters laterally.
**tangential p.**, a radiographic projection with the central ray on a tangent to an organ or part.
**thalamocortical p's**, see under *fiber*.
**Towne's p.**, a radiographic projection of the head in which the central ray enters obliquely through the frontal bone, yielding a view of facial structures and the occipital bone; it is an anteroposterior half-axial projection.
**tunnel p.**, a posteroanterior projection in which the knee is flexed 40 to 50 degrees with the patient prone and the foot supported; the central ray is perpendicular to the lower leg for a view of the intercondylar fossa of the femur.
**verticosubmental p.**, a radiographic projection in which the central ray passes from the vertex of the head to the base of the chin, for visualization of the mandible, the base of the skull, and the nasal region.
**Waters' p.**, a radiographic projection of the anterior head, used for viewing the maxillary sinuses and sphenoid bone; the central ray enters at an angle through the chin.
**West Point p.**, a rare type of radiographic projection for evaluation of an unstable or repeatedly dislocating shoulder that may have a subtle condition such as the Hill-Sachs lesion. The patient lies prone with the affected arm abducted and the forearm hanging off the table; the central ray enters in the scapular region at an angle from the rear to visualize scapular and shoulder structures.

**pro·kary·on** (pro-kar′e-on) [*pro-* + *karyon*] 1. nuclear material that is scattered in the cytoplasm of the cell, rather than bounded by a membrane; found in some unicellular organisms, such as bacteria. 2. prokaryote.

**pro·karyo·sis** (pro″kar-e-o′sis) [*pro-* + *karyo-* + *-osis*] the state of not having a true nucleus, the nuclear membrane being absent and the nuclear material being either scattered in the cytoplasm of the cell or collected in a nucleoid region; a characteristic of bacteria. Cf. *eukaryosis.*

**Pro·karyo·tae** (pro-kar″e-o′te) [*pro-* + Gr. *karyon* nucleus] Procaryotae.

**pro·kary·ote** (pro-kar′e-ōt) [*pro-* + Gr. *karyon* nut, kernel] any member of the kingdom Procaryotae. Prokaryotes are cellular organisms lacking a true nucleus and nuclear membrane. Their nuclear material consists of a single double-stranded DNA molecule, not associated with basic proteins. The microorganisms, comprising the bacteria and blue-green bacteria (formerly blue-green algae), are predominantly unicellular but may have filamentous, mycelial, or colonial forms. All (except the Mollicutes and Archaeobacteria) have a true cell wall containing peptidoglycan, and all reproduce by cell fission. See also *Procaryotae* Cf. *eukaryote.*

**pro·kary·ot·ic** (pro″kar-e-ot′ik) pertaining to a prokaryon or to a prokaryote or to prokaryosis.

**Pro·ke·ta·zine** (pro-ke′tə-zēn) trademark for preparations of carphenazine maleate.

**Pro·kine** (pro′kīn) trademark for a preparation of sargramostim.

**pro·la·bi·um** (pro-la′be-əm) [*pro-* + *labium*] the prominent central part of the upper lip.

**pro·lac·tin (PRL, Prl)** (pro-lak′tin) [*pro-* + L. *lac* milk] [MeSH: Prolactin] a hormone of molecular weight 23,000, with 198 amino acids, secreted by special cells of the adenohypophysis, which stimulates and sustains lactation in postpartum mammals, the mammary glands having been prepared by other hormones, including estrogens, progesterone, growth hormone, corticosteroids, and insulin. It also stimulates formation of "milk" in the crop sac of birds such as pigeons and doves (an action formerly used for bioassay), is luteotropic in certain mammals, and has many other effects, including essential roles in the maintenance of immune system functions. Called also *lactogen, lactotropin, luteotropin, mammotropin,* and *galactopoietic, lactation, lactogenic,* or *luteotropic hormone.*

**pro·lac·ti·no·ma** (pro-lak″tĭ-no′mə) [MeSH: Prolactinoma] a pituitary adenoma made up of lactotrophs that secretes excessive amounts of prolactin; this may delay puberty in either sex, cause galactorrhea-amenorrhea syndrome in women, or decrease libido and fertility in men. Called also *prolactin cell adenoma, prolactin-secreting adenoma, lactotrope adenoma,* and *lactotroph adenoma.*

**pro·lac·to·lib·er·in** (pro-lak″to-lib′ər-in) [*prolactin* + *-liberin*] prolactin-releasing hormone.

**pro·lac·to·stat·in** (pro-lak″to-stat′in) [*prolactin* + *-statin*] prolactin-inhibiting hormone.

**pro·lam·in** (pro-lam′in, pro′lə-min) any of a group of globular proteins found mainly in cereals; they are soluble in 70–80 per cent alcohol but insoluble in water and absolute alcohol and contain high levels of glutamic acid and proline. Examples are gliadin (found in wheat and rye) and zein (found in corn). Called also *alcohol-soluble protein.*

**pro·lan** (pro′lən) a name formerly given to the gonadotropic principle of human pregnancy urine, responsible for the biologic pregnancy tests.

**pro·lapse** (pro-laps′) [L. *prolapsus; pro* before + *labi* to fall] [MeSH: Prolapse] 1. the falling down, or sinking, of a part or viscus; called also *procidentia* and *ptosis.* 2. to undergo such displacement.
**anal p., p. of anus,** protrusion of modified anal skin through the anal orifice.
**p. of the cord,** premature expulsion of the umbilical cord in labor before the fetus is delivered.
**frank p.,** prolapse of the uterus in which the vagina is inverted and hangs from the vulva.
**p. of the iris,** protrusion of the iris through a wound in the cornea.
**mitral valve p. (MVP),** redundancy or hooding of mitral valve leaflets so that they prolapse into the left atrium, often causing mitral regurgitation; see *mitral valve prolapse syndrome,* under *syndrome.* Called also *floppy mitral valve.*
**Morgagni's p.,** chronic inflammatory hyperplasia of the mucosa and submucosa of the sacculus laryngis.
**rectal p., p. of rectum,** protrusion of the rectal mucous membrane through the anus in varying degree, classified as *incomplete* or *partial* with no displacement of anal sphincter muscle, *complete with displacement* of anal sphincter muscle, *complete with no displacement* of anal muscles but usually with herniation of bowel, and *internal complete (concealed)* with intussusception of the rectosigmoid and upper portion of the rectum into the lower rectum.
**p. of uterus,** downward displacement of the uterus so that the cervix is within the vaginal orifice *(first-degree p.),* the cervix is outside the orifice *(second-degree p.),* or the entire uterus is outside the orifice *(third-degree p.).*

**pro·lap·sus** (pro-lap′səs) [L.] prolapse.

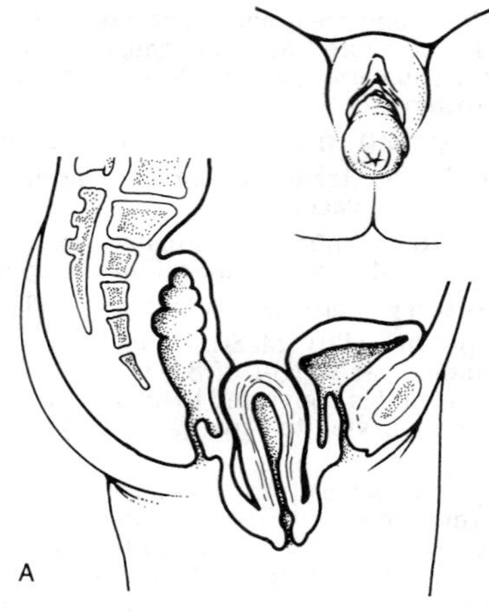


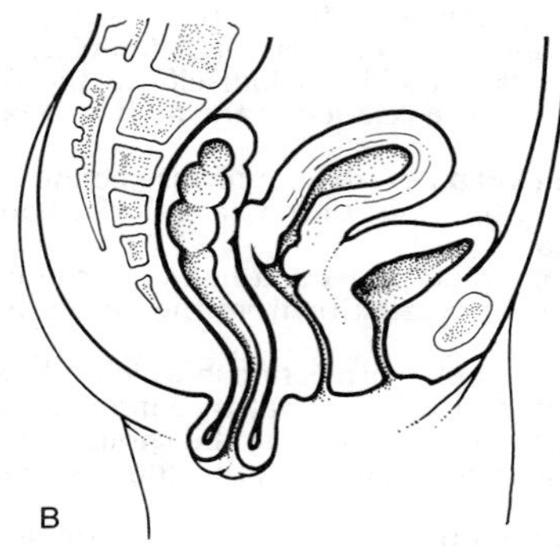


*(A),* Prolapse of uterus; *(B),* prolapse of rectum.

**p. a′ni,** prolapse of anus.
**p. rec′ti,** prolapse of rectum.
**p. u′teri,** prolapse of uterus.

**Pro·las·tin** (pro-las′tin) trademark for a preparation of alpha$_1$-proteinase inhibitor (human).

**Pro·lene** (pro′lēn) trademark for a preparation of polypropylene.

**pro·lep·sis** (pro-lep′sis) the return of a paroxysm before the expected time.

**pro·lep·tic** (pro-lep′tik) occurring prior to the usual time; said of a periodic disease whose paroxysms return at successively shorter intervals.

**Pro·leu·kin** (pro-loo′kin) trademark for a preparation of aldesleukin.

**pro·leu·ko·cyte** (pro-loo′ko-sīt) old term for a precursor of a leukocyte; the term was not adopted by any classification scheme of white cell morphological development.

**pro·li·dase** (pro′lĭ-dās) X-Pro dipeptidase.

**pro·li·dase de·fi·cien·cy** an autosomal recessive aminoacidopathy due to deficiency of X-Pro dipeptidase; defective cleavage of imino acid–containing peptides results in urinary excretion of imidodipeptides. Clinical manifestations are variable, but include chronic skin lesions, impaired motor or cognitive development, frequent infections, and skeletal abnormalities.

**pro·lif·er·ate** (pro-lif′ər-āt) to grow by the reproduction of similar cells.

**pro·lif·er·a·tion** (pro-lif″ə-ra′shən) [L. *proles* offspring + *ferre* to bear] the reproduction or multiplication of similar forms, especially of cells and morbid cysts. See also *hyperplasia* and *hypertrophy.*
**fibroplastic p.,** an overgrowth of collagenous connective tissue involving many organs of the body, as occurs in systemic lupus erythematosus, scleroderma, and other collagen diseases.

**pro·lif·er·a·tive** (pro-lif′ər-ə-tiv) characterized by proliferation.

**pro·lif·er·ous** (pro-lif′ər-əs) proliferative.

**pro·lif·ic** (pro-lif′ik) [L. *prolificus*] fruitful; productive.

**pro·lig·er·ous** (pro-lig′ər-əs) [L. *proles* offspring + *gerere* to bear] producing offspring.

**pro·lin·ase** (pro′lĭ-nās) Pro-X dipeptidase.

**pro·line** (pro′lēn) [MeSH: Proline] a nonessential amino acid, 2-pyrrolidinecarboxylic acid, discovered by Fischer in 1901; it is a major constituent of collagen (see *tropocollagen*). Symbols Pro and P. See also table at *amino acid.*

**pro·line de·hy·dro·gen·ase** (pro′lēn de-hi′dro-jən-ās) [EC 1.5.99.8] an enzyme of the oxidoreductase class that catalyzes the dehydrogenation of proline to form $\Delta^1$-pyrroline 5-carboxylate, using ubiquinone as an electron acceptor. The enzyme is a flavoprotein (FAD) of the mitochondrial membrane and the reaction is the initial step in the degradation of proline to glutamate. Deficiency of the enzyme, an autosomal recessive trait, is the cause of hyperprolinemia Type I. Called also *proline oxidase.*

**pro·line di·pep·ti·dase** (pro′lēn di-pep′tĭ-dās) X-Pro dipeptidase.

**pro·lin·emia** (pro″lĭ-ne′me-ə) hyperprolinemia.

**pro·line ox·i·dase** (pro′lēn ok′sĭ-dās) [MeSH: Proline Oxidase] proline dehydrogenase.

**pro·line ra·ce·mase** (pro′lēn ra′sə-mās) [EC 5.1.1.4] an enzyme of the isomerase class that catalyzes the interconversion of L- and D-proline.

**Pro·lix·in** (pro-lik′sin) trademark for preparations of fluphenazine hydrochloride.

**Pro·loid** (pro′loid) trademark for a preparation of thyroglobulin (def. 2).

**Pro·lu·ton** (pro-lu′ton) trademark for preparations of progesterone.

**pro·lyl** (pro′ləl) the acyl radical of proline.

**pro·lyl di·pep·ti·dase** (pro′ləl di-pep′tĭ-dās) Pro-X dipeptidase.

**pro·lyl 3-hy·drox·y·lase** (pro′ləl hi-drok′sə-lās) an enzyme of the oxidoreductase class that catalyzes the hydroxylation at the 3 position of specific proline residues in nascent procollagen chains. The enzyme requires $Fe^{2+}$, ascorbate, and $\alpha$-ketoglutarate for activity. In EC nomenclature, called *procollagen-proline, 3-dioxygenase.*

**pro·lyl 4-hy·drox·y·lase** (pro′ləl hi-drok′sə-lās) an enzyme of the oxidoreductase class that catalyzes the hydroxylation at the 4 position of specific proline residues in nascent procollagen chains. The enzyme requires $Fe^{2+}$, ascorbate, and $\alpha$-ketoglutarate for activity, and the reaction is necessary for thermal stability of the collagen triple helical structure. The enzyme is a tetramer comprising $2\alpha$ and $2\beta$ chains; the $\beta$ chain in monomeric form is the enzyme protein disulfide-isomerase (q.v.). In EC nomenclature, called *procollagen-proline dioxygenase.*

**pro·lym·pho·cyte** (pro-lim′fo-sīt) a developmental form in the lymphocytic series (q.v.), intermediate between the lymphoblast and lymphocyte.

**pro·man·ide** (pro′mə-nīd) glucosulfone sodium.

**pro·mas·ti·gote** (pro-mas′tĭ-gōt) [*pro-* + *mastigote*] any of the bodies representing the morphological (leptomonad) stage in the life cycle of certain trypanosomatid protozoa resembling the typical adult form of members of the genus *Leptomonas,* in which the elongate or pear-shaped cell has a central nucleus and at the anterior end a kinetoplast and a basal body from which arises a single long, slender flagellum. Cf. *amastigote, choanomastigote, epimastigote, opisthomastigote,* and *trypomastigote.*

**pro·ma·zine hy·dro·chlo·ride** (pro′mə-zēn) [USP] a phenothiazine derivative used as an antipsychotic agent, as an antiemetic, and as an analgesic- and anesthetic-potentiating agent, administered orally, intramuscularly, and intravenously.

**pro·mega·karyo·cyte** (pro-meg″ə-kar′e-o-sīt) a precursor in the thrombocytic series, a large cell intermediate between the megakaryoblast and the megakaryocyte.

**pro·meg·a·lo·blast** (pro-meg′ə-lo-blast) the earliest developmental form in the abnormal red cell maturation sequence occurring in vitamin $B_{12}$ and folic acid deficiencies; it corresponds to the pronormoblast, but differs from it by its larger size, abundant basophilic cytoplasm, and reticulated, unclumped nuclear chromatin. Several nucleoli are usually present.

**pro·meta·phase** (pro-met′ə-fās) the phase of mitosis which generally begins with the disintegration of the nuclear membrane. When this has occurred, a more fluid zone is noted in the center of the cell, in which the chromosomes move freely and in apparent disorder, making their way toward the equator.

**pro·meth·a·zine hy·dro·chlo·ride** (pro-meth′ə-zēn) [USP] a phenothiazine derivative having marked antihistaminic activity as well as sedative and antiemetic actions; used to provide bedtime, surgical, and obstetrical sedation, to potentiate the action of central depressants, and to manage nausea and vomiting associated with surgery, pregnancy, and motion sickness, administered orally, intramuscularly, and intravenously.

**pro·meth·es·trol di·pro·pi·o·nate** (pro-meth′əs-trol) an orally effective, synthetic, nonsteroidal estrogenic agent, having actions and uses similar to those of diethylstilbestrol (q.v.). Called also *methestrol dipropionate.*

**pro·me·thi·um** (pro-me′the-əm) [MeSH: Promethium] the radioactive metallic chemical element of atomic number 61, atomic weight 147, and symbol Pm.

**pro·mine** (pro′mēn) a substance widely distributed in animal cells, characterized by its ability to promote cell division and growth. Cf. *retine.*

**prom·i·nence** (prom′ĭ-nəns) a protrusion or projection; for names of specific anatomical structures, see under *prominentia.*
**Ammon's scleral p.,** a prominence on the globe of the eye of the fetus.
**frontonasal p.,** an expansive facial prominence in the embryo that develops into the forehead and bridge of the nose. Formerly called *frontonasal process.*
**mandibular p.,** the ventral prominence formed by bifurcation of the mandibular (first pharyngeal) arch in the embryo, which unites ventrally with its fellow to form the lower jaw. Formerly called *mandibular process.*
**maxillary p.,** the dorsal prominence formed by bifurcation of the mandibular (first pharyngeal) arch in the embryo, which joins with the ipsilateral median nasal prominence in the formation of the upper jaw. Formerly called *maxillary process.*
**nasal p., lateral,** the more lateral of the two limbs of the horseshoe-shaped elevation bounding a nasal pit in the embryo, which participates in formation of the side and wing of the nose. Formerly called *lateral nasal process.*
**nasal p., medial, nasal p., median,** the more central of the two limbs of the horseshoe-shaped elevation bounding a nasal pit in the embryo, which participates with the ipsilateral maxillary process in forming half of the upper jaw. Formerly called *medial* or *median nasal process.*
**tubal p.,** torus tubarius.

**prom·i·nen·tia** (prom″ĭ-nen′shə) gen. and pl. *prominen′tiae* [L.] [TA] prominence: a general term for a small protrusion on another structure or part.
**p. cana′lis facia′lis** [TA], prominence of facial canal: an elongated elevation on the medial wall of the tympanic cavity, just inferior to the prominence of the lateral semicircular canal and superior and posterior to the vestibular window.
**p. cana′lis semicircula′ris latera′lis** [TA], prominence of lateral semicircular canal: a large rounded prominence on the upper portion of the medial wall of the tympanic cavity, between the vestibular window and the mastoid antrum.
**p. laryn′gea** [TA], laryngeal prominence: a subcutaneous prominence on the front of the neck produced by the thyroid cartilage of the larynx; called also *Adam's apple.*
**p. mallea′ris membra′nae tym′pani, p. mallea′ris membra′nae tympa′nicae** [TA], **p. malleola′ris membra′nae tym′pani,** mallear prominence of tympanic membrane: a small projection at the upper extremity of the stria mallearis, formed by the lateral process of the malleus. Called also *short process of malleus.*
**p. spira′lis** [TA], spiral prominence: a prominence on the external wall of the cochlear duct, separating the stria vascularis from the external spiral sulcus.
**p. styloi′dea** [TA], styloid prominence: an irregular nodule on the posterior portion of the floor of the tympanic cavity, corresponding to the base of the styloid process.

**prom·i·nen·tiae** (prom″ĭ-nen′she-e) [L.] genitive and plural of *prominentia.*

**pro·mono·cyte** (pro-mon′o-sīt) a precursor in the monocytic series, being a cell intermediate in development between the monoblast and monocyte.

**prom·on·to·ri·um** (prom″on-tor′e-əm) pl. *promonto′ria* [L.] [TA] promontory: a projecting eminence or process.
**p. os′sis sa′cri** [TA], promontory of sacrum: the prominent anterior border of the pelvic surface of the body of the first sacral vertebra.
**p. tym′pani** [TA], promontory of tympanic cavity: the prominence on the medial wall of the tympanic cavity, formed by the first turn of the cochlea.

**prom·on·to·ry** (prom′on-tor″e) a projecting eminence or process; for names of specific anatomical structures see under *promontorium.*

**pro·mo·ter** (pro-mo′tər) 1. a segment of DNA usually occurring upstream from a gene coding region and acting as a controlling element in the expression of that gene; it serves as a recognition signal for an RNA polymerase and marks the site of initiation of transcription. 2. a substance in a catalyst which increases the rate of activity of the latter. Cf. *protector.* 3. a type of epigenetic carcinogen that promotes neoplastic growth only after initiation by another substance; called also *cocarcinogen.*

**pro·mo·tion** (prə-mo'shən) the activity of a promoter or the results of such activity.

**pro·my·elo·cyte** (pro-mi'ə-lo-sīt) [MeSH: Granulocytes] a precursor in the granulocytic series, being a cell intermediate in development between a myeloblast and myelocyte, and containing a few, as yet undifferentiated, cytoplasmic granules. Called also *premyelocyte* and *progranulocyte.*

**pro·nate** (pro'nāt) to assume or place in a prone position; see *pronation.*

**pro·na·tion** (pro-na'shən) [L. *pronatio*] [MeSH: Pronation] the act of assuming the prone position, or the state of being prone. Applied to the hand, the act of turning the palm posteriorly (or inferiorly when the forearm is flexed), performed by medial rotation of the forearm. Applied to the foot, a combination of eversion and abduction movements taking place in the tarsal and metatarsal joints and resulting in lowering of the medial margin of the foot, hence of the longitudinal arch. Cf. *supination.*

**pro·na·to·flex·or** (pro-na"to-flek'sor) both pronator and flexor.

**pro·na·tor** (pro-na'tor) [L.] a muscle that serves to pronate; see *pronation.*

**prone** (prōn) [L. *pronus* inclined forward] lying face downward; see also *pronation.* Called also *procumbent.*

**pro·neph·ron** (pro-nef'ron) pronephros.

**pro·neph·ros** (pro-nef'ros) pl. *proneph'roi* [*pro-* + Gr. *nephros* kidney] the primordial kidney; a vestigial excretory structure or its rudiments developing in the embryo at four weeks, before the mesonephros. Although nonfunctional, its duct is later used by the mesonephros, which arises caudal to it.

**Pro·nes·tyl** (pro-nes'təl) trademark for preparations of procainamide hydrochloride.

**pro·net·a·lol** (pro-net'ə-lol) pronethalol.

**pro·neth·a·lol** (pro-neth'ə-lol) a beta-adrenergic blocking agent having the same actions as propranolol (q.v.). Called also *nethalide* and *pronetalol.*

**prong** (prong) a conical projection.
**nasal p's,** nasal cannula.

**pro·no·grade** (pro'no-grād) [L. *pronus* bent downward + *gradi* to walk] characterized by walking with the body approximately horizontal, such as the quadrupeds. Cf. *orthograde.*

**pro·nom·e·ter** (pro-nom'ə-tər) a goniometer for the forearm.

**pro·nor·mo·blast** (pro-nor'mo-blast) [MeSH: Erythroblasts] a term now often considered a synonym of *proerythroblast;* sometimes more specifically one in a course of normal erythrocyte maturation, as opposed to a *promegaloblast.*

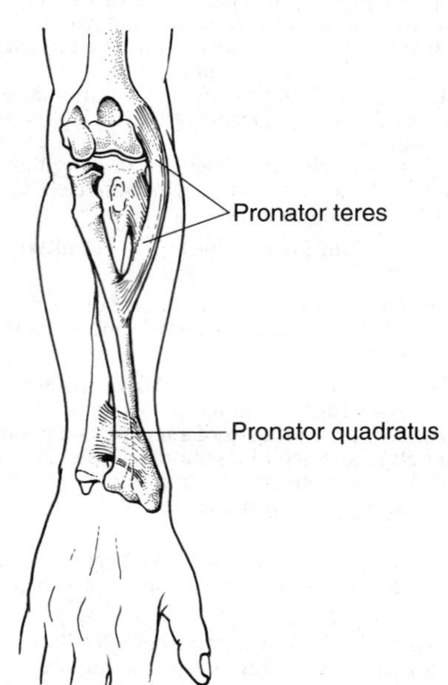


Pronators contracted, forearm and hand pronated.

**Pron·to·sil** (pron'to-sil) trademark for the forerunner of the sulfonamide drugs, first prepared in 1932 and no longer used therapeutically. Called also *P. flavum* and *P. rubrum.*

**pro·nu·cle·us** (pro-noo'kle-əs) the precursor of a nucleus.
**female p.,** the haploid nucleus of the fully mature oocyte, which loses its nuclear envelope and liberates its chromosomes to meet in synapsis with those similarly derived from the male pronucleus.
**male p.,** the nuclear material of the head of a spermatozoon after it has penetrated the oocyte and acquired a pronuclear membrane.

**pro-opio·mel·a·no·cor·tin (POMC)** (pro-o"pe-o-mel"ə-no-kor'tin) [*pro-* + endogenous *opio*ids + *melano*cyte stimulating hormone + *cor*ticotropin + *-in*] [MeSH: Pro-Opiomelanocortin] the 31,000 dalton prohormone that is the precursor of adrenocorticotropic hormone, the lipotropins, the melanocyte-stimulating hormones, and the endorphins, all of which are produced by posttranslational proteolytic cleavage in cell types that produce these hormones.

**pro·ot·ic** (pro-ot'ik) [*pro-* + *otic*] preauricular.

**Pro·pa·drine** (pro'pə-drēn) trademark for preparations of phenylpropanolamine hydrochloride.

**pro·pa·fe·none hy·dro·chlo·ride** (pro"pə-fe'nōn) [USP] a sodium channel blocker that acts on the Purkinje fibers and myocardium, used in the treatment of life-threatening arrhythmias; administered orally.

**prop·a·ga·tion** (prop"ə-ga'shən) reproduction.

**prop·a·ga·tive** (prop'ə-ga"tiv) pertaining to or concerned in propagation.

**pro·pane** (pro'pān) [MeSH: Propane] a hydrocarbon of the methane series, $CH_3CH_2CH_3$, which is a constituent of natural gas and crude petroleum, and occurs as a colorless flammable gas with a characteristic odor.

**pro·pan·i·did** (pro-pan'ĭ-did) [MeSH: Propanidid] a short-acting anesthetic, derived from eugenol; administered intravenously.

**pro·pa·no·ic ac·id** (pro"pə-no'ik) systematic name for propionic acid.

**pro·pan·the·line bro·mide** (pro-pan'thə-lēn) an anticholinergic, which inhibits gastrointestinal hypermotility and hyperacidity; used especially as adjunctive therapy in the treatment of peptic ulcer, administered orally, intravenously, and intramuscularly.

**pro·par·a·caine hy·dro·chlo·ride** (pro-par'ə-kān) [USP] an anesthetic, applied topically to the conjunctiva.

**pro·pene** (pro'pēn) propylene.

**2-pro·pene·ni·trile** (pro"pēn-ni'trīl) acrylonitrile.

**pro·pe·nyl** (pro-pe'nəl) a three-carbon radical with one double bond between two of the carbons, $CH_3CH{=}CH{-}$.

**pro·pep·tone** (pro-pep'tōn) hemialbumose.

**pro·pep·ton·uria** (pro-pep'to-nu're-ə) hemialbumosuria.

**pro·per·din** (pro'pər-din) [MeSH: Properdin] a nonimmunoglobulin gamma globulin component of the alternative pathway of complement activation; it complexes with C3b and stabilizes alternative pathway C3 and C5 convertases (C3bBb and $C3b_nBb$). Called also *factor P.*

**pro·peri·to·ne·al** (pro"pər-ĭ-to-ne'əl) situated between the parietal peritoneum and the abdominal wall; preperitoneal.

**prop·er·ty** (prop'ər-te) a characteristic quality, ability, capability, or function.
**colligative p.,** any of the properties of solutions that depend only on the concentration of osmotically active particles: boiling point elevation, freezing point depression, osmotic pressure, and vapor pressure lowering.

**pro·phage** (pro'fāj) [*pro-* + *phage*] the latent stage of a phage in a lysogenic bacterium, in which the viral genome becomes inserted into a specific portion of the host chromosome and is duplicated each cell generation.

**pro·phase** (pro'fāz) [MeSH: Prophase] the first stage in cell reduplication. In mitosis, the stage during which the chromosomes become visible (because of supercoiling of DNA), the cell nucleus starts to lose its identity, and the centrioles begin to migrate. In meiosis, the prophase of the first division consists of five stages: leptotene, zygotene, pachytene, diplotene, and diakinesis. In the second meiotic division, prophase resembles that in mitotic division. See *meiosis* and *mitosis.*

**pro·phen·py·rid·amine** (pro"fən-pī-rid'ə-mēn) pheniramine.

**pro·phy·lac·tic** (pro"fə-lak'tik) [Gr. *prophylaktikos*] 1. tending to ward off or prevent something, particularly disease. 2. pertaining to prophylaxis. 3. an agent that tends to ward off disease. 4. a device for preventing sexually transmitted disease and/or conception, particularly a condom.

**pro·phy·lax·is** (pro"fə-lak'sis) [Gr. *prophylassein* to keep guard be-

fore] intervention aimed at the prevention of disease; called also *preventive treatment, prophylactic treatment,* and *protective therapy.*
**causal p.,** removal of the cause of a disease.
**chemical p.,** chemoprophylaxis.
**collective p.,** the protection of the community from infection.
**dental p.,** oral p.
**drug p.,** chemoprophylaxis.
**gametocidal p.,** the use of drugs, such as primaquine, to destroy the gametocytes of malaria.
**individual p.,** the prevention of infection in an individual.
**mechanical p.,** prevention of the transmission of venereal disease by mechanical means (e.g., a condom).
**oral p.,** cleansing the teeth in the dental office, including removal of plaque, materia alba, calculus, and stains from the exposed and unexposed surfaces of the teeth by scaling and polishing of the teeth, as a preventive measure for the control of local irritational factors. Called also *dental p.*

**Pro·phyl·lin** (pro-fil′in) trademark for a preparation of chlorophyllin copper complex and sodium propionate.

**pro·pi·cil·lin** (pro″pĭ-sil′in) levopropylcillin potassium.

**pro·pid·ium io·dide** stain for nucleic acids

**pro·pio·lac·tone** (pro″pe-o-lak′tōn) [MeSH: Propiolactone] a disinfectant effective against gram-positive, gram-negative, and acid-fast bacteria, fungi, and viruses. It is also used to prepare inactivated vaccines because it destroys the nucleic acid core of viruses but does not damage the capsid. Called also *betapropiolactone.*

**pro·pi·o·ma·zine hy·dro·chlo·ride** (pro″pe-o-ma′zēn) a phenothiazine derivative, used to provide bedtime, perioperative, and obstetrical sedation and as an antiemetic during labor, administered intramuscularly and intravenously.

**pro·pi·o·nate** (pro′pe-o-nāt) any salt of propionic acid.

**Pro·pi·on·i·bac·te·ri·a·ceae** (pro″pe-on″e-bak-tēr″e-a′se-e) [MeSH: Propionibacteriaceae] a family of bacteria closely related to the actinomycetes, consisting of gram-positive, asporogenous, anaerobic or aerotolerant, branching or regular rods or filaments. The organisms are inhabitants of the skin and respiratory and intestinal tracts, and are sometimes found in soft tissue infections. It includes the genera *Eubacterium* and *Propionibacterium.*

**Pro·pi·on·i·bac·te·ri·um** (pro″pe-on″e-bak-tēr′e-əm) [*pro-* + Gr. *piōn* fat + *baktērion* little rod] [MeSH: Propionibacterium] a genus of bacteria of the family Propionibacteriaceae, made up of nonspore-forming, anaerobic or aerotolerant, gram-positive rods. The organisms, found as saprophytes in humans, animals, and dairy products, occasionally cause soft tissue infections.
**P. ac′nes,** a species that is a normal inhabitant of the skin and a frequent contaminant of anaerobic cultures. It is a potential pathogen associated with chronic infections in the blood and bone marrow. Called also *Corynebacterium acnes* and *C. parvum.*
**P. freudenrei′chii,** a species isolated from dairy products and important in the manufacture of cheese. Some authorities recognize the subspecies *freudenreichii, globosum,* and *shermanii.*
**P. granulo′sum,** a species isolated from the intestinal tract and abscesses of humans. Called also *Corynebacterium granulosum.*
**P. jense′nii,** a species isolated from dairy products and silage, occasionally found in infections.
**P. propio′nicum,** *Arachnia propionicum.*

**pro·pi·on·i·bac·te·ri·um** (pro″pe-on″ĭ-bak-tēr′e-əm) pl. *propionibacte′ria* [MeSH: Propionibacterium] an organism of the genus Propionibacterium.

**pro·pi·on·ic ac·id** (pro″pe-on′ik) a three-carbon saturated fatty acid that can be fermented by several species of bacteria; in mammals it can be converted to the thioester propionyl CoA, a metabolic intermediate.

**pro·pi·on·ic·ac·i·de·mia** (pro″pe-on″ik-as″ĭ-de′me-ə) 1. an autosomal recessive aminoacidopathy characterized by an excess of propionic acid in the blood and urine, with ketosis, acidosis, hyperglycinemia, hyperglycinuria, and often neurologic complications. The disorder is caused by deficiency of propionyl-CoA carboxylase activity due to defects in either subunit of the carboxylase; the term sometimes denotes also deficiency of this enzyme due to multiple carboxylase deficiency (q.v.). 2. excess of propionic acid in the blood.

**pro·pi·o·nyl** (pro′pe-ə-nəl) the acyl radical of propionic acid; the thioester it forms with coenzyme A, propionyl CoA, is an intermediate in the degradation of some amino acids and in the oxidation of odd number chain length fatty acids.

**pro·pi·o·nyl-CoA car·boxy·lase** (pro′pe-ə-nəl ko-a′ kahr-bok′sə-lās) [EC 6.4.1.3] an enzyme of the ligase class that catalyzes the carboxylation of propionyl CoA to form methylmalonyl CoA; the reaction is part of the route by which three-carbon compounds from some amino acids and from odd numbered fatty acids are used as fuels. The enzyme is an oligomer comprising $4\alpha$ and $4\beta$ chains and requires a biotin cofactor. Deficiency of enzyme activity due to a defect in either chain, an autosomal recessive trait, causes propionicacidemia; see also *multiple carboxylase deficiency,* under *carboxylase.*

**pro·plas·ma·cyte** (pro-plaz′mə-sīt) a precursor in the plasmacytic series, being a cell intermediate between the plasmablast and the plasma cell.

**pro·plas·min** (pro-plaz′min) plasminogen.

**Pro·plast** (pro′plast) [MeSH: Proplast] trademark for an alloplastic material that is a porous composite of vitreous carbon fibers and polytef, used for submucosal implantation.

**pro·po·fol** (pro′po-fol) [MeSH: Propofol] an anesthetic and sedative used for either induction of anesthesia, sedation only, or general anesthesia for procedures lasting less than one hour; administered intravenously.

**pro·por·tion** (prə-por′shən) [L. *proportio*] the relation of one part to the whole.
**mutant p.,** in genetics, the proportion of all cases of a given phenotype that arise through new mutation rather than by inheritance. Determined by the mutation rate (q.v.) and the fitness of the mutant phenotype.

**pro·pos·i·tus** (pro-poz′ĭ-təs) gen. and pl. *propo′siti* [L. "the one on display"] 1. proband. 2. more specifically the first proband to be ascertained (index case).

**pro·poxy·caine hy·dro·chlo·ride** (pro-pok′sĭ-kān) [USP] a local anesthetic, used for infiltration and block anesthesia.

**pro·poxy·phene** (pro-pok′sĭ-fēn) [MeSH: Propoxyphene] an analgesic, structurally related to methadone. Called also *dextropropoxyphene.* See also *levopropoxyphene napsylate.*
**p. hydrochloride** [USP], the hydrochloride salt of propoxyphene, used as an analgesic to provide relief in mild to moderate pain, administered orally.
**p. napsylate** [USP], the napsylate salt of propoxyphene, used the same as the hydrochloride salt.

**pro·pran·o·lol** (pro-pran′ə-lol) [MeSH: Propranolol] a beta-adrenergic blocking agent, which decreases cardiac rate and output, reduces blood pressure, and is effective in the prophylaxis of migraine.
**p. hydrochloride** [USP], the hydrochloride salt of propranolol, used as an antiarrhythmic, and also as an antihypertensive, in the management of hypertrophic aortic stenosis, and in conjunction with an alpha-adrenergic blocking agent in the symptomatic treatment of inoperable pheochromocytoma. It is also effective in the prophylaxis of migraine and in preventing fatal recurrences of cardiac failure. Administered orally or intravenously.

**pro·pri·e·tary** (pro-pri′ə-tar-e) a proprietary medicine; "any chemical, drug, or similar preparation used in the treatment of diseases, if such article is protected against free competition as to name, product, composition, or process of manufacture by secrecy, patent, trademark, or copyright, or by any other means."

**pro·prio·cep·tion** (pro″pre-o-sep′shən) [MeSH: Proprioception] perception mediated by proprioceptors or proprioceptive tissues.

**pro·prio·cep·tive** (pro″pre-o-sep′tiv) receiving stimuli within the tissues of the body, as within muscles and tendons. See *proprioceptor.*

**pro·prio·cep·tor** (pro″pre-o-sep′tor) sensory nerve terminals found in muscles, tendons, and joint capsules, which give information concerning movements and position of the body; sometimes the receptors in the labyrinth are also considered proprioceptors. See *exteroceptor, interoceptor,* and *receptor,* def. 3.

**pro·prio·spi·nal** (pro″pre-o-spi′nəl) pertaining wholly to the spinal cord; said of ascending and descending nerve fibers that interconnect segments of the spinal cord.

**pro·pro·tein** (pro-pro′tēn) a precursor of a protein that is converted into the active protein by proteolysis or glycosylation.

**prop·tom·e·ter** (prop-tom′ə-tər) exophthalmometer.

**prop·to·sis** (prop-to′sis) exophthalmos.

**Pro·pul·sid** (pro-pul′sid) trademark for a preparation of cisapride.

**pro·pul·sion** (pro-pul′shən) [*pro-* + *pulsion*] 1. tendency to fall forward in walking. 2. festination.

**pro·pyl** (pro′pəl) the univalent chemical radical, $CH_3CH_2CH_2$—, from propane.
**p. gallate** [NF], an antioxidant, used in pharmaceutical preparations.

**prop·y·lene** (prop′ə-lēn) chemical name: propene. A gaseous hydrocarbon, $CH_3CH{=}CH_2$, of the olefin series.
**p. glycol** [USP], 1,2-propanediol, a clear, colorless, viscous liquid used as a humectant and solvent in pharmaceutical preparations.

**p. carbonate** [NF], a clear, colorless, mobile liquid used as a solvent in oral and topical pharmaceutical preparations.

**pro·pyl·hex·e·drine** (pro″pəl-hek′sə-drēn) [USP] an adrenergic compound, used as a vasoconstrictor to decongest nasal mucosa, administered by inhalation.

**pro·pyl·io·done** (pro″pəl-i′o-dōn) [USP] [MeSH: Propyliodone] a radiopaque medium, used in bronchography, administered intratracheally.

**pro·pyl·par·a·ben** (pro″pəl-par′ə-bən) [NF] an antifungal agent, used as a preservative in pharmaceutical preparations.

**pro·pyl·thio·ura·cil** (pro″pəl-thi″o-u′rə-sil) [USP] [MeSH: Propylthiouracil] a thyroid inhibitor, used in the treatment of hyperthyroidism, particularly to prepare patients for thyroid surgery and to maintain those who are poor surgical risks, administered orally.

**pro re na·ta** (pro re na′tə) [L.] according to circumstances. Abbreviated p.r.n.

**pro·re·nin** (pro′re-nin) the inactive precursor of renin, stored in the juxtaglomerular cells of the kidney and activated by cleavage to renin.

**pro·ren·nin** (pro-ren′in) prochymosin.

**Pro·ro·cen·trum** (pro″ro-sen′trəm) [*L. prora* prow + *centrum* center] a genus of plantlike, marine and freshwater protozoa (order Dinoflagellida, class Phytomastigophorea), which like other dinoflagellates produce discoloration of the water (red tide) when present in vast numbers.

**pror·sad** (pror′səd) [L. *prorsum* forward] in an anterior direction.

**pro·ru·bri·cyte** (pro-roo′brĭ-sīt) basophilic erythroblast.

**Pros·car** (pros′kahr) trademark for a preparation of finasteride.

**pro·scil·lar·i·din** (pro-sil-ar′ĭ-din) [MeSH: Proscillaridin] a cardiac glycoside obtained from squill, composed of a molecule of rhamnose linked to a steroid base, and having the same actions and uses as digitalis; administered orally and intravenously.

**pro·se·cre·tin** (pro″se-kre′tin) a hypothetical precursor of secretin, thought to be contained in epithelial cells of the duodenum and jejunum and to be converted into secretin on hydrolysis with acids.

**pro·sec·tion** (pro-sek′shən) a carefully prepared dissection for demonstration of anatomic structure.

**pro·sec·tor** (pro-sek′tor) [L.] one who dissects anatomical subjects for demonstration.

**pros·en·ceph·a·lon** (pros″ən-sef′ə-lon) [*pros-* + *encephalon*] [MeSH: Prosencephalon] 1. [TA] the part of the brain developed from the anterior of the three primary vesicles of the embryonic neural tube; it comprises the diencephalon and telencephalon. 2. the most anterior of the three primary brain vesicles in the embryo, later dividing into the telencephalon and the diencephalon. Called also *forebrain.*

**pros(o)-** [Gr. *prosō* forward] a prefix meaning forward, or anterior.

**Proso·bran·chi·a·ta** (pro″so-brang″ke-a′tə) Streptoneura.

**proso·cele** (pros′o-sēl) prosocoele.

**proso·coele** (pros′o-sēl) [*proso-* + *-coele*] the foremost cavity of the brain; the ventricular cavity of the prosencephalon.

**proso·de·mic** (pros″o-dem′ik) [*proso-* + Gr. *dēmos* people] pertaining to or denoting a disease transmitted directly from person to person rather than spread generally (as by a contaminated water supply).

**pros·o·dy** (pros′o-de) [Gr. *prosodos* a solemn procession] the variation in stress, pitch, and rhythm of speech by which different shades of meaning are conveyed.

**proso·gas·ter** (pros′o-gas″tər) [*proso-* + Gr. *gastēr* stomach] foregut.

**proso·pag·no·sia** (pros″o-pag-no′se-ə) [*prosop-* + *agnosia*] a form of visual agnosia characterized by an inability to recognize familiar faces, or even one's own face in a mirror, which occurs as a result of bilateral damage to the medioinferior occipital lobes along the medioventral surfaces of the temporal lobes. Called also *face* or *facial agnosia.*

**proso·pec·ta·sia** (pros″o-pək-ta′zhə) [*prosop-* + *ectasia*] oversize of the face.

**Pro·so·pis** (pro-so′pis) the mesquites, a genus of shrubs of the family Leguminosae, found in the southwestern United States and other arid regions of the Americas. *P. juliflo′ra* L. is the source of mesquite gum that is used medicinally; its beans contain a toxin that can cause fatal neurotoxicity in ruminants.

**proso·pla·sia** (pros″o-pla′shə) [*proso-* + *-plasia*] 1. abnormal differentiation of tissue. 2. development into a higher level of organization or of function.

**prosop(o)-** [Gr. *prosōpon* face] a combining form denoting relationship to the face.

**pros·o·po·an·os·chi·sis** (pros″o-po-ə-nos′ĭ-kis) [*prosopo-* + *ana-* + *-schisis*] oblique facial cleft.

**pros·o·pop·a·gus** (pros″o-pop′ə-gəs) [*prosopo-* + *-pagus*] asymmetrical conjoined twins in which the parasite is attached to the face elsewhere than at the jaw.

**pros·o·po·ple·gia** (pros″o-po-ple′jə) [*prosopo-* + *-plegia*] facial paralysis.

**pros·o·pos·chi·sis** (pros″o-pos′kĭ-sis) [*prosopo-* + *-schisis*] facial cleft, def. 2.

**pros·o·po·ster·no·dy·mus** (pros″o-po-ster″no-di′məs) [*prosopo-* + *sterno-* + *-didymus*] conjoined twins joined face to face and sternum to sternum.

**pros·o·po·tho·ra·cop·a·gus** (pros″o-po-thor″ə-cop′ə-gəs) [*prosopo-* + *thoraco-* + *-pagus*] symmetrical conjoined twins united in the frontal plane, the fusion extending from the oral region through the thorax.

**pros·ta·cy·clin** (pros″tə-si′klin) a prostaglandin, $PGI_2$, synthesized by endothelial cells lining the cardiovascular system; it is the most potent known inhibitor of platelet aggregation and a powerful vasodilator and thus is a physiologic antagonist of thromboxane $A_2$. It is used as an inhibitor of platelet aggregation. When used pharmaceutically, its nonproprietary name is *epoprostenol.*

**pros·ta·cy·clin syn·thase** (pros″tə-si′klin sin′thās) prostaglandin-I synthase.

**pros·ta·glan·din** (pros″tə-glan′din) [*prostate gland* + *-in* because they were originally thought to originate in the prostate] any of a group of components derived from unsaturated 20-carbon fatty acids, primarily arachidonic acid, via the cyclooxygenase pathway; they are potent mediators of numerous different physiologic processes. The abbreviation for prostaglandin is PG; specific compounds are designated by adding a letter to indicate the type of ring structure and a numerical subscript to indicate the number of double bonds in the hydrocarbon skeleton (e.g., $PGE_2$, etc.). Most naturally occurring prostaglandins have two double bonds and are synthesized from arachidonic acid by the pathway shown in the illustration. The 1 series and 3 series are produced by the same pathway starting with fatty acids that have one fewer or one more double bond than arachidonic acid. The subscript $\alpha$ or $\beta$ indicates the three-dimensional configuration of alcoholic groups attached to the ring structures ($\alpha$ denotes a substituent below the plane of the ring, $\beta$, above the plane). The naturally occurring PGF's all have the $\alpha$ configuration. Prostaglandins act in the cells in which they are synthesized and surrounding cells, and their actions and effects vary with concentration, hormonal environment, and cell type.
**p. $D_2$ ($PGD_2$),** the major prostaglandin produced by mast cells; it is a mediator of immediate hypersensitivity synthesized and released in response to binding of immunoglobulin E to receptors on the mast cell, and its effects include vasodilation and contraction of nonvascular smooth muscle.
**p. $E_1$ ($PGE_1$),** the analogue of $PGE_2$ having one double bond; many of its effects, including vasodilation, are similar to those of $PGE_2$, but unlike the latter it inhibits platelet aggregation; it is used pharmaceutically and called *alprostadil* as a vasodilator in neonates with congenital heart disease.
**p. $E_2$ ($PGE_2$),** an important prostaglandin produced in the renal medulla, gastrointestinal mucosa, and other tissues; it causes renal vasodilation and inhibition of renal tubular sodium resorption, inhibition of gastric secretion, and either contraction or relaxation of smooth muscle (depending on the tissue). It is also released by macrophages and modulates several inflammatory responses; it increases vascular permeability, increases pain sensitivity, is pyrogenic, and suppresses lymphocyte transformation, release of mediators from mast cells, and cell-mediated cytotoxicity. $PGE_2$ produced by some tumors causes hypercalcemia by stimulation of bone resorption by osteoclasts. When used pharmaceutically its nonproprietary name is *dinoprostone.*
**p. $F_{2\alpha}$ ($PGF_{2\alpha}$),** a stable prostaglandin formed from $PGH_2$ or $PGE_2$; it stimulates the contraction of uterine and bronchial smooth muscle and produces vasoconstriction in some vessels. As a pharmaceutical, its nonproprietary name is *dinoprost.*
**p. $F_{2\alpha}$ tromethamine,** dinoprost tromethamine.
**p. $G_2$ ($PGG_2$),** a prostaglandin cyclic endoperoxide formed from arachidonic acid by incorporation of two oxygen molecules, catalyzed by the cyclooxygenase activity of prostaglandin endoperoxide synthase; it is an unstable intermediate and is converted rapidly and spontaneously to $PGH_2$.
**p. $H_2$ ($PGH_2$),** a prostaglandin cyclic endoperoxide sometimes formed from $PGG_2$ by the peroxidase reaction of prostaglandin endoperoxide synthase, although the synthase is not required; it is an unstable intermediate that can be converted to several important prostaglandins and thromboxanes.

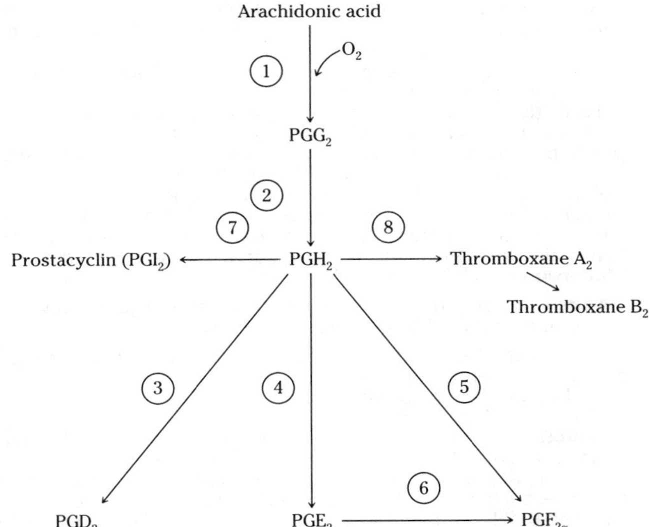


KEY TO ENZYMES (Circled Numbers)

1. Prostaglandin synthase (cyclooxygenase activity)
2. Prostaglandin synthase (peroxidase activity)
3. Prostaglandin-$H_2$ D-isomerase
4. Prostaglandin-$H_2$ E-isomerase
5. Endoperoxide reductase
6. Prostaglandin-$E_2$ 9-reductase
7. Prostacyclin synthase
8. Thromboxane synthase

Cyclooxygenase pathway of prostaglandin and thromboxane synthesis.

**p. $I_2$ ($PGI_2$),** prostacyclin.

**pros·ta·glan·din-D syn·thase** (pros″tə-glan′din sin′thās) [EC 5.3.99.2] an enzyme of the isomerase class that catalyzes the conversion of the intermediate prostaglandin $H_2$ ($PGH_2$) to prostaglandin $D_2$ ($PGD_2$). The enzyme requires glutathione. See illustration at *prostaglandin.* Called also *endoperoxide-D-isomerase* and *prostaglandin-$H_2$ D-isomerase.*

**pros·ta·glan·din en·do·per·ox·ide syn·thase** (pros″tə-glan′din en″do-pər-ok′sīd sin′thās) [EC 1.14.99.1] an enzyme of the oxidoreductase class that has both cyclooxygenase and peroxidase activities, which together catalyze the first three reactions in the synthesis of prostaglandins and thromboxanes from arachidonic acid. Its cyclooxygenase activity catalyzes the first two reactions, each of which adds a molecule of oxygen to arachidonic acid, to form the intermediate $PGG_2$; its peroxidase activity catalyzes the conversion of $PGG_2$ to the intermediate $PGH_2$, from which are formed the prostaglandins and thromboxanes. See illustration at *prostaglandin.*

**pros·ta·glan·din-$E_2$ re·duc·tase** (pros″tə-glan′din re-duk′tās) [EC 1.1.1.189] an enzyme of the oxidoreductase class that catalyzes the reduction of prostaglandin $E_2$ to prostaglandin $F_{2\alpha}$. It can also act on a variety of similar prostaglandin derivatives with 9-keto or 15-keto groups, reducing them to the corresponding hydroxy compounds. See also illustration at *prostaglandin.*

**pros·ta·glan·din-E syn·thase** (pros″tə-glan′din sin′thās) [EC 5.3.99.3] an enzyme of the isomerase class that catalyzes the conversion of the intermediate prostaglandin $H_2$ ($PGH_2$) to prostaglandin $E_2$ ($PGE_2$). The enzyme requires glutathione. See also illustration at *prostaglandin.* Called also *endoperoxide-E-isomerase* and *prostaglandin-$H_2$ E-isomerase.*

**pros·ta·glan·din-$H_2$ D-isom·er·ase** (pros″tə-glan′din i-som′ər-ās) prostaglandin-D synthase.

**pros·ta·glan·din-$H_2$ E-isom·er·ase** (pros″tə-glan′din i-som′ər-ās) prostaglandin-E synthase.

**pros·ta·glan·din-I syn·thase** (pros″tə-glan′din sin′thās) [EC 5.3.99.4] an enzyme of the isomerase class that catalyzes the conversion of the prostaglandin intermediate prostaglandin $H_2$ ($PGH_2$) to prostacyclin ($PGI_2$). The enzyme acts predominantly in the endothelium of blood vessel walls. See also illustration at *prostaglandin.* Called also *prostacyclin synthase.*

**pros·ta·glan·din syn·thase** (pros″tə-glan′din sin′thās) prostaglandin endoperoxide synthase.

**pros·ta·noid** (pros′tə-noid) any of a group of complex fatty acids derived from arachidonic acid, being 20 carbons in length with an internal five- or six-carbon ring; examples are the prostaglandins, prostanoic acid, and the thromboxanes.

**Pros·taph·lin** (pros-taf′lin) trademark for preparations of oxacillin sodium.

**pros·ta·ta** (pros′tə-tə) [L] [TA] prostate.

**pros·ta·tal·gia** (pros″tə-tal′jə) [*prostate* + *-algia*] pain in the prostate.

**pros·ta·tauxe** (pros″tə-tawk′se) prostatomegaly.

**pros·tate** (pros′tāt) [Gr. *prostates* one who stands before, from *pro* before + *histanai* to stand] [MeSH: Prostate] a gland in the male which surrounds the neck of the bladder and the urethra. It consists of a median lobe and two lateral lobes, and is made up partly of glandular matter, whose ducts empty into the prostatic portion of the urethra, and partly of muscular fibers that encircle the urethra. The prostate contributes to the seminal fluid a secretion containing acid phosphatase, citric acid, and proteolytic enzymes that account for the liquefaction of the coagulated semen. Called also *prostata* [TA], *glandula prostatica*, and *prostate gland.*

**pros·ta·tec·to·my** (pros″tə-tek′tə-me) [*prostate* + *-ectomy*] [MeSH: Prostatectomy] surgical removal of the prostate or of a part of it.
**perineal p.,** removal of the prostate through an incision in the perineum.
**radical p.,** removal of the prostate with its capsule, seminal vesicles, ductus deferens, some pelvic fasciae, and sometimes pelvic lymph nodes; performed via either the retropubic or the perineal route.
**retropubic prevesical p.,** removal of the prostate through a suprapubic incision but without entering the urinary bladder.
**suprapubic transvesical p.,** removal of the prostate through an incision above the pubis and through the urinary bladder.
**transurethral p.,** transurethral resection of the prostate; see under *resection.*

**pros·ta·tel·co·sis** (pros″tə-təl-ko′sis) [*prostate* + *helcosis*] ulceration of the prostate.

**pros·tat·ic** (pros-tat′ik) pertaining to the prostate.

**pros·tat·i·co·ves·i·cal** (pros-tat″ĭ-ko-ves′ĭ-kəl) pertaining to the prostate and the bladder.

**pros·tat·i·co·ve·sic·u·lec·to·my** (pros-tat″ĭ-ko-və-sik″u-lek′tə-me) excision of the prostate and seminal vesicles.

**pros·ta·tism** (pros′tə-tiz-əm) a symptom complex resulting from compression or obstruction of the urethra, due most commonly to nodular hyperplasia of the prostate (see under *hyperplasia*). Symptoms include diminution in caliber and force of the urinary stream, hesitancy in initiating voiding, inability to end urination abruptly (with postvoiding dribbling), a sensation of incomplete bladder emptying, and occasionally urinary retention.
**vesical p.,** a condition of retention of the urine resembling that of prostatic disease, but existing in the absence of any affection of the prostate.

**pros·ta·tisme** (pros-tə-tēzm′) prostatism.
**p. sans prostate′,** the symptoms of prostatic obstruction without enlargement of the prostate.

**pros·ta·ti·tic** (pros″tə-ti′tik) pertaining to prostatitis.

**pros·ta·ti·tis** (pros″tə-ti′tis) [MeSH: Prostatitis] inflammation of the prostate.

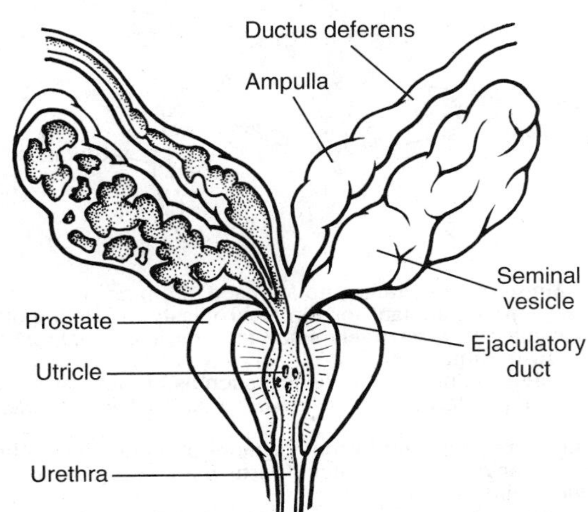


Prostate and seminal vesicles.

**allergic p., eosinophilic p.,** a condition seen in patients with certain allergies, characterized by diffuse infiltration of the prostate by eosinophils, with the development of small foci of fibrinoid necrosis.
**nonspecific granulomatous p.,** prostatitis characterized histologically by focal or diffuse infiltration of the tissues by peculiar, large, pale macrophages.

**pros·ta·to·cys·ti·tis** (pros″tə-to-sis-tiʹtis) [*prostate* + *cysto-* + *-itis*] inflammation of the neck of the bladder (prostatic urethra) and the bladder cavity.

**pros·ta·to·cys·tot·o·my** (pros″tə-to-sis-totʹə-me) [*prostate* + *cysto-* + *-tomy*] surgical incision of the bladder and prostate.

**pros·ta·to·dyn·ia** (pros″tə-to-dinʹe-ə) [*prostate* + *-odynia*] prostatalgia.

**pros·ta·tog·ra·phy** (pros″tə-togʹrə-fe) radiography of the prostate.

**pros·tato·lith** (pros-tatʹo-lith) a prostatic calculus.

**pros·ta·to·li·thot·o·my** (pros″tə-to-lĭ-thotʹə-me) incision of the prostate for the removal of calculus.

**pros·ta·to·meg·a·ly** (pros″tə-to-megʹə-le) [*prostate* + *-megaly*] hypertrophy of the prostate.

**pros·ta·tom·e·ter** (pros″tə-tomʹə-tər) [*prostate* + *-meter*] an instrument for measuring the prostate.

**pros·tat·o·my** (pros-tatʹə-me) prostatotomy.

**pros·ta·tor·rhea** (pros″tə-to-reʹə) [*prostate* + *-rrhea*] a catarrhal discharge from the prostate.

**pros·ta·tot·o·my** (pros″tə-totʹə-me) [*prostate* + *-tomy*] surgical incision of the prostate.

**pros·ta·to·ve·sic·u·lec·to·my** (pros″tə-to-və-sik″u-lekʹtə-me) excision of the prostate and seminal vesicles.

**pros·ta·to·ve·sic·u·li·tis** (pros″tə-to-və-sik″u-liʹtis) inflammation of the prostate and seminal vesicles.

**pro·ster·na·tion** (pro″stər-naʹshən) camptocormia.

**pros·the·ca** (pros-theʹkə) pl. *prostheʹcae* [Gr. *prosthēkē* appendage] 1. an appendage of a prokaryotic cell that forms a narrow extension and is enclosed by the cell wall. 2. a movable mandibular appendage in certain insects.

**pros·the·ses** (pros-theʹsēz) [Gr.] [MeSH: Prosthesis] plural of *prosthesis.*

**pros·the·sis** (pros-theʹsis) pl. *prostheʹses* [Gr. "a putting to"] [MeSH: Prosthesis] an artificial substitute for a missing body part, such as an arm or leg, eye or tooth, used for functional or cosmetic reasons, or both.
**Angelchik p.,** a C-shaped silicone device that wraps around the distal esophagus for treatment of reflux esophagitis or during laparotomy.
**antireflux p.,** a ring-shaped device that is placed around the esophagus above the stomach and below the diaphragm for treatment of gastroesophageal reflux and hiatal hernia.

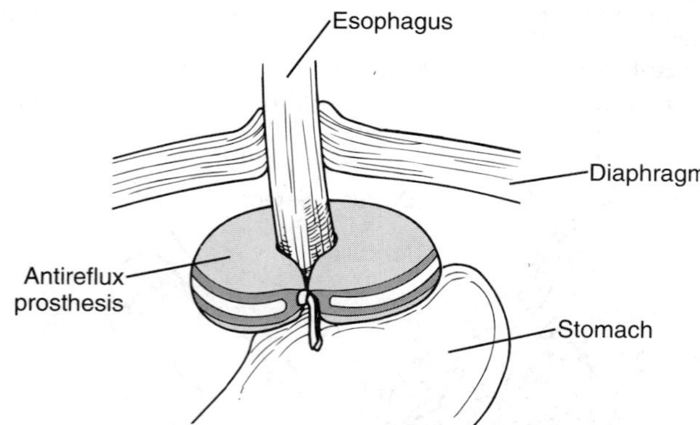


**Austin Moore p.,** a metallic implant used in hip arthroplasty.
**Charnley's p.,** an implant for hip arthroplasty consisting of an acetabular cup and a relatively small femoral head component that form a low-friction joint.
**cleft palate p.,** a prosthetic device, such as an obturator, used to correct cleft palate. See also *speech-aid p.,* and *artificial palate,* under *palate.*
**dental p.,** a replacement for one or more of the teeth or other oral structure, ranging from a single tooth to a complete denture. See also *bridge* and *denture.*
**heart valve p.,** artificial cardiac valve; see under *valve.*
**maxillofacial p.,** a prosthetic replacement for those regions in the maxilla, mandible, and face that are missing or defective because of surgical intervention, trauma, pathology, or development malformations. See also under *prosthetics.*
**ocular p.,** 1. an artificial eye; see under *eye.* 2. any other aid to vision, e.g., eyeglasses or occluders.
**palatal lift p.,** a type of speech-aid prosthesis sometimes used to aid in closure in cases of velopharyngeal insufficiency.
**penile p.,** a semirigid rod or inflatable device implanted in the penis to provide an erection in men with organic impotence.
**Robinson p.,** a type of stainless steel prosthetic stapes.
**speech-aid p.,** a device designed to close a cleft of the hard or soft palate and to substitute for structures used for normal speech. Called also *artificial palate, obturator,* and *prosthetic speech aid.*
**Thompson p.,** a Vitallium implant used in hip arthroplasty.

**pros·thet·ic** (pros-thetʹik) serving as a substitute; pertaining to the use or application of prostheses.

**pros·thet·ics** (pros-thetʹiks) the field of knowledge relating to prostheses, their design, use, etc.
**dental p., denture p.,** prosthodontics.
**facial p.,** maxillofacial p.
**maxillofacial p.,** that branch of prosthodontics concerned with anatomic, functional, and cosmetic reconstruction by means of synthetic substitutes of those regions of the maxilla, mandible, and face that have been damaged, absent, or malformed due to illness, injury, congenital defects, or surgical intervention. Called also *facial p.* See also under *prosthesis.*

**pros·the·tist** (prosʹthə-tist) [Gr. *prosthetes* one who adds] a person skilled in prosthetics and practicing its application in individual cases.

**pros·thi·on (PR)** (prosʹthe-on) [Gr. *prosthios* foremost] a craniometric landmark located at the point of the maxillary alveolar process that projects most anteriorly in the midline of the maxilla; used for measuring upper facial height and in determining the gnathic index.

**pros·tho·don·tia** (pros″tho-donʹshə) prosthodontics.

**pros·tho·don·tics** (pros″tho-donʹtiks) [*prosthesis* + Gr. *odous* tooth] [MeSH: Prosthodontics] that branch of dentistry pertaining to the restoration and maintenance of oral function, comfort, appearance, and health of the patient by the replacement of missing teeth and contiguous tissues with artificial substitutes. Called also *dental prosthetics, denture prosthetics, prosthetic dentistry,* and *prosthodontia.*

**pros·tho·don·tist** (pros″tho-donʹtist) a dentist who specializes in prosthodontics.

**Pros·tho·gon·i·mus** (pros″tho-gonʹĭ-məs) a genus of trematodes. *P. macrorʹchis* parasitizes chickens, turkeys, and other birds.

**pros·tho·ker·a·to·plas·ty** (pros″tho-kerʹə-to-plas″te) [*prosthesis* + *kerato-* + *-plasty*] surgical replacement of corneal tissue (as in cataract) by an inert transparent prosthesis.

**Pro·stig·min** (pro-stigʹmin) trademark for preparations of neostigmine.

**Pros·tin E2** (prosʹtin) trademark for preparations of dinoprostone.

**Pros·tin F2 Alpha** (prosʹtin) trademark for preparations of dinoprost tromethamine.

**Pros·tin VR** (prosʹtin) trademark for a preparation of alprostadil.

**pros·tra·tion** (pros-traʹshən) [L. *prostratio*] extreme exhaustion or powerlessness.
**heat p.,** heat exhaustion.
**nervous p.,** neurasthenia.

**pro·tac·tin·i·um** (pro″tak-tinʹe-əm) [MeSH: Protactinium] a radioactive metallic chemical element occurring along with radium in pitchblende, carnotite, and other minerals; atomic weight, 231; atomic number, 91; symbol Pa.

**pro·tal** (proʹtəl) congenital; first; dating from the beginning.

**Pro·tal·ba** (pro-talʹbə) trademark for preparations of protoveratrine A.

**pro·tal·bu·mose** (pro-talʹbu-mōs) a primary proteose.

**pro·ta·mine** (proʹtə-mēn) [*prot-* + *amine*] any of a class of basic proteins of low molecular weight, occurring in combination with nucleic acids in the sperm of salmon and certain other fish and having the property of neutralizing heparin.
**p. sulfate** [USP], a purified mixture of simple protein principles obtained from the sperm or testes of suitable species of fish; it has the property of neutralizing heparin, and is used as an antidote to overdosage with heparin, administered intravenously.

**pro·tan** (proʹtan) 1. pertaining to protanomaly or protanopia. 2. a person with protanomaly or protanopia.

**pro·ta·nom·al** (pro″tə-nomʹəl) a person with protanomaly.

**pro·ta·nom·a·lous** (pro″tə-nom′ə-ləs) pertaining to or characterized by protanomaly.

**pro·ta·nom·a·ly** (pro″tə-nom′ə-le) [*prot-* + *anomaly*] a type of anomalous trichromasy in which the first, red-sensitive, cones have decreased sensitivity; therefore a greater than normal proportion of lithium red light to thallium green light is required to match a fixed sodium yellow light.

**pro·ta·nope** (pro′tə-nōp) an individual exhibiting protanopia.

**pro·ta·no·pia** (pro″tə-no′pe-ə) [*prot-* + *an-*[1] + *-opia*] a dichromasy characterized by retention of the sensory mechanism for two hues only (blue and yellow) of the normal 4-primary quota, and lacking that for red and green and their derivatives, with loss of luminance and shift of brightness and hue curves toward the short-wave end of the spectrum, as in twilight vision.

**pro·ta·nop·ic** (pro″tə-nop′ik) pertaining to or characterized by protanopia.

**pro·ta·nop·sia** (pro″tə-nop′se-ə) protanopia.

**Pro·ta·phane NPH** (pro′tə-fān) trademark for preparations of isophane insulin suspension.

**Pro·tea** (pro′te-ə) [L.] a genus of trees of the family Proteaceae; many species grow in wet and warm regions and several are medicinal. *P. melli′fera* L. is the sugar protea, which is made into a syrup used for coughs and pulmonary disorders.

**pro·te·an** (pro′te-ən) [Gr. *Prōteus* an ocean deity able to appear in many different forms] assuming different shapes; changeable in form.

**pro·te·ase** (pro′te-ās) endopeptidase.

**pro·tec·tant** (pro-tek′tənt) protective.

**pro·tec·tin** (pro-tek′tin) a membrane-bound protein, CD59, present in many types of cells; it binds homologous complement factors C8 and C9 and prevents insertion of the membrane attack complex into the membrane, thereby protecting normal bystander cells from lysis after complement activation in nearby bacteria or immune complexes. Called also *membrane inhibitor of reactive lysis.*

**pro·tec·tive** (pro-tek′tiv) [L. *protegere* to cover over] 1. affording defense or immunity. 2. an agent that affords defense against a deleterious influence, such as a substance applied to the skin *(skin p.)* to avoid the effects of the sun's rays *(solar p.)* or other noxious influences; called also *screen.*

**pro·tec·tor** (pro-tek′tər) a substance in a catalyst which prolongs the rate of activity in the latter. Cf. *promotor.*

**LATS p.,** an immunoglobulin found in the serum of patients with Graves' disease that neutralizes the capacity of thyroid tissue to bind LATS (long-acting thyroid stimulator); it interferes with the binding of thyrotropin to the human thyroid cell membrane.

**Pro·te·eae** (pro-te′e-e) in some systems of classification, a tribe of gram-negative, facultatively anaerobic, rod-shaped bacteria of the family Enterobacteriaceae, made up of the genera *Morganella, Proteus,* and *Providencia.*

**pro·tein** (pro′tēn) [Gr. *prōtos* first] any of a group of complex organic compounds which contain carbon, hydrogen, oxygen, nitrogen, and usually sulfur, the characteristic element being nitrogen. Proteins, the principal constituents of the protoplasm of all cells, are of high molecular weight and consist essentially of combinations of $\alpha$-amino acids in peptide linkages. Twenty different amino acids are commonly found in proteins, and each protein has a unique genetically defined amino acid sequence which determines its specific shape and function. Their roles include enzymatic catalysis, transport and storage, coordinated motion, nerve impulse generation and transmission, control of growth and differentiation, immunity, and mechanical suppport.

## Protein

**p. A,** staphylococcal p. A.

**AA p.,** amyloid A p.

**acute phase p.,** any of the non-antibody proteins found in increased amounts in serum during the acute phase response; they include C-reactive protein, serum amyloid A protein, fibrinogen, and $\alpha$1-acid glycoprotein.

**AL p.,** amyloid light chain p.

**alcohol-soluble p.,** prolamin.

**amyloid A p.,** a pathological fibrillar low-molecular-weight protein occurring in reactive systemic amyloidosis and familial Mediterranean fever; it is antigenically related to the high-molecular-weight serum amyloid A (SAA) protein. Called also *AA p.* See also *amyloid* (def. 3).

**amyloid light chain p.,** a pathological fibrillar low-molecular-weight protein occurring in immunocyte-derived amyloidosis; it is structurally and immunologically similar to the variable region of either the kappa chains or the lambda chains of immunoglobulins. Called also *AL p.* See also *amyloid* (def. 3).

**bactericidal permeability increasing p. (BPI),** a cationic 59-kD antibacterial protein occurring in neutrophil granules; it causes phospholipase activation and phospholipid degradation and increases the permeability of the bacterial cell membrane.

**bacterial p.,** a protein formed by bacterial activity.

**bacterial cellular p.,** a protein that forms part of the substance of a bacterium.

**Bence Jones p.,** an abnormal plasma or urinary protein, consisting of monoclonal immunoglobulin light chains, excreted in some plasma cell dyscrasias and characterized by its unusual solubility properties: on heating it precipitates at 50°–60°C and redissolves at 90°–100°C, and on cooling it again precipitates and redissolves. See *M component,* under *component.*

**binding p.,** 1. any protein able to specifically and reversibly bind other substances, such as ions, sugars, nucleic acids, or amino acids; they are believed to function in transport. 2. transport p.

**bone Gla p.,** osteocalcin.

**bone morphogenetic p.,** a noncollagenous factor, believed to be a protein, that occurs in demineralized bone and stimulates osteogenesis.

**p. C,** a vitamin K–dependent plasma protein that, when activated by thrombin, inhibits the clotting cascade at the levels of factor V and factor VIII by enzymatic cleavage of the activated forms of these clotting factors; it also enhances fibrinolysis. Deficiency of protein C results in recurrent venous thrombosis. The activated form is abbreviated APC.

**CAD p.,** a protein containing catalytic sites for three enzyme activities: carbamoyl-phosphate synthase (glutamine-hydrolyzing) [EC 6.3.5.5], aspartate carbamoyltransferase [EC 2.1.3.2], and dihydroorotase [EC 3.5.2.3]. The enzyme activities catalyze the first three reactions of pyrimidine biosynthesis.

**carrier p.,** 1. a protein which, when coupled to hapten *in vivo* or *in vitro,* renders the hapten capable of eliciting an immune response. See *hapten.* 2. carrier (def. 6).

**cationic p's,** antimicrobial cationic proteins occurring in the primary (azurophilic) granules of neutrophils. They have low molecular weights, are rich in arginine, and appear to inhibit microbial growth. They presumably include the previously characterized substances termed *leukin* and *phagocytin.*

**C4 binding p.,** a complement system regulatory protein that inhibits activation of the classical pathway; it both accelerates decay of the classical pathway C3 convertase by binding to C4b and displacing C2a and is also a cofactor for factor I–mediated cleavage of C4b.

**coagulated p.,** an insoluble form which certain proteins assume when denatured at their isoelectric point by heat, alcohol, ultraviolet rays, or other agents.

**complement control p. (CCP),** any of a superfamily of proteins involved in complement regulation, encoded in a closely linked gene cluster, and having one or more stretches of a common short consensus repeat encoding a 60 amino acid domain. Included are factor H, C4 binding protein, decay accelerating factor, membrane cofactor protein, and several complement receptors. Called also *regulator of complement activation.*

**complete p.,** a protein composed of amino acids in appropriate proportion to each other so that when it is the sole source of protein, the amino acids can all be used by the body; it is therefore more valuable for nutrition than is the partial protein (q.v.).

**compound p., conjugated p.,** one in which the protein is linked to a nonprotein (prosthetic) group other than as a salt. Included are nucleoproteins, glycoproteins, lipoproteins, metalloproteins, chromoproteins, hemoproteins, and phosphoproteins. Cf. *simple p.*

**constitutive p's,** proteins produced in fixed amounts, regardless of the organism's need for them.

**cord p's,** the proteins of blood from the umbilical cord.

**C-reactive p. (CRP),** a globulin that forms a precipitate with the somatic C-polysaccharide of the pneumococcus in vitro; the most predominant of the acute phase proteins.

**cystic fibrosis transmembrane regulator p.,** cystic fibrosis transmembrane conductance regulator.

**denatured p.**, see *protein denaturation,* under *denaturation.*
**derived p.**, derivatives of the protein molecule formed by hydrolytic changes, including coagulated proteins, proteoses, peptones, and peptides.
**encephalitogenic p.**, myelin basic p.
**fibrillar p., fibrous p.**, one that is insoluble in water or dilute salt solution, having extensive secondary structure, such as $\alpha$-helix or $\beta$-pleated sheet structure; included are the principal structural proteins of the body, such as collagens, elastins, keratins, actin, and myosin. Cf. *globular p.*
**fusion p.**, a protein produced by a recombinant DNA construct engineered such that the coding region of one gene is linked distal to the 5′ end of another gene and within its coding region, placing expression of both genes under regulatory control of the second, usually well characterized, gene.
**G p.**, any of a family of similar heterotrimeric proteins of the intracellular portion of the plasma membrane that bind activated receptor complexes and, through conformational changes and cyclic binding and hydrolysis of GTP, directly or indirectly effect alterations in channel gating and so couple cell surface receptors to intracellular responses. Some G proteins are named for their activities, e.g., $G_s$ stimulates and $G_i$ inhibits enzyme activity.
**glial fibrillary acidic p. (GFAP)**, the protein forming the glial filaments of the astrocytes; it is used as an immunohistochemical marker of these cells. It also occurs in radial glia and occasionally in peripheral neuroglia.
**globular p.**, any of the group of simple proteins soluble in water or dilute salt solution, their polypeptide chains coiled into a globular shape; they constitute most of the proteins in the body, including albumins, globulins, histones, and protamines. Cf. *fibrous p.*
**GM activator p.**, sphingolipid activator p.
**GTPase-activating p.**, a protein that stimulates the GTPase activity of a GTP-binding protein, resulting in the conversion of the protein to its inactive form.
**GTP-binding p.**, any of a number of regulatory proteins, including the G proteins and the monomeric *small GTP-binding proteins,* in which the exchange of GDP for GTP induces a conformational change to produce an active state, while the hydrolysis of GTP to GDP produces an inactive state. GTP-binding proteins act as switches that couple cell-surface receptor activation with intracellular processes such as protein synthesis.
**guanyl-nucleotide-binding p.**, G p.
**heat shock p.**, any of a group of prokaryotic and eukaryotic proteins first identified as being synthesized in response to hyperthermia, hypoxia, or other stresses and believed to enable cells to recover from these stresses, perhaps by enabling recovery of gene expression. Many have been found to be molecular chaperones (q.v.) and these are synthesized abundantly regardless of stress.
**immune p.**, immunoglobulin.
**incomplete p.**, a protein having a ratio of amino acids different from that of the average body protein, and therefore less valuable for nutrition than is the complete protein (q.v.). Called also *partial p.*
**insoluble p.**, a substance left behind after the other proteins have been extracted from a cell.
**iron-sulfur p.**, a group of proteins, including ferredoxins and adrenodoxin, that function in electron transport; they contain iron-sulfur centers of the form $Fe_2S_2Cys_4$ or $Fe_4S_4Cys_4$, where Cys denotes a cysteine residue; the iron atoms undergo reversible transitions between the +2 and +3 oxidation states.
**leukocyte adhesion p. (LAP)**, $\beta_2$ integrin.
**M p.**, 1. a type-specific protein, consisting of two protein chains in a coiled structure, located on the surface of the cell wall of *Streptococcus pyogenes;* it is responsible for adhesion of the bacterium to host epithelial cells and mediates virulence by diminishing activation of the alternative pathway, thereby inhibiting phagocytosis. 2. a permease involved in the transport of $\beta$-galactosides across the cell membrane of *Escherichia coli.* 3. matrix p.
**maintenance p.**, the smallest amount of protein upon which the normal conditions of the body can be maintained.
**major basic p. (MBP)**, a cationic 10- to 15-kD protein occurring in eosinophilic granules and having cytotoxic activity against many parasites; it can also induce tissue injury in allergic and inflammatory diseases and, because it induces injury to the bronchial epithelium, is linked to asthma.
**matrix p.**, a nonglycosylated protein occurring between the nucleocapsid and envelope layers of certain viruses, such as orthomyxoviruses, and playing a role in the assembly of the virus particle. Called also *M p.*
**membrane p.**, one found in association with the cell membrane, either attached to (extrinsic or peripheral) or inserted in (intrinsic or integral) the membrane; possible roles include enzyme, receptor for a hormone or other molecule, and mediator of active or passive transport of lipid-insoluble substances across the membrane.
**membrane cofactor p. (MCP)**, a transmembrane protein, CD46, found in most blood cells, endothelial and epithelial cells, and fibroblasts; it restricts the turnover of complement by acting as a cofactor for factor I–mediated catabolism of C3b and C4b.
**membrane transport p.**, one facilitating the transport of one or more specific substances across the plasma membrane; see also *transport p.*
**myelin basic p. (MBP)**, a basic protein (MW 18,000) that constitutes about 30 per cent of myelin proteins; elevated levels of MBP occur in acute exacerbation of multiple sclerosis and acute cerebral infarction. Immunization of laboratory animals with MBP produces encephalomyelitis by inducing T cell activity that leads to demyelination and lymphoid infiltration. Called also *encephalitogenic p.*
**myeloma p.**, any of the pathological immunoglobulin proteins or fragments, such as M component and Bence-Jones protein, secreted by myeloma cells.
**native p.**, unchanged animal or vegetable protein, especially as it occurs in foods.
**parathyroid hormone–like p., parathyroid hormone–related p.**, see under *peptide.*
**partial p.**, incomplete p.
**plasma p's**, the hundreds of different proteins present in blood plasma, including transport proteins such as albumin, transferrin, and haptoglobin; fibrinogen and other coagulation factors; complement components; immunoglobulins; enzyme inhibitors; precursors of substances such as angiotensin and bradykinin; and many others.
**plasma p. fraction**, see under *fraction.*
**prion p. (PrP)**, a 33–35 kD protein of uncertain function, in humans coded for by a gene on the short arm of chromosome 20. The 27–30 kD protease-resistant core is the functional, and perhaps only, component of prions; several isoforms have been identified and are responsible for prion disease. Extracellular prion protein aggregates into rod-shaped structures that resemble amyloid.
**proteolipid p. (PLP)**, a hydrophobic protein that is the major constituent of myelin in the central nervous system. Defective synthesis of PLP results in Pelizaeus-Merzbacher disease. Called also *lipophilin.*
**R p.**, any of a group of similar proteins, so named for their rapid electrophoretic mobility relative to intrinsic factor (IF), that avidly bind ingested or circulating cobalamins or analogues and travel with them to the duodenum, where proteolytic digestion frees the vitamin to bind IF. Called also *cobalophilin* and *haptocorrin.*
**racemized p.**, protein so changed by chemical or other agents, usually dilute alkali, that its optical activity is lowered and it becomes more resistant to enzymatic hydrolysis. Acid hydrolysis of a racemized protein shows inactivation (racemization) of several of its constituent amino acids.
**recombinant p.**, a protein obtained by introducing recombinant DNA into a heterologous host (microorganism or yeast cell) and causing it to produce the gene product.
**retinol binding p. (RBP)**, an $\alpha$-globulin synthesized and secreted by the liver. It binds retinol and transthyretin in a 1:1:1 ratio; the complex solubilizes retinol and protects it from glomerular filtration and renal excretion while transporting it to the peripheral tissues.
**p. S**, a vitamin K–dependent plasma protein that inhibits blood clotting by serving as a cofactor for activated protein C. Not to be confused with *S p.*
**S p.**, see *vitronectin.* Not to be confused with *protein S.*
**S-100 p.**, a protein occurring in the central nervous system and in Schwann cells and satellite cells of ganglia; because it is present in tumors only of neural origin, it has been used to help determine the histological origins of some neoplasms.
**SAA p.**, serum amyloid A p.
**serum p's**, proteins of blood serum, i.e., all the plasma proteins except fibrinogen.
**serum amyloid A p.**, a high-molecular-weight protein antigenically related to amyloid A protein; it is an acute phase reactant and apparently suppresses antibody responses. Called also *SAA p.*
**silver p., mild**, see under *silver.*
**silver p., strong**, see under *silver.*
**simple p.**, one that contains only amino acids on complete hydrolysis. Cf. *conjugated p.*
**sphingolipid activator p. (SAP)**, any of a group of non-enzymatic lysosomal proteins that stimulate the actions of specific lysosomal hydrolases by binding and solubilizing their sphingolipid substrates. *SAP-1* is a glycoprotein that binds sulfatide, ganglioside $GM_1$, and ceramide trihexoside, activating cerebroside sulfatase, lysosomal $\beta$-galactosidase, and $\alpha$-galactosidase activities, respectively. Deficiency of SAP-1, an autosomal recessive trait, results in a disorder considered to be a form of juvenile metachromatic leukodystrophy. *SAP-2* is a glycoprotein necessary for the hydrolysis of ganglioside $GM_2$ via activation of hexosaminidases A and B; deficiency of SAP-2 results in $GM_2$ gangliosidosis, variant AB.
**staphylococcal p. A**, a *Staphylococcus aureus* cell wall protein that binds immunoglobulin G molecules and circulating immune com-

plexes and is used as a selective immunoadsorbent in biochemical research and in the treatment of idiopathic thrombocytopenic purpura.

**Tamm-Horsfall p.**, see under *mucoprotein.*

**transport p.**, a protein that binds to a substance and provides a transport system for it, either in the plasma or across a plasma membrane (see *facilitated diffusion,* under *diffusion*). Some are specific for one substance, such as a hormone, and others bind to several different substances. The term is sometimes used specifically for proteins that bind other proteins. Called also *carrier, translocase,* and *transporter.*

**uncoupling p.**, a protein that occurs in the inner membrane of the mitochondria of brown adipose tissue, important in nonshivering thermogenesis; it dissipates the proton gradient created by the respiratory chain, thus uncoupling oxidation from phosphorylation so that production of heat occurs instead of phosphorylation of ADP to ATP. Called also *thermogenin.*

**whole p.**, protein which has not been split.

**zinc finger p.**, any of a class of nucleic acid–binding proteins that also contain one or more zinc-binding domains (tandemly repeated, highly conserved stretches of 28 nucleotides). The class is named for the fingerlike secondary and tertiary structures formed in the zinc-binding regions of the molecules; individual proteins appear to be involved in transcriptional regulation and in RNA transport.

**pro·tein·a·ceous** (pro″tēn-a′shəs) pertaining to or of the nature of a protein.

**pro·tein·ase** (pro′tēn-ās) endopeptidase.

**pro·tein di·sul·fide-isom·er·ase** (pro′tēn di-sul′fīd-i-som′ə-rās) [EC 5.3.4.1] an enzyme of the isomerase class that catalyzes the rearrangement of disulfide bonds within proteins during folding. It is a monomer identical to one of the subunits of prolyl 4-hydroxylase (q.v.). Called also *disulfide isomerase.*

**pro·tein·emia** (pro″tēn-e′me-ə) hyperproteinemia.

**Bence Jones p.**, the presence of Bence Jones protein in serum.

**pro·tein-glu·ta·mine γ-glu·ta·myl·trans·fer·ase** (pro′tēn gloo′tə-mēn gloo″tə-məl-trans′fər-ās) [EC 2.3.2.13] an enzyme of the transferase class that creates crosslinks within and between fibrin molecules, transferring the glutamyl portion of glutamine side chains to the amino group of lysine side chains: protein-glutamine + lysine-protein = protein-glutamyl lysine-protein + $NH_3$. The resultant polymerization of fibrin is an important part of blood clotting. It is the activated form of coagulation factor XIII (coagulation factor XIIIa). Called also *transglutaminase.*

**pro·tein·ic** (pro-tēn′ik) pertaining to protein.

**pro·tein ki·nase** (pro′tēn ki′nās) [EC 2.7.1.37] an enzyme of the transferase class that catalyzes the phosphorylation of serine, threonine, or tyrosine groups in enzymes and other proteins, using ATP as a phosphate donor. Specific protein kinases, usually named for their substrates, regulate by phosphorylation enzymes catalyzing key reactions in processes such as glycogen turnover, cholesterol biosynthesis, and amino acid transformations. Others create the caseins secreted in milk.

**p. k. A,** cAMP-dependent protein kinase.

**p. k. C,** any of a family of protein kinase isozymes, occurring in numerous tissues, that catalyze the phosphorylation of specific serine or threonine residues of a variety of intracellular proteins, altering their activities. The enzymes are activated via receptor binding by the hormones, growth factors, and other agents that cause increases in intracellular calcium and cleavage of phosphoinositides; some isozymes require calcium and phospholipid for activity, which is enhanced by diacylglycerol. The enzyme is involved in several types of cellular signal transduction and has been shown to play a role in platelet activation and in the inhibition of some peptide hormone receptors and to be a binding site for phorbol esters and other tumor promoters, as well as having numerous other roles and substrates, only some of which are known.

**cAMP-dependent p. k., cyclic AMP–dependent p. k.,** see under *C.*

**pro·tein·o·chrome** (pro-tēn′o-krōm) [*protein* + *-chrome*] any one of a series of coloring matters formed by the action of bromine or chlorine on tryptophan.

**pro·tein·og·e·nous** (pro″tēn-oj′ə-nəs) formed by or from a protein.

**pro·tein·ol·o·gy** (pro″tēn-ol′ə-je) [*protein* + *-logy*] the scientific study of proteins or of the protein status of the body.

**pro·tein·o·sis** (pro″tēn-o′sis) the accumulation of excess protein in the tissues.

**alveolar p.**, pulmonary alveolar p.

**lipid p.**, an autosomal recessive disorder of lipid metabolism characterized by the deposition of hyaline material in the skin and mucosa of the mouth, pharynx, hypopharynx, and larynx, resulting in prolonged hoarseness, often from birth, due to infiltration of the vocal cords. Skin lesions are first manifested as recurrent pustules or bullae on the face and distal exposed surfaces of the arms and legs, which heal and leave white varioliform scars, and later by waxy yellow ivory papules, nodules, or verrucoid plaques primarily located on the face, eyelids, nape, hands, fingers, elbows, and knees. Called also *hyalinosis cutis et mucosae, lipoproteinosis,* and *Urbach-Wiethe disease.*

**pulmonary alveolar p.**, a chronic lung disease characterized by dyspnea, productive cough, chest pain, weakness, weight loss, and hemoptysis, and by the filling of the distal alveoli with a bland, eosinophilic, probably endogenous, proteinaceous material that prevents ventilation of affected areas.

**tissue p.**, see *amyloidosis.*

**pro·tein phos·pha·tase** (pro′tēn fos′fə-tās) phosphoprotein phosphatase.

**p. p. 1,** a specific phosphoprotein phosphatase (q.v.) that catalyzes the dephosphorylation of several enzymes involved in the regulation of glycogen metabolism; phosphorylase kinase, glycogen phosphorylase *a,* and glycogen synthase *b.* The enzyme activity encompasses activities formerly assigned to the individual enzymes [phosphorylase] phosphatase and [glycogen-synthase-D] phosphatase.

**pro·tein-ty·ro·sine ki·nase** (pro′tēn ti′ro-sēn ki′nās) [EC 2.7.1.112] [MeSH: Protein-Tyrosine Kinase] any of a group of enzymes of the transferase class that catalyze the phosphorylation of tyrosine residues in specific membrane vesicle–associated proteins. The enzyme activity is present in certain membrane proteins and is a product of some oncogenes. The reaction plays a role in the control of cell growth.

**pro·tein-ty·ro·sine-phos·pha·tase** (pro′tēn ti′ro-sēn fos′fə-tās) [EC 3.1.3.48] [MeSH: Protein-Tyrosine-Phosphatase] any of a group of enzymes of the hydrolase class that catalyze the removal of phosphate groups from tyrosine residues of proteins. The enzyme activity modulates that of the protein-tyrosine kinases and thus may decrease or inhibit cell growth and tumorigenesis.

**pro·tein·uria** (pro″te-nu′re-ə) [MeSH: Proteinuria] the presence of an excess of serum proteins in the urine; called also *albuminuria.*

**accidental p.**, adventitious p.

**adventitious p.**, that which is not due to a kidney disease; called also *accidental* or *false p.*

**athletic p.**, functional proteinuria occurring in athletes; effort p.

**Bence Jones p.**, the presence in the urine of Bence Jones protein.

**cardiac p.**, proteinuria caused by cardiac disease.

**colliquative p.**, proteinuria which is at first mild, but increases suddenly and markedly during convalescence; it is seen in several systemic and renal diseases.

**dietetic p., digestive p.**, that produced by the use of certain foods.

**effort p.**, functional proteinuria occurring as a result of vigorous and prolonged exercise of the lower limbs; called also *athletic p.*

**emulsion p.**, proteinuria in which the turbidity does not disappear on filtration, heating, or adding acid; seen in puerperal eclampsia.

**enterogenic p.**, that due to intestinal decomposition.

**essential p.**, a form of functional proteinuria which is not associated with or followed by renal disease; it includes effort and orthostatic proteinuria.

**false p.**, adventitious p.

**febrile p.**, proteinuria due to fever.

**functional p.**, any proteinuria which is not truly pathologic, such as the transient proteinurias of pregnancy or of adolescence; also known variously as *intermittent, paroxysmal, physiologic,* and *transient p.*

**globular p.**, proteinuria due to renal excretion of red blood cells and dependent on blood in the urine.

**gouty p.**, functional proteinuria, with excessive secretion of uric acid.

**hematogenous p., hemic p.**, a variety due to abnormal condition of the blood, as in some intoxications.

**intermittent p.**, functional p.
**intrinsic p.**, true p.
**light-chain p.**, increased urinary excretion of light-chain fragments of immunoglobulins, as in Fanconi syndrome.
**lordotic p.**, postural proteinuria due to lordotic deformity of the spine.
**mixed p.**, true proteinuria occurring concurrently with adventitious proteinuria.
**nephrogenous p.**, that caused by renal disease; called also *renal p.*
**orthostatic p.**, a form of functional proteinuria, usually seen between the ages of ten and twenty, which occurs on standing erect and disappears on lying down.
**overflow p.**, that due to hemoglobin, myoglobin, or immunoglobulin loss into the urine, not usually associated with glomerular or tubular disease.
**palpatory p.**, temporary proteinuria produced by bimanual palpation of the kidneys.
**paroxysmal p.**, functional p.
**physiologic p.**, functional p.
**postrenal p.**, proteinuria which has arisen at some point beyond the uriniferous tubule, such as the renal pelvis, ureter, bladder, prostate, or urethra.
**postural p.**, proteinuria related to body position, as orthostatic and lordotic proteinuria.
**prerenal p.**, proteinuria due primarily to a disease other than one of the kidney, such as heart disease, liver disease, fever, hyperthyroidism.
**pretuberculous p.**, proteinuria seen in early stages of tuberculosis.
**pseudo-p.**, adventitious p.
**pyogenic p.**, that due to the absorption of pus cells or exudates, as in pneumonia, septic processes, etc.
**regulatory p.**, proteinuria or the transitory elimination of protein after excessive physical exercise, etc.
**renal p.**, nephrogenous p.
**residual p.**, persistence of protein in the urine after an attack of acute nephritis.
**serous p.**, true p.
**transient p.**, functional p.
**true p.**, that which is characterized by the discharge with the urine of some of the protein elements of the blood; called also *intrinsic p.* and *serous p.*

**pro·tein·uric** (pro″tēn-u′rik) pertaining to or marked by proteinuria.

**pro·teo·clas·tic** (pro″te-o-klas′tik) [*protein* +Gr. *klasis* breakage] splitting up proteins or the protein molecule.

**pro·teo·gly·can** (pro″te-o-gli′kan) any of a group of polysaccharide-protein conjugates occurring primarily in the matrix of connective tissue and cartilage, composed mainly of polysaccharide chains, particularly glycosaminoglycans, as well as minor protein components. Individual subunits consist of a polypeptide backbone to which many glycosaminoglycan chains are covalently linked; large aggregates resembling bottle brushes are formed when many such subunits are attached via small proteins to long hyaluronic acid chains.

**Pro·te·og·ly·pha** (pro″te-og′lĭ-fə) Proteroglypha.

**pro·teo·lip·id** (pro″te-o-lip′id) 1. a conjugated protein having a lipid component that is soluble in some nonpolar solvents, but insoluble in aqueous solutions. 2. a hydrophobic protein, which may or may not have a lipid component, that is soluble in some nonpolar solvents.

**pro·te·ol·y·sis** (pro″te-ol′ĭ-sis) [*protein* + *-lysis*] the splitting of proteins by hydrolysis of the peptide bonds with formation of smaller polypeptides; the process may be catalyzed by proteolytic enzymes, by acids, or by bases.

**pro·teo·lyt·ic** (pro″te-o-lit′ik) 1. pertaining to, characterized by, or promoting proteolysis. 2. an enzyme that promotes proteolysis.

**pro·te·ome** (pro′te-ōm) [*prote*in + geno*me*] the complete set of proteins produced from the information encoded in a genome.

**pro·teo·meta·bol·ic** (pro″te-o-met″ə-bol′ik) pertaining to proteometabolism.

**pro·teo·me·tab·o·lism** (pro″te-o-mə-tab′ə-liz-əm) the metabolism of protein.

**Pro·teo·my·ces** (pro″te-o-mi′sēz) Trichosporon.

**pro·teo·pec·tic** (pro″te-o-pek′tik) proteopexic.

**pro·teo·pep·sis** (pro″te-o-pep′sis) [*protein* + Gr. *pepsis* digestion] the digestion of protein.

**pro·teo·pep·tic** (pro″te-o-pep′tik) digesting protein; pertaining to the digestion of protein.

**pro·teo·pex·ic** (pro″te-o-pek′sik) fixing protein within the organism.

**pro·teo·pexy** (pro′te-o-pek″se) [*protein* + *-pexy*] the fixation of proteins within the organism.

**pro·te·ose** (pro′te-ōs) [*protein* + *-ose*] a secondary protein derivative or a mixture of split products formed by a hydrolytic cleavage of the protein molecule more complete than that which occurs with the primary protein derivatives, but not so complete as that which forms amino acids. The *primary* proteoses are precipitated by half saturation with ammonium sulfate, the *secondary,* by full saturation.

**pro·te·os·uria** (pro″te-o-su′re-ə) the presence of proteose in the urine.

**pro·ter** (pro′tər) [Gr. *proteros* front] the anterior daughter organism after transverse division of a ciliate protozoan; cf. *opisthe.*

**Pro·ter·o·glypha** (pro″tər-o-glif′ə) a group of venomous snakes that have small stationary fangs which are grooved rather than hollow and so must be held in the wound if the poison is to reach the deeper tissues. Examples are the Indian cobra and the Sonoran coral snake. Called also *Ankyloproglypha* and *Proteoglypha.*

**pro·te·uria** (pro″te-u′re-ə) proteinuria.

**pro·te·uric** (pro″te-u′rik) proteinuric.

**Pro·te·us** (pro′te-əs) [Gr. *Prōteus* an ocean deity able to appear in many different forms] [MeSH: Proteus] a genus of gram-negative, facultatively anaerobic, rod-shaped bacteria of the family Enterobacteriaceae, made up of actively motile, pleomorphic organisms. Colonies exhibit the swarming phenomenon. The organisms are found in fecal material, especially in patients treated with oral antibiotics, and are potential pathogens, associated with urinary tract infections, bacteremia, and abdominal and wound infections.
**P. hydro′philus,** *Aeromonas hydrophila.*
**P. incon′stans,** a former species that has been classified as a separate genus, *Providencia. P. inconstans* subgroup *A* comprises *P. alcalifaciens; P. inconstans* subgroup *B* comprises *P. stuartii.*
**P. melanovo′genes,** *Aeromonas hydrophila.*
**P. mira′bilis,** the species most frequently isolated from human clinical material, also found in soil and sewage. It is a leading cause of urinary tract infections and can cause pneumonia in debilitated or immunocompromised patients; see also Proteus *pneumonia,* under *pneumonia.*
**P. morga′nii,** *Morganella morganii.*
**P. myxofa′ciens,** a species found as a pathogen of gypsy moth larvae, not present in human clinical specimens.
**P. pen′neri,** a species found in human clinical specimens. It ferments maltose, but is negative for ornithine decarboxylase and indole.
**P. rett′geri,** *Providencia rettgeri.*
**P. vulga′ris,** a widespread species found in fecal matter, sewage, and soil. It is a common cause of cystitis and pyelonephritis and is associated with eye and ear infections, pleuritis, peritonitis, and suppurative abscesses. In debilitated or immunocompromised patients it can cause pneumonia (see Proteus *pneumonia,* under *pneumonia*). The species has many serotypes. The Ox antigens (Ox-2, Ox-19, Ox-K) react with antibodies formed in rickettsial infections and are used in the Weil-Felix reaction for the diagnosis of typhus, scrub typhus, and Rocky Mountain spotted fever. See plate accompanying *bacterium.*
**P. zen′keri,** *Kurthia zopfii.*

**Pro·te·us syn·drome** (pro′te-əs) [Gr. *Prōteus* an ocean deity able to appear in many different forms] see under *syndrome.*

**pro·te·us** (pro′te-əs) pl. *pro′tei* [MeSH: Proteus] an organism of the genus *Proteus.*

**pro·thal·lus** (pro-thal′əs) the independent, free-living gametophyte generation of ferns and related lower vascular plants.

**pro·thi·pen·dyl hy·dro·chlo·ride** (pro-thi′pən-dəl) an antihistaminic and sedative, $C_{16}H_{19}N_3S{\cdot}HCl{\cdot}H_2O$.

**pro·throm·bin** (pro-throm′bin) [*pro-* + *thrombo-* + *-in* chemical suffix] [MeSH: Prothrombin] factor II; see under *coagulation factors,* at *factor.*

**pro·throm·bin·ase** (pro-throm′bin-āse) 1. the complex formed between activated coagulation factor X and calcium, phospholipid, and modified factor V; it can cleave and activate prothrombin to thrombin. 2. sometimes specifically the active enzyme center of the complex, activated factor X (Xa).

**pro·throm·bi·no·gen·ic** (pro-throm″bĭ-no-jen′ik) promoting the production of prothrombin (coagulation factor II).

**pro·throm·bi·no·pe·nia** (pro-throm″bĭ-no-pe′ne-ə) hypoprothrombinemia.

**pro·thy·mo·cyte** (pro-thi′mo-sīt) a term applied to the lymphoid precursor cell of thymocytes.

**pro·tio·dide** (pro-ti′o-dīd) that one of the series of iodides of the same base which contains the smallest amount of iodine.

**pro·ti·re·lin** (pro-ti′rə-lin) [MeSH: Protirelin] thyrotropin-releasing hormone (def. 2).

**pro·tist** (pro′tist) any member of the kingdom Protista; a single-celled organism.
**eukaryotic p.,** the higher protists, comprising those organisms having a true nucleus. See *Protista.*
**higher p.,** eukaryotic p's.
**lower p.,** prokaryotic p's.
**prokaryotic p.,** the lower protists, comprising those organisms lacking a true nucleus. See *Monera.*

**Pro·tis·ta** (pro-tis′tə) [Gr. *prōtista* the very first, from *prōtos* first] in some systems of classification, a kingdom comprising both animal-like and plantlike unicellular organisms with distinct nuclei, i.e., the eukaryotes, including protozoa, algae (except blue-green algae or bacteria), and certain intermediate forms. In some other systems, Protista includes only the protozoa. Cf. *Monera.*

**pro·ti·um** (pro′te-əm) the mass one isotope of hydrogen, symbol $^1H$; ordinary, or light, hydrogen. See *hydrogen.* Cf. *deuterium* and *tritium.*

**prot(o)-** [Gr. *prōtos* first] 1. a combining form meaning first or primitive. 2. in chemistry, a prefix denoting the member of a series of compounds with the lowest proportion of the element or radical to which it is affixed.

**pro·to·al·bu·mose** (pro″to-al′bu-mōs) a primary proteose.

**pro·to·anem·o·nin** (pro″to-ə-nem′o-nin) a toxic, irritating antibiotic substance that results from enzymatic breakdown of ranunculin after certain plants of the family Ranunculaceae are eaten by an animal; toxic effects include potentially fatal ventricular fibrillation and respiratory failure. As an antibiotic it is active against a variety of gram-positive and gram-negative bacteria. It sometimes breaks down further to form anemonin.

**pro·to·bi·ol·o·gy** (pro″to-bi-ol′ə-je) [*proto-* + *bio-* + *-logy*] the science which deals with the forms of life more minute than bacteria, such as viruses.

**pro·to·blast** (pro′to-blast) [*proto-* + *-blast*] 1. a cell with no cell wall; an embryonic cell. 2. the nucleus of an oocyte. 3. a blastomere from which a particular organ or part develops.

**pro·to·blas·tic** (pro″to-blas′tik) pertaining to a protoblast.

**pro·to·bro·chal** (pro″to-bro′kəl) [*proto-* + Gr. *brochos* mesh] denoting the first stage in the development of an ovary.

**Pro·to·cal·liph·o·ra** (pro″to-kə-lif′ə-rə) a genus of flies whose larvae feed on nesting birds.

**pro·to·cary·on** (pro″to-kar′e-on) [*proto-* + *karyon*] a cell nucleus formed of a single karyosome in a network of linin.

**pro·to·cat·e·chu·ic ac·id** (pro″to-kat″ə-choo′ik) 3,4-dihydroxybenzoic acid, a catabolite of epinephrine.

**pro·to·chlo·ride** (pro″to-klor′id) that one of a series of chlorides of the same element which contains the least amount of chlorine.

**pro·to·chlo·ro·phyll** (pro″to-klor′ə-fəl) a substance in plant tissue which is changed by the action of light into chlorophyll.

**pro·to·chon·dral** (pro″to-kon′drəl) pertaining to the protochondrium or to centers of chondrification.

**pro·to·chon·dri·um** (pro″to-kon′dre-əm) [*proto-* + Gr. *chondros* cartilage] the basophil substance developed from precartilage which constitutes the intermediate stage in cartilage formation.

**Pro·to·cil·i·a·ta** (pro″to-sil″e-a′tə) [*proto-* + *ciliate*] in former systems of classification, a subclass of ciliate protozoa, the members of which have been assigned to the subphylum Opalinata.

**Pro·to·coc·ci·di·i·da** (pro″to-kok″sĭ-di′ĭ-də) [*proto-* + Gr. *kokkos* berry] an order of parasitic protozoa (subclass Coccidia, class Sporozoea) found in invertebrates, the life cycle of which involves gametogony and sporogony.

**pro·to·col** (pro′to-kol) 1. an explicit, detailed plan of an experiment, procedure, or test. 2. the original notes made on a necropsy, experiment, or case of disease.
**Balke p., Balke-Ware p.,** a procedure for assessing cardiovascular health using a graded treadmill exercise test in which the treadmill speed is held constant and its slope increased, with the incremental increases in work so closely spaced as to approach continuity.
**Bruce p.,** a procedure for assessing cardiovascular health using uphill treadmill walking in a graded exercise test; each interval is at a specific load level for three minutes and is followed by another at a prescribed incremental increase in treadmill speed and slope.
**Ellestad p.,** a procedure for assessing cardiovascular health using a graded treadmill exercise test; over six stages the treadmill speed is incrementally raised five times and its slope is raised once.
**modified Bruce p.,** an alteration in the Bruce protocol so that the treadmill is initially horizontal rather than uphill, with the first few intervals increasing the treadmill slope only.
**Naughton p.,** a procedure for assessing cardiovascular health using a graded treadmill exercise test; the selected treadmill speed remains constant through the test but the treadmill slope is raised at the end of each two-minute increment.

**pro·to·cone** (pro′to-kōn) [*proto-* + Gr. *kōnos* cone] the principal mesiolingual cusp of the upper molar of man and certain mammals, such as the opossum and dog.

**pro·to·co·nid** (pro″to-ko′nid) [*proto-* + Gr. *kōnos* cone + *-id*] the mesiobuccal cusp of the lower molars of primitive mammals and man, being greatly modified in many higher mammals and completely disappearing in some.

**pro·to·co·op·er·a·tion** (pro″to-ko-op″ər-a′shən) 1. symbiosis in which both populations (or individuals) gain from the association but are able to survive without it. 2. the tendency of animals to cluster in groups and thereby to mutually facilitate the survival of individual organisms.

**pro·to·cop·ro·por·phyr·ia** (pro″to-kop″ro-por-fir′e-ə) variegate porphyria.

**pro·to·di·a·stol·ic** (pro″to-di″ə-stol′ik) pertaining to early diastole, i.e., immediately following the second heart sound.

**pro·to·du·o·de·num** (pro″to-doo″o-de′nəm) the first or proximal portion of the duodenum, extending from the pylorus to the duodenal papilla, and developed embryonically from the foregut.

**pro·to·elas·tose** (pro″to-e-las′tōs) hemielastin.

**pro·to·fi·bril** (pro″to-fi′bril) the first elongated unit appearing in the process of formation of any type of fiber.

**pro·to·gas·ter** (pro′to-gas″tər) [*proto-* + *gaster*] archenteron.

**pro·to·glob·u·lose** (pro″to-glob′u-lōs) a primary product formed in the digestion of globulin.

**pro·to·go·no·cyte** (pro″to-go′no-sīt) [*proto-* + *gonocyte*] one of the two cells resulting from division of the zygote; in certain lower forms this constitutes the primordial germ cell from which all gametes derive.

**pro·to·heme** (pro″to-hēm) a heme in which the porphyrin is protoporphyrin; an example is *protoheme IX,* the heme found in hemoglobin.

**pro·to·he·min** (pro″to-he′min) protoheme in which the iron atom is oxidized to the +3 oxidation state.

**pro·to·io·dide** (pro″to-i′o-dīd) protiodide.

**pro·to·ky·lol hy·dro·chlo·ride** (pro″to-ki′lol) an adrenergic used as a bronchodilator for the treatment of bronchospasm associated with bronchial asthma, pulmonary emphysema, bronchitis, and bronchiectasis, administered orally.

**Pro·to·mas·tig·i·da** (pro″to-mas-tij′ĭ-də) [*proto-* + Gr. *mastix* whip] Kinetoplastida.

**pro·tom·e·ter** (pro-tom′ə-tər) exophthalmometer.

**Pro·to·mo·na·di·na** (pro″to-mo″nə-di′nə) [*proto-* + Gr. *monas* unit] Kinetoplastida.

**pro·ton** (pro′ton) [Gr. *prōton,* from *prōtos* first] [MeSH: Protons] an elementary particle of positive charge which forms the nucleus of the ordinary hydrogen atom of mass 1; along with neutrons, protons form the nuclei of atoms of all other elements. The proton is the unit of positive electricity; it has one quantum of charge ($1.6 \times 10^{-19}$ coulomb), equivalent to the electron but of opposite polarity, and its mass is $1.67 \times 10^{-27}$ kilogram, approximately that of the hydrogen ion. Symbol p.

**pro·to·neph·ron** (pro″to-nef′ron) pronephros.

**pro·to·neph·ros** (pro″to-nef′ros) pronephros.

**pro·to·ni·trate** (pro″to-ni′trāt) that one of several nitrates of the same base which contains the least amount of nitric acid.

**pro·to·on·co·gene** (pro″to-ong′ko-jēn) a normal cellular gene that with alteration, such as by mutation, DNA rearrangement, or nearby insertion of viral DNA, becomes an active oncogene; most proto-oncogenes are believed to normally function in cell growth and differentiation. See also *oncogene.*

**Pro·to·pam** (pro′to-pam) trademark for preparations of pralidoxime.

**pro·to·path·ic** (pro″to-path′ik) [*proto-* + *path-* + *-ic*] primary; idiopathic. See *protopathic sensibility,* under *sensibility.*

**pro·to·pec·tin** (pro″to-pek′tin) any of the precursor polysaccharides from which are derived pectins; they occur in a variety of plants, in the fruits, roots, leaves, and stems.

**pro·to·phyl·lin** (pro″to-fil′in) a colorless substance which is changed into chlorophyll by the action of air or carbon dioxide.

**Pro·to·phy·ta** (pro″to-fi′tə) [*proto-* + Gr. *phyton* plant] in former systems of classification, the lowest division of the plant kingdom, consisting of the algae and variously defined to include also the blue-green algae, yeasts, fungi, lichens, bacteria, or viruses.

**pro·to·pine** (pro'to-pin) 1. an alkaloid from *Eschscholtzia californica,* the California poppy, and many other plants; it is an anodyne and hypnotic. 2. a poisonous alkaloid from various species of perennial herbs of the genus *Dicentra.*

**pro·to·pla·sia** (pro-to-pla'se-ah) primary formation of tissue.

**pro·to·plasm** (pro'to-plaz-əm) [*proto-* + *-plasm*] the viscid, translucent, polyphasic colloid with water as the continuous phase that makes up the essential material of all plant and animal cells. It is composed mainly of nucleic acids, proteins, lipids, carbohydrates, and inorganic salts. The protoplasm surrounding the nucleus is known as the *cytoplasm* and that composing the nucleus is the *nucleoplasm.*
**granular p.,** protoplasm having granular inclusions.
**superior p.,** endoplasmic reticulum.

**pro·to·plas·mat·ic** (pro″to-plaz-mat'ik) protoplasmic.

**pro·to·plas·mic** (pro″to-plaz'mik) pertaining to or consisting of protoplasm.

**pro·to·plast** (pro'to-plast) [*proto-* + *-plast*] [MeSH: Protoplasts] a bacterial, yeast, or fungal cell that results after complete removal of the rigid cell wall, which forms a membrane-bound cell into a spherical shape that is dependent for its integrity on an isotonic or hypertonic medium. Cf. *spheroplast.*

**pro·to·por·phyr·ia** (pro″to-por-fir'e-ə) EPP; an autosomal dominant disorder seen in both humans and cattle; there is partial deficiency of ferrochelatase, with increased levels of protoporphyrin in the erythrocytes, plasma, liver, and feces. Photosensitive skin changes vary widely, ranging from a burning or pruritic sensation to erythema, plaquelike edema, and wheals. It is classified as an erythropoietic or erythrohepatic form of porphyria depending on whether the latter form is used in a given system. Called also *erythropoietic porphyria* and *erythrohepatic porphyria.*

**pro·to·por·phy·rin** (pro″to-por'fə-rin) the porphyrin produced by oxidation of the methylene bridge of protoporphyrinogen. Protoporphyrin IX is the only naturally occurring isomer; it is an intermediate in heme biosynthesis, combining with ferrous iron to form protoheme IX, the heme prosthetic group of hemoglobin. It is accumulated and excreted excessively in the feces in protoporphyria and variegate porphyria.
**free erythrocyte p.,** FEP; protoporphyrin free in the blood rather than incorporated into erythrocytes; most is actually bound to zinc as zinc protoporphyrin. The amount increases greatly in iron-deficiency anemia, lead poisoning, and protoporphyria.
**zinc p.,** free erythrocyte protoporphyrin that is bound to zinc.

**pro·to·por·phy·rin·o·gen** (pro″to-por″fə-rin'ə-jən) a porphyrinogen (q.v.) in which two pyrrole rings each have one methyl and one propionate side chain and the other two pyrrole rings each have one methyl and one vinyl side chain. Fifteen isomers are possible but only one, type IX, occurs naturally, produced by oxidative decarboxylation of coproporphyrinogen; it is an intermediate in heme biosynthesis.

**pro·to·por·phy·rin·o·gen ox·i·dase** (pro″to-por″fə-rin'ə-jən ok'sĭ-dās) [EC 1.3.3.4] an enzyme of the oxidoreductase class that catalyzes the oxidation of protoporphyrinogen IX to protoporphyrin IX, the penultimate step in heme and porphyrin synthesis. Deficiency of the enzyme, an autosomal dominant trait, causes variegate porphyria.

**pro·to·por·phy·rin·uria** (pro″to-por″fə-rĭ-nu're-ə) the presence of protoporphyrin in the urine.

**pro·to·pro·te·ose** (pro″to-pro'te-ōs) a primary proteose.

**pro·to·salt** (pro'to-sawlt) that one of a series of salts of the same base which contains the smallest amount of the substance combining with the base.

**Pro·to·spi·ru·ra** (pro″to-spi-roo'rə) a genus of nematodes of the family Spiruridae. *P. gra'cilis* is found in the stomachs of cats.

**pro·to·spore** (pro'to-spor) the first product of progressive cleavage, a multinucleate mass of cytoplasm surrounded by cleavage planes.

**pro·to·sto·ma** (pro″to-sto'mə) blastopore.

**pro·to·stome** (pro'to-stōm) [*proto-* + Gr. *stoma* mouth] an individual of the Protostomia.

**Pro·to·sto·mia** (pro″to-sto'me-ə) a series of the Eucoelomata, including the mollusks, annelids, and arthropods, in all of which the mouth arises from the blastopore.

**Pro·to·stron·gy·li·dae** (pro″to-stron-jil'ĭde) a family of nematodes that includes the genera *Cystocaulus, Muellerius, Neostrongylus, Parelaphostrongylus,* and *Protostrongylus.* Several species are lungworms that infect sheep, goats, and other mammals.

**Pro·to·stron·gy·lus** (pro″to-stron'jə-ləs) a genus of nematode lungworms of the family Protostrongylidae. *P. rufes'cens* causes hoose or verminous bronchitis in sheep, goats, deer, and rabbits.

**pro·to·sul·fate** (pro″to-sul'fāt) that one of several sulfates of the same base which contains the smallest proportion of sulfate ion.

**Pro·to·the·ca** (pro″to-the'kə) [*proto-* + Gr. *thēkē* sheath] [MeSH: Prototheca] a genus of ubiquitous yeastlike organisms generally considered to be achloric algae, occurring as a spherical, ovoid, or elliptical cell containing several thick-walled autospores. *P. wickerha'mii* and *P. zop'fii* cause protothecosis in humans and domestic animals.

**pro·to·the·co·sis** (pro″to-the-ko'sis) [*proto-* + *theca* + *-osis*] infection of humans or domestic animals by organisms of the genus *Prototheca,* especially *P. wickerhamii* or *P. zopfii,* varying from cutaneous and subcutaneous lesions to systemic invasion involving several internal organs; in cows it may be manifested as mastitis. It may occur as an opportunistic infection or as a result of traumatic implantation of the pathogen into the tissues.

**Pro·to·the·ria** (pro″to-the're-ə) [*proto-* + Gr. *thērion* beast, animal] in some systems of classification, a subclass of the Mammalia, including the order Monotremata, the egg-laying mammals.

**pro·to·troph** (pro'to-trōf) [*proto-* + Gr. *trophē* nourishment] a prototrophic organism.

**pro·to·troph·ic** (pro″to-trof'ik) having the same growth factor requirements as the ancestral or prototype strain; said of microbial mutants.

**pro·tot·ro·py** (pro-tot'rə-pe) proton tautomerism. Cf. *anionotropy.*

**Pro·to·tu·ni·ca·tae** (pro″to-too″nĭ-ka'te) in fungal taxonomy, a series of the subphylum Ascomycotina, consisting of those having a prototunicate ascus. Orders in this series that contain human pathogens are Eurotiales and Onygenales.

**pro·to·type** (pro'to-tīp) [*proto-* + *type*] 1. the original type or form after which other types or forms are developed. 2. in microbiology, the standard reference strain to which other strains are compared.

**pro·to·ver·a·trine** (pro″to-ver'ə-trēn) an ester alkaloid obtained from the liliaceous plant *Veratrum album* L. It occurs in two forms, designated A and B, both of which have antihypertensive properties. Protoveratrine A is said to be more active than the B form; the two are usually administered in combination.

**pro·to·ver·te·bra** (pro″to-ver'tə-brə) 1. somite. 2. the caudal half of a somite that forms most of a vertebra.

**pro·tox·ide** (pro-tok'sid) that one of a series of oxides of the same metal which contains the smallest amount of oxygen.

**Pro·to·zoa** (pro″to-zo'ə) [*proto-* + Gr. *zoon* animal] [MeSH: Protozoa] a subkingdom (formerly a phylum) comprising the simplest organisms of the animal kingdom, consisting of unicellular organisms that range in size from submicroscopic to macroscopic; most are free living, but some lead commensalistic, mutualistic, or parasitic existences. According to newer classifications, Protozoa is divided into seven phyla: Sarcomastigophora, Labyrinthomorpha, Apicomplexa, Microspora, Acetospora, Myxozoa, and Ciliophora. Cf. *Metazoa.*

**pro·to·zoa** (pro″to-zo'ə) [MeSH: Protozoa] plural of *protozoon.*

**pro·to·zo·a·cide** (pro″to-zo'ə-sīd) destructive to protozoa; an agent destructive to protozoa.

**pro·to·zo·al** (pro″to-zo'əl) protozoan, def. 2.

**pro·to·zo·an** (pro″to-zo'ən) 1. any individual of the Protozoa; called also *protozoon.* 2. of or pertaining to the Protozoa; called also *protozoal.*

**pro·to·zo·ia·sis** (pro″to-zo-i'ə-sis) any disease caused by protozoa.

**pro·to·zo·ol·o·gy** (pro″to-zo-ol'ə-je) the study of protozoa.

**pro·to·zo·on** (pro″to-zo'on) pl. *protozo'a* [*proto-* + Gr. *zōon* animal] protozoan, def. 1.

**pro·to·zo·o·phage** (pro″to-zo'o-fāj) [*protozoa* + *-phage*] a cell which has a phagocytic action on protozoa.

**pro·to·zo·o·sis** (pro″to-zo-o'sis) protozoiasis.

**pro·trac·tion** (pro-trak'shən) [L. *protrahere* to drag forth] 1. drawing out or lengthening. 2. extension or protrusion. 3. a condition in which the teeth or other maxillary or mandibular structures are situated anterior to their normal position.
**mandibular p.,** 1. the protrusive movement of the mandible initiated by the lateral and medial pterygoid muscles acting simultaneously. Cf. *mandibular retraction.* 2. a facial anomaly in which the gnathion lies anterior to the orbital plane.
**maxillary p.,** a facial anomaly in which the subnasion is anterior to the orbital plane.

**pro·trac·tor** (pro-trak'tor) [*pro-* + L. *trahere* to draw] an instrument for extracting bits of bone, bullets, or other foreign material from wounds.

**pro·trans·glu·tam·i·nase** (pro-tranz″gloo-tam′ĭ-nās) [MeSH: Factor XIII] the proenzyme of protein-glutamine γ-glutamyltransferase (transglutaminase). It is the inactive precursor form of coagulation factor XIII.

**pro·trip·ty·line hy·dro·chlo·ride** (pro-trip′tə-lēn) [USP] a tricyclic antidepressant of the dibenzocycloheptadiene class; it is also used in the treatment of attention-deficit/hyperactivity disorder and of cataplexy associated with narcolepsy. Administered orally.

**pro·tru·sio** (pro-troo′ze-o) [L.] the state of being thrust forward; projection.
**p. aceta′buli,** arthrokatadysis.

**pro·tru·sion** (pro-troo′zhən) [L. *protrudere* to push forward] the state of being thrust forward or laterally, as in masticatory movements of the mandible.
**bimaxillary p.,** the projection of both the maxilla and the mandible beyond normal limits in relation to the cranial base.
**bimaxillary dentoalveolar p.,** the positioning of the entire dentition forward with respect to the facial profile.
**disk p.,** herniation of an intervertebral disk.
**intrapelvic p.,** arthrokatadysis.

**pro·tryp·sin** (pro-trip′sin) trypsinogen.

**pro·tu·ber·ance** (pro-too′bər-əns) [*pro-* + L. *tuber* bulge] a projecting part, or prominence; an apophysis, process, or swelling.
**p. of chin,** protuberantia mentalis.
**laryngeal p.,** prominentia laryngea.
**mental p.,** protuberantia mentalis.
**occipital p., external,** protuberantia occipitalis externa.
**occipital p., internal,** protuberantia occipitalis interna.
**occipital p., transverse,** torus occipitalis.
**palatine p.,** torus palatinus.
**tubal p.,** torus tubarius.

**pro·tu·ber·an·tia** (pro-too″bər-an′shə) gen. and pl. *protuberan′tiae* [L., from *pro-* + *tuber* bulge] [TA] protuberance: a projecting part, or prominence.
**p. menta′lis** [TA], mental protuberance: a more or less distinct and triangular prominence on the anterior surface of the body of the mandible, on or near the median line.
**p. occipita′lis exter′na** [TA], external occipital protuberance: a prominence at the center of the outer surface of the squama of the occipital bone which gives attachment to the ligamentum nuchae.
**p. occipita′lis inter′na** [TA], internal occipital protuberance: the projection of bone at the midpoint of the cruciform eminence, on the internal surface of the squama of the occipital bone, sometimes presenting as a ridge (*crista occipitalis interna*).

**pro-UK** prourokinase.

**pro·uro·ki·nase (pro-UK)** (pro″ur-o-ki′nās) the single chain proenzyme cleaved by plasmin to form u-plasminogen activator (urokinase); it is found circulating in plasma and urine. Although it is inactive in plasma, it is slowly activated in the presence of fibrin clots, which it lyses via fibrin-dependent plasminogen activation. It resembles t-plasminogen activator in having both a higher specific thrombolytic activity and better fibrin specificity than does u-plasminogen activator, and it has been used for therapeutic thrombolysis. Called also *single chain urokinase-type plasminogen activator.*

**Pro·vell** (pro-vel′) trademark for a preparation of protoveratrines A and B.

**Pro·ven·til** (pro-ven′til) trademark for preparations of albuterol.

**pro·ven·tric·u·lus** (pro″vən-trik′u-ləs) [*pro-* + *ventriculus*] [MeSH: Proventriculus] 1. the glandular first portion of the stomach of birds, in which food from the crop is mixed with peptic enzymes and passed to the gizzard. 2. the portion of the foregut in certain invertebrates, e.g., some insects, which may function as a gizzard or as a valve into the stomach.

**Pro·vera** (pro-ver′ə) trademark for preparations of medroxyprogesterone acetate.

**pro·ver·te·bra** (pro-ver′tə-brə) protovertebra.

**Pro·vi·den·cia** (prov″ĭ-den′shə) [*Providence,* Rhode Island] [MeSH: Providencia] a genus of gram-negative, facultatively anaerobic, motile, rod-shaped bacteria of the family Enterobacteriaceae, occurring in normal urine and feces. The organisms are potential pathogens associated with urinary tract and secondary tissue infections. It was formerly classified as a species of the genus *Proteus (P. inconstans).*
**P. alcalifa′ciens,** a species that does not ferment trehalose or *myo*-inositol; isolated especially from stools of children with diarrhea. Called also *Proteus inconstans* subgroup A.
**P. rett′geri,** a species isolated from human clinical specimens and from chicken feces, a possible cause of nosocomial infections. Called also *Proteus rettgeri.*
**P. stuar′tii,** a species that ferments trehalose and *myo*-inositol. It causes nosocomial infections and is a major agent in burn infections. Called also *Proteus inconstans* subgroup B.

**pro·vi·rus** (pro-vi′rəs) the genome of an animal virus integrated (by crossing over) into the chromosome of the host cell, and thus replicated in all of its daughter cells. It can be activated, spontaneously or by induction, to produce a complete virus; it can also cause transformation of the host cell.

**pro·vi·sion·al** (prə-vizh′ən-əl) formed or performed for temporary purposes; temporary.

**pro·vi·ta·min** (pro-vi′tə-min) a precursor of a vitamin.
**p. A,** usually β-carotene; however, the term is sometimes used more broadly to denote any of the provitamin A carotenoids.
**p. $D_2$,** ergosterol.
**p. $D_3$,** 7-dehydrocholesterol.

**prov·o·ca·tion** (prov″ə-ka′shən) challenge (def. 3).
**bronchial p.,** see under *challenge.*
**inhalational p.,** see under *challenge.*

**pro·voc·a·tive** (pro-vok′ə-tiv) stimulating the appearance of a sign, reflex, reaction, or therapeutic effect.

**Pro·wa·zek's bodies** (pro-vaht′səks) [Stanislas Joseph Matthias von *Prowazek,* German zoologist, 1875–1915] see under *body.*

**Pro·wa·zek-Greeff bodies** (pro-vaht′sək-grāf) [S. J. M. von *Prowazek;* Carl Richard *Greeff,* German ophthalmologist, 1862–1938] trachoma b′s.

**Pro-X di·pep·ti·dase** (di-pep′tĭ-dās″) [EC 3.4.13.8] a dipeptidase that catalyzes the cleavage of an N-terminal proline or another imino acid from imidodipeptides. Called also *prolinase* and *prolyl dipeptidase.*

**prox·e·mics** (prok-se′miks) the study of the effects of spatial distance between persons interacting with each other, and of their orientation toward each other.

**prox·i·mad** (prok′sĭ-mad) toward the proximal end or in a proximal direction.

**prox·i·mal** (prok′sĭ-məl) [L. *proximus* next] nearest; closer to any point of reference: opposed to *distal.*

**prox·i·ma·lis** (prok″sĭ-ma′lis) [L.] [TA] proximal; a term denoting proximity to the point of origin or attachment of an organ or part.

**prox·i·mate** (prok′sĭ-māt) [L. *proximatus* drawn near] immediate or nearest.

**prox·i·mo·atax·ia** (prok″sĭ-mo-ə-tak′se-ə) ataxia affecting the proximal part of an extremity, as the arm, forearm, thigh, or leg.

**prox·i·mo·buc·cal** (prok″sĭ-mo-buk′əl) pertaining to the proximal and buccal surfaces of a posterior tooth.

**prox·i·mo·la·bi·al** (prok″sĭ-mo-la′be-əl) pertaining to the proximal and labial surfaces of an anterior tooth.

**prox·i·mo·lin·gual** (prok″sĭ-mo-ling′gwəl) pertaining to the proximal and lingual surfaces of a tooth.

**Pro·zac** (pro′zak) trademark for a preparation of fluoxetine hydrochloride.

**pro·zo·nal** (pro′zo-nəl) 1. situated before a sclerozone. 2. pertaining to a prozone.

**pro·zone** (pro′zōn) [*pro-* + *zone*] in an agglutination or precipitation reaction, the zone of relatively high antibody concentrations within which no reaction occurs. As the antibody concentration is lowered below the prozone, the reaction occurs. This phenomenon may be due simply to antibody excess (see *precipitin reaction,* under *reaction*), or it may be due to blocking antibody or to nonspecific inhibitors in serum. Called also *prezone.*

**PrP** prion protein.

**PRPP** phosphoribosylpyrophosphate.

**PRU** peripheral resistance unit.

**pru·i·nate** (proo′ĭ-nāt) [L. *pruina* hoarfrost] having the appearance of being covered with hoarfrost.

**Pru·let** (proo′lət) trademark for a preparation of oxyphenisatin acetate.

**Pru·nel·la** (proo-nel′ə) a genus of herbs of the family Labiatae, native to Europe and Asia. *P. vulga′ris* L. is called heal-all or self-heal and is astringent and tonic.

**Pru·nus** (proo′nəs) [L. "plum-tree"] a genus of trees and shrubs of the family Rosaceae, including many that are cultivated for their fruit; the seeds or pits of many varieties contain cyanogenetic compounds such as amygdalin and may cause fatal cyanide poisoning in animals if eaten in large quantities. *P. amyg′dalus* Batsch. (called also *P. commu′nis* L.) is the almond (q.v.). *P. seroti′na* Ehrh. is the wild cherry and *P. virginia′na* is the choke cherry (see under *cherry*).

The pits of *P. armeni'aca* (the apricot) and *P. per'sica* (the peach) yield persic oil (see under *oil*).

**pru·rig·i·nous** (proo-rij'ĭ-nəs) of the nature of or tending to cause prurigo.

**pru·ri·go** (proo-ri'go) [L. "the itch"] [MeSH: Prurigo] a name applied to several itchy skin eruptions of unknown cause, in which the characteristic lesion (prurigo papule) is dome-shaped with a small transient vesicle on top, followed by crusting or lichenification; specific types are usually indicated by a modifying term.
**p. ag'ria,** a severe, chronic pruriginous dermatosis characterized chiefly by hard excoriated prurigo papules and lichenification. Called also *p. ferox.*
**Besnier's p., p. of Besnier,** atopic dermatitis.
**Besnier's p. of pregnancy,** p. gestationis of Besnier.
**p. chro'nica multifor'mis,** a pruriginous dermatosis characterized by the presence of prurigo papules, patches of lichenification and eczematization, enlarged regional lymph nodes, and eosinophilia.
**p. estiva'lis,** a papular dermatosis regarded as a form of polymorphous light eruption, usually occurring in childhood during the summer months, and sometimes improving or resolving after puberty. Called also *summer p. of Hutchinson.*
**p. fe'rox,** p. agria.
**p. gestatio'nis, p. gestationis of Besnier,** an extremely pruritic condition of unknown etiology occurring in the third trimester of pregnancy characterized by the development of tiny crust-covered excoriated papules mainly on the extensor surfaces of the limbs but also found on the upper trunk and other areas of the body, and leaving postinflammatory residua on resolution of the lesions. It tends to clear after delivery, and occasionally recurs with subsequent pregnancies. Called also *Besnier's p. of pregnancy.*
**p. of Hebra,** p. mitis.
**melanotic p.,** a form associated with primary biliary cirrhosis in women, characterized by reticulated hyperpigmentation and intense itching.
**p. mi'tis,** an extremely pruritic, chronic pruriginous dermatosis beginning in early childhood, characterized by excoriations, lichenification, and eczematization that become progressively more pronounced, and accompanied by enlarged glands and associated constitutional symptoms. The condition may be the same as papular urticaria. Called also *p. of Hebra.*
**nodular p.,** a chronic, intensely pruritic form of neurodermatitis, usually occurring in women, located chiefly on the extremities, especially on the anterior thighs and legs, and characterized by the presence of single or multiple, pea-sized or larger, firm, and erythematous or brownish nodules that become verrucous or fissured.
**p. sim'plex,** a form in which the prurigo papules are present in various stages of development, especially on the trunk and extensor surfaces of the extremities in middle-aged persons, and usually occur in crops.
**summer p. of Hutchinson,** 1. p. estivalis. 2. hydroa vacciniforme.

**pru·rit·ic** (proo-rit'ik) pertaining to or characterized by pruritus.

**pru·rit·o·gen·ic** (proo″rit-o-jen'ik) capable of causing or tending to cause pruritus.

**pru·ri·tus** (proo-ri'təs) [L. from *prurire* to itch] [MeSH: Pruritus] 1. an unpleasant cutaneous sensation that provokes the desire to rub or scratch the skin to obtain relief. Called also *itching.* 2. any of various conditions marked by this sensation, the specific site or type being indicated by a modifying term. See also *itch.*
**p. a'ni,** intense chronic itching in the anal region.
**aquagenic p.,** pruritus and other skin sensations, such as burning, lasting for 30 minutes to two hours after contact with water, without the overt skin changes seen in aquagenic urticaria. The etiology is usually unknown, although it is sometimes seen accompanying polycythemia vera and in other cases it may be familial. A similar condition is seen in elderly women but lasts only 10 to 20 minutes and is relieved by emollients.
**p. hiema'lis,** xerotic eczema.
**p. scro'ti,** intense itching in the scrotal area.
**senile p., p. seni'lis,** an itching in the aged, possibly due to dryness of the skin occurring as a result of decreased sweat and sebum secretion, or bathing too frequently, or both.
**uremic p.,** generalized itching associated with chronic renal failure and not attributable to other internal or skin disease.
**p. vul'vae,** intense itching of the external genitals of the female, as in lichen sclerosus.

**Prus·sak's fibers, pouch, space** (proo͞'sahks) [Alexander *Prussak,* Russian otologist, 1839–1897] see under *fiber,* and see *recessus superior membranae tympanicae.*

**prus·si·ate** (prus'e-āt) cyanide.

**prus·sic ac·id** (prus'ik) hydrogen cyanide.

**PS** phosphatidylserine; pulmonary stenosis.

**ps** abbreviation for *per second.*

**PSA** prostate-specific antigen.

**psal·te·ri·al** (sal-tēr'e-əl) pertaining to the psalterium.

**psal·te·ri·um** (sal-tēr-e-əm) [L.; Gr. *psaltērion* harp] 1. commissura fornicis. 2. the omasum.

**Psal·y·do·lyt·ta** (sal″ĭ-do-lit'ə) a genus of blister beetles (family Meloidae). *P. fus'ca* and *P. substriga'ta* of Africa produce a severe vesicular dermatitis.

**psamm(o)-** [Gr. *psammos* sand] a combining form meaning sandlike or denoting relationship to sand.

**psam·mo·car·ci·no·ma** (sam″o-kahr″sĭ-no'mə) [*psammo-* + *carcinoma*] carcinoma containing calcareous matter.

**psam·mo·ma** (sam-o'mə) [*psamm-* + *-oma*] 1. any tumor that contains psammoma bodies. 2. psammomatous meningioma.

**psam·mo·ma·tous** (sam-o'mə-təs) characterized by the presence of or containing psammoma bodies.

**psam·mous** (sam'əs) sandy.

**psau·os·co·py** (saw-os'kə-pe) [Gr. *psauein* to touch + *-scopy*] a method of physical examination done by passing the ball of the index finger back and forth lightly over the margin of an abnormal area. Over the pathological area the finger seems to encounter greater resistance and the skin seems more tense and less supple.

**$P_{450}$SCC** cholesterol monooxygenase (side-chain-cleaving).

**psel·a·phe·sia** (sel-ə-fe'zhə) [Gr. *psēlaphēsis* touching] touch, def. 1.

**psel·lism** (sel'iz-əm) [Gr. *psellisma* stammer] stuttering.

**pseud·agraph·ia** (soo″də-graf'e-ə) echographia.

**pseud·al·bu·mi·nu·ria** (soo″dəl-bu″mĭ-nu're-ə) adventitious proteinuria.

**Pseu·dal·les·che·ria** (so͞od″al-əs-kēr'e-ə) [MeSH: Pseudallescheria] a genus of fungi of the family Microascaceae.
**P. boy'dii,** a widely distributed saprobic species commonly isolated from mycetoma and other fungal infections; its perfect (sexual) stage is *Scedosporium apiospermum.* Formerly called *Allescheria boydii.*

**pseu·dal·les·che·ri·a·sis** (so͞od″əl-es-kə-ri'ə-sis) infection with *Pseudallescheria boydii;* clinical manifestations are highly variable, the most common being eumycotic mycetoma and pulmonary infection. Formerly called *allescheriasis* and *allescheriosis.*

**Pseud·am·phis·to·mum** (so͞od″am-fis'to-məm) [*pseud-* + *amphi-* + Gr. *stoma* mouth] a genus of trematodes of the family Opisthorchiidae; called also *Pseudoamphistomum. P. trunca'tum* is found in the bile ducts of cats, dogs, seals, deer, and occasionally humans in Europe and India and causes a condition resembling opisthorchiasis.

**pseud·an·gi·na** (sood″an-ji'nə) pseudoangina.

**pseud·an·ky·lo·sis** (sood″ang-kə-lo'sis) pseudoankylosis.

**pseud·aphia** (sood-a'fe-ə) [*pseud-* + Gr. *haphē* touch + *-ia*] paraphia.

**pseud·ar·thro·sis** (sood″ahr-thro'sis) [*pseud-* + *arthrosis*] [MeSH: Pseudarthrosis] a pathologic entity characterized by deossification of a weight-bearing long bone, followed by bending and pathologic fracture, with inability to form normal callus leading to existence of the "false joint" that gives the condition its name.

**Pseu·dech·is** (soo-dek'is) [*pseud-* + Gr. *echis* viper] a genus of venomous Australian snakes of the family Elapidae. *P. porphyria'cus,* is the Australian blacksnake. See table at *snake.*

**pseud·en·ceph·a·lus** (sood″ən-sef'ə-ləs) [*pseud-* + Gr. *enkephalos* brain] a fetus with a vascular tumor in place of the brain.

**pseud·es·the·sia** (sood″əs-the'zhə) [*pseud-* + *esthesia*] 1. synesthesia. 2. a sensation felt without any external stimulus.

**pseud(o)-** [Gr. *pseudēs* false] combining form signifying false or spurious.

**pseu·do·ac·an·tho·sis** (soo″do-ak″an-tho'sis) [*pseudo-* + *acanthosis*] a condition clinically resembling acanthosis.
**p. ni'gricans,** a benign form of acanthosis nigricans associated with obesity; the obesity is sometimes associated with endocrine disturbance.

**pseu·do·aceph·a·lus** (soo″do-a-sef'ə-ləs) [*pseudo-* + *acephalus*] in asymmetrical conjoined twins, a parasitic twin, apparently headless, but with a rudimentary cranium contained in the more developed twin.

**pseu·do·ag·glu·ti·na·tion** (soo″do-ə-gloo″tĭ-na'shən) rouleau formation.

**pseu·do·agraph·ia** (soo″do-ə-graf'e-ə) echographia.

**pseu·do·al·bu·mi·nu·ria** (soo″do-al-bu″mĭ-nu′re-ə) adventitious proteinuria.

**pseu·do·al·leles** (soo″do-ə-lēlz′) [*pseudo-* + *allele*] genes that are seemingly allelic but can eventually be shown to have distinct but closely linked loci.

**pseu·do·al·lel·ic** (soo″do-ə-lel′ik) pertaining to pseudoalleles; seemingly allelic but located at different sites on homologous chromosomes.

**pseu·do·al·le·lism** (soo″do-al′ə-liz-əm) the possession of pseudoalleles.

**pseu·do·al·ve·o·lar** (soo″do-al-ve′o-lər) simulating an alveolar structure.

**Pseu·do·am·phis·to·mum** (soo″do-əm-fis′to-məm) *Pseudamphistomum.*

**pseu·do·ana·phy·lac·tic** (soo″do-an″ə-fə-lak′tik) pertaining to pseudoanaphylaxis.

**pseu·do·ana·phy·lax·is** (soo″do-an″ə-fə-lak′sis) [*pseudo-* + *anaphylaxis*] anaphylactoid reaction.

**pseu·do·ane·mia** (soo″do-ə-ne′me-ə) [*pseudo-* + *anemia*] marked pallor with no clinical or hematological evidence of anemia.
**p. angiospas′tica,** a form due to vasoconstriction.

**pseu·do·an·eu·rysm** (soo″do-an′u-riz-əm) dilatation of a vessel, sometimes with tortuosity, giving the appearance of an aneurysm. Called also *false* or *spurious aneurysm* and *pulsating hematoma.*

**pseu·do·an·gi·na** (soo″do-an-ji′nə) [*pseudo-* + *angina*] false angina; a syndrome occurring in nervous individuals, marked by precordial pain, fatigue, and lassitude, without evidence of organic disease of the heart. See *angina pectoris vasomotoria.*

**pseu·do·an·ky·lo·sis** (soo″do-ang″kə-lo′sis) fibrous ankylosis.

**pseu·do·an·odon·tia** (soo″do-an″o-don′shə) [*pseudo-* + *anodontia*] a condition characterized by the presence of multiple unerupted permanent teeth.

**pseu·do·an·tag·o·nist** (soo″do-an-tag′ə-nist) a muscle which by flexing a joint enhances the effect of another muscle crossing that joint to act on a more distant one.

**pseu·do·ap·o·plexy** (soo″do-ap′o-plek″se) [*pseudo-* + *apoplexy*] a condition resembling apoplexy, but without cerebral hemorrhage.

**pseu·do·ap·pen·di·ci·tis** (soo″do-ə-pen″dĭ-si′tis) a condition with symptoms simulating appendicitis, sometimes hysterical and sometimes of syphilitic origin, but without affection of the appendix.
**p. zooparasi′tica,** a condition in which parasites are present in the vermiform appendix.

**pseu·do·ar·thro·sis** (soo″do-ahr-thro′sis) pseudarthrosis.

**pseu·do·ath·e·to·sis** (soo″do-ath″ə-to′sis) movements of the fingers elicited when the patient closes his eyes and extends his arms, associated with impairment of joint position sense.

**pseu·do·at·ro·pho·der·ma col·li** (soo″do-at″ro-fo-der′mə ko′li) a skin disease characterized by papillomatous, depigmented, glossy lesions on the sides of the neck; the depigmented areas resemble vitiligo. It probably differs from confluent reticulated papillomatosis chiefly in its location.

**pseu·do·bac·il·lus** (soo″do-bə-sil′əs) an exceedingly small, rodlike poikilocyte, resembling a microorganism.

**pseu·do·bac·te·ri·um** (soo″do-bak-tēr′e-əm) [*pseudo-* + *bacterium*] a cell that resembles a bacterium.

**pseu·do·bas·e·dow** (soo″do-baz′ə-do) basedoid.

**pseu·do·bron·chi·ec·ta·sis** (soo″do-brong″ke-ek′tə-sis) a condition in which a bronchiectasis-like pattern appears in the bronchogram of partially atelectatic pulmonary segments when the larger bronchi have become shortened and broadened in outline; these reversible changes do not indicate destruction of the bronchial walls.

**pseu·do·bul·bar** (soo″do-bul′bər) apparently, but not really, due to a bulbar lesion.

**pseu·do·car·ti·lage** (soo″do-kahr′tĭ-ləj) chondroid tissue.

**pseu·do·car·ti·lag·i·nous** (soo″do-kahr″tĭ-laj′ĭ-nəs) composed of a substance resembling cartilage.

**pseu·do·cast** (soo′do-kast) a false cast: a form of urinary sediment resembling true casts, but being an accidental formation, taking the shape of casts by adherence to mucous threads, cotton fibers, etc.

**pseu·do·cele** (soo′do-sēl) cavum septi pellucidi.

**pseu·do·ceph·a·lo·cele** (soo″do-sef′ə-lo-sēl) an encephalocele that is not congenital, but due to disease or injury of the skull.

**pseu·do·chan·cre** (soo″do-shang′kər) an indurated lesion resembling or simulating chancre.
**p. re′dux,** a gummatous recurrence at the site of a primary syphilitic lesion.

**pseu·do·cho·le·cys·ti·tis** (soo″do-ko″le-sis-ti′tis) a syndrome resembling cholecystitis but occurring as an allergic response to eating certain foods.

**pseu·do·cho·lin·es·ter·ase (PCE)** (soo″do-ko″lin-es′tər-ās) [MeSH: Pseudocholinesterase] cholinesterase.

**pseu·do·chrom·es·the·sia** (soo″do-krōm″əs-the′zhə) [*pseudo-* + *chrom-* + *esthesia*] a synesthesia in which certain sounds induce sensations of color.

**pseu·do·chro·mid·ro·sis** (soo″do-kro″mid-ro′sis) [*pseudo-* + *chromidrosis*] the presence of pigment on the skin caused by the action of pigment-producing bacteria.

**pseu·do·chro·mo·some** (soo″do-kro′mo-sōm) rodlike Golgi bodies of the spermatocytes.

**pseu·do·chy·lo·tho·rax** (soo″do-ki″lo-tho′raks) chyliform effusion.

**pseu·do·chy·lous** (soo″do-ki′ləs) resembling chyle, but containing no fat. Cf. *chyliform.*

**pseu·do·clo·nus** (soo″do-klo′nəs) a short-lived clonic response.

**pseu·do·co·arc·ta·tion** (soo″do-ko″ahrk-ta′shən) an imprecise term used to refer to a condition radiographically resembling coarctation, but without compromise of the lumen of the affected structure, such as a "kinked aorta" (which is possibly an aortic arch anomaly).
**p. of the aorta,** an uncommon congenital anomaly of the arch of the aorta that simulates coarctation radiographically but does not produce occlusion of the vessel.

**pseu·do·coele** (soo′do-sēl) [*pseudo-* + *cele*[2]] cavum septi pellucidi.

**pseu·do·coe·lom** (soo″do-se′lom) in zoology, a body cavity between the mesoderm and endoderm; a persistent blastocoele.

**pseu·do·coel·o·mate** (soo″do-sēl′o-māt) 1. having a pseudocoelom. 2. an animal having a pseudocoelom, as the aschelminths.

**pseu·do·col·loid** (soo″do-kol′oid) a mucoid substance sometimes found in ovarian cysts.

**pseu·do·col·o·bo·ma** (soo″do-kol″o-bo′mə) a line or scar on the iris giving the appearance of a coloboma.

**pseu·do·coma** (soo″do-co′mə) locked-in syndrome.

**pseu·do·cop·u·la·tion** (soo″do-cop″u-la′shən) exchange of gametes by close contact between male and female but without intromission, as in frogs.

**pseu·do·cor·pus lu·te·um** (soo″do-kor′pəs loo-te′əm) a maturing graafian follicle which does not rupture but retains its ovum and then becomes luteinized.

**pseu·do·cow·pox** (soo″do-kou′poks) 1. paravaccinia, def. 1. 2. milker's nodules, def. 1.

**pseu·do·cox·al·gia** (soo″do-kok-sal′jə) osteochondrosis of the capitular epiphysis of the femur.

**pseu·do·cri·sis** (soo′do-kri″sis) [*pseudo-* + *crisis*] a false crisis; a sudden but temporary abatement of fever.

**pseu·do·croup** (soo″do-kro͞op′) laryngismus stridulus.

**pseu·do·cy·a·nin** (soo″do-si′ə-nin) pseudoisocyanin.

**pseu·do·cy·e·sis** (soo″do-si-e′sis) [*pseudo-* + *cyesis*] false pregnancy.

**pseu·do·cy·lin·droid** (soo″do-sə-lin′droid) a shred of mucin in the urine resembling a cylindroid; sometimes of spermatic origin.

**pseu·do·cyst** (soo′do-sist) [*pseudo-* + *cyst*] 1. an abnormal or dilated cavity resembling a true cyst but not lined with epithelium. Called also *adventitious* or *false cyst.* 2. a cystic collection of fluid and necrotic debris whose walls are formed by the pancreas and other surrounding organs. It occurs as a complication of acute pancreatitis, and may subside spontaneously or become secondarily infected and develop into an abscess. Cf. *phlegmon* (def. 2). 3. a cluster of small, comma-shaped forms of *Toxoplasma gondii* (bradyzoites), perhaps containing thousands of organisms, enclosed by an irregular wall, and representing a resting stage, as opposed to the active, motile stage *(tachyzoite)*; pseudocysts are found in the tissues, especially muscles and the brain, in chronic (latent) toxoplasmosis. Called also *tissue cyst.*
**adrenal p.,** a cyst of the adrenal gland with no epithelial or endothelial lining, often with thick, irregular walls; it results from adrenal hemorrhage or develops within an adrenal neoplasm. Predisposing factors include trauma to the neck, infection, bleeding diathesis, embolism, aneurysm, or, in infants, anoxia.
**p's of lung,** cystic disease of lung.

**pancreatic p.,** see *pseudocyst,* def. 2.
**pararenal p.,** urinoma.
**pulmonary p's,** cystic disease of lung.

**pseu·do·de·men·tia** (soo″do-də-men′shə) a disorder resembling dementia but that is not due to organic brain disease and is potentially reversible by treatment; usually due to depression or other psychiatric disorder.
**depressive p.,** dementia syndrome of depression; the term is discouraged as technically incorrect because the cognitive deficits are now believed to be real, if reversible.

**pseu·do·dex·tro·car·dia** (soo″do-deks″tro-kahr′de-ə) a condition in which the heart is displaced to the right, but the ventricles are not inverted nor are the great vessels transposed.

**pseu·do·di·a·be·tes** (soo″do-di″ə-be′tēz) impaired glucose tolerance due to subclinical diabetes.
**uremic p. mellitus,** impaired glucose tolerance in chronic renal failure.

**pseu·do·diph·the·ria** (soo″do-dif-the′re-ə) any of a group of infections resembling diphtheria but not caused by *Corynebacterium diphtheriae.* Called also *diphtheroid* and *Epstein's disease.*

**pseu·do·dis·ease** (soo′do-dĭ-zēz″) an occult disease that would never become apparent to a patient during his or her lifetime without the use of diagnostic testing.

**pseu·do·di·ver·tic·u·lum** (soo″do-di″vər-tik′u-ləm) herniation of the esophageal or intestinal mucosa and submucosa through a tear in the muscular coat. Called also *false diverticulum.*

**pseu·do·dom·i·nant** (soo″do-dom′ĭ-nənt) quasidominant.

**pseu·do·dys·en·tery** (soo″do-dis′ən-ter″e) a condition marked by the symptoms of dysentery, but due to some local irritation and not to the organisms of dysentery.

**pseu·do·ede·ma** (soo″do-ə-de′mə) a puffy state resembling edema.

**pseu·do·em·bry·on·ic** (soo″do-em″bre-on′ik) apparently, but not truly, embryonic.

**pseu·do·em·phy·se·ma** (soo″do-em″fĭ-ze′mə) a condition resembling emphysema, but due to temporary blocking of the bronchial tubes.

**pseu·do·en·ceph·a·lo·ma·la·cia** (soo″do-ən-sef″ə-lo-mə-la′shə) polioencephalomalacia.

**pseu·do·en·do·me·tri·tis** (soo″do-en″do-mə-tri′tis) a condition simulating endometritis, in which there are changes in the blood vessels, hyperplasia of the stroma and glands, and atrophy.

**pseu·do·eo·sin·o·phil** (soo″do-e″o-sin′o-fil) a neutrophilic leukocyte with granules showing a predilection for acid dyes.

**pseu·do·ephed·rine** (soo″do-ə-fed′rin) one of the stereoisomers of ephedrine, having less pressor action and fewer central stimulant effects than ephedrine.
**p. hydrochloride** [USP], the hydrochloride salt of pseudoephedrine, used as a nasal decongestant and as a bronchodilator, administered orally.
**p. sulfate** [USP], the sulfate salt of pseudoephedrine, having the same actions and uses as the hydrochloride salt.

**pseu·do·epi·lepsy** (soo″do-ep′ĭ-lep-se) pseudoseizure.

**pseu·do·epiph·y·sis** (soo″do-ə-pif′ə-sis) an accessory bone at the distal and the proximal ends of the second metacarpal bone.

**pseu·do·es·the·sia** (soo″do-əs-the′zhə) pseudesthesia.

**pseu·do·ex·fo·li·a·tion** (soo″do-eks″fo-le-a′shən) exfoliation syndrome.

**pseu·do·exo·pho·ria** (soo″do-ek″so-for′e-ə) [*pseudo-* + *exophoria*] an outward tendency of the visual axis excited by diminishing the activity of the accommodative centers.

**pseu·do·ex·stro·phy** (soo″do-ek′strə-fe) a developmental anomaly marked by the characteristic musculoskeletal defects of exstrophy of the bladder but with no major defect of the urinary tract.

**pseu·do·far·cy** (soo′do-fahr″se) lymphangitis epizootica.

**pseu·do·fluc·tu·a·tion** (soo″do-fluk″choo-a′shən) a movement resembling fluctuation, such as is sometimes seen on tapping lipomas or muscular tissue.

**pseu·do·fol·lic·u·li·tis** (soo″do-fə-lik″u-li′tis) [*pseudo-* + *folliculitis*] a bacterial disorder, usually caused by *Staphylococcus aureus,* occurring chiefly in the beards of men of African descent, occurring especially in the submandibular region of the neck. The characteristic lesions are erythematous papules, sometimes pustules, containing buried hairs whose tips can easily be freed up; in contrast to sycosis barbae, which is most often seen in bearded men, pseudofolliculitis affects exclusively those who shave. Called also *barber's itch* and *p. barbae.*

**pseu·do·frac·ture** (soo″do-frak′chər) a condition seen in a radiograph of a bone as a thickening of the periosteum and formation of new bone over what looks like an incomplete fracture.

**pseu·do·gan·gli·on** (soo″do-gang′gle-on) a thickening of a nerve simulating a ganglion.
**Bochdalek's p.,** plexus dentalis superior.
**Cloquet's p.,** see under *ganglion.*
**Valentin's p.,** intumescentia tympanica.

**pseu·do·gene** (soo″do-jēn) [*pseudo-* + *gene*] [MeSH: Pseudogenes] a DNA sequence that is similar to an active gene in base sequence but is not transcribed.

**pseu·do·ges·ta·tion** (soo″do-jes-ta′shən) false pregnancy.

**pseu·do·geus·es·the·sia** (soo″do-gōōs″es-the′zhə) [*pseudo-* + Gr. *geusis* taste + *esthesia*] pseudogeusia.

**pseu·do·geu·sia** (soo″do-goo′zhə) [*pseudo-* + Gr. *geusis* taste + *-ia*] a synesthesia in which taste is experienced in association with a stimulus of a different modality.

**pseu·do·glan·ders** (soo″do-glan′dərz) 1. epizootic lymphangitis. 2. melioidosis.

**pseu·do·glan·du·lar** (soo″do-glan′du-lər) resembling a gland; see under *phase.*

**pseu·do·gli·o·ma** (soo″do-gli-o′mə) a condition resembling glioma, a membrane being produced behind the lens because of failure of the posterior vascular sheath of the lens to atrophy, or because of its replacement by connective tissue.

**pseu·do·glob·u·lin** (soo″do-glob′u-lin) one of a class of globulins characterized by being soluble in water in the absence of neutral salts and thus not a true globulin (euglobulin); see also under *globulin.*

**pseu·do·glot·tic** (soo″do-glot′ik) pertaining to the pseudoglottis.

**pseu·do·glot·tis** (soo″do-glot′is) 1. rima vestibuli. 2. neoglottis.

**pseu·do·glu·co·sa·zone** (soo″do-gloo-kōs′ə-zōn) a crystalline substance sometimes developed in normal urine in testing for glucose.

**pseu·do·gon·or·rhea** (soo″do-gon″ə-re′ə) nongonococcal urethritis.

**pseu·do·gout** (soo′do-gout) [*pseudo-* + *gout*] calcium pyrophosphate deposition disease, particularly the acute and subacute forms.

**pseu·do·graph·ia** (soo″do-graf′e-ə) [*pseudo-* + *graph-* + *-ia*] the production of meaningless written symbols imitating letters, the written equivalent of jargon aphasia.

**pseu·do·gyn·e·co·mas·tia** (soo″do-jin″ə-ko-mas′te-ə) an excess of adipose tissue in the male breast with no increase in glandular tissue.

**pseu·do·hal·lu·ci·na·tion** (soo″do-hə-loo″sĭ-na′shən) 1. an image perceived to be occurring externally but which the subject knows to be generated within the mind. 2. a hallucination which is perceived as unreal.

**pseu·do·hau·stra·tion** (soo″do-haw-stra′shən) a false appearance of normal sacculation of the wall of the colon, the radiographic appearance being produced by edematous islands of mucosa regularly spaced between deep areas of ulceration in the muscle layers.

**pseu·do·hel·minth** (soo″do-hel′minth) [*pseudo-* + *helminth*] something that resembles an endoparasitic worm.

**pseu·do·hem·ag·glu·ti·na·tion** (soo″do-he″mə-gloo″tĭ-na′shən) rouleau formation.

**pseu·do·he·ma·tu·ria** (soo″do-he″mə-tu′re-ə) the presence in the urine of pigments that give it a pink or red color, but with no detectable hemoglobin or blood cells.

**pseu·do·he·mo·phil·ia** (soo″do-he″mo-fil′e-ə) von Willebrand's disease.

**pseu·do·he·mop·ty·sis** (soo″do-he-mop′tĭ-sis) spitting of blood which comes from some source other than the lungs or bronchial tubes.

**pseu·do·he·red·i·tary** (soo″do-hə-red′ĭ-tar″e) occurring in successive generations because of imposition of the same environmental factors and not because of genetic transmission.

**pseu·do·her·maph·ro·dism** (soo″do-hər-maf′ro-diz-əm) pseudohermaphroditism.

**pseu·do·her·maph·ro·dite** (soo″do-hər-maf′ro-dīt) an individual with pseudohermaphroditism.
**female p.,** an individual with female pseudohermaphroditism. Called also *female intersex.*
**male p.,** an individual with male pseudohermaphroditism. Called also *male intersex.*

**pseu·do·her·maph·ro·dit·ism** (soo″do-hər-maf′ro-dit-iz″əm) [MeSH: Pseudohermaphroditism] a condition in which an individual is genetically and gonadally of one sex but has significant secondary sex characters of the opposite sex, often with ambiguous external genitalia. See also *intersexuality* and *hermaphroditism.* Called also *androgynism* and *spurious* or *false hermaphroditism.*
**female p.,** a form in which the affected individual is genetically female and has female gonads (ovaries) but has significant male secondary sex characters. Called also *androgynism* and *gynandrism.*
**male p.,** a form in which the affected individual is genetically male and has male gonads (testes) but has significant typically female morphological characteristics.

**pseu·do·her·nia** (soo″do-her′ne-ə) an inflamed sac or gland simulating strangulated hernia.

**pseu·do·het·ero·to·pia** (soo″do-het″ər-o-to′pe-ə) displacement of gray or white matter of the brain or cord, produced by unskillful manipulation during autopsy.

**pseu·do·hy·dro·ceph·a·lus** (soo″do-hi″dro-sef′ə-ləs) abnormally large appearance of a normal-sized head, due to smallness of the face and body, as in Silver's syndrome.

**pseu·do·hy·dro·ne·phro·sis** (soo″do-hi″dro-nə-fro′sis) a paranephritic cyst.

**pseu·do·hy·os·cy·amine** (soo″do-hi″o-si′ə-min) norhyoscyamine.

**pseu·do·hypa·cu·sis** (soo″do-hīp-ə-ku′sis) [*pseudo-* + *hyp-* + *acusis*] functional hearing loss.

**pseu·do·hy·per·ka·le·mia** (soo″do-hi″pər-kə-le′me-ə) a laboratory artifact in which serum potassium is elevated when plasma potassium is normal. It occurs in the presence of thrombocytosis or leukocytosis, most commonly in myeloproliferative disorders, because blood clotting causes the release of potassium from platelets and leukocytes.

**pseu·do·hy·per·ten·sion** (soo″do-hi″pər-ten′shən) a falsely elevated blood pressure reading by sphygmomanometry, occurring particularly in elderly patients, caused by loss of compliance of the arterial walls.

**pseu·do·hy·per·tri·cho·sis** (soo″do-hi″pər-trĭ-ko′sis) persistence after birth of the fine hair present during fetal life, owing to inability of the skin to throw it off.

**pseu·do·hy·per·tri·glyc·er·i·de·mia** (soo″do-hi″pər-tri-glis″ə-ri-de′me-ə) false elevation of blood triglyceride levels, usually due to an artifact of testing.

**pseu·do·hy·per·troph·ic** (soo″do-hi″pər-trof′ik) characterized by apparent, but not real, hypertrophy.

**pseu·do·hy·per·tro·phy** (soo″do-hi-per′tro-fe) false hypertrophy; increase of size without true hypertrophy.
**muscular p.,** an increase in the size of a muscle which is not due to enlargement of muscle fibers but to infiltration of the muscle with other tissue, e.g., fat.

**pseu·do·hy·pha** (soo″do-hi′fə) a string of cells resulting from the building of the blastoconidia, without the cytoplasmic connection of a true hypha; seen in some yeasts.

**pseu·do·hy·po·al·dos·ter·on·ism** (soo″do-hi″po-al-dos′tər-ōn-iz-əm) [MeSH: Pseudohypoaldosteronism] 1. a hereditary disorder of infancy characterized by severe salt and water depletion and other signs of aldosterone deficiency, even though normal or elevated amounts of aldosterone are secreted. Causes include aldosterone receptor defects and renal dysfunction. Some affected infants outgrow the need for dietary salt supplements in early childhood. 2. the endocrine abnormality associated with sodium-losing nephropathy, usually due to chronic pyelonephritis, seen primarily in adults. See also *Gordon's syndrome,* under *syndrome.*

**pseu·do·hy·po·na·tre·mia** (soo″do-hi″po-nə-tre′me-ə) a decreased serum sodium concentration that does not correspond to a real hypotonic disorder, i.e., the serum osmolality is normal. It occurs when hyperlipidemia increases the serum non-water volume or hyperproteinemia increases the serum non-sodium solute.

**pseu·do·hy·po·para·thy·roi·dism** (soo″do-hi″po-par″ə-thi′roi-diz-əm) [MeSH: Pseudohypoparathyroidism] a hereditary condition clinically resembling hypoparathyroidism, but caused by inability to respond to rather than deficiency of parathyroid hormone. The major cause is defective G proteins required for signal transduction; in some cases, there is an associated inability to respond to other hormones that require the same G protein types. It is characterized by hypocalcemia and hyperphosphatemia, and is commonly associated with short stature, obesity, short metacarpals, and ectopic calcification.

**pseu·do·hy·po·phos·pha·ta·sia** (soo″do-hi″po-fos″fə-ta′zhə) a condition resembling hypophosphatasia, characterized by osteopathy of the skull and long bones, muscular hypotonia, hypercalcemia, and increased urinary excretion of phosphoethanolamine. It is distinguished by normal alkaline phosphatase activity.

**pseu·do·hy·po·thy·roi·dism** (soo″do-hi″po-thi′roi-diz-əm) inability to use thyroxine in tissue cells, despite normal thyroid function, leading to development of symptoms and certain stigmata of hypothyroidism.

**pseu·do·ic·ter·us** (soo″do-ik′tər-əs) pseudojaundice.

**pseu·do·in·farc·tion** (soo″do-in-fahrk′shən) the simulation in the electrocardiographic pattern of myocardial infarction, due to disorders other than coronary artery disease.

**pseu·do·in·ti·ma** (soo″do-in′tĭ-mə) in a blood vessel graft or vascular prosthesis, a new layer on the intimal surface that consists of cells other than endothelial cells, such as plasma proteins or collagen. Cf. *neointima.*

**pseu·do·iso·chro·mat·ic** (soo″do-i″so-kro-mat′ik) seemingly of the same color throughout: applied to solutions for testing color blindness, containing two pigments which will be distinguished by the normal eye, but not by the color blind. Cf. *anisochromatic.*

**pseu·do·iso·cy·a·nin** (soo″do-i″so-si′ə-nin) an orange metachromatic dye used for the selective demonstration of insulin in pancreatic islet beta cells.

**pseu·do·jaun·dice** (soo″do-jawn′dis) skin discoloration caused by blood changes and not due to liver disease, as in carotenemia. Called also *pseudoicterus.*

**pseu·do·ker·a·tin** (soo″do-ker′ə-tin) false keratin, found in the skin and the nervous system.

**pseu·do·la·mel·lar** (soo″do-lə-mel′ər) resembling lamellae.

**pseu·do·leu·ke·mia** (soo″do-loo-ke′me-ə) an obsolete term for a group of conditions resembling one another in showing enlargement of the lymph glands and in characteristics which resemble the conditions present in leukemia, but without leukemic blood findings. The group included Hodgkin's disease, multiple myeloma, agnogenic myeloid metaplasia, and several other conditions.

**pseu·do·li·thi·a·sis** (soo″do-lĭ-thi′ə-sis) a condition with symptoms of spasm resembling biliary colic.

**pseu·do·lo·gia** (soo″do-lo′jə) [*pseudo-* + *log-* + *-ia*] lying; falsehood.
**p. fantas′tica,** a tendency to tell extravagant and fantastic falsehoods centered about the storyteller, who often comes to believe in and may act on them.

**pseu·do·lux·a·tion** (soo″do-lək-sa′shən) partial dislocation of a bone.

**pseu·do·lym·pho·ma** (soo″do-lim-fo′mə) [*pseudo-* + *lymphoma*] [MeSH: Pseudolymphoma] a group of disorders having a benign course but exhibiting clinical and histologic features suggestive of malignant lymphoma. Called also *lymphocytoma.*
**Spiegler-Fendt p.,** lymphocytoma cutis.

**Pseu·do·lynch·ia** (soo″do-linch′e-ə) a genus of parasitic flies of the family Hippoboscidae. *P. canarien′sis* (called also *P. mari′rah*), parasitizes pigeons and spreads to them a type of malaria, and is also a vector of the protozoon *Haemoproteus columbae.*

**pseu·do·mal·func·tion** (soo″do-mal-fungk′shən) in cardiac pacing terminology, apparent pacemaker malfunction actually due to an artifact, such as mechanical errors in electrocardiographic analysis.

**pseu·do·ma·lig·nan·cy** (soo″do-mə-lig′nən-se) [*pseudo-* + *malignancy*] any of several types of tumors exhibiting benign clinical behavior but having a distinctly malignant microscopic appearance; see also *pseudolymphoma* and *pseudomelanoma.*

**pseu·do·mam·ma** (soo″do-mam′ə) a structure resembling a nipple, or even a complete breast, sometimes found on ovarian dermoids.

**pseu·do·ma·nia** (soo″do-ma′ne-ə) [*pseudo-* + *-mania*] 1. false or pretended mental disorder. 2. a mental disorder in which the patient admits to crimes of which he is innocent.

**pseu·do·mega·co·lon** (soo″do-meg′ə-ko″lon) dilatation of the colon in adults. Cf. *megacolon.*

**pseu·do·mel·a·no·ma** (soo″do-mel″ə-no′mə) [*pseudo-* + *melanoma*] a benign melanotic lesion resembling a superficial spreading melanoma occurring at the site of an incompletely removed melanocytic nevus.

**pseu·do·mel·a·no·sis** (soo″do-mel″ə-no′sis) a staining of the tissue after death with pigments from the blood.

**pseu·do·me·lia** (soo″do-me′le-ə) [*pseudo-* + *-melia*] phantom limb.

**pseu·do·mem·brane** (soo″do-mem′brān) false membrane.

**pseu·do·mem·bra·nelle** (soo″do-mem′brə-nel) [*pseudo-* + *membranelle*] 1. a membranelle-like organelle, composed of a group of complex kinetofragments, representing a modified frange in certain ciliate protozoa. Called also *pavé.* 2. loosely, any of various membranelle-like ciliary complexes seen in protozoa.

**pseu·do·mem·bra·nous** (soo″do-mem′brə-nəs) marked by or pertaining to a *pseudomembrane.*

**pseu·do·men·in·gi·tis** (soo″do-men″in-ji′tis) meningism.

**pseu·do·men·stru·a·tion** (soo″do-men″stroo-a′shən) uterine discharge unattended with endometrial changes of menstruation, usually occurring in newborn babies.

**pseu·do·met·he·mo·glo·bin** (soo″do-met-he″mo-glo′bin) former name for *methemalbumin.*

**pseu·do·mo·nad** (soo″do-mo′nad) any member of the genus *Pseudomonas.*

**Pseu·do·mo·na·da·ceae** (soo″do-mo″nə-da′se-e) [MeSH: Pseudomonadaceae] a family of bacteria consisting of gram-negative, aerobic, straight or curved rods that are motile with polar flagella, occurring in soil and fresh and salt water. It contains the genera *Pseudomonas, Xanthomonas,* and *Zoogloea.*

**Pseu·do·mo·na·da·les** (soo″do-mo″nə-da′lēz) an order of bacteria used in some systems of classification to denote those organisms that possess polar flagella; cf. *Eubacteriales.*

**Pseu·do·mo·na·di·neae** (soo″do-mo″nə-di′ne-e) in former systems of classification, a suborder of Pseudomonadales, made up of bacteria containing pigments.

**Pseu·do·mo·nas** (soo″do-mo′nəs) [*pseudo-* + Gr. *monas* unit, from *monos* single] [MeSH: Pseudomonas] a genus of gram-negative bacteria of the family Pseudomonadaceae, consisting of straight or curved rods that are motile by polar flagella. The genus comprises several hundred species, including many of uncertain status. Most species are strict aerobes and some produce pigments. The organisms are usually saprophytic, being found in soil, water, and decomposing matter; some are pathogenic for plants and animals.
**P. acido′vorans,** a widespread species that is an occasional opportunistic pathogen.
**P. aerugino′sa,** the type species of the genus; it produces pyocyanin and fluorescein, which give the color to the "blue pus" observed in certain infections, and it produces a variety of toxins and enzymes. It is a major cause of nosocomial infection, such as *P. aeruginosa* pneumonia (q.v.), especially in young, debilitated, or immunocompromised patients, or severe, even fatal infections of the urinary tract, wounds, abscesses, or the bloodstream. It may also cause eye infections in those who use contact lenses. Called also *Bacillus pyocyaneus, P. polycolor,* and *P. pyocyanea.*
**P. alcali′genes,** an occasionally opportunistic species found in water reservoirs and recovered from clinical specimens of blood, urine, respiratory tract, and abscesses. It has been associated with empyema and eye infections.
**P. cepa′cia,** former name for *Burkholderia cepacia.*
**P. diminu′ta,** a species isolated from waters of streams and ditches and from clinical specimens.
**P. eisenber′gii,** *P. putida.*
**P. fluores′cens,** a fluorescent species that is an environmental contaminant and occasionally an opportunistic pathogen for humans, causing infections of the urinary tract, wounds, and the bloodstream. It also occurs as a contaminant of blood and blood products used for transfusion, sometimes causing fatal shock.
**P. mal′lei,** former name for *Burkholderia mallei.*
**P. maltophi′lia,** *Xanthomonas maltophilia.*
**P. mendoci′na,** a nonpathogenic species isolated from soil, water, and urine.
**P. paucimobi′lis,** a species isolated from clinical specimens and environmental sources that may be an opportunistic pathogen.
**P. pertucino′gena,** a species that produces pertucin. Called also *Bordetella pertussis,* Phase IV.
**P. picket′tii,** former name for *Ralstonia picketii.*
**P. polyco′lor,** *P. aeruginosa.*
**P. pseudoalcali′genes,** a species isolated from water reservoirs and clinical specimens that is sometimes associated with infection.
**P. pseudomal′lei,** former name for *Burkholderia pseudomallei.*
**P. pu′tida,** a fluorescent species that is a common inhabitant of soil, water, and plants. It is frequently isolated from clinical specimens, and is occasionally an opportunistic pathogen. Called also *P. eisenbergii.*
**P. putrefa′ciens,** a species of wide distribution that causes spoilage in marine foods, butter, and meats. It has been recovered from clinical specimens, occasionally associated with infection.
**P. pyocya′nea,** *P. aeruginosa.*
**P. pyrroci′nia,** a species that produces pyrrolnitrin.
**P. reptili′vora,** a species which is pathogenic for lizards.
**P. sep′tica,** a species which causes a disease of caterpillars.
**P. stani′eri,** *P. stutzeri.*
**P. stut′zeri,** a widespread species often recovered from clinical specimens. It is an occasional opportunistic pathogen, particularly in drug addicts. Called also *P. stanieri.*
**P. syncya′nea,** a species isolated from blue milk, which produces the blue pigment responsible for its color.
**P. testostero′ni,** a widespread species found in soil and isolated from clinical specimens.
**P. thoma′sii,** former name for a biovar of *Ralstonia pickettii.*
**P. vesicula′ris,** a species isolated from water and clinical specimens. It has been associated with genitourinary tract infections. Called also *Corynebacterium vesiculare.*

**pseu·do·mo·nil·e·thrix** (soo″do-mo-nil′ə-thriks) a condition, inherited as an autosomal dominant trait, in which the hairs exhibit irregularly spaced nodal swellings, the internodal areas being normal; cf. *monilethrix.*

**Pseu·do·mo·nil·ia** (soo″do-mo-nil′e-ə) former name for *Candida.*

**pseu·do·mor·phine** (soo″do-mor′fin) a compound occurring in opium and prepared by the oxidation of morphine; called also *dehydromorphine.*

**pseu·do·mo·tor** (soo″do-mo′tər) dyskinetic.

**pseu·do·mu·cin** (soo″do-mu′sin) a substance resembling mucin found in ovarian cysts.

**pseu·do·mu·ci·nous** (soo″do-mu′sĭ-nəs) pertaining to pseudomucin.

**pseu·do·my·ia·sis** (soo″do-mi-i′ə-sis) the presence of fly maggots in the digestive tract due to ingestion; if present in large numbers, they may cause diarrhea and other symptoms.

**pseu·do·my·o·pia** (soo″do-mi-o′pe-ə) [*pseudo-* + *myopia*] defective vision resembling myopia, caused by spasm of the ciliary muscle or by failure of relaxation of accommodation.

**pseu·do·myx·o·ma** (soo″do-mik-so′mə) a condition in which mucinous cells implant throughout the peritoneal cavity and secrete gelatinous mucinous material. Called also *p. peritonei.*
**p. peritone′i,** the presence in the peritoneal cavity of mucoid matter from a ruptured ovarian cyst or a ruptured mucocele of the appendix; called also *hydrops spurius.*

**pseu·do·nar·cot·ic** (soo″do-nahr-kot′ik) sedative and apparently, but not directly, narcotic.

**pseu·do·neo·plasm** (soo″do-ne′o-plaz-əm) [*pseudo-* + *neoplasm*] pseudotumor.

**pseu·do·neu·ri·tis** (soo″do-no͞o-ri′tis) [*pseudo-* + *neuritis*] a hyperemic condition of the optic papilla, occurring as a congenital anomaly.

**pseu·do·neu·ro·ma** (soo″do-no͞o-ro′mə) false neuroma.

**pseu·do·neu·ro·no·pha·gia** (soo″do-no͞o-ro″no-fa′jə) a false appearance of phagocytosis of nerve cells; cf. *satellitosis.*

**Pseu·do·no·car·dia** (soo″do-no-kahr′de-ə) [Gr. *pseudes* false + *nocardia*] in former systems of classification, a genus of bacteria of the family Nocardiaceae, order Actinomycetales, characterized by aerial hyphae that grow by budding. The organisms have now been assigned to other genera.

**pseu·do·nu·cle·o·lus** (soo″do-noo-kle′o-ləs) [*pseudo-* + *nucleolus*] karyosome.

**pseu·do·nys·tag·mus** (soo″do-nis-tag′məs) end-position nystagmus.

**pseu·do·ob·struc·tion** (soo″do-ob-struk′shən) a condition simulating obstruction.
**intestinal p.-o.,** a condition characterized by constipation, colicky pain, and vomiting, but without evidence of organic obstruction apparent at laparotomy.

**pseu·do·ochro·no·sis** (soo″do-o-kro′no-sis) a condition resembling ochronosis, but not caused by a disorder of metabolism.

**pseu·do·op·to·gram** (soo″do-op′to-gram) an optogram in which the rods strip off from the illuminated spot and only the cones remain.

**pseu·do·os·teo·ma·la·cia** (soo″do-os″te-o-mə-la′shə) rachitic contraction of the pelvis.

**pseu·do·pap·il·lary** (soo″do-pap′ĭ-lar″e) having a pattern that resembles the growth of papillae but results from necrosis of cells distant from the blood supply, with the preserved cells forming fingerlike projections.

**pseu·do·pap·il·le·de·ma** (soo″do-pap″ĭ-lə-de′mə) [*pseudo-* + *papilledema*] anomalous elevation of the optic disk.

**pseu·do·pa·ral·y·sis** (soo″do-pə-ral′i-sis) false paralysis: apparent loss of muscular power, without true paralysis, marked by defective coordination of movements or by repression of movement on account of pain.

**Parrot's p., syphilitic p.,** pseudoparalysis of one or more of the extremities in infants caused by syphilitic osteochondritis of an epiphysis.

**pseu·do·para·ple·gia** (soo″do-par″ə-ple′jə) spurious paralysis of the lower limbs, as in malingering or conversion disorder.

**pseu·do·par·a·site** (soo″do-par′ə-sīt) any object resembling or mistaken for a parasite.

**pseu·do·pa·ren·chy·ma** (soo″do-pə-reng′kĭ-mə) a mass of hyphae fused together to form a tissuelike structure.

**pseu·do·pa·re·sis** (soo″do-pə-re′sis) a hysterical or other nonorganic condition simulating paresis.

**pseu·do·pe·lade** (soo″do-pe′lād) [*pseudo-* + *pelade*] an uncommon type of alopecia characterized by the asymptomatic development of a distinctive cicatricial patchy alopecia in adults.

**pseu·do·pel·lag·ra** (soo″do-pə-lag′rə) a condition in alcoholics now recognized as identical to pellagra.

**pseu·do·pep·tone** (soo″do-pep′tōn) ovomucoid.

**pseu·do·peri·car·di·al** (soo″do-per″ĭ-kahr′de-əl) seemingly, but not actually, arising from the pericardium.

**pseu·do·peri·to·ni·tis** (soo″do-per″ĭ-to-ni′tis) peritonism.

**pseu·do·per·ox·i·dase** (soo-do-pər-ok′sĭ-dās) any of a class of substances, including hemoglobin, that act like peroxidase, catalyzing a reduction-oxidation reaction between hydrogen peroxide and a variety of organic compounds.

**pseu·do·pha·kia** (soo″do-fa′ke-ə) a condition in which the degenerated crystalline lens is replaced by mesodermal tissue.
**p. adipo′sa,** a condition in which the crystalline lens is replaced by a mass of fatty tissue.
**p. fibro′sa,** replacement of the crystalline lens by a mass of connective tissue that represents hyperplasia of both the anterior and posterior vascular sheaths of the lens.

**pseu·do·pha·ko·do·ne·sis** (soo″do-fak″o-do-no′sis) [*pseudo* + *phakos* + Gr. *donein* to shake] movement of an implanted artificial lens.

**pseu·do·phak·os** (soo″do-fak′əs) [*pseudo-* + Gr. *phakos* lentil-shaped object] an implantable artificial lens used in the treatment of cataracts.

**pseu·do·pho·tes·the·sia** (soo″do-fo″tes-the′zhə) photism.

**Pseu·do·phyl·lid·ea** (soo″do-fĭ-lid′e-ə) an order of cestodes in which the scolex typically has two opposing sucking organs. It includes the family Diphyllobothriidae.

**pseu·do·phyl·lid·e·an** (soo″do-fĭ-lid′e-ən) pertaining to or caused by tapeworms of the order Pseudophyllidea.

**pseu·do·plasm** (soo′do-plaz-əm) a new growth which disappears spontaneously.

**pseu·do·plas·mo·di·um** (soo″do-plaz-mo′de-əm) [*pseudo-* + *plasmodium*] a multinucleate plasmodium-like body formed by aggregation of myxamebae without fusion of their protoplasm.

**pseu·do·ple·gia** (soo″do-ple′jə) [*pseudo-* + *-plegia*] hysterical paralysis or pseudoparalysis.

**pseu·do·pneu·mo·nia** (soo″do-noo-mo′ne-ə) a condition marked by the symptoms of pneumonia, but without any lesions in the lungs.

**pseu·do·po·dia** (soo″do-po′de-ə) [L.] [MeSH: Pseudopodia] plural of *pseudopodium.*

**pseu·do·po·di·o·spore** (soo″do-po′de-o-spor) [*pseudopodium* + *spore*] amebula, def. 2.

**pseu·do·po·di·um** (soo″do-po′de-əm) pl. *pseudopo′dia* [L., from *pseudo-* + Gr. *pous* foot] a temporary cytoplasmic extrusion by means of which an ameba or other ameboid organism or cell moves about or engulfs food. Pseudopodia are of four types: axopodia, filopodia, lobopodia, and reticulopodia.

**pseu·do·po·lio·my·eli·tis** (soo″do-po″le-o-mi″ə-li′tis) a poliomyelitis-like disease caused by an enterovirus other than poliovirus.

**pseu·do·poly·cy·the·mia** (soo″do-pol″e-si-the′me-ə) 1. stress polycythemia. 2. relative polycythemia.

**pseu·do·poly·me·lia** (soo″do-pol″e-me′le-ə) an illusory sensation that may be referred to many extreme portions of the body, including the nose, nipples, and glans penis, as well as the hands and feet.
**paresthetic p.,** sensations of pseudopolymelia in the form of paresthesias.

**pseu·do·pol·yp** (soo″do-pol′ip) a hypertrophied tab of mucous membrane resembling a polyp, but caused by ulceration surrounding and sometimes undermining a portion of intact mucosa; frequently observed in chronic inflammatory diseases, such as ulcerative colitis. Called also *hyperplastic, inflammatory,* or *regenerative polyp.*

**pseu·do·pol·y·po·sis** (soo″do-pol″ĭ-po′sis) the occurrence of numbers of pseudopolyps in the colon and rectum, as the result of long-standing inflammation.

**pseu·do·preg·nan·cy** (soo″do-preg′nən-se) [MeSH: Pseudopregnancy] 1. false pregnancy. 2. the premenstrual stage of the endometrium; so called because it resembles the endometrium just before implantation of the blastocyst.

**pseu·do·prog·na·thism** (soo″do-prog′nə-thiz-əm) protruding mandible resembling prognathism but due to altered tooth alignment, resulting from malocclusion.

**pseu·do·pro·tein·uria** (soo″do-pro″te-nu′re-ə) adventitious proteinuria.

**pseu·do·pseu·do·hy·po·para·thy·roid·ism** (soo″do-soo″do-hi″po-par″ə-thi′roi-diz-əm) [MeSH: Pseudopseudohypoparathyroidism] an incomplete form of pseudohypoparathyroidism characterized by the same constitutional features but by normal levels of calcium and phosphorus in the serum.

**pseu·do·pter·yg·i·um** (soo″do-tər-ij′e-əm) a conjunctival scar attached to the cornea, superficially resembling a true pterygium, but usually not firmly adherent to the underlying tissue.

**pseu·do·pto·sis** (soo″do-to′sis) [*pseudo-* + *ptosis*] decrease in the size of the palpebral aperture.

**pseu·do·pty·al·ism** (soo″do-ti′əl-iz-əm) accumulation and drooling of saliva due to dysphagia.

**pseu·do·pu·ber·ty** (soo″do-pu′bər-te) development of secondary sex characters and accessory reproductive organs without pubertal levels of gonadotropins and gonadotropin-releasing hormone, most often as a result of the release of steroid hormones by an adrenocortical or gonadal tumor; it may be either isosexual or contrasexual.
**precocious p.,** appearance of some secondary sex characters before the normal age of puberty but without maturation of the gonads.

**pseu·do·ra·bies** (soo″do-ra′bēz) [MeSH: Pseudorabies] a highly contagious viral disease caused by a herpesvirus and primarily affecting the central nervous system. It is endemic in pigs; older pigs usually have a mild respiratory infection but piglets often have convulsions and die. It sometimes spreads to cattle, dogs, cats, and other mammals, in which its characteristics include sudden onset, severe pruritus, late paralysis, convulsions, and death within three to four days. Called also *Aujeszky's disease* or *itch, mad itch,* and *infectious bulbar paralysis.*

**pseu·do·re·ac·tion** (soo″do-re-ak′shən) a false or deceptive reaction; a skin reaction in intradermal tests which is not due to the specific protein used in the test but to the protein of the medium employed in producing the toxin.

**pseu·do·re·duc·tion** (soo″do-re-duk′shən) the apparent halving of the chromosome number by synapsis.

**pseu·do·ret·in·i·tis pig·men·to·sa** (soo″do-ret″in-i′tis pig″mən-to′sə) pigmentary degeneration of the retina mimicking retinitis pigmentosa, but arising from intrauterine viral infections, vascular lesions, and other causes.

**pseu·do·rheu·ma·tism** (soo″do-roo′mə-tiz-əm) a condition resembling rheumatic fever, due to some nonrheumatic disease, as gonorrhea.

**pseu·do·rick·ets** (soo″do-rik′əts) renal osteodystrophy.

**pseu·do·rin·der·pest** (soo″do-rin′dər-pest) peste des petits ruminants.

**pseu·do·ro·sette** (soo″do-ro-zet′) a radial cluster of tumor cells encircling a small blood vessel; called also *perivascular pseudorosette.*

**pseu·do·sar·co·ma** (soo″do-sahr-ko′mə) [*pseudo-* + *sarcoma*] sarcomatoid transformation of a carcinoma histologically resembling a sarcoma; cf. *carcinosarcoma.*

**pseu·do·sar·co·ma·tous** (soo″do-sahr-ko′mə-təs) mimicking sarcoma; used of both benign and malignant lesions that histologically resemble sarcoma.

**pseu·do·scar·la·ti·na** (soo″do-skahr″lə-te′nə) a febrile condition with an eruption like that of scarlet fever, but due to septic poisoning.

**pseu·do·scle·re·ma** (soo″do-sklə-re′mə) adiponecrosis subcutanea neonatorum.

**pseu·do·scle·ro·sis** (soo″do-sklə-ro′sis) [*pseudo-* + *sclerosis*] a condition with the symptoms but without the lesions of multiple sclerosis.
**Strümpell-Westphal p., Westphal-Strümpell p.,** Wilson's disease.

**pseu·do·scro·tum** (soo″do-skro′təm) a solid partition with a median raphe, resembling the scrotum in the male, obliterating the opening into the vagina of a female pseudohermaphrodite.

**pseu·do·sei·zure** (soo″do-se′zhər) an attack resembling an epileptic seizure but having purely psychological causes; it lacks the electroencephalographic characteristics of epilepsy and the patient may be able to stop it by an act of will. Called also *pseudoepilepsy.*

**pseud·os·mia** (soo-doz′me-ə) [*pseudo-* + *osm-*[1] + *-ia*] a sensation of odor without the appropriate stimulus.

**pseu·do·so·lu·tion** (soo″do-so-loo′shən) solutions which do not act according to the usual physical laws of solutions; the term is sometimes applied to colloidal systems.

**pseu·do·sto·ma** (soo″do-sto′mə) [*pseudo-* + *stoma*] an apparent communication between silver-stained endothelial cells.

**pseu·do·stra·bis·mus** (soo″do-strə-bis′məs) apparent strabismus due to an overhanging epicanthus which narrows the visible width of the sclera medial to the iris.

**pseu·do·stro·phan·thin** (soo″do-stro-fan′thin) a poisonous glycoside from the African shrub *Strophanthus hispidus.*

**pseu·do·ta·bes** (soo″do-ta′bēz) [*pseudo-* + *tabes*] any neuropathy with symptoms like those of tabes dorsalis.
**diabetic p.,** a form of diabetic neuropathy characterized by sensory loss, ataxia, and ulceration in the lower limbs; sometimes it includes lancinating pains in the legs, joint deformities, and Argyll Robertson pupils. Called also *diabetic tabes.*
**pupillotonic p.,** Adie's syndrome.

**pseu·do·tet·a·nus** (soo″do-tet′ə-nəs) persistent muscular contractions resembling tetanus but not associated with the presence of *Clostridium tetani.*

**pseu·do·thrill** (soo′do-thril) a condition that simulates a true thrill.

**pseu·do·tox·in** (soo″do-tok′sin) a poisonous extract from belladonna leaves.

**pseu·do·tra·cho·ma** (soo″do-trə-ko′mə) a disease of the eye and lids resembling trachoma.

**pseu·do·tris·mus** (soo″do-tris′məs) a motor disorder of the mouth with symptoms similar to those of trismus.

**pseu·dot·ro·pine** (soo-dot′rə-pēn) a dark-brown, syrupy, liquid base, a decomposition product of tropine.

**pseu·do·trun·cus ar·te·ri·o·sus** (soo″do-trung′kəs ahr-tēr″e-o′səs) the most severe form of tetralogy of Fallot with associated pulmonary atresia in which outflow is through a single major vessel, the aorta, accompanied by the remnant of the atretic pulmonary artery.

**pseu·do·tu·ber·cle** (soo″do-too′bər-kəl) a tubercle resembling that of tuberculosis, but not due to the tubercle bacillus.

**pseu·do·tu·ber·cu·lo·ma** (soo″do-too-bər″ku-lo′mə) a tumor resembling in structure a tuberculoma.

**pseu·do·tu·ber·cu·lo·sis** (soo″do-too-ber″ku-lo′sis) [*pseudo-* + *tuberculosis*] any of various animal diseases resembling tuberculosis but caused by pathogens other than the tubercle bacillus; caseous swellings resembling tubercular nodules (pseudotubercles) form in organs throughout the body, and there may be fever and diarrhea with a fatal outcome. See *caseous lymphadenitis* and *yersiniosis* (def. 3).

**pseu·do·tu·mor** (soo″do-too′mər) an enlargement that resembles a tumor; it may result from inflammation, accumulation of fluid, or other causes, and may or may not regress spontaneously. Called also *pseudoneoplasm* and *false tumor.*
**p. ce′rebri,** a condition caused by venous sinus occlusion and cerebral edema associated with a number of pathologic conditions, marked by raised intracranial pressure with normal cerebrospinal fluid, headache, nausea, vomiting, and papilledema, but without neurological signs except occasional abducens paralysis. Called also *benign intracranial hypertension.*
**inflammatory p.,** a general term for a tumorlike mass representing an inflammatory reaction, occurring in a variety of organs and composed of granulation tissue with leukocyte infiltration.
**orbital p.,** a distinctive, chronic inflammatory reaction in the orbital tissues of the eye, of unknown etiology, that may closely resemble a neoplasm and often becomes bilateral. Symptoms include exophthalmos and congestion of the lids with edema. When limitation of ocular motility also occurs, it is sometimes called *orbital myositis.*

**pseu·do·ty·phus** (soo″do-ti′fəs) a disease of Sumatra resembling scrub typhus (tsutsugamushi disease).

**pseu·do·ure·mia** (soo″do-u-re′me-ə) uremia-like symptoms occurring in acute glomerulonephritis and in hypertensive vascular disease (hypertensive encephalopathy).

**pseu·do·uri·dine** (soo′do-ūr′ĭ-dēn) [MeSH: Pseudouridine] 5-ribosyluracil, an unusual nucleotide occurring in transfer RNA; it is produced by posttranscriptional isomerization of uridine and differs from uridine in having the linkage between the 5-carbon of uracil and the 1-carbon of ribose. Symbol ψ.

**pseu·do·vac·u·ole** (soo″do-vak′u-ōl) a round space within certain red blood cells that contains an animal microorganism.

**pseu·do·ven·tri·cle** (soo″do-ven′trĭ-kəl) cavum septi pellucidi.

**pseu·do·ver·ti·go** (soo″do-vər′tĭ-go) any dizziness or other form of lightheadedness that resembles vertigo but does not involve a sense of rotation. Among many possible causes are hyperventilation, orthostatic hypotension, and panic disorder.

**pseu·do·voice** (soo′do-vois) the vocal sounds produced under proper training after laryngectomy; see also *esophageal speech.*

**pseu·do·vom·it·ing** (soo″do-vom′it-ing) regurgitation of matter from the stomach without expulsive effort.

**pseu·do·xan·thine** (soo″do-zan′thēn) 1. a compound from muscle tissue or nucleic acids. 2. a compound from uric acid.

**pseu·do·xan·tho·ma elas·ti·cum** (soo″do-zan-tho′mə e-las′tĭ-kəm) [MeSH: Pseudoxanthoma Elasticum] a rare, progressive disorder with autosomal recessive and dominant forms, usually appearing after puberty with skin, eye, and cardiovascular manifestations, most of which result from basophilic degeneration of elastic tissue. Symptoms include small yellow cutaneous macules and papules that merge to form plaques, mainly in flexural areas; lax, inelastic, redundant skin; angioid streaks in the retina; arterial insufficiency in the lower extremities; premature calcification of peripheral arteries; reduced arterial pulses; symptoms of coronary insufficiency, hypertension, and mitral valve prolapse; and gastrointestinal and other hemorrhages. Called also *nevus elasticus.*

**psi** pounds per square inch.

**psi·co·fur·a·nine** (si″ko-fūr′ə-nēn) a nucleoside antibiotic produced by *Streptomyces hygroscopicus* that has antibacterial and antitumor activity.

**psi·lo·cin** (si′lo-sin) a hallucinogenic compound found in some species of *Psilocybe;* its chemical structure and activity are similar to psilocybin.

**Psi·lo·cy·be** (si″lo-si′be) a genus of mushrooms of the family Strophariaceae, native to the southern United States and Mexico; several species are sources of psilocybin and psilocin and are consumed in some North American Indian cultures as part of religious ceremonies.

**psi·lo·cy·bin** (si″lo-si′bin) a hallucinogenic crystalline compound with indole characteristics, isolated from mushrooms of the genus *Psilocybe,* especially *P. mexicana* Heim.

**psit·ta·cine** (sit′ə-sīn) [Gr. *psittakos* parrot] [MeSH: Psittacines] of or relating to parrots, parakeets, and related birds. See also *psittacosis.*

**psit·ta·co·sis** (sit″ə-ko′sis) [Gr. *psittakos* parrot + *-osis*] 1. an acute or chronic respiratory and systemic disease of wild and domestic birds, caused by infection with *Chlamydia psittaci;* it was originally seen in psittacine birds and is transmissible to humans and other animals. Called also *chlamydiosis.* 2. human infection by *Chlamydia psittaci,* generally acquired by inhalation of dried bird excreta containing the pathogen; it may also be acquired by handling feathers or tissues of infected birds, through an open skin lesion, or from the bite of an infected bird. It may be asymptomatic, have mild influenzalike symptoms, or manifest as a severe, highly fatal pneumonia. Called also *parrot disease* or *fever* and *ornithosis.*

**PSM** presystolic murmur.

**PSMA** prostate-specific membrane antigen.

**pso·as** (so′as) see under *musculus.*

**pso·dy·mus** (sŏ′dĭ-məs) [*psoas* + *-didymus*] conjoined twins with two heads and trunks, but single at and below the loins.

**pso·itis** (so-i′tis) [*psoas* + *-itis*] inflammation of a psoas muscle or of its sheath.

**psor·a·len** (sor′ə-lən) 1. any of a group of photosensitizing constituents of plants such as *Ammi majus* or *Psoralea corylifolia;* they include methoxsalen and trioxsalen and may be ingredients of perfumes or drugs. See also *phototoxic dermatitis,* under *dermatitis.* 2. any of the plants that contain one of these substances.

**Psor·con** (sor′kon) trademark for a preparation of diflorasone diacetate.

**psor·en·ter·itis** (sor-en″tər-i′tis) [Gr. *psōros* scabby + *enteritis*] a condition of the intestinal mucosa thought to be peculiar to cholera, marked by loss of villi and a granular debris in the surface mucous sheath.

**Pso·rer·ga·tes** (sor″ər-ga′tēz) a genus of parasitic mites; *P. o′vis* causes pruritus and dermatitis in sheep. Called also *Psorobia.*

**pso·ri·as·i·form** (so″re-as′ĭ-form) resembling psoriasis.

**pso·ri·a·sis** (sə-ri′ə-sis) [Gr. *psōriasis*] [MeSH: Psoriasis] a common chronic, squamous dermatosis with polygenic inheritance and a fluctuating course. Principal histological findings are Munro microabscesses and spongiform pustules; also seen are rounded, circumscribed, erythematous, dry, scaling patches of various sizes, covered by grayish white or silvery white, umbilicated, and lamellar scales, usually on extensor surfaces, nails, scalp, genitalia, and the lumbosacral region. Central clearing and coalescence of the lesions produce lesions of diverse shapes, including annular or circinate, discoid or nummular, figurate, and gyrate.
**annular p., p. annula′ris, p. annula′ta,** see *psoriasis.*
**arthritic p., p. arthropa′thica, p. artho′pica,** psoriatic arthritis.
**Barber's p.,** localized pustular p.
**p. bucca′lis,** a rare form of psoriasis affecting the oral mucosa.
**circinate p., p. circina′ta,** see *psoriasis.*
**discoid p., p. discoi′dea,** see *psoriasis.*
**erythrodermic p.,** a severe generalized erythrodermic condition usually developing in chronic forms of psoriasis, e.g., as a reaction to topical therapy or as a result of ultraviolet exposure, or rarely occurring as the initial manifestation of psoriasis, which may be characterized by massive exfoliation of the skin and serious systemic illness associated with abnormalities of temperature and cardiovascular regulation. Called also *erythroderma psoriaticum* and *exfoliative p.*
**exfoliative p.,** erythrodermic p.
**p. figura′ta, figurate p.,** see *psoriasis.*
**flexural p.,** inverse p.
**follicular p.,** a form of psoriasis characterized by the presence of prominent follicularly oriented papules, involving mainly the thighs in adults, principally in females, and the trunk in children; in the latter, the lesions extend to form large plaques. Older lesions show nucleated cells in the openings of the hair follicles, along with other epidermal and dermal changes.
**p. gutta′ta, guttate p.,** a form of psoriasis seen primarily in children and young adults, especially following streptococcal infections, and characterized by the abrupt appearance of small droplike lesions over much of the skin surface, generally involving the trunk and proximal extremities.
**p. gyra′ta, gyrate p.,** see *psoriasis.*
**inverse p.,** a seborrheic dermatitis–like form of psoriasis in which the lesions are moist and erythematous with a minimal amount of greasy, soft scales, and occur in a flexural distribution with involvement of the intertriginous folds of the axillae and inguinal region, of the inframammary, intergluteal, and perianal skin, and of the palms, soles, and nails. Called also *flexural p., seborrheic p., seborrhiasis,* and *volar p.*
**p. invetera′ta,** a form with confluent lesions and with thickening and hardening of the skin.
**p. lin′guae,** a rare form of psoriasis affecting the mucosa of the tongue.
**nummular p., p. nummula′ris,** see *psoriasis.*
**p. ostra′cea, ostraceous p.,** psoriasis in which the lesions form thick, tough patches covered with scales, giving them a resemblance to the outside of an oyster shell. Called also *p. rupioides.*
**palmar p.,** a patchy hyperkeratotic form of psoriasis chiefly involving the contact points of the volar surfaces of the palms and fingers, which is thought to be related to local physical or chemical injury, thus representing the Koebner phenomenon; the same changes are less common on the soles.
**p. of palms and soles,** see *inverse p., palmar p.,* and *localized pustular p.*
**pustular p., generalized,** a severe, acute, generalized, sometimes fatal, erythematous pustular eruption in patients with mild to moderate psoriasis or in those with psoriatic arthritis or exfoliative p., which is accompanied by high fever, leukocytosis, hypocalcemia, arthralgia, malaise, and other systemic symptoms. Called also *von Zumbusch's* or *Zumbusch's p.*
**pustular p., localized,** a sterile eruption of pustules superimposed on discrete erythematous plaques involving the volar skin of the hands or feet, or both, usually in the presence of psoriasis at other sites, which may also involve the paronychial skin, and associated with swelling, erythema, and local discomfort. Called also *Barber's p., pustulosis palmaris et plantaris,* and *palmoplantar pustulosis.* Cf. *pustulosis palmaris et plantaris,* def. 2.
**p. rupioi′des,** p. ostracea.
**seborrheic p.,** inverse p.
**volar p.,** 1. inverse p. 2. palmar p. 3. see *localized pustular p.*
**von Zumbusch's p.,** generalized pustular p.
**p. vulga′ris,** psoriasis.
**Zumbusch's p.,** generalized pustular p.

**pso·ri·at·ic** (so″re-at′ik) 1. pertaining to, affected with, or of the nature of, psoriasis. 2. a person affected with psoriasis.

**Pso·ro·bia** (so-ro′be-ə) *Psorergates.*

**Pso·roph·o·ra** (sə-rof′o-rə) a genus of large, annoying mosquitoes of the tribe Aedini, subfamily Culicinae; their larvae prey on the larvae of other mosquitoes. Some species, particularly *P. ferox′* and *P. lut′zii,* act as carrier hosts of the eggs of *Dermatobia hominis.*

**psor·oph·thal·mia** (sor″of-thal′me-ə) [Gr. *psōrophthalmia*] a form of ulcerative marginal blepharitis.

**Pso·rop·tes** (sə-rop′tēz) a genus of mites of the family Psoroptidae, the cause of psoroptic mange (q.v.). *P. cuni′culi* infests the ears of rabbits and goats; *P. e′qui* infests horses; and *P. o′vis* (called also *P. bo′vis*) causes sheep scab in sheep and scabies in cattle and horses.

**pso·rop·tic** (sə-rop′tik) pertaining to or caused by *Psoroptes.*

**Pso·rop·ti·dae** (so-rop′tĭ-de) a family of parasitic long-legged mites, many of which cause mange in various animal species. Genera include *Chorioptes, Otodectes,* and *Psoroptes.*

**PSP** phenolsulfonphthalein.

**PSRO** Professional Standards Review Organization.

**PSVT** paroxysmal supraventricular tachycardia.

**psy·chal·ga·lia** (si″kəl-ga′le-ə) psychalgia.

**psy·chal·gia** (si-kal′jə) [*psych-* + *-algia*] 1. pain, usually in the head and perceived as being of emotional origin, that may accompany intolerable ideas, obsessions, or hallucinations; called also *algopsychalia* and *psychic pain.* 2. psychogenic pain; see also *pain disorder,* under *disorder.*

**psy·chal·gic** (si-kal′jik) pertaining to or characterized by psychalgia.

**psy·chas·the·nia** (si″kəs-the′ne-ə) [*psych-* + *asthenia*] *(obs.)* a term used by Janet to cover all psychoneuroses not classified as hysteria; it mainly included what would now be called anxiety disorders.

**psy·cha·tax·ia** (si″kə-tak′se-ə) a disordered mental condition marked by confusion and inability to concentrate.

**psy·che** (si′ke) [Gr. *psychē* the organ of thought and judgment] 1. the human faculty for thought, judgment, and emotion; the mental life, including both conscious and unconscious processes; the mind in its totality, as distinguished from the body. 2. the soul or self.

**psy·che·del·ic** (si″kə-del′ik) [*psyche* + Gr. *dēlos* manifest, evident] 1. pertaining to or characterized by hallucinations, distortions of perception and awareness, and sometimes psychotic-like behavior. 2. a drug that produces such effects.

**psy·chi·at·ric** (si″ke-at′rik) pertaining to or within the purview of psychiatry.

**psy·chi·a·trist** (si-ki′ə-trist) [MeSH: Psychiatry] a physician who specializes in psychiatry.

**psy·chi·a·try** (si-ki′ə-tre) [*psych-* + *-iatry*] [MeSH: Psychiatry] that branch of medicine which deals with the study, treatment, and prevention of mental disorders.
**addiction p.,** a subspecialty concerned with the diagnosis and treatment of addiction and other problems related to substance use.
**administrative p.,** that concerned with the organization and management of mental health programs and facilities, including public and private hospitals, clinics, and centers.
**biological p.,** that which emphasizes biochemical, neurological, and pharmacological causes and treatment approaches.
**community p.,** the branch of psychiatry concerned with the detection, prevention, and treatment of mental disorders as they develop within psychosocial, cultural, or geographical areas, with emphasis given to environmental factors.
**consultation liaison p.,** that which connects psychiatry with other areas of medicine, bringing a psychosocial approach to the biological treatment of organic illness. Called also *liaison p.*
**cross-cultural p., cultural p.,** the study of mental illness and mental health among different societies, nations, and cultures; called also *transcultural p.*
**descriptive p.,** psychiatry based on the study of observable symptoms and behavioral phenomena, rather than underlying psychodynamic processes; cf. *dynamic p.*
**dynamic p.,** psychiatry based on the study of the unconscious mechanisms, conflicts, and other emotional processes that motivate and underlie human behavior, rather than the more observable behaviors themselves; cf. *descriptive p.*
**existential p.,** that based on the existential philosophy of Kierkegaard, Heidegger, Jaspers, and others, holding the view that a person takes responsibility for his own existence.
**forensic p.,** psychiatry which deals with the legal aspects of mental disorders.
**geriatric p.,** geropsychiatry.
**industrial p.,** that concerned with the diagnosis and prevention of mental illness in the work setting, including aspects of absenteeism, accident proneness, personnel policies, occupational fatigue, substance abuse, vocational adjustment, retirement, interpersonal relations, and related phenomena.

**liaison p.**, consultation liaison p.
**military p.**, the study and treatment of psychiatric problems done under the auspices of military organizations such as induction centers, training facilities, and military hospitals; it includes emergency and nonemergency treatment for active-duty and retired military personnel and their dependents.
**occupational p.**, industrial p.
**orthomolecular p.**, that based on the theory that psychiatric illnesses are due to disturbances in the molecular environment of the brain and can be cured by restoration of optimal concentrations of substances normally present in the body, such as vitamins *(orthomolecular therapy)*.
**preventive p.**, that broadly concerned with the amelioration, control, and limitation of psychiatric disability. It is often categorized as *primary*—measures to prevent a disorder; *secondary*—therapeutic measures to limit a disorder; and *tertiary*—measures and intervention to reduce impairment or disability following a disorder.
**social p.**, that concerned with the cultural, ecologic, and sociologic facts that engender, precipitate, intensify, prolong, or otherwise complicate maladaptive patterns of behavior and their treatment.
**transcultural p.**, cross-cultural p.

**psy·chic** (si'kik) pertaining to the psyche or to the mind; mental.

**psych(o)-** [Gr. *psychē* the mind, reason] a combining form denoting relationship to the psyche, or to the mind.

**psy·cho·acous·tics** (si″ko-ə-ko͞os'tiks) [MeSH: Psychoacoustics] a branch of psychophysics involving the study of the relationship between acoustic stimuli and behavior.

**psy·cho·ac·tive** (si″ko-ak'tiv) affecting the mind or behavior, as psychoactive substances.

**psy·cho·an·a·lep·tic** (si″ko-an″ə-lep'tik) [*psycho-* + *analeptic*] exerting a stimulating effect upon the mind.

**psy·cho·anal·y·sis** (si″ko-ə-nal'ĭ-sis) [MeSH: Psychoanalysis] 1. a theory of human mental phenomena and behavior (Freud). 2. a method of investigation into the contents of the mind. 3. a therapeutic technique based on Freud's theory, focusing on the influence of such unconscious forces as repressed impulses, internal conflicts, and childhood trauma on the mental state. The therapist elicits from patients past emotional experiences and their role in influencing current mental life, so as to delineate the conflicts and mechanisms by which their pathologic mental state has been produced and furnish hints for psychotherapeutic procedures; the method employs free association, recall and interpretation of dreams, and interpretation of transference and resistance phenomena.

**psy·cho·an·a·lyst** (si″ko-an'ə-list) a practitioner of psychoanalysis.

**psy·cho·an·a·lyt·ic** (si″ko-an″ə-lit'ik) pertaining to psychoanalysis.

**psy·cho·au·di·to·ry** (si″ko-aw'dĭ-tor″e) pertaining to the conscious and intelligent perception of sound.

**psy·cho·bi·o·log·i·cal** (si″ko-bi″o-loj'ĭ-kəl) pertaining to psychobiology.

**psy·cho·bi·ol·o·gist** (si″ko-bi-ol'ə-jist) a practitioner of psychobiology.

**psy·cho·bi·ol·o·gy** (si″ko-bi-ol'ə-je) 1. a field of study examining the relationship between brain and mind, studying the effect of biological influences, including biochemical, neurological, and pharmacological factors, on psychological functioning or mental processes. Called also *biopsychology*. 2. Adolf Meyer's school of psychiatric thought, in which the human being is viewed as an integrated unit, incorporating psychological, social, and biological functions, with behavior a function of the total organism.

**psy·cho·ca·thar·sis** (si″ko-kə-thahr'sis) [*psycho-* + *catharsis*] catharsis (def. 2).

**psy·cho·chem·is·try** (si″ko-kem'is-tre) the science that deals with the relationship between chemistry and psychologic processes.

**psy·cho·chrome** (si'ko-krōm) [*psycho-* + *-chrome*] a subjective mental association between any bodily sensation and some particular color.

**psy·cho·chrom·es·the·sia** (si″ko-krōm″əs-the'zhə) chromesthesia.

**psy·cho·cor·ti·cal** (si″ko-kor'tĭ-kəl) [*psycho-* + *cortical*] pertaining to the mind and to the cortex of the brain as the site of mental functions.

**psy·cho·cu·ta·ne·ous** (si″ko-ku-ta'ne-əs) pertaining to the relations between mental or emotional factors and skin disorders.

**psy·cho·di·ag·no·sis** (si″ko-di″əg-no'sis) the use of psychological methods of assessment in the diagnosis of psychiatric disorders.

**psy·cho·di·ag·nos·tics** (si″ko-di″əg-nos'tiks) psychodiagnosis.

**Psy·cho·di·dae** (si-ko'dĭ-de) [MeSH: Psychodidae] a family of flies, the owl flies or sandflies, of the order Diptera, characterized by small size, long legs, and abundant hair on both wings and body. It includes the genera *Lutzomyia, Phlebotomus,* and *Psychodopygus.*

**psy·cho·dom·e·ter** (si″ko-dom'ə-tər) an instrument for measuring the rate of mental processes.

**psy·cho·dom·e·try** (si″ko-dom'ə-tre) [*psycho-* + Gr. *hodos* way + *-metry*] measurement of the rate of mental processes.

**Psy·cho·do·py·gus** (si″ko-do-pi'gəs) [Gr. *psychē* butterfly + *pygē* rump] a genus of sandflies of the family Psychodidae. *P. wellcomei* is a vector of *Leishmania viannia braziliensis,* an etiologic agent of cutaneous and mucocutaneous leishmaniasis.

**psy·cho·dra·ma** (si″ko-drah'mə) [MeSH: Psychodrama] a form of group psychotherapy in which patients dramatize their own or assigned life situations in order to achieve insight into personalities, relationships, conflicts, and emotional problems, and to alter faulty behavior patterns.

**psy·cho·dy·nam·ics** (si″ko-di-nam'iks) [*psycho-* + *dynamics*] the interplay of conscious and unconscious motivational forces, such as wishes, drives, emotions, conflict, and defense mechanisms, that gives rise to the expression of mental processes, as in attitudes, behavior, or symptoms.

**psy·cho·dys·lep·tic** (si″ko-dis-lep'tik) [*psycho-* + Gr. *dys-* bad + *lēpsis* a taking hold] inducing a dreamlike or delusional state of mind.

**psy·cho·gal·va·nom·e·ter** (si″ko-gal″və-nom'ə-tər) an instrument for determining changes in skin resistance to electric current applied to electrodes on the skin.

**psy·cho·gen·e·sis** (si″ko-jen'ə-sis) [*psycho-* + *-genesis*] 1. mental development. 2. production of a symptom or illness by psychic factors.

**psy·cho·gen·ic** (si″ko-jen'ik) [*psycho-* + *-genic*] produced or caused by psychological factors. See also *psychosomatic.*

**psy·cho·ger·i·at·rics** (si″ko-jer″e-at'riks) geropsychiatry.

**psy·cho·gog·ic** (si″ko-goj'ik) increasing intrapsychic tensions and acting as a stimulant.

**psy·cho·gram** (si'ko-gram) [*psycho-* + *-gram*] 1. psychograph. 2. a visual sensation associated with a mental idea, as of a certain number which appears visualized when it is thought of.

**psy·cho·graph** (si'ko-graf) [*psycho-* + *-graph*] 1. a chart for recording graphically the personality traits of an individual. 2. a written description of the mental functioning of an individual.

**psy·cho·ki·ne·sis** (si″ko-kĭ-ne'sis) [*psycho-* + *-kinesis*] the postulated direct influence of volitional action on a physical object, or the influence of mind on matter without the intermediation of physical force.

**psy·cho·lag·ny** (si'ko-lag″ne) [*psycho-* + Gr. *lagneia* lust] the experiencing of sexual enjoyment from imagining or thinking of sexual acts.

**psy·cho·lep·sy** (si'ko-lep″se) [*psycho-* + Gr. *lēpsis* a taking hold, a seizure] a sudden, intense lowering of mood level, usually of short duration, in individuals with unstable psychic tension.

**psy·cho·lin·guis·tics** (si″ko-ling-gwis'tiks) [MeSH: Psycholinguistics] the study of psychological aspects of language acquisition, processing, and production, on the part of both the producer and the receiver.

**psy·cho·log·ic, psy·cho·log·i·cal** (si″ko-loj'ik, si″ko-loj'ĭ-kəl) pertaining to psychology.

**psy·chol·o·gist** (si-kol'ə-jist) [MeSH: Psychology] a qualified specialist in psychology.

**psy·chol·o·gy** (si-kol'ə-je) [*psycho-* + *-logy*] [MeSH: Psychology] that branch of science which deals with the mind and mental processes, especially in relation to human and animal behavior.
**abnormal p.**, the study of mental disorders and behavior disturbances.
**analytic p., analytical p.**, the system of psychology founded by Carl Gustav Jung, based on the concepts of the collective unconscious and the complex.
**animal p.**, the study of the mental activity of animals.
**behavioristic p.**, see *behaviorism.*
**child p.**, the study of the development of the mind of the child.
**clinical p.**, the use of psychologic knowledge and techniques in the treatment of persons with mental, emotional, behavior, and developmental disorders.
**cognitive p.**, that branch of psychology which deals with how the human mind receives and interprets impressions and ideas.
**community p.**, the application of psychological principles to the

study and support of the mental health of individuals in their social context.
**comparative p.,** the study of behavior using a comparison of species as a source of knowledge.
**criminal p.,** the study of the mentality, the motivation, and the social behavior of criminals.
**depth p.,** the study of unconscious mental processes.
**developmental p.,** the study of changes in behavior that occur through the life span.
**dynamic p.,** psychology that stresses the causes of and motivations for behavior.
**environmental p.,** study of the effects of the physical and social environment on behavior.
**experimental p.,** the study of mental operations and behaviors by the employment of controlled laboratory procedures.
**gestalt p.,** see *gestaltism.*
**individual p.,** Alfred Adler's psychological theory that stresses the role of compensation for feelings of inferiority as the source of psychological and interpersonal problems.
**physiologic p., physiological p.,** the branch of psychology that studies the relationship between physiologic and psychologic processes.
**social p.,** psychology that focuses on social interaction, on the ways in which actions of others influence the behavior of an individual.

**psy·chom·e·ter** (si-kom'ə-tər) an instrument used in psychometry.

**psy·cho·me·tri·cian** (si″ko-mə-trish'ən) a person skilled in psychometry.

**psy·cho·met·rics** (si″ko-met'riks) [MeSH: Psychometrics] psychometry.

**psy·chom·e·try** (si-kom'ə-tre) [*psycho-* + *-metry*] systematic measurement of mental processes and behavioral acts.

**psy·cho·mo·tor** (si″ko-mo'tor) pertaining to motor effects of cerebral or psychic activity.

**psy·cho·neu·ral** (si″ko-noor'əl) relating to the totality of neural events initiated by a sensory input and leading to storage, to discrimination, or to an output of any kind.

**psy·cho·neu·ro·en·do·cri·nol·o·gy** (si″ko-noor″o-en″do-krĭ-nol'ə-je) [*psycho-* + *neuroendocrinology*] the study of the effects of the nervous and endocrine system on emotional processes.

**psy·cho·neu·ro·sis** (si″ko-noo͡-ro'sis) [*psycho-* + *neuro-* + *-osis*] 1. *(obs.)* Freud's term for neuroses such as hysteria, obsessions, and phobias originating in childhood experiences; cf. *actual neurosis,* under *neurosis.* 2. neurosis.

**psy·chon·o·my** (si″kon-o'me) [*psycho-* + Gr. *nomos* law] the science of the laws of mental activity.

**psy·cho·path** (si'ko-path) former term for a person with antisocial personality disorder (see under *personality*).

**psy·cho·path·ic** (si″ko-path'ik) pertaining to psychopathy, particularly to antisocial behavior or antisocial personality disorder.

**psy·cho·pa·thol·o·gy** (si″ko-pə-thol'ə-je) [*psycho-* + *pathology*] [MeSH: Psychopathology] 1. the pathology of mental disorders; the branch of medicine which deals with the causes and nature of mental disease. 2. abnormal, maladaptive behavior or mental activity.

**psy·chop·a·thy** (si-kop'ə-the) [*psycho-* + *-pathy*] older term for a mental disorder, sometimes specifically *antisocial personality disorder.*

**psy·cho·phar·ma·col·o·gy** (si″ko-fahr″mə-kol'ə-je) [MeSH: Psychopharmacology] 1. the study of the action of drugs on psychological functions and mental states. 2. the use of drugs to modify psychological functions and mental states.

**psy·cho·phys·i·cal** (si″ko-fiz'ĭ-kəl) pertaining to the mind and its relation to physical manifestations.

**psy·cho·phys·ics** (si″ko-fiz'iks) [*psycho-* + *physics*] [MeSH: Psychophysics] the science dealing with the quantitative relationships between the characteristics or patterns of physical stimuli and the resultant sensations.

**psy·cho·phys·io·log·ic** (si″ko-fiz″e-o-loj'ik) [*psycho-* + *physiologic*] 1. psychosomatic. 2. pertaining to psychophysiology (physiologic psychology).

**psy·cho·phys·i·ol·o·gy** (si″ko-fiz″e-ol'ə-je) [MeSH: Psychophysiology] physiologic psychology.

**psy·cho·ple·gic** (si″ko-ple'jik) an agent that lessens cerebral activity or excitability.

**psy·cho·sen·so·ri·al** (si″ko-sən-sor'e-əl) psychosensory.

**psy·cho·sen·so·ry** (si″ko-sen'sə-re) pertaining to the conscious perception of sensory impulses to the mind and to sensation.

**psy·cho·ses** (si-ko'sēz) plural of *psychosis.*

**psy·cho·sex·u·al** (si″ko-sek'shoo-əl) pertaining to the mental or emotional aspects of sex or sexuality.

**psy·cho·sine** (si'ko-sēn) [MeSH: Psychosine] a cerebroside derivative lacking its fatty acyl chain; it is sphingosine linked via its 1-hydroxyl group to a monosaccharide group.

**psy·cho·sis** (si-ko'sis) pl. *psycho'ses* [*psych-* + *-osis*] 1. a mental disorder characterized by gross impairment in reality testing as evidenced by delusions, hallucinations, markedly incoherent speech, or disorganized and agitated behavior, usually without apparent awareness on the part of the patient of the incomprehensibility of his behavior; called *psychotic disorder* in DSM-IV. 2. the term is also used in a more general sense to refer to mental disorders in which mental functioning is sufficiently impaired as to interfere grossly with the patient's capacity to meet the ordinary demands of life. Historically, the term has been applied to many conditions, e.g., manic-depressive psychosis, that were first described in psychotic patients, although many patients with the disorder are not judged psychotic.
**acute delusional p.,** bouffée délirante.
**affective p.,** one in which a disturbance in mood is the prominent characteristic; see *mood disorder,* under *disorder.*
**alcoholic p's,** psychoses associated with alcohol use and involving organic brain damage, a category that includes alcohol withdrawal delirium, Korsakoff's syndrome, alcohol hallucinosis, and alcoholic paranoia (concurrent paranoia and alcoholism).
**bipolar p.,** see under *disorder.*
**brief reactive p.,** see *brief psychotic disorder.*
**depressive p.,** older term for a psychosis characterized by severe depression; now more commonly described as a form of major depressive disorder.
**drug p.,** any psychosis associated with drug use.
**functional p.,** a psychosis for which organic disease or dysfunction cannot be found to play a causative role.
**Korsakoff's p.,** see under *syndrome.*
**manic p.,** the manic phase of bipolar disorder.
**manic-depressive p.,** former name for bipolar disorder; see *bipolar disorders* (def. 2), under *disorder.*
**organic p.,** a psychotic disorder with a known or presumed organic etiology.
**postpartum p.,** a psychotic episode occurring in the postpartum period.
**prison p.,** any psychosis for which a prison environment has been a precipitating factor.
**schizoaffective p.,** see under *disorder.*
**senile p.,** depressive or paranoid delusions or hallucinations or other mental disorders due primarily to degeneration of the brain in old age, as in senile dementia.
**toxic p.,** a psychosis due to the ingestion of toxic agents (e.g., alcohol, opium) or to the presence of toxins within the body.
**unipolar p.,** a mood disorder characterized by recurrent major depressive episodes.

**psy·cho·so·cial** (si″ko-so'shəl) pertaining to or involving both psychic and social aspects.

**psy·cho·so·mat·ic** (si″ko-so-mat'ik) [*psycho-* + *somat-* + *-ic*] pertaining to the mind-body relationship; having bodily symptoms of psychic, emotional, or mental origin; called also *psychophysiologic.* See also under *disorder.*

**psy·cho·so·mi·met·ic** (si-ko″so-mi-met'ik) psychotomimetic.

**psy·cho·stim·u·lant** (si″ko-stim'u-lənt) 1. producing a transient increase in psychomotor activity. 2. a drug that produces such effects, such as caffeine, methylphenidate, or the amphetamines.

**psy·cho·sur·gery** (si″ko-sər'jər-e) [MeSH: Psychosurgery] brain surgery performed for treatment of psychiatric disorders; called also *psychiatric surgery* and *functional neurosurgery.*

**psy·cho·sur·gi·cal** (si″ko-sər'jĭ-kəl) pertaining to psychosurgery.

**psy·cho·tech·nics** (si″ko-tek'niks) [*psycho-* + Gr. *technē* art] the employment of psychological methods in studying sociological and other problems.

**psy·cho·ther·a·peu·tics** (si″ko-ther″ə-pu'tiks) psychotherapy.

**psy·cho·ther·a·py** (si″ko-ther'ə-pe) [*psycho-* + *therapy*] [MeSH: Psychotherapy] treatment of mental disorders and behavioral disturbances using verbal and nonverbal communication, including such psychological techniques as support, suggestion, persuasion, reeducation, reassurance, and insight, in order to alter maladaptive patterns of coping, relieve emotional disturbance, and encourage personality growth. It is usually contrasted with therapies involving physical interventions, such as drug or convulsive therapies. See also under *therapy.*
**brief p.,** any of numerous forms of psychotherapy limited to a preagreed number of sessions, generally 10 to 20, or termination date;

**Selected Brief Psychotherapy Methods**

Brief dynamic psychotherapy (BDP)
Brief psychotherapy for stress-response syndromes (BPSRS)
Cognitive-behavioral therapy (CBT)
Dialectical behavior therapy (DBT)
Interpersonal psychotherapy (IPT)
Short-term anxiety-provoking psychotherapy (STAPP)
Short-term dynamic psychotherapy (STDP)
Supportive-expressive (SE) psychotherapy
Time-limited psychotherapy (TLP)
Time-limited dynamic psychotherapy (TLDP)

most types are active and directive, and many are oriented toward a specific problem or symptom. See table.

**existential p.,** that based on the existential philosophy of Kierkegaard, Heidegger, Jaspers, etc., in which the emphasis is on present interactions and feeling experiences rather than on rational thinking.

**group p.,** see under *therapy.*

**interpersonal p.,** a form of brief psychotherapy that treats mood disorders by addressing interpersonal problems, emphasizing that the mood disorder is a medical illness and focusing on healing current relationships in a specific problem area in the here and now.

**psychoanalytic p.,** psychoanalysis, def. 3.

**supportive p.,** that aimed at reinforcing a patient's defenses, relieving immediate crises or acute disequilibria, reducing symptoms to a premorbid level, and promoting the healthy aspects of the patient, without probing emotional conflicts or trying to alter the basic personality. Specific methods include advice; guidance; reassurance; desensitization; art, music, or dance therapy; and occupational therapy.

**psy·chot·ic** (si-kot′ik) 1. pertaining to, characterized by, or caused by psychosis. 2. a person exhibiting psychosis.

**psy·chot·o·gen·ic** (si-kot″o-jen′ik) 1. producing a state of psychosis. 2. a drug that produces such effects.

**psy·choto·mi·met·ic** (si-kot″o-mi-met′ik) [*psychosis* + *-mimetic*] pertaining to, characterized by, or producing manifestations resembling those of a psychosis, e.g., visual hallucinations, distortion of perception, and schizophrenia-like behavior; applied to a drug that produces these effects.

**psy·cho·trop·ic** (si″ko-trop′pik) [*psycho-* + *-tropic*] exerting an effect upon the mind; capable of modifying mental activity; usually applied to drugs that affect the mental state.

**psychr(o)-** [Gr. *psychros* cold] a combining form denoting relationship to cold.

**psy·chro·al·gia** (si″kro-al′jə) a painful feeling of cold. Cf. *cryesthesia* and *crymodynia.*

**psy·chro·es·the·sia** (si″kro-əs-the′zhə) [*psychro-* + *esthsia*] a state in which a part of the body, though objectively warm when touched, is experienced as being cold.

**psy·chrom·e·ter** (si-krom′ə-tər) [*psychro-* + *-meter*] an apparatus for measuring atmospheric moisture by the difference in reading of two thermometers, one with a dry bulb and one with a wet bulb.

**sling p.,** an instrument in which the thermometers are swung through the air to facilitate evaporation from the wet bulb.

**psy·chro·phile** (si′kro-fīl) an organism which grows best at low temperatures.

**psy·chro·phil·ic** (si″kro-fil′ik) [*psychro-* + *-philic*] fond of cold; said of bacteria that grow in the cold, often growing best between 15° and 20° C. See also *mesophilic* and *thermophilic.*

**psy·chro·phore** (si′kro-for) [*psychro-* + *-phore*] a double-lumen catheter for applying cold to the urethra.

**psyl·li·um** (sil′e-əm) [MeSH: Psyllium] a plant of the genus *Plantago. Blond p.* is *P. ovata* and *Spanish p.* is *P. psyllium.*

**PT** prothrombin time.

**Pt** symbol for *platinum.*

**PTA** [MeSH: Factor XI] plasma thromboplastin antecedent (factor XI; see under *coagulation factors,* at *factor*).

**ptar·mic** (tahr′mik) [Gr. *ptarmikos* making to sneeze] relating to or producing spasmodic sneezing.

**ptar·mus** (tahr′məs) [Gr. *ptarmos*] spasmodic sneezing.

**PTC** [MeSH: Factor IX] plasma thromboplastin component (factor IX; see *coagulation factors,* under *factor*); phenylthiocarbamide.

**PteGlu** pteroylglutamate or pteroylglutamic acid; see *folic acid.*

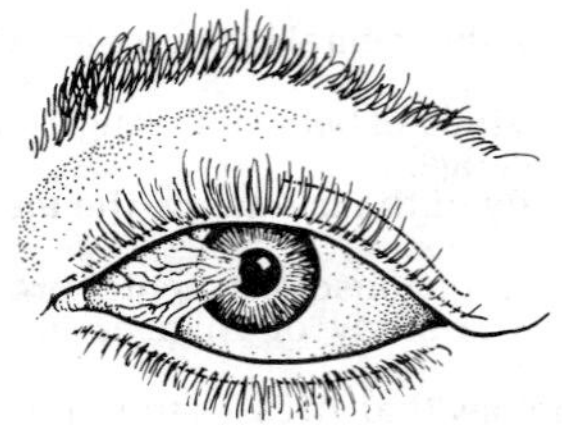

Pterygium.

**PTEN** pentaerythritol tetranitrate.

**pter·i·dine** (ter′ĭ-dēn) a bicyclic aromatic nitrogenous compound or the class of compounds containing such a ring structure. Most naturally occurring pteridine derivatives are pterins.

**Pte·ri·di·um** (tə-rid′e-əm) a genus of ferns. *P. aquili′num* L. Kuhn (Polypodia′ceae) is the bracken. See also *bracken poisoning,* under *poisoning.*

**pter·in** (ter′in) [Gr. *pteron* wing] the 2-amino, 4-hydroxy derivative of pteridine; the term is also used to denote the class of compounds containing such a ring structure, such as tetrahydrobiopterin or folic acid. Pterins are so named because they were first identified in the wings of butterflies.

**pte·ri·on** (tēr′e-on) [Gr. *pteron* wing] [TA] a point at the junction of the frontal, parietal, temporal, and greater wing of the sphenoid bone; about 3 cm posterior to the external angular process of the orbit.

**pter·nal·gia** (tər-nal′jə) [Gr. *pterna* heel + *-algia*] calcaneodynia.

**pte·ro·ic ac·id** (tə-ro′ik) a constituent of folic acid consisting of *p*-aminobenzoic acid linked to a substituted pteridine by a methylene bridge.

**pter·o·yl·glu·ta·mate** (ter″o-əl-gloo′tə-māt) an anionic form of pteroylglutamic (folic) acid. Abbreviated PteGlu. See *folic acid.*

**pter·o·yl·glu·tam·ic ac·id** (ter″o-əl-gloo-tam′ik) folic acid. Abbreviated PteGlu.

**pter·o·yl·poly·glu·ta·mate** (ter″o-əl-pol″e-gloo′tə-māt) any of the folate compounds having more than one glutamate residue; it is the usual form in which folates are stored in foods and in body tissues.

**pte·ryg·i·um** (tə-rij′e-əm) pl. *ptery′gia* [Gr. *pterygion* wing] [MeSH: Pterygium] a winglike structure, applied especially to an abnormal triangular fold of membrane, in the interpalpebral fissure, extending from the conjunctiva to the cornea, being immovably united to the cornea at its apex, firmly attached to the sclera throughout its middle portion, and merged with the conjunctiva at its base.

**p. col′li,** a congenital condition in which a thick fold of skin extends from the mastoid region to the acromion on the lateral aspect of the neck; it occurs in association with various genetic syndromes, such as Turner's syndrome and Noonan's syndrome. Called also *webbed neck.*

**congenital p.,** epitarsus.

**pter·y·goid** (ter′ĭ-goid) [Gr. *pterygōdēs* like a wing] shaped like a wing.

**pter·y·go·man·dib·u·lar** (ter″ĭ-go-man-dib′u-lər) pertaining to the pterygoid process and the mandible.

**pter·y·go·max·il·lary** (ter″ĭ-go-mak′sĭ-lar-e) pertaining to a pterygoid process and the maxilla.

**pter·y·go·pal·a·tine** (ter″ĭ-go-pal′ə-tīn) pertaining to a pterygoid process and to the palate bone; in anatomy it is sometimes interchangeable with the term *sphenopalatine.*

**PTFE** polytetrafluoroethylene; see *polytef.*

**PTH** parathyroid hormone.

**Pthir·us** (thir′əs) *Phthirus.*

**pto·maine** (to′mān, to-mān′) [Gr. *ptōma* carcass] any of several toxic bases formed by decarboxylation of an amino acid, often by bacterial action, such as cadaverine, muscarine, neurine, ptomatropine, or putrescine.

**pto·mat·ro·pine** (to-mat′ro-pēn) [*ptomaine* + *atropine*] a poison from putrid sausages and the viscera of corpses of those dead from typhoid fever; it has effects somewhat like those of atropine.

**ptosed** (tōst) affected with ptosis; prolapsed.

**pto·sis** (to′sis) [Gr. *ptōsis* fall] 1. prolapse. 2. drooping of the upper eyelid from paralysis of the third nerve or from sympathetic innervation.

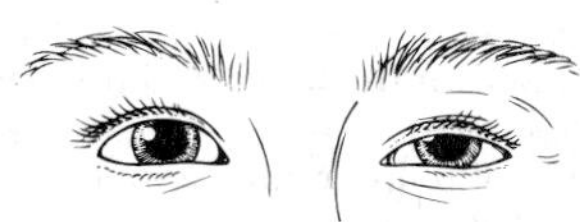

Ptosis of the left eyelid.

**p. adipo'sa, false p.,** an apparent ptosis caused by a fold of skin and fat hanging down below the border of the eyelid.
**Horner's p.,** moderate ptosis of an eye, with retraction of the eyeball, miosis, and flushing of the affected side of the face, due to lesions of the cervical sympathetic nerves; see also *Horner's syndrome,* under *syndrome.* Called also *p. sympathetica.*
**p. lipomato'sis,** ptosis produced by lipoma of the eyelid.
**morning p.,** waking p.
**p. sympathe'tica,** Horner's syndrome; see under *syndrome.*
**waking p.,** temporary paralysis of the upper lid on awakening from sleep.

**-ptosis** [Gr. *ptōsis* fall] a word termination indicating downward displacement.

**ptot·ic** (tot'ik) pertaining to or affected with ptosis.

**PTSD** posttraumatic stress disorder.

**PTT** partial thromboplastin time; activated partial thromboplastin time.

**pty·al·a·gogue** (ti-al'ə-gog) [*ptyalo-* + *-agogue*] sialagogue.

**pty·a·lec·ta·sis** (ti"ə-lek'tə-sis) [*ptyalo-* + *ectasis*] 1. operative dilatation of a salivary duct. 2. dilatation of one of the ducts of the salivary glands.

**pty·a·lin** (ti'ə-lin) [Gr. *ptyalon* spittle] $\alpha$-amylase occurring in saliva.

**pty·a·lism** (ti'ə-liz-əm) [Gr. *ptyalismos*] excessive flow of saliva. Called also *hyperptyalism, hypersalivation, polysialia, ptyalorrhea, salivation, sialism, sialismus,* and *sialorrhea.*

**pty·a·lize** (ti'ə-līz) to increase or stimulate the secretion of saliva.

**ptyal(o)-** [Gr. *ptyalon* saliva] a combining form denoting relationship to saliva. See also words beginning *sial(o)-.*

**pty·alo·cele** (ti-al'o-sēl) [*ptyalo-* + *-cele*[1]] a cystic tumor containing saliva.
**sublingual p.,** ranula.

**pty·al·o·gen·ic** (ti"ə-lo-jen'ik) [*ptyalo-* + *-genic*] formed from or by the action of saliva.

**pty·a·log·ra·phy** (ti"ə-log'rə-fe) [*ptyalo-* + *-graphy*] sialography.

**pty·a·lo·li·thi·a·sis** (ti"ə-lo-lĭ-thi'ə-sis) [*ptyalo-* + *lith-* + *-iasis*] sialolithiasis.

**pty·a·lo·li·thot·o·my** (ti"ə-lo-lĭ-thot'ə-me) sialolithotomy.

**pty·a·lor·rhea** (ti"ə-lo-re'ə) [*ptyalo-* + *-rrhea*] ptyalism.

**pty·oc·ri·nous** (ti-ok'rĭ-nəs) [Gr. *ptyon* a winnowing shovel, or fan + *krinein* to separate] elaborating secretion in the form of granules which are eventually extruded; said of unicellular glands, as goblet cells, which secrete in this way. Cf. *diacrinous.*

**Pu** symbol for *plutonium.*

**pu·bar·che** (pu-bahr'ke) the beginning of puberty, signalled by growth of the pubic hair.

**pu·ber·al** (pu'bər-əl) pubertal.

**pu·ber·tal** (pu'bər-təl) [L. *puber* of marriageable age] pertaining to or characteristic of puberty; called also *puberal.*

**pu·ber·tas** (pu-ber'təs) [L.] puberty.
**p. prae'cox,** precocious puberty.

**pu·ber·ty** (pu'bər-te) [L. *pubertas*] [MeSH: Puberty] the period during which the secondary sex characteristics begin to develop and the capability of sexual reproduction is attained.
**precocious p.,** onset of sexual maturation at an earlier age than normal, defined as two standard deviations below the mean, or before age 8 in girls and 9 in boys. It is usually hormonal *(central precocious p.),* but occasionally it occurs in otherwise normal children *(constitutional precocious p.)* Called also *sexual precocity* and *pubertas praecox.*
**precocious p., central,** precocious puberty due to premature hypothalamic-pituitary-gonadal maturation; it is always isosexual and involves not only development of secondary sex characters but also development of the gonads. Increases in height and weight and osseous maturation are accelerated, and early closing of the epiphyses leads to short stature. Cf. *precocious pseudopuberty,* under *pseudopuberty.* Called also *true precocious p.*
**precocious p., constitutional,** that occurring in otherwise normal children generally with a family history of early onset of puberty. The age range for such individuals overlaps the upper range for those with idiopathic precocious puberty.
**precocious p., contrasexual,** precocious puberty in which secondary sex characters of the opposite sex are developed; called also *heterosexual precocious p.*
**precocious p., gonadotropin-dependent,** precocious pseudopuberty.
**precocious p., heterosexual,** contrasexual precocious p.
**precocious p., idiopathic,** central precocious puberty in which no underlying causative lesion can be found; it affects mainly females and is usually sporadic, although there is a hereditary form whose occurrence is confined largely to males.
**precocious p., incomplete,** the premature maturation of certain secondary sex characters, most commonly breast development and the growth of pubic and axillary hair, without development of other signs of puberty.
**precocious p., isosexual,** precocious puberty in which sex characters are consistent with the sex of the individual.
**precocious p., neurogenic,** central precocious puberty that is caused by a lesion of the central nervous system, such as tumor, congenital defect, or trauma.
**precocious p., true,** central precocious p.

**pu·bes** (pu'bēz) gen. *pu'bis* [L.] 1. pubic hairs; the hairs covering the pubic region. 2. hypogastrium.

**pu·bes·cence** (pu-bes'əns) the state of being pubescent.

**pu·bes·cent** (pu-bes'ənt) [L. *pubescens* becoming hairy] 1. reaching sexual maturation; see *puberty.* 2. covered with down or lanugo.

**pu·bic** (pu'bik) pertaining to or situated near the pubes, the os pubis, or the pubic region.

**pu·bio·plas·ty** (pu'be-o-plas"te) a plastic operation on the pubes.

**pu·bi·ot·o·my** (pu"be-ot'ə-me) [*pubis* + *-tomy*] surgical separation of the pubic bone lateral to the median line.

**pu·bis** (pu'bis) [L., gen. of *pubes*] TA alternative for *os pubis.* See illustration at *skeleton.*

**pu·bo·coc·cyg·e·al** (pu"bo-kok-sij'e-əl) pertaining to the pubis and coccyx or to the musculus pubococcygeus.

**pu·bo·coc·cy·ge·us** (pu"bo-kok-sij'e-əs) pertaining to the pubis and coccyx; see under *musculus.*

**pu·bo·fem·o·ral** (pu"bo-fem'ə-rəl) pertaining to the os pubis and femur.

**pu·bo·pros·tat·ic** (pu"bo-pros-tat'ik) pertaining to the os pubis and prostate.

**pu·bo·rec·tal** (pu"bo-rek'təl) pertaining to the pubis and rectum or to the musculus puborectalis.

**pu·bo·rec·ta·lis** (pu"bo-rek-ta'lis) pertaining to the pubis and rectum; see under *musculus.*

**pu·bo·tib·i·al** (pu"bo-tib'e-əl) pertaining to the pubes and tibia.

**pu·bo·ves·i·cal** (pu"bo-ves'ĭ-kəl) vesicopubic.

**PUBS** percutaneous umbilical blood sampling.

**pu·den·da** (pu-den'də) [L.] plural of *pudendum.*

**pu·den·dal** (pu-den'dəl) pertaining to the pudendum.

**pu·den·dum** (pu-den'dəm) pl. *puden'da* [L., from *pudere* to be ashamed] the external genitalia of humans, especially of the female; see also *p. femininum.*
**p. femini'num** [TA], female pudendum: that portion of the female genitalia comprising the mons pubis, labia majora, labia minora, vestibule of the vagina, bulb of the vestibule, greater and lesser vestibular glands, and vaginal orifice. Commonly used to denote the entire external female genitalia (i.e., to include the clitoris and urethra as well). Called also *p. muliebre;* cf. *vulva.*
**p. mulie'bre,** p. femininum.

**pu·dic** (pu'dik) [L. *pudicus*] pertaining to the pudendum.

**pu·er·ile** (pu'ər-il) [L. *puerilis; puer* child] pertaining to childhood or to children; childish.

**pu·er·pera** (pu-er'pər-ə) [L. *puer* child + *parere* to bring forth, to bear] a woman who has just given birth to an infant.

**pu·er·per·al** (pu-er'pər-əl) [L. *puerperalis*] pertaining to the puerperium.

**pu·er·per·al·ism** (pu-er'pər-əl-iz-əm) a disease condition incident to childbirth.

**pu·er·per·ant** (pu-er'pər-ənt) puerpera.

**pu·er·pe·ri·um** (pu"ər-pēr'e-əm) [L.] [MeSH: Puerperium] the period from the end of the third stage of labor until involution of the uterus is complete, usually lasting 3 to 6 weeks.

**PUFA** polyunsaturated fatty acid.

**puff** (puf) [A.S. *pyffan*] 1. a short, blowing, auscultation sound. 2. in genetics, any of the regions of the giant chromosomes of certain

insects at which disorganized arrangement and most of RNA synthesis occurs.
**chromosome p's,** active loci of RNA and DNA synthesis in the giant salivary gland chromosomes of insects.

**puff·er** (puf′ər) puffer fish.

**puf·fer fish** (puf′ər fish) any of several species of marine fish of the order Tetraodontidae, which when disturbed can inflate themselves to a spherical shape. Their flesh contains tetrodotoxin and can cause fatal poisoning. Called also *puffer.*

**puff·ing** (puf′ing) enlargement in giant polytene chromosomes of insect larval organs; these chromosome puffs are repositories of RNA and DNA synthesis.

**pu·gil, pu·gil·lus** (pu′jil; pu-jil′əs) [L. *pugillus*] a handful.

**Pu·lex** (pu′leks) [L. "flea"] a genus of fleas which are parasitic on man, dogs, cats, and badgers.
**P. cheo′pis,** *Xenopsylla cheopis.*
**P. duge′si,** *P. irritans.*
**P. ir′ritans,** the common flea or human flea, which is parasitic on the skin of humans and various domestic animals; its bite produces itching.
**P. pe′netrans,** *Tunga penetrans;* see *chigoe.*

**pu·lex** (pu′leks) pl. *pu′lices* [L.] a flea of the genus *Pulex.*

**Pul·heems** (pul′hēmz) a system of medical classification for recording the physical and mental status of recruits in the British armed services, representing: P, physical capacity; U, upper limbs; L, lower limbs; H, hearing (acuity); EE, eyesight (visual acuity); M, mental capacity; S, stability (emotional).

**pu·lic·i·cide** (pu-lis′ĭ-sīd) [*pulex* + *-cide*] an agent destructive to fleas.

**Pu·lic·i·dae** (pu-lis′ĭ-de) a family of the Siphonaptera which includes most of the fleas. Four genera are important to man: *Ctenocephalides, Hoplopsyllus, Pulex,* and *Xenopsylla.*

**pull** (pool) 1. to strain a muscle. 2. the injury sustained in a muscle strain.

**pull-through** (pool′throo) the surgical pulling of one segment of intestine through a segment distal to it. See under *operation,* and see *ileoanal pull-through anastomosis,* under *anastomosis.*

**pul·lu·late** (pul′u-lāt) to germinate.

**pul·lu·la·tion** (pul″u-la′shən) [L. *pullulare* to sprout] the act or process of budding, as in yeast, or of sprouting; germination.

**Pul·mi·cort** (pul′mĭ-kort) trademark for a preparation of budesonide in powdered form.

**pul·mo** (pool′mo) gen. *pulmo′nis,* pl. *pulmo′nes* [L.] [TA] lung.
**p. dex′ter** [TA], right lung; see *lung.*
**p. sinis′ter** [TA], left lung; see *lung.*

**pulmo-** [L. *pulmo* lung] a combining form denoting relationship to the lungs; see also words beginning *pulmon(o)-.*

**pul·mo·aor·tic** (pool″mo-a-or′tik) aorticopulmonary.

**pul·mo·gram** (pool′mo-gram) a radiograph of the lungs.

**Pul·mo·lite** (pul′mo-līt″) trademark for a kit for the preparation of technetium Tc 99m albumin aggregated.

**pul·mo·lith** (pool′mo-lith) [*pulmo-* + *-lith*] pneumolith.

**pul·mo·nal** (pool′mo-nəl) pulmonary (def. 1).

**pul·mo·nary** (pool′mo-nar″e) [L. *pulmonarius*] 1. pertaining to the lungs. Called also *pneumonic* and *pulmonic.* 2. pulmonic (def. 2).

**Pul·mo·nata** (pul″mə-na′tə) an order of snails and slugs of the subclass Euthyneura, including genera with lungs or respiratory sacs. Many are intermediate hosts of trematodes and other pathogens. Its suborders include Basommatophora and Stylommatophora.

**pul·mo·nec·to·my** (pool″mo-nek′tə-me) pneumonectomy.

**pul·mo·nes** (pəl-mo′nes) [L.] 1. plural of *pulmo.* 2. [TA] the right and left lungs.

**pul·mon·ic** (pəl-mon′ik) 1. pulmonary. 2. pertaining to the pulmonary artery.

**pul·mo·ni·tis** (pool″mo-ni′tis) pneumonitis.

**pulmon(o)-** [L. *pulmo,* gen. *pulmonis* lung] a combining form denoting relationship to the lungs; see also words beginning *pulmo-.*

**pul·mo·no·he·pat·ic** (pool″mə-no-hə-pat′ik) pertaining to or communicating with the lungs and the liver; hepatopulmonary.

**pul·mo·nol·o·gist** (pool″mə-nol′ə-jist) an individual skilled in pulmonology.

**pul·mo·nol·o·gy** (pool″mo-nol′ə-je) the science concerned with the anatomy, physiology, and pathology of the lungs.

**pul·mo·no·per·i·to·ne·al** (pool″mə-no-per″ĭ-to-ne′əl) pertaining to or communicating with the lungs and the peritoneum.

**pulp** (pulp) [L. *pulpa* flesh] any soft, juicy animal or vegetable tissue, such as the dental pulp or splenic pulp.
**coronal p.,** pulpa coronalis.
**dead p.,** necrotic p.
**dental p.,** pulpa dentis.
**devitalized p.,** necrotic p.
**digital p.,** the mass of tissue forming the soft cushion on the palmar or plantar surface of the distal phalanx of a finger or toe.
**enamel p.,** stellate reticulum.
**exposed p.,** dental pulp which, through trauma or disease, has become exposed to the external environment.
**mummified p.,** the dry, shriveled pulp seen in dry gangrene.
**necrotic p., nonvital p.,** dental pulp which has been deprived of its blood and nerve supply and is no longer composed of living tissue, with or without bacterial invasion, as evidenced by its insensitivity to stimulation by electricity, heat, cold, or trauma. Called also *dead p.* and *devitalized p.* See also *gangrenous pulp necrosis,* under *necrosis.*
**putrescent p.,** a necrotic pulp which has been invaded by putrefactive microorganisms and is characterized by a particularly foul odor.
**radicular p.,** pulpa radicularis.
**red p., p. of spleen, splenic p.,** pulpa splenica.
**tooth p.,** pulpa dentis.
**vertebral p.,** nucleus pulposus disci intervertebralis.
**vital p.,** a dental pulp which is characterized by vascularity and sensation; one that is not necrotic.
**white p.,** noduli lymphoidei splenici; see under *nodulus.*

**pul·pa** (pul′pə) gen. and pl. *pul′pae* [L. "flesh"] [TA] pulp: any soft, juicy tissue.
**p. corona′lis** [TA], coronal pulp; the portion of the dental pulp in the crown portion of the pulp cavity.
**p. den′tis** [TA], dental pulp: the richly vascularized and innervated connective tissue of mesodermal origin contained in the central cavity of a tooth and delimited by the dentin, and having formative, nutritive, sensory, and protective functions. The portion within the tooth chamber proper is the *p. coronalis,* and that within the root is the *p. radicularis.* Called also *endodontium* and *tooth pulp.*
**p. liena′lis,** TA alternative for *p. splenica.*
**p. radicula′ris** [TA], radicular pulp; the portion of the dental pulp in the root canal of a tooth.
**p. sple′nica** [TA], splenic pulp: the dark, reddish-brown substance that fills up the interspaces of the sinuses of the spleen; called also *pulp of spleen, p. lienalis* [TA alternative], and *red pulp.*

**pul·pal** (pul′pəl) pertaining to the pulp.

**pul·pal·gia** (pəl-pal′je-ə) pain in the pulp of a tooth.

**pul·pec·to·my** (pəl-pek′tə-me) [*pulp* + *-ectomy*] [MeSH: Pulpectomy] root canal therapy consisting of complete extirpation of the dental pulp from the pulp. Called also *dental pulp extirpation.*

**pul·pit·i·des** (pəl-pit′ĭ-dēz) [MeSH: Pulpitis] plural of *pulpitis;* applied to all types of pulp inflammation collectively.

**pul·pi·tis** (pəl-pi′tis) pl. *pulpi′tides* [*pulp* + *-itis*] [MeSH: Pulpitis] inflammation of the dental pulp, usually due to bacterial infection in dental caries, tooth fracture, or other conditions causing exposure of the pulp to bacterial invasion. Chemical irritants, thermal factors, hyperemic changes, and other factors may also cause pulpitis.
**anachoretic p.,** that caused by bacteria circulating in the blood stream, which settle at sites of pulpal inflammation resulting from a chemical or mechanical injury.
**closed p.,** that characterized by the absence of a direct communication between the dental pulp and the oral environment.
**hyperplastic p.,** a chronic productive type of pulpitis usually occurring in teeth with large carious lesions; it is characterized by proliferation of the dental pulp tissue, filling the cavity with a pedunculated or sessile, pinkish red, fleshy mass.
**open p.,** that characterized by the presence of a direct communication between the dental pulp and the oral environment.

**pulp·less** (pulp′ləs) without pulp; having the pulp removed.

**pul·pot·o·my** (pəl-pot′ə-me) [*pulp* + *-tomy*] [MeSH: Pulpotomy] root canal therapy consisting of partial excision of the dental pulp. Called also *pulp amputation.*

**pul·py** (pul′pe) soft or pultaceous.

**pul·sate** (pul′sāt) to beat rhythmically, as the heart.

**pul·sa·tile** (pul′sə-tīl) characterized by a rhythmical pulsation.

**pul·sa·tion** (pəl-sa′shən) [L. *pulsatio*] a throb or rhythmical beat, as of the heart.
**expansile p.,** a pulsation that expands with each beat of the pulse; it reflects an increase in volume of a mass, usually an aneurysm.
**suprasternal p.,** arterial pulsation in the region of the suprasternal

notch, due to dilatation and/or elongation of the aortic arch or to aneurysm.

**pul·sa·tor** (pul′sa-tor) an apparatus for maintaining respiration.
**Bragg-Paul p.,** a pulsator consisting of an air bag placed around the patient's chest and abdomen and rhythmically inflated and deflated by an electric pump.

**pulse** (puls) [L. *pulsus* stroke] [MeSH: Pulse] 1. the rhythmic expansion of an artery, palpable with the finger. See also *pulse rate,* under *rate,* and *beat.* 2. any rhythmic expansion, such as a venous pulse. 3. a brief surge, as of current or voltage.
**abdominal p.,** the pulse over the abdominal aorta.
**abrupt p.,** quick p.
**allorhythmic p.,** irregular p.
**alternating p.,** pulsus alternans.
**anacrotic p.,** one in which the ascending limb of the tracing shows a transient drop in amplitude, or a notch.
**anadicrotic p.,** one in which the ascending limb of the tracing has two waveforms separated by a notch, signifying a transient drop in amplitude.
**anatricrotic p.,** one in which the ascending limb of the tracing shows three small additional waves or notches.
**arterial pressure p.,** pressure p.
**atrial liver p.,** a presystolic pulse corresponding to the atrial venous pulse, sometimes occurring in tricuspid stenosis.
**atrial venous p., atriovenous p.,** a venous pulse in the neck having an accentuated a wave during atrial systole, owing to increased force of contraction of the right atrium; a characteristic of tricuspid stenosis.
**biferious p., bisferious p.,** pulsus bisferiens.
**bounding p.,** strong p.
**bigeminal p.,** a pulse in which beats occur as two in rapid succession separated from the following pair by a longer interval; it is usually related to regularly occurring ventricular premature beats.
**brachial p.,** one felt over the brachial artery at the inner aspect of the elbow.
**cannonball p.,** Corrigan's p.
**capillary p.,** Quincke's p.
**carotid p.,** the pulse in the carotid artery; tracings of it can be used in timing the phases of the cardiac cycle.
**catacrotic p.,** one in which the descending limb of the tracing has a notch.
**catadicrotic p.,** one in which the descending limb of the tracing has a notch between two small additional waveforms.
**catatricrotic p.,** one in which the descending limb of the tracing has two notches between three small waveforms.
**centripetal venous p.,** an abnormal venous pulse caused by a systolic volume expansion that passes from the arteries through the capillaries and venules into the larger veins.
**collapsing p.,** Corrigan's p.
**Corrigan's p.,** a jerky pulse with a full expansion, followed by a sudden collapse, occurring in aortic regurgitation. Called also *cannonball, collapsing, pistol-shot, trip-hammer,* or *water-hammer p.*
**coupled p.,** bigeminal p.
**dicrotic p.,** a pulse whose tracing has two peaks instead of the usual one, the second one coming during diastole as an exaggeration of the dicrotic wave. See also *anacrotic p.* and *catadicrotic p.*
**dorsalis pedis p.,** one felt on the dorsum of the foot between the first and second metatarsal bones; in 8 to 10 per cent of the population it cannot be detected.
**dropped-beat p.,** intermittent p.
**entoptic p.,** the subjective sensation of seeing in the dark a flash of light at each heart beat.
**epigastric p.,** abdominal p.
**febrile p.,** a type of pulse that is both strong and quick, seen in fever.
**femoral p.,** one felt over the femoral artery in the femoral triangle.
**filiform p.,** thready p.
**formicant p.,** low-tension p.
**frequent p.,** one faster in rate than normal; called also *pulsus frequens* and *quick p.*
**full p.,** strong p.
**funic p.,** the arterial tide in the umbilical cord.
**gate p.,** an electrical pulse that serves as a control signal for a gate (q.v.).
**hard p.,** high-tension p.
**high-tension p.,** one characterized by a gradual impulse, long duration, slow subsidence, and a firm, cordy state of the artery between the beats.
**infrequent p.,** slow p.
**intermittent p.,** one in which various beats are dropped. Called also *dropped-beat p.*
**irregular p.,** one in which the beats occur at irregular intervals. Called also *allorhythmic p.*
**jerky p.,** a type of pulse that is both quick and strong; called also *sharp p.* and *vibrating p.*
**jugular p.,** a venous pulse seen or felt over the internal jugular vein.
**Kussmaul's p.,** paradoxical p.
**labile p.,** a pulse that is normal when the patient is resting but increased by sitting, standing, or exercise.
**low-tension p.,** a pulse with sudden onset, short duration, low amplitude, and quick decline, easily obliterated by pressure. Called also *formicant* or *soft p.* and *pulsus formicans, mollis, parvus,* or *vacuus.*
**monocrotic p.,** one in which the tracing has just one waveform per beat of the artery.
**nail p.,** the pulsation of blood under the nails; sometimes demonstrated by the onychograph.
**paradoxical p.,** a pulse that markedly decreases in size during inspiration, as that which often occurs in constrictive pericarditis. Called also *Kussmaul's p.* or *sign* and *pulsus paradoxus.*
**paradoxical p., reversed,** a rise in arterial pressure during inspiration, seen in hypertrophic obstructive cardiomyopathy and some cases of tricuspid insufficiency and atrioventricular dissociation.
**pistol-shot p.,** Corrigan's p.
**plateau p.,** a pulse which is slowly rising and sustained.
**polycrotic p.,** one whose tracing shows secondary pulse waves; see *dicrotic p.* and *tricrotic p.*
**popliteal p.,** one palpated in the popliteal fossa, most easily detected when the patient is lying prone with the knee flexed about 45 degrees.
**posterior tibial p.,** one felt over the posterior tibial artery just posterior to the medial malleolus on the inner aspect of the ankle.
**pressure p.,** the arterial pulse caused directly by systole; see also *blood pressure,* under *pressure.* Called also *arterial pressure p.*
**quadrigeminal p.,** one with a pause after every fourth beat.
**quick p.,** 1. one that strikes the finger smartly and leaves it quickly; called also *pulsus celer* and *abrupt* or *short p.* 2. frequent p.
**Quincke's p.,** alternate blanching and flushing of the skin that may be elicited in several ways, e.g., by observing the nail bed or skin at the root of the nail while pressing on the end of the nail. Caused by pulsation of subpapillary arteriolar and venous plexuses, it is sometimes seen in aortic insufficiency and other disorders, but may occur in normal persons under certain conditions. It was originally thought to be due to pulsation of the capillaries, hence the name *capillary p.* Called also *Quincke's sign.*
**radial p.,** that felt over the radial artery.
**respiratory p.,** one observed normally in the superficial cervical veins after rapid exercise or at other times of increased respiration.
**retrosternal p.,** a venous pulse perceptible just above the suprasternal notch.
**Riegel's p.,** a pulse which is diminished in size during expiration.
**running p.,** a pulse with small irregular excursions.
**sharp p.,** jerky p.
**short p.,** quick p., def. 1.
**slow p.,** one with less than the usual number of pulsations per minute. Called also *infrequent* or *vagus p.* and *pulsus tardus.*
**soft p.,** low-tension p.
**strong p.,** a forcible pulse of high amplitude; see also *high-tension p.* Called also *bounding, full,* or *tense p.* and *pulsus fortis, magnus,* or *plenus.*
**tense p.,** strong p.
**thready p.,** one that is very fine and scarcely perceptible. Called also *filiform p.* and *pulsus filiformis.*
**tricrotic p.,** one in which the tracing shows three expansions of the artery in one beat. See also *anatricrotic p.* and *catatricrotic p.*
**trigeminal p.,** one with a pause after every third beat.
**trip-hammer p.,** Corrigan's p.
**unequal p.,** a pulse in which some of the beats are strong and others weak.
**vagus p.,** slow p.
**venous p.,** the pulsation which occurs in a vein, usually observed at the right jugular vein just above the sternoclavicular junction.

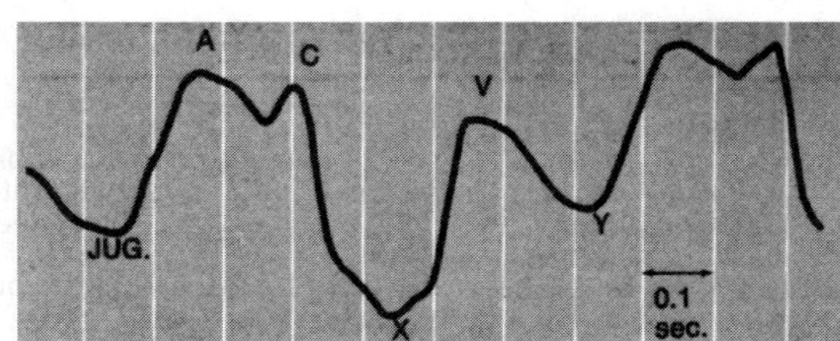


Normal jugular venous pulse: *A,* a positive wave due to contraction of the right atrium; *C,* a positive deflection due to bulging of the tricuspid valve toward the atria at the onset of ventricular contraction; *X,* a negative deflection due to atrial relaxation; *V,* a positive deflection due to filling of the right atrium against the closed tricuspid valve during ventricular contraction; *Y,* a negative deflection due to emptying of the right atrium upon ventricular relaxation.

**vermicular p.**, a small rapid pulse giving to the finger a sensation of wormlike movement.
**vibrating p.**, jerky p.
**water-hammer p.**, Corrigan's p.
**wiry p.**, a small, tense pulse.

**pul·sion** (pul'shən) a pushing forward, or outward or to either side.

**pul·sus** (pul'səs) pl. *pul'sus* [L., from *pellere* to beat] pulse.
**p. abdomina'lis**, abdominal pulse.
**p. alter'nans**, alternating pulse: a pulse in which there is regular alternation of weak and strong beats without changes in cycle length, usually indicative of serious myocardial disease.
**p. bife'riens, p. bisfe'riens**, a pulse with two strong systolic peaks separated by a midsystolic dip, usually seen in pure aortic regurgitation and aortic regurgitation with stenosis. Called also *biferious* or *bisferious pulse* and *p. biferiens*.
**p. bige'minus**, bigeminal pulse.
**p. ce'ler**, quick pulse.
**p. dif'ferens**, inequality of the pulse observable at corresponding sites on either side of the body.
**p. filifor'mis**, thready pulse.
**p. for'micans**, low-tension pulse.
**p. for'tis**, strong pulse.
**p. fre'quens**, frequent pulse.
**p. irregula'ris perpe'tuus**, irregular pulse.
**p. mag'nus**, strong pulse.
**p. mag'nus et ce'ler**, one that is both strong and quick; see *febrile pulse* and *jerky pulse*.
**p. mol'lis**, low-tension pulse.
**p. paradox'us**, paradoxical pulse.
**p. par'vus**, low-tension pulse.
**p. par'vus et tar'dus**, a slow pulse that is also low-tension.
**p. ple'nus**, strong pulse.
**p. tar'dus**, slow pulse.
**p. trige'minus**, trigeminal pulse.
**p. va'cuus**, low-tension pulse.
**p. veno'sus**, venous pulse.

**pul·ta·ceous** (pəl-ta'shəs) [L. *pultaceus*] like a pulp or poultice.

**pulv.** abbreviation for L. *pulvis* powder.

**pul·ver·iza·tion** (pul″vər-ĭ-za'shən) [L. *pulvis* powder] the reduction of any substance to powder.

**pul·ver·u·lent** (pəl-ver'u-lənt) [L. *pulverulentus*] powdery; dustlike.

**pul·vi·nar** (pəl-vi'nər) [L. "a cushioned seat"] the prominent, cushion-like mass of nuclei that forms the medial portion of the posterior extremity of the thalamus, which partly overhangs the rostral colliculus and its brachium and is separated inferiorly from the geniculate body by the brachium of the rostral colliculus; it receives fibers from other thalamic nuclei and gives off widespread cortical projections. It is thought by some to be related to language functions. In official terminology, called *pulvinar thalami*.
**p. tha'lami** [TA], official terminology for *pulvinar*.
**p. tu'nicae inter'nae segmen'ti arteria'lis anastomo'sis arteriove'nae glomerifor'mis**, the wall of the internal coat of the arterial segment of the anastomosis arteriovenosa glomeriformis, consisting of three to six layers of contractile glomus cells. Called also *p. tunicae intimae segmenti arterialis anastomosis arteriovenae glomeriformis*.

**pul·vi·nate** (pul'vĭ-nāt) [L. *pulvinus* cushion] shaped like a cushion.

**pul·vis** (pul'vis) [L.] powder.

**pu·mex** (pu'məks) [L.] pumice.

**pum·ice** (pum'is) [USP] a substance of volcanic origin, consisting chiefly of complex silicates of aluminum, potassium, and sodium, occurring as a very light, hard, rough, porous, grayish powder; used in dentistry as an abrasive or polishing agent, the effect achieved depending on the particle size.

**pump** (pump) 1. an apparatus for drawing or forcing fluids or gases. 2. to draw or force fluids or gases.
**acid p.**, proton p.
**air p.**, a pump for exhausting or forcing in air.
**blood p.**, a machine used to propel blood through the tubing of extracorporeal circulation devices, designed to do so without damaging blood constituents, particularly the erythrocytes. See also *centrifugal p.* and *roller p.*
**breast p.**, a manual or electric pump for abstracting milk from the breast.
**calcium p.**, the mechanism of active transport of calcium ($Ca^{2+}$) across a membrane, as of the sarcoplasmic reticulum of muscle cells, against a concentration gradient; the mechanism is driven by the hydrolysis of ATP by the membrane-bound enzyme $Ca^{2+}$-ATPase.
**cardiac balloon p.**, intra-aortic balloon p.
**centrifugal p.**, a blood pump in which centrifugal force generated by cones or impellers rotating in a closed unit returns the blood to the patient.
**electrogenic p.**, a protein channel pump in which the ion exchange is not one-to-one and hyperpolarization results on one side of the membrane. Cf. *sodium-potassium p.*
**infusion p.**, a device for injecting a measured amount of fluid during a specific interval of time.
**infusion-withdrawal p.**, a pump for the simultaneous injection and withdrawal of fluid at the same rate.
**insulin p.**, an externally worn pump that can supply insulin to subcutaneous tissues through a plastic tube; a large bolus is infused before every meal and a continuous basal rate of insulin is maintained at other times. Called also *continuous subcutaneous insulin infusion*.
**intra-aortic balloon p. (IABP)**, a pump used in intra-aortic balloon counterpulsation (q.v.).
**Lindbergh p.**, a perfusion apparatus by means of which an organ removed from the body may be kept alive indefinitely.
**muscle p.**, compression of veins by the contraction of skeletal muscles, forcing blood towards the heart against the flow of gravity; seen particularly in the deep veins of the lower limbs. Called also *venous p.*
**$Na^+$-$K^+$ p.**, sodium p.
**peristaltic p.**, a pump that moves liquid through tubing by alternate contractions and relaxations on the tubing.
**proton p.**, a system for transporting protons across cell membranes, often exchanging them for other positively charged ions; it may be driven by energy supplied by ATP metabolism, light, or a flow of electrons. See also *H+,K+-ATPase*.
**roller p.**, a blood pump in which flow is maintained by the compression of the tubing containing the blood between a continuously moving roller and a curved back plate.
**sodium p., sodium-potassium p.**, the mechanism of active transport by which gradients of the ions sodium ($Na^+$) and potassium ($K^+$) are formed across the cell membrane; using the energy generated by the $Na^+$,$K^+$-ATPase, sodium is extruded from the cell and potassium is brought in. The gradients are necessary for protein biosynthesis, maintenance of osmotic equilibrium, propagation of nerve impulses, and secondary transport of some molecules (e.g., glucose) across cell membranes. Called also *Na+-K+p.*
**stomach p.**, a pump for removing the contents from the stomach.
**venous p.**, muscle p.

**pump-oxy·gen·a·tor** (pump-ok″sĭ-jə-na'tər) an apparatus, usually extracorporeal, comprising an arterial pump and blood oxygenator plus filters and traps, for saturating blood with oxygen and perfusing the body tissue; used for cardiopulmonary bypass during cardiac surgery.

**punch** (punch) an instrument for indenting, perforating, or excising a disk or segment of tissue or other material.
**biopsy p.**, an instrument used to remove a small amount of skin or other tissue; see also *punch biopsy*, under *biopsy*.
**kidney p., Murphy's kidney p.**, see *Murphy's test*, under *tests*.
**pin p.**, an instrument for perforating a metal backing to receive the pins for fastening artificial teeth.
**plate p.**, a punch for cutting out parts of an artificial dental plate.
**rubber dam p.**, an instrument for punching holes in a rubber dam in order to permit passage of the dam over the crowns of teeth.

**punch·drunk** (punch'drunk) boxer's dementia.

**punched-out** (puncht'out) having the appearance of substance or tissue having been removed with a punch.

**punc·ta** (punk'tə) [L.] plural of *punctum*.

**punc·tal** (punk'təl) [L. *punctum*, q.v.] pertaining to the punctum lacrimale.

**punc·tate** (punk'tāt) [L. *punctum* point] resembling or marked with points or dots.

**punc·ti·form** (punk'tĭ-form) [*punctum* + *form*] 1. like a point; located in a point. 2. in bacteriology, denoting very minute colonies.

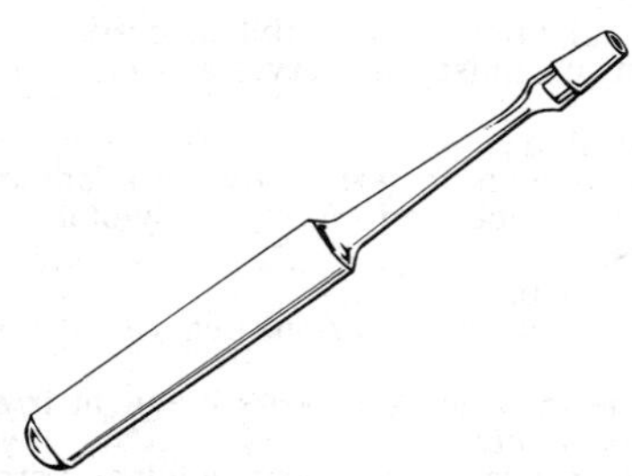

Biopsy punch.

**punc·to·graph** (punk'to-graf) [*punctum* + *-graph*] an instrument for the radiographic localization of foreign bodies in the tissues.

**punctuation** (punk″choo-a'shən) small points or dots.
**Schüffner's p.,** Schüffner's dots.

**punc·tum** (pungk'təm) pl. *punc'ta* [L.] an extremely small spot, or point; used in anatomical nomenclature as a general term to designate an extremely small area, or point of projection.
**p. cae'cum,** blind spot; see under *spot.*
**imperforate p.,** congenital atresia of the punctum lacrimale, resulting in epiphora; it is particularly common in small breeds of dogs and in pigs.
**p. lacrima'le** [TA], lacrimal point: the opening on the lacrimal papilla of an eyelid, near the medial angle of the eye, into which tears from the lacrimal lake drain to enter the lacrimal canaliculi.
**p. lu'teum,** macula lutea.
**p. ossificatio'nis,** centrum ossificationis.
**p. ossificatio'nis prima'rium,** centrum ossificationis primarium.
**p. ossificatio'nis secunda'rium,** centrum ossificationis secundarium.
**p. prox'imum,** near point.
**p. remo'tum,** far point.
**punc'ta vasculo'sa,** minute red spots marking the cut surface of the white substance of the brain, produced by blood from divided vessels.

**punc·tum·e·ter** (pəngk-tum'ə-tər) [*punctum* + *-meter*] an instrument for measuring the range of accommodation.

**punc·ture** (pungk'chər) [L. *punctura*] [MeSH: Punctures] 1. the act of piercing or penetrating with a pointed object or instrument. 2. a wound so made.
**Bernard's p.,** puncture of the brain of an experimental animal at a specific point of the floor of the fourth ventricle to cause diabetes *(puncture diabetes)* and glycosuria. Called also *diabetic p.*
**Blom-Singer p.,** tracheoesophageal p.
**cisternal p.,** puncture of the cisterna cerebellomedullaris through the posterior atlanto-occipital membrane for the purpose of withdrawing cerebrospinal fluid; called also *intracisternal p.* and *suboccipital p.*
**cranial p.,** cisternal p.
**diabetic p.,** Bernard's p.
**exploratory p.,** puncture of a cavity or tumor and removal of some portion of the contents for examination.
**heat p.,** elevation of the temperature of the animal body produced by puncturing the base of the brain.
**intracisternal p.,** cisternal p.
**Kronecker's p.,** in experimental medicine, puncture of the inhibitory nerve center of the heart by means of a long fine needle.
**lumbar p.,** the withdrawal of fluid from the subarachnoid space in the lumbar region, usually between the third and fourth lumbar vertebrae, for diagnostic or therapeutic purposes. Called also *spinal p., thecal p., rachiocentesis,* and *spinal tap.*
**spinal p.,** lumbar p.
**splenic p.,** puncture of the spleen to obtain a specimen of splenic tissue for examination or to measure portal pressure.
**sternal p.,** removal of bone marrow from the manubrium of the sternum through an appropriate needle.
**suboccipital p.,** cisternal p.
**thecal p.,** lumbar p.
**tracheoesophageal p.,** a one-way plastic valve placed in a surgically-created tracheoesophageal fistula to restore speech after laryngectomy. Called also *Blom-Singer p.*
**transethmoidal p.,** a technique for obtaining postmortem biopsy specimens of the brain, using a trocar inserted through the nostril.
**ventricular p.,** puncture of a cerebral ventricle for the purpose of withdrawing fluid.

**pun·gent** (pun'jənt) [L. *pungens* pricking] sharp or biting; somewhat acrid.

**Pun·nett square** (pun'ət) [Reginald Crundall *Punnett,* English geneticist, 1875–1967] see *checkerboard.*

**Pun·ti·us** (pun'te-əs) a genus of fresh-water fish.
**P. java'nicus,** a species placed in fresh-water ponds in certain areas of the world, because it eliminates the weeds necessary for the propagation of mosquitoes.

**PUO** *p*yrexia of *u*nknown *o*rigin.

**pu·pa** (pu'pə) [L. "a doll"] [MeSH: Pupa] the second stage in the development of an insect, between the larva and the imago.

**pu·pal** (pu'pəl) pertaining to a pupa.

**pu·pil** (pu'pil) [L. *pupilla* girl] [MeSH: Pupil] pupilla. Symbol P.
**Adie's p.,** tonic p.
**Argyll Robertson p.,** one which is miotic and which responds to accommodation effort, but not to light.
**artificial p.,** one made by iridectomy.

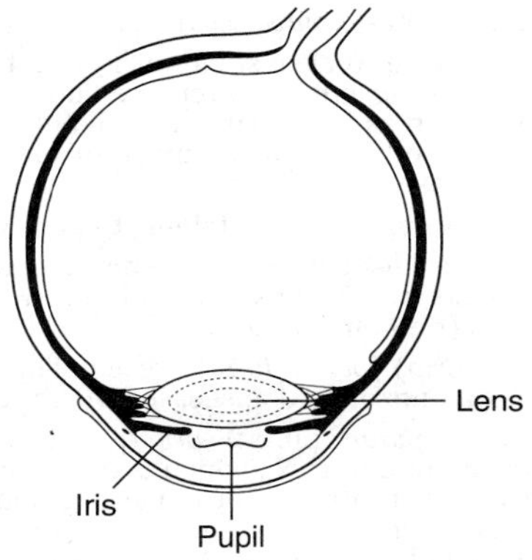

**Behr's p.,** contralateral dilatation of the pupil in lesions of the optic tract.
**bounding p.,** a pupil which shows alternating dilatation and contraction.
**Bumke's p.,** dilation of the pupil after a psychic stimulus.
**cat's-eye p.,** one with a narrow vertical aperture.
**cornpicker's p's,** dilated pupils resulting from exposure to dust from jimsonweed (which contains stramonium) in the cornfield.
**fixed p.,** a pupil which does not react either to light or on convergence, or in accommodation.
**Hutchinson's p.,** a condition of the pupils in which one is dilated and the other not.
**keyhole p.,** a pupil with a coloboma or a sector iridectomy on one side of the margin.
**Marcus Gunn p.,** the abnormal pupil noted with Marcus Gunn's pupillary phenomenon.
**myotonic p.,** tonic p.
**pinhole p.,** one which is extremely contracted.
**skew p's,** a condition in which one of the ocular axes deviates upward and the other downward.
**stiff p.,** Argyll Robertson p.
**tonic p.,** a usually unilateral condition of the eye in which the affected pupil is larger than the other, responds to accommodation and convergence in a slow, delayed fashion, and reacts to light only after prolonged exposure to dark or light. Called also *Adie's p., myotonic p.,* and *pupillotonia.* See also *Adie's syndrome,* under *syndrome.*

**pu·pil·la** (pu-pil'ə) pl. *pupil'lae* [L. "girl"] [TA] pupil: the opening at the center of the iris of the eye, through which light enters the eye. See also *iris.*

**pu·pil·lary** (pu'pĭ-lar-e) pertaining to the pupil.

**pu·pil·la·to·nia** (pu″pil-ə-to'ne-ə) tonic pupil.

**Pu·pil·li·dae** (pu-pil'ĭ-de) a family of small to minute terrestrial snails and slugs of the suborder Stylommatophora, commonly found in moist wooded regions in North America; it includes the genus *Chondrina.*

**pupill(o)-** [L. *pupilla,* q.v.] a combining form denoting relationship to the pupil.

**pu·pil·lo·graph** (pu-pil'o-graf) [*pupillo-* + *-graph*] an instrument that detects responses of the pupil of the eye.

**pu·pil·lom·e·ter** (pu″pĭ-lom'ə-tər) [*pupillo-* + *-meter*] an instrument for measuring the width or diameter of the pupil; called also *coreometer.*

**pu·pil·lom·e·try** (pu″pĭ-lom'ə-tre) measurement of the diameter or width of the pupil of the eye; called also *coreometry.*

**pu·pil·lo·mo·tor** (pu″pĭ-lo-mo'tər) pertaining to the movement of the pupil.

**pu·pil·lo·ple·gia** (pu″pĭ-lo-ple'jə) [*pupillo-* + *-plegia*] tonic pupil.

**pu·pil·lo·scope** (pu-pil'o-skōp) 1. an instrument for observing the pupil and its reactions. 2. retinoscope.

**pu·pil·los·co·py** (pu″pĭ-los'kə-pe) [*pupillo-* + *-scopy*] retinoscopy.

**pu·pil·lo·sta·tom·e·ter** (pu-pil″o-stə-tom'ə-tər) [*pupillo-* + Gr. *statos* placed + *-meter*] an instrument for measuring the distance between the pupils.

**pu·pil·lo·to·nia** (pu″pĭ-lo-to'ne-ə) tonic pupil.

**pure** (pūr) [L. *purus*] free from mixture with or contamination by other materials; a reagent is *chemically pure* when it contains no other chemicals that might interfere with its action.

**pur·ga·tion** (pər-ga'shən) [L. *purgatio*] emptying of the bowels, as by a medicine; called also *catharsis* and *evacuation.*

**pur·ga·tive** (pur'gə-tiv) [L. *purgativus*] cathartic (defs. 1 and 2).

**purge** (purj) [L. *purgare* to cleanse, to purify] 1. to relieve of fecal matter. 2. to cleanse or purify, to remove undesirable substances from something, such as from marrow in an autologous bone marrow transplant or food from the stomach or intestines. 3. a purgative remedy or dose.

**pu·ric** (pu'rik) 1. purulent. 2. pertaining to purine.

**pu·ri·fi·ca·tion** (pūr"ĭ-fĭ-ka'shən) the separating of foreign or contaminating elements from a substance of interest.
**affinity p.**, that carried out by means of affinity chromatography.

**pu·ri·form** (pu'rĭ-form) [*pus* + *form*] resembling pus; the term is applied to the contents of cold abscesses which resemble pus.

**pu·rine** (pu'rēn) [L. *purum* pure + *urine*] a colorless crystalline heterocyclic compound, $C_5H_4N_4$, which is not found free in nature, but is variously substituted to produce a group of compounds known as *purines* or *purine bases* (see illustration at *base*), of which uric acid is a metabolic end product. The purine bases include adenine and guanine, which are constituents of nucleic acids, and hypoxanthine and xanthine.
**amino p.**, aminopurine.
**methyl p's**, alkaloids formed from purines by substituting methyl groups, usually in positions 1, 3, 7. The principal ones are caffeine, theobromine, and theophylline.

**pu·rin·emia** (pu"rĭ-ne'me-ə) the presence of purine bases in the blood.

**pu·rin·emic** (pu"rĭ-ne'mik) pertaining to or characterized by purinemia.

**pu·rine-nu·cleo·side phos·phor·y·lase** (pu'rēn noo'kle-o-sīd fos-for'ə-lās) [EC 2.4.2.1] [MeSH: Purine-Nucleoside Phosphorylase] an enzyme of the transferase class that catalyzes the cleavage of purine nucleosides to form purines and ribose 1-phosphates in the degradation of nucleotides and nucleic acids. Absence of activity, an autosomal recessive trait, results in defective cell-mediated immunity.

**Pu·rine·thol** (pu'rēn-thol) trademark for a preparation of mercaptopurine.

**pu·rino·lyt·ic** (pu"rin-o-lit'ik) [*purine* + *-lytic*] splitting up purines.

**pu·rin·om·e·ter** (pu"rin-om'ə-tər) [*purine* + *-meter*] an apparatus for estimating the quantity of purine bodies in the urine.

**Pur·kin·je's cells, fibers,** etc. (pər-kin'jēz) [Jan Evangelista *Purkinje*, Czech physiologist, 1787–1869] see under *cell, fiber, figure, network, phenomenon, system,* and *vesicle* and see *stratum neuronorum piriformium.*

**Pur·kin·je-San·son mirror images** (pər-kin'je-sah-saw') [J. E. *Purkinje;* Louis Joseph *Sanson,* French physician, 1790–1841] see under *image.*

**pu·ro·hep·a·ti·tis** (pu"ro-hep"ə-ti'tis) [*pus* + *hepatitis*] hepatic abscess.

**pu·ro·mu·cous** (pu"ro-mu'kəs) consisting of or containing pus and mucus; mucopurulent.

**pu·ro·my·cin** (pūr"o-mi'sin) [MeSH: Puromycin] an antibiotic produced by *Streptomyces alboniger,* which has been used experimentally as an antineoplastic because of its ability to inhibit protein synthesis; it also has trypanosomicidal and amebicidal activity and was formerly used in the treatment of African trypanosomiasis and amebic dysentery.

**pur·ple** (pur'pəl) 1. a color between blue and red. 2. a substance of this color used as a dye or indicator.
**bromcresol p.**, an indicator, dibromo-*o*-cresolsulfonphthalein, used in the determination of hydrogen ion concentration, being yellow at 5.2 and purple at 6.8. Written also *bromocresol p.*
**visual p.**, rhodopsin.

**Pur·pu·ra** (pur'pu-rə) [MeSH: Purpura] a genus of marine snails of the family Muricidae. Some species furnish a purple dye and others contain the neurotoxin purpurine or murine.

**pur·pu·ra** (pur'pu-rə) [L. "purple"] [MeSH: Purpura] 1. any of a group of conditions characterized by ecchymoses or other small hemorrhages in the skin, mucous membranes, or serosal surfaces; possible causes include blood disorders, vascular abnormalities, and trauma. 2. any of several conditions similar to the traditional purpura group, which may be caused by decreased platelet counts, platelet abnormalities, vascular defects, or reactions to drugs.
**allergic p., anaphylactoid p.**, Schönlein-Henoch p.
**p. annula'ris telangiecto'des,** a rare purpuric eruption, commonly beginning on the lower extremities and becoming generalized, the original punctate erythematous lesions coalescing to form an annular or serpiginous pattern; involution is gradual, sometimes followed by atrophy and loss of hair in the area. Called also *Majocchi's p.* or *disease.*
**brain p.**, a hemorrhagic encephalopathy resembling acute necrotizing hemorrhagic encephalomyelitis, but without the inflammatory or necrotic changes of that disorder. It is marked by small pericapillary hemorrhages in the white matter of the brain, with adjacent demyelination and destruction of the axons; clinical manifestations include stupor and coma. The etiology is uncertain, but it is sometimes secondary to viral pneumonia or arsenical intoxication. Called also *pericapillary encephalorrhagia.*
**fibrinolytic p., p. fibrinoly'tica,** purpura secondary to and accompanied by increased fibrinolytic activity of the blood.
**p. ful'minans,** a form of nonthrombocytopenic purpura, observed mainly in children, usually following an infectious disease such as scarlet fever, and characterized by fever, shock, anemia, and sudden and rapidly spreading symmetrical skin hemorrhages of the lower extremities, often associated with extensive intravascular thromboses and gangrene.
**p. hemorrha'gica,** 1. idiopathic thrombocytopenic p. 2. an acute, usually fatal disease of horses that may occur after a respiratory tract infection; characteristics include subcutaneous edema and petechiae around the head with tachycardia.
**Henoch's p.**, a variety of Schönlein-Henoch purpura characterized by acute visceral symptoms such as vomiting, diarrhea, abdominal distention, hematuria, and renal colic, and without articular symptoms. Called also *p. nervosa.*
**Henoch-Schönlein p.**, Schönlein-Henoch p.
**idiopathic p.**, idiopathic thrombocytopenic p.
**itching p.**, a recurrent, pruritic, eruptive hemorrhagic dermatosis, usually seen in males, manifested as erythematous macules with punctate purpura beginning on the legs and spreading to the trunk, upper extremities, and in severe cases the large flexural areas. It is usually seen in the spring and summer, and it clears spontaneously. Called also *disseminated pruritic angiodermatitis.*
**Majocchi's p.**, p. annularis telangiectodes.
**malignant p.**, meningococcal meningitis.
**p. nervo'sa,** Henoch's p.
**p. of newborn,** a form of thrombocytopenia observed soon after birth, presumed in certain instances to be due to the passage of anti-platelet factors across the placenta.
**nonthrombocytopenic p.**, purpura without any decrease in the platelet count of the blood. Called also *p. simplex.*
**palpable p.**, the characteristic lesion of cutaneous necrotizing venulitis: an erythematous lesion that does not blanch when the skin is pressed.
**psychogenic p.**, painful bruising syndrome; the term is sometimes used more narrowly to denote only those cases without evidence of sensitivity to erythrocytes.
**p. rheuma'tica,** Schönlein p.
**Schönlein p.**, Schönlein-Henoch purpura with articular and dermatological symptoms but without gastrointestinal symptoms. Called also *p. rheumatica, rheumatocelis,* and *Schönlein disease.*
**Schönlein-Henoch p.**, a form of nonthrombocytopenic purpura, sometimes a type of hypersensitivity vasculitis and sometimes of unknown cause, usually seen in children and associated with a variety of clinical symptoms including urticaria and erythema, arthropathy and arthritis, gastrointestinal symptoms, and renal involvement. Called also *allergic p., anaphylactoid p.,* and *Schönlein-Henoch syndrome.*
**p. seni'lis,** dark purplish red ecchymoses occurring on the forearms and back of the hands in the elderly. See also *steroid p.*
**p. sim'plex,** nonthrombocytopenic p.
**steroid p.**, bizarre-shaped broad hemorrhages beneath the skin of the back of the forearms, hands, or shins caused by attrition of dermal and vascular connective tissue due to long-term treatment with adrenocortical steroid hormones. It is identical with purpura senilis in appearance.
**thrombocytopenic p.**, any form of purpura in which the platelet count is decreased; it may be either *primary (idiopathic)* or *secondary.*
**thrombocytopenic p., idiopathic, thrombocytopenic p., primary,** thrombocytopenic purpura not directly associated with any definable systemic disease, although it often follows a systemic infection; the cause is thought to be an IgG immunoglobulin that acts as an antibody against platelets, causing ecchymoses, petechiae, and other bleeding. There are both an acute and a chronic form: the *acute form* has a sudden onset, is more common in children, and usually resolves spontaneously within a few months; the *chronic form* has a slower onset, is more common in adults, and may be recurrent.
**thrombocytopenic p., secondary,** thrombocytopenic purpura occurring as a consequence of a primary hematologic disease such as leukemia, or an underlying systemic nonhematologic entity.
**thrombocytopenic p., thrombotic,** a form of thrombotic microangiopathy characterized by thrombocytopenia with thromboses in terminal arterioles and capillaries; other symptoms include hemolytic anemia, azotemia, fever, and bizarre neurological manifestations. Some authorities consider it identical to the hemolytic uremic syndrome. Called also *microangiopathic* or *microangiopathic hemolytic anemia* and *Moschcowitz's disease.*

**thrombopenic p.,** thrombocytopenic p.

**pur·pu·ric** (pər-pu′rik) of the nature of, pertaining to, or affected with purpura.

**pur·pu·ric ac·id** (pər-pu′rik) an imino-condensation product of alloxan, found in Weidel's test for uric acid. See also *murexide,* and *Weidel's test* (1), under *tests.*

**pur·pu·rin** (pur′pu-rin) 1. a glycoside from madder root that has been used as a nuclear stain. 2. uroerythrin. 3. purpurine.

**pur·pu·rine** (pur′pu-rēn) 1. a neurotoxic substance derived from the median zone of the hypobranchial or purple gland of gastropods of the genus *Purpura,* thought to be an ester or a mixture of esters of choline; the substance is called *murexine* when derived from snails of the genus *Murex.* 2. purpurin.

**pur·pu·rin·uria** (pur″pu-rĭ-nu′re-ə) the presence of uroerythrin in the urine.

**pur·pu·rog·e·nous** (pur″pu-roj′ə-nəs) [L. *purpura* purple + *-genous*] producing visual purple (rhodopsin).

**purr** (pur) a low vibratory murmur.

**purr·ing** (pur′ing) having a tremulous quality, like the purr of a cat.

**pur·shi·a·nin** (pər-shi′ə-nin) a brown, oily liquid glycoside mixture from *Rhamnus purshiana* D.C. (Rhamnaceae), having laxative action.

**Pur·ti·lo's syndrome** (pər-til′ōz) [David T. *Purtilo,* American physician, 20th century] X-linked lymphoproliferative syndrome; see under *syndrome.*

**Purt·scher's disease (angiopathic retinopathy)** (poor′cherz) [Otmar *Purtscher,* German ophthalmologist, 1852–1927] see under *disease.*

**pu·ru·lence** (pu′roo-ləns) [L. *purulentia*] the condition or fact of being purulent.

**pu·ru·len·cy** (pu′roo-len″se) purulence.

**pu·ru·lent** (pu′roo-lənt) [L. *purulentus*] consisting of or containing pus; associated with the formation of or caused by pus.

**pu·ru·loid** (pu′roo-loid) resembling pus; puriform.

**pus** (pus) pl. *pu′ra,* gen. *pu′ris* [L.] a liquid inflammation product made up of cells (leukocytes) and a thin protein-rich fluid called liquor puris.
**anchovy sauce p.,** the brownish pus seen in amebic abscess of the liver.
**blue p.,** pus with a bluish tint, seen in certain suppurative infections, the color occurring as a result of the presence of a bacterial pigment (pyocyanin) produced by *Pseudomonas aeruginosa.*
**burrowing p.,** pus which is not walled off but may extend between fascial planes for considerable distances.
**cheesy p.,** thick, nearly solid pus.
**curdy p.,** pus mixed with cheesy flakes.
**green p.,** pus having a greenish tint.
**laudable p., p. laudan′dum,** a term once applied to a creamy yellow, inodorous pus, secreted by a healthy granulating surface, and regarded as indicative of less danger than other varieties.
**sanious p.,** bloody pus, often ichorous and ill smelling.

**pus·tu·la** (pus′tu-lə) pl. *pus′tulae* [L.] pustule.

**pus·tu·lar** (pus′tu-lər) pertaining to or of the nature of a pustule; consisting of pustules.

**pus·tu·la·tion** (pus″tu-la′shən) the formation of pustules.

**pus·tule** (pus′tūl) [L. *pustula*] a visible collection of pus within or beneath the epidermis, often in a hair follicle or sweat pore.
**malignant p.,** see *cutaneous anthrax,* under *anthrax.*
**multilocular p.,** a pustule with several compartments, indicating origin from a spongiotic vesicle within the epidermis rather than from infection arising in a follicle or sweat pore, or beneath the epidermis.
**simple p.,** unilocular p.
**spongiform p., spongiform p. of Kogoj,** a focal subcorneal area of epidermal spongiosis lined with edematous epidermal cells and containing neutrophils in the intercellular spaces, which is a cardinal sign of active psoriasis, and found also in other dermatologic conditions such as seborrheic dermatitis and Reiter's disease. Cf. *Munro microabscess.*
**unilocular p.,** one consisting of a single cavity filled with pus, suggesting origin within a follicle or sweat pore or from beneath the epidermis, rather than within it; called also *simple p.*

**pus·tu·lo·sis** (pus″tu-lo′sis) a condition marked by an outbreak of pustules.
**p. palma′ris et planta′ris, palmoplantar p.,** 1. localized pustular psoriasis. 2. a pustular eruption similar to localized pustular psoriasis except that psoriasis is not present.
**p. vaccinifor′mis acu′ta, p. variolifor′mis acu′ta,** Kaposi's varicelliform eruption.

**pu·ta·men** (pu-ta′mən) [L. "shell"] [TA] [MeSH: Putamen] the larger, darker and more lateral part of the lentiform nucleus, separated from the lateral globus pallidus by the lateral medullary lamina.

**Put·nam-Da·na syndrome** (put′nəm-da′nə) [James Jackson *Putnam,* American neurologist, 1846–1918; Charles Loomis *Dana,* American neurologist, 1852–1935] see *subacute combined degeneration of spinal cord,* under *degeneration.*

**pu·tre·fac·tion** (pu″trə-fak′shən) [L. *putrefactio*] enzymic decomposition, especially of proteins, with the production of foul-smelling compounds, such as hydrogen sulfide, ammonia, and mercaptans. Cf. *fermentation.*

**pu·tre·fac·tive** (pu″trə-fak′tiv) pertaining to or of the nature of putrefaction.

**pu·tre·fy** (pu′trə-fi) to decompose, with the production of foul-smelling compounds; a term applied especially to the decomposition of proteins and organic matter.

**pu·tres·cence** (pu-tres′əns) partial or complete rottenness.

**pu·tres·cent** (pu-tres′ənt) [L. *putrescens* decaying] rotting; undergoing putrefaction.

**pu·tres·cine** (pu-tres′in) [MeSH: Putrescine] chemical name: tetramethylene-diamine. A polyamine first found in decaying animal tissues but now known to occur in almost all tissues and in cultures of certain bacteria. It is formed by decarboxylation of ornithine and is itself a precursor of spermidine.

**pu·trid** (pu′trid) [L. *putridus*] characterized by putrefaction; rotten or corrupt.

**Puus·epp's reflex** (poos′eps) [Lyudvig Martinovich *Puusepp,* Estonian neurosurgeon, 1875–1942] see under *reflex.*

**PUVA** psoralen plus ultraviolet A.

**PVC** 1. polyvinyl chloride. 2. postvoiding cystogram. 3. premature ventricular contraction; see *ventricular premature complex,* under *complex.* 4. pulmonary venous congestion.

**PVL** periventricular leukomalacia.

**PVP** polyvinylpyrrolidone.

**PVP-I** povidone-iodine.

**PVS** persistent vegetative state.

**PWA** person with AIDS.

**PWM** pokeweed mitogen.

**py·ar·thro·sis** (pi″ahr-thro′sis) [*pyo-* + *arthr-* + *-osis*] acute suppurative arthritis.

**Pyc·nan·the·mum** (pik-nan′thə-məm) [Gr. *pyknos* dense + *anthemon* bloom] the mountain mints, a genus of American herbs of the family Labiatae; they are aromatic and carminative and resemble pennyroyal or spearmint in taste and smell.

**pyc·nid·ium** (pik-nid′e-əm) a flask-shaped or spherical fruiting body whose inner wall is lined with conidiogenous cells.

**pycn(o)-** for words thus beginning, see those beginning *pykn(o)-.*

**py·elec·ta·sia** (pi″ə-lək-ta′zhə) pyelectasis.

**py·elec·ta·sis** (pi″ə-lek′tə-sis) [*pyel-* + *ectasis*] dilatation of the renal pelvis.

**py·el·ic** (pi-el′ik) pertaining to the pelvis of the kidney.

**py·elit·ic** (pi″ə-lit′ik) pertaining to or affected with pyelitis.

**py·eli·tis** (pi″ə-li′tis) [*pyel-* + *-itis*] [MeSH: Pyelitis] inflammation of the pelvis of the kidney. It is attended by pain and tenderness in the loins, irritability of the bladder, remittent fever, bloody or purulent urine, diarrhea, vomiting, and a peculiar pain on flexion of the thigh. See also *pyelonephritis.*
**calculous p.,** that which is caused by calculi.
**p. cys′tica,** pyelitis with the formation of multiple submucosal cysts.
**defloration p.,** pyelitis in women after the first sexual intercourse, as a result of infection following rupture of the hymen.
**encrusted p.,** pyelitis with ulcers which are encrusted with urinary salts.
**p. glandula′ris,** pyelitis with conversion of transitional mucosal into cylindrical epithelium, with formation of glandular acini.
**p. granulo′sa,** pyelitis marked by the presence of exuberant granulations.
**p. gravida′rum,** inflammation of the kidney and ureter occurring in pregnancy.
**hematogenous p.,** pyelitis in which the infection comes from the blood.
**hemorrhagic p.,** that which is attended with hemorrhage.
**suppurative p.,** a form with development of pus which causes abscess of the kidney, or pyonephrosis.
**urogenous p.,** pyelitis in which the infection comes from the urine.

**pyel(o)-** [Gr. *pyelos* pelvis] combining form denoting relationship to the renal pelvis.

**py·elo·cali·ec·ta·sis** (pi″ə-lo-kal″e-ek′tə-sis) [*pyelo-* + *caliectasis*] dilatation of the kidney pelvis and calices.

**py·elo·cys·ti·tis** (pi″ə-lo-sis-ti′tis) [*pyelo-* + *cyst-* + *-itis*] inflammation of the renal pelvis and of the bladder.

**py·elo·flu·o·ros·co·py** (pi″ə-lo-floo-ros′kə-pe) examination of the renal pelvis by means of the fluoroscope.

**py·elo·gram** (pi′ə-lo-gram) [*pyelo-* + *-gram*] a radiograph of the kidney and ureter, especially showing the pelvis of the kidney.
**dragon p.,** bizarre forms in the pyelogram seen in polycystic kidney.

**py·elo·graph** (pi′ə-lo-graf) pyelogram.

**py·elog·ra·phy** (pi″ə-log′rə-fe) [*pyelo-* + *-graphy*] radiography of the renal pelvis and ureter after the structures have been filled with a contrast solution.
**air p.,** pneumopyelography.
**antegrade p.,** that in which the contrast medium is introduced by percutaneous needle puncture into the renal pelvis.
**ascending p.,** retrograde p.
**p. by elimination,** intravenous p.
**excretion p.,** intravenous p.
**intravenous p.,** pyelography in which an intravenous injection is made of a contrast medium which passes quickly into the urine.
**lateral p.,** pyelography in which the patient lies in lateral position with his questionable side next to the film.
**respiration p.,** pyelography with a diphasic film showing the kidney under several phases of the respiratory cycle.
**retrograde p.,** pyelography in which the contrast fluid is injected into the renal pelvis through the ureter.
**wash-out p.,** that in which the radiograph is taken after the kidneys have been filled with a contrast solution and then "washed-out" by water diuresis; this procedure increases the contrast between a normal and a malfunctioning kidney.

**py·elo·il·eo·cu·ta·ne·ous** (pi″ə-lo-il″e-o-ku-ta′ne-əs) pertaining to the renal pelvis, ileum, and skin; see under *anastomosis.*

**py·elo·in·ter·sti·tial** (pi″ə-lo-in″tər-stish′əl) pertaining to the interstitial tissue of the renal pelvis.

**py·elo·li·thot·o·my** (pi″ə-lo-lĭ-thot′ə-me) [*pyelo-* + *lithotomy*] the operation of excising a renal calculus from the pelvis of the kidney.

**py·elom·e·try** (pi″ə-lom′ə-tre) [*pyelo-* + *-metry*] the measurement by tracings of the waves of contraction and relaxation of the renal pelvis, recorded by changes of pressure through a ureteral catheter.

**py·elo·ne·phri·tis** (pi″ə-lo-nə-fri′tis) [*pyelo-* + *nephr-* + *-itis*] [MeSH: Pyelonephritis] inflammation of the kidney and its pelvis because of bacterial infection; it begins in the interstitium and rapidly extends to involve the tubules, glomeruli, and blood vessels.
**acute p.,** pyelonephritis of sudden onset characterized by fever, shaking chills, pain in the costovertebral region or flanks, and symptoms of bladder inflammation.
**chronic p.,** pyelonephritis attributed to cicatricial effects of a previous infection or to recurring or progressive infection. Typically, it is of insidious onset, and occasionally may lead to chronic renal insufficiency.
**emphysematous p.,** a rare, life-threatening complication of acute pyelonephritis, seen in diabetics, in which gas produced by lactose-fermenting bacteria collects within the parenchyma of the kidney, resulting in necrosis.
**contagious bovine p.,** an inflammatory condition of cattle due to infection of the kidneys and urinary tract with *Corynebacterium renale*; characteristics include painful swollen kidneys and thickened inflamed walls throughout the urinary tract with hematuria and pyuria. Other domestic animals occasionally suffer from a similar condition.
**p. of pregnancy,** a renal infection during pregnancy characterized by dilatation of the renal pelvis and the ureters; some degree of ureteric obstruction may be caused by the gravid uterus.
**xanthogranulomatous p.,** a form of chronic pyelonephritis characterized by enlargement and loss of function in the kidney, thickening and adhesion of the perirenal tissue and capsule, destruction of parenchymal tissue, the presence of calculi, and the accumulation of foam cells, granulomas, and abscesses in the medulla. It is frequently associated with infection by *Proteus* spp.

**py·elo·ne·phro·sis** (pi″ə-lo-nə-fro′sis) [*pyelo-* + *nephr-* + *-osis*] any disease of the kidney and its pelvis.

**py·elop·a·thy** (pi″ə-lop′ə-the) [*pyelo-* + *-pathy*] any disease of the renal pelvis.

**py·elo·phle·bi·tis** (pi″ə-lo-flə-bi′tis) [*pyelo-* + *phleb-* + *-itis*] inflammation of the veins of the renal pelvis.

**py·elo·plas·ty** (pi′ə-lo-plas″te) [*pyelo-* + *-plasty*] a plastic operation on the pelvis of the kidney.

**py·elos·co·py** (pi″ə-los′kə-pe) [*pyelo-* + *-scopy*] observation of the kidney pelvis under the fluoroscope after intravenous or retrograde injection of a contrast medium.

**py·elos·to·my** (pi″ə-los′tə-me) [*pyelo-* + *-stomy*] surgical formation of an opening into the renal pelvis to temporarily divert the urine from the ureter.

**py·elot·o·my** (pi″ə-lot′ə-me) [*pyelo-* + *-tomy*] incision of the pelvis of the kidney.

**py·elo·ure·ter·ec·ta·sis** (pi″ə-lo-u-re″tər-ek′tə-sis) dilatation of a renal pelvis and a ureter.

**py·elo·ure·ter·og·ra·phy** (pi″ə-lo-u-re″tər-og′rə-fe) pyelography.

**py·elo·ure·ter·ol·y·sis** (pi″ə-lo-u-re″tər-ol′ə-sis) [*pyelo-* + *uretero-* + *-lysis*] the surgical freeing of fibrous bands or adhesions near the junction of the renal pelvis and ureter.

**py·elo·ure·tero·plas·ty** (pi″ə-lo-u-re′tər-o-plas″te) ureteropyeloplasty.

**py·elo·ve·nous** (pi″ə-lo-ve′nəs) pertaining to the kidney pelvis and renal veins.

**py·em·e·sis** (pi-em′ə-sis) [*pyo-* + *-emesis*] vomiting of purulent matter.

**py·e·mia** (pi-e′me-ə) [*pyo-* + *-emia*] a general septicemia in which secondary foci of suppuration occur and multiple abscesses are formed. The condition is marked by fever, chills, sweating, jaundice, and abscesses in various parts of the body. Called also *metastatic infection.*
**arterial p.,** a form due to the dissemination of septic emboli from the heart.
**cryptogenic p.,** that in which the source of infection is unidentified.
**otogenous p.,** that which originates from inflammation in the ear.
**portal p.,** suppurative pylephlebitis.
**tick p.,** a condition seen in lambs in the British Isles up to the age of three months, in which the bite of the tick *Ixodes ricinus* becomes infected by *Staphylococcus aureus*, sometimes with septicemia or bacteremia that can be fatal.

**py·e·mic** (pi-e′mik) pertaining to or marked by pyemia.

**Py·e·mo·tes** (pi″ə-mo′tez) a genus of parasitic mites; formerly called *Pediculoides. P. ventrico′sus* parasitizes the larvae of insects and is found in the straw of cereals; it can cause a vesiculopapular dermatitis called *grain itch* in humans.

**py·en·ceph·a·lus** (pi″en-səf′ə-ləs) [*py-* + *enkephalos* brain] brain abscess.

**py·e·sis** (pi-e′sis) suppuration.

**py·gal** (pi′gəl) gluteal.

**py·gal·gia** (pi-gal′jə) [*pygo-* + *-algia*] pain in the buttocks.

**pyg·ma·li·on·ism** (pig-ma′le-on-iz″əm) [*Pygmalion,* a Greek sculptor who fell in love with a statue he had carved] the falling in love with an object made by oneself.

**pyg(o)-** [Gr. *pygē* rump] a combining form denoting relationship to the buttocks.

**py·go·amor·phus** (pi″go-ə-mor′fəs) asymmetrical conjoined twins in which the parasite is an amorphous mass attached to the sacral region of the more developed twin.

**py·go·did·y·mus** (pi″go-did′ĭ-məs) [*pygo-* + *-didymus*] a fetus with double hips and pelvis.

**py·gom·e·lus** (pi-gom′ə-ləs) [*pygo-* + Gr. *melos* limb] a fetus with a supernumerary limb or limbs attached to or near the buttock.

**py·gop·a·gus** (pi-gop′ə-gəs) [*pygo-* + *-pagus*] conjoined twins consisting of two nearly complete individuals joined at the sacrum so that the two components are back to back.
**p. parasi′ticus,** asymmetrical conjoined twins in which the parasitic twin is attached to the sacral region of the more developed twin.

**py·gop·a·gy** (pi-gop′ə-je) the condition of being a pygopagus.

**py·go·style** (pi′go-stīl) a flat bone at the end of the vertebral column of birds, representing the union of several vertebrae and serving as a site of attachment for the tail feathers. Called also *plowshare bone.*

**py·ic** (pi′ik) of or pertaining to pus.

**pyk·nic** (pik′nik) [Gr. *pyknos* thick] having a short, thick, stocky build.

**pykn(o)-** [Gr. *pyknos* thick, frequent] a combining form meaning thick, compact, or frequent. Also *pycn(o)-.*

**pyk·no·cyte** (pik″no-sīt) a distorted and contracted, occasionally spiculed erythrocyte normally occurring in small numbers in the full-term infant, but in greater numbers in hemolytic disorders.

**pyk·no·cy·to·sis** (pik″no-si-to′sis) conspicuous increases in the numbers of pyknocytes in the blood.

**pyk·no·dys·os·to·sis** (pik″no-dis″os-to′sis) an autosomal recessive symptom complex consisting of dwarfism, osteopetrosis, partial agenesis of terminal digits of hands and feet, cranial anomalies, frontal and occipital bossing, and hypoplasia of the angle of the mandible.

**pyk•no•ep•i•lep•sy** (pik″no-ep′ĭ-lep″se) former name for absence epilepsy.

**pyk•nom•e•ter** (pik-nom′ə-tər) [*pykno-* + *-meter*] an instrument for determining the specific gravity of fluids.

**pyk•nom•e•try** (pik-nom′ə-tre) measurement by the pyknometer.

**pyk•no•mor•phic** (pik″no-mor′fik) pyknomorphous.

**pyk•no•mor•phous** (pik″no-mor′fəs) [*pykno-* + *morph-* + *-ous*] having the stainable elements compactly arranged; a term applied to certain nerve cells.

**pyk•no•phra•sia** (pik″no-fra′zhə) [*pykno-* + Gr. *phrasis* speech + *-ia*] thickness of speech.

**pyk•no•plas•son** (pik″no-plas′on) [*pykno-* + *plasson*] the protoplasm of a non-nucleated cell in its unexpanded form. Cf. *chasmatoplasson.*

**pyk•no•sis** (pik-no′sis) [Gr. *pyknōsis* condensation] a thickening, especially degeneration of a cell in which the nucleus shrinks in size and the chromatin condenses to a solid, structureless mass or masses.

**pyk•not•ic** (pik-not′ik) [Gr. *pyknōtikos*] 1. serving to close the pores. 2. pertaining to pyknosis.

**Pyle's disease** (pīlz) [Edwin *Pyle,* American physician, 1891–1961] metaphyseal dysplasia; see under *dysplasia.*

**pyle-** [Gr. *pylē* gate] a combining form denoting relationship to the portal vein.

**py•le•phle•bec•ta•sis** (pi″le-flə-bek′tə-sis) [*pyle-* + *phlebectasis*] dilatation of the portal vein.

**py•le•phle•bi•tis** (pi″le-flə-bi′tis) [*pyle-* + *phlebitis*] inflammation of the portal vein; it usually results from intestinal disease.
**adhesive p.,** pylethrombophlebitis.
**suppurative p.,** pylephlebitis with pyemia; called also *portal pyemia.*

**py•le•throm•bo•phle•bi•tis** (pi″le-throm″bo-flə-bi′tis) [*pyle-* + *thrombophlebitis*] thrombosis and inflammation of the portal vein.

**py•le•throm•bo•sis** (pi″le-throm-bo′sis) thrombosis of the portal vein.

**py•lic** (pi′lik) [Gr. *pylē* gate] portal (def. 2).

**py•lon** (pi′lon) a temporary artificial leg.

**py•lo•ral•gia** (pi″lo-ral′jə) [*pylor-* + *-algia*] pain in the region of the pylorus.

**py•lo•rec•to•my** (pi″lo-rek′tə-me) [*pylor-* + *-ectomy*] excision of the pylorus.

**py•lo•ric** (pi-lor′ik) pertaining to the pylorus or to the pyloric part of the stomach (pars pylorica ventriculi).

**py•lo•ri•ste•no•sis** (pi-lor″ĭ-stə-no′sis) pyloric stenosis.

**py•lo•ri•tis** (pi″lor-i′tis) inflammation of the pylorus.

**pylor(o)-** [L. *pylorus,* q.v.] a combining form denoting relationship to the pylorus.

**py•lo•ro•di•o•sis** (pi-lo″ro-di-o′sis) [*pyloro-* + Gr. *diōsis* pushing asunder] dilation of a stricture of the pylorus with the finger.

**py•lo•ro•du•o•de•ni•tis** (pi-lor″o-du″o-de-ni′tis) inflammation of the pyloric and duodenal mucosa.

**py•lo•ro•gas•trec•to•my** (pi-lo″ro-gas-trek′tə-me) excision of the pylorus.

**py•lo•ro•my•ot•o•my** (pi-lor″o-mi-ot′ə-me) the operation for congenital stenosis of the pylorus, performed by longitudinally incising the thickened serosa and muscularis down to the mucosa; called also *Fredet-Ramstedt operation.*

**py•lo•ro•plas•ty** (pi-lor′o-plas″te) [*pyloro-* + *-plasty*] incision of the pylorus and reconstruction of the pyloric channel to relieve pyloric obstruction or to accelerate gastric emptying after truncal or selective vagotomy in treatment of duodenal ulcer.
**double p.,** posterior pyloromyotomy combined with the Heineke-Mikulicz pyloroplasty.
**Finney p.,** reconstruction of the pyloric channel by means of a longitudinal incision through the pylorus and adjacent walls of the stomach and duodenum and the establishment of an inverted U-shaped anastomosis between the stomach and duodenum.
**Heineke-Mikulicz p.,** reconstruction of the pyloric channel by incising the pylorus longitudinally and suturing the incision transversely.

**py•lo•ros•co•py** (pi″lor-os′kə-pe) [*pyloro-* + *-scopy*] inspection of the pylorus with an endoscope.

**py•lo•ro•spasm** (pi-lor′o-spaz″əm) [*pyloro-* + *spasm*] spasm of the pylorus or of the pyloric portion of the stomach.
**congenital p.,** spasm of the pylorus in infants due to prenatal conditions.
**reflex p.,** pylorospasm due to extragastric conditions.

**py•lo•ro•ste•no•sis** (pi-lor″o-stə-no′sis) pyloristenosis.

**py•lo•ros•to•my** (pi″lor-os′to-me) [*pyloro-* + *-stomy*] surgical formation of an opening through the abdominal wall into the stomach near the pylorus.

**py•lo•rot•o•my** (pi″lor-ot′o-me) [*pyloro-* + *-tomy*] surgical incision of the pylorus.

**py•lo•rus** (pi-lor′əs) [Gr. *pyloros,* from *pylē* gate + *ouros* guard] [TA] [MeSH: Pylorus] the distal aperture of the stomach surrounded by a strong band of circular muscle, and through which the stomach contents are emptied into the duodenum. It is variously used to mean pyloric part of the stomach, pyloric antrum, pyloric canal, pyloric opening, and pyloric sphincter.

**py(o)-** [Gr. *pyon* pus] a combining form denoting relationship to pus.

**pyo•ar•thro•sis** (pi″o-ahr-thro′sis) acute suppurative arthritis.

**pyo•blen•nor•rhea** (pi″o-blen″o-re′ə) suppurative blennorrhea.

**pyo•ca•lix** (pi″o-ka′liks) the presence of pus in a calix of the renal pelvis.

**pyo•cele** (pi′o-sēl) [*pyo-* + *-cele*[1]] distention of a cavity or tube with pus due to retention; as an accumulation of pus in the scrotum.

**pyo•ce•lia** (pi″o-se′le-ə) [*pyo-* + *celi-* + *-ia*] pus in the abdominal cavity.

**pyo•ceph•a•lus** (pi″o-sef′ə-ləs) [*pyo-* + *-cephalus*] brain abscess.

**pyo•che•zia** (pi″o-ke′ze-ə) [*pyo-* + Gr. *chezein* to defecate + *-ia*] presence of pus in the feces.

**pyo•cin** (pi′o-sin) [*pyo-* + *-cin* from L. caedere to kill] a protein bacteriocin produced by certain strains of *Pseudomonas aeruginosa.*

**pyo•coc•cic** (pi″o-kok′sik) pertaining to or produced by pus-forming cocci.

**pyo•coc•cus** (pi″o-kok′əs) any pus-forming coccus.

**pyo•col•po•cele** (pi″o-kol′po-sēl) [*pyo-* + *colpo-* + *-cele*[1]] a tumor of the vagina containing pus.

**pyo•col•pos** (pi″o-kol′pos) [*pyo-* + Gr. *kolpos* vagina] a collection of pus within the vagina.

**pyo•cy•an•ic** (pi″o-si-an′ik) pertaining to blue pus, or to *Pseudomonas aeruginosa (P. pyocyanea).*

**pyo•cy•a•nin** (pi″o-si′ə-nin) [*pyo-* + *cyan-* + *-in* chemical suffix] a blue-green pigment produced by *Pseudomonas aeruginosa;* it gives the color to blue pus.

**pyo•cy•a•no•gen•ic** (pi″o-si″ə-no-jen′ik) producing pyocyanin.

**pyo•cy•a•no•sis** (pi″o-si″ə-no′sis) any disease due to infection with *Pseudomonas aeruginosa (P. pyocyanea).*

**pyo•cyst** (pi′o-sist) [*pyo-* + *cyst*] a cyst containing pus.

**pyo•cys•tis** (pi″o-sis′tis) pus in the urinary bladder.

**pyo•der•ma** (pi″o-der′mə) [*pyo-* + *derma*] [MeSH: Pyoderma] any purulent skin disease. Called also *pyodermia.*
**chancriform p., p. chancrifor′me faci′ei,** an eroded, ulcerated, nodular, solitary lesion with a rolled edge, closely resembling a syphilitic chancre, and generally occurring in association with regional lymphadenopathy. The lesion, which usually involutes and heals with scarring, is most often located on the face, especially near the eyes, although some genital lesions have been reported.
**p. facia′le,** an acute, localized skin disease occurring on the face of young women and preadolescent girls, usually in the absence of acne, and characterized by the presence of intense erythema and the development of numerous abscesses and cysts, with the for-

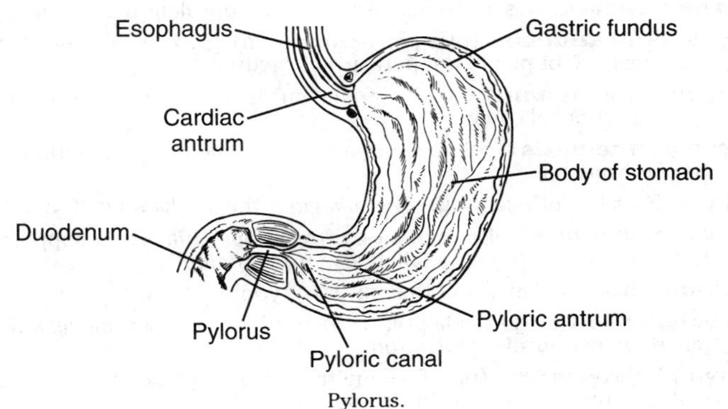

Pylorus.

mation of sinus tracts between deep-seated lesions, which may heal with severe scarring if untreated.
**p. gangreno′sum,** a rapidly evolving, idiopathic, chronic debilitating skin disease that usually accompanies a systemic disease, especially chronic ulcerative colitis, and is characterized by irregular, boggy, blue-red ulcers with undermined borders surrounding purulent necrotic bases.
**juvenile p.,** a skin disease of unknown etiology seen in puppies, particularly shorthaired breeds; characteristics include pustular lesions of the skin of the face, head, and sometimes other parts of the body with fever and lymphadenopathy. The commonly seen submandibular lymphadenopathy gives the disease its nickname *puppy strangles.* Called also *juvenile cellulitis.*
**malignant p.,** a destructive, progressive ulcerative and suppurative skin disease located predominantly on the head and neck region and trunk, which may develop spontaneously or at the site of trauma and enlarge peripherally, and sometimes associated with neurological disturbances.
**p. ve′getans,** see under *dermatitis.*

**pyo·der·mia** (pi″o-der′me-ə) pyoderma.

**pyo·fe·cia** (pi″o-fe′se-ə) pus in the feces.

**pyo·gen·e·sis** (pi″o-jen′ə-sis) [*pyo-* + *-genesis*] the formation of pus; pyopoiesis.

**pyo·gen·ic** (pi″o-jen′ik) producing pus; pyopoietic.

**py·og·e·nous** (pi-oj′ə-nəs) caused by pus.

**pyo·he·mia** (pi″o-he′me-ə) pyemia.

**pyo·he·mo·tho·rax** (pi″o-he″mo-thor′aks) [*pyo-* + *hemothorax*] a collection of pus and blood in the pleural space.

**pyo·hy·dro·ne·phro·sis** (pi″o-hi″dro-nə-fro′sis) the accumulation of pus and urine in the kidney.

**py·oid** (pi′oid) [*pyo-* + *-oid*] 1. resembling pus. 2. a puslike substance from raw or granulating surfaces, but free from bacteria and nontoxic.

**pyo·me·tra** (pi″o-me′trə) [*pyo-* + *metra*] an accumulation of pus within the uterus.

**pyo·me·tri·tis** (pi″o-mə-tri′tis) purulent inflammation of the uterus.

**pyo·me·tri·um** (pi″o-me′tre-əm) pyometra.

**pyo·my·o·ma** (pi″o-mi-o′mə) a leiomyoma that has undergone suppuration.

**pyo·myo·si·tis** (pi″o-mi″o-si′tis) [*pyo-* + *myositis*] an acute bacterial infection of skeletal muscle, usually seen in the tropics, especially in Africa and less often in South America and Asia, which occurs spontaneously without other foci of infection. It is most commonly caused by *Staphylococcus aureus,* and is characterized by suppuration followed by abscess formation within the fascial covering of the affected muscle(s). Called also *spontaneous bacterial myositis* and *tropical p.*
**tropical p.,** pyomyositis.

**pyo·ne·phri·tis** (pi″o-nə-fri′tis) purulent inflammation of the kidney.

**pyo·neph·ro·li·thi·a·sis** (pi″o-nef″ro-lĭ-thi′ə-sis) [*pyo-* + *nephrolithiasis*] the presence of stones and pus in the kidney.

**pyo·neph·ro·sis** (pi″o-nə-fro′sis) [*pyo-* + *nephrosis*] suppurative destruction of the parenchyma of the kidney, with total or almost complete loss of renal function. Called also *nephropyosis.*

**pyo·ne·phrot·ic** (pi″o-nə-frot′ik) pertaining to or characterized by pyonephrosis.

**pyo·ova·ri·um** (pi″o-o-va′re-əm) abscess of an ovary.

**Pyo·pen** (pi′o-pen) trademark for a preparation of carbenicillin disodium.

**pyo·peri·car·di·tis** (pi″o-per″ĭ-kahr-di′tis) purulent pericarditis.

**pyo·peri·car·di·um** (pi″o-per″ĭ-kahr′de-əm) [*pyo-* + *pericardium*] the presence of pus in the pericardial cavity.

**pyo·peri·to·ne·um** (pi″o-per″ĭ-to-ne′əm) [*pyo-* + *peritoneum*] pus in the peritoneal cavity.

**pyo·peri·to·ni·tis** (pi″o-per″ĭ-to-ni′tis) purulent inflammation of the peritoneum.

**pyo·pha·gia** (pi″o-fa′jə) [*pyo-* + *-phagia*] the swallowing of pus.

**py·oph·thal·mia** (pi″of-thal′me-ə) [*py-* + *ophthalmia*] a suppurative condition of the eye; called also *pyophthalmitis.*

**py·oph·thal·mi·tis** (pi″of-thəl-mi′tis) pyophthalmia.

**pyo·phy·lac·tic** (pi″o-fi-lak′tik) [*pyo-* + *phylactic*] serving as a defense against purulent infection.

**pyo·phy·so·me·tra** (pi″o-fi″so-me′trə) [*pyo-* + *physo-* + *metra*] a collection of pus and gas in the uterus.

**pyo·pla·nia** (pi″o-pla′ne-ə) [*pyo-* + Gr. *planē* wandering] extension of pus from one part to another.

**pyo·pneu·mo·cho·le·cys·ti·tis** (pi″o-noo″mo-ko″le-sis-ti′tis) [*pyo-* + *pneumo-* + *cholecyst* + *-itis*] distention of the gallbladder with pus and gas.

**pyo·pneu·mo·cyst** (pi″o-noo′mo-sist) [*pyo-* + *pneumo-* + *cyst*] a cyst containing pus and gas.

**pyo·pneu·mo·hep·a·ti·tis** (pi″o-noo″mo-hep″ə-ti′tis) abscess of the liver with pus and gas in the abscess cavity.

**pyo·pneu·mo·peri·car·di·um** (pi″o-noo″mo-per″ĭ-kahr′de-əm) [*pyo-* + *pneumo-* + *pericardium*] the presence of pus and gas or air in the pericardial cavity.

**pyo·pneu·mo·peri·to·ne·um** (pi″o-noo″mo-per″ĭ-to-ne′əm) the presence of pus and gas in the peritoneal cavity.

**pyo·pneu·mo·peri·to·ni·tis** (pi″o-noo″mo-per″ĭ-to-ni′tis) [*pyo-* + *pneumo-* + *peritonitis*] peritonitis with the presence of pus and gas in the peritoneal cavity.

**pyo·pneu·mo·tho·rax** (pi″o-noo″mo-thor′aks) [*pyo-* + *pneumothorax*] a collection of pus and air or gas in the pleural cavity. Called also *pneumoempyema* and *pneumopyothorax.*

**pyo·poi·e·sis** (pi″o-poi-e′sis) [*pyo-* + *-poiesis*] the formation of pus; pyogenesis.

**pyo·poi·et·ic** (pi″o-poi-et′ik) producing pus; pyogenic.

**py·op·ty·sis** (pi-op′tĭ-sis) [*pyo-* + Gr. *ptysis* spitting] spitting of purulent matter.

**pyo·py·elec·ta·sis** (pi″o-pi″ə-lek′tə-sis) [*pyo-* + *pyelectasis*] dilatation of the renal pelvis with purulent fluid.

**py·or·rhea** (pi″o-re′ə) [*pyo-* + *-rrhea*] 1. periodontitis (def. 1). 2. marginal periodontitis.
**p. alveola′ris,** marginal periodontitis.
**Schmutz p.,** marginal periodontitis.

**py·or·rhe·al** (pi″o-re′əl) pertaining to or characterized by periodontitis or marginal periodontitis.

**pyo·ru·bin** (pi″o-roo′bin) a bright-red, water-soluble, nonfluorescent pigment produced by some strains of *Pseudomonas aeruginosa.*

**pyo·sal·pin·gi·tis** (pi″o-sal″pin-ji′tis) [*pyo-* + *salping-* + *-itis*] purulent salpingitis.

**pyo·sal·pin·go·ooph·o·ri·tis** (pi″o-sal-ping″go-o″of-ə-ri′tis) inflammation of the ovary and oviduct, with the formation and accumulation of pus.

**pyo·sal·pin·go·oo·the·ci·tis** (pi″o-sal-ping″go-o″o-the-si′tis) pyosalpingo-oophoritis.

**pyo·sal·pinx** (pi″o-sal′pinks) [*pyo-* + *salpinx*] a collection of pus in an oviduct.

**pyo·scle·ro·sis** (pi″o-sklə-ro′sis) an inflammatory, purulent sclerosis.

**pyo·sep·ti·ce·mia** (pi″o-sep″tĭ-se′me-ə) pyemia combined with septicemia.

**pyo·sper·mia** (pi″o-sper′me-ə) [*pyo-* + *sperm-* + *-ia*] presence of pus in the semen.

**pyo·stat·ic** (pi″o-stat′ik) [*pyo-* + *-static*] 1. arresting suppuration. 2. an agent that arrests the formation of pus.

**pyo·sto·ma·ti·tis** (pi″o-sto″mə-ti′tis) [*pyo-* + *stomatitis*] a suppurative inflammation of the mouth.
**p. ve′getans,** a variant of dermatitis vegetans involving the oral mucosa, sometimes occurring in association with ulcerative colitis and other gastrointestinal disturbances. The primary lesions are miliary abscesses with a tendency to form groups and become proliferative, soft, red, folded, and verrucous, sometimes spreading over the entire oral cavity. They may remain confined to the mouth or may coexist with typical dermatitis vegetans.

**pyo·tho·rax** (pi″o-tho′raks) [*pyo-* + *thorax*] empyema (def. 2).

**pyo·um·bil·i·cus** (pi″o-əm-bil′ĭ-kəs) infection of the umbilicus.

**pyo·ura·chus** (pi″o-u′rə-kəs) the presence of pus in the urachus.

**pyo·ure·ter** (pi″o-u-re′tər) [*pyo-* + *ureter*] an accumulation of pus in a ureter.

**pyo·ve·sic·u·lo·sis** (pi″o-və-sik″u-lo′sis) an accumulation of pus in the seminal vesicles.

**pyo·xan·thine** (pi″o-zan′thin) a brownish red pigment derivable by oxidation from pyocyanin.

**pyo·xan·those** (pi″o-zan′thōs) [*pyo-* + Gr. *xanthos* yellow] a yellow pigment produced by the oxidation of pyocyanin in blue pus when exposed to air.

**pyr·a·brom** (pir′ə-brom) an antihistaminic, $C_{24}H_{30}BrN_7O_3$.

**py·ra·cin** (pi′rə-sin) a derivative of pyridoxine.

**Pyr·a·lis** (pir'ə-lis) a genus of widely distributed small moths. *P. farina'lis* is a meal moth that acts as a host for parasites such as tapeworms of the genus *Hymenolepis.*

**pyr·a·mid** (pir'ə-mid) [Gr. *pyramis*] a pointed or cone-shaped structure or part; called also *pyramis* [TA]. The term is often used alone to indicate the pyramid of the medulla oblongata.
**p. of cerebellum,** pyramis vermis.
**p. of Ferrein,** pars radiata lobuli corticalis renis.
**p's of kidney,** pyramides renales; see under *pyramis.*
**Lalouette's p.,** lobus pyramidalis glandulae thyroideae.
**p. of light,** see under *cone.*
**Malacarne's p.,** the posterior end of the pyramid of the vermis.
**p's of Malpighi,** pyramides renales; see under *pyramis.*
**p. of medulla oblongata,** pyramis medullae oblongatae.
**petrous p.,** pars petrosa ossis temporalis.
**renal p's,** pyramides renales; see under *pyramis.*
**p. of temporal bone,** pars petrosa ossis temporalis.
**p. of thyroid,** lobus pyramidalis glandulae thyroideae.
**p. of tympanum,** eminentia pyramidalis.
**p. of vermis,** pyramis vermis.
**p. of vestibule,** pyramis vestibuli.

**py·ram·i·dal** (pĭ-ram'ĭ-dəl) [L. *pyramidalis*] shaped like a pyramid; see also under *tract.*

**py·ram·i·da·le** (pĭ-ram″ĭ-da'le) [L.] os triquetrum.

**py·ram·i·da·lis** (pĭ-ram″ĭ-da'lis) [L.] pyramidal; see under *musculus.*

**py·ram·i·des** (pĭ-ram'ĭ-dēz) [Gr.] plural of *pyramis.*

**py·ram·i·dot·o·my** (pĭ″ram-ĭ-dot'ə-me) section of the pyramidal tract.

**pyr·a·mis** (pir'ə-mis) pl. *pyra'mides* [Gr.] [TA] pyramid; in anatomical nomenclature, a part or structure resembling a pyramid.
**p. bul'bi,** TA alternative for *p. medullae oblongatae.*
**pyra'mides Malpi'ghii,** pyramides renales.
**p. medul'lae oblonga'tae** [TA], pyramid of medulla oblongata: either of two rounded masses, one on either side of the anterior median fissure of the medulla oblongata, composed of motor fibers (pyramidal tract) from the cerebral cortex to the spinal cord and medulla oblongata. Called also *p. bulbi* [TA alternative].
**pyra'mides rena'les** [TA], **pyra'mides rena'les [Malpi'ghii],** renal pyramids: the conical masses that make up the medullary substance of the kidney; they contain the loops of Henle, the collecting ducts, and the arteriolae rectae renis.
**p. ver'mis** [TA], pyramid of vermis: the part of the vermis of the cerebellum between the tuber vermis and the uvula.
**p. vesti'buli** [TA], pyramid of vestibule: the triangular-shaped anterior end of the vestibular crest.

**py·ran** (pi'ran) a heterocyclic compound, the ring structure that forms the basis of the pyranoses.

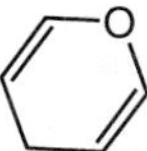


**pyr·a·nose** (pir'ə-nōs) any sugar containing a pyran ring structure, a cyclic form that ketoses and aldoses may take in solution. See also individual sugars, e.g., *glucopyranose.*

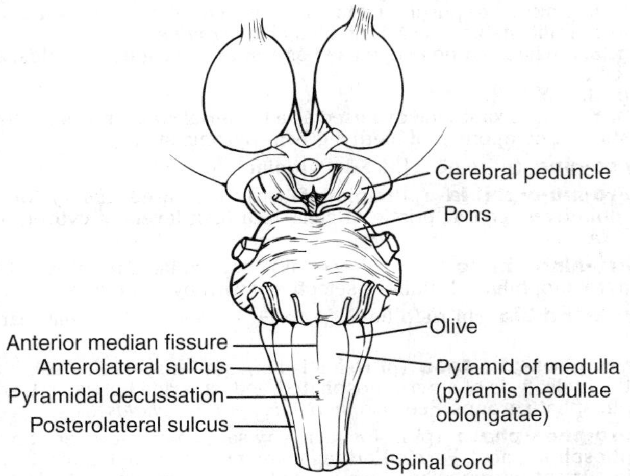


Pyramis medullae oblongatae (pyramid of medulla) in an anterior (inferior) view of the brain stem.

**py·ran·o·side** (pĭ-ran'o-sīd) a glycoside in which the sugar is in pyranose configuration.

**py·ran·tel** (pĭ-ran'təl) [MeSH: Pyrantel] a broad-spectrum anthelmintic, effective against pinworms and roundworms in humans, domestic animals, and horses; it acts as a depolarizing neuromuscular blocking agent, producing spastic paralysis of the parasite. Usually seen as the pamoate salt.
**p. pamoate** [USP], the pamoate salt of pyrantel, used in humans, dogs, cats, and horses for treatment of ascariasis and enterobiasis, administered orally.
**p. tartrate,** the tartrate salt of pyrantel, having the same actions as the pamoate salt.

**py·ran·yl** (pi'ran-əl) the radical $C_5H_5O-$, derived from pyran by removal of hydrogen.

**py·ra·thi·a·zine hy·dro·chlo·ride** (pir″ə-thi'ə-zēn) an antihistamine.

**pyr·a·zin·amide** (pir″ə-zin'ə-mīd) [USP] [MeSH: Pyrazinamide] an antibacterial derived from nicotinic acid, used as a tuberculostatic, administered orally.

**py·ra·zine** (pĭ'rə-zēn) an aromatic compound comprising a six-membered ring with nitrogen atoms at positions 1 and 4; it is a component of the folates and of the isoalloxazine ring system of flavins.

**pyr·az·o·lone** (pir-az'o-lōn) any of a class of nonsteroidal anti-inflammatory agents that have been used in the treatment of arthritis and other musculoskeletal and joint disorders.

**py·rec·tic** (pi-rek'tik) [Gr. *pyrektikos* feverish] 1. febrile. 2. pyrogen.

**py·rene** (pi'rēn) a carcinogenic polycyclic hydrocarbon, $C_{16}H_{10}$, used in biochemical research.

**Py·re·no·chae·ta** (pi″rə-no-ke'tə) a genus of Fungi Imperfecti of the form-class Coelomycetes, widely found on plants and in the soil. *P. ro'meroi* has been isolated from cases of eumycotic mycetoma.

**py·re·noid** (pi'rə-noid) [Gr. *pyrēn* fruit stone + *-oid*] one of the proteinaceous refringent bodies found closely associated with the chloroplasts of most phytoflagellates; involved in the synthesis and storage of polysaccharide.

**py·re·nol·y·sis** (pi″rə-nol'ĭ-sis) [Gr. *pyrēn* fruit stone + *-lysis*] the breaking down of the nucleolus of a cell.

**py·re·ther·a·py** (pi″rə-ther'ə-pe) [Gr. *pyr* fever + *therapy*] pyretotherapy.

**py·reth·rin** (pi-reth'rin) either of two esters, *pyrethrin I* and *pyrethrin II,* found in the flowers of certain species of *Chrysanthemum,* used alone or in combination with piperonyl butoxide as an insecticide and topical pediculicide. See also *pyrethrum extract,* under *extract.*

**py·reth·roid** (pi-reth'roid) any of a group of growth regulators, analogous to insect juvenile hormones, that interfere with the development of insect larvae; used in the control of insects that are harmful in the adult stage.

**py·re·thron** (pi'rə-thron) a neutral ester from pyrethrum.

**Py·re·thrum** (pi-re'thrəm) [MeSH: Pyrethrum] former genus name applied to certain plants of genus *Chrysanthemum* that are sources of pyrethrins.

**py·re·thrum** (pi-re'thrəm) [Gr. *pyrethron*] [MeSH: Pyrethrum] the species of *Chrysanthemum* that contain pyrethrins.

**py·ret·ic** (pi-ret'ik) [Gr. *pyretos* fever] 1. febrile. 2. pyrogen.

**pyret(o)-** [Gr. *pyretos* fever] a combining form denoting relationship to fever.

**py·ret·o·gen** (pi-ret'o-jən) pyrogen.

**py·re·to·gen·e·sis** (pi″rə-to-jen'ə-sis) [*pyreto-* + *-genesis*] the origin and causation of fever.

**py·re·to·ge·net·ic** (pi″rə-to-jə-net'ik) pyrogenic.

**py·re·to·gen·ic** (pi″rə-to-jen'ik) pyrogenic.

**py·re·tog·e·nous** (pi″rə-toj'ə-nəs) 1. caused by high body temperature. 2. pyrogenic.

**py·re·tog·ra·phy** (pi″rə-tog'rə-fe) [*pyreto-* + *-graphy*] a description of fever.

**py·re·tol·o·gy** (pi″rə-tol'ə-je) [*pyreto-* + *-logy*] the sum of what is known regarding fevers; the science of fevers.

**py·re·tol·y·sis** (pi″rə-tol'ĭ-sis) [*pyreto-* + *-lysis*] 1. reduction of fever. 2. lysis which is hastened by fever.

**py·re·to·ther·a·py** (pi″rə-to-ther'ə-pe) [*pyreto-* + *therapy*] 1. treatment of a disease by raising the patient's temperature, especially by means of injecting fever-producing vaccines. 2. the treatment of fever.

**py·re·to·ty·pho·sis** (pi″rə-to-ti-fo′sis) [*pyreto-* + Gr. *typhōsis* delirium] the delirium of fever.

**py·rex·ia** (pi-rek′se-ə) pl. *pyrex′iae* [Gr. *pyressein* to be feverish] fever.
**Pel-Ebstein p.**, see under *fever.*

**py·rex·i·al** (pi-rek′se-əl) febrile.

**py·rex·i·o·gen·ic** (pi-rek″se-o-jen′ik) pyrogenic.

**Pyr·i·ben·za·mine** (pir″ĭ-ben′zə-mēn) trademark for preparations of tripelennamine.

**pyr·i·dine** (pir′ĭ-dēn) a toxic, colorless, liquid hydrocarbon comprising a substituted benzene ring, $C_5H_5N$, usually derived from coal tar; it is used as a laboratory and industrial intermediate.

**Py·rid·i·um** (pi-rid′e-əm) trademark for preparations of phenazopyridine hydrochloride.

**pyr·i·do·stig·mine bro·mide** (pir″ĭ-do-stig′mēn) [USP] [MeSH: Pyridostigmine Bromide] a cholinergic, used in the treatment of myasthenia gravis and as an antidote for nondepolarizing muscle relaxants, such as curariform drugs, administered orally and parenterally.

**pyr·i·dox·al** (pir″ĭ-dok′səl) [MeSH: Pyridoxal] one of the forms of vitamin $B_6$ (q.v.).
**p. phosphate,** pyridoxal phosphorylated at the hydroxymethyl group of C-5; it is the prosthetic group of many enzymes involved in amino acid transformations.

**pyr·i·dox·amine** (pir″ĭ-doks′ə-mēn) [MeSH: Pyridoxamine] one of the three active forms of vitamin $B_6$.

**pyr·i·dox·ic ac·id** (pir″ĭ-dok′sik) [MeSH: Pyridoxic Acid] oxidation product of pyridoxal, the principal urinary excretion product of vitamin $B_6$.

**pyr·i·dox·ine** (pēr″ĭ-dok′sēn) [MeSH: Pyridoxine] one of the forms of vitamin $B_6$ (q.v.).
**p. hydrochloride** [USP], the hydrochloride salt of pyridoxine, used in the prophylaxis and treatment of vitamin $B_6$ deficiency. It has also been used in neuromuscular and neurological diseases, in dermatoses, and in the management of nausea and vomiting of pregnancy and irradiation sickness.

**pyr·i·form** (pir′ĭ-form) piriform.

**py·ril·amine** (pə-ril′ə-mēn) [MeSH: Pyrilamine] an ethylenediamine derivative with antihistaminic, sedative, and hypnotic actions.
**p. maleate** [USP], the maleate salt of pyrilamine, used as an antihistaminic and as a sedative and hypnotic; administered orally.
**p. tannate,** the tannate salt of pyrilamine, used as an antihistaminic in combination antihistamine-decongestant preparations; administered orally.

**pyr·i·meth·amine** (pir″ĭ-meth′ə-mēn) [USP] [MeSH: Pyrimethamine] a folic acid antagonist, used as an antimalarial, especially for suppressive prophylaxis, and also used concomitantly with a sulfonamide in the treatment of toxoplasmosis, administered orally.

**py·rim·i·dine** (pə-rim′ĭ-dēn) an organic compound, a metadiazine, $C_4H_4N_2$, which is the fundamental form of the pyrimidine bases. These are mostly oxy or amino derivatives, for example, 2,4-dioxypyrimidine is uracil, 2-oxy-4-aminopyrimidine is cytosine, and 2,4-dioxy-5-methylpyrimidine is thymine. Some of these are constituents of nucleic acid (uracil, thymine, and cytosine). See illustration at *base.*

**py·rim·i·dine-nu·cleo·side phos·phor·y·lase** (pə-rim′ĭ-dēn noo′kle-o-sīd″ fos-for′ə-lās) [EC 2.4.2.2] an enzyme of the transferase class that catalyzes the cleavage of pyrimidine nucleosides to form pyrimidines and ribose 1-phosphates in the degradation of nucleotides and nucleic acids.

**pyr·i·thi·amine** (pir″ĭ-thi′ə-mēn) [MeSH: Pyrithiamine] a synthetic compound which by metabolic competition can cause symptoms of thiamine deficiency.

**pyr(o)-** [Gr. *pyr* fire] 1. a combining form denoting relationship to fire or heat. 2. in chemistry, a prefix meaning produced by heating. 3. in inorganic chemistry, a prefix indicating a dimeric acid anhydride, e.g., pyrophosphoric acid.

**py·ro·bo·rate** (pi-ro-bor′āt) any salt of pyroboric acid.

**py·ro·bo·ric ac·id** (pi″ro-bor′ik) a dimer of boric acid, $H_2B_4O_7$, produced by heating boric acid. Called also *tetraboric acid.*

**py·ro·cat·e·chin** (pi″ro-kat′ə-kin) pyrocatechol.

**py·ro·cat·e·chol** (pi″ro-kat′ə-kol) a compound comprising the aromatic portion in the synthesis of endogenous catecholamines; it is obtained by distilling catechu, etc., or produced synthetically, and has been used as a topical antiseptic and as a reagent. Called also *catechol* and *pyrocatechin.*

**py·ro·dex·trin** (pi″ro-dek′strin) dextrin.

**py·ro·gal·lic ac·id** (pi″ro-gal′ik) pyrogallol.

**py·ro·gal·lol** (pi″ro-gal′ol) [MeSH: Pyrogallol] a poisonous acid, derived from gallic acid, and used externally as an antimicrobial and irritant; it is also used as a reagent. Called also *pyrogallic acid.*

**py·ro·gen** (pi′ro-jən) [*pyro-* + *-gen*] a fever-producing substance. Called also *pyretogen, pyretic,* and *pyrectic.*
**bacterial p.,** a fever-producing agent of bacterial origin; endotoxin.
**endogenous p.,** fever-producing subtances produced by the macrophages or other cells in response to infection or to events inducing cell-mediated immunity; included are interleukin-1 and tumor necrosis factor.
**exogenous p's,** fever-producing agents of external origin, e.g., bacterial endotoxins and other microbial products, antigen-antibody complexes, viruses and synthetic polynucleotides, incompatible blood and blood products, and androgen breakdown products such as etiocholanone; the action is mediated by endogenous pyrogen.
**leukocytic p.,** interleukin-1.

**py·ro·ge·net·ic** (pi″ro-jə-net′ik) pyrogenic.

**py·ro·gen·ic** (pi″ro-jen′ik) [*pyro-* + *-genic*] causing fever. Called also *febricant, febrifacient, pyretogenic, pyretogenous,* and *pyrogenetic.*

**py·rog·e·nous** (pi-roj′ə-nəs) pyrogenic.

**py·ro·glob·u·lin** (pi″ro-glob′u-lin) [*pyro-* + *globulin*] a monoclonal immunoglobulin that precipitates irreversibly upon heating to 56°C (as opposed to Bence Jones proteins, which precipitate but redissolve on cooling).

**py·ro·glob·u·lin·emia** (pi″ro-glob″u-lin-e′me-ə) the presence of pyroglobulin in the blood, occurring most frequently in multiple myeloma, Waldenström's macroglobulinemia, and other lymphoproliferative disorders but also occasionally without known associated disease.

**py·ro·glu·ta·mate** (pi″ro-gloo′tə-māt) 5-oxoproline.

**py·ro·glu·tam·ic ac·id** (pi″ro-gloo-tam′ik) 5-oxoproline.

**py·ro·glu·tam·ic·ac·id·uria** (pi″ro-gloo-tam″ik-as″ĭ-du′re-ə) 5-oxoprolinuria.

**py·ro·lag·nia** (pi″ro-lag′ne-ə) [*pyro-* + Gr. *lagneia* lust] sexual gratification from witnessing or making fires.

**py·ro·lig·ne·ous** (pi″ro-lig′ne-əs) [*pyro-* + *ligneous*] pertaining to the destructive distillation of wood.

**Py·ro·lite** (pi′ro-līt) trademark for a kit for the preparation of technetium Tc 99m (pyro- and trimeta-) phosphates.

**py·rol·y·sis** (pi-rol′ĭ-sis) [*pyro-* + *-lysis*] decomposition of organic substances under the influence of a rise in temperature.

**Py·ro·lyte** (pi′ro-līt) trademark for a type of pyrolytic carbon.

**py·ro·ma·nia** (pi″ro-ma′ne-ə) [*pyro-* + *-mania*] [DSM-IV] an impulse control disorder characterized by the compulsion to set or watch fires in the absence of monetary or other gain, the act being preceded by tension or arousal and resulting in pleasure or relief.
**erotic p.,** pyrolagnia.

**py·rom·e·ter** (pi-rom′ə-tər) [*pyro-* + *-meter*] an instrument for measuring the intensity of heat, especially for very high temperatures which cannot be measured with a mercury thermometer.

**py·rone** (pi′rōn) a principle found in opium, from which several other constituents are derived by substitution.

**py·ro·nin** (pi′ro-nin) any of several basic xanthene dyes ranging from pink-red to purple-red in color, used as histological stains and as specific stains for RNA. Spelled also *pyronine.*
**p. B,** a basic xanthene dye used as a stain for bacteria, molds, and RNA.
**p. G,** p. Y.
**p. Y,** a basic xanthene dye used as a bacterial stain and as the RNA-staining component of methyl green–pyronin stain.

**py·ro·nine** (pi′ro-nēn) [MeSH: Pyronine] pyronin.

**py·ro·nin·o·phil·ia** (pi″ro-nin″o-fil′e-ə) increased affinity for pyronin dyes, characteristic of cells with high levels of cytoplasmic RNA.

**py·ro·nino·phil·ic** (pi″ro-nin″o-fil′ik) 1. pertaining to or exhibiting pyroninophilia. 2. staining selectively with pyronin dyes.

**py·ro·pho·bia** (pi″ro-fo′be-ə) [*pyro-* + *-phobia*] abnormal fear of fire.

**py·ro·phos·pha·tase** (pi″ro-fos′fə-tās) any enzyme that catalyzes the hydrolysis of a pyrophosphate bond, cleaving between the two phosphate groups. See also *inorganic pyrophosphatase.*

**py·ro·phos·phate** (pi″ro-fos′fāt) any salt, anion, or ester of pyrophosphoric acid. Formed during many metabolic reactions, it is an important intermediate because its large free energy of hydrolysis makes the reactions essentially irreversible. The symbol $PP_i$ denotes the uncombined form.

**py·ro·phos·pho·ki·nase** (pi″ro-fos″fo-ki′nās) a term used in the recommended names of the diphosphotransferases.

**py·ro·phos·pho·ric ac·id** (pi″ro-fos-for′ik) the ester-linked dimeric form of phosphoric acid, $H_4P_2O_7$. See also *phosphoric acid.*

**py·ro·phos·pho·trans·fer·ase** (pi″ro-fos″fo-trans′fər-ās) diphosphotransferase.

**py·ro·poi·ki·lo·cy·to·sis** (pi″ro-poi″kĭ-lo-si-to′sis) presence in the blood of numerous bizarre-shaped heat-sensitive poikilocytes.
**hereditary p.,** an autosomal recessive blood disorder in which there are many different types of heat-sensitive poikilocytes and erythrocyte fragments, with severe hemolytic anemia. It resembles severe hereditary elliptocytosis, but there are few if any elliptocytes.

**py·ro·sis** (pi-ro′sis) [Gr. *pyrōsis* burning] heartburn.

**py·rot·ic** (pi-rot′ik) [Gr. *pyrōtikos*] caustic; burning.

**py·roxy·lin** (pi-rok′sə-lin) [*pyr-* + Gr. *xylon* wood] [USP] a product of the action of a mixture of nitric and sulfuric acids on cotton, consisting chiefly of cellulose tetranitrate; a necessary ingredient of collodion. Called also *guncotton, soluble guncotton,* and *nitrocellulose.*

**pyr·ro·caine hy·dro·chlo·ride** (pir′o-kān) a local anesthetic used in dentistry to produce infiltration and nerve block anesthesia.

**pyr·role** (pēr′ol) a toxic, basic heterocyclic compound, or its substituted derivatives; it is obtained in the destructive distillation of various animal substances and used in the manufacture of pharmaceuticals.

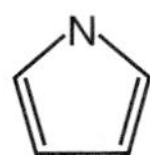


**pyr·rol·i·dine** (pĭ-rol′ĭ-din) a simple base, tetramethylene imine, $(CH_2)_4NH$, which may be obtained from tobacco or prepared from pyrrole.

**pyr·ro·line** (pir′o-lēn) pyrrole in which one of the two double bonds has been hydrogenated.
**$\Delta^1$-p. 5-carboxylate,** a carboxy derivative of pyrroline that acts as an intermediate in the degradation and synthesis of proline.

**1-pyr·ro·line-5-car·box·y·late de·hy·dro·gen·ase** (pir′o-lēn kahr-bok′sə-lāt de-hi′dro-jən-ās) [EC 1.5.1.12] an enzyme of the oxidoreductase class that catalyzes the dehydrogenation of $\Delta^1$-pyrroline 5-carboxylate to glutamate, using $NAD^+$ as an electron acceptor; the reaction is a step in the degradation of proline and excess ornithine. The enzyme can also oxidize the 3-hydroxy derivative of $\Delta^1$-pyrroline 5-carboxylate to form 4-hydroxyglutamate. Deficiency of the enzyme, an autosomal recessive trait, is the cause of hyperprolinemia, type II.

**pyr·ro·line-5-car·box·y·late re·duc·tase** (pir′o-lēn kahr-bok′sə-lāt re-duk′tās) [EC 1.5.1.2] an enzyme of the oxidoreductase class that catalyzes the irreversible reduction of $\Delta^1$-pyrroline 5-carboxylate to proline, using NADPH (or NADH) as an electron donor; the reaction is the final step in the biosynthesis of proline from glutamate or ornithine. The enzyme may also reduce the 3-hydroxy analog of pyrroline 5-carboxylate to form hydroxyproline.

**pyr·ro·line 5-car·boxy·late syn·thase** (pir′o-lēn kahr-bok′sə-lāt sin′thās) a mitochondrial enzyme activity that catalyzes the conversion of glutamate to $\Delta^1$-pyrroline 5-carboxylate, an intermediate in the synthesis of proline. ATP is hydrolyzed in the reaction and NADPH is the electron donor.

**pyr·ro·liz·i·dine** (pĭ-ro-liz′ĭ-dēn) any of a group of alkaloids found in various plants, causing hepatotoxic syndromes in ruminants. Included are jacobine, monocrotaline, retrorsine, senecifoline, and senecine.

**pyr·rol·ni·trin** (pir-ol-ni′trin) [MeSH: Pyrrolnitrin] an antifungal antibiotic isolated from *Pseudomonas pyrrocinia,* effective against *Trichophyton* species.

**pyr·ro·lo·por·phyr·ia** (pir″ə-lo-por-fir′e-ə) acute intermittent porphyria.

**py·ru·vate** (pi′roo-vāt) a salt, ester, or anionic form of pyruvic acid. In biochemistry, the term is used interchangeably with pyruvic acid, even though pyruvate technically refers to the negatively charged ion. Pyruvate is the end product of glycolysis, and it in turn may be converted to lactate or acetyl CoA or to ethanol (as in yeasts).

**py·ru·vate car·box·y·lase** (pi′roo-vāt kahr-bok′sə-lās) [EC 6.4.1.1] [MeSH: Pyruvate Carboxylase] an enzyme of the ligase class that catalyzes the irreversible carboxylation of pyruvate to form oxaloacetate. The enzyme is a mitochondrial protein containing a biotin prosthetic group, requiring $Mg^{2+}$ or $Mn^{2+}$ and acetyl CoA, and occurs in liver but not in muscle. The reaction is necessary for gluconeogenesis from lactate or amino acids forming pyruvate and also provides four-carbon compounds for the tricarboxylic acid cycle. Deficiency of the enzyme, an autosomal recessive trait, causes severe psychomotor retardation and lactic acidosis in infants; there is a particularly severe, rapidly fatal form, in which hyperammonemia, citrullinemia, and hyperlysinemia are also present.

**py·ru·vate de·car·box·y·lase** (pi′roo-vāt de″kahr-bok′sə-lās) [EC 4.1.1.1] [MeSH: Pyruvate Decarboxylase] 1. an enzyme of the lyase class that catalyzes the decarboxylation of 2-keto acids to form aldehydes, part of the anaerobic fermentation pathway that produces ethanol and $CO_2$ from glucose. The enzyme occurs in yeast and requires thiamine pyrophosphate as a cofactor. 2. formerly, used to describe the enzyme now properly called *pyruvate dehydrogenase (lipoamide).*

**py·ru·vate de·hy·dro·gen·ase com·plex** (pi′roo-vāt de-hi′dro-jən-ās kom′pleks) [MeSH: Pyruvate Dehydrogenase Complex] see under *complex.*

**py·ru·vate de·hy·dro·gen·ase (lip·o·am·ide)** (pi′roo-vāt de-hi′dro-jən-ās lip″o-am′īd) [EC 1.2.4.1] an enzyme of the oxidoreductase class that is a component of the multienzyme pyruvate dehydrogenase complex (q.v.). The enzyme catalyzes the oxidative decarboxylation of pyruvate, forming acetyl bound to the cofactor thiamine pyrophosphate; the acetyl is subsequently transferred to lipoamide to form acetyldihydrolipoamide, an intermediate in the overall reaction catalyzed by the complex. Deficiency of the enzyme causes lacticacidemia, ataxia, psychomotor retardation, and sometimes lactic acidosis.

**[py·ru·vate de·hy·dro·gen·ase (lip·o·am·ide)] ki·nase** (pi′roo-vāt de-hi′dro-jən-ās lip″o-am′īd ki′nās) [EC 2.7.1.99] an enzyme of the transferase class that catalyzes the phosphorylation of the decarboxylase component of the pyruvate dehydrogenase complex, inactivating the complex. It is inhibited by pyruvate and ADP.

**[py·ru·vate de·hy·dro·gen·ase (lip·o·am·ide)]-phos·pha·tase** (pi′roo-vāt de-hi′dro-jən-ās lip″o-am′īd fos′fə-tās) [EC 3.1.3.43] an enzyme of the hydrolase class that catalyzes the dephosphorylation of the pyruvate dehydrogenase complex, which activates the complex. Deficiency of the enzyme causes metabolic acidosis with high levels of lactic, pyruvic, and free fatty acids in serum.

**py·ru·vate ki·nase (PK)** (pi′roo-vāt ki′nās) [MeSH: Pyruvate Kinase] an enzyme of the transferase class that catalyzes the transfer of high energy phosphate from phospho*enol*pyruvate to ADP to yield ATP and pyruvate; it is one of two reactions generating ATP in the Embden-Meyerhof pathway (see illustration at *pathway*) and a key regulatory site in this pathway. The enzyme has three distinct isozymes. Deficiency of pyruvate kinase activity in erythrocytes, an autosomal recessive trait, results in hemolytic anemia.

**py·ru·vate ki·nase (PK) deficiency** deficiency of the erythrocytic isozyme of pyruvate kinase, the most common glycolytic enzyme defect in the Embden-Meyerhof pathway; deficient product (ATP) causes chronic hemolytic anemia of widely variable severity. PK deficiency is an autosomal recessive trait and has no distinguishing clinical features from the other hemolytic disorders.

**py·ru·ve·mia** (pi″roo-ve′me-ə) increased pyruvic acid in the blood.

**py·ru·vic ac·id** (pi-roo′vik) [MeSH: Pyruvic Acid] $\alpha$-ketopropionic acid, $CH_3COCOOH$, the end product of the Embden-Meyerhof pathway of glucose metabolism, also produced by the catabolism of several amino acids. Pyruvate can be converted to acetyl coenzyme A, which can enter the tricarboxylic acid cycle for aerobic production of energy or be used for fatty acid synthesis. Energy can be obtained anaerobically by conversion of pyruvate to lactate (which occurs in mammalian muscle tissue) or to ethanol, small organic acids, and many other compounds (microbial fermentations). Pyruvate can also be converted to oxaloacetate, the first step in gluconeogenesis.

**6-py·ru·voyl·tet·ra·hy·drop·ter·in syn·thase** (pi-roo″vo-əl-tet″rə-hi-drop′tər-in sin′thās) an enzyme catalyzing the rate-limiting reaction in the synthesis of tetrahydrobiopterin from guanosine triphosphate. Deficiency of the enzyme, an autosomal recessive trait, causes malignant hyperphenylalaninemia.

**pyr·vin·i·um pam·o·ate** (pir-vin′e-əm) [USP] an anthelmintic that acts by preventing the uptake of exogenous glucose and is administered orally in the treatment of enterobiasis.

**Py·thi·a·ceae** (pith″e-a′se-e) a family of aquatic moldlike organisms of the order Peronosporales, consisting mainly of plant parasites with some saprobes, having an intracellular mycelium and sporangia born singly on branching sporangiophores; it includes a genus pathogenic for animals, *Pythium.*

**pyth·i·o·sis** (pith″e-o′sis) infection by *Pythium insidiosum,* primarily affecting horses and mules but also seen in dogs and cattle, in India, Indonesia, Europe, and the southern United States; characteristics include formation of subcutaneous abscesses that enlarge until the overlying skin is destroyed, leaving large raw surfaces. It is often confused with cutaneous habronemiasis because of the close clinical similarity between the two conditions. Called also *bur-*

*satti, bursautee, hyphomycosis destruens equi, leeches,* and *swamp cancer.*

**Py·thi·um** (pith'e-əm) [Gr. *pythein* to make rot] [MeSH: Pythium] a genus of root-parasitic moldlike organisms of the family Pythiaceae, having filamentous sporangia and smooth-walled spherical oogonia. *P. insidio'sum* causes pythiosis in horses, mules, and other animals.

**py·tho·gen·e·sis** (pi″tho-jen'ə-sis) [Gr. *pythein* to rot + *-genesis*] the origination of a process of decay or decomposition.

**py·tho·gen·ic** (pi″tho-jen'ik) [Gr. *pythein* to rot + *-genic*] causing decay or decomposition.

**py·thog·e·nous** (pi-thoj'ə-nəs) caused by putrefaction or filth.

**py·u·ria** (pi-u're-ə) [*pyo-* + *-uria*] [MeSH: Pyuria] the presence of pus in the urine.
**miliary p.,** the presence in the urine of miliary bodies consisting of pus cells, blood cells, and epithelium.

**PZI** protamine zinc insulin; see under *insulin.*

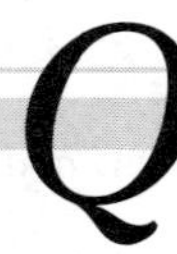

**Q** symbol for *ubiquinone.*

***Q*** symbol for *electric charge, heat,* and *reaction quotient.*

**$Q_{10}$** symbol for *temperature coefficient* and *ubiquinone.*

**$\dot{Q}$** symbol for *rate of blood flow.*

**q** symbol for the long arm of a chromosome.

**q.** abbreviation for L. *qua'que,* each, every.

***q*** symbol for *electric charge, ubiquinone,* and (in statistics) the probability of an alternative event occurring where *p* is the probability of the specified event and $q = 1 - p$. Cf. *p.*

**Q an·gle** [Q for *quadriceps*] see under *angle.*

**q.d.** abbreviation for L. *qua'que di'e,* every day.

**Q fe·ver** (ku fe'vər) [Q for *query;* so called because the etiologic agent was unknown when it was first reported in Queensland, Australia, in 1935] [MeSH: Q Fever] see under *fever.*

**q.h.** abbreviation for L. *qua'que ho'ra,* every hour.

**q.i.d.** abbreviation for L. *qua'ter in di'e,* four times a day.

**q.l.** abbreviation for L. *quan'tum li'bet,* as much as desired.

**QNS** abbreviation for *Queen's Nursing Sister* (of Queen's Institute of District Nursing).

**qns** abbreviation for *quantity not sufficient.*

**q.p.** abbreviation for L. *quan'tum pla'ceat,* as much as desired.

**q.q.h.** abbreviation for L. *qua'que quar'ta ho'ra,* every four hours.

**Qq.hor.** abbreviation for L. *qua'que ho'ra,* every hour.

**$QS_2$** symbol for *electromechanical systole.*

**q.s.** abbreviation for L. *quan'tum sa'tis,* sufficient quantity.

**q-sort** (ku'sort) [MeSH: Q-Sort] a technique of personality assessment in which the subject (or an observer) indicates the degree to which a standardized set of descriptive statements applies to the subject.

**q.suff.** abbreviation for L. *quan'tum suf'ficit,* as much as suffices.

**Quaa·lude** (kwa'lo͞od) trademark for a preparation of methaqualone.

**quack** (kwak) [from *quacksalver*] one who fraudulently misrepresents his ability and experience in the diagnosis and treatment of disease or the effects to be achieved by the treatment he offers.

**quack·ery** (kwak'ər-e) [MeSH: Quackery] the fraudulent misrepresentation of one's ability and experience in the diagnosis and treatment of disease or of the effects to be achieved by the treatment offered.

**quack·sal·ver** (kwak-sal'vər) [Dutch "salve peddler"] one claiming special merit for treatment with his medications and salves.

**Quad·ra·moid** (kwod'rə-moid) trademark for an oral suspension of trisulfapyrimidines.

**quad·ran·gle** (kwod'rang-gəl) 1. quadrilateral. 2. a dental instrument having four angulations in the shank connecting the handle, or shaft, with the working portion of the instrument, known as the blade, or nib. Cf. *binangle, monangle,* and *triple-angle.*

**quad·ran·gu·lar** (kwod-rang'gu-lər) [*quadri-* + *angular*] having four angles.

**quad·rant** (kwod'rənt) [L. *quadrans* quarter] 1. one quarter of a circle; that portion of the circumference of a circle that subtends an angle of 90 degrees. 2. any one of four corresponding parts or quarters, as of the abdominal surface, the field of vision, the dentition, or the tympanic membrane.

**quad·ran·tal** (kwod-ran'təl) resembling or affecting a quadrant.

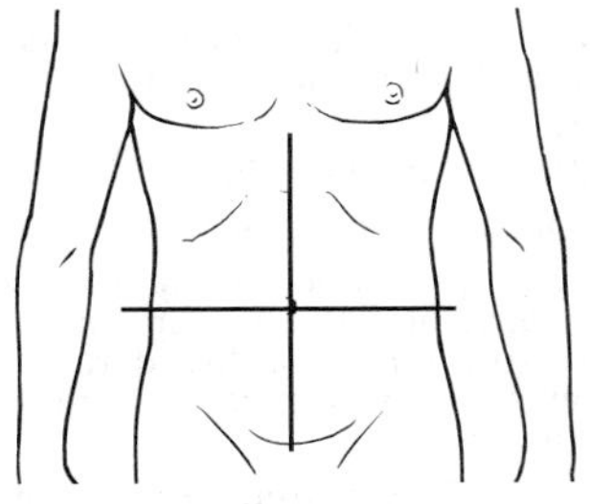

Quadrants of the abdomen.

**quad·rant·an·o·pia** (kwod″rənt-ə-no'pe-ə) [*quadrant* + *an-* neg. + *-opia*] hemianopia in one fourth of the visual field, bounded by a vertical and a horizontal radius. Called also *tetartanopia* and *quadrant hemianopia.*

**quad·rant·an·op·sia** (kwod″rənt-ə-nop'se-ə) quadrantanopia.

**quad·ran·tec·to·my** (kwod″rən-tek'tə-me) a form of partial mastectomy involving en bloc excision of tumor in one quadrant of breast tissue, as well as the pectoralis major muscle fascia and overlying skin.

**quad·rate** (kwod'rāt) [L. *quadratus* squared] square or squared; four sided.

**quad·ra·ti·pro·na·tor** (kwod-ra″tĭ-pro-na'tor) musculus pronator quadratus.

**quad·ra·tus** (kwod-ra'təs) [L.] squared; four sided.

**quadr(i)-** [L. *quattuor* four, in combination, *quadri-*] a prefix signifying four, or fourfold.

**qua·dri·ba·sic** (kwod″rĭ-ba'sik) having four replaceable atoms of hydrogen.

**qua·dri·ceps** (kwod'rĭ-seps) [*quadri-* + L. *caput* head] four headed; possessing four heads. See under *musculus.*

**qua·dri·ceps·plas·ty** (kwod'rĭ-seps-plas″te) plastic repair of a ruptured quadriceps femoris muscle.

**qua·dri·cus·pid** (kwod″rĭ-kus'pid) [*quadri-* + *cuspid*] 1. having four cusps; said of a tooth, or of a semilunar (aortic or pulmonary) valve with four cusps. 2. a tooth with four cusps.

**qua·dri·den·tate** (kwod″rĭ-den'tāt) forming four coordinate covalent bonds in a chelate.

**qua·dri·dig·i·tate** (kwod″rĭ-dij'ĭ-tāt) tetradactylous.

**quad·ri·gem·i·nal** (kwod″rĭ-jem'ĭ-nəl) [L. *quadrigeminus*] 1. fourfold, or in four parts; forming a group of four. 2. pertaining to the corpora quadrigemina.

**quad·ri·gem·i·nus** (kwod″rĭ-jem'ĭ-nəs) [L.] quadrigeminal.

**quad·ri·gem·i·ny** (kwod″rĭ-jem'ə-ne) [*quadri-* + L. *geminus* twin] 1. occurrence in fours. 2. the occurrence of a quadrigeminal pulse.

**quad·ri·lat·er·al** (kwod″rĭ-lat'ər-əl) [*quadri-* + *lateral*] 1. having four sides. 2. a figure that has four sides; called also *quadrangle.* 3. a postulate with four parts.

**Celsus' q.**, "Notae vero inflammationis sunt quattuor, rubor et tumor, cum calore et dolore." There are in fact four signs of inflammation—redness, swelling, heat, and pain.

**quad·ri·loc·u·lar** (kwod″ri-lok'u-lər) [*quadri-* + *locular*] having four cells, cavities, or chambers.

**quad·rip·a·ra** (kwod-rip'ə-rə) [*quadri-* + *para*] a woman who has had four pregnancies which resulted in viable offspring; also written *para IV.*

**quad·ri·pa·re·sis** (kwod″rĭ-pə-re'sis) tetraparesis.

**quad·ri·par·tite** (kwod″rĭ-pahr'tīt) having four parts or divisions.

**quad·ri·ple·gia** (kwod″rĭ-ple'jə) [*quadri-* + *-plegia*] [MeSH: Quadriplegia] paralysis of all four limbs; called also *tetraplegia.*

**quad·ri·po·lar** (kwod″rĭ-po'lər) having four poles, as a cell.

**quad·ri·sect** (kwod'rĭ-sekt) [*quadri-* + L. *secare* to cut] to cut into four parts.

**quad·ri·sec·tion** (kwod″rĭ-sek'shən) [*quadri-* + *section*] division into four parts.

**quad·ri·tu·ber·cu·lar** (kwod″rĭ-too-ber'ku-lər) having four tubercles or cusps.

**quad·ri·va·lent** (kwod″rĭ-va'lənt) tetravalent.

**quad·ru·ped** (kwod'roo-pəd) [*quadri-* + L. *pes* foot] 1. four footed. 2. an animal having four feet.

**quadrupl.** abbreviation for L. *quadruplica'to,* four times as much.

**quad·rup·let** (kwod-ro͞op'lət) [L. *quadrupulus* fourfold] [MeSH: Quadruplets] one of four offspring produced in one gestation period.

**qua·le** (kwa'le) the quality of a thing; especially the quality of a sensation or other conscious process.

**qual·i·ta·tive, qual·i·tive** (kwahl'ĭ-ta″tiv, kwahl'ĭ-tiv) [L. *qualitativus*] pertaining to quality.

**qual·i·ty** (kwahl'ĭ-te) in radiology, the ability of a particular form or type of ionizing radiation to penetrate matter.

**Quant's sign** (quahnts) [C.A.J. *Quant,* Dutch physician, early 20th century] see under *sign.*

**quan·ta** (kwahn'tə) [L.] plural of *quantum.*

**quan·tal** (kwahn'təl) 1. of or relating to quanta. 2. denoting an all-or-none response, one for which partial responses are undetectable or are not measured, or a procedure (a quantal assay) in which such a response is measured.

**quan·tile** (kwahn'tīl) [*quantity* + *-ile* (by analogy with *quartile, percentile,* etc.)] any of the values that divide the range of an observed or theoretical probability distribution into a given number of equal, ordered parts; examples are the median, quartiles, and percentiles. Each value divides the range into two specified parts, with the part below the value corresponding to a prescribed fraction *p* and the part above to $1 - p$.

**quan·tim·e·ter** (kwahn-tim'ə-tər) [L. *quantus* how much + *-meter*] an apparatus for measuring the quantity of x-rays generated by a tube.

**quan·ti·ta·tive** (kwahn'tĭ-ta"tiv) [L. *quantitativus*] 1. denoting or expressing a quantity. 2. relating to the proportionate quantities or to the amount of the constituents of a compound.

**quan·ti·ty** (kwahn'tĭ-te) 1. a characteristic, as of energy or mass, susceptible of precise physical measurement. 2. a measurable amount.

**quan·tum** (kwahn'təm) pl. *quan'ta* [L. "as much as"] a unit of energy under the quantum theory. It is h$\nu$, in which h is Planck's constant, $6.626 \times 10^{-34}$ joule second, and $\nu$ is the frequency of vibration with which the energy is associated. See *quantum theory,* under *theory.*

**q. of light,** a quantity of light (radiant energy) equivalent to the frequency of the light times $6.626 \times 10^{-34}$ joule second.

**quan·tum li·bet** (kwahn'təm li'bət) [L.] as much as desired.

**quan·tum sat·is** (kwahn'təm sat'is) [L.] a sufficient quantity.

**quan·tum suf·fi·cit** (kwahn'təm suf'ĭ-sit) [L.] as much as suffices.

**quar·an·tine** (kwor'ən-tēn) [Ital. *quarantina,* from L. *quadraginta* forty] [MeSH: Quarantine] 1. restriction of freedom of movement of apparently well individuals who have been exposed to infectious disease, which is imposed for the usual maximal incubation period of the disease *(quarantine period).* Cf. *surveillance,* def. 2. 2. a period (originally of 40 days' duration) of detention of vessels, vehicles, or travelers coming from infected or suspected ports or places. 3. the place where persons are detained for inspection. 4. to detain or isolate on account of suspected contagion.

**quart** (kwort) [L. *quartus* fourth] the fourth part of a gallon (946 mL).

**quar·tan** (kwor'tən) [L. *quartanus,* pertaining to the fourth] recurring every 72 hours (fourth day, counting the day of the previous paroxysm). See *malaria.*

**quar·ter** (kwor'tər) the part of a horse's hoof lying between the heel and the toe.

**false q.,** a cleft from top to bottom of the quarter of a horse's hoof.

**quar·tile** (kwor'tīl) [L. *quartilis* pertaining to a fourth, from *quartus* fourth] any of the three values that divide the range of a probability distribution into four parts of equal probability; i.e., the 1st, 2nd, and 3rd quartiles are the 25th, 50th, and 75th percentiles.

**quar·tip·a·ra** (kwor-tip'ə-rə) quadripara.

**quar·ti·sect** (kwor'tĭ-sәkt) [L. *quartus* fourth + *secare* to cut] to cut into four parts.

**quar·ti·ster·nal** (kwor"tĭ-ster'nəl) [L. *quartus* fourth + *sternum* sternum] pertaining to the fourth sternebra, or the bony segment of the sternum opposite the fourth intercostal space.

**quartz** (kworts) [MeSH: Quartz] a crystalline form of silica; workers inhaling excessive amounts of its dust may suffer from silicosis. Called also *rock crystal.*

**Quar·zan** (kwahr'zan) trademark for a preparation of clidinium bromide.

**quasi-** [L. *quasi* as if, as though] a prefix meaning almost, seemingly, or resembling.

**qua·si·dip·loid** (kwah"zĭ-dip'loid) [*quasi-* + *diploid*] 1. having two sets of chromosomes but with an abnormal distribution. In tissue cell cultures, a chromosome of one pair may be missing and may be replaced by an extra chromosome from another pair. 2. an organism or cell that is quasidiploid.

**qua·si·dom·i·nance** (kwah"zĭ-dom'ĭ-nəns) [*quasi-* + *dominance*] the mimicking of dominant inheritance by the direct transmission, generation to generation, of a recessive trait, produced by mating of a recessive homozygote and a heterozygote, the proportion of affected offspring thus resembling that in dominant inheritance.

**qua·si·dom·i·nant** (kwah"zĭ-dom'ĭ-nənt) pertaining to or exhibiting quasidominance.

**quas·sa·tion** (kwah-sa'shən) [L. *quassatio*] the crushing of drugs, or their reduction to small pieces.

**Quas·sia** (kwosh'ə) [after *Quassi,* 18th century black slave of Surinam who used it] a genus of tropical trees of the family Simaroubaceae whose wood is used as an antipyretic. *Q. ama'ra* L. is Surinam quassia, a source of medicinal quassia.

**quas·sia** (kwosh'ə) 1. any of various tropical trees of the genera *Picrasma* and *Quassia.* 2. the dried, bitter heartwood of *Picrasma excelsa* (Jamaica quassia) or *Quassia amara* (Surinam quassia); it has been used as an enema for seatworms.

**quas·sin** (kwah'shin) the major bitter principle, $C_{22}H_{30}O_6$, of quassia.

**Quat., quat.** abbreviation for L. *quat'tuor,* four.

**qua·ter in die** (kwah'ter in de'a) [L.] four times a day.

**qua·ter·nary** (kwah'tər-nar"e, kwah-ter'nar-e) [L. *quaternarius,* from *quattuor* four] 1. fourth in order. 2. containing four elements or groups.

**Qua·tre·fages' angle** (kah"trə-fahzh'əz) [Jean Louis Armand de *Quatrefages* de Bréau, French naturalist, 1810–1892] parietal angle.

**qua·ze·pam** (kwah'zə-pam) [USP] a benzodiazepine used as a sedative and hypnotic in the treatment of insomnia; administered orally.

**Queck·en·stedt's sign (phenomenon, test)** (kwek'ən-shtets") [Hans Heinrich Georg *Queckenstedt,* German physician, 1876–1918] see under *sign.*

**Quel·i·cin** (kwel'ĭ-sin) trademark for a preparation of succinylcholine chloride.

**quench·ing** (kwench'ing) 1. extinguishing, suppressing, or diminishing a physical property, as the rapid chilling of a hot metal by plunging it into cold liquid. 2. in biochemistry, decrease of fluorescence from an excited molecule by interference that reduces the fluorescence intensity, such as deexcitation of the fluorescent molecule by collision with other molecules, absorption of fluorescent emission by the surrounding medium, or a decrease or shift in wavelength of fluorescence due to chemical interaction of the fluorescent molecule with other molecules. 3. in liquid scintillation counting, interference with generation or propagation of light energy from the sample, decreasing the counting efficiency of the detector. 4. the termination of secondary and subsequent ionizations in a detector to give it time to become sensitive again.

**fluorescence q.,** a technique for measuring the primary interaction of antigen and antibody by determination of the amount of light absorbed by bound antigen from fluorescent-labeled antibody exposed to ultraviolet light.

**Quénu's hemorrhoidal plexus** (ka-nūz') [Eduard André Victor Alfred *Quénu,* French surgeon, 1852–1933] see under *plexus.*

**Qué·nu-Mu·ret sign** (ka-nu' mu-ra') [E. A. V. A. *Quénu;* Paul Louis *Muret,* French surgeon, born 1878] see under *sign.*

**Quer·cus** (kwer'kəs) [L.] the oaks, a genus of large leaf-bearing, hardwood trees of the family Fagaceae. *Q. al'ba* (the white oak) and other species make the excrescence called the nutgall (q.v.). White oak bark is medicinal (see under *bark*). Oaks have gallic and tannic acids in their leaves and acorns, making those parts poisonous to livestock.

**Quer·vain** (kār-vă') see *de Quervain.*

**Ques·tran** (kwes'tran) trademark for a preparation of cholestyramine resin.

**Quey·rat's erythroplasia** (ka-rahz') [Louis Auguste *Queyrat,* French dermatologist, 1856–1933] see under *erythroplasia.*

**Quib·ron** (kwib'ron) trademark for preparations of theophylline and guaifenesin.

**Quick's test** (kwik) [Armand James *Quick,* American physician, 1894–1978] see under *test.*

**quick** (kwik) 1. rapid. 2. alive. 3. pregnant and able to feel the fetal movements.

**quick·en·ing** (kwik'ən-ing) the first recognizable movements of the fetus, appearing usually from the sixteenth to the twentieth week of pregnancy.

**quick·lime** (kwik'līm) calcium oxide.

**quick·sil·ver** old name for *mercury.*

**quid·ding** (kwid'ing) a condition in horses in which food is taken into the mouth, repeatedly chewed, and then expelled; it may be caused by injuries to the mouth, disorders of the teeth or gums, paralysis of the muscles of mastication, or some other condition causing inability to swallow.

**Quide** (kwīd) trademark for a preparation of piperacetazine.

**quil·la·ia** (kwĭ-la′yə) the dried inner bark of *Quillaja saponaria,* formerly used in medicine for its local irritant action. Its chief constituent is quillaic acid, and it is used in the manufacture of saponin, shampoos, and detergents. Called also *soap bark, soap tree bark,* and *quillay bark.*

**Quil·la·ja** (kwĭ-la′yə) [Sp. Am. *quillai*] a genus of trees of the family Rosaceae. *Q. sapona′ria* Molina is a species native to South America that is a source of quillaia.

**quin·a·crine hy·dro·chlo·ride** (kwin′ə-krin) an antimalarial, antiprotozoal, and anthelmintic, used especially for suppressive therapy of malaria and in the treatment of giardiasis and tapeworm infestations, administered orally. Called also *chinacrine hydrochloride* and *mepacrine hydrochloride.*

**Quin·a·glute** (kwin′ə-glo͞ot) trademark for a preparation of quinidine gluconate.

**quin·al·bar·bi·tone** (kwin″əl-bahr′bĭ-tōn) secobarbital.

**quin·al·dic ac·id** (kwin-al′dik) a catabolite of tryptophan that is excreted in the urine. Called also *quinaldinic acid.*

**quin·al·din·ic ac·id** (kwin″əl-din′ik) quinaldic acid.

**quin·a·pril hy·dro·chlo·ride** (kwin′ə-pril″) an angiotensin-converting enzyme inhibitor used alone or in combination with a thiazide diuretic for the treatment of hypertension; administered orally.

**Quin·cke's edema (disease) pulse (sign)** (kwing′kəz) [Heinrich Irenaeus *Quincke,* German physician, 1842–1922] see *angioedema* and see under *pulse.*

**Quin·e·prox** (kwin′ə-proks) trademark for a preparation of hydroxychloroquine sulfate.

**quin·eth·a·zone** (kwin-eth′ə-zōn) a sulfonamide derivative that has a different chemical structure from but the same pharmacological actions as the thiazide diuretics, used in the treatment of hypertension and edema; administered orally.

**quin·ic ac·id** (kwin′ik) [MeSH: Quinic Acid] a compound found in cinchona bark and in many plants. Called also *kinic acid.*

**Quin·i·dex** (kwin′ĭ-deks) trademark for a preparation of quinidine sulfate.

**quin·i·dine** (kwin′ĭ-dēn) [MeSH: Quinidine] the dextrorotatory isomer of quinine obtained from various species of *Cinchona* and their hybrids, and from *Remijia pedunculata,* or prepared from quinine. It has cardiac depressant activity, and is as potent an antimalarial as quinine but is rarely used for the latter effect except in those having an idiosyncrasy to quinine.
**q. gluconate** [USP], the gluconate salt of quinidine, having the same actions as the base; used in the treatment of certain cardiac arrhythmias, administered intravenously and intramuscularly.
**q. polygalacturonate,** a salt of quinidine, having actions and uses the same as the other salts of quinidine; administered orally.
**q. sulfate** [USP], the sulfate salt of quinidine, used for the treatment of cardiac arrhythmias; administered orally.

**qui·nine** (kwin′in, kwin-ēn′, kwi′nīn) [L. *quinina*] [MeSH: Quinine] an alkaloid of cinchona, which suppresses the asexual erythrocytic forms of all malarial parasites and has a slight effect on the gametocytes of *Plasmodium vivax* and *P. malariae* but none on those of *P. falciparum.* Once widely used to prevent and control malaria, it has been largely replaced by less toxic and more effective synthetic antimalarials, and is now used chiefly (usually in the form of one of its soluble salts) in the treatment of falciparum malaria resistant to other antimalarials. Quinine also has analgesic, antipyretic, mild oxytocic, cardiac depressant, and sclerosing properties, and it decreases the excitability of the motor endplate.
**q. and urea hydrochloride,** a double salt of quinine and urea hydrochloride, which has been used to produce sclerosing, thrombosis, and obliteration of internal hemorrhoids and varicose veins, and as a local anesthetic.
**q. dihydrochloride,** the dihydrochloride salt of quinine, having the same actions and uses as the base; administered intravenously.
**q. ethylcarbonate,** a white crystalline compound formed by the action of ethyl chlorocarbonate on quinine; it has been used like quinine sulfate.
**q. hydrochloride,** a white salt resembling the sulfate in taste and uses.
**q. sulfate** [USP], the dihydrate sulfate salt of quinine, having the same actions and uses as the base, and also used to prevent nocturnal cramps in the legs and feet; administered orally.

**qui·nin·ism** (kwin′ĭ-niz″əm) cinchonism.

**quin·o·line** (kwin′o-lēn) a tertiary amine or alkaloid derivable from quinine, coal tar, and various other sources, which has antiseptic, antipyretic, and antiperiodic properties.

**quin·o·lin·ic ac·id** [MeSH: Quinolinic Acid] a cyclic, nitrogen-containing, dicarboxylic compound for which a class of glutamate receptors has an affinity; it may play a role in neurodegenerative disorders.

**quin·o·lone** (kwin′o-lōn) [MeSH: Quinolones] any of a group of synthetic antibacterial agents that includes nalidixic acid, cinoxacin, rosoxacin, and the fluorinated 4-q's.
**fluorinated 4-q.,** fluoroquinolone.

**qui·none** (kwi-nōn′, kwin′ōn) any of a group of highly conjugated aromatic diketones, usually in the *ortho* or *para* configuration, derived from benzene or from multiple ring hydrocarbons such as anthracene or naphthalene; they are subclassified on the basis of ring structure (e.g., anthraquinone or benzoquinone), are mild oxidizing agents, and are usually colored yellow, red, or orange. The term is often used specifically to denote benzoquinone (q.v.), particularly 1,4-benzoquinone.

**quin·o·noid** (kwin′o-noid) resembling a quinone or containing a quinone (particularly a benzoquinone) ring structure.

**Quin·o·ra** (kwin′o-rə) trademark for a preparation of quinidine sulfate.

**Quinq.** abbreviation for L. *quin′que,* five.

**quin·que·cus·pid** (kwing″kwə-kus′pid) [L. *quinque* five + *cuspid*] 1. having five cusps. 2. a tooth with five cusps.

**quin·que·tu·ber·cu·lar** (kwing″kwə-too-ber′ku-lər) having five tubercles or cusps.

**quin·que·va·lent** (kwing″kwə-va′lənt) pentavalent.

**quin·qui·na** (kin-ke′nə) cinchona.

**quin·sy** (kwin′ze) [Gr. *kynanche* sore throat] peritonsillar abscess.

**quint-** [L. *quintus* fifth] a prefix signifying five or fifth.

**Quint.** abbreviation for L. *quin′tus,* fifth.

**quin·tan** (kwin′tan) [L. *quintanus* of the fifth] recurring every fifth day, as a fever.

**quin·tes·sence** (kwin-tes′əns) [*quint-* + *essence*] the highly concentrated extract of any substance.

**quin·tile** (kwin′tīl) [L. *quintilis* pertaining to a fifth, from *quintus* fifth] any of the four values that divide the range of a probability distribution into five parts of equal probability, i.e., the 1st, 2nd, 3rd, and 4th quintiles are the 20th, 40th, 60th, and 80th percentiles.

**quin·tip·a·ra** (kwin-tip′ə-rə) [*quint-* + *para*] a woman who has had five pregnancies which resulted in viable offspring; also written para V.

**quin·ti·ster·nal** (kwin″tĭ-ster′nəl) [*quint-* + *sternal*] denoting the fifth bony portion of the sternum, or the part above the xiphoid process and adjacent to the fifth intercostal space.

**Quin·ton-Scrib·ner shunt** (kwin′tən skrib′nər) [Wayne E. *Quinton,* American nephrologist, 20th century: Belding H. *Scribner,* American nephrologist, born 1921] see under *shunt.*

**quin·tup·let** (kwin-tup′lət) [L. *quintuplex* five-fold] [MeSH: Quintuplets] one of five offspring produced in one gestation period.

**quis·qual·ic ac·id** (kwis-kwah′lik) [MeSH: Quisqualic Acid] an excitotoxin found in the *Quisqualus* nut; it has actions and experimental uses similar to those of kainic acid.

**quit·tor** (kwit′or) a fistulous sore on the quarters or the coronet of a horse's foot.
**simple q.,** local inflammation resulting in a slough, with formation of pus immediately above the hoof.
**skin q.,** a painful ulcer of the skin above the hoof.
**subhorny q.,** inflammation from the coronary band to beneath the hoof, with pus formation in the sensitive tissue.
**tendinous q.,** quittor in which inflammation extends into the tendons of the leg and the ligaments of the joint.

**quo·ad vi·tam** (kwo′ad vi′tam) [L.] so far as life is concerned.

**Quo·tane** (kwo′tān) trademark for preparations of dimethisoquin hydrochloride.

**Quotid.** abbreviation for L. *quotid′ie,* daily.

**quo·tid·i·an** (kwo-tid′e-ən) [L. *quotidianus* daily] recurring every day; applied to the type of fever caused by certain forms of malarial parasites.

**quo·tient** (kwo′shənt) a number obtained as the result of division; a number indicating how many times one number is contained in another.
**achievement q.,** a percentage statement of the extent to which a child has progressed in learning in proportion to his ability. Abbreviated AQ.
**albumin q.,** the amount of albumin in the blood plasma divided by the amount of albumin present in the blood.
**caloric q.,** the quotient obtained by dividing the heat evolved (ex-

pressed in calories) by the oxygen consumed (expressed in milligrams) in a metabolic process.
**D q.,** the ratio of glucose to nitrogen in the urine.
**growth q.,** that part of the entire food energy that is used for growth.
**intelligence q.,** the measure of intelligence obtained by dividing the patient's mental age, as ascertained by the Binet test, by his chronological age and multiplying the result by 100. Abbreviated IQ.
**protein q.,** the number obtained by dividing the quantity of globulin in the blood plasma by the quantity of albumin.
**reaction q.,** for a balanced chemical equation, the product of the concentrations of the reaction products, each raised to the power equal to the coefficient of the product in the equation, divided by the concentrations of the reactants, each raised to the power equal to its coefficient. For the equation $aA + bB + \ldots = rR + sS + \ldots$,

$$Q = \frac{[R]^r[S]^s}{[A]^a[B]^b}.$$

At equilibrium the reaction quotient equals the equilibrium constant.
**respiratory q.,** the ratio of the volume of carbon dioxide given off by the body tissues to the volume of oxygen absorbed by them; usually equal to the corresponding volumes given off and taken up by the lungs. Abbreviated RQ.

**q.v.** abbreviation for L. *quan'tum vis,* as much as you please, and for *quod vi'de,* which see.

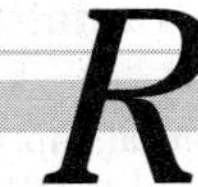

# R

**R** symbol for *rate, expiratory exchange ratio, resistance, respiration, rhythm, right, roentgen, rough* (colony), *Rankine scale, Réaumur scale,* and *Behnken's unit;* chemical symbol for an organic *radical.*

**R.** abbreviation for L. *remo'tum,* far.

***R*** symbol for *resistance* and the *gas constant.*

***R*-** [L. *rectus* right] a stereodescriptor used to specify the absolute configuration of compounds having asymmetric carbon atoms. The four different substituents at the asymmetric carbon atom are ranked according to the Cahn-Ingold-Prelog sequence rules; then, looking at the molecule with the lowest ranking substituent pointing directly away from the viewer, if the other three substituents are in clockwise order going from highest to lowest ranked, the configuration is *R;* otherwise *S.* Example: L-threonine is (2*S*:3*R*)-2-amino-3-hydroxybutanoic acid.

℞ symbol for L. *re'cipe,* take. See *prescription.*

**$R_A$, $R_{AW}$** airway resistance.

**$R_e$** Reynolds' number.

***$R_f$*** in paper or thin-layer chromatography, the distance moved by a solute spot from the origin expressed as a fraction of the distance moved by the solvent front.

**r** symbol for *ring chromosome* and *drug resistance;* former symbol for *roentgen,* officially replaced by R.

***r*** symbol for *correlation coefficient, distance, radius,* and *drug resistance.*

***$r_s$*** symbol for *Spearman's rank correlation coefficient.*

***ρ*** rho, the seventeenth letter of the Greek alphabet; symbol for *correlation coefficient* (of a population), *mass density* and *electric charge density.*

**Ra** symbol for *radium.*

**Rab·A·vert** (rāb'ə-vert") trademark for a preparation of purified chick embryo cell vaccine.

**rab·bet·ing** (rab'ət-ing) impaction of the denticulated broken surfaces of a fractured bone.

**rab·bit** (rab'it) [MeSH: Rabbits] any of a variety of short-tailed, long-eared burrowing mammals of the family Leporidae, originally Old World but introduced into many New World areas where it has often become a pest; it is used extensively in laboratory medicine.
**Watanabe heritable hyperlipidemic (WHHL) r.,** a mutant strain of rabbits that have a genetic deficiency of low-density lipoprotein (LDL) receptors similar to that occurring in human familial hypercholesterolemia; they are used in studies of lipoprotein metabolism and atherogenesis.

**rab·bit·pox** (rab'it-poks) an acute eruptive skin disease of rabbits, caused by a virus closely related to the vaccinia virus; it is often fatal.

**rab·e·la·i·sin** (rab"ə-la'ĭ-sin) a poisonous glycoside from *Rabelaisia philippinensis,* a plant of the Philippine Islands: a heart stimulant.

**rab·id** (rab'id) [L. *rabidus*] infected with rabies.

**ra·bies** (ra'bēz, ra'be-ēz) [L. *rabere* to rage] [MeSH: Rabies] an acute infectious disease of the central nervous system affecting almost any mammal, including humans, caused by a rhabdovirus. It is usually spread by contamination with virus-laden saliva of bites from infected animals, although aerosol infection can occur via the respiratory route, transplantation, or ingestion of infected tissues. Important animal vectors include the dog, cat, vampire bat, mongoose, skunk, wolf, raccoon, and fox. The incubation period in both humans and animals is highly variable, depending on the size of the inoculum and the site of the bite, being shorter after a bite near the brain than after one farther away. Symptoms usually include paresthesia, pain, or a burning sensation at the site of inoculation; periods of hyperexcitability, hallucinations, delirium, and bizarre behavior alternating with periods of calmness and lucidity; painful spasms of pharyngeal and laryngeal muscles, hypersalivation, and fearfulness provoked by attempts to drink or even by the sight of fluids (hydrophobia); convulsions; meningismus; paralysis; and coma. Recovery is rare, with death usually associated with progressive respiratory depression and cardiorespiratory failure. Formerly called *hydrophobia.*
**dumb r.,** paralytic r.
**furious r.,** a stage or form of rabies in which excessive motor activity is prominent.
**paralytic r.,** a stage or form of rabies in which the most prominent symptom is ascending paralysis. Called also *dumb r.*

**ra·bi·form** (ra'bĭ-form) resembling rabies.

**Rab·son-Men·den·hall syndrome** (rab'sən men'dən-hawl) [S. M. *Rabson,* American physician, 20th century; E. N. *Mendenhall,* American physician, 20th century] see under *syndrome.*

**race** (rās) 1. an ethnic stock, or division of humankind; in a narrower sense, a national or tribal stock; in a still narrower sense, a genealogic line of descent; a class of persons of a common lineage. In genetics, races are considered as populations having different distributions of gene frequencies. 2. a class or breed of animals; a group of individuals having certain characteristics in common, owing to a common inheritance; a subspecies.

**ra·ce·mase** (ra'sə-mās) a term used in the names of some enzymes of the subclass racemases and epimerases [EC 5.1] to denote those that catalyze inversion of the configuration around the asymmetric carbon atom in a substrate having only one center of asymmetry; thus, racemers are interconverted. Cf. *epimerase.*

**ra·ce·mate** (ra'sə-māt) an equimolecular mixture of two enantiomorphic isomers, being optically inactive in solution because of the presence of the same number of dextro- and levorotatory molecules. In the solid state it may have the properties of a loosely bound molecular compound. Called also *racemic form, racemic mixture,* or *racemic modification.*

**ra·ce·mic** (ra-se'mik) made up of two enantiomorphic isomers and therefore optically inactive.

**ra·ce·mi·za·tion** (ra"sə-mĭ-za'shən) the transformation of one half of the molecules of an optically active compound into molecules which possess exactly the opposite (mirror-image) configuration, with complete loss of rotatory power because of the statistical balance between equal numbers of dextro- and levorotatory molecules. Cf. *mutarotation.*

**rac·e·mose** (ras'ə-mōs) [L. *racemosus*] resembling a bunch of grapes on its stalk.

**ra·ceph·e·drine hy·dro·chlo·ride** (ra-sef'ə-drēn) the racemic form of ephedrine hydrochloride, used as a sympathomimetic.

**rac·er** (ra'sər) any of several species of fast-moving colubrid snakes.
**black r.,** blacksnake, def. 2.

**ra·chi·al** (ra'ke-əl) spinal (def. 2).

**ra·chi·al·gia** (ra"ke-al'jə) rachiodynia.

**ra·chi·cen·te·sis** (ra"ke-sən-te'sis) [*rachi-* + *-centesis*] lumbar puncture.

**ra·chid·i·al** (ra-kid'e-əl) spinal (def. 2).

**ra·chid·i·an** (ra-kid'e-ən) spinal (def. 2).

**ra·chi·graph** (ra'ke-graf) [*rachi-* + *-graph*] an instrument for recording the outlines of the spine and back.

**ra·chil·y·sis** (ra-kil'ĭ-sis) [*rachi-* + *-lysis*] mechanical treatment of a curved vertebral column by combined traction and pressure.

**rachi(o)-** [Gr. *rhachis* spine] a combining form denoting relation to the spine.

**ra·chio·camp·sis** (ra"ke-o-kamp'sis) [*rachio-* + Gr. *kampsis* curve] curvature of the spinal column.

**ra·chio·cen·te·sis** (ra"ke-o-sən-te'sis) [*rachio-* + *-centesis*] lumbar puncture.

**ra·chio·chy·sis** (ra"ke-ok'ĭ-sis) [*rachio-* + Gr. *chysis* a pouring] the effusion of a fluid within the vertebral canal.

**ra·chio·cy·pho·sis** (ra"ke-o-si-fo'sis) kyphosis.

**ra·chi·odyn·ia** (ra"ke-o-din'e-ə) [*rachio-* + *-odynia*] pain in the vertebral column. Called also *rachialgia.* Cf. *spondylodynia.*

**ra·chio·ky·pho·sis** (ra"ke-o-ki-fo'sis) kyphosis.

**ra·chi·om·e·ter** (ra"ke-om'ə-tər) [*rachio-* + *-meter*] an instrument for measuring curvatures of the vertebral column.

**ra·chio·my·eli·tis** (ra"ke-o-mi"ə-li'tis) [*rachio-* + *myelitis*] myelitis (def. 1).

**ra·chi·op·a·gus** (ra"ke-op'ə-gəs) [*rachio-* + *pagus*] symmetrical conjoined twins united back to back in the sagittal plane, fusion being limited to the upper trunk and cervical region.

**ra·chi·op·a·thy** (ra"ke-op'ə-the) [*rachio-* + *-pathy*] spondylopathy.

**ra·chio·sco·li·o·sis** (ra"ke-o-sko"le-o'sis) lateral curvature of the spine.

**ra·chio·tome** (ra'ke-o-tōm) an instrument for cutting the vertebrae.

**ra·chi·ot·o·my** (ra"ke-ot'ə-me) [*rachio-* + *-tomy*] incision of a vertebra, or of the vertebral column.

**ra·chip·a·gus** (ra-kip'ə-gəs) [*rachi-* + *-pagus*] conjoined twins joined at the vertebral column.

**ra·chis** (ra'kis) [Gr. *rhachis* spine] columna vertebralis.

**ra·chis·chi·sis** (ra-kis'kĭ-sis) [*rachi-* + *-schisis*] congenital fissure of the vertebral column; see also *spina bifida.* Called also *schistorachis* and *spondyloschisis.*
**r. partia'lis,** merorachischisis.
**r. poste'rior,** spina bifida.
**r. tota'lis,** fissure of the entire vertebral column; called also *holorachischisis.* See also *spina bifida.*

**ra·chit·ic** (ra-kit'ik) pertaining to or affected with rickets.

**ra·chi·tis** (ra-ki'tis) [Gr. *rachitis*] 1. rickets. 2. spondylitis.
**r. feta'lis anula'ris,** the formation before birth of anular thickenings on the long bones.
**r. feta'lis microme'lica,** deficient longitudinal growth of the bones of the fetus.

**rach·i·tism** (rak'ĭ-tiz"əm) a tendency to rickets.

**ra·chit·o·gen·ic** (rə-kit"o-jen'ik) causing rickets.

**rach·i·tome** (rak"ĭ-tōm) rachiotome.

**ra·chit·o·my** (rə-kit'ə-me) rachiotomy.

**ra·cial** (ra'shəl) pertaining to a particular race.

**rac·lo·pride** (rak'lo-prīd) an antipsychotic compound related to sulpiride; used investigationally.
**r. C 11** [USP], raclopride in which a portion of the molecules have been labeled at the *o*-methyl position with $^{11}C$; administered intravenously.

**RAD** right axis deviation.

**rad** [acronym for *r*adiation *a*bsorbed *d*ose] 1. a unit of measurement of the absorbed dose of ionizing radiation; it corresponds to an energy transfer of 100 ergs per gram of any absorbing material (including tissues). The biological effect of 1 rad varies with the kind of radiation the tissue is exposed to. 2. abbreviation for *radian.*

**rad.** abbreviation for L. *ra'dix,* root.

**ra·dec·to·my** (ra-dek'tə-me) [*radix* + *-ectomy*] root amputation.

**Rad·for·dia** (rad-for'de-ə) a genus of mites of the family Myobiidae; *R. ensi'fera* is found on laboratory rats and sometimes causes severe pruritus with alopecia.

**ra·di·a·bil·i·ty** (ra"de-ə-bil'ĭ-te) the property of being radiable.

**ra·di·a·ble** (ra'de-ə-bəl) capable of being penetrated by radiation, especially by x-rays.

**ra·di·ad** (ra'de-ad) toward the radius or radial side of the forearm.

**ra·di·al** (ra'de-əl) [L. *radialis*] 1. pertaining to the radius of the forearm or to the radial (lateral) aspect of the arm as opposed to the ulnar (medial) aspect. 2. pertaining to a radius. 3. radiating; spreading outward from a common center.

**ra·di·a·lis** (ra"de-a'lis) [L., from *radius,* q.v.] [TA] radial; a general term denoting relationship to the radius or to the radial aspect of the forearm

**ra·di·an** (ra'de-ən) [from *radius*] a unit of plane angle equal to the angle subtended to the center of a circle by an arc whose length is equal to the radius of the circle. One radian equals $360°/2\pi$ or approximately 57.295°. Abbreviated rad.

**ra·di·ant** (ra'de-ənt) [L. *radians*] 1. diverging from a common center. 2. emitting radiation or heat. 3. transmitted by radiation.

**ra·di·ate** (ra'de-āt) [L. *radiare, radiatus*] 1. to diverge or spread from a common point. 2. arranged in a radiating manner.

**ra·di·a·ther·my** (ra-di"ə-ther'me) short wave diathermy.

**ra·di·a·tio** (ra-de-a'she-o) pl. *radiatio'nes* [L., from *radiare* to furnish with spokes] a radiation or radiating structure; used in anatomical nomenclature to designate a collection of nerve fibers connecting different portions of the brain.
**r. acus'tica** [TA], acoustic radiation: a fiber tract arising in the medial geniculate nucleus and passing laterally in the sublenticular portion of the internal capsule to terminate in the transverse temporal gyri of the temporal lobe; the radiation provides reciprocal connections and forms part of the caudal peduncle of the thalamus.
**r. cor'poris callo'si** [TA], radiation of corpus callosum: the projection of fibers from the corpus callosum to all parts of the neopallium.
**r. op'tica** [TA], optic radiation: a fiber tract that begins at the lateral geniculate body, passes laterally through the pars retrolentiformis of the internal capsule, follows the lateral wall of the lateral ventricle, and finally projects posteriorly to end in the striate area on the medial surface of the occipital lobe on either side of the calcarine sulcus; the radiation provides reciprocal connections and forms part of the posterior thalamic peduncle. Called also *geniculocalcarine tract, occipitothalamic radiation,* and *radiation of Gratiolet.*
**r. tha'lami ante'rior** [TA], anterior thalamic radiation: the group of thalamocortical fibers of the anterior limb of the internal capsule connecting the medial and anterior thalamic nuclei and the cortex of the frontal lobe.
**r. tha'lami centra'lis** [TA], central thalamic radiation: the group of thalamocortical fibers of the posterior limb of the internal capsule, presumably carrying general sensory impulses from the ventral thalamic nuclei to the postcentral gyrus. Called also *superior thalamic radiation.*
**r. tha'lami infe'rior** [TA], inferior thalamic radiation: the smallest of the four thalamic peduncles; it connects the medial geniculate body with certain areas of the cortex of the temporal lobe, forming one of the principal components of the ansa peduncularis. Called also *pedunculus thalamicus inferior* and *inferior peduncle of thalamus.*
**r. tha'lami poste'rior** [TA], posterior thalamic radiation: the group of thalamocortical fibers of the retrolentiform part of the internal capsule connecting the cortices of the occipital and parietal lobes and the caudal parts of the thalamus.

**ra·di·a·tion** (ra"de-a'shən) [L. *radiatio,* q.v.] [MeSH: Radiation] 1. divergence from a common center. 2. a structure made up of divergent elements, as one of the fiber tracts in the brain; for official names of specific structures, see under *radiatio.* 3. energy transmitted by waves through space or through some medium; usually referring to electromagnetic radiation when used without a modifier. By extension, a stream of particles, such as electrons, neutrons, protons, or alpha particles.
**acoustic r.,** radiatio acustica.
**adaptive r.,** evolution from a generalized, primitive species to diverse, specialized species, each adapted to a distinct mode of life.
**α-r., alpha r.,** see under *ray.*
**annihilation r.,** radiation produced by the collision and annihilation of a particle and its antiparticle, especially the two 0.511 MeV gamma ray photons produced by the annihilation of a positron and an electron.
**auditory r.,** radiatio acustica.
**background r.,** radiation arising from radioactive material other than that directly under consideration or study. Background radiation due to cosmic rays and natural radioactivity in the environment is always present; additional background radiation may be due to the presence of other radioactive material in the vicinity, or radioactive components of building materials, etc.
**beta r., β-r.,** see under *ray.*
**braking r.,** bremsstrahlung.
**Cerenkov r.,** visible light emitted by a high-speed charged particle moving through a transparent medium at a speed greater than the speed of light in that medium.
**r. of corpus callosum,** radiatio corporis callosi.
**corpuscular r's,** radiations consisting of streams of subatomic particles, such as protons, deuterons, electrons, positrons, and neutrons.
**electromagnetic r.,** see under *wave.*
**gamma r., γ-r.,** see under *ray.*
**r. of Gratiolet,** radiatio optica.
**heterogeneous r.,** radiation consisting of a beam of particles of various energies, or having different frequencies, or containing different types of particles.
**homogeneous r.,** radiation consisting of an extremely narrow band of frequencies or a beam of monoenergetic particles of a single type.
**interstitial r.,** energy emitted by radium, radon, or some other radiopharmaceutical inserted directly into the tissue; see *interstitial radiotherapy,* under *radiotherapy.*
**ionizing r.,** corpuscular or electromagnetic radiation capable of producing ionization, directly or indirectly, in its passage through matter.
**mitogenetic r., mitogenic r.,** specific energy allegedly given off by a cell undergoing mitosis.
**monochromatic r.,** radiation having a single wavelength.
**monoenergetic r.,** radiation of a given type, as of alpha, beta, or gamma rays, in which all particles or photons originate with and have the same energy.
**occipitothalamic r., optic r.,** radiatio optica.
**photochemical r.,** that part of the radiant spectrum which produces chemical changes.
**pyramidal r.,** the projection of fibers from the cerebral cortex to the pyramidal tract of the medulla oblongata.
**tegmental r.,** fibers radiating laterally from the red nucleus.
**thalamic r's,** the four two-way radiations of thalamocortical fibers that connect the dorsal thalamus with many parts of the cerebral cortex; they form a major portion of the internal capsule and the corona radiata. See terms beginning *radiatio thalami,* under *radiatio.* Called also *thalamic peduncles.*
**thalamic r., anterior,** radiatio thalami anterior.
**thalamic r., caudal,** radiatio thalami inferior.
**thalamic r., central,** radiatio thalami centralis.
**thalamic r., inferior,** radiatio thalami inferior.
**thalamic r., posterior,** radiatio thalami posterior.
**thalamic r., superior,** radiatio thalami centralis.

**thalamostriate r.**, the extension of fibers from the thalamus and hypothalamus to the corpus striatum.
**thalamotemporal r.**, radiatio acustica.
**r's of thalamus**, thalamic r's.
**white r.**, bremsstrahlung, def. 1.

**ra·di·a·ti·o·nes** (ra-de-a″she-o′nēz) [L.] plural of *radiatio*.

**rad·i·cal** (rad′ĭ-kəl) [L. *radicalis*] 1. directed to the cause; directed to the root or source of a morbid process, as radical surgery. 2. a group of atoms which enters into and goes out of chemical combination without change, and which forms one of the fundamental constituents of a molecule. Organic radicals are symbolized R.
**acid r.**, 1. the electronegative element which combines with hydrogen to form an acid. 2. all of an acid except the hydroxyl group.
**alcohol r.**, all of the alcohol molecule except the hydrogen atom of the —OH group; an alkoxy radical.
**color r.**, chromophore.
**free r.**, a radical that carries an unpaired electron; such radicals are extremely reactive, with a very short half-life ($10^{-5}$ second or less in an aqueous solution).

**rad·i·ces** (rad′ĭ-sēz) [L.] plural of *radix*.

**ra·dic·i·form** (ra-dis′ĭ-form) [*radix* + *form*] shaped like a root; shaped like the root of a tooth.

**rad·i·cle** (rad′ĭ-kəl) [L. *radicula*] any one of the smallest branches of a vessel or nerve. Called also *radicula* and *ramulus*.

**rad·i·cot·o·my** (rad″ĭ-kot′ə-me) rhizotomy.

**ra·dic·u·la** (rə-dik′u-lə) [L.] radicle.

**ra·dic·u·lal·gia** (rə-dik″u-lal′jə) pain due to disease of the spinal nerve roots.

**ra·dic·u·lar** (rə-dik′u-lər) of or pertaining to a radix or root.

**ra·dic·u·lec·to·my** (rə-dik″u-lek′tə-me) [*radicula* + *-ectomy*] excision of a rootlet, especially resection of spinal nerve roots.

**ra·dic·u·li·tis** (rə-dik″u-li′tis) [*radicula* + *-itis*] [MeSH: Radiculitis] inflammation of the root of a spinal nerve, especially of that portion of the root which lies between the spinal cord and the intervertebral canal. Called also *radicular neuritis*.

**ra·dic·u·lo·gan·gli·o·ni·tis** (rə-dik″u-lo-gang″gle-o-ni′tis) inflammation of the posterior spinal nerve roots and their ganglia.

**ra·dic·u·lo·med·ul·lary** (rə-dik″u-lo-med′u-lar″e) pertaining to or affecting the nerve roots and the spinal cord.

**ra·dic·u·lo·me·nin·go·my·eli·tis** (rə-dik″u-lo-mə-ning″go-mi″ə-li′tis) meningomyeloradiculitis.

**ra·dic·u·lo·my·elop·a·thy** (rə-dik″u-lo-mi″ə-lop′ə-the) myeloradiculopathy.

**ra·dic·u·lo·neu·ri·tis** (rə-dik″u-lo-n o͞o-ri′tis) acute idiopathic polyneuritis.

**ra·dic·u·lo·neu·rop·a·thy** (rə-dik″u-lo-no͞o-rop′ə-the) disease of the nerve roots and nerve.

**ra·dic·u·lop·a·thy** (rə-dik″u-lop′ə-the) disease of the nerve roots.
**cervical r.**, radiculopathy of cervical nerve roots, often manifesting as neck or shoulder pain.
**spondylotic caudal r.**, compression of the cauda equina due to encroachment upon a congenitally small spinal canal by spondylosis, resulting in pseudoclaudication or more profound neural disorders of the lower limbs.

**ra·di·ec·to·my** (ra″de-ek′tə-me) [*radix* + *-ectomy*] root amputation.

**ra·dii** (ra′de-i) [L.] genitive and plural of *radius*.

**radio-** [L. *radius*, q.v.] 1. a combining form denoting relationship *(a)* to the radius (def. 2), or *(b)* to radiant energy, rays, or ionizing radiation. 2. in chemistry, a combining form denoting a radioactive isotope of the element to which it is affixed, e.g., radiocarbon, radiogold.

**ra·dio·ac·tin·i·um** (ra″de-o-ak-tin′e-əm) a substance formed by the disintegration of actinium.

**ra·dio·ac·tive** (ra″de-o-ak′tiv) having the property of radioactivity.

**ra·dio·ac·tiv·i·ty** (ra″de-o-ak-tiv′ĭ-te) [MeSH: Radioactivity] the quality of emitting or the emission of corpuscular or electromagnetic radiations consequent to nuclear disintegration, a natural property of all chemical elements of atomic number above 83, and possible of induction in all other known elements.
**artificial r., induced r.**, radioactivity produced by bombarding an element with high velocity particles, as the radioactivity of synthetic nuclides.

**ra·dio·al·ler·go·sor·bent** (ra″de-o-al″ər-go-sor′bənt) denoting a radioimmunoassay technique for the measurement of specific IgE antibody to a variety of allergens; see under *tests*.

**ra·dio·au·to·gram** (ra″de-o-aw′to-gram) autoradiograph.

**ra·dio·au·to·graph** (ra″de-o-aw′to-graf) autoradiograph.

**ra·dio·au·tog·ra·phy** (ra″de-o-aw-tog′rə-fe) autoradiography.

**ra·dio·bi·cip·i·tal** (ra″de-o-bi-sip′ĭ-təl) pertaining to the radius and the biceps muscle of the arm.

**ra·dio·bi·o·log·i·cal** (ra″de-o-bi″ə-loj′ĭ-kəl) pertaining to radiobiology: concerning cellular and tissue response to irradiation.

**ra·dio·bi·ol·o·gist** (ra″de-o-bi-ol′ə-jist) one who devotes his studies to radiobiology.

**ra·dio·bi·ol·o·gy** (ra″de-o-bi-ol′ə-je) [MeSH: Radiobiology] that branch of science which is concerned with the effect of light and of ultraviolet and ionizing radiations upon living tissue or organisms.

**ra·dio·cal·ci·um** (ra″de-o-kal′se-əm) any of several radioactive isotopes of calcium. The isotopes $^{45}$Ca, with a half-life of 163 days and emitting beta particles of energy 0.255 MeV, and $^{47}$Ca, with a half-life of 4.54 days and emitting beta particles of energy 1.98 and 0.67 MeV and gamma rays of energy 1.30, 0.81, and 0.49 MeV, have been used as tracers in the study of calcium metabolism.

**ra·dio·car·bon** (ra″de-o-kahr′bon) a radioactive isotope of carbon, such as $^{11}$C or $^{14}$C.

**ra·dio·car·ci·no·gen·e·sis** (ra″de-o-kahr″sĭ-no-jen′ə-sis) cancer formation caused by exposure to radiation.

**ra·dio·car·dio·gram** (ra″de-o-kahr′de-o-gram) the graphic record obtained by radiocardiography.

**ra·dio·car·di·og·ra·phy** (ra″de-o-kahr″de-og′rə-fe) 1. the graphic recording of the variation with time of the concentration, in a selected chamber of the heart, of a radioactive isotope, usually injected intravenously. 2. radioelectrocardiography.

**ra·dio·car·pal** (ra″de-o-kahr′pəl) pertaining to the radius and carpus.

**ra·dio·car·pus** (ra″de-o-kahr′pəs) musculus flexor carpi radialis.

**ra·dio·chem·is·try** (ra″de-o-kem′is-tre) [MeSH: Radiochemistry] the branch of chemistry which treats of radioactive materials.

**ra·dio·che·mo·ther·a·py** (ra″de-o-ke-mo-ther′ə-pe) chemoradiotherapy.

**ra·dio·chro·ism** (ra″de-o-kro′iz-əm) [*radio-* + Gr. *chroa* color] the capacity of a substance to absorb certain radioactive and x-rays.

**ra·dio·col·loids** (ra″de-o-kol′oids) radioisotopes in pure form in solution, which tend to behave more like colloids than solutes.

**ra·dio·cur·a·ble** (ra″de-o-kūr′ə-bəl) curable by radiation therapy.

**ra·dio·cys·ti·tis** (ra″de-o-sis-ti′tis) acute or chronic inflammatory tissue changes in the urinary bladder caused by ionizing radiation.

**ra·di·ode** (ra′de-ōd) an instrument for the therapeutic application of a radioactive source.

**ra·dio·dense** (ra′de-o-dens″) radiopaque.

**ra·dio·den·si·ty** (ra″de-o-den′sĭ-te) radiopacity.

**ra·dio·der·ma·ti·tis** (ra″de-o-der″mə-ti′tis) [MeSH: Radiodermatitis] a cutaneous inflammatory reaction occurring as a result of exposure to biologically effective levels of ionizing radiation.

**ra·dio·di·ag·no·sis** (ra″de-o-di″əg-no′sis) diagnosis by means of x-rays and radiographs.

**ra·dio·di·ag·nos·tics** (ra″de-o-di″əg-nos′tiks) the art of x-ray diagnosis.

**ra·dio·dig·i·tal** (ra″de-o-dij′ĭ-təl) pertaining to the radius and to the fingers.

**ra·di·odon·tics** (ra″de-o-don′tiks) dental radiology.

**ra·di·odon·tist** (ra″de-o-don′tist) dental radiologist.

**ra·dio·ecol·o·gy** (ra″de-o-e-kol′ə-je) the science dealing with the effects of radiation on species of plants and animals in natural communities or ecosystems.

**ra·dio·elec·tro·car·dio·gram** (ra″de-o-e-lek″tro-kahr′de-o-gram″) the graphic recording obtained by radioelectrocardiography.

**ra·dio·elec·tro·car·di·o·graph** (ra″de-o-ə-lek″tro-kahr′de-o-graf″) a device for transmission of electrocardiographic signals in radioelectrocardiography.

**ra·dio·elec·tro·car·di·og·ra·phy** (ra″de-o-e-lek″tro-kahr″de-og′rə-fe) electrocardiography in which impulses are beamed by radio from the subject to a receiver close to or at a distance from the subject.

**ra·dio·el·e·ment** (ra″de-o-el′ə-mənt) any chemical element having radioactive properties.

**ra·dio·en·ceph·a·lo·gram** (ra″de-o-ən-sef′ə-lo-gram″) the graphic record obtained by radioencephalography.

**ra·dio·en·ceph·a·log·ra·phy** (ra″de-o-ən-sef″ə-log′rə-fe) 1. REG; the study of the passage of an injected tracer through the cerebral blood vessels as revealed by an external scintillation counter. 2. the recording of changes in the electric potential of the brain without direct attachment between the recording apparatus and the subject, the impulses being beamed by radio waves from the subject to the receiver.

**ra·dio·epi·der·mi·tis** (ra″de-o-ep″ĭ-dər-mi′tis) radiodermatitis.

**ra·dio·epi·the·li·tis** (ra″de-o-ep″ĭ-the-li′tis) radiodermatitis.

**ra·dio·fre·quen·cy** (ra″de-o-fre′kwən-se) radio frequency.

**ra·dio·gen·e·sis** (ra″de-o-jen′ə-sis) the production of rays or radioactivity.

**ra·di·o·gen·ic** (ra″de-o-jen′ik) [*radio-* + *-genic*] produced by irradiation.

**ra·dio·gold** (ra′de-o-gōld″) one of the radioactive isotopes of gold, particularly $^{198}$Au. See *gold Au 198,* under *gold.*

**ra·dio·gram** (ra′de-o-gram″) radiograph.

**ra·dio·graph** (ra′de-o-graf″) a film produced by radiography.
**bite-wing r.,** a type of dental radiograph that reveals the crowns, necks, coronal thirds of the roots of both the upper and lower teeth, and the dental arches, produced on dental x-ray film that has a central protruding tab or wing on which the teeth close to hold the film in position (bite-wing film).
**cephalometric r.,** a radiograph of the head, including the mandible, in full lateral view; used for making cranial measurements. Called also *cephalogram.*
**lateral oblique jaw r.,** a radiograph of the mandible that unilaterally reveals the mandible from symphysis to condyle.
**lateral ramus r.,** a radiograph of the mandibular ramus and condyle.
**lateral skull r.,** a radiograph of the sinuses and lateral aspects of the skeletal structures of the cranium.
**maxillary sinus r.,** Waters' view r.
**panoramic r.,** a type of extraoral body-section radiograph on which the maxilla and the mandible are depicted on a single film. Called also *orthopantograph.*
**submental vertex r., submentovertex r.,** the radiograph made from a submentovertex projection.
**Waters' projection r., Waters' view r.,** the radiograph made from Waters' projection.

**ra·dio·graph·ic** (ra″de-o-graf′ik) pertaining to or produced by radiography.

**ra·di·og·ra·phy** (ra″de-og′rə-fe) [*radio-* + *-graphy*] [MeSH: Radiography] the making of film records (radiographs) of internal structures of the body by passage of x-rays or gamma rays through the body to act on specially sensitized film. Formerly called *roentgenography.*
**body section r.,** tomography.
**digital r.,** a technique in which x-ray absorption is quantified by the assignment of a number to the amount of x-rays reaching the detector; the information is entered into a computer and manipulated to produce an optimal image.
**double-contrast r.,** mucosal relief r.
**electron r.,** a technique in which a latent electron image is produced on clear plastic by passing x-ray photons through a gas with a high atomic number; this image is then developed into a black-and-white picture.
**mass r.,** examination by x-rays of the general population or of large groups of the population.
**miniature r., mass,** the use of miniature x-ray film in mass radiography.
**mucosal relief r.,** radiography of the mucosa of the gastrointestinal tract in a double-contrast examination; called also *double-contrast r.*
**neutron r.,** that in which a narrow beam of neutrons from a nuclear reactor is passed through tissues, especially useful in visualizing bony tissue.
**panoramic r.,** pantomography.
**selective r.,** radiography of certain segments of the population, chosen on some specific basis such as symptoms.
**serial r.,** the taking of several exposures of a selected area at arbitrary intervals.
**spot-film r.,** the making of localized instantaneous radiographs during the course of a fluoroscopic examination, see also *spot film,* under *film.*

**ra·dio·hu·mer·al** (ra″de-o-hu′mər-əl) pertaining to the radius and humerus.

**ra·dio·im·mu·ni·ty** (ra″de-o-ĭ-mu′nĭ-te) a condition of decreased sensitivity to radiation sometimes produced by repeated irradiation.

**ra·dio·im·mu·no·as·say** (ra″de-o-im″u-no-as′a) [MeSH: Radioimmunoassay] a highly sensitive and specific assay method that uses the competition between radiolabeled and unlabeled substances in an antigen-antibody reaction to determine the concentration of the unlabeled substance; it can be used to determine antibody concentrations or to determine the concentration of any substance against which specific antibody can be produced. Abbreviated RIA.

**ra·dio·im·mu·no·de·tec·tion** (ra″de-o-im″u-no-de-tek′shən) [MeSH: Radioimmunodetection] immunodetection by means of the specific interaction of radiolabeled antibody with antigen, as the use of labeled antibody to detect elevated levels of a specific antigen in the diagnosis of certain cancers.

**ra·dio·im·mu·no·dif·fu·sion** (ra″de-o-im″u-no-dĭ-fu′zhən) immunodiffusion conducted with radioisotope-labeled antibodies or antigens.

**ra·dio·im·mu·no·elec·tro·pho·re·sis** (ra″de-o-im″u-no-e-lek″tro-fə-re′sis) immunoelectrophoresis in which a radiolabeled antigen or antibody is located within a specific precipitin arc using autoradiography.

**ra·dio·im·mu·no·im·ag·ing** (ra″de-o-im″u-no-im′ə-jing) imaging in which a radiolabled antibody is introduced into the body to react specifically with its appropriate antigen and thus enable a structure or system of interest to be visualized, as by scintigraphy (immunoscintigraphy).

**ra·dio·im·mu·no·pre·cip·i·ta·tion** (ra″de-o-im″u-no-pre-sip″ĭ-ta′shən) see under *assay.*

**ra·dio·im·mu·no·scin·tig·ra·phy** (ra″de-o-im″u-no-sin-tig′rə-fe) immunoscintigraphy.

**ra·dio·im·mu·no·sor·bent** (ra″de-o-im″u-no-sor′bənt) denoting a radioimmunoassay technique for measuring IgE in samples of serum; see under *tests.*

**ra·dio·io·dine** (ra″de-o-i′o-dīn) any of the nine radioactive isotopes of iodine; $^{131}$I, $^{125}$I, and $^{123}$I are the most commonly used in the diagnosis and treatment of both benign and malignant disease of the thyroid gland and in the scintiscanning of such organs as the lung, liver, and kidney. Called also *radioactive iodine.*

**ra·dio·iron** (ra″de-o-i′ərn) any radioactive isotope of iron; see *iron 55* and *iron 59.*

**ra·dio·iso·tope** (ra″de-o-i′sə-tōp) an isotope which is radioactive; one having an unstable nucleus and emitting characteristic radiation during its decay to a stable form. Radioisotopes have important diagnostic and therapeutic uses in clinical medicine and research. See also *radiopharmaceutical* and *radiotherapy.*
**carrier-free r.,** see *carrier-free.*

**ra·dio·la·bel** (ra′de-o-la″bəl) 1. radioactive label. 2. to incorporate such a radioactive label into a compound.

**ra·dio·lab·eled** (ra″de-o-la′bəld) marked by incorporation of a radioisotope. See also *radioactive tracer,* under *tracer.*

**ra·dio·le·sion** (ra″de-o-le′zhən) a lesion caused by exposure to radiation.

**ra·dio·li·gand** (ra″de-o-li′gand, rad″de-o-lig′and) a radiolabeled substance, e.g., an antigen, used in the quantitative measurement of an unlabeled substance by its binding reaction to a specific antibody or other receptor site.

**ra·di·o·log·ic, ra·di·o·log·i·cal** (ra″de-o-loj′ik, ra″de-o-loj′ĭ-kəl) pertaining to radiology.

**ra·di·ol·o·gist** (ra″de-ol′ə-jist) a physician who specializes in the use of x-rays and other forms of radiation in the diagnosis and treatment of disease.
**dental r.,** a dentist who specializes in dental radiology. Called also *radiodontist.*

**ra·di·ol·o·gy** (ra″de-ol′ə-je) [*radio-* + *-logy*] [MeSH: Radiology] that branch of the health sciences dealing with radioactive substances and radiant energy and with the diagnosis and treatment of disease by means of both ionizing (e.g., x-rays) and nonionizing (e.g., ultrasound) radiations.
**dental r., oral r.,** the branch of radiology dealing primarily with orofacial structures. Called also *radiodontics.*
**interventional r.,** the branch of radiology concerned with providing diagnosis and treatment of disease by a variety of percutaneous procedures performed under the guidance of radiologic imaging.

**ra·dio·lu·cen·cy** (ra″de-o-loo′sən-se) the property of being radiolucent.

**ra·dio·lu·cent** (ra″de-o-loo′sənt) [*radio-* + L. *lucēre* to shine] permitting the passage of x-rays or other forms of radiant energy with little attenuation; radiolucent areas appear dark on the exposed film.

**ra·di·o·lus** (ra-de′o-ləs) [L., dim. of *radius* ray] a probe, staff, or sound.

**ra·di·om·e·ter** (ra″de-om′ə-tər) an instrument for detecting and measuring radiant energy.

**ra·dio·mi·crom·e·ter** (ra″de-o-mi-krom′ə-tər) [*radio-* + *micro-* +

*-meter*] a sensitive radiometer for detecting minute amounts of radiant energy.

**ra·dio·mi·met·ic** (ra″de-o-mi-met′ik) [*radio-* + *-mimetic*] exerting effects similar to those of ionizing radiation.

**ra·dio·mus·cu·lar** (ra″de-o-mus′ku-lər) going from the radial artery or nerve to the muscles.

**ra·dio·mu·ta·tion** (ra″de-o-mu-ta′shən) change in the character of cells caused by exposure to radiation.

**ra·dio·ne·cro·sis** (ra″de-o-nə-kro′sis) destruction of tissue caused by radiation; called also *radiation necrosis.*

**ra·dio·neu·ri·tis** (ra″de-o-no͞o-ri′tis) neuritis resulting from excessive exposure to ionizing radiation.

**ra·di·o·ni·tro·gen** (ra″de-o-ni′trə-jən) any radioactive isotope of nitrogen; see also *nitrogen 13.*

**ra·dio·nu·clide** (ra″de-o-noo′klīd) a radioactive nuclide; one that disintegrates with the emission of corpuscular or electromagnetic radiations.

**ra·dio-opac·i·ty** (ra″de-o-o-pas′ĭ-te) radiopacity.

**ra·di·opac·i·ty** (ra″de-o-pas′ĭ-te) the property of being radiopaque.

**ra·di·opaque** (ra″de-o-pāk′) [*radio-* + *opaque*] not penetrable by x-rays or other forms of radiant energy; radiopaque areas appear light or white on the exposed film.

**ra·dio·par·en·cy** (ra″de-o-par′ən-se) radiolucency.

**ra·dio·par·ent** (ra″de-o-par′ənt) radiolucent.

**ra·dio·pa·thol·o·gy** (ra″de-o-pə-thol′ə-je) pathology having to do with the effects of radiation on tissues.

**ra·dio·phar·ma·ceu·ti·cal** (ra″de-o-fahr″mə-soo′tĭ-kəl) a radioactive pharmaceutical, nuclide, or other chemical used for diagnostic or therapeutic purposes.

**ra·dio·phar·ma·cy** (ra″de-o-fahr′mə-se) the preparation of radioactive pharmaceuticals and radionuclides.

**ra·dio·pho·bia** (ra″de-o-fo′be-ə) [*radio-* + *-phobia* ] irrational anxiety about the damaging effects of x-rays and sources of radiation.

**ra·dio·phos·pho·rus** (ra″de-o-fos′fə-rəs) either of two radioactive isotopes of phosphorus, $^{32}$P and $^{33}$P. See *phosphorus 32; chromic phosphate P 32,* under *phosphate;* and *sodium phosphate P 32.*

**ra·dio·pho·tog·ra·phy** (ra″de-o-fo-tog′rə-fe) photography of the fluorescent image produced by an x-ray beam.

**ra·dio·phy·lax·is** (ra″de-o-fə-lak′sis) the modifying effect of a small dose of radiation on the reaction to a large subsequent radiation.

**ra·dio·phys·ics** (ra″de-o-fiz′iks) the physics of radiology.

**ra·dio·po·tas·si·um** (ra″de-o-po-tas′e-əm) a radioactive isotope of potassium; see *potassium 42.*

**ra·dio·po·ten·ti·a·tion** (ra″de-o-po-ten″she-a′shən) the action of a drug in enhancing the effect of irradiation.

**ra·dio·prax·is** (ra″de-o-prak′sis) [*radio-* + *praxis*] use of rays of light, electricity, etc., in treatment of disease.

**ra·dio·pro·tec·tant** (ra″de-o-pro-tek′tənt) 1. providing protection against the toxic effects of ionizing radiation. 2. radioprotector.

**ra·dio·pro·tec·tor** (ra″de-o-pro-tek′tər) an agent that provides protection against the toxic effects of ionizing radiation.

**ra·dio·pul·mo·nog·ra·phy** (ra″de-o-pul″mə-nog′rə-fe) a rapid method for estimation of ventilation of localized lung areas, based on measurement of variation in intensity of low-voltage x-rays passed through the lungs during breathing.

**ra·dio·re·ac·tion** (ra″de-o-re-ak′shən) a bodily reaction, especially a skin reaction, to radiation.

**ra·dio·re·cep·tor** (ra″de-o-re-sep′tor) 1. a receptor for the stimuli that are excited by radiant energy, such as light or heat. 2. a receptor that can bind to either a radioligand or an unlabeled ligand; see also *radioreceptor assay*, under *assay.*

**ra·dio·re·sis·tance** (ra″de-o-re-zis′təns) resistance, as of tissue or cells, to the injurious effects of radiation.

**ra·dio·re·sis·tant** (ra″de-o-re-zis′tənt) exhibiting the property of radioresistance.

**ra·di·os·co·py** (ra″de-os′kə-pe) [*radio-* + *-scopy*] fluoroscopy.

**ra·dio·sen·si·bil·i·ty** (ra″de-o-sen″sĭ-bil′ĭ-te) radiosensitivity.

**ra·dio·sen·si·tive** (ra″de-o-sen′sĭ-tiv) sensitive to radiant energy, as x-ray or other radiations; said of skin, tumor tissue, etc.

**ra·dio·sen·si·tive·ness** (ra″de-o-sen′sĭ-tiv-nəs) radiosensitivity.

**ra·dio·sen·si·tiv·i·ty** (ra″de-o-sen″sĭ-tiv′ĭ-te) sensitivity, as of the skin or other tissue, to radiant energy, such as x-ray or other radiations.

**ra·dio·sen·si·ti·zer** (ra″de-o-sen′sĭ-ti″zər) a chemotherapeutic agent used to enhance the effect of radiation therapy.

**ra·dio·so·di·um** (ra″de-o-so′de-əm) a radioactive isotope of sodium; see *sodium 22* and *sodium 24.*

**ra·dio·ste·re·os·co·py** (ra″de-o-ster″e-os′kə-pe) [*radio-* + *stereo-* + *-scopy*] the inspection of the interior organs by means of x-rays.

**ra·dio·stron·ti·um** (ra″de-o-stron′she-əm) a radioactive isotope of strontium, four of medical importance being the isotopes $^{85}$Sr, $^{87m}$Sr, $^{89}$Sr, and $^{90}$Sr. See also individual isotopes under *strontium.*

**ra·dio·sul·fur** (ra″de-o-sul′fər) a radioactive isotope of sulfur. See *sulfur 35.*

**ra·dio·sur·gery** (ra″de-o-sər′jər-e) [MeSH: Radiosurgery] surgery in which tissue destruction is by means of ionizing radiation rather than surgical incision; the radiation may be from an implant or an external source.
**stereotactic r., stereotaxic r.,** stereotactic surgery in which lesions are produced by ionizing radiation.

**ra·dio·tel·em·e·try** (ra″de-o-təl-em′ə-tre) the determination of measurement of various factors, the specific data being transmitted by radio waves from the object of measurement to the recording apparatus.

**ra·dio·than·a·tol·o·gy** (ra″de-o-than″ə-tol′ə-je) [*radio-* + *thanato-* + *-logy*] the study of the effect of radiant energy on dead tissue.

**ra·dio·ther·a·peu·tics** (ra″de-o-ther″ə-pu′tiks) 1. the body of knowledge comprising the available information regarding the therapeutic use of ionizing radiation. 2. radiotherapy.

**ra·dio·ther·a·pist** (ra″de-o-ther′ə-pist) a specialist in radiotherapy.

**ra·dio·ther·a·py** (ra″de-o-ther′ə-pe) [*radio-* + *therapy*] [MeSH: Radiotherapy] the treatment of disease by ionizing radiation. Called also *irradiation* and *radiation therapy.*
**extended field r.,** see under *irradiation.*
**external beam r.,** treatment by radiation emitted from a source located at a distance from the body; called also *beam therapy* and *external beam therapy.*
**hemibody r.,** see under *irradiation.*
**high-voltage r.,** radiotherapy in which the radiation has a voltage of over 300 KV. See *orthovoltage r., supervoltage r.,* and *megavoltage r.*
**hyperfractionated r.,** hyperfractionation.
**interstitial r.,** that administered with the radioactive element contained in devices (e.g., needles or wire) inserted directly into the tissues.
**intracavitary r.,** that in which the radioactive element is introduced into a natural body cavity.
**inverted Y field r.,** see under *irradiation.*
**involved field r.,** see under *irradiation.*
**mantle field r.,** see under *irradiation.*
**megavoltage r.,** radiotherapy in which the radiation has voltage of 1000 KV or more.
**neoadjuvant r.,** radiotherapy used as neoadjuvant therapy (q.v.) for cancer. Called also *preoperative r.*
**orthovoltage r.,** radiotherapy in which the radiation has voltage between 140 and 400 KV.
**preoperative r.,** neoadjuvant r.
**supervoltage r.,** radiotherapy in which the radiation has voltage between 400 and 1000 KV.

**ra·di·ot·o·my** (ra″de-ot′ə-me) [*radio-* + *-tomy*] tomography.

**ra·dio·tox·emia** (ra″de-o-tok-se′me-ə) toxemia produced by radiation or a radioactive substance.

**ra·dio·tra·cer** (ra″de-o-tra′sər) radioactive tracer.

**ra·dio·trans·par·en·cy** (ra″de-o-trans-par′ən-se) radiolucency.

**ra·dio·trans·par·ent** (ra″de-o-trans-par′ənt) radiolucent.

**ra·di·o·trop·ic** (ra″de-o-trop′ik) influenced by radiation.

**ra·di·ot·ro·pism** (ra″de-ot′ro-piz-əm) a tropism with regard to radiation.

**ra·dio·ul·nar** (ra″de-o-ul′nər) pertaining to the radius and ulna.

**ra·di·sec·to·my** (ra″de-sek′tə-me) [*radix* + *-ectomy*] root amputation.

**rad·ish** (rad′ish) 1. any of various plants of the genus *Raphanus.* 2. the edible root of *Raphanus sativus.*

**ra·di·um** (ra′de-əm) [so called from its radiant quality] [MeSH: Radium] a rare radioactive element in the uranium decay series. It has an atomic weight of 226, an atomic number of 88, and a half-life of 1600 years. It is found mainly in pitchblende and undergoes spontaneous disintegration with formation of a gas called radon (half-life = 3.85 days). In this process it emits alpha particles. Radon (alpha emitter) on deposit in solid form disintegrates into a series of decay products: radium A (half-life = 3 minutes), radium B (half-life = 26.7 minutes), and radium C (half-life = 19.5 minutes). The beta particles and gamma radiations used in clinical therapy originate from radium B and C. With radium in a sealed container and the same number of atoms of each decay product disintegrating per second, radium and its decay products are in equilibrium. In this state, the formation of beta particles and gamma rays reaches its maximum. In clinical gamma-ray therapy, shielding off of the beta particles can be accomplished by a metallic container, e.g., of gold or platinum. A glass wall container permits irradiation with beta particles as well as gamma rays.

**ra•di•us** (ra′de-əs) gen. and pl. *ra′dii* [L. "spoke" (of a wheel)] [MeSH: Radius] 1. a line segment from the center to the circumference of a circle or the surface of a sphere; the length of such a segment. Symbol *r.* 2. [TA] the bone on the outer or thumb side of the forearm, articulating proximally with the humerus and ulna and distally with the ulna and carpus; see Plate 45.

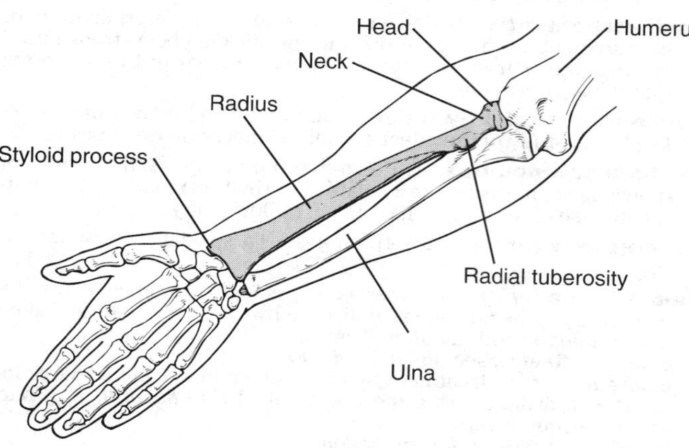


Radius.

**r. cur′vus,** Madelung's deformity.
**r. fix′us,** a straight line from the hormion to the inion.
**ra′dii len′tis** [TA], radii of lens: imaginary lines extending from the midpoint of the axis of the lens of the eye to the capsule of the lens.
**ra′dii medulla′res** [TA], medullary radii: the cortical extensions of bundles of tubules from the renal pyramids.
**van der Waals r.,** the distance at which there is a balance between van der Waals attractive and repulsive forces in the formation of chemical bonds.

**ra•dix** (ra′diks) gen. *ra′dicis,* pl. *ra′dices* [L.] [TA] root: a general term for the most inferior part, or a part by which a structure is anchored, as the portion of a hair, nail, or tooth that is buried in the tissues, or the part of a nerve adjacent to the center to which it is connected.

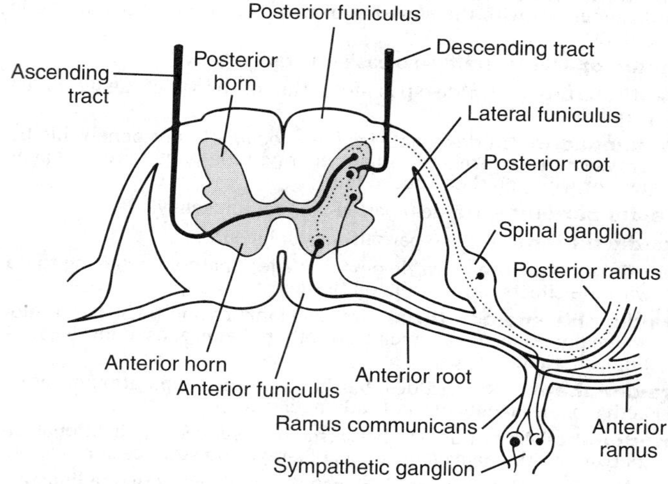


Diagram of a horizontal section of the spinal cord, with posterior and anterior roots and a spinal nerve.

## Radix

Descriptions are given on TA terms, and include anglicized names of specific roots.

**r. ante′rior an′sae cervica′lis,** r. superior ansae cervicalis.
**r. ante′rior ner′vi spina′lis** [TA], anterior root of spinal nerve: the motor division of each spinal nerve, attached centrally to the spinal cord and joining peripherally with the corresponding posterior (sensory) root to form the nerve before it emerges through the intervertebral foramen. It conveys motor fibers to skeletal muscle and contains preganglionic autonomic fibers at thoracolumbar and sacral levels. There are 31 anterior and 31 posterior roots: 8 cervical, 12 thoracic, 5 lumbar, 5 sacral, and 1 coccygeal. Called also *ventral* or *motor root of spinal nerve, r. ventralis nervi spinalis,* and *r. motoria nervi spinalis* [TA alternative].
**r. ar′cus ver′tebrae,** pediculus arcus vertebralis.
**r. basa′lis ante′rior ve′nae basa′lis commu′nis,** anterior basal root of common basal vein: a venous root draining the anterior basal segment of the right lung and emptying into the common basal vein.
**r. cli′nica** [TA], clinical root: that portion of a tooth below the clinical crown, being attached to the gingiva or alveolus.
**r. cochlea′ris ner′vi vestibulocochlea′ris,** the central continuation of the cochlear nerve from the spiral ganglion, passing dorsal to the inferior cerebellar peduncle to enter the brain; called also *r. inferior nervi vestibulocochlearis.*
**r. crania′lis ner′vi accesso′rii** [TA], cranial root of accessory nerves: any of the nerve roots originating from the nucleus ambiguus and emerging from the side of the medulla oblongata below the roots of the vagus nerve; they then unite with the spinal portion in the jugular foramen. Their constituent fibers then form the internal branch, which joins the vagus nerve and is distributed to the soft palate, constrictors of the pharynx, and the larynx. Called also *pars vagalis nervi accessorii* [TA alternative].
**r. den′tis** [TA], root of tooth: the portion of a tooth which is covered by cementum, proximal to the neck of the tooth and ordinarily embedded in the dental alveolus; called also *anatomical root.*
**r. dorsa′lis ner′vi spina′lis,** r. posterior nervi spinalis.
**r. facia′lis,** nervus canalis pterygoidei.
**r. infe′rior an′sae cervica′lis** [TA], inferior root of ansa cervicalis: a strand of filaments connecting the ansa cervicalis with branches of the second and third cervical nerves; called also *r. posterior ansae cervicalis* and *posterior root of ansa cervicalis.*
**r. infe′rior ner′vi vestibulocochlea′ris,** r. cochlearis nervi vestibulocochlearis.
**r. interme′dia gan′glii pterygopala′tini,** TA alternative for *nervus petrosus major.*
**r. latera′lis ner′vi media′ni** [TA], lateral root of median nerve: the fibers contributed to the median nerve by the lateral cord of the brachial plexus.
**r. latera′lis trac′tus op′tici** [TA], lateral root of optic tract: fibers from the optic tract that enter the lateral geniculate body.
**r. lin′guae** [TA], root of tongue: the portion of the tongue posterior to the sulcus terminalis, being attached inferiorly to the hyoid bone, and directed posteriorly and superiorly.
**r. media′lis ner′vi media′ni** [TA], medial root of median nerve: the fibers contributed to the median nerve by the medial cord of the brachial plexus.
**r. media′lis trac′tus op′tici** [TA], medial root of optic tract: fibers from the optic tract that enter the superior colliculus and the pretectal region.
**r. mesente′rii** [TA], root of mesentery: the line of attachment of the mesentery to the posterior abdominal wall, extending from the duodenojejunal flexure at the left of the second lumbar vertebra diagonally downward to the upper border of the right sacroiliac articulation.

**r. moto'ria ner'vi spina'lis,** TA alternative for *r. anterior nervi spinalis.*

**r. moto'ria ner'vi trige'mini** [TA], motor root of trigeminal nerve: the smaller of the two roots by which the trigeminal nerve is attached to the side of the pons; it contains proprioceptive as well as motor fibers, and continues deep to the trigeminal ganglion to join the mandibular nerve.

**r. nasa'lis,** TA alternative for *r. nasi.*

**r. na'si** [TA], root of nose: the upper portion of the nose, which is attached to the frontal bone. Called also *r. nasalis* [TA alternative].

**r. nasocilia'ris gan'glii cilia'ris,** TA alternative for *r. sensoria ganglii ciliaris.*

**r. oculomoto'ria gan'glii cilia'ris,** TA alternative for *r. parasympathica ganglii ciliaris.*

**r. parasympa'thica gan'glii cilia'ris** [TA], parasympathetic root of ciliary ganglion: a short collection of fibers passing from the inferior branch of the oculomotor nerve to the posterior inferior portion of the ciliary ganglion; it contains preganglionic parasympathetic fibers for the sphincter papillae and the ciliary muscle. Called also *r. oculomotoria ganglii ciliaris* [TA alternative], *ramus nervi oculomotorii ad ganglion ciliare* [TA alternative], and *motor, short,* or *oculomotor root of ciliary ganglion.*

**r. parasympa'thica gan'glii o'tici,** TA alternative for *nervus petrosus minor.* NOTE: when considering the ganglia of the pars parasympathica, this is the preferred term in the official nomenclature.

**r. parasympa'thica ganglio'rum pelvico'rum** [TA], parasympathetic root of pelvic ganglia: *origin,* sacral plexus—S3–S4; *distribution,* leaving the sacral plexus, they enter the inferior hypogastric plexus and supply the pelvic organs; *modality,* preganglionic parasympathetic and visceral afferent. Called also *nervi splanchnici pelvici* [TA alternative] and *pelvic splanchnic nerves.*

**r. parasympa'thica gan'glii pterygopalati'ni,** TA alternative for *nervus petrosus major.* NOTE: when considering the ganglia of the pars parasympathica, this is the preferred term in the official nomenclature.

**r. parasympa'thica gan'glii sublingua'lis, r. parasympa'thica gan'glii submandibula'ris,** TA alternative for *chorda tympani.* NOTE: when considering the ganglia of the pars parasympathica, this is the preferred term in the official nomenclature.

**r. pe'nis** [TA], root of penis: the proximal, attached portion of the penis, consisting of the diverging crura of the corpora cavernosa and the bulb.

**r. pi'li,** root of hair: the proximal portion of a hair embedded in the hair follicle.

**ra'dices plex'us brachia'lis** [TA], roots of brachial plexus: the anterior branches of the four lower cervical spinal nerves and the first thoracic nerve, which combine to form the trunks of the brachial plexus; see *rami ventrales nervorum cervicalium* and *rami ventrales nervorum thoracicorum,* under *ramus.*

**r. poste'rior an'sae cervica'lis,** r. inferior ansae cervicalis.

**r. poste'rior ner'vi spina'lis** [TA], posterior root of spinal nerve: the sensory division of each spinal nerve, attached centrally to the spinal cord and joining peripherally with the anterior (motor) root to form the nerve before it emerges through the intervertebral foramen: each posterior root bears a spinal ganglion and conveys sensory fibers to the spinal cord. There are 31 anterior and 31 posterior nerve roots: 8 cervical, 12 thoracic, 5 lumbar, 5 sacral, and 1 coccygeal. Called also *dorsal* or *sensory root of spinal nerves, r. dorsalis nervi spinalis,* and *r. sensoria nervi spinalis* [TA alternative].

**r. pulmo'nis** [TA], root of lung: the attachment of either lung, comprising the structures entering and emerging at the hilum; called also *pedicle of lung* and *pediculus pulmonis.*

**r. senso'ria gan'glii cilia'ris** [TA], sensory root of ciliary ganglion: sensory fibers from the cornea, iris, ciliary body, and choroid that pass through the ciliary ganglion to the nasociliary nerve. Called also *r. nasociliaris ganglii ciliaris* [TA alternative], *ramus communicans nervi nasociliaris cum ganglio ciliari,* [TA alternative], and *long* or *nasociliary root of ciliary ganglion.*

**r. senso'ria gan'glii o'tici,** TA alternative for *rami ganglionares nervi mandibularis ad ganglion oticum.*

**r. senso'ria gan'glii pterygopalati'ni,** TA alternative for *rami ganglionares nervi maxillaris ad ganglion pterygopalatinum.*

**r. senso'ria gan'glii submandibula'ris,** TA alternative for *rami ganglionares nervi lingualis ad ganglion submandibulare.*

**r. senso'ria ner'vi spina'lis,** TA alternative for *r. posterior nervi spinalis.*

**r. senso'ria ner'vi trige'mini** [TA], sensory root of trigeminal nerve: the larger of the two roots by which the trigeminal nerve is attached to the side of the pons. It contains sensory fibers and expands into a large flat ganglion (the trigeminal ganglion) which gives rise to the ophthalmic, maxillary, and mandibular nerves.

**r. spina'lis ner'vi accesso'rii** [TA], spinal root of accessory nerve: any of the nerve roots originating from the gray matter of the spinal cord and emerging from the side of the cord as far down as a level between the third and seventh cervical nerves; they then form a trunk that ascends in the vertebral canal, passes through the foramen magnum, and unites with the cranial portion in the jugular foramen. The constituent fibers then form the external branch, which supplies the sternocleidomastoid and trapezius muscles. Called also *pars spinalis nervi accessorii* [TA alternative].

**r. supe'rior an'sae cervica'lis** [TA], superior root of ansa cervicalis: fibers of the first or second cervical nerve, descending in company with the hypoglossal nerve, connecting it with the ansa cervicalis and helping supply the infrahyoid muscles. Called also *r. anterior ansae cervicalis* and *anterior root of ansa cervicalis.*

**r. supe'rior ner'vi vestibulocochlea'ris,** r. vestibularis nervi vestibulocochlearis.

**r. sympathe'tica gan'glii cilia'ris, r. sympa'thica gan'glii cilia'ris** [TA], sympathetic root of ciliary ganglion: postganglionic fibers from the superior cervical ganglion, derived from the internal carotid plexus, to the ciliary ganglion, for distribution by the short ciliary nerves to the dilator muscle of the pupil, orbital muscle and tarsal muscles, and blood vessels of the eyeball. Called also *ramus sympatheticus ganglii ciliaris* [TA alternative] and *ramus sympathicus ganglii ciliaris.*

**r. sympa'thica gang'lii pterygopalati'ni,** TA alternative for *nervus petrosus profundus.* NOTE: when considering the ganglia of the pars parasympathica, this is the preferred term in the official nomenclature.

**r. un'guis,** root of nail: the proximal portion of the nail, situated in the sulcus of the matrix of the nail.

**r. ventra'lis ner'vi spina'lis,** r. anterior nervi spinalis.

**r. vestibula'ris ner'vi vestibulocochlea'ris,** vestibular root of vestibulocochlear nerve: the central continuation of the vestibular nerve from the vestibular ganglion, entering the brain, just lateral to the intermediate nerve and in front of the inferior cerebellar peduncle. Called also *r. superior nervi vestibulocochlearis* and *superior root of vestibulocochlear nerve.*

**ra·don** (ra'don) [MeSH: Radon] a heavy, colorless, gaseous, radioactive element, symbol Rn, atomic weight 222, atomic number 86, obtained by the breaking up of radium, and used in radiotherapy. $^{219}$Rn is a radioactive isotope of the actinium radioactive series. $^{220}$Rn is a radioactive isotope of the thorium radioactive series.

**Ra·do·vi·ci's sign** (rah-do-ve'sez) [André *Radovici,* French physician, 20th century] see *palm-chin reflex,* under *reflex.*

**RAE** right atrial enlargement; see *atrial enlargement,* under *enlargement.*

**Rae·der's syndrome, paratrigeminal syndrome** (ra'dərz) [Johan Georg *Raeder,* Norwegian ophthalmologist, 1889–1956] see under *syndrome.*

**raf·fi·nose** (raf'ĭ-nōs) [MeSH: Raffinose] a nonreducing trisaccharide occurring abundantly in sugar beets and other plants; it is composed of galactose linked $\alpha$-(1,6) to glucose, which is linked $\beta$-(1,2) to fructose. Formerly called *melitose.*

**ra·fox·a·nide** (rə-fok'sə-nīd) [MeSH: Rafoxanide] a salicylanilide anthelmintic used in cattle and sheep.

**rage** (rāj) [MeSH: Rage] a state of violent anger.

**sham r.,** an outburst of behavior in a decorticated animal, resembling fear or anger; a similar phenomenon may be observed in humans with insulin-induced hypoglycemia or carbon monoxide poisoning.

**rag·o·cyte** (rag'o-sīt) [*Ragg* (*r*heumatoid serum *agg*lutinator + *-cyte*] a polymorphonuclear leukocyte with cytoplasmic inclusions of ingested aggregated IgG, rheumatoid factor, fibrin, and complement, found in the joints in rheumatoid arthritis. Called also *RA cell.*

**rag·weed** (rag'wēd) any of various species of plants of the genus *Ambrosia* whose pollen can cause hay fever.

**rag·wort** (rag'wərt) any of various poisonous plants of the genus *Senecio.*

**Rah·nel·la** (rə-nel'ə) [Otto *Rahn,* German-American microbiologist] a genus of gram-negative, facultatively anaerobic, rod-shaped bacteria of the family Enterobacteriaceae, occurring in fresh water and occasionally isolated from human clinical specimens. The type species is *R. aqua'tilis.*

**ra·i·gan** (ra'ĭ-gan) [Chinese] dried mushrooms of the species *Omphalia lapidescens,* an anthelmintic used in Chinese medicine.

**Rail·li·e·tia** (ri-le'te-ə) [Louis-Joseph Alcide *Railliet,* French biologist, 1852–1930] a genus of parasitic mites; *R. au'ris* is found in the ears of cattle and sometimes causes ulceration.

**Rail·li·e·ti·na** (ri″le-ə-ti'nə) [L.-J. A. *Railliet*] a genus of tapeworms of the family Davaineidae, many species of which infect birds, domestic fowl, and mammals. *R. asia'tica, R. celeben'sis, R. demararien'sis (Taenia demarariensis), R. formosa'na, R. loechesa'lavezi,* and *R. madagascarien'sis (Taenia madagascariensis)* (the Madagascar tapeworm) have been reported from human infections.

**rail·li·e·ti·ni·a·sis** (ri″le-ə-tĭ-ni'ə-sis) infection with a parasite of the genus *Raillietina.*

**Rai·ney's tube, tubule** (ra'nēz) [George *Rainey,* English anatomist, 1801–1884] sarcocyst.

**RAIU** radioactive iodine uptake.

**rak·ing** (ra'king) gathering, moving, scraping, or loosening, as with a rake.
**back r.,** extraction of impacted feces from the rectum of an animal.

**rale** (rahl) [MeSH: Respiratory Sounds] a discontinuous sound (q.v.) consisting of a series of short nonmusical noises, heard primarily during inhalation; called also *crackle.*
**amphoric r.,** a coarse, musical, and tinkling rale caused by the splashing of fluid in a cavity connected with a bronchus. Called also *bottle sound.*
**atelectatic r.,** a nonpathologic rale that is dissipated by deep breathing or coughing and is best observed at the margin of a lung. This type is frequently heard in those who breathe feebly and superficially, when on deep inspiration the moist walls of the unexpanded alveoli are suddenly forced apart by the entering air; after a few deep inspirations these rales are lost. Called also *marginal* or *border r.*
**border r.,** atelectatic r.
**bubbling r.,** a moist rale heard when air passes through areas of bronchi that contain mucus.
**cavernous r.,** a hollow and metallic rale caused by the alternate expansion and contraction of a pulmonary cavity during respiration.
**cellophane r.,** one resembling the rustling of cellophane, heard in interstitial pulmonary fibrosis.
**clicking r.,** a small, sticky moist rale heard in inspiration, caused by the passage of air through secretions in the smaller bronchi.
**consonating r.,** a clear, ringing sound produced in bronchial tubes that are surrounded by consolidation tissues.
**crackling r.,** subcrepitant r.
**crepitant r.,** a very fine rale, resembling the sound produced by rubbing a lock of hair between the fingers or by particles of salt thrown on fire; heard at the end of inspiration. Called also *crepitus.*
**dry r.,** originally, a rale with a whistling or squeaking quality produced by the presence of viscid secretions in the bronchial tubes or by spastic contraction of the tube walls. Because it seemed contradictory to refer to such a rale as "dry," the term is now more often used to describe fine crackles associated with many types of interstitial lung disease, including idiopathic pulmonary fibrosis.
**gurgling r.,** a very coarse type of bubbling rale.
**guttural r.,** a rale produced in the throat.
**marginal r.,** atelectatic r.
**metallic r.,** consonating r.
**moist r.,** any of numerous rales produced by the presence of liquid in the bronchial tubes.
**mucous r.,** bubbling r.
**subcrepitant r.,** a fine, moist rale heard in conditions that are associated with liquid in the smaller tubes; called also *crackling r.*
**tracheal r.,** a rale produced in the trachea.
**vesicular r.,** crepitant r.

**Ral·gro** (ral'gro) trademark for a preparation of zeranol.

**ral·ox·i·fene hy·dro·chlo·ride** (ral-ok'sĭ-fēn) a selective estrogen receptor modulator that has estrogenlike effects on bone, increasing bone mineral density, and lipid metabolism, decreasing total and LDL cholesterol, but not on breast and uterine tissue; used for the prevention of postmenopausal osteoporosis, administered orally.

**Ral·sto·nia** (rawl-sto'ne-ə) a genus of gram-negative rod-shaped bacteria of the family Pseudomonadaceae, formerly included in group II of the genus *Pseudomonas.*
**R. picket'tii,** the type species, isolated from numerous clinical and environmental sources and a potential human pathogen. One biovar, a strain formerly called *P. thomasii,* has been isolated from contaminated intravenous fluids and identified as the cause of nosocomial infections of the blood and urinary and respiratory tracts. Formerly called *Pseudomonas pickettii* and *Burkholderia pickettii.*

**ra·mal** (ra'məl) pertaining to a ramus; branching.

**Ra·man effect** (rah'mahn) [Sir Chandrasekhara Venkata *Raman,* Indian physicist, 1888–1970; winner of the Nobel prize for physics in 1930] see under *effect.*

**RAMC** Royal Army Medical Corps.

**ra·mi** (ra'mi) [L.] genitive and plural of *ramus.*

**Ra·mi·bac·te·ri·um** (ra″me-bak-tēr'e-əm) [L. *ramus* branch + *bacterium*] in former systems of classification, a genus of bacteria of the family Lactobacillaceae, made up of nonsporulating, anaerobic, gram-positive, rod-shaped organisms. These organisms are now assigned to the genus *Eubacterium.*

**ram·i·cot·o·my** (ram″ĭ-kot'ə-me) [*ramus* + *-tomy*] ramisection.

**ram·i·fi·ca·tion** (ram″ĭ-fĭ-ka'shən) [*ramus* + L. *facere* to make] 1. distribution in branches. 2. a branch or set of branches. 3. the manner of branching.

**ram·i·fy** (ram'ĭ-fi) [*ramus* + L. *facere* to make] 1. to branch; to diverge in various directions. 2. to traverse in branches.

**ra·mi·pril** (rə-mi'pril) [MeSH: Ramipril] an angiotensin-converting enzyme inhibitor used as an antihypertensive, administered orally.

**rami·sec·tion** (ram″ĭ-sek'shən) [*ramus* + *section*] the operation of cutting one or more of the rami communicantes of the sympathetic nervous system; called also *ramicotomy, ramisectomy,* and *sympathetic ramisection.*

**ram·i·sec·to·my** (ram″ĭ-sek'tə-me) ramisection.

**ram·itis** (ram-i'tis) [*ramus* + *-itis*] inflammation of a ramus.

**Ramm·stedt** (rahm'shtet) see *Ramstedt.*

**ra·mol·lisse·ment** (rah″mo-lēs-maw') [Fr.] softening.

**Ra·mon's flocculation test** (rah-mawz') [Gaston *Ramon,* French bacteriologist 1886–1963] see under *test.*

**Ram·ond's sign** (rah-mawz') [Louis *Ramond,* French internist, 1879–1952] see under *point* and *sign.*

**Ra·món y Ca·jal** (rah-mōn'e-kah-hahl') Santiago. Spanish physician and histologist, 1852–1934; co-winner, with Camillo Golgi, of the Nobel prize for medicine or physiology in 1906 for describing the terminal branches of neurons, developing a method of staining nerve tissues, and discovering the structure of the nervous system.

**ra·mose** (ra'mos) [L. *ramus* branch] branching; having many branches.

**ram·part** (ram'pahrt) a broad, encircling embankment.
**maxillary r.,** a ridge or mound of epithelial cells seen in that portion of the jaw of the embryo which is to become the alveolar border.

**Ram·say Hunt paralysis, syndrome** (ram'se-hunt) [James *Ramsay Hunt,* American neurologist, 1872–1937] see *dyssynergia cerebellaris progressiva;* see *juvenile paralysis agitans (of Hunt),* under *paralysis;* and see under *syndrome.*

**Rams·den's eyepiece** (ramz'dənz) [Jesse *Ramsden,* English instrument maker and optician, 1735–1800] see under *eyepiece.*

**Ram·stedt operation** (rahm'shtet) [Conrad *Ramstedt,* German surgeon, 1867–1963] see *Fredet-Ramstedt operation,* under *operation.*

**ram·u·lus** (ram'u-ləs) pl. *ra'muli* [L., dim. of *ramus*] radicle.

**ra·mus** (ra'məs) gen. and pl. *ra'mi* [L.] [TA] a branch: a general term for a smaller structure given off by a larger one, or into which the larger structure, such as a blood vessel or nerve, divides.

Descriptions are give on TA terms, and include anglicized names of specific branches.

**r. accesso'rius arte'riae menin'geae me'diae** [TA], accessory branch of middle meningeal artery: a branch arising from the middle meningeal artery, or directly from the maxillary artery, and entering the middle cranial fossa through the foramen ovale to supply the trigeminal ganglion, walls of the cavernous sinus, and neighboring dura mater.

**r. acetabula'ris arte'riae circumflex'ae fe'moris media'lis** [TA], acetabular branch of medial circumflex femoral artery: a branch of the medial circumflex artery of the thigh, distributed to the head of the femur and to the acetabulum. Called also *acetabular artery* and *r. acetabuli arteriae circumflexae femoris medialis.*

**r. acetabula'ris arte'riae obturato'riae** [TA], acetabular branch of obturator artery: a branch distributed to the hip joint; called also *acetabular artery* and *arteria acetabuli.*

**r. aceta'buli arte'riae circumflex'ae fe'moris media'lis,** r. acetabularis arteriae circumflexae femoris medialis.

**r. acromia'lis arte'riae suprascapula'ris** [TA], acromial branch of suprascapular artery: a branch distributed to the acromion process; called also *r. acromialis arteriae transversae scapulae.*

**r. acromia'lis arte'riae thoracoacromia'lis** [TA], acromial branch of thoracoacromial artery: a branch distributed to the deltoid muscle and acromion process.

**r. acromia'lis arte'riae transver'sae sca'pulae,** r. acromialis arteriae suprascapularis.

**r. al'bus ner'vi spina'lis,** r. communicans albus nervi spinalis.

**ra'mi alveola'res superio'res anterio'res ner'vi maxilla'ris** [TA], anterior superior alveolar branches of maxillary nerve: branches from the infraorbital nerve that innervate the incisor and canine teeth of the upper jaw, help form the superior dental plexus, and give terminal twigs to the floor of the nose; modality, general sensory.

**r. alveola'ris supe'rior me'dius ner'vi maxilla'ris** [TA], middle superior alveolar branch of maxillary nerve: a branch from the infraorbital nerve that innervates the premolar teeth of the upper jaw by way of the superior dental plexus; modality, general sensory.

**ra'mi alveola'res superio'res posterio'res ner'vi maxilla'ris** [TA], posterior superior alveolar branches of maxillary nerve: branches that innervate the maxillary sinus, cheek, gums, and molar and premolar teeth of the upper jaw; they form part of the superior dental plexus; modality, general sensory.

**rami anastomo'tici,** rami communicantes (def. 2).

**r. anastomo'ticus arte'riae lacrima'lis cum arte'ria menin'gea me'dia** [TA], a branch of the lacrimal artery that anastomoses with the meningeal artery.

**r. anastomo'ticus arte'riae menin'geae me'diae cum arte'ria lacrima'li** [TA], a branch of the middle meningeal artery that is distributed to the orbit and anastomoses with the recurrent meningeal branch of the lacrimal artery.

**r. ante'rior arte'riae obturato'riae** [TA], anterior branch of obturator artery: a branch that passes forward around the medial margin of the obturator foramen, on the obturator membrane, and is distributed to the obturator and adductor muscles.

**r. ante'rior arte'riae pancreaticoduodena'lis inferio'ris** [TA], anterior branch of inferior pancreaticoduodenal artery: a branch that passes in front of the head of the pancreas and then ascends to anastomose with the anterior superior pancreaticoduodenal artery; it supplies the head of the pancreas and adjoining parts of the duodenum.

**r. ante'rior arte'riae recurren'tis ulna'ris** [TA], anterior branch of ulnar recurrent artery: a branch that helps supply the pronator teres and brachialis muscles and runs to the front of the medial epicondyle, supplying the elbow joint and adjacent structures.

**r. ante'rior arte'riae rena'lis** [TA], anterior branch of renal artery: a branch supplying the anterior, superior, and inferior segments of the kidney.

**r. ante'rior arte'riae thyroi'deae superio'ris,** r. glandularis anterior arteriae thyroideae superioris.

**r. ante'rior duc'tus hepa'tici dex'tri** [TA], the anterior branch of the right hepatic duct.

**r. ante'rior ner'vi auricula'ris mag'ni** [TA], anterior branch of great auricular nerve; a branch distributed to the skin of the face over the parotid gland; modality, general sensory.

**ra'mi anterio'res nervo'rum cervica'lium** [TA], anterior branches of cervical nerves: eight nerve branches of which the upper four form the cervical plexus and the lower four form most of the brachial plexus; see also *r. anterior nervi spinalis.* Called also *rami ventrales nervorum cervicalium* [TA alternative].

**r. ante'rior ner'vi coccy'gei** [TA], anterior branch of coccygeal nerve: a branch of the last spinal nerve, emerging from the sacral hiatus and contributing to the coccygeal plexus; called also *r. ventralis nervi coccygei* [TA alternative].

**r. ante'rior ner'vi cuta'nei antebra'chii media'lis** [TA], anterior branch of medial cutaneous nerve of forearm: a branch that innervates the skin of the front and medial aspect of the forearm; modality, general sensory.

**ra'mi anterio'res nervo'rum lumba'lium** [TA], anterior branches of lumbar nerves: the anterior branches of the five lumbar spinal nerves; the upper four form the lumbar plexus, and the fifth and a part of the fourth form part of the sacral plexus. Called also *rami ventrales nervorum lumbalium* [TA alternative].

**r. ante'rior ner'vi obturato'rii** [TA], anterior branch of obturator nerve: a branch that supplies the gracilis and the adductor longus and brevis muscles and the pectineus, and occasionally gives off a branch to the skin of the medial side of the thigh and leg; modality, motor and general sensory.

**ra'mi anterio'res nervo'rum sacra'lium** [TA], anterior branches of sacral nerves: branches of the five sacral spinal nerves; the upper four emerge from the sacrum through the anterior foramina and contribute to the sacral plexus, and the fifth emerges through the sacral hiatus and, with a communication from the fourth, contributes to the coccygeal plexus. Called also *rami ventrales nervorum sacralium* [TA alternative].

**r. ante'rior ner'vi spina'lis** [TA], anterior branch of spinal nerve: the anterior and usually larger of the two branches into which each spinal nerve divides almost as soon as it emerges from the intervertebral foramen; the anterior branches supply anterior and lateral parts of the trunk and all parts of the limbs.

**ra'mi anterio'res nervo'rum thoracico'rum,** TA alternative for *nervi intercostales.*

**r. ante'rior sul'ci latera'lis ce'rebri** [TA], anterior branch of lateral cerebral sulcus: a branch that runs forward a short distance into the inferior frontal gyrus.

**anterior rami of thoracic nerves,** nervi intercostales.

**r. ante'rior ve'nae pulmona'lis dex'trae superio'ris,** TA alternative for *vena anterior lobi superioris pulmonis dextri.*

**r. ante'rior ve'nae pulmona'lis sinis'trae superio'ris,** TA alternative for *vena anterior lobi superioris pulmonis sinistri.*

**r. apica'lis arte'riae pulmona'lis dex'trae,** arteria segmentalis apicalis pulmonis dextri.

**r. apica'lis arte'riae pulmona'lis sinis'trae,** arteria segmentalis apicalis pulmonis sinistri.

**r. apica'lis ve'nae pulmona'lis dex'trae superio'ris,** TA alternative for *vena apicalis lobi superioris pulmonis dextri.*

**r. apicoposte'rior ve'nae pulmona'lis sinis'trae superio'ris,** TA alternative for *vena apicoposterior lobi superioris pulmonis sinistri.*

**r. articula'ris** [TA], articular branch: any of the branches of a mixed (afferent or efferent) peripheral nerve supplying a joint and its associated structures.

**ra'mi articula'res arte'riae descenden'tis genicula'ris** [TA], articular branches of descending genicular artery: branches that pass downward in the vastus medialis muscle and help supply the knee joint. Called also *rami articulares arteriae genus descendentis.*

**ra'mi articula'res arte'riae ge'nus descenden'tis,** rami articularis arteriae descendentis genicularis.

**r. ascen'dens arte'riae circumflex'ae fe'moris latera'lis** [TA], ascending branch of lateral circumflex femoral artery: a branch that runs upward along the trochanteric line of the femur and between the gluteus medius and minimus muscles, and anastomoses with branches of the superior gluteal artery. It helps supply the upper thigh muscles.

**r. ascen'dens arte'riae circumflex'ae fe'moris media'lis** [TA], ascending branch of medial circumflex femoral artery: a branch that ascends in front of the quadratus femoris muscle to the trochanteric fossa, and there anastomoses with gluteal arteries.

**r. ascen'dens arte'riae circumflex'ae i'lium profun'dae** [TA], ascending branch of deep circumflex iliac artery: a branch leaving the deep circumflex iliac artery near the anterior superior iliac spine, rising between and distributing to the transversus abdominis and internal oblique muscles.

**r. ascen'dens arte'riae segmenta'lis anterio'ris pulmo'nis dex'tri** [TA], ascending branch of anterior segmental artery of right lung: one of the branches of the anterior segmental artery that supply the anterior segment of the superior lobe of the right lung.

**r. ascen'dens arte'riae segmenta'lis ante'rioris pulmo'nis sinis'tri** [TA], ascending branch of anterior segmental artery of left lung: one of the branches of the anterior segmental artery that supply the anterior segment of the superior lobe of the left lung.

**r. ascen'dens arte'riae segmenta'lis posterio'ris pulmo'nis dex'tri** [TA], ascending branch of posterior segmental artery of right lung: one of the branches of the posterior segmental artery that supply the posterior segment of the superior lobe of the right lung.

**r. ascen'dens arte'riae segmenta'lis posterio'ris pulmo'nis sinis'tri** [TA], ascending branch of posterior segmental artery of left lung: one of the branches of the posterior segmental artery that supply the posterior segment of the superior lobe of the left lung.

**r. ascen'dens ra'mi superficia'lis arte'riae transver'sae col'li** [TA], the ascending branch of the superficial branch of the transverse cervical artery.

**r. ascen'dens sul'ci latera'lis ce'rebri** [TA], ascending branch of lateral cerebral sulcus: a branch that runs superiorly a short distance into the inferior frontal gyrus.

**r. atria'lis anastomo'ticus ra'mi circumflex'i arte'riae corona'riae sinis'trae** [TA], atrial anastomotic branch of circumflex branch of left coronary artery: a branch of the circumflex branch of the left coronary artery that passes the interatrial septum to anastomose with the right coronary artery; called also *atrial anastomotic artery* and *anastomotic atrial artery.*

**ra'mi atria'les arte'riae corona'riae dex'trae** [TA], atrial branches of right coronary artery: branches of the right coronary artery, consisting of anterior and lateral branches chiefly distributed to the right atrium, and usually a single posterior branch distributed to the right and left atria.

**ra'mi atria'les ra'mi circumflex'i arte'riae corona'riae sinis'trae** [TA], atrial branches of circumflex branch of left coronary artery: branches distributed to the left atrium, consisting of anterior, lateral, and posterior groups.

**r. atria'lis interme'dius arte'riae corona'riae dex'trae** [TA], intermediate atrial branch of right coronary artery: a branch of the right coronary artery arising opposite to the marginal branch and ascending to over the right atrium; called also *right intermediate atrial artery.*

**r. atria'lis interme'dius ra'mi circumflex'i arte'riae corona'riae sinis'tri** [TA], intermediate atrial branch of circumflex branch of left coronary artery: a branch that distributes along the left atrium above the coronary sulcus; called also *left intermediate atrial artery.*

**ra'mi atrioventricula'res ra'mi circumflex'i arte'riae corona'riae sinis'trae** [TA], atrioventricular branches of circumflex branch of left coronary artery: small recurrent branches distributed to the atria and ventricles.

**ra'mi auricula'res anterio'res arte'riae tempora'lis superficia'lis** [TA], anterior auricular branches of superficial temporal artery: branches that supply the lateral aspect of the pinna and the external acoustic meatus. Called also *anterior auricular arteries.*

**r. auricula'ris arte'riae auricula'ris posterio'ris** [TA], auricular branch of posterior auricular artery: a branch supplying the pinna and adjacent skin.

**r. auricula'ris arte'riae occipita'lis** [TA], auricular branch of occipital artery: an inconstant branch of the occipital artery that helps supply the medial aspect of the pinna.

**r. auricula'ris ner'vi va'gi** [TA], auricular branch of vagus nerve: a branch arising from the superior ganglion of the vagus, innervating the cranial surface of the auricle, the floor of the external acoustic meatus, and the adjacent part of the tympanic membrane; modality, general sensory.

**r. autono'micus** [TA], autonomic branch: any of the branches of the parasympathetic or sympathetic nerves of the autonomic nervous system; called also *r. visceralis.*

**r. basa'lis ante'rior arte'riae pulmona'lis dex'trae,** arteria segmentalis basalis anterior pulmonis dextri.

**r. basa'lis ante'rior arte'riae pulmona'lis sinis'trae,** arteria segmentalis basalis anterior pulmonis sinistri.

**r. basa'lis ante'rior ve'nae basa'lis commu'nis,** TA alternative for *vena basalis anterior.*

**r. basa'lis latera'lis arte'riae pulmona'lis dex'trae,** arteria segmentalis basalis lateralis pulmonis dextri.

**r. basa'lis latera'lis arte'riae pulmona'lis sinis'trae,** arteria segmentalis basalis lateralis pulmonis sinistri.

**r. basa'lis media'lis arte'riae pulmona'lis dex'trae,** arteria segmentalis basalis medialis pulmonis dextri.

**r. basa'lis media'lis arte'riae pulmona'lis sinis'trae,** arteria segmentalis basalis medialis pulmonis sinistri.

**r. basa'lis poste'rior arte'riae pulmona'lis dex'trae,** arteria segmentalis basalis posterior pulmonis dextri.

**r. basa'lis poste'rior arte'riae pulmona'lis sinis'trae,** arteria segmentalis basalis posterior pulmonis sinistri.

**r. basa'lis tento'rii arte'riae caro'tidis inter'nae** [TA], basal tentorial branch of internal carotid artery: a twig from the cavernous part of the internal carotid artery that supplies the base of the tentorium; called also *r. tentorii basalis arteriae carotidis internae.*

**ra'mi bronchia'les anterio'res ner'vi va'gi,** see *rami bronchiales nervi vagi.*

**ra'mi bronchia'les aor'tae thora'cicae,** rami bronchiales partis thoracicae aortae.

**ra'mi bronchia'les arte'riae thora'cicae inter'nae** [TA], bronchial branches of internal thoracic artery: small, variable branches of the internal thoracic artery, with distribution to the bronchi and trachea. Called also *anterior bronchial arteries.*

**r. bronchia'lis eparteria'lis,** eparterial bronchus.

**ra'mi bronchia'les hyparteria'les,** hyparterial bronchi.

**ra'mi bronchia'les ner'vi va'gi** [TA], branches of the vagus that supply the bronchi and the pulmonary vessels, both directly and by way of the anterior and posterior parts of the pulmonary plexus; there are two or three short anterior branches and numerous longer posterior branches; modality, parasympathetic, and visceral afferent.

**ra'mi bronchia'les par'tis thora'cicae aor'tae** [TA], bronchial branches of thoracic part of aorta: branches arising from the thoracic aorta to supply the bronchi and lower trachea, and passing along the posterior sides of the bronchi to ramify about the respiratory bronchioles; distributed also to adjacent lymph nodes, pulmonary vessels, and pericardium, and to part of the esophagus. Called also *bronchial arteries* or *arteriae bronchiales.*

**ra'mi bronchia'les posterio'res ner'vi va'gi,** see *rami bronchiales nervi vagi.*

**ra'mi bronchia'les segmento'rum,** intrasegmental bronchial branches: smaller branches arising from the segmental bronchi.

**ra'mi bucca'les ner'vi facia'lis** [TA], buccal branches of facial nerve: branches that innervate the zygomatic, levator labii superioris, buccinator, and orbicularis oris muscles; modality, motor and general sensory.

**ra'mi calca'nei arte'riae tibia'lis posterio'ris** [TA], calcaneal branches of posterior tibial artery: branches that arise from the posterior tibial artery and are distributed to the medial aspect and back of the heel.

**ra'mi calca'nei latera'les ner'vi sura'lis** [TA], lateral calcaneal branches of sural nerve: branches that innervate the skin on the back of the leg and the lateral side of the foot and heel; modality, general sensory.

**ra'mi calca'nei media'les ner'vi tibia'lis** [TA], medial calcaneal branches of tibial nerve: branches supplying the medial side of the heel and of the posterior part of the sole; modality, general sensory.

**ra'mi calca'nei ramo'rum malleola'rium latera'lium arte'riae fibula'ris** [TA], calcaneal branches of lateral malleolar branches of fibular artery: branches distributed to the lateral aspect and back of the heel. Called also *rami calcanei ramorum malleolarium lateralium arteriae peroneae* [TA alternative].

**ra'mi calca'nei ramo'rum malleola'rium latera'lium arte'riae perone'ae,** TA alternative for *rami calcanei ramorum malleolarium lateralium arteriae fibularis.*

**r. calcari'nus arte'riae occipita'lis media'lis** [TA], calcarine branch of medial occipital artery: a branch that supplies the calcarine fissure.

**ra'mi cap'sulae inter'nae** [TA], branches of internal capsule: small branches of the anterior choroidal artery that supply the internal capsule.

**ra'mi capsula'res arte'riae rena'lis** [TA], capsular branches of renal artery: branches that supply the renal capsule.

**ra'mi cardi'aci cervica'les inferio'res ner'vi va'gi** [TA], inferior cardiac branches of the vagus nerve: branches (sometimes called cervicothoracic) arising from the vagi and from the recurrent laryngeal nerves at the thoracic inlet, and joining cervicothoracic sympathetic cardiac nerves, the combined nerves passing to the cardiac plexus; modality, parasympathetic and visceral afferent.

**ra'mi cardi'aci cervica'les superio'res ner'vi va'gi** [TA], superior cervical cardiac branches of vagus nerve: variable branches arising from the vagus in the cervical region and usually joining the cervical sympathetic cardiac nerves. The conjoined nerves then descend in front of, or behind, the arch of the aorta to the cardiac plexus; modality, parasympathetic and visceral afferent.

**ra'mi cardi'aci thora'cici** [TA], thoracic cardiac branches: branches of the second through fourth or fifth thoracic ganglia of the sympathetic trunk, supplying the heart and having a sympathetic (accelerator) modality as well as a visceral afferent one (chiefly for pain). Called also *thoracic cardiac nerves* and *nervi cardiaci thoracici.*

**ra'mi cardi'aci thora'cici ner'vi va'gi** [TA], thoracic cardiac branches of the vagus nerve: branches which arise in the thorax from the right and left vagus and left recurrent laryngeal nerves. They go directly to the posterior walls of the atria, to the coronary plexuses, and to the anterior pulmonary plexuses.

**ra'mi caroticotympa'nici arte'riae caro'tidis inter'nae,** arteriae caroticotympanicae.

**r. carpa'lis dorsa'lis arte'riae radia'lis** [TA], dorsal carpal branch of radial artery: a branch running medially deep to the extensor tendons, and helping form the dorsal carpal rete.

**r. carpa'lis dorsa'lis arte'riae ulna'ris** [TA], dorsal carpal branch of ulnar artery: a variable branch of the ulnar artery that runs laterally deep to the tendons of the ulnar muscles of the wrist, helping to form the dorsal carpal rete.

**r. carpa'lis palma'ris arte'riae radia'lis** [TA], palmar carpal branch of radial artery: a branch that passes medially behind the flexor tendons on the palmar aspect of the wrist and forms a network with a corresponding branch of the ulnar artery.

**r. carpa'lis palma'ris arte'riae ulna'ris** [TA], palmar carpal branch of ulnar artery: a branch that passes laterally behind the flexor tendons on the palmar aspect of the wrist and forms a network with a corresponding branch of the radial artery.

**r. car'peus dorsa'lis arte'riae radia'lis,** r. carpalis dorsalis arteriae radialis.

**r. car'peus dorsa'lis arte'riae ulna'ris,** r. carpalis dorsalis arteriae ulnaris.

**r. car'peus palma'ris arte'riae radia'lis,** r. carpalis palmaris arteriae radialis.

**r. car'peus palma'ris arte'riae ulna'ris,** r. carpalis palmaris arteriae ulnaris.

**ra'mi cau'dae nu'clei cauda'ti arte'riae choroi'deae anterio'ris** [TA], small branches of the anterior choroidal artery that supply the tail of the caudate nucleus.

**r. cau'dae nu'clei cauda'ti arte'riae communican'tis posterio'ris,** a branch of the posterior communicating artery that supplies the tail of the caudate nucleus.

**ra'mi cauda'ti par'tis transver'sae,** r. lobi caudati partis transversae venae portae hepatis.

**ra'mi celi'aci ner'vi va'gi,** rami coeliaci nervi vagi.

**ra'mi centra'les anteromedia'les arte'riae ce'rebri anterio'ris,** the anteromedial central branches of the precommunical part of the anterior cerebral artery.

**r. cervica'lis ner'vi facia'lis,** TA alternative for *r. colli nervi facialis.*

**r. chiasma'ticus arte'riae communican'tis posterio'ris** [TA], a branch of the posterior communicating artery that supplies the optic chiasm.

**ra'mi choroi'dei posterio'res latera'les arte'riae ce'rebri posterio'ris** [TA], the lateral choroid branches of the posterior cerebral artery that supply the lateral ventricle.

**ra'mi choroi'dei posterio'res media'les arte'riae ce'rebri posterio'ris** [TA], medial choroid branches of posterior cerebral artery: branches that supply the choroid plexuses of the third ventricle.

**ra'mi choroi'dei ventri'culi latera'lis** [TA], small branches of the anterior choroidal artery that supply the choroid plexus of the lateral ventricle.

**r. choroi'deus ventri'culi quar'ti arte'riae inferio'ris posterio'ris cerebel'li** [TA], a branch of the posterior inferior cerebellar artery that supplies the choroid plexus of the fourth ventricle.

**ra'mi choroi'dei ventri'culi ter'tii** [TA], small branches of the anterior choroidal artery that supply the third ventricle.

**r. cingula'ris arte'riae callosomargina'lis** [TA], the cingular branch of the callosomarginal branch (artery) of the anterior cerebral artery.

**r. circumflex'us arte'riae corona'riae sinis'trae** [TA], circumflex branch of left coronary artery: a branch that curves around to the back of the left ventricle in the coronary sulcus, supplying the left ventricle and left atrium. Called also *circumflex artery.*

**r. circumflex'us fibula'ris arte'riae tibia'lis posterio'ris** [TA], fibular circumflex branch of posterior tibial artery: a branch that winds laterally around the neck of the fibula, helping supply the soleus muscle and contributing to the anastomosis around the knee joint; called also *r. circumflexus peronealis arteriae tibialis posterioris* [TA alternative].

**r. circumflex'us peronea'lis arte'riae tibia'lis posterio'ris,** TA alternative for *r. circumflexus fibularis arteriae tibialis posterioris.*

**r. clavicula'ris arte'riae thoracoacromia'lis** [TA], clavicular branch of thoracoacromial artery: a vessel that passes medially to supply the subclavius muscle.

**ra'mi cliva'les** [TA], clival branches: twigs from the cerebral part of the internal carotid artery that supply the clivus.

**ra'mi clu'nium inferio'res,** nervi clunium inferiores.

**ra'mi clu'nium media'les,** nervi clunium medii.

**ra'mi clu'nium superio'res,** nervi clunium superiores.

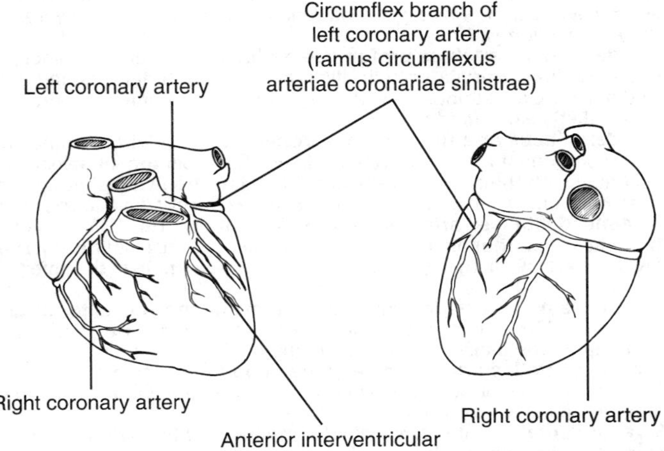


Ramus circumflexus arteriae coronariae sinistrae (circumflex branch of left coronary artery, or circumflex artery), shown on the anterior, or sternocostal, *(left)* and diaphragmatic *(right)* surfaces of the heart.

**r. cochlea'ris arte'riae labyrinthi'nae, r. cochlea'ris arte'riae vestibulocochlea'ris** [TA], cochlear branch of vestibulocochlear artery: a branch that supplies the cochlea. Called also *cochlear artery.*

**ra'mi coeli'aci ner'vi va'gi** [TA], celiac branches of vagus nerve: branches that arise from both the anterior and posterior vagal trunks and join the celiac plexus; modality, parasympathetic and visceral afferent. Called also *celiac nerves* and *rami celiaci nervi vagi.*

**r. co'licus arte'riae ileoco'licae** [TA], colic branch of ileocolic artery: a branch that passes upward on the ascending colon and anastomoses with the right colic artery; called also *arteria ascendens ileocolica* and *ascending ileocolic artery.*

**r. collatera'lis arteria'rum intercosta'lium posterio'rum** [TA], collateral branch of posterior intercostal arteries: a branch helping supply the thoracic wall, arising from the posterior intercostal arteries near the angle of the rib and running forward in the lower part of the corresponding intercostal space.

**r. col'li ner'vi facia'lis** [TA], cervical branch of facial nerve: a branch lying deep to and innervating the platysma muscle; modality, motor. Called also *r. cervicalis nervi facialis* [TA alternative].

**ra'mi communican'tes,** 1. communicating branches between two nerves; in official terminology called *rami communicantes nervorum spinalium.* 2. branches connecting two arteries. Called also *rami anastomotici.*

**r. commu'nicans al'bus ner'vi spina'lis** [TA], white communicating branch of spinal nerve: one of the two types of communicating nerve branches between a sympathetic ganglion and a spinal nerve; the white type are largely myelinated, send impulses from the spinal nerves to and through the ganglia, and are located mainly in the thoracic and upper lumbar region. Called also *r. albus nervi spinalis.* Cf. *r. communicans griseus nervi spinalis.*

**r. commu'nicans arte'riae fibula'ris** [TA], communicating branch of fibular artery: a communicating branch between the fibular and the posterior tibial arteries, distributed to the interosseous membrane and supramalleolar region. Called also *r. communicans arteriae peroneae* [TA alternative].

**r. commu'nicans arte'riae perone'ae,** TA alternative for *r. communicans arteriae fibularis.*

**r. commu'nicans cochlea'ris ner'vi vestibula'ris** [TA], cochlear communicating branch of vestibular nerve: a branch of the vestibular nerve that unites with the cochlear nerve.

**r. commu'nicans fibula'ris ner'vi fibula'ris commu'nis** [TA], fibular or sural communicating branch of common fibular nerve: a small branch arising from the common fibular nerve, either with the lateral cutaneous sural nerve or separately; distally it joins the medial sural cutaneous nerve to form the sural nerve. Called also *r. communicans peroneus nervi peronei communis* [TA alternative].

**r. commu'nicans gri'seus ner'vi spina'lis** [TA], gray communicating branch of spinal nerve: one of the two types of communicating nerve branches between a sympathetic ganglion and a spinal nerve; these branches carry postganglionic impulses back to the spinal nerves and then to the periphery, supplying blood vessels, sweat glands, and smooth muscles. Called also *r. griseus nervi spinalis.* Cf. *r. communicans albus nervi spinalis.*

**ra'mi communican'tes ner'vi auriculotempora'lis cum ner'vo facia'li** [TA], communicating branches of auriculotemporal nerve with facial nerve: branches containing sensory fibers from the auriculotemporal nerve that join the facial nerve within the parotid gland, to be distributed with branches of the latter.

**r. commu'nicans ner'vi facia'lis cum ner'vo glossopharyn'geo** [TA], communicating branch of facial nerve with glossopharyngeal nerve: a branch that interconnects the glossopharyngeal nerve and the facial nerve after emergence of the latter from the stylomastoid foramen.

**r. commu'nicans ner'vi glossopharyn'gei cum chor'da tym'pani** [TA], communicating branch of glossopharyngeal nerve with chorda tympani: a small branch that interconnects the glossopharyngeal nerve and the chorda tympani.

**r. commu'nicans ner'vi glossopharyn'gei cum ner'vo auriculotempora'li** [TA], communicating branch of glossopharyngeal nerve with auriculotemporal nerve: a branch carrying postganglionic parasympathetic fibers from the glossopharyngeal nerve to the auriculotemporal nerve for distribution to the parotid gland.

**r. commu'nicans ner'vi glossopharyn'gei cum ra'mo auricula'ri ner'vi va'gi** [TA], communicating branch of glossopharyngeal nerve with auricular branch of vagus nerve: a small branch connecting the glossopharyngeal nerve with the auricular branch of the vagus nerve.

**r. commu'nicans ner'vi glossopharyn'gei ra'mo menin'geo ner'vi va'gi** [TA], communicating branch of glossopharyngeal nerve with meningeal branch of vagal nerve: a branch that carries autonomic fibers destined for the meninges from the glossopharyngeal nerve to the meningeal branch of the vagal nerve.

**r. commu'nicans ner'vi interme'dii cum ner'vo va'go** [TA], communicating branch of intermediate nerve with vagus nerve: a branch of the intermediate nerve that communicates with the vagus nerve.

**r. commu'nicans ner'vi interme'dii cum plex'u tympa'nico** [TA], communicating branch of intermediate nerve with tympanic plexus: a branch of the intermediate nerve that communicates with the tympanic plexus.

**r. commu'nicans ner'vi lacrima'lis cum ner'vo zygoma'tico** [TA], communicating branch of lacrimal nerve with zygomatic nerve: a branch that carries parasympathetic postganglionic fibers originating in the pterygopalatine ganglion and destined for the lacrimal gland.

**r. commu'nicans ner'vi laryn'gei inferio'ris cum ra'mo laryn'geo inter'no,** communicating branch of inferior laryngeal nerve with internal laryngeal branch: a small branch interconnecting the inferior laryngeal nerve with the internal branch of the superior laryngeal nerve, behind or in the posterior cricoarytenoid muscle.

**r. commu'nicans ner'vi laryn'gei superio'ris cum ner'vo laryn'geo inferio're,** communicating branch of superior laryngeal nerve with inferior laryngeal nerve: a small branch interconnecting the internal branch of the superior laryngeal nerve with the inferior laryngeal nerve, behind or in the posterior cricoarytenoid muscle. Called also *Galen's nerve.*

**r. commu'nicans ner'vi lingua'lis cum chor'da tym'pani,** communicating branch of lingual nerve with chorda tympani: the chorda tympani as it joins the lingual nerve in the infratemporal fossa medial to the lateral pterygoid muscle; modality, parasympathetic and special sensory.

**ra'mi communican'tes ner'vi lingua'lis cum ner'vo hypoglos'so** [TA], communicating branches of lingual nerve with hypoglossal nerve: plexiform terminal branches interconnecting the lingual and hypoglossal nerves just in front of the hyoglossus muscle.

**r. commu'nicans ner'vi media'ni cum ner'vo ulna'ri** [TA], communicating branch of median nerve with ulnar nerve: a small branch across the flexor digitorum profundus muscle, connecting the median with the ulnar nerve.

**r. commu'nicans cum ner'vo nasocilia'ri,** radix sensoria ganglii ciliaris.

**r. commu'nicans ner'vi nasocilia'ris cum gan'glio cilia'ri,** TA alternative for *radix sensoria ganglii ciliaris.*

**ra'mi communican'tes nervo'rum spina'lium** [TA], communicating branches of spinal nerves: branches connecting spinal nerves with sympathetic ganglia, each spinal nerve receiving a gray communicating ramus, and the thoracic and upper lumbar spinal nerves having in addition a white communicating ramus. Called also *rami communicantes.*

**r. commu'nicans ner'vi va'gi cum ner'vo glossopharyn'geo** [TA], communicating branch of vagus nerve with glossopharyngeal nerve; see *r. communicans nervi glossopharyngei cum ramo auriculari nervi vagi.*

**r. commu'nicans perone'us ner'vi perone'i commu'nis,** TA alternative for *r. communicans fibularis nervi fibularis communis.*

**r. commu'nicans ulna'ris ner'vi radia'lis** [TA], ulnar communicating branch of radial nerve: a small branch in the hand that interconnects the most medial dorsal digital nerve from the superficial branch of the radial nerve with the adjacent most lateral dorsal digital nerve from the dorsal branch of the ulnar nerve.

**r. co'ni arterio'si arte'riae corona'riae dex'trae** [TA], conus arteriosus branch of right coronary artery: the first ventricular branch of the right coronary artery, which supplies the conus arteriosus, and anastomoses with the left conus artery (branch) of the anterior interventricular branch of the left coronary artery; called also *conal* or *conus artery, right conus artery,* and *third conus artery.*

**r. co'ni arterio'si arte'riae corona'riae sinis'trae** [TA], conus arteriosus branch of left coronary artery: a small branch of the anterior interventricular branch of the left coronary artery, which supplies the conus arteriosus, and anastomoses with the right conus artery (branch) of the right coronary artery; called also *conal* or *conus artery* and *left conus artery.*

**ra'mi cor'poris amygdaloi'dei** [TA], small branches of the anterior choroidal artery that supply the amygdaloid body.

**r. cor'poris callo'si dorsa'lis arte'riae occipita'lis media'lis** [TA], a branch of the middle occipital artery that supplies the dorsum of the corpus callosum.

**ra'mi cor'poris genicula'ti latera'lis** [TA], small branches of the anterior choroidal artery that supply the lateral geniculate body.

**r. costa'lis latera'lis arte'riae thora'cicae inter'nae** [TA], lateral costal branch of internal thoracic artery: an occasional branch passing inferolaterally behind the ribs, supplying ribs and costal cartilages, and anastomosing with the posterior intercostal arteries.

**r. cricothyroi'deus arte'riae thyroi'deae superio'ris** [TA], cricothyroid branch of superior thyroid artery: a vessel running medially over the cricothyroid muscle, toward the cricothyroid ligament, and anastomosing with its fellow of the opposite side. Called also *cricothyroid artery.*

**r. cuta'neus** [TA], cutaneous branch: a branch of a mixed (afferent or efferent) peripheral nerve innervating a region of the skin.

**r. cuta'neus ante'rior abdomina'lis ner'vi intercosta'lis** [TA], anterior abdominal cutaneous branch of intercostal nerve: a branch from the intercostal nerve that contributes to innervation of the skin in the anteriomedial abdominal region. Its modality is general sensory.

**ra'mi cuta'nei anterio'res ner'vi femora'lis** [TA], anterior cutaneous branches of femoral nerve: branches that innervate the skin on the front and medial aspect of the thigh and patella and contribute to the subsartorial and patellar plexuses; modality, general sensory.

**r. cuta'neus ante'rior ner'vi iliohypogas'trici** [TA], anterior cutaneous branch of iliohypogastric nerve: a branch that runs forward between the internal and external oblique muscles and innervates the skin over the pubis; modality, general sensory.

**r. cuta'neus ante'rior pectora'lis ner'vi intercosta'lis** [TA], anterior pectoral cutaneous branch of intercostal nerve: a branch from the intercostal nerve that contributes to innervation of the skin in the anteriomedial thoracic region; in the breast region it sends further branches (see *rami mammarii mediales rami cutanei anterioris pectoralis nervi intercostalis*). Its modality is general sensory.

**ra'mi cuta'nei cru'ris media'les ner'vi saphe'ni** [TA], medial crural cutaneous branches of saphenous nerve: branches distributed by the saphenous nerve to the skin of the medial aspect of the leg; modality, general sensory.

**r. cuta'neus latera'lis abdomina'lis ner'vi intercosta'lis** [TA], lateral abdominal cutaneous branch of intercostal nerve: a branch from the intercostal nerve that, through its anterior and posterior subdivisions, innervates the skin of the lateral and posterior body wall; it has a general sensory modality.

**r. cuta'neus latera'lis arteria'rum intercosta'lium posterio'rum** [TA], lateral cutaneous branch of posterior intercostal arteries: a branch arising from the posterior intercostal arteries, supplying the anterolateral thoracic wall. The branches of the third through fifth give off small mammary branches.

**r. cuta'neus latera'lis ner'vi iliohypogas'trici** [TA], lateral cutaneous branch of iliohypogastric nerve: a nerve branch distributed to the skin over the side of the buttock; modality, general sensory.

**r. cuta'neus latera'lis pectora'lis ner'vi intercosta'lis** [TA], lateral pectoral cutaneous branch of intercostal nerve: a branch from the intercostal that, through its anterior and posterior subdivisions, innervates the skin of the lateral and posterior body wall; it has a general sensory modality. Those of the fourth through sixth anterior thoracic branches send further branches (see *rami mammarii laterales rami cutanei lateralis pectoralis nervi intercostalis*).

**r. cuta'neus latera'lis ra'mi dorsa'lis arteria'rum intercosta'lium posterio'rum** [TA], lateral cutaneous branch of dorsal branch of posterior intercostal arteries: a branch that supplies the posterolateral aspect of the thorax. The branches of the third through fifth arteries give off small mammary branches.

**r. cuta'neus media'lis ra'mi dorsa'lis arteria'rum intercosta'lium posterio'rum** [TA], medial cutaneous branch of dorsal branch of posterior intercostal arteries: a branch that supplies the skin adjacent to the vertebral column.

**r. cuta'neus ner'vi obturato'rii** [TA], cutaneous branch of obturator nerve: a variable branch arising from the anterior branch of the obturator nerve, forming part of the subsartorial plexus, and supplying the skin of the medial aspect of the thigh and leg; modality, general sensory.

**r. cuta'neus poste'rior ra'mi posterio'ris ner'vi thora'cici** [TA], posterior cutaneous branch of dorsal branch of thoracic nerve: cutaneous branches of either of the two divisions of a dorsal branch; see *r. lateralis rami posterior nervi thoracici* and *r. medialis rami posterior nervi thoracici.*

**r. deltoi'deus arte'riae profun'dae bra'chii** [TA], deltoid branch of deep brachial artery: a branch distributed to the brachialis and deltoid muscles, anastomosing with the posterior circumflex humeral artery; called also *deltoid artery.*

**r. deltoi'deus arte'riae thoracoacromia'lis** [TA], deltoid branch of thoracoacromial artery: a branch of the thoracoacromial artery descending with the cephalic vein and helping to supply the deltoid and pectoralis major muscles; called also *deltoid artery of thoracoacromial.*

**ra'mi denta'les arte'riae alveola'ris inferio'ris** [TA], dental branches of inferior alveolar artery: branches arising from the inferior alveolar artery in the mandibular canal and supplying the inferior teeth.

**ra'mi denta'les arteria'rum alveola'rium superio'rum anterio'rum** [TA], dental branches of anterior superior alveolar arteries: branches that supply the incisor and canine teeth.

**ra'mi denta'les arte'riae alveola'ris superio'ris posterio'ris** [TA], dental branches of posterior superior alveolar artery: branches that supply the molar and premolar teeth.

**ra'mi denta'les inferio'res plex'us denta'lis inferio'ris** [TA], inferior dental branches of inferior dental plexus: branches that innervate the lower teeth; modality, general sensory.

**ra'mi denta'les superio'res plex'us denta'lis superio'ris** [TA], superior dental branches of superior dental plexus: branches that innervate the teeth of the upper jaw; modality, general sensory.

**r. descen'dens arte'riae circumflex'ae fe'moris latera'lis** [TA], descending branch of lateral circumflex femoral artery: a branch passing from the lateral circumflex artery (sometimes directly from the deep femoral) to the knee, and supplying the thigh muscles.

**r. descen'dens arte'riae occipita'lis** [TA], descending branch of occipital artery: a branch that arises from the occipital artery on the obliquus capitis superior muscle and divides into superficial and deep branches, supplying the trapezius and deep neck muscles.

**r. descen'dens arte'riae segmenta'lis anterio'ris pulmo'nis dex'tri** [TA], descending branch of anterior segmental artery of right lung: one of the branches of the anterior segmental artery that supply the anterior segment of the superior lobe of the right lung.

**r. descen'dens arte'riae segmenta'lis anterio'ris pulmo'nis sinis'tri** [TA], descending branch of anterior segmental artery of left lung: one of the branches of the anterior segmental artery that supply the anterior segment of the superior lobe of the left lung.

**r. descen'dens arte'riae segmenta'lis posterio'ris pulmo'nis dex'tri** [TA], ascending branch of posterior segmental artery of right lung: one of the branches of the posterior segmental artery that supply the posterior segment of the superior lobe of the right lung.

**r. descen'dens arte'riae segmenta'lis posterio'ris pulmo'nis sinis'tri** [TA], descending branch of posterior segmental artery of left lung: one of the branches of the posterior segmental artery that supply the posterior segment of the superior lobe of the left lung.

**r. descen'dens ra'mi superficia'lis arte'riae transver'sae col'li** [TA], descending branch of the superficial branch of the transverse cervical artery.

**r. dex'ter arte'riae hepa'ticae pro'priae** [TA], right branch of proper hepatic artery: the right of the two branches into which the proper hepatic artery normally divides; it supplies the right lobe of the liver and a branch, the cystic artery, to the gallbladder.

**r. dex'ter ve'nae por'tae he'patis** [TA], right branch of portal vein of liver: a branch distributed to the right lobe of the liver.

**r. digas'tricus ner'vi facia'lis** [TA], digastric branch of facial nerve: a branch that innervates the posterior belly of the digastric muscle; modality, motor; called also *digastric nerve*.

**r. diplo'icus arte'riae supraorbita'lis** [TA], diploic branch of supraorbital artery: a small branch arising as the artery passes through the supraorbital notch and supplying the diploe of the frontal bone and the lining of the frontal sinus.

**r. dorsa'lis arteria'rum intercosta'lium posterio'rum** [TA], dorsal branch of posterior intercostal arteries: a branch arising from a posterior intercostal artery, passing backward with the dorsal branch of the corresponding intercostal nerve to supply the posterior thoracic wall; it has a spinal branch and a medial and a lateral cutaneous branch.

**ra'mi dorsa'les arte'riae intercosta'lis supre'mae** [TA], dorsal branches of highest intercostal artery: the dorsal branches arising from the first and second posterior intercostal arteries, which stem from the highest intercostal artery. Their distribution is similar to that of the other posterior intercostals; see *r. dorsalis arteriarum intercostalium posteriorum*.

**r. dorsa'lis arteria'rum lumba'lium** [TA], dorsal branch of lumbar arteries: the larger of the two branches into which each lumbar artery (four or five) divides; it supplies lumbar back muscles and gives off a spinal branch.

**r. dorsa'lis arte'riae subcosta'lis** [TA], dorsal branch of subcostal artery: a branch supplying back muscles, its distribution being similar to that of the dorsal branches of the lower posterior intercostal arteries.

**ra'mi dorsa'les lin'guae arte'riae lingua'lis** [TA], dorsal lingual branches of lingual artery: branches of the lingual artery arising beneath the hyoglossus muscle and supplying the tonsil and the back of the tongue.

**ra'mi dorsa'les nervo'rum cervica'lium,** TA alternative for *rami posteriores nervorum cervicalium*.

**r. dorsa'lis ner'vi coccy'gei,** TA alternative for *r. posterior nervi coccygei*.

**ra'mi dorsa'les nervo'rum lumba'lium,** TA alternative for *rami posteriores nervorum lumbalium*.

**ra'mi dorsa'les nervo'rum sacra'lium,** TA alternative for *rami posteriores nervorum sacralium*.

**r. dorsa'lis ner'vi spina'lis,** TA alternative for *r. posterior nervi spinalis*.

**ra'mi dorsa'les nervo'rum thoracico'rum,** TA alternative for *rami posteriores nervorum thoracicorum*.

**r. dorsa'lis ner'vi ulna'ris** [TA], dorsal branch of ulnar nerve: a large cutaneous branch that arises from the ulnar nerve and passes down the distal portion of the forearm to the medial side of the back of the hand, where it divides usually into three, sometimes four, dorsal digital nerves; modality, general sensory.

**r. dorsa'lis ve'nae intercosta'lis, r. dorsa'lis ve'nae intercosta'lis posterio'ris** [TA], dorsal branch of posterior intercostal vein: a branch corresponding to the dorsal branch of the posterior intercostal artery *(r. dorsalis arteriarum intercostalium posteriorum)*.

**ra'mi duodena'les arte'riae pancreaticoduodena'lis superio'ris anterio'ris** [TA], duodenal branches of anterior superior pancreaticoduodenal artery: vessels that supply the duodenum.

**ra'mi duodena'les arte'riae pancreaticoduodena'lis superio'ris posterio'ris** [TA], duodenal branches of posterior superior pancreaticoduodenal artery: vessels supplying the duodenum.

**ra'mi epididyma'les arte'riae testicula'ris** [TA], epididymal branches of testicular artery: they are distributed to the epididymis.

**ra'mi epiplo'ici arte'riae gastroepiplo'icae dex'trae,** rami omentales arteriae gastro-omentalis dextrae.

**ra'mi epiplo'ici arte'riae gastroepiplo'icae sinis'trae,** rami omentales arteriae gastro-omentalis sinistrae.

**ra'mi esophagea'les aor'tae thora'cicae,** rami oesophageales partis thoracicae aortae.

**ra'mi esophagea'les arte'riae gas'tricae sinis'trae,** rami oesophageales arteriae gastricae sinistrae.

**ra'mi esophagea'les arte'riae thyroi'deae inferio'ris,** rami oesophageales arteriae thyroideae inferioris.

**ra'mi esophagea'les par'tis thora'cicae aor'tae,** rami oesophageales partis thoracicae aortae.

**ra'mi esopha'gei ner'vi laryn'gei recurren'tis,** rami oesophagei nervi laryngei recurrentis.

**r. exter'nus ner'vi accesso'rii** [TA], external branch of accessory nerve: the branch of the eleventh cranial accessory nerve that originates from the spinal roots of the nerve; it sends muscular branches to supply the sternocleidomastoid and trapezius muscles.

**r. exter'nus ner'vi laryn'gei superio'ris** [TA], external branch of superior laryngeal nerve: the smaller of the two branches into which the superior laryngeal nerve divides, descending under cover of the sternothyroid muscle and innervating the cricothyroid and the inferior constrictor of the pharynx; modality, motor.

**ra'mi faucia'les ner'vi lingua'lis,** rami isthmi faucium nervi lingualis.

**r. femora'lis ner'vi genitofemora'lis** [TA], femoral branch of genitofemoral nerve: a branch arising by division of the genitofemoral nerve above the inguinal ligament; entering the femoral sheath, it turns forward and supplies the skin of the femoral triangle; modality, general sensory. Called also *nervus lumboinguinalis*.

**r. fronta'lis anteromedia'lis arte'riae callosomargina'lis** [TA], the anteromedial frontal branch of the callosomarginal branch (artery) of the anterior cerebral artery.

**r. fronta'lis arte'riae menin'geae me'diae** [TA], frontal branch of middle meningeal artery: a branch lodged in grooves on the sphenoid and parietal bones, and supplying the dura mater of the front of the brain. A part of it is sometimes enclosed in a bony canal.

**r. fronta'lis arte'riae tempora'lis superficia'lis** [TA], frontal branch of superficial temporal artery: a tortuous terminal branch that supplies the forehead and frontal scalp.

**r. fronta'lis posteromedia'lis arte'riae callosomargina'lis** [TA], the posteromedial frontal branch of the callosomarginal branch (artery) of the anterior cerebral artery.

**ra'mi gangliona'res ner'vi lingua'lis ad gan'glion submandibula're** [TA], ganglionic branches of lingual nerve to submandibular ganglion: branches which interconnect the lingual nerve and the submandibular ganglion, and by which the ganglion is suspended from the nerve; they carry preganglionic fibers that derive from the chorda tympani and synapse in the submandibular ganglion, and postganglionic fibers. Called also *radix sensoria ganglii submandibularis* [TA alternative] and *motor* or *sensory root of submandibular ganglion*.

**ra'mi gangliona'res ner'vi mandibula'ris ad gan'glion o'ticum** [TA], ganglionic branches of mandibular nerve to otic ganglion: branches of the mandibular nerve that communicate with the otic ganglion. Called also *radix sensoria ganglii otici* [TA alternative].

**ra'mi gangliona'res ner'vi maxilla'ris ad gan'glion pterygopalati'num** [TA], ganglionic branches of maxillary nerve to pterygopalatine ganglion: fibers connecting the maxillary nerve to the pterygopalatine ganglion. Called also *radix sensoria ganglii pterygopalatini* [TA alternative] and *sensory root of pterygopalatine ganglion*.

**ra'mi gangliona'res trigemina'les** [TA], **ra'mi gangliona'res trige'mini,** branches to trigeminal ganglion: short branches from the cavernous part of the internal carotid artery that supply the trigeminal ganglion.

**ra'mi gas'trici anterio'res trun'ci vaga'lis anterio'ris** [TA], anterior gastric branches of anterior vagal trunk: branches arising from the anterior trunk of the vagus near the cardiac end of the stomach, innervating the anterior aspect of the lesser curvature and the anterior surface of the stomach almost to the pylorus; modality, parasympathetic and visceral afferent.

**ra'mi gas'trici arte'riae gastroepiplo'icae dex'trae,** rami gastrici arteriae gastro-omentalis dextrae.

**ra'mi gas'trici arte'riae gastroepiplo'icae sinis'trae,** rami gastrici arteriae gastro-omentalis sinistrae.

**ra'mi gas'trici arte'riae gastroomenta'lis dex'trae** [TA], gastric branches of right gastro-omental artery: vessels that supply both surfaces of the stomach; called also *rami gastrici arteriae gastroepiploicae dextrae.*

**ra'mi gas'trici arte'riae gastroomenta'lis sinis'trae** [TA], gastric branches of left gastro-omental artery: vessels that supply both surfaces of the stomach; called also *rami gastrici arteriae gastroepiploicae sinistrae.*

**ra'mi gas'trici ner'vi va'gi,** see *rami gastrici anteriores trunci vagalis anterioris* and *rami gastrici posteriores trunci vagalis posterioris.*

**ra'mi gas'trici posterio'res trun'ci vaga'lis posterio'ris** [TA], posterior gastric branches of posterior vagal trunk: branches arising from the posterior vagal trunk near the cardiac end of the stomach, and innervating the cardiac orifice and fundus, the posterior aspect of the lesser curvature, and the posterior surface of the stomach to the pyloric antrum; modality, parasympathetic and visceral afferent.

**r. genita'lis ner'vi genitofemora'lis** [TA], genital branch of genitofemoral nerve: a branch arising from the genitofemoral nerve above the inguinal ligament; entering the inguinal canal through the deep ring, it supplies the cremaster and continues to the skin of the scrotum or of the labium majus, and that of the adjacent area of the thigh; modality, general sensory and motor. Called also *nervus spermaticus externus.*

**ra'mi gingiva'les inferio'res plex'us denta'lis inferio'ris** [TA], inferior gingival branches of inferior dental plexus: branches originating from the inferior dental plexus and innervating the gingivae of the lower jaw; modality, general sensory.

**ra'mi gingiva'les ner'vi menta'lis** [TA], gingival branches of mental nerve: branches that innervate the gums; modality, general sensory.

**ra'mi gingiva'les superio'res plex'us denta'lis superio'ris** [TA], superior gingival branches of superior dental plexus: branches arising from the superior dental plexus and innervating the gingivae of the upper jaw; modality, general sensory.

**r. glandula'ris ante'rior arte'riae thyroi'deae superio'ris** [TA], anterior branch of the superior thyroid artery: a branch principally supplying the anterior surface of the thyroid gland, and anastomosing with the artery of the opposite side.

**ra'mi glandula'res arte'riae facia'lis** [TA], **ra'mi glandula'res arte'riae maxilla'ris exter'nae,** glandular branches of facial artery: branches given off to the submandibular gland by the facial artery as it passes over the lateral surface of the gland.

**ra'mi glandula'res arte'riae thyroi'deae inferio'ris,** glandular branches of the inferior thyroid artery.

**ra'mi glandula'res arte'riae thyroi'deae superio'ris,** glandular branches of the superior thyroid artery.

**ra'mi glandula'res gan'glii submandibula'ris,** glandular branches of submandibular ganglion: short branches running from the submandibular ganglion to innervate the submandibular gland, bearing postganglionic parasympathetic (secretory) fibers from this ganglion and sympathetic fibers that are postganglionic from the superior cervical ganglion. Called also *submaxillary nerves.*

**r. glandula'ris latera'lis arte'riae thyroi'deae superio'ris** [TA], lateral branch of superior thyroid artery: a branch distributed to the lateral surface of the thyroid gland.

**r. glandula'ris poste'rior arte'riae thyroi'deae superio'ris** [TA], posterior glandular branch of the superior thyroid artery: a branch distributed mainly to the medial and lateral surfaces of the thyroid gland; it anastomoses with the inferior thyroid artery.

**ra'mi glo'bi pal'lidi** [TA], small branches of the anterior choroidal artery that supply the globus pallidus.

**ra'mi glutea'les inferio'res,** nervi clunium inferiores.

**ra'mi glutea'les media'les,** nervi clunium medii.

**ra'mi glutea'les superior'res,** nervi clunium superiores.

**r. gri'seus ner'vi spina'lis,** r. communicans griseus nervi spinalis.

**ra'mi helici'ni arte'riae uteri'nae** [TA], helicine branches of uterine artery: the exceedingly tortuous terminal branches of the uterine artery in the uterine muscle. Called also *helicine arteries.*

**ra'mi hepa'tici trun'ci vaga'lis anterio'ris** [TA], hepatic branches of anterior vagal trunk: branches (sometimes only one) arising from the anterior vagal trunk, contributing to the hepatic plexus, and helping innervate the liver, gallbladder, pancreas, pylorus, and duodenum; modality, parasympathetic and visceral afferent.

**r. hypothala'micus arte'riae communican'tis posterio'ris** [TA], a branch of the posterior communicating artery that supplies the hypothalamus.

**r. ilea'lis arte'riae ileoco'licae** [TA], ileal branch of ileocolic artery: a branch that passes upward and to the left of the lower ileum and anastomoses with the end of the superior mesenteric artery.

**r. ili'acus arte'riae iliolumba'lis** [TA], iliac branch of iliolumbar artery: one of the two branches into which the iliolumbar artery divides in the iliac fossa; it supplies the iliacus muscle and sends a large nutrient branch to the ilium.

**r. infe'rior ner'vi oculomoto'rii** [TA], inferior branch of oculomotor nerve: the branch of the oculomotor nerve that innervates the medial and inferior rectus and inferior oblique muscles of the eyeball and, via the motor root of the ciliary ganglion and then the short ciliary nerves, supplies the sphincter pupillae and ciliary muscles; modality, motor and parasympathetic.

**ra'mi inferio'res ner'vi transver'si col'li** [TA], inferior branches of transverse nerve of neck: the more inferior of the branches that arise from the transverse cervical nerve near the anterior border of the sternocleidomastoid muscle, innervating skin and subcutaneous tissue in the anterior cervical region; modality, general sensory.

**r. infe'rior os'sis is'chii,** r. ossis ischii.

**r. infe'rior os'sis pu'bis** [TA], inferior ramus of pubic bone: the short flattened bar of bone that projects from the body of the pubic bone in a posteroinferolateral direction to meet the ramus of the ischium.

**r. infe'rior ra'mi profun'di arte'riae glu'teae superio'ris** [TA], inferior branch of deep branch of superior gluteal artery: the lower division of the deep branch of the superior gluteal artery, accompanied by the superior gluteal artery, accompanied by the superior gluteal nerve and helping supply the gluteus medius, gluteus minimus, and tensor fasciae latae muscles and the hip joint and ilium.

**r. infrahyoi'deus arte'riae thyroi'deae superio'ris** [TA], infrahyoid branch of superior thyroid artery: a vessel running along the inferior border of the hyoid bone, supplying the infrahyoid region, and anastomosing with its fellow of the opposite side.

**r. infrapatella'ris ner'vi saphe'ni** [TA], infrapatellar branch of saphenous nerve: a branch running inferolaterally from the saphenous nerve to the patellar plexus; modality, general sensory.

**ra'mi inguina'les arte'riae puden'dae exter'nae profun'dae** [TA], inguinal branches of deep external pudendal artery: branches arising from the deep external pudendal arteries and supplying the inguinal region.

**ra'mi intercosta'les anterio'res arte'riae thora'cicae inter'nae** [TA], **ra'mi intercosta'les arte'riae mamma'riae inter'nae,** anterior intercostal branches of internal thoracic artery: twelve branches, two in each of the upper six intercostal spaces, that supply the intercostal spaces and the pectoralis major muscle. Within each space both branches run laterally, the upper anastomosing with the posterior intercostal artery, the lower with the collateral branch of that artery.

**ra'mi intergangliona'res trun'ci sympa'thici** [TA], interganglionic branches of sympathetic trunk: the branches that interconnect the ganglia of the sympathetic trunk.

**r. inter'nus ner'vi accesso'rii** [TA], internal branch of accessory nerve: the branch that continues from the cranial roots of the nerve, carrying motor fibers that are distributed by branches of the vagus to the soft palate, pharyngeal constrictors, and larynx.

**r. inter'nus ner'vi laryn'gei superio'ris** [TA], internal branch of superior laryngeal nerve: the larger of the two branches of the superior laryngeal nerve, which innervates the mucosa of the epiglottis, base of the tongue, and larynx; modality, general sensory.

**r. interventricula'ris ante'rior arte'riae corona'riae sinis'trae** [TA], anterior interventricular branch of left coronary artery: the branch of the left coronary artery that runs to the apex of the heart in the anterior interventricular sulcus, supplying the ventricles and most of the interventricular septum; called also *anterior interventricular artery.*

**r. interventricula'ris poste'rior arte'riae corona'riae dex'trae** [TA], posterior interventricular branch of right coronary artery: a branch running toward the apex of the heart in the posterior interventricular sulcus, supplying the diaphragmatic surface of the ventricles and part of the interventricular septum.

**ra'mi interventricula'res septa'les arte'riae corona'riae dex'trae** [TA], interventricular septal branches of right coronary artery: numerous relatively small branches of the posterior interventricular branch of the right coronary artery that supply about one-third of the posterior of the interventricular septum. Called also *posterior interventricular septal arteries* and *posterior septal arteries.*

**ra'mi interventricula'res septa'les arte'riae corona'riae sinis'trae** [TA], interventricular septal branches of left coronary artery: branches of the anterior interventricular branch of the left coronary artery that supply about the ventral two-thirds of the anterior interventricular septum; called also *anterior interventricular septal arteries* and *anterior septal arteries.*

**ischial r.,** r. ossis ischii.

**ischiopubic r., r. ischiopu'bicus** [TA], the inferior ramus of the pubis and the adjacent part of the ramus of the ischium, considered as a unit.

**r. of ischium,** r. ossis ischii.

**ra'mi isth'mi fau'cium ner'vi lingua'lis** [TA], branches from the lingual nerve to the isthmus of the fauces; modality, general sensory. Called also *rami fauciales nervi lingualis.*

**r. of jaw,** r. mandibulae.

**ra'mi labia'les anterio'res arte'riae puden'dae exter'nae profun'dae** [TA], anterior labial branches of deep external pudendal artery: branches that arise from the deep external pudendal artery and supply the labium majus; called also *anterior labial arteries of vulva* and *arteriae labiales anteriores vulvae.*

**ra′mi labia′les ner′vi menta′lis** [TA], labial branches of mental nerve: branches of the mental nerve that innervate the lower lip; modality, general sensory.

**ra′mi labia′les posterio′res arte′riae puden′dae inter′nae** [TA], posterior labial branches of internal pudendal artery: two branches arising from the internal pudendal artery in the anterior part of the ischiorectal fossa, helping to supply the ischiocavernosus and bulbospongiosus muscles, and supplying the labium majus and labium minus. Called also *posterior labial arteries of vulva* and *arteriae labiales posteriores vulvae.*

**ra′mi labia′les superio′res ner′vi infraorbita′lis** [TA], superior labial branches of infraorbital nerve: branches of the infraorbital nerve that are distributed to mucous membranes of the mouth and skin of the upper lip; modality, general sensory.

**ra′mi laryngopharyn′gei gan′glii cervica′lis superio′ris** [TA], laryngopharyngeal branches of superior cervical ganglion: branches from the superior cervical ganglion to the larynx and walls of the pharynx; modality, sympathetic.

**ra′mi latera′les arteria′rum centra′lium anterolatera′lium,** lateral branches of anterolateral central arteries: branches supplied by the middle cerebral artery, supplying the basal nuclei of the brain and its internal capsule. Called also *lateral striate arteries.*

**r. latera′lis arte′riae pulmona′lis dex′trae,** arteria segmentalis lateralis pulmonis dextri.

**r. latera′lis duc′tus hepa′tici sinis′tri** [TA], the lateral branch of the left hepatic duct.

**r. latera′lis interventricula′ris anterio′ris arte′riae corona′riae sinis′trae** [TA], lateral branch of the anterior interventricular branch of the left coronary artery.

**r. latera′lis na′si arte′riae facia′lis** [TA], lateral nasal branch of the facial artery: a branch supplying the ala and dorsum of the nose.

**r. latera′lis ner′vi supraorbita′lis** [TA], lateral branch of supraorbital nerve: a branch of the supraorbital nerve that supplies the frontal sinus, upper eyelid, and skin and subcutaneous tissue of the forehead and scalp laterally as far as the temporal region; modality, general sensory.

**r. latera′lis ra′mi posterio′ris ner′vi cervica′lis** [TA], lateral branch of posterior branch of cervical nerve: the lateral branch that arises from the posterior branch of a cervical nerve and supplies adjacent muscles.

**r. latera′lis ra′mi posterio′ris ner′vi lumba′lis** [TA], lateral branch of posterior branch of lumbar nerve: a branch that runs inferolaterally from the posterior branch of each lumbar nerve and innervates adjacent muscle; these branches have upper terminal branches that constitute the superior cluneal nerves and innervate the skin of the buttock.

**r. latera′lis ra′mi posterio′ris ner′vi sacra′lis** [TA], lateral branch of posterior branch of sacral nerve: a branch that arises from the posterior branch of one of the three upper sacral nerves and supplies the posterior gluteal skin.

**r. latera′lis ra′mi posterio′ris ner′vi thora′cici** [TA], lateral branch of posterior branch of thoracic nerve: the lateral of the terminal divisions of the posterior branch; it supplies first its corresponding levator costae muscle and then the longissimus thoracis and iliocostalis thoracis muscles. The lower branches pierce the latissimus dorsi and supply the skin of the back.

**ra′mi liena′les arte′riae liena′lis,** TA alternative for *rami splenici arteriae splenicae.*

**r. lingua′lis ner′vi facia′lis** [TA], lingual branch of facial nerve: an inconstant branch of the facial nerve sometimes arising together with the stylohyoid branch, and helping to supply the styloglossal and glossopalatine muscles; modality, motor.

**ra′mi lingua′les ner′vi glossopharyn′gei** [TA], lingual branches of glossopharyngeal nerve: branches of the glossopharyngeal nerve that innervate the posterior third of the tongue; modality, general and special sensory.

**ra′mi lingua′les ner′vi hypoglos′si** [TA], lingual branches of hypoglossal nerve: branches of the hypoglossal nerve that innervate the intrinsic and extrinsic muscles of the tongue; modality, motor.

**ra′mi lingua′les ner′vi lingua′lis** [TA], lingual branches of lingual nerve: branches that innervate the anterior two-thirds of the tongue, adjacent areas of the mouth, and the gums; modality, general and special sensory.

**r. lingula′ris arte′riae pulmona′lis sinis′trae,** arteria lingularis.

**r. lingula′ris infe′rior arte′riae pulmona′lis sinis′trae,** arteria lingularis inferior.

**r. lingula′ris supe′rior arte′riae pulmona′lis sinis′trae,** arteria lingularis superior.

**r. lingula′ris ve′nae pulmona′lis sinis′trae superio′ris,** vena lingularis.

**ra′mi lo′bi cauda′ti par′tis transver′sae ve′nae por′tae he′patis** [TA], caudate branches of transverse part of hepatic portal vein: the branches of the left branch of the portal vein that drain the caudate lobe of the liver.

**ra′mi lo′bi inferio′ris arte′riae pulmona′lis dex′trae,** arteriae lobares inferiores pulmonis dextri.

**ra′mi lo′bi inferio′ris arte′riae pulmona′lis sinis′trae,** arteriae lobares inferiores pulmonis sinistri.

**r. lo′bi me′dii arte′riae pulmona′lis dex′trae,** arteria lobaris media pulmonis dextri.

**r. lo′bi me′dii ve′nae pulmona′lis dex′trae superio′ris,** vena lobi medii pulmonis dextri.

**ra′mi lo′bi superio′ris arte′riae pulmona′lis dex′trae,** arteriae lobares superiores pulmonis dextri.

**ra′mi lo′bi superio′ris arte′riae pulmona′lis sinis′trae,** arteriae lobares superiores pulmonis sinistri.

**r. lumba′lis arte′riae iliolumba′lis** [TA], lumbar branch of iliolumbar artery: a branch that arises from the iliolumbar artery in the iliac fossa and ascends to supply the psoas and quadratus lumborum muscles, sending a spinal branch through the intervertebral foramen just above the sacrum.

**ra′mi malleola′res latera′les arte′riae fibula′ris** [TA], lateral malleolar branches of fibular artery: branches that supply the lateral aspect of the ankle and give off calcaneal branches to the lateral aspect and back of the heel; called also *rami malleolares laterales arteriae peroneae* [TA alternative].

**ra′mi malleola′res latera′les arte′riae perone′ae,** TA alternative for *rami malleolares laterales arteriae fibularis.*

**ra′mi malleola′res media′les arte′riae tibia′les posterio′ris** [TA], medial malleolar branches of posterior tibial artery: vessels supplying the area of the medial malleolus and giving off calcaneal branches to the medial aspect and back of the heel.

**ra′mi mamma′rii latera′les arte′riae thora′cicae latera′lis** [TA], lateral mammary branches of lateral thoracic artery: branches that supply the mammary gland.

**ra′mi mamma′rii latera′les ra′mi cuta′nei latera′lis arte′riarum intercosta′lium posterio′rium** [TA], lateral mammary branches of lateral cutaneous branch of posterior intercostal arteries: branches that arise from the third, fourth, and fifth posterior intercostal arteries.

**ra′mi mamma′rii latera′les ra′mi cuta′nei latera′lis pectora′lis ner′vi intercosta′lis** [TA], the lateral mammary branches of the lateral pectoral cutaneous branch of the intercostal nerve: modality, general sensory.

**ra′mi mamma′rii media′les ra′mi cuta′nei anterio′ris pectora′lis ner′vi intercosta′lis** [TA], the medial mammary branches of the anterior pectoral cutaneous branch of the intercostal nerve; modality, general sensory.

**ra′mi mamma′rii media′les ra′mi perforan′tium arte′riae thora′cicae inter′nae** [TA], medial mammary branches of perforating branch of internal thoracic artery: branches that arise from the second, third, and fourth perforating branches of the internal thoracic artery and help supply the mammary gland.

**r. mandi′bulae** [TA], ramus of mandible: a quadrilateral process projecting superiorly from the posterior part of either side of the mandible. Called also *r. of jaw.*

**r. margina′lis dex′ter arte′riae corona′riae dex′trae** [TA], right marginal branch of right coronary artery: a branch that passes toward the apex of the heart along the acute margin of the heart and ramifies over the right ventricle; called also *right marginal artery.*

**r. margina′lis mandibula′ris ner′vi facia′lis** [TA], marginal mandib-

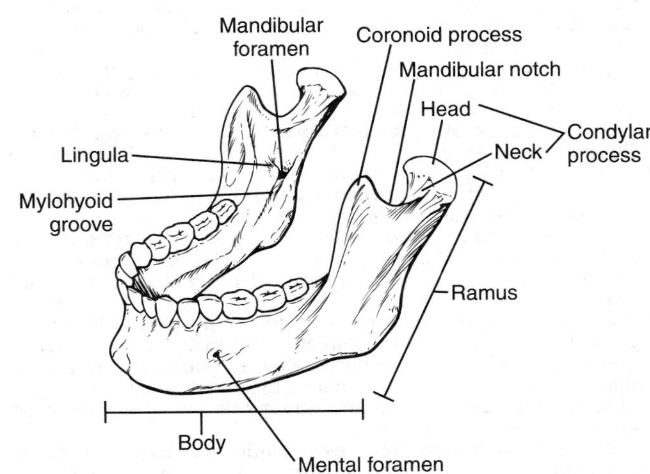


Ramus mandibulae (ramus of mandible), which together with the corpus mandibulae (body of mandible) compose the mandible.

ular branch of facial nerve: a branch of the facial nerve that runs forward from the front of the parotid gland along the border of the mandible, deep to the platysma and depressor anguli oris muscles, supplying the latter and the risorius, depressor labii inferioris, and mentalis muscles; modality, motor.

**r. margina'lis sinis'ter ra'mi circumflex'i arte'riae corona'riae sinis'trae** [TA], left marginal branch of circumflex branch of left coronary artery: a branch that follows the left margin of the heart and supplies the left ventricle. Called also *left marginal artery.*

**r. margina'lis tento'rii arter'iae caro'tidis inter'nae** [TA], tentorial marginal branch of internal carotid artery: a twig from the cavernous part of the internal carotid artery that supplies the margin of the tentorium; called also *r. tentorii marginalis arteriae carotidis internae.*

**ra'mi mastoi'dei arte'riae auricula'ris posterio'ris** [TA], mastoid branches of posterior auricular artery: branches that supply the mastoid cells.

**r. mastoi'deus arte'riae occipita'lis** [TA], mastoid branch of occipital artery: a branch that enters the cranial cavity through the mastoid foramen and supplies the dura mater, diploe, and mastoid cells. Called also *mastoid artery.*

**r. mea'tus acus'tici inter'ni arte'riae basila'ris,** arteria labyrinthina.

**ra'mi media'les arteria'rum centra'lium anterolatera'lium,** medial branches of anterolateral central artery: branches supplied by the middle cerebral artery, supplying the anterior lenticular and caudate nuclei and internal capsule. Called also *medial striate arteries.*

**r. media'lis arte'riae pulmona'lis dex'trae,** arteria segmentalis medialis pulmonis dextri.

**r. media'lis duc'tus hepa'tici sinis'tri** [TA], the medial branch of the left hepatic duct.

**r. media'lis ner'vi supraorbita'lis** [TA], medial branch of supraorbital nerve: a nerve branch that supplies the frontal sinus, upper eyelid, and skin and subcutaneous tissue of the forehead and adjacent scalp as far back as the parietal bone; modality, general sensory.

**r. media'lis ra'mi posterio'ris ner'vi cervica'lis** [TA], medial branch of posterior branch of cervical nerve: the medial branch that arises from the posterior branch of a cervical nerve and supplies muscle, periosteum, ligaments, and joints; all except the first and sometimes the sixth through eighth have an eventual cutaneous distribution.

**r. media'lis ra'mi posterio'ris ner'vi lumba'lis** [TA], medial branch of posterior branch of lumbar nerve: a branch of the posterior branch of each lumbar nerve, mainly innervating deep muscle but also helping supply ligaments, periosteum, and joints.

**r. media'lis ra'mi posterio'ris ner'vi sacra'lis** [TA], medial branch of posterior branch of sacral nerve: a branch arising from the posterior branch of one of the three upper sacral nerves and innervating the multifidus muscle.

**r. media'lis ra'mi posterio'ris ner'vi thora'cici** [TA], medial branch of posterior branch of thoracic nerve: one of the terminal divisions of the posterior branch of the thoracic nerve, supplying periosteum, ligaments, and joints. Those of the upper thoracic nerves supply the skin of the back and those of the lower nerves supply primarily the erector spinae muscle.

**ra'mi mediastina'les aor'tae thora'cicae,** rami mediastinales partis thoracicae aortae.

**ra'mi mediastina'les arte'riae thora'cicae inter'nae** [TA], mediastinal branches of internal thoracic artery: branches that supply areolar tissue, pericardium, lymph nodes, and the thymus in the anterior and superior mediastina. Called also *anterior mediastinal arteries* and *arteriae mediastinales anteriores.*

**ra'mi mediastina'les par'tis thora'cicae aor'tae** [TA], mediastinal branches of thoracic part of aorta: small vessels supplying connective tissue and lymph nodes in the posterior mediastinum.

**ra'mi medulla'res latera'les arte'riae inferio'ris posterio'ris cerebel'li** [TA], lateral medullary branches of posterior inferior cerebellar artery: the branch supplies the undersurface of the hemisphere of the cerebellum and anastomoses with the anterior inferior cerebellar and superior cerebellar branches of the basilar artery.

**ra'mi medulla'res media'les arte'riae inferio'ris posterio'ris cerebel'li** [TA], medial medullary branches of posterior inferior cerebellar artery, ramifying on the cerebellar vermis between the hemispheres.

**r. membra'nae tym'pani ner'vi auriculotempora'lis** [TA], branch to tympanic membrane of auriculotemporal nerve: a branch given to the tympanic membrane by the nerve of the external acoustic meatus, a branch of the auriculotemporal nerve; modality, general sensory.

**r. menin'geus accesso'rius arte'riae menin'geae me'diae,** r. accessorius arteriae meningeae mediae.

**r. menin'geus ante'rior arte'riae ethmoida'lis anterio'ris** [TA], anterior meningeal branch of anterior ethmoidal artery; a branch that supplies the dura mater. Called also *arteria meningea anterior* and *anterior meningeal artery.*

**r. menin'geus ante'rior arte'riae vertebra'lis,** see *rami meningei arteriae vertebralis.*

**r. menin'geus arte'riae caro'tidis inter'nae** [TA], meningeal branch of internal carotid artery: a twig from the cavernous part of the internal carotid artery that supplies the meninges of the anterior cranial fossa.

**r. menin'geus arte'riae occipita'lis** [TA], meningeal branch of occipital artery: one or more variable branches of the occipital artery that enter the posterior fossa and supply the dura mater.

**ra'mi menin'gei arte'riae vertebra'lis** [TA], meningeal branches of vertebral artery: branches, anterior and posterior, arising from the vertebral artery in the foramen magnum, and ramifying in the posterior cranial fossa to supply the dura mater, including the falx cerebelli and bone.

**r. menin'geus ner'vi mandibula'ris** [TA], meningeal branch of mandibular nerve: a branch that arises from the trunk of the mandibular nerve, re-enters the cranium through the foramen spinosum, accompanies the middle meningeal artery to supply the dura mater, and also helps innervate the mucous membrane of the mastoid air cells. Called also *nervus spinosus* [TA alternative].

**r. menin'geus ner'vi maxilla'ris** [TA], meningeal branch of maxillary nerve: a branch arising from the maxillary nerve in the middle cranial fossa, accompanying the middle meningeal artery, and supplying the dura mater; modality, general sensory. Called also *meningeal nerve* and *nervus meningeus medius.*

**r. menin'geus ner'vi spina'lis** [TA], meningeal branch of spinal nerve: the small branch of each spinal nerve that re-enters the intervertebral foramen to supply the dura mater, vertebral column, and associated ligaments. Called also *r. recurrens nervi spinalis* [TA alternative].

**r. menin'geus ner'vi va'gi** [TA], meningeal branch of vagus nerve: a branch that arises in the jugular foramen from the superior ganglion of the vagus nerve, innervating dura mater of the posterior cranial fossa.

**r. menin'geus poste'rior arte'riae vertebra'lis,** see *rami meningei arteriae vertebralis.*

**r. menin'geus recur'rens arte'riae lacrima'lis** [TA], recurrent meningeal branch of the lacrimal artery: a branch that anastomoses with a branch of the meningeal artery between the internal and external carotid arteries.

**r. menin'geus recur'rens ner'vi ophthal'mici** [TA], tentorial branch of ophthalmic nerve: a branch that arises from the ophthalmic nerve close to its origin from the trigeminal ganglion, turning back to innervate the dura mater of the tentorium cerebelli and falx cerebri; modality, general sensory. Called also *r. tentorius nervi ophthalmici* [TA alternative].

**r. menta'lis arte'riae alveola'ris inferio'ris** [TA], mental branch of inferior alveolar artery: a branch arising from the inferior alveolar artery in the mandibular canal, which leaves the canal at the mental foramen, supplies the chin, and anastomoses with its fellow of the opposite side and with the submental and inferior labial arteries. Called also *mental artery* and *arteria mentalis.*

**ra'mi menta'les ner'vi menta'lis** [TA], mental branches of mental nerve: branches that innervate the skin of the chin; modality, general sensory.

**r. muscula'ris** [TA], muscular branch: a branch of a peripheral nerve or vessel that supplies muscle.

**ra'mi muscula'res arte'riae vertebra'lis** [TA], muscular branches of vertebral artery: branches of the transverse part of the vertebral artery that supply the deep muscles of the neck and anastomose with the descending branch of the occipital artery and the deep cervical artery.

**ra'mi muscula'res ner'vi axilla'ris** [TA], muscular branches of axillary nerve: branches that innervate the deltoid and teres minor muscles; modality, motor.

**ra'mi muscula'res ner'vi femora'lis** [TA], muscular branches of femoral nerve: branches that innervate the anterior thigh muscles; modality, motor.

**ra'mi muscula'res ner'vi fibula'ris profun'di** [TA], muscular branches of deep fibular nerve: branches that innervate the tibialis anterior, extensor hallucis longus, extensor digitorum longus, and peroneus tertius muscles; modality, motor. Called also *rami musculares nervi peronei profundi* [TA alternative].

**ra'mi muscula'res ner'vi fibula'ris superficia'lis** [TA], muscular branches of superficial fibular nerve: branches that innervate the peroneus longus and peroneus brevis muscles; modality, motor; called also *rami musculares nervi peronei superficialis* [TA alternative].

**ra'mi muscula'res nervo'rum intercosta'lium** [TA], muscular branches of intercostal nerves: branches that supply numerous muscles of the lateral and ventral regions of the thorax and abdomen.

**ra'mi muscula'res ner'vi ischia'dici,** muscular branches of the sciatic nerve: branches innervating the muscles of the thigh.

**ra'mi muscula'res ner'vi media'ni** [TA], muscular branches of median nerve: branches that innervate most of the flexor muscles on the front of the forearm and most of the short muscles of the thumb; modality, motor.

**ra'mi muscula'res ner'vi musculocuta'nei** [TA], muscular branches of musculocutaneous nerve: branches that innervate the coracobrachialis, biceps, and brachialis muscles; modality, motor and general sensory.

**ra'mi muscula'res ner'vi perone'i profun'di,** TA alternative for *rami musculares nervi fibularis profundi.*

**ra'mi muscula'res ner'vi perone'i superficia'lis,** TA alternative for *rami musculares nervi fibularis superficialis.*

**ra'mi muscula'res ner'vi radia'lis** [TA], muscular branches of radial nerve: branches that innervate the triceps, anconeus, brachioradialis, and extensor carpi radialis muscles; a branch to the brachialis muscle is probably sensory; modality, motor and sensory.

**ra'mi muscula'res ner'vi tibia'lis** [TA], muscular branches of tibial nerve: branches that supply muscles of the back of the leg; modality, motor.

**ra'mi muscula'res ner'vi ulna'ris** [TA], muscular branches of ulnar nerve: branches that innervate the flexor carpi ulnaris muscle and the ulnar half of flexor digitorum profundus; modality, motor.

**ra'mi muscula'res plex'us lumba'lis,** muscular branches of the lumbar plexus: branches that innervate the quadratus lumborum, psoas minor, psoas major, and iliacus muscles.

**ra'mi muscula'res ra'mi anterio'ris ner'vi obturato'rii** [TA], muscular branches of anterior branch of obturator nerve: branches arising from the anterior ramus of the obturator nerve and innervating the gracilis and adductor longus muscles, usually the adductor brevis, and often the pectineus; modality, motor.

**ra'mi muscula'res ra'mi exter'ni ner'vi accesso'rii** [TA], muscular branches of external branch of accessory nerve: the branches of the external branch of the accessory nerve that supply the sternocleidomastoid and trapezius muscles.

**ra'mi muscula'res ra'mi posterio'ris ner'vi obturato'rii** [TA], muscular branches of posterior branch of obturator nerve: branches arising from the posterior ramus of the obturator nerve and innervating the obturator externus and adductor brevis muscles, and sometimes the adductor magnus; modality, motor.

**r. mus'culi stylopharyn'gei ner'vi glossopharyn'gei** [TA], stylopharyngeal branch of glossopharyngeal nerve: a branch that supplies the stylopharyngeal muscle; modality, motor.

**r. mylohyoi'deus arte'riae alveola'ris inferio'ris** [TA], mylohyoid branch of inferior alveolar artery: a branch that descends with the mylohyoid nerve in the mylohyoid sulcus to supply the floor of the mouth.

**ra'mi nasa'les anterio'res latera'les arte'riae ethmoida'lis anterio'ris** [TA], anterior lateral nasal branches of anterior ethmoidal artery; branches that supply twigs to the lateral wall and septum of the nose.

**r. nasa'lis exter'nus ner'vi ethmoida'lis anterio'ris** [TA], external nasal branch of anterior ethmoidal nerve: a branch that is essentially a continuation, or terminal branch, of the anterior ethmoidal nerve, innervating the skin of the dorsal part of the nose; modality, general sensory.

**ra'mi nasa'les exter'ni ner'vi infraorbita'lis** [TA], external nasal branches of infraorbital nerve: they innervate the skin of the side of the nose; modality, general sensory.

**ra'mi nasa'les inter'ni latera'les ner'vi ethmoida'lis anterio'ris** [TA], lateral internal nasal branches of anterior ethmoidal nerve: branches arising from the internal nasal branches of the anterior ethmoidal nerve and innervating the mucosa of the lateral wall of the nasal cavity; modality, general sensory.

**ra'mi nasa'les inter'ni media'les ner'vi ethmoida'lis anterio'ris** [TA], medial internal nasal branches of anterior ethmoidal nerve: branches arising from the internal nasal branches of the anterior ethmoidal nerve and supplying the nasal septum; modality, general sensory.

**ra'mi nasa'les inter'ni ner'vi ethmoida'lis anterio'ris** [TA], internal nasal branches of anterior ethmoidal nerve: the medial and lateral branches that innervate the nasal septum and the mucous membrane of the lateral wall of the nasal cavity; modality, general sensory.

**ra'mi nasa'les inter'ni ner'vi infraorbita'lis** [TA], internal nasal branches of infraorbital nerve: branches that innervate the mobile septum of the nose; modality, general sensory.

**ra'mi nasa'les ner'vi ethmoida'lis anterio'ris,** nasal branches of anterior ethmoidal nerve: the internal and external nasal branches of the anterior ethmoidal nerve, and their subdivisions.

**ra'mi nasa'les posterio'res inferio'res ner'vi palati'ni majo'ris** [TA], inferior posterior nasal branches of greater palatine nerve: nerve branches of the maxillary nerve, usually branches of the greater palatine nerve, that supply the middle and inferior nasal meatus and inferior conchae; modality, general sensory.

**ra'mi nasa'les posterio'res superio'res latera'les ner'vi maxilla'ris** [TA], lateral superior posterior nasal branches of maxillary nerve: branches that supply the superior and middle nasal conchae and the posterior ethmoidal sinuses; modality, general sensory.

**ra'mi nasa'les posterio'res superio'res media'les ner'vi maxilla'ris** [TA], medial superior posterior nasal branches of maxillary nerve: nerve branches, usually branches of the nasopalatine nerve, that supply the nasal septum; modality, general sensory.

**r. ner'vi oculomoto'rii arte'riae communican'tis posterio'ris** [TA], oculomotor nerve branch of posterior communicating artery: the branch that supplies the oculomotor nerve.

**r. ner'vi oculomoto'rii ad gan'glii cilia're,** TA alternative for *r. parasympathica ganglii ciliaris.*

**r. no'di atrioventricula'ris arte'riae corona'riae dex'trae** [TA], atrioventricular nodal branch of right coronary artery: a branch of the right coronary artery usually arising opposite the origin of the posterior interventricular artery and inserting into the atrioventricular node. Called also *atrioventricular nodal artery.*

**r. no'di atrioventricula'ris ra'mi circumflex'i arte'riae corona'riae sinis'trae** [TA], atrioventricular nodal branch of circumflex branch of left coronary artery: a branch of the left coronary artery occasionally found supplying the atrioventricular node.

**r. no'di sinuatria'lis arte'riae corona'riae dex'trae** [TA], sinoatrial nodal branch of right coronary artery: a branch of the right coronary artery that supplies the right atrium, encircles the base of the superior vena cava, and inserts into the sinoatrial node. Called also *nodal artery, sinoatrial* or *sinuatrial nodal artery,* and *sinus node artery.*

**r. no'di sinuatria'lis ra'mi circumflex'i arte'riae corona'riae sinis'trae** [TA], sinoatrial nodal branch of circumflex branch of left coronary artery: a branch of the left coronary artery occasionally found supplying the sinoatrial node.

**ra'mi nu'clei ru'bri** [TA], small branches of the anterior choroidal artery that supply the red nucleus.

**ra'mi nucleo'rum hypothalamico'rum** [TA], small branches of the anterior choroidal artery that supply the hypothalamic nuclei.

**r. obturato'rius ra'mi pu'bici arte'riae epigas'tricae inferio'ris** [TA], obturator branch of inferior epigastric artery: a vessel connecting the pubic branches of the inferior epigastric and the obturator arteries. The obturator artery is sometimes replaced by an accessory obturator that arises from the inferior epigastric artery by way of this communication.

**r. occipita'lis arte'riae auricula'ris posterio'ris** [TA], occipital branch of posterior auricular artery: a branch distributed to the epicranial muscle.

**ra'mi occipita'les arte'riae occipita'lis** [TA], occipital branches of occipital artery: a medial and a lateral branch of the occipital artery, distributed to the scalp and, through the meningeal branch, to the dura mater.

**r. occipita'lis ner'vi auricula'ris posterio'ris** [TA], occipital branch of posterior auricular nerve: a branch supplying the occipital belly of the occipitofrontalis muscle; modality, motor.

**r. occipitotempora'lis arte'riae occipita'lis media'lis** [TA], occipitotemporal branch of middle occipital artery: a branch that supplies the occipital and temporal areas of the cerebral cortex.

**ra'mi oesophagea'les aor'tae thora'cicae,** rami oesophageales partis thoracicae aortae.

**ra'mi oesophagea'les arte'riae gas'tricae sinis'trae** [TA], esophageal branches of left gastric artery: branches that supply the esophagus; called also *inferior esophageal arteries* and *rami esophageales arteriae gastricae sinistrae.*

**ra'mi oesophagea'les arte'riae thyroi'deae inferio'ris** [TA], esophageal branches of inferior thyroid artery: branches that supply the esophagus; called also *rami esophageales arteriae thyroideae inferioris.*

**ra'mi oesophagea'les ganglio'rum thora'cicorum** [TA], esophageal branches of thoracic ganglia: sympathetic nerve branches from the thoracic ganglia, helping to innervate the thoracic and abdominal esophagus.

**ra'mi oesophagea'les par'tis thora'cicae aor'tae** [TA], esophageal branches of thoracic part of aorta: branches, usually two, that arise from the front of the aorta to supply the esophagus; called also *rami esophageales partis thoracicae aortae.*

**ra'mi oesopha'gei ner'vi laryn'gei recurren'tis** [TA], esophageal branches of recurrent laryngeal nerve: branches that help innervate the esophagus; modality, visceral afferent and general sensory; called also *rami esophagei nervi laryngei recurrentis.*

**ra'mi omenta'les arte'riae gastroomenta'lis dex'trae** [TA], omental branches of right gastro-omental artery: branches that supply the greater omentum.

**ra'mi omenta'les arte'riae gastroomenta'lis sinis'trae** [TA], omental branches of left gastro-omental artery; branches that supply the stomach and greater omentum.

**r. orbita'lis arte'riae menin'geae me'diae** [TA], the orbital branch of the middle meningeal artery.

**ra'mi orbita'les gan'glii pterygopalati'ni, ra'mi orbita'les ner'vi maxilla'ris** [TA], orbital branches of pterygopalatine ganglion: branches passing from the pterygopalatine ganglion through the inferior orbital fissure to supply the orbital periosteum and the ethmoidal and sphenoidal sinuses; modality, general sensory and parasympathetic.

**r. orbitofronta′lis media′lis arte′riae ce′rebri anterio′ris,** TA alternative for *arteria frontobasalis medialis.*

**r. os′sis is′chii** [TA], ramus of ischium: the flattened bar of bone that projects from the inferior end of the body of the ischium in an anterosuperomedial direction to meet the inferior ramus of the pubis. It forms part of the border of the obturator foramen. Called also *r. inferior ossis ischii.*

**r. os′sis pu′bis,** see *r. inferior ossis pubis* and *r. superior ossis pubis.*

**r. ova′ricus arte′riae uteri′nae** [TA], ovarian branch of uterine artery: the terminal branch of the uterine artery, which supplies the ovary and anastomoses with the ovarian artery.

**r. palma′ris ner′vi media′ni** [TA], palmar branch of median nerve: a branch arising from the median nerve in the lower part of the forearm and supplying the skin of the outer part of the palm; modality, general sensory.

**r. palma′ris ner′vi ulna′ris** [TA], palmar branch of ulnar nerve: a branch arising from the ulnar nerve in the lower part of the forearm, supplying the cutaneous structures of the medial part of the palm; modality, general sensory.

**r. palma′ris profun′dus arte′riae ulna′ris** [TA], deep palmar branch of ulnar artery: a branch that accompanies the deep palmar branch of the ulnar nerve and joins the radial artery to form the deep palmar arch.

**r. palma′ris superficia′lis arte′riae radia′lis** [TA], superficial palmar branch of radial artery: a branch arising from the radial artery in the lower part of the forearm and supplying the thenar eminence.

**ra′mi palpebra′les inferio′res ner′vi infraorbita′lis** [TA], inferior palpebral branches of infraorbital nerve: branches that supply the skin and conjunctiva of the lower eyelid; modality, general sensory.

**ra′mi palpebra′les ner′vi infratrochlea′ris** [TA], palpebral branches of infratrochlear nerve: branches that help supply the eyelids; modality, general sensory.

**ra′mi pancrea′tici arte′riae liena′lis,** TA alternative for *rami pancreatici arteriae splenicae.*

**ra′mi pancrea′tici arte′riae pancreaticoduodena′lis superio′ris anterio′ris** [TA], pancreatic branches of the anterior superior pancreaticoduodenal artery: vessels that supply the pancreas.

**ra′mi pancrea′tici arte′riae pancreaticoduodena′lis superio′ris posterio′ris** [TA], pancreatic branches of posterior superior pancreaticoduodenal artery: vessels that supply the pancreas.

**ra′mi pancrea′tici arte′riae sple′nicae** [TA], pancreatic branches of splenic artery: branches that supply the pancreas, arising from the splenic artery during its tortuous course along the superior border of the body of the pancreas. Called also *rami pancreatici arteriae lienalis* [TA alternative].

**r. parieta′lis arte′riae menin′geae me′diae** [TA], parietal branch of middle meningeal artery: a vessel that arises in the middle cranial fossa, grooves the temporal and parietal bones, and supplies the posterior dura mater.

**r. parieta′lis arte′riae occipita′lis media′lis** [TA], the branch of the middle occipital artery that supplies the parietal lobe.

**r. parieta′lis arte′riae tempora′lis superficia′lis** [TA], parietal branch of superficial temporal artery: the posterior terminal branch of the superficial temporal artery, supplying the scalp in the parietal region.

**ra′mi parieta′les par′tis abdomina′lis aor′tae,** parietal branches of the abdominal part of the aorta, comprising the inferior phrenic and the lumbar arteries.

**ra′mi parieta′les par′tis thora′cicae aor′tae,** parietal branches of the thoracic part of the aorta, supplying the thoracic wall.

**ra′mi parietooccipita′les arte′riae ce′rebri anterio′ris** [TA], parietooccipital branches of anterior cerebral artery: vessels originating in the postcommunical part of the anterior cerebral artery and supplying the parietal lobe and sometimes the occipital lobe.

**r. parietooccipita′lis arte′riae occipita′lis media′lis** [TA], parietooccipital branch of medial occipital artery: a vessel that supplies the cortex of the medial surface of the hemisphere up to the area of the parietooccipital sulcus.

**r. paroti′deus arte′riae auricula′ris posterio′ris** [TA], parotid branch of the posterior auricular artery: a branch supplying the parotid gland.

**r. paroti′deus arte′riae tempora′lis superficia′lis** [TA], parotid branch of superficial temporal artery: a branch supplying the parotid gland and the temporomandibular joint.

**ra′mi paroti′dei ner′vi auriculotempora′lis** [TA], parotid branches of auriculotemporal nerve: branches that bear postganglionic fibers from the otic ganglion to the parotid gland; modality, parasympathetic.

**ra′mi paroti′dei ve′nae facia′lis** [TA], parotid branches of facial vein: small veins from the substance of the parotid gland which follow the parotid duct and open into the facial vein; called also *anterior parotid veins.*

**ra′mi pectora′les arte′riae thoracoacromia′lis** [TA], pectoral branches of thoracoacromial artery: branches that descend between the pectoralis major and minor muscles, supplying these muscles and the mammary gland.

**ra′mi peduncula′res arte′riae ce′rebri poste′rioris** [TA], the branches of the posterior cerebral artery that supply the cerebral peduncles.

**ra′mi perforan′tes ar′cus palma′ris profun′dus** [TA], perforating branches of deep palmar arch: vessels connecting the palmar metacarpal arteries and deep palmar arch with the dorsal metacarpal arteries, between the bases of the metacarpal bones and in the interosseous spaces.

**r. per′forans arte′riae fibula′ris** [TA], perforating branch of fibular artery: a branch passing forward from the fibular artery where the interosseous membrane and the tibiofibular syndesmosis are continuous and descending to supply the syndesmosis and the ankle joint.

**ra′mi perforan′tes arteria′rum metatarsea′rum planta′rium** [TA], perforating branches of plantar metatarsal arteries: vessels connecting the plantar metatarsal arteries with the dorsal metatarsal arteries through the interosseous spaces.

**ra′mi perforan′tes arte′riae thora′cicae inter′nae** [TA], perforating branches of internal thoracic artery: six branches, one in each of the upper six intercostal spaces, supplying the pectoralis major muscle and adjacent skin; the second, third, and fourth branches give off mammary branches.

**ra′mi pericardi′aci aor′tae thora′cicae,** rami pericardiaci partis thoracicae aortae.

**r. pericardi′acus ner′vi phre′nici** [TA], pericardiac branch of phrenic nerve: a branch arising from the phrenic or accessory phrenic nerve and supplying the pericardium; modality, general sensory.

**ra′mi pericardi′aci par′tis thora′cicae aor′tae** [TA], pericardiac branches of thoracic part of aorta: small branches from the aorta distributed to the surface of the pericardium.

**ra′mi peridenta′les arte′riae alveola′ris inferio′ris** [TA], peridental branches of inferior alveolar artery: branches arising from the inferior alveolar artery in the mandibular canal and supplying the roots and pulp of the teeth.

**ra′mi peridenta′les arte′riae alveola′ris superio′ris posterio′ris** [TA], peridental branches of posterior superior alveolar artery: branches arising from the posterior superior alveolar artery and supplying the maxillary gingivae.

**ra′mi perinea′les ner′vi cuta′nei fe′moris posterio′ris** [TA], perineal branches of posterior femoral cutaneous nerve: branches arising from the posterior femoral cutaneous nerve at the lower margin of the gluteus maximus muscle and innervating the skin of the external genitalia; modality, general sensory.

**r. petro′sus arte′riae menin′geae me′diae** [TA], **r. petro′sus superficia′lis arte′riae menin′geae me′diae,** petrosal branch of middle meningeal artery: a branch that arises in the region of the petrous part of the temporal bone, entering the hiatus for the greater petrosal nerve and anastomosing with the stylomastoid artery.

**ra′mi pharyngea′les arte′riae pharyn′geae ascenden′tis** [TA], pharyngeal branches of ascending pharyngeal artery: irregular vessels supplying the pharynx.

**ra′mi pharyngea′les arte′riae thyroi′deae inferio′ris** [TA], pharyngeal branches of inferior thyroid artery: vessels that supply the pharynx.

**r. pharyn′geus arte′riae cana′lis pterygoi′dei** [TA], pharyngeal branch of artery of pterygoid canal: a branch lying medial to the pterygopalatine ganglion.

**ra′mi pharyn′gei arte′riae pharyn′geae ascenden′tis,** rami pharyngeales arteriae pharyngeae.

**ra′mi pharyn′gei arte′riae thyroi′deae inferio′ris,** rami pharyngeales arteriae thyroideae inferioris.

**r. pharyn′geus gan′glii pterygopalati′ni,** nervus pharyngeus.

**ra′mi pharyn′gei ner′vi glossopharyn′gei** [TA], pharyngeal branches of glossopharyngeal nerve: branches innervating the mucous membrane of the oropharynx, with a general sensory modality.

**ra′mi pharyn′gei ner′vi laryn′gei recurren′tis** [TA], pharyngeal branches of recurrent laryngeal nerve: small nerve branches that innervate the inferior constrictor muscle of the pharynx.

**r. pharyn′geus ner′vi va′gi** [TA], pharyngeal branch of vagus nerve: any of several branches that innervate the pharyngeal muscles and mucosa and have motor and general sensory modalities.

**ra′mi phrenicoabdomina′les ner′vi phre′nici** [TA], phrenicoabdominal branches of phrenic nerve: branches of the phrenic or accessory phrenic nerve that supply the diaphragm and contribute to the celiac plexus; modality, general sensory and motor.

**r. planta′ris profun′dus arte′riae dorsa′lis pe′dis,** arteria plantaris profunda.

**ra′mi ad pon′tem arte′riae basila′ris,** arteriae pontis.

**r. poste′rior arte′riae obturato′riae** [TA], posterior branch of obturator artery: a branch passing backward around the lateral margin of the obturator foramen, on the obturator membrane, supplying muscles around the ischial tuberosity and giving off an acetabular branch.

**r. poste'rior arte'riae pancreaticoduodena'lis inferio'ris** [TA], posterior branch of inferior pancreaticoduodenal artery: a branch that ascends behind the head of the pancreas, which it sometimes pierces, and anastomoses with the posterior superior pancreaticoduodenal artery; it supplies the head of the pancreas and adjoining parts of the duodenum.

**r. poste'rior arte'riae recurren'tis ulna'ris** [TA], posterior branch of ulnar recurrent artery: a branch running to the back of the medial epicondyle, supplying the elbow joint and neighboring muscles.

**r. poste'rior arte'riae rena'lis** [TA], posterior branch of renal artery: a branch supplying the posterior segment of the kidney.

**r. poste'rior arte'riae thyroi'deae superio'ris,** r. glandularis posterior arteriae thyroideae superioris.

**r. poste'rior duc'tus hepa'tici dex'tri** [TA], the posterior branch of the right hepatic duct.

**r. poste'rior ner'vi auricula'ris mag'ni** [TA], posterior branch of great auricular nerve: a branch, formed by division of the great auricular nerve, that innervates the skin over the mastoid process and the back of the external ear; modality, general sensory.

**ra'mi posterio'res nervo'rum cervica'lium** [TA], posterior branches of cervical nerves: branches of the eight cervical spinal nerves, further subdividing into lateral and medial branches (see *r. lateralis rami posterior nervi cervicalis* and *r. medialis rami posterior nervi cervicalis*). Called also *rami dorsales nervorum cervicalium* [TA alternative].

**r. poste'rior ner'vi coccy'gei** [TA], posterior branch of coccygeal nerve: a branch of the last spinal nerve, helping to innervate the skin over the coccyx. Called also *r. dorsalis nervi coccygei* [TA alternative].

**r. poste'rior ner'vi cuta'nei antebra'chii media'lis** [TA], posterior branch of medial antebrachial cutaneous nerve: a branch that innervates the skin of the posteromedial and medial aspects of the forearm; modality, general sensory.

**ra'mi posterio'res nervo'rum lumba'lium** [TA], posterior branches of the five lumbar spinal nerves; they subdivide into lateral and medial branches (see *r. lateralis rami posterioris nervi lumbalis* and *r. medialis rami posterioris nervi lumbalis*). Called also *rami dorsales nervorum lumbalium* [TA alternative].

**r. poste'rior ner'vi obturato'rii** [TA], posterior branch of obturator nerve: a branch that descends to innervate the knee joint, giving muscular branches to the obturator externus, adductor magnus, and sometimes the adductor brevis muscle; modality, general sensory and motor.

**ra'mi posterio'res nervo'rum sacra'lium** [TA], posterior branches of sacral nerves: branches of the five sacral spinal nerves, emerging from the sacrum through the posterior foramina; they subdivide into medial and lateral branches (see *r. medialis rami posterioris nervi sacralis* and *r. lateralis rami posterioris nervi sacralis*). Called also *rami dorsales nervorum sacralium* [TA alternative].

**r. poste'rior ner'vi spina'lis** [TA], posterior branch of spinal nerve: the posterior and usually smaller of the two branches into which each spinal nerve divides almost as soon as it emerges from the intervertebral foramen; the posterior branches supply the skin, muscles, joints, and bone of the posterior part of the neck and trunk. Most of these branches further subdivide into a medial and a lateral portion. Called also *r. dorsalis nervi spinalis* [TA alternative].

**ra'mi posterio'res nervo'rum thoracico'rum** [TA], posterior branches of thoracic nerves: branches of the twelve thoracic spinal nerves; they subdivide into lateral and medial and posterior cutaneous branches; see *r. lateralis rami posterioris nervi thoracici, r. medialis rami posterioris nervi thoracici,* and *r. cutaneus posterior rami posterioris nervi thoracici.* Called also *rami dorsales nervorum thoracicorum* [TA alternative].

**r. poste'rior sul'ci latera'lis ce'rebri** [TA], posterior branch of lateral cerebral sulcus: the part of the lateral cerebral sulcus that runs obliquely posteriorly between the temporal and the parietal lobes.

**r. poste'rior ve'nae pulmona'lis dex'trae superio'ris,** TA alternative for *vena posterior lobi superioris pulmonis dextri.*

**r. poste'rior ventri'culi sinis'tri ra'mi circumflex'i arte'riae corona'riae sinis'trae** [TA], posterior left ventricular branch of circumflex branch of left coronary artery: an interventricular continuation of the circumflex branch; there may be two or three vessels. Called also *r. ventriculi sinistri posterior.*

**r. posterolatera'lis dex'ter arte'riae corona'riae dex'trae** [TA], an inconstant branch of the right coronary artery.

**r. profun'dus arte'riae circumflex'ae fe'moris media'lis** [TA], deep branch of medial circumflex femoral artery: a branch ascending toward the trochanteric fossa, and anastomosing with gluteal branches.

**r. profun'dus arte'riae glu'teae superio'ris** [TA], deep branch of superior gluteal artery: a branch passing forward between the gluteus medius and minimus muscles, and dividing into superior and inferior branches.

**r. profun'dus arte'riae planta'ris media'lis** [TA], deep branch of medial plantar artery: a branch that supplies the anteromedial aspect of the sole, anastomosing with the medial three plantar metatarsal arteries.

**r. profun'dus arte'riae transver'sae cer'vicis,** TA alternative for *r. profundus arteriae transversae colli.*

**r. profun'dus arte'riae transver'sae col'li** [TA], deep branch of transverse cervical artery: a branch that descends to supply medial and deep back muscles; sometimes replaced by an artery stemming directly from the subclavian artery *(arteria dorsalis scapularis).* Called also *descending* or *dorsal scapular artery, arteria scapularis descendens,* and *arteria scapularia dorsalis.*

**r. profun'dus ner'vi planta'ris latera'lis** [TA], deep branch of lateral plantar nerve: a branch that accompanies the lateral plantar artery on its medial side and the plantar arch, innervating the interossei, the second, third, and fourth lumbrical, and the adductor hallucis muscles, and some articulations; modality, general sensory.

**r. profun'dus ner'vi radia'lis** [TA], deep branch of radial nerve: a branch arising from the radial nerve and winding laterally around the radius to the back of the forearm, supplying the supinator, extensor digitorum, extensor digiti minimi, and extensor carpi ulnaris muscles, and often the extensor carpi radialis brevis muscle. Its continuation, the posterior interosseous nerve, supplies distal forearm muscles and the carpal and intercarpal joints; modality, motor.

**r. profun'dus ner'vi ulna'ris** [TA], deep branch of ulnar nerve: the deep branch that is accompanied by the deep palmar branch of the ulnar artery, rounds the hook of the hamate bone, and follows the deep palmar arch beneath the flexor tendons, supplying the wrist joint, the interossei, third and fourth lumbrical, and adductor pollicis muscles, and usually the deep head of the flexor pollicis brevis muscle; modality, general sensory and motor.

**ra'mi prosta'tici arte'riae vesica'lis inferio'ris** [TA], prostatic branches of inferior vesical artery: branches that supply the prostate and communicate with corresponding vessels on the opposite side.

**ra'mi pterygoi'dei arte'riae maxilla'ris** [TA], **ra'mi pterygoi'dei arte'riae maxilla'ris inter'nae,** pterygoid branches of maxillary artery: branches that supply the pterygoid muscles.

**pubic r., inferior,** r. inferior ossis pubis.

**pubic r., superior,** r. superior ossis pubis.

**r. pu'bicus arte'riae epigas'tricae inferio'ris** [TA], pubic branch of inferior epigastric artery: a branch that arises from the inferior epigastric artery near the deep inguinal ring and descends on the back of the pubis, anastomosing through an obturator branch with the pubic branch of the obturator artery.

**r. pu'bicus arte'riae obturato'riae** [TA], pubic branch of obturator artery: a branch that ascends on the pelvic surface of the ilium, anastomosing with its fellow of the other side and with the pubic branch of the inferior epigastric artery.

**r. of pubis,** see *r. inferior ossis pubis* and *r. superior ossis pubis.*

**r. of pubis, ascending,** r. superior ossis pubis.

**r. of pubis, descending,** r. inferior ossis pubis.

**ra'mi pulmona'les plex'us pulmona'lis** [TA], pulmonary branches of pulmonary plexus: branches of the anterior and posterior pulmonary plexuses that accompany the blood vessels and bronchi into the lungs; modality, sympathetic and visceral afferent.

**ra'mi pulmona'les thora'cici ganglio'rum thoracico'rum** [TA], pulmonary thoracic branches of thoracic ganglia: branches from the second to the fourth, fifth, or sixth thoracic ganglia to the posterior pulmonary plexus, sometimes going on to follow intercostal arteries to the hilum of the lung.

**r. recur'rens ner'vi spina'lis,** TA alternative for *r. meningeus nervi spinalis.*

**r. rena'lis ner'vi splanch'nici mino'ris** [TA], renal branch of lesser splanchnic nerve: a branch from the lesser splanchnic nerve to the aorticorenal ganglion; modality, sympathetic preganglionic fibers and visceral afferent.

**ra'mi rena'les ner'vi va'gi** [TA], **ra'mi rena'les plex'us coeli'aci,** renal branches of vagus nerve: branches passing from the vagal trunks via the celiac plexus to the kidney; modality, parasympathetic and visceral afferent.

**ra'mi sacra'les latera'les arte'riae sacra'lis media'nae** [TA], lateral sacral branches of median sacral artery: branches that anastomose with the lateral sacral arteries laterally.

**r. saphe'nus arte'riae descenden'tis ge'nus** [TA], saphenous branch of descending genicular artery: a vessel that accompanies the saphenous nerve between the sartorius and gracilis muscles on the medial side of the knee, supplying the skin and anastomosing with the medial inferior genicular artery.

**ra'mi scrota'les anterio'res arte'riae puden'dae exter'nae profun'dae** [TA], anterior scrotal branches of deep external pudendal artery: branches arising from the deep external pudendal artery and supplying the anterior scrotal region in the male; called also *anterior scrotal arteries* and *arteriae scrotales anteriores.*

**ra'mi scrota'les posterio'res arte'riae puden'dae inter'nae** [TA], posterior scrotal branches of internal pudendal artery; two branches arising from the internal pudendal artery in the anterior part of the ischiorectal fossa, helping to supply the ischiocavernosus and bulbospongiosus muscles, and distributed to the scrotum. Called also *posterior scrotal arteries* and *arteriae scrotales posteriores.*

**ra'mi septa'les anterio'res arte'riae ethmoida'lis anterio'ris** [TA], anterior septal branches of anterior ethmoidal artery; twigs of the posterior lateral nasal branch that supply the lateral wall and septum of the nose.

**ra'mi septa'les posterio'res arte'riae sphenopalati'nae** [TA], posterior septal branches of sphenopalatine artery: branches that anastomose with the ethmoidal arteries.

**r. sep'ti na'si arte'riae labia'lis superio'ris** [TA], nasal septum branch of superior labial artery: a branch that ramifies on the lower and front part of the nasal septum.

**r. sinis'ter arte'riae hepa'ticae pro'priae** [TA], left branch of proper hepatic artery: a branch that supplies the left lobe of the liver.

**r. sinis'ter ve'nae por'tae he'patis** [TA], left branch of portal vein of liver: a branch distributed to the left lobe of the liver.

**r. si'nus caro'tici ner'vi glossopharyn'gei** [TA], branch of glossopharyngeal nerve to carotid sinus: a branch that supplies the pressoreceptors and chemoreceptors of the carotid sinus and carotid body with visceral afferent fibers.

**r. si'nus caverno'si arte'riae caro'tidis inter'nae** [TA], a twig from the cavernous part of the internal carotid artery that supplies the walls of the cavernous sinus.

**ra'mi spina'les arte'riae cervica'lis ascenden'tis** [TA], spinal branches of ascending cervical artery: branches that help supply the vertebral canal.

**r. spina'lis arte'riae iliolumba'lis** [TA], spinal branch of iliolumbar artery; a branch that passes through the intervertebral foramen between the fifth lumbar vertebra and the sacrum to help supply the contents of the vertebral canal.

**ra'mi spina'les arteria'rum intercosta'lium posterio'rum** [TA], spinal branches of posterior intercostal arteries: branches that arise from the dorsal branches of the posterior intercostal arteries and enter the vertebral canal through the vertebral foramina to supply the vertebrae, spinal cord, and meninges.

**ra'mi spina'les arte'riae intercosta'lis supre'mae** [TA], spinal branches of highest intercostal artery: vessels arising from the dorsal branches of the first and second posterior intercostal arteries, entering intervertebral foramina with the corresponding two spinal nerves to help supply the contents of the vertebral canal.

**r. spina'lis arteria'rum lumba'lium** [TA], spinal branch of lumbar arteries: a branch arising from the dorsal branch of the lumbar arteries and entering an intervertebral foramen with the spinal nerve to help supply the contents of the vertebral canal.

**ra'mi spina'les arteria'rum sacra'lium latera'lium** [TA], spinal branches of lateral sacral arteries: vessels arising from the two lateral sacral arteries and entering the pelvic sacral foramina to help supply the contents of the vertebral canal.

**r. spina'lis arte'riae subcosta'lis** [TA], spinal branch of subcostal artery: a spinal branch corresponding to those arising from the dorsal branches of the posterior intercostal arteries; it enters the vertebral canal to help supply the contents of the canal.

**ra'mi spina'les arte'riae vertebra'lis** [TA], spinal branches of vertebral artery: branches of the transverse part of the vertebral artery; they supply the spinal cord and its meninges, the vertebral bodies, and the intervertebral disks; called also *arteries of Adamkiewicz* and *spinal arteries.*

**r. spina'lis ra'mi dorsa'lis arteria'rum intercosta'lium posterio'rum** [TA], spinal branch of dorsal branch of posterior intercostal arteries: one of the two branches into which the dorsal branch of a posterior intercostal artery divides, passing through the intervertebral foramen with the corresponding spinal nerve to help supply the contents of the vertebral canal.

**r. spina'lis ve'nae intercosta'lis, r. spina'lis ve'nae intercosta'lis posterio'ris** [TA], spinal branch of posterior intercostal vein: a vessel, the vena comitans of the arterial spinal branch, that emerges from the vertebral canal and contributes to the dorsal branch of each posterior intercostal vein.

**ra'mi sple'nici arte'riae sple'nicae** [TA], splenic branches of splenic artery: the terminal branches of the splenic artery, which follow the trabeculae; called also *rami lienales arteriae lienalis* [TA alternative].

**r. stape'dius arte'riae auricula'ris posterio'ris** [TA], stapedial branch of posterior auricular artery: a variable branch supplying the stapedius muscle and tendon.

**ra'mi sterna'les arte'riae thora'cicae inter'nae** [TA], sternal branches of internal thoracic artery: branches that supply the sternum and the transversus thoracis muscle.

**ra'mi sternocleidomastoi'dei arte'riae occipita'lis** [TA], sternocleidomastoid branches of occipital artery: branches of the occipital artery, usually an upper and a lower, that supply the sternocleidomastoid and adjacent muscles. Called also *sternocleidomastoid artery* and *arteria sternocleidomastoidea.*

**r. sternocleidomastoi'deus arte'riae thyroi'deae superio'ris** [TA], sternocleidomastoid branch of superior thyroid artery: a branch that arises from the superior thyroid artery, but sometimes directly from the external carotid artery, passing across the carotid sheath to supply the middle portion of the sternocleidomastoid muscle.

**r. stylohyoi'deus ner'vi facia'lis** [TA], stylohyoid branch of facial nerve: a branch that arises from the facial nerve just below the base of the skull to innervate the stylohyoid muscle; modality, motor.

**ra'mi subendocardia'les** [TA], subendocardial branches: small ramifications of the conducting system of the heart (Purkinje fibers), which form a plexus in the papillary muscles and ventricles. Called also *Purkinje network* and *subendocardial terminal network.*

**ra'mi subscapula'res arte'riae axilla'ris** [TA], subscapular branches of axillary artery: branches that supply the subscapularis muscle.

**ra'mi substan'tiae ni'grae** [TA], small branches of the anterior choroidal artery that supply the substantia nigra.

**ra'mi substan'tiae perfora'tae anterio'ris** [TA], small branches of the anterior choroidal artery that supply the anterior perforated substance.

**r. superficia'lis arte'riae circumflex'ae fe'moris media'lis** [TA], superficial branch of medial circumflex femoral artery: a branch passing between the quadratus femoris and the proximal border of the adductor magnus and anastomosing with the inferior gluteal, lateral circumflex femoral, and first perforating arteries.

**r. superficia'lis arte'riae glu'teae superio'ris** [TA], superficial branch of superior gluteal artery: a branch that ramifies to supply the gluteus maximus muscle.

**r. superficia'lis arte'riae planta'ris media'lis** [TA], superficial branch of medial plantar artery: a branch that supplies the medial side of the great toe.

**r. superficia'lis arte'riae transver'sae cer'vicis,** TA alternative for *r. superficialis arteriae transversae colli.*

**r. superficia'lis arte'riae transver'sae col'li** [TA], superficial branch of transverse cervical artery: a branch that arises from the transverse cervical artery at the anterior border of the levator scapulae muscle, it has ascending and descending branches that supply the levator scapulae, trapezius, and splenius muscles. Called also *arteria cervicalis superficialis* [TA alternative].

**r. superficia'lis ner'vi planta'ris latera'lis** [TA], superficial branch of lateral plantar nerve: a branch that arises from the lateral plantar nerve at the lateral border of the quadratus plantae muscle and passes forward, dividing into a lateral part that innervates skin of the lateral side of the sole and little toe, joints of the toe, and the flexor digiti minimi brevis muscle, and a medial part, a common plantar digital nerve, that gives two proper plantar digital nerves to the adjacent sides of the fourth and fifth toes; modality, general sensory.

**r. superficia'lis ner'vi radia'lis** [TA], superficial branch of radial nerve: the continuation of the radial nerve that accompanies the radial artery in the forearm, winds dorsalward, supplies the lateral side of the back of the hand, and divides into dorsal digital nerves that supply the skin of the dorsal surface and adjacent surfaces of the thumb, index, and middle fingers, and sometimes the radial side of the ring finger; modality, general sensory.

**r. superficia'lis ner'vi ulna'ris** [TA], superficial branch of ulnar nerve: the branch of the ulnar nerve in the hand that supplies the palmaris brevis muscle and divides into a proper palmar digital nerve for the medial side of the little finger, a common palmar digital nerve giving off two proper nerves to supply adjacent sides of the little and fourth fingers, and sometimes palmar digital nerves also for the adjacent sides of the third and fourth fingers; modality, general sensory and motor.

**r. supe'rior lo'bi inferio'ris arte'riae pulmona'lis dex'trae,** arteria segmentalis superior pulmonis dextra.

**r. supe'rior lo'bi inferio'ris arte'riae pulmona'lis sinis'trae,** arteria segmentalis superior pulmonis sinistri.

**r. supe'rior ner'vi oculomoto'rii** [TA], superior branch of oculomotor nerve: the upper and smaller of the two branches of the oculomotor nerve, which supplies the superior rectus muscle and, terminally, the levator palpebrae superioris; modality, motor.

**ra'mi superio'res ner'vi transver'si col'li** [TA], superior branches of transverse cervical nerve: the upper of the branches that arise from the transverse cervical nerve near the anterior border of the sternocleidomastoid muscle, innervating skin and subcutaneous tissue in the anterior cervical region; modality, general sensory.

**r. supe'rior os'sis is'chii,** a name formerly given to what is now considered the lower part of the body of the ischium (corpus ossis ischii).

**r. supe'rior os'sis pu'bis** [TA], superior ramus of pubic bone: the bar of bone projecting from the body of the pubic bone in a postero-superolateral direction to the iliopubic eminence, and forming part of the acetabulum. Called also *superior pubic r.*

**r. supe'rior ra'mi profun'di arte'riae glu'teae superio'ris** [TA], superior branch of deep branch of superior gluteal artery: the upper division of the deep branch of the superior gluteal artery, extending as far as the anterior superior iliac spine and helping supply the gluteus medius, gluteus minimus, and tensor fasciae latae muscles.

**r. supe'rior ve'nae pulmona'lis dex'trae inferio'ris,** TA alternative for vena superior lobi inferioris pulmonis dextri.

**r. supe'rior ve'nae pulmona'lis sinis'trae inferio'ris,** TA alternative for vena superior lobi inferioris pulmonis sinistri.

**r. suprahyoi'deus arte'riae lingua'lis** [TA], suprahyoid branch of lingual artery: a branch passing along the upper border of the hyoid bone, supplying suprahyoid muscles and anastomosing with its fellow of the other side.

**r. sympathe'ticus gan'glii cilia'ris,** radix sympathica ganglii ciliaris.

**r. sympa'thicus gan'glii cilia'ris,** radix sympathica ganglii ciliaris.

**r. sympa'thicus ad gan'glion submandibula're,** sympathetic branch to submandibular ganglion: a branch bearing sympathetic fibers, postganglionic from the superior cervical ganglion and derived from a plexus on the facial artery, to the submandibular ganglion, for distribution to the submandibular gland.

**ra'mi tempora'les anterio'res arte'riae occipita'lis latera'lis** [TA], anterior temporal branches of lateral occipital artery: branches that supply the cortex of the anterior part of the temporal lobe.

**ra'mi tempora'les interme'dii media'les arte'riae occipita'lis latera'lis** [TA], intermediate branches of lateral occipital artery: branches that supply the cortex of the mediate and intermediate part of the temporal lobe.

**ra'mi tempora'les ner'vi facia'lis** [TA], temporal branches of facial nerve: terminal branches of the facial nerve that innervate the anterior and superior auricular muscles, the frontal belly of the occipitofrontal muscle, and the orbicularis oculi and corrugator muscles; modality, motor.

**ra'mi tempora'les posterio'res arte'riae occipita'lis latera'lis** [TA], posterior temporal branches of lateral occipital artery: branches that supply the posterior part of the temporal lobe.

**ra'mi tempora'les superficia'les ner'vi auriculotempora'lis** [TA], superficial temporal branches of auriculotemporal nerve: branches to the skin of the scalp in the temporal region; modality, general sensory.

**r. tento'rii basa'lis arte'riae caro'tidis inter'nae,** r. basalis tentorii arteriae carotidis internae.

**r. tento'rii margina'lis arte'riae caro'tidis inter'nae,** r. marginalis tentorii arteriae carotidis internae.

**r. tento'rii ner'vi ophthal'mici,** TA alternative for *r. meningeus recurrens nervi ophthalmici.*

**ra'mi thala'mici arte'riae ce'rebri posterio'ris,** branches of the postcommunical part of the posterior cerebral artery that supply the thalamus.

**r. thala'micus arte'riae communican'tis posterio'ris,** a branch of the posterior communicating artery that supplies the thalamus.

**ra'mi thy'mici arte'riae thora'cicae inter'nae** [TA], thymic branches of internal thoracic artery: branches distributed to the thymus gland in the anterior mediastinum; called also *thymic arteries* and *arteriae thymicae.*

**r. thyrohyoi'deus an'sae cervica'lis** [TA], thyrohyoid branch of ansa cervicalis: a branch from the superior root of the ansa cervicalis, innervating the thyrohyoid muscle; modality, motor.

**r. tonsil'lae cerebel'li arte'riae inferio'ris posterio'ris cerebel'li** [TA], tonsillar branch of posterior inferior cerebellar artery: a branch that ascends upward from the posterior inferior cerebellar artery to the tonsil of the cerebellum to supply the dentate nucleus of the cerebellum.

**r. tonsilla'ris arte'riae facia'lis** [TA], **r. tonsilla'ris arte'riae maxilla'ris exter'ni,** tonsillar branch of facial artery: a vessel ascending from the facial artery on the pharynx to supply the tonsil and the root of the tongue.

**ra'mi tonsilla'res ner'vi glossopharyn'gei** [TA], tonsillar branches of glossopharyngeal nerve: branches that supply the mucosa over the palatine tonsil and the adjacent portion of the soft palate; modality, general sensory.

**ra'mi tonsilla'res nervo'rum palatino'rum mino'rum** [TA], tonsillary branches of lesser palatine nerves: branches that innervate the palatine tonsils.

**ra'mi trachea'les arte'riae thora'cicae inter'nae** [TA], the tracheal branches of internal thoracic artery.

**ra'mi trachea'les arte'riae thyroi'deae inferio'ris** [TA], tracheal branches of inferior thyroid artery: vessels supplying the trachea.

**ra'mi trachea'les ner'vi laryn'gei recurren'tis** [TA], **ra'mi trachea'les ner'vi recurren'tis,** tracheal branches of recurrent laryngeal nerve: branches distributed to the tracheal mucosa; modality, general sensory.

**ra'mi trac'tus op'tici** [TA], small branches of the anterior choroid artery that supply the optic tract.

**r. transver'sus arte'riae circumflex'ae fe'moris latera'lis** [TA], transverse branch of lateral circumflex femoral artery: a branch that pierces the vastus lateralis muscle, turning around the femur to anastomose with the transverse branch of the medial circumflex femoral artery and with other arteries, deep to the gluteus maximus muscle.

**r. transver'sus arte'riae circumflex'ae fe'moris media'lis,** transverse branch of medial circumflex femoral artery: a branch that passes between the quadratus femoris and adductor magnus muscles, supplying them, and then turning around the femur to anastomose with the transverse branch of the lateral circumflex femoral artery and with other arteries, deep to the gluteus maximus muscle.

**ra'mi trigemina'les et trochlea'res,** a twig from the cavernous portion of the internal carotid artery that supplies the trigeminal and trochlear nerves.

**ra'mi tuba'les arte'riae ova'ricae,** rami tubarii arteriae ovaricae.

**r. tuba'lis arte'riae uteri'nae,** r. tubarius arteriae uterinae.

**r. tuba'lis plex'us tympa'nici,** r. tubarius plexus tympanici.

**ra'mi tuba'rii arte'riae ova'ricae** [TA], tubal branches of ovarian artery: branches distributed to the uterine tubes.

**r. tuba'rius arte'riae uteri'nae** [TA], tubal branch of uterine artery: a branch that supplies the uterine tube and the round ligament. Called also *r. tubalis arteriae uterinae.*

**r. tuba'rius plex'us tympa'nici** [TA], tubal branch of tympanic plexus: a branch given to the auditory tube from the tympanic plexus; modality, general sensory. Called also *r. tubalis plexus tympanici* [TA alternative].

**ra'mi tu'beris cine'rei** [TA], small branches of the anterior choroidal artery that supply the tuber cinereum.

**ra'mi urete'rici arte'riae duc'tus deferen'tis** [TA], ureteral branches of artery of ductus deferens: branches that supply the lower portion of the ureter.

**ra'mi urete'rici arte'riae ova'ricae** [TA], ureteral branches of ovarian artery: branches distributed to the ureter.

**ra'mi urete'rici arte'riae rena'lis** [TA], ureteral branches of renal artery: branches that supply the upper portion of the ureter.

**ra'mi urete'rici arte'riae testicula'ris** [TA], ureteral branches of testicular artery: branches distributed to the ureter.

**ra'mi vagina'les arte'riae recta'lis me'diae** [TA], a branch of the middle rectal artery that supplies the vagina.

**ra'mi vagina'les arte'riae uteri'nae** [TA], vaginal branches of uterine artery: two median longitudinal vessels formed by anastomosis of branches of the uterine and vaginal arteries, one of which descends in front of and the other behind the vagina. Called also *arteriae azygoi vaginae* and *azygous arteries of vagina.*

**ra'mi ventra'les nervo'rum cervica'lium,** TA alternative for *rami anteriores nervorum cervicalium.*

**r. ventra'lis ner'vi coccy'gei,** TA alternative for *r. anterior nervi coccygei.*

**ra'mi ventra'les nervo'rum lumba'lium,** TA alternative for *rami anteriores nervorum lumbalium.*

**ra'mi ventra'les nervo'rum sacra'lium,** TA alternative for *rami anteriores nervorum sacralium.*

**r. ventra'lis ner'vi spina'lis,** r. anterior nervi spinalis.

**ra'mi ventra'les nervo'rum thoracico'rum,** TA alternative for *nervi intercostales.*

**ventral rami of thoracic nerves,** nervi intercostales.

**r. ventri'culi sinis'tri poste'rior,** ramus posterior ventriculi sinistri rami circumflexi arteriae coronariae sinistrae.

**ra'mi vestibula'res arte'riae labyrinthi'nae** [TA], vestibular branches of labyrinthine artery: vessels supplying the vestibule of the ear. Called also *vestibular arteries.*

**r. viscera'lis,** r. autonomicus.

**ra'mi viscera'les par'tis abdomina'lis aor'tae,** visceral branches of the abdominal aorta, comprising the celiac trunk and the superior and inferior mesenteric, renal, testicular, and ovarian arteries.

**ra'mi viscera'les par'tis thora'cicae aor'tae,** visceral branches of the thoracic part of the aorta, supplying the lungs, bronchi, esophagus, and pericardium.

**ra'mi zygoma'tici ner'vi facia'lis** [TA], zygomatic branches of facial nerve: branches that cross the zygomatic bone and innervate the orbicularis oculi muscle; modality, motor.

**r. zygomaticofacia'lis ner'vi zygoma'tici** [TA], zygomaticofacial branch of zygomatic nerve: a branch that passes from the lateral wall of the orbit, piercing the zygomatic bone to supply overlying skin; modality, general sensory.

**r. zygomaticotempora'lis ner'vi zygoma'tici** [TA], zygomaticotemporal branch of zygomatic nerve: a branch that passes from the lateral wall of the orbit, piercing the zygomatic bone to innervate skin of the anterior temporal region; modality, general sensory.

**ran·cid** (ran′sid) [L. *rancidus*] having a musty, rank taste or smell; applied to fats that have undergone decomposition, with the liberation of fatty acids.

**ran·cid·i·fy** (ran-sid′ĭ-fi) to decompose, with the liberation of fatty acids; a term applied especially to the decomposition of fats.

**ran·cid·i·ty** (ran-sid′ĭ-te) the quality of being rancid.

**Ran·dall's plaques** (ran′dəlz) [Alexander *Randall,* American urologist, 1883–1951] see under *plaque.*

**ran·dom** (ran′dom) [Old French *randon* violence] pertaining to a chance-dependent process, particularly one that occurs according to a known probability distribution.

**ran·dom·iza·tion** (ran″dom-i-za′shən) assignment of experimental subjects to treatment groups according to some known probability distribution governed by chance, so that the distribution of subjects within each group should vary only by chance.

**range** (rānj) 1. the difference between the upper and lower limits of a variable or of a series of values. 2. an interval in which values sampled from a population, or the values in the population itself, are known to lie. 3. the geographic region in which a given species is found.
**r. of accommodation,** the alteration in the refractive state of the eye produced by accommodation. It is the difference in diopters between the refraction by the eye adjusted for its far point and that when adjusted for its near point. Called also *amplitude of accommodation.*
**r. of audibility,** see under *limit.*
**interquartile r.,** the difference between the data values at the 75th and 25th percentiles, encompassing the middle 50 percent of the data.
**r. of motion,** the range, measured in degrees of a circle, through which a joint can be extended and flexed. See also under *exercise.*
**normal r., r. of normal,** see *reference values,* under *value.*

**ran·i·my·cin** (ran-ĭ-mi′sin) an antibacterial antibiotic derived from a variant of *Streptomyces lincolnensis.*

**ra·nine** (ra′nīn) [L. *raninus,* from *rana* frog] 1. pertaining to a frog. 2. ranular. 3. sublingual.

**ra·ni·ti·dine hy·dro·chlo·ride** (ra-ni′tĭ-dēn) [USP] an antagonist to histamine $H_2$ receptors, used to inhibit gastric acid secretion in the treatment of gastric and duodenal ulcer, gastroesophageal reflux, and conditions that cause gastric hypersecretion; administered orally.

**rank** (rangk) 1. in statistics, the position of a sample observation (or population value) in the sequence of sample values (or population values) arranged in order, usually from lowest to highest. 2. to place in such an order.

**Ranke's angle** (rahng′kez) [Hans Rudolph *Ranke,* Dutch anatomist, 1849–1887] see under *angle.*

**Ranke's complex, stages** (rahng′kəz) [Karl Ernst von *Ranke,* German internist, 1870–1926] see *primary complex,* under *complex,* and see under *stage.*

**ran·u·la** (ran′u-lə) [L., dim. of *rana* frog] [MeSH: Ranula] a form of retention cyst of the floor of the mouth, usually due to obstruction of the ducts of the submaxillary or sublingual glands, presenting a slowly enlarging painless deep burrowing mucocele of one side of the mouth. Called also *sublingual cyst* and *sublingual ptyalocele.*
**plunging r.,** a rare type of ranula that has become invasive and penetrates into the mylohyoid muscle, the submental region, or the submandibular region.
**pancreatic r.,** a retention cyst of the pancreatic duct.

**ran·u·lar** (ran′u-lər) pertaining to or of the nature of a ranula.

**Ra·nun·cu·la·ceae** (rə-nung″ku-la′se-e) a family of flowering plants, most of which contain the glycoside ranunculin; when the plants are eaten, the ranunculin breaks down to form the lethal toxin protoanemonin. Genera include *Aconitum, Actaea, Anemone, Cimicifuga, Clematis, Delphinium, Helleborus, Hydrastis,* and *Ranunculus.*

**ra·nun·cu·lin** (rə-nung′ku-lin) a glycoside found in most plants of the family Ranunculaceae; when the plants are eaten, enzymes in animals convert ranunculin to protoanemonin, a toxin that can be lethal.

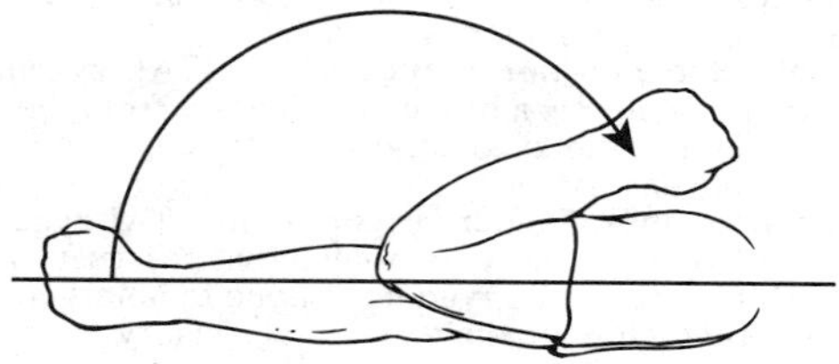
Range of motion of the elbow joint.

**Ra·nun·cu·lus** (rə-nung′ku-ləs) the crowfoots and buttercups, a genus of plants of the family Ranunculaceae. Some species are poisonous to humans and livestock, since they contain the glycoside ranunculin, which when ingested is enzymatically broken down into highly toxic protoanemonin.

**Ran·vier's crosses, nodes, segment (internode), tactile disks** (rahn-ve-āz′) [Louis Antoine *Ranvier,* French pathologist, 1835–1922] see under *cross, disk,* and *node,* and see *internodal segment* under *segment.*

**RAO** right anterior oblique.

**Ra·oult's law** (rah-o͞olz′) [François Marie *Raoult,* French physical chemist, 1830–1901] see under *law.*

**rape**[1] (rāp) [L. *rapere* to seize] [MeSH: Rape] nonconsensual sexual penetration of an adolescent or adult, obtained by force or threat, or in cases in which the victim is not capable of consent.

**rape**[2] (rāp) [L. *rapum*] [MeSH: Rape] *Brassica napus,* an edible plant whose seeds are the source of rapeseed oil.

**ra·pha·nia** (rə-fa′ne-ə) [Gr. *raphanos* radish] poisoning of humans or livestock by seeds of the wild radish, *Raphanus raphanistrum.*

**ra·phae** (ra′fe) plural of *raphe.*

**Ra·phan·us** (rə-fan′əs) [L., from Gr. *raphanos* radish] the radishes, a genus of plants of the family Cruciferae native to Europe and Asia. *R. raphanis′trum* is the wild radish, whose seeds contain a mustard oil glycoside and are poisonous to humans and livestock (see *raphania*). *R. sati′vus* is cultivated for food.

**ra·phe** (ra′fe) gen. *raphēs* pl. *ra′phae* [Gr. *rhaphē*] [TA] a seam; a general term for the line of union of the halves of various symmetrical parts.
**abdominal r.,** linea alba.
**amniotic r.,** the line of junction of the amniotic folds in the amnion of those vertebrates in which it is formed by folding.
**r. anococcy′gea, anococcygeal r.,** corpus anococcygeum.
**r. cor′poris callo′si, r. of corpus callosum,** see *stria longitudinalis medialis corporis callosi* and *stria longitudinalis lateralis corporis callosi.*
**lateral palpebral r.,** r. palpebralis lateralis.
**median r. of medulla oblongata, r. media′na medul′lae oblonga′tae,** r. medullae oblongatae.
**median r. of neck, posterior,** ligamentum nuchae.
**median r. of perineum,** r. perinei.
**median r. of pons, r. media′na ponti′na,** r. pontis.
**r. medul′lae oblonga′tae** [TA], raphe of medulla oblongata: a median line at the union of the two lateral halves of the medulla oblongata which continues into the dorsal part of the pons; called also *median r. of medulla oblongata* and *r. mediana medullae oblongatae.*
**r. pala′ti** [TA], palatine raphe: a narrow whitish streak at the midline of the roof of the mouth (both the hard and soft palates), extending from the incisive papilla to the tip of the uvula; it may present as a ridge in front and as a groove posteriorly.
**r. palpebra′lis latera′lis,** a thin horizontal band of connective tissue extending from the external angle of the rima palpebralis to the lateral margin of the orbit.
**r. pe′nis** [TA], a narrow dark streak or ridge continuous posteriorly with the raphe scroti and extending forward for a variable distance along the midline on the under side of the penis; in the newborn it may extend to the tip of the glans.
**r. perinea′lis, r. perine′i** [TA], perineal raphe: a ridge along the median line of the perineum that runs forward from the anus; in the male, it is continuous with the raphe of the scrotum and raphe of the penis. Called also *median r. of perineum.*
**r. pharyn′gis** [TA], raphe of pharynx: a more or less distinct band of connective tissue extending downward from the base of the skull along the posterior wall of the pharynx in the median plane, and giving attachment to the constrictor muscles of the pharynx.
**r. pon′tis** [TA], raphe of pons: a median line at the union of the two lateral halves of the pons, which is a continuation of the raphe of the medulla oblongata into the dorsal part of the pons; called also *median r. of pons* and *r. mediana pontina.*
**r. pterygomandibula′ris** [TA], pterygomandibular raphe: a tendinous line between the buccinator and the constrictor pharyngis superior muscles, from which the middle portions of both muscles originate.
**scrotal r., r. scrota′lis,** r. scroti.
**r. scro′ti** [TA], raphe of scrotum: a ridge along the surface of the scrotum in the median line, dividing it into nearly equal lateral parts.

**ra·phes** (ra′fēz) genitive singular of *raphe.*

**Rap·pa·port Classification** (rap′ə-port) [Henry *Rappaport,* American pathologist, born 1913] see under *classification.*

**rap·port** (rah-por') [Fr.] a relation of harmony and accord between two persons, as between patient and physician.

**rap·ture of the deep** popular name for *nitrogen narcosis.*

**rar·e·fac·tion** (rar″ə-fak'shən) [L. *rarefactio*] the condition of being or becoming less dense; diminution in density and weight, but not in volume.

**RAS** renal artery stenosis; renin-angiotensin system.

**rash** (rash) a temporary eruption on the skin, as in urticaria; a drug eruption or viral exanthem.
**brown-tail r.,** see under *dermatitis.*
**butterfly r.,** butterfly, def. 3.
**caterpillar r.,** see *insect dermatitis,* under *dermatitis.*
**diaper r.,** see under *dermatitis.*
**drug r.,** drug eruption.
**heat r.,** miliaria rubra.
**hydatid r.,** an urticarial eruption which sometimes follows tapping or rupture of a hydatid cyst.
**nettle r.,** urticaria in domestic animals as an allergic reaction to nettles.
**wandering r.,** benign migrating glossitis.

**Rash·kind balloon atrial septostomy** (rash'kind) [W. J. *Rashkind,* American surgeon, 20th century] see under *septostomy.*

**ra·sion** (ra'zhən) [L. *rasio*] the grating of drugs with a file.

**Ras·mus·sen's aneurysm** (rahs'moo͝-sənz) [Fritz Waldemar *Rasmussen,* Danish physician, 1834–1877] see under *aneurysm.*

**rasp** (rasp) 1. a coarse file used in surgery. Called also *raspatory* and *xyster.* 2. to file with this instrument.

**ras·pa·to·ry** (ras'pə-to-re) [L. *raspatorium*] rasp (def. 1).

**rasp·ber·ry** (raz'ber-e) 1. either *Rubus iridaeus* or *R. strigosus.* 2. the fruit of either *R. iridaeus* or *R. strigosus,* used as a flavoring agent. See also under *juice* and *syrup.*

**RAST** radioallergosorbent test.

**Ras·tel·li operation** (rahs-tel'e) [Gian Carlo *Rastelli,* Italian cardiovascular surgeon, 1933–1970] see under *operation.*

**rat** (rat) [MeSH: Rats] any of numerous small rodents of the genus *Rattus* and related genera of the family Muridae; many are aggressive and omnivorous pests found about human habitations. Rats not only cause great economic loss but are vectors of human disease; they harbor at least eleven species of intestinal parasites that are transmissible to humans, such as tapeworms, roundworms, and trichinae, and they are reservoirs for the infective agents of plague, typhus, Weil's disease, and rat-bite fever. Albino mutants of *R. norvegicus* are used as laboratory animals.
**albino r.,** white r.
**BB r.,** a strain that serves as a model of type I diabetes mellitus.
**black r.,** *Rattus rattus,* the European black rat and the one most commonly responsible for transmitting plague to man by means of its flea *(Xenopsylla cheopis).*
**brown r.,** *Rattus norvegicus;* also called the barn rat, gray rat, Norway rat, sewer rat, and wharf rat. It is larger than the black rat, has a brownish gray color, and short ears and tail.
**fa/fa r.,** a rat homozygous for the *fa* gene; such rats are genetically obese, hyperphagic, and hyperinsulinemic, with normal intravenous but abnormal oral glucose tolerance. Used as an experimental model of insulin resistance associated with glucose intolerance.
**Fischer 344 r.,** an inbred strain of albino laboratory rats developed in 1920; used particularly in cancer research.
**Holtzman r.,** a strain of albino rat descended originally from S–D strain which originated from Wistar Institute sometime before 1929.
**Long-Evans r.,** a strain of rat, developed at the University of Rochester, characterized by a brownish to black color of the head and shoulders.
**multimammate r.,** see under *mouse.*
**pack r.,** wood r.
**Sprague-Dawley r.,** a strain of albino rat developed by the Sprague-Dawley Animal Company, widely used in experimental work because of its calmness and ease of handling.
**white r.,** an albino form of *Rattus rattus* or of *R. norvegicus* which is much used as a laboratory animal.
**Wistar r.,** a strain of albino rat developed at the Wistar Institute but which has spread so widely to other institutions that there is probably marked dilution of the strain.
**wood r.,** a rat of the genus *Neotoma,* also known as *brush rat, mountain rat, pack r.,* or *trade rat.* These rats are hosts of fleas and ticks.
**Zucker r.,** a mutant strain of laboratory rats existing as a lean phenotype (genotype Fa/Fa or Fa/fa) and a genetically obese phenotype (genotype fa/fa); the obese Zucker rat is used as an experimental model of juvenile onset obesity.

**rate** (rāt) [L. *rata,* from *ratus* calculated] 1. the amount of change of a physical quantity or number of occurrences of an event per unit time. 2. in epidemiology and demography, the frequency of an event in a specified population; correctly applied only to fractions for which all of the cases contributing to the numerator are also counted in the denominator and for which the denominator is the entire population at risk. Rates are often multiplied by a factor to give the number of events per 1000, 10,000, or 100,000 population. 3. more generally, a term sometimes used to denote some measured quantity with respect to another. Symbol R.

## Rate

**adjusted r.,** a fictitious summary rate statistically adjusted to remove the effect of a demographic or other influential variable such as age or sex, thus permitting unbiased comparison between groups having different underlying compositions with respect to these variables. Called also *standardized r.* Cf. *crude r.* and *specific r.*
**attack r.,** in the analysis of acute outbreaks of disease, the proportion of persons who are exposed to the disease during the outbreak who do become ill.
**basal metabolic r.,** an expression of the rate at which oxygen is utilized by the body cells, or the calculated equivalent heat production by the body, in a fasting subject at complete rest. Abbreviated BMR. See also *basal metabolism,* under *metabolism.*
**birth r.,** a rate in which the numerator is the number of live births in a geographic area in a defined period, usually one year. The denominator of the *crude birth rate* is the average total population or the midyear population in the area during the period. Specific birth rates for subsets of the population may also be calculated, e.g., an *age-specific birth rate,* limited to the population of females of a defined age range.
**case r.,** attack r.
**case fatality r.,** the proportion of persons contracting a disease who die of that disease: the numerator is the number of deaths caused by a disease and the denominator is the number of diagnosed cases of the disease. Called also *case fatality ratio, fatality r.,* and *lethality r.*
**circulation r.,** the amount of blood pumped through the body by the heart per unit time; usually expressed in milliliters or liters per minute.
**crude r.,** one giving the total number of events occurring in an entire population over a period of time, without reference to any of the individuals or subgroups within the population. Cf. *adjusted r.* and *specific r.*
**cumulative incidence r.,** the proportion of an initially disease-free population developing a disease over a fixed interval, calculated by cumulating the proportions developing the disease within short subintervals.
**death r.,** a rate expressing the number of deaths in a population at risk. The *crude death rate* is the ratio of the number of deaths in a geographic area in one year divided by the average or midyear population in the area during the year. An *age-specific death rate* is the ratio of the number of deaths occurring in a specified age group in one year to the average or midyear population of that group. A *cause-specific death rate* is the ratio of the number of deaths due to a specified cause in one year to the average or midyear total population. Called also *mortality r.*
**DEF r.,** an expression of dental caries experience in deciduous teeth: calculated by adding number of decayed primary teeth requiring filling *(D),* decayed primary teeth requiring extraction *(E),* and primary teeth successfully filled *(F);* missing primary teeth are not included in the calculation.
**DMF r.,** an expression of the condition of the teeth based on the number of teeth decayed, missing, indicated for removal and of those filled or bearing restorations: calculated by adding the number of carious permanent teeth requiring filling *(D),* carious permanent teeth requiring extraction *(Mr),* permanent teeth previously extracted because of caries *(Mp),* and permanent teeth filled *(F)* Number of DMF teeth per child of a specific age or age group is calculated by the formula:

$$\frac{\text{D + Mr + Mp + F}}{\text{number of children examined}} = \text{DMF.}$$

**dose r.,** the amount of any agent administered per unit of time.

**erythrocyte sedimentation r. (ESR),** the rate at which erythrocytes precipitate out from a well-mixed specimen of venous blood, measured by the distance the top of the column of erythrocytes falls in a given time interval under specified conditions; an increase in rate is usually due to elevated levels of plasma proteins, especially fibrinogen and immunoglobulins, which decrease the zeta potential on erythrocytes by dielectric shielding and thus promote rouleau formation. It is increased in monoclonal gammopathy, hypergammaglobulinemia due to inflammatory disease, hyperfibrinogenemia, active inflammatory disease, and anemia. The traditional methods of calculating ESR are the *Westergren method* and the *Wintrobe method.* See also *zeta sedimentation ratio* under *ratio.*

**fatality r.,** 1. the death rate in a specific group of persons simultaneously affected by some event, such as a natural disaster. 2. case fatality r.

**fertility r.,** a measure of fertility in a defined population over a specified period of time, usually one year; particularly the *general fertility r.*, but also including more specific rates such as those for females of a given parity or a particular decade in age or that describing the completed rate for females who have finished childbearing.

**fetal death r.,** the ratio of the number of fetal deaths in one year to the total number of both live births and fetal deaths in that year. Cf. *fetal death ratio.*

**five-year survival r.,** an expression of the number of survivors with no trace of disease five years after each has been diagnosed or treated for the same disease.

**flow r.,** flow (def. 2).

**general fertility r.,** the most widely used measure of fertility; the number of live births in a geographic area in a year per 1000 women of childbearing age, which is usually defined as age 15 to 44 years.

**glomerular filtration r. (GFR),** the quantity of glomerular filtrate formed per unit time in all nephrons of both kidneys, equal to the inulin clearance; usually measured clinically by the endogenous creatinine clearance.

**growth r.,** an expression of the increase in size of an organic object per unit time, calculations usually being made as to both the absolute and the relative increment.

**heart r.,** the number of contractions of the ventricles of the heart per unit of time (usually a minute). It usually corresponds to the pulse rate, but occasionally some of the contractions of the left ventricle fail to produce peripheral pulse waves, so that the rate of the pulse at the wrist is less than that of the heart.

**incidence r.,** the probability of developing a particular disease during a given period of time; the numerator of the rate is the number of new cases during the specified time period and the denominator is the population at risk during the period. Cf. *prevalence r.*

**infant mortality r.,** the ratio of the number of deaths in one year of children less than one year of age to the number of live births in that year.

**lethality r.,** case fatality r.

**maternal mortality r.,** a rate in which the numerator is the number of maternal deaths ascribed to puerperal causes in one year; the number of live births in that year is often used as the denominator although to make a true rate the denominator should be the number of pregnancies (live births and fetal deaths). Called also *puerperal mortality r.*

**maximal midexpiratory flow r., maximum midexpiratory flow r.,** maximum midexpiratory f.

**morbidity r.,** a rate in which the numerator is a number of cases of a disease and the denominator is the number of people at risk for the disease; it can denote either of the more precise terms *incidence r.* and *prevalence r.*

**mortality r.,** death r.

**mutation r.,** the number of mutations at a given locus per gamete per generation. See also *mutant proportion,* under *proportion.*

**neonatal mortality r.,** the ratio of the number of deaths in one year of children less than 28 days of age to the number of live births in that year.

**oocyst r.,** the percentage of wild female mosquitoes found to contain oocysts in the midgut.

**output exposure r.,** in radiology, the exposure to radiation at a specified point per unit of time, usually expressed in roentgens per minute.

**parasite r.,** the percentage of persons, in a particular age group or area, in whom parasites, especially malarial parasites, can be found.

**peak expiratory flow r. (PEFR),** see under *flow.*

**perinatal mortality r.,** the ratio of the number of the sum of fetal deaths after 28 or more weeks of gestation (stillbirths) and deaths of infants less than 7 days of age in one time period and population to the sum of the number of live births and fetal deaths after 28 or more weeks of gestation (stillbirths) in that same time period and population.

**postneonatal mortality r.,** the ratio of the number of deaths in a given year of children between the 28th day of life and the first birthday relative to the difference between the number of the live births and neonatal deaths in that year; the denominator is sometimes simplified, less correctly, to the number of live births. The ratio is sometimes approximated as the difference between the infant mortality rate and the neonatal mortality rate.

**prevalence r.,** the number of people in a population who have a disease or other condition at a given time: the numerator of the rate is the number of existing cases of the condition at a specified time and the denominator is the total population. Time may be a point or a defined interval; if unspecified it is traditionally the former. Cf. *incidence r.*

**puerperal mortality r.,** maternal mortality r.

**pulse r.,** the rate of pulsation noted in a peripheral artery per minute, normally from 50 to 100.

**relative survival r.,** a statistical comparison between the rate of patients in a cohort surviving for a certain length of time and the survival rate of a comparable group in the general population.

**respiration r.,** the number of breaths per minute, usually measured by movements of the chest.

**secondary attack r.,** the attack rate in a closed exposed group, such as a household. The index case, which brings the group to the attention of the investigator, and also other initial cases occurring too early to be related to the index case are excluded from both the numerator and the denominator when possible.

**sedimentation r.,** the rate at which a sediment is deposited in a given volume of solution, especially when subjected to the action of a centrifuge; see also *erythrocyte sedimentation r.*

**sickness r.,** morbidity r.

**slew r.,** the rate of change of the voltage between the positive and negative peaks on the electrogram, or the rate of change in the steepest portion if the electrogram is monophasic.

**specific r.,** a rate that applies to a specific demographic subgroup, e.g., individuals of a specific age, sex, or race, giving the total number of events in relation only to that subgroup. Cf. *adjusted r.* and *crude r.*

**sporozoite r.,** the percentage of wild female mosquitoes found to contain sporozoites in the glands.

**standardized r.,** adjusted r.

**stillbirth r.,** fetal death r.

**Westergren sedimentation r.,** Westergren method.

---

**Rath·ke's column, duct, fold,** etc. (raht'kez) [Martin Heinrich *Rathke,* German anatomist, 1793–1860] see under *column, cyst, duct, fold,* and *pouch,* see *craniopharyngioma,* and see *trabeculae cranii,* under *trabecula.*

**rat·i·cide** (rat'ĭ-sīd) an agent destructive to rats.

**ra·tio** (ra'she-o) [L.] an expression of the quantity of one substance or entity in relation to that of another; the relationship between two quantities expressed as the quotient of one divided by the other.

**A-G r., albumin-globulin r.,** the ratio of albumin to globulin in the blood serum, plasma, or the urine in various types of renal or liver disease. It is being replaced by quantitiative measurement of specific serum proteins.

**arm r.,** a figure expressing the relation of the length of the longer arm of a mitotic chromosome to that of the shorter arm.

**Blackburne-Peel r.,** the ratio of the perpendicular distance between the tibial and patellar articular surfaces to the length of the patellar articular surface with the knee in 30° of flexion; it is equal to 0.8 in the normal knee.

**body-weight r.,** body weight in grams divided by stature in centimeters.

**cardiothoracic r.,** the ratio of the transverse diameter of the heart to the internal diameter of the chest at its widest point just above the level of the dome of the diaphragm, a rough guide to cardiac enlargement, being normally less than 0.5.

**case fatality r.,** see under *rate.*

**concentration r.,** the ratio of the average concentration of a solid in the urine to its concentration in the blood.

**conduction r.,** in cardiac physiology, the ratio of atrial to ventricular depolarizations, measured as the ratio of P waves to QRS complexes in the electrocardiogram; it is normally 1:1.

**critical r.**, any of a class of tests of statistical significance in which a parameter is divided by its standard error; e.g., used on Student's *t*-test, the critical ratio is the difference between two means divided by the standard error of that difference. The larger the ratio, the more likely the difference is significant.
**cross-product r.**, odds r.
**curative r.**, therapeutic r.
**expiratory exchange r.**, respiratory exchange r.
**extraction r.**, the extent to which the plasma concentration of a substance is reduced as the blood flows through a clearing organ; calculated by the formula

$$E = \frac{C_A - C_V}{C_A},$$

where E is the extraction rate, $C_A$ is the inflow plasma concentration, and $C_V$ is the outflow plasma concentration.
***F*-r.**, the variance between the means of several groups relative to the variance within the groups; used in the *F*-test (q.v.) in the analysis of variance (ANOVA).
**fetal death r.**, the ratio of fetal deaths in one year to the number of live births in that year. Cf. *fetal death rate.*
**grid r.**, in radiology, the ratio of the height of the lead strips to the width of the interspacing of a grid.
**hand r.**, the ratio of the length of the hand to its width.
**holdaway r.**, a means of expressing the relationship of the pogonion and the lower incisor to the nasion-basion plane; used in radiographic cephalometric diagnosis.
**Insall-Salvati r.**, the ratio of the length of the ligamentum patellae to the height of the patella, equal to approximately 1 in the normal knee.
**karyoplasmic r.**, nucleocytoplasmic r.
**ketogenic-antiketogenic r.**, the proportion between substances that form glucose in the body and those that form fatty acids.
**lecithin-sphingomyelin r., L/S r.**, the ratio of lecithin to sphingomyelin concentration in the amniotic fluid, used to predict the degree of pulmonary maturity of the fetus and thus the risk of respiratory difficulties for the newborn.
**likelihood r.**, 1. an index of diagnostic marker tests, the odds of a disease given a specified test value relative to the odds of the disease in the study population. It can be calculated for either a positive or a negative test, the former (LR+) being the ratio of the sensitivity to the false-positive error rate and the latter (LR−) being the ratio of the false-negative error rate to the specificity. Depending on how it is written, it can be viewed either as a risk ratio or an odds ratio. 2. see under *test.*
**mendelian r.**, an expression of the occurrence of distinctly contrasted mendelian characters in succeeding generations of hybrid offspring.
**nucleocytoplasmic r., nucleoplasmic r.**, the ratio of nuclear to cytoplasmic volume.
**nutritive r.**, the ratio between the digestible protein and the digestible fats and carbohydrates in a ration in stock feeding.
**odds r.**, the ratio of the probability of occurrence of one event to that of its alternative; it is often used in epidemiological analysis as it closely approximates relative risk.
**proportionate mortality r. (PMR)**, 1. the ratio of the number of deaths from a particular cause to the total number of deaths in the same time period. 2. in occupational epidemiology, the ratio of observed deaths due to a specific cause in an occupational cohort to the expected deaths due to that cause, as determined by the proportion of deaths from the cause in the general population or comparison population, multiplied by 100. Cf. *standardized mortality r.*
**respiratory exchange r.**, the ratio of carbon dioxide output to oxygen uptake in respiration. Symbol R. Called also *expiratory exchange r.*
**risk r.**, relative risk.
**sex r.**, the proportion of one sex to the other; by tradition the number of males in a population to the number of females, usually stated as the number of males per 100 females.
**signal-to-noise r.**, the ratio between the amplitude of a signal being measured and that of the noise (q.v.).
**standardized morbidity r. (SMR)**, a ratio like a standardized mortality ratio except that cases of disease rather than deaths are the observed data.
**standardized mortality r. (SMR)**, the ratio of the number of observed deaths in a study population to the number of expected deaths in that population. The expected deaths are calculated by classifying the study group by demographic variables such as age, sex, or race; computing the expected deaths for each class by multiplying the number of individuals in the study group in that class by the class-specific death rate in a standard reference population; and adding the expected deaths in all classes. Cf. *proportionate mortality r.,* def 2.
**stimulation r. (SR)**, see *lymphocyte proliferation test* under *tests.*
**therapeutic r.**, the fraction of the minimal lethal dose of a drug that is therapeutically effective; called also *curative r.*
**urea excretion r.**, the ratio of the number of milligrams of urea in the urine excreted in one hour to the number of milligrams in 100 mL of blood; the normal ratio is 50.
**ventilation-perfusion r.**, the ratio of oxygen received in the pulmonary alveoli to the flow of blood through the corresponding alveolar capillaries.
**zeta sedimentation r. (ZSR)**, a measurement comparable to the erythrocyte sedimentation rate, except that it is unaffected by anemia. The packed-cell volume *(zetacrit)* of a blood specimen is calculated by centrifuging the specimen in a *Zetafuge,* a specially designed instrument that produces controlled cycles of compaction and dispersion and allows rouleaux to form and sediment rapidly. The zetacrit divided into the true hematocrit gives the zeta sedimentation ratio.

**ra·tion** (ră'shən, ra'shən) [L. *ratio* proportion] a fixed allowance of food or drink per day or other unit of time.
**basal r.**, a ration giving the required energy, but lacking in one or more vitamins.

**ra·tion·al** (ră'shən-əl) [L. *rationalis* reasonable] based upon reason; characterized by possession of one's reason.

**ra·tio·nale** (ră"shən-al') [L.] a rational exposition of principles; the logical basis of a procedure.

**ra·tion·al·iza·tion** (ră"shən-əl-ĭ-za'shən) [MeSH: Rationalization] an unconscious defense mechanism by which one justifies, by an incorrect application of reason, attitudes and behavior that would otherwise be unacceptable.

**rat-tails** (rat'tālz) a swollen condition of the hair papillae over the flexor tendons of a horse's legs, due to filth and bacteria.

**rat·tler** (rat'lər) rattlesnake.

**rat·tle·snake** (rat'əl-snāk) any of the New World pit vipers of the genera *Crotalus* and *Sistrurus,* having a series of cornified interlocking segments at the tip of the tail; when disturbed they vibrate the tail to produce the characteristic rattling or buzzing sound. See table at *snake.*
**eastern diamondback r.**, *Crotalus adamanteus,* a venomous snake found along the Eastern Seaboard and Gulf Coast of the United States.
**ground r.**, 1. massasauga. 2. pygmy r.
**Massasauga r.**, massasauga.
**Mojave r.**, *Crotalus scutula'tus scutula'tus,* a poisonous species found in the southwestern United States.
**prairie r.**, *Crotalus viridis viridis,* a venomous snake found in the prairies and plains of the midwestern United States.
**pygmy r.**, *Sistrurus miliarius,* a small venomous species found in the southeastern United States.
**timber r.**, *Crotalus horridus,* a venomous yellowish-brown snake found from the East Coast of the United States west into Texas.
**western diamondback r.**, *Crotalus atrox,* a venomous snake found in the southwestern United States and northern Mexico.

**Rat·tus** (rat'əs) a genus of small rodents, including several common species of rats. *R. norve'gicus* is the brown rat and *R. rat'tus* is the black rat.

**Rau's apophysis, process** (rouz) [Johann J. *Rau* (Ravius), Dutch anatomist, 1668–1719] processus anterior mallei.

**Rau·ber's layer** (rou'bərz) [August Antinous *Rauber,* German-born anatomist in Estonia, 1841–1917] see under *layer.*

**Rau-Sed** (rou'sed) trademark for a preparation of reserpine.

**Rau·ser·pa** (raw-ser'pə) trademark for a preparation of rauwolfia serpentina.

**Rau·wi·loid** (rou'wĭ-loid) trademark for preparations of alseroxylon.

**Rau·wol·fia** (rou-wool'fe-ə) [Leonhard *Rauwolf,* 16th century German botanist] [MeSH: Rauwolfia] a large genus of tropical trees and shrubs of the family Apocyanaceae. Many species provide alkaloids of medical interest, such as reserpine, and have long been used medicinally in South America, Africa, and Asia.
**R. serpenti'na**, (L.) Benth. ex Kurz, a small shrub native to India and elsewhere in Asia, containing many alkaloids, particularly reserpine and rescinnamine; its dried root is the medicinal substance called *rauwolfia serpentina.*

**rau·wol·fia** (rou-wool'fi-ə) [MeSH: Rauwolfia] 1. any member of the genus *Rauwolfia.* 2. the medicinal dried root or an extract of the dried root of *Rauwolfia.*
**r. serpenti'na** [USP], the dried root of *Rauwolfia serpentina,* sometimes with fragments of rhizome and aerial stem bases attached; used as an antihypertensive. It is also used as a sedative and tranquilizer.
**r. serpenti'na, powdered** [USP], rauwolfia serpentina reduced to a very fine powder adjusted, if necessary, to contain between 0.15 and 0.20 per cent of reserpine-rescinnamine group alkaloids.

**Rau·zide** (rou'zīd) trademark for preparations of rauwolfia serpentina with bendroflumethiazide.

**RAV** Rous-associated virus.

**Ra·vi·us** (ra've-əs) see *Rau.*

**Rax·ar** (rak'ahr) trademark for a preparation of grepafloxacin hydrochloride.

**ray** (ra) [L. *radius* spoke] 1. a line emanating from a center. 2. a more or less distinct portion of radiant energy (light or heat), proceeding in a specific direction (used in the plural as a general term for any form of radiant energy, whether vibratory or particulate). 3. one of the individual elements of the hand plate at the distal end of the limb of an early embryo, foretelling development of a digital ray. 4. any of various marine elasmobranch fishes with flattened bodies and narrow tails. See also *stingray.*
**actinic r.**, a light ray which produces chemical changes. In general, light rays become more actinic as one passes from the red through the spectrum to the violet and even into the ultraviolet.
**α-r's,** alpha r's.
**alpha r's,** high-speed helium nuclei which have been ejected from radioactive substances. Owing to their high velocity (one tenth that of light) their kinetic energy is so great that a single alpha particle produces a microscopic flash of light when it hits a spinthariscope; when it hits another atom (as of nitrogen) it may cause it to disintegrate.
**anode r's,** positive r's.
**astral r.**, one of the rays of an aster. Called also *polar r.*
**β-r's, beta r's,** electrons ejected from radioactive substances with velocities which may be as high as 0.98 of the velocity of light.
**cathode r's,** negative particles of electricity streaming out in a vacuum tube at right angles to the surface of the cathode and away from it irrespective of the position of the anode. They move in a straight line unless deflected by a magnet. By striking on solids they generate x-rays. See also *electron stream.*
**central r.**, the straight line passing through the center of the radiation source and the center of the final beam-limiting diaphragm.
**characteristic r's,** x-rays emitted as a result of the rearrangement of electrons in the inner shells of atoms, as when electrons are ejected from the inner shells by high-speed bombarding electrons or when an orbital electron is captured by the nucleus during radioactive decay; the wavelengths of the rays produced depend on the element and the energy levels involved. Cf. *characteristic fluorescent r's.*
**characteristic fluorescent r's,** secondary rays emitted as a result of the rearrangement of electrons in the inner shells of atoms; identical with characteristic rays (q.v.) except that characteristic rays are caused by the bombardment of the x-ray tube target by electrons, whereas characteristic fluorescent rays are caused by primary ray photon bombardment of an absorbing material.
**chemical r.**, actinic r.
**convergent r.**, a ray which is approaching a focus; it may be produced by passage through a convex lens or by reflection from a concave mirror.
**δ-r's, delta r's,** secondary beta rays produced in a gas by the passage of alpha particles.
**digital r.**, a digit of the hand or foot and the corresponding portion of the metacarpus or metatarsus, considered as a continuous structural unit.
**direct r.**, primary reinforcer
**divergent r's,** rays coming from a source nearer than infinity, or a pencil or bundle of light rays directed away from a focus after passing through a concave lens or after being reflected from a convex mirror.
**dynamic r's,** rays that are active physically or therapeutically.
**fluorescent r's,** characteristic fluorescent r's.
**γ-r's, gamma r's,** electromagnetic radiation of short wavelengths emitted by the nucleus of an atom during a nuclear reaction. They consist of high energy photons, have no mass and no electric charge, and travel with the speed of light and are usually associated with beta rays.
**glass r's,** the rays formed in an x-ray tube by the cathode rays striking the glass wall of the tube, so called to distinguish them from the x-rays originating at the anticathode.
**grenz r's,** very soft x-rays with a wavelength of about 20 nm, lying between x-rays and ultraviolet rays in the electromagnetic spectrum.
**hard r's,** x-rays of short wavelength, high energy, and great penetrative power.
**heat r's,** see *radiant heat,* under *heat.*
**incident r.**, see *reflection,* def. 2, and *refraction,* def. 2.
**indirect r's,** rays formed at the surface of the glass of the cathode ray tube.
**infrared r's,** radiations just beyond the red end of the visible spectrum; their wavelengths range between 0.75 and 1000 μm; see *infrared.*
**infra roentgen r's,** grenz r's.
**intermediate r's,** wavelengths between the ultraviolet and the x-rays.
**luminous r's,** the visible rays of the spectrum.
**medullary r's,** radii medullares.
**necrobiotic r's,** short ultraviolet rays which kill living cells.
**parallel r's,** rays which come from a source at an infinite distance; divergent rays may be made parallel by means of a convex lens or a concave mirror.
**polar r.**, astral r.
**positive r's,** streams of positively charged atoms traveling at high speed from the anode of a partially evacuated tube under the influence of an applied voltage.
**primary r's,** rays coming directly from a source, such as a radioactive substance or an x-ray tube, without interactions with matter.
**reflected r.**, see *reflection,* def. 2.
**refracted r.**, see *refraction,* def. 2.
**roentgen r's,** x-r's.
**Sagnac r's,** secondary beta rays formed when gamma rays are reflected from a metal surface.
**scattered r's,** secondary rays whose direction has been changed by interaction with matter in their passage through a substance. See also *scattering.*
**secondary r's,** rays generated by the interaction of primary rays with matter.
**soft r's,** x-rays of long wavelength, low energy, and little penetrative power.
**ultraviolet r's,** those invisible rays of the spectrum which are beyond the violet rays; their wavelengths range between 4 and 400 nm; see *ultraviolet.*
**W r's,** intermediate r's.
**x-r's,** electromagnetic vibrations of short wavelengths (approximately 0.01 to 10 nm) or corresponding quanta (wave mechanics), produced when electrons moving at high velocity impinge on various substances, especially heavy metals; they are commonly generated by passing a current of high voltage (10,000 volts or more) through a Coolidge tube. They can penetrate most substances to some extent, some more readily than others, and to affect a photographic plate; this enables their use for *radiography.* They can also cause certain substances to fluoresce, making *fluoroscopy* possible. Because of the high energy of their quanta, they strongly ionize tissue through which they pass by means of the photoelectrons, both primary and secondary, that they liberate; this enables their use in treating various pathological conditions (see *radiotherapy*). Formerly called *roentgen r's.*

**Ray·mond's apoplexy** (ra-mawz') [Fulgence *Raymond,* French neurologist, 1844–1910] see under *apoplexy.*

**Ray·mond-Cés·tan syndrome** (ra-maw'ses-tah') [F. *Raymond;* Raymond *Céstan,* French neurologist, 1872–1934] see under *syndrome.*

**Ray·naud's disease (gangrene), phenomenon, sign** (ra-nōz') [Maurice *Raynaud,* French physician, 1834–1881] see under *disease* and *phenomenon,* and see *acrocyanosis.*

**ra·zox·ane** (ra-zok'sān) [MeSH: Razoxane] an antineoplastic that may reduce the cardiac toxicity of doxorubicin and related antitumor anthracyclines when given in conjunction with those drugs.

**Rb** symbol for *rubidium.*

**RBBB** right bundle branch block; see *bundle branch block,* under *block.*

**RBC** red blood cell; red blood [cell] count (see *blood count,* under *count*).

**RBC IT** red blood cell iron turnover.

**RBD** REM sleep behavior disorder.

**RBE** relative biological effectiveness; see under *effectiveness.*

**RBP** retinol binding protein.

**RCA** 1. right coronary artery. 2. regulator of complement activation.

**RCM** Royal College of Midwives.

**RCN** Royal College of Nursing.

**RCOG** Royal College of Obstetricians and Gynaecologists.

**RCP** Royal College of Physicians.

**rcp** reciprocal translocation.

**RCS** Royal College of Surgeons.

**RCU** red cell utilization.

**RCVS** Royal College of Veterinary Surgeons.

**RD** reaction of degeneration; see under *reaction.*

**rd** abbreviation for *rutherford.*

**RDA** recommended dietary allowance; right displacement of the abomasum.

**RDE** receptor-destroying enzyme.

**RE** radium emanation (see *radon*); right eye; retinol equivalent.

**Re** symbol for *rhenium*.

**re-** [L.] a prefix meaning back or again.

**re·ab·sorb** (re″əb-sorb′) to absorb again; to undergo or to subject to reabsorption (q.v.); to resorb.

**re·ab·sorp·tion** (re″ab-sorp′shən) 1. the act or process of absorbing again, as the selective absorption by the kidneys of substances (glucose, proteins, sodium, etc.) already secreted into the renal tubules, and their return to the circulating blood. 2. resorption.

**re·act** (re-akt′) 1. to respond to a stimulus. 2. to enter into chemical action.

**re·ac·tance** (re-ak′təns) the part of electric impedance that arises from inductors and capacitors. It is a part of the impedance of electric current flow in an alternating current electric circuit. Symbol *X*.

**re·ac·tant** (re-ak′tənt) an original substance entering into a chemical reaction.

**acute phase r.**, see under *protein*.

**re·ac·tion** (re-ak′shən) [*re-* + L. *agere* to act] 1. opposite action, or counteraction. 2. response. 3. the phenomena caused by the action of chemical agents; a chemical process in which one substance is transformed into another substance or substances. For named reactions not defined here, see under *test*. 4. in psychology, the mental and/or emotional state elicited in response to any particular situation.

## Reaction

**acetic acid r.**, Rivalta's r.

**acid r.**, 1. one in which an acid participates. 2. a surplus of hydrogen ions in a solution or a pH below 7.0. 3. any test by which a surplus of hydrogen ions is recognized, such as the reddening of blue litmus.

**acrosome r.**, a sequence of structural changes that occur in spermatozoa when in the vicinity of an oocyte in the oviduct or uterine tube, and that are believed to facilitate entry of a spermatozoon into the oocyte: the outer membrane of the acrosome fuses at multiple points with the overlying plasma membrane of the sperm head, creating openings through which the enzymes of the acrosome are liberated.

**acute situational r., acute stress r.**, a transient, self-limiting acute emotional reaction to severe psychological stress; it is variably defined as comprising one or more of the following DSM-IV categories: *adjustment disorder, brief reactive psychosis, acute stress disorder,* and *posttraumatic stress disorder.* Called also *transient situational disturbance*.

**adjustment r.**, see under *disorder*.

**alarm r.**, the physiologic effects in response to acute stress, fright, or rage (increased blood pressure and cardiac output, increased blood flow to skeletal muscles, decreased flow to the viscera, increased rate of glycolysis and blood glucose concentration), mediated by sympathetic nervous system discharge and release of adrenal medullary hormones; called also *fight-or-flight r.* See also *stress r.*

**alkaline r.**, 1. the presence in a solution of more hydroxyl ions than hydrogen ions, i.e., a pH greater than 7.0. 2. any test by which such a solution is recognized, such as the bluing of red litmus.

**allergic r.**, hypersensitivity r.; used particularly to denote a type I hypersensitivity r.

**allograft r.**, the rejection of an allogeneic graft by a normal host; called also *homograft r.*

**alpha-naphthol r.**, Molisch's test (defs. 2, 3).

**anamnestic r.**, see under *response*.

**anaphylactic r.**, anaphylaxis.

**anaphylactoid r.**, a reaction resembling generalized anaphylaxis but not caused by IgE-mediated allergic reaction, instead being due to nonimmunologic degranulation of mast cells with release of the pharmacological mediators involved in anaphylaxis. Called also *anaphylactoid shock*.

**anaplerotic r.**, a reaction restoring the concentration of crucial intermediates that have been depleted in cellular function.

**anniversary r.**, abnormal behavior, symptoms, illness, or dreams occurring on the anniversary of a disturbing event.

**antibody-mediated cytotoxic hypersensitivity r.**, type II hypersensitivity r.

**antibody-mediated hypersensitivity r.**, 1. type II hypersensitivity r. 2. occasionally, any hypersensitivity reaction in which antibodies are the primary mediators, as contrasted with those mediated by T lymphocytes; included are *types I, II,* and *III hypersensitivity r's.*

**antigen-antibody r.**, the reversible binding of antigen to homologous antibody brought about by the formation of weak bonds between antigenic determinants on antigen molecules and antigen binding sites on immunoglobulin molecules. Certain effects, e.g., precipitation and agglutination reactions and viral neutralization, result from the binding itself; other effects, e.g., complement activation and opsonization, result from conformational changes that occur in immunoglobulin molecules with antigen binding and enable them to interact with complement proteins and Fc receptors on phagocytes.

**antiglobulin r.**, the agglutination of particles (usually erythrocytes) that have been (1) sensitized by the adsorption of soluble antigen, (2) treated with antibody to that antigen, and (3) treated with antiserum to the serum globulin of the animal species that produced the antibody.

**anxiety r.**, a reaction characterized by abnormal apprehension or uneasiness; see also *anxiety disorders,* under *disorder*.

**Arias-Stella r.**, changes in the cells of the endometrial epithelium consisting chiefly of bizarre-shaped hyperchromatic enlarged nuclei associated with a loss of cellular polarity; cytoplasmic vacuolization is occasionally present. The changes are thought to be associated with the presence of chorionic tissue in an intrauterine or extrauterine site, and are seen in some cases of ectopic pregnancy.

**Arthus r.**, the development of an inflammatory lesion, with induration, erythema, edema, hemorrhage, and necrosis, a few hours after intradermal injection of antigen into a previously sensitized animal producing precipitating antibody; it is classed as a type III hypersensitivity reaction in the Gell and Coombs classification of immune responses. The lesion results from the precipitation of antigen-antibody complexes, which causes complement activation and the release of complement fragments that are chemotactic for neutrophils; large numbers of neutrophils infiltrate the site and cause tissue destruction by release of lysosomal enzymes. Called also *Arthus phenomenon*.

**Arthus-type r.**, any pathologic process involving the same mechanism as the Arthus reaction, i.e., deposition of immune complexes and complement activation, as in immune complex disease.

**associative r.**, a reaction in which the response is withheld until the idea presented has suggested an associated idea.

**axon r., axonal r.**, the series of changes in a neuron following the severing of its axon, including central chromatolysis with displacement of the nucleus; called also *axonal, Nissl,* or *retrograde degeneration*.

**Bekhterev's (Bechterew's) r.**, in cases of tetany, the minimum of electric current needed to arouse muscular contraction needs to be diminished at every interruption or change of density in order to prevent tetanic contraction.

**Bence Jones r.**, the precipitation of protein by heat followed by its redissolving on boiling and being precipitated again on cooling.

**Berthelot r.**, the reaction of ammonia with Berthelot's reagent to form phenol-indophenol, a stable, deep blue product; used in colorimetric methods for ammonia and urea.

**Bittorf's r.**, in renal colic the pain produced by squeezing the testicle or pressing the ovary radiates to the kidney.

**biuret r.**, biuret ($H_2N$—CO—NH—CO—$NH_2$) forms a chelate having an intense violet-red color with the $Cu^{2+}$ ion in alkaline solution; the same reaction also occurs with tripeptides and polypeptides, but not with dipeptides or amino acids and is used in colorimetric methods for total protein.

**Bordet-Gengou r.**, complement fixation.

**cadaveric r.**, total loss of electrical response in the affected muscles in familial periodic paralysis.

**Cannizzaro's r.**, the reaction which certain aldehydes may undergo in concentrated alkali; one molecule of the aldehyde is reduced to the corresponding alcohol and another molecule is simultaneously oxidized to the salt of a carboxylic acid.

**capsular r.**, the reaction of the capsular substance of bacteria with a homologous antibody.

**carbamino r.**, alpha-amino acids unite with $CO_2$ in the presence of alkalis or alkaline earths to form salts of carbamino-carboxylic acids. This reaction is used in studying the course of protein digestion. See *formol titration,* under *method*.

**Casoni's r.**, see *Casoni's intradermal test,* under *test*.

**cell-mediated hypersensitivity r.**, type IV hypersensitivity r.

**chromaffin r.**, the taking on of a deep brown color by tissue of the adrenal medulla or other types that contain the catecholamines epinephrine and norepinephrine, within 12 hours after it is placed in a dichromate solution; this can be used to detect pheochromocytomas and other tumors that produce catecholamines. See also *chromaffin cells,* under *cell.*

**cockade r.,** the reaction of a sensitized guinea pig to intradermal injection of tuberculin; it consists of a large papule with a necrotic, hemorrhagic center.

**complement fixation r.,** see under *fixation.*

**conglutination r.,** a characteristic agglutination reaction obtained by a mixture of conglutinin, cells (e.g., bacteria or red cells), fresh complement, and a cell-specific immune serum from which the agglutinins have been removed by absorption. See *conglutinin.*

**consensual r.,** 1. crossed reflex. 2. an involuntary action that accompanies a voluntary action.

**conversion r.,** see under *disorder.*

**cross r.,** the interaction of an antigen with an antibody formed against a different antigen with which the first antigen shares identical or closely related antigenic determinants.

**cutaneous r.,** a positive reaction indicating immunity or hypersensitivity in a skin test. Called also *skin r., cutireaction,* and *dermoreaction.*

**cytotoxic hypersensitivity r.,** type II hypersensitivity r.

**Dale r.,** an in vitro test for anaphylactic sensitization in the guinea pig: a small amount of the antigen added to a tissue bath in which is immersed the excised uterine horn (smooth muscle) of an anaphylactically sensitized guinea pig causes contraction of the sensitized uterine muscle. Called also *Schultz-Dale r.* NOTE: Schultz employed intestinal muscle; Dale used uterine muscle from virgin guinea pigs.

**defense r.,** see under *mechanism.*

**r. of degeneration,** the reaction to electric stimulation of muscles whose nerves have degenerated. It consists of a loss of response to a faradic stimulus in a muscle, and to galvanic and faradic stimulus in a nerve. Galvanic irritability of the muscle is increased. Abbreviated Ea. R. (Ger. *Entartungs-Reaktion*) and RD.

**delayed hypersensitivity r.,** a reaction of cell-mediated immunity, named in contrast to immediate hypersensitivity reactions because its onset is 24 to 72 hours after the antigenic challenge; the term is usually used to denote the subset of type IV hypersensitivity reactions (Gell and Coombs classification) involving cytokine release and macrophage activation, as opposed to direct cytolysis, but can be used more broadly, even sometimes being used synonymously with *type IV hypersensitivity r.* The classic delayed hypersensitivity reaction is the tuberculin reaction observed in skin testing.

**depressive r.,** depression; the term is sometimes used to denote specific types of depression, such as reactive depression, or any of various mood disorders in which depression plays the predominant role.

**desmoplastic r.,** see *desmoplastic.*

**diazo r.,** Ehrlich's diazo r.

**Dick r.,** see under *test.*

**digitonin r.,** the formation of a precipitate on treating a sterol, such as cholesterol or ergosterol, with digitonin; employed to define cholesterol esters which do not precipitate in total serum cholesterol determinations.

**displacement r.,** a chemical reaction in which a reactant displaces a functional group from a substrate and becomes bound in the position formerly occupied by the leaving group; see also *displacement.*

**dissociative r.,** see under *disorder.*

**dopa r.,** the reaction by which dopa is changed into melanin under the influence of monophenol monooxygenase.

**downgrading r.,** a lepra reaction, similar in appearance to the reversal ("upgrading") reaction, representing a deterioration in the immune response to *Mycobacterium leprae* with worsening of the clinical symptoms of leprosy and an increased index of *M. leprae* in the tissues; it may be seen during antileprosy treatment in those in whom *M. leprae* has become drug resistant or in those with poor compliance with the chemotherapeutic regimen.

**egg yellow r.,** a yellow foam appearing in Ehrlich's diazo reaction before the addition of ammonia; believed to indicate acute pneumonia.

**Ehrlich's aldehyde r.,** urobilinogen reacts with *p*-dimethylaminobenzene to form a red-colored substance; used for semiquantitative determination of urobilinogen in urine and feces.

**Ehrlich's diazo r.,** a reaction of a pure pink or red color resulting from the action of diazotized sulfanilic acid and ammonia upon certain aromatic substances, e.g., urobilinogen, found in the urine in some conditions. This reaction has diagnostic value in hepatic disease, typhoid fever, and measles and prognostic value in tuberculosis.

**erythrocyte sedimentation r.,** see under *rate.*

**r. of exhaustion,** reaction to electric stimulation seen in conditions of exhaustion. In it the reaction normally produced by a certain current can be reproduced only by an increase in the current.

**Felix-Weil r.,** Weil-Felix test.

**Fernandez r.,** see *lepromin test,* under *test.*

**Feulgen r.,** a specific histochemical reaction for DNA (deoxyribonucleic acid): after acid hydrolysis at 60°C, tissue sections are stained in Schiff's reagent; DNA stains magenta.

**fight-or-flight r.,** alarm r.

**foreign body r.,** a granulomatous inflammatory reaction evoked by the presence of an exogenous material in the tissues, a characteristic feature of which is the formation of foreign body giant cells.

**fuchsinophil r.,** certain substances when stained with fuchsin retain the stain on being treated with picric acid alcohol.

**graft-versus-host r.,** see under *disease.*

**Grignard's r.,** see under *reagent.*

**group r.,** see under *agglutination.*

**Gruber's r., Gruber-Widal r.,** Widal's test.

**hemagglutination-inhibition r.,** the inhibition by antibodies of viral agglutination of red cells.

**hemiopic pupillary r.,** reaction in certain cases of hemianopia in which the stimulus of light thrown upon one side of the retina causes the iris to contract, while light thrown on the other side arouses no response. Called also *Wernicke's r.*

**Henle's r.,** a staining dark brown of the cells of the adrenal medulla on treatment with chromium salts.

**Herxheimer's r.,** Jarisch-Herxheimer r.

**homograft r.,** allograft r.

**hunting r.,** periods of vasoconstriction alternating with periods of vasodilatation in a finger or other part exposed to temperatures below 15°C, as if the body were hunting for an equilibrium point of skin temperature.

**hypersensitivity r.,** one in which the body mounts an exaggerated or inappropriate immune response to a substance either foreign or perceived as foreign, resulting in local or general tissue damage. Such reactions are usually classified as types I–IV on the basis of the Gell and Coombs classification (q.v.).

**type I,** that occurring within minutes when a sensitized individual is reexposed to antigen, resulting from interaction of IgE and the antigen; clinical manifestations can range from localized dermatitis, urticaria, or angioedema to allergic rhinitis or asthma to systemic anaphylaxis. The first exposure to the antigen induces the production of IgE antibodies that bind to receptors on mast cells and basophils. Upon subsequent exposure the antigen cross-links receptor-bound IgE molecules, triggering production and release of a diverse array of mediators (see table) that act on other cells, producing symptoms such as bronchospasm, edema, mucous secretion, and inflammation. Called also *immediate hypersensitivity r.*

**type II,** tissue or cell damage resulting from the interaction of antibodies and antigens on cell surfaces; specific IgG or IgM against cell surface or extracellular matrix antigens or cell surface receptors binds and causes damage at the site of binding by any of several mechanisms involving either complement activation and lysis or opsonization mediated by receptors for Fc or C3b leading to phagocytosis and destruction by macrophages and neutrophils. Examples of disorders caused by such tissue damage include myasthenia gravis, hemolytic anemia, Goodpasture's syndrome, and Rh incompatibility and transfusion reactions. Called also antibody-mediated hypersensitivity r. and *cytotoxic hypersensitivity r.*

**type III,** local or general inflammatory response due to formation of circulating antigen-antibody complexes and their deposition in tissues; the complexes activate complement and other inflammatory mediators, initiating processes including increased vascular permeability, stimulation of mast cell degranulation and neutrophil chemotaxis and accumulation, and ag-

**Mediators of Immediate Hypersensitivity**

| Mediator | Actions |
|---|---|
| *Preformed—Released from Storage Vesicles* | |
| Histamine | Increased vascular permeability<br>Smooth muscle contraction |
| ECF-A | Chemotactic for eosinophils |
| Lysosomal enzymes | Tissue damage and repair<br>Activation of kinin system |
| Heparin | Anticoagulant |
| NCF | Chemotactic for neutrophils |
| Serotonin | Increased vascular permeability |
| *Newly Formed—Produced upon Stimulation* | |
| SRS-A (leukotrienes $LTC_4$, $LTD_1$, $LTE_4$) | Smooth muscle contraction<br>Increased vascular permeability |
| Prostaglandins ($PGD_2$) | Smooth muscle contraction |
| HETE, HHT | Chemotactic for eosinophils |
| PAF | Platelet aggregation<br>Platelet mediator release |

ECF-A, eosinophil chemotactic factor of anaphylaxis; NCF, neutrophil chemotactic factor; SRS-A, slow reacting substance of anaphylaxis; HETE, hydroxyeicosatetraenoic acid; HHT, hydroxyheptadecatrienoic acid; PAF, platelet activating factor.

gregation of platelets, and resulting in tissue damage. Ensuing diseases, called also *immune complex diseases,* can be roughly classified as being due to persistent infection, to autoimmunity, or to inhalation of antigenic material; examples include serum sickness, Arthus reaction, subacute bacterial endocarditis, systemic lupus erythematosus, and farmer's lung. Called also *immune complex–mediated hypersensitivity r.*

**type IV,** a reaction of cell-mediated immunity, the immune response being initiated by antigen-specific T lymphocytes; in contrast to the reactions of immediate hypersensitivity, reactions take one or more days to develop and can be transferred by lymphocytes but not by serum. Reactions are mediated by T lymphocytes both through release of cytokines and through direct cytolysis. In the former mechanism, release of vasoactive and chemotactic cytokines is triggered by contact between the T cells and specific antigens on antigen-presenting cells; the cytokines attract and activate non–antigen-specific monocytes and macrophages, resulting in local erythema and induration, and leading to granuloma formation and necrosis if the eliciting stimulus cannot be eliminated. A common example is the tuberculin reaction elicited in skin testing for tuberculosis. In direct cytolysis, sometimes called *cell-mediated cytotoxicity,* cytotoxic T lymphocytes interact with foreign antigens presented by class I MHC molecules on cell surfaces, causing lysis of these foreign cells, as in allograft rejection. Type IV reactions can be induced by intracellular parasites, such as certain viruses, mycobacteria, and fungi, foreign tissue, tumor cells, soluble proteins, and haptens. The term is often equated with *delayed hypersensitivity reaction,* although the latter is sometimes restricted to cytokine-mediated reactions (as contrasted with direct cytolysis). Called also *cell-mediated* or *T cell–mediated hypersensitivity r.*

**id r.,** a sterile secondary skin eruption occurring in sensitized patients as a result of circulation of allergenic products from a primary site of infection; the morphology and site of the lesion vary.

**r. of identity,** a reaction pattern seen in double diffusion in two dimensions: the precipitin lines between the antigen wells and the antiserum well stop at their point of intersection, indicating that the antigen samples are identical. See also *r. of nonidentity* and *r. of partial identity.*

**immediate hypersensitivity r.,** 1. type I hypersensitivity r. 2. occasionally, any hypersensitivity reaction mediated by antibodies and developing rapidly, generally in minutes to hours (i.e., *type I, II,* or *III hypersensitivity r.*), as distinguished from those mediated by T lymphocytes and macrophages and generally requiring 24 to 72 hours to develop (*type IV hypersensitivity r's,* sometimes called *delayed hypersensitivity r's*).

**immune r.,** see under *response.*

**immune complex–mediated hypersensitivity r.,** type III hypersensitivity r.

**intracutaneous r., intradermal r.,** the reaction to an intracutaneous injection of antigen in a skin test.

**Jaffe r.,** creatinine when treated with picric acid in strongly alkaline solution gives an intense red color.

**Jarisch-Herxheimer r.,** a transient, short-term immunologic reaction commonly seen following antibiotic treatment of early and later stages of syphilis and less often in other diseases, such as borreliosis, brucellosis, typhoid fever, and trichinellosis, which is manifested by fever, chills, headache, myalgias, and exacerbation of cutaneous lesions. The reaction has been attributed to liberation of endotoxin-like substances or of antigens from the killed or dying microorganisms, but its exact pathogenesis is unclear. Called also *Herxheimer's r.*

**johnin r.,** a skin reaction like the tuberculin reaction, produced by filtrates of cultures of *Mycobacterium paratuberculosis* (see *johnin*); used in the diagnosis of Johne's disease in cattle.

**Jolly's r.,** failure of response to faradic stimulation in a muscle, the power of voluntary contraction as well as the response to galvanic stimulation being retained.

**Jones-Mote r.,** a weak type IV hypersensitivity reaction to protein antigens associated with basophil infiltration, occurring on challenge a few days after priming with a protein antigen in aqueous solution or in Freund's incomplete adjuvant. Called also *cutaneous basophil hypersensitivity.*

**Koch's r.,** see under *phenomenon.*

**late phase r.,** an IgE-mediated immune reaction occurring 5 to 8 hours after exposure to antigen, after the wheal and flare reactions of immediate hypersensitivity have diminished; it is characterized by inflammation, with accumulation of neutrophils, basophils, eosinophils, and $CD4^+$ T lymphocytes, pruritis, and minor cellular infiltration. Prostaglandins are not formed. Inflammation subsides after reaching a maximum around 24 hours after exposure.

**lengthening r.,** the elongation of the extensor muscles which permits flexion of a limb.

**lepra r.,** an acute or subacute hypersensitivity state occurring during the course of anti-leprosy treatment or in untreated leprosy categories, involving two types of immunological reactions, one a delayed hypersensitivity reaction (see *reversal r's*) and the other an immune complex reaction (see *erythema nodosum leprosum*).

**lepromin r.,** see under *test.*

**leukemic r., leukemoid r.,** a peripheral blood picture resembling that of leukemia or indistinguishable from it on the basis of morphologic appearance alone, with leukocytosis of varying degrees and increased numbers of immature cells in circulation. It may be seen with infections such as tuberculosis, brucellosis, toxoplasmosis, staphylococcal infections, and streptococcal infections; with inflammatory disorders such as glomerulonephritis, rheumatoid arthritis, liver failure, and diabetic acidosis; with tumors and granulomatous infiltration of bone marrow; and with intoxications such as eclampsia, severe burns, and mercury poisoning.

**Liebermann-Burchard r.,** see under *test.*

**Loeb's decidual r.,** the presence of a glass bead or other irritant causes the formation of a small deciduoma in the uterine mucosa when corpora lutea are developing normally.

**Lohmann r.,** an easily reversible reaction occurring in muscle, in which the high-energy phosphate bond of ATP is transferred to creatine, forming creatine phosphate; the reaction is catalyzed by creatine kinase.

**Machado r., Machado-Guerreiro r.,** see under *test.*

**manic-depressive r.,** former name for bipolar disorder; see *bipolar disorders* (def. 2), under *disorder.*

**Mantoux r.,** see under *test.*

**Marchi's r.,** failure of the degenerated myelin sheath of a nerve to become discolored when treated with osmic acid.

**Mazzotti r.,** the set of adverse reactions, which may be severe or rarely life-threatening, that accompany the administration of diethylcarbamazine in onchocerciasis, most commonly an intensely pruritic rash, but sometimes also systemic manifestations such as fever, malaise, lymph node swelling, eosinophilia, arthralgias, tachycardia, and hypotension; if numerous microfilariae are present in the eyes, blindness may occur. See also *Mazzotti test,* under *test.*

**Mitsuda r.,** see *lepromin test,* under *test.*

**mixed agglutination r.,** agglutination of a mixture of different cell types by antibody directed against an antigenic determinant present on all of the cells.

**mixed leukocyte r., mixed lymphocyte r.,** see under *culture.*

**Molisch's r.,** see under *test.*

**Moloney r.,** see under *test.*

**Montenegro r.,** see *leishmanin test,* under *test.*

**mouse tail r.,** stiffening of the tail in rats and mice following the administration of a small dose of morphine.

**myasthenic r.,** progressively diminished response of a muscle to repeated electric stimuli.

**Nagler's r.,** the formation of an opaque zone around colonies of *Clostridium perfringens* on egg yolk agar, produced by the action of a diffusible lecithinase.

**near-point r.,** constriction of the pupil when the gaze is fixed on a near point.

**Neill-Mooser r.,** a reaction in laboratory animals produced by inoculation with rickettsiae of murine typhus. The inflammatory exudate of the scrotal swelling contains large mononuclear cells filled with rickettsiae.

**Neufeld's r.,** when pneumococci and other capsulated microorganisms are mixed with specific immune serum there occurs in addition to agglutination a swelling (Ger. *quellung*) of the capsules of the organisms, owing to the binding of antibody with the capsular polysaccharide; called also *capsular swelling* and *quellung r.*

**neurotonic r.,** muscular contraction persisting after the stimulus which produced it has ceased.

**neutral r.,** the presence of an equal number of $H^+$ and $OH^-$ ions in a solution, i.e., a pH of 7.0.

**Ninhydrin r.,** see *triketohydrindene hydrate test,* under *test.*

**r. of nonidentity,** a reaction pattern seen in double diffusion in two dimensions: the precipitin lines between the antigen wells and the antiserum well cross, indicating that the antigen samples have no antigenic determinants in common. See also *r. of identity* and *r. of partial identity.*

**obsessive-compulsive r.,** see under *disorder.*

**Oestreicher's r.,** xanthydrol r.

**orbicularis r.,** orbicularis pupillary reflex.

**oxidation-reduction r.,** redox r.

**pain r.,** dilatation of the pupil on a feeling of pain.

**parallergic r.,** see *parallergy.*

**r. of partial identity,** a reaction pattern seen in double diffusion in two dimensions: one of the precipitin lines between the antigen wells and the antiserum well stops at the point of intersection, whereas the other continues past it, indicating that the antigen samples have some, but not all, antigenic determinants in common. See also *r. of identity* and *r. of nonidentity.*

**PAS r.,** periodic acid–Schiff r.

**passive cutaneous anaphylaxis r.,** passive cutaneous anaphylaxis.

**passive cutaneous Arthus r.,** a variation of the Arthus reaction in which a nonimmune host is inoculated with large quantities of precipitating antibody intravenously, followed by local cutaneous inoculation of antigen.

**Pasteur's r.,** see under *effect.*

**Paul-Bunnell r.**, see under *test.*

**periodic acid–Schiff r.**, a tissue section is exposed to periodic acid, which oxidizes hydroxyl groups on adjacent carbon atoms or adjacent hydroxyl groups and amino groups to aldehydes, and then is stained with Schiff's reagent, which forms an additional product with aldehydes to produce a red or magenta reaction product; used to test for glycogen, epithelial mucins, neutral polysaccharides, and glycoproteins; called also *PAS r.*

**peroxidase r.**, the appearance of deep-blue granules in leukocytes of marrow origin when stained with Goodpasture's stain, distinguishing them from cells of lymphatic origin.

**Pfeiffer's r.**, see under *phenomenon.*

**phobic r.**, phobic disorder; see *phobia.*

**photochemical r.**, photoreaction.

**Pirquet r.**, see under *test.*

**polymerase chain r. (PCR)**, a rapid technique for in vitro amplification of specific DNA or RNA sequences, allowing small quantities of short sequences to be analyzed without cloning: oligonucleotide primers are annealed to single-stranded nucleotide sequences, which are copied by polymerase; the number of copies is geometrically amplified by repeated cycles of annealing and copying.

**Porter-Silber r.**, the reaction of the dihydroxyacetone side chain of certain 17-hydroxycorticosteroids (Porter-Silber chromogens) with phenylhydrazine in acid, which produces a yellow color; an index of adrenocortical function now largely supplanted by immunoassay techniques.

**Prausnitz-Küstner r.**, a type I hypersensitivity reaction produced in a nonatopic subject by intradermal injection of serum from an atopic subject followed 12 or more hours later by an injection of antigen into the same site; the presence of specific IgE antibody in the transferred serum results in a classic wheal and flare reaction to the antigen. Once the standard method of demonstrating IgE, this test is no longer used because of the risk of transmitting serum hepatitis and because serum IgE can now be measured by in vitro assays, e.g., RAST and RIST.

**precipitin r.**, the formation of an insoluble precipitate by reaction of antigen and antibody; it occurs only with multivalent antigens and is dependent on electrolyte concentration, pH, temperature, and the relative concentrations of antigen and antibody, the amount of precipitate formed increasing to a maximum and then decreasing as the relative antigen concentration is increased.

**prozone r.**, see *prozone.*

**pseudoallergic r.**, a clinical state exhibiting what appear to be the signs and symptoms of an immediate hypersensitivity reaction, but with no evidence for an immunologic mechanism.

**psychotic depressive r.**, psychosis characterized by depressed mood resulting from a specific event, usually in a patient without prior history of severe depression; the condition has been incorporated into major depressive disorder.

**quellung r.** [Ger. "swelling"], Neufeld's r.

**redox r.**, one in which there is transfer of electrons from an electron donor (the reducing agent) to an electron acceptor (the oxidizing agent).

**reversal r.**, a lepra reaction usually occurring during chemotherapy in borderline leprosy representing a type IV (delayed) hypersensitivity reaction with "upgrading" of cell-mediated immunity to *Mycobacterium leprae,* which tends to move the disease toward the tuberculoid pole. It is chiefly characterized by erythema, edema, and tenderness of preexisting quiescent lesions, the appearance of new lesions, neuritis with nerve damage, fever, adenopathy, and elevation of the leukocyte count. See also *downgrading r.*

**reverse passive Arthus r.**, the reaction produced when precipitating antibody is inoculated into a skin site in an experimental animal followed in 30 minutes to 2 hours by inoculation of the homologous antigen, either intravenously or intracutaneously at the same site. Thus the usual anatomical locations of precipitating antibody and antigen in an Arthus reaction are reversed.

**reversible r.**, a chemical reaction which occurs in either direction, depending on conditions; a reaction in which the products react to re-form the reactants.

**Rivalta's r.**, a reaction for distinguishing fluids of transudation and exudation, utilizing acetic acid.

**Russo r.**, a reaction of the urine of typhoid patients on adding 4 drops of a solution of methylene blue to 15 mL of urine. In the first stage of typhoid, the urine becomes light green; at the height of the disease, an emerald color; and during the decline, a bluish color.

**Schick r.**, see under *test.*

**Schultz-Charlton r.**, when scarlet fever antitoxin or scarlet fever convalescent serum is injected into an area of the skin showing a bright red rash, a blanching of the skin at the site of the injection occurs. Serum from scarlet fever patients does not produce this reaction.

**Schultz-Dale r.**, see *Dale r.*

**second-set r.**, see under *phenomenon.*

**Selivanoff's (Seliwanow's) r.**, see under *test.*

**serological r., serum r.**, seroreaction.

**serum sickness–like r.**, see *serum sickness,* under *sickness.*

**shortening r.**, the shortening that succeeds the lengthening reaction when a limb is brought back into the extended position.

**Shwartzman r., generalized,** a generalized reaction following two intravenous injections of endotoxin separated by 24 hours; it is characterized by widespread hemorrhages, bilateral cortical necrosis of the kidneys, and a marked fall in leukocyte and platelet counts and usually results in death of the animal.

**Shwartzman r., localized,** a localized cutaneous reaction consisting of vascular necrosis, petechial hemorrhages, and leukocyte infiltration that occurs at the site of an original subcutaneous injection of endotoxin approximately 24 hours after an intravenous injection of the same or another endotoxin given at a site other than the original injection site.

**skin r.**, cutaneous r.

**startle r.**, the various psychophysiological phenomena, including involuntary motor and autonomic reactions, evidenced by an individual in reaction to a sudden, unexpected stimulus, as a loud noise.

**Straus' r.**, when material containing virulent glanders bacilli is inoculated into the peritoneal cavity of male guinea pigs, scrotal lesions develop; called also *Straus' phenomenon.*

**stress r.**, any of the biological reactions to adverse stimuli, physical, mental, or emotional, internal or external, that tend to disturb the organism's homeostasis; should these compensating reactions, physiological or psychological, be inadequate or inappropriate, they may lead to disorders. See *alarm r.* and *acute stress r.;* see *general adaptation syndrome,* under *syndrome;* and see *acute stress disorder, adjustment disorder,* and *posttraumatic stress disorder,* under *disorder.*

**sympathetic stress r.**, alarm r.

**T cell–mediated hypersensitivity r.**, type IV hypersensitivity r.

**tendon r.**, see under *reflex.*

**toxin-antitoxin r.**, the antigen-antibody reaction between a toxin and antitoxin.

**transfusion r.**, any symptoms due to agglutination or hemolysis of the recipient's blood cells when blood for transfusion is incorrectly matched (see *crossmatching*), or when the recipient has a hypersensitivity reaction to some element of the donor blood.

**trigger r.**, see under *action.*

**tuberculin r.**, the presence of induration or vesiculation as a delayed reaction at the site of a tuberculin test, a positive result. See also under *test.*

**Turnbull's blue r.**, blue-black coloration produced when tissue containing chemically active iron is treated with potassium ferrocyanide and hydrochloric acid.

**upgrading r.**, see *reversal r.*

**vestibular pupillary r.**, dilatation of the pupils arising from stimulation of the external auditory canal.

**Voges-Proskauer r.**, see under *test.*

**von Pirquet's r.**, Pirquet test.

**Weil-Felix r.**, see under *test.*

**Wernicke's r.**, hemiopic pupillary r.

**wheal and erythema r., wheal and flare r.**, the characteristic local cutaneous reaction consisting of an elevated, blanched wheal surrounded by a spreading "flare" of erythema that occurs within a few minutes at the site of a minor nonpenetrating skin injury and also in response to administration of allergen to an atopic individual; it is caused by release of histamine from mast cells.

**white-graft r.**, an immune reaction to a tissue graft, e.g., a skin graft, as a result of which the grafted tissue does not become vascularized due to rapid rejection.

**Widal's r.**, see under *test.*

**xanthydrol r.**, when tissue from a uremic patient is fixed in a solution of xanthydrol in glacial acetic acid, a large deposit of xanthydrol occurs in the tissue.

**zed r.**, a reaction which appears in infants in cases of starvation after the starvation is relieved; it consists of a slight gain in weight, elevation of temperature, and the appearance of watery stools containing a large number of cells.

**re·ac·tion·for·ma·tion** (re-ak′shən for-ma′shən) an unconscious defense mechanism in which a person assumes an attitude that is the reverse of a wish or impulse that he harbors.

**re·ac·ti·vate** (re-ak′tĭ-vāt) to make active again; especially the restoring of the activity to immune serum that has had its activity destroyed.

**re·ac·ti·va·tion** (re-ak″tĭ-va′shən) the restoration of activity to something that has been inactivated.
**r. of serum,** restoration of immunological activity to serum by adding fresh complement.

**re·ac·ti·va·tor** (re-ak′tĭ-va-tor) an agent that restores activity.
**cholinesterase r.,** an agent that restores the activity of acetylcholinesterase that has been inactivated by an organophosphate compound; see *pralidoxime.*

**re·ac·tiv·i·ty** (re″ak-tiv′ĭ-te) 1. the process or property of reacting. 2. in electroencephalography, the capability of alternation of a given pattern of electrical activity upon sensory stimulation or other physiological change.

**re·ac·to·gen·ic** (re-ak″to-jen′ik) [*reaction* + *-genic*] causing an excessive local or systemic reaction; said of vaccine.

**Re·ac·trol** (re-ak′trol) trademark for a preparation of clemizole hydrochloride.

**read·ing** (rēd′ing) [MeSH: Reading] understanding of written or printed symbols representing words.
**lip r., speech r.,** the understanding of speech through observation of the movement of the lips of the speaker. Called also *visual hearing.*

**re·a·gent** (re-a′jənt) [*re-* + *agent*] a substance employed to produce a chemical reaction so as to detect, measure, produce, etc., other substances.
**amino-acid r.,** a 0.5 per cent solution of sodium $\beta$-naphthoquinone-4-sulfonate freshly prepared.
**arsenic–sulfuric acid r.,** Rosenthaler's r.
**Benedict's r.,** any of several alkaline copper sulfate solutions used for Benedict's test for glucose.
**Berthelot's r.,** an alkaline solution of phenol and hypochlorite, used in the Berthelot reaction.
**Bial's r.,** orcinol 1.5 g, fuming hydrochloric acid 500 g, ferric chloride (10 per cent) 20–30 drops.
**biuret r.,** any of various alkaline copper sulfate solutions containing a variety of stabilizers, used in the biuret reaction (q.v.).
**Bogg's r.,** dissolve 25 g of phosphotungstic acid in 125 mL of water. Dilute 25 mL of concentrated hydrochloric acid to 100 mL. Mix the two solutions.
**diazo r.,** a reagent consisting of two solutions which are mixed just prior to the test in the proportion of 25 mL of solution *A* to 0.75 mL of *B*. Solution *A:* sulfanilic acid, 1 g; distilled water, 1000 mL. Solution *B:* sodium nitrite, 0.5 g: distilled water, 100 mL.
**Ehrlich's aldehyde r.,** 4 g of paradimethylaminobenzaldehyde in a mixture of 80 mL of concentrated hydrochloric acid and 380 mL of ethyl alcohol.
**Ehrlich's diazo r.,** Solution *A:* dissolve 5 g of sodium nitrite in 1 L of distilled water. Solution *B:* dissolve 5 g of sulfanilic acid and 50 mL of hydrochloric acid in 1 L of distilled water. For use mix 1 part of *A* with 50 to 100 parts of *B.*
**Fouchet's r.,** 1.0 g ferric chloride and 25.0 g trichloroacetic acid dissolved in water to make 100 mL; see *Fouchet's test,* under *test.*
**general r.,** a reagent that indicates the general class of bodies to which a substance belongs.
**Gies' biuret r.,** see under *test.*
**Grignard's r.,** any of several compounds of magnesium with an organic radical and a halogen; these reagents undergo reactions with many substances producing important products.
**Lloyd's r.,** an especially fine preparation of fuller's earth obtained by elutriation; used to absorb alkaloids from solutions.
**Millon's r.,** see under *test.*
**Mörner's r.,** a solution of 1 volume of formalin, 45 volumes of distilled water, 55 volumes of concentrated sulfuric acid; used as a test for tyrosine. See under *tests.*
**Nessler's r.,** an aqueous solution of 5 per cent of potassium iodide, 2.5 per cent of mercury bichloride, and 16 per cent of potassium hydroxide; used as a test for ammonia.
**Ninhydrin r.,** trademark for a preparation of triketohydrindene hydrate (q.v.).
**Rosenthaler's r.,** *(for alkaloids),* 1 part of potassium arsenate in 100 parts of concentrated sulfuric acid.
**Schiff's r.,** a reagent for testing for the presence of aldehydes, prepared by dissolving 0.25 g of fuchsin in 1 liter of water and decolorizing by passing sulfur dioxide into it. In the presence of aldehyde the blue color is restored.
**Scott-Wilson r.,** add 90 g sodium hydroxide in solution to 5 g mercuric cyanide in solution, then add 1.45 g silver nitrate solution with constant stirring.
**splenic r.,** any drug or stimulus which causes the spleen to contract.

**re·a·gin** (re′ə-jin) [*reagent* + *-in*] 1. the antibody that mediates type I hypersensitivity reactions; in humans, IgE. 2. former name for the serum antibody detected by the Wassermann test.

**re·a·gin·ic** (re″ə-jin′ik) pertaining to reagin.

**re·al·gar** (re′al-gahr″) [Arabic *rahj al-ghar* powder of the mine] arsenic disulfide, $As_2S_2$: a pigment.

**ream·er** (rēm′ər) in root canal therapy, an engine-driven or hand-operated instrument for canal enlargement, consisting of a serrated triangular shaft twisted into a loosely spiraled form.

**re·at·tach·ment** (re″ə-tach′mənt) 1. joining together parts that have been separated. 2. the recementing of a dental crown or other prosthesis. 3. embedding of new periodontal ligament fibers into new cementum and the attachment of gingival epithelium to tooth surface previously denuded by disease.

**Ré·au·mur's scale, thermometer** (ra″o-mūrz′) [René Antoine Feschault de *Réaumur,* French naturalist, 1683–1757] see under *scale* and *thermometer.*

**re·base** (re-bās′) to refit a denture by means of the replacement of the denture base material without changing the occlusal relations of the teeth.

**re·bound** (re′bound) a reversed response on the withdrawal of a stimulus; see also under *phenomenon* and *tenderness.*
**heparin r.,** the return of anticoagulant activity following the complete neutralization of heparin in a patient's blood by protamine.
**REM r.,** the phenomenon in which a subject deprived of REM (rapid eye movement) sleep for a prolonged period will, on being permitted to sleep undisturbed, compensate by having increased REM sleep.

**re·cal·ci·fi·ca·tion** (re-kal″sĭ-fĭ-ka′shən) the restoration of calcium salts to the bodily tissues.

**re·call** [MeSH: Recall] 1. (re-kawl′) to remember or recollect. 2. (re′kawl) the process of bringing information back into consciousness.

**re·can·al·iza·tion** (re-kan″ə-lĭ-za′shən) formation of new canals or paths, especially blood vessels, through an obstruction such as a clot. Called also *canalization.*

**re·ca·pit·u·la·tion** (re″kə-pit″u-la′shən) see under *theory.*

**re·cei·ver** (re-sēv′ər) 1. a vessel for collecting a gas or a distillate. 2. the portion of an apparatus by which electric energy is converted into signals which may be seen or heard.

**re·cep·tac·u·lum** (re″səp-tak′u-ləm) pl. *receptac′ula* [L., from *recipere* to receive] a receptacle or container; that which serves for receiving or containing something.
**r. chy′li,** cisterna chyli.
**r. gan′glii petro′si,** fossula petrosa.
**r. Pecquet′i,** cisterna chyli.

**re·cep·tor** (re-sep′tər) [L. *recipere* to receive, accept] 1. a molecular structure within a cell or on the surface characterized by (1) selective binding of a specific substance and (2) a specific physiologic effect that accompanies the binding, e.g., membrane receptors for peptide hormones, neurotransmitters, antigens, complement fragments, and immunoglobulins, and nuclear receptors for steroid hormones. 2. a sensory nerve terminal that responds to stimuli of various kinds; classified in various ways including by the type of stimulus (see *chemoreceptor, mechanoreceptor, photoreceptor,* and *thermoreceptor*) and by the location in the body (see *exteroceptor, interoceptor,* and *proprioceptor*).
**adrenergic r's,** postulated sites on effector organs innervated by postganglionic adrenergic fibers of the sympathetic nervous system, classified as $\alpha$-adrenergic and $\beta$-adrenergic receptors according to their reaction to norepinephrine and epinephrine, respectively, and to certain blocking and stimulating agents. Called also *adrenoceptor* and *adrenoreceptor.*
**$\alpha$-adrenergic r's,** adrenergic receptors that respond to norepinephrine and to such blocking agents as phenoxybenzamine hydrochloride and phentolamine. Called also *alpha receptors.*
**$\beta$-adrenergic r's,** adrenergic receptors that respond to epinephrine and to such blocking agents as propranolol; they are of two types: $\beta_1$ (lipolysis and cardiostimulation) and $\beta_2$ (bronchodilation and vasodilation). Called also *beta r's.*
**alpha r's,** $\alpha$-adrenergic r's.
**$\gamma$-aminobutyric acid r's,** a type of membrane receptor that bind the neurotransmitter $\gamma$-aminobutyric acid to facilitate its inhibitory effect on postsynaptic cells. There are two types: the more common *GABA A receptors* are ligand-gated chloride channels that attenuate postsynaptic potentials on neuron bodies and dendrites and inhibit the release of neurotransmitters at nerve terminals; the less common *GABA B receptors* include G proteins and activate cellular coupling systems to either open potassium channels, prevent the opening of calcium channels, or inhibit the production of cyclic adenosine monophosphate. Called also *GABA r's.*
**B cell antigen r's,** monomeric IgM, IgD, and (on memory cells only)

IgG that is attached to the cell membrane of B lymphocytes and which, in conjunction with T cell help, triggers B cell activation on contact with antigen.

**beta r's,** $\beta$-adrenergic r's.

**cell-surface r.,** membrane r.

**cholinergic r's,** cell-surface receptors that bind the neurotransmitter acetylcholine and mediate its action on postjunctional cells, including parasympathetic autonomic effector cells, sympathetic and parasympathetic autonomic ganglion cells, striated muscle, and certain central neurons; they are commonly divided into two classes, *muscarinic r's* and *nicotinic r's.* Called also *cholinoceptors.*

**cold r.,** a cutaneous thermoreceptor particularly sensitive to temperatures between 15°and 35°C. See also *paradoxical cold response,* under *response.*

**complement r's,** cell-surface receptors for products of complement reactions, with roles including recognition of pathogens, phagocytosis, adhesion, and clearance of immune complexes. At least nine types exist, with the best characterized being CR1–4, which bind C3 fragments already bound to a surface. Other complement receptors are named according to ligand (e.g., C5a receptor)

**CR1,** CD35 or C3b receptor; a membrane glycoprotein specific for C3b and C4b and expressed on erythrocytes and many other cell types including neutrophils, monocytes, T and B lymphocytes, and eosinophils; its roles include inhibition of C3 convertases, stimulation of phagocytosis of complement-coated particles and microorganisms, and clearance of immune complexes from the circulation.

**CR2,** CD21 or C3d receptor; a single-chain membrane glycoprotein present on B lymphocytes, follicular dendritic cells, and certain epithelial cells; it is specific for complement fragments iC3b and C3dg, produced by cleavage of bound C3b by factor I and is involved in B lymphocyte activation. CR2 is the Epstein-Barr virus receptor and also binds interferon-$\alpha$.

**CR3,** glycoprotein Mac-1.

**CR4,** a $\beta_2$ integrin (CD11c/CD18) expressed on monocytes, macrophages, neutrophils, and NK cells that binds to inactivated C3b (iC3b) and to the fragment C3dg and also mediates leukocyte adhesion. It is involved in both Fc receptor–mediated and Fc-independent phagocytosis. It comprises an $\alpha$ and a $\beta$ chain; the latter is common also to CR3. Called also *glycoprotein p150,95* and *p150,95.*

**contact r.,** mechanoreceptor.

**cutaneous r.,** any of the various types of sense organs found in the dermis or epidermis, usually a mechanoreceptor, thermoreceptor, or nociceptor; see also *exteroceptor.*

**cytokine r's,** transmembrane proteins that bind cytokines via extracellular domains, acting to convert an extracellular signal to an intracellular one; they are divided into five families on the basis of sequence homologies and folding motifs.

**distance r.,** teleceptor.

**estrogen r.,** a type of nuclear receptor consisting of a cellular regulatory protein that binds estrogens, found on nearly all cell types, but particularly in estrogen-sensitive tissues such as the uterus and breast. Cytoplasmic levels are measured in surgically removed breast carcinoma; high levels indicate that a positive response to endocrine therapy is likely.

**Fc r's,** specific cell-surface receptors for antigen-antibody complexes or aggregated immunoglobulins that bind a site in the Fc portion of the immunoglobulin molecule and may exhibit specificity for particular immunoglobulin classes. Fc receptors are found on B cells, K cells, macrophages, neutrophils, and eosinophils, and, during some developmental stages, on T cells; those on K cells, macrophages, and neutrophils bind to opsonizing antibodies bound to antigens and trigger phagocytosis of the antigen.

**GABA r's,** $\gamma$-aminobutyric acid r's.

**gustatory r.,** a receptor for taste, located in the taste cell of a taste bud.

**$H_1$ r's, $H_2$ r's,** see *histamine.*

**hair follicle r's,** rapidly adapting receptors that surround the roots of hair follicles.

**homing r.,** a cell-surface molecule that directs tissue- or organ-specific attachment of that cell; specifically, one of the surface proteins of lymphocytes that mediate their attachment to a particular type of vascular enothelium.

**IgE r's,** membrane receptors for immunoglobulin E (IgE) on mast cells and basophils; the IgE molecules are bound by a site in the Fc region leaving their antigen-binding sites exposed; binding of a multivalent antigen that cross-links the receptors triggers release of mediators of immediate hypersensitivity.

**insulin r's,** specific membrane receptors for insulin found on target cells. When insulin binds to a receptor, either the receptor protein kinase is activated, leading to the activation of other protein kinases within the cell, or the occupied receptors move to coated pits and are endocytosed; in the latter case, in addition to the effects mediated by kinases, a few effects may depend on degradation products.

**joint r.,** any of several mechanoreceptors that occur in joint capsules and respond to deep pressure and to other stimuli such as stress or change in position.

**low-density lipoprotein (LDL) r's,** specific receptors for LDL found in coated pits on the surface of mammalian cells. The coated pits are internalized forming coated vesicles from which LDL receptors are recycled back to the plasma membrane while LDL particles are transferred to lysosomes where they are degraded releasing free cholesterol, phospholipids, and amino acids. Genetic defects in LDL receptors are responsible for familial hypercholesterolemia.

**membrane r.,** a receptor located on or in the membrane of a cell; called also *cell-surface r.*

**muscarinic r's,** cholinergic r's that are stimulated by the alkaloid muscarine and blocked by atropine; they are found on autonomic effector cells and on central neurons in the thalamus and cerebral cortex. Three types may be distinguished on the basis of pharmacologic specificity and five types on the basis of molecular structure; a number of differing nomenclatures have been applied to these types.

**muscle r.,** a mechanoreceptor found in a muscle or tendon; see *muscle spindle* under *spindle* and *Golgi tendon organ* under *organ.*

**$N_1$-r's,** nicotinic receptors that are preferentially blocked by hexamethonium; they occur on autonomic ganglion cells.

**$N_2$-r's,** nicotinic receptors that are preferentially blocked by decamethonium; they occur on striated muscle.

**nicotinic r's,** cholinergic receptors that are stimulated initially and blocked at high doses by the alkaloid nicotine and blocked by tubocurarine; they are found on autonomic ganglion cells, on striated muscle, and on spinal central neurons. See *$N_1$-r's* and *$N_2$-r's.*

**nonadapting r.,** a mechanoreceptor, such as a nociceptor, that responds to stimulation with a continual steady discharge and little or no accommodation over time.

**nuclear r.,** a receptor located in the nucleus of a cell, responding to substances that can cross the cell membrane without passing through the transducing systems of the membrane; steroid hormones, thyroid hormones, and vitamin metabolites such as retinoids and calcitriol bind to nuclear receptors.

**olfactory r.,** a chemoreceptor in the nasal epithelium that is sensitive to stimulation, giving rise to the sensation of odors.

**opiate r., opioid r.,** any of a number of types of receptors for opiates and opioids; at least seven different types are postulated at different locations in the body, grouped into three major classes ($\delta$, $\kappa$, and $\mu$) according to the specific substances they bind and to the specific physiological effect(s) (e.g. analgesia, respiratory depression, or a psychotomimetic effect) that binding causes or inhibits. See accompanying table.

**orphan r.,** a protein identified as a putative receptor on the basis of structural homology with a known class of receptors but without identification of possible ligands or evidence of function.

**paciniform r's,** see under *corpuscle.*

**pain r.,** nociceptor.

**pressure r.,** slowly adapting r.

**rapidly adapting r.,** a mechanoreceptor that responds quickly to stimulation but that rapidly accommodates and stops firing if the stimulus remains constant. Examples are Meissner's corpuscles, pacinian corpuscles, and Golgi-Mazzoni corpuscles.

**sensory r.,** receptor (def. 2).

**slowly adapting r.,** a mechanoreceptor that responds slowly to stimulation and continues firing as long as the stimulus continues. Examples are Merkel's disks and Ruffini's corpuscles.

**steroid r., steroid hormone r.,** a type of nuclear receptor consisting of a protein of high molecular weight, found in the target tissue of a given steroid hormone.

**stretch r.,** a sense organ in a muscle or tendon that responds to elongation; see *Golgi tendon organ* under *organ* and *muscle spindle* under *spindle.*

**tactile r.,** a mechanoreceptor for the sense of touch; called also *touch r.*

**T cell antigen r. (TCR),** the characteristic marker of T lymphocytes, consisting of two polypeptide chains linked by a disulfide bridge. Two forms exist: TCR-1, composed of $\alpha$ and $\beta$ chains and occurring on helper and cytotoxic T cells, and the much less common TCR-2, composed of $\gamma$ and $\delta$ chains and occurring on certain T cells of the gut and epidermis; both forms are associated with the CD3 molecule. The TCR has a constant and a variable (antibody-binding) portion and recognizes (1) specific foreign antigens and (2) self MHC antigens; both must be seen simultaneously to trigger T cell activation.

**thermal r.,** thermoreceptor.

**touch r.,** tactile r.

**vibration r.,** a rapidly adapting receptor sensitive to vibrations.

**visual r.,** photoreceptor.

**volume r's,** postulated receptors which respond to increased plasma extracellular fluid volume and stimulate corrective measures.

**warmth r.,** a cutaneous thermoreceptor particularly sensitive to temperature between 30° and 45°C.

**re·cess** (re'ses) a small empty space or hollow; for specific anatomic structures not found here, see under *recessus.* See also *cavity, pocket,* and *pouch.*

**accessory r. of elbow,** recessus sacciformis articulationis cubiti.

**acetabular r.,** fossa acetabuli.

**Opioid Receptor Classes**

| Class / *Subclass* | Endogenous Ligand | Action |
|---|---|---|
| delta ($\delta$) | leu-enkephalin | *Increase in:* feeding, growth hormone release; *Decrease in:* dopamine release |
| $\delta_1$ | | Supraspinal analgesia |
| $\delta_2$ | | Supraspinal and spinal analgesia |
| kappa ($\kappa$) | | *Increase in:* feeding, psychotomimesis, sedation; *Decrease in:* gastrointestinal motility |
| $\kappa_1$ | dynorphin A; dynorphin B; $\alpha$-neoendorphin | Supraspinal analgesia; *Increased in:* diuresis |
| $\kappa_2$ | | |
| $\kappa_3$ | | Supraspinal analgesia |
| mu ($\mu$) | met-enkephalin; $\beta$-endorphin | *Increase in:* feeding, sedation |
| $\mu_1$ | | Supraspinal analgesia; *Decrease in:* acetylcholine release |
| $\mu_2$ | | Spinal analgesia; *Increase in:* growth hormone release; *Decrease in:* dopamine release, gastrointestinal motility, respiratory function |

**anterior r. of tympanic membrane,** recessus anterior membranae tympanicae.
**aorticomediastinal r.,** a small space between the ramifications of the left pulmonary artery and descending thoracic aorta, into which tissue of the left lung intrudes.
**azygoesophageal r.,** a small space between the azygos vein and the esophagus, into which tissue of the lower lobe of the right lung intrudes.
**azygomediastinal r.,** a small space between the azygos vein and mediastinum, into which tissue of the right lung intrudes.
**chiasmatic r.,** recessus opticus.
**facial r.,** a roughly triangular depression on the surface of the temporal bone, bounded on two sides by the facial nerve and with an apex at the external genu of the facial nerve. Called also *suprapyramidal r.*
**Hyrtl's r.,** recessus epitympanicus.
**infundibular r.,** recessus infundibuli.
**infundibuliform r.,** recessus pharyngeus.
**r. of interpeduncular fossa, anterior,** the portion of the interpeduncular fossa that passes under the corpora mammillaria; called also *Tarin's r.* and *Tarin's space.*
**r. of interpeduncular fossa, posterior,** the portion of the interpeduncular fossa that slightly undermines the anterior margin of the pons.
**laryngopharyngeal r.,** recessus piriformis.
**lateral r. of fourth ventricle,** recessus lateralis ventriculi quarti.
**lateral r. of nasopharynx,** recessus pharyngeus.
**r. of lesser omental cavity,** recessus splenicus.
**optic r.,** recessus supraopticus.
**paracolic r's,** sulci paracolici.
**r. of pelvic mesocolon,** recessus intersigmoideus.
**pharyngeal r., middle,** bursa pharyngealis.
**phrenicohepatic r's,** see *recessus subhepatici, recessus subphrenici,* and *recessus hepatorenalis.*
**pineal r.,** recessus pinealis.
**pleural r's,** recessus pleurales.
**posterior r. of tympanic membrane,** recessus posterior membranae tympanicae.
**Reichert's r.,** recessus cochlearis vestibuli.
**retroannular r.,** a deep groove formed by the cell membrane immediately behind the annulus of spermatozoa of some species.
**r. of Rosenmüller,** recessus pharyngeus.
**sacciform r. of articulation of elbow,** recessus sacciformis articulationis cubiti.
**saccular r.,** recessus sphericus vestibuli.
**sphenoethmoidal r.,** recessus spheno-ethmoidalis.
**subhepatic r's,** recessus subhepatici.
**subphrenic r's,** recessus subphrenici.
**superior r. of tympanic membrane,** recessus superior membranae tympanicae.
**supraoptic r.,** recessus supraopticus.
**suprapineal r.,** recessus suprapinealis.
**suprapyramidal r.,** facial r.
**supratonsillar r.,** fossa supratonsillaris.
**Tarin's r.,** anterior r. of interpeduncular fossa.
**triangular r.,** a small triangular recess sometimes found on the anterior wall of the third ventricle of the brain, with its base below the anterior commissure and its sides formed by the converging columns of the fornix.
**r's of Tröltsch,** see *recessus membranae tympani anterior* and *recessus membranae tympani posterior.*
**tubotympanic r.,** see under *canal.*
**utricular r.,** recessus ellipticus vestibuli.
**r's of vestibule,** see *recessus cochlearis vestibuli, recessus ellipticus vestibuli,* and *recessus sphericus vestibuli.*

**re·ces·sion** (re-sesh'ən) [L. *recedere* to draw back or away] the drawing away of a tissue or part from its normal position.
**angle r.,** recession of the angle of the anterior chamber of the eye; see also under *glaucoma.*
**gingival r.,** the drawing back of the gingivae from the necks of the teeth with exposure of root surfaces.
**r. of ocular muscle,** surgical displacement of the insertion of an ocular muscle posteriorly; done to weaken the stronger muscle in strabismus.

**re·ces·sive** (re-ses'iv) 1. tending to recede; not exerting a ruling or controlling influence; in genetics, incapable of expression unless the responsible allele is carried by both members of a pair of homologous chromosomes. 2. a recessive allele or trait.

**re·ces·sus** (re-ses'əs) pl. *reces'sus* [L.] [TA] a recess, *cavity, pocket,* or *pouch.*
**r. ante'rior membra'nae tympa'nicae** [TA], anterior recess of tympanic membrane: a pocket in the tympanic membrane formed by the tunica mucosa between the anterior mallear fold and the anterior superior part of the pars tensa of the membrane, ending blindly above.
**r. cochlea'ris vesti'buli** [TA], cochlear recess of vestibule: a small depressed area on the medial wall of the vestibule of the ear, situated just below the posterior end of the crista vestibuli, and perforated with foramina through which nerve fibers pass to the posterior portion of the ductus cochlearis. Called also *Reichert's recess.*
**r. costodiaphragma'ticus pleura'lis** [TA], costodiaphragmatic recess of pleura: the pleural recess situated at the junction of the costal and diaphragmatic pleurae; called also *sinus phrenicocostalis.*
**r. costomediastina'lis pleura'lis** [TA], costomediastinal recess of pleura: a wedge-shaped space, not completely filled with lung tissue, along the line at which the costal pleura meets the mediastinal pleura in front; called also *sinus costomediastinalis pleurae.*
**r. duodena'lis infe'rior** [TA], inferior duodenal recess: a pocket in

the peritoneum on the left side of the ascending portion of the duodenum, bounded by the inferior duodenal fold.
**r. duodena'lis supe'rior** [TA], **r. duodenojejuna'lis,** superior duodenal recess: a peritoneal pocket behind the superior duodenal fold.
**r. ellip'ticus vesti'buli** [TA], elliptical recess of the vestibule: an oval depressed area in the roof and medial wall of the vestibule of the inner ear, situated above and behind the crista and pierced by 25 to 30 small foramina through which nerves come from the internal acoustic meatus to the utricle, which occupies the depression. Called also *r. utricularis vestibuli* [TA alternative].
**r. epitympa'nicus** [TA], epitympanic recess: the portion of the tympanic cavity above the level of the tympanic membrane, containing the greater part of the incus and the upper half of the malleus. Called also *attic, epitympanum, epitympanic space,* and *Hyrtl's recess.*
**r. hepatorena'lis** [TA], hepatorenal recess: a peritoneal pouch between the liver and the kidney.
**r. ileocaeca'lis infe'rior** [TA], inferior ileocecal recess: a peritoneal pocket situated behind the ileocecal fold, above the vermiform appendix below the ileum, and medial to the cecum; also spelled *r. ileocecalis inferior.*
**r. ileocaeca'lis supe'rior** [TA], superior ileocecal recess: a peritoneal pocket situated behind and below the vascular cecal fold, above the ileum and medial to the lower end of the ascending colon; also spelled *r. ileocecalis superior.*
**r. ileoceca'lis infe'rior,** r. ileocaecalis inferior.
**r. ileoceca'lis supe'rior,** r. ileocaecalis superior.
**r. infe'rior bur'sae omenta'lis** [TA], inferior omental recess: the lower portion of the omental bursa, including its extension down into the great omentum. It is bounded in front by the posterior wall of the stomach, and behind by the pancreas, the transverse colon and its mesocolon, the left suprarenal gland, and part of the left kidney.
**r. infundibula'ris,** TA alternative for *r. infundibuli.*
**r. infundi'buli** [TA], infundibular recess: a funnel-shaped depression in the anterior part of the floor of the third ventricle of the brain, within the infundibulum of the hypophysis. Called also *r. infundibularis* [TA alternative].
**r. intersigmoi'deus** [TA], intersigmoidal recess: a shallow peritoneal pocket running downward and to the left at the base of the sigmoid mesocolon.
**r. latera'lis ventri'culi quar'ti** [TA], lateral recess of fourth ventricle: a narrow, curved prolongation of the cavity of the fourth ventricle of the brain, extending laterally onto the dorsal surface of the inferior cerebellar peduncle; it contains a lateral prolongation of the choroid plexus and provides for the passage of cerebrospinal fluid into the subarachnoid space.
**r. liena'lis,** TA alternative for *r. splenicus.*
**r. membra'nae tym'pani ante'rior,** r. anterior membranae tympanicae.
**r. membra'nae tym'pani poste'rior,** r. posterior membranae tympanicae.
**r. membra'nae tym'pani supe'rior,** r. superior membranae tympanicae.
**r. op'ticus,** recessus supraopticus.
**r. paraco'lici,** sulci paracolici.
**r. paraduodena'lis** [TA], paraduodenal recess: a pocket occasionally found in the peritoneum behind a fold containing a branch of the left colic artery.
**r. pharyn'geus** [TA], **r. pharyn'geus [Rosenmül'leri],** pharyngeal recess: a wide, slitlike lateral extension in the wall of the nasopharynx, cranial and dorsal to the pharyngeal orifice of the auditory tube; called also *Rosenmüller's cavity* or *fossa.*
**r. phrenicohepa'tici,** see *r. subhepatici, r. subphrenici,* and *r. hepatorenalis.*
**r. phrenicomediastina'lis pleura'lis** [TA], phrenicomediastinal recess of pleura: the pleural recess situated at the line of junction of the diaphragmatic and mediastinal pleurae.
**r. pinea'lis** [TA], pineal recess: an extension of the third ventricle into the stalk of the pineal body.
**r. pirifor'mis** [TA], piriform recess: a pear-shaped fossa in the wall of the laryngeal pharynx lateral to the arytenoid cartilage and medial to the lamina of the thyroid cartilage. Called also *piriform sinus.*
**r. pleura'les** [TA], pleural recesses: the spaces where the different portions of the pleura join at an angle and which are never completely filled by lung tissue; see *r. costodiaphragmaticus pleuralis, r. costomediastinalis pleuralis,* and *r. phrenicomediastinalis pleuralis.* Called also *sinus pleurae.*
**r. pneumatoente'ricus,** either of the paired embryonic excavations alongside the dorsal mesogastrium, the right one sometimes persisting as the infracardiac bursa.
**r. poste'rior membra'nae tympa'nicae** [TA], posterior recess of tympanic membrane: a pocket in the tympanic membrane formed by the tunica mucosa between the posterior mallear fold and the posterior superior part of the pars tensa of the membrane, ending blindly above.
**r. retrocaeca'lis** [TA], retrocecal recess: a peritoneal pocket extending upward behind the cecum and sometimes behind the colon; also spelled *r. retrocecalis.*
**r. retroceca'lis,** r. retrocaecalis.
**r. retroduodena'lis** [TA], retroduodenal recess: an occasional peritoneal pocket extending behind the horizontal and ascending parts of the duodenum.
**r. saccifor'mis articulatio'nis cu'biti** [TA], sacciform recess of articulation of elbow: the distal bulging of the articular capsule of the elbow joint, situated between the incisura radialis ulnae and the circumferentia articularis radii.
**r. saccifor'mis articulatio'nis radioulna'ris dista'lis** [TA], sacciform recess of distal radioulnar articulation: a bulging of the synovial membrane of the articular capsule of the distal radioulnar joint, which extends proximally between the radius and ulna beyond the point of their articular surfaces.
**r. saccula'ris vesti'buli,** TA alternative for *r. sphericus vestibuli.*
**r. sphenoethmoida'lis** [TA], sphenoethmoidal recess: the most superior and posterior part of the nasal cavity, above the superior nasal concha, into which the sphenoidal sinus opens.
**r. sphe'ricus vesti'buli** [TA], spherical recess of vestibule: a circular depressed area in the anteroinferior portion of the medial wall of the vestibule of the inner ear. It is pierced by 12 to 15 small foramina through which nerves come from the internal acoustic meatus to the saccule, which occupies the depression. Called also *r. saccularis vestibuli* [TA alternative].
**r. sple'nicus** [TA], splenic recess: an extension of the omental bursa to the left behind the gastrosplenic ligament almost to the spleen; called also *r. lienalis* [TA alternative].
**r. subhepa'tici** [TA], subhepatic recesses: peritoneal pockets located beneath the liver.
**r. subphre'nici** [TA], subphrenic recesses: peritoneal pockets located beneath the diaphragm.
**r. subpopli'teus** [TA], subpopliteal recess: a prolongation of the synovial tendon sheath of the popliteus muscle outside the knee joint into the popliteal space; called also *bursa musculi poplitei.*
**r. supe'rior membra'nae tympa'nicae** [TA], superior recess of tympanic membrane: a recess in the tympanic membrane formed by the tunica mucosa between the neck of the malleus and the pars flaccida of the membrane, and ending blindly below. Called also *Prussak's pouch* or *space.*
**r. supe'rior bur'sae omenta'lis** [TA], superior omental recess: a rather long, narrow peritoneal pocket leading from the vestibule upward toward the liver, between the inferior vena cava on the right, the esophagus on the left, the gastrohepatic ligament in front, and the diaphragm behind.
**r. supraop'ticus** [TA], supraoptic recess: a depression in the floor of the third ventricle of the brain, between the chiasma behind and the lamina terminalis in front. Called also *r. opticus* and *optic recess.*
**r. suprapinea'lis** [TA], suprapineal recess: the posterior extension of the third ventricle of the brain above and around the pineal body.
**r. utricula'ris vesti'buli, r. utri'culi vestibula'ris,** TA alternative for *r. ellipticus vestibuli.*

**re·cid·i·va·tion** (re-sid″ĭ-va′shən) relapse, recurrence, or repetition, as of a disease or condition or of a pattern of behavior, particularly a criminal act.

**re·cid·i·vism** (re-sid′ĭ-viz-əm) a tendency to relapse into a previous condition, disease, or pattern of behavior, particularly a return to criminal behavior.

**re·cid·i·vist** (re-sid′ĭ-vist) [Fr. *récidiviste,* from L. *recidere* to fall back] one who tends to relapse, especially a person who tends to return to criminal habits after treatment or punishment.

**rec·i·pe** (res′ĭ-pe) 1. [L.] take; used at the head of a physician's prescription, and usually indicated by the symbol ℞. See *prescription.* 2. a formula for the preparation of a specific combination of ingredients.

**re·cip·i·ent** (re-sip′e-ənt) one who receives, as blood in transfusion, or a tissue or organ graft.
**universal r.,** a person thought to be able to receive blood of any "type" without agglutination of the donor cells.

**re·cip·ro·ca·tion** (re-sip″ro-ka′shən) [L. *reciprocare* to move backward and forward] 1. to give and receive in exchange; the complementary interaction of two distinct entities. 2. in dentistry, the means by which one part of a removable partial denture framework is made to counter the effect created by another part of the framework.

**re·cir·cu·la·tion** (re-sər″ku-la′shən) in hemodialysis, circulation of part of the blood from the venous line to the arterial line, thus reducing concentration gradients across the dialyzer membranes, which reduces the efficiency of dialysis.

**Reck·ling·hau·sen's canals, disease, disease of bone** (rek′ling-hou″zenz) [Friedrich Daniel von *Recklinghausen,* German pathologist, 1833–1910] see under *canal,* and see *neurofibromatosis 1,* under *neurofibromatosis,* and *osteitis fibrosa cystica.*

**Reck·ling·hau·sen-Ap·ple·baum disease** (rek'ling-hou-zen-ahp'əl-boum) [F.D. von *Recklinghausen;* L. *Applebaum,* German physician, 20th century] hemochromatosis.

**re·cog·ni·tion** (rek"og-nĭ'shən) 1. the act of recognizing or state of being recognized. 2. antigen recognition; the interaction of immunologically competent cells with antigen that begins with the binding of the antigen to specific antigen receptors on B and T lymphocytes and results in an immune response directed against the antigen.

**re·coil** (re-koil') 1. to pull back quickly, such as towards a resting position upon removal of a strong opposing force. 2. (re'koil) a pulling back quickly.
**elastic r.,** the ability of a stretched elastic object or organ, such as the lung or bladder, to return to its resting position. See also *elastance.*

**re·com·bi·nant** (re-kom'bĭ-nənt) a cell or an individual with a new combination of genes not found together in either parent; usually applied to linked genes.
**r. DNA,** see under *DNA.*
**hGH-r.,** growth hormone recombinant; see *growth hormone,* under *hormone.*

**re·com·bi·na·tion** (re"kom-bĭ-na'shən) 1. the reunion, in the same or a different arrangement, of formerly united elements which have become separated. 2. in genetics, the formation of new combinations of genes as a result of crossing over between homologous chromosomes.
**bacterial r.,** in bacterial genetics, the process of producing a new gene by any of several processes, e.g., the sexual union of two parents, molecular crossing over between two DNA chains, or transformation.

**Re·com·bi·vax HB** (re-kom'bĭ-vaks") a trademark for a preparation of hepatitis B vaccine (recombinant).

**re·com·pres·sion** (re"kəm-presh'ən) the restoration of pressure, especially the return to conditions of normal pressure after exposure to greatly diminished atmospheric pressure.

**re·con·sti·tu·tion** (re"kon-stĭ-too'shən) 1. a type of regeneration in which a new organ forms by the rearrangement of tissues rather than from new formation at an injured surface. 2. the restoration to original form of a substance previously altered for preservation and storage, as the restoration to a liquid state of blood serum or plasma that has been dried and stored.

**re·con·struc·tion** (re"kən-struk'shən) 1. the act or process of reassembling or re-forming from constituent parts. 2. surgical restoration of function of a part, such as with a bypass or plastic surgery.
**aortic r.,** restoration of function to a damaged aorta, as by bypass or aortoplasty.
**arterial r.,** restoration of arterial blood supply to a part, as by a bypass, arterioplasty, or endarterectomy.
**image r. from projections,** radiography in which two- or three-dimensional images of an object are reconstructed from a set of mathematical projections, as in transverse axial tomography.
**venous r.,** restoration of venous drainage of a part, as by a graft or phleboplasty.

**re·con·tour** (re-kon'to͞or) 1. to give new shape or contour to. 2. in dentistry, to change the contour of a crown or a complete or partial denture.

**rec·ord** (rek'ord) 1. a permanent or long-lasting account of something (as on film, in writing, etc). 2. see *registration.*
**chew-in r., functional,** 1. a record of the natural chewing movements of the mandible made on the occlusion rim by the teeth or scribing studs. 2. a record of movements of the mandible made on the occluding surface of the opposing occlusion rim by the teeth or scribing studs; produced by simulated chewing movements. 3. a record of lateral and protrusive movements of the mandible made on the occlusal surface of the occlusion rim by the teeth or scribing studs on an opposing rim; produced during simulated movements of bruxism.
**face-bow r.,** a registration by means of a face-bow of the position of the hinge axis and/or the condyles; used to orient the maxillary cast to the opening and closing axis of the articulator.
**interocclusal r.,** a record of the positional relation of the teeth or jaws to each other, made on occlusal surfaces of occlusion rims or teeth in a plastic material which hardens, such as plaster of Paris, wax, or zinc oxide and eugenol paste.
**interocclusal r., centric,** a record of the centric jaw position (relation).
**interocclusal r., eccentric,** a record of a jaw relation other than the centric relation.
**interocclusal r., lateral,** a record of a lateral eccentric jaw position.
**interocclusal r., protrusive,** a record of a protruded eccentric jaw position.
**jaw relation r.,** a registration of any positional relationship of the mandible in reference to the maxillae; these records may be of any of the many vertical, horizontal, or orientation relations.
**maxillomandibular r.,** a record of the relation of the mandible to the maxillae. Called also *maxillomandibular registration.*
**occluding centric relation r.,** a registration of centric relation made at the established occlusal vertical dimension.
**problem-oriented r. (POR),** an approach to patient care record keeping that focuses on those specific health problems of the patient that require immediate attention and on the structuring of a cooperative health care plan designed to cope with the identified problems. The components basic to the POR are: *the data base,* which provides information obtained from the variety of sources required for each patient regardless of diagnosis or presenting problems; *the problem list,* which contains those major problems currently needing attention and serves as the basis of a plan of care; *the plan,* which specifies what is to be done with regard to each problem; *the progress notes,* which document the observations, assessments, nursing care plans, physician's orders, etc., of all health care personnel directly involved in the care of the patient. See also *SOAP.*
**profile r.,** a record showing the sagittal outline form or profile of the face.
**protrusive r.,** a registration of a forward position of the mandible with reference to the maxillae.
**terminal jaw relation r.,** a record of the relationship of the mandible to the maxilla made at the vertical relation of occlusion and at the centric position.

**rec·re·ment** (rek'rə-mənt) [L. *recrementum*] the saliva or other material which, after secretion, is reabsorbed into the blood.

**rec·re·men·ti·tious** (rek"rə-mən-tĭ'shəs) of the nature of a recrement.

**re·cru·des·cence** (re"kroo-des'əns) [L. *recrudescere* to become sore again] the recurrence of symptoms after a temporary abatement. See *relapse.* The chief distinction between a recrudescence and a relapse is the time interval, a recrudescence occurring after some days or weeks, a relapse after some weeks or months.

**re·cru·des·cent** (re"kroo-des'ənt) [L. *recrudescens*] breaking out afresh.

**re·cruit·ment** (re-kro͞ot'mənt) 1. the gradual increase to a maximum in a reflex when a stimulus of unaltered intensity is prolonged. 2. in audiology, an abnormally large increase in the perceived loudness of a sound caused by a slight increase in its intensity. 3. in muscle physiology, the orderly increase in number of activated motor units with increasing strength of voluntary muscle contractions. See also *recruitment pattern.*

**Rect.** abbreviation for L. *rectifica'tus,* rectified.

**rec·tal** (rek'təl) pertaining to the rectum.

**rec·tal·gia** (rek-tal'jə) [*rect-* + *-algia*] proctalgia.

**rec·tec·to·my** (rek-tek'tə-me) [*rect-* + *-ectomy*] proctectomy.

**rec·ti·fi·ca·tion** (rek"tĭ-fĭ-ka'shən) [L. *rectificatio*] 1. the act of making straight, pure, or correct. 2. redistillation of a liquid to purify it. 3. conversion of alternating current to direct current.
**spontaneous r.,** a transverse lie which rectifies itself before labor begins.

**rec·ti·fied** (rek"tĭ-fīd) refined; made straight; converted to direct current (DC).

**rec·ti·fi·er** (rek'tĭ-fi"ər) a device for obtaining a direct (unidirectional) current from an alternating current.
**thermionic r.,** a rectifier consisting of an electric valve in which the electrons are supplied by a heated electrode.

**rec·tis·chi·ac** (rek-tis'ke-ak) pertaining to the rectum and the ischium.

**rec·ti·tis** (rek-ti'tis) proctitis.

**rect(o)-** [L. *rectum*] a combining form designating relationship to the rectum. See also words beginning *proct(o)-.*

**rec·to·ab·dom·i·nal** (rek"to-ab-dom'ĭ-nəl) pertaining to the rectum and abdomen.

**rec·to·cele** (rek'to-sēl) [*recto-* + *-cele*[1]] hernial protrusion of part of the rectum into the vagina; called also *proctocele.*

**rec·to·coc·cy·ge·al** (rek"to-kok-sij'e-əl) pertaining to the rectum and the coccyx.

**rec·to·coc·cy·ge·us** (rek"to-kok-sij'e-əs) [L.] rectococcygeal; see under *musculus.*

**rec·to·coc·cy·pexy** (rek"to-kok'sĭ-pek-se) proctococcypexy.

**rec·to·co·li·tis** (rek"to-ko-li'tis) proctocolitis.

**rec·to·cu·ta·ne·ous** (rek"to-ku-ta'ne-əs) pertaining to the rectum and the skin.

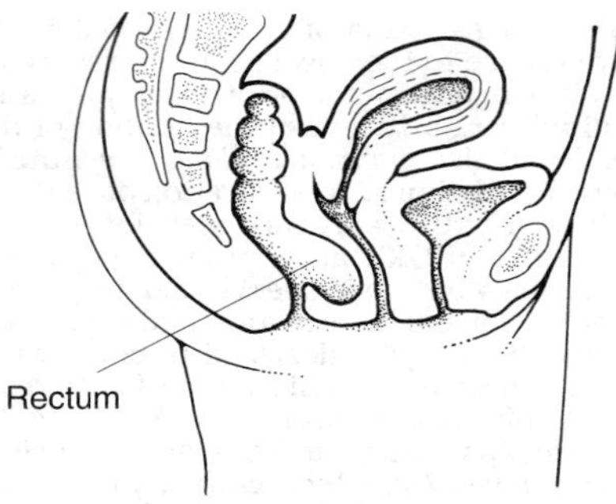

Rectocele.

**rec·to·cys·tot·o·my** (rek″to-sis-tot′ə-me) proctocystotomy.

**rec·to·la·bi·al** (rek″to-la′be-əl) pertaining to or communicating with the rectum and a labium majus, as a rectolabial fistula.

**rec·to·peri·ne·or·rha·phy** (rek″to-per″ĭ-ne-or′ə-fe) proctoperineorrhaphy.

**rec·to·pexy** (rek′to-pek″se) proctopexy.

**rec·to·plas·ty** (rek′to-plas″te) proctoplasty.

**rec·to·ro·mano·scope** (rek″to-ro-man′ə-skōp) proctosigmoidoscope.

**rec·to·ro·ma·nos·co·py** (rek″to-ro-mə-nos′kə-pe) [*recto-* + L. *romanum* sigmoid + *-scopy*] proctosigmoidoscopy.

**rec·tor·rha·phy** (rek-tor′ə-fe) [*recto-* + *-rrhaphy*] proctorrhaphy.

**rec·to·scope** (rek′to-skōp) proctoscope.

**rec·tos·co·py** (rek-tos′kə-pe) proctoscopy.

**rec·to·sig·moid** (rek″to-sig′moid) the rectum and sigmoid colon.

**rec·to·sig·moi·dec·to·my** (rek″to-sig″moi-dek′tə-me) excision of the rectum and sigmoid.

**rec·to·ste·no·sis** (rek″to-stə-no′sis) proctostenosis.

**rec·tos·to·my** (rek-tos′tə-me) proctostomy.

**rec·to·tome** (rek′to-tōm) proctotome.

**rec·tot·o·my** (rek-tot′ə-me) proctotomy.

**rec·to·ure·thral** (rek″to-u-re′thrəl) pertaining to or communicating with the rectum and urethra, as a rectourethral fistula.

**rec·to·uter·ine** (rek″to-u′tər-in) pertaining to the rectum and the uterus.

**rec·to·vag·i·nal** (rek″to-vaj′ĭ-nəl) pertaining to or communicating with the rectum and vagina, as a rectovaginal fistula.

**rec·to·ves·i·cal** (rek″to-ves′ĭ-kəl) pertaining to or communicating with the rectum and urinary bladder, as a rectovesical fistula. Called also *vesicorectal.*

**rec·to·ves·tib·u·lar** (rek″to-vəs-tib′u-lər) pertaining to or communicating with the rectum and the vestibule of the vagina, as a rectovestibular fistula.

**rec·to·vul·var** (rek″to-vul′vər) pertaining to or communicating with the rectum and vulva, as a rectovulvar fistula.

**Rec·tules** (rek′tūlz) trademark for a preparation of chloral hydrate.

**rec·tum** (rek′təm) [L. "straight"] [TA] [MeSH: Rectum] the distal portion of the large intestine, beginning anterior to the third sacral vertebra as a continuation of the sigmoid and ending at the anal canal; called also *intestinum rectum.*

**rec·tus** (rek′təs) [L.] straight; a general term denoting a straight structure, as a muscle (see entries beginning *musculus rectus*).

**re·cum·bent** (re-kum′bənt) lying down.

**re·cu·per·a·tion** (re-koo″pər-a′shən) [L. *recuperatio*] the recovery of health and strength.

**re·cur·rence** (re-kur′əns) [L. *re-* again + *currere* to run] [MeSH: Recurrence] the return of symptoms after a remission; see also *relapse* and *recrudescence.*

**re·cur·rent** (re-kur′ənt) [L. *recurrens* returning] 1. running back, or toward the source. 2. returning after remissions.

**re·cur·va·tion** (re″kər-va′shən) [L. *recurvatio*] a backward bending or curvature.

**red** (red) [L. *rubrum*] 1. one of the primary colors produced by the longest waves of the visible spectrum. 2. a red dye or stain.
**alizarin r.,** the sodium salt of alizarin monosulfonate.
**alizarin r. S, alizarin water-soluble r.,** sodium alizarinsulfonate.
**aniline r.,** basic fuchsin.
**basic r. 2,** safranin O.
**basic r. 9,** rosaniline.
**bordeaux r.,** cerasine.
**bromphenol r.,** an indicator, dibromphenolsulfonphthalein, used in determining hydrogen ion concentration, being yellow at pH 5.2 and red at pH 6.8. Written also *bromophenol r.*
**carmine r.,** a stain derived from carmine.
**cerasine r.,** Sudan III.
**chlorophenol r.,** a pH indicator with a range of 5.2 (yellow) to 6.8 (red).
**Congo r.,** an odorless, dark red or reddish brown powder which decomposes on exposure to acid fumes. It is used as a diagnostic aid in amyloidosis, and has been used as an antihemolytic and detoxicant. See also under *tests.*
**cotton r.,** safranin O.
**cotton r. B, cotton r. C,** Congo r.
**cotton r. 4 B,** benzopurpurine 4 B.
**cresol r.,** an indicator, ortho-cresol-sulfonphthalein, used in the determination of the hydrogen ion concentration. It has a pH range of 7.2 to 8.8, being yellow at 7.2 and red at 8.8.
**dianil r. 4 C, dianin r. 4 B,** benzopurpurine 4 B.
**direct r.,** Congo r.
**direct r. 4 B,** benzopurpurine 4 B.
**fast r. B** or **P,** cerasine.
**indigo r., indoxyl r.,** a coloring matter produced by heating an aqueous solution of indoxyl to 130°C.
**magdala r.,** a basic dye used for staining connective tissue. It is a mixture of monoamino- and diamino-naphthosafranins.
**methyl r.,** a dye, used as an indicator in the determination of hydrogen ion concentration; it has a pH range of 4.4 to 6, being red at 4.4 and yellow at 6.
**naphthaline r.,** magdala r.
**neutral r.,** a basic red fluorochrome dye used as a pH indicator with a range of 6.8 (red) to 8 (yellow) and as a stain in the supravital staining of blood.
**oil r.,** Sudan III.
**oil r. IV,** scarlet r.
**oil r. O,** a red diazo dye that is more soluble in fat than in water or alcohols; used as a stain for neutral fats.
**phenol r.,** phenolsulfonphthalein.
**provisional r.,** a colored lipin obtained from rhodopsin.
**scarlet r.,** a red fat-soluble azo dye, used as a biological stain for fats; it has some power to stimulate the proliferation of cells, and has been used to enhance wound healing. Called also *oil r. IV, ponceau 3B, scarlet R, scharlach R,* and *Sudan IV.*
**scarlet r. sulfonate,** the sodium salt of azo-benzene-disulfonic acid azobeta-naphthol; used for the same purpose as scarlet red.
**senitol r.,** a dye with a highly selective germicidal action on staphylococci; it is also used to sensitize photographic plates to red rays of light.
**Sudan r.,** magdala r.
**toluylene r.,** neutral r.
**tony r.,** Sudan III.
**trypan r.,** an acid azo dye used as a vital stain and which possesses some trypanocidal activity.
**vital r.,** a dye which is introduced directly into the circulation by venipuncture for the purpose of estimating the volume of the blood in the body by determining the concentration of the dye in the blood plasma.

**re·de·cus·sate** (re″de-kus′āt) to form a secondary decussation.

**red·foot** (red′foot) a fatal condition of unknown etiology affecting newborn lambs, in which the sensitive lamina of the feet become exposed owing to detachment of the overlying horn.

**re·dia** (re′de-ə) pl. *re′diae* [named after F. *Redi,* Italian naturalist, 1626–1698] a larval stage of certain trematode parasites, which develops in the body of a snail host and gives rise to daughter rediae, or to the cercariae.

**re·dif·fer·en·ti·a·tion** (re″dif-ər-en″she-a′shən) the return of a dedifferentiated tissue or part to its original or another more or less similar condition.

**Redig. in pulv.** abbreviation for L. *rediga′tur in pul′verem,* let it be reduced to powder.

**Red. in pulv.** abbreviation for L. *reduc′tus in pul′verem,* reduced to powder.

**red·in·te·gra·tion** (red-in″tə-gra′shən) [L. *redintegrare* to make whole again] 1. the restoration or repair of a lost or damaged part. 2. that type of psychic process in which a part of a complex stimulus revokes the complete reaction that was previously made to the complex stimulus as a whole. 3. reintegration (def. 2).

**re·dis·lo·ca·tion** (re″dis-lo-ka′shən) dislocation recurring after reduction.

**Red·i·sol** (red′ĭ-sol) trademark for a preparation of crystalline vitamin $B_{12}$; see *cyanocobalamin.*

**re·dox** (re′doks) oxidation-reduction.

**re·dresse·ment** (rə-dres-maw′) [Fr.] 1. a second or repeated dressing. 2. correction of a deformity.

**red tide** (red tīd) contamination of water with toxic species of *Gonyaulax.*

**re·duce** (re-do͞os′) [*re-* + L. *ducere* to lead] 1. to restore to the normal place or relation of parts, as to *reduce* a fracture. 2. in chemistry, to submit to reduction. 3. to decrease in weight.

**re·duced** (re-do͞ost′) 1. returned to the proper place or position, as a *reduced* fracture. 2. restored to a metallic form, as *reduced* iron. 3. altered by a chemical change involving a gain of electrons.

**re·du·ci·ble** (re-doo′sĭ-bəl) permitting of reduction; capable of being reduced.

**re·duc·tant** (re-duk′tənt) the electron donor in an oxidation-reduction (redox) reaction.

**re·duc·tase** (re-duk′tās) a term used in the recommended names of some enzymes of the oxidoreductase class [EC 1], usually denoting those catalyzing reactions physiologically important solely for reduction of a metabolite.
**5α-r.,** an enzyme that catalyzes the irreversible reduction of testosterone to dihydrotestosterone with NADPH as the hydrogen donor. Deficiency of the enzyme, with resultant deficiency in dihydrotestosterone, is an autosomal recessive condition characterized by male pseudohermaphroditism, prepubertal ambiguous or female-type external genitalia (usually some form of perineal hypospadias), and some masculinization at puberty without gynecomastia.

**re·duc·tion** (re-duk′shən) [L. *reductio*] 1. the correction of a fracture, dislocation, or hernia. 2. in chemistry, the addition of hydrogen to a substance, or more generally, the gain of electrons.
**r. of chromosomes,** the passing of the members of a chromosome pair to the daughter cells during meiosis, each daughter cell receiving half the diploid number.
**closed r.,** the manipulative reduction of a fracture or dislocation without incision.
**r. en masse,** reduction of a strangulated hernia included within its sac, so that the strangulation is not relieved.
**open r.,** reduction of a fracture or dislocation after incision into the site.
**weight r.,** the lessening of one's body weight by a specific regimen which is especially designed for that purpose.

**re·du·pli·ca·tion** (re″doo-plĭ-ka′shən) [L. *reduplicatio*] 1. a doubling back. 2. the recurrence of paroxysms of a double type. 3. a doubling of parts, connected at some point, the extra part being usually a mirror image of the other.

**re·du·vi·id** (re-du′vĭ-id) belonging to the family Reduviidae.

**Re·du·vi·i·dae** (re″du-vi′ĭ-de) a family of winged hemipterous insects of the suborder Heteroptera, including various biting species called cone-nose bugs, kissing bugs, and assassin bugs. Many inflict painful bites on humans and other mammals; some species transmit Chagas' disease. Genera include *Eratyrus, Eutriatoma, Melanolestes, Panstrongylus, Reduvius* (type genus), *Rhodnius,* and *Triatoma.*

**Re·du·vi·us** (re-du′ve-us) a genus of hemipterous blood-sucking insects. *R. persona′tus* has a painful bite that may cause nausea, urticaria, or other allergic symptoms.

**Re·dux** (re′duks) trademark for a preparation of dexfenfluramine hydrochloride.

**red·wa·ter** (red′waw-tər) 1. bovine babesiosis. 2. bacillary hemoglobinuria.

**Reed's cells** (rēdz) [Dorothy *Reed,* American pathologist, 1874–1964] Reed-Sternberg cells.

**Reed-Hodg·kin disease** (rēd-hoj′kin) [D. *Reed;* Thomas *Hodgkin,* English physician, 1798–1866] Hodgkin's disease.

**Reed-Stern·berg cells** (rēd-stərn′bərg) [D. *Reed;* Carl von *Sternberg,* Austrian pathologist, 1872–1935] [MeSH: Reed-Sternberg Cells] see under *cell.*

**reef** (rēf) an infolding or tuck of tissue, as a tuck made in plication.

**re·en·try** (re-en′tre) reexcitation of a region of cardiac tissue by a single impulse, continuing for one or more cycles and sometimes resulting in ectopic beats or tachyarrhythmias. It can exist over either an anatomical or a functional area of slowed impulse conduction and requires also refractoriness of tissue to stimulation and an area of unidirectional block to conduction. See also *reflection* and *reentrant mechanism,* under *mechanism.*
**anatomical r.,** reentry in which the block to conduction is an anatomical obstacle; it is usually described by the ring model.
**anisotropic r.,** reentry that is functional in not occurring around an anatomical obstacle but whose functional properties are conferred by the inherent structural anisotropy of the cardiac muscle fibers; thus it has qualities of both functional and anatomical reentry.
**atrial r.,** reentry in which the entire reentrant circuit lies within one or both atria, excluding the sinus node.
**functional r.,** reentry in which the block to conduction is due to functional heterogeneity of the electrophysiological properties of regions of cardiac tissue; it is usually described by the leading circle model.
**intra-atrial r.,** atrial r.
**reflected r.,** reflection, def. 4.
**sinus nodal r.,** reentry in which impulses traverse a reentrant circuit within or near the sinus node before being conducted to the rest of the heart.

**Rees' test** (rēs) [George Owen *Rees,* English physician, 1813–1889] see under *test.*

**re·fect** (re-fekt′) to induce refection.

**re·fec·tion** (re-fek′shən) [L. *reficere* to restore] recovery; repair: applied specifically to the ability of the flora of the cecum of rats to synthesize vitamins of the B group from deficient diets and supply them to the host animal.

**re·fec·tious** (re-fek′shəs) capable of causing, or pertaining to, refection.

**re·fine** (re-fīn′) to purify or free from foreign matter.

**re·flect·ed** (re-flek′təd) turned or bent back; mirrored.

**re·flec·tion** (re-flek′shən) [L. *reflexus,* past participle of *reflectere* to bend back] 1. a turning or bending back; a bending back upon its course. 2. in physics, the turning back of a ray of light, sound, or heat when it strikes against a surface that it does not penetrate. The ray before reflection is known as the *incident ray;* after reflection, it is the *reflected ray.* 3. an image produced by this process. 4. a special form of reentry in which an impulse crosses a narrow area of diminished responsiveness to excite distal tissue, pauses long enough for repolarization of proximal tissue, and returns, retracing its pathway and reexciting the same fibers in reverse rather than traversing a circuit. If the returning impulse is strong enough, a seesaw movement of current can result, causing tachyarrhythmias.
**pericardial r.,** a point or line of folding along which the lamina visceralis pericardii serosi (visceral pericardium) becomes the lamina parietalis pericardii serosi (parietal pericardium).

**re·flec·tor** (re-flek′tor) a device for reflecting light or sound.
**dental r.,** a mouth mirror used to reflect light on the field of action during a dental operation or examination.

**re·flex** (re′fleks) [L. *reflexus,* past participle of *reflectere* to bend back] [MeSH: Reflex] 1. reflected. 2. a reflected action or movement; the sum total of any particular involuntary activity. See *reflex arc* and *reflex action.* 3. a reflection or a reflected image of an object.

## Reflex

**abdominal r's,** contractions of the abdominal muscles on scratching of the abdominal wall.
**abdominocardiac r.,** any reflex in the heart produced by stimulating the abdominal sympathetic nerves. See also *Livierato's sign,* under *sign.*
**Abrams' heart r.,** contraction of the myocardium, with reduction in the area of cardiac dullness, which results when the skin of the precordial region is irritated. It is observed with the fluoroscope.
**accommodation r.,** the coordinated changes that occur when the eye adapts itself for near vision; they are constriction of the pupil, convergence of the eyes, and increased convexity of the lens.
**Achilles tendon r.,** triceps surae r.
**acoustic r.,** contraction of the stapedius muscle in response to intense sound. Called also *cochleostapedial r.* and *stapedial r.*
**acquired r.,** conditioned response.
**adductor r. of foot,** Hirschberg's sign.
**adductor r. of thigh,** on tapping the tendon of the adductor magnus with the thigh in abduction, contraction of the adductors results.

**allied r's,** reflexes in which two afferent stimuli use the same common pathway or produce effects on two synergistic muscles.

**anal r.,** contraction of the anal sphincter on scratching or other irritation of the skin of the anus.

**ankle r.,** triceps surae r.

**antagonistic r's,** reflex movements occurring not in the muscle which has been stretched but in its antagonist.

**anticus r.,** Piotrowski's sign.

**antigravity r's,** reflexes that keep the antigravity muscles in extension to hold the body upright.

**Aschner's r.,** oculocardiac r.

**atriopressor r.,** rise in arterial blood pressure (vasoconstriction) attributed to a change of pressure in the right atrium and great veins.

**attention r. of pupil,** alteration of size in the pupil when the attention is suddenly fixed; called also *Piltz's r.*

**attitudinal r's,** those reflexes having to do with the position of the body, primarily controlled by input from receptors in the utriculus; called also *statotonic r's.*

**audito-oculogyric r.,** a turning of both eyes in the direction of a sudden sound.

**auditory r.,** any reflex caused by stimulation of the auditory (vestibulocochlear) nerve, especially momentary closure of both eyes produced by a sudden sound.

**auricle r.,** involuntary movement of the auricle of the ear produced by auditory stimuli (more pronounced in some other animals than in humans).

**auriculocervical nerve r.,** Snellen's r.

**auriculopalpebral r.,** Kisch's r.

**autonomic r.,** a response of smooth muscle, glands, and conducting tissue of the heart, which alters the functional state of the innervated organ.

**axon r.,** a reflex resulting from a stimulus applied to one branch of a nerve which sets up an impulse that moves centrally to the point of division of the nerve where it is reflected down the other branch to the effector organ.

**Babinski's r.,** dorsiflexion of the big toe on stimulating the sole of the foot; normal in infants but in others a sign of a lesion in the central nervous system, particularly in the pyramidal tract. Called also *Babinski's phenomenon* or *sign* and *toe phenomenon* or *sign.*

**Babkin r.,** pressure by the examiner's thumbs on the palms of both hands of the infant results in opening of the infant's mouth; it is elicited in many newborn infants, normal and abnormal, except when lethargic or comatose.

**Bainbridge r.,** rise in pressure in, or increased distention of, the large somatic veins or the right atrium, results in acceleration of the heart beat.

**bar r.,** a pathological reflex in which movement of one leg is followed by similar movements of the other leg when the patient is recumbent; indicative of a lesion, often a tumor, in the prefrontal area.

**Barkman's r.,** contraction of the rectus abdominis muscle on the same side after stimulation of the skin just below one of the nipples.

**baroreceptor r.,** the reflex responses to stimulation of baroreceptors of the carotid sinus and aortic arch, regulating blood pressure by controlling heart rate, strength of heart contractions, and diameter of blood vessels.

**basal joint r.,** finger-thumb r.

**Bechterew's r.,** Bekhterev's r.

**behavior r.,** conditioned response.

**Bekhterev's r.,** 1. Bekhterev's deep r. 2. hypogastric r. 3. nasal r. 4. paradoxical pupillary r.

**Bekhterev's deep r.,** with corticospinal tract lesions, if the toes and foot are passively flexed in a plantar direction and then released, they will flex in a dorsal direction and the knees and hip will also flex.

**Bekhterev-Mendel r.,** Mendel-Bekhterev r.

**Bezold r., Bezold-Jarisch r.,** a cardiovascular reflex occurring upon stimulation of chemoreceptors, primarily in the left ventricle, by certain antihypertensive alkaloids and similar substances; afferent vagal fibers carry the impulses to the medulla oblongata, after which impulses carried back by efferent vagal fibers cause reflex bradycardia and hypotension.

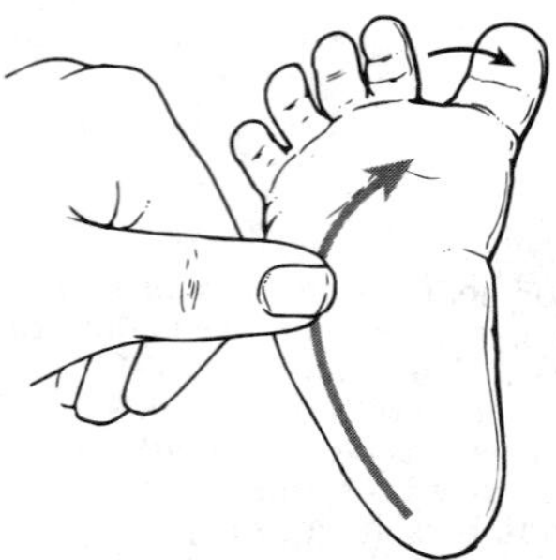

Babinski reflex.

**biceps r.,** contractions of the biceps muscle of the arm when its tendon is tapped; this reflex is normal but when greatly increased it indicates the same disease as increased knee jerk.

**bladder r.,** the reflex contracting and emptying of the bladder in response to filling, the first step in the micturition reflex; it can be voluntarily inhibited by impulses from the brain in patients with normal neurological function.

**blink r.,** 1. corneal r. (def. 1). 2. blink responses considered together.

**brachioradialis r.,** tapping on the lower end of the radius produces flexion of the forearm.

**Brain's r.,** an extension of the hemiplegic flexed arm when the patient assumes the quadrupedal position; called also *quadrupedal extensor r.*

**brain stem r's,** reflexes regulated at the level of the brain stem, such as pupillary, pharyngeal, and cough reflexes and the control of respiration. Their prolonged absence is one criterion of brain death.

**bregmocardiac r.,** pressure upon the bregmatic fontanelle slows the action of the heart.

**Brissaud's r.,** contraction of the tensor muscle of fascia lata on tickling the sole.

**Brudzinski's r.,** see under *sign.*

**bulbocavernosus r.,** bulbospongiosus r.

**bulbomimic r.,** in coma from apoplexy, pressure on the eyeball causes contraction of the facial muscles on the side opposite to the lesion; in coma from toxic causes, the reflex occurs on both sides. Called also *facial r.* and *Mondonesi's r.*

**bulbospongiosus r.,** contraction of the bulbospongiosus muscle in response to a tap on the dorsum of the penis; called also *penile* or *virile r.*

**carotid sinus r.,** pressure on, or in, the carotid artery at the level of its bifurcation causing reflex slowing of the heart rate; this reflex originates in the wall of the sinus of the internal carotid artery. See *carotid sinus syndrome,* under *syndrome.*

**cat's eye r.,** see under *amaurosis.*

**cerebral cortex r.,** Haab's r.

**Chaddock's r.,** stimulation below the external malleolus produces extension of the great toe; it occurs in lesions of the pyramidal tract.

**chain r.,** a series of reflexes, each serving as a stimulus to the next one, representing a complete activity.

**chin r.,** jaw r.

**choked r.,** in fluoroscopy, absence of movement of the retinal illumination on reaching the point of reversal.

**ciliary r.,** the movement of the pupil in accommodation.

**ciliospinal r.,** painful stimulation of the skin of the neck, face, or another body part dilates the ipsilateral pupil. Called also *Parrot's sign.*

**clasp-knife r.,** see under *rigidity.*

**closed loop r.,** a reflex, such as a stretch reflex, in which the stimulus (such as muscle stretch) decreases when it receives feedback from the response mechanism.

**cochleo-orbicular r., cochleopalpebral r.,** contraction of the orbicularis palpebrarum muscle when a sharp, sudden noise is made close to the ear; does not occur in total deafness from labyrinthine disease.

**cochleopupillary r.,** a reaction of the iris (contraction of the pupil followed by dilatation) to a loud sound.

**cochleostapedial r.,** acoustic r.

**cold pressor r.,** immersion of the hand in ice water for several minutes causes vasoconstriction, tachycardia, and transient hypertension due to activation of the sympathetic nervous system.

**concealed r.,** one elicited by a stimulus but concealed by a more dominant reflex elicited by the same stimulus.

**conditioned r.,** see under *response.*

**conjunctival r.,** closure of the eyelid when the conjunctiva is touched.

**consensual r.,** crossed r.

**consensual light r.,** stimulation of one eye by light produces a reflex response in the opposite pupil.

**convergency r.,** convergence of the visual axes with fixation on a near point.

**convulsive r.,** one in which several muscles contract convulsively without coordination.

**coordinated r.,** one in which several muscles react so as to produce an orderly and useful movement.

**corneal r.,** 1. irritation of the cornea results in reflex closure of the lids; called also *blink r., eyelid closure r.,* and *lid r.* 2. reflection of light from the cornea.

**corneomandibular r.,** movement of the lower jaw toward the side opposite the eye whose cornea is lightly touched, the mouth being open.

**corneomental r.,** unilateral wrinkling of the muscles of the chin when pressure is applied to the cornea.

**corneopterygoid r.**, corneomandibular r.
**coronary r.**, the reflex that controls the caliber of the coronary blood vessels.
**cough r.**, the sequence of events initiated by the sensitivity of the lining of the airways and mediated by the medulla as a consequence of impulses transmitted by the vagus nerve, resulting in coughing, i.e., the clearing of the passageways of foreign matter.
**cranial r.**, any reflex whose paths are connected directly with the brain.
**cremasteric r.**, stimulation of the skin on the front and inner side of the thigh retracts the testis on the same side. The presence of this reflex indicates integrity of the first lumbar nerve segment of the spinal cord or its root; absence indicates damage of the first lumbar nerve segment or its root or lesion of the corticospinal tract. Cf. *Geigel's r.* and *hypogastric r.*
**crossed r.**, a response on the side of the body opposite to the side being stimulated, such as the consensual light reflex or the crossed adductor reflex.
**crossed adductor r.**, adduction of one leg when an attempt is made to elicit the quadriceps jerk on the opposite side.
**crossed extension r.**, reflex extension of a limb or body part in response to a flexion reflex in the contralateral part.
**cuboidodigital r.**, Mendel-Bekhterev r.
**cutaneous pupillary r.**, ciliospinal r.
**dartos r.**, vermicular contractions of the dartos muscle when a cold or stroking stimulus is applied to the perineum; called also *scrotal r.*
**dazzle r.**, a reflex by which a strong light shining on the eyes causes an immediate closing of the eyelids which lasts as long as the stimulus.
**deep r.**, tendon r.
**defecation r.**, rectal r.
**delayed r.**, a reflex which occurs some time after the stimulus provoking it has been received.
**depressor r.**, a response to stimulation resulting in decreased motor activity.
**digital r.**, Hoffmann's sign (def. 2).
**direct light r.**, when a ray of light is thrown upon the retina through the pupil there is immediate contraction of the sphincter iridis, reducing the size of the pupillary aperture.
**diving r.**, a reflex involving cardiovascular and metabolic adaptations to conserve oxygen occurring in animals during diving into water; observed in reptiles, birds, and mammals, including man.
**doll's eye r.**, when the head is rotated laterally, the eyes deviate synergistically in the opposite direction; assessed in premature infants and the comatose to test for integrity of function of the oculomotor nerves and brain stem. Called also *Cantelli's sign* and *doll's eye sign.*
**dorsal r.**, contraction of the back muscles in response to stimulation of the skin over the erector spinae muscle; called also *erector spinae r.*
**dorsocuboidal r.**, Mendel-Bekhterev r.
**elbow r.**, triceps r.
**embrace r.**, Moro's r.
**emergency light r.**, excessive stimulation of the retina by light produces contraction of the pupils, closure of the eyelids, and lowering of the eyebrows.
**enterogastric r.**, inhibition of gastric motility when irritants enter the duodenum.
**epigastric r.**, contraction of the abdominal muscles caused by stimulating the skin of the epigastrium or over the fifth and sixth intercostal spaces near the axilla.
**Erben's r.**, slowing down of the pulse upon bending the head and trunk strongly forward, due to vagal excitability, called also *Erben's phenomenon* or *sign.*
**erector spinae r.**, dorsal r.
**Escherich's r.**, see under *sign.*
**esophagosalivary r.**, excessive salivation due to irritation of the esophagus, as by a tumor or gastroesophageal reflux; called also *Roger's r.*
**external auditory meatus r.**, Kisch's r.
**eyeball compression r., eyeball-heart r.**, oculocardiac r.
**eyelid closure r.**, 1. corneal r. (def. 1). 2. conjunctival r.
**facial r.**, bulbomimic r.
**faucial r.**, reflex vomiting caused by irritation of the fauces, cf. *pharyngeal r.*
**femoral r.**, Remak's r.
**finger-thumb r.**, passive flexion of the metacarpophalangeal joint of one of the fingers causes flexion of the basal joint and extension of the terminal joint of the thumb; called also *basal joint r.* and *Mayer's r.*
**flexion r.**, a reflex that results in movement of a limb or part toward the body, often in response to a painful stimulus; it may cause a crossed extension reflex in the contralateral body part.
**flexor r., paradoxical,** dorsiflexion of the great toe or of all the toes when the deep muscles of the calf are pressed upon, seen in cases of pyramidal tract disease; called also *Gordon's r.*
**fontanelle r.**, Grünfelder's r.
**foveal r.**, the dotlike reflex of light caused by the foveola retinae, seen during ophthalmoscopy.
**front-tap r.**, a tap on the skin muscles of the extended leg contracts the gastrocnemius.
**fundus r.**, red r.
**fusion r.**, the reflex which tends to merge the images on the two retinas into a single impression.
**gag r.**, pharyngeal r.
**gastrocolic r.**, an increase in intestinal and colonic peristaltic activity following entrance of food into the empty stomach.
**gastroileal r.**, an increase in ileal motility and opening of the ileocecal valve when food enters the empty stomach.
**gastropancreatic r.**, an increase in pancreatic secretion induced by distention of the corpus of the stomach; it is mediated by the vagus nerve.
**Gault's cochleopalpebral r.**, cochleopalpebral r.
**Geigel's r.**, a reflex in the female corresponding to the cremasteric reflex in the male; i.e., on stroking of the inner anterior aspect of the upper thigh there is a contraction of the muscular fibers at the upper edge of Poupart's ligament; cf. *hypogastric r.* Called also *inguinal r.*
**Gifford's r., Gifford-Galassi r.**, orbicularis pupillary r.
**gluteal r.**, a stroke over the skin of the buttock contracts the glutei muscles.
**Gordon's r.**, flexor r., paradoxical.
**grasp r., grasping r.**, a reflex consisting of a grasping motion of the fingers or of the toes in response to stimulation; normal in infancy, but in later life indicative of a frontal lobe lesion.
**Grünfelder's r.**, dorsal flexion of the great toe with a fanwise spreading of the other toes elicited by continued pressure at the corner of the posterior lateral fontanelle; normal in infants but a sign of middle ear disease in older children.
**gustolacrimal r.**, syndrome of crocodile tears.
**H-r.**, a monosynaptic reflex elicited by stimulating a nerve, particularly the tibial nerve, with an electric shock. See also *H wave.*
**Haab's r.**, bilateral pupillary contraction when the patient sits in a darkened room, and without accommodation or convergence directs attention to a bright object already within the field of vision. Called also *cerebral cortex r.*
**heart r.**, Abrams' heart r.
**heel-tap r.**, a reflex occurring in disease of the pyramidal tract and consisting of fanning and plantar flexion of the toes produced by tapping the patient's heel.
**hepatojugular r.**, incorrect term for *hepatojugular reflux.*
**Hering-Breuer r.**, the nervous mechanism that tends to limit respiratory excursions. Stimuli from the sensory endings in the lungs and perhaps in other parts passing up the vagi tend to limit both inspiration and expiration in ordinary breathing.
**Hirschberg's r.**, see under *sign.*
**Hoffmann's r.**, Hoffmann's sign (def. 2).
**Hughes' r.**, virile r. (def. 2).
**hypochondrial r.**, sudden inspiration caused by quick pressure beneath the lower border of the ribs.
**hypogastric r.**, contraction of the muscles of the lower abdomen on stroking the skin of the inner surface of the thigh; cf. *cremasteric r.* and *Geigel's r.* Called also *Bekhterev's r.*
**ileogastric r.**, inhibition of gastric motility by distention of the ileum.
**inborn r.**, unconditioned response.
**indirect r.**, crossed r.
**infraspinatus r.**, tapping a spot over the shoulder blade on a line bisecting the angle formed by the spine of the bone and its inner border causes outward rotation of the arm and straightening of the elbow.
**inguinal r.**, Geigel's r.
**interscapular r.**, a stimulus applied between the scapulae contracts the scapular muscles; called also *scapular r.*
**intestinointestinal r.**, when a part of the intestine becomes overdistended or its mucosa becomes excessively irritated, activity in other parts of the intestine is inhibited as long as the distention persists.
**inverted radial r.**, a flexion of the fingers without movement of the forearm, produced by tapping the lower end of the radius; it indicates disease of the fifth cervical segment of the spinal cord associated with damage of the pyramidal tract below that level.
**iris contraction r.**, pupillary r.
**ischemic r.**, the elevation of arterial pressure in response to cerebral ischemia.
**jaw r., jaw jerk r.**, closure of the mouth caused by a downward blow on the lower jaw while it hangs passively open. It is seen only rarely in health, but is very noticeable in lesions of the corticospinal tract. Called also *jaw jerk, chin r.,* and *mandibular r.*
**Joffroy's r.**, twitching of the gluteal muscles on pressure against the buttocks in spastic paralysis.
**Juster r.**, extension of the fingers instead of flexion on stimulation of the palm.

**juvenile r.,** a glistening white reflection from the smooth surface of the retina in young people.
**Kehrer's r., Kisch's r.,** closure of the eye as a result of tactile or thermal stimulation of the deepest part of the external auditory meatus and tympanum.
**knee jerk r.,** patellar r.
**Kocher's r.,** contraction of the abdominal muscle on compression of the testicle; called also *testicular compression r.*
**labyrinthine r's,** vestibular r's.
**lacrimal r.,** secretion of tears elicited by touching or otherwise irritating the conjunctiva or the cornea.
**Landau r.,** when an infant is held in the prone position, the entire body forms a convex upward arc; gentle pressure on the head or gravity flexes the neck and hip, reversing the arc.
**laryngeal r.,** a type of cough reflex in which irritation of the fauces and larynx causes cough.
**laughter r.,** laughter brought on by tickling.
**let-down r.,** the ejection or release of milk from the alveoli of the breast into the ducts, caused by a combination of neurogenic and hormonal reflexes involving the hormone oxytocin and, to a lesser extent, vasopressin; called also *milk ejection r.* and *milk let-down r.*
**lid r.,** corneal r. (def. 1).
**Liddell and Sherrington r.,** stretch r.
**light r.,** 1. cone of light. 2. a circular spot of light seen reflected from the retina with the retinoscopic mirror. 3. pupillary r. (def. 1).
**lip r.,** a reflex movement of the lips of sleeping babies which occurs on tapping near the angle of the mouth.
**local r.,** a reflex whose arc does not pass through the spinal cord, such as occurs in the enteric nervous system. See also *intramural plexus,* under *plexus.*
**Lovén r.,** general vasodilatation of an organ when its afferent nerve is stimulated; this secures a maximal supply of blood to the organ, together with a general rise of blood pressure.
**lumbar r.,** dorsal r.
**Lust's r.,** see under *phenomenon.*
**McCarthy's r.,** supraorbital r.
**McCormac's r.,** patelloadductor r.
**McDowall r.,** a decrease in systemic blood pressure following vagotomy, due to abolishment of the afferent impulses from the atria, which normally induce vasoconstriction.
**macular r.,** in ophthalmoscopy, an annular reflection of light surrounding the macula retina.
**Magnus and de Kleijn neck r's,** extension of both ipsilateral limbs, or one, or part of a limb, and increase of tonus on the side to which the chin is turned when the head is rotated to the side, and flexion with loss of tonus on the side to which the occiput points; a sign of decerebrate rigidity except in infants. See also *tonic neck r.*
**mandibular r.,** jaw r.
**Marinesco-Radovici r.,** palm-chin r.
**mass r.,** in severe injury of the spinal cord, stimulation below the level of the lesion produces flexion reflexes of the lower extremity, evacuation of the bowels and bladder, and sweating of the skin below the level of the lesion. Called also *Riddoch's mass r.*
**Mayer's r.,** finger-thumb r.
**Mendel's r., Mendel's dorsal r. of foot,** Mendel-Bekhterev r.
**Mendel-Bekhterev r.,** percussion of the dorsum of the foot normally causes dorsal flexion of the second to fifth toes; in certain organic nervous conditions it causes plantar flexion of the toes. Called also *Bekhterev-Mendel r., cuboidodigital r., dorsocuboidal r., Mendel's r., Mendel's dorsal r. of foot,* and *tarsophalangeal r.*
**micturition r.,** any of the reflexes necessary for effortless evacuation of urine and subconscious maintenance of continence: vesical contraction following distention of the bladder, vesical contraction evoked by urethral flow, vesical contraction evoked by proximal urethral distention, relaxation of the urethra resulting from running liquid in the urethra, distention of the bladder resulting in relaxation of the external sphincter, relaxation of the proximal urethral smooth muscle by distention of the bladder, and vesical contraction related to running liquid through the urethra.
**milk ejection r., milk let-down r.,** let-down r.
**Mondonesi's r.,** bulbomimic r.
**Morley's peritoneocutaneous r.,** when any of the cerebrospinal nerve endings in the peritoneum or subperitoneal tissues are irritated, pain will be referred to the corresponding segmental skin area.
**Moro's r., Moro embrace r.,** flexion of an infant's thighs and knees, fanning and then clenching of the fingers, with arms first thrown outward then brought together as if in an embrace, produced by a sudden stimulus such as the table being struck next to the child, or by sudden extension of the neck when the head is allowed to fall backward or the child is pulled up by both hands from a lying position and then let go. It is seen normally in infants up to 3 to 4 months of age. Called also *embrace r.* and *startle r.*
**muscular r.,** stretch r.
**myenteric r.,** peristaltic r.

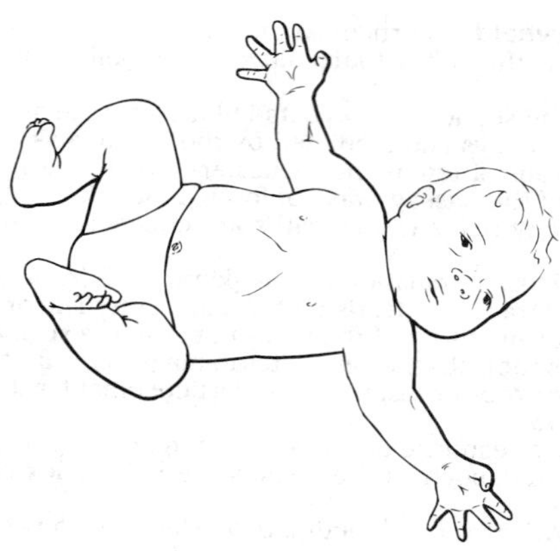

Moro's reflex.

**myopic r.,** Weiss' r.
**myotatic r.,** stretch r.
**nasal r.,** tickling of the mucosa of the nasal cavity produces contraction of the facial muscles on the same side of the face; called also *Bekhterev's r.*
**nasolabial r.,** sudden retroversion of the head, stretching of the back, retroversion of the arms at the shoulder, extension and pronation of the forearms, and extension and adduction of the legs, elicited by a slight vertical sweeping motion touching the tip of the nose; it frequently occurs in healthy infants, and disappears around the fifth month of age.
**nasomental r.,** contraction of the mentalis muscle on tapping the side of the nose with a percussion hammer.
**neck r's,** reflex adjustments in trunk posture and limb position caused by stimulation of proprioceptors in the neck joints and muscles when the head is turned; this tends to maintain a constant orientation between the head and the body.
**neck righting r.,** rotation of the trunk in the direction in which the head of the supine infant is turned; this reflex is absent or decreased in infants with spasticity.
**nociceptive r's,** reflexes initiated by painful stimuli.
**obliquus r.,** stimulation of the skin below Poupart's ligament contracts a part of the external oblique muscle.
**oculoauricular r.,** slight flattening of the pinna of one ear against the skull when the eyes deviate strongly to the opposite side. Absence on one side indicates facial nerve palsy at or proximal to the stylomastoid foramen.
**oculocardiac r.,** a slowing of the rhythm of the heart following compression of the eyes. A slowing of from 5 to 13 beats per minute is normal; one of from 13 to 50 or more is exaggerated; one of from 1 to 5 is diminished. If ocular compression produces acceleration of the heart, the reflex is called *inverted.* Called also *Aschner's r.* or *phenomenon.*
**oculocephalogyric r.,** the reflex by which the movements of the eye, the head, and the body are directed in the interest of visual attention.
**oculopharyngeal r.,** rapid deglutition together with spontaneous closing of the eyes in response to irritation of the conjunctiva.
**oculopupillary r.,** stimulation of the cornea or of the eyelid results in dilation and then contraction of both pupils; called also *oculosensory r.* and *trigeminus r.*
**oculosensory r.,** oculopupillary r.
**oculovagal r.,** pressure on the eyeball induces ectopic atrioventricular beats or rhythm.
**open loop r.,** a reflex, such as a flexion reflex, in which the stimulus causes activity that it does not further control and that does not give it feedback.
**Oppenheim's r.,** dorsiflexion of the big toe on stroking downward along the medial side of the tibia, seen in pyramidal tract disease.
**opticofacial winking r.,** closure of the lids when an object is brought suddenly into the field of vision.
**orbicularis r.,** orbicularis pupillary r.
**orbicularis oculi r.,** normal contraction of the orbicularis oculi muscle, with resultant closing of the eye, on percussion at the outer aspect of the supraorbital ridge, over the glabella, or around the margin of the orbit.
**orbicularis pupillary r.,** unilateral contraction of the pupil, followed by dilatation after closure or attempted closure of eyelids that are forcibly held apart. Called also *Galassi's pupillary, orbicularis,* or *Westphal-Piltz phenomenon* and *Gifford's, Gifford-Galassi,* or *Westphal's pupillary r.*
**orienting r.,** the response of an animal to an unexpected or novel

stimulus or alteration of a stimulus; it involves adjustments of head, body, or sensory organs to pay close attention to the stimulus. In higher vertebrates including humans it is mediated at the brain stem level. Called also *orienting response.*

**palatal r., palatine r.,** stimulation of the palate causes swallowing; called also *swallowing r.*

**palmar r.,** flexion of the fingers in response to scratching of the palm.

**palm-chin r., palmomental r.,** twitching of the chin produced by stimulating (scratching) the palm; called also *Marinesco-Radovici r.* and *Radovici's sign.*

**paradoxical pupillary r.,** 1. reversed pupillary r. 2. dilatation of the pupil on exposure to light; sometimes seen in conditions such as tabes dorsalis. Called also *Bekhterev's r.* and *paradoxical pupillary phenomenon.*

**patellar r.,** contraction of the quadriceps and extension of the leg when the patellar ligament is tapped; called also *knee jerk, quadriceps jerk,knee jerk r.,* and *quadriceps r.*

**patelloadductor r.,** crossed adduction of the thigh produced by tapping the quadriceps tendon as in the patellar reflex; called also *McCormac's r.*

**pathologic r.,** one which is not normal, but is the result of a pathologic condition, and may serve as a sign of disease.

**pectoral r.,** the subject's arm is placed half way between adduction and abduction and the examiner's finger in the muscle tendon near the humerus: a sharp blow of the finger elicits adduction and slight internal rotation.

**penile r., penis r.,** bulbospongiosus r.

**perianal r.,** anal r.

**periosteal r.,** contraction of a muscle after tapping of a nearby bone that lies just below the surface of the skin; see *radial r., tibioadductor r.* and *ulnar r.*

**peristaltic r.,** when a portion of the intestine is irritated or distended, the area just proximal contracts and the area just distal relaxes.

**peritoneointestinal r.,** inhibition of motility of the stomach and intestine resulting from retroperitoneal irritation or hemorrhage.

**pharyngeal r.,** contraction of the constrictor muscle of the pharynx elicited by touching the back of the pharynx; called also *gag r.*

**phasic r.,** coordinated r.

**Philippson's r.,** excitation of the knee extensor in one leg induced by inhibition in the knee extensor of the other leg.

**pilomotor r.,** the production of goose flesh on stroking the skin; trichographism.

**Piltz's r.,** attention r. of pupil.

**placing r.,** flexion followed by extension of the leg when the infant is held erect and the dorsum of the foot is drawn along the under edge of a table top; it is obtainable in the normal infant up to the age of six weeks.

**plantar r.,** irritation of the sole contracts the toes; cf. *Babinski's r.*

**platysmal r.,** contraction of the pupil upon nipping of the platysma.

**pollicomental r.,** palm-chin r.

**postural r.,** a reflex which consists of some assumption of posture.

**pressor r.,** a reflex that increases the blood pressure.

**Preyer's r.,** auricle r.

**proprioceptive r.,** a reflex that is initiated by a stimulus to a proprioceptor.

**psychic r.,** a reflex aroused by a stored-up impression of memory, such as the secretion of saliva at the sight or thought of good-tasting food.

**psychocardiac r.,** increase in the pulse rate on recalling an individual emotional experience.

**psychogalvanic r.,** galvanic skin response.

**pulmonocoronary r.,** reflex vasoconstriction of the coronary arteries, mediated by the vagus nerves, such as with a pulmonary embolism.

**pupillary r.,** 1. contraction of the pupil on exposure of the retina to light. Called also *light r.* 2. any reflex involving the iris, changing the size of the pupil in response to a stimulus, e.g., change in illumination, change in point of fixation, sudden loud noise, or emotional stimulus.

**Puusepp's r.,** abduction of the little toe on stimulating the posterior external part of the sole of the foot; indicative of lesions of the extrapyramidal and pyramidal tracts.

**quadriceps r.,** patellar r.

**quadrupedal extensor r.,** Brain's r.

**radial r.,** flexion of the forearm, following tapping on the lower end of the radius; when the fingers flex as well, it indicates hyperreflexia.

**rectal r.,** the process by which the accumulation of feces in the rectum excites defecation; called also *defecation r.*

**rectoanal inhibitory r.,** relaxation of the internal anal sphincter in response to increased pressure in the rectum; it can be tested by inflating a balloon in the lumen. It is absent in cases of congenital megacolon.

**red r.,** a luminous red appearance seen upon the retina during retinoscopy; called also *fundus r.*

**regional r.,** segmental r.

**Remak's r.,** plantar flexion of the first three toes and sometimes of the foot, with extension of the knee on stroking of the upper anterior surface of the thigh, a sign of a spinal cord lesion; called also *femoral r.*

**renointestinal r.,** inhibition of motility of the intestine resulting from renal irritation.

**renorenal r.,** a reflex pain or anuria in a sound kidney in cases in which the other kidney is diseased.

**retrobulbar pupillary r.,** slight dilation of the pupil, which contracts under light stimulation and then dilates while the light stimulation is still present.

**reversed pupillary r.,** any abnormal *pupillary r.* opposite to that which occurs normally; e.g., stimulation of the retina by light dilates the pupil. Called also *paradoxical pupillary r.* or *phenomenon.*

**Riddoch's mass r.,** mass r.

**righting r.,** the ability to assume optimal position when there has been a departure from it.

**Roger's r.,** esophagosalivary r.

**rooting r.,** a reflex in the newborn in which stimulation of the side of the cheek or the upper or lower lip causes the infant to turn his mouth and face to the stimulus.

**Rossolimo's r.,** on tapping the plantar surface of the toes, plantar flexion of the toes occurs when there are lesions of the pyramidal tract.

**Ruggeri's r.,** acceleration of the pulse following strong convergence of the eyeballs toward something very close to the eyes; it indicates sympathetic excitability.

**Saenger's r.,** see under *sign.*

**scapular r.,** interscapular r.

**scapulohumeral r.,** adduction with outward rotation of the humerus produced by percussing along the inner edge of the scapula.

**Schäffer's r.,** dorsiflexion of the great toe on pinching the Achilles tendon at its middle third; seen in organic hemiplegia.

**scratch r.,** a spinal reflex by which an itch or other irritation of the skin causes a nearby body part to move over and briskly rub the affected area.

**scrotal r.,** dartos r.

**segmental r.,** a reflex controlled by a single segment or region of the spinal cord.

**senile r.,** a gray reflection from the pupil of aged people due to hardening of the lens.

**sexual r.,** the reflex of erection and ejaculation produced by stimulation of the genitals.

**shot-silk r.,** shot-silk retina.

**simple r.,** a reflex involving a single muscle.

**skin r.,** a reflex occurring on stimulation of the skin.

**skin pupillary r.,** ciliospinal r.

**Snellen's r.,** unilateral congestion of the ear upon stimulation of the distal end of the divided great auricular nerve; called also *auriculocervical nerve r.*

**sole r.,** plantar r.

**somatointestinal r.,** inhibition of intestinal motility when the skin over the abdomen is stimulated.

**spinal r.,** any reflex whose arc is connected with a center in the spinal cord.

**stapedial r.,** acoustic r.

**startle r.,** 1. Moro's r. 2. see under *reaction.*

**static r.,** any of the reflexes for maintenance of position and righting of the body, such as the *postural reflex, righting reflex,* or *vestibular reflexes.*

**statotonic r's,** attitudinal r's.

**stepping r.,** 1. movements of progression elicited when the infant is held upright and inclined forward with the soles of the feet touching a flat surface; it is obtainable in the normal infant up to the age of six weeks. 2. extension of the hind leg of a dog when the plantar surface of the foot is pressed.

**Stookey's r.,** with the leg semiflexed at the knee, the tendons of the semimembranosus and the semitendinosus muscles are tapped: flexion of the leg results.

**stretch r.,** reflex contraction of a muscle in response to passive longitudinal stretching; called also *Liddell and Sherrington r.* and *myotatic r.* See also *muscle spindle,* under *spindle.*

**Strümpell's r.,** leg movement with adduction of the foot produced by stroking the thigh or abdomen.

**sucking r.,** sucking movements of the mouth elicited by the touching of an object to an infant's lips.

**superficial r.,** any withdrawal reflex elicited by noxious or tactile stimulation of the skin, cornea, or mucous membrane, including the corneal reflex, pharyngeal reflex, cremasteric reflex, etc.

**supinator longus r.,** brachioradialis r.

**supraorbital r.,** contraction of the orbicularis oculi muscle on tapping the supraorbital nerve; called also *McCarthy's r.*

**suprapatellar r.**, with the subject's leg extended the index finger of the examiner is crooked above the patella and is struck; the result is a kick-back of the patella.
**suprapubic r.**, stroking the abdomen above Poupart's ligament causes deviation of the linea alba toward the side that is stroked.
**supraumbilical r.**, epigastric r.
**swallowing r.**, palatal r.
**tapetal light r.**, the glowing of eyes in the dark, as occurs in some carnivorous animals.
**tarsophalangeal r.**, Mendel-Bekhterev r.
**tendon r.**, involuntary contraction of a muscle after brief stretching caused by percussion of its tendon; tendon reflexes include the biceps reflex, triceps reflex, quadriceps reflex, and others. Called also *deep r.* and *tendon jerk* or *reaction*.
**testicular compression r.**, Kocher's r.
**threat r.**, sudden closure of the eyes at a sign of danger.
**Throckmorton's r.**, a variation of the Babinski reflex elicited by percussion of the metatarsophalangeal region in the dorsum of the foot.
**tibioadductor r.**, tapping of the tibia on the inner side of the leg results either in homolateral adduction of the leg or crossed adduction from side to side.
**toe r.**, strong flexion of the great toe flexes all the muscles of the lower extremity in pathologic states accompanied by hyperreflexia.
**tonic r.**, 1. one in which an appreciable period of time passes between muscle contraction and relaxation. 2. a reflex which maintains the reflex contractions that are the basis of posture and attitude.
**tonic neck r.**, a reflex in the newborn consisting of extension of the arm and sometimes of the leg on the side to which the head is forcibly turned, with flexion of the contralateral limbs; cf. *Magnus and de Kleijn neck r's.*
**trained r.**, conditioned response.
**triceps r.**, contraction of the belly of the triceps muscle and slight extension of the arm when the tendon of the muscle is tapped directly, with the arm flexed and fully supported and relaxed. Called also *elbow r.* or *jerk*.
**triceps surae r.**, plantar flexion of the foot caused by a twitchlike contraction of the triceps surae muscle, elicited by a tap on the Achilles tendon preferably while the patient kneels on a bed or chair, the feet hanging free over the edge; called also *Achilles jerk, ankle jerk, triceps surae jerk, Achilles tendon r.,* and *ankle r.*
**trigeminus r.**, oculopupillary r.
**ulnar r.**, tapping of the styloid process of the ulna results in pronation of the hand.
**unconditioned r.**, see under *response*.
**urinary r.**, micturition r.
**vagus r.**, abnormal sensitiveness to pressure over the course of the vagus nerve.
**vascular r., vasopressor r.**, vasoconstriction with a rise in blood pressure caused by neural stimulation.
**vertebra prominens r.**, pressure upon the last cervical vertebra of an animal reduces the tone of all four limbs.
**vesical r.**, bladder r.
**vesicointestinal r.**, inhibition of intestinal motility due to irritation of the bladder.
**vestibular r's**, the reflexes for maintaining the position of the eyes and body in relation to changes in orientation of the head; the neural pathways are complex, traveling from the vestibular nerve to the vestibular nuclei and thence to the involved muscles of the eye and body; cf. *static r.*

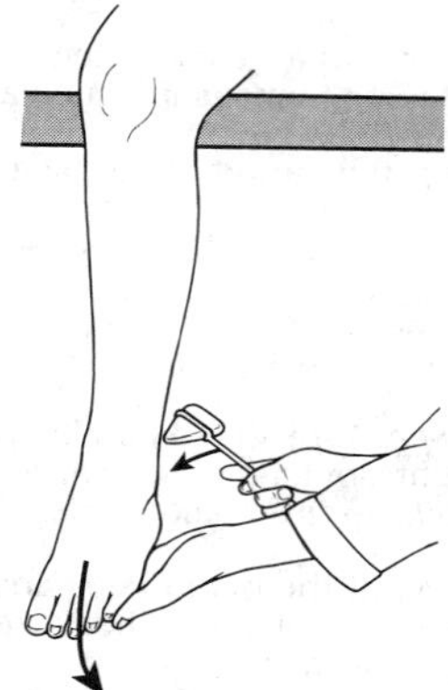

Triceps surae reflex.

**vestibulo-ocular r.**, nystagmus or deviation of the eyes in response to stimulation of the vestibular system by angular acceleration or deceleration or when the caloric test is performed (irrigation of the ears with warm or cool water or air). See *caloric test* and *harmonic acceleration test*, under *test*.
**virile r.**, 1. bulbospongiosus r. 2. in the flaccid penis, a sudden reflexive downward jerk elicited by pulling upward the foreskin or glans penis. Called also *Hughes' r.*
**visceral r.**, that in which the stimulus is set up by some state of an internal organ.
**viscerocardiac r.**, reflex alteration in cardiac rhythm or contractility caused by visceral excitation.
**visceromotor r.**, contraction of abdominal muscles (abdominal rigidity) over a diseased viscus.
**viscerosensory r.**, a response or reaction to pressure on some part of the body due to disease of some internal organ.
**viscerotrophic r.**, degeneration of any peripheral tissue as a result of chronic inflammation of any of the viscera.
**vomiting r.**, vomiting due to reflexive stimulation of muscles of the gastrointestinal tract and throat, allowing their contents to be forcibly expelled; it is mediated by centers in the medulla oblongata and can be set in motion by many different stimuli such as touching the back of the pharynx. See also *pharyngeal reflex*.
**von Mering r.**, relaxation of overlying abdominal muscles following ingestion of food.
**water-silk r.**, shot-silk retina.
**Weiss' r.**, a curved reflection seen with the ophthalmoscope on the fundus of the eye to the nasal side of the disk; believed to be indicative of myopia.
**Westphal's pupillary r., Westphal-Piltz r.**, orbicularis pupillary r.
**withdrawal r.**, a nociceptive reflex in which a body part is quickly moved away from a painful stimulus.
**zygomatic r.**, lateral motion of the lower jaw to the percussed side on percussion over the zygoma.

**re·flex·o·gen·ic** (re-flek″so-jen′ik) [*reflex* + *-genic*] 1. producing or increasing reflex action. 2. resulting from a reflex action.

**re·flex·og·e·nous** (re″flek-soj′ə-nəs) reflexogenic.

**re·flexo·graph** (re-flek′so-graf) [*reflex* + *-graph*] an instrument for graphically recording a reflex.

**re·flex·ol·o·gy** (re″flek-sol′ə-je) the science or study of reflexes.

**re·flex·om·e·ter** (re″flek-som′ə-tər) [*reflex* + *-meter*] an instrument for measuring the force necessary to produce myotatic contraction.

**re·flexo·phil** (re-flek′so-fil) [*reflex* + *-phil*] characterized by exaggerated activity of reflexes.

**re·flexo·ther·a·py** (re-flek″so-ther′ə-pe) [MeSH: Reflexotherapy] reflex therapy.

**re·flux** (re′fləks) [*re-* + *flux*] a backward or return flow. Cf. *regurgitation* (def. 1).
**duodenogastric r.**, reflux of the contents of the duodenum into the stomach; it may occur normally, especially during fasting.
**duodenogastroesophageal r.**, gastroesophageal r.
**gastroesophageal r.**, reflux of the stomach and duodenal contents into the esophagus, which may sometimes occur normally, particularly in the distended stomach postprandially, or as a chronic pathological condition (see *reflux esophagitis*, under *esophagitis*). Called also *esophageal ring*.
**hepatojugular r.**, distention of the jugular vein induced by pressure over the liver; it suggests insufficiency of the right heart; sometimes incorrectly called *hepatojugular reflex*.
**intrarenal r.**, reflux of urine into the renal parenchymal tissue.
**urethrovesiculo-differential r.**, the passage of a liquid, sperm, or injected substance from the posterior urethra into the genital system.
**valvular r.**, backflow of blood past a venous valve in the lower limb due to venous insufficiency.
**venous r.**, any reflux of blood in the veins, usually of the lower limbs, due to venous insufficiency.
**vesicoureteral r., vesicoureteric r.**, the passage of urine from the bladder back into a ureter; called also *vesicoureteral regurgitation*.

**re·fract** (re-frakt′) [L. *refringere* to break apart] 1. to cause to deviate. 2. to ascertain errors of ocular refraction.

**re·frac·ta do·si** (re-frak′tə do′si) [L.] in repeated and divided doses.

**re·frac·tile** (re-frak′til) capable of refracting.

**re·frac·tion** (re-frak′shən) 1. the act or process of refracting; specifically the determination of the refractive errors of the eye and their correction by glasses. 2. the deviation of light in passing obliquely from one medium to another of different density. The deviation occurs at the surface of junction of the two mediums, which is known as the refracting surface. The ray before refraction is called the *incident ray;* after refraction it is the *refracted ray.* The point of junction of the incident and the refracted ray is known as the *point of incidence.* The angle between the incident ray and a line perpendicular to the refracting surface at the point of incidence is known as the *angle of incidence;* that between the refracted ray and this perpendicular is called the *angle of refraction.* The sine of the angle of incidence divided by the sine of the angle of refraction gives the *relative index of refraction.*
**double r.,** that in which the incident ray is divided into two refracted rays, so as to produce a double image. Double refraction is produced by Iceland spar. See *Nicol prism,* under *prism.*
**dynamic r.,** the normal accommodation of the eye which is being continually exerted without conscious effort.
**ocular r.,** the refraction of light produced by the mediums of the normal eye and resulting in the focusing of images upon the retina.
**static r.,** the refraction of the eye when its accommodation is paralyzed.

**re·frac·tion·ist** (re-frak′shən-ist) one skilled in determining the refracting power of the eyes and correcting refractive defects.

**re·frac·tive** (re-frak′tiv) pertaining to or subserving a process of refraction; having the power to refract.

**re·frac·tiv·i·ty** (re″frak-tiv′ĭ-te) the quality of being refractive; the power or ability to refract.

**re·frac·tom·e·ter** (re″frak-tom′ə-tər) [*refraction* + *-meter*] 1. an instrument for measuring the refractive power of the eye. 2. an instrument for determining the indexes of refraction of various substances, particularly for determining the strength of lenses of spectacles.

**re·frac·tom·e·try** (re″frak-tom′ə-tre) [MeSH: Refractometry] the measurement of refractive power with the refractometer.

**re·frac·tor** (re-frak′tər) a device for retinoscopic examination of the eye to determine its refractive power.

**re·frac·to·ry** (re-frak′tə-re) [L. *refractorius*] resistant to treatment. See also *resistance.*

**re·frac·ture** (re-frak′chər) the operation of breaking over again a bone which has been fractured and has united with a deformity; called also *anaclasis.*

**re·fran·gi·bil·i·ty** (re-fran″jĭ-bil′ĭ-te) susceptibility to being refracted; the quality of being refrangible.

**re·fran·gi·ble** (re-fran′jĭ-bəl) susceptible to being refracted.

**re·fresh** (re-fresh′) 1. to freshen. 2. to denude a wound of epithelium to enhance tissue repair.

**re·frig·er·a·tion** (re-frij″ər-a′shən) [MeSH: Refrigeration] cooling.

**re·frin·gent** (re-frin′jənt) refractive.

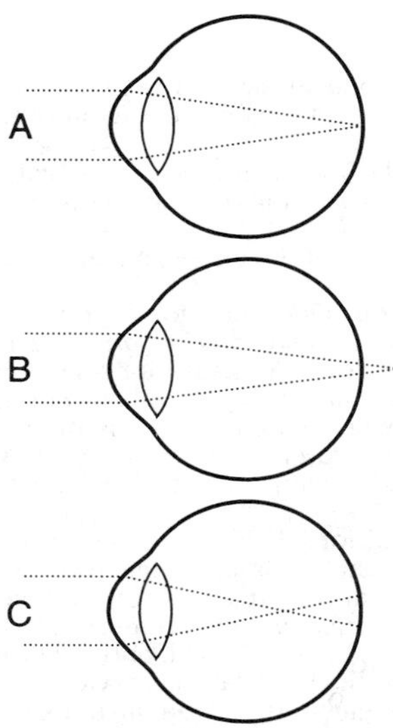

Refraction by the eye in *(A)* emmetropia; *(B)* hyperopia; and *(C)* myopia.

**Ref·sum's disease (syndrome)** (ref′soomz) [Sigvald Bernhard *Refsum,* Norwegian physician, born 1907] see under *disease.*

**re·fu·sion** (re-fu′zhən) [L. *refusio*] the return of blood to the circulation after temporary removal or stoppage of flow.

**REG** radioencephalography.

**re·gain·er** (re-gān′ər) space regainer; a space maintainer that pushes back teeth that have crowded the edentulous area. See also under *maintainer* and *retainer.*
**space r.,** regainer.

**re·gain·er-main·tain·er** (re-gān′ər mān-tān′ər) an orthodontic appliance combining the characteristics of a space regainer and a maintainer.

**re·gen·er·a·tion** (re-jen″ər-a′shən) [*re-* + *generation*] [MeSH: Regeneration] the natural renewal of a structure, as of a lost tissue or part.
**epimorphic r.,** epimorphosis.
**guided tissue r.,** treatment of the tissue of an accidental or surgical wound using microporous membranes as barriers to undesirable types of cells so that only the desired types of cells can enter the wound and regenerate.
**morphallactic r.,** morphallaxis.

**reg·i·men** (rej′ĭ-mən) [L. "guidance"] a strictly regulated scheme of medication, diet, exercise, or other activity designed to achieve certain ends. See also *method, technique, therapy,* and *treatment.*

**re·gio** (re′je-o) pl. *regio′nes* [L. "a space enclosed by lines"] [TA] region: general anatomical nomenclature for an area on the surface of the body within defined boundaries.

## Regio

Descriptions are given on TA terms, and include anglicized names of specific regions.

**r.′nes abdomina′les** [TA], abdominal regions: the various anatomical regions of the abdomen including the right and left hypochondriac, lateral, and inguinal regions, and the epigastric, umbilical, and pubic regions. Called also *abdominal zones.* See illustration under *abdomen.*

**r. ana′lis** [TA], anal region: the portion of the perineal region surrounding the anus; called also *anal triangle.*

**r. antebrachia′lis** [TA], antebrachial region; see *r. antebrachii anterior* and *r. antebrachii posterior.*

**r. antebrachia′lis ante′rior,** TA alternative for *r. antebrachii anterior.*

**r. antebrachia′lis poste′rior,** TA alternative for *r. antebrachii posterior.*

**r. antebra′chii ante′rior** [TA], anterior region of forearm: the anterior, or palmar, region of the forearm; called also *r. antebrachialis anterior* [TA alternative].

**r. antebra′chii poste′rior** [TA], posterior antebrachial region: the posterior, or dorsal, region of the forearm; called also *r. antebrachialis posterior* [TA alternative].

**r. auricula′ris** [TA], auricular region: the surface region of the head about the ear.

**r. axilla′ris** [TA], axillary region: the region of the thorax around the fossa axillaris.

**r. brachia′lis** [TA], brachial region: see *r. brachii anterior* and *r. brachii posterior.*

**r. brachia′lis ante′rior,** TA alternative for *r. brachii anterior.*

**r. brachia′lis poste′rior,** TA alternative for *r. brachii posterior.*

**r. bra′chii ante′rior** [TA], anterior region of arm: the anterior region of the arm; called also *r. brachialis anterior* [TA alternative] and *anterior brachial region.*

**r. bra′chii poste′rior** [TA], posterior region of arm: the posterior region of the arm; called also *r. brachialis posterior* [TA alternative] and *posterior brachial region.*

**r. bucca'lis** [TA], buccal region: the region of the cheek.

**r. calca'nea** [TA], heel region: the region of the foot overlying the calcaneus.

**r.'nes ca'pitis** [TA], the various anatomical regions of the head, including the frontal, parietal, occipital, temporal, auricular, mastoid, and facial regions.

**r. carpa'lis** [TA], carpal region: see *r. carpalis anterior* and *r. carpalis posterior.*

**r. carpa'lis ante'rior** [TA], anterior region of wrist: the anterior aspect of the wrist; called also *anterior carpal region.*

**r. carpa'lis poste'rior** [TA], posterior region of wrist: the posterior aspect of the wrist; called also *posterior carpal region.*

**r.'nes cervica'les** [TA], the various anatomical regions of the neck, including the anterior, lateral, and posterior cervical regions and the sternocleidomastoid region; called also *regiones colli* and *cervical regions.*

**r. cervica'lis ante'rior** [TA], anterior cervical region: the region of the neck anterior to the sternocleidomastoid muscle, subdivided into the submandibular, carotid, muscular, and submental triangles. Called also *r. colli anterior, trigonum cervicale anterius* [TA alternative], *trigonum colli anterius* [TA alternative], and *anterior cervical triangle.*

**r. cervica'lis latera'lis** [TA], lateral cervical region: the region of the neck lateral to the regio sternocleidomastoidea (posterior to the sternocleidomastoid muscle); called also *r. colli lateralis, lateral region of neck, trigonum cervicale posterius* [TA alternative], and *trigonum colli laterale* [TA alternative].

**r. cervica'lis poste'rior** [TA], posterior cervical region: the region of the neck posterior to the regio cervicalis lateralis. Called also *r. nuchalis, nuchal region, posterior region of neck,* and *r. colli posterior* [TA alternative].

**r.'nes col'li,** regiones cervicales.

**r. col'li ante'rior,** r. cervicalis anterior.

**r. col'li latera'lis,** regio cervicalis lateralis.

**r. col'li poste'rior,** TA alternative for *r. cervicalis posterior.*

**r. cox'ae** [TA], hip region: the region of the lower limb overlying the hip joint.

**r. crura'lis ante'rior,** r. cruris anterior.

**r. crura'lis poste'rior,** r. cruris posterior.

**r. cru'ris** [TA], leg region: the lower leg, including the regio cruris anterior, the regio cruris posterior, the regio talocruralis anterior, and the regio talocruralis posterior.

**r. cru'ris ante'rior** [TA], the anterior region of the leg; called also *r. cruralis anterior* and *anterior crural region.*

**r. cru'ris poste'rior** [TA], the posterior region of the leg; called also *r. cruralis posterior* and *posterior crural region.*

**r. cubita'lis** [TA], cubital region: the area of the arm about the elbow.

**r. cubita'lis ante'rior** [TA], anterior cubital region: the anterior region around the elbow.

**r. cubita'lis poste'rior** [TA], posterior cubital region: the posterior or dorsal region around the elbow.

**r. deltoi'dea** [TA], deltoid region: the surface region overlying the deltoid muscle.

**r.'nes dorsa'les** [TA], regions of back: the various anatomical regions of the back, including the vertebral, sacral, scapular, infrascapular, and lumbar regions. Called also *regiones dorsi* [TA alternative] and *dorsal regions.*

**r. dorsa'lis ma'nus** [TA], back of hand: the hand surface opposite the palm.

**r. dorsa'lis pe'dis,** TA alternative for *dorsum pedis.*

**r.'nes dor'si,** TA alternative for *regiones dorsales.*

**r. epigas'trica,** TA alternative for *epigastrium.*

**r. facia'lis** [TA], the facial region, which includes the various anatomical regions of the face: the orbital, nasal, parotid, oral, mental, infraorbital, buccal, and zygomatic regions.

**r. femora'lis,** r. femoris.

**r. femora'lis ante'rior,** r. femoris anterior.

**r. femora'lis poste'rior,** r. femoris posterior.

**r. fe'moris** [TA], femoral region: the region overlying the femur. Called also *r. femoralis.*

**r. fe'moris ante'rior** [TA], the anterior region of the thigh; called also *r. femoralis anterior.*

**r. fe'moris poste'rior** [TA], the posterior region of the thigh; called also *r. femoralis posterior.*

**r. fronta'lis** [TA], frontal region: the surface region of the head overlying the frontal bone; the forehead.

**r. genua'lis ante'rior,** r. genus anterior.

**r. genua'lis poste'rior,** r. genus posterior.

**r. ge'nus** [TA], knee region: the region of the lower limb overlying the knee joint, comprising the *regio genus anterior* and the *regio genus posterior.*

**r. ge'nus ante'rior** [TA], the anterior region about the knee; called also *r. genualis anterior.*

**r. ge'nus poste'rior** [TA], the posterior region about the knee, including the popliteal fossa; called also *r. genualis posterior.*

**r. glutea'lis** [TA], gluteal region: the region overlying the gluteal muscles.

**r. hypochondri'aca** [TA], TA alternative for *hypochondrium.*

**r. hypogas'trica,** hypogastrium.

**r. hypothala'mica ante'rior,** area hypothalamica rostralis.

**r. hypothala'mica dorsa'lis,** area hypothalamica dorsalis.

**r. hypothala'mica interme'dia,** area hypothalamica intermedia.

**r. hypothala'mica latera'lis,** area hypothalamica lateralis.

**r. hypothala'mica poste'rior,** area hypothalamica posterior.

**r. inframamma'ria** [TA], inframammary region: the region of the anterior aspect of the thorax situated inferior to either mamma and superior to the inferior border of the twelfth rib.

**r. infraorbita'lis** [TA], infraorbital region: the region inferior to the eye, adjacent to the regio nasalis.

**r. infrascapula'ris** [TA], infrascapular region: the region of the back inferior to the scapula and lateral to the inferior thoracic vertebrae.

**r. infratempora'lis,** fossa infratemporalis.

**r. inguina'lis,** TA alternative for *inguen.*

**r. latera'lis,** lateral region: TA alternative for *latus.*

**r. lumba'lis** [TA], **r. lumba'ris,** lumbar region: the region of the back lying lateral to the lumbar vertebrae; see also *lumbus.*

**r. mamma'ria** [TA], mammary region: the region of the anterior aspect of the thorax, around the mammary gland.

**r. ma'nus** [TA], hand region: the region of the upper limb distal to the antebrachial region and comprising the various regions of the hand and wrist.

**r. mastoi'dea** [TA], mastoid region: the region of the head on either side roughly corresponding to the outline of the mastoid process of the temporal bone.

**r.'nes mem'bri inferio'ris** [TA], the various anatomical regions of the lower limb, including the gluteal, hip, femoral, knee, leg, and foot regions.

**r.'nes mem'bri superio'ris** [TA], the various anatomical regions of the upper limb; including the deltoid, brachial, cubital, antebrachial, and hand regions.

**r. menta'lis** [TA], mental region: the region of the chin.

**r. metacarpa'lis** [TA], metacarpal region: the region of the surface of the hand overlying the metacarpals.

**r. metatarsa'lis** [TA], metatarsal region: the region of the foot overlying the metatarsals.

**r. nasa'lis** [TA], nasal region: the region of the face about the nose.

**r. nucha'lis,** r. cervicalis posterior.

**r. occipita'lis** [TA], : the surface region of the head overlying the occipital bone.

**r. olfacto'ria,** pars olfactoria cavitatis nasi.

**r. ora'lis** [TA], oral region: the region of the face about the mouth.

**r. orbita'lis** [TA], orbital region: the region of the face about the eye; called also *ocular region.*

**r. palma'ris,** TA alternative for *palma.*

**r. parieta'lis** [TA], parietal region: the surface region of the head on either side roughly corresponding to the outline of the parietal bone.

**r. parotideomasseter'ica** [TA], parotideomasseteric region: the region of the face on either side, about the parotid gland and masseter muscle.

**r. pectora'lis** [TA], pectoral region: the aspect of the thorax, or chest, bounded by the pectoralis major muscle, and including the lateral pectoral, mammary, and inframammary regions.

**r.'nes pectora'les,** regiones thoracicae anteriores et laterales.

**r. pectora'lis latera'lis** [TA], lateral pectoral region: the region of the anterior thorax lateral to the pectoral region, bounded by the axillary region and the hypochondrium.

**r. pe'dis** [TA], foot region: the region of the lower limb distal to the leg region *(regio cruris),* comprising the various regions of the ankle and foot.

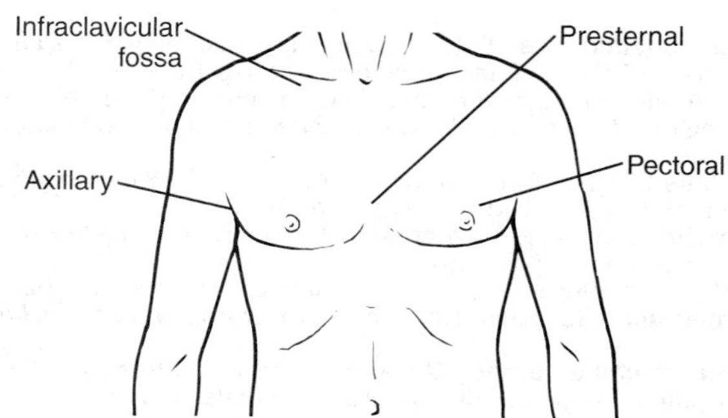


Regiones pectorales (pectoral regions).

**r. perinea'lis** [TA], perineal region: the region overlying the pelvic outlet, including the anal and urogenital regions.
**r. planta'ris,** TA alternative for *planta.*
**r.'nes pleuropulmona'les,** pleuropulmonary regions: one-half of the thoracic cavity excluding the mediastinum.
**r. presterna'lis** [TA], presternal region: the region of the chest superficial to the sternum.
**r. pu'bica** [TA], TA alternative for *hypogastrium.*
**r. respirato'ria,** pars respiratoria cavitatis nasi.
**r. retromalleola'ris latera'lis** [TA], lateral retromalleolar region: the region posterior to the lateral malleolus of the fibula.
**r. retromalleola'ris media'lis** [TA], medial retromalleolar region: the region posterior to the medial malleolus of the tibia.
**r. sacra'lis** [TA], sacral region: the region of the back overlying the sacrum.
**r. scapula'ris** [TA], scapular region: the region of the back overlying the scapula.
**r. sternocleidomastoi'dea** [TA], sternocleidomastoid region: the region of the neck overlying the sternocleidomastoid muscle.
**r. su'rae** [TA], **r. sura'lis,** sural region: the region on the posterior aspect of the leg around the calf; see *sura.*
**r. talocrura'lis ante'rior** [TA], anterior talocrural region: the anterior aspect of the lower limb between the leg and foot; called also *anterior ankle region.*
**r. talocrura'lis poste'rior** [TA], posterior talocrural region: the posterior aspect of the lower limb between the leg and foot; called also *posterior ankle region.*
**r. tarsa'lis** [TA], ankle region: the region overlying the tarsal bones.
**r. tempora'lis** [TA], temporal region: the surface region of the head on either side roughly corresponding to the outline of the temporal bone.
**r.'nes thora'cicae anterio'res et latera'les** [TA], anterior and lateral thoracic regions: the various regions of the chest, including the presternal, pectoralis, mammary, inframammary, and axillary regions, infraclavicular and axillary fossae, and clavipectoral trigone. Called also *regiones pectorales.*
**r. umbilica'lis,** TA alternative for *umbilicus* (def. 2).
**r. urogenita'lis** [TA], urogenital region: the portion of the perineal region surrounding the urogenital organs. Called also *genitourinary region* and *urogenital triangle.*
**r. vertebra'lis** [TA], vertebral region: the middle region of the back, overlying the vertebral column.
**r. zygoma'tica** [TA], zygomatic region: the region of the face on either side, about the zygomatic bone.

**re·gion** (re'jən) a plane area with more or less definite boundaries; for names of specific regions not listed here, see under *regio.*
**abdominal r's,** regiones abdominales.
**r. of accommodation,** the space including all points to which the eye can be adjusted by accommodation.
**AN r.,** see *nodus atrioventricularis.*
**anal r.,** regio analis.
**ankle r.,** regio tarsalis.
**ankle r., anterior,** regio talocruralis anterior.
**ankle r., posterior,** regio talocruralis posterior.
**antebrachial r.,** regio antebrachialis.
**anterior r. of arm,** regio brachii anterior.
**anterior r. of forearm,** regio antebrachii anterior.
**anterior r. of knee,** regio genus anterior.
**anterior r. of leg,** regio cruris anterior.
**anterior r. of neck,** regio cervicalis anterior.
**anterior r. of wrist,** regio carpalis anterior.
**auricular r.,** regio auricularis.
**axillary r.,** regio axillaris.
**r's of back,** regiones dorsales.
**basilar r.,** the base of the skull.
**brachial r.,** regio brachialis.
**brachial r., anterior,** regio brachii anterior.
**brachial r., posterior,** regio brachii posterior.
**Broca's r.,** see under *convolution.*
**buccal r.,** regio buccalis.
**calcaneal r.,** calx.
**carpal r.,** regio carpalis.
**carpal r., anterior,** regio carpalis anterior.
**carpal r., posterior,** regio carpalis posterior.
**cervical r's,** regiones cervicales.
**cervical r., anterior,** regio cervicalis anterior.
**cervical r., lateral,** regio cervicalis lateralis.
**cervical r., posterior,** regio cervicalis posterior.
**ciliary r.,** the part of the eye occupied by the ciliary body and its adjuncts.
**constant (C) r.,** the C-terminal portion of an immunoglobulin heavy ($C_H$) or light ($C_L$) chain, comprising one homology region in light chains and three or four in heavy chains, that has a constant amino acid sequence for chains of a single type produced by one individual. Constant regions vary among the heavy chain classes and subclasses (isotypic variation) and among individuals (allotypic variation).
**crural r., anterior,** regio cruris anterior.
**crural r., posterior,** crural region, posterior.
**cubital r.,** regio cubitalis.
**cubital r., anterior,** regio cubitalis anterior.
**cubital r., posterior,** regio cubitalis posterior.
**deltoid r.,** regio deltoidea.
**dorsal r's,** regiones dorsales.
**dorsal r. of foot,** dorsum pedis.
**dorsal lip r.,** the mesodermal tissue around the dorsal lip of the blastopore of an amphibian; an analogous region in the human embryo is the organizer which by induction initiates and controls early development.
**encephalic r.,** lamina alaris.
**epigastric r.,** epigastrium.
**external r.,** see *regio lateralis.*
**extrapolar r.,** that region of the body which lies outside the influence of the poles in electrotherapy.
**Fab r.,** see *Fab.*
**facial r.,** regio facialis.
**Fc r.,** see *Fc.*
**femoral r.,** regio femoris.
**foot r.,** foot region.
**frontal r.,** regio facialis.
**genitourinary r.,** regio urogenitalis.
**gluteal r.,** regio glutealis.
**hand r.,** regio manus.
**heel r.,** regio calcanea.
**hinge r.,** a short flexible region between the $C_H1$ and $C_H2$ domains of immunoglobulin heavy chains which allows each of the Fab regions (the "arms" of the Y-shaped immunoglobulin molecule) to move independently as necessary to bind to antigens.
**hip r.,** regio coxae.
**homogeneously staining r's (HSR),** long unbanded regions on chromosomes created by gene amplification; they are tumor markers indicative of solid neoplasms with poor prognosis.
**homology r's,** regions of immunoglobulin heavy and light chains containing about 110 amino acid residues and forming compact globular domains stabilized by one intrachain disulfide bond; they have a high degree of sequence homology and similar three-dimensional structure. Each variable region ($V_H$ and $V_L$) of heavy and light chains and the light chain constant region ($C_L$) are coextensive with a single homology region. Heavy chain constant regions are composed of three (in $\gamma$, $\delta$, and $\alpha$ chains) or four (in $\mu$ and $\epsilon$ chains) homology regions, $C_H1$, $C_H2$, $C_H3$, and $C_H4$, and a hinge region separating $C_H1$ and $C_H2$.
**hypervariable r's,** regions a few amino acids in length within immunoglobulin heavy and light chain variable regions at which the amino acid sequence is extremely variable; there are three in light chains and four in heavy chains. They contain most of the amino acid residues forming the antigen binding site.
**hypochondriac r.,** hypochondrium.
**hypogastric r.,** hypogastrium.
**hypothalamic r., anterior,** area hypothalamica rostralis.
**hypothalamic r., dorsal,** area hypothalamica dorsalis.
**hypothalamic r., intermediate,** area hypothalamica intermedia.
**hypothalamic r., lateral,** area hypothalamica lateralis.
**hypothalamic r., posterior,** area hypothalamica posterior.
**I r.,** that part of the mouse major histocompatibility complex (H-2 complex) containing the immune response genes.
**iliac r.,** inguen.
**infraclavicular r.,** fossa infraclavicularis.
**inframammary r.,** regio inframammaria.
**infraorbital r.,** regio infraorbitalis.
**infrascapular r.,** regio infrascapularis.
**infratemporal r.,** fossa infratemporalis.
**infundibulotubular r.,** area hypothalamica intermedia.
**inguinal r.,** inguen.

**knee r.**, regio genus.
**lateral r.**, latus[2].
**lateral r. of neck**, regio cervicalis lateralis.
**leg r.**, regio cruris.
**lumbar r.**, 1. regio lumbalis. 2. see *regio lateralis.*
**mammary r.**, regio mammaria.
**mammillary r.**, regio hypothalamica posterior.
**mastoid r.**, regio mastoidea.
**mental r.**, regio mentalis.
**metacarpal r.**, regio metacarpalis.
**metatarsal r.**, regio metatarsalis.
**motor r.**, see under *area.*
**mylohyoid r.**, the region on the lingual surface of the mandible to which the mylohyoid muscle is attached.
**N r.**, see *nodus atrioventricularis.*
**r. of nape**, regio cervicalis posterior.
**nasal r.**, regio nasalis.
**NH r.**, see *nodus atrioventricularis.*
**nuchal r.**, regio cervicalis posterior.
**occipital r.**, regio occipitalis.
**ocular r.**, regio orbitalis.
**olfactory r.**, pars olfactoria cavitatis nasi.
**opticostriate r.**, nuclei basales; see under *nucleus.*
**oral r.**, regio oralis.
**orbital r.**, regio orbitalis.
**palmar r.**, regio palmaris; see *palma.*
**parietal r.**, regio parietalis.
**pectoral r.**, regio pectoralis.
**pectoral r., lateral,** regio pectoralis lateralis.
**perineal r.**, regio perinealis.
**pleuropulmonary r's,** regiones pleuropulmonales.
**posterior r. of arm,** regio brachii posterior.
**posterior r. of forearm,** regio posterior antebrachii.
**posterior r. of knee,** regio genus posterior.
**posterior r. of leg,** crural region, posterior.
**posterior r. of neck,** regio cervicalis posterior.
**posterior r. of wrist,** regio carpalis posterior.
**precordial r.**, a part of the anterior surface of the body covering the heart and the epigastric fossa or pit of the stomach.
**prefrontal r.**, see under *area.*
**preoptic r.**, 1. area hypothalamica rostralis. 2. the part of the anterior hypothalamic region ventral to the optic chiasm, containing the medial and lateral preoptic nuclei.
**presternal r.**, regio presternalis.
**presumptive r.**, an area of the blastula which has been proved under normal conditions to develop into a specific organ or type of tissue.
**pretectal r.**, area pretectalis.
**pubic r.**, hypogastrium.
**respiratory r.**, pars respiratoria cavitatis nasi.
**retromalleolar r., lateral,** regio retromalleolaris lateralis.
**retromalleolar r., medial,** regio retromalleolaris medialis.
**rolandic r.**, primary somatomotor area.
**sacral r.**, regio sacralis.
**scapular r.**, regio scapularis.
**sensory r's,** primary receiving areas.
**sternocleidomastoid r.**, regio sternocleidomastoidea.
**subauricular r.**, fossa retromandibularis.
**supraclavicular r.**, the region superior to the clavicle.
**supraoptic r.**, the part of the anterior hypothalamic region dorsal to the optic chiasm, containing the paraventricular, supraoptic, and anterior hypothalamic nuclei.
**sural r.**, regio surae.
**talocrural r., anterior,** regio talocruralis anterior.
**talocrural r., posterior,** regio talocruralis posterior.
**temporal r.**, regio temporalis.
**trabecular r.**, the region of the embryonic skull from which the sphenoid bone is developed.

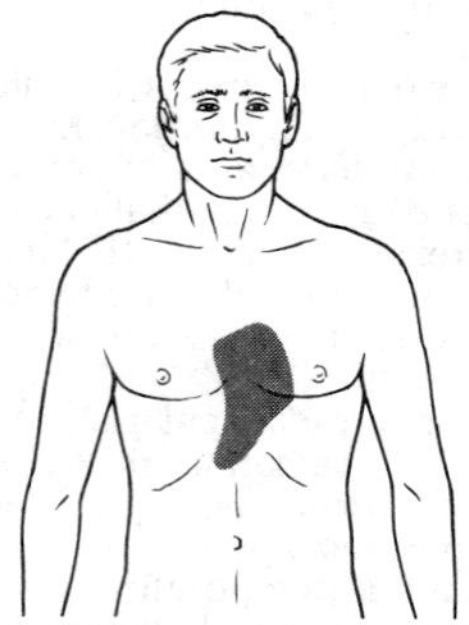
Precordial region.

**umbilical r.**, umbilicus (def. 2).
**urogenital r.**, regio urogenitalis.
**variable (V) r.**, the N-terminal portion, composing one homology region, of an immunoglobulin heavy ($V_H$) or light ($V_L$) chain that varies in amino acid sequence among chains of a single type. The antigen binding sites of immunoglobulin molecules are formed by parts of the $V_H$ and $V_L$ regions; thus the $V_H$ and $V_L$ amino acid sequences determine the antigenic specificity of the antibody molecule. Although variable regions vary among antibodies of different specificity (idiotype variation), all of the immunoglobulins produced by a single clone of plasma cells (a clonotype) have the same variable regions but may have different constant regions.
**vertebral r.**, regio vertebralis.
**vestibular r.**, the lowest and the movable portion of the nose; see *vestibulum nasi.*
**zygomatic r.**, regio zygomatica.

**re·gion·al** (re'jən-əl) pertaining to, limited to, or affecting a certain region or regions.

**re·gi·o·nes** (re″je-o'nēz) [L.] plural of *regio.*

**reg·is·trant** (rej'is-trənt) a nurse who is listed on the books of a registry as available for duty.

**reg·is·trar** (rej'is-trahr) 1. an official keeper of records. 2. in British hospitals, a resident specialist who acts as assistant to the chief or attending specialist.

**reg·is·tra·tion** (rej″is-tra'shən) in dentistry, the making of a record of the jaw relations present, or of those desired, in order to transfer them to an articulator to facilitate proper construction of a dental prosthesis.
**maxillomandibular r.**, see under *record.*

**reg·is·try** (rej'is-tre) [MeSH: Registries] 1. an office where a nurse may have his or her name listed as being available for duty. 2. a central agency for the collection of pathologic material and related clinical, laboratory, x-ray, and other data in a specified field of pathology, so organized that the data can be properly processed and made available for study.

**Reg·i·tine** (rej'ĭ-tēn) trademark for a preparation of phentolamine.

**Reg·lan** (reg'lan) trademark for preparations of metoclopramide hydrochloride.

**Reg·o·nol** (reg'o-nōl) trademark for preparations of pyridostigmine bromide.

**re·gres·sion** (re-gresh'ən) [L. *regressio* a return] 1. a return to a former or earlier state. 2. a subsidence of symptoms or of a disease process. 3. in biology, the tendency in successive generations toward the mean; see *Galton's law of regression,* under *law.* 4. a return to earlier, especially to infantile, patterns of thought or behavior, a characteristic of many mental disorders also exhibited by normal persons in many situations, e.g., feelings of helplessness and dependency in a patient with a serious physical illness. 5. a functional relationship between the mean value of a random variable and the corresponding values of one or more variables identified by the experimenter (the independent variables).
**linear r.**, the statistical procedure for fitting a straight regression line to observed data, usually by minimizing the sum of the squared deviations of the observed values of the dependent variable from the regression line *(least-squares regression).*
**logistic r.**, a multivariate statistical method used for modeling the probability of occurrence of a dichotomous outcome as a function of multiple independent variables; it always yields a probability between 0 and 1.
**multiple r.**, a form of linear regression or other regression method analyzing the effects of multiple independent variables simultaneously.

**re·gres·sive** (re-gres'iv) going back; subsiding; characterized by regression.

**Reg·ro·ton** (reg'ro-ton) trademark for preparations of chlorthalidone and reserpine.

**reg·u·lar** (reg'u-lər) [L. *regularis; regula* rule] normal or conforming to rule; occurring at proper or fixed intervals.

**reg·u·la·tion** (reg″u-la'shən) [L. *regula* rule] 1. the act of adjusting or state of being adjusted to a certain standard. 2. in biology, the adaptation of form or behavior of an organism to changed conditions. 3. the power to form a whole embryo from stages before the gastrula.

**reg·u·la·tor** (reg'u-la″tər) something that regulates.
**r. of complement activation (RCA),** complement control protein.
**cystic fibrosis transmembrane conductance r., cystic fibrosis transmembrane r. (CFTR),** an abnormal protein found in the gene for cystic fibrosis, consisting of a single peptide chain with 1480 amino acids; it causes abnormal chloride channels in cell membranes of the respiratory epithelium, pancreas, salivary glands, sweat glands, intestines, and reproductive tract.

**re·gur·gi·tant** (re-gur′jĭ-tənt) [*re-* + L. *gurgitare* to flood] flowing back or in the opposite direction from normal.

**re·gur·gi·ta·tion** (re-gur″jĭ-ta′shən) [*re-* + L. *gurgitare* to flood] 1. flow in the opposite direction from normal, as the backward flowing of blood into the heart or between heart chambers. See also *reflux*. 2. vomiting.
**aortic r. (AR),** the backflow of blood from the aorta into the left ventricle, owing to insufficiency of the aortic semilunar valve; it may be chronic or acute.
**mitral r. (MR),** the backflow of blood from the left ventricle into the left atrium, owing to insufficiency of the mitral valve; it may be acute or chronic, and is usually due to mitral valve prolapse, rheumatic heart disease, or a complication of cardiac dilatation.
**pulmonic r. (PR),** the backflow of blood from the pulmonary artery into the right ventricle, owing to insufficiency of the pulmonic semilunar valve.
**tricuspid r. (TR),** the backflow of blood from the right ventricle into the right atrium, owing to imperfect functioning (insufficiency) of the tricuspid valve.
**valvular r.,** regurgitation of the blood through the orifices of the heart valves owing to imperfect closing of the valves; see *aortic, mitral, pulmonic,* and *tricuspid r.*
**vesicoureteral r.,** see under *reflux.*

**re·ha·bil·i·ta·tion** (re″hə-bil″ĭ-ta′shən) [L. *rehabilitare* to rehabilitate] [MeSH: Rehabilitation] 1. the restoration of normal form and function after injury or illness. 2. the restoration of the ill or injured patient to optimal functional level in the home and community in relation to physical, psychosocial, vocational, and recreational activity.

**re·ha·bil·i·tee** (re″hə-bil′ĭ-te) the subject of rehabilitation.

**re·hy·dra·tion** (re″hi-dra′shən) the restoration of water or of fluid content to a body or to a substance which has become dehydrated; see also *oral rehydration therapy,* under *therapy.*

**Rei·chel's cloacal duct** (ri′kelz) [Friedrich Paul *Reichel,* German obstetrician, 1858–1934] see under *duct.*

**Rei·chert's canal,** etc. (ri′kərts) [Karl Bogislaus *Reichert,* German anatomist, 1811–1883] see under *canal, cartilage, recess, scar,* and *substance.*

**Reich·stein** (rīk′shtīn) Tadeus. Polish-born Swiss organic chemist, born 1897; co-winner, with Edward Calvin Kendall and Philip Showalter Hench, of the Nobel prize for medicine or physiology in 1950 for his research on the structure and biological effects of the hormones of the adrenal cortex.

**Reid's base line** (rēdz) [Robert William *Reid,* Scottish anatomist, 1851–1939] see *base line,* under *line.*

**Reif·en·stein's syndrome** (ri′fən-stīnz) [Edward Conrad *Reifenstein* Jr., American endocrinologist, 1908–1975] see under *syndrome.*

**Reil's band,** etc. (rīlz) [Johann Christian *Reil,* German anatomist, 1759–1813] see under *ribbon* and see , *lobus insularis,* and *trigonum lemnisci.*

**re·im·plan·ta·tion** (re″im-plan-ta′shən) replantation of tissue or a structure, such as a tooth, in the site from which it was previously lost or removed.

**re·in·fec·tion** (re″in-fek′shən) a second infection by the same pathogenic agent, or a second infection of an organ such as the kidney by a different pathogenic agent.

**re·in·force·ment** (re″in-fors′mənt) in behavioral science, the presentation of a stimulus following a response that increases the frequency of subsequent responses; see *positive r.* and *negative r.*
**continuous r.,** a schedule of reinforcement in which each response results in a reward.
**covert r.,** that in which behavioral frequency is increased by imagined rather than physical reward.
**negative r.,** presentation of an unpleasant, undesirable event that strengthens responses leading to its removal or termination.
**partial r.,** any of several schedules of reinforcement (q.v.) in which a response yields a reward only at certain times or after certain numbers of responses.
**positive r.,** presentation of a desirable event that strengthens future occurrences of the behavior that preceded it.
**r. of reflex,** the increasing of a reflex response by causing the patient to perform some mental or physical concentration while the reflex is being elicited.

**re·in·forc·er** (re″in-for′sər) any stimulus that produces reinforcement.
**negative r.,** an unpleasant, undesirable event strengthening responses leading to its removal or termination.
**positive r.,** a pleasant, desirable event strengthening responses preceding its occurrence.
**primary r.,** a stimulus having an inherent effect on behavior, generally one affecting a biological process, e.g., sleeping or eating.
**secondary r.,** a stimulus that acquires its effects on behavior only through association with a primary reinforcer.

**re·in·fu·sate** (re″in-fu′sāt) fluid for reinfusion into the body, usually after being subjected to a treatment process.

**re·in·fu·sion** (re″in-fu′zhən) infusion of body fluid that has previously been withdrawn from the same individual, e.g., reinfusion of ascitic fluid after ultrafiltration.

**Rein·ke's crystalloids (crystals), edema, space** (rīn′kez) [Friedrich Berthold *Reinke,* German anatomist, 1862–1919] see under *crystalloid, edema,* and *space.*

**re·in·ner·va·tion** (re″in-ər-va′shən) restoration of nerve function to a part from which it was lost; it may occur spontaneously or be achieved by nerve grafting.

**re·in·oc·u·la·tion** (re″in-ok″u-la′shən) an inoculation that follows a previous one with the same virus.

**re·in·te·gra·tion** (re″in-tə-gra′shən) 1. biological integration after a state of disruption. 2. restoration of harmonious mental function after disintegration of the personality in mental illness. Called also *redintegration.*

**re·in·tu·ba·tion** (re″in-too-ba′shən) intubation performed after extubation.

**re·in·ver·sion** (re″in-ver′zhən) restoration to its normal place of an inverted organ, especially restoration of an inverted uterus.

**re·in·vo·ca·tion** (re″in-vo-ka′shən) reactivation.

**Reis·sei·sen's muscles** (rīs′i-senz) [Franz Daniel *Reisseisen,* German anatomist, 1773–1828] see under *muscle.*

**Reiss·ner's fiber, membrane** (rīs′nerz) [Ernst *Reissner,* German anatomist, 1824–1878] see under *fiber,* and see *paries vestibularis ductus cochlearis.*

**Rei·ter's syndrome (disease)** (ri′tərz) [Hans *Reiter,* German physician, 1881–1969] see under *syndrome.*

**re·it·er·a·ture** (re-it″ər-ə-tu′re) [L.] repeat or renew, as a prescription.

**re·jec·tion** (re-jek′shən) an immune response against grafted tissue that may result in failure of the graft to survive; called also *graft r.*
**acute r., acute cellular r.,** the classic type of graft rejection, occurring 1 to 3 weeks after transplantation or following a cessation of immunosuppressive therapy and resulting primarily from the cell-mediated immune response of the recipient against incompatible HLA antigens; it is manifested histologically as extensive infiltration of the graft by mononuclear cells, primarily small lymphocytes, accompanied by edema and interstitial hemorrhage.
**cellular r.,** acute r.
**chronic r.,** a gradual progressive loss of function of the transplanted organ occurring months or years after transplantation.
**first-set r.,** see under *phenomenon.*
**graft r.,** see *rejection.*
**hyperacute r.,** graft rejection occurring immediately after transplantation and resulting from the presence of preformed, circulating cytotoxic antibodies against antigens (often non-HLA antigens) on the graft. Antigen-antibody complexes on vascular endothelium initiate an Arthus-type (type III) reaction in which complement activation results in infiltration by neutrophils, endothelial injury, and occlusion of capillaries with fibrin-platelet thrombi; adequate blood flow to the graft is never established.
**second-set r.,** see under *phenomenon.*

**re·ju·ve·nes·cence** (re-joo″və-nes′əns) [*re-* + L. *juvenescere* to become young] a renewal of youth or of strength and vigor.

**Re·la** (re′lə) trademark for a preparation of carisoprodol.

**Rel·a·fen** (rel′ə-fen) trademark for a preparation of nabumetone.

**re·lapse** (re-laps′) [L. *relapsus*] the return of a disease after its apparent cessation. Cf. *recrudescence.*
**intercurrent r.,** a relapse occurring before the temperature has reached a normal level.
**rebound r.,** return of some of the symptoms of a disease on cessation of treatment, applied especially to the relapse of patients with rheumatoid arthritis on withdrawal of cortisone or ACTH (Hench).

**re·la·tion** (re-la′shən) [L. *relatio* a carrying back] the condition or state of one object or entity when considered in connection with another.
**acentric r.,** eccentric jaw r.
**buccolingual r.,** the position of a tooth or space in the dental arch in relation to the tongue and the cheek.
**centric r., centric jaw r.,** the position of the mandible, obtained principally by operator guidance, in which the condyles are in the rearmost uppermost position in the fossae of the temporomandibular joint. Called also *median retruded r., terminal hinge position,* and *true centric.*

**dynamic r's,** those existing between two objects or entities when one or both of them are moving or constantly changing, as the relation between the mandible and the maxilla.
**eccentric r., eccentric jaw r.,** any relation of the mandible to the maxillae other than the centric relation; called also *acentric r.* and *eccentric position.*
**eccentric jaw r., acquired,** an eccentric relation of the mandible to the maxilla that is assumed in order to bring the teeth into centric occlusion.
**Frank-Starling r.,** Starling's law of the heart.
**jaw r.,** any relation of the mandible to the maxilla, variously designated as centric, eccentric, median, occlusal, protrusive, and the like. Called also *maxillomandibular r.*
**lateral occlusal r.,** the relation of the mandible to the maxilla when the lower jaw is in a position to either side of centric relation.
**length-tension r.,** the relationship between the tension placed on a resting muscle, or preload, and the length of that muscle; see *Starling's law of the heart,* under *law.*
**maxillomandibular r.,** jaw r.
**median jaw r.,** the relation between the maxilla and the mandible when the lower jaw is in the median sagittal plane, without being displaced to either side; ideally, median and centric relations should coincide.
**median retruded jaw r.,** centric r.
**object r's,** the emotional bonds formed between one person and another, as contrasted with interest in and love for oneself and usually described as the capacity for love for and appropriate reaction to others.
**occlusal r.,** see under *position.*
**posterior border jaw r.,** see under *position.*
**protrusive jaw r.,** an occlusal position in which the mandible is protruded. See also *prognathism.*
**rest jaw r.,** rest position.
**ridge r.,** the positional relation of the mandibular ridge to the maxillary ridge.
**static r's,** those existing between two objects or entities when neither one of them is moving or changing in any way.
**unstrained jaw r.,** that maintained when a state of balanced tonus exists among all the muscles involved, being achieved without undue or unnatural force and causing no distortion of the tissues of the temporomandibular joints.

**re·lax·ant** (re-lak'sənt) [L. *relaxare* to loosen] 1. lessening or reducing tension. 2. an agent that lessens tension.
**muscle r.,** an agent that specifically aids in reducing muscle tension, as those acting at the polysynaptic neurons of motor nerves (e.g., meprobamate) or at the myoneural junction (curare and related compounds); see also *myoneural blocking agent,* under *agent.*

**re·lax·a·tion** (re″lak-sa'shən) [MeSH: Relaxation] 1. a lessening of tension. 2. a mitigation of pain.
**isometric r.,** relaxation of a muscle without shortening.
**isovolumetric r., isovolumic r.,** see under *period.*

**re·lax·in** (re-lak'sin) [MeSH: Relaxin] a water-soluble polypeptide (molecular weight approx. 8000) extractable from the corpus luteum of pregnancy; it produces relaxation of the pubic symphysis and dilation of the uterine cervix in certain animal species. Its role in the human pregnant female is uncertain.

**re·li·a·bil·i·ty** (re-li″ə-bil'ĭ-te) 1. the tendency of a system to be resistant to failure. 2. precision (def. 2).

**re·lief** (re-lēf') [L. *relevatio*] 1. the mitigation or removal of pain or distress. 2. the reduction or elimination of undesirable pressure or force from a specific area under a denture base. See also under *chamber,* and *space.* 3. a thin lining of adhesive or hard baseplate wax in the master cast beneath lingual bar connectors or bar portions of the lingual plates, areas where major connectors will contact thin tissue, and beneath framework extension onto bridge areas for attachment of resin bases, which correspond accurately to the tissue topography. See also *blockout.*

**re·lieve** (re-lēv') [L. *relevare* to lighten] to mitigate or remove pain or distress.

**re·line** (re-līn') to resurface the tissue side of a denture with new base material in order to achieve a more accurate fit.

**re·lux·a·tion** (re″lək-sa'shən) redislocation.

**REM** rapid eye movements (see also under *sleep*).

**rem** (rem) [*r*oentgen-*e*quivalent–*m*an] the quantity of any ionizing radiation which has the same biological effectiveness as 1 rad of x-rays; 1 rem = 1 rad × RBE (relative biological effectiveness).

**Re·mak's ganglion** (ra'mahks) [Robert *Remak,* German neurologist, 1815–1865] see under *ganglion.*

**Re·mak's paralysis, reflex, symptom (sign)** (ra'mahks) [Ernst Julius *Remak,* German neurologist, 1848–1911] see under *paralysis, reflex,* and *symptom.*

**re·me·di·al** (rə-me'de-əl) [L. *remedialis*] curative, acting as a remedy.

**rem·e·dy** (rem'ə-de) [L. *remedium*] anything that cures, palliates, or prevents disease.
**concordant r's,** a homeopathic term for remedies of similar action, but of dissimilar origin.
**inimic r's,** a homeopathic term for remedies whose actions are antagonistic.
**tissue r's,** the twelve remedies which, according to the biochemical school of homeopathy, form the mineral bases of the body.

**rem·i·fen·ta·nil hy·dro·chlo·ride** (rem″ĭ-fen'tə-nil) a short-acting opioid analgesic, used as an anesthesia adjunct.

**Re·mij·ia** (re-mij'e-ə) a genus of shrubs of the family Rubiaceae. *R. peduncula'ta* Flueck. is a source of cuprea bark, which contains cinchona alkaloids.

**re·min·er·al·i·za·tion** (re-min″ər-əl-ĭ-za'shən) the restoration of mineral elements, as of calcium salts to bones or teeth.

**re·mis·sion** (re-mish'ən) [L. *remissio*] a diminution or abatement of the symptoms of a disease; also the period during which such diminution occurs.

**re·mit·tence** (re-mit'əns) temporary abatement, without actual cessation, of symptoms.

**re·mit·tent** (re-mit'ənt) [L. *remittere* to send back] having periods of abatement and of exacerbation.

**rem·nant** (rem'nənt) something remaining; a residue; a vestige.
**acroblastic r.,** the peripheral part of the acroblast which recedes into the protoplasm of the spermatid and later disintegrates.
**chylomicron r's,** partially metabolized chylomicrons that have lost most of their triglycerides via degradation in muscle and adipose tissue but retain their cholesteryl esters; they reenter the bloodstream and are taken up into hepatic cells via receptor-mediated endocytosis. Within the liver, they are digested and their cholesteryl esters cleaved to generate free cholesterol.

**re·mod·el·ing** (re-mod'əl-ing) reorganization or renovation of an old structure.
**bone r.,** absorption of bone tissue and simultaneous deposition of new bone; in normal bone the two processes are in dynamic equilibrium.

**re·mo·ti·va·tion** (re-mo″tĭ-va'shən) any of various group therapy techniques used with long-term, withdrawn patients in mental hospitals to stimulate their communication, vocational, and social skills and interest in their environment.

**ren** (ren) gen. *re'nis* pl. *re'nes,* [L.] [TA] kidney (q.v.): either of the two organs in the lumbar region that excrete the urine.
**r. mo'bilis,** hypermobile kidney.
**r. ungulifor'mis,** horseshoe kidney.

**Re·nac·i·din** (re-nas'ĭ-din) trademark for a preparation of hemiacidrin.

**re·nal** (re'nəl) [L. *renalis*] pertaining to the kidney; called also *nephric.*

**Re·naut's bodies** (rĕ-nōz') [Joseph Louis *Renaut,* French physician, 1844–1917] see under *body.*

**ren·cu·lus** (ren'ku-ləs) pl. *ren'culi* [L.] renal lobe; see *lobi renales,* under *lobus.*

**Ren·du-Os·ler-Web·er syndrome** (ron-du' ōs'lər va'bər) [Henri Jules Louis Marie *Rendu,* French physician, 1844–1902; Sir William *Osler,* Canadian physician, 1849–1919; Frederick Parkes *Weber,* British physician, 1863–1962] hereditary hemorrhagic telangiectasia.

**re·nes** (re'nēz) [L.] plural of *ren.*

**Ren·ese** (rə-nēs') trademark for preparations of polythiazide.
**R.-R,** trademark for a fixed combination of polythiazide and reserpine.

**re·nic·u·lus** (rə-nik'u-ləs) pl. *renic'uli* [L.] renal lobe; see *lobi renales,* under *lobus.*

**ren·i·form** (ren'ĭ-form) [*ren-* + *form*] shaped like a kidney.

**re·nin** (re'nin) [EC 3.4.23.15] [MeSH: Renin] an enzyme of the hydrolase class that catalyzes cleavage of the leucine-leucine bond in angiotensinogen to generate angiotensin I. The enzyme is synthesized as inactive prorenin in the kidney and released into the blood in the active form in response to various metabolic stimuli. Not to be confused with *rennin* (chymosin).
**big r.,** prorenin.

**re·nin·ism** (re'nin-iz″əm) a condition marked by overproduction of renin; see also *hyperreninemia..*
**primary r.,** a syndrome of hypertension, hypokalemia, hyperaldosteronism, and elevated plasma renin activity, due to proliferation of juxtaglomerular cells.

**reni·pel·vic** (ren″ĭ-pel′vik) pertaining to the pelvis of the kidney.

**reni·por·tal** (ren″ĭ-por′təl) [*ren-* + *portal*] pertaining to the portal system of the kidneys.

**ren·net** (ren′ət) a commercial preparation of chymosin (rennin), used to make cheeses and rennet custards.

**ren·nin** (ren′in) chymosin.

**ren(o)-** [L. *ren* kidney] a combining form denoting relationship to a kidney.

**re·no·cor·ti·cal** (re″no-kor′tĭ-kəl) pertaining to the cortex of a kidney.

**re·no·cu·ta·ne·ous** (re″no-ku-ta′ne-əs) pertaining to the kidneys and skin.

**re·no·cys·to·gram** (re″no-sis′to-gram) renogram.

**re·no·gas·tric** (re″no-gas′trik) pertaining to the kidney and stomach; nephrogastric.

**Re·no·graf·in** (re″no-graf′in) trademark for preparations of diatrizoate sodium and diatrizoate meglumine.

**re·no·gram** (re′no-gram) a graphic record of kidney function produced by externally monitoring the level of radioactivity in the bladder as a radiopharmaceutical agent enters it from the kidney via the ureters; called also *renocystogram.*

**re·nog·ra·phy** (re-nog′rə-fe) [*reno-* + *-graphy*] radiography of the kidney.

**re·no·in·tes·ti·nal** (re″no-in-tes′tĭ-nəl) pertaining to the kidney and intestine.

**re·no·med·ul·lary** (re″no-med′u-lar″e) [*reno-* + *medullary*] pertaining to the medulla of the kidney.

**re·nop·a·thy** (re-nop′ə-the) [*reno-* + *-pathy*] nephropathy.

**re·no·pri·val** (re″no-pri′vəl) pertaining to, characterized by, or resulting from deprivation of kidney function.

**Re·no·quid** (re′no-kwid) trademark for a preparation of sulfacytine.

**re·no·troph·ic** (re″no-trof′ik) having the ability to increase kidney size.

**re·no·trop·ic** (re″no-trop′ik) having a special affinity for kidney tissue.

**re·no·vas·cu·lar** (re″no-vas′ku-lər) [*reno-* + *vascular*] pertaining to or affecting the blood vessels of the kidney.

**Re·no·vist** (re″no-vist′) trademark for preparations of diatrizoate sodium and diatrizoate meglumine.

**Ren·shaw cells** (ren′shaw) [Birdsey *Renshaw,* American neurophysiologist, 20th century] see under *cell.*

**ren·ule** (ren′ūl) an area of the kidney supplied by a branch of the renal artery, usually consisting of three or four medullary pyramids and their corresponding cortical substance.

**re·nun·cu·lus** (re-nung′ku-ləs) renal lobe; see *lobi renales,* under *lobus.*

**Reo·Pro** (re′o-pro″) trademark for a preparation of abciximab.

**Reo·vi·ri·dae** (re″o-vir′ĭ-de) [MeSH: Reoviridae] the reoviruses: a family of RNA viruses having a nonenveloped icosahedral virion 60–80 nm in diameter; virions have two protein shells, the particle with the outer shell removed being referred to as the core. The genome consists of 10 to 12 structural segments of linear double-stranded RNA (total MW 12–20 × $10^6$, 10–27 kbp depending on the genus). Virions contain 10–12 structural proteins, including a transcriptase, and are resistant to heat but sensitive to lipid solvents. Replication and assembly occur in the cytoplasm. Transmission is by the fecal-oral route, by fomites, or by arthropod vectors. Vertebrate pathogens are included in the genera *Orthoreovirus, Orbivirus, Rotavirus, Coltivirus,* and *Aquareovirus.* Other genera contain arthropod and plant pathogens.

**reo·vi·rus** (re′o-vi″rəs) [*r*espiratory and *e*nteric *o*rphan + *virus*] 1. any virus belonging to the family Reoviridae. 2. any virus belonging to the genus *Orthoreovirus.*

**re·ox·i·da·tion** (re-ok″sĭ-da′shən) the act of taking up oxygen again, as by hemoglobin.

**re·ox·y·gen·a·tion** (re-ok″sĭ-jə-na′shən) in radiobiology, the phenomenon in which hypoxic (and thus radioresistant) tumor cells become more exposed to oxygen (and thus more radiosensitive) by coming into closer proximity to capillaries after death and loss of other tumor cells due to previous irradiation.

**Rep.** abbreviation for L. *repeta′tur,* let it be repeated.

**rep** (rep) [*r*oentgen *e*quivalent *p*hysical] an unofficial unit of the amount of radiation of any kind which yields an amount of energy transferred to the tissue equal to that transferred by 1 roentgen of hard x- or γ-radiation (200 V or greater); it is approximately 93 ergs per gram of water or soft tissue.

**re·pair** (re-pār′) the physical or mechanical restoration of damaged or diseased tissues by the growth of healthy new cells or by surgical apposition.

**re·pa·ten·cy** (re-pa′tən-se) [*re-* + *patency*] reestablishment of the opening in a part or vessel which has been closed.

**re·peat** (rə-pēt′) something done or occurring more than once, particularly over and over.
**long terminal r's (LTR),** identical nucleotide sequences occurring at each end of a proviral genome or a transposon and believed to be essential for integration of the molecule into host DNA; an LTR is several hundred nucleotides long and contains a short, inverted, repeated sequence at each of its own ends. Many also contain elements regulating the expression of the DNA they surround.

**re·peat·a·bil·i·ty** (re-pēt″ə-bil′ĭ-te) precision (def. 2).

**re·pel·lent** (re-pel′ənt) [L. *repellere* to drive back] able to repel or drive off; also an agent so acting, as *insect repellent.*

**re·pel·ler** (re-pel′ər) an instrument used in labor of animals to push back the fetus until the head and limbs can be properly placed for normal delivery.

**re·per·co·la·tion** (re″pər-ko-la′shən) [*re-* + *percolation*] a second or repeated percolation with the same materials.

**re·per·cus·sion** (re″pər-kush′ən) [L. *repercussio* rebound] 1. the driving in of an eruption or the scattering of a swelling. 2. ballottement.

**re·per·cus·sive** (re″pər-kus′iv) 1. causing or pertaining to repercussion. 2. an agent causing repercussion; a repellent.

**re·per·fu·sion** (re″pər-fu′zhən) [MeSH: Reperfusion] restoration of blood flow to an area or part that was temporarily ischemic.

**re·pe·ta·tur** (re″pe-ta′tūr) [L.] let it be repeated.

**re·place·ment** (re-plās′ment) 1. substitution; see also *replacement therapy,* under *therapy.* 2. arthroplasty.
**joint r.,** arthroplasty.
**total joint r.,** see under *arthroplasty.*

**re·plan·ta·tion** (re″plan-ta′shən) [MeSH: Replantation] the replacement of an organ or other structure, such as a digit, limb, or tooth, to the site from which it was previously lost or removed; called also *reimplantation.*

**re·plen·ish·er** (re-plen′ish-ər) an agent that restores what has been lost, used up, or is lacking.

**re·ple·tion** (re-ple′shən) [L. *repletio*] the condition of being full.

**rep·li·case** (rep′lĭ-kās) 1. an RNA-directed RNA polymerase. 2. more generically, any enzyme that replicates nucleic acids, i.e., a DNA or RNA polymerase.

**rep·li·ca·tion** (rep″lĭ-ka′shən) [L. *replicatio* a fold backwards] 1. a turning back of a part so as to form a duplication. 2. repetition of an experiment to ensure accuracy. 3. the process of duplicating or reproducing, as the replication of an exact copy of a polynucleotide strand of DNA or RNA.
**DNA r.,** the production of multiple identical copies of a DNA molecule by unwinding the two strands of the double helix and forming new complementary strands thereto.
**semiconservative r.,** a term used to characterize the mode in which DNA is replicated, to wit, each daughter molecule has one newly synthesized strand and one strand from the parent molecule.

**rep·li·con** (rep′lĭ-kon) [MeSH: Replicon] a unit of DNA that contains an initiation point and a termination point and is capable of self-replication. A bacterial chromosome or plasmid consists of a single replicon, while a mammalian chromosome may contain 30,000 to 40,000 replicon units.

**Re·poise** (re-poiz′) trademark for preparations of butaperazine.

**re·po·lar·iza·tion** (re-po″lər-ĭ-za′shən) the reestablishment of polarity, especially the return of cell membrane potential to resting potential after depolarization. See also *potassium channel* and *sodium channel,* under *channel.*
**early r.,** a normal variant of the usually isoelectric ST segment in which the segment is elevated at its J point; it is seen mostly in children, young adults, and black men.

**re·po·si·tion·ing** (re″pə-zish′ən-ing) the replacing of a structure or part to its normal site.
**jaw r.,** the changing of any relative position of the mandible to the maxilla, usually by altering the occlusion of the natural or artificial teeth.
**muscle r.,** surgical replacement of a muscle attachment into a more acceptable functional position.

**re·pos·i·tor** (re-poz′ĭ-tor) an instrument used in returning a displaced organ, especially the uterus, to the normal position.

**re·pos·i·to·ry** (re-poz′ĭ-tor-e) a place where something is stored; used in pharmacology to refer to the injection, usually intramuscularly, of a long-acting drug, which is slowly absorbed and is therefore prolonged in its action.

**re·pres·sion** (re-presh′ən) [MeSH: Repression] 1. the act of restraining, inhibiting, or suppressing. 2. in psychiatry, an unconscious defense mechanism in which unacceptable ideas, fears, and impulses are thrust out or kept out of consciousness. 3. gene r.
**coordinate r.**, parallel diminution of the concentrations of the several enzymes of a metabolic pathway, resulting from increases in the level of repressor.
**endproduct r.**, enzyme r.
**enzyme r.**, interference, usually by the endproduct of a pathway, with synthesis of the enzymes of that pathway.
**gene r.**, the inhibition of gene transcription of an operon; in prokaryotes the mechanism involves binding of the operon by a repressor, sometimes also requiring the binding of a corepressor or absence of an inducer. The end result is frequently a decrease in the level of an enzyme.

**re·pres·sor** (re-pres′or) [L. "a restrainer"] in genetics, a substance produced by a regulator gene which acts through the cytoplasm to prevent initiation by the operator gene of protein synthesis by the operon.

**re·pro·duc·i·bil·i·ty** (re″-pro-doo″sĭ-bil′ĭ-te) precision (def. 2).

**re·pro·duc·tion** (re″pro-duk′shən) [*re-* + L. *productio* production] [MeSH: Reproduction] 1. the production of offspring by organized bodies. 2. the creation of a similar object or situation; duplication; replication.
**asexual r.**, reproduction without the fusion of sexual cells, as by fission or budding.
**bisexual r.**, see *sexual r.*
**cytogenic r.**, reproduction in which the new individual proceeds from a single germ cell or zygote.
**sexual r.**, reproduction by the fusion of a female sexual cell with a male sexual cell *(bisexual r., amphigony, gamogenesis, syngamy)* or by the development of an unfertilized egg *(unisexual r., parthenogenesis).*
**somatic r.**, reproduction in which the new individual proceeds from a multicellular fragment produced by fission or budding.
**unisexual r.**, see *sexual r.*

**re·pro·duc·tive** (re″pro-duk′tiv) subserving or pertaining to the production of offspring.

**re·pro·ter·ol hy·dro·chlo·ride** (re″pro-ter′ōl) a bronchodilator, $C_{18}H_{23}N_5O_5 \cdot HCl$.

**rep·til·ase** (rep′til-ās) [MeSH: Reptilase] an enzyme from Russell's viper venom that clots fibrinogen and can be used to determine blood coagulation time.

**rep·tile** (rep′tīl) [MeSH: Reptiles] any member of the class Reptilia.

**Rep·til·ia** (rep-til′e-ə) a class of aquatic or terrestrial, cold-blooded vertebrates, including snakes, lizards, turtles, alligators, and crocodiles, as well as the extinct dinosaurs, which have bodies covered with horny scales or plates and breathe by means of lungs; most lay eggs outside of the body.

**re·pul·lu·la·tion** (re-pul″u-la′shən) [*re-* + *pullulation*] renewed growth by sprouting.

**re·pul·sion** (re-pul′zhən) [L. *re-* back + *pellere* to drive] 1. the act of driving apart or away; a force which tends to drive two bodies apart. It is the opposite of attraction. 2. in genetics, occurrence on opposite chromosomes in a double heterozygote of the two mutant alleles of interest. Cf. *coupling.*

**RES** reticuloendothelial system.

**re·up·take** (re-up′tāk) reabsorption of a previously secreted substance.

**re·sa·zu·rin** (re-sa′zu-rin) a quinone-imine compound used as a pH indicator with a pH range of 3.8 (orange) to 6.5 (violet). It is also used as an indicator of redox potential, turning from blue (oxidized) to pink (partially reduced) to colorless (fully reduced).

**re·scin·na·mine** (re-sin′ə-min) an alkaloid obtained from *Rauwolfia serpentina* and other species of *R.;* used as an antihypertensive and also as a tranquilizer.

**res·cue** (res′ku) salvage.

**re·sect** (re-sekt′) to remove part or all of an organ or tissue.

**re·sec·ta·ble** (re-sek′tə-bəl) capable of being resected; lending itself to resection.

**re·sec·tion** (re-sek′shən) [L. *resectio*] removal of a portion or all of an organ or other structure. Called also *excision* and *ectomy.*
**gastric r.**, gastrectomy.
**Girdlestone r.**, removal of the femoral head and neck in cases of severe hip infection.
**root r.**, apicoectomy.
**sleeve r.**, see under *lobectomy.*
**submucous r.**, a formerly common technique for correction of a deviated nasal septum: the mucous membrane is opened and a portion of the underlying tissue is excised and repositioned or replaced.
**transurethral r. of bladder tumor (TURBT),** removal of a tumor of the urinary bladder by means of a cystoscope passed through the urethra.
**transurethral r. of the prostate (TURP), transurethral prostatic r.,** resection of the prostate by means of a cystoscope passed through the urethra.
**wedge r.**, removal of a triangular-shaped segment of tissue.

**re·sec·to·scope** (re-sek′to-skōp) an instrument with a wide-angle telescope and an electrically activated wire loop for transurethral removal or biopsy of lesions of the bladder, prostate, or urethra.

**re·sec·tos·co·py** (re″sək-tos′kə-pe) resection or biopsy of lesions by means of the resectoscope.

**re·ser·pine** (rə-sər′pēn) [USP] [MeSH: Reserpine] an alkaloid isolated from the root of *Rauwolfia serpentina* (L.) Benth. ex Kurz (Apocyanaceae) and other species of *R.;* used as an antihypertensive, and also as a sedative, administered orally and intramuscularly.

**Res·er·poid** (res′ər-poid) trademark for a preparation of reserpine.

**re·serve** (re-zerv′) 1. to hold back for future use. 2. a supply, beyond that ordinarily used, which may be utilized in an emergency.
**alkali r., alkaline r.,** the amount of conjugate base components of the blood buffers; since bicarbonate is the most important of these conjugate bases, the blood bicarbonate is often considered to be equivalent.
**cardiac r.**, the potential ability of the heart to perform a wide range of work beyond that required under basal conditions, depending on changing demands of various physiological or pathological states; usually expressed as a percentage increase above normal.
**contractile r.**, the additional amount of contractility that can be elicited from abnormally contracting ventricular wall segments by application of a suitable stimulus.
**renal r.**, the increase in glomerular filtration rate that is seen for 2 to 4 hours after intake of a high-protein meal.

**re·ser·voir** (rez′ər-vwahr) [Fr. *réservoir,* from *réserver* to reserve] 1. a place or cavity for storage. 2. cisterna. 3. an alternate or passive host or carrier that harbors pathogenic organisms, without injury to itself, and serves as a source from which other individuals can be infected. Called also *reservoir host* or *r. of infection.*
**chromatin r.**, karyosome.
**continent ileal r.**, an intra-abdominal pouch having a volume of at least 500 mL and a valve; it maintains continence of feces and is emptied by a catheter when full. See also *Kock pouch.*
**ileoanal r.**, a pouch for the retention of feces, formed by suturing together multiple limbs of ileum and connected to the anus by a short conduit of ileum; done in conjunction with colectomy and ileoanal anastomosis to provide for continent elimination of feces in the management of ulcerative colitis.

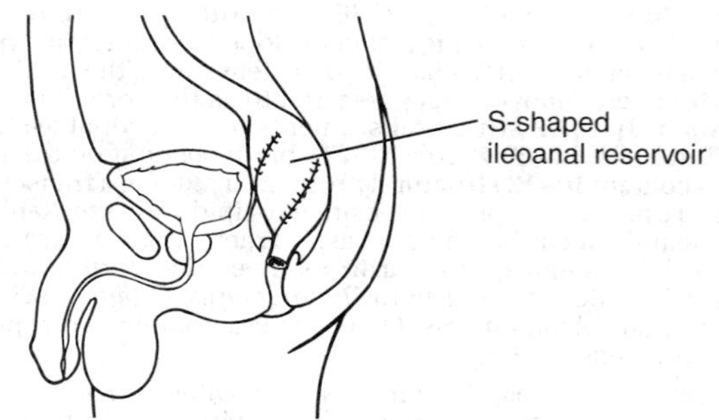


**r. of infection,** reservoir, def. 3.
**Ommaya r.**, a device implanted beneath the galea aponeurotica for instillation of medication or removal of fluid through a catheter positioned in a lateral ventricle of the brain.
**Pecquet's r.**, cisterna chyli.

**re·shap·ing** (re-shāp′ing) a restoration or change of shape, as of a crown, bridge, or denture.

**res·i·dent** (rez′ĭ-dənt) a graduate and licensed physician receiving training in a specialty in a hospital.

**re·sid·ua** (re-zid′u-ə) [L.] plural of *residuum.*

**re·sid·u·al** (re-zid′u-əl) [L. *residuus*] remaining or left behind.

**res·i·due** (rez'ĭ-doo) [L. *residuum,* from *re-* back + *sidere* to sit] 1. a remainder; that which remains after the removal of other substances. 2. in biochemistry, the portion of a molecule that remains after it has lost some of its components, as an amino acid residue, which loses a water molecule when it is joined to another amino acid.
**day r.,** the thoughts, feelings, and ideas related to the events of the day that appear in or shape the contents of the dreams that night.

**re·sid·u·um** (re-zid'u-əm) pl. *resid'ua* [L.] 1. a residue or remainder. 2. in coccidian protozoa, the material remaining after completion of different stages in the life cycle of the parasite. Called also *residual body.*
**gastric r.,** the contents of the stomach during the interdigestive period, as in the morning before eating.

**re·sil·ience** (rə-zil'yəns) [L. *resilire* to leap back] 1. the property of being able to return to the original form after distortion, as by bending, compressing, or stretching. 2. the ability to recover readily from an illness. 3. resiliency.

**re·sil·ien·cy** (rə-zil'yən-se) 1. resilience. 2. a measure of the energy required to stress an object to the proportional limit (see under *limit*).

**re·sil·i·ent** (re-zil'yənt) [L. *resiliens*] elastic; returning to its former shape or size after distortion.

**res·in** (rez'in) [L. *resina*] a mixture of carboxylic acids, essential oils, and terpenes, occurring as exudations on various trees and shrubs or produced synthetically. Resins are highly combustible semisolids or amorphous solids that are insoluble in water, while some are soluble in ethanol and others in carbon tetrachloride, ether, and volatile oils. Most are soft and sticky, but harden after exposure to cold.
**acrylic r's,** a class of thermoplastic resins, ethylene derivatives containing a vinyl group, produced by polymerization of acrylic or methacrylic acid or their derivatives; used in the fabrication of medical prostheses and dental restorations and appliances.
**activated r.,** self-curing r.
**anion exchange r.,** see *ion exchange r.*
**A-stage r.,** resole.
**autopolymer r.,** self-curing r.
**azure A carbacrylic r.,** azuresin.
**carbacrylamine r's,** a mixture of 87.5 per cent of cation exchangers, carbacrylic resin, and potassium carbacrylic resin, with 12.5 per cent of the anion exchanger, polyaminemethylene resin; used to increase fecal excretion of sodium in the treatment of edema.
**cation exchange r.,** see *ion exchange r.*
**cholestyramine r.** [USP], a strongly basic anion exchange resin in the chloride form, consisting of styrene-divinylbenzene copolymer with quaternary ammonium functional groups, having an affinity for bile acids, which it binds into an insoluble complex that is excreted in the feces, resulting in elimination of bile acids from the enterohepatic circulation and in increased oxidation of cholesterol to bile acids; administered orally for the relief of pruritus associated with cholestasis occurring in partial biliary obstruction and as adjunctive therapy to diet in the management of patients with elevated cholesterol due to primary type II hyperlipoproteinemia (patients with pure hypercholesterolemia).
**cold-curing r.,** self-curing r.
**composite r.,** resin matrix composite.
**copolymer r.,** one produced by the concurrent and joint polymerization of two or more different monomers or polymers.
**C-stage r.,** resite.
**cyanoacrylate r.,** a resin based on alkyl 2-cyanoacrylates, used in surgical sutures and periodontal dressings.
**direct filling r.,** a resin or a composite, usually an acrylic, that is inserted directly into the prepared cavity and allowed to polymerize at the temperature in the mouth.
**epoxy r.,** a thermosetting resin based on reactivity of the epoxide group, which is characterized by toughness, adhesibility, chemical resistance, dielectric properties, and dimensional stability; several modified types are used as denture base material. Inhalation of its vapors can cause *epoxy resin lung,* a form of hypersensitivity pneumonitis.
**heat-curing r.,** one that requires the use of heat to effect its polymerization.
**ion exchange r.,** a high molecular weight, insoluble polymer of simple organic compounds with the ability to exchange its attached ions for other ions in the surrounding solution. They are classified as *(a) cation* or *anion exchange resins,* depending on which ions the resin exchanges, and *(b) carboxylic, sulfonic,* etc., depending on the nature of the active groups. *Cation exchange resins* are used to restrict intestinal sodium absorption in edematous states; *anion exchange resins* are used as antacids in the treatment of ulcers.
**ionomer r.,** a copolymer of ethylene and a vinyl monomer with an acid group to form a transparent resilient thermoplastic material; used in flasks, bottles, and tubing.
**light-activated r., light-cured r.,** one whose polymerization is activated by exposure to light; dental resins are usually activated by blue light (wavelength 400–500 nm).
**podophyllum r.** [USP], a powdered mixture of resins removed from podophyllum by percolation with alcohol and subsequent precipitation upon addition of acidified water; used as a topical caustic in the treatment of laryngeal papillomas, condyloma acuminatum, and other epitheliomas, as a 25 per cent dispersion in compound benzoin tincture, or as a solution in alcohol. Formerly used as a cathartic. Called also *podophyllin.* See also *podophyllotoxin.*
**polyamine-methylene r.,** a polyethylene polyamine methylene substituted resin of diphenylol dimethylmethane and formaldehyde in basic form; because of its exchange-resin action it has been used as a gastric antacid.
**quick-cure r.,** self-curing r.
**self-curing r.,** any resin that can be polymerized by the addition of an activator and a catalyst without the use of external heat; used in dental restorations and repairs. Called also *activated r., autopolymer r., cold-curing r.,* and *quick-cure r.*
**styrene r.,** polystyrene.
**synthetic r.,** an amorphous, organic, semisolid or solid material produced from low-molecular-weight organic compounds by polymerization or condensation.
**thermoset r., thermosetting r.,** a resin that after its initial hardening reaction remains rigid or solid when cooled and reheated; several are used in dentistry. A common example is epoxy resin.
**vinyl r.,** a thermoplastic resin, an ethylene derivative containing the vinyl radical, $CH_2{=}CH{-}$.

**Res·i·nat** (rez'ĭ-nat) trademark for preparations of polyamine-methylene resin.

**res·i·noid** (rez'ĭ-noid) 1. resembling a resin. 2. a substance resembling a resin. 3. a dry therapeutic precipitate prepared from a vegetable tincture.

**res·i·nous** (rez'ĭ-nəs) [L. *resinosus*] of the nature of a resin.

**re·sis·tance** (re-zis'təns) [L. *resistere* to stand back] 1. opposition, or counteracting force. 2. in psychiatry, conscious or unconscious defenses that prevent material in the unconscious, as repressed thoughts, from coming into awareness. 3. the natural ability of an organism to resist microorganisms or toxins produced in disease. 4. the opposition to the flow of electrical current between two points of a circuit; it is the voltage drop between the two points divided by the current flow, expressed in ohms. Symbol R or *R.*
**airway r.,** the opposition of the tracheobronchial tree to air flow: the mouth-to-alveoli pressure difference divided by the air flow. Symbol $R_A$ or $R_{AW}$.
**androgen r.,** resistance of target organs to the action of androgens, resulting in any of a spectrum of defects from normal-appearing phenotypes in which men may have normal genitalia but infertility due to *incomplete* and *complete androgen resistance.*
**androgen r., complete,** an extreme form of male pseudohermaphroditism due to androgen resistance. The individual is phenotypically female but is of XY chromosomal sex; there may be rudimentary uterus and tubes, but the gonads are typically testes, which may be abdominal or inguinal in position. Called also *androgen insensitivity syndrome, feminizing testes syndrome, Morris syndrome, testicular feminization,* and *testicular feminization syndrome.*
**androgen r., incomplete,** forms manifested by any of various degrees of ambiguous genitalia less than in complete androgen resistance, such as a male phenotype with hypospadias and a small vaginal pouch, a hooded phallus, or a bifid scrotum that may or may not contain gonads. Called also *incomplete testicular feminization.*
**drug r.,** the ability of a microorganism to withstand the effects of a drug that are lethal to most members of its species. Primary drug resistance refers to initial infection by a resistant organism; secondary drug resistance to resistance that develops during the course of therapy. Microbial resistance to a drug can be symbolized by the superscript R, *R,* r, or *r* attached to the name of the drug.
**electrical r.,** resistance (def. 4).
**environmental r.,** the sum of the physical and biologic factors that prevent a species from reproducing at its maximum rate.
**insulin r.,** impairment of normal biologic responses to insulin, which may result from abnormalities in the beta-cell products, binding of insulin to antagonists such as anti-insulin antibodies, defects in or reduced numbers of receptors, or defects in the insulin action cascade in the target cell. It can also be caused by excessive quantities of growth hormone, adrenocortical steroids, or some other regulators, or by chronic hyperinsulinemia secondary to hyperphagia. Incidence is increased with conditions such as obesity, diabetes mellitus, acromegaly, uremia, and certain rare, possibly genetic, autoimmune disorders.
**internal r.,** the electrical resistance within a voltage source, e.g., a battery, power supply, or generator.
**multidrug r., multiple drug r.,** a phenomenon seen in some malignant cell lines: cells that have developed natural resistance to a single cytotoxic compound are also resistant to structurally unrelated chemotherapy agents.

**peripheral vascular r.**, total peripheral r.
**pleiotropic drug r.**, multidrug r.
**pulmonary vascular r.**, the vascular resistance of the pulmonary circulation, equal to the difference between the mean pulmonary arterial pressure and the left atrial filling pressure divided by the cardiac output.
**total peripheral r.**, the vascular resistance of the systemic circulation: the difference between the mean arterial pressure and central venous pressure divided by the cardiac output. Called also *peripheral vascular r.*
**total pulmonary r.**, pulmonary vascular r.
**vascular r.**, the opposition to blood flow in a vascular bed; it is the pressure drop across the bed divided by the blood flow, conventionally expressed in peripheral resistance units or in dyne sec $cm^{-5}$. Symbol R or *R*.
**venous r.**, resistance to blood flow by a vein; under normal conditions it depends largely on extrinsic factors such as compression by surrounding structures. Thrombi often but not always cause an increase in resistance.

**res•ite** (res'īt) an insoluble, infusible cross-linked form produced by further reaction of resole under heat.

**res•ole** (res'ōl) a thermosetting resin in the uncured, unformed state, consisting primarily of partially condensed phenol alcohols.

**res•o•lu•tion** (rez″o-loo'shən) [L. *resolutum,* from *resolvere* to unbind] 1. the subsidence of a pathologic state, as the subsidence of an inflammation, or the softening and disappearance of a swelling. 2. the perception as separate of two adjacent objects or points. In microscopy, it is the minimal distance at which two adjacent objects can be distinguished as separate. The resolving power of an instrument depends on the wavelength of the radiation used and the numerical aperture of the system; it is expressed in microns distance or lines per millimeter.

**re•solve** (re-zolv') [L. *resolvere*] 1. to restore to the normal state after some pathologic process. 2. to separate a thing into its component parts.

**re•sol•vent** (re-zol'vənt) [L. *resolvens* dissolving] 1. promoting resolution or the dissipation of a pathologic growth. 2. an agent that promotes resolution.

**res•o•nance** (rez'o-nəns) [L. *resonare* to echo] 1. the prolongation and intensification of sound produced by transmission of its vibrations to a cavity, especially a sound elicited by percussion. See also *dullness* and *flatness.* 2. a vocal sound as heard in auscultation. 3. mesomerism.
**amphoric r.**, a sound heard upon percussion or auscultation, resembling that produced by blowing over the mouth of an empty bottle, as in amphoric respiration. See also *cavernous voice,* under *voice.* Called also *amphoric murmur.*
**bandbox r.**, the extremely resonant sound elicited by percussion in cases of emphysema of the lungs. Called also *bandbox sound.*
**cough r.**, a peculiar auscultatory sound elicited by coughing.
**cracked-pot r.**, a peculiar sound elicited by percussion over a pulmonary cavity that communicates with a bronchus. Called also *cracked-pot sound.*
**electron paramagnetic r., electron spin r.**, in spectrometry, a measure of electron spin as an indication of the presence and extent of activity of free radicals in an organic reaction. Abbreviated EPR or ESR.
**hydatid r.**, a peculiar sound heard in the combined auscultation and percussion of a hydatid cyst.
**nuclear magnetic r.**, a measure, by means of applying an external magnetic field to a solution in a constant radio frequency field, of the magnetic moment of atomic nuclei to determine the structure of organic compounds. This technique is used in magnetic resonance imaging (q.v.).
**osteal r.**, the sound elicited by percussion over a bony structure.
**skodaic r.**, increased percussion resonance at the upper part of the chest, with flatness below it; heard above a large pleural effusion or area of consolidation. Called also *Skoda's sign* or *tympany* and *skodaic tympany.*
**tympanic r.**, tympanitic r. (def. 2).
**tympanitic r.**, 1. the peculiar sound elicited by percussing a tympanitic abdomen. 2. the drumlike reverberation of a cavity full of air; called also *tympanic r.*
**vesicular r.**, vesicular breath sounds; see under *sound.*
**vesiculotympanitic r.**, a resonance, heard upon auscultation, that is partly vesicular and partly tympanitic. Called also *wooden r.*
**vocal r. (VR)**, the sound of ordinary speech as heard through the chest wall.
**whispering r.**, whispered pectoriloquy.
**wooden r.**, vesiculotympanitic r.

**res•o•nant** (rez'o-nənt) giving a vibrant sound on percussion.

**res•o•na•tor** (rez'o-na″tor) an instrument used to intensify sounds. In electricity, an electrical circuit in which oscillations of a certain frequency are set up by oscillations of the same frequency in another circuit.

**re•sorb** (re-sorb', re-zorb') to take up or absorb again; to undergo resorption.

**re•sor•cin** (rə-sor'sin) resorcinol.

**re•sor•ci•nism** (rə-sor'sĭ-niz″əm) chronic poisoning by resorcinol, resulting in methemoglobinemia, paralysis, and damage to the capillaries, kidneys, heart, and nervous system.

**re•sor•ci•nol** (rə-sor'sĭ-nol) [USP] a bactericidal, fungicidal, keratolytic, exfoliative, and antipruritic agent, used especially as a topical keratolytic in the treatment of acne and other dermatoses, such as seborrheic dermatitis. Called also *resorcin.*
**r. monoacetate** [USP], the monoacetate salt of resorcinol, used topically as an antiseborrheic and keratolytic.

**re•sorp•tion** (re-sorp'shən) [L. *resorbere* to swallow again] 1. the loss of substance through physiologic or pathologic means, such as loss of dentin and cementum of a tooth, or of the alveolar process of the mandible or maxilla. 2. reabsorption of fluid.
**bone r.**, a type of bone loss (resorption) due to osteoclastic activity.
**idiopathic r.**, resorption of calcified tissues without apparent cause.
**root r.**, resorption in which cementum or dentin is lost from the root of a tooth owing to cementoclastic or osteoclastic activity in conditions such as trauma of occlusion or neoplasms.
**tooth r., external,** resorption of calcified dental tissue, beginning on the external surface of the root and extending to the cementum, dentin, and eventually into the root canal. See also *internal tooth r.,* def. 1.
**tooth r., internal,** 1. an unusual form of tooth resorption beginning centrally in a tooth, and apparently initiated by inflammatory hyperplasia of the pulp, characterized by a pink hued area on the crown showing the hyperplastic vascular pulp tissue filling the resorbed area. Called also *chronic perforating hyperplasia* and *pink tooth of Mummery.* 2. external tooth resorption that ramifies into the dentin.
**tubular r.**, resorption by renal tubular cells of elements of the fluid filtered at the glomerulus.

**res•pir•a•ble** (rə-spir'ə-bəl) 1. suitable for respiration. 2. small enough to be inhaled, such as an irritating particle.

**res•pi•ra•tion** (res″pĭ-ra'shən) [L. *respiratio*] [MeSH: Respiration] 1. the exchange of oxygen and carbon dioxide between the atmosphere and the cells of the body. The process includes *ventilation* (inspiration and expiration), the diffusion of oxygen from pulmonary alveoli to the blood and of carbon dioxide from the blood to the alveoli, and the transport of oxygen to and carbon dioxide from the body cells. Symbol R. 2. ventilation (def. 2). 3. the exergonic metabolic processes in living cells by which molecular oxygen is taken in, organic substances are oxidized, free energy is released, and carbon dioxide, water, and other oxidized products are given off by the cell; called also *cell r.*
**abdominal r.**, respiration maintained by contribution of the diaphragm and respiratory muscles. Cf. *thoracic r.*
**aerobic r.**, the oxidative transformation of certain substrates into secretory products, the released energy being used in the process of assimilation.
**amphoric r.**, respiration characterized by amphoric resonance, heard over pulmonary cavities or pneumothorax.
**anaerobic r.**, a form of respiration in which energy is released from chemical reactions in which free oxygen takes no part.
**artificial r.**, any artificial method of ventilation in which air is forced into and out of the lungs of a person who has stopped breathing. It may be either mechanical (see *mechanical ventilation*) or done as an emergency procedure with no mechanical equipment. The most effective nonmechanical emergency technique is the *mouth-to-mouth method;* other less used techniques are the *Holger Nielsen method, Schafer method,* and *Silvester method* (see under *method*). Called also *artificial* or *assisted ventilation.*
**asthmoid r.**, wheezing respiration like that of bronchial asthma.
**Biot's r.**, breathing characterized by irregular periods of apnea alternating with periods in which four or five breaths of identical depth are taken; seen in patients with increased intracranial pressure. Called also *Biot's breathing* or *sign.*
**bronchial r.**, bronchial breath sounds; see under *sound.*
**bronchocavernous r.**, breath sounds intermediate in character between bronchial and cavernous, heard over a lung cavity with solidified lung tissue adjacent to it.
**bronchovesicular r.**, bronchovesicular breath sounds; see under *sound.*
**cavernous r.**, cavernous breath sounds; see under *sound.*
**cell r.**, respiration, def. 2.
**Cheyne-Stokes r.**, breathing characterized by rhythmic waxing and waning of the rate and depth of respiration, with regularly recurring periods of apnea; seen especially in coma resulting from affection of the nervous centers.
**cogwheel r.**, a form with a peculiar jerky inspiration; the expiratory

and inspiratory sounds are not continuous but are split into two or more separate sounds. Called also *interrupted r.* and *jerky r.*
**collateral r.**, see under *ventilation.*
**controlled diaphragmatic r.**, the intentional use of abdominal respiration for the purpose of limiting the motion of the apices of the lung.
**costal r.**, thoracic r.
**diaphragmatic r.**, that which is mainly performed by the diaphragm.
**divided r.**, respiration marked by a pause between the inspiratory and expiratory sounds.
**electrophrenic r.**, artificial respiration induced by electric stimulation of the phrenic nerve to produce rhythmic contractions of the diaphragm, done to provide ventilatory support in patients with diaphragmatic paralysis. Abbreviated EPR. Called also *diaphragmatic* or *phrenic pacing.*
**external r.**, the exchange of gases between the lungs and the blood. Cf. *internal r.*
**fetal r.**, gaseous interchange through the placenta.
**forced r.**, deliberate hyperventilation.
**internal r.**, the exchange of gases between the body cells and the blood; cf. *external r.* Called also *tissue r.*
**interrupted r.**, cogwheel r.
**jerky r.**, cogwheel r.
**Kussmaul's r., Kussmaul-Kien r.**, a pattern of deep and rapid respiration, seen particularly in metabolic acidosis. Called also *air hunger.*
**paradoxical r.**, respiration in which all or part of a lung is deflated during inspiration and inflated during expiration, as with flail chest or paralysis of the diaphragm.
**periodic r.**, Cheyne-Stokes r.
**puerile r.**, that in which the breathing sounds are more intense than those of normal adult respiration and resemble those of childhood.
**suppressed r.**, respiration without any appreciable sound, as may occur in extensive consolidation of the lung, or pleuritic effusion.
**thoracic r.**, respiration performed by the intercostal and other thoracic muscles. Cf. *abdominal r.* Called also *costal r.*
**tissue r.**, internal r.
**tubular r.**, bronchial breath sounds; see under *sound.*
**vesicular r.**, vesicular breath sounds; see under *sound.*
**vesiculocavernous r.**, cavernous breath sounds with a vesicular quality, indicating a cavity surrounded by healthy lung tissue.
**vicarious r.**, increased action in one lung when that of the other lung is diminished.

**res•pi•ra•tor** (res′pĭ-ra″tor) [MeSH: Ventilators, Mechanical] ventilator (def. 2).
**cuirass r.**, see under *ventilator.*
**Drinker r.**, a type of negative-pressure ventilator consisting of a metal tank enclosing the body of the patient with the head outside. It was formerly in wide use, but its use has now decreased in favor of less cumbersome cuirass and jacket ventilators. Called also *tank ventilator* and, popularly, *iron lung.*
**Engström r.**, a volume-controlled, piston-operated respirator with a sine wave airflow pattern.

**res•pi•ra•to•ry** (res′pĭ-rə-tor″e) [*re-* + L. *spirare* to breathe] pertaining to respiration. Called also *pneumatic.*

**res•pi•rom•e•ter** (res″pĭ-rom′ə-tər) an instrument for determining the character of the respiratory movements.

**re•sponse** (re-spons′) [L. *respondere* to answer, reply] an action or movement due to the application of a stimulus. Called also *reaction.*
**acute phase r.**, a group of physiologic processes occurring soon after the onset of infection, trauma, inflammatory processes, and some malignant conditions. The most prominent change is a dramatic increase of acute phase proteins, especially C-reactive protein, in the serum. Also seen are fever, increased vascular permeability, and a variety of metabolic and pathologic changes.
**anamnestic r.**, secondary immune r.
**autoimmune r.**, an immune response against an autoantigen.
**blink r's**, compound muscle action potentials evoked in the orbicularis oculi muscles by stimulation of the skin innervated by the supraorbital nerve. An early response (the $R_1$ wave) occurs on the same side as the stimulation and a later response (the $R_2$ wave) occurs on both sides along with a twitch of both orbicularis oculi muscles. Called also *blink reflexes.*
**booster r.**, secondary immune r.
**cold r., paradoxical**, an inappropriate sensation of cold due to response of some cold receptors to contact with an object having a temperature above 45°C.
**conditioned r.**, a response evoked by a conditioned stimulus; one occurring to a stimulus that was incapable of evoking it before conditioning.
**decremental r., decrementing r.**, a progressive decrease in amplitude of successive M waves upon repetitive nerve stimulation (q.v.); it may indicate impaired neuromuscular transmission, neuropathy, myopathy, or motor neuron disease. Cf. *incrementing r.*
**F r.**, F waves (def. 2); see under *wave.*
**galvanic skin r.**, the alteration in electrical resistance of the skin associated with sympathetic nerve discharge.
**immune r.**, any response of the immune system to an antigenic stimulus, including antibody production, cell-mediated immunity, and immunologic tolerance. The responses causing tissue injury are generally classified into the types described by the Gell and Coombs classification (q.v.).
**immune r., primary**, the immune response occurring on the first exposure to an antigen. After a lag or latent period of from 3 to 14 days depending on the antigen, specific antibodies appear in the blood. There is a peak of IgM production lasting several days followed immediately by a peak of IgG production. Antibody production ceases after several weeks, but memory cells remain in circulation.
**immune r., secondary**, the immune response occurring on the second and subsequent exposures to an antigen; compared to a primary response, the lag period is shorter, the peak antibody titer is higher and lasts longer, IgG production predominates, the antibodies produced have a higher affinity for the antigen, and a much smaller dose of the antigen is required to initiate the response. Called also *anamnestic r.* and *booster r.*
**incremental r.**, the progressive increase in amplitude of successive M waves upon repetitive nerve stimulation (q.v.); excessive increase is pathologic. Cf. *decrementing r.*
**M r.**, see under *wave.*
**orienting r.**, see under *reflex.*
**relaxation r.**, a group of physiologic changes that cause decreased activity of the sympathetic nervous system and consequent relaxation after stimulation of certain regions of the hypothalamus. They are the opposite of the alarm reaction and may be self-induced through techniques such as meditation and biofeedback.
**reticulocyte r.**, increase in the formation of reticulocytes in response to a bone marrow stimulus, such as that provided by administration of a hematinic.
**triple r. (of Lewis)**, a physiologic reaction of the skin to stroking with a blunt instrument: first a red line develops at the site of stroking, owing to the release of histamine or a histamine-like substance, then a flare develops around the red line due to vasodilation, and finally a wheal is formed as a result of local edema.
**unconditioned r.**, a response elicited spontaneously by an unconditioned stimulus; an unlearned response, i.e., one that occurs naturally. Called also *inborn* or *unconditioned reflex.*

**rest** (rest) [MeSH: Rest] 1. repose after exertion. 2. a fragment of embryonic tissue that has been retained within the adult organism; called also *embryonic, epithelial,* and *fetal r.* 3. that part of a removable partial denture that rests on the abutment tooth, and thus prevents movement of the denture and helps in providing occlusal support.
**aberrant r.**, choristoma.
**adrenal r's**, glandulae suprarenales accessoriae.
**bed r.**, confinement of a patient to bed.
**carbon r.**, the amount of carbon in the deproteinized blood.
**cingulum r.**, lingual r.
**embryonic r., epithelial r., fetal r.**, see *rest,* def. 2.
**incisal r.**, a metallic part or extension of a removable partial denture that rests on the prepared incisal edge of an anterior abutment tooth.
**lingual r.**, a metallic part or extension of a removable partial denture that rests on the prepared lingual surface of an anterior abutment tooth and thus provides support or indirect retention. Called also *cingulum r.*
**Malassez r.**, the remaining cells of the root sheath in the periodontal ligament, which persist and sometimes form an epithelial network and occasionally develop into a dental cyst.
**occlusal r.**, a rest placed on the occlusal surface of a posterior tooth for transmitting occlusal stresses parallel to its long axis and holding the clasp in its predetermined position; a component of removable partial dentures. Called also *occlusal stop.*
**precision r.**, a prefabricated, rigid, metallic extension of a fixed or removable partial denture, consisting of two closely fitted interlocking parts, the insert of which fits into a box-type rest or keyway (female) portion of the attachment in the cast restoration of a tooth.
**recessed r.**, a rigid extension of a partial denture which contacts a definite seat prepared in the surface of a tooth.
**semiprecision r.**, a denture rest, sometimes supplemented by a spring-loaded plunger or clip, which fits into a seat in an abutment tooth that has been specially deepened to provide added retention. See also under *attachment.*
**suprarenal r's**, glandulae suprarenales accessoriae.
**surface r.**, a rigid extension of a partial denture which contacts the unaltered extracoronal surface of a tooth.
**Walthard's cell r's**, see under *islet.*

**rest•bite** (rest′bīt) the relation of the teeth when the jaw is at rest.

**re•ste•no•sis** (re″stə-no′sis) recurrent stenosis, especially of a valve of the heart, after surgical correction of the primary condition.

**false r.**, stenosis recurring after failure to divide either commissure of the cardiac valve beyond the area of incision of the papillary muscles.
**true r.**, restenosis occurring after complete opening of one or both of the commissures of the cardiac valve involved.

**re·sten·ot·ic** (re″stə-not′ik) pertaining to or characterized by restenosis.

**res·ti·form** (res′tĭ-form) [L. *restis* rope + *form*] shaped like a rope.

**res·ti·tu·tion** (res″tĭ-too′shən) [L. *restitutio*] 1. an active process of restoration. 2. the spontaneous realignment of the fetal head with the fetal body, after delivery of the head.

**res·to·ra·tion** (res″tə-ra′shən) [L. *restaurare* to review, rebuild] 1. the act of renewing, rebuilding, or reconstructing. 2. the return to a previous state or condition, as of health. 3. the process of replacing by artificial means a missing, damaged, or diseased tooth or teeth or any part thereof. See also *prosthetic r.* and *restorative dentistry,* under *dentistry.* 4. the act of re-forming the contours of parts of teeth destroyed by lesions or injury, thereby restoring their functional properties.
**buccal r.**, the replacement, usually with silver alloy, gold, or plastic, of the buccal portion of a posterior tooth lost through caries or injury.
**cusp r.**, restoration of the summit of a cusp or the incisal edge of a tooth, done for functional or cosmetic reasons.
**facial r.**, the replacement, usually with silver alloy, gold, or acrylic resin, of the facial portion of a posterior tooth lost through caries or injury.
**prosthetic r.**, 1. the replacement of a lost or absent body part with an artificial structure, such as the use of an inlay, crown, bridge, or partial or complete denture, or other appliance to replace lost tooth structure, teeth, or oral tissue or structure 2. any appliance, such as an inlay, crown, bridge, or partial or complete denture, used to replace lost tooth structure, teeth, or oral tissue or structure.

**Res·tor·il** (res′tə-ril″) trademark for a preparation of temazepam.

**re·straint** (re-strānt′) the forcible confinement or control of a subject, as of a violently psychotic or irrational person.

**re·stric·tion** (re-strik′shən) 1. anything that limits; also, a limitation. 2. see *restriction endonuclease,* under *endonuclease.*
**intrauterine growth r. (IUGR),** birth weight below the tenth percentile for gestational age for infants in a given population; classified as *symmetric* or *proportionate* (both weight and length below normal) and *asymmetric* or *disproportionate* (weight below normal, length normal). Called also *intrauterine growth retardation.*
**MHC r.**, the phenomenon of certain cell-cell interactions in the immune response occurring only between MHC haploidentical cells. Helper T cells are activated by antigen only when the antigen is "seen" in conjunction with self class II MHC antigens (Ia antigens in mice, HLA-DR antigens in humans) as is the case when antigen is presented by macrophages. Cytotoxic T cells are activated by and kill only cells displaying foreign antigens (e.g., viral antigens or tumor antigens) plus self class I MHC antigens (K or D antigens in mice, HLA-A, -B, or -C antigens in humans).

**re·sub·limed** (re″səb-līmd′) subjected to repeated processes of sublimation.

**re·sul·tant** (re-zul′tənt) any of the products of a chemical reaction.

**re·su·pi·na·tion** (re″soo-pĭ-na′shən) [L. *resupinare* to turn on the back] 1. the act of turning upon the back or dorsum. 2. the position of one lying upon the back.

**re·sus·ci·ta·tion** (re-sus″ĭ-ta′shən) [L. *resuscitare* to revive] [MeSH: Resuscitation] the restoration to life or consciousness of one apparently dead; it includes such measures as artificial respiration and cardiac massage.
**cardiopulmonary r. (CPR),** the artificial substitution of heart and lung action as indicated for cardiac arrest or apparent sudden death resulting from electric shock, drowning, respiratory arrest, and other causes. The two major components of CPR are artificial respiration and closed chest cardiac massage; see Plate 44.

**re·sus·ci·ta·tor** (re-sus′ĭ-ta″tor) an apparatus for initiating respiration in cases of asphyxia.
**cardiopulmonary r.**, an apparatus that simultaneously assists the patient's breathing and applies external cardiac massage.

**re·su·ture** (re-soo′chər) secondary suture.

**re·tain·er** (re-ta′nər) 1. a device for retaining or keeping something in position. 2. the part of a denture that unites the abutment tooth with the suspended portion of the bridge, such as an inlay, partial crown, or complete crown. 3. an orthodontic device for maintaining in position the teeth and jaws. 4. any form of clasp, attachment, or other device used for the fixation or stabilization of a prosthetic appliance. 5. the portion of a fixed prosthesis attaching a pontic to the abutment teeth.
**continuous bar r.**, continuous clasp.

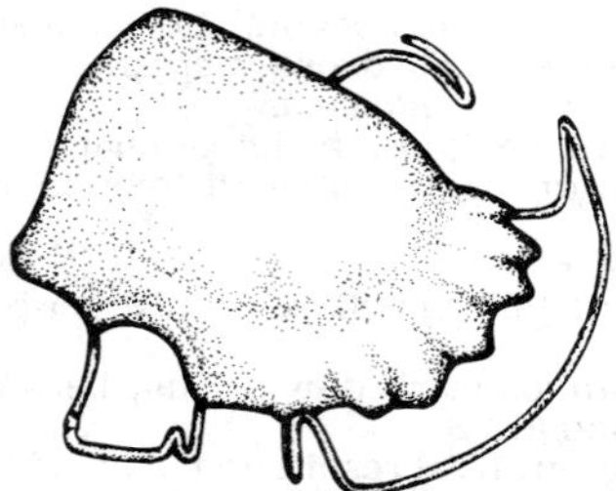

Hawley retainer.

**direct r.**, a clasp or attachment applied to an abutment tooth, by which a removable partial denture is maintained in position.
**Hawley r.**, an orthodontic appliance consisting of a removable palatal wire and an acrylic biteplate resting against the palate, used to stabilize teeth after their movement or as a basis for tooth movement by providing anchorage for other attachments. Called also *Hawley appliance.*
**indirect r.**, a part of a removable partial denture that assists the direct retainers in preventing displacement of distal-extension denture bases by functioning through lever action on the opposite side of the fulcrum line.
**matrix r.**, a mechanical device designed to engage the ends of a matrix band or strip and to tighten the matrix around the tooth.
**space r.**, an orthodontic appliance that retains the space created by premature loss of a tooth or the space to be filled by an erupting tooth. See also under *maintainer* and *regainer.*

**re·tar·date** (re-tahr′dāt) older term for a mentally retarded person.

**re·tar·da·tion** (re″tahr-da′shən) [L. *retardare* to slow down, impede] delay; hindrance; delayed development.
**intrauterine growth r.**, see under *restriction.*
**mental r.** [DSM-IV], a mental disorder characterized by significantly subaverage general intellectual functioning associated with impairments in adaptive behavior and manifested during the developmental period. It is classified on the basis of severity as *mild, moderate, severe,* and *profound;* a fifth subgroup, *borderline intellectual functioning,* is sometimes included.
**mental r., borderline** [DSM-IV], borderline intellectual functioning.
**mental r., mild** [DSM-IV], that in which IQ is between 50–55 and 70; the person can develop social and communication skills during the preschool period, has minimal sensorimotor impairment, by the late teens can acquire academic skills up to the sixth grade level, and usually achieves social and vocational skills adequate for minimal self-support.
**mental r., moderate** [DSM-IV], that in which IQ is between 35–40 and 50–55; the person may talk or learn to communicate but has poor social awareness and only fair motor development, is unlikely to progress to the second grade level in academic skills, but can profit from vocational training and with moderate supervision can perform personal care.
**mental r., profound** [DSM-IV], that in which IQ is less than 20–25; the person has limited sensorimotor development, may achieve very limited self-care, and requires a highly structured environment with constant supervision.
**mental r., severe** [DSM-IV], that in which IQ is between 20–25 and 35–40; the person has poor motor development and minimal speech in the preschool period, may learn to talk by the late teens, can be trained in elementary hygiene skills, and as an adult may learn to perform simple work under close supervision.
**psychomotor r.**, generalized slowing of mental and physical activity, as is common in depression and in catatonic schizophrenia.

**retch·ing** (rech′ing) a strong involuntary effort to vomit.

**re·te** (re′te) pl. *re′tia* [L. "net"] a general term used in anatomical nomenclature to designate a network, especially of arteries or veins. See also *net, network,* and *plexus.*
**r. acromia′le** [TA], acromial rete or network: a network formed by ramification of the acromial branch of the thoracoacromial artery on the acromion process.
**r. arterio′sum** [TA], arterial network: an anastomotic network formed by arteries just before they become arterioles or capillaries.
**r. arterio′sum der′midis,** arterial network of dermis: the arterial portion of the deep vascular plexus, found in the skin at the boundary between the dermis and the tela subcutanea. Called also *r. cutaneum* and *cutaneous arterial network.*
**r. arterio′sum subpapilla′re,** subpapillary network: the arterial portion of the superficial vascular plexus, found in the skin at the boundary between the papillary and reticular layers. Called also *r. subpapillare.*

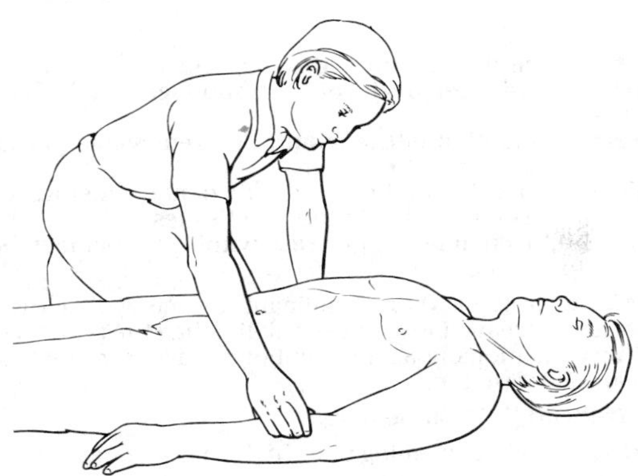

1. Place victim supine on a hard, flat surface.

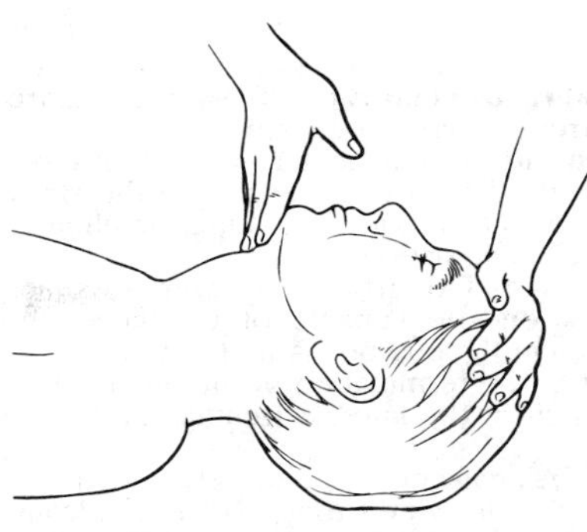

2. To open the airway, place one hand under the victim's chin and the other on top of the head. Tilt the head backward by lifting up on the chin and pushing down on the top of the head.

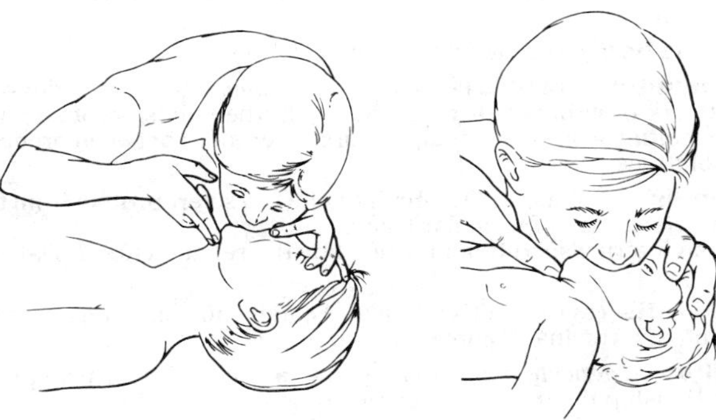

3. While keeping the head tilted and the chin raised, pinch the nostrils with the thumb and index finger. Take a deep breath, place your lips tightly around the victim's mouth, and give two quick breaths. The lungs may also be inflated by covering the victim's mouth and blowing through the nose or, if a tracheostomy is present, by blowing through the stoma. In infants, cover both the mouth and nose with your mouth and use only small puffs from your cheeks.

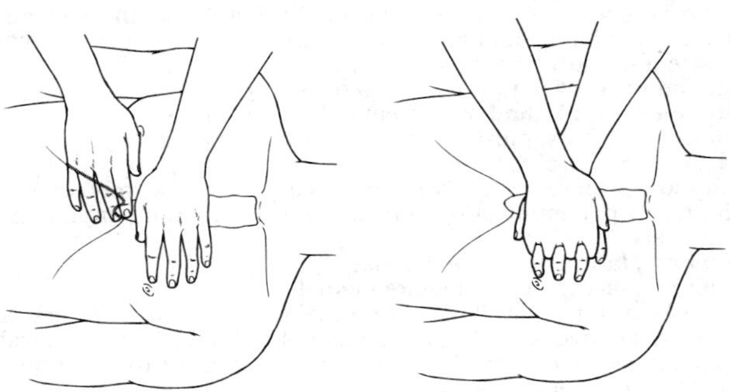

4. To locate the correct point on the sternum for chest compression, locate the notch where the ribs and sternum come together. Place the middle finger on the notch and the index finger next to it. Place the heel of the other hand on the sternum, next to the index finger of the first hand. Then place the heel of the first hand on top of the hand whose heel is resting on the sternum. For children one to eight years of age, the pressure of only one hand is sufficient.

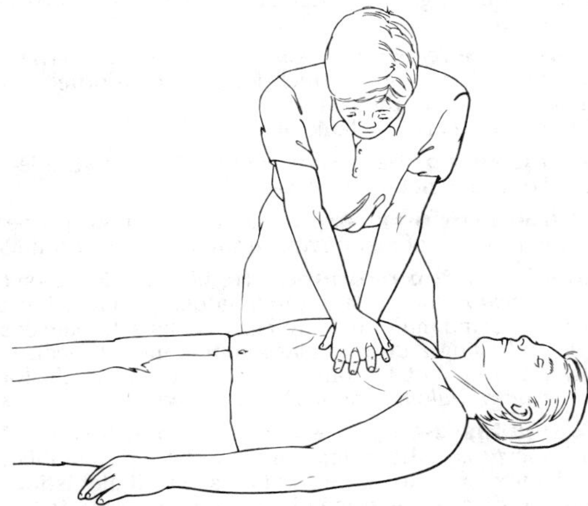

5. Compress the chest with the arms straight and the elbows locked and the shoulders positioned directly over the hands. The sternum should be depressed 4–5 cm (1.5–2 in) in older children and adults, 2.5–4 cm (1–1.5 in) in children aged one to eight years. Perform 15 compressions. A single rescuer should continue a cycle of two breaths and 15 compressions. The carotid pulse and breathing should be assessed every one to three minutes.

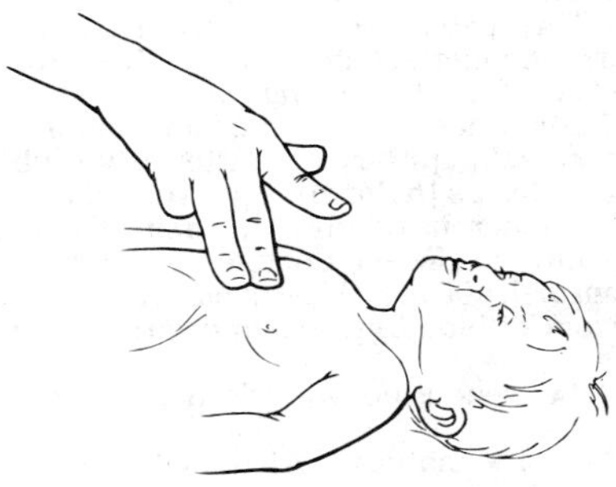

6. Only moderate pressure on the middle third of the sternum, using the tips of two or three fingers, should be used for chest compression in infants. The compression distance should be 1.3–2.5 cm (0.5–1 in).

**PLATE 44—**TECHNIQUE OF RESUSCITATION BY CLOSED CARDIAC MASSAGE

**articular r.,** r. vasculosum articulare.
**articular cubital r., articular r. of elbow,** r. articulare cubiti.
**articular r. of knee,** r. articulare genus.
**r. articula're cu'biti** [TA], articular network of elbow: an arterial network formed on the posterior aspect of the elbow by the posterior ulnar recurrent, inferior and superior ulnar collateral, and interosseous recurrent arteries.
**r. articula're ge'nus** [TA], articular network of knee: an extensive arterial network on the capsule of the knee joint, supplying branches to the contiguous bones and joints. It is formed by the genicular arteries, the termination of the deep femoral artery, the descending branch of the lateral circumflex artery, and the tibial recurrent artery.
**r. calca'neum** [TA], calcaneal rete or network: an arterial network on the posterior and lower surfaces of the calcaneus, receiving branches from the calcaneal branches of the fibular artery and the lateral malleolar branches of the fibular artery.
**r. cana'lis hypoglos'si,** plexus venosus canalis hypoglossi.
**carpal r., dorsal,** r. carpale dorsale.
**r. carpa'le dorsa'le** [TA], **r. car'pi dorsa'le,** dorsal carpal network: an arterial rete formed by the dorsal radial carpal and dorsal ulnar carpal arteries and giving off the second, third, and fourth dorsal metacarpal arteries to the dorsum of the hand and the second, third, and fourth fingers. Called also *dorsal* or *posterior carpal arch.*
**r. cuta'neum,** r. arteriosum dermidis.
**dorsal venous r. of foot,** r. venosum dorsale pedis.
**dorsal venous r. of hand,** r. venosum dorsale manus.
**r. fora'minis ova'lis,** plexus venosus foraminis ovalis.
**r. of Haller, r. Halle'ri,** r. testis.
**r. lymphocapilla're** [TA], lymphocapillary network: any of the closed, freely communicating networks formed by the lymphocapillary vessels.
**malleolar r., lateral,** r. malleolare laterale.
**malleolar r., medial,** r. malleolare mediale.
**r. malleola're latera'le** [TA], lateral malleolar rete or network: a small arterial network on the lateral malleolus, formed by the lateral anterior malleolar artery, the perforating branch of the peroneal artery, and the lateral tarsal artery.
**r. malleola're media'le** [TA], medial malleolar rete or network: a small arterial network on the medial malleolus, formed by the medial anterior malleolar artery and branches from the posterior tibial artery.
**malpighian r.,** stratum germinativum.
**r. mira'bile** [TA], 1. a vascular network formed by division of an artery or a vein into a large number of smaller vessels that subsequently reunite into a single vessel; in the human this occurs only in the arterioles that supply the glomeruli of the kidney. 2. arterial anastomosis of the brain occurring between the external and internal carotid arteries as a result of longstanding thrombosis of the internal carotid arteries.
**r. ole'crani,** r. articulare cubiti.
**r. ova'rii,** a homologue of the rete testis, developed in the early female fetus, but vestigial in the adult.
**r. of patella, r. patel'lae,** r. patellare.
**r. patella're** [TA], patellar rete or network: a network of arterial branches surrounding the patella and derived from the various arteries of the knee. Called also *r. patellae.*
**plantar r., plantar venous r.,** r. venosum plantare.
**r. subpapilla're, subpapillary r.,** r. arteriosum subpapillare.
**r. tes'tis** [TA], **r. tes'tis [halle'ri],** a network of channels, formed by the straight seminiferous tubules, traversing the mediastinum testis and draining into the efferent ductules; called also *r. of Haller.*
**r. vasculo'sum articula're** [TA], articular vascular network: an anastomotic network of blood vessels in or around a joint; called also *articular r.*
**r. veno'sum** [TA], venous network: an anastomotic network of small veins.
**r. veno'sum dorsa'le ma'nus** [TA], dorsal venous network of hand: a venous network on the back of the hand, formed by the dorsal metacarpal veins.
**r. veno'sum dorsa'le pe'dis** [TA], dorsal venous network of foot: a superficial network of anastomosing veins on the dorsum of the foot proximal to the transverse venous arch, draining into the great and the small saphenous veins.
**r. veno'sum planta're** [TA], plantar venous network: a thick venous network in the subcutaneous tissue of the sole of the foot. Called also *plantar venous rete* and *plantar cutaneous venous network.*

**re·ten·tion** (re-ten'shən) [L. *retentio,* from *retentare* to hold firmly back] 1. the act or process of keeping in possession, or of holding in place or position. 2. the persistent keeping within the body of matter normally excreted. 3. in cavity preparation, the prevention of displacement of a restoration. 4. in orthodontic therapy, the period during which the patient is wearing an appliance(s) to maintain and stabilize the teeth in the position into which they were moved.
**denture r.,** the holding in proper position in the mouth of a removable denture. See *direct r.* and *indirect r.*
**direct r.,** denture retention through the use of attachments or clasps that resist removal from the abutment teeth. See under *retainer.*
**indirect r.,** retention in the mouth of a removable partial denture by means of an indirect retainer.
**surgical r.,** retention in the mouth of a dental prosthesis by means of attachments embedded in the oral tissues.
**r. of urine,** accumulation of urine within the bladder because of inability to urinate.

**ret·e·plase** (ret'əplās) recombinant plasminogen activator; a mutant of alteplase having a longer half-life than the parent compound, used investigationally as a thrombolytic agent in the treatment of myocardial infarction.

**re·tia** (re'te-ə) [L.] plural of *rete.*

**re·ti·al** (re'te-əl) pertaining to or of the nature of a rete; cf. *reticular.*

**re·tic·u·la** (rə-tik'u-lə) [L.] plural of *reticulum.*

**re·tic·u·lar** (rə-tik'u-lər) [L. *reticularis*] 1. pertaining to or resembling a net, network, or reticulum. 2. pertaining to the reticulum of a ruminant.

**re·tic·u·lat·ed** (rə-tik'u-lāt″əd) reticular.

**re·tic·u·la·tion** (rə-tik″u-la'shən) [L. *reticulum* a net] in radiology, a network of wrinkles or corrugations in the emulsion of an x-ray film resulting from sharp temperature differences between processing solutions.

**re·tic·u·lin** (rə-tik'u-lin) [MeSH: Reticulin] a scleroprotein from the connective fibers of reticular tissue.
**r. M,** an internal secretion produced by the reticuloendothelial system.

**re·tic·u·li·tis** (rə-tik″u-li'tis) [*reticul-* + *-itis*] inflammation of the reticulum of a ruminant animal.

**reticul(o)-** [L. *reticulum* dim. of *rete* net] a combining form denoting a relationship to a reticulum or to a reticular structure.

**re·tic·u·lo·cyte** (rə-tik'u-lo-sīt″) [*reticulo-* + *-cyte*] [MeSH: Reticulocytes] an immature erythrocyte showing a basophilic reticulum under vital staining.

**re·tic·u·lo·cy·to·gen·ic** (rə-tik″u-lo-si″to-jen'ik) causing the formation of reticulocytes.

**re·tic·u·lo·cy·to·pe·nia** (rə-tik″u-lo-si″to-pe'ne-ə) [*reticulocyte* + *-penia*] a decrease in the number of reticulocytes in the blood.

**re·tic·u·lo·cy·to·sis** (rə-tik″u-lo-si-to'sis) an increase in the number of reticulocytes in the peripheral blood.

**re·tic·u·lo·en·do·the·li·al** (rə-tik″u-lo-en″do-the'le-əl) pertaining to tissues having both reticular and endothelial attributes; see under *system.*

**re·tic·u·lo·en·do·the·li·o·sis** (rə-tik″u-lo-en″do-the-le-o'sis) [*reticuloendothelium* + *-osis*] [MeSH: Reticuloendotheliosis] hyperplasia of reticuloendothelial tissue.
**leukemic r.,** hairy cell leukemia.

**re·tic·u·lo·en·do·the·li·um** (rə-tik″u-lo-en″do-the'le-əm) the tissue of the reticuloendothelial system.

**re·tic·u·lo·his·tio·cy·tary** (rə-tik″u-lo-his″te-o-si'tər-e) pertaining to or composed of histiocytes of the reticuloendothelial system.

**re·tic·u·lo·his·ti·o·cy·to·ma** (re-tik″u-lo-his″te-o-si-to'mə) [*reticulo-* + *histiocytoma*] a granulomatous proliferation of lipid-laden histiocytes and multinucleated giant cells with pale eosinophilic cytoplasm having a ground glass appearance. It occurs in two clinically different but histologically indistinguishable forms, *reticulohistiocytic granuloma* and *multicentric reticulohistiocytosis.*

**re·tic·u·lo·his·ti·o·cy·to·sis** (rə-tik″u-lo-his″te-o-si-to'sis)[*reticulo-* + *histiocytosis*] the formation of multiple reticulohistiocytomas.
**multicentric r.,** one of the two types of reticulohistiocytoma, a rare systemic disease seen mainly in women, characterized by polyarthritis of the hands and large joints with nodular swellings in the skin, bone, and mucous and synovial membranes and sometimes soft cystic ganglialike swellings over the extensor and flexor surfaces of the wrists; there may be evidence of internal malignancy. It may become quiescent, leaving only crippling arthropathy and disfigured skin, or it may progress to multiple organ involvement and eventual death. Called also *lipid* or *lipoid dermatoarthritis.*

**re·tic·u·loid** (rə-tik'u-loid) 1. resembling reticulosis. 2. a condition resembling reticulosis.
**actinic r.,** chronic photodermatitis with sensitivity to a broad spectrum of radiation, usually occurring in older men; it first occurs on sun-exposed areas as a scaly pruritic erythema, often spreading and leading to thick plaques, furrows, and leonine facies. Lesions are characterized histologically by a polymorphous dermal infiltrate that resembles lymphoma.

**re·tic·u·lo·nod·u·lar** (rə-tik″u-lo-nod'u-lər) said of a pattern that is reticular and contains nodules, such as a lung with asbestosis or any of various kinds of pneumonia.

**re·tic·u·lo·pe·nia** (rə-tik″u-lo-pe′ne-ə) [*reticulo-* + *-penia*] reticulocytopenia.

**re·tic·u·lo·peri·car·di·tis** (rə-tik″u-lo-per″ĭ-kahr-di′tis) inflammation of the reticulum and pericardium of a ruminant.
**traumatic r.,** traumatic pericarditis (def. 2).

**re·tic·u·lo·peri·the·li·um** (rə-tik″u-lo-per″ĭ-the′le-əm) [*reticulo-* + *peri-* + *thelium*] retoperithelium.

**re·tic·u·lo·peri·to·ni·tis** (rə-tik″u-lo-per″ĭ-tə-ni′tis) inflammation of the reticulum and peritoneal cavity of a ruminant.
**traumatic r.,** inflammation following perforation of the wall of the reticulum by an ingested foreign object such as metallic debris; it is often benign, but if the object pierces another organ, serious complications may arise. See also *traumatic pericarditis* (def. 2). Called also *hardware disease.*

**re·tic·u·lo·pi·tu·i·cyte** (rə-tik″u-lo-pĭ-too′ĭ-sīt) see *pituicyte.*

**re·tic·u·lo·po·di·um** (rə-tik″u-lo-po′de-əm) reticulopo′dia [*reticulo-* + Gr. *pous* foot] a filamentous pseudopodium with interconnected branches. Cf. *axopodium, filopodium,* and *lobopodium.* Called also *rhizopodium.*

**re·tic·u·lo·ru·men** (rə-tik″u-lo-ru′mən) the reticulum and rumen considered as a unit.

**re·tic·u·lo·ru·mi·nal** (rə-tik″u-lo-roo′mĭ-nəl) pertaining to the rumen and reticulum. Called also *ruminoreticular.*

**re·tic·u·lo·sis** (rə-tik″u-lo′sis) [*reticul-* + *-osis*] an abnormal increase in cells derived from or related to reticuloendothelial cells, such as that seen in leukemia and lymphoma.
**familial hemophagocytic r., familial histiocytic r.,** histiocytic medullary r.
**histiocytic medullary r.,** a fatal hereditary disorder transmitted as an autosomal recessive trait, characterized by anemia, granulocytopenia, thrombocytopenia, intense phagocytosis of red blood cells, diffuse proliferation of histiocytes of various organs, and enlargement of the liver, spleen, and lymph nodes. Called also *familial hemophagocytic r., familial histiocytic r.,* and *Omenn's syndrome.*
**inflammatory r.,** granulomatous meningoencephalitis.
**lipomelanic r.,** dermatopathic lymphadenopathy.
**malignant midline r., midline malignant r.,** polymorphic r.
**pagetoid r.,** a usually solitary skin lesion of long duration and slow growth characterized histologically by large numbers of abnormal mononuclear cells infiltrating the epidermis with an underlying reactive mixed dermal infiltrate, which is considered by some authorities to represent an indolent, epidermotropic form of cutaneous T cell lymphoma. Called also *Woringer-Kolopp disease* or *syndrome.*
**polymorphic r.,** a form of angiocentric immunoproliferative lesion involving midline structures of the nose and face; called also *malignant midline r.* and *midline malignant r.*

**re·tic·u·lo·the·li·um** (rə-tik″u-lo-the′le-əm) the retothelium.

**re·tic·u·lum** (rə-tik′u-ləm) pl. *retic′ula* [L., dim. of *rete* net] [MeSH: Reticulum] 1. a network, especially a protoplasmic network in cells, as the flattened double membrane sheets of the endoplasmic reticulum. 2. reticular tissue. 3. the second stomach of a ruminant; its mucous membranes are covered with many small pockets. Called also *honeycomb.*
**agranular r.,** see *endoplasmic r.*
**Chiari's r.,** Chiari's network.
**Ebner's r.,** a network of cells in the seminiferous tubules.
**endoplasmic r.,** an ultramicroscopic organelle of nearly all cells of higher plants and animals, consisting of a more or less continuous system of membrane-bound cavities that ramify throughout the cytoplasm of a cell. Two forms have been distinguished: *rough* or *granular r.* (chromidial substance, ergastoplasm), which bears large numbers of ribosomes on the outer surface of its membrane and is basophilic, and *smooth* or *agranular r.,* which contains no ribosomes and has no distinctive staining properties. Called also *superior protoplasm.*
**granular r.,** see *endoplasmic r.*
**reti′cula lie′nis,** trabeculae splenicae.
**sarcoplasmic r.,** a special form of agranular reticulum found in the sarcoplasm of striated muscle and comprising a system of smooth-surfaced tubules forming a plexus around each myofibril.
**stellate r.,** the soft, middle part of the enamel organ of a developing tooth, the cells being separated by an increase in the gelatinous intercellular substance that forces the cells apart without breaking the intercellular connections, giving them a stellate appearance and providing protection later for the enamel-forming cells.
**r. trabecula′re** [TA], a trabeculum of loose fibers found at the iridocorneal angle between the anterior chamber of the eye and the venous sinus of the sclera; the aqueous humor filters through the spaces between the fibers into the sinus and passes into the bloodstream. The reticulum is divided into a corneoscleral part and a uveal part. Called also *Hueck's ligament, ligamentum pectinatum anguli iridocornealis, pectinate ligament, pectinate ligament of iris,* and *trabecular meshwork.*

**re·ti·form** (re′tĭ-form, ret′ĭ-form) [*rete* + *form*] resembling a network.

**Ret·in-A** (ret′in-a) trademark for preparations of tretinoin.

**ret·i·na** (ret′ĭ-nə) [L.] [TA] [MeSH: Retina] the innermost of the three tunics of the eyeball, surrounding the vitreous body and continuous posteriorly with the optic nerve. It is divided into the *pars optica,* which rests upon the choroid, the *pars ciliaris,* which rests upon the ciliary body, and the *pars iridica,* which rests upon the posterior surface of the iris. The pars optica is subdivided into an outer, pigmented layer *(pars pigmentosa)* and an inner, transparent layer *(pars nervosa).* The pars nervosa is divided into nine layers, as follows (see illustration): (1) the internal limiting membrane; (2) the nerve fiber layer; (3) the layer of ganglion cells; (4) the inner plexiform layer; (5) the inner nuclear layer; (6) the outer plexiform layer; (7) the outer nuclear layer; (8) the external limiting membrane; (9) the layer of rods and cones. The layer of rods and cones is the percipient part of the retina, responding to visual stimuli by a photochemical reaction; it is connected with the nerve fiber layer by nerve fibers that join to form the optic nerve. In the center of the posterior part of the retina is the *macula lutea,* the most sensitive portion of the retina, with the fovea centralis at its center. About 0.25 cm inside the fovea is the point of entrance of the optic nerve and the central artery of the retina; at this point the retina is incomplete and forms the blind spot.

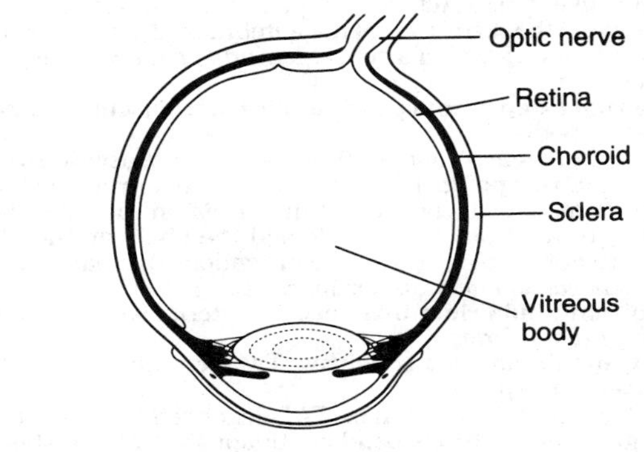


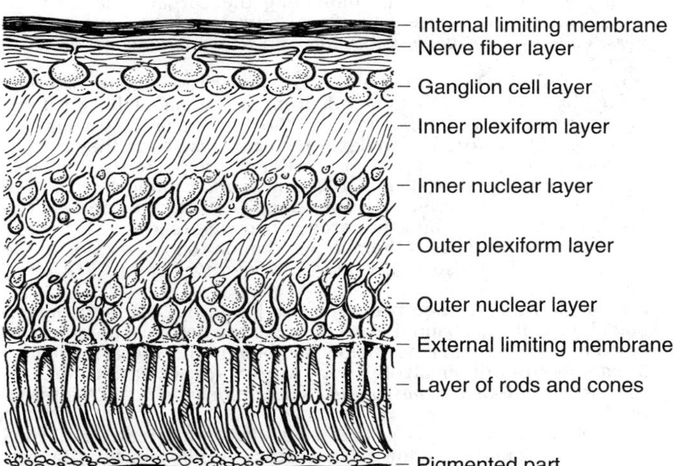


Schematic representation of the optic part of the retina.

**coarctate r.,** a funnel-shaped condition of the retina caused by a fluid exudation between the retina and the choroid.
**detached r., detachment of r.,** separation of the inner layers of the retina (neural retina) from the pigment epithelium; called also *ablatio retinae* and *amotio retinae.*
**leopard r.,** see under *fundus.*
**shot-silk r.,** an opalescent effect, as of changeable silk, sometimes seen in the retinas of young persons. Called also *shot-silk phenomenon* or *reflex* and *watered-silk r.*
**tessellated r., tigroid r.,** see under *fundus.*
**watered-silk r.,** shot-silk r.

**ret·i·nac·u·lum** (ret″ĭ-nak′u-ləm) pl. *retina′cula* [L. "a rope, cable"] 1. [TA] a structure that retains an organ or tissue in place. 2. an instrument or device for retracting tissues during surgery. See *tenaculum.*

**r. of arcuate ligament,** r. ligamenti arcuati.

**r. cap'sulae articula'ris cox'ae,** one of the longitudinal folds of the cervical portion of the articular capsule of the hip.

**r. cauda'le** [TA], caudal retinaculum: a fibrous band that extends from the tip of the coccyx to the adjacent skin and thus forms the foveola coccygea; called also *ligamentum caudale integumenti communis.*

**r. cos'tae ul'timae,** ligamentum lumbocostale.

**retina'cula cu'tis** [TA], bands of connective tissue attaching the corium to the subcutaneous tissue.

**extensor r. of foot, inferior,** r. musculorum extensorum inferius pedis.

**extensor r. of foot, superior,** r. musculorum extensorum superius pedis.

**extensor r. of hand,** r. musculorum extensorum manus.

**r. extenso'rum ma'nus,** r. musculorum extensorum manus.

**flexor r. of foot,** r. musculorum flexorum pedis.

**flexor r. of hand,** r. musculorum flexorum manus.

**r. flexo'rum ma'nus,** r. musculorum flexorum manus.

**r. ligamen'ti arcua'ti,** retinaculum of arcuate ligament: a band of converging fibers passing from the convex lower margin of the arcuate popliteal ligament to the head of the fibula.

**r. musculo'rum extenso'rum infe'rius pe'dis** [TA], inferior extensor retinaculum of foot: a thickened band of the fascia cruris passing from each malleolus across the front of the ankle joint, there crossing the other and passing onto the dorsum of the foot; called also *ligamentum cruciatum cruris.*

**r. musculo'rum extenso'rum ma'nus** [TA], extensor retinaculum of muscles of hand: the distal part of the antebrachial fascia, overlying the extensor tendons; called also *r. extensorum manus* and *ligamentum carpi dorsale.*

**r. musculo'rum extenso'rum pe'dis infe'rius,** r. musculorum extensorum inferius pedis.

**r. musculo'rum extenso'rum pe'dis supe'rius, r. musculo'rum extenso'rum supe'rius pe'dis** [TA], superior extensor retinaculum of foot: the thickened lower portion of the fascia on the front of the leg, attached to the tibia on one side and the fibula on the other, and serving to hold in place the extensor tendons that pass beneath it; called also *ligamentum transversum cruris.*

**r. musculo'rum fibula'rium infe'rius,** TA alternative for *r. musculorum peroneorum inferius.*

**r. musculo'rum fibula'rium supe'rius,** TA alternative for *r. musculorum peroneorum superius.*

**r. musculo'rum flexo'rum ma'nus** [TA], flexor retinaculum of muscles of hand: a heavy fibrous band continuous with the distal part of the antebrachial fascia, completing the carpal canal through which pass the tendons of the flexor muscles of the hand and fingers; called also *r. flexorum manus* and *ligamentum carpi transversum.*

**r. musculo'rum flexo'rum pe'dis** [TA], flexor retinaculum of foot: a strong band of fascia that extends from the medial malleolus down onto the calcaneus. It holds in place the tendons of the tibialis posterior, flexor digitorum, and flexor hallucis muscles as they pass to the sole of the foot, and gives protection to the posterior tibial vessels and tibial nerve. Called also *ligamentum laciniatum.*

**r. musculo'rum peroneo'rum infe'rius** [TA], inferior peroneal retinaculum: a fibrous band that arches over the tendons of the peroneal muscles and holds them in position on the lateral side of the calcaneus; called also *r. musculorum fibularium inferius* [TA alternative].

**r. musculo'rum peroneo'rum supe'rius** [TA], superior peroneal retinaculum: a fibrous band that arches over the peroneal tendons and helps to hold them in place below and behind the lateral malleolus; it extends from the malleolus downward and backward to the calcaneus. Called also *r. musculorum fibularium superius* [TA alternative].

**r. patel'lae latera'le** [TA], lateral patellar retinaculum: a fibrous membrane from the tendon of the vastus lateralis muscle, attached to the lateral margin of the patella and then along the side of the patellar ligament, and inserted into the tibia as far distal as the fibularcollateral ligament; it also blends with the iliotibial tract of the fascia lata. Called also *lateral patellar ligament.*

**r. patel'lae media'le** [TA], medial patellar retinaculum: a fibrous membrane from the tendon of the vastus medialis muscle, attached to the medial margin of the patella and then along the side of the patellar ligament, and inserted into the tibia as far distal as the tibial collateral ligament.

**patellar r., lateral,** r. patellae laterale.

**patellar r., medial,** r. patellae mediale.

**peroneal r., inferior,** r. musculorum peroneorum inferius.

**peroneal r., superior,** r. musculorum peroneorum superius.

**r. ten'dinum,** a tendinous restraining structure, such as an annular ligament.

**r. ten'dinum musculo'rum extenso'rum,** r. musculorum extensorum manus.

**r. ten'dinum musculo'rum extenso'rum infe'rius,** r. musculorum extensorum inferius pedis.

**r. ten'dinum musculo'rum extenso'rum supe'rius,** r. musculorum extensorum superius pedis.

**r. ten'dinum musculo'rum flexo'rum,** r. musculorum flexorum manus.

**retina'cula un'guis,** structures homologous to the retinacula cutis, attaching the nail to underlying tissue.

**Weitbrecht's r.,** retinacular fibers attached to the neck of the femur.

**ret·i·nal** (ret'ĭ-nəl) 1. pertaining to the retina. 2. the aldehyde of retinol, derived from absorbed dietary carotenoids or esters of retinol, and having vitamin A activity. In the retina, retinal combines with opsins of rods (scotopsins) and cones (photopsins), functioning as the prosthetic group in the resulting visual pigments rhodopsin and the iodopsins.

**11-*cis* r.,** a retinal isomer that combines with opsins to form photoreceptive molecules, in the rods combining with scotopsin to form rhodopsin and in the cones combining with photopsins to form several iodopsins. In the presence of light, it is converted to the all-*trans* isomer.

**all-*trans* r.,** a retinal isomer formed from the 11-*cis* isomer upon bleaching of the photoreceptor proteins of the retina by light; the isomer dissociates from the opsins and is reconverted to the 11-*cis* isomer in the dark to renew the visual cycle.

**ret·i·nal isom·er·ase** (ret'ĭ-nəl i-som'ər-ās) [EC 5.2.1.3] an enzyme of the isomerase class that catalyzes the interconversion of the all-*trans* and 11-*cis* isomers of retinal. The reaction regenerates 11-*cis* retinal in the visual cycle.

**ret·i·nal re·duc·tase** (ret'ĭ-nəl re-duk'tās) older name for an enzyme activity now known to be *alcohol dehydrogenase (NAD(P)$^+$).*

**ret·ine** (ret'ēn) a substance stated to be widely distributed in animal cells, which is characterized by its ability to retard cell division and growth. Cf. *promine.*

**ret·i·ni·tis** (ret"ĭ-ni'tis) [MeSH: Retinitis] inflammation of the retina; used in the older ophthalmologic literature to denote impairment of sight, perversion of vision, edema, and exudation into the retina, and occasionally by hemorrhages into the retina.

**actinic r.,** retinitis due to exposure to actinic light rays.

**r. albuminu'rica,** that which is associated with kidney disease. Cf. *arteriosclerotic retinopathy* and *hypertensive retinopathy.*

**apoplectic r.,** that which is characterized by extravasations of blood within the retina.

**azotemic r.,** retinitis due to nitrogenous waste products in renal disease.

**central angiospastic r.,** central serous retinopathy.

**r. circina'ta, circinate r.,** circinate retinopathy.

**Coats' r.,** exudative retinopathy.

**cytomegalovirus r.,** opportunistic infection of the retina by cytomegalovirus, seen in patients with immunodeficiency; symptoms include retinal necrosis and hemorrhage, leading to blindness.

**diabetic r.,** see under *retinopathy.*

**disciform r.,** disciform macular degeneration.

**exudative r.,** see under *retinopathy.*

**gravidic r.,** inflammation of the retina occurring along with the albuminuria of pregnancy.

**hypertensive r.,** see under *retinopathy.*

**Jacobson's r.,** syphilitic r.

**Jensen's r.,** retinochoroiditis juxtapapillaris.

**leukemic r.,** see under *retinopathy.*

**metastatic r.,** retinitis caused by the location of septic emboli in the retinal vessels.

**nephritic r.,** renal retinopathy.

**r. pigmento'sa,** a group of diseases, frequently hereditary, marked by progressive loss of retinal response (as elicited by the electroretinogram), retinal atrophy, attenuation of the retinal vessels, and clumping of the pigment, with contraction of the field of vision. It may be transmitted as a dominant, recessive, or X-linked trait and is sometimes associated with other genetic defects.

**r. pigmento'sa si'ne pigmen'to,** retinitis pigmentosa without clumping of pigment.

**r. proli'ferans, proliferating r.,** a condition sometimes resulting from intraocular hemorrhage, with neovascularization and the formation of fibrous tissue bands extending into the vitreous from the surface of the retina; retinal detachment is sometimes a sequel.

**r. puncta'ta albes'cens,** a type of retinal disorder in which there is a diffusion of white spots on the retina.

**renal r.,** see under *retinopathy.*

**r. sclopeta'ria,** a severe traumatic retinal lesion, as from the impact of a bullet.

**serous r., simple r.,** simple inflammation of the superficial layers of the retina.

**solar r.,** retinitis due to excessive exposure to sunlight.

**r. stella'ta,** stellate retinopathy.

**striate r.,** a form marked by the presence of gray or yellowish streaks just behind the retinal vessels.

**suppurative r.**, retinitis due to pyemic infection.
**syphilitic r., r. syphili'tica,** retinitis complicating syphilitic iritis.
**uremic r.**, retinitis occurring in uremia.

**ret·i·no·blas·to·ma** (ret″ĭ-no-blas-to'mə) [*retina* + *blastoma*] [MeSH: Retinoblastoma] a malignant congenital blastoma, occurring in both hereditary and sporadic forms, composed of tumor cells arising from the retinoblasts, appearing in one or both eyes in children under 5 years of age, and usually diagnosed initially by a bright white or yellow pupillary reflex (leukokoria). Called also *glioma retinae.*
**endophytic r., r. endo'phytum,** a retinoblastoma that begins in the inner layers of the retina and spreads toward the center of the globe; called also *glioma endophytum.*
**exophytic r., r. exo'phytum,** a retinoblastoma that begins in the outer layers of the retina and spreads away from the center of the globe; called also *glioma exophytum.*

**ret·i·no·cho·roid** (ret″ĭ-no-kor'oid) pertaining to the retina and the choroid.

**ret·i·no·cho·roi·di·tis** (ret″ĭ-no-kor-oi-di'tis) chorioretinitis.
**r. juxtapapilla'ris,** a condition seen in young healthy subjects marked by a small inflammatory area on the fundus close to the papilla; called also *Jensen's retinitis* or *retinochoroiditis.*
**toxoplasmic r.**, see under *chorioretinitis.*

**ret·i·no·cy·to·ma** (ret″ĭ-no-si-to'mə) a rare benign variant of retinoblastoma composed of viable cells with substantial photoreceptor differentiation and often fleurettes; vision is often normal. Called also *retinoma.*

**ret·i·no·di·al·y·sis** (ret″ĭ-no-di-al'ĭ-sis) [*retina* + *dialysis*] disinsertion of the retina; detachment of the retina at its peripheral insertion.

**ret·i·no·graph** (ret'ĭ-no-graf) a photograph of the retina.

**ret·i·nog·ra·phy** (ret″ĭ-nog'rə-fe) photography of the retina.

**ret·i·no·ic ac·id** (ret″ĭ-no'ik) an oxidized derivative of retinol, formed by carboxylation of the aldehyde group of retinal (q.v.). It is believed to be the form of vitamin A that plays a role in the development and growth of bone and in the maintenance of normal epithelial structures. In pharmacology, the term is often used alone to mean the all-*trans* isomer (tretinoin); the 13-*cis* isomer is usually called isotretinoin.

**ret·i·noid** (ret'ĭ-noid) 1. resembling the retina. 2. retinol, retinal, or any structurally similar natural derivative or synthetic compound; the latter need any not have vitamin A activity.

**ret·i·nol** (ret'ĭ-nol) a 20-carbon primary alcohol occurring as several isomers; it is the form of vitamin A (vitamin $A_1$) found in mammals. Most dietary sources occur as esters of retinol, also the predominant forms for storage and transport; the de-esterified alcohol can be converted to the metabolically active forms retinal and retinoic acid.

**ret·i·nol de·hy·dro·gen·ase** (ret'ĭ-nol de-hi'dro-jən-ās) [EC 1.1.1.105] an enzyme of the oxidoreductase class that catalyzes the reversible oxidation of retinol to retinal, using $NAD^+$ as an electron acceptor.

**ret·i·nol *O*-fat·ty-ac·yl·trans·fer·ase** (ret'ĭ-nol fat'e a″səl-trans'fər-ās) [EC 2.3.1.76] an enzyme of the transferase class that catalyzes the esterification of retinol with long chain fatty acids (particularly palmitic acid) derived from acyl coenzyme A molecules; the reaction occurs in the intestinal mucosa, creating retinyl esters for transport and storage.

**ret·i·no·ma** (ret″ĭ-no'mə) retinocytoma.

**ret·i·no·ma·la·cia** (ret″ĭ-no-mə-la'shə) [*retina* + *malacia*] softening of the retina.

**ret·i·no·pap·il·li·tis** (ret″ĭ-no-pap″ĭ-li'tis) inflammation of the retina and the optic papilla.

**ret·i·nop·a·thy** (ret″ĭ-nop'ə-the) [*retina* + *-pathy*] 1. retinitis. 2. retinosis.
**AIDS-associated r.**, HIV-associated r.
**arteriosclerotic r.**, sclerosis of retinal arterioles marked by increased tortuosity, attenuation, copper-wire appearance, perivascular sheathing, nipping at arteriovenous crossings, small, scattered hemorrhaging, and small, white, well-defined exudates with no surrounding edema.
**background r., background diabetic r.,** diabetic retinopathy characterized by progression of microaneurysms, intraretinal punctate hemorrhages, yellow exudates, cotton-wool spots, and sometimes macular edema that can compromise vision.
**central angiospastic r.**, central serous r.
**central disk-shaped r.**, disciform macular degeneration.
**central serous r.**, a usually self-limiting condition marked by acute localized detachment of the neural retina or retinal pigment epithelium in the region of the macula, with hypermetropia; called also *central angiospastic retinitis* or *retinopathy.*
**circinate r.**, a condition marked by a circle of white spots enclosing the macular area, leading to complete foveal blindness; called also *retinitis circinata* or *circinate retinitis.*
**diabetic r.**, retinopathy associated with diabetes mellitus. A less serious type is called *background retinopathy;* a type that often progresses to blindness is called *progressive retinopathy.* Called also *diabetic retinitis.*
**exudative r.**, a condition marked by masses of white or yellowish exudate in the posterior part of the fundus oculi, with deposit of cholesterin and blood debris from retinal hemorrhage, and leading to destruction of the macula and blindness. Called also *exudative retinitis,* and *Coats' disease* or *retinitis.*
**hemorrhagic r.**, retinopathy marked by profuse hemorrhaging in the retina, occurring in diabetes, occlusion of the central vein, and hypertension.
**HIV-associated r.**, a usually asymptomatic microangiopathy affecting the retina, seen in human immunodeficiency virus infection; it is manifested by transient cotton-wool spots, and occasionally hemorrhages, microaneurysms, and other lesions of the microvasculature. Called also *retinal microvasculopathy* and *AIDS-associated r.*
**hypertensive r.**, that associated with essential or malignant hypertension; changes may include irregular narrowing of the retinal arterioles, hemorrhages in the nerve fiber layers and the outer plexiform layer, exudates and cotton-wool patches, a lipid star in the macula, arteriosclerotic changes, and, in malignant hypertension, papilledema. Called also *hypertensive retinitis.* See also *renal r.* and *stellate r.*
**leukemic r.**, a condition occurring in leukemia, with paleness of the fundus resulting from infiltration of the retina and choroid with leukocytes, and swelling of the disk with blurring of its margin.
**r. of prematurity,** a bilateral retinopathy typically occurring in premature infants treated with high concentrations of oxygen, characterized by vascular dilatation, proliferation, and tortuosity, edema, and retinal detachment, with ultimate conversion of the retina into a fibrous mass that can be seen as a dense retrolental membrane; usually, growth of the eye is arrested and may result in microphthalmia, and blindness may occur. Called also *retrolental fibroplasia* and *Terry's syndrome.*
**pigmentary r.**, see *retinitis pigmentosa.*
**proliferative r., proliferative diabetic r.,** diabetic retinopathy characterized by neovascularization of the retina and optic disk (which may project into the vitreous), proliferation of fibrous tissue, vitreous hemorrhage, and eventually retinal detachment with blindness.
**Purtscher's angiopathic r.**, Purtscher's disease.
**renal r.**, a retinopathy associated with renal and hypertensive disorders, and presenting the same symptoms as hypertensive retinopathy; called also *renal retinitis.* See also *stellate r.*
**stellate r.**, a retinopathy not associated with hypertensive, renal, or arteriosclerotic disorders, but presenting the same symptoms as hypertensive retinopathy; called also *stellate retinitis.* See also *renal r.*

**ret·i·nos·chi·sis** (ret″ĭ-nos'kĭ-sis) [*retina* + *-schisis*] splitting of the retina: in the *juvenile form* the splitting occurs in the nerve fiber layer, and in the *adult form* in the external plexiform layer. The disorder is usually more benign and slowly progressive than retinal detachment.

**ret·i·no·scope** (ret'ĭ-no-skōp″) an instrument for performing retinoscopy; called also *skiascope.*

**ret·i·nos·co·py** (ret″ĭ-nos'kə-pe) [*retina* + *-scopy*] an objective method for investigating, diagnosing, and evaluating refractive errors of the eye, by projection of a beam of light into the eye and observation of the movement of the illuminated area on the retina surface and of the refraction by the eye of the emergent rays. Called also *pupilloscopy, skiascopy, skiametry, shadow test,* and *umbrascopy.*

**ret·i·no·sis** (ret″ĭ-no'sis) [*retina* + *-osis*] a general term for degenerative, noninflammatory conditions of the retina.

**ret·i·no·top·ic** (ret″ĭ-no-top'ik) relating to the organization of the visual pathways and visual area of the brain.

**ret·i·no·tox·ic** (ret″ĭ-no-tok'sik) exerting a toxic or deleterious effect upon the retina.

**ret·i·nyl** (ret'ĭ-nəl) pertaining to or derived from retinol.

**ret·i·nyl-pal·mi·tate es·ter·ase** (ret'ĭ-nəl pal'mĭ-tāt es'tər-ās) [EC 3.1.1.21] an enzyme of the hydrolase class that catalyzes the cleavage of palmitic acid from the corresponding retinyl ester to form the free alcohol retinol. The reaction occurs in the intestinal lumen and in the liver in the metabolism of vitamin A.

**reti·so·lu·tion** (ret″ĭ-sə-loo'shən) [*rete* + *solution*] dissolution of the Golgi apparatus.

**reti·sper·sion** (ret″ĭ-sper'shən) [L. *rete* net + *spargere* to throw about] migration of the Golgi apparatus from its normal position to the periphery of the cell.

**re·to·peri·the·li·um** (re″to-per″ĭ-the′le-əm) [*rete* + *peri-* + *thelium*] the layer of cells covering a reticular framework.

**Re·tor·ta·mo·nad·i·da** (re-tor″tə-mo-nad′ĭ-də) an order of parasitic intestinal flagellate protozoa (class Zoomastigophorea, subphylum Mastigophora), characterized by the presence of two to four flagella, one of which is turned posteriorly and associated with a ventral cytosomal region; Golgi apparatus and mitochondria are absent. Representative genera include *Chilomastix* and *Retortamonas.*

**Re·tor·tam·o·nas** (re″tor-tam′o-nas) [L. *retortus* bent back + Gr. *monas* unit, from *monos* single] a genus of biflagellate nonpathogenic parasitic intestinal protozoa (order Retortamonadida, class Zoomastigophorea), found in various insects, amphibians, reptiles, and mammals, and characterized by the presence of two anterior flagella, one of which extends posteriorly and trails from the body.

**re·to·thel** (re′to-thel) reticuloendothelial.

**re·to·the·li·al** (re″to-the′le-əl) pertaining to the retothelium; containing reticulum cells.

**re·to·the·li·um** (re″to-the′le-əm) [*rete* + *thelium*] the layer of cells covering a reticular tissue.

**re·trac·tile** (re-trak′til) [L. *retractilis*] susceptible of being drawn back.

**re·trac·tion** (re-trak′shən) [L. *retrahere* to draw back] 1. the act of drawing back; the condition of being drawn back. 2. distal movement of teeth, usually accomplished with an orthodontic appliance.
**clot r.,** the drawing away of a blood clot from the wall of a vessel, a stage of wound healing caused by contraction of platelets.
**gingival r.,** the displacement of the marginal gingiva away from a tooth.
**mandibular r.,** 1. drawing back or retracting the mandible, accomplished by contraction of the middle and posterior parts of the temporal muscles and the suprahyoid muscle. 2. the condition of the mandible in which it lies posterior to the orbital plane. Cf. *mandibular protraction.*

**re·trac·tor** (re-trak′tor) 1. an instrument for maintaining operative exposure by separating the edges of a wound and holding back underlying organs and tissues; many shapes, sizes, and styles are available. 2. any retractile muscle.
**Emmet's r.,** a self-retaining vaginal speculum.
**Moorehead's r.,** one for retracting the lips, cheeks, or margins of a surgical wound. It fits over the crown of the head and is provided with metal buttons, to which shields (or retractors) of desired shapes or sizes may be attached.

**re·trad** (re′trad) [L. *retro* backward] toward a posterior or dorsal part.

**re·triev·al** (re-tre′vəl) in psychology, the process of obtaining memory information from wherever it has been stored.

**retr(o)-** [L. *retro* backward] a prefix meaning backward, or located behind.

**ret·ro·ac·tion** (ret″ro-ak′shən) action in a reversed direction; reaction.

**ret·ro·au·ric·u·lar** (ret″ro-aw-rik′u-lər) postauricular.

**ret·ro·buc·cal** (ret″ro-buk′əl) pertaining to the posterior part of the mouth near the cheek.

**ret·ro·bul·bar** (ret″ro-bul′bər) [*retro-* + *bulbar*] 1. posterior or inferior to the medulla oblongata. 2. posterior to the eyeball.

**ret·ro·cal·ca·neo·bur·si·tis** (ret″ro-kal-ka″ne-o-bər-si′tis) achillobursitis.

**ret·ro·cer·vi·cal** (ret″ro-ser′vĭ-kəl) posterior to the cervix uteri.

**ret·ro·ces·sion** (ret″ro-sesh′ən) [L. *retrocessio*] a going backward; backward displacement; specifically a dropping backward of the entire uterus.

**ret·ro·coch·le·ar** (ret″ro-kok′le-ər) 1. posterior to the cochlea. 2. denoting the eighth cranial nerve and cerebellopontine angle as opposed to the cochlea.

**ret·ro·col·lic** (ret″ro-kol′ik) 1. nuchal. 2. torticollar.

**ret·ro·col·lis** (ret″ro-kol′is) [*retro-* + *collum*] spasmodic torticollis in which the head is drawn directly backward.

**ret·ro·cru·ral** (ret″ro-kroo′rəl) situated at the back of the leg, or crus.

**ret·ro·cur·sive** (ret″ro-kur′siv) [*retro-* + L. *currere* to run] marked by stepping backward.

**ret·ro·de·vi·a·tion** (ret″ro-de″ve-a′shən) any displacement backwards; a general term that includes retroversion, retroflexion, and other deviations. Called also *retrodisplacement* and *retroposition.*

**ret·ro·dis·place·ment** (ret″ro-dis-plās′mənt) retrodeviation.

**ret·ro·fill·ing** (ret″ro-fil′ing) a method of root canal therapy in which the canal is filled from the apex, which has been surgically exposed; zinc-free silver alloy is the most commonly used filling material. Called also *reverse filling* and *root-end filling.*

**ret·ro·flexed** (ret′ro-flekst) [*retro-* + L. *flexus* bent] bent posteriorly; in a state of retroflexion.

**ret·ro·flex·ion** (ret″ro-flek′shən) [*retro-* &plus *flexion*] the bending of an organ or part so that its top is turned posteriorly; particularly, the bending posteriorly of the body of the uterus toward the cervix, resulting in a sharp angle at the point of bending.

**ret·ro·gas·se·ri·an** (ret″ro-gə-sēr′e-ən) pertaining to the sensory (posterior) root of the trigeminal (gasserian) ganglion.

**ret·ro·gna·thia** (ret″ro-nath′e-ə) [*retro-* + *gnath-* + *-ia*] retrusion of the mandible. Called also *retrognathism.*

**ret·ro·gnath·ic** (ret″ro-nath′ik) pertaining to or characterized by retrognathia.

**ret·ro·gnath·ism** (ret″ro-nath′iz-əm) [MeSH: Retrognathism] retrognathia.

**ret·ro·grade** (ret′ro-grād) [*retro-* + L. *gradi* to step] 1. moving backward or against the usual direction of flow. 2. degenerating, deteriorating, or catabolic.

**ret·rog·ra·phy** (ret-rog′rə-fe) [*retro-* + *-graphy*] mirror writing.

**ret·ro·gres·sion** (ret″ro-gresh′ən) [*retro-* + L. *gressus* course] degeneration; deterioration; regression; return to an earlier, less complex condition.

**ret·ro·in·fec·tion** (ret″ro-in-fek′shən) infection of the mother by the fetus.

**ret·ro·jec·tion** (ret″ro-jek′shən) [*retro-* + L. *jacere* to throw] irrigation of a cavity by injection of fluid.

**ret·ro·lab·y·rin·thine** (ret″ro-lab″ə-rin′thēn) posterior to a labyrinth.

**ret·ro·lis·the·sis** (ret″ro-lis′thə-sis) [*retr-* + Gr. *olisthanein* to slip] retrospondylolisthesis.

**ret·ro·mo·lar** (ret″ro-mo′lər) behind a molar.

**ret·ro·mor·pho·sis** (ret″ro-mor-fo′sis) [*retro-* + *morphosis*] retrograde metamorphosis.

**ret·ro·peri·to·ne·al** (ret″ro-per″ĭ-to-ne′əl) external to or posterior to the peritoneum.

**ret·ro·peri·to·ne·um** (ret″ro-per″ĭ-to-ne′əm) spatium retroperitoneale.

**ret·ro·peri·to·ni·tis** (ret″ro-per″ĭ-to-ni′tis) inflammation in the retroperitoneal space.

**ret·ro·pha·ryn·ge·al** (ret″ro-fə-rin′je-əl) 1. pertaining to the retropharynx. 2. posterior to the pharynx.

**ret·ro·phar·yn·gi·tis** (ret″ro-far″in-ji′tis) inflammation of the posterior part of the pharynx.

**ret·ro·phar·ynx** (ret″ro-far′inks) the posterior part of the pharynx.

**ret·ro·pla·cen·tal** (ret″ro-plə-sen′təl) posterior to the placenta.

**ret·ro·pla·sia** (ret″ro-pla′zhə) [*retro-* + *-plasia*] retrograde metaplasia; degeneration of a tissue or cell into a more primitive type.

**ret·ro·posed** (ret′ro-pōzd) [*retro-* + L. *positus* placed] displaced backward or posteriorly.

**ret·ro·po·si·tion** (ret″ro-pə-zish′ən) retrodeviation.

**ret·ro·pul·sion** (ret″ro-pul′shən) [*retro-* + *pulsion*] 1. a driving back. 2. a tendency to walk backward involuntarily, seen in some varieties of parkinsonism; called also *opisthoporeia* and *backward progression.* 3. an abnormal gait in which the body is bent backward.

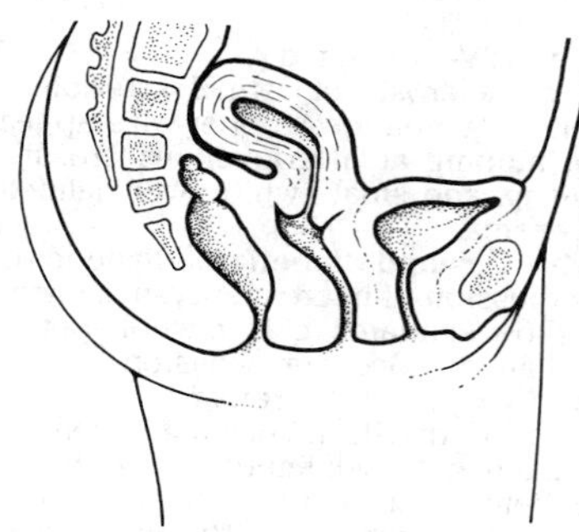

Retroflexion of uterus.

**ret·ror·sine** (ret'ror-sin) a poisonous pyrrolizidine alkaloid found in various species of *Senecio,* causing seneciosis in ruminants.

**ret·ro·sig·moid·al** (ret″ro-sig-moi'dəl) posterior to the sigmoid sinus.

**ret·ro·spon·dy·lo·lis·the·sis** (ret″ro-spon″də-lo-lis-the'sis) posterior displacement of one vertebral body on the subjacent body.

**ret·ro·stal·sis** (ret″ro-stahl'sis) reversed or backward peristaltic action.

**ret·ro·ster·nal** (ret″ro-ster'nəl) [*retro-* + *sternal*] situated or occurring posterior to the sternum.

**ret·ro·sym·phys·i·al** (ret″ro-sim-fiz'e-əl) posterior to the symphysis pubis.

**ret·ro·uter·ine** (ret″ro-u'tər-in) [*retro-* + *uterine*] posterior to the uterus.

**ret·ro·ver·sio·flex·ion** (ret″ro-vər″se-o-flek'shən) retroversion combined with retroflexion.

**ret·ro·ver·sion** (ret″ro-ver'zhən) [*retro-* + *version* ] the tipping of an entire organ in a posterior direction; particularly, the tipping back of the entire uterus in relation to the pelvic axis.

**ret·ro·vert·ed** (ret″ro-ver'təd) in a condition of retroversion.

**ret·ro·ves·i·cal** (ret″ro-ves'ĭ-kəl) posterior to the urinary bladder.

**Ret·ro·vir** (ret'ro-vir) trademark for a preparation of zidovudine.

**Ret·ro·vi·ri·dae** (ret″ro-vir'ĭ-de) [MeSH: Retroviridae] the retroviruses: a family of RNA viruses having a virion 80–100 nm in diameter consisting of a lipid-containing envelope with peplomers, surrounding an icosahedral capsid. The genome consists of two identical molecules of polyadenylated positive-sense single-stranded RNA; the monomers are connected at the 5′ end by hydrogen bonds and each has a molecular weight of approximately $3 \times 10^6$ and a size of 3.5–9 kb, depending on the genus. Viruses contain seven major polypeptides, including a reverse transcriptase, and are resistant to ultraviolet light but sensitive to lipid solvents and detergents. Replication is unique: genomic RNA serves as a template for DNA synthesis via reverse transcriptase; complementary DNA is synthesized from viral DNA and integrated into the host cell DNA, where it is used for transcription. Assembly occurs by budding through the plasma membrane. Most retroviruses are oncogenic. Included in this family are the mammalian type B and type C retroviruses, avian type C retroviruses, type D retroviruses, the BLV-HTLV retroviruses, *Lentivirus,* and *Spumavirus.*

**ret·ro·vi·rus** (ret'ro-vi″rəs) [MeSH: Retroviridae] any virus belonging to the family Retroviridae.
**avian type C r's,** a genus having the same virion morphology as the mammalian type C retroviruses and causing infection and malignancies in birds.
**BLV-HTLV r's,** a genus similar in morphology and replication to the type C retroviruses; organisms have a long latency and cause B and T cell leukemia and lymphoma and neurologic disease. Included in this genus are bovine leukemia virus, human T-lymphotropic virus 1 and 2, and simian T-lymphotropic virus.
**mammalian Type B r's,** a genus having a characteristic dense core 40–60 nm in diameter enclosed by a membranous envelope 90–120 nm in diameter with prominent surface spikes; capsid assembly occurs in the cytoplasm prior to budding from the plasma membrane. It contains a single species, mouse mammary tumor virus.
**mammalian type C r's,** a widely distributed genus having a dense, centrally located core within a lipoprotein envelope covered with barely visible spikes; replication occurs at the inner surface of the plasma membrane at the same time as budding.
**type D r's,** a genus whose virion lacks surface spikes; included here are species pathogenic for Old World primate and sheep.

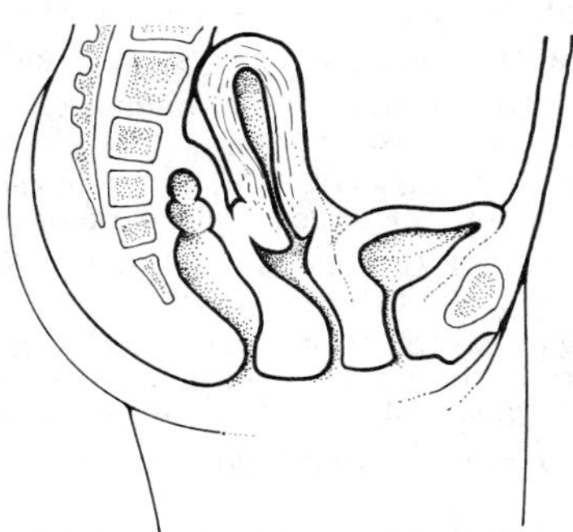

Retroversion of uterus.

**re·tru·sion** (re-troo'zhən) [L. *re-* back + *trudere* to shove] 1. the state of being located posterior to the normal position, such as the mandible or a tooth displaced in the line of occlusion. 2. the backward movement of the mandible. 3. the pressing backward of the teeth.

**Rett syndrome** (ret) [Andreas *Rett,* Austrian physician, 20th century] [MeSH: Rett Syndrome] see under *syndrome.*

**re·turn** (re-tərn') a coming back.
**venous r.,** the flow of blood into the heart from the peripheral vessels.

**Ret·zi·us' fibers, space (cavity), veins** (ret'ze-oos) [Anders Adolf *Retzius,* Swedish anatomist, 1796–1860] see under *fiber* and *vein,* and see *spatium retropubicum.*

**Ret·zi·us' foramen, lines (striae, stripes)** (ret'ze-oos) [Magnus Gustav *Retzius,* Swedish anatomist, 1842–1919] see *apertura lateralis ventriculi quarti,* and see *incremental lines,* under *line.*

**Reuss' color charts (tables)** (rois) [August Ritter von *Reuss,* Austrian ophthalmologist, 1841–1924] see under *chart.*

**re·vac·ci·na·tion** (re″vak-sĭ-na'shən) a second vaccination.

**re·vas·cu·lar·iza·tion** (re-vas″ku-lər-ĭ-za'shən) 1. the restoration of blood supply, as after a wound. 2. the restoration of an adequate blood supply to a part, such as with a bypass (q.v.) using a vascular graft or prosthesis.

**re·ve·hent** (rə-ve'hənt) carrying back; said of veins and arteries.

**re·ver·ber·a·tion** (re-vər″bə-ra'shən) [L. *reverberare* to cause to rebound] duration of neuronal activity well beyond an initial stimulus due to transmission of impulses along branches of nerves arranged in a circle, permitting positive feedback; it occurs in the brain and perhaps elsewhere and is thought to be related to processes such as learning, memory, and habituation. See also *reverberating circuit,* under *circuit.*

**Re·ver·din's graft, needle** (rĕ-ver-daz') [Jacques Louis *Reverdin,* Swiss surgeon, 1842–1929] see *epidermic graft,* under *graft,* and see under *needle.*

**re·ver·sal** (re-ver'səl) a turning or change in the opposite direction.
**r. of gradient,** a changing of direction of the fecal stream due to an area of irritation causing local spasticity of the intestine with higher tonus than that of the proximal area.

**re·verse tran·scrip·tase** (re-vərs' tran-skrip'tās) RNA-directed DNA polymerase.

**re·ver·si·ble** (re-vər'sĭ-bəl) capable of going through a series of changes in either direction, forward or backward, as a reversible chemical reaction.

**re·ver·sion** (re-vər'zhən) [*re-* + *version*] 1. a returning to a previous condition; regression. 2. in genetics, the mutation of a mutant phenotype so that the original function is restored; the term denotes mutation of the DNA such that the parental base sequence is regained (reverse mutation), but can be used to describe production of an altered base sequence that nevertheless encodes the original amino acid or masking of the first alteration by a second via suppression (q.v.).
**antigenic r.,** a change in the antigenic structure of adult cells to that of immature cells, as in certain tumors.
**true r.,** reversion occurring via reverse mutation.

**Rev·ex** (rev'eks) trademark for a preparation of nalmefene hydrochloride.

**Re·vil·liod's sign** (rĕ-ve-yōz') [Jean Léonard Adolphe *Revilliod,* Swiss physician, 1835–1919] see under *sign.*

**re·vi·ves·cence** (re″vi-ves'əns) [L. *revivescere* to revive] the renewal of vital activities.

**re·viv·i·fi·ca·tion** (re-viv″ĭ-fĭ-ka'shən) [*re-* + *vivi-* + *facere* to make] 1. restoration to life or consciousness. 2. refreshing of diseased surfaces to promote their union.

**rev·o·lute** (rev'o-lo͞ot) turned back or curled back.

**re·vul·sion** (re-vul'shən) [L. *revulsio;* from *re-* back + *vellere* to draw] the drawing of blood from one part to another, as occurs in counterirritation.

**Rex·ed's laminae** (rek″sedz) [B. *Rexed,* 20th century] see under *lamina.*

**Reye's syndrome** (rīz) [Ralph Douglas Kenneth *Reye,* Australian physician, 20th century] [MeSH: Reye's Syndrome] see under *syndrome.*

**Reye-John·son syndrome** (ri-jon'sən) [R.D.K. *Reye;* George Magnus *Johnson,* American physician, born 1935] Reye's syndrome.

**Rey·nals** (ra-nahlz') see *Duran-Reynals.*

**Rey·nolds' number** (ren'əldz) [Osborne *Reynolds,* Irish physicist, 1842–1912] see under *number.*

**Rez·i·pas** (rez′ĭ-pas) trademark for a preparation of para-aminosalicylic acid.

**Rez·u·lin** (rez′u-lin) trademark for a preparation of troglitazone.

**RF** rheumatoid factor.

**RFA** right frontoanterior (position of the fetus).

**RfD** reference dose.

**RFLP** restriction fragment length polymorphism; see under *polymorphism.*

**RFP** right frontoposterior (position of the fetus).

**RFPS(Glasgow)** Royal Faculty of Physicians and Surgeons of Glasgow.

**RFT** right frontotransverse (position of the fetus).

**RGN** Registered General Nurse (Scotland).

**Rh** symbol for *rhodium.*

**$Rh_{null}$** symbol for a rare blood type in which all Rh factors are lacking; see also *Rh-null syndrome,* under *syndrome.*

**Rh antibody, blood group, factor** [from *Rhesus* monkeys, whose blood was found to contain the factor in 1940] see under *antibody, blood group,* and *factor.*

**Rhab·di·a·soi·dea** (rab″do-ə-soi′de-ə) [MeSH: Rhabdiasoidea] in some classifications, a superfamily of phasmids, including the genus *Strongyloides.*

**rhab·dit·ic** (rab-dit′ik) pertaining or belonging to *Rhabditis,* or to the Rhabditoidea.

**Rhab·di·ti·dae** (rab-dit′ĭ-de) a family of nematodes that contains both free-living and parasitic species. Genera of medical or veterinary interest include *Rhabditis* and *Strongyloides.*

**rhab·dit·i·form** (rab-dit′ĭ-form) rhabdoid.

**Rhab·di·tis** (rab-di′tis) [Gr. *rhabdos* rod] a genus of minute phasmid nematodes of the superfamily Rhabditoidea, family Rhabditidae, living mostly in damp earth, and as an accidental parasite in humans and domestic animals.
**R. ho′minis,** a species found in human feces.
**R. intestina′lis,** a species found in human feces.
**R. niel′lyi,** a species found as an accidental parasite on human skin.
**R. pel′lio,** a species found in the human genitourinary tract.
**R. strongyloi′des,** a species that usually lives in decaying vegetable matter but may invade broken skin of humans and other animals, causing rhabditic dermatitis.

**rhab·di·toid** (rab′dĭ-toid) rhabdoid.

**Rhab·di·toi·dea** (rab″dĭ-toi′de-ə) [MeSH: Rhabditoidea] a superfamily of phasmids, some members of which are free-living and others parasitic to plants and animals; it includes the genera *Rhabditis* and *Strongyloides.*

**rhabd(o)-** [Gr. *rhabdos* rod] a combining form meaning rod-shaped or denoting relationship to a rod.

**rhab·doid** (rab′doid) [*rhabdo-* + *-oid*] resembling a rod; rod-shaped.

**rhab·do·myo·blast** (rab″do-mi′o-blast″) [*rhabdo-* + *myoblast*] a pathologic type of myoblast that is typically rounded at one part and narrowed at another so that it is spindle-shaped or racket-shaped; it has an eccentric nucleus, eosinophilic cytoplasm, and sometimes cross striations resembling those of striated muscle. It is the prototypic cell of rhabdomyosarcoma.

**rhab·do·myo·blas·tic** (rab″do-mi″o-blas′tik) pertaining to a rhabdomyoblast.

**rhab·do·myo·blas·to·ma** (rab″do-mi″o-blas-to′mə) [*rhabdo-* + *myo-* + *blastoma*] rhabdomyosarcoma.

**rhab·do·myo·chon·dro·ma** (rab″do-mi″o-kon-dro′mə) [*rhabdo-* + *myo-* + *chondroma*] a benign mesenchymoma containing striated muscle and cartilaginous elements.

**rhab·do·my·ol·y·sis** (rab″do-mi-ol′ĭ-sis) [*rhabdo-* + *myo-* + *-lysis*] [MeSH: Rhabdomyolysis] disintegration or dissolution of muscle, associated with excretion of myoglobin in the urine.
**exertional r.,** 1. that due to intense, prolonged physical exertion, with symptoms often resembling those elicited by exercise in persons with occlusive arterial disease. 2. severe muscular soreness and recumbency in an animal during exercise, either after it does unusually strenuous exercise or when it returns to heavy exercise after a prolonged rest; symptoms include heavy sweating, rapid pulse, and stiffness of gait, sometimes with myoglobinuria. See also *azoturia* (def. 2) and *capture myopathy.*

**rhab·do·my·o·ma** (rab″do-mi-o′mə) [*rhabdo-* + *myoma*] [MeSH: Rhabdomyoma] a benign tumor derived from striated muscle. The cardiac form is considered to be a hamartoma and is often associated with tuberous sclerosis; the extracardiac form is a true neoplasm and is often divided into fetal and adult forms on the basis of the degree of cellular differentiation, distribution, patient age, and other factors.

**rhab·do·myo·myx·o·ma** (rab″do-mi″o-mik-so′mə) [*rhabdo-* + *myo-* + *myxoma*] a benign mesenchymoma containing striated muscle cell and myxoid elements.

**rhab·do·myo·sar·co·ma** (rab″do-mi″o-sahr-ko′mə) [*rhabdo-* + *myo-* + *sarcoma*] [MeSH: Rhabdomyosarcoma] a highly malignant tumor of striated muscle derived from primitive mesenchymal cells and exhibiting differentiation along rhabdomyoblastic lines, including but not limited to the presence of cells with recognizable cross striations. It occurs in three forms: *pleomorphic r., alveolar r.,* and *embryonal r.* Called also *rhabdomyoblastoma* and *rhabdosarcoma.*
**alveolar r.,** a type containing dense proliferations of small round cells among fibrous septa that form alveoli; it occurs mainly in adolescents and young adults and affects muscles of the extremities, trunk, orbit, and elsewhere.
**botryoid r.,** see under *sarcoma.*
**embryonal r.,** the most common form of rhabdomyosarcoma, containing alternating loosely cellular areas having myxoid stroma and densely cellular areas having spindle cells; it occurs mainly in infants and young children and affects the head and neck, lower genitourinary tract, pelvis, and extremities. A subtype is sarcoma botryoides.
**orbital r.,** rhabdomyosarcoma in the orbit and surrounding structures, usually superior to the globe; the most common types are embryonal and alveolar. It may affect patients of any age and is the most common primary malignant orbital tumor in children.
**paratesticular r.,** a tumor of the spermatic cord, usually seen in boys under age 15, presenting as a scrotal mass that may grow rapidly; most cases are embryonal rhabdomyosarcomas.
**pleomorphic r.,** a type seen in skeletal muscles, usually in the extremities of adults, possibly representing dedifferentiation of skeletal muscle cells; the cells are large and have bizarre hyperchromatic nuclei.
**r. of prostate,** a variety of embryonal rhabdomyosarcoma seen mainly in the prostates of young men; it is large and fleshy and may grow fast, filling the pelvis.

**Rhab·do·ne·ma** (rab″do-ne′mə) *Rhabditis.*

**rhab·dos** (rab′dos) [Gr. "rod"] a straight cytopharyngeal apparatus with walls supported by nematodesmata and sometimes containing toxicysts; it is characteristic of the lower ciliate protozoa. Cf. *cyrtos.*

**rhab·do·sar·co·ma** (rab″do-sahr-ko′mə) rhabdomyosarcoma.

**rhab·do·sphinc·ter** (rab″do-sfingk′tər) [*rhabdo-* + *sphincter*] a sphincter consisting of striated muscle fibers.
**intrinsic r.,** slow-twitch muscle fibers within the wall of the urethra, part of the musculus sphincter urethrae.

**Rhab·do·vi·ri·dae** (rab″do-vir′ĭ-de) [MeSH: Rhabdoviridae] the rhabdoviruses: a family of RNA viruses having a bullet- or rod-shaped virion 130–430 × 45–100 nm consisting of a lipid-containing envelope, with large G-protein peplomers, surrounding a helical nucleocapsid. The genome consists of a single molecule of negative-sense single-stranded RNA (MW 3.5–4.6 × $10^6$, size 11–15 kb). Viruses contain four or five major polypeptides, including a transcriptase, and are sensitive to lipid solvents, detergents, and proteolytic enzymes. Replication occurs in the cytoplasm and assembly is by budding on the plasma membrane or intracytoplasmic membranes. Transmission is by biologic or mechanical vectors. Vertebrate pathogens are included in the genera *Vesiculovirus, Lyssavirus,* and *Ephemerovirus*; at least six serogroups of viruses that infect animals and a large number of ungrouped viruses have not yet been assigned to genera.

**rhab·do·vi·rus** (rab′do-vi″rəs) [*rhabdo-* + *virus*] [MeSH: Rhabdoviridae] any virus of the family Rhabdoviridae.

**rhachi-** for words beginning thus, see those beginning *rachi-.*

**rha·co·ma** (ra-ko′mə) [Gr. *rhakōma* rags] a pendulous scrotum.

**rhae·bo·cra·nia** (re″bo-kra′ne-ə) [Gr. *rhaibos* crooked + *crani-* + *-ia*] torticollis, or wryneck.

**rhae·bo·sce·lia** (re″bo-se′le-ə) [Gr. *rhaibos* crooked + *skelos* leg + *-ia*] genu varum (bowleg), or genu valgum (knock knee).

**rhae·bo·sis** (re-bo′sis) [Gr. *rhaibos* crooked + *-osis*] crookedness of the legs or of any normally straight part.

**rhag·a·des** (rag′ə-dēz) [pl. of Gr. *rhagas* rent] fissures, cracks, or fine linear scars in the skin, especially such lesions around the mouth or other regions subjected to frequent movement.

**rha·gad·i·form** (rə-gad′ĭ-form) [*rhagades* + *form*] resembling rhagades.

**rhag·io·crine** (raj′e-o-krīn) [Gr. *rhax* grape + *krinein* to separate] denoting colloid vacuoles in the cytoplasm of gland cells that represent a stage in the development of secretory granules.

**rhag·i·on·id** (raj″e-on′id) a fly of the family Rhagionidae.

**Rhag·i·on·i·dae** (raj″e-on′ĭ-de) the snipe flies, a family of biting flies; the genera *Spaniopsis, Suragina,* and *Symphoromyia* contain species that are vicious biters.

**rham·nose** (ram′nōs) [MeSH: Rhamnose] a methylpentose structurally derived from mannose (6-deoxymannose); the L- isomer occurs naturally as a component of many plant glycosides and of lipopolysaccharides of some gram-negative bacteria.

**rham·no·side** (ram′no-sīd) a glycoside that on hydrolysis yields rhamnose.

**Rham·nus** (ram′nəs) [L.; Gr. *rhamnos* a kind of prickly shrub] [MeSH: Rhamnus] a genus of trees and shrubs of the family Rhamnaceae, often with a purgative bark and fruit. Among them are *R. cathar′tica* L., or buckthorn, *R. purshia′na* D.C., the source of cascara sagrada, and *R. fran′gula* L. *R. califor′nica* L., California buckthorn or coffee tree, has been used in rheumatism. *R. cro′ceus* Nutt. is a species of buckthorn with edible red fruit, the excessive use of which tinges the skin red.

**rha·pha·nia** (rə-fa′ne-ə) raphania.

**rha·phe** (ra′fe) [Gr. *rhaphē*] raphe.

**Rha·zes** (ra′zes) [Ar. Abu Bakr Mohammad Ibn Zakariya *Razi,* c. 845 to c. 930] a Persian physician distinguished for his clinical practice and scholarship. He published the first known monograph distinguishing smallpox and measles *(Liber de variolis et morbillis);* and his students made a posthumous compilation of his writings on medicine and surgery *(Liber continens, The Comprehensive Book),* which was a standard textbook in western Europe for more than 600 years.

**rhe** (re) [Gr. *rheos* current] in the CGS system, the unit of fluidity; it is the reciprocal of the unit of viscosity and is expressed as 1/poise or 1/centipoise.

**rheg·ma** (reg′mə) [Gr. *rhēgma*] 1. tear. 2. fracture.

**rheg·ma·tog·e·nous** (reg″mə-toj′ə-nəs) arising from a rhegma, as rhegmatogenous detachment of the retina.

**rhe·ni·um** (re′ne-əm) [MeSH: Rhenium] a chemical element, atomic number 75, atomic weight 186.2, symbol Re.
**r. 186,** a radioactive isotope of rhenium, atomic mass 186, having a half-life of 3.78 days and emitting beta particles (1.077, 0.933 MeV) and gamma rays (0.137, 0.632, 0.768 MeV); in the form of a colloid suspension it has been injected into joints for synoviorthesis.
**r. 188,** a radioactive isotope of rhenium. atomic mass 188, having a half-life of 16.9 hours and emitting beta particles (2.12, 1.96 MeV) and gamma rays (0.155 MeV).

**rheo-** [Gr. *rheos* current] a combining form denoting relationship to an electric current, or to a flow, as of fluids.

**rheo·base** (re′o-bās) [*rheo-* + *base*] the minimal electric current of infinite duration necessary to produce a twitch in a muscle.

**rhe·og·ra·phy** (re-og′rə-fe) the recording of flow of a fluid.
**light reflection r.,** a type of photoplethysmography used to assess deep venous thrombosis; the diode and sensor are placed on the medial surface of the calf over the vein to be tested.

**rhe·ol·o·gy** (re-ol′ə-je) [MeSH: Rheology] the science of the deformation and flow of matter, such as the flow of blood through the heart and blood vessels.

**Rheo·mac·ro·dex** (re″o-mak′ro-deks) trademark for a preparation of dextran 40.

**rhe·om·e·ter** (re-om′ə-tər) [*rheo-* + *-meter*] galvanometer.

**rheo·nome** (re′o-nōm) [*rheo-* + Gr. *nemein* to distribute] an apparatus for determining the effect of irritation on a nerve.

**rheo·scope** (re′o-skōp) [*rheo-* + *-scope*] an instrument for detecting the presence of an electric current.

**rheo·stat** (re′o-stat) [*rheo-* + *-stat*] an appliance for regulating the resistance and thus controlling the amount of current entering an electric circuit.

**rhe·os·to·sis** (re″os-to′sis) [*rheo-* + *ostosis*] a condition of hyperostosis marked by the presence of streaks in the bones; see also *melorheostosis.*

**rheo·ta·chyg·ra·phy** (re″o-tə-kig′rə-fe) [*rheo-* + *tachy-* + *-graphy*] the recording of the variation in the electromotive action of muscles.

**rheo·tax·is** (re″o-tak′sis) [*rheo-* + *-taxis*] the orientation of an organism in a stream of liquid, with its long axis parallel with the direction of fluid flow.
**negative r.,** rheotaxis with movement of the organism in the same direction as that of the liquid.
**positive r.,** rheotaxis with movement of the organism in the opposite direction to that of the liquid.

**rhe·ot·ro·pism** (re-ot′ro-piz-əm) rheotaxis.

**rhe·sus (Rh)** (re′səs) rhesus monkey.

**Rhe·um** (re′əm) the rhubarbs, a genus of plants of the family Polygonaceae, some species of which are cathartic.
**R. rhapon′ticum,** L., the common edible garden rhubarb; its leaves are rich in oxalates and can cause oxalate poisoning in humans and other animals.
**R. officina′le,** Baill., a species that is the source of a cathartic fluid extract or aromatic tincture used medicinally; see *aromatic rhubarb tincture,* under *tincture.*

**rheum, rheu·ma** (ro͞om) [Gr. *rheuma* flux] a watery discharge.

**rheu·ma·tal·gia** (roo″mə-tal′jə) chronic rheumatic pain.

**rheu·mat·ic** (roo-mat′ik) [Gr. *rheumatikos*] pertaining to or affected by rheumatism.

**rheu·ma·tid** (roo′mə-tid) any skin lesion or eruption etiologically associated with rheumatism.

**rheu·ma·tism** (roo′mə-tiz-əm) [L. *rheumatismus;* Gr. *rheumatismos*] any of a variety of disorders marked by inflammation, degeneration, or metabolic derangement of the connective tissue structures of the body, especially the joints and related structures, including muscles, bursae, tendons, and fibrous tissue. It is attended by pain, stiffness, or limitation of motion of these parts. Rheumatism confined to the joints is classified as arthritis.
**articular r., acute,** rheumatic fever.
**articular r., chronic,** see *rheumatoid arthritis,* under *arthritis,* and *osteoarthritis.*
**Besnier's r.,** chronic arthrosynovitis.
**cerebral r.,** acute rheumatic fever marked by chorea, delirium, convulsions, and coma.
**desert r.,** primary coccidioidomycosis.
**gonorrheal r.,** acute articular rheumatism associated with gonorrheal urethritis, and frequently producing ankylosis of the joints.
**r. of the heart,** involvement of the heart by the rheumatic fever process.
**Heberden's r.,** rheumatism of the finger joint, marked by the formation of nodosities.
**inflammatory r.,** rheumatic fever.
**muscular r.,** fibrositis.
**palindromic r.,** a condition in which there are repeated episodes of arthritis and periarthritis without fever and without producing irreversible changes in the joints.
**Poncet's r.,** tuberculous arthritis.
**subacute r.,** a mild but protracted form of rheumatism.
**tuberculous r.,** see under *arthritis.*

**rheu·ma·tis·mal** (roo″mə-tiz′məl) pertaining to or of the nature of rheumatism.

**rheu·ma·to·gen·ic** (roo″mə-to-jen′ik) [*rheumatism* + *-genic*] producing or causing rheumatism.

**rheu·ma·toid** (roo′mə-toid) [*rheumatism* + *-oid*] 1. resembling rheumatism. 2. associated with rheumatoid arthritis.

**rheu·ma·tol·o·gist** (roo″mə-tol′ə-jist) a specialist in rheumatic conditions.

**rheu·ma·tol·o·gy** (roo″mə-tol′ə-je) [MeSH: Rheumatology] the branch of medicine dealing with rheumatic disorders, their causes, pathology, diagnosis, treatment, etc.

**rheu·ma·to·sis** (roo″mə-to′sis) any disorder attributed to rheumatic origin.

**Rheu·ma·trex** (roo′mə-treks″) trademark for preparations of methotrexate.

**rheu·mic** (roo′mik) pertaining to a rheum or flux.

**rhex·is** (rek′sis) [Gr. *rhēxis* a breaking forth, bursting] the rupture of an organ or vessel.

**rhi·go·sis** (rĭ-go′sis) [Gr. *rhigōsis* a shivering] the ability to feel cold; see *temperature sense,* under *sense.*

**rhi·got·ic** (rĭ-got′ik) pertaining to rhigosis.

**rhi·nal** (ri′nəl) [*rhin-* + *-al*[1]] nasal.

**rhi·nal·gia** (ri-nal′jə) [*rhin-* + *-algia*] pain in the nose. Called also *rhinodynia.*

**rhi·nal·ler·go·sis** (ri″-nal-ər-go′sis) [*rhin-* + *allergy* + *-osis*] allergic rhinitis.

**rhi·nede·ma** (ri″nə-de′mə) [*rhin-* + *edema*] edema of the nose.

**rhi·nen·ce·pha·lia** (ri″nən-sə-fa′le-ə) rhinocephaly.

**rhin·en·ceph·a·lon** (ri″nən-sef′ə-lon) [*rhin-* + *encephalon*] 1. a term generally applied to certain parts of the brain previously thought to be concerned entirely with olfactory mechanisms, including the olfactory nerves, bulbs, tracts, and subsequent connections (all olfactory in function) and the limbic system (not primarily olfactory in function); it is homologous with the olfactory portions of the brain in lower animals. Called also *olfactory brain* and *smell* *brain.* 2. a term formerly used in official terminology to designate the area of the brain comprising the substantia perforata anterior, stria diagonalis (Broca), area subcallosa, and gyrus paraterminalis. 3. one of the portions of the telencephalon in the embryo.

**rhi·nen·ceph·a·lus** (ri″nən-sef′ə-ləs) rhinocephalus.

**rhin·i·on** (rin′e-on) [Gr., dim. of *rhis*] a cephalometric landmark located at the lower end of the suture between the nasal bones.

**rhi·nism** (ri′niz-əm) rhinolalia.

**rhi·ni·tis** (ri-ni′tis) [*rhin-* + *-itis*] [MeSH: Rhinitis] inflammation of the mucous membrane of the nose.
**acute r., acute catarrhal r.,** an acute congestion of the mucous membrane of the nose, marked by dryness, followed by increased mucous secretion from the membrane, impeded respiration through the nose, and pain. Called also *coryza.*
**allergic r.,** a general term used to denote any allergic reaction of the nasal mucosa; it may occur perennially *(nonseasonal allergic r.)* or seasonally *(hay fever).*
**allergic r., nonseasonal,** allergic rhinitis that may occur continuously or intermittently all year round; it is caused by an allergen to which the individual is more or less always exposed, such as house dust, danders, and food, and is characterized by sudden attacks of sneezing, swelling of the nasal mucosa with a profuse watery discharge, itching of the eyes, and lacrimation. Called also *atopic* or *perennial r.* Cf. *hay fever.*
**allergic r., seasonal,** hay fever.
**anaphylactic r.,** allergic r.
**atopic r.,** nonseasonal allergic r.
**atrophic r.,** a chronic form of rhinitis that is nonallergic and noninfectious, marked by wasting of the mucous membrane and the glands. In the early stages there are small dry areas with crusting, either with viscid secretions or without secretions (see *r. sicca*). In later stages the nasal passages become enlarged and have a foul smell, progressing to ozena (q.v.). It is sometimes the result of trauma, and vascular damage by radiation therapy, environmental irritants, and disease has also been implicated.
**atrophic r. of swine,** a disease of young swine caused by severe persistent inflammation of the nasal mucosa; severe cases may result in marked atrophy of the turbinate bones and lateral displacement of the snout. The primary inflammatory reaction may be caused by a variety of agents, including a virus. See also *inclusion body r.*
**r. caseo′sa,** rhinitis with a caseous, gelatinous, fetid discharge.
**chronic r.,** long-term inflammation of nasal mucous membranes, manifested as either *hypertrophic rhinitis* or *atrophic rhinitis.*
**fibrinous r.,** membranous r.
**gangrenous r.,** a gangrenelike inflammation of the nasal mucosa. See also *cancrum nasi.*
**hypertrophic r.,** a form of rhinitis that is nonallergic and noninfectious, and in which the mucous membrane thickens and swells. See also *vasomotor r.*
**inclusion body r.,** mucopurulent rhinitis and sinusitis of young pigs due to infection with a cytomegalovirus; severe cases may be marked by atrophy of the turbinate bones (see *atrophic r. of swine*) and distortion of the snout, sneezing, stunting of growth, and, histologically, by the presence of inclusion bodies in scrapings of the nasal mucous membranes.
**r. medicamento′sa,** rhinitis that is nonallergic and noninfectious and is caused by rebound vasodilation after prolonged or excessive use of vasoconstricting nasal sprays or drops.
**membranous r.,** chronic rhinitis with the formation of a false membrane, as in nasal diphtheria. Called also *fibrinous r.* and *pseudomembranous r.*
**necrotic r.,** suppuration, necrosis, and swelling of the nose of a pig due to infection by *Fusobacterium necrophorum* that enters through a wound. Called also *bullnose.*
**perennial r.,** nonseasonal allergic r.
**porcine inclusion body r.,** inclusion body r.
**pseudomembranous r.,** membranous r.
**r. sic′ca,** atrophic rhinitis without secretions.
**syphilitic r.,** a variety caused by syphilis, and marked by ulceration, caries of the nasal bone, and a fetid discharge.
**tuberculous r.,** a variety due to tuberculosis, and attended with ulceration, caries of the nasal bone, and ozena.
**vasomotor r.,** 1. a form of hypertrophic rhinitis with symptoms similar to those of allergic rhinitis; transient changes in vascular tone and permeability are brought on by such stimuli as chilling, fatigue, anger, and anxiety. 2. any type of allergic or nonallergic rhinitis not caused by an infectious agent.

**rhin(o)-** [Gr. *rhis,* gen. *rhinos* nose] a combining form denoting relationship to the nose, or a noselike structure.

**rhi·no·an·tri·tis** (ri″no-ən-tri′tis) [*rhino-* + *antritis*] inflammation of the nasal cavity and the antrum of Highmore. Called also *nasoantritis.*

**rhi·no·by·on** (ri-no′be-on) [*rhino-* + Gr. *byein* to plug] a nasal tampon.

**rhi·no·can·thec·to·my** (ri″no-kan-thek′tə-me) rhinommectomy.

**rhi·no·cele** (ri′no-sēl) rhinocoele.

**rhi·no·ceph·a·lus** (ri″no-sef′ə-ləs) a fetus exhibiting rhinocephaly.

**Rhi·no·ceph·a·lus an·nu·la·tus** (ri″no-sef′ə-ləs an″u-la′təs) *Boophilus annulatus.*

**rhi·no·ceph·a·ly** (ri″no-sef′ə-le) [*rhino-* + *-cephaly*] a developmental anomaly characterized by the presence of a proboscis-like nose superior to eyes that are partially or completely fused into one.

**rhi·no·chei·lo·plas·ty** (ri″no-ki′lo-plas″te) [*rhino-* + *cheiloplasty*] plastic surgery of the nose and lip.

**Rhi·no·clad·i·el·la** (ri″no-klad″e-el′ə) a genus of imperfect fungi of the form-class Hyphomycetes, form-family Dematiaceae. *R. aquasper′sa* causes chromoblastomycosis.

**rhi·no·coele** (ri′no-sēl) [*rhino-* + *-coele*] the ventricle of the olfactory lobe of the brain.

**Rhi·no·cort** (ri′no-kort) trademark for a preparation of budesonide in liquid solution for inhalation.

**rhi·no·dyn·ia** (ri″no-din′e-ə) [*rhin-* + *-odynia*] rhinalgia.

**rhi·no·en·to·moph·tho·ro·my·co·sis** (ri″no-en″to-mof″thə-ro-mi-ko′sis) the usual form of entomophthoromycosis conidiobolae, marked by development of large polyps in the subcutaneous tissues of the nose and paranasal sinuses; orbital involvement with unilateral blindness may follow. Sometimes, especially in weak or immunocompromised patients, it can spread to the central nervous system and cause fatal rhinocerebral zygomycosis. Called also *rhinofacial zygomycosis.*

**Rhi·noes·trus** (ri-nes′trəs) a genus of flies of the family Oestridae whose larvae occur in the nasal passages of horses in Europe, Asia, and Africa; they may deposit larvae in the human eye.

**rhi·nog·e·nous** (ri-noj′ə-nəs) [*rhino-* + *-genous*] arising in the nose.

**rhi·no·ky·pho·sis** (ri″no-ki-fo′sis) [*rhino-* + *kyphosis*] the presence of an abnormal hump in the ridge of the nose.

**rhi·no·la·lia** (rhi″no-la′le-ə) [*rhino-* + *lal-* + *-ia*] altered speech due to some abnormality of nasal structures; see *hypernasality* and *hyponasality.* Called also *rhinism* and *rhinophonia.*
**r. aper′ta,** hypernasality.
**r. clau′sa,** hyponasality.
**open r.,** hypernasality.

**rhi·no·lar·yn·gi·tis** (ri″no-lar″in-ji′tis) inflammation of the mucous membrane of the nose and larynx.

**rhi·no·lar·yn·gol·o·gy** (ri″no-lar″in-gol′ə-je) [*rhino-* + *laryngology*] a branch of otorhinolaryngology that focuses on the nose and larynx and their diseases.

**rhi·no·lith** (ri′no-lith) [*rhino-* + *-lith*] a nasal stone or concretion. Called also *nasal calculus.*

**rhi·no·li·thi·a·sis** (ri″no-lĭ-thi′ə-sis) the presence of rhinoliths in the nose.

**rhi·nol·o·gist** (ri-nol′ə-jist) a specialist in rhinology.

**rhi·nol·o·gy** (ri-nol′ə-je) [*rhino-* + *-logy*] the medical specialty that deals with the nose and its diseases.

**rhi·no·ma·nom·e·ter** (ri″no-mə-nom′ə-tər) [*rhino-* + *manometer*] a manometer used in rhinomanometry; called also *nasomanometer.*

**rhi·no·ma·nom·e·try** (ri″no-mə-nom′ə-tre) measurement of the airflow and pressure within the nose during respiration; nasal resistance or obstruction can be calculated from the data obtained.

**rhi·nom·e·ter** (ri-nom′ə-tər) [*rhino-* + *-meter*] an instrument for measuring the nose and nasal cavities.

**rhi·nom·mec·to·my** (ri″no-mek′tə-me) [*rhin-* + Gr. *omma* eye + *ectomy*] excision of the inner canthus of the eye.

**rhi·no·my·co·sis** (ri″no-mi-ko′sis) fungal infection of the nasal mucosa.

**rhi·no·ne·cro·sis** (ri″no-nə-kro′-sis) necrosis of the nasal bones.

**rhi·no·nem·me·ter** (ri″no-nem′ə-tər) a device for measuring nasal air flow rates. Cf. *pneumotachometer.*

**rhi·no·path·ia** (ri″no-path′e-ə) rhinopathy.
**r. vasomoto′ria,** vasomotor rhinitis.

**rhi·nop·a·thy** (ri-nop′ə-the) [*rhino-* + *-pathy*] any disease of the nose.

**rhi·no·pha·ryn·ge·al** (ri″no-fə-rin′je-əl) nasopharyngeal.

**rhi·no·phar·yn·gi·tis** (ri″no-far″in-ji′tis) nasopharyngitis.

**rhi·no·pha·ryn·go·cele** (ri″no-fə-ring′go-sēl) an aerocele of the nasopharynx.

**rhi·no·pha·ryn·go·lith** (ri″no-fə-ring′go-lith) [*rhino-* + *pharyngo-* + *-lith*] calculus of the nasal pharynx.

**rhi·no·phar·ynx** (ri″no-far′inks) pars nasalis pharyngis.

**rhi·no·pho·nia** (ri″no-fo′ne-ə) [*rhino-* + *phon-* + *-ia*] rhinolalia.

**rhi·no·phy·co·my·co·sis** (ri″no-fi″ko-mi-ko′sis) rhinoentomophthoromycosis.

**rhi·no·phy·ma** (ri″no-fi′mə) [*rhino-* + *phyma*] [MeSH: Rhinophyma] a manifestation of severe rosacea involving the lower half of the nose and sometimes spreading to adjacent cheek areas, usually seen in men, and characterized by thickened, lobulated overgrowth of the sebaceous glands and epithelial connective tissue.

**rhi·no·plas·tic** (ri″no-plas′tik) pertaining to rhinoplasty.

**rhi·no·plas·ty** (ri′no-plas″te) [*rhino-* + *-plasty*] [MeSH: Rhinoplasty] a plastic surgical operation on the nose, either reconstructive, restorative, or cosmetic.
**Carpue's r.,** Indian r.
**English r.,** that in which a nose is formed out of flaps from the cheeks.
**Indian r.,** the reconstruction of a nose by a flap of skin taken from the forehead, with its pedicle at the root of the nose; called also *Carpue's operation.*
**Joseph r.,** an operation for modification of the shape of the nose by resection of the dorsal osteocartilaginous hump with a saw.
**Italian r.,** tagliacotian r.
**tagliacotian r.,** the reconstruction of a nose by a flap of skin taken from the arm, the flap remaining attached to the arm until union has taken place; called also *Italian* or *tagliacotian operation.*

**rhi·no·pneu·mo·ni·tis** (ri″no-noo″mo-ni′tis) [*rhino-* + *pneumonitis*] inflammation of the nasal and pulmonary mucous membranes.
**equine viral r.,** a highly contagious disease of horses caused by a herpesvirus; characteristics include mild respiratory infection in young animals and abortion in mares exposed for the first time; in the latter it is called *equine virus abortion.*

**rhi·no·poly·pus** (ri″no-pol′ĭ-pəs) nasal polyp.

**rhi·nor·rha·gia** (ri″no-ra′je-ə) [*rhino-* + *-rrhagia*] epistaxis.

**rhi·nor·rha·phy** (ri-nor′ə-fe) [*rhino-* + *-rrhaphy*] an operation for epicanthus performed by excising a fold of skin from the nose and closing the opening with sutures.

**rhi·nor·rhea** (ri″no-re′ə) [*rhino-* + *-rrhea*] the free discharge of a thin nasal mucus.
**cerebrospinal fluid r.,** discharge of cerebrospinal fluid through the nose; see also *cerebrospinal fluid fistula.*

**rhi·no·sal·pin·gi·tis** (ri″no-sal-pin-ji′tis) [*rhino-* + *salpingitis*] inflammation of the nasal mucosa and the eustachian tube.

**rhi·no·scle·ro·ma** (ri″no-sklə-ro′mə) [*rhino-* + *scleroma*] [MeSH: Rhinoscleroma] a granulomatous disease in which hard patches or nodules form on the nose and nasopharynx, thought to be due to *Klebsiella rhinoscleromatis*; it occurs in Egypt, Eastern Europe, and Central and South America.

**rhi·no·scope** (ri′no-skōp) [*rhino-* + *-scope*] an instrument used in nasal examinations; various types of specula and endoscopes may be used. Called also *nasoscope.*

**rhi·no·scop·ic** (ri″no-skop′ik) pertaining to rhinoscopy.

**rhi·nos·co·py** (ri-nos′kə-pe) examination of the nasal passages with a rhinoscope.
**anterior r.,** rhinoscopy of anterior nasal structures through the nares.
**median r.,** examination of superior structures in the nasal cavity, such as the openings of the ethmoid cells, by means of a long nasal speculum.
**posterior r.,** rhinoscopy of posterior nasal structures through the nasopharynx.

**rhi·no·si·nu·si·tis** (ri″no-si″nə-si′tis) [*rhino-* + *sinus* + *-itis*] inflammation of the paranasal sinuses; called also *nasosinusitis.*

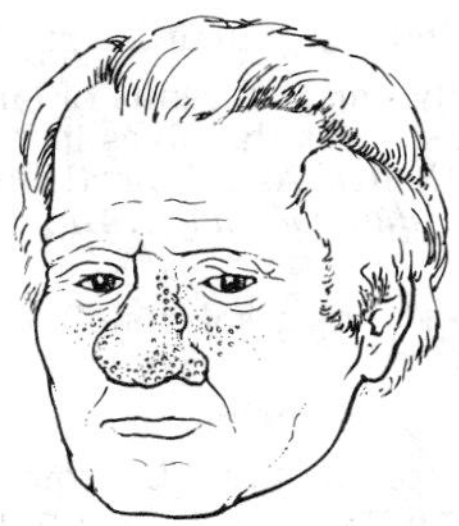
Rhinophyma.

**rhi·no·spo·rid·i·o·sis** (ri″no-spor-id″e-o′sis) [*rhino-* + Gr. *sporidion* dim. of *sporos* seed] [MeSH: Rhinosporidiosis] a chronic, localized granulomatous fungal infection with *Rhinosporidium seeberi*, seen in humans and other animals, affecting mucocutaneous tissues, usually of the nose but sometimes elsewhere in the body; characterized by polyps, papillomas, and other wartlike lesions.

**Rhi·no·spo·rid·i·um see·beri** (ri″no-spor-id′e-əm se′bər-i) the as yet unisolated organism, presumably a fungus, that causes rhinosporidiosis.

**rhi·no·ste·no·sis** (ri′no-stə-no′sis) narrowing of a nasal passage.

**rhi·not·o·my** (ri-not′ə-me) [*rhino-* + *-tomy*] incision into the nose.

**rhi·no·tra·che·itis** (ri″no-tra″ke-i′tis) [*rhino-* + *tracheitis*] inflammation of the nasal mucous membranes and trachea.
**feline r., feline viral r.,** the feline respiratory disease complex when it is caused by feline herpesvirus 1, usually manifesting as an acute febrile infection of the upper respiratory tract and conjunctivae in kittens, with a mucopurulent discharge from the eyes and nose, photophobia, coughing, and sneezing.
**infectious r., infectious bovine r.,** an acute, infectious, febrile, disease of cattle, caused by bovine herpesvirus 1 and marked by inflammation and ulceration of the upper respiratory tract, which may be followed by pneumonia, coughing, profuse discharge from the eyes and nose, excessive salivation, anorexia, and, in pregnant cows, abortion.

**rhi·no·vi·ral** (ri″no-vi′rəl) pertaining to or caused by rhinoviruses.

**Rhi·no·vi·rus** (ri′no-vi″rəs) [*rhino-* + *virus*] [MeSH: Rhinovirus] a genus of viruses of the family Picornaviridae that infect the upper respiratory tract and cause the common cold. Over 100 antigenically distinct types infect humans; bovine and equine rhinoviruses have also been isolated.

**rhi·no·vi·rus** (ri′no-vi″rəs) [MeSH: Rhinovirus] any virus belonging to the genus *Rhinovirus.*

**Rhi·pi·cen·tor** (ri″pĭ-sen′tor) [Gr. *rhipis* fan + *kentein* to prick or stab] a genus of ticks. The bite of *R. bicor′nis (Ixodes bicornis),* a Mexican tick that infests the cougar, may cause a high fever in the human adult and may kill a child.

**Rhi·pi·ceph·a·lus** (ri″pĭ-sef′ə-ləs) [Gr. *rhipis* fan + *-cephalus*] a genus of cattle ticks of the family Ixodidae, species of which transmit *Babesia,* causing bovine babesiosis and other diseases.
**R. appendicula′tus,** the brown tick; it transmits *Theileria parva,* the cause of East Coast fever in African cattle.
**R. bur′sa,** a species that transmits *Babesia ovis,* which causes icterohematuria in sheep.
**R. capen′sis,** an African species found on cattle and horses, which may transmit *Theileria parva,* the cause of East Coast fever.
**R. decolora′tus,** a species regarded as the transmitter of *Borrelia theileri,* the cause of tickborne relapsing fever, of *Rickettsia conorii,* causing tickborne typhus, and of bovine anaplasmosis in some parts of Africa.
**R. evert′si,** an African species found on horses and cattle; it may transmit *Theileria parva* and *Rickettsia conorii.*
**R. sangui′neus,** the brown dog tick, a species found on many domestic animals; it transmits *Rickettsia rickettsii,* the cause of Rocky Mountain spotted fever; *R. conorii,* the cause of tickborne typhus and Boutonneuse fever in humans; *Ehrlichia canis,* the cause of canine ehrlichiosis; and various species of *Babesia.*
**R. si′mus,** the black pitted tick, a species that transmits *Theileria parva,* the cause of East Coast fever.

**rhitid(o)-** for words beginning thus, see those beginning *rhytid(o)–.*

**rhiz(o)-** [Gr. *rhiza* root] a combining form denoting relationship to a root.

**rhi·zo·blast** (ri′zo-blast) [*rhizo-* + *-blast*] flagellar rootlet.

**Rhi·zoc·to·nia** (ri-zok-to′ne-ə) [MeSH: Rhizoctonia] a genus of imperfect fungi of the form-class Hyphomycetes. *R. legumini′cola* contains the mycotoxin slofromine and sometimes contaminates clover hay, causing slobbers (q.v.) in farm animals.

**rhi·zo·don·tro·py** (ri″zo-don′trə-pe) [*rhizo-* + *odont-* + *-tropy*] 1. the act of rotating a tooth root. 2. the act of attaching an artificial crown to a tooth root by means of a pivot.

**rhi·zo·don·try·py** (ri″zo-don′trĭ-pe) [*rhizo-* + *odont-* + Gr. *trephination*] surgical perforation of a tooth root to provide a channel of egress for a confined fluid.

**Rhi·zog·ly·phus** (ri-zog′lĭ-fəs) a genus of mites; *R. parasi′ticus* lives on the ground in India and causes sore feet in tea plantation workers.

**rhi·zoid** (ri′zoid) [*rhiz-* + *-oid*] 1. rootlike; resembling a root. 2. a filamentous rootlike structure of fungi and certain algae that extends into the substrate. See Plate 29.

**rhi·zoi·dal** (ri-zoi′dəl) rhizoid, def. 1.

**rhi·zol·y·sis** (ri-zol'ə-sis) percutaneous radiofrequency rhizotomy.

**Rhi·zo·mas·tig·i·da** (ri″zo-mas-tij'ĭ-də) [*rhizo-* + Gr. *mastix* whip] in former systems of classification, an order of zooflagellates characterized by the presence of one to many flagella and pseudopodia occurring simultaneously or at different times in the trophozoite.

**rhi·zome** (ri'zōm) [Gr. *rhizōma* root stem] the subterraneous root stock of a plant.

**rhi·zo·mel·ic** (ri-zo-mel'ik) [*rhizo-* + *mel-* + *-ic*] pertaining to or involving the hip joint and shoulder joint.

**rhi·zo·me·nin·go·my·eli·tis** (ri″zo-mə-ning″go-mi″ə-li'tis) meningomyeloradiculitis.

**Rhi·zo·mu·cor** (ri″zo-mu'kor) [*rhizo-* + L. *mucor* bread mold] a genus of saprobic fungi of the family Mucoraceae, having few, poorly developed rhizoids. *R. pusil'lus* sometimes causes mucormycosis or opportunistic infections in humans; in other animals it is a more common pathogen and is a major cause of bovine mycotic infection.

**rhi·zo·plast** (ri'zo-plast) [*rhizo-* + *-plast*] flagellar rootlet.

**Rhi·zop·o·da** (ri-zop'ə-də) [*rhizo-* + Gr. *pous* foot] 1. a superclass of protozoa (subphylum Sarcodina, phylum Sarcomastigophora), comprising the amebae, which move about and acquire food by means of filopodia, lobopodia, or reticulopodia, or by protoplasmic flow without production of discrete pseudopodia. The majority are free-living in soil and water, but some are parasitic and pathogenic in humans. It comprises eight classes: Lobosea, Acarpomyxea, Acrasea, Eumycetozoea, Plasmodiophorea, Filosea, Granuloreticulosa, and Xenophyophorea. 2. Sarcodina.

**rhi·zo·po·di·um** (ri″zo-po'de-əm) pl. *rhizopo'dia* [*rhizo-* + Gr. *pous* foot] reticulopodium.

**Rhi·zo·pus** (ri'zo-pəs) [*rhizo-* + Gr. *pous* foot] [MeSH: Rhizopus] a genus of fungi of the family Mucoraceae, characterized by sporangiophores that arise from nodes at the point where the rhizoids are formed and by a hemispherical columella; it is widespread as a saprobe and a facultative parasite of fruits and vegetables. *R. ory'zae* (called also *R. arrhi'zus*) is the most common cause of mucormycosis in humans and occasionally infects other animals. *R. rhizopodifor'mis* (called also *M. rhizopodiformis*) also causes human mucormycosis and is an important cause of bovine gastritis, bovine mycotic abortion, and porcine gastric diseases.

**rhi·zot·o·my** (ri-zot'ə-me) [*rhizo-* + *-tomy*] [MeSH: Rhizotomy] interruption of a cranial or spinal nerve root; see also *neurolysis* (def. 4).
**anterior r.**, division of the anterior or motor spinal nerve roots.
**chemical r.**, rhizotomy by injection of a neurolytic chemical such as glycerol or phenol adjacent to the nerve root; see also *glycerol r.* and *chemical neurolysis.*
**dorsal r.**, posterior r.
**glycerol r.**, chemical rhizotomy of the trigeminal or spinal nerves by injection of glycerol; see also *chemical neurolysis.*
**percutaneous r.**, trigeminal rhizotomy not involving brain surgery, such as glycerol rhizotomy or percutaneous radiofrequency rhizotomy.
**percutaneous radiofrequency r.**, trigeminal rhizotomy in which radio waves are used to destroy part of the trigeminal ganglion.
**posterior r.**, division of the posterior or sensory spinal nerve roots; done for relief of intractable pain. Called also *dorsal r.*
**retrogasserian r.**, trigeminal r.
**trigeminal r.**, destruction of part of the sensory root of the trigeminal nerve above the trigeminal ganglion, or of the ganglion itself, for the relief of trigeminal neuralgia. The most common surgical techniques used are Dandy's operation and the Frazier-Spiller operation; nonsurgical techniques include percutaneous radiofrequency rhizotomy and glycerol rhizotomy. Called also *retrogasserian r.*

**rho** (ro) [P, ρ] the seventeenth letter of the Greek alphabet.
**Spearman's r.**, Spearman's rank correlation coefficient.

**rho·da·mine** (ro'də-mēn) [*rhod-* + *amine*] any of a group of red fluorescent dyes used to label proteins in various immunofluorescence techniques.
**r. B**, a basic red fluorescent dye used in dyeing paper, as a reagent for heavy metals, and as a stain in immunofluorescence techniques; used as a component of the Truant auramine-rhodamine stain.

**rho·da·nate** (ro'də-nāt) a salt of rhodanic acid.

**rho·dan·ic ac·id** (ro-dan'ik) 1. thiocyanic acid. 2. rhodanine.

**rho·da·nine** (ro'də-nēn) [MeSH: Rhodanine] a reagent that gives colored products with aldehydes and ketones.

**rho·di·um** (ro'de-əm) [Gr. *rhodon* rose] [MeSH: Rhodium] a hard and rare metal of the platinum group; atomic number, 45; atomic weight, 102.905; symbol, Rh.

**Rhod·ni·us** (rod'ne-əs) [MeSH: Rhodnius] a genus of South American insects of the family Reduviidae. *R. prolix'us* is a species that transmits *Trypanosoma cruzi,* the etiologic agent of Chagas' disease.

**rhod(o)-** [Gr. *rhodon* rose] a combining form meaning red.

**Rho·do·coc·cus** (ro″do-kok'əs) [*rhodo-* + *coccus*] [MeSH: Rhodococcus] a genus of nocardioform actinomycete bacteria, consisting of nonmotile, gram-positive, aerobic, chemo-organotrophic organisms that form a mycelium that breaks up into bacillary and coccal forms. They are widely distributed, occurring especially in soil and the manure of herbivores; some species are pathogenic for humans and other animals.
**R. bronchia'lis**, a species that forms rough brown colonies with coalescing filaments, isolated from the sputum of patients with pulmonary disease.
**R. e'qui**, a species that forms smooth, shiny, orange to red colonies with elemental hyphae, found in soil and herbivore dung and in the intestinal tracts of cows, horses, sheep, and pigs; it causes bronchopneumonia in foals and can infect immunocompromised humans. See also *R. equi pneumonia,* under *pneumonia.* Called also *Corynebacterium equi.*

**Rho·do·den·dron** (ro″də-den'drən) a genus of shrubs and trees found in the Northern Hemisphere; they contain andromedotoxin and have caused poisoning in sheep.

**rho·do·gen·e·sis** (ro″do-jen'ə-sis) [*rhodo-* + *-genesis*] the restoration of the purple tint to rhodopsin after it has become bleached by the action of light.

**rho·do·phy·lac·tic** (ro″do-fi-lak'tik) tending to preserve or restore rhodopsin; pertaining to rhodophylaxis.

**rho·do·phy·lax·is** (ro″do-fi-lak'sis) [*rhodo-* + *phylaxis*] the ability of the retinal epithelium to regenerate rhodopsin.

**rho·dop·sin** (ro-dop'sin) [*rhodo-* + *opsin*] [MeSH: Rhodopsin] visual purple: a photosensitive purple-red chromoprotein in the retinal rods that is bleached and activated by light, producing stimulation of the retinal sensory endings as it is formed and degraded in the visual cycle (see illustration at *cycle*). It is a conjugated protein containing an 11-*cis* retinal prosthetic group linked to opsin.

**rho·dop·sin ki·nase** (ro-dop'sin ki'nās) an enzyme that phosphorylates activated rhodopsin, enabling it to bind arrestin and thus inhibiting its binding to transducin; the reaction occurs in the deactivation of activated rhodopsin during the visual cycle.

**Rho·do·tor·u·la** (ro″do-tor'u-lə) [MeSH: Rhodotorula] a genus of yeastlike imperfect fungi of the form-family Cryptococcaceae. *R. glu'tinis* is a nonpathogenic species from the air, potatoes, and the skin in seborrhea. *R. ru'bra* is a skin contaminant that occasionally causes opportunistic infections in humans.

**rho·do·tox·in** (ro″do-tok'sin) a poisonous compound from the flowers and leaves of various shrubs and trees, such as *Rhododendron;* it is also found in honey from *Rhododendron* flowers.

**RhoGAM** (ro'gam) trademark for a preparation of $Rh_o$(D) immune globulin.

**rhomb·en·ceph·a·lon** (rom″ben-sef'ə-lon) [Gr. *rhombos* rhomb + *enkephalos* brain] [MeSH: Rhombencephalon] 1. [TA] the part of the brain developed from the posterior of the three primary brain vesicles of the embryonic neural tube; it comprises the metencephalon (cerebellum and pons) and myelencephalon (medulla oblongata). 2. the most caudal of the three primary brain vesicles in the embryo, later dividing into the metencephalon and myelencephalon. Called also *hindbrain.*

**rhom·bo·coele** (rom'bo-sēl) ventriculus terminalis medullae spinalis.

**rhom·boid** (rom'boid) [Gr. *rhombos* rhomb + *-oid*] having a shape similar to a rectangle that has been skewed to one side so that the angles are oblique.
**Michaelis' r.**, a diamond-shaped area over the posterior aspect of the pelvis formed by the dimples of the posterior superior spines of the ilia, the lines formed by the gluteal muscles, and the groove at the distal end of the vertebral column.

**rhom·bo·mere** (rom'bo-mēr) neuromere (def. 1).

**Rhom·bo·mys** (rom'bo-mis) a genus of large rodents. *R. opi'mus* is the great gerbil, a species that lives in colonies in deserts from the Middle East and Central Asia to northwestern India; it is a common reservoir for *Leishmania major,* the cause of wet cutaneous leishmaniasis.

**rhon·chal, rhon·chi·al** (rong'kəl, rong'ke-əl) pertaining to, or of the nature of, a rhonchus.

**rhon·chi·al** (rong'ke-əl) rhonchal.

**rhon·chus** (rong'kəs) pl. *rhon'chi* [L., from Gr. *rhonchos* a snoring sound] [MeSH: Respiratory Sounds] a continuous sound (q.v.) consisting of a dry, low-pitched, snorelike noise, produced in the throat

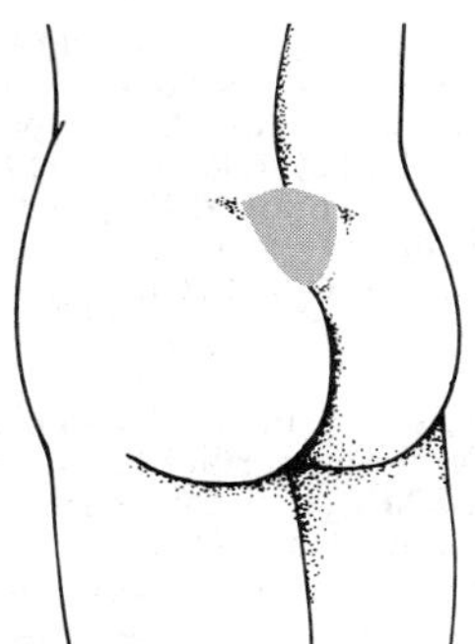

Michaelis' rhomboid.

or bronchial tube due to a partial obstruction such as by secretions. Sometimes called *sonorous r.* (q.v.).
**sibilant r.**, wheeze (def. 1).
**sonorous r.**, a term sometimes used in place of *rhonchus* to distinguish it from a *wheeze* or *sibilant rhonchus.*
**whistling r.**, wheeze (def. 1).

**Rho·pa·lo·psyl·lus** (ro″pə-lo-sil′əs) a genus of fleas. *R. cavi′cola* is the South American cavy flea, which transmits *Pasteurella pestis.*

**rhop·try** (rōp′tre) [Gr. *rhopalon* club] either of the electron-dense, paired, tubular, saccular, or club-shaped organelles arising anteriorly and extending toward the posterior end of the body of apicocomplexans, forming part of the apical complex. Called also *toxoneme.*

**rho·ta·cism** (ro′tə-sizm) a speech disorder consisting of imperfect pronunciation of the *r* sound. Called also *pararhotacism.*

**rhu·barb** (roo′bahrb) [MeSH: Rhubarb] 1. any of various members of the genus *Rheum.* 2. the dried rhizome and root of *Rheum officinale,* used in fluidextract or aromatic tincture as a cathartic. See *aromatic rhubarb tincture,* under *tincture.*

**r-HuEPO** recombinant human erythropoietin; see *epoetin.*

**Rhus** (rus) [L., gen. *rhois*] a genus of vines and shrubs of the family Anacardiaceae, many of them poisonous. Some species contain urushiol, a highly allergenic oleoresin mixture, and contact with them produces a severe dermatitis *(rhus dermatitis)* in sensitive persons. The most important toxic species are *R. ra′dicans* L. (poison ivy), *R. diversilo′ba* L. (western poison oak), *R. quercifo′lia* (eastern poison oak), and *R. ver′nix* L. (poison sumac). Extracts of the leaves and twigs of these plants (see *poison ivy extract* and *poison oak extract,* under *extract*) have been used in the prophylaxis and treatment of dermatitis associated with these species. Called also *Toxicodendron.*

**rhus** (rus) any member of the genus *Rhus.* See also *rhus dermatitis,* under *dermatitis.*

**rhythm** (rith′əm) [L. *rhythmus;* Gr. *rhythmos*] a measured movement; the recurrence of an action or function at regular intervals.
**accelerated atrioventricular (AV) junctional r.**, a cardiac rhythm in which increased rhythmicity of the atrioventricular junction causes it to initiate a series of ectopic impulses, usually occurring at a rate of 70 to 130 beats per minute.
**accelerated idioventricular r.**, a rapid ventricular rhythm, approximately 60 to 110 beats per minute; it usually results from premature beats or an escape rhythm generated by slowing of the sinus pacemaker or acceleration of a ventricular pacemaker.
**alpha r.**, a uniform rhythm of waves in the normal electroencephalogram, showing an average frequency of 10 per second; see *alpha waves* under *wave.* Called also *Berger r.* and *alpha activity.*
**atrial escape r.**, a cardiac dysrhythmia occurring when sustained suppression of sinus impulse formation causes other atrial foci to act as cardiac pacemakers.
**atrioventricular (AV) junctional r.**, the heart rhythm that results when the atrioventricular junction acts as pacemaker.
**atrioventricular (AV) junctional escape r.**, a cardiac rhythm of four or more AV junctional escape beats at a rate below 60 beats per minute, the impulses originating in the AV junction due to absence of normal impulse generation by or conduction from the sinus node or atria.
**atrioventricular (AV) nodal r.**, atrioventricular (AV) junctional r.
**Berger r.**, alpha r.
**beta r.**, a rhythm in the electroencephalogram consisting of waves smaller than those of the alpha rhythm, having an average frequency of 25 per second; see *beta waves* under *wave.* Called also *beta activity.*
**biologic r.**, the established regularity with which certain phenomena recur in living organisms.
**circadian r.**, the regular recurrence in cycles of approximately 24 hours from one stated point to another, as certain biological activities which occur at that interval, regardless of constant darkness or other conditions of illumination.
**circus r.**, circus movement, def. 2.
**coupled r.**, heart beats occurring in pairs, the second beat of the pair usually being a ventricular premature beat; see also *bigeminal pulse* and *bigeminy.*
**delta r.**, rhythm on the electroencephalogram consisting of delta waves (q.v.). Called also *delta activity.*
**ectopic r.**, a heart rhythm initiated by a focus outside the sinoatrial node.
**escape r.**, a heart rhythm initiated by lower centers when the sinoatrial node fails to initiate impulses, its rhythmicity is depressed, or its impulses are completely blocked.
**gallop r.**, an auscultatory finding of three *(triple r.)* or four *(quadruple r.)* heart sounds; the extra sounds occur in diastole and are related either to atrial contraction ($S_4$ gallop), to early rapid filling of a ventricle ($S_3$ gallop), or to concurrence of both events (summation gallop).
**gamma r.**, a rhythm of waves in the electroencephalogram having a frequency of 50 per second.
**idioventricular r.**, a sustained series of impulses propagated by an independent pacemaker within the ventricles, with a rate of 20 to 50 beats per minute. See also *accelerated idioventricular r.*
**infradian r.**, the regular recurrence in cycles of more than 24 hours from one stated point to another, as certain biologic activities which occur at such intervals, regardless of conditions of illumination.
**isochronal r.**, a rhythm of ciliary beats in which all the cilia beat simultaneously; see *ciliary beat,* under *beat.*
**junctional r.**, atrioventricular junctional r.
**junctional escape r.**, atrioventricular junctional escape r.
**metachronal r.**, a rhythm of ciliary beats in which successive cilia in each row start their beats sequentially, producing a wavelike movement; see *ciliary beat,* under *beat.*
**mu r.**, a pattern of rapid activity sometimes seen on an electroencephalogram over the central regions during wakefulness; waves have rounded electropositive and pointed electronegative components and are of little diagnostic significance.
**nodal r.**, atrioventricular junctional r.
**nyctohemeral r.**, a day and night rhythm.
**pendulum r.**, alternation in the rhythm of the heart sounds in which the diastolic sound is equal in time, character, and loudness to the systolic sound, the beat of the heart resembling the tick of a watch.
**quadruple r.**, the gallop rhythm cadence produced when all four heart sounds, $S_1$ to $S_4$, recur in successive cardiac cycles. Cf. *triple r.* and *summation gallop.*
**reciprocal r.**, a cardiac dysrhythmia established by a sustained reentrant mechanism in which impulses traveling back toward the atria through the atrioventricular junction also travel forward to reexcite the ventricles; thus each cycle contains a reciprocal beat, with two ventricular contractions.
**reciprocating r.**, a cardiac dysrhythmia in which an impulse initiated in the atrioventricular node travels both up toward the atria and down toward the ventricles, followed by cycles of bidirectional propagation of the impulse that alternately initiate from the impulses traveling up toward the atria and those traveling down toward the ventricles.
**reentrant r.**, an abnormal cardiac rhythm resulting from a reentry circuit.
**sinoatrial r.**, sinus r.
**sinus r.**, normal heart rhythm originating in the sinoatrial node.
**supraventricular r.**, any cardiac rhythm originating above the ventricles, either normally in the sinoatrial node or abnormally elsewhere in the atria or in the atrioventricular node. Cf. *supraventricular arrhythmia.*
**theta r.**, rhythm on the electroencephalogram consisting of theta waves (q.v.). Called also *theta activity.*
**triple r.**, the gallop rhythm cadence produced when three heart sounds recur in successive cardiac cycles, due to the presence of either a third or a fourth heart sound. Cf. *quadruple r.*
**ultradian r.**, the regular recurrence in cycles of less than 24 hours from one stated point to another, as certain biologic activities which occur at such intervals, regardless of conditions of illumination.
**ventricular r.**, 1. idioventricular r. 2. any cardiac rhythm controlled by a focus within the ventricles.

**rhyth·meur** (rith-mer′) a device for making rhythmic interruptions of the current in an x-ray machine.

**rhyth·mi·cal** (rith′mĭ-kəl) characterized by rhythm.

**rhyth·mic·i·ty** (rith-mis′ĭ-te) 1. the state of being rhythmical. 2. automaticity, def. 2.

**rhyt·i·dec·to·my** (rit″ĭ-dek′tə-me) plastic surgery to eliminate wrinkles from the facial skin by excising loose or redundant tissue; popularly called *face-lift.* Called also *rhytidoplasty.*

**rhytid(o)-** a combining form denoting relationship to wrinkles. Also *rhitid(o)-.*

**rhyt·i·do·plas·ty** (rit′ĭ-do-plas″te) [MeSH: Rhytidoplasty] rhytidectomy.

**rhyt·i·do·sis** (rit″ĭ-do′sis) [Gr. *rhytidōsis; rhytis* wrinkle] a wrinkling of the cornea.

**RIA** radioimmunoassay.

**rib** (rib) [MeSH: Ribs] 1. costa (def. 1). 2. something resembling this bone.
**abdominal r's, asternal r's,** costae spuriae.
**bicipital r.,** an anomalous rib resulting from fusion of the anterior part of the seventh cervical vertebra with the first thoracic rib.
**cervical r.,** costa cervicalis.
**false r's,** costae spuriae.
**floating r's,** costae fluitantes.
**slipping r.,** a rib whose attaching cartilage is repeatedly dislocated.
**spurious r's,** costae spuriae.
**sternal r's,** costae verae.
**Stiller's r.,** an abnormally movable tenth rib.
**true r's,** costae verae.
**vertebral r's,** costae fluitantes.
**vertebrocostal r's,** the upper three false ribs of either side, articulating with the vertebrae and connected by cartilage to the costal cartilage of the ipsilateral seventh rib.
**vertebrosternal r's,** costae verae.
**Zahn's r's,** lines of Zahn.

**ri·ba·vi·rin** (ri″bə-vi′rin) [USP] [MeSH: Ribavirin]a synthetic nucleoside resembling guanosine; used as a broad-spectrum antiviral in the treatment of severe viral pneumonia caused by respiratory syncytial virus, particularly in high-risk infants with underlying conditions such as cardiopulmonary disease. Administered by aerosol.

**Rib·bert's theory** (rib′ərts) [Moritz Wilhelm Hugo *Ribbert,* German pathologist, 1855–1920] see under *theory.*

**rib·bon** (rib′ən) a band-like structure.
**r. of Reil,** the rostral part of the lemniscus medialis.
**synaptic r.,** 1. a dense lamella surrounded by a halo of synaptic vesicles, found at a right angle to the apex of the synaptic ridge in the outer plexiform layer of the retina. 2. a similar structure found in varying numbers in the cytoplasm of the hair cells of the ear.

**Ribes' ganglion** (rēbz) [François *Ribes,* French surgeon, 1765–1845] see under *ganglion.*

**ri·bi·tol** (ri′bĭ-tol) [MeSH: Ribitol] a sugar alcohol formed by reduction of the carbonyl group of ribose; it is a constituent of a class of teichoic acids.

**ri·bo·fla·vin** (ri′bo-fla″vin) [MeSH: Riboflavin] 1. vitamin $B_2$, a heat-stable, water-soluble flavin comprising a substituted isoalloxazine ring system linked to ribitol. It serves as a component of two coenzymes, FAD and FMN, of flavoproteins, which function as electron carriers in oxidation-reduction processes. It occurs in milk, organ meats, eggs, leafy green vegetables, whole grains and enriched cereals and breads, and various algae, and is an essential nutrient for man, the requirement being related to body size, metabolic rate, and growth rate. Deficiency of the vitamin is known as ariboflavinosis (q.v.). 2. [USP] a standardized preparation of riboflavin, used in the treatment and prophylaxis of riboflavin deficiency; administered orally and parenterally.
**r. 5′-phosphate,** flavin mononucleotide.
**r. 5′-phosphate sodium** [USP], a preparation of the sodium salt of riboflavin 5′-phosphate, administered orally or parenterally in the treatment of dietary riboflavin deficiency.

**ri·bo·fla·vin ki·nase** (ri″bo-fla′vin ki′nās) [EC 2.7.1.26] an enzyme of the transferase class that catalyzes the phosphorylation of riboflavin to form flavin mononucleotide (FMN), a cofactor for electron transfer reactions.

**ri·bo·nu·cle·ase** (ri″bo-noo′kle-ās) [EC 3.1] any nuclease specifically catalyzing the cleavage of phosphate ester linkages in ribonucleic acids; the ribonucleases are grouped as those cleaving internal bonds (endoribonucleases) and those cleaving at termini (exoribonucleases).
**r. I,** pancreatic r.
**pancreatic r.** [EC 3.1.27.5], an endoribonuclease isolated from the pancreas of ruminants and used extensively in studies of enzyme mechanics and in molecular biology research; it catalyzes cleavage specifically of terminal pyrimidine nucleoside 3′-phosphate residues. Called also *r. I, RNase, RNase I,* and *RNase A.*

**ri·bo·nu·cle·ic ac·id** (ri″bo-noo-kle′ik) RNA; the nucleic acid in which the sugar is ribose, constituting the genetic material in the RNA viruses and playing a role in the flow of genetic information. Ribosyl moieties are linked via phosphate groups attached to their 5′ and 3′ hydroxyl groups to form the backbone of a linear polymer, with purine and pyrimidine bases attached to the sugars as side chains. The characteristic bases adenine (A), uracil (U), cytosine (C), and guanine (G) are specified by the presence of thymine (T), A, G, and C, respectively, in the gene being transcribed. Many RNA molecules contain bases modified by posttranscriptional processing (methylation, deamination, isomerization), and some contain secondary structure such as base pairing between self-complementary sequences, which stabilizes specific conformations. For specific types of RNA, see under *RNA.*

**ri·bo·nu·cleo·pro·tein** (ri″bo-noo″kle-o-pro′tēn) a substance composed of both protein and ribonucleic acid. Abbreviated RNP.
**small nuclear r. (snRNP),** a ribonucleoprotein in which the RNA component is a small nuclear RNA; several snRNPs, designated U1 through U10 for their high uracil content, have been identified and at least some play key roles in RNA splicing.

**ri·bo·nu·cleo·side** (ri″bo-noo′kle-o-sīd) a nucleoside in which the purine or pyrimidine base is combined with ribose.

**ri·bo·nu·cleo·side di·phos·phate re·duc·tase** (ri″bo-noo′kle-o-sīd″ di-fos′fāt re-duk′tās) [EC 1.17.4.1] [MeSH: Ribonucleoside Diphosphate Reductase] an enzyme of the oxidoreductase class that catalyzes the formation of 2′-deoxyribonucleotides from the corresponding ribonucleoside diphosphates using NADPH as the ultimate electron donor. The deoxyribonucleoside diphosphates are used in DNA synthesis. Called also *ribonucleotide reductase.*

**ri·bo·nu·cleo·tide** (ri″bo-noo′kle-o-tīd) a nucleotide in which the purine or pyrimidine base is combined with ribose.

**ri·bo·nu·cleo·tide re·duc·tase** (ri″bo-noo′kle-o-tīd″ re-duk′tās) ribonucleoside diphosphate reductase.

**ri·bo·py·ra·nose** (ri″bo-pir′ə-nōs) ribose occurring in the cyclic pyranose configuration; it is the usual form in solution although not in ribonucleic acids.

**ri·bose** (ri′bōs) [MeSH: Ribose] an aldopentose found in riboflavin and ribonucleic acid (RNA) as well as in free ribonucleosides and ribonucleotides.
**r. 5-phosphate,** a phosphorylated form of ribose occurring as an intermediate in the pentose phosphate pathway and in the synthesis of nucleotides.

**ri·bose-5-phos·phate isom·er·ase** (ri′bōs fos′fāt i-som′ər-ās) [EC 5.3.1.6] an enzyme of the isomerase class that catalyzes the interconversion of ribulose 5-phosphate and ribose 5-phosphate. The reaction is part of the pentose phosphate pathway and is important in ribose metabolism.

**ri·bose-phos·phate py·ro·phos·pho·ki·nase** (ri′bōs fos′fāt pi″ro-fos″fo-ki′nās) [EC 2.7.6.1] [MeSH: Ribose-Phosphate Pyrophosphokinase] an enzyme of the transferase class that catalyzes the phosphorylation of ribose 5-phosphate to form phosphoribosylpyrophosphate, the initial reactant in purine and pyrimidine nucleotide biosynthesis. Enhanced enzyme activity, an X-linked recessive trait, leads to increased purine synthesis and causes primary gout. Called also *phosphoribosylpyrophosphate synthetase.*

**ri·bo·some** (ri′bo-sōm) [MeSH: Ribosomes] a large molecular structure having two dissociable subunits that is the site of protein synthesis (see *translation*). The two subunits together contain 4 different ribosomal RNA (rRNA) chains and about 70 different proteins. Ribosomes found in the cytosol of eukaryotes have a molecular weight of 4.5 million and a sedimentation coefficient of 80S; the subunits have coefficients of 60S and 40S. Ribosomes found in prokaryotes and mitochondria are smaller (70S) and also differ from eukaryotic ribosomes in their sensitivity to certain antibiotics.

**ri·bo·syl** (ri′bo-səl) a glycosyl radical formed from ribose by removal of the anomeric hydroxyl group.

**5-ri·bo·syl·ura·cil** (ri″bo-səl-ūr′ĭ-sil) pseudouridine.

**Ri·bot's law** (re-bōz′) [T. *Ribot,* French neurologist, 19th century] see under *law.*

**ri·bo·thy·mi·dine** (ri″bo-thi′mĭ-dēn) the ribosyl analogue of thymidine, a rare base found in small amounts in transfer RNA.

**ri·bo·vi·rus** (ri′bo-vi″rəs) RNA virus.

**ri·bu·lose** (ri′bu-lōs) a ketopentose isomeric with ribose and occurring in phosphorylated form *(ribose 5-phosphate)* as an intermediate in the pentose phosphate pathway.

**ri·bu·lose-phos·phate 3-epim·er·ase** (ri′bu-lōs fos′fāt ə-pim′ər-ās) [EC 5.1.3.1] an enzyme of the isomerase class that catalyzes the interconversion of ribulose 5-phosphate and xylulose 5-phosphate. The reaction is a part of the pentose phosphate pathway.

**RIC** Royal Institute of Chemistry.

**rice** (rīs) [MeSH: Rice] 1. *Oryza sativa.* 2. the seed or grain of *O. sativa,* which consists mainly of starch and is used as a food and a dusting powder.
**r. polishings,** the pericarp and germ layers of rice; they are a rich source of thiamine but are removed in the production of white rice.

**Rich·ards** (rich'ərdz) Dickinson Woodruff, Jr. American physician, 1895–1973; co-winner, with Werner Theodor Otto Forssmann and André Frédéric Cournand, of the Nobel prize for medicine or physiology in 1956 for research on pathologic changes in the circulatory system and for developing cardiac catheterization.

**Ri·chards-Run·dle syndrome** (rich'ərdz-run'dəl) [B.W. *Richards,* British physician, 20th century; A.T. *Rundle,* British physician, 20th century] see under *syndrome.*

**Ri·chet** (re-sha') Charles Robert. French physiologist, 1850–1935; winner of the Nobel prize for medicine or physiology in 1913 for his research on anaphylaxis.

**Ri·chet's aneurysm** (re-shāz') [Didier Dominique Alfred *Richet,* French surgeon, 1816–1891] a fusiform aneurysm.

**Rich·ner-Han·hart syndrome** (rik'nər-hahn'hahrt) [Hermann *Richner,* Swiss physician, born 1908; Ernst *Hanhart,* Swiss physician, 1891–1973] tyrosinemia, type II.

**Rich·ter's hernia** (rik'tərz) [August Gottlieb *Richter,* German surgeon, 1742–1812] see under *hernia.*

**Rich·ter's syndrome** (rik'tərz) [Maurice Nathaniel *Richter,* American pathologist, 20th century] see under *syndrome.*

**Rich·ter-Mon·ro line** (rik'tər-mon-ro') [A.G. *Richter;* Alexander *Monro* (Secundus), Scottish anatomist and surgeon, 1733–1817] Monro-Richter line.

**ri·cin** (ri'sin) [MeSH: Ricin] a phytotoxin found in the seeds of the castor oil plant *(Ricinus communis)* and used in the synthesis of immunotoxins; ingestion causes ricinism.

**ri·cin·ism** (ri'sĭ-niz-əm) poisoning of humans or animals by inhalation or ingestion of ricin; characterized by superficial inflammation of the respiratory mucosa with hemorrhages into the lungs, or edema and hemorrhage of the gastrointestinal tract.

**ri·cin·ole·ic ac·id** (ri"sin-o-le'ik) 1. an unsaturated 18-carbon fatty acid constituting 80 per cent of the fatty acid content of castor oil. 2. a mixture of fatty acids obtained by hydrolysis of castor oil and used as a spermicide in some contraceptive creams and jellies.

**Ric·i·nus** (ris'ĭ-nəs) [L.] [MeSH: Ricinus] a genus of plants of the family Euphorbiaceae. *R. commu'nis* is the castor bean or castor oil plant, which yields castor oil but whose seed (the castor bean) contains the phytotoxin ricin and causes ricinism in humans and other animals.

**rick·ets** (rik'əts) [thought to be a corruption of Gr. *rhachitis* a spinal complaint] [MeSH: Rickets] an interruption in the development and mineralization of the growth plate of bone, with radiographic abnormalities, osteomalacia, bone pain, fatigability, growth retardation, and often hypotonia, convulsions, and tetany. Biochemical abnormalities include hypocalcemia, elevated serum alkaline phosphatase, hypophosphatemia, and decreased intestinal absorption of calcium and phosphorus. It is caused by a variety of defects in vitamin D, calcium, and phosphorus homeostasis, including dietary deficiencies or malabsorption, primary disorders of bone matrix, and acquired or inherited metabolic and hormonal abnormalities. See also *osteomalacia.*

**adult r.,** osteomalacia.

**anticonvulsant r.,** rickets occurring in children receiving long-term anticonvulsant therapy; the drugs induce vitamin D deficiency (frequently compounded by dietary insufficiency of the vitamin) and hypocalcemia, hypophosphatemia, and secondary hyperparathyroidism by increasing the rate of conversion of the vitamin to inactive metabolites.

**autosomal dominant vitamin D–resistant r.,** a form of familial hypophosphatemic rickets clinically similar to X-linked hypophosphatemia, but showing autosomal dominant inheritance.

**familial hypophosphatemic r.,** any of several inherited disorders of proximal renal tubular function causing phosphate loss, hypophosphatemia, and skeletal deformities, including rickets and osteomalacia. See *X-linked hypophosphatemia, hypophosphatemic bone disease,* and *hereditary hypophosphatemic r. with hypercalciuria.*

**fetal r.,** achondroplasia.

**hepatic r.,** rickets associated with hepatic disease, believed to result from inadequate absorption of vitamin D.

**hereditary hypophosphatemic r. with hypercalciuria,** a form of familial hypophosphatemic rickets inherited as an autosomal trait; hypophosphatemia is accompanied by elevated levels of serum 1,25-dihydroxyvitamin D, increased intestinal absorption of calcium and phosphate, and hypercalciuria, indicating a defect in renal tubular function distinct from that of X-linked hypophosphatemia.

**hypophosphatemic r.,** any of a group of disorders characterized by rickets associated with hypophosphatemia, resulting from dietary phosphorus deficiency *(antacid-induced osteomalacia)* or due to defects in renal tubular function, either hereditary *(familial hypophosphatemic rickets)* or acquired. While skeletal deformities (e.g., bowed legs, short stature) are present, neither hypocalcemia, myopathy, nor tetany occur, and serum parathyroid hormone is normal.

**oncogenous r.,** oncogenous osteomalacia occurring in children.

**pseudodeficiency r.,** vitamin D–dependent r. type I and type II.

**pseudovitamin D–deficiency r.,** vitamin D–dependent r., type I; the term is sometimes used to denote types I and II collectively.

**refractory r.,** vitamin D–resistant r.

**renal r.,** older name for *renal osteodystrophy.*

**scurvy r.,** rachitic changes in the skeleton associated with infantile scurvy.

**vitamin D–dependent r., type I,** an autosomal recessive disorder of rickets with myopathy, hypocalcemia, moderate hypophosphatemia, secondary hyperparathyroidism, and subnormal serum concentrations of 1,25-dihydroxyvitamin D. The disorder can be overcome by high doses of vitamin D or physiologic doses of calcitriol; the defect is reduced or absent calcidiol 1-monooxygenase activity.

**vitamin D–dependent r., type II,** an autosomal recessive disorder similar to type I but with elevated serum concentrations of 1,25-dihydroxyvitamin D. The disorder cannot be overcome by high levels of vitamin D or its metabolites and is believed to be due to end organ refractoriness to the active metabolite, owing to defective receptor binding, absence of the receptors, or post-receptor defects. Multiple variants exist, subdivided as those with or without alopecia.

**vitamin D–refractory r.,** vitamin D–resistant r.

**vitamin D–resistant r.,** 1. X-linked hypophosphatemia. 2. any of a group of disorders characterized by rickets but not responding to high doses of vitamin D; most are forms of familial hypophosphatemic rickets.

**rick·ett·se·mia** (rik"ət-se'me-ə) the presence of rickettsiae in the blood.

**Rick·ett·sia** (rĭ-ket'se-ə) [Howard Taylor *Ricketts,* American pathologist, 1871–1910] [MeSH: Rickettsia] a genus of bacteria of the tribe Rickettsieae, family Rickettsiaceae, order Rickettsiales, made up of small rod-shaped to coccoid, often pleomorphic microorganisms. The cells have typical cell walls, possess no flagella, are gram-negative, and multiply only inside host cells. They occur intracytoplasmically or free in the lumen of the gut in lice, fleas, ticks, and mites, by which they are transmitted to man and other animals. The various species contain the organisms causing typhus fevers, spotted fevers and scrub typhus (tsutsugamushi disease).

**R. akamu'shi,** *R. tsutsugamushi.*

**R. a'kari,** the etiologic agent of rickettsialpox, transmitted by the mite *Allodermanyssus sanguineus* from the reservoir of infection in house mice.

**R. austra'lis,** the etiologic agent of North Queensland tick typhus, transmitted from infected marsupials by Ixodes ticks.

**R. burne'tii,** *Coxiella burnetii.*

**R. ca'nis,** *Ehrlichia canis.*

**R. cono'rii,** the etiologic agent of boutonneuse fever, transmitted by the bites of various species of ixodid ticks, including those of the genera *Rhipicephalus, Amblyomma, Haemaphysalis,* and *Hyalomma.* The principal animal reservoirs are dogs and rodents.

**R. diapo'rica,** *Coxiella burnetii.*

**R. moo'seri,** *R. typhi.*

**R. murico'la,** *R. typhi.*

**R. nippo'nica, R. orienta'lis,** *R. tsutsugamushi.*

**R. pedi'culi,** *Bartonella quintana.*

**R. prowaze'kii,** the etiologic agent of epidemic typhus and the recrudescent infection Brill-Zinsser disease. The organisms are transmitted from man to man via the louse *Pediculus humanus* var. *corporis* and from flying squirrels to man by fleas and lice.

**R. quinta'na,** *Bartonella quintana.*

**R. rickett'sii,** the etiologic agent of Rocky Mountain spotted fever, transmitted by *Dermacentor, Rhipicephalus, Haemaphysalis, Amblyomma* and *Ixodes* ticks from a natural reservoir in rodents, dogs, and foxes. Called also *Dermacentroxenus rickettsii.*

**R. sennet'su,** *Ehrlichia sennetsu.*

**R. sibi'rica,** the etiologic agent of Siberian tick typhus, which is transmitted from infected rodents by *Ixodes* ticks.

**R. tsutsugamu'shi,** the etiologic agent of scrub typhus, transmitted by larval mites of the genus *Trombicula,* including *T. akamushi* and *T. deliensis,* from rodent reservoirs of infection. Called also *R. akamushi, R. nipponica,* and *R. orientalis.*

**R. ty'phi,** the etiologic agent of murine typhus, transmitted from infected rats to humans chiefly by rat fleas. Called also *Dermacentroxenus typhi, R. mooseri, R. muricola,* and *R. typhi (mooseri).*

**R. ty'phi (moo'seri),** *R. typhi.*

**R. wolhy'nica,** *Bartonella quintana.*

**rick·ett·sia** (rĭ-ket'se-ə) pl. *rickett'siae* [MeSH: Rickettsia] any scotobacterium of the order Rickettsiales.

**Rick·ett·si·a·ceae** (rĭ-ket"se-a'se-e) [MeSH: Rickettsiaceae] a family of bacteria of the order Rickettsiales, made up of small rod-shaped, ellipsoidal, coccoid, or diplococcus-shaped, often pleomorphic microorganisms often occurring intracellularly in arthropods, by which they are transmitted to man and other animals, causing disease. It includes three tribes, Ehrlichieae, Rickettsieae, and Wolbachieae.

**Rick·ett·siae** (rĭ-ket′se-e) Rickettsieae.

**rick·ett·siae** (rĭ-ket′se-e) plural of *rickettsia*.

**rick·ett·si·al** (rĭ-ket′se-əl) caused by rickettsiae.

**Rick·ett·si·a·les** (rĭ-ket″se-a′lēz) [MeSH: Rickettsiales] an order of bacteria, class Scotobacteria, division Gracilicutes, kingdom Procaryotae, comprising small, gram-negative, rod-shaped or coccoid, often pleomorphic microorganisms occurring as elementary bodies that typically multiply only inside the cells of the host. Found as parasites in both vertebrates and invertebrates, which may serve as vectors, they may be pathogenic for both man and other animals. The order includes the families Anaplasmataceae, Bartonellaceae, and Rickettsiaceae.

**rick·ett·si·al·pox** (rĭ-ket′se-əl-poks″) a mild self-limited febrile disease caused by *Rickettsia akari,* transmitted to humans by the mite *Allodermanyssus sanguineus,* an ectoparasite of the house mouse, and characterized principally by the presence of an escharlike primary cutaneous lesion, generalized papulovesicular rash, headache, and backache. Called also *Kew Gardens fever.*

**rick·ett·si·ci·dal** (rĭ-ket″sĭ-si′dəl) destructive to rickettsiae.

**Rick·ett·si·eae** (rik″et-si′e-e) [MeSH: Rickettsieae] a tribe of bacteria of the family Rickettsiaceae, order Rickettsiales, made up of small pleomorphic, most intracellular organisms, which are classified in three genera, *Coxiella, Rickettsia,* and *Bartonella.* They occur as parasites in arthropods and cause disease in vertebrate hosts. Pathogenic species fall generally into four groups, based upon immunologic characterization (Weil-Felix reaction): I, classic typhus (epidemic typhus, Brill-Zinsser disease, murine typhus); II, spotted fever (Rocky Mountain spotted fever, oriental spotted fever, Flinders island spotted fever, boutonneuse fever, rickettsialpox, Siberian tick typhus, Queensland tick typhus); III, scrub typhus (tsutsugamushi disease); and IV, miscellaneous organisms (Q fever and trench fever). Called also *Rickettsiae.* See also *typhus.*

**rick·ett·si·o·sis** (rĭ-ket″se-o′sis) infection with rickettsiae.
**canine r.,** see under *ehrlichiosis.*

**rick·ett·sio·stat·ic** (rĭ-ket″se-o-stat′ik) inhibiting the growth and activity of rickettsiae.

**Ri·co·le·sia** (ri″ko-le′zhə) [*R*ickettsia + J. D. W. A. *Coles*] a genus of bacteria of uncertain status of the order Chlamydiales, reported to be the cause of keratoconjunctivitis in cattle, goats, fowl, and swine.

**ric·tal** (rik′təl) pertaining to a fissure.

**ric·tus** (rik′təs) [L.] 1. a fissure or cleft. 2. a gaping, as of the mouth.

**RID** radial immunodiffusion; see *single radial diffusion,* under *diffusion.*

**Rid·au·ra** (rid-aw′rə) trademark for a preparation of auranofin.

**Rid·doch's mass reflex** (rid′oks) [George *Riddoch,* British neurologist, 1888–1947] see under *reflex.*

**Rid·e·al-Walk·er coefficient, method (test)** (rid′e-əl-wah′kər) [Samuel *Rideal,* English chemist, 1863–1929; J.T. Ainslie *Walker,* English chemist, 1868–1930] see *phenol coefficient,* under *coefficient,* and see under *method.*

**ridge** (rij) a projection or projecting structure; see also *carina, crest* and *crista.*
**alveolar r.,** the bony ridge of the maxilla or mandible which contains the alveoli.
**alveolar r., residual,** the bony ridge remaining after disappearance of the alveoli from the alveolar process following removal or loss of the teeth. Called also *edentulous r.* and *residual r.*
**basal r.,** cingulum (def. 3).
**bicipital r., anterior,** crista tuberculi minoris.
**bicipital r., external,** crista tuberculi majoris.
**bicipital r., internal,** crista tuberculi minoris.
**bicipital r., outer, bicipital r., posterior,** crista tuberculi majoris.
**buccocervical r., buccogingival r.,** a ridge or prominence on the buccal surface above the cementoenamel junction of posterior teeth.
**bulbar r's,** spiral endocardial thickenings in the bulbus cordis that fuse to form the bulbar septum, separating the bulbus cordis into aortic and pulmonary trunks.
**cerebral r's of cranial bones,** variable ridges on the inner surface of the cranium, corresponding to the sulci of the brain.
**deltoid r.,** tuberositas deltoidea humeri.
**dental r.,** any linear elevation on the crown of a tooth named according to the surface on which it is located, such as buccal or lingual, or in recognition of some other characteristic.
**dermal r's,** cristae cutis.

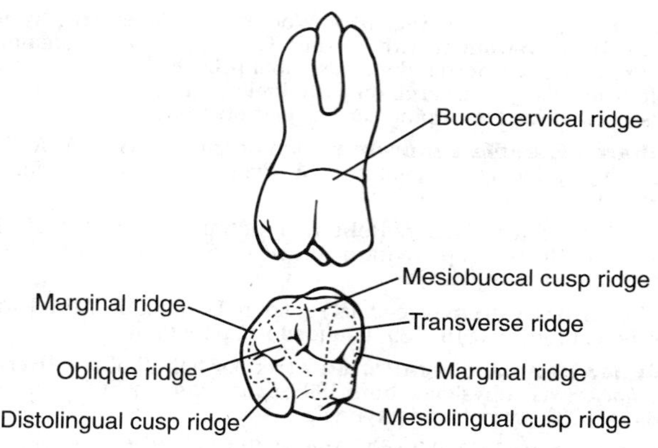


Dental ridges in a maxillary molar.

**edentulous r.,** alveolar r., residual.
**epicondylic r., lateral,** crista supraepicondylaris lateralis humeri.
**epicondylic r., medial,** crista supraepicondylaris medialis humeri.
**epipericardial r.,** a ventral ridge separating the ventral ends of the pharyngeal (branchial) arches in the embryo from the pericardial swelling.
**gastrocnemial r.,** a ridge on the posterior surface of the femur, giving attachment to the gastrocnemius muscle.
**genital r., germ r.,** the more medial portion of the urogenital ridge, which gives rise to the ovary or testis. Called also *genital fold.*
**gluteal r. of femur,** tuberositas glutea femoris.
**healing r.,** an indurated ridge that normally forms deep to the skin along the length of a healing wound and extends about 1 cm. on each side of the wound.
**r. of humerus,** tuberositas deltoidea humeri.
**incisal r.,** that portion of the crown of an anterior tooth that makes up the actual incisal portion.
**interarticular r. of head of rib,** crista capitis costae.
**interosseous r. of fibula,** margo interosseus fibulae.
**interosseous r. of radius,** margo interosseus radii.
**interosseous r. of tibia,** margo interosseus tibiae.
**interosseous r. of ulna,** margo interosseus ulnae.
**intertrochanteric r.,** crista intertrochanterica.
**interureteric r.,** plica interureterica.
**linguocervical r., linguogingival r.,** cingulum (def. 3).
**longitudinal r. of hard palate,** the part of the palatine raphe that is on the hard palate.
**Mall's r.,** pulmonary r.
**mammary r.,** milk line.
**r. of mandibular neck,** a blunt, smooth ridge passing obliquely downward and forward from the mandibular condyle on the medial surface of the mandibular neck and ramus, serving as their buttress.
**marginal r.,** crista marginalis.
**mesonephric r.,** the more lateral portion of the urogenital ridge, which gives rise to the mesonephros.
**middle r. of femur,** linea pectinea.
**milk r.,** see under *line.*
**mylohyoid r.,** linea mylohyoidea mandibulae.
**r. of neck of rib,** crista colli costae.
**r. of nose,** agger nasi.
**oblique r.,** 1. an elevated crest of variable prominence, comprised jointly of the triangular ridge of the distobuccal cusp and the distal ridge of the mesiolingual cusp, coursing obliquely across the occlusal surface of the maxillary molars to link the apices of the distobuccal and the mesiolingual cusps. 2. tuberositas masseterica.
**oblique r's of scapula,** lineae musculares scapulae.
**palatine r's, transverse,** plicae palatinae transversae.
**Passavant's r.,** see under *bar.*
**pectoral r.,** crista tuberculi majoris.
**pharyngeal r.,** Passavant's bar.
**pterygoid r.,** crista infratemporalis.
**pulmonary r.,** a ridge along the common cardinal vein in the embryo, which develops into the pleuropericardial membrane.
**radial r. of wrist,** eminentia carpi radialis.
**residual r.,** alveolar r., residual.
**rete r's,** the inward projections of the epidermis into the dermis at the dermoepidermal junction, as seen histologically in vertical sections. Called also *rete pegs.*
**rough r. of femur,** linea aspera.
**semicircular r. of parietal bone, inferior,** linea temporalis inferior ossis parietalis.
**semicircular r. of parietal bone, superior,** linea temporalis superior ossis parietalis.
**skin r's,** cristae cutis.

**sphenoid r.**, crista sphenoidalis.
**sublingual r.**, frenulum linguae.
**superciliary r.**, arcus superciliaris.
**supinator r.**, crista musculi supinatoris.
**supplemental r.**, an abnormal ridge on the surface of a tooth.
**supracondylar r. of humerus, lateral,** crista supraepicondylaris lateralis humeri.
**supracondylar r. of humerus, medial,** crista supraepicondylaris medialis humeri.
**supraepicondylar r. of humerus, lateral,** crista supraepicondylaris lateralis humeri.
**supraepicondylar r. of humerus, medial,** crista supraepicondylaris medialis humeri.
**supraorbital r.**, arcus superciliaris.
**suprarenal r.**, a caudal projection of the dorsal portion of the pleuroperitoneal membrane of the embryo, in which the adrenal cortex develops.
**synaptic r.**, a wedge-shaped projection in the retina of a cone pedicle or of a rod spherule, on either side of which lie the horizontal cells whose dendrites are inserted into the ridge.
**taste r's,** papillae foliatae.
**tentorial r.**, a ridge on the inner surface of the cranium just superior to the groove for the transverse sinus, to which the tentorium is attached.
**transverse r.**, crista transversalis.
**transverse r's of sacrum,** lineae transversae ossis sacri.
**transverse r's of vaginal wall,** rugae vaginales.
**trapezoid r.**, linea trapezoidea.
**triangular r.**, crista triangularis.
**tubercular r. of sacrum,** crista sacralis mediana.
**ulnar r. of wrist,** eminentia carpi ulnaris.
**urethral r.**, carina urethralis vaginae.
**urogenital r.**, a longitudinal ridge or fold in the embryo, lateral to the root of the dorsal mesentery, which later subdivides longitudinally into the mesonephric and genital ridges.
**wolffian r.**, mesonephric r.

**rid·gel** (rid'jəl) ridgling.

**ridg·ing** (rij'ing) in plastic surgery, a visible line or ridge at the margin of an area that has been surgically planed; occasionally encountered when beveling at the junction of treated and untreated areas has not been performed.

**ridg·ling** (rij'ling) an animal, especially a horse, with one or both testes undescended.

**Rid·ley's sinus** (rid'lēz) [Humphrey *Ridley,* English anatomist, 1653–1708] sinus circularis.

**Rie·chert-Mun·din·ger apparatus, technique** (re'kərt-moon'ding-ər) [T. *Riechert,* German neurosurgeon, 20th century; F. *Mundinger,* German neurosurgeon, born 1924] see under *apparatus* and *technique.*

**Rie·del's lobe, thyroiditis (disease, struma)** (re'delz) [Bernhard Moritz Carl Ludwig *Riedel,* German surgeon, 1846–1916] see under *lobe* and *thyroiditis.*

**Rie·der's cell leukemia, lymphocyte (cell)** (re'dərz) [Hermann *Rieder,* German roentgenologist, 1858–1932] see under *leukemia* and *lymphocyte.*

**Rie·gel's pulse** (re'gəlz) [Franz *Riegel,* German physician, 1843–1904] see under *pulse.*

**Rie·ger's anomaly, syndrome** (re'gərz) [Herwigh *Rieger,* German ophthalmologist, 1898–1986] see under *anomaly* and *syndrome.*

**Riehl's melanosis** (rēlz) [Gustav *Riehl,* Austrian dermatologist, 1855–1943] see under *melanosis.*

**Ries·man's sign** (rēs'mənz) [David *Riesman,* American physician, 1867–1940] see under *sign.*

**Rieux's hernia** (re-yooz') [Léon *Rieux,* French surgeon, 19th century] retrocecal hernia.

**RIF** right iliac fossa.

**rif·a·bu·tin** (rif″ə-bu'tin) [USP] [MeSH: Rifabutin] an antibacterial derived from rifamycin S, used for the prevention of disseminated *Mycobacterium avium* complex (MAC) disease in patients with advanced human immunodeficiency virus infection; administered orally.

**Rif·a·din** (rif'ə-din) trademark for a preparation of rifampin.

**Rif·a·mate** (rif'ə-māt) trademark for a preparation of rifampin and isoniazid.

**rif·a·mide** (rif'ə-mīd) a semisynthetic antibacterial antibiotic derived from rifamycin B, having the actions of the other rifamycins; it has been used in the treatment of respiratory infections due to gram-positive cocci and in biliary tract infections due to gram-negative and gram-positive organisms. See also *rifamycin.*

**rif·am·pi·cin** (rif'am-pĭ-sin) the international nonproprietary name for rifampin.

**rif·am·pin** (rif'am-pin) [USP] [MeSH: Rifampin] a semisynthetic derivative of rifamycin SV, having the antibacterial actions of the rifamycin (q.v.) group of antibiotics; administered orally. Called also *rifampicin.*

**rif·a·my·cin** (rif″ə-mi'sin) any of a family of antibiotics biosynthesized by a strain of *Streptomyces mediterranei,* effective against a broad spectrum of bacteria, including gram-positive cocci, some gram-negative bacilli, and *Mycobacterium tuberculosis* and certain other mycobacteria. The five components are designated A, B, C, D, and E; rifamycins O, S, and SV are derivatives of the B component, and AG and X are derivatives of the O component. In the United States the rifamycins are used only for the initial treatment and retreatment of pulmonary tuberculosis and for treatment of asymptomatic nasopharyngeal carriers of *Neisseria meningitidis;* they have been used in other countries to treat various infectious diseases due to susceptible organisms, such as leprosy, gonorrhea, and biliary tract and respiratory infections.

**Rift Val·ley fever** (rift-val'e) [*Rift Valley,* Kenya, where it was first described in 1931] [MeSH: Rift Valley Fever] see under *fever.*

**Riga-Fede disease** (re'gah-fa'da) [Antonio *Riga,* Italian physician, 1832–1919; Francesco *Fede,* Italian pediatrician, 1832–1913] see under *disease.*

**Riggs' disease** (rigz) [John Mankey *Riggs,* American dentist, 1810–1885] marginal periodontitis.

**right-hand·ed** (rīt han'dəd) using the right hand preferentially, or more skillfully than the left, in voluntary motor acts. See also *handedness* and *laterality.*

**ri·gid·i·ty** (rĭ-jid'ĭ-te) [L. *rigiditas; rigidus* stiff] stiffness or inflexibility, chiefly that which is abnormal or morbid; rigor.
**cadaveric r.**, rigor mortis.
**catatonic r.**, maintenance of a rigid posture in spite of attempts to be moved, characteristic of catatonic schizophrenia.
**clasp-knife r.**, an exaggerated stretch reflex of skeletal muscles seen in spasticity and decerebrate rigidity, resembling the opening of a penknife or clasp knife; there is increased resistance to the extensors (induced by passive flexion of a joint), which suddenly gives way on exertion of further pressure. Called also *clasp-knife effect, phenomenon, reflex,* or *spasticity.*
**cogwheel r.**, rigidity of a muscle that gives way in a series of little jerks upon being passively stretched, analogous to the ratcheting movement when a spring-loaded rod drops into the successive notches of a cog. Called also *cogwheel phenomenon* or *sign* and *Negro's phenomenon* or *sign.*
**congenital articular r.**, rigid or deformed joints in newborn calves or lambs; a hereditary variety is seen among Charolais cattle, and a type acquired in utero is part of the Akabane virus disease. Called also *congenital arthrogryposis.*
**decerebrate r.**, the posture produced in an experimental animal by decerebration (q.v.), marked by rigid extension of the legs. In humans it occurs as a result of lesions of the upper part of the brain stem or of severe bilateral lesions of the cerebrum and is manifested as a posture of lying in rigid extension with arms internally rotated at the shoulders and pronated; elbows, knees, and hips rigidly extended; and fingers, ankles, and toes flexed. Cf. *antigravity reflex.*
**hemiplegic r.**, rigidity of the paralyzed limbs in hemiplegia.
**lead-pipe r.**, diffuse muscular rigidity resembling the resistance to bending of a thin-walled metal pipe; seen in parkinsonism.
**mydriatic r.**, orbicularis pupillary reflex.
**paratonic r.**, an intermittent abnormal increase in resistance to passive movement in a comatose patient.
**postmortem r.**, rigor mortis.

**rig·or** (rig'or,ri'gor) [L.] 1. a chill. 2. rigidity.
**acid r.**, coagulation of the protein of muscle produced by acids.
**calcium r.**, arrest of cardiac muscle in full contraction, caused by an excess of calcium.
**heat r.**, rigidity of muscles induced by heat.
**r. mor'tis,** the stiffening of a dead body, accompanying the depletion of adenosine triphosphate in the muscle fibers.
**water r.**, a condition of rigor in a muscle caused by immersing it in water.

**Ri·ley-Day syndrome** (ri'le-da) [Conrad Milton *Riley,* American pediatrician, born 1913; Richard Lawrence *Day,* American pediatrician, born 1905] dysautonomia.

**Ri·ley-Smith syndrome** (ri'le-smith) [Harris Dewitt *Riley,* Jr., American pediatrician, born 1925; William Robert *Smith,* American physician, born 1931] see under *syndrome.*

**ril·u·zole** (ril'u-zōl) a compound used in the treatment of amyotrophic lateral sclerosis; it prolongs survival time but does not improve muscular strength or neurologic function.

**rim** (rim) a border, or edge.

**bite r.,** occlusion r.
**occlusion r., record r.,** a border constructed on temporary or permanent denture bases for the purpose of recording the maxillomandibular relation and for positioning the teeth. Called also *bite-block, bitelock,* and *bite r.*

**ri·ma** (ri'mə) gen. and pl. *ri'mae* [L.] [TA] anatomical nomenclature for a cleft, crack, or similar opening.
**r. a'ni, r. clu'nium,** crena analis.
**r. glot'tidis** [TA], fissure of glottis: the elongated opening between the true vocal cords and between the arytenoid cartilages. It consists of an intercartilaginous part and an intermembranous part; see *pars intercartilaginea rimae glottidis* and *pars intermembranacea rimae glottidis.*
**intercartilaginous r.,** pars intercartilaginea rimae glottidis.
**intermembranous r.,** pars intermembranacea rimae glottidis.
**r. o'ris** [TA], oral fissure: the longitudinal opening of the mouth, between the lips.
**r. palpebra'rum** [TA], palpebral fissure: the longitudinal opening between the eyelids.
**r. puden'di** [TA], pudendal fissure: the cleft between the labia majora in which the urethra and vagina open.
**r. vesti'buli** [TA], fissure of vestibule: the space between the right and left vestibular folds of the larynx.
**r. vul'vae,** r. pudendi.

**Rim·ac·tane** (rim-ak'tān) trademark for a preparation of rifampin.

**ri·mae** (ri'me) [L.] genitive and plural of *rima.*

**ri·mal** (ri'məl) pertaining to a rima.

**ri·man·ta·dine hy·dro·chlo·ride** (ri-man'tə-dēn) an antiviral agent that has been used in the prophylaxis of influenza type A.

**ri·mex·o·lone** (rĭmek'səlōn") [USP] a corticosteroid used as a topical anti-inflammatory in the treatment of postoperative inflammation following eye surgery and in the treatment of anterior uveitis.

**Rim·i·fon** (rim'ĭ-fon) trademark for a preparation of isoniazid.

**rim·i·ter·ol hy·dro·bro·mide** (rim"ĭ-ter'ōl) an adrenergic used as a bronchodilator.

**rim·ose** (rim'ōs) [L. *rima* crack] marked by cracks and fissures.

**rim·u·la** (rim'u-lə) pl. *ri'mulae* [L.] a minute fissure, especially of the spinal cord or brain.

**RIND** reversible ischemic neurologic deficit.

**rin·der·pest** (rin'dər-pest) [Ger. *Rinder* cattle + *pest* plague] [MeSH: Rinderpest] a disease of cattle, which sometimes affects sheep and swine and is caused by a paramyxovirus; symptoms are fever and croupous, ulcerative diphtheritic lesions of the gastrointestinal tract. Called also *cattle plague.*

**Rind·fleisch's folds** (rint'flīsh-əz) [Georg Eduard *Rindfleisch,* German physician, 1836–1908] see under *fold.*

**ring** (ring) [from Old English *hring;*] 1. any annular or circular organ or area; for names of specific anatomical structures, see under *anulus.* See also *circle* and *circulus.* 2. in chemistry, a collection of atoms united in a continuous or closed chain.
**abdominal r., deep,** anulus inguinalis profundus.
**abdominal r., external,** anulus inguinalis superficialis.
**abdominal r., internal,** anulus inguinalis profundus.
**abdominal r., superficial,** anulus inguinalis superficialis.
**Albl's r.,** a ring-shaped shadow observed in a radiograph of the skull, caused by an aneurysm of a cerebral artery.
**amnion r.,** the attached margin of the amnion about the umbilicus of the fetus.
**annular r's,** round or oval opacities surrounding a translucent area in a radiograph of the lung, indicative of cavitation in pulmonary tuberculosis. Called also *pleural rings.*
**apical r.,** polar r.
**atrial r.,** the ring surrounding the opening between the atrium and ventricle of the primitive vertebrate heart; represented in the mammalian heart by the atrioventricular node.
**atrioventricular r's, atrioventricular valve r's,** see *anulus fibrosus dexter/sinister cordis.*
**Balbiani's r's,** a series of loops of the chromonemata of polytene chromosomes, similar in nature to chromosome puffs and in appearance to lampbrush chromosomes.
**Bandl's r.,** pathologic retraction r.; see *retraction r.*
**benzene r.,** the closed hexagon of carbon atoms in benzene ($C_6H_6$), from which the different benzene compounds are derived by replacement of the hydrogen atoms.

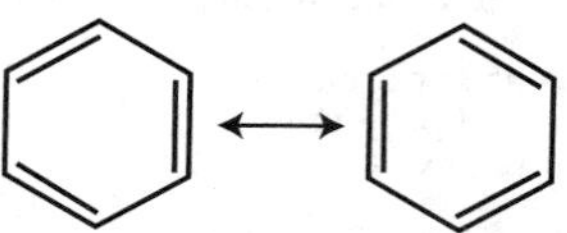

Benzene ring structure represented as a hybrid of two possible ring structures; sometimes called a resonance hybrid.

**Bickel's r.,** Waldeyer's tonsillar r.
**Cabot's r's,** Cabot's ring bodies; see under *body.*
**Cannon's r.,** in the radiograph after a barium meal, a narrow area or focal contraction at the mid-third of the transverse colon, representing the junction of the primitive midgut and hindgut and marking an area of overlap between the superior and inferior nerve plexuses.
**carbocyclic r.,** a chemical ring that includes only carbon atoms.
**cardiac lymphatic r.,** anulus lymphaticus cardiae.
**Carpentier r.,** a semi-rigid prosthetic ring used in annuloplasty to restore competence to a regurgitant cardiac valve.
**casting r.,** 1. a cylinder used as a container for the investment and mold during the process of casting. 2. refractory flask.
**ciliary r.,** orbiculus ciliaris.
**circumaortic venous r.,** see under *collar.*
**common tendinous r.,** anulus tendineus communis.
**conjunctival r.,** anulus conjunctivae.
**constriction r.,** a contracted area of the uterus, allegedly possible at any level, occurring where the resistance of the uterine contents is slight, as over a depression in the contour of the fetal body, or below the presenting part. Cf. *retraction r.*
**contact r.,** the wound inflicted at the site of entrance of a bullet on the surface of the body.
**contraction r.,** see *constriction r.* and *retraction r.*
**coronary r.,** see under *band.*
**crural r.,** anulus femoralis.
**Döllinger's tendinous r.,** thickening of Descemet's membrane, forming an elastic ring around the limbus.
**Duran r.,** a flexible prosthetic ring used in annuloplasty to restore competence to a regurgitant cardiac valve.
**esophageal r.,** an annular constriction of the lower esophagus, usually at the junction of the esophageal and gastric mucosa. Called also *Schatzki's r.*
**femoral r.,** anulus femoralis.
**fibrocartilaginous r. of tympanic membrane,** anulus fibrocartilagineus membranae tympani.
**fibrous r., interpubic,** discus interpubicus.
**fibrous r's of heart,** see anulus fibrosus dexter/sinister cordis.
**fibrous r. of intervertebral disk,** anulus fibrosus disci intervertebralis.
**Fleischer r.,** an incomplete annular pigmented line at the base of the cone in keratoconus.
**Fleischer-Strümpell r.,** Kayser-Fleischer r.
**germ r.,** the proliferating marginal zone of the early blastoderm that is about to become the lips of the blastopore.
**glaucomatous r.,** a light yellowish ring around the optic disk in glaucoma, indicating atrophy of the choroid.

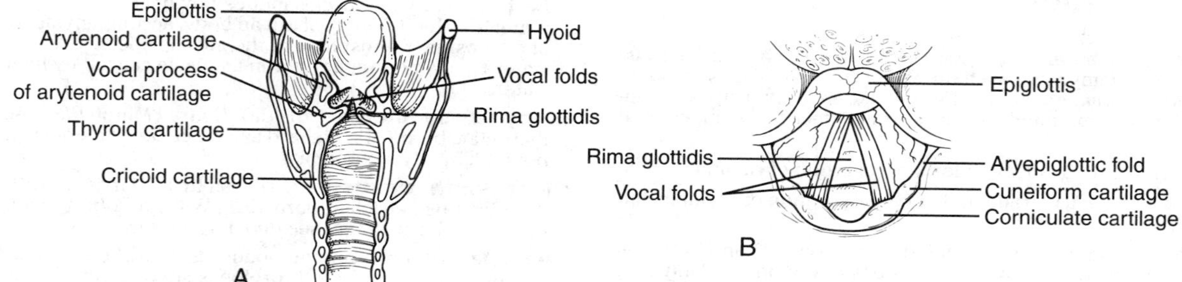


Rima glottidis in *(A)* coronal section showing posterior view of anterior wall of larynx; *(B)* laryngoscopic view.

**heterocyclic r.**, a chemical ring that includes atoms of different elements.
**homocyclic r.**, a chemical ring in which all the members are atoms of the same element.
**inguinal r., deep,** anulus inguinalis profundus.
**inguinal r., external,** anulus inguinalis superficialis.
**inguinal r., internal,** anulus inguinalis profundus.
**inguinal r., superficial,** anulus inguinalis superficialis.
**r. of iris, greater,** anulus iridis major.
**r. of iris, lesser,** anulus iridis minor.
**isocyclic r.**, homocyclic r.
**Kayser-Fleischer r.**, a golden brown or green discoloration at the level of Descemet's membrane in the limbic region of the cornea seen in Wilson's disease and other liver disorders.
**Landolt's r's,** broken rings used in testing of visual acuity, the width of the ring and the break in its continuity each being one-fifth of its overall diameter; the observer is to identify the orientation of the break, with the ability to identify a break subtending 1 minute of arc corresponding to 20/20 vision.
**Liesegang r's,** 1. see under *phenomenon.* 2. concentric laminations due to deposition of calcium, such as occur within some tumors or other lesions.
**Löwe's r.**, a ring in the visual field caused by the macula retinae.
**Lower's r's,** see anulus fibrosus dexter/sinister cordis.
**lymphoid r.**, Waldeyer's tonsillar r.
**Maxwell's r.**, a ring resembling Löwe's, but smaller and fainter.
**mitral r., mitral valve r.**, see *anulus fibrosus dexter/sinister cordis.*
**neonatal r.**, see *neonatal line,* under *line.*
**Ochsner's r.**, a circular mucosal thickening at the opening of the pancreatic duct into the common bile duct.
**periosteal bone r.**, see under *collar.*
**pleural r's,** annular r's.
**polar r.**, an electron-dense, annular, anterior thickening of the pellicle of apicocomplexan protozoa, occurring at some stage in the life cycle, and forming part of the apical complex. Called also *apical r.*
**retraction r.**, a ringlike thickening and indentation occurring in normal labor at the junction of the isthmus and corpus uteri, delineating the upper contracting portion and the lower dilating portion *(physiologic retraction r.),* or a persistent retraction ring in abnormal or prolonged labor that obstructs expulsion of the fetus *(pathologic retraction r.).* Cf. *constriction r.*
**right/left fibrous r. of heart,** see *anulus fibrosus dexter/sinister cordis.*
**pelvic r.**, pelvis ossea.
**Schatzki's r.**, esophageal r.
**Schwalbe's r., Schwalbe's anterior border r.**, a circular ridge composed of collagenous fibers surrounding the outer margin of Descemet's membrane (lamina limitans posterior corneae).
**scleral r.**, a white ring seen adjacent to the optic disk in ophthalmoscopy when the retinal pigment epithelium and choroid do not extend to the disk.
**sewing r.**, a cloth-covered ring surrounding an artificial cardiac valve and used for securing the valve in position.
**signet r.**, ring form.
**Soemmering's r.**, 1. a doughnut-shaped remnant of lens behind the pupil, occurring after cataract surgery or secondary to trauma as a result of contact between the anterior capsule and the posterior capsule, which traps varying amounts of lens substance peripherally; called also *Soemmering's ring cataract.* 2. a developmental cataract in which the primary lens cells fail to develop or are absorbed during intrauterine disease. Later developing subcapsular cells, having no fetal nucleus around which to grow, form doughnut-shaped ring cataracts.
**tracheal r's,** cartilagines tracheales.
**tricuspid r., tricuspid valve r.**, see *anulus fibrosus dexter/sinister cordis.*
**tympanic r.**, anulus tympanicus.
**umbilical r.**, anulus umbilicalis.
**vascular r.**, any of various developmental anomalies in which the aortic arches encircle the trachea and esophagus, sometimes compressing them.
**r. of Vieussens,** limbus fossae ovalis.
**Vossius' r.**, a ring of pigment on the lens caused by pressure of the pupillary margin against the lens following a contusion.
**Waldeyer's tonsillar r.**, the circular series of lymphoid tissue formed by the lingual, pharyngeal, and faucial tonsils. Called also *Bickel's r.* and *lymphoid r.*
**Zinn's r.**, anulus tendineus communis.

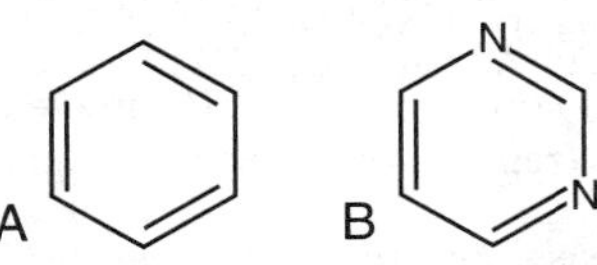


*(A),* Benzene, having a homocyclic ring structure; *(B),* pyrimidine, having a heterocyclic ring structure.

**ring-bone** (ring'bōn) exostosis involving the first or second phalanx of the horse, resulting in lameness if the articular surfaces are affected.
**low r.-b.**, buttress foot.

**Ring·er's injection, irrigation (mixture, solution)** (ring'ər z) [Sydney *Ringer,* English physiologist, 1835–1910] see under *injection* and *irrigation.*

**ring·womb** (ring'wōōm) failure of the cervix of a ewe to dilate during parturition, usually resulting in the death of the lamb in utero.

**ring·worm** (ring'wərm) popular name for tinea (in humans) or dermatophytosis (in other animals); so called because of the ring-shaped configuration of the lesions.
**r. of the beard,** tinea barbae.
**black-dot r.**, one of two common types of tinea capitis; this type is due usually to *Trichophyton tonsurans* but occasionally to *T. violaceum,* and is manifested as multiple areas of alopecia studded with black dots representing infected hairs broken off at or below the surface of the scalp. See also *gray-patch r.*
**r. of the body,** tinea corporis.
**r. of the face,** tinea faciale.
**r. of the foot,** tinea pedis.
**gray-patch r.**, one of two common types of tinea capitis; this type is usually caused by *Microsporum audouinii* but may sometimes be caused by *M. canis, M. ferugineum,* or *M. gypseum,* and is manifested by multiple gray scaly lesions, stubs of broken hairs, and minimal inflammatory response; it is benign and resolves spontaneously. See also *black-dot r.*
**r. of the groin,** tinea cruris.
**r. of the hand,** tinea manus.
**honeycomb r.**, favus.
**r. of the nails,** tinea unguium.
**Oriental r.**, tinea imbricata.
**r. of the scalp,** tinea capitis.
**Tokelau r.**, tinea imbricata.

**Rinne's test** (rin'əz) [Heinrich Adolf *Rinne,* German otologist, 1819–1868] see under *test.*

**Ri·o·lan's anastomosis, arch,** etc. (re″o-lahz′) [Jean *Riolan,* French physician and physiologist, 1580–1657] see under *anastomosis, arch, bone, muscle, nosegay,* and *ossicle.*

**Ri·o·pan** (ri'o-pan) trademark for preparations of magaldrate.

**RIPA** radioimmunoprecipitation assay.

**RIPHH** Royal Institute of Public Health and Hygiene.

**Ris·don approach** (riz'don) [E. Fulton *Risdon,* Canadian plastic surgeon, 1880–1968] see under *approach.*

**risk** (risk) [Fr. *risque,* from L. *resecare* to cut off] [MeSH: Risk] a danger or hazard, the probability of suffering harm or other unfavorable outcome.
**attributable r.**, the amount or proportion of incidence of disease or death (or risk of disease or death) in individuals exposed to a specific risk factor that can be attributed to exposure to that factor; the difference in the risk for unexposed versus exposed individuals. The term is sometimes incorrectly used to denote *population attributable r.*
**competing r.**, an event that removes a subject from being at risk for the outcome under study; e.g., death from automobile accident is a competing risk that removes a subject from the risk of heart disease.
**empiric r.**, the probability that a trait will occur or recur in a family, based solely on experience rather than on knowledge of the causative mechanism. See also *genetic r.*
**genetic r.**, the probability that a trait will occur or recur in a family, based on knowledge of its pattern of genetic transmission. See also *empiric r.*
**population attributable r.**, in a total population, the proportion of a disease incidence, or risk of the disease, that can be attributed to exposure to a specific risk factor; the difference between the risk in the total population and the risk in the unexposed group.
**relative r.**, for a disease, death, or other outcome, the ratio of the incidence rate among individuals with a given risk factor to the incidence rate among those without it.

**Ris·ley's prism** (riz'lēz) [Samuel Doty *Risley,* American ophthalmologist, 1845–1920] see under *prism.*

**Ris·per·dal** (ris'pər-dal) trademark for a preparation of risperidone.

**ris·per·i·done** (ris-per'ĭdōn) [MeSH: Risperidone] a benzisoxazole derivative used as an antipsychotic agent, administered orally. Its mechanism of action is unknown, but its activity may result from a combination of dopamine and serotonin antagonism.

**Ris·ser jacket** (ris′ər) [Joseph C. *Risser,* American orthopedic surgeon, 1892–1942] see under *jacket.*

**RIST** radioimmunosorbent test; see under *tests.*

**ris·to·ce·tin** (ris″to-se′tin) [MeSH: Ristocetin] an antibiotic substance produced by the fermentation of *Nocardia lurida;* formerly used in treatment of severe staphylococcal infections resistant to other antibiotics.

**ri·sus** (ri′səs) [L.] laughter.
**r. cani′nus,** r. sardonicus.
**r. sardo′nicus,** a grinning expression produced by spasm of the facial muscles; see *sardonic.*

**Rit·a·lin** (rit′ə-lin) trademark for preparations of methylphenidate hydrochloride.

**Rit·gen maneuver (method)** (rit′gen) [Ferdinand August Marie Franz von *Ritgen,* German gynecologist, 1787–1867] see under *maneuver.*

**rit·o·drine hy·dro·chlor·ide** (rit′o-drēn) [USP] a $beta_2$-adrenergic agent used as a smooth muscle (uterine muscle) relaxant to delay uncomplicated premature labor; administered orally and intravenously.

**ri′to′na′vir** (ri-to′nə-vir) [MeSH: Ritonavir] a protease inhibitor active against the human immunodeficiency virus, causing the formation of immature, noninfectious viral particles, used in the treatment of human immunodeficiency virus infection and acquired immunodeficiency syndrome; administered orally.

**Rit·ter's disease** (rit′ərz) [Gottfried *Ritter* von Rittershain, German physician, 1820–1883] staphylococcal scalded skin syndrome.

**rit·u·al** (rich′u-əl) in psychiatry, behavior performed compulsively to relieve anxiety, as in obsessive-compulsive disorder.

**ri·val·ry** (ri′vəl-re) a state of competition or antagonism.
**binocular r., retinal r.,** the apparent alternate displacement of two figures when viewed together, there being no fusion into a continuous picture of the images of the two eyes.
**sibling r.,** competition between siblings for the love, affection, and attention of one or both parents or for other recognition or gain.

**Ri·val·ta's reaction (test)** (rĭ-vahl′təz) [Fabio *Rivalta,* Italian pathologist, late 19th century] see under *reaction.*

**ri·vi·ni·an** (rĭ-vin′e-ən) named for A.Q. *Rivinus.*

**Ri·vi·nus ducts (canals), gland,** etc. (rĭ-ve′nəs) [Augustus Quirinus *Rivinus,* German anatomist and botanist, 1652–1723] see *ductus sublinguales minores, glandula sublingualis, incisura tympanica,* and *pars flaccida membranae tympanicae.*

**ri·vus** (ri′vəs) pl. *ri′vi* [L.] a brook, or little stream.
**r. lacrima′lis** [TA], the pathway by which the tears reach the lacrimal lake from the excretory ductules of the lacrimal gland.

**riz·i·form** (riz′ĭ-form) resembling grains of rice.

**RLF** retrolental fibroplasia; see *retinopathy of prematurity,* under *retinopathy.*

**RLL** right lower lobe; see *lobus inferior pulmonis dextri.*

**RMA** right mentoanterior (position of the fetus).

**RML** right middle lobe; see *lobus medius pulmonis dextri.*

**RMP** right mentoposterior (position of the fetus).

**RMT** right mentotransverse (position of the fetus).

**RN** Registered Nurse.

**Rn** symbol for *radon.*

**RNA** [MeSH: RNA] ribonucleic acid.
**ambisense RNA,** negative-sense RNA that functions not only as a template for the transcription of complementary RNA but also as a template for protein synthesis.
**antisense RNA,** an RNA molecule transcribed off the coding, rather than the template, strand of DNA, so that it is complementary to the sense (messenger) RNA; formation of a duplex between the sense and antisense RNA molecules blocks transcription and also subjects both molecules to double strand–specific nucleases.
**complementary RNA (cRNA),** viral RNA that is transcribed from negative-sense RNA and serves as a template for protein synthesis.
**heterogeneous nuclear RNA (hnRNA),** in eukaryotes, a diverse group of long primary transcripts formed in the nucleus, many of which will be processed to messenger RNA molecules by splicing followed by transport to the cytoplasm.
**messenger RNA (mRNA),** RNA molecules, usually 400 to 10,000 bases long, that serve as templates for protein synthesis (translation); in eukaryotes they have characteristic posttranscriptional modifications, the 5′-cap and poly A tail. The base sequence of an mRNA transcript completely specifies the corresponding polypeptide amino acid sequence.
**negative-sense RNA,** viral RNA that has a base sequence complementary to that of mRNA; during replication it serves as a template for the transcription of viral complementary RNA, which in turn serves as a template for protein synthesis.
**positive-sense RNA,** viral RNA that has the same base sequence as mRNA; during replication, it functions as mRNA and serves as a template for protein synthesis.
**ribosomal RNA (rRNA),** the most abundant form of RNA; together with proteins it forms the ribosomes, playing a structural role and also a role in ribosomal binding of mRNA and tRNAs. Individual chains are conventionally designated by their sedimentation coefficients. In eukaryotes, four large chains exist, synthesized in the nucleolus and constituting about 50 per cent of the ribosome.
**small nuclear RNA (snRNA),** an abundant class of eukaryotic RNA found in the nucleus, usually less than 300 nucleotides long but excluding ribosomal or transfer RNA of this size; most occur as ribonucleoproteins and they appear to play a role in processing of heterogeneous nuclear RNA.
**transfer RNA (tRNA),** small RNA molecules, 73–93 nucleotides, occurring in cells in 20 or more varieties and functioning in translation; each variety carries a specific amino acid to a site specified by an RNA codon, binding to amino acid, ribosome, and to the codon via an anticodon region. All have numerous modified bases and extensive secondary structure; see also illustration.

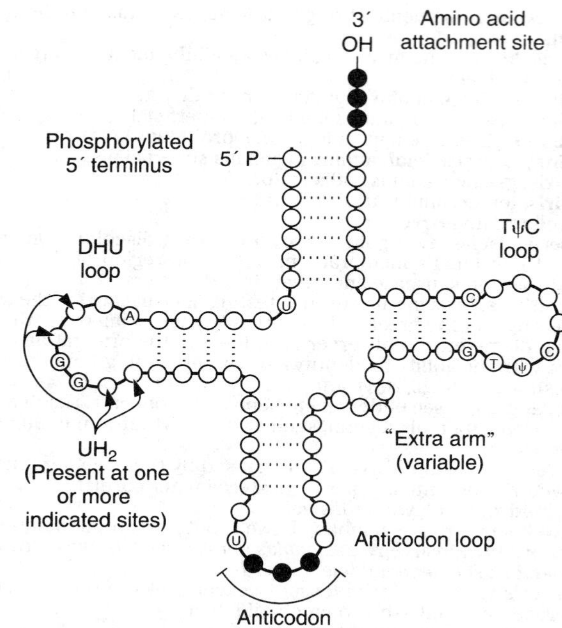

Schematic diagram of features common to transfer RNA molecules, depicting the anticodon and amino acid attachment regions. Dotted lines between chains represent hydrogen-bonded base pairs. The characteristic cloverleaf is formed by the hairpin and loop structures that result from intrachain hydrogen bonding.

**RNA-di·rect·ed DNA po·lym·er·ase** (dĭ-rek′təd pə-lim′ər-ās) [EC 2.7.7.49] [MeSH: RNA-Directed DNA Polymerase] an enzyme of the transferase class that catalyzes the template-directed, step by step addition of deoxyribonucleotides to the 3′ end of a DNA or RNA primer or growing DNA chain, using a single-stranded RNA template. The enzyme occurs in retroviruses and the DNA is an intermediate in the formation of progeny RNA from the original virion RNA. See also *retrovirus.* Called also *reverse transcriptase.*

**RNA-di·rect·ed RNA po·lym·er·ase** (dĭ-rek′təd pə-lim′ər-ās) [EC 2.7.7.48] an enzyme of the transferase class that catalyzes the template-directed step by step addition of ribonucleotides to the 3′ end of a growing RNA chain, using a single-stranded RNA template. The reaction is important for transcription, and in some cases replication, of RNA in most RNA viruses except retroviruses.

**RNA nu·cleo·tid·yl·trans·fer·ase** (noo″kle-o-tīd″əl-trans′fər-ās) older name for an RNA polymerase.

**RNA po·lym·er·ase** (pə-lim′ər-ās) 1. a general term denoting any enzyme catalyzing the template-directed incorporation of ribonucleotides into an RNA chain; see *DNA-directed RNA polymerase* and *RNA-directed RNA polymerase.* 2. DNA-directed RNA polymerase.

**RNA rep·li·case** (rep′lĭ-kās) [MeSH: RNA Replicase] RNA-directed RNA polymerase.

**RNase** ribonuclease, sometimes used specifically to denote pancreatic ribonuclease.
**R. I,** pancreatic ribonuclease.

**R. A,** pancreatic ribonuclease.

**RNP** ribonucleoprotein.

**ROA** right occipitoanterior (position of the fetus).

**roach** (rōch) cockroach.

**roar·ing** (ror′ing) a rough sound on inspiration and sometimes on expiration by a horse, usually due to obstruction in the respiratory tract or laryngeal hemiplegia.

**Ro·ba·late** (ro′bə-lāt) trademark for preparations of dihydroxyaluminum aminoacetate.

**Ro·bax·in** (ro-bak′sin) trademark for preparations of methocarbamol.

**Ro·bax·i·sal** (ro-bak′sĭ-sal) trademark for a preparation of methocarbamol.

**Rob·bins** (rob′inz) Frederick Chapman. American pediatrician, born 1916; co-winner, with John Franklin Enders and Thomas Huckle Weller, of the Nobel prize in medicine or physiology for 1954 for the discovery that viruses (specifically, poliomyelitis viruses) can be grown in tissue culture and thereby be isolated and studied, making possible the production of vaccines.

**ro·ben·i·dine hy·dro·chlo·ride** (ro-ben′ĭ-dēn) a compound related to guanidine, formerly used as a coccidiostat for poultry.

**Ro·bert's ligament** (ro-bārz′) [César Alphonse *Robert,* French surgeon, 1801–1862] see under *ligament.*

**Rob·erts** (rob′ərts) Richard J. American biochemist, born 1944. Co-winner, with Phillip A. Sharp, of the Nobel prize for medicine or physiology in 1993 for his discoveries about the structure of genes and the transmission of genetic information.

**Rob·erts' syndrome** (rob′ərts) [John Bingham *Roberts,* American surgeon, 1852–1924] see under *syndrome.*

**Rob·ert·son's sign** (rob′ərt-sənz) [William Egbert *Robertson,* American physician, 1869–1956] see under *sign.*

**Ro·bin's anomalad, syndrome** (ro-baz′) [Pierre *Robin,* French pediatrician, 1867–1950] Pierre Robin syndrome.

**ro·bin** (ro′bin) a phytotoxin found in the bark of the tree *Robinia pseudacacia,* which has caused poisoning of livestock.

**Ro·bin·ia** (ro-bin′e-ə) a genus of North American shrubs and trees of the family Leguminosae. *R. pseudaca′cia* is the black locust or black acacia tree, whose bark contains the phytotoxin robin and has caused poisoning in livestock.

**Rob·i·now's syndrome (dwarfism)** (rob′ĭ-nouz) [Meinhard *Robinow,* American physician, born 1909] see under *syndrome.*

**Rob·in·son's circle** (rob′in-sənz) [Frederick Byron *Robinson,* American anatomist, 1857–1910] see under *circle.*

**Ro·bi·nul** (ro′bĭ-nəl) trademark for preparations of glycopyrrolate.

**Ro·bi·son ester** (ro′bĭ-sən) [Robert *Robison,* British chemist, 1884–1941] glucose 6-phosphate.

**Ro·bi·tus·sin** (ro″bĭ-tus′in) trademark for preparations of guaifenesin.

**Rob·son's line, point, position** (rob′sənz) [Sir Arthur William Mayo *Robson,* London surgeon, 1853–1933] see under *line, point,* and *position.*

**ro·bust** (ro-bust′) in statistics, a somewhat imprecise term that is applied to a procedure that is relatively insensitive to violations of the assumptions on which it is based or to procedures that are based on weaker (more easily satisfied) assumptions, e.g., nonparametric tests.

**Ro·cal·trol** (ro′kal-trōl) trademark for a preparation of calcitriol.

**Ro·ceph·in** (ro-sef′in) trademark for a preparation of ceftriaxone sodium.

**Ro·cha·li·maea** (ro″kə-li-me′ə) [Henrique da *Rocha-Lima,* French physician in Germany, born 1879] see *Bartonella.*

**Ro·cher's sign** (ro-shārz′) [Henri Gaston Louis *Rocher,* French surgeon, born 1876] see under *sign.*

**Ro·chon-Du·vi·gneaud's syndrome** (ro-shaw′doo-ve-nyōz′) [André *Rochon-Duvigneaud,* French ophthalmologist, late 19th century] superior orbital fissure syndrome.

**ro·cu·ro·ni·um bro·mide** (ro″ku-ro′ne-um) a nondepolarizing neuromuscular blocking agent, structurally related to and less potent than vecuronium, used as an adjunct in general anesthesia to facilitate endotracheal intubation and as a skeletal muscle relaxant during surgery or mechanical ventilation; administered intravenously.

**rod** (rod) 1. a straight, slim mass of substance. 2. retinal r.
**Auer r's,** see under *body.*
**Corti's r's,** pillar cells.
**Cotrel-Dubousset r.,** a rigid contoured rod used in Cotrel-Dubousset instrumentation.
**enamel r's,** the approximately parallel rods or prisms forming the enamel of teeth. They are enclosed in a sheath of organic matter (the enamel rod sheath, or prism sheath) and are embedded in the interprismatic or cement substance.
**Harrington r.,** a rigid, contoured metal rod used in Harrington instrumentation.
**r's of Heidenhain,** the rodlike cells of the renal tubules.
**Knodt r.,** a rigid, contoured rod used in Knodt instrumentation.
**König's r's,** a series of steel bars each of which gives a note of certain pitch when struck.
**Luque r.,** a rigid, contoured stainless steel rod used in Luque instrumentation.
**Maddox r's,** a set of parallel cylindrical glass rods used in testing for heterophoria. The rods, placed before the eye, distort the image of a point source of light into a long streak perpendicular to the axis of the rods, interfere with fusion, and break up binocular vision.
**Meckel's r.,** Meckel's cartilage.
**muscle r.,** myofibril.
**olfactory r.,** the slender apical portion of an olfactory bipolar neuron, a modified dendrite, extending as a cylindrical process from the nucleus to surface of the epithelium.
**retinal r.,** a visual cell that serves night vision and detection of motion. The synaptic terminal is a rounded spherule; the dendritic inner and outer segments are long and cylindrical; the membranous disks contain rhodopsin and are free saccules completely enclosed by the outer cell membrane. There are about 120 million rods in the retina—none in the foveola, the greatest concentration about 20 degrees away from the fovea, and a gradually decreasing density approaching the retinal periphery. Called also *rod* and *rod cell.* See also *retinal cone,* under *cone,* and *visual cell,* under *cell.*

**Rod·bell** (Rod′bel) Martin. American physiologist, born 1925. Co-winner with Alfred G. Gilman of the Nobel prize for medicine or physiology in 1994 for his research into the role of G proteins in cell responses to environmental signals.

**ro·dent** (ro′dənt) [L. *rodere* to gnaw] [MeSH: Rodentia] any mammal of the order *Rodentia.*

**Ro·den·tia** (ro-den′shə) [MeSH: Rodentia] the rodents, an order of mammals characterized by large chisel-shaped incisors in the upper and lower jaws; it includes the rats, mice, and squirrels. Numerous species serve as reservoirs for infectious diseases.

**ro·den·ti·cide** (ro-den′tĭ-sīd) 1. destructive to rodents. 2. any agent for destroying rodents.
**anticoagulant r.,** an anticoagulant that kills rodents by causing massive hemorrhaging; such substances can usually also kill other mammals or humans that accidentally ingest them. Most are derivatives of indanedione or warfarin. See table.

**ro·den·tine** (ro-den′tīn) pertaining to a rodent.

**roent·gen** (rent′gən) [Wilhelm Konrad *Röntgen*] the international unit of x- or $\gamma$-radiation. It is the quantity of x- or $\gamma$-radiation such that the associated corpuscular emission per 0.001293 gram of dry air (1 $cm^3$ at 0°C and 760 mm Hg) produces in air ions carrying 1 electrostatic unit of electrical charge of either sign. Symbol R.

**roent·gen rays** (rent′gen) [Wilhelm Konrad *Röntgen,* German physicist, 1845–1923, who discovered the rays in 1895 and won the Nobel prize in physics in 1901] see under *ray.*

**roent·geno·graph** (rent′gən-o-graf) radiograph.

**roent·geno·graph·ic** (rent″gən-o-graf′ik) radiographic.

**roent·gen·og·ra·phy** (rent″gən-og′rə-fe) [*roentgen* + *-graphy*] radiography.

**roent·gen·ol·o·gist** (rent″gən-ol′ə-jist) radiologist.

**roent·gen·ol·o·gy** (rent″gən-ol′ə-je) radiology.

**roent·geno·scope** (rent-gen′o-skōp) fluoroscope.

**roent·gen·os·co·py** (rent″gən-os′kə-pe) fluoroscopy.

**Ro·fer·on-A** (ro-fēr′on) trademark for a preparation of interferon alfa-2a.

**Ro·gaine** (ro′gān) trademark for a preparation of minoxidil.

**Anticoagulant Rodenticides**

| | |
|---|---|
| Brodifacoum | Difenacoum |
| Bromadiolone | Diphenadione (diphaenone) |
| Chlorophacinone | Pindone |
| Coumachlor | Valone |
| Coumafuryl | Warfarin |
| Coumatetralyl | |

**Ro·ger's disease, reaction, symptom** (ro-zhăz') [Henri Louis *Roger,* French physician, 1809–1891] see under *disease* and *symptom.*

**Ro·ger's reflex** (ro-zhăz') [Georges Henri *Roger,* French physiologist, 1860–1946] esophagosalivary reflex.

**Röhl's marginal corpuscles** (rerlz) [Wilhelm *Röhl,* German physician, 1881–1929] see under *corpuscle.*

**Ro·ki·tan·sky's diverticulum, hernia, pelvis** (ro″kĭ-tahn'skēz) [Karl Freiherr von *Rokitansky,* Czech pathologist in Austria, 1804–1878] see *massive hepatic necrosis,* under *necrosis,* see *spondylolisthetic pelvis,* under *pelvis,* and see under *diverticulum.*

**Ro·ki·tan·sky-Cush·ing ulcers** (ro″kĭ-tahn'ske-koosh'ing) [K.F. von *Rokitansky;* Harvey Williams *Cushing,* American surgeon, 1869–1939] see under *ulcer.*

**Ro·ki·tan·sky-Kü·ster-Hau·ser syndrome** (ro″kĭ-tahn'ske-ke'stər-hou'zər) [K.F. von *Rokitansky;* Hermann *Küster,* German gynecologist, early 20th century; G.A. *Hauser,* Swiss physician, 20th century] Mayer-Rokitansky-Küster-Hauser syndrome.

**ro·lan·dic** (ro-lan'dik) described by or named in honor of Luigi *Rolando;* see under *angle* and *area.*

**Ro·lan·do's angle, cells,** etc. (ro-lahn'dōz) [Luigi *Rolando,* Italian anatomist, 1773–1831] see under *angle, cell,* and *line;* see *motor area,* under *area;* and see *substantia gelatinosa cornu posterioris medullae spinalis, sulcus centralis cerebri,* and *tuberculum trigeminale.*

**role** (rōl) [MeSH: Role] the behavior pattern that an individual presents to others.
**gender r.,** the public expression of gender; the image projected by a person that identifies their maleness or femaleness, which need not correspond to their gender identity (q.v.).

**ro·li·tet·ra·cy·cline** (ro-lĭ-tet″rə-si'klin) [MeSH: Rolitetracycline] a semisynthetic broad-spectrum antibiotic of the tetracycline group, used as an antibacterial, administered intravenously or intramuscularly.
**r. nitrate,** a salt of rolitetracycline, having the same actions and uses as the base.

**roll** (rōl) a cylindrical structure.
**iliac r.,** a mass shaped like a sausage, located in the left iliac fossa and produced by a collection of feces or by induration of the walls of the sigmoid fossa.
**scleral r.,** see under *spur.*

**Rol·ler's nucleus** (rol'ərz) [Christian Friedrich Wilhelm *Roller,* German neurologist, 1802–1878] sublingual nucleus.

**roll·er** (rōl'ər) a small cylinder of rolled cotton, linen, or flannel for surgical use.

**Rol·le·ston's rule** (rol'əs-tənz) [Sir Humphrey Davy *Rolleston,* English physician, 1862–1944] see under *rule.*

**Rol·let's stroma** (rol'ets) [Alexander *Rollet,* Austrian physiologist, 1834–1903] see under *stroma.*

**Rol·let's syndrome** (ro-lāz') [J. *Rollet,* French physician, 20th century] orbital apex syndrome; see under *syndrome.*

**Ro·ma·ña's sign** (ro-mahn'yəz) [Cecilio *Romaña,* Argentine physician in Brazil, 20th century] see under *sign.*

**Ro·mano-Ward syndrome** (ro-mah'no-word) [C. *Romano,* Italian physician, born 1923; O.C. *Ward,* Irish physician, 20th century] see under *syndrome.*

**ro·mano·scope** (ro-man'o-skōp) [L. *romanum* the sigmoid + *-scope*] sigmoidoscope.

**Ro·ma·nov·sky's (Ro·ma·now·sky's) stain (method)** (ro″mah-nof'skēz) [Dimitri Leonidovich *Romanovsky* (or *Romanowsky*), Russian physician, 1861–1921] see under *stain.*

**Ro·maz·i·con** (ro-maz'ĭ-kon) trademark for a preparation of flumazenil.

**Rom·berg's disease (trophoneurosis), sign, spasm, test** (rom'bərgz) [Moritz Heinrich *Romberg,* German physician, 1795–1873] see *facial hemiatrophy,* under *hemiatrophy,* and see under *sign, spasm,* and *test.*

**rom·berg·ism** (rom'bərg-izm) [M.H. *Romberg*] Romberg's sign.

**Ro·mil·ar** (ro'mĭ-lahr) trademark for preparations of dextromethorphan hydrobromide.

**Rom·me·laere's sign** (rom-ə-lārz') [Guillaume *Rommelaere,* Belgian physician, 1836–1916] see under *sign.*

**Rom·ney Marsh disease** (rom'ne mahrsh) [*Romney Marsh,* England, where it was first reported] struck.

**Ron·do·my·cin** (ron″do-mi'sin) trademark for a preparation of methacycline hydrochloride.

**ron·geur** (raw-zhur') [Fr. "gnawing, biting"] a forcepslike instrument for cutting tough tissue, particularly bone.

**Ro·ni·a·col** (ro-ni'ə-kol) trademark for preparations of nicotinyl alcohol.

**ro·nid·a·zole** (ro-nid'ə-zōl) [MeSH: Ronidazole] a veterinary antiprotozoal and antimicrobial used to treat histomoniasis and swine dysentery.

**Rön·ne's nasal step** (rərn'ez) [Henning Kristian Trappaud *Rönne,* Danish ophthalmologist, 1878–1947] see under *step.*

**ron·nel** (ron'əl) an organophosphorus insecticide, effective against flies, roaches, screw worms, and cattle grub.

**Rönt·gen** (rent'gen) Wilhelm Conrad (1845–1923). German physicist, born at Lennep (Rhineland). For his discovery of x-rays in 1895, while experimenting with a cathode ray tube, he received the first Nobel prize for physics in 1901.

**Rood method** (rood) [Margaret *Rood,* American physical therapist, 20th century] see under *method.*

**roof** (rōōf) a covering structure; see also *tectum* and *tegmen.*
**r. of fourth ventricle,** tegmen ventriculi quarti.
**r. of lateral ventricle,** the superior covering of a lateral ventricle, formed by parts of the corpus callosum and its tapetum as well as the tail of the caudate nucleus and the stria terminalis.
**r. of mouth,** palatum.
**r. of nasal cavity,** the superior surface of the cavity, formed by portions of the sphenoid, ethmoid, frontal, and nasal bones; it is narrow anteriorly and wider posteriorly.
**nasopharyngeal r., r. of nasopharynx,** fornix pharyngis.
**r. of orbit,** paries superior orbitae.
**r. of skull,** calvaria.
**r. of third ventricle,** the tela choroidea ventriculi tertii and the ependyma, which form the superior covering structures of the third ventricle.
**r. of tympanic cavity,** paries tegmentalis cavitatis tympani.
**r. of tympanum,** 1. tegmen tympani. 2. paries tegmentalis cavitatis tympani.

**room** (rōōm) an enclosed place in a building, set apart for specific purposes such as the performance of procedures.
**anechoic r.,** see under *chamber.*
**delivery r.,** a hospital room to which an obstetrical patient is taken for delivery.
**intensive therapy r.,** old term for *intensive care unit.*
**labor r.,** predelivery r.
**operating r.,** a room in a hospital equipped and used for surgical operations.
**postdelivery r.,** a recovery room for the care of obstetric patients immediately after delivery.
**predelivery r.,** a hospital room where an obstetric patient remains during the first stage of labor, i.e., from the time the pains begin until she is ready for delivery; called also *labor r.*
**recovery r.,** a hospital unit adjoining operating or delivery rooms, with special equipment and personnel for the care of postoperative or postpartum patients until they may safely be returned to general nursing care in their own rooms or wards.

**room·ing-in** (rōōm'ing-in) the practice of keeping a newly born infant in a crib near the mother's bed, instead of in a nursery, during the hospital stay.

**root** (rōōt) 1. radix. 2. the lowermost part of a plant or other structure.
**anatomical r.,** the portion of a tooth that is covered by cementum; see *radix dentis.*
**r's of ansa cervicalis,** see *radix superior ansae cervicalis* and *radix inferior ansae cervicalis.*
**anterior r. of ansa cervicalis,** radix superior ansae cervicalis.
**anterior r. of spinal nerve,** radix anterior nervi spinalis.
**anterior r. of zygomatic process of temporal bone,** a short thick continuation of the inferior border of the zygomatic process, extending medially to the articular tubercle.

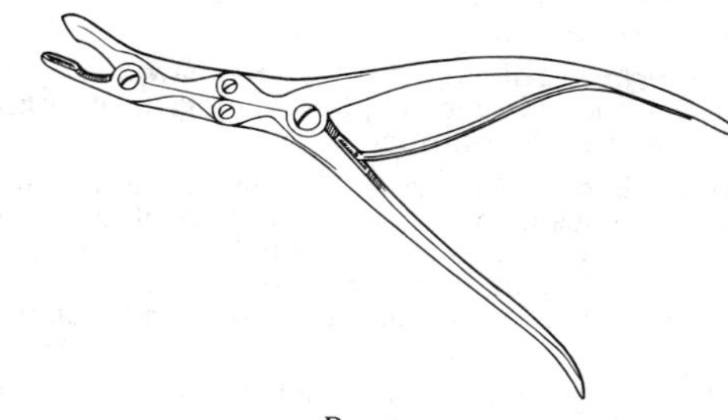

Rongeur.

**r. of aorta, aortic r.**, the dense fibrous area that encircles the aortic valve and constitutes the junction between the aortic vestibule of the left ventricle and the aorta.
**r. of arch of vertebra**, pediculus arcus vertebrae.
**belladonna r.**, the dried root of *Atropa belladonna,* which contains various anticholinergic alkaloids; called also *deadly nightshade r.* See *belladonna.*
**bitter r.**, gentian.
**r's of brachial plexus**, radices plexus brachialis.
**clinical r.**, radix clinica.
**r. of clitoris**, crus clitoridis.
**cochlear r. of vestibulocochlear nerve**, radix cochlearis nervi vestibulocochlearis.
**cranial r. of accessory nerve**, radix cranialis nervi accessorii.
**deadly nightshade r.**, belladonna r.
**dorsal r. of spinal nerve**, radix posterior nervi spinalis.
**facial r., r. of facial nerve**, a motor nerve root consisting of fibers passing from the nucleus of the facial nerve to the facial colliculus, and from there through the ventral surface of the lower part of the pons, where the sensory root (the nervus intermedius) joins it to form the facial nerve.
**r. of hair**, radix pili.
**inferior r. of ansa cervicalis**, radix inferior ansae cervicalis.
**inferior r. of vestibulocochlear nerve**, radix cochlearis nervi vestibulocochlearis.
**lateral r. of median nerve**, radix lateralis nervi mediani.
**lateral r. of optic tract**, radix lateralis tractus optici.
**licorice r.**, glycyrrhiza.
**lingual r.**, that root of a posterior tooth, especially a maxillary molar, which is situated nearest the tongue.
**long r. of ciliary ganglion**, radix sensoria ganglii ciliaris.
**r. of lung**, radix pulmonis.
**mandrake r.**, podophyllum.
**medial r. of median nerve**, radix medialis nervi mediani.
**medial r. of optic tract**, radix medialis tractus optici.
**motor r. of ciliary ganglion**, radix parasympathica ganglii ciliaris.
**motor r. of mandibular nerve**, a small root that emerges from the trigeminal ganglion and combines with the corresponding sensory root to form the mandibular nerve.
**motor r. of spinal nerve**, radix anterior nervi spinalis.
**motor r. of submandibular ganglion**, rami ganglionares nervi lingualis ad ganglion submandibulare.
**motor r. of trigeminal nerve**, radix motoria nervi trigemini.
**r. of nail**, radix unguis.
**nasociliary r. of ciliary ganglion**, radix sensoria ganglii ciliaris.
**nerve r's**, the anterior and posterior roots of the spinal nerves; see *radix anterior nervi spinalis* and *radix posterior nervi spinalis.* Called also *spinal r's.*
**nerve r., motor**, radix posterior nervi spinalis.
**nerve r., sensory**, radix anterior nervi spinalis.
**r. of nose**, radix nasi.
**oculomotor r. of ciliary ganglion**, radix parasympathica ganglii ciliaris.
**orizaba jalap r.**, ipomea.
**orris r.**, orris (def. 2).
**r. of otic ganglion**, the preganglionic fibers of the lesser petrosal nerve.
**palatine r.**, that root of a maxillary molar tooth which is situated nearest the palate.
**parasympathetic r. of ciliary ganglion**, radix parasympathica ganglii ciliaris.
**parasympathetic r. of otic ganglion**, nervus petrosus minor.
**parasympathetic r. of pterygopalatine ganglion**, nervus petrosus major.
**parasympathetic r. of sublingual ganglion, parasympathetic r. of submandibular ganglion**, chorda tympani.
**physiological r.**, the portion of a tooth proximal to the gingival crevice, or embedded in the dental alveolus.
**pleurisy r.**, *Asclepias tuberosa.*
**posterior r. of ansa cervicalis**, radix inferior ansae cervicalis.
**posterior r. of spinal nerve**, radix posterior nervi spinalis.
**posterior r. of zygomatic process of temporal bone**, a continuation of the superior border of the zygomatic process, extending above the external acoustic meatus and ending continuous with the supramastoid crest.
**puccoon r., red r.**, sanguinaria.
**retained r.**, 1. a tooth root, or part of a root, remaining in the soft tissue or in bone following trauma, extensive tooth decay, or incomplete extraction. 2. a tooth root intentionally retained to prevent resorption of the alveolar process.
**sensory r. of ciliary ganglion**, radix sensoria ganglii ciliaris.
**sensory r. of mandibular nerve**, a large root that emerges from the trigeminal ganglion and combines with the corresponding motor root to form the mandibular nerve.
**sensory r. of otic ganglion**, rami ganglionares nervi mandibularis ad ganglion oticum.
**sensory r. of pterygopalatine ganglion**, rami ganglionares nervi maxillaris ad ganglion pterygopalatinum.
**sensory r. of spinal nerve**, radix posterior nervi spinalis.
**sensory r. of submandibular ganglion**, rami ganglionares nervi lingualis ad ganglion submandibulare.
**sensory r. of trigeminal nerve**, radix sensoria nervi trigemini.
**short r. of ciliary ganglion**, radix parasympathica ganglii ciliaris.
**spinal r's**, nerve r's.
**spinal r. of accessory nerve**, radix spinalis nervi accessorii.
**r's of spinal nerves**, nerve r's.
**superior r. of ansa cervicalis**, radix superior ansae cervicalis.
**superior r. of vestibulocochlear nerve**, radix vestibularis nervi vestibulocochlearis.
**sympathetic r. of ciliary ganglion**, radix sympathica ganglii ciliaris.
**sympathetic r. of pterygopalatine ganglion**, nervus petrosus profundus.
**r. of tongue**, radix linguae.
**r. of tooth**, radix dentis.
**ventral r. of spinal nerve**, radix anterior nervi spinalis.
**vestibular r. of vestibulocochlear nerve**, radix vestibularis nervi vestibulocochlearis.

**root·let** (ro͞ot′lət) a small root or rootlike structure or a division of such a structure.
**flagellar r.**, one of the delicate striated fibrils of the flagellar root system that arise from the basal body and run deep into the cytoplasm, perhaps serving as anchoring organelles or having a skeletal function. They occur most commonly in phytoflagellate protozoa, and were formerly thought to connect the basal body to the nucleus of the cell. Called also *rhizoblast* and *rhizoplast.*
**r's of spinal nerve**, fila radicularia nervi spinalis.

**ROP** right occipitoposterior (position of the fetus).

**ro·ri·din** (ro′rĭ-din) any of several trichothecene mycotoxins found in species of *Stachybotrys,* especially *S. alternans,* causing stachybotryotoxicosis.

**Ror·schach test** (ror′shahk) [Hermann *Rorschach,* Swiss psychiatrist, 1884–1922] [MeSH: Rorschach Test] see under *test.*

**Ro·sa** (ro′zə) the roses, a genus of flowering, usually prickly, plants of the family Rosaceae. *R. al′ba* L., *R. centifo′lia* L., *R. damasce′na* Mill., and *R. gal′lica* L. have flowers that yield rose oil.

**ro·sa·cea** (ro-za′she-ə) a chronic hyperemic disease of the skin, usually involving the middle third of the face, characterized by persistent erythema and often by telangiectasia with acute episodes of edema, papules, and pustules, and usually affecting both men and women, although the most severe cases (see *rhinophyma* and see *rosacea keratitis,* under *keratitis)* are usually seen in men. Called also *acne rosacea.*
**granulomatous r.**, rosacea in which discrete papules occur on the medial and lateral facial areas of the face as well as periorally; on diascopy the lesions appear as yellowish brown nodules, and as noncaseating epithelioid cell granulomas histologically. Called also *granulomatous r., lupoid r.,* and *micronodular* or *rosacea-like tuberculid.*
**lupoid r.**, granulomatous r.
**papular r.**, granulomatous r.

**ro·sac·ic ac·id** (ro-zas′ik) uroerythrin.

**Ro·sai-Dorf·man disease** (ro′zi dorf′mən) [Juan *Rosai,* American pathologist, 20th century; Ronald F. *Dorfman,* American pathologist, 20th century] see under *disease.*

**ro·sa·mi·cin** (ro″zə-mi′sin) a macrolide antibiotic, derived from *Micromonospora rosaria,* having a broad spectrum of antibacterial activity against gram-positive bacteria and some activity against gram-negative bacteria; the butyrate, propionate, sodium phosphate, and stearate salts have antibacterial activity similar to that of the base.

**ro·san·i·line** (ro-zan′ĭ-lin) a basic dye derived from triphenylmethane, occurring as reddish brown crystals, which is soluble in acids and alcohol and slightly soluble in water. It is used, usually as the hydrochloride, in the preparation of other dyes and as a component of basic fuchsin.

**ro·sa·ry** (ro′zə-re) a structure resembling a string of beads.
**rachitic r.**, rachitic beads; see under *bead.*
**scorbutic r.**, scorbutic beads; see under *bead.*

**Rose's position** (ro′zəz) [Frank Atcherly *Rose,* British surgeon, 1873–1935] see under *position.*

**rose** (rōz) [L. *rosa*] 1. any plant of the genus *Rosa.* 2. a dark pink or light red color.
**r. bengal**, a dye, the dichlor- or the tetrachlorerythrosin, $NaO{\cdot}(C_6HI_2{\cdot}O)_2C{\cdot}C_6H_2Cl_2{\cdot}COONa$.
**r. bengal sodium I 131** [USP], rose bengal in which a portion of the molecules contain radioiodine ($^{131}I$); it has been used as a radioactive tracer in liver function studies.

**ro·se·in** (ro′ze-in) fuchsin.

**rose·ma·ry** (rōz′mar-e) *Rosmarinus officinalis.*

**Ro·sen·bach's sign** (ro′zən-bahks) [Ottomar *Rosenbach,* German physician, 1851–1907] see under *sign.*

**Ro·sen·berg-Berg·strom syndrome** (ro′zən-bərg-bərg′strəm) [Alan L. *Rosenberg,* American physician, 20th century; Lavonne *Bergstrom,* American physician, 20th century] see under *syndrome.*

**Ro·sen·berg-Chu·tor·i·an syndrome** (ro′zən-bərg-choo-tor′e-ən) [Roger N. *Rosenberg,* American physician, 20th century; Abe Milton *Chutorian,* American physician, born 1929] see under *syndrome.*

**Ro·sen·mül·ler's organ,** etc. (ro′zən-me″lərz) [Johann Christian *Rosenmüller,* German anatomist, 1771–1820] see *epoöphoron, plica lacrimalis,* and *recessus pharyngeus.*

**Ro·sen·thal's canal** (ro′zən-tahlz) [Isidor *Rosenthal,* German physiologist, 1836–1915] canalis spiralis modioli.

**Ro·sen·thal syndrome** (ro′zen-thawl) [Robert Louis *Rosenthal,* American hematologist, born 1923] see under *syndrome.*

**Ro·sen·thal's test** (ro′zən-thawlz) [Sanford Morris *Rosenthal,* American physician, 20th century] see under *test.*

**Ro·sen·thal's vein** (ro′zən-tahlz) [Friedrich Christian *Rosenthal,* German anatomist, 1779–1829] vena basalis.

**ro·se·o·la** (ro-ze′o-lə, ro″ze-o′lə) [L.] 1. a rose-colored rash, as may be seen in measles, syphilis, and certain other exanthematous diseases. 2. exanthema subitum.
**r. infan′tum,** exanthema subitum.
**syphilitic r.,** macular syphilid.

**Ro·se·o·lo·vi·rus** (ro″ze-o′lo-vi″əs) [*roseola* + *virus*] a genus of viruses of the subfamily Betaherpesvirinae (family Herpesviridae), containing the single species human herpesvirus 6, the etiologic agent of exanthema subitum.

**ro·sette** (ro-zet′) [Fr. "little rose"] a structure, formation, or part occurring in a loosely attached cluster resembling a rose, such as *(a)* the clusters of polymorphonuclear leukocytes around a globule of lysed nuclear material, observed in a test for systemic lupus erythematosus; *(b)* a figure formed by the chromosomes in an early stage of mitosis; *(c)* a unique glandular complex present near the oral area of certain ciliate protozoa, the function of which is unclear; or *(d)* the symmetrical segmenter stage of certain malarial plasmodia, especially *Plasmodium malariae.*
**E r.,** see under *assay.*
**EAC r.,** see under *assay.*
**ependymal r.,** glandlike structures consisting of tumor cells with epithelial features and having long, slender processes extending into a lumen; seen in ependymoma.
**Flexner-Wintersteiner r.,** a cell formation found in retinoblastoma and certain other ophthalmic tumors, with columnar cells radiating out from a clear central core and separated from it by a membrane; spokes like those of a wheel may also be seen, representing rods and cones.
**Homer Wright r.,** a circular or spherical grouping of dark tumor cells around a pale, eosinophilic, central area that contains neurofibrils but lacks a lumen; seen in some medulloblastomas, neuroblastomas, and retinoblastomas or other ophthalmic tumors.

**ro·sin** (roz′in) the solid resin obtained from *Pinus palustris* Mill. (Pinaceae) and other species of pine, occurring as sharply angular, translucent, amber-colored fragments, frequently covered with yellow dust, and containing about 90 per cent resin. It has been widely used in the preparation of plasters and ointments, as well as chewing gums, varnishes, and polishes; usage has declined because it is a common cause of contact allergy.

**Ros·ma·ri·nus** (ros″mə-ri′nəs) [L. "sea-dew"] a genus of plants of the family Labiatae. *R. officina′lis* L. is rosemary, a species native to southern Europe and Turkey that is the source of the spice rosemary and of rosemary oil.

**ro·sox·a·cin** (ro-soks′ə-sin) a broad-spectrum quinolone antibacterial agent, administered orally.

**Ross** (ros) Sir Ronald. British physician and protozoologist, 1857–1932; winner of the Nobel prize for medicine or physiology in 1902 for his demonstration of the life history of the malarial parasite *Plasmodium* in the stomach of the *Anopheles* mosquito and its transmission by the bite of the female anopheline mosquito.

**Ross' black spores** (ros′əz) [Sir Ronald *Ross*] see under *spore.*

**Ross' bodies** (ros′əz) [Edward Halford *Ross,* English pathologist, 1875–1928] see under *body.*

**Ross·bach's disease** (ros′bahks) [Michael Josef *Rossbach,* German physician, 1842–1894] hyperchlorhydria.

**Ros·so·li·mo's reflex (sign)** (ros″o-le′mōz) [Gregorij Ivanovich *Rossolimo,* Russian neurologist, 1860–1928] see under *reflex.*

**Ros·tan's asthma** (ros-tahz′) [Louis Léon *Rostan,* Paris physician, 1790–1866] cardiac asthma.

**ros·tel·lum** (ros-tel′əm) pl. *rostel′la* [L. "little beak"] a small protuberance or beak, especially the fleshy protuberance of the scolex of a tapeworm, which may or may not bear hooks.

**ros·tra** (ros′trə) plural of *rostrum.*

**ros·trad** (ros′trad) 1. toward a rostrum; situated nearer the rostrum in relation to a specific point of reference. 2. cephalad.

**ros·tral** (ros′trəl) [L., *rostralis,* from *rostrum* beak] 1. pertaining to or resembling a rostrum; having a rostrum or beak. 2. toward a rostrum or beak. 3. in human anatomy, toward the oral and nasal region, which may mean superior (for areas of the spinal cord) or anterior (for brain areas).

**ros·tra·lis** (ros-tra′lis) [L., from *rostrum,* beak] [TA] rostral.

**ros·trate** (ros′trāt) [L. *rostratus* beaked] having a beaklike process.

**ros·tri·form** (ros′trĭ-form) [*rostrum* + *form*] shaped like a beak.

**ros·trum** (ros′trəm) pl. *ros′trums* or *ros′tra* [L. "beak"] [TA] a general term in anatomic nomenclature for a beaklike appendage or part.
**r. cor′poris callo′si** [TA], rostrum of corpus callosum: the anterior and lower end of the corpus callosum.
**r. sphenoida′le** [TA], sphenoidal rostrum: the prominent ridge on the inferior surface of the sphenoid bone that articulates with a deep depression between the wings of the vomer.

**ROT** right occipitotransverse (position of the fetus).

**Rot** see *Roth.*

**rot** (rot) 1. decay, def. 1. 2. liver r.
**Barcoo r.,** desert sore.
**fleece r.,** dermatitis in sheep resulting from prolonged skin wetness, accompanied by matted wool and exudation; it is often a precursor of cutaneous myiasis.
**foot r.,** inflammation with interdigital dermatitis and mild to severe necrosis of the hoof of an animal, caused by a bacterial infection; in cattle and sheep it is exacerbated in wet or cold weather or soggy pastures, and in pigs it usually follows trauma. See *foot r. of cattle, foot r. of pigs,* and *foot r. of sheep.*
**foot r., benign,** foot rot of sheep that is mainly confined to the skin between the digits; lameness is less severe than with virulent foot rot. Called also *scald* and *foot scald.*
**foot r., bovine,** foot r. of cattle.
**foot r., contagious,** virulent foot r.
**foot r., ovine,** foot r. of sheep.
**foot r., porcine,** foot r. of pigs.
**foot r., strawberry,** dermatophilosis in sheep.
**foot r., virulent,** foot rot of sheep with chronic necrosis of the hoof and underlying dermis, destruction and eventual detachment of the hoof, lameness, and recumbency. The cause is usually a combined infection with *Fusobacterium necrophorum* and *Bacteroides nodosus,* and it is worse in wet or cold weather or in a soggy pasture. Called also *contagious foot r.*
**foot r. of cattle,** inflammation of the foot of a cow or bull, with dermatitis between the digits, lameness, fever, swelling of the coronet, and necrotic foul-smelling material around the lesion. It is thought to be caused by infection with *Fusobacterium necrophorum.* Called also *bovine foot r., foul in the foot, interdigital necrobacillosis,* and *pododermatitis.*
**foot r. of pigs,** a noncontagious foot infection of pigs, usually caused by *Fusobacterium necrophorum* or *Corynebacterium pyogenes* that invades through lesions on lateral digits of the hind legs, often after trauma such as from living in a pen with a hard or abrasive floor. Abscess formation is followed by lameness and sometimes permanent foot deformity. Called also *porcine foot r.*
**foot r. of sheep,** infection of the hooves of sheep with *Fusobacterium necrophorum* or *Bacteroides nodosus.* There are two varieties, *benign foot r.* and *contagious* or *virulent foot r.*
**liver r.,** a form of fascioliasis seen in cattle and sheep, and occasionally humans, characterized by fibrosis of the liver with anemia and weight loss; severe cases can be fatal. The infecting fluke is *Fasciola hepatica.* Called also *rot.*
**pizzle r., sheath r.,** enzootic balanoposthitis.

**ro·tab·la·tion** (ro″tab-la′shən) an atherectomy technique in which a rotating bur is inserted through a catheter into an artery; the bur rotates and debulks atherosclerotic plaque. Called also *rotational ablation* or *atherectomy.*

**Ro·ta·hal·er** (ro′tə-hāl″ər) trademark for a type of dry powder inhaler that delivers single doses of medication.

**ro·tam·e·ter** (ro-tam′ə-tər) a flow-rate meter of variable area with a rotating float in a tapered tube, used for measuring the flow of gases in administering an anesthetic.

**ro·ta·ry** (ro′tə-re) marked by or produced by rotation.

**ro·tate** (ro′tāt) to turn around an axis; to twist.

**ro·ta·tion** (ro-ta′shən) [L. *rotare* to turn] [MeSH: Rotation] 1. the process of turning around an axis; movement of a body about its

axis, called the *axis of rotation*. 2. the turning of the fetal head through 90 degrees during labor so that the long diameter of the head corresponds with the long diameter of the pelvic outlet. It should occur naturally, but if it does not the rotation may be accomplished manually or instrumentally by the obstetrician. See also *maneuver*. 3. a turning around a central axis without undergoing any displacement from the axis. See also *hinge movement*, under *movement*. 4. a procedure whereby a malturned tooth is turned into its normal position. 5. malposition due to an abnormal turning of a tooth around its longitudinal axis.
**molecular r.,** the figure obtained by multiplying the specific rotation by the molecular weight and dividing by 100.
**optical r.,** the quality of certain optically active substances whereby the plane of polarized light is changed, so that it is rotated in an arc the length of which is characteristic of the substance.
**specific r.,** the arc through which a substance of specified concentration rotates the plane of polarization in a specified light path, as observed in a polarimeter.
**van Ness r.,** fusion of the knee joint and rotation of the ankle to function as the knee; done to correct a congenitally missing femur.
**wheel r.,** torsion (def. 3).

**ro·ta·tion·plas·ty** (ro-ta″shən-plas′te) the moving of a rotation flap over a defect.

**ro·ta·tor** (ro′ta-tər) 1. causing rotation. 2. a muscle that rotates a body part; see *musculi rotatores*.

**ro·ta·to·ry** (ro″tə-tor′e) occurring in or caused by rotation.

**Ro·ta·vi·rus** (ro′tə-vi″rəs) [L. *rota* wheel + *virus*] [MeSH: Rotavirus] the rotaviruses, a genus of viruses of the family Reoviridae that have a wheellike appearance; they are transmitted by the fecal-oral route and cause acute infantile gastroenteritis and diarrhea in young children and many animal species. There are six antigenic groups (A–F). See Plate 55.

**Ro·ta·Shield** (ro′tə-shēld) trademark for a preparation ofrotavirus vaccine live oral.

**ro·ta·vi·ral** (ro′tə-vi″rəl) pertaining to or caused by rotaviruses.

**ro·ta·vi·rus** (ro′tə-vi″rəs) [L. *rota* wheel + *virus*] [MeSH: Rotavirus] any member of the genus *Rotavirus*.

**Rotch's sign** (roch′əs) [Thomas Morgan *Rotch*, American physician, 1849–1914] see under *sign*.

**ro·te·none** (ro′tə-nōn) [MeSH: Rotenone] a poisonous compound from the dried roots and other parts of plants of the genera *Derris* and *Lonchocarpus;* used as an insecticide and scabicide.

**ro·texed** (ro′tekst) rotated and bent to one side.

**ro·tex·ion** (ro-tek′shən) act of rotating and flexing; also the state of being rotated and flexed.

**Roth's disease** (rōts) [Vladimir Karlovich *Roth* (or *Rot*), Russian neurologist, 1848–1916] meralgia paresthetica.

**Roth's spots, vas aberrans** (rōts) [Moritz *Roth*, Swiss physician, 1839–1915] see under *spot*, and see *ductuli aberrantes*.

**Roth-Bern·hardt disease** (rōt-bern′hahrt) [V. K. *Roth;* Martin *Bernhardt*, German neurologist, 1844–1915] meralgia paraesthetica.

**Ro·the·ra's test** (roth′ər-ahz) [Arthur Cecil Hamel *Rothera*, Australian biochemist, 1880–1915] see under *test*.

**Roth·ia** (roth′e-ə) [Genevieve D. *Roth*, American bacteriologist, 20th century] a genus of bacteria of the family Actinomycetaceae, order Actinomycetales, made up of aerobic, gram-positive, nonacid-fast, nonspore-forming organisms occurring in coccoid, diphtheroid, and branched filament forms.
**R. dentocario′sa,** a species found in the oral cavity of man and other primates, particularly in plaque and calculus deposits on the teeth and in carious material. Called also *Actinomyces dentocariosus*.

**Roth·mann-Ma·kai syndrome** (rot′mahn-maw′koi) [Max *Rothmann*, German pathologist, 1868–1915; Endre *Makai*, Hungarian surgeon, 20th century] see under *syndrome*.

**Roth·mund-Thom·son syndrome** (rot′moond-tom′son) [August von *Rothmund*, Jr., German physician, 1830–1906; Mathew Sidney *Thomson*, English dermatologist, 1894–1969] see under *syndrome*.

**Ro·tor's syndrome** (ro-tōrz′) [Arturo B. *Rotor*, Filipino physician, 20th century] see under *syndrome*.

**ro·tox·amine** (ro-toks′ə-mēn) the *l*-isomer of carbinoxamine, having antihistaminic potency about twice that of the racemic form.
**r. tartrate,** the tartrate salt of rotoxamine, having the same actions as the base; used in the treatment of allergic disorders, administered orally.

**rott·le·ra** (rot′lər-ə) kamala (def. 2).

**rott·ler·in** (rot′lər-in) a toxic anthelmintic dye obtained from the kamala tree, *Mallotus philippinensis;* called also *mallotoxin*.

**rouge** (rōōzh) a fine red powder composed of iron oxide ($Fe_2O_3$), usually in cake form but sometimes impregnated on paper or cloth; used in dentistry as a polishing agent for restorations of gold and precious metal alloys.

**Rou·get's bulb** (roo-zhāz′) [Antoine D. *Rouget*, French physiologist, 19th century] bulb of the ovary.

**Rou·get's cell, muscle** (roo-zhāz′) [Charles Marie Benjamin *Rouget*, French physiologist and anatomist, 1824–1904] see *pericyte*, and see under *muscle*.

**rough** (ruf) not smooth; having an irregular surface.

**rough·age** (ruf′əj) indigestible material such as fibers, cellulose, etc., in the diet.

**Roug·non-Heb·er·den disease** (rōōn-yaw′heb′ər-dən) [Nicholas François *Rougnon* de Magny, French physician, 1727–1799; William *Heberden*, Sr., English physician, 1710–1801] angina pectoris.

**rou·leau** (roo-lo′) pl. *rouleaux′* [Fr. "roll"] an abnormal group of red blood cells adhering together like a roll of coins.

**round·worm** (round′wərm) nematode.

**Rous** (rous) Francis Peyton. American pathologist, 1879–1970; co-winner, with Charles Brenton Huggins, of the Nobel prize for medicine or physiology in 1966 for his discovery of tumor-inducing viruses in 1910.

**Rous sarcoma, test** (rous) [Francis Peyton *Rous*] see under *sarcoma* and *test*.

**Rous·sy-De·je·rine syndrome** (roo-se′ dĕ-zhĕ-rēn′) [Gustave *Roussy*, French pathologist, 1874–1948; Joseph Jules *Dejerine*, French neurologist, 1849–1917] thalamic syndrome.

**Rous·sy-Lé·vy syndrome (hereditary areflexic dystasia)** (roo-se′ la-ve′) [Gustave *Roussy;* Gabrielle *Lévy*, French neurologist, 1886–1935] see under *syndrome*.

**Rou·vière's node** (roo-vyārz′) [Henri *Rouvière*, French anatomist and embryologist, 1875–1952] see under *node*.

**Roux-en-Y (anastomosis, operation)** (roo-en-wi, Fr. roo″ahn-e-grek′) [César *Roux*, Swiss surgeon, 1857–1926] see under *anastomosis*.

**Ro·vi·ghi's sign** (ro-ve′gēz) [Alberto *Rovighi*, Italian physician, 1856–1919] see under *sign*.

**Rov·sing's procedure, sign, syndrome** (rov′singz) [Niels Thorkild *Rovsing*, Danish surgeon, 1862–1927] see under *procedure*, *sign*, and *syndrome*.

**Ro·wa·sa** (row-a′sə) trademark for a preparation of mesalamine.

**Rox·a·nol** (rok′sə-nol) trademark for a preparation of morphine sulfate.

**rox·ar·sone** (rok-sahr′sōn) [USP] an arsenical used in veterinary practice for the treatment of coccidiosis and necrotic enteritis in poultry and for the treatment of swine dysentery.

**Rox·i·co·done** (rok-se-ko′dōn) trademark for a preparation of oxycodone hydrochloride.

**RPF** renal plasma flow.

**R Ph** abbreviation for Registered Pharmacist.

**RPLND** retroperitoneal lymph node dissection; see under *lymphadenectomy*.

**rpm** revolutions per minute.

**RPS** renal pressor substance.

**RQ** respiratory quotient.

**RRA** Registered Record Administrator.

**-rrhage** [Gr. *rhegnynai* to burst forth.] a word termination denoting abnormal or excessive flow. Also, *-rrhagia*.

**-rrhagia** see *-rrhage*.

**-rrhaphy** [Gr. *rhaphē* suture] a word termination denoting suture or operative repair.

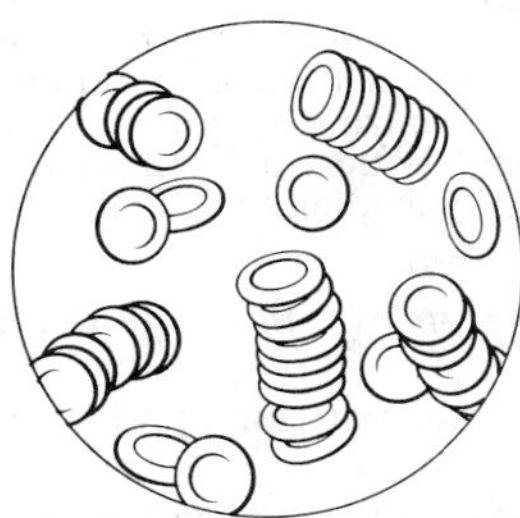

Human red blood cells arranged in rouleaux.

**-rrhea** [Gr. *rhoia* flow] a word termination denoting flow or discharge.

**-rrhexis** [Gr. *rhēxis* from *rhēgnynai* to burst] a word termination denoting the action or process of breaking, rupturing, or splitting.

**-rrhoea** see *-rrhea.*

**rRNA** ribosomal RNA; see under *RNA.*

**RSA** right sacroanterior (position of the fetus).

**RScA** right scapuloanterior (position of the fetus).

**RSCN** Registered Sick Children's Nurse.

**RScP** right scapuloposterior (position of the fetus).

**RSM** Royal Society of Medicine.

**RSNA** Radiological Society of North America.

**RSP** right sacroposterior (position of the fetus).

**RST** right sacrotransverse (position of the fetus).

**RSTMH** Royal Society of Tropical Medicine and Hygiene.

**RSV** Rous sarcoma virus; respiratory syncytial virus.

**RTA** renal tubular acidosis.

**RTF** resistance transfer factor.

**Ru** symbol for *ruthenium.*

**RU-486** mifepristone.

**rub** (rub) 1. to move something over a surface with friction. 2. the action of such movement. 3. friction r.
**friction r.,** an auscultatory sound caused by the rubbing together of two serous surfaces, as in a pericardial rub or pleural friction rub; called also *rub.*
**pericardial r., pericardial friction r.,** a scraping or grating noise heard with the heart beat, usually a to-and-fro sound, associated with pericarditis or other pathological condition of the pericardium.
**pleural r., pleural friction r.,** a rub produced by friction between the visceral and costal pleurae. Called also *pleuritic r.*
**pleuritic r.,** pleural r.

**Ru·barth's disease** (roo'bahrts) [Sven *Rubarth,* Swedish veterinarian, 20th century] hepatitis contagiosa canis; see under *hepatitis.*

**rub·ber** (rub'ər) 1. an elastic material made from the milky latex of any of various trees of the genera *Hevea* and *Ficus.* 2. a synthetic product resembling this material.
**polysulfide r.,** an elastomeric synthetic rubber used in dentistry as an impression material for fixed partial prosthodontic structures, inlays for single quadrants, and dental impressions.

**ru·be·fa·cient** (roo"bə-fa'shənt) [*ruber* + *-facient*] 1. reddening the skin. 2. an agent that reddens the skin by producing active or passive hyperemia.

**ru·bel·la** (roo-bel'ə) [L. from *rubellus* reddish, from *ruber* red] [MeSH: Rubella] an acute, usually benign, infectious disease caused by a togavirus and most often affecting children and nonimmune young adults, in which the virus enters the respiratory tract via droplet nuclei and spreads to the lymphatic system. It is characterized by a slight cold, sore throat, and fever, followed by enlargement of the postauricular, suboccipital, and cervical lymph nodes, and the appearance of a fine pink rash that begins on the head and spreads to become generalized. Transplacental infection of the fetus as a result of maternal infection in the first trimester can cause death of the conceptus or severe developmental abnormalities in the newborn infant (see *congenital rubella syndrome,* under *syndrome*). Called also *German measles* and *three-day measles.* In French and Spanish the word *rubeola* is used for this disease.

**Ru·bens flap** (roo'bənz) [Peter Paul *Rubens,* Flemish painter, 1577–1640] see under *flap.*

**ru·be·o·la** (roo-be'o-lə, roo-be-o'lə) [dim. of L. *rubeus* red] 1. measles. 2. French and Spanish term for *rubella.*

**ru·be·o·sis** (roo"be-o'sis) redness.
**r. i'ridis,** a condition characterized by a new formation of vessels and connective tissue on the surface of the iris, frequently seen in diabetics *(r. i'ridis diabe'tica)* and following occlusion of the central retinal vein or artery. It gives rise to severe intractable glaucoma.
**r. re'tinae,** a name proposed for a condition characterized by formation of new vessels in front of the optic papilla in retinitis proliferans, seen in nondiabetics, as well as in diabetics *(r. re'tinae diabe'tica),* and usually leading to retinal detachment.

**ru·ber** (roo'bər) [L.] red.

**ru·bes·cent** (roo-bes'ənt) [L. *rubescere* to become red] reddish; becoming red.

**Ru·bex** (roo'beks) trademark for a preparation of doxorubicin hydrochloride.

**ru·bid·i·um** (roo-bid'e-əm) [L. *rubidus* red] [MeSH: Rubidium] a rare metallic alkaline element; atomic number, 37; atomic weight, 85.47; symbol, Rb.
**r. 82,** a radioactive isotope of rubidium, atomic mass 82, having a half-life of 1.273 minutes; it decays by positron emission (3.15 MeV) and is used as a tracer in positron emission tomography.
**r. and ammonium bromide,** a substance, $RbBr + 3NH_4Br$, used like potassium bromide.
**r. chloride Rb 82** [USP], the chloride salt of $^{82}Rb$, used for positron emission tomography in the diagnosis of cardiac disease; administered intravenously.

**ru·bid·o·my·cin** (roo-bid'o-mi"sin) daunorubicin.

**ru·big·i·nous, ru·big·i·nose** (roo-bij'ĭ-nəs, roo-bij'ĭ-nōs) [L. *rubigo* rust] having a rusty, brownish color; said of sputum.

**Ru·bin's test** (roo'binz) [Isidor Clinton *Rubin,* American physician, 1883–1958] see under *test.*

**ru·bin** (roo'bin) fuchsin.

**Ru·bin·stein's syndrome** (roo'bin-stīnz) [Jack Herbert *Rubinstein,* American pediatrician, born 1925] see under *syndrome.*

**Ru·bin·stein-Tay·bi syndrome** (roo'bin-stīn-ta'be) [J.H. *Rubinstein;* Hooshang *Taybi,* American radiologist, born 1919] [MeSH: Rubinstein-Taybi Syndrome] see under *syndrome.*

**Ru·bi·vi·rus** (roo'bĭ-vi"rəs) [L. *rubeus* red + *virus*] [MeSH: Rubivirus] rubella virus; a genus of viruses of the family Togaviridae containing the causative agent of rubella.

**Ru·bu·la·vi·rus** (roo'bu-ləvi"rəs) [L. *rubula inflans* mumps] a genus of viruses of the subfamily Paramyxovirinae (family Paramyxoviridae) containing a number of species that cause disease in humans and other animals.

**Rub·ner's law, test** (roob'nərz) [Max *Rubner,* German physiologist, 1854–1932] see under *law* and *test.*

**ru·bor** (roo'bor) [L.] redness, one of the cardinal signs of inflammation.

**Ru·bra·tope-57** (roo'brə-tōp) trademark for a preparation of cyanocobalamin Co 57.

**ru·bra·tox·in** (roo'brətok"sin) a mycotoxin found in *Penicillium purpurogenum* and *P. rubrum,* which contaminate corn and can cause hepatotoxicity in livestock.

**ru·bri·blast** (roo'brĭ-blast) proerythroblast.

**ru·bric** (roo'bric) red; specifically, pertaining to the red nucleus.

**ru·bri·cyte** (roo'brĭ-sīt) [L. *rubrum* red + *-cyte*] polychromatophilic erythroblast.

**ru·bro·spi·nal** (roo"bro-spi'nəl) pertaining to the red nucleus and the spinal cord.

**ru·bro·tha·lam·ic** (roo"bro-thə-lam'ik) pertaining to the red nucleus and the thalamus.

**Ru·bus** (roo'bəs) [L.] a genus of prickly plants of the family Rosaceae, including brambles, raspberries, and blackberries. The root barks of several species of blackberry are tonic and astringent, and have been used in diarrhea. *R. idae'us* L. and *R. strigo'sus* Michx. are varieties of raspberry (q.v.).

**ruc·tus** (ruk'təs) [L.] eructation.

**Rud's syndrome** (roodz) [Einar *Rud,* Danish physician, born 1892] see under *syndrome.*

**ru·di·ment** (roo'dĭ-mənt) 1. primordium. 2. a structure that has remained undeveloped, or one with little or no function at present but which was functionally developed earlier either in the individual or in its phylogenetic ancestors.
**lens r.,** see under *placode.*
**r. of vaginal process,** vestigium processus vaginalis.

**ru·di·men·ta·ry** (roo"dĭ-men'tə-re) 1. imperfectly developed. 2. vestigial.

**ru·di·men·tum** (roo"dĭ-men'təm) pl. *rudimen'ta* [L. "a first beginning"] 1. primordium. 2. a vestigial structure.
**r. processus vaginalis,** vestigium processus vaginalis.

**Ru·di·mi·cro·spo·rea** (roo"dĭ-mi"kro-spor'e-ə) [*rudiment* + *micro-* + *spore*] a class of protozoa (phylum Microspora) found as hyperparasites of gregarines in annelids, the spores of which have a simple extrusion apparatus consisting of a polar cap and a thick polar tube extending backward from the cap, bending laterally and terminating in an infundibulum; a polaroplast and posterior vacuole are absent. It comprises one order: Metchnikovellida.

**rue** (roo) [L. *Ruta*] 1. *Ruta graveolens.* 2. any of various plants that resemble *R. graveolens.*
**African r.,** *Peganum harmala.*

**Ru·fen** (roo'fən) trademark for preparations of ibuprofen.

**Ruf·fi·ni's corpuscle (brush, cylinder, ending, organs)** (roo-fe'nēz) [Angelo *Ruffini,* Italian anatomist, 1864–1929] see under *corpuscle.*

**ru·fous** (roo'fəs) [L. *rufus* red] erythristic.

**ru·ga** (roo'gə) pl. *ru'gae* [L.] a ridge, wrinkle, or fold, as of mucous membrane.
**rugae gas'tricae,** rugae of stomach.
**ru'gae palati'nae, palatine rugae,** plicae palatinae transversae.
**rugae of stomach,** large folds of the mucous membrane of the stomach, occurring especially in the corpus, which are seen when the stomach is empty or undistended.
**rugae of vagina, ru'gae vagina'les** [TA], small transverse folds of the mucous membrane of the vagina extending outward from the columns.
**ru'gae vesi'cae bilia'ris,** TA alternative for *plicae mucosae vesicae biliaris.*

**ru·gae** (roo'je) [L.] plural of *ruga.*

**Rug·ge·ri's reflex (sign)** (roo-jār'ēz) [Ruggero *Ruggeri,* Italian physician, 1823–1905] see under *reflex.*

**ru·gine** (roo-zhēn') a raspatory.

**ru·gi·tus** (roo'jĭ-təs) [L. "roaring"] rumbling in the intestines caused by movement of flatus; see *borborygmus.*

**ru·gose** (roo'gōs) [L. *rugosus*] characterized by wrinkles.

**ru·gos·i·ty** (roo-gos'ĭ-te) [L. *rugositas*] 1. the condition of being wrinkled. 2. a fold, wrinkle, or ruga.

**ru·gous** (roo'gəs) [L. *rugosus*] rugose.

**Ru·ka·vi·na type familial amyloid polyneuropathy (syndrome)** (roo-kah-vi'nah) [John G. *Rukavina,* American physician, 20th century] Indiana type familial amyloid polyneuropathy; see under *polyneuropathy.*

**RUL** right upper lobe; see *lobus superior pulmonis dextri.*

**rule** (ro͞ol) [L. *regula*] a statement of conditions commonly observed in a given situation, or a statement of a prescribed course of action to obtain a result. Cf. *law.*
**Allen's r.,** the extended body parts of warm-blooded species (tail, ears, and limbs) are relatively shorter in the colder regions of a species range than in the warmer.
**Arey's r.,** the total length of an embryo or fetus in inches, for the first five months, equals the numerical sum of the number of the previous lunar months since conception; for the last five lunar months, it equals the product of the number of the month multiplied by 2.
**Bartholomews' r. of fourths,** if the uterine fundus is one-fourth of the way from the pubic symphysis to the umbilicus, the pregnancy is of two months' duration; one-half of the way, three months' duration; three-quarters of the way, four months' duration; at the umbilicus, five months' duration. The fundus then rises one-quarter of the way to the ensiform process each month until the ninth, when it sinks to the level it occupied at eight months.
**Bastedo's r.,** the dose of a drug for a child is obtained by multiplying the adult dose by the child's age in years, adding 3 to the product, and dividing the sum by 30.
**Bergmann's r.,** the body size of geographic races of warm-blooded species is smaller in the warmer parts of the species range than in the colder parts of the range.
**r. of bigeminy,** bigeminy tends to be self-perpetuating because the premature complexes both precipitate and are caused by long cardiac cycles.
**Budin's r.,** a bottle-fed baby should not take more than 10 per cent of its own weight of cow's milk per day.
**Cahn-Ingold-Prelog sequence r's,** in chemistry, a set of rules used to determine the absolute configuration of chiral molecules by assigning priority rankings to the atoms attached to a chiral center. Atoms directly attached to the chiral center are ranked in order of decreasing atomic number; if these are alike then the groups incorporating the atoms are ranked using the site of difference nearest the chiral center, with identical groups ranked on the basis of their nearest neighbors. Multiple bonds are treated as if the atoms of the bond are replicated once for each extra bond. Isotopes are ranked by descending atomic mass. See also *E-, Z-, R-,* and *S-.*
**Clark's r.,** the dose of a drug for a child is obtained by multiplying the adult dose by the weight of the child in pounds and dividing the result by 150.
**Cowling's r.,** the dose of a drug for a child is obtained by multiplying the adult dose by the age of the child at his next birthday and dividing by 24.
**delivery date r.,** Nägele's r.
**dermatomal r.,** the theory that visceral pain is referred to the dermatomes supplied by the posterior roots through which the visceral afferent impulses reach the spinal cord.
**Durham r.,** a definition of criminal responsibility from a 1954 federal court of appeals case, Durham vs. United States; the court held that "an accused is not criminally responsible if his unlawful act was the product of mental disease or mental defect." In 1972 the same court reversed itself and adopted the American Law Institute formulation (see under *formulation*).
**Fried's r.,** the dose of a drug for an infant less than 2 years old is obtained by multiplying the child's age in months by the adult dose and dividing the result by 150.
**Goodsall's r.,** a guide to classification of anal fistulas; those with external openings in the posterior half of the perianal area usually originate in the posterior half of the anus and those with external openings in the anterior perineum usually originate in the anterior quadrant of the anus.
**Haase's r.,** the total length of an embryo or fetus in centimeters, for the first five months, equals the square of the number of lunar months since conception; for the last five months it equals the product of the number of the month multiplied by 5.
**Hardy-Weinberg r.,** see under *law.*
**Hudson's lactone r.,** molecular optical rotation of a carbohydrate or its derivatives is given as the sum of the rotation contributions at each asymmetric center. Certain other empirical conclusions may also be drawn from existing data.
**Jackson's r.,** see under *law.*
**Liebermeister's r.,** in febrile tachycardia, the pulse beats increase at the rate of about eight per minute to every degree centigrade of temperature.
**Lossen's r.,** in hemophilia, only women transmit the condition, only men inherit it.
**McDonald's r.,** the length in centimeters of the abdominal contour from the upper margin of the pubic symphysis to the fundus of the uterus, divided by 3.5, gives the duration of pregnancy in lunar months; applicable only after the sixth month of pregnancy.
**M'Naghten r.,** a definition of criminal responsibility formulated in 1843 by English judges questioned by the House of Lords as a result of the acquittal of Daniel M'Naghten on grounds of insanity. It holds that "to establish a defense on the ground of insanity, it must be clearly proved that, at the time of committing the act, the party accused was laboring under such a defect of reason, from disease of the mind, as not to know the nature and quality of the act he was doing, or, if he did know it, he did not know he was doing what was wrong" and further that a defendant who "labors under partial delusions only and is not in other respects insane . . . must be considered in the same situation as to responsibility as if the facts with respect to which the delusion exists were real." These rules are still used in many American jurisdictions.
**Nägele's r.,** to predict the first day of labor and confinement, subtract three months from one year after the first day of the last menstruation and add seven days.
**r. of nines,** a method of estimating the extent of body surface that has been burned in an adult; the body surface is divided into sections of 9 per cent or multiples of 9 per cent. See accompanying table. For children the Lund-Browder classification may be used.
**octet r.,** when atoms combine to form molecules, they tend to share or transfer electrons until eight (four pairs) are in the valence shell of each atom.
**phase r.,** a heterogeneous chemical system of *p* coexistent phases and *c* variable components has $c - p + 2$ degrees of freedom or variations of phase, i.e., the sum of its coexistent phases and its possible changes of phase exceeds the number of its components by 2.
**Pitres' r.,** see under *law.*
**Rolleston's r.,** the ideal systolic pressure for an adult is the figure represented by 100 plus half the age in years.
**van't Hoff's r.,** the velocity of chemical reactions is increased twofold or more for each rise of 10°C in temperature; it is generally true when temperatures approximate those under which the reaction normally occurs. Called also *van't Hoff's law.* See also *temperature coefficient,* under *coefficient.*
**Weinberg's r.,** the total number of dizygotic twins in any population

**Rule of Nines**

| Region | Percentage of Body Surface |
|---|---|
| Head and neck | 9% |
| Anterior trunk | 18% |
| Posterior trunk | 18% |
| Left arm | 9% |
| Right arm | 9% |
| Left leg | 18% |
| Right leg | 18% |
| Genitalia and perineum | 1% |

is twice the number of twins of different sex, and the sum of these subtracted from the total number of all twins gives the number of monozygotic twins.

**Young's r.,** the dose of a drug for a child is obtained by multiplying the adult dose by the age in years and dividing the result by the sum of the child's age plus 12.

**ru·men** (roo'mən) [MeSH: Rumen] the first stomach of a ruminant, consisting of a huge sac lined by a mucous membrane, with several subdivisions, where partially chewed food is stored prior to rumination. Called also *paunch.*

**ru·men·i·tis** (roo″mə-ni'tis) inflammation of the rumen.

**ru·men·ot·o·my** (roo″mə-not'ə-me) [*rumen* + *-tomy*] surgical incision of the rumen of an animal to remove a foreign body or impacted food or to evacuate gases.

**ru·mi·nal** (roo'mĭ-nəl) pertaining to the rumen.

**ru·mi·nant** (roo'mĭ-nənt) [MeSH: Ruminants] 1. any of the suborder Ruminantia (order Artiodactyla), hoofed mammals that have four stomachs (the *rumen, reticulum, omasum,* and *abomasum*), through which the food passes in digestion. It includes cattle, sheep, goats, deer, and antelopes. 2. chewing the cud.

**Ru·mi·nan·tia** (roo″mĭ-nan'she-ə) the ruminants, a suborder of mammals of the order Artiodactyla.

**ru·mi·na·tion** (roo″mĭ-na'shən) [L. *ruminare* to think over] 1. in ruminants, the casting up of food (called *cud*) out of the rumen and chewing of it a second time; called also *cudding.* 2. in humans, the regurgitation of food after almost every meal, part of it being vomited and the rest swallowed: a condition sometimes seen in infants *(rumination disorder)* or in mentally retarded individuals. 3. meditation.

**ru·mi·na·tive** (roo'mĭ-nə″tiv) characterized by rumination; constantly dwelling on certain topics or ideas.

**Ru·mi·no·coc·cus** (roo″mĭ-no-kok'əs) [L. *ruminalis* of the rumen + *coccus*] a genus of anaerobic, gram-positive bacteria of the family Peptococcaceae, occurring as spherical to elongated cocci, which are involved in the fermentation of cellulose in the rumens of cattle and sheep.

**ru·mi·no·re·tic·u·lar** (roo″mĭ-no-rə-tik'u-lər) reticuloruminal.

**rump** (rump) the buttock or gluteal region.

**Rum·pel-Leede phenomenon (sign, test)** (room'pəl-lēd) [Theodor *Rumpel,* German physician, 1862–1923; Carl Stockbridge *Leede,* American physician, 1882–1964] see under *phenomenon.*

**Run·dles-Falls syndrome** (run'dəlz-fawlz) [Ralph Wayne *Rundles,* American internist, born 1911; Harold Francis *Falls,* American ophthalmologist and geneticist, born 1909] hereditary sideroblastic anemia.

**runt** (runt) a young animal with growth retardation.

**Run·yon classification, group** (run'yən) [Ernest H. *Runyon,* American microbiologist, 20th century] see under *classification.*

**ru·pia** (roo'pe-ə) [Gr. *rhypos* filth] thick, dark, raised, lamellated, adherent crusts on the skin somewhat resembling oyster shells, as in late recurrent secondary syphilis.

**ru·pi·al** (roo'pe-əl) pertaining to or resembling rupia.

**ru·pi·oid** (roo'pe-oid) resembling rupia.

**rup·ture** (rup'chər) [MeSH: Rupture] 1. forcible tearing or disruption of tissue. 2. to forcibly disrupt tissue. 3. hernia.

**defense r.,** a breaking down of the body's defense against infection, such as is seen when silica particles inhaled by a worker break down the resistance against tuberculosis.

**Rus·co·ni's anus** (roo-sko'nēz) [Mauro *Rusconi,* Italian biologist, 1776–1849] the blastopore.

**Rush** (rush) Benjamin (1745–1813). American physician and statesman, born in Philadelphia; he was the first professor of chemistry at the College of Philadelphia and wrote the first American book on chemistry. Rush was a Surgeon General in the Continental Army and physician to Pennsylvania Hospital, where he introduced clinical instruction; he was the founder of the Philadelphia Dispensary (the first in America), founder of the Philadelphia College of Physicians, and professor of the Institutes of Medicine (i.e., physiology and pathology) and Clinical Medicine at the University of Pennsylvania. Rush was the first American to investigate mental illness, to write on cholera infantum, and to notice focal infection in teeth; he was a founder of experimental physiology; and he also wrote on alcoholism, personal hygiene, and public health and on the great yellow fever epidemic in Philadelphia (1793). Rush's views on that epidemic (that it originated locally and was not imported) and his treatment of the sufferers (excessive purging and blood letting) caused controversy and lawsuits.

**rush** (rush) a powerful wave of contractile activity that travels long distances down the small intestine; it is caused by intense irritation or unusual distention. Called also *peristaltic reflex.*

**Rus·sell's bodies** (rus'əlz) [William *Russell,* Scottish physician, 1852–1940] see under *body.*

**Rus·sell's dwarf, syndrome (dwarfism)** (rus'əlz) [Alexander *Russell,* British pediatrician, 20th century] see under *dwarf* and see *Silver-Russell syndrome,* under *syndrome.*

**Rus·sell effect** (rus'əl) [William James *Russell,* English chemist, 1830–1909] see under *effect.*

**Russell traction** (rus'əl) [R. Hamilton *Russell,* Australian surgeon, 1860–1933] see under *traction.*

**Rus·sell's viper, viper venom** (rus'əlz) [Patrick *Russell,* English physician in Syria, 1727–1805] see under *viper* and *venom.*

**Rus·sell-Sil·ver syndrome (dwarf·ism)** (rus'əl-sil'vər) [A. *Russell;* Henry K. *Silver,* American pediatrician, born 1918] Silver-Russell syndrome.

**Rus·so's reaction (test)** (roo'sōz) [Mario *Russo,* Italian physician, late 19th century] see under *reaction.*

**Rust's disease, phenomenon (sign), syndrome** (roosts) [Johann Nepomuk *Rust,* Austrian surgeon, 1775–1840] see under *disease, phenomenon,* and *syndrome.*

**rust** (rust) 1. iron oxide or hydroxide, forming a reddish deposit on metallic iron where the latter has been exposed to moisture; also a similar deposit on other metals that have been exposed to dampness. 2. a fungus of the order Uredinales, members of which cause the plant disease also called rust. 3. a fungal disease of plants, caused by members of the class Uredinales and characterized by the formation of spots on their skin that resemble the rust of metals.

**rut** (rut) [L. *rugitus* roaring] 1. the period or season of heightened sexual activity in some male mammals that coincides with the season of estrus in the females. 2. estrus.

**Ru·ta** (roo'tə) a genus of strong-scented flowering herbs of the family Rutaceae, native to Europe and Asia. *R. graveo'lens* is rue, a species whose leaves contain oil that is an irritant poison.

**ru·the·ni·um** (roo-the'ne-əm) [MeSH: Ruthenium] a rare, very hard metallic element; symbol, Ru; atomic weight, 101.07; atomic number, 44.

**Ruth·er·ford's theory** (ruth'ər-fordz) [William *Rutherford,* Scottish physiologist, 1839–1899] frequency theory

**ruth·er·ford** (ruth'ər-ford) [Sir Ernest *Rutherford,* British physicist, 1871–1937] the unit representing one million disintegrations of radioactive matter per second. Abbreviated rd.

**ru·ti·do·sis** (roo″tĭ-do'sis) rhytidosis.

**ru·tin** (roo'tin) [MeSH: Rutin] a bioflavonoid (q.v.) obtained from buckwheat and other plants.

**Ru·val·ca·ba's syndrome** (roo″vahl-ka'bahz) [R.H. *Ruvalcaba,* American physician, born 1934] see under *syndrome.*

**Ruysch's glomeruli, membrane,** etc. (roish'əz) [Frederic *Ruysch,* Dutch anatomist, 1638–1731] see *glomeruli renis* and *lamina choroidocapillaris,* and see under *muscle* and *tube.*

**ruysch·ian membrane** (roi'she-an) [Frederic *Ruysch*] see under *membrane.*

**RV** residual volume.

**RVA** rabies vaccine adsorbed.

**RVAD** right ventricular assist device.

**RVH** right ventricular hypertrophy; see *ventricular hypertrophy,* under *hypertrophy.*

**Rye classification** (ri) [*Rye,* New York, where a conference in 1965 adopted the classification] see under *classification.*

**rye** (ri) [MeSH: Rye] 1. *Secale cereale.* 2. the seed of *S. cereale,* which is used as food and can grow a fungus that is the source of ergot.

**spurred r.,** see *ergot,* def. 1.

**Ryle's tube** (rīlz) [John Alfred *Ryle,* British physician, 1889–1950] see under *tube.*

**Ryth·mol** (rith'mol) trademark for a preparation of propafenone hydrochloride.

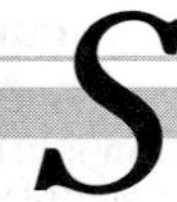

**S** symbol for *sulfur, sacral vertebrae* (S1 through S5), *siemens, smooth* (colony), *spherical lens, substrate,* and *Svedberg unit.*

**S.** abbreviation for L. *sig'na,* mark; see *prescription* and *signature,* def. 1.

***S*** symbol for *entropy.*

**S-** [L. *sinister* left] a stereodescriptor used to specify the absolute configuration of compounds having asymmetric carbon atoms. See *R-*.

**$S_1$** first heart sound; see under *sound.*

**$S_2$** second heart sound; see under *sound.*

**$S_3$** third heart sound; see under *sound* and see *gallop rhythm* under *rhythm.*

**$S_4$** fourth heart sound; see under *sound* and see *gallop rhythm* under *rhythm.*

**$S_f$** Svedberg flotation unit.

**s** symbol for *second.*

**s.** abbreviation for L. *sinis'ter* (left) and *semis (half).*

**s̄** abbreviation for L. *si'ne,* without.

***s*** symbol for *sample standard deviation.*

**$s^{-1}$** reciprocal second; $ms^{-1}$ is equivalent to m/s.

**Σ** the Greek capital letter sigma; used in mathematics to indicate a sum;

$$\sum_{i=1}^{n} x_i = x_1 + x_2 + x_3 + \ldots + x_n.$$

***σ*** sigma, the eighteenth letter of the Greek alphabet; symbol for *standard deviation.*

**SA** sinoatrial.

**S.A.** abbreviation for L. *secun'dum ar'tem,* according to art.

**Sa·bin's vaccine** (sa'binz) [Albert Bruce *Sabin,* Russian-born American virologist 1906–1993] live oral poliovirus vaccine; see under *vaccine.*

**Sa·bin-Feld·man syndrome** (sa'bin-feld'mən) [A. B. *Sabin;* Henry Alfred *Feldman,* American epidemiologist, born 1914] see under *syndrome.*

**sab·i·nism** (sab'ĭ-niz-əm) poisoning by savin.

**sab·i·nol** (sab'ĭ-nol) a terpene alcohol from the evergreen shrub *Juniperus sabina* L. which is the chief constituent of savin oil; see also *savin.*

**Sab·ou·raud's dextrose agar** (sah-boo-rōz') [Raymond Jacques Adrien *Sabouraud,* French dermatologist, 1864–1938] see under *culture medium.*

**Sab·ou·rau·di·tes** (sab"oo-ro-di'tēz) *Microsporum.*

**Sa·bril** (sa'bril) trademark for a preparation of vigabatrin.

**sab·u·lous** (sab'u-ləs) [L. *sabulosus; sabulum* sand] gritty or sandy.

**sa·bur·ra** (sə-bur'ə) [L.] foulness of the stomach, mouth, or teeth.

**sa·bur·ral** (sə-bur'əl) [L. *saburra* sand] pertaining to or of the nature of sordes, or of foulness of the stomach.

**sac** (sak) [L. *saccus;* Gr. *sakkos*] a baglike organ or structure; see also *pouch, saccus,* and *saccule.*
**abdominal s.,** a serous sac in the embryo which develops into the abdominal cavity.
**air s.,** 1. in birds, one of the air-filled cavities connected with the air passages of the lungs and usually with cavities in the bones; they assist in respiration and lower the body's specific gravity. Domestic fowl have one or two unpaired sacs and three symmetrically arranged pairs including cranial, thoracic, and abdominal pairs. 2. (in plural) sacculi alveolares.
**allantoic s.,** the dilated portion of the allantois which becomes a part of the placenta in many mammals.
**alveolar s's,** sacculi alveolares.
**amniotic s.,** the sac formed by the amnion; popularly known as the *bag of waters.*
**anal s.,** in carnivores, either of two sacs found between the internal and external anal sphincters, lined with sebaceous glands and in some species with apocrine glands.
**aneurysmal s.,** the chamber of a sacculated aneurysm.
**aortic s.,** the homologue in mammalian embryos of the ventral aorta, from which arise the series of aortic arches.
**chorionic s.,** the chorion of a mammal.
**conjunctival s.,** saccus conjunctivalis.
**dental s.,** a concentric layer of connective tissue in which the enamel organ and dental papilla are embedded, which completely surrounds the developing tooth after the epithelial attachment that connects the enamel organ with the dental lamina disintegrates. Called also *sacculus dentis.*
**embryonic s.,** blastocyst.
**enamel s.,** the enamel organ during the stage in which its outer layer forms a sac enclosing the whole dental germ.
**endolymphatic s.,** saccus endolymphaticus.
**epiploic s.,** omental bursa.
**gestation s.,** the extraembryonic membranes that envelop the embryo or fetus; in man, the fused amnion and chorion.
**greater s. of peritoneum,** the peritoneum of the peritoneal cavity proper.
**heart s.,** pericardium.
**hernial s.,** the pouch of peritoneum enclosing a hernia.
**Hilton's s.,** sacculus laryngis.
**lacrimal s.,** saccus lacrimalis.
**lesser s. of peritoneal cavity,** omental bursa.
**Lower's s's,** the bulbus inferior venae jugularis and bulbus superior venae jugularis.
**omental s.,** omental bursa.
**pericardial s.,** pericardium.
**pleural s.,** cavitas pleurae.
**serous s.,** the sac made up of the pleura, pericardium, and peritoneum.
**splenic s.,** recessus splenicus.
**tear s.,** saccus lacrimalis.
**vitelline s.,** yolk s.
**yolk s.,** the extraembryonic membrane that connects with the midgut; at the end of the fourth week of development it expands into the pear-shaped *umbilical vesicle* connected to the body of the embryo by the long narrow *yolk stalk.* In marsupial and placental mammals, it produces a complete vitelline circulation in the early embryo and then undergoes regression; in oviparous vertebrates, it encloses the yolk mass, breaks down yolk, and makes it available to the developing organism. In human embryos it does not serve a primary nutritive function, but it is the first hematopoietic organ of the embryo. Called also *vitelline s.*

**sac·brood** (sak'brōōd) an infectious disease of the larvae of bees, caused by a virus.

**sac·cade** (sə-kād') [Fr. "jerking"] [MeSH: Saccades] the series of involuntary, abrupt, rapid, small movements or jerks of both eyes simultaneously in changing the point of fixation on a visualized object, such as the series of jumps the eyes make in scanning a line of print. See also *saccadic movement* under *movement.*

**sac·cad·ic** (sə-kad'ik) pertaining to a saccade.

**sac·cate** (sak'āt) [L. *saccatus*] 1. shaped like a sac. 2. contained in a sac.

**sac·cha·rate** (sak'ə-rāt) a salt of a saccharide.

**sac·char·eph·i·dro·sis** (sak"ər-ef"ĭ-dro'sis) [*sacchar-* + Gr. *ephidrōsis* sweating] the discharge of sugar in the sweat.

**sac·char·ic ac·id** (sə-kar'ik) older term used for (1) glucaric acid and (2) any dicarboxylic sugar acid.

**sac·cha·ride** (sak'ə-rīd) one of a series of carbohydrates, including the sugars. The saccharides are divided into monosaccharides, oligosaccharides, and polysaccharides, according to the number of monosaccharide groups ($C_nH_{2n}O_{n-1}$) composing them.

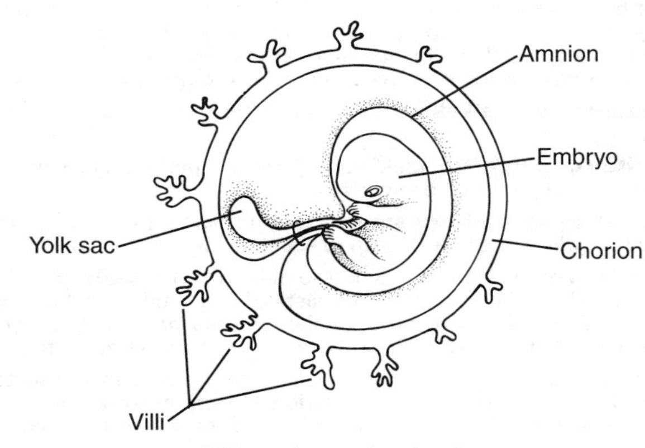

Yolk sac (six week embryo).

**sac·char·i·fi·ca·tion** (sə-kar″ĭ-fĭ-ka′shən) [*sacchar-* + L. + *facere* to make] conversion of starch into sugar.

**sac·cha·rim·e·ter** (sak″ə-rim′ə-tər) [*sacchar-* + *-meter*] a device for estimating the proportion of sugar in a solution. It may be either a polarimeter, a hydrometer, or a closed container in which the volume of $CO_2$ produced by fermentation may be assayed.

**sac·cha·rin** (sak′ə-rin) [NF] [MeSH: Saccharin] a white crystalline compound, several hundred times sweeter than sucrose; used as a sweetening agent in pharmaceutical preparations.
**s. calcium** [USP], the calcium salt of saccharin, used as a non-nutritive sweetener when sugar is contraindicated.
**s. sodium** [USP], the sodium salt of saccharin, used like the calcium salt.

**sac·cha·rine** (sak′ə-rīn) [Gr. *sakcharon* sugar] sugary; having a sweet taste.

**sac·char·i·nol** (sə-kar′ĭ-nol) saccharin.

**sac·cha·ri·num** (sak″ə-ri′nəm) saccharin.

**sacchar(o)-** [L. *saccharum,* from Gr. *sakcharon* sugar] a combining form denoting relationship to sugar.

**sac·cha·ro·co·ria** (sak″ə-ro-kor′e-ə) abhorrence of sugar.

**sac·cha·ro·lyt·ic** (sak″ə-ro-lit′ik) [*saccharo-* + *-lytic*] capable of breaking the glycosidic bonds in saccharides.

**sac·cha·ro·me·ta·bol·ic** (sak″ə-ro-met″ə-bol′ik) pertaining to the metabolism of sugar.

**sac·cha·ro·me·tab·o·lism** (sak″ə-ro-mə-tab′o-liz-əm) [*saccharo-* + *metabolism*] the metabolism of sugar.

**sac·cha·rom·e·ter** (sak″ə-rom′ə-tər) saccharimeter.

**Sac·cha·ro·my·ces** (sak″ə-ro-mi′sēz) [*saccharo-* + Gr. *mykēs* fungus] [MeSH: Saccharomyces] a genus of yeasts, fungi of the family Saccharomycetaceae. Many species formerly put in this genus have now been classified elsewhere.
**S. al′bicans, S. an′ginae,** former names for *Candida albicans.*
**S. baya′nus,** *S. pastorianus.*
**S. carlsbergen′sis,** a species used in microbiological assay in measuring vitamin $B_6$ in the urine, and in the brewing of beer; it has been implicated in a few cases of mycosis of the stomach.
**S. cerevi′siae,** brewers' yeast or bakers' yeast, a species with oval or spherical cells, used for alcoholic fermentation and leavening in bread; it occasionally causes lung disease.
**S. dairen′sis,** a species with oval or elliptical cells that produces a fermentation in milk; called also *S. galacticolus.*
**S. ellipsoi′deus,** a species that forms elliptical cells that are solitary or in branching chains; it causes alcoholic fermentation in wines.
**S. exi′guus,** a form in beer yeast, whose cells are elliptical and solitary, or in branching chains; it causes late fermentation in beer.
**S. fra′gilis,** a species that is sometimes part of the normal flora of the human throat and gastrointestinal tract but can also cause opportunistic infection.
**S. galacti′colus,** *S. dairensis.*
**S. glu′tinis,** *Rhodotorula glutinis.*
**S. granulomato′sus,** *Cryptococcus neoformans.*
**S. guttula′tus,** *Saccharomycopsis guttulatus.*
**S. hanse′nii,** *Debaryomyces hansenii.*
**S. mesente′ricus,** *Candida mesenterica.*
**S. mycoder′ma,** *Candida vini.*
**S. neofor′mans,** *Cryptococcus neoformans.*
**S. pastoria′nus,** a species from fermenting wine and beer; it has been implicated in a few cases of mycosis of the stomach. Called also *S. bayanus.*

**sac·cha·ro·my·ces** (sak″ə-ro-mi′sēz) pl. *saccharomyce′tes* [MeSH: Saccharomyces] An organism of the genus *Saccharomyces.*

**Sac·cha·ro·my·ce·ta·ceae** (sak″ə-ro-mi″sə-ta′se-e) a family of fungi of the order Endomycetales, including unicellular yeasts that reproduce sexually by formation of ascospores; it includes the genera *Hansenula, Saccharomyces,* and *Saccharomyccopsis.*

**sac·cha·ro·my·ce·tes** (sak″ə-ro-mi-se′tēz) plural of *saccharomyces.*

**sac·cha·ro·my·cet·ic** (sak″ə-ro-mi-set′ik) pertaining to or due to the presence of saccharomycetes.

**sac·cha·ro·my·ce·tol·y·sis** (sak″ə-ro-mi″sə-tol′ĭ-sis) [*saccharomycetes* + *-lysis*] the splitting up of saccharomycetes.

**Sac·cha·ro·my·cop·sis** (sak″ə-ro-mi-kop′sis) [MeSH: Saccharomycopsis] a genus of perfect yeasts of the family Saccharomycetaceae. *S. guttula′tus* (formerly called *Saccharomyces guttulatus*) is found in the intestines of herbivores and can cause enteritis.

**sac·cha·ro·pine** (sak′ə-ro-pēn″) an intermediate in the metabolism of lysine, formed by condensation of lysine and α-ketoglutarate; it accumulates abnormally in some disorders of lysine degradation.

**sac·cha·ro·pine de·hy·dro·gen·ase (NAD⁺, L-glu·ta·mate-form·ing)** (sak′ə-ro-pēn″ de-hi′dro-jən-ās gloo′tə-māt form′ing) [EC 1.5.1.9] an enzyme activity that catalyzes oxidative cleavage of saccharopine to form α-aminoadipate semialdehyde and glutamate, using $NAD^+$ as an electron acceptor. The reaction is the second step in the major route of lysine degradation; the enzyme activity is part of the bifunctional enzyme α-aminoadipic semialdehyde synthase (q.v.). The enzyme activity is absent in hyperlysinemia and the variant saccharopinuria.

**sac·cha·ro·pine de·hy·dro·gen·ase (NADP⁺, L-ly·sine-form·ing)** (sak′ə-ro-pēn″ de-hi′dro-jən-ās li′sēn form′ing) [EC 1.5.1.8] an enzyme activity that catalyzes the condensation of L-lysine and α-ketoglutarate to form saccharopine, using NADPH as an electron donor. The reaction is the initial step in the major route of lysine degradation; the enzyme activity is part of the bifunctional enzyme α-aminoadipic semialdehyde synthase (q.v.). The enzyme activity is absent in hyperlysinemia and substantially reduced in the variant saccharopinuria. Usually called *lysine ketoglutarate reductase.*

**sac·cha·ro·pin·emia** (sak″ə-ro-pĭ-ne′me-ə) an excess of saccharopine in the blood, as in hyperlysinemia or saccharopinuria.

**sac·cha·ro·pin·uria** (sak″ə-ro-pĭ-nu′re-ə) 1. excretion of saccharopine in the urine. 2. a variant form of hyperlysinemia due to partial deficiency of α-aminoadipic semialdehyde synthase activity; the activity of saccharopine dehydrogenase ($NAD^+$, L-glutamate-forming) is absent, but substantial saccharopine dehydrogenase ($NADP^+$, L-lysine-forming) activity is retained. It is clinically similar to hyperlysinemia but with higher urinary saccharopine and lower lysine.

**sac·ci** (sak′si) genitive and plural of *saccus.*

**Sac·cha·rum** (sak′ə-rəm) a genus of plants of the family Gramineae. *S. officina′rum* L. is sugar cane, a major commercial source of sugar (sucrose).

**sac·ci·form** (sak′sĭ-form) [*saccus* +*form*] shaped like a sac or bag.

**sac·cu·lar** (sak′u-lər) shaped like a sac.

**sac·cu·lat·ed** (sak′u-lāt″əd) [L. *sacculatus*] characterized by sacculation or by the presence of saccules.

**sac·cu·la·tion** (sak″u-la′shən) 1. a sacculus, or pouch. 2. the quality of being sacculated, or pursed out with little pouches.
**s's of colon,** haustra coli.

**sac·cule** (sak′ūl) [L. *sacculus*] sacculus.
**air s's, alveolar s's,** sacculi alveolares.
**laryngeal s., s. of larynx,** sacculus laryngis.

**sac·cu·li** (sak′u-li) [L.] genitive and plural of *sacculus.*

**sac·cu·li·tis** (sak″u-li′tis) inflammation of a small sac or saccule.
**anal s.,** inflammation of the anal sacs, usually accompanied by an infection.

**sac·cu·lo·coch·le·ar** (sak″u-lo-kok′le-ər) pertaining to the sacculus and cochlea.

**sac·cu·lus** (sak′u-ləs) gen. and pl. *sac′culi* [L., dim. of *saccus*] 1. a little pouch or sac. 2. [TA] saccule: the smaller of the two divisions of the membranous labyrinth within the vestibule; it communicates with the cochlear duct by way of the ductus reuniens.
**sac′culi alveola′res,** alveolar saccules: the spaces into which the alveolar ducts open distally, and with which the alveoli communicate; called also *alveolar sacs.*

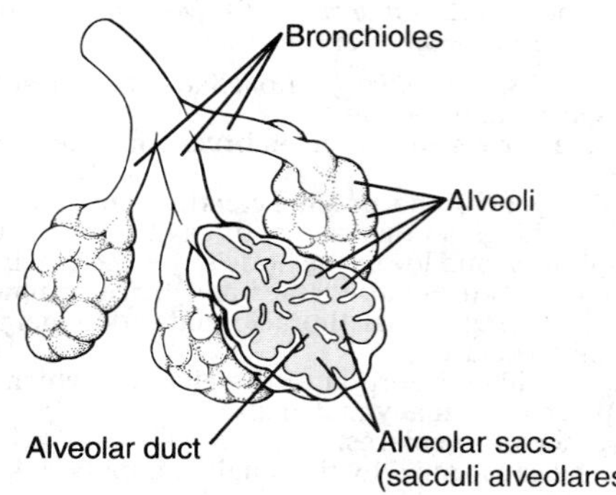


**sacculi of Beale,** periluminal; hepatic duct; entrapped in benign sclerotic processes, e.g. sclerosing cholangitis.
**s. den′tis,** dental sac.
**s. laryn′gis** [TA], laryngeal saccule: a diverticulum extending upward from the front of the laryngeal ventricle, between the vestibular fold medially and the thyroarytenoid muscle and thyroid cartilage laterally; called also *appendage* or *appendix of ventricle of*

*larynx, appendix ventriculi laryngis, Hilton's sac,* and *laryngeal pouch* or *saccule.*

**sac·cus** (sak'əs) gen. and pl. *sac'ci* [L.; Gr. *sakkos*] [TA] sac: general anatomical nomenclature for a saclike or pouchlike structure.
**s. an'ticus,** one of the four pouches in the fetal middle ear, later developing into the anterior recess of the tympanic membrane.
**s. conjunctiva'lis** [TA], conjunctival sac: the potential space, lined by conjunctiva, between the eyelids and the eyeball.
**s. endolympha'ticus** [TA], endolymphatic sac: the blind, flattened cerebral end of the endolymphatic duct. Called also *Böttcher's space.*
**s. lacrima'lis** [TA], lacrimal sac: the dilated upper end of the nasolacrimal duct.
**s. me'dius,** one of the four pouches in the fetal middle ear, later subdividing to form the epitympanum and the region of the petrous part of the temporal bone.
**s. pos'ticus,** one of the four pouches in the fetal middle ear, later developing into the round window, oval window, and sinus tympani.
**s. profun'dus perine'i** [TA], deep perineal pouch: the region superior (deep) to the perineal membrane and extending into the pelvis; called also *spatium profundum perinei* [TA alternative] and *deep perineal space.*
**s. subcuta'neus perine'i** [TA], subcutaneous perineal pouch: a potential space between the membranous layer of the perineal subcutaneous tissue and the superficial layer of the fascia of the perineal muscles.
**s. supe'rior,** one of the four pouches in the fetal middle ear, later developing into the posterior recess of the tympanic membrane, part of the mastoid process, and the space below the incus.

**SACH** solid ankle cushion heel; see under *foot.*

**Sachs' disease** (saks) [Bernard Parney *Sachs,* American neurologist, 1858–1944] see *Tay-Sachs disease,* under *disease.*

**sa·crad** (sa'krad) toward the sacrum, or sacral aspect.

**sa·cral** (sa'krəl) [L. *sacralis*] pertaining to or situated near the sacrum.

**sa·cral·gia** (sa-kral'jə) [*sacr-* + *-algia*] pain in the sacrum.

**sa·cral·iza·tion** (sa″krəl-ĭ-za'shən) anomalous fusion of the fifth lumbar vertebra to the first segment of the sacrum, so that the sacrum consists of six segments.

**sa·crar·thro·gen·ic** (sa″krahr-thro-jen'ik) [*sacr-* + *arthro-* + *-genic*] resulting from disease of a sacral joint.

**sa·crec·to·my** (sa-krek'tə-me) [*sacr-* + *-ectomy*] excision or resection of the sacrum.

**sac·ri·fice** (sak'rĭ-fīs) to kill an experimental animal.

**sacr(o)-** [L. *sacrum,* q.v.] a combining form denoting relationship to the sacrum.

**sa·cro·an·te·ri·or** (sa″kro-an-te're-or) having the sacrum directed forward; see under *position.*

**sa·cro·coc·cy·ge·al** (sa″kro-kok-sij'e-əl) pertaining to or located in the region of the sacrum and coccyx.

**sa·cro·coc·cyx** (sa″kro-kok'siks) the sacrum and coccyx together.

**sa·cro·cox·al·gia** (sa″kro-kok-sal'jə) pain in the sacroiliac joint.

**sa·cro·cox·itis** (sa″kro-kok-si'tis) [*sacro-* + *coxa* + *-itis*] inflammation of the sacroiliac joint.

**sa·cro·dyn·ia** (sa″kro-din'e-ə) [*sacro-* + *-odynia*] pain in the sacral region.

**sa·cro·il·i·ac** (sa″kro-il'e-ak) pertaining to the sacrum and ilium; denoting the joint or articulation between the sacrum and ilium and the ligaments associated therewith.

**sa·cro·il·i·itis** (sa″kro-il″e-i'tis) inflammation (arthritis) in the sacroiliac joint.

**sa·cro·lis·the·sis** (sa″kro-lis-the'sis) the condition in which the sacrum lies anterior to the fifth lumbar vertebra.

**sa·cro·lum·bar** (sa″kro-lum'bər) [*sacro-* + *lumbar*] pertaining to the sacrum and the loin.

**sa·cro·peri·ne·al** (sa″kro-per″ĭ-ne'əl) pertaining to the sacrum and the perineum.

**sa·cro·pos·te·ri·or** (sa″kro-pos-te're-or) having the sacrum directed backward; see under *position.*

**sa·cro·prom·on·to·ry** (sa″kro-prom'ən-tor-e) the promontory of the sacrum.

**sa·cro·sci·at·ic** (sa″kro-si-at'ik) pertaining to the sacrum and the ischium.

**sa·cro·spi·nal** (sa″kro-spi'nəl) [*sacro-* + *spinal*] pertaining to the sacrum and the spine, or vertebral column.

**sac·ro·spi·nous** (sa″kro-spi'nəs) sacrospinal.

**sa·crot·o·my** (sa-krot'ə-me) [*sacro-* + *-tomy*] the operation of cutting into the lower end of the sacrum.

**sa·cro·trans·verse** (sa″kro-trans-vərs') relating to the direction of the fetal sacrum in breech presentation; see under *position.*

**sa·cro·uter·ine** (sa″kro-u'tər-in) pertaining to the sacrum and the uterus.

**sa·cro·ver·te·bral** (sa″kro-ver'tə-brəl) pertaining to the sacrum and the vertebral column.

**sa·crum** (sa'krəm) [L. "sacred"] [MeSH: Sacrum] the triangular bone just below the lumbar vertebrae; see *os sacrum* [TA]. See illustration.
**assimilation s.,** see *assimilation pelvis,* under *pelvis.*
**scimitar s.,** a congenitally deformed sacrum shaped like a scimitar, usually accompanied by other defects such as anorectal or neural anomalies.
**tilted s.,** a condition marked by separation of the sacroiliac joint and forward displacement of the sacrum.

**sac·to·sal·pinx** (sak″to-sal'pinks) [Gr. *saktos* stuffed + *salpinx*] dilatation of the inflamed uterine tube by retained secretions.

**SAD** seasonal affective disorder.

**sad·dle** (sad'əl) 1. a support whose shape fits the contour of the object resting upon it. 2. a saddle-shaped structure or part. 3. denture base s.
**denture base s.,** that part of a complete or partial denture which rests upon the basal seat and to which the teeth are attached. Called also *saddle.* See also *denture base,* under *base.*

**sa·dism** (sa'diz-əm, sad'iz-əm) [Comte Donatien Alphonse François, Marquis de *Sade,* French novelist, 1740–1814] [MeSH: Sadism] the act or instance of gaining pleasure from inflicting physical or psychological pain on another; the term is usually used to denote *sexual s.*
**anal s.,** in freudian theory, the destructive and aggressive manifestations of anal erotism, such as aggressiveness, selfishness, and stinginess.
**oral s.,** in freudian theory, a sadistic form of oral erotism manifested by fantasies of chewing, biting, or otherwise using the mouth, lips, or teeth aggressively or destructively.
**phallic s.,** in freudian theory, the aggressive and destructive tend-

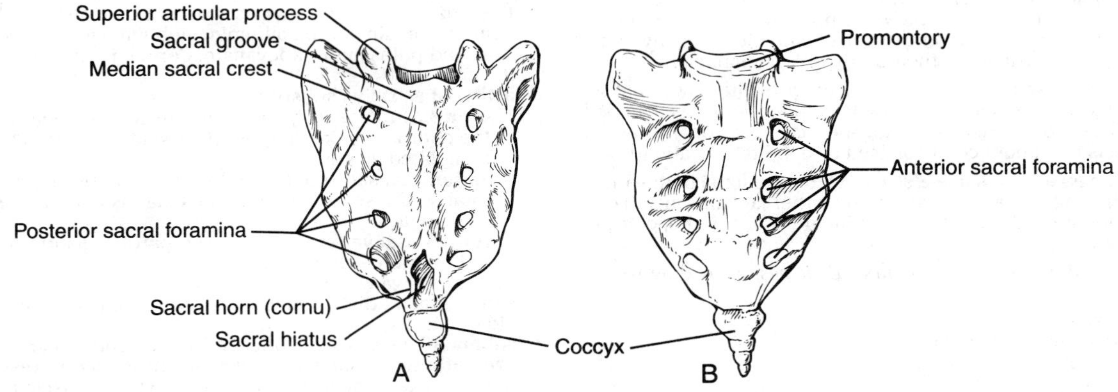


Doral *(A)* and pelvic *(B)* surfaces of the sacrum.

encies associated with the childhood phallic stage of development, stemming from the child's interpretation of sexual intercourse as aggressive and violent.
**sexual s.** [DSM-IV], a paraphilia in which sexual gratification is derived from hurting, humiliating, or otherwise inflicting physical or psychological suffering on another.

**sa·dist** (sa'dist) one who practices sadism.

**sa·dis·tic** (sə-dis'tik) pertaining to or characterized by sadism.

**sa·do·ma·so·chism** (sa"do-mas'ə-kiz-əm) a state characterized by both sadistic and masochistic tendencies.

**sa·do·ma·so·chis·tic** (sa"do-mas"ə-kis'tik) characterized by both sadism and masochism.

**SADS** Schedule for Affective Disorders and Schizophrenia.

**St. John's wort** (sānt jonz wort) [NF] any of various species of the genus *Hypericum; H. perforatum* is the medicinal herb, which is used as a mild antidepressant, sedative, and anxiolytic; it is also used topically for inflammation of the skin, contusions, myalgia, and first-degree burns.

**Sae·misch's operation (section), ulcer** (sa'mish-əz) [Edwin Theodor *Saemisch,* German ophthalmologist, 1833–1909] see under *operation,* and see *ulcus serpens corneae.*

**Saeng·er's macula** (sāng'erz) [Max *Saenger,* German obstetrician in Prague, 1853–1903] see *macula gonorrhoeica.*

**Saeng·er's sign (reflex)** (sāng'erz) [Alfred *Saenger,* German neurologist, 1861–1921] see under *sign.*

**Saethre-Chot·zen syndrome** (sa'trə-kot'zən) [Haakon *Saethre,* Norwegian psychiatrist, 20th century; F. *Chotzen,* German psychiatrist, 20th century] Chotzen's syndrome.

**Saff** (saf) trademark for a preparation of safflower oil.

**Saf·flor** (saf'lor) trademark for a preparation of safflower oil.

**saf·flow·er** (saf'low-ər) *Carthamus tinctorius.*

**safranin O** (saf'rə-nin) a basic red aniline dye used as a nuclear stain and as a counterstain in Gram's method. Spelled also *safranine O.*

**saf·role** (saf'rol) [MeSH: Safrole] a methylene ether obtained from sassafras oil, formerly used as an anodyne and flavoring but now restricted because it is carcinogenic.

**saf·ro·sin** (saf'ro-sin) bluish eosin.

**sage** (sāj) *Salvia officinalis,* an herb whose leaves contain a volatile oil and are sudorific, carminative, and astringent; the dried leaves are used as an antisecretory agent in hyperhidrosis, sialorrhea, pharyngitis, and bronchitis.

**sag·it·tal** (saj'ĭ-təl) [L. *sagittalis; sagitta* arrow] 1. shaped like or resembling an arrow; straight. 2. situated in the plane of the sagittal suture or parallel to it; said of an anteroposterior plane or section parallel to the median plane of the body.

**sag·it·ta·lis** (saj"ĭ-ta'lis) [TA] sagittal: a general term denoting a structure situated in the plane of or parallel to the sagittal suture.

**sa·go** (sa'go) a starch mainly derived from the pith of various species of palm, chiefly of the genus *Sagus.*

**Sah·li's method** (zah'lēz) [Herman *Sahli,* Swiss physician, 1856–1933] acid hematin method.

**Saint's triad** (sānts) [Charles Frederick Morris *Saint,* South African radiologist, 20th century] see under *triad.*

**Sa·ka·ti-Ny·han syndrome** (sah'kah-te-ni'han) [Nadia *Sakati,* American pediatrician, 20th century; William Leo *Nyhan,* American pediatrician, born 1926] acrocephalopolysyndactyly, type III.

**Sak·mann** (zahk'mahn) Bert. German cell physiologist, born 1942. Co-winner with Erwin Neher of the Nobel prize for medicine or physiology in 1991 for their work on cellular communications involving electrical signals, particularly their study of ion channels.

**Sak·se·naea** (sak"sə-ne'ə) a genus of fungi of the family Saksenaeaceae, characterized by coenocytic hyphae and flask-shaped sporangia. *S. vasifor'mis* is a soil saprobe that occasionally causes mucormycosis in immunocompromised or debilitated patients.

**Sak·se·naea·ceae** (sak"sən-e-a'se-e) a family of fungi of the order Mucorales, having sporangia that may be either lageniform and columellate or lobate and acolumellate; it includes one pathogenic genus, *Saksenaea.*

**S.A.L.** abbreviation for L. *secun'dum ar'tis le'ges,* according to the rules of art.

**sal** (sal) [L.] salt.
**s. ammoniac,** ammonium chloride.
**s. diure'ticum,** potassium acetate.
**s. so'da,** sodium carbonate.
**s. vola'tile,** ammonium carbonate.

**Sala's cells** (sah'lahz) [Luigi *Sala,* Italian zoologist, 1863–1930] see under *cell.*

**Sal·a·gen** (sal'ə-jən) trademark for a preparation of pilocarpine hydrochloride.

**sal·a·man·der** (sal"ə-man'dər) [Gr. *salamandra* a kind of lizard] [MeSH: Urodela] any member of the order Caudata, tailed amphibians often used in experiments.

**sal·a·man·der·in** (sal"ə-man'dər-in) a poisonous base from the skin of a species of salamander.

**sal·an·tel** (sal'ən-təl) a veterinary anthelmintic.

**sal·a·zo·sul·fa·pyr·i·dine** (sal"ə-zo-sul"fə-pir'ĭ-dēn) sulfasalazine.

**sal·bu·ta·mol** (sal-bu'tə-mol) INN for albuterol.

**sal·i·cyl·amide** (sal"ĭ-səl-am'īd) an amide of salicylic acid used as an analgesic and antipyretic, administered orally.

**sal·i·cyl·an·i·lide** (sal"ĭ-səl-an'ĭ-līd) any of several compounds usually prepared by the interaction of salicylic acid and aniline; some are anthelmintics and others are topical antifungal agents. See *bromsalans, closantel, niclosamide, oxyclozanide,* and *rafoxanide.*

**sal·i·cyl·ate** (sal"ĭ-sil'āt, sə-lis'ə-lāt) a salt, ester of salicylic acid (e.g., methyl salicylate), or salicylate ester of an organic acid (e.g., aspirin, acetylsalicylic acid); such compounds have analgesic, antipyretic, and anti-inflammatory activity; they act by inhibiting prostaglandin synthesis.

**sal·i·cyl·at·ed** (sal'ĭ-sil"āt-əd) containing or impregnated with salicylic acid.

**sal·i·cyl·a·zo·sul·fa·pyr·i·dine** (sal"ĭ-sil"ə-zo-sul"fə-pir'ĭ-dēn) sulfasalazine.

**sal·i·cyl·emia** (sal"ĭ-sə-le'me-ə) [*salicylate* + *-emia*] the presence of salicylate in the blood.

**sal·i·cyl·ic** (sal"ĭ-sil'ik) pertaining to the radical salicyl.

**sal·i·cyl·ic ac·id** (sal'ĭ-sil'ik) [USP] orthohydroxybenzoic acid, obtained from the bark of the white willow and wintergreen leaves, and also prepared synthetically; it has bacteriostatic, fungicidal, and keratolytic actions; its salts, the salicylates, are used as analgesics.

**sal·i·cyl·ism** (sal'ĭ-sil"iz-əm) the commonly occurring toxic effects of excessive dosage with salicylic acid or its salts, usually marked by tinnitus, nausea, and vomiting.

**sal·i·cyl·sul·fon·ic ac·id** (sal"ĭ-səl-sul-fon'ik) sulfosalicylic acid.

**sal·i·cyl·ur·ic ac·id** (sal"ĭ-səl-ūr'ik) the glycine conjugate of salicylic acid, a form in which salicylates are excreted in the urine.

**sal·i·fi·a·ble** (sal'ĭ-fi"ə-bəl) [*sal* + L. *fieri* to become] capable of combining with acids so as to form salts.

**sal·i·fy** (sal'ĭ-fi) to convert into a salt.

**sa·lim·e·ter** (sə-lim'ə-tər) [*sal* + *-meter*] a hydrometer for ascertaining the concentration of saline solutions.

**sa·line** (sa'lēn, sa'līn) [L. *salinus; sal* salt] salty; of the nature of a salt; containing a salt or salts.
**physiological s.,** an isotonic aqueous solution of NaCl for temporarily maintaining living cells.

**sal·i·nom·e·ter** (sal"ĭ-nom'ə-tər) an instrument (hydrometer) for direct reading of the salt content of a liquid.

**sal·i·no·my·cin** (sal"in-o-mi'sin) an antibiotic produced by *Streptomyces albus*; used as a coccidiostat in poultry.

**sa·li·va** (sə-li'və) [L.] [MeSH: Saliva] the clear, alkaline, somewhat viscid secretion from the parotid, submaxillary, sublingual, and smaller mucous glands of the mouth. It serves to moisten and soften the food, keeps the mouth moist, and contains α-amylase, a digestive enzyme which converts starch into maltose. The saliva also contains mucin, serum albumin, globulin, leukocytes, epithelial debris, and potassium thiocyanate. Certain toxins frequently occur in it.
**artificial s.,** saliva substitute.
**chorda s.,** submaxillary saliva produced in response to stimulation of the chorda tympani nerve, less viscid and turbid than that of the unstimulated gland.
**ganglionic s.,** saliva obtained by irritating the submaxillary gland.
**lingual s.,** the secretion of Ebner's glands and other serous glands of the tongue.
**parotid s.,** saliva produced by the parotid gland; thinner and less viscid than the other varieties.
**ropy s.,** saliva which is highly viscid.
**sublingual s.,** that produced by the sublingual gland, the most viscid of all.
**submaxillary s.,** that produced by the submaxillary gland.
**sympathetic s.,** submaxillary saliva produced in response to stimulation of its sympathetic nerve supply; more viscid and turbid than that of the unstimulated gland.

**sal·i·vant** (sal'ĭ-vənt) provoking a flow of saliva.

**sa·li·va·ria** (sal″ĭ-var'e-ə) in some systems of classification, a group or section comprising those trypanosomes in which the developmental cycle is completed in the salivary glands (anterior station) of the vector and transmission is usually by inoculation through the hypopharynx. The group includes the subgenera *Duttonella, Nannomonas,* and *Trypanozoon.* Cf. *stercoraria.*

**sal·i·var·i·an** (sal″ĭ-var'e-ən) pertaining to or caused by trypanosomes of the salivaria group or section.

**sal·i·vary** (sal'ĭ-var-e) [L. *salivarius*] pertaining to the saliva.

**sal·i·vate** (sal'ĭ-vāt) to produce an excessive flow of saliva.

**sal·i·va·tion** (sal″ĭ-va'shən) [L. *salivatio*] [MeSH: Salivation] 1. the secretion of saliva. 2. ptyalism.

**sal·i·va·tor** (sal'ĭ-va″tor) an agent that causes salivation.

**sal·i·va·to·ry** (sal'ĭ-və-to″re) causing salivation.

**Salk vaccine** (sawk) [Jonas Edward *Salk,* American physician and virologist, 1914–1995] see under *vaccine.*

**Sal·kow·ski's test** (sahl-kof'skēz) [Ernst Leopold *Salkowski,* German physiologic chemist, 1844–1923] see under *test.*

**sal·met·er·ol xin·a·fo·ate** (sal-met'ər-ol) a bronchodilator used for maintenance treatment of asthma and prevention of exercise-induced bronchospasm; administered by inhalation.

**sal·min** (sal'min) a toxic substance derived from the sperm of salmon.

**Sal·mo·nel·la** (sal″mo-nel'ə) [Daniel Elmer *Salmon,* American pathologist, 1850–1914] [MeSH: Salmonella] a genus of gram-negative, facultatively anaerobic bacteria of the family Enterobacteriaceae, made up of nonspore-forming rods, usually motile with peritrichous flagella. They utilize citrate as a sole carbon source and generally ferment glucose but not sucrose or lactose. The genus is separated into species or serotypes on the basis of O (somatic), Vi (capsular), and H (flagellar) antigens (Kauffman-White scheme). The somatic antigen is the basis for separation into serogroups not contained in another group. Agglutination tests with pooled (polyvalent) antisera for groups A through E and Vi antigen can detect 95 per cent of the serotypes isolated from humans and lower animals; approximately 2400 serotypes that cause illness in humans have been identified. The H antigen of *Salmonella* is biphasic, designated as phase 1 (specific) or phase 2 (nonspecific). Serotypes are identified by antigenic formulae, taking the general form O antigen: phase 1⇄ phase 2, in which the O antigens are designated by numerals, the phase 1 antigens by lowercase letters, and the phase 2 antigens by numerals. Clinical laboratories frequently report salmonellae as one of three species, differentiated on the basis of serologic and biochemical reactions: *S. typhi, S. choleraesuis,* and *S. enteritidis;* the last contains all serotypes except the first two (Ewing scheme). Numerous strains familiarly named as species are thus designated as serotypes of *S. enteritidis.* For taxonomic purposes the salmonellae are grouped in five subgenera on the basis of biochemical characteristics and are separated into species on the basis of antigenic reactions. The subgenera and selected representative serovars are: subgenus I (containing most serotypes), *S. choleraesuis, S. hirschfeldii, S. typhi, S. paratyphi-A, S. schottmuelleri, S. typhimurium, S. enteritidis,* and *S. gallinarum;* subgenus II, *S. salamae;* subgenus III, *S. ariyonae;* subgenus IV, *S. houtenae;* and subgenus V, *S. bongor.* The genus contains pathogenic species causing enteric fevers (typhoid and paratyphoid), septicemias, and gastroenteritis. The most frequent clinical manifestation is food poisoning. *Salmonella* species are widely distributed in lower animals, frequently producing disease.
**S. abor'tus e'qui,** *S. enteritidis* serotype *abortus equi.*
**S. abor'tus o'vis,** *S. enteritidis* serotype *abortus ovis.*
**S. ago'na,** *S. enteritidis* serotype *agona.*
**S. arizo'nae,** a species originally found in reptiles, which also occurs in fowl and other domestic animals, and has been isolated from dried egg powder and other food sources. Ingestion of contaminated food produces gastroenteritis and enteric fever (salmonellosis); the organisms can also cause bacteremias and local infections. The organisms may ferment lactose rapidly. The members of this species are frequently classified in a separate genus, *Arizona.*
**S. bon'gor,** the type species of subgenus V.
**S. choleraesu'is,** a group C species, pathogenic for man and animals. It is found as a secondary invader in hog cholera and has been associated with paratyphoid, gastroenteritis, and septicemia in humans. Called also *Bacterium choleraesuis* and *S. suipestifer.* See also *suipestifer.*
**S. choleraesu'is** var. **ku'zendorf,** a strain associated with paratyphoid gastroenteritis; seen with increasing frequency in the United States.
**S. choleraesu'is** var. **typhisu'is,** a strain pathogenic for pigs that may infect humans.
**S. dub'lin,** *S. enteritidis* serotype *dublin.*
**S. enteri'tidis,** a species containing group A, B, C, and D serotypes, occurring frequently in humans and animals. It comprises more than 1500 different serotypes, known also by their individual names, which may produce paratyphoid fever, septicemia, and gastroenteritis. Called also *Gärtner bacillus.*
**S. enteri'tidis** serotype **abor'tus e'qui,** a group B serotype causing infectious abortion in mares; not found in other animals. Called also *S. abortus equi.*
**S. enteri'tidis** serotype **abor'tus o'vis,** a group B serotype causing abortion in sheep.
**S. enteri'tidis** serotype **ago'na,** a group B serotype sometimes isolated in the United States. Called also *S. agona.*
**S. enteri'tidis** serotype **dub'lin,** a group C serotype frequently isolated from cattle, sheep, and pigs in the United States and northern Europe; it causes septicemia, enteritis, and abortion.
**S. enteri'tidis** serotype **gallina'rum,** a group $D_1$ serotype, the causative agent of fowl typhoid; it has little or no pathogenicity for humans. It is nonmotile and contains somatic O antigen but no H antigen. Called also *S. gallinarum.*
**S. enteri'tidis** serotype **hei'delberg,** a group B serotype frequently isolated in the United States. Called also *S. heidelberg.*
**S. enteri'tidis** serotype **hirschfel'dii,** a group C serotype, closely related to strains of *S. choleraesuis;* it is the etiologic agent of human paratyphoid fever in parts of Asia, Africa, and northeastern Europe and is reported as an important cause of illness and death in Guyana. Called also *S. hirschfeldii* and *S. paratyphi C.*
**S. enteri'tidis** serotype **infan'tis,** a group C serotype sometimes isolated in the United States. Called also *S. infantis.*
**S. enteri'tidis** serotype **new'port,** a group C serotype, one of the most common types isolated in the United States. Called also *S. newport.*
**S. enteri'tidis** serotype **paraty'phi A,** a group A serotype causing mild paratyphoid fever in humans; it is one of the most frequent causes of the disease in India. Called also *S. paratyphi* and *S. paratyphi A.*
**S. enteri'tidis** serotype **pullo'rum,** the causative agent of pullorum disease in chickens; serologically identical with *S. enteritidis* serotype *gallinarum.* Called also *S. pullorum.*
**S. enteri'tidis** serotype **schottmuel'leri,** a group B serotype, the most common cause of paratyphoid fever in the northern United States and northern Europe. Some strains also infect animals. Called also *S. paratyphi B* and *S. schottmuelleri.*
**S. enteri'tidis** serotype **sen'dai,** a group D serotype found in Japan and the Far East.
**S. enteri'tidis** serotype **typhimu'rium,** a group B serotype, a parasite of rats and mice, a serotype frequently isolated in the United States and northern Europe; the most frequent agent of food poisoning, it also causes paratyphoid fever, and recurrent fevers and diarrhea are seen in immunocompromised patients. Called also *S. typhimurium.*
**S. gallina'rum,** *S. enteritidis* serotype *gallinarum.*
**S. hei'delberg,** *S. enteritidis* serotype *heidelberg.*
**S. hirschfel'dii,** *S. enteritidis* serotype *hirschfeldii.*
**S. hou'tenae,** the type species of subgenus IV.
**S. infan'tis,** *S. enteritidis* serotype *infantis.*
**S. morga'ni,** *Morganella morganii.*
**S. new'port,** *S. enteritidis* serotype *newport.*
**S. paraty'phi,** *S. enteritidis* serotype *paratyphi A.*
**S. paraty'phi A,** *S. enteritidis* serotype *paratyphi A.*
**S. paraty'phi B,** *S. enteritidis* serotype *schottmuelleri.*
**S. paraty'phi C,** *S. enteritidis* serotype *hirschfeldii.*
**S. pullo'rum,** *S. enteritidis* serotype *pullorum.*
**S. sala'mae,** the type species of subgenus II, a group D serotype originally isolated in Dar-es-Salaam, Tanzania. Called also *Dar es Salaam bacterium.*
**S. schottmuel'leri,** *S. enteritidis* serotype *schottmuelleri.*
**S. sen'dai,** *S. enteritidis* serotype *sendai.*
**S. suipes'tifer,** *S. choleraesuis.*
**S. ty'phi,** a group D serotype, a strict parasite of humans and the cause of typhoid fever. Strains containing the Vi (virulence) antigen are designated V strains; those that have partially lost Vi antigen, V-W strains; and those that do not contain Vi antigen, W strains. The species is also subdivided into phage types on the basis of susceptibility to empirically numbered bacteriophages. The organism is transmitted by water or food contaminated by human excreta. Called also *typhoid bacillus.* Formerly called *Bacillus typhi, Bacillus typhosus, Eberthella typhi,* and *S. typhosa.*
**S. typhimu'rium,** *S. enteritidis* serotype *typhimurium.*
**S. typhisu'is,** *S. choleraesuis* var. *typhisuis.*
**S. typho'sa,** *S. typhi.*

**sal·mo·nel·la** (sal″mo-nel'ə) pl. *salmonel'lae* [MeSH: Salmonella] A bacterium of the genus *Salmonella.*

**sal·mo·nel·lal** (sal″mo-nel'əl) caused by salmonellae.

**Sal·mo·nel·leae** (sal″mo-nel'e-e) in some systems of classification, a tribe of gram-negative, facultatively anaerobic, rod-shaped bacteria of the family Enterobacteriaceae, made up of the genera *Arizona, Citrobacter,* and *Salmonella.*

**sal·mo·nel·lo·sis** (sal″mo-nəl-o′sis) any disease caused by infection with a species of *Salmonella;* in humans it is most often manifested as food poisoning with acute gastroenteritis, vomiting, diarrhea, and rarely septicemia, or as typhoid or paratyphoid fever. Recurrent fevers and diarrhea with more serious gastrointestinal symptoms are seen in immunocompromised patients. Salmonellal infections also cause abortions in horses and sheep and diarrhea and fowl typhus in chickens.

**sal·o·coll** (sal′o-kol) phenocoll salicylate, $C_2H_5O{\cdot}C_6H_4{\cdot}NH{\cdot}CO{\cdot}CH_2{\cdot}NH_2{\cdot}C_6H_4(OH)CO_2H$, a crystalline salt used as an antirheumatic.

**sa·lol** (sa′lol) phenyl salicylate.

**sal·pin·gec·to·my** (sal″pin-jek′tə-me) [*salping-* + *-ectomy*] surgical removal of the uterine tube; called also *tubectomy.*

**sal·pin·gem·phrax·is** (sal″pin-jəm-frak′sis) [*salping-* + *emphraxis*] obstruction of the auditory tube.

**sal·pin·gi·an** (sal-pin′je-ən) pertaining to the auditory or to the uterine tube.

**sal·pin·gi·on** (sal-pin′je-on) a point at the apex of the petrous bone on its lower surface.

**sal·pin·git·ic** (sal″pin-jit′ik) pertaining to or characterized by salpingitis.

**sal·pin·gi·tis** (sal″pin-ji′tis) [*salping-* + *-itis*] [MeSH: Salpingitis] 1. inflammation of the uterine tube. 2. inflammation of the auditory tube.
**chronic interstitial s.,** inflammation of the uterine tube associated with infiltration of mucosa, connective tissue, and muscle with lymphocytes and plasma cells.
**eustachian s.,** salpingitis, def. 2.
**hemorrhagic s.,** inflammation of the uterine tube associated with rupture of a blood vessel and effusion of blood.
**hypertrophic s.,** pachysalpingitis.
**s. isth′mica nodo′sa,** inflammation and nodular thickening of parts of both uterine tubes, usually of the isthmic and proximal ampullary portions; tubal epithelium is found within the myosalpinx or beneath the serosa, resulting from diverticula from the tubal lumen. Called also *nodular s.*
**mural s.,** pachysalpingitis.
**nodular s.,** s. isthmica nodosa.
**parenchymatous s.,** pachysalpingitis.
**s. pro′fluens,** inflammation of the uterine tube, with accumulation in its lumen of fluid that ultimately escapes.
**pseudofollicular s.,** inflammation of the uterine tube characterized by agglutination of its walls, causing a formation of saccules.
**purulent s.,** inflammation of the uterine tube attended with suppuration; called also *pyosalpingitis.*
**tuberculous s.,** infection of the uterine tube by the tubercle bacillus, *Mycobacterium tuberculosis.*

**salping(o)-** [Gr. *salpinx* tube] a combining form denoting relationship to a tube, specifically to the uterine or to the auditory tube.

**sal·pin·go·cele** (sal-ping′go-sēl) [*salpingo-* + *-cele*[2]] hernial protrusion of a uterine tube.

**sal·pin·gog·ra·phy** (sal″ping-gog′rə-fe) [*salpingo-* + *-graphy*] radiography of the uterine tubes after the injection of an opaque medium.

**sal·pin·go·li·thi·a·sis** (sal-ping″go-lĭ-thi′ə-sis) the presence of calcareous deposits in the wall of the uterine tubes.

**sal·pin·gol·y·sis** (sal″ping-gol′ĭ-sis) surgical lysis of adhesions involving the uterine tubes.

**sal·pin·go-ooph·o·rec·to·my** (sal-ping″go-o″of-ə-rek′tə-me) surgical removal of a uterine tube and ovary. Called also *ovariosalpingectomy, oophorosalpingectomy,* and *tubo-ovariotomy.*

**sal·pin·go-ooph·o·ri·tis** (sal-ping″go-o″of-ə-ri′tis) inflammation of a uterine tube and ovary.

**sal·pin·go-ooph·oro·cele** (sal-ping″go-o-of′ə-ro-sēl) hernia containing a uterine tube and ovary.

**sal·pin·go-oo·the·ci·tis** (sal-ping″go-o″o-the-si′tis) [*salpingo-* + *oothec-* + *-itis*] salpingo-oophoritis.

**sal·pin·go-oo·the·co·cele** (sal-ping″go-o″o-the′ko-sēl) [*salpingo-* + *ootheco-* + *-cele*[2]] salpingo-oophorocele.

**sal·pin·go-ovar·i·ec·to·my** (sal-ping″go-o-var″e-ek′tə-me) salpingo-oophorectomy.

**sal·pin·go-ovar·i·ot·o·my** (sal-ping″go-o-var″e-ot′o-me) salpingo-oophorectomy.

**sal·pin·go·peri·to·ni·tis** (sal-ping″go-per″ĭ-to-ni′tis) inflammation of the peritoneum covering the uterine tube.

**sal·pin·go·pexy** (sal-ping′go-pek″se) [*salpingo-* + *-pexy*] operative fixation of the uterine tube.

**sal·pin·go·pha·ryn·ge·al** (sal-ping″go-fə-rin′je-əl) pertaining to the auditory tube and the pharynx.

**sal·pin·go·plas·ty** (sal-ping′go-plas″te) [*salpingo-* + *-plasty*] plastic repair of the uterine tube; called also *tuboplasty.*

**sal·pin·gor·rha·phy** (sal″ping-gor′ə-fe) [*salpingo-* + *-rrhaphy*] suture of the fallopian tube.

**sal·pin·gos·co·py** (sal″ping-gos′kə-pe) visual inspection of a tube.

**sal·pin·go·sto·mat·o·my** (sal-ping″go-sto-mat′ə-me) [*salpingo-* + *stoma* + *-tomy*] surgical resection of a portion of the uterine tube, with creation of a new abdominal ostium.

**sal·pin·go·sto·mato·plas·ty** (sal-ping″go-sto-mat′o-plas″te) salpingostomatomy.

**sal·pin·gos·to·my** (sal″ping-gos′tə-me) [*salpingo-* + *-stomy*] [MeSH: Salpingostomy] 1. formation of an opening or fistula into a uterine tube. 2. surgical restoration of the patency of a uterine tube.

**sal·pin·got·o·my** (sal″ping-got′ə-me) [*salpingo-* + *-tomy*] surgical incision of a uterine tube.

**sal·pinx** (sal′pinks) [Gr.] 1. a tube. 2. TA alternative for *tuba uterina.*
**s. auditi′va,** tuba auditiva.
**s. uteri′na,** tuba uterina.

**sal·sa·late** (sal′sə-lāt) [USP] the salicylate ester of salicylic acid, which hydrolyzes in vivo to form salicylate; used for treatment of osteoarthritis and rheumatoid arthritis, administered orally.

**salt** (sawlt) [L. *sal;* Gr. *hals*] 1. sodium chloride, or common salt. 2. any compound of a base and an acid; any compound of an acid some of whose replaceable hydrogen atoms have been substituted. 3. in the plural, a saline purgative. See *magnesium sulfate* (Epsom s.), *sodium sulfate* (Glauber's s.), and *potassium sodium tartrate* (Preston's, Rochelle, or Seignette's s.).
**acid s.,** any salt in which the combining power of the acid is not completely exhausted.
**basic s.,** any salt with more than the normal proportion of the basic elements.
**bile s's,** glycine or taurine conjugates of bile acids that are formed in the liver and excreted in the bile; they are powerful detergents that disperse fat globules in the intestine, enabling fats to be digested and absorbed.
**bone s's,** the crystalline salts deposited in the organic matrix (principally collagen fibers) of bone, composed chiefly of calcium and phosphate.
**buffer s.,** a salt, such as sodium bicarbonate and sodium phosphate, the anion of which functions as a conjugate base in a buffer system.
**Carlsbad s.,** a mixture of sodium sulfate, potassium sulfate, sodium chloride, and sodium bicarbonate, used as a purgative.
**diuretic s.,** potassium acetate.
**double s.,** any salt in which the two hydrogen atoms of a dibasic acid have been replaced by two separate metals or basic radicals, as in potassium ammonium tartrate.
**Epsom s.,** magnesium sulfate.
**Glauber's s.,** sodium sulfate.
**halide s., haloid s.,** any binary compound of a metal or basic radical with a halogen—i.e., chlorine, iodine, bromine, fluorine.
**neutral s., normal s.,** any salt which is neither acidic nor basic in reaction.
**oral rehydration s's (ORS),** a solution of glucose, sodium chloride, potassium chloride, and either trisodium citrate or sodium bicarbonate used in oral rehydration therapy (q.v.).
**Preston's s., Rochelle s., Seignette's s.,** potassium sodium tartrate.
**smelling s's,** aromatized ammonium carbonate: stimulant and restorative.
**Wurster's s's,** the univalent oxidation products of the aromatic *p*-diamines. They are free radicals which may polymerize in a sufficiently concentrated solution and at low temperatures or in the solid state.

**sal·ta·tion** (sal-ta′shən) [L. *saltatio* from *saltare* to jump] 1. the action of leaping. 2. the jerky dancing or leaping that sometimes occurs in chorea. 3. saltatory conduction. 4. in genetics, an abrupt variation in species; a mutation. 5. sudden increases or changes in the course of an illness; called also *saltatory progression.*

**sal·ta·to·ri·al, sal·ta·to·ric** (sal″tə-tor′e-əl, sal″tə-tor′ik) saltatory.

**sal·ta·to·ry** (sal′tə-tor″e) pertaining to or characterized by saltation; see also under *evolution* and *spasm.*

**Sal·ter's lines** (sawl′tərz) [Sir Samuel James A. *Salter,* English dentist, 1825–1897] Owen's lines; see under *line.*

**salt·ing in** (sawl′ting in) dissolving proteins by raising the salt concentration; certain proteins that are insoluble in pure water dissolve when small amounts of neutral salt are added.

**salt·ing out** (sawl′ting out) precipitation of proteins by raising the salt concentration; any soluble protein will precipitate out of solution if enough neutral salt is added.

**salt·pe·ter** (sawlt-pe′tər) [L. *salpetra* or *sal petrae*] potassium nitrate.
**Chile s.,** sodium nitrate.

**sa·lu·bri·ous** (sə-loo′bre-əs) [L. *salubris*] conducive to health; wholesome.

**sal·ure·sis** (sal″u-re′sis) [*sal* + *-uresis*] the excretion of sodium and chloride ions in the urine.

**sal·uret·ic** (sal″u-ret′ik) 1. pertaining to, characterized by, or promoting saluresis. 2. an agent that promotes saluresis.

**Sal·u·ron** (sal′u-ron) trademark for a preparation of hydroflumethiazide.

**sal·u·tary** (sal′u-tar″e) [L. *salutaris*] favorable to the preservation or restoration of health.

**Sal·u·ten·sin** (sal″u-ten′sin) trademark for a preparation of hydroflumethiazide with reserpine.

**Sal·u·ten·sin-Demi** (sal″u-ten′sin-dem′e) trademark for a preparation of hydroflumethiazide with reserpine.

**sal·vage** (sal′vəj) [Fr.] pertaining to therapeutic measures taken late in the treatment process after other measures have failed. Called also *rescue.*

**sal·var·san** (sal′vər-sən) arsphenamine.

**salve** (sav) a thick ointment or cerate; see *ointment.*

**Sal·via** (sal′ve-ə) [L.] a genus of plants of the family Labiatae. *S. officina′lis* L. is the medicinal herb sage (q.v.). *S. reflex′a* L. is mintweed, an Australian plant rich in nitrates, which can cause fatal nitrite poisoning in ruminants.

**Sal·yr·gan** (sal′ər-gən) trademark for a preparation of mersalyl.

**Salz·mann's nodular corneal dystrophy** (sahlts′mahnz) [Maximilian *Salzmann,* Austrian-born ophthalmologist in Germany, 1862–1954] see under *dystrophy.*

**sam·an·dar·i·dine** (sam″ən-dar′ĭ-din) an alkaloid, from the skin of various salamanders; less poisonous than samandarine.

**sam·an·da·rine** (sə-man′də-rin) a poisonous alkaloid from the skin of various salamanders.

**sa·mar·i·um** (sə-mar′e-əm) [MeSH: Samarium] a very rare, metallic element; symbol, Sm; atomic number, 62; atomic weight, 150.35.
**s. 153,** a radioactive isotope of samarium, atomic mass 153, having a half life of 46.70 hours and emitting beta particles (0.81, 0.71, 0.64 MeV) and gamma rays (0.103, 0.070 MeV); it has been used in synoviorthesis and in the palliation of bone pain caused by metastatic disease.

**SAMHSA** Substance Abuse and Mental Health Services Agency.

**Sam·bu·cus** (sam-boo′kus) the elders, a genus of flowering berry-producing trees of Europe and North America. The most common species are *S. canaden′sis* L. of North America and *S. ni′gra* L. (Caprifoliaceae). Their berries (elderberries) contain a volatile oil that has been used to treat wounds, burns, and ulcers and as a laxative and diuretic; animals eating large amounts may have toxic reactions and diarrhea.

**sam·ple** (sam′pəl) [L. *exemplum* example] 1. a representative part taken to typify the whole. 2. a subset of a population that is selected for inclusion in a research study.
**random s.,** a sample chosen from a population in such a way that each choice is independent of the other choices and every member of the population has a fixed and determinate probability of being chosen (usually an equal probability).
**stratified s.,** that in which the population is first divided into multiple mutually exclusive groups or strata prior to choosing the sample; the most common form uses random samples, so that the term is often used to denote a *stratified random s.*
**stratified random s.,** a stratified sample in which random samples are chosen within each stratum. Sometimes called *stratified s.*

**sam·pling** (sam′pling) the selection or making of a sample.
**chorionic villus s. (CVS),** a procedure used for prenatal diagnosis at 9 to 12 weeks' gestation (7 to 10 weeks after fertilization). One method is aspiration of fetal tissue for analysis by catheter through the cervix from the villous chorion (chorion frondosum), under ultrasonic guidance. Another method is insertion of a needle, guided by ultrasonography, through the mother's abdominal and uterine walls into the uterine cavity. Spelled also *chorionic villous sampling.* Called also *chorionic villus biopsy.*
**percutaneous umbilical blood s.,** PUBS; cordocentesis.

**Samp·son's cyst** (samp′sənz) [John Albertson *Sampson,* American gynecologist, 1873–1946] chocolate cyst.

**Sam·u·els·son** (sam′u-əl-sən) Bengt Ingemar. Swedish biochemist, born 1934; co-winner, with Sune Bergström and John Robert Vane, of the Nobel prize for medicine or physiology in 1982 for their discovery of prostaglandins and related substances.

**san·a·tive** (san′ə-tiv) [L. *sanare* to heal] having a tendency to heal; curative.

**san·a·to·ri·um** (san″ə-tor′e-əm) [L. *sanatorius* conferring health, from *sanare* to cure] 1. old term for an establishment for the treatment of sick persons, such as a private hospital for convalescents or those who are not extremely ill, particularly an establishment for the open-air treatment of tuberculous patients. 2. a health resort in a hot region.

**san·a·to·ry** (san′ə-tor″e) [L. *sanatorius*] conducive to health; salubrious.

**Sanc·to·ri·us** (sank-tor′e-əs) [It. Santorio Santorio, 1561–1636] an Italian physician, professor of medicine at Padua, who devised several instruments of precision (e.g., a clinical thermometer and a pulse clock), and made quantitative experiments on basal metabolism or "insensible perspiration."

**sanc·tu·ary** (sangk′cho͞o-ar″e) an area in the body where a drug tends to collect and to escape metabolic breakdown.

**sand** (sand) small, gritty particles, usually of some mineral such as silica.
**brain s.,** sand bodies.

**san·dal·wood** (san′dəl-wood) [L. *santalum*] 1. *Santalum album.* 2. the fragrant wood of *S. album* or other trees of the genera *Santalum* and *Fusanus,* which yields santal oil (see under *oil*). 3. the dried heartwood of the leguminous tree *Pterocarpus santalinus,* used as a coloring agent.

**sand crack** (sand krak) see under *crack.*

**San·ders' disease** (san′dərz) [Murray *Sanders,* American bacteriologist, born 1910] epidemic keratoconjunctivitis.

**sand·fly** (sand′fli) [MeSH: Psychodidae] 1. any of various two-winged flies of the families Heleidae, Simuliidae, and Psychodidae. 2. more specifically, any fly of the genus *Phlebotomus.*

**Sand·hoff disease** (sahnd′hof) [K. *Sandhoff,* German biochemist, 20th century] [MeSH: Sandhoff Disease] see under *disease.*

**San·di·fer's syndrome** (san′dĭ-fər) [Paul *Sandifer,* British radiologist, 20th century] see under *syndrome.*

**Sand·im·mune** (san′dim-ūn) trademark for a preparation of cyclosporine.

**San·do·glob·u·lin** (san″do-glob′u-lin) trademark for a preparation of immune globulin.

**San·do·sta·tin** (san′do-stat″in) trademark for a preparation of octreotide acetate.

**San·dril** (san′dril) trademark for preparations of reserpine.

**Sand·ström's bodies, glands** (zahnt′strermz) [Ivar Victor *Sandström,* Swedish anatomist, 1852–1889] see *parathyroid glands,* under *gland* and *glandulae thyroideae accessoriae.*

**Sand·with's bald tongue** (sand′withs) [Fleming Mant *Sandwith,* British physician, 1853–1918] see under *tongue.*

**sane** (sān) [L. *sanus*] of sound mind; compos mentis.

**San·fi·lip·po's syndrome** (san-fĭ-lip′ōz) [Sylvester J. *Sanfilippo,* American pediatrician, 20th century] see under *syndrome.*

**San·ger** (sang′ər) Frederick. English biochemist, born 1918; winner of the Nobel prize for chemistry in 1958 for isolating and identifying the amino acid components of the insulin molecule and creating a method to identify the order of amino acids in more complicated protein molecules.

**Sän·ger** see *Saenger.*

**sangui-** [L. *sanguis* blood] a combining form denoting relationship to blood; see also terms beginning with *hemat(o)-* and *hem(o)-.*

**san·guic·o·lous** (sang-gwik′ə-ləs) [*sangui-* + L. *colere* to dwell] inhabiting or living in the blood.

**san·gui·fa·cient** (sang″gwi-fa′shənt) [*sangui-* + *-facient*] hematopoietic.

**san·guif·er·ous** (sang-gwif′ər-əs) [*sangui-* + *-ferous*] 1. containing blood. 2. circulatory (def. 3).

**san·gui·fi·ca·tion** (sang-gwĭ-fĭ-ka′shən) hematopoiesis.

**san·gui·mo·tor** (sang″gwĭ-mo′tər) [*sangui-* + *motor*] circulatory (def. 2).

**san·gui·na·ria** (sang″gwĭ-nar′e-ə) the dried rhizome and root of the bloodroot, *Sanguinaria canadensis,* a perennial herb, used as an ingredient of compound white pine syrup. It was formerly used as an expectorant and externally in the treatment of chronic eczema and cancer of the skin. It contains several alkaloids, e.g., sanguinarine.

**san·gui·na·rine** (sang″gwĭ-na′rēn) an alkaloid obtained from sanguinaria and other species of the same family, including *Argemone mexicana;* see also *epidemic dropsy.*

**san·guine** (sang′gwin) [L. *sanguineus; sanguis* blood] 1. plethoric (def. 2). 2. see under *temperament.*

**san·guin·e·ous** (sang-gwin′e-əs) 1. plethoric (def. 2). 2. hemic.

**san·guin·o·lent** (sang-gwin′ə-lənt) [L. *sanguinolentus*] of a bloody tinge.

**san·gui·no·pu·ru·lent** (sang″gwĭ-no-pu′roo-lənt) containing both blood and pus.

**san·gui·nous** (sang′gwi-nəs) 1. plethoric (def. 2). 2. hemic.

**san·gui·re·nal** (sang″gwĭ-re′nəl) [*sangui-* + *renal*] pertaining to the blood and the kidneys.

**san·guis** (sang′gwis) [L.] TA alternative for *haema;* see *blood.*

**san·guiv·o·rous** (sang-gwiv′ə-rəs) [*sangui-* + L. *vorare* to eat] hematophagous.

**sa·ni·es** (sa′ne-ēz) [L.] a fetid, ichorous discharge from a wound or ulcer, containing serum, pus, and blood.

**sa·nio·pu·ru·lent** (sa″ne-o-pu′roo-lənt) partly sanious and partly purulent.

**sa·nio·se·rous** (sa″ne-o-se′rəs) partly sanious and partly serous.

**sa·ni·ous** (sa′ne-əs) [L. *saniosus*] of the nature of sanies.

**san·i·tar·i·an** (san″ĭ-tar′e-ən) a person who is expert in matters of sanitation and public health.

**san·i·tar·i·um** (san″ĭ-ta′re-əm) [L.] an institution for the promotion of health. The word was originally coined to designate the institution established by the Seventh Day Adventists at Battle Creek, Michigan, to distinguish it from institutions providing care for mental or tuberculous patients.

**san·i·tary** (san′ĭ-tar″e) [L. *sanitarius*] pertaining to health or promoting or conducive to health; usually used in reference to an environment that is clean, i.e., without an agent that is deleterious to health.

**san·i·ta·tion** (san″ĭ-ta′shən) [L. *sanitas* health] [MeSH: Sanitation] the establishment of environmental conditions favorable to health.

**san·i·ti·za·tion** (san″ĭ-tĭ-za′shən) the process of making or the quality of being made sanitary; see *sanitize.*

**san·i·tize** (san′ĭ-tīz) to clean and sterilize, as eating or drinking utensils.

**san·i·ty** (san′ĭ-te) [L. *sanitas* soundness] soundness, especially soundness of mind.

**San Joa·quin Val·ley fever (disease)** (san wah-kēn′) [*San Joaquin Valley,* California, where the disease is particularly prominent] primary coccidioidomycosis.

**San·o·rex** (san′ə-reks) trademark for a preparation of mazindol.

**San·sert** (san′sərt) trademark for a preparation of methysergide maleate.

**San·som's sign** (san′səmz) [Arthur Ernest *Sansom,* English physician, 1838–1907] see under *sign.*

**San·son's images** (sah-sawz′) [Louis Joseph *Sanson,* French physician, 1790–1841] Purkinje's images; see under *image.*

**San·ta·lum** (san′tə-ləm) a genus of trees of the family Santalaceae. *S. al′bum* L. and other species are called sandalwood and yield santal oil (sandalwood oil).

**san·ta·lum** (san′tə-ləm) sandalwood.
**s. ru′brum,** sandalwood, def. 3.

**San·ta·vu·ori's disease (syndrome)** (sahn″tah-vwo′rēz) [Pirkko *Santavuori,* Finnish physician, 20th century] Haltia-Santavuori disease; see under *disease.*

**San·ta·vu·ori-Hal·tia disease (syndrome)** (sahn″tah-vwo′re-hahl′te-ah) [P. *Santavuori;* M. *Haltia,* Finnish physician, 20th century] Haltia-Santavuori disease; see under *disease.*

**san·ton·i·ca** (san-ton′ĭ-kə) [L.] 1. *Artemisia maritima.* 2. the dried unexpanded flower heads of *A. maritima,* the source of santonin; formerly used as an anthelmintic and stomachic.

**san·to·nin** (san′to-nin) [MeSH: Santonin] a lactone, which may be obtained from the unexpanded flower heads of *Artemisia maritima* L. (Compositae), santonica, or other species of *A.;* used as an anthelmintic against *Ascaris lumbricoides.*

**San·to·ri·ni's cartilage,** etc. (sahn″to-re′nēz) [Giovanni Domenico *Santorini,* Italian anatomist, 1681–1737] see *cartilago corniculata, ductus pancreaticus accessorius, incisura cartilaginis meatus acustici, ligamentum cricopharyngeum, musculus risorius, papilla duodeni major, plexus prostaticus,* and *tuberculum corniculatum.*

**sap** (sap) the natural juice of a living organism or tissue.
**cell s.,** hyaloplasm, def. 1.
**nuclear s.,** karyolymph.

**sa·phe·na** (sə-fe′nə) [L.; Gr. *saphēnēs* manifest] any of the three venae saphenae; see *vena.*

**saph·e·nec·to·my** (saf″ə-nek′tə-me) [*saphena* + *-ectomy*] excision of a saphenous vein.

**saph·en·og·ra·phy** (saf″ən-og′rə-fe) phlebography of the great saphenous vein after injection of contrast medium at the ankle.

**sa·phe·nous** (sə-fe′nəs) pertaining to or associated with a vena saphena.

**sap·id** (sap′id) [L. *sapidus*] having or imparting an agreeable taste.

**sa·po** (sa′po) [L. "soap"] soap.
**s. mol′lis,** soft soap.
**s. mol′lis medicina′lis,** green soap.
**s. vi′ridis,** green soap.

**sa·pog·e·nin** (sə-poj′ə-nin) a compound resulting from the decomposition of saponin.

**sa·po·na·ceous** (sa″po-na′shəs) [L. *sapo* soap] of a soapy quality or nature.

**Sa·po·na·ria** (sa″po-nar′e-ə) a genus of plants of the family Caryophyllaceae. *S. officina′lis* is soapwort, whose root contains saponin and sapotoxin and was formerly used in skin diseases; livestock eating the plant may get enteritis with diarrhea.

**sa·po·na·tus** (sa″po-na′təs) [L., from *sapo* soap] charged or mixed with soap.

**sa·pon·i·fi·ca·tion** (sə-pon″ĭ-fĭ-ka′shən) [L. *sapo* soap + *facere* to make] the act or process of converting fats into soaps and glycerol by heating with alkalis. In chemistry, the term now denotes hydrolysis of an ester by an alkali, resulting in the production of a free alcohol and an alkali salt of the ester acid.

**sap·o·nin** (sap′o-nin) any of a group of glycosides found in plants such as *Quillaja saponaria* and *Saponaria officinalis;* they form a durable foam when their watery solutions are shaken and can dissolve red blood cells even in high dilutions. Their aglycone is sapogenin.
**cholan s's,** a group of saponins that on hydrolysis yield sterol-like compounds.
**triterpenoid s's,** a group of saponins that on hydrolysis yield 1,2,7-trimethyl naphthalene.

**sap·o·phore** (sap′o-for) [L. *sapor* taste + *-phore*] the group of atoms in the molecule of a compound that gives the substance its characteristic taste.

**sap·o·tal·ene** (sap′o-tal″ēn) a hydrocarbon, formed by the reduction of sapogenin.

**sa·po·tox·in** (sa″po-tok′sin) any of various toxic saponins found in such plants as *Agave lechuguilla, Phytolacca americana, Quillaja saponaria,* and *Saponaria officinalis.* Livestock consuming these plants may suffer from enteritis or gastroenteritis with diarrhea that can be fatal.

**Sap·pey's fibers, ligament, veins** (sah-pāz′) [Marie Philibert Constant *Sappey,* French anatomist, 1810–1896] see under *fiber* and *ligament,* and see *venae paraumbilicales.*

**sap·phism** (saf′iz-əm) [*Sappho,* Greek poetess, about 600 B.C.] homosexuality between women; lesbianism.

**sapr(o)-** [Gr. *sapros* rotten] a combining form meaning rotten or putrid, or designating relationship to decay or to decaying material.

**sa·probe** (să′prōb) [*sapro-* + Gr. *bios* life] an organism, usually referring to a fungus, that feeds on dead or decaying organic matter. Cf. *saprophyte.*

**sa·pro·bic** (sə-pro′bik) pertaining to or of the nature of a saprobe.

**Sap·ro·leg·nia** (sap″ro-leg′ne-ə) [*sapro-* + Gr. *legnon* border] a genus of partially saprobic aquatic moldlike organisms of the order Saprolegniales; they can cause parasitic disease in fish and amphibians.

**Sap·ro·leg·ni·a·les** (sap″ro-leg″ne-a′lēz) an order of mostly saprobic funguslike organisms of the class Oomycetes, having an extensive mycelial thallus without cross walls. Genera include *Saprolegnia* and *Achlya.* They are commonly called "water molds," although some inhabit soil.

**sap·ro·no·sis** (sap″ro-no′sis) a disease caused by organisms of the environment.

**sa·proph·i·lous** (sə-prof′ĭ-ləs) [*sapro-* + *-phil* + *-ous*] saprophytic.

**sap·ro·phyte** (sap′ro-fīt) [*sapro-* + *-phyte*] an organism that lives on dead or decaying plant or animal material; said especially of plants or so-called plantlike organisms, such as certain protozoa and bacteria. Fungi with this characteristic are called *saprobes.* See also *autophyte* and *saprozoic.*

**sap·ro·phyt·ic** (sap″ro-fit′ik) 1. pertaining to or of the nature of a saprophyte. 2. saprozoic.

**sap·ro·zo·ic** (sap″ro-zo′ik) [*sapro-* + *zoic*] having a type of nutrition involving uptake of organic materials in dissolved form obtained from dead or decaying plant or animal matter; said of animals or so-called animal-like organisms (e.g., certain protozoa). Called also *saprophytic.* Cf. *holozoic* and *saprophytic.*

**sa·quin·a·vir mes·y·late** (sə-kwin′-ə-vir) a protease inhibitor active against the human immunodeficiency virus, causing the formation of immature, noninfectious viral particles, used in the treatment of human immunodeficiency virus infection and acquired immunodeficiency syndrome; administered orally.

**sar·al·a·sin ac·e·tate** (sər-al′ə-sin) an angiotensin-II antagonist, used as an antihypertensive in the treatment of severe hypertension and in the diagnosis of renin-dependent hypertension.

**Sar·ci·na** (sahr′sĭ-nə) [L. "package," "bundle"] [MeSH: Sarcina] a genus of spherical, gram-positive bacteria of the family Micrococcaceae, occurring in cubical packets of eight or more cells. They are strict anaerobes found in soil and on grains and occasionally in clinical specimens.

**sar·ci·na** (sahr′sĭ-nə) pl. *sar′cinae* [MeSH: Sarcina] 1. a spherical bacterium occurring predominantly in cubical packets of eight cells as a consequence of failure of daughter cells to separate following cell division in three planes. 2. an organism of the genus *Sarcina.*

**sarc(o)-** [Gr. *sarx, sarkos* flesh] a combining form denoting relationship to flesh.

**sar·co·blast** (sahr′ko-blast) [*sarco-* + *-blast*] myoblast.

**sar·co·car·ci·no·ma** (sahr″ko-kahr″sĭ-no′mə) carcinosarcoma.

**sar·co·cele** (sahr′ko-sēl) [*sarco-* + *-cele*[1]] any fleshy swelling or tumor of the testis.

**sar·co·cyst** (sahr′ko-sist) [*sarco-* + *cyst*] 1. a protozoan of the genus *Sarcocystis.* 2. one of the elongated, fusiform, cylindrical, membrane-bound hyaline bodies containing the numerous crescentic or banana-shaped, uninucleate trophozoites (Rainey's corpuscles) of the protozoan *Sarcocystis,* found in the muscles of those with sarcocystosis. Called also *Miescher's tube* or *tubule, Rainey's tube* or *tubule,* and *sarcosporidian cyst.*

**sar·co·cys·tin** (sahr″ko-sis′tin) a toxin obtained from species of *Sarcocystis.*

**Sar·co·cys·tis** (sahr″ko-sis′tis) [*sarco-* + Gr. *kystis* bladder] [MeSH: Sarcocystis] a genus of coccidian protozoa (suborder Eimeriina, order Eucoccidiida) that are parasitic in birds, reptiles, and many mammalian species, including humans and occur as elongated cylindrical bodies (sarcocysts) in the host's muscles. They have an obligatory two-host life cycle, with sexual reproduction in the definitive host (a carnivore) and asexual reproduction, including schizogony and sarcocyst formation, in the intermediate host. Infection is transmitted by ingestion of the sporocysts in the feces passed by infected animals (see *sarcocystosis*).
**S. boviho′minis,** a species for which cattle are the specific intermediate hosts and humans the definitive hosts; it causes intestinal sarcocystosis in the latter. Together with *S. suihominis,* formerly considered to be a single species, *S. hominis (Isospora hominis).*
**S. ho′minis,** see *S. bovihominis* and *S. suihominis.*
**S. lindeman′ni,** a species causing human infection, most cases of which are asymptomatic, although it may cause polymyositis sometimes associated with eosinophilia.
**S. suiho′minis,** a species for which swine are the specific intermediate hosts and humans the definitive hosts; it causes intestinal sarcocystosis in the latter. Together with *S. bovihominis,* formerly considered to be a single genus, *S. hominis (Isospora hominis).*

**sar·co·cys·to·sis** (sahr″ko-sis-to′sis) [MeSH: Sarcocystosis] infection with protozoa of the genus *Sarcocystis,* which in humans is usually asymptomatic or manifested either by muscle cysts associated with myositis or myocarditis or by intestinal infection. It is usually transmitted by the eating of raw or undercooked beef or pork containing sporocysts of the parasites or by ingestion of sporocysts from the feces of an infected animal, usually in contaminated soil. Heavy infections in cattle and other animals may be associated with anorexia, emaciation, fever, nervousness, lameness, hypersalivation, anemia, and abortion. Called also *sarcosporidiasis* and *sarcosporidiosis.*

**Sar·co·di·na** (sahr″ko-di′nə) [Gr. *sarkōdēs* fleshlike] [MeSH: Sarcodina] a subphylum of protozoa (phylum Sarcomastigophora), the organisms of which alter their body shape and move about and acquire food by extension of cytoplasmic organelles (pseudopodia) of various types, or by protoplasmic flow without producing discrete pseudopodia. Some have flagella during developmental or other temporary stages. The body of some sarcodines is naked, while in others an external or internal test or skeleton is present. It comprises two superclasses: Rhizopoda, some members of which are pathogenic for humans, and Actinopoda; the former has been used as a synonym of Sarcodina.

**sar·co·dine** (sahr′ko-dīn) 1. pertaining to the subphylum Sarcodina. 2. any individual protozoan of the subphylum Sarcodina. Called also *sarcodinian.*

**sar·co·din·i·an** (sahr″ko-din′e-ən) sarcodine.

**sar·co·en·chon·dro·ma** (sahr″ko-en″kon-dro′mə) chondrosarcoma.

**sar·co·gen·ic** (sahr″ko-jen′ik) [*sarco-* + *-genic*] forming muscle.

**sar·co·hy·dro·cele** (sahr″ko-hi′dro-sēl) sarcocele combined with hydrocele.

**sar·coid** (sahr′koid) [*sarc-* + *-oid*] 1. sarcoidosis. 2. a sarcomalike tumor. 3. fleshlike.
**Boeck's s., s. of Boeck,** sarcoidosis.
**Darier-Roussy s.,** a form of sarcoidosis characterized by the large size of the nodules and their subcutaneous location.
**equine s.,** a common wartlike benign cutaneous tumor of horses, caused by an unidentified virus.
**Schaumann's s.,** sarcoidosis.
**Spiegler-Fendt s.,** lymphocytoma cutis.

**sar·coi·do·sis** (sahr″koi-do′sis) [*sarcoid* + *-osis*] [MeSH: Sarcoidosis] a chronic, progressive, systemic granulomatous reticulosis of unknown etiology, characterized by hard tubercles (q.v.) in almost any organ or tissue, including the skin, lungs, lymph nodes, liver, spleen, eyes, and small bones of the hands and feet. Laboratory findings may include hypercalcemia and hypergammaglobulinemia; there is usually low or absent reactivity to tuberculin, and in active cases, a positive Kveim reaction. The acute form has an abrupt onset and a high spontaneous remission rate, whereas the chronic form, insidious in onset, is progressive. Called also *sarcoid, Besnier-Boeck disease, Boeck's disease* or *sarcoid,* and *Schaumann's disease, sarcoid,* or *syndrome.*
**cardiac s.,** involvement of the heart in sarcoidosis, with lesions ranging from a few asymptomatic, microscopic granulomas to widespread infiltration of the myocardium by large masses of sarcoid tissue, often leading to arrhythmias, heart block, mitral regurgitation, or sudden death.
**muscular s.,** sarcoidosis involving the skeletal muscles, with sarcoid tubercles, interstitial inflammation with fibrosis, and disruption and atrophy of the muscle fibers.

**sar·co·lem·ma** (sahr″ko-lem′ə) [*sarco-* + *-lemma*] [MeSH: Sarcolemma] the delicate plasma membrane which invests every striated muscle fiber.

**sar·co·lem·mic** (sahr″ko-lem′ik) pertaining to or of the nature of sarcolemma.

**sar·co·lem·mous** (sahr″ko-lem′əs) sarcolemmic.

**L-sar·co·ly·sin** (sahr″ko-li′sin) melphalan.

**sar·co·ma** (sahr-ko′mə) pl. *sarcomas, sarco′mata* [*sarc-* + *-oma*] [MeSH: Sarcoma] any of a group of tumors usually arising from connective tissue, although the term now includes some of epithelial origin; most are malignant. Many types have prefixes denoting the type of tissue or structure involved; see *chondrosarcoma, fibrosarcoma, lymphosarcoma, melanosarcoma, myxosarcoma, osteosarcoma, rhabdomyosarcoma,* and so on.
**adipose s.,** liposarcoma.
**alveolar soft part s.,** a well-circumscribed, slow growing, painless, highly metastatic malignant neoplasm of unknown cell origin, characterized by a distinctive alveolar pattern and occurring predominantly in the extremities, head, and neck of young adults.
**ameloblastic s.,** see under *fibrosarcoma.*
**avian s.,** any of a group of rare sarcomas of fowls, transmitted by retroviruses related to avian leukosis virus; the earliest known one was the Rous sarcoma. Called also *chicken s.*
**botryoid s., s. botryoi′des,** a variety of embryonal rhabdomyosarcoma, arising in submucosal tissue, presenting grossly as a polypoid grapelike structure, and found most often in young children or infants in the upper vagina, cervix uteri, or neck of the urinary bladder.
**chicken s.,** avian s.
**chloromatous s.,** chloroma.
**chondroblastic s.,** the chondroblastic form of osteosarcoma.
**clear cell s. of kidney,** a malignant kidney tumor similar to Wilms' tumor but with a poorer prognosis; its cells have pale or clear cytoplasm and are arranged uniformly in vascularized nests. It often metastasizes to bone.
**embryonal s.,** Wilms' tumor.
**endometrial stromal s.,** a pale, polypoid, fleshy, malignant tumor of the endometrial stroma, usually arising from the uterine fundus.
**epithelioid s.,** a rare, frequently metastatic tumor consisting of lobulated masses of spindle and epithelioid cells surrounding a necrotic center; it usually arises in the deep soft tissues of the distal extremities in young adults, particularly males.

**Ewing's s.,** a highly malignant, metastatic, primitive small round cell tumor of bone, usually occurring in the diaphyses of long bones, ribs, and flat bones of children or adolescents. It is characterized by saucerization of the cortex, patchy, permeative destruction, and often a large soft tissue mass; the most common symptoms include pain, swelling, leukocytosis, and fever. Called also *Ewing's tumor.*
**fascial s.,** a sarcoma arising in the fasciae about the joints, especially in the lower extremities.
**fibroblastic s.,** the fibroblastic form of osteosarcoma.
**fowl s.,** chicken s.
**giant cell s.,** 1. a form of giant cell tumor of bone (q.v.) that arises malignant de novo, rather than transforming to malignancy. 2. sarcoma characterized by large anaplastic (giant) cells.
**granulocytic s.,** chloroma.
**hemangioendothelial s.,** hemangiosarcoma.
**Hodgkin's s.,** Hodgkin's disease, lymphocyte depletion type.
**idiopathic multiple pigmented hemorrhagic s.,** Kaposi's s.
**immunoblastic s. of B cells,** large cell, immunoblastic lymphoma composed predominantly of B cells.
**immunoblastic s. of T cells,** large cell, immunoblastic lymphoma made up predominantly of T cells.
**Jensen's s.,** a malignant tumor in mice transmissible to healthy mice by transplanting a small portion of the tumor. Called also *Jensen's tumor.*
**Kaposi's s.,** a multicentric, malignant neoplastic vascular proliferation characterized by bluish-red cutaneous nodules, usually on the legs, toes, or feet, that slowly increase in size and number and spread to more proximal sites. The tumors have endothelium-lined channels and vascular spaces mixed with aggregates of spindle-shaped cells; they may remain confined to skin and subcutaneous tissue, but widespread visceral involvement may occur. Kaposi's sarcoma is endemic in certain parts of Central Africa and Central and Eastern Europe, and a virulent and disseminated form occurs in immunocompromised patients. Human herpesvirus 8 has been implicated in its etiology. Called also *multiple idiopathic hemorrhagic s.* and *idiopathic multiple pigmented hemorrhagic s.*
**Kupffer cell s.,** hepatic angiosarcoma.
**leukocytic s.,** leukosarcoma.
**lymphatic s.,** diffuse lymphoma.
**melanotic s.,** malignant melanoma.
**mixed cell s.,** malignant mesenchymoma.
**multiple idiopathic hemorrhagic s.,** Kaposi's s.
**multipotential primary s. of bone,** small-cell osteosarcoma.
**osteoblastic s.,** the osteoblastic form of osteosarcoma.
**osteogenic s.,** osteosarcoma.
**parosteal s.,** see under *osteosarcoma.*
**polymorphous s.,** malignant mesenchymoma.
**pseudo–Kaposi s.,** unilateral subacute to chronic dermatitis, often with postinflammatory hyperpigmentation, occurring in association with underlying arteriovenous fistula, which closely resembles Kaposi's sarcoma both clinically and histologically.
**reticulum cell s.,** histiocytic lymphoma.
**reticulum cell s. of the brain,** former name for *primary central nervous system lymphoma.*
**Rous s.,** a type of avian sarcoma transmitted by a retrovirus; it metastasizes freely and is sometimes highly lethal. Experimental inoculation into other fowls produces similar growths. This was the first sarcoma known to be caused by a virus.
**soft tissue s.,** a general term for a malignant tumor derived from extraskeletal connective tissue, including fibrous, fat, smooth muscle, nerve, vascular, histiocytic, and synovial tissue, with almost all lesions originating from primitive mesoderm. Tumors arising in Schwann cells are also included.
**spindle cell s.,** 1. any sarcoma composed of spindle-shaped cells; cf. *rhabdomyosarcoma.* 2. a type of soft tissue sarcoma whose cells are spindle-shaped; it is usually resistant to radiation therapy and may be of either high or low grade malignancy.
**synovial s.,** synoviosarcoma.
**telangiectatic s.,** a sarcoma that develops a rich vascular network; the endothelial cells may be mistaken for the neoplastic element.

**sar·co·ma·gen·ic** (sahr″ko-mə-jen′ik) causing sarcoma. See also cancerigenic.

**Sar·co·mas·ti·goph·o·ra** (sahr″ko-mas″tĭ-gof′ə-rə) [*sarco-* + Gr. *mastix* whip + *phoros* bearing] [MeSH: Sarcomastigophora] a phylum comprising protozoa that typically possess an endosome nucleus characterized by a ring of nuclear chromatin around a central chromatin-free region, and are motile by means of flagella, pseudopodia, or both types of locomotor organs. The phylum includes the subphyla Mastigophora (flagellates), Sarcodina (amebae), and Opalinata (opalinids).

**sar·co·ma·ta** (sahr-ko′mə-tə) plural of *sarcoma.*

**sar·co·ma·toid** (sahr-ko′mə-toid) resembling sarcoma.

**sar·co·ma·to·sis** (sahr″ko-mə-to′sis) a condition characterized by the formation of sarcomas.

**sar·co·ma·tous** (sahr-ko′mə-təs) pertaining to or of the nature of sarcoma.

**sar·co·mere** (sahr′ko-mēr) [*sarco-* + *-mere*] [MeSH: Sarcomeres] the contractile unit of myofibrils; sarcomeres are repeating units, delimited by the Z bands along the length of the myofibril. See Plate 35.

**sar·co·neme** (sahr′ko-nēm) [*sarco-* + Gr. *nēma* thread] microneme.

**sar·co·pe·nia** (sahr″ko-pe′ne-ə) [*sarco-* + *-penia*] age-related reduction in skeletal muscle mass in the elderly.

**Sar·coph·a·ga** (sahr-kof′ə-gə) [*sarco-* + Gr. *phagein* to eat] a genus of gray flesh flies of the family Sarcophagidae. The larvae of several species have been found in wounds, ulcers, nasal passages, and sinuses of humans and other animals. The most important species is *S. haemorrhoida′lis.* Other species are *S. carna′ria, S. fuscicau′da, S. dux, S. nificor′nis,* and *S. rubicor′nis.*

**Sar·co·phag·i·dae** (sahr″ko-faj′ĭ-de) the flesh flies, a family of insects of the order Diptera; genera *Sarcophaga* (type genus) and *Wohlfahrtia* produce myiasis in humans and other animals.

**sar·co·plasm** (sahr′ko-plaz″əm) [*sarco-* + *-plasm*] the interfibrillary matter of the striated muscles; the substance in which the fibrillae of the muscle fiber are embedded.

**sar·co·plas·mic** (sahr″ko-plaz′mik) composed of or containing sarcoplasm; see also under *reticulum.*

**sar·co·plast** (sahr′ko-plast) [*sarco-* + *-plast*] an interstitial cell of a muscle, itself capable of being transformed into a muscle.

**sar·co·poi·et·ic** (sahr″ko-poi-et′ik) [*sarco-* + Gr. *poiein* to make] producing flesh or muscle.

**Sar·cop·syl·la** (sahr″kop-sil′ə) *Tunga.*

**Sar·cop·tes** (sahr-kop′tēz) [*sarco-* + Gr. *koptein* to cut] a genus of mites of the family Sarcoptidae. *S. scabie′i,* the itch mite of humans, produces scabies. Varieties of *S. scabiei* cause mange of domestic animals, including pigs, horses, cows, and dogs.

**sar·cop·tic** (sahr-kop′tik) of, relating to, or caused by *Sarcoptes.*

**Sar·cop·ti·dae** (sahr-kop′tĭ-de) a family of acarid mites; genera of medical and veterinary interest include *Notoedres* and *Sarcoptes.*

**sar·cop·ti·do·sis** (sahr-kop″tĭ-do′sis) infestation with *Sarcoptes.*

**sar·co·sine** (sahr′ko-sēn) [MeSH: Sarcosine] an amino acid occurring as an intermediate in the metabolism of choline in the kidney and liver; it is normally not detectable in human blood or urine.

**sar·co·sine de·hy·dro·gen·ase** (sahr′ko-sēn de-hi′dro-jən-ās) [EC 1.5.99.1] a mitochondrial enzyme of the oxidoreductase class that catalyzes the oxidative demethylation of sarcosine to form glycine; electrons are transferred via its flavin (FAD) cofactor to electron transfer flavoprotein. Folate is also a cofactor. The reaction occurs in the inner mitochondrial membrane in liver and kidney; deficiency of the enzyme, an autosomal recessive trait, results in sarcosinemia.

**sar·co·si·ne·mia** (sahr″ko-sĭ-ne′me-ə) 1. an autosomal recessive aminoacidopathy caused by deficiency of sarcosine dehydrogenase and characterized by accumulation and excretion of sarcosine; it is probably benign but may be associated with neurologic abnormalities. 2. accumulation of sarcosine in the blood, usually resulting from defects in sarcosine dehydrogenase or electron transfer flavoprotein, or from severe folate deficiency. Called also *hypersarcosinemia.*

**sar·co·si·nu·ria** (sahr″ko-sĭ-nu′re-ə) excretion of sarcosine in the urine.

**sar·co·sis** (sahr-ko′sis) [*sarco-* + *-osis*] abnormal increase of flesh.

**Sar·co·spo·rid·ia** (sahr″ko-spor-id′e-ə) in former systems of classification, an order of sporozoan protozoa that included the genus *Sarcocystis.*

**sar·co·spo·rid·i·a·sis** (sahr″ko-spor″ĭ-di′ə-sis) sarcocystosis.

**sar·co·spo·rid·i·o·sis** (sahr″ko-spor-id″e-o′sis) sarcocystosis.

**sar·cos·to·sis** (sahr″kos-to′sis) [*sarco-* + *ostosis*] ossification of fleshy tissues.

**sar·co·style** (sahr′ko-stīl) [*sarco-* + Gr. *stylos* column] 1. a myofibril. 2. a bundle of myofibrils; called also *column of Kolliker* and *muscle column.*

**sar·cot·ic** (sahr-kot′ik) [Gr. *sarkōtikos*] 1. promoting the growth of flesh. 2. pertaining to sarcosis.

**sar·co·tu·bules** (sahr″ko-too′būlz) membrane-limited structures that extend throughout the sarcoplasm and form a closely meshed canalicular network around each myofibril.

**sar·cous** (sahr′kəs) pertaining to flesh or to muscular tissues.

**sar·don·ic** (sahr-don′ik) [Gr. *sardonios* Sardinian, substituted for *sardanios* bitter because of the facial distortion supposedly caused by eating a poisonous Sardinian herb] denoting a kind of spasmodic or tetanic grin or involuntary smile, as *risus sardonicus.*

**sar·gra·mos·tim** (sahr-gram′o-stim) [USP] granulocyte-macrophage colony-stimulating factor developed by recombinant technology that acts as a hematopoietic stimulant, used as an adjuvant to myelosuppressive cancer chemotherapy and to promote myeloid engraftment in bone marrow transplantation.

**sa·rin** (zah-rēn′) an organophosphorus compound that is a potent cholinesterase inhibitor and is used as a nerve gas; symptoms of poisoning include bronchial constriction, convulsions, and often death. See also *organophosphorus compound poisoning,* under *poisoning.*

**Sa·ro·tham·nus** (sa″ro-tham′nəs) [Gr. *saron* broom + *thamnos* shrub] *Cytisus.*

**Sar·ra·ce·nia** (sar″ə-se′ne-ə) [Michel *Sarrazin,* Canadian physician and naturalist, 1659–1734] a genus of plants of the family Sarraceniaceae. *S. purpu′rea* L. is the most common pitcher plant of North America; the secretion of its pitcher contains digestant enzymes and is a stimulant, diuretic, and laxative.

**sar·sa** (sahr′sə) gen. *sar′sae* [L.; Sp. *zarza* briar] sarsaparilla.

**sar·sa·pa·ril·la** (sahr″sə-pə-ril′ə, sas″pə-ril′ə) [L.; Sp. "briar vine"] 1. any of various plants of the genus *Smilax.* 2. the dried root of any of various species of *Smilax,* used as a flavoring agent in beverages, and in the treatment of psoriasis. It contains sarsasapogenin, a precursor in the manufacture of compounds in the pregnane series. Called also *sarsa.*

**sar·sa·sapo·gen·in** (sahr″sə-sap″o-jen′in) a steroid sapogenin from sarsaparilla, used in the synthesis of hormones of the pregnane series.

**Sas·sa·fras** (sas′ə-fras) [L.] a genus of trees of the family Lauraceae. *S. albi′dum* Nutt. (called also *S. varifo′lia* and *S. officina′le*) is a North American tree whose root contains sassafras oil, the source of the beverage root beer.

**sat·el·lite** (sat′ə-līt) [L. *satelles* companion] 1. a subservient smaller body that is under the influence of a larger one. 2. a vein that closely accompanies an artery, such as the brachial. 3. a minor, or attendant, lesion situated near a larger one. 4. a globoid mass of chromatin attached at the secondary constriction to the ends of the short arms of acrocentric autosomes. 5. exhibiting satellitism. 6. the posterior of a pair of gregarines undergoing syzygy.
**bacterial s.,** satellite colony.
**centriolar s.,** one of the small dense, amorphous bodies associated with the centrioles, which serve as nucleation sites for polymerization of tubulin to form microtubules.
**chromosomal s.,** satellite (def. 3).
**nucleolar s.,** a small mass of chromatin found next to the nucleolar membrane in most nerve cells of the female; sex chromatin.

**sat·el·li·tism** (sat′ə-li-tiz-əm) 1. the presence or formation of satellites. 2. the phenomenon in which certain bacterial species grow more vigorously in the immediate vicinity of colonies of other unrelated species (e.g., *Haemophilus influenzae* near a colony of staphylococci), owing to the production of an essential metabolite by the latter species.
**platelet s.,** a phenomenon sometimes seen in blood that has been anticoagulated with ethylenediaminetetraacetic acid (EDTA), in which platelets surround or adhere to leukocytes.

**sat·el·li·to·sis** (sat″ə-li-to′sis) accumulation of neuroglial cells about neurons; seen whenever neurons are damaged.

**sa·ti·e·ty** (sə-ti′ə-te) [L. *satietas*] 1. sufficiency. 2. full gratification of appetite or thirst, with abolition of the desire to eat or drink.

**sa·tra·tox·in** (sa″trə-tok′sin) any of several trichothecene mycotoxins found in species of *Stachybotrys,* especially *S. alternans,* causing stachybotryotoxicosis.

**Sat·tler's layer** (sat′lərz) [Hubert *Sattler,* Austrian ophthalmologist, 1844–1928] see under *layer.*

**sa·tu·mo·mab** (sə-tu′mo-mab) a monoclonal antibody specific to colorectal and ovarian adenocarcinomas; see *indium In III satumomab pendetide.*

**sat·u·rat·ed** (sach′ər-āt-əd) 1. of a chemical compound, having all the chemical affinities satisfied; i.e., no double or triple bonds are present. The term is most commonly used for carbon-carbon bonds, as in saturated fatty acids. 2. of a solution, containing as much solute as may be dissolved under stated conditions.

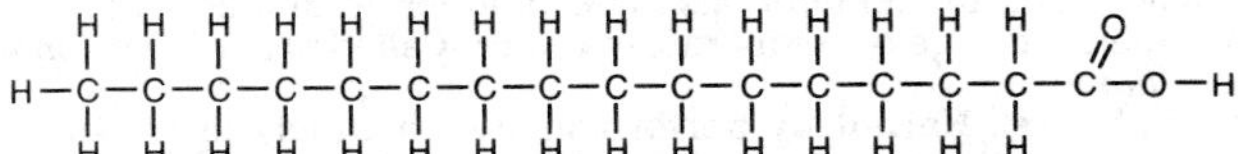

Palmitic acid, a common saturated fatty acid.

**sat·u·ra·tion** (sach″ə-ra′shən) [L. *saturatio*] 1. the act of saturating or condition of being saturated. 2. in radiotherapy, the delivery of a maximum tolerable tissue dose within a short time period and then maintenance of this biologic effect for an extended period of time by additional smaller fractional doses.
**oxygen s.,** a measure of the degree to which oxygen is bound to hemoglobin, usually measured by a pulse oximeter, given as a percentage calculated by dividing the maximum oxygen capacity into the actual oxygen content and multiplying by 100.
**transferrin s.,** the percentage of transferrin bound to iron in a serum sample, calculated by the formula

$$\frac{\text{serum iron}}{\text{total iron-binding capacity (TIBC)}} \times 100;$$

used in the evaluation of patients with iron deficiency or overload.

**sat·ur·nine** (sat′ər-nīn) [L. *saturninus; saturnus* lead] pertaining to or produced by lead; having the dull, heavy properties associated with lead.

**sat·ur·nism** (sat′ər-niz-əm) [L. *saturnus* lead] lead poisoning.

**sat·y·ri·a·sis** (sat″ĭ-ri′ə-sis) [Gr. *satyros* satyr + *-iasis*] abnormal, excessive, insatiable sexual desire in the male. Cf. *nymphomania.*

**sat·y·ro·ma·nia** (sat″ĭ-ro-ma′ne-ə) [Gr. *satyros* satyr + *-mania*] satyriasis.

**sau·cer** (saw′sər) a rounded, shallow depression.
**auditory s.,** see under *placode.*

**sau·cer·iza·tion** (saw″sər-ĭ-za′shən) 1. the excavation of tissue to form a shallow shelving depression usually performed to facilitate drainage from infected areas of bone. 2. the shallow, saucer-like depression on the upper surface of a vertebra which has suffered a compression fracture.

**Saun·ders' disease, sign** (sawn′dərz) [Edward Watt *Saunders,* American physician, 1854–1927] see under *disease* and *sign.*

**Saus·sure's hygrometer** (so-sūrz′) [Horace Bénédict de *Saussure,* Swiss physicist, 1740–1799] see under *hygrometer.*

**sav·in** (sav′in) [L. *sabina*] *Juniperus sabina,* whose fresh tops are the source of savin oil; a preparation of the young twigs was formerly used as a diuretic.

**saw** (saw) a cutting instrument with a cutting or serrated edge.
**Adams' s.,** a small straight saw with a long handle, for osteotomy.
**amputating s.,** one for use in performing amputations.
**bayonet s.,** a surgical bone saw used for the excision of the nasal dorsal hump.
**Butcher's s.,** an amputating saw with a blade that can be set at various angles.
**chain s.,** one in which the teeth are set on links, the saw being moved by pulling one or the other handle.
**crown s.,** a form of trephine.
**Farabeuf's s.,** a saw the blade of which can be set at any desired angle.
**Gigli's wire s.,** a flexible wire with saw teeth.
**Hey's s.,** a small saw for enlarging orifices in bones.
**hole s.,** a trephine.
**separating s.,** a saw for separating teeth.
**Shrady's s., subcutaneous s.,** a saw for bone work operated through a fenestrated cannula which has been introduced alongside the bone by a trocar.

**saw pal·met·to** (saw pal-met′to) 1. a small creeping palm of the southeastern United States, *Serenoa repens.* 2. [NF] the partially dried, ripe fruit of the saw palmetto, used for urination problems associated with benign prostatic hypertrophy.

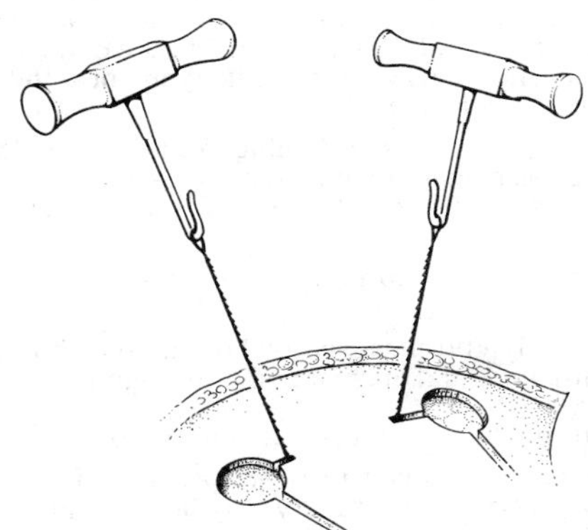

Gigli's wire saw as used in removing segment of the skull.

**saxi·tox·in** (sak″sĭ-tok′sin) [MeSH: Saxitoxin] a powerful, heat-stable, low molecular weight neurotoxin synthesized and secreted by certain dinoflagellates, such as species of *Gonyaulax;* it accumulates in the tissues of bivalve mollusks feeding on the dinoflagellates, and may cause a severe toxic reaction in those who eat the mollusks. See also *shellfish poisoning,* under *poisoning.* Called also *shellfish poison.*

**Sayre's apparatus** (sa′ərz) [Lewis Albert *Sayre,* American surgeon, 1820–1900] see under *apparatus.*

**SB** sinus bradycardia.

**Sb** symbol for *antimony* (L. *stibium*).

**SBE** subacute bacterial endocarditis; see *infective endocarditis,* under *endocarditis.*

**SC** secretory component; closure of semilunar valves; subcutaneous.

**Sc** symbol for *scandium.*

**scab** (skab) 1. a crust formed on the surface of a wound. 2. to become covered with a crust or scab. 3. scabies in domestic animals.
**foot s.,** sheep s.
**head s.,** any acariasis of the head, especially the sarcoptic scab of the head of sheep.
**sheep s.,** psoroptic mange in sheep, the most common type of mange in that species, caused by the mite *Psoroptes ovis,* which infests the skin at the base of the hairs. A scab forms, which later detaches along with the wool; open sores may lead to infection, emaciation, and even death.

**sca·bet·ic** (skə-bet′ik) scabietic.

**sca·bi·cide** (ska′bĭ-sīd) 1. destructive to *Sarcoptes scabiei;* used in the treatment of scabies. 2. an agent for destroying *Sarcoptes scabiei.*

**sca·bies** (ska′bēz) [L., from *scabere* scratch] [MeSH: Scabies] 1. a contagious dermatitis of humans and various wild and domestic animals caused by the mite *Sarcoptes scabiei;* the egg-laying female mite digs into the upper layer of the epidermis and makes raised sinuous burrows (cuniculi), which then cause a papular eruption accompanied by intense pruritus sometimes associated with eczema from scratching and secondary bacterial infection. Called also *seven-year itch* (in humans) and *sarcoptic mange* (in other animals). 2. psoroptic mange in cattle and horses caused by *Psoroptes ovis.*
**crusted s.,** Norwegian s.
**Norwegian s.,** a rare, severe form with an unusually heavy mite infestation, seen especially in senile, mentally retarded, or immunocompromised patients, those with poor sensation, or those with severe systemic disease, thought to represent an abnormal host immune response to the mites. It is characterized by crusting dermatitis of the hands and feet with subungual horny debris, erythematous scaling plaques on the neck, scalp, and trunk that may become generalized, and usually lymphadenopathy and eosinophilia. Called also *crusted s.*

**sca·bi·et·ic** (ska″be-et′ik) pertaining to or affected with scabies.

**SCAD de·fi·cien·cy** short-chain acyl-CoA dehydrogenase deficiency; see under *acyl-CoA dehydrogenase.*

**sca·la** (ska′lə) pl. *sca′lae* [L. "staircase"] a stairlike structure; applied especially to various passages of the cochlea.
**s. of Löwenberg, s. me′dia,** ductus cochlearis.
**s. tym′pani** [TA], the perilymph-filled part of the cochlea that is continuous with the scala vestibuli at the helicotrema, is separated from other cochlear structures by the spiral lamina and the basilar membrane of the cochlear duct, and ends blindly near the fenestra cochleae. Called also *tympanic canal of cochlea.*
**s. vesti′buli** [TA], the perilymph-filled part of the cochlea that begins in the vestibule, is separated from other cochlear structures by the spiral lamina and Reissner's membrane of the cochlear duct, and becomes continuous with the scala tympani at the helicotrema. Called also *vestibular canal.*

**sca·lar** (ska′lər) [L. *scalaris* pertaining to a ladder or staircase] 1. a quantity that has magnitude only (as opposed to also having direction), such as mass or temperature. Cf. *vector.* 2. pertaining to a scalar.

**sca·lar·i·form** (skə-lar′ĭ-form) [*scalar* + *form*] resembling the rungs of a ladder.

**scald** (skawld) 1. a burn caused by hot liquid or hot, moist vapor. 2. to burn with hot liquid or steam. 3. interdigital dermatitis. 4. benign foot rot.
**foot s.,** 1. interdigital dermatitis. 2. benign foot rot.

**scale**[1] (skāl) [L. *scala,* usually pl. *scalae,* a series of steps] a scheme or device by which some property may be evaluated or measured, such as a linear surface bearing marks at regular intervals, representing certain predetermined units.
**absolute s., absolute temperature s.,** 1. one with its zero at absolute zero (−273.15°C, −459.67°F). 2. Kelvin s.
**Apgar s.,** see under *score.*
**Baumé's s.,** a scale for expressing the specific gravity of liquids, based on the extent to which the liquid is lighter or heavier than water.
**binary s.,** dichotomous s.
**Borg s.,** a numerical scale for assessing dyspnea, from 0 representing no dyspnea to 10 as maximal dyspnea.
**Brazelton behavioral s.,** a method for assessing infant behavior by its responses to environmental stimuli.
**Brief Psychiatric Rating S.,** BPRS; a rating scale for assessing psychopathology on the basis of a small number, usually 16 to 24, items encompassing psychosis, depression, and anxiety symptoms.
**Cattell Infant Intelligence S.,** a test of general motor and cognitive development, assessed by performance of tasks, in the first 18 months of life.
**Celsius s.,** a temperature scale on which 0° is officially 273.15 kelvins and 100° is 373.15 kelvins; abbreviated *C* or *Cel.* Before 1948 (and still, unofficially) the degree Celsius (°C) was called the degree centigrade (symbol °C) with 0° at the freezing point of fresh water and 100° at the boiling point, at normal atmospheric pressure (760 mm Hg). See also *kelvin* and Appendix 3 for Celsius-Fahrenheit, Fahrenheit-Celsius equivalents.
**centigrade s.,** 1. one in which the interval between two fixed points is divided into 100 equal units. 2. Celsius s.
**Charrière s.,** French s.
**Clark's s.,** a scale used in denoting the hardness of water, based on the number of grains of calcium carbonate per imperial gallon.
**Columbia Mental Maturity S.,** a test of specific kinds of mental function and general abilities, suitable for children (ages 3 to 12) with no speech or with limited physical capabilities, such as those with cerebral palsy.
**continuous s.,** an interval scale in which the intervals can be broken into finer and finer gradations, e.g., blood glucose or weight scales.
**Defensive Functioning S.,** a scale comprising defense mechanisms used to prevent or allay anxiety.
**dichotomous s.,** a nominal scale (q.v.) with two categories.
**dimensional s.,** interval s.
**Dunfermline s.,** a scheme used in denoting the nutritional status of children: 1, superior condition; 2, passable condition; 3, requiring supervision; 4, requiring medical treatment.
**Fahrenheit s.,** a temperature scale, obsolescent but still commonly, unofficially used in the United States, in which the interval between Fahrenheit's two original fixed points, which are the lowest temperature attainable by a freezing mixture of ice and salt (0°) and the normal temperature of the human body (96° originally), is divided into 96 degrees (96 having 10 factors besides itself and 1); fresh water freezes at about 32° and boils at about 212° under average atmospheric pressure. See *Celsius s.* and Appendix 3 for Celsius-Fahrenheit, Fahrenheit-Celsius equivalents.
**French s.,** a scale used for denoting the size of catheters, sounds, and other tubular instruments; one French unit (symbol F) is 0.33 mm in diameter, so that an 18 French or 18F needle has a diameter of 6 mm.
**Gaffky s.,** a scale used in denoting the prognosis in tuberculosis, based on the number of tubercle bacilli in the sputum. Called also *Gaffky table.*
**Glasgow Coma S.,** a standardized system for assessing response to stimuli in a neurologically impaired patient; reactions are given a numerical value in three categories (eye opening, verbal responsiveness, and motor responsiveness), and the three scores are then added together. The lowest values are the worst clinical scores.
**Glasgow Outcome S.,** a scale used to describe outcome after serious head injury, based on the general level of social functioning regained. Patients are assigned to one of five categories: good recovery, moderately disabled, severely disabled, vegetative, or dead.
**Global Assessment of Functioning (GAF) s.,** a rating of psychiatric status from 1 (lowest level of functioning) to 100 (highest level), assessing psychological, social, and occupational functioning; widely used in studies of treatment effectiveness.
**gray s.,** see under *ultrasonography.*
**Hamilton Depression Rating S.,** one designed to score the severity of depression on the basis of a semistructured interview eliciting depression-related symptoms.
**homigrade s.,** a temperature scale in which 0° represents the melting point of ice (0°C, 32°F), 100°, normal human temperature (37°C, 98.6°F), and 270° the boiling point of water.
**hydrometer s.,** a scale used for expressing the specific gravity of liquids.
**interval s.,** one used to classify data in which the values have intrinsic order and all intervals have an inherent and equal distance between, e.g., age or temperature scales. Called also *dimensional s.* Cf. *ratio s.*
**Karnofsky s., Karnofsky performance s.,** a widely used performance scale, assigning scores ranging from 0 for a nonfunctional or dead patient to 100 for one with completely normal functioning.

**Kelvin s.,** an absolute temperature scale whose unit of measurement, the kelvin, is equivalent to the degree Celsius, the ice point therefore being at 273.15 kelvins.
**nominal s.,** the weakest qualitative, not quantitative or ordered, classification of the samples into separate categories so that each possible result belongs to only one category, with the categories not able to be ordered relative to each other, e.g., one dealing with religion or sex and not size, weight, or temperature. Cf. *ordinal s.*
**nonlinear s.,** one in which the divisions corresponding to the steps are unequal, e.g., a scale with divisions showing logarithmic or exponential growth or change.
**ordinal s.,** a scale used to classify data into qualitative ordered categories, e.g., defining socioeconomic status as low, medium, or high; the values have a distinct order but intervals are created arbitrarily and lack an intrinsic numerical equality.
**performance s.,** a scale that measures a patient's ability to function, serving as a prognostic indicator of seriousness of disease or disability. The most widely used scale is the Karnofsky scale.
**ranked s.,** a scale in which the adjacent categories are arranged according to a progressively ascending or descending magnitude, as an ordinal scale or interval scale.
**Rankine s.,** an absolute scale on which the unit of measurement corresponds with that of the Fahrenheit scale, so that the ice point is at 491.67 degrees Rankine (°R).
**ratio s.,** an interval scale (q.v.) with a true zero point, e.g., mass, length, or income; thus ratios between values can be meaningfully defined.
**Réaumur s.,** a temperature scale with the ice point at 0 degrees and the normal boiling point of water at 80 degrees Rankine (°R).
**Social and Occupational Functioning Assessment S.,** SOFAS; one that describes the level of an individual's social and occupational functioning, either present or past; unlike the GAF scale, it is not directly influenced by the severity of the individual's psychological symptoms.
**temperature s.,** a scale used for expressing the degree of heat, based on absolute zero as a reference point (absolute scale), or with a certain value arbitrarily assigned to such temperatures as the ice point and boiling point of water under certain stipulated conditions, the range between and beyond them being divided into a designated number of identical units.
**visual analog s.,** one that enables a patient to indicate the perceived level of intensity of a symptom (e.g., of pain) by locating its position on a line representing a range from least intensity to greatest intensity.
**Wechsler Adult Intelligence S. (WAIS),** a group of tests for assessment of intellectual functioning in adults.
**Wechsler Intelligence S. for Children (WISC),** a group of tests for assessment of intellectual functioning in children ages 5 to 15.

**scale[2] (skāl)** [Old Fr. *escale* shell, husk] 1. a thin, compacted, flaky fragment, such as a delicate plate of bone or enamel or a bit of dried horny epidermis. 2. a thin fragment of tartar or other concretion on the surface of a tooth. 3. to remove calcareous deposits from the teeth and from beneath the gingival margin with an instrument.
**adhesive s.,** one not readily sloughed, as in lupus erythematosus.

**sca·lene** (ska'lēn) [Gr. *skalēnos* uneven] 1. uneven; unequally three-sided. 2. pertaining to one of the scalene muscles (see terms beginning *musculus scalenus*).

**sca·le·nec·to·my** (ska″lə-nek'tə-me) [*scalenus* + *-ectomy*] the surgical resecting of a scalenus muscle.

**sca·le·not·o·my** (ska″lə-not'ə-me) [*scalenus* + *-tomy*] sectioning of the scalene muscles to restrict respiratory activity of the upper thorax and thus induce apical rest; formerly used in treatment of pulmonary tuberculosis.

**sca·le·nus** (ska-le'nəs) [L.; Gr. *skalēnos*] uneven (scalene); see under *musculus.*

**sca·ler** (ska'lər) 1. a dental instrument used in removing calculus from tooth surfaces. See also *scaling.* 2. an electronic instrument for rapid counting of radiation-induced pulses emitted from a Geiger counter or other radiation detectors.
**chisel s.,** periodontal chisel.
**deep s.,** one of several types of scalers designed for removal of subgingival deposits from the teeth.
**double-ended s.,** one with blades on both sides of the handle, one blade for the right side, the other for the left.
**hoe s.,** one made with different angular relationships of shank and handle, but with the blade bent at a 99° angle, and the flattened termination surface beveled at an angle of 45°, used for planing and smoothing root surfaces.
**sickle s.,** a scaler that removes tenacious supragingival or subgingival deposits; it has a sickle-like blade with flattened sides and a trapezoidal cross section.
**superficial s.,** one of several types of scalers designed for removal of supragingival deposits from the teeth.
**ultrasonic s.,** an ultrasonic instrument with a tip for supplying high-frequency vibrations, used to remove adherent deposits from the teeth and bits of inflamed tissue from the walls of the gingival crevice.

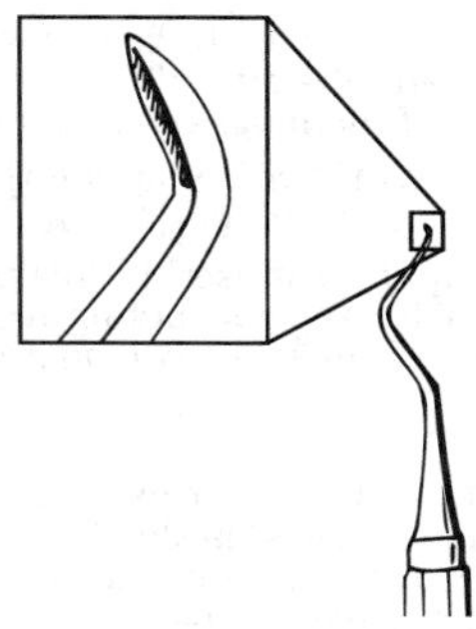

Scaler.

**scal·ing** (skāl'ing) removal of plaque and calculus from the surface of a tooth by means of a scaler.
**deep s.,** removal of plaque and calculus from the surface of a tooth apical to the gingival margin, usually accumulated in periodontal pockets. Called also *subgingival s.* and *root s.*
**root s.,** deep s.
**subgingival s.,** deep s.
**ultrasonic s.,** removal of debris, plaque, and calculus from the surface of the teeth with an ultrasonic scaler.

**scalp** (skalp) [MeSH: Scalp] that part of the skin of the head, exclusive of the face and ears, which normally is covered with hair.
**double s.,** thinning of the bones of the scalp in young sheep, usually because of an inadequate diet; called also *cappie.*
**gyrate s.,** cutis verticis gyrata.

**scal·pel** (skal'pəl) [L. *scalpellum*] a small surgical knife with a straight handle and, usually, a blade with a convex edge.

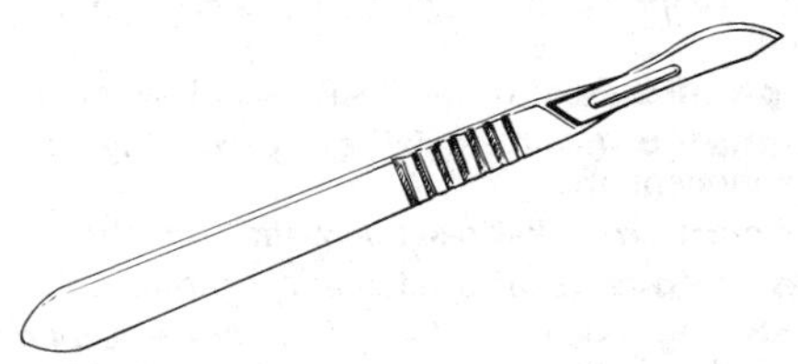

Scalpel.

**scal·pri·form** (skal'prĭ-form) shaped like a chisel.

**sca·ly** (ska'le) [L. *squamosus*] 1. scalelike. 2. characterized by scales.

**scam·mo·nia** (skə-mo'ne-ə) scammony.

**scam·mo·ny** (skam'ə-ne) [L. *scammonium, scammonia*] 1. *Convolvulus scammonia.* 2. the dried root of *C. scammonia,* which contains a gummy resinous exudate that has anthelmintic and cathartic properties. 3. any of various other plants resembling *C. scammonia.*
**Mexican s.,** ipomea.

**scan** (skan) 1. to examine or map the body, or one or more organs or regions of it, by gathering information with a sensing device. 2. the data or image so obtained, often designated according to the organ under examination, as *brain scan, kidney scan, thyroid scan,* etc. 3. shortened form of *scintiscan.*
**A-s.,** display on a cathode ray tube of ultrasonic echoes, in which one axis represents the time required for return of the echo and the other corresponds to the strength of the echo.
**B-s.,** display on a cathode ray tube of ultrasonic echoes, in which the position of a bright dot on the tube corresponds to the time elapsed and the brightness of the spot to the strength of the echo; movement of the transducer across the skin surface yields a two-dimensional cross-sectional display.
**CAT s., CT s.,** computerized axial tomography; see under *tomography.*
**Meckel s.,** a technetium-99m pertechnetate gastric-mucosa scan used to demonstrate ectopic gastric mucosa, particularly in Meckel's diverticulum.
**M-mode s.,** the image obtained using M-mode echocardiography, showing the motion (M) over time of a monodimensional ("icepick") section of the heart.
**ventilation-perfusion s., V/Q s.,** a scintigraphic technique for demonstrating perfusion defects in normally ventilated areas of the lung

in the diagnosis of pulmonary embolism, consisting of the imaging of the distribution of an inhaled radionuclide followed by the imaging of the perfusion of the lungs by an injected radionuclide.

**scan·di·um** (skan′de-əm) [MeSH: Scandium] a very rare metallic element; symbol, Sc; atomic number, 21; atomic weight, 44.956.

**scan·ner** (skan′ər) equipment used for making scans or scanning.
**EMI s.**, an instrument for reconstructing tomographic images for display on a cathode ray tube; see *computerized axial tomography*, under *tomography*.
**scintillation s.**, scintiscanner.

**scan·ning** (skan′ing) 1. the act of examining visually, as a small area or different isolated areas, in detail. 2. the act of examining with a sensing device, as to perform a scan. 3. scanning speech.
**infarct avid s.**, see under *scintigraphy*.
**MUGA s., multiple gated acquisition s.**, equilibrium radionuclide angiocardiography.
**radioisotope s.**, production of a two-dimensional record or image representing the gamma rays emitted by a radioactive isotope concentrated in a specific tissue of the body, such as the brain or thyroid gland.
**thallium s.**, see *thallium-201 myocardial perfusion scintigraphy*, under *scintigraphy* and *thallium stress test*, under *tests*.

**sca·nog·ra·phy** (skan-og′rə-fe) a method of making radiographs by the use of a narrow slit beneath the tube in such a manner that only a line or sheet of x-rays is employed and the x-ray tube moves over the object so that all the rays of the central beam pass through the part being radiographed at the same angle.

**scan·sion** (skan′shən) scanning speech.

**Scan·zo·ni's maneuver (operation)** (skahn-tso′nēz) [Friedrich Wilhelm *Scanzoni*, German obstetrician, 1821–1891] see under *operation*.

**sca·pha** (ska′fə) [L. "a skiff"] [TA] the long curved depression that separates the helix from the anthelix; called also *scaphoid fossa* and *fossa helicis*.

**sca·phi·on** (ska′fe-on) [Gr. *skaphion* a small bowl or basin] basis cranii externa.

**scaph(o)-** [Gr. *skaphē* skiff or light boat] a combining form meaning boat-shaped.

**scapho·ce·pha·lia** (skaf″o-sə-fa′le-ə) scaphocephaly.

**scapho·ce·phal·ic** (skaf″o-sə-fal′ik) pertaining to or characterized by scaphocephaly.

**scapho·ceph·a·lism** (skaf″o-sef′ə-liz-əm) scaphocephaly.

**scapho·ceph·a·lous** (skaf″o-sef′ə-ləs) scaphocephalic.

**scapho·ceph·a·ly** (skaf″o-sef′ə-le) [*scapho-* + *-cephaly*] a condition in which the skull is abnormally long and narrow, as a result of premature closure of the sagittal suture, with heavy centers of ossification in the line of the suture; usually accompanied by inflammation and atrophy of the optic papillae and by mental retardation. Called also *sagittal synostosis*.

**scapho·hy·dro·ceph·a·lus** (skaf″o-hi″dro-sef′ə-ləs) hydrocephalus in which the head assumes a boatlike shape.

**scapho·hy·dro·ceph·a·ly** (skaf″o-hi″dro-sef′ə-le) scaphohydrocephalus.

**scaph·oid** (skaf′oid) [*scaph-* + *-oid*] shaped like a boat; navicular. Used especially in reference to the most lateral bone in the proximal row of carpal bones; see *os scaphoideum*.

**scaph·oid·itis** (skaf″oi-di′tis) inflammation of the scaphoid bone.
**tarsal s.**, 1. inflammation involving the navicular (scaphoid) bone of the tarsus. 2. Köhler's bone disease (def. 1).

**scapho·lu·nate** (skaf″ə-loo′nāt) pertaining to the scaphoid and lunate bones.

**Scap·to·co·sa** (skap″to-ko′sə) a genus of wolf spiders (family Lycosidae). *S. rapto′ria* is a Brazilian species whose powerful hemolytic venom causes necrotic arachnidism.

**scap·u·la** (skap′u-lə) pl. *scap′ulae* [L.] [TA] [MeSH: Scapula] the flat, triangular bone in the back of the shoulder; the shoulder blade. See Plate 45.
**alar s., s. ala′ta**, winged s.
**elevated s.**, Sprengel's deformity.
**Graves' s.**, scaphoid s.
**scaphoid s.**, a scapula in which the vertebral border is more or less concave.
**winged s.**, a scapula having a prominent vertebral border.

**scap·u·lal·gia** (skap″u-lal′jə) pain in the scapular region.

**scap·u·lar** (skap′u-lər) of or pertaining to the scapula.

**scap·u·lary** (skap′u-lar″e) a shoulder bandage, with the appearance of a pair of suspenders or braces, to hold in place a body bandage or girdle.

**scap·u·lec·to·my** (skap″u-lek′tə-me) [*scapula* + *-ectomy*] surgical removal or resection of the scapula.

**scap·u·lo·an·te·ri·or** (skap″u-lo-an-tēr′e-or) denoting a position of the fetus in transverse lie, with the scapula directed anteriorly.

**scap·u·lo·cla·vic·u·lar** (skap″u-lo-klə-vik′u-lər) pertaining to the scapula and the clavicle.

**scap·u·lo·dyn·ia** (skap″u-lo-din′e-ə) [*scapula* + *-odynia*] pain in the region of the shoulder.

**scap·u·lo·hu·mer·al** (skap″u-lo-hu′mər-əl) pertaining to the scapula and the humerus.

**scap·u·lo·per·o·ne·al** (skap″u-lo-per-o-ne′əl) pertaining to or involving both the scapula and the fibula or outer calf.

**scap·u·lo·pexy** (skap′u-lo-pek″se) [*scapula* + *-pexy*] surgical fixation of the scapula.

**scap·u·lo·pos·te·ri·or** (skap″u-lo-pos-tēr′e-or) denoting a position of the fetus in transverse lie, with the scapula directed posteriorly.

**sca·pus** (ska′pəs) pl. *sca′pi* [L.] shaft: general anatomical nomenclature for a shaftlike structure.
**s. pe′nis**, corpus penis.
**s. pi′li**, hair shaft.

**scar** (skahr) [Gr. *eschara* the scab or eschar on a wound caused by burning] [MeSH: Cicatrix] 1. a mark remaining after the healing of a wound or other morbid process; called also *cicatrix*. 2. any of various manifestations of an earlier event.
**apical s.**, a translucent area of bone commonly found around the apex of a tooth after root canal therapy or other endodontic treatment.
**hypertrophic s.**, one formed by exuberant cicatrization, giving it the appearance of a keloid but without the latter's tendency to progressive extension or to recurrence after excision.
**Reichert's s.**, an area over the implanting blastocyst of some species, consisting of a fibrinous membrane in place of the decidual tissue.
**white s. of ovary**, corpus albicans, def. 1.

**scar·i·fi·ca·tion** (skar″ĭ-fĭ-ka′shən) [L. *scarificatio*, Gr. *skariphismos* a scratching up] production in the skin of many small, superficial scratches or punctures, as for the introduction of smallpox vaccine. The term is sometimes used erroneously for scarring.

**scar·i·fi·ca·tor** (skar′ĭ-fĭ-ka″tər) scarifier.

**scar·i·fi·er** (skar′ĭ-fi″ər) an instrument bearing one or more sharp points, used in scarification.

**scar·la·ti·na** (skahr″lə-te′nə) [L. "scarlet"] scarlet fever; see under *fever*.
**s. angino′sa**, scarlet fever associated with painful pharyngitis, with tonsillar enlargement or peritonsillar abscess.
**puerperal s.**, a scarlet rash sometimes seen in puerperal fever.

**scar·lat·i·nal** (skahr-lat′ĭ-nəl) pertaining to or due to scarlatina (scarlet fever).

**scar·lat·i·nel·la** (skahr-lat″ĭ-nel′ə) Dukes' disease.

**scar·la·tin·i·form** (skahr″lə-tin′ĭ-form) resembling scarlet fever, especially the skin eruption of scarlet fever; scarlatinoid.

**scar·lat·i·noid** (skahr-lat′ĭ-noid) scarlatiniform.

**scar·let** (skahr′lət) 1. bright red tinged with orange or yellow. 2. a scarlet dye.
**Biebrich s., water-soluble**, an azo dye used as a plasma stain.
**s. G**, Sudan III.
**s. R**, scarlet red.

**Scar·pa's fascia**, etc. (skahr′pahz) [Antonio *Scarpa*, Italian anatomist and surgeon, 1747–1832] see under *fascia* and *foramen;* see *posterior staphyloma* under *staphyloma;* and see *cornu superius marginis falciformis, fascia cremasterica, ganglion vestibulare, membrana tympani secundaria, nervus nasopalatinus*, and *trigonum femorale*.

**SCAT** sheep cell agglutination test.

**Scat·chard plot** (skach′ərd) [George *Scatchard*, American chemist, 1892–1973] see under *plot*.

**scat(o)-** [Gr. *skōr*, gen. *skatos* dung] a combining form denoting relation to dung, or fecal matter; see also words beginning *skat(o)-*.

**sca·tol** (ska′tōl) skatole.

**scato·lo·gia** (skat″ah-lo′jə) scatology, def. 2.
**telephone s.**, a paraphilia in which sexual arousal or activity is linked to the placing of obscene phone calls.

**scato·log·ic** (skat″o-loj′ik) pertaining to fecal matter, or to scatology.

**sca·tol·o·gy** (skah-tol′ə-je) [*scato-* + *-logy*] 1. the study and analysis of the feces, as for diagnostic purposes. 2. a preoccupation with feces, filth, or obscenities.

**sca·to·ma** (skə-to′mə) [*scat-* + *-oma*] stercoroma.

**sca·toph·a·gy** (skə-tof′ə-je) [*scato-* + *-phagy*] the eating of excrement.

**sca·tos·co·py** (skə-tos′kə-pe) [*scato-* + *-scopy*] inspection of the feces.

**scat·ter** (skat′ər) the change in energy or momentum of radiation or particles (e.g., photons or x-rays) produced by interaction with the medium through which the rays or particles pass. See also *backscatter.*

**scat·ter·gram** (skat′ər-gram) scatterplot.

**scat·ter·ing** (skat′ər-ing) a change in direction of a photon or subatomic particle as the result of a collision or interaction.
**Compton s.,** modified scattering; the deflection of an incident photon by interaction with a free electron or an orbital electron of much lower energy than the photon; the photon is deflected from its original path and gives up part of its energy to displace the electron.
**Thomson s.,** unmodified scattering; deflection of a photon by interaction with an atom with no loss of energy by the photon.

**scat·ter·plot** (skat′ər-plot) a plot in rectangular coordinates of paired observations of two random variables, each observation plotted as one point on the graph; the scatter or clustering of points provides an indication of the relationship between the two variables. Called also *scatter diagram* or *scattergram.*

**scat·u·la** (skat′u-lə) [L. "parallelepiped"] an oblong paper box for powders or pills.

**scav·en·ger** (skav′ən-jər) a substance that influences the course of a chemical reaction by ready combination with free radicals.

**ScD** Doctor of Science.

**ScDA** abbreviation for L. *scapulodextra anterior* (right scapuloanterior; a presentation of the fetus).

**ScDP** abbreviation for L. *scapulodextra posterior* (right scapuloposterior; a presentation of the fetus).

**Sce·do·spo·ri·um** (se-do-spor′e-əm) a genus of Fungi Imperfecti of the form-class Hyphomycetes, form-family Moniliaceae; its perfect (sexual) stage is *Pseudallescheria. S. apiosper′mum* is the anamorph of *P. boydii,* a major cause of eumycotic mycetoma. *S. infla′tum* has been isolated from several cases of osteomyelitis. Formerly called *Monosporium.*

**sce·lal·gia** (sə-lal′jə) [Gr. *skelos* leg + *-algia*] pain in the leg.

**scelo·tyr·be** (sel″o-tər′be) [Gr. *skelos* leg + *tyrbē* disorder] spastic paralysis of the legs.

**Scha·cho·wa's spiral tubes** (shah-ko′vəz) [Seraphina *Schachowa,* Russian histologist in Switzerland, 19th century] tubuli renales.

**Scha·fer's method** (sha′fərz) [Sir Edward Albert Sharpey-*Schafer,* English physiologist, 1850–1935] see under *respiration, artificial.*

**Schä·fer's syndrome** (sha′fərz) [Erich *Schäfer,* German physician, born 1897] see under *syndrome.*

**Schäf·fer's reflex** (shāf′ərz) [Max *Schäffer,* German neurologist, 1852–1923] see under *reflex.*

**Schal·ly** (shahl′e) Andrew Victor. Lithuanian-born American biochemist, born 1926; co-winner, with Roger Charles Louis Guillemin and Rosalyn Sussman Yalow, of the Nobel prize for medicine or physiology in 1977 for the discovery of releasing factors, low-molecular-weight polypeptides secreted by the hypothalamus that regulate the release of hormones by the pituitary gland.

**Scham·berg's disease (dermatosis)** (shahm′bərgz) [Jay Frank *Schamberg,* American dermatologist, 1870–1934] see under *disease.*

**Schanz's disease, syndrome** (shahnts′ez) [Alfred *Schanz,* German orthopedist, 1868–1931] see under *disease* and *syndrome.*

**schar·lach R** (shahr′lak) scarlet red.

**Schat·zki's ring** (shaht′skēz) [Richard *Schatzki;* German-born American radiologist, 1901–1992] see *esophageal ring,* under *ring.*

**Schau·dinn's fluid** (shou′dinz) [Fritz Richard *Schaudinn,* German bacteriologist, 1871–1906] see under *fluid.*

**Schau·mann's bodies, disease, sarcoid, syndrome** (shou′mahnz) [Jörgen *Schaumann,* Swedish dermatologist, 1879–1953] see under *body,* and see *sarcoidosis.*

**Schau·ta's operation** (shou′təz) [Friedrich *Schauta,* Austrian gynecologist, 1849–1919] see under *operation.*

**SChE** serum cholinesterase; see *cholinesterase.*

**Sche·de's operation** (sha′dəz) [Max *Schede,* German surgeon, 1844–1902] see under *operation.*

**sched·ule** (sked′ūl) [MeSH: Appointments and Schedules] a formal list, plan of procedure, or timetable.
**S. for Affective Disorders and Schizophrenia,** SADS; a semistructured interview administered by a professional and designed to yield diagnostic information about current and lifetime incidences of affective disorders and schizophrenia.
**Diagnostic Interview S.,** DIS; a structured interview, administered by trained nonclinicians, assessing lifetime as well as current occurrence of symptoms of a variety of mental disorders; diagnoses are aided by computer algorithms.
**Gesell developmental s.,** a test of the developmental status of infants that includes assessment of motor development, adaptive behavior, language development, and personal-social behavior.
**s. of reinforcement,** a series of rules governing the delivery or nondelivery of reinforcement; it may occur after every response (continuous reinforcement) or not (partial reinforcement). In partial reinforcement, delivery may occur after predetermined amounts of time (*intervals*) or numbers of responses (*ratios*), either of these being unvarying (*fixed*) or changing (*variable*), e.g., a *fixed-interval s.* or a *variable ratio s.*

**Scheibe's deafness** (shi′bəz) [A. *Scheibe,* American physician, born 1875] see under *aplasia* and *deafness.*

**Scheie's syndrome** (shāz) [Harold Glendon *Scheie,* American ophthalmologist, 1909–1990] see under *syndrome.*

**Schei·ner's experiment** (shi′nərz) [Christoph *Scheiner,* German astronomer, 1575–1650] see under *experiment.*

**sche·ma** (ske′mə) [Gr. *schēma* form, shape] a plan, outline, or arrangement.

**sche·mat·ic** (ske-mat′ik) serving as a diagram or model.

**Sche·pel·mann's sign** (sha′pəl-mahnz) [Emil *Schepelmann,* German physician, 20th century] see under *sign.*

**sche·ro·ma** (ske-ro′mə) xerophthalmia.

**Scheu·er·mann's disease, kyphosis** (shoi′ər-mahnz) [Holger Werfel *Scheuermann,* Danish surgeon, 1877–1960] osteochondrosis of the vertebrae; see *osteochondrosis.*

**Schick's sign, test (reaction)** (shiks) [Béla *Schick,* Hungarian pediatrician in the United States, 1877–1967] see under *sign* and *test.*

**Schief·fer·deck·er's symbiosis, theory** (she′fər-dek″ərz) [Paul *Schiefferdecker,* German anatomist, 1849–1931] see under *theory.*

**Schiff's biliary cycle** (shifs) [Moritz *Schiff,* German physiologist, 1823–1896] see under *cycle.*

**Schiff's reagent** (shifs) [Hugo (Ugo) *Schiff,* German chemist in Italy, 1834–1915] see under *reagent.*

**Schil·der's disease (encephalitis)** (shil′dərz) [Paul Ferdinand *Schilder,* Austrian neurologist in the United States, 1886–1940] see under *disease.*

**Schil·ler's test** (shil′ərz) [Walter *Schiller,* Austrian pathologist in the United States, 1887–1960] see under *test.*

**Schil·ling's leukemia** (shil′ingz) [Victor Theodor Adolf Georg *Schilling,* German hematologist, 1883–1960] acute monocytic leukemia.

**Schil·ling test** (shil′ing) [Robert Frederick *Schilling,* American hematologist, born 1919] [MeSH: Schilling Test] see under *test.*

**Schim·mel·busch's disease** (shim′əl-boosh′əz) [Curt *Schimmelbusch,* German surgeon, 1860–1895] cystic disease of the breast; see under *disease.*

**schin·dy·le·sis** (skin″də-le′sis) [Gr. *schindylēsis* a splintering] [TA] a form of articulation in which a thin plate of one bone is received into a cleft in another, as in the articulation of the perpendicular plate of the ethmoid bone with the vomer. Called also *wedge-and-groove joint.*

**Schi·øtz's tonometer** (she-ets′ez) [Hjalmar *Schiøtz,* Norwegian physician, 1850–1927] see under *tonometer.*

**Schir·mer's syndrome** (shir′mərz) [Rudolf *Schirmer,* German ophthalmologist, 1831–1896] see under *syndrome.*

**-schisis** [Gr. *schisis* cleft] combining form denoting a cleft or cleavage.

**schis·ta·sis** (skis′tə-sis) a splitting; specifically, a congenital defect consisting of a cleft or fissure of the body, as schistocormia, schistomelia, schistosomia.

**schist(o)-** [Gr. *schistos* split] a combining form meaning split or cleft.

**schis·to·ce·lia** (shis″, skis″to-se′le-ə) schistocoelia.

**schis·to·ceph·a·lus** (shis″, skis″to-sef′ə-ləs) [*schisto-* + *-cephalus*] a fetus with cranium bifidum.

**schis·to·coe·lia** (shis″, skis″to-se′le-ə) [*schisto-* + *coel-* + *-ia*] congenital fissure of the abdomen.

**schis·to·cor·mia** (shis″, skis″to-kor′me-ə) [*schisto-* + Gr. *kormos* trunk + -*ia*] a developmental anomaly characterized by a cleft condition of the trunk.

**schis·to·cor·mus** (shis″, skis″to-kor′məs) a fetus exhibiting schistocormia.

**schis·to·cys·tis** (shis″to-sis′tis) [*schisto-* + *cystis*] fissure of the bladder.

**schis·to·cyte** (shis′, skis′to-sīt) a fragment of an erythrocyte, commonly observed in the blood in hemolytic anemias; called also *helmet cell* and *schizocyte.*

**schis·to·cy·to·sis** (shis″, skis″to-si-to′sis) the accumulation of schistocytes in the blood; called also *schizocytosis.*

**schis·to·me·lia** (shis″, skis″to-me′le-ə) [*schisto-* + *-melia*] a developmental anomaly characterized by a cleft condition of a limb.

**schis·tom·e·lus** (shis-, skis-tom′ə-ləs) a fetus exhibiting schistomelia.

**schis·to·pro·so·pia** (shis″, skis″to-pro-so′pe-ə) [*schisto-* + *prosop-* + *-ia*] a developmental anomaly characterized by fissure of the face; schizoprosopia.

**schis·to·pros·o·pus** (shis″, skis″to-pros′o-pəs) a fetus exhibiting schistoprosopia.

**schis·tor·a·chis** (shis-, skis-tor′ə-kis) [*schisto-* + *rachis*] rachischisis.

**schis·to·sis** (shis-, skis-to′sis) [*schist* a form of slate + *-osis*] pneumoconiosis in slate workers.

**Schis·to·so·ma** (shis″, skis″to-so′mə) [*schisto-* + Gr. *sōma* body] [MeSH: Schistosoma] a genus of trematodes of the family Schistosomatidae; the blood flukes; called also *Bilharzia.*
**S. bo′vis,** a species found in the portal system of sheep and cattle in Iraq, Africa, and certain islands in the Mediterranean.
**S. haemato′bium,** a common parasite in North Africa, other parts of the Mediterranean littoral, and the Arabian peninsula. The adult worms are found in the veins, especially those of the vesical plexus, producing irritability of the bladder, hematuria, and dysentery. The parasites enter the body through the skin of persons coming in contact with infested waters, the invertebrate hosts being small snails of the genus *Bulinus,* including the subgenus *Physopsis.* Called also *Bilharzia haematobia* and, formerly, *Distoma haematobium* and *D. capense.*

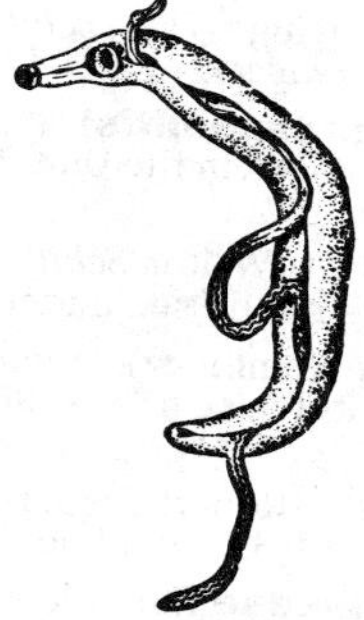

*Schistosoma haematobium,* male carrying female in gynecophoral canal (×6).

**S. in′dicum,** a species occurring in cattle, sheep, goats, and other ruminants in India, Zimbabwe, and Zambia.
**S. intercala′tum,** a species found in the veins of humans, horses, and ruminants in west central Africa; it causes schistosomiasis intercalatum by penetrating the skin of persons coming in contact with infested water. The proven transmitting hosts are certain snails of the genus *Bulinus.*
**S. japo′nicum,** a species found in the veins of humans and other animals in Japan, China, the Philippines, Taiwan, and Indonesia; it causes schistosomiasis japonica by penetrating the skin of persons coming in contact with infested waters. The usual transmitting hosts are small snails of the genus *Oncomelania.*
**S. manso′ni,** a species found in the veins of humans and other animals in Egypt and elsewhere in Africa as well as in South America and the West Indies; it causes schistosomiasis mansoni by penetrating the skin of persons coming in contact with infested waters. The transmitting hosts are planorbid snails, especially those of the genus *Biomphalaria.*
**S. mat′theei,** a species found in the portal mesenteric vein of sheep, goats, game animals, monkeys, and rarely man in South Africa.
**S. mekon′gi,** a species found in Laos and Cambodia that differs from *S. japonicum* chiefly in requiring a different intermediate host.
**S. spinda′le,** a species parasitic in water buffalo, cattle, sheep, and goats in India, Malaysia, Indonesia, Zambia, and South Africa.

**schis·to·so·ma·ci·dal** (shis″, skis″to-so″mə-si′dəl) schistosomicidal.

**schis·to·so·ma·cide** (shis″, skis″to-so′mə-sīd) schistosomicide.

**schis·to·so·mal** (shis″, skis″to-so′məl) pertaining to or caused by *Schistosoma.* Called also *bilharzial.*

**Schis·to·so·ma·ti·dae** (shis″, skis″tə-so-mat′ĭ-de) [MeSH: Schistosomatidae] a family of trematodes, including the genera *Schistosoma, Heterobilharzia,* and *Trichobilharzia.*

**Schis·to·so·ma·ti·um** (shis″, skis″to-so-ma′she-əm) a genus of blood flukes of the family Schistosomatidae. *S. douthit′ti* is found in the hepatic portal veins of the meadow mouse.

**schis·to·some** (shis′, skis′to-sōm) an individual of the genus *Schistosoma.*

**schis·to·so·mia** (shis″, skis″to-so′me-ə) [*schisto-* + *soma* + *-ia*] a developmental anomaly characterized by a fissure of the abdomen, with lower limbs rudimentary or lacking.

**schis·to·so·mi·a·sis** (shis″, skis″to-so-mi′ə-sis) [MeSH: Schistosomiasis] infection with flukes of the genus *Schistosoma;* called also *bilharziasis* and *bilharziosis.*
**cutaneous s.,** cercarial dermatitis.
**eastern s.,** s. japonica.
**genitourinary s.,** urinary s.
**s. haemato′bia,** urinary s.
**hepatic s.,** the chronic form of s. mansoni and japonica in which the liver is involved. Ova of the parasites lodge in the hepatic portal venules, stimulating an inflammatory reaction with pipestem fibrosis; portal venous destruction leads to portal hypertension.
**s. intercala′tum,** an endemic intestinal disease of west central Africa due to infection by flukes of the species *Schistosoma intercalatum,* with abdominal pain, diarrhea in which the stools may contain blood and mucus, hyperplasia of the mucosa of the rectal valves, inflammation of the rectal walls, and sometimes polyposis.
**intestinal s.,** the chronic form of schistosomiasis mansoni and japonica in which the intestinal tract is involved. Most of those infected are asymptomatic but some have intermittent diarrhea and blood and mucus in the stools.
**s. japo′nica,** infection by flukes of the species *Schistosoma japonicum.* The acute infection in its early stages produces a serum sickness–like illness (see *Katayama fever,* under *fever*). Chronic effects of infection, which may be very severe, are caused by fibrosis around the eggs deposited by the parasite in the liver, lungs, and central nervous system.
**Manson's s., s. manso′ni,** infection with flukes of the species *Schistosoma mansoni,* which live mainly in the inferior and superior mesenteric veins but migrate to deposit their eggs in venules, primarily of the large intestine. Eggs lodging in the liver may lead to peripheral fibrosis, hepatosplenomegaly, and ascites. Called also *Manson's disease.*
**Oriental s.,** s. japonica.
**pulmonary s.,** schistosomiasis in which migrating cercariae cause a type of pneumonia, and the ova, and sometimes the adult worms, cause embolization of pulmonary arterioles. Allergic pneumonia, allergic asthma, and emphysema may occur.
**urinary s., vesical s.,** infection with *Schistosoma haematobium,* involving the urinary tract and causing cystitis and hematuria; called also *endemic hematuria, genitourinary s.,* and *s. haematobia.*
**visceral s.,** infection with *Schistosoma mansoni* or *S. japonicum,* as opposed to urinary schistosomiasis.

**schis·to·so·mi·ci·dal** (shis″, skis″to-so″mĭ-si′dəl) destructive to schistosomes; called also *schistosomacidal.*

**schis·to·so·mi·cide** (shis″, skis″to-so′mĭ-sīd) an agent that destroys schistosomes; called also *schistosomacide.*

**schis·to·so·mu·lum** (shis″, skis″to-som′u-ləm) *schistoso′mula.* a stage in the life cycle of a schistosome occurring just after it has penetrated human skin as a cercaria; it loses its tail and becomes physiologically modified in order to be capable of anaerobic metabolism in the bloodstream.

**Schis·to·so·mum** (shis″, skis″to-so′məm) *Schistosoma.*

**schis·to·so·mus** (shis″, skis″to-so′məs) a fetus with schistosomia.

**schis·to·ster·nia** (shis″, skis″to-ster′ne-ə) [*schisto-* + *stern-* + *-ia*] cleft sternum.

**schis·to·tho·rax** (shis″, skis″to-thor′aks) [*schisto-* + *thorax*] thoracoschisis.

**schis·to·tra·che·lus** (shis″, skis″to-trə-ke′ləs) [*schisto-* + *trachēlos* neck] a fetus with a fissure of the neck.

**schiz·am·ni·on** (skiz-am′ne-ən) [*schiz-* + *amnion*] an amnion formed by cavitation over or in the inner cell mass, as occurs in human development.

**schiz·ax·on** (skiz-ak′son) an axon which is divided into two equal, or nearly equal, branches.

**schiz·en·ce·phal·ic** (skiz″ən-sə-fal′ik) having abnormal clefts in the brain substance; see under *porencephaly*.

**schiz·en·ceph·a·ly** (skiz″ən-sef′ə-le) [*schiz-* + Gr. *enkephalos* brain] schizencephalic porencephaly.

**schiz(o)-** [Gr. *schizein* to divide] a combining form meaning divided, or denoting relationship to division.

**schizo·af·fec·tive** (skiz″o-ə-fek′tiv) pertaining to or exhibiting features of both schizophrenic and mood disorders (mania and depression).

**Schizo·blas·to·spo·ri·on** (skiz″o-blas″to-spor′e-on) a former genus of Fungi Imperfecti whose species have now been classified in other genera.

**schizo·ce·pha·lia** (skiz″o-sə-fa′le-ə) a developmental anomaly characterized by a longitudinal fissure of the head.

**schizo·cyte** (skiz′o-sīt) schistocyte.

**schizo·cy·to·sis** (skiz″o-si-to′sis) schistocytosis.

**schizo·gen·e·sis** (skiz″o-jen′ə-sis) [*schizo-* + *-genesis*] reproduction by fission.

**schi·zog·e·nous** (skĭ-zog′ə-nəs) reproducing by fission.

**schi·zog·o·ny** (skĭ-zog′ə-ne) [*schizo-* + Gr. *gonē* seed] a form of asexual reproduction characteristic of certain sarcodines and sporozoa in which daughter cells are produced by multiple fission of the nucleus of the parasite (schizont) followed by segmentation of the cytoplasm to form separate masses around each smaller nucleus. Called also *agametogeny* and *agamogenesis*. See also *gametogony, merogony,* and *sporogony*.

**schizo·gy·ria** (skiz″o-ji′re-ə) a condition in which the cerebral convolutions are marked by wedge-shaped cracks.

**schiz·oid** (skiz′oid, skit′soid) 1. characterized by or resulting from excessive shyness, sensitivity, social withdrawal, and introversion; see under *personality*. 2. a term used loosely to refer to any of a variety of characteristics related to schizophrenia, including schizophrenia-like traits said to indicate a predisposition to schizophrenia as well as any disorder other than schizophrenia either occurring in a relative of a schizophrenic or occurring more commonly than average in families of schizophrenics.

**schizo·ki·ne·sis** (skiz″o-kĭ-ne′sis) the condition in which, when an overt specific conditioned response has been extinguished, concomitant nonspecific responses continue to be elicited by the stimulus.

**schizo·my·cete** (skiz″o-mi-sēt′) any organism or species belonging to the Schizomycetes; a bacterium.

**Schizo·my·ce·tes** (skiz″o-mi-se′tēz) [*schizo-* + Gr. *mykēs* fungus] a former taxonomic class comprising the bacteria, consisting of unicellular organisms that commonly multiply by cell division. As originally proposed, it included eight orders, Actinomycetales, Chlamydiales, Cytophagales, Mycoplasmatales, Myxobacteriales, Rhodospirillales, Rickettsiales, and Spirochaetales.

**schiz·ont** (skiz′ont) [*schizo-* + Gr. *ōn, ontos* being] the multinucleate stage or form in the development of certain sarcodines and sporozoa during schizogony. See also *meront* and *segmenter*.

**schi·zon·ti·cide** (skĭ-zon′tĭ-sīd) an agent that destroys schizonts.

**schizo·nych·ia** (skiz″o-nik′e-ə) [*schizo-* + *onych-* + *-ia*] splitting of the nails.

**schizo·pha·sia** (skiz″o-fa′zhə) word salad; see under *W*.

**schizo·phre·nia** (skiz″o-fre′ne-ə, skit″so-fre′ne-ə) [*schizo-* + *phren* + *-ia*] [MeSH: Schizophrenia] [DSM-IV] a mental disorder or heterogeneous group of disorders (the schizophrenias or schizophrenic disorders) comprising most major psychotic disorders and characterized by disturbances in form and content of thought (loosening of associations, delusions, and hallucinations), mood (blunted, flattened, or inappropriate affect), sense of self and relationship to the external world (loss of ego boundaries, dereistic thinking, and autistic withdrawal), and behavior (bizarre, apparently purposeless, and stereotyped activity or inactivity). The definition and clinical application of the concept of schizophrenia have varied greatly. The DSM-IV criteria emphasize marked disorder of thought (delusions, hallucinations, or other thought disorder accompanied by disordered affect or behavior), deterioration from a previous level of functioning, and chronicity (duration of more than 6 months), thus excluding from this classification conditions referred to by others as acute, borderline, simple, or latent schizophrenia. Originally called *dementia praecox* and characterized as a psychosis with adolescent onset and a chronic course ending in deterioration. The term schizophrenia was introduced by Bleuler because neither early onset nor terminal deterioration is an essential feature; he emphasized the splitting and lack of personality integration seen in the disorder.

**acute s.,** acute schizophrenic episode; a condition characterized by acute onset of schizophrenic symptoms; since DSM-IV defines schizophrenia as a chronic disorder, such conditions must now be classified in another psychotic syndrome, such as schizophreniform disorder, brief psychotic disorder, or schizoaffective disorder.

**ambulatory s.,** mild schizophrenia sufficiently well compensated so that the patient can maintain himself in the community without hospitalization.

**borderline s.,** older term for *latent s.*

**catatonic s.** [DSM-IV], a type of schizophrenia characterized by marked psychomotor disturbance, including some combination of motoric immobility (stupor, catalepsy), excessive motor activity, extreme negativism, mutism, echolalia, echopraxia, and peculiarities of voluntary movement such as posturing, mannerisms, grimacing, or stereotyped behaviors.

**childhood s.,** schizophrenia-like symptoms with onset before puberty, characterized by autistic, withdrawn behavior, failure to develop an identity separate from the mother's, and gross developmental immaturity, a category that formerly included all types of childhood "psychosis" including symbiotic psychosis and infantile autism. DSM-IV, taking the position that there is no clear relationship between these disorders and adolescent and adult schizophrenia and other psychotic disorders, calls them pervasive developmental disorders.

**disorganized s.** [DSM-IV], a type that is characterized by frequent incoherence, marked loosening of associations, or grossly disorganized behavior and flat or grossly inappropriate affect and that does not meet the criteria for the catatonic type; associated features include extreme social withdrawal, grimacing, mannerisms, mirror gazing, inappropriate giggling, and other unusual behavior. Called also *hebephrenia* and *hebephrenic s.*

**hebephrenic s.,** disorganized s.

**latent s.,** a type of schizophrenia characterized by clear symptoms of schizophrenia but no history of a psychotic schizophrenic episode; it includes conditions that have been called ambulatory, borderline, prepsychotic, pseudoneurotic, and pseudopsychopathic schizophrenia in which has there has been no acute psychotic episode. Patients described by these terms do not fit the DSM-IV definition of schizophrenia; most would be classified as having schizotypal personality disorder.

**paranoid s.** [DSM-IV], a type of schizophrenia characterized by preoccupation with one or more systematized delusions or with frequent auditory hallucinations but without disorganized speech, disorganized or catatonic behavior, or flat or inappropriate affect.

**prepsychotic s.,** latent s.

**process s.,** a subset of schizophrenias assumed (like the original concept of dementia praecox) to have endogenous origin and poor prognosis as compared to other cases, termed reactive schizophrenia, that are assumed to be caused by predisposing or precipitating environmental factors and to have a better prognosis; called also *schizophrenic process*.

**pseudoneurotic s.,** a form characterized by all-pervasive anxiety and a wide variety of neurotic symptoms that initially mask underlying psychotic tendencies, which may be manifest as occasional, brief psychotic episodes. It is often considered to be more of a personality disorder; see also *schizotypal personality disorder,* under *personality*.

**pseudopsychopathic s.,** a term applied to patients in whom antisocial, impulsive, or sociopathic tendencies initially mask underlying psychotic tendencies typical of schizophrenia. It is often considered to be more of a personality disorder; see *schizotypal personality disorder,* under *personality*.

**reactive s.,** a subset of schizophrenias assumed to be caused by predisposing or precipitating environmental factors and to have a more favorable prognosis than process schizophrenia.

**residual s.** [DSM-IV], a type of schizophrenia characterized by a history of one or more episodes of schizophrenia with prominent psychotic symptoms, current lack of such symptoms, but continuing presence of other schizophrenic symptoms, such as blunted or inappropriate affect, social withdrawal, eccentric behavior, illogical thinking, or loosening of associations.

**schizoaffective s.,** see under *disorder*.

**simple s.,** a form characterized by gradual, insidious loss of drive, social withdrawal, and emotional apathy, but without prominent psychotic features. It is often considered to be a form of personality disorder; see *schizotypal personality disorder,* under *personality*.

**undifferentiated s.** [DSM-IV], a type of schizophrenia characterized by the presence of prominent psychotic symptoms but not classifiable as catatonic, disorganized, or paranoid.

**schizo·phren·ic** (skiz″o-fren′ik) 1. pertaining to or characterized by schizophrenia. 2. a person affected with schizophrenia.

**schizo·phren·i·form** (skiz″o-fren′ĭ-form) resembling schizophrenia.

**Schizo·phy·ceae** (skiz″o-fi′se-e) [*schizo-* + Gr. *phykos* seaweed] Cyanobacteria.

**Schiz·oph·yl·lum** (skiz-of'ĭ-ləm) [MeSH: Schizophyllum] a genus of fungi of the subphylum Basidiomycotina, order Aphyllophorales. *S. commu'ne* has been isolated from human infections, including maxillary sinusitis.

**schizo·pro·so·pia** (skiz"o-pro-so'pe-ə) ununited fissure of the face, as in cleft lip or cleft palate; schistoprosopia.

**Schizo·py·ren·i·da** (skiz"o-pĭ-ren'ĭ-də) [*schizo-* + Gr. *pyrēn* fruit stone] [MeSH: Schizopyrenida] an order of cylindrical, monopodial, typically uninucleate ameboid protozoa (subclass Gymnamoebia, class Lobosea), some species of which exhibit temporary flagellate stages during their life cycle. Representative genera include *Naegleria* and *Vahlkampfia*.

**schizo·tho·rax** (skiz"o-thor'aks) thoracoschisis.

**schizo·to·nia** (skiz"o-to'ne-ə) [*schizo-* + *ton-* + *-ia*] division of the influx of tone to the muscles, so that, for instance, the flexor groups of the arm become hypertonic, while in the leg the extensors become hypertonic.

**schizo·trich·ia** (skiz"o-trik'e-ə) [*schizo-* + *trich-* + *-ia*] splitting of the hairs at the ends.

**Schizo·tryp·a·num** (skiz"o-trip'ə-nəm) [*schizo-* + Gr. *trypanon* borer] in some systems of classification: *(a)* a subgenus of stercorarian trypanosomes comprising *Trypanosoma cruzi;* and *(b)* a genus of trypanosomes comprising the etiologic agent of Chagas' disease when it is considered genically distinct from *T.*, in which case the agent is known as *S. cruzi.*

**schizo·ty·pal** (skiz"o-ti'pəl, skit"so-ti'pəl) exhibiting eccentricities in behavior and communication style, and decreased ability to form social relationships, similar to those of schizophrenia but less severe. See under *personality.*

**schizo·zo·ite** (skiz"o-zo'īt) [*schizo-* + *zo-* + *-ite*[1]] merozoite.

**Schlat·ter's disease (sprain)** (shlaht'ərz) [Carl *Schlatter,* Swiss surgeon, 1864–1934] see *Osgood-Schlatter disease,* under *disease.*

**Schlat·ter-Os·good disease** (shlaht'ər-oz'good) [C. *Schlatter;* Robert Bayley *Osgood,* American orthopedist, 1873–1956] see *Osgood-Schlatter disease,* under *disease.*

**Schlemm's canal, ligaments** (shlemz) [Friedrich S. *Schlemm,* German anatomist, 1795–1858] see *sinus venosus sclerae,* and under *ligament.*

**Schlep·per** (shlep'ər) [Ger. *Schlepper,* hauler, tractor, tugboat] carrier (def. 7).

**Schle·sin·ger's sign (phenomenon)** (shla'sing-ərz) [Hermann *Schlesinger,* Austrian physician, 1866–1934] see under *sign.*

**Schlich·ter test** (shlik'tər) [Jakub G. *Schlichter,* American internist, born 1912] see *serum bactericidal activity test,* under *test.*

**Schlös·ser's treatment** (shler'serz) [Karl *Schlösser,* German ophthalmologist, 1857–1925] see under *treatment.*

**Schluss·ko·ag·u·lum** (shloos"ko-ag'u-ləm) [Ger.] the clot that closes the gap made in the uterine lining by the implanting blastocyst; called also *closing coagulum.*

**Schmidt's diet, syndrome** (shmits) [Adolf *Schmidt,* German physician, 1865–1918] see under *diet* and *syndrome.*

**Schmidt's syndrome** (shmits) [Martin Benno *Schmidt,* German pathologist, 1863–1949] see under *syndrome.*

**Schmidt-Lan·ter·man incisures (clefts), segment** (shmit'lahn'ter-mahn") [Henry D. *Schmidt,* American anatomist, 1823–1888; A. J. *Lanterman,* American anatomist at Strasbourg, late 19th century] see *incisures of Lanterman,* under *incisure,* and *medullary segment,* under *segment.*

**Schmin·cke tumor** (shming'kə) [Alexander *Schmincke,* German pathologist, 1877–1953] lymphoepithelioma.

**Schmitz bacillus** (shmits) [Karl Eitel Friedrich *Schmitz,* German physician, born 1889] *Shigella dysenteriae* type 2.

**Schmorl's body, disease, nodule** (shmorlz) [Christian Georg *Schmorl,* German pathologist, 1861–1932] see under *body, disease,* and *nodule.*

**Schna·bel's caverns** (shnah'bəlz) [Isidor *Schnabel,* Austrian ophthalmologist, 1842–1908] see under *cavern.*

**schnauz·krampf** (shnouts'krahmpf) [Ger. *schnauze* snout, muzzle + *krampf* cramp] a facial grimace resembling pouting; observed in some catatonic patients.

**Schnei·der's carmine** (shni'dərz) [Franz Coelestin *Schneider,* German chemist, 1813–1897] see under *carmine.*

**schnei·de·ri·an membrane** (shni-de're-ən) [Conrad Victor *Schneider,* German physician, 1614–1680] see *tunica mucosa nasi* and see under *carcinoma.*

**Schoe·ma·ker's line** (shoo'mah-kərz) [Jan *Schoemaker,* Dutch surgeon, 1871–1940] see under *line.*

**Scholz's disease** (shōlts'əz) [Willibald Oscar *Scholz,* German neurologist, born 1889] see under *disease.*

**Schön's theory** (shernz) [Wilhelm *Schön,* German ophthalmologist, 1848–1917] see under *theory.*

**Schön·bein's test** (shern'bīnz) [Christian Friedrich *Schönbein,* German chemist, 1799–1868] see under *test.*

**Schön·lein's purpura (disease)** (shern'līnz) [Johann Lukas *Schönlein,* German physician, 1793–1864] purpura rheumatica.

**Schön·lein-Hen·och purpura (syndrome)** (shern'līn-hen'ōk) [J. L. *Schönlein;* Eduard Heinrich *Henoch,* German pediatrician, 1820–1910] see under *purpura.*

**Schott·mül·ler's disease** (shot'me-lər) [Hugo *Schottmüller,* German physician, 1867–1936] paratyphoid.

**schra·dan** (shra'dan) octamethyl pyrophosphoramide.

**Schre·ger's lines (bands, striae, zones)** (shra'gərz) [Christian Heinrich Theodor *Schreger,* Danish anatomist, 1768–1833] see under *line.*

**Schrei·ber's maneuver** (shri'bərz) [Julius *Schreiber,* German physician, 1849–1932] see under *maneuver.*

**Schroe·der's disease** (shrər'dərz) [Robert *Schroeder,* German gynecologist, 1884–1959] see under *disease.*

**Schroe·der's test** (shrer'dərz) [Woldemar von *Schroeder,* German physician, 1850–1898] see under *test.*

**Schroe·der van der Kolk's law** (shrer'dər vahn dār kolks) [Jacob Ludwig Conrad *Schroeder van der Kolk,* Dutch physiologist, 1797–1862] see under *law.*

**Schrön's granule** (shrernz) [Otto von *Schrön,* German pathologist in Italy, 1837–1917] see under *granule.*

**Schrön-Much granules** (shrern-mook) [Otto von *Schrön;* Hans Christian *Much,* German physician, 1880–1932] Much's granules.

**Schu·chardt's incision** (shoo'kahrts) [Karl August *Schuchardt,* German surgeon, 1856–1901] paravaginal incision.

**Schüff·ner's dots (granules, stippling)** (shēf'nərz) [Wilhelm August Paul *Schüffner,* German pathologist, 1867–1949] see under *dot.*

**Schül·ler's disease (syndrome)** (shēl'ərz) [Artur *Schüller,* Austrian neurologist, 1874–1958] see *Hand-Schüller-Christian disease,* under *disease,* and see *osteoporosis circumscripta cranii.*

**Schül·ler-Chris·tian disease (syndrome)** (shēl'ər-kris'chən) [Artur *Schüller;* Henry A. *Christian,* American physician, 1876–1951] Hand-Schüller-Christian d.

**Schultz's syndrome (angina)** (shoolt'səz) [Werner *Schultz,* German internist, 1878–1947] agranulocytosis.

**Schultz-Charl·ton reaction (phenomenon, test)** (shoolts-kahrl'ton) [Werner *Schultz;* Willy *Charlton,* German physician, born 1889] see under *reaction.*

**Schultz-Dale reaction** (shoolts-dāl) [W. *Schultz;* Sir Henry Hallett *Dale,* English physiologist and pharmacologist, 1875–1968] see under *reaction.*

**Schult·ze's cells, tract** (shoolt'səz) [Max Johann Sigismund *Schultze,* German biologist, 1825–1874] see *olfactory cells,* under *cell,* and *fasciculus interfascicularis.*

**Schult·ze's fold** (shoolt'səz) [Bernhard Sigismund *Schultze,* German gynecologist, 1827–1919] see under *fold.*

**Schult·ze's sign** (shoolt'səz) [Friedrich *Schultze,* German physician, 1848–1934] Chvostek's sign; see under *sign.*

**Schult·ze-Chvos·tek sign** (shoolt'sə-kvos'tek) [Friedrich *Schultze;* Franz *Chvostek,* Austrian surgeon, 1835–1884] Chvostek's sign.

**Schumm's test** (shoomz) [Otto *Schumm,* German chemist, early 20th century] see under *test.*

**Schütz's fasciculus (bundle, tract)** (shēt'səz) [Hugo *Schütz,* German neurologist, early 20th century] see *fasciculus longitudinalis dorsalis,* under *fasciculus.*

**Schwa·bach's test** (shvah'bahks) [Dagobert *Schwabach,* German otologist, 1846–1920] see under *test.*

**Schwal·be's corpuscles,** etc. (shvahl'bəz) [Gustav Albert *Schwalbe,* German anatomist, 1844–1917] see under *corpuscle, fissure, foramen, nucleus, ring, sheath,* and *space.*

**Schwann's cell, membrane (sheath), nucleus, substance** (shvahnz) [Theodor *Schwann,* German anatomist and physiologist, 1810–1882] see under *cell* and *nucleus,* and see *neurilemma.*

**schwan·ni·tis** (shwah-ni'tis) schwannosis.

**schwan·no·gli·o·ma** (shwah"no-gli-o'mə) schwannoma.

**schwan·no·ma** (shwah-no'mə) 1. a neoplasm originating from Schwann cells (of the myelin sheath) of neurons; the two types are

neurilemomas and neurofibromas. Called also *schwannoglioma* and *Schwann cell tumor.* 2. neurilemoma.
**acoustic s.,** see under *neuroma.*
**granular cell s.,** see under *tumor.*

**schwan·no·min** (shwah-no'min) merlin.

**schwan·no·sis** (shwah-no'sis) hypertrophy of the sheaths of Schwann.

**Schwartz-Jam·pel syndrome** (shworts-jam'pəl) [Oscar *Schwartz,* American pediatrician, born 1919; Robert Steven *Jampel,* American ophthalmologist, born 1926] see under *syndrome.*

**Schwartz-Jam·pel-Aber·feld syndrome** (shworts-jam'pəl-a'bər-feld) [O. *Schwartz;* R.S. *Jampel;* D.C. *Aberfeld,* British physician, 20th century] see under *syndrome.*

**Schwart·ze's sign** (shvahrt'zəz) [Hermann Hugo Rudolf *Schwartze,* German otologist, 1837–1910] see under *sign.*

**Schwarz activator, appliance** (shvahrtz) [Arthur Martin *Schwarz,* Austrian orthodontist, born 1887] see *bow activator,* under *activator,* and see under *appliance.*

**Schwe·di·au·er** (shva'de-ou"ər) see *Swediaur.*

**Schweig·ger-Sei·del sheath** (shvi'gər-si'dəl) [Franz *Schweigger-Seidel,* German physiologist, 1834–1871] see under *sheath.*

**Schwen·in·ger-Buz·zi anetoderma** (shven'in-gər-boots'e) [Ernst *Schweninger,* German physician, 1850–1924; Fausto *Buzzi,* German dermatologist, late 19th century] see under *anetoderma.*

**SCI** spinal cord injury.

**scia-** for other words beginning thus, see also those beginning *skia-.*

**Sci·an·na blood group** (se-ah'nah) [from the name of the propositus family first reported on in the 1960s] see under *blood group.*

**sci·at·ic** (si-at'ik) [L. *sciaticus;* Gr. *ischiadikos*] 1. pertaining to or located near the sciatic nerve or vein; ischiadic; ischiatic. 2. ischial.

**sci·at·i·ca** (si-at'ĭ-kə) [L.] [MeSH: Sciatica] a syndrome characterized by pain radiating from the back into the buttock and into the lower extremity along its posterior or lateral aspect, and most commonly caused by protrusion of a low lumbar intervertebral disk; the term is also used to refer to pain anywhere along the course of the sciatic nerve. Called also *Cotugno's disease, sciatic neuralgia,* and *sciatic neuritis.*

**SCID** severe combined immunodeficiency.

**sci·ence** (si'əns) [L. *scientia* knowledge] [MeSH: Science] 1. the systematic observation of natural phenomena for the purpose of discovering laws governing those phenomena. 2. the body of knowledge accumulated by such means.
**applied s.,** that concerned with the application of discovered laws to the matters of everyday living.
**behavioral s.,** the interdisciplinary study of the behavior of man and lower animals for the purpose of understanding man as an individual and social being; it involves principally psychology, sociology, and anthropology, but also political science and other social sciences.
**pure s.,** that concerned solely with the discovery of unknown laws relating to particular facts.

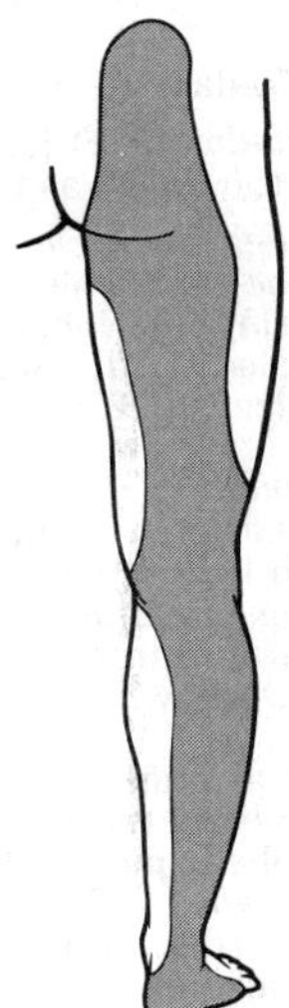

Distribution of pain in sciatica.

**sci·en·tist** (si'ən-tist) one learned in science, especially one active in some particular field of investigation.

**sci·er·opia** (si-ər-o'pe-ə) [Gr. *skieros* shady + *-opia*] visual defect in which objects appear in a shadow.

**scil·la** (sil'ə) [L.] squill.

**scil·la·bi·ose** (sil"ə-bi'ōs) a disaccharide obtained by acid hydrolysis of scillaren A.

**scil·la·ren** (sil'ə-rən) a mixture of cardioactive glycosides, scillaren A and B, from fresh squill.

**scil·lir·o·side** (sil'ir-o-sīd) a cardiac glycoside that is the active principle in red squill (q.v.); in small amounts it causes convulsions and in larger amounts cardiac arrest.

**scil·lism** (sil'iz-əm) poisoning of humans or other animals by squill.

**scil·lit·ic** (sil'it-ik) squillitic.

**scim·i·tar** (sim'ĭ-tahr) [Persian *shimshir*] 1. a sword used in the Middle East that curves to one side. 2. shaped like such a sword.

**scin·ti·gram** (sin'tĭ-gram) the graphic record obtained by scintigraphy.

**scin·ti·graph·ic** (sin"tĭ-graf'ik) pertaining to scintigraphy.

**scin·tig·ra·phy** (sin-tig'rə-fe) the production of two-dimensional images of the distribution of radioactivity in tissues after the internal administration of radionuclide, the images being obtained by a scintillation camera.
**acute infarct s.,** infarct avid s.
**exercise thallium s.,** thallium-201 scintigraphy performed in conjunction with an exercise stress test; see *thallium stress test,* under *tests.*
**gated blood pool s.,** equilibrium radionuclide angiocardiography.
**infarct avid s.,** that performed following myocardial infarction to confirm infarction as well as detect, localize, and quantify regions of myocardial necrosis. A radiotracer that concentrates in these regions, usually technetium $^{99m}$Tc pyrophosphate, is administered intravenously and images are obtained with a gamma camera. For maximal sensitivity, the study is performed between 24 and 72 hours after infarction.
**myocardial perfusion s.,** that performed using a radiotracer that traverses the myocardial capillary system and enters myocardial cells; after the radionuclide, usually thallium 201, is introduced into the bloodstream, regional myocardial blood flow and cell viability are assessed using immediate and delayed images. Scintigraphy is frequently combined with an exercise stress test in the diagnosis of coronary artery disease. See also *thallium-201 myocardial perfusion s.* and *thallium stress test,* under *tests.*
**technetium Tc 99m pyrophosphate s.,** infarct avid s.
**thallium-201 myocardial perfusion s.,** the most common type of myocardial perfusion scintigraphy; the radionuclide used is thallium 201 in the form of thallous chloride. It is most frequently performed in conjunction with exercise stress tests in the diagnosis of coronary artery disease, but is sometimes performed on resting patients to detect transient ischemia or myocardial infarction. See also *thallium stress test,* under *tests.*

**scin·til·la·tion** (sin"tĭ-la'shən) [L. *scintilla* spark] 1. an emission of sparks. 2. a subjective visual sensation, as of seeing sparks. 3. a particle emitted in disintegration of a radioactive element.

**scin·ti·pho·to·graph** (sin"tĭ-fo'to-graf) scintigram.

**scin·ti·pho·tog·ra·phy** (sin"tĭ-fo-tog'rə-fe) scintigraphy.

**scin·tis·can** (sin'tĭ-skan) a two-dimensional representation (map) of the radiation emitted by a radioisotope, revealing its varying concentration in specific tissues of the body, such as the brain, kidney, or thyroid gland.

**scin·ti·scan·ner** (sin"tĭ-skan'ər) the system of equipment used in the making of a scintiscan.

**sci·op·o·dy** (ski-op'ə-de) unusually large feet, especially in children.

**scirrh(o)-** [Gr. *skirrhos* hard] a combining form meaning hard, or denoting relationship to a hard cancer or scirrhous carcinoma.

**scir·rhoid** (skir'oid) [*scirrho-* + *-oid*] resembling scirrhous carcinoma.

**scir·rho·ma** (skĭ-ro'mə) [*scirrho-* + *-oma*] scirrhous carcinoma.

**scir·rhoph·thal·mia** (skir"of-thal'me-ə) [*scirrho-* + *ophthalm-* + *-ia*] scirrhous carcinoma of the eye.

**scir·rhous** (skir'əs) [L. *scirrhosus*] pertaining to or of the nature of a hard cancer; see also under *carcinoma.*

**scir·rhus** (skir'əs) [Gr. *skirrhos*] scirrhous carcinoma.

**scis·sion** (sizh'ən) [L. *scindere* to split] fission; splitting. In chemistry, the splitting of a molecule into two or more simpler molecules.

**scis·sors** (siz'ərz) a cutting instrument with two opposed shearing blades.

**canalicular s.**, delicate scissors with one of the blades probe pointed; used in slitting the lacrimal canal.
**cannula s.**, scissors used in slitting a canal lengthwise.
**craniotomy s.**, strong F-shaped shears for use in opening the fetal head.
**Fox s.**, delicate, fine-pointed scissors designed to gain access to interproximal areas for the removal of small tissue tabs or slight soft tissue deformities during gingivoplasty or gingivectomy.
**Liston's s.**, scissors for cutting plaster-of-Paris bandages.
**Smellie's s.**, short, strong-bladed scissors with external cutting edges, used in craniotomy.

**scis·sors-bite** (siz'erz-bīt') see under *bite.*

**Sciu·ri·dae** (syoo'rĭ-de) [MeSH: Sciuridae] the squirrel family, a family of rodents usually having long bushy tails and strong hind legs; there are both tree-dwelling and ground-dwelling genera. Genera of public health interest include *Ammospermophilus, Cynomys, Marmota,* and *Spermophilus.*

**ScLA** abbreviation for L. *scapulolaeva anterior* (left scapulo-anterior; a presentation of the fetus).

**SCLC** small cell lung carcinoma (or cancer).

**scle·ra** (sklēr'ə) gen. and pl. *scle'rae* [L.; Gr. *skleros* hard] [TA] [MeSH: Sclera] the tough white outer coat of the eyeball, covering approximately the posterior five-sixths of its surface, and continuous anteriorly with the cornea and posteriorly with the external sheath of the optic nerve.

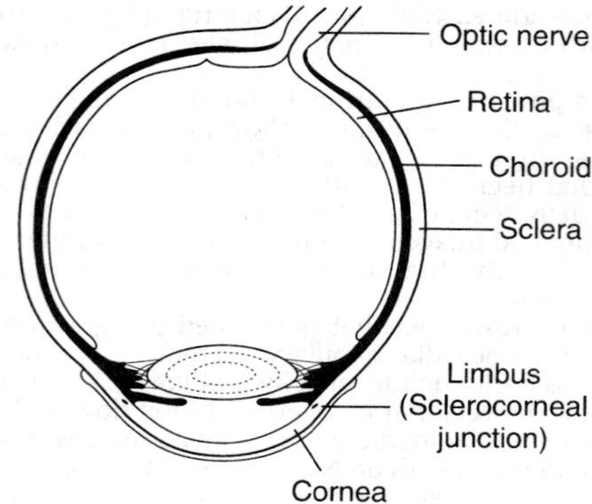


**blue s.**, a condition of unusual blueness of the sclera; it is normal in infants, but is also a prominent feature of osteogenesis imperfecta, and is seen in certain other abnormalities.

**scle·rad·e·ni·tis** (sklēr"ad-ə-ni'tis) [*sclero-* + *aden-* + *-itis*] inflammation and hardening of a gland.

**scle·ral** (sklēr'əl) pertaining to the sclera.

**scle·ra·ti·tis** (sklēr"ə-ti'tis) scleritis.

**scle·ra·tog·e·nous** (sklēr"ə-toj'ə-nəs) sclerogenous.

**scle·rec·ta·sia** (sklēr"ək-ta'zhə) [*scler-* + *ectasia*] a bulging out of the sclera.

**scle·rec·ta·sis** (sklə-rek'tə-sis) sclerectasia.

**scle·rec·to·iri·dec·to·my** (sklə-rek"to-ir"ĭ-dek'tə-me) [*sclerectomy* + *iridectomy*] the operation of excision of a portion of the sclera and of the iris for glaucoma; called also *Lagrange's operation.*

**scle·rec·to·iri·do·di·al·y·sis** (sklə-rek"to-ir"ĭ-do-di-al'ĭ-sis) [*sclera* + *-ectomy* + *irido-* + *dialysis*] sclerectomy and iridodialysis.

**scle·rec·tome** (sklə-rek'tōm) an instrument for performing sclerectomy.

**scle·rec·to·my** (sklə-rek'tə-me) [*sclero-* + *ectomy*] excision of the sclera by scissors (Lagrange's operation), by punch (Holth's operation), or by trephining (Elliot's operation).

**scle·re·de·ma** (sklēr"ə-de'mə) [*scler-* + *edema*] diffuse, symmetrical, wooden-like, nonpitting induration of the skin of unknown etiology, typically beginning on the face, head, or neck and spreading progressively to involve the shoulders, arms, thorax, and sometimes extracutaneous sites, and usually preceded by any of various infectious processes, especially a staphylococcal infection. It occurs in association with diabetes mellitus in most cases, predominantly in females, and usually resolves spontaneously in 6 months to 2 years. Called also *Buschke's s.,* and although the disorder is not restricted to adults, it is called also *s. adultorum,* and sometimes, erroneously, *sclerema adultorum.*
**s. adulto'rum, Buschke's s.,** scleredema.
**s. neonato'rum,** sclerema.

**scle·re·ma** (sklə-re'mə) [*scler-* + (ed)*ema*] a severe, sometimes fatal, disorder of adipose tissue occurring chiefly in preterm, sick, or debilitated infants suffering from a serious underlying illness, manifested by diffuse, rapidly progressive, nonpitting induration of the involved tissue, causing the skin to become cold, yellowish white, mottled, boardlike, and inflexible. Called also *s. adiposum, s. neonatorum, Underwood's disease,* and sometimes, erroneously, *s. neonatorum.*
**s. adipo'sum,** sclerema.
**s. adulto'rum,** scleredema.
**s. neonato'rum,** sclerema.

**scle·ren·ce·pha·lia** (sklēr"ən-sə-fa'le-ə) sclerencephaly.

**scle·ren·ceph·a·ly** (sklēr"ən-sef'ə-le) [*sclero* + Gr. *enkephalos*] sclerosis of the brain.

**scle·ri·a·sis** (sklə-ri'ə-sis) [Gr. *sklēriasis*] a hardened state of an eyelid.

**scle·ri·rit·o·my** (sklēr"ĭ-rit'ə-me) [*scler-* + *iritomy*] incision of the sclera and iris in anterior staphyloma.

**scle·ri·tis** (sklə-ri'tis) [*scler-* + *-itis*] [MeSH: Scleritis] inflammation of the sclera; it may be superficial *(episcleritis)* or deep, the latter form causing bulging and thinning of the sclera. It may occur alone or with keratitis or uveitis.
**annular s.**, scleritis occurring in a ring around the limbus of the cornea.
**anterior s.**, inflammation of the sclera adjoining the limbus of the cornea.
**brawny s.**, a virulent, usually bilateral scleritis involving a thickening of the periphery of the cornea; called also *gelatinous s.*
**s. necro'ticans, necrotizing s.**, scleromalacia.
**nodular s.**, that marked by localized dark blue patches in the anterior portion of the sclera, resulting from the choroid being visible through a translucent sclera.
**posterior s.**, scleritis involving the posterior sclera, the vagina bulbi, and the underlying retina and choroid.

**scler(o)-** [Gr. *sklēros* hard] a combining form meaning hard, often used especially to denote relationship to the sclera.

**scle·ro·ad·i·pose** (sklēr"o-ad'ĭ-pōs) composed of fibrous and fatty tissue.

**scle·ro·blas·te·ma** (sklēr"o-blas-te'mə) [*sclero-* + *blastema*] the embryonic tissue which takes part in the formation of bone.

**scle·ro·blas·tem·ic** (sklēr"o-blas-te'mik) pertaining to the scleroblastema.

**scle·ro·cho·roi·di·tis** (sklēr"o-ko"roi-di'tis) inflammation of the sclera and the choroid coat, resulting in atrophy of both coats and protrusion of the former.
**s. ante'rior,** a form involving the anterior portions of the sclera and causing anterior staphyloma.
**s. poste'rior,** a condition seen in progressive myopia in which posterior staphyloma occurs in the region of the optic disk.

**scle·ro·con·junc·ti·val** (sklēr"o-kon"jənk-ti'vəl) pertaining to the sclera and conjunctiva.

**scle·ro·con·junc·ti·vi·tis** (sklēr"o-kən-junk"tĭ-vi'tis) inflammation of the sclera and the conjunctiva.

**scle·ro·cor·nea** (sklēr"o-kor'ne-ə) the sclera and the cornea considered as forming a single coat or layer.

**scle·ro·cor·ne·al** (sklēr"o-kor'ne-əl) pertaining to the sclera and the cornea.

**scle·ro·dac·tyl·ia** (sklēr"o-dak-til'e-ə) sclerodactyly.

**scle·ro·dac·ty·ly** (sklēr"o-dak'tə-le) [*sclero-* + Gr. *daktylos* finger] localized scleroderma of the digits, as in acrosclerosis.

**scle·ro·der·ma** (sklēr"o-der'mə) [*sclero-* + *derma*] chronic hardening and thickening of the skin, which may be a finding in several different diseases, occurring in a localized or focal form and as a systemic disease. Called also *dermatosclerosis.*
**circumscribed s.**, 1. localized s. 2. morphea.
**diffuse s.**, see *systemic s.*
**generalized s.**, see *systemic s.*
**linear s.**, a form of localized scleroderma characterized by bandlike lesions of induration with hyper- and hypopigmentation and atrophy of the skin, underlying subcutaneous tissue, muscle, and bone. When it involves the frontal or frontoparietal area of the forehead and the scalp the lesion is known as *en coup de sabre.* Called also *linear morphea.*
**localized s.**, 1. scleroderma confined to the skin and subcutaneous tissue or secondarily involving the musculoskeletal system. It occurs in three forms: morphea, linear scleroderma, and en coup de sabre. Called also *circumscribed s.* Cf. *systemic s.* 2. morphea.
**systemic s.**, a systemic disorder of the connective tissue characterized by induration and thickening of the skin, by abnormalities involving both the microvasculature *(telangiectasia)* and larger vessels *(Raynaud's phenomenon),* and by fibrotic degenerative changes

in various body organs, including the heart, lungs, kidneys, and gastrointestinal tract. It may remain confined to the face and hands for long periods or may be progressive and spread diffusely to become generalized. Called also *systemic sclerosis.* See also *CREST syndrome.*

**scle·ro·der·ma·tous** (sklēr″o-der′mə-təs) pertaining to or characterized by scleroderma.

**scle·ro·des·mia** (sklēr″o-des′me-ə) [*sclero-* + *desm-* + *-ia*] hardening of ligaments.

**scle·ro·gen·ic** (sklēr″o-jen′ik) sclerogenous.

**scle·rog·e·nous** (sklə-roj′ə-nəs) [*sclero-* + *-genous*] producing sclerosis or sclerous tissue.

**scle·ro·gum·ma·tous** (sklēr″o-gum′ə-təs) composed of fibrous and gummatous tissue.

**scle·roid** (sklēr′oid) [*sclero-* + *-oid*] having a hard texture.

**scle·ro·iri·tis** (sklēr″o-i-ri′tis) inflammation of the sclera and of the iris.

**scle·ro·ker·a·ti·tis** (sklēr″o-ker″ə-ti′tis) inflammation of the sclera and of the cornea.

**scle·ro·ker·a·to·iri·tis** (sklēr″o-ker″ə-to-i-ri′tis) inflammation of the sclera, cornea, and iris.

**scle·ro·ker·a·to·sis** (sklēr″o-ker″ə-to′sis) sclerokeratitis.

**scle·ro·ma** (sklə-ro′mə) [Gr. *sklērōma* induration] a hardened patch or induration, especially of the nasal or laryngeal tissues. See also *laryngoscleroma, pharyngoscleroma,* and *rhinoscleroma.*
**s. respirato′rium,** rhinoscleroma.

**scle·ro·ma·la·cia** (sklēr″o-mə-la′shə) [*sclero-* + *malacia*] degeneration and thinning (softening) of the sclera, occurring in patients with rheumatoid arthritis; called also *scleromalacia perforans.*

**scle·ro·mere** (sklēr′o-mēr) [*sclero-* + *-mere*] 1. any segment or metamere of the skeletal system. 2. the caudal half of a sclerotome (def. 3).

**scle·ro·mu·cin** (sklēr″o-mu′sin) a slimy, active principle from ergot.

**scle·ro·myx·ede·ma** (sklēr″o-mik″sə-de′mə) [*sclero-* + *myxedema*] 1. lichen myxedematosus. 2. a term sometimes used to refer to lichen myxedematosus associated with scleroderma, producing, especially on the face, exaggerated furrowing of the skin.

**scle·ro·nych·ia** (sklēr″o-nik′e-ə) [*sclero-* + *onych-* + *-ia*] a simultaneous thickening and dryness of the nails.

**scle·ro·nyx·is** (sklēr″o-nik′sis) [*sclero-* + *nyxis*] surgical puncture of the sclera.

**scle·ro-ooph·o·ri·tis** (sklēr″o-o-of″ə-ri′tis) sclerosing inflammation of an ovary.

**scle·ro-oo·the·ci·tis** (sklēr″o-o″o-the-si′tis) sclero-oophoritis.

**scle·roph·thal·mia** (sklēr″of-thal′me-ə) [*sclero-* + *-ophthalmia*] the condition in which, from imperfect differentiation of the sclera and cornea, the periphery of the cornea is opaque and only the central part remains clear.

**scle·ro·pro·tein** (sklēr″o-pro′tēn) [*sclero-* + *protein*] a simple protein which is characterized by its insolubility and fibrous structure, and which usually serves a supportive or protective function in the body; called also *albuminoid.*

**scle·ro·sal** (sklə-ro′səl) sclerous.

**scle·ro·sant** (sklə-ro′sənt) sclerosing agent.

**scle·rose** (sklə-rōs′) to undergo sclerosis; to harden.

**sclé·rose en plaques** (skla-rōz′ ahn plahk) [Fr.] multiple sclerosis.

**scle·ros·ing** (sklə-rōs′ing) causing or undergoing sclerosis.

**scle·ro·sis** (sklə-ro′sis) [Gr. *sklērōsis* hardness] [MeSH: Sclerosis] an induration or hardening, such as hardening of a part from inflammation, increased formation of connective tissue, or disease of the interstitial substance.
**amyotrophic lateral s.,** a motor neuron disease marked by progressive degeneration of the neurons that give rise to the corticospinal tract and of the motor cells of the brain stem and spinal cord, resulting in a deficit of upper and lower motor neurons; it usually ends fatally within two to three years. Called also *Lou Gehrig disease* and *Charcot's syndrome.*
**anterolateral s.,** sclerosis of the ventral and lateral columns of the spinal cord, leading to spastic paraplegia; called also *ventrolateral s.*
**arterial s., arteriocapillary s.,** arteriosclerosis.
**arteriolar s.,** arteriolosclerosis.
**bone s.,** eburnation.
**combined s.,** subacute combined degeneration of the spinal cord; see under *degeneration.*
**concentric s.,** Baló's disease.
**dentinal s.,** regressive alteration in tooth substance with calcification of the dentinal tubules, usually caused by trauma, abrasion, or normal aging processes, and producing translucent zones (transparent dentin).
**diaphyseal s.,** diaphyseal dysplasia.
**diffuse s.,** sclerosis that affects large areas of the brain and spinal cord.
**diffuse cerebral s.,** the infantile form of metachromatic leukodystrophy; see under *leukodystrophy.*
**diffuse systemic s.,** see *systemic scleroderma,* under *scleroderma.*
**disseminated s.,** multiple s.
**endocardial s.,** see under *fibroelastosis.*
**Erb's s.,** primary lateral s.
**familial centrolobar s.,** Pelizaeus-Merzbacher disease.
**focal s.,** multiple s.
**focal glomerular s.,** the occurrence of focal sclerosing lesions of the renal glomeruli, marked by proteinuria, hematuria, hypertension, and the nephrotic syndrome; it may be idiopathic or secondary to other diseases, including heroin-abuse nephropathy, chronic interstitial nephritis, and malignancies. Exacerbations and remissions may occur, most often in children; progression to renal failure occurs at a variable and unpredictable rate. Called also *focal segmental glomerulosclerosis.*
**gastric s.,** linitis plastica.
**glomerular s.,** glomerulosclerosis.
**hippocampal s.,** loss of neurons in the hippocampal region with gliosis, sometimes seen with epilepsy. Called also *mesial temporal s.*
**hyperplastic s.,** a form of arteriosclerosis seen in small arteries and arterioles as a subintimal thickening of the wall of the vessel.
**insular s.,** multiple s.
**lateral s.,** a motor neuron disease consisting of degeneration of the lateral columns of the spinal cord, leading to spastic paraplegia. See *amyotrophic lateral s.* and *primary lateral s.*
**lobar s.,** presence of narrow, scar-distorted convolutions over a large area (lobe) of the surface of the cerebral hemispheres; seen frequently in cerebral palsy.
**medial calcific s.,** Mönckeberg's arteriosclerosis.
**mesial temporal s.,** hippocampal s.
**miliary s.,** sclerosis occurring in minute spots.
**Mönckeberg's s.,** see under *arteriosclerosis.*
**multiple s. (MS),** a disease in which there are foci of demyelination of various sizes throughout the white matter of the central nervous system, sometimes extending into the gray matter. Typically, the symptoms of lesions of the white matter are weakness, incoordination, paresthesias, speech disturbances, and visual complaints. The course of the disease is usually prolonged, so that the term *multiple* also refers to remissions and relapses that occur over a period of many years. The etiology is unknown. Called also *disseminated s., focal s., insular s.,* and *sclérose en plaques.*
**Pelizaeus-Merzbacher s.,** see under *disease.*
**peritoneal s.,** sclerosing peritonitis.
**posterior s., posterior spinal s.,** tabes dorsalis.
**posterolateral s.,** subacute combined degeneration of spinal cord; see under *degeneration.*
**primary lateral s.,** a form of motor neuron disease in which the degenerative process is limited to the corticospinal pathways. Called also *Erb's s.*
**progressive systemic s.,** see *systemic scleroderma,* under *scleroderma.*
**renal arteriolar s.,** arteriosclerosis involving chiefly the renal arterioles, resulting in contracted kidney.
**subendocardial s.,** endocardial fibroelastosis.
**systemic s.,** see under *scleroderma.*
**tuberous s.,** an autosomal dominant disease characterized principally by the presence of hamartomas of the brain (tubers), retina (phakomas), and viscera, mental retardation, seizures, and adenoma sebaceum, and often associated with other skin lesions, including subungual fibromas, vitiliginous patches, shagreen patches, and café-au-lait spots. Called also *Bourneville's disease* and *epiloia.*
**unicellular s.,** the development of bands of fibrous material between the cells of a gland.
**valvular s.,** fibrous thickening of a cardiac valve, especially the mitral valve.
**vascular s.,** arteriosclerosis.
**venous s.,** phlebosclerosis.
**ventrolateral s.,** anterolateral s.

**scle·ro·skel·e·ton** (sklēr″o-skel′ə-ton) [*sclero-* + *skeleton*] those parts of the bony skeleton that are formed by the ossification of ligaments, tendons, or fasciae.

**scle·ro·ste·no·sis** (sklēr″o-stə-no′sis) [*sclero-* + *stenosis*] induration or hardening combined with contraction.

**Scle·ros·to·ma** (sklə-ros′to-mə) *Strongylus.*
**S. duodena′le,** *Ancylostoma duodenale.*
**S. syn′gamus,** *Syngamus trachea.*

**scle·ros·to·my** (sklə-ros′tə-me) [*sclero-* + *-stomy*] [MeSH: Sclerostomy] the surgical creation of an opening through the sclera; it is usually performed in the treatment of glaucoma.

**scle·ro·ther·a·py** (sklĕr″o-ther′ə-pe) [MeSH: Sclerotherapy] the injection of a chemical irritant (see *sclerosing agent*) into a vein to produce inflammation and eventual fibrosis and obliteration of the lumen, done for the treatment of hemorrhoids, varicose veins, or esophageal varices.

**scle·ro·tia** (sklə-ro′she-ə) plural of *sclerotium.*

**scle·rot·ic** (sklə-rot′ik) 1. hard, or hardening; affected with sclerosis. 2. scleral.

**scle·rot·i·ca** (sklə-rot′ĭ-kə) [L. *scleroticus;* Gr. *sklēros* hard] sclera.

**scle·rot·ic ac·id** (sklə-rot′ik) an acid found in ergot, of which it is one of the active principles.

**scle·rot·i·co·cho·roid·itis** (sklə-rot″ĭ-ko-kor″oid-i′tis) sclerochoroiditis.

**Scle·ro·tin·ia** (sklĕr″o-tin′e-ə) a genus of fungi of the family Sclerotiniaceae, which includes many pathogens of plants. Its imperfect (sexual) stage is *Monilia.*

**Scle·ro·tin·i·a·ceae** (sklĕr″o-tin-e-a′she-e) a family of fungi of the order Helotiales; it includes the genus *Sclerotinia.*

**scle·ro·tin·ic acid** (sklĕr″o-tin′ik) sclerotic acid.

**scle·ro·ti·tis** (sklĕr″o-ti′tis) scleritis.

**scle·ro·ti·um** (sklə-ro′she-əm) [L. *sclerotica* hard] 1. in fungi, a hard mass of intertwined mycelia, usually with pigmented walls resistant to adverse environmental conditions; it will germinate to produce new hyphae under favorable conditions or in response to a chemical stimulus from a prospective host. 2. in certain protozoa, a multinucleate hard cyst into which the plasmodium divides in response to adverse environmental conditions, such as desiccation; sclerotia will germinate and fuse together to produce a new plasmodium under favorable conditions.

**scle·ro·tome** (sklĕr′o-tōm) [*sclero-* + *-tome*] 1. an instrument used in the incision of the sclera. 2. the area of a bone innervated from a single spinal segment. 3. one of the paired masses of mesenchymal tissue, separated from the ventromedial part of a somite, which develop into vertebrae and ribs.

**scle·rot·o·my** (sklə-rot′ə-me) [*sclero-* + *-tomy*] surgical incision of the sclera.
**anterior s.,** the surgical opening of the anterior chamber of the eye, chiefly done for the relief of glaucoma.
**posterior s.,** an opening made into the vitreous through the sclera, as for detached retina or the removal of a foreign body.

**scle·rous** (sklĕr′əs) hard; indurated.

**scle·ro·zone** (sklĕr′o-zōn) [*sclero-* + *zone*] any surface on a bone giving attachment to the muscles from a given myotome.

**ScLP** abbreviation for L. *scapulolaeva posterior* (left scapuloposterior; a presentation of the fetus).

**SCM** State Certified Midwife.

**sco·le·ces** (sko′lə-sēz) [L.] plural of *scolex.*

**sco·le·ci·a·sis** (sko″lə-si′ə-sis) [*scoleco-* + *-iasis*] the condition caused by the presence of larvae of moths or butterflies in the body.

**sco·lec·i·form** (sko-les′ĭ-form) resembling a scolex.

**scoleco-** [Gr. *skōlēx,* gen. *skōlēkos* worm] a combining form denoting relationship to a worm.

**sco·le·coid** (sko′lə-koid) [Gr. *skōlekoeidēs* vermiform] 1. resembling a worm. 2. resembling a scolex; hydatid.

**sco·le·col·o·gy** (sko″lə-kol′ə-je) [*scoleco-* + *-logy*] helminthology.

**sco·lex** (sko′leks) pl. *sco′leces, sco′lices* [Gr. *skōlēx* worm] the attachment (or holdfast) organ of a tapeworm, generally considered the anterior, or cephalic, end.

**sco·li·ces** (sko′lĭ-sēz) plural of *scolex.*

**scolio-** [Gr. *skolios* twisted] a combining form meaning twisted or crooked.

**sco·lio·ky·pho·sis** (sko″le-o-ki-fo′sis) [*scolio-* + *kyphosis*] combined lateral (scoliosis) and posterior (kyphosis) curvature of the spine.

**sco·lio·ra·chit·ic** (sko″le-o-rə-kit′ik) affected with scoliosis and rickets.

**sco·li·o·si·om·e·try** (sko″le-o-se-om′ə-tre) [*scoliosis* + *-metry*] measurement of curvatures, especially those of the vertebral column.

**sco·li·o·sis** (sko″le-o′sis) [Gr. *skoliōsis* curvation] [MeSH: Scoliosis] an appreciable lateral deviation in the normally straight vertical line of the spine. Cf. *kyphosis* and *lordosis.*

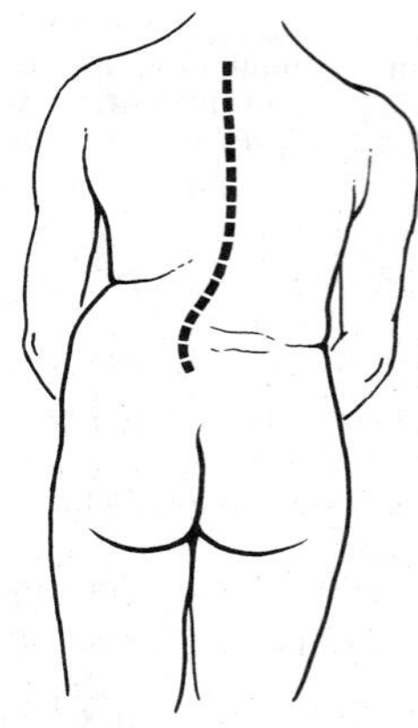

Scoliosis.

**Brissaud's s.,** sciatic s.
**cicatricial s.,** that which is due to a cicatricial contraction following caries or necrosis.
**coxitic s.,** scoliosis in the lumbar region caused by hip disease.
**empyematic s.,** that which is caused by empyema.
**habit s.,** scoliosis due to improper posture.
**inflammatory s.,** that which is due to vertebral disease.
**ischiatic s.,** that which is due to hip disease.
**myopathic s.,** paralytic s.
**ocular s., ophthalmic s.,** scoliosis attributed to tilting of the head on account of astigmatism or muscle imbalance.
**osteopathic s.,** that which is caused by disease of the vertebrae.
**paralytic s.,** lateral curvature of the spinal column due to muscle paralysis; called also *myopathic s.*
**rachitic s.,** spinal curvature due to rickets.
**rheumatic s.,** that which is due to rheumatism of the dorsal muscles.
**sciatic s.,** a list of the lumbar part of the spine away from the affected side in sciatica; called also *Brissaud's s.*
**static s.,** that which is due to difference in the length of the legs.

**sco·li·o·som·e·ter** (sko″le-o-som′ə-tər) an apparatus for measuring curves, especially those of the spinal column.

**sco·li·ot·ic** (sko″le-ot′ik) [Gr. *skoliōtos* looking askew] pertaining to or characterized by scoliosis.

**sco·lio·tone** (sko′le-o-tōn) an apparatus for the forcible correction of scoliosis.

**Sco·lo·pen·dra** (sko″lo-pen′drə) [Gr. *skolops* anything pointed] a genus of venomous centipedes (class Chilopoda). The bite of some large species may produce a severe local inflammation attended with pain, glandular enlargement, vomiting, headache, vertigo, and fever. *S. he′ros* and *S. mor′sitans* are American species; *S. gigan′tea* is a tropical species.

**sco·lop·sia** (sko-lop′se-ə) [Gr. *skolops* anything pointed] a suture between two bones that allows motion of one on the other.

**scom·broid** (skom′broid) 1. of or pertaining to the suborder Scombroidea. 2. a fish of the suborder Scombroidea. See also under *poisoning.*

**Scom·broi·dea** (skom-broi′de-ə) a suborder of larger, bony, marine fish having oily flesh, including tunas, bonitos, mackerels, albacores, and skipjacks. The flesh of these fish may contain a toxic histamine-like substance and, if ingested, can cause scombroid poisoning.

**scom·bro·tox·ic** (skom″bro-tok′sik) pertaining to or caused by scombrotoxin.

**scom·bro·tox·in** (skom″bro-tok′sin) the histaminelike toxin formed in scombroid fish by bacterial action; it causes scombroid poisoning.

**scoop** (skōōp) a spoonlike instrument for evacuating cavities.
**Mules's s.,** a form of curet used in eye operations.

**sco·pa·fun·gin** (sko″pə-fun′jin) an antibacterial and antifungal antibiotic derived from a variant of *Streptomyces hygroscopicus.*

**sco·pa·rin** (sko-pa′rin) a diuretic principle found in scoparius.

**sco·pa·ri·us** (sko-pa′re-əs) the tops of *Cytisus scoparius,* or broom; they contain the alkaloid sparteine and the principle scoparin, and are diuretic, purgative, and emetic. Scoparius is also abused by being smoked for its euphoric properties. Called also *spartium.*

**-scope** [Gr. *skopein* to view, examine] a word termination denoting an instrument for examining or observing.

**sco·po·la** (sko-po'lə) the dried rhizome and larger roots of *Scopolia carniolica,* which contains the same constituents as belladonna and is used as an anticholinergic.

**sco·po·lag·nia** (sko″po-lag'ne-ə) [Gr. *skopein* to view + *lagneia* lust] scopophilia.

**sco·pol·a·mine** (sko-pol'ə-mēn) [MeSH: Scopolamine] an anticholinergic alkaloid, derived from several solanaceous plants, including *Atropa belladonna, Hyoscyamus niger, Datura* species, and *Scopolia* species. It has effects on the autonomic nervous system similar to those of atropine. Called also *hyoscine.*
**s. hydrobromide** [USP], the trihydrate salt of scopolamine, used as a cerebral sedative, administered orally or subcutaneously, and as a cycloplegic and mydriatic, applied topically to the conjunctiva.
**s. methylbromide,** methscopolamine bromide.

**Sco·po·lia** (sko-po'le-ə) [Johann-Antoni *Scopoli,* Italian physician, 1723–1788] a genus of plants of the family Solanaceae. *S. carnio 'lica atropoi'des* Jacq., a European species, and *S. japo'nica* and *S. lu'rida,* Asian species, have properties like those of hyoscyamus and belladonna.

**sco·pom·e·ter** (sko-pom'ə-tər) [Gr. *skopein* to examine + *-meter*] an instrument for measuring the turbidity of solutions, i.e., the density of a precipitate.

**sco·pom·e·try** (sko-pom'ə-tre) measurement of the optical density of a precipitate to determine the amount of a substance in suspension.

**sco·po·phil·ia** (sko-po-fil'e-ə) [Gr. *skopein* to view + *-philia*] 1. voyeurism; the derivation of sexual pleasure from looking at another's genital organs *(active s.).* 2. exhibitionism; the desire to be looked at by others *(passive s.).*

**sco·po·pho·bia** (sko″po-fo'be-ə) [Gr. *skopein* to view + *-phobia*] irrational fear of being seen.

**scop·to·phil·ia** (skop″to-fil'e-ə) scopophilia.

**scop·to·pho·bia** (skop″to-fo'be-ə) scopophobia.

**scop·u·la** (skop'u-lə) [L. "small brush"] an aboral organelle of peritrichous protozoa comprising a field of kinetosomes and immobile cilia, which may function as a holdfast organ or may be the origin of the stalk.

**Scop·u·lar·i·op·sis** (skop″u-lar″e-op'sis) a genus of Fungi Imperfecti of the family Moniliaceae. *S. brevicau'lis* sometimes causes onychomycosis and other forms of scopulariopsosis. Formerly called *Acaulium.*

**scop·u·lar·i·op·so·sis** (skop″u-lar″e-op-so'sis) infection with a fungus of the genus *Scopulariopsis;* it usually takes the form of onychomycosis caused by *S. brevicaulis,* but other infections such as fungus balls and pneumonia have also been seen.

**-scopy** [Gr. *skopein* to examine] word termination denoting the act of examining.

**scor·bu·tic** (skor-bu'tik) [L. *scorbuticus*] pertaining to or affected with scurvy.

**scor·bu·ti·gen·ic** (skor-bu″tĭ-jen'ik) causing scurvy.

**scor·bu·tus** (skor-bu'təs) [L.] scurvy.

**scor·di·ne·ma** (skor″dĭ-ne'mə) [Gr. *skordinēma*] yawning and stretching with a feeling of lassitude, occurring as a preliminary symptom of some infectious diseases.

**score** (skor) a rating, usually expressed numerically, based on achievement or the degree to which certain qualities or conditions are present.
**APACHE s.,** [*a*cute *p*hysiological *a*ssessment and *c*hronic *h*ealth *e*valuation] a widely-used method for assessing severity of illness in acutely ill patients in intensive care units, taking into account a variety of routine physiological parameters.
**Apgar s.,** a numerical expression of the condition of a newborn infant, usually determined at 60 seconds after birth, being the sum of points gained on assessment of the heart rate, respiratory effort, muscle tone, reflex irritability, and color. Cf. *recovery s.*
**Bishop s.,** a score for estimating the prospects of induction of labor in a primigravida, arrived at by evaluating the extent of cervical dilatation, effacement, the station of the fetal head, consistency of the cervix, and the cervical position in relation to the vaginal axis.
**Gleason s.,** see under *grade.*
**lod s.,** "*lo*garithm of the *od*ds" score, which measures the likelihood of two genes being within measurable genetic or recombinational distance of each other.
**recovery s.,** a number expressing the condition of an infant at various intervals, which should be stipulated, greater than 1 minute after birth, based on the same features assessed by the Apgar score at 60 seconds after birth.
**standard s.,** *z* value.
**stroke s.,** any of various scoring systems that seek to characterize a patient's clinical state following a stroke.
***z* s.,** see under *value.*

**scor·ings** (skor'ings) small transverse lines caused by increased density of bone, seen in radiographs at the metaphysis of growing bones, and due to temporary cessation of growth.

**scor·pi·on** (skor'pe-ən) [MeSH: Scorpions] any arthropod of the order Scorpionida.
**bark s.,** any of various species of *Centruroides.*
**black s.,** *Euscorpius italicus,* a species found in southern Europe and North Africa.
**whip s.,** any arachnid of the order Pedipalpa.

**Scor·pi·o·nes** (skor-pe-o'nēz) Scorpionida.

**Scor·pi·on·ida** (skor-pe-on'ĭ-də) the scorpions, an order of arachnids with elongated bodies, usually found in tropical or subtropical climates; many have venomous stings on their erectile tails. Important genera include *Buthus, Centruroides, Euscorpius,* and *Tityus.* Called also *Scorpiones.*

**scor·pi·on·ism** (skor'pe-ən-iz″əm) poisoning by scorpion stings.

**scot(o)-** [Gr. *skotos* darkness] a combining form denoting relationship to darkness.

**Sco·to·bac·te·ria** (sko″to-bak-tēr'e-ə) [*scoto-* + *bacteria*] a class of bacteria of the division Gracilicutes, kingdom Procaryotae, made up of gram-negative organisms that do not derive energy from light (nonphototrophic metabolism). It contains aerobic and anaerobic rods and cocci, including the medically important families Spirochaetaceae, Spirosomaceae, Pseudomonadaceae, Enterobacteriaceae, Vibrionaceae, Bacteroidaceae, Neisseriaceae, Legionellaceae, Pasteurellaceae, and Veillonellaceae and the orders Rickettsiales and Chlamydiales.

**sco·to·bac·te·ri·um** (sko″to-bak-tēr'e-əm) 1. an individual organism of the class Scotobacteria. 2. a bacterium capable of growing in the dark.

**sco·to·chro·mo·gen** (sko″to-kro'mo-jən) [*scoto-* + *chromo-* + *-gen*] a microorganism whose pigmentation develops in the dark as well as in the light; specifically, a member of Runyon Group II of the nontuberculous mycobacteria, but applicable also to many other organisms. See also *nontuberculous mycobacteria,* under *mycobacterium.*

**sco·to·chro·mo·gen·ic** (sko″to-kro″mo-jen'ik) pertaining to or characterized by scotochromogenicity.

**sco·to·chro·mo·ge·nic·i·ty** (sko″to-kro″mo-jə-nis'ĭ-te) the property of forming pigment in the dark, the coloration occurring irrespective of exposure to light.

**sco·to·din·ia** (sko″to-din'e-ə) [*scoto-* + Gr. *dinos* whirl] dizziness with blurring of vision and headache. Called also *apoplectic vertigo* and *tenebric vertigo.*

**sco·to·ma** (sko-to'mə) pl. *scoto'mata* [Gr. *skotōma*] [MeSH: Scotoma] 1. an area of lost or depressed vision within the visual field, surrounded by an area of less depressed or of normal vision. 2. mental s.
**absolute s.,** an area within the visual field in which perception of light is entirely lost.
**annular s.,** a circular area of depressed vision in the visual field, surrounding the point of fixation.
**arcuate s.,** a scotoma arising at or near the blind spot and arching inferiorly or superiorly toward the nasal field, following the paths of the retinal nerve fibers.
**aural s., s. au'ris,** loss of ability to perceive auditory stimuli coming from a certain direction.
**Bjerrum's s.,** a further development of Seidel's scotoma, the sickle-shaped defect contiguous to the blind spot extending above and below the fixation point and encircling it more or less completely.
**cecocentral s.,** centrocecal s.
**central s.,** an area of depressed vision corresponding with the point of fixation and interfering with or entirely abolishing central vision.
**centrocecal s.,** a horizontal oval defect in the field of vision situated between and embracing both the point of fixation and the blind spot.
**color s.,** an isolated area of depressed or defective vision for color in the visual field.
**flittering s.,** teichopsia.
**hemianopic s.,** depressed or lost vision affecting half of the central visual field. Cf. *hemianopia.*
**mental s.,** in psychiatry, a figurative blind spot in a person's psychological awareness, the patient being unable to gain insight into and to understand his mental problems; lack of insight. See also *scotomization.*
**motile s's,** floating opacities, not true scotomata, occurring in the vitreous, muscae volitantes being an example of such a defect.

**negative s.**, a scotoma appearing as a blank spot in the visual field; the patient is unaware of it, and it is detected only by examination.
**paracentral s.**, an area of depressed vision situated near the point of fixation.
**peripapillary s.**, an area of depressed vision in the visual field near that corresponding with the optic disk.
**peripheral s.**, an area of depressed vision distant from the point of fixation, toward the periphery of the visual field.
**physiologic s.**, that area of the visual field corresponding with the optic disk, in which the photosensitive receptors are absent.
**positive s.**, a scotoma subjectively perceived as a black spot in the visual field, and of which the patient is aware.
**relative s.**, an area of the visual field in which perception of light is only diminished, or the loss is restricted to light of certain wavelengths.
**ring s.**, annular s.
**scintillating s.**, teichopsia.
**Seidel's s.**, a further development of an arcuate scotoma, which extends at either or both ends, the concavity of the prolongation always being directed toward the fixation point.

**sco·to·ma·graph** (sko-to'mə-graf) [*scotoma* + *-graph*] an instrument for recording a scotoma.

**sco·to·ma·ta** (sko-to'mə-tə) plural of *scotoma.*

**sco·tom·a·tous** (sko-tom'ə-təs) pertaining to or affected with scotoma.

**sco·tom·e·ter** (sko-tom'ə-tər) [*scotoma* + *-meter*] an instrument for diagnosing and measuring scotomata.
**Bjerrum's s.**, campimeter.

**sco·tom·e·try** (sko-tom'ə-tre) the measurement of isolated areas of depressed vision (scotomata) within the visual field.

**sco·to·phil·ia** (sko"to-fil'e-ə) [*scoto-* + *-philia*] nyctophilia.

**sco·to·pho·bia** (sko"to-fo'be-ə) [*scoto-* + *-phobia*] irrational fear of darkness.

**sco·to·pia** (sko-to'pe-ə) [*scot-* + *-opia*] night vision; see also *dark adaptation.*

**sco·top·ic** (sko-top'ik) pertaining to scotopia.

**sco·top·sin** (sko-top'sin) the opsin of the rods of the retina that combines with 11-*cis* retinal to form rhodopsin. See illustration at *visual cycle,* under *cycle.*

**sco·tos·co·py** (sko-tos'kə-pe) [*scoto-* + *scopy*] retinoscopy.

**scours** (skourz) diarrhea in animals other than humans.
**black s.**, acute dysentery in cattle, accompanied by intestinal hemorrhage producing a dark color of the feces; the etiology is unknown. See also *bloody s.* and *winter dysentery.*
**bloody s.**, swine dysentery.
**calf s.**, see under *diarrhea.*
**peat s.**, molybdenum poisoning in grazing cattle.
**weanling pig s.**, 1. postweaning diarrhea. 2. coliform gastroenteritis.
**white s.**, neonatal diarrhea in calves, lambs, and foals during the first few days after birth, usually caused by enteropathogenic strains of *Escherichia coli* and less often by other bacteria or viruses; marked by fever, dehydration, and depression, with fetid light-colored feces that may be bloodstained late in the disease.
**winter s.**, see under *dysentery.*

**scr** scruple.

**scra·pie** (skra'pe) [MeSH: Scrapie] the first of the prion diseases to be recognized, occurring in sheep and goats and characterized by severe pruritus, muscular incoordination, and increasing debility, ending in death.

**scratch** (skrach) 1. to scrape or rub a surface lightly with the nails or with a sharp or jagged instrument, particularly to relieve itching. 2. a slight wound. 3. to make shallow cuts on a surface. 4. to make a thin grating sound.
**Means-Lerman s.**, a systolic grating sound heard in the second left intercostal space during expiration in hypertension; it is due to friction between the pleural and pericardial surfaces.

**scratch·es** (skrach'əz) greasy heel.

**screen** (skrēn) 1. a structure resembling a curtain or partition, used as a protection or shield, e.g., against excessive radiation exposure; see under *shield.* 2. a large flat surface upon which light rays are projected. 3. an agent that affords defense against a deleterious influence; called also *protectant* and *protective.* 4. to examine by fluoroscopy (Great Britain). 5. to separate well individuals in a population from those who have an undiagnosed disease, defect, or other pathologic condition or who are at high risk, by means of tests, examinations, or other procedures. See also *screening.*
**Bjerrum s.**, tangent s.
**fluorescent s.**, a sheet of cardboard, paper, or glass coated with suitable material, which fluoresces visibly, as calcium tungstate, used as an intensifying screen in radiography; as the chief part of a fluoroscope; as a substitute for a fluoroscope in a darkened room.
**intensifying s.**, a thin sheet of celluloid or other substance coated with a finely divided substance which fluoresces under the influence of x-rays and intended to be used in close contact with the emulsion of a photographic plate or film for the purpose of reinforcing the image.
**oral s.**, vestibular s.
**skin s.**, a substance applied to the skin to protect it from the effects of the sun's rays or other noxious agents.
**solar s., sun s.**, sunscreen.
**tangent s.**, a large square of black cloth, stretched on a frame, hung from a roller, and having a central mark for fixation; used with a campimeter to map the field of vision. Called also *Bjerrum s.*
**vestibular s.**, an acrylic resin removable orthodontic appliance that covers the labial or buccal surface of one or both dental arches, fitting between the oral mucosa and the teeth; used to treat oral habits and to stimulate tooth movement. Called also *oral s.* and *oral shield.*

**screen·ing** (skrēn'ing) 1. examination or testing of a group of individuals to separate those who are well from those who have an undiagnosed disease or defect or who are at high risk. 2. fluoroscopy (Great Britain).
**antibody s.**, a method of determining the presence and amount of anti-HLA antibodies in the serum of a potential allograft recipient: aliquots of the recipient's serum are mixed with a panel of leukocytes from well-characterized cell donors and complement is added. Reaction between the recipient's pre-existing antibody and specific antigen in the donor cells leads to cell lysis; the percentage of different cells lysed provides a rough measure of the sensitization of the recipient (referred to as the *panel reactive antibody*).
**mass s.**, that performed on or made available to an entire population.
**multiphasic s., multiple s.**, that in which various diagnostic procedures are employed during the same screening program.
**prescriptive s.**, that performed for the early detection of disease or disease precursors in apparently well individuals so that health care can be provided early in the course of the disease or before the disease becomes manifest.

**screw** (skroo) a solid cylinder with a helical thread on its exterior surface, used to hold two objects together.
**pedicle s.**, a screw that goes into the pedicle of a vertebral arch, often in the lumbar region, used in various types of instrumentation.

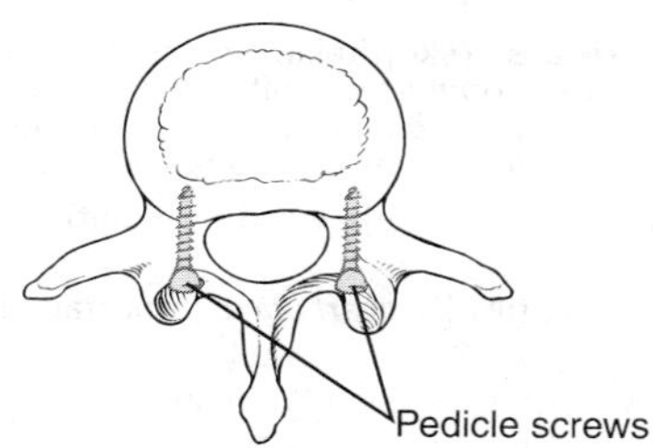


**screw·worm** (skroo'wərm) the larva of *Cochliomyia hominivorax.*

**Scrib·ner shunt** (skrib'nər) [Belding H. *Scribner,* American nephrologist, born 1921] Quinton-Scribner shunt.

**scro·bic·u·late** (skro-bik'u-lāt) [L. *scrobiculatus*] marked with pits or cavities.

**scro·bic·u·lus** (scro-bik'u-ləs) [L. "little trench," "pit"] fossula.
**s. cor'dis**, fossa epigastrica.

**scrof·u·la** (skrof'u-lə) [L. "brood sow"] former name for tuberculous cervical lymphadenitis. See also *scrofuloderma.*

**scrof·u·lo·der·ma** (skrof"u-lo-dər'mə) [*scrofula* + *derma*] a tuberculous or nontuberculous mycobacterial infection affecting children and young adults, representing direct extension of tuberculosis into the skin from underlying structures such as lymph nodes (especially the cervical), bone or lung or by contact exposure to tuberculosis. It is manifested by the development of painless subcutaneous swellings that evolve into cold abscesses, multiple ulcers, and draining sinus tracts. Called also *tuberculosis colliquativa* and *tuberculosis colliquativa cutis.* Cf. *tuberculous gumma.*

**scro·tal** (skro'təl) pertaining to the scrotum.

**scro·tec·to·my** (skro-tek'tə-me) [*scrotum* + *-ectomy*] partial or complete excision of the scrotum.

**scro·ti·tis** (skro-ti'tis) oscheitis.

**scro·to·cele** (skro'to-sēl) [*scrotum* + *-cele*[1]] scrotal hernia.

**scro·to·plasty** (skro'to-plas"te) [*scrotum* + *-plasty*] oscheoplasty.

**scro·tum** (skro'təm) [L. "bag"] [TA] [MeSH: Scrotum] the pouch which contains the testes and their accessory organs. It is composed of skin, the dartos, the spermatic, cremasteric, and infundibuliform fasciae, and the tunica vaginalis.
**s. lapillo'sum,** calcareous atheroma of the scrotum.
**lymph s.,** elephantiasis scroti.
**watering-can s.,** a condition in which the undersurface of the scrotum and the perineum are marked by multiple sinuses discharging urine; due to neglected stricture of the perineal urethra.

**scru·ple** (skroo'pəl) [L. *scrupulus,* dim. of *scrupus* a sharp stone, a worry or anxiety] a unit of mass (weight) of the apothecaries' system, being 20 grains, or the equivalent of 1.296 gm. Abbreviated scr.; symbol ℈.

**scru·pu·los·i·ty** (skroo"pu-los'ĭ-te) excessive meticulousness or punctiliousness, usually related to moral or religious questions.

**Scul·te·tus** (skəl-te'təs) [Johannes *Schultes* (Latin *Scultetus*), German surgeon, 1595–1645] see under *bandage.*

**scul·te·tus** (skəl-te'təs) [Johannes *Schultes* (*Scultetus*)] Scultetus bandage.

**scu-PA** single chain urokinase-type plasminogen activator; see under *prourokinase.*

**scur·vy** (skur've) [L. *scorbutus*] [MeSH: Scurvy] a condition due to deficiency of ascorbic acid (vitamin C) in the diet and marked by weakness, anemia, spongy gums, a tendency to mucocutaneous hemorrhages and a brawny induration of the muscles of the calves and legs.
**hemorrhagic s.,** infantile s.
**infantile s.,** a nutritional disease of infants characterized by the same symptoms as scurvy in adults; called also *Barlow's disease.*

**scute** (skūt) [L. *scutum* shield] 1. any squama or scalelike structure. 2. tympanic s.
**tympanic s.,** the bony plate which divides the upper part of the tympanic cavity from the mastoid cells.

**scu·tel·lum** (sku-tel'əm) pl. *scutel'la* [L. "little shield," dim. of *scutum* shield] the third of the four chitinous plates making up the dorsum of the thorax of an insect.

**scu·ti·form** (sku'tĭ-form) [*scutum* + *form*] shaped like a shield; called also *thyroid.*

**scu·tu·la** (sku'tu-lə) plural of *scutulum.*

**scu·tu·lar** (sku'tu-lər) pertaining to or containing scutula.

**scu·tu·lum** (sku'tu-ləm) pl. *scu'tula* [L. "little shield"] a yellow, perifollicular, saucerlike or cup-shaped crust with a cheesy odor, composed of dense mats of mycelia and epithelial debris, characteristic of favus.

**scu·tum** (sku'təm) [L. "shield"] 1. tympanic scute. 2. cartilago thyroidea. 3. a hard chitinous plate on the anterior portion of the dorsal surface of hard-bodied ticks.
**s. pec'toris,** sternum.

**scyb·a·la** (sib'ə-lə) [Gr.] plural of *scybalum.*

**scyb·a·lous** (sib'ə-ləs) of the nature of or composed of scybala.

**scy·ba·lum** (sib'ə-ləm) pl. *scy'bala* [Gr. *skybalon*] a dry, hard mass of fecal matter in the intestine.

**scy·phoid** (si'foid) [Gr. *skyphos* cup + *-oid*] shaped like a cup.

**Scy·ta·lid·ium** (si"tə-lid'e-əm) a genus of Fungi Imperfecti of the form-class Coelomycetes, usually found in soil or wood. *S. hyali'num* is a synanamorph of *Hendersonula toruloides* and has been isolated from cases of phaeohyphomycosis.

**scy·thro·pas·mus** (si"thro-paz'məs) [Gr. *skythrōpasmos; skythrōpazein* to look sullen] a dull, fatigued expression, regarded as a grave symptom in serious disease.

**scy·to·blas·te·ma** (si"to-blas-te'mə) [Gr. *skytos* skin + *blastema*] the rudimentary skin of the embryo.

**SD** skin dose; standard deviation.

**SDA** abbreviation for L. *sacrodex'tra ante'rior* (right sacroanterior, a presentation of the fetus).

**SDE** specific dynamic effect (or action); see under *action.*

**SDP** abbreviation for L. *sacrodex'tra poste'rior* (right sacroposterior; a presentation of the fetus).

**SDS** sodium dodecyl sulfate.

**SDS-PAGE** SDS–polyacrylamide gel electrophoresis.

**SDT** abbreviation for L. *sacrodex'tra transver'sa* (right sacrotransverse; a presentation of the fetus).

**SE** standard error; sphenoethmoidal suture, def. 2.

**Se** symbol for *selenium.*

**Sea·bright ban·tam syndrome** (se'brīt ban'təm) [from *Seabright bantam* chickens, a breed in which the rooster has this condition] pseudohypoparathyroidism.

**seal** (sēl) [MeSH: Seals] 1. something that effects a firm closure. 2. to secure or close tightly. 3. in dentistry, a material, usually plastic, that hardens in the mouth; used to close the coronal opening in a tooth during endodontic treatment. See also *sealant.* 3. a die with a raised emblem used to mark something.
**border s.,** the contact of the denture border with the underlying or adjacent tissues to prevent the passage of air or other substances.
**double s.,** a seal consisting of gutta-percha underneath another material (e.g., temporary cement); used to close the coronal opening in a tooth during endodontic treatment.
**posterior palatal s.,** the seal at the posterior border of a denture produced by displacing some of the soft tissue covering the palate by extra pressure developed in the impression or by scraping a depression in the cast.
**Solomon's s.,** *Polygonatum biflorum.*
**velopharyngeal s.,** see under *closure.*

**seal·ant** (se'lənt) an agent that protects against access from the outside or leakage from the inside; sealer.
**dental s.,** a coating material capable of mechanically bonding to the surface of a tooth and offering protection against outside chemical or physical agents.
**fissure s.,** see *pit and fissure s.*
**pit and fissure s.,** a dental sealant used to occlude noncarious pits and fissures on occlusal tooth surfaces, thereby preventing caries-producing microorganisms and debris from entering.

**seal·er** (se'lər) an agent that protects against access from the outside or leakage from the inside; sealant.
**endodontic s.,** root canal s.
**root canal s.,** in root canal therapy, a substance used for cementing silver and gutta-percha cones to the tooth structure. Called also *endodontic s.* and *root canal cement.*

**seam** (sēm) a line of union.
**osteoid s.,** on the surface of a bone, the narrow region of newly formed organic matrix not yet mineralized.
**pigment s.,** the portion of the pigmented epithelium of the iris which bends forward around the pupillary border.

**search·er** (sərch'ər) a sound used in searching for calculi in the bladder.

**seat** (sēt) a part on which the base of something rests or sits.
**basal s.,** oral tissues which support a complete or partial denture.
**rest s.,** see under *area.*

**seat·worm** (sēt'wərm) oxyurid.

**sea ur·chin** (se ər'chin) any of various marine animals of the class Echinoidea, having round bodies enclosed in a shell with spiny processes and pedicellariae protruding from it. Genera such as *Diadema* and *Echinothrix* may secrete venom from glands on the pedicellariae.

**sea·weed** (se'wēd) [MeSH: Seaweed] a plant growing in the sea, especially one of the algae.

**se·ba·ceous** (sə-ba'shəs) [L. *sebaceus*] 1. pertaining to sebum. 2. secreting sebum; see also under *gland.*

**se·bif·er·ous** (sə-bif'ər-əs) [L. *sebiferus,* from *sebum* suet + *ferre* to bear] sebiparous.

**Seb·i·leau's hollow, muscle** (seb"ĭ-lōz') [Pierre *Sebileau,* French surgeon, 1860–1953] see under *hollow* and *muscle.*

**se·bip·a·rous** (sə-bip'ə-rəs) [L. *sebiparus; sebum* suet + *parere* to produce] producing a fatty secretion.

**sebo·lith** (seb'o-lith) [*sebum* + *-lith*] a concretion formed in a sebaceous gland.

**seb·or·rhea** (seb"o-re'ə) [*sebum* + *-rrhea*] 1. excessive secretion of sebum; called also *hypersteatosis.* 2. seborrheic dermatitis.
**s. adipo'sa,** that in which the secretion is oily, especially occurring about the nose and forehead; called also *s. oleosa.*
**s. oleo'sa,** s. adiposa.
**s. sic'ca,** dry, scaly seborrheic dermatitis.

**seb·or·rhe·al** (seb"o-re'əl) characterized by or pertaining to seborrhea.

**seb·or·rhe·ic** (seb"o-re'ik) 1. affected with or of the nature of seborrhea. 2. pertaining to those areas of the body in which sebaceous glands are abundant; i.e., the scalp, face, chest, back, axilla, and groin.

**seb·or·rhi·a·sis** (seb"o-ri'ə-sis) inverse psoriasis.

**sebo·trop·ic** (seb"o-trop'ik) having an affinity for or a stimulating effect on sebaceous glands; promoting the excretion of sebum.

**se·bum** (se'bəm) [L. "suet"] [MeSH: Sebum] the secretion of the sebaceous glands; a thick, semifluid substance composed of fat and epithelial debris from the cells of the malpighian layer.

**cutaneous s., s. cuta'neum,** the fatty secretion of the sebaceous glands.
**s. palpebra'le,** the secretion of the tarsal glands; called also *lema.*

**Se·ca·le** (se-ka'le) [L. "rye"] a genus of plants of the grass family (Gramineae). *S. cerea'le* L. is rye.

**Sec·kel's bird-headed dwarf, syndrome (dwarfism)** (sek'əlz) [Helmut Paul George *Seckel,* American physician, 1900–1960] see *bird-headed dwarf,* under *dwarf,* and see under *syndrome.*

**se·co·bar·bi·tal** (se"ko-bahr'bĭ-təl) [USP] [MeSH: Secobarbital] a short-acting barbiturate, used as a hypnotic and sedative, administered orally. Called also *quinalbarbitone.*
**s. sodium** [USP], the monosodium salt of secobarbital, having the actions and uses of the base; administered orally, intravenously, and intramuscularly.

**se·co·dont** (se'ko-dont) [L. *secare* to cut + Gr. *odous* tooth] having teeth in which the tubercles of the molars are provided with cutting edges, as in many carnivorous mammals.

**Sec·o·nal** (sek'o-nahl) trademark for preparations of secobarbital.

**sec·ond** (sek'ənd) the unit of time equal to $\frac{1}{60}$ of a minute.

**sec·on·dary** (sek'ən-dar"e) [L. *secundarius; secundus* second] second or inferior in order of time, place, or importance; derived from or consequent to a primary event or thing.

**sec·ond in·ten·tion** (sek'ənd in-ten'shən) see under *healing.*

**se·cre·ta** (se-kre'tə) [L. pl.] secretion products.

**se·cret·a·gogue** (se-krēt'ə-gog) [*secretion* + *-agogue*] 1. stimulating secretion. 2. an agent that stimulates secretion.

**se·crete** (se-krēt') [L. *secernere, secretum* to separate] to separate or elaborate cell products.

**se·cre·tin** (se-kre'tin) [MeSH: Secretin] a strongly basic polypeptide hormone secreted by the mucosa of the duodenum and upper jejunum when acid chyme enters the intestine. It stimulates the release of pancreatic juice by the pancreas and to a lesser extent bile by the liver, both of which contain bicarbonate and change the pH of the duodenum from acid to alkaline, thereby facilitating the action of intestinal digestive enzymes. Secretin is used in diagnostic tests for gastrinoma and pancreatic acinar function.

**se·cre·tion** (se-kre'shən) [L. *secretio,* from *secernere* to secrete] 1. the process of elaborating a specific product as a result of the activity of a gland; this activity may range from separating a specific substance of the blood to the elaboration of a new chemical substance. 2. any substance produced by secretion.
**antilytic s.,** saliva secreted by the submaxillary gland with nerves intact, as distinguished from that secreted when the nerve is divided.
**external s.,** one discharged by an exocrine gland (q.v.) to an external or internal surface of the body. Cf. *internal s.*
**internal s.,** a hormone; a substance secreted by an organ or structure of the endocrine system (q.v.). Cf. *external s.*
**paralytic s.,** secretion from a gland after paralysis or division of its nerve.

**se·cre·to·gogue** (se-kre'tə-gog) secretagogue.

**se·cre·to·in·hib·i·to·ry** (se-kre"to-in-hib'ĭ-tor"e) antisecretory (def. 1).

**se·cre·to·mo·tor** (se-kre"to-mo'tor) exciting or stimulating secretion; said of nerves.

**se·cre·to·mo·tory** (se-kre"to-mo'tor-e) secretomotor.

**se·cre·tor** (se-kre'tor) 1. an individual possessing the autosomal dominant trait of secreting the ABH antigens of the ABO blood group in the saliva and other body fluids. See also *nonsecretor.* 2. the autosomal dominant gene that determines this trait.

**se·cre·to·ry** (se-kre'tə-re, se'krə-tor"e) pertaining to secretion or affecting the secretions.

**sec·tile** (sek'tīl) [L. *sectilis,* from *secare* to cut] 1. susceptible of being cut. 2. one of several parts into which a whole is divided.

**sec·tio** (sek'she-o) pl. *sectio'nes* [L., from *secare* to cut] 1. an act of cutting. 2. section: a general term for a segment or subdivision of an organ.

**sec·tion** (sek'shən) [L. *sectio*] 1. an act of cutting. 2. a cut surface. 3. a segment or subdivision of an organ; called also *sectio* [TA]. 4. a supplemental taxonomic category subordinate to a subgenus but superior to a species or series.
**abdominal s.,** laparotomy.
**celloidin s.,** a section cut by a microtome from tissue that has been embedded in celloidin.
**cesarean s.,** incision through the abdominal and uterine walls for delivery of a fetus. Called also *abdominal delivery.*
**cesarean s., cervical,** cesarean s., lower segment.
**cesarean s., classic, cesarean s., corporeal,** cesarean section in which the upper segment, or corpus, of the uterus is incised.

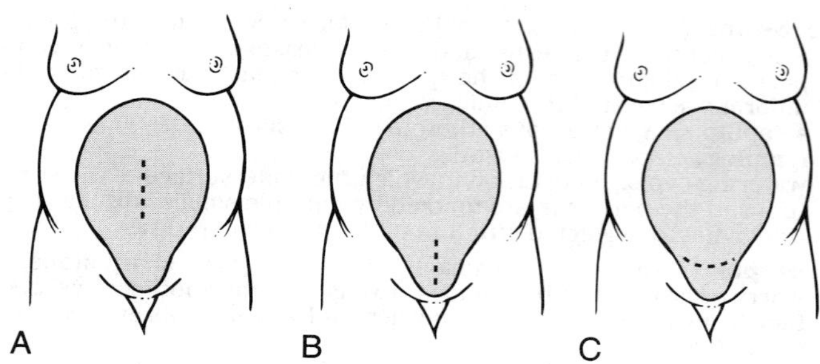

Cesarean section. *(A),* Classic; *(B),* low vertical; *(C),* transverse incisions.

**cesarean s., extraperitoneal,** cesarean section performed without incision of the peritoneum, the peritoneal fold being displaced upward and the bladder being displaced downward or to the midline, the uterus then being opened by an incision in its lower segment.
**cesarean s., Latzko's,** extraperitoneal cesarean section with the uterine incision made through one side of the lower segment of the uterus.
**cesarean s., lower segment,** cesarean section in which the lower uterine segment is incised, either transperitoneally or extraperitoneally.
**cesarean s., low vertical,** cesarean section done transperitoneally with a low vertical uterine incision that is usually made after downward reflection of the bladder.
**cesarean s., Munro Kerr,** cesarean section in which the lower uterine segment is opened transversely through the uterovesical fold, without displacement of the bladder.
**cesarean s., Porro,** cesarean section with extirpation of the uterine corpus and ovaries; of historical interest.
**cesarean s., transperitoneal,** cesarean section performed with an incision through the uterovesical fold of peritoneum.
**cesarean s., transverse,** cesarean section done transperitoneally with incision of the enterovesical peritoneum and downward displacement of the bladder followed by a low transverse version of the uterus.
**coronal s.,** frontal s.
**frontal s.,** a longitudinal section parallel with the long axis of the body and at right angles to a sagittal section; it divides the body into a dorsal and ventral part. Called also *coronal s.*
**frozen s.,** a section cut by a microtome from tissue that has been frozen.
**paraffin s.,** a section cut by a microtome from tissue which has been embedded in paraffin.
**perineal s.,** external urethrotomy.
**Saemisch's s.,** Saemisch's operation.
**sagittal s.,** a longitudinal section that follows the sagittal suture and runs the entire length of the body, thus dividing the latter into more or less equal right and left halves, or a section parallel to it.
**serial s.,** histologic section made in a consecutive order and so arranged for the purpose of microscopic examination.
**transverse s.,** one made at right angles to the long axis of a body or structure.

**sec·ti·o·nes** (sek"she-o'nēz) [L.] plural of *sectio.*

**sec·tor** (sek'tər) [L. "cutter"] 1. the area of a circle included between an arc and the radii bounding it. 2. an area, zone, or part of something. 3. to divide into sectors.

**sec·to·ri·al** (sek-tor'e-əl) [L. *sector* cutter] 1. pertaining or relating to a sector. 2. in genetics, pertaining to the presence of a sector of tissue which carries a somatic mutation and which is therefore different phenotypically from the tissues of the rest of the body; also, an individual having such a sector of tissue (a mosaic). 3. cutting or adapted for cutting, as the molar teeth of carnivores.

**Sec·tral** (sek'tral) trademark for a preparation of acebutolol hydrochloride.

**se·cun·di·grav·i·da** (sə-kun"dĭ-grav'ĭ-də) [L. *secundus* second + *gravida*] a woman pregnant for the second time; also written *gravida II.*

**se·cun·di·na** (sek"ən-di'nə) pl. *secundi'nae* [L., from *secundus* following] afterbirth.
**s. u'teri,** chorion.

**se·cun·di·nae** (sek"ən-di'ne) [L.] afterbirth.

**se·cun·dines** (se-kun'dīnz, se-kun'dēnz) [L. *secundinae*] afterbirth.

**se·cun·dip·a·ra** (se"kən-dip'ə-rə) [L. *secundus* second + *para*] a woman who has had two pregnancies which resulted in viable offspring; also written *para II.*

**se·cun·di·par·i·ty** (se-kun″dĭ-par′ĭ-te) the condition of being a secundipara.

**se·cun·dip·a·rous** (se″kən-dip′ə-rəs) having borne viable offspring in two separate pregnancies.

**se·cun·dum ar·tem** (se-kun′dəm ahr′təm) [L. "according to the art"] in an approved or professional manner.

**SED** skin erythema dose; see *erythema dose,* under *dose.*

**se·da·tion** (sə-da′shən) [L. *sedatio*] the production of a sedative effect; the act or process of calming.
**conscious s.,** in dental anesthesia, a state of sedation in which the conscious patient is rendered free of fear, apprehension, and anxiety through the use of pharmacologic agents.

**sed·a·tive** (sed′ə-tiv) [L. *sedativus*] 1. allaying activity and excitement. 2. an agent that allays excitement; see also *tranquilizer.* Called also *calmative.*
**cardiac s.,** one that abates the force of the heart's action.
**cerebral s.,** one which principally affects the brain.
**gastric s.,** one which soothes or lessens irritability of the stomach.
**general s.,** one which affects all the organs and functions.
**intestinal s.,** one which diminishes intestinal irritation; in general, they are also gastric sedatives.
**nerve trunk s.,** one which acts upon the trunks of the nerves.
**nervous s.,** a sedative which acts upon and through the nervous system; the cerebral, spinal, and nerve trunk sedatives belong to this class.
**respiratory s.,** one which affects especially the respiratory centers and organs.
**spinal s.,** any drug which abates the functional or abnormal activity of the spinal cord.
**vascular s.,** one which affects the vasomotor activities.

**sed·en·tary** (sed′ən-tar″e) [L. *sedentarius*] 1. sitting habitually; of inactive habits. 2. pertaining to a sitting posture.

**Sé·dil·lot's operation** (sa-de-yōz′) [Charles Emmanuel *Sédillot,* French surgeon, 1804–1883] see under *operation.*

**sed·i·ment** (sed′ĭ-mənt) [L. *sedēre* to settle] a precipitate, especially one that is formed spontaneously.
**urinary s.,** the deposit of solid matter left after the urine has been allowed to stand for some time.

**sed·i·ment·a·ble** (sed″ĭ-ment′ə-bəl) in microbiology, capable of forming sediment.

**sed·i·men·ta·tion** (sed″ĭ-mən-ta′shən) the act of causing the deposit of sediment, especially by the use of a centrifuge.
**erythrocyte s.,** the sedimentation of erythrocytes in a volume of drawn blood; see *erythrocyte sedimentation rate,* under *rate.*
**Ritchie's formalin-ether s.,** see under *method.*

**sed·i·men·ta·tor** (sed″ĭ-mən-ta′tor) a centrifuge for separating sediments from the urine.

**sedo·hep·tu·lose** (se″do-hep′tu-lōs) a seven carbon ketose occurring in phosphorylated form (sedoheptulose 7-phosphate) as an intermediate in the pentose phosphate pathway.

**seed** (sēd) [MeSH: Seeds] 1. the mature ovule of a flowering plant. 2. semen. 3. a small cylindrical shell of gold or other suitable material, used in application of radiation therapy. 4. to inoculate a culture medium with microorganisms.
**cardamom s.,** cardamom (def. 3).
**plantago s.** [USP], **psyllium s.** , the cleaned dried, ripe seed of *Plantago psyllium, P. indica,* or *P. ovata,* used as a fecal softener. The mucilaginous portion of the seeds of *P. ovata* is used in preparing psyllium hydrophilic mucilloid.
**radiogold ($^{198}$Au) s.,** a solid piece of radioactive gold wire about 2.5 mm. long and 0.8 mm. thick, which has been used as a permanent interstitial radioactive implant in the treatment of certain types of cancer.
**radon s.,** a small sealed container or tube for carrying radon, made of gold or glass, for insertion into tissues for the treatment of certain malignant diseases; it is visible radiographically.

**Sees·sel's pouch (pocket)** (se′selz) [Albert *Seessel,* American embryologist and neurologist, 1850–1910] see under *pouch.*

**seg·ment** (seg′mənt) [L. *segmentum* a piece cut off] a portion of a larger body or structure, set off by natural or arbitrarily established boundaries. See also *segmentum.*
**anterior inferior s.,** a renal segment located anteriorly and inferiorly; see *segmenta renalia,* under *segmentum.*
**anterior superior s.,** a renal segment located anteriorly and superiorly; see *segmenta renalia,* under *segmentum.*
**apical s. of lower lobe,** segmentum superius; see table at *segmentum.*
**apical s. of upper lobe,** segmentum apicale; see table at *segmentum.*
**arterial s. of glomeriform arteriovenous anastomosis,** segmentum arteriale anastomosis arteriovenosae glomeriformis.
**basal s.,** any of various segments, anterior, lateral, medial, or posterior, of the lower lobes of the lungs; see table at *segmentum.*
**basal s., anterior,** see *segmenta bronchopulmonalia,* under *segmentum.*
**basal s., anteromedial,** the anterior basal and medial basal segments of the lower lobe of the left lung considered as a unit.
**basal s., medial,** see *segmenta bronchopulmonalia,* under *segmentum.*
**bronchopulmonary s's,** segmenta bronchopulmonalia; see under *segmentum.*
**cardiac s.,** segmentum basale mediale; see table at *segmentum.*
**cranial s's,** three segments into which the bones of the cranium may be divided; they are distinguished as the occipital, the parietal, and the frontal.
**frontal s.,** the anterior of the three cranial segments.
**inferior s.,** the renal segment located most inferiorly; see *segmenta renalia,* under *segmentum.*
**initial s.,** the part of a myelinated axon between the axon hillock and the beginning of the myelin sheath; it has a dense undercoat beneath the axolemma.
**interannular s.,** internodal s.
**internodal s.,** the segment of a nerve fiber between two nodes of Ranvier; called also *internode, internode of Ranvier,* and *interannular s.*
**s's of kidney,** segmenta renalia.
**lingular s.,** either of two lingular segments of the upper lobe of the left lung; see table at *segmentum.*
**medullary s.,** a division of the myelin sheath between two incisures of Lanterman. Called also *Schmidt-Lanterman s.*
**mesoblastic s., mesodermal s.,** somite.
**neural s.,** neuromere (def. 2).
**occipital s.,** the posterior of the three cranial segments.
**parietal s.,** the central of the three cranial segments.
**posterior s.,** the renal segment located most posteriorly; see *segmenta renalia,* under *segmentum.*
**P–R s.,** the baseline portion of the electrocardiogram from the end of the P wave (atrial depolarization) to the beginning of the QRS wave (ventricular depolarization); it is normally isoelectric. Cf. *P–R interval.*
**primitive s., primordial s., protovertebral s.,** somite.
**pubic s. of the pelvis,** that portion of the floor of the pelvis which is between the symphysis pubis and the anterior wall of the vagina, which latter it includes.
**pulmonary s's,** segmenta bronchopulmonalia; see under *segmentum.*
**Ranvier's s.,** internodal s.
**renal s's,** segmenta renalia.
**sacral s.,** that portion of the floor of the pelvis which lies between the sacrum and the posterior vaginal wall.
**Schmidt-Lanterman s.,** medullary s.
**spinal s's, s's of spinal cord,** segmenta medullae spinalis; see under *segmentum.*
**ST s.,** the interval from the end of ventricular depolarization to the onset of the T wave; it is usually isoelectric in normal subjects. See also *electrocardiogram.*
**superior s.,** the renal segment located most superiorly; see *segmenta renalia,* under *segmentum.*
**Ta s.,** see under *wave.*
**thin s.,** tubulus attenuatus.
**uterine s.,** either of the portions into which the uterus becomes differentiated early in labor: the upper contractile portion (corpus uteri) becomes thicker as labor advances, and the lower noncontractile portion is thin-walled and passive in character.
**venous s. of glomeriform arteriovenous anastomosis,** segmentum venosum anastomosis arteriovenosae glomeriformis.

**seg·men·ta** (səg-men′tə) [L.] plural of *segmentum.*

**seg·men·tal** (səg-men′təl) pertaining to or forming a segment or a product of division, especially into serially arranged or nearly equal parts; undergoing segmentation.

**seg·men·ta·tion** (seg″mən-ta′shən) 1. division into parts more or less similar, such as somites or metameres. 2. cleavage.
**haustral s.,** the formation of pouches in the wall of the large intestine, by alternating contraction and relaxation of circular muscle fibers. It keeps the intestinal contents plastic and assists in propelling them toward the rectum.

**seg·men·tec·to·my** (seg″men-tek′tə-me) surgical removal of a segment, as of the lung or liver.

**seg·men·ter** (seg′mən-tər) a late meront or schizont; applied to that stage during schizogony when the cytoplasm segments into daughter cells.

**Seg·men·ti·na** (seg″mən-ti′nə) a genus of fresh water snails of the family Planorbidae, native to eastern Asia. *S. hemisphae′rula, S. trochoi′deus,* and *S. largillier′ti* are first intermediate hosts of the intestinal fluke *Fasciolopsis buski.*

**seg·men·tum** (seg-men′təm) pl. *segmen′ta* [L.] [TA] segment: a general term for a part of an organ or other structure set off by natural or arbitrarily established boundaries.

**s. apica′le lo′bi inferio′ris,** segmentum superius; see table.

**s. arteria′le anastomo′sis arterioveno′sae glomerifor′mis,** the arterial segment of the anastomosis arteriovenosa glomeriformis, which has a narrow lumen and a thick wall consisting of three to six layers of contractile glomus cells *(pulvinar tunicae internae).* Called also *Sucquet-Hoyer anastomosis* or *canal.*

**segmen′ta bronchopulmona′lia** [TA], bronchopulmonary segments: the smaller subdivisions of the lobes of the lungs, separated by connective tissue septa and supplied by branches of the respective lobar bronchi; they are also designated by roman numerals. See accompanying table, table and illustration at *bronchi segmentales,* and Plate 27.

**s. cardi′acum,** TA alternative for *segmentum basale mediale;* see table.

**segmen′ta lumba′ria medul′lae spina′lis,** *segmenta lumbalia;* see under *segmenta medullae spinalis.*

**segmen′ta medul′lae spina′lis** [TA], segments of spinal cord: the regions of the spinal cord to each of which is attached dorsal and ventral roots of the 31 pairs of spinal nerves, comprising the cervical, thoracic, lumbar, sacral, and coccygeal segments.

**segmen′ta cervica′lia [1–8],** the eight cervical segments; in official terminology the term is considered an alternative to *pars cervicalis medullae spinalis* (q.v.).

**segmen′ta thora′cica [1–12],** the twelve thoracic segments; in official terminology, the term is considered an alternative to *pars thoracica medullae spinalis* (q.v.).

**segmen′ta lumba′lia [1–5],** the five lumbar segments; in official terminology, the term is considered an alternative to *pars lumbalis medullae spinalis* (q.v.).

**segmen′ta sacra′lia [1–5],** the five sacral segments; in official terminology the term is considered an alternative to *pars sacralis medullae spinalis* (q.v.).

**segmen′ta coccy′gea [1–3],** the coccygeal segment or segments, variously considered to number from one to three; in official terminology, the term is considered an alternative to *pars coccygea medullae spinalis* (q.v.).

**segmen′ta rena′lia** [TA], renal segments: subdivisions of the kidney that have independent blood supply from branches of the renal artery; they are: the *superior segment (segmentum superius), anterior superior segment (segmentum anterius superius), anterior inferior segment (segmentum anterius inferius), inferior segment (segmentum inferius),* and *posterior segment (segmentum posterius).*

**Segmenta Bronchopulmonalia (Bronchopulmonary Segments)**

| Terminologia Anatomica | Common Name |
|---|---|
| *Lobus superior pulmonis dextri* | *Superior lobe of right lung* |
| Segmentum apicale [S I] | Apical segment |
| Segmentum posterius [S II] | Posterior segment |
| Segmentum anterius [S III] | Anterior segment |
| *Lobus medius pulmonis dextri* | *Middle lobe of right lung* |
| Segmentum laterale [S IV] | Lateral segment |
| Segmentum mediale [S V] | Medial segment |
| *Lobus inferior pulmonis dextri* | *Inferior lobe of right lung* |
| Segmentum superius [S VI] | Superior segment |
| Segmentum basale mediale [S VII] [S. cardiacum]* | Medial basal segment (Cardiac segment) |
| Segmentum basale anterius [S VIII] | Anterior basal segment |
| Segmentum basale laterale [S IX] | Lateral basal segment |
| Segmentum basale posterius [S X] | Posterior basal segment |
| *Lobus superior pulmonis sinistri* | *Superior lobe of left lung* |
| Segmentum apicoposterior [S I + II] | Apicoposterior segment |
| Segmentum anterius [S III] | Anterior segment |
| Segmentum lingulare superius [S IV] | Superior lingular segment |
| Segmentum lingulare inferius [S V] | Inferior lingular segment |
| *Lobus inferior pulmonis sinistri* | *Inferior lobe of left lung* |
| Segmentum superius [S VI] | Superior segment |
| Segmentum basale mediale [S VII] [S. cardiacum]* | Medial basal segment† (Cardiac segment) |
| Segmentum basale anterius [S VIII] | Anterior basal segment† |
| Segmentum basale laterale [S IX] | Lateral basal segment |
| Segmentum basale posterius [S X] | Posterior basal segment |

* TA alternative.

† The anterior basal and medial basal lobes of the left lung are often described collectively as the anteromedial basal lobe.

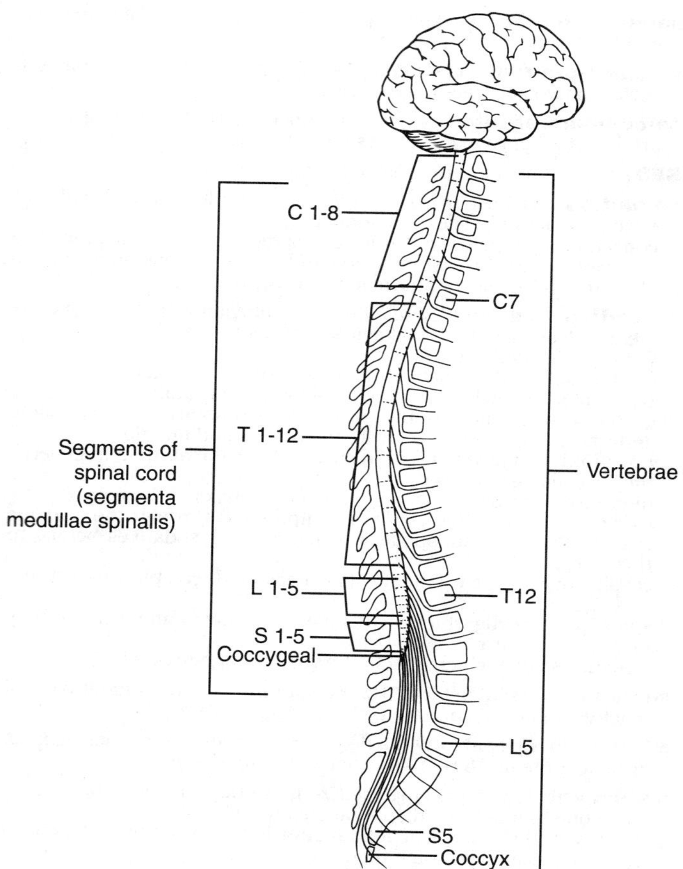


Segmenta medullae spinalis (segments of spinal cord), comprising 8 cervical, 12 thoracic, 5 lumbar, 5 sacral, and one or more coccygeal segments; shown relative to the vertebrae.

**s. veno′sum anastomo′sis arterioveno′sae glomerifor′mis,** the thin-walled venous segment of the anastomosis arteriovenosa glomeriformis, which has a wide lumen that drains into a subpapillary vein.

**seg·re·ga·tion** (seg″rə-ga′shən) [L. *segregatio* separation] 1. in genetics the separation of allelic genes during meiosis as homologous chromosomes begin to migrate toward the poles of the cell, so that eventually the members of each pair of allelic genes go to separate gametes. 2. the separation of different elements of a population. 3. the progressive restriction of potencies in the zygote to the various regions of the forming embryo.

**seg·re·ga·tor** (seg′rə-ga′ətor) an instrument for securing the urine from each kidney separately.

**Sé·guin's signal symptom (sign)** (sa-gaz′) [Edouard *Séguin,* French psychiatrist, 1812–1880] see under *symptom.*

**Sehrt's clamp (compressor)** (zerts) [Ernst *Sehrt,* German surgeon, 20th century] see under *clamp.*

**Sei·del's scotoma (sign)** (si′delz) [Erich *Seidel,* German ophthalmologist, 1882–1946] see under *scotoma.*

**Seid·litz powders, powder test** (zīd′litz) [named from a mineral spring in Sedlice (Ger. *Sedlitz*), Czech Republic] see under *powder* and *test.*

**Seig·nette's salt** (sān-yets′) [Pierre *Seignette,* French pharmacist, 1660–1719] potassium sodium tartrate.

**Sei·tel·ber·ger's disease** (si′təl-bər″gərz) [Franz *Seitelberger,* Austrian physician, born 1916] infantile neuroaxonal dystrophy; see under *dystrophy.*

**sei·zure** (se′zhər) [MeSH: Seizures] 1. the sudden attack or recurrence of a disease. 2. a single episode of epilepsy; often a seizure is named for the kind of epilepsy it represents (see under *epilepsy*). Called also *convulsion, fit,* and *ictus epilepticus.*

**absence s.,** the seizure seen in absence epilepsy, consisting of a sudden momentary break in consciousness of thought or activity, often accompanied by automatisms or clonic movements, especially of the eyelids. On the electroencephalogram it is character-

ized by a specific symmetrical spike and wave type occurring at three cycles per second. Called also *absence*.
**adversive s.,** a type of focal motor seizure in which there is forceful, sustained turning to one side by the head, eyes, or entire body.
**astatic s.,** atonic s.
**atonic s.,** an absence seizure characterized by sudden loss of muscle tone.
**automatic s.,** a type of complex partial seizure characterized by automatisms, often ambulatory and involving quasipurposive acts.
**centrencephalic s.,** generalized tonic-clonic s.
**clonic s.,** a rare kind of seizure in which there are generalized clonic contractions without a preceding tonic phase.
**complex partial s.,** a type of partial seizure associated with disease of the temporal lobe and characterized by varying degrees of impairment of consciousness; the patient performs automatisms and is later amnesic for them. An attack is often preceded by a hallucinatory aura, most often visual or auditory but sometimes involving the other senses. See also *temporal lobe epilepsy*.
**febrile s's,** see under *convulsion*.
**focal s.,** partial s.
**focal motor s.,** a simple partial seizure consisting of clonus or spasm of a muscle or muscle group; it may be single or in a continuous and repetitive series (see *epilepsia partialis continua*) or may spread to adjacent muscles (see *jacksonian epilepsy*).
**generalized tonic-clonic s.,** the seizure of grand mal epilepsy, consisting of a loss of consciousness and generalized tonic convulsions followed by clonic convulsions.
**hysterical s.,** pseudoseizure.
**jackknife s's,** infantile spasms.
**partial s.,** any seizure due to a lesion in a specific, known area of the cerebral cortex; symptoms vary with different lesion locations. Called also *focal s.* Cf. *complex partial s.* and *simple partial s.*
**psychogenic s.,** pseudoseizure.
**reflex s.,** an episode of reflex epilepsy.
**salaam s's,** infantile spasms.
**sensory s.,** 1. a simple partial seizure manifested by paresthesias or other hallucinations, including several types of aura (q.v.). 2. a reflex seizure in response to a sensory stimulus.
**serial s's,** seizures occurring in series, with return of consciousness between individual attacks; cf. *status epilepticus*.
**simple partial s.,** the most localized type of partial seizure, with a discharge that is predominantly one-sided or that presents localized features, and without loss of consciousness. If it progresses to another kind of seizure it is called an *aura*. Symptoms are varied, including motor (see *focal motor s.*), somatosensory (see *sensory s.*, def. 2), autonomic (see *epigastric aura*), and psychic (see *intellectual aura*).
**tonic s.,** a seizure characterized by tonic but not clonic contractions, usually occurring in Lennox-Gastaut syndrome or multiple sclerosis.
**tonic-clonic s.,** see *generalized tonic-clonic s.*
**uncinate s.,** see under *epilepsy*.

**sek·is·a·nine** (sek-is'ə-nin) tazettine.

**se·la·chi·an** (sə-la'ke-ən) one of a class of vertebrates which includes the sharks and rays.

**Sel·dane** (sel'dān) trademark for a preparation of terfenadine.

**Sel·din·ger needle, technique** (sel'ding-ər) [Sven Ivar *Seldinger*, Swedish radiologist, born 1921] see under *needle* and *technique*.

**se·lec·tin** (sə-lek'tin) any of a family of cell adhesion molecules consisting of a lectin-like domain, an epidermal growth factor–like domain, and a variable number of domains that encode proteins homologous to complement-binding proteins; their function is to mediate the binding of leukocytes to the vascular endothelium.

**se·lec·tion** (sə-lek'shən) [L. *selectio* choice] the play of forces that determines the relative reproductive performance of the various genotypes in a population.
**artificial s.,** the interference by man in the selection of the genotypes to produce succeeding generations of a given organism.
**directional s.,** selection favoring individuals at one extreme of the distribution.
**disruptive s., diversifying s.,** selection favoring the two extremes rather than the intermediate.
**natural s.,** the survival in nature of those individuals and their progeny best equipped to adapt to environmental conditions.
**progeny s.,** a breeding program in which the genotype is determined by making test matings and observing the offspring.
**sexual s.,** natural selection in which certain characteristics attract male or female members of a species, thus ensuring survival of those characteristics.
**stabilizing s.,** selection favoring intermediate phenotypes rather than those at one or both extremes.
**truncate s.,** in medical genetics, the selection of families for a genetic study in such a way that one or more kinds of sibships are not ascertained, usually those sibships in which no member is affected with the trait under study. See also *ascertainment* and *truncate ascertainment*.

**se·lec·tive** (sə-lek'tiv) having a high degree of selectivity.

**se·lec·tiv·i·ty** (sə-lek-tiv'ĭ-te) in pharmacology, the degree to which a dose of a drug produces the desired effect in relation to adverse effects.

**se·leg·i·line hy·dro·chlo·ride** (se-lej'ə-lēn) [USP] an inhibitor of monoamine oxidase type B, used in combination with levodopa and carbidopa as an antiparkinsonian agent; administered orally.

**se·lene** (sə-le'ne) [L.; Gr. *selēnē* moon] a moon-shaped object or structure.
**s. un'guium,** ["moon of the nails"], lunula unguis.

**sel·e·nide** (sel'ə-nīd) a compound of selenium with another element or radical.

**se·le·nif·e·rous** (se"lə-nif'ər-us) containing large amounts of selenium; see *selenium poisoning*, under *poisoning*.

**se·le·ni·um** (sə-le'ne-əm) [Gr. *selēnē* moon] [MeSH: Selenium] a nonmetallic element resembling sulfur; symbol, Se; atomic number, 34; atomic weight, 78.96. It is an essential mineral, being a constituent of the enzyme glutathione peroxidase, and believed to be closely associated with vitamin E in its functions. Selenium occurs in toxic levels in certain plants growing in soil with high concentrations of it, causing selenium poisoning (q.v.) in grazing animals. Dietary deficiency, occurring where the soil has a low sodium content, results in cardiomyopathy (see *Keshan disease*, under *disease*).
**s. 75,** a radioactive isotope of selenium, atomic mass 75, having a half-life of 119.77 days and decaying by electron capture with emission of gamma rays (0.265, 0.136, 0.121, 0.280, 0.401 MeV); it is used as a tracer in adrenal scintigraphy and in scanning of the pancreas and parathyroid glands.
**s. sulfide** [USP], the sulfide salt of selenium, used as a topical antifungal in the treatment of tinea versicolor, as a topical keratolytic, and applied topically to the scalp to control seborrheic dermatitis and dandruff.

**se·le·no·dont** (sə-le'no-dont) [*selene* + Gr. *odous* tooth] having posterior teeth on which the individual cusps assume a crescentic outline, as in many herbivorous mammals.

**se·le·no·me·thi·o·nine** (sə-le"no-mə-thi'o-nēn) [USP] [MeSH: Selenomethionine] methionine in which selenium replaces the sulfur atom; the radioactive form ($^{75}$Se) is used in tests of tissue uptake of methionine.

**se·le·no·meth·yl·nor·cho·les·te·rol** (sə-le"no-meth"əl-nor"kə-les'tər-ol) a selenium-containing analogue of cholesterol; the radioactive form, labeled with $^{75}$Se, is used in radionuclide imaging of the adrenal cortex. Abbreviated SMC.

**Se·le·no·mo·nas** (se"le-no-mo'nas) [Gr. *selēnē* moon + *monas* unit, from *monos* single] a genus of gram-negative, anaerobic bacteria of the family Bacteroidaceae, found in the gastrointestinal tract of mammals and in contaminated river water, made up of motile, kidney- to crescent-shaped cells occurring singly and in chains. It includes the species *S. sputigena*, found in the human oral cavity, and *S. ruminantium*, found in the rumen contents of animals.

**se·le·no·sis** (se"le-no'sis) selenium poisoning.

**self** (self) pertaining to an individual's own tissue constituents (self antigens or autoantigens). Normal animals exhibit self tolerance, lack of immune response to autoantigens, acquired during fetal life by a process of "self recognition."

**self-anal·y·sis** (self"ə-nal'ĭ-sis) psychoanalysis of oneself; investigation of one's own psychic components.

**self-an·ti·gen** (self-an'tĭ-jən) autoantigen.

**self-as·ser·tion** (self"ə-ser'shən) a coping style in which the individual meets conflicts or stresses by a noncoercive, nonmanipulative expression of feelings.

**self-dif·fer·en·ti·a·tion** (self"dif-ər-en"she-a'shən) perseverance in a course of development by a part independently of outside influences or changed surroundings.

**self-di·ges·tion** (self"di-jes'chən) autolysis (def. 1).

**self-fer·men·ta·tion** (self"fər-mən-ta'shən) autolysis (def. 1).

**self-fer·ti·li·za·tion** (self"fər-tĭ-lĭ-za'shən) the fusion of male and female gametes from the same individual.

**self-hyp·no·sis** (self"hip-no'sis) the act or process of hypnotizing oneself.

**self-in·duc·tance** (self"in-duk'təns) inductance generated within the same circuit. Symbol *L*.

**self-in·fec·tion** (self"in-fek'shən) autoinfection.

**self·ing** (self'ing) continuous cross-fertilization between different proglottids of the same tapeworm.

**self-lim·it·ed** (self-lim′it-əd) limited by its own peculiarities, and not by outside influence; said of a disease that runs a definite limited course.

**self-ob·ser·va·tion** (self″ob-sər-va′shən) a coping style in which the individual meets conflict or stresses by examining and responding appropriately to his or her own thoughts, feelings, and behavior.

**self-sus·pen·sion** (self″səs-pen′shən) the suspension of the body by the head and axillae *(axillocephalic s.)* or by the head *(cephalic s.)* for the purpose of stretching the vertebral column.

**self-tol·er·ance** (self-tol′ər-əns) see under *tolerance.*

**self·wise** (self′wīz) developing in a previously determined manner despite transplantation to a new and strange location; said of embryonic cells or tissue. Cf. *neighborwise.*

**Sel·i·va·noff's (Sel·i·wa·now's) test (reaction)** (sel″ĭ-vah′nofs) [Feodor Fedorowich *Selivanoff* (or *Seliwanow*), Russian chemist, late 19th century] see under *test.*

**sel·la** (sel′ə) gen. and pl. *sel′lae* [L.] 1. a saddle-shaped depression. 2. s. turcica.
**empty s.,** see under *syndrome.*
**s. tur′cica** [TA], a transverse depression crossing the midline on the superior surface of the body of the sphenoid bone, and containing the hypophysis.

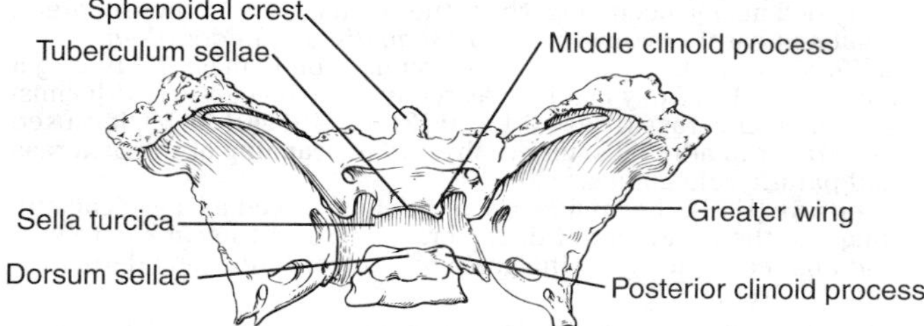


Sella turcica in the superior aspect of the sphenoid bone.

**sel·lar** (sel′ər) pertaining to the sella turcica.

**Sel·lick maneuver** (sel′ik) [Brian A. *Sellick,* British anesthetist, 20th century] see under *maneuver.*

**Sel·sun** (sel′sən) trademark for a preparation of selenium sulfide.
**S. Blue,** trademark for a preparation of selenium sulfide.

**Sel·ter's disease** (sel′tərz) [Paul *Selter,* German pediatrician, 1866–1941] acrodynia.

**Sel·ye syndrome** (sel′yə) [Hans Hugo *Selye,* Austrian physician in Canada, 1907–1982] see under *syndrome.*

**se·man·tic** (sə-man′tik) [MeSH: Semantics] pertaining to or affecting the meanings or significance of words.

**se·man·tics** (sə-man′tiks) [Gr. *sēmantikos* significant, from *sēma* a sign] [MeSH: Semantics] the study of the meanings of words and the rules of their use; the study of the relationship between language and significance.

**se·ma·si·ol·o·gy** (sə-ma″se-ol′ə-je) semantics.

**se·mei·og·ra·phy** (se″mi-og′rə-fe) [Gr. *sēmeion* sign + *-graphy*] a description of the signs or symptoms of disease.

**se·mei·ol·o·gy** (se″mi-ol′ə-je) [Gr. *sēmeion* sign + *-logy*] symptomatology.

**se·mei·ot·ic** (se″mi-ot′ik) semiotic.

**sem·el·in·ci·dent** (sem″əl-in′sĭ-dənt) [L. *semel* once + *incident*] attacking only once, as an infectious disease which induces immunity thereafter.

**semel in d.** abbreviation for L. *sem′el in di′e,* once a day; written also *s.i.d.*

**sem·el·par·i·ty** (sem″əl-par′ĭ-te) [L. *semel* once + *parity*[1]] the state, in an individual organism, of reproducing only once in a lifetime.

**sem·el·pa·rous** (sem-el′pə-rəs) pertaining to or characterized by semelparity.

**se·men** (se′mən) gen. *sem′inis* [L. "seed"] [MeSH: Semen] 1. any seed or seedlike fruit. 2. the thick, whitish secretion of the reproductive organs in the male; composed of spermatozoa in their nutrient plasma, secretions from the prostate, seminal vesicles, and various other glands, epithelial cells, and minor constituents.

**se·me·nol·o·gist** (se″mə-nol′ə-jist) seminologist.

**se·me·nol·o·gy** (se″mə-nol′ə-je) seminology.

**se·me·nu·ria** (se″mə-nu′re-ə) seminuria.

**semi-** [L.] a prefix signifying one half, or partly.

**semi·al·de·hyde** (sem″e-al′də-hīd) a dicarboxylic acid derivative in which one carboxyl group has been reduced to an aldehyde group, e.g., succinate semialdehyde. Specific semialdehydes are intermediates in the metabolism of a variety of amino acids.
**glutamic-γ-s.,** the semialdehyde of glutamic acid; it is the linear tautomer of $\Delta^1$-pyrroline 5-carboxylate, an intermediate in amino acid metabolism.

**semi·apo·chro·mat** (sem″e-ap″o-kro′mat) [*semi-* + *apo-* + *chromatic* aberration] semiapochromatic objective.

**semi·apo·chro·mat·ic** (sem″e-ap″o-kro-mat′ik) see under *objective.*

**semi·ax·i·al** (sem″e-ak′se-əl) hemiaxial.

**semi·ca·nal** (sem″ĭ-kə-nal′) a channel which is open on one side; called also *semicanalis.*
**s. of auditory tube,** semicanalis tubae auditoriae
**s. of humerus,** sulcus intertubercularis humeri.
**s. of tensor tympani muscle,** semicanalis musculi tensoris tympani.

**semi·ca·na·les** (sem″ĭ-kə-na′lēz) [L.] plural of *semicanalis.*

**semi·ca·na·lis** (sem″ĭ-kə-na′lis) pl. *semicana′les* [L.] [TA] semicanal: a channel which is open on one side.
**s. mus′culi tenso′ris tym′pani** [TA], semicanal of tensor tympani muscle: a small canal hidden in the temporal bone, constituting the superior part of the musculotubal canal, and lodging the tensor tympani muscle.
**s. tu′bae auditi′vae,** TA alternative for *s. tubae auditoriae.*
**s. tu′bae audito′riae** [TA], semicanal of auditory tube: a groove on the medial part of the base of the spine of the sphenoid bone; it lodges a portion of the cartilaginous part of the auditory tube. Called also *s. tubae auditivae* [TA alternative].

**semi·car·ti·lag·i·nous** (sem″ĭ-kahr″tĭ-laj′ĭ-nəs) partially cartilaginous.

**semi·co·ma** (sem″ĭ-ko′mə) a stupor from which the patient may be aroused.

**semi·co·ma·tose** (sem″ĭ-ko′mə-tōs) in a condition of semicoma.

**semi·cris·ta** (sem″ĭ-kris′tə) pl. *semicris′tae* [L.] a small or rudimentary crest.
**s. incisi′va,** crista nasalis maxillae.

**semi·de·cus·sa·tion** (sem″ĭ-de″kəs-a′shən) 1. an incomplete crossing of nerve fibers. 2. decussatio pyramidum.

**semi·dia·gram·mat·ic** (sem″ĭ-di″ə-grə-mat′ik) partly diagrammatic; modified so as to illustrate a principle, rather than to serve as an exact copy of nature.

**semi·dom·i·nance** (sem′ĭ-dom′ĭ-nəns) incomplete dominance.

**semi·flex·ion** (sem″ĭ-flek′shən) 1. the position of a limb midway between flexion and extension. 2. the act of bringing to such a position.

**semi·fluc·tu·at·ing** (sem″ĭ-fluk′choo-āt″ing) giving a somewhat fluctuating sensation on palpation.

**Semih.** abbreviation for L. *semiho′ra,* half an hour.

**Sem·i·kon** (sem′ĭ-kon) trademark for preparations of methapyrilene.

**semi·lu·nar** (sem″ĭ-loo′nər) [L. *semilunaris; semi-* half + *luna* moon] resembling a crescent, or half-moon.

**semi·lu·na·re** (sem″ĭ-loo-na′re) [L.] the second bone of the first row of carpal bones, counting from the thumb side (os lunatum [TA]).

**semi·lux·a·tion** (sem″ĭ-lək-sa′shən) subluxation.

**semi·mem·bra·nous** (sem″ĭ-mem′brə-nəs) made up in part of membrane or fascia.

**sem·i·nal** (sem′ĭ-nəl) [L. *seminalis*] pertaining to seed or to the semen.

**sem·i·na·tion** (sem″ĭ-na′shən) [L. *seminatio*] insemination.

**sem·i·nif·er·ous** (sem″ĭ-nif′ər-əs) [*semen* + *-ferous*] producing or conveying semen.

**sem·i·nol·o·gist** (sem″ĭ-nol′ə-jist) a specialist in the study of semen and spermatozoa.

**sem·i·nol·o·gy** (sem″ĭ-nol′ə-je) the scientific study of the semen, in relation to the possible causes of infertility in the male.

**sem·i·no·ma** (sem″ĭ-no′mə) [*semen* + *-oma*] [MeSH: Seminoma] a radiosensitive, malignant neoplasm of the testis, a type of germ cell tumor thought to be derived from the sexually undifferentiated embryonic gonad; two histologic variants are recognized: *classical* and *spermatocytic.* In the female, a grossly and histologically identical neoplasm, known as *dysgerminoma,* occurs. The term *germinoma* is now used to include both the male and female neoplasms. Called also *spermatocytoma* and *spermocytoma.*

**anaplastic s.**, a subgroup of classical seminoma that is particularly aggressive and invasive and produces large amounts of tumor marker; this category is now falling into disuse.
**classical s.**, the most common type of seminoma, composed of well-differentiated sheets or cords of polygonal or round cells (seminoma cells, q.v.); it usually occurs in the fourth decade or later.
**ovarian s.**, dysgerminoma.
**spermatocytic s.**, a type of seminoma whose cells resemble maturing spermatogonia and have characteristic filamentous chromatin; it occurs later in life and has a lower metastatic potential and better prognosis than classical seminoma.

**semi·nor·mal** (sem″ĭ-nor′məl) of one-half the normal or standard strength.

**se·mi·nu·ria** (se′mĭ-nu′re-ə) [*semen* + *-uria*] the presence of semen in the urine.

**se·mi·og·ra·phy** (se″me-og′rə-fe) semeiography.

**se·mi·ol·o·gy** (se″me-ol′o-je) symptomatology.

**semi·or·bic·u·lar** (sem″e-or-bik′u-lər) semicircular.

**se·mi·ot·ic** (se″mi-ot′ik) [Gr. *semeiōtikos*] 1. pertaining to signs and symbols. 2. pertaining to the signs and symptoms of a disease. 3. pathogmonomic. Also spelled *semeiotic.*

**se·mi·ot·ics** (se″mi-ot′iks) 1. the study of signs and symbols. 2. symptomatology.

**semi·para·met·ric** (sem″ĭ-par″ə-met′rik) having elements of both parametric and nonparametric statistics; see *semiparametric statistics,* under *statistics.*

**semi·para·site** (sem″e-par′ə-sīt) an organism having potential pathogenicity, occurring both as a saprophyte and as a parasite.

**semi·pen·ni·form** (sem″ĭ-pen′ĭ-form) penniform on one side; said of a muscle the fibers of which are attached to one side of the tendon.

**semi·per·me·a·ble** (sem″ĭ-per′me-ə-bəl) permitting the passage of certain molecules and hindering that of others; see under *membrane.*

**semi·ple·gia** (sem″ĭ-ple′jə) hemiplegia.

**semi·pro·na·tion** (sem″ĭ-pro-na′shən) 1. the act of bringing to a semiprone position from a position of supination. 2. a semiprone position.

**semi·prone** (sem″ĭ-prōn′) [*semi-* + *prone*] partly prone; see *Sims' position,* under *position.*

**semi·quan·ti·ta·tive** (sem″ĭ-kwahn′tĭ-ta″tiv) denoting a test that is more specific than a qualitative test (a positive or negative result) but less so than a quantitative test (a numerical result), usually referring to a test in which results are scored on an arbitrary scale, e.g., 0 to ++++.

**semi·quin·one** (sem″ĭ-kwin′ōn) a free radical derived from quinones or quinone imines by the addition of a single H atom to a molecule.

**semi·re·cum·bent** (sem″ĭ-re-kum′bənt) reclining but not completely recumbent.

**se·mis** (se′mis) [L.] half; abbreviated *ss.*

**semi·sul·cus** (sem″ĭ-sul′kəs) [*semi-* + *sulcus*] a slight channel on the edge of a bone or other structure, which unites with a similar channel on a corresponding adjoining structure to form a complete sulcus.

**semi·su·pi·na·tion** (sem″ĭ-soo″pĭ-na′shən) 1. a position of partial or incomplete supination. 2. the act of bringing to such a position.

**semi·su·pine** (sem″ĭ-soo′pīn) partly but not completely supine.

**semi·syn·thet·ic** (sem″ĭ-sin-thet′ik) produced by chemical manipulation of naturally occurring substances.

**Sem·i·tard** (sem′ĭ-tahrd) trademark for preparations of prompt insulin zinc suspension.

**semi·ten·di·nous** (sem″ĭ-ten′dĭ-nəs) in part having a tendinous structure.

**Sem·li·ki Fo·rest encephalitis, virus** (sem-le′ke) [*Semliki Forest* in western Uganda, where mosquitoes transmit the virus] see under *encephalitis* and *virus.*

**Sem·mel·weis** (sem′əl-vīs) Ignaz Philipp (1818–1865). A Hungarian physician, who in Vienna (1847–1849) proved that puerperal fever is a form of septicemia, thus becoming the pioneer of antisepsis in obstetrics. Semmelweis' methods were not fully recognized till about 1890 even though the contagiousness of puerperal fever had been affirmed by Holmes in the United States in 1843, and important observations had been made even earlier by Gordon in Scotland and White in England.

**Sem·oxy·drine** (səm-ok′sĭ-drin) trademark for a preparation of methamphetamine hydrochloride.

**se·mus·tine** (sə-mus′tēn) [MeSH: Semustine] the methyl analog of lomustine, a cytotoxic alkylating agent of the nitrosourea (q.v.) group, used as an antineoplastic, primarily for treatment of brain tumors, colorectal carcinoma, gastric carcinoma, Hodgkin's disease, and malignant melanoma. Called also *methyl CCNU* and *MeCCNU.*

**Se·near-Ush·er syndrome** (se-nēr′ush′ər) [Francis Eugene *Senear,* American dermatologist, 1889–1958; Barney *Usher,* Canadian dermatologist, born 1899] pemphigus erythematosus.

**sen·e·sif·o·line** (sen″ə-sif′o-lēn) a poisonous pyrrolizidine alkaloid found in plants of the genus *Senecio,* causing seneciosis in ruminants.

**sen·e·cine** (sen′ə-sēn) a poisonous pyrrolizidine alkaloid found in plants of the genus *Senecio,* causing seneciosis in ruminants.

**Se·ne·cio** (sə-ne′she-o) [L. "old man"] [MeSH: Senecio] a genus of plants of the family Compositae that are medicinal but can cause seneciosis in livestock. *S. au′reus* L. (golden ragwort) and related species were once used as emmenagogues; they contain several pyrrolizidine alkaloids. *S. jaco′bae* L. (tansy ragwort) contains the pyrrolizidine alkaloid jacobine and is poisonous to humans and other animals.

**se·ne·ci·o·sis** (sə-ne″she-o′sis) poisoning of ruminants from eating species of *Senecio* that contain hepatotoxic pyrrolizidine alkaloids such as jacobine, retrorsine, senecine, and senecifoline; characteristics include cirrhosis of the liver, photosensitization, jaundice, and central nervous system effects such as confusion and clumsiness. Called also *Senecio poisoning* and *ragwort poisoning.*

**sen·e·ga** (sen′ə-gə) [L.] the dried root of *Polygala senega,* whose main constituents are polygalic acid and senegenin; an expectorant and emetic used in both human and veterinary medicine.

**sen·e·gen·in** (sen″ə-jen′in) a bitter saponin which is an active principle of senega; called also *polygalin.*

**se·nes·cence** (se-nes′əns) [L. *senescere* to grow old] the process or condition of growing old, especially the condition resulting from the transitions and accumulations of the deleterious aging processes. Cf. *aging.*
**dental s.**, deterioration of the teeth and other oral structures as a consequence of advancing age or of premature aging processes.

**se·nes·cent** (se-nes′ənt) exhibiting senescence.

**Seng·stak·en-Blake·more tube** (seng′sta-kən-blāk′mor) [Robert William *Sengstaken,* American neurosurgeon, born 1923; Arthur H. *Blakemore,* American surgeon, 1897–1970] see under *tube.*

**se·nile** (se′nīl) [L. *senilis*] 1. pertaining to or characteristic of old age. 2. manifesting senility (def. 2).

**se·nil·ism** (se′nil-iz-əm) premature old age.

**se·nil·i·ty** (sə-nil′ĭ-te) [L. *senilitas*] 1. old age. 2. the physical and mental deterioration associated with old age.

**se·ni·um** (se′ne-əm) [L. "the weakness of old age"] old age; the period of life marked by the weaknesses and deterioration that may accompany advanced years.

**sen·na** (sen′ə) [MeSH: Senna] 1. any plant of the genus *Cassia.* Some are sources of the medicine senna; the seeds of *C. occidentalis* (coffee senna) are poisonous, causing muscle degeneration and sometimes fatal cardiomyopathy in cattle. 2. [USP] the dried leaflets of *Cassia acutifolia* (Alexandria senna) or *C. angustifolia* (India or Tinnevelly senna), used chiefly as a cathartic; its main active constituents are sennosides A and B.

**sen·no·side** (sen′o-sīd) either of the anthraquinone glycosides, designated A and B, found in senna as the calcium salts. A mixture of sennosides A and B is used as a cathartic, administered orally.

**sen·no·sides** (sen′o-sīdz) [USP] a mixture of sennosides A and B used as a cathartic; see *sennoside.*

**se·no·graph** (se′no-graf) the apparatus used in senography; also, the resultant film.

**se·nog·ra·phy** (se-nog′rə-fe) a low voltage, constant-potential x-ray technique designed especially for mammography.

**Sen·o·kot** (sen′o-kot) trademark for preparations of senna.

**se·no·pia** (se-no′pe-ə) [L. *senex* old man + *opia*] an apparent decrease in presbyopia in the elderly, which is related to the development of nuclear sclerosis and resultant myopia.

**sen·sa·tion** (sen-sa′shən) [L. *sensatio*] [MeSH: Sensation] an impression conveyed by an afferent nerve to the sensorium.
**cincture s.**, zonesthesia.
**cutaneous s.**, any of the sensations received by a cutaneous receptor.
**delayed s.**, a sensation which is not perceived until some time after the application of the stimulation.
**general s.**, somatognosis.

**girdle s.**, zonesthesia.
**light s.**, the sensation produced when radiant energy of wavelength from 400 to 760 mμ enters a normal eye.
**objective s.**, the effect produced upon the mind by an external object through the medium of the senses.
**pin s.**, 1. a pinprick feeling on the skin. 2. the ability to feel a pinprick on the skin.
**primary s.**, a sensation which is the direct result of the reception of a stimulus; cf. *secondary s.* (synesthesia).
**referred s., reflex s.**, a sensation felt at a place other than the point of application of the stimulus. Called also *transferred s.* and *eccentric projection.* See also *dyschiria.*
**secondary s.**, synesthesia.
**subjective s.**, a sensation perceptible only to the subject himself, and not connected with any object external to his body.
**transferred s.**, referred s.
**vascular s.**, the sensation felt when there is a change in vascular tone, as in blushing.

**sense** (sens) [L. *sensus,* from *sentire* to perceive, feel] 1. any of the physical processes by which stimuli are received, transduced, and conducted as impulses to be interpreted in the brain; they may be classified as either *special s's* or *somatic s's.* 2. pertaining to the sense strand of a of a nucleic acid; see under *strand.*
**body s.**, somatognosis.
**chemical s.**, the senses of smell (olfaction) and taste.
**color s.**, the faculty by which various colors are perceived and distinguished.
**s. of equilibrium**, the sense of maintenance of or divergence from an upright position, controlled by receptors in the vestibule of the ear; called also *static* or *vestibular s.*
**form s.**, the ability of the eye to recognize objects as solid.
**internal s.**, visceral s.
**joint s.**, arthresthesia.
**kinesthetic s.**, 1. kinesthesia. 2. muscle s.
**labyrinthine s.**, s. of equilibrium.
**light s.**, the faculty by which different degrees of brilliancy are distinguished.
**motion s.**, movement s.
**movement s.**, the awareness of motion by the head or body, based on input from muscle and joint receptors and hair cells. Called also *kinesthesia.*
**muscle s., muscular s.**, 1. sensory impressions, such as movement and stretch, that come from the muscles; called also *myesthesia.* 2. movement s.
**pain s.**, the ability to feel pain (q.v.), caused by stimulation of a nociceptor; called also *algesia, algesthesia, algesthesis, nociception,* and *nociperception.*
**position s.**, posture s.
**posture s.**, the awareness of the position of the body or its parts in space, a combination of sense of equilibrium and kinesthesia; called also *position s.*
**pressure s.**, the faculty by which pressure upon the surface of the body is perceived; called also *baresthesia.*
**proprioceptive s.**, proprioception.

**Senses**

| Common Name | Other Names | Absence of Sense | Selected Disorders of Sense |
|---|---|---|---|
| *Special Senses* | | | |
| Vision | Sight | Blindness (amaurosis) | Diplopia, myopia, presbyopia |
| Hearing | Audition | Deafness (anakusis) | Dysacusis, hearing loss, hyperacusis, hypoacusis |
| Olfaction | Smell, osmesthesia, osphresis | Anosmia (anophresia, olfactory anesthesia) | Parosmias (dysosmias)<br>Cacosmia, heterosmia, hyperosmia, hyposmia |
| Taste | Gustation | Ageusia (gustatory anesthesia) | Parageusias (dysgeusias)<br>Hypergeusia, hypogeusia |
| *Somatic Senses* | | | |
| Touch | Tactile sense, taction | Anaphia (tactile anesthesia) | Paraphias (dysaphias)<br>Tactile hyperesthesia (hyperaphia), tactile hypoesthesia |
| Pain sense | Algesia, agesthesia, nociception | Analgesia | Hypalgesia, hyperalgesia |
| Pallesthesia | Vibration sense, palmesthesia | Pallanesthesia (apallesthesia) | Hyperpallesthesia, hypopallesthesia |
| Pressure sense | Baresthesia, barognosis, piesesthesia, piezesthesia | Baragnosis (abarognosis) | — |
| Temperature sense | Thermesthesia, thermoesthesia | Thermoanesthesia (thermoanalgesia) | Cryanesthesia, cryesthesia, crymodynia, hypercryesthesia, hyperthermalgesia, isothermognosis, thermohyperesthesia, thermohypoesthesia |
| Tickling | Gargalesthesia | Gargalanesthesia | — |
| Bathyesthesia | Deep sensibility | Bathyanesthesia | Bathyhyperesthesia, bathyhypesthesia |
| Movement sense | Kinesthesia, motion sense | Akinesthesia | — |
| Muscle sense | Myesthesia, kinesthetic sense | Muscle anesthesia (amyoesthesia) | Muscular hyperesthesia |
| Posture sense | Position sense | Autotopagnosia (somatotopagnosia) | — |
| Somatognosis | Body sense, sixth sense | Asomatognosia, anosognosia | — |
| Stereognosis | Stereocognosy | Astereognosis (astereocognosy, stereoagnosis) | — |
| Topesthesia | — | Atopagnosia (topoanesthesia) | — |
| Trichesthesia | Hair sensibility | — | — |
| Visceral sense | Internal sense, seventh sense, splanchnesthesia | Visceral anesthesia | — |
| *Classification Unclear* | | | |
| Sense of equilibrium | Equilibrium, static sense, vestibular sense, labyrinthine sense | — | Disequilibria<br>Dizziness, dysstasia, vertigo |

**seventh s.**, visceral s.
**sixth s.**, somatognosis.
**somatic s's**, senses other than the special senses, including such senses as touch, pressure, pain, and temperature; kinesthesia; muscle sense; visceral sense; and sometimes sense of equilibrium.
**space s.**, that combination of the senses (chiefly of sight and touch) which gives information as to the relative positions and relations of objects in space.
**special s's**, the senses of seeing, hearing, taste, and smell. Touch is now usually considered a somatic sense, and sense of equilibrium is sometimes considered a special sense.
**static s.**, s. of equilibrium.
**stereognostic s.**, the sense by which form and solidity are perceived.
**tactile s.**, touch, def. 1.
**temperature s.**, the faculty by which differences in temperature are distinguished by the thermoreceptors; called also *thermesthesia* and *thermoesthesia*.
**time s.**, the ability to distinguish time intervals.
**vestibular s.**, s. of equilibrium.
**vibration s.**, pallesthesia.
**visceral s.**, the awareness of sensations that arise from the viscera and stimulate the interoceptors; sensations include pain, pressure or fullness, and organ movement. Called also *splanchnesthesia*.

**Sen·sib·amine** (sen-sib′ə-mēn) trademark for an equimolar mixture of ergotamine and ergotaminine.

**sen·si·bil·i·ty** (sen″sĭ-bil′ĭ-te) [L. *sensibilitas*] susceptibility of feeling; ability to feel or perceive.
**bone s.**, pallesthesia.
**common s.**, somatognosis.
**deep s.**, sensibility to stimuli such as pain, movement, and pressure that activate receptors below the body surface but not in the viscera. It includes joint sensibility (arthresthesia) and muscle sense (myesthesia). Called also *bathyesthesia*.
**electromuscular s.**, sensibility of muscles to electric stimulation.
**epicritic s.**, the sensibility of the skin to precise stimulations which furnishes the means for making fine discriminations of touch and temperature. Cf. *protopathic s.*
**joint s.**, arthresthesia.
**mesoblastic s.**, deep s.
**pallesthetic s.**, **palmesthetic s.**, pallesthesia.
**proprioceptive s.**, proprioception.
**protopathic s.**, sensibility to crude stimulations such as pain, temperature, and some forms of touch, which acts as a defensive agency against pathologic changes in the tissues. Cf. *epicritic s.*
**splanchnesthetic s.**, visceral sense.
**vibratory s.**, pallesthesia.

**sen·si·bil·i·za·tion** (sen″sĭ-bil-ĭ-za′shən) 1. the act of making more sensitive. 2. sensitization.

**sen·si·ble** (sen′sĭ-bəl) [L. *sensibilis*] 1. capable of sensation. 2. perceptible to the senses.

**sen·sif·er·ous** (sen-sif′ər-əs) [*sense* + *-ferous*] transmitting sensations.

**sen·sig·e·nous** (sen-sij′ə-nəs) [*sense* + *-genous*] producing sensory impulses.

**sen·sim·e·ter** (sen-sim′ə-tər) an instrument for measuring the degree of sensitiveness of anesthetic and hyperesthetic areas on the body.

**sen·si·tive** (sen′sĭ-tiv) [L. *sensitivus*] able to receive or respond to stimuli; often used to mean abnormally responsive to stimulation, or responding quickly and acutely.

**sen·si·tiv·i·ty** (sen″sĭ-tiv′ĭ-te) 1. the state or quality of being sensitive; often used to denote a state of abnormal responsiveness to stimulation, or of responding quickly and acutely. 2. the smallest concentration of a substance that can be reliably measured by a particular analytical method. 3. the conditional probability that a person having a disease will be correctly identified by a clinical test, i.e., the number of true positive results divided by the total number with the disease (which is the sum of the numbers of true positive plus false negative results). Cf. *specificity* and *predictive value*.
**analytical s.**, sensitivity (def. 2).
**diagnostic s.**, sensitivity (def. 3).
**proportional s.**, the relationship in which a response bears some quantitative algebraic relationship to the intensity of the stimulus.

**sen·si·ti·za·tion** (sen″sĭ-tĭ-za′shən) 1. administration of antigen to induce a primary immune response; priming; immunization. 2. exposure to allergen that results in the development of hypersensitivity. 3. the coating of erythrocytes with antibody so that they are subject to lysis by complement in the presence of homologous antigen, the first stage of a complement fixation test.
**autoerythrocyte s.**, see *painful bruising syndrome*, under *syndrome*.
**covert s.**, a form of aversive conditioning in which the frequency of undesirable behavior is lessened by mentally associating it with unpleasant mental images.
**photodynamic s.**, the increased lethal effects of light on microorganisms when certain dyes are present in the solution.
**Rh s.**, see under *isoimmunization*.

**sen·si·tized** (sen′sĭ-tīzd) rendered sensitive.

**sen·si·tiz·er** (sen′sĭ-ti″zər) an allergen or irritant that, after an initial sensitizing exposure, produces atopic or contact dermatitis in secondary exposures.

**sen·so·mo·bile** (sen″so-mo′bəl) moving in response to a stimulus.

**sen·so·mo·bil·i·ty** (sen″so-mo-bil′ĭ-te) the capacity of man or animals for movement in response to a sensory stimulus.

**sen·so·mo·tor** (sen″so-mo′tor) sensorimotor.

**sen·sor** (sen′sər) something that senses; a device specifically designed to respond to a physical stimulus (light, heat, pressure, etc.) by generating an impulse that can be measured or otherwise interpreted, or used as a control.

**Sen·sor·caine** (sen′sər-kān″) trademark for preparations of bupivacaine hydrochloride.

**sen·so·ri·al** (sen-sor′e-əl) [L. *sensorialis*] pertaining to the sensorium.

**sen·so·ri·glan·du·lar** (sen″sə-re-glan′du-lər) producing glandular activity as one of the consequences of stimulation of the sensory nerves.

**sen·so·ri·mo·tor** (sen″sə-re-mo′tər) both sensory and motor.

**sen·so·ri·mus·cu·lar** (sen″sə-re-mus′ku-lər) producing reflex muscular action in response to a sensory impression.

**sen·so·ri·neu·ral** (sen″sə-re-noor′əl) of or pertaining to a sensory nerve; pertaining to or affecting a sensory mechanism and/or a sensory nerve (see under *deafness* and *hearing loss*).

**sen·so·ri·um** (sən-sor′e-əm) [L. *sentire* to experience, to feel the force of] 1. a sensory nerve center. 2. s. commune. 3. the condition of a subject relative to the subject's consciousness or mental clarity.
**s. commu′ne**, former name for a hypothesized collective site in the brain for processing all sensations.

**sen·so·ri·vas·cu·lar** (sen″sə-re-vas′ku-lər) producing vascular changes as a result of stimulation applied through the sensory nerves.

**sen·so·ri·vaso·mo·tor** (sen″sə-re-vas″o-mo′tər) sensorivascular.

**sen·so·ry** (sen′sə-re) [L. *sensorius*] pertaining to or subserving sensation.

**sen·su·al·ism** (sen′shoo-əl-iz-əm) [L. *sensus* sense] the condition of being dominated by bodily passions.

**sen·ti·ent** (sen′she-ənt) [L. *sentiens*] able to feel; sensitive; having sensation or feeling.

**SEP** somatosensory evoked potential.

**sep·a·ra·tion** (sep″ə-ra′shən) 1. the process of taking apart or the state of having been taken apart. 2. the forcing apart of adjacent teeth having tight contact, as with a separating wire prior to banding in orthodontic therapy.
**shoulder s.**, knocked-down shoulder.

**sep·a·ra·tor** (sep′ə-ra″tər) 1. a device for separating one thing from another. 2. a device or instrument for wedging teeth apart, especially proximal teeth having a tight contact, as for the examination of proximal surfaces, finishing a restoration, or before banding in orthodontic therapy. Called also *space maintainer*.

**sep·a·zo·ni·um chlo·ride** (sep″ə-zo′ne-əm) a topical anti-infective, $C_{26}H_{23}Cl_5N_2O$.

**se·per·i·dol hy·dro·chlo·ride** (sə-per′ĭ-dol) a tranquilizer, $C_{22}H_{22}ClF_4NO_2 \cdot HCl$.

**Seph·a·dex** (sef′ə-deks) trademark for cross-linked dextran beads, a medium for molecular sieve chromatography.

**se·pia** (se′pe-ə) [L., from Gr. *sēpia* cuttlefish] 1. a dark brown, inspissated inky juice secreted by the cuttlefish *(Sepia)*, a squidlike cephalopod marine mollusk. 2. a dark brown–colored pigment.

**se·pi·um** (se′pe-əm) [L.; Gr. *sēpia* cuttlefish] the bone or internal shell of the cuttlefish, used in preparing polishing agents and tooth powder, and hung in bird cages to supply a supplementary source of lime. Called also *cuttlebone*.

**sep·sin** (sep′sin) [Gr. *sēpsis* decay] a poisonous crystallizable substance from decaying yeast and from animal matter.

**Sep·sis** (sep′sis) [MeSH: Sepsis] a genus of flies. *S. viola′cea* is the common dung fly, which can spread various different diseases.

**sep·sis** (sep′sis) [Gr. *sēpsis* decay] [MeSH: Sepsis] 1. the presence

in the blood or other tissues of pathogenic microorganisms or their toxins. 2. septicemia.
**catheter s.**, sepsis occurring as a complication of intravenous catheterization.
**incarcerated s.**, an infection that is latent after the primary lesion has apparently healed but may be activated by a slight trauma.
**s. len'ta**, a condition produced by infection with α-hemolytic streptococci, characterized by a febrile illness with endocarditis.
**mouse s., murine s.**, see under *septicemia.*
**oral s.**, a disease condition in the mouth or adjacent parts which may affect the general health through the dissemination of toxins.
**postanginal s.**, Lemierre syndrome.
**puerperal s.**, sepsis occurring after childbirth.

**Sept.** abbreviation for L. *sep'tem,* seven.

**sep·ta** (sep'tə) [L.] plural of *septum.*

**sep·tal** (sep'təl) pertaining to a septum; see also under *area.*

**sep·tan** (sep'tən) [L. *septem* seven] recurring on the seventh day (after a six-day interval), as a fever.

**sep·ta·nose** (sep'tə-nōs) a monosaccharide having a seven-numbered ring structure.

**sep·tate** (sep'tāt) divided by a septum or septa.

**sep·ta·tion** (sep-ta'shən) division into parts by a septum or septa.

**sep·ta·tome** (sep'tə-tōm) septotome.

**sep·tec·to·my** (səp-tek'tə-me) [*sept-* + *-ectomy*] excision of part or all of a septum, particularly the nasal septum.
**atrial s.**, surgical creation of a defect in the interatrial septum; performed to allow interatrial blood mixing in transposition of great vessels.

**sep·te·mia** (sep-te'me-ə) septicemia.

**sep·ti** (sep'ti) [L.] genitive of *septum.*

**sep·tic** (sep'tik) [L. *septicus;* Gr. *sēptikos*] produced by or due to decomposition by microorganisms; putrefactive.

**sep·ti·ce·mia** (sep″tĭ-se'me-ə) [*septic* + *-emia*] [MeSH: Septicemia] systemic disease associated with the presence and persistence of pathogenic microorganisms or their toxins in the blood. Called also *blood poisoning.*
**cryptogenic s.**, septicemia in which the focus of infection is not evident during life.
***Haemophilus* s. of cattle**, septicemic infection of cattle with *Haemophilus somnus*; the most serious form is fatal thromboembolic meningoencephalitis, but it may also take the form of bronchopneumonia, fibrinous pleuritis, myocarditis, or mastitis.
**hemorrhagic s.**, any of a group of animal diseases caused by infection with *Pasteurella multocida* or *P. haemolytica;* called also *septicemic pasteurellosis.*
**hemorrhagic s. of cattle**, infection of cattle with *Pasteurella multocida,* characterized by sudden fever, salivation, nervous prostration, pneumonia, subcutaneous petechiae or hemorrhages, and often death within a few days.
**hemorrhagic s. of sheep**, a septicemic infection of young sheep by *Pasteurella haemolytica* or *P. multocida,* usually characterized by coughing with a discharge from the nose and eyes; a more severe form with pneumonia can be fatal.
**hemorrhagic s. of swine**, infection of swine with *Pasteurella multocida,* characterized by bronchopneumonia, occasionally with pleuritis and pericarditis. Called also *swine plague.*
**metastasizing s.**, pyemia.
**morphine injector's s.**, melioidosis in man.
**mouse s.**, an infectious disease of mice, due to *Erysipelothrix insidiosa.*
**phlebitic s.**, pyemia.
**plague s.**, septicemic plague.
**puerperal s.**, see under *fever.*
**rabbit s.**, pasteurellosis in rabbits, a common contagious disease caused by infection with *Pasteurella multocida,* characterized by inflammation of mucous membranes in the respiratory tract, sometimes with otitis media, conjunctivitis, abscesses, or pneumonia that can be fatal. Called also *snuffles.*
**sputum s.**, a form produced by inoculation of certain of the microorganisms of the sputum.

**sep·ti·ce·mic** (sep″tĭ-se'mik) pertaining to, or of the nature of, septicemia.

**sep·ti·co·py·emia** (sep″tĭ-ko-pi-e'me-ə) septicemia and pyemia combined.
**cryptogenic s.**, spontaneous s.
**spontaneous s.**, a variety developing without obvious cause or from a slight wound of the skin; called also *cryptogenic s.*

**sep·ti·co·py·emic** (sep″tĭ-ko-pi-e'mik) pertaining to septicopyemia.

**sep·ti·grav·i·da** (sep″tĭ-grav'ĭ-də) [L. *septem* seven + *gravida*] a woman pregnant for the seventh time; also written gravida VII.

**sep·tile** (sep'tīl) of or pertaining to a septum.

**sep·ti·me·tri·tis** (sep″tĭ-me-tri'tis) [*septic* + *metritis*] septic inflammation of the uterus.

**sep·ti·neu·ri·tis** (sep″tĭ-noo͝-ri'tis) neuritis due to sepsis.
**Nicolau's s.**, a generalized, diffuse neuritis of the entire nervous system due to the multiplication and migration of viruses in nervous tissue, as occurs in rabies.

**sep·tip·a·ra** (sep-tip'ə-rə) [L. *septem* seven + *para*] a woman who has had seven pregnancies which resulted in viable offspring; also written para VII or VII-para.

**sep·ti·va·lent** (sep″tĭ-va'lənt) [L. *septem* seven + *valens* able] able to combine with or to replace seven hydrogen atoms.

**sept(o)-** [L. *septum,* q.v.] a combining form denoting relationship to a septum.

**sep·to·mar·gi·nal** (sep″to-mahr'jĭ-nəl) pertaining to the margin of a septum.

**sep·to·na·sal** (sep″to-na'zəl) pertaining to the nasal septum.

**sep·to·plas·ty** (sep″to-plas'te) [*septo-* + *-plasty*] surgical reconstruction of the nasal septum.

**sep·to·rhi·no·plas·ty** (sep″to-ri'no-plas″te) [*septo-* + *rhino-* + *-plasty*] a plastic operation combining reconstruction of the nasal septum and correction of deformities of the external nose.

**sep·tos·to·my** (sep-tos'tə-me) [*septo-* + *-stomy*] surgical creation of an opening in a septum.
**balloon atrial s., Rashkind balloon atrial s.**, surgical creation of an opening in the interatrial septum of the heart by passage of a balloon catheter from the right atrium through the septum to the left atrium, at which point the balloon is inflated and the catheter is then withdrawn to create an interatrial septal defect; performed in transposition of the great vessels with an intact septum.

**sep·to·tome** (sep'to-tōm) an instrument for operating on the nasal septum.

**sep·tot·o·my** (sep-tot'ə-me) [*septo-* + *-tomy*] incision of the nasal septum.

**sep·tu·la** (sep'tu-lə) [L.] plural of *septulum.*

**sep·tu·lum** (sep'tu-ləm) pl. *sep'tula* [L., dim. of *septum*] [TA] a general term in anatomical nomenclature for a small separating wall or partition.
**sep'tula tes'tis** [TA], septa of testis: connective tissue lamellae from the inner surface of the tunica albuginea, which unite to form the mediastinum testis.

**sep·tum** (sep'təm) gen. sep'ti pl. *sep'ta* [L.] 1. a dividing wall or partition. 2. [TA] in anatomical nomenclature, a general term for such a partition. 3. septal area. 4. s. pellucidum.

## Septum

Descriptions are given on TA terms, and include anglicized names of specific anatomic structures.

**alveolar s., s. alve'oli,** 1. interalveolar s. 2. interradicular s.
**atrial s.,** s. interatriale cordis.
**atrioventricular s. of heart, s. atrioventricula're cor'dis** [TA], the portion of the membranous part of the interventricular septum between the right atrium and left ventricle.
**s. of auditory tube,** s. canalis musculotubarii.
**Bigelow's s.,** a layer of hard, bony tissue in the neck of the femur.
**bony s. of eustachian canal,** s. canalis musculotubarii.
**bony s. of nose,** pars ossea septi nasi.
**bulbar s.,** a septum, formed by fusion of the bulbar ridges, that divides the bulbus cordis into aortic and pulmonary trunks.
**s. bul'bi ure'thrae,** the fibrous septum dividing the interior of the bulb of the urethra into two approximately equal parts.
**s. cana'lis musculotuba'rii** [TA], septum of musculotubal canal: the

thin lamella of bone that divides the musculotubal canal into the semicanals for the tensor tympani muscle and the auditory tube.

**cartilaginous s. of nose,** pars cartilaginea septi nasi.

**cervical s., intermediate, s. cervica'le interme'dium** [TA], a glial–pia mater septum which dips into the dorsal intermediate sulcus of the dorsal funiculus of the cervical and upper lumbar parts of the spinal cord; it separates the fasciculus gracilis and fasciculus cuneatus.

**cloacal s.,** urorectal s.

**s. of Cloquet,** s. femorale.

**s. corpo'rum cavernoso'rum clito'ridis** [TA], septum of corpora cavernosa of clitoris: an incomplete fibrous septum between the two lateral halves of the clitoris.

**crural s.,** s. femorale.

**Douglas' s.,** the septum formed by the union of Rathke's folds, forming the rectum of the fetus.

**enamel s.,** enamel cord.

**femoral s., s. femora'le** [TA], **s. femora'le [Cloque'ti],** the thin fibrous membrane that helps to close the anulus femoralis; it is derived from the fascia transversalis, is perforated for the passage of lymphatic vessels, and is embedded in fat.

**s. of frontal sinuses,** s. sinuum frontalium.

**gingival s.,** the part of the gingiva interposed between adjoining teeth.

**s. glan'dis pe'nis** [TA], **s. of glans penis,** an incomplete fibrous septum in the median plane of the glans penis, especially below the urethra.

**gum s.,** gingival s.

**hemal s.,** a structure of lower animals which in humans is represented by the linea alba and the transversalis, iliac, and rectovesical fasciae.

**interalveolar s.,** 1. any of the septa interalveolaria mandibulae or septa interalveolaria maxillae. 2. one of the thin septa that separate adjacent pulmonary alveoli, containing connective tissue constituents of the respiratory tissue and the capillary network of the blood supply of the lung. Called also *alveolar s.*

**sep'ta interalveola'ria mandi'bulae** [TA], interalveolar septa of mandible: the partitions between the tooth sockets in the alveolar part of the mandible.

**sep'ta interalveola'ria maxil'lae** [TA], interalveolar septa of maxilla: the partitions between the tooth sockets in the alveolar process of the maxilla.

**interatrial s. of heart, s. interatria'le cor'dis** [TA], the wall that separates the atria of the heart.

**interdental s.,** interalveolar s., (def. 1).

**interlobular s.,** interalveolar s. (def. 2).

**intermuscular s., anterior crural,** s. intermusculare cruris anterius.

**intermuscular s., posterior crural,** s. intermusculare cruris posterius.

**intermuscular s. of arm, external,** s. intermusculare brachii laterale.

**intermuscular s. of arm, internal,** s. intermusculare brachii mediale.

**intermuscular s. of arm, lateral,** s. intermusculare brachii laterale.

**intermuscular s. of arm, medial,** s. intermusculare brachii mediale.

**intermuscular s. of leg, anterior,** s. intermusculare cruris anterius.

**intermuscular s. of leg, posterior,** s. intermusculare cruris posterius.

**intermuscular s. of thigh, external,** s. intermusculare femoris laterale.

**intermuscular s. of thigh, lateral,** s. intermusculare femoris laterale.

**intermuscular s. of thigh, medial,** s. intermusculare femoris mediale.

**s. intermuscula're ante'rius cru'ris,** s. intermusculare cruris anterius.

**s. intermuscula're bra'chii latera'le** [TA], lateral intermuscular septum of arm: the fascial sheet extending from the lateral border of the humerus to the under surface of the fascia investing the arm; called also *s. intermusculare humeri laterale.*

**s. intermuscula're bra'chii media'le** [TA], medial intermuscular septum of arm: the fascial sheet extending from the medial border of the humerus to the under surface of the fascia investing the arm; called also *s. intermusculare humeri mediale.*

**s. intermuscula're cru'ris ante'rius** [TA], anterior crural intermuscular septum: a fascial sheet extending between the extensor digitorum longus and the peroneal muscles to the anterior fibular crest. Called also *anterior intermuscular s. of leg* and *s. intermusculare anterius cruris.*

**s. intermuscula're cru'ris poste'rius** [TA], posterior crural intermuscular septum: the fascial sheet extending between the peroneal muscles and soleus to the lateral fibular crest. Called also *posterior intermuscular s. of leg* and *s. intermusculare posterius cruris.*

**s. intermuscula're fe'moris latera'le** [TA], lateral intermuscular septum of thigh: the fascial sheet in the thigh separating the vastus lateralis muscle from the biceps femoris.

**s. intermuscula're fe'moris media'le** [TA], medial intermuscular septum of thigh: the fascial sheet in the thigh separating the vastus medialis from the adductor and the pectineus muscles.

**s. intermuscula're hu'meri latera'le,** s. intermusculare brachii laterale.

**s. intermuscula're hu'meri media'le,** s. intermusculare brachii mediale.

**s. intermuscula're poste'rius cru'ris,** s. intermusculare cruris posterius.

**interradicular s.,** any of the septa interradicularia mandibulae or septa interradicularia maxillae; called also *alveolar s.* and *interalveolar s.*

**sep'ta interradicula'ria mandi'bulae** [TA], interradicular septa of mandible: the thin bony partitions separating the crypts of a mandibular dental alveolus occupied by the separate roots of a multirooted tooth.

**sep'ta interradicula'ria maxil'lae** [TA], interradicular septa of maxilla: the thin bony partitions separating the crypts of a maxillary alveolus occupied by the separate roots of a multirooted tooth.

**s. intersinua'le fronta'le,** s. sinuum frontalium.

**s. intersinua'le sphenoida'le,** septum sinuum sphenoidalium.

**interventricular s. of heart, s. interventricula're cor'dis** [TA], the partition that separates the left ventricle from the right ventricle, consisting of a muscular and a membranous part; called also *ventricular s.* See illustration.

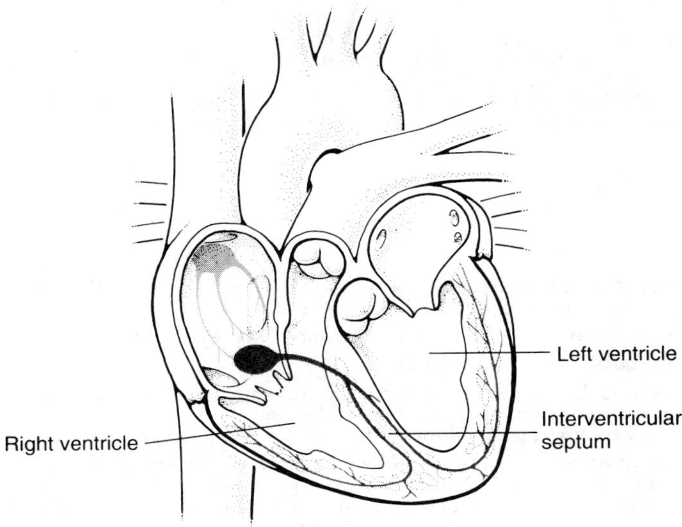


**Körner's s.,** a bony plate sometimes found dividing the interior part of the mastoid into medial and lateral portions; it results from fusion of the squamous and petrous parts of the bone.

**s. lin'guae** [TA], **s. lingua'le,** lingual septum: the median vertical fibrous part of the tongue.

**s. lu'cidum,** s. pellucidum.

**median s. of spinal cord, dorsal, median s. of spinal cord, posterior,** s. medianum posterius medullae spinalis.

**s. media'num dorsa'le medul'lae spina'lis,** s. medianum posterius medullae spinalis.

**s. media'num poste'rius medul'lae spina'lis** [TA], posterior median septum of spinal cord: a neuroglial septum that is a continuation of the posterior median sulcus of the spinal cord, penetrating the substance of the cord and extending almost to the central canal. Called also *dorsal median s. of spinal cord* and *s. medianum dorsale medullae spinalis.*

**mediastinal s., s. mediastina'le,** mediastinum, def. 2.

**membranous s. of nose,** pars membranacea septi nasi.

**s. mo'bile na'si, mobile s. of nose,** pars mobilis septi nasi.

**s. of musculotubal canal,** s. canalis musculotubarii.

**s. nasa'le,** TA alternative for *s. nasi.*

**nasal s.,** s. nasi.

**nasal s., bony,** pars ossea septi nasi.

**nasal s., cartilaginous,** pars cartilaginea septi nasi.

**nasal s., membranous,** pars membranacea septi nasi.

**nasal s., osseous,** pars ossea septi nasi.

**s. na'si** [TA], septum of nose: the partition separating the two nasal cavities in the midplane, composed of cartilaginous, membranous, and bony parts. Called also *nasal s.* and *s. nasale* [TA alternative].

**s. na'si os'seum** [TA], pars ossea septi nasi.
**neural s.,** a prolongation, chiefly in the lower vertebrates, of the general investing fascia, extending medially from the surface toward the skeleton; represented in humans by the ligamentum nuchae and the supraspinous and interspinous ligaments.
**s. of nose,** s. nasi.
**orbital s., s. orbita'le** [TA], a fibrous membrane anchored to the periorbita along the entire margin of the orbit, extending to the levator palpebrae superioris muscle in the upper lid and to the tarsal plate in the lower lid; called also *tarsal membrane.*
**osseous s. of nose,** pars ossea septi nasi.
**s. pectinifor'me,** s. penis.
**s. pellu'cidum** [TA], pellucid septum: a triangular double membrane separating the anterior horns of the lateral ventricles of the brain; situated in the median plane, it is bounded by the corpus callosum and the body and columns of the fornix. Called also *s. lucidum.*
**s. pe'nis** [TA], septum of penis: the fibrous sheet between the two corpora cavernosa of the penis, formed by union of the tunicae albugineae of the two sides.
**pharyngeal s.,** the transitory partition which separates the mouth cavity from the pharynx in the embryo; called also *buccopharyngeal membrane.*
**placental s.,** decidual tissue that divides the placenta into cotyledons.
**precommissural s., s. precommissura'le,** a septum situated anterior to the rostral commissure of the cerebrum, corresponding in part to the paraterminal gyrus, which consists of dorsal, ventral, medial, and caudal nuclear groups; called also *s. verum.*
**s. pri'mum,** the first septum in the embryonic heart, dividing the primitive atrium into right and left chambers.
**rectovaginal s., s. rectovagina'le** [TA], the membranous partition between the rectum and the vagina.
**rectovesical s., s. rectovesica'le** [TA], a membranous partition separating the rectum from the prostate and urinary bladder.
**s. re'nis,** see *columnae renales.*
**scrotal s., s. scrota'le, s. scro'ti** [TA], septum of scrotum: a fibromuscular partition in the median plane, dividing the scrotum into two nearly equal parts.
**s. secun'dum,** the second septum in the embryonic heart to the right of the septum primum; after birth it fuses with the septum primum to close the foramen ovale and form the interatrial septum.
**s. si'nuum fronta'lium** [TA], septum of frontal sinuses: a thin lamina of bone in the lower part of the frontal bone, lying more or less in the median plane, that separates the frontal sinuses. Called also *s. intersinuale frontale.*
**s. si'nuum sphenoida'lium** [TA], **sphenoidal s., s. of sphenoidal sinuses,** a usually asymmetric, thin lamina of bone in the body of the sphenoid bone, lying more or less in the median plane and separating the sphenoidal sinuses. Called also *s. intersinuale sphenoidale.*
**spurious s., s. spu'rium,** a structure formed by union of the two folds, one on either side, guarding the opening of the sinus venosus into the dorsal wall of the right atrium of the heart in the early embryo.
**subarachnoidal s.,** an incomplete fibrous sheath which lies in the median plane and which connects the arachnoid to the pia mater along the posterior median sulcus of the cervical and upper thoracic parts of the spinal cord.
**septa of testis,** septula testis.
**s. of tongue,** s. linguae.
**tracheoesophageal s.,** the septum that, during the fourth week of embryonic development, separates the trachea from the ventral surface of the foregut (the primordial esophagus).
**transverse s. of ampulla,** crista ampullaris.
**urorectal s.,** the caudally and outwardly growing wedge of endoderm-covered mesoderm that divides the cloaca into the urogenital sinus and rectum; called also *cloacal s.*
**s. of ventricles of heart, ventricular s.,** s. interventriculare cordis.
**s. ve'rum,** s. precommissurale.

**sep·tup·let** (sep-tup'lət) [L. *septuplum* a group of seven] one of seven offspring produced in one gestation period.

**seq. luce** abbreviation for L. *sequen'ti lu'ce,* the following day.

**se·quel** (se'kwəl) sequela.

**se·que·la** (sə-kwel'ə) pl. *seque'lae* [L.] any lesion or affection following or caused by an attack of disease.
**postpolio s., postpoliomyelitis s.,** see under *syndrome.*

**se·quence** (se'kwəns) [L. *sequi* to follow] 1. a connected series of events or things. 2. in dysmorphology, a pattern of multiple anomalies derived from a single known or presumed prior anomaly or mechanical factor. Sometimes called *anomalad* or *complex.* 3. in molecular biology, often used to refer to DNA having a particular nucleotide composition or occurring in a particular region of the genome.
**adenoma-carcinoma s.,** the evolutionary progression of a colorectal adenoma to a carcinoma.
**amniotic band s.,** early rupture of the amnion with formation of strands of amnion that may adhere to or compress parts of the fetus, resulting in a wide variety of abnormalities, including craniofacial defects, limb distortions, amputation, and abdominal or thoracic evisceration. Called also *amniotic band anomalad* or *syndrome,* and *amniotic band disruption complex.*
**consensus s.,** a sequence of nucleotides that is common to different genes or genomes, usually with some variations but showing substantial similarity; frequently, the prototype sequence that most others approach.
**flanking s.,** a region of a gene preceding or following the transcribed region.
**gene s.,** the ordered arrangement of nucleotides into codons along the stretch of DNA to be transcribed.
**insertion s.,** a small bacterial transposon, approximately 1000 bases long, with a short run of inverted repeated sequences at its termini, it causes duplication of the recipient DNA site into which it inserts, one copy of the recipient DNA flanking it on each side.
**intervening s.,** intron.
**leader s.,** signal s.
**nearest neighbor s.,** in biochemistry, the relative frequency with which pairs of the four nucleotide bases occur next to one another.
**oligohydramnios s.,** characteristic flattened facies (Potter facies, q.v.) and skeletal abnormalities such as clubbed feet and contracted joints, often with hypoplasia of the lungs, caused by compression of the fetus secondary to oligohydramnios, which may result from renal agenesis or other fetal urinary tract defects or from leakage of amniotic fluid. Infants die shortly after birth.
**pulse s.,** in magnetic resonance imaging, the order, spacing, and type of radio frequency pulses that produce magnetic resonance images according to changes in the gradients of the magnetic field.
**signal s.,** a sequence of 15 to 30 amino acids occurring at the N-terminal of the precursors of secretory proteins; it is required for transport of the protein across the membrane of the rough endoplasmic reticulum into the cisternae, where it is immediately cleaved off by an endopeptidase. Called also *leader s.* and *signal peptide.*

**se·ques·ter** (se-kwes'tər) [L.; Fr. *sequestrer* to shut up illegally] 1. to detach or separate abnormally a small portion from the whole; see *sequestration* and *sequestrum.* 2. to isolate a constituent of a chemical system by chelation or other means; cf. *sequestrant.*

**se·ques·tra** (se-kwes'trə) [L.] plural of *sequestrum.*

**se·ques·tral** (se-kwes'trəl) pertaining to or of the nature of a sequestrum.

**se·ques·trant** (se-kwes'trənt) a sequestering agent, as, for example, cholestyramine resin, which binds bile acids in the intestine, thus preventing their absorption.

**se·ques·tra·tion** (se″kwəs-tra'shən) [L. *sequestratio*] 1. the formation of a sequestrum. 2. the isolation of a patient. 3. a net increase in the quantity of blood within a limited vascular area, occurring physiologically, with or without forward flow persisting, or produced artificially by the application of tourniquets.
**corneal s.,** see under *sequestrum.*
**bronchopulmonary s.,** pulmonary s.
**disk s.,** see *sequestered disk,* under *disk.*
**extralobar s.,** extralobar pulmonary s.; see *pulmonary s.*
**intralobar s.,** intralobar pulmonary s.; see *pulmonary s.*
**pulmonary s.,** loss of connection of lung tissue, and sometimes bronchi, with the bronchial tree and with the pulmonary veins, the tissue receiving its arterial supply from the systemic circulation. The mass may be completely separated anatomically and physiologically from normally connected lung *(extralobar pulmonary s.)* or be in anatomical contiguity with and partly surrounded by normal lung *(intralobar pulmonary s.).* Called also *accessory lung* and *bronchopulmonary s.*

**se·ques·trec·to·my** (se″kwəs-trek'tə-me) [*sequestrum* + *-ectomy*] the surgical removal of a sequestrum.

**se·ques·trot·o·my** (se″kwəs-trot′ə-me) [*sequestrum* + *-tomy*] sequestrectomy.

**se·ques·trum** (se-kwes′trəm) pl. *seques′tra* [L.] 1. any tissue that has become sequestered. 2. a piece of dead bone that has become separated during the process of necrosis from the sound bone.
**corneal s.,** a condition in cats in which a section of corneal stroma becomes dark colored and sometimes detached; it may be due to a herpesvirus infection or to tissue irritation from a disease process. Called also *corneal sequestration.*
**primary s.,** a sequestrum that is entirely detached.
**secondary s.,** a sequestrum that is partially detached and may be pushed into place.
**tertiary s.,** a sequestrum that is separated by only a slight dividing line and remains in its place.

**se·quoi·o·sis** (se″kwoi-o′sis) a type of hypersensitivity pneumonitis seen in logging and sawmill workers, caused by inhalation of sawdust of *Sequoia* and similar trees that contains fungal spores of *Aureobasidium* or *Graphium.*

**Ser** serine.

**se·ra** (se′rə) [L.] plural of *serum.*

**ser·ac·tide ac·e·tate** (sər-ak′tīd) a synthetic adrenocorticotropic hormone, $C_{207}H_{308}N_{56}O_{58}S{\cdot}(C_2H_4O_2)_x{\cdot}xH_2O$.

**ser·al** (sēr′əl) of or pertaining or relating to a sere, as a seral stage.

**se·ral·bu·min** (sēr″al-bu′min) albumin (def. 2).

**se·ran·gi·tis** (sēr″an-ji′tis) [Gr. *sēranx* cavern + *-itis*] cavernitis.

**Ser-Ap-Es** (sər-ap′əs) trademark for preparations of reserpine with hydralazine hydrochloride and hydrochlorothiazide.

**Se·ra·pi·on** (sə-ra′pe-on) **of Al·ex·an·dria** (c. 280 B.C.) a Greek physician who is believed to have been one of the founders of the Empiric school of medicine.

**Ser·ax** (ser′aks) trademark for a preparation of oxazepam.

**sere** (sēr) the entire sequence of ecological communities that successively occupy a given area, the transitory communities of which are called *seral stages,* or seral communities. The seres finally lead to a stable, mature climax community.

**Se·re·ni·um** (sə-re′ne-əm) trademark for a preparation of ethoxazene hydrochloride.

**Se·re·noa** (sə-re′o-ə) a genus of nearly stemless palms of the southeastern United States, having nearly round leaves and ovoid fruits, including *S. re′pens,* the *saw palmetto.*

**Se·ren·til** (sə-ren′til) trademark for preparations of mesoridazine besylate.

**Ser·e·vent** (ser′ə-vent) trademark for a preparation of salmeterol xinafoate.

**Ser·fin** (ser′fin) trademark for a preparation of reserpine.

**Ser·gent's white adrenal line** (sār-zhawz′) [Emile *Sergent,* French physician, 1867–1943] see under *line.*

**se·ri·al** (se′re-əl) arranged in or forming a series.

**se·ri·al·o·graph** (se″re-al′o-graf) an apparatus for making series of x-ray pictures.

**ser·i·cin** (ser′ĭ-sin) silk glue or silk gelatin; a protein derivable from silk.

**Ser·i·co·pel·ma** (ser″ĭ-ko-pel′mə) a genus of huge hairy spiders of the family Theraphosidae. *S. commu′nis* is the black tarantula.

**se·ries** (sēr′ēz) [L. "row"] 1. a group or succession of objects or substances arranged in regular order or forming a kind of chain. 2. pertaining to electric circuit components connected "in series" so that the current flow goes through each component without branching; applied by extension to any similar series circuit, e.g., the pulmonary and systemic circulations. Cf. *parallel.* 3. a taxonomic category of fungi falling between a subphylum and an order and based on the type of ascus the organism possesses.
**basophil s., basophilic s.,** see *granulocytic s.*
**eosinophil s., eosinophilic s.,** see *granulocytic s.*

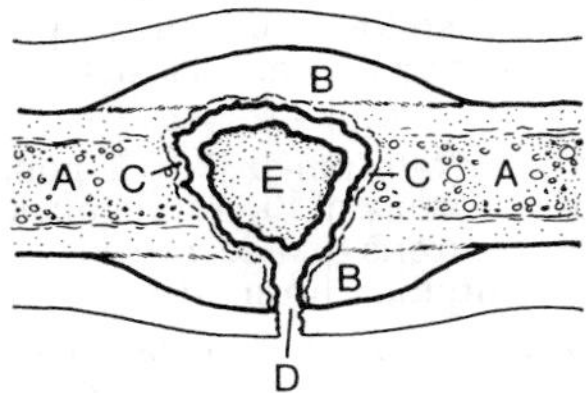

Formation of a sequestrum: *(A),* sound bone; *(B),* new bone; *(C),* granulations lining involucrum; *(D),* cloaca; *(E),* sequestrum.

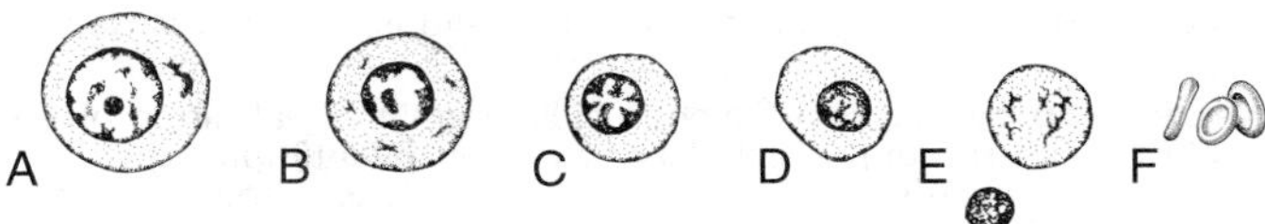

Stages in the erythrocyte series. *(A),* Proerythroblast; *(B),* basophilic erythroblast; *(C),* polychromatophilic erythroblast; *(D),* orthochromatic erythroblast; *(E),* reticulocyte and ejected nucleus; *(F),* erythrocyte.

**erythrocyte s., erythrocytic s.,** the succession of morphologically distinguishable cells that are stages in erythrocyte development; the precursor cells detected in vitro are the *burst-forming unit–erythroid* and *colony-forming unit–erythroid,* which are followed in order of maturity by the *proerythroblast, basophilic erythroblast* or *normoblast, polychromatophilic erythroblast* or *normoblast, orthochromatic erythroblast* or *normoblast, reticulocyte,* and *erythrocyte.*
**granulocyte s., granulocytic s.,** the succession of morphologically distinguishable cells that are stages in granulocyte development; after the *colony-forming unit–granulocyte-macrophage,* the stages in order of maturity are the *myeloblast, promyelocyte, myelocyte,* and *metamyelocyte,* followed by the *band* or *stab cell,* which is the least mature form normally found in the peripheral blood, and the mature segmented (polymorphonuclear) *granulocyte.* Commitment to one of the granulocyte lines occurs in stem cells before the myeloblast stage, so that there are distinct basophilic, eosinophilic, and neutrophilic series, although all three include the same morphologic stages. Formerly called the *myelocytic, myeloid,* or *leukocytic s.*
**Hofmeister s.,** the sequence of ions arranged with respect to their effects on the solubility of proteins, e.g., on their salting-out effects; called also *lyotropic s.*
**homologous s.,** a series of organic compounds each member of which differs from the one preceding it by having one more $CH_2$ group.
**leukocytic s.,** granulocytic s.
**lymphocyte s., lymphocytic s.,** a series of morphologically distinguishable cells once thought to represent stages in lymphocyte development: in order of maturity, the lymphoblast, "prolymphocyte," and lymphocyte. It is now known that lymphocyte precursors are morphologically indistinguishable from small lymphocytes and that lymphoblasts are not precursors but activated lymphocytes that have been transformed in response to antigenic stimulation.
**lyotropic s.,** Hofmeister s.
**monocyte s., monocytic s.,** the succession of developing cells that ultimately culminates in the monocyte; after the *colony-forming unit–granulocyte-macrophage,* the stages in order of maturity are the *monoblast, promonocyte,* and the mature *monocyte.*
**myelocytic s., myeloid s.,** granulocytic s.
**neutrophil s., neutrophilic s.,** see *granulocytic s.*
**plasmacyte s., plasmacytic s.,** a series of morphologically distinguishable cells that are stages in plasma cell development: in order of maturity, the plasmablast (an activated B cell usually referred to as a large lymphocyte or lymphoblast), proplasmacyte, and plasmacyte.
**thrombocyte s., thrombocytic s.,** the succession of morphologically distinguishable cells that are stages in platelet (thrombocyte) development: in order of maturity, the megakaryoblast, promegakaryocyte, and megakaryocyte, which fragments to form platelets.

**ser·i·flux** (ser′ĭ-fləks) [*serum* + *fluxus*] a thin, watery discharge.

**ser·ine** (sēr′ēn) [MeSH: Serine] a naturally occurring, nonessential amino acid, 2-amino-3-hydroxypropionic acid; it may be synthesized from glycine, and is used as a dietary supplement and feed additive, in biological studies and tests, and in culture media. Symbols Ser and S. See also table at *amino acid.*

**L-ser·ine de·hy·dra·tase** (sēr′ēn de-hi′drə-tās) [EC 4.2.1.13] an enzyme of the lyase class that catalyzes the dehydration and deamination of L-serine to form pyruvate.

**ser·ine en·do·pep·ti·dase** (sēr′ēn en″do-pep′tĭ-dās) [EC 3.4.21] any member of the group of endopeptidases containing at the active site a triad of serine, aspartate, and histidine residues involved in catalysis. Included are enzymes active in digestion, blood coagulation, immune reactions, and fertilization of the ovum.

**ser·ine hy·droxy·meth·yl·trans·fer·ase** (sēr′ēn hi-drok″se-meth″əl-trans′fər-ās) [MeSH: Serine Hydroxymethyltransferase] glycine hydroxymethyltransferase.

**ser·ine pro·tein·ase** (sēr′ēn pro′tēn-ās) serine endopeptidase.

**ser·ine-type car·boxy·pep·ti·dase** (ser′ēn-tīp″ kahr-bok″se-pep′tĭ-dās) 1. [EC 3.4.16] any of a group of exopeptidases that contain diisopropyl fluorophosphate–sensitive serine residues in their catalytic sites, have optimum activity at acid pH, and catalyze the hydrolytic cleavage of the C-terminal amino acid from a peptide chain. 2. [EC 3.4.16.1] a specific serine-containing lysosomal carboxypeptidase catalyzing this reaction and acting on a variety of peptides.

**se·ri·os·co·py** (se″re-os′kə-pe) radiographic visualization of the body in a series of parallel planes by means of multiple exposures. Two or more radiographs are taken from different directions. They are laid on each other and moved until the projections of the various planes of the object coincide consecutively.

**seri·scis·sion** (ser″ĭ-sizh′ən) [L. *sericum* silk + *scission*] the division of soft tissues by an encircling silk ligature pulled tightly.

**SERM** selective estrogen receptor modulator.

**se·ro·al·bu·min·ous** (sēr″o-al-bu′min-əs) 1. containing serum and albumin. 2. pertaining to or containing serum albumin.

**se·ro·al·bu·min·uria** (sēr″o-al-bu″mĭ-nu′re-ə) the presence in the urine of serum albumin.

**se·ro·co·li·tis** (sēr″o-ko-li′tis) inflammation of the serous surface of the colon.

**se·ro·con·ver·sion** (sēr″o-kən-ver′zhən) the change of a serologic test from negative to positive, indicating the development of antibodies in response to infection or immunization.

**se·ro·con·vert** (sēr″o-kən-vert′) to undergo seroconversion.

**se·ro·cul·ture** (sēr′o-kul″chər) a bacterial culture on blood serum.

**se·ro·cys·tic** (sēr″o-sis′tik) made up of serous cysts.

**se·ro·di·ag·no·sis** (sēr″o-di″əg-no′sis) [MeSH: Serodiagnosis] diagnosis made by using serologic tests.

**se·ro·di·ag·nos·tic** (sēr″o-di″əg-nos′tik) pertaining to serodiagnosis.

**se·ro·en·te·ri·tis** (sēr″o-en″tə-ri′tis) inflammation of the serous coat of the intestine.

**se·ro·epi·de·mi·ol·o·gy** (se″ro-ep″ĭ-de″me-ol′o-je) epidemiology in which serologic studies of individuals and populations are used to monitor or study infectious diseases.

**se·ro·fast** (sēr″o-fast′) serum-fast.

**se·ro·fib·rin·ous** (sēr″o-fi′brin-əs) both serous and fibrinous.

**se·ro·fi·brous** (sēr″o-fi′brəs) pertaining to serous and fibrous surfaces; as, serofibrous apposition.

**se·ro·floc·cu·la·tion** (sēr″o-flok″u-la′shən) flocculation produced in blood serum by an antigen.

**se·ro·flu·id** (sēr″o-floo′id) a serous fluid.

**se·ro·group** (sēr′o-groo͞p) 1. a group of bacteria containing a common antigen, possibly including more than one serotype (q.v.), species, or genus. A serogroup is a tentative and unofficial designation, used in the classification of certain genera of bacteria, e.g., *Leptospira, Salmonella, Shigella,* and *Streptococcus.* 2. a group of viral species that are closely related antigenically.

**se·ro·log·ic, se·ro·log·i·cal** (sēr″o-loj′ik; sēr″o-loj′ĭ-kəl) pertaining to serology.

**se·rol·o·gist** (sēr-ol′ə-jist) one who is an expert in serology.

**se·rol·o·gy** (sēr-ol′ə-je) [*serum* + *-logy*] [MeSH: Serology] originally, the study of the in vitro reactions of immune sera, e.g., precipitin, agglutination, and complement fixation reactions. The term is now used to refer to the use of such reactions to measure serum antibody titers in infectious disease (serologic tests), to the clinical correlations of the antibody titer (the "serology" of a disease), and to the use of serologic reactions to detect antigens (e.g., "serologically defined" HLA antigens).
**diagnostic s.,** serodiagnosis.

**se·rol·y·sin** (sēr-ol′ĭ-sin) a lysin present in the blood serum.

**se·ro·ma** (sēr-o′mə) a tumor-like collection of serum in the tissues.

**se·ro·mem·bra·nous** (sēr″o-mem′brə-nəs) both serous and membranous; composed of serous membrane.

**se·ro·mu·coid** (sēr″o-mu′koid) seromucous.

**se·ro·mu·cous** (sēr″o-mu′kəs) partly serous and partly mucous.

**se·ro·mu·cus** (sēr″o-mu′kəs) a secretion which is part serum and part mucus.

**se·ro·mus·cu·lar** (sēr″o-mus′ku-lər) pertaining to the serous and muscular coats of the intestine.

**Sero·my·cin** (ser′o-mi″sin) trademark for preparations of cycloserine.

**se·ro·my·ot·o·my** (se″ro-mi-ot′ə-me) a cutting into the serosal and muscular layers of the wall of an organ.

**se·ro·neg·a·tive** (sēr″o-neg′ə-tiv) serologically negative; showing negative results on serological examination; showing a lack of antibody.

**se·ro·neg·a·tiv·i·ty** (sēr″o-neg″ə-tiv′ĭ-te) the state of being seronegative, or of showing negative results on serological examination.

**se·ro·peri·to·ne·um** (sēr″o-per″ĭ-to-ne′əm) the presence of free fluid in the peritoneum; ascites.

**se·ro·phil·ic** (sēr″o-fil′ik) a term used to describe a bacterium whose growth is enhanced in the presence of serum.

**se·ro·plas·tic** (sēr″o-plas′tik) serofibrinous.

**se·ro·pneu·mo·tho·rax** (sēr″o-noo″mo-thor′aks) hydropneumothorax.

**se·ro·pos·i·tive** (sēr″o-poz′ĭ-tiv) serologically positive; showing positive results on serological examination; showing a high level of antibody.

**se·ro·pos·i·tiv·i·ty** (sēr″o-poz″ĭ-tiv′ĭ-te) the state of being seropositive, or of showing positive results on serologic examination.

**se·ro·prog·no·sis** (sēr″o-prog-no′sis) the prognosis of a disease based on the results of serologic tests.

**se·ro·pu·ru·lent** (sēr″o-pu′roo-lənt) both serous and purulent.

**se·ro·pus** (sēr′o-pus″) serum mingled with pus.

**se·ro·re·ac·tion** (sēr″o-re-ak′shən) serological reaction; a reaction demonstrating a specific antibody or antigen in serum.

**se·ro·re·lapse** (sēr″o-re′laps) a definite rise in serological titer occurring after treatment.

**se·ro·re·sis·tance** (sēr″o-re-zis′təns) failure of the serological titer to fall satisfactorily after treatment.

**se·ro·re·sis·tant** (sēr″o-re-zis′tənt) pertaining to seroresistance; showing a seropositive reaction to a pathogen after treatment.

**se·ro·re·ver·sal** (sēr″o-re-ver′səl) a fall in serological titer after treatment.

**se·ro·re·ver·sion** (se″ro-re-ver′zhən) spontaneous or induced conversion from a seropositive to a seronegative state.

**se·ro·sa** (sēr-o′sə, sēr-o′zə) 1. any serous membrane (tunica serosa). 2. chorion.

**se·ro·sal** (sēr-o′səl) pertaining to or composed of serosa.

**se·ro·sa·mu·cin** (sēr-o″sə-mu′sin) a protein resembling mucin, found in inflammatory ascitic exudates.

**se·ro·san·guin·e·ous** (sēr″o-sang-gwin′e-əs) pertaining to or containing both serum and blood.

**se·ro·se·rous** (sēr″o-sēr′əs) pertaining to two or more serous membranes.

**se·ro·si·tis** (sēr″o-si′tis) pl. *serosi′tides* [*serous membrane* + *-itis*] [MeSH: Serositis] inflammation of a serous membrane.
**infectious avian s.,** a septicemic disease of ducklings and geese, characterized by fibrinous peritonitis, pericarditis, and airsacculitis, and caused by *Pasteurella anatipestifer.* Called also *new duck disease* in ducklings and *goose influenza* in geese.
**multiple s.,** polyserositis.

**se·ros·i·ty** (sēr-os′ĭ-te) the quality possessed by serous fluids.

**se·ro·sur·vey** (sēr″o-sur′va) a population survey using a serologic test to screen for exposure and immunity to an infectious disease.

**se·ro·sy·no·vi·al** (sēr″o-sĭ-no′ve-əl) both serous and synovial.

**se·ro·syn·o·vi·tis** (sēr″o-sin″o-vi′tis) synovitis with effusion of serum.

**se·ro·ther·a·py** (sēr″o-ther′ə-pe) [*serum* + Gr. *therapy*] the treatment of disease by the injection of immune serum or antitoxin.

**se·ro·tho·rax** (sēr″o-thor′aks) hydrothorax.

**ser·o·ton·er·gic** (ser″o-tōn-er′jik) serotoninergic.

**sero·to·nin** (ser″o-to′nin) [MeSH: Serotonin] a monoamine vasoconstrictor, synthesized in the intestinal chromaffin cells or in central or peripheral neurons and found in high concentrations in many body tissues, including the intestinal mucosa, pineal body, and central nervous system. Produced enzymatically from tryptophan by hydroxylation and decarboxylation, it has many physiologic properties, such as inhibition of gastric secretion, stimulation of smooth muscle, serving as a central neurotransmitter, and being a precursor of melatonin. It is also found in animal species from coelenterates to vertebrates, in bacteria, and in many plants. Called also *5-hydroxytryptamine.*

**sero·to·nin·er·gic** (ser″o-to″nin-er′jik) 1. containing or activated by serotonin, as the neurons of the raphe nuclei of the brain stem. 2. of or pertaining to neurons that secrete serotonin, which, in turn, stimulates release of pituitary hormones. Called also *serotonergic.*

**se·ro·type** (sēr′o-tīp″) 1. the type of a microorganism as determined by the kinds and combinations of constituent antigens present in the cell. 2. to distinguish organisms on the basis of their constituent antigens. 3. a taxonomic subdivision of bacteria based

on the kinds and combinations of constituent antigens present in the cell, or a formula expressing the antigenic analysis on which such a subdivision is based. Called also *serovar.* See also *serogroup.*
**heterologous s.,** a related but not identical serotype.
**homologous s.,** an identical serotype.

**se·rous** (sēr′əs) [L. *serosus*] 1. pertaining to or resembling serum. 2. producing or containing serum, as a serous gland or cyst.

**se·ro·vac·ci·na·tion** (sēr″o-vak″sĭ-na′shən) injection of serum combined with bacterial vaccination to produce passive immunity by the former and active immunity by the latter.

**se·ro·var** (sēr′o-var) serotype.

**Ser·pa·sil** (ser′pə-sil) trademark for preparations of reserpine.

**Ser·pen·tes** (ser′pen-tēz) *Ophidia.*

**ser·pig·i·nous** (sər-pij′ĭ-nəs) [L. *serpere* to creep] having a wavy or much indented margin, as a lesion in noduloulcerative cutaneous syphilis.

**ser·pin** (sər′pin) any of a superfamily of inhibitors of serine proteinase occurring in plasma and tissues, all being strongly homologous single-chain glycoproteins, $M_r$ approximately 60,000, and having a specific, highly ordered tertiary structure with a mobile reaction center, although individual serpins are highly specific for particular proteinases. Among their targets are serine proteinases involved in coagulation, complement activation, fibrinolysis, inflammation, and tissue remodeling. The serpins include alpha$_1$-antitrypsin, antithrombin III, $\alpha_2$-antiplasmin, C1 inhibitor, heparin cofactor II, and plasminogen activator inhibitor 1 (PAI-1). Called also *serine proteinase inhibitor.*

**ser·rat·ed** (ser′āt-ed) [L. *serratus,* from *serra* saw] having a sawlike edge.

**Ser·ra·tia** (sə-ra′she-ə) [Serafino *Serrati,* Italian physicist, 18th century] [MeSH: Serratia] a genus of gram-negative, facultatively anaerobic bacteria of the family Enterobacteriaceae, consisting of motile, peritrichously flagellated rods, sometimes capsulated. Most strains produce white, pink, or red pigments. The organisms occur on plants, in soil, and in water. Many species are opportunistic pathogens, causing infections of the endocardium, blood, wounds, and urinary and respiratory tracts in immunocompromised patients.
**S. liquefa′ciens,** a nonpigmented species sometimes found in clinical specimens as an opportunistic pathogen; it is ornithine decarboxylase positive. Called also *S. proteamaculans.*
**S. marces′cens,** the most frequently isolated species, with red-pigmented varieties, occurring in water, soil, and food and in clinical specimens; it is ornithine decarboxylase positive. It is an opportunistic pathogen, causing nosocomial bacteremia, endocarditis, and pneumonia in immunocompromised patients. See also *Serratia pneumonia,* under *pneumonia.*
**S. odori′fera,** a species with a characteristic musty, potato-like odor, occasionally isolated from plants or food and rarely found as an opportunistic pathogen.
**S. plymu′thica,** a species with pigmented strains that is lysine decarboxylase negative and ornithine decarboxylase negative, reported in human sputum.
**S. proteama′culans,** *S. liquefaciens.*
**S. rubidae′a,** a species with pigmented strains that is ornithine decarboxylase negative, found in ripe coconuts; strains have been isolated rarely from human patients.

**ser·ra·tion** (sə-ra′shən) [L. *serratio*] 1. a structure or formation with teeth like those of a saw. 2. the condition of being serrated. 3. on an electrodiagnostic recording, part of an abnormal wave that has several changes in direction without crossing the baseline.

**ser·ra·tus** (sə-ra′təs) [L.] serrated.

**serre·fine** (sār-fēn′) [Fr.] a small spring forceps for compressing bleeding vessels.

**Serres' angle, glands** (sārz) [Antoine Etienne Reynaud Augustin *Serres,* French physiologist, 1786–1868] see *metafacial angle,* under *angle,* and *Epstein's pearls,* under *pearl.*

**ser·ru·late** (ser′u-lāt) [L. *serrulatus*] marked or bordered with small serrations or projections.

**Ser·to·li's cell, column** (ser-to′lēz) [Enrico *Sertoli,* Italian histologist, 1842–1910] see under *cell* and *column.*

**ser·tra·line hy·dro·chlo·ride** (sər′trə-lēn) a selective serotonin reuptake inhibitor used as an antidepressant; administered orally.

**se·rum** (sēr′əm) pl. *serums* or *se′ra* [L. "whey"] 1. the clear portion of any body fluid; the clear fluid moistening serous membranes. 2. blood s. 3. antiserum.
**active s.,** a serum that contains complement.
**anticomplementary s.,** a serum which interferes with or destroys the activity of complement.
**antilymphocyte s. (ALS),** antiserum derived from animals that have been immunized against human lymphocytes, a powerful nonspecific immunosuppressive agent that causes destruction of circulating lymphocytes.
**antipneumococcus s.,** type-specific horse or rabbit antiserum used effectively to treat pneumococcal pneumonia before the advent of antibiotics.
**antirabies s.** [USP], antiserum obtained from the blood serum or plasma of animals (generally horses) immunized with rabies vaccine; used for postexposure prophylaxis against rabies. Rabies immune globulin is used instead (because of its lower incidence of adverse reactions), if available.
**antitetanic s. (A.T.S.),** tetanus antitoxin.
**antitoxic s.,** antitoxin.
**articular s.,** synovia.
**bacteriolytic s.,** serum containing a bacteriolysin capable of inducing complement-dependent lysis of a bacterium.
**blood s.,** the clear liquid that separates from the blood when it is allowed to clot completely. It is therefore blood plasma from which fibrinogen has been removed in the process of clotting.
**blood s., glycerin,** blood serum containing glycerin.
**blood s., Loeffler's, Löffler's blood s.,** see *Loeffler coagulated serum medium* under *culture medium.*
**blood grouping s's** [USP], preparations containing particular antibodies against red cell antigens, used for blood typing. Those most commonly used are the anti-A and anti-B blood grouping serums, used to determine ABO blood types, and the anti-Rh blood grouping serums (anti-D, anti-C, anti-E, anti-c, and anti-e), used to determine Rh blood types.
**convalescence s., convalescent s., convalescents' s.,** blood serum from a patient convalescing from an infectious disease, formerly used as a prophylactic injection in such diseases as measles, scarlet fever, or whooping cough.
**despeciated s.,** a heterologous antiserum treated to remove some of the species-specific proteins so that it is less likely to cause anaphylaxis.
**foreign s.,** heterologous s., def. 1.
**heterologous s.,** 1. serum obtained from an animal belonging to a species different from that of the recipient. 2. serum prepared from an animal immunized by an organism differing from that against which it is to be used.
**homologous s.,** 1. serum obtained from an animal belonging to the same species as the recipient. 2. serum prepared from an animal immunized by the same organism against which it is to be used.
**hyperimmune s.,** antiserum with an especially high antibody titer produced by repeated antigen injections.
**immune s.,** antiserum.
**inactivated s.,** serum which has been heated, usually at 56°C for 30 minutes, to destroy the lytic activity of contained complement components.
**leukocyte typing s.** [USP], a preparation of serum derived from blood or plasma obtained from animals or from human donors and containing antibody for the identification of HLA antigens; used for in vitro histocompatibility testing.
**lymphatolytic s.,** serum which destroys lymphatic tissues, such as the spleen and lymph glands.
**monovalent s.,** antiserum containing antibodies against only one of several strains or species of microorganisms or only one of a group of antigens.
**normal s.,** serum from a normal untreated animal.
**pericardial s.,** pericardial fluid.
**polyvalent s.,** antiserum containing antibodies to a group of two or more strains or species of microorganism or to a group of two or more antigens.
**pooled s.,** the mixed serum from a number of individuals.
**pregnancy s.,** blood serum taken from pregnant women.
**Sclavo's s.,** a specific anti-anthrax serum that may be used against human anthrax.
**specific s.,** monovalent s.
**truth s.,** a misnomer for the drugs sometimes employed in narcoanalysis, especially amobarbital sodium and thiopental sodium; the agent used is not a serum and its use does not guarantee truthfulness.

**se·ru·mal** (sēr-oo′məl) pertaining to or formed from serum.

**se·rum-fast** (sēr′əm-fast) resistant to the destructive effect of serum; said of bacteria.

**se·rum·uria** (sēr″əm-u′re-ə) albuminuria.

**Serv.** abbreviation for L. *ser′va,* keep, preserve.

**Ser·ve·tus** (ser-ve′təs) Michael (Sp. *Miguel Serveto,* 1511–1553) Spanish theologian in France and Austria who also wrote, among other subjects, on geography, astrology, and medicine. His *Christianismi restitutio* (1553) contains the first printed description of the lesser circulation. Servetus was burned at the stake in Geneva for heresy the same year and most copies of his book were burned, although three copies survived.

**ser·vo·mech·a·nism** (ser″vo-mek′ə-niz-əm) a control system in which feedback is used to control errors in another system. The term is also applied to biological systems, such as the mechanism that controls the diameter of the pupil of the eye according to the amount of incident light.

**ser·yl** (sēr'əl, ser'əl) the acyl radical of serine.

**Ser·zone** (sər'zōn) trademark for a preparation of nefazodone hydrochloride.

**ses·a·me** (ses'ə-me) [L. *sesamum;* Gr. *sēsamon*] 1. *Sesamum indicum.* 2. the seeds of *S. indicum,* used as a demulcent and laxative; they yield sesame oil.

**ses·a·moid** (ses'ə-moid) [L. *sesamoides;* Gr. *sēsamon* sesame + *eidos* form] 1. denoting a small nodular bone embedded in a tendon or joint capsule. 2. a sesamoid bone. See under *bone.*

**ses·a·moi·di·tis** (ses"ə-moi-di'tis) inflammation of the sesamoid bones and surrounding structures of a horse's foot.

**Ses·a·mum** (ses'ə-məm) [L.] a genus of herbs of the family Pedaliaceae, native to hot regions of Africa and Asia. *S. in'dicum* L. is sesame, the source of sesame oil.

**sesqui-** [L. *sesqui* a half more] a prefix meaning one and a half.

**sesquih.** abbreviation for L. *sesquiho'ra,* an hour and a half.

**ses·qui·ho·ra** (ses"kwe-hor'ə) [L.] an hour and a half.

**ses·qui·ox·ide** (ses"kwe-ok'sid) a compound of three parts of oxygen with two of another element.

**ses·qui·sul·fate** (ses"kwe-sul'fāt) a sulfate containing three parts of sulfuric acid united with two of another element.

**ses·qui·sul·fide** (ses"kwe-sul'fīd) a sulfide containing three parts of sulfur united with two of another element.

**ses·sile** (ses'il) [L. *sessilis*] attached by a base; not pedunculated or stalked.

**Ses·sin·ia** (sə-sin'e-ə) the coconut beetles, a genus of blister beetles (family Meloidae), found on various Pacific islands.

**ses·ta·mibi** (ses"tə-mib'e) a compound comprising six substituted isocyanide (isonitrile) chains; as a complex with radiolabeled technetium (Tc 99m) it is used in studies of myocardial perfusion and thyroid and parathyroid imaging. See table at *technetium.*

**set** (set) 1. to align bones or bone fragments, as in reducing a fracture. 2. in psychology, a readiness to perceive or respond in a certain way because of past experience, requirements of a task, etc.
**phalangeal s.,** a surgical office procedure for correction of deformities of the lesser toes, involving incision to reach the bony joint and manipulation for proper positioning.

**se·ta** (se'tə) pl. *se'tae* [L.] 1. bristle. 2. any bristle-like structure, such as the multicellular stalk of certain plants.

**se·ta·ceous** (se-ta'shəs) [L. *setaceus; seta* bristle] slender and rigid, like a bristle.

**Se·ta·ria** (se-tar'e-ə) [MeSH: Setaria] 1. a large genus of grasses found in Europe and North America, often used for forage or hay. *S. sphacela'ta* and other species contain oxalates and can cause oxalate poisoning in livestock that eat large amounts of them. 2. a genus of nematodes of the superfamily Filarioides. *S. equi'na* is found in the abdominal cavities of horses, other equids, buffalo, cattle, and sometimes humans. *S. labiatopapillo'sa* (or *S. cer'vi*) is found in the peritoneal cavities of cattle and various game animals in Africa.

**set-fast** (set'fast) azoturia (def. 2).

**se·tif·er·ous** (se-tif'ər-əs) [*seta* + *-ferous*] bearing bristles; covered with bristles.

**se·tig·er·ous** (se-tij'ər-əs) [*seta* + L. *gerere* to carry] setiferous.

**se·ton** (se'ton) [Fr. *seton;* L. *seta* bristle] a thread of silk, linen, or other finely drawn material for passage through a sinus, fistula, or epithelial tract, often to serve as a guide for subsequent dilatation with instruments of larger diameter.

**set-point** (set'point) the target value of a controlled variable that is maintained physiologically by bodily control mechanisms for homeostasis, e.g., the point at which body temperature is controlled by the hypothalamic thermostat. Written also *set point.*

**Set·te·gast's projection** (set'ə-gasts) [H. *Settegast,* German radiologist, 20th century] see under *projection.*

**set·up** (set'əp) 1. organization or arrangement. 2. the arrangement of teeth on a trial denture base.
**diagnostic s.,** a procedure involving dissection of teeth from a plaster model and repositioning of the teeth in desired positions to aid in case analysis preliminary to constructing an orthodontic appliance.

**Se·ver's disease** (se'vərz) [James Warren *Sever,* American orthopedic surgeon, 1878–1964] see under *disease.*

**Sev·in** (sev'in) trademark for a preparation of carbaril.

**se·vo·flu·rane** (se"vo-floo'rān) an inhalation anesthetic used for the induction and maintenance of general anesthesia.

**sew·age** (soo'əj) [MeSH: Sewage] the used water supply of a community, consisting of an aqueous suspension of human and animal excreta and other waste materials from structures inhabited by humans; the contents of sewers.
**activated s.,** sewage mixed with activated sludge.
**domestic s.,** sewage from dwellings, business buildings, factories, or institutions.
**septic s.,** sewage undergoing anaerobic bacterial decomposition.

**sex** (seks) [L. *sexus*] [MeSH: Sex] 1. the distinction between male and female, found in most species of animals and plants, based on the type of gametes produced by the individual or the category into which the individual fits on the basis of that criterion. Ova are produced by the female and spermatozoa by the male; the union of these distinctive germ cells being the prerequisite for the production of a new individual in sexual reproduction. 2. see gender identity, under *identity.* 3. sexual intercourse. 4. to determine whether an individual is male or female.
**chromosomal s.,** sex as determined by the presence of the XX (female) or the XY (male) genotype in somatic cells, and without regard to phenotypic manifestations; called also *genetic s.*
**endocrinologic s.,** sex determined by gender-specific hormonal patterns. See also *phenotypic s.*
**genetic s.,** chromosomal s.
**genital s.,** phenotypic s.
**gonadal s.,** that part of the phenotypic sex that is determined by the gonadal tissue present, whether ovarian or testicular.
**morphological s.,** that part of the phenotypic sex that is determined by the morphology of the external genitals.
**nuclear s.,** the sex as determined on the basis of the presence or absence of sex chromatin in somatic cells, its presence normally indicating the XX (female) genotype, and its absence the XY (male) genotype.
**phenotypic s., somatic s.,** the phenotypic manifestations of sex such as presence of genital organs and secondary sex characters, under endocrine influences; see also *endocrinologic sex, gonadal sex,* and *morphological sex.*

**sex-con·di·tioned** (seks"kən-dish'ənd) see under *gene.*

**sex·dig·i·tate** (seks-dij'ĭ-tāt) [L. *sex* six + *digitate*] having six fingers on the hand or six toes on the foot.

**sex·duc·tion** (seks-suk'shən) F-duction.

**sex-in·flu·enced** (seks-in'floo-ənst) see under *gene.*

**sex·iv·a·lent** (sek-siv'ə-lənt) hexavalent.

**sex-lim·it·ed** (seks-lim'it-əd) see under *gene.*

**sex-linked** (seks'linkt) see under *gene.*

**sex·ol·o·gy** (seks-ol'ə-je) the study of sex and sexual relations and their evolutionary, physiological, developmental, and sociological aspects.

**sex·op·a·thy** (seks-op'ə-the) paraphilia.

**sex·tan** (seks'tən) [L. *sextanus* of the sixth] recurring every sixth day; said of fevers.

**sex·ti·grav·i·da** (seks"tĭ-grav'ĭ-də) [L. *sextus* sixth + *gravida*] a woman pregnant for the sixth time; also written gravida VI.

**sex·tip·a·ra** (seks-tip'ə-rə) [L. *sextus* sixth + *para*] a woman who has had six pregnancies which resulted in viable offspring; also written para VI or VI-para.

**sex·tup·let** (seks-tup'lət) [L. *sextus* sixth] one of six offspring produced in one gestation period.

**sex·u·al** (sek'shoo-əl) [L. *sexualis*] 1. pertaining to, characterized by, involving, or endowed with sex, sexuality, the sexes, or the sex organs and their functions. 2. characterized by the property of maleness or femaleness. 3. pertaining to reproduction involving both male and female gametes. 4. implying or symbolizing erotic desires or activity.

**sex·u·al·i·ty** (sek"shoo-al'ĭ-te) [MeSH: Sexuality] 1. the characteristic quality of the male and female reproductive elements. 2. the constitution of an individual in relation to sexual attitudes or activity.
**infantile s.,** in freudian theory, the erotic life of infants and children, encompassing the oral, anal, and phallic stages of psychosexual development.

**sex·u·al·iza·tion** (sek"shoo-al-ĭ-za'shən) the endowing of an object or function with sexual significance or instinct, as occurs with various body parts during development; it may also occur indirectly and unconsciously for seemingly unrelated events or objects.

**Sey·der·helm's solution** (si'dər-helmz) [Richard *Seyderhelm,* German physician, 1888–1940] see under *solution.*

**Sé·za·ry cell, syndrome (erythroderma)** (sa-zah-re′) [Albert *Sézary,* French dermatologist, 1880–1956] see under *cell* and *syndrome.*

**SFEMG** single fiber electromyography.

**SGOT** serum glutamic-oxaloacetic transaminase; see *aspartate transaminase.*

**SGPT** serum glutamic-pyruvic transaminase; see *alanine transaminase.*

**SH** serum hepatitis; see *hepatitis B.*

**shad·ow** (shad′o) 1. an attenuated image of an actual object, as a faded or colorless erythrocyte. 2. a figure or image created by the interruption of light or other rays, such as the representation on a radiograph of radiopaque structures.
**bat's wing s.,** a radiographic shadow that radiates through both lungs from the hilar region toward the periphery, leaving a clear zone at the apices, periphery, and bases.
**heart s.,** cardiac silhouette.
**Purkinje s.,** see under *figure.*

**shad·ow-cast·ing** (shad″o-kast′ing) a technique for increasing the visibility of ultramicroscopic specimens under the microscope by applying a coating of chromium, gold, or other metal.

**shaft** (shaft) a long slender part, such as the diaphysis of a long bone.
**s. of femur,** corpus ossis femoris.
**s. of fibula,** corpus fibulae.
**hair s.,** the major portion of a hair, designating especially the portion that extends beyond the surface of the skin.
**s. of humerus,** corpus humeri.
**s. of metacarpal bone,** corpus ossis metacarpi.
**s. of metatarsal bone,** corpus ossis metatarsi.
**s. of penis,** corpus penis.
**s. of phalanx of hand,** corpus phalangis manus.
**s. of phalanx of foot,** corpus phalangis pedis.
**s. of radius,** corpus radii.
**s. of rib,** corpus costae.
**s. of tibia,** corpus tibiae.
**s. of ulna,** corpus ulnae.

**sha·green** (shah-gren′) 1. a type of untanned leather covered with granulations. 2. the rough skin of various types of sharks. 3. said of a type of human skin lesion that has a rough, nevoid surface and resembles shark skin.

**shakes** (shāks) a vernacular term for the cold paroxysm of intermittent fever.
**hatter's s.,** popular name for a type of mercury poisoning seen among fur hat workers.
**kwaski s.,** a condition seen in children who, having been severely malnourished, suffer rhythmic twitches and shaking a week or two after introduction of a better diet. The condition disappears within a few weeks.
**spelter s.,** metal fume fever seen among brass-founders.
**Teflon s.,** polymer fume fever.

**sham-feed·ing** (sham-fēd′ing) sham feeding; see under *feeding.*

**shank** (shangk) 1. leg (def. 1). 2. crus (def. 2).

**shap·ing** (shāp′ing) an operant conditioning technique used in behavior therapy in which new behavior is produced by providing reinforcement for progressively closer approximations of the final desired behavior. Called also *successive approximation.*

**shark** (shahrk) [MeSH: Sharks] any of numerous elasmobranch fishes, usually found in the ocean; some are carnivorous and predatory and may attack humans. See also *shark liver oil* and *elasmobranch poisoning.*
**Greenland s.,** *Somniosus microcephalus.*
**soupfin s.,** *Galeorhinus zyopterus,* so called because its fin is used for soup by the Chinese.

**Sharp** (shahrp) Phillip A. British biochemist, born 1943. Co-winner, with Richard J. Roberts, of the Nobel prize for medicine or physiology in 1993 for his discoveries about the structure of genes and the transmission of genetic information.

**Shar·pey's fibers** (shahr′pēz) [William *Sharpey,* Scottish anatomist and physiologist, 1802–1880] see under *fiber.*

**Sha·ver's disease** (sha′vərz) [Cecil Gordon *Shaver,* Canadian physician, born 1901] bauxite pneumoconiosis.

**shear** (shēr) 1. an applied force that tends to cause an opposite but parallel sliding motion of the planes of an object. 2. the strain resulting from such force.

**sheath** (shēth) [L. *vagina;* Gr. *thēkē*] a tubular structure enclosing or surrounding some organ or part.
**arachnoid s.,** the continuation of the arachnoidea mater around the optic nerve, forming part of the internal sheath of the optic nerve.
**bulbar s.,** vagina bulbi.
**carotid s., carotid s. of cervical fascia,** vagina carotica fasciae cervicalis.
**caudal s.,** a tubular cytoplasmic structure at the base of the nucleus in the early spermatid.
**chordal s.,** notochordal s.
**common s. of tendons of peroneal muscles,** vagina communis tendinum musculorum fibularium.
**common s. of testis and spermatic cord,** fascia spermatica interna.
**crural s.,** femoral s.
**dentinal s.,** Neumann s.
**dural s.,** vagina externa nervi optici.
**enamel prism s., enamel rod s.,** a sheath of organic tissue completely or partially surrounding each enamel prism. Called also *prism s.* and *rod s.*
**external s. of optic nerve,** vagina externa nervi optici.
**s. of eyeball,** vagina bulbi.
**fascial s. of prostate,** the sheath, derived from the rectovesical fascia, which surrounds the prostate.
**female s.,** vagina (def. 2).
**femoral s.,** the fascial covering of the proximal portion of the femoral vessels, derived from the intra-abdominal fascia; the most medial portion of the sheath, separated by a septum, forms the canalis femoralis. Called also *crural s.*
**fibrous s's of fingers,** vaginae fibrosae digitorum manus.
**fibrous s. of optic nerve,** vagina externa nervi optici.
**fibrous s. of spermatozoon,** the fibrous sheath surrounding the principal piece of the tail of a spermatozoon.
**fibrous s. of tendon,** vagina fibrosa tendinis.
**fibrous s's of toes,** vaginae fibrosae digitorum pedis.
**s. of Henle,** endoneurium.
**Hertwig s., s. of Hertwig,** root s., def. 1.
**inner s. of optic nerve, internal s. of optic nerve,** vagina interna nervi optici.
**s. of Key and Retzius,** endoneurium.
**lamellar s.,** perineurium.
**masculine s.,** utriculus prostaticus.
**Mauthner's s.,** axolemma.
**medullary s.,** myelin s.
**mitochondrial s.,** the sheath of circumferentially oriented mitochondria arranged end to end, which surrounds the middle piece of a spermatozoon and is thought to control the movements of the tail.
**mucous s's,** bursa synovialis and vaginae synoviales.
**mucous s., intertubercular,** septum intermusculare cruris anterius.
**mucous s. of tendon,** vagina synovialis tendinis.
**mucous s's of tendons of fingers,** vaginae synoviales digitorum manus.
**mucous s's of tendons of toes,** vaginae synoviales digitorum pedis.
**myelin s.,** the cylindrical covering on the axons of some neurons; it consists of concentric layers of myelin, formed in the peripheral nervous system by the plasma membrane of Schwann cells, and in the central nervous system by oligodendrocytes. It is interrupted at intervals along its length by gaps known as nodes of Ranvier. Myelin is an electrical insulator that serves to speed the conduction of nerve impulses. See also *myelinated nerve fibers,* under *fiber.* Called also *medullary s.*
**nerve s.,** myelin s.
**Neumann s., s. of Neumann,** an area of interface between peri- and intertubular dental structures. Called also *dentinal s.*
**neurilemmal s.,** neurilemma.
**notochordal s.,** an elastic sheath surrounding the notochord.
**s's of optic nerve,** the internal and external meningeal sheaths of the optic nerve within the orbit, continuous with the meninges of the brain. See *vagina externa nervi optici* and *vagina interna nervi optici.*
**outer s. of optic nerve,** vagina externa nervi optici.
**periarterial lymphatic s., periarterial lymphoid s. (PALS),** any of the sheaths of lymphatic tissue that make up the white pulp of the spleen.
**perinephric s.,** the sheath of fascia investing the kidney.
**perivascular s.,** a pia glial membrane which accompanies blood vessels into the brain.
**pial s.,** the continuation of the pia mater around the optic nerve, forming part of the internal sheath of the optic nerve.
**s. of plantar tendon of long peroneal muscle,** vagina plantaris tendinis musculi fibularis longi.
**prism s.,** enamel prism s.
**rectus s., s. of rectus abdominis muscle,** vagina musculi recti abdominis.
**rod s.,** enamel prism s.
**root s.,** 1. an epithelial extension of the cervical loop of the enamel organ, consisting of the inner and outer enamel epithelium, and directing the number and morphological growth of the roots. It is bordered externally by the dental sac and internally by developing cementum and root dentin, and ultimately becomes the epithelial

diaphragm. Called also *Hertwig's s.* and *s. of Hertwig.* 2. the epithelial portion of the hair follicle, divided into the inner root sheath and the outer root sheath, which gives rise to the sebaceous glands.
**Scarpa's s.,** fascia cremasterica.
**Schwalbe's s.,** the thin envelope of an elastic fiber.
**s. of Schwann,** neurilemma.
**Schweigger-Seidel s.,** a spindle-shaped thickening in the walls of the second portion of the arterial branches forming the penicilli in the spleen; see *sheathed artery,* under *artery.* Called also *ellipsoid.*
**spiral s.,** a heavily staining filament winding around the axial filament of the middle piece of a spermatozoon.
**s. of styloid process,** vagina processus styloidei.
**synovial s., intertubercular,** vagina synovialis intertubercularis.
**synovial s. of bicipital groove,** vagina synovialis intertubercularis.
**synovial s. of intertubercular groove,** vagina synovialis intertubercularis.
**synovial s. of tendon,** vagina synovialis tendinis.
**synovial s. of tendons of foot,** vaginae synoviales digitorum pedis.
**tendinous s's of flexor muscles of fingers,** vaginae fibrosae digitorum manus.
**tendinous s's of flexor muscles of toes,** vaginae fibrosae digitorum pedis.
**tendinous s. of leg,** fascia cruris.
**tendinous s. of long peroneal muscle, plantar,** vagina plantaris tendinis musculi fibularis longi.
**tendon s.,** vagina tendinis.
**tendon s. of anterior tibial muscle,** vagina tendinis musculi tibialis anterioris.
**tendon s's of long extensor muscles of toes,** vaginae tendinum musculi extensoris digitorum longi pedis.
**tendon s's of long flexor muscles of toes,** vaginae tendinum musculi flexoris digitorum longi pedis.
**tendon s. of posterior tibial muscle,** vagina tendinis musculi tibialis posterioris.

**Shee·han's syndrome** (she'anz) [Harold Leeming *Sheehan,* English pathologist, born 1900] see *postpartum pituitary necrosis,* under *necrosis.*

**sheep-pox** (shēp-poks) a contagious disease of sheep caused by a poxvirus, which is characterized by fever, systemic disturbances, and widespread skin lesions on non-woolbearing areas or where the hair is not long; it is usually more severe, often fatal, in younger animals. Called also *ovine smallpox* and *variola ovina.*

**sheet** (shēt) 1. a rectangular piece of cotton, linen, etc., for a bed covering. 2. any structure resembling such a covering.
**β s., beta s., β pleated s., beta pleated s.,** pleated s.
**draw s.,** a folded sheet placed under a patient in bed so that it may be withdrawn without lifting the patient.
**drip s.,** a wet sheet from which the water is wrung out and which is then wrapped around a patient standing in a tub of water.
**pleated s.,** a secondary structure occurring in many proteins, consisting of several polypeptide chains running in the same direction (a parallel pleated sheet) or in alternating directions (an antiparallel pleated sheet) and joined by hydrogen bonds between the imino hydrogen of each peptide bond and the carbonyl oxygen of a peptide bond in the next chain over. Called also *β structure, β s.,* and *β pleated s.*
**secretory s.,** the simplest form of multicellular gland, consisting of secreting cells alone, e.g., the surface epithelium of the mammalian gastric mucosa.

**shelf** (shelf) a broad, flat surface, normal or abnormal, in the body.
**buccal s.,** the surface of the mandible from the residual alveolar ridge or the alveolar ridge to the external oblique line in the region of the lower buccal vestibule; it is covered with cortical bone.
**dental s.,** the shelflike epithelial invagination formed by the dental ridge, beneath which the dental papillae are formed.
**mesocolic s.,** the transverse mesocolon and the great omentum taken together.
**palatine s.,** see *lateral palatine process* and *median palatine process,* under *process.*

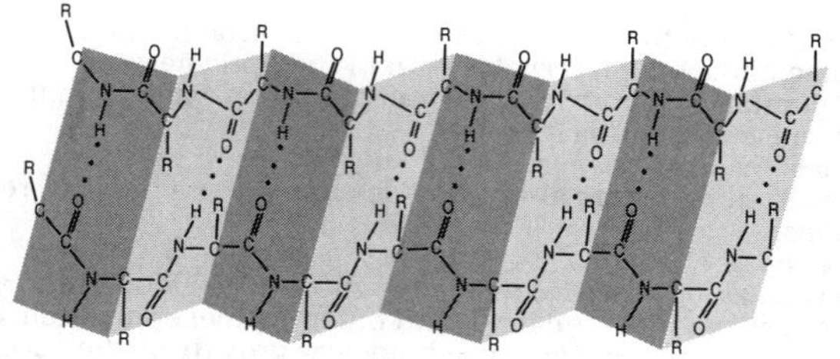

Diagram of a portion of a pleated sheet structure formed by interstrand hydrogen bonding between two polypeptide regions.

**shel·lac** (shə-lak') a product of lac from India, produced on various plants by an insect, *Laccifer lacca* Kerr (Coccidae); sometimes used in dentistry and surgery, and in coating confections and medicinal tablets.

**Shen·ton's line (arch)** (shen'tənz) [Edward Warren Hine *Shenton,* English radiologist, 1872–1955] see under *line.*

**Shep·herd's fracture** (shep'ərds) [Francis John *Shepherd,* Canadian surgeon, 1851–1929] see under *fracture.*

**Sher·man plate** (shər'mən) [Harry Mitchell O'Neill *Sherman,* American surgeon, 1854–1921] see under *plate.*

**Sher·ring·ton** (sher'ing-tən) Sir Charles Scott. English physiologist, 1857–1952; co-winner, with Baron Adrian of Cambridge, of the Nobel prize for medicine or physiology in 1932 for their work on the function of the neuron and particularly for his studies of reflex action and neurophysiology.

**Sher·ring·ton's law** (sher'ing-tənz) [Sir Charles Scott *Sherrington*] see under *law.*

**Shib·ley's sign** (shib'lēz) [Gerald Spencer *Shibley,* American physician, 1890–1981] see under *sign.*

**shield** (shēld) any protecting structure.
**Buller's s.,** a watch glass fitted over the unaffected eye to guard it from infection from the affected eye.
**embryonic s.,** the double-layered disk from which the embryo proper develops; see *embryonic disc,* under *disc.*
**eye s.,** a covering for the eyes to protect them from light or injury.
**lead s.,** in radiology, a lead barrier for protecting personnel from radiation.
**nipple s.,** a cover to protect the nipple of a nursing woman.
**oral s.,** see under *screen.*

**shift** (shift) a change, as of position or status.
**chloride s.,** the exchange of chloride ($Cl^-$) and bicarbonate ($HCO_3^-$) between the plasma and the red blood cells; it takes place whenever $HCO_3^-$ is generated or decomposed within the red cells. Called also *Hamburger phenomenon* or *interchange.*
**Doppler s.,** the magnitude of the change in frequency caused by the Doppler effect.
**s. to the left,** an increase in the percentage of neutrophils that have only one or two lobes, seen in some bacterial infections. See *Arneth count,* under *count.*
**Purkinje s.,** see under *phenomenon.*
**s. to the right,** an increase in the percentage of neutrophils with 5 or more lobes, seen most often in cobalamine and folate deficiencies. See *Arneth count,* under *count.*
**antigenic s.,** a sudden, major change in the antigenicity of a virus, seen especially in influenza viruses, resulting from the recombination of the genomes of two virus strains; it is associated with pandemics because hosts do not have immunity to the new strain. Cf. *antigenic drift,* under *drift.*

**Shi·ga's bacillus, toxin** (she'gahz) [Kiyoshi *Shiga,* Japanese physician, 1870–1957] see *Shigella dysenteriae* type 1, and see under *toxin.*

**Shi·gel·la** (shĭ-gel'ə) [Kiyoshi *Shiga*] [MeSH: Shigella] a genus of gram-negative, facultatively anaerobic, rod-shaped bacteria of the family Enterobacteriaceae, made up of nonmotile bacilli that cannot utilize citrate as a sole carbon source and that ferment carbohydrates with acid but no gas production. The genus consists of four species, differentiated by biochemical reactions: *S. dysenteriae* (subgroup A), *S. flexneri* (subgroup B), *S. boydii* (subgroup C), and *S. sonnei* (subgroup D). Their normal habitat is the intestinal tract of humans and higher monkeys; all species cause dysentery. See also *shigellosis.*
**S. ambi'gua,** *S. dysenteriae* type 2.
**S. arabinotar'da type A,** *S. dysenteriae* type 3.
**S. arabinotar'da type B,** *S. dysenteriae* type 4.
**S. boy'dii,** a species that causes acute diarrheal disease in humans, especially in tropical regions. It has 15 serological types; all ferment mannitol but not lactose.
**S. ceylonen'sis,** *S. sonnei.*
**S. dysente'riae,** a highly pathogenic species that causes severe dysentery, separable into 10 serologic types; it does not ferment lactose or mannitol. *S. dysenteriae* type 1, the classic Shiga bacillus, produces a potent neurotoxin and causes epidemic dysentery, which can be fatal in children. *S. dysenteriae* type 2, the Schmitz bacillus, is serologically related to *Escherichia coli* type 0112; it is the cause of occasional epidemic diarrheal disease in humans and among captive chimpanzees. The other numbered types of dysentery bacilli include the parashiga, the Large-Sachs, and the arabinotarda groups. Formerly called *Bacillus dysenteriae* and *Bacterium dysenteriae.*
**S. etou'sae,** *S. boydii* type 7.
**S. flexne'ri,** a species that causes severe dysentery. It has six serotypes and two variants (X and Y); type 2 produces an enterotoxin.

The organisms ferment mannitol but not lactose. Called also *S. paradysenteriae* and *Flexner's bacillus.*
**S. new'castle,** *S. flexneri* type 6.
**S. paradysente'riae,** *S. flexneri.*
**S. parashi'gae,** a name formerly given to a group of non-mannitol-fermenting dysentery bacilli serologically differentiable from the Shiga bacillus (now *S. dysenteriae* type 1); also known as the Large-Sachs group of parashiga bacilli, they are now known as *S. dysenteriae,* types 3 to 7.
**S. schmit'zii,** *S. dysenteriae* type 2.
**S. shi'gae,** *S. dysenteriae* type 1.
**S. son'nei,** the least pathogenic species, causing a milder but frequently encountered form of bacillary dysentery; organisms are serologically homogeneous, but two antigens, designated I and II, occur in varying proportions. Called also *Sonne-Duval bacillus* and, formerly, *Bacterium sonnei.*

**shi·gel·la** (shĭ-gel'ə) pl. *shigel'lae* [MeSH: Shigella] a bacterium of the genus *Shigella.*

**shi·gel·lo·sis** (shĭ'gəl-o'sis) any condition produced by infection with organisms of the genus *Shigella,* such as bacillary dysentery (see under *dysentery*).

**shik·i·mene** (shik'ĭ-mēn) sikimin.

**shin** (shin) 1. the crest or anterior edge of the tibia. 2. the anterior aspect of the leg below the knee.
**bucked s's,** sore s's.
**cucumber s.,** a tibia which is curved with the concavity forward.
**saber s.,** a tibia with a marked anterior convexity as seen in congenital syphilis, yaws, and osteitis deformans.
**sore s's,** periostitis of the large metacarpal or metatarsal bone of the horse.

**shin·gles** (shing'gəlz) [L. *cingulus*] herpes zoster.

**shiv·er** (shiv'ər) 1. a slight chill or tremor. 2. to tremble, as from a chill.

**shiv·er·ing** (shiv'ər-ing) [MeSH: Shivering] involuntary trembling or quivering of the body caused by contraction or twitching of the muscles, a physiologic method of heat production in man and other mammals.

**SHML** sinus histiocytosis with massive lymphadenopathy; see *Rosai-Dorfman disease,* under *disease.*

**shock** (shok) [MeSH: Shock] 1. a sudden disturbance of mental or physical equilibrium. 2. a condition of profound hemodynamic and metabolic disturbance characterized by failure of the circulatory system to maintain adequate perfusion of vital organs. It may result from inadequate blood volume (hypovolemic shock); inadequate cardiac function (cardiogenic shock); or inadequate vasomotor tone (neurogenic shock and septic shock).
**anaphylactic s.,** see *anaphylaxis.*
**anaphylactoid s.,** see under *reaction.*
**burn s.,** shock resulting from the loss of plasma into a burn wound.
**cardiac s.,** cardiogenic s.
**cardiogenic s.,** shock resulting from primary failure of the heart in its pumping function, as in myocardial infarction, severe cardiomyopathy, or mechanical obstruction or compression of the heart; clinical characteristics are similar to those of hypovolemic shock.
**deferred s., delayed s.,** shock occurring a considerable time after the injury is received.
**diastolic s.,** the cardiac impulse which strikes the palpating hand in early diastole.
**electric s.,** the immediate effects produced by the passage of an electric current through any part of the body, e.g., painful stimulation of nerves or tetanic contractions of muscles.
**endotoxic s., endotoxin s.,** septic shock due to release of endotoxins by gram-negative bacteria.
**hematogenic s.,** hypovolemic s.
**hemorrhagic s.,** hypovolemic shock resulting from hemorrhage.
**histamine s.,** a reaction resembling anaphylactic shock produced in experimental animals by histamine injection.
**hypoglycemic s.,** 1. insulin s. 2. a hypoglycemic reaction resulting from severe adrenocortical insufficiency, especially during fasting.
**hypovolemic s.,** shock resulting from insufficient blood volume for the maintenance of adequate cardiac output, blood pressure, and tissue perfusion. Without modification the term refers to absolute hypovolemic shock caused by acute hemorrhage or excessive fluid loss. Relative hypovolemic shock refers to a situation in which the blood volume is normal but insufficient because of widespread vasodilation as in neurogenic shock or septic shock. Clinical characteristics include hypotension; hyperventilation; cold, clammy, cyanotic skin; a weak and rapid pulse; oliguria; and mental confusion, combativeness, or anxiety. Called also *hematogenic* or *oligemic s.*
**insulin s.,** a hypoglycemic reaction to overdosage of insulin, a skipped meal, or strenuous exercise in an insulin-dependent diabetic; early symptoms are tremor, irritability, dizziness, cool moist skin, hunger, and tachycardia; if untreated it can progress to coma (see *diabetic coma*) and convulsions. Called also *hypoglycemic s.*
**irreversible s.,** a condition in which the changes produced cannot be corrected by treatment, and death is inevitable.
**neurogenic s.,** shock resulting from neurogenic vasodilation, which can be produced by cerebral trauma or hemorrhage, spinal cord injury, deep general or spinal anesthesia, or toxic central nervous system depression.
**oligemic s.,** hypovolemic s.
**osmotic s.,** exposure of cells to an extremely hypotonic environment, which results in rupture of the plasma membrane and loss of cell contents, except for cells that have a rigid cell wall, which prevents rupture of the plasma membrane.
**pleural s.,** a hypotensive condition sometimes following thoracentesis, characterized by cyanosis, pallor, dilated pupils, and disturbance of pulse and respiration.
**postoperative s.,** a state of shock following a surgical operation.
**secondary s.,** shock appearing one or more hours after injury; delayed shock.
**septic s.,** shock associated with overwhelming infection, most commonly infection with gram-negative bacteria, although it may be produced by other bacteria, viruses, fungi, and protozoa. It is thought to result from the action of endotoxins or other products of the infectious agent on the vascular system causing large volumes of blood to be sequestered in the capillaries and veins; activation of the complement and kinin systems and the release of histamine, cytokines, prostaglandins, and other mediators may be involved. Clinical characteristics include initial chills and fever, warm flushed skin, increased cardiac output, and a lesser degree of hypotension than with hypovolemic shock; if therapy is ineffective, it may progress to the clinical picture associated with hypovolemic shock.
**serum s.,** anaphylactic shock resulting from administration of foreign serum to a sensitized individual.
**shell s.,** term used during World War I and later for *posttraumatic stress disorder.*
**spinal s.,** the loss of spinal reflexes after injury of the spinal cord, which affects the muscles innervated by the cord segments situated below the site of the lesion.
**surgical s.,** shock that occurs during or after surgical operation.
**testicular s.,** the effect of a sharp blow upon the testes.
**traumatic s.,** any shock produced by trauma.
**vasogenic s.,** shock caused by marked vasodilation.

**shoe** (shoo) [MeSH: Shoes] a covering or appliance for the foot.
**Charlier's s.,** a special type of horseshoe that allows the sole and the frog to come to the ground exactly as in the unshod foot.

**Shope papilloma** (shōp) [Richard Edwin *Shope,* American pathologist, 1902–1966] see *rabbit fibroma,* under *fibroma* and *rabbit papilloma,* under *papilloma.*

**short·sight·ed·ness** (short-sīt'əd-nəs) myopia.

**shot-com·pres·sor** (shot-kəm-pres'ər) see under *compressor.*

**shot·ty** (shot'e) like shot; resembling the pellets used in shotgun cartridges.

**shoul·der** (shōl'dər) [MeSH: Shoulder] the junction of the arm and trunk; also that part of the trunk which is bounded at the back by the scapula. See also *regio deltoidea.*
**drop s.,** depression of one shoulder below the level of the other.
**frozen s.,** adhesive capsulitis.
**knocked-down s.,** separation or dislocation of the shoulder at the acromioclavicular joint occurring in athletes. Called also *shoulder separation.*
**loose s.,** a condition seen in progressive muscular atrophy in which, when attempts to lift the patient by grasping the upper arms at their sides are made, the arms move up but the trunk remains behind.
**slipped s.,** suprascapular paralysis.
**stubbed s.,** sprain of the shoulder joint occurring in athletes.

**shoul·der-blade** (shōl'dər-blād) the scapula.

**shoul·der slip** (shōl'dər slip) suprascapular paralysis.

**show** (sho) the appearance of blood as a forerunner of labor or menstruation.

**Shprint·zen syndrome** (shprint'sən) [Robert J. *Shprintzen,* American geneticist, 20th century] see under *syndrome.*

**Shra·dy's saw** (shra'dēz) [George Frederick *Shrady,* American surgeon, 1837–1907] see under *saw.*

**Shrap·nell's membrane** (shrap'nəlz) [Henry Jones *Shrapnell,* English anatomist and Army surgeon, 1761–1841] pars flaccida membranae tympanicae.

**shrink·age** (shring'kəj) a reduction in size, extent, or quantity.
**casting s.,** the decrease in volume of a metal dental cast as it cools and hardens.
**polymerization s.,** the decrease in volume of dental resin as polymerization occurs.

**shud·der** (shud′ər) 1. an involuntary or convulsive quiver or shake. 2. in a pulse tracing, the graphic representation of a thrill.

**Shul·man's syndrome** (shool′mənz) [Lawrence Edward *Shulman*, American rheumatologist, born 1919] eosinophilic fasciitis.

**shunt** (shunt) 1. to turn to one side; to divert or bypass. 2. a passage or anastomosis between two natural channels, especially between blood vessels; it may be formed either physiologically (e.g., to bypass a thrombosis), or by a structural anomaly. 3. a surgically created anastomosis. 4. the operation of forming such an anastomosis.
**arteriovenous s.,** 1. direct passage of blood from an artery to a vein. 2. a U-shaped plastic tube inserted between an artery and a vein (usually between the radial artery and cephalic vein), bypassing the capillary network, a formerly common means of arteriovenous access (q.v.).
**Blalock-Taussig s.,** see under *operation.*
**Buselmeier s.,** a modification of the Quinton-Scribner shunt in which the Silastic tube is implanted under the skin, with two ports projecting through the skin.
**cardiovascular s.,** an abnormality of blood flow between the sides of the heart or between the systemic and pulmonary circulation; see *left-to-right s.* and *right-to-left s.*
**Denver s.,** a modification of the LeVeen peritoneovenous shunt that includes a manual pump mechanism for ascitic fluid.
**Glenn s.,** see under *operation.*
**hexose monophosphate s.,** pentose phosphate pathway.
**left-to-right s.,** diversion of blood from the left side of the heart to the right side or from the systemic to the pulmonary circulation through an anomalous opening such as a septal defect or patent ductus arteriosus.
**LeVeen peritoneovenous s.,** a surgically implanted subcutaneous plastic tube for continuous shunting of ascites fluid from the peritoneal cavity to the jugular vein; a pressure-activated valve buried in the abdominal wall ensures one-way flow.
**Linton s.,** splenorenal s.
**lumboperitoneal s.,** a communication between the lumbar subarachnoid space and the peritoneum by means of a plastic tube with an in-line pressure-flow regulator; created to permit drainage of cerebrospinal fluid for relief of communicating hydrocephalus.
**mesocaval s.,** a portosystemic shunt between the superior mesenteric vein and the inferior vena cava, done for the treatment of esophageal varices in portal hypertension.
**pentose s.,** pentose phosphate pathway.
**peritoneovenous s.,** LeVeen peritoneovenous s.
**portacaval s.,** a portosystemic shunt between the portal vein and vena cava, done for treatment of portal hypertension.
**portosystemic s.,** a surgically created shunt that connects the portal and systemic circulations, such as a mesocaval, portacaval, or splenorenal shunt for treatment of portal hypertension. Called also *portosystemic anastomosis.*
**postcaval s.,** portacaval s.
**Potts s.,** see under *operation.*
**Quinton-Scribner s.,** an arteriovenous shunt for hemodialysis, consisting of an external cannula composed of a U-shaped Silastic tube with Teflon tips; it is inserted between the radial artery and the cephalic vein.
**reversed s.,** right-to-left s.
**right-to-left s.,** diversion of blood from the right side of the heart to the left side or from the pulmonary to the systemic circulation through an anomalous opening such as a septal defect or patent ductus arteriosus; called also *reversed s.*
**Scribner s.,** Quinton-Scribner s.
**splenorenal s.,** removal of the spleen with anastomosis of the splenic vein to the left renal vein; done for the treatment of esophageal varices in portal hypertension. Called also *Linton s.*
**splenorenal s., distal,** anastomosis of the distal splenic vein to the inferior vena cava with preservation of the spleen; done for the treatment of esophageal varices in portal hypertension. Called also *Warren s.*
**Thomas s.,** an arteriovenous shunt for hemodialysis, consisting of a Silastic cannula with Dacron cuffs inserted between the femoral artery and femoral vein.
**Torkildsen's s.,** ventriculocisternal s.
**transjugular intrahepatic portosystemic s. (TIPS),** percutaneous creation of a shunt between the hepatic and portal veins within the liver followed by placement of an expandable stent in the tract created, performed by a transjugular route under radiologic guidance; done for the treatment of bleeding esophageal varices.
**ventriculoatrial s.,** the surgical creation of a communication between a cerebral ventricle and a cardiac atrium by means of a plastic tube with an in-line pressure-flow regulator, to permit drainage of cerebrospinal fluid for relief of hydrocephalus.
**ventriculocisternal s.,** an obsolete procedure in which a communication is surgically established between a lateral ventricle and the cisterna magna for drainage of cerebrospinal fluid in hydrocephalus; of historic interest. Called also *Torkildsen's s.* or *operation* and *ventriculocisternostomy.*
**ventriculoperitoneal s.,** the most common shunting procedure for the relief of hydrocephalus, consisting of the creation of a channel between a cerebral ventricle and the peritoneum by means of plastic tubing.
**ventriculopleural s.,** a communication between a cerebral ventricle

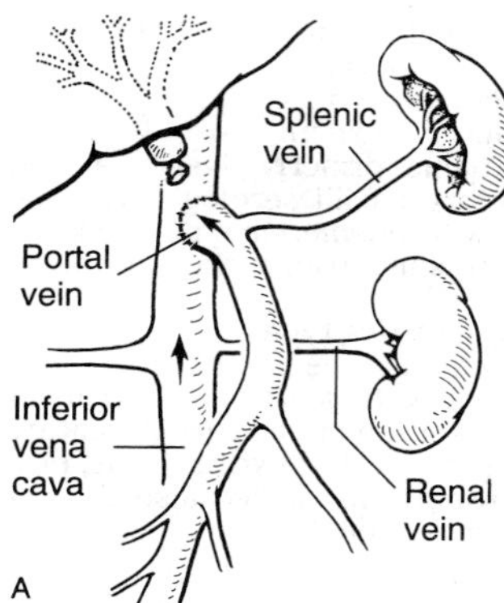


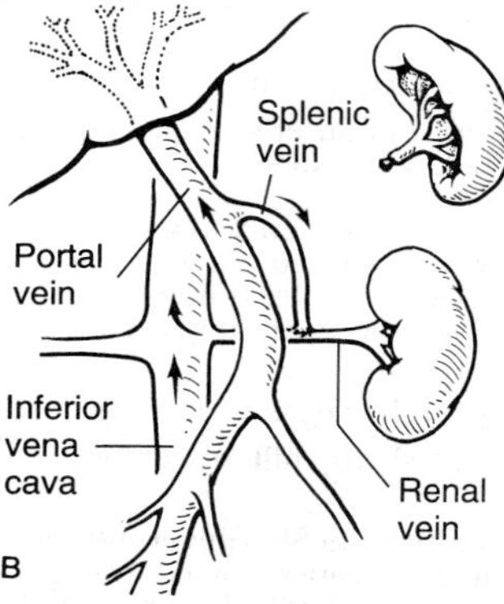


Shunts diverting portal venous blood flow from the liver. *(A),*Portacaval shunt; *(B),* splenorenal shunt.

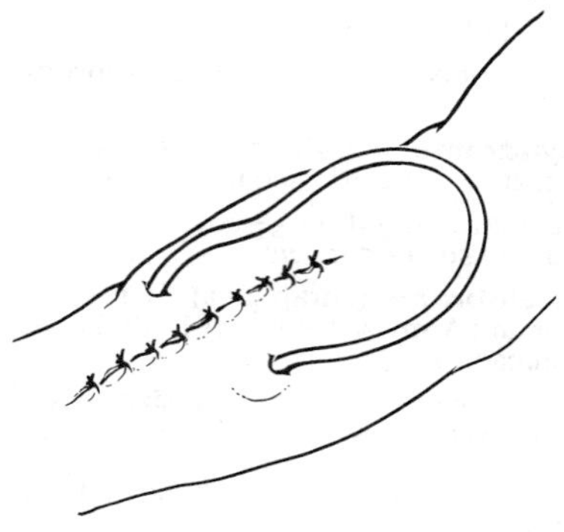

Arteriovenous shunt.

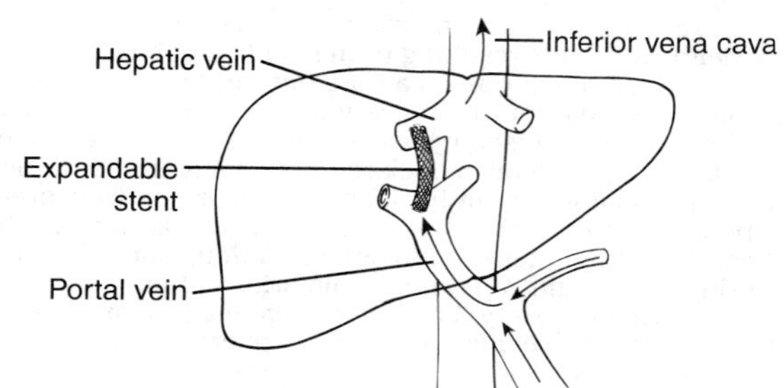


Transjugular intrahepatic portosystemic shunt.

and the pleural cavity by means of a plastic tube with an in-line pressure-flow regulator, done for the relief of hydrocephalus.
**ventriculovenous s.,** creation of a communication between a cerebral ventricle and the internal jugular vein by means of a plastic tube with an in-line pressure-flow regulator, to permit drainage of cerebrospinal fluid for relief of hydrocephalus.
**Warren s.,** distal splenorenal s.
**Waterston s.,** see under *operation.*

**shut·tle** (shut'əl) [A.S. *scytel* a dart] in biochemistry, a mechanism for the transport of electrons or an organic group, or both, across a membrane.
**glycerol phosphate s.,** a cyclic mechanism for transferring electrons from cytosolic NADH to the mitochondrial electron transport chain and thus to oxygen, acting by means of enzyme-catalyzed redox reactions that interconvert glycerol 3-phosphate and dihydroxyacetone phosphate. It occurs primarily in white fibers of striated muscle and nervous tissue. See also illustration.
**malate-aspartate s.,** a mechanism for transferring electrons into mitochondria from the cytosol of red fibers of skeletal muscle, heart, and the brain, involving cytosolic and mitochondrial forms of the enzymes malate dehydrogenase and aspartate transaminase, and two transmembrane carriers. Electrons from cytosolic NADH are used to reduce oxaloacetate to malate, which enters the mitochondrial matrix and donates electrons to $NAD^+$, becoming reoxidized to oxaloacetate. To return to the cytosol, oxaloacetate is first transaminated to form aspartate, which can traverse the membrane; once in the cytosol it is deaminated to oxaloacetate.

**Shwach·man syndrome** (shwahk'mən) [Harry *Shwachman,* American pediatrician, 1910–1986] see under *syndrome.*

**Shwach·man-Di·a·mond syndrome** (shwahk'mən-di'ə-mond) [Harry *Shwachman;* Louis Klein *Diamond,* American pediatrician, born 1902] see under *syndrome.*

**Shwartz·man reaction (phenomenon)** (shwahrts'mən) [Gregory *Shwartzman,* Russian bacteriologist in the United States, 1896–1965] see under *reaction.*

**Shy-Drager syndrome** (shi-dra'gər) [George Milton *Shy,* American neurologist, 1919–1967; Glenn A. *Drager,* American neurologist, born 1917] [MeSH: Shy-Drager Syndrome] see under *syndrome.*

**Shy-Ma·gee syndrome** (shi-mə-gee') [G. M. *Shy;* Kenneth Raymond *Magee,* American physician, born 1926] central core disease.

**SI** 1. Système International d'Unités, or International System of Units. See also *SI unit,* under *unit.* 2. stimulation index; see *lymphocyte proliferation test,* under *tests.*

**Si** symbol for *silicon.*

**SIADH** syndrome of inappropriate antidiuretic hormone.

**si·al·a·den** (si-al'ə-dən) [Gr. *sial-* + Gr. *adēn* gland] a salivary gland.

**si·al·ad·e·nec·to·my** (si″əl-ad″ə-nek'tə-me) sialoadenectomy.

**si·al·ad·e·ni·tis** (si″əl-ad″ə-ni'tis) [MeSH: Sialadenitis] inflammation of a salivary gland.
**chronic nonspecific s.,** an inflammatory disease of the major salivary glands, characterized by intermittent swelling that may lead to fibrous degeneration, resulting from obstruction of the salivary ducts by calculi, foreign bodies, tumors, or scar formation, with subsequent bacterial invasion.

**si·al·ad·e·nog·ra·phy** (si″əl-ad″ə-nog'rə-fe) radiography of the salivary glands and ducts.

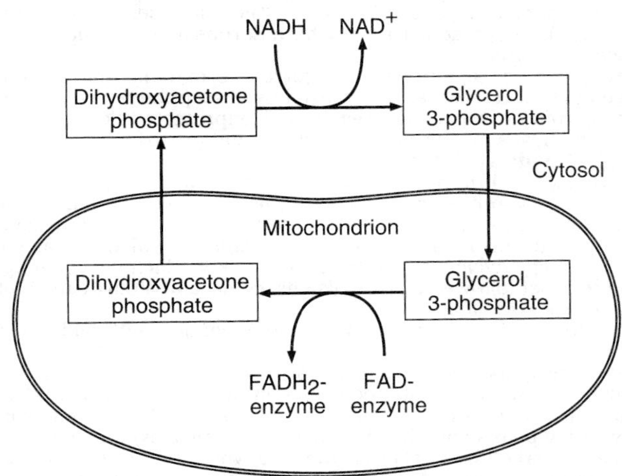


Glycerol phosphate shuttle.

**si·al·ad·e·no·ma** (si″əl-ad″ə-no'mə) a benign tumor of the salivary glands.
**s. papilli'ferum,** a benign exophytic papillomatous lesion of the salivary glands, usually occurring in the hard palate or buccal mucosa of male adults; it appears to originate from the superficial portion of the salivary gland excretory duct.

**si·al·ad·e·nop·athy** (si″al-ad″ən-op'ə-the) [*sial-* + *adeno-* + *-pathy*] sialadenosis.
**benign lymphoepithelial s.,** see under *lesion.*

**si·al·ad·e·no·sis** (si″əl-ad″ə-no'sis) [*sial-* + *adenosis*] a disease of a salivary gland; see also *sialadenitis.* Called also *sialadenopathy.*

**si·al·ad·e·not·o·my** (si″əl-ad″ə-not'ə-me) sialoadenotomy.

**si·a·la·gog·ic** (si″ə-lə-goj'ik) promoting the flow of saliva.

**si·al·a·gogue** (si-al'ə-gog) [*sial-* + *-agogue*] an agent that promotes the flow of saliva. Called also *ptyalagogue.*

**si·a·late** (si'ə-lāt) any salt of a sialic acid.

**si·al·ec·ta·sia** (si″əl-ek-ta'zhə) dilatation of a salivary duct.

**si·al·ic** (si-al'ik) [Gr. *sialikos*] 1. pertaining to the saliva. 2. pertaining to sialic acid.

**si·al·ic ac·id** (si-al'ik) an *N*-acyl derivative of neuraminic acid, e.g., *N*-acetylneuraminic acid; sialic acids occur in many polysaccharides, glycoproteins, and glycolipids in animals and bacteria.

**si·al·i·dase** (si-al'ĭ-dās) 1. an enzyme of the hydrolase class that catalyzes the cleavage of glucosidic linkages between a sialic acid residue and a hexose or hexosamine residue at the nonreducing terminal of oligosaccharides in glycoproteins, glycolipids, and proteoglycans. Deficiency of the enzyme, an autosomal recessive trait, causes sialidosis; enzyme activity is also lacking in galactosialidosis. In EC nomenclature, called *exo-α-sialidase.* 2. the enzyme with this activity specifically cleaving sialic acid–containing gangliosides; it is deficient in mucolipidosis IV. Called also *neuraminidase.*

**si·al·i·do·sis** (si-al″ĭ-do'sis) an autosomal recessive disorder due to a deficiency of sialidase, occurring as two types with differing manifestations. *Type I* is of adolescent or adult onset and is characterized by myoclonus, ocular cherry red spot with progressive loss of visual acuity, and storage of sialyloligosaccharides. *Type II* is additionally characterized by somatic abnormalities, coarse facies, and dysostosis multiplex. It occurs as several variants of increasing severity with earlier age of onset; that of infantile onset is characterized also by visceromegaly and mental retardation, and the congenital form is additionally characterized by ascites, hydrops fetalis, facial edema, inguinal hernias, and early death. Cases of a juvenile form have been shown to be galactosialidosis (q.v.)

**si·a·line** (si'ə-lin) [L. *sialinus*] salivary.

**si·al·ism, si·al·is·mus** (si'əl-iz-əm, si″əl-iz'məs) [Gr. *sialismos*] ptyalism.

**si·a·li·tis** (si″ə-li'tis) 1. sialadenitis. 2 inflammation of a salivary duct.

**sial(o)-** [Gr. *sialon* saliva] combining form denoting relationship to *(a)* saliva or to the salivary glands or *(b)* sialic acid.

**si·a·lo·ad·e·nec·to·my** (si″ə-lo-ad″ə-nek'tə-me) [*sialo-* + *aden-* + *-ectomy*] excision of a salivary gland.

**si·a·lo·ad·e·ni·tis** (si″ə-lo-ad″ə-ni'tis) sialadenitis.

**si·a·lo·ad·e·not·o·my** (si″ə-lo-ad″ə-not'ə-me) [*sialo-* + *adeno-* + *-tomy*] incision and drainage of a salivary gland.

**si·alo·aer·oph·a·gy** (si″ə-lo-ār-of'ə-je) [*sialo-* + *aero-* + *-phagy*] excessive swallowing of saliva and air.

**si·alo·an·gi·ec·ta·sis** (si″ə-lo-an″je-ek'tə-sis) [*sialo-* + *angi-* + *ectasis*] dilatation of the salivary ducts.

**si·alo·an·gi·itis** (si″ə-lo-an″je-i'tis) inflammation of the salivary ducts. Called also *sialodochitis* and *sialoductitis.*

**si·alo·an·gi·og·ra·phy** (si″ə-lo-an″je-og'rə-fe) radiography of the ducts of the salivary glands after injection of radiopaque material.

**si·alo·an·gi·tis** (si″ə-lo-an-ji'tis) sialoangiitis.

**si·alo·cele** (si'ə-lo-sēl″) [*sialo-* + *-cele*[1]] a salivary cyst or tumor.

**si·a·lo·da·cry·o·ad·e·ni·tis** (si″ə-lo-dak″re-o-ad″əni'tis) severe inflammation of the salivary and lacrimal glands in rats, caused by a coronavirus. Characteristics include exophthalmos, facial swelling, and redness around the eyes. It is usually self-limiting, but severe forms can lead to blindness.

**si·alo·do·chi·tis** (si″ə-lo-do-ki'tis) sialoangiitis.

**si·alo·do·cho·plas·ty** (si″ə-lo-do'ko-plas″te) [*sialo-* + Gr. *dochos* receptacle + *-plasty*] plastic operation on the salivary ducts.

**si·alo·duc·ti·tis** (si″ə-lo-dək-ti'tis) sialoangiitis.

**si·alo·gas·trone** (si″ə-lo-gas'trōn) a substance in saliva reputed to inhibit gastric secretion and motility.

**si·a·log·e·nous** (si″ə-loj′ə-nəs) [*sialo-* + *-genous*] producing saliva.

**si·alo·gly·co·con·ju·gate** (si-al″o-gli″ko-kon-ju′gət) a compound comprising a sialic acid residue in glycosidic linkage with a glycoconjugate; most of the sialic acid in body fluids and tissues is so complexed.

**si·alo·gog·ic** (si″ə-lo-goj′ik) sialagogic.

**si·alo·gogue** (si-al′o-gog) sialagogue.

**si·alo·gram** (si-al′o-gram) [*sialo-* + *-gram*] a radiograph produced by sialography.

**si·alo·graph** (si-al′o-graf) sialogram.

**si·a·log·ra·phy** (si″ə-log′rə-fe) [*sialo-* + *-graphy*] [MeSH: Sialography] radiographic demonstration of the salivary ducts by means of the injection of substances opaque to x-radiation.

**si·alo·lith** (si-al′o-lith) [*sialo-* + *-lith*] [MeSH: Salivary Gland Calculi] a calcareous concretion or calculus in the salivary ducts or glands, involving most commonly the submaxillary gland and its duct, less frequently the parotid and sublingual glands and their ducts, and seldom the minor salivary glands. Called also *salivary calculus* and *salivary stone.*

**si·alo·li·thi·a·sis** (si″ə-lo-lĭ-thi′ə-sis) [*sialo-* + *lithiasis*] a condition characterized by the presence of sialoliths. Called also *ptyalolithiasis.*

**si·alo·li·thot·o·my** (si″ə-lo-lĭ-thot′ə-me) [*sialolith* + *-tomy*] incision of a salivary gland or duct for the removal of a calculus.

**si·al·o·ma** (si″ə-lo′mə) a salivary tumor.

**si·alo·meta·pla·sia** (si″ə-lo-met″ə-pla′zhə) metaplasia of the salivary glands.
**necrotizing s.,** a benign inflammatory condition of the minor salivary glands, simulating mucoepidermoid and squamous cell carcinoma. Histological findings usually show lobular necrosis and ductal and glandular metaplasia.

**si·alo·mu·cin** (si″ə-lo-mu′sin) a mucin whose carbohydrate groups contain a sialic acid.

**si·alo·pha·gia** (si′ə-lo-fa′jə) [*sialo-* + *-phagia*] excessive swallowing of saliva.

**si·a·lor·rhea** (si″ə-lo-re′ə) [*sialo-* + *-rrhea*] [MeSH: Sialorrhea] ptyalism.

**si·a·los·che·sis** (si″ə-los′kə-sis) [*sialo-* + Gr. *schesis* suppression] suppression of the salivary secretion.

**si·a·lo·se·mei·ol·o·gy** (si″ə-lo-se″mi-ol′ə-je) [*sialo-* + *semeiology*] analysis of the saliva as a means of determining the physiologic status of the patient, especially in regard to metabolic processes.

**si·alo·sis** (si″ə-lo′sis) [*sial-* + *-osis*] 1. the flow of saliva. 2. ptyalism.

**si·alo·ste·no·sis** (si″ə-lo-stə-no′sis) [*sialo-* + *stenosis*] stenosis, or narrowing, of a salivary duct.

**si·alo·sy·rinx** (si″ə-lo-si′rinks) [*sialo-* + *syrinx*] 1. a salivary fistula. 2. a syringe for washing out the salivary ducts, or a drainage tube for the salivary ducts.

**si·al·yl·ol·i·go·sac·cha·ride** (si-al″əl-ol″ĭ-go-sak′ə-rīd) any of the oligosaccharides to which are attached one or more sialic acid residues; they accumulate when the sialidase specific for oligosaccharides and glycoproteins is deficient, as in sialidosis and galactosialidosis.

**si·al·yl·trans·fer·ase** (si-al″əl-trans′fər-ās) a term used in the recommended names of some enzymes of the transferase class that catalyze the formation of sialylglycoconjugates via transfer of the sialic acid group from CMP to one of several glycoconjugate acceptors.

**sib** (sib) [A. S. *sib* kin] 1. a blood relative; one of a group of persons, all of whom are descendants of a common ancestor. 2. sibling.

**sib·i·lant** (sib′ĭ-lənt) [L. *sibilans* hissing] 1. having a shrill, hissing, or whistling character. 2. a consonant sound produced with a hiss, such as *s, sh, z,* or *zh.*

**sib·ling** (sib′ling) [A. S. *sib* kin + *ling* a diminutive] [MeSH: Nuclear Family] any of two or more offspring of the same parents; a brother or sister. Called also *sib.*

**si·bor·ox·ime** (si″bo-rok′sēm) a compound which, complexed with technetium 99m, constitutes a BATO that has been used in brain imaging; see table at *technetium.*

**sib·ship** (sib′ship) 1. relationship by blood. 2. a group of persons, all of whom are descendants of a common ancestor, commonly used as the basis of study to determine genetic influences. 3. a group of siblings.

**Sib·son's aponeurosis (fascia),** etc. (sib′sənz) [Francis *Sibson,* English physician, 1814–1876] see under *furrow, groove,* and *notch,* and see *membrana suprapleuralis, musculus scalenus minimus,* and *vestibule of aorta.*

**Si·card's syndrome** (se-kahrz′) [Jean Athanase *Sicard,* Paris neurologist, 1872–1929] Collet's syndrome.

**sic·cant** (sik′ənt) [L. *siccare* to dry] drying.

**sic·co·la·bile** (sik″o-la′bīl) altered or destroyed by drying.

**sic·co·sta·bile** (sik″o-sta′bīl) not altered by drying.

**sic·cus** (sik′əs) [L.] dry.

**sick** (sik) 1. not in good health; afflicted by disease; ill. 2. affected with nausea.

**sick bay** (sik ba) hospital and dispensary quarters on a naval vessel or station.

**sick·le·mia** (sik-le′me-ə) sickle cell anemia.

**sick·ling** (sik′ling) the development of sickle cells in the blood, as in sickle cell anemia.

**sick·ness** (sik′nəs) disease.
**aerial s.,** air s.
**African horse s.,** an infectious disease of horses and mules caused by orbivirus; it is endemic in most of sub-Saharan Africa but has also been found in Europe and the Middle East. Four types are distinguished: the *respiratory type* (fever, dyspnea, copious fluid discharge, and usually a fatal inhalation pneumonia), the *cardiac type* (edema of the head with widespread petechiae, often but not always fatal), the *mixed cardiac and respiratory type,* and a mild type called *horse s. fever.* Called also *pestis equorum* and *equine plague.*
**African sleeping s.,** see under *trypanosomiasis.*
**air s.,** sickness due to change in air pressure and to the movements experienced in an airplane, marked by nausea, salivation, and cold sweats.
**altitude s.,** the condition resulting from difficulty in adjusting to diminished oxygen pressure at high altitudes. It may take the form of mountain sickness (q.v.), high-altitude pulmonary edema, or cerebral edema. Called also *high altitude s.*
**athletes' s.,** weakness, blurred vision, nausea, and headache, following a short period of intense physical exercise.
**aviation s.,** air s.
**balloon s.,** a condition similar to mountain sickness occurring during balloon ascents.
**bay s.,** Haff disease.
**bush s.,** enzootic marasmus in New Zealand due to cobalt deficiency.
**caisson s.,** decompression s.
**car s.,** nausea and malaise produced by the motion of trains or automobiles or other vehicles.
**compressed-air s.,** decompression s.
**decompression s.,** joint pains, respiratory manifestations, skin lesions, and neurologic signs occurring in aviators flying at high altitudes or in persons who have been breathing compressed air in caissons or diving apparatus if air pressure is reduced too rapidly. Called also *caisson s.* or *disease, compressed-air s., divers' palsy,* and *divers' paralysis.*
**gall s.,** anaplasmosis.
**Gambian horse s.,** a fatal type of nagana seen in horses throughout central Africa, caused by *Trypanosoma congolense.*
**Gambian sleeping s.,** see under *trypanosomiasis.*
**grass s.,** a usually fatal disease of horses occurring after they have been put to graze on grass, usually between May and July; characteristics include dysphagia, severe diarrhea, dehydration, interrupted peristalsis, and priapism. It was first observed in Scotland but has now spread across northern Europe and elsewhere. Called also *grass disease.*
**green tobacco s.,** a transient, recurrent form of nicotine poisoning seen in tobacco harvesters, caused by absorption of dissolved nicotine from wet tobacco leaves through unprotected skin; symptoms include headache, dizziness, vomiting, and prostration.
**high-altitude s.,** altitude s.
**horse s.,** see *African horse s.* and *Gambian horse s.*
**Jamaican vomiting s.,** a type of poisoning seen in Jamaica and nearby areas of the West Indies, due to ingestion of damaged or unripe fruit of the akee tree *(Blighia sapida),* which contains the toxins hypoglycine A and B; characteristics include vomiting of acute onset followed by convulsions, coma, and often death. Called also *akee poisoning.*
**lambing s.,** a condition of ewes almost identical with milk fever of cows.
**laughing s.,** pseudobulbar paralysis.
**milk s.,** acute, often fatal poisoning in humans who drink milk, or eat milk products or meat, from cattle or sheep that were poisoned by eating plants containing tremetol (see *trembles*); the human disease is marked by weakness, anorexia, vomiting, constipation, and sometimes muscular tremors. Called also *milk poisoning.*

**morning s.,** the nausea of early pregnancy.
**motion s.,** sickness caused by motion experienced in any kind of travel, such as sea sickness, train sickness, car sickness, and air sickness.
**mountain s.,** a type of high altitude sickness caused by exposure to altitude high enough to cause hypoxia, occurring as a result of decreased atmospheric pressure with consequent lowering of arterial oxygen content. It occurs as acute, subacute, and chronic forms. The subacute and chronic forms can be cured by descent to a lower altitude. Called also *mountain disease.*
**mountain s., acute,** a type that appears a few hours after exposure to high altitude, characterized by fatigue, dizziness, breathlessness, headache, nausea, vomiting, insomnia, impairment of mental capacity, and prostration. Called also *Acosta's disease.*
**mountain s., chronic,** a type characterized by loss of tolerance to hypoxia in a previously acclimatized person, with secondary polycythemia. It occurs in two types: an *emphysematous* type in which dyspnea is the dominant symptom and bronchitis, laryngitis, and cyanosis are often present; and an *erythremic* type in which there is an erythremic color that becomes cyanotic on mild exertion, with fatigue, headache, episodic stupor, paresthesias, anorexia, nausea, vomiting, and decreased visual acuity. Called also *Andes disease* and *Monge's disease.*
**mountain s., subacute,** a type milder than the chronic form and similar clinically to the acute form except for being persistent and amenable to cure by a descent in altitude.
**radiation s.,** a condition resulting from exposure to a whole-body dose of over 1 gray of ionizing radiation and characterized by the symptoms of the acute radiation syndrome (q.v.). Its severity varies with the dose level.
**railroad s.,** transit tetany.
**Rhodesian sleeping s.,** see under *trypanosomiasis.*
**salt s.,** enzootic marasmus in Florida.
**sea s.,** nausea and malaise caused by the motion of a ship.
**serum s.,** a hypersensitivity reaction to the administration of foreign serum or serum proteins characterized by fever, urticaria, arthralgia, edema, and lymphadenopathy. It is caused by the formation of circulating antigen-antibody complexes that are deposited in tissues and trigger tissue injury mediated by complement and polymorphonuclear leukocytes. Serum sickness is classed with the Arthus reaction and other immune complex diseases as a type III hypersensitivity reaction (Gell and Coombs classification). Although serum sickness is now rare because of the replacement of most animal-derived antisera with human immune globulins, an identical illness *(serum sickness–like reaction* or *syndrome)* can be produced by hypersensitivity reactions to penicillin and other drugs.
**sleeping s.,** a disease characterized by increasing drowsiness and lethargy, caused by a protozoal infection, such as African trypanosomiasis, or by a viral infection, such as lethargic encephalitis, St. Louis encephalitis, or eastern or western encephalomyelitis.
**space s.,** space adaptation syndrome.
**stiff s.,** bovine ephemeral fever.
**sweating s.,** a febrile, tickborne illness affecting African cattle, especially calves, due to a toxin produced by *Hyalomma truncatum,* and characterized by the presence of moist eczematous lesions of the mucous membranes. Called also *tick toxicosis.*
**three-day s.,** bovine ephemeral fever.
**turning s.,** an unusual form of bovine theileriasis in which *Theileria parva* invades the central nervous system, causing either acute attacks of spinning followed by unconsciousness or chronic circling and incoordination.
**veld s., veldt s.,** heartwater.
**vomiting s.,** Jamaican vomiting s.
**x-ray s.,** radiation s.

**Sid blood group** (sid) [from part of the name of the English propositus first reported on in the 1960s] see under *blood group.*

**s.i.d.** abbreviation for L. *sem'el in di'e,* once a day; written also *semel in d.*

**side** (sīd) the lateral (right or left) portion or aspect of the body or a structure.
**balancing s.,** the segment of a denture or dental arch on the side opposite to that toward which the mandible is moved. The term pertains to occlusion and bears no relation to masticatory activity. Called also *nonfunctioning s.*
**functioning s.,** working s.
**nonfunctioning s.,** balancing s.
**working s.,** the segment of a denture or dental arch on the same side as that toward which the mandible is moved. The term pertains to occlusion and bears no relation to masticatory activity. Called also *functioning s.*

**side-bone** (sīd'bōn) a condition of horses marked by ossification of the lateral cartilages of the third phalanx of the foot.

**side ef·fect** (sīd' ə-fekt″) a consequence other than the one(s) for which an agent or measure is used, as the adverse effects produced by a drug, especially on a tissue or organ system other than the one sought to be benefited by its administration.

**sid·er·in·uria** (sid″ər-ĭ-nu're-ə) [*sidero-* + *-uria*] excretion of iron in the urine.

**sider(o)-** [Gr. *sidēros* iron] a combining form denoting relationship to iron.

**sid·ero·blast** (sid'ər-o-blast″) a normoblast that contains granules of iron in the form of ferritin in its cytoplasm and stains with Prussian blue.
**ringed s.,** an abnormal sideroblast containing many iron granules in its mitochondria in a ring shape around the periphery of the nucleus, as seen in sideroblastic anemia.

**sid·ero·cyte** (sid'ər-o-sīt″) an erythrocyte containing granules of ferritin in its cytoplasm.

**sid·ero·der·ma** (sid″ər-o-der'mə) bronzed coloration of the skin from the deposition of iron derived from degenerated hemoglobin.

**sid·ero·fi·bro·sis** (sid″ər-o-fi-bro'sis) fibrosis of the spleen marked by iron-containing deposits.

**sid·ero·my·cin** (sid″ər-o-mi'sin) any of a class of antibiotics structurally related to hydroxamic acid that inhibit bacterial growth by interfering with iron uptake. Sideromycins are synthesized by certain species of actinomycetes.

**sid·ero·pe·nia** (sid″ər-o-pe'ne-ə) [*sidero-* + *-penia*] iron deficiency.

**sid·ero·pe·nic** (sid″ər-o-pe'nik) pertaining to or characterized by iron deficiency.

**sid·ero·phage** (sid'ər-o-fāj″) a macrophage laden with phagocytosed iron-containing particles.

**sid·ero·phil** (sid'ər-o-fil) 1. siderophilous. 2. a siderophilous tissue or structure.

**sid·er·oph·il·in** (sid″ər-of'ĭ-lin) transferrin.

**sid·er·oph·i·lous** (sid″ər-of'ĭ-ləs) [*sidero-* + Gr. *philein* to love] having a tendency to absorb iron.

**sid·ero·phone** (sid'ər-o-fōn) [*sidero-* + Gr. *phōnē* voice] an instrument for detecting, by a telephone-like arrangement, the presence of iron splinters in the eyeball.

**sid·ero·phore** (sid'ər-o-for″) [*sidero-* + *-phore*] 1. a substance that binds iron. 2. a macrophage containing hemosiderin. 3. a compound produced by certain species of mycobacteria and enterobacteria that chelates iron and facilitates its uptake by the cell.

**sid·ero·scope** (sid'ər-o-skōp) [*sidero-* + *-scope*] a magnet or other appliance for determining the presence of metallic iron as a foreign body in the eye.

**sid·er·o·sil·i·co·sis** (sid″ər-o-sil″ĭ-ko'sis) a type of mixed dust pneumoconiosis consisting of siderosis with silicosis, due to the inhalation of dust containing particles of iron ore and silica. Called also *silicosiderosis.*

**sid·er·o·sis** (sid″ər-o'sis) [MeSH: Siderosis] 1. a benign type of pneumoconiosis caused by the inhalation of iron particles; it usually becomes serious only when combined with silicosis (see *siderosilicosis*). Called also *pneumoconiosis siderotica* and *pulmonary s.* 2. hyperferremia. 3. the deposit of iron in tissues; see also hemochromatosis and hemosiderosis.
**Bantu s.,** a form of siderosis observed among the Bantu people of southern Africa; it was formerly thought to be always caused by use of cast iron vessels for cooking and food storage, but in some families a hereditary susceptibility has been found.
**s. bul'bi,** the deposit of an iron pigment within the eyeball.
**s. conjuncti'vae,** a rust brown or yellowish discoloration of the conjunctiva due to the presence of an iron foreign body; the condition may also be seen in hemochromatosis.
**hepatic s.,** the deposit of an abnormal quantity of iron in the liver; see also under *hemosiderosis.*
**nutritional s.,** excessive iron in the blood due to a diet very high in iron and low in protein and calories.
**pulmonary s.,** siderosis (def. 1).
**urinary s.,** presence of hemosiderin granules in the urine.

**sid·er·ot·ic** (sid″ər-ot'ik) pertaining to or characterized by siderosis.

**sid·er·ous** (sid'ər-əs) containing iron.

**side·wind·er** (sīd'wīnd-ər) *Crotalus ceras'tes,* a pale-colored venomous rattlesnake found in desert areas of the southwestern United States.

**SIDS** sudden infant death syndrome.

**Sie·gert's sign** (ze'gertz) [Ferdinand *Siegert,* German pediatrician, 1865–1946] see under *sign.*

**Sie·gle's otoscope** (ze'gəlz) [Emil *Siegle*, German otologist, 1833–1900] see under *otoscope.*

**sie·mens** (se'mənz) the SI unit of conductance or of admittance; it is the conductance of one ampere per volt in a body with one ohm resistance. Formerly called *mho* because conductance in siemens is the reciprocal of resistance in ohms. Symbol S.

**Sie·mer·ling's nucleus** (ze'mer-lingz) [Ernst *Siemerling*, German neurologist and psychiatrist, 1857–1931] see under *nucleus.*

**sieve** (siv) a device having pores or perforations of uniform size used for separating objects or particles of different sizes.
**molecular s.,** a crystalline substance having uniform pores of molecular size that adsorbs smaller but not larger molecules; used in chemical separation.

**sie·vert** (se'vərt) the SI unit of radiation absorbed dose equivalent, defined as that producing the same biologic effect in a specified tissue as 1 gray of high-energy x-rays; 1 sievert equals 100 rem. Abbreviated Sv.

**Sig.** abbreviation for L. *signe'tur,* let it be labeled.

**sigh** (si) [L. *suspirium*] an audible and prolonged inspiration, followed by an audible expiration.

**sight** (sīt) [A.S. *sihth*] vision (defs. 1 and 2).
**day s.,** nyctalopia, or night blindness.
**far s., long s.,** hyperopia.
**near s.,** myopia.
**night s.,** hemeralopia, or day blindness.
**old s.,** presbyopia.
**second s.,** senopia.
**short s.,** myopia.

**sig·ma·tism** (sig'mə-tiz-əm) the incorrect, difficult, or too frequent use of the *s* sound. See also *lisping.* Called also *parasigmatism.*

**sig·moid** (sig'moid) [Gr. *sigmoeidēs*, from the letter *sigma* + *eidos* form] [MeSH: Sigmoid] 1. shaped like the letter S or the letter C. 2. the sigmoid colon.

**sig·moid·ec·to·my** (sig″moi-dek'tə-me) excision of the sigmoid colon; called also *sigmoid colectomy.*

**sig·moid·itis** (sig″moi-di'tis) inflammation of the sigmoid colon.

**sig·moido·pexy** (sig-moi'do-pek″se) [*sigmoid* + *-pexy*] suspension of the sigmoid colon, usually performed for treatment of rectal prolapse.

**sig·moido·proc·tos·to·my** (sig-moi″do-prok-tos'tə-me) the creation of an artificial opening between the sigmoid colon and the rectum; also, the opening so created.

**sig·moido·rec·tos·to·my** (sig-moi″do-rək-tos'tə-me) sigmoidoproctostomy.

**sig·moido·scope** (sig-moi'do-skōp) [*sigmoid* + *-scope*] a rigid or flexible endoscope with appropriate illumination for examining the sigmoid colon.

**sig·moid·os·co·py** (sig″moi-dos'kə-pe) [MeSH: Sigmoidoscopy] inspection of the sigmoid colon through a sigmoidoscope.

**sig·moido·sig·moi·dos·to·my** (sig-moi″do-sig-moi-dos'tə-me) the operative formation of an anastomosis between two portions of the sigmoid colon; also, the opening so created.

**sig·moid·os·to·my** (sig″moi-dos'tə-me) [*sigmoid* + *-stomy*] 1. formation of an artificial opening from the body surface into the sigmoid colon. 2. the opening produced by this procedure.

**sig·moid·ot·o·my** (sig″moi-dot'ə-me) operative incision into the sigmoid colon.

**sig·moido·ves·i·cal** (sig-moi″do-ves'ĭ-kəl) pertaining to or communicating with the sigmoid colon and the urinary bladder, as a sigmoidovesical fistula.

**Sig·mund's glands** (zig'moonts) [Karl Ludwig *Sigmund*, Austrian physician, 1810–1883] see under *gland.*

**sign** (sīn) [L. *signum*] an indication of the existence of something; any objective evidence of a disease, i.e., such evidence as is perceptible to the examining physician, as opposed to the subjective sensations (symptoms) of the patient.

## Sign

For terms not found here, see also under *phenomenon, reflex, symptom,* and *syndrome.*

**Aaron's s.,** a sensation of pain or distress in the epigastric or precordial region on pressure over McBurney's point in appendicitis.
**Abadie's s.,** 1. [Charles *Abadie*] spasm of the levator palpebrae superioris muscle; a sign of Graves' disease. 2. [Jean *Abadie*] insensibility of the Achilles tendon to pressure; seen in tabes dorsalis.
**accessory s.,** any nonpathognomonic sign of disease.
**air-cushion s.,** Klemm's s.
**Allis' s.,** relaxation of the fascia between the crest of the ilium and the greater trochanter: a sign of fracture of the neck of the femur.
**Amoss' s.,** in painful flexure of the spine, the patient, when rising to a sitting posture from lying in bed, does so by supporting himself with his hands placed far behind him in the bed.
**André Thomas s.,** 1. if during the finger to nose test, the patient is directed to raise his arm over his head and is then suddenly ordered to let it fall to his head, the arm will rebound; seen in disease of the cerebellum. Cf. *rebound phenomenon.* 2. pinching of the trapezius muscle causes gooseflesh above the level of a spinal cord lesion.
**Anghelescu's s.,** inability to bend the spine while lying on the back so as to rest on the head and heels alone, seen in tuberculosis of the vertebrae.
**antecedent s.,** any precursory indication of an attack of disease.
**anterior drawer s.,** see under *test.*
**anterior tibial s.,** tibialis s.
**anticus s.,** Piotrowski's s.
**Argyll Robertson pupil s.,** see under *pupil.*
**Arroyo's s.,** asthenocoria.
**assident s.,** accessory s.
**Auenbrugger's s.,** a bulging of the epigastrium, due to extensive pericardial effusion.
**Auspitz s.,** the appearance of multiple fine bleeding points when a scale is removed from a psoriatic plaque, caused by thinning of the epidermis over the dermal papillae.
**Babinski's s.,** 1. loss or lessening of the Achilles tendon reflex in sciatica: this distinguishes it from hysteric sciatica. 2. a misnomer for Babinski's reflex. 3. in hemiplegia, the contraction of the platysma muscle in the healthy side is more vigorous than on the affected side, as seen in opening the mouth, whistling, blowing, etc. 4. when a hemiplegic patient is lying with arms crossed upon the chest, and makes an effort to sit up, the thigh on the paralyzed side is flexed upon the pelvis and the heel is lifted from the ground, while on the healthy side the limb does not move. 5. when the paralyzed forearm is placed in supination, it turns over to pronation: seen in organic paralysis. Called also *pronation s.*
**Babinski's toe s.,** Babinski's reflex.
**Baccelli's s.,** aphonic pectoriloquy.
**Baillarger's s.,** inequality of the pupils in general paresis.
**Ballance's s.,** resonance of right flank when the patient lies on the left side; said to be present in splenic rupture.
**Ballet's s.,** external ophthalmoplegia, with loss of all voluntary eye movements, the pupillary movements and reflex eye movements persisting; seen in Graves' disease and hysteria.
**Bamberger's s.,** 1. allochiria. 2. presence of signs of consolidation at the angle of the scapula, which disappear when the patient leans forward; a sign of pericardial effusion.
**banana s.,** a flattened and curved, bananalike shape of the cerebellar hemispheres seen in axial section in sonography of the fetal skull; a sign of the Arnold-Chiari deformity.
**Bárány's s.,** caloric test; see under *test.*
**Bard's s.,** in organic nystagmus the oscillations of the eye increase as the patient's attention follows the finger moved alternately from one side to the other; but in congenital nystagmus the oscillations disappear in like condition.
**Barré's s.,** contraction of the iris is retarded in mental deterioration.
**Barré's pyramidal s.,** the patient lies face down and the legs are flexed at the knee; he is unable to hold the legs in this vertical position if there is disease of the pyramidal tracts.
**Bastian-Bruns' s.,** see under *law.*
**Battle's s.,** discoloration over the skin of the mastoid region of the skull, in the line of the posterior auricular artery, the ecchymosis first appearing near the tip of the mastoid process; seen in fracture of the base of the skull.
**Becker's s.,** see under *phenomenon.*
**Béclard's s.,** a sign of the maturity of the fetus consisting of a center of ossification in the lower epiphysis of the femur.
**Beevor's s.,** 1. a sign of functional paralysis consisting of inability of the patient to inhibit the antagonistic muscles. 2. upward deviation

of the umbilicus on attempting to lift the head, caused by contraction of the upper but not the lower abdominal muscles and indicative of a spinal cord lesion in the region of the lower thoracic vertebrae.

**Bekhterev's s.,** 1. see under *reflex.* 2. paralysis of the facial muscles for automatic movements.

**Bell's s.,** see under *phenomenon.*

**Berger's s.,** an irregularly shaped or elliptical pupil in the early stages of tabes dorsalis, paralytic dementia, and certain paralyses.

**Bergman's s.,** in urologic radiography, *(a)* the ureter is dilated immediately below a neoplasm, rather than collapsed as below an obstructing stone and *(b)* the ureteral catheter tends to coil in this dilated portion of the ureter.

**Bethea's s.,** when the examiner, standing behind the patient, places his fingertips on the upper surfaces of corresponding ribs high in the patient's axillae, unilateral impairment of chest expansion is indicated by less respiratory movement of the ribs on the side affected. Called also *Bethea's method.*

**Bezold's s.,** an inflammatory swelling below the apex of the mastoid process; evidence of mastoiditis.

**Biederman's s.,** a dark red color (instead of the normal pink) of the anterior pillars of the throat, seen in some patients with syphilis.

**Biernacki's s.,** analgesia of the ulnar nerve in general paresis and tabes dorsalis.

**Biot's s.,** see under *respiration.*

**Bird's s.,** a definite zone of dullness with absence of the respiratory sounds in hydatid disease of the lung.

**Bjerrum's s.,** see under *scotoma.*

**Blatin's s.,** hydatid thrill.

**Blumberg's s.,** pain on abrupt release of steady pressure (rebound tenderness) over the site of a suspected abdominal lesion; seen in peritonitis.

**Boas' s.,** see under *point.*

**Bonnet's s.,** pain on thigh adduction in sciatica.

**Bordier-Fränkel s.,** Bell's phenomenon.

**Borsieri's s.,** when the fingernail is drawn along the skin in early stages of scarlet fever, a white line is left which quickly turns red; called also *Borsieri's line.*

**Boston's s.,** Graefe's s.

**Bouillaud's s.,** permanent retraction of the chest in the precordial region; a sign of adherent pericardium.

**bowler hat s.,** a shadow resembling a bowler hat, seen on a radiograph of the colon; it represents the filling defect of either a sessile polyp on the inferior wall or a diverticulum.

**Boyce's s.,** a gurgling sound heard on pressure by the hand on the side of the neck, in diverticulum of the esophagus.

**Bozzolo's s.,** a visible pulsation of the arteries within the nostrils; said to indicate aneurysm of the thoracic aorta.

**Bragard's s.,** with the knee stiff, the lower extremity is flexed at the hip until the patient experiences pain; the foot is then dorsiflexed. Increase of pain points to disease of the nerve root.

**Branham's s.,** bradycardia produced by digital closure of an artery proximal to an arteriovenous fistula.

**Braunwald s.,** occurrence of a weak pulse instead of a strong one immediately after a premature ventricular contraction.

**Braxton Hicks' s.,** see under *contraction.*

**Broadbent's s.,** a retraction seen on the left side of the back, near the eleventh and twelfth ribs, related to pericardial adhesion.

**Broadbent's inverted s.,** pulsations synchronizing with ventricular systole on the posterior lateral wall of the chest in gross dilatation of the left atrium.

**Brockenbrough's s.,** occurrence of a weak pulse instead of a strong one immediately after a premature ventricular contraction; indicative of idiopathic hypertrophic subaortic stenosis.

**Brodie's s.,** a black spot on the glans penis, a sign of gangrene due to urinary extravasation into the corpus spongiosum.

**broken straw s.,** a sharply angulated spindle cell resembling a broken straw; characteristic of the spindle cell form of embryonal rhabdomyosarcoma.

**Brown's s.,** blanching of the tympanic membrane and of the area behind it, seen with pneumatic pressure on the membrane; it indicates presence of a vascular tumor or other lesion in the middle ear.

**Brown-Séquard's s.,** see under *syndrome.*

**Brudzinski's s.,** 1. in meningitis, flexion of the neck usually results in flexion of the hip and knee; called also *neck s.* 2. in meningitis, when passive flexion of the lower limb on one side is made, a similar movement will be seen in the opposite limb; called also *contralateral s.*

**Brunati's s.,** the appearance of opacities in the cornea during the course of pneumonia or typhoid fever.

**Bruns' s.,** see under *syndrome.*

**Bryant's s.,** lowering of the axillary folds in dislocation of the shoulder.

**Burton's s.,** lead line.

**Cantelli's s.,** doll's eye reflex.

**Carabelli's s.,** see under *cusp.*

**cardinal s's (of inflammation),** dolor, calor, rubor, tumor, and functio laesa; see *inflammation.*

**cardiorespiratory s.,** a change in the normal pulse-respiration ratio from 4:1 to 2:1; seen in infantile scurvy.

**Carman's s., Carman-Kirklin s., Carman-Kirklin meniscus s.,** meniscus s.

**Carnett's s.,** a test for parietal tenderness: the abdomen is palpated while the patient holds the anterior abdominal muscles tense; the tense muscles prevent the examiner's fingers from coming in contact with the underlying viscera and any tenderness elicited over them will be parietal in location. Tenderness elicited over relaxed muscles may be either parietal or intra-abdominal in origin; that present with relaxed muscles and absent with tense muscles is due to a subparietal lesion and its cause is inside the abdomen; that found with both relaxed and tensed muscles is due to an anterior parietal lesion and its cause is outside the abdominal cavity.

**Carvallo's s.,** in tricuspid regurgitation, augmentation of the pansystolic murmur by inspiration.

**Cegka's s.,** invariability of the cardiac dullness during the different phases of respiration; a sign of adherent pericardium.

**Chaddock's s.,** see under *reflex.*

**Chadwick's s.,** a dark bluish or purplish-red and congested appearance of the vaginal mucosa, an indication of pregnancy.

**Charcot's s.,** the raising of the eyebrow in peripheral facial paralysis, and the lowering of the same part in facial contraction.

**Cheyne-Stokes s.,** see under *respiration.*

**Chilaiditi's s.,** hepatoptosis (def. 2).

**Chvostek's s., Chvostek-Weiss s.,** spasm of the facial muscles elicited by tapping the facial nerve in the region of the parotid gland; seen in tetany. Called also *Schultze's s.* and *Schultze-Chvostek s.*

**Claude's hyperkinesis s.,** reflex movements of paretic muscles elicited by painful stimuli.

**clavicular s.,** a tumefaction on the inner third of the right clavicle; seen in congenital syphilis. Called also *Higouménaki's s.*

**Cleeman's s.,** creasing of the skin just above the patella, indicative of fracture of the femur with overriding of fragments.

**Codman's s.,** in rupture of the supraspinatus tendon, the arm can be passively abducted without pain, but when support of the arm is removed and the deltoid contracts suddenly, pain occurs again.

**cogwheel s.,** see under *rigidity.*

**coiled spring s.,** a concentric ring pattern of the mucosa of the intestine, seen on barium enema examination in a variety of diseases, including posttraumatic hematoma of the duodenum, acute appendicitis, intussusception of the appendix, mucocele, endometriosis of the appendix, and carcinoma.

**Cole's s.,** deformity of the duodenal contour as seen in the radiograph, a sign of the presence of duodenal ulcer.

**colon cutoff s.,** a radiographic sign of appendiceal perforation or colonic spasm, consisting of absence of gas and feces in the right lower quadrant, reflex dilatation of the transverse colon, and sharp cutoff of gas at the hepatic flexure.

**commemorative s.,** any sign of a previous disease.

**Comolli's s.,** a sign of scapular fracture consisting of the appearance in the scapular region, shortly after the accident, of a triangular swelling reproducing the shape of the body of the scapula.

**complementary opposition s.,** Grasset-Gaussel-Hoover s.

**contralateral s.,** Brudzinski's s., def. 2.

**Coopernail's s.,** ecchymosis on the perineum and scrotum or labia: a sign of fracture of the pelvis.

**Cope's s.,** psoas s.

**Corrigan's s.,** 1. see under *line.* 2. see under *pulse.*

**coughing s.,** Huntington's s.

**Courvoisier's s.,** see under *law.*

**Cowen's s.,** when light is shone into one pupil, there is jerky constriction of the contralateral pupil in Graves' disease.

**crescent s.,** meniscus s.

**Crichton-Browne's s.,** tremor of the outer angles of the eyes and of the labial commissures in the earlier stages of general paresis.

**Crowe's s.,** axillary freckling seen in neurofibromatosis.

**Cullen's s.,** a bluish discoloration of the skin around the umbilicus sometimes associated with intraperitoneal hemorrhage, especially following rupture of the uterine tube in ectopic pregnancy. A similar discoloration is seen in acute hemorrhagic pancreatitis.

**Dalrymple's s.,** one manifestation of Graves' orbitopathy, consisting of retraction of the eyelids so that the palpebral opening is abnormally wide. See also *Stellwag's s.*

**D'Amato's s.,** in pleural effusion, the location of dullness is altered from the vertebral area in the sitting position to the heart region when the patient assumes a lateral position on the side opposite the effusion.

**Darier's s.,** urtication and itching occurring on rubbing the lesions of urticaria pigmentosa.

**Dawbarn's s.,** in acute subacromial bursitis, when the arm hangs by the side palpation over the bursa causes pain, but when the arm is abducted this pain disappears.

**Dejerine's s.,** aggravation of symptoms of radiculitis produced by coughing, sneezing, and straining at stool.

**Delbet's s.,** in aneurysm of the main artery of a limb, if the nutrition of the part distal to the aneurysm is maintained, although the pulse may have disappeared, the collateral circulation is sufficient.

**Demarquay's s.,** fixation or lowering of the larynx during phonation and deglutition; a sign of syphilis of the trachea.

**Demianoff's s.,** with the patient in dorsal decubitus position, extreme pain when the attempt is made to lift an extended leg above ten degrees, a sign of a lesion in the erector spinae muscles of the lumbar region. Cf. *Lasègue's s.*

**de Musset's s.,** Musset's s.

**Dennie's s.,** Morgan's line.

**Desault's s.,** a sign of intracapsular fracture of the femur, consisting of alteration of the arc described by rotation of the great trochanter, which normally describes the segment of a circle, but in this fracture rotates only as the apex of the femur as it rotates about its own axis.

**d'Espine's s.,** in the normal person, on auscultation over the spinous processes, pectoriloquy ceases at the bifurcation of the trachea, and in infants opposite the seventh cervical vertebra. If pectoriloquy is heard lower than this, it indicates enlargement of the bronchial lymph nodes.

**Dew's s.,** in diaphragmatic hydatid abscess beneath the right cupola, the area of resonance moves caudally with the patient on hands and knees.

**Dixon Mann's s.,** Mann's s.

**doll's eye s.,** see under *reflex.*

**Dorendorf's s.,** fullness of the supraclavicular groove on one side in aneurysm of the aortic arch.

**double bubble s.,** the appearance on the radiograph of the abdomen of two foci of gas, one in the stomach and the other in the duodenum; a sign of duodenal obstruction. The same sign, in this case consisting of the stomach and duodenum distended by fluid, may be observed in the fetus by ultrasonography.

**drawer s's,** see under *test.*

**Drummond's s.,** a whiff heard at the open mouth during respiration in cases of aortic aneurysm.

**DTP s.** ***(distal tingling on percussion),*** Tinel's s.

**Dubois' s.,** shortness of the little finger in congenital syphilis.

**Duchenne's s.,** the sinking in of the epigastrium on inspiration in paralysis of the diaphragm or in certain cases of hydropericardium.

**Duckworth's s.,** see under *phenomenon.*

**Dugas' s.,** see under *test.*

**Dupuytren's s.,** 1. a crackling sensation on pressure over a sarcomatous bone. 2. in congenital dislocation of the head of the femur, there is a free up-and-down movement of the head of the bone.

**Duroziez's s.,** see under *murmur.*

**E s.,** reversed three s.

**echo s.,** 1. a percussion sound resembling an echo which is heard over a hydatid cyst. 2. the repetition of the last word or clause of a sentence, seen in certain brain diseases; echolalia.

**Elliot's s.,** 1. induration of the edge of a syphilitic skin lesion. 2. a scotoma extending from the blind spot and made up of numerous points or spots.

**Ely's s.,** see under *test.*

**Enroth's s.,** abnormal fullness of the eyelids, a manifestation of Graves' orbitopathy.

**Erben's s.,** see under *reflex.*

**Erichsen's s.,** when the iliac bones are sharply pressed toward each other pain is felt in sacroiliac disease but not in hip disease.

**Escherich's s.,** in tetany, percussion of the inner surface of the lips or tongue produces contraction of the lips, tongue, and masseter muscles. Called also *Escherich's reflex.*

**Eustace Smith's s.,** Smith's s.

**Ewart's s.,** bronchial breathing and dullness on percussion at the lower angle of the left scapula in pericardial effusion.

**Ewing s.,** tenderness at the upper inner angle of the orbit: a sign of obstruction of the outlet of the frontal sinus.

**external malleolar s.,** Chaddock's reflex.

**fabere s.,** see *Patrick's test,* under *test.*

**facial s.,** Chvostek's s.

**Fajersztajn's crossed sciatic s.,** in sciatica, when the leg is flexed, the hip can also be flexed, but not when the leg is held straight; flexing the sound thigh with the leg held straight causes pain on the affected side.

**fan s.,** spreading apart of the toes following the stroking of the sole of the foot; it forms part of the Babinski reflex.

**fat pad s.,** distention and displacement of the fat adjacent to a joint capsule, usually in the elbow or knee, visible on a radiograph when the joint is flexed; a sign of a fracture within the joint that involves little or no bone displacement.

**Federici's s.,** on auscultation of the abdomen, the cardiac sounds can be heard in cases of intestinal perforation with gas in the peritoneal cavity.

**figure three s.,** a pair of bulges in the wall of the aortic arch, one above and one below the aortic knuckle, seen on a radiograph and signifying coarctation of the aorta. See also *reversed three s.* Called also *three s.*

**Filipovitch's s., Filipowicz's s.,** the yellow discoloration of prominent parts of the palms and soles in typhoid fever; called also *palmoplantar s.*

**flag s.,** dyspigmentation of the hair occurring as a band of light hair, seen in children who have recovered from kwashiorkor.

**floating tooth s.,** on radiographic examination of the mandible, erosion of the bony alveoli around the teeth so that they seem to be floating in space; it occurs in some forms of histiocytosis X.

**flush-tank s.,** the passage of a large amount of urine and the coincident temporary disappearance of a lumbar swelling; a sign of hydronephrosis.

**forearm s.,** Léri's s.

**formication s.,** Tinel's s.

**Fränkel's s.,** excessive range of passive movement of the hip joint, indicating diminished tone of the surrounding musculature in tabes dorsalis.

**Friedreich's s.,** diastolic collapse of the cervical veins due to adherent pericardium.

**Froment's paper s.,** flexion of the distal phalanx of the thumb when a sheet of paper is held between the thumb and index finger; a sign of a lesion of the ulnar nerve.

**Gaenslen's s.,** with the patient in the supine position, the knee and hip of one leg are held in flexed position by the patient, while the other leg, hanging over the edge of the table, is pressed down by the examiner to produce hyperextension of the hip: pain occurs on the affected side in lumbosacral disease.

**Galeazzi s.,** in congenital dislocation of the hip, apparent shortening of the femur, as shown by the difference of knee levels with the knees and hips flexed at right angles with the patient lying on a flat table.

**Gauss' s.,** an increase in uterine mobility seen early in pregnancy.

**Gianelli's s.,** Tournay's s.

**Gilbert's s.,** opsiuria indicative of hepatic cirrhosis.

**Glasgow's s.,** a systolic sound in the brachial artery in latent aneurysm of the aorta.

**Goggia's s.,** in health, the fibrillary contraction produced by striking and then pinching the brachial biceps extends throughout the whole muscle: in debilitating disease, such as typhoid fever, the contraction is local.

**Goldstein's s.,** wide space between the great toe, and the adjoining toe seen in cretinism and Down's syndrome.

**Goldthwait's s.,** the patient lying supine, his leg is raised by the examiner with one hand, the other hand being placed under the patient's lower back; leverage is then applied to the side of the pelvis. If pain is felt by the patient before the lumbar spine is moved, the lesion is a sprain of the sacroiliac joint. If pain does not appear until after the lumbar spine moves, the lesion is in the sacroiliac or lumbosacral articulation.

**Goodell's s.,** softening of the cervix uteri as a sign of pregnancy.

**Gordon's s.,** finger phenomenon (def. 1).

**Gorlin's s.,** the ability to touch the tip of the nose with the tongue, frequently a sign of Ehlers-Danlos syndrome.

**Gottron's s.,** 1. a cutaneous sign pathognomonic of dermatomyositis, consisting of symmetrical macular violaceous erythema, with or without edema, overlying the dorsal aspect of the interphalangeal joints of the hands, olecranon processes, patellas, and medial malleoli. 2. see under *papule.*

**Gowers' s.,** 1. abrupt intermittent oscillation of the iris under the influence of light; seen in certain stages of tabes dorsalis. 2. a sign of pseudohypertrophic muscular dystrophy; to stand from the supine position, the patient rolls to the prone position, kneels, and raises himself to a standing position by pushing with his hands against shins, knees, and thighs. Called also *Gowers' maneuver* or *phenomenon.*

**Graefe's s.,** failure of the upper lid to move downward promptly and evenly with the eyeball in looking downward; instead it moves tardily and jerkingly, a manifestation of Graves' orbitopathy. Called also *Boston's s.* and *von Graefe's s.*

**Grancher's s.,** equality of pitch between expiratory and inspiratory murmurs; a sign of obstruction to expiration.

**Granger's s.,** if in the radiograph of an infant two years old or less, the anterior wall of the lateral sinus is visible, extensive destruction of the mastoid is indicated.

**Grasset's s., Grasset-Bychowski s.,** Grasset's phenomenon.

**Grasset-Gaussel-Hoover s.,** when a recumbent patient with hemiparesis attempts to lift the paretic limb, there is greater downward pressure on the examiner's hand with the sound limb than is observed in the test with a normal person.

**Grey Turner's s.,** Turner's s.

**Griesinger's s.,** edematous swelling behind the mastoid process; seen in thrombosis of the transverse sinus.

**Griffith's s.,** lower lid lag on upward gaze, a manifestation of Graves' orbitopathy.

**Grocco's s.,** 1. see under *triangle.* 2. extension of the liver dullness to the left of the midspinal line, indicating enlargement of the organ.

**Gubler's s.,** see under *tumor.*

**Guilland's s.,** brisk flexion at the hip and knee joint when the contralateral quadriceps muscle is pinched; a sign of meningeal irritation.

**Gunn's s.,** 1. Gunn's crossing s. 2. Marcus Gunn's pupillary phenomenon. 3. see under *syndrome.*

**Gunn's crossing s.,** a crossing of an artery over a vein in the fundus of the eye, indicative of essential hypertension.

**Gunn's pupillary s.,** Marcus Gunn's pupillary phenomenon.

**Guyon's s.,** the ballottement and palpation of a floating kidney.

**Hahn's s.,** persistent rotation of the head from side to side in cerebellar disease of childhood.

**Hall's s.,** a tracheal diastolic shock felt in aneurysm of the aorta.

**halo s.,** a halo effect produced in the radiograph of the fetal head between the subcutaneous fat and the cranium; said to be indicative of intrauterine death of the fetus.

**Hamman's s.,** a precordial crunching, clicking, or knocking sound, synchronous with each heart beat, heard on auscultation in such conditions as acute mediastinitis, pneumomediastinum, and pneumothorax. Called also *Hamman's murmur.*

**harlequin s.,** reddening of the lower half of the laterally recumbent body and blanching of the upper half, due to temporary vasomotor disturbance in newborn infants.

**Hatchcock's s.,** tenderness on running the finger toward the angle of the jaw in mumps.

**Haudek's s.,** a projecting shadow in radiographs of penetrating gastric ulcer, due to settlement of bismuth in pathologic niches of the stomach wall; called also *Haudek's niche.*

**Hawkins s.,** in fractures of the talar neck, a radiolucent zone beneath the subchondral plate of the head of the talus, indicative of disuse osteoporosis; its absence reflects increased risk of talar avascular necrosis.

**Heberden's s's,** see under *node.*

**Hefke-Turner s.,** a widening and change in contour of the normal obturator x-ray shadow, indicative of pathologic condition of the hip joint; called also *obturator s.*

**Hegar's s.,** softening of the lower segment of the uterus, an indication of pregnancy.

**Heilbronner's s.,** see under *thigh.*

**Heim-Kreysig s.,** a depression of the intercostal spaces occurring along with the cardiac systole in adherent pericarditis.

**Helbing's s.,** medialward curving of the Achilles tendon as viewed from behind; seen in flatfoot.

**Hennebert's s.,** rotatory nystagmus when positive or negative pressure is applied to the tympanic membrane, indicative of labyrinthitis with leakage of perilymph; positive pressure (air compression) causes nystagmus toward the affected side, and negative pressure (air rarefaction) causes nystagmus away from the affected side.

**Hennings' s.,** an angular deformity of the angulus of the stomach, in which it assumes a Gothic arch shape; a sign of chronic gastric ulcer. Called also *Gothic arch formation.*

**Higouménaki's s.,** clavicular s.

**Hill's s.,** disproportionate femoral systolic hypertension, seen in aortic regurgitation and certain other conditions involving increased stroke volume.

**Hirschberg's s.,** adduction, inversion, and slight plantar flexion of the foot on stroking the inner aspect (not the sole) of the foot from the great toe to the heel; called also *adductor reflex of foot.*

**Hitzelberger's s.,** anesthesia of medial, posterior, or superior areas of the external auditory canal caused by an acoustic neuroma that is pressing against the facial nerve.

**Hochsinger's s.,** see under *phenomenon.*

**Hoehne's s.,** absence of uterine contractions during delivery despite repeated injections of oxytocics, regarded as a sign of rupture of the uterus.

**Hoffmann's s.,** 1. see under *phenomenon.* 2. in hemiplegia, a sudden nipping of the nail of the index, middle, or ring finger will produce flexion of the terminal phalanx of the thumb and of the second and third phalanges of some other finger; called also *digital reflex* and *Hoffmann's reflex.*

**Holmes' s.,** rebound phenomenon.

**Homans' s.,** pain on passive dorsiflexion of the foot; a sign of thrombosis of deep calf veins.

**Hoover's s.,** 1. in the normal state or in genuine paralysis, if the patient, lying on a flat surface, is directed to press the leg against the surface, there will be a lifting movement in the other leg; this phenomenon is absent in hysteria and malingering. 2. movement of the costal margins toward the midline in inspiration, occurring bilaterally in pulmonary emphysema and unilaterally in conditions causing flattening of the diaphragm, such as pleural effusion and pneumothorax.

**Hope's s.,** double heart beat in aortic aneurysm.

**Horn's s.,** pain produced by traction on the right spermatic cord in acute appendicitis.

**Horner's s.,** Spalding's s.

**Horsley's s.,** if there is a difference in the temperature in the two axillae, the higher temperature will be on the paralyzed side.

**Howship-Romberg s.,** pain passing down the inner side of the thigh to the knee due to pressure on the obturator nerve by an obturator hernia.

**Hoyne's s.,** a sign elicited in paralytic or nonparalytic poliomyelitis: with the patient in the supine position, his head falls back when his shoulders are elevated.

**Hueter's s.,** the absence of the transmission of osseous vibration in cases of fracture with fibrous material interposed between the fragments.

**Huntington's s.,** the patient is recumbent, with his legs hanging over the edge of a table, and is told to cough. If the coughing produces flexion of the thigh and extension of the leg in the paralyzed limb, it indicates that the paralysis is due to an upper motor neuron lesion.

**Hutchinson's s.,** 1. interstitial keratitis and a dull-red discoloration of the cornea in congenital syphilis. 2. see under *tooth.* 3. see under *triad.*

**hyperkinesis s.,** Claude's hyperkinesis s.

**interossei s.,** Souques' phenomenon.

**Jendrassik's s.,** paralysis of the extraocular muscles, one manifestation of Graves' orbitopathy.

**jugular s.,** Queckenstedt's s.

**Kanavel's s.,** a point of maximum tenderness in the palm 1 inch proximal to the base of the little finger in infection of tendon sheath.

**Kantor's s.,** string s. (def. 1).

**Karplus' s.,** a modification of the vocal resonance, in which, on auscultation over a pleural effusion, the vowel *u* spoken by the patient is heard as *a.*

**Keen's s.,** increased diameter of the leg at the malleoli in Pott's fracture of the fibula.

**Kehr's s.,** severe pain in the left shoulder in some cases of rupture of the spleen.

**Kellock's s.,** increase of the vibration of the ribs on sharp percussion with the right hand, the left hand being placed firmly on the thorax under the nipple; a sign of pleural effusion.

**Kelly's s.,** if the ureter is teased with an artery forceps, it will contract like a snake or worm.

**Kerandel's s.,** deep hyperesthesia accompanied by pain, often retarded, after some slight blow upon a bony projection of the body; seen in African trypanosomiasis.

**Kergaradec's s.,** uterine souffle.

**Kernig's s.,** a sign of meningitis: the patient can easily and completely extend the leg when in dorsal decubitus position but not when in the sitting posture or when lying with the thigh flexed upon the abdomen.

**Kerr's s.,** alteration of the texture of the skin below the somatic level in lesions of the spinal cord.

**Kestenbaum's s.,** a decrease in number of arterioles traversing the optic disk margin as a criterion for optic atrophy.

**Kleist's s.,** the fingers of the patient when gently elevated by the fingers of the examiner will hook into the examiner's fingers; indicative of frontal and thalamic lesions.

**Klemm's s.,** in the radiograph in chronic appendicitis, there is often an indication of tympanites in the right lower quadrant.

**Klippel-Weil s.,** flexion and adduction of the thumb when the patient's flexed fingers are quickly extended by the examiner; indicative of pyramidal tract disease.

**Knies' s.,** unequal dilatation of the pupils, one manifestation of Graves' orbitopathy.

**Kocher's s.,** a sign of Graves' orbitopathy: the examiner places one hand on a level with the patient's eyes and then lifts it higher; the patient's upper lid springs up more quickly than the eyeball does.

**Koplik's s.,** see under *spot.*

**Kreysig's s.,** Heim-Kreysig s.

**Krisovski's s., Krisowski's s.,** cicatricial lines radiating from the mouth in congenital syphilis.

**Kussmaul's s.,** 1. distention of the jugular veins on inspiration, seen in constrictive pericarditis and mediastinal tumor. 2. paradoxical pulse.

**Küstner's s.,** a cystic tumor on the median line anterior to the uterus in cases of ovarian dermoids.

**Lafora's s.,** picking of the nose regarded as an early sign of cerebrospinal meningitis.

**Langoria's s.,** relaxation of the extensor muscles of the thigh; a symptom of intracapsular fracture of the femur.

**Lasègue's s.,** in sciatica, flexion of the hip is painful when the knee is extended, but painless when the knee is flexed. This distinguishes the disorder from disease of the hip joint. Cf. *Demianoff's s.*

**Laugier's s.**, a condition in which the styloid process of the radius and of the ulna are on the same level; seen in fracture of the lower part of the radius.

**leg s.**, 1. Schlesinger's s. 2. Neri's s.

**Leichtenstern's s.**, in cerebrospinal meningitis, tapping lightly any bone of the extremities causes the patient to wince suddenly.

**lemon s.**, scalloping of the frontal bones giving the skull a lemon-shaped configuration in axial section in sonography of the fetal skull during the second trimester of pregnancy; a sign of the Arnold-Chiari deformity.

**Lennhoff's s.**, a furrow appearing on deep inspiration below the lowest rib and above an echinococcus cyst of the liver.

**Léri's s.**, passive flexion of the hand and wrist of the affected side in hemiplegia shows no normal flexion at the elbow.

**Leser-Trélat s.**, sudden appearance and rapid increase in size and number of seborrheic keratoses, which may be a sign of internal malignancy, especially of the gastrointestinal tract.

**Lhermitte's s.**, the development of sudden, transient, electric-like shocks spreading down the body when the patient flexes the head forward; seen mainly in multiple sclerosis but also in compression and other disorders of the cervical cord.

**Lichtheim's s.**, in some types of motor aphasia the patient cannot speak but can indicate with fingers the number of syllables in a word being thought of. Called also *Dejerine-Lichtheim phenomenon.*

**ligature s.**, in hematuria, the development of ecchymoses in the distal part of a limb to which a ligature has been applied.

**Linder's s.**, with the patient recumbent or sitting with outstretched legs, passive flexion of the head will cause pain in the leg or the lumbar region in sciatica.

**Livierato's s.**, vasoconstriction when the abdominal sympathetic nerve is irritated by striking the anterior abdomen along the xiphoumbilical line.

**Lloyd's s.**, a symptom of renal calculus, consisting of pain in the loin on deep percussion over the kidney, even when pressure causes no pain.

**Lucas' s.**, distention of the abdomen in the early stages of rickets.

**Ludloff's s.**, swelling and ecchymosis at the base of Scarpa's triangle together with inability to raise the thigh when in a sitting posture, a sign of traumatic separation of the epiphysis of the greater trochanter.

**Lust's s.**, see under *phenomenon.*

**McBurney's s.**, tenderness at a point two-thirds the distance from the umbilicus to the anterior superior spine of the ilium; indicative of appendicitis. See also under *point.*

**Macewen's s.**, on percussion of the skull behind the junction of the frontal, temporal, and parietal bones, there is a more resonant note than normal in internal hydrocephalus and cerebral abscess. Called also *cracked-pot sound* and *cranial cracked-pot sound.*

**McGinn-White s.**, a Q wave and late inversion of the T wave in lead III, low ST intervals and T waves in lead II, and inverted T waves in chest leads $V_2$ and $V_3$, the electrocardiographic evidence of right ventricular dilatation due to massive pulmonary embolism, plus the clinical signs of acute cor pulmonale.

**McMurray s.**, see under *test.*

**Magendie's s., Magendie-Hertwig s.**, skew deviation.

**Magnan's s.**, formication.

**Mahler's s.**, a steady increase of pulse rate without corresponding elevation of temperature; seen in thrombosis.

**Maisonneuve's s.**, marked hyperextensibility of the hand; a symptom of Colles' fracture.

**Mann's s.**, with Graves' orbitopathy, the two eyes appear not to be on the same level. Called also *Dixon Mann's s.*

**Mannkopf's s.**, increase in the frequency of the pulse on pressure over a painful spot; not present in simulated pain.

**Marcus Gunn's pupillary s.**, see under *phenomenon.*

**Marfan's s.**, a red triangle at the tip of a coated tongue indicates typhoid fever; a rarely observed phenomenon.

**Marie's s.**, tremor of the body or extremities in Graves' disease and other types of hyperthyroidism.

**Marie-Foix s.**, withdrawal of lower leg on transverse pressure of tarsus or forced flexion of toes when the leg is incapable of voluntary movement.

**Marinesco's s.**, Marinesco's succulent hand; see under *hand.*

**Mean's s.**, Kocher's s.

**Meltzer's s.**, loss of the normal second sound, heard on auscultation of the heart after swallowing; symptomatic of occlusion or contraction of the lower part of the esophagus.

**Mendel-Bekhterev s.**, see under *reflex.*

**meniscus s.**, the radioscopic appearance of a crescentic shadow made by the crater of a gastric ulcer: when the convexity of the crescent points outward the ulcer is on the lesser curvature; when the convexity points downward the ulcer is distal to the angular incisure. Called also *Carman's s., Carman-Kirklin s.,* and *crescent s.*

**Mennell's s.**, an examining thumb is placed over the posterosuperior spine of the sacrum and then made to slide, first outward and then inward. If on pressure over the former point tenderness is detected, it is due to a sensitive deposit in the structures of the gluteal aspect of the posterosuperior spine. If the tenderness is over the inner point, it is probable that the superior ligaments of the sacroiliac joint are strained and sensitive. If the tenderness is increased by pressure backward on the anterosuperior aspect of the ilium and decreased by pulling forward the crest from behind, this is positive proof that it is caused by the sensitive ligaments.

**Mercedes-Benz s.**, shadows shaped like the logo of the Mercedes-Benz automobile, seen on radiographs of the gallbladder; they indicate the presence of gas-filled fissures within gallstones, although the gallstones themselves may not be visible.

**Mexican hat s.**, a shadow resembling a large-brimmed Mexican hat, seen on a radiograph of the colon; it represents the filling defect caused by a pedunculated polyp on the inferior wall.

**Minor's s.**, the method of rising from a sitting position characteristic of the patient with sciatica; he supports himself on the healthy side, placing one hand on the back, bending the affected leg and balancing on the healthy leg.

**Mirchamp's s.**, when a sapid substance, such as vinegar, is applied to the mucous membrane of the tongue, a painful reflex secretion of saliva in the gland about to be affected is indicative of sialadenitis, e.g., mumps.

**Möbius' s., Moebius' s.**, inability to keep the eyeballs converged due to insufficiency of the internal rectus muscles; a manifestation of Graves' orbitopathy.

**Morquio's s.**, the patient lying supine resists all attempts to raise the trunk to a sitting posture until the legs are passively flexed; noticed in epidemic poliomyelitis.

**Moschcowitz's s.**, see under *test.*

**Mosler's s.**, sternal tenderness in acute myeloblastic leukemia.

**moulage s.**, a waxy cast appearance of bowel segments, a radiographic sign of celiac disease.

**Müller's s.**, a sign of aortic insufficiency consisting of pulsation of the uvula and redness of the tonsils and velum palati, occurring synchronously with the action of the heart.

**Munson's s.**, abnormal bulging of the lower lid when the patient rolls his eyes downward, caused by abnormal curvature of the cornea (keratoconus).

**Murphy's s.**, a sign of gallbladder disease consisting of interruption of the patient's deep inspiration when the physician's fingers are pressed deeply beneath the right costal arch, below the hepatic margin.

**Musset's s.**, rhythmical jerking movement of the head; seen in cases of aortic aneurysm and aortic insufficiency.

**Myerson's s.**, ready induction of blepharospasm when the frontalis muscle is tapped, a sign of Parkinson's disease.

**neck s.**, Brudzinski's s. (def. 1).

**Negro's s.**, cogwheel rigidity.

**Neri's s.**, 1. a sign of organic hemiplegia, consisting in the spontaneous bending of the knee of the affected side as the leg is passively lifted, the patient being in the dorsal position. 2. with the patient standing, forward bending of the trunk will cause flexion of the knee on the affected side in lumbosacral and iliosacral lesions.

**niche s.**, Haudek's s.

**Nicoladoni's s.**, Branham's s.

**Nikolsky's s.**, ready separation of the outer layer of the epidermis from the basal layer with sloughing of the skin produced by minor trauma, such as by exerting a sliding or rubbing pressure on the area involved, which may occur in pemphigus and in other conditions such as certain hereditary blistering skin diseases, scalded skin syndrome, adult toxic epidermal necrolysis, and thermal burns.

**Ober's s.**, see under *test.*

**objective s.**, one that can be seen, heard, or felt by the diagnostician; called also *physical s.*

**obturator s.**, 1. hypogastric or adductor pain elicited by passive internal rotation of the flexed thigh, due to contact between an inflammatory process and the internal obturator muscle; a sign of appendicitis. 2. Hefke-Turner s.

**Oliver's s.**, tracheal tugging; see under *tugging.*

**Oppenheim's s.**, see under *reflex.*

**orbicularis s.**, in hemiplegia, inability to close the eye on the paralyzed side without closing the other.

**Ortolani's s.**, the presence of a palpable click in and out as the hip is reduced by abduction and dislocated by adduction in congenital dislocation of the hip; called also *Ortolani's click.*

**Osler's s.**, small, painful, erythematous swellings (Osler's nodes) in the skin of the hands and feet, pathognomonic of subacute bacterial endocarditis.

**palmoplantar s.**, Filipovitch's s.

**Parkinson's s.**, see under *facies.*
**Parrot's s.**, 1. ciliospinal reflex. 2. bony nodes on the outer table of the skull of infants with congenital syphilis, so that it has a hot cross bun or buttock shape; called also *Parrot's nodes, hot cross bun skull,* and *natiform skull.*
**Pastia's s.**, see under *line.*
**patent bronchus s.**, the radiologic finding of an unobstructed bronchus supplying a collapsed lung, lobe, or segment.
**Patrick's s.**, see under *test.*
**Pende's s.**, André Thomas s.
**Perez's s.**, a friction sound heard over the sternum when the patient raises and drops his arms; a sign of mediastinal tumor or of aneurysm of the arch of the aorta.
**peroneal s.**, Lust's phenomenon.
**Pfuhl's s.**, inspiration increases the force of flow in paracentesis in the case of subphrenic abscess, but lessens it in the case of pyopneumothorax. This distinction is lost when the diaphragm is paralyzed.
**physical s.**, objective s.
**Piltz's s.**, 1. attention reflex of pupil; see under *reflex.* 2. orbicularis pupillary reflex.
**Pins' s.**, Ewart's s.
**Piotrowski's s.**, percussion of the anterior tibialis muscle produces dorsal flexion and supination of the foot. When this reflex is excessive it indicates organic disease of the central nervous system. Called also *anticus s.* or *reflex.*
**Piskacek's s.**, asymmetrical enlargement of the corpus uteri due to enlargement of the pregnant uterus in the cornual region, usually over the site of implantation.
**Pitres' s.**, hypoesthesia of the scrotum and testes in tabes dorsalis.
**pivot shift s.**, see under *phenomenon.*
**placental s.**, implantation bleeding.
**Plummer's s.**, inability to step up onto a chair or to walk up steps, seen in Graves' disease and other forms of hyperthyroidism.
**Pool-Schlesinger s.**, Schlesinger's s.
**Porter's s.**, tracheal tugging; see under *tugging.*
**posterior drawer s.**, see under *test.*
**Potain's s.**, 1. extension of percussion dullness over the arch of the aorta, in dilatation of the aorta, from the manubrium to the third costal cartilage on the right-hand side. 2. timbre métallique.
**Prehn's s.**, elevation and support of the scrotum will relieve the pain in epididymo-orchitis, but not in torsion of the testicle.
**Prévost's s.**, conjugate deviation of the head and eyes, the eyes looking toward the affected hemisphere and away from the palsied extremities; seen in hemiplegia.
**pronation s.**, 1. Babinski's s. (def. 5). 2. pronation of the forearm caused by passive flexion, seen in hemiplegia; called also *Strümpell's s.*
**pseudo-Babinski's s.**, in poliomyelitis the Babinski reflex is modified so that only the big toe is extended, because all the foot muscles except the dorsiflexors of the big toe are paralyzed.
**pseudo-Graefe's s.**, slow descent of the upper lid on looking down, and quick ascent on looking up; seen in conditions other than Graves' disease.
**psoas s.**, flexion of or pain on hyperextension of the hip due to contact between an inflammatory process and the psoas muscle; a sign often seen in appendicitis. Called also *Cope's s.*
**puddle s.**, in examination for ascites, a method for detecting free fluid in the abdominal cavity. The patient lies prone for five minutes, then rises to his hands and knees. While the examiner lightly flicks a finger against one flank, a Bowles stethoscope is moved slowly from the most dependent part of the abdomen to the flank. That part of the ventral abdomen containing the fluid "puddle" shows a loss of high-frequency vibration, which will be detected as soon as the edge of the fluid is reached, indicating the amount of fluid.
**pyramid s., pyramidal s.**, any sign pointing to disease of the pyramidal tract.
**Quant's s.**, a T-shaped depression in the occipital bone, sometimes seen in rickets.
**Queckenstedt's s.**, when the veins in the neck are compressed on one or both sides, in healthy persons there is a rapid rise in the pressure of the cerebrospinal fluid, which returns quickly to normal when pressure is taken off the neck. When there is a block in the vertebral canal the pressure of the cerebrospinal fluid is affected little or not at all by this maneuver. Called also *Queckenstedt's phenomenon* or *test.*
**Quénu-Muret s.**, in aneurysm, the main artery of the limb is compressed and then a puncture is made at the periphery; if blood flows, the collateral circulation is probably established.
**Quincke's s.**, see under *pulse.*
**radialis s.**, inability to close the fist without marked dorsal extension of the wrist, seen in hemiplegia; called also *Strümpell's s.*
**Radovici's s.**, palm-chin reflex.
**Ramond's s.**, rigidity of the erector spinae muscle indicative of pleurisy with effusion; the rigidity relaxes when the effusion becomes purulent.
**Raynaud's s.**, acrocyanosis.
**Remak's s.**, see under *symptom.*
**reservoir s.**, the ability of a patient to produce cerebrospinal fluid rhinorrhea at will by moving the head, indicating presence of a fistula with pooling in a paranasal sinus.
**reversed three s.**, a pair of indentations, one on either side of the aortic knuckle, seen on barium contrast imaging of the esophagus and representing mirror images of a figure three sign; it signifies coarctation of the aorta. Called also *E s.*
**Revilliod's s.**, orbicularis s.
**Riesman's s.**, 1. Snellen's s. 2. softening of the eyeball in diabetic coma.
**Robertson's s.**, 1. fibrillary contraction of the pectoralis muscle over the cardiac area in approaching death from heart disease. 2. absence of pupillary dilatation on pressure over alleged painful areas in malingering. 3. in ascites, fullness and tension in the patient's flanks, felt by the examiner with the patient supine.
**Rocher's s.**, in torsion of the testis, the epididymis cannot be distinguished from the body of the testis, whereas in epididymitis the body of the testis can be felt in the enlarged crescent of the epididymis.
**Romaña's s.**, unilateral ophthalmia with palpebral edema, conjunctivitis, and swelling of regional lymph glands as a sign of Chagas' disease.
**Romberg's s.**, swaying of the body or falling when standing with the feet close together and the eyes closed; the result of loss of joint position sense, seen in tabes dorsalis and other diseases affecting the posterior columns. Called also *rombergism, Brauch-Romberg symptom,* and *Romberg-Howship symptom;* see also *Romberg test,* under *test.*
**Rommelaere's s.**, an abnormally small proportion of normal phosphates and of sodium chloride in the urine in cancerous cachexia.
**rope s.**, acute angulation between chin and larynx, due to weakness of hyoid muscles, noted in bulbar poliomyelitis.
**Rosenbach's s.**, 1. absence of the abdominal skin reflex in inflammatory disease of the intestines. 2. absence of the abdominal skin reflex in pinching the skin of the abdomen on the paralyzed side in hemiplegia.
**Rossolimo's s.**, see under *reflex.*
**Rotch's s.**, dullness on percussion of the right fifth intercostal space, a sign of pericardial effusion.
**Rovighi's s.**, a fremitus felt on percussion and palpation of a superficial hepatic hydatid cyst.
**Rovsing's s.**, pressure on the left side over the point corresponding to McBurney's point will elicit the typical pain at McBurney's point in appendicitis.
**Ruggeri's s.**, see under *reflex.*
**Rumpel-Leede s.**, see under *phenomenon.*
**Rust's s.**, see under *phenomenon.*
**Saenger's s.**, a light reflex of the pupil that has ceased returns after a short stay in the dark; observed in cerebral syphilis but not in tabes dorsalis.
**Sansom's s.**, 1. marked increase of the area of dullness in the second and third intercostal spaces, due to pericardial effusion. 2. a rhythmical murmur heard with a stethoscope applied to the lips in aneurysm of the thoracic aorta.
**Saunders' s.**, on wide opening of the mouth there take place in children associated movements of the hand consisting of opening of the hand and extension and separation of the fingers; called also *mouth-and-hand synkinesia.*
**Schepelmann's s.**, in dry pleurisy, the pain is increased when the patient bends his body toward the normal side, whereas in intercostal neuralgia it is increased by bending toward the affected side.
**Schick's s.**, stridor heard on expiration in an infant with tuberculosis involving the bronchial glands.
**Schlesinger's s.**, in tetany, if the patient's leg is held at the knee joint and flexed strongly at the hip joint, there will follow within a short time an extensor spasm at the knee joint, with extreme supination of the foot. Called also *Pool's* or *Schlesinger's phenomenon.*
**Schultze's s., Schultze-Chvostek s.**, Chvostek's s.
**Schwartze's s.**, a pink blush behind the tympanic membrane, sometimes seen in otosclerosis because of hyperemia of the mucous membrane around the promontory.
**scimitar s.**, on a radiograph of the chest, a scimitar-shaped shadow to the right of the lower border of the heart, representing the anomalous vein of the scimitar syndrome.
**Séguin's s.**, Séguin's signal symptom; see under *symptom.*
**Seidel's s.**, see under *scotoma.*
**setting-sun s.**, downward deviation of the eyes, so that each iris appears to "set" beneath the lower lid, with white sclera exposed between it and the upper lid; indicative of intracranial pressure (hemorrhage or meningoependymitis), hydrocephalus, or pineal tumor.
**Shibley's s.**, in the presence of consolidation of the lung or a collection of fluid in the pleural cavity, all spoken vowels are heard through the stethoscope as "ah."

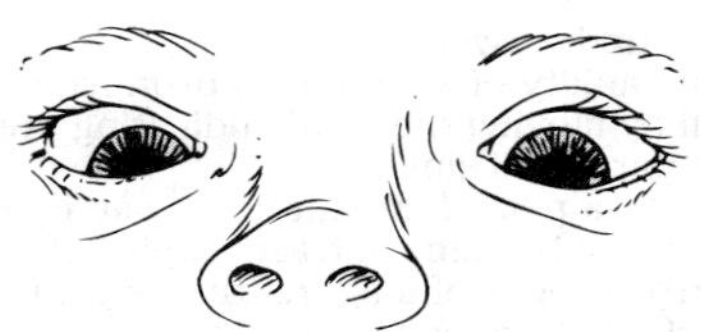

Setting-sun sign.

**Siegert's s.,** in Down's syndrome, the little fingers are short and curved inward.

**Silex's s.,** furrows radiating from the mouth in congenital syphilis.

**Simon's s.,** 1. [C. E. *Simon*] retraction or fixation of the umbilicus during inspiration. 2. [J. *Simon*] absence of the usual correlation between the movements of the diaphragm and thorax; seen in beginning meningitis.

**Sisto's s.,** constant crying as a sign of congenital syphilis in infancy.

**Skoda's s.,** skodaic resonance.

**Smith's s.,** a murmur heard in cases of enlarged bronchial glands on auscultation over the manubrium with the patient's head thrown back.

**Snellen's s.,** the bruit heard with a stethoscope over the closed eye in Graves' disease; see also *Graves' orbitopathy,* under *orbitopathy.*

**Soto-Hall s.,** with the patient flat on his back, on flexion of the spine beginning at the neck and going downward, pain will be felt at the site of the lesion in back abnormalities.

**Souques' s.,** 1. when the patient seated in a chair is suddenly thrown back, the lower extremities do not extend normally or otherwise attempt to counteract the loss of balance; it indicates advanced striatal disease. 2. see under *phenomenon.*

**Spalding's s.,** in the x-ray film of the fetus in utero, overriding of the bones of the vault of the skull indicates death of the fetus.

**spinal s.,** tonic contraction of the spinal muscles on the diseased side in pleurisy.

**spine s.,** disinclination to flex the spine anteriorly on account of pain; seen in poliomyelitis.

**square root s.,** in constrictive pericarditis, the diastolic level of the right ventricular pressure curve is initially normal but rapidly rises abnormally.

**stairs s.,** difficulty in descending a stairway in tabes dorsalis.

**Stellwag's s.,** a sign of Graves' orbitopathy: infrequent and incomplete blinking accompanied by Dalrymple's sign (retraction of the upper eyelids producing apparent widening of the palpebral opening).

**Sternberg's s.,** sensitiveness to palpation of the muscles of the shoulder girdle in pleurisy.

**Stewart-Holmes s.,** rebound phenomenon.

**Stierlin's s.,** absence of the normal shadow on a radiographic image of the colon after a barium enema, due to an indurating or ulcerating process such as tuberculosis of the cecum or colon.

**Strauss' s.,** increase of fat following the use of fatty foods in chylous ascites.

**string s.,** 1. in radiography of the colon, a stringlike configuration of contrast material through a filling defect; called also *Kantor's s.* 2. the stringing out of tubules, observed on pulling the tissues of an intact testis or one in which there is active spermatogenesis, a phenomenon which is prevented by the fibrosis and hyalinization about the tubules when the testis is atrophic.

**string of beads s.,** a series of round shadows resembling a string of beads or pearls, seen on a radiograph of the small intestine, indicating bubbles of trapped gas surrounded by the fluid of an obstructed and distended bowel.

**Strümpell's s.,** 1. tibialis s. 2. radialis s. 3. pronation s. (def. 2).

**Strunsky's s.,** a sign for detecting lesions of the anterior arch of the foot. The examiner grasps the toes and flexes them suddenly. This procedure is painless in the normal foot, but causes pain if there is inflammation of the anterior arch.

**Suker's s.,** deficient complementary fixation in lateral eye rotation, one manifestation of Graves' orbitopathy.

**Sumner's s.,** on gentle palpation of the iliac fossa, a slight increase in tonus of the abdominal muscles may indicate appendicitis, stone in the ureter or kidney, or a twisted pedicle of an ovarian cyst.

**swinging flashlight s.,** Marcus Gunn's pupillary phenomenon.

**Tay's s.,** see *cherry-red spot,* under *spot.*

**Theimich's lip s.,** a protrusion or pouting of the lips elicited by tapping the orbicularis oris muscle.

**Thomas' s.,** 1. [Hugh Owen *Thomas*] the flexion deformity seen in a hip in the Thomas test. 2. [André *Thomas*] André Thomas s.

**Thomson's s.,** Pastia's lines.

**Thornton's s.,** severe pain in the region of the flanks in nephrolithiasis.

**three s.,** figure three s.

**Throckmorton's s.,** see under *reflex.*

**tibialis s.,** dorsal flexion of the foot when the thigh is drawn up toward the body; seen in spastic paralysis of the lower limb. Called also *Strümpell's s.* or *phenomenon* and *anterior tibial s.*

**Tinel's s.,** a tingling sensation in the distal end of a limb when percussion is made over the site of a divided nerve. It indicates a partial lesion or the beginning regeneration of the nerve. Called also *DTP s., formication s.,* and *distal tingling on percussion.*

**toe s.,** Babinski's reflex.

**Tournay's s.,** unilateral dilatation of the pupil of the abducting eye on extreme lateral fixation.

**Traube's s.,** a loud sound like a pistol shot heard in auscultation over the femoral arteries in aortic regurgitation. Called also *pistol-shot sound.*

**Trendelenburg's s.,** Trendelenburg's test (def. 2).

**trepidation s.,** patellar clonus.

**Tresilian's s.,** a reddish appearance in Stensen's duct in mumps.

**Trimadeau's s.,** if the dilatation above an esophageal stricture is conic, the stricture is fibrous; if cup shaped, the stricture is malignant.

**Troisier's s.,** signal node.

**Trousseau's s.,** 1. see under *phenomenon.* 2. tache cérébrale.

**Turner's s.,** discoloration (bruising) and induration of the skin of the costovertebral angle caused by extravasation of blood in acute hemorrhagic pancreatitis.

**Turyn's s.,** in sciatica, if the patient's great toe is bent dorsally, pain will be felt in the gluteal region.

**twin peak s.,** a sonographic sign of dichorionic twinning consisting of a triangular zone whose echotexture is similar to that of the placenta, wider at the chorionic surface of the placenta and tapering to a point within the intertwin membrane.

**Unschuld's s.,** a tendency to cramp in the calves of the legs; a nonspecific early indication of diabetes.

**Vanzetti's s.,** in sciatica the pelvis is always horizontal in spite of scoliosis, but in other lesions with scoliosis the pelvis is inclined.

**vein s.,** a bluish cord along the midaxillary line formed by the swollen junction of the thoracic and superficial epigastric vein; seen in tuberculosis involving the bronchial glands and in superior vena cava obstruction.

**vital s's,** the pulse, respiration, and temperature.

**von Graefe's s.,** Graefe's s.

**Wartenberg's s.,** 1. a sign of ulnar palsy, consisting of a position of abduction assumed by the little finger. 2. reduction or absence of the pendulum movements of the arm in walking; seen in patients with cerebellar disease.

**Weber's s.,** see under *syndrome.*

**Wegner's s.,** a broadened, discolored appearance of the epiphyseal line in infants who have died from congenital syphilis.

**Weill's s.,** absence of expansion in the subclavicular region of the affected side in infantile pneumonia.

**Wernicke's s.,** hemiopic pupillary reaction.

**Westermark's s.,** transient clearing (avascularity) of the normal radiologic shadow of pulmonary tissue distal to a pulmonary embolism.

**Westphal's s.,** loss of the knee jerk in tabes dorsalis.

**Widowitz's s.,** protrusion of the eyeballs and sluggish movements of the eyeballs and eyelids seen in diphtheritic paralysis.

**Wilder's s.,** an early sign of Graves' orbitopathy, consisting of a slight twitch of the eyeball when it changes its movement from adduction to abduction or vice versa.

**Williamson's s.,** markedly diminished blood pressure in the leg as compared with that in the arm on the same side; seen in pneumothorax and pleural effusion.

**Wimberger's s.,** symmetrical erosions of the proximal tibia seen radiographically in infants with congenital syphilis.

**Winterbottom's s.,** enlargement of posterior cervical lymph nodes in African trypanosomiasis.

**Wood's s.,** relaxation of the orbicularis muscle, fixation of the eyeball, and divergent strabismus, indicative of profound anesthesia.

**sig·na** (sig'nə) [L.] mark, or write; abbreviated S. or sig. on prescriptions. See *prescription.*

**sig·na·ture** (sig'nə-chər) [L. *signatura*] 1. that part of a prescription which gives directions to the patient for taking of medicine; abbreviated S. or sig. See *prescription.* 2. any characteristic feature of a substance formerly regarded as an indication of its medicinal virtues: thus, the eyelike mark on the flower of the euphrasia was supposed to show its usefulness in eye diseases; the liver-like shape of the leaf of liverwort pointed to its use in hepatic diseases; the yellow color of saffron indicated its use in jaundice.

**sig·nif·i·cant** (sig-nif'ĭ-kənt) in statistics, probably resulting from something other than chance.

**sign·ing** (sīn'ing) dactylology.

**Sig. n. pro.** abbreviation for L. *sig'na nom'ine pro'prio,* label with the proper name.

**sig·ua·te·ra** (sig"wə-ta'rə) [Sp.] ciguatera.

**si·ki·mi** (se'ke-me) [Japanese] *Illicium religiosum.*

**sik·i·min** (sik'ĭ-min) a poisonous hydrocarbon found in the leaves of *Illicium religiosum.* Called also *shikimene.*

**sik·im·i·tox·in** (sik-im"ĭ-tok'sin) a poisonous substance found in *Illicium religiosum* (sikimi).

**sil·a·fil·con A** (sil"ə-fil'kon) a hydrophilic contact lens material.

**sil·a·fo·con A** (sil"ə-fo'kon) a hydrophobic contact lens material.

**Si·lain** (si'lān) trademark for preparations of simethicone.

**Si·las·tic** (sĭ-las'tik) trademark for polymeric silicone substances that have the properties of rubber but are biologically inert; used in surgical prostheses.

**sil·den·a·fil cit·rate** (sil-den'ə-fil") a phosphodiesterase inhibitor that relaxes the smooth muscle of the penis, thereby facilitating blood flow to the corpus cavernosum; used to treat erectile dysfunction in impotence therapy.

**si·lence** (si'lens) [L. *silēre* to be quiet] a state of being silent.
**electrical s.,** in electroencephalography and electromyography, absence of measurable electrical activity in tissue.
**electrocerebral s. (ECS),** electrical silence in the cerebral cortex. Temporary silence may occur with overdoses of depressant drugs such as barbiturates and benzodiazepines, with hypothermia, or with cardiogenic shock. Permanent silence is one of the criteria for a diagnosis of brain death. Called also *electrocerebral inactivity.*

**si·lent** (si'lənt) 1. noiseless. 2. producing no detectable signs or symptoms.

**Si·lex's sign** (se'leks-əz) [Paul *Silex,* German ophthalmologist, 1858–1929] see under *sign.*

**si·lex** (si'leks) [L. "flint"] a refined form of silica powder, which may be mixed with water or a mouthwash solution to form a fine abrasive paste for polishing metal castings.

**Silf·ver·skiöld's syndrome** (sil'vər-sherldz) [Nils G. *Silfverskiöld,* Swedish orthopedist, 1888–1957] see under *syndrome.*

**sil·hou·ette** (sil"ə-wet') [Fr.] the outline or contour of a thing.
**cardiac s.,** the contour of the heart appearing on radiographs of the chest.
**cardiopericardial s.,** the contour of the heart and pericardium appearing on radiographs of the chest.
**cardiovascular s.,** the contour of the heart and great vessels appearing on radiographs of the chest.

**sil·i·ca** (sil'ĭ-kə) [L. *silex* flint] $SiO_2$, silicon dioxide or silicic anhydride, occurring in nature as agate, sand, amethyst, chalcedony, cristobalite, flint, quartz, and tridymite. It is one of the major constituents of dental porcelain and a common filler in resin composites; in granular form it serves as a dental abrasive and polishing agent. See also *silicosis.*

**sil·i·cate** (sil'ĭ-kāt) [L. *silicus*] a salt of any of the silicic acids.

**sil·i·ca·to·sis** (sil"ĭ-kə-to'sis) pneumoconiosis caused by the inhalation of the dust of silicates, particularly aluminum silicate and magnesium silicate (e.g., asbestos, fuller's earth, kaolin, mica, or talc). See *asbestosis,* and see other types under *pneumoconiosis.*

**si·lic·ea** (sĭ-lis'e-ə) a homeopathic preparation of silica.

**si·li·ceous, si·li·cious** (sĭ-lish'əs) containing silica or a compound of silicon.

**si·lic·ic ac·id** (sĭ-lik'ik) [MeSH: Silicic Acid] the molecular species $Si(OH)_4$ occurring in hydrated forms of silica, e.g., silica gel.

**sil·i·co·an·thra·co·sis** (sil"ĭ-ko-an"thrə-ko'sis) anthracosilicosis.

**sil·i·co·flu·o·ride** (sil"ĭ-ko-floor'īd) fluorosilicate.

**sil·i·con** (sil'ĭ-kon) [L. *silex* flint] [MeSH: Silicon] a nonmetallic element occurring in nature as silica (s. *dioxide);* symbol, Si; atomic number, 14; atomic weight, 28.086.
**s. carbide,** a compound produced by the reaction of silicon and carbon at extremely high temperature; it ranks next to diamond in hardness and is used in dentistry as an abrasive and refractory.
**s. dioxide,** silica.
**s. dioxide, colloidal** [NF], a submicroscopic fumed silica prepared by the vapor-phase hydrolysis of a silicon compound; used as a tablet diluent and as a suspending and thickening agent.
**s. fluoride,** $SiF_4$, a colorless gas sometimes fatal to workers in superphosphate factories.

**sil·i·cone** (sil'ĭ-kōn) any of a large group of organic compounds comprising alternating silicon and oxygen atoms linked to organic radicals; uses have included wetting agents and surfactants, sealants, coolants, surgical membranes, implants, and dental impression materials.

**sil·i·co·pro·tein·o·sis** (sil"ĭ-ko-pro"tēn-o'sis) a rapidly fatal pneumoconiosis occurring several weeks to months after massive exposure to silica dust, characterized by the presence of proteinaceous fluid in the air spaces.

**sil·i·co·sid·er·o·sis** (sil"ĭ-ko-sid"ər-o'sis) siderosilicosis.

**sil·i·co·sis** (sil"ĭ-ko'sis) [*silica* + *-osis*] [MeSH: Silicosis] pneumoconiosis due to the inhalation of the dust of stone, sand, or flint containing silica, with formation of generalized nodular fibrotic changes in both lungs. Since many common minerals contain silica, there are numerous different types of silicosis. Called also *pneumosilicosis* and *grinders' disease.*
**infective s.,** silicotuberculosis.

**Sil·i·cote** (sil'ĭ-kōt) trademark for preparations of dimethicone.

**sil·i·cot·ic** (sil"ĭ-kot'ik) pertaining to or characterized by silicosis.

**sil·i·co·tu·ber·cu·lo·sis** (sil"ĭ-ko-too-ber"ku-lo'sis) [MeSH: Silicotuberculosis] tuberculous infection of the silicotic lung; called also *infective silicosis* and *tuberculosilicosis.*

**sil·i·qua** (sil'ĭ-kwə) [L.] a pod, or husk.
**s. oli'vae,** amiculum olivare.

**sil·i·quose** (sil'ĭ-kwōs) pertaining to or resembling a pod or husk.

**silk** (silk) the protein filament produced by the larvae of various insects; braided, degummed silk obtained from the cocoons of the silkworm *Bombyx mori* is used as a nonabsorbable suture material.
**virgin s.,** silk from which the adhesive protein sericin has not been removed; used as a suture material in ophthalmic microsurgery.

**silk·worm** (silk'wərm) [MeSH: Silkworms] the larva of *Bombyx mori.*

**si·lox·ane** (si-lok'sān) any of a group of silica-based polymers occurring as greases, resins, oily liquids, plastics, and artifical rubber; see also *polysiloxane.*

**Sil·va·dene** (sil'və-dēn) trademark for a preparation of silver sulfadiazine.

**Sil·ver's syndrome** (sil'vərz) [Henry K. *Silver,* American pediatrician, born 1918] Silver-Russell syndrome.

**Sil·ver-Rus·sell syndrome (dwarfism)** (sil'vər-rus'əl) [H.K. *Silver;* Alexander *Russell,* British pediatrician, 20th century] see under *syndrome.*

**sil·ver** (sil'vər) [L. *argentum*] [MeSH: Silver] a white, soft, malleable, and ductile metal; symbol, Ag; atomic number, 47; atomic weight, 107.870. Its compounds are extensively used in medicine and in x-ray and photographic films; metallic silver is used in surgery and in the manufacture of instruments. In dentistry, it is used chiefly in prostheses, in alloys such as amalgam, in soldering, to neutralize the color imparted by copper in alloys, and as points to obliterate the root canal.
**s. chloride,** an insoluble white salt, AgCl, that darkens in light.
**colloidal s.,** a silver preparation in which the silver exists as free ions to only a small extent. See *mild protein s.,* and *strong protein s.*
**s. iodide, colloidal,** silver iodide in solution rendered stable by gelatin, an antiseptic for treating inflammations of mucous membranes.
**methenamine s.,** see under *methenamine.*
**mild s. protein,** a preparation containing 19–23 per cent of silver, rendered colloidal by the presence of, or combination with, protein; it is used as a topical anti-infective in various rectal, ocular, vaginal, urethral, otic, nasal, and pharyngeal infections.
**s. nitrate** [USP], a powerful germicide, $AgNO_3$, used as an antiseptic, applied topically to the conjunctiva as a prophylactic against ophthalmia neonatorum, and also used as an antiseptic and astringent, especially in infections of the skin and mucous membranes. It has also been used to purify drinking water.
**s. nitrate, fused, s. nitrate, molded,** toughened s. nitrate.
**s. nitrate, toughened** [USP], a compound prepared by fusing silver nitrate with hydrochloric acid, sodium chloride, or potassium nitrate, occurring as white crystalline masses molded into pencils or cones, and containing 94.5 per cent of silver nitrate; used as a caus-

tic and applied topically after being dipped in water. Called also *lunar caustic, fused silver nitrate,* and *molded silver nitrate.*
**strong s. protein,** a compound of silver and protein containing 7.5–8.5 per cent of silver; an active germicide with a local irritant and astringent effect. It may cause argyria.
**s. sulfadiazine** [USP], the silver derivative of sulfadiazine, having bactericidal activity against many gram-positive and gram-negative organisms, as well as being effective against yeasts; used as a topical anti-infective for the prevention and treatment of wound sepsis in patients with second- and third-degree burns.

**Sil·ver·man's needle** (sil'vər-mənz) [Irving *Silverman,* American surgeon, born 1904] see under *needle.*

**Sil·ver·man's syndrome** (sil'vər-mənz) [Frederic Noah *Silverman,* American pediatrician, born 1914] Currarino-Silverman syndrome.

**Sil·ves·tri·ni-Cor·da syndrome** (sil-vəs-tre'ne-kor'də) [R. *Silvestrini,* Italian physician, 20th century; L. *Corda,* Italian physician, 20th century] see under *syndrome.*

**Sil·vi·us** (sil've-əs) a genus of Australian biting flies of the family Tabanidae.

**Si·ly·bum** (sil'ĭ-bəm) a genus of thistles, including *S. maria'num,* the milk thistle.

**Sim·a·ru·ba** (sim"ə-roo'bə) a genus of tropical American trees of the family Simaroubaceae; several species are medicinal. The root bark of *S. ama'ra* Aubl. is a bitter tonic and astringent, and has been used in amebiasis; its active principle is simarubidin.

**sim·a·ru·bi·din** (sim"ə-roo'bĭ-din) the active principle of the bark and wood of *Simaruba amara;* used experimentally in canine amebiasis.

**si·ma·zine** (si'mə-zēn) [MeSH: Simazine] an herbicide used in gardens; it is toxic to ruminants, causing liver and kidney damage and neurotoxicity that can be fatal.

**si·meth·i·cone** (sĭ-meth'ĭ-kōn) [MeSH: Simethicone] a mixture of dimethicones and silicon dioxide, with a molecular weight between 14,000 and 21,000, occurring as a translucent, gray, viscous fluid. It is administered orally as an antifoaming agent in gastroscopy, and is also used as an antiflatulent and as a releasing agent in pharmaceutical preparations. Called also *dimethicone* or *activated dimethicone.* It is used in veterinary medicine in the treatment and prevention of bloat in cattle.

**si·mi·lia si·mi·li·bus cu·ran·tur** (sĭ-mĭ'le-ə sĭ-mĭ'lĭ-bəs ku-ran'tər) [L. "likes are cured by likes"] the doctrine which lies at the foundation of homeopathy; namely, that a disease is cured by those remedies which produce effects resembling the disease itself.

**si·mil·li·mum** (sĭ-mil'ĭ-məm) [L. "likest"] the homeopathic remedy which most exactly reproduces the symptoms of any disease.

**Sim·monds' disease (syndrome)** (sim'əndz) [Morris *Simmonds,* German physician, 1855–1925] see *panhypopituitarism.*

**Si·mon's septic factor, sign** (si'mənz) [Charles Edmund *Simon,* American physician, 1866–1927] see under *factor* and see *Simon's sign* (def. 1), under *sign.*

**Si·mon's sign** (si'mənz) [Sir John *Simon,* English surgeon, 1816–1904] see under *sign.*

**Si·mo·nart's thread (band)** (se"mo-nahrz') [Pierre Joseph Cécilien *Simonart,* Belgian obstetrician, 1817–1847] see under *thread.*

**Si·mo·nea fol·li·cu·lo·rum** (sĭ-mo'ne-ə fə-lik"u-lor'əm) *Demodex folliculorum.*

**Si·mons' disease** (ze'monz) [Arthur *Simons,* German physician, 20th century] partial lipodystrophy.

**sim·ple** (sim'pəl) [L. *simplex*] 1. neither compound nor complex; single. 2. an old term for any herb with real or supposed medicinal virtues.

**Sim·plex·vi·rus** (sim'pleks-vi"rəs) [herpes *simplex* + *virus*] [MeSH: Simplexvirus] the herpes simplex virus group; a genus of ubiquitous viruses of the subfamily Alphaherpesvirinae (family Herpesviridae) that infect both humans and animals, including herpes simplex viruses 1 and 2, bovine herpesvirus 2, and herpesvirus B.

**Simp·son's forceps** (simp'sənz) [Sir James Young *Simpson,* Scottish obstetrician, 1811–1870] see under *forceps.*

**Sims' position, speculum** (simz) [James Marion *Sims,* American gynecologist, 1813–1883] see under *position* and *speculum.*

**sim·ul** (sim'əl) [L.] at the same time as.

**sim·u·la·tion** (sim"u-la'shən) [L. *simulatio*] 1. an imitation or pretense. 2. the act of counterfeiting a disease; malingering. 3. the mimicking of one disease by another.
**Monte Carlo s.,** see under *method.*

**sim·u·la·tor** (sim"u-la'tor) something that simulates, such as an apparatus that simulates conditions that will be encountered in real life.

**Si·mu·li·i·dae** (si"mu-le'ĭ-de) [MeSH: Simuliidae] a family of small flies of the suborder Nematocera, characterized by a humped back and short stubbed antennae of 10 or 11 segments. It contains approximately 600 species, known variously as black flies, buffalo gnats, or turkey gnats. The females of several species are vicious biters of humans and other animals.

**Si·mu·li·um** (si-mu'le-əm) a genus of flies of the family Simuliidae, found in many parts of the world; many bite animals and humans and transmit disease-producing organisms. *S. amazo'nicum* is a vector of *Mansonella ozzardi* in Brazil and Guyana. *S. arc'ticum* is found in Alaska. *S. columbaczen'se,* a species in southern Europe, has caused fatal anemia in animals. *S. damno'sum* is an intermediate host of *Onchocerca volvulus* in Africa. *S. metal'licum* and *S. ochra'ceum* transmit *O. volvulus* in Mexico. *S. pecua'rium,* the buffalo gnat, is a terrible scourge to horses and cattle. *S. venus'tum* is widely distributed in North America and Denmark.

**si·mul·tag·no·sia** (si"məl-tag-no'zhah) simultanagnosia.

**si·mul·tan·ag·no·sia** (si"məl-tān"əg-no'zhah) impaired purposeful search of a complex visual display, reflecting a difficulty in integrating the parts as a whole; called also *simultagnosia.*

**SIMV** synchronized intermittent mandatory ventilation; see under *ventilation.*

**sim·va·stat·in** (sim"və-stat'in) [USP] an antihyperlipidemic agent that acts as a competitive inhibitor of hydroxymethylglutaryl-CoA reductase, used to lower blood lipid levels in hypercholesterolemia; administered orally.

**si·nal** (si'nəl) pertaining to a sinus; sinusal.

**sin·al·bin** (sin-al'bin) a glycoside found in white (or yellow) mustard; animals eating large quantities of these plants, especially the seeds, may develop fatal gastroenteritis.

**Sin·a·pis** (sin'ə-pis) former genus name for the mustards, plants now classified in genus *Brassica. S. al'ba* is now called *B. alba* and *S. ni'gra* is now called *B. nigra.*

**sin·ca·lide** (sin'kə-līd) [USP] the synthetic C-terminal octapeptide of cholecystokinin, used to stimulate gallbladder contraction in gallbladder function testing and cholecystography; administered intravenously.

**sin·cip·i·tal** (sin-sip'ĭ-təl) pertaining to the sinciput.

**sin·ci·put** (sin'sĭ-pət) [L.] [TA] forehead: the anterior and superior part of the head.

**Sind·bis fever, virus** (sind'bis) [*Sindbis,* Egypt, village where the fever was observed in the 1950's] see under *fever* and *virus.*

**sin·e·fun·gin** (sin"ə-fun'jin) an antifungal antibiotic derived from *Streptomyces griseolus.*

**Sin·e·quan** (sin'ə-kwahn) trademark for a preparation of doxepin hydrochloride.

**sin·ew** (sin'u) the tendon of a muscle.
**weeping s.,** an encysted ganglion, chiefly on the back of the hand, containing synovial fluid.

**sing.** abbreviation of L. *singulo'rum,* of each.

**sin·gle blind** (sing'gəl blīnd) pertaining to a clinical trial or other experiment in which subjects do not know which treatment they are receiving.

**Sin·gu·lair** (sing"gu-lar') trademark for a preparation of montelukast sodium.

**sin·gul·ta·tion** (sing"gəl-ta'shən) a hiccup.

**sin·gul·tous** (sing-gul'təs) affected with hiccup.

**sin·gul·tus** (sing-gul'təs) [L.] hiccup.

**sin·i·grin** (sin'ĭ-grin) potassium myronate, a glycoside found in black or brown mustard *(Brassica nigra)* and horseradish *(Armoracia lapathifolia),* from which allyl isothiocyanate is derived. Animals eating large quantities of these plants, especially their seeds, can develop fatal gastroenteritis.

**si·nis·ter** (sĭ-nis'tər) [L.] [TA] left: a term denoting the left hand one of two similar structures, or the one situated on the left side of the body.

**si·nis·trad** (sĭ-nis'trad) to or toward the left.

**sin·is·tral** (sin'is-trəl) [L. *sinistralis*] 1. pertaining to the left side. 2. a left-handed person.

**sin·is·tral·i·ty** (sin"is-tral'ĭ-te) the preferential use, in voluntary motor acts, of the left member of the major paired organs of the body, as the left ear, eye, hand, and foot.

**sin·is·trau·ral** (sin"is-traw'rəl) [*sinistr-* + *aural*[1]] hearing better with the left ear.

**sinistr(o)-** [L. *sinister* left] a combining form meaning left, or denoting relationship to the left side.

**sin·is·tro·car·dia** (sin″is-tro-kahr′de-ə) [*sinistro-* + Gr. *kardia* heart] displacement of the heart leftward in the thorax.

**sin·is·tro·cer·e·bral** (sin″is-tro-ser′ə-brəl) pertaining to or situated in the left cerebral hemisphere.

**sin·is·troc·u·lar** (sin″is-trok′u-lər) [*sinistro-* + *ocular*] left eyed; having the left eye the dominant eye.

**sin·is·troc·u·lar·i·ty** (sin″is-trok″u-lar′ĭ-te) the state of having the left eye the dominant eye.

**sin·is·tro·gy·ra·tion** (sin″is-tro-ji-ra′shən) [*sinistro-* + *gyration*] a turning to the left, as a movement of the eye or the plane of polarization.

**sin·is·tro·man·u·al** (sin″is-tro-man′u-əl) [*sinistro-* + *manual*] left-handed.

**sin·is·trop·e·dal** (sin″is-trop′ə-dəl) [*sinistro-* + *pedal*] using the left foot in preference to the right.

**sin·is·tro·tor·sion** (sin″is-tro-tor′shən) [*sinistro-* + *torsion*] a twisting toward the left; said mainly of the eye.

**sino-** [L. *sinus,* q.v.] combining form denoting relationship to a sinus.

**si·no·atri·al** (si″no-a′tre-əl) pertaining to the sinus venosus (sinus of venae cavae) and the atrium of the heart; called also *sinuatrial.*

**si·no·bron·chi·tis** (si″no-brong-ki′tis) [*sino-* + *bronchitis*] chronic paranasal sinusitis with recurrent bronchitis.

**si·nog·ra·phy** (si-nog′rə-fe) [*sino-* + *-graphy*] radiography of the sinuses or of a pathologic sinus.

**si·nom·e·nine** (si-nom′ə-nin) a toxic crystalline alkaloid from the root of *Sinomenium acutum,* structurally related to thebaine. Called also *coculine* and *cucoline.*

**Si·no·me·ni·um** (si″no-me′ne-əm) a genus of plants of the family Menispermaceae. *S. acu′tum* (Thumb.) Rehd. Wils. is a species native to eastern Asia whose root is a source of the toxic alkaloid sinomenine.

**Si non val.** abbreviation for L. *si non va′leat,* if it is not enough.

**si·no·pul·mo·nary** (si″no-pul′mə-nar″e) involving the paranasal sinuses and the lungs.

**si·no·spi·ral** (si″no-spi′rəl) pertaining to the sinus venosus and having a spiral course; said of certain bundles of cardiac muscle fibers. See also under *fiber.*

**si·no·ven·tric·u·lar** (si″no-vən-trik′u-lər) pertaining to the sinus venosus (sinus of venae cavae) and the ventricle of the heart.

**sin·ter** (sin′tər) [Ger.] 1. a chemical sedimentary rock deposited by mineral springs, especially one containing silica or calcium carbonate. 2. to transform a powder into a solid mass by heating below the melting point under specific conditions of pressure and decreased surface area.

**Sin·trom** (sin′trom) trademark for a preparation of acenocoumarol.

**sin·u·ate** (sin″u-āt) having a wavy margin.

**sinu·at·ri·al** (sin″u-a′tre-əl) sinoatrial.

**sin·u·ous** (sin′u-əs) [L. *sinuosus*] bending in and out; winding.

**si·nus** (si′nəs) pl. *si′nus* or *sinuses* [L. "a hollow"] 1. [TA] a cavity, or channel; in anatomical nomenclature, a general term for such spaces, including venous sinuses and paranasal sinuses. 2. an abnormal channel or fistula permitting the escape of pus.

## Sinus

Descriptions are given on TA terms, and include anglicized names of specific sinuses.

**accessory s's of the nose,** s. paranasales.

**air s.,** an air-containing space within the substance of a bone.

**anal s's, s. ana′les** [TA], furrows, with pouchlike recesses at the lower end, separating the rectal columns; called also *s. rectales* and *crypts of Morgagni.*

**anterior s's, s. anterio′res,** s. ethmoidales anteriores.

**s. of anterior chamber,** the narrow space at the edge of the anterior chamber of the eye, between the border of the cornea and the root of the iris.

**s. aor′tae** [TA], aortic sinus: a dilatation between the aortic wall and each of the semilunar cusps of the aortic valve; from two of these sinuses the coronary arteries take origin. Called also *Petit's s., s. of Morgagni,* and *s. of Valsalva.*

**Arlt's s.,** s. of Maier.

**articular s. of atlas,** fovea dentis atlantis.

**articular s. of atlas, superior,** fovea articularis superior atlantis.

**articular s. of axis, anterior,** facies articularis anterior axis.

**articular s. of vertebrae, inferior,** see *facies articulares inferiores vertebrarum.*

**s. of atlas, anterior,** fovea dentis atlantis.

**basilar s.,** plexus basilaris.

**s. of Bochdalek,** hiatus pleuroperitonealis.

**branchial s.,** an abnormal opening between a pharyngeal groove and its corresponding pharyngeal pouch, homologous with an ancestral gill slit.

**Breschet's s.,** s. sphenoparietalis.

**s. caro′ticus** [TA], **carotid s.,** the dilated portion of the internal carotid artery, situated above the division of the common carotid artery into its two main branches, or sometimes on the terminal portion of the common carotid artery, containing in its wall pressoreceptors that are stimulated by changes in blood pressure. Called also *bulbus caroticus.*

**s. caverno′sus** [TA], **cavernous s.,** either of two sinuses of the dura mater, irregularly shaped and located at either side of the body of the sphenoid bone, extending from the medial end of the superior orbital fissure in front to the apex of the petrous temporal bone behind. Each sinus receives the corresponding superior ophthalmic vein, superficial middle cerebral vein, and the sphenoparietal sinus, and communicates with the opposite cavernous sinus and with the transverse sinuses and internal jugular vein by way of the petrosal sinuses. Each cavernous sinus commonly comprises one or more main venous channels and contains the internal carotid artery and abducent nerve.

**cervical s.,** a temporary depression caudal to the embryonic hyoid arch, containing the succeeding pharyngeal arches; it is overgrown by the second pharyngeal arch (hyoid arch) and closes off as the cervical vesicle.

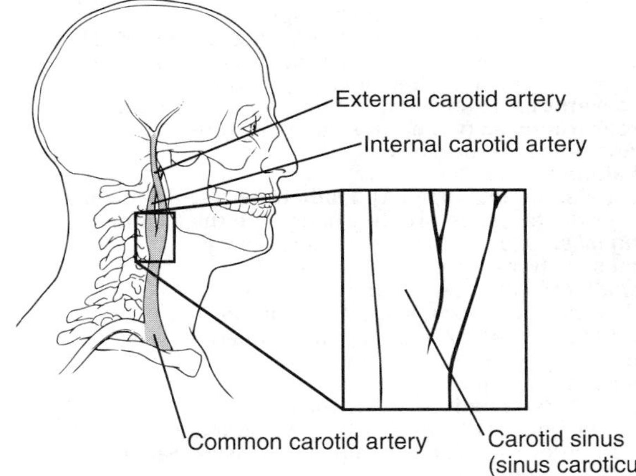


**circular s., s. circula′ris,** the venous ring around the hypophysis formed by the two cavernous and the anterior and posterior intercavernous sinuses; called also *Ridley's s.*

**s. circula′ris i′ridis,** s. venosus sclerae.

**coccygeal s.,** a pilonidal sinus situated just over or close to the tip of the coccyx. Called also *sacrococcygeal s.*

**s. condylo′rum fe′moris,** fossa intercondylaris femoris.

**s. corona′rius** [TA], **coronary s.,** the terminal portion of the great cardiac vein, which lies in the coronary sulcus between the left atrium and ventricle, and empties into the right atrium between the orifice of the inferior vena cava and the atrioventricular orifice.

**cortical s's,** lymph sinuses in the cortex of a lymph node, which arise from the marginal sinuses and continue into the medullary sinuses; called also *intermediate s's.*

**costal s's of sternum,** incisurae costales sterni.

**costodiaphragmatic s.,** recessus costodiaphragmaticus pleuralis.

**costomediastinal s. of pleura, s. costomediastina′lis pleu′rae,** recessus costomediastinalis pleuralis.

**costophrenic s.,** recessus costodiaphragmaticus pleuralis.
**cranial s's,** s. durae matris.
**Cuvier's s's,** common cardinal veins.
**dermal s.,** a congenital sinus tract extending from the surface of the body, between the bodies of two adjacent lumbar vertebrae, to the spinal canal.
**s's of dura mater, s. du'rae ma'tris** [TA], large venous channels forming an anastomosing system between the layers of the dura mater encephali. They are devoid of valves, do not collapse when drained, and in some parts contain numerous trabeculae. They drain the cerebral veins and some diploic and meningeal veins into the veins of the neck. Those at the base of the skull also drain most of the blood from the orbit. In some places they communicate with superficial veins by small emissary vessels. Called also *cranial s's, s. venosi durales,* and *venous s's of dura mater.*
**dural s's,** s. durae matris.
**s. epididy'midis** [TA], **s. of epididymis,** a long, slitlike serous pocket between the upper part of the testis and the overlying epididymis.
**Eternod's s.,** a loop of vessels connecting the vessels of the chorion with those in the underside of the yolk sac.
**ethmoid s's, ethmoidal s's,** sinus ethmoidales.
**ethmoidal s's, anterior,** s. ethmoidales anteriores.
**ethmoidal s's, middle,** s. ethmoidales medii.
**ethmoidal s's, posterior,** s. ethmoidales posteriores.
**s. ethmoida'les,** cellulae ethmoidales.
**s. ethmoida'les anterio'res,** cellulae ethmoidales anteriores.
**s. ethmoida'les me'dii,** cellulae ethmoidales mediae.
**s. ethmoida'les posterio'res,** cellulae ethmoidales posteriores.
**Forssell's s.,** a smooth space in the wall of the stomach surrounded by folds of the mucosa; seen on radiographic examination.
**s. fronta'lis** [TA], frontal sinus: one of the paired irregular shaped paranasal sinuses located in the frontal bone deep to the superciliary arch, separated from its fellow of the opposite side by a bony septum; it communicates by way of the nasofrontal duct with the middle meatus of the nasal cavity on the same side.
**Guérin's s.,** a diverticulum behind Guérin's fold.
**Huguier's s.,** a depression in the tympanum between the fenestra ovalis and the fenestra rotunda.
**s. intercaverno'sus ante'rior** [TA], the anterior of the two sinuses of the dura mater connecting the two cavernous sinuses, passing anterior to the infundibulum of the hypophysis.
**s. intercaverno'sus poste'rior** [TA], the posterior of the two sinuses of the dura mater connecting the two cavernous sinuses, passing posterior to the infundibulum of the hypophysis.
**intercavernous s., anterior,** s. intercavernosus anterior.
**intercavernous s., posterior,** s. intercavernosus posterior.
**intermediate s's,** cortical s's.
**s. of kidney,** s. renalis.
**lacteal s's, s. lacti'feri** [TA], **lactiferous s's,** enlargements in the lactiferous ducts just before they open onto the mammary papilla.
**laryngeal s., s. of larynx,** ventriculus laryngis.
**lateral s.,** s. transversus durae matris.
**s. liena'lis,** TA alternative for *s. splenicus.*
**longitudinal s., inferior,** s. sagittalis inferior.
**longitudinal s., superior,** s. sagittalis superior.
**lunate s. of radius,** incisura ulnaris radii.
**lunate s. of ulna,** incisura radialis ulnae.
**lymph s's, lymphatic s's,** irregular tortuous spaces within lymphoid tissue (nodes) through which a continuous stream of lymph passes, to enter the efferent lymphatic vessels. See also *cortical s's, marginal s's,* and *medullary s's.*
**s. of Maier,** a slight diverticulum from the upper part of the lacrimal sac, into which the lacrimal canaliculi open, either together or separately; called also *Arlt's s.*
**marginal s's,** 1. marginal lakes; see under *lake.* 2. bowl-shaped lymph sinuses separating the capsule from the cortical parenchyma of a lymph node, and from which lymph flows into the cortical sinuses; called also *subcapsular s's.* 3. see *s. marginalis.*
**s. margina'lis** [TA], marginal sinus: any of the variably developed veins that connect the occipital sinus with the vertebral venous plexuses.
**mastoid s's,** cellulae mastoideae.
**s. maxilla'ris** [TA], **s. maxilla'ris [Highmo'ri],** maxillary sinus: one of the paired paranasal sinuses, located in the body of the maxilla on either side and communicating with the middle meatus of the nasal cavity on the same side. Called also *antrum of Highmore.*
**maxillary s.,** s. maxillaris.
**s. me'dii,** s. ethmoidales medii.
**medullary s's,** lymph sinuses in the medulla of a lymph node, which divide the lymphoid tissue into a number of medullary cords.
**Meyer's s., s. Mey'eri,** a small depression in the floor of the external auditory canal just in front of the tympanic membrane.
**middle s's,** s. ethmoidales medii.
**middle s. of atlas,** fovea dentis atlantis.
**s. of Morgagni,** 1. see *s. anales.* 2. sinus aortae. 3. ventriculus laryngis.
**mucous s's of male urethra,** lacunae urethrales.
**oblique s. of pericardium, s. obli'quus pericar'dii** [TA], a recess of serous pericardium that passes upward behind the left atrium and between the left and right pulmonary veins.
**occipital s., s. occipita'lis** [TA], one of the sinuses of the dura mater; it begins in right and left branches, the marginal sinuses, and passes upward along the attached margin of the cerebellar falx to end in the confluence of the sinuses.
**oral s.,** stomodeum.
**s. paranasa'les** [TA], paranasal sinuses: the mucosa-lined air cavities in the cranial bones which communicate with the nasal cavity, including the ethmoidal, frontal, maxillary, and sphenoidal sinuses.

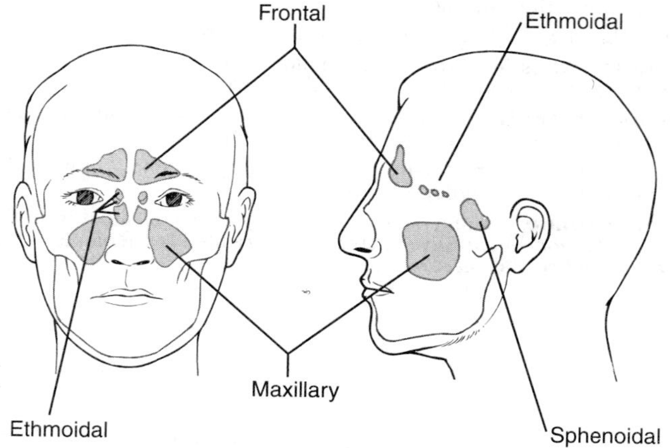


Sinus paranasales (paranasal sinuses).

**parasinoidal s's,** lacunae laterales.
**pericardial s.,** an enlarged blood-filled portion of the hemocoelom surrounding the heart in many invertebrates with open circulatory systems, such as arthropods. Called also *pericardium.*
**s. pericar'dii,** s. transversus pericardii.
**peroneal s. of tibia,** incisura fibularis tibiae.
**Petit's s.,** s. aortae.
**petrosal s., inferior,** s. petrosus inferior.
**petrosal s., superior,** s. petrosus superior.
**s. petrosquamo'sus** [TA], **petrosquamous s.,** an inconstant sinus, one of the sinuses of the dura mater; it runs along the petrosquamous fissure, connecting posteriorly with the transverse sinus and anteriorly with the retromandibular vein.
**s. petro'sus infe'rior** [TA], inferior petrosal sinus: one of the sinuses of the dura mater, arising from the cavernous sinus and running along the line of the petrooccipital synchondrosis to the superior bulb of the internal jugular vein.
**s. petro'sus supe'rior** [TA], superior petrosal sinus: one of the sinuses of the dura mater, arising at the cavernous sinus, passing along the attached margin of the cerebellar tentorium, and draining into the transverse sinus.
**phrenicocostal s., s. phrenicocosta'lis,** recessus costodiaphragmaticus pleuralis.
**pilonidal s.,** a suppurating sinus containing a tuft of hair, occurring chiefly in the coccygeal region *(coccygeal sinus),* but also seen in other regions of the body. It is usually the result of repeated friction that has caused hairs to penetrate the skin. Called also *piliferous cyst, pilonidal cyst,* and *pilonidal fistula.*
**piriform s.,** recessus piriformis.
**s. pleu'rae, pleural s's,** recessus pleurales.
**pleuroperitoneal s.,** hiatus pleuroperitonealis.
**s. pocula'ris,** utriculus prostaticus.
**posterior s's, s. posterio'res,** s. ethmoidales posteriores.
**s. poste'rior cavita'tis tympa'nicae** [TA], posterior sinus of tympanic cavity: a groove in the posterior wall of the tympanic cavity inferior to the pyramidal eminence.
**s. precervica'lis,** the depression at the side of the neck, produced in the developing embryo by the growth of the pharyngeal (branchial) arches.
**prostatic s., s. prosta'ticus** [TA], the posterolateral recess between the seminal colliculus and the wall of the urethra.
**s. of pulmonary trunk,** s. trunci pulmonalis.
**pyriform s.,** recessus piriformis.

**rectal s's, s. recta'les,** s. anales.
**s. rec'tus** [TA], straight sinus: one of the sinuses of the dura mater, situated in the line of union of the cerebral falx and the cerebellar tentorium, formed by the junction of the great cerebral vein and the inferior sagittal sinus, and commonly ending in the opposite transverse sinus at the confluence of the sinuses.
**renal s., s. rena'lis** [TA], a cavity within the substance of the kidney, occupied by the renal pelvis, calices, vessels, nerves, and fat.
**s. reu'niens,** the sinus venosus of the embryonic heart into which empty all the veins that go to the heart.
**rhomboid s. of Henle,** ventriculus terminalis medullae spinalis.
**Ridley's s.,** s. circularis.
**Rokitansky-Aschoff s's,** small outpouchings of the mucosa of the gallbladder extending through the lamina propria and the muscular layer.
**sacrococcygeal s.,** coccygeal s.
**sagittal s., inferior,** s. sagittalis inferior.
**sagittal s., superior,** s. sagittalis superior.
**s. sagitta'lis infe'rior** [TA], inferior sagittal sinus: one of the sinuses of the dura mater; it is small and situated in the posterior half of the lower concave border of the falx cerebri, and it opens into the upper end of the straight sinus. Called also *inferior longitudinal s.*
**s. sagitta'lis supe'rior** [TA], superior sagittal sinus: one of the sinuses of the dura mater; it begins in front of the crista galli and extends backward in the convex border of the falx cerebri. Near the internal occipital protuberance it ends in a variable way in the confluence of the sinuses. It receives the superior cerebral veins, communicates with the lateral lacunae of adjacent dura mater, and is partially invaginated by arachnoidal granulations. Called also *superior longitudinal s.*
**semilunar s. of tibia,** incisura fibularis tibiae.
**sigmoid s., s. sigmoi'deus** [TA], either of two sinuses of the dura mater, continuations of the transverse sinuses; each curves downward from the tentorium cerebelli to become continuous with the superior bulb of the internal jugular vein.
**sphenoid s., sphenoidal s.,** s. sphenoidalis.
**s. sphenoida'lis** [TA], sphenoidal sinus: one of the paired paranasal sinuses, located in the anterior part of the body of the sphenoid bone and communicating with the superior meatus of the nasal cavity on the same side; it is separated from its fellow on the opposite side by a septum.
**sphenoparietal s., s. sphenoparieta'lis** [TA], either of two sinuses of the dura mater, each beginning at a meningeal vein next to the apex of the small wing of the sphenoid bone and draining into the anterior part of the cavernous sinus. Called also *Breschet's s.*
**s. of spleen, splenic s., s. sple'nicus** [TA], a dilated venous sinus not lined by ordinary endothelial cells, found in the splenic pulp; called also *s. lienalis* [TA alternative].
**straight s.,** s. rectus.
**subarachnoidal s's,** cisternae subarachnoideae.
**subcapsular s's,** marginal s's (def. 2.)
**tarsal s., s. tar'si** [TA], the space between the calcaneus and talus, containing the interosseous ligament; called also *tarsal canal.*
**tentorial s.,** s. rectus.
**terminal s.,** a vein which encircles the vascular area in the blastoderm.
**tonsillar s.,** fossa tonsillaris.
**s. tonsilla'ris,** TA alternative for *fossa tonsillaris.*
**transverse s. of dura mater,** s. transversus durae matris.
**transverse s. of pericardium,** s. transversus pericardii.
**s. transver'sus du'rae ma'tris** [TA], transverse sinus of dura mater: either of two large sinuses of the dura mater that begin in a variable fashion at the confluence of the sinuses near the internal occipital protuberance. Each follows the attached margin of the tentorium cerebelli to the petrous temporal bone, where it becomes the sigmoid sinus. At their origin in the confluence, the right and left sinuses communicate with each other, and with the superior sagittal sinus and the straight sinus.
**s. transver'sus pericar'dii** [TA], transverse sinus of pericardium: a passage behind the aorta and pulmonary trunk and in front of the atria; it is lined by serous pericardium.
**traumatic s.,** a sinus due to trauma.
**s. trun'ci pulmona'lis** [TA], sinus of pulmonary trunk: a slight dilatation between the wall of the pulmonary trunk and each of the semilunar cusps of the pulmonary trunk valve.
**s. tym'pani** [TA], tympanic sinus: a deep fossa in the posterior part of the tympanic cavity; it is bounded superiorly by the eminentia pyramidalis and inferiorly by the subiculum promontorii, and it opens anteriorly into the fossula fenestrae cochleae.
**s. of tympanic cavity, posterior,** s. posterior cavi tympani.
**s. un'guis,** the space underlying the advancing free edge of the fingernail or toenail.
**urogenital s., s. urogenita'lis,** an elongated sac formed by division of the cloaca in the early embryo, communicating with the mesonephric ducts and bladder, and forming the vestibule, urethra, and vagina in the female and some of the urethra in the male.
**uterine s's,** venous channels in the wall of the uterus in pregnancy.
**s. of Valsalva,** s. aortae.
**s. of venae cavae, s. vena'rum cava'rum** [TA], the portion of the right atrium bounded medially by the interatrial septum and laterally by the crista terminalis, and into which the superior and inferior venae cavae empty; it is often called the sinus venosus because it develops from that embryonic structure.
**s. veno'sus,** 1. [TA] venous sinus: the common venous receptacle in the embryonic heart, attached to the posterior wall of the primordial atrium; it receives the umbilical and vitelline veins and the common cardinal veins (ducts of Cuvier). 2. venous s. (def. 1). 3. s. venarum cavarum.
**s. veno'si dura'les,** s. durae matris.
**s. veno'sus scle'rae** [TA], venous sinus of sclera: a circular channel at the junction of the sclera and cornea, which is the main pathway for elimination of aqueous humor from the eye. Called also *Schlemm's canal.*
**venous s.,** 1. a large vein or channel for the circulation of venous blood, such as one of the sinuses of the dura mater. 2. s. venosus (def. 1).
**venous s's of dura mater,** s. durae matris.
**venous s. of sclera,** s. venosus sclerae.
**s. ventri'culi,** Forssell's s.

**si·nus·al** (si'nə-səl) pertaining to a sinus.

**si·nus·itis** (si"nə-si'tis) [MeSH: Sinusitis] inflammation of a sinus, usually a paranasal sinus; it may be purulent or nonpurulent, acute or chronic. Types are named for the sinus involved.
**ethmoid s.,** inflammation of an ethmoidal sinus; called also *ethmoiditis.*
**frontal s.,** inflammation of a frontal sinus.
**infectious s. of turkeys,** a common, sometimes highly fatal respiratory disease of turkeys and game birds, caused by pleuropneumonia-like organisms (q.v.) and marked by swelling below the eyes and sneezing; called also *airsac disease.*
**maxillary s.,** inflammation of a maxillary sinus; called also *antritis.*
**sphenoid s.,** inflammation of a sphenoidal sinus; called also *sphenoiditis.*

**si·nus·oid** (si'nə-soid) [*sinus* + *-oid*] 1. resembling a sinus. 2. vas sinusoideum.

**si·nus·oi·dal** (si"nə-soi'dəl) 1. located in a sinusoid or affecting the circulation in the region of a sinusoid; used especially to denote the location of vascular resistance in portal hypertension. 2. shaped like or pertaining to a sine wave.

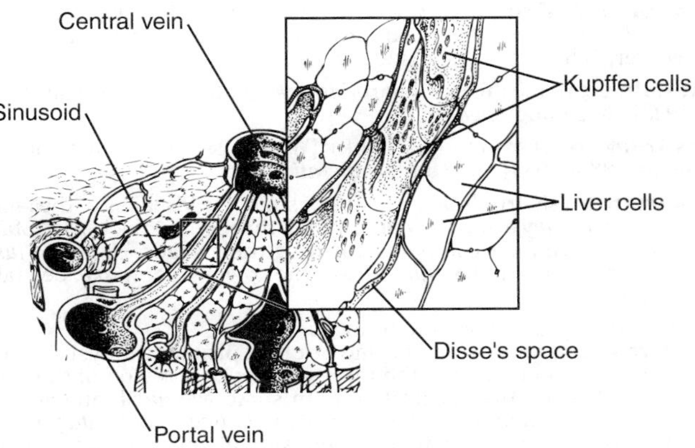

Sinusoids in a schematic view of a portion of a hepatic lobule.

**si·nus·ot·o·my** (si″nə-sot′ə-me) [*sinus* + *-tomy*] incision into a sinus.

**si·nu·spi·ral** (si″nu-spi′rəl) sinospiral.

**si·nu·ven·tric·u·lar** (si″nu-vən-trik′u-lər) sinoventricular.

**Si op. sit** abbreviation for L. *si o′pus sit,* if it is necessary.

**si·phon** (si′fən) [Gr. *siphōn* tube] a bent tube with two arms of unequal length, used to transfer liquids from a higher to a lower level by the force of atmospheric pressure.
**s. caro′ticum** [TA], **carotid s.,** the innermost section of the petrosal part of the internal carotid artery just before the artery enters the cranial cavity.

**si·phon·age** (si′fon-əj) the use of the siphon, as in gastric lavage or in draining the bladder.

**Si·pho·na ir·ri·tans** (si-fo′nə ir′ĭ-təns) *Haematobia irritans.*

**Si·pho·nap·tera** (si″fo-nap′tər-ə) [Gr. *siphon* tube + *apteros* wingless] the fleas, an order of laterally compressed, highly chitinized and sclerotized small wingless blood-sucking ectoparasites of mammals and birds. More than 800 species have been described, grouped in six or more families. See also *flea.*

**Si·phun·cu·la·ta** (si-fun″ku-la′tə) Anoplura.

**Si·phun·cu·li·na** (si-fun″ku-li′nə) a genus of dipterous insects of the family Chloropidae. *S. funi′cola* is the common eye fly of India, where it spreads conjunctivitis and trachoma.

**Sip·ple's syndrome** (sip′əl) [John H. *Sipple,* American physician, born 1930] multiple endocrine neoplasia, type IIA; see under *neoplasia.*

**Sip·py diet** (sip′e) [Bertram Welton *Sippy,* American physician, 1866–1924] see under *diet.*

**si·qua** (si′kwə) [coined from L. *sidentis altitudinis quadratio,* the square of the sitting height] Pirquet's unit for calculating the area of the absorptive surface of the intestine; it is the square of the sitting height (in centimeters).

**si·reno·me·lia** (si″rən-o-me′le-ə) [Gr. *seirēn* siren + *-melia*] apodal symmelia.

**si·ren·om·e·lus** (si″rən-om′ə-ləs) [Gr. *seirēn* siren + *melos* limb] a fetus with sirenomelia; called also *apus, sympus apus,* and *sireniform fetus.*

**sir·i·a·sis** (sir-i′ə-sis) [Gr. *seiriasis* a disease produced by the heat of the sun] sunstroke.

**sir·up** (sir′əp) syrup.

**-sis** [Gr. suffix of action] a word termination denoting an action, process, or condition. Appears most commonly in the suffixes *-asis, -esis, -iasis,* and *-osis.*

**SISI** short increment sensitivity index; see under *index.*

**siso·mi·cin** (sis″o-mi′sin) [MeSH: Sisomicin] an aminoglycoside antibiotic derived from *Micromonospora inyoensis,* closely related to the $C_{1a}$ component of the gentamicin complex; it is bactericidal for many gram-negative and some gram-positive organisms, having a range of activity similar to that of gentamicin.
**s. sulfate** [USP], the sulfate salt of sisomicin, used in the treatment of infections caused by susceptible gram-negative organisms; administered intravenously or intramuscularly.

**sis·so·rex·ia** (sis″o-rek′se-ə) a tendency of the spleen to accumulate blood corpuscles.

**sis·ter** (sis′tər) the nurse in charge of a hospital ward (Great Britain).

**Sis·ter Mary Jo·seph's nodule** (sis′tər mar′e jo′səfs) [*Sister Mary Joseph* Dempsey, American Roman Catholic nun and medical worker, 1856–1929] see under *nodule.*

**Sis·to's sign** (sēs′tōz) [Genaro *Sisto,* Argentine pediatrician, 1870–1923] see under *sign.*

**Sis·trunk operation** (sis′trənk) [Walter *Sistrunk,* American surgeon, 1880–1933] see under *operation.*

**Sis·tru·rus** (sis-troo′rəs) a genus of small rattlesnakes of the family Crotalidae; they are widely distributed throughout the United States and have symmetrical plates covering their heads. *S. catena′tus* is the massasauga and *S. milia′rius* is the *pygmy rattlesnake.* See table at *snake.*

**site** (sīt) a place, position, or locus.
**active s.,** that part of an enzyme or other protein catalyst at which the reaction occurs; it is the three-dimensional region of the molecule that binds the substrate and in some way facilitates its conversion to a reaction product. See also *binding s.* and *catalytic s.*
**allosteric s.,** a specific site on a multi-subunit enzyme that is not the substrate binding site but that when reversibly bound by an effector induces a conformational change in the enzyme, altering its catalytic properties.
**antigen-binding s., antigen-combining s.,** the region of the immunoglobulin molecule that binds to antigens; there is one such site on each of the two Fab regions of each immunoglobulin monomer.
**binding s.,** in an enzyme or other protein, the three-dimensional configuration of specific groups on specific amino acids that binds particular compounds such as substrates or effectors, with high affinity and specificity.
**catalytic s.,** in an enzyme, the portion of the active site that converts the substrate to a reaction product or otherwise interacts with it. Cf. *binding s.*
**combining s.,** antigen-binding s.
**immunologically privileged s's,** regions of the body that are not normally accessible to effector cells of the immune system and thus sites where allograft rejection does not occur and tumors escape immune surveillance, e.g., the meninges of the brain and the anterior chamber of the eye.
**operator s.,** a site adjacent to the structural genes in the operon, believed to be the site on the DNA to which repressor molecules are bound, thereby inhibiting the synthesis of mRNA by the genes in the adjacent operon.
**restriction s.,** a base sequence in a DNA segment recognized by a particular restriction endonuclease.
**sequence-tagged s. (STS),** a short length (100–1000 base pairs) of DNA that can be detected by polymerase chain reaction.
**splice s.,** the nucleotides in an exon that span the junction where an intron was removed from DNA; those formerly 5′ to the intron form the splice donor site, while those 3′ constitute the splice acceptor site.

**sit(o)-** [Gr. *sitos* food] a combining form denoting relationship to food.

**Si·to·phi·lus** (si-tof′ĭ-lus) a genus of weevils. *S. grana′rius* is the wheat weevil, which feeds on and lays eggs in kernels of grain; hypersensitivity to it causes miller's lung.

**si·to·pho·bia** (si″to-fo′be-ə) [*sito-* + *-phobia*] irrational fear of eating or of food.

**si·tos·ter·ol** (si-tos′tər-ol) 1. a generic term for a group of closely related natural plant sterols, the individual compounds being designated by Greek letters, and sometimes subscript numerals, as $\alpha_1$, $\alpha_2$, $\alpha_3$, $\beta$, and $\gamma$, on the basis of differing characteristics. 2. a pharmaceutical preparation consisting of $\beta$-sitosterol and related plant sterols, used as an anticholesterolemic agent.

**si·tos·ter·ol·emia** (si-tos″tər-ol-e′me-ə) excessive levels of sitosterols in the blood, especially $\beta$-sitosterol, absorbed from dietary vegetables due to an unknown intestinal defect. A rare form is associated with xanthomatosis, with tuberous and tendon xanthomas appearing in childhood. Written also *$\beta$-sitosterolemia.*

**si·to·tax·is** (si″to-tak′sis) sitotropism.

**si·to·tox·in** (si″to-tok′sin) any basic food poison, especially that generated in a cereal food by a plant microorganism.

**si·to·tox·ism** (si″to-tok′siz-əm) [*sito-* + *tox-* + *-ism*] food poisoning.

**si·tot·ro·pism** (si-tot′ro-piz-əm) [*sito-* + *tropism*] response of living cells to the presence of nutritive elements.

**sit·u·a·tion** (sich″o͞o-a′shən) the combination of factors with which an individual is confronted. In psychology, the total sum of physical, psychological, and sociocultural factors that act on a person and influence his behavior.

**si·tus** (si′təs) pl. *si′tus* [L.] site, or position.
**s. inver′sus vis′cerum,** lateral transposition of the viscera of the thorax and abdomen; a familial pattern and consanguineous parents have been reported. Complete transposition of the viscera in the absence of other defects is structurally sound, but see *dextrocardia, levocardia,* and *Kartagener's syndrome.*
**s. perver′sus,** dislocation of any viscus.
**s. so′litus,** the normal position of the viscera.
**s. transver′sus,** s. inversus viscerum.

**SIV** [MeSH: SIV] simian immunodeficiency virus.

**Si vir. perm.** abbreviation for L. *si vi′res permit′tant,* if the strength will permit.

**Sjö·gren's syndrome (disease)** (shər′grenz) [Henrik Samuel Conrad *Sjögren,* Swedish ophthalmologist, born 1899] see under *syndrome.*

**Sjö·gren-Lars·son syndrome** (shər′grən-lahr′sən) [Karl Gustaf Torsten *Sjögren,* Swedish physician, born 1896; Tage Konrad Leopold *Larsson,* Swedish physician, born 1905] see under *syndrome.*

**skat·ole** (skat′ōl) [Gr. *skōr,* gen. *skatos* dung] [MeSH: Skatole] a crystalline amine, with a strong characteristic odor, from human feces. It is produced by the decomposition of proteins in the intestine and directly from the amino acid tryptophan by decarboxylation.

**ska·tox·yl** (skə-tok′sil) an oxidation product of skatole, found in the urine in certain cases of disease of the large intestine.

**skein** (skān) spireme.
**Holmgren's s's, test s's,** skeins of colored worsted used in Holmgren's test of color perception.

**ske·lal·gia** (ske-lal′jə) [Gr. *skelos* leg + *-algia*] pain in the leg.

**ske·las·the·nia** (ske″ləs-the′ne-ə) [Gr. *skelos* leg + *asthenia*] weakness of the legs.

**Ske·lax·in** (skə-laks′in) trademark for a preparation of metaxalone.

**skel·e·tal** (skel′ə-təl) pertaining to the skeleton.

**skel·e·tin** (skel′ə-tin) any of a number of gelatinous substances occurring in invertebrate tissue, and including chitin, sericin, spongin, etc.

**skel·e·ti·za·tion** (skel″ə-tĭ-za′shən) 1. extreme emaciation. 2. the removal of the soft parts from the skeleton.

**skel·e·tog·e·nous** (skel″ə-toj′ə-nəs) producing skeletal or bony structures.

**skel·e·tog·e·ny** (skel″ə-toj′ə-ne) the formation of the skeleton; the origin and development of the skeleton.

**skel·e·tog·ra·phy** (skel″ə-tog′rə-fe) [*skeleton* + *-graphy*] a description of the skeleton.

**skel·e·tol·o·gy** (skel″ə-tol′ə-je) [*skeleton* + *-logy*] the sum of what is known regarding the skeleton.

**skel·e·ton** (skel′ə-tən) [Gr. "a dried body, mummy"] [MeSH: Skeleton] the hard framework of the animal body, especially the bony framework of the body of higher vertebrate animals; the bones of the body collectively. See illustration. See also *endoskeleton, exoskeleton,* and *splanchnoskeleton.*
**appendicular s., s. appendicula′re** [TA], the bones of the upper and lower limbs.
**axial s., s. axia′le** [TA], the bones of the cranium, vertebral column, ribs, and sternum.
**cardiac s.,** the fibrous or fibrocartilaginous framework that supports and gives attachment to the cardiac muscle fibers and valves, and the roots of the aorta and pulmonary trunk; it includes the anuli fibrosi cordis, left and right fibrous trigones, membranous part of the interventricular septum, and the infundibular tendon. Called also *fibrous s. of heart.*
**fibrous s. of heart,** cardiac s.
**s. of heart,** cardiac s.
**s. mem′bri inferio′ris li′beri,** pars libera membri inferioris.
**s. mem′bri superio′ris li′beri,** pars libera membri superioris.
**thoracic s., s. thora′cicus,** s. thoracis.
**s. thora′cis** [TA], skeleton of thorax: the skeletal framework enclosing the thorax, consisting of the thoracic vertebrae and intervertebral disks, the ribs and costal cartilages, and the sternum; called also *compages thoracis, rib cage,* and *thoracic cage.*
**visceral s.,** that portion of the skeleton which protects the viscera, as the sternum, ribs, and os coxae.

**skel·e·to·pia** (skel″ə-to′pe-ə) [*skeleton* + Gr. *topos* place] the position of an organ in relation to the skeleton.

**skel·e·to·py** (skel′ə-to″pe) skeletopia.

**Skene's glands (ducts, tubules)** (skēnz) [Alexander Johnston Chalmers *Skene,* American gynecologist, 1838–1900] see *ductus para-urethrales urethrae femininae.*

**ske·ni·tis** (ske-ni′tis) inflammation of the ductus paraurethrales (Skene's glands).

**ske·no·scope** (ske′no-skōp) [*Skene's* glands + *-scope*] an endoscope for examining Skene's glands.

**skew** (sku) 1. deviating from a straight line; slanting. 2. asymmetric or antisymmetric. 3. of a probability distribution, not symmetric about the mean.

**skew·foot** (sku′foot) a general term for any deformity of the foot in which its forepart deviates toward the midline; see *metatarsus varus* and *talipes varus.*

**skew·ness** (sku′nəs) of a probability distribution, lack of symmetry about the mean, or any measure of the lack of symmetry.

**skia-** [Gr. *skia* shadow] a combining form denoting reference to shadows, especially of internal structures as produced by x-rays.

**skia·gram** (ski′ə-gram) [*skia-* + *-gram*] a radiograph.

**skia·graph** (ski′ə-graf) radiograph.

**ski·ag·ra·phy** (ski-ag′rə-fe) radiography.

**ski·am·e·try** (ski-am′ə-tre) retinoscopy.

**skia·scope** (ski′ə-skōp) retinoscope.

**ski·as·co·py** (ski-as′kə-pe) [*skia-* + *-scopy*] retinoscopy.

**Skil·lern's fracture** (skil′ərnz) [Penn Gaskell *Skillern,* American surgeon, born 1882] see under *fracture.*

**skim·ming** (skim′ing) the removing of floating matter from a liquid.
**plasma s.,** the action of red cells in flowing blood which leaves a zone near the wall of a vessel that is relatively free of cells.

**skin** (skin) [MeSH: Skin] the outer integument or covering of the body, consisting of the dermis and the epidermis, and resting upon the subcutaneous tissues; called also *cutis* [TA]. See accompanying illustration.
**alligator s.,** see *ichthyosis.*
**bronzed s.,** bronze-colored skin, as seen in Addison's disease and hemochromatosis.
**collodion s.,** see under *baby,* and see *ichthyosis.*
**crocodile s.,** see *ichthyosis.*
**elastic s.,** Ehlers-Danlos syndrome.
**farmers' s.,** actinic elastosis.
**fish s.,** see *ichthyosis.*
**glossy s.,** a condition occurring secondary to neuritis in which the skin, usually on an extremity, becomes erythematous and then assumes a grayish, shiny ivory-like appearance, and may be associated with alopecia, fissuring, and ulceration; nails on the affected part become ridged. Called also *atrophoderma neuriticum.*
**India rubber s.,** Ehlers-Danlos syndrome.
**lax s., loose s.,** cutis laxa.
**marble s.,** cutis marmorata.
**piebald s.,** a term applied to the appearance of the skin in partial albinism or vitiligo.
**porcupine s.,** see *ichthyosis.*
**sailors' s.,** actinic elastosis.
**shagreen s.,** a large connective tissue nevus often occurring in children in association with tuberous sclerosis, presenting as a skin-colored or yellowish, elevated, knobby plaque resembling shark or pig skin, which is predominantly located on the back, especially on the lumbosacral region. Called also *peau de chagrin* and *shagreen patch.*

**skin·fold** (skin′fōld) the layer of skin and subcutaneous fat raised by pinching the skin and letting the underlying muscle fall back to the bone; measurements of skinfold thickness (most often taken over the biceps or triceps muscles, above the iliac crest, or below the scapula) are used to estimate the percentage of body fat. See also *triceps skinfold thickness,* under *thickness.*

**Skin·ner box** (skin′ər) [Burrhus Frederic *Skinner,* American psychologist, 1904–1990] see under *box.*

**Skin·ner classification** (skin′ər) [C.N. *Skinner,* American dentist, early 20th century] see under *classification.*

**Ski·o·dan** (ski′o-dan) trademark for preparations of methiodal sodium.

**skler(o)-** for words beginning thus, see those beginning *scler(o)-.*

**Sklow·sky's symptom** (slov′skēz) [E. L. *Sklowsky,* German physician, 20th century] see under *symptom.*

**Sko·da's sign, tympany** (sko′dahz) [Josef *Skoda,* Czech-born physician in Austria, 1805–1881] skodaic resonance.

**sko·da·ic** (sko-da′ik) named for Josef *Skoda;* see under *resonance.*

**skole-** for words beginning thus, see those beginning *scole-.*

**sko·pom·e·ter** (sko-pom′ə-tər) an instrument for measuring color, cloudiness, and other optical phenomena of liquids without using standards for comparison.

**skot(o)-** for words beginning thus, see those beginning *scot(o)-.*

**SKSD** streptokinase-streptodornase.

**skull** (skul) [MeSH: Skull] the skeleton of the head, including the cranium and the mandible. See illustration.
**cloverleaf s.,** kleeblattschädel.
**hot cross bun s.,** 1. Parrot's sign (def. 2). 2. caput quadratum.
**lacuna s.,** craniolacunia.
**maplike s.,** a skull marked by irregular tracings resembling outlines on a map; seen in x-ray films of the cranial bones in Hand-Schüller-Christian disease.
**natiform s.,** 1. Parrot's sign (def. 2). 2. caput quadratum.
**steeple s., tower s.,** oxycephaly.
**West's lacuna s., West-Engstler's s.,** a honeycomb appearance of the skull in radiographs, associated with spina bifida or meningocele and occasionally with encephalocele.

**sl** abbreviation for *slyke.*

**SLA** abbreviation for L. *sacrolaeva anterior* (left sacroanterior, a presentation of the fetus).

**SLAC** scapholunate advanced collapse.

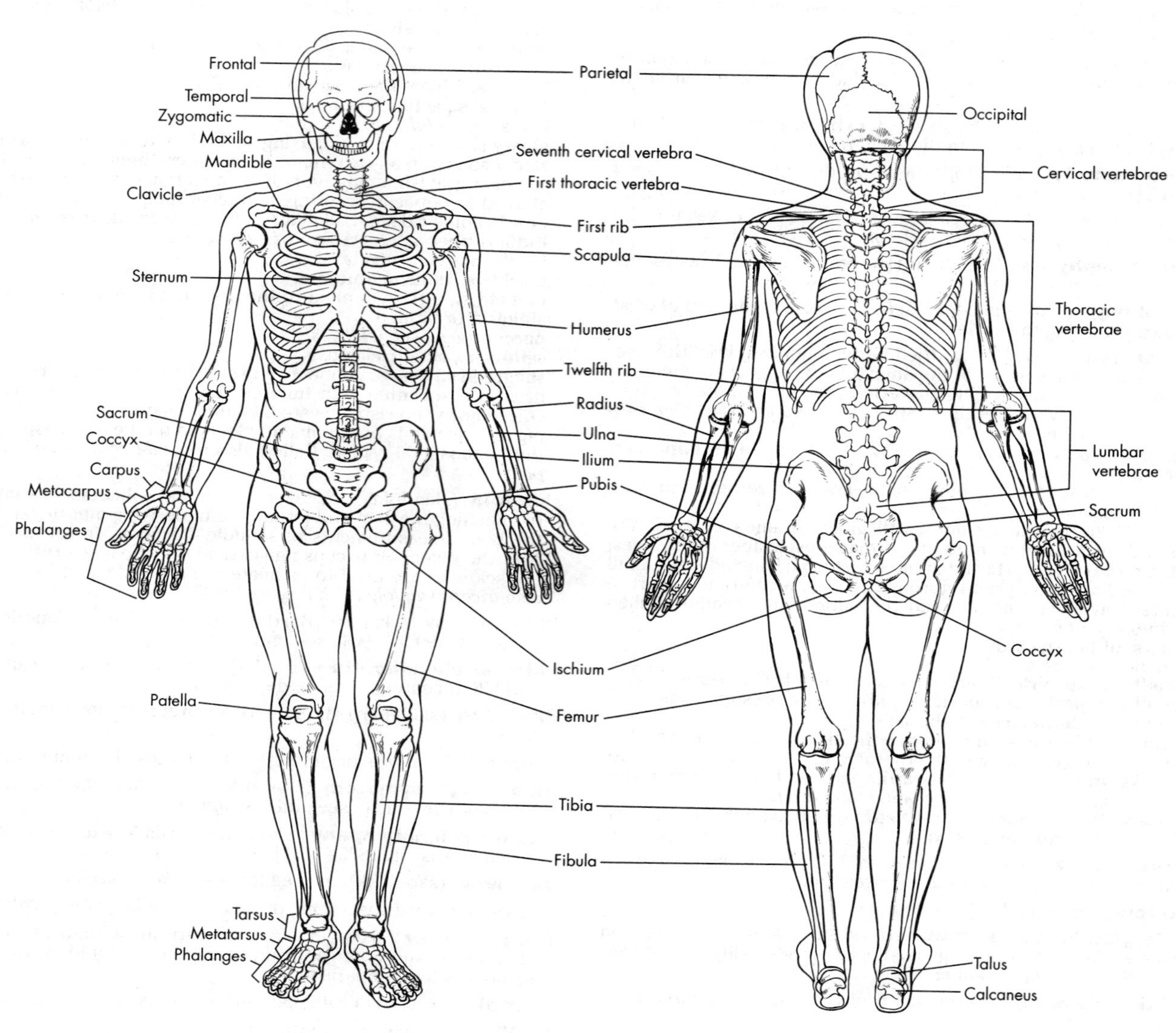


**PLATE 45—**ANTERIOR AND POSTERIOR VIEWS OF THE HUMAN SKELETON

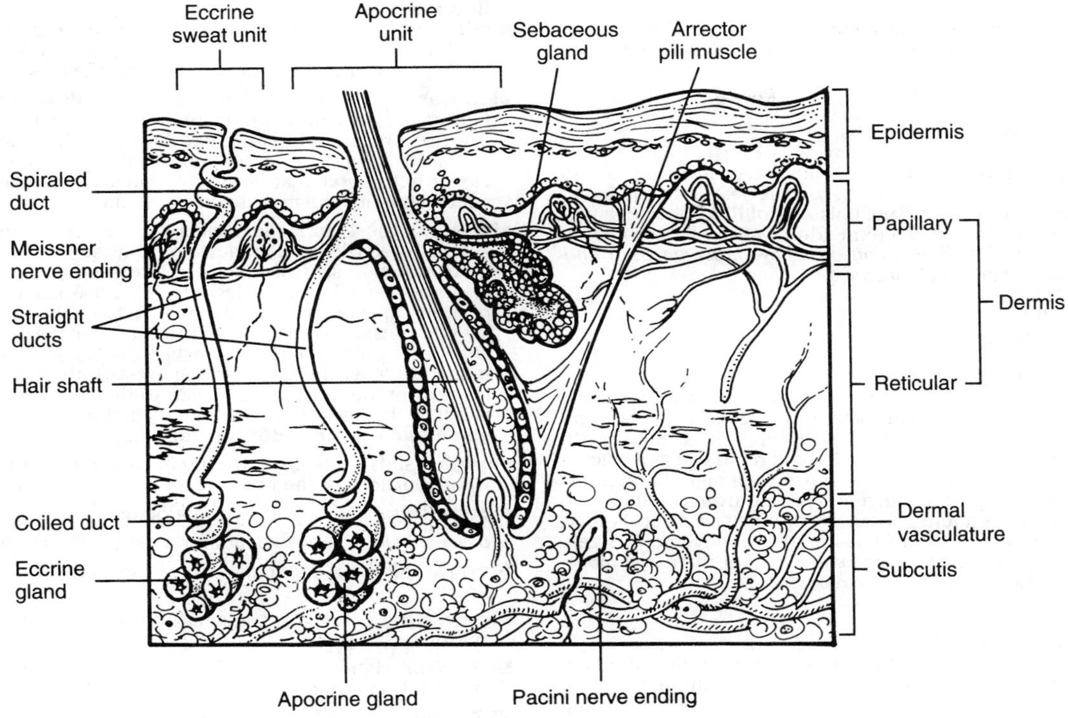


Cross section of the skin.

**slaf·ra·mine** (slaf′rə-mēn) a sialogogic mycotoxin found in *Rhizoctonia leguminicola,* which causes slobbers (q.v.) in livestock.

**slant** (slant) 1. a sloping surface of agar in a test tube. 2. a slant culture.

**SLE** systemic lupus erythematosus.

**sleep** (slēp) [MeSH: Sleep] a period of rest for the body and mind, during which volition and consciousness are in partial or complete abeyance and the bodily functions partially suspended. Sleep has also been described as a behavioral state marked by a characteristic immobile posture and diminished but readily reversible sensitivity to external stimuli. Sleep is divisible into two types: *NREM* (non–rapid eye movement) *s.* and *REM* (rapid eye movement) *s.*

**active s.,** REM s.

**D s.,** REM s.

**deep s.,** NREM s.

**desynchronized s.,** REM s.

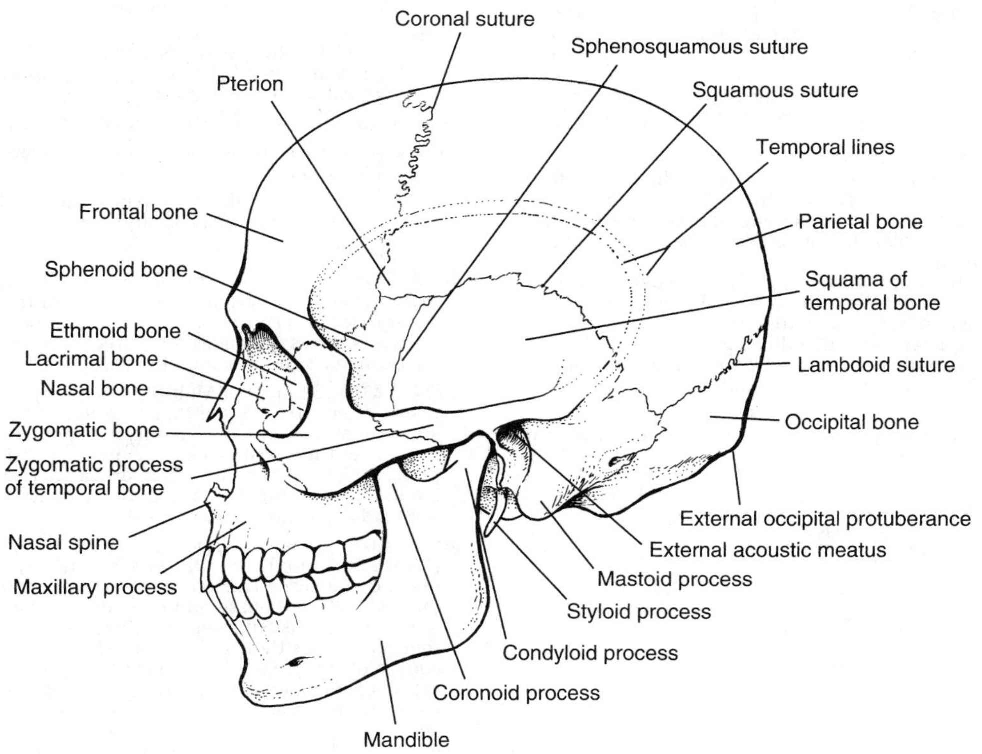


Lateral view of the skull.

**dreaming s.,** REM s.
**electric s.,** loss of voluntary movement and presence of general anesthesia induced by the application to the head of a rapidly interrupted electric current.
**electrotherapeutic s.,** electrosleep.
**fast wave s.,** REM s.
**non–rapid eye movement s.,** NREM s.
**NREM s.,** the dreamless period of sleep, consisting of four stages of succeeding depth, during which the brain waves are slow and of high voltage, and autonomic activities, such as heart rate and blood pressure, are low and regular. Brief episodes of REM sleep occur at intervals during this type of sleep; in adults, about 80 per cent of sleep is NREM sleep. Called also *non–rapid eye movement s., orthodox s., slow wave s.,* and *synchronized s.*
**orthodox s.,** NREM s.
**paradoxical s.,** REM s.
**paroxysmal s.,** narcolepsy.
**quiet s.,** NREM s.
**rapid eye movement s.,** REM s.
**REM s.,** the period of sleep during which the brain waves are fast and of low voltage, and autonomic activities, such as heart rate and respiration, are irregular. This type of sleep is associated with dreaming, mild involuntary muscle jerks, and rapid eye movements (REM). It usually occurs three to four times each night at intervals of 80 to 120 minutes, each occurrence lasting from 5 minutes to more than an hour. In adults, about 20 per cent of sleep is REM sleep and 80 per cent is NREM (non–rapid eye movement) sleep. Called also *desynchronized s., paradoxical s.,* and *rapid eye movement s.* See also *REM rebound,* under *rebound.*
**S s.,** NREM s.
**slow wave s.,** NREM s.
**synchronized s.,** NREM s.
**twilight s.,** a condition of analgesia and amnesia, produced by hypodermic administration of morphine and scopolamine. In this state the patient, although responding to pain, does not retain it in memory. Formerly widely used in obstetrics.

**sleep·talk·ing** (slēp′tawk-ing) somniloquism.

**sleep·walk·ing** (slēp′wawk-ing) somnambulism.

**slee·py·grass** (sle′pe-gras) *Stipa viridula.*

**slice** (slīs) in tomography, a cross-sectional plane of the body selected for imaging.

**slide** (slīd) a glass plate on which objects are placed for microscopic examination.

**sling** (sling) 1. a bandage or suspensory for supporting all or part of the body. 2. an anatomical configuration in which a long narrow structure passes underneath another structure and holds it up; it may be normal, anomalous, or surgically-induced.
**Glisson's s.,** a leather collar applied around the neck and under the chin to which is attached an extension apparatus over a pulley at the head of the patient's bed: for applying extension to the vertebral column.
**mandibular s.,** a structure suspending the mandible, formed by the medial pterygoid and masseter muscles and aiding in mandibulomaxillary articulation.
**pterygomasseteric s.,** mandibular s.
**pulmonary artery s.,** a rare cardiac anomaly in which the left pulmonary artery arises aberrantly from the right pulmonary artery and lies between the trachea and esophagus; it is frequently characterized by respiratory obstruction. See also *pulmonary sling syndrome,* under *syndrome.*
**suburethral s.,** a support constructed surgically from muscle, ligament, or synthetic material that elevates the bladder from underneath in the treatment of stress incontinence.
**vaginal wall s.,** a support constructed using a vaginal wall graft in order to provide urethral resistance to increased intra-abdominal pressure and stabilize the base of the bladder in the treatment of stress incontinence.

**slit** (slit) 1. a long narrow opening or incision. 2. to make a long narrow opening or incision.

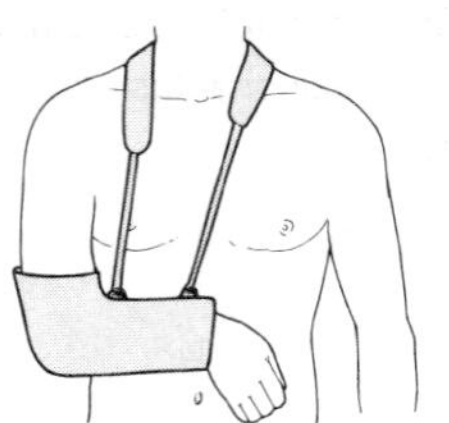
Sling.

**filtration s's,** slit pores.
**gill s.,** a long narrow opening from the pharynx to the exterior of the body of many aquatic animals, such as fishes and salamanders, through which water is drawn to bathe the gills.

**slob·bers** (slob′ərz) 1. dermatitis of the dewlap in domestic rabbits, caused by continuous dribbling of liquids from feeding devices. 2. a toxic reaction in cattle and horses in the United States, with excessive salivation, lacrimation, and diarrhea, caused by eating clover hay contaminated with the fungus *Rhizoctonia leguminicola,* which contains the mycotoxin slaframine.

**slope** (slōp) 1. an inclined plane; a surface which is neither horizontal nor vertical. 2. to deviate from the horizontal and from the vertical plane; said of a surface intersecting the horizontal at an angle between 1 and 90 degrees. 3. a mathematical means of expressing the position of a line relative to the horizontal and vertical axes, expressed as the ratio of the change in vertical distance to the change in horizontal distance when the line is traversed.
**lower ridge s.,** the slope of the crest of the mandibular residual ridge from the third molar region to its most anterior aspect in relation to the lower border of the mandible as viewed in profile.
**mandibular anteroposterior ridge s.,** lower ridge s.

**slough** (sluf) 1. necrotic tissue in the process of separating from viable portions of the body. 2. to shed or cast off.

**slough·ing** (sluf′ing) the formation or separation of a slough.

**Slow-Fe** (slo′fe′) trademark for a preparation of ferrous sulfate.

**Slow-K** (slo′ka′) trademark for a preparation of potassium chloride.

**Slow-Mag** (slo′mag′) trademark for a preparation of magnesium chloride.

**SLP** abbreviation for L. *sacrolaeva posterior* (left sacroposterior, a presentation of the fetus).

**SLT** abbreviation for L. *sacrolaeva transversa* (left sacrotransverse, a presentation of the fetus).

**Slu·der's method, neuralgia (syndrome)** (sloo′dərz) [Greenfield *Sluder,* American laryngologist, 1865–1925] see under *method* and *neuralgia.*

**sludge** (sluj) a suspension of solid or semisolid particles in a fluid which itself may or may not be a truly viscous fluid.
**activated s.,** sludge from aerated sewage, consisting mainly of aerobic bacteria (e.g., *Sphaerotilus, Zoogloea*), protozoa (e.g., *Opercularia, Vorticella*), yeasts, and molds. Further treatment consists of anaerobic digestion. A portion serves as inoculum for a succeeding batch of screened and sedimented raw sewage.

**sludg·ing** (sluj′ing) the settling out of solid particles from solution.
**s. of blood,** intravascular agglutination.

**slug** (slug) general term for any of numerous terrestrial gastropods closely related to the snails but having a rudimentary or absent shell; they are divided between the subclasses Euthyneura and Streptoneura. Some are intermediate hosts of parasitic trematodes.

**slur·ry** (slur′e) a watery mixture or suspension of insoluble matter.

**Sly syndrome** (sli) [William S. *Sly,* American physician, born 1932] see under *syndrome.*

**slyke** (slīk) a unit of buffer value, named after D.D. Van Slyke, a pioneer in buffering analysis; abbreviated sl.

**Sm** symbol for *samarium.*

**SMA 6/60** [Sequential Multiple Analyzer] trademark for an automated chemistry system that determines the concentrations of six substances in serum in 60 minutes and reports the results in a fixed sequence; the substances measured are creatinine or glucose, urea nitrogen, chloride, carbon dioxide, sodium, and potassium.

**SMA 12/60** [Sequential Multiple Analyzer] trademark for an automated chemistry system that determines the concentrations of 12 substances in serum in 60 minutes and reports the results in a fixed sequence; the substances measured are calcium, inorganic phosphorus, glucose, urea nitrogen, uric acid, cholesterol, total protein, albumin, total bilirubin, alkaline phosphatase, lactate dehydrogenase, and aspartate transaminase.

**small·pox** (smawl′poks) [compared to "great pox" (syphilis)] [MeSH: Smallpox] variola: an acute, highly contagious, often fatal infectious disease caused by an orthopoxvirus characterized by a biphasic febrile course and distinctive progressive skin eruptions. Vaccination has succeeded in eradicating smallpox worldwide; therefore, since there are no animal vectors of the disease, the only source of the virus is in medical laboratories. One clinical classification of smallpox comprised hemorrhagic, flat, ordinary, and modified varieties, each of which were subdivided into types. See also *variola major* and *variola minor.*
**flat s.,** a severe variety of smallpox in which the lesions do not pro-

ject above the skin surface, and depending upon the density of the rash are of three types: confluent, semiconfluent, and discrete. Called also *malignant s.*
**fulminant s.,** hemorrhagic s.
**hemorrhagic s.,** a severe and highly fatal variety of smallpox in which hemorrhages occur in the skin and mucous membranes before the onset of the rash (early type) or after the rash appears (late type). Called also *fulminant s.*
**malignant s.,** flat s.
**modified s.,** a variety of smallpox occurring in previously vaccinated, partially immune individuals in which all signs and symptoms are less severe than in other varieties of smallpox; depending on whether the rash is present and its density, this variety is divided into four types: that in which no rash occurs (variola sine eruptione), and confluent, discrete, and semiconfluent. Called also *varioloid.*
**ordinary s.,** the most common variety of smallpox, in which after an incubation period and a prodrome of high fever, chills, myalgia, and malaise, petechial reddish spots appear on the oral mucosa followed by a raised macular cutaneous rash that usually starts on the forehead and spreads to become generalized. The lesions evolve to become papules and vesicles, umbilicate, crust, and scab, leaving small depressed, depigmented scars (pock marks); depending upon the density of the rash, the lesions are of three types: confluent, discrete, and semiconfluent.
**ovine s.,** sheep-pox.

**SMC** selenomethylnorcholesterol.

**smear** (smēr) a specimen for microscopic study prepared by spreading the material across the glass slide.
**Pap s., Papanicolaou s.,** see under *test.*

**smeg·ma** (smeg'mə) [Gr. *smēgma* soap] [MeSH: Smegma] the secretion of sebaceous glands, especially the cheesy secretion, consisting principally of desquamated epithelial cells, found chiefly beneath the prepuce.
**s. embryo'num,** vernix caseosa.

**smeg·ma·lith** (smeg'mə-lith) [*smegma* + *-lith*] a calcareous concretion in the smegma.

**smeg·mat·ic** (smeg-mat'ik) pertaining to or composed of smegma.

**smell** (smel) [MeSH: Smell] 1. olfaction. 2. odor.

**smell-brain** (smel'brān) rhinencephalon, def. 1.

**Smel·lie's method, scissors** (smel'ēz) [William *Smellie,* British obstetrician, 1697–1763] see under *scissors* and see *Mauriceau maneuver,* under *maneuver.*

**smi·la·cin** (smi'lə-sin) [Gr. *smilakinos* pertaining to smilax] a poisonous glycoside, from sarsaparilla.

**smi·la·gen·in** (smi"lə-jen'in) a steroid precursor from several species of *Smilax;* used in the manufacture of compounds of the pregnane series.

**Smi·lax** (smi'laks) [L., Gr. "bindweed"] a genus of climbing plants of the family Liliaceae. Several species are called sarsaparilla and are sources of the flavoring sarsaparilla; some have a starchy root that was formerly used as food; and some are sources of smilagenin.

**Smith** (smith) Hamilton Othanel. American microbiologist, born 1931; co-winner, with Werner Arber and Daniel Nathans, of the Nobel prize for medicine or physiology in 1978 for his work on restriction enzymes.

**Smith's dislocation, fracture** (smiths) [Robert William *Smith,* Irish surgeon, 1807–1873] see under *dislocation* and *fracture.*

**Smith's operation** (smiths) [Henry *Smith,* English surgeon in India, 1862–1948] see under *operation.*

**Smith's sign** (smiths) [Eustace *Smith,* English physician, 1835–1914] see under *sign.*

**Smith-Lem·li-Opitz syndrome** (smith-lem'le-o'pits) [David W. *Smith,* American pediatrician, 1926–1981; Luc *Lemli,* American physician, 20th century; John Marius *Opitz,* American pediatrician, born 1935] [MeSH: Smith-Lemli-Opitz Syndrome] see under *syndrome.*

**Smith-Strang disease** (smith-strang) [Allan J. *Smith,* British physician, 20th century; Leonard Birnie *Strang,* British physician, born 1925] see under *disease.*

**Smith-Pe·ter·sen nail** (smith-pa'tər-sen) [Marius Nygaard *Smith-Petersen,* American orthopedic surgeon, 1886–1953] see under *nail.*

**smog** (smog) [MeSH: Smog] a mixture of smoke and fog; a colloid system in which the disperse phase consists of a mixture of gas and moisture and the dispersion medium is air.

**smoke** (smōk) [MeSH: Smoke] a colloid system in which one or more solids is dispersed in a gas or vapor.

**SMON** subacute myelo-opticoneuropathy.

**SMR** standardized morbidity ratio; standardized mortality ratio.

**smut** (smut) 1. any fungus of the order Ustilaginales. 2. contamination of cereal grass (wheat, oats, rye, corn) by one of these fungi, particularly of the genera *Tilletia, Ustilago,* or *Urocystis.* Ingestion of contaminated seeds causes poisoning in humans and livestock; see *ergotism* and *ustilaginism.*
**corn s.,** a smut of *Zea mays* caused by *Ustilago maydis;* ingestion of the infected seeds cause ustilaginism.
**rye s.,** ergot (def. 1).
**wheat s.,** smut on wheat caused by *Tilletia tritici*; ingestion causes glomerulonephritis in livestock.

**S.N.** abbreviation for L. *secun'dum natu'ram,* according to nature.

**Sn** symbol for *tin* [L. *stannum*].

**sn-** [for *s*tereospecific *n*umbering] a chemical prefix used to indicate stereoisomers of glycerol derivatives: the glycerol chain is numbered as if it were derived from L-glyceraldehyde. This provides an unambiguous numbering. The enantiomer is obtained by reversing the numbering. For example *sn*-glycerol 1-phosphate is the same as L-glycerol 1-phosphate; the enantiomer D-glycerol 1-phosphate is the same as L-glycerol 3-phosphate or *sn*-glycerol 3-phosphate. See D-.

**snail** (snāl) [MeSH: Snails] general term for any of numerous gastropods that have external spiral shells; they are divided between the subclasses Euthyneura and Streptoneura. Many snails in tropical countries are intermediate hosts of parasitic trematodes; the miracidium of the parasite develops into a cercaria in the body of the snail. Cf. *slug.*

**snake** (snāk) [MeSH: Snakes] 1. a limbless reptile of the suborder Ophidia, some of which are poisonous. See table. 2. any of various worms that resemble members of Ophidia.
**black s.,** blacksnake.
**brown s.,** a venomous elapid snake of Australia and New Guinea belonging to the genus *Demansia.*
**cabbage s.,** see *Mermithidae.*
**colubrid s.,** colubrid, def. 1.
**coral s.,** any of various venomous snakes of the genera *Micrurus* and *Micruroides;* called also *harlequin s.*
**coral s., Arizona,** *Micruroides euryxanthus.*
**coral s., Eastern,** a subspecies of *Micrurus fulvius* found in the Southeastern United States.
**coral s., Sonoran,** *Micruroides euryxanthus.*
**coral s., Texas,** a subspecies of *Micrurus fulvius* found in Texas and nearby areas.
**crotalid s.,** crotalid, def. 1.
**elapid s.,** elapid, def. 1.
**hair s.,** see *Gordius.*
**harlequin s.,** coral s.
**poisonous s's,** 1. venomous s's. 2. snakes that contain poison, either in venom glands or in other organs or tissues.
**sea s.,** a snake of the family Hydrophiidae.
**tiger s.,** *Notechis scutatus,* a very venomous elapid Australian snake whose body is chiefly brown with dark bands.
**venomous s's,** snakes that secrete substances (venoms) capable of producing a deleterious effect on either the blood (see *hemotoxin*) or the nervous system (see *neurotoxin*); the venom is injected into the body of the victim by the snake's bite. Called also *poisonous s's, thanatophidia,* and *toxicophidia.*
**viperine s.,** true viper.

**snake·root** (snāk'ro͞ot) 1. any plant of the genus *Asarum.* 2. any of certain other plants, such as *Polygala senega,* formerly used as remedies for snakebite.
**Canadian s.,** *Asarum canadense.*
**seneca s., senega s.,** *Polygala senega.*

**SNAP** sensory nerve action potential.

**snap** (snap) a short sharp sound.
**mitral opening s.,** an opening snap caused by abnormal movement of the mitral valve, usually due to mitral stenosis.
**opening s.,** a short, sharp sound occurring in early diastole, caused by abrupt halting at its maximal opening of an abnormal atrioventricular valve; usually indicative of a stenotic valve that is still pliable.
**tricuspid opening s.,** an opening snap caused by abnormal movement of the tricuspid valve, usually due to valvular stenosis.

**snare** (snār) a wire loop or noose for removing polyps and tumors by encircling them at the base and closing the loop.

**Sned·don's syndrome** (sned'ənz) [Ian Bruce *Sneddon,* English dermatologist, born 1915] see under *syndrome.*

**Sned·don-Wil·kin·son disease** (sne'dən-Wil'kin-sən) [I. B. *Sneddon;* Darrell Sheldon *Wilkinson,* English dermatologist, 20th century] subcorneal pustular dermatosis.

**sneeze** (snēz) 1. to expel air forcibly and spasmodically through

**Important Venomous Snakes**

| Family | Type of Fangs | Common Names | Type of Venom | Distribution | Remarks |
|---|---|---|---|---|---|
| Colubridae | Rear, immovable, grooved | Colubrids | Mostly mild | Warm parts of both hemispheres | Over 1000 species, the few poisonous ones not dangerous |
| | | Boomslang | Hemorrhagin | South Africa | Arboreal, timid |
| Elapidae | Front, immovable, grooved | Elapids | Predominantly neurotoxin | Mostly in Old World | Over 150 species, very poisonous |
| | | Cobras | Mostly neurotoxin | Africa, India, Asia, Philippines, Celebes | Spitting cobra in Africa aims at eyes |
| | | Kraits | Strong neurotoxin | India, Southeast Asia, Indonesia | Sluggish, often buried in dust |
| | | Mambas | Neurotoxin | Tropical West Africa | Arboreal |
| | | Blacksnake | Neurotoxin | Australia | Large snake, wet terrain |
| | | Copperhead | Neurotoxin | Australia, Tasmania, Solomons | Damp environment |
| | | Brown snake | Neurotoxin | Australia, New Guinea | Slender |
| | | Tiger snake | Strong neurotoxin | Australia | Dry environment, aggressive, very dangerous |
| | | Death adder | Neurotoxin | Australia, New Guinea | Sandy terrain |
| | | Coral snakes | Neurotoxin | United States, tropical America | About 26 species, 2 in southern United States |
| Hydrophiidae | Front, immovable, hollow | Sea snakes | Some mild, others very toxic | Tropical, Indian and Pacific Oceans | Rudder-like tail, gentle, over 50 species |
| Viperidae | Front, movable, hollow | True vipers; viperines; viperids | Predominantly hemotoxin | Entirely in Old World | About 50 species |
| | | European viper | Hemotoxin | Europe (rare), North Africa, Near East | Dry rocky country |
| | | Russell's viper | Hemotoxin | Southeast Asia, Java, Sumatra | Mostly open terrain, deadly |
| | | Sand vipers | Hemotoxin | Northern Sahara | Buried in sand |
| | | Puff adder | Hemotoxin | Arabia, Africa | Open terrain, sluggish |
| | | Gaboon viper | Neurotoxin and hemotoxin | Tropical West Africa | Forests, deadly |
| | | Rhinoceros viper | Hemotoxin | Tropical Africa | Wet forests |
| Crotalidae | Front, movable, hollow | Pit vipers; crotalids; crotalines | Predominantly hemotoxin | Old and New Worlds; none in Africa | Over 80 species, pit between eye and nostril |
| | | Habu viper | Neurotoxin | Warmer parts of East Asia, Ryukyu Islands | Caves and dry rocky country |
| | | Rattlesnakes | Predominantly hemotoxin | North, Central, and South America | South American form neurotoxic |
| | | Bushmaster | Hemotoxin | Central and South America | Wet forests, large |
| | | Fer-de-lance | Hemotoxin | Central America, Northern South America, few West Indies | Common on plantations |
| | | Palm vipers | Hemotoxin | Southern Mexico, Central and South America | Arboreal, small, greenish, bites face |
| | | Copperhead | Hemotoxin | United States | Dry stony terrain |
| | | Water moccasin | Hemotoxin | Southeast United States to Texas | Swamps |
| | | Asiatic pit vipers | Hemotoxin | Southeast Asia, Taiwan | Most arboreal |

the nose and mouth. 2. an involuntary, sudden, violent, and audible expulsion of air through the mouth and nose. Called also *sternutation.*

**sneeze·weed** (snēz′wēd) *Helenium.*

**Snell** (snel) George Davis. American geneticist, born 1903; co-winner, with Jean Baptiste Gabriel Dausset and Baruj Benacerraf, of the Nobel prize for medicine or physiology in 1980 for their work on the major histocompatibility complex and the genetic control of immune responses.

**Snell's law** (snelz) [Willebrord van Roijen *Snell,* Dutch astronomer and mathematician, 1591–1626] see under *law.*

**Snel·len's chart,** etc. (snel′ənz) [Hermann *Snellen,* Dutch ophthalmologist, 1834–1908] see under *chart, eye, sign, test,* and *test type.*

**SNM** Society of Nuclear Medicine.

**snore** (snor) 1. rough, noisy breathing during sleep, due to vibration of the uvula and soft palate; called also *stertor.* 2. to produce such sounds during sleep.

**snout** (snout) the long, specialized upper lip and apex of the nose seen in pigs and certain other animals.

**snow** (sno) [MeSH: Snow] a freezing or frozen mixture consisting of discrete particles or crystals.

**carbon dioxide s.**, solid carbon dioxide, formed by rapid evaporation of liquid carbon dioxide; it gives a temperature of about −79°C (−110°F). It has been used in cryotherapy to freeze the skin, thus producing local anesthesia and arrest of blood flow, and, in the form of a slush, as an escharotic to destroy certain skin lesions such as warts or moles.

**snow·blind·ness** (sno′blīnd-nəs) temporary loss of sight due to injury to superficial cells of the cornea caused by ultraviolet rays of the sun reinforced by those reflected by snow.

**snRNA** small nuclear RNA; see under *RNA.*

**snRNP** small nuclear ribonucleoprotein; see under *ribonucleoprotein.*

**SNS** sympathetic nervous system.

**snuff** (snuf) a medicinal or errhine powder to be inhaled through the nose.

**snuf·fles** (snuf′əlz) 1. a catarrhal discharge from the nasal mucous membrane in infants, generally in congenital syphilis. 2. rabbit septicemia.

**SO** the spheno-occipital synchondrosis.

***SOAP*** a device for conceptualizing the process of recording the progress notes in the *problem-oriented record* (see under *record*): *S* indicates subjective data obtained from the patient and others close to him; *O* designates objective data obtained by observation, physical examination, diagnostic studies, etc.; *A* refers to assessment of the patient's status through analysis of the problem, possible interaction of the problems, and changes in the status of the problems; *P* designates the plan for patient care.

**soap** (sōp) [L. *sapo*] [MeSH: Soaps] any compound of one or more fatty acids, or their equivalents, with an alkali. Soap is detergent and is much employed in liniments, enemas, and in making pills. It is also a mild aperient, antacid, and antiseptic.
**carbolic s.**, a disinfectant soap containing 10 per cent of phenol.
**curd s.**, sapo domesticus.
**green s.** [USP], a potassium soap made by the saponification of vegetable oils, excluding coconut oil and palm kernel oil, without the removal of glycerin. It is the chief ingredient of green soap tincture (q.v.). Called also *medicinal soft s., sapo mollis medicinalis,* and *soft s.*
**hexachlorophene liquid s.** [USP], a solution of hexachlorophene in a 10 to 13 per cent solution of potassium soap, used as a topical anti-infective and detergent.
**medicinal soft s.**, green s.
**potash s.**, green s.
**soft s.**, 1. a liquid soap made from potash and some oil; called also *potash s.* and *sapo mollis.* 2. green s.
**superfatted s.**, a soap having an excess of fat over that necessary to neutralize all the alkali.
**zinc s.**, a soap containing zinc oxide or zinc sulfate; for use as an ointment or plaster.

**soap·stone** (sōp′stōn) the solid stony form in which talc (q.v.) is found in nature. Called also *steatite.*

**Soave operation** (so-ah′va) [F. *Soave*, Italian pediatric surgeon, 20th century] see under *operation.*

**SOB** shortness of breath.

**so·cia** (so′she-ə) [L. "a comrade, associate"] a detached part or exclave of an organ.
**s. paro′tidis,** accessory parotid gland.

**so·cial·iza·tion** (so″shəl-ĭ-za′shən) [MeSH: Socialization] the process by which society integrates the individual, and the individual learns to behave in socially acceptable ways.

**so·cio·acu·sis** (so″se-o-ə-ku′sis) noise-induced hearing loss due to prolonged exposure to high levels of noise. Cf. *boilermakers' deafness.*

**so·cio·bio·log·ic, so·cio·bio·log·i·cal** (so″se-o-bi″o-loj′ik; so″se-o-bi″o-loj′ĭ-kəl) pertaining to sociobiology.

**so·cio·bi·ol·o·gist** (so″se-o-bi-ol′ə-jist) an individual trained in sociobiology.

**so·cio·bi·ol·o·gy** (so″se-o-bi-ol′ə-je) the branch of theoretical biology which proposes that all animal (including human) behavior has a biological basis, which is controlled by the genes; the study of the biological basis of behavior.

**so·ci·o·gen·ic** (so″se-o-jen′ik) arising from or imposed by society.

**so·ci·ol·o·gist** (so″se-ol′ə-jist) an individual trained in sociology.

**so·ci·ol·o·gy** (so″se-ol′ə-je) [L. *socius* fellow + *-logy*] [MeSH: Sociology] the science dealing with social relations and phenomena.

**so·ci·om·e·try** (so″se-om′ə-tre) [L. *socius* fellow + *-metry*] the branch of sociology concerned with the measurement of human social behavior.

**so·cio·path** (so′se-o-path″) a previously used term for a person exhibiting antisocial personality disorder.

**so·cio·path·ic** (so″se-o-path′ik) pertaining to antisocial behavior or to antisocial personality disorder.

**so·ci·op·a·thy** (so″se-op′ə-the) former term for antisocial personality disorder (see under *personality*).

**so·cio·ther·a·py** (so″se-o-ther′ə-pe) any treatment emphasizing socioenvironmental and interpersonal rather than intrapsychic factors.

**sock·et** (sok′ət) 1. a hollow or depression, into which a corresponding part fits. 2. gomphosis.
**dry s.**, a condition sometimes occurring after tooth extraction, particularly after traumatic extraction, resulting in a dry appearance of the exposed bone in the socket, due to disintegration or loss of the blood clot. It is basically a focal osteomyelitis without suppuration and is accompanied by severe pain (alveolalgia) and foul odor. Called also *alveolar osteitis* and *alveolitis sicca dolorosa.*
**eye s.**, orbita.
**tooth s's,** dental alveoli.

**so·da** (so′də) a term loosely applied to sodium bicarbonate (baking s.), sodium hydroxide (caustic s.), or sodium carbonate (washing s.).
**baking s., bicarbonate of s.**, sodium bicarbonate.
**caustic s.**, sodium hydroxide.
**chlorinated s.**, a mixture of sodium chloride and sodium hypochlorite.
**s. lime** [NF], calcium hydroxide with sodium or potassium hydroxide, or both; used as adsorbent of carbon dioxide in equipment for metabolism tests, inhalant anesthesia, or oxygen therapy.
**washing s.**, sodium carbonate.

**so·dio·cit·rate** (so″de-o-sit′rāt) a compound containing sodium and a salt of citric acid.

**so·dio·tar·trate** (so″de-o-tahr′trāt) a compound containing sodium and a salt of tartaric acid.

**so·di·um** (so′de-əm) gen. *so′dii* [L. *na′trium,* gen. *na′trii*] [MeSH: Sodium] a soft, silver white, alkaline metallic element; symbol, Na; atomic number, 11; atomic weight, 22.990; specific gravity, 0.971. With a valence of 1, it has a strong affinity for oxygen and other nonmetallic elements. Sodium provides the chief cation of the extracellular body fluids. See also *sodium pump,* under *pump.* The salts of sodium are the most widely used salts in medicine. (NOTE: For sodium salts not listed below, see the name of the active ingredient.)

## Sodium

**s. 22,** a radioactive isotope of sodium, atomic mass 22, having a half-life of 2.60 years and decaying by positron emission (0.545, 1.83 MeV) with electron capture and emission of gamma rays (1.275 MeV). It has been used in the determination of body sodium space and total exchangeable sodium.
**s. 24,** a radioactive isotope of sodium, atomic mass 24, having a half-life of 14.66 hours and emitting beta particles (1.389, 4.17 MeV) and gamma rays (1.369, 2.754 MeV); it has been used in the determination of sodium space and total exchangeable sodium.
**s. acetate** [USP], the trihydrate sodium salt of acetic acid, used as a source of sodium ions in solutions for hemodialysis and peritoneal dialysis. It has also been used as a systemic and urinary alkalizer, diuretic, and expectorant.
**s. acetate C 11** [USP], sodium acetate in which a portion of the molecules have been labeled with carbon 11, used as a tracer in positron emission tomography in the study of cardiac metabolism; administered intravenously.
**s. acid phosphate,** s. biphosphate.
**s. alginate** [NF], a purified carbohydrate product extracted from brown seaweeds with dilute alkali; used as a suspending agent. It is also used for its emulsifying, stabilizing, thickening, and water-binding qualities in foods, medicines, and cosmetics.

**s. alizarinsulfonate,** a yellow-brown or orange-yellow powder used as a stain in microscopy, as a reagent for aluminum, as an acid-base indicator, and in the determination of fluorine. Called also *alizarin red S* and *alizarin water-soluble red.*

**s. antimonyltartrate,** antimony sodium tartrate.

**s. arsenate,** $Na_2HAsO_4$, an odorless, amorphous white powder used when effects of arsenic are desired.

**s. ascorbate** [USP], the monosodium salt of ascorbic acid, $C_6H_7NaO_6$, used in the preparation of parenteral dosage forms of ascorbic acid.

**s. aurothiomalate,** INN for gold sodium thiomalate; see under *gold.*

**s. benzoate** [NF], the sodium salt of benzoic acid, $C_7H_5NaO_2$, used as an antifungal preservative in pharmaceutical preparations and foods. It may also be used as a test for liver function, administered orally or intravenously.

**s. bicarbonate** [USP], the monosodium salt of carbonic acid, $NaHCO_3$, used as an electrolyte replenisher and systemic alkalizer, administered by intravenous injection or infusion. It is also administered orally as a gastric antacid and urinary alkalizer, and is applied topically in solution to wash the nose, mouth, or vagina, and as a cleansing enema; sometimes used in solution as a dressing for minor burns. Called also *baking soda* and *bicarbonate of soda.*

**s. biphosphate,** the monohydrate monosodium salt of phosphoric acid, $NaH_2PO_4 \cdot H_2O$, given orally with sodium phosphate as an antihypercalcemic; orally and rectally with sodium phosphate as a cathartic; and orally as a urinary acidifier.

**s. bisulfite,** the monosodium salt of sulfurous acid, $HNaO_3S$, used as an antioxidant in pharmaceutical preparations.

**s. borate** [NF], the sodium salt of boric acid, $Na_2B_4O_7$, used as an alkalizing agent in pharmaceutical preparations. It has also been used for its weak antibacterial and mild astringent properties in lotions, gargles, and mouthwashes. Called also *borax, s. pyroborate,* and *s. tetraborate.*

**s. bromide,** a sedative, used occasionally in the management of grand mal seizures. See also *bromide* and *brominism.*

**s. calcium edetate, s. calciumedetate,** edetate calcium disodium.

**s. caprylate,** the sodium salt of caprylic acid, used as a topical antifungal in the treatment of cutaneous mycotic infections.

**s. carbonate** [NF], the disodium salt of carbonic acid, used as an alkalizing agent in pharmaceutical preparations. Called also *sal soda* and *washing soda.*

**s. caseinate,** casein-sodium.

**s. cellulose phosphate,** an ion exchange resin used in the treatment of recurrent calcium phosphate renal calculi; see under *cellulose.*

**s. chloride,** common table salt: a mineral soluble in water and found widely distributed over the earth, such as in sea water. It is a necessary constituent of the body and consequently of the diet, making up over 90 per cent of the inorganic constituents of the blood serum, and is the principal salt involved in maintaining osmotic tension of blood and tissues. It is used in medicine [USP] for many purposes, such as in the preparation of isotonic and physiologic saline solutions; as a fluid and electrolyte replenisher; as an isotonic vehicle for drugs; as an antihypercalcemic; as an antidote to silver nitrate poisoning, administered by intravenous infusion; as a topical anti-inflammatory; to irrigate wounds and body cavities; as an enema to flush the colon and promote evacuation; as a mucolytic, administered by inhalation; and as a topical osmotic agent in ophthalmology. Also used widely as a food preservative and seasoning.

**s. chromate,** the disodium salt of chromic acid; it is toxic and has a variety of industrial uses. See also *s. chromate Cr 51.*

**s. chromate Cr 51** [USP], sodium chromate prepared using the radioactive isotope chromium 51; used as a biological tracer to tag erythrocytes and estimate red cell or whole blood volume as well as for red cell survival time demonstrations and sequestration studies, and for the diagnosis of gastrointestinal bleeding. Labeled platelets are used for platelet survival studies.

**s. citrate** [USP], the trisodium salt of citric acid, used as an anticoagulant for blood or plasma that is to be fractionated or for blood that is to be stored. It is also administered orally as a urinary alkalizer.

**s. cyanide,** an extremely poisonous compound, NaCN, occurring as white granules or fused pieces, used for various industrial processes and to fumigate fruit trees. See also *cyanide poisoning,* under *poisoning.*

**s. dodecyl sulfate (SDS),** the more usual name for sodium lauryl sulfate when used as an anionic detergent to solubilize proteins.

**s. fluoride** [USP], a dental caries prophylactic, NaF, occurring as a white powder; used in the fluoridation of water and applied topically to the teeth.

**s. fluoride F 18** [USP], sodium fluoride in which a portion of the molecules are labeled with $^{18}F$.

**s. fluoroacetamide,** a sodium salt related chemically to sodium fluoroacetate, also used as a rodenticide and causing poisoning similar to fluoroacetate poisoning in many mammals.

**s. fluoroacetate,** the sodium salt of fluoroacetic acid, a toxin found in the South African tree *Dichapetalum cymosum* and used as a rodenticide. It is poisonous to humans and many other mammals; see *fluoroacetate poisoning,* under *poisoning.*

**s. fluosilicate,** s. silicofluoride.

**s. folate,** a water-soluble compound used in various anemias and in sprue.

**s. glutamate,** the monosodium salt of L-glutamic acid, used in treatment of encephalopathies associated with hepatic disease. It is also used to enhance the flavor of foods and tobacco. See also *Chinese restaurant syndrome,* under *syndrome.*

**s. glycocholate,** a salt with a pH of 6.6; used as a laboratory reagent.

**s. hyaluronate,** the sodium salt of hyaluronic acid, a highly viscous, high molecular weight, viscoelastic compound injected into the anterior or posterior chamber during surgical procedures on the eye; used as an adjunct to maintain the shape of the eye, manipulate and separate tissues by hydraulic pressure, and to protect intraocular structures from trauma.

**s. hydrate,** s. hydroxide.

**s. hydroxide** [NF], a caustic alkali, NaOH, used as an alkalizing agent in pharmaceutical preparations. Called also *caustic soda* and *s. hydrate.*

**s. hypochlorite,** the sodium salt of hypochlorous acid, NaClO, having germicidal and disinfectant properties.

**s. hyposulfite,** s. thiosulfate.

**s. iodide** [USP], a binary haloid, NaI, used in various conditions as a source of iodine. It is also used as an expectorant.

**s. iodide I 123,** sodium iodide labeled with $^{123}I$, available in several dosage forms: *sodium iodide I 123 capsules* [USP] and *sodium iodide I 123 solution* [USP]. It is used in thyroid uptake tests and thyroid imaging; administered orally or intravenously.

**s. iodide I 125,** sodium iodide labeled with $^{125}I$; administered orally or intravenously as a tracer in tests of thyroid functioning and in thyroid imaging.

**s. iodide I 131,** sodium iodide labeled with $^{131}I$, available in several dosage forms: *sodium iodide I 131 capsules* [USP] and *sodium iodide I 131 solution* [USP]. It is used as a tracer in thyroid uptake tests and thyroid imaging and is used in the treatment of hyperthyroidism and thyroid carcinoma; administered orally or intravenously.

**s. ipodate,** ipodate sodium.

**s. lactate** [USP], the sodium salt of racemic or inactive lactic acid, used intravenously in one-sixth molar solution as a fluid and electrolyte replenisher to combat acidosis.

**s. lauryl sulfate** [NF], an anionic surfactant, used as a wetting agent, emulsifying aid, and detergent in various cosmetic and dermatologic preparations, and as an ingredient of toothpastes. Called also *irium.* See also *s. dodecyl sulfate.*

**s. metabisulfite** [NF], an antioxidant, $Na_2S_2O_5$, used in pharmaceutical preparations.

**s. monofluorophosphate** [USP], a dental caries prophylactic, applied topically to the teeth.

**s. morrhuate,** morrhuate sodium.

**s. nitrate,** a compound, $NaNO_3$, formerly used as a diuretic and in treatment of dysentery, but now used as a reagent, in fertilizers, and in certain industrial processes; it is sometimes responsible for nitrite poisoning in livestock. Called also *Chile saltpeter.*

**s. nitrite** [USP], an antidote for cyanide poisoning, $NaNO_2$; it reduces hemoglobin to methemoglobin, which has a greater affinity for cyanide than does cytochrome oxidase. It is also used in the relief of the pain of angina pectoris, Raynaud's disease, asthma, and such conditions as lead colic and spastic colitis.

**s. nitroferricyanide,** s. nitroprusside.

**s. nitroprusside** [USP], an antihypertensive used in the treatment of hypertensive crisis and to produce controlled hypotension during surgery, administered by intravenous infusion. It is also used as a reagent and testing solution. Called also *s. nitroferricyanide.*

**s. para-aminosalicylate,** aminosalicylate sodium.

**s. perborate,** a compound, $NaBO_3 \cdot 4H_2O$, prepared by interaction of boric acid or sodium borate with sodium or hydrogen peroxide. It is an antiseptic, used in 2 per cent solution as a mouthwash and in a 10–20 per cent powder in dentifrices.

**s. pertechnetate Tc 99m** [USP], official nomenclature for *technetium 99m pertechnetate.*

**s. phosphate, dibasic** [USP], the heptahydrate monosodium salt of phosphoric acid, given orally as a cathartic, orally and rectally with sodium biphosphate as a cathartic, and orally with sodium biphosphate as an antihypercalcemic.

**s. phosphate, dried,** the anhydrous salt, $NaHPO_4 \cdot xH_2O$, dried at 105°C for four hours; used as an oral cathartic.

**s. phosphate, effervescent,** a dry granular mixture of citric acid, dried sodium phosphate, tartaric acid, and sodium bicarbonate; used as an oral cathartic.

**s. phosphate, exsiccated,** dried s. phosphate.

**s. phosphate, monobasic** [USP], the monohydrate, dihydrate, or anhydrous monosodium salt of phosphoric acid; used in buffer solutions, as a urinary acidifier, and as a source of phosphorus in hypophosphatemia, often in combination with potassium phosphate.

**s. phosphate P 32** [USP], sodium phosphate labeled with radiophosphorus ($^{32}P$); used in the treatment of polycythemia vera, chronic myelocytic leukemia, and chronic lymphocytic leukemia, in the localization of certain tumors, and in the palliation of metastatic skeletal disease; administered orally or intravenously.

**s. phytate,** the sodium salt of phytic acid; a calcium chelating agent.

**s. polyphosphate,** disodium salt of polyphosphoric acid; a pharmaceutic aid, $(NaPO_3)_n$.

**s. polystyrene sulfonate** [USP], a cation-exchange resin prepared in the sodium form, each gram of which exchanges 110–135 mg of potassium, calculated on the anhydrous basis; used as an antihyperkalemic, administered orally and rectally.

**potassium s. tartrate,** see under *potassium.*

**s. propionate** [NF], the sodium salt of propionic acid, having antifungal properties; used alone or in combination with calcium propionate or other agents as a preservative to inhibit mold production in bakery and dairy products and other foods and in pharmaceuticals. It is also used as a topical antifungal in the treatment of various mycoses.

**s. pyroborate,** s. borate.

**s. pyrophosphate,** a compound, $Na_4P_2O_7$, produced by heating sodium phosphate at a red heat; used in detergents.

**s. salicylate** [USP], the monosodium salt of salicylic acid, $C_7H_5NaO_3$, used as an analgesic, antipyretic, and antirheumatic; administered orally.

**s. silicofluoride,** a white, granular powder which is toxic in high concentrations. It is sometimes added to water to produce 0.7 to 1 part per million of fluorine, to prevent dental caries and is sometimes used in insecticides. Called also *s. fluosilicate.*

**s. stearate** [NF], a mixture of sodium stearate, sodium palmitate, and small amounts of the sodium salts of other fatty acids; used as a stiffening and emulsifying agent in pharmaceutical preparations.

**s. stibocaptate,** INN for *stibocaptate.*

**s. sulfate** [USP], the decahydrate disodium salt of sulfuric acid, used as an antihypercalcemic and antidote to barium poisoning, administered by intravenous infusion. It is also used orally as a cathartic or laxative and has been applied topically as a lymphagogue for infected wounds. Called also *Glauber's salt.*

**s. sulfite, anhydrous, s. sulfite, exsiccated,** a fairly stable compound, $Na_2SO_3$, occurring as small white crystals or powder; used as a reagent.

**s. tetraborate,** s. borate.

**s. tetradecyl sulfate,** an anionic surfactant with sclerosing properties; used as a wetting agent and in the treatment of varicose veins and hemorrhoids.

**s. thiamylal,** thiamylal sodium.

**s. thiosulfate** [USP], a compound used intravenously as an antidote to cyanide poisoning; also used in solution as a foot bath to prevent ringworm infection at swimming pools and public shower-baths, topically in tinea versicolor, and in measuring the volume of extracellular body fluid and the renal glomerular filtration rate. It was formerly used in the treatment of arsenic poisoning.

**s. trimetaphosphate,** the trisodium salt of metaphosphoric acid; a pharmaceutic aid, $Na_3P_3O_9$.

---

**so·do·ku** (so'do-koo) [Japanese *so* rat + *doku* poison] the spirillary form of rat-bite fever (see under *fever*).

**sod·o·my** (sod'ə-me) [after the city of *Sodom*] 1. anal intercourse. 2. old term for any form of homosexuality; sometimes extended to refer to any of numerous paraphilias.

**Soem·mer·ing's spot** (sərm'ər-ingz) [Samuel Thomas von *Soemmering,* German anatomist, 1755–1830] see under *ring* and *swelling,* and see *macula luteae.*

**SOFAS** Social and Occupational Functioning Assessment Scale.

**sof·ten·ing** (sof'en-ing) malacia (def. 1).

**s. of the brain,** encephalomalacia.

**colliquative s.,** see under *necrosis.*

**green s.,** malacia in which there is green pus present.

**hemorrhagic s.,** a hemorrhagic infarct of the brain; see also *cerebral infarction.*

**mucoid s.,** myxomatous degeneration.

**pyriform s.,** yellow s.

**red s.,** 1. hemorrhagic infarct. 2. hemorrhagic s.

**s. of the stomach,** gastromalacia; softening of the stomach walls due to an extremely acidic condition of its contents, a condition usually seen after death.

**white s.,** an area of white-colored necrosis in the brain occurring in the late stages of cerebral infarction.

**yellow s.,** an area of yellow-colored necrosis in the brain occurring in the late stages of cerebral infarction.

**Soh·val-Sof·fer syndrome** (so'vahl-sof'ər) [Arthur R. *Sohval,* American internist, 1904–1985; Louis J. *Soffer,* American internist, born 1904] see under *syndrome.*

**Sol.** solution.

**sol** (sol) [*sol*ution] a colloid system in which the dispersion medium is liquid or gas; the latter is usually called an *aerosol.*

**metal s.,** a colloidal dispersion of a metal in a liquid. Such dispersions often have catalytic properties similar to those of enzymes, and are therefore sometimes called inorganic enzymes.

**So·la·na·ceae** (so″lə-na'se-e) a large family of widely distributed herbs, shrubs, and trees, having great economic importance, and including many poisonous and medicinal species. *Atropa, Capsicum, Datura, Duboisia, Hyoscyamus, Nicotiana, Scopolia,* and *Solanum* are important genera.

**so·la·na·ceous** (so″lə-na'shəs) of or pertaining to the family Solanaceae.

**so·lan·drine** (so-lan'drin) pseudohyoscyamine.

**so·la·nine** (so'lə-nēn) [MeSH: Solanine] a steroidal glycoalkaloid found in several species of *Solanum,* such as the nightshades and the green spots on potatoes; in humans and other animals it causes erythrolysis, central nervous system depression, and often fatal respiratory failure.

**so·la·noid** (so'lə-noid) [*solanum* + *-oid*] resembling a raw potato in texture.

**So·la·num** (so-la'nəm) [L. "nightshade"] a large genus of plants of the family Solanaceae. It includes the potato, tomato, eggplant, several of the nightshades, and many poisonous and medicinal species. *S. carolinen'se* L. is a North American species poisonous to humans and other animals. *S. dimidia'tum, S. fastigia'tum,* and *S. kweben'se* cause crazy cow syndrome respectively in the United States, Brazil, and South Africa. *S. malacox'ylon* is a South American species that causes enzootic calcinosis in ruminants.

**so·lap·sone** (so-lap'sōn) an antibacterial derivative of dapsone, having actions similar to those of the parent compound but less toxic; used as a leprostatic, administered orally and intramuscularly. Called also *solasulfone.*

**so·lar** (so'lər) [L. *solaris*] 1. pertaining to the sun. 2. denoting the great sympathetic plexus and its principal ganglia (especially the celiac); so called because of their radiating nerves.

**so·la·ri·um** (so-lar'e-əm) [L.] a room especially designed to allow exposure to light of the sun or to artificial light.

**so·la·sul·fone** (so″lə-sul'fōn) solapsone.

**So·la·tene** (so'lə-tēn) trademark for a preparation of beta carotene.

**sol·a·tion** (sol-a'shən) the conversion of a gel into a sol.

**sold·er** (sod'ər) [L. *solidatio* making solid, fastening] 1. a fusible metal or alloy of metals used to unite pieces of metals with higher fusion temperatures. 2. to fasten together pieces of metal through the use of fusible metals or alloys of metal.

**sole** (sōl) [L. *solea; planta*] 1. planta. 2. the inferior surface of a horse's hoof.

**solen(o)-** [Gr. *sōlēn* a channel, gutter, pipe] a combining form denoting relationship to a pipe or gutter; tubular or grooved.

**So·le·nog·ly·pha** (so″lə-nog'lĭ-fə) [*soleno-* + Gr. *glyphein* to cut out with a knife] a group of venomous snakes with fangs that are hollow like a hypodermic needle and that normally fold back against the roof of the mouth but can be erected for striking and piercing. Examples are the massasauga and the rattlesnakes.

**so·le·noid** (so'lə-noid) [Gr. *sōlēnoeidēs* pipe-shaped, from *sōlēn* pipe] 1. a coil of insulated wire in which a magnetic field is produced by a flow of electric current. 2. a coil surrounding a movable iron core that is pulled in when the coil is energized. It can be used to perform some mechanical work, such as opening a valve, or as a switch.

**so·le·no·nych·ia** (so″lə-no-nik′e-ə) [*soleno-* + *onychia*] dystrophia unguis mediana canaliformis.

**So·le·no·po·tes** (so″lə-no-po′tēz) [*soleno-* + Gr. *pōtēs* a drinker] a genus of sucking lice (order Anoplura); *S. capilla′tus* is found on cattle.

**So·le·nop·sis** (so″lə-nop′sis) the fire ants, a genus of stinging ants (family Formicidae), which may attack humans, inflicting painful burning stings and causing local or systemic reactions. *S. gemina′ta* is indigenous to the United States. *S. saevis′sima rich′teri* is a viciously aggressive South American species that has now gained a foothold in North America.

**sol·fer·i·no** (sol″fər-e′no) fuchsin.

**Sol·ga·nal** (sol′gə-nəl″) trademark for a preparation of aurothioglucose.

**sol·id** (sol′id) [L. *solidus*] 1. not fluid or gaseous. 2. not hollow. 3. a substance or tissue not fluid or gaseous.
**color s.,** a three-dimensional geometrical body, devised to show the relation of all hues and brightnesses, including black, white, and grays, in their various modes.

**Sol·i·da·go** (sol″ĭ-da′go) [L.] the goldenrods, a genus of composite-flowered plants (family Compositae). *S. virgau′rea* L., of Europe and North America, is aromatic and diuretic. Certain other species are toxic or deadly to livestock.

**sol·i·dism** (sol′ĭ-diz-əm) the fundamental theory of Asclepiades and Themison, opposed to humoralism and pneumatism. Solidism is a development of atomism that made possible a new classification for disease: either the atoms were too distant and the bodily pores too lax, or the atoms too close and the pores too tight.

**sol·ip·sism** (sōl′ip-siz-əm) [L. *solus* alone + *ipse* self] the belief that the world exists only in the mind of the individual, or that it consists solely of the individual himself and his own experiences.

**sol·ip·sis·tic** (sōl″ip-sis′tik) pertaining to or characterized by solipsism.

**sol·lu·nar** (sōl-lu′nər) [L. *sol* sun + *luna* moon] pertaining to or caused by the sun and moon.

**sol·pu·gid** (sol-pu′jid) an individual of the order Solpugida.

**Sol·pu·gida** (sol″pu-jid′ə) the jointed spiders, a family of hairy spiders that are differentiated from other spiders by having a segmented abdomen more broadly joined to the cephalothorax; solpugids can inflict deep painful bites and are found mainly in desert, tropical, and subtropical areas.

**sol·u·bil·i·ty** (sol″u-bil′ĭ-te) [MeSH: Solubility] the quality or fact of being soluble; susceptibility of being dissolved.

**sol·u·ble** (sol′u-bəl) [L. *solubilis*] susceptible of being dissolved.

**Solu-Cor·tef** (sol″u-kor′tef) trademark for a preparation of hydrocortisone sodium succinate.

**Sol·u·rex** (sol′u-reks″) trademark for preparations of dexamethasone.

**so·lute** (sol′ūt) a substance dissolved in a solvent; a solution consists of a solute and a solvent.

**so·lu·tio** (so-loo′she-o) [L., from *solvēre* to dissolve] solution.

**so·lu·tion** (sə-loo′shən) [L. *solutio*] 1. a homogeneous mixture of one or more substances (solutes) dispersed molecularly in a sufficient quantity of dissolving medium (solvent). The solute may be gas, liquid, or solid; the solvent is usually liquid, but may be solid, as in a solid solution of copper in silver (sterling silver). In pharmacology, a liquid preparation containing one or several soluble chemical substances usually dissolved in water and not, for various reasons, falling into another category. 2. the process of dissolving. 3. a loosening or separation.

## Solution

**acetic acid otic s.** [USP], a solution of glacial acetic acid in a nonaqueous solvent; used topically to treat otitis externa caused by *Pseudomonas, Candida,* and *Aspergillus.*
**Albright's s.,** one consisting of 75 g of sodium citrate, 25 g of potassium citrate, 140 g of citric acid, and 1000 mL of water; used in the treatment of renal tubular acidosis.
**alcoholic s.,** a solution in which alcohol is used as the solvent.
**aluminum acetate topical s.** [USP], an astringent solution prepared from aluminum subacetate topical solution by the addition of glacial acetic acid and water; used as a gargle or mouthwash and applied to the skin as a wet dressing, diluted with 10 to 40 parts water. Called also *Burow's s.*
**aluminum subacetate topical s.** [USP], a solution containing aluminum sulfate, acetic acid, precipitated calcium carbonate, and water, used topically on the skin and mucous membranes as an astringent. It is also used as a topical antiseptic and as a wet dressing in various skin diseases.
**amaranth s.,** a clear, vivid red solution of amaranth in purified water, used as a coloring agent in pharmaceutical preparations.
**amaranth s., compound,** a solution composed of amaranth solution, caramel, alcohol, and purified water; used as a coloring agent in pharmaceutical preparations.
**aminoacetic acid sterile s.,** a sterile, aqueous solution containing 95 to 105 per cent of the labeled amount of aminoacetic acid; used as a nutrient.
**ammonia s., dilute,** a colorless, transparent, alkaline liquid, containing 9 to 10 percent of ammonia; used as a pharmaceutic necessity. Called also *ammonia water* or *diluted ammonium hydroxide s.*
**ammonia s., strong** [NF], a colorless, transparent, strongly alkaline liquid containing 27–31 per cent ammonia; used as a solvent and as a source of ammonia in pharmaceutical preparations.
**ammonium acetate s.,** a clear, colorless liquid, containing ammonium acetate, which has been used as a diaphoretic and diuretic.
**ammonium citrate s., alkaline,** a preparation of dibasic ammonium citrate and strong ammonia solution; used in tests for zinc.
**ammonium hydroxide s., diluted,** ammonia s., dilute.
**ammonium hydroxide s., stronger,** ammonia s., strong.
**anisotonic s.,** a solution having tonicity differing from that of the standard of reference.
**anticoagulant citrate dextrose s.** [USP], a solution of citric acid, sodium citrate, and dextrose in water for injection, used as an anticoagulant in the preservation of whole blood.
**anticoagulant citrate phosphate dextrose s.** [USP], a solution containing citric acid, sodium citrate, sodium biphosphate, and dextrose in water for injection; used for preservation of whole blood or red cells for up to 21 days. Called also *CPD s.*
**anticoagulant citrate phosphate dextrose adenine s.** [USP], a solution consisting of anticoagulant citrate phosphate dextrose solution and adenine; used for the preservation of whole blood or red cells for up to 35 days. Called also *CPDA-1 s.* and *CPD-adenine s.*
**anticoagulant heparin s.** [USP], a sterile solution of heparin solution in sodium chloride injection, used as an anticoagulant in the preservation of whole blood.
**anticoagulant sodium citrate s.** [USP], a solution of sodium citrate in water for injection, used for the storage of whole blood, and for the preparation of citrated human plasma.
**antipyrine and benzocaine otic s.** [USP], a solution of antipyrine and benzocaine in glycerin instilled into the ear canal for relief of pain and inflammation in acute otitis media and as an adjunct in cerumen removal.
**antipyrine, benzocaine, and phenylephrine hydrochloride otic s.** [USP], a solution of antipyrine, benzocaine, and phenylephrine hydrochloride in a suitable nonaqueous solvent; instilled into the ear canal for relief of pain and inflammation in acute otitis media.
**aqueous s.,** a solution in which water is used as the solvent.
**arsenious acid s.,** a clear, colorless, odorless liquid, with an acid reaction, containing arsenic trioxide.
**Benedict's s.,** sodium citrate, sodium carbonate, and copper sulfate water solution. Its normal blue color changes to yellow, orange, or red in the presence of a reducing sugar such as glucose. It is used in urinalysis.
**Bouin's s.,** see under *fluid.*
**buffer s.,** a solution which resists appreciable change in its hydrogen ion concentration when acid or alkali is added to it.
**Burow's s.,** aluminum acetate topical s.
**calcium hydroxide topical s.** [USP], a clear, colorless liquid with an alkaline reaction, containing at least 140 mg of calcium hydroxide per 100 mL at 25°C (77°F); used in preparing various astringent formulations for topical application to the skin and mucous membranes. It has also been used internally as an antacid and has been added to infant formulas to decrease the curd size formed from cow's milk. Called also *lime water.*
**carbamide peroxide topical s.** [USP], a solution of carbamide peroxide in anhydrous glycerin, used as a cerumen-softening agent and as a dental cleanser and anti-inflammatory.
**carbol-fuchsin topical s.** [USP], a dark purple solution containing,

in each 1000 mL, basic fuchsin (3 g), phenol (45 g), resorcinol (100 g), acetone (50 mL), alcohol (100 mL), and purified water; used as a local antifungal in the treatment of dermatophytosis, tinea, and other skin infections. Called also *Castellani's paint.*

**cardioplegic s.,** a cold solution injected into the aortic root or coronary ostia to induce cardiac arrest and protect the heart from damage during open heart surgery; it is usually potassium in either a buffered electrolyte solution or blood.

**carmine s.,** a deep red, rather viscous liquid, compounded of carmine, diluted ammonia solution, glycerin, and water; used as a coloring agent.

**Carnoy's s.,** an acid fixative used for studying the cell nucleus and chromosomes, composed of: 3 parts absolute ethanol, 5 parts saturated picric acid, 5 parts 40 per cent formaldehyde (formalin), and 1 part glacial acetic acid.

**centinormal s.,** hundredth-normal s.

**cochineal s.,** a dark, purplish red fluid with a slightly aromatic odor, compounded of cochineal, potassium carbonate, alum, potassium bitartrate, glycerin, and water; used as a coloring agent.

**colloid s., colloidal s.,** imprecise term for a *colloidal system;* see *colloid,* def. 2.

**contrast s.,** a solution of a substance opaque to the x-ray, used to facilitate radiographic visualization of some organ or structure in the body.

**CPD s.,** anticoagulant citrate phosphate dextrose s.

**CPDA-1 s., CPD-adenine s.,** anticoagulant citrate phosphate dextrose adenine s.

**cresol s., compound, cresol s., saponated,** a mixture of cresol, vegetable oil, potassium hydroxide, alcohol, and water, and containing, in each 100 mL, 46 to 52 mL of cresol; used as a disinfectant, chiefly to sterilize instruments, dishes, utensils, and other inanimate objects.

**crystal violet s.,** gentian violet topical s.

**Czapek-Dox s.,** Czapek-Dox agar; see under *culture medium.*

**Dakin's s., Dakin's s., modified,** diluted sodium hypochlorite s.

**decimolar s.,** a solution having one-tenth the concentration of a molar solution.

**decinormal s.,** tenth-normal s.

**desonide and acetic acid otic s.,** a solution of desonide and acetic acid used topically for the treatment of superficial external auditory canal infections accompanied by inflammation.

**dexamethasone sodium phosphate ophthalmic s.** [USP], a sterile aqueous solution of dexamethasone sodium phosphate, instilled into the conjunctival sac in the treatment of inflammatory and allergic conditions and into the otic canal for the treatment of superficial external auditory canal infections accompanied by inflammation.

**diatrizoate sodium s.** [USP], a solution of diatrizoate sodium in purified water, or a solution of diatrizoic acid in purified water prepared with the aid of sodium hydroxide; used orally as a diagnostic radiopaque medium in radiography of the gastrointestinal tract.

**disclosing s.,** a solution used for the purpose of making something apparent, such as one to be painted on the surface of a tooth in order to stain, and thus render visible, foreign matter or bacterial plaque.

**double-normal s.,** a solution having double the strength of a normal solution: designated 2 N.

**Drabkin's s.,** an aqueous solution containing 1.0 g sodium bicarbonate, 0.05 g potassium cyanide, and 0.20 g potassium ferricyanide per liter; used to lyse red cells and convert hemoglobin to cyanmethemoglobin in hemoglobinometry.

***dl*-ephedrine hydrochloride s.,** racephedrine hydrochloride s.

**Farrant's s.,** a mounting preparation used in bacteriological work, containing glycerin, water, arsenious acid solution, and gum arabic.

**Fehling's s.,** an alkaline copper sulfate solution similar to Benedict's reagent.

**ferric subsulfate s.,** a reddish-brown, almost odorless, aqueous solution of basic ferric sulfate, used as an astringent.

**fiftieth-normal s.,** a solution having one-fiftieth the strength of a normal solution: designated N/50 or 0.02 N.

**fixative s.,** see *fixative.*

**Flemming's s.,** a solution for hardening histological specimens, consisting of chromium trioxide, osmium tetroxide, glacial acetic acid, and water.

**Fonio's s.,** a solution of magnesium sulfate in water, used as a diluent for blood platelets.

**formaldehyde s.** [USP], a solution of formaldehyde in water, containing not less than 37 per cent of formaldehyde; used as a disinfectant. Called also *formalin* and *formol.*

**formol-Zenker s.,** a fixing solution consisting of Zenker's solution and formaldehyde solution.

**Fowler's s.,** potassium arsenite s.

**gelatin s., special intravenous,** a 5 or 6 per cent sterile, pyrogen-free solution of gelatin in isotonic sodium chloride solution; used as a plasma volume expander.

**gentian violet topical s.** [USP], a purple liquid with a slight odor of alcohol, containing gentian violet, alcohol, and purified water, applied topically to the skin and mucous membranes in infections associated with gram-positive bacteria and molds. Called also *crystal violet s.* and *methylrosaniline chloride s.*

**Gilson's s.,** a fixative solution consisting of mercury bichloride, nitric acid, glacial acetic acid, 70 per cent alcohol, and water.

**gold s.,** any of a variety of gold compounds available for medicinal purposes with differences in their physical properties and clinical effectiveness, e.g., aurothioglucose, gold sodium thiomalate, and gold sodium thiosulfate.

**Gowers' s.,** a solution of sodium sulfate, glacial acetic acid, and water, used for the dilution of blood prior to counting red blood cells with a hemocytometer.

**Gram's s.,** see under *stain.*

**gram molecular s.,** molar s.

**half-normal s.,** a solution having half the strength of a normal solution; designated N/2.

**Hamdi's s.,** a solution for preserving histological specimens, consisting of sodium sulfate, salt, glycerin, and water.

**Hayem's s.,** a solution of mercury bichloride, sodium chloride, and sodium sulfate, used in diluting blood prior to counting red blood cells with a hemocytometer.

**heparin lock flush s.** [USP], a sterile preparation of heparin sodium injection with sufficient sodium chloride to make it isotonic with blood, used to maintain patency of indwelling intravascular devices designed for intermittent injection or infusion therapy or blood sampling.

**hundredth-normal s.,** a solution having one-hundredth the strength of a normal solution; designated N/100 or 0.01 N.

**hydrogen dioxide s.,** hydrogen peroxide topical s.

**hydrogen peroxide topical s.** [USP], a solution containing 2.5–3.5 g hydrogen peroxide per 100 mL; used as a topical anti-infective to the skin and mucous membranes.

**hydroxypropyl methylcellulose ophthalmic s.** [USP], a sterile solution containing 85–115 per cent hydroxypropyl methylcellulose; applied topically to the conjunctiva to protect the cornea during certain ophthalmic procedures and to lubricate the cornea.

**hyperbaric s.,** a solution having a greater specific gravity than a standard of reference, such as one used for spinal anesthesia having a specific gravity greater than that of the spinal fluid, causing it to migrate downward and produce anesthesia below the level of injection.

**hypobaric s.,** a solution having a specific gravity less than that of a standard of reference, such as one used for spinal anesthesia having a specific gravity less than that of the spinal fluid, causing it to migrate upward and produce anesthesia above the level of injection.

**indium In 111 chloride s.** [USP], a solution of indium 111 in dilute hydrochloric acid, used for the radiolabeling of proteins such as monoclonal antibodies.

**iodine s., compound, iodine s., strong** [USP], a transparent, deep brown liquid, with the odor of iodine, consisting of iodine and potassium iodide in purified water, containing 4.5–5.5 g of iodine and 9.5–10.5 g of potassium iodide per 100 mL; used as a source of iodine in preparation for thyroid surgery, administered orally. Called also *Lugol's s.*

**iodine topical s.** [USP], transparent, reddish brown liquid, with the odor of iodine, consisting of iodine and sodium iodide in purified water, each 100 mL of which contains 1.8 to 2.2 g of iodine and 2.1 to 2.6 g of sodium iodide; used as a topical anti-infective.

**isobaric s.,** a solution having the same specific gravity as a standard of reference, such as one used for spinal anesthesia having a specific gravity the same as that of the spinal fluid, causing it to remain and produce anesthesia at the level of injection.

**Kaiserling's s.,** 1. *for fixation:* formalin 400 mL, water 2000 mL, potassium nitrate 30 g, potassium acetate 60 g. 2. *for restoring color:* alcohol 80 per cent. 3. *for preservation:* potassium acetate 200 g, glycerol 400 mL, sodium arsenate 100 g, water 2000 mL.

**Labarraque's s.,** sodium hypochlorite solution, diluted with an equal volume of water.

**lactulose s.** [USP], an aqueous solution prepared from lactulose concentrate, consisting principally of lactulose, with small quantities of lactose and galactose and traces of other related sugars; used to reduce blood ammonia levels in the treatment of hepatic encephalopathy, administered orally.

**Lang's s.,** see under *fluid.*

**Lange's s.,** a solution of colloidal gold.

**lime s., sulfurated,** sulfurated lime topical s.

**liver s.,** a brownish liquid prepared from mammalian livers and containing the soluble thermostable fraction which stimulates hematopoiesis in patients with pernicious anemia. Called also *liquid liver extract.*

**Locke's s.,** a solution of sodium chloride, calcium chloride, potassium chloride, sodium bicarbonate, and dextrose; used in physiological experiments to keep the mammalian heart beating.

**Locke's s., citrated,** a solution of sodium chloride, potassium chloride, calcium chloride, and sodium citrate in distilled water, with pH adjusted to 7.4.

**Locke-Ringer's s.,** a test solution containing sodium chloride, potassium chloride, calcium chloride, magnesium chloride, sodium bicarbonate, dextrose, and water.

**Lugol's s.,** strong iodine s.

**Magendie's s.,** a solution for parenteral use containing morphine sulfate.

**magnesium citrate oral s.** [USP], a colorless to slightly yellow, clear, effervescent liquid, with a sweet, acidulous taste and a lemon flavor, which consists of magnesium carbonate, anhydrous citric acid, syrup, talc, lemon oil, potassium bicarbonate, and purified water; used as a cathartic.

**methoxsalen topical s.** [USP], a preparation containing 9.2 to 10.8 mg of methoxsalen per mL; used in conjunction with exposure to ultraviolet light to facilitate repigmentation in idiopathic vitiligo, and also as a suntan accelerator and sun protectant.

**methylcellulose ophthalmic s.** [USP], a sterile solution of methylcellulose, applied topically to protect the cornea during certain ophthalmic procedures and to lubricate the cornea.

**methylrosaniline chloride s.,** gentian violet topical s.

**molal s.,** a solution containing 1 mole of solute dissolved in 1000 g of solvent.

**molar s.,** a solution each liter of which contains 1 mole of solute per liter of solution: designated M/1 or 1 M. The concentration of other solutions may be expressed in relation to that of molar solutions as tenth-molar (M/10 or 0.1 M), etc.

**molecular disperse s.,** a solution in which the dispersed particles have a diameter of about 0.1 picometer.

**Monsel's s.,** ferric subsulfate s.

**Nessler's s.,** see under *reagent.*

**normal s.,** a solution each liter of which contains 1 gram equivalent weight of the dissolved substance: designated N/1 or 1 N.

**normal saline s., normal salt s.,** physiological salt s.

**normobaric s.,** isobaric s.

**ophthalmic s.,** a sterile solution, essentially free from foreign particles and suitably compounded and dispensed, for instillation into the eye.

**Orth's s.,** a solution for fixing histological specimens, consisting of Müller's fluid and formaldehyde solution.

**Perenyi's s.,** an embryological fixing solution, consisting of 10 per cent solution of nitric acid, alcohol, and 0.5 per cent solution of chromic acid.

**physiological salt s., physiological sodium chloride s.,** an aqueous solution of sodium chloride having an osmolality similar to that of blood serum.

**pituitary s., pituitary s., posterior,** posterior pituitary injection.

**potassium arsenite s.,** a solution formerly used to treat chronic myelogenous leukemia and chronic dermatitis in humans and emphysema, nonparasitic dermatitis, and cough in other animals. Called also *Fowler's s.*

**potassium citrate and citric acid oral s.** [USP], a solution of potassium citrate and citric acid monohydrate in an aqueous medium, providing approximately 2 mmole potassium per mL and used as an electrolyte replenisher.

**povidone-iodine topical s.** [USP], a reddish brown, transparent solution of povidone-iodine and water, applied topically as an anti-infective.

**racephedrine hydrochloride s.,** a clear, colorless solution with a camphoraceous odor and taste, compounded of racephedrine hydrochloride, chlorobutanol, and Ringer's solution, each 100 mL of which contains between 930 mg and 1.07 g of racephedrine; used as an adrenergic.

**Randall's s.,** a solution consisting of the acetate, bicarbonate, and citrate salts of potassium; used especially in the treatment of potassium deficiency, administered orally.

**Ringer's s.,** see under *irrigation.*

**Ringer's s., lactated,** see under *injection.*

**Ruge's s.,** a solution of glacial acetic acid, 40 per cent formaldehyde solution, and water; used as a stain.

**saline s., salt s.,** a solution of sodium chloride, or common salt, in purified water.

**saturated s.,** a solution in which the solvent has taken up all of the dissolved substance that it can hold in solution.

**Schällibaum's s.,** a solution of celloidin and oil of cloves used in histological work to attach paraffin sections to slides.

**sclerosing s.,** a solution of an irritant substance for injection into a vein to produce obliteration of the vein, or into a hernia to induce fibrous formation and obliteration of the sac.

**seminormal s.,** half-normal s.

**Seyderhelm's s.,** a colloidal mixture of Congo red and trypan blue, for staining urinary sediment.

**Shohl's s.,** a solution containing 140 g citric acid and 98 g hydrated crystalline salt of sodium citrate in distilled water to make 1000 mL; used to correct electrolyte imbalance in the treatment of renal tubular acidosis.

**silver nitrate s., ammoniacal,** an ammonium compound of silver nitrate; used as an antiseptic and in the detection and prevention of dental caries. Because of inflammatory and necrotic tissue reaction, its use has now declined.

**sodium chloride s.,** see under *irrigation.*

**sodium fluoride and orthophosphoric acid s.,** a solution containing 90 to 110 per cent of the labeled amount of fluoride ion; used as a dental caries prophylactic, applied topically to the teeth.

**sodium hypochlorite s.** [USP], a clear, pale, greenish yellow liquid with the odor of chlorine, containing 4–6 per cent sodium hypochlorite; used as a disinfectant for utensils, etc., but not suitable for application to wounds. It has also been used as a deodorant and bleaching agent.

**sodium hypochlorite s., diluted,** a colorless to light yellow liquid with a faint odor of chlorine, compounded of sodium hypochlorite solution, sodium bicarbonate, and water, each 100 mL containing 450 to 500 mg of sodium hypochlorite; used as a topical anti-infective. It is also used for wound irrigation, and has been used to irrigate the urinary bladder. Called also *Dakin's fluid, Dakin's s., modified Dakin's s.,* and *surgical s. of chlorinated soda.* See also *Carrel's treatment,* under *treatment.*

**solid s.,** a crystalline phase of solution that is homogeneous but has several different chemical components, whose molecules are randomly distributed on the points of the space lattice. See also under *alloy.*

**sorbitol s.** [USP], a clear, colorless, syrupy liquid with a sweet taste, consisting essentially of D-sorbitol with a small quantity of mannitol and other isomeric polyhydric alcohols; used as a flavored humectant in pharmaceutic preparations.

**standard s.,** one which contains in each liter a definitely stated amount of reagent; usually expressed in terms of normality (equivalent weights of solute per liter of solution) or molarity (moles of solute per liter of solution).

**sulfurated lime topical s.** [USP], a solution compounded of 165 g lime, 250 g sublimed sulfur, and 1000 mL water, boiled until the mixture is reduced to 1000 mL; used in diluted form as a topical antiparasitic fungicide, and keratolytic.

**supersaturated s.,** an unstable solution that contains more of the solute than it can permanently hold.

**surgical s. of chlorinated soda,** diluted sodium hypochlorite s.

**susa s.,** a decalcifying solution composed of mercury bichloride, sodium chloride, trichloroacetic acid, glacial acetic acid, formaldehyde solution, and water.

**TAC s.,** a solution of tetracaine, epinephrine, and cocaine, used as a local anesthetic in the emergency treatment of uncomplicated lacerations.

**tenth-normal s.,** one having one-tenth the strength of a normal solution: designated N/10 or 0.1 N.

**test s's,** standard solutions (in purity and concentration) of specified chemical substances used in performing certain test procedures.

**thousandth-normal s.,** a solution having one-thousandth the strength of a normal solution: designated N/1000 or 0.001 N.

**Toison's s.,** a fluid used in diluting blood for the counting of the erythrocytes, consisting of gentian violet, sodium chloride, sodium sulfate, glycerin, and water. Called also *Toison's fluid.*

**Tyrode's s.,** a modified Locke's solution containing magnesium.

**Vleminckx's s.,** sulfurated lime topical s..

**volumetric s.,** one which contains a specific quantity of solute per stated unit of volume; see also *standard s.*

**Zenker's s.,** a fixative solution consisting of mercury bichloride, potassium dichromate, glacial acetic acid, and water.

**Ziehl's s.,** see *Ziehl-Neelson carbolfuchsin,* under *stain.*

**solv.** abbreviation for L. *sol've,* dissolve.

**sol·va·ble** (sol'və-bəl) soluble.

**sol·vate** (sol'vāt) a compound of one or more molecules of a solvent with the ions or with the molecules of a dissolved substance.

**sol·va·tion** (sol-va'shən) chemical combination of a solvent with the solute.

**sol·vent** (sol'vənt) [L. *solvere* to dissolve] 1. dissolving; effecting a solution. 2. a substance, usually a liquid, that dissolves or that is capable of dissolving; the component of a solution that is present in greater amount. Cf. *solute.*

**sol·vol·y·sis** (sol-vol'ĭ-sis) a general term for double decomposition reactions of the type of hydrolysis, ammonolysis, and sulfolysis.

**So·ma** (so'mə) trademark for preparations of carisoprodol.

**so·ma** (so'mə) [Gr. *sōma* body] 1. the body as distinguished from the mind. See *corpus.* 2. the body tissue as distinguished from the germ cells. 3. cell body.

**so·mal** (so'məl) somatic.

**som·a·lin** (som'ə-lin) a cardioactive glycoside from plants of the genus *Adenium.*

**so·man** (so'man) an organophosphorus compound that is a potent cholinesterase inhibitor and is used as a nerve gas; symptoms of poisoning include bronchial constriction, convulsions, and often death. See also *organophosphorus compound poisoning,* under *poisoning.*

**so·ma·plasm** (so'mə-plaz-əm) somatoplasm.

**som·as·the·nia** (sōm"əs-the'ne-ə) [*soma* + *asthenia*] a condition of bodily weakness, poor appetite and sleep, and inability to maintain a normal active life without easy exhaustion.

**so·ma·tal·gia** (so"mə-tal'jə) [*somato-* + *-algia*] bodily pain.

**so·mat·as·the·nia** (so"mat-əs-the'ne-ə) somasthenia.

**so·mat·es·the·sia** (so"mat-əs-the'zhə) [*somato-* + *esthesia*] 1. somatic sense. 2. somatognosis.

**so·mat·es·thet·ic** (so"mat-əs-thet'ik) pertaining to somatesthesia (somatognosis).

**so·mat·ic** (so-mat'ik) [Gr. *sōmatikos*] 1. pertaining to or characteristic of the soma or body. 2. pertaining to the body wall in contrast to the viscera.

**so·mat·i·co·splanch·nic** (so-mat"ĭ-ko-splank'nik) somaticovisceral.

**so·mat·i·co·visc·er·al** (so-mat"ĭ-ko-vis'ər-əl) pertaining to the body proper and viscera.

**so·ma·tist** (so'mə-tist) one who believes that mental disorders are of physical origin and are based on bodily lesions.

**so·ma·ti·za·tion** (so"mə-tĭ-za'shən) in psychiatry, the conversion of mental experiences or states into bodily symptoms.

**somat(o)-** [Gr. *sōma,* gen. *sōmatos* body] a combining form denoting relationship to the body.

**so·mato·chrome** (so-mat'o-krōm) [*somato-* + *-chrome*] any neuron that has cytoplasm completely surrounding the nucleus and easily stainable Nissl bodies.

**so·ma·to·cri·nin** (so"mə-to-kri'nin) growth hormone–releasing hormone.

**so·mato·derm** (so-mat'o-dərm) [*somato-* + *-derm*] somatic layer.

**so·ma·to·did·y·mus** (so"mə-to-did'ĭ-məs) conjoined twins exhibiting somatodymia.

**so·ma·to·dym·ia** (so"mə-to-dim'e-ə) [*somato-* + Gr. *didymos* twin + *-ia*] a developmental anomaly in which conjoined twins have their trunks fused into one.

**so·mato·form** (so-mat'o-form) [*somato-* + L. *forma* form] denoting physical symptoms that can not be attributed to organic disease and appear to be of psychic origin.

**so·ma·to·gen·e·sis** (so"mə-to-jen'ə-sis) [*somato-* + *-genesis*] the formation or emergence of bodily structure out of hereditary sources; the formation of somatoplasm out of germ plasm.

**so·ma·to·ge·net·ic** (so-mat"o-jə-net'ik) 1. pertaining to somatogenesis. 2. somatogenic.

**so·ma·to·gen·ic** (so"mə-to-jen'ik) [*somato-* + *-genic*] originating in the cells of the body, as a disease process; opposed to psychogenic.

**so·ma·tog·no·sis** (so"mə-tog-no'sis) [*somato-* + Gr. *gnōsis* recognition] the general feeling of the existence of one's body and of the functioning of the organs. Called also *cenesthesia, somatesthesia, somesthesia,* and *body* or *sixth sense.*

**so·mato·gram** (so-mat'o-gram) [*somato-* + *-gram*] a radiograph of the body.

**so·ma·to·lib·er·in** (so"mə-to-lib'ər-in) [*somatotropin* + *-liberin*] growth hormone–releasing hormone.

**so·ma·tol·o·gy** (so"mə-tol'o-je) [*somato-* + *-logy*] the sum of what is known regarding the body; the study of the anatomy and physiology of the body.

**so·ma·to·mam·mo·tro·pin** (so"mə-to-mam'o-tro"pin) a family of hormones, including growth hormone and prolactin, produced by the anterior pituitary, and human placental lactogen, produced by the placenta.
**chorionic s.,** human placental lactogen.

**so·ma·to·me·din** (so"mə-to-me'din) any of several peptides formed in the liver and other tissues and found in plasma, complexed with binding proteins; they stimulate cellular growth and replication, particularly in bone and muscle, as second messengers in the somatotropic actions of growth hormone and also have insulin-like biological activities. Two such peptides have been isolated, insulin-like growth factors I and II (q.v.).
**s. A,** former name for *insulin-like growth factor II.*
**s. C,** former name for *insulin-like growth factor I.*

**so·ma·to·meg·a·ly** (so"mə-to-meg'ə-le) [*somato-* + *-megaly*] gigantism.

**so·ma·tom·e·try** (so"mə-tom'ə-tre) [*somato-* + *-metry*] measurement of the body.

**so·ma·top·a·gus** (so"mə-top'ə-gəs) [*somato-* + *-pagus*] somatodidymus.

**so·ma·to·path·ic** (so"mə-to-path'ik) [*somato-* + *path-* + *-ic*] pertaining to or characterized by somatopathy.

**so·ma·top·a·thy** (so"mə-top'ə-the) [*somato-* + *-pathy*] a bodily disorder as distinguished from a mental one.

**so·ma·to·phre·nia** (so"mə-to-fre'ne-ə) [*somato-* + *phren-* + *-ia*] exaggeration or imagination of bodily ills.

**so·mato·plasm** (so-mat'o-plaz-əm) [*somato-* + *-plasm*] the protoplasm of the body cells as distinguished from that of the germ cells. Cf. *germ plasm.*

**so·ma·to·pleu·ral** (so"mə-to-ploor'əl) pertaining to the somatopleure.

**so·mato·pleure** (so-mat'o-ploor) [*somato-* + Gr. *pleura* side] the embryonic body wall, formed by ectoderm and somatic mesoderm.

**so·ma·to·psy·chic** (so"mə-to-si'kik) [*somato-* + *psychic*] pertaining to both body and mind; relating to the effects of the body on the mind.

**so·ma·tos·chi·sis** (so"mə-tos'kĭ-sis) [*somato-* + *-schisis*] a developmental anomaly characterized by a fissure of the trunk.

**so·ma·tos·co·py** (so"mə-tos'kə-pe) [*somato-* + *-scopy*] viewing or examination of the body.

**so·ma·to·sen·sory** (so"mə-to-sen'sə-re) pertaining to sensations received in the skin and deep tissues.

**so·ma·to·sex·u·al** (so"mə-to-sek'shoo-əl) [*somato-* + *sexual*] pertaining to the physical manifestations of sexual development.

**so·ma·to·splanch·no·pleur·ic** (so"mə-to-splank"no-ploor'ik) pertaining to the somatopleure and the splanchnopleure.

**so·ma·to·stat·in (SS)** (so"mə-to-stat'in) [*somato*tropin + *-statin*] [MeSH: Somatostatin] any of several cyclic tetradecapeptides elaborated primarily by the median eminence of the hypothalamus and by the delta cells of the pancreatic islets; they inhibit release of growth hormone, thyrotropin, and corticotropin by the adenohypophysis, of insulin and glucagon by the pancreas, of gastrin by the gastric mucosa, of secretin by the intestinal mucosa, and of renin by the kidney. Called also *growth hormone release–inhibiting hormone* and *somatotropin release–inhibiting hormone.*

**so·ma·to·stat·i·no·ma** (som"ə-to-stat"ĭ-no'mə) [MeSH: Somatostatinoma] a rare type of tumor that secretes somatostatin; most are islet cell tumors associated with diabetes mellitus or abnormal glucose tolerance, but some are found in the duodenum.

**so·ma·to·ther·a·py** (so"mə-to-ther'ə-pe) [*somato-* + *therapy*] biological treatment of mental disorders, such as by electric shock or drug therapy.

**so·ma·to·to·nia** (so"mə-to-to'ne-ə) [*somato-* + *ton-* + *-ia*] a temperament type characterized by love of physical adventure, boundless energy, boldness, aggressiveness, and need for exercise and activity; the behavioral counterpart of mesomorphy.

**so·ma·to·top·ag·no·sia** (so"mə-to-tōp"ag-no'zhə) [*somato-* + *top-* + *agnosia*] autotopagnosia.

**so·ma·to·top·ic** (so"mə-to-top'ik) related to particular areas of the body; describing the organization of the motor area of the brain, control of the movement of different parts of the body being centered in specific regions of the cortex.

**so·ma·to·trid·y·mus** (so″mə-to-trid′ĭ-məs) [*somato-* + *tri-* + *-didymus*] a fetus with three trunks.

**so·mato·trope** (so-mat′o-trōp) somatotroph.

**so·mato·troph** (so-mat′o-trōf) an acidophil of the adenohypophysis that stains preferentially with orange G and secretes growth hormone. Called also *somatotrope cell, somatotroph cell,* and *alpha acidophil.*

**so·ma·to·troph·ic** (so″mə-to-trōf′ik) somatotropic.

**so·ma·to·tro·phin** (so′mə-to-tro″fin) growth hormone.

**so·ma·to·trop·ic** (so″mə-to-trop′ik) [*somato-* + *-tropic*] 1. having an affinity for or stimulating the body or the body cells; also having an influence on the body. 2. having a stimulating effect on body nutrition and growth. 3. having the properties of a growth hormone (somatotropin).

**so·ma·to·tro·pin** (so′mə-to-tro″pin) [MeSH: Somatotropin] growth hormone.

**so·mato·type** (so-mat′o-tīp) [*somato-* + *type*] [MeSH: Somatotypes] a particular category of body build, determined on the basis of certain physical characteristics. See *ectomorph, endomorph,* and *mesomorph.*

**so·mato·typ·ing** (so-mat′o-tīp″ing) a method of studying objectively the physical types of individuals.

**so·mato·ty·py** (so-mat′o-ti″pe) the determination of the type of body build.

**so·mat·ro·pin** (so-mat′ro-pin) [MeSH: Somatropin] growth hormone.

**-some** [Gr. *soma* body] a word termination denoting a body.

**so·mes·the·sia** (so″mes-the′zhə) somatognosis.

**so·mes·thet·ic** (so″mes-thet′ik) pertaining to somatognosis (somesthesia).

**SOMI** sternal-occipital-mandibular immobilizer.

**-somia** [Gr. *sōma* body + *-ia*] word termination denoting a condition of the body.

**so·mite** (so′mīt) [MeSH: Somites] one of the paired, blocklike masses of mesoderm, arranged segmentally alongside the neural tube of the embryo, forming the vertebral column and segmental musculature; called also *mesoblastic,mesodermic, primitive, primordial,* or *protovertebral segment.*

**som·nam·bu·lance** (som-nam′bu-ləns) somnambulism.

**som·nam·bu·la·tion** (som-nam″bu-la′shən) somnambulism.

**som·nam·bu·lism** (som-nam′bu-liz-əm) [*somn-* + L. *ambulare* to walk] [MeSH: Somnambulism] rising out of bed and walking about or performing other complex motor behavior during an apparent state of sleep, usually occurring in the first third of the night and lasting a few minutes to a half hour. The individual is relatively unresponsive, not alert, not easily awakened, and usually amnesic for the episode later. Called also *noctambulation, sleepwalking,* and *somnambulance.* See also *sleepwalking disorder,* under *disorder.*

**som·nam·bu·list** (som-nam′bu-list) a person who walks in his sleep.

**somn(i)-** [L. *somnus* sleep] a combining form denoting relationship to sleep.

**som·ni·fa·cient** (som″nĭ-fa′shənt) [*somni-* + *-facient*] 1. causing sleep; hypnotic. 2. an agent that induces sleep.

**som·nif·er·ous** (som-nif′ər-əs) [*somni-* + *-ferous*] inducing or causing sleep.

**som·nif·ic** (som-nif′ik) somniferous.

**som·nil·o·quence** (som-nil′o-kwəns) somniloquism.

**som·nil·o·quism** (som-nil′o-kwiz-əm) [*somni-* + L. *loqui* to speak] talking during sleep.

**som·nil·o·quist** (som-nil′o-kwist) one who talks in his sleep.

**som·nil·o·quy** (som-nil′o-kwe) somniloquism.

**Som·ni·o·sus** (som″ne-o′səs) a genus of sharks. *S. microce′phalus* is the Greenland shark, a species with a small head, weak jaws, and small teeth whose muscle tissue is poisonous, causing elasmobranch poisoning in humans and other animals.

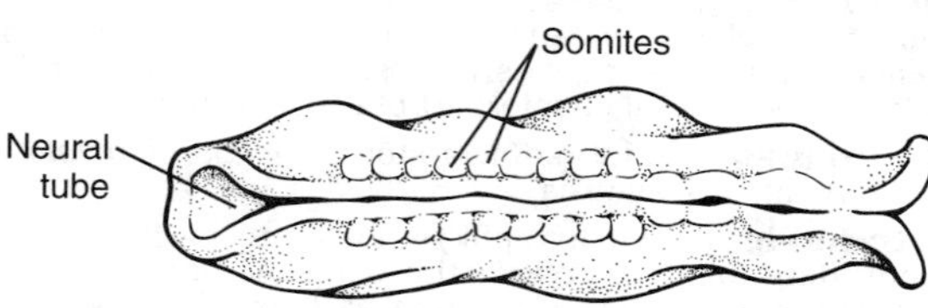

Somites in a 22 day embryo.

**som·no·cin·e·ma·to·graph** (som″no-sin″ə-mat′o-graf) [*somnus* + *cinematograph*] an apparatus for recording movements made during sleep.

**som·no·lence** (som′nə-ləns) [L. *somnolentia* sleepiness] drowsiness or sleepiness, particularly in excess.

**som·no·lent** (som′nə-lənt) [L. *somnolentus*] affected with somnolence; sleepy.

**som·no·len·tia** (som″nə-len′shə) [L.] 1. drowsiness, or somnolence. 2. sleep drunkenness.

**Som·nos** (som′nos) trademark for preparations of chloral hydrate.

**So·mo·gyi phenomenon (effect), unit** (so′mo-je) [Michael *Somogyi,* American biochemist, 1883–1971] see under *phenomenon* and *unit.*

**son·ant** (so′nənt) voiced.

**so·nar·og·ra·phy** (so″nər-og′rə-fe) ultrasonic scanning that provides a two-dimensional image corresponding to clear sections of acoustic interfaces in tissues.

**sonde** (sond) [Fr.] sound.
**s. coudé** (koo-da′) [Fr. "bent sound"], a catheter with an elbow, or sharp, beaklike bend, near the end.

**sone** (sōn) a unit of loudness, being the loudness of a simple tone of 1,000 cycles per second, 40 decibels above a listener's threshold.

**son·i·cate** (son′ĭ-kāt) 1. to expose to sound waves; to disrupt bacteria by exposure to high-frequency sound waves. 2. the products of such disruption.

**son·i·ca·tion** (son″ĭ-ka′shən) [MeSH: Sonication] exposure to sound waves; disruption of bacteria by exposure to high-frequency sound waves.

**Son·ne dysentery** (son′ə) [Carl Olaf *Sonne,* Danish bacteriologist, 1882–1948] see under *dysentery.*

**sono·gram** (son′o-gram) a record or display obtained by ultrasonic scanning.

**sono·graph·ic** (son″o-graf′ik) ultrasonographic.

**so·nog·ra·phy** (sə-nog′rə-fe) ultrasonography.

**sono·lu·cen·cy** (son″o-loo′sən-se) the property of being sonolucent.

**so·no·lu·cent** (so″no-loo′sənt) in ultrasonography, permitting the passage of ultrasound waves without reflecting them back to their source (without giving off echoes).

**so·no·rant** (sə-nor′ənt) voiced.

**so·no·rous** (sə-no′rəs, son′ə-rəs) [L. *sonorus*] resonant; sounding.

**so·phis·ti·ca·tion** (sə-fis″tĭ-ka′shən) [Gr. *sophistikos* deceitful] the adulteration of food or medicine.

**So·pho·ra** (so-fo′rə) [Arabic *sofara*] a genus of trees and shrubs of the family Leguminosae. The root and seed of *S. tomento′sa* are used in India to arrest choleraic vomiting. *S. secundiflo′ra* is the mescal bean, one of the North American plants called *locoweed.*

**so·por** (so′por) [L.] unnaturally deep or profound sleep.

**so·po·rif·er·ous** (so″por-if′ər-əs) [*sopor* + *-ferous*] inducing deep or profound slumber.

**sop·o·rif·ic** (sop″o-rif′ik, so″po-rif′ik) [*sopor* + L. *facere* to make] 1. causing or inducing profound sleep. 2. a drug or other agent which induces sleep.

**so·por·ous** (so′por-əs) associated or affected with coma or profound slumber.

**S. op. s.** abbreviation for L. *si o′pus sit,* if it is necessary.

**So·ran·us** (so-ran′us) **of Ephe·sus** [2nd century A.D.] a Greek physician of the Methodist school; he studied in Alexandria and practiced in Rome. His writings on obstetrics, gynecology, and pediatrics survive.

**sorb** (sorb) to attract and retain substances by absorption or adsorption.

**sor·be·fa·cient** (sor″bə-fa′shənt) [*sorb* + *-facient*] 1. promoting absorption. 2. an agent that promotes absorption.

**sor·bent** (sor′bənt) an agent that sorbs.

**sor·bic ac·id** (sor′bik) [MeSH: Sorbic Acid] 2,4-hexadienoic acid, a compound found in berries of the mountain ash *Sorbus aucuparia* and in many other plants; it inhibits the growth of yeasts and molds and is used as an antimicrobial preservative.

**sor·bi·tan** (sor′bĭ-tən) a generic name for an anhydride of sorbitol, whose fatty acids are surfactants (*s. monolaurate* [NF], *s. monooleate* [NF], *s. monopalmitate* [NF], *s. monostearate* [NF], *s. sesqui-*

*oleate* [NF], *s. trioleate* [NF], *s. tristearate*). See also *polysorbate*. Called also *sorbitol anhydride*.

**sor·bi·tol** (sor'bĭ-tol) [MeSH: Sorbitol] 1. a six-carbon sugar alcohol formed by reduction of the carbonyl group of glucose and occurring naturally in a variety of fruits. It is a precursor of the fructose in seminal plasma and is also found in lens deposits in diabetes mellitus. 2. [NF] an official preparation used as a sweetening agent and tablet excipient in pharmaceutical preparations and, in a 50 per cent solution, as an intravenous osmotic diuretic. Called also *glucitol*.

**sor·bi·tol de·hy·dro·gen·ase** (sor'bĭ-tol de-hi'dro-jən-ās) L-iditol 2-dehydrogenase.

**Sor·bi·trate** (sor'bĭ-trāt) trademark for a preparation of isosorbide dinitrate.

**Sor·da·ri·a·ceae** (sor"də-re-a'se-e) a family of fungi of the order Sordariales; it includes the genera *Neurospora* and *Chaetomium*.

**Sor·da·ri·a·les** (sor-da"re-a'lēz) an order of perfect fungi of the subphylum Ascomycotina, series Unitunicatae, characterized by inoperculate asci; most are saprobes. It includes the family Sordariaceae.

**sor·des** (sor'dēz) [L. "filth"] dirt; debris; especially the encrustations and accumulations of food, epithelial matter, and bacteria collected on the teeth and lips during a prolonged fever.
**s. gas'tricae,** undigested food, mucus, etc., in the stomach.

**sore** (sor) 1. a popular term for almost any lesion of the skin or mucous membranes. 2. painful.
**bay s.,** chiclero ulcer.
**bed s.,** decubitus ulcer.
**canker s.,** recurrent aphthous stomatitis.
**chrome s.,** chrome ulcer.
**cold s.,** herpes febrilis.
**desert s.,** a type of phagedenic ulcer seen in South Africa and Australia characterized initially by papulovesicular lesions on the extremities, especially on the backs of the hands, forearms, knees, and shins that rupture and form painful, crusted purulent ulcers. It probably represents an infected ulcer from some previously neglected lesion. Called also *Barcoo rot, veldt s.,* and numerous local names.
**hard s.,** chancre (def. 1).
**mixed s.,** see under *chancre*.
**pressure s.,** decubitus ulcer.
**saddle s.,** see under *gall*.
**soft s.,** chancroid.
**summer s's,** cutaneous habronemiasis.
**veldt s.,** desert s.
**venereal s.,** any sore that accompanies or manifests a venereal disease, especially a chancroid.

**sore·head** (sōr'hed) elaeophoriasis.

**So·ret band, effect (phenomenon)** (so-ra') [Charles *Soret*, French physicist, 1854–1904] see under *band* and *effect*.

**sore throat** (sor thrōt) 1. pharyngitis. 2. faucitis.
**clergyman's s. t.,** hypertrophic pharyngitis after speaking at length, as in a clergyman or other public speaker. Called also *dysphonia clericorum*.
**epidemic streptococcal s. t.,** streptococcal pharyngitis.
**septic s. t.,** streptococcal pharyngitis.
**spotted s. t.,** follicular tonsillitis.
**streptococcal s. t.,** see under *pharyngitis*.
**ulcerated s. t.,** gangrenous pharyngitis.

**Sor·ghum** (sōr'gum) a genus of grasses (family Graminae); several species are sources of the syrup called sorghum. Three species, *S. halepen'se* (Johnson grass), *S. sudanen'se* (Sudan grass), and *S. vulga're* (also called *S. bi'color*) are commonly used as fodder for cattle and horses but contain cyanogenetic compounds and when eaten fresh can cause cyanide poisoning. Johnson grass and Sudan grass cause hay fever in susceptible humans.

**so·ri** (so'ri) plural of *sorus*.

**So·ria·tane** (so're-ə-tān) trademark for a preparation of acitretin.

**sorp·tion** (sorp'shən) [L. *sorbere* to suck in] the process or state of being sorbed; absorption or adsorption.

**Sors·by's syndrome** (sorz'bēz) [Arnold *Sorsby*, British ophthalmologist, 1900–1980] see under *syndrome*.

**sort·er** (sor'tər) a device for sorting.
**fluorescence-activated cell s. (FACS),** an automated instrument that separates cell populations labeled with fluorescent antibodies or other fluorescent labels. The sample stream is broken up into droplets which are electrostatically charged and deflected into different collecting tubes depending on the measured fluorescence of the droplets.

**so·rus** (so'rəs) pl. *so'ri* [Gr. *sōros* heap] a mass, group, or cluster of spores, sporangia, or reproductive bodies occurring in certain plants, fungi, and protozoa.

**S.O.S.** abbreviation for L. *si o'pus sit,* if it is necessary.

**So·ta·cor** (so'te-kor") trademark for a preparation of sotalol hydrochloride.

**so·ta·lol hy·dro·chlo·ride** (so'tə-lol) a non-cardioselective beta-adrenergic blocking agent similar in action to propranolol, used in the treatment of angina pectoris, hypertension, and life-threatening cardiac arrhythmias; administered orally.

**So·to-Hall sign** (so"to-hawl') [Ralph *Soto-Hall*, American surgeon, 20th century] see under *sign*.

**So·tos' syndrome** (so'tōs) [Juan Fernandez *Sotos*, American pediatrician, born 1927] see under *syndrome*.

**souf·fle** (soo'fəl) [Fr. "a puff"; L. *sufflare* to blow] a soft, blowing, auscultatory sound; called also *bruit de soufflet*.
**cardiac s.,** any cardiac or vascular murmur of a blowing quality.
**funic s., funicular s.,** a hissing souffle synchronous with the fetal heart sounds, and supposed to be produced in the umbilical cord.
**mammary s.,** a functional cardiac murmur with a blowing sound, heard over the breasts in late pregnancy and during lactation; it may be either restricted to systole or continuous.
**placental s.,** a souffle supposed to be produced by the blood current in the placenta.
**splenic s.,** a sound said to be sometimes audible over a diseased spleen.
**umbilical s.,** funic s.
**uterine s.,** a sound made by the blood within the arteries of the gravid uterus.

**sound** (sound) [L. *sonus*] [MeSH: Sound] 1. the effect produced on the organ of hearing and its central connections by the vibrations of air or other media. 2. mechanical radiant energy, the motion of particles of the material medium through which it travels (gas, liquid, or solid) being longitudinal along the line of transmission; such energy, of frequency between 8 and 20,000 cycles per second, provides the stimulus for the subjective sensation of hearing. 3. an instrument to be introduced into a cavity to detect a foreign body or to dilate a stricture. 4. a noise, normal or abnormal, heard within the body; for other sounds see under *bruit, fremitus, murmur,* and *rale*.

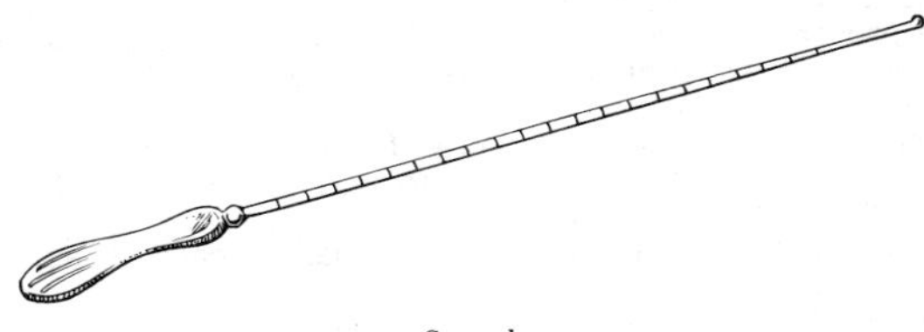

Sound.

**adventitious s's,** abnormal auscultatory sounds heard over the lungs, such as rales, rhonchi, or any of the abnormal types of resonance; they are usually characterized as either *continuous s's* or *discontinuous s's*. Cf. *breath s's*.
**aortic ejection s.,** an ejection sound due to abnormality of structure or function of the aortic valve or aorta.
**aortic second s.,** the audible vibrations related to the closure of the aortic valve. Symbol $A_2$. See also *second heart s.*
**atrial s.,** fourth heart s.
**auscultatory s's,** sounds heard on auscultation, such as heart sounds, Korotkoff sounds, breath sounds, or adventitious sounds.
**bandbox s.,** see under *resonance*.
**bellows s.,** to-and-fro murmur.
**bottle s.,** amphoric rale.
**breath s's,** auscultatory sounds heard in relation to the patient's breathing; they are usually listened for over a lung or a bronchus. Types include *bronchial, bronchovesicular, vesicular,* and *cavernous breath sounds*. Cf. *adventitious sounds*.
**breath s's, bronchial,** breath sounds with a high pitch like that of blowing through a tube. In healthy persons they are heard over the normal manubrium sterni on auscultation during respiration. When heard elsewhere they are pathologic and may indicate areas of adjacent consolidated or compressed lung. Called also *bronchial breathing* and *bronchial* or *tubular respiration*.
**breath s's, bronchovesicular,** breath sounds intermediate between bronchial and vesicular, with inspiration and expiration being of similar duration and quality. They are heard normally near the anterior part of the first two intercostal spaces and on the back between the scapulae. When heard over the lung they usually indicate an area of partial consolidation. Called also *bronchovesicular respiration*.
**breath s's, cavernous,** abnormal breath sounds marked by a peculiar prolonged hollow resonance, usually due to an underlying cavity in the lung. Called also *cavernous respiration*.
**breath s's, vesicular,** low-pitched sounds heard on auscultation

over the normal lung during ventilation. Called also *vesicular resonance.*
**cardiac s's,** heart s's.
**continuous s's,** adventitious sounds that last longer than 0.2 sec; they include wheezes and rhonchi.
**cracked-pot s.,** 1. see under *resonance.* 2. Macewen's sign.
**cranial, cracked-pot s.,** Macewen's sign.
**discontinuous s's,** adventitious sounds that last less than 0.2 sec and come in a series; the most common kind are rales (crackles).
**ejection s's,** high-pitched clicking sounds occurring shortly after the first heart sound, at the time of maximal opening of the semilunar valves; seen in patients with abnormalities of these valves or dilatations of the aortic or pulmonary arteries. The sounds may be described as aortic or pulmonic and vascular or valvular. Called also *ejection clicks.*
**entotic s's,** sounds that originate within the ear, such as tinnitus.
**esophageal s.,** a long, flexible sound for exploring the esophagus.
**first s., first heart s.,** the heart sound occurring during closure of the mitral and tricuspid valves; it is dull, firm, prolonged, and is heard as a "lubb" sound. It begins with an inaudible, low-frequency vibration (M) occurring at the onset of ventricular systole, followed by two intense, high-frequency vibratory bursts associated with mitral and tricuspid valve closure ($M_1$ and $T_1$, respectively), and ending with several variable low-intensity vibrations. Splitting of $M_1$ and $T_1$ is not usually discernible in normal adults. Abbreviated $S_1$.
**flapping s.,** the peculiar sound made by the closure of the heart valves.
**fourth s., fourth heart s.,** the heart sound associated with atrial contraction, occurring during the presystolic phase of diastole. It is rarely audible in normal hearts but when accentuated is usually called an $S_4$ gallop. Abbreviated $S_4$. See also *gallop rhythm,* under *rhythm.*
**friction s.,** see under *rub.*
**heart s's,** the sounds heard over the cardiac region in auscultation, which are produced by the functioning of the heart. The first and second are normally audible as the "lubb-dupp"sound, the third is normally audible only in youth, and the fourth is normally inaudible. See also individual sounds and see entries under *gallop* and *gallop rhythm,* under *rhythm.*
**hippocratic s's,** succussion s's.
**Korotkoff s's,** sounds heard during auscultatory determination of blood pressure, produced by sudden distention of the artery, the walls of which were previously relaxed because of the proximally placed pneumatic cuff.
**lacrimal s.,** a sound of small caliber for use in the lacrimal canal.
**Le Fort s.,** a sound with a screw tip for attachment of a filiform, used to pass through tight urethral strictures.
**metallic s.,** a sound having a metallic quality heard especially over cavities in the chest.
**muscle s.,** the sound heard over a muscle when in a condition of contraction.
**nonejection systolic s.,** midsystolic click.
**percussion s.,** any sound obtained by percussion.
**pericardial friction s.,** see under *rub.*
**physiological s's,** sounds heard when the auditory canals are plugged, caused by the rush of blood through blood vessels in or near the inner ear and by adjacent muscles in continuous low frequency vibration.
**pistol-shot s.,** Traube's sign.
**pulmonic ejection s.,** an ejection sound due to abnormality of structure or function of the pulmonary valve or artery.
**pulmonic second s.,** the audible vibrations related to the closure of the pulmonary valve; abbreviated $P_2$. See also *second heart s.*
**respiratory s's,** breath s's.
**second s., second heart s.,** the heart sound occurring during closure of the two semilunar valves at the beginning of diastole, and heard as a "dupp"sound. It consists of two sharp, high frequency vibrations representing closure of the aortic ($A_2$) then pulmonary ($P_2$) valves; the sounds are generally merged on expiration but split on inspiration in normal adults. Abbreviated $S_2$.
**$S_3$ gallop s.,** see under *gallop.*
**$S_4$ gallop s.,** see under *gallop.*
**shaking s.,** succussion s.
**speech s.,** one of the minimal elements of a spoken language, such as a consonant or vowel. See also *phoneme.*
**subjective s.,** phonism.
**succussion s's,** splashing sounds heard on succussion over a distended stomach and in hydropneumothorax. Called also *hippocratic s's.*
**systolic ejection s's,** ejection s's.
**third s., third heart s.,** the heart sound associated with low frequency vibrations of the ventricular walls during rapid ventricular filling in early diastole. It is normally detected only in youthful patients unless accentuated due to cardiac disease; it is then usually called an $S_3$ gallop. Abbreviated $S_3$. See also *gallop rhythm,* under *rhythm.*
**tick-tack s's,** the heart sounds of a pendulum rhythm.
**to-and-fro s.,** see under *murmur.*
**urethral s.,** a long, slim, slightly conical instrument of steel for exploring and dilating the urethra.
**valvular ejection s.,** an ejection sound resulting from abnormality of one or both semilunar valves. Cf. *vascular ejection s.*
**vascular ejection s.,** an ejection sound resulting from abnormality of the pulmonary artery or aorta without abnormality of either semilunar valve. Cf. *valvular ejection s.*
**voice s's,** auscultatory sounds heard over the lungs or airways when the patient speaks; increased resonance indicates consolidation or an airless lung underlying an effusion. Types include *bronchophony, egophony, laryngophony, pectoriloquy, tracheophony,* and *cavernous voice.*
**water-wheel s.,** bruit de moulin.
**white s.,** that produced by a mixture of all frequencies of mechanical vibration perceptible as sound.
**Winternitz's s.,** a double-current catheter.
**xiphisternal crunching s.,** a peculiar sound, of unknown origin, frequently heard (20 per cent of healthy men) over the lower sternum and xiphoid process.

**Souques's phenomenon, sign** (soo'kəz) [Alexandre Achille *Souques,* French neurologist, 1860–1944] see under *phenomenon* and *sign.*

**South·ern blot technique (blot analysis, blot hybridization, blot test)** (Suth'ərn) [E. M. *Southern,* British biologist, 20th century] see under *technique.*

**sow·dah** (sou'dah) [Ar. "black"] the typical cutaneous manifestation of onchocerciasis in Yemen and Saudi Arabia, usually limited to one or both lower limbs, characterized by black pigmentation, thickening, and roughness of the skin, edema, intense pruritus, papules, and regional lymphadenopathy. Similar cases have been reported from the Sudan and West Africa.

**Soxh·let's apparatus** (soks'lets) [Franz Ritter von *Soxhlet,* German chemist, 1848–1926] see under *apparatus.*

**soya** (soi'yə) see *soybean.*

**soy·bean** (soi'bēn) [MeSH: Soybeans] the bean of the leguminous plant, *Glycine max.* It contains little starch and is rich in protein.

**sp.** abbreviation for L. *spir'itus,* spirit.

**SP-40,40** clusterin.

**space** (spās) 1. a delimited area. 2. an actual or potential cavity of the body; called also *spatium* [TA]. 3. the expanse of the universe beyond the earth and its atmosphere.

## Space

For descriptions of specific anatomic structures not listed here, see under *spatium*

**apical s.,** the region between the wall of the alveolus and the apex of the root of a tooth.
**axillary s.,** axilla.
**Blessig's s's,** see under *cyst.*
**Bogros' s.,** a region bounded by the peritoneum above and the fascia transversalis below, in which the lower part of the external iliac artery can be found without cutting the peritoneum; called also *retroinguinal s.*
**Böttcher's s.,** saccus endolymphaticus.
**Bowman's s.,** capsular s.
**bregmatic s.,** fonticulus anterior.
**buccal s.,** a tissue space lateral to the buccopharyngeal fascia, between the buccinator and masseter muscles; it contains the buccal fat pad, Stensen's duct, and the facial artery.
**Burns' s.,** fossa jugularis, def. 1.
**capsular s.,** a narrow chalice-shaped cavity between the glomerular and the capsular epithelium of the glomerular capsule of the kidney; called also *Bowman's s.*

**carotid s., carotid bundle s.,** the potential space within the carotid sheath, extending from the base of the skull to the superior mediastinum.

**cartilage s's,** the spaces in hyaline cartilage which contain the cartilage cells.

**cathodal dark s.,** Crookes' s.

**cell s's,** the spaces in the ground substance of connective tissue enclosing the connective tissue corpuscles.

**chyle s's,** the central lymphatic spaces of the villi of the intestine.

**circumlental s.,** see *spatia zonularia,* under *spatium.*

**Colles' s.,** a space under the perineal fascia containing the transversus perinei, ischiocavernosus, and bulbocavernosus muscles, the posterior scrotal or labial vessels and nerves, and the bulbous portion of the urethra.

**complemental s.,** portions of the pleural cavity that are not occupied by lung tissue, such as the triangular spaces below the lower borders of the lungs and irregular spaces about the heart.

**corneal s's,** the spaces between the lamellae of the substantia propria of the cornea which contain corneal cells and tissue fluid; called also *interlamellar s's.*

**Cotunnius' s.,** the space within the membranous labyrinth.

**Crookes' s.,** a dark space at the cathode of a nearly exhausted x-ray tube through which a current is being passed; called also *cathodal dark s.*

**cupular s.,** pars cupularis recessus epitympanici.

**Czermak's s's,** spatia interglobularia; see under *spatium.*

**danger s.,** a subdivision of the spatium retropharyngeum, lying in the midline between the alar fascia and the prevertebral fascia and extending from the base of the skull to the level of the diaphragm; so called because it provides a route by which infection of the pharynx can spread to the mediastinum. Called also *prevertebral s.*

**dead s.,** 1. space remaining after closure of surgical or other wounds, permitting the accumulation of blood or serum and resultant delay in healing. 2. see *anatomic dead s.* and *physiologic dead s.*

**dead s., alveolar,** the difference between physiologic dead space and anatomic dead space, representing the space in alveoli occupied by air that does not participate in oxygen–carbon dioxide exchange (see *alveolar ventilation,* under *>ventilation*). It varies in different parts of the lungs and under different conditions.

**dead s., anatomic,** those portions of the airway, from the nose and mouth to the terminal bronchioles, in which exchange of oxygen and carbon dioxide does not occur. Cf. *physiologic dead s.*

**dead s., physiologic,** the anatomic dead space plus the alveolar dead space; it reflects nonuniformity of ventilation and perfusion in different parts of the lung.

**dead s., respiratory,** the part of either the anatomic or the physiologic dead space that represents a volume of air that does not take part in alveolar ventilation.

**s's in dentin,** spatia interglobularia.

**s's of Disse,** small spaces which separate the sinusoids of the liver from the liver cells and which carry the lymph of the liver.

**Douglas' s.,** excavatio recto-uterina.

**epicerebral s.,** the potential space between the brain and the pia mater.

**epidural s.,** spatium epidurale.

**episcleral s.,** spatium episclerale.

**epispinal s.,** the potential space between the substance of the spinal cord and the pia mater.

**epitympanic s.,** recessus epitympanicus.

**escapement s's,** spaces which permit the escape of material being comminuted between the occlusal surfaces of the teeth, provided by the cusps and ridges, sulci and developmental ridges of the teeth, and the embrasures between the teeth.

**extradural s.,** spatium epidurale.

**extraperitoneal s.,** spatium extraperitoneale.

**s's of Fontana,** spatia anguli iridocornealis; see under *spatium.*

**freeway s.,** interocclusal distance.

**globular s's of Czermak,** spatia interglobularia.

**H. s.,** Holzknecht's s.

**haversian s.,** canalis nutricius.

**Henke's s.,** a space containing connective tissue between the vertebral column and the pharynx and esophagus.

**His' perivascular s's,** perivascular s's.

**Holzknecht's s.,** the middle one of the three clear lung fields in the radiograph of the chest in oblique projection when the rays pass from the left posteriorly to the right anteriorly; called also *H. s., prevertebral s.,* and *retrocardiac s.*

**iliocostal s.,** the area between the twelfth rib and the crest of the ilium.

**infrahyoid s's,** the potential spaces in the neck just inferior to the hyoid bone, including the anterior visceral and retropharyngeal spaces.

**interarytenoid s.,** pars intercartilaginea rimae glottidis.

**intercostal s.,** spatium intercostale.

**intercristal s.,** 1. all of the area within the inner membrane of a mitochondrion. 2. the clefts between the inward extensions of the mitochondrial membrane space.

**intercrural s.,** fossa interpeduncularis.

**interdental s.,** interproximal s.

**interfascial s.,** spatium episclerale.

**interglobular s's (of Owen),** spatia interglobularia.

**interlamellar s's,** corneal s's.

**interocclusal s.,** interocclusal distance (clearance).

**interosseous s's of metacarpus,** spatia interossea metacarpi.

**interosseous s's of metatarsus,** spatia interossea metatarsi.

**interpeduncular s.,** fossa interpeduncularis.

**interpleural s.,** mediastinum, def. 2.

**interproximal s., interproximate s.,** the space between the proximal surfaces of adjoining teeth; sometimes used to designate especially the space between the proximal surfaces of adjoining teeth that is gingival to the area of contact *(septal s.).* Cf. *embrasure.*

**interradicular s.,** 1. the space between roots. 2. in dentistry, the entire extent of the space between the roots of a tooth, from apex to base.

**interseptal s.,** a space between the two folds uniting to form the spurious septum in the heart of the early embryo.

**intervaginal s.,** spatium episclerale.

**intervaginal s's of optic nerve,** spatia intervaginalia nervi optici.

**intervillous s.,** the space of the placenta into which the chorionic villi project and through which maternal blood circulates.

**s's of iridocorneal angle,** spatia anguli iridocornealis.

**Kiernan's s's,** the triangular spaces bounded by invaginated Glisson's capsule between the liver lobules, containing the larger interlobular branches of the portal vein, hepatic artery, and hepatic duct.

**Kiesselbach's s.,** see under *area.*

**Kretschmann's s.,** a depressed area in the recessus epitympanicus, below Prussak's space.

**Larrey's s's,** intervals between those parts of the diaphragm which are attached to the ribs and that which is attached to the sternum.

**leeway s.,** see *Nance's leeway s.*

**Lesshaft's s.,** a rhomboid space found in some persons between the external oblique muscle in front, the latissimus dorsi behind, the serratus posticus above, and the internal oblique below; frequently the site of pointing of an abscess, or occurrence of a hernia. Called also *Lesshaft's* or *Grynfeltt's triangle.*

**lymph s.,** any space in tissue occupied by lymph.

**Magendie's s's,** subarachnoid spaces between the pia and arachnoid, corresponding to the principal sulci of the brain.

**mandibular s.,** a tissue space formed by splitting of the superficial layer of the cervical fascia at the inferior border of the mandible, containing the anterior part of the ramus of the mandible and adjacent structures.

**Marie's quadrilateral s.,** see *quadrilateral s. of Marie.*

**marrow s.,** cavitas medullaris.

**masticator s.,** a potential space of the neck anterior and lateral to the pharyngomaxillary space, formed by splitting of the superficial layer of the deep cervical fascia and containing the muscles of mastication, the ramus and posterior part of the mandible, branches of the mandibular nerve, and the maxillary artery and its branches.

**Meckel's s.,** cavum trigeminale.

**mediastinal s.,** mediastinum, def. 2.

**medullary s.,** cavitas medullaris.

**midpalmar s.,** the palmar space lying between the middle metacarpal bone and the radial side of the hypothenar eminence.

**mitochondrial membrane s.,** a narrow space between the inner and outer membranes of a mitochondrion, including its inward projections between the cristae.

**Mohrenheim's s.,** a groove on the deltoid muscle for the cephalic vein and a branch of the acromiothoracic artery.

**Nance's leeway s.,** the amount by which the space occupied by the deciduous canine and first and second deciduous molars exceeds that occupied by the canine and premolar teeth of the permanent dentition, usually averaging 1.7 mm on each side of the dental arch.

**Nuel's s's,** 1. outer tunnel. 2. cuniculus medius.

**palmar s.,** a large fascial space in the hand, divided by a fibrous septum into the midpalmar space and the thenar space.

**paraglottic s.,** a laryngeal space bounded inferiorly by the conus elasticus, medially by the quadrangular membrane, posteriorly by the mucosa of the piriform fossa, and anterolaterally by the thyroid cartilage.

**parapharyngeal s.,** pharyngomaxillary s.

**parasinoidal s's,** lacunae laterales.

**Parona's s.,** a space between the pronator quadratus muscle and the deep flexor tendons in the forearm, about 5 cm. above the wrist, in direct continuity with the tendon sheaths and the midpalmar space.

**parotid s.,** a potential space within the parotid fascia, containing the parotid gland.

**perforated s., anterior,** substantia perforata rostralis.

**perforated s., posterior,** substantia perforata posterior.
**periaxial s.,** a fluid-filled cavity surrounding the nuclear bag and myotubule regions of a muscle spindle.
**perichoroidal s.,** spatium perichoroideum.
**perilymphatic s.,** spatium perilymphaticum.
**perineal s., deep,** saccus profundus perinei.
**perineal s., superficial,** compartimentum superficiale perinei.
**perineuronal s.,** the extracellular compartment surrounding nerve cells of the central nervous system; its histologic appearance as a space is an artefact.
**perinuclear s.,** see under *cisterna.*
**peripharyngeal s.,** spatium peripharyngeum.
**periplasmic s.,** a zone between the plasma membrane and the outer membrane of the cell wall of gram-negative bacteria.
**perisinusoidal s's,** s's of Disse.
**peritonsillar s.,** a potential space of the neck bounded by the palatine tonsil, the superior constrictor muscle of the pharynx, and the anterior and posterior faucial arches.
**perivascular s's,** spaces (often only potential) that surround blood vessels for a short distance as they enter the brain; their inner wall is formed by a prolongation of a membrane like the arachnoid, and the outer wall by a continuation of the pia; the intervening channel communicates with the subarachnoid space. Called also *His' perivascular s's* and *Virchow-Robin s's.*
**perivitelline s.,** a space between the ovum and the zona pellucida; in the ovum of some animals, a fluid-filled space separating the fertilization membrane from the surface of the egg.
**pharyngeal s., lateral,** spatium lateropharyngeum.
**pharyngeal mucosal s.,** a potential space of the neck on the airway side of the buccopharyngeal fascia, extending from the base of the skull to the level of the cricoid cartilage and containing muscles, the torus tubarius, salivary glands, and mucosal and lymphoid tissue.
**pharyngomaxillary s.,** a potential space of the neck bounded by the buccopharyngeal fascia, the internal pterygoid muscle, and the prevertebral fascia, forming a cone with its base at the sphenoid bone and its apex at the hyoid bone; it is divided by the styloid process into anterior and posterior compartments, the latter containing the carotid sheath and cranial nerves IX–XII. Called also *parapharyngeal s.* and *lateral pharyngeal s.*
**phrenocostal s.,** the space between the outer edge of the diaphragm and the costal surface.
**pleural s.,** cavitas pleuralis.
**pneumatic s.,** a portion of bone occupied by air-containing cells; applied especially to spaces in the bones of the head constituting the paranasal sinuses.
**Poiseuille's s.,** that part of the lumen of a tube where no flow of liquid occurs, as next to the wall of a blood vessel, where the red cells are virtually motionless and constitute a layer over which the inner layers of liquid slide.
**popliteal s.,** fossa poplitea.
**pre-epiglottic s.,** a fat-filled laryngeal space bounded superiorly by the vallecula and hyoepiglottic ligament, posteriorly by the epiglottis and quadrangular membrane, and anteriorly by the thyrohyoid membrane and thyroid cartilage.
**preperitoneal s.,** spatium retropubicum.
**preputial s.,** the space between the prepuce and the glans penis.
**pretracheal s.,** anterior visceral s.
**prevertebral s.,** 1. a potential space between the prevertebral fascia and the bodies of the vertebrae, attached to the transverse process of the vertebrae, and extending from the base of the skull to the coccyx; it contains muscles, nerves, the vertebral artery and vein, and the vertebral bodies. 2. danger s. 3. Holzknecht's s.
**prevesical s.,** spatium retropubicum.
**prezonular s.,** portion of the eyeball anterior to the zonula ciliaris, occupied by the aqueous humor.
**proximal s., proximate s.,** interproximal s.
**Prussak's s.,** recessus superior membranae tympanicae.
**quadrilateral s. of Marie,** a space in the cerebral hemisphere bounded externally by the cortex, medially by the internal capsule, and anteriorly and posteriorly by the insula, which Marie thought important in speech function.
**Reinke's s.,** a potential space between the vocal ligament and the overlying mucosa; inflammation results in Reinke's edema.
**relief s.,** the space between the slightly elevated lingual bar type of major connector and the underlying soft tissue that allows for a minor degree of settling of a removable partial denture, without impinging on the structure over which the bar passes.
**retrobulbar s.,** the space lying behind the fascia of the bulb of the eye, containing the eye muscles and the ocular vessels and nerves.
**retrocardiac s.,** Holzknecht's s.
**retroesophageal s.,** spatium retropharyngeum.
**retroinguinal s.,** Bogros' s.
**retromylohyoid s.,** the part of the alveolingual sulcus just lingual to the retromolar pad, and posterior to the lingual tuberosity.
**retro-ocular s.,** retrobulbar s.
**retroperitoneal s.,** spatium retroperitoneale.
**retropharyngeal s.,** 1. spatium retropharyngeum. 2. retrovisceral s.
**retropubic s.,** spatium retropubicum.
**retrovisceral s.,** a subdivision of the spatium retropharyngeum lying between the pretracheal and prevertebral layers of the deep cervical fascia. Called also *retropharyngeal s.*
**Retzius s.,** 1. spatium perilymphaticum. 2. spatium retropubicum.
**Schwalbe's s's,** spatia intervaginalia nervi optici.
**semilunar s.,** see *Traube's semilunar s.*
**septal s.,** that portion of the interproximal space gingival to the contact area of adjacent teeth in a dental arch.
**subarachnoid s.,** spatium subarachnoideum.
**subchorial s.,** see under *lake.*
**subdural s.,** spatium subdurale.
**subepicranial s.,** the potential space between the epicranius muscle and the pericranium; it is traversed by small arteries which supply the pericranium and by the emissary veins connecting the intracranial venous sinuses with the superficial veins of the scalp.
**subgingival s.,** gingival crevice.
**sublingual s.,** the superior part of the submandibular space, containing the sublingual gland and loose connective tissue surrounding the tongue.
**submandibular s.,** a potential space of the neck bounded by the oral mucosa and tongue anteriorly and medially; the superficial layer of the deep cervical fascia laterally, and the hyoid bone inferiorly; it comprises two spaces, the sublingual and submaxillary spaces, divided by the mylohyoid muscle.
**submaxillary s.,** the inferior part of the submandibular space; see *trigonum submandibulare.*
**submental s.,** the medial part of the submaxillary space; see *trigonum submentale.*
**subphrenic s.,** the space between the diaphragm and subjacent abdominal organs.
**subumbilical s.,** the somewhat triangular space within the body cavity just inferior to the umbilicus.
**suprahyoid s's,** the potential spaces of the neck and pharyngeal region superior to the hyoid bone, including the pharyngomaxillary and submandibular spaces.
**suprasternal s.,** fossa jugularis, def. 1.
**Tarin's s.,** anterior recess of interpeduncular fossa; see under *recess.*
**Tenon's s.,** spatium episclerale.
**thenar s.,** the palmar space lying between the middle metacarpal bone and the tendon of the flexor pollicis longus.
**thiocyanate s.,** a quantitative expression of the space occupied by the extracellular fluid in the body, computed after intravenous injection of sodium thiocyanate.
**thyrohyal s.,** the depressed space between the thyroid cartilage and hyoid bone in front.
**Traube's semilunar s.,** an area on the left anterior inferior part of the thorax, over which the air in the stomach produces a vesiculotympanitic sound.
**Tröltsch's s's,** see *recessus membranae tympani anterior* and *recessus membranae tympani posterior.*
**Virchow-Robin s's,** perivascular s's.
**visceral s.,** a potential space between the pretracheal fascia and the prevertebral fascia, extending from the hyoid bone to the mediastinum and containing the lower pharynx, larynx, trachea, esophagus, thyroid, great vessels, and areolar tissue. It is subdivided into the *anterior visceral, posterior visceral (retrovisceral),* and *visceral vascular* or *carotid spaces.*
**visceral s., anterior,** a potential space in the neck surrounded by the pretracheal layer of the deep cervical fascia; it contains the thyroid gland, the esophagus, and the trachea. Called also *pretracheal s.*
**visceral s., posterior,** spatium retropharyngeum.
**visceral vascular s.,** carotid s.
**Westberg's s.,** the space between the pericardium and the beginning of the aorta.
**yolk s.,** the space formed by retraction of the vitellus of the ovum from the zona pellucida.
**Zang's s.,** fossa supraclavicularis minor.
**zonular s's,** spatia zonularia.

**spac·er** (spās'ər) on a metered dose inhaler, a chamber between the inhaler canister and the patient's mouth where droplets of medication can slow down and evaporate so that there is less direct impact on the oropharynx.

**Spal·ding's sign** (spawl'dingz) [Alfred Baker *Spalding*, American obstetrician and gynecologist, 1874–1942] see under *sign.*

**Spal·lan·za·ni's law** (spahl"ahn-tsah'nēz) [Lazaro *Spallanzani*, Italian anatomist, 1729–1799] see under *law.*

**spal·la·tion** (spaw-la'shən) splintering; the process of breaking into small bits; see *spallation products,* under *product.*

**span** (span) 1. a measurement of reach or extent. 2. the distance in a fully extended hand between the tips of the thumb and little finger. 3. the distance between the tips of the fingers when the arms are extended.

**Span·i·op·sis** (span"e-op'sis) a genus of blood-sucking flies of the family Rhagionidae found in Australia.

**Span·ish wind·lass** (span'ish wind'ləs) see under *windlass.*

**span(o)-** [Gr. *spanos* scarce] a combining form meaning scanty or scarce.

**spar** (spahr) a nonmetallic, rather lustrous mineral.
**Iceland s.,** a crystalline form of calcium carbonate, usually found in Iceland, and used in making Nicol prisms.

**spar·flox·a·cin** (spahr-flok'sə-sin) a broad-spectrum antimicrobial agent administered orally.

**spar·ga·no·sis** (spahr"gə-no'sis) [MeSH: Sparganosis] infection with migrating spargana (tapeworm larvae), which invade the subcutaneous tissues, causing inflammation and fibrosis that resembles cellulitis.

**spar·ga·num** (spahr'gə-nəm) pl. *spar'gana* [Gr. *sparganon* swaddling clothes] [MeSH: Sparganum] the larval stage (plerocercoid) of certain cestodes, especially of the genera *Diphyllobothrium* and *Spirometra,* which may migrate in the subcutaneous tissues of humans and other animals and cause sparganosis.

**Spar·ine** (spahr'ēn) trademark for preparations of promazine hydrochloride.

**spar·te·ine** (spahr'tēn) [L. *spartium* broom] [MeSH: Sparteine] a poisonous alkaloid obtained from the legumes *Cytisus scoparius* (broom), *Lupinus luteus* (yellow lupin bean), *L. niger* (black lupin bean), and *Anagyris foetida* (Mediterranean stinkbush). See *lupinosis* and *broom poisoning.*
**s. sulfate,** the pentahydrate sulfate salt of sparteine, used as an oxytocic for the induction of labor and stimulation of hypotonic or subnormal uterine contractions. Formerly used as a substitute for digitalis.

**spar·ti·um** (spahr'she-əm) [Gr. *sparton*] scoparius.

**spasm** (spaz'əm) [L. *spasmus;* Gr. *spasmos*] [MeSH: Spasm] 1. a sudden, violent, involuntary contraction of a muscle or a group of muscles, attended by pain and interference with function, producing involuntary movement and distortion. 2. a sudden but transitory constriction of a passage, canal, or orifice.
**s. of accommodation,** spasm of the ciliary muscles, producing excess of accommodation for near objects.
**athetoid s.,** a spasm in which the affected member makes movements like those of athetosis.
**Bell's s.,** facial s.
**bronchial s.,** bronchospasm.
**cadaveric s.,** rigor mortis causing movements of the limbs.
**canine s.,** risus sardonicus.
**carpopedal s.,** spasm of the hand or foot, or of the thumbs and great toes, seen in tetany.
**clonic s.,** a spasm consisting of clonic contractions.
**cynic s.,** risus sardonicus.
**dancing s.,** saltatory s.
**diffuse esophageal s.,** strong, uncoordinated, nonpropulsive contractions of the esophagus evoked by deglutition, especially in the elderly; on barium radiography, the esophageal lumen appears as an irregular series of concentric narrowings, or a spiral coil (curling). Called also *esophageal dysrhythmia* or *s., esophagism, esophagospasm, dysphagia nervosa,* and *dysphagia spastica.*
**esophageal s.,** diffuse esophageal s.
**facial s.,** tonic spasm of the muscles supplied by the facial nerve, either involving the entire side of the face or confined to a limited region around the eye. Called also *Bell's s., histrionic s., convulsive* or *facial tic, mimetic convulsion,* and *mimic convulsion* or *tic.*
**fixed s.,** permanent rigidity of a muscle or set of muscles.
**glottic s.,** laryngospasm.
**habit s.,** see under *tic.*
**hemifacial s.,** facial spasm confined to one side.
**histrionic s.,** facial s.
**infantile s's, infantile massive s's,** a syndrome of severe myoclonus appearing in the first 18 months of life and associated with general cerebral deterioration; it is marked by severe flexion spasms of the head, neck, and trunk and extension of the arms and legs. Called also *jackknife seizures* or *spasms, salaam convulsions, seizures,* or *spasms,* and *West's syndrome.*
**inspiratory s.,** spasmodic contraction of the muscles of inspiration.
**intention s.,** muscular spasm occurring on attempting voluntary movement.
**jackknife s's,** infantile s's.
**lock s.,** a firm tonic spasm that seems to lock the fingers together, as in writers' cramp and in similar affections.
**malleatory s.,** malleation.
**massive s.,** a spasm characterized by contraction of most of the body musculature. Cf. *seizure* and *infantile massive s.*
**mixed s.,** a spasm in which there are both extensor and flexor movements.
**mobile s.,** athetosis.
**myopathic s.,** that which accompanies a disease of the muscles.
**nictitating s.,** winking s.
**nodding s.,** spasmus nutans.
**phonatory s.,** spasm of the tensors of the vocal cords, which interferes with speech. See also *dysphonia spastica.*
**progressive torsion s.,** dystonia musculorum deformans.
**respiratory s.,** spasm of the muscles of respiration.
**retrocollic s's,** retrocollis.
**Romberg's s.,** trismus.
**rotatory s.,** intermittent spasm of the splenius muscle causing rotation of the head; cf. *vetrocollis* and *torticollis.*
**salaam s's,** infantile s's.
**saltatory s.,** clonic spasm of the muscles of the legs, producing a peculiar jumping or springing motion, seen in conditions such as Gilles de la Tourette's syndrome, saltatory chorea, and the jumping diseases. Called also *Bamberger's disease, dancing spasm,* and *saltatory tic.*
**tetanic s., tonic s.,** tetanus, def. 2.
**tonoclonic s.,** a convulsive twitching of the muscles.
**torsion s.,** spasm marked by a twisting or turning of the body, especially of the pelvis, as in dystonia musculorum deformans.
**toxic s.,** that which is due to a poison.
**winking s.,** spasmodic twitching of the orbicularis palpebrarum muscle and of the eyelid.
**writers' s.,** writers' cramp.

**spasm(o)-** [Gr. *spasmos* spasm] a combining form denoting relationship to a spasm.

**spas·mod·ic** (spaz-mod'ik) [Gr. *spasmōdēs*] of the nature of a spasm.

**spas·mo·gen** (spaz'mo-jən) [*spasmo-* + *-gen*] a substance that produces or causes spasms.

**spas·mo·gen·ic** (spaz"mo-jen'ik) relating to the production of or causing spasms.

**spas·mo·lyg·mus** (spaz"mo-lig'məs) [*spasmo-* + Gr. *lygmos* hiccup] hiccup.

**spas·mol·y·sant** (spaz-mol'ĭ-zənt) 1. relieving or relaxing spasms. 2. an agent that relieves spasm.

**spas·mol·y·sis** (spaz-mol'ĭ-sis) the elimination or checking of spasm.

**spas·mo·lyt·ic** (spaz"mo-lit'ik) checking spasms; antispasmodic.

**spas·mo·phile** (spaz'mo-fīl) spasmophilic.

**spas·mo·phil·ic** (spaz"mo-fil'ik) marked by a tendency to spasms.

**spas·mus** (spaz'məs) [L.] spasm.
**s. nu'tans,** nodding of the head accompanied by nystagmus, seen in infants and young children; called also *nodding spasm.*

**spas·tic** (spas'tik) [Gr. *spastikos*] 1. of the nature of or characterized by spasms. 2. hypertonic, so that the muscles are stiff and the movements awkward; see *cerebral palsy,* under *palsy,* and *spastic paraplegia,* under *paraplegia.*

**spas·tic·i·ty** (spas-tis'ĭ-te) the state of being spastic; see *spastic* (def. 2).
**clasp-knife s.,** see under *rigidity.*
**inherited periodic s.,** an autosomal recessive muscle disorder seen in adult cattle; upon arising, for a few seconds to 30 minutes the animal is unable to flex the hindlimbs or walk and may have limb tremors. Called also *stretches.*

**spa·tia** (spa'she-ə) [L.] plural of *spatium.*

**spa·tial** (spa'shəl) pertaining to space.

**spa·ti·um** (spa'she-əm) pl. *spa'tia* [L.] [TA] space: a general anatomical term for an actual or potential delimited area or open region.
**spa'tia an'guli i'ridis [Fonta'nae], spa'tia an'guli iridocornea'lis** [TA], spaces of the iridocorneal angle: the spaces between the fibers

of the pectinate ligament through which communication is effected between the anterior chamber and the canal of Schlemm. Called also *Fontana's spaces.*
**s. epidura'le** [TA], epidural space: the space between the dura mater and the walls of the vertebral canal, containing venous plexuses and fibrous and alveolar tissue. Called also *cavitas epiduralis, epidural cavity, s. extradurale* [TA alternative], *extradural space,* and *s. peridurale* [TA alternative].
**s. episclera'le** [TA], episcleral space: the space between the bulbar fascia and the eyeball; called also *s. intervaginale, s. interfasciale [Tenoni], intervaginal space,* and *Tenon's space.*
**s. extradura'le,** TA alternative for *s. epidurale.*
**s. extraperitonea'le** [TA], extraperitoneal space: the thin space between the abdominal walls and the transverse fascia occupied by the extraperitoneal fascia.
**s. intercosta'le** [TA], intercostal space: the space intervening between two adjacent ribs.
**s. interfascia'le [Teno'ni],** s. episclerale.
**spa'tia interglobula'ria,** interglobular spaces: numerous small irregular spaces on the outer surface of the dentin in the root of a tooth. Called also *Czermak's spaces, globular spaces of Czermak,* and *interglobular spaces (of Owen).*
**spa'tia interos'sea metacar'pi** [TA], interosseous spaces of the metacarpus: the four spaces between the metacarpal bones.
**spa'tia interos'sea metatar'si** [TA], interosseous spaces of metatarsus: the four spaces between the metatarsal bones.
**s. intervagina'le,** s. episclerale.
**spa'tia intervagina'lia ner'vi op'tici,** intervaginal spaces of optic nerve: the subdural or subarachnoid spaces between the internal and external sheaths of the optic nerve; called also *Schwalbe's space.*
**s. lateropharyn'geum** [TA], lateral pharyngeal space: the part of the spatium peripharyngeum that is lateral to the pharynx.
**s. leptomenin'geum,** TA alternative for *s. subarachnoideum.*
**s. perichoroidea'le, s. perichoroi'deum** [TA], perichoroidal space: any of the spaces between the laminae of the nonvascular layer of the choroid nearest the sclera.
**s. peridura'le,** TA alternative for *s. epidurale.*
**s. perilympha'ticum** [TA], perilymphatic space: the fluid-filled space separating the membranous from the osseous labyrinth; called also *Retzius space.*
**s. peripharyn'geum** [TA], peripharyngeal space: the space around the pharynx, which is filled with areolar tissue; it is subdivided into the *s. lateropharyngeum* and the *s. retropharyngeum.*
**s. profun'dum perine'i,** TA alternative for *saccus profundus perinei.*
**s. retroperitonea'le** [TA], retroperitoneal space: the space between the posterior parietal peritoneum and the posterior abdominal wall, containing the kidneys, suprarenal glands, ureters, duodenum, ascending and descending colon, pancreas, and the large vessels and nerves. Called also *retroperitoneum.*
**s. retropharyn'geum** [TA], retropharyngeal space: the part of the spatium peripharyngeum that lies just behind the prevertebral layer of the deep cervical fascia, extending from the base of the skull to the level of the second thoracic vertebra. It is subdivided into the *retrovisceral space* (also called the *retropharyngeal space*) and the *prevertebral* or *danger space.* Called also *retroesophageal space* and *posterior visceral s.*
**s. retropu'bicum** [TA], retropubic space: the extraperitoneal space between the inferior aspect of the apex of the bladder, and the transversalis fascia and the posterosuperior aspect of the pubic symphysis, extending along the sides of the bladder to the lateral ligaments and limited inferiorly by the puboprostatic ligaments.

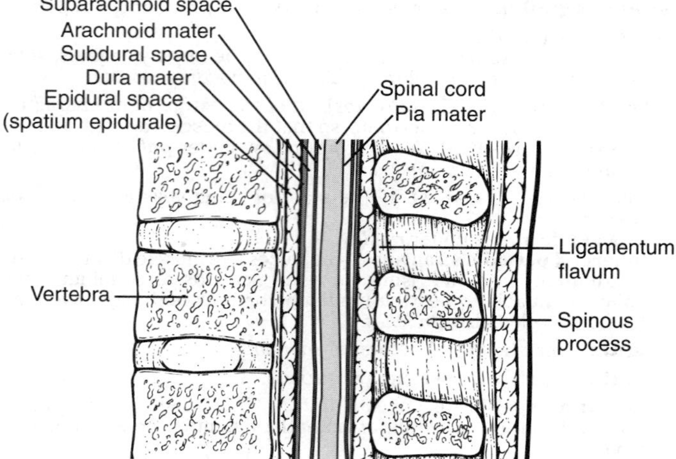


Spatium epidurale (epidural space) relative to the spinal cord and meninges, in a sagittal section of the vertebral column.

**s. subarachnoi'deum** [TA], subarachnoid space: the space between the arachnoidea mater and the pia mater, containing cerebrospinal fluid and bridged by delicate trabeculae; called also *cavitas subarachnoidea, subarachnoid cavity,* and *s. leptomeningeum* [TA alternative].
**s. subdura'le** [TA], subdural space: a narrow fluid-containing space, often only a potential space, between the dura mater and the arachnoid; called also *subdural cavity.*
**s. superficia'le perine'i,** TA alternative for *compartimentum superficiale perinei.*
**spa'tia zonula'ria** [TA], zonular spaces: the lymph-filled interstices between the fibers of the zonula ciliaris, communicating with the posterior chamber of the eye; called also *Petit's canal.*

**spat·u·la** (spach'ə-lə) [L.] 1. a flat, blunt, usually flexible instrument, used for spreading plasters and for mixing ointments and masses. 2. a spatulate structure.
**s. mal'lei,** umbo membranae tympani.

**spat·u·lar** (spach'ə-lər) spatulate, def. 1.

**spat·u·late** (spach'ə-lāt) 1. having a flat blunt end. 2. to mix or manipulate with a spatula. 3. to make a longitudinal incision in the cut end of a tubular structure and spread it open in order to increase the size of the opening for anastomosis.

**spat·u·la·tion** (spach"ə-la'shən) the mixing of combined materials to a homogeneous mass by repeatedly scraping them up and smoothing out the mass on a flat surface with a spatula.

**spav·in** (spav'in) 1. any of various enlargements of the tarsus of equines, usually medially and distal to the tibiotarsal articulation and involving the metatarsals. 2. bone s.
**blood s.,** a spavin consisting of dilatation of either or both of the medial metatarsal veins or the saphenous veins, forming a soft enlargement on the dorsomedial surface of the tarsus.
**bog s.,** a spavin consisting of distention of the synovial capsule of the tibiotarsal joint.
**bone s.,** a spavin consisting of osteoperiostitis or arthritis of the intertarsal or tarsometatarsal articulations, commonly followed by exostosis and ankylosis; locations include anterior, posterior, and high. See also *occult s.* Called also *spavin.*
**occult s.,** a bone spavin that lacks visible radiographic exostoses, with the lesion confined to the joint surfaces between two bones.

**spav·ined** (spav'ind) affected with spavin.

**spay** (spa) to castrate a female animal, usually by oophorohysterectomy.

**SPCA** [MeSH: Factor VII] serum prothrombin conversion accelerator (factor VII; see under *coagulation factors,* at *factor*).

**Spear·man's rank correlation coefficient (rho)** (spēr'mənz) [Charles Edward *Spearman,* British psychologist, 1863–1945] see under *coefficient.*

**spear·mint** (spēr'mint) 1. any of various species of mint. *Mentha spicata* (called also *M. viridis*) is common spearmint and *M. cardiaca* is Scotch spearmint. 2. the dried leaves and flowering tops of *M. spicata* or *M. cardiaca,* used as a flavoring agent and source of spearmint oil.

**spe·cial·ism** (spĕ'shəl-iz-əm) [MeSH: Specialism] limitation of practice or study to a particular branch of medicine or surgery.

**spe·cial·ist** (spĕ'shəl-ist) [MeSH: Specialism] a physician whose practice is limited to a particular branch of medicine or surgery, especially one who, by virtue of advanced training, is certified by a specialty board as being qualified to so limit his practice.
**clinical nurse s., nurse s.,** see under *nurse.*

**spe·cial·iza·tion** (spĕ"shəl-ĭ-za'shən) in medicine, medical practice limited to some special branch of medicine or surgery.

**spe·cial·ty** (spĕ'shəl-te) the field of practice of a specialist.

**spe·ci·a·tion** (spe"se-a'shən) the evolutionary formation of new species, or the process of such formation.

**spe·cies** (spe'shēz, spe'sēz) [L.] a taxonomic category subordinate to a genus (or subgenus), and superior to a subspecies or variety, composed of individuals possessing common characters distinguishing them from other categories of individuals of the same taxonomic level. In taxonomic nomenclature, species are designated by the genus name followed by a Latin or latinized adjective or noun.
**concordant s.,** see under *xenograft.*
**diovulatory s.,** a species of animal, the females of which ordinarily discharge two ova in one ovulatory cycle.
**discordant s.,** see under *xenograft.*
**fugative s.,** a species of plant or animal that inhabits or grows in a region for only a short period of time.
**monovulatory s.,** a species of animal, the females of which usually discharge only one ovum in any one ovulatory cycle.

**polyovulatory s.**, a species of animal, the females of which normally discharge several (3–16) ova at each ovulatory cycle.
**type s.**, in bacteriology, the species that characterizes a genus, usually the first species validly described in the genus, but it may be one arbitrarily designated as such for classification purposes.

**spe·cies-spe·cif·ic** (spe″sēz-spə-sif′ik) 1. characteristic of a particular species. 2. having a characteristic effect on, or interaction with, cells or tissues of members of a particular species; said of an antigen, drug, or infective agent.

**spe·cif·ic** (spə-sif′ik) [L. *specificus*] 1. pertaining to a species. 2. produced by a single kind of microorganism. 3. restricted in application, effect, etc., to a particular structure, function, etc. 4. a remedy specially indicated for any particular disease. 5. in immunology, pertaining to the special affinity of antigen for the corresponding antibody.

**spec·i·fic·i·ty** (spes″ĭ-fis′ĭ-te) 1. the quality or state of being specific. 2. the conditional probability that a person not having a disease will be correctly identified by a clinical test, i.e., the number of true negative results divided by the total number of those without the disease (which is the sum of the numbers of true negative plus false positive results). Cf. *sensitivity* and *predictive value.*
**diagnostic s.**, specificity (def. 2).
**neuronal s.**, the invariance of the locations, trajectories, and spatial arrangement of neurons in all members of the same species.

**spec·i·men** (spes′ĭ-mən) 1. a sample or part of a thing, or of several things, taken to show or to determine the character of the whole, as a specimen of urine. 2. a preparation of tissue for pathological examination or of a normal tissue, organ, or organism for study of its structure.
**corrosion s.**, a preparation of an organ, such as the liver, by injection of certain of its structures, as the arteries and veins, and chemical digestion of surrounding substance.

**SPECT** single-photon emission computed tomography.

**spec·ta·cles** (spek′tə-kəlz) [L. *spectacula; spectare* to see] a pair of lenses in a frame to assist vision; see also *glasses* and *lens.*
**compound s.**, spectacles fitted with extra colored glasses, or extra lenses, to be used as occasion requires.
**decentered s.**, spectacles with lenses formed from eccentric portions of two convex lenses.
**divided s.**, bifocal glasses.
**industrial s.**, protective s.
**Masselon's s.**, spectacles with an attachment for keeping the upper lid raised in cases of paralytic ptosis.
**mica s.**, spectacles of sheet mica used to protect the eye from foreign bodies.
**pantoscopic s.**, bifocal glasses.
**periscopic s.**, spectacles with either menisci or concavoconvex lenses, with the concave surfaces toward the eyes; they allow the eyes considerable latitude of motion.
**prismatic s.**, spectacles with prismatic lenses for correcting muscular defects.
**protective s.**, spectacles designed to protect the eyes rather than to correct defective vision; the spectacles may have side shields, plastic or hardened lenses, or lenses that protect against ultraviolet or infrared rays.
**pulpit s.**, spectacles containing the lenses in the lower segments of the glasses only.
**safety s.**, protective s.
**stenopeic s.**, spectacles fitted with metal plates, having each a small central aperture.
**tinted s.**, spectacles of a glass so colored as to protect the eyes from the effects of too bright light.
**wire frame s.**, a kind of spectacles of wire gauze worn to protect the eye from the entrance of foreign bodies.

**spec·ti·no·my·cin** (spek″tĭ-no-mi′sin) [MeSH: Spectinomycin] an antibiotic, derived from *Streptomyces spectabilis,* that has moderate antibacterial activity against many gram-positive and gram-negative organisms, but is especially effective against *Neisseria gonorrhoeae.* It is also used in veterinary medicine in bacterial enteritis and coccidiosis of dogs.
**s. hydrochloride** [USP], the pentahydrate dihydrochloride salt of spectinomycin, having the same actions as the base; used in the treatment of acute gonorrheal urethritis and proctitis in the male and acute gonorrheal cervicitis and proctitis in the female when due to susceptible strains of *Neisseria gonorrhoeae.*

**spec·tra** (spek′trə) plural of *spectrum.*

**spec·tral** (spek′trəl) pertaining to a spectrum; performed by means of a spectrum.

**spec·trin** (spek′trin) [MeSH: Spectrin] a contractile protein attached to glycophorin at the cytoplasmic surface of the cell membrane of erythrocytes, important in the maintenance of cell shape.

**spectro-** [L. *spectrum* image] a combining form denoting relationship to a spectrum or to an image.

**Spec·tro·bid** (spek′tro-bid″) trademark for a preparation of bacampicillin hydrochloride.

**spec·tro·col·or·im·e·ter** (spek″tro-kul″ər-im′ə-tər) [*spectro-* + *colorimeter*] an ophthalmospectroscope using a source of light from a selected wavelength of the spectrum to detect color blindness for one color.

**spec·tro·flu·o·rom·e·ter** (spek″tro-flo͞o-rom′ə-tər) an optical instrument for analysis of fluorescence spectra.

**spec·tro·graph** (spek′tro-graf) [*spectro-* + *-graph*] an instrument for photographing spectra on a sensitive photographic plate.
**mass s.**, mass spectrometer.

**spec·trom·e·ter** (spek-trom′ə-tər) [*spectro-* + *-meter*] 1. an instrument for measuring the index of refraction by measuring the external angle of a prism of the substance. 2. a spectroscope for measuring the wavelengths of rays of a spectrum.
**infrared s.**, a device that analyzes the chemical composition of a substance either by passing infrared light through a specimen and characterizing its absorption spectrum or by measuring the amount of infrared light emitted by excited atoms or molecules in a specimen; infrared light is emitted or absorbed in a given band in proportion to the concentration of the molecule characterized by the band.
**mass s.**, an analytical instrument which identifies a substance by sorting a stream of electrified particles (ions) according to their mass; the sorting is most commonly done as follows: when the stream of charged particles enters a magnetic field, the particles are deflected into semicircular paths varying with their mass and charge components, ultimately striking a photographic plate or photomultiplier tube sensor. Called also *mass spectrograph.*
**Mossbauer s.**, an instrument that detects small changes in interaction between an atomic nucleus and its environment caused by changes in temperature, pressure, and chemical state; used in chemical-physical research with applications in medicine.

**spec·trom·e·try** (spek-trom′ə-tre) the determination of the wavelengths or frequencies of the lines in a spectrum.

**spec·tro·pho·to·flu·o·rom·e·ter** (spek″tro-fo″to-flo͞o-rom′ə-tər) an analytical instrument combining the techniques of spectrophotometry and fluorescence analysis.

**spec·tro·pho·tom·e·ter** (spek″tro-fo-tom′ə-tər) [*spectro-* + *photometer*] an apparatus for estimating the quantity of coloring matter in solution by the quantity of light absorbed (as indicated by the spectrum) in passing through the solution. Cf. *colorimeter.*
**absorption s.**, an analytical instrument for comparing the absorption of radiation of a given wavelength against a standard to identify a sample material.

**spec·tro·pho·tom·e·try** (spek″tro-fo-tom′ə-tre) [MeSH: Spectrophotometry] the use of the spectrophotometer.

**spec·tro·po·lar·im·e·ter** (spek″tro-po″lər-im′ə-tər) a combined spectroscope and polariscope for determining optical rotation.

**spec·tro·scope** (spek′tro-skōp) [*spectro-* + *-scope*] an instrument for developing and analyzing spectra.

**spec·tro·scop·ic** (spek″tro-skop′ik) of, pertaining to, or performed by, the spectroscope.

**spec·tros·co·py** (spek-tros′kə-pe) [*spectro-* + *-scopy*] the propagation and analysis of spectra; examination by means of a spectroscope.
**infrared s.**, examination by means of an infrared spectrometer, to study systems or molecules by examining their interactions with infrared radiation.

**spec·trum** (spek′trəm) pl. *spec′tra* [L. "image"] 1. a charted band of wavelengths of electromagnetic vibrations obtained by refraction and diffraction. See *invisible s.* and *visible s.* 2. by extension, a measurable range of activity, such as the range of bacteria affected by an antibiotic *(antibacterial s.)* or the complete range of manifestations of a disease.
**absorption s.**, the spectrum afforded by light which has passed through various gaseous media, each gas absorbing those rays of which its own spectrum is composed.
**action s.**, the range of wavelength of incident light producing a response in the material under study (e.g., the inactivation of an enzyme); also, a graph plotting the magnitude of the response as a function of the wavelength of the incident light.
**antibacterial s.**, see *spectrum,* def. 2.
**broad-s.**, effective against a wide range of microorganisms; said of an antibiotic.
**chemical s.**, that part of the spectrum which includes the ultraviolet or actinic rays.
**chromatic s.**, that portion of the range of wavelengths of electromagnetic vibrations (from 770 to 390 nm) which gives rise to the sensation of color (red to violet) to the normally perceptive eye; coincident with the visible spectrum.
**color s.**, chromatic s.

**continuous s.**, one in which absorption lines are not developed.
**continuous x-ray s.**, bremsstrahlung, def. 1.
**diffraction s.**, a spectrum formed by the passage of light through a diffraction grating.
**electromagnetic s.**, the continuous range of electromagnetic energy from cosmic rays to electric waves, including gamma, x-, and ultraviolet rays, visible light, infrared waves, and radio waves.
**fortification s.**, a form of migraine aura characterized by scintillating or zigzag bands of colored light forming the edge of an area of teichopsia. Called also *fortification figures.*
**gaseous s.**, one which is afforded by an incandescent gas.
**invisible s.**, that made up of vibrations of wavelengths less than 390 nm (ultraviolet, grenz rays, x-rays, and gamma rays) and between 770 and 12,000 nm (infrared).
**ocular s.**, afterimage.
**prismatic s.**, one produced by the passage of light through a prism.
**solar s.**, that portion of the range of wavelengths of electromagnetic vibrations emanating from the sun, including the visible (chromatic, or color) spectrum and small portions of the infrared and ultraviolet radiations at either extreme.
**visible s.**, that portion of the range of wavelengths of electromagnetic vibrations (from 770 to 390 nm) which is capable of stimulating specialized sense organs and is perceptible as light.
**x-ray s.**, the spectrum of a heterogeneous beam of x-rays produced by a suitable grating, generally a crystal.

**spec·u·lum** (spek'u-ləm) pl. *spec'ula* [L. "mirror"] an instrument that exposes the interior of a passage or cavity of the body by enlarging the opening.
**Bozeman's s.**, a bivalve speculum the blades of which remain parallel when separated.
**Brinkerhoff's s.**, a rectal speculum consisting of a conical tube having a closed extremity, but provided with a sliding bar on the side which provides an opening.
**Cook's s.**, a three-pronged rectal speculum.
**duck-billed s.**, a form of two-valved vaginal speculum.
**eye s.**, an appliance for keeping the eyelids apart.
**Fergusson's s.**, a cylindrical vaginal speculum made of silvered glass.
**Graves' s.**, a type of two-valved vaginal speculum.
**Kelly's s.**, a rectal speculum tubular in shape and fitted with an obturator; called also *Kelly's sphincteroscope.*
**Martin's s., Martin and Davy s.**, a rectal speculum consisting of a conical cylinder with an obturator.
**Mathews' s.**, a four-pronged rectal speculum.
**Sims' s.**, a double duck-billed vaginal speculum.
**stop s.**, an eye speculum with an appliance for controlling the degree to which its branches spread.

**Spee's curve (curvature)** (shpāz) [Ferdinand Graf von *Spee,* German embryologist, 1855–1937] see under *curve.*

**speech** (spēch) [MeSH: Speech] the utterance of vocal sounds conveying ideas. Cf. *phonation.*
**alaryngeal s.**, esophageal s.
**cerebellar s.**, speech seen with cerebellar lesions, varying from jerky or scanning to explosive. See also *scanning s.* and *explosive s.*
**cleft palate s.**, dysphasia due to a cleft palate, often characterized by hypernasality, difficulty with fricatives, and other problems due to the velopharyngeal insufficiency.
**clipped s.**, speech in which the words are slurred over and uncompleted; called also *scamping s.* and *slurred s.*
**echo s.**, echolalia.
**esophageal s.**, a method of speech used after laryngectomy, with sound produced by vibration of the column of air in the esophagus against the contracting cricopharyngeal sphincter.
**explosive s.**, speech uttered with more force than necessary; see also *cerebellar s.*
**mirror s.**, a speech abnormality in which the order of syllables in a sentence is reversed.
**plateau s.**, speech which is characterized by a level, monotonous, unvaried pitch.
**pressured s.**, logorrhea.
**scamping s.**, clipped s.
**scanning s.**, 1. slurring, monotonous speech sometimes seen in multiple sclerosis. 2. staccato s.
**slurred s.**, clipped s.
**staccato s.**, speech in which each syllable is uttered separately; seen in multiple sclerosis.
**telegraphic s.**, speech consisting of only certain prominent words and lacking modifiers, articles, and other ancillary words. It is typical of children around age two but in older persons it is a form of agrammatism.

**Spe·mann** (shpa'mahn) Hans. German zoologist, 1869–1941; winner of the Nobel prize for medicine or physiology in 1935 for investigating the organizer effect in embryonic development.

**Spe·mann's induction** (shpa'mahnz) [Hans *Spemann*] see under *induction.*

**Spence's tail** (spen'səz) [James *Spence,* Scottish surgeon, 19th century] see under *tail.*

**Speng·ler's fragments** (shpeng'lərz) [Carl *Spengler,* Swiss physician, 1860–1937] see under *fragment.*

**Spens' syndrome** (spenz) [Thomas *Spens,* Scottish physician, 1769–1842] Adams-Stokes syndrome; see under *syndrome.*

**sperm** (sperm) [Gr. *sperma* seed] 1. the semen or testicular secretion. 2. spermatozoon.
**muzzled s.**, spermatozoa which are unable to adhere to the ovum.

**sper·ma** (sper'mə) semen.

**sper·ma·ceti** (sper"mə-set'e) [Gr. *sperma* seed + *kētos* whale] a waxy substance obtained from the head of the sperm whale, *Physeter macrocephalus,* occurring as white, somewhat translucent, slightly unctuous masses, having a crystalline fracture and a pearly luster; used in the preparation of ointment bases, such as cold cream and rose water ointment.
**synthetic s.**, cetyl esters wax.

**sper·ma·cra·sia** (sper"mə-kra'zhə) [*sperm-* + *akrasia* ill mixture] deficiency of spermatozoa in the semen.

**sper·mag·glu·ti·na·tion** (sper"mə-gloo"tĭ-na'shən) the agglutination of spermatozoa.

**sper·ma·te·li·o·sis** (sper"mə-te"le-o'sis) spermiogenesis.

**sper·mat·em·phrax·is** (sper"mat-əm-frak'sis) [*spermat-* + *emphraxis*] obstruction to the discharge of semen.

**sper·mat·ic** (spər-mat'ik) [L. *spermaticus;* Gr. *spermatikos*] pertaining to the semen; seminal.

**sper·mat·i·cide** (spər-mat'ĭ-sīd) spermicide.

**sper·ma·tid** (sper'mə-tid) [MeSH: Spermatids] a cell derived from a secondary spermatocyte by fission, and developing into a spermatozoon; called also *spermatoblast.*

**sper·ma·tin** (sper'mə-tin) an albuminoid substance derived from the semen; it is related to mucin and to nucleoalbumin.

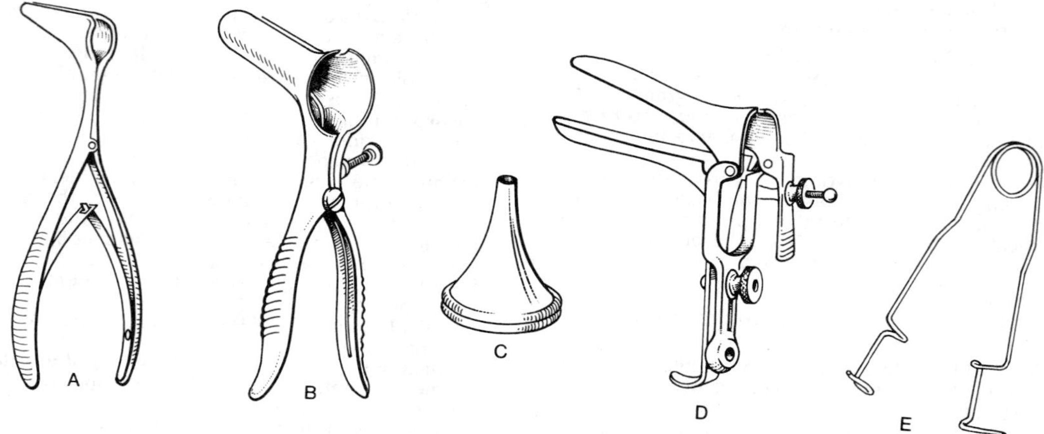

Specula. *(A),* Nasal speculum; *(B),* rectal speculum; *(C),* speculum for otoscope; *(D),* vaginal duckbill speculum; *(E),* eye speculum.

**sper·ma·tism** (sper′mə-tiz-əm) [Gr. *spermatismos*] the production or discharge of semen.

**sper·ma·ti·tis** (sper″mə-ti′tis) deferentitis.

**spermat(o)-** [Gr. *sperma,* gen. *spermatos* seed] a combining form denoting relationship to seed, specifically to the male generative element; also *sperm(o)-.*

**sper·ma·to·blast** (sper′mə-to-blast″) [*spermato-* + *-blast*] [MeSH: Spermatids] a term originally applied to the supporting cells of Sertoli, but now used with the same meaning as *spermatid.*

**sper·ma·to·cele** (sper′mə-to-sēl″) [*spermato-* + *-cele*[1]] [MeSH: Spermatocele] a cystic distention of the epididymis or the rete testis containing spermatozoa.

**sper·ma·to·ce·lec·to·my** (spər-mat″o-sə-lek′tə-me) [*spermatocele* + *-ectomy*] excision of a spermatocele.

**sper·ma·to·ci·dal** (sper″mə-to-si′dəl) spermicidal.

**sper·ma·to·cyst** (sper′mə-to-sist″) [*spermato-* + *cyst*] 1. a seminal vesicle. 2. a spermatocele.

**sper·ma·to·cys·tec·to·my** (sper″mə-to-sis-tek′tə-me) [*spermatocyst* + *-ectomy*] excision of the seminal vesicles.

**sper·ma·to·cys·ti·tis** (sper″mə-to-sis-ti′tis) inflammation of a seminal vesicle.

**sper·ma·to·cys·tot·o·my** (sper″mə-to-sis-tot′ə-me) [*spermatocyst* + *-tomy*] incision of the seminal vesicles.

**sper·ma·to·cy·tal** (sper″mə-to-si′təl) pertaining to a spermatocyte.

**sper·ma·to·cyte** (sper′mə-to-sīt″) [*spermato-* + *-cyte*] [MeSH: Spermatocytes] the parent cell of a spermatid.
**primary s.,** a cell derived from a spermatogonium and dividing into two secondary spermatocytes; called also *spermiocyte.*
**secondary s.,** one of the two cells into which a primary spermatocyte divides, and which in turn gives origin to spermatids; called also *prespermatid.*

**sper·ma·to·cy·to·gen·e·sis** (sper″mə-to-si″to-jen′ə-sis) the first stage of formation of spermatozoa in which the spermatogonia develop into spermatocytes and then into spermatids.

**sper·ma·to·cy·to·ma** (sper″mə-to-si-to′mə) seminoma.

**sper·ma·to·gen·e·sis** (sper″mə-to-jen′ə-sis) [*spermato-* + *-genesis*] [MeSH: Spermatogenesis] the process of formation of spermatozoa, including spermatocytogenesis and spermiogenesis.

**sper·ma·to·gen·ic** (sper″mə-to-jen′ik) [*spermato-* + *-genic*] producing semen or spermatozoa.

**sper·ma·tog·e·nous** (sper″mə-toj′ə-nəs) spermatogenic.

**sper·ma·tog·e·ny** (sper″mə-toj′ə-ne) spermatogenesis.

**sper·ma·to·gone** (sper′mə-to-gōn″) spermatogonium.

**sper·ma·to·go·nia** (sper″mə-to-go′ne-ə) [MeSH: Spermatogonia] plural of *spermatogonium.*

**sper·ma·to·go·ni·um** (sper″mə-to-go′ne-əm) pl. *spermatogo′nia* [*spermato-* + Gr. *gonē* generation] an undifferentiated germ cell of a male, originating in a seminiferous tubule and dividing into two primary spermatocytes; called also *spermatophore, spermatospore,* and *spermospore.*

**sper·ma·toid** (spər′mə-toid) [*spermato-* + *-oid*] resembling a spermatozoon.

**sper·ma·tol·o·gy** (sper′mə-tol′ə-je) [*spermato-* + *-logy*] the sum of what is known regarding the semen.

**sper·ma·tol·y·sin** (sper″mə-tol′ĭ-sin) a specific lysin produced by injecting an animal with spermatozoa; spermatotoxin.

**sper·ma·tol·y·sis** (sper′mə-tol′ĭ-sis) [*spermato-* + *-lysis*] destruction or solution of spermatozoa.

**sper·ma·to·lyt·ic** (sper″mə-to-lit′ik) pertaining to, characterized by, or causing spermatolysis.

**sper·ma·to·path·ia** (sper″mə-to-path′e-ə) [*spermato-* + *path-* + *-ia*] a morbid condition of the semen.

**sper·ma·top·a·thy** (sper″mə-top′ə-the) spermatopathia.

**sper·ma·to·phore** (sper′mə-to-for″) [*spermato-* + *-phore*] [MeSH: Spermatogonia] 1. a capsule, containing several spermatozoa, extruded by some of the lower animals. 2. spermatogonium.

**sper·ma·to·poi·et·ic** (sper″mə-to-poi-et′ik) [*spermato-* + Gr. *poiētikos* creative, productive] subserving or promoting the secretion of semen.

**sper·ma·tor·rhea** (sper′mə-to-re′ə) [*spermato-* + *-rrhea*] involuntary, too frequent, and excessive discharge of semen without copulation.

**sper·ma·tos·che·sis** (sper″mə-tos′kə-sis) [*spermato-* + Gr. *schesis* check] suppression of the secretion of semen.

**sper·mato·spore** (spər-mat′o-spor) [*spermato-* + *spore*] spermatogonium.

**sper·ma·to·tox·in** (sper″mə-to-tok′sin) a toxin destructive to spermatozoa; especially a cytotoxic antibody produced by injecting an animal with spermatozoa.

**sper·ma·tox·in** (sper″mə-tok′sin) spermatotoxin.

**sper·ma·to·zoa** (sper″mə-to-zo′ə) [Gr.] [MeSH: Spermatozoa] plural of *spermatozoon.*

**sper·ma·to·zo·al** (sper″mə-to-zo′əl) pertaining to spermatozoa.

**sper·ma·to·zo·i·cide** (sper″mə-to-zo′ĭ-sīd) spermicide.

**sper·ma·to·zoid** (sper′mə-to-zoid) [*spermatozoon* + *-oid*] 1. spermatozoon. 2. the male germ cell in plants.

**sper·ma·to·zo·on** (sper″mə-to-zo′on) pl. *spermatozo′a* [*spermato-* + Gr. *zōon* animal] a mature male germ cell, the specific output of the testes. It is the generative element of the semen which serves to fertilize the ovum, and contains the genetic information to be transmitted to the zygote by the male. It consists of a head (or nucleus), a neck, a middle piece, and a tail with an end piece. Spermatozoa, formed in the seminiferous tubules, are derived from spermatogonia, which first develop into spermatocytes, which, in turn, undergo meiosis to produce spermatids; the spermatids then differentiate into spermatozoa. Called also *sperm.*

**sper·ma·tu·ria** (sper″mə-tu′re-ə) [*spermato-* + *-uria*] seminuria.

**sper·mec·to·my** (spər-mek′tə-me) excision of a portion of the spermatic cord.

**sper·mi·a·tion** (sper″me-a′shən) the freeing of mature spermatozoa from the Sertoli cells.

**sper·mi·ci·dal** (sper″mĭ-si′dəl) [*sperm* + L. *caedere* to kill] destructive to spermatozoa.

**sper·mi·cide** (sper′mĭ-sīd) an agent that is destructive to spermatozoa.

**sper·mid** (sper′mid) spermatid.

**sper·mi·dine** (sper′mĭ-din) [MeSH: Spermidine] a polyamine, first found in human semen but now known to occur in almost all tissues, in association with nucleic acids; it is formed from putrescine and is itself a precursor of spermine.

**sper·mi·duct** (sper′mĭ-dukt″) [*sperm* + *duct*] the ejaculatory duct and vas deferens together.

**sper·mine** (sper′min) [MeSH: Spermine] a polyamine, first found in human semen but now known to occur in almost all tissues in association with nucleic acids, being formed from spermidine.

**spermi(o)-** see *spermat(o)-.*

**sper·mio·cyte** (sper′me-o-sīt″) [*spermio-* + *-cyte*] [MeSH: Spermatocytes] primary spermatocyte.

**sper·mio·gen·e·sis** (sper″me-o-jen′ə-sis) the second stage in the formation of spermatozoa in which the spermatids transform into spermatozoa.

**sper·mio·go·ni·um** (sper″me-o-go′ne-əm) spermatogonium.

**sper·mio·gram** (sper′me-o-gram) a diagram of the various cells formed during the development of the sperm.

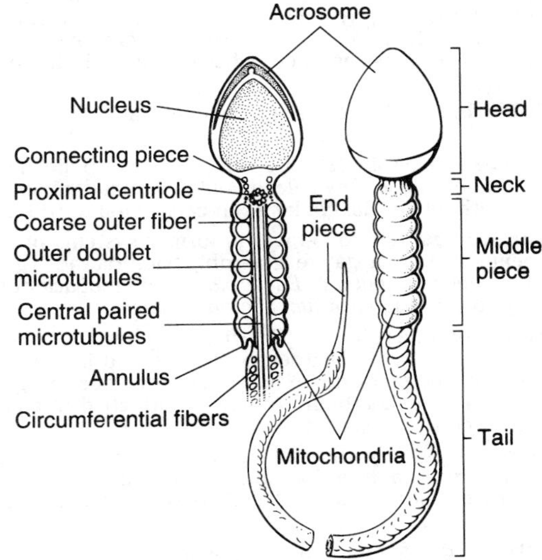


Human spermatozoon: side view (in cross section) and flat view.

**sper·mio·te·le·o·sis** (sper″me-o-te″le-o′sis) [*spermio-* + *tele-*[1] + *-osis*] the progressive development of the spermatogonium through the successive changes necessary for becoming a mature spermatozoon.

**sper·mio·te·le·ot·ic** (sper″me-o-te″le-ot′ik) [*spermio-* + Gr. *teleiōtikos* perfective] pertaining to or characteristic of spermioteleosis.

**sperm(o)-** see *spermat(o)-*.

**sper·mo·blast** (sper′mo-blast) [*spermo-* + *-blast*] spermatid.

**sper·mo·cy·to·ma** (sper″mo-si-to′mə) seminoma.

**sper·mo·lith** (sper′mo-lith) [*spermo-* + *-lith*] a calculus in the spermiduct.

**sper·mol·y·sin** (spər-mol′ĭ-sin) spermatolysin.

**sper·mol·y·sis** (spər-mol′ĭ-sis) spermatolysis.

**sper·mo·lyt·ic** (sper″mo-lit′ik) spermatolytic.

**sper·mo·neu·ral·gia** (sper″mo-nōō-ral′jə) [*spermo-* + *neur-* + *-algia*] neuralgic pain in the spermatic cord.

**Sper·moph·i·lus** (spər-mof′ĭ-ləs) a genus of ground squirrels (family Sciuridae) that harbor organisms transmissible to humans. *S. bee′cheyi* is a species of California that is often infected with plague; also, it and the species *S. mol′lis* of Utah and *S. orego′nus* of Oregon are natural reservoirs of *Francisella tularensis.* Formerly called *Citellus.*

**sper·mo·phle·bec·ta·sia** (sper″mo-fleb″ək-ta′zhə) [*spermo-* + *phleb-* + *ectasia*] varicosity of the spermatic veins.

**sper·mo·plasm** (sper′mo-plaz-əm) [*spermo-* + *-plasm*] the protoplasm of the spermatids.

**sper·mo·sphere** (sper′mo-sfēr) [*spermo-* + *sphere*] a group or mass of spermatids formed by the segmentation of a secondary spermatocyte.

**sper·mo·spore** (sper′mo-spor) spermatogonium.

**sper·mo·tox·ic** (sper″mo-tok′sik) destructive to spermatozoa.

**sper·mo·tox·in** (sper″mo-tok′sin) spermatotoxin.

**Sper·ry** (sper′e) Roger Wolcott. American psychobiologist, born 1913; co-winner, with David Hunter Hubel and Tolsten Nils Wiesel, of the Nobel prize for medicine or physiology in 1981 for his studies of functional specialization of the cerebral hemispheres.

**SPF** specific-pathogen free, a term applied to animals reared for use in laboratory experiments, and known to be free of specific pathogenic microorganisms.

**sp gr** specific gravity.

**sph** spherical or spherical lens.

**sphac·e·late** (sfas′ə-lāt) to become gangrenous.

**sphac·e·la·tion** (sfas″ə-la′shən) gangrene.

**sphac·e·lism** (sfas′ə-liz-əm) [Gr. *sphakelismos*] necrosis.

**sphac·e·lous** (sfas′ə-ləs) gangrenous.

**sphac·e·lus** (sfas′ə-ləs) [L.; Gr. *sphakelos*] 1. a mass of gangrenous tissue. 2. gangrene.

**Sphae·ria** (sfe′re-ə) a former genus of fungi whose species have been reclassified. *S. sinen′sis* is now called *Cordyceps sinensis.*

**Sphae·ri·a·les** (sfe′re-a′lēz) [MeSH: Sphaeriales] an order of perfect fungi of the subphylum Ascomycotina, series Unitunicatae, characterized by inoperculate asci. Many fungi formerly in this order have now been assigned elsewhere, such as in the order Sordariales.

**sphaer(o)-** for words beginning thus, see also those beginning *spher(o)-*.

**Sphae·roi·des** (sfe-roi′dēz) a genus of marine puffer fish of the family Tetraodontidae. Their flesh contains tetrodotoxin, and consumption without special cooking can cause fatal tetrodotoxism.

**Sphae·ro·pho·rus** (sfe-ro′fə-rəs) in former systems of classification, a genus of gram-negative anaerobic bacteria the organisms of which have been assigned to *Bacteroides* and *Fusobacterium.*
**S. necro′phorus,** *Fusobacterium necrophorum.*

**Sphae·ro·ti·lus** (sfe-ro′tĭ-ləs) [Gr. *sphaira* sphere + *tilos* anything shredded] a genus of sheathed bacteria found in polluted fresh waters and in sludge, made up of straight rods occurring singly or in chains in a thin sheath and frequently attached to a substrate. The type species is *S. na′tans.*

**Sphe·ci·dae** (sfe′sĭ-de) the solitary wasps, a family of flying insects of the order Hymenoptera that have a long thin body and delicate wings; many species can sting. Members of this family live in comparative isolation.

**sphen·eth·moid** (sfən-eth′moid) sphenoethmoid.

**sphe·ni·on** (sfe′ne-on) pl. *sphe′nia* [Gr. *sphēn* wedge + *on* neuter ending] the cranial point at the sphenoid angle of the parietal bone.

**sphen(o)-** [Gr. *sphēn* wedge] a combining form denoting relationship to the sphenoid bone or to a wedge, or meaning wedge-shaped.

**sphe·no·bas·i·lar** (sfe″no-bas′ĭ-lər) pertaining to the sphenoid bone and the basilar part of the occipital bone. Cf. *spheno-occipital.*

**sphe·noc·cip·i·tal** (sfe″nok-sip′ĭ-təl) spheno-occipital.

**sphe·no·ceph·a·lus** (sfe″no-sef′ə-ləs) a fetus exhibiting sphenocephaly.

**sphe·no·ceph·a·ly** (sfe″no-sef′ə-le) [*spheno-* + *-cephaly*] a developmental anomaly characterized by a wedge-shaped appearance of the head.

**sphe·no·eth·moid** (sfe″no-eth′moid) denoting the curved plate of bone anterior to the lesser wing of the sphenoid bone.

**sphe·no·fron·tal** (sfe″no-fron′tal) pertaining to the sphenoid and frontal bones.

**sphe·noid** (sfe′noid) [*sphen-* + *-oid*] 1. wedge-shaped. 2. pertaining to the sphenoid bone.

**sphe·noi·dal** (sfe-noi′dəl) sphenoid.

**sphe·noi·di·tis** (sfe″noi-di′tis) sphenoid sinusitis.

**sphe·noi·dos·to·my** (sfe″noi-dos′tə-me) [*sphenoid* + *-ostomy*] operative removal of the anterior wall of the sphenoidal sinus.

**sphe·noi·dot·o·my** (sfe″noi-dot′ə-me) incision into the sphenoidal sinus.

**sphe·no·ma·lar** (sfe″no-ma′lər) sphenozygomatic.

**sphe·no·max·il·lary** (sfe″no-mak′sĭ-lar″e) pertaining to the sphenoid bone and the maxilla.

**sphe·no·oc·cip·i·tal** (sfe″no-ok-sip′ĭ-təl) pertaining to the sphenoid and occipital bones.

**sphe·nop·a·gus** (sfe-nop′ə-gəs) [*spheno-* + *-pagus*] symmetrical conjoined twins fused at the sphenoid bone at the base of the skull.

**sphe·no·pal·a·tine** (sfe″no-pal′ə-tin) pertaining to or in relation with the sphenoid and palatine bones; in anatomy it is sometimes interchangeable with the term *pterygopalatine.*

**sphe·no·pa·ri·e·tal** (sfe″no-pə-ri′ə-təl) pertaining to the sphenoid and parietal bones.

**sphe·no·pe·tro·sal** (sfe″no-pə-tro′səl) pertaining to the sphenoid bone and the petrous part of the temporal bone.

**sphe·nor·bi·tal** (sfe-nor′bĭ-təl) pertaining to the sphenoid bone and the orbits.

**sphe·no·squa·mo·sal** (sfe″no-skwə-mo′səl) pertaining to the sphenoid bone and the squamous portion of the temporal bone.

**sphe·no·tem·po·ral** (sfe″no-tem′pə-rəl) pertaining to the sphenoid and temporal bones.

**sphe·not·ic** (sfe-not′ik) [*spheno-* + *otic*] denoting a fetal bone which becomes that part of the sphenoid which is adjacent to the carotid groove.

**sphe·no·tur·bi·nal** (sfe″no-tur′bĭ-nəl) sphenoid and turbinate, as the sphenoturbinal bone (*concha sphenoidalis* [TA]).

**sphe·no·vo·mer·ine** (sfe″no-vo′mər-in) pertaining to the sphenoid and to the vomer.

**sphe·no·zy·go·mat·ic** (sfe″no-zi″go-mat′ik) pertaining to the sphenoid and zygomatic bones.

**sphere** (sfēr) [Gr. *sphaira* sphere] a three dimensional round body; called also *globe.*
**attraction s.,** centrosphere, def. 1.
**embryotic s.,** the morula.
**segmentation s.,** 1. the morula. 2. a blastomere.
**vitelline s., yolk s.,** the morula.

**sphe·ri·cal** (sfēr′ĭ-kəl) [Gr. *sphairikos*] pertaining to a sphere; sphere-shaped.

**spher(o)-** [Gr. *sphaira* a ball or globe] a combining form meaning round, or denoting relationship to a sphere.

**sphe·ro·cyl·in·der** (sfēr-o-sil′in-dər) a combined spherical and cylindrical lens.

**sphe·ro·cyte** (sfēr′o-sīt) [*sphero-* + *-cyte*] [MeSH: Spherocytes] a small, globular, completely hemoglobinated erythrocyte without the usual central pallor, found characteristically in hereditary spherocytosis but also observed in acquired hemolytic anemia.

**sphe·ro·cyt·ic** (sfēr″o-sit′ik) characterized by the presence of spherocytes.

**sphe·ro·cy·to·sis** (sfēr″o-si-to′sis) the presence of spherocytes in the blood; called also *microspherocytosis.*
**hereditary s.,** a congenital, usually autosomal dominant form of

spherocytosis with hemolytic anemia, abnormal fragility of erythrocytes, jaundice, and splenomegaly; it is the most common form of hereditary anemia among people of European descent. Called also *congenital hemolytic* or *spherocytic anemia; chronic familial, congenital familial,* or *congenital hemolytic icterus; chronic acholuric* or *familial acholuric jaundice;* and *Minkowski-Chauffard syndrome.*

**sphe·roid** (sfēr′oid) [*sphero-* + *-oid*] [MeSH: Spheroids] a globular body, or one resembling a sphere.

**sphe·roi·dal** (sfēr-oi′dəl) having the form or shape of a sphere.

**sphe·roi·din** (sfēr-oi′din) [*Sphaeroides* a genus of puffer fish] a toxic fraction from tetrodotoxin.

**sphe·ro·lith** (sfēr′o-lith) [*sphero-* + *-lith*] any of the minute spherical deposits found in the kidney tissue of the newborn; they are probably uratic deposits.

**sphe·rom·e·ter** (sfēr-om′ə-tər) [*sphero-* + *-meter*] an instrument for measuring the curvature of a surface.

**sphe·ro·pha·kia** (sfēr″o-fa′ke-ə) [*sphero* + *phak-* + *ia*] a developmental defect in which a smaller, more spherical optic lens than normal is formed, with partial or complete aplasia of the zonule.

**Spher·oph·o·rous** (sfēr-of′ə-rəs) *Sphaerophorus.*

**sphe·ro·plast** (sfēr′o-plast) [MeSH: Spheroplasts] a bacterial, yeast, or fungal cell that results after partial removal of the rigid cell wall, which forms a membrane-bound cell with a spherical shape that is dependent for its integrity on an isotonic or hypertonic medium. Cf. *protoplast,* def. 3.

**sphe·ro·sper·mia** (sfēr″o-sper′me-ə) [*sphero-* + *sperm-* + *-ia*] a round, tailless spermatozoon.

**sphe·rule** (sfēr′ūl) [L. *sphaerula* little ball] 1. a small sphere. 2. a spherical multinucleate cell of the parasitic stage of *Coccidioides immitis,* in which endospores are developed.
**s's of Fulci,** numerous spherical red bodies seen in the spinal cord in inflammatory conditions of the cord.
**rod s.,** the pear-shaped ending of a retinal rod cell, which synapses with the bipolar and horizontal cells in the outer plexiform layer.

**sphe·ru·lin** (sfēr′u-lin) a skin test antigen prepared from spherule-endospore phase *Coccidioides immitis* organisms, which detects almost all persons who are coccidioidin-positive, as well as a group of coccidioidin-negative persons with previous *C. immitis* exposure. Cf. *coccidioidin.*

**sphinc·ter** (sfingk′tər) [L.; Gr. *sphinktēr* that which binds tight] a ringlike band of muscle fibers that constricts a passage or closes a natural orifice; called also *musculus sphincter* [TA].
**anal s., external,** musculus sphincter ani externus.
**anal s., internal,** musculus sphincter ani internus.
**s. a′ni,** see *musculus sphincter ani externus* and *musculus sphincter ani internus.*
**s. of Boyden,** a superior choledochal sphincter encircling the common bile duct just proximal to the duodenum.
**cardiac s., cardioesophageal s.,** muscle fibers about the opening of the esophagus into the stomach.
**cornual s.,** tubal s.
**cricopharyngeal s.,** pars cricopharyngea musculi constrictoris pharyngis inferioris.
**esophageal s., lower,** LES; gastroesophageal s.
**esophageal s., upper,** UES; the upper 3–5 cm of the esophagus, including the cricopharyngeal muscle, which prevents the aspiration of air from the pharynx into the esophagus.
**gastroesophageal s.,** the terminal few centimeters of the esophagus, which prevents reflux of gastric contents into the esophagus; see also *esophagogastric junction,* under *junction.*
**Giordano's s.,** musculus sphincter ductus choledochi.
**Glisson's s.,** musculus sphincter ampullae hepatopancreaticae.
**Henle's s.,** muscle fibers surrounding the prostatic urethra.
**hepatic s.,** a thickened portion of the muscular coat of the hepatic veins near their entrance into the inferior vena cava.
**s. of hepatopancreatic ampulla,** musculus sphincter ampullae hepatopancreaticae.
**Hyrtl's s.,** an incomplete band or thickening of the muscle fibers in the rectum a few inches above the anus in the upper part of the rectal ampulla; called also *rectal s.*
**inguinal s.,** a ring of muscle fibers around the spermatic cord at the internal opening of the inguinal canal.
**s. i′ridis,** musculus sphincter pupillae.
**Lütkens' s.,** a thickening of the muscle fibers in the neck of the gallbladder.
**Nélaton's s.,** an occasional and often incomplete band of muscle fibers about the rectum at the level of the prostate.
**O'Beirne's s.,** circular muscle fibers in the wall of the large intestine at the junction of the sigmoid colon and rectum.
**s. o′culi,** musculus orbicularis oculi.
**s. of Oddi,** 1. the sheath of muscle fibers investing the associated bile and pancreatic passages as they traverse the wall of the duodenum; the combination of the musculus sphincter ductus choledochi and the musculus sphincter ampullae hepatopancreaticae. Called also *Oddi's muscle.* 2. musculus sphincter ampullae hepatopancreaticae.
**s. o′ris,** musculus orbicularis oris.
**palatopharyngeal s.,** a transverse band of muscle fibers in the posterior wall of the pharynx, derived from the superior constrictor or palatopharyngeal muscle, which contracts during swallowing to form Passavant's bar; it also contracts during speech in persons with cleft palate.

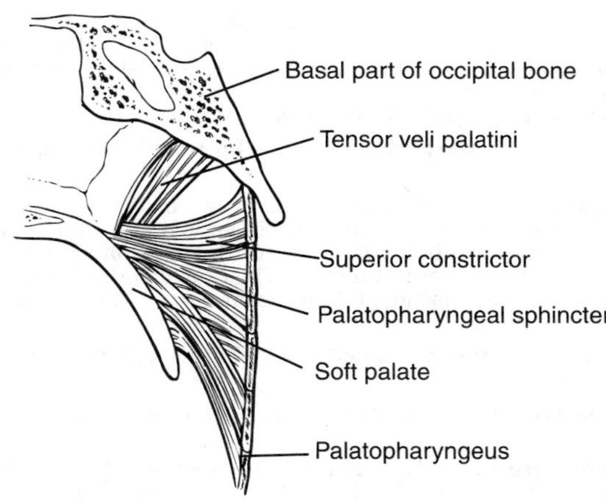


Palatopharyngeal sphincter shown in a sagittal view of the soft palate and adjoining pharyngeal wall. The levator veli palatini has been removed for clarity.

**pharyngoesophageal s.,** a region of higher muscular tone at the pharyngoesophageal junction, involved in movements of swallowing.
**precapillary s.,** a smooth muscle fiber encircling a true capillary where it originates from the arterial capillary, which can open and close the capillary entrance.
**prepyloric s.,** a band of muscle fibers in the wall of the stomach proximal to the pyloric sphincter.
**s. pupil′lae,** musculus sphincter pupillae.
**pyloric s.,** a thickening of the circular muscle of the stomach around its opening into the duodenum; called also *musculus sphincter pyloricus* [TA].
**rectal s.,** Hyrtl's s.
**tubal s.,** an encircling band of muscle fibers at the junction of the uterine tube and the uterus.
**s. ure′thrae,** musculus sphincter urethrae.
**s. vagi′nae,** the musculus bulbospongiosus in the female.
**s. vesi′cae,** musculus sphincter vesicae urinariae.

**sphinc·ter·al** (sfingk′tər-əl) pertaining to a sphincter.

**sphinc·ter·al·gia** (sfingk″tər-al′jə) [*sphincter* + *-algia*] pain in a sphincter muscle, as of the anus.

**sphinc·ter·ec·to·my** (sfingk″tər-ek′tə-me) [*sphincter* + *-ectomy*] excision of any sphincter, such as the sphincter iridis.

**sphinc·ter·ic** (sfingk-ter′ik) pertaining to a sphincter.

**sphinc·ter·is·mus** (sfingk″tər-iz′məs) spasm of the sphincter ani.

**sphinc·ter·itis** (sfingk″tər-i′tis) inflammation of a sphincter, particularly of the sphincter of Oddi.

**sphinc·ter·ol·y·sis** (sfingk″tər-ol′ĭ-sis) [*sphincter* + *lysis*] the operation of separating the iris from the cornea in anterior synechia.

**sphinc·tero·plas·ty** (sfingk′tər-o-plas″te) [*sphincter* + *-plasty*] surgical repair of a defective sphincter.

**sphinc·tero·scope** (sfingk′tər-o-skōp″) [*sphincter* + *-scope*] a speculum for inspecting the anal sphincter.
**Kelly's s.,** see under *speculum.*

**sphinc·ter·os·co·py** (sfingk″tər-os′kə-pe) inspection of a sphincter.

**sphinc·tero·tome** (sfingk′tər-o-tōm″) an instrument for cutting a sphincter.

**sphinc·ter·ot·o·my** (sfingk″tər-ot′ə-me) [*sphincter* + *-tomy*] division of a sphincter.
**internal s.,** incision of the internal anal sphincter.

**sphin·ga·nine** (sfing′gə-nēn) a dihydroxy derivative of sphingosine and similarly a common component of sphingolipids in mammals.

**sphingo-** [Gr. *sphingein* to bind fast] a combining form denoting relationship to sphingosine or a sphingolipid.

**sphin·go·ga·lac·to·side** (sfing″go-gə-lak′to-sīd) a substance composing part of the material characteristic of the spleen in Gaucher's disease.

**sphin·go·in** (sfing′go-in) a leukomaine from the substance of the brain.

**sphin·go·lip·id** (sfing″go-lip′id) a lipid in which the backbone is sphingosine or a related base; the basic unit is a ceramide (q.v.) which is attached via its 1-hydroxyl group to a polar head group. The sphingolipids include sphingomyelins, cerebrosides, and gangliosides.

**sphin·go·lip·i·do·sis** (sfing″go-lip″ĭ-do′sis) [*sphingolipid* + *-osis*] 1. any lysosomal storage disease characterized by abnormal storage of sphingolipids. 2. Niemann-Pick disease. Called also *sphingolipodystrophy.*
**cerebral s.,** neuronal ceroid lipofuscinosis.

**sphin·go·lipo·dys·tro·phy** (sfing″go-lip″o-dis′trə-fe) sphingolipidosis.

**sphin·go·my·e·lin** (sfing″go-mi′ə-lin) any of the group of sphingolipids in which the head group is phosphorylated choline, making them sphingophospholipids; they are the only phospholipids not derived from glycerol in humans. They occur in membranes, primarily in nervous tissue, and are accumulated abnormally in Niemann-Pick disease.

**sphin·go·my·e·lin·ase** (sfing″go-mi′ə-lin-ās) sphingomyelin phosphodiesterase.

**sphin·go·my·eli·no·sis** (sfing″go-mi″ə-lin-o′sis) Niemann-Pick disease.

**sphin·go·my·e·lin phos·pho·di·es·ter·ase** (sfing″go-mi′ə-lin fos″fo-di-es′tər-ās) [EC 3.1.4.12] [MeSH: Sphingomyelin Phosphodiesterase] an enzyme of the hydrolase class that catalyzes the cleavage of sphingomyelin to ceramide and phosphorylated choline in the major pathway for sphingomyelin degradation. Deficiency of the enzyme, an autosomal recessive trait, causes Niemann-Pick disease. Called also *sphingomyelinase.*

**sphin·go·phos·pho·lip·id** (sfing″go-fos″fo-lip′id) a phospholipid derived from sphingosine or a related base; in higher animals, the most abundant are the sphingomyelins.

**sphin·go·sine** (sfing′go-sēn) [MeSH: Sphingosine] an amino alcohol with a long unsaturated hydrocarbon chain; sphingosine and its derivative sphinganine are the major bases of the sphingolipids in mammals.

**sphin·go·sine *N*-ac·yl·trans·fer·ase** (sfing′go-sēn a″səl-trans′fər-ās) [EC 2.3.1.24] an enzyme of the transferase class that catalyzes the transfer of a fatty acyl group from an acyl (usually stearoyl) coenzyme A to sphingosine to form a ceramide. The reaction occurs in microsomes as a step in the synthesis of sphingolipids.

**sphyg·mic** (sfig′mik) [Gr. *sphygmikos*] pertaining to the pulse.

**sphygm(o)-** [Gr. *sphygmos* pulse] a combining form denoting relationship to the pulse.

**sphyg·mo·chro·no·graph** (sfig″mo-kro′no-graf) [*sphygmo-* + *chronograph*] a form of self-registering sphygmograph.

**sphyg·mo·dy·na·mom·e·ter** (sfig″mo-di″nə-mom′ə-tər) [*sphygmo-* + *dynamometer*] an instrument for determining the force of the pulse.

**sphyg·mo·gram** (sfig′mo-gram) [*sphygmo-* + *gram*] the record or tracing made by a sphygmograph; it consists of a curve having a sudden rise *(primary elevation),* followed by a sudden fall, after which there is a gradual descent marked by a number of secondary elevations. Called also *pulse curve.*

**sphyg·mo·graph** (sfig′mo-graf) [*sphygmo-* + *graph*] an instrument for registering the movements, form, and force of the arterial pulse.

**sphyg·mo·graph·ic** (sfig″mo-graf′ik) pertaining to the sphygmograph.

**sphyg·mog·ra·phy** (sfig-mog′rə-fe) the production of pulse tracings with the sphygmograph.

**sphyg·moid** (sfig′moid) [*sphygm-* + *-oid*] resembling a pulse.

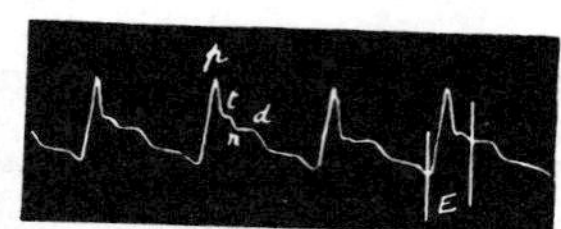


Radial sphygmogram from a healthy person: *p,* percussion wave; *t,* tidal or predicrotic wave; *n,* dicrotic or aortic notch; *d,* dicrotic wave; *E,* the sphygmic period, during which the semilunar valves are open.

**sphyg·mol·o·gy** (sfig-mol′ə-je) [*sphygmo-* + *-logy*] the sum of what is known regarding the pulse.

**sphyg·mo·ma·nom·e·ter** (sfig″mo-mə-nom′ə-tər) an instrument for measuring blood pressure in the arteries. There are many forms of the instrument, each named for the person who devised it, as *Riva-Rocci s., Faught's s., Erlanger's s., Janeway's s., Mosso's s., Rogers' s., Stanton's s., Tychos s.*

**sphyg·mom·e·ter** (sfig-mom′ə-tər) [*sphygmo-* + *-meter*] an instrument for measuring the force and frequency of the pulse.

**sphyg·mo·met·ro·graph** (sfig″mo-met′ro-graf) an apparatus for recording the maximal and minimal arterial blood pressures.

**sphyg·mo·met·ro·scope** (sfig″mo-met′ro-skōp) an instrument for taking the blood pressure by the auscultatory method.

**sphyg·mo·os·cil·lom·e·ter** (sfig″mo-os″ĭ-lom′ə-tər) a form of sphygmomanometer in which the disappearance and reappearance of the pulse are indicated by an oscillating needle.

**sphyg·mo·pal·pa·tion** (sfig″mo-pal-pa′shən) the act of palpating or feeling the pulse.

**sphyg·mo·phone** (sfig′mo-fōn) [*sphygmo-* + Gr. *phōnē* sound] an apparatus for rendering audible the vibrations of the pulse.

**sphyg·mo·ple·thys·mo·graph** (sfig″mo-plə-thiz′mo-graf) a plethysmograph which traces a record of the pulse, together with the curve of fluctuation of volume.

**sphyg·mo·scope** (sfig′mo-skōp) [*sphygmo-* + *-scope*] a device for rendering the pulse beat visible.
**Bishop's s.,** an apparatus for measuring the blood pressure, especially the diastolic pressure.

**sphyg·mos·co·py** (sfig-mos′kə-pe) examination of the pulse.

**sphyg·mo·sys·to·le** (sfig″mo-sis′tə-le) [*sphygmo-* + *systole*] that part of the sphygmogram that corresponds to the systole of the heart.

**sphyg·mo·to·nom·e·ter** (sfig″mo-to-nom′ə-tər) [*sphygmo-* + *tonometer*] an instrument for measuring the elasticity of the arterial walls.

**sphyg·mo·vis·co·sim·e·try** (sfig″mo-vis″ko-sim′ə-tre) [*sphygmo-* + *viscosimetry*] measurement of the blood pressure and the viscosity of the blood.

**spi·ca** (spi′kə) [L. "ear of wheat"] a figure-of-8 bandage with turns that cross one another usually at the shoulder or hip; see under *bandage.*

**spic·u·lar** (spik′u-lər) pertaining to a spicule.

**spic·ule** (spik′ūl) [L. *spiculum*] a sharp, needle-like body.

**spic·u·lum** (spik′u-ləm) pl. *spic′ula* [L.] spicule.

**spi·der** (spi′dər) [MeSH: Spiders] 1. any arachnid of the order Araneae, usually characterized by a body in two parts: the cephalothorax, which has eight legs attached, and the abdomen. Some species have venomous bites. Cf. *arachnidism.* 2. a spider-like nevus; see *vascular s.*
**arterial s.,** vascular s.
**banana s.,** *Heteropoda venatoria,* a large tropical spider, sometimes found outside the Tropics in shipments of fruit such as bananas; its bite is painful but not serious.
**bird s.,** any of various members of the family Theraphosidae, large hairy tropical spiders reputed to sometimes catch and eat small birds.
**black widow s.,** *Latrodectus mactans,* a species found in the United States, whose bite causes pain and sometimes death.
**brown s.,** *Loxosceles laeta,* the species whose bite causes loxoscelism in South America.
**brown recluse s.,** *Loxosceles reclusa,* the species whose bite causes loxoscelism in North America.
**cat-headed s.,** *Mastophora gasteracanthoides,* a venomous spider of Peru, Chile, and Argentina whose bite causes necrotic spots on vineyard workers.
**comb-footed s.,** any member of the family Theridiidae.
**European wolf s.,** European tarantula.
**funnel-web s.,** any spider of the Australian genus *Atrax.* Six species have venomous bites, and the bite of *A. robustus* has caused human deaths.
**hobo s.,** *Tegenaria agrestis.*
**jointed s.,** any member of the family Solpugida.
**lynx s.,** *Peucetia viridans,* a species that squirts a corrosive spray that produces painful burns in the eye of its prey.
**tree funnel-web s.,** *Atrax formidabilis,* an Australian spider with a venomous bite.
**vascular s.,** a telangiectasis with a round red central portion and branching radiations resembling the profile of a spider, caused by dilatation and ramification of superficial cutaneous arteries. The lesions may occur singly or in large numbers, and may be nevoid or

acquired; they are often associated with pregnancy or liver disease. See also *vascular nevus,* under *nevus.* Called also *arterial s., nevus araneus,* and *spider angioma, nevus,* or *telangiectasia.*

**wandering s.,** *Ctenus ferus,* a South American species with a painful bite. Severe reactions may involve weakness, irregular heartbeat, breathing difficulties, and temporary blindness; in young children deaths have occurred.

**wolf s.,** any spider of the family Lycosidae.

**Spie·ghel's line** (shpe'gelz) [Adriaan van der *Spieghel* (L. *Spigelius*), Flemish anatomist, 1578–1625] linea semilunaris.

**Spie·gler-Fendt sarcoid** (shpe'gler-fent) [E. *Spiegler;* Heinrich *Fendt,* Austrian dermatologist, 1860–1908] lymphocytoma cutis.

**Spiel·mey·er-Vogt disease** (shpēl'mi-ər-fōkt) [Walter *Spielmeyer,* German physician, 1879–1935; Heinrich *Vogt,* German physician, early 20th century] Vogt-Spielmeyer disease; see under *disease.*

**spi·ge·li·an** (spi-je'le-ən) named for Adriaan van der *Spieghel,* as spigelian line (linea semilunaris) or *spigelian* lobe (lobus caudatus).

**spike** (spīk) a sharp upward deflection in a curve, such as the main deflection of the oscillographic tracing of the action potential wave, the following smaller wave being called the *after-potential.* See also under *potential.*

**end-plate s's,** the biphasic type of end-plate activity.

**Spi·lan·thes** (spi-lan'thēz) [Gr. *spilos* spot + Gr. *anthos* flower] a genus of composite-flowered plants (family Compositae). *S. acmel'la* Murr., the Para cress of tropical America and Asia, is a mosquito larvicide and was formerly used as a remedy for toothache.

**spill·way** (spil'wa) embrasure.

**spin** (spin) the angular momentum of a nucleus or electron.

**spi·na** (spi'nə) gen. and pl. *spi'nae* [L.] 1. [TA] spine: general anatomical nomenclature for a thornlike process or projection. 2. columna vertebralis.

**s. bi'fida,** a developmental anomaly characterized by defective closure of the vertebral arch, through which the spinal cord and meninges may protrude *(s. bifida cystica)* or may not *(s. bifida occulta).* Cf. *rachischisis.* Called also *hydrocele spinalis* and *cleft spine.*

**s. bi'fida ante'rior,** a defect of closure on the anterior surface of the vertebral canal, often associated with defective development of the abdominal and thoracic viscera.

**s. bi'fida aper'ta,** s. bifida manifesta.

**s. bi'fida cys'tica,** spina bifida in which there is protrusion through the defective vertebral arch of a cystic swelling involving the meninges (meningocele), spinal cord (myelocele), or both (meningomyelocele).

**s. bi'fida manifes'ta,** spina bifida with detectable external manifestations; it includes all types of spina bifida cystica and a few types of spina bifida occulta. Called also *s. bifida aperta.*

**s. bi'fida occul'ta,** spina bifida in which there is a defect of the vertebral arch without protrusion of the spinal cord or meninges.

**s. bi'fida poste'rior,** a defect of closure on the posterior surface of the vertebral canal.

**s. fronta'lis,** s. nasalis ossis frontalis.

**s. he'licis** [TA], spine of helix: a small, forward-projecting cartilaginous process on the anterior portion of the helix at about the junction of the helix and its crus, just above the tragus.

**s. ili'aca ante'rior infe'rior** [TA], anterior inferior iliac spine: a blunt bony process projecting forward from the lower part of the anterior margin of the ilium, just above the acetabulum.

**s. ili'aca ante'rior supe'rior** [TA], anterior superior iliac spine: a blunt bony projection on the anterior border of the ilium, forming the anterior end of the iliac crest.

**s. ili'aca poste'rior infe'rior** [TA], posterior inferior iliac spine: a blunt bony projection from the posterior border of the ilium, corresponding to the posterior lower extremity of the facies auricularis and the posterior upper extremity of the incisura ischiadica major.

**s. ili'aca poste'rior supe'rior** [TA], posterior superior iliac spine: a blunt bony projection on the posterior border of the ilium, forming the posterior end of the iliac crest.

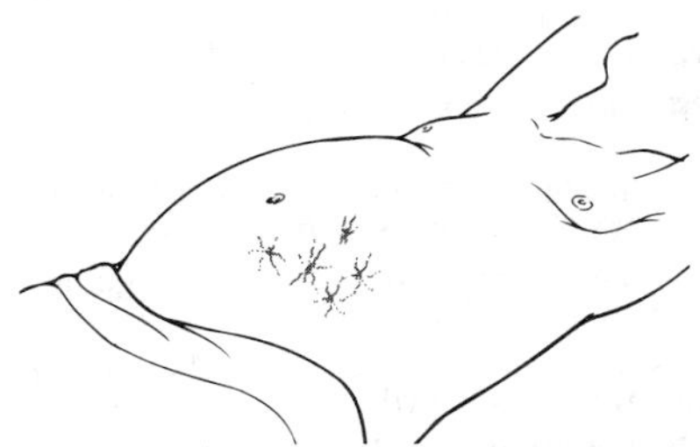

Vascular spiders on the abdomen in pregnancy.

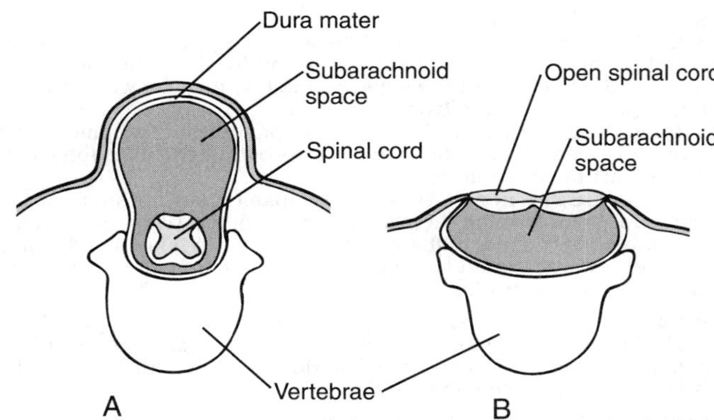


Two types of spina bifida cystica shown in transverse section through the spinal column. *(A),* Meningocele, characterized by protrusion of the meninges; *(B),* a form of myelocele characterized by myeloschisis and protrusion of the defective spinal cord.

**s. intercondyloi'dea,** eminentia intercondylaris.

**s. ischia'dica** [TA], **s. ischia'lis,** spine of ischium: a strong process of bone projecting backward and medialward from the posterior border of the ischium, on a level with the lower border of the acetabulum and serving to separate the major and minor ischiadic notches. Called also *ischial spine.*

**s. mea'tus,** s. suprameatica.

**s. menta'lis,** mental spine: any of the small bony projections (usually four in number) located on the internal surface of the mandible, near the lower end of the midline, serving for attachment of the genioglossal and geniohyoid muscles. Called also *genial apophysis.*

**s. nasa'lis ante'rior maxil'lae** [TA], anterior nasal spine of maxilla: the sharp anterosuperior projection at the anterior extremity of the nasal crest of the maxilla.

**s. nasa'lis os'sis fronta'lis** [TA], nasal spine of frontal bone: a rough and somewhat irregular process of bone projecting downward and forward from the front part of the inferior surface of the pars nasalis of the frontal bone and fitting between the nasal bones and the ethmoid bone; called also *s. frontalis.*

**s. nasa'lis poste'rior os'sis palati'ni** [TA], posterior nasal spine of palatine bone: a small, sharp, backward-projecting bony spine forming the medial posterior angle of the horizontal plate of the palatine bone; called also *nasal spine of palatine bone.*

**s. os'sis sphenoida'lis** [TA], spine of sphenoid bone: a small bony process projecting inferiorly from the inferior aspect of the greater wing of the sphenoid bone where the wing projects into the angle between the petrous and squamous portions of the temporal bone; it is just posterior to the foramen spinosum and serves for attachment of the sphenomandibular and pterygospinous ligaments. Called also *s. angularis.*

**spi'nae palati'nae** [TA], palatine spines: ridges which are laterally placed on the inferior surface of the maxillary part of the hard palate, separating the palatine sulci.

**s. sca'pulae** [TA], spine of scapula: a triangular plate of bone attached by one edge to the back of the scapula, its tip being at the vertebral border of the scapula; it passes laterally toward the shoulder joint and at its base bears the acromion.

**s. suprameata'lis,** TA alternative for *s. suprameatica.*

**s. suprame'atica** [TA], suprameatal spine: a pointed process that sometimes projects from the temporal bone, just above and at the back of the external acoustic meatus. Called also *Henle's spine* or *spine of Henle* and *s. suprameatalis* [TA alternative].

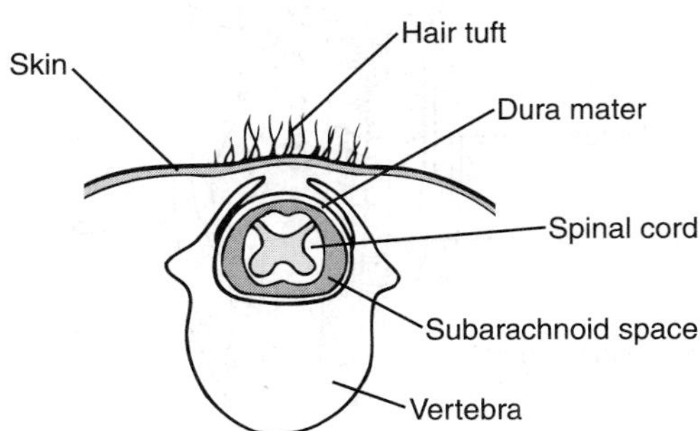


Spina bifida occulta in a transverse section through the spinal column.

**s. ti'biae,** tuberositas tibiae.
**s. trochlea'ris** [TA], trochlear spine: a spicule of bone on the anteromedial part of the orbital surface of the frontal bone for attachment of the trochlea of the superior oblique muscle; when absent, it is represented by the trochlear fovea.
**s. tympa'nica ma'jor** [TA], greater tympanic spine: a spine of the temporal bone forming the anterior edge of the tympanic notch (deficient part of tympanic sulcus).
**s. tympa'nica mi'nor** [TA], lesser tympanic spine: a spine of the temporal bone forming the posterior edge of the tympanic notch.
**s. vento'sa,** a true dactylitis occurring mostly in infants and young children, characterized by enlargement of the fingers or toes, with caseation, sequestration, and sinus formation.

**spi·nal** (spi'nəl) [L. *spinalis*] 1. pertaining to a spine. 2. pertaining to the vertebral column; called also *rachial, rachidial,* and *rachidian.* 3. pertaining to the spinal cord's functioning independently from the brain; see under *animal* and *reflex.*

**spi·nae** (spi'ne) [L.] genitive and plural of *spina.*

**spi·na·lis** (spi-na'lis) [L.] spinal.

**spi·nant** (spi'nənt) any agent that acts directly upon the spinal cord, increasing its reflex activity.

**spi·nate** (spi'nāt) [L. *spinatus*] having thorns; shaped like a thorn.

**spin·dle** (spin'dəl) 1. the fusiform figure occurring in the cell nucleus during the metaphase of mitosis, composed of microtubules radiating from the centrioles and connecting the chromosomes at their centromeres. Called also *achromatic s., mitotic s.,* and *nuclear s.* 2. a type of fusiform brain wave occurring on the electroencephalogram in groups at a frequency of about 14 per second, usually while the patient is falling asleep. 3. muscle s.
**aortic s.,** the dilated part of the aorta just below the isthmus; called also *His' s.*
**Axenfeld-Krukenberg s.,** Krukenberg's s.
**Bütschli's nuclear s.,** spindle (def. 1).
**central s.,** the bundle of fibers in the axial part of the spindle of an amphiaster.
**cleavage s.,** any spindle formed during cleavage of the zygote.
**enamel s's,** clublike structures in the inner third of the dental enamel, believed to be terminals of protoplasmic processes of the odontoblasts that have passed across the dentinoenamel junction.
**His' s.,** aortic s.
**Krukenberg's s.,** a vertical spindle-shaped, brownish-red opacity on the posterior surface of the cornea.
**mitotic s.,** spindle (def. 1).
**muscle s.,** a fusiform end organ found between skeletal muscle fibers and acting as a mechanoreceptor; the muscle spindles are arranged in parallel with muscle fibers, and respond to passive stretch of the muscle but cease to discharge if the muscle contracts isotonically, thus signaling muscle length. The muscle spindle is the receptor responsible for the stretch or myotatic reflex. Called also *neuromuscular s.*
**neuromuscular s.,** muscle s.
**neurotendinous s.,** Golgi tendon organ.
**nuclear s.,** spindle (def. 1).
**sleep s's,** bursts of activity at frequencies of about 14 per second, seen on the electroencephalogram in light or early sleep.
**tendon s.,** Golgi tendon organ.
**urine s's,** spindle-shaped, urine-filled segments of the ureter due to incomplete occlusion of the ureter during peristalsis.

**spine** (spīn) [MeSH: Spine] 1. a thornlike process or projection; called also *spina* [TA]. 2. columna vertebralis. 3. bar, def. 5.

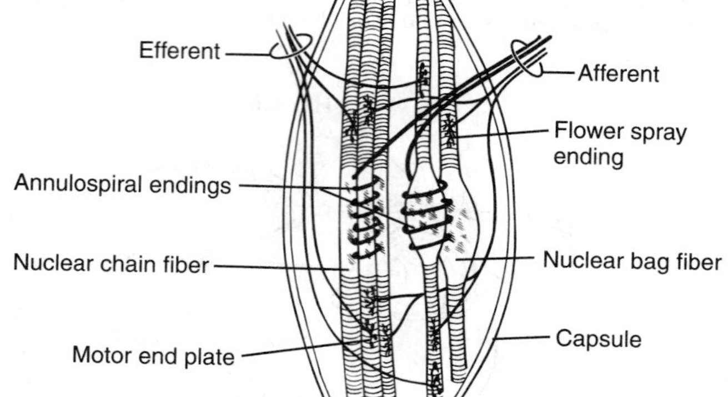

Diagrammatic cross-section of a muscle spindle showing the intrafusal fibers and afferent and efferent endings.

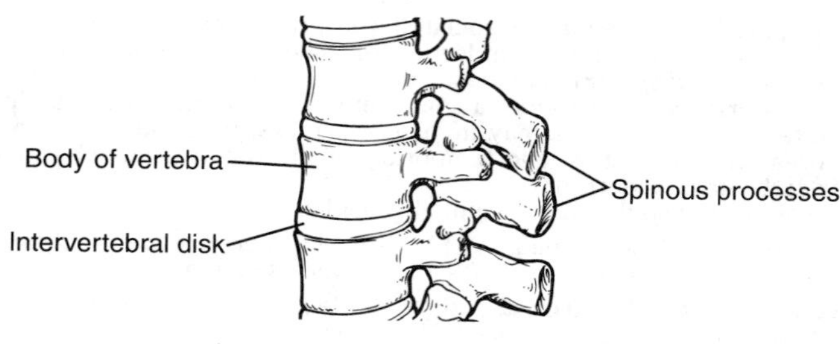

Kissing spines.

**alar s., angular s.,** spina ossis sphenoidalis.
**bamboo s.,** the rigid spine produced by ankylosing spondylitis; so called because of the radiographic appearance caused by lipping of the vertebral margins.
**basilar s.,** tuberculum pharyngeum.
**Civinini's s.,** processus pterygospinosus.
**cleft s.,** spina bifida.
**dendritic s.,** gemmule, def. 2.
**dorsal s.,** columna vertebralis.
**frontal s.,** spina nasalis ossis frontalis.
**s. of greater tubercle of humerus,** crista tuberculi majoris.
**s. of helix,** spina helicis.
**hemal s.,** a ventral projection from the hemal arch, which is attached to the underside of certain vertebral centra in lower vertebrates.
**Henle's s., s. of Henle,** spina suprameatica.
**iliac s.,** any of four bony projections on the ilium; see terms beginning *spina iliaca.*
**iliac s., anterior inferior,** spina iliaca anterior inferior.
**iliac s., anterior superior,** spina iliaca anterior superior.
**iliac s., posterior inferior,** spina iliaca posterior inferior.
**iliac s., posterior superior,** spina iliaca posterior superior.
**iliopectineal s.,** eminentia iliopubica.
**intercondyloid s.,** eminentia intercondylaris.
**ischial s., s. of ischium,** spina ischiadica.
**kissing s's,** a condition in which the spinous processes of adjacent vertebra are in contact; called also *Baastrup's disease* or *syndrome.*
**s. of lesser tubercle of humerus,** crista tuberculi minoris.
**s. of maxilla,** spina nasalis anterior maxillae.
**meatal s.,** spina suprameatica.
**mental s., external,** protuberantia mentalis.
**nasal s., anterior,** spina nasalis anterior maxillae.
**nasal s., posterior,** spina nasalis posterior ossis palatini.
**nasal s. of frontal bone,** spina nasalis ossis frontalis.
**nasal s. of palatine bone,** spina nasalis posterior ossis palatini.
**nasal s. of palatine bone, posterior,** spina nasalis posterior ossis palatini.
**neural s.,** processus spinosus vertebrae.
**obturator s.,** crista obturatoria.
**occipital s., external,** protuberantia occipitalis externa.
**occipital s., internal,** protuberantia occipitalis interna.
**peroneal s. of os calcis,** trochlea fibularis calcanei.
**pharyngeal s.,** tuberculum pharyngeum.
**poker s.,** the ankylosed spine produced by rheumatoid spondylitis; so called because of its rigidity.
**s. of pubic bone, s. of pubis,** tuberculum pubicum ossis pubis.
**rigid s.,** poker s.
**sciatic s.,** spina ischiadica.
**s. of sphenoid bone, sphenoidal s.,** spina ossis sphenoidalis.
**suprameatal s.,** spina suprameatica.
**s. of tibia, tibial s.,** tuberositas tibiae.
**trochanteric s., greater,** labium laterale lineae asperae femoris.
**trochanteric s., lesser,** labium mediale lineae asperae femoris.
**tympanic s., anterior, tympanic s., greater,** spina tympanica major.
**tympanic s., lesser, tympanic s., posterior,** spina tympanica minor.
**typhoid s.,** a painful condition of the spine due to osteomyelitis of the vertebrae following typhoid fever.
**s. of vertebra,** processus spinosus vertebrae.

**Spi·nel·li's operation** (spe-nel'ēz) [Pier Giuseppe *Spinelli,* Italian gynecologist, 1862–1929] see under *operation.*

**Spin·hal·er** (spin'hāl-ər) trademark for a type of dry powder inhaler that delivers single doses of medication.

**spi·nif·u·gal** (spi-nif'u-gəl) [*spina* + *-fugal*] going, conducting, or moving away from the spinal cord.

**spi·nip·e·tal** (spi-nip'ə-təl) [*spina* + *-petal*] tending, conducting, or moving toward the spinal cord.

**spinn·bar·keit** (spin'bahr-kīt) [Ger.] the formation of a thread by mucus from the cervix uteri when spread onto a glass slide and drawn out by a coverglass; the time at which it can be drawn to the maximum length usually precedes or coincides with the time of ovulation.

**spi·no·bul·bar** (spi″no-bul′bər) pertaining to the spinal cord and the medulla oblongata.

**spi·no·cel·lu·lar** (spi″no-sel′u-lər) containing, made up of, or marked by prickle cells.

**spi·no·cer·e·bel·lar** (spi″no-ser″ə-bel′ər) pertaining to the spinal cord and the cerebellum.

**spi·no·cer·e·bel·lum** (spi″no-ser″ə-bel′əm) [*spino-* + *cerebellum*] [TA] the portion of the cerebellum serving as the primary site of termination of the major spinocerebellar afferents, roughly corresponding to the vermis; therefore, the term is sometimes equated with paleocerebellum, which is the anatomical division of the cerebellum comprising predominantly the vermis of the anterior lobe, as well as the pyramis, uvula, and paraflocculus. Cf. *vestibulocerebellum* and *pontocerebellum.*

**spi·no·cor·ti·cal** (spi″no-kor′tĭ-kəl) corticospinal.

**spi·no·cos·tal·is** (spi″no-kos-ta′lis) the serratus posterior superior and inferior muscles together.

**spi·no·gal·van·iza·tion** (spi″no-gal″vən-ĭ-za′shən) galvanization of the spinal cord, performed by moving the anode slowly up and down the spine.

**spi·no·gle·noid** (spi″no-gle′noid) pertaining to the spine of the scapula and the glenoid cavity.

**spi·no·gram** (spi′no-gram) a radiograph of the spine or of the spinal cord.

**spi·nop·e·tal** (spi-nop′ə-təl) spinipetal.

**spi·nose** (spi′nōs) spinous.

**spi·no·tec·tal** (spi″no-tek′təl) tectospinal.

**spi·no·tha·lam·ic** (spi″no-thə-lam′ik) pertaining to or extending between the spinal cord and the thalamus.

**spi·nous** (spi′nəs) [L. *spinosus*] 1. like a spine; acanthoid. 2. pertaining to a spine or to a spinelike process.

**spin·ther·ism** (spin′thər-iz-əm) [Gr. *spinthērizein* to emit sparks] synchysis scintillans.

**spin·ther·om·e·ter** (spin″thər-om′ə-tər) [Gr. *spinthēr* spark + *-meter*] an apparatus for measuring the changes which occur in the vacuum of the x-ray tube, and hence the penetrating power of the rays.

**spin·ther·o·pia** (spin″thər-o′pe-ə) [Gr. *spinthēr* spark + *-opia*] synchysis scintillans.

**spin·tom·e·ter** (spin-tom′ə-tər) spintherometer.

**spip·e·rone** (spip′ə-rōn) [MeSH: Spiperone] a tranquilizer, $C_{23}H_{26}FN_3O_2$, used in treatment of schizophrenia.

**spir.** abbreviation for L. *spir′itus,* spirit.

**spir·a·cle** (spir′ə-kəl) [L. *spirare* to breathe] a breathing orifice of arthropods; an accessory opening for the intake of water in the respiratory system of cartilaginous fish.

**spir·ad·e·no·ma** (spīr″ad-ə-no′mə) [*spir-*[1] + *adenoma*] a benign tumor of the sweat glands, particularly of the coil portion.
**eccrine s.,** a benign, solitary, deep-seated nodule arising from the coil portion of an eccrine gland; it is covered by normal appearing skin and may be accompanied by paroxysmal pain.

**spi·ral** (spi′rəl) [L. *spiralis* from *spira;* Gr. *speira*] 1. winding about a center like a coil or the thread of a screw; called also *helical.* 2. a winding structure. See also *coil* and *helix.*
**Curschmann's s's,** coiled mucinous fibrils sometimes found in the sputum in bronchial asthma. Cf. *Laënnec's pearls.*
**Herxheimer's s's,** see under *fiber.*
**Perroncito's s's,** see under *apparatus.*

**spir·a·my·cin** (spir″ə-mi′sin) [MeSH: Spiramycin] a macrolide antibiotic produced by *Streptomyces ambofaciens;* administered orally.

**spi·reme** (spi′rēm) [Gr. *speirēma* coil] the threadlike, continuous or segmented figure formed by the chromosome material during the prophase of mitosis or meiosis. Called also *skein.*

**spi·ril·la** (spi-ril′ə) [L., dim. of *spira* coil] plural of *spirillum.*

**Spi·ril·la·ceae** (spi″ril-a′se-e) in former systems of classification, a family of spiral and curved bacteria that included the genera *Spirillum* and *Campylobacter.*

**spi·ril·le·mia** (spi″ril-e′me-ə) [*spirilla* + *-emia*] the presence of spirilla in the blood.

**spi·ril·li·ci·dal** (spi-ril″ĭ-si′dəl) destroying spirilla.

**spi·ril·li·cide** (spi-ril′ĭ-sīd) [*spirilla* + *-cide*] 1. destroying spirilla. 2. an agent that destroys spirilla.

**spi·ril·lol·y·sis** (spi″rĭ-lol′ĭ-sis) [*spirilla* + *-lysis*] the breaking up of or destruction of spirilla.

**spi·ril·lo·sis** (spi″rĭ-lo′sis) any disease condition attended or marked by the presence of spirilla in the body.

**spi·ril·lo·trop·ic** (spi″rĭ-lo-trop′ik) having an affinity for spirilla.

**spi·ril·lot·ro·pism** (spi″rĭ-lot′ro-piz-əm) [*spirilla* + *tropism*] the property of having an affinity for spirilla.

**Spi·ril·lum** (spi-ril′əm) [L., dim. of *spira* coil] [MeSH: Spirillum] a genus of spiral and curved bacteria of the family Spirillaceae, consisting of short, rigid, helical cells with bipolar flagella. The organisms are motile and microaerophilic or aerobic; they are found in fresh and salt waters that contain organic matter.
**S. mi′nus,** a species of uncertain status that is a normal parasite of the nasopharynx of rats and mice; it is the etiologic agent of the spirillary form of rat-bite fever.

**spi·ril·lum** (spi-ril′əm) pl. *spiril′la* [L., dim. of *spira* coil] [MeSH: Spirillum] any organism of the genus *Spirillum.*
**s. of Finkler and Prior,** *Vibrio metschnikovii.*
**s. of Vincent,** *Treponema vincentii.*

**spir·it** (spir′it) [L. *spiritus*] 1. any volatile or distilled liquid. 2. a solution of a volatile material in alcohol.
**ammonia s., aromatic** [USP], **s. of ammonia, aromatic,** a preparation compounded of ammonia, ammonium carbonate, strong ammonia solution, lemon oil, lavender oil, myristica oil, alcohol, and purified oil; used as a respiratory stimulant in syncope, weakness, or threatened faint. In veterinary medicine, it is used as a respiratory and circulatory stimulant, and sometimes as a carminative and antacid.
**benzaldehyde s.,** a mixture of benzaldehyde, alcohol, and distilled water; used as a flavoring agent.
**camphor s.** [USP], a solution of camphor and alcohol, used topically as a local irritant. It was formerly used for the treatment of diarrhea, and in hysteria and nervous excitement.
**orange s., compound,** an alcoholic preparation containing orange, lemon, coriander, and anise oils; used as a flavoring agent.
**peppermint s.** [USP], a preparation of peppermint, peppermint oil, and alcohol, used as a digestive aid and flavor. Called also *essence of peppermint.*
**proof s.,** a product containing 50 per cent by volume of ethanol.
**s's of turpentine,** turpentine oil.

**spir(o)-**[1] [Gr. *speira* coil] a combining form denoting relationship to a coil or spiral.

**spir(o)-**[2] [L. *spirare* to breathe] a combining form denoting relationship to the breath or to breathing.

**Spi·ro·cer·ca** (spi″ro-ser′kə) a genus of nematodes of the superfamily Spiruroidea. *S. lu′pi* (called also *S. sanguinolen′ta*) infests the walls of the aorta, esophagus, and stomach of canines and felines, forming large nodules; see *spirocercosis.*

**spi·ro·cer·co·sis** (spi″ro-sər-ko′sis) infestation of the esophagus or aorta of a canine or feline with *Spirocerca lupi,* which forms large nodules that sometimes obstruct the lumen and sometimes undergo transformation into a sarcoma.

**Spi·ro·chae·ta** (spi″ro-ke′tə) [Gr. *speira* coil + *chaitē* hair] [MeSH: Spirochaeta] a genus of bacteria of the family Spirochaetaceae, made up of large (up to 500 μm long) free-living organisms, found in hydrogen sulfide–containing mud, sewage, and polluted water. Most organisms formerly in this genus have been assigned to other genera. The type species is *S. plica′tilis.*

**Spi·ro·chae·ta·ceae** (spi″ro-ke-ta′se-e) [MeSH: Spirochaetaceae] a family of bacteria of the order Spirochaetales consisting of slender, undulating, motile organisms, 6 to 500 μm in length, occurring in the form of spirals with one or more complete turns in the helix. It contains the genera *Borrelia, Spirochaeta,* and *Treponema.*

**Spi·ro·chae·ta·les** (spi″ro-ke-ta′lēz) [MeSH: Spirochaetales] an order of bacteria comprising the families Spirochaetaceae and Leptospiraceae, the members of which are free-living, commensal, or parasitic, with some species being pathogenic.

**spi·ro·che·tal** (spi″ro-ke′təl) pertaining to or caused by spirochetes.

**spi·ro·chete** (spi′ro-kēt) [*spiro-*[1] + Gr. *chaitē* hair] 1. a spiral bacterium; a general term for any microorganism of the order Spirochaetales. 2. an organism of the genus *Spirochaeta.*
**Dutton's s.,** *Borrelia duttonii.*

**spi·ro·che·te·mia** (spi″ro-ke-te′me-ə) [*spirochete* + *-emia*] the presence of spirochetes in the blood.

**spi·ro·che·ti·ci·dal** (spi″ro-ke″tĭ-si′dəl) [*spirochete* + L. *caedere* to kill] destructive to spirochetes.

**spi·ro·che·ti·cide** (spi″ro-ke′tĭ-sīd) an agent that causes the destruction of spirochetes.

**spi·ro·che·tog·e·nous** (spi″ro-ke-toj′ə-nəs) caused by spirochetes.

**spi·ro·che·tol·y·sin** (spi″ro-ke-tol′ĭ-sin) a substance which causes lysis of spirochetes.

**spi·ro·che·tol·y·sis** (spi″ro-ke-tol′ĭ-sis) [*spirochete* + *-lysis*] the destruction of spirochetes by lysis.

**spi·ro·che·to·lyt·ic** (spi″ro-ke″to-lit′ik) pertaining to, characterized by, or causing spirochetolysis.

**spi·ro·che·to·sis** (spi″ro-ke-to′sis) infection with spirochetes.
**s. arthri′tica,** spirochetosis in which there is rheumatoid involvement of the joints.
**avian s.,** fowl s.
**bronchopulmonary s.,** hemorrhagic bronchitis.
**fowl s.,** a septicemic disease of fowls caused by the spirochete *Borrelia anserina,* and spread by the fowl tick *Argas persicus;* symptoms include fever, anorexia, diarrhea, and neurologic problems ranging from mild incoordination to convulsions, sometimes with paralysis and death.
**rabbit s.,** see under *syphilis.*

**spi·ro·che·tu·ria** (spi″ro-ke-tu′re-ə) [*spirochete* + *-uria*] the presence of spirochetes in the urine.

**spi·ro·gram** (spi′ro-gram) [*spiro-*[2] + *-gram*] a tracing or graph of respiratory movements. Called also *pneumatogram* and *pneumogram.*

**spi·ro·graph** (spi′ro-graf) [*spiro-*[2] + *-graph*] an instrument for registering the respiratory movements. See also *spirometer.* Called also *pneumatograph* and *pneumograph.*

**spi·rog·ra·phy** (spi-rog′rə-fe) the graphic measurement of breathing, including breathing movements and breathing capacity. See also *spirometry.* Called also *pneumography.*

**spi·roid** (spi′roid) resembling a spiral.

**spi·ro·in·dex** (spi″ro-in′deks) [*spiro-*[2] + *index*] the value obtained by dividing the vital capacity by the height of the individual.

**spi·ro·lac·tone** (spi″ro-lak′tōn) any of a group of compounds bearing 17$\alpha$-propionic acid as gamma-lactone with 17$\beta$-hydroxyl, capable of opposing the action of sodium-retaining steroids on renal transport of sodium and potassium. Three such compounds have been studied. The first contains angular methyl groups at $C_{13}$ and $C_{10}$, and is 3-(3-keto-17$\beta$-hydroxy-4-androsten-17$\alpha$-yl)-propionic acid-$\gamma$-lactone; the second, without the angular methyl group at $C_{10}$, is more potent; and the third (spironolactone), with a thioacetyl group at $C_7$, is highly active orally.

**spi·ro·ma** (spi-ro′mə) spiradenoma.

**spi·rom·e·ter** (spi-rom′ə-tər) [*spiro-*[2] + *-meter*] an instrument for measuring the air inhaled into and exhaled from the lungs, such as in pulmonary function tests.

**Spi·ro·me·tra** (spi″ro-me′trə) [*spiro-*[1] + Gr. *metra* womb, uterus] [MeSH: Spirometra] a genus of tapeworms of the family Diphyllobothriidae, parasites of fish-eating cats, dogs, and birds. Infection in humans is caused by eating inadequately cooked fish.
**S. erinaceieuropae′i,** a species parasitic in man, dogs, and cats.
**S. mansonoi′des,** a species parasitic in dogs and cats, especially bobcats, which may cause diarrhea and anemia; infection with the larvae may cause sparganosis in man.

**spi·ro·met·ric** (spi″ro-met′rik) pertaining to spirometry or the spirometer.

**spi·rom·e·try** (spi-rom′ə-tre) [MeSH: Spirometry] the measurement of the breathing capacity of the lungs, such as in pulmonary function tests. See also *spirography.*
**bronchoscopic s.,** bronchospirometry.
**incentive s.,** a maneuver in which sustained maximal inspiration is performed by the patient with the encouragement of visual feedback until predicted inspiratory reserve volume is achieved.

**Spi·ro·ne·ma** (spi″ro-ne′mə) [Gr. *speira* coil + *nēma* thread] in former systems of classification, a genus of bacteria made up of organisms now assigned to the genus *Treponema.*

**spir·o·no·lac·tone** (spi″ro-no-lak′tōn) [USP] [MeSH: Spironolactone] a synthetic 17-spirolactone steroid that is a competitive antagonist of aldosterone and blocks the aldosterone-dependent exchange of sodium and potassium in the distal tubule, thus increasing the excretion of sodium and water and decreasing the excretion of potassium; used in the treatment of edema due to congestive heart failure or hepatic or renal disease, in the treatment of hypokalemia, in the management of primary hyperaldosteronism, and, usually in combination with other drugs, in the treatment of hypertension.

**Spi·rop·tera** (spi-rop′tər-ə) a genus of nematodes of the family Habronematidae. *S. neoplas′tica* causes gastric carcinoma in rats.

**Spi·ro·schau·din·nia** (spi″ro-shaw-din′e-ə) in former systems of classification, a genus of bacteria made up of organisms now assigned to the genera *Borrelia* and *Treponema.*

**spi·ro·scope** (spi′ro-skōp) [*spiro-*[2] + *-scope*] an apparatus for respiration exercises by which the patient can see the amount of water displaced in a given time and thus gauge his respiratory capacity.

**spi·ros·co·py** (spi-ros′kə-pe) the use of the spiroscope.

**Spi·ru·roi·dea** (spi″roo-roi′de-ə) [MeSH: Spiruroidea] a superfamily of phasmid nematodes, including the families Gnathostomatidae, Physalopteridae, and Thelaziidae.

**spis·sat·ed** (spis′āt-əd) [L. *spissatus*] inspissated: thickened by evaporation.

**spis·si·tude** (spis′ĭ-tood) [L. *spissitudo*] the state or quality of being inspissated.

**Spitz nevus** (spits) [Sophie *Spitz,* American pathologist, born 1910] spindle and epithelioid cell nevus.

**Spitz·ka's nucleus, tract** (spits′kəz) [Edward Charles *Spitzka,* New York neurologist, 1852–1914] see *Perlia's nucleus,* under *nucleus,* and see *tractus posterolateralis.*

**Spitz·ka-Lis·sau·er tract (column)** (spits′kə-lis′ou-ər) [E. C. *Spitzka;* Heinrich *Lissauer,* German neurologist, 1861–1891] tractus posterolateralis.

**splanch·nap·o·phys·e·al** (splank″nap-o-fiz′e-əl) pertaining to a splanchnapophysis.

**splanch·na·poph·y·sis** (splank″nə-pof′ĭ-sis) [*splanchno-* + *apophysis*] a skeletal element, like the lower jaw, connected with the alimentary canal.

**splanch·nec·to·pia** (splan″nək-to′pe-ə) [*splanchno-* + *-ectopia*] displacement of a viscus.

**splanch·nes·the·sia** (splank″nəs-the′zhə) [*splanchno-* + *esthesia*] visceral sense.

**splanch·nes·thet·ic** (splank″nəs-thet′ik) pertaining to splanchnesthesia.

**splanch·nic** (splank′nik) [Gr. *splanchnikos;* L. *splanchnicus*] pertaining to the viscera.

**splanch·ni·cec·to·my** (splank″nĭ-sek′tə-me) [*splanchnic* + *-ectomy*] resection of one or more of the splanchnic nerves for the treatment of hypertension or intractable pain.

**splanch·ni·cot·o·my** (splank″nĭ-kot′ə-me) [*splanchnic* + *-otomy*] splanchnicectomy.

**splanchn(o)-** [Gr. *splanchnos* viscus] a combining form denoting relationship to a viscus, or to the splanchnic nerve.

**splanch·no·blast** (splank′no-blast) [*splanchno-* + *-blast*] the primordium or anlage of any viscus.

**splanch·no·cele** (splank′no-sēl) [*splanchno-* + *-cele*[1]] hernial protrusion of a viscus.

**splanch·no·coele** (splank′no-sēl) [*splanchno-* + *-coele*] that portion of the embryonic body cavity, or coelom, from which are developed the abdominal, pericardial, and pleural cavities; called also *pleuroperitoneal cavity.*

**splanch·no·cra·ni·um** (splank″no-kra′ne-əm) viscerocranium.

**splanch·no·derm** (splank′no-dərm) splanchnopleure.

**splanch·no·di·as·ta·sis** (splank″no-di-as′tə-sis) [*splanchno-* + *diastasis*] separation of a viscus; displacement of a viscus.

**splanch·nog·ra·phy** (splank-nog′rə-fe) [*splanchno-* + *-graphy*] the descriptive anatomy of the viscera.

**splanch·no·lith** (splank′no-lith) [*splanchno-* + *-lith*] an intestinal calculus or concretion.

**splanch·nol·o·gy** (splank-nol′ə-je) [*splanchno-* + *-logy*] the scientific study of the viscera of the body; applied also to the body of knowledge relating thereto.

**splanch·no·meg·a·lia** (splank″no-mə-ga′le-ə) splanchnomegaly.

**splanch·no·meg·a·ly** (splank″no-meg′ə-le) [*splanchno-* + *-megaly*] visceromegaly.

**splanch·no·mic·ria** (splank″no-mik′re-ə) [*splanchno-* + *micr-* + *-ia*] abnormal smallness of the viscera.

**splanch·nop·a·thy** (splank-nop′ə-the) [*splanchno-* + *-pathy*] disease of the abdominal viscera.

**splanch·no·pleu·ral** (splank″no-ploor′əl) pertaining to the splanchnopleure.

**splanch·no·pleure** (splank′no-ploor) [*splanchno-* + Gr. *pleura* side] the layer formed by the union of the splanchnic mesoderm with endoderm; from it are developed the muscles and the connective tissue of the digestive tube. Called also *splanchnoderm.*

**splanch·no·scle·ro·sis** (splank″no-sklə-ro′sis) [*splanchno-* + *sclerosis*] induration of the viscera.

**splanch·nos·co·py** (splank-nos′kə-pe) [*splanchno-* + *-scopy*] inspection of the viscera by endoscopy.

**splanch·no·skel·e·ton** (splank″no-skel′ə-tən) [*splanchno-* + *skeleton*] the totality of the skeletal structures connected with the viscera, especially the bony structure that forms within certain organs of animals, as in the gills, tongue, eye, penis, etc.

**splanch·no·so·mat·ic** (splank″no-so-mat′ik) [*splanchno-* + *somatic*] pertaining to the viscera and the body proper.

**splanch·not·o·my** (splank-not′o-me) [*splanchno-* + *-tomy*] the anatomy or dissection of the viscera.

**splanch·no·tribe** (splank′no-trīb) [*splanchno-* + Gr. *tribein* to crush] an instrument for crushing the intestine and so closing its lumen.

**S-plasty** in plastic surgery, a technique for distributing the contractile forces of wound healing in more than one direction by making an S-shaped incision, instead of a straight line, in areas where skin is loose.

**splay·foot** (spla′foot) flatfoot; talipes valgus.

**splay·leg** (spla′leg) myofibrillar hypoplasia.

**spleen** (splēn) [Gr. *splēn;* L. *splen*] [MeSH: Spleen] a large glandlike but ductless organ situated in the upper part of the abdominal cavity on the left side and lateral to the cardiac end of the stomach. Called also *splen* [TA] and *lien* [TA alternative]. It is of a flattened oblong shape and about 125 mm long, the largest structure in the lymphoid system; it has a purple color and a pliable consistency, and is distinguished by two types of tissue: red pulp and white pulp (see under *pulp*). It disintegrates the red blood cells and sets free the hemoglobin, which the liver converts into bilirubin; gives rise to new red blood cells during fetal life and in the newborn; serves as a reservoir of blood, produces lymphocytes and plasma cells, and has other important functions, the full scope of which is not entirely determined.
**accessory s.,** splen accessorius.
**bacon s.,** a spleen with areas of amyloid degeneration, giving its cut surfaces the appearance of fried bacon.
**cyanotic s.,** a contracted form of spleen due to passive congestion.
**diffuse waxy s.,** amyloid degeneration of the spleen involving especially the coats of the venous sinuses and the reticulum of the organ.
**enlarged s.,** splenomegaly.
**flecked s. of Feitis,** multiple necroses of the spleen, characterized by nonembolic multiple areas of anemic necrosis.
**floating s.,** a spleen displaced and preternaturally movable; called also *wandering s.*
**Gandy-Gamna s.,** siderotic splenomegaly.
**lardaceous s.,** waxy s.
**movable s.,** floating s.
**porphyry s.,** a spleen which is the seat of nodular infiltration.
**sago s.,** a spleen having on its cut surface the appearance of grains of sago; due to amyloid infiltration.
**speckled s.,** flecked s. of Feitis.
**wandering s.,** floating s.
**waxy s.,** a spleen affected with amyloid degeneration; called also *lardaceous s.*

**splen** (splen) [Gr. *splēn*] [TA] a large glandlike but ductless organ situated in the upper part of the abdominal cavity; see *spleen.* Called also *lien* [TA alternative].
**s. accesso′rius** [TA], accessory spleen: a connected or detached outlying portion, or exclave, of the spleen; called also *lien accessorius* [TA alternative], *splenculus, spleneolus, splenulus,* and *splenunculus.*

**sple·nal·gia** (sple-nal′jə) [*splen-* + *-algia*] neuralgic pain in the spleen.

**splen·at·ro·phy** (splen-at′rə-fe) atrophy of the spleen.

**sple·nauxe** (sple-nawk′se) [*splen-* + Gr. *auxē* increase] splenomegaly.

**splen·cer·a·to·sis** (splen″ser-ə-to′sis) splenokeratosis.

**splen·cu·lus** (spleng′ku-ləs) [L. "little spleen"] splen accessorius.

**sple·nec·ta·sis** (sple-nek′tə-sis) [*splen-* + *ectasis*] splenomegaly.

**sple·nec·to·mize** (sple-nek′tə-mīz) to remove the spleen.

**sple·nec·to·my** (sple-nek′tə-me) [*splen-* + *-etomy*] [MeSH: Splenectomy] excision or extirpation of the spleen.

**sple·nec·to·pia** (sple″nek-to′pe-ə) [*splen-* + *ectopia*] displacement of the spleen; wandering or floating spleen.

**sple·nec·to·py** (sple-nek′tə-pe) splenectopia.

**sple·nel·co·sis** (sple″nəl-ko′sis) [*splen-* + *elcosis*] ulceration of the spleen.

**sple·ne·mia** (sple-ne′me-ə) [*splen-* + *-emia*] congestion of the spleen with blood.

**sple·nem·phrax·is** (sple″nəm-frak′sis) [*splen-* + *emphraxis*] congestion of the spleen.

**sple·ne·o·lus** (sple-ne′o-ləs) splen accessorius.

**sple·ni·al** (sple′ne-əl) pertaining to the splenium corporis callosi or to the splenius muscle.

**splen·ic** (splen′ik) [Gr. *splēnikos;* L. *splenicus*] pertaining to the spleen; lienal.

**splen·ic·ter·us** (splen-ik′tər-əs) [*splen-* + *icterus*] inflammation of the spleen associated with jaundice.

**splen·i·form** (splen′ĭ-form) resembling the spleen.

**splen·i·ser·rate** (splen″ĭ-ser′āt) pertaining to the splenius and the serratus muscles.

**sple·ni·tis** (sple-ni′tis) [*splen-* + *-itis*] inflammation of the spleen, a condition usually produced by pyemia. It is attended by enlargement of the organ with pus, and is marked by much local pain.
**spodogenous s.,** that due to accumulation of foreign particles in the spleen.

**sple·ni·um** (sple′ne-um) [L.; Gr. *splēnion*] 1. a bandlike structure. 2. a bandage or compress. 3. s. corporis callosi.
**s. cor′poris callo′si** [TA], the posterior rounded end of the corpus callosum; it conveys visual information between the two cerebral hemispheres.

**splen(o)-** [Gr. *splēn* spleen] a combining form denoting relationship to the spleen.

**sple·no·blast** (sple′no-blast) the cell from which a splenocyte develops.

**sple·no·cele** (sple′no-sēl) [*spleno-* + *-cele*[1]] hernia of the spleen.

**sple·no·cer·a·to·sis** (sple″no-ser″ə-to′sis) splenokeratosis.

**sple·no·clei·sis** (sple″no-kli′sis) [*spleno-* + Gr. *kleisis* closure] irritation of the surface of the spleen to induce the development of new fibrous tissue.

**sple·no·col·ic** (sple″no-kol′ik) [*spleno-* + *colic* (def. 1)] pertaining to the spleen and colon.

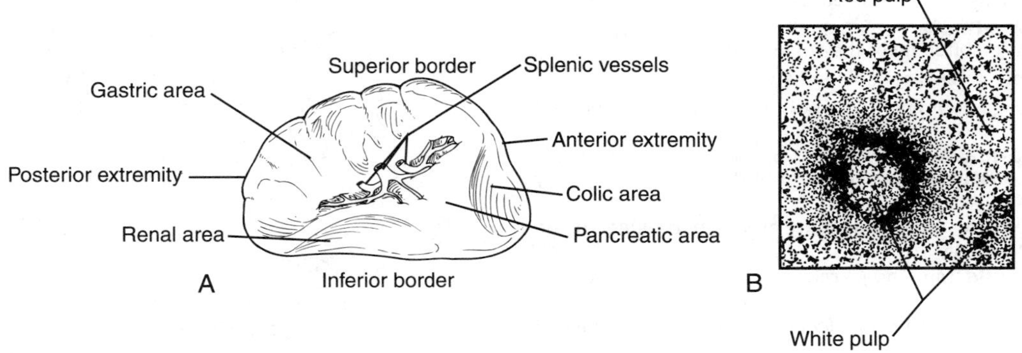


Spleen. *(A),* visceral surface; *(B),* section, showing the red and white pulp.

**sple·no·cyte** (sple′no-sīt) the monocyte characteristic of the spleen.

**sple·no·dyn·ia** (sple″no-din′e-ə) [*spleno-* + *-odynia*] pain in the spleen.

**sple·nog·e·nous** (sple-noj′ə-nəs) arising in or formed by the spleen.

**sple·no·gram** (sple′no-gram) 1. a radiograph of the spleen. 2. a differential count of the cells found in a stained preparation of material obtained by splenic puncture.

**sple·nog·ra·phy** (sple-nog′rə-fe) [*spleno-* + *-graphy*] 1. radiography of the spleen. 2. a description of the spleen.

**sple·no·hep·a·to·me·ga·lia** (sple″no-hep″ə-to-me-ga′le-ə) splenohepatomegaly.

**sple·no·hep·a·to·meg·a·ly** (sple″no-hep″ə-to-meg′ə-le) [*spleno-* + *hepato-* + *-megaly*] enlargement of the spleen and liver.

**sple·noid** (sple′noid) [*spleno-* + *-oid*] resembling the spleen.

**sple·no·ker·a·to·sis** (sple″no-ker″ə-to′sis) [*spleno-* + *kerat-* + *-osis*] hardening of the spleen.

**sple·no·lap·a·rot·o·my** (sple″no-lap″ə-rot′ə-me) laparosplenotomy.

**sple·nol·o·gy** (sple-nol′ə-je) [*spleno-* + *-logy*] the sum of knowledge regarding the spleen, its functions and diseases.

**sple·no·lym·phat·ic** (sple″no-lim-fat′ik) pertaining to the spleen and lymph nodes.

**sple·nol·y·sin** (sple-nol′ĭ-sin) [*spleno-* + *-lysin*] a lysin destructive to splenic tissue.

**sple·nol·y·sis** (sple-nol′ĭ-sis) destruction of spleen tissue.

**sple·no·ma** (sple-no′mə) pl. *splenomas* or *spleno′mata* [*spleno-* + *-oma*] a tumor of the spleen.

**sple·no·ma·la·cia** (sple″no-mə-la′shə) [*spleno-* + *-malacia*] abnormal softness of the spleen; softening of the spleen.

**sple·no·med·ul·lary** (sple″no-med′u-lar″e) of or pertaining to the spleen and bone marrow.

**sple·no·me·ga·lia** (sple″no-mə-ga′le-ə) splenomegaly.

**sple·no·meg·a·ly** (sple″no-meg′ə-le) [*spleno-* + *-megaly*] [MeSH: Splenomegaly] enlargement of the spleen.
**congestive s.,** enlargement of the spleen occurring secondary to portal hypertension, with ascites, anemia, thrombocytopenia, leukopenia, and episodic hemorrhage from the gastrointestinal tract. Called also *Banti's disease* and *splenic anemia.*
**Egyptian s.,** that caused by *Schistosoma mansoni.*
**Gaucher's s.,** see under *disease.*
**hemolytic s.,** that associated with any disorder causing increased degradation of erythrocytes, such as hereditary spherocytosis.
**infectious s., infective s.,** splenomegaly associated with an infection.
**myelophthisic s.,** enlargement of the spleen marked by decrease in myeloid tissue and by fibrosis.
**siderotic s.,** splenomegaly characterized by marked fibrosis with deposit of iron and calcium (Gamna nodules); called also *Gandy-Gamna disease.*
**spodogenous s.,** enlargement of the spleen attributed to accumulation of erythrocytes in the organ.
**thrombophlebitic s.,** Opitz's disease.
**tropical s.,** 1. visceral leishmaniasis. 2. malarial hyperreactive spleen syndrome.

**sple·nom·e·try** (sple-nom′ə-tre) determination of the size of the spleen.

**sple·no·my·elog·e·nous** (sple″no-mi″ə-loj′ə-nəs) formed in the spleen and bone marrow; splenomedullary.

**sple·no·my·elo·ma·la·cia** (sple″no-mi″ə-lo-mə-la′shə) [*spleno-* + *myelo-* + *-malacia*] softening of the spleen and bone marrow.

**sple·non·cus** (sple-nong′kəs) splenoma.

**sple·no·neph·ric** (sple″no-nef′rik) pertaining to the spleen and the kidney.

**sple·no·neph·rop·to·sis** (sple″no-nef″rop-to′sis) [*spleno-* + *nephro-* + *-ptosis*] downward displacement of the spleen and kidney on the same side.

**sple·no·pan·cre·at·ic** (sple″no-pan″kre-at′ik) pertaining to the spleen and the pancreas.

**sple·no·pa·rec·ta·sis** (sple″no-pə-rek′tə-sis) [*spleno-* + *parectasis*] splenomegaly.

**sple·nop·a·thy** (sple-nop′ə-the) [*spleno-* + *-pathy*] any disease of the spleen.

**sple·no·pexy** (sple′no-pek″se) [*spleno-* + *-pexy*] surgical fixation of a mobile spleen.

**sple·no·phren·ic** (splen-o-fren′ik) [*spleno-* + *-phren-* + *-ic*] pertaining to the spleen and diaphragm.

**sple·no·por·tog·ra·phy** (sple″no-por-tog′rə-fe) splenic portography.

**sple·nop·to·sia** (sple″nop-to′se-ə) splenoptosis.

**sple·nop·to·sis** (sple″nop-to′sis) [*spleno-* + *-ptosis*] prolapse or downward displacement of the spleen.

**sple·no·re·nal** (sple″no-re′nəl) pertaining to the spleen and kidney, or to splenic and renal veins.

**sple·nor·rha·gia** (sple″no-ra′jə) [*spleno-* + *-rrhagia*] hemorrhage from the spleen.

**sple·nor·rha·phy** (sple-nor′ə-fe) [*spleno-* + *-rrhaphy*] surgical repair of the spleen.

**sple·no·sis** (sple-no′sis) [MeSH: Splenosis] a condition in which multiple implants of splenic tissue are present throughout the peritoneal cavity.

**sple·not·o·my** (sple-not′ə-me) [*spleno-* + *-tomy*] surgical incision of the spleen.

**sple·no·tox·in** (sple″no-tok′sin) a toxin produced by or acting on the spleen.

**sple·nu·lus** (splĕ′nu-ləs) pl. *sple′nuli* [L.] splen accessorius.

**sple·nun·cu·lus** (sple-nung′ku-ləs) splen accessorius.

**splic·ing** (spli′sing) [Middle Dutch *splissen*] 1. the attachment of individual DNA molecules to each other, as in the production of chimeric genes. 2. RNA s.
**alternative s.,** the splicing of RNA at variable positions on the primary transcript as a function of the type of tissue or of the developmental stage, removing varying introns to yield distinct mRNA's that encode specific proteins; it is a mechanism for developmental regulation and for tissue specificity.
**RNA s.,** the removal (splicing out) of introns from a primary transcript and the subsequent joining (splicing together) of exons in the production of a mature RNA molecule.

**splint** (splint) [MeSH: Splints] 1. an appliance, either rigid or flexible, used to hold in position a displaced or movable part or to keep in place and protect an injured part. See also *orthosis.* 2. the act of fastening or confining with such an appliance. 3. to fasten or confine with such an appliance. 4. see *splinting,* def. 2. 5. an exostosis on the splint bone of a horse; see also *splints.*
**abutment s.,** adjacent tooth restorations that have been rigidly united at their proximal contact areas to form a single abutment with multiple roots.
**airplane s.,** a static orthosis that holds the arm in abduction at the level of the shoulder; used following burns in the axillary region and for short periods following surgery to the shoulder or brachial plexus.
**anchor s.,** a splint for fracture of the jaw, with metal loops fitting over the teeth and held together by a rod.
**Anderson s.,** a splint for external internal fixation of fractures: two or more long screws, Kirschner wire, or nails are inserted through the tissues into the bone above and below the fracture; each group of screws, wires or nails is attached to an external plate and the plates are joined by an adjustable screw.
**Angle's s.,** a splint for fracture of the mandible.
**anti-boutonnière s.,** boutonnière s.

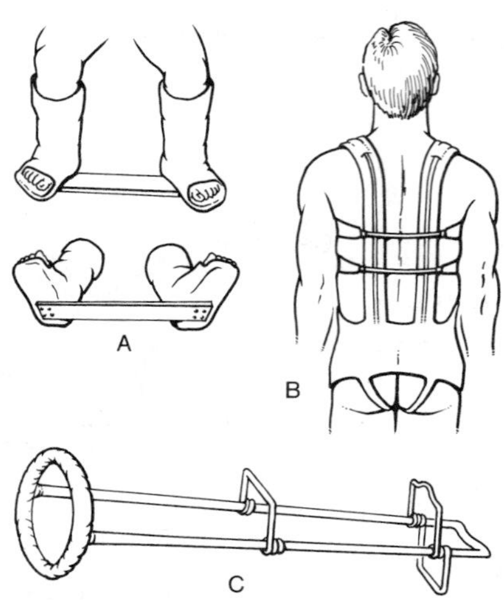

Splints: *(A),* Denis Browne splint; *(B),* Taylor splint; *(C),* Thomas knee splint.

**anti–swan neck s.,** swan neck s.
**anti–ulnar deviation s.,** ulnar deviation s.
**Asch s.,** a splint used in operations on the nose.
**Balkan s.,** see under *frame.*
**banjo traction s.,** a dynamic orthosis to aid extension of the fingers using a banjo-shaped steel bar attached to the fingers with rubber bands and plastic rings.
**boutonnière s.,** a dynamic splint designed to limit or correct boutonnière deformities; it encourages palmar displacement of the lateral tendons of the fingers, causing them to act as flexors and stabilize the proximal interphalangeal joints.
**cap s.,** a plastic or metallic fracture or stabilization appliance designed to cover the crowns of the teeth and usually cemented in place.
**coaptation s's,** small splints adjusted about a fractured limb for the purpose of producing coaptation of fragments.
**Cramer's s.,** a flexible wire splint consisting of parallel stout wires between which smaller wires are stretched like the rungs of a ladder.
**Denis Browne s.,** a splint consisting of a pair of metal foot splints joined by a cross bar; used in talipes equinovarus. See illustration.
**dynamic s.,** see under *orthosis.*
**Essig-type s.,** a stainless steel wire passed labially and lingually around a segment of the dental arch and held in position by individual ligature wires around the contact areas of the teeth; used to stabilize fractured or repositioned teeth.
**fracture s.,** 1. a device fabricated of metal or plastic and used to fix segments in the treatment of fractures or facial deformities. 2. a plastic material contoured to the lingual and buccal-labial aspects of the teeth and fixed with wire or cement.
**Frejka pillow s.,** Frejka pillow.
**functional s.,** dynamic orthosis.
**Gilmer's s.,** a stainless steel wire fastening for holding the lower teeth to the upper ones in fracture of the mandible.
**Gunning's s.,** an interdental splint used in treating fractured mandible or maxilla.
**Hodgen s.,** one similar to the Thomas splint with only half a ring; used for fracture of the femur below the upper third.
**interdental s.,** one for fracture of the jaws, held in place by wires passed around the teeth.
**Keller-Blake s.,** a hinged half-ring modification of the Thomas splint for fracture of the femur.
**Kingsley s.,** one used for jaw fractures, consisting of a baseplate adapted to the upper dental arch, with stout metal arms extending out through the mouth and curving backward along the sides of the cheeks to provide fixation to the head cap.
**Kirschner-Eimer s.,** an external splint used in veterinary medicine for fixation of a long bone fracture, consisting of transverse pins driven into the bone above and below the fracture and an external clamp to hold the pins (and thus the bone fragments) in position.
**Kirschner wire s.,** see under *wire.*
**knuckle bender s.,** a dynamic splint used to release extension contractures of the metacarpophalangeal joints; the splint maintains the knuckles in a flexion angle just smaller than where pain begins; over time, the joint tissues yield and stretch and the splint is readjusted.
**labial s.,** an appliance of plastic or metal, or both, made to conform to the outer aspect of the dental arch; used in the management of jaw and facial injuries.
**lingual s.,** one similar to the labial splint, but conforming to the inner aspect of the dental arch.
**Liston's s.,** a simple straight splint, often made of wood with padding, adapted to the side of the leg and body and used for fractures of the femur.
**lively s.,** dynamic orthosis.
**opponens s.,** see under *orthosis.*
**plaster s.,** a splint composed of gauze impregnated with plaster of Paris.
**plastic s.,** pneumatic orthosis.
**resting s.,** static orthosis.
**Roger Anderson s.,** Anderson s.
**shin s's,** strain of the flexor digitorum longus muscle occurring in athletes, marked by pain along the shin bone.
**Stader s.,** a splint used in veterinary medicine for external-internal fixation of fractures, consisting of a metal bar that bridges the fracture and has steel pins at each end for insertion into the bone; the ends of the fractured bone are drawn together by adjusting screws.
**static s.,** see under *orthosis.*
**swan neck s.,** a dynamic splint designed to limit or correct swan-neck deformities; it restricts extension of the proximal interphalangeal joints but permits full flexion.
**Taylor s.,** see under *brace.*
**therapeutic s.,** dynamic orthosis.
**Thomas s.,** a knee-ankle-foot orthosis consisting of two rigid rods attached to an ovoid ring that fits around the thigh; used in emergencies or for transporting patients, or combined with other apparatus to provide traction. See illustration.
**Toronto s.,** a splinting catheter for use in the ureter after plastic operation.
**ulnar deviation s.,** a dynamic splint designed to restrict or correct ulnar deviation; metacarpophalangeal flexion is reduced but otherwise hand function is possible.
**wrist cock-up s.,** a dynamic splint that stabilizes and immobilizes a subluxated wrist, alleviating pain in normal hand functions.

**splin·ter** (splin'tər) 1. a small slender fragment, as a piece of fractured bone. 2. to break into small fragments.

**splint·ing** (splint'ing) 1. treatment by use of a splint. 2. in dentistry, the application of a fixed restoration to join two or more teeth into a single rigid unit. 3. rigidity of muscles occurring as a means of avoiding pain caused by movement of a part.

**splints** (splints) [MeSH: Splints] development of exostoses, sometimes with inflammation, of the splint bones of horses.

**split·ting** (split'ing) 1. the division of a single object into two or more objects or parts. 2. in psychoanalytic theory, a primitive defense mechanism in which "objects" (persons) possessing a natural mix of positive and negative attributes are perceived as being either "all good" or "all bad." Characteristic of very young children, it is also seen in patients with borderline personality disorder and sometimes in those with other personality disorders or psychoses.
**fixed s. of $S_2$,** abnormal splitting of the second heart sound in which the gap between the aortic and pulmonic components does not vary with the phases of respiration. It is heard in patients with atrial septal defects.
**s. of heart sounds,** the presence of two components in the first or second heart sound complexes; used chiefly to denote the separation of the elements of the second sound, with the first component heard normally corresponding to aortic valve closure (aortic second sound) and the second to pulmonic valve closure (pulmonic second sound). The gap between the two components normally varies with the phases of respiration.
**reversed s. of $S_2$,** altered splitting of the second heart sound such that the order of the components is reversed; pulmonic valve closure precedes aortic valve closure. It occurs when left-sided ejection is delayed or left-sided systole is prolonged.
**sagittal s. of mandible,** intraoral osteotomy of the ascending mandibular ramus and posterior body of the mandible in the sagittal plane for correction of prognathism, retrognathism, or open bite; an alternative procedure confines the split to the body of the mandible.
**wide s. of $S_2$,** altered splitting of the second heart sound in which the gap between the aortic and pulmonic valve closures is increased, usually due to hemodynamic or electrical abnormalities that cause delay of the pulmonic second sound.

**spod(o)-** [Gr. *spodos* ashes] a combining form denoting relation to waste materials.

**spo·dog·e·nous** (spo-doj'ə-nəs) [*spodo-* + *-genous*] pertaining to or caused by waste materials in an organ.

**spon·dee** (spon'de) [L. *spondeum* of a libation] any word of two syllables having equal stress on each syllable (e.g., pancake); used in tests of speech reception threshold.

**spon·dy·lal·gia** (spon"dĭ-lal'jə) spondylodynia.

**spon·dyl·ar·thri·tis** (spon"dəl-ahr-thri'tis) [*spondyl-* + *arthritis*] arthritis of the spine.
**s. ankylopoie'tica,** ankylosing spondylitis.

**spon·dyl·ar·throc·a·ce** (spon"dəl-ahr-throk'ə-se) [*spondyl-* + *arthr-* + Gr. *kakē* badness] tuberculosis of the vertebrae.

**spon·dyl·ar·throp·a·thy** (spon"dil-ahr-throp'əthe) spondyloarthropathy.

**spon·dyl·ex·ar·thro·sis** (spon"dəl-eks"ahr-thro'sis) [*spondyl-* + Gr. *exarthrōsis* dislocation] dislocation of a vertebra.

**spon·dy·lit·ic** (spon"də-lit'ik) pertaining to or characterized by spondylitis.

**spon·dy·li·tis** (spon"də-li'tis) [MeSH: Spondylitis] inflammation of the vertebrae; called also *rachitis.*
**s. ankylopoie'tica, s. ankylo'sans,** ankylosing s.
**ankylosing s.,** a form of degenerative joint disease that affects the spine. It is a systemic illness of unknown etiology, affecting young persons predominantly, and producing pain and stiffness as a result of inflammation of the sacroiliac, intervertebral, and costovertebral joints; paraspinal calcification, with ossification and ankylosis of the spinal joints, may cause complete rigidity of the spine and thorax. Called also *Bekhterev's arthritis* or *disease, Bekhterev's s.; Marie-Strümpell s.* or *disease; Strümpell-Marie disease; rheumatoid* or *rhizomelic s.; s. deformans;* and *rhizomelic spondylosis.*
**Bekhterev's (Bechterew's) s., s. defor'mans,** ankylosing s.
**hypertrophic s.,** spondylitis with evidence of hypertrophic changes in the vertebrae.
**s. infectio'sa,** inflammation of the vertebrae caused by a specific pathogen.

**Kümmell's s.,** see under *disease.*
**Marie-Strümpell s.,** ankylosing s.
**muscular s.,** a morbid condition of the spine resulting from muscular weakness and not a true inflammation.
**post-traumatic s.,** Kümmell's disease.
**rheumatoid s., rhizomelic s.,** ankylosing s.
**traumatic s.,** spondylitis occurring as a result of injury to the vertebrae.
**s. tuberculo'sa, tuberculous s.,** tuberculosis of the spine.
**s. typho'sa,** inflammation of the vertebrae following typhoid fever.

**spon·dy·li·ze·ma** (spon″də-li-ze′mə) [*spondyl-* + Gr. *izēmia* depression] downward displacement of a vertebra in consequence of the destruction or softening of the one below it.

**spondyl(o)-** [Gr. *spondylos* vertebra] combining form denoting relationship to a vertebra, or to the spinal column.

**spon·dy·lo·ar·throp·a·thy** (spon″də-lo-ahr-throp′ə-the) disease of the joints of the spine.
**seronegative s's,** a general term comprising a number of degenerative joint diseases having common clinical, immunologic, pathologic, and radiographic features, including synovitis of the peripheral joints, enthesopathy, bony ankylosis of the large peripheral joints, lack of rheumatoid factor, and, in many cases, a positive status for the HLA antigen HLA-B27. Included in this group are *enteropathic arthritis, psoriatic arthritis, ankylosing spondylitis,* and *Reiter's syndrome.*

**spon·dy·loc·a·ce** (spon″də-lok′ə-se) [*spondylo-* + Gr. *kakē* badness] tuberculosis of the vertebrae.

**spon·dy·lo·di·dym·ia** (spon″də-lo-di-dim′e-ə) [*spondylo-* + Gr. *didymos* twin + *-ia*] union of conjoined twins by the vertebrae.

**spon·dy·lod·y·mus** (spon″də-lod′ĭ-məs) vertebrodidymus.

**spon·dy·lo·dyn·ia** (spon″də-lo-din′e-ə) [*spondyl-* + *-odynia*] pain in a vertebra. Called also *spondylalgia.* Cf. *rachiodynia.*

**spon·dy·lo·lis·the·sis** (spon″də-lo-lis-the′sis) [*spondyl-* + *olisthe* + *-sis*] [MeSH: Spondylolisthesis] forward displacement (olisthy) of one vertebra over another, usually of the fifth lumbar over the body of the sacrum, or of the fourth lumbar over the fifth, usually due to a developmental defect in the pars interarticularis.
**congenital s.,** dysplastic s.
**degenerative s.,** that caused by long-standing instability due to progressive degeneration of the spinal joints, usually accompanied by rotation of the affected disk.
**dysplastic s.,** that resulting from congenital anomalies of the lumbosacral junction, allowing the fifth lumbar vertebra to slip forward on the first sacral vertebra. Called also *congenital s.*
**isthmic s.,** that accompanied by a lesion of the pars interarticularis, divided into three subtypes on the basis of the type of lesion: *lytic* (stress fracture of the pars interarticularis), *elongated* (elongation of the pars interarticularis due to continuous cracking and healing), and *acute fracture.*
**pathological s.,** that due to alterations in the structure of the pedicle, the pars articularis, or the articular processes caused by bone disease.
**traumatic s.,** that due to acute fracture of the facets, pedicle, or lamina, rather than of the pars interarticularis.

**spon·dy·lo·lis·thet·ic** (spon″də-lo-lis-thet′ik) pertaining to or caused by spondylolisthesis.

**spon·dy·lol·y·sis** (spon″də-lol′ĭ-sis) [*spondylo-* + *-lysis*] [MeSH: Spondylolysis] dissolution of a vertebra; a condition marked by platyspondylia, aplasia of the vertebral arch, and separation of the pars interarticularis.

**spon·dy·lo·ma·la·cia** (spon″də-lo-mə-la′shə) softening of vertebrae.
**s. trauma'tica,** Kümmell's disease.

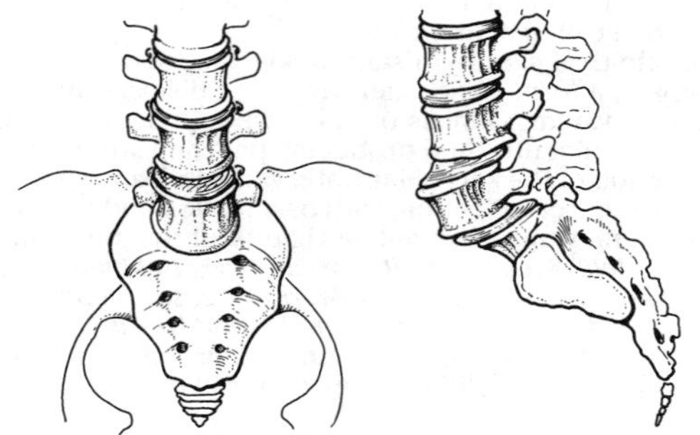
Spondylolisthesis of the fifth lumbar vertebra over the sacrum.

**spon·dy·lop·a·thy** (spon″də-lop′ə-the) [*spondylo-* + *-pathy*] any disorder of the vertebrae; called also *rachiopathy.*
**traumatic s.,** Kümmell's disease.

**spon·dy·lop·to·sis** (spon″də-lop-to′sis) spondylolisthesis.

**spon·dy·lo·py·o·sis** (spon″də-lo-pi-o′sis) [*spondylo-* + *pyo-* + *-sis*] suppuration of a vertebra or of vertebrae.

**spon·dy·los·chi·sis** (spon″dĭ-los′kĭ-sis) [*spondylo-* + *-schisis*] rachischisis.

**spon·dy·lo·sis** (spon″də-lo′sis) 1. ankylosis of a vertebral joint. 2. a general term for degenerative spinal changes due to osteoarthritis.
**cervical s.,** degenerative joint disease affecting the cervical vertebrae, intervertebral disks, and surrounding ligaments and connective tissue, sometimes with pain or paresthesia radiating down the arms as a result of pressure on the nerve roots.
**s. chro'nica ankylopoie'tica,** ankylosing spondylitis.
**lumbar s.,** degenerative joint disease affecting the lumbar vertebrae and intervertebral disks, causing pain and stiffness, sometimes with sciatic radiation due to nerve root pressure by associated protruding disks or osteophytes.
**rhizomelic s.,** ankylosing spondylitis.
**s. uncovertebra'lis,** cervical spondylosis affecting the uncinate process of a vertebra.

**spon·dy·lo·syn·de·sis** (spon″də-lo-sin-de′sis) [*spondylo-* + *syndesis*] spinal fusion.

**spon·dy·lot·ic** (spon″də-lot′ik) pertaining to or due to spondylosis.

**spon·dy·lot·o·my** (spon″də-lot′ə-me) [*spondylo-* + *-tomy*] rachitomy.

**spon·dy·lous** (spon′də-ləs) pertaining to a vertebra; vertebral.

**sponge** (spunj) [L., Gr. *spongia*] [MeSH: Porifera] 1. the elastic fibrous skeleton of certain marine animals; used mainly as an absorbent. 2. an absorbent pad of gauze or other material.
**Bernays' s.,** compressed disks of cotton that expand under moisture, used in treatment of epistaxis.
**fibrin s.,** a spongy form of fibrin, used as a hemostatic.
**gelatin s.,** a spongy form of denatured gelatin used as a hemostatic, especially when wet with thrombin.
**gelatin s., absorbable** [USP], a sterile, absorbable, water-insoluble gelatin-base sponge; used as a local hemostatic.

**spon·ge·itis** (spun″je-i′tis) spongiitis.

**spon·gi·form** (spun′jĭ-form) [*spongi-* + *form*] resembling a sponge.

**spon·gi·itis** (spun″je-i′tis) inflammation of the corpus spongiosum of the penis; periurethritis.

**spongi(o)-** [L., *spongia* sponge] a combining form meaning like a sponge, or denoting relationship to a sponge.

**spon·gio·blast** (spun′je-o-blast) [*spongio-* + *-blast*] 1. any of the embryonic epithelial cells, developed about the neural tube, which become transformed, some into neuroglial and some into ependymal cells. 2. amacrine cell; see under *cell.*

**spon·gio·blas·to·ma** (spən″je-o-blas-to′mə) any tumor containing spongioblasts; considered to be one of the neuroepithelial tumors. See *gliosarcoma, glioblastoma,* and *polar s.*
**s. multifor'me,** see under *glioblastoma.*
**polar s., s. pola're,** a rare malignant brain tumor seen from childhood to young adulthood, characterized by palisades of unipolar spongioblasts; sites may be either cerebral or cerebellar. Called also *piloid astrocytoma* and *unipolar s.*
**unipolar s., s. unipola're,** polar s.

**spon·gio·cyte** (spun′je-o-sīt″) 1. a neuroglial cell. 2. a type of cell with spongy vacuolated protoplasm found in the adrenal cortex.

**spon·gio·cy·to·ma** (spun″je-o-si-to′mə) spongioblastoma.

**spon·gi·oid** (spun′je-oid) [*spongi-* + *-oid*] resembling a sponge in structure or appearance.

**spon·gi·o·plasm** (spun′je-o-plaz-əm) [*spongio-* + *-plasm*] a network of fibrils pervading the cell substance; seen in histological specimens following the use of certain fixatives.

**spon·gio·sa** (spun″je-o′sə) [L.] spongy; sometimes used alone to mean the substantia spongiosa ossium.

**spon·gio·sa·plas·ty** (spun″je-o″sə-plas′te) autoplasty of the substantia spongiosa ossium to potentiate formation of new bone or to cover bone defects.

**spon·gi·o·sis** (spun″je-o′sis) intercellular edema of the spongy layer (malpighian layer) of the skin.

**spon·gio·si·tis** (spun″je-o-si′tis) inflammation of the corpus spongiosum of the penis.

**spon·gi·ot·ic** (spun″je-ot′ik) pertaining to or characterized by spongiosis.

**spon·gy** (spun′je) of a spongelike appearance or texture.

**spon·ta·ne·ous** (spon-ta′ne-əs) [L. *spontaneus*] 1. voluntary; instinctive. 2. occurring without external influence.

**Spon·tin** (spon′tin) trademark for a lyophilized preparation of ristocetins A and B.

**spool** (spo͞ol) a tubular surgical instrument around which suture material is usually wound.

**spoon** (spo͞on) 1. a metallic instrument with an oval bowl to which a handle is attached. 2. spoon excavator.
**Daviel's s.**, an instrument used in removing the crystalline lens from the eye.
**sharp s.**, a surgical instrument consisting of a spoon with sharp edges for scraping away granulations.
**Volkmann's s.**, sharp s.

**spo·rad·ic** (spə-rad′ik) [from Gr. *sperein* to sow seed] neither endemic nor epidemic; occurring occasionally in a random or isolated manner.

**spo·ran·gia** (spə-ran′je-ə) plural of *sporangium.*

**spo·ran·gi·al** (spə-ran′je-əl) pertaining to a sporangium.

**spo·ran·gio·phore** (spə-ran′je-o-for) [*sporangium* + *-phore*] a specialized hypha that gives rise to a sporangium.

**spo·ran·gio·spore** (spə-ran′je-o-spor) a spore contained in a sporangium.

**spo·ran·gi·um** (spə-ran′je-əm) pl. *sporan′gia* [*spore* + Gr. *angeion* vessel] a fungal or protozoal cell that produces spores internally (sporangiospores) by the process called *progressive cleavage.* See also Plate 29.

**Spo·ra·nox** (spor′ə-noks) trademark for a preparation of itraconazole.

**spo·ra·tion** (spo-ra′shən) sporulation.

**spore** (spor) [L. *spora,* Gr. *spora* seed] [MeSH: Spores] 1. a refractile, oval body formed within bacteria, especially genera of the family Bacillaceae *(Bacillus, Clostridium, Desulfotomaculum, Sporolactobacillus, Sporosarcina),* which is regarded as a resting stage during the life history of the cell, and is characterized by its resistance to environmental changes. Called also *bacterial s.* 2. the reproductive element, produced sexually or asexually, of one of the lower organisms, such as protozoa, fungi, algae, etc. See *asexual s., sexual s.,* and *sporulation.*
**asexual s.**, a spore produced without a sexual process, such as in an imperfect fungus; see *aleuriospore, chlamydospore, conidium, endospore,* and *zoospore.*
**bacterial s.**, see *spore,* def. 1.
**black s's of Ross**, pigmented malarial oocysts in the stomach wall of a mosquito.
**resting s.**, a spore that has thick walls and remains dormant for a long period, usually to survive adverse conditions, after which it can germinate.
**sexual s.**, a spore produced by a sexual process, such as in a perfect fungus; see *ascospore, basidiospore, oospore,* and *zygospore.*
**swarm s.**, a spore made up of numerous active motile individuals; a zoospore.

**spo·ri·ci·dal** (spor″ĭ-si′dəl) [*spore* + L. *caedere* to kill] destroying spores.

**spo·ri·cide** (spor′ĭ-sīd) an agent that destroys spores.

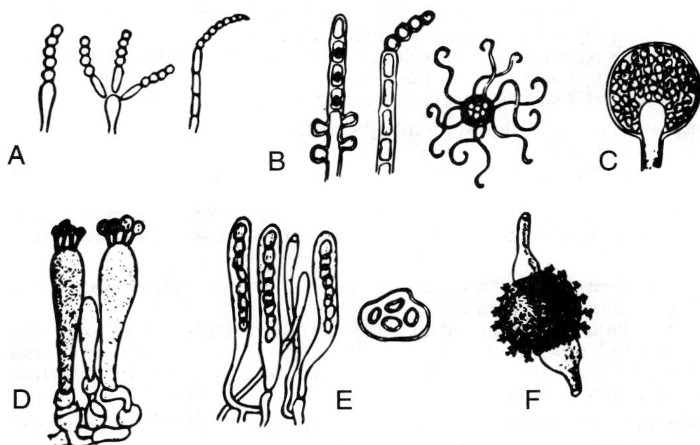

Various types of spores in fungi: *(A),* conidiospores; *(B),* chlamydospores; *(C),* sporangiospores; *(D),* basidiospores; *(E),* ascospores; *(F),* zygospores.

**spo·ri·des·min** (spor″ĭ-des′min) a poison isolated from the fungus *Pithomyces chartarum;* it causes facial eczema and liver damage in sheep and cattle in New Zealand and Australia.

**Spo·rid·i·a·les** (spə-rid″e-a′lēz) in some systems of classification, an order of perfect fungi of the subphylum Basidiomycotina, including part of what others call order Ustilaginales. It contains the genera *Filobasidiella* and *Filobasidium.*

**spo·rif·er·ous** (spə-rif′ər-əs) [*spore* + *-ferous*] producing or bearing spores; called also *sporiparous.*

**spo·rip·a·rous** (spə-rip′ə-rəs) [*spore* + *-parous*] sporiferous.

**spor(o)-** [Gr. *sporos* seed] a combining form denoting relationship to a spore.

**spo·ro·ag·glu·ti·na·tion** (spor″o-ə-gloo″tĭ-na′shən) agglutination of spores in the diagnosis of sporotrichosis.

**spo·ro·blast** (spor′o-blast) [*sporo-* + *-blast*] 1. an immature coccidian sporocyst. 2. a mass of spore-forming cells within a pansporoblastic membrane.

**Spo·rob·o·lo·my·ces** (spə-rob″ə-lo-mi′sēz) a genus of Fungi Imperfecti of the form-class Hyphomycetes; several species have been isolated from human infections.

**spo·ro·cyst** (spor′o-sist) [*sporo-* + *cyst*] 1. any cyst, envelope, or sac containing spores or reproductive cells. 2. a germinal saclike stage in the life cycle of digenetic trematodes produced by metamorphosis of a miracidium and giving rise to rediae. 3. a stage in the life cycle of certain coccidian protozoa contained within an oocyst, produced by a sporoblast, and giving rise to sporozoites.

**spo·ro·do·chi·um** (spor″o-do′ke-əm) a cushion-shaped mass of hyphae covered with conidiophores.

**spo·ro·duct** (spor′o-dəkt) [*sporo-* +*duct*] a tubelike structure through which spores of certain sporozoans and some fungi pass to the outside of the cell.

**spo·ro·gen·e·sis** (spor″o-jen′ə-sis) [*sporo-* + *genesis*] sporulation (def. 1).

**spo·ro·gen·ic** (spor″o-jen′ik) pertaining to or characterized by sporulation. Called also *sporogenous.*

**spo·rog·e·nous** (spə-roj′ə-nəs) sporogenic.

**spo·rog·e·ny** (spə-roj′ə-ne) [*sporo-* + *-geny*] sporulation (def. 1).

**spo·rog·o·ny** (spə-rog′ə-ne) [*sporo-* + Gr. *goneia* generation] 1. sporulation (def. 1). 2. in protozoa, sporulation involving multiple fission of a sporont (schizogony), resulting in the production of sporocysts (if present in the life cycle) and sporozoites.

**spo·ront** (spor′ont) [*sporo-* + Gr. *ōn, ontos* being] a zygote of coccidian protozoa enclosed within an oocyst, which undergoes sporogony to produce sporoblasts, each of which forms a sporocyst containing sporozoites.

**spo·ro·phore** (spor′o-for) [*sporo-* + *-phore*] that part of an organism that supports the spores.

**spo·ro·phyte** (spor′o-fīt) [*sporo-* + *-phyte*] the diploid or asexual stage in the alternation of generations (metagenesis) in plants.

**spo·ro·plasm** (spor′o-plaz-əm) [*sporo-* + *-plasm*] 1. the protoplasm of spores. 2. the central dinucleate mass of cytoplasm of certain protozoa that leaves the spore through the polar tube as an amebula to infect the host.

**spo·ro·plas·mic** (spor″o-plaz′mik) pertaining to or of the nature of sporoplasm.

**Spo·ro·thrix** (spor′o-thriks) a genus of Fungi Imperfecti of the form-class Hyphomycetes, form-family Moniliaceae. *S. schen′ckii* (formerly called *Sporotrichum schenckii*) causes sporotrichosis. Many other species, including *S. car′nis,* cause the formation of white mold on meat in cold storage.

**spo·rot·ri·chin** (spə-rot′rĭ-kin) a derivative of *Sporothrix schenckii* used as a skin test in the diagnosis of sporotrichosis.

**spo·ro·tri·cho·sis** (spor″o-trĭ-ko′sis) [*sporo-* + *trich-* + *-osis*] [MeSH: Sporotrichosis] a chronic fungal infection in humans and other animals due to *Sporothrix schenckii;* in most species it is characterized by nodular lesions of the cutaneous and subcutaneous tissues and adjacent lymphatics that suppurate and ulcerate. It is acquired by fungal implantation into the skin by trauma or through an abrasion, or by inhalation into the lungs. The infection may remain localized or may be disseminated by the bloodstream to involve the osteoarticular and musculoskeletal tissues, viscera, mucous membranes, central nervous system, eye, or genitourinary system.

**spo·ro·tri·chot·ic** (spor″o-tri-kot′ik) 1. pertaining to or caused by fungi of the genus *Sporothrix.* 2. pertaining to sporotrichosis.

**Spo·rot·ri·chum** (spə-rot′rĭkəm) [*sporo-* + Gr. *thrix* hair] [MeSH: Sporotrichum] a genus of soil-inhabiting Fungi Imperfecti of the form-class Hyphomycetes, form-family Moniliaceae; it formerly also included those now in the genus *Sporothrix.*

**Spo·ro·zoa** (spor″o-zo′ə) [*sporo-* + Gr. *zōon* animal] 1. Sporozoea. 2. in some former systems of classification, a subphylum and in others a class of protozoa, the members of which have been assigned to four phyla: Apicomplexa, Acetospora, Microspora, and Myxozoa. The organisms in the last three phyla form spores; many of the Apicomplexa do not. 3. Apicomplexa.

**spo·ro·zoa** (spor″o-zo′ə) plural of *sporozoon.*

**spo·ro·zo·an** (spor″o-zo′ən) [*sporo-* + Gr. *zōon* animal] 1. any protozoan of the phyla Apicomplexa (especially those of the class Sporozoea), Ascetospora, Microspora, and Myxozoa. Called also *sporozoon.* 2. pertaining or relating to protozoa of the phyla Apicomplexa, Ascetospora, Microspora, and Myxozoa.

**Spo·ro·zoea** (spor″o-ze′ə) [MeSH: Sporozoea] a class of homoxenous or heteroxenous parasitic protozoa (phylum Apicomplexa) having a conoid (if present) forming a complete cone; both sexual and asexual phases; oocysts generally containing infective sporozoites that result from sporogeny; flagella in microgametes of some groups; and pseudopods (if present) used for feeding only. Locomotion of mature organisms is by means of body flexion, gliding, or undulation of longitudinal ridges on the body surface. It comprises three subclasses: Gregarinia, Coccidia, and Piroplasmia. Called also *Sporozoa.*

**spo·ro·zo·ite** (spor″o-zo′īt) [*sporo-* + *zo-* + *-ite*] the elongate, nucleated, motile infective stage resulting from sporogony in gregarine and coccidian protozoa. In malaria, the sporozoites of *Plasmodium* spp. are liberated from the oocysts in the mosquito, accumulate in the vector's salivary glands, and are transferred to the definitive host by the bite of the infected mosquito.

**spo·ro·zo·on** (spor″o-zo′on) pl. *sporozo′a* [*sporo-* + Gr. *zōon* animal] sporozoan, def. 1.

**spo·ro·zo·o·sis** (spor″o-zo-o′sis) infection with a protozoon of the class *Sporozoea.*

**sport** (sport) a mutation; lusus naturae.

**spor·u·lar** (spor′u-lər) pertaining to a spore.

**spor·u·la·tion** (spor″u-la′shən) 1. the formation of spores. Called also *sporogenesis, sporogeny,* and *sporogony.* 2. the liberation of spores.

**spor·ule** (spor′ūl) 1. a small spore. 2. spore.

**spot** (spot) a circumscribed area or place distinguished by its color; called also *loculus, macula* and *tache.*
**acoustic s's,** the maculae sacculi and maculae utriculi.
**ash-leaf s.,** see under *macule.*
**Bitot's s's,** superficial, foamy gray, triangular spots on the conjunctiva, consisting of keratinized epithelium; they are associated with vitamin A deficiency. See also *xerosis conjunctivae.*
**blind s.,** 1. discus nervi optici. 2. mental scotoma.
**blue s.,** 1. [pl.] maculae ceruleae. 2. mongolian s.
**Brushfield's s's,** small white spots on the periphery of the iris, usually crescentic, with the concavity outward, frequently but not exclusively seen in children with Down syndrome.
**café au lait s's,** (kah-fa′o-la′) [Fr.] pigmented macules of a distinctive light brown color, like coffee with milk, as in neurofibromatosis and Albright's syndrome.
**Carleton's s's,** sclerosed spots in the bones in gonorrheal disease.
**Cayenne pepper s's,** red angiomatous puncta within or on the border of the lesions of Schamberg's disease.
**cherry-red s.,** a red circular area (the choroid) surrounded by gray-white retina, seen through the fovea centralis of the eye in the infantile and sometimes in the late infantile form of neuronal ceroid lipofuscinosis; called also *Tay's s.* or *sign.*
**Christopher's s's,** Maurer's dots; see under *dot.*
**chromatin s.,** sex chromatin.
**cold s.,** 1. see *temperature s's.* 2. an area of a strand of DNA that has a particularly low tendency for recombination.
**cotton-wool s's,** white or gray soft-edged opacities in the retina composed of cytoid bodies; seen in hypertensive retinopathy, lupus erythematosus, and numerous other conditions. Called also *cotton-wool exudates* or *patches.*
**cribriform s's,** maculae cribrosae.
**deaf s.,** see under *point.*
**De Morgan's s's,** cherry angiomas.
**embryonic s.,** see under *disc.*
**epigastric s.,** a point of tenderness exactly over the xiphoid process.
**eye s.,** 1. the rudiment of an eye in the embryo. 2. eyespot.
**flame s's,** flame-shaped hemorrhages in the nerve fiber layer of the retina.
**focal s.,** the part of the target of an x-ray tube which is bombarded by the focused electron stream when the tube is energized.
**Fordyce's s's,** see under *granule.*
**Forschheimer s's,** a fleeting exanthem consisting of discrete rose spots on the soft palate, which may coalesce into a red blush and may extend over the fauces; sometimes seen in rubella just prior to the onset of the skin rash.
**germinal s.,** the nucleolus of an oocyte (ovum).
**hot s.,** 1. see *temperature s's.* 2. the sensitive area of a neuroma. 3. an area of increased density on an x-ray or thermographic film. 4. an area of a strand of DNA that has a particularly high tendency for recombination.
**hypnogenetic s.,** any superficial area the stimulation of which will bring on sleep.
**Koplik's s's,** small, irregular, bright red spots on the buccal and lingual mucosa, with a minute bluish white speck in the center of each; seen in the prodromal stage of measles. Called also *Koplik's sign.*
**lance-ovate s.,** ash-leaf macule.
**light s.,** cone of light.
**liver s.,** 1. senile lentigo. 2. (in plural) tinea versicolor.
**Mariotte's s.,** blind s.
**Maurer's s's,** see under *dot.*
**Maxwell's s.,** macula luteae.
**mental blind s.,** mental scotoma.
**milk s's,** 1. whitish spots of fibrous thickening seen on the visceral layer of the pericardium in postmortem examination. 2. dense masses of macrophages in the omentum.
**milky s's,** aggregations of macrophages in the subserous connective tissue of the pleura and peritoneum.
**mongolian s.,** a congenital melanocytic nevus manifested by a flat, smooth, bluish gray to gray-brown macular patch(es), most often located on the central lumbosacral area, occurring especially in dark-skinned people including those of East Asian ancestry, and usually disappearing before 5 years of age. Called also *blue* or *sacral s.* and *mongolian macula.* See also *nevus of Ito* and *nevus of Ota.*
**pain s's,** spots on the skin where alone the sense of pain can be produced by a stimulus.
**pelvic s's,** round or oval shadows often seen on fluoroscopic examination in the region of the inferior spine of the ilium and the horizontal ramus of the pubic bone.
**rose s's,** an eruption of rose-colored macules developing especially on the skin of the abdomen and thighs in the early stage of typhoid fever. Called also *typhoid s's.*
**Roth's s's,** round or oval white spots consisting of coagulated fibrin seen in the retina in a number of diseases in which a vascular insult resulting in hemorrhage is followed by healing.
**sacral s.,** mongolian s.
**shin s's,** diabetic dermopathy on the shins.
**Soemmering's s.,** macula luteae.
**soldier's s's,** milk s's, def. 1.
**spongy s.,** zona vasculosa.
**Stephen's s's,** Maurer's dots.
**Tardieu's s's,** spots of ecchymosis under the pleura following death by suffocation.
**Tay's s.,** cherry-red s.
**temperature s's,** hot and cold spots: spots on the skin normally anesthetic to pain and pressure and sensitive respectively to heat and cold; they are arranged in lines, often somewhat curved, and show the peculiar arrangement of the end-organ with respect to the temperature sense.
**tendinous s's,** maculae albidae.
**Trousseau's s.,** tache cérébrale.
**typhoid s's,** rose s's.
**warm s's,** minute areas in the skin that are peculiarly sensitive to temperatures above body temperature; see *temperature s's.*
**yellow s.,** macula luteae.

**sprain** (sprān) [MeSH: Sprains and Strains] a joint injury in which some of the fibers of a supporting ligament are ruptured but the continuity of the ligament remains intact.
**rider's s.,** sprain of the adductor longus muscle of the thigh, resulting from strain in riding horseback.
**Schlatter's s.,** Osgood-Schlatter disease.

**spray** (spra) a liquid minutely divided or nebulized as by a jet of air or steam.
**needle s.,** a water spray administered through a device having needle-sized jets.
**pepper s.,** an aerosolized form of oleoresins from capsicum, highly irritant to the skin and mucous membranes; used similarly to tear gas.

**spread·er** (spred′ər) an instrument for distributing something over a broader area.
**root canal filling s.,** in root canal therapy, a hand-operated, smooth, pointed, tapered metal instrument used to compress filling material laterally against the walls of the canal to make room for insertion of additional cones.

**Spren·gel's deformity** (shpreng′gəlz) [Otto Gerhard Karl *Sprengel,* German surgeon, 1852–1915] see under *deformity.*

**spring** (spring) 1. a piece of resilient metal, such as a hardened

coiled steel wire, that will return to its original shape after bending. 2. a resilient wire attached to a denture or other appliance.
**auxiliary s.,** a short piece of wire attached to an orthodontic appliance to serve as a lever to apply force to a tooth or teeth.
**bow s.,** a loop spring with the shape of a labial bow; used in a removable orthodontic appliance to move teeth.
**closed s.,** one having both ends attached.
**coil s.,** a spiral winding of fine resilient wire; attached to orthodontic appliances to open or to close spaces between teeth.
**finger s.,** a finger-shaped stainless steel wire spring; used interproximally as an open spring in removable orthodontic appliances.
**Kesling s.,** a tooth-spacing spring used to gain separation between the teeth to facilitate band placement in fitting orthodontic appliances.
**loop s.,** a closed orthodontic spring having a variety of different shapes, from that of a hairpin to that of a bow.
**open s.,** one having free ends; in orthodontic appliances, one having only one end anchored in the active plate.
**paddle s.,** a paddle-shaped wire spring used in removable orthodontic appliances; it is activated by bending it toward the tooth.
**separating s.,** one placed between the teeth to obtain separation.
**uprighting s.,** a coiled spring used for uprighting teeth in orthodontic therapy.
**Z s.,** a spring bent in the form of a Z with a coil loop at each end, used to move an individual tooth or groups of teeth buccally or labially.

**Sprinz-Du·bin syndrome** (sprints-doo′bin) [Helmuth *Sprinz,* German-born American pathologist, born 1911; Isidore Nathan *Dubin,* American pathologist, born 1913] Dubin-Johnson syndrome.

**Sprinz-Nel·son syndrome** (sprints-nel′sun) [H. *Sprinz;* R.S. *Nelson,* American physician, 20th century] Dubin-Johnson syndrome.

**sprue** (sproo) 1. a chronic form of malabsorption syndrome occurring in both tropical and nontropical forms; called also *catarrhal dysentery.* 2. in a dental casting, an opening in the investment through which the molten alloy or metal can reach the mold space after the wax has been eliminated.
**celiac s.,** see under *disease.*
**collagenous s.,** a rare, often fatal condition resembling celiac sprue but not responsive to dietary gluten withdrawal, characterized by extensive deposition of collagen in the lamina propria of the colon.
**nontropical s.,** celiac disease.
**refractory s.,** 1. malabsorption and flat jejunal mucosa, signs of celiac disease, which do not respond to withdrawal of dietary gluten. 2. celiac disease in which initial responsiveness to gluten withdrawal deteriorates with time; it is often characterized by persistent absence of villi in the proximal mucosa and malabsorption even during the initial period of clinical responsiveness. Called also *unclassified s.*
**tropical s.,** a malabsorption syndrome occurring in the tropics and subtropics. Malabsorption usually leads to protein malnutrition, and anemia due to folic acid deficiency is common. Administration of antibiotics (especially tetracycline) and folic acid usually results in remission. Called also *stomatitis intertropica* and *stomatitis tropica.*
**unclassified s.,** refractory s.

**Spt.** abbreviation for L. *spir′itus,* spirit.

**Spu·ma·vi·ri·nae** (spu″mə-vir-i′ne) the foamy viruses: a former subfamily of the Retroviridae, containing the genus *Spumavirus.*

**Spu·ma·vi·rus** (spu′mə-vi″rəs) [L. *spuma* foam + *virus*] [MeSH: Spumavirus] foamy viruses; a genus of nonpathogenic viruses of the family Retroviridae, having characteristic virion morphology with a central condensed core and prominent surface spikes, named for the foamy appearance of infected cells in culture caused by extensive vacuolation. Capsid assembly occurs in the cytoplasm prior to budding through the plasma membrane. Organisms induce persistent, asymptomatic infection in humans, primates, cats, cattle, and hamsters.

**spu·ma·vi·rus** (spu′mə-vi″rəs) [MeSH: Spumavirus] 1. any virus of the subfamily Spumavirinae. 2. any virus belonging to the genus *Spumavirus.*

**spur** (spur) 1. a spiked object or other type of goad; called also *calcar.* 2. in dentistry, a piece of metal projecting from a plate, band, or other dental appliance.
**calcaneal s.,** a bone excrescence on the lower surface of the calcaneus which frequently causes pain on walking.
**calcarine s.,** calcar avis.
**s. of malleus,** on the head of the malleus, a projection on the inferior margin of the facet for the incus; called also *cog tooth of malleus.*
**Morand's s.,** calcar avis.
**occipital s.,** an abnormal process of bone on the occipital bone behind the posterior process of the atlas.
**olecranon s.,** an abnormal process of bone at the insertion of the triceps muscle.
**scleral s.,** the posterior lip of the venous sinus of the sclera to which most of the fibers of the trabecular reticulum of the iridocorneal angle and the meridional fibers of the ciliary muscle are attached; called also *scleral roll.*

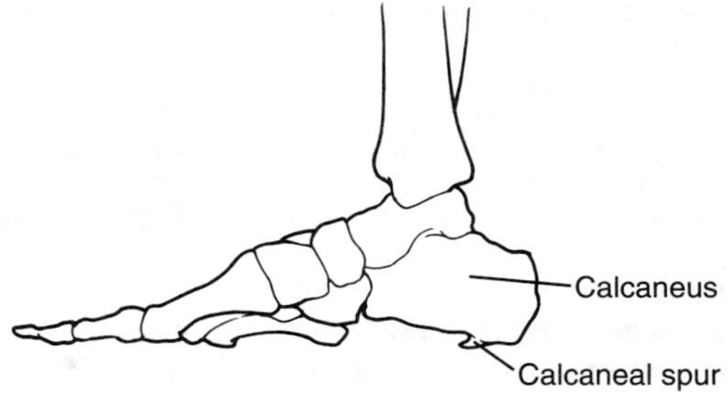


**spu·ri·ous** (spu′re-əs) [L. *spurius*] simulated; not genuine; false.

**Spur·way's syndrome** (spər′wāz) [John *Spurway,* English physician, late 19th century] osteogenesis imperfecta (type I); see under *osteogenesis.*

**spu·tum** (spu′təm) [L.] [MeSH: Sputum] matter ejected from the lungs, bronchi, and trachea, through the mouth. Called also *expectoration.*
**s. aerogino′sum,** sputum discolored green by overgrowth of *Pseudomonas aeruginosum.*
**albuminoid s.,** a yellowish, frothy sputum of persons from whom large amounts of pleural fluid have been withdrawn; believed to be due to pulmonary edema.
**s. cruen′tum,** bloody sputum.
**globular s.,** nummular s.
**green s.,** sputum that has a greenish tint due to a bile pigment, as in certain types of jaundice. Called also *icteric s.*
**icteric s.,** green s.
**nummular s.,** sputum in rounded disks, shaped somewhat like coins.
**prune juice s.,** dark reddish brown, bloody sputum, seen in lung conditions such as certain forms of pneumonia, cancer, or gangrene.
**rusty s.,** sputum stained with blood or blood pigments, as in pneumococcal pneumonia.

**SQ** subcutaneous.

**squa·lane** (skwah′lān) [NF] a saturated hydrocarbon obtained by hydrogenation of squalene from fish oil and used as an oleaginous vehicle in pharmaceuticals.

**squa·lene** (skwa′lēn) [first isolated from *Squalus,* a genus of sharks] [MeSH: Squalene] an unsaturated, symmetrical, 30-carbon triterpene intermediate formed in the biosynthesis of cholesterol and all other cyclic triterpenes. It can be isolated from shark and other fish oils and some plants.

**squa·ma** (skwa′mə) pl. *squa′mae* [L.] [TA] a general term in anatomical nomenclature for a scale or platelike structure.
**s. alveola′ris,** alveolar cell, type I.
**s. of frontal bone, s. fronta′lis** [TA], frontal squama: the broad, curved portion of the frontal bone, situated superior to the supraorbital margin and forming the forehead.
**mental s., external,** protuberantia mentalis.
**occipital s.,** squama occipitalis.
**occipital s., superior,** os interparietale.
**s. occipita′lis** [TA], squamous part of occipital bone: the largest of the four parts of the occipital bone, extending from the posterior edge of the foramen magnum to the lambdoid suture, its external surface bearing the external occipital protuberance and nuchal lines.
**perpendicular s.,** s. frontalis.
**temporal s., s. of temporal bone, s. tempora′lis,** pars squamosa ossis temporalis.

**squa·mate** (skwa′māt) [L. *squamatus,* from *squama* scale] scaly; having or resembling scales.

**squa·ma·ti·za·tion** (skwa″mə-tĭ-za′shən) the transformation of cells of other types into squamous cells; squamous metaplasia.

**squame** (skwām) [L. *squama*] a scale or scalelike substance.

**squa·mo·cel·lu·lar** (skwa″mo-sel′u-lər) [*squama* + *cellular*] having squamous cells.

**squa·mo·fron·tal** (skwa″mo-fron′təl) pertaining to the squama frontalis.

**squa·mo·mas·toid** (skwa″mo-mas′toid) pertaining to the squamous and mastoid portions of the temporal bone.

**squa·mo-oc·cip·i·tal** (skwa″mo-ok-sip′ĭ-təl) pertaining to the squama occipitalis.

**squa·mo·pa·ri·e·tal** (skwa″mo-pə-ri′ə-təl) pertaining to the pars squamosa ossis temporalis and the parietal bone.

**squa·mo·pe·tro·sal** (skwa″mo-pə-tro′səl) pertaining to the squamous and petrous portions of the temporal bone.

**squa·mo·sa** (skwa-mo′sə) [L.] scaly, or platelike; see *pars squamosa.*

**squa·mo·sal** (skwa-mo′səl) squamous.

**squa·mo·so·pa·ri·e·tal** (skwa-mo″so-pə-ri′ə-təl) squamoparietal.

**squa·mo·sphe·noid** (skwa″mo-sfe′noid) sphenosquamosal.

**squa·mo·tem·po·ral** (skwa″mo-tem′pə-rəl) pertaining to the squamous portion of the temporal bone.

**squa·mous** (skwa′məs) [L. *squamosus* scaly] scaly, or platelike.

**squa·mo·zy·go·mat·ic** (skwa″mo-zi″go-mat′ik) pertaining to the squamous portions of the temporal bone and the zygomatic bone.

**square** (skwār) a plane figure with four equal sides and four right angles.
**Punnett s.,** checkerboard.

**squat·ting** (skwaht′ing) a position of flexion of the knees and hips, the buttocks being lowered to the level of the heels. It is sometimes adopted by the parturient at delivery. Children with certain types of cyanotic cardiac defects, particularly those with tetralogy of Fallot, frequently adopt the position.

**squeeze** (skwēz) subjection to pressure; compression.
**tussive s.,** the compression of the lung in coughing, which is said to force material from the alveoli and smaller air passages into the bronchi.

**squill** (skwil) [L. *scilla;* Gr. *skilla*] 1. any of various plants of the genus *Urginea,* particularly *U. maritima* or *U. indica.* 2. the fleshy inner scales of the bulb of *U. maritima* or *U. indica;* a distinction is made between those with white bulbs *(white squill)* and those with red bulbs *(red squill).* Called also *scilla.*
**red s.,** 1. a variety of *Urginea maritima* that has red bulbs. 2. the fleshy inner scales of the bulb of this plant, a source of the cardiac glycoside scilliroside; it can cause convulsions or cardiac arrest and is used as a rodenticide.
**white s.,** 1. a variety of *Urginea maritima* that has white bulbs. 2. the fleshy inner scales of the bulb of this plant, a source of the cardiac glycosides glucoscillaren A, scillaren A, and proscillaridin A, as well as other principles; it has been used as a diuretic, emetic, expectorant, and cardiotonic.

**squil·lit·ic** (skwĭ-lit′ik) [L. *scilliticus;* Gr. *skillitikos*] pertaining to or containing squill; called also *scillitic.*

**squint** (skwint) strabismus; for types of squint not entered here, see under *strabismus.*
**accommodative s.,** esotropia.
**comitant s., concomitant s.,** concomitant strabismus.
**convergent s.,** esotropia.
**divergent s.,** exotropia.
**upward and downward s.,** hypertropia.

**squir·rel** (skwər′əl) [MeSH: Sciuridae] any of numerous species of rodents of the family Sciuridae; several are reservoirs of plague and other diseases.
**antelope s.,** any squirrel of the genus *Ammospermophilus.*
**ground s.,** any of several ground-dwelling members of the genus *Spermophilus,* found in many northern regions of the world, sometimes reservoirs of plague.
**Russian ground s.,** *Spermophilus citellus* and other species found in northern Europe and Siberia, which are sometimes reservoirs of plague.

**SR** stimulation ratio; see *lymphocyte proliferation test* under *test.*

**Sr** symbol for *strontium.*

**sr** abbreviation for *steradian.*

**SRBC** sheep red blood cell.

**SRF** skin reactive factor.

**SRH** somatotropin-releasing hormone.

**SRIF** somatotropin release–inhibiting factor.

**SRN** State Registered Nurse (England and Wales).

**SRS-A** [MeSH: SRS-A] slow-reacting substance of anaphylaxis.

**SRT** speech reception threshold; speech recognition threshold.

**SS** somatostatin.

**ss.** abbreviation for L. *se′mis,* one half.

**Ssa·ba·ne·jew-Frank operation** (sah-bah′nĕ-yev-frahngk′) [Ivan *Ssabanejew,* Russian surgeon, late 19th century; Rudolf *Frank,* Vienna surgeon, 1862–1913] see under *operation.*

**SSD** source-skin distance.

**ssDNA** single-stranded DNA.

**SSPE** subacute sclerosing panencephalitis.

**SSRI** selective serotonin reuptake inhibitor.

**ssRNA** single-stranded RNA.

**SSS** sick sinus syndrome, specific soluble substance.

**s.s.s.** abbreviation for L. *stra′tum su′per stra′tum,* layer upon layer.

**S.S.V.** abbreviation for L. *sub sig′no vene′ni,* under a poison label.

**ST** sinus tachycardia.

**S.T. 37** trademark for a solution of hexylresorcinol.

**St** stoke.

**St.** abbreviation for L. *stet,* let it stand; or *stent,* let them stand.

**sta·bi·late** (sta′bĭ-lāt) a population of microorganisms preserved in a genetically stable and viable condition (as by freeze-drying or low temperature); distinguished from a strain that may be maintained by subculture.

**sta·bile** (sta′bil, sta′bīl) [L. *stabilis* stable, abiding] not moving; stationary; resistant to chemical change; opposed to *labile.*
**heat s.,** thermostabile.

**sta·bil·i·ty** (stə-bil′ĭte) the quality of maintaining a constant character in the presence of forces which threaten to disturb it; resistance to change.
**dimensional s.,** the resistance of a material to change in its shape or measurements.

**sta·bil·iza·tion** (sta″bil-ĭ-za′shən) the creation of a stable state.

**sta·ble** (sta′bəl) not moving, fixed, firm; resistant to change.

**stac·ca·to** (stə-kah′to) [Ital. "detached"] said of speech delivered in a quick, jerky manner, with an interval between each two syllables. See also *staccato speech,* under *speech.*

**stachy·bot·ry·o·tox·i·co·sis** (stak″e-bot″re-o-tok″sĭ-ko′sis) mycotoxicosis in livestock caused either by eating contaminated feed or by sleeping on contaminated bedding containing fungi of the genera *Stachybotrys* or *Myrothecium,* especially *S. alternans,* or *M. verrucaria,* which contain roridins, satrotoxins, and verrucarins. It has been seen in France, southeastern Europe, Brazil, and Russia. Initial symptoms include fever, diarrhea, and incoordination; continued exposure can lead to hemorrhaging in various organs, sometimes followed by coma and death. Humans working in contaminated areas have occasionally also been affected.

**Stachy·bot·rys** (stak″e-bot′ris) [MeSH: Stachybotrys] a genus of Fungi Imperfecti of the order Moniliales. *S. alter′nans* (called also *S. at′ra* or *S. charta′rum*), which has been found contaminating animal feed and bedding, contains roridins, satratoxins, and verrucarins, which cause stachybotryotoxicosis in livestock and occasionally humans.

**stac·tom·e·ter** (stak-tom′ə-tər) [Gr. *staktos* oozing out in drops + *-meter*] an instrument for measuring drops.

**Sta·der splint** (sta′dər) [Otto *Stader,* American veterinary surgeon, 20th century] see under *splint.*

**Sta·de·ri·ni's nucleus** (stah′də-re″nēz) [Rutilio *Staderini,* Italian anatomist, late 19th century] nucleus intercalatus.

**sta·di·um** (sta′de-əm) pl. *sta′dia* [L.; Gr. *stadion* course] stage, def. 1.
**s. ac′mes,** the height of a disease.
**s. augmen′ti,** s. incrementi.
**s. calo′ris,** hot stage.
**s. decremen′ti, s. defervescen′tiae,** defervescent stage.
**s. fluorescen′tiae,** eruptive stage.
**s. fri′goris,** cold stage.
**s. incremen′ti,** the period of increase in the intensity of a disease; the stage of development of fever.
**s. invasio′nis,** incubation period.
**s. sudo′ris,** sweating stage.

**Sta·dol** (sta′dol) trademark for preparations of butorphanol tartrate.

**staff** (staf) 1. a wooden rod or rodlike structure. 2. a grooved director used as a guide for the knife in lithotomy. 3. the professional personnel of a hospital. 4. band cell.
**s. of Aesculapius,** a rod or staff with a snake entwined around it, commonly appearing in the ancient representations of Aesculapius, the god of medicine. It is the symbol of medicine and is the official emblem of the American Medical Association.
**attending s.,** the corps of attending physicians and surgeons of a hospital.
**consulting s.,** the corps of physicians and surgeons attached to a hospital who do not visit regularly, but may be consulted by members of the attending staff.

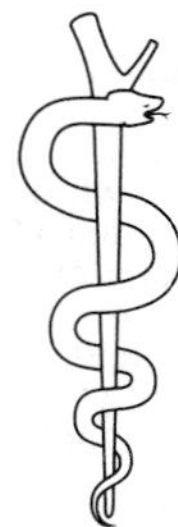

Staff of Aesculapius.

**house s.,** the resident physicians and surgeons of a hospital.
**s. of Wrisberg,** a slight mounding up of the mucosa over Wrisberg's cartilage (cartilago cuneiformis) in the larynx.

**stage** (stāj) 1. a period or distinct phase in the course of a disease, the life history of an organism, or any biological process. See also *staging.* 2. the platform of a microscope on which a slide is placed for viewing of the specimen.
**algid s.,** a condition characterized by a flickering pulse, subnormal temperature, and varied nervous symptoms.
**amphibolic s.,** the stage of an infectious disease between the acme and the decline in which the diagnosis is uncertain.
**anal s.,** in psychoanalytic theory, the second stage of psychosexual development, occurring between the ages of 1 and 3 years, during which the infant's activities, interests, and concerns are on the anal zone; it is preceded by the oral stage and followed by the phallic stage.
**asexual s.,** anamorph.
**bell s.,** the third stage of odontogenesis, a time of morphodifferentiation and histodifferentiation in which the enamel organ changes in shape from a cap to a bell that has four distinct layers.
**cap s.,** the second stage of odontogenesis, a time of proliferation characterized by formation of the enamel cap in the tooth germ and organization of the dental cells into three layers.
**Carnegie s.,** a numbered stage of human embryonic development defined by anatomical characteristics such as the appearance of the developing limbs.
**cold s.,** the chill or rigor period of an intermittent fever such as malaria; called also *stadium frigoris.*
**defervescent s.,** the period of decrease in severity of a disease or fever. Called also *stadium decrementi.*
**eruptive s.,** that period during the course of an eruptive fever or exanthem when the rash is present. Called also *stadium fluorescentiae.*
**expulsive s.,** the stage of labor during which the child is being expelled from the uterus; the second stage of labor.
**s. of fervescence,** pyrogenetic s.
**first s.,** (of labor), the earliest stage of labor, ending with dilatation of the os uteri.
**fourth s.,** (of labor), a name sometimes applied to the immediate postpartum period.
**genital s.,** in psychoanalytic theory, the last stage in psychosexual development, occurring during puberty, during which the person can achieve sexual gratification from genital-to-genital contact and is capable of a mature relationship with a person of the opposite sex; it follows the latency stage.
**hot s.,** the period of pyrexia in an intermittent fever such as malaria; called also *stadium caloris.*
**imperfect s.,** anamorph.
**incubative s.,** incubation period.
**knäuel s.,** spireme.
**lamina-bud s.,** the first stage of odontogenesis, characterized by initial formation of the tooth bud and development of dental lamina.
**latency s.,** 1. the incubation period of any infectious disorder. 2. the quiescent period following an active period in certain infectious diseases, during which the pathogen remains dormant for a variable length of time before again initiating signs of active disease. 3. in psychoanalytic theory, the period of relative quiescence in psychosexual development, lasting from age 5 or 6 years to adolescence, during which interest in persons of the opposite sex ceases and the child tends to associate mainly with persons of his own sex; it is preceded by the phallic stage and followed by the genital stage.
**mechanical s.,** a platform of a microscope by which the specimen being viewed can be moved in either of two mutually perpendicular directions.
**oral s.,** in psychoanalytic theory, the earliest stage of psychosexual development, lasting from birth to about 18 months, during which the oral zone is the center of the infant's needs, expression, and pleasurable erotic experiences; it is followed by the anal stage.
**perfect s.,** teleomorph.
**phallic s.,** in psychoanalytic theory, the third stage in psychosexual development, lasting from age 2 or 3 years to 5 or 6 years, during which sexual interest, curiosity, and pleasurable experiences are centered on the penis in boys and the clitoris in girls; it is preceded by the anal stage and followed by the latency stage.
**placental s.,** third s.
**preeruptive s.,** 1. the stage after infection and before eruption. 2. the period of tooth development, before tooth eruption, characterized by growth of the coronal portion of the tooth, prior to the beginning of the growth of the root.
**premenstrual s.,** the condition of the uterine mucosa after ovulation and the formation of a corpus luteum.
**prodromal s.,** the period of early symptoms of a disease occurring after the incubation period and just before the appearance of the characteristic symptoms of the disease; called also *prodromal period.*
**progestational s.,** the secretory stage of the endometrial cycle immediately preceding menstruation or implantation of the ovum.
**proliferative s.,** the phase of the uterine mucosa following the first stage of rest: the mucosa shows hypertrophy of the glands and increase of the lining epithelium.
**pyretogenic s., pyrogenetic s.,** the stage of invasion of a febrile attack.
**Ranke's s's,** the hypothesis that tuberculosis of the lungs develops in three stages: (1) the primary focus, (2) generalized spread of the tubercle bacillus, and (3) isolated organ tuberculosis, chiefly of the lungs.
**rest s.,** the stage of the uterine mucosa immediately following the completion of menstruation.
**resting s.,** the stage of a cell or its nucleus when no mitotic changes are going on; interphase.
**ring s.,** see under *form.*
**second s.,** (of labor), period during which the infant is expelled from the uterus and vagina.
**seral s.,** any of the individual transitional series of communities of an ecological sere, which finally leads to a stable, mature climax community. Called also *seral community.*
**sexual s.,** teleomorph.
**s's of sleep,** see *NREM sleep,* under *sleep.*
**stepladder s.,** an early stage of enteric fever; so called from the peculiar form of the temperature curve.
**sweating s.,** the final stage of a malarial paroxysm, marked by sweating.
**third s.,** (of labor), the period following expulsion of the infant and ending with expulsion of the placenta and membranes from the uterus.
**transitional pulp s.,** a condition of the dental pulp in which chronic inflammatory cells are present but not in sufficient quantities to constitute a typical inflammatory exudate, usually resulting from abrasion, attrition, caries, periodontal disease, or a reaction to a restorative procedure.
**ugly duckling s.,** a development stage in the mixed dentition when the upper central and lateral incisors may be flared, with the crowns

**Erickson's Eight Stages of Man**

| Psychosexual stage | Approximate age | Crisis |
|---|---|---|
| Oral-sensory | Birth to 18 mo. | Trust/mistrust |
| Anal-muscular | 18 mo. to 3 years | Autonomy/shame, self-doubt |
| Genital-locomotor control | 3 to 5 years | Initiative/guilt |
| Latency | 5 to 13 years | Industry, competence/inferiority, failure |
| Puberty | 13 to 21 years | Identity/role confusion |
| Genitality (young adulthood) | 21 to 40 years | Intimacy/isolation |
| Productivity (adulthood) | 40 to 60 years | Generativity/self-absorption, stagnation |
| Maturity | 60 years to death | Integrity, self-worth/despair |

distally and with diastema present before the maxillary canine teeth erupt.
**vegetative s.**, resting s.

**stag·gers** (stag′ərz) 1. incoordination in animals. 2. a form of vertigo occurring in decompression sickness.
**blind s.**, 1. any of various syndromes in animals characterized by wandering, unsteady gait, and lack of awareness of the surroundings. 2. acute selenium poisoning; see under *poisoning.* 3. gid.
**grass s.**, 1. locoism. 2. lactation tetany.
**paspalum s.**, a temporary type of paspalism seen in livestock that eat seeds of paspalum grasses contaminated with an ergot; characteristics include tremors and ataxia.
***Phalaris* s.**, head nodding, incoordination, and sometimes convulsions in ruminants grazing on certain species of *Phalaris* (canary grass). The etiology is unknown, but it occurs more often in cool weather when the grass is growing rapidly.
**rye grass s.**, 1. a neurotoxic disease seen in ruminants in North America, Europe, Australia, and New Zealand after they eat the rye grass *Lolium perenne* when it is contaminated by an endophytic fungus; characteristics include head nodding, incoordination, limb stiffness, and opisthotonos, all of which soon subside if the animals stop eating the grass. 2. a neurotoxic disease resembling the mycotoxic disease, seen in sheep in Australia and South Africa after they eat the rye grass *Lolium rigidum* when its seed galls are carrying a nematode infected with species of *Corynebacterium.* Characteristics include tremor, ataxia, seizures, nystagmus, and opisthotonos, often ending fatally.
**sleepy s., stomach s.**, forage poisoning.
***Zamia* s., zamia s.**, the neurotoxic effects seen in ruminants after they eat seeds or leaves of zamias or other cycads; characteristics include ataxia of the hind limbs that may progress to paralysis.

**stag·ing** (stāj′ing) 1. the determination of distinct phases or periods in the course of a disease, the life history of an organism, or any biological process. 2. the classification of neoplasms according to the extent of the tumor; see *TNM s.*
**TNM s.**, staging of tumors according to three basic components: primary tumor (T), regional nodes (N), and metastasis (M). Adscripts are used to denote size and degree of involvement; for example, 0 indicates undetectable, and 1, 2, 3, and 4 a progressive increase in size or involvement. Thus a tumor may be described as T1N2M0.

**Stahr's gland** (shtahrz) [Hermann *Stahr,* German anatomist and pathologist, 1868–1947] see under *gland.*

**stain** (stān) 1. any dye, reagent, or other material used in producing coloration, such as a substance used in coloring tissues or microorganisms for microscopical study. For specific stains, see Stains and Staining Methods below. 2. a superficial discoloration, or an artificially colored spot in the skin.
**acid s.**, a stain which is acid in reaction and more readily colors the protoplasm of cells.
**basic s.**, a stain which is basic in reaction and shows an affinity for the nuclei of cells.
**contrast s.**, material used to color an unstained portion of a tissue after another portion has been stained with another dye.
**counter s.**, see *counterstain.*
**differential s.**, one that facilitates differentiation of various elements in a specimen.
**electron s's**, substances containing heavy atoms, such as osmic tetroxide, uranyl, and lead ions, which, under certain conditions, act as "electron stains," comparable to histologic stains, by combining selectively with certain regions of the specimen; used in the visualization of the ultrastructure.
**heavy-metal s.**, any of the elements of high atomic weight often used as stains in electron microscopy.
**lipoid s.**, a stain made from any fatlike, or lipid, substance e.g., Sudan III.
**metachromatic s.**, a stain that colors certain cell constituents a color different from that of the stain itself.
**neutral s.**, a combination of an acid and a basic stain for staining neutrophil tissues.
**nuclear s.**, a stain which has a special affinity for the nuclei of cells.
**plasmatic s., plasmic s.**, a stain which colors the tissue uniformly throughout.
**port-wine s.**, a persistent dark red to purple nevus flammeus that grows proportionately with the affected child and is usually found on the face. Initially it is macular, but the surface may develop angiomatous overgrowths with time. Port-wine stains occur in association with other congenital abnormalities, such as the Klippel-Trénaunay and Sturge-Weber syndromes. Called also *port-wine mark* or *nevus.*
**protoplasmic s.**, a stain which has a special affinity for the protoplasm of cells.
**selective s.**, a stain which has a special affinity for a certain tissue element, staining it more vividly than, or to the exclusion of, other elements of the same specimen.
**tumor s.**, an area of increased density in a radiograph due to collection of contrast material in distorted and abnormal vessels, prominent in the capillary and venous phase of arteriography, and presumed to indicate neoplasm.

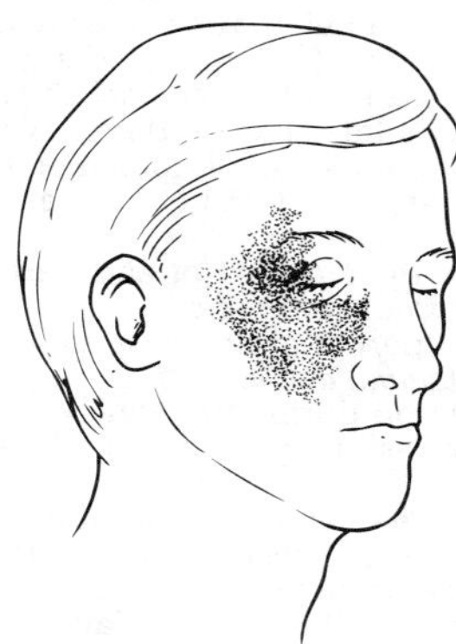

Port-wine stain.

## Stains and Staining Methods

Listing some of the preparations and methods commonly employed in histologic and pathologic technique *(arranged alphabetically).* For other stains, see under *blue, red,* etc.

**Achúcarro's s.**, a silver-tannin stain for impregnating connective tissue.
**acid-fast s.**, a staining procedure for demonstrating acid-fast microorganisms. See *Kinyoun carbolfuchsin s.* and *Ziehl-Neelsen s.*
**acid fuchsin s.**, a diffuse stain containing acid fuchsin and diluted hydrochloric acid in purified water, for demonstrating axons and as a component of connective tissue stains.
**Albert's diphtheria s.**, a stain containing toluidine blue and methyl (or malachite) green. Following treatment with iodine solution, the metachromatic granules appear black, the bars dark green to black, and the remainder of the diphtheria bacillus a light green.
**alum-carmine s.**, a preparation of ordinary alum and carmine.
**Alzheimer s.**, a methylene blue and eosin polychrome stain for demonstrating Negri bodies.
**Anthony capsule s.**, a method of demonstrating the capsules of bacteria. A smear of a milk culture is air dried, or a smear is mixed with milk and dried. The slide is stained with crystal violet and washed with copper sulfate. The capsule appears unstained against a purple background; the cells are deeply stained.
**auramine-rhodamine s.**, Truant auramine-rhodamine s.
**azan s.**, Heidenhain's modification of Mallory's triple stain.
**basic fuchsin s.**, a stain containing basic fuchsin in distilled water.
**Benda's s.**, a method for demonstrating nerve tissue.
**Bensley's neutral gentian orange G s.**, a preparation used for demonstrating secretion granules.
**Best's carmine s.**, a stain for demonstrating glycogen.
**Bethe's method**, a method of fixing methylene blue stains of nerve fibers.
**Bielschowsky's method**, a method for demonstrating axons and neurofibrils using an ammoniacal silver stain.
**Bodian method**, a method of staining nerve fibers and nerve endings with colloidal silver.
**Bowie s.**, a stain used to demonstrate the slightly basophilic cytoplasm and the specific granules of juxtaglomerular cells.
**Cajal method**, a method of staining astrocytes by a gold chloride–mercuric chloride compound.
**Cajal's double method**, a method of demonstrating ganglion cells.
**carbolfuchsin s.**, a stain for microorganisms containing basic fuch-

sin with dilute phenol as a mordant. It is also used as a counterstain for *Legionella pneumophila* following other routine stains. Stained cells appear pink to red.

**carbol–gentian violet s.**, a solution containing gentian violet and carbolic acid.

**Castaneda's s.**, a method of demonstrating rickettsiae. A smear is air dried and treated with methylene blue, then counterstained with safranin O, washed, and air dried. Rickettsiae appear blue against red cellular elements.

**Ciaccio's s.**, a stain for demonstrating lipids.

**Cox's modification of Golgi's corrosive sublimate method**, a method for staining ganglion cells.

**Davenport's s.**, a stain for demonstrating various elements of nerve tissue, dependent upon the special affinity of nerve cells and their processes for silver.

**Delafield's hematoxylin** [USP], a preparation of hematoxylin, alcohol, ammonia alum, water, glycerin, and methanol, used as a nuclear stain.

**Dieterle's s.**, a silver impregnation method for staining *Legionella* and other organisms. Slides are sensitized in uranyl nitrate, treated with gum mastic, incubated in silver nitrate, and developed in a solution of hydroquinone, sodium sulfite, acetone, formaldehyde, pyridine, and gum mastic. Cells stain black on a yellow-tan background.

**Ehrlich's acid hematoxylin**, a preparation of hematoxylin, used as a nuclear stain.

**Ehrlich's neutral s.**, a mixture of methylene blue and acid fuchsin, used to stain blood corpuscles.

**Ehrlich's triacid s.**, a stain containing acid fuchsin, orange G, and methyl green; used for demonstrating various formed elements in the blood.

**F method, F-staining method**, chromosomes are treated with phosphate buffer, rinsed and stored for 60–72 hours in saline citrate solution, then fixed in methanol-acetic acid, and stained by the Feulgen method.

**Feulgen method**, a method of demonstrating chromatin and deoxyribonucleic acid (DNA).

**Fite's method**, a staining method used for acid-fast bacilli. Tissue sections are deparaffinized in 2:1 xylene and peanut oil, then stained with Ziehl-Nielsen carbolfuchsin, decolorized with acid alcohol, and counterstained with methylene blue.

**Fontana's s.**, a method of staining spirochetes by silver impregnation, using ammoniacal silver nitrate solution.

**Fontana-Masson s.**, an ammoniacal silver nitrate stain for melanin and argentaffin material; used in the diagnosis of melanoma, pheochromocytoma, and carcinoid tumors.

**Giemsa s.**, a solution containing azure II-eosin, azure II, glycerin, and methanol; used for staining protozoan parasites such as *Plasmodium* and *Trypanosoma,* for *Chlamydia,* for differential staining of blood smears, and for viral inclusion bodies. Stained elements appear pink to purple to blue.

**Gimenez s.**, a method for staining *Chlamydia* and other rickettsiae and *Legionella.* Smears are stained with carbol–basic fuchsin solution, washed, and counterstained with malachite green. Cells appear red against a greenish background.

**Golgi's mixed method**, a method of staining nerve cells and all of their processes; historically of very great importance.

**Gomori's s's**, stains used for histological demonstration of enzymes, especially phosphatases and lipases in sections; also methods for demonstration of connective tissue fibers and secretion granules. Called also *Gomori-Takamatsu s's.*

**Gomori-Takamatsu s's**, Gomori's s's.

**Gomori-Wheatley s.**, trichrome s.

**Gomori's methenamine silver s.**, methenamine silver s.

**Goodpasture's s.**, a method for demonstrating the peroxidase reaction.

**Gram's method, Gram s.**, an empirical staining procedure devised by Gram in which microorganisms are stained with crystal violet, treated with 1:15 dilution of Lugol's iodine, decolorized with ethanol or ethanol-acetone, and counterstained with a contrasting dye, usually safranin. Those microorganisms that retain the crystal violet stain are said to be gram-positive, and those that lose the crystal violet stain by decolorization but stain with the counterstain are said to be gram-negative.

**Grimelius' argyrophil method**, a method for demonstrating granule-containing cells such as APUD cells. Incubation in a buffered silver nitrate solution is followed by reduction in a hydroquinone and sodium sulfite solution; reactive cell granules appear black.

**Grocott-Gomori methenamine–silver nitrate s.**, a method for demonstrating actinomycetes and fungi in tissue. Sections are treated with chromic acid, stained with methenamine-silver nitrite solution, and counterstained with light green solution. Cells appear brown against a green background.

**Hale's iron s.**, a stain used on substances with a high acid polysaccharide content because of the ability of polyanionic polysaccharides to bind polyvalent cations. Its main component is colloidal iron ($Fe^{3+}$).

**Harris' hematoxylin**, a nuclear stain.

**Harris' method**, a method for demonstrating Negri bodies.

**Heidenhain's iron hematoxylin s.**, an important cytological method for the demonstration of most cellular structures: nuclei, chromosomes, centrioles, fibrils, mitochondria, cilia, etc.

**hemalum s.**, a nuclear stain containing hematoxylin and alum, widely used, especially in combination with eosin.

**hematoxylin-eosin s.**, a mixture of hematoxylin in distilled water and aqueous eosin solution, employed also universally for routine examination of tissues; numerous variations are employed in execution of the stain.

**hematoxylin-eosin-azure II**, Maximow's method for the staining of blood-forming organs.

**Hiss capsule s.**, a method of demonstrating bacterial capsules. Smears are treated with crystal violet, heated, and rinsed with copper sulfate solution. Capsules appear as pale blue halos around deep blue to purple cells.

**Hortega method**, a method of demonstrating microglia, employing ammoniacal silver carbonate.

**India ink capsule s.**, a method of demonstrating cell capsules, especially of *Cryptococcus neoformans.* The smear is mixed with India ink, covered with a coverglass, and examined microscopically. Capsules appear as a clear halo around the cells against a black background.

**iron hematoxylin method**, a staining procedure in which the sections are treated with an iron salt, stained with hematoxylin, and differentiated with the same iron salt.

**Janus green B**, a stain used supravitally for the demonstration of mitochondria.

**Jenner's method**, a method for demonstrating blood corpuscles.

**Kinyoun carbolfuchsin s.**, a stain for acid-fast organisms. A heat-fixed smear is treated with carbolfuchsin solution. The slide is washed with water, decolorized with acid alcohol, and counterstained with methylene blue. Acid-fast organisms appear red against a blue background.

**Leifson flagella s.**, a method for demonstrating bacterial flagella. Smears are air dried, treated with alcoholic pararosaniline–tannic acid solution, and washed. Flagella are visible against a clear background.

**Leishman's s.**, a mixture of methylene blue and eosin for staining blood cells and certain parasites.

**Levaditi's method**, a method for demonstrating *Treponema pallidum* in sections, employing reduced silver.

**lithium-carmine s.**, a diffuse stain used intravitally for the demonstration of macrophages.

**Löffler's alkaline methylene blue s.**, a simple stain used especially for demonstrating granules in *Corynebacterium diphtheriae.* Methylene blue made alkaline with potassium hydroxide is applied to a smear briefly and the slide washed. Granules appear deep blue in lighter blue cells.

**Lorrain Smith s.**, Nile blue sulfate staining fatty acids blue and neutral fat pink.

**Lugol's iodine s.**, a solution (Lugol's iodine) of potassium iodide and iodine in water, containing 5 per cent iodine; used as a stain for protozoa in wet mounts.

**Luxol fast blue s.**, trademark for a group of dyes used in histology as stains for complex lipids, particularly myelin; they have a marked affinity for phospholipids, lecithin, and cephalin.

**Macchiavellos s.**, a rickettsial stain, used especially for *Chlamydia.* The heat-fixed smear is stained with basic fuchsin, decolorized in citric acid, and counterstained with methylene blue. Rickettsiae stain red against a blue background.

**Mallory's acid fuchsin, orange G, and aniline blue s.**, a stain for demonstrating connective tissue and secretion granules. Called also *Mallory's triple s.*

**Mallory's phloxine–methylene blue s.**, a stain used in histology to demonstrate connective tissue.

**Mallory's phosphotungstic acid–hematoxylin s.**, a stain used for demonstrating nuclear and cytoplasmic detail and connective tissue fibers.

**Mallory's triple s.**, Mallory's acid fuchsin, orange G, and aniline blue s.

**Marchi's method**, a method of demonstrating degenerated nerve fibers, the tissue first being fixed in a solution containing potassium bichromate, which prevents the normal myelinated fibers from staining with osmic acid.

**Masson s.**, a trichrome stain for connective tissue.

**Maximow's method**, hematoxylin-eosin-azure II.

**May's spore s.**, a method of staining the spores of bacteria in which they are treated with 5 per cent chromic acid, then with ammonia, stained with hot carbol-fuchsin, decolorized with dilute sulfuric acid, and counterstained with methylene blue. The spores appear red, the vegetative cells blue.

**May-Grünwald s.,** an alcoholic neutral mixture of methylene blue and eosin.

**Mayer's hemalum,** an aqueous solution of hematein, alum, thymol, and 90 per cent alcohol.

**Mayer's mucihematein,** a specific stain for mucin.

**methenamine silver s.,** 1. *(for argentaffin cells)* a methenamine silver solution used together with gold chloride, sodium thiosulfate, and a safranin O counterstain; argentaffin granules are black while granules of mast cells remain red. 2. *(for fungi)* Grocott-Gomori methenamine–silver nitrate s.

**methyl green-pyronin s.,** a solution of methyl green and pyronin (usually pyronin Y) used as a differential stain for DNA and RNA: DNA is stained blue-green by methyl green and RNA is stained red by pyronin.

**methyl violet s.,** an aniline dye used as a bacteriological stain.

**methylene blue,** an aniline dye much used as a staining agent; prepared in a saturated solution (7 per cent) in absolute alcohol, which is diluted for use.

**Michaelis' s.,** a mixture of alcoholic solution of methylene blue and a solution of eosin in acetone; used for demonstrating blood corpuscles.

**Milligan's trichrome s.,** a differential stain for connective tissue and smooth muscle. Nuclei and muscle appear magenta; collagen appears green or blue, depending on whether fast green or aniline blue is used as a counterstain; and red blood cells appear orange to orange red.

**neutral red,** an important supravital stain for the demonstration of vacuoles in cells, and especially of the vacuome.

**Nissl's method,** a method employed in the study of nerve cell bodies.

**Pal's modification of Weigert's myelin sheath s.,** a method for the study of myelinated nerves, the specimen being treated for several weeks in a solution containing potassium bichromate.

**Papanicolaou's s.,** a method of staining smears of various body secretions, from the respiratory, digestive or genitourinary tract, for the examination of exfoliated cells, to detect the presence of a malignant process. See also *Papanicolaou test,* under *tests.*

**Pappenheim's s.,** the original methyl green–pyronin staining method, used to differentiate between basophilic granules of erythrocytes and nuclear fragments.

**PAS s.,** periodic acid–Schiff s.

**Perdrau's method,** a modification of Bielschowsky's method for staining collagen and reticulin.

**periodic acid–Schiff (PAS) s.,** see under *reaction.*

**Perls' s.,** see under *test.*

**peroxidase s.,** see Goodpasture's s.

**phosphotungstic acid–hematoxylin s.,** see *Mallory's phosphotungstic acid–hematoxylin s.*

**polychrome methylene blue,** a stain for demonstrating plasma cells and mast cells, employing potassium carbonate and methylene blue.

**quinacrine fluorescent method,** chromosomes are exposed to quinacrine derivatives, after which they fluoresce, the degree of fluorescence varying from one chromosome segment to another; the resultant fluorescent patterns (Q bands) are characteristic for each chromosome. Called also *Q method.*

**Ranson's pyridine silver s.,** a stain used for demonstrating nerve cells and their processes.

**resorcin-fuchsin s.,** Weigert's resorcin-fuchsin s.

**reverse Giemsa method,** a method in which the reciprocal (R-bands) of the banding pattern seen in the Giemsa method for chromosomes is obtained; called also *R method.*

**Romanovsky's (Romanowsky's) s.,** the prototype of the many eosin-methylene blue stains for blood smears and malarial parasites, including Giemsa stain, Leishman's stain, and Wright's stain.

**Seller's s.,** a combination of alcoholic solutions of methylene blue and basic fuchsin which stains Negri bodies a bright red against a purplish-pink background; used in rapid diagnosis of rabies.

**Sternheimer-Malbin s.,** a stain used in urinalysis which has ready affinity for hyaline casts, epithelial casts, red cells, bladder epithelial nuclei, nuclei of vaginal epithelium, and trichomonads, staining each a different color.

**Sudan black B fat s.,** a stain used to demonstrate *Legionella* and fat vacuoles in bacterial cells. A heat-fixed smear is treated with Sudan black B, cleared with xylol, and counterstained with safranin. Fat vacuoles stain blue-black; bacterial cells stain pink.

**T method, T-staining method,** a method for staining only the terminal ends of chromosomes by means of either Giemsa stain or acridine orange; it results in bands (T bands) of dark violet (Giemsa) or fiery orange (acridine orange).

**tetrachrome s.,** a stain combining eosin Y, methylene blue, azur A, and methylene violet, in methyl alcohol.

**trichrome s.,** a rapid staining method which adequately demonstrates structural details of the various intestinal protozoa. The solution is as follows: chromotrope 2R 0.6 g, light green SF 0.3 g, phosphotungstic acid 0.7 g, acetic acid 1.00 mL, and distilled water 100.00 mL. Called also *Gomori-Wheatley s.*

**Truant auramine-rhodamine s.,** a method for demonstrating mycobacteria. A smear is heat fixed, stained with auramine-rhodamine solution, decolorized, counterstained with potassium permanganate, and examined under ultraviolet light; acid-fast organisms glow with a yellow-orange color.

**Unna's alkaline methylene blue,** a strongly alkaline solution of methylene blue which is valuable for staining plasma cells.

**Unna-Pappenheim s.,** a variation of methyl green–pyronin stain, used to detect plasma cells and demonstrate nucleoproteins.

**van Gieson's solution of trinitrophenol and acid fuchsin,** a stain for connective tissue, consisting of acid fuchsin and aqueous solution of trinitrophenol.

**Verhoeff's s.,** a stain for demonstrating elastic tissue.

**Verhoeff-van Gieson s.,** a histopathological stain for demonstrating elastic fibers.

**von Kossa's s.,** a silver nitrate stain for bone mineral.

**Warthin-Starry silver s.,** a method for staining *Bartonella* and spirochetes. A smear is air-dried, immersed in absolute ethanol, washed in distilled water, and incubated in 2 per cent silver nitrate. The cover glass is then developed in a mixture of silver nitrate, gelatin, glycerol, agar, and hydroquinone. Organisms appear black on a light background.

**Wayson s.,** a method used to demonstrate polar staining. A smear is treated with a mixture of basic fuchsin and methylene blue with phenol, washed with water, and dried. It is used especially to demonstrate *Yersinia pestis* in specimens from tissues and lymph nodes.

**Weigert's fibrin s.,** a method, many variations of which have been used in both fixation and staining; stains gram-positive bacteria as well as fibrin.

**Weigert's iron hematoxylin s.,** a simple method for staining most nuclear and cytoplasmic constituents.

**Weigert's myelin sheath method,** a method of demonstrating the myelin sheath of nerve cell processes.

**Weigert's neuroglia fiber s.,** a complicated method for demonstrating fibrous glia, which works best on human material.

**Weigert's resorcin-fuchsin s.,** a method for the demonstration of elastic fibers.

**Weil's s.,** a method for staining myelin sheaths.

**Wirtz-Conklin spore s.,** a smear is heated with malachite green, rinsed, then counterstained with safranin. Spores appear green in red-stained cells.

**Wright's s.,** a mixture of eosin and methylene blue, used for demonstrating blood corpuscles and malarial parasites.

**Ziehl-Neelsen s.,** a stain for acid-fast organisms. A heat-fixed smear is flooded with carbolfuchsin, heated for 5 minutes, cooled, and washed. The slide is decolorized with acid alcohol, washed, and counterstained with methylene blue. Acid-fast organisms appear red against a blue background.

**Ziehl-Neelsen carbolfuchsin,** a mixture of basic fuchsin, alcohol, liquefied phenol, and purified water.

---

**stain·ing** (stān′ing) [MeSH: Staining] 1. the artificial coloration of a substance, such as the introduction or application of material to facilitate examination of tissues, microorganisms, or other cells under the microscope. For various methods, see under *stain.* 2. modification of the color of the teeth or denture base to achieve a more lifelike appearance.

**bipolar s.,** staining at the two poles only, or staining differently at the two poles.

**differential s.,** staining with a substance for which different bacteria or different elements of the bacteria or specimen being stained show varying affinities, resulting in their differentiation.

**double s.,** staining with two different dyes which have an affinity for different tissue elements.

**fluorescent s.,** the coloration of tissues with a fluorescent dye.

**intravital s.,** vital s.

**multiple s.,** staining with several different dyes to facilitate identification of different tissue elements.

**negative s.,** staining of the background and not the organism, to facilitate the microscopical study of bacteria.

**polar s.,** staining in which the ends of the rod stain deeply while the central portion of the organism is nearly or quite unstained, as in the pasteurellas.

**postvital s.,** staining that occurs after death of a tissue which has been previously stained by vital methods.
**preagonal s.,** vital s.
**relief s.,** a method of staining that colors the background and leaves the cells uncolored.
**simple s.,** staining with a single substance, such as the staining of microorganisms with a single dye.
**substantive s.,** the coloration of tissues by direct absorption of dyes in which they are immersed.
**supravital s.,** staining of living tissue removed from the body, but before cessation of the chemical life of the cells.
**telomeric s., terminal s.,** differential staining of chromosomes to stain chromosome telomeric regions, consisting of pretreatment with a heated salt solution before treatment with buffered Giemsa stain or acridine orange; only the telomeric regions of the chromosomes retain the stain.
**triple s.,** staining with three different dyes to facilitate identification of the different elements.
**vital s.,** staining of a tissue by a dye which is introduced into a living organism and which, by virtue of affinity for certain tissues, will stain those tissues; called also *intravital s.*

**stal·ag·mom·e·ter** (stal″əg-mom′ə-tər) [Gr. *stalagmos* dropping + *-meter*] an instrument for measuring surface tension by determining the exact number of drops in a given quantity of a liquid.

**stalk** (stawk) an elongated, more or less slender anatomical structure resembling the stem of a plant; see also *peduncle* and *pedunculus.*
**allantoic s.,** the more slender tube interposed in most mammals between the urogenital sinus and the allantoic sac. It is the precursor of the umbilical cord. Called also *connecting s.*
**body s.,** a bridge of mesoderm connecting the caudal end of the young embryo with the chorion and eventually giving passage to the allantois with its important accompanying blood vessels; it is the precursor of the allantoic stalk.
**cerebellar s.,** any of the cerebellar peduncles.
**connecting s.,** allantoic s.
**hypophysial s.,** infundibulum neurohypophyseos.
**infundibular s.,** 1. infundibulum neurohypophyseos. 2. see under *stem.*
**neural s.,** infundibulum neurohypophyseos.
**optic s.,** a slender structure attaching the optic vesicle to the brain wall in the early embryo.
**pineal s.,** habenula, def. 2.
**pituitary s.,** infundibulum neurohypophyseos.
**s's of thalamus,** see under *peduncle.*
**yolk s.,** the narrow tube connecting the yolk sac (umbilical vesicle) with the midgut of the early embryo, which becomes partly incorporated into the embryo and usually undergoes complete obliteration, but occasionally persists in the embryo, and, rarely, is found in the adult as a diverticulum from the small intestine *(ileal* or *Meckel's diverticulum).* Called also *omphalomesenteric duct, umbilical duct,* and *vitelline duct.*

**stal·li·my·cin hy·dro·chlo·ride** (stal″ĭ-mi′sin) an antibacterial administered in the form of a topical ointment.

**sta·men** (sta′mən) the structure of a flower which bears the male gamete, or pollen.

**stam·i·na** (stam′ĭ-nə) [L.] vigor or endurance.

**stam·mer·ing** (stam′ər-ing) a speech disorder marked by involuntary pauses; sometimes used synonymously with *stuttering,* especially in Great Britain.

**Stam·no·so·ma** (stam″no-so′mə) [Gr. *stamnos* jar + *sōma* body] a genus of flukes. *S. arma′tum* and *S. formosa′num* are parasites of birds, but experimental human infections have been reported.

**stance** (stans) the posture and general bodily orientation of a person standing. Cf. *gait.*

**stan·dard** (stan′dərd) something established as a measure or model to which other similar things should conform.

**stan·dard·iza·tion** (stan″dərd-ĭ-za′shən) 1. the bringing of any preparation to a specified standard as to quality or ingredients. 2. the formulation of standards for a substance or for a procedure.

**stan·dard·ize** (stan′dərd-īz) to compare with or conform to a standard; to establish standards.

**stand·still** (stand′stil) suspension of activity or movement.
**atrial s.,** cardiac arrhythmia in which there is a pause in atrial contraction, as occurs secondary to sinus arrest or sinoatrial block, the ventricle continuing to respond to its own pacemaker.
**cardiac s.,** cessation of contraction of the myocardium.
**sinus s.,** see under *arrest.*
**ventricular s.,** cardiac arrhythmia in which there is an absence of ventricular contraction.

**Stan·ford-Bi·net test** (stan′fərd-be-na′) [*Stanford* University, where test was revised for use in the U.S.; Alfred *Binet,* French physiologist and psychologist, 1857–1911] [MeSH: Stanford-Binet Test] see under *test.*

**Stan·ley** (stan′le) Wendell Meredith. American biochemist, 1904–1971; co-winner, with James Batcheller Sumner and John Howard Northrop, of the Nobel prize for chemistry in 1946 for isolating virus crystals and for isolating nucleic acid from crystallized virus.

**Stan·ley bacillus** (stan′le) [*Stanley,* England, where it was first isolated] see under *bacillus.*

**Stan·ley Kent** see *Kent.*

**stan·nic** (stan′ik) containing tin as a quadrivalent element.
**s. chloride,** a caustic liquid used as a mordant in dyemaking and for various other purposes; it is toxic and corrosive if inhaled or spilled on the skin.
**s. oxide,** a compound found in nature as the mineral cassiterite, or produced through a reaction between tin and concentrated nitric acid at high temperatures. Used as a polishing agent for glass, metals, and especially to produce a high polish on metallic dental restorations. Called also *tin oxide.*

**stan·nif·er·ous** (stan-if′ər-əs) [*stannum* + *-ferous*] containing tin.

**stan·no·sis** (stan-o′sis) benign pneumoconiosis due to the inhalation of tin oxide; it is symptomless unless accompanied by silicosis.

**stan·nous** (stan′əs) containing tin as a bivalent element.
**s. chloride,** tin chloride, $SnCl_2$, used in the anhydrous and dihydrated forms as a reagent and, as the dihydrate, as a pharmaceutic aid.
**s. fluoride** [USP], a compound, $SnF_2$, applied topically to the teeth as a dental caries prophylactic.
**s. pyrophosphate,** $Sn_2P_2O_7$, a diagnostic aid used in bone imaging.

**stan·num** (stan′əm) [L.] tin (symbol Sn).

**stan·o·lone** (stan′o-lōn) [MeSH: Stanolone] a semisynthetic form of dihydrotestosterone, having the same actions and uses as testosterone. It is used for its anabolic and antineoplastic actions in inoperable breast cancer and in postoperative metastatic breast cancer.

**stan·o·zo·lol** (stan′o-zo-lol″) [USP] [MeSH: Stanozolol] an androgenic anabolic steroid, used orally, especially to increase hemoglobin levels in some patients with aplastic (congenital and idiopathic) anemia.

**sta·pe·dec·to·my** (sta″pə-dek′tə-me) [*stapes* + *-ectomy*] excision of the stapes.

**sta·pe·di·al** (sta-pe′de-əl) pertaining to the stapes.

**sta·pe·di·ol·y·sis** (sta-pe″de-ol′ĭ-sis) stapes mobilization.

**sta·pe·dio·plas·ty** (sta-pe″de-o-plas′te) stapedectomy followed by replacement with a prosthetic stapes, done to correct hearing loss due to otosclerosis.

**sta·pe·dio·te·not·o·my** (sta-pe″de-o-tə-not′ə-me) the cutting of the tendon of the stapedius muscle.

**sta·pe·dio·ves·tib·u·lar** (sta-pe″de-o-vəs-tib′u-lər) pertaining to the stapes and vestibule.

**sta·pe·dot·o·my** (sta″pə-dot′ə-me) the surgical creation of a small opening in the footplate of the stapes.

**sta·pes** (sta′pēz) gen. *stape′dis* [L. "stirrup"] [TA] [MeSH: Stapes] the innermost of the auditory ossicles, shaped somewhat like a stirrup; it articulates by its head with the incus, and its base is inserted into the fenestra vestibuli. Called also *stirrup.*

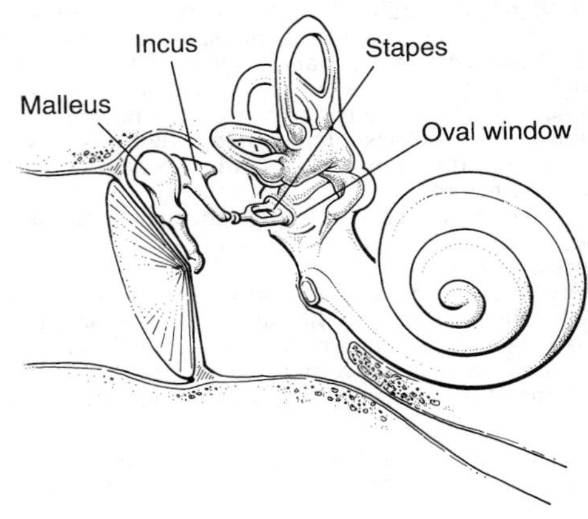


**Staph·cil·lin** (staf-sil′in) trademark for preparations of methicillin sodium.

**staph·i·sa·gria** (staf″ĭ-sa′gre-ə) [Gr. *staphis* raisin + *agrios* wild] the seeds of *Delphinium staphisagria,* which were formerly used as a topical parasiticide; the plant and its seeds are poisonous and narcotic, containing numerous alkaloids such as delphinine, delphinoidine, delphisine, and staphisagrine.

**staph·i·sa·grine** (staf″ĭ-sa′grin) a poisonous alkaloid found in the seeds of *Delphinium staphisagria.*

**staph·yl·ede·ma** (staf″əl-ə-de′mə) [*staphyl-* + *edema*] an enlargement or swollen state of the uvula.

**staph·y·line** (staf′ə-līn) 1. botryoid. 2. uvular.

**staph·y·lin·id** (staf″ə-lin′id) 1. pertaining to or due to beetles of the family Staphylinidae. 2. a beetle of the family Staphylinidae.

**Staph·y·lin·i·dae** (staf″ə-lin′ĭ-de) the rove beetles, a family of beetles that feed on decaying animal or vegetable matter; some species produce an irritating substance that causes blistering.

**staph·y·li·nus** (staf″ə-li′nəs) [L.] uvular.

**sta·phyl·i·on** (stə-fil′e-on) [Gr. "little grape"] an encephalometric landmark on the posterior edge of the hard palate at the median line.

**staph·y·li·tis** (staf″ə-li′tis) uvulitis.

**staphyl(o)-** [Gr. *staphylē* a bunch of grapes] a combining form denoting resemblance to a bunch of grapes, used especially to denote relationship to the uvula or to staphylococci.

**staph·y·lo·coc·cal** (staf″ə-lo-kok′əl) pertaining to or caused by staphylococci.

**staph·y·lo·coc·ce·mia** (staf″ə-lo-kok-se′me-ə) [*staphylococcus* + *-emia*] a condition in which staphylococci are present in the blood; septicemia caused by staphylococci.

**staph·y·lo·coc·ci** (staf″ə-lo-kok′si) plural of *staphylococcus.*

**staph·y·lo·coc·cic** (staf″ə-lo-kok′sik) staphylococcal.

**staph·y·lo·coc·cin** (staf″ə-lo-kok′sin) a bacteriocin produced by certain strains of *Staphylococcus aureus.*

**staph·y·lo·coc·co·sis** (staf″ə-lo-kok-o′sis) infection caused by staphylococci; see *staphylococcal endocarditis, impetigo, parotitis,* and *pneumonia,* and see *staphylococcal scalded skin syndrome,* under *syndrome.*

**Staph·y·lo·coc·cus** (staf″ə-lo-kok′əs) [Gr. *staphylē* bunch of grapes + *kokkos* berry] [MeSH: Staphylococcus] a genus of gram-positive, facultatively anaerobic bacteria of the family Micrococcaceae, order Eubacteriales, consisting of cocci, usually unencapsulated, 0.5 to 1.5 μm in diameter. The organisms occur singly, in pairs, and in irregular clusters, and are nonsporogenous and nonmotile. They are potential pathogens, causing local lesions and serious opportunistic infections.
**S. al′bus,** *S. aureus.*
**S. au′reus,** a species comprising the yellow-pigmented, coagulase-positive pathogenic forms of the genus, causing serious suppurative infections and systemic disease, such as *impetigo bullosa, staphylococcal pneumonia,* and *staphylococcal scalded skin syndrome.* This species also produces toxins that cause food poisoning and toxic shock syndrome. Called also *S. pyogenes.*
**S. epider′midis,** a coagulase-negative species that ferments glucose and produces colonies that are usually white. It is commonly found on normal skin, but many strains are pathogens or secondary invaders in diseases such as abscesses, infected wounds, the peritonitis seen in peritoneal dialysis, and subacute bacterial endocarditis.
**S. haemoly′ticus,** a coagulase-negative variety sometimes occurring on human skin and mucous membranes; it may be associated with infections of wounds, the urinary tract, and the conjunctiva, and with septicemia; its pathogenicity is not certain.
**S. ho′minis,** a coagulase-negative variety commonly occurring on human skin; it may be associated with infections of wounds, the urinary tract, and the conjunctiva, and with septicemia; its pathogenicity is not certain.
**S. hy′icus,** a species that infects pigs through wounds in the skin and causes greasy pig disease.
**S. pyo′genes,** *S. aureus.*
**S. saprophy′ticus,** a coagulase-negative species that ferments glucose weakly; they are usually harmless commensals but are occasionally pathogenic, causing urinary tract infections.
**S. si′mulans,** a coagulase-negative species isolated from certain human infections of the urinary tract, wounds, and occasionally other sites.

**staph·y·lo·coc·cus** (staf″ə-lo-kok′əs) pl. *staphylococ′ci* [MeSH: Staphylococcus] An organism of the genus *Staphylococcus.*

**staph·y·lo·der·ma** (staf″ə-lo-der′mə) cutaneous pyogenic infection by staphylococci.

**staph·y·lo·ede·ma** (staf″ə-lo-ə-de′mə) staphyledema.

**staph·y·lo·ki·nase** (staf″ə-lo-ki′nās) a bacterial kinase produced by certain strains of staphylococci, which can activate plasminogen in the blood of various species of animals.

**staph·y·lol·y·sin** (staf″ə-lol′ə-sin) a principle with hemolytic activity produced by staphylococci.
**α s., alpha s.,** a hemolysin produced by pathogenic staphylococci which lyses both sheep and rabbit erythrocytes at 37°C and has leukocidin activity.
**β s., beta s.,** a hot-cold hemolysin produced by staphylococci which lyses sheep but not rabbit erythrocytes in the cold following preliminary incubation at 37°C.
**δ s., delta s.,** a hemolysin produced by pyogenic staphylococci which lyses red cells from man and several other species; it differs immunologically from the α and β staphylolysins, and is both dermonecrotic and lethal.
**ε s., epsilon s.,** a hemolysin formed almost exclusively by nonpathogenic, coagulase-negative strains of staphylococci.
**γ s., gamma s.,** a hemolysin produced by staphylococci which is similar to, but serologically distinguishable from, the α staphylolysin.

**staph·y·lo·ma** (staf″ə-lo′mə) [Gr. *staphylōma* a defect in the eye inside the cornea] protrusion of the cornea or sclera lined with uveal tissue, resulting from inflammation.
**annular s.,** staphyloma of the sclera in the ciliary region, extending around the margin of the cornea.
**anterior s.,** scleral or corneal staphyloma in the anterior part of the eye.
**ciliary s.,** scleral staphyloma in the part covered by the ciliary body.
**s. cor′neae, corneal s.,** 1. ectasia of the cornea with adherent uveal tissue; called also *projecting s.* 2. staphyloma formed by an iris which has protruded through a wound in the cornea.
**s. cor′neae racemo′sum,** staphyloma corneae (def. 2) in which there are a number of perforations from which small portions of iris protrude.
**equatorial s.,** scleral staphyloma occurring in the equatorial region of the eye.
**intercalary s.,** that which occurs in the rim of sclera anterior to the insertion of the ciliary body.
**posterior s., s. posti′cum,** backward bulging of the sclera at the posterior pole of the eye; called also *Scarpa's s.*
**projecting s.,** s. corneae.
**retinal s.,** a forward bulging of the retina.
**Scarpa's s.,** posterior s.
**scleral s.,** protrusion of the contents of the eyeball at a point where the sclera has become too thin.
**uveal s.,** protrusion of the uvea through a ruptured sclera.

**staph·y·lom·a·tous** (staf″ə-lom′ə-təs) pertaining to or resembling staphyloma.

**staph·y·lon·cus** (staf″ə-long′kəs) [*staphylo-* + Gr. *onkos* mass] a tumor or swelling of the uvula.

**staph·y·lo·phar·yn·gor·rha·phy** (staf″ə-lo-far″in-gor′ə-fe) [*staphylo-* + *pharyngo-* + *-rrhaphy*] the stitching of the halves of the velum palatini to the posterior wall of the pharynx.

**staph·y·lo·plas·ty** (staf′ə-lo-plas″te) [*staphylo-* + *-plasty*] plastic repair of the soft palate and uvula. See also *palatoplasty.*

**staph·y·lop·to·sia** (staf″ə-lop-to′se-ə) uvuloptosis.

**staph·y·lop·to·sis** (staf″ə-lop-to′sis) uvuloptosis.

**staph·y·lor·rha·phy** (staf″ə-lor′ə-fe) palatorrhaphy.

**staph·y·los·chi·sis** (staf″ə-los′kĭ-sis) [*staphylo-* + *-schisis*] bifid uvula.

**staph·y·lo·tome** (staf′ə-lo-tōm) [Gr. *staphylotomon*] uvulotome.

**staph·y·lot·o·my** (staf″ə-lot′ə-me) [*staphylo-* + *-tomy*] 1. uvulotomy. 2. excision of a staphyloma.

**staph·y·lo·tox·in** (staf″ə-lo-tok′sin) any of the several toxins produced by *Staphylococcus aureus;* see *staphylococcal toxin,* under *toxin.*

**stap·ling** (sta′pling) the act or process of fastening with staples.
**gastric s.,** gastric partitioning.

**star** (stahr) 1. a symmetrical, round geometrical figure with five or more points radiating out from a center. 2. any structure resembling such a figure.
**daughter s.,** amphiaster.
**dental s.,** a marking on the incisor teeth of horses, first appearing in the lower central incisors at about the age of eight years; used in judging a horse's age.
**lens s's,** starlike lines formed within the lens of the eye by fibers which pass from the anterior to the posterior surface.
**mother s.,** monaster.
**polar s's,** the starlike figures of the amphiaster.
**s's of Verheyen,** venae stellatae renis.

**Winslow's s's,** whorls of capillary vessels from which arise the vorticose veins of the choroid coat of the eye.

**starch** (stahrch) [A. S. *stercan* to stiffen] [MeSH: Starch] 1. any of a group of polysaccharides of the general formula $(C_6H_{10}O_5)_n$, composed of a long-chain polymer of glucose in the form of amylose and amylopectin; it is the chief storage form of energy reserve (carbohydrates) in plants. 2. [NF] a preparation consisting of the granules separated from the mature grain of corn or wheat, or from potato tubers, occurring as irregular, angular, white masses or fine powder; used as a dusting powder and as a filler, binder, and disintegrant in pharmaceutical preparations.
**s. glycerite,** a preparation of starch, benzoic acid, purified water, and glycerin; used as an emollient in pharmaceutical preparations intended for external use.
**pregelatinized s.** [NF], starch processed to rupture all or part of the granules in the presence of water, and subsequently dried; it occurs as a moderately coarse to fine, white to off-white powder and is used as a tablet excipient in pharmaceutical preparations.
**soluble s.,** starch partially hydrolyzed with hydrochloric acid so that it is water soluble; usually amylodextrin.

**starch phos·phor·y·lase** (stahrch fos-for'ə-lās) see *phosphorylase.*

**Star·gardt's disease (macular degeneration)** (shtahr'gahrts) [Karl Bruno *Stargardt,* German ophthalmologist, 1875–1927] see under *disease.*

**Star·ling's hypothesis, law** (stahr'lingz) [Ernest Henry *Starling,* English physiologist, 1866–1927] see under *curve, hypothesis,* and *law.*

**Starr-Ed·wards valve** (stahr-ed'wərdz) [Albert *Starr,* American surgeon, born 1926; M.L. *Edwards,* American physician, born 1906] see under *valve.*

**start·er** (stahr'tər) a culture of microorganisms used to initiate fermentation, as in dairy products.

**stas·i·mor·phia** (stas″ĭ-mor'fe-ə) stasimorphy.

**stas·i·mor·phy** (stas″ĭ-mor'fe) [Gr. *stasis* standing + *morphē* form] deformity or abnormality of shape in any organ, due to arrest of development.

**sta·sis** (sta'sis) [Gr. "a standing still"] 1. a stoppage or diminution of the flow of blood or other body fluid in any part. 2. a state of equilibrium among opposing forces.
**ileal s.,** abnormal delay in the passage of the intestinal contents through the ileum; it is usually associated with dilatation of the ileum.
**intestinal s.,** any condition in which normal passage of intestinal content is impaired; it may be due to mechanical obstruction or impaired intestinal motility.
**papillary s.,** papilledema.
**pressure s.,** stoppage of the circulation caused by undue pressure on a part.
**urinary s.,** stoppage of the flow or discharge of urine, which may occur at any level of the urinary tract.
**venous s.,** cessation or impairment of venous flow, such as with venous insufficiency; see also *stasis ulcer,* under *ulcer.* Called also *phlebostasis* and *venostasis.*

**-stasis** [Gr. "a standing still"] a word termination indicating the maintenance of (or maintaining) a constant level; preventing increase or multiplication.

**stat.** abbreviation for L. *sta'tim,* immediately.

**-stat** [Gr. *-states* one who causes to stand, from *histanai* to cause to stand] a word termination denoting an agent that inhibits growth without killing, or a device that maintains something in a steady state.

**state** (stāt) [L. *status*] 1. condition or situation; see also *status.* 2. the crisis, or the turning point of an attack of disease.
**acute confusional s.,** older term for *delirium.*
**alpha s.,** the state of relaxation and peaceful awakefulness, associated with prominent alpha brain wave activity.
**anelectrotonic s.,** the condition occurs in a nerve near the anode during the passage of a continuous current.
**anxiety s.,** the condition of experiencing undue anxiety, as in anxiety disorders. It was temporarily the official replacement for the term *anxiety neurosis.*
**asexual s.,** anamorph.
**borderline s.,** a diagnostic term used when it is difficult to determine which of two states are indicated by the presenting symptoms, generally for a state that has some characteristics of psychosis but in which the patient has some contact with reality.
**carrier s.,** see *carrier,* def. 1.
**catelectrotonic s.,** the condition of a nerve near the cathode during the passage of an electric current.
**central excitatory s.,** a condition in which there is stored up in a reflex center of the spinal cord a number of stimuli which do not reveal themselves in reflex response.
**correlated s.,** dynamic equilibrium.
**de-efferented s.,** locked-in syndrome.
**dreamy s.,** a state of altered consciousness lasting for a few minutes and accompanied by hallucinations; associated with temporal lobe lesions. See also *temporal lobe epilepsy,* under *epilepsy,* and *petit mal status,* under *status.*
**excited s.,** the condition of a nucleus, atom, or molecule produced by the addition of energy to the system as the result of absorption of photons or of inelastic collisions with other particles or systems.
**ground s.,** the condition of lowest energy of a nucleus, atom, or molecule, as opposed to the excited state.
**hypercoagulable s.,** a pathologic condition of hypercoagulability of the blood.
**hypnagogic s.,** that state of semiconsciousness which immediately precedes falling asleep.
**hypnopompic s.,** that state of semiconsciousness which immediately precedes complete awakening from sleep.
**imperfect s.,** anamorph.
**inotropic s.,** cardiac contractility.
**local excitatory s.,** the condition of a nerve produced by an ineffectual stimulus.
**metastable s.,** 1. an excited state with an unusually long lifetime, ranging from $10^{-6}$ second to several minutes. 2. an intermediate state between the ground and excited states, requiring additional energy before decay to the ground state can occur.
**oxidation s.,** see under *number.*
**perfect s.,** teleomorph.
**persistent vegetative s.,** a condition of profound nonresponsiveness in the wakeful state caused by brain damage at whatever level and characterized by a nonfunctioning cerebral cortex, the absence of any discernible adaptive response to the external environment, akinesia, mutism, and inability to signal; the electroencephalogram may be isoelectric or show abnormal activity.
**plastic s., pluripotent s.,** the state of parts of the zygote or very early embryo in which they may develop into any adult tissue or part.
**refractory s.,** a condition of subnormal excitability of muscle and nerve following excitation.
**resting s.,** the physiological condition achieved by complete bed rest for a period of at least one hour, a condition required in a number of different tests of various body functions.
**sexual s.,** teleomorph.
**singlet s.,** the excited state occurring when one electron of a pair is excited to a higher energy level without changing its spin; it is unstable and can decay to either a ground state or a triplet state.
**steady s.,** dynamic equilibrium.
**triplet s.,** the excited state resulting when an electron is activated by absorbing a photon, moves to an outer orbital of higher energy, with the electron spin parallel to that of the other unpaired electron; it is a long-lived state that cannot decay to a ground state unless the spin changes again.
**twilight s.,** a temporary absence of consciousness in which the patient may perform certain acts involuntarily and without remembrance of them afterward. Examples are complex partial seizures, absence seizures, and dreamy states.

**stath·mo·ki·ne·sis** (stath″mo-ki-ne'sis) a state of arrested mitosis, or pseudometaphase, as that induced by subjecting cells to the action of an agent such as colchicine, which destroys the fibrillar structure of cell spindles and thus permits the calculation of mitosis time.

**stat·ic** (stat'ik) [Gr. *statikos* causing to stand, from *histanai* to cause to stand] 1. at rest; in equilibrium; not in motion. 2. not dynamic.

**-static** [Gr. *statikos* causing to stand, from *histanai* to cause to stand] a word termination meaning inhibiting, or denoting an agent that inhibits, or pertaining to the maintenance of a constant level.

**stat·ics** (stat'iks) that phase of mechanics which deals with the action of forces and systems of forces on bodies at rest.

**sta·tim** (sta'tim) [L.] immediately, at once. Abbreviated *stat.*

**-statin** [Gr. *stasis* a standing still] a word termination denoting cessation or inhibition; used in names of hormones.

**sta·tion** (sta'shən) [L. *statio,* from *stare* to stand still] 1. a position or location. 2. the location of the presenting part of the fetus in the birth canal, designated as −5 to −1 according to the number of centimeters the part is above an imaginary plane passing through the ischial spines, 0 when at the plane, and +1 to +5 according to the number of centimeters the part is below the plane. 3. the location of the presenting part of the fetus in the birth canal with the long axis of the birth canal divided into thirds above and below the plane of the ischial spines; the location is designated as −3 to −1 when the part is above the plane, 0 when it is at the plane, and +1 to +3 when it is below the plane. 4. a specified site to which the sick and wounded are brought.

**anterior s.**, see *salivaria.*
**posterior s.**, see *stercoraria.*

**sta·tion·ary** (sta'shən-ar"e) [L. *stationarius*] not subject to variations or to changes of place.

**sta·tis·tic** (stə-tis'tik) [back formation from *statistics*] 1. an item of numerical data. 2. a value summarizing, representing, or characterizing some aspect of a sample or the population from which the sample was drawn.

**sta·tis·tics** (stə-tis'tiks) [Ger. *Statistik* originally "political science of state affairs," from L. *status* state] [MeSH: Statistics] 1. a collection of numerical data. 2. a discipline devoted to the collection, analysis, and interpretation of numerical data using the theory of probability, concerned particularly with methods for drawing inferences about characteristics of a population from examination of a random sample.
**bayesian s.**, a somewhat controversial statistical methodology that, unlike conventional statistics, which treats population parameters as fixed (though unknown) values, treats parameters as random variables with a specified probability distribution, termed the prior (or *a priori*) distribution. Bayes' theorem is then used to convert the probability distribution of an observable statistic (treated as a conditional probability for a given parameter value) to a conditional probability distribution of the parameter values for a given value of the observable statistic. This distribution is termed the posterior (or *a posteriori*) distribution because it assigns a probability to each parameter value that depends on the observed data. The controversial point is the prior distribution, which represents a subjective opinion of the experimenter as to the *a priori* credibility of the various parameter values; for example, in estimating the probability of the presence of a particular disease given a positive test result, the prior distribution represents the experimenter's judgment of the prevalence of the disease in the population under study.
**descriptive s.**, that measuring and describing characteristics of groups, without drawing inferences about the population in general.
**inferential s.**, that generalizing conclusions from sample data, using theories of probability to estimate population parameters.
**nonparametric s.**, a statistical methodology that can be used on data without making the assumption that the data are drawn from a population with a normal or other specified distribution. See also under *test.*
**parametric s.**, statistical methodology that depends upon assumptions about the distribution of the data, e.g., that the data approximate a normal distribution and are homoscedastic.
**semiparametric s.**, statistical methodology that combines both parametric and nonparametric elements; used for estimating population parameters when a function is unknown, e.g. the distribution function of a random variable that has not been observed.
**vital s.**, the data, usually collected by governmental bodies, detailing the rates of birth, death, disease, marriage, and divorce in a population.

**stato·acous·tic** (stat"o-ə-ko͞os'tik) pertaining to balance and hearing.

**stato·co·nia** (stat"o-ko'ne-ə) [Gr. *statos* standing + *konos* dust] plural of *statoconium.*

**stato·co·ni·um** (stat"o-ko'ne-əm) [TA] one of the minute calciferous granules within the gelatinous statoconic membrane surmounting the acoustic maculae *(membrana statoconiorum macularum).* Called also *otolith, otolite, otoconium,* and *ear crystal.*

**stato·lith** (stat'o-lith) 1. statoconium. 2. a solid or semisolid body occurring in the statocyst of animals.

**stat·o·lon** (stat'o-lon) an antiviral agent derived from *Penicillium stoloniferum,* which inhibits the multiplication of certain picornaviruses and arboviruses.

**sta·tom·e·ter** (stə-tom'ə-tər) exophthalmometer.

**stat·u·ral** (stach'o͞o-rəl) pertaining to stature.

**sta·ture** (stach'oor) [L. *statura*] the height or tallness of a person standing.

**sta·tus** (sta'təs) [L.] state; particularly used in reference to a morbid condition.
**absence s.**, a type of petit mal status that lasts for several hours and has few stereotyped or abnormal movements.
**s. asthma'ticus**, a particularly severe episode of asthma that does not respond adequately to ordinary therapeutic measures and may require hospitalization.
**s. calci'fames**, calcium hunger.
**s. chore'icus**, a severe and persistent form of chorea.
**complex partial s.**, status epilepticus consisting of a series of complex partial seizures without return to full consciousness in between. Called also *psychomotor s.*
**s. convulsi'vus**, s. epilepticus (def. 1).
**s. criba'lis, s. cribro'sus**, a sievelike condition of the brain due to dilatation of the perivascular lymph spaces.
**s. cri'ticus**, a severe and persistent form of tabetic crises.
**s. dysmyelina'tus, s. dysmyelinisa'tus**, Hallervorden-Spatz syndrome.
**s. dysra'phicus**, faulty closure of the embryonic neural tube resulting in faulty formation of midline adult structures, such as the vertebral column, sternum, breasts, and palate; called also *arrhaphia.*
**s. epilep'ticus**, 1. a continuous series of generalized tonic-clonic seizures without return to consciousness, a life-threatening emergency. Called also *convulsive s. epilepticus.* 2. any prolonged series of similar seizures without return to full consciousness between them; the two major types are *convulsive s. epilepticus,* which is life-threatening, and *nonconvulsive s. epilepticus,* which is serious but not usually life-threatening.
**s. epilepticus, convulsive**, s. epilepticus (def. 1).
**s. epilepticus, nonconvulsive**, status epilepticus that does not include generalized tonic-clonic seizures; see *complex partial s., petit mal s.,* and *epilepsia partialis continua.*
**s. epilepticus, tonic-clonic**, s. epilepticus (def. 1).
**s. hemicra'nicus**, s. migrainosus.
**s. lacuna'ris, s. lacuno'sus**, a condition of the brain marked by numerous small infarcts *(lacunes)* or losses of substance.
**s. lympha'ticus**, developmentally normal hyperplasia of lymphoid tissue and the thymus, formerly thought to be an important cause of sudden death (by airway obstruction) in infants; called also *s. thymicolymphaticus,* and *s. thymicus.*
**s. marmora'tus**, a usually congenital condition marked by excessive myelinization of the nerve fibers of the corpus striatum, as in Vogt's syndrome; called also *état marbré.*
**s. migraino'sus**, a state marked by constantly recurring attacks of migraine; called also *s. hemicranicus.*
**performance s.**, ability of a patient to function as measured by a performance scale.
**petit mal s.**, any of a variety of clinical disorders with symptoms ranging from momentary interruption of consciousness to longer-lasting spells of loss of motor control. They have a distinctive pattern on the electroencephalogram, with spike and wave discharges at three cycles per second.
**s. prae'sens**, the condition of a patient at the time of observation.
**psychomotor s.**, complex partial s.
**simple partial s.**, epilepsia partialis continua.
**s. thymicolympha'ticus, s. thy'micus**, s. lymphaticus.
**s. thy'micus**, s. lymphaticus
**s. verruco'sus**, a wartlike appearance of the cerebral cortex, produced by disorderly arrangement of the neuroblasts so that the formation of fissures and sulci is irregular and unpredictable.
**s. vertigino'sus**, prolonged vertigo.

**Staub-Trau·gott effect (test)** (shtoub-trou'got) [Hans *Staub,* Swiss internist, 1890–1967; Carl *Traugott,* German internist, born 1885] see under *effect* and *phenomenon.*

**Stauf·fer syndrome** (staw'fər) [Maurice H. *Stauffer,* American gastroenterologist, 20th century] see under *syndrome.*

**stau·ri·on** (staw're-on) [Gr., dim. of *stauros* cross] a point at the crossing of the median and transverse palatine sutures.

**stau·ro·ple·gia** (staw"ro-ple'jə) [Gr. *stauros* cross + *-plegia*] alternate hemiplegia.

**staves·acre** (stāvz-a'kər) 1. *Delphinium staphisagria.* 2. staphisagria.

**stav·u·dine** (stav'u-dēn) [MeSH: Stavudine] a nucleoside analogue of thymidine that inhibits human immunodeficiency virus (HIV) replication, used in the treatment of HIV infection in patients who have previously received prolonged treatment with zidovudine; administered orally.

**stax·is** (stak'sis) [Gr. "a dripping"] hemorrhage.

**stay** (sta) 1. a narrow structure that gives support. 2. bar, def. 5.
**frog s.**, bar, def. 5.
**s. of white line**, adminiculum lineae albae.

**STD** sexually transmitted disease.

**STE** subperiosteal tissue expander.

**steal** (stēl) diversion of something from its normal course, usually refering to blood flow in occlusive arterial disease.
**subclavian s.**, in occlusive disease of the subclavian artery, a reversal of blood flow in the ipsilateral vertebral artery from the basilar artery to the subclavian artery beyond the point of occlusion; this may deprive the brain of blood and cause the subclavian steal syndrome.

**ste·a·ral·de·hyde** (ste"ə-ral'də-hīd) a long-chain, aliphatic free aldehyde found in plasmalogens, giving the so-called plasmal reaction upon direct treatment of the tissue with Schiff's reagent.

**ste·a·rate** (ste'ə-rāt) any salt (soap), ester, or anionic form of stearic acid.

**ste·a·ric ac·id** (ste-ar'ik) [*stear-* + *-ic*] 1. a saturated 18-carbon fatty acid occurring in most fats and oils, particularly the oils of

land animals and fats of tropical plants; stearic and palmitic acids are the two most common saturated fatty acids in body fluids. See also table at *fatty acid.* 2. [NF] a preparation containing a mixture of stearic and palmitic acids, prepared by hydrogenation of fats and oils that are derived from edible sources unless the preparation is for external use only; used as a tablet and capsule lubricant and as an emulsifying and solubilizing agent.
**purified s. a.** [NF], a preparation containing a mixture of stearic acid and palmitic acids, which together constitute at least 96 per cent of the total, with at least 90 per cent of the total being stearic acid; it is prepared by hydrogenation of fats and oils that are derived from edible sources, unless the mixture is for external use only, and is used like stearic acid.

**ste·ar·i·form** (ste-ar′ĭ-form) fatlike.

**ste·a·rin** (ste′ə-rin) tristearin.

**stear(o)-** [Gr. *stear,* gen. *steatos* fat] combining forms denoting relationship to fat.

**ste·a·rop·tene** (ste″ə-rop′tən) [*stearo-* + Gr. *ptēnos* volatile] the more solid component of a volatile oil, cf. *eleoptene.*

**ste·a·ro·yl** (stēr′o-əl) the acyl radical of stearic acid.

**ste·a·ro·yl-CoA de·sat·u·rase** (ste-ar′o-əl ko-a′ de-sach′u-rās) [EC 1.14.99.5] [MeSH: Stearoyl-CoA Desaturase] an enzyme activity of the oxidoreductase class that catalyzes the desaturation of stearoyl coenzyme A to form oleoyl coenzyme A. It is part of a complex in the endoplasmic reticulum that also includes a flavoprotein (FAD), cytochrome $b_5$, and cytochrome-$b_5$ reductase. Called also *acyl CoA desaturase.*

**ste·ar·rhea** (ste″ə-re′ə) [*stearo-* + *-rrhea*] steatorrhea.

**ste·a·tite** (ste′ə-tīt) soapstone.

**ste·a·ti·tis** (ste″ə-ti′tis) [*steato-* + *-itis*] [MeSH: Steatitis] 1. inflammation of adipose tissue. See also *panniculitis.* 2. yellow fat disease.
**nutritional s.,** yellow fat disease.

**steat(o)-** stear(o)-.

**ste·ato·cele** (ste-at′o-sēl) [*steato-* + *-cele*[1]] a fatty mass formed within the scrotum.

**ste·a·to·cys·to·ma** (ste″ə-to-sis-to′mə) an epithelial cyst.
**s. mul′tiplex,** an autosomal dominant disorder chiefly affecting males at birth or presenting about the time of puberty, characterized by the development of numerous flesh-colored to yellow epidermal cysts, especially involving the skin of the sternum, the proximal extremities, and the scrotum in males. The cysts typically have an intricately infolded thin epidermal lining, without a granular layer, incorporating abortive hair follicles and at times sebaceous, eccrine, or apocrine structures, and contain lanugo hair and an oily material.

**ste·a·tog·e·nous** (ste″ə-toj′ə-nəs) lipogenic.

**ste·a·to·hep·a·ti·tis** (ste″ə-to-hep″ə-ti′tis) [*steato-* + *hepatitis*] fatty liver in alcoholics; see under *liver.*
**nonalcoholic s.,** NASH; an inflammatory disease of the liver of uncertain pathogenesis and histologically resembling alcoholic hepatitis, but occurring in nonalcoholic patients, most often obese women with non–insulin-dependent diabetes mellitus; clinically it is generally asymptomatic or mild, but fibrosis or cirrhosis may result.

**ste·a·tol·y·sis** (ste″ə-tol′ĭ-sis) [*steato-* + *-lysis*] lipolysis.

**ste·a·to·lyt·ic** (ste″ə-to-lit′ik) lipolytic.

**ste·a·to·ma** (ste″ə-to′mə) pl. *steato′mata* or *steatomas* [*steat-* + *-oma*] 1. a lipoma. 2. a fatty mass retained within a sebaceous gland.

**ste·a·to·ma·to·sis** (ste″ə-to-mə-to′sis) 1. lipomatosis. 2. steatocystoma multiplex.

**ste·a·tom·ery** (ste″ə-tom′ər-e) [*steato-* + Gr. *mēros* thigh] a deposit of fat on the outer aspect of the thighs and buttocks.

**ste·a·to·ne·cro·sis** (ste″ə-to-nə-kro′sis) fat necrosis.

**ste·a·to·pyg·ia** (ste″ə-to-pij′e-ə) [*steato-* + *pyg-* + *-ia*] excessive fatness of the buttocks, usually seen in women.

**ste·a·top·y·gous** (ste″ə-top′ĭ-gəs) pertaining to or characterized by steatopygia.

**ste·a·tor·rhea** (ste″ə-to-re′ə) [*steato-* + *-rrhea*] excessive amounts of fats in the feces, as in malabsorption syndromes.
**idiopathic s.,** celiac disease.

**ste·a·to·sis** (ste″ə-to′sis) fatty degeneration.
**s. cardi′aca,** cardiomyoliposis.
**macrovesicular s.,** fatty change in which a single large droplet occupies most of the cell, displacing the cytoplasm and nucleus to a ring around the droplet. Cf. *microvesicular s.*
**microvesicular s.,** fatty change in which numerous small lipid droplets are present in the cytoplasm. Cf *macrovesicular s.*

**stech·i·ol·o·gy** (stek″e-ol′ə-je) stoichiology.

**stech·i·om·e·try** (stek″e-om′ə-tre) stoichiometry.

**Stec·lin** (stek′lin) trademark for preparations of tetracycline.

**Steele-Ri·chard·son-Ol·szew·ski syndrome** (stēl-rich′ərd-sən-ol-shev′ske) [John C. *Steele,* Canadian physician, 20th century; John Clifford *Richardson,* Canadian neurologist, born 1909; Jerzy *Olszewski,* Polish-born Canadian neurologist, 1913–1966] see under *syndrome.*

**Steell's murmur** (stēlz) [Graham *Steell,* English physician, 1851–1942] Graham Steell's murmur; see under *murmur.*

**stef·fi·my·cin** (stef-ĭ-mi′sin) an antibacterial with antiviral properties, produced by *Streptomyces steffisburgensis* var. *steffisburgensis.*

**steg·no·sis** (steg-no′sis) [Gr. *stegnōsis* obstruction] constriction; stenosis.

**steg·not·ic** (steg-not′ik) pertaining to, characterized by, or promoting stegnosis; astringent.

**Steg·o·my·ia** (steg″o-mi′yə) [Gr. *stegos* roof + *myia* fly] a subgenus of mosquitoes of the genus *Aedes,* native to various Pacific islands. *S. argen′teus, S. cal′opus* and *S. fascia′tus* are old names for *Aedes aegypti.*

**Stein's test** (stīnz) [Stanislav Aleksandr Fyodorovich von *Stein,* Russian otologist, late 19th century] see under *test.*

**Stein-Lev·en·thal syndrome** (stīn-lev′ən-thahl) [Irving Freiler *Stein,* Sr., American gynecologist, born 1887; Michael Leo *Leventhal,* American obstetrician and gynecologist, 1901–1971] polycystic ovary syndrome; see under *syndrome.*

**Stein·brock·er's syndrome** (stīn′brok-ərz) [Otto *Steinbrocker,* American physician, 20th century] shoulder-hand syndrome.

**Steind·ler operation** (stīnd′lər) [Arthur *Steindler,* American orthopedic surgeon, 1878–1959] see under *operation.*

**Stei·ner's syndrome** (shti′nerz) [L. *Steiner,* German physician, early 20th century] Curtius' syndrome.

**Stei·nert's disease** (shti′nerts) [Hans *Steinert,* German physician, early 20th century] myotonic dystrophy; see under *dystrophy.*

**Stein·mann pin** (shtīn′mahn) [Fritz *Steinmann,* Swiss surgeon, 1872–1932] see under *pin.*

**Stein·stras·se** (shtīn′shtrah-sə) [Ger. "stone street"] urinary tract obstruction due to fragments of calculi that become lodged in the ureter after extracorporeal shock wave lithotripsy.

**Stel·a·zine** (stel′ə-zēn) trademark for preparations of trifluoperazine hydrochloride.

**stel·la** (stel′ə) pl. *stel′lae* [L.] star.
**s. len′tis hyaloi′dea,** the posterior pole of the crystalline lens.
**s. len′tis iri′dica,** the anterior pole of the crystalline lens.

**stel·late** (stel′āt) [L. *stellatus*] shaped like a star; arranged in a roset, or in rosets.

**stel·lec·to·my** (stə-lek′tə-me) removal of the stellate ganglion; done for the relief of pain.

**Stel·lite** (stel′it, stel′īt) trademark for any of a group of nonferrous, very hard, noncorrosive alloys composed chiefly of cobalt and chromium, with or without small amounts of other metals added. Used especially in the manufacture of cutting tools such as surgical instruments.

**stel·lu·la** (stel′u-lə) pl. *stel′lulae* [L., dim. of *stella*] little star.
**stel′lulae vasculo′sae winslow′ii,** Winslow's stars.
**stellulae of Verheyen, stel′lulae verhey′enii,** venae stellatae renis.

**Stell·wag's sign** (shtel′vahks) [Carl von Carion *Stellwag,* Austrian ophthalmologist, 1823–1904] see under *sign.*

**stem** (stem) a stalklike supporting structure; see also *peduncle.*
**brain s.,** brainstem; see under *B.*
**infundibular s.,** 1. the inferior part of the infundibulum hypothalami, which contains the neural connections of the pituitary gland and is continuous with the tuber cinereum.

**stem bro·me·lain** (stem bro′mə-lān) [EC 3.4.22.32] see *bromelain.*

**Sten·der dish** (sten′dər) [Wilhelm P. *Stender,* German manufacturer, 19th century] see under *dish.*

**sten·i·on** (sten′e-on) pl. *sten′ia* [Gr. *stenos* narrow + *-on* neuter ending] an encephalometric landmark, the craniometrical point situated at each end of the smallest transverse diameter of the head in the temporal region.

**Ste·no** (ste′no) see *Stensen.*

**sten(o)-** [Gr. *stenos* narrow] a combining form meaning contracted or narrow.

**steno·breg·mat·ic** (sten″o-breg-mat′ik) [*steno-* + *bregmatic*] having the superior and anterior portion of the head narrowed.

**steno·ce·pha·lia** (sten″o-sə-fa′le-ə) stenocephaly.

**steno·ceph·a·lous** (sten″o-sef′ə-ləs) having a narrow head.

**steno·ceph·a·ly** (sten″o-sef′ə-le) [*steno-* + *-cephaly*] excessive narrowness of the head.

**steno·cho·ria** (sten″o-kor′e-ə) [*steno-* + Gr. *chōros* space] stenosis, or narrowing.

**steno·co·ri·a·sis** (sten″o-kə-ri′ə-sis) [*steno-* + *core-* + *-iasis*] contraction of the pupil of the eye.

**steno·cro·ta·phia** (sten″o-kro-ta′fe-ə) [*steno-* + *crotaphion* + *-ia*] narrowness of the temporal region.

**steno·crot·a·phy** (sten″o-krot′ə-fe) stenocrotaphia.

**steno·pe·ic** (sten″o-pe′ik) [*sten-* + Gr. *opē* opening] having a narrow slit or opening, as stenopeic spectacles.

**ste·no·sal** (stə-no′səl) stenotic.

**ste·nosed** (stə-nōzd′) narrowed or constricted.

**ste·no·sis** (stə-no′sis) pl. *steno′ses* [Gr. *stenōsis*] an abnormal narrowing of a duct or canal; called also *arctation, coarctation,* and *stricture.*

**aortic s. (AS),** narrowing of the orifice of the aortic valve or of the supravalvular or subvalvular regions; see also *supravalvular aortic s.* and *subvalvular aortic s.*

**aortic s., subvalvular,** subaortic s.

**aortic s., supravalvular,** a rare form of aortic stenosis occurring above the aortic valve, usually caused by a complete circumferential fibrous ring of constricting tissue at the level of the sinus of Valsalva. See also *Williams syndrome,* under *syndrome.*

**caroticovertebral s.,** atherosclerotic stenosis of the cervical portions of the vertebral arteries, resulting in cerebral ischemia.

**cicatricial s.,** stenosis caused by the contraction of a cicatrix.

**gastric s., infantile hypertrophic,** congenital hypertrophy and hyperplasia of the musculature of the pyloric sphincter, occurring within the first few weeks of life and leading to partial obstruction of the gastric outlet.

**granulation s.,** stenosis or narrowing caused by the deposit of granulations or by their contraction.

**infundibular s.,** stenosis below the pulmonary valve, within the infundibulum (conus arteriosus) of the right ventricle of the heart.

**infundibular s., subpulmonic,** infundibular s.

**mitral s.,** a narrowing of the left atrioventricular orifice (mitral orifice).

**mitral s., buttonhole,** mitral stenosis in which adhesion and shortening of the mitral cusps produces a diaphragmatic slit resembling a buttonhole; called also *fishmouth mitral s.*

**mitral s., fishmouth,** buttonhole mitral s.

**postdiphtheritic s.,** stenosis of the larynx or trachea following diphtheria.

**pulmonary s. (PS),** narrowing of the opening between the pulmonary artery and the right ventricle, usually at the level of the valve leaflets.

**pyloric s.,** obstruction of the pyloric orifice of the stomach; it may be congenital as in hypertrophic pyloric stenosis, or acquired due to peptic ulceration or prepyloric carcinoma.

**pyloric s., hypertrophic,** narrowing of the pyloric canal by muscular hypertrophy and mucosal edema, occurring chiefly in infants, and marked by nausea, vomiting, epigastric pain, anorexia, weight loss, dehydration, and hypochloremic alkalosis; in infants there are a palpable pyloric mass and visible peristalsis.

**renal artery s. RAS,** narrowing of one or both renal arteries, caused by atherosclerosis or by fibrous dysplasia or hyperplasia, so that renal function is impaired; increased renin release by the affected kidney causes renovascular hypertension, and bilateral stenosis may result in chronic renal failure.

**spinal s.,** narrowing of the vertebral canal, nerve root canals, or intervertebral foramina of the lumbar spine caused by encroachment of bone upon the space; symptoms are caused by compression of the cauda equina and include pain, paresthesias, and neurogenic claudication. The condition may be either congenital or due to spinal degeneration. See also *spinal compression* under *compression.*

**subaortic s.,** aortic stenosis due to an obstructive lesion in the left ventricle below the aortic valve, causing a pressure gradient across the obstruction within the ventricle.

**subaortic s., idiopathic hypertrophic,** a form of hypertrophic cardiomyopathy, in which the left ventricle is hypertrophied (commonly with disproportionate involvement of the interventricular septum) and the cavity is small; it is marked by obstruction to left ventricular outflow. Called also *muscular subaortic s.*

**subaortic s., muscular,** idiopathic hypertrophic subaortic s.

**subglottic s.,** stenosis of the trachea below the glottis. A congenital form results in neonatal stridor or laryngotracheitis, often requiring tracheotomy but resolving with age. An acquired form is caused by repeated intubations.

**tricuspid s. (TS),** narrowing or stricture of the tricuspid orifice of the heart.

**valvular s.,** stenosis affecting any of the valves of the heart; see *aortic s., mitral s., pulmonary s.,* and *tricuspid s.*

**steno·ther·mal** (sten″o-ther′məl) stenothermic.

**steno·ther·mic** (sten″o-ther′mik) [*steno-* + *therm-* + *-ic*] capable of development only within a narrow range of temperature, e.g., a bacterial culture.

**steno·tho·rax** (sten″o-thor′aks) [*steno-* + *thorax*] abnormal narrowness of the chest.

**ste·not·ic** (stə-not′ik) [Gr. *stenotēs* narrowness] pertaining to or characterized by stenosis; abnormally narrowed.

**Sten·sen's canal, duct,** etc. (sten′sənz) [Niels *Stensen* (Nicolaus Steno), Danish physician, anatomist in Italy, 1638–1686] see under *experiment* and *plexus,* and see *canalis incisivum, ductus parotideus,* and *foramen incisivum.*

**Stent graft, mass** (stent) [Charles R. *Stent,* English dentist, late 19th century] see under *mass* and see *inlay graft* under *graft.*

**stent** (stent) [from Charles R. *Stent,* English dentist, died 1901] [MeSH: Stents] 1. a mold for keeping a skin graft in place, made of Stent's mass or some acrylic or dental compound. 2. a slender rod-like or threadlike device used to provide support for tubular structures that are being anastomosed, or to induce or maintain their patency. See also *endoprosthesis.*

**Palmaz s.,** an intravascular stent made of rigid wire mesh; it is introduced by a guidewire and then expanded into place by a balloon.

**intravascular s.,** a metal wire or tube introduced into a stenotic blood vessel to create and maintain luminal patency; it may be self-expanding or balloon-expandable.

**step** (step) one of a series of footrests on different levels, or a structure resembling it.

**Rönne's nasal s.,** a steplike defect in the nasal side of the visual field; seen in glaucoma.

**ste·pha·ni·al** (stə-fa′ne-əl) pertaining to the stephanion.

**ste·pha·ni·on** (stə-fa′ne-ən) [Gr. *stephanos* crown + *-on* neuter ending] the point on the side of the cranium at which the coronal suture meets the superior temporal line.

**Ste·phano·fi·la·ria** (stef″ə-no-fī-lar′e-ə) a genus of nematodes of the superfamily Filarioidea. *S. stile′si* causes stephanofilariasis in cattle in the United States.

**steph·a·no·fi·la·ri·a·sis** (stef″ə-no-fil″ə-ri′ə-sis) a chronic skin disease of cattle in certain parts of the United States, due to infestation with the nematode *Stephanofilaria stilesi;* called also *filarial* or *verminous dermatitis* and *stephanofilarosis.*

**steph·a·no·fil·a·ro·sis** (stef″ə-no-fil″ə-ro′sis) stephanofilariasis.

**Steph·a·nu·ri·dae** (stef″ə-nu′rĭ-de) a family of nematodes that includes the genus *Stephanurus.*

**Steph·a·nu·rus** (stef″ə-nu′rəs) a genus of nematode parasites of the family Stephanuridae. *S. denta′tus* is parasitic in the urinary tract and occasionally other organs in pigs.

**ste·ra·di·an** (stə-ra′de-ən) [Gr. *ster-* solid + *radian*] the unit of measurement of solid angles, equivalent to the angle subtended at the center of a sphere by an area on its surface equal to the square of its radius. A full sphere subtends $4\pi$ steradians. Abbreviated sr.

**Ster·ane** (ster′ān) trademark for preparations of prednisolone.

**Ster·a·pred** (ster′ə-pred″) trademark for preparations of prednisone.

**sterc(o)-** [L. *stercus* dung] a combining form denoting relationship to feces.

**ster·co·bi·lin** (stər″ko-bi′lin) [*sterco-* + *bilin*] a bile pigment derivative, formed by air oxidation of stercobilinogen, which is in turn derived by reduction of bilirubin; it is a brown-orange-red pigmentation contributing to the color of feces and urine.

**ster·co·bi·lin·o·gen** (stər″ko-bi-lin′o-jən) a bilirubin metabolite and precursor of stercobilin, formed by reduction of urobilinogen.

**ster·co·lith** (stər′ko-lith) [*sterco-* + *-lith*] fecalith.

**ster·co·ra·ceous** (stər″kə-ra′shəs) [L. *stercoraceus*] fecal.

**ster·co·ral** (stər′kə-rəl) fecal.

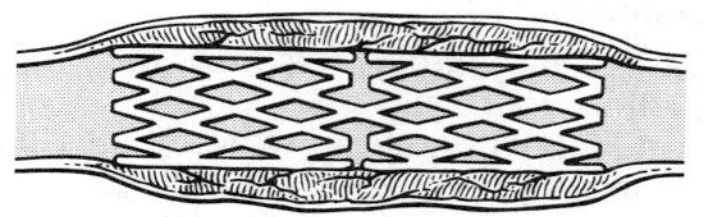

Expanded intraluminal stent within a vessel.

**ster·co·ra·ria** (stər″kə-rar′e-ə) in some systems of classification, a group or section comprising those trypanosomes in which the developmental cycle is completed in the hindgut (posterior station) of the vector and transmission is by fecal contamination during biting of the host by the vector. The group includes the subgenera *Megatrypanum, Herpetosoma,* and *Schizotrypanum.* Cf. *salivaria.*

**ster·co·rar·i·an** (stər″kə-rar′e-ən) pertaining to or caused by trypanosomes of the stercoraria group or section.

**ster·co·ro·lith** (stər′kə-ro-lith) stercolith.

**ster·co·ro·ma** (stər″kə-ro′mə) a large accumulation of fecal matter forming a tumor-like mass in the rectum; called also *coproma, fecaloma,* and *scatoma.*

**ster·co·rous** (stər′kə-rəs) [L. *stercorosus*] fecal.

**Ster·cu·lia** (stər-ku′le-ə) a large genus of mostly tropical trees and shrubs of the family Sterculiaceae, named for the stercorous (manurelike) odor of certain species. Some species have edible seeds and others are medicinal. *S. u′rens* and other species yield the gummy exudate called *karaya gum. S. ape′tala* is a Panamanian species whose hairs may be very irritating.

**ster·cu·lia** (stər-ku′le-ə) any plant of the genus *Sterculia.*

**ster·cus** (stər′kəs) pl. *ster′cora* [L.] feces.

**stere** (stēr) [Gr. *stereos* solid] a cubic meter.

**stereo-** [Gr. *stereos* solid] a combining form meaning solid, having three dimensions, or firmly established.

**ster·eo·ag·no·sis** (ster″e-o-ag-no′sis) astereognosis.

**ster·eo·an·es·the·sia** (ster″e-o-an″es-the′zhə) inability to identify by touch the form, size, weight, and texture of objects, owing to cortical disease or an interruption of nerve tracts. Cf. *astereognosis.*

**ster·eo·ar·throl·y·sis** (ster″e-o-ahr-throl′ĭ-sis) [*stereo-* + *arthro-* + *-lysis*] operative formation of a movable new joint in cases of bony ankylosis.

**ster·eo·aus·cul·ta·tion** (ster″e-o-aws″kəl-ta′shən) auscultation by means of two phonendoscopes each on different parts of the chest. One tube of each instrument is placed in the ears, the other tube of each being closed with the fingers.

**ster·eo·blas·tu·la** (ster″e-o-blas′tu-lə) a solid blastula, all of whose cells reach the external surface.

**ster·eo·cam·pim·e·ter** (ster″e-o-kam-pim′ə-tər) [*stereo-* + *campimeter*] an instrument for studying unilateral central scotomas and defects in the central retinal area.

**ster·eo·chem·i·cal** (ster″e-o-kem′ĭ-kəl) pertaining to stereochemistry, or to the space relations of the atoms of a molecule.

**ster·eo·chem·is·try** (ster″e-o-kem′is-tre) that chemical theory which supposes an arrangement of the atoms of certain molecules in three-dimensional spaces; that branch of chemistry which treats of the space relations between atoms.

**ster·eo·cil·i·um** (ster″e-o-sil′e-əm) pl. *stereocil′ia* [*stereo-* + *cilium*] A nonmotile protoplasmic filament on the free surface of a cell; found on hair cells of the inner ear and on pseudostratified epithelial cells of the male epididymis. Cf. *kinocilium.*

**ster·eo·cine·flu·o·rog·ra·phy** (ster″e-o-sin″ə-flo͞o-rog′rə-fe) photographic recording by motion picture camera of x-ray images produced by stereofluoroscopy, affording three-dimensional visualization.

**ster·eo·cog·no·sy** (ster″e-o-kog′no-se) stereognosis.

**ster·eo·en·ceph·a·lo·tome** (ster″e-o-ən-sef′ə-lo-tōm″) a guiding instrument used in stereoencephalotomy.

**ster·eo·en·ceph·a·lot·o·my** (ster″e-o-ən-sef″ə-lot′ə-me) [*stereo-* + *encephalo-* + *-tomy*] stereotaxic surgery.

**ster·eo·flu·o·ros·co·py** (ster″e-o-flo͞o-ros′kə-pe) stereoscopic fluoroscopy.

**ster·e·og·no·sis** (ster″e-og-no′sis) [*stereo-* + Gr. *gnōsis* knowledge] [MeSH: Stereognosis] 1. the faculty of perceiving and understanding the form and nature of objects by the sense of touch. 2. perception by the senses of the solidity of objects.

**ster·e·og·nos·tic** (ster″e-og-nos′tik) pertaining to stereognosis.

**ster·eo·gram** (ster′e-o-gram) 1. a stereoscopic radiograph. 2. a stereoscopic drawing.

**ster·eo·graph** (ster′e-o-graf) stereogram.

**ster·eo·iso·mer** (ster″e-o-i′so-mər) [MeSH: Stereoisomerism] one of a group of compounds having a stereoisomeric relationship.

**ster·eo·iso·mer·ic** (ster″e-o-i″so-mer′ik) pertaining to or exhibiting stereoisomerism.

**ster·eo·isom·er·ism** (ster″e-o-i-som′ər-iz-əm) [*stereo-* + *isomerism*] [MeSH: Stereoisomerism] the relationship between two or more isomers that have the same structure (the same linkages between atoms) but different configurations (spatial arrangements) in contrast to constitutional isomerism in which the isomers have different structures. Stereoisomers are further classified into *enantiomers,* those having molecules that are mirror images of each other, and *diastereomers,* those that do not. An older classification used the subdivisions optical and geometric isomerism (q.v.), which did not include all forms of stereoisomerism. Called also *configurational, stereochemical,* or *spatial isomerism.*

**ster·e·ol·o·gy** (ster″e-ol′ə-je) the study of the three-dimensional properties of objects usually seen in two dimensions.

**ster·e·om·e·ter** (ster″e-om′ə-tər) [*stereo-* + *-meter*] an instrument for performing stereometry.

**ster·e·om·e·try** (ster″e-om′ə-tre) the measurement of the cubic or solid contents of a solid body, or of the capacity of a hollow space.

**ster·eo·oph·thal·mo·scope** (ster″e-o-of-thal′mo-skōp) binocular ophthalmoscope.

**Ster·eo·or·thop·ter** (ster″e-o-or-thop′tər) trademark for a mirror-reflecting instrument used to correct strabismus.

**ster·eo·pho·rom·e·ter** (ster″e-o-fo-rom′ə-tər) [*stereo-* + *phorometer*] a phorometer with a stereoscopic attachment.

**ster·eo·pho·to·mi·cro·graph** (ster″e-o-fo″to-mi′kro-graf) a stereoscopic photograph of a microscopical subject.

**ster·eo·plasm** (ster′e-o-plaz-əm) [*stereo-* + *-plasm*] the more solid portions of protoplasm.

**ster·e·op·sis** (ster″e-op′sis) [*stereo-* + Gr. *opsis* vision] stereoscopic vision.

**ster·eo·ra·di·og·ra·phy** (ster″e-o-ra″de-og′rə-fe) the making of a radiograph giving an impression of depth as well as of width and height.

**ster·eo·ra·di·om·e·try** (ster″e-o-ra″di-om′ə-tre) measurement of the solid dimensions of a radiopaque object from its stereoscopic radiographs.

**ster·eo·sal·pin·gog·ra·phy** (ster″e-o-sal″ping-gog′rə-fe) salpingography in which an impression of depth is achieved.

**ster·eo·scope** (ster′e-o-skōp″) [*stereo-* + *-scope*] an instrument for producing the appearance of solidity and relief by combining the images of two pictures of an object seen from slightly dissimilar viewpoints.

**ster·eo·scop·ic** (ster″e-o-skop′ik) having the effect of a stereoscope; giving to objects seen a solid or three-dimensional appearance.

**ster·eo·ski·ag·ra·phy** (ster″e-o-ske-ag′rə-fe) stereoradiography.

**ster·eo·spe·cif·ic** (ster″e-o-spə-sif′ik) exhibiting marked specificity for one of several stereoisomers of a substrate or reactant; said of enzymes or of synthetic organic reactions.

**ster·eo·tac·tic** (ster″e-o-tak′tik) [*stereo-* + L. *tactus* touch] 1. characterized by precise positioning in space; said especially of discrete areas of the brain that control specific functions. 2. pertaining to types of brain surgery that use a system of three-dimensional coordinates to locate the site to be operated on. 3. thigmotactic.

**ster·eo·tax·ic** (ster″e-o-tak′sik) 1. stereotactic. 2. thigmotactic.

**ster·eo·tax·is** (ster″e-o-tak′sis) 1. stereotactic surgery. 2. thigmotaxis.

**ster·eo·taxy** (ster″e-o-tak′se) stereotactic surgery.

**ster·eo·trop·ic** (ster″e-o-trop′ik) thigmotropic.

**ster·e·ot·ro·pism** (ster″e-ot′rə-piz-əm) [*stereo-* + *tropism*] thigmotropism.

**ster·eo·ty·py** (ster′e-o-ti″pe) [*stereo-* + Gr. *typos* type] the persistent repetition of senseless acts or words, frequently occurring in disorders such as autistic disorder and schizophrenia.

**Ste·re·um** (ste′re-əm) a genus of bracken fungi of the order Aphyllophorales, including some species causing tree and wood rot.

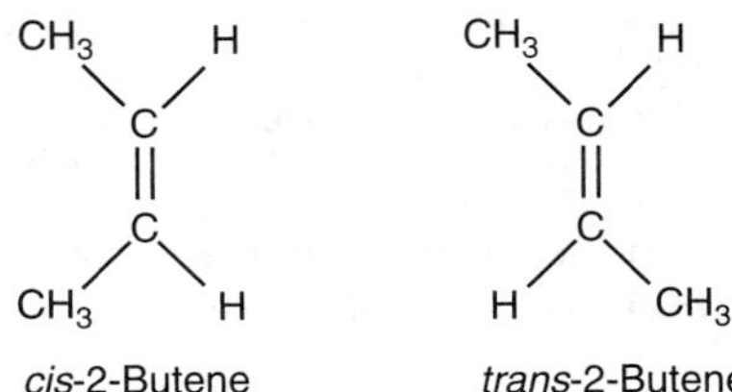


Stereoisomerism, exemplified by a pair of *cis-trans* diastereomers.

**ste•ric** (ste'rik) pertaining to the arrangement of atoms in space; pertaining to stereochemistry.

**ste•rig•ma** (ste-rig'mə) pl. *sterig'mata* [Gr. *stērigma* support] 1. the narrow stalk at the end of a basidium that gives rise to basidiospores. 2. metula.

**ste•rig•ma•to•cys•tin** (ste-rig"mə-to-sis'tin) a mycotoxin produced by *Aspergillus versicolor*, which sometimes contaminates corn; it is hepatotoxic and carcinogenic.

**Ste•rig•ma•to•cys•tis** (ste-rig"mə-to-sis'tis) former name for *Aspergillus*.

**ster•i•lant** (ster'ĭ-lənt) a sterilizing agent, i.e., an agent that destroys microorganisms.

**ster•ile** (ster'il) [L. *sterilis*] 1. unable to produce offspring; called also *barren*. 2. aseptic.

**ste•ril•i•ty** (stə-ril'ĭ-te) [L. *sterilitas*] 1. inability to produce offspring, i.e. either to conceive *(female s.)* or to induce conception *(male s.)*. Cf. *infertility*. 2. asepsis.
**absolute s.**, complete and irremediable inability to produce offspring.
**female s.**, inability of the female to conceive as a result of a structural or functional defect in the reproductive organs.
**male s.**, inability of the male to fertilize the ovum as a result of failure to produce living spermatozoa *(aspermatogenic s.)*, an abnormality in spermatozoa production *(dysspermatogenic s.)*, or some cause other than inability to produce live, normal spermatozoa *(normospermatogenic s.)*.
**one-child s.**, inability to produce further offspring after having produced one.
**primary s.**, 1. inability to produce offspring because of the absence of some factor essential for reproduction. 2. sterility in which no offspring has ever been produced.
**relative s.**, infertility.
**secondary s.**, 1. inability to produce further offspring after having conceived or induced conception. See *one-child s.* and *two-child s.* 2. inability to produce offspring resulting from a noncongenital defect.
**two-child s.**, inability to produce further offspring after having produced two.

**ster•i•li•za•tion** (ster"ĭ-lĭ-za'shən) [MeSH: Sterilization] 1. the complete destruction or elimination of all living microorganisms, accomplished by physical methods (dry or moist heat), chemical agents (ethylene oxide, formaldehyde, alcohol), radiation (ultraviolet, cathode), or mechanical methods (filtration). 2. any procedure by which an individual is made incapable of reproduction, as by castration, vasectomy, or salpingectomy.
**eugenic s.**, the process of rendering a person incapable of reproduction because the offspring would probably be undesirable types or because the parent is incapable of rearing the child responsibly.
**fractional s.**, **intermittent s.**, destruction of microbial viability by successive application of the procedure at intervals, to allow spores to develop into vegetative forms, which are more easily destroyed.

**ster•i•lize** (ster'ĭ-līz) 1. to render sterile; to free from microorganisms. 2. to render incapable of reproduction.

**ster•i•liz•er** (ster'ĭ-līz"ər) an apparatus used for the destruction of microorganisms; see *sterilization*.

**Ster•i•sil** (ster'ĭ-sil) trademark for a preparation of hexetidine.

**ster•nad** (ster'nad) toward the sternum, or sternal aspect.

**ster•nal** (ster'nəl) [L. *sternalis*] pertaining to the sternum.

**ster•nal•gia** (stər-nal'jə) [*stern-* + *-algia*] pain in the sternum; called also *sternodynia*.

**Stern•berg's disease, giant cells, sign** (shtern'bərgz) [Carl von *Sternberg*, Austrian pathologist, 1872–1935] see *Hodgkin's disease*, under *disease*, see *Reed-Sternberg cells*, under *cell*, and see under *sign*.

**Stern•berg-Reed cells** (shtern'berg-rēd) [Carl von *Sternberg;* Dorothy *Reed*, American pathologist, 1874–1964] see *Reed-Sternberg cells*, under *cell*.

**ster•ne•bra** (stər'ne-brə) pl. *ster'nebrae* [*sternum* + *vertebrae*] any of the segments of the developing sternum in the embryo, which later fuse to form the corpus sterni.

**Ster•nee•dle** (stər'ne-dəl) trademark for a controlled-depth, multiple puncture apparatus used in the diagnosis of tuberculosis. See *Sterneedle tuberculin test*, under *test*.

**ster•nen** (stər'nən) pertaining to the sternum alone.

**stern(o)-** [L. *sternum*, q.v.] a combining form denoting relationship to the sternum.

**ster•no•cla•vic•u•lar** (stər"no-klə-vik'u-lər) pertaining to the sternum and clavicle.

**ster•no•cla•vic•u•la•ris** (stər"no-klə-vik"u-lar'is) [L.] sternoclavicular.

**ster•no•clei•dal** (stər"no-kli'dəl) [*sterno-* + *cleid-* + *-al*[1]] sternoclavicular.

**ster•no•clei•do•mas•toid** (stər"no-kli"do-mas'toid) pertaining to the sternum, clavicle, and mastoid process.

**ster•no•cos•tal** (stər"no-kos'təl) [*sterno-* + *costal*] pertaining to the sternum and ribs.

**ster•nod•y•mus** (stər-nod'ĭ-məs) [*sterno-* + *didymus*] thoracopagus.

**ster•no•dyn•ia** (ster"no-din'e-ə) sternalgia.

**ster•no•go•ni•om•e•ter** (stər"no-go"ne-om'ə-tər) an instrument for measuring the sternal angle.

**ster•no•hy•oid** (stər"no-hi'oid) pertaining to the sternum and to the hyoid bone.

**ster•noid** (stər'noid) resembling the sternum.

**ster•no•mas•toid** (stər"no-mas'toid) pertaining to the sternum and the mastoid process of the temporal bone.

**ster•nop•a•gus** (stər-nop'ə-gəs) [*sterno-* + *-pagus*] thoracopagus.

**ster•no•peri•car•di•al** (stər"no-per"ĭ-kahr'de-əl) pertaining to the sternum and the pericardium.

**ster•no•scap•u•lar** (stər"no-skap'u-lər) pertaining to the sternum and the scapula.

**ster•nos•chi•sis** (stər-nos'kĭ-sis) [*sterno-* + *-schisis*] cleft sternum.

**Ster•no•sto•ma** (stər"no-sto'mə) a genus of mites that infest the trachea and bronchi of wild and domestic birds and cause respiratory difficulty.

**ster•no•thy•roid** (stər"no-thi'roid) pertaining to the sternum and to the thyroid cartilage or gland.

**ster•not•o•my** (stər-not'ə-me) [*sterno-* + *-tomy*] the operation of cutting through the sternum.
**median s.**, incision through the midline of the sternum, done to gain access to thoracic organs and other structures.

**ster•no•tra•che•al** (stər"no-tra'ke-əl) [*sterno-* + *tracheal*] pertaining to the sternum and to the trachea.

**ster•no•try•pe•sis** (stər"no-tri-pe'sis) [*sterno-* + *trypesis*] surgical perforation of the sternum.

**ster•no•ver•te•bral** (stər"no-vər'tə-brəl) pertaining to the sternum and vertebrae.

**ster•no•xi•phop•a•gus** (stər"no-zi-fop'ə-gəs) [*sterno-* + *xipho-* + *-pagus*] a type of thoracopagus in which conjoined twins are united in the region of the xiphoid process of the sternum.

**ster•num** (stər'nəm) [L., from Gr. *sternon*] [TA] [MeSH: Sternum] a longitudinal unpaired plate of bone forming the middle of the anterior wall of the thorax; it articulates above with the clavicles and along its sides with the cartilages of the first seven ribs. It consists of three portions: the manubrium, the body, and the xiphoid process.

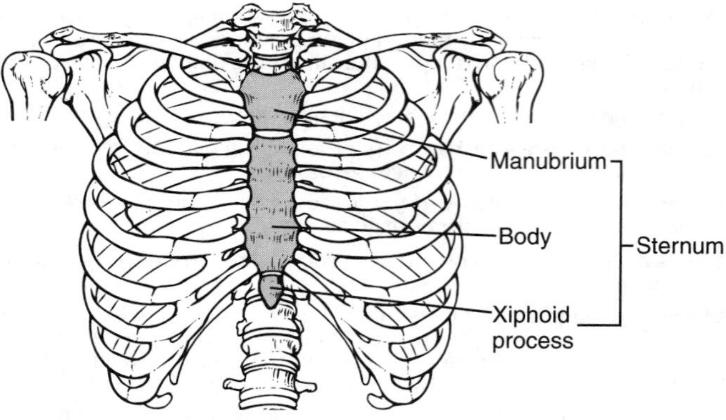


**cleft s.**, a developmental defect in which the sternum is longitudinally fissured as a result of incomplete fusion of the cartilaginous sternal bars. Called also *sternoschisis, schistosternia,* and *sternal cleft.*

**ster•nu•ta•tion** (stər"nu-ta'shən) [L. *sternutatio*] sneeze (def. 2).

**ster•nu•ta•tor** (stər'nu-ta"tər) a gas or other substance that causes sneezing.

**ster•nu•ta•to•ry** (stər-nu'tə-tor"e) [L. *sternutatorius*] 1. producing or causing sneezing. 2. an agent that causes sneezing.

**stern·zel·len** (shtern'tsel-en) [Ger. "star cells"] Kupffer's cells.

**ster·oid** (ster'oid) any of a group of lipids that contain a hydrogenated cyclopentanoperhydrophenanthrene ring system. Some of the substances included in this group are progesterone, adrenocortical hormones, the gonadal hormones, cardiac aglycones, bile acids, sterols (such as cholesterol), toad poisons, saponins, and some of the carcinogenic hydrocarbons.
**adrenal cortical s., adrenocortical s.,** corticosteroid.
**anabolic s.,** any of a group of synthetic derivatives of testosterone having pronounced anabolic properties and relatively weak androgenic properties; they are used clinically mainly to promote growth and repair of body tissues in senility, debilitating illness, and convalescence.
**gonadal s.,** sex s.
**ovarian s.,** a gonadal steroid produced by the ovary, such as an estrogen or a progestational agent.
**sex s.,** a steroid hormone produced by a gonad, such as an estrogen, androgen, or progestational agent. Called also *gonadal s.*

**ster·oid 11β-mono·oxy·gen·ase** (ster'oid mon"o-ok'sə-jən-ās) [EC 1.14.15.4] an enzyme of the oxidoreductase class that catalyzes the NADPH-dependent hydroxylation of steroids at the 11 position as a step in the synthesis of steroid hormones. The enzyme is a mitochondrial cytochrome P-450 acting as a terminal oxidase in an electron transport chain that also includes adrenodoxin and a flavoprotein. Deficiency of the enzyme, an autosomal recessive trait, is called 11β-hydroxylase deficiency and causes congenital adrenal hyperplasia (type IV). The enzyme may include the enzyme activities of corticosterone 18-monooxygenase (q.v.). Called also *11β-hydroxylase.*

**ster·oid 17α-mono·oxy·gen·ase** (ster'oid mon"o-ok'sə-jən-ās) [EC 1.14.99.9] an enzyme of the oxidoreductase class that catalyzes the hydroxylation of steroids at the 17 position. The enzyme is a microsomal cytochrome P-450 that accepts electrons from NADPH via a flavoprotein. The reactions catalyzed are steps in the synthesis of steroid hormones, including cortisol, androgens, and estrogens. Deficiency of the enzyme, an autosomal recessive trait, is called 17α-hydroxylase deficiency and causes congenital adrenal hyperplasia (type V). The enzyme also possesses 17α-hydroxyprogesterone aldolase activity. Called also *17α-hydroxylase.*

**ster·oid 21-mono·oxy·gen·ase** (ster'oid mon"o-ok'sə-jən-ās) [EC 1.14.99.10] [MeSH: Steroid 21-Monooxygenase] an enzyme of the oxidoreductase class that catalyzes the NADPH-dependent hydroxylation of steroids at the 21 position. The enzyme is a microsomal cytochrome P-450, requires a flavoprotein for reducing equivalents, and is part of the steroid hormone synthesis system. Deficiency of the enzyme, an autosomal recessive trait, inhibits conversion of 17-hydroxyprogesterone to 11-deoxycortisol; it is called 21-hydroxylase deficiency (q.v.) and causes congenital adrenal hyperplasia (type III). Called also *21-hydroxylase.*

**ste·roi·do·gen·e·sis** (stə-roi"do-jen'ə-sis) the biosynthesis of steroids, as by the adrenal glands and gonads.

**ste·roi·do·gen·ic** (stə-roi'do-jen'ik) producing or giving rise to steroids.

**ster·oid sul·fa·tase** (ster'oid sul'fə-tās) steryl-sulfatase.

**ster·ols** (ster'olz) [*stereo-* + *-ol*] [MeSH: Sterols] steroids with long (8–10 carbons) aliphatic side-chains at position 17 and at least one alcoholic hydroxyl group, usually at position 3. They have lipid-like solubility. Examples are cholesterol and ergosterol.

**ster·ol O-ac·yl·trans·fer·ase** (ster'ol a"səl-trans'fər-ās) [EC 2.3.1.26] an enzyme of the transferase class that catalyzes the transfer of acyl groups from acyl coenzyme A to cholesterol to form cholesteryl esters, a step in the metabolism of cholesterol. Called also *acyl CoA:cholesterol acyltransferase* and *cholesterol acyltransferase.*

**ster·ol es·ter·ase** (ster'ol es'tər-ās) [EC 3.1.1.13] an enzyme of the hydrolase class that catalyzes the cleavage of cholesterol and other sterol esters and triglycerides. Deficiency of the lysosomal enzyme causes the allelic autosomal recessive disorders Wolman's disease and cholesteryl ester storage disease. Called also *acid lipase* and *cholesterol esterase.*

**ster·tor** (stər'tor) [L.] snore (def. 1).
**hen-cluck s.,** a respiration sound like a hen's cluck in cases of post-pharyngeal abscess.

**ster·to·rous** (stər'tə-rəs) characterized by snoring (stertor).

**ster·yl-sul·fa·tase** (ster'əl sul'fə-tās) [EC 3.1.6.2] a microsomal enzyme of the hydrolase class that catalyzes the cleavage of the sulfate group from sulfated sterols. Deficiency of the enzyme, an X-linked trait, causes X-linked ichthyosis. Called also *steroid sulfatase.*

**steth·acous·tic** (steth"ə-koos'tik) heard with the stethoscope.

**steth·al·gia** (steth-al'jə) 1. thoracalgia (def. 1). 2. pectoralgia (def. 1).

**steth(o)-** [Gr. *stēthos* chest] a combining form denoting relationship to the chest.

**stetho·cyr·to·graph** (steth"o-sir'to-graf) [*stetho-* + *cyrto-* + *-graph*] an instrument for measuring and recording the curves of the chest. Called also *stethokyrtograph.*

**stetho·go·ni·om·e·ter** (steth"o-go"ne-om'ə-tər) [*stetho-* + *goniometer*] an apparatus for measuring the curvature of the chest.

**stetho·graph** (steth'o-graf) [*stetho-* + *-graph*] an instrument for recording movements of the chest.

**steth·og·ra·phy** (steth-og'rə-fe) [*stetho-* + *-graphy*] use of the stethograph to record movements of the chest.

**stetho·kyr·to·graph** (steth"o-kir'to-graf) stethocyrtograph.

**steth·om·e·ter** (steth-om'ə-tər) [*stetho-* + *-meter*] an instrument for measuring the circular dimension or expansion of the chest. Called also *thoracometer.*

**stetho·my·itis** (steth"o-mi-i'tis) stethomyositis.

**stetho·my·o·si·tis** (steth"o-mi"o-si'tis) [*stetho* + *myo-* + *-itis*] inflammation of the muscles of the chest.

**stetho·pa·ral·y·sis** (steth"o-pə-ral'ĭ-sis) paralysis of the chest muscles.

**stetho·phone** (steth'o-fōn) [*stetho-* + Gr. *phōnē* voice] 1. an instrument designed to transmit stethoscopic sounds so that many persons can hear them simultaneously. 2. a term proposed as a more accurate name for stethoscope.

**stetho·pho·nom·e·ter** (steth"o-fo-nom'ə-tər) [*stetho-* + *phono-* + *-meter*] an instrument for measuring the intensity of auscultatory sounds.

**stetho·poly·scope** (steth"o-pol'ĭ-skōp) [*stetho-* + *poly-* + *-scope*] a stethoscope for the simultaneous use of several persons.

**stetho·scope** (steth'o-skōp) [*stetho-* + *-scope*] [MeSH: Stethoscopes] an instrument of various form, size, and material for performing mediate auscultation. By means of this instrument the respiratory, cardiac, pleural, arterial, venous, uterine, fetal, intestinal, and other sounds are conveyed to the ear of the observer.
**binaural s.,** one with two adjustable branches, designed for use with both ears.
**Cammann's s.,** a binaural stethoscope.
**DeLee-Hillis obstetric s.,** a stethoscope worn on the head of the examiner, used for listening to the fetal heart.
**differential s.,** one by means of which sounds at two different portions of the body may be compared.
**electronic s.,** an electronic amplifier of sounds within the body; selective controls permit tuning for low or high frequency tones. An auxiliary output permits the recording or viewing of audio patterns.
**esophageal s.,** one which is positioned within the esophagus to transmit heart and respiratory sounds.
**Leff s.,** one for listening to the fetal heart.

**stetho·scop·ic** (steth"o-skop'ik) pertaining to or performed by means of the stethoscope.

**steth·os·co·py** (steth-os'kə-pe) examination by means of the stethoscope.

**stetho·spasm** (steth'o-spaz-əm) spasm of the chest muscles.

**Ste·vens-John·son syndrome** (ste'vənz-jon'sən) [Albert Mason *Stevens,* American pediatrician, 1884–1945; Frank Chambliss *Johnson,* American pediatrician, 1894–1934] [MeSH: Stevens-Johnson Syndrome] see under *syndrome.*

**Ste·wart-Holmes sign** (stoo'ərt-hōmz) [Purves *Stewart,* English

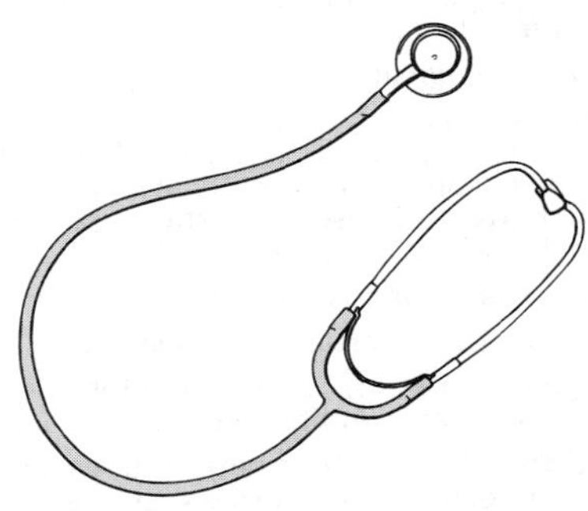

Stethoscope.

physician, 1869–1949; Eric Gordon *Holmes,* English neurologist, 1876–1965] rebound phenomenon.

**Ste·wart-Treves syndrome** (stoo′ərt-trēvz) [Fred Waldorf *Stewart,* American physician, born 1894; Norman *Treves,* American physician, 20th century] see under *syndrome.*

**sthe·nia** (sthe′ne-ə) [*sthen-* + *-ia*] a condition of strength and activity.

**sthen·ic** (sthen′ik) active; strong.

**sthen(o)-** [Gr. *sthenos* strength] a combining form denoting relationship to strength.

**sthen·om·e·try** (sthen-om′ə-tre) [*stheno-* + *-metry*] the measurement of bodily strength.

**STI** systolic time intervals.

**stib·i·al·ism** (stib′e-əl-iz-əm) [L. *stibium* antimony] antimony poisoning.

**stib·i·at·ed** (stib′e-āt″əd) containing antimony.

**stib·i·um** (stib′e-əm) [L.] antimony.

**stibo·cap·tate** (stib″o-kap′tāt) [BAN] a trivalent antimony compound, used as an antischistosomal, administered intramuscularly. Called also *antimony sodium dimercaptosuccinate* and *sodium stibocaptate.*

**stibo·phen** (stib′o-fən) a trivalent antimony compound, used as an anthelmintic, chiefly in the treatment of schistosomiasis due to *Schistosoma mansoni, S. haematobium,* and *S. japonicum.* It is now rarely used because of its toxicity.

**Stick·er's disease** (shtik′ərz) [Georg *Sticker,* German hygienist, 1860–1960] erythema infectiosum.

**Stick·ler's syndrome** (stik′lərz) [Gunnar B. *Stickler,* American physician, 20th century] hereditary progressive arthro-ophthalmopathy.

**Stie·da's disease, fracture** (shte′dahz) [Alfred *Stieda,* German surgeon, 1869–1945] see *Pellegrini's disease,* under *disease,* and see under *fracture.*

**Stie·da's process** (shte′dahz) [Ludwig *Stieda,* German anatomist, 1837–1918] processus posterior tali.

**Stier·lin's sign** (shtēr′linz) [Eduard *Stierlin,* German surgeon, 1878–1919] see under *sign.*

**stiff·ness** (stif′nəs) a quality of rigidity or inflexibility; see also *ankylosis.*

**chamber s.,** a term used for elastance when describing the cardiac ventricles.

**sti·fle** (sti′fəl) [MeSH: Stifle] stifle joint.

**stig·ma** (stig′mə) pl. *stig′mas* or *stig′mata* [Gr. "mark"] 1. any mental or physical mark or peculiarity which aids in the identification or in the diagnosis of a condition. 2. a mark, spot, or pore on the surface of an organ or organism. 3. follicular s. 4. in botany, the uppermost part of a pistil, which secretes a moist, sticky substance to trap and hold the pollen that reaches it. 5. an eyespot of chromatophore-bearing protozoa, such as certain euglenoids, comprising a dark pigmented mass that functions in light detection by shielding the photoreceptor cells from specific wavelengths. 6. a distinguishing personal trait that is perceived as or actually is physically, socially, or psychologically disadvantageous. 7. in the plural, gill slits around the pharynx in urochordates, through which pass respiratory and feeding currents. 8. in the plural, purpuric or hemorrhagic lesions of the hands and/or feet, which resemble crucifixion wounds.

**follicular s.,** a spot on the surface of an ovary where the vesicular follicle will rupture and permit passage of the ovum during ovulation. Called also *macula folliculi.*

**Giuffrida-Ruggieri s.,** abnormal shallowness of the glenoid fossa.

**malpighian s's,** the points where the smaller veins enter into the larger veins of the spleen.

**stig·mal** (stig′məl) stigmatic.

**stig·mas·te·rol** (stig-mas′tə-rol) [MeSH: Stigmasterol] an unsaturated plant sterol initially isolated from Calabar bean *(Physostigma)* and also occurring in other plant fats such as soybean oil, rape seed oils, and cocoa butter; it is used as a starting material in the manufacture of synthetic progesterone.

**stig·ma·ta** (stig′mə-tə) [Gr.] plural of *stigma.*

**stig·mat·ic** (stig-mat′ik) pertaining to a stigma.

**stig·ma·tism** (stig′mə-tiz-əm) 1. the condition due to or marked by stigmata. 2. the accurate rendition of points by a lens system.

**stig·ma·ti·za·tion** (stig″mə-tĭ-za′shən) 1. the act or process of developing or being identified as possessing one or more stigmata. 2. the act or process of negatively labeling or characterizing another. 3. stigmatism (def. 1).

**stig·ma·tom·e·ter** (stig″mə-tom′ə-tər) [*stigma* + *-meter*] an instrument for testing the refraction of the eye by retinoscopy and for direct ophthalmoscopy.

**stig·ma·to·phil·ia** (stig-mə-to-fil′e-ə) [Gr. *stigma* mark made by a pointed instrument + *-philia*] a paraphilia in which sexual excitement depends on piercing or tattooing the body.

**stil·baz·i·um io·dide** (stil-baz′e-əm) an anthelmintic, reported to be effective against roundworms, threadworms, and whipworms.

**Stil·bel·la·ceae** (stil-bə-la′se-e) a family of Fungi Imperfecti of the form-order Moniliales, including the genus *Dendrodochium.*

**stil·bene** (stil′bēn) an unsaturated hydrocarbon that is the nucleus of diethylstilbestrol and related compounds; it is used in the manufacture of dyes and optical bleaches.

**stil·bes·trol** (stil-bes′trol) diethylstilbestrol.

**Sti·le·sia** (sti-le′zhə) a genus of cestodes of the family Anoplocephalidae. *S. globipuncta′ta* is found in the small intestines of ruminants; heavy infestations can be fatal.

**sti·let** (sti-let′) [Fr. *stilette*] stylet.

**sti·lette** (sti-let′) [Fr.] stylet.

**Still's disease** (stilz) [Sir George Frederick *Still,* English physician, 1868–1941] see under *disease.*

**Still-Chauf·fard syndrome** (stil-sho-fahr′) [Sir G. F. *Still;* Anatole Marie Emile *Chauffard,* French physician, 1855–1932] Chauffard's syndrome.

**still·birth** (stil′birth) the delivery of a dead child; see *fetal death,* under *death.*

**still·born** (stil′born) born dead.

**Stil·ler's rib** (stil′ərz) [Berthold *Stiller,* Hungarian physician, 1837–1922] see under *rib.*

**Stil·ling's canal,** etc. (shtil′ingz) [Benedict *Stilling,* German anatomist, 1810–1879] see *canalis hyaloideus* and *nucleus thoracicus posterior* and see under *fiber* and *fleece.*

**Stil·ling's syndrome** (shtil′ingz) [Jakob *Stilling,* German ophthalmologist, 1842–1915] Duane's syndrome; see under *syndrome.*

**Stil·ling-Türk-Du·ane syndrome** (shtil′ing-tērk-dwān) [J. *Stilling;* Siegmund *Türk,* Swiss ophthalmologist, late 19th century; Alexander *Duane,* American ophthalmologist, 1858–1926] Duane's syndrome; see under *syndrome.*

**Stil·phos·trol** (stil-fos′trōl) trademark for a preparation of diethylstilbestrol diphosphate.

**sti·lus** (sti′ləs) pl. *sti′li* [L.] stylus.

**Stim·ate** (stim′āt) trademark for a preparation of desmopressin acetate.

**Stim·son's meth·od** (stim′sənz) [Lewis A. *Stimson,* American surgeon, 1844–1917] see under *method.*

**stim·u·lant** (stim′u-lənt) [L. *stimulans*] 1. producing stimulation; especially producing stimulation by causing tension on muscle fiber through the nervous tissue. 2. an agent or remedy that produces stimulation.

**central s.,** a stimulant of the central nervous system.

**cerebral s.,** one which exalts the functional activities of the brain.

**diffusible s.,** one which acts promptly and strongly, but transiently.

**general s.,** one which acts upon the whole body.

**local s.,** one which affects only, or mainly, that part to which it is applied.

**nervous s.,** one which acts mainly upon the nerve centers; a cerebral or a spinal stimulant.

**spinal s.,** one which acts upon and through the spinal cord.

**topical s.,** local s.

**uterine s.,** an agent which stimulates uterine contraction or menstruation.

**vascular s., vasomotor s.,** one which affects the vasomotor centers.

**stim·u·late** (stim′u-lāt) to excite to functional activity.

**stim·u·la·tion** (stim″u-la′shən) [L. *stimulatio,* from *stimulare* to goad] the act or process of stimulating; the condition of being stimulated.

**areal s.,** stimulation of an extended portion of a sense organ.

**audio-visual-tactile s.,** the simultaneous rhythmic excitation of the receptors for the senses of hearing, sight, and touch.

**functional electrical s. (FES),** the application of an electrical current by means of a prosthesis, some parts of which may be implanted, to stimulate and restore partial function to muscle disabled by neurological lesions.

**nonspecific s.,** stimulation of a sense organ by a modality other than the usual one, such as when pressure or an electric current stimulates the retina.

**paradoxical s.,** application of a warm object to one of the cold spots of the body produces a sensation of cold.

**paraspecific s.**, nonspecific s.
**punctual s.**, excitation of a sense organ by stimulation at a single point.
**repetitive nerve s.**, repeated supramaximal stimulation of a motor nerve while recording the M wave of its muscle to note any changes in the wave. Types of responses include the *decrementing response, incrementing response, postactivation exhaustion,* and *postactivation facilitation.*
**transcutaneous electrical nerve s. (TENS), transcutaneous nerve s. (TNS),** electrical stimulation of nerves for relief of pain, either by electrodes attached to the skin or by an apparatus manually held against the skin; the stimulus interferes with neural transmission of pain signals and thus has an analgesic effect.

**stim·u·la·tor** (stim'u-la"tər) 1. any agent that excites functional activity. 2. in electrodiagnosis, an instrument that applies pulses of current to stimulate a nerve, muscle, or area of the central nervous system.
**Bimler s.**, see under *appliance.*
**electronic s.**, stimulator (def. 2).
**human thyroid adenylate cyclase s's (HTACS),** thyroid-stimulating immunoglobulins.
**long-acting thyroid s. (LATS),** the original name given to thyroid-stimulating immunoglobulins, referring to a mouse bioassay in which thyroid stimulation by this substance peaks later than that induced by thyroid-stimulating hormone.

**stim·u·li** (stim'u-li) plural of *stimulus.*

**stim·u·lon** (stim'u-lon) a viral antigen postulated to have anti-interferon activity and which therefore promotes the multiplication of other viruses.

**stim·u·lus** (stim'u-ləs) pl. *stim'uli* [L. "goad"] any agent, act, or influence that produces functional or trophic reaction in a receptor or in an irritable tissue.
**adequate s.**, a stimulus of the specific form of energy to which the receptor is most sensitive; called also *homologous s.*
**aversive s.**, one which, when applied following the occurrence of a response, decreases the strength of that response on later occurrences.
**chemical s.**, a chemical substance capable of exciting a response in an organism mediated through specialized nerve endings.
**conditioned s.**, a stimulus that acquires the capacity to evoke a particular response by repeated pairing with another stimulus that is naturally capable of eliciting the response (*unconditioned s.*).
**discriminative s.**, a stimulus, associated with reinforcement, which exerts control over a particular form of behavior; the subject discriminates between closely related stimuli and responds positively only in the presence of that stimulus.
**electric s.**, a galvanic, induced, or other electric current or shock as applied to a responsive tissue.
**eliciting s.**, any stimulus, conditioned or unconditioned, which elicits a response.
**heterologous s.**, one which produces an effect or sensation when applied to any part of a nerve tract.
**heterotopic s.**, a stimulus to heart contraction arising elsewhere than in the sinoatrial node, the normal pacemaker of the heart.
**homologous s.**, adequate s.
**liminal s.**, threshold s.
**maximal s.**, a stimulus of just sufficient intensity to cause the maximal amplitude of the evoked potential; see also *supramaximal s.*
**mechanical s.**, a stimulant application of mechanical force, as in friction or pinching.
**patterned s.**, a photic stimulus consisting of a checkerboard or other pattern of alternating light and dark areas, used to elicit visual evoked potentials.
**reinforcing s.**, reinforcer.
**subliminal s.**, subthreshold s.
**subthreshold s.**, one well below the threshold.
**supraliminal s.**, suprathreshold s.
**supramaximal s.**, a stimulus more intense than a maximal one; used in electrodiagnostic studies to ensure that the evoked potential stays at its maximum level.
**suprathreshold s.**, one well above the threshold.
**threshold s.**, a stimulus that is just strong enough to elicit a response; see also *threshold* (defs. 1 and 2).
**unconditioned s.**, any stimulus naturally capable of eliciting a specific response.

**sting** (sting) [MeSH: Bites and Stings] 1. an injury caused by the venom of a plant or animal (biotoxin) introduced into the individual or with which he has come in contact, together with the mechanical trauma caused by the organ responsible for its introduction. 2. the organ used to inflict such injury.
**Irukandji s.**, see under *syndrome.*

**sting·er** (sting'er) colloquial term for pain, paresthesia, and transient weakness and numbness of the upper extremity caused by neurapraxia of the brachial plexus or a cervical nerve root.

**sting·ray** (sting'ra) any of various rays having sharp barbed venomous spines near the base of the tail; different species vary from a few centimeters to several meters in length. Stinging causes cardiovascular symptoms such as vasoconstriction and bradycardia.

**Sti·pa** (sti'pə) a genus of grasses (family Gramineae). *S. viri'dula* is sleepygrass, a species found in the southwestern United States that is poisonous to cattle and horses and is said to be a powerful narcotic, diuretic, sudorific, and cardiac poison.

**stipe** (stīp) [L. *stipes* tree trunk] in botany, a stalk, especially that of a mushroom or seaweed or the stem of a fern frond.

**stip·pling** (stip'ling) [Dutch *stippelen* to keep spotting] 1. the appearance of fine light or dark dots, or a spotted appearance. 2. the appearance of the retina as if dotted with light and dark points. 3. punctate basophilia. 4. gingival s.
**epiphyseal s.**, the radiographic appearance of punctate opacities in the epiphyses, representing foci of calcification; seen in chondrodysplasia punctata.
**gingival s.**, a condition in which the gingiva presents a minutely lobulated surface, like that of an orange peel, which is a normal adaptive process of the gingiva and its absence or reduction indicates gingival disease.
**malarial s.**, the finely granular appearance often seen in stained erythrocytes that harbor tertian malarial parasites; see *Maurer's s.* and *Schüffner's s.*
**Maurer's s.**, malarial stippling with Maurer's dots.
**Schüffner's s.**, malarial stippling with Schüffner's dots.

**sti·ro·fos** (sti'ro-fos) a veterinary insecticide.

**stir·pi·cul·tur·al** (stir"pĭ-kul'chər-əl) pertaining to stirpiculture.

**stir·pi·cul·ture** (stir'pĭ-kul"chər) [L. *stirps* stock + *culture*] the systematic attempt at improving a stock by attention to the laws of breeding.

**stir·rup** (stər'əp) 1. a structure or device resembling the stirrup of a saddle, or the portion of an apparatus on which to rest the feet. 2. the stapes.
**Finochietto's s.**, an apparatus for exerting skeletal traction in leg fractures, with a U-shaped steel band passed over the posterior process of the calcaneus and fixed by a cross bar, from which traction is applied.

**stitch** (stich) 1. suture (def. 2). 2. suture (def. 3). 3. a popular term for a severe, sudden pain, generally at the costal margin on one side.

**sto·chas·tic** (sto-kas'tik) [Gr. *stochastikos* conjecturing] pertaining to a random process, used particularly to refer to a time series of random variables.

**stoe·chi·ol·o·gy** (stek"e-ol'ə-je) stoichiology.

**Stoerk's blennorrhea** (shtərks) [Carl *Stoerk,* Austrian laryngologist, 1832–1899] see under *blennorrhea.*

**stoi·chi·ol·o·gy** (stoi"ke-ol'ə-je) [Gr. *stoicheion* element + *-logy*] the science of elements, especially the physiology of the cellular elements of tissues.

**stoi·chi·om·e·try** (stoi"ke-om'ə-tre) [Gr. *stoicheion* element + *-metry*] the study of the numerical relationships of chemical elements and compounds and the mathematical laws of chemical changes; the mathematics of chemistry.

**stoke** (stōk) a unit of kinematic viscosity, being that of fluid with a viscosity of 1 poise and a density of 1 gram per cubic centimeter. Abbreviated St.

**Stokes' amputation (operation)** (stōks) [Sir William *Stokes,* Irish surgeon, 1839–1900] Gritti-Stokes amputation.

**Stokes' collar, law, syndrome** (stōks) [William *Stokes,* Irish physician, 1804–1878] see under *collar* and *law* and see *Adams-Stokes syndrome,* under *syndrome.*

**Stokes-Ad·ams attack, syndrome (syncope)** (stōks-ad'əmz) [William *Stokes; Robert Adams,* Irish physician, 1791–1875] see *Adams-Stokes attack,* under *attack* and *Adams-Stokes syndrome,* under *syndrome.*

**Stok·vis-Tal·ma syndrome** (stok'vis-tahl'mah) [B.J.E. *Stokvis;* Sape *Talma,* Dutch physician, 1847–1918] enterogenous cyanosis.

**sto·lon** (sto'lon) [L. *stolo,* gen. *stolonis* shoot] a runner that can develop roots and a stem; in fungi an aerial hypha that forms rhizoids and an aerial mycelium when it contacts the surface of the substrate. See Plate 29.

**sto·ma** (sto'mə) pl. *sto'mas* or *sto'mata* [Gr. "mouth"] 1. any minute pore, orifice, or opening on a free surface. 2. the opening established in the abdominal wall by colostomy, ileostomy, or a similar operation. 3. the opening between two portions of the intestine in an anastomosis.

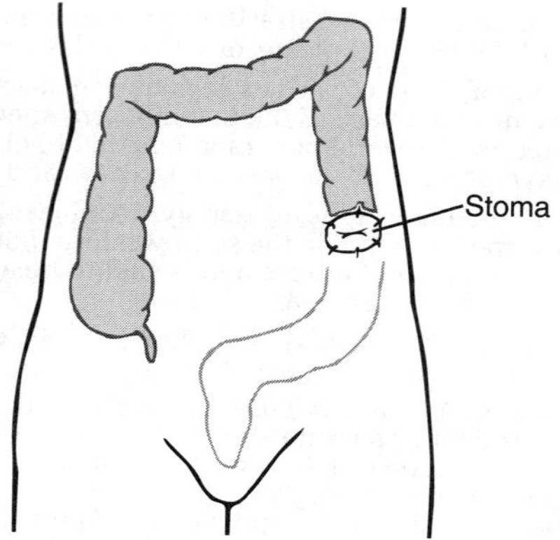

Stoma resulting from a descending colostomy.

**sto·mac·a·ce** (sto-mak′ə-se) [Gr. *stoma* mouth + *kakē* badness] ulcerative stomatitis.

**stom·ach** (stum′ək) [L. *stomachus;* Gr. *stomachos*] [MeSH: Stomach] 1. gaster. 2. in ruminants, any of four expansions of the alimentary canal between the esophagus and the duodenum; the first three, the *rumen, reticulum,* and *omasum,* are called *forestomachs,* and the fourth, the *abomasum,* is analogous to the stomach of a nonruminant. 3. the midgut of an invertebrate.
**aberrant umbilical s.,** an umbilical structure containing gastric mucosa.
**bilocular s.,** hourglass s.
**cardiac s.,** the portion of the stomach close to the esophagus.
**cascade s.,** an atypical form of hourglass stomach, characterized radiographically by a drawing up of the posterior wall; an opaque medium first fills the upper sac and then cascades into the lower sac.
**cup-and-spill s.,** a radiographic finding in which the barium remains for a time in the gastric fundus, before spilling over into the main cavity of the stomach, as a result of pressure by a distended colon.
**dumping s.,** a complication that sometimes follows partial gastrectomy and gastroenterostomy, in which food is emptied rapidly from the stomach into the jejunum through the new opening, producing weakness, sweating, palpitation, and varying degrees of syncope. See *dumping syndrome,* under *syndrome.*
**hourglass s.,** a stomach more or less completely and permanently divided into two parts, so that it resembles an hourglass in shape; the deformity is due to scarring which complicates chronic gastric ulcer.
**leather bottle s.,** linitis plastica.
**miniature s.,** Pavlov's s.
**Pavlov's s.,** a portion of the stomach of a dog isolated from communication with the rest of the stomach and opening on to the abdominal wall through a fistula; used in studying gastric secretion.
**sclerotic s.,** linitis plastica.
**thoracic s.,** a stomach which is situated or drawn up above the level of the diaphragm; i.e., that part of the stomach which has herniated through the diaphragmatic hiatus.
**trifid s.,** a stomach with two constrictions, producing three pouches.
**upside-down s.,** thoracic s.
**waterfall s.,** cascade s.
**watermelon s.,** a vascular anomaly of the gastric antrum, consisting of dilated and thrombosed capillaries and veins, which form lines in the antrum that radiate toward the pylorus and resemble the stripes on a watermelon.

**stom·a·chal** (stum′ə-kəl) gastric.

**stom·a·chal·gia** (stum″ə-kal′jə) gastrodynia.

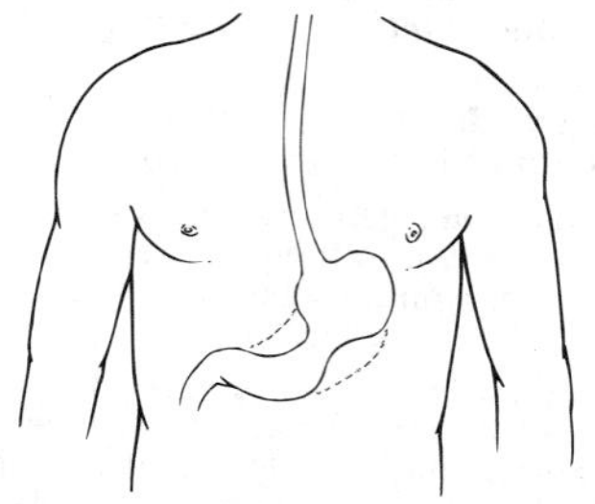
Hourglass stomach.

**sto·mach·ic** (sto-mak′ik) [L. *stomachicus;* Gr. *stomachikos*] 1. gastric. 2. a medicine which promotes the functional activity of the stomach.

**stom·a·cho·dyn·ia** (stum″ə-ko-din′e-ə) [*stomach* + *-odynia*] gastrodynia.

**sto·ma·de·um** (sto″mə-de′əm) stomodeum.

**sto·mal** (sto′məl) pertaining to a stoma or stomata.

**sto·mal·gia** (sto-mal′jə) stomatalgia.

**sto·ma·ta** (sto′mə-tə) [Gr.] plural of *stoma.*

**sto·ma·tal** (sto′mə-təl) pertaining to stomata.

**sto·ma·tal·gia** (sto″mə-tal′jə) pain in the mouth; called also *stomatodynia.*

**sto·mat·ic** (sto-mat′ik) pertaining to the mouth.

**sto·ma·tit·i·des** (sto″mə-tit′ĭ-dēz) [MeSH: Stomatitis] plural of *stomatitis.* A general term applied collectively to inflammatory conditions of the oral mucosa.

**sto·ma·ti·tis** (sto″mə-ti′tis) pl. *stomatit′ides* [*stomato-* + *-itis*] [MeSH: Stomatitis] inflammation of the oral mucosa, due to local or systemic factors, which may involve the buccal and labial mucosa, palate, tongue, floor of the mouth, and the gingivae.
**allergic s.,** stomatitis caused by exposure to allergens or as a manifestation of an allergic condition. See also *s. venenata.*
**angular s.,** perlèche.
**s. aphtho′sa, aphthous s.,** recurrent aphthous s.
**s. arsenica′lis,** stomatitis due to arsenic poisoning.
**bismuth s.,** stomatitis due to bismuth poisoning, characterized by a thin blue-black line in the marginal gingivae *(bismuth line),* pigmentation of the buccal mucosa, sore tongue, metallic taste, and a burning sensation of the mouth. Called also *bismuth gingivitis.*
**bovine papular s.,** a mild disease of young cattle, caused by a poxvirus, with oral lesions resembling those of foot-and-mouth disease.
**catarrhal s.,** transitory inflammation of the oral mucosa, sometimes with gingivitis, erythema, swelling, and occasionally epithelial desquamation; believed to be caused by the oral bacterial flora.
**contact s.,** s. venenata.
**denture s.,** inflammation of the oral mucosa seen in some patients with new dentures or with old, ill-fitting ones, caused by *Candida albicans*; characterized by redness, swelling, and pain of mucosa that is in contact with the denture. Called also *chronic atrophic candidiasis* and *denture sore mouth.*
**erythematopultaceous s.,** uremic s.
**s. exanthema′tica,** stomatitis secondary to an exanthematous disease.
**fusospirochetal s.,** necrotizing ulcerative gingivostomatitis.
**gangrenous s.,** noma (def. 1).
**gonococcal s.,** gonorrheal s.
**gonorrheal s.,** gonorrhea of the oral cavity, usually transmitted by orogenital contact, characterized by a linear or flattened eruption associated with redness, itching, and burning of the mucosa. Called also *gonococcal s.*
**herpetic s.,** herpes simplex involving the oral mucosa and lips, characterized by the formation of yellowish vesicles that rupture and produce ragged painful ulcers covered by a gray membrane and surrounded by an erythematous halo. Called also *vesicular s.*
**infectious s.,** a general term for a usually mild infection of the oral mucosa, beginning with a circumscribed red, itchy area.
**s. intertro′pica,** stomatitis associated with tropical sprue.
**lead s.,** the oral manifestations of lead poisoning, including the *lead line,* a bluish line along the free gingival margin, pigmentation of the mucosa in contact with the teeth, metallic taste, excessive salivation, and swelling of the salivary glands.
**s. medicamento′sa,** stomatitis due to an allergic reaction to drugs, ingested, absorbed through the skin or mucosa, or given by hypodermic injection. Principal symptoms include vesicles, erosion, ulcers, erythema, purpura, angioedema, burning, and itching. See also *s. venenata.*
**membranous s.,** infection of the oral mucosa, accompanied by the formation of a false membrane.
**mercurial s., mercury s.,** stomatitis due to mercury poisoning; symptoms include necrotic and ulcerative lesions and discoloration similar to lead lines of the gingivae, soreness of gums, strong metallic taste, foul breath, ptyalism, and necrosis of the alveolar process.
**mycotic s.,** thrush, def. 1.
**necrotic s.,** calf diphtheria in the oral cavity.
**s. nicoti′na,** a condition believed to be a variant of oral leukoplakia, seen in smokers of tobacco, particularly heavy pipe smokers. Characteristics include grayish white nodules or papules on the palate with a red spot in the center of each, representing dilated orifices of accessory palatal salivary glands; thickening, keratinization, and epithelial wrinkling with development of fissures and cracks may occur in later stages. Called also *smokers' palate* or *patches.*
**nonspecific s.,** inflammation of the oral mucosa occurring in asso-

ciation with other conditions, such as menstruation, diabetes, or uremia.
**recurrent aphthous s.,** a recurrent disease of unknown etiology, characterized by the appearance on the oral mucosa of one or more small round or oval ulcers that are covered by a grayish fibrinous exudate and surrounded by a bright red halo. The lesions usually persist for 7 to 14 days and then heal without scarring. A severe form is known as *periadenitis mucosa necrotica recurrens.* Called also *aphthae, aphthous s.,* and *canker sore.*
**s. scarlati'na,** a condition of the oral mucosa seen in scarlatina (scarlet fever), characterized in the early stages by fiery red coloration, congestion, and exudate of the throat, and by strawberry tongue and raspberry tongue in the later stages.
**s. scorbu'tica,** stomatitis associated with vitamin C deficiency, characterized by red swollen gums, gingival ulcers and gangrene, periodontal destruction, loose teeth, hemorrhage from the dental pulp, hypoplasia of the dental enamel, arrest of dentin formation, and exaggerated sensitivity of the oral mucosa to irritants. See also *scurvy.*
**syphilitic s.,** stomatitis due to systemic syphilis.
**tropical s.,** see under *sprue.*
**ulcerative s.,** stomatitis characterized by the appearance of shallow ulcers on the cheeks, tongue, and lips. Called also *stomacace* and *stomatocace.*
**ulcerative s. of sheep,** contagious ecthyma.
**uremic s.,** the oral manifestation of uremia, consisting of azotemic odor of the breath, erythema, exudation, ulcerations, pseudomembrane formation, and burning sensations. Called also *erythematopultaceous s.*
**s. venena'ta,** an allergic condition of the oral mucosa resulting from contact with a substance to which the patient is sensitized, including cosmetics, dentifrices, mouthwashes, and dental materials, as well as drugs applied topically; inflammation and edema of the mucosa accompanied by burning and sometimes itching are the principal symptoms. Called also *contact s.* See also *s. medicamentosa.*
**vesicular s.,** 1. herpetic s. 2. a viral infection in swine, cattle, and horses, caused by a rhabdovirus and characterized by vesicular eruptions on the oral mucosa. There may also be vesicles in swine on the snout and interdigital spaces, in cattle on the udder and teats, and in horses on the coronary band. It must be distinguished from foot-and-mouth disease.
**Vincent's s.,** acute necrotizing ulcerative gingivitis.

**stomat(o)-** [Gr. *stoma,* gen. *stomatos* mouth] a combining form denoting relationship to the mouth or to the ostium uteri. Also, *stom(o)-.*

**sto·ma·toc·a·ce** (sto″mə-tok′ə-se) [*stomato-* + Gr. *kakē* badness] ulcerative stomatitis.

**sto·ma·to·cyte** (sto′mə-to-sīt) an abnormal erythrocyte in which a slit or mouthlike area replaces the normal circle of pallor, usually due to edema. See also *stomatocytosis.*

**sto·ma·to·cy·to·sis** (sto″mə-to-si-to′sis) the presence of stomatocytes in the blood, as seen in liver disease, Rh null syndrome, a rare congenital type of hemolytic anemia, and a few other conditions. Called also *hydrocytosis.*

**sto·ma·to·dyn·ia** (sto″mə-to-din′e-ə) [*stomat-* + *-odynia*] stomatalgia.

**sto·ma·to·dys·o·dia** (sto″mə-to-dis-o′de-ə) [*stomato-* + Gr. *dysōdia* stench] halitosis.

**sto·ma·to·gen·e·sis** (sto″mə-to-jen′ə-sis) [*stomato-* + *genesis*] a morphologic process seen in ciliate protozoa in which all oral structures and associated organelles are formed or existing ones are replaced.

**sto·ma·to·glos·si·tis** (sto″mə-to-glos-i′tis) inflammation involving the oral mucous membranes and the tongue, occurring in nutritional disorders such as pellagra, beriberi, vitamin B complex deficiency, and in infections, etc.

**sto·ma·tog·nath·ic** (sto″mə-tog-nath′ik) [*stomato-* + *gnathic*] denoting the mouth and jaws collectively.

**sto·ma·tog·ra·phy** (sto″mə-tog′rə-fe) [*stomato-* + *-graphy*] a description of the mouth.

**sto·ma·to·la·lia** (sto″mə-to-la′le-ə) [*stomato-* + *lal-* + *-ia*] hyponasality.

**sto·ma·to·log·i·cal** (sto″mə-to-loj′ĭ-kəl) pertaining to stomatology.

**sto·ma·tol·o·gist** (sto″mə-tol′ə-jist) an expert in stomatology.

**sto·ma·tol·o·gy** (sto″mə-tol′ə-je) [*stomato-* + *-logy*] the branch of medical science concerning the mouth and its diseases, functions, and structure; called also *oralogy.* See also *dentistry.*

**sto·ma·to·ma·la·cia** (sto″mə-to-mə-la′she-ə) [*stomato-* + *malacia*] excessive or abnormal softness of the oral structures.

**sto·ma·to·me·nia** (sto″mə-to-me′ne-ə) [*stomato-* + *men-*+ *-ia*] bleeding from the mucous membrane of the mouth at the time of menstruation.

**sto·mat·o·my** (sto-mat′ə-me) [*stoma-* + *-tomy*] surgical incision of the ostium uteri.

**sto·ma·to·my·co·sis** (sto″mə-to-mi-ko′sis) [*stomato-* + *mycosis*] any oral disease due to a fungus.

**sto·ma·top·a·thy** (sto″mə-top′ə-the) [*stomato-* + *-pathy*] any pathological condition of the mouth.

**sto·ma·to·plas·tic** (sto″mə-to-plas′tik) pertaining to stomatoplasty.

**sto·ma·to·plas·ty** (sto′mə-to-plas″te) [*stomato-* + *-plasty*] plastic repair of defects of or reconstruction of the mouth.

**sto·ma·tor·rha·gia** (sto″mə-to-ra′jə) [*stomato-* + *-rrhagia*] hemorrhage from the mouth.
**s. gingiva'rum,** hemorrhage from the gingivae.

**sto·ma·tos·chi·sis** (sto″mə-tos′kĭ-sis) [*stomato-* + *-schisis*] cleft lip.

**sto·ma·to·scope** (sto-mat′o-skōp) [*stomato-* + *-scope*] an instrument used in inspecting the mouth.

**sto·ma·tot·o·my** (sto″mə-tot′ə-me) stomatomy.

**sto·men·ceph·a·lus** (sto″mən-sef′ə-ləs) stomocephalus.

**sto·mi·on** (sto′me-ən) [Gr. *stomion,* dim. of *stoma* mouth] a cephalometric landmark, being the midpoint in the oral fissure when the lips are closed.

**stom(o)-** see *stomat(o)-.*

**sto·mo·ceph·a·lus** (sto″mo-sef′ə-ləs) [*stomo-* + *-cephalus*] a fetus with a rudimentary head and jaws, so that the skin hangs in folds about the mouth.

**sto·mo·de·al** (sto″mo-de′əl) pertaining to the stomodeum.

**sto·mo·de·um** (sto″mo-de′əm) [*stomo-* + Gr. *hodaios* pertaining to a way] an invagination of the surface ectoderm of the embryo during the fourth week, at the point where later the mouth is formed.

**sto·mos·chi·sis** (sto-mos′kĭ-sis) [*stomo-* + *-schisis*] cleft lip.

**Sto·mox·ys** (sto-mok′sis) a genus of flies of the family Muscidae. *S. bouffar'di* transmits trypanosomes to goats in South America. *S. cal'citrans* is the stable fly, a common pest that bites humans and livestock and transmits many diseases, such as anthrax, infectious anemia, surra, and tetanus.

**-stomy** (sto′me) [Gr. *stoma* mouth] a word termination denoting the surgical creation of an artificial opening into a hollow organ (colostomy, tracheostomy) or a new opening between two such structures (gastroenterostomy, pyeloureterostomy); also denoting the opening so created.

**stone** (stōn) 1. calculus. 2. a unit of weight in Great Britain, the equivalent of 14 pounds (avoirdupois), or about 6.34 kg (metric). 3. an abrading instrument or tool, such as one used for sharpening instruments.
**bladder s.,** vesical calculus.
**blue s.,** cupric sulfate.
**chalk s.,** articular calculus.
**dental s.,** a very strong dental plaster composed chiefly of the $\alpha$-hemihydrate of gypsum, used for construction of casts of the oral structures.
**infection s.,** struvite calculus.
**kidney s.,** renal calculus.
**pulp s.,** denticle, def. 2.
**salivary s.,** sialolith.
**skin s's,** calcareous nodules in the skin.
**tear s.,** dacryolith.
**vein s.,** phlebolith.
**womb s.,** uterine calculus.

**Stook·ey's reflex** (stook′ēz) [Byron Polk *Stookey,* American neurologic surgeon, 1887–1966] see under *reflex.*

**stool** (stōōl) feces.
**bilious s.,** yellowish or brownish feces, turning darker on exposure, that are characteristic of bilious diarrhea.
**caddy s.,** dark, sandy feces seen in yellow fever.
**fatty s.,** feces containing fat; seen in diseases of the pancreas and in malabsorption syndromes.
**lienteric s.,** feces containing much undigested food.
**mucous s.,** feces containing a large amount of mucus; seen in intestinal inflammation or mucous colitis.
**pea soup s.,** the characteristic liquid evacuation of typhoid fever.
**pipe-stem s.,** feces shaped like a pipe stem, seen in stricture of the lower rectum.
**ribbon s.,** long flattened feces seen in lower rectal stricture.
**rice-water s's,** the characteristic and diagnostic watery, light gray to clear diarrhea of cholera, containing flecks of mucous material, epithelial cells, and many cholera vibrios.

**sago-grain s.,** feces seen in amebiasis, consisting of diarrhea containing small flecks of blood-stained mucus.
**silver s.,** silver- colored feces due to a mixture of melena and white fatty feces, seen in tropical sprue and in children with diarrhea who are given sulfonamides, and is indicative of biliary tract obstruction.
**spinach s.,** dark green feces, the color of cooked spinach, resulting from the use of calomel in infants.

**stop** (stop) 1. to come to a halt. 2. to cease, discontinue, or arrest. 3. any device that serves to prevent further progression or advancement. 4. plosive.
**centric s.,** facies approximalis dentis.
**glottal s.,** a speech sound made by closure of the glottis and then an explosive release.
**occlusal s.,** see under *rest.*

**sto·rax** (stor'aks) [L. *storax, styrax,* from Gr. *styrax*] [USP] a balsam from the trunk of *Liquidambar orientalis* Mill (Levant s.), a tree of western Asia, or of *L. styraciflua* L. (American s.) of North America, used as an ingredient of compound benzoin tincture (see under *tincture*). It has been used as an expectorant and topical parasiticide. Called also *styrax.*

**stor·i·form** (stor'ĭ-form) [L. *storea, storia* a rush mat + *form*] denoting a matted, irregularly whorled pattern, somewhat resembling that of a straw mat; said of the microscopic appearance of dermatofibromas.

**storm** (storm) crisis (def. 2).
**thyroid s., thyrotoxic s.,** see under *crisis.*

**Storm van Leeu·wen chamber** (storm vahn la'vən) [William *Storm van Leeuwen,* Dutch pharmacologist, 1882–1933] see under *chamber.*

**Stox·il** (stok'sil) trademark for a preparation of idoxuridine.

**STP** 1. standard temperature and pressure: 0°C and 760 mm Hg. 2. slang term for the hallucinogen 2,5-dimethoxy-4-methamphetamine (DOM).

**stra·bis·mal** (strə-biz'məl) strabismic.

**stra·bis·mic** (strə-biz'mik) pertaining to or of the nature of strabismus.

**stra·bis·mol·o·gy** (strə"biz-mol'ə-je) the study of strabismus.

**stra·bis·mom·e·ter** (strə"biz-mom'ə-tər) [*strabismus* + *-meter*] an apparatus for measuring strabismus; called also *ophthalmotropometer* and *strabometer.*

**stra·bis·mom·e·try** (strə"biz-mom'ə-tre) [*strabismus* + *-metry*] measurement of the amount of strabismus; called also *ophthalmotropometry* and *strabometry.*

**stra·bis·mus** (strə-biz'məs) [Gr. *strabismos* a squinting] [MeSH: Strabismus] deviation of the eye which the patient cannot overcome. The visual axes assume a position relative to each other different from that required by the physiological conditions. The various forms of strabismus are spoken of as tropias, their direction being indicated by the appropriate prefix, as *cyclo*tropia, *eso*tropia, *exo*tropia, *hyper*tropia, and *hypo*tropia. Called also *cast, heterotropia, manifest deviation,* and *squint.*
**absolute s.,** that which occurs at all distances of the fixation point; called also *constant s.*
**accommodative s.,** that which is due to excessive or deficient accommodative effort.
**alternating s., bilateral s., binocular s.,** that which affects each eye alternately.
**comitant s., concomitant s.,** that which is due to faulty insertion of the eye muscles, resulting in the same amount of deviation in whatever direction the eyes are looking, because the squinting eye follows the movements of the other eye; called also *muscular s.* and *concomitant squint.*
**constant s.,** absolute s.
**convergent s.,** esotropia.
**cyclic s.,** intermittent strabismus that recurs at regular intervals.
**s. deor'sum ver'gens,** that in which the visual axis of the squinting eye falls below the fixation point.
**divergent s.,** exotropia.
**external s.,** exotropia.
**incomitant s.,** nonconcomitant s.
**intermittent s.,** that which occurs only at intervals.
**internal s.,** esotropia.
**kinetic s.,** strabismus due to spasm of the muscles controlling ocular movements.
**latent s.,** that which occurs only when one eye is occluded.
**manifest s.,** strabismus that is evident in binocular vision.
**mechanical s.,** that due to pressure or traction on the eye, as by a tumor, producing deflection.
**monocular s., monolateral s.,** unilateral s.
**muscular s.,** concomitant s.
**noncomitant s., nonconcomitant s.,** that in which the amount of deviation of the squinting eye varies according to the direction in which the eyes are turned; called also *incomitant s.*
**nonparalytic s.,** concomitant strabismus that is not due to paralysis of the extraocular muscles.
**paralytic s.,** that which is due to paralysis of an eye muscle.
**s. sur'sum ver'gens,** that in which the visual axis of the squinting eye lies above the fixation point.
**unilateral s., uniocular s.,** strabismus affecting only one eye.
**vertical s.,** strabismus in which the deviation of the visual axis is in the vertical plane; see *hypertropia* and *hypotropia.*

**stra·bom·e·ter** (strə-bom'ə-tər) strabismometer.

**stra·bom·e·try** (strə-bom'ə-tre) strabismometry.

**strabo·tome** (strab'o-tōm) a knife for performing strabotomy.

**stra·bot·o·my** (strə-bot'ə-me) [Gr. *strabos* squinting + *-tomy*] the cutting of the tendon of a muscle of the eye in treatment of strabismus.

**Stra·chan's syndrome** (strawnz) [William Henry Williams *Strachan,* British physician, 1857–1921] see under *syndrome.*

**Stra·chan-Scott syndrome** (strawn-skot) [W.H.W. *Strachan;* Sir Henry Harold *Scott,* British physician, 1874–1956] Strachan's syndrome.

**strah·len** (strah'lən) [Ger. "streaming," "ray"] a large locomotor organelle resembling an axopodium; seen in protozoa of the subclass Piroplasmia.

**strain** (strān) [MeSH: Sprains and Strains] 1. to overexercise; to use to an extreme and harmful degree. 2. excessive effort or undue exercise. 3. an overstretching or overexertion of some part of the musculature. 4. to filter or subject to colation. 5. change in the size or shape of a body as the result of an externally applied force; expressed as the fractional or percentage change in dimension resulting from the application of stress (q.v.). 6. a group of organisms within a species or variety, characterized by some particular quality, as rough or smooth strains of bacteria.
**cell s.,** cells derived from a primary culture or cell line by the selection and cloning of cells having specific properties.
**heterologous s.,** a strain of microorganisms different from the strain originally isolated, tested, etc.
**high-jumper's s.,** strain of the rotator muscles of the thigh occurring in high jumpers.
**homologous s.,** a strain of microorganisms similar to the strain originally isolated, tested, etc.
**reference s.,** a strain of bacteria or other microorganisms used as a standard of reference, which appears to meet the criteria of the type strain but is not officially accepted as a neotype.
**resistant s.,** a strain of organisms that is resistant to the effects of the agents, such as antibiotics or insecticides, used to control them.
**R s.,** the rough strain that results from bacterial dissociation; R colonies have a dull, uneven surface and irregular border, the growth in fluid media tends to flake out, no capsules are seen, and the culture tends to be less virulent.
**S s.,** the smooth strain that results from bacterial dissociation. The S colonies have a smooth surface and an unbroken border, growth in fluid media tends to be diffuse; capsules, if present at all, are found in this strain, and the culture tends to be more virulent.
**Vi s.,** a strain of bacteria, especially *Salmonella typhi,* that contains the Vi (virulence) antigen of Felix.
**wild-type s.,** the strain used as a standard for a given species or variety of organism, usually presumed to be the type found in nature. See also *wild type,* under *type.*

**strain·er** (strān'ər) an apparatus for straining.

**strait** (strāt) a narrow passageway.
**pelvic s., inferior,** apertura pelvis inferior.
**pelvic s., superior,** apertura pelvis superior.

**strait·jack·et** (strāt'jak"ət) informal name for *camisole.*

**stra·mo·ni·um** (strə-mo'ne-əm) [MeSH: Stramonium] 1. *Datura stramonium.* 2. the dried leaf and flowering or fruiting tops of *Datura stramonium;* used like belladonna and in the treatment of asthma. Called also *thorn apple.*

**strand** (strand) a thread or fiber or a structure resembling one.
**antisense s.,** the strand of a double-stranded nucleic acid that is complementary to the sense strand, in DNA being thus the template strand on which the mRNA is synthesized. Cf. *sense s.* See also *antisense RNA.*
**Billroth's s's,** trabeculae splenici.
**coding s.,** sense s.
**lateral enamel s.,** lateral dental lamina.
**sense s.,** the strand of a double-stranded nucleic acid that encodes the product; in DNA it is the strand that encodes the RNA, having thus the same base sequence except changing T for U in the RNA. Called also *coding s.* Cf. *antisense s.*
**template s.,** antisense s.

**stran·gal·es·the·sia** (strang″gəl-əs-the′zhə) [Gr. *strangalizein* to choke + *esthsia*] zonesthesia.

**stran·gle** (strang′gəl) [L. *strangulare*] choke (def. 1).

**stran·gles** (strang′gəlz) 1. in horses, an infectious disease characterized by a mucopurulent inflammation of the respiratory mucous membrane, with lymph node abscesses, and caused by *Streptococcus equi.* Called also *equine* or *horse distemper.* 2. in pigs, infection of the lymph nodes of the neck and pharynx with heavily encapsulated abscesses.
**bastard s.,** a usually fatal complication of strangles in horses involving spread of abscesses to organs such as the lungs, brain, or lymph nodes of the trunk.
**puppy s.,** juvenile pyoderma.

**stran·gu·lat·ed** (strang′gu-lāt′əd) [L. *strangulatus*] congested by reason of constriction or hernial stricture, with compromise of the blood supply; see *hernia.*

**stran·gu·la·tion** (strang″gu-la′shən) [L. *strangulatio*] 1. choke (def. 2). 2. arrest of the circulation in a part, due to compression. See *hemostasis* (def. 2).

**stran·gu·ria** (strang-gu′re-ə) strangury.

**stran·gu·ry** (strang′gu-re) [Gr. *stranx* drop + *ouron* urine] slow and painful discharge of the urine, due to spasm of the urethra and bladder.

**strap** (strap) 1. a band or strip, such as a strap muscle. 2. a band of adhesive tape used in attaching parts to each other; see also *strapping.* 3. to bind down tightly.
**Montgomery s's,** straps made of lengths of adhesive tape, used to secure dressings that must be changed frequently. Called also *Montgomery's tapes.*

**strap·ping** (strap′ing) the application of strips of adhesive tape, one overlapping the other, to cover and exert pressure upon an extremity or other area of the body; see Plate 46, and see also *bandaging.*
**Gibney's s.,** see under *bandage.*

**Stras·bur·ger's cell plate** (shtrahs′boorg-ərz) [Eduard Adolf *Strasburger,* German botanist, 1844–1912] midbody.

**stra·ta** (stra′tə) [L.] plural of *stratum.*

**strat·i·fi·ca·tion** (strat″ĭ-fĭ-ka′shən) [L. *stratum* layer + *facere* to make] disposal in layers.

**strat·i·fied** (strat′ĭ-fīd) disposed in layers.

**strat·i·form** (strat′ĭ-form) [*stratum* + *-form*] having the form of strata.

**stra·tig·ra·phy** (strə-tig′rə-fe) [*stratum* + *-graphy*] tomography.

**stra·tum** (stra′təm) pl. *stra′ta* [L.] [TA] a general term in anatomical nomenclature for a sheetlike mass of substance; see also *layer* and *lamina.*

## Stratum

Descriptions are given on TA terms, and include anglicized names of specific terms.

**s. adamanti′num,** dental enamel.
**s. basa′le,** basal layer: the deepest layer of the endometrium, which contains the blind ends of the uterine glands; the cells of this layer undergo minimal change during the sexual cycle.
**s. basa′le epider′midis,** basal layer of epidermis: the deepest stratum of the epidermis, composed of a single layer of deeply basophilic cells. See figure at *epidermis* and see also *s. germinativum.* Called also *s. cylindricum epidermidis.*
**cerebral s. of retina, s. cerebra′le re′tinae,** pars nervosa retinae.
**s. cine′reum,** s. griseum superficiale colliculi superioris.
**circular s. of tympanic membrane,** s. circulare membranae tympanicae.
**s. circula′re gas′tris,** s. circulare tunicae muscularis gastris.

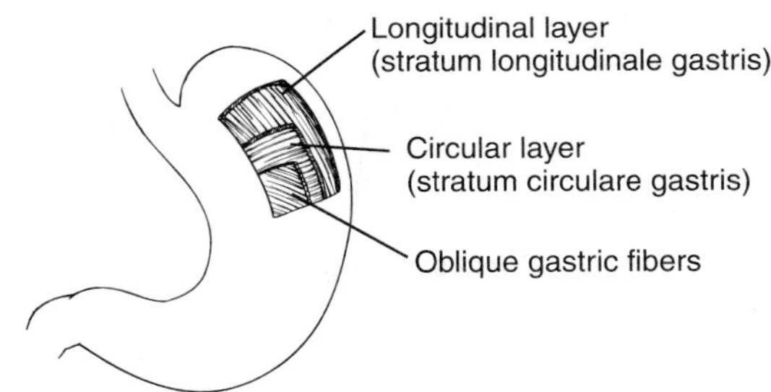


Layers (strata) of the muscular tunic of stomach.

**s. circula′re membra′nae tympa′nicae,** circular layer of tympanic membrane: the inner part of the fibrous stratum of the membrane, consisting of circularly coursing fibers deep to the mucous layer of the tympanic membrane; it is best developed near the periphery.
**s. circula′re tu′nicae muscula′ris co′li** [TA], circular layer of muscular coat of colon: the inner layer of circularly coursing fibers in the muscular coat of the colon.
**s. circula′re tu′nicae muscula′ris gas′tris** [TA], circular layer of muscular coat of stomach: the layer of circularly coursing fibers in the muscular coat of the stomach. Called also *s. circulare tunicae muscularis ventriculi.*
**s. circula′re tu′nicae muscula′ris intesti′ni ten′uis** [TA], circular layer of muscular coat of small intestine: the inner layer of circularly coursing fibers in the muscular coat of the small intestine.
**s. circula′re tu′nicae muscula′ris rec′ti** [TA], circular layer of muscular coat of rectum: the inner layer of circularly coursing fibers in the muscular coat of the rectum.
**s. circula′re tu′nicae muscula′ris ventri′culi,** s. circulare tunicae muscularis gastris.
**s. circula′re ventri′culi,** stratum circulare tunicae muscularis gastris.
**stra′ta colli′culi rostra′lis, stra′ta colli′culi superio′ris,** see *strata grisea et alba colliculi superioris.*
**s. compac′tum,** compact layer: the layer of the endometrium nearest the surface, which contains the necks of the uterine glands; together with the stratum spongiosum, it forms the *stratum functionale* (q.v.).
**s. cor′neum epider′midis,** horny layer of epidermis: the outermost layer of the epidermis, consisting of cells that are dead and desquamating. See figure at *epidermis.*
**s. cor′neum un′guis,** horny layer of nail: the outer, compact layer of the nail; called also *nail plate.*
**s. cuta′neum membra′nae tympa′nicae,** cutaneous layer of tympanic membrane: a very thin form of skin that constitutes the lateral layer of the tympanic membrane.
**s. cylin′dricum epider′midis,** s. basale epidermidis.
**s. ebo′ris,** dentinum.
**s. exter′num tu′nicae muscula′ris duc′tus deferen′tis,** the outer layer of fibers in the muscular coat of the ductus deferens.
**s. exter′num tu′nicae muscula′ris ure′teris,** the outer layer of fibers in the muscular coat of the ureter.
**s. exter′num tu′nicae muscula′ris ves′icae urina′riae,** the outer layer of fibers in the muscular coat of the urinary bladder.
**s. fibro′sum cap′sulae articula′ris,** TA alternative for *membrana fibrosa capsulae articularis.*
**s. fibro′sum vagi′nae ten′dinis** [TA], the fibrous layer of a tendon sheath.
**fibrous s. of tympanic membrane,** the middle layer of the membrane, consisting of radiating fibers externally *(stratum radiatum)* and circular fibers internally *(stratum circulare).* Called also *fibrous layer of tympanic membrane* and *lamina propria membranae tympanicae.*
**s. functiona′le,** functional layer: the stratum compactum and stratum spongiosum considered together (i.e., all of the endometrium except for the stratum basale), the cells of which are cast off at menstruation and at parturition. It is known as the *decidua* during pregnancy. Called also *pars functionalis.*
**s. gangliona′re ner′vi op′tici,** ganglionic layer of optic nerve; see under *layer.*
**s. gangliona′re re′tinae,** s. ganglionicum retinae.
**ganglionic s. of optic nerve,** see under *layer.*
**ganglionic s. of retina, s. ganglio′nicum re′tinae** [TA], the layer of the nervous part of the retina that contains the bipolar cells; see also *retina.* Called also *ganglionic layer of retina* and *s. ganglionare retinae.*
**s. germinati′vum, s. germinati′vum epider′midis [Malpi′ghii],** germinative layer: the stratum basale epidermidis and the stratum spinosum epidermidis considered as a single layer. The term is also sometimes used to designate only the stratum basale epidermidis. Called also *germinative layer of epidermis, malpighian layer* or *rete, mucous layer,* and *s. malpighii.*
**s. germinati′vum un′guis,** germinative layer of nail: the lower layer

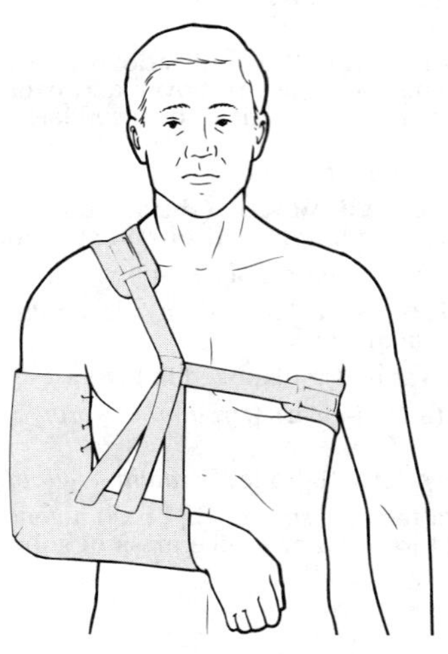

Strapping for acromioclavicular dislocation

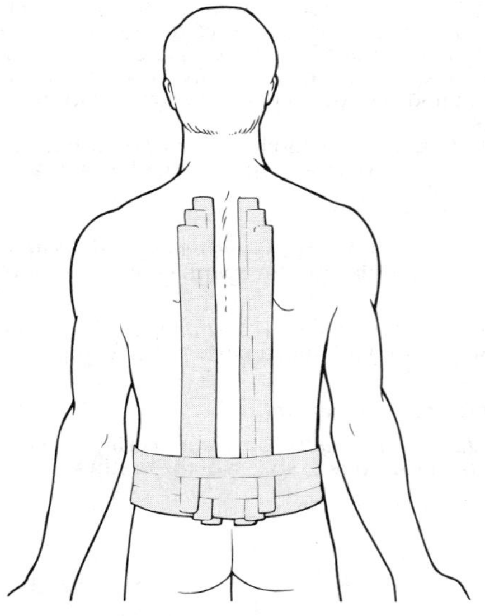

Strapping of the trunk to prevent rotation and flexion

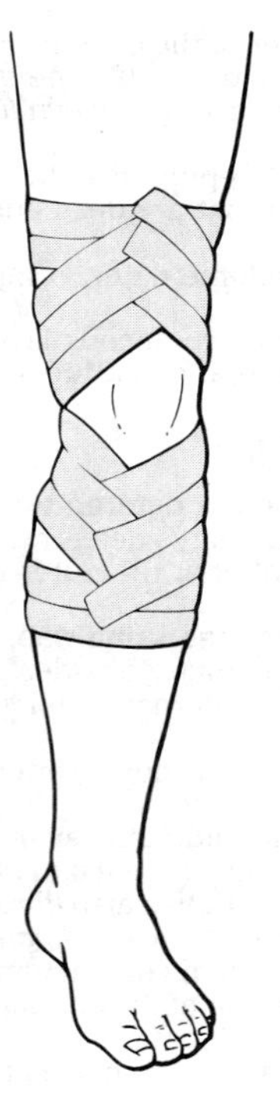

Knee strapping

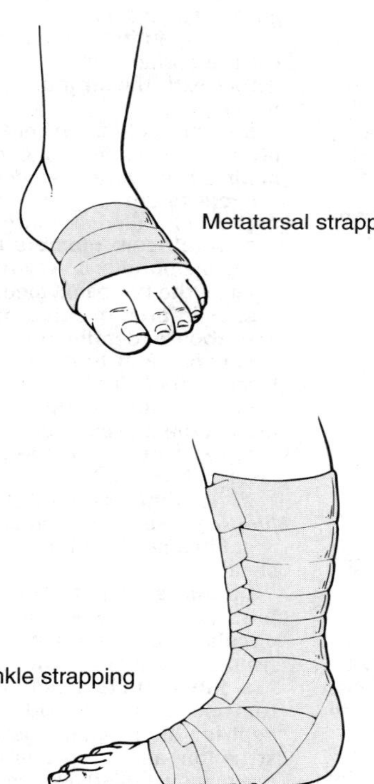

Metatarsal strapping

Ankle strapping

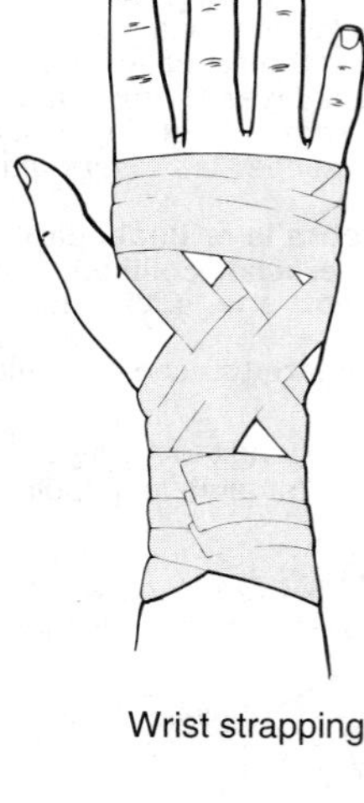

Wrist strapping

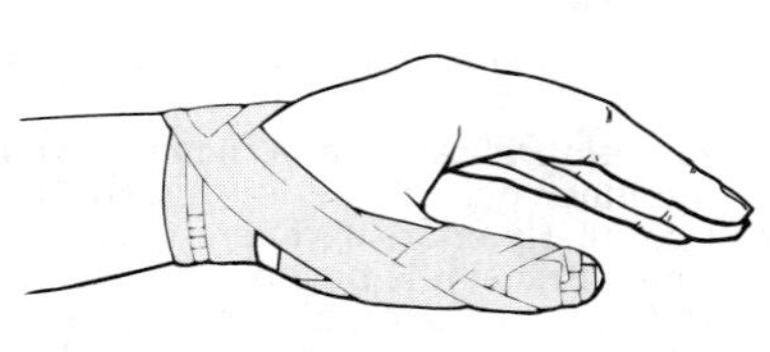

Sprained thumb strapping

**PLATE 46**—VARIOUS TYPES OF STRAPPING

of the nail, from which the nail grows; it is continuous with the stratum basale and stratum spinosum of the epidermis. Called also *nail plate.*

**s. granulo'sum cerebel'li** [TA], granular layer of cerebellum: the deep layer of the cortex of the cerebellum; it contains many small neurons (granule cells) and is separated from the molecular layer by the Purkinje cell layer.

**s. granulo'sum epider'midis,** granular layer of epidermis: the layer of the epidermis between the stratum lucidum epidermidis and the stratum spinosum epidermidis. See figure at *epidermis.* See also *s. corneum epidermidis.*

**s. granulo'sum folli'culi oo'phori vesiculo'si,** s. granulosum folliculi ovarici vesiculosi.

**s. granulo'sum folli'culi ova'rici vesiculo'si, s. granulo'sum ova'rii,** granular layer of follicle of ovary: the layer of follicle cells lining the theca of a vesicular ovarian follicle.

**stra'ta gri'sea et al'ba colli'culi rostra'lis,** strata grisea et alba colliculi superioris.

**stra'ta gri'sea et al'ba colli'culi superio'ris,** gray and white layers of superior colliculus: the four deepest layers of the colliculus (layers IV–VII), two gray and two white, consisting of nerve cells of various types; the intermediate gray and white layers are the main afferent area of the colliculus, and the deep gray and white layers are the main efferent area of the colliculus. See also *layers of superior colliculus.*

**s. gri'seum interme'dium colli'culi superio'ris** [TA], intermediate gray layer of superior colliculus: the outer gray layer of the gray and white layers of the superior colliculus; it is Layer IV of the colliculus. See *strata grisea et alba colliculi superioris.*

**s. gri'seum profun'dum colli'culi superio'ris** [TA], deep gray layer of superior colliculus: the inner gray layer of the gray and white layers of the superior colliculus; it is Layer VI of the colliculus. See *strata grisea et alba colliculi superioris.*

**s. gri'seum superficia'le colli'culi superio'ris** [TA], superficial gray layer of superior colliculus: a layer containing many small multipolar nerve cells which synapse with neurons from the overlying zonal layer and the underlying optic layer; it is Layer II of the colliculus. Called also *s. cinereum.*

**s. interme'dium,** the layer of cells of the enamel organ of a tooth just peripheral to the ameloblastic layer.

**s. lacuno'sum,** the fibrous layer situated between the stratum radiatum and the stratum moleculare of the hippocampus, consisting chiefly of a dense fiber layer in association with Schaffer collaterals, axons ascending from the alveus, and axons and collaterals ascending from neurons of the stratum oriens.

**s. lemnis'ci,** the strata (grisea et alba) colliculi superioris considered as a single layer.

**s. longitudina'le gas'tris,** s. longitudinale tunicae muscularis gastris.

**s. longitudina'le tu'nicae muscula'ris co'li** [TA], longitudinal layer of muscular coat of colon: the outer layer of the muscular coat of the colon, consisting of longitudinally coursing fibers; it is thick in the regions of the three teniae coli and very thin between them.

**s. longitudina'le tu'nicae muscula'ris gas'tris** [TA], longitudinal layer of muscular coat of stomach: the layer of longitudinally coursing fibers in the muscular coat of the stomach. Called also *s. longitudinale tunicae muscularis ventriculi.*

**s. longitudina'le tu'nicae muscula'ris intesti'ni ten'uis** [TA], longitudinal layer of muscular coat of small intestine: the outer layer of the muscular coat of the small intestine, consisting of longitudinally coursing fibers.

**s. longitudina'le tu'nicae muscula'ris rec'ti** [TA], longitudinal layer of muscular tunic of rectum: the outer layer of the muscular coat of the rectum, consisting of longitudinally coursing fibers.

**s. longitudina'le tu'nicae muscula'ris ventri'culi,** s. longitudinale tunicae muscularis gastris.

**s. longitudina'le ventri'culi,** s. longitudinale tunicae muscularis gastris.

**s. lu'cidum epider'midis,** clear layer of epidermis: the clear translucent layer of the epidermis, just beneath the stratum corneum epidermidis. See figure at *epidermis.* See also *s. corneum epidermidis.*

**s. lu'cidum hippocam'pi,** the cellular (as opposed to dendritic) segment of the stratum pyramidalis of the hippocampus; cf. *s. radiatum hippocampi.*

**s. malpi'ghii,** s. germinativum.

**s. me'dium tu'nicae muscula'ris duc'tus deferen'tis,** the middle layer of the muscular coat of the ductus deferens.

**s. me'dium tu'nicae muscula'ris ure'teris,** the middle layer of the muscular coat of the ureter.

**s. me'dium tu'nicae muscula'ris ve'sicae urina'riae,** the middle layer of the muscular coat of the urinary bladder.

**s. medulla're interme'dium colli'culi superio'ris** [TA], intermediate white layer of superior colliculus: the outer white layer of the gray and white layers of the superior colliculus; it is Layer V of the colliculus. See *strata grisea et alba colliculi superioris.*

**s. medulla're profun'dum colli'culi superio'ris** [TA], deep white layer of superior colliculus: the inner white layer of the gray and white layers of the superior colliculus; it is Layer VII of the colliculus. See *strata grisea et alba colliculi superioris.*

**s. molecula're cerebel'li** [TA], molecular layer of cerebellum: the superficial layer of the cortex of the cerebellum, containing a relatively small number of stellate neurons, and separated from the granular layer by the Purkinje cell layer; called also *plexiform layer of cerebellum* and *s. plexiforme cerebelli.*

**s. molecula're hippocam'pi,** the most superficial layer of the hippocampus, in which the apical dendrites of the pyramidal cells terminate.

**s. muco'sum membra'nae tympa'nicae,** mucous layer of tympanic membrane: the inner layer of the tympanic membrane, continuous with the mucosa lining the tympanic cavity.

**mucous s. of tympanic membrane,** s. mucosum membranae tympanicae.

**s. nervo'sum re'tinae** [TA], pars nervosum retinae.

**neuroepithelial s. of retina, s. neuroepithelia'le re'tinae,** neuroepithelial layer of retina; see under *layer.*

**s. neurono'rum pirifor'mium,** s. purkinjense cerebelli.

**s. op'ticum colli'culi superio'ris** [TA], optic layer of superior colliculus: a layer of white fibers below the superficial gray layer and above the intermediate gray layer; many of its fibers are from the optic tract and it contains a few other large neurons.

**s. o'riens hippocam'pi** [TA], oriens layer of hippocampus: one of the layers of the hippocampus, lying between the alveus and the stratum pyramidalis; it is composed of neurons with ascending axons (basket cells), the ramifications of the basal dendrites of the pyramidal cells, and their axon collaterals.

**s. papilla're co'rii,** TA alternative for *s. papillare dermidis.*

**s. papilla're cu'tis, s. papilla're der'midis** [TA], papillary layer of dermis: the outer layer of the dermis, characterized by the presence of ridges or papillae protruding into the epidermis. Called also *papillary layer of corium* and *s. papillare corii* [TA alternative].

**pigmented s. of ciliary body,** see under *layer.*

**pigmented s. of iris,** see under *layer.*

**pigmented s. of retina,** pars pigmentosa retinae.

**s. pigmen'ti bul'bi o'culi,** pars pigmentosa retinae.

**s. pigmen'ti cor'poris cilia'ris,** pigmented layer of ciliary body; see under *layer.*

**s. pigmen'ti i'ridis,** pigmented layer of iris; see under *iris.*

**s. pigmento'sum re'tinae** [TA], pars pigmentosa retinae.

**s. plexifor'me cerebel'li,** s. moleculare cerebelli.

**s. purkinjen'se cerebel'li** [TA], Purkinje cell layer: the layer of Purkinje neurons situated between the external molecular layer and the internal granular layer of the cerebellar cortex; considered by some to be the deepest layer of the molecular layer. Called also *Purkinje layer, stratum neuronorum piriformium* and *piriform neuronal layer.*

**s. pyramida'le hippocam'pi** [TA], pyramidal layer of hippocampus: a well-defined double layer of pyramidal cells in the hippocampus; their dendrites extend from the stratum oriens to the stratum moleculare.

**radiate s. of tympanic membrane,** s. radiatum membranae tympanicae.

**s. radia'tum hippocam'pi** [TA], the superficial part of the pyramidal cell layer of the hippocampus, the bulk of which is formed by apical dendrites together with their axons and a few pyramidal cells.

**s. radia'tum membra'nae tympa'nicae,** radiate layer of tympanic membrane: the outer part of the fibrous stratum of the membrane, consisting of fibers radiating outward from the manubrium of the malleus to pass into the fibrocartilaginous ring.

**s. reticula're co'rii,** TA alternative for *s. reticulare dermidis.*

**s. reticula're cu'tis,** s. reticulare dermidis.

**s. reticula're der'midis** [TA], reticular layer of dermis: the inner layer of the dermis, consisting chiefly of dense fibrous tissue. Called also *proper coat of corium* or *dermis, reticular layer of corium, s. reticulare corii* [TA alternative], *s. reticulare cutis,* and *tunica propria corii.*

**s. spino'sum epider'midis,** spinous layer of epidermis: the layer of the skin between the stratum granulosum epidermidis and the stratum basale epidermidis characterized by the presence of prickle cells. See figure at *epidermis,* and see also *s. germinativum.* Called also *prickle cell layer.*

**s. spongio'sum,** spongy layer: the middle layer of the endometrium, which contains the tortuous portions of the uterine glands; together with the stratum compactum, it forms the *stratum functionale* (q.v.).

**s. submuco'sum,** the inner layer of the myometrium, which is in contact with the endometrium; called also *s. subvasculare.*

**submucous s. of bladder,** tela submucosa vesicae urinariae.

**submucous s. of colon,** tela submucosa intestini crassi.

**submucous s. of rectum,** tela submucosa recti.
**submucous s. of small intestine,** tela submucosa intestini tenuis.
**submucous s. of stomach,** tela submucosa gastris.
**s. subsero'sum,** the outer layer of the myometrium, which is in contact with the serous coat of the uterus.
**s. subvascula're,** s. submucosum.
**s. supravascula're,** the layer of the myometrium that lies between the stratum vasculare and the stratum subserosum.
**s. synovia'le cap'sulae articula'ris,** TA alternative for *membrana synovialis capsulae articularis.*
**s. synovia'le vagi'nae ten'dinis** [TA], the synovial layer of a tendon sheath.
**s. vascula're,** the middle layer of the myometrium, forming most of its bulk, and composed of circular and spiral fibers.
**s. zona'le colli'culi superio'ris** [TA], zonal layer of superior colliculus: the most external layer of the superior colliculus (Layer I), containing myelinated and unmyelinated fibers primarily from the occipital lobe.
**s. zona'le tha'lami,** zonal layer of thalamus: a layer of myelinated fibers covering the superior aspect of the dorsal thalamus.

**Straus' reaction (phenomenon, test)** (strous) [Isidore *Straus,* French physician, 1845–1896] see under *reaction.*

**Strauss' sign** (shtrous) [Hermann *Strauss,* German physician, 1868–1944] see under *sign.*

**streak** (strēk) a line, stria, striation, or stripe.
**angioid s's,** red to black irregular bands observed in the ocular fundus running outward from the region of the optic disk, which are seen in certain conditions, including pseudoxanthoma elasticum, osteitis deformans, and sickle-cell anemia. The lesions are thought to represent ruptures in Bruch's membrane.
**fatty s.,** a small, flat, yellow-gray area, composed mainly of cholesterol-laden macrophages, within an artery; possibly an early stage of atherosclerosis.
**germinal s.,** primitive s.
**Knapp's s's,** lines resembling blood vessels seen occasionally in the retina after hemorrhage.
**medullary s.,** the neural groove.
**meningitic s.,** tache cérébrale.
**Moore's lightning s's,** vertical flashes of light resembling lightning, sometimes seen on the peripheral side of the field of vision when the eyes are moved; a benign condition.
**primitive s.,** a faint white trace at the caudal end of the embryonic disc, formed by the movement of cells at the beginning of mesoderm formation; it provides the earliest evidence of the embryonic axis.

**stream** (strēm) a current or flow of water or other fluid.
**axial s.,** see under *current.*
**blood s.,** bloodstream; see under *B.*
**electron s.,** a stream of negatively charged particles (electrons) moving from cathode to anode across a potential difference in a low-pressure gas tube or a vacuum tube.
**hair s's,** flumina pilorum.

**stream·ing** (strēm'ing) the movement of a current in a fluid.
**cytoplasmic s., protoplasmic s.,** cyclosis.

**streb·lo·mi·cro·dac·ty·ly** (streb″lo-mi″kro-dak'tə-le) [Gr. *streblos* twisted + *mikros* small + *daktylos* finger] streptomicrodactyly.

**strength** (strength) intensity or power.
**electric field s.,** electric intensity.
**fatigue s.,** the maximum stress at which a material will withstand cyclic loading for a given period.
**ionic s.,** a quantity proportional to the amount of electrostatic interaction between ions in solution; equal to

$$\frac{1}{2}\sum_i c_i Z_i^2,$$

where $c_i$ is the molar concentration of the *i*th species, and $Z_i$ the ionic charge. Symbol *I.*
**muscle s.,** the greatest force that can be put forth by a muscle; it is measured with either isometric, isokinetic, or isotonic exercises.
**yield s.,** an amount of deforming stress just above the elastic limit, when a substance begins to be permanently changed in shape.

**streph·eno·po·dia** (stref″ə-no-po'de-ə) [*streph-* + Gr. *en* in + *pous* foot] talipes varus.

**streph·exo·po·dia** (stref″ək-so-po'de-ə) [*streph-* + Gr. *exō* out + *pous* foot] talipes valgus.

**streph(o)-** [Gr. *strephein* to twist] a combining form meaning twisted.

**strepho·po·dia** (stref″o-po'de-ə) talipes equinus.

**strepho·sym·bo·lia** (stref″o-sim-bo'le-ə) [*strepho-* + *symbol* + *-ia*] 1. a disorder of perception in which objects seem reversed, as in a mirror. 2. a type of dyslexia in which letters are perceived as in a mirror; it begins with confusion between similar but oppositely oriented letters (b-d, q-p) and there may be a tendency to reverse direction in reading.

**strep·i·tus** (strep'ĭ-təs) [L.] a noise; a sound heard on auscultation.

**strepo·gen·in** (strep″o-jen'in) a factor present in casein and certain other proteins which is essential to optimal growth of animals.

**strep·ta·mine** (strep'tə-mēn″) one of the fractions derived from the degradation of streptomycin.

**Strep·tase** (strep'tās) trademark for a preparation of streptokinase.

**strep·tav·i·din** (strep-tav'ĭ-din) a bacterial protein used as a probe in immunologic and biochemical assays because of its great affinity and specificity for biotin; it is frequently part of an indirect system in which specific substrates are biotinylated and then visualized by binding streptavidin to which is linked an easily detected compound, such as a fluorochrome.

**strep·ti·ce·mia** (strep″tĭ-se'me-ə) streptococcemia.

**strep·ti·dine** (strep'tĭ-dīn) one of the fractions derived from degradation of streptomycin, the other fraction being streptobiosamine.

**strept(o)-** [Gr. *streptos* twisted] a combining form meaning twisted.

**strep·to·bac·il·li** (strep″to-bə-sil'i) plural of *streptobacillus.*

**Strep·to·bac·il·lus** (strep″to-bə-sil'əs) [*strepto-* + *bacillus*] [MeSH: Streptobacillus] a genus of facultatively anaerobic, gram-negative, rod-shaped bacteria of uncertain affiliation, made up of organisms that may be highly pleomorphic, varying from single rods with central swelling to chains or filaments resembling strings of beads. Serum, ascitic fluid, or blood is required for growth. The organisms are found in the throat and nasopharynx of wild and laboratory rats, and they may cause rat-bite fever in humans. The genus contains a single species, *S. (Haverhillia) moniliformis.*
**S. monilifor'mis,** the single species of the genus. Called also *Haverhillia multiformis.*

**strep·to·bac·il·lus** (strep″to-bə-sil'əs) pl. *streptobacil'li* [MeSH: Streptobacillus] a bacterium of the genus *Streptobacillus.*

**strep·to·bio·sa·mine** (strep″to-bi-o'sə-mēn) a disaccharide containing streptose and *N*-methyl-L-glucosamine, a product of the acid hydrolysis of streptomycin in which it is linked glycosidally to streptidine.

**strep·to·cer·ci·a·sis** (strep″to-sər-ki'ə-sis) infection with *Mansonella streptocerca,* whose microfilariae produce a pruritic rash resembling that in onchocerciasis; transmitted by midges of the genus *Culicoides,* it occurs in Central Africa.

**Strep·to·coc·ca·ceae** (strep″to-kok-a'se-e) [MeSH: Streptococcaceae] a family of gram-positive, facultative anaerobic cocci, which are usually nonmotile, and occur in pairs, chains, or tetrads. It includes the genera *Aerococcus, Gemella, Leuconostoc, Pediococcus,* and *Streptococcus.*

**strep·to·coc·cal** (strep″to-kok'əl) pertaining to or caused by a streptococcus.

**strep·to·coc·ce·mia** (strep″to-kok-se'me-ə) [*streptococcus* + *-emia*] the presence of streptococci in the blood.

**strep·to·coc·ci** (strep″to-kok'si) plural of *streptococcus.*

**strep·to·coc·cic** (strep″to-kok'sik) streptococcal.

**strep·to·coc·ci·cide** (strep″to-kok'sĭ-sīd) an agent that is destructive to streptococci.

**strep·to·coc·col·y·sin** (strep″to-kŏ-kol'ĭ-sin) streptolysin.

**strep·to·coc·co·sis** (strep″to-kŏ-ko'sis) infection with streptococci.

**Strep·to·coc·cus** (strep″to-kok'əs) [*strepto-* + Gr. *kokkos* berry] [MeSH: Streptococcus] a genus of gram-positive, facultatively anaerobic cocci occurring in pairs or chains, assigned to the family

Streptococcaceae. Streptococci are cytochrome-, oxidase-, and catalase-negative organisms that are nonmotile, nonsporeforming, and homofermentative. The genus consists of four groups: the *pyogenic* group, the *viridans* group, the *enterococcus* group, and the *lactic* group. The first group includes the β-hemolytic human and animal pathogens, the second includes α-hemolytic, potentially pathogenic organisms occurring as normal flora in the human upper respiratory tract, the third group includes organisms with variable hemolysis that are normal flora of the intestinal tract, and the fourth group includes saprophytic forms associated with the souring of milk. Streptococci are classified according to patterns of hemolysis on blood agar, antigenic composition, and physiologic and biochemical characteristics. See also *hemolytic streptococcus,* under *streptococcus,* and *Lancefield classification,* under *classification.*
**S. acidomi'nimus,** an α-hemolytic species with no group-specific antigen, found in the bovine vagina and in raw milk; it occasionally causes human infection.
**S. agalac'tiae,** a β-hemolytic or nonhemolytic species of group B, found in raw milk; it causes mastitis in cattle and is associated with human infection in infants. Called also *S. mastitidis.*
**S. anaero'bius,** *Peptostreptococcus anaerobius.*
**S. angino'sus,** a species that includes streptococci of both group F and group G. β-Hemolytic strains are found in several human sources and in abscesses. The α-hemolytic and nonhemolytic species *(streptococcus MG)* are associated with primary atypical pneumonia.
**S. a'vium,** *Enterococcus avium.*
**S. bo'vis,** an α-hemolytic or nonhemolytic species, one of the nonenterococcus group D streptococci. It is found in the bovine alimentary tract and sometimes in human feces; sometimes associated with human endocarditis.
**S. cremo'ris,** an α-hemolytic or nonhemolytic species of group N, which is one of the lactic group. It occurs in dairy products; its action on milk results in the production of buttermilk.
**S. epide'micus,** former name for *S. pyogenes,* thought to be disease-specific for epidemic infection of the upper respiratory tract.
**S. e'qui,** β-hemolytic streptococci of group C, the specific etiologic agent of strangles in horses; it is nonpathogenic for man.
**S. equi'nus,** an α-hemolytic species of the viridans group, which is one of the nonenterococcus group D streptococci. It is found in the alimentary tract of the horse, and is sometimes associated with human infection.
**S. equisi'milis,** a β-hemolytic species of group C, occurring in the upper respiratory tract of humans and animals. It is sometimes associated with erysipelas and puerperal fever.
**S. erysipe'latis,** *S. pyogenes.*
**S. faeca'lis,** *Enterococcus faecalis.*
**S. fae'cium,** *Enterococcus faecium.*
**S. foe'tidus,** *Peptostreptococcus anaerobius.*
**S. hemoly'ticus,** *S. pyogenes.*
**S. lac'ticus, S. lac'tis,** an α-hemolytic or nonhemolytic, nonpathogenic species of group N, which is one of the lactic group. It is found in dairy products and is commonly responsible for the souring of milk.
**S. lanceola'tus,** *Peptostreptococcus lanceolatus.*
**S. masti'tidis,** *S. agalactiae.*
**S. mi'cros,** *Peptostreptococcus micros.*
**S. mi'tis,** an α-hemolytic species of the viridans group, which has no specific group antigen. It is found in the normal human upper respiratory tract and has been associated with subacute bacterial endocarditis.
**S. mu'tans,** a group K species of the viridans group with variable hemolysis. It has been implicated in the formation of dental caries.
**S. pneumo'niae,** an α-hemolytic species with no specific group antigen. It is the most common cause of lobar pneumonia; it also causes numerous other serious acute pyogenic disorders, e.g., meningitis, septicemia, empyema, and peritonitis. There are many serotypes, distinguished on the basis of the specificity of the capsular polysaccharides. See plate accompanying *bacterium,* and see also *pneumococcus polysaccharide,* under *polysaccharide.* Called also *Diplococcus pneumoniae.*
**S. pyo'genes,** a species of β-hemolytic, toxigenic pyogenic streptococci comprising group A of the Lancefield classification, separable into numbered serotypes on the basis of the specificity and combination of the M, R, and T antigens, and causing septic sore throat, scarlet fever, rheumatic fever, puerperal sepsis, acute glomerulonephritis, and other conditions in man. Called also *S. hemolyticus* and *S. scarlatinae.*
**S. saliva'rius,** a group K streptococcus with variable hemolysis, making up a part of the normal flora of the upper respiratory tract, and occasionally associated with apical abscesses of the teeth and the subacute form of bacterial endocarditis.
**S. san'guis,** an α-hemolytic species of the viridans group, tentatively identified with group H. It is found in humans in dental plaque, in blood, and in subacute bacterial endocarditis.
**S. scarlati'nae,** *S. pyogenes.*
**S. su'is,** a β-hemolytic species of group D, found in young pigs suffering from bacteremia and in asymptomatic older pigs; infection takes various forms, including streptococcal meningitis.
**S. thermo'philus,** an α-hemolytic species of the viridans group, found in milk and milk products.
**S. u'beris,** an α-hemolytic or nonhemolytic species with no specific group antigen, found in milk and bovine sources, and occasionally associated with human infections.
**S. vi'ridans,** a former species name for α-hemolytic streptococci, especially those strains found in human disease; see *hemolytic streptococcus,* under *streptococcus.*
**S. zooepide'micus,** β-hemolytic streptococci of group C, commonly causing pyogenic disease in lower animals and known as "animal pyogenes"; it is rarely found in man.

**strep·to·coc·cus** (strep"to-kok'əs) pl. *streptococ'ci* [MeSH: Streptococcus] An organism of the genus *Streptococcus.*
**alpha s., alpha-hemolytic s.,** see *hemolytic s.*
**anhemolytic s.,** nonhemolytic s.
**beta s., beta-hemolytic s.,** see *hemolytic s.*
**gamma s.,** nonhemolytic s.
**group A, B, C (etc.) streptococci,** a classification of β-hemolytic streptococci based on cell-wall carbohydrate antigens; see *Lancefield classification,* under *classification.*
**hemolytic s.,** any streptococcus capable of hemolyzing red blood cells or of producing a zone of hemolysis about the colonies on blood agar. The great majority of streptococci found in pathologic processes belong to this type. The hemolytic streptococci have been classified as the *alpha* (α-hemolytic) or *viridans type,* which produces about the colony on blood agar a zone of greenish discoloration considerably smaller than the clear zone produced by the beta type (see also *viridans s.*); and the *beta* (β-hemolytic) *type,* which produces a clear zone of hemolysis immediately surrounding the colony on blood agar. On immunological grounds, the β-hemolytic streptococci may be divided according to the presence of specific antigenic carbohydrates in the cell wall (C-substance) into Lancefield groups A through T. Those causing human infection are found primarily in groups A through G. See *Lancefield classification,* under *classification.*
**indifferent s.,** nonhemolytic s.
**s. MG,** any of a strain of biochemically and antigenically homogeneous, nonhemolytic streptococci of group F agglutinated by the sera of patients with mycoplasmal pneumonia.
**nonhemolytic s.,** any streptococcus that does not cause a change in the medium when cultured on blood agar. Called also *gamma s.* and *indifferent s.*
**viridans s.,** any of a group of α-hemolytic streptococci that have no defined group antigens, found as part of the normal flora of the respiratory tract; streptococci of this group cause dental caries and bacterial endocarditis. See also *hemolytic s.*

**strep·to·dor·nase** (strep"to-dor'nās) [*strepto*coccus + *d*eoxyribo*n*ucle*ase*] a deoxyribonuclease produced by hemolytic streptococci.

**strep·to·du·o·cin** (strep"to-doo'o-sin) an antibiotic compound consisting of approximately equal parts of dihydrostreptomycin sulfate and streptomycin sulfate.

**strep·to·gen·in** (strep"to-jen'in) a growth-stimulating factor for certain microorganisms and laboratory animals, found in protein hydrolysates. Since a large number of peptides have streptogenin activity, they may serve simply as an accessible source of amino acids.

**strep·to·he·mol·y·sin** (strep"to-he-mol'ĭ-sin) streptolysin.

**strep·to·ki·nase** (strep"to-ki'nās) [*strepto*coccus + *kinase*] [MeSH: Streptokinase] a protein produced by β-hemolytic streptococci; although it has no intrinsic enzymatic activity, it binds plasminogen and causes cleavage of that molecule to plasmin. It is used as a thrombolytic agent.
**s.-streptodornase (SKSD),** a mixture of the proteins streptokinase and streptodornase produced by hemolytic streptococci; used topically on surface lesions and by instillation in closed body cavities to remove clotted blood or fibrinous or purulent accumulations; also used as a skin test antigen in evaluating generalized cell-mediated immunodeficiency.

**strep·tol·y·sin** (strep-tol'ĭ-sin) [*strepto*coccus + hemo*lysin*] an exotoxin produced by certain strains of streptococci, particularly those of group A, that lyses red blood cells.
**s. O,** an oxygen-labile and antigenic hemolysin produced by most group A streptococci and by some of groups C and G. It is inactive in the oxidized state but is readily activated by treatment with mild reducing agents, such as sulfite.
**s. S,** an oxygen-stable and nonantigenic hemolysin and leukocidin produced by many strains of group A streptococci. It is sensitive to treatment with heat or acid, but is not inactivated by oxygen.

**strep·to·mi·cro·dac·ty·ly** (strep"to-mi"kro-dak'tə-le) [*strepto-* + *micro-* + Gr. *daktylos* finger] camptodactyly in which the little fingers only are involved.

**Strep·to·my·ces** (strep″to-mi′sēz) [*strepto-* + Gr. *mykēs* fungus] [MeSH: Streptomyces] a genus of fungus-like bacteria of the family Streptomycetaceae, order Actinomycetales, consisting of aerobic, nonacid-fast organisms that form a nonfragmented aerial mycelium. The genus is separable into several hundred different species, usually soil forms but occasionally parasitic on plants and animals. Most species produce pigments. More than half of the antibiotics of practical value, including the aminoglycosides, the tetracyclines, and the macrolides, are produced from species of *Streptomyces.*
**S. al′bus,** a species that produces the antibiotic salinomycin.
**S. ambofa′ciens,** a species that produces ambomycin, azotomycin, duazomycin, and spiramycin.
**S. antibio′ticus,** a species that produces the antibiotic oleandomycin.
**S. aureofa′ciens,** a species that produces the antibiotic partricin.
**S. azu′reus,** a species that produces the antibiotic thiostrepton.
**S. bambergien′sis,** a species that is a source of bambermycins.
**S. cinnamonen′sis,** a species that produces the antibiotic monensin.
**S. coeruleoru′bidus,** a species that produces the antineoplastic antibiotic daunorubicin.
**S. ederen′sis,** a species that is a source of bambermycins.
**S. eryth′reus,** a species that is the source of the antibiotic erythromycin.
**S. fra′diae,** a species that produces neomycin.
**S. geysirien′sis,** a species that is a source of bambermycins.
**S. ghanaen′sis,** a species that is a source of bambermycins.
**S. grise′olus,** a species that produces the antibiotic sinefungin.
**S. gri′seus,** a species that produces streptomycin.
**S. hygrosco′picus,** a species that includes a variant that produces the antibiotic scopafungin.
**S. kanamyce′ticus,** a species that produces kanamycin.
**S. kitasoen′sis,** a species that is the source of the antibiotic kitasamycin.
**S. lasalien′sis,** a species that produces the antibiotic lasalocid.
**S. lincolnen′sis,** a species that produces the antibiotic lincomycin.
**S. ni′veus,** a species that produces the antibiotic novobiocin.
**S. noboritoen′sis,** a species that produces the antibiotic hygromycin.
**S. nodo′sus,** a species some strains of which produce amphotericin B.
**S. noga′later,** a species including a variant that produces the antineoplastic substance nogalamycin.
**S. nour′sei,** a species that produces the antibiotic nystatin.
**S. orchida′ceus,** a species that is the source of cycloserine.
**S. orienta′lis,** a species that is the source of vancomycin.
**S. paraguayen′sis,** a pathogenic species of uncertain status.
**S. peuce′tius,** a species that produces the antineoplastic antibiotics daunorubicin and doxorubicin.
**S. rimo′sus,** a species containing a variant, *S. rimo′sus* var. *paromomyci′nus,* that produces the antibiotic paromomycin.
**S. somalien′sis,** a species commonly found in Africa, North and South America, Israel, and India, causing actinomycotic mycetoma in which the granules in the discharged pus are white to yellow.
**S. specta′bilis,** a species from which the antibiotic spectinomycin is derived.
**S. tenebra′rius,** a species that produces nebramycin, the antibiotic complex from which tobramycin is derived.
**S. tsukubaen′sis,** a species that produces the macrolide tacrolimus.
**S. vina′ceus,** a species that produces vitamin $B_{12}$. Called also *Actinomyces vinaceus.*

**Strep·to·my·ce·ta·ceae** (strep″to-mi″se-ta′se-e) [MeSH: Streptomycetaceae] a family of bacteria of the order Actinomycetales. It consists of the genera *Streptomyces, Streptoverticillium, Sporichthya,* and *Microellobosporia.* The only genus containing clinically important organisms is *Streptomyces.*

**strep·to·my·cin** (strep″to-mi′sin) [MeSH: Streptomycin] the first of the aminoglycoside antibiotics to be isolated, derived from *Streptomyces griseus;* it is effective against a wide variety of aerobic gram-negative bacilli and some gram-positive bacteria, including mycobacteria. Its use is now limited because of the emergence of resistant strains.
**s. sulfate** [USP], the sesquisulfate salt of streptomycin, used as a tuberculostatic in combination with other antituberculosis agents, and for the treatment of certain nontuberculous infections due to susceptible organisms, including plague, tularemia and (in combination with other drugs) brucellosis, granuloma inguinale, chancroid, and bacterial endocarditis; administered intramuscularly.

**strep·to·my·co·sis** (strep″to-mi-ko′sis) infection with bacteria of the genus *Streptomyces.*

**Strep·to·neu·ra** (strep″to-noor′ə) a subclass of gastropods, including snails found in salt water and occasionally fresh water habitats. A number of primary or intermediate hosts for trematodes and other pathogens are in this group in the order Mesogastropoda. A second order is the marine-dwelling Neogastropoda. Called also *Prosobranchiata.*

**strep·to·sep·ti·ce·mia** (strep″to-sep″tĭ-se′me-ə) septicemia due to a streptococcus.

**strep·to·thri·cin** (strep″to-thri′sin) an antibiotic substance active against both gram-negative and gram-positive bacteria; it was the first antibiotic isolated, but was found to be too toxic for systemic use.

**Strep·to·thrix** (strep′to-thriks) [*strepto-* + Gr. *thrix* hair] former name for a genus of sheathed bacteria found in fresh water and activated sludge.
**S. bo′vis,** *Dermatophilus congolensis.*
**S. farci′ni,** *Nocardia farcinica.*
**S. nocar′dii,** *Nocardia farcinica.*

**strep·to·zo·cin** (strep″to-zo′sin) [MeSH: Streptozocin] an antineoplastic antibiotic of the nitrosourea (q.v.) group, derived from *Streptomyces achromogenes* or produced by synthesis; used principally in the treatment of islet-cell tumors of the pancreas and also other endocrine tumors including gastrinomas associated with Zollinger-Ellison syndrome and glucagon-secreting alpha cell tumors of the pancreas.

**strep·to·zo·to·cin** (strep″to-zo-to′sin) streptozocin.

**stress** (stres) [MeSH: Stress] 1. forcibly exerted influence; pressure. 2. force per unit area, which may cause strain (q.v.) on an object. 3. in dentistry, the pressure of the upper teeth against the lower in mastication. 4. a state of physiological or psychological strain caused by adverse stimuli, physical, mental, or emotional, internal or external, that tend to disturb the functioning of an organism and which the organism naturally desires to avoid; see also *stress reaction,* under *reaction.* 5. the stimuli that elicit such a state or stress reactions.

**stress-break·er** (stres′brāk-ər) a device built into a removable partial denture that relieves the abutment teeth from excessive occlusal loads and stresses. Two basic types are recognized: one consisting of a movable joint between the direct retainer and the denture base *(hinge s.)* and the other consisting of a flexible connection between the direct retainer and the denture base or using a movable joint between two major connectors. Called also *stress divider* and *stress equalizer.*

**stretch·er** (strech′ər) a portable couchlike or bedlike structure for carrying the sick or injured. Called also *litter.*

**stretch·es** (strech′əz) inherited periodic spasticity.

**stria** (stri′ə) pl. *stri′ae* [L. "a furrow, groove"] 1. a band, line, streak, or stripe. 2. [TA] a general term for such longitudinal collections of nerve fibers in the brain.
**acoustic striae,** striae medullares ventriculi quarti.
**stri′ae albican′tes,** see *striae atrophicae.*
**striae of Amici,** Z band; see under *band.*
**stri′ae atro′phicae,** linear, depressed, atrophic, pinkish or purplish, scarlike lesions that later become white *(striae albicantes, lineae albicantes),* occurring on the abdomen, breasts, buttocks, and thighs. They are due to weakening of the elastic tissues, and are associated with pregnancy *(striae gravidarum),* excessive obesity, rapid growth during puberty and adolescence, Cushing's syndrome, or topical or prolonged treatment with corticosteroids. Called also *striae distensae, lineae atrophicae,* and *linear atrophy.*
**auditory striae,** striae medullares ventriculi quarti.
**Baillarger's external s.,** s. laminae granularis internae.
**Baillarger's inner s., Baillarger's internal s.,** s. laminae pyramidalis internae.
**Baillarger's outer s.,** s. laminae granularis internae.
**stri′ae cilia′res,** slight dark ridges running parallel with each other from the teeth of the ora serrata of the retina to the valleys between the ciliary processes.
**s. diagona′lis** [TA], **s. diagona′lis (Bro′ca),** diagonal band: a band of nerve fibers that forms the caudal zone of the anterior perforated substance where it adjoins the optic tract, which is continuous caudolaterally with the periamygdaloid area and rostromedially passes above the optic chiasm to blend with the paraterminal gyrus; called also *band of Broca, bandaletta diagonalis (Broca), Broca's diagonal band,* and *diagonal band of Broca.*
**stri′ae disten′sae,** striae atrophicae.
**external s. of Baillarger,** s. laminae granularis internae.
**s. of external granular layer,** s. laminae granularis externae.
**s. of Gennari,** see under *line.*
**stri′ae gravida′rum,** see *striae atrophicae.*
**inner s. of Baillarger, internal s. of Baillarger,** s. laminae pyramidalis internae.
**s. of internal granular layer,** s. laminae granularis internae.
**s. of internal pyramidal layer,** s. laminae pyramidalis internae.
**Kaes' s., Kaes-Bekhterev s.,** Kaes-Bekhterev layer.
**Knapp's striae,** see under *streak.*

**s. la′minae granula′ris exter′nae** [TA], stria of external granular layer: a band of tangentially oriented nerve fibers in the external granular layer of the cerebral cortex.
**s. la′minae granula′ris inter′nae** [TA], stria of internal granular layer: a band of tangentially oriented white nerve fibers in the internal granular layer of the cerebral cortex. In the region of the calcarine sulcus, this stria is thick and highly visible and here is known as the *line of Gennari* (see also *striate cortex,* under *cortex*). Called also *external band, line, stria,* or *stripe of Baillarger.* See also *s. laminae pyramidalis internae.*
**s. la′minae molecula′ris** [TA], **s. la′minae plexifor′mis,** stria of molecular layer: a band of tangentially oriented myelinated nerve fibers in the molecular layer of the cerebral cortex.
**s. la′minae pyramida′lis inter′nae** [TA], stria of internal pyramidal layer: a band of tangentially oriented white nerve fibers in the internal pyramidal layer of the cerebral cortex; called also *internal band, line, stria,* or *stripe of Baillarger.* See also *s. laminae granularis internae.*
**s. of Lanci,** s. longitudinalis medialis corporis callosi.
**Langhans′ s.,** cytotrophoblast.
**Liesegang′s striae,** see under *phenomenon.*
**longitudinal s. of corpus callosum, lateral,** s. longitudinalis lateralis corporis callosi.
**longitudinal s. of corpus callosum, medial,** s. longitudinalis medialis corporis callosi.
**s. longitudina′lis latera′lis cor′poris callo′si** [TA], lateral longitudinal stria of corpus callosum: one of two slender bands of myelinated fibers which form longitudinal ridges in the indusium griseum on the superior aspect of each half of the corpus callosum.
**s. longitudina′lis media′lis cor′poris callo′si** [TA], medial longitudinal stria of corpus callosum: one of two slender bands of myelinated fibers which form longitudinal ridges in the indusium griseum on the superior aspect of each half of the corpus callosum.
**s. mallea′ris membra′nae tym′pani, s. mallea′ris membra′nae tympa′nicae** [TA], **s. malleola′ris membra′nae tym′pani,** mallear stria of tympanic membrane: a nearly vertical radial band seen on the outer surface of the tympanic membrane; it extends from the umbo upward to the prominentia mallearis and is caused by the manubrium mallei.
**stri′ae medulla′res acus′ticae, stri′ae medulla′res fos′sae rhomboi′deae,** striae medullares ventriculi quarti.
**s. medulla′ris tha′lami** [TA], medullary stria of thalamus: a fiber bundle that arises from the subcallosal and paraterminal gyri, the preoptic area, and amygdaloid area, and runs backward along the junction of the dorsal and medial surfaces of the thalamus to reach the habenular nucleus.
**stri′ae medulla′res ventri′culi quar′ti** [TA], medullary striae of fourth ventricle: bundles of white fibers coursing transversely across the floor of the fourth ventricle; they arise from the arcuate nuclei, pass dorsally close to the midline, and after having reached the fourth ventricle finally enter the inferior cerebellar peduncle. Called also *striae medullares fossae rhomboideae.*
**medullary s. of corpus striatum, lateral,** lamina medullaris lateralis corporis striati.
**medullary s. of corpus striatum, medial,** lamina medullaris medialis corporis striati.
**medullary striae of fourth ventricle, medullary striae of rhomboid fossa,** striae medullares ventriculi quarti.
**medullary s. of thalamus,** 1. s. medullaris thalami. 2. see *laminae medullares thalami.*
**meningitic s.,** tache cérébrale.
**s. of molecular layer,** s. laminae molecularis.
**Nitabuch′s s.,** see under *layer.*
**stri′ae olfacto′riae** [TA], olfactory striae: the radiating fibers of the olfactory tract, which diverge into a lateral and a medial band at the olfactory trigone and border the anterior perforated substance; the bands are covered by the lateral and medial olfactory gyri, respectively. See also *intermediate olfactory s.*
**s. olfacto′ria latera′lis** [TA], see *striae olfactoriae.*
**s. olfacto′ria media′lis** [TA], see *striae olfactoriae.*
**olfactory striae,** see *striae olfactoriae* and *intermediate olfactory s.*
**olfactory s., intermediate,** a small band of fibers that pass from the center of the olfactory trigone to penetrate the anterior perforated substance; its presence is variable. See also *striae olfactoriae.*
**olfactory striae, lateral,** stria olfactoria lateralis.
**olfactory s., medial,** stria olfactoria medialis.
**outer s. of Baillarger,** s. laminae granularis internae.
**Retzius′ parallel striae,** incremental lines.
**Rohr′s s.,** a layer of fibrin in the developing placenta, within the intervillous space at the fetal-maternal junction.
**Schreger′s striae,** lines of Schreger.
**s. termina′lis** [TA], terminal stria: a band of fibers along the lateral margin of the ventricular surface of the thalamus, covering the thalamostriate vein and, following the course of the vein, marking the line of separation between the thalamus and the caudate nucleus; it extends from the region of the interventricular foramen to the temporal horn of the lateral ventricle, carrying fibers from the amygdaloid nuclei to the septal, hypothalamic, and thalamic areas. Cf. *ventral amygdalofugal tract,* under *tract.*
**transverse striae of corpus callosum,** transverse bands of fibers on the upper surface of the corpus callosum.
**s. vascula′ris duc′tus cochlea′ris** [TA], vascular stria of cochlear duct: a layer of vascular tissue consisting of epithelial cells, mesothelial cells, and probably some neuroectoderm; it covers the outer wall of the cochlear duct and is thought to secrete the endolymph.
**Wickham′s striae,** pale grayish dots or lines forming a network on the surface of the papules, characteristic of lichen planus.

**striae** (stri′e) [L.] plural of *stria.*

**stri•a•tal** (stri-a′təl) pertaining to the corpus striatum.

**stri•ate** (stri′āt) striated.

**stri•at•ed** (stri′āt-əd) [L. *striatus*] striped; marked by striae.

**stri•a•tion** (stri-a′shən) 1. the quality of being marked by stripes or striae. 2. a streak or scratch.
**tabby cat s., tigroid s.,** a striation or marking on muscle tissue that has undergone marked fatty degeneration; seen especially in degenerated heart muscle.

**stri•a•to•ni•gral** (stri″ə-to-ni′grəl) projecting from the corpus striatum to the substantia nigra.

**stri•a•tum** (stri-a′təm) [L., neuter of *striatus* striped] 1. striped, or grooved. 2. corpus striatum. 3. neostriatum.

**stric•ture** (strik′chər) [L. *strictura*] stenosis.
**annular s.,** a stricture which encircles the lumen of a tubular structure.
**bridle s.,** a fold of membrane stretched across a canal, and partially closing it.
**cicatricial s.,** see under *stenosis.*
**contractile s.,** one which may be mechanically dilated, but which soon returns to its contracted condition; called also *recurrent s.*
**false s., functional s.,** spasmodic s.
**Hunner′s s.,** stricture of the ureter due to local inflammation of the wall of the ureter.
**irritable s.,** one through which the passage or attempted passage of an instrument produces pain.
**organic s., permanent s.,** a stricture due to a structural change in or about a canal.
**recurrent s.,** contractile s.
**spasmodic s., spastic s.,** one that is due to muscular spasm; called also *false s., functional s.,* and *temporary s.*
**temporary s.,** spasmodic s.

**stric•ture•plas•ty** (strik′chər-plas″te) surgical enlargement of the caliber of a constricted bowel segment by means of longitudinal incision and transverse suturing of the stricture. See illustration.

**stric•tur•iza•tion** (strik″chər-ĭ-za′shən) the process of decreasing in caliber or of becoming constricted.

**stric•turo•plas•ty** (strik′chər-o-plas″te) strictureplasty.

**stric•turo•tome** (strik′chər-o-tōm″) a knife for cutting strictures.

**stric•tur•ot•o•my** (strik″chər-ot′ə-me) incision of a stricture.

**stri•dent** (stri′dənt) characterized by stridor; shrill and harsh in sound. Called also *stridulous.*

**stri•dor** (stri′dər) [L.] a harsh, high-pitched respiratory sound such as the inspiratory sound often heard in acute laryngeal obstruction. Cf. *laryngismus stridulus.*

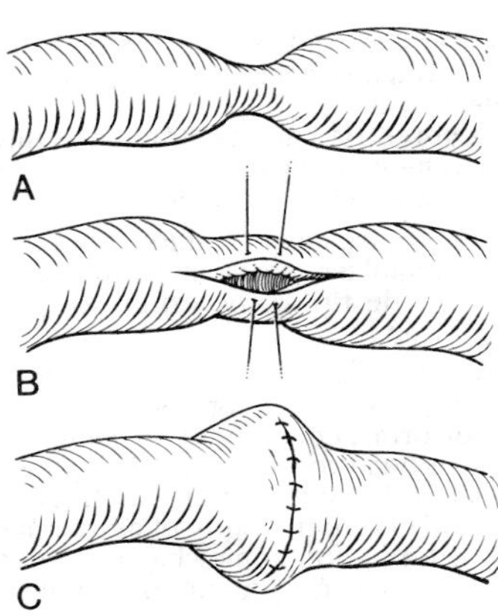

Strictureplasty. *(A),* Stricture; *(B),* longitudinal incision; *(C),* transverse closure.

**congenital laryngeal s.,** stridor and dyspnea of the newborn due to an indrawing or infolding of a congenitally flabby epiglottis and aryepiglottic folds (laryngomalacia) during inspiration; the condition is usually outgrown in two years.
**laryngeal s.,** stridor due to laryngeal obstruction; see also *congenital laryngeal s.*
**s. serra'ticus,** a sound like that made by filing a saw, caused by respiration through a tracheostomy tube.

**strid·u·lous** (strid'u-ləs) [L. *stridulus*] strident.

**strike** (strīk) cutaneous myiasis (def. 1).
**blowfly s.,** cutaneous blowfly myiasis.
**body s.,** cutaneous myiasis on the back of an animal.
**breech s., crotch s., crutch s.,** cutaneous myiasis in the breech region of an animal. Called also *tail s.*
**fly s.,** cutaneous blowfly myiasis.
**pizzle s.,** cutaneous myiasis around the external genitals (particularly the prepuce) of a male animal.
**poll s.,** cutaneous myiasis on the poll of an animal, either at a wound site (see *wound myiasis*) or in an area with folds of skin.
**tail s.,** breech s.
**wound s.,** see under *myiasis.*

**string·halt** (string'hawlt) myoclonus of the hind leg of a horse, causing a gait in which the leg is suddenly raised and then stamped on the ground. Called also *spring hock.*

**strio·cel·lu·lar** (stri″o-sel'u-lər) [*stria* + *cellular*] composed of striated muscle fibers and cells.

**strio·cer·e·bel·lar** (stri″o-ser″ə-bel'ər) pertaining to or affecting both the corpus striatum and the cerebellum, as striocerebellar tremor.

**strio·mo·tor** (stri″o-mo'tər) pertaining to or affecting neurons supplying skeletal muscle.

**strio·mus·cu·lar** (stri″o-mus'ku-lər) pertaining to or composed of striated muscle.

**strio·ni·gral** (stri″o-ni'grəl) striatonigral.

**strip** (strip) 1. a thin, narrow, comparatively long piece of material. 2. to express the contents from a canal, such as a blood vessel, by running the finger along it. 3. to excise lengths of large veins and competent tributaries by subcutaneous dissection and the use of a stripper. 4. to reduce the mesiodistal width of teeth, usually done to make space to align crowded segments. 5. to remove metal from the inside of a crown electrochemically in order to increase the inside diameter.
**abrasive s.,** a strip of linen or polymer film having abrasive material such as silica or garnet bonded to one side; used for polishing and contouring of the proximal surface of a tooth or denture.
**linen s.,** an abrasive strip with a linen backing.

**stripe** (strīp) a streak or stria.
**Baillarger's external s.,** stria laminae granularis internae.
**Baillarger's inner s., Baillarger's internal s.,** stria laminae pyramidalis internae.
**Baillarger's outer s., external s. of Baillarger,** stria laminae granularis internae.
**s. of Gennari,** see under *line.*
**Hensen's s.,** a band near the middle of the under surface of the membrana tectoria of the ear.
**inner s.,** in the outer zone of the renal medulla, the part next to the inner zone and away from the cortex; it contains thin descending and thick ascending limbs of the loop of Henle.
**inner s. of Baillarger, internal s. of Baillarger,** stria laminae pyramidalis internae.
**Mees's s's,** diagonal white stripes on the fingernails in arsenic poisoning.
**outer s.,** in the outer zone of the renal medulla, the part next to the cortex; it contains thick descending and thick ascending limbs of the loop of Henle.
**outer s. of Baillarger,** stria laminae granularis internae.
**s's of Retzius,** incremental lines.
**Vicq d'Azyr's s.,** Kaes-Bekhterev layer.

**strip·per** (strip'ər) a surgical instrument for excision of veins, consisting of a flexible stainless steel cable with a stripping cup or disk at one end and a guide tip at the other; a rigid type of external stripper is also utilized.

**stro·bi·la** (stro-bi'lə) pl. *strobi'lae* [L., from Gr. *strobilos* anything twisted up] 1. the chain of proglottids constituting the bulk of the body of adult tapeworms; considered by some to include the entire body, including the head, neck, and proglottids. 2. The chain of individuals produced by strobilation, such as the series of buds produced at the oral end of the body of certain jellyfish, which during the process of formation somewhat resemble a pile of plates; each bud is released to form an immature, free-swimming jellyfish.

**stro·bile** (stro'bīl) strobila.

**stro·bi·loid** (stro'bĭ-loid) resembling a row of tapeworm segments.

**stro·bi·lus** (stro-bi'ləs) [L., from Gr. *strobilos* anything twisted up] strobila.

**stro·bo·scope** (stro'bo-skōp) [Gr. *strobos* whirl + *-scope*] an instrument by which the successive phases of animal movements may be studied; motion may appear to come to rest. See also *laryngostroboscope.*

**stro·bo·scop·ic** (stro″bo-skop'ik) pertaining to the stroboscope.

**stroke** (strōk) 1. a sudden and severe attack; called also *ictus.* 2. stroke syndrome. 3. a pulsation.
**back s.,** the recoil of the ventricles at the time the blood is forced into the aorta.
**completed s.,** stroke syndrome reflecting the infarction of the vascular territory that is put at risk by a stenosis or occlusion of a feeding vessel.
**developing s.,** s. in evolution.
**effective s.,** the part of a ciliary beat in which the cilium stiffens and moves forward.
**embolic s.,** stroke syndrome due to cerebral embolism; onset of symptoms is usually sudden, reflecting abrupt loss of blood flow to the region of the occluded artery.
**s. in evolution,** a preliminary, unstable stage of stroke syndrome in which the blockage is present but the syndrome has not progressed to the stage of completed stroke.
**heat s.,** a condition caused by exposure to excessive heat, natural or artificial, and marked by dry skin, vertigo, headache, thirst, nausea, and muscular cramps; body temperature may be dangerously elevated, contrasting with heat exhaustion in which the body temperature may be subnormal. Called also *heat apoplexy* and *thermoplegia.* Cf. *sunstroke.*
**heat s., exertional,** heat stroke resulting from the production of heat by skeletal muscle during exercise faster than it can be dissipated by thermoregulatory mechanisms; it is usually accompanied by lactic acidosis.
**ischemic s.,** stroke syndrome caused by ischemia of an area of the brain.
**light s.,** a fatal narcosis produced in sensitized mice by exposure to light.
**lightning s.,** loss of consciousness and shock with burns, frequently fatal, caused by lightning.
**paralytic s.,** stroke syndrome that produces paralysis.
**recovery s.,** the part of a ciliary beat in which the cilium becomes flexible and bends.
**sun s.,** see *sunstroke.*
**thrombotic s.,** stroke syndrome due to cerebral thrombosis, most often superimposed on a plaque of atherosclerosis; onset of symptoms ranges from minutes to days after the obstruction.

**stro·ma** (stro'mə) pl. *stro'mata* [Gr. *strōma* anything laid out for lying or sitting upon] the matrix or supporting tissue of an organ, as distinguished from its *parenchyma* or functional element.
**s. of cornea,** substantia propria corneae.
**s. gan'glii** [TA], **s. ganglio'nicum,** stroma of ganglion: the endoneurial stroma that permeates the capsule of a neural ganglion and surrounds and supports the neuronal and axonal components of the ganglion.
**s. glan'dulae thyroi'deae** [TA], stroma of thyroid gland: the tissue that forms the framework of the thyroid gland.
**s. i'ridis** [TA], **s. of iris,** the soft mass of connective tissue fibers that make up the major portion of the iris.
**s. ova'rii** [TA], **s. of ovary,** the fibrous tissue and smooth muscle composing the framework of the ovary.
**Rollet's s.,** the part of an erythrocyte left after removal of the hemoglobin.
**s. of thyroid gland,** s. glandulae thyroideae.
**vitreous s., s. vit'reum** [TA], the framework of firmer material making up the vitreous body of the eye, and enclosing within its meshes the more fluid portion (humor vitreus).

**stro·mal** (stro'məl) pertaining to or resembling stroma.

**stro·mat·ic** (stro-mat'ik) stromal.

**stro·ma·tin** (stro'mə-tin) a protein constituent of the stroma of erythrocytes.

**stro·ma·tog·e·nous** (stro″mə-toj'ə-nəs) [*stroma* + *-genous*] originating in the stroma or connective tissue of an organ.

**stro·ma·tol·y·sis** (stro″mə-tol'ĭ-sis) [*stroma* + *-lysis*] destruction of the stroma of a cell, especially that of a red blood cell.

**stro·ma·to·sis** (stro″mə-to'sis) adenomyosis in which the invading endometrial substance is stromal and not glandular; stromal adenomyosis.

**Stro·mey·er's cephalhematocele** (shtro'mi-ərz) [Georg Friedrich Ludwig *Stromeyer,* German surgeon, 1804–1876] see under *cephalhematocele.*

**stro·muhr** (shtro'moor) [Ger. "stream clock"] an instrument for measuring the velocity of the blood flow; specifically one invented by Ludwig in 1867. It was superseded by the flowmeter. See also *thermostromuhr.*

**Strong's bacillus** (strongz) [Richard Pearson *Strong,* American physician, 1872–1948] *Shigella flexneri.*

**stron·gy·li** (stron'jə-li) plural of *strongylus.*

**stron·gy·li·a·sis** (stron"jə-li'ə-sis) strongylosis.

**stron·gy·lid** (stron'jə-lid) 1. of or pertaining to the superfamily Strongyloidea. 2. strongylus.

**Stron·gyl·i·dae** (stron-jil'ĭ-de) a family of nematodes of the superfamily Strongyloidea; many are intestinal parasites in mammals, including humans. Genera of medical or veterinary interest include *Chabertia, Oesophagodontus, Oesophagostomum, Strongylus, Ternidens,* and *Triodontophorus.*

**Stron·gy·loi·dea** (stron"jə-loi'de-ə) [MeSH: Strongyloidea] a superfamily of phasmids, including the hookworms and related bursate nematodes. It comprises the families Ancylostomidae, Strongylidae, Trichostrongylidae, Metastrongylidae, and Syngamidae.

**Stron·gy·loi·des** (stron"jə-loi'dēz) [MeSH: Strongyloides] a genus of phasmid nematodes belonging to the family Rhabditidae, superfamily Rhabditoidea, widely distributed as intestinal parasites of mammals. In some systems of classification, included in the superfamily Rhabdiasoidea.
**S. intestina'lis,** *S. stercoralis.*
**S. papillo'sus,** a species found in cows, pigs, sheep, goats, rabbits, and rats.
**S. ranso'mi,** a species found in pigs.
**S. rat'ti,** a species found in rats.
**S. stercora'lis,** a species occurring widely in tropical and subtropical countries, the cause of strongyloidiasis in humans and domestic animals. Called also *Anguillula intestinalis, Anguillula stercoralis,* and *S. intestinalis.*

**stron·gy·loi·di·a·sis** (stron"jə-loi-di'ə-sis) [MeSH: Strongyloidiasis] infection of humans or domestic animals with *Strongyloides stercoralis.* The female worm and her larvae inhabit the mucosa and submucosa of the small intestine (see *intestinal s.*), and the larvae expelled in the feces develop in the soil and can penetrate skin on contact. They later are carried in the bloodstream to the lungs (see *pulmonary s.*), and from there they travel to the intestine via the trachea and esophagus. Massive infections are occasionally seen in immunocompromised patients and those treated with corticosteroids or certain other agents. An endogenous cycle of development may occur, allowing infections to persist for many years.
**intestinal s.,** the stage of human strongyloidiasis in which the worms are in the intestines, causing ulceration and diarrhea; in some persons infection is subclinical for decades.
**pulmonary s.,** the stage of human strongyloidiasis in which the worms are in the lungs, causing coughing, wheezing, and dyspnea; it occasionally progresses to sepsis or meningitis that can be fatal. Initial invasion from the bloodstream into the alveoli may be accompanied by hemorrhage and hemoptysis.

**stron·gy·loi·do·sis** (stron"jə-loi-do'sis) strongyloidiasis.

**stron·gy·lo·sis** (stron"jə-lo'sis) infection of a horse or other equid with worms of the genus *Strongylus.*

**Stron·gy·lus** (stron'jə-ləs) [Gr. *strongylos* round] [MeSH: Strongylus] a genus of parasitic nematodes of the family Strongylidae; several species infect horses and other equids.
**S. edenta'tus,** a species found in horses.
**S. equi'nus,** a species parasitic in the intestines of horses; called also *palisade worm.*
**S. fila'ria,** *Dictyocaulus filaria.*
**S. gibso'ni,** *Mecistocirrus digitatus.*
**S. gi'gas,** *Dioctophyma renale.*
**S. longevagina'tus,** *Metastrongylus elongatus.*
**S. micru'rus,** *Dictyocaulus viviparus.*
**S. paradox'us,** *Metastrongylus elongatus.*
**S. rena'lis,** *Dioctophyma renale.*
**S. sub'tilis,** *Trichostrongylus colubriformis.*
**S. vulga'ris,** a species that causes verminous aneurysm in equines.

**stron·gy·lus** (stron'jə-ləs) pl. *stron'gyli* [MeSH: Strongylus] An individual organism of the genus *Strongylus.*

**stron·ti·um** (stron'she-əm) [*Strontian,* Scotland] [MeSH: Strontium] a dark yellowish metal: symbol, Sr; atomic number, 38; atomic weight, 87.62. See also *radiostrontium.*
**s. 85,** a radioactive isotope of strontium, atomic mass 85, having a half-life of 64.84 days and decaying by electron capture with emission of gamma rays (0.514 MeV); it is used in the form of the chloride or nitrate salt as a radioactive tracer in bone imaging.
**s. 87m,** a metastable radioactive isotope of strontium, atomic mass 87, having a half-life of 2.80 hours and decaying with emission of gamma rays (0.388 MeV); it is used in the form of the chloride or nitrate salt as a radioactive tracer in bone imaging.
**s. 89,** a radioactive isotope of strontium, atomic mass 89, having a half-life of 50.55 days; it decays by beta emission (1.488 MeV) and is used as a radiation source in radiation therapy.
**s. 90,** a radioactive isotope of strontium, atomic mass 90, having a half-life of 28.5 years; it decays by emission of beta particles and forms yttrium 90 (q.v.) as a daughter product. It is used as a source of beta radiation in the treatment of a variety of benign ophthalmologic conditions.
**s. chloride Sr 89** [USP], the chloride salt of strontium 89, a calcium analogue that concentrates in areas of increased osteogenesis; used as a local radiation source for palliative treatment of bone pain in patients with metastatic bone lesions; administered intravenously.

**stron·ti·ure·sis** (stron"she-u-re'sis) the elimination of strontium from the body by way of the urine.

**stron·ti·uret·ic** (stron"she-u-ret'ik) pertaining to, characterized by, or promoting strontiuresis.

**stro·phan·thi·din** (stro-fan'thĭ-din) [MeSH: Strophanthidin] an aglycone obtained by hydrolysis of glycosides from *Strophanthus kombé.*

**stro·phan·thin** (stro-fan'thin) a glycoside or a mixture of steroidal glycosides obtained from *Strophanthus kombé,* occurring as a white or yellowish white powder; it is a cardioactive poison.
**G-s., s.-G,** ouabain.

**Stro·phan·thus** (stro-fan'thəs) [Gr. *strophos* a twisted band + *anthos* flower] a genus of shrubs, trees, and woody vines of the family Apocynaceae, found mostly in tropical Africa; several species are poisonous. *S. gra'tus* (Wall. & Hock.) Baill. yields ouabain; *S. his'pidus* DC. yields onaye and pseudostrophanthin; and *S. kom'bé* Oliv. yields strophanthidin and strophanthin.

**Stro·pha·ri·a·ceae** (strə-fa"re-a'se-e) a family of mushrooms (order Agaricales). Several genera are edible, and the genus *Psilocybe* is hallucinogenic.

**stropho·ceph·a·lus** (strof"o-sef'ə-ləs) a fetus exhibiting strophocephaly.

**stropho·ceph·a·ly** (strof"o-sef'ə-le) [Gr. *strophos* a twisted band + *-cephaly*] a developmental anomaly characterized by distortion of the head and face.

**stropho·so·mus** (strof"o-so'məs) [Gr. *strophos* a twisted band + *sōma* body] a celosomus, especially in chicks, in which the extremities are reflexed onto the back with the distal ends resting on the head.

**stroph·u·lus** (strof'u-ləs) [L.] papular urticaria.

**struck** (struk) a usually fatal enterotoxemia of calves, lambs, and piglets, caused by *Clostridium perfringens* type C, occurring chiefly in the winter and spring and characterized by hemorrhagic enteritis and peritonitis. Called also *hemorrhagic enterotoxemia* and *Romney Marsh disease.*

**struc·tur·al** (struk'chər-əl) pertaining to or affecting the structure.

**struc·ture** (struk'chər) [L. *struere* to build] the components and their manner of arrangement in constituting a whole.
**antigenic s.,** (of microorganisms), the mosaic of individual antigens present in cells of a microorganism.
**$\beta$ s.,** pleated sheet.
**covalent s.,** primary s.
**denture-supporting s's,** the tissues, either the teeth or residual ridges, or both, which serve as the foundation for removable partial or complete dentures.
**fine s.,** ultrastructure.
**primary s.,** the amino acid sequence of a polypeptide chain or the base sequence of a nucleic acid strand. Called also *covalent s.*
**quaternary s.,** the geometric arrangement of the subunits of a macromolecule.
**secondary s.,** aspects of the three-dimensional structure of macromolecules that have a regular geometric pattern, e.g., $\alpha$ helix or $\beta$ sheet regions in proteins, double helix regions in nucleic acids, or the cloverleaf structure of transfer RNAs.
**tertiary s.,** the three dimensional structure of a monomeric macromolecule or of a subunit of a multimeric macromolecule.

**stru·ma** (stroo'mə) [L.] goiter.
**s. aberra'ta,** aberrant goiter.
**cast iron s.,** Riedel's thyroiditis.
**s. colloi'des,** colloid goiter.
**s. endothora'cica,** intrathoracic goiter.
**s. fibro'sa,** fibrous goiter.
**s. follicula'ris,** parenchymatous goiter.
**s. gelatino'sa,** colloid goiter.
**Hashimoto's s.,** see under *disease.*
**ligneous s.,** Riedel's thyroiditis.
**s. lymphomato'sa,** Hashimoto's disease.
**s. nodo'sa,** multinodular goiter.
**s. ova'rii,** a rare teratoid tumor of the ovary composed almost entirely of thyroid tissue, with large follicles containing abundant colloid; occasionally there are symptoms of hyperthyroidism.

**s. parenchymato'sa,** parenchymatous goiter.
**Riedel's s.,** see under *thyroiditis.*

**stru•mec•to•my** (stroo-mek'tə-me) [*struma* + *-ectomy*] surgical removal of a goiter.
**median s.,** thyroidectomy.

**stru•mi•tis** (stroo-mi'tis) thyroiditis.

**Strüm•pell's disease, sign** (shtrēm'pəlz) [Adolf von *Strümpell,* German physician, 1853–1925] see under *disease* and *sign.*

**Strüm•pell-Leich•ten•stern encephalitis disease** (shtrēm' pəl-līk'tən-shtərn) [A. von *Strümpell;* Otto *Leichtenstern,* German physician, 1845–1900] hemorrhagic encephalitis.

**Strüm•pell-Ma•rie disease** (shtrēm'pəl-mah-re') [A. von *Strümpell;* Pierre *Marie,* French physician, 1853–1940] rheumatoid spondylitis.

**Strüm•pell-West•phal pseudosclerosis** (shtrēm'pəl-vest'fahl) [A. von *Strümpell;* Carl Friedrich Otto *Westphal,* German neurologist, 1833–1890] Wilson's disease; see under *disease.*

**Strun•sky's sign** (strun'skēz) [Max *Strunsky,* American orthopedic surgeon, 1873–1957] see under *sign.*

**Struth•ers' ligament** (struth'ərz) [Sir John *Struthers,* Scottish anatomist, 1823–1899] see under *ligament.*

**stru•vite** (stroo'vīt) [Baron Heinrich Christian Gottfried von *Struve,* German-born Russian diplomat, 1772–1851] a hard crystalline form of magnesium ammonium phosphate, a common type of urinary calculus.

**strych•nine** (strik'nīn) [MeSH: Strychnine] an extremely poisonous alkaloid obtained chiefly from *Strychnos nux-vomica* and other species of *S.,* which causes excitation of all portions of the central nervous system by blocking postsynaptic inhibition of neural impulses. See also *strychninism.*

**strych•nin•ism** (strik'nin-iz-əm) chronic strychnine poisoning. Symptoms include increased acuity of hearing, vision, touch, taste, and smell, followed by tonic convulsions and vomiting; in severe cases, it may culminate in respiratory paralysis and death.

**strych•nino•ma•nia** (strik″nin-o-ma'ne-ə) [*strychnine* + *-mania*] mental aberration due to strychnine poisoning.

**strych•nism** (strik'niz-əm) poisoning by strychnine.

**Strych•nos** (strik'nos) [Gr. "nightshade"] a genus of tropical trees of the family Loganiaceae whose seeds contain strychnine and other toxic alkaloids. *S. nux-vo'mica* L. has seeds called *nux vomica. S. igna'tii* has seeds called *St. Ignatius' beans.*

**STS** serologic test for syphilis; Society of Thoracic Surgeons.

**Stu•dent's *t*-test** (stoo'dənts) [*"Student,"* pseudonym of William Sealy Gossett, British mathematician, 1876–1937] see *t-test,* under *test.*

**study** (stud'e) 1. an examination or procedure. 2. a research project; see also *clinical trial,* under *trial.*
**barium s.,** a radiographic examination of the gastrointestinal tract using barium as a contrast agent; cf. *barium enema* and *double-contrast examination.*
**blind s.,** see *blind.*
**cardiac electrophysiologic s.,** see *cardiac electrophysiology* under *electrophysiology.*
**case s.,** one that identifies and samples individuals with a particular disease or condition, noting characteristics of the disease or condition and persons afflicted. Case studies are often used to call attention to new diseases or to diseases entering new populations.
**case-cohort s.,** an epidemiologic study in which samples of cases and surviving noncases of the condition being studied are drawn from the same cohort of a cohort study. The cases and noncases are matched for duration of survival and their histories are compared.
**case-control s.,** retrospective s.
**cohort s.,** prospective s.
**cross-sectional s.,** one employing a single point of data collection for each participant or system being studied; used for examining phenomena expected to be static through the period of interest. Cf. *longitudinal s.*
**ecological s.,** a statistical study exploring hypotheses by comparing groups, rather than individuals, e.g., comparing rates of breast cancer and levels of fat intake by country.
**longitudinal s.,** one in which participants, processes, or systems are studied over time, with data being collected at multiple intervals. The two main types are *prospective s.* and *retrospective s.* Cf. *cross-sectional s.*
**nerve conduction s's,** electroneurography.
**nested case-control s.,** a case-control study nested within a cohort study: a population is identified and baseline data obtained and stored; after following the cohort for some time, a case-control study is performed using the small percentage of people who develop the disease, with controls selected as a sample of those surviving members without disease who were at risk at the time of occurrence of each case. Baseline data can be analyzed solely for this small subset of the original population, and recall bias and other hazards of case-control studies are avoided.
**prospective s.,** a longitudinal epidemiologic study in which the groups of individuals (cohorts) are selected on the basis of factors that are to be examined for their effects on outcomes, e.g., the effect of exposure to a specific risk factor on the eventual development of a particular disease, and are then followed over a period of time to determine the incidence rates of the outcomes in question in relation to the original factors. Called also *cohort s.* "Prospective" usually implies a cohort selected in the present and followed into the future, but the cohort method can also be applied to existing longitudinal historical data, such as insurance or medical records: a cohort is identified and classified as to exposure to some factor at some date in the past and followed up to the present to determine incidence rates of the outcome. This is called a historical prospective study, prospective study of past data, or retrospective cohort study. Cf. *retrospective s.*
**retrospective s.,** a longitudinal epidemiologic study in which participating individuals are classified as either having (cases) or lacking (controls) some outcome and their histories are examined for the presence of specific factors possibly associated with that outcome. Cases and controls are often matched with respect to certain demographic or other variables but need not be. As compared to prospective studies, retrospective studies suffer from drawbacks: although they can measure the odds ratio, which often approximates relative risk, they cannot reveal true incidence rates or attributable risk. Also, large biases can be introduced both in the selection of controls and in the recall of past exposure to risk factors. The advantage of the retrospective study is its small scale, usually short time for completion, and its applicability to rare diseases, which would require study of very large cohorts in prospective studies. See also *prospective s.*

**stump** (stump) the distal end of the limb left after amputation.
**conical s.,** a cone-shaped amputation stump produced as a result of undue retraction of the muscles.

**stun** (stun) to knock senseless; to render unconscious by a blow or other force.

**stun•ning** (stun'ing) loss of function, analogous to unconsciousness.
**myocardial s.,** temporarily impaired myocardial function, resulting from a brief episode of ischemia, that persists for some period after reperfusion. Cf. *myocardial hibernation.*

**stunt** (stunt) to retard the growth of.

**stupe** (stōōp) [L. *stupa* oakum] a cloth, sponge, or the like, for external application, charged with hot water, wrung out nearly dry, and then made irritant or otherwise medicated.

**stu•pe•fa•cient** (stoo″pə-fa'shənt) [L. *stupefacere* to make senseless] 1. inducing stupor. 2. an agent that induces stupor.

**stu•pe•fac•tive** (stoo″pə-fak'tiv) producing narcosis or stupor.

**stu•por** (stoo'pər) [L.] 1. a lowered level of consciousness manifested by the subject's responding only to vigorous stimulation. See also *consciousness* 2. in psychiatry, a disorder marked by greatly reduced responsiveness, inattentiveness to the environment, and inaction.
**benign s.,** a condition of inattentiveness, inaction, and unresponsiveness from which recovery is likely; the term is often used to denote such symptoms occurring in the depressive phase of bipolar disorder, although it is now recognized that this condition has a poor prognosis and is more correctly termed a malignant stupor.
**catatonic s.,** the extreme decrease in reactivity to the environment and in spontaneous activity characteristic of catatonic schizophrenia.
**epileptic s.,** stupor following an epileptic convulsion; called also *postconvulsive s.*
**malignant s.,** one from which recovery is unlikely; see also *benign s.*
**postconvulsive s.,** epileptic s.

**stu•por•ous** (stoo'pər-əs) affected with or characterized by stupor.

**stupp** (stup) a poisonous kind of soot which accumulates in the condensers of mercury smelters; it contains metallic mercury in a finely divided condition.

**stur•dy** (stur'de) gid.

**Sturge's syndrome** (stər'jəz) [William Allen *Sturge,* British physician, 1850–1919] Sturge-Weber syndrome.

**Sturge-Kal•is•cher-Web•er syndrome** (stərj-kah'lish-ər-va'bər) [W.A. *Sturge;* Siegfried *Kalischer,* German physician, late 19th century; Frederick Parkes *Weber,* British physician, 1863–1962] Sturge-Weber syndrome.

**Sturge-Web·er syndrome** (stərj-va′bər) [W.A. *Sturge;* F.P. *Weber*] [MeSH: Sturge-Weber Syndrome] see under *syndrome.*

**Sturm's conoid, interval** (shtoormz) [Johann Christoph *Sturm,* German mathematician and physician, 1635–1703] see under *conoid,* and see *focal interval,* under *interval.*

**stut·ter·ing** (stut′ər-ing) [MeSH: Stuttering] a speech disorder involving three factors: (1) dysfluency with repetition of words and parts of words, prolongations of sounds, interjections of sounds or words, and long pauses; (2) listener reaction, considering the dysfluency to be abnormal or unacceptable; and (3) the speaker's reaction to the dysfluency and to the listener's reaction, with a self-conception as a stutterer. See also *stammering.*
**urinary s.,** stuttering urination.

**sty** (sti) pl. *sties.* Stye.

**sty·co·sis** (sti-ko′sis) the presence of calcium sulfate in the organs of the body, especially in the lymph nodes.

**stye** (sti) [L. *hordeolum*] hordeolum.
**meibomian s.,** one involving a meibomian gland, usually draining through the conjunctival surface of the lid.
**zeisian s.,** one involving a gland of Zeis, occurring on the surface of the skin at the edge of the lid.

**style** (stīl) 1. the way in which something is done or said. 2. stylet.
**coping s.,** defense mechanism.

**sty·let** (sti′lət) [L. *stilus;* Gr. *stylos* pillar] 1. a wire run through a catheter or cannula to render it stiff or to remove debris from its lumen. 2. a slender probe.

**sty·li·form** (sti′lĭ-form) [*stilo-* + *form*] long and pointed; styloid.

**sty·lis·cus** (sti-lis′kəs) [L., from Gr. *styliskos* rod] a slender cylindrical tent.

**styl(o)-** [L. *stilus* a stake, pole] a combining form denoting resemblance to a stake or pole, used especially to denote relationship to the styloid process of the temporal bone.

**sty·lo·hy·al** (sti″lo-hi′əl) stylohyoid.

**sty·lo·hy·oid** (sti″lo-hi′oid) pertaining to the styloid process of the temporal bone and to the hyoid bone.

**sty·loid** (sti′loid) [*styl-* + *-oid*] resembling a pillar; long and pointed; styliform.

**sty·loid·itis** (sti″loi-di′tis) inflammation of tissues around the styloid process of the temporal bone.

**sty·lo·man·dib·u·lar** (sti″lo-man-dib′u-lər) pertaining to the styloid process of the temporal bone and the mandible.

**sty·lo·mas·toid** (sti″lo-mas′toid) pertaining to the styloid process of the temporal bone and the mastoid process.

**sty·lo·max·il·lary** (sti″lo-mak′sĭ-lar″e) pertaining to the styloid process of the temporal bone and to the maxilla.

**Sty·lom·ma·to·pho·ra** (sti-lom″ə-tof′ə-rə) a suborder of the order Pulmonata, including land snails and slugs. Families of medical importance include Helicellidae, Helicidae, and Pupillidae.

**sty·lo·my·loid** (sti″lo-mi′loid) [*stylo-* + Gr. *mylē* mill + *-oid*] pertaining to the styloid process of the temporal bone and to the region of the lower molar teeth.

**sty·lo·po·di·um** (sti″lo-po′de-əm) see *limb.*

**sty·lo·staph·y·line** (sti″lo-staf′ə-līn) pertaining to the styloid process of the temporal bone and the velum palatinum.

**sty·los·teo·phyte** (sti-los′te-o-fīt) a pillar-shaped exostosis.

**sty·lo·stix·is** (sti″lo-stik′sis) [*stylo-* + Gr. *stixis* pricking] acupuncture.

**sty·lus** (sti′ləs) [L. *stilus*] 1. a stylet. 2. a pencil-shaped medicinal preparation, as a stick of caustic.

**sty·ma·to·sis** (sti″mə-to′sis) [Gr. *styma* priapism] priapism with a bloody discharge.

**styp·sis** (stip′sis) [Gr. *stypsis* contraction] 1. astringency; astringent action. 2. treatment by astringents.

**styp·tic** (stip′tik) [Gr. *styptikos*] 1. astringent; arresting hemorrhage by means of an astringent quality. 2. an astringent and hemostatic remedy.
**chemical s.,** one which arrests hemorrhage by causing coagulation through chemical action.
**mechanical s.,** one which acts by causing coagulation mechanically, as a pledget of cotton.
**vascular s.,** one which acts by producing contraction of injured or divided blood vessels of small caliber.

**Styp·ven** (stip′vən) trademark for a preparation of Russell's viper venom; used as a hemostatic agent. See also under *tests.*

**Sty·rax** (sti′raks) a genus of shrubs and trees the family Styracaceae, most of which are native to Indonesia, Malaysia, or Thailand; various species are sources of the medicinal substance benzoin.

**sty·rax** (sti′raks) storax.

**sty·rene** (sti′rēn) an unsaturated oily liquid hydrocarbon used in the manufacture of plastic, synthetic rubber, resins, as a dental filling component, and in drug manufacturing; it polymerizes spontaneously to form polystyrene. It is an irritant, toxic, possibly carcinogenic, and releases carbon monoxide on burning. Called also *cinnamene, cinnamol, styrol, styrolene,* and *vinyl benzene.*

**sty·rol** (sti′rol) styrene.

**sty·ro·lene** (sti′ro-lēn) styrene.

**su.** abbreviation for L. *su′mat,* let him take.

**sub-** [L. *sub* under] 1. a prefix meaning under, near, almost, partial, moderately, or subordinate. 2. in chemistry, a prefix denoting a basic compound or a compound containing less of an element or radical than another compound of the same elements.

**sub·ab·dom·i·nal** (sub″ab-dŏm′nəl) situated inferior to the abdomen.

**sub·ab·dom·i·no·peri·to·ne·al** (sub″ab-dom″ĭ-no-per″ĭ-to-ne′əl) subperitoneal.

**sub·ac·e·tab·u·lar** (sub″as-ə-tab′u-lər) situated below the acetabulum.

**sub·ac·e·tate** (səb-as′ə-tāt) any basic acetate.

**sub·ac·id** (səb-as′id) somewhat acid.

**sub·a·cid·i·ty** (sub″ə-sid′ĭ-te) deficient acidity.

**sub·acro·mi·al** (sub″ə-kro′me-əl) situated below or beneath the acromion.

**sub·acute** (sub″ə-kūt′) somewhat acute; between acute and chronic.

**sub·al·i·men·ta·tion** (sub″al-ĭ-mən-ta′shən) hypoalimentation.

**sub·anal** (səb-a′nəl) situated inferior to the anus.

**sub·ap·i·cal** (səb-ap′ĭ-kəl) situated inferior to an apex.

**sub·apo·neu·rot·ic** (sub″ap-o-noo͝-rot′ik) situated beneath an aponeurosis.

**sub·arach·noid** (sub″ə-rak′noid) situated or occurring between the arachnoid and the pia mater.

**sub·ar·cu·ate** (səb-ahr′ku-āt) [*sub-* + *arcuate*] somewhat arched or bent.

**sub·are·o·lar** (sub″ə-re′ə-lər) beneath an areola, particularly the areola of the breast.

**sub·as·trag·a·lar** (sub″əs-trag′ə-lər) situated or occurring inferior to the astragalus (talus).

**sub·astrin·gent** (sub″ə-strin′jənt) moderately astringent.

**sub·at·loi·de·an** (sub″at-loi′de-ən) situated inferior to the atlas.

**sub·atom·ic** (sub″ə-tom′ik) of or pertaining to the constituent parts of an atom as considered under the theory of the nuclear atom; occurring within an atom; smaller than an atom.

**sub·au·ral** (səb-aw′rəl) situated inferior to the ear.

**sub·au·ra·le** (sub″aw-ra′le) an anthropometric landmark, the lowest point on the inferior border of the ear lobule when the subject is looking straight ahead.

**sub·au·ric·u·lar** (sub″aw-rik′u-lər) inferior to the pinna (auricle) of the ear.

**sub·ax·i·al** (səb-ak′se-əl) inferior to an axis.

**sub·ax·il·lary** (səb-ak′sĭ-lar″e) inferior to the axilla, or armpit.

**sub·ba·sal** (səb-ba′səl) inferior to a base.

**sub·bra·chi·al** (səb-bra′ke-əl) relating to the brachium colliculi caudalis.

**sub·bra·chy·ce·phal·ic** (sub″bra-ke-sə-fal′ik) somewhat brachycephalic; having a cephalic index of 78 to 79.

**sub·cal·ca·re·ous** (sub″kal-kar′e-əs) slightly calcareous.

**sub·cal·car·ine** (səb-kal′kər-īn) inferior to the calcarine fissure.

**sub·cap·su·lar** (səb-kap′su-lər) situated beneath a capsule.

**sub·cap·su·lo·peri·os·te·al** (səb-kap″su-lo-per″e-os′te-əl) beneath the capsule and the periosteum of a joint.

**sub·car·bo·nate** (səb-kahr′bo-nāt) any basic carbonate.

**sub·ca·ri·nal** (sub″kə-ri′nəl) situated below the carina tracheae.

**sub·car·ti·lag·i·nous** (sub″kahr-tĭ-laj′ĭ-nəs) 1. situated beneath a cartilage. 2. partly cartilaginous.

**sub·cen·tral** (səb-sen′trəl) located deep to the center.

**sub·cep·tion** (səb-sep′shən) perception below the level of awareness.

**sub·chlo·ride** (səb-klor′īd) that chloride of any series which contains the smallest proportion of chlorine.

**sub·chon·dral** (səb-kon′drəl) beneath a cartilage.

**sub·chor·dal** (səb-kor′dəl) 1. below the notochord. 2. below the vocal folds (cords).

**sub·cho·ri·on·ic** (sub″kor-e-on′ik) situated beneath the chorion.

**sub·cho·roi·dal** (sub″ko-roi′dəl) beneath the choroid.

**sub·chron·ic** (sub-kron′ik) between chronic and subacute.

**sub·class** (sub′klas) a taxonomic category sometimes established, subordinate to a class and superior to an order.

**sub·cla·vi·an** (səb-kla′ve-ən) situated inferior to the clavicle, as the subclavian artery.

**sub·cla·vic·u·lar** (sub″klə-vik′u-lər) subclavian.

**sub·clin·i·cal** (səb-klin′ĭ-kəl) without clinical manifestations; said of the early stage(s) of an infection or other disease or abnormality before symptoms and signs become apparent or detectable by clinical examination or laboratory tests, or of a very mild form of an infection or other disease or abnormality. See also under *infection.*

**sub·clone** (sub′klōn) 1. the progeny of a mutant cell arising in a clone. 2. each new DNA population produced by cleaving DNA from a clonal population into fragments and cloning each fragment.

**sub·con·junc·ti·val** (sub″kən-jənk-ti′vəl) situated or occurring beneath the conjunctiva.

**sub·con·scious** (səb-kon′shəs) 1. imperfectly or partially conscious. 2. a term formerly used to include the preconscious and unconscious.

**sub·con·scious·ness** (səb-kon′shəs-nəs) the state of being partially conscious.

**sub·cor·a·coid** (səb-kor′ə-koid) situated inferior to the coracoid process.

**sub·cor·tex** (səb-kor′təks) that part of the brain substance which underlies the cortex.

**sub·cor·ti·cal** (səb-kor′tĭ-kəl) situated beneath the cortex.

**sub·cos·tal** (səb-kos′təl) situated inferior to a rib.

**sub·cos·ta·lis** (sub″kos-ta′lis) pl. *subcosta′les* [L.] subcostal.

**sub·cra·ni·al** (səb-kra′ne-əl) beneath the cranium.

**sub·crep·i·tant** (səb-krep′ĭ-tənt) pertaining to a rale that is slightly more coarse than a crepitant rale; see under *rale.*

**sub·crep·i·ta·tion** (sub″krep-ĭ-ta′shən) the sound of a subcrepitant rale.

**sub·cul·ture** (sub′kəl-chər) 1. a culture of bacteria derived from another culture. 2. the act of preparing a fresh culture from an existing one.

**sub·cu·ta·ne·ous** (sub″ku-ta′ne-əs) beneath the skin. Abbreviated SQ.

**sub·cu·tic·u·lar** (sub″ku-tik′u-lər) situated beneath the epidermis; subepidermal.

**sub·cu·tis** (səb-ku′tis) [*sub-* + *cutis*] subcutaneous tissue (tela subcutanea [TA]).

**sub·de·lir·i·um** (sub″də-lēr′e-əm) partial or mild delirium.

**sub·del·toid** (səb-del′toid) beneath the deltoid muscle.

**sub·den·tal** (səb-den′təl) [*sub-* + *dental*] beneath the teeth.

**sub·di·a·phrag·mat·ic** (sub″di-ə-frag-mat′ik) subphrenic.

**sub·di·vi·sion** (sub′dĭ-vĭ″zhən) in the classification of plants and fungi, a taxonomic category inferior to a division but superior to a class; equivalent to the subphylum of animal taxonomy.

**sub·dor·sal** (səb-dor′səl) situated inferior to the dorsal region.

**sub·duct** (səb-dukt′) [L. *subducere* to lead down] to depress or draw down; see *subduction.*

**sub·duc·tion** (səb-duk′shən) infraduction.

**sub·du·ral** (səb-doo′rəl) situated between the dura mater and the arachnoid.

**sub·en·do·car·di·al** (sub″ən-do-kahr′de-əl) beneath the endocardium.

**sub·en·do·the·li·al** (sub″ən-do-the′le-əl) situated beneath an endothelium.

**sub·en·do·the·li·um** (sub″ən-do-the′le-əm) Debove's membrane.

**sub·ep·en·dy·mal** (sub″ep-en′dĭ-məl) situated beneath the ependyma.

**sub·ep·en·dy·mo·ma** (sub″ep-en″dĭ-mo′mə) an ependymoma in which there is a diffuse proliferation of subependymal fibrillary astrocytes among the ependymal tumor cells. A few are malignant and others cause obstructive hydrocephalus, but many are clinically silent and are discovered only at autopsy.

**sub·epi·car·dial** (sub″ep-ĭ-kahr′de-əl) situated below the epicardium.

**sub·epi·der·mal, sub·epi·der·mic** (sub″ep-ĭ-der′məl, sub″ep-ĭ-der′mik) beneath the epidermis; subcuticular.

**sub·epi·glot·tic** (sub″ep-ĭ-glot′ik) below the epiglottis.

**sub·epi·the·li·al** (sub″ep-ĭ-the′le-əl) situated beneath an epithelium.

**su·ber·i·tin** (soo-ber′ĭ-tin) [*Suberites,* a marine sponge (from L. *suber* cork) + chemical suffix *-in*] a toxic substance derived from the marine sponge, *Suberites domunculus,* which, when injected into dogs, produces intestinal hemorrhages and respiratory distress.

**su·ber·o·sis** (soo″bə-ro′sis) [L. *suber* cork + *-osis*] a type of hypersensitivity pneumonitis seen in those who work with cork, caused by inhalation of moldy cork dust containing spores of various species of *Penicillium;* called also *cork handler's disease.*

**sub·fam·i·ly** (səb′fam-ĭ-le) a taxonomic category sometimes established, subordinate to a family and superior to a tribe or genus.

**sub·fas·cial** (səb-fash′əl) situated beneath a fascia.

**sub·fer·tile** (səb-fer′til) characterized by less than normal fertility.

**sub·fer·til·i·ty** (sub″fər-til′ĭ-te) the state of being less than normally fertile; relative sterility.

**Sub fin. coct.** abbreviation for L. *sub fi′nem coctio′nis,* toward the end of boiling.

**sub·fo·li·ar** (səb-fo′le-ər) pertaining to a subfolium.

**sub·fo·li·um** (səb-fo′le-əm) [*sub-* + *folium*] any of the elementary divisions of a cerebellar folium.

**sub·fron·tal** (sub-frun′təl) situated or extending underneath the frontal lobe.

**sub·ga·le·al** (səb-ga′le-əl) situated beneath the galea aponeurotica.

**sub·gal·late** (səb-gal′āt) a basic gallate.

**sub·gem·mal** (səb-jem′əl) [*sub-* + *gemma*] situated under a taste bud or other bud.

**sub·ge·nus** (səb′je-nəs) a taxonomic category between a genus and a species.

**sub·ger·mi·nal** (səb-jər′mĭ-nəl) below or under the germ.

**sub·gin·gi·val** (səb-jin′jĭ-vəl) beneath the gingiva.

**sub·gle·noid** (səb-gle′noid) situated inferior to the glenoid cavity of the scapula.

**sub·glos·sal** (səb-glos′əl) sublingual.

**sub·glos·si·tis** (sub″glos-i′tis) [*sub-* + *gloss-* + *-itis*] inflammation of the lower surface of the tongue.

**sub·glot·tic** (səb-glot′ik) infraglottic.

**sub·glot·tis** (sub-glot′is) cavitas infraglottica.

**sub·gran·u·lar** (səb-gran′u-lər) somewhat granular.

**sub·gron·da·tion** (sub″gron-da′shən) [Fr.] a type of depressed skull fracture, with depression of one fragment of bone beneath another.

**sub·gy·rus** (səb-ji′rəs) any gyrus that is partly concealed or covered by another or by others.

**sub·he·pat·ic** (sub″hə-pat′ik) situated inferior to the liver.

**sub·hu·mer·al** (səb-hu′mər-əl) inferior to or beneath the humerus.

**sub·hy·a·loid** (səb-hi′ə-loid) situated or occurring beneath the hyaloid membrane.

**sub·hy·oid** (sub-hi′oid) situated inferior to the hyoid bone.

**sub·hy·oi·de·an** (sub″hi-oi′de-ən) subhyoid.

**sub·ic·ter·ic** (sub″ik-ter′ik) somewhat jaundiced.

**su·bic·u·lar** (sə-bik′u-lər) of or pertaining to a subiculum, particularly the subiculum cornu ammonis (gyrus parahippocampalis).

**su·bic·u·lum** (sə-bik′u-ləm) [L., from *subicere* to raise, lift] [TA] an underlying or supporting structure.
**s. cor′nu ammo′nis, s. hippocam′pi,** gyrus parahippocampalis.
**s. promonto′rii cavita′tis tym′pani** [TA], **s. promonto′rii cavita′tis tympa′nicae,** subiculum of promontory of tympanic cavity: a ridge of bone bounding the tympanic sinus inferiorly.

**sub·il·i·ac** (səb-il′e-ak) inferior to the ilium.

**sub·il·i·um** (səb-il′e-əm) the most inferior portion of the ilium.

**sub·in·flam·ma·tion** (sub″in-flə-ma′shən) a slight or mild inflammation.

**sub·in·flam·ma·to·ry** (sub″in-flam′ə-tor″e) pertaining to or causing only mild inflammation.

**sub·in·ti·mal** (səb-in′tĭ-məl) beneath the intima of a vessel.

**sub·in·trance** (səb-in′trans) recurrence of a paroxysm after a shorter period than usual.

**sub·in·trant** (səb-in′trənt) [L. *subintrans* entering by stealth] 1. beginning before the completion of a previous cycle or paroxysm; anticipating. 2. characterized by recurrence at lessening intervals.

**sub·in·vo·lu·tion** (sub″in-vo-loo′shən) incomplete involution; failure of a part to return to its normal size and condition after enlargement due to functional activity, as subinvolution of the uterus after delivery of a baby.
**chronic s. of uterus,** a diffuse, symmetrical uterine enlargement commonly associated with painless menorrhagia and occurring soon after pregnancy.

**sub·io·dide** (səb-i′o-dīd) that iodide of any series which contains the smallest proportion of iodine.

**sub·ja·cent** (səb-ja′sənt) [*sub-* + L. *jacere* to lie] lying just beneath or underneath.

**sub·ject**[1] (səb-jekt′) [L. *subjectare* to throw under] to cause to undergo, or submit to; to render subservient.

**sub·ject**[2] (sub′jəkt) [L. *subjectus* cast under] a person or animal which has been the object of treatment, observation, or experiment.

**sub·jec·tive** (səb-jek′tiv) [L. *subjectivus*] pertaining to or perceived only by the affected individual; not perceptible to the senses of another person.

**sub·jec·to·scope** (səb-jek′to-skōp) [*subjective* + *-scope*] an instrument used in the study of subjective visual sensations.

**sub·ju·gal** (səb-joo′gəl) situated inferior to the zygomatic bone.

**sub·la·tio** (səb-la′she-o) [L.] sublation.
**s. re′tinae,** detachment of the retina.

**sub·la·tion** (səb-la′shən) [L. *sublatio*] a lifting up, or elevation.

**sub·le·sion·al** (səb-le′zhən-əl) performed or occurring beneath a lesion.

**sub·le·thal** (səb-le′thəl) not quite fatal; insufficient to cause death.

**sub·li·mate** (sub′lĭ-māt) [L. *sublimare* to elevate] 1. a substance obtained or prepared by sublimation. 2. to divert consciously unacceptable instinctual drives into personally and socially acceptable channels through a mechanism operating outside of and beyond conscious awareness.
**corrosive s.,** mercury bichloride.

**sub·li·ma·tion** (sub″lĭ-ma′shən) [MeSH: Sublimation] 1. the direct change of state from solid to vapor. 2. an unconscious defense mechanism in which consciously unacceptable instinctual drives are diverted into personally and socially acceptable channels.

**Sub·li·maze** (sub′lĭ-māz) trademark for a preparation of fentanyl citrate.

**sub·lime** (səb-līm′) [L. *sublimare* to elevate] to volatilize a solid body by heat and then to collect it in a purified form as a solid or powder.

**sub·lim·i·nal** (səb-lim′ĭ-nəl) [*sub-* + *liminal*] below the limen, or threshold, of sensation.

**sub·li·mis** (səb-li′mis) [L.] superficial.

**sub·lin·gual** (səb-ling′gwəl) beneath the tongue; called also *hypoglossal* and *subglossal.*

**sub·lin·gui·tis** (sub″ling-gwi′tis) inflammation of the sublingual gland.

**sub·lobe** (sub′lōb) a division of a lobe; a lobule.

**sub·lob·u·lar** (səb-lob′u-lər) situated beneath a lobule.

**sub·lux·ate** (səb-luk′sāt) to partially dislocate.

**sub·lux·a·tion** (sub″lək-sa′shən) [*sub-* + *luxation*] an incomplete or partial dislocation.
**atlantoaxial s.,** a complication of rheumatoid arthritis of the cervical spine; degeneration of the atlas and axis cause malalignment and cervical myelopathy.
**s. of lens,** partial dislocation of lens of the eye.
**Volkmann's s.,** a type of tuberculous arthritis marked by flexion contracture of the knee, external rotation of the leg, valgus position of the knee, and bending of the upper third of the tibia.

**sub·lym·phe·mia** (sub″lim-fe′me-ə) lymphocytopenia.

**sub·mam·ma·ry** (səb-mam′ə-re) situated or occurring beneath or deep to a mammary gland. Called also *inframammary.*

**sub·man·dib·u·lar** (sub″man-dib′u-lər) below the mandible.

**sub·mar·gi·nal** (səb-mahr′jĭ-nəl) situated inferior to or beneath a margin.

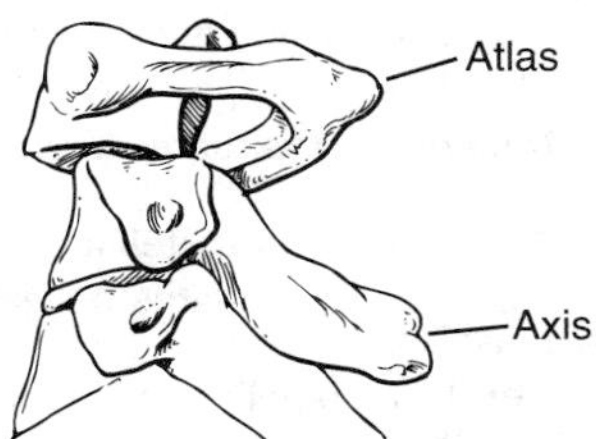


Atlantoaxial subluxation with forward displacement of the atlas on the axis.

**sub·max·il·la** (sub″mak-sil′ə) [*sub-* + *maxilla*] the mandible.

**sub·max·il·lar·itis** (səb-mak″sĭ-lər-i′tis) inflammation of the submaxillary gland.

**sub·max·il·lary** (səb-mak″sĭ-lar′e) situated inferior to or beneath the maxilla. Called also *inframaxillary.*

**sub·me·di·al** (səb-me′de-əl) submedian.

**sub·me·di·an** (səb-me′de-ən) beneath or near the middle; submedial.

**sub·mem·bra·nous** (səb-mem′brə-nəs) partly membranous.

**sub·men·tal** (səb-men′təl) [*sub-* + *mental*[2]] situated inferior to the chin.

**sub·men·to·ver·tex** (sub-ment″to-ver′təks) proceeding from underneath the chin toward the vertex of the head.

**sub·mer·sion** (səb-mər′zhən) [*sub-* + L. *mergere* to dip] the act of placing or the condition of being under the surface of a liquid.

**sub·meta·cen·tric** (sub″met-ə-sen′trik) having the centromere more or less equidistant from the center of the chromosome and one end, so that one arm is shorter than the other. Cf. *acrocentric* and *metacentric.*

**sub·mi·cro·scop·ic, sub·mi·cro·scop·i·cal** (səb-mi″kro-skop′ik, sub″mi-kro-skop′ĭ-kəl) too small to be visible under the light microscope.

**sub·mor·phous** (səb-mor′fəs) neither amorphous nor perfectly crystalline.

**sub·mu·co·sa** (sub″mu-ko′sə) the layer of areolar tissue situated beneath the mucous membrane; see the terms beginning *tela submucosa,* under *tela.*

**sub·mu·co·sal** (sub″mu-ko′səl) pertaining to the submucosa, or situated beneath the mucous membrane.

**sub·mu·cous** (səb-mu′kəs) situated or performed beneath the mucous membrane.

**sub·nar·cot·ic** (sub″nahr-kot′ik) moderately narcotic.

**sub·na·sal** (səb-na′zəl) situated inferior to the nose.

**sub·na·sa·le** (sub″na-sa′le) an anthropometric landmark situated at the point at which the nasal septum merges, with the upper lip in the median plane. Called also *subnasion.*

**sub·na·sion** (səb-na′ze-on) subnasale.

**sub·na·tant** (səb-na′tənt) 1. situated below or at the bottom of something. 2. the liquid phase situated below another liquid or a solid phase, having a greater density than the upper layer.

**sub·neu·ral** (səb-no͞o′rəl) situated beneath a nerve, as a subneural apparatus.

**sub·ni·trate** (səb-ni′trāt) a basic nitrate.

**sub·nor·mal** (səb-nor′məl) below or less than normal; characterized by qualities, such as intelligence, lower than the level usually observed.

**sub·nor·mal·i·ty** (sub″nor-mal′ĭ-te) the state of being subnormal.

**sub·no·to·chor·dal** (sub″no-to-kor′dəl) situated beneath the notochord.

**sub·nu·cle·us** (səb-noo′kle-əs) a partial or secondary nucleus into which a large nerve nucleus may be split up.

**sub·nu·tri·tion** (sub″noo-trĭ′shən) malnutrition.

**sub·oc·cip·i·tal** (sub″ok-sip′ĭ-təl) situated inferior to the occiput.

**sub·or·bi·tal** (səb-or′bĭ-təl) infraorbital.

**sub·or·der** (sub′or-dər) a taxonomic category sometimes established, subordinate to an order and superior to a family.

**sub·ox·ide** (səb-ok′sīd) that oxide in any series which contains the smallest proportion of oxygen.

**sub·pap·il·lary** (səb-pap′ĭ-lar-e) underlying the stratum papillare of the skin, as the subpapillary layer.

**sub·pap·u·lar** (səb-pap′u-lər) indistinctly papular.

**sub·par·a·lyt·ic** (sub″par-ə-lit′ik) partially paralytic.

**sub·pa·ri·e·tal** (sub″pə-ri′ə-təl) situated inferior to a parietal bone, lobe, etc.

**sub·pa·tel·lar** (sub″pə-tel′ər) infrapatellar.

**sub·pec·tor·al** (səb-pek′tər-əl) situated beneath or inferior to the pectoral region or muscles.

**sub·pel·vi·peri·to·ne·al** (səb-pel″vĭ-per″ĭ-to-ne′əl) situated beneath the pelvic peritoneum.

**sub·peri·car·di·al** (sub″pər-ĭ-kahr′de-əl) beneath the pericardium.

**sub·peri·os·te·al** (sub″pər-e-os′te-əl) situated beneath the periosteum.

**sub·peri·os·teo·cap·su·lar** (sub″pər-e-os″te-o-kap′su-lər) subcapsuloperiosteal.

**sub·peri·to·ne·al** (sub″pər-ĭ-to-ne′əl) situated beneath or deep to the peritoneum, as a subperitoneal abscess.

**sub·peri·to·neo·ab·dom·i·nal** (sub″pər-ĭ-to-ne″o-əb-dom′ĭ-nəl) subperitoneal.

**sub·peri·to·neo·pel·vic** (sub″pər-ĭ-to-ne″o-pel′vik) occurring beneath the peritoneum of the pelvis.

**sub·pha·ryn·ge·al** (sub″fə-rin′je-əl) situated inferior to the pharynx.

**sub·phren·ic** (səb-fren′ik) situated inferior to the diaphragm; subdiaphragmatic.

**sub·phy·lum** (səb-fi′ləm) pl. *subphy′la*. A taxonomic category sometimes established, subordinate to a phylum and superior to a class.

**sub·pi·al** (səb-pi′əl) situated beneath the pia mater.

**sub·pla·cen·ta** (sub″plə-sen′tə) the decidua basalis.

**sub·pleu·ral** (səb-ploor′əl) situated beneath the pleura.

**sub·pre·pu·tial** (sub″pre-pu′shəl) situated beneath the prepuce.

**sub·pu·bic** (səb-pu′bik) situated or performed inferior to the pubic arch.

**sub·pul·mo·nary** (səb-pul′mo-nar″e) situated or occurring below the lung, between the lung and the diaphragm.

**sub·pul·pal** (səb-pul′pəl) below the dental pulp.

**sub·py·ram·i·dal** (sub″pĭ-ram′ĭ-dəl) below a pyramid, as the subpyramidal fossa.

**sub·rec·tal** (səb-rek′təl) inferior to the rectum.

**sub·ret·i·nal** (səb-ret′ĭ-nəl) below the retina.

**sub·scapho·ceph·a·ly** (sub″skaf-o-sef′ə-le) the condition of being moderately scaphocephalic.

**sub·scap·u·lar** (səb-skap′u-lər) situated inferior to the scapula.

**sub·scle·ral** (səb-skler′əl) located or occurring beneath the sclera.

**sub·scle·rot·ic** (sub″sklə-rot′ik) 1. subscleral. 2. partly sclerosed.

**sub·scrip·tion** (səb-skrip′shən) that part of a prescription which gives the directions for compounding the ingredients; see *prescription.*

**sub·se·ro·sa** (sub″sēr-o′sə) a layer of tissue situated beneath a serous membrane. Called also *tela subserosa.*

**sub·se·rous** (səb-sēr′əs) situated beneath a serous membrane.

**sub·sib·i·lant** (səb-sib′ĭ-lənt) having a muffled, whistling sound.

**sub·son·ic** (səb-son′ik) infrasonic.

**sub·spec·ial·ty** (səb-spesh′əl-te) a branch of medicine subordinate to a specialty, as gastroenterology is a subspecialty of internal medicine.

**sub·spe·cies** (sub′spe-sēz) a taxonomic category subordinate to a species, whose members differ morphologically from other members of the species but remain capable of interbreeding with them; a variety or race.

**sub·spi·na·le** (sub″spi-na′le) the deepest midline point on the maxilla on the concavity between the anterior nasal spine and the prosthion. Called also *point A.*

**sub·spi·nous** (səb-spi′nəs) situated inferior to a spinous process.

**sub·sple·ni·al** (səb-sple′ne-əl) beneath the splenium of the corpus callosum.

**sub·stage** (sub′stāj) that part of the microscope which is situated beneath the stage.

**sub·stance** (sub′stəns) [L. *substantia*] 1. matter with a particular set of characteristics; material. 2. the material constituting an organ or body; called also *substantia* [TA]. 3. psychoactive s.

**α-s.,** old name for *reticular s.*
**adamantine s. of tooth,** enamelum.
**alpha s.,** old name for *reticular s.*
**arborescent white s. of cerebellum,** arbor vitae cerebelli.
**β-s., beta s.,** old name for *Heinz bodies,*
**black s.,** substantia nigra.
**blood group s's,** see under *antigen.*
**blood group specific s's A, B, and AB** [USP], a sterile, isotonic solution of the polysaccharide–amino acid complexes that are capable of neutralizing the anti-A and the anti-B isoagglutinins of group O blood. Specific substance A is usually isolated from hog gastric mucin, and specific substance B usually from the glandular portion of horse gastric mucosa. Used for the immunization of plasma donors in the production of reagents for *in vitro* diagnosis.
**cement s., cementing s.,** material which serves to hold together the different components of a tissue, as the intercellular substance in endothelium or the interprismatic substance in tooth enamel.
**central gelatinous s. of spinal cord,** substantia gelatinosa centralis medullae spinalis.
**chromidial s.,** granular endoplasmic reticulum.
**chromophil s.,** Nissl bodies.
**colloid s.,** a jelly-like material formed in colloid degeneration.
**compact s. of bones,** substantia compacta ossium.
**controlled s.,** any of the drugs regulated under the Controlled Substances Act (see under *C*).
**cortical s. of bone,** substantia corticalis ossium.
**cortical s. of cerebellum,** cortex cerebelli.
**cortical s. of kidney,** cortex renalis.
**cortical s. of lens,** cortex lentis.
**cortical s. of lymph node,** cortex nodi lymphoidei.
**depressor s.,** a substance that tends to decrease activity or blood pressure.
**gelatinous s. of posterior horn of spinal cord,** substantia gelatinosa cornu posterioris medullae spinalis.
**gray s.,** substantia grisea.
**gray s., central,** substantia grisea centralis.
**gray s. of spinal cord,** substantia grisea medullae spinalis.
**ground s.,** the amorphous gel-like material in which connective tissue cells and fibers are embedded.
**H s.,** H antigen (def. 2).
**I s.,** an inhibitory substance which appears in the synapses of the vertebrate central nervous system, which seems generally to act as a hypopolarizer of the postsynaptic junction.
**interfibrillar s. of Flemming, interfilar s.,** hyaloplasm, def. 1.
**intermediate s. of spinal cord, central,** substantia intermedia centralis medullae spinalis.
**intermediate s. of spinal cord, lateral,** substantia intermedia lateralis medullae spinalis.
**interprismatic s.,** a cementing substance occupying the space between the round or polygonal enamel prisms; it is softer and more plastic than the enamel prism itself.
**interspongioplastic s.,** hyaloplasm, def. 1.
**interstitial s.,** ground s.
**intertubular s. of tooth, ivory s. of tooth,** dentinum.
**s. of lens,** substantia lentis.
**medullary s.,** 1. substantia alba. 2. the soft, marrow-like substance of the interior of an organ; see under *medulla.*
**medullary s. of bone,** medulla ossium.
**medullary s. of bone, red,** medulla ossium rubra.
**medullary s. of bone, yellow,** medulla ossium flava.
**medullary s. of kidney,** medulla renalis.
**medullary s. of lymph node,** medulla nodi lymphoidei.
**metachromatic s.,** fine particles seen in erythrocytes, especially after supravital staining.
**müllerian inhibiting s.,** antimüllerian hormone.
**Nissl's s.,** Nissl bodies.
**no-threshold s's,** those substances in the blood which are excreted into the urine in proportion to their absolute amount in the blood. Cf. *threshold s's.*
**onychogenic s.,** the nail-forming substance which occurs in parallel fibrils in the nail matrix.
**organ-forming s's,** specialized materials that become segregated in definite blastomeres, thus bringing about a mosaic type of development.
**s. P,** a peptide composed of 11 amino acids, present in nerve cells scattered throughout the body and in special endocrine cells in the gut; it increases the contractions of gastrointestinal smooth muscle and causes vasodilatation, it is one of the most potent vasoactive substances known, and it seems to be a sensory neurotransmitter mediating pain, touch, and temperature.
**pellagra-preventing s.,** a dietary substance which will prevent or abolish pellagra.
**perforated s., anterior,** substantia perforata anterior.
**perforated s., interpeduncular, perforated s., posterior,** substantia perforata posterior.
**perforated s., rostral,** substantia perforata anterior.

**periaqueductal gray s., periventricular gray s.,** substantia grisea centralis.
**prelipid s.,** degenerated nerve tissue which has not yet been converted into fat.
**pressor s.,** any substance that tends to increase blood pressure.
**proper s. of tooth,** dentinum.
**psychoactive s.,** any chemical compound that affects the mind or mental processes; used particularly for drugs used therapeutically in psychiatry, the major classes being the antipsychotics, antidepressants, anxiolytics-sedatives, and mood-stabilizing drugs, but also sometimes used to include other classes of mind-altering substances such as drugs of abuse and some toxins.
**red s. of spleen,** pulpa splenica.
**Reichert's s.,** substantia innominata.
**reticular s.,** 1. formatio reticularis. 2. the netlike mass seen in erythrocytes after vital staining.
**reticular s. of mesencephalon,** formatio reticularis mesencephali.
**Rolando's gelatinous s.,** substantia gelatinosa cornu posterioris medullae spinalis.
**Rollett's secondary s.,** the transparent material lying in narrow zones on each side of Krause's membranes.
**sarcous s.,** the substance composing the sarcous element of muscle.
**second visceral s. of spinal cord,** substantia visceralis secundaria medullae spinalis.
**slow-reacting s. of anaphylaxis,** an inflammatory agent released by mast cells in the anaphylactic reaction; it induces slow, prolonged contraction of certain smooth muscles and is a potent bronchoconstrictor and an important mediator of allergic bronchial asthma. It is composed of a mixture of leukotrienes $C_4$, $D_4$, and $E_4$. Abbreviated SRS-A.
**specific soluble s. (SSS),** the polysaccharide capsular material of pneumococci *(Streptococcus pneumoniae),* which exhibits type-specific antigenic differences.
**spongy s. of bone,** substantia spongiosa ossium.
**threshold s's,** those substances in the blood, such as glucose, which are excreted into the urine only when their concentration in plasma exceeds a certain value.
**thromboplastic s.,** a general term for any material with procoagulant activity. Called also *zymoplastic s.*
**tigroid s.,** Nissl bodies.
**trabecular s. of bone,** substantia spongiosa ossium.
**transmitter s.,** neurotransmitter.
**white s.,** substantia alba.
**white s. of cerebellum,** corpus medullare cerebelli.
**white s. of spinal cord,** substantia alba medullae spinalis.
**zymoplastic s.,** thromboplastic s.

**sub·stan·tia** (səb-stan′she-ə) pl. *substan′tiae* [L.] substance: general anatomical nomenclature for material of which a tissue, organ, or body is composed. Called also *matter.*
**s. adamanti′na den′tis,** dental enamel.
**s. al′ba** [TA], white substance: the white nervous tissue, constituting the conducting portion of the brain and spinal cord; it is composed mostly of myelinated nerve fibers arranged in anterior, posterior, and lateral funiculi. Called also *white matter of nervous system.*
**s. al′ba medul′lae spina′lis** [TA], the white substance of the spinal cord, consisting of long myelinated nerve fibers arranged in parallel longitudinal bundles.
**s. cine′rea,** s. grisea.
**s. compac′ta os′sium** [TA], compact substance of bone: bone substance which is dense and hard; called also *compact bone.*
**s. cortica′lis len′tis,** cortex lentis.
**s. cortica′lis lymphoglan′dulae,** cortex nodi lymphoidei.

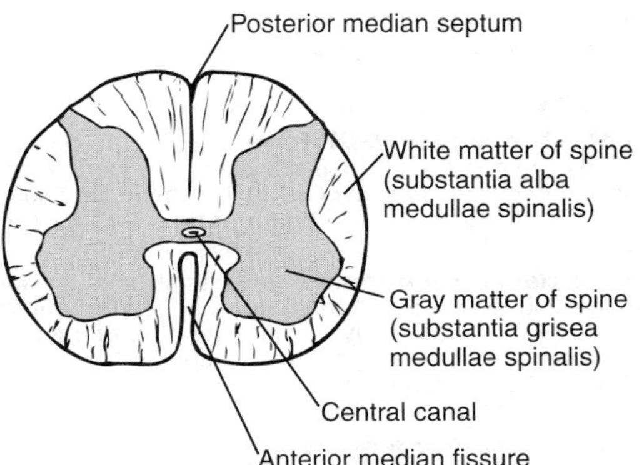


Transverse section of the spinal cord in the lumbar region, showing the fibrous arrangement of the substantia alba medullae spinalis (spinal white matter) and the central substantia grisea medullae spinalis (spinal gray matter).

**s. cortica′lis os′sium** [TA], cortical substance of bone: the substance comprising the hard outer layer of a bone.
**s. cortica′lis re′nis,** cortex renalis.
**s. ebur′nea den′tis,** dentinum.
**s. ferrugi′nea,** locus coeruleus.
**s. gelatino′sa centra′lis medul′lae spina′lis** [TA], central gelatinous substance of spinal cord: the zone of gelatinous-appearing substance consisting chiefly of neuroglia but also containing a few nerve fibers and cells, that encircles the central canal of the spinal cord and is surrounded by the central intermediate gray substance.
**s. gelatino′sa cor′nu posterio′ris medul′lae spina′lis** [TA], gelatinous substance of posterior horn of spinal cord: gelatinous-appearing material in Rexed's laminae II and III of the posterior column of the spinal cord, consisting chiefly of Golgi type II neurons and some larger nerve cells.
**s. gelatino′sa Rolan′di,** s. gelatinosa cornu posterioris medullae spinalis.
**s. glandula′ris pro′statae,** glandular substance of prostate: tissue composed of branched tubuloalveolar glands, outgrowths of the tunica mucosa of the urethra, which terminate in excretory ducts opening into the male urethra; it is enclosed in muscular substance and permeated by muscular strands. Called also *corpus glandulare prostatae.*
**s. gri′sea** [TA], gray substance: the gray nervous tissue composed of nerve cell bodies, unmyelinated nerve fibers, and supportive tissue. See also *Rexed's laminae,* under *lamina.* Called also *gray matter of nervous system.*
**s. gri′sea centra′lis** [TA], periaqueductal gray substance: diffuse collections of small cells immediately surrounding the ependymal lining of the third ventricle of the brain, around the cerebral aqueduct, and in the floor of the fourth ventricle. Called also *central* or *periventricular gray substance* and *s. grisea periaqueductalis.*
**s. gri′sea medul′lae spina′lis** [TA], gray substance of spinal cord: it contains fewer myelinated fibers but more nerve cell bodies, unmyelinated nerve fibers, and blood vessels than the white substance.
**s. gri′sea periaqueducta′lis,** s. grisea centralis.
**s. hyali′na,** the more fluid interstitial part of the protoplasm of a cell. Cf. *s. opaca.*
**s. innomina′ta** [TA], nerve tissue immediately inferior to the anterior perforated substance, and anterior to the globus pallidus and ansa lenticularis. Also known as the *s. innominata of Reichert* or *of Reil.*
**s. innominata of Reichert, s. innominata of Reil,** s. innominata.
**s. interme′dia centra′lis medul′lae spina′lis** [TA], central intermediate substance of spinal cord: the gray substance that makes up the gray commissure of the spinal cord.
**s. interme′dia latera′lis medul′lae spina′lis** [TA], lateral intermediate substance of spinal cord: the gray substance of the spinal cord that intervenes between the central intermediate substance, the intermediate column, and the anterior and posterior columns.
**s. intertubula′ris den′tis,** dentinum.
**s. len′tis** [TA], substance of lens: the fibrous material making up the bulk of the lens of the eye.
**s. medulla′ris lymphoglan′dulae,** medulla nodi lymphoidei.
**s. medulla′ris re′nis,** medulla renalis.
**s. metachromaticogranula′ris,** old name for *Heinz bodies.*
**s. muscula′ris pro′statae** [TA], muscular substance of prostate: the muscular stroma of the prostate, which is intimately blended with the fibrous capsule and permeates the glandular substance; called also *musculus prostaticus.*
**s. ni′gra** [TA], black substance: the layer of gray substance that separates the posterior parts of the cerebral peduncles (tegmentum mesencephali) from the anterior parts; it includes a posterior compact part with many pigmented cells *(pars compacta)* and an anterior reticular part whose cells contain little pigment *(pars reticularis).*
**s. opa′ca,** the reticulum of the protoplasm of a cell. Cf. *s. hyalina.*
**s. os′sea den′tis,** cementum.
**s. perfora′ta ante′rior** [TA], anterior perforated substance: an area on the base of the brain anterior to each optic tract, containing numerous perforations through which small branches of the anterior and middle cerebral arteries are transmitted to deeper structures. Called also *olfactory area, s. perforata rostralis,* [TA alternative] and *rostral perforated substance.*
**s. perfora′ta interpeduncula′ris, s. perfora′ta poste′rior** [TA], posterior perforated substance: the floor of the interpeduncular fossa, between the cerebral peduncles, which is pierced by central branches of the posterior cerebral artery; called also *interpeduncular perforated substance.*
**s. perfora′ta rostra′lis,** TA alternative for *s. perforata anterior.*
**s. pro′pria cor′neae** [TA], proper substance of cornea: the fibrous, tough, and transparent main part of the cornea, between the anterior and the posterior limiting lamina; called also *stroma of cornea.*
**s. pro′pria scle′rae** [TA], proper substance of sclera: the chief part of the sclera, lying between the lamina fusca and the episcleral lamina, composed of dense bands of fibrous tissue, mostly parallel with

the surface, and crossing each other in all directions. It is structurally continuous with the substantia propria corneae.
**s. reticula'ris,** formatio reticularis.
**s. reticulofilamento'sa,** reticular substance.
**s. spongio'sa os'sium** [TA], spongy substance of bone: bone substance made up of thin intersecting lamellae, usually found internal to compact bone; called also *cancellated* or *cancellous bone, spongy bone, trabecular substance,* and *s. trabecularis ossium* [TA alternative].
**s. trabecula'ris os'sium,** TA alternative for *s. spongiosa ossium.*
**s. viscera'lis secunda'ria medul'lae spina'lis** [TA], second visceral substance of spinal cord: the gray substance lying ventral to the central intermediate substance.

**sub·ster·nal** (səb-stər'nəl) situated beneath or inferior to the sternum. Called also *infrasternal.*

**sub·ster·no·mas·toid** (sub"stər-no-mas'toid) beneath or inferior to the sternocleidomastoid muscle.

**sub·stit·u·ent** (səb-stich'u-ənt) 1. a substitute; especially an atom, radical, or group substituted for another in a compound. 2. of or pertaining to such an atom, radical, or group.

**sub·sti·tute** (sub'stĭ-tōōt) [L. *substitutus,* past participle of *substituere* to substitute] a material which may be used in place of another.
**blood s., plasma s.,** a fluid which may be used instead of whole blood or plasma for replacement of circulating fluid in the body.
**saliva s.,** a solution, such as methylcellulose and mouthwash in distilled water, used to lubricate the oral tissues in xerostomia.

**sub·sti·tu·tion** (sub"stĭ-too'shən) 1. the act of putting one thing in the place of another, especially the chemical replacement of one element or radical by some other. 2. a defense mechanism, operating unconsciously, in which an unattainable or unacceptable goal, emotion, or object is replaced by one that is attainable or acceptable.
**creeping s. of bone,** the formation of new bone on the surfaces of necrotic trabeculae by osteoblasts, occurring after the revascularization of an area that has been disrupted by fracture, as at the head of the femur after fracture of the neck has disrupted the blood supply to the head of the bone.

**sub·sti·tu·tive** (sub"tĭ-too'tiv) effecting a change or substitution.

**sub·strate** (sub'strāt) 1. a substance upon which an enzyme acts. Symbol S. 2. a neutral substance containing a nutrient solution. 3. a surface upon which a different material is deposited or adhered, usually in a coating or layer.
**renin s.,** angiotensinogen.

**sub·stra·tum** (səb-stra'təm) [L.] 1. a substrate. 2. a lower layer or stratum.

**sub·struc·ture** (sub'strək-chər) 1. a structure that provides a foundation for another structure. 2. a basic underlying or supporting part of an organ or structure. Called also *infrastructure.* 3. implant s.
**implant s.,** a metal framework implanted beneath the mucoperiosteum, in contact with bone, that retains, supports, and stabilizes the superstructural part of an implant denture. Called also *implant framework* and *implant infrastructure.*

**sub·sul·cus** (səb-sul'kəs) a sulcus concealed by another.

**sub·sul·fate** (səb-sul'fāt) a basic sulfate.

**sub·syl·vi·an** (səb-sil've-ən) situated deep in the lateral sulcus (fissure of Sylvius).

**sub·ta·lar** (səb-ta'lər) [*sub-* + *talar*] inferior to the talus, as the subtalar joint.

**sub·tar·sal** (səb-tahr'səl) situated inferior to the tarsus.

**sub·telo·cen·tric** (səb-tel"o-sen'trik) having the centromere almost, but not quite, at the telocentric position.

**sub·tem·por·al** (səb-tem'por-əl) infratemporal.

**sub·te·ni·al** (səb-te'ne-əl) situated beneath a taenia.

**sub·ten·to·ri·al** (səb"ten-to're-əl) situated beneath the tentorium of the cerebellum.

**sub·ter·mi·nal** (səb-tər'mĭn-əl) situated near an end or extremity.

**sub·te·tan·ic** (sub"tə-tan'ik) mildly tetanic.

**sub·tha·lam·ic** (sub"thə-lam'ik) 1. situated below the thalamus. 2. pertaining to the subthalamus.

**sub·thal·a·mus** (səb-thal'ə-məs) [TA] a large ovoid mass in the anterior part of the diencephalon interposed between the dorsal thalamus, hypothalamus, and tegmentum of the mesencephalon; it contains the nuclei of the lateral and medial geniculate bodies, subthalamic and reticular nuclei, zona incerta, and nuclei of areae H (Forel's fields). Some authorities consider this to be part of the thalamus and refer to it as the *ventral thalamus.*

**sub·tile** (sut'əl) [L. *subtilis*] keen and acute.

**sub·til·in** (sub'til-in) an antibiotic substance isolated from strains of the soil bacteria *Bacillus subtilis,* which is chiefly effective against gram-positive bacteria and certain acid-fast bacilli.

**sub·til·i·sin** (səb-til'ĭ-sin) a proteolytic enzyme isolated from strains of the soil bacteria *Bacillus subtilis,* which catalyzes the hydrolysis of certain peptide bonds; analysis has shown it to be composed of 274 amino acid residues.

**sub·tle** (sut'əl) [L. *subtilis*] 1. very fine. 2. subtile.

**sub·to·tal** (sub-to'təl) less than complete, often something that is not much less than complete.

**sub·tra·pe·zi·al** (sub"trə-pe'ze-əl) situated beneath or inferior to the trapezius muscle.

**sub·tribe** (sub'trīb) a taxonomic category sometimes established, subordinate to a tribe and superior to a genus.

**sub·tro·chan·ter·ic** (sub"tro-kan-ter'ik) situated inferior to a trochanter.

**sub·troch·le·ar** (səb-trok'le-ər) situated inferior to a trochlea.

**sub·tu·ber·al** (səb-too'bər-əl) situated beneath or inferior to a tuber.

**sub·tym·pan·ic** (sub"tim-pan'ik) 1. infratympanic. 2. having a somewhat tympanic quality.

**sub·um·bil·i·cal** (sub"əm-bil'ĭ-kəl) situated inferior to the umbilicus.

**sub·un·gual** (səb-ung'gwəl) [*sub-* + *ungual*] situated beneath a nail; hyponychial.

**sub·ure·thral** (sub"u-re'thrəl) situated or occurring beneath the urethra.

**sub·vag·i·nal** (səb-vaj'ĭ-nəl) situated under a sheath, or inferior to the vagina.

**sub·ver·te·bral** (səb-vər'tə-brəl) situated on the anterior side of the vertebral column.

**sub·vit·ri·nal** (səb-vit'rĭ-nəl) situated beneath the vitreous.

**sub·vo·lu·tion** (sub"vo-loo'shən) [*sub-* + L. *volvere* to turn] the operation of reversing a flap; especially the operation of dissecting and turning up a pterygium, so that the outer or cutaneous surface comes in contact with the raw surface of the dissection. It is done to prevent readhesion.

**sub·wak·ing** (səb-wāk'ing) intermediate between waking and sleeping.

**sub·zo·nal** (səb-zo'nəl) situated beneath or inferior to a zone, as below the zona pellucida.

**sub·zy·go·mat·ic** (sub"zi-go-mat'ik) situated inferior to the zygomatic arch.

**suc·ca·gogue** (suk'ə-gog) [*succus* + *-agogue*] 1. inducing glandular secretion. 2. an agent that stimulates glandular secretion.

**suc·ce·da·ne·ous** (suk"sə-da'ne-əs) 1. pertaining to a succedaneum. 2. coming after or replacing something else.

**suc·ce·da·ne·um** (suk"sə-da'ne-əm) [L. *succedaneus* taking another's place] a medicine or material that may be substituted for another of like properties.

**suc·cen·tu·ri·ate** (suk"sən-tu're-āt) [L. *succenturiare* to substitute] accessory; serving as a substitute.

**suc·ci·mer** (suk'sĭ-mər) [MeSH: Succimer] DMSA; a chelating agent that is an analogue of dimercaprol, administered orally in the treatment of heavy metal poisoning; a complex with technetium 99m is used as a diagnostic aid in renal function testing. See table at *technetium.*

**suc·ci·nate** (suk'sĭ-nāt) any salt, ester, or anionic form of succinic acid.
**s. semialdehyde,** γ-hydroxybutyric acid.

**suc·ci·nate-CoA li·gase (GDP-form·ing)** (suk'sĭ-nāt-ko-a' li'gās) [EC 6.2.1.4] an enzyme of the ligase class that catalyzes the cleavage of succinate from succinyl CoA, using the energy so generated to form GTP from GDP. The reaction is part of the tricarboxylic acid cycle (see illustration at *cycle*). Called also *succinyl CoA synthetase.*

**suc·ci·nate de·hy·dro·gen·ase** (suk'sĭ-nāt de-hi'dro-jən-ās) [EC 1.3.99.1] [MeSH: Succinate Dehydrogenase] an enzyme of the oxidoreductase class that catalyzes the oxidation of succinate to fumarate, using a variety of hydrogen acceptors. An iron-containing flavoprotein, it is a component of succinate dehydrogenase (ubiquinone), an enzyme complex of the tricarboxylic acid cycle.

**suc·ci·nate de·hy·dro·gen·ase (ubiq·ui·none)** (suk'sin-āt de-hi'dro-jən-ās u-bik'win-ōn") [EC 1.3.5.1] an enzyme of the oxidoreductase class that catalyzes the oxidation of succinate to fumarate, using ubiquinone as an electron acceptor. It occurs in mitochondria as a membrane-bound complex, an iron-containing flavoprotein

(FAD) with an associated iron-sulfur protein. The reaction is part of the tricarboxylic acid cycle (see illustration at *cycle*).

**suc·ci·nate-semi·al·de·hyde de·hy·dro·gen·ase** (suk′sĭ-nāt sem″e-al′də-hīd de-hi′dro-jən-ās) [EC 1.2.1.24] an enzyme of the oxidoreductase class that catalyzes the oxidation of 4-hydroxybutyric acid to succinate. The reaction is the final step in the inactivation of γ-aminobutyric acid (GABA); when enzyme activity is deficient, increased levels of GABA and 4-hydroxybutyric acid can be detected in urine, plasma, and cerebrospinal fluid.

**suc·cin·ic ac·id** (sək-sin′ik) 1,4-butanedioic acid, an intermediate in the tricarboxylic acid cycle (q.v.).

**suc·cin·ic semi·al·de·hyde de·hy·dro·gen·ase de·fi·cien·cy** (suk-sin′ik sem″e-al′də-hīd de-hi′dro-jən-ās) an autosomal recessive aminoacidopathy caused by deficiency of the enzyme succinate semialdehyde dehydrogenase. The resulting increase in γ-aminobutyric acid and γ-hydroxybutyric acid causes mental retardation, hypotonia, and ataxia. Called also γ- or 4-hydroxybutyricaciduria.

**suc·ci·ni·mide** (sək-sin′ĭ-mīd) 1. an organic compound comprising a pyrrole ring with two carbonyl substitutions. 2. any of a class of anticonvulsants with such a basic structure, including ethosuximide, methsuximide, and phensuximide.

**Suc·ci·ni·mo·nas** (suk″sĭ-nĭ-mo′nas) [L. *acidum succinicum* succinic acid + Gr. *monas* unit, from *monos* single] a genus of gram-negative, anaerobic bacteria of the family Bacteroidaceae, made up of motile, short, straight rods with rounded ends that produce large amounts of succinic acid, found in the rumen contents of cattle. The genus contains a single species, *S. amyloly′tica.*

**Suc·ci·ni·vib·rio** (suk″sĭ-nĭ-vib′re-o) [L. *acidum succinicum* succinic acid + *vibrio*] a genus of gram-negative, anaerobic bacteria of the family Bacteroidaceae, made up of motile curved rods with pointed ends, found in the rumen contents of cattle and sheep. The genus contains a single species, *S. dextrinosol′vens.*

**suc·ci·nyl** (suk′sĭ-nəl) an acyl radical of succinic acid.

**suc·ci·nyl·ac·e·to·ac·e·tate** (suk″sin-əl-ə-se″to-as′ə-tāt) a compound formed by reduction of fumarylacetoacetate; it occurs at elevated levels in tyrosinemia, type I, due to the deficiency of fumarylacetoacetase. It is readily decarboxylated to succinylacetone (q.v.); both compounds can cause hepatorenal damage.

**suc·ci·nyl·ac·e·tone** (suk″sin-əl-as′ə-tōn) the compound formed by decarboxylation of succinylacetoacetate, occurring at elevated levels in tyrosinemia, type I, and believed to cause the characteristic hepatorenal damage. It competitively inhibits porphobilinogen synthase by being a structural analog of δ-aminolevulinic acid, secondarily inhibits other enzymes of tyrosine metabolism, and is structurally similar to maleic acid, an inhibitor of renal tubular function.

**suc·ci·nyl·cho·line chlo·ride** (suk″sĭ-nəl-ko′lēn) [USP] a neuromuscular blocking agent that produces skeletal muscle relaxation by blocking transmission at the myoneural junction; used for its muscle relaxant action during shock therapy and such procedures as endotracheal intubation and endoscopy, and as an adjunct to surgical anesthesia, administered intravenously and intramuscularly.

**suc·ci·nyl CoA** (suk′sĭ-nəl ko-a′) succinyl coenzyme A.

**suc·ci·nyl CoA syn·the·tase** (suk′sĭ-nəl ko-a′ sin′thə-tās) succinate-CoA ligase (GDP-forming).

**suc·ci·nyl co·en·zyme A** (suk″sĭ-nəl-ko-en′zīm) the succinate monothioester of coenzyme A, a high energy intermediate formed in the tricarboxylic acid cycle (q.v.). It is also a precursor in the synthesis of porphyrins.

**suc·ci·nyl·di·hy·dro·lipo·am·ide** (suk″sĭ-nəl-di-hi″dro-lip″o-am′īd) succinyl bound to lipoamide, an intermediate in the reaction catalyzed by the α-ketoglutarate dehydrogenase complex.

**suc·ci·nyl·sul·fa·thi·a·zole** (suk″sĭ-nəl-sul″fə-thi′ə-zōl) a sulfonamide used as an antibacterial in patients undergoing gastrointestinal surgery and in the treatment of gastrointestinal infections due to susceptible organisms, administered orally.

**suc·cor·rhea** (suk″o-re′ə) [*succus* + *-rrhea*] an excessive flow of a juice or secretion, as in ptyalism.

**suc·cus** (suk′əs) pl. *suc′ci* [L.] any fluid derived from living tissue; used in anatomical nomenclature as a general term for a bodily secretion or a fluid derived from body tissue; called also *juice.*
**s. cera′si,** cherry juice.
**s. ente′ricus,** intestinal juice: the liquid secreted by the glands in the wall of the small intestine.
**s. gas′tricus,** gastric juice: the liquid secretion of the glands of the stomach.
**s. pancrea′ticus,** pancreatic juice: the liquid secretion of the exocrine pancreas, which is discharged into the duodenum.
**s. prosta′ticus,** the secretion of the prostate gland, which contributes to formation of the semen.
**s. ru′bi idae′i,** raspberry juice.

**suc·cus·sion** (sə-kush′ən) [L. *succussio* a shaking from beneath, earthquake] shaking of the body during an examination; a splashing sound is indicative of the presence of fluid and air in a body cavity.
**hippocratic s.,** succussion to elicit a splashing sound in the chest; see *succussion sounds,* under *sound.*

**suck·le** (suk′əl) to derive or to provide nourishment by feeding at the breast.

**Su·cos·trin** (sə-kos′trin) trademark for a preparation of succinylcholine chloride.

**Suc·quet-Hoy·er anastomosis (canal)** (su-ka′hoy′ər) [J.P. *Sucquet,* French anatomist, 1840–1870; Heinrich Friedrich *Hoyer,* Polish anatomist, 1834–1907] segmentum arteriale anastomosis arteriovenae glomeriformis.

**su·cral·fate** (soo-kral′fāt) [USP] [MeSH: Sucralfate] a complex of aluminum and a sulfated polysaccharide, used as a gastrointestinal antiulcerative; administered orally.

**su·cra·lose** (soo′krə-lōs) [NF] a chlorinated derivative of sucrose, used as a sweetening agent.

**su·crase** (soo′krās) [MeSH: Sucrase] an enzyme of the hydrolase class that catalyzes the cleavage of the glycosidic bond in the disaccharides sucrose and maltose to yield their component sugars. The enzyme occurs complexed with α-dextrinase in the brush border of the intestinal mucosa; deficiency of enzyme complex activity, an autosomal recessive trait, called sucrase-isomaltase deficiency, is a form of disaccharide intolerance. In EC nomenclature called *sucrose α-glucosidase.*

**su·crase-iso·mal·tase de·fi·cien·cy** (soo′krās i-so-mawl′tās) a disaccharidase deficiency in which deficient activity of the sucrase-isomaltase complex of the intestinal mucosa results in malabsorption of sucrose and starch dextrins; it is characterized by watery, osmotic-fermentative diarrhea, sometimes leading to dehydration and malnutrition, manifest in infancy *(congenital sucrose intolerance).* While sucrase activity is always absent, α-dextrinase (isomaltase) activity may be either greatly reduced or relatively normal. See also *disaccharide intolerance,* under *intolerance.*

**su·crate** (soo′krāt) a compound of a substance with sucrose.

**su·cro·clas·tic** (soo″kro-klas′tik) [*sucrose* + *-clastic*] splitting of sugar.

**su·crose** (soo′krōs) [Fr. *sucre* sugar] [MeSH: Sucrose] 1. a nonreducing disaccharide obtained from sugar cane *(Saccharum officinarum),* sugar beet *(Beta vulgaris),* and sorghum; it is composed of glucose and fructose linked via their anomeric carbons. It is used extensively as a food and a sweetener. 2. [NF] an official preparation used as a sweetening agent, tablet excipient, lozenge basis, and suspending and viscosity increasing agent.
**s. octaacetate** [NF], a white, almost odorless, hygroscopic powder, having an intensely bitter taste; used as an alcohol denaturant.

**su·crose α-glu·co·si·dase** (soo′krōs gloo-kōs′ĭ-dās) EC nomenclature for *sucrase.*

**su·cros·emia** (soo″kro-se′me-ə) the presence of sucrose in the blood.

**su·cros·uria** (soo″kro-su′re-ə) the presence of sucrose in the urine.

**suc·tion** (suk′shən) [L. *sugere* to suck] [MeSH: Suction] aspiration of gas or fluid by mechanical means.
**post-tussive s.,** a sucking sound heard over a lung cavity just after a cough.
**Wangensteen s.,** see under *tube.*

**suc·to·ri·al** (sək-tor′e-əl) fitted for performing suction.

**Su·da·fed** (soo′də-fed) trademark for preparations of pseudoephedrine hydrochloride.

**su·da·men** (soo-da′mən) pl. *suda′mina* [L., from *sudare* to sweat] a whitish vesicle caused by the retention of sweat in the sudorific ducts or the layers of the epidermis. In the plural *(sudamina),* an eruption of such vesicles, known as *miliaria crystallina.*

**su·dam·i·nal** (soo-dam′ĭ-nəl) pertaining to or resembling sudamina.

**Su·dan** (soo-dan′) [MeSH: Sudan] a group of azo compounds used as stains for fats.
**S. I,** a yellow fat-soluble azo dye, chemical name 1-phenylazo-2-naphthol; it is an irritant and suspected carcinogen.
**S. II,** an orange fat-soluble azo dye, chemical name 1-[2,4-xylylazo]-2-naphthol used in biological staining of fats; it is an irritant and suspected carcinogen.
**S. III,** chemical name: 1-(*p*-phenylazophenylazo)-2-naphthol. A red fat-soluble azo dye; an important stain for the demonstration of neutral fats.

**S. IV,** scarlet red.
**S. black B,** a black, fat-soluble diazo dye, used as a stain for fats.
**S. G,** S. III.
**S. yellow G,** a brown powder used as a stain for fats.

**su·dano·phil** (soo-dan′o-fil) an element that stains readily with Sudan.

**su·dano·phil·ia** (soo-dan″o-fil′e-ə) [*sudan* + *-philia*] affinity for Sudan stain.

**su·dano·phil·ic** (soo-dan″o-fil′ik) staining readily with Sudan.

**su·dan·oph·i·lous** (soo″dən-of′ĭ-ləs) sudanophilic.

**su·da·tion** (soo-da′shən) [L. *sudatio*] sweating.

**Su·deck's atrophy (disease)** (soo′deks) [Paul Hermann Martin *Sudeck,* German surgeon, 1866–1938] see *post-traumatic osteoporosis,* under *osteoporosis.*

**Su·deck-Le·riche syndrome** (soo′dek-lə-rēsh′) [P. H. M. *Sudeck;* René *Leriche,* French surgeon, 1879–1955] see under *syndrome.*

**su·do·gram** (soo′do-gram) [L. *sudor* sweat + *-gram*] a graphic representation of the areas of the body on which sweating is present.

**su·do·mo·tor** (soo″do-mo′tər) [L. *sudor* sweat + *motor*] stimulating the sweat glands.

**su·do·re·sis** (soo″do-re′sis) diaphoresis.

**su·do·rif·er·ous** (soo″do-rif′ər-əs) [L. *sudor* sweat + *-ferous*] 1. conveying sweat. 2. sudoriparous.

**su·do·rif·ic** (soo″do-rif′ik) [L. *sudorificus*] diaphoretic.

**su·do·rip·a·rous** (soo″do-rip′ə-rəs) [L. *sudor* sweat + *parere* to produce] secreting or producing sweat.

**SUDS** sudden unexplained death syndrome; see under *syndrome.*

**su·et** (soo′ət) [L. *sevum*] the fat from the abdominal cavity of a ruminant animal, especially the sheep or ox; used in the preparation of cerates and ointments and as an emollient. The preparation employed in pharmacy is the internal fat of the abdomen of the sheep.
**prepared s.,** the internal fat of the abdomen of the sheep purified by melting and straining.

**Su·fen·ta** (soo-fen′tə) trademark for a preparation of sufentanil.

**su·fen·ta·nil cit·rate** (soo-fen′tə-nil) [USP] an opioid analgesic derived from fentanyl, used as an analgesic adjunct in the maintenance of general anesthesia and as a primary agent for induction and maintenance of general anesthesia in selected patients undergoing major surgery; administered intravenously.

**suf·fo·cant** (suf′ə-kənt) an agent that causes suffocation.

**suf·fo·ca·tion** (suf″ə-ka′shən) [L. *suffocatio*] asphyxiation.

**suf·fu·sion** (sə-fu′zhən) [L. *suffusio*] 1. the process of overspreading, or diffusion. 2. the condition of being moistened or of being permeated through, as by blood.

**sug·ar** (shoog′ər) any of a class of sweet, water-soluble, crystallizable carbohydrates, which are the monosaccharides and smaller oligosaccharides; often used specifically for sucrose. In animals, they are the chief source of energy and their derivatives are universal constituents of structural materials (e.g., glycosaminoglycans, cellulose).
**s. alcohol,** see under *alcohol.*
**amino s.,** a sugar in which an amino group substituent has replaced a hydroxyl group; the amino sugars and their acyl derivatives are constituents of a variety of polysaccharides, glycoproteins, and glycolipids.
**anhydrous s.,** anhydrosugar.
**beet s.,** sucrose derived from the root of the beet.
**blood s.,** glucose.
**burnt s.,** caramel.
**cane s.,** sucrose obtained from sugar cane.
**compressible s.** [NF], a preparation which contains 95–98 per cent sucrose and which may contain starch, dextrin, and invert sugar; used as a sweetening agent and tablet excipient in pharmaceutical preparations.
**confectioner's s.** [NF], sucrose ground together with corn starch to a fine powder, containing 95–97 per cent sucrose; used as a sweetening agent and tablet excipient in pharmaceutical preparations.
**deoxy s.,** a sugar in which one or more carbon atoms have been reduced, thus losing their hydroxyl groups.
**diabetic s.,** the glucose found in the urine in diabetes mellitus.
**invert s.,** a mixture of equal amounts of dextrose and fructose obtained by hydrolysing sucrose; used in solution as a parenteral nutrient.
**reducing s.,** any sugar that can act as a reducing agent in an alkaline solution; included are all monosaccharides and di- or oligosaccharides in which at least one anomeric carbon is a free aldehyde or keto group.
**simple s.,** a monosaccharide.
**threshold s.,** the lower limit of hyperglycemia at which glucose appears in the urine.

**sug·ges·ti·bil·i·ty** (səg-jes″tĭ-bil′ĭ-te) a condition of enhanced susceptibility to suggestion.

**sug·ges·ti·ble** (səg-jes′tĭ-bəl) highly susceptible to suggestion.

**sug·ges·tion** (səg-jes′chən) [L. *suggestio*] [MeSH: Suggestion] 1. the act of offering an idea for action or for consideration of action. 2. an idea so offered. 3. in psychiatry, the process of causing uncritical acceptance of an idea.
**hypnotic s.,** a suggestion imparted to a person in the hypnotic state, by which he is induced to alter perceptions or memory or to perform actions.
**posthypnotic s.,** implantation in the mind of a subject during hypnosis of a suggestion to be acted upon after recovery from the hypnotic state.

**sug·gil·la·tion** (sug″jĭ-la′shən) [L. *suggillatio*] 1. a bruise or ecchymosis. 2. a mark of postmortem lividity.

**su·i·cide** (soo′ĭ-sīd) [L. *sui* of himself + *-cide*] [MeSH: Suicide] the taking of one's own life.
**psychic s.,** the termination of one's own life without employment of physical agents.

**su·i·ci·dol·o·gy** (soo″ĭ-sīd-ol′ə-je) [*suicide* + *-logy*] the study of the causes and prevention of suicide.

**su·id** (soo′id) porcine.

**suint** (swint) a fat-like substance derivable from sheep's wool, from which anhydrous lanolin is prepared. Called also *suint de laine.*

**su·i·pes·ti·fer** (soo″ĭ-pes′tĭ-fər) a group of salmonellae *(Salmonella choleraesuis* var. *kuzendorf, S. choleraesuis* var. *typhisuis, S. enteritidis* serotype *hirschfeldii)* causing paratyphoid gastroenteritis in humans and pigs.

**Sui·pox·vi·rus** (soo′ĭ-poks″vi′rəs) [L. *sus,* gen. *suis* pig + *poxvirus*] [MeSH: Suipoxvirus] swinepox virus; a genus of viruses of the subfamily Chordopoxvirinae (family Poxviridae) that cause swinepox in piglets.

**suit** (so͞ot) an outer garment covering the entire body.
**antiblackout s., anti-G s.,** G s.
**antishock s.,** pneumatic antishock garment.
**G s.,** a garment worn by pilots, designed to increase their ability to withstand ill effects of the acceleratory forces experienced in certain aerial maneuvers.

**Su·ker's sign** (soo′kərz) [George Franklin *Suker,* American ophthalmologist, 20th century] see under *sign.*

**Sul·am·yd** (sul′am-id) trademark for a preparation of sulfacetamide.

**Su·lar** (soo′lahr) trademark for a preparation of nisoldipine.

**sul·bac·tam** (səl-bak′təm) [MeSH: Sulbactam] a $\beta$-lactamase inhibitor.
**s. sodium** [USP], the sodium salt of sulbactam; a $\beta$-lactamase inhibitor used to increase the antibacterial activity of penicillins and cephalosporins against $\beta$-lactamase–producing organisms.

**sul·ben·ox** (səl-ben′ox) a veterinary growth stimulant.

**sul·cate** (sul′kāt) [L. *sulcatus*] furrowed or marked with sulci.

**sul·ca·tion** (səl-ka′shən) the formation of sulci; the state of being marked by sulci.

**sul·ci** (sul′si) [L.] genitive and plural of *sulcus.*

**sul·ci·form** (sul′sĭ-form) formed like a groove.

**sul·con·a·zole ni·trate** (səl-kon′ə-zōl) [USP] a broad-spectrum antifungal, applied topically in the treatment of tinea pedis, tinea corporis, tinea cruris, and tinea versicolor, and in the treatment of *Candida albicans* infections.

**sul·cu·lus** (sul′ku-ləs) pl. *sul′culi* [L.] a small or minute sulcus.

**sul·cus** (sul′kəs) gen. and pl. *sul′ci* [L.] 1. a groove, trench, or furrow. 2. [TA] a general term for such a depression, especially one of those on the surface of the brain, separating the gyri. See also *fissure.* 3. a linear depression or valley in the occlusal surface of a tooth, the sloping sides of which meet at an angle.

## Sulcus

Descriptions are given on TA terms, and include anglicized names of specific sulci.

**alveolabial s.,** the furrow between the dental arch and the lips.
**alveolingual s.,** the depression between the dental arch and the tongue.
**s. ampulla′ris** [TA], **ampullary s.,** a transverse groove on the membranous ampulla of each semicircular duct, for the ampullary branch of the pars vestibularis nervi octavi.
**angular s.,** incisura angularis gastris.
**anterolateral s. of medulla oblongata,** s. anterolateralis medullae oblongatae.
**anterolateral s. of spinal cord,** s. anterolateralis medullae spinalis.
**s. anterolatera′lis medul′lae oblonga′tae** [TA], anterolateral sulcus of medulla oblongata: a longitudinal sulcus on the anterior surface of the medulla oblongata, lateral to the pyramid, from which emerge the fibers of the hypoglossal nerve. Called also *anterolateral groove of medulla oblongata, ventrolateral s. of medulla oblongata,* and *s. ventrolateralis medullae oblongatae.*
**s. anterolatera′lis medul′lae spina′lis** [TA], anterolateral sulcus of spinal cord: the longitudinal groove on the anterolateral surface of the spinal cord, from which the anterior nerve roots emerge; it separates the anterior and lateral funiculi. Called also *anterolateral groove of spinal cord, ventrolateral s. of spinal cord,* and *s. ventrolateralis medullae spinalis.*
**s. anthe′licis transver′sus,** transverse sulcus of anthelix: the depression on the medial surface of the pinna corresponding to the lower crus of the anthelix.
**aortic s., s. aor′ticus,** groove for aorta.
**s. arte′riae menin′geae me′diae** [TA], sulcus for middle meningeal artery: either of two grooves in the parietal bone for branches of the meningeal artery; one, posterior to the coronal suture, lodges the frontal branch, and the other, anterior to the mastoid angle, lodges the parietal branch.
**s. arte′riae occipita′lis** [TA], sulcus for occipital artery: the groove just medial to the mastoid notch on the temporal bone, lodging the occipital artery. Called also *occipital groove.*
**s. arte′riae subcla′viae** [TA], sulcus for subclavian artery: a transverse groove on the cranial surface of the first rib, just posterior to the anterior scalene tubercle; it lodges the subclavian artery; called also *subclavian s.* and *s. subclavius.*
**s. arte′riae tempora′lis me′diae** [TA], sulcus for middle temporal artery: a nearly vertical groove running just superior to the external acoustic meatus on the external surface of the squamous part of the temporal bone; it lodges the middle temporal artery.
**s. arte′riae vertebra′lis atlan′tis** [TA], sulcus for vertebral artery of atlas: the groove on the cranial surface of the posterior arch of the atlas; it lodges the vertebral artery and the first spinal nerve.
**arterial sulci, sul′ci arteria′les,** sulci arteriosi.
**sul′ci arterio′si** [TA], arterial sulci: grooves on the internal surfaces of the cranial bones for the meningeal arteries; called also *arterial grooves.*
**atrioventricular s.,** s. coronarius cordis.
**s. for auditory tube,** semicanalis tubae auditoriae.
**s. of auricle, posterior, s. auri′culae poste′rior,** s. posterior auriculae.
**s. of auricular branch of vagus nerve,** s. canaliculi mastoidei.
**s. auricula′ris poste′rior,** s. posterior auriculae.
**basilar s. of occipital bone,** s. sinus petrosi inferioris ossis occipitalis.
**basilar s. of pons, s. basila′ris pon′tis** [TA], the anteromedian groove in the pons, lodging the basilar artery.
**bicipital s., lateral,** s. bicipitalis lateralis.
**bicipital s., medial,** s. bicipitalis medialis.
**bicipital s., radial,** s. bicipitalis lateralis.
**bicipital s., ulnar,** s. bicipitalis medialis.
**s. bicipita′lis latera′lis** [TA], lateral bicipital sulcus: a longitudinal groove on the lateral side of the arm which marks the limit between the lateral border of the biceps muscle and the brachialis; called also *lateral* or *radial bicipital groove, radial bicipital s.,* and *s. bicipitalis radialis* [TA alternative].
**s. bicipita′lis media′lis** [TA], medial bicipital sulcus: a longitudinal groove on the medial side of the arm which marks the limit between the medial border of the biceps muscle and the brachialis; called also *medial* or *ulnar bicipital groove, s. bicipitalis ulnaris* [TA alternative], and *ulnar bicipital s.*
**s. bicipita′lis radia′lis,** TA alternative for *s. bicipitalis lateralis.*
**s. bicipita′lis ulna′ris,** TA alternative for *s. bicipitalis medialis.*
**bulbopontine s., s. bulboponti′nus** [TA], a transverse groove in front and on each side of the pons that demarcates it from the medulla oblongata, which is occupied by the abducent, facial, and vestibulocochlear nerves. Called also *medullopontine s.*
**calcaneal s., s. calca′nei** [TA], a rough, deep groove on the upper surface of the calcaneus, between the medial and the posterior articular surfaces and giving attachment to the interosseous talocalcaneal ligament.
**calcarine s., s. calcari′nus** [TA], a sulcus on the medial surface of the occipital lobe, separating the cuneus from the lingual gyrus; called also *calcarine fissure.*
**callosal s.,** s. corporis callosi.
**callosomarginal s.,** s. cinguli.
**s. canali′culi mastoi′dei,** a small groove in the petrous portion of the temporal bone leading to the mastoid canaliculus.
**s. caro′ticus os′sis sphenoida′lis** [TA], **carotid s.,** the groove on the side of the body of the sphenoid bone that lodges the internal carotid artery and the cavernous sinus.
**carpal s., s. car′pi** [TA], a broad deep groove on the volar surface of the carpal bones, which transmits the flexor tendons and the median nerve into the palm of the hand.
**central cerebral s., central s. of cerebrum,** s. centralis cerebri.
**central s. of insula,** s. centralis insulae.
**s. centra′lis ce′rebri** [TA], central sulcus of cerebrum: a relatively deep, nearly vertical sulcus on the cerebral hemisphere, which separates the frontal from the parietal lobe.
**s. centra′lis in′sulae** [TA], central sulcus of insula: a deep, oblique furrow which divides the insula into a larger anterior and a smaller posterior part.
**cerebral sulci, sul′ci cerebra′les,** sulci cerebri.
**sul′ci ce′rebri** [TA], **sulci of cerebrum,** cerebral sulci: the furrows between the cerebral gyri.
**chiasmatic s., s. chias′matis,** s. prechiasmaticus.
**cingulate s., s. cingula′tus,** s. cinguli.
**s. cin′guli** [TA], **s. of cingulum,** cingulate sulcus: a long, irregularly shaped sulcus on the medial surface of a hemisphere, which separates the cingulate gyrus below from the medial frontal gyrus and the paracentral lobule above. At its posterior end it turns up to form a marginal part between the precuneus and the paracentral lobule.
**circular s. of insula, s. circula′ris in′sulae** [TA], a fissure that almost surrounds the insula (lobus insularis) and separates it from the opercula.
**collateral s., s. collatera′lis** [TA], a longitudinal sulcus on the inferior surface of the cerebral hemisphere between the fusiform gyrus and the hippocampal gyrus; called also *collateral fissure.*
**s. col′li mandi′bulae,** the shallow groove between the ridge of the mandibular neck and the line of attachment of the sphenomandibular ligament.
**s. corona′rius cor′dis** [TA], **coronary s. of heart,** a groove on the external surface of the heart, separating the atria from the ventricles; portions of it are occupied by the major arteries and veins of the heart; called also *atrioventricular groove.*
**s. cor′poris callo′si** [TA], **s. of corpus callosum,** a sulcus encircling the convex aspect of the corpus callosum at the bottom of the longitudinal cerebral fissure.
**s. cos′tae** [TA], **costal s.,** a sulcus that follows the inferior and internal surface of a rib anteriorly from the tubercle, gradually becoming less distinct; it lodges the intercostal vessels and nerves.
**costal s., inferior,** s. costae.
**s. cru′ris he′licis** [TA], **s. of crus of helix,** a transverse sulcus on the medial surface of the pinna, corresponding to the crus helicis on the lateral surface.
**cuboid s.,** s. tendinum musculorum peroneorum calcanei.
**sul′ci cu′tis** [TA], sulci of skin: the fine depressions on the surface of the skin between the dermal ridges. Called also *skin furrows.*
**dorsolateral s. of medulla oblongata,** s. posterolateralis medullae oblongatae.
**dorsolateral s. of spinal cord,** s. posterolateralis medullae spinalis.
**s. dorsolatera′lis medul′lae oblonga′tae,** s. posterolateralis medullae oblongatae.

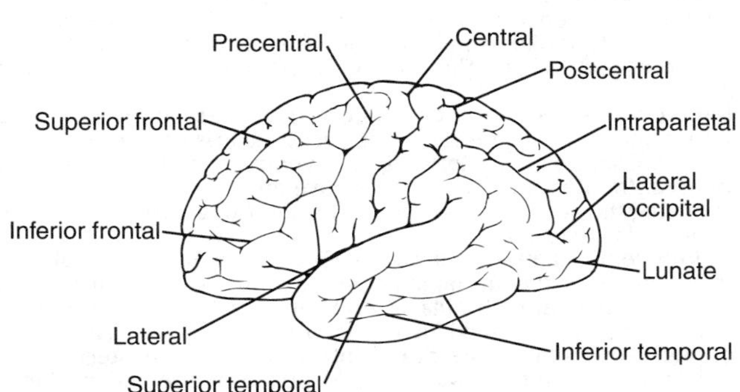

Sulci cerebri (cerebral sulci), showing some major sulci on the superolateral surface of the left cerebral hemisphere.

**s. dorsolatera'lis medul'lae spina'lis,** s. posterolateralis medullae spinalis.

**ethmoidal s. of nasal bone, s. ethmoida'lis os'sis nasa'lis** [TA], a groove that extends the entire length of the posteromedial surface of the nasal bone and lodges the external nasal branch of the anterior ethmoid nerve.

**s. of eustachian tube,** semicanalis tubae auditoriae.

**fimbriodentate s., s. fimbriodenta'tus** [TA], a shallow groove between the medial parts of the dentate gyrus and fimbria hippocampi.

**frontal s., inferior,** s. frontalis inferior.

**frontal s., superior,** s. frontalis superior.

**s. fronta'lis infe'rior** [TA], inferior frontal sulcus: a short longitudinal sulcus that separates the inferior and middle frontal gyri.

**s. fronta'lis supe'rior** [TA], superior frontal sulcus: a longitudinal sulcus that separates the middle and superior frontal gyri.

**gingival s., s. gingiva'lis** [TA], a shallow V-shaped space around the tooth, bounded by the tooth surface on one side and the epithelium lining the free margin of the gingiva on the other; considered by some authorities to be the same as the gingival crevice.

**gluteal s., s. glutea'lis** [TA], a curved transverse groove or fold on the posterior aspect of the upper thigh, separating the upper part of the thigh from the nates (buttocks); called also *gluteal fold* or *furrow.*

**s. for greater petrosal nerve,** s. nervi petrosi majoris.

**s. of habenula, s. habe'nulae,** s. habenularis.

**habenular s., s. habenula'ris** [TA], a groove separating the trigonum habenulae from the upper surface of the thalamus.

**s. ha'muli pterygoi'dei** [TA], sulcus of pterygoid hamulus: a smooth groove on the lateral surface of the medial pterygoid plate of the sphenoid bone, in the angle at the base of the pterygoid hamulus; it lodges the tendon of the tensor veli palatini muscle.

**Harrison's s.,** see under *groove.*

**hippocampal s., s. hippocampa'lis** [TA], **s. hippocam'pi,** the sulcus that extends from the splenium of the corpus callosum almost to the tip of the temporal lobe, and forms the medial boundary of the hippocampal gyrus; called also *hippocampal fissure.*

**horizontal s. of cerebellum,** fissura horizontalis cerebelli.

**hypothalamic s., s. hypothala'micus** [TA], **s. hypothala'micus [Monro'i],** a shallow curved sulcus on the wall of the third ventricle, extending from the interventricular foramen to the cerebral aqueduct.

**s. for inferior petrosal sinus of occipital bone,** s. sinus petrosi inferioris ossis occipitalis.

**s. for inferior petrosal sinus of temporal bone,** s. sinus petrosi inferioris ossis temporalis.

**infraorbital s. of maxilla, s. infraorbita'lis maxil'lae** [TA], a groove in the orbital surface of the maxilla, commencing near the middle of the posterior edge of the surface and running anteriorly for a short distance to become continuous with the infraorbital canal.

**infrapalpebral s., s. infrapalpebra'lis** [TA], the furrow below the lower eyelid.

**interarticular s. of calcaneus,** s. calcanei.

**interarticular s. of talus,** s. tali.

**sul'ci interloba'res ce'rebri** [TA], interlobar sulci of cerebrum: the sulci that separate the lobes of the brain from each other.

**intermediate s. of spinal cord, dorsal, intermediate s. of spinal cord, posterior,** s. intermedius posterior medullae spinalis.

**s. interme'dius dorsa'lis medul'lae spina'lis,** s. intermedius posterior medullae spinalis.

**s. interme'dius gas'tricus,** a slight groove in the stomach about 2.5 cm from the duodenopyloric junction.

**s. interme'dius poste'rior medul'lae spina'lis** [TA], posterior intermediate sulcus of spinal cord: a longitudinal sulcus in the cervical and upper thoracic parts of the spinal cord between the fasciculus gracilis and the fasciculus cuneatus. Called also *dorsal intermediate s. of spinal cord* and *s. intermedius dorsalis medullae spinalis.*

**interparietal s.,** s. intraparietalis.

**intertubercular s. of humerus, s. intertubercula'ris hu'meri** [TA], a longitudinal groove on the anterior surface of the humerus, lying between the tubercula above and between the cristae tuberculi farther down, and lodging the tendon of the long head of the biceps muscle.

**interventricular s., anterior,** s. interventricularis anterior.

**interventricular s., inferior,** s. interventricularis posterior.

**interventricular s., posterior,** s. interventricularis posterior.

**interventricular s. of heart,** the groove dividing the two ventricles, comprising the sulcus interventricularis anterior and the sulcus interventricularis posterior.

**s. interventricula'ris ante'rior** [TA], anterior interventricular sulcus: a groove on the sternocostal surface of the heart marking the position of the interventricular septum and the line of separation between the ventricles; called also *anterior interventricular groove.*

**s. interventricula'ris infe'rior,** s. interventricularis posterior.

**s. interventricula'ris poste'rior** [TA], posterior interventricular sulcus: a groove on the diaphragmatic surface of the heart marking the position of the interventricular septum and the line of separation between the ventricles; called also *inferior interventricular groove.*

**intraparietal s., s. intraparieta'lis** [TA], an irregular sulcus on the convex surface of the parietal lobe of the cerebrum and between the inferior and superior parietal lobuli; called *Pansch's fissure.*

**Jacobson's s.,** 1. s. promontorii cavitatis tympani. 2. sulcus tympanicus ossis temporalis.

**labiodental s.,** the arched groove in the embryo which separates off the anterior part of the mandibular process, thus helping to form the lower lip.

**lacrimal s. of lacrimal bone,** s. lacrimalis ossis lacrimalis.

**lacrimal s. of maxilla, s. lacrima'lis maxil'lae** [TA], a groove directed inferiorly and somewhat posteriorly on the nasal surface of the body of the maxilla, just anterior to the large opening into the maxillary sinus; it is converted into the nasolacrimal canal by the lacrimal bone and inferior nasal concha.

**s. lacrima'lis os'sis lacrima'lis** [TA], lacrimal sulcus of lacrimal bone: a deep vertical groove on the anterior part of the lateral surface of the lacrimal bone, which with the maxilla forms the fossa for the lacrimal sac.

**lateral cerebral s., lateral s. of cerebrum,** s. lateralis cerebri.

**lateral s. of crus cerebri,** lateral s. of mesencephalon.

**lateral s. for lateral sinus of occipital bone,** s. sinus transversi.

**lateral s. for lateral sinus of parietal bone,** s. sinus sigmoidei ossis parietalis.

**lateral s. of medulla oblongata, anterior,** s. anterolateralis medullae oblongatae.

**lateral s. of medulla oblongata, posterior,** s. posterolateralis medullae oblongatae.

**lateral s. of mesencephalon,** s. lateralis mesencephali.

**lateral s. for sigmoidal part of lateral sinus,** s. sinus sigmoidei ossis temporalis.

**lateral s. of spinal cord, anterior,** s. ventrolateralis medullae spinalis.

**lateral s. of spinal cord, posterior,** s. dorsolateralis medullae spinalis.

**s. latera'lis ce'rebri** [TA], lateral cerebral s.: a deep cleft beginning at the anterior perforated substance, extending laterally between the temporal and frontal lobes, and turning posteriorly between the temporal and parietal lobes. It divides into posterior, ascending, and anterior branches. Called also *s. Sylvii, fissure* or *fossa of Sylvius,* and *sylvian fissure* or *fossa.*

**s. latera'lis mesence'phali** [TA], lateral sulcus of mesencephalon: a longitudinal groove on the side of the mesencephalon, separating the crus cerebri from the tegmentum. Called also *lateral s. of crus cerebri.*

**s. latera'lis pedun'culi ce'rebri,** s. lateralis mesencephali.

**s. for lesser petrosal nerve,** s. nervi petrosi minoris.

**s. li'mitans fos'sae rhomboi'deae** [TA], sulcus limitans of rhomboid fossa, a longitudinal groove on the lateral side of the medial eminence, extending the entire length of the floor of the fourth ventricle.

**s. limitans of insula,** s. circularis insulae.

**s. lim'itans ventriculo'rum ce'rebri,** sulcus limitans of cerebral ventricles: a groove midway on the inner surface of each lateral wall of the neural tube, which separates it into a dorsal, alar plate and a ventral, basal plate.

**longitudinal s. of heart, anterior,** s. interventricularis anterior.

**longitudinal s. of heart, posterior,** s. interventricularis posterior.

**lunate s., s. luna'tus** [TA], a small semilunar furrow sometimes seen on the lateral surface of the occipital lobe of the cerebrum; this sulcus is conspicuous in the brain of certain apes and was called by Reidinger *Affenspalte* [Ger. "ape fissure"].

**mallear s. of temporal bone,** a groove that runs obliquely downward and forward across the inner aspect of the anterior tympanic ring, which lodges the anterior process of the malleus, chorda tympani, and anterior tympanic artery at birth. Called also *malleolar s. of temporal bone.*

**malleolar s. of fibula,** s. malleolaris fibulae.

**malleolar s. of temporal bone,** mallear s. of temporal bone.

**malleolar s. of tibia,** s. malleolaris tibiae.

**s. malleola'ris fi'bulae** [TA], malleolar sulcus of fibula: a groove on the posterior surface of the lateral malleolus of the fibula, which lodges the tendons of the peroneal muscles.

**s. malleola'ris ti'biae** [TA], malleolar sulcus of tibia: a short longitudinal groove on the posterior surface of the medial malleolus of the tibia, which lodges the tendons of the posterior tibial muscle and the long flexor muscle of the toes.

**mandibular s.,** s. colli mandibulae.

**s. of mastoid canaliculus,** s. canaliculi mastoidei.

**s. ma'tricis un'guis, s. of matrix of nail,** the cutaneous fold in which the proximal part of the nail is embedded.

**medial s. of crus cerebri, medial s. of mesencephalon,** s. nervi oculomotorii.

**median s. of fourth ventricle,** s. medianus ventriculi quarti.

**median s. of medulla oblongata, dorsal, median s. of medulla oblongata, posterior,** s. medianus posterior medullae oblongatae.

**median s. of spinal cord, dorsal, median s. of spinal cord, posterior,** s. medianus posterior medullae spinalis.

**median s. of tongue,** s. medianus linguae.

**s. media'nus dorsa'lis medul'lae oblonga'tae,** s. medianus posterior medullae oblongatae.

**s. media'nus dorsa'lis medul'lae spina'lis,** s. medianus posterior medullae spinalis.

**s. media'nus lin'guae** [TA], median sulcus of tongue: a shallow groove on the dorsal surface of the tongue in the midline.

**s. media'nus poste'rior medul'lae oblonga'tae** [TA], posterior median sulcus of medulla oblongata: a narrow groove present only in the closed part of the medulla oblongata, separating the two fasciculi graciles; it is the continuation of the posterior median sulcus of the spinal cord. Called also *dorsal* or *posterior median fissure of medulla oblongata, dorsal median s. of medulla oblongata,* and *s. medianus dorsalis medullae oblongatae.*

**s. media'nus poste'rior medul'lae spina'lis** [TA], posterior median sulcus of spinal cord: a shallow vertical groove on the posterior median surface of the spinal cord, separating the two posterior funiculi; the posterior median septum extends out from it. Called also *dorsal* or *posterior median fissure of spinal cord, dorsal median s. of spinal cord,* and *s. medianus dorsalis medullae spinalis.*

**s. media'nus ventri'culi quar'ti** [TA], median sulcus of fourth ventricle: a median groove in the floor of the fourth ventricle.

**medullopontine s.,** s. bulbopontinus.

**meningeal sulci,** sulci arteriosi.

**mentolabial s., s. mentolabia'lis** [TA], the depression between the lower lip and the chin. Called also *mentolabial furrow.*

**s. for middle temporal artery,** s. arteriae temporalis mediae.

**s. of Monro,** s. hypothalamicus.

**s. mus'culi flexo'ris hal'lucis lon'gi calca'nei,** s. tendinis musculi flexoris hallucis longi calcanei.

**s. mus'culi flexo'ris hal'lucis lon'gi ta'li,** s. tendinis musculi flexoris hallucis longi tali.

**s. mus'culi peronae'i os'sis cuboi'dei,** s. tendinis musculi fibularis longi.

**s. mus'culi subcla'vii** [TA], sulcus for subclavian muscle: a groove on the inferior surface of the clavicle into which the subclavian muscle is inserted by muscle fibers; called also *subclavian groove.*

**mylohyoid s. of mandible, s. mylohyoi'deus mandi'bulae** [TA], a groove on the medial surface of the ramus of the mandible, passing downward and forward from the foramen mandibulae and lodging the mylohyoid artery and nerve.

**nasal s., posterior,** meatus nasopharyngeus.

**nasolabial s., s. nasolabia'lis** [TA], the depression between the nose and the upper lip.

**s. ner'vi oculomoto'rii** [TA], oculomotor sulcus: a longitudinal groove on the medial surface of the anterior part of the cerebral peduncle that lodges the oculomotor nerve; called also *s. oculomotorius, medial s. of crus cerebri,* and *medial s. of mesencephalon.*

**s. ner'vi petro'si majo'ris** [TA], sulcus for greater petrosal nerve: a small groove sometimes present on the anterior surface of the petrous part of the temporal bone (the floor of the middle cranial fossa), running anteromedially from the hiatus of the facial canal to the foramen lacerum, and lodging the greater petrosal nerve; called also *groove for greater petrosal nerve.*

**s. ner'vi petro'si mino'ris** [TA], sulcus for lesser petrosal nerve: a small groove on the anterior surface of the petrous part of the temporal bone (the floor of the middle cranial fossa), running anteromedially just lateral to the sulcus of the greater petrosal nerve, and lodging the lesser petrosal nerve. Called also *groove for lesser petrosal nerve, innominate canaliculus,* and *Arnold's canal.*

**s. ner'vi radia'lis** [TA], sulcus for radial nerve: a broad oblique groove on the posterior surface of the humerus for the radial nerve and the deep brachial artery; called also *radial groove, spiral s.,* and *s. spiralis.*

**s. ner'vi spina'lis** [TA], sulcus for spinal nerve: the groove on the upper surface of each transverse process of a cervical vertebra, extending from the foramen transversarium lateralward and separating the anterior and posterior tubercles. It lodges the ventral branch of a cervical nerve.

**s. ner'vi ulna'ris** [TA], sulcus for ulnar nerve: a shallow vertical groove on the posterior surface of the medial epicondyle of the humerus for the ulnar nerve; called also *groove of ulnar nerve* or *ulnar groove.*

**nymphocaruncular s., nymphohymeneal s.,** a groove between either labium minus and the carunculae hymenales.

**obturator s. of pubis, s. obturato'rius os'sis pu'bis** [TA], a groove that obliquely crosses the inferior surface of the superior ramus of the pubis, giving passage to the obturator vessels and nerve.

**occipital s., anterior,** s. occipitalis anterior.

**occipital sulci, lateral,** sulci occipitales laterales.

**occipital sulci, superior,** sulci occipitales superiores.

**occipital s., transverse,** s. occipitalis transversus.

**s. for occipital artery,** s. arteriae occipitalis.

**s. occipita'lis ante'rior,** anterior occipital sulcus: a variable, vertically disposed furrow on the convex surface of the cerebrum, which by some is taken as the line of division between the parietal and the occipital lobes.

**sul'ci occipita'les latera'les,** lateral occipital sulci: horizontal furrows that divide the lateral occipital gyri into upper and lower portions.

**sul'ci occipita'les superio'res,** superior occipital sulci: irregular sulci associated with the superior occipital gyri.

**s. occipita'lis transver'sus** [TA], transverse occipital sulcus: a vertical sulcus in back of the gyrus angularis, which may help to form the anterior boundary of the occipital lobe or may lie within it.

**occipitotemporal s., s. occipitotempora'lis** [TA], a longitudinal sulcus on the inferior surface of the temporal lobe that separates the inferior temporal gyrus.

**oculomotor s., s. oculomoto'rius, s. for oculomotor nerve,** s. nervi oculomotorii.

**s. olfacto'rius lo'bi fronta'lis** [TA], olfactory sulcus of frontal lobe: a straight parasagittal sulcus on the inferior surface of the frontal lobe, lodging the olfactory bulb and tract, and separating the gyrus rectus from the gyri orbitales.

**s. olfacto'rius na'si** [TA], olfactory sulcus of nose: a shallow sulcus on the wall of the nasal cavity, passing upward from the level of the anterior end of the middle concha just above the agger nasi to the lamina cribrosa.

**olfactory s. of frontal lobe,** s. olfactorius lobi frontalis.

**olfactory s. of nose,** s. olfactorius nasi.

**optic s.,** s. prechiasmaticus.

**orbital sulci of frontal lobe, sul'ci orbita'les lo'bi fronta'lis** [TA], irregular sulci between the orbital gyri of the frontal lobe.

**palatine sulci of maxilla,** sulci palatini maxillae.

**palatine s. of maxilla, greater,** s. palatinus major maxillae.

**palatine s. of palatine bone, greater,** s. palatinus major ossis palatini.

**palatinovaginal s., s. palatinovagina'lis** [TA], the groove on the vaginal process of the pterygoid process of the sphenoid bone that participates in formation of the palatinovaginal canal.

**s. palati'nus ma'jor maxil'lae** [TA], greater palatine sulcus of maxilla: the sulcus on the nasal surface of the maxilla which, along with the corresponding one on the perpendicular plate of the palatine bone, forms the canal for the greater palatine nerve.

**s. palati'nus ma'jor os'sis palati'ni** [TA], greater palatine sulcus of palatine bone: a vertical groove on the maxillary surface of the perpendicular plate of the palatine bone; it articulates with the maxilla to form the canal for the greater palatine nerve.

**sul'ci palati'ni maxil'lae** [TA], palatine sulci of maxilla: the laterally placed furrows, between the palatine spines on the inferior surface of the hard palate, that lodge the palatine vessels and nerves. Called also *palatine grooves of maxilla.*

**paracolic sulci, sul'ci paraco'lici** [TA], small, shallow, and variable peritoneal pockets situated lateral to the descending colon; called also *recessus paracolici.*

**paraglenoid sulci of hip bone, sul'ci paraglenoida'les os'sis cox'ae,** slight grooves, anterior and inferior to the auricular surface of the ilium, that serve for attachment of the ventral and interosseous sacroiliac ligaments.

**parietooccipital s., s. parietooccipita'lis** [TA], a sulcus in the medial surface of each cerebral hemisphere, running upward from the calcarine sulcus and marking the boundary between the cuneus and precuneus, and also between the parietal and occipital lobes. Called also *parietooccipital fissure.*

**parolfactory s., anterior,** a sulcus on the medial surface of the cerebral hemisphere, between the area parolfactoria behind and the inferior frontal gyrus in front.

**parolfactory s., posterior,** a curved sulcus on the medial surface of the cerebral hemisphere, below the splenium of the corpus callosum and between the gyrus paraterminalis and the area parolfactoria.

**petrobasilar s.,** s. sinus petrosi inferioris ossis temporalis.

**petrosal s. of occipital bone, inferior,** s. sinus petrosi inferioris ossis occipitalis.

**petrosal s. of temporal bone, inferior,** s. sinus petrosi inferioris ossis temporalis.

**petrosal s. of temporal bone, posterior,** s. sinus petrosi inferioris ossis temporalis.

**petrosal s. of temporal bone, superior,** s. sinus petrosi superioris.

**s. petro'sus infe'rior os'sis occipita'lis,** s. sinus petrosi inferioris ossis occipitalis.

**s. petro'sus infe'rior os'sis tempora'lis,** s. sinus petrosi inferioris ossis temporalis.

**s. petro'sus supe'rior os'sis tempora'lis,** s. sinus petrosi superioris.

**polar s.,** any of the small fissures which surround the posterior end of the calcarine sulcus.

**pontobulbar s.,** s. bulbopontinus.

**pontopeduncular s.,** the sulcus that separates the pons from the mesencephalon (as represented by the cerebral peduncles).

**s. popli'teus fe'moris** [TA], popliteal sulcus of femur: a smooth, well-marked groove separated from the lateral condyle by a prominent lip and extending superiorly and posteriorly to the posterior extremity of the lateral condyle; it lodges the tendon of the popliteal muscle.

**postcentral s., s. postcentra'lis** [TA], a sulcus on the superolateral surface of the cerebrum, separating the postcentral gyrus from the remainder of the parietal lobe.

**postclival s.,** see under *fissure.*

**s. poste'rior auri'culae** [TA], posterior sulcus of auricle: the slight depression on the pinna that separates the anthelix from the antitragus. Called also *s. auriculae posterior* and *s. auricularis posterior.*

**posterointermediate s. of spinal cord,** s. intermedius posterior medullae spinalis.

**posterolateral s. of medulla oblongata,** s. posterolateralis medullae oblongatae.

**posterolateral s. of spinal cord,** s. posterolateralis medullae spinalis.

**s. posterolatera'lis medul'lae oblonga'tae** [TA], posterolateral sulcus of medulla oblongata: an upward extension of the posterolateral sulcus of the spinal cord; it gives attachment to the fibers of the glossopharyngeal, vagus, and accessory nerves. Called also *posterolateral groove of medulla oblongata, dorsolateral s. of medulla oblongata,* and *s. dorsolateralis medullae oblongatae.*

**s. posterolatera'lis medul'lae spina'lis** [TA], posterolateral sulcus of spinal cord: a longitudinal sulcus on the posterolateral surface of the spinal cord; it gives entrance to the posterior nerve roots and separates the lateral and posterior funiculi. Called also *posterolateral groove of spinal cord, dorsolateral s. of spinal cord,* and *s. dorsolateralis medullae spinalis.*

**postnodular s.,** fissura dorsolateralis cerebelli.

**postpyramidal s.,** fissura secunda cerebelli.

**precentral s., s. precentra'lis** [TA], a vertical sulcus on the convex surface of a cerebral hemisphere, separating the precentral gyrus from the remainder of the frontal lobe.

**prechiasmatic s., s. prechiasma'ticus** [TA], **s. prechias'matis,** a furrow on the superior surface of the sphenoid bone, located just anterior to the tuberculum sellae; it lodges the optic chiasm. Called also *chiasmatic s., s. chiasmatis, optic groove,* and *optic s.*

**preclival s.,** fissura prima cerebelli.

**prepyramidal s.,** see under *fissure.*

**prerolandic s.,** s. precentralis.

**s. promonto'rii cavita'tis tym'pani** [TA], a groove in the surface of the promontory of the tympanic cavity, lodging the tympanic nerve.

**s. of pterygoid hamulus,** s. hamuli pterygoidei.

**pterygoid s. of pterygoid process,** s. pterygopalatinus processus pterygoidei.

**pterygopalatine s. of palatine bone,** s. palatinus major ossis palatini.

**pterygopalatine s. of pterygoid process,** s. pterygopalatinus processus pterygoidei.

**s. pterygopalati'nus proces'sus pterygoi'dei,** pterygopalatine sulcus of pterygoid process: a small groove on the inferior surface of the vaginal process of the medial pterygoid plate of the sphenoid bone, forming part of the wall of the vomerovaginal canal.

**s. pulmona'lis** [TA], **pulmonary s.,** a large vertical groove in the posterior part of the thoracic cavity, one on either side of the bodies of the vertebrae posterior to the level of their ventral surface, lodging the posterior, bulky portion of the lung.

**radial s. of humerus, s. of radial nerve,** s. nervi radialis.

**Reil's s.,** s. circularis insulae.

**s. retrooliva'ris** [TA], retroolivary groove: a groove running longitudinally across the posterolateral surface of the upper medulla oblongata just behind the olive; it is the forward continuation of the sulcus posterolateralis medullae oblongatae.

**rhinal s., s. rhina'lis** [TA], a fissure on the inferior surface of the hemisphere, separating the anterior part of the parahippocampal gyrus from the rest of the temporal lobe.

**sagittal s.,** s. sinus sagittalis superioris.

**s. scle'rae** [TA], **scleral s., sclerocorneal s.,** the groove at the junction of the sclera and cornea.

**s. of semicanal of humerus,** s. intertubercularis humeri.

**semilunar s. of radius,** incisura ulnaris radii.

**sigmoid s., s. of sigmoid sinus,** s. sinus sigmoidei.

**s. for sigmoid sinus of occipital bone,** s. sinus sigmoidei ossis occipitalis.

**s. for sigmoid sinus of parietal bone,** s. sinus sigmoidei ossis parietalis.

**s. for sigmoid sinus of temporal bone,** s. sinus sigmoidei ossis temporalis.

**s. sigmoi'deus os'sis tempora'lis,** s. sinus sigmoidei ossis temporalis.

**s. si'nus petro'si inferio'ris os'sis occipita'lis** [TA], sulcus for inferior petrosal sinus of occipital bone: the groove in the floor of the posterior cranial fossa at the line of junction between the basilar part of the occipital and the petrous portion of the temporal bone; it lodges the inferior petrosal sinus. Called also *s. petrosus inferior ossis occipitalis.*

**s. si'nus petro'si inferio'ris os'sis tempora'lis** [TA], sulcus for inferior petrosal sinus of temporal bone: a groove on the posteromedial edge of the internal surface of the petrous portion of the temporal bone, which, with a corresponding groove on the adjacent basilar part of the occipital bone, lodges the inferior petrosal sinus. Called also *s. petrosus inferior ossis temporalis.*

**s. si'nus petro'si superio'ris** [TA], sulcus for superior petrosal sinus: a small posterolaterally directed sulcus that runs along the internal surface of the petrous part of the temporal bone on the angle separating the posterior and middle cranial fossae; it lodges the superior petrosal sinus. Called also *s. petrosus superior ossis temporalis.*

**s. si'nus sagitta'lis supe'rioris** [TA], sulcus for superior sagittal sinus: a groove on the internal surface of the frontal, parietal, and occipital bones that lodges the superior sagittal sinus; called also *sagittal groove* and *sagittal s.*

**s. si'nus sigmoi'dei,** sulcus for sigmoid sinus: an S-shaped sulcus beginning on the internal surface of the posteroinferior edge of the parietal bone and continuous with the lateral end of the sulcus of the transverse sinus; it passes onto the internal surface of the mastoid part of the temporal bone, where it bends inferiorly and medially to continue onto the lateral portion of the occipital bone, ending at the jugular foramen. It lodges the sigmoid sinus.

**s. si'nus sigmoi'dei os'sis occipita'lis** [TA], sulcus for sigmoid sinus of occipital bone: the portion of the sulcus of the sigmoid sinus found on the occipital bone.

**s. si'nus sigmoi'dei os'sis parieta'lis** [TA], sulcus for sigmoid sinus of parietal bone: a short groove on the internal surface of the posteroinferior angle of the parietal bone, continuous with both the sulcus for the sigmoid sinus on the temporal bone and the sulcus for the transverse sinus on the occipital bone; it lodges the superior part of the sigmoid sinus. Called also *s. transversus ossis parietalis.*

**s. si'nus sigmoi'dei os'sis tempora'lis** [TA], sulcus for sigmoid sinus of temporal bone: the portion of the sulcus of the sigmoid sinus found on the temporal bone; called also *s. sigmoideus ossis temporalis.*

**s. si'nus transver'si** [TA], sulcus for transverse sinus: a wide groove that passes horizontally, lateralward, and anteriorly from the internal occipital protuberance to the parietal bone, where it becomes continuous with the sulcus of the sigmoid sinus; it lodges the transverse sinus. Called also *s. transversus ossis occipitalis.*

**sulci of skin,** sulci cutis.

**s. of spinal nerve,** s. nervi spinalis.

**spiral s.,** 1. see *s. spiralis externus* and *s. spiralis internus.* 2. s. nervi radialis.

**spiral s., external,** s. spiralis externus.

**spiral s., internal,** s. spiralis internus.

**spiral s. of humerus,** s. nervi radialis.

**s. spira'lis,** 1. see *s. spiralis externus* and *s. spiralis internus.* 2. s. nervi radialis.

**s. spira'lis exter'nus** [TA], external spiral sulcus: a concavity within the cochlear duct immediately above the basilar crest.

**s. spira'lis inter'nus** [TA], internal spiral sulcus: the C-shaped concavity within the cochlear duct formed by the limbus laminae spiralis and its tympanic and vestibular labia along the edge of the osseous spiral lamina.

**subclavian s.,** 1. s. arteriae subclaviae. 2. groove for subclavian artery. 3. s. musculi subclavii. 4. s. venae subclaviae.

**s. for subclavian artery,** 1. s. arteriae subclaviae. 2. see under *groove.*

**subclavian s. of lung,** groove for subclavian artery.

**s. for subclavian muscle,** s. musculi subclavii.

**s. for subclavian vein,** s. venae subclaviae.

**s. subcla'vius,** 1. s. arteriae subclaviae. 2. groove for subclavian artery. 3. s. musculi subclavii. 4. s. venae subclaviae.

**s. subcla'vius pulmo'nis,** groove for subclavian artery.

**subparietal s., s. subparieta'lis** [TA], a sulcus on the medial surface of a cerebral hemisphere, above the splenium of the corpus callosum, separating the precuneus from the cingulate gyrus.

**s. for superior petrosal sinus,** s. sinus petrosi superioris.

**supra-acetabular s., s. supraacetabula'ris** [TA], supra-acetabular groove: a sulcus located posterosuperior to the margin of the acetabulum, which is the site of attachment of the reflexed head of the rectus femoris muscle.

**supraorbital s.,** foramen supraorbitale.

**suprapalpebral s., s. suprapalpebra'lis** [TA], the furrow above the upper eyelid.

**suprasplenial s.,** s. subparietalis.

**s. Syl'vii,** fossa lateralis cerebralis.

**s. ta'li** [TA], **s. of talus,** a transverse groove on the inferior surface of the talus, between the medial and the posterior articular surface, which helps to form the sinus tarsi.

**temporal s., inferior, temporal s., middle,** s. temporalis inferior.

**temporal s., superior,** s. temporalis superior.
**temporal s., transverse,** s. temporalis transversus.
**s. tempora'lis infe'rior** [TA], inferior temporal sulcus: a longitudinal sulcus on the lateral surface of the temporal lobe, separating the middle and the inferior temporal gyri.
**s. tempora'lis supe'rior** [TA], superior temporal sulcus: a longitudinal sulcus on the lateral surface of a cerebral hemisphere, passing posteriorly from the temporal pole, separating the superior and the middle temporal gyri and ending in the gyrus angularis.
**s. tempora'lis transver'sus** [TA], transverse temporal sulcus: an irregularly vertical sulcus in the part of the temporal lobe that lies within the lateral sulcus; sometimes occurring as a pair.
**s. ten'dinis mus'culi fibula'ris lon'gi** [TA], sulcus for tendon of long fibular muscle: a deep groove on the inferior surface of the cuboid bone, which in certain foot positions lodges the tendon of the peroneus longus muscle; called also *s. tendinis musculi peronei longi* [TA alternative].
**s. ten'dinis mus'culi flexo'ris hal'lucis lon'gi calca'nei** [TA], sulcus for tendon of flexor hallucis longus of calcaneus: a groove on the inferior surface of the sustentaculum tali of the calcaneus, lodging the tendon of the flexoris hallucis longus muscle; called also *s. musculi flexoris hallucis longi calcanei.*
**s. ten'dinis mus'culi flexo'ris hal'lucis lon'gi ta'li** [TA], sulcus for tendon of flexor hallucis longus of talus: the sagittal groove on the posterior surface of the body of the talus that transmits the tendon of the flexor hallucis longus muscle; called also *s. musculi flexoris hallucis longi tali.*
**s. ten'dinis mus'culi perone'i lon'gi,** TA alternative for *s. tendinis musculi fibularis longi.*
**s. ten'dinum musculo'rum fibula'rium calca'nei,** TA alternative for *s. tendinum musculorum peroneorum calcanei.*
**s. ten'dinum musculo'rum peroneo'rum calca'nei** [TA], sulcus for tendons of peroneus muscles: a slight groove on the inferior part of the lateral surface of the calcaneus, lodging the tendons of the peroneus longus and brevis muscles; called also *s. tendinum musculorum fibularium calcanei* [TA alternative].
**s. for tendon of flexor hallucis longus muscle of calcaneus,** s. tendinis musculi flexoris hallucis longi calcanei.
**s. for tendon of flexor hallucis longus muscle of talus,** s. tendinis musculi flexoris hallucis longi tali.
**s. for tendon of long fibular muscle, s. for tendon of peroneus longus muscle,** s. tendinis musculi fibularis longi.
**s. for tendons of peroneus muscles,** s. tendinum musculorum peroneorum calcanei.
**terminal s. of heart, terminal s. of right atrium,** s. terminalis cordis.
**terminal s. of tongue,** s. terminalis linguae.
**s. termina'lis a'trii dex'tri, s. termina'lis cor'dis** [TA], terminal sulcus of heart: a shallow groove on the external surface of the right atrium of the heart between the superior and inferior venae cavae; it represents the junction of the sinus venosus with the primitive atrium in the embryo, and corresponds to a ridge on the internal surface, the crista terminalis. Called also *terminal s. of right atrium.*
**s. termina'lis lin'guae** [TA], terminal sulcus of tongue: a more or less distinct groove on the tongue, extending from the foramen cecum anteriorly and lateralward to the margin of the tongue on either side, and dividing the dorsum of the tongue from the root. It is marked by a row of vallate papillae.
**s. of tongue,** see *s. medianus linguae* and *s. terminalis linguae.*
**transverse s. of anthelix,** s. anthelicis transversus.
**transverse s. of occipital bone,** s. sinus transversi.
**transverse s. of parietal bone,** s. sinus sigmoidei ossis parietalis.
**s. for transverse sinus,** s. sinus transversi.
**transverse s. of temporal bone,** s. sinus sigmoidei ossis temporalis.
**s. transver'sus os'sis occipita'lis,** s. sinus transversi.
**s. transver'sus os'sis parieta'lis,** s. sinus sigmoidei ossis parietalis.
**s. tu'bae auditi'vae,** TA alternative for *s. tubae auditoriae.*
**s. tu'bae audito'riae** [TA], sulcus for auditory tube: a groove on the medial part of the base of the spine of the sphenoid bone; it lodges a portion of the cartilaginous part of the auditory tube. Called also *s. tubae auditivae* [TA alternative] and *groove for auditory tube.*
**Turner's s.,** s. intraparietalis.
**s. tympa'nicus os'sis tempora'lis** [TA], tympanic sulcus of temporal bone: a narrow groove in the medial part of the external acoustic meatus of the temporal bone, into which the tympanic membrane fits; it is deficient above. Called also *Jacobson's s.*
**s. for ulnar nerve,** s. nervi ulnaris.
**s. for umbilical vein,** s. venae umbilicalis.
**s. valle'culae,** a groove in the inferior cerebellum that separates the uvula vermis from the tonsils.
**sulci for veins,** sulci venosi.
**s. for vena cava, s. ve'nae ca'vae** [TA], a groove on the upper part of the posteroinferior surface of the liver, separating the right lobe from the caudate lobe and lodging the inferior vena cava; called also *fossa venae cavae.*
**s. ve'nae subcla'viae** [TA], sulcus for subclavian vein: a transverse groove on the cranial surface of the first rib, just anterior to the anterior scalene tubercle; it lodges the subclavian vein.
**s. ve'nae umbilica'lis,** sulcus for umbilical vein: the impression on the visceral surface of the liver in the fetus, which lodges the umbilical vein.
**sul'ci veno'si** [TA], **venous sulci,** grooves on the internal surfaces of the cranial bones for the meningeal veins; called also *venous grooves.*
**ventral s. of spinal cord,** fissura mediana anterior medullae spinalis.
**s. ventra'lis medul'lae spina'lis,** fissura mediana anterior medullae spinalis.
**ventrolateral s. of medulla oblongata,** s. anterolateralis medullae oblongatae.
**ventrolateral s. of spinal cord,** s. anterolateralis medullae spinalis.
**s. ventrolatera'lis medul'lae oblonga'tae,** s. anterolateralis medullae oblongatae.
**s. ventrolatera'lis medul'lae spina'lis,** s. anterolateralis medullae spinalis.
**vermicular s.,** a fissure between the vermis and the hemisphere of the cerebellum.
**s. for vertebral artery of atlas,** s. arteriae vertebralis atlantis.
**vertical s.,** s. precentralis.
**s. vo'meris** [TA], vomeral sulcus: the cleft in the inferior half on the anterior border of the vomer that receives the inferior border of the septal cartilage of the nose. Called also *vomeral groove.*
**vomerovaginal s., s. vomerovagina'lis** [TA], the groove on the vaginal process of the pterygoid process of the sphenoid bone that helps form the vomerovaginal canal.
**s. of wrist,** s. carpi.

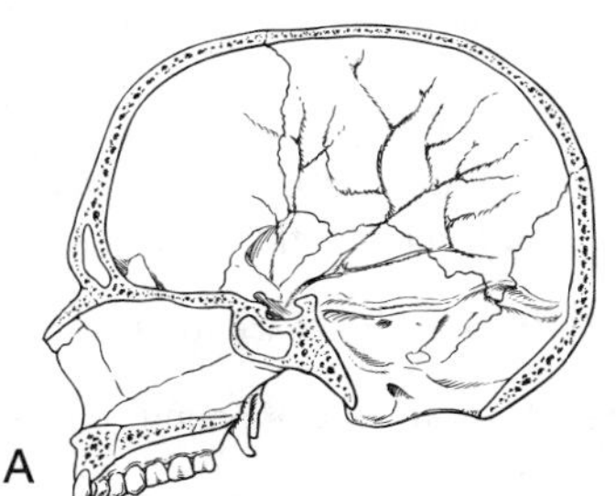


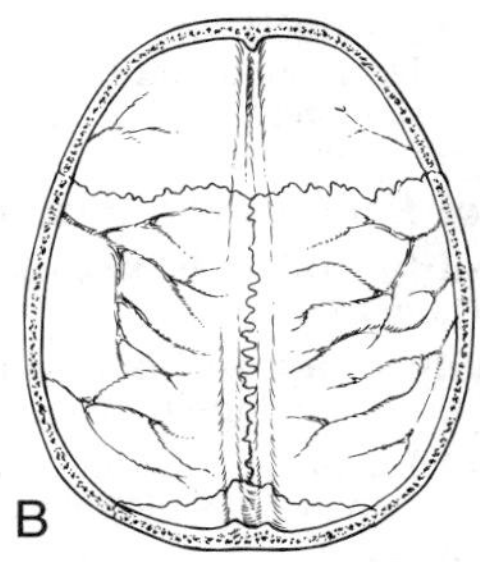


Sulci venosi (venous grooves) seen in *(A),* lateral view of the internal surface of the cranium; *(B),* internal surface of the calvaria (skull cap).

**sul·fa·benz·a·mide** (sul″fə-ben′zə-mīd) [USP] a sulfonamide antibacterial having properties similar to those of sulfamethoxazole; used topically in combination with sulfacetamide and sulfathiazole in the treatment of vaginal bacteriosis.

**sul·fa·cet·a·mide** (sul″fə-set′ə-mīd) [MeSH: Sulfacetamide] a sulfonamide which has been used in the treatment of urinary tract infections.
**s. sodium** [USP], the sodium salt monohydrate of sulfacetamide, applied topically to the conjunctiva in the treatment of sulfonamide-responsive eye infections.

**sul·fa·chlor·pyr·id·a·zine** [sul″fə-klor″pir-id′ə-zēn] [USP] [MeSH: Sulfachlorpyridazine] a sulfonamide used as an antibacterial in the treatment of veterinary enteric infections.

**sulf·ac·id** (səlf-as′id) thio acid.

**sul·fa·cy·tine** (sul″fə-si′tēn) a short-acting sulfonamide, used orally in the treatment of acute urinary tract infections when due to susceptible strains of *Escherichia coli, Klebsiella-Enterobacter* group, *Staphylococcus aureus, Proteus mirabilis,* and *P. vulgaris.*

**sul·fa·di·a·zine** (sul″fə-di′ə-zēn) [USP] [MeSH: Sulfadiazine] a sulfonamide frequently used in combination with other sulfonamides in the treatment of infections due to susceptible organisms, including meningitis caused by *Haemophilus influenzae,* chancroid, acute urinary tract infections, early manifestations of lymphogranuloma venereum, and falciparum malaria caused by chloroquine-resistant plasmodia. It is administered orally.

**s. silver,** the silver derivative of sulfadiazine, used as a topical antibacterial to prevent wound sepsis in the treatment of second and third degree burns.

**s. sodium** [USP], the monosodium salt of sulfadiazine, having the same actions and uses as the base; administered subcutaneously and intravenously.

**sul•fa•di•me•thox•ine** (sul″fə-di″mə-thok′sēn) [MeSH: Sulfadimethoxine] a long-acting sulfonamide, used as an antibacterial in a variety of infections; administered orally.

**sul•fa•di•me•tine** (sul″fə-di′mə-tēn) sulfisomidine.

**sul•fa•di•mi•dine** (sul″fə-di′mĭ-dēn) sulfamethazine.

**sul•fa•dox•ine** (sul″fə-dok′sēn) [MeSH: Sulfadoxine] a long-acting sulfonamide which has been used in the treatment of leprosy and falciparum malaria.

**sul•fa•eth•i•dole** (sul″fə-eth′ĭ-dōl) a short-acting sulfonamide used principally as a urinary antiseptic, administered orally.

**sul•fa•fu•ra•zole** (sul″fə-fu′rə-zōl) sulfisoxazole.

**sul•fa•guan•i•dine** (sul″fə-gwahn′ĭ-dēn) [MeSH: Sulfaguanidine] a sulfonamide used as an antibacterial in the treatment of gastrointestinal infections, especially bacillary dysentery; administered orally.

**sul•fa•lene** (sul′fə-lēn) [MeSH: Sulfalene] a long-acting sulfonamide used as an antibacterial, especially in the treatment of urinary tract infections.

**sul•fa•mer•a•zine** (sul″fə-mer′ə-zēn) [MeSH: Sulfamerazine] a readily absorbed antibacterial substance usually used in combination with other sulfonamides. Called also *sulfamethyldiazine.*

**sul•fa•me•ter** (sul′fə-me″tər) [MeSH: Sulfameter] a long-acting sulfonamide used as an antibacterial, especially in the treatment of acute and chronic urinary tract infections; administered orally.

**sul•fa•meth•a•zine** (sul″fə-meth′ə-zēn) [USP] [MeSH: Sulfamethazine] a sulfonamide used as an antibacterial in a variety of infections in the United States, usually used in combination with other sulfonamides. It is administered orally. Called also *sulfadimidine.*

**sul•fa•meth•i•zole** (sul″fə-meth′ĭ-zōl) [MeSH: Sulfamethizole] a compound used as an antibacterial agent mainly in the treatment of infections of the urinary tract. Called also *sulfamethylthiadiazole.*

**sul•fa•meth•ox•a•zole** (sul″fə-məth-ok′sə-zōl) [USP] [MeSH: Sulfamethoxazole] a sulfonamide used as an antibacterial, especially for the prophylaxis and treatment of acute urinary tract infections and of pyodermata and infections of wounds and soft tissues, administered orally.

**sul•fa•meth•oxy•py•rid•a•zine** (sul″fə-məth-ok′se-pi-rid′ə-zēn) [MeSH: Sulfamethoxypyridazine] a compound used as an antibacterial agent in the treatment of infections of the urinary tract and other infections.

**sul•fa•meth•yl•di•a•zine** (sul″fə-meth″əl-di′ə-zēn) sulfamerazine.

**sul•fa•meth•yl•thi•a•di•a•zole** (sul″fə-meth″əl-thi″ə-di′ə-zōl) sulfamethizole.

**Sul•fa•mez•a•thine** (sul″fə-mez′ə-thēn) trademark for a preparation of sulfamethazine.

**sul•fam•i•do** (səl-fam′ĭ-do) one of a group of compounds containing an aminosulfone group, $SO_2 \cdot NH_2$.

**sul•fam•i•do•chry•soi•dine** (səl-fam″ĭ-do-krĭ-soi′dēn) a compound, the hydrochloride salt of which *(Prontosil)* was the forerunner of the sulfonamide drugs.

**sul•fam•ine** (səl-fam′in) the univalent radical, $—SO_2NH_2$.

**Sul•fa•my•lon** (sul″fə-mi′lon) trademark for preparations of mafenide.

**sul•fa•nil•amide** (sul″fə-nil′ə-mīd) a potent antibacterial compound, the first of the sulfonamides discovered. Formerly used in the treatment of various infections, it has been replaced by more effective and less toxic derivatives, and by antibiotics.

**sul•fan•i•late** (səl-fan′ĭ-lāt) a salt of sulfanilic acid.

**sul•fa•nil•ic ac•id** (sul″fə-nil′ik) a white crystalline compound whose diazotized form (diazobenzenesulfonic acid) is used in Ehrlich's diazo reaction.

**sul•fa•ni•tran** (sul″fə-ni′tran) an antibacterial sulfonamide and coccidiostat for poultry.

**sul•fa•nu•ria** (sul″fə-nu′re-ə) anuria resulting from the use of sulfonamide drugs.

**sul•fa•pyr•i•dine** (sul″fə-pir′ĭ-dēn) [USP] [MeSH: Sulfapyridine] an antibacterial compound used as an oral suppressant for dermatitis herpetiformis. It was formerly used in the treatment of pneumonia and streptococcal infections.

**sul•fa•quin•ox•a•line** (sul″fə-kwin-ok′sə-lēn) [USP] [MeSH: Sulfaquinoxaline] a sulfonamide used as a coccidiostat for poultry; administered orally or as a feed additive.

**sul•fa•sal•a•zine** (sul″fə-sal′ə-zēn) [USP] [MeSH: Sulfasalazine] an antibacterial sulfonamide derivative used orally in the treatment of mild to moderate ulcerative colitis, as adjunctive therapy in severe ulcerative colitis due to susceptible organisms, and in the treatment of rheumatoid arthritis; administered orally. Called also *salazosulfapyridine* and *salicylazosulfapyridine.*

**Sul•fa•sux•i•dine** (sul″fə-suk′sĭ-dēn) trademark for preparations of succinylsulfathiazole.

**sul•fa•tase** (sul′fə-tās) 1. a term used in the recommended and trivial names for the sulfuric ester hydrolases [EC 3.1.6], which catalyze the cleavage of inorganic sulfate from sulfate esters to form alcohols. 2. arylsulfatase.

**multiple s. deficiency,** an autosomal recessive lysosomal storage disease in which a deficiency of at least nine lysosomal and microsomal sulfatases leads to accumulation of sulfate-containing glycolipids, mucopolysaccharides, and steroids. The disorder generally presents as metachromatic leukodystrophy and later also shows features of mucopolysaccharidoses, variably combining phenotypic features of the specific enzymatic defects. Neurologic deterioration is rapid. Called also *mucosulfatidosis.*

**sul•fate** (sul′fāt) [L. *sulphas*] any salt of sulfuric acid.

**acid s.,** one in which only one half of the hydrogen of the sulfuric acid is replaced; a bisulfate.

**basic s.,** one in which the normal sulfate of the base is combined with a hydroxide of the same base; a subsulfate.

**conjugated s's,** aromatic substances, such as phenol, skatoxyl, and indoxyl, which occur in the urine along with mineral sulfates.

**cupric s.** [USP], the pentahydrate sulfate salt of copper, $CuSO_4 \cdot 5H_2O$, a powerful emetic; used orally as an antidote to phosphorus poisoning. Topical application of a 1 per cent solution is used in the treatment of phosphorus burns of the skin. It is also used as a catalyst with iron in the treatment of iron deficiency anemia. In 1:1,000,000 concentration it is used to prevent growth of algae in ponds, reservoirs, and swimming pools. Called also *blue vitriol, copper sulfate,* and *bluestone.*

**ethereal s's,** conjugated s's.

**mineral s's,** sulfates in the urine which are combinations of sulfuric acid with mineral substances such as sodium, potassium, calcium, and magnesium.

**neutral s., normal s.,** one in which all the hydrogen of the sulfuric acid is replaced.

**preformed s's,** mineral s's.

**sul•fat•emia** (sul″fə-te′me-ə) the presence of sulfates in the blood.

**Sul•fa•thal•i•dine** (sul″fə-thal′ĭ-dēn) trademark for phthalylsulfathiazole.

**sul•fa•thi•a•zole** (sul″fə-thi′ə-zōl) a compound once widely used as an antibacterial agent but replaced by less toxic sulfonamides and antibiotics.

**sul•fa•tide** (sul′fə-tīd) any of the cerebrosides esterified with a sulfate residue at the C-6 of the sugar; they are found largely in the medullated nerve fibers, and may accumulate in the white matter of the brain in metachromatic leukodystrophy.

**sul•fa•tion** (sul-fa′shən) addition of a sulfate group to a molecule.

**sul•faz•a•met** (səl-faz′ə-met) a veterinary sulfonamide antibacterial.

**sulf•he•mo•glo•bin** (sulf″he-mo-glo′bin) [MeSH: Sulfhemoglobin] sulfmethemoglobin.

**sulf•he•mo•glo•bin•emia** (sulf″he-mo-glo″bin-e′me-ə) [MeSH: Sulfhemoglobinemia] the presence of sulfmethemoglobin in the blood; the most significant symptom is cyanosis. It usually results from excessive exposure to sulfur-containing drugs or other chemicals.

**sulf•hy•drate** (səlf-hi′drāt) the $HS^-$ anion or a salt containing this ion.

**sulf•hy•dryl** (səlf-hi′drəl) the univalent radical, —SH.

**sul•fide** (sul′fīd) any binary compound of sulfur; a compound of sulfur with another element or radical or base.

**sul•fin•ic ac•id** (səl-fin′ik) an organic compound containing an $—SO_2H$ group bonded to a carbon atom.

**sul•fin•py•ra•zone** (sul″fin-pi′rə-zōn) [USP] [MeSH: Sulfinpyrazone] a sulfoxide analogue of phenylbutazone, used as a uricosuric agent in treatment of gout; administered orally. It also prolongs platelet survival and inhibits platelet adherence to subendothelial cells and prostaglandin synthesis and has been studied as an antithrombotic agent.

**sul·fi·nyl** (sul′fĭ-nəl) the bivalent radical, —SO—.

**sul·fi·som·i·dine** (səl-fĭ-som′ĭ-dēn) [MeSH: Sulfisomidine] a structural isomer of sulfamethazine used as an antibacterial agent in the treatment of systemic and urinary tract infections. Called also *sulfadimetine.*

**sul·fi·sox·a·zole** (sul″fə-sok′sə-zōl) [USP] [MeSH: Sulfisoxazole] a short-acting sulfonamide used as an antibacterial in the treatment of a wide variety of infections, administered orally. Called also *sulfafurazole.*
**s. acetyl** [USP], a tasteless derivative of sulfisoxazole having the same actions and uses as the base; usually used in infants and children; administered orally.
**s. diolamine,** the diethanolamine salt of sulfisoxazole having the same actions and uses as the base; administered intramuscularly and intravenously. It is also used in the topical treatment of susceptible eye infections.

**sul·fite** (sul′fīt) [L. *sulfis*] any salt of sulfurous acid.

**sul·fite ox·i·dase** (sul′fīt ok′sĭ-dās) [EC 1.8.3.1] an enzyme of the oxidoreductase class that catalyzes the final reaction in the degradation of sulfur-containing amino acids, oxidizing sulfite to sulfate; it also oxidizes and detoxifies sulfite and sulfur dioxide from exogenous sources. It is a mitochondrial molybdoenzyme that transfers electrons to cytochrome *c* via its $b_5$ heme. Deficiency of enzyme activity, due to defect in the enzyme protein or to molybdenum cofactor deficiency (q.v.), results in progressive neurologic abnormalities, lens dislocation, and mental retardation.

**sulf·met·he·mo·glo·bin** (sulf″mət-he′mo-glo″bin) hemoglobin with a sulfur atom on one of its porphyrin rings, so that it is ineffective for transporting oxygen and has a green color; see *sulfhemoglobinemia.* Called also *sulfhemoglobin.*

**sulf(o)-** [*sulfur*] a prefix used in naming chemical compounds, indicating the presence of divalent sulfur or of the group $SO_2OH$.

**sul·fo·bro·mo·phthal·ein so·di·um** (sul″fo-bro″mo-thal′ēn) a water-soluble triphenylmethane derivative bound by plasma proteins and excreted by the liver, used to test the functional capacity of the liver.

**sul·fo·con·ju·ga·tion** (sul″fo-kon″jə-ga′shən) the formation of conjugated sulfates; see under *sulfate.*

**sul·fo·cy·a·nate** (sul″fo-si′ə-nāt) thiocyanate.

**sul·fo·cy·an·ic ac·id** (sul″fo-si-an′ic) thiocyanic acid.

**sul·fo·gel** (sul′fo-jel) a gel in which sulfuric acid is the medium instead of water.

***N*-sul·fo·glu·cos·amine sul·fo·hy·dro·lase** (sul″fo-gloo-kōs′ə-mēn sul″fo-hi′dro-lās) [EC 3.10.1.1] an enzyme of the hydrolase class that catalyzes the cleavage of sulfate groups from the amino groups of sulfated glucosamine residues. The enzyme may be identical with *heparan N-sulfatase* (q.v.).

**sul·fo·hy·drate** (sul″fo-hi′drāt) sulfhydrate.

**sul·fo·lip·id** (sul″fo-lip′id) any lipid carrying a sulfate residue on its polar head group, usually a sphingolipid or steroid derivative.

**sul·fo·litho·cho·lyl·gly·cine** (sul″fo-lith″o-ko″ləl-gli′sēn) a bile salt, the sulfate ester at C-3 of lithocholylglycine.

**sul·fo·litho·cho·lyl·tau·rine** (sul″fo-lith″o-ko″ləl-taw′rēn) a bile salt, the sulfate ester at C-3 of lithocholyltaurine.

**sul·fol·y·sis** (səl-fol′ĭ-sis) [*sulfo-* + *-lysis*] a double decomposition, similar to hydrolysis, but in which sulfuric acid takes the place of water.

**sul·fo·mu·cin** (sul″fo-mu′sin) a mucin containing sulfated carbohydrate groups.

**sul·fon·amide** (səl-fon′ə-mīd) the chemical group $SO_2NH_2$. The sulfonamides, or sulfa drugs, are derivatives of sulfanilamide, which competitively inhibit folic acid synthesis in microorganisms, and are bacteriostatic against gram-positive cocci (streptococci and pneumococci), gram-negative cocci (meningococci and gonococci), gram-negative bacilli (*Escherichia coli* and shigellae), and a wide variety of other bacteria. Sulfonamides have been largely supplanted by more effective and less toxic antibiotics.

**sul·fon·am·i·de·mia** (sul″fōn-am″ĭ-de′me-ə) the presence of a sulfonamide compound in the blood.

**sul·fon·am·i·do·cho·lia** (sul″fōn-am″ĭ-do-ko′le-ə) the presence of a sulfonamide compound in the bile.

**sul·fon·am·i·do·ther·a·py** (sul″fōn-am″ĭ-do-ther′ə-pe) treatment with sulfonamide compounds.

**sul·fon·am·i·du·ria** (sul″fōn-am″ĭ-du′re-ə) the presence of a sulfonamide compound in the urine.

**sul·fo·nate** (sul′fo-nāt) a salt, ester, or anion of a sulfonic acid.

**sul·fone** (sul′fōn) 1. the radical $SO_2$. 2. any compound containing two hydrocarbon radicals attached to the radical $SO_2$, especially dapsone (4,4′-sulfonylbisbenzenamine) and its derivatives, which are potent antibacterials effective against many gram-positive and gram-negative organisms, and are widely used as leprostatics.

**sul·fon·ic** (səl-fon′ik) indicating chemical compounds containing the monovalent $—SO_2OH$ or $—SO_3H$ radical.

**sul·fon·ic ac·id** (səl-fon′ik) an organic compound having the formula $RSO_2OH$; used in synthesizing dyes and phenols.

**Sul·fon·sol** (səl-fon′sol) trademark for a preparation of trisulfapyrimidines oral suspension; see under *suspension.*

**sul·fo·nyl** (sul′fo-nəl) the bivalent radical, $—SO_2—$.

**sul·fo·nyl·urea** (sul″fə-nil-u-re′ə) any of a class of compounds that exert hypoglycemic activity by stimulating the islet tissue to secrete insulin; used to control hyperglycemia in type 2 diabetics who cannot be treated solely by diet and exercise.

**sul·fo·pro·tein** (sul″fo-pro′tēn) any of a series of albumins containing loosely combined sulfur.

**sul·fo·sa·lic·yl·ate** (sul″fo-sə-lis′ĭ-lāt) a salt, anion, or ester of sulfosalicylic acid.

**sul·fo·sal·i·cyl·ic ac·id** (sul″fo-sal″ĭ-sil′ik) a protein precipitant used in qualitative tests for protein in urine and cerebrospinal fluid. See under *method.* Called also *salicylsulfonic acid.*

**Sul·fose** (sul′fōs) trademark for preparations of trisulfapyrimidines.

**sul·fo·sol** (sul′fo-sol) a sol in which sulfuric acid is the dispersion medium.

**sul·fo·trans·fer·ase** (sul″fo-trans′fər-ās) [EC 2.8.2] any member of a sub-subclass of enzymes of the transferase class that catalyze the transfer of a sulfate group.

**sul·fox·i·da·tion** (səl-fok″sĭ-da′shən) the addition of an oxygen atom to the sulfur atom of an organic compound of the form R—S—R or R—R—S to form a sulfoxide; in the liver, it is an important reaction, mediated by hepatic microsomal enzymes, in the metabolism of sulfur-containing compounds.

**sul·fox·ide** (səl-fok′sīd) 1. the bivalent radical =SO. 2. any compound consisting of two organic radicals attached to the =SO radical.

**sul·fox·ism** (səl-fok′siz-əm) sulfuric acid poisoning.

**sul·fox·one so·di·um** (səl-fok′sōn) an antibacterial derivative of dapsone having actions similar to those of the parent compound, occurring as a white to pale yellow powder; used primarily as a leprostatic in the treatment of lepromatous and tuberculoid leprosy, administered orally.

**sul·fur** (sul′fər) gen. *sul′furis* [L.] [MeSH: Sulfur] a nonmetallic element existing in many allotropic forms; symbol, S; atomic number, 16; atomic weight, 32.064. It occurs in protein, being a constituent of the amino acids cysteine and methionine. Sulfur is a laxative and diaphoretic and is used in diseases of the skin; it formerly was used for a variety of other medicinal purposes.
**s. 35,** a radioactive isotope of sulfur, atomic mass 35, having a half-life of 87.51 days and decaying by emission of beta particles (0.167 MeV); it has been used in the determination of extracellular fluid volume; administered intravenously.
**colloidal s.,** sulfur in a state of extremely fine division.
**s. dioxide** [NF], a colorless, nonflammable, water soluble gas, $SO_2$, with a strong, irritating odor; used as an antioxidant in pharmaceutical preparations. It is also an important air pollutant, irritating to the eyes and respiratory tract, usually the product of incomplete combustion of coal, oil, and gasoline. Dry sulfur dioxide is often used to kill fleas, mosquitoes, flies, rats, and other vermin. Called also *sulfurous anhydride.*
**flowers of s.,** sublimed s.
**s. hydride,** $H_2S$, a poisonous gas having the smell of rotten eggs.
**s. lo′tum,** washed s.
**s. monochloride,** a lacrimating war gas, $S_2Cl_2$.
**precipitated s.** [USP], a very fine, pale yellow, amorphous or microcrystalline powder, containing not less than 99.5 per cent sulfur, obtained by adding acid to a solution containing a polysulfide and a thiosulfate; used topically as a scabicide, and also used in various dermatologic formulations for its antiparasitic, antifungal, and keratolytic effects.
**roll s.,** sulfur melted and cast in the form of rods or cylinders.
**sublimed s.** [USP], a fine yellow powder, containing not less than 99.5 per cent sulfur, obtained by subliming elemental sulfur and condensing the vapor. It is used topically as a scabicide and parasiticide. Called also *flores sulfuris* and *flowers of sulfur.*
**washed s.,** sublimed sulfur purified by washing with water.

**sul·fu·rat·ed** (sul′fu-rāt″əd) combined or charged with sulfur.

**sul·fu·ra·tor** (sul′fu-ra″tor) an apparatus for applying fumes of sulfur dioxide, used for disinfecting.

**sul·fu·ret·ted** (sul′fu-ret″əd) sulfurated.

**sul·fur·ic ac·id** (səl-fūr′ik) a strong mineral acid, $H_2SO_4$, that is a strong oxidizing agent and is extremely corrosive to skin and mucous membranes; concentrated sulfuric acid can cause severe skin burns.

**sul·fu·rize** (sul′fu-rīz) to cause to combine with sulfur.

**sul·fur·ous ac·id** (səl-fūr′əs) the chemical species $H_2SO_3$, which is formed in aqueous solutions of sulfur dioxide, $SO_2$; its salts are sulfites.

**sul·fur·trans·fer·ase** (sul″fər-trans′fər-ās) [EC 2.8.1] any member of the sub-subclass of enzymes of the transferase class that catalyze the transfer of sulfur atoms.

**sul·fu·ryl** (sul′fu-rəl) the radical $SO_2$.

**sul·fy·dryl** (səl-fi′drəl) sulfhydryl.

**sul·iso·ben·zone** (səl-i″so-ben′zōn) [USP] a sunscreen that absorbs ultraviolet light in the UVA range.

**sul·in·dac** (səl-in′dak) [USP] [MeSH: Sulindac] a nonsteroidal anti-inflammatory, analgesic, and antipyretic used in the treatment of osteoarthritis, rheumatoid arthritis, ankylosing spondylitis, acute painful shoulder, and acute gouty arthritis.

**Sul·la** (sul′ə) trademark for a preparation of sulfameter.

**sul·lage** (sul′əj) sewage.

**Sul·li·van's test** (sul′ĭ-vənz) [Michael Xavier *Sullivan*, American physician, 1875–1963] see under *test*.

**sulph-** for words beginning thus, see those beginning *sulf-*.

**sul·pi·ride** (sul′pĭ-rīd) [MeSH: Sulpiride] an antidepressant and antipsychotic, used in the treatment of schizophrenia and other psychoses; administered orally and intramuscularly.

**Sul-Span·sion** (səl-span′shən) trademark for a preparation of sulfaethidole.

**sul·thi·ame** (səl-thi′ām) a carbonic anhydrase inhibitor used as an anticonvulsant in the treatment of all forms of epilepsy except petit mal.

**Sulz·ber·ger-Gar·be syndrome** (sulz′bər-gər-gahr′be) [Marion Baldur *Sulzberger*, American dermatologist, born 1895; William *Garbe*, Canadian dermatologist, born 1908] exudative discoid and lichenoid dermatitis.

**sum.** abbreviation for L. *su′mat*, let him take; or *sumen′dum*, to be taken.

**su·mac** (soo′mak) any of various species of *Rhus*.
**poison s., swamp s.,** *Rhus vernix*.

**su·ma·trip·tan suc·ci·nate** (soo″mə-trip′tan) a selective serotonin antagonist used in the acute treatment of migraine headache; administered subcutaneously and orally.

**sum·ma·tion** (sə-ma′shən) [L. *summa* total] the accumulative effects of a number of stimuli applied to a muscle, nerve, or reflex arc.
**central s.,** the condition in which successive subliminal stimuli accumulate in a reflex center until they finally produce a reflex discharge.

**sum·mit** (sum′it) [L. *summus*, superlative of *superus*] apex.
**s. of bladder,** apex vesicae.

**Sum·ner** (sum′nər) James Batcheller, 1887–1955; co-winner, with Wendell Meredith Stanley and John Howard Northrop, of the Nobel prize for chemistry in 1946 for isolating and crystallizing an enzyme, urease, and showing it to be a protein.

**Sum·ner's sign** (sum′nərz) [Franklin W. *Sumner*, British surgeon, 20th century] see under *sign*.

**Su·my·cin** (soo-mi′sin) trademark for preparations of tetracycline hydrochloride.

**sun·burn** (sun′bərn) [MeSH: Sunburn] injury to the skin, with erythema, tenderness, and sometimes blistering, following excessive exposure to sunlight, and produced by ultraviolet rays, which are not filtered out by clouds or water.

**sun·down·ing** (sun′doun-ing) the appearance of confusion, agitation, and other severely disruptive behavior coupled with inability to remain asleep, occurring solely or markedly worsening at night; sometimes seen in older patients with dementia or other mental disorders.

**Sun·Dare** (sun′dār) trademark for preparations of cinoxate.

**sun·screen** (sun′skrēn) [MeSH: Sunscreening Agents] a substance applied to the skin to protect it from the effects of the sun's rays; sunscreens act by absorbing ultraviolet radiation or by reflecting the incident light. Called also *solar screen* or *sun screen*.

**sun·stroke** (sun′strōk) [MeSH: Sunstroke] insolation, or thermic fever; a condition produced by exposure to the sun, and marked by convulsions, coma, and a high temperature of the skin. Cf. *heat exhaustion* and *heat stroke*.

**super-** [L. *super* above] a prefix meaning above, more than normal, excessive, or next above in rank. Cf. *hyper-*.

**su·per·ab·duc·tion** (soo″pər-əb-duk′shən) extreme or excessive abduction.

**su·per·ac·id** (soo″pər-as′id) excessively acid.

**su·per·acid·i·ty** (soo″pər-ə-sid′ĭ-te) excessive acidity.

**su·per·acro·mi·al** (soo″pər-ə-kro′me-əl) supra-acromial.

**su·per·ac·tiv·i·ty** (soo″pər-ak-tiv′ĭ-te) activity greater than normal; hyperactivity.

**su·per·acute** (soo″pər-ə-kūt′) extremely acute.

**su·per·al·i·men·ta·tion** (soo″pər-al″ĭ-mən-ta′shən) therapeutic treatment by excessive feeding beyond the requirements of the appetite, employed in wasting diseases; called also *gavage*.

**su·per·al·ka·lin·i·ty** (soo″pər-al″kə-lin′ĭ-te) excessive alkalinity.

**su·per·an·ti·gen** (soo″pər-an′tĭ-jən) any of a group of powerful antigens occurring in various bacteria and viruses that binds outside of the normal T cell receptor site and is able to react with multiple T cell receptor molecules of a given $\beta$ chain variable element, regardless of their $\alpha$ chain sequence, thus activating T cells nonspecifically. Included are staphylococcal enterotoxins and toxins causing toxic shock syndrome and exfoliative dermatitis.

**su·per·au·ra·le** (soo″pər-aw-ra′le) an anthropometric landmark, the highest point on the superior border of the helix of the ear.

**su·per·car·bon·ate** (soo″pər-kahr′bon-āt) bicarbonate.

**su·per·cen·tral** (soo″pər-sen′trəl) above or superior to a center.

**su·per·cil·ia** (soo″pər-sil′e-ə) [L., pl. of *supercilium*] [TA] the hairs growing on the transverse elevation at the junction of the forehead and the upper lid of either eye; called also *eyebrow*.

**su·per·cil·i·ary** (soo″pər-sil′e-ar-e) pertaining to the eyebrow.

**su·per·cil·i·um** (soo″pər-sil′e-əm) pl. *superci′lia* [L.] [TA] the transverse elevation at the junction of the forehead and the upper eyelid; see *eyebrow* (def. 1), and see also *supercilia*.

**su·per·class** (soo′pər-klas) a taxonomic category sometimes established, subordinate to a phylum and superior to a class.

**su·per·coil** (soo′pər-koil) 1. the process of forming a superhelix in a DNA molecule. 2. superhelix. 3. a shape assumed by chromosomes when they have attained their maximum length during interphase, resembling a "zig-zag" pattern with broad turns.

**su·per·dis·ten·tion** (soo″pər-dis-ten′shən) excessive distention.

**su·per·duct** (soo″pər-dukt′) [*super-* + *duct*] to carry up or elevate.

**su·per·duc·tion** (soo″pər-duk′shən) supraduction.

**su·per·ego** (soo″pər-e′go) [*super-* + *ego*] [MeSH: Superego] in psychoanalytic theory, the aspect of the personality acting as a monitor and evaluator of ego functioning, comparing it with an ideal standard (see *ego ideal*, under *ideal*) and including psychic functions expressed as social attitudes, self-criticism, and a concept of right and wrong (conscience or morality). Cf. *ego* and *id*[1].

**su·per·ex·tend·ed** (soo″pər-ək-stend′əd) extended beyond the normal.

**su·per·ex·ten·sion** (soo″pər-ək-sten′shən) excessive extension.

**su·per·fam·i·ly** (soo″pər-fam′ĭ-le) 1. a taxonomic category sometimes established, subordinate to an order and superior to a family. 2. any of a group of proteins having similarities such as areas of structural homology and believed to descend from the same ancestral gene; e.g., integrins or immunoglobulins.

**su·per·fe·cun·da·tion** (soo″pər-fe″kən-da′shən) [*super-* + *fecundation*] fertilization of two or more ova during the same ovulatory cycle by separate coital acts.

**su·per·fe·ta·tion** (soo″pər-fe-ta′shən) [*super-* + *fetation*] [MeSH: Superfetation] the fertilization and subsequent development of an ovum when a fetus is already present in the uterus, a result of fertilization of ova during different ovulatory cycles and yielding fetuses of different ages.

**su·per·fi·cial** (soo″pər-fish′əl) [L. *superficialis*] pertaining to or situated near the surface.

**su·per·fi·ci·a·lis** (soo″pər-fish″e-a′lis) [TA] superficial; a term used to designate a structure situated closer than another to the surface of the body.

**su·per·fi·ci·es** (soo″pər-fish′e-ēz) [L.] an outer surface.

**su·per·flex·ion** (soo″pər-flek′shən) extreme or excessive flexion.

**su·per·func·tion** (soo″pər-funk′shən) excessive activity of an organ or structure; hyperfunction.

**su·per·gen·u·al** (soo″pər-jen′u-əl) superior to the knee.

**su·per·group** (soo′per-groop) an unofficial designation for a group of viral serogroups that are related antigenically.

**su·per·he·lix** (soo″pər-he′liks) a tertiary conformation that may be adopted by a DNA molecule with constrained ends, such as a plasmid; the molecule is over- or underwound, with the axis of the helix twisted upon itself. In prokaryotes, such a conformation is believed to be important in the control of replication, transcription, recombination, and other processes; in eukaryotes its purpose is poorly understood.
**negative s.**, one in which the DNA axis twists in the direction opposite that of the normal helical turns, causing underwinding of the helix; it is believed to be the physiological state of many DNA molecules.
**positive s.**, one in which the DNA axis twists with the direction of the normal helical turns, causing overwinding of the helix.

**su·per·im·preg·na·tion** (soo″pər-im″preg-na′shən) [*super-* + *impregnation*] superfetation.

**su·per·in·duce** (soo″pər-in-doos′) to induce or bring on in addition to some already existing condition.

**su·per·in·fec·tion** (soo″pər-in-fek′shən) [MeSH: Superinfection] a new infection occurring in a patient having a preexisting infection, such as bacterial superinfection in viral respiratory disease or infection of a chronic hepatitis B carrier with hepatitis D virus. Superinfection can complicate the course of antimicrobial therapy when the new infection is by organisms resistant to the drugs in use.

**su·per·in·vo·lu·tion** (soo″pər-in″vo-loo′shən) prolonged involution of the uterus after delivery, to a size much smaller than the normal, occurring in nursing mothers. Called also *hyperinvolution.*

**su·pe·ri·or** (soo-pe′re-or) [L. "upper"; neut. *superius*] 1. situated above, or directed upward. 2. [TA] a term used in reference to a structure occupying a position nearer the vertex.

**su·per·ja·cent** (soo″pər-ja′sənt) located immediately above; overlying.

**su·per·lac·ta·tion** (soo″pər-lak-ta′shən) hyperlactation.

**su·per·lat·tice** (soo′pər-lat″is) in a solid solution, an arrangement of atoms or molecules consisting of a lattice in which the different kinds of atoms or molecules have well-defined, regular locations with respect to each other.

**su·per·le·thal** (soo″pər-le′thəl) more than sufficient to cause death.

**su·per·me·di·al** (soo″pər-me′de-əl) superomedial.

**su·per·mo·til·i·ty** (soo″pər-mo-til′ĭ-te) excessive motility.

**su·per·na·tant** (soo″pər-na′tənt) [*super-* + L. *natare* to swim] 1. situated above or on top of something. 2. the overlying liquid after precipitation of a solid component of a system.

**su·per·nate** (soo′pər-nāt) supernatant, def. 2.

**su·per·nor·mal** (soo″pər-nor′məl) more than normal.

**su·per·nu·mer·ary** (soo″pər-noo′mər-ar″e) [L. *supernumerarius*] in excess of the regular or normal number.

**su·per·nu·tri·tion** (soo″pər-noo-trĭ′shən) excessive nutrition.

**su·per·oc·cip·i·tal** (soo″pər-ok-sip′ĭ-təl) supraoccipital.

**su·pero·lat·er·al** (soo″pər-o-lat′ər-əl) superior and at the side.

**su·pero·me·di·al** (soo″pər-o-me′de-əl) situated superior to the middle.

**su·per·ov·u·la·tion** (soo″pər-ov″u-la′shən) [MeSH: Superovulation] extraordinary acceleration of ovulation, producing a greater than normal number of ova, usually as a result of the administration of exogenous gonadotropins.

**su·per·ox·ide** (soo″pər-ok′sīd) any compound containing the highly reactive superoxide radical, $O_2^-$, which is produced by reduction of molecular oxygen in many biological oxidations; this highly toxic free radical is continuously removed by the enzyme superoxide dismutase.

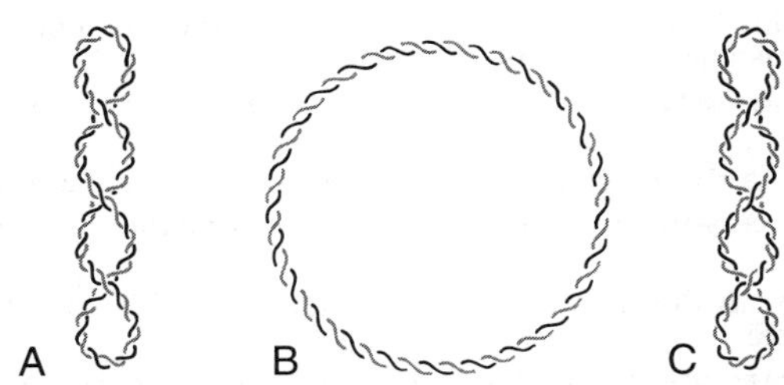

*(A),* Positive superhelix; *(B),* relaxed circle; *(C),* negative superhelix.

**su·per·ox·ide dis·mu·tase** (soo″pər-ok′sīd dis-mu′tās) [EC 1.5.1.1] [MeSH: Superoxide Dismutase] an enzyme of the oxidoreductase class that catalyzes the reduction of superoxide anions to hydrogen peroxide, protecting cells against dangerous levels of superoxide.

**su·per·par·a·site** (soo″pər-par′ə-sīt) 1. a parasite involved in superparasitism. 2. hyperparasite.

**su·per·par·a·sit·ism** (soo″pər-par′ə-sit″iz-əm) 1. infestation with more parasites of one species than the host can support or bring to maturity. 2. hyperparasitic.

**su·per·phos·phate** (soo″pər-fos′fāt) any acid phosphate, especially calcium superphosphate (see *calcium phosphate, monobasic*).

**su·per·re·gen·e·ra·tion** (soo″pər-re-jen″ə-ra′shən) the development of superfluous tissue, organs, or parts as a result of regeneration.

**su·per·salt** (soo′pər-sawlt) any salt obtained by reaction with an excess of acid; a persalt or acid salt.

**su·per·sat·u·rate** (soo″pər-sach′ər-āt) to add more of an ingredient than can be held in solution permanently.

**su·per·scrip·tion** (soo″pər-skrip′shən) [L. *superscriptio*] the sign ℞ before a prescription; see *prescription.*

**su·per·se·cre·tion** (soo″pər-sə-kre′shən) excessive secretion.

**su·per·sen·si·tiv·i·ty** (soo″pər-sen″sĭ-tiv′ĭ-te) abnormally increased sensitivity.
**disuse s.**, increased activity of a neural pathway following chronic exposure to an antagonist drug caused by changes in postsynaptic receptors.

**su·per·sen·si·ti·za·tion** (soo″pər-sen″sĭ-tĭ-za′shən) hypersensitization.

**su·per·soft** (soo″pər-soft′) extremely soft; applied to x-rays of extremely long wavelengths, large absorption coefficients, and low penetrating power.

**su·per·son·ic** (soo″pər-son′ik) [*super-* + L. *sonus* sound] 1. having a speed greater than the velocity of sound, that is, faster than approximately one-fifth mile per second (or 720 miles an hour) in air. 2. ultrasonic.

**su·per·son·ics** (soo″pər-son′iks) the general science relating to phenomena associated with speed greater than the velocity of sound.

**su·per·sphe·noid** (soo″pər-sfe′noid) superior to the sphenoid bone.

**su·per·struc·ture** (soo′pər-struk″chər) 1. any structure built on something else. 2. the overlying or visible portion of a structure. 3. implant s.
**implant s.**, a removable denture retained, supported, and stabilized by an abutment post protruding from the substructure of an implanted framework.

**su·per·vas·cu·lar·iza·tion** (soo″pər-vas″ku-lər-ĭ-za′shən) in radiotherapy, the relative increase in vascularity that occurs when tumor cells are destroyed so that the remaining tumor cells are better supplied by the (uninjured) capillary stroma.

**su·per·ven·tion** (soo″pər-ven′shən) the development of some condition in addition to an already existing one.

**su·per·ver·sion** (soo″pər-ver′zhən) sursumversion.

**su·per·vis·or** (soo′pər-vīz″ər) an individual who oversees the activities of others, such as a nurse who oversees the nursing activities in a specific ward or department of a hospital.

**su·per·vi·ta·min·o·sis** (soo″pər-vi″tə-min-o′sis) hypervitaminosis.

**su·per·vol·tage** (soo′pər-vōl″təj) in radiotherapy, voltage in the range of 500 kilovolts, as contrasted with orthovoltage (140 to 400 kilovolts) and megavoltage (greater than 1 megavolt).

**su·pi·nate** (soo′pĭ-nāt) to assume or place in a supine position.

**su·pi·na·tion** (soo″pĭ-na′shən) [L. *supinatio*] [MeSH: Supination] the act of assuming the supine position, or the state of being supine. Applied to the hand, the act of turning the palm forward (anteriorly) or upward, performed by lateral rotation of the forearm. Applied to the foot, it generally implies movements resulting in raising of the medial margin of the foot, hence of the longitudinal arch. Cf. *pronation.*

**su·pi·na·tor** (soo′pĭ-na-tər) 1. a muscle that serves to supinate. 2. musculus supinator.

**su·pine** (soo′pīn) [L. *supinus* lying on the back, face upward] lying with the face upward; see also *supination.*

**sup·port** (sə-port′) 1. a structure that bears the weight of some-

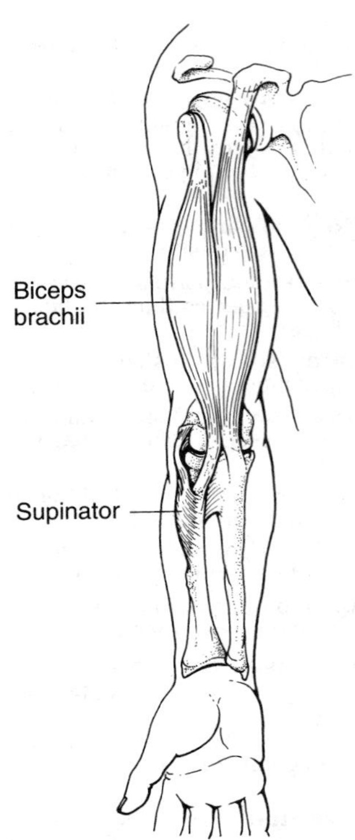


Supinators contracted, forearm, hand supinated.

thing else. 2. a mechanism or arrangement that helps keep something else functioning. 3. the foundation upon which a denture rests.

**sup·port·ive** (sə-por′tiv) providing support or aid. See also *supportive treatment,* under *treatment.*

**sup·pos·i·to·ry** (sə-poz′ĭ-tor-e) [L. *suppositorium*] a medicated mass adapted for introduction into the rectal, vaginal, or urethral orifice of the body; suppository bases are solid at room temperature but melt or dissolve at body temperature. Commonly used bases are cocoa butter, glycerinated gelatin, hydrogenated vegetable oils, polyethylene glycols of various molecular weights, and fatty acid esters of polyethylene glycol.
**glycerin s.** [NF], a suppository made up of a mixture of glycerin and sodium stearate; used as a rectal evacuant.

**Sup·pre·lin** (sə-pre′lin) trademark for a preparation of histrelin acetate.

**sup·pres·sant** (sə-pres′ənt) 1. inducing suppression. 2. an agent that stops secretion, excretion, or normal discharge.

**sup·pres·sion** (sə-presh′ən) [L. *suppressus,* past participle of *supprimere* to hold back] 1. the act of holding back or checking. 2. sudden stoppage or inhibition, as of a secretion, excretion, normal discharge, or other function. 3. in psychiatry, conscious inhibition of an unacceptable impulse or idea as contrasted with repression, which is unconscious. 4. in genetics, masking of the phenotypic expression of a mutation by the occurrence of a second (suppressor) mutation at a different site from the first; the organism appears to be reverted but is in fact doubly mutant. Cf. *reversion,* def. 2. 5. inhibition of the erythrocytic stage of *Plasmodium* to prevent clinical attacks of malaria; used for prophylaxis. 6. cortical inhibition of perception of objects in all or part of the visual field of one eye during binocular vision.
**bone marrow s.,** suppression of bone marrow activity, resulting in reduction in the number of platelets, red cells, and white cells, such as in aplastic anemia. See also *bone marrow failure,* under *failure.* Called also *myelophthisis* and *myelosuppression.*
**overdrive s.,** transient suppression of automaticity in a cardiac pacemaker following a period of stimulation by a more rapidly discharging pacemaker, proportional to the rate and duration of the dominating pacemaker. See also *overdrive pacing,* under *pacing.*

**sup·pu·rant** (sup′u-rənt) [L. *suppurans*] 1. characterized by suppuration. 2. an agent that causes suppuration.

**sup·pu·ra·tion** (sup″u-ra′shən) [*sub-* + L. *puris* pus] [MeSH: Suppuration] the formation of pus; the act of becoming converted into and discharging pus.
**alveodental s.,** periodontitis with the formation of pus.

**sup·pu·ra·tive** (sup′u-ra″tiv) producing pus, or associated with suppuration.

**supra-** [L. "above"] a prefix signifying above or over.

**su·pra-acro·mi·al** (soo″prə-ə-kro′me-əl) above or over the acromion.

**su·pra-anal** (soo″prə-a′nəl) situated superior to the anus.

**su·pra-au·ric·u·lar** (soo″prə-aw-rik′u-lər) superior to the ear.

**su·pra-ax·il·lary** (soo″prə-ak′sĭ-lar″e) superior to the axilla.

**su·pra·buc·cal** (soo″prə-buk′əl) superior to the buccal region.

**su·pra·bulge** (soo′prə-bəlj″) the surface or the crown of a tooth sloping toward the occlusal surface from the height of contour or survey line. Cf. *infrabulge.*

**su·pra·ca·ri·nal** (soo″prə-kə-ri′nəl) situated above the carina tracheae.

**su·pra·cer·e·bel·lar** (soo″prə-ser-ə-bel′ər) superior to or over the cerebellum.

**su·pra·cho·roid** (soo″prə-kor′oid) superior to or over the choroid.

**su·pra·cho·roi·dea** (soo″prə-ko-roi′de-ə) lamina suprachoroidea.

**su·pra·cil·i·ary** (soo″prə-sil′e-ar″e) superciliary.

**su·pra·cla·vic·u·lar** (soo″prə-klə-vik′u-lər) superior to the clavicle.

**su·pra·cla·vic·u·la·ris** (soo″prə-klə-vik″u-lar′is) [L.] supraclavicular.

**su·pra·clu·sion** (soo″prə-kloo′zhən) the condition in which the occluding surface of a tooth extends beyond the normal occlusal plane. Called also *overeruption* and *supraocclusion.*

**su·pra·con·dy·lar** (soo″prə-kon′də-lər) superior to a condyle or condyles.

**su·pra·con·dy·loid** (soo″prə-kon′də-loid) supracondylar.

**su·pra·cos·tal** (soo″prə-kos′təl) superior to or over a rib or ribs.

**su·pra·cot·y·loid** (soo″prə-kot′ə-loid) superior to the acetabulum.

**su·pra·cra·ni·al** (soo″prə-kra′ne-əl) on the superior surface of the cranium.

**su·pra·di·a·phrag·mat·ic** (soo″prə-di″ə-frag-mat′ik) situated superior to the diaphragm.

**su·pra·duc·tion** (soo″prə-duk′shən) [*supra-* + L. *duction*] 1. the upward rotation of an eye around its horizontal axis. 2. the upward rotation of one eye independent of the other by a basedown prism in testing for vertical divergence. See also *sursumversion.* Called also *superduction, sursumduction, supravergence,* and *sursumvergence.*

**su·pra·epi·con·dy·lar** (soo″prə-ep″ĭ-kon′də-lər) superior to an epicondyle.

**su·pra·epi·troch·le·ar** (soo″prə-ep″ĭ-trok′le-ər) superior to the medial epicondyle of the humerus.

**su·pra·gle·noid** (soo″prə-gle′noid) superior to the glenoid cavity.

**su·pra·glot·tic** (soo″prə-glot′ik) 1. superior to the glottis. 2. pertaining to the supraglottis.

**su·pra·glot·tis** (soo″prə-glot′is) the area of the pharynx above the glottis as far as the epiglottis.

**su·pra·glot·ti·tis** (soo″prə-glŏ-ti′tis) inflammation of supraglottic structures in the larynx, often as a result of infection with *Haemophilus influenzae* type B. Types range from a benign variety lasting a few days to a virulent form with edema that obstructs the airway.

**su·pra·he·pat·ic** (soo″prə-hə-pat′ik) superior to the liver.

**su·pra·hy·oid** (soo″prə-hi′oid) situated superior to the hyoid bone.

**su·pra·in·gui·nal** (soo″prə-ing′gwĭ-nəl) superior to the inguinal region, or groin.

**su·pra·in·tes·ti·nal** (soo″prə-in-tes′tĭ-nəl) superior to the intestine.

**su·pra·lim·i·nal** (soo″prə-lim′ĭ-nəl) above the limen of sensation; more than just perceptible.

**su·pra·lum·bar** (soo″prə-lum′bahr) superior to the loin or lumbar region.

**su·pra·mal·le·o·lar** (soo″prə-mə-le′o-lər) above a malleolus.

**su·pra·mam·ma·ry** (soo″prə-mam′ə-re) superior to a mammary gland.

**su·pra·man·dib·u·lar** (soo″prə-man-dib′u-lər) superior to the mandible.

**su·pra·mar·gi·nal** (soo″prə-mahr′jĭ-nəl) above a margin.

**su·pra·mas·toid** (soo″prə-mas′toid) superior to the mastoid portion of the temporal bone.

**su·pra·max·il·lary** (soo″prə-mak′sĭ-lar″e) superior to the maxilla.

**su·pra·max·i·mal** (soo″prə-mak′sĭ-məl) above the maximum.

**su·pra·me·a·tal** (soo″prə-me-a′təl) above a meatus.

**su·pra·men·tal** (soo″prə-men′təl) above the chin.

**su·pra·men·ta·le** (soo″prə-mən-ta′le) in radiographic cephalometry, the most posterior midline point in the concavity between the infradentale and pogonion, determined on the lateral head film.

**su·pra·na·sal** (soo″prə-na′səl) superior to the nose.

**Sup·rane** (soo′prān) trademark for a preparation of desflurane.

**su·pra·nor·mal** (soo″prə-nor′məl) greater than normal; present or occurring in excess of normal amounts or values.

**su·pra·nu·cle·ar** (soo″prə-noo′kle-ər) situated or occurring superior to or on the cortical side or surface of a nucleus in the nervous system; see also under *paralysis.*

**su·pra·oc·cip·i·tal** (soo″prə-ok-sip′ĭ-təl) above or in the superior portion of the occiput.

**su·pra·oc·clu·sion** (soo″prə-ŏ-kloo′zhən) supraclusion.

**su·pra·oc·u·lar** (soo″prə-ok′u-lər) superior to the eye.

**su·pra·omo·hy·oid** (soo″prə-o″mo-hi′oid) superior to the omohyoid muscle.

**su·pra·op·ti·mal** (soo″prə-op′tĭ-məl) greater than optimal.

**su·pra·op·ti·mum** (soo″prə-op′tĭ-məm) a condition or quantity exceeding the optimum.

**su·pra·or·bi·tal** (soo″prə-or′bĭ-təl) superior to the orbit.

**su·pra·pa·tel·lar** (soo″prə-pə-tel′ər) superior to the patella.

**su·pra·pel·vic** (soo″prə-pel′vik) above the pelvis.

**su·pra·phar·ma·co·log·ic** (soo″prə-fahr″mə-ko-loj′ik) much greater than the usual therapeutic dose or pharmacologic concentration of a drug.

**su·pra·phys·i·o·log·i·cal** (soo″prə-fiz″e-o-loj′ĭ-kəl) [*supra-* + *physiological*] said of an abnormal or artificially created state in which a naturally occurring substance is at a concentration greater than that occurring naturally.

**su·pra·pon·tine** (soo″prə-pon′tīn) above or in the upper part of the pons.

**su·pra·pu·bic** (soo″prə-pu′bik) above or over the pubic arch.

**su·pra·re·nal** (soo″prə-re′nəl) [*supra-* + *renal*] 1. superior to a kidney. 2. adrenal (def. 1).

**su·pra·re·nal·ec·to·my** (soo″prə-re″nəl-ek′tə-me) adrenalectomy.

**su·pra·re·nal·ism** (soo″prə-re′nəl-iz-əm) adrenalism.

**su·pra·re·nal·op·a·thy** (soo″prə-re″nəl-op′ə-the) [*suprarenal* + *-pathy*] adrenalopathy.

**Su·pra·ren·in** (soo″prə-ren′in) trademark for a preparation of epinephrine.

**su·pra·re·no·gen·ic** (soo″prə-re″no-jen′ik) adrenogenous.

**su·pra·re·nop·a·thy** (soo″prə-re-nop′ə-the) adrenalopathy.

**su·pra·re·no·trop·ic** (soo″prə-re″no-trop′ik) adrenotropic.

**su·pra·scap·u·lar** (soo″prə-skap′u-lər) above or on the upper part of the scapula.

**su·pra·scle·ral** (soo″prə-sklēr′əl) on the outer surface of the sclera.

**su·pra·sel·lar** (soo″prə-sel′ər) superior to the sella turcica.

**su·pra·sep·tal** (soo″prə-sep′təl) superior to a septum.

**su·pra·spi·nal** (soo″prə-spi′nəl) above or upon a spine.

**su·pra·spi·nous** (soo″prə-spi′nəs) 1. supraspinal. 2. superior to a spinous process.

**su·pra·sta·pe·di·al** (soo″prə-stə-pe′de-əl) superior to the stapes.

**su·pra·ster·nal** (soo″prə-ster′nəl) superior to the sternum.

**su·pra·syl·vi·an** (soo″prə-sil′ve-ən) superior to the sylvian fissure.

**su·pra·tem·po·ral** (soo″prə-tem′pə-rəl) situated superior to the temporal bone, fossa, or region.

**su·pra·ten·to·ri·al** (soo″prə-tən-tor′e-əl) superior to the tentorium of the cerebellum.

**su·pra·tho·rac·ic** (soo″prə-thə-ras′ik) superior to the thorax.

**su·pra·ton·sil·lar** (soo″prə-ton′sĭ-lər) superior to a tonsil.

**su·pra·troch·le·ar** (soo″prə-trok′le-ər) superior to a trochlea.

**su·pra·tym·pan·ic** (soo″prə-tim-pan′ik) above the tympanum.

**su·pra·um·bil·i·cal** (soo″prə-əm-bil′ĭ-kəl) superior to the umbilicus.

**su·pra·vag·i·nal** (soo″prə-vaj′ĭ-nəl) 1. superior to or outside a sheath. 2. above the vagina.

**su·pra·val·var** (soo″prə-val′vər) above a valve, particularly the aortic or pulmonary valve.

**su·pra·ven·tric·u·lar** (soo″prə-vən-trik′u-lər) situated or occurring above the ventricles, especially in an atrium or atrioventricular node.

**su·pra·ver·gence** (soo″prə-ver′jəns) [*supra-* + *vergence*] disjunctive reciprocal movement of the eyes in which one eye rotates upward while the other one remains still; called also *sursumvergence.*

**su·pra·ver·sion** (soo″prə-ver′zhən) [*supra-* + *version*] 1. malocclusion in which a tooth or other maxillary or mandibular structure extends farther away from the alveolus than normal, the occluding surfaces of the teeth extending beyond the normal occlusal line. 2. sursumversion.

**su·pra·ves·i·cal** (soo″prə-ves′ĭ-kəl) [*supra-* + *vesical*] above the urinary bladder.

**su·pra·vi·tal** (soo″prə-vi′təl) denoting a staining method in which the dye is added to a medium of cells already removed from the living organism.

**Su·prax** (soo′praks) trademark for a preparation of cefixime.

**su·pra·xi·phoid** (soo″prə-zi′foid) superior to the xiphoid process.

**su·pra·zy·go·mat·ic** (soo″prə-zi″go-mat′ik) situated above the zygomatic bone.

**su·pro·fen** (soo-pro′fən) [USP] [MeSH: Suprofen] a prostaglandin inhibitor having anti-inflammatory activity; applied topically to the conjunctiva to inhibit miosis during ophthalmic surgery.

**su·ra** (soo′rə) [TA] calf: the fleshy mass formed chiefly by the gastrocnemius muscle on the posterior aspect of the leg below the knee. See also *regio surae.*

**Su·ra·gi·na** (soo-rə-ji′nə) a genus of flies of the family Rhagionidae. *S. lon′gipes* of Mexico is a vicious biter.

**su·ral** (soo′rəl) pertaining to the calf of the leg.

**sur·al·i·men·ta·tion** (sur″al-ĭ-mən-ta′shən) superalimentation.

**su·ra·min so·di·um** (soo′rə-min) an antitrypanosomal and antifilarial agent, used in the prophylaxis and treatment of African trypanosomiasis and in the treatment of onchocerciasis (for which use it has largely been replaced by ivermectin); it also suppresses growth of and hormone production by adrenocortical cells and is used in the treatment of inoperable, metastasizing adrenocortical cancer.

**surd** (sərd) [L. *surdus*] voiceless.

**sur·ex·ci·ta·tion** (sur″ek-si-ta′shən) [L. *super* over + *excitation*] excessive excitation.

**sur·face** (sur′fəs) the outer part or external aspect of an object; called *facies* in official anatomical nomenclature. For anatomical surfaces not listed here, see under *facies.*

**alveolar s. of maxilla,** arcus alveolaris maxillae.

**anterior s.,** 1. that surface which in humans is toward the front of the body (on or nearest the ventral aspect; *facies anterior* [TA]), or toward the head in quadrupeds. 2. in dentistry, the proximal surface of any tooth that is closest to the midline of the dental arch.

**anterior s. of adrenal gland,** facies anterior glandulae suprarenalis.

**anterior s. of body of maxilla,** facies anterior corporis maxillae.

**anterior s. of heart,** facies sternocostalis cordis.

**anterior s. of kidney,** facies anterior renis.

**anterior s. of manubrium and gladiolus,** planum sternale.

**anterior s. of pancreas,** see *facies anteroinferior* and *facies anterosuperior corporis pancreatis.*

**anterior s. of sacral bone,** facies pelvica ossis sacri.

**anterior s. of scapula,** facies costalis scapulae.

**anterior s. of stomach,** paries anterior gastris.

**anterior s. of suprarenal gland,** facies anterior glandulae suprarenalis.

**anteroinferior s. of body of pancreas,** facies anteroinferior corporis pancreatis.

**anterolateral s. of humerus,** facies anterolateralis humeri.

**anteromedial s. of humerus,** facies anteromedialis humeri.

**anterosuperior s. of body of pancreas,** facies anterosuperior corporis pancreatis.

**approximal s.,** facies approximalis dentis.

**articular s.,** that surface of a bone or cartilage which forms a joint with another (*facies articularis* [TA]).

**articular s. of acetabulum,** facies lunata acetabuli.

**articular s. of atlas, inferior,** facies articularis inferior atlantis.

**articular s. of atlas, superior,** facies articularis superior atlantis.
**articular s. of head of fibula,** facies articularis capitis fibulae.
**articular s. of head of rib,** facies articularis capitis costae.
**articular s. of sacral bone, lateral,** facies auricularis ossis sacri.
**articular s. of tubercle of rib,** facies articularis tuberculi costae.
**auricular s. of ilium,** facies auricularis ossis ilii.
**auricular s. of sacrum,** facies auricularis ossis sacri.
**axial s.,** any surface parallel with an axis; in dentistry, any surface of a tooth that is parallel with its long axis, including the buccal, distal, labial, lingual, and medial surfaces.
**basal s.,** that surface of a denture the detail of which is determined by the impression and which rests upon the supporting tissues of the mouth. Called also *foundation s.* and *impression s.*
**buccal s.,** facies buccalis dentis.
**cerebral s. of greater wing,** facies cerebralis alae majoris.
**cerebral s. of parietal bone,** facies interna ossis parietalis.
**condyloid s. of tibia,** facies articularis superior tibiae.
**contact s.,** facies approximalis dentis.
**costal s. of lung,** facies costalis pulmonis.
**costal s. of scapula,** facies costalis scapulae.
**diaphragmatic s.,** the surface of an organ of the thoracic or abdominal cavity that is directed toward the diaphragm (*facies diaphragmatica* [TA]).
**diaphragmatic s. of heart,** facies diaphragmatica cordis.
**diaphragmatic s. of lung,** facies diaphragmatica pulmonis.
**distal s.,** 1. that surface of a structure that is farther from a point of reference. 2. facies distalis dentis.
**dorsal s.,** the aspect of a structure that is toward the back of the body. In humans, synonymous with posterior surface (*facies posterior* [TA]). In quadrupeds, the superior aspect. Cf. *ventral s.*
**dorsal s. of scapula,** facies posterior scapulae.
**extensor s.,** the aspect of a joint of a limb (such as the knee or the elbow) on the side toward which the movement of extension is directed.
**external s. of cranial base,** basis cranii externa.
**facial s.,** facies vestibularis dentis.
**flexor s.,** the aspect of a joint of a limb (such as the knee or the elbow) on the side toward which the movement of flexion is directed.
**foundation s.,** basal s.
**impression s.,** basal s.
**incisal s.,** the cutting edges of the anterior teeth, the incisors and canines, which come into contact with those of the opposite teeth during the act of protrusive occlusion, in which they assume an edge-to-edge relationship. See also *facies occlusalis dentis.*
**inferior s.,** that surface which is lower (directed away from the head, in humans) (*facies inferior* [TA]).
**inferior s. of heart,** facies diaphragmatis cordis.
**inferior s. of tongue,** facies inferior linguae.
**infratemporal s. of body of maxilla,** facies infratemporalis corporis maxillae.
**interlobar s. of lung,** facies interlobaris pulmonis.
**labial s.,** facies labialis dentis.
**lateral s.,** 1. a surface nearer to or directed toward the side of the body (*facies lateralis* [TA]). 2. in dentistry, the proximal surface of an incisor or canine tooth that is farthest from the midline of the dental arch.
**lateral s. of zygomatic bone,** facies lateralis ossis zygomatici.
**left s. of heart,** see *facies pulmonis cordis.*
**lingual s.,** facies lingualis dentis.
**masticatory s.,** 1. occlusal s., working. 2. facies occlusalis dentis.
**maxillary s. of greater wing,** facies maxillaris alae majoris.
**maxillary s. of perpendicular plate of palatine bone,** facies maxillaris laminae perpendicularis ossis palatini.
**medial s.,** 1. a surface nearer to or directed toward the median plane of the body; for official anatomical nomenclature, see terms beginning with *facies medialis,* under *facies.* 2. facies mesialis dentis.
**mediastinal s. of lung,** facies mediastinalis pulmonis.
**mesial s.,** facies mesialis dentis.

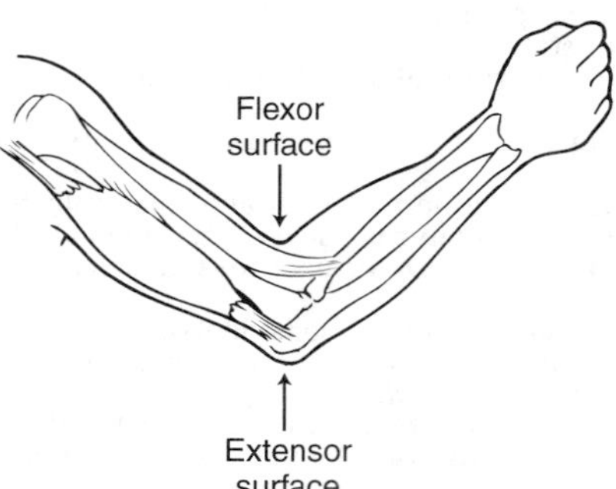


**morsal s's,** the occlusal surfaces of the mandibular and maxillary teeth which make contact in centric occlusion.
**nasal s. of body of maxilla,** facies nasalis corporis maxillae.
**nasal s. of horizontal plate of palatine bone,** facies nasalis laminae horizontalis ossis palatini.
**nasal s. of perpendicular plate of palatine bone,** facies nasalis laminae perpendicularis ossis palatini.
**occlusal s., working,** the occlusal surfaces of the teeth engaged in the masticatory activities; called also *masticatory s.* and *facies masticatoria dentis.*
**occlusal s. of teeth,** 1. facies occlusalis dentis. 2. see *incisal s.* and *occlusal s., working.*
**oral s.,** facies lingualis dentis.
**orbital s. of body of maxilla,** facies orbitalis corporis maxillae.
**orbital s. of frontal bone,** facies orbitalis ossis frontalis.
**orbital s. of greater wing,** facies orbitalis alae majoris.
**orbital s. of zygomatic bone,** facies orbitalis ossis zygomatici.
**palatal s.,** facies palatalis dentis.
**palatine s. of horizontal plate of palatine bone,** facies palatina laminae horizontalis ossis palatini.
**pelvic s. of sacrum,** facies pelvica ossis sacri.
**polished s.,** one that is smoothed to a fine finish; in dentistry, that portion of the surface of a denture that is usually polished, including the palatal surface, and the buccal and lingual surfaces of the teeth.
**posterior s.,** 1. that surface which in humans is toward the back of the body (on or nearest the dorsal aspect; *facies posterior* [TA]), or toward the tail in quadrupeds. 2. in dentistry, the surface of any tooth that is farthest from the midline of the dental arch.
**posterior s. of adrenal gland,** facies posterior glandulae suprarenalis.
**posterior s. of body of pancreas,** facies posterior corporis pancreatis.
**posterior s. of kidney,** facies posterior renis.
**posterior s. of sacral bone,** facies dorsalis ossis sacri.
**posterior s. of scapula,** facies posterior scapulae.
**posterior s. of stomach,** paries posterior gastris.
**posterior s. of suprarenal gland,** facies posterior glandulae suprarenalis.
**proximal s., proximate s.,** 1. any surface nearer to a point of reference. 2. facies approximalis dentis.
**pulmonary s. of heart,** facies pulmonalis cordis.
**renal s. of adrenal gland, renal s. of suprarenal gland,** facies renalis glandulae suprarenalis.
**right s. of heart,** see *facies pulmonalis cordis.*
**sacropelvic s. of ilium,** facies sacropelvica ossis ilii.
**sternocostal s. of heart,** facies sternocostalis cordis.
**subocclusal s.,** a portion of the surface of a tooth that is directed toward but does not make contact with the occlusal surface of its opposite number in the other jaw.
**superior s.,** that surface which is upper or higher (toward the head, in humans; *facies superior* [TA]).
**symphysial s. of pubic bone,** facies symphysialis ossis pubis.
**temporal s. of frontal bone,** facies temporalis ossis frontalis.
**temporal s. of greater wing,** facies temporalis alae majoris.
**temporal s. of zygomatic bone,** facies temporalis ossis zygomatici.
**tentorial s.,** the portion of the cerebral surface that is in contact with the tentorium cerebelli.
**ventral s.,** 1. in humans, the anterior surface. 2. In quadrupeds, the surface that is lower, or on or nearest the abdominal aspect. Cf. *dorsal s.*
**ventral s. of scapula,** facies costalis scapulae.
**vestibular s.,** facies vestibularis dentis.

**sur·fac·tant** (sər-fak′tənt) 1. surface-active agent. 2. in pulmonary physiology, a mixture of phospholipids (chiefly lecithin and sphingomyelin) secreted by the alveolar type II cells into the alveoli and respiratory air passages, which reduces the surface tension of pulmonary fluids and thus contributes to the elastic properties of pulmonary tissue.

**Sur·fak** (sur′fak) trademark for a preparation of docusate calcium.

**sur·geon** (sur′jən) [L. *chirurgio;* Fr. *chirurgien*] 1. a physician who specializes in surgery. 2. the senior medical officer of a military unit.
**acting assistant s.,** contract s.
**barber s.,** formerly a barber who was authorized to practice minor surgery, including bloodletting.
**contract s.,** in the U.S. Army a physician or dentist engaged for temporary service in the medical department; called also *acting assistant s.*
**s. general,** 1. the chief of medical services in one of the armed forces. 2. the chief medical officer of the United States Public Health Service, or of a state public health agency.
**house s.,** a surgeon who is an employee of a hospital and available there when on duty.
**post s.,** the surgeon of an established army post.

**sur·gery** (sur′jər-e) [L. *chirurgia,* from Gr. *cheir* hand + *ergon* work] [MeSH: Surgery] 1. the branch of medicine that treats diseases, injuries, and deformities by manual or operative methods. 2. the work performed by a surgeon; see also *method, operation, procedure,* and *technique.* 3. the place in a hospital or doctor's or dentist's office where surgery is performed. 4. in Great Britain, a room or office where a doctor sees and treats patients.

**abdominal s.,** surgery of the abdominal viscera.

**ambulatory s.,** an operative procedure, performed either in a hospital or in a freestanding facility, that does not require an overnight stay in a hospital.

**antiseptic s.,** surgery done using antiseptic principles; see also *aseptic s.*

**aseptic s.,** surgery performed with aseptic techniques (q.v.).

**aural s.,** the surgical treatment of diseases of the ear.

**bench s.,** surgery performed on an organ that has been removed from the body, after which it is reimplanted.

**cardiac s.,** surgery of the heart.

**cineplastic s.,** creation of a skin-lined tunnel through a muscle adjacent to the stump of an amputated limb, to permit use of the muscle in operating a prosthesis.

**clinical s.,** the study of surgical disease by symptomatic analysis, examination, and observation.

**conservative s.,** surgery designed to preserve, or to remove with minimal risk, diseased or injured organs, tissues, or extremities. Cf. *radical s.*

**cosmetic s.,** that department of plastic surgery which deals with procedures designed to improve the patient's appearance by plastic restoration, correction, removal of blemishes, etc.

**cytoreductive s.,** debulking.

**dental s.,** oral and maxillofacial s.

**dentofacial s.,** that branch of the healing arts which deals with the surgical and adjunctive treatment of diseases, injuries, and defects involving the face and structures of the mouth.

**functional endoscopic sinus s. (FES),** endoscopic surgery of the paranasal sinuses to correct problems causing sinus infection.

**general s.,** that which deals with surgical problems of all kinds, rather than those in a restricted area, or in a surgical specialty such as neurosurgery.

**major s.,** surgery that is particularly difficult or hazardous.

**maxillofacial s.,** oral and maxillofacial s.

**minimal access s., minimally invasive s.,** surgery done with only a small incision or no incision at all, such as through a cannula with a laparoscope or endoscope.

**minor s.,** surgery restricted to the management of minor problems and injuries.

**Mohs' s.,** see under *technique.*

**open heart s.,** surgery that involves incision into one or more chambers of the heart.

**operative s.,** the operative or mechanical aspect of surgery; that which deals with manual and manipulative methods or procedures.

**oral s.,** oral and maxillofacial s.

**oral and maxillofacial s.,** that branch of dental practice that deals with the diagnosis and the surgical and adjunctive treatment of diseases, injuries, and defects of the human mouth and dental structures. Called also *maxillofacial s.* and formerly *dental s.* and *oral s.*

**orthognathic s.,** surgery to correct deformities of the jaw; see also *surgical orthodontics,* under *orthodontics.*

**orthopedic s.,** that branch of surgery which deals with the correction of deformities of the musculoskeletal system; orthopedics.

**plastic s.,** surgery concerned with the restoration, reconstruction, correction, or improvement in the shape and appearance of body structures that are defective, damaged, or misshapen by injury, disease, or growth and development.

**psychiatric s.,** psychosurgery.

**radical s.,** surgery designed to extirpate all areas of locally extensive disease and adjacent zones of lymphatic drainage; cf. *conservative s.* Called also *radical operation.*

**reconstructive s.,** plastic s.

**sonic s.,** the use of focused ultrasonic waves to produce precisely circumscribed alterations within tissues at predetermined sites.

**stereotactic s., stereotaxic s.,** any of several techniques for the production of sharply circumscribed lesions in specific tiny areas of pathologic tissue in deep-seated structures of the central nervous system. The site to be worked on is localized with three-dimensional coordinates; precise images, obtained usually with computed tomography or magnetic resonance imaging may be compared with those in a stereotactic atlas. An arc guidance system is used to direct the electrode or other lesion-producing instrument; methods of producing lesions include heat, cold, x-rays, and ultrasound. See also *stereotactic technique,* under *technique.* Called also *stereoencephalotomy, stereotaxy,* and *stereotactic neurosurgery.*

**structural s.,** surgery devoted to the correction of morphologic abnormalities.

**veterinary s.,** the surgery of domestic animals.

**video-assisted thoracic s., video-assisted thoracoscopic s.,** the use of a thoracoscope and other video assistive devices as well as instruments inserted through trocars for thoracic surgery; because of the smaller incisions, it has a lower morbidity rate than traditional open thoracic surgery.

**sur·gi·cal** (sur'jĭ-kəl) of, pertaining to, or correctable by surgery.

**Sur·gi·cel** (sur'jĭ-sel) trademark for an absorbable knitted fabric prepared by controlled oxidation of cellulose, used as a hemostatic agent to control intraoperative hemorrhage when other conventional methods are impractical or ineffective.

**Sur·i·tal** (sur'ĭ-təl) trademark for preparations of sodium thiamylal.

**sur·ma** (sər'mə) a lead sulfide traditionally applied to the eyelids in India for cosmetic and medical purposes; it can cause lead poisoning.

**Sur·mon·til** (sur'mon-til) trademark for a preparation of trimipramine maleate.

**Sur·van·ta** (sər-van'tə) trademark for a preparation of beractant.

**sur·ra** (soor'ə) [Marathi *sūra* wheezing] trypanosomiasis of domestic animals, e.g., equines, camels, elephants, pigs, goats, and dogs, caused by *Trypanosoma evansi,* usually transmitted by tabanid flies; common signs include fever, anemia, edema, progressive emaciation and weakness, and death. It occurs in East Asia, the Middle East, North Africa, and Central and South America; in the latter regions it is usually seen in horses, is spread by vampire bats as well as flies, and is called *murrina* or *derrengadera.*

**sur·ro·gate** (sur'o-gət) [L. *surrogatus* substituted] substitute; one put into the place of another.

**sur·sum·duc·tion** (sur″səm-duk'shən) supraduction.

**sur·sum·ver·gence** (sur″səm-ver'jəns) supravergence.

**sur·sum·ver·sion** (sur″səm-ver'zhən) [L. *sursum* upward + *version*] binocular conjugate upward rotation of both eyes; called also *supraversion* and *superversion.*

**su·ru·çu·cu** (soo″roo-soo'koo) bushmaster.

**sur·veil·lance** (sər-vāl'əns) 1. watching or monitoring. 2. a procedure used instead of quarantine to control the spread of infectious disease, involving close supervision during the incubation period of possible contacts of individuals exposed to an infectious disease.

**epidemiologic s.,** the ongoing and systematic collection, analysis, and interpretation of data about a disease or health condition; used in planning, implementing, and evaluating public health programs. It may be *passive,* requiring those parties responsible for reporting disease to do so on their own, or *active,* providing visits or other monitoring to those parties to ensure that information is obtained.

**immune s., immunological s.,** a hypothesized monitoring function by which the immune system protects against cancer; according to the theory, tumor cells constantly arise throughout life by malignant transformation of normal cells but almost all are recognized and destroyed by the immune system, only a few somehow escaping or circumventing immune surveillance to grow and become clinically detectable cancers.

**sus·cep·ti·bil·i·ty** (sə-sep″tĭ-bil'ĭ-te) the state of being readily affected or acted upon; diminished immunity to a disease, especially an infection.

**differential s.,** nonhomogeneity in response by the various regions of an embryo when subjected to a diffusely applied injurious agent.

**sus·cep·ti·ble** (sə-sep'tĭ-bəl) 1. capable of impression; readily acted on. 2. not having immunity to an infectious disease and thus at risk of infection.

**sus·lik** (so͞os'lik) [MeSH: Sciuridae] Russian ground squirrel.

**sus·pen·op·sia** (sus″pən-op'se-ə) [L. *suspensio* wavering + *-opsia*] a condition of frequently occurring momentary suppression of attention in the visual cortex to impulses arising in the central retinal areas.

**sus·pen·si·om·e·ter** (səs-pen″se-om'ə-tər) nephelometer.

**sus·pen·sion** (səs-pen'shən) [L. *suspensio*] 1. a condition of temporary cessation, as of animation, of pain, or of any vital process. 2. a preparation of a finely divided drug intended to be incorporated (suspended) in some suitable liquid vehicle before it is used, or already incorporated in such a vehicle. 3. attachment of an organ or other body part to a supporting structure, as of the uterus or bladder in the correction of a hernia or relapse.

**colloid s.,** a colloid system; see *colloid,* def. 2. Sometimes used specifically for a sol in which the dispersed phase is solid and the particles are large enough to settle out of solution.

**corticotropin zinc hydroxide injectable s.** [USP], a sterile suspension of corticotropin with prolonged action, adsorbed on zinc hydroxide; administered intramuscularly for diagnostic testing of adrenocortical function and to stimulate adrenal cortex activity.

**dexamethasone ophthalmic s.** [USP], a suspension of dexamethasone in an aqueous medium, applied topically to the conjunctiva in the treatment of inflammatory and allergic conditions.

**propyliodone s., sterile,** a sterile suspension of propyliodone in wa-

ter for injection, containing 47.5 to 52.5 per cent of propyliodone and a suitable suspending or dispersing agent; used as a radiopaque medium in bronchography, administered intratracheally.
**propyliodone injectable oil s.** [USP], a suspension of propyliodone in peanut oil; used as a radiopaque medium in bronchography, administered intratracheally.
**selenium sulfide detergent s.,** an aqueous, stabilized suspension of selenium sulfide containing a suitable dispersing agent, buffer, and detergent, used as an antiseborrheic shampoo to control seborrheic dermatitis and dandruff.
**trisulfapyrimidines oral s.** [USP], a suspension of sulfadiazine, sulfamerazine, and sulfamethazine, used as an antibacterial in various sulfonamide-responsive infections.

**sus·pen·soid** (səs-pen′soid) lyophobic colloid.

**sus·pen·so·ri·us** (sus″pən-sor′e-əs) [L.] suspensory.

**sus·pen·so·ry** (səs-pen′sor-e) [L. *suspensorius*] 1. serving to hold up a part. 2. a ligament, bone, muscle, sling, or bandage which serves to hold up a part.

**Sus-Phrine** (sus′frin) trademark for a preparation of epinephrine.

**sus·ten·tac·u·lar** (sus″tən-tak′u-lər) [L. *sustentare* to support] 1. pertaining to a sustentaculum. 2. serving to support.

**sus·ten·tac·u·lum** (sus″tən-tak′u-ləm) pl. *sustentac′ula* [L.] a support.
**s. lie′nis,** ligamentum splenorenale.
**s. ta′li** [TA], **s. of talus,** a process of the calcaneus which supports the talus.

**sus·to** (soos′to) [Sp. "fright, shock"] a culture-specific syndrome seen in Latin America consisting of symptoms attributed to a severe fright that causes the soul to leave the body. It is characterized by anxiety, sadness, altered sleep and eating habits, and somatic symptoms such as headache, stomachache, muscle aches, and diarrhea.

**Suth·er·land** (suth′ər-lənd) Earl Wilbur, Jr. American pharmacologist, 1915–1974; winner of the Nobel prize for medicine or physiology in 1971 for isolation of cyclic AMP in the formation of ATP.

**su·ti·ka** (su′tik-ə) a disease of pregnant women of Eastern India and Bangladesh, marked by digestive troubles and fever during pregnancy, with progressive pernicious anemia occurring after delivery.

**su·ti·lains** (soo′tĭ-lāns) a substance containing proteolytic enzymes derived from *Bacillus subtilis,* occurring as a cream-colored powder; used as a proteolytic agent for débridement of wounds.

**Sut·ton's disease** (sut′ənz) [Richard Lightburn *Sutton,* Jr., American dermatologist, born 1908] granuloma fissuratum.

**Sut·ton's nevus (disease)** (sut′ənz) [Richard Lightburn *Sutton,* American dermatologist, 1878–1952] see *periadenitis mucosa necrotica recurrens,* and see *halo nevus,* under *nevus.*

**Sut·to·nel·la** (sut″ə-nel′ə) a genus of gram-negative, nonmotile, aerobic or facultatively anaerobic rod-shaped bacteria that are normal inhabitants of the human oropharynx. Certain organisms formerly assigned to the genus *Kingella* are included here.
**S. indolo′genes,** a species isolated from eye infections and endocarditis; called also *Kingella indologenes.*

**su·tu·ra** (soo-tu′rə) pl. *sutu′rae* [L. "a seam"] [TA] suture: a type of fibrous joint in which the apposed bony surfaces are so closely united by a thin layer of fibrous connective tissue that no movement can occur; found only in the skull. Called also *s. vera* and *true suture.*
**s. corona′lis** [TA], coronal suture: the line of junction of the frontal bone with the two parietal bones.
**sutu′rae crania′les, sutu′rae cra′nii** [TA], cranial sutures: the sutures between the various bones of the skull, named generally for the specific components participating in their formation.
**s. denta′ta,** s. serrata.
**s. ethmoidolacrima′lis** [TA], ethmoidolacrimal suture: the vertical line of junction, on the medial wall of the orbit, between the lacrimal bone and the orbital plate of the ethmoid bone; called also *lacrimoethmoidal suture.*
**s. ethmoidomaxilla′ris** [TA], ethmoidomaxillary suture: the line of junction between the orbital lamina of the ethmoid bone and the orbital surface of the maxilla.
**s. fronta′lis,** frontal suture: the usually transient line of junction between the right and left halves of the frontal bone. The inferior part may persist in the adult, in which case it is called the *metopic suture* (sutura frontalis persistens [TA]).
**s. fronta′lis meto′pica,** TA alternative for *s. frontalis persistens.*
**s. fronta′lis persis′tens** [TA], the name given to the inferior part of the frontal suture when it persists in the adult; called also *s. frontalis metopica* [TA alternative] and *metopic s.*
**s. frontoethmoida′lis** [TA], frontoethmoidal suture: the line of junction in the anterior cranial fossa between the frontal bone and the cribriform plate of the ethmoid bone.
**s. frontolacrima′lis** [TA], frontolacrimal suture: the line of junction between the upper edge of the lacrimal bone and the orbital part of the frontal bone.

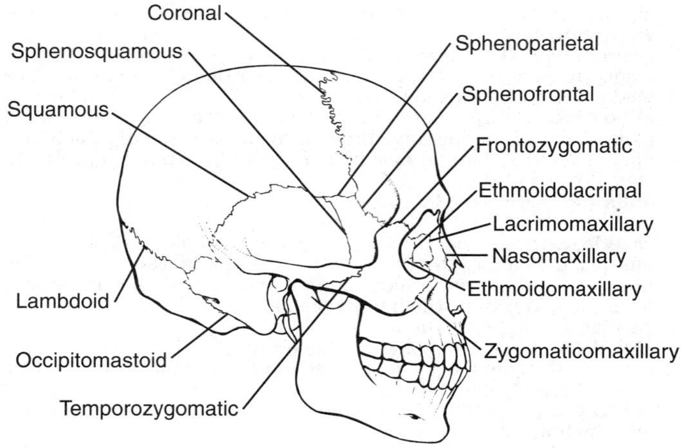


Suturae cranii (cranial sutures).

**s. frontomaxilla′ris** [TA], frontomaxillary suture: the line of junction between the frontal bone and the frontal process of the maxilla.
**s. frontonasa′lis** [TA], frontonasal suture: the line of junction between the frontal and the two nasal bones; called also *nasofrontal suture.*
**s. frontozygoma′tica** [TA], frontozygomatic suture: the line of junction between the zygomatic bone and the zygomatic process of the frontal bone; called also *zygomaticofrontal suture.*
**s. harmo′nia,** s. plana.
**s. incisi′va** [TA], incisive suture: an indistinct suture sometimes seen extending laterally from the incisive fossa to the space between the canine tooth and the lateral incisor, indicating the line of fusion between the premaxilla and the maxilla.
**s. infraorbita′lis,** TA alternative for *s. zygomaticomaxillaris.*
**s. intermaxilla′ris** [TA], intermaxillary suture: the line of junction between the maxillary bones of either side, just inferior to the anterior nasal spine.
**s. internasa′lis** [TA], internasal suture: the line of junction between the two nasal bones.
**s. lacrimoconcha′lis** [TA], lacrimoconchal suture: the line of junction between the lacrimal bone and the inferior nasal concha.
**s. lacrimomaxilla′ris** [TA], lacrimomaxillary suture: a suture on the inner wall of the orbit, between the lacrimal bone and the maxilla.
**s. lambdoi′dea** [TA], lambdoid suture: the line of junction between the occipital and parietal bones, shaped like the Greek letter lambda.
**s. limbo′sa** [TA], limbous suture: a type of squamous suture in which there is interlocking of the beveled surfaces of the bones.
**s. nasofronta′lis,** s. frontonasalis.
**s. nasomaxilla′ris** [TA], nasomaxillary suture: the line of junction between the lateral edge of the nasal bone and the frontal process of the maxilla.
**s. occipitomastoi′dea** [TA], occipitomastoid suture: an extension of the lambdoid suture between the occipital bone and the posterior edge of the mastoid portion of the temporal bone.
**s. palati′na media′na** [TA], median palatine suture: the line of junction between the horizontal part of the palatine bones of either side.
**s. palati′na transver′sa** [TA], transverse palatine suture: the line of junction between the palatine processes of the maxillae and the horizontal parts of the palatine bones.
**s. palatoethmoida′lis** [TA], palatoethmoidal suture: the line of junction between the orbital process of the palatine bone and the orbital lamina of the ethmoid bone.
**s. palatomaxilla′ris** [TA], palatomaxillary suture: the suture in the floor of the orbit, between the orbital processes of the palatine bone and the orbital portion of the maxilla.
**s. parietomastoi′dea** [TA], parietomastoid suture: the line of junction between the posterior inferior angle of the parietal bone and the mastoid process of the temporal bone.
**s. pla′na** [TA], flat suture: a type of suture in which there is simple apposition of the contiguous surfaces, with no interlocking of the edges of the participating bones. Called also *false suture.*
**s. sagitta′lis** [TA], sagittal suture: the line of junction between the two parietal bones.
**s. serra′ta** [TA], serrated suture: a type of suture in which the participating bones are united by interlocking processes resembling the teeth of a saw.
**s. sphenoethmoida′lis** [TA], sphenoethmoidal suture: the line of junction between the body of the sphenoid bone and the orbital lamina of the ethmoid bone.
**s. sphenofronta′lis** [TA], sphenofrontal suture: a long suture joining

the orbital part of the frontal bone to the greater and lesser wings of the sphenoid bone on either side of the skull.

**s. sphenomaxilla'ris** [TA], sphenomaxillary suture: a suture occasionally seen between the pterygoid process of the sphenoid bone and the maxilla.

**s. sphenoorbita'lis,** sphenoorbital suture: the line or junction between the orbital process of the palatine bone and the body of the sphenoid bone.

**s. sphenoparieta'lis** [TA], sphenoparietal suture: the line of junction between the greater wing of the sphenoid bone and the parietal bone.

**s. sphenosquamo'sa** [TA], sphenosquamous suture: the line of junction between the greater wing of the sphenoid bone and the squamous part of the temporal bone.

**s. sphenovomera'lis** [TA], **s. sphenovomeria'na,** sphenovomerine suture: the line of junction between the vaginal processes of the medial pterygoid plates of the sphenoid and the ala of the vomer.

**s. sphenozygoma'tica** [TA], sphenozygomatic suture: the line of junction between the greater wing of the sphenoid bone and the zygomatic bone.

**s. squamomastoi'dea** [TA], squamomastoid suture: a suture existing early in life between the squamous and mastoid portions of the temporal bone. Called also *s. squamosomastoidea.*

**s. squamo'sa** [TA], squamous suture: a type of suture formed by overlapping of the broad beveled edges of the participating bones.

**s. squamo'sa cra'nii** [TA], squamous suture of cranium: the suture between the squamous part of the temporal bone and the parietal bone.

**s. squamosomastoi'dea,** s. squamomastoidea.

**s. temporozygoma'tica** [TA], temporozygomatic suture: the line of junction between the zygomatic process of the temporal bone and the temporal process of the zygomatic bone.

**s. ve'ra,** sutura.

**s. zygomaticomaxilla'ris** [TA], zygomaticomaxillary suture: the line of junction between the zygomatic bone and the zygomatic process of the maxilla.

**su·tur·al** (soo'chə-rəl) of or pertaining to a suture.

**su·tur·a·tion** (soo"chə-ra'shən) the act or process of suturing.

**su·ture** (soo'chər) [L. *sutura* a seam] [MeSH: Sutures] 1. sutura. 2. a loop of thread, catgut, or similar material used to secure apposition of the edges of a surgical or accidental wound; called also *stitch.* See Plate 47. 3. to unite the edges of a wound using such loops; called also *stitch.* 4. the material used in thus closing a wound; see *absorbable s.* and *nonabsorbable s.*

## Suture

For descriptions of specific anatomic structures not listed here, see under *sutura.*

**absorbable s.,** a surgical suture that closes a wound and later either is digested by proteolytic enzymes derived from inflammatory cells or is hydrolyzed by water.

**absorbable surgical s.** [USP], a sterile absorbable suture made of collagen derived from healthy mammals or from a synthetic polymer, available in various diameters and tensile strengths; it may be treated to modify its resistance to absorption, impregnated with a suitable antimicrobial agent, and colored.

**Albert's s.,** a form of Czerny's suture in which the first row of stitches is passed through the entire thickness of the intestine.

**Appolito's s.,** Gély's s.

**apposition s.,** a superficial suture used for bringing together the cutaneous edges of a wound.

**approximation s.,** a deep suture for bringing together the deep tissues of a wound.

**arcuate s.,** sutura coronalis.

**atraumatic s.,** a suture fused into the end of a small eyeless needle.

**basilar s.,** fissura spheno-occipitalis.

**Bell's s.,** a form of lock-stitch in which the needle is passed from within outward alternately on the two edges of the wound.

**biparietal s.,** sutura sagittalis.

**bolster s.,** a suture the ends of which are tied over a tiny roll of gauze or a piece of rubber tubing, in order to lessen the pressure on the skin.

**bony s.,** sutura.

**bregmatomastoid s.,** sutura parietomastoidea.

**Bunnell's s.,** a figure-of-eight zigzag suture used for tendon repair.

**buried s.,** one that is placed deep in the tissues and concealed by the skin.

**button s.,** one in which the stitch is passed through a button-like disk to prevent the suture material from cutting through the skin.

**catgut s.,** see *surgical gut,* under *gut.*

**chain s.,** a continuous suture in which each loop of thread is caught by the next adjacent loop.

**circular s.,** one that is applied to the entire circumference of a hollow viscus to secure closure, or to a portion of a visceral wall to achieve inversion of the enclosed circular area.

**coaptation s.,** apposition s.

**cobblers' s.,** one made with suture material threaded through a needle at each end.

**Connell s.,** a U-shaped continuous s. used in intestinal anastomosis, the stitches being placed parallel to and about 4 mm from the edge of the wound, and passing through all the layers of the bowel. See Plate 47.

**continuous s.,** one in which a continuous, uninterrupted length of material is used to approximate the cut edges of one or more layers of tissues.

**coronal s.,** sutura coronalis.

**cranial s's,** suturae cranii.

**Cushing s.,** a continuous inverting suture used for closing the seromuscular layers in surgery of the gastrointestinal tract. See Plate 47.

**Czerny's s.,** 1. an intestinal suture in which the thread is passed through the mucous membrane alone. 2. a method of uniting a ruptured tendon by splitting one of the ends and suturing the other end into the slit.

**Czerny-Lembert s.,** a combination of Czerny and Lembert sutures in circular enterorrhaphy.

**dentate s.,** sutura serrata.

**double-button s.,** a form of stitch in which the suture material is passed deep across the edges of the wound, between two buttons placed on the surface of the skin, one on either side of the suture line.

**Dupuytren's s.,** a continuous Lembert suture.

**ethmoidomaxillary s.,** sutura ethmoidomaxillaris.

**everting s.,** a method by which the approximated edges of a wound are turned outward; formed by encircling with the needle a larger amount of tissue at the depth of the wound than at the periphery. See Plate 47.

**false s.,** sutura plana.

**figure-of-eight s.,** one in which the thread follows the contours of the figure 8.

**flat s.,** sutura plana.

**frontal s.,** 1. sutura frontalis. 2. sutura frontalis persistens.

**frontoethmoidal s.,** sutura frontoethmoidalis.

**frontolacrimal s.,** sutura frontolacrimalis.

**frontomaxillary s.,** sutura frontomaxillaris.

**frontonasal s.,** sutura frontonasalis.

**frontoparietal s.,** sutura coronalis.

**frontosphenoid s.,** sutura sphenofrontalis.

**frontozygomatic s.,** sutura frontozygomatica.

**furrier's s.,** a method of stitching intestinal wounds by piercing first one margin of the incision and then the other from within outward; overlying sutures are placed through the seromuscular layers to reinforce the closure and prevent leakage.

**Gaillard-Arlt s.,** a suture used in correction of entropion.

**Gély's s.,** a continuous suture for repair of intestinal wounds, made by a thread with a needle at each end, and consisting of a series of cross-stitches closing the wound.

**glover's s.,** lock-stitch s.

**s. of Goethe,** sutura incisiva.

**Gussenbauer's s.,** a figure-of-eight suture used in repairing a rent of the intestine.

**Halsted s.,** a modification of the Lembert suture, consisting of a stitch parallel to the wound on one side, with the two free ends of the material emerging on the other side, where they are tied. See Plate 47.

**harelip s.,** a figure-of-eight suture used in the correction of cleft lip.

**hemostatic s's,** sutures used to control oozing of blood from raw areas.

**incisive s.,** sutura incisiva.

**infraorbital s.,** sutura zygomaticomaxillaris.

**intermaxillary s.,** sutura intermaxillaris.

**internasal s.,** sutura internasalis.

**interparietal s.,** sutura sagittalis.

**interrupted s.,** a noncontinuous suture; one in which each stitch is made with a separate piece of material.

**intradermic s.,** a suture applied parallel with the edges of the wound, but within the layers of the skin, usually a continuous stitch.

**inverting s.,** a seromuscular stitch used in intestinal anastomosis

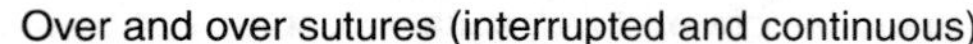



Over and over sutures (interrupted and continuous)

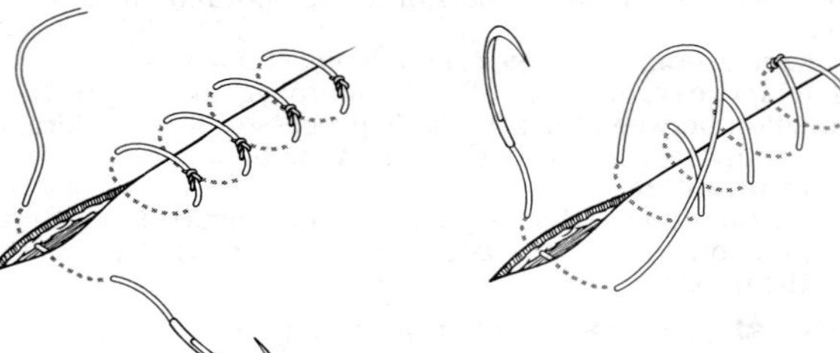

Subcuticular suture (interrupted and continuous)

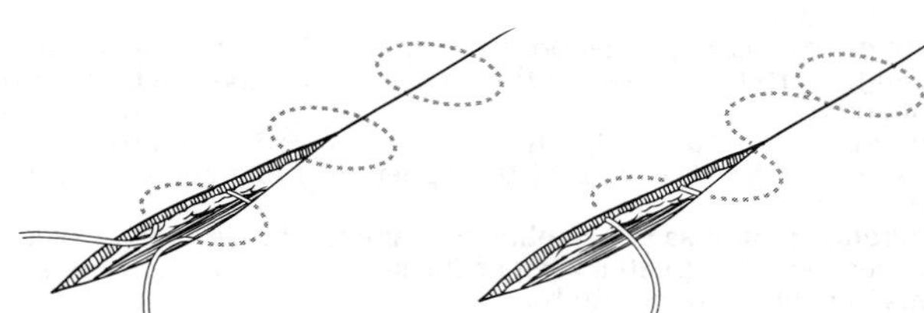

Horizontal mattress sutures (interrupted and continuous)

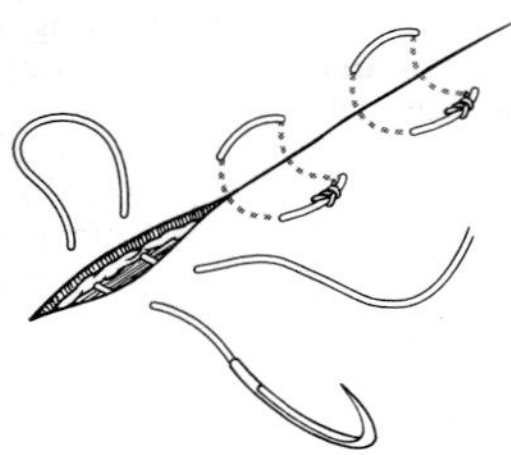

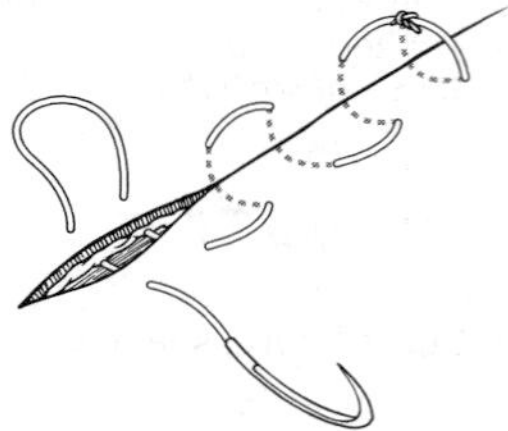

Vertical mattress sutures (interrupted and continuous)

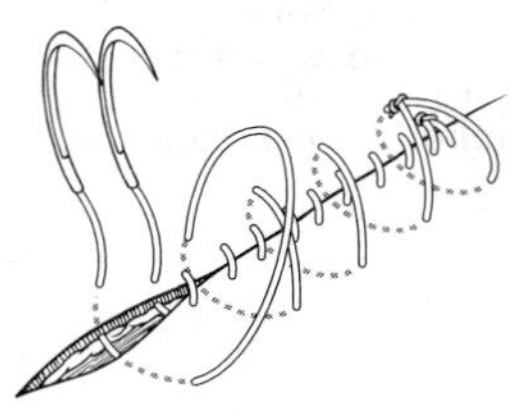

Lembert sutures (interrupted and continuous)

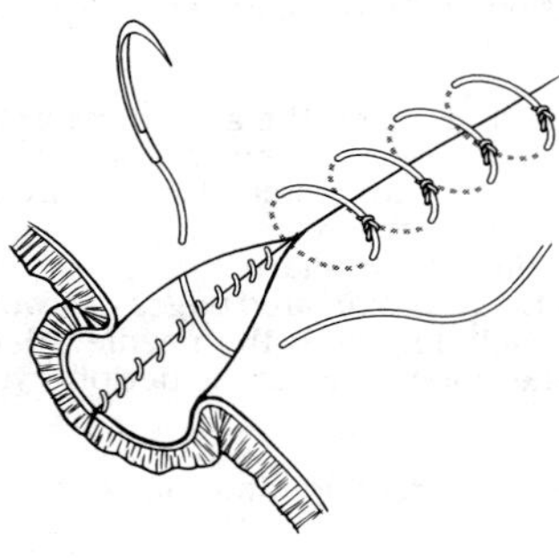

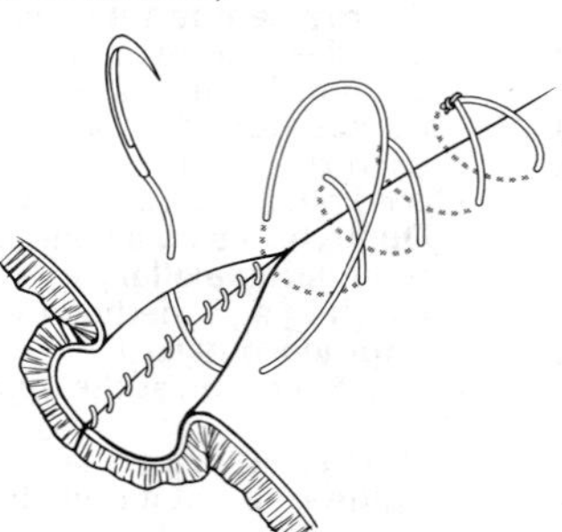

Cushing suture

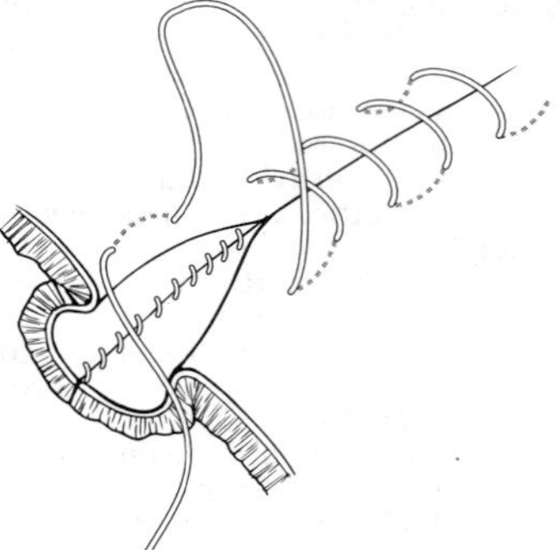

Everting suture

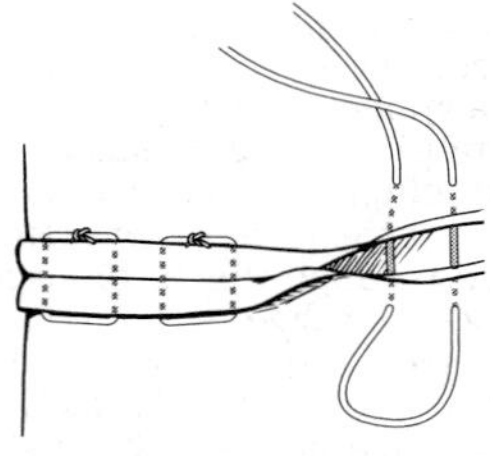

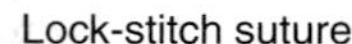

Lock-stitch suture

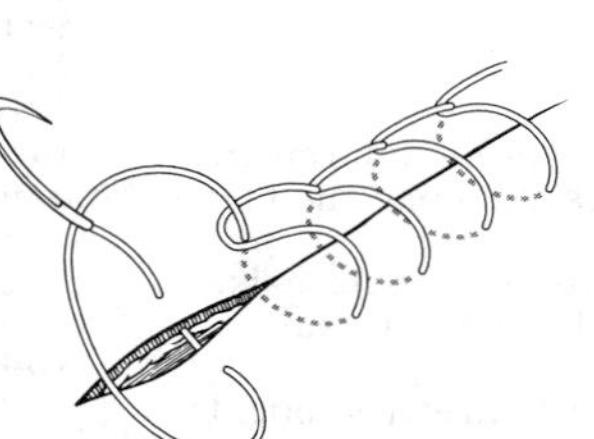

Halsted suture

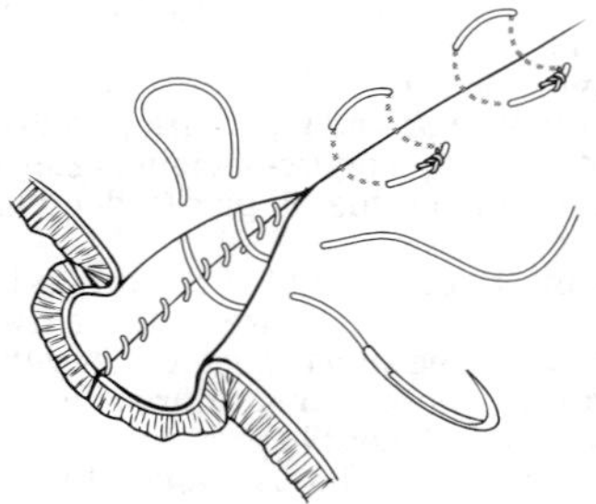

Connell suture

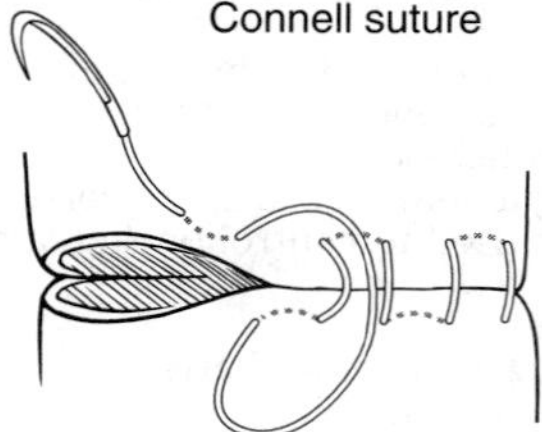

Purse-string suture

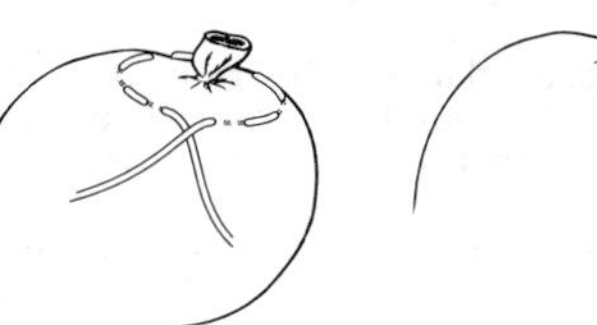

**PLATE 47—**VARIOUS TYPES OF SUTURES

to appose and invert the serosal surfaces of the two segments, as in the Cushing or Lembert suture.

**jugal s.,** sutura sagittalis.

**lacrimoconchal s.,** sutura lacrimoconchalis.

**lacrimoethmoidal s.,** sutura ethmoidolacrimalis.

**lacrimomaxillary s.,** sutura lacrimomaxillaris.

**lambdoid s.,** sutura lambdoidea.

**Le Dentu's s.,** for a divided tendon: two stitches are passed on each side, right and left, and are tied in front; a third is taken from right to left above and below the cut and is tied on one side.

**Le Fort's s.,** for a divided tendon: a single loop is passed above the cut, entering at one side, coming out and going in at the front; it is then passed below the cut at each side, coming out in front, and is there tied.

**Lembert s.,** an inverting suture commonly used in gastrointestinal surgery: the needle is inserted about 2.5 mm lateral to the incision, through the serous and muscular tunics but not the submucosa, and brought out near the edge of the incision, then inserted near the edge on the opposite side and brought out at the more distant point, without having entered the lumen of the gut. It may be either interrupted or continuous. See Plate 47.

**limbous s.,** sutura limbosa.

**lock-stitch s.,** a continuous hemostatic suture used in intestinal surgery: the needle is passed through all layers of the bowel and the loop of suture material is made to fall over the point of emergence of the needle, which comes up through the loop, forming a self-locking stitch when the strand is pulled taut. See Plate 47.

**longitudinal s.,** sutura sagittalis.

**loop s.,** interrupted s.

**mammillary s., mastoid s.,** sutura occipitomastoidea.

**mattress s., horizontal,** a method in which the stitches are made parallel with the edges of the wound, the suture material crossing deeply from one side to the other. See Plate 47.

**mattress s., right-angle,** mattress s., vertical.

**mattress s., vertical,** a method in which the stitches are made at right angles to the edges of the wound, taking both deep and superficial bites of tissue, the latter achieving more exact apposition of the cutaneous margins. See Plate 47.

**metopic s.,** sutura frontalis persistens.

**nasofrontal s.,** sutura frontonasalis.

**nasomaxillary s.,** sutura nasomaxillaris.

**nerve s.,** neurorrhaphy.

**nonabsorbable s.,** material for closing wounds which is not absorbed in the body, e.g., silk, cotton, and stainless steel, or synthetic material such as nylon.

**nonabsorbable surgical s.** [USP], a strand of material resistant to the action of living mammalian tissue, available in various diameters and tensile strengths. There are three types: *Class I* is composed of monofilament, twisted, or braided silk or synthetic fibers; if there is a coating, it does not significantly affect the thickness. *Class II* is composed of cotton or linen fibers or of coated natural or synthetic fibers having a coating that significantly affects the thickness but not the strength. *Class III* is monofilament or multifilament wire.

**occipital s.,** sutura lambdoidea.

**occipitomastoid s.,** sutura occipitomastoidea.

**occipitoparietal s.,** sutura lambdoidea.

**occipitosphenoidal s.,** fissura spheno-occipitalis.

**over-and-over s.,** a method in which equal bites of tissue are taken on each side of the wound; it may be either interrupted or continuous. See Plate 47.

**palatine s., anterior,** sutura incisiva.

**palatine s., median, palatine s., middle,** sutura palatina mediana.

**palatine s., transverse,** sutura palatina transversa.

**palatoethmoidal s.,** sutura palato-ethmoidalis.

**palatomaxillary s.,** sutura palatomaxillaris.

**Pancoast's s.,** a form of tongue-and-groove suture; see *plastic s.*

**Paré's s.,** the use of strips of cloth applied along the edges of a wound, and then stitched together to bring the margins of the wound into apposition.

**parietal s.,** sutura sagittalis.

**parietomastoid s.,** sutura parietomastoidea.

**parietooccipital s.,** sutura lambdoidea.

**petrobasilar s., petrosphenobasilar s.,** synchondrosis petro-occipitalis.

**petrosphenooccipital s. of Gruber,** fissura petro-occipitalis.

**petrosquamous s.,** fissura petrosquamosa.

**plastic s.,** a method in which a tongue is cut in one lip of the wound and a groove in the other, the tongue and groove then being stitched together, and the ends of the thread tied over a roll of adhesive plaster.

**premaxillary s.,** sutura incisiva.

**presection s.,** a stitch or series of stitches placed in the tissues before an incision is made.

**primary s.,** prompt surgical closure of a wound.

**purse-string s.,** a continuous suture placed around a circular opening that is to be inverted; commonly used for the stump of the appendix or a hernia sac. See Plate 47.

**quilt s., quilted s.,** a continuous mattress suture.

**relaxation s.,** any suture placed to close a wound but so formed that it may be loosened in order to relieve the tension should it become too great.

**retention s.,** a reinforcing suture for abdominal wounds, utilizing exceptionally strong material like braided silk or stainless steel, and including a large amount of tissue in each stitch; intended to relieve pressure on the primary suture line and prevent postoperative wound disruption or evisceration.

**rhabdoid s.,** sutura sagittalis.

**sagittal s.,** sutura sagittalis.

**secondary s.,** 1. delayed closure of an operative or accidental wound, usually because of the presence or expectation of infection. 2. resuture of an operative wound following disruption.

**seroserous s.,** a suture which apposes two serous surfaces.

**serrated s.,** sutura serrata.

**shotted s.,** one in which the two ends of the suture wire are passed through a split or perforated lead shot, which is then compressed.

**Sims' s.,** a shotted suture.

**s's of skull,** suturae cranii.

**sphenoethmoidal s.,** 1. sutura sphenoethmoidalis. 2. a craniometric landmark, being the most superior point of the sutura sphenoethmoidalis. Called also *point SE.* Abbreviated SE.

**sphenofrontal s.,** sutura sphenofrontalis.

**sphenomaxillary s.,** sutura sphenomaxillaris.

**sphenooccipital s.,** fissura sphenooccipitalis.

**sphenoorbital s.,** sutura sphenoorbitalis.

**sphenoparietal s.,** sutura sphenoparietalis.

**sphenopetrosal s.,** synchondrosis petro-occipitalis.

**sphenosquamous s., sphenotemporal s.,** sutura sphenosquamosa.

**sphenovomerine s.,** sutura sphenovomeralis.

**sphenozygomatic s.,** sutura sphenozygomatica.

**squamomastoid s., squamosomastoid s.,** sutura squamomastoidea.

**squamosoparietal s.,** sutura squamosa cranii.

**squamososphenoid s.,** sutura sphenosquamosa.

**squamous s.,** sutura squamosa.

**squamous s. of cranium,** sutura squamosa cranii.

**subcuticular s.,** a method of skin closure involving placement of stitches in the subcuticular tissues parallel with the line of the wound; continuous or interrupted sutures may be used. See Plate 47.

**superficial s.,** one that is placed through the superficial fascia only.

**temporal s.,** sutura squamosa cranii.

**temporozygomatic s.,** sutura temporozygomatica.

**tongue-and-groove s.,** plastic s.

**transverse s. of Krause,** sutura zygomaticomaxillaris.

**true s.,** sutura.

**uninterrupted s.,** continuous s.

**zygomaticofrontal s.,** sutura frontozygomatica.

**zygomaticomaxillary s.,** sutura zygomaticomaxillaris.

**zygomaticotemporal s.,** sutura temporozygomatica.

**sux·a·me·tho·ni·um chlo·ride** (suk″sə-mə-tho′ne-əm) succinylcholine chloride.

**Sux-Cert** (suk′sərt) trademark for preparations of succinylcholine chloride.

**Su·zanne's gland** (su-zahnz′) [Jean Georges *Suzanne,* French physician, late 19th century] see under *gland.*

**SV** stroke volume; sinus venosus; simian virus.

**SV40** simian virus 40.

**Sv** sievert.

**SVC** superior vena cava.

**sved·berg** (sfed′bərg) Svedberg unit.

**Sved·berg unit, flotation unit** (sfed'bərg) [Theodor *Svedberg,* Swedish chemist, 1884–1971, inventor of the ultracentrifuge and winner of the Nobel prize for chemistry in 1926 for his work on disperse systems] see under *unit.*

**SVT** supraventricular tachycardia.

**swab** (swahb) a wad of cotton or other absorbent material firmly attached to the end of a wire or stick, used for applying medication, removing material, collecting bacteriological material, etc.

**swad·dler** (swahd'lər) a wrapping for an infant's body.
**silver s.,** a swaddler composed of polyester laminated on the inside surface with a thin layer of aluminum, used to prevent hypothermia in the newborn.

**swage** (swāj) 1. to shape metal by hammering or by adapting it to a die. 2. to fuse suture material to a needle, especially an eyeless needle. 3. a tool or form, often one of a pair, for shaping metal by pressure.

**swag·er** (swāj'ər) a device or apparatus for shaping metal to a desired form by using simultaneous pressures from various angles.

**Swain·so·na** (swān'sə-nə) the Darling peas, a genus of Australian legumes related to *Astragalus*; they contain a chemical that inhibits mannosidase activity and causes mannosidosis with potentially fatal neurological symptoms (similar to those of loco poisoning) in livestock grazing on them for extended periods.

**swal·low·ing** (swahl'o-ing) the taking in of a substance through the mouth and pharynx, past the cricopharyngeal constriction through the esophagus and into the stomach. The oral phase is a voluntary act, whereas the remainder is a reflex act mediated by an integrating swallowing center in the medulla oblongata. Called also *deglutition.*

**swarm·ing** (swawr'ming) spreading in a swarm; a term applied to bacteria, especially *Proteus* species, which spread over the surface of the colony.

**sway·back** (swa'bak) [MeSH: Swayback] 1. abnormal downward curvature of the spinal column in the dorsal region in horses. 2. see *lordosis.* 3. enzootic ataxia.

**sweat** (swet) [MeSH: Sweat] 1. the liquid secreted by the sweat glands (glandulae sudoriferae), having a salty taste and a pH that varies from 4.5 to 7.5. Sweat produced by the eccrine sweat glands is clear with a faint characteristic odor, and contains water, sodium chloride, and traces of albumin, urea, and other compounds; its composition varies with many factors, e.g., fluid intake, external temperature and humidity, and some hormonal activity. Sweat produced by the larger, deeper, apocrine sweat glands of the axillae contains, in addition, organic material which on bacterial decomposition produces an offensive odor. Called also *perspiration.* Cf. *diaphoresis.* 2. to secrete this fluid.
**bloody s.,** hematidrosis.
**blue s.,** chromhidrosis in which the sweat has a blue color; it may occur in copper workers.
**fetid s.,** bromhidrosis.
**green s.,** a greenish sweating seen among workers in copper.
**night s.,** sweating during sleep, a symptom frequently occurring in tuberculosis and acquired immune deficiency syndrome.
**phosphorescent s.,** phosphorescent perspiration, sometimes observed in miliaria and after the eating of phosphorescent fish.

**sweat·ing** (swet'ing) [MeSH: Sweating] the secretion of sweat. Called also *perspiration, diaphoresis,* and *sudoresis.*
**gustatory s.,** auriculotemporal syndrome.

**Swe·di·aur's disease** (sva'dyour) [François Xavier *Swediaur* (or *Schwediauer*), Austrian physician, 1748–1824] see under *disease.*

**swee·ney** (swe'ne) suprascapular paralysis.

**swee·ny** (swe'ne) suprascapular paralysis.

**Sweet's syndrome** (swēts) [Robert Douglas *Sweet,* English dermatologist, 20th century] [MeSH: Sweet's Syndrome] acute febrile neutrophilic dermatosis.

**swell·head** (swel'hed) 1. lechuguilla fever. 2. big head, def. 2.

**swell·ing** (swel'ing) 1. a transient abnormal enlargement or increase in volume of a body part or area not caused by proliferation of cells. See also *tumor* (def. 1). Called also *turgescence, tumescence,* and *tumefaction.* 2. an eminence, or elevation.
**arytenoid s.,** an eminence on each side of the embryonic laryngeal orifice that presages the future larynx.
**blennorrhagic s.,** swelling of the knee in gonorrheal synovitis.
**Calabar s's,** edematous areas, up to several centimeters in diameter, appearing suddenly on various portions of the body, and lasting only 2 or 3 days; fever, pruritus, and urticaria may occur. It is caused by infection with *Loa loa.* Called also *ambulant edema* and *Calabar edema.*
**capsular s.,** the development of a swollen appearance of capsulated pneumococci on exposure to type-specific antibody, due to the binding of antibody with capsular polysaccharide; called also *Neufeld's reaction.*
**cloudy s.,** a term formerly applied to an early stage of toxic degenerative changes, especially in the protein constituents of organs in infectious diseases. The tissues appear swollen, parboiled, and opaque, but revert to normal when the cause is removed. At the cellular level, it is characterized by slight swelling of the cell and granularity and cloudiness of the cytoplasm.
**fugitive s.,** an extremely short-lived swelling.
**genital s.,** labioscrotal s.
**glassy s.,** amyloid degeneration.
**hunger s.,** edematous swellings in wet beriberi.
**Kamerun s's,** Calabar s's.
**labial s.,** the primordium of a labium majus.
**labioscrotal s.,** an elevation on each side of the embryonic phallus that becomes either a labial (labia majora) or a scrotal swelling. Called also *genital s.*
**lingual s., lingual s., lateral,** distal tongue bud.
**scrotal s.,** the primordium of one-half of the scrotum.
**Soemmering's crystalline s.,** annular edema of the lower portion of the lens capsule after the removal of a cataractous lens.
**tropical s's,** Calabar s's.
**tympanic s.,** intumescentia tympanica.

**Swen·son's operation** (swen'sənz) [Orvar *Swenson,* American surgeon, born 1909] see under *operation.*

**Swift's disease** (swifts) [H. *Swift,* Australian physician, 1858–1937] acrodynia.

**Swift-Feer disease** (swift-fār) [H. *Swift;* Emil *Feer*-Sulzer, Swiss pediatrician, 1864–1955] acrodynia.

**swine·pox** (swīn-poks) an acute infectious, eruptive disease of piglets, marked by lesions of the skin of the abdomen, flanks, and head, caused by a poxvirus; it is usually mild but occasionally serious or fatal.

**switch** (swich) 1. a transfer, shift, or change. 2. a device that makes or breaks an electric circuit.
**class s.,** the mechanism by which a B cell or plasma cell switches from production of IgM to production of IgG, IgA, or IgE. See *immunoglobulin genes,* under *gene.*
**isotype s.,** the mechanism by which a B cell changes from the production of one isotype to another in response to stimulation by various cytokines.

**Swy·er syndrome** (swi'ər) [Gerald Isaac MacDonald *Swyer,* British endocrinologist, born 1917] 46,XY gonadal dysgenesis.

**Swy·er-James syndrome** (swi'ər-jāmz) [Paul R. *Swyer,* English physician in Canada, born 1921; G. C. W. *James,* American physician, 20th century] see under *syndrome.*

**sy·ceph·a·lus** (si-sef'ə-ləs) syncephalus.

**sych·nu·ria** (sik-nu're-ə) [Gr. *sychnos* frequent + *-uria*] pollakiuria.

**sy·co·si·form** (si-ko'sĭ-form) resembling sycosis.

**sy·co·sis** (si-ko'sis) [Gr. *sykōsis,* from *sykon* fig] 1. a disease marked by inflammation of the hair follicles, especially of the beard. 2. a kind of ulcer on the eyelids.
**s. bar'bae,** bacterial folliculitis involving the bearded region, usually caused by *Staphylococcus aureus,* in which the primary lesion is a pinhead-sized pustule, pierced by a hair, which may, if neglected, lead to impetiginization and crust formation and become chronic. Called also *barber's itch, folliculitis barbae,* and *s. vulgaris.* See also *pseudofolliculitis.*
**lupoid s.,** a chronic, scarring form of deep sycosis barbae, characterized by a slowly enlarging patch with follicular papulopustules in the active, advancing border, and healing in the central area leaving scars.
**s. nu'chae,** dermatitis papillaris capillitii.
**s. tar'si,** blepharitis.
**s. vulga'ris,** s. barbae.

**Syd·en·ham's chorea, cough** (sid'ən-hamz) [Thomas *Sydenham,* English physician, sometimes called "the English Hippocrates," 1624–1689] see under *chorea.*

**syl·vat·ic** (səl-vat'ik) sylvan; pertaining to, located in, or living in the woods. See under *plague.*

**Syl·vest's disease** (səl-vests') [Ejnar *Sylvest,* Norwegian physician, 1880–1931] epidemic pleurodynia.

**syl·vi·an** (sil've-ən) 1. described by or named for Franciscus *Sylvius* (François de la Böe). 2. described by or named for Jacobus *Sylvius.*

**Syl·vi·us** (sil've-əs) Jacobus. (Fr. *Jacques Dubois,* 1478–1555), French physician. Confusion exists as to whether some terms ascribed to Franciscus Sylvius should be ascribed instead to this man, particularly the aqueductus mesencephali and related terms.

**Syl·vi·us' angle, fissure,** etc. (sil've-əs) [Franciscus *Sylvius* (François de la Böe), Dutch physician, anatomist, and physiologist, 1614–

1672] see under *angle,* and see *aqueductus mesencephali, fossa lateralis cerebri, cavum septi pellucidi, sulcus lateralis cerebri,* and *valvula venae cavae inferioris.* Cf. Jacobus *Sylvius.*

**Sym·a·dine** (sim'ə-dēn) trademark for a preparation of amantadine hydrochloride.

**sym·bal·lo·phone** (sim-bal'o-fōn) [*syn-* + *ballein* to throw + *phōnē* sound] a special type of double stethoscope making possible the comparison of sounds and detection of their direction.

**sym·bi·ol·o·gy** (sim″bi-ol'ə-je) the scientific study of symbiosis and symbiotic organisms.

**sym·bi·on** (sim'bi-on) symbiont.

**sym·bi·on·ic** (sim-bi-on'ik) pertaining to or characterized by symbiosis.

**sym·bi·ont** (sim'bi-ont, sim'be-ont) [*syn-* + Gr. *bioun* to live] an organism which lives in a state of symbiosis.

**sym·bi·o·sis** (sim″bi-o'sis) pl. *symbio'ses* [Gr. *symbiōsis*] [MeSH: Symbiosis] 1. in parasitology, the living together or close association of two dissimilar organisms, each of the organisms being known as a *symbiont.* The association may be beneficial to both (mutualism), beneficial to one without effect on the other (commensalism), beneficial to one and detrimental to the other (parasitism), detrimental to one without effect on the other (amensalism), or detrimental to both (synnecrosis). 2. in psychiatry, a mutually reinforcing relationship between two persons who are dependent on each other; a normal characteristic of the relationship between the mother and infant child.
**antagonistic s., antipathetic s.,** an association between two organisms which is to the disadvantage of one of them; parasitism.
**conjunctive s.,** association between two different organisms, with bodily union between them.
**constructive s.,** an association between two organisms which is of benefit to the physiologic processes of one of them.
**disjunctive s.,** symbiosis without actual union of the organisms.

**sym·bi·ote** (sim'bi-ōt) symbiont.

**sym·bi·ot·ic** (sim″bi-ot'ik) associated in symbiosis; living together.

**sym·bleph·a·ron** (sim-blef'ə-ron) [*syn* + Gr. *blepharon* eyelid] an adhesion between the tarsal conjunctiva and the bulbar conjunctiva.
**anterior s.,** attachment of the lid to the eyeball by fibrous bands.
**posterior s.,** adhesion between the lid and the eyeball extending into the fornix.
**total s.,** adhesion of the entire conjunctival surface between the lid and the eyeball.

**sym·bleph·a·rop·ter·yg·i·um** (sim-blef″ə-ro-tər-ij'e-əm) a combination of symblepharon and pterygium; a form of symblepharon in which the lid is joined to the eyeball by a cicatricial band resembling a pterygium.

**sym·bol** (sim'bəl) [Gr. *symbolon,* from *symballein* to interpret] 1. something, particularly an object, representing something else. 2. in chemistry, a letter or combination of letters representing an atom or a group of atoms. 3. in psychoanalytic theory, a representation or perception that replaces unconscious mental content.
**phallic s.,** in psychoanalysis, any pointed or upright object which may represent the phallus or penis.

**sym·bo·lia** (sim-bo'le-ə) ability to recognize the nature of objects by their distinctive forms.

**sym·bol·ism** (sim'bəl-iz-əm) [MeSH: Symbolism] 1. the act or process of representing something by a symbol. 2. in psychoanalytic theory, a mechanism of unconscious thinking characterized by substitution of a symbol for a repressed or threatening impulse or object, which is often of a sexual nature, so as to avoid censorship by the superego.

**sym·bol·iza·tion** (sim″bəl-ĭ-za'shən) an unconscious defense mechanism in which one idea or object comes to represent another because of similarity or association between them.

**sym·brachy·dac·tyl·ia** (sim-brak″e-dak-til'e-ə) symbrachydactyly.

**sym·brachy·dac·tyl·ism** (sim-brak″e-dak'təl-iz-əm) symbrachydactyly.

**sym·brachy·dac·ty·ly** (sim-brak″e-dak'tə-le) [Gr. *syn* together + *brachys* short + *daktylos* finger] a condition in which the fingers or toes are short and adherent; webbed fingers or toes.

***sym*-di·chlo·ro·meth·yl ether** (sim-di-klor″o-meth'əl e'thər) bis(chloromethyl)ether.

**Syme's amputation** (sīmz) [James *Syme,* Scottish surgeon, 1799–1870] see under *amputation.*

**sym·e·lus** (sim'ə-ləs) symmelus.

**Sy·ming·ton's body** (si'ming-tonz) [Johnson *Symington,* Scottish anatomist, 1851–1924] the anococcygeal body; see under *body.*

**sym·me·lia** (sĭ-me'le-ə) [*syn-* + *-melia*] a developmental anomaly characterized by an apparent fusion of the lower limbs. There may be three feet *(tripodial s.),* two feet *(dipodial s.),* one foot *(monopodial s.),* or no feet *(apodal s.* or *sirenomelia).*

**sym·me·lus** (sim'ə-ləs) a fetus exhibiting symmelia.

**Sym·mers' disease** (sim'ərz) [Douglas *Symmers,* American physician, 1879–1952] nodular lymphoma.

**Sym·mers' fibrosis** (sim'ərz) [William St. Clair *Symmers,* Irish pathologist, 1863–1937] pipestem fibrosis.

**Sym·me·trel** (sim'ə-trəl) trademark for a preparation of amantadine hydrochloride.

**sym·met·ri·cal** (sĭ-met'rĭ-kəl) [Gr. *symmetrikos*] pertaining to or exhibiting symmetry; in chemistry, denoting compounds which contain atoms or groups at equal intervals in the molecule.

**sym·me·try** (sim'ə-tre) [Gr. *symmetria; syn* with + *metron* measure] the similar arrangement in form and relationships of parts around a common axis, or on each side of a plane of the body.
**bilateral s.,** the configuration of an irregularly shaped body (as the human body or that of higher animals) which can be divided by a longitudinal plane into halves that are mirror images of each other.
**helical s.,** an arrangement of capsomers seen in viruses with a rodlike or filamentous capsid, in which subunits form a coiled structure, with each subunit forming bonds with the subunit in each of the adjoining turns to provide stability.
**icosahedral s.,** an arrangement of viral subunits in which the structure of the viral capsid is characterized by symmetry having the rotation axes of a regular polygon with 20 triangular surfaces (icosahedron); each face contains several subunits, the total number of subunits in the capsid being a multiple of 60.

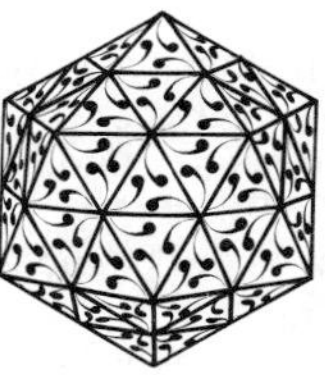

Icosahedral symmetry, the 20 faces of the figure each divided into 12 subunits (represented by apostrophes), for a total of 240 subunits.

**inverse s.,** correspondence as between an object and its mirror image, in which one side of one object corresponds to the opposite side of another.
**radial s.,** symmetry in which the body parts are arranged regularly around a central axis.

**sym·pa·thec·to·mize** (sim″pə-thek'tə-mīz) to subject to sympathectomy.

**sym·pa·thec·to·my** (sim″pə-thek'tə-me) [*sympathetic* + *-ectomy*] [MeSH: Sympathectomy] the transection or other interruption of any part of the sympathetic nervous pathways. Operations may be named according to the location of the nerve, ganglion, or plexus operated on, as *cervical, dorsal, lumbar,* or *thoracolumbar s.,* or in reference to the diaphragm, as *subdiaphragmatic, supradiaphragmatic,* or *transdiaphragmatic s.*
**chemical s.,** suppression of the activity of the sympathetic nervous system by appropriate drugs.

**sym·pa·the·tec·to·my** (sim″pə-thə-tek'tə-me) sympathectomy.

**sym·pa·thet·ic** (sim″pə-thet'ik) [Gr. *sympathētikos*] 1. pertaining to, caused by, or exhibiting sympathy. 2. pertaining to the sympathetic nervous system or one of its nerves; see under *system.*

**sym·pa·thet·i·co·mi·met·ic** (sim″pə-thet″ĭ-ko-mi-met'ik) [*sympathetic* + *-mimetic*] sympathomimetic.

**sym·pa·thet·i·co·to·nia** (sim″pə-thet″ĭ-ko-to'ne-ə) sympathicotonia.

**sym·pa·theto·blast** (sim″pə-thet'o-blast) sympathoblast.

**sym·path·ic** (sim-path'ik) sympathetic.

**sym·path·i·cec·to·my** (sim-path″ĭ-sek'tə-me) sympathectomy.

**sym·path·i·co·blast** (sim-path'ĭ-ko-blast″) sympathoblast.

**sym·path·i·co·blas·to·ma** (sim-path″ĭ-ko-blas-to'mə) a neuroblastoma arising in one of the ganglia of the sympathetic nervous system; called also *sympathicogonioma, sympathoblastoma,* and *sympathogonioma.*

**sym·path·i·co·go·ni·o·ma** (sim-path″ĭ-ko-go″ne-o'mə) sympathicoblastoma.

**sym·path·i·co·lyt·ic** (sim-path″ĭ-ko-lit'ik) sympatholytic.

**sym·path·i·co·mi·met·ic** (sim-path″ĭ-ko-mi-met'ik) sympathomimetic.

**sym·path·i·cop·a·thy** (sim-path″ĭ-kop′ə-the) any disease due to disorder of the sympathetic nervous system.

**sym·path·i·co·to·nia** (sim-path″ĭ-ko-to′ne-ə) a condition in which the sympathetic nervous system dominates the general functioning of the body organs, characterized by vascular spasm, heightened blood pressure, dermographic formation of goose flesh, and activity of the ciliospinal reflex. Called also *sympatheticotonia.*

**sym·path·i·co·ton·ic** (sim″path″ĭ-ko-ton′ik) pertaining to or characterized by sympathicotonia.

**sym·path·i·co·trip·sy** (sim-path″ĭ-ko-trip′se) [*sympathetic ganglion* + *-tripsy*] the surgical crushing of a nerve, ganglion, or plexus of the sympathetic nervous system.

**sym·path·i·co·trope** (sim-path′ĭ-ko-trōp) sympathicotropic (def. 2).

**sym·path·i·co·trop·ic** (sim-path″ĭ-ko-trop′ik) [*sympathetic* + *-tropic*] 1. having an affinity for the sympathetic nervous system. 2. an agent that has an affinity for or exerts its principal effect upon the sympathetic nervous system.

**sym·pa·thism** (sim′pə-thiz-əm) suggestibility.

**sym·patho·ad·re·nal** (sim″pə-tho-ə-dre′nəl) 1. pertaining to the sympathetic nervous system and the adrenal medulla. 2. involving the sympathetic nervous system and the adrenal glands, such as the effects of the alarm reaction.

**sym·patho·blast** (sim-path′o-blast″) [*sympathetic* + *-blast*[1]] a pluripotential cell in the embryo that will develop into a sympathetic nerve cell or a chromaffin cell; called also *sympathetoblast, sympathicoblast,* and *sympathetic neuroblast.*

**sym·patho·blas·to·ma** (sim″pə-tho-blas-to′mə) sympathicoblastoma.

**sym·pa·tho·gone** (sim′pə-tho-gōn″) sympathogonium.

**sym·pa·tho·go·nia** (sim″pə-tho-go′ne-ə) sing. *sympathogo′nium* [*sympathetic* + Gr. *gonē* seed] undifferentiated embryonic cells which develop into sympathetic cells.

**sym·pa·tho·go·ni·o·ma** (sim″pə-tho-go″ne-o′mə) sympathicoblastoma.

**sym·pa·tho·go·ni·um** (sim″pə-tho-go′ne-əm) singular of *sympathogonia.*

**sym·pa·tho·lyt·ic** (sim″pə-tho-lit′ik) [*sympathetic* + *-lytic*] 1. opposing the effects of impulses conveyed by adrenergic postganglionic fibers of the sympathetic nervous system. 2. an agent that opposes the effects of impulses conveyed by adrenergic postganglionic fibers of the sympathetic nervous system; called also *antiadrenergic.*

**sym·pa·tho·mi·met·ic** (sim″pə-tho-mi-met′ik) [*sympathetic* + *-mimetic*] 1. mimicking the effects of impulses conveyed by adrenergic postganglionic fibers of the sympathetic nervous system. 2. an agent that produces effects similar to those of impulses conveyed by adrenergic postganglionic fibers of the sympathetic nervous system. Called also *adrenergic.*

**sym·pa·thy** (sim′pə-the) [Gr. *sympatheia*] 1. compassion for another person's thoughts, feelings, and experiences; cf. *empathy.* 2. an influence produced in any organ by disease, disorder, or other change in another part. 3. a relation which exists between people or things such that change in the state of one is reflected in the other.

**sym·pec·to·thi·ene** (sim-pek″to-thi′ēn) ergothioneine.

**sym·pec·to·thi·on** (sim-pek″to-thi′on) ergothioneine.

**sym·pex·ion** (sim-pek′se-on) pl. *sympex′ia* [Gr. *sympēxis* condensation, coagulation + *-on* neuter ending] a concretion.

**sym·pha·lan·gia** (sim″fə-lan′je-ə) [*syn-* + *phalang-* + *-ia*] congenital end-to-end fusion of contiguous phalanges of a digit, usually associated with other deformity of the hand or foot.

**sym·phal·an·gism** (sim-fal′ən-jiz-əm) symphalangia.

**sym·phor·i·car·pus** (sim″for-ĭ-kahr′pəs) [Gr. *symphorein* to bear together + *karpos* fruit] a homeopathic preparation of the fruit of *Symphoricarpos racemosus,* or snowberry, a shrub of North America.

**Sym·pho·ro·my·ia** (sim″for-o-mi′yə) a genus of flies (snipe flies) of the family Rhagionidae, some of which are severe biters of man and animals.

**sym·phyo·ceph·a·lus** (sim″fe-o-sef′ə-ləs) [*syn-* + Gr. *phyein* to grow + *-cephalus*] a twin fetus joined at the head.

**sym·phys·e·al** (sim-fiz′e-əl) pertaining to a symphysis.

**sym·phys·e·or·rha·phy** (sim-fiz″e-or′ə-fe) symphysiorrhaphy.

**sym·phy·ses** (sim′fĭ-sēz) [Gr.] plural of *symphysis.*

**sym·phys·i·al** (sim-fiz′e-əl) symphyseal.

**sym·phys·ic** (sim-fiz′ik) characterized by abnormal fusion of adjacent parts.

**sym·phys·i·ol·y·sis** (sim-fiz″e-ol′ĭ-sis) [*symphysis* + *-lysis*] separation or slipping of symphyses, especially the symphysis pubis.

**sym·phys·i·or·rha·phy** (sim-fiz″e-or′ə-fe) [*symphysis* + *-rrhaphy*] suture of a divided symphysis.

**sym·phys·io·tome** (sim-fiz′e-o-tōm) a knife used in performing symphysiotomy.

**sym·phys·i·ot·o·my** (sim-fiz″e-ot′ə-me) [*symphysis* + *-tomy*] [MeSH: Symphysiotomy] the division of the fibrocartilage of the symphysis pubis, in order to facilitate delivery, by increasing the diameter of the pelvis.

**sym·phy·sis** (sim′fĭ-sis) pl. *sym′physes* [Gr. "a growing together, natural junction"] [TA] a type of cartilaginous joint in which the apposed bony surfaces are firmly united by a plate of fibrocartilage; called also *fibrocartilaginous joint.*
**s. intervertebra′lis** [TA], intervertebral symphysis: the union between the vertebral bodies, consisting of the anterior and posterior longitudinal ligaments, and the intervertebral disks.
**s. mandi′bulae** [TA], mandibular symphysis: the line of fusion in the median plane of the mandible that marks the union of the two halves of the mandible; called also *s. mentalis* and *s. menti.*
**s. manubriosterna′lis** [TA], manubriosternal symphysis: the joint uniting the manubrium with the body of the sternum, which begins as a synchondrosis *(synchondrosis manubriosternalis)* and later becomes a symphysis.
**s. menta′lis, s. men′ti,** s. mandibulae.
**s. os′sium pu′bis,** s. pubica.
**s. pu′bica** [TA], **s. pu′bis,** pubic symphysis: the joint formed by union of the bodies of the pubic bones in the median plane by a thick mass of fibrocartilage; called also *s. ossium pubis.*
**s. sacrococcy′gea, sacrococcygeal s.,** articulatio sacrococcygea.
**sacroiliac s.,** articulatio sacroiliaca.

**sym·phy·so·dac·ty·ly** (sim″fĭ-so-dak′tə-le) [Gr. *symphysis* a growing together + *daktylos* finger] fusion of the fingers or toes.

**Sym·phy·tum** (sim′fĭ-təm) [L.; Gr. *symphyton*] a genus of plants of the family Boraginaceae. *S. officina′le* L. is comfrey, a species native to Europe and North America whose roots and leaves are demulcent and astringent.

**sym·phy·tum** (sim′fĭ-təm) a demulcent and astringent homeopathic preparation of *Symphytum officinale.*

**sym·plasm** (sim′plaz-əm) tissue in which there is no cellular structure.

**sym·plas·mat·ic** (sim″plaz-mat′ik) marked by union of protoplasm.

**sym·plast** (sim′plast) symplasm.

**sym·plex** (sim′pleks) a chemical compound in which a high molecular substance is bound by residual valencies; included are activators, adsorbents, hemoglobin, and toxin-antitoxin.

**sym·po·dia** (sim-po′de-ə) [*syn-* + *pod-* + *-ia*] symmelia.

**sym·po·di·al** (sim-po′de-əl) said of a pattern of growth of conidiogenous cells in which after a spore breaks off at an apex the following apex and spore appear slightly farther back and to the side.

**sym·pod·u·la** (sim-pod′u-lə) a conidiogenous cell that grows in a sympodial pattern.

**sym·port** (sim′port) a mechanism of transporting two compounds simultaneously across a cell membrane in the same direction, one compound being transported down a concentration gradient, the other against a gradient. Cf. *antiport* and *cotransport.*

**symp·tom** (simp′təm) [L. *symptoma;* Gr. *symptōma* anything that has befallen one] any subjective evidence of disease or of a patient's condition, i.e., such evidence as perceived by the patient; a noticeable change in a patient's condition indicative of some bodily or mental state. See also *sign.*
**abstinence s's,** substance withdrawal.
**accessory s.,** any symptom not necessarily characteristic of the patient's disease.
**Anton's s.,** see under *syndrome.*
**assident s.,** accessory s.
**Bárány's s.,** 1. in disturbances of equilibrium of the vestibular apparatus, the direction of the fall is influenced by changing the position of the patient's head. 2. caloric test; see under *test.*
**Bonhoeffer's s.,** loss of normal muscle tonus in chorea.
**Brauch-Romberg s.,** Romberg's sign.
**Buerger's s.,** in thromboangiitis obliterans, the pain in the affected leg when the patient is lying down is relieved only by lying with the leg hung over the side of the bed.
**cardinal s.,** 1. a symptom of greatest significance to the physician, establishing the identity of the illness. 2. [pl.] the symptoms shown in the pulse, temperature, and respiration.

**Castellani-Low s.,** a fine tremor of the tongue seen in sleeping sickness.
**characteristic s.,** a symptom that is almost universally associated with a particular disease or condition.
**Colliver's s.,** a peculiar twitching, tremulous, or convulsive movement of the limbs, face, jaw, and sometimes of the entire body, seen in the preparalytic stage of poliomyelitis.
**concomitant s.,** a symptom not essential to a disease, but which may have an accessory value in its diagnosis.
**constitutional s.,** a symptom which is indicative of or due to disorder of the whole body.
**conversion s.,** symbolic representation of psychic conflict by alteration or absence of a voluntary motor or sensory function suggesting a neurological or general medical condition but not fully explained by either, and neither intentionally produced nor feigned.
**crossbar s. of Fraenkel,** blocking of the peristaltic wave on the lesser curvature of the stomach at the site of an ulcer, on fluoroscopy of the stomach.
**deficiency s.,** a symptom caused by a lack of something necessary for normal bodily functioning, such as an enzyme, vitamin, or hormone. See also *deficiency.*
**delayed s.,** one which does not appear for some time after the occurrence of the causes which produce it.
**direct s.,** one which is directly caused by the disease.
**dissociation s.,** see under *anesthesia.*
**Epstein's s.,** a symptom seen in nervous infants, consisting of failure of the upper lid to move downward, giving the child a frightened expression.
**equivocal s.,** a symptom which may be produced by several different diseases.
**factitious s.,** one produced intentionally, usually by the patient; cf. *induced s.*
**general s.,** constitutional s.
**guiding s.,** characteristic s.
**Haenel s.,** in tabes there is a lack of sensation on pressure over the eyeballs.
**halo s.,** the seeing of colored rings around an individual light source; indicative of glaucoma.
**incarceration s.,** periodically recurring symptoms of displaced kidney, such as nephralgia, gastralgia, and severe collapse; called also *Dietl's crisis.*
**indirect s.,** a symptom which points to a condition that may or may not be due to a particular disease or lesion.
**induced s.,** one produced intentionally; cf. *factitious s.*
**labyrinthine s's,** the symptoms of disease of the inner ear.
**Liebreich's s.,** a symptom of red-green color blindness in which light effects appear red and shadows green.
**local s.,** one due to local disease or to a particular lesion.
**localizing s's,** symptoms that indicate the location of a lesion.
**Magendie's s.,** skew deviation.
**Magnan's s.,** formication.
**negative s.,** one in which a characteristic of normal health is diminished or absent in disease, such as the flat affect or alogia of schizophrenia.
**objective s.,** one that is obvious to the senses of the observer; see *sign.*
**Oehler's s.,** coldness and pallor of the feet in intermittent claudication.
**pathognomonic s.,** one that establishes with certainty the diagnosis of the disease.
**precursory s., premonitory s.,** signal s.
**presenting s.,** the symptom or group of symptoms of which the patient complains the most or from which he seeks relief.
**rainbow s.,** halo s.
**rational s.,** subjective s.
**reflex s.,** a symptom occurring in a part remote from that which is affected by the disease.
**Remak's s.,** either polyesthesia or a prolongation of the lapse of time before a painful impression is perceived, seen in tabes dorsalis.
**Roger's s.,** a temperature below the normal in the third stage of tuberculous meningitis.
**Séguin's signal s.,** the involuntary contraction of the muscles just before an epileptic attack.
**signal s.,** a sensation, aura, or other subjective experience that gives warning of the approach of an epileptic or other seizure.
**Sklowsky's s.,** when light pressure with the index finger is made upon the healthy skin near, and then over, a vesicle in varicella, the wall of the vesicle easily collapses and the contents are discharged.
**static s.,** an unchanging symptom.
**subjective s.,** one that is perceptible to the patient only.
**sympathetic s.,** one due to sympathy, as when pain or other disorder affects a part when some other part is the seat of the disease proper.
**Trendelenburg's s.,** a waddling gait due to paralysis of the gluteal muscles; see also *Trendelenburg's test* (def. 2).
**Wernicke's s.,** hemiopic pupillary reaction.
**withdrawal s's,** substance withdrawal.

**symp·to·mat·ic** (simp″to-mat′ik) [Gr. *symptōmatikos*] 1. pertaining to or of the nature of a symptom. 2. indicative (of a particular disease or disorder). 3. exhibiting the symptoms of a particular disease but having a different cause. 4. directed at the allaying of symptoms, as symptomatic treatment.

**symp·tom·a·tol·o·gy** (simp″təm-ə-tol′ə-je) 1. that branch of medicine which treats of symptoms; the systematic discussion of symptoms. 2. the combined symptoms of a disease.

**symp·to·ma·to·lyt·ic** (simp″to-mat″o-lit′ik) [*symptom* + *-lytic*] causing the disappearance of symptoms.

**symp·to·mo·lyt·ic** (simp″to-mo-lit′ik) symptomatolytic.

**symp·to·sis** (simp-to′sis) [*syn-* + *-ptosis*] the gradual wasting of the whole body or of any organ.

**sym·pus** (sim′pəs) [Gr. *syn* together + *pous* foot] symmelus.
**s. a′pus,** sirenomelus.
**s. di′pus,** a fetus with dipodial symmelia.
**s. mo′nopus,** a fetus with monopodial symmelia.

**Syms' tractor** (simz) [Parker *Syms,* American surgeon, 1860–1933] see under *tractor.*

**syn-** [Gr. *syn* with, together] a prefix signifying union or association.

**Syn·a·cort** (sin′ə-kort″) trademark for preparations of hydrocortisone.

**syn·a·del·phus** (sin″ə-del′fəs) [*syn-* + *-adelphus*] conjoined twins with a single body and eight limbs.

**syn·ae·ti·on** (sin-e′te-on) [Gr. *synaitios* being a joint cause] the secondary or cooperative cause of a disease.

**Syn·a·lar** (sin′ə-lahr) trademark for preparations of fluocinolone acetonide.

**syn·al·bu·min** (sin″al-bu′min) a postulated competitive inhibitor of insulin, an insulin B chain bound to albumin; its significance in human diabetes mellitus is unknown.

**syn·al·gia** (sin-al′jə) [*syn-* + *-algia*] referred pain.

**syn·al·gic** (sin-al′jik) pertaining to or affected by referred pain.

**syn·ana·morph** (sin-an′ə-morf″) [*syn-* + *anamorph*] any of two or more anamorphs having the same teleomorph.

**syn·an·thrin** (sin-an′thrin) inulin.

**syn·aph·y·men·i·tis** (sin-af″ĭ-mən-i′tis) conjunctivitis.

**syn·apse** (sin′aps) [Gr. *synapsis* a conjunction, connection] [MeSH: Synapses] the site of functional apposition between neurons, at which an impulse is transmitted from one neuron to another, usually by a chemical neurotransmitter (e.g., acetylcholine, norepinephrine, etc.) released by the axon terminal of the excited (presynaptic) cell. The neurotransmitter diffuses across the synaptic cleft to bind with receptors on the postsynaptic cell membrane, and thereby effects electrical changes in the postsynaptic cell which result in depolarization (excitation) or hyperpolarization (inhibition). Synapses also occur at sites of apposition between nerve endings and effector organs (e.g., the neuromuscular junction). A few synapses in the central nervous system are electrical synapses (q.v.). In official terminology called *synapsis.*
**axoaxonic s.,** one between the axon of one neuron and the axon of another neuron.

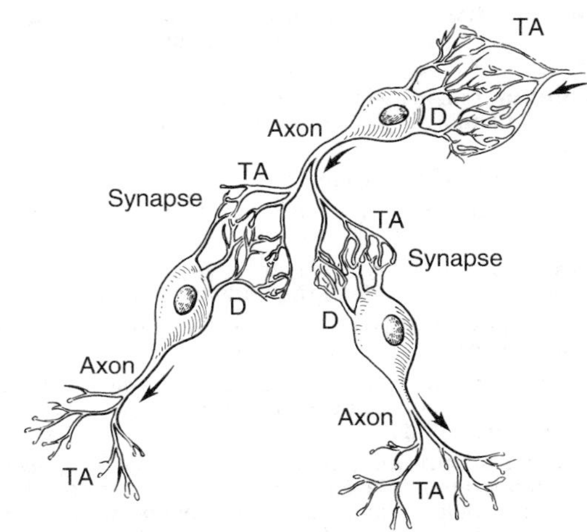

Diagram of three synapses. Nerve impulse is indicated by arrows, showing that the direction of passage is from the terminal arborization *(TA)* or nerve endings of the axon of one neuron to the dendrites *(D)* of another neuron.

**axodendritic s.**, one between the axon of one neuron and dendrites of another.
**axodendrosomatic s.**, one between the axon of one neuron and the dendrites and body (soma) of another, as in motoneurons.
**axosomatic s.**, one between the axon of one neuron and the body (soma) of another.
**chemical s.**, the usual type of synapse seen in vertebrates, in which the impulse is carried by a neurotransmitter. Cf. *electrical s.*
**dendrodendritic s.**, a rare type of synapse involving transmission from a dendrite of one cell to a dendrite of another.
**electrical s.**, a point of lateral contact (other than a synapse) between nerve fibers, across which impulses are conducted directly through the nerve membranes from one fiber to the other; it is common in invertebrates but in vertebrates it has been found at only a few central nervous system sites. Cf. *chemical s.* Called also *ephapse.*
**electrotonic s.**, see *gap junction,* under *junction.*
**en passant s.**, synaptic contact between non-terminal parts of axons; seen in coelenterates and among certain special cells in the central nervous system of vertebrates. Cf. *bouton en passant.*
**loop s.**, one having a relatively long area of contact of fiber membranes; seen in many invertebrates.

**syn·ap·sis** (sĭ-nap′sis) [Gr. "conjunction"] 1. the pairing off in point-for-point association of homologous chromosomes from the male and female pronuclei during the early prophase of meiosis. 2. [TA] official terminology for *synapse.*

**syn·ap·tene** (sĭ-nap′tēn) zygotene.

**syn·ap·tic** (sĭ-nap′tik) 1. pertaining to or affecting a synapse. 2. pertaining to synapsis.

**syn·ap·tol·o·gy** (sin″ap-tol′ə-je) that branch of neurology which deals with the synaptic correlations of the nervous system.

**syn·ap·to·some** (sin-ap′to-sōm″) [MeSH: Synaptosomes] any of the membrane-bound sacs that break away from axon terminals at a synapse after brain tissue has been homogenized in sugar solution; it contains synaptic vessels and mitochondria.

**Syn·a·rel** (sin′ə-rel) trademark for a preparation of nafarelin acetate.

**syn·ar·thro·dia** (sin″ahr-thro′de-ə) [*syn-* + Gr. *arthrōdia* joint] synarthrosis.

**syn·ar·thro·di·al** (sin″ahr-thro′de-əl) pertaining to a synarthrosis.

**syn·ar·thro·phy·sis** (sin-ahr″thro-fi′sis) [*syn-* + *arthro-* + *physis* growth] any ankylosing process; progressive ankylosis of joints.

**syn·ar·thro·ses** (sin″ahr-thro′sēz) [Gr.] plural of *synarthrosis.*

**syn·ar·thro·sis** (sin″ahr-thro′sis) pl. *synarthro′ses* [*syn-* + *arthrosis*] [TA] a bony junction that is immovable and is connected by solid connective tissue; the two types are the fibrous joint *(junctura fibrosa)* and the cartilaginous joint *(junctura cartilaginea).*

**syn·ath·re·sis** (sin″əth-re′sis) synathroisis.

**syn·ath·roi·sis** (sin″əth-roi′sis) [*syn-* + Gr. *athroisis* collection] local hyperemia or congestion.

**syn·can·thus** (sin-kan′thəs) [*syn-* + *canthus*] adhesion of the eyeball to the orbital structures.

**syn·cary·on** (sin-kar′e-on) synkaryon.

**syn·ce·lom** (sin-se′lom) the perivisceral cavities of the body considered as one structure, including the pleural, cardiac, and peritoneal cavities, and tunica vaginalis.

**Syn·ceph·a·las·trum** (sin-sef″ə-las′trəm) a genus of fungi of the order Mucorales. *S. racemo′sum* has been found in cases of mucormycosis.

**syn·ceph·a·lus** (sin-sef′ə-ləs) [*syn-* + *-cephalus*] conjoined twins with one head and a single face with four ears, two on the back of the head.

**syn·che·sis** (sin′ke-sis) synchysis.

**syn·chi·lia** (sin-ki′le-ə) [*syn-* + *chil-* + *-ia*] congenital adhesion of the lips.

**syn·chi·ria** (sin-ki′re-ə) [*syn-* + *chir-* + *-ia*] dyschiria in which a stimulus applied to one side of the body is referred to both sides.

**syn·cho·lia** (sin-ko′le-ə) [*syn-* + *chol-* + *-ia*] the secretion of substances of exogenous origin in the bile.

**syn·chon·drec·to·my** (sin″kon-drek′tə-me) [*synchondrosis* + *-ectomy*] surgical excision of a synchondrosis, especially of the symphysis of the pubic bone.

**syn·chon·dro·se·ot·o·my** (sin″kon-dro″se-ot′ə-me) [*synchondrosis* + *-tomy*] an operation for exstrophy of the bladder done by cutting through the sacroiliac ligaments and forcibly drawing together the pelvic bones; called also *Trendelenburg's operation.*

**syn·chon·dro·sis** (sin″kon-dro′sis) pl. *synchondro′ses* [Gr. *synchondrōsis* a growing into one cartilage] [TA] a union between two bones formed by either hyaline cartilage or fibrocartilage; it is usually temporary, the intervening cartilage being converted into bone before adult life.
**s. arycornicula′ta**, the cartilaginous union between the upper end of the arytenoid cartilage and the base of the corniculate cartilage.
**costoclavicular s.**, ligamentum costoclaviculare.
**synchondro′ses crania′les, synchondro′ses cra′nii** [TA], synchondroses of skull: the cartilaginous junctions between certain bones of the cranium. Called also *cranial synchondroses.*
**s. intersphenoida′lis**, intersphenoidal synchondrosis: the cartilaginous union of the two halves of the body of the sphenoid bone in the fetus.
**intraoccipital s., anterior**, s. intraoccipitalis anterior.
**intraoccipital s., posterior**, s. intraoccipitalis posterior.
**s. intraoccipita′lis ante′rior** [TA], anterior intraoccipital synchondrosis: the cartilaginous union of the pars basilaris with the partes laterales of the occipital bone in the newborn.
**s. intraoccipita′lis poste′rior** [TA], posterior intraoccipital synchondrosis: the cartilaginous union of the squama with the partes laterales of the occipital bone in the newborn.
**s. manubriosterna′lis** [TA], manubriosternal synchondrosis: the joint uniting the manubrium with the body of the sternum, which begins as a synchondrosis and later becomes a symphysis *(symphysis manubriosternalis).*
**neurocentral s.**, junctio neurocentralis.
**s. petrooccipita′lis** [TA], petrooccipital synchondrosis: the plate of cartilage in the petro-occipital fissure which helps to unite the basilar portion of the occipital bone and the petrous portion of the temporal bone.
**pubic s., s. pu′bis**, symphysis pubica.
**sacrococcygeal s.**, articulatio sacrococcygea.
**s's of skull**, synchondroses cranii.
**sphenobasilar s.**, s. sphenooccipitalis.
**s. sphenoethmoida′lis** [TA], sphenoethmoidal synchondrosis: the cartilaginous union between the body of the sphenoid and the labyrinth of the ethmoid bone.
**sphenooccipital s.**, 1. s. sphenooccipitalis. 2. in cephalometric radiology, the uppermost point of the synchondrosis spheno-occipitalis. Called also *point SO.* Abbreviated SO.
**s. sphenooccipita′lis** [TA], sphenooccipital synchondrosis: the cartilaginous union of the anterior end of the basilar portion of the occipital bone with the posterior surface of the body of the sphenoid bone.
**s. sphenopetro′sa** [TA], sphenopetrosal synchondrosis: the cartilaginous union of the inferior border of the greater wing of the sphenoid bone with the petrous portion of the temporal bone in the sphenopetrosal fissure.
**s. sterna′lis** [TA], sternal synchondrosis: the cartilaginous union between the manubrium and the body of the sternum.
**s. sternocosta′lis cos′tae pri′mae** [TA], sternocostal synchondrosis of first rib: the articulation between the sternum and the first rib, in which the costal cartilage is united directly to the sternum.
**s. xiphisterna′lis** [TA], xiphisternal synchondrosis: the joint between the xiphoid process and the body of the sternum; called also *xiphisternal joint.*

**syn·chon·drot·o·my** (sin″kon-drot′ə-me) [*synchondrosis* + *-tomy*] the division of the symphysis pubis or of any other synchondrosis.

**syn·cho·ri·al** (sin-kor′e-əl) sharing a common placenta; said of multiple fetuses.

**syn·chro·nia** (sin-kro′ne-ə) 1. synchronism. 2. the formation of parts or tissues at the usual time. Cf. *heterochronia* (def. 1).

**syn·chro·nism** (sin′kro-niz-əm) occurrence at the same time; called also *synchronia* and *synchrony.*

**syn·chro·nous** (sin′kro-nəs) [*syn-* + *chron-* + *-ous*] occurring at the same time; cf. *heterochronic* and *metachronous.*

**syn·chro·ny** (sin′krə-ne) 1. the simultaneous occurrence of two events. 2. the linkage of two events by a fixed time interval. 3. synchronism.
**atrioventricular (AV) s.**, in the heart, the physiological condition of atrial electrical activity followed by ventricular electrical activity, with the interval between being that necessary for impulse conduction from atria to ventricles.
**bilateral s.**, the occurrence of a secondary synchronous discharge at a location in the brain exactly contralateral to a discharge caused by a lesion.

**syn·chro·tron** (sin′kro-tron) [MeSH: Synchrotrons] a machine for accelerating charged particles (electrons, protons) in circular orbits, by simultaneously manipulating the strength of the magnetic field and the frequency of the accelerating voltage. It combines features of the cyclotron and betatron and will produce 70 million volts.

**syn·chy·sis** (sin′kĭ-sis) [Gr. "a mixing together"] a softening or fluid condition of the vitreous body of the eye.
**s. scintil′lans**, cholesterol crystals in the vitreous that develop as a

degenerative change following inflammation or other ocular diseases.

**syn·ci·ne·sis** (sin″si-ne′sis) synkinesis.

**syn·cli·nal** (sin-kli′nəl) [Gr. *synklinein* to lean together] bent or inclined together.

**syn·clit·ic** (sin-klit′ik) pertaining to or marked by synclitism.

**syn·clit·i·cism** (sin-klit′ĭ-siz-əm) synclitism.

**syn·clit·ism** (sin′klit-iz-əm) [Gr. *synklinein* to lean together] 1. parallelism between the planes of the fetal head and those of the pelvis. 2. normal, synchronous maturation of the nucleus and cytoplasm of blood cells. Cf. *asynclitism.* Called also *syncliticism.*

**syn·clo·nus** (sin′klo-nəs) [*syn-* + *clonus*] 1. muscular tremor, or the successive clonic contraction of various muscles together. 2. any disease characterized by muscular tremors.
**s. beribe′rica,** muscular tremors associated with beriberi.

**syn·co·pal** (sing′kə-pəl) pertaining to or characterized by syncope.

**syn·co·pe** (sing′kə-pe) [Gr. *synkopē*] [MeSH: Syncope] a temporary suspension of consciousness due to generalized cerebral ischemia; a faint or swoon.
**Adams-Stokes s.,** see under *syndrome.*
**cardiac s.,** sudden loss of consciousness, with momentary or no premonitory symptoms, due to cerebral anemia caused by obstructions to cardiac output or arrhythmias such as ventricular asystole, extreme bradycardia, or ventricular tachycardia.
**carotid sinus s.,** see under *syndrome.*
**convulsive s.,** syncope with convulsive movements that are milder than those seen in epilepsy.
**cough s.,** tussive s.
**digital s.,** a sudden temporary loss of strength in the fingers.
**laryngeal s.,** tussive s.
**micturition s.,** brief loss of consciousness during or immediately after micturition, associated with rising from bed at night to urinate; it may be a form of orthostatic hypotension.
**postural s.,** that resulting from orthostatic hypotension.
**Stokes-Adams s.,** Adams-Stokes syndrome
**stretching s.,** syncope associated with stretching the arms upward with the spine extended.
**swallow s.,** syncope associated with swallowing, a disorder of atrioventricular conduction mediated by the vagus nerve.
**tussive s.,** brief loss of consciousness associated with vigorous and explosive paroxysms of coughing, usually seen in men; called also *cough s., laryngeal s.,* and *laryngeal vertigo.*
**vasodepressor s., vasovagal s.,** vasovagal attack.

**syn·cop·ic** (sin-kop′ik) syncopal.

**syn·cre·tio** (sin-kre′she-o) [L.] a growing together or adhesion, as between inflamed serous surfaces in contact.

**Syn·cu·rine** (sin′ku-rēn) trademark for a preparation of decamethonium bromide.

**syn·cy·tial** (sin-sish′əl) of, pertaining to, or producing a syncytium.

**syn·cyt·i·ol·y·sin** (sin″sit-e-ol′ĭ-sin) a lysin destructive to the syncytium; formed in the blood of an animal into which matter from the placenta of another animal has been injected.

**syn·cyt·i·o·ma** (sin-sit″e-o′mə) syncytial endometritis.
**s. malig′num,** choriocarcinoma.

**syn·cyt·io·tox·in** (sin-sit″e-o-tok′sin) a toxin that has a specific action on the placenta.

**syn·cyt·io·tropho·blast** (sin-sit″e-o-trof′o-blast) 1. the outer syncytial layer of the trophoblast; called also *syntrophoblast.* 2. syncytiotrophoblastic cell.

**syn·cyt·io·tropho·blas·tic** (sin-sit″e-o-trof″o-blas′tik) pertaining to or of the nature of the syncytiotrophoblast.

**syn·cy·ti·um** (sin-sish′e-əm) a multinucleate mass of protoplasm produced by the merging of cells.

**syn·cy·toid** (sin′sĭ-toid) resembling a syncytium.

**syn·dac·tyl·ia** (sin″dak-til′e-ə) syndactyly.

**syn·dac·ty·lism** (sin-dak′tə-liz-əm) syndactyly.

**syn·dac·ty·lous** (sin-dak′tə-ləs) pertaining to or characterized by syndactyly.

**syn·dac·ty·lus** (sin-dak′tə-ləs) an individual exhibiting syndactyly.

**syn·dac·ty·ly** (sin-dak′tə-le) [*syn-* + Gr. *daktylos* finger] [MeSH: Syndactyly] an autosomal dominant trait, the most common congenital anomaly of the hand or foot, marked by persistence of the webbing between adjacent digits, so they are more or less completely attached.
**complete s.,** syndactyly in which the connection extends from the base of the involved digits to the tip.
**complicated s.,** syndactyly in which the bones or nails of the involved digits are fused.

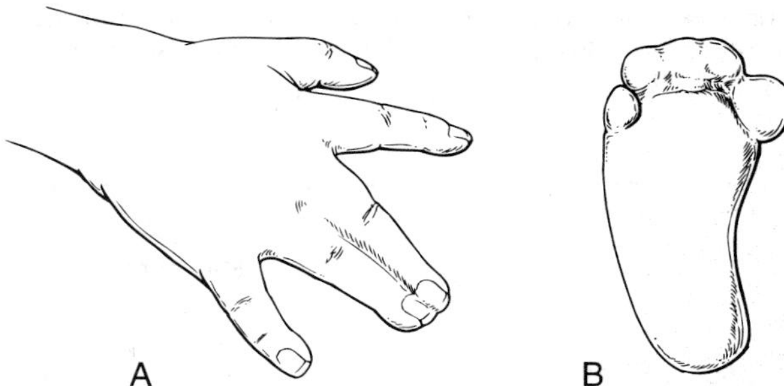

Syndactyly of the hand *(A)* and foot *(B)*.

**double s.,** syndactyly involving three digits (two webs).
**partial s.,** syndactyly in which the connecting web extends only part way up from the base of the involved digits.
**simple s.,** syndactyly in which the connecting web consists only of skin.
**single s.,** syndactyly involving two digits (a single web).
**triple s.,** syndactyly involving four digits (three webs).

**syn·dec·to·my** (sin-dek′tə-me) peritectomy.

**syn·del·phus** (sin-del′fəs) synadelphus.

**syn·de·sis** (sin′də-sis, sin-de′sis) [*syn-* + *-desis*] 1. arthrodesis. 2. synapsis.

**syn·des·mec·to·my** (sin″dəz-mek′tə-me) [*syndesm-* + *-ectomy*] excision or resection of a ligament.

**syn·des·mec·to·pia** (sin″dəz-mək-to′pe-ə) [*syndesm-* + *ectopia*] unusual situation of a ligament.

**syn·des·mi·tis** (sin″dez-mi′tis) [*syndesm-* + *-itis*] 1. inflammation of a ligament or ligaments. 2. conjunctivitis.
**s. metatar′sea,** inflammation of the metatarsal ligaments occurring during strenuous marches; called also *march tumor.*

**syndesm(o)-** [Gr. *syndesmos* band or ligament] a combining form denoting relationship to connective tissue, particularly the ligaments.

**syn·des·mo·cho·ri·al** (sin″dəz-mo-kor′e-əl) a type of placentation, occurring in ruminants, characterized by limited destruction of the endometrial epithelium.

**syn·des·mog·ra·phy** (sin″dəz-mog′rə-fe) [*syndesmo-* + *-graphy*] a description of the ligaments.

**syn·des·mo·lo·gia** (sin″dəz-mo-lo′jə) arthrologia.

**syn·des·mol·o·gy** (sin″dəz-mol′ə-je) [*syndesmo-* + *-logy*] arthrology.

**syn·des·mo-odon·toid** (sin-dez″mo-o-don′toid) the posterior of the two atloaxoid articulations formed between the anterior surface of the transverse ligaments and the back of the odontoid process.

**syn·des·mo·pexy** (sin-dez′mo-pek″se) [*syndesmo-* + *-pexy*] the operative fixation of a dislocation by reattachment of the ligaments.

**syn·des·mo·phyte** (sin-dez′mo-fīt) [*syndesmo-* + *-phyte*] an osseous excrescence, or bony outgrowth, from a ligament.

**syn·des·mo·plas·ty** (sin-dez′mo-plas″te) [*syndesmo-* + *-plasty*] plastic operation on a ligament.

**syn·des·mor·rha·phy** (sin″dəz-mor′ə-fe) [*syndesmo-* + *-rrhaphy*] suture or repair of ligaments.

**syn·des·mo·sis** (sin″dəz-mo′sis) pl. *syndesmo′ses* [Gr. *syndesmos* band] [TA] a type of fibrous joint in which the intervening fibrous connective tissue forms an interosseous membrane or ligament.
**s. dentoalveola′ris** [TA], dentoalveolar syndesmosis: one of the fibrous joints by which a tooth is held in its socket. Called also gomphosis [TA alternative].
**s. radioulna′ris** [TA], radioulnar syndesmosis: the fibrous union of the radius and ulna, which consists of the interosseous membrane of the forearm and the oblique cord of the elbow; called also *articulatio radioulnaris* and *radioulnar articulation.*
**s. tibiofibula′ris** [TA], tibiofibular syndesmosis: inferior tibiofibular articulation: a firm fibrous union formed at the distal ends of the tibia and fibula between the fibular notch of the tibia and a roughened triangular surface on the fibula, which frequently contains a synovial prolongation of the cavity of the talocrural articulation. Called also *articulatio tibiofibularis.*
**s. tympanostapedia′lis** [TA], tympanostapedial syndesmosis: the connection of the base of the stapes with the secondary membrane in the fenestra vestibuli; see also *ligamentum anulare stapediale.*

**syn·des·mot·o·my** (sin″dəz-mot′ə-me) [*syndesmo-* + *-tomy*] the dissection or cutting of a ligament.

**syn·drome** (sin'drōm) [Gr. *syndromē* concurrence] [MeSH: Syndrome] a set of symptoms which occur together; the sum of signs of any morbid state; a symptom complex. In genetics, a pattern of multiple malformations thought to be pathogenetically related.

## Syndrome

For terms not found here, see also under *disease.*

**Aarskog s., Aarskog-Scott s.,** an X-linked syndrome characterized by ocular hypertelorism, anteverted nostrils, broad upper lip, peculiar scrotal "shawl" above the penis, and small hands. Called also *faciogenital dysplasia* and *faciodigitogenital s.*

**Aase s.,** a familial syndrome characterized by mild growth retardation, hypoplastic anemia, variable leukocytopenia, triphalangeal thumbs, narrow shoulders, and late closure of fontanels, and occasionally by cleft lip, cleft palate, retinopathy, and web neck. A recessive mode of inheritance has been suggested.

**abstinence s.,** substance withdrawal.

**achalasia-addisonian s.,** Allgrove's s.

**Achard s.,** arachnodactyly associated with receding mandible and joint laxity limited to the hands and feet.

**Achard-Thiers s.,** masculinization with hirsutism and adult-onset diabetes mellitus in postmenopausal women resulting from overproduction of adrenocortical androgens.

**acquired immune deficiency s., acquired immunodeficiency s.,** an epidemic, transmissible retroviral disease due to infection with human immunodeficiency virus (HIV), manifested in severe cases as profound depression of cell-mediated immunity, and affecting certain recognized risk groups, including homosexual or bisexual males, intravenous drug abusers, hemophiliacs and other blood transfusion recipients, sexual contacts of individuals with HIV infection, and newborn infants of mothers infected with the virus. The criteria established by the Centers for Disease Control and Prevention for the diagnosis of AIDS (CDC/AIDS) comprise: the presence of reliably diagnosed disease that is at least moderately indicative of an underlying defect in cell-mediated immunity (e.g., Kaposi sarcoma in an individual less than 60 years of age, or pneumocystis pneumonia or other life-threatening opportunistic infection), occurring in the absence of known causes of underlying immunodeficiency or of any other host defense defects reported to be associated with that disease (e.g., iatrogenic immunosuppression or lymphoreticular malignancies) or the presence of any of the following in an HIV-infected person: a CD4+ T lymphocyte count of less than 200/mL or a CD4+ T lymphocyte percentage of less than 14 per cent, pulmonary tuberculosis, invasive cervical cancer, or recurrent pneumonia. See also *AIDS-related complex,* under *complex.*

**acute brain s.,** older term for *delirium.*

**acute chest s.,** a complex of symptoms seen in patients with sickle cell disease, often due to a bacterial infection or to infarction of lung tissue; characteristics include severe chest pain, dyspnea, tachypnea, fever, excessive leukocytosis, pulmonary edema, and sometimes petechiae on the chest or conjunctivae as well as fat emboli. Death may result from severe pulmonary complications.

**acute nephritic s.,** the sudden onset of hematuria, proteinuria, diminished urine production, azotemia, hypertension, and edema; the clinical manifestation of acute glomerulonephritis.

**acute organic brain s.,** older term for *delirium.* It is occasionally used more generally to denote the acute form of an organic mental syndrome.

**acute radiation s.,** a syndrome caused by exposure to a whole-body dose of over 1 gray of ionizing radiation. Symptoms, whose severity and time of onset depend on the size of the dose, include erythema, nausea and vomiting, fatigue, diarrhea, fever, petechiae, bleeding from the mucous membranes, reduction in the number of lymphocytes, granulocytes, and platelets, gastrointestinal hemorrhage, epilation, hypotension, tachycardia, and dehydration; death may occur within hours or weeks of exposure.

**acute respiratory distress s. (ARDS),** fulminant pulmonary interstitial and alveolar edema, which usually develops within a few days after the initiating trauma, thought to result from alveolar injury that has led to increased capillary permeability. Called also *adult respiratory distress s.* and *shock lung.*

**acute retinal necrosis s.,** necrotizing retinitis occurring with uveitis, retinal periarteritis, vasculitis, and hyalitis, and marked by retinal vascular narrowing and obstruction, exudates from the peripheral retina, patches of vitreous opacification, and severe loss of vision, and often accompanied by retinal detachment. The etiology is viral.

**Adair Dighton's s.,** osteogenesis imperfecta (type I).

**Adams-Stokes s.,** episodic cardiac arrest and syncope due to failure of normal and escape pacemakers, with or without ventricular fibrillation; it is the principal clinical manifestation of severe heart block. Called also *Adams-Stokes syncope, Morgagni-Adams-Stokes s.,* and *Stokes-Adams s.* or *syncope.*

**addisonian s.,** the complex of symptoms resulting from adrenocortical insufficiency; see *Addison's disease,* under *disease.*

**addisonian-achalasia s.,** Allgrove's s.

**Adie's s.,** a syndrome consisting of a pathological pupil reaction (tonic pupil), the most important element of which is a myotonic condition on accommodation; the pupil on the affected side contracts on near vision more slowly than does the pupil on the opposite side, and it also dilates more slowly. The affected pupil does not usually react to direct or indirect light, but it may do so in an abnormal fashion. Certain tendon reflexes are absent or diminished, usually the patellar reflexes, but there are no motor or sensory disturbances, nor demonstrable changes indicative of disease of the nervous system. Called also *Holmes-Adie s.*

**adiposogenital s.,** adiposogenital dystrophy.

**adrenogenital s.,** a general term for the group of syndromes in which inappropriate masculinization or feminization, sometimes with precocious puberty, results from disorders of adrenal function that also affect gonadal steroidogenesis; it includes congenital adrenal hyperplasia and tumors of the adrenal cortex.

**adult respiratory distress s. (ARDS),** acute respiratory distress s.

**AEC s.,** Hay-Wells s.

**afferent loop s.,** chronic partial obstruction of the proximal loop of duodenum and jejunum after partial gastrectomy and gastrojejunostomy, resulting in duodenal distention, pain, and nausea following ingestion of food.

**aglossia-adactylia s.,** hypoglossia-hypodactyly s.

**Ahumada-del Castillo s.,** galactorrhea-amenorrhea syndrome with low gonadotropin secretion.

**Aicardi's s.,** a syndrome affecting female infants, characterized by agenesis of the corpus callosum, large discrete areas of chorioretinopathy, spasms and tonic seizures, and mental retardation.

**akinetic-rigid s.,** muscular rigidity with varying degrees of slowness of movement; seen in parkinsonism and disorders of the basal ganglia.

**Alagille s.,** an autosomal dominant syndrome of neonatal jaundice, cholestasis with peripheral pulmonic stenosis, and occasionally septal defects or patent ductus arteriosus, due to paucity or absence of intrahepatic bile ducts; it is characterized by unusual facies and ocular, vertebral, and nervous system abnormalities.

**Alajouanine's s.,** symmetric lesions of the sixth and seventh cranial nerves with bilateral facial paralysis and bilateral lateral rectus palsy of the eyeball, associated with bilateral clubfoot. Cf. *Möbius' s.*

**Albright's s., Albright-McCune-Sternberg s.,** polyostotic fibrous dysplasia, patchy dermal pigmentation, and endocrine dysfunction. Called also *McCune-Albright s.*

**Aldrich's s.,** Wiskott-Aldrich s.

**Alezzandrini's s.,** unilateral tapetoretinal degeneration followed by facial vitiligo and poliosis on the same side, sometimes associated with deafness.

**"Alice in Wonderland" s.,** a delusional state manifested by depersonalization, alteration in the sense of the passage of time, distorted perception of objects, hallucinations, and other delusions or illusions. It may be associated with schizophrenia, epilepsy, migraine, diseases of the parietal lobe, hypnagogic states, or the use of hallucinogenic drugs.

**Allemann's s.,** the association of double kidney and clubbed fingers, sometimes associated with facial asymmetry and degeneration of various motor nerves.

**Allgrove's s.,** glucocorticoid deficiency with achalasia and alacrima; inherited as an autosomal recessive trait; called also *achalasia-addisonian s., addisonian-achalasia s.,* and *triple-A s.*

**Alport's s.,** a hereditary disorder characterized by progressive sensorineural hearing loss, progressive pyelonephritis or glomerulonephritis, and, occasionally, ocular defects. It is transmitted as an autosomal dominant or X-linked trait.

**Alström s.,** an autosomal recessive syndrome of retinitis pigmentosa with nystagmus and early loss of central vision, deafness, obesity, and diabetes mellitus.

**amnesic s., amnestic s., amnestic-confabulatory s.,** a mental disorder characterized by impaired memory with anterograde and sometimes retrograde amnesia in a normal state of consciousness; i.e., the syndrome does not include the impaired memory seen in dementia or delirium. There may be disorientation, confabulation, and lack of insight into the memory deficit. The most common cause is thiamine deficiency from chronic alcohol abuse *(Wernicke-Korsakoff syndrome),* but it may also result from any pathological process causing bilateral damage to parts of the medial temporal lobe or diencephalon, such as the hippocampal formations, mammillary bodies, or dorsal medial nuclei of the thalamus. Other causes include head trauma, brain tumors, infarction, cerebral hypoxia, carbon monoxide poisoning, and herpes simplex encephalitis. Called also *dysmnesic s.*

**amniotic band s.,** see under *sequence.*

**amniotic infection s. of Blane,** a syndrome in which fetal sepsis follows swallowing and at times aspiration of contaminated amniotic fluid.

**amyostatic s.,** Wilson's disease.

**Andersen's s.,** bronchiectasis, cystic fibrosis of the pancreas, and vitamin A deficiency.

**Andrade's s.,** Portuguese type familial amyloid polyneuropathy.

**androgen insensitivity s.,** complete androgen resistance; see under *resistance.*

**Angelman's s.,** an autosomal recessive syndrome characterized by jerky puppetlike movements, frequent laughter, mental and motor retardation, peculiar open-mouthed facies, and seizures. It can be caused by a deletion on chromosome 15 inherited from the mother; the same deletion inherited from the father causes Prader-Willi syndrome.

**Angelucci s.,** excitable temperament, palpitation, and vasomotor disturbance in patients with vernal conjunctivitis.

**angular gyrus s.,** a syndrome resulting from an infarction or other lesion of the angular gyrus on the dominant side; symptoms may include alexia or agraphia or may feature the symptoms of Gerstmann's syndrome.

**ankyloblepharon–ectodermal dysplasia–clefting s.,** Hay-Wells s.

**anorexia-cachexia s.,** a systemic response to conditions such as cancer or the acquired immunodeficiency syndrome, resulting from a poorly understood relationship between anorexia and cachexia, manifested by malnutrition, weight loss, muscular weakness, acidosis, and toxemia. The anorexia may be caused by a severe metabolic disturbance that contributes to development of cachectic wasting, which in turn reinforces anorexia by release from the tumor of a humoral product that stimulates the satiety center in the hypothalamus.

**anterior abdominal wall s.,** continuous pain in the anterior abdominal wall, affecting either the left or right lower quadrant or the superior margins of the upper quadrant area; etiology unknown.

**anterior chamber cleavage s.,** a term for several types of mesenchymal dysgenesis affecting neural crest derivatives in the iris, trabecula, and cornea. In ascending severity these disorders are: *Axenfeld's anomaly, Axenfeld's syndrome, Rieger's anomaly,* and *Rieger's syndrome.*

**anterior cord s.,** anterior spinal artery s.

**anterior cornual s.,** muscular atrophy due to lesions of the anterior horns of the spinal cord. Cf. *spinal muscular atrophy.*

**anterior interosseous s.,** a complex of symptoms caused by a lesion of the anterior interosseous nerve, usually resulting from fracture or laceration but sometimes resulting from compression, with pain in the proximal forearm and weakness of the muscles innervated by the nerve.

**anterior spinal artery s.,** injury to the ventral spinal cord caused by blockage of the anterior spinal artery and infarction of the areas it supplies. Below the level of the lesion complete paralysis, hypalgesia, and hypesthesia occur but there is relative preservation of the posterior sensations of touch, position, and vibration.

**anterior tibial compartment s.,** rapid swelling, increased tension, pain, and ischemic necrosis of the muscles of the anterior tibial compartment of the leg; the skin becomes glossy, erythematous, and edematous as the necrosis occurs. The cause is unknown, but usually there is a history of excessive exertion.

**anticholinergic s.,** the central and peripheral effects produced by overdosage or abnormal reaction to clinical dosage of anticholinergic drugs, e.g., atropine, phenothiazines, antihistamines, and tricyclic antidepressants; signs and symptoms include anxiety, delirium, disorientation, hallucinations, seizures, tachycardia, hyperpyrexia, mydriasis, vasodilation, gastric and urinary retention, and decreased salivary, sweat, bronchial, and nasopharyngeal secretions.

**antiphospholipid-antibody s.,** a multisystem inflammatory disorder characterized by the presence of circulating antiphospholipid antibodies and by thrombosis and vascular occlusion, spontaneous abortion, thrombocytopenia, valvular heart disease, and other less frequent symptoms.

**Anton's s., Anton-Babinski s.,** a form of anosognosia in which the patient denies, and often is unaware of, the existence of clinically demonstrable blindness and may resort to confabulation to hide it; it may be the result of denial (q.v.) or of bilateral infarctions of the occipital lobes.

**anxiety s.,** the physical symptoms accompanying anxiety, such as palpitation of the heart, rapid and shallow respiration, sweating, pallor, and a feeling of panic.

**aortic arch s.,** any of a group of disorders leading to occlusion of the arteries arising from the aortic arch; causes include atherosclerosis, arterial embolism, syphilitic or tuberculous arteritis, and other conditions. See also *Takayasu's arteritis,* under *arteritis.*

**Apert's s.,** acrocephalosyndactyly.

**argentaffinoma s.,** the most common type of carcinoid syndrome, in which the tumor arises from the argentaffin cells of the gastrointestinal tract.

**Arnold-Chiari s.,** see under *malformation.*

**Arnold's nerve reflex cough s.,** a reflex cough due to irritation of the area supplied by Arnold's nerve (the auricular branch of the vagus nerve); this area is the posterior and inferior portion of the external auditory canal and the posterior half of the tympanic membrane.

**arthropathy-camptodactyly s.,** a rare autosomal recessive disorder characterized by arthropathy associated with congenital flexion contractures of the fingers and synovial and tendon abnormalities, and by constrictive pericarditis.

**Ascher s.,** blepharochalasis occurring with goiter (adenoma of the thyroid) and redundancy of the mucous membrane and submucous tissue of the upper lip.

**Asherman's s.,** persistent amenorrhea and secondary sterility due to intrauterine adhesions and synechiae, usually occurring as a result of uterine curettage.

**Asherson's s.,** a syndrome of dysphagia due to neuromuscular incoordination and achalasia of the cricopharyngeal sphincter muscle during the third stage of swallowing. It causes diversion of liquids into the air passages, precipitating paroxysms of coughing. Called also *cricopharyngeal achalasia s.*

**Asperger's s.** [DSM-IV], a pervasive developmental disorder resembling autistic disorder, being characterized by severe impairment of social interactions and by restricted interests and behaviors, but lacking the delays in development of language, cognitive function, and self-help skills that additionally define autistic disorder. It may be equivalent to a high-functioning form of autistic disorder.

**asplenia s.,** Ivemark's s.

**ataxia-telangiectasia s.,** ataxia-telangiectasia; see under *ataxia.*

**auriculotemporal s.,** redness and sweating on the cheek in connection with eating, seen in lesions of the parotid gland or the auriculotemporal nerve. Called also *Frey's s.* and *gustatory sweating s.*

**autoerythrocyte sensitization s.,** painful bruising s.

**autoimmune polyendocrine-candidiasis s.,** polyglandular autoimmune s., type I.

**Avellis' s.,** a syndrome in which a brain stem lesion limits vagal innervation unilaterally, resulting in ipsilateral paralysis of the vocal cord and soft palate and loss of sensitivity to pain and temperature in the contralateral leg, trunk, arm, and neck, and in the skin over the scalp; called also *ambiguospinothalamic paralysis* and *Avellis' paralysis.*

**Axenfeld's s.,** Axenfeld's anomaly accompanied by glaucoma and defective development of the corneoscleral trabecular meshwork and other angle structures. See also *anterior chamber cleavage s.*

**Ayerza's s.,** pulmonary hypertension with dilatation of the pulmonary arteries, related to disease of the lungs; cf. *plexogenic pulmonary arteriopathy.*

**Baastrup's s.,** kissing spines.

**Babinski's s.,** the association of cardiac and arterial disorders with chronic syphilitic meningitis, tabes dorsalis, paralytic dementia, and other late syphilitic manifestations.

**Babinski-Fröhlich s.,** adiposogenital dystrophy.

**Babinski-Nageotte s.,** a syndrome due to multiple lesions affecting the medullary pyramid and sensory tracts, the cerebellar peduncle, and the reticular formation, and marked by contralateral hemiplegia and hemianesthesia (usually only of the pain and temperature senses), ipsilateral hemiasynergia, hemiataxia, and Horner's syndrome.

**Babinski-Vaquez s.,** Babinski's s.

**bacterial overgrowth s.,** stasis s.

**BADS s.,** a syndrome of *b*lack locks, oculocutaneous *a*lbinism, and *d*eafness of the *s*ensorineural type; see *oculocutaneous albinism.*

**Bäfverstedt's s.,** lymphocytoma cutis.

**Balint's s.,** cortical paralysis of visual fixation, optic ataxia, and disturbance of visual attention, with preservation of spontaneous and reflex eye movements. Bilateral parietooccipital lesions are seen, often after cardiac onset.

**Baller-Gerold s.,** an autosomal recessive syndrome characterized by craniosynostosis and radial aplasia. Called also *craniosynostosis–radial aplasia s.*

**ballooning mitral valve s., ballooning posterior leaflet s.,** mitral valve prolapse s.

**Bannayan-Zonana s.,** a rare autosomal dominant syndrome characterized by hemangiomas of the trunk, cutaneous lipomas, macrocephaly, and swelling of the abdomen with angiomas.

**Bannwarth's s.**, the European term for the meningopolyneuritis that may occur in Lyme disease.

**Bardet-Biedl s.**, an autosomal recessive disorder characterized by mental retardation, pigmentary retinopathy, obesity, polydactyly, and hypogonadism; cf. *Laurence-Moon s.* and *Biemond s., II.*

**Barlow's s.**, mitral valve prolapse s.

**Barraquer-Simons' s.**, partial lipodystrophy.

**Barré-Guillain s.**, acute idiopathic polyneuritis.

**Barrett's s.**, peptic ulcer of the lower esophagus, often with stricture, due to the presence of columnar-lined epithelium, which may contain functional mucous cells, parietal cells, or chief cells, in the esophagus instead of normal squamous cell epithelium. It is sometimes premalignant, followed by esophageal adenocarcinoma. Called also *Barrett's esophagus.*

**Bart's s.**, a form of epidermolysis bullosa dystrophica inherited as an autosomal dominant trait, characterized by congenital localized absence of the skin with blister formation as a result of mechanical trauma and nail dystrophy.

**Bartter's s.**, hypertrophy and hyperplasia of the juxtaglomerular cells, producing hypokalemic alkalosis and hyperaldosteronism, characterized by absence of hypertension in the presence of markedly increased plasma renin concentrations, and by insensitivity to the pressor effects of angiotensin. It usually affects children, may be hereditary, and may be associated with other anomalies such as mental retardation and short stature. Called also *juxtaglomerular cell hyperplasia.*

**basal cell nevus s.**, an autosomal dominant syndrome characterized by the development in early life of numerous basal cell carcinomas, occurring in association with abnormalities of the skin (especially an unusual erythematous pitting edema of the hands and feet), bone, nervous system, eyes, and reproductive tract. Called also *Gorlin's s., Gorlin-Goltz s., nevoid basal cell carcinoma s.,* and *nevoid basalioma s.*

**basilar artery s.**, vertebrobasilar insufficiency.

**Bassen-Kornzweig s.**, abetalipoproteinemia.

**battered-child s.**, unexplained or inappropriately explained physical trauma and other manifestations of severe, repeated physical abuse of children, usually by a parent or other caretaker.

**Bazex's s.**, eczematous and psoriasiform lesions on the ears, nose, cheeks, hands, feet, and knees in patients with carcinomas of the upper respiratory and digestive tracts. Called also *paraneoplastic acrokeratosis.*

**Beals' s.**, see *congenital contractural arachnodactyly,* under *arachnodactyly.*

**Bearn-Kunkel s., Bearn-Kunkel-Slater s.**, lupoid hepatitis.

**Beckwith's s., Beckwith-Wiedemann s.**, a congenital autosomal dominant syndrome with variable expressivity characterized by exomphalos, macroglossia, and gigantism, often associated with visceromegaly, adrenocortical cytomegaly, and dysplasia of the renal medulla. Called also *EMG s.* and *exomphalos-macroglossia-gigantism s.*

**Behçet's s.**, a chronic inflammatory disorder involving the small blood vessels, which is of unknown etiology, and is characterized by recurrent aphthous ulceration of the oral and pharyngeal mucous membranes and the genitalia, skin lesions, severe uveitis, retinal vasculitis, and optic atrophy. It frequently also involves the joints, gastrointestinal system, and central nervous system.

**Benedikt's s.**, a syndrome consisting of ipsilateral oculomotor paralysis, contralateral hyperkinesia, contralateral tremor and paresis of the arm and leg, and ipsilateral ataxia; caused by lesions that damage the third nerve and involve the nucleus ruber and corticospinal tract. Called also *tegmental mesencephalic paralysis* and *tegmental s.*

**Berardinelli-Seip s.**, total lipodystrophy.

**Bernard's s., Bernard-Horner s.**, Horner's s.

**Bernard-Sergent s.**, addisonian crisis.

**Bernard-Soulier s. (BSS)**, an autosomal recessive disorder characterized by giant platelets with membranes lacking glycoprotein Ib, the probable receptor for plasma von Willebrand's factor; this keeps the platelets from binding the factor, which is necessary for their adhesion to the subendothelial surfaces of blood vessels. Symptoms include mild to moderate mucocutaneous and visceral hemorrhaging, purpura, and prolonged bleeding time. Called also *giant platelet s.* See also *thrombasthenia* and *von Willebrand's disease.*

**Bernheim's s.**, right heart failure due to left ventricular hypertrophy with bulging of the interventricular septum that causes obstruction to flow from the right atrium to ventricle, altering ventricular filling and capacity.

**Bertolotti's s.**, sacralization of the fifth lumbar vertebra together with sciatica and scoliosis.

**Biemond s., II**, an autosomal recessive disorder characterized by iris coloboma, obesity, mental retardation, hypogonadism, and postaxial polydactyly; cf. *Bardet-Biedl s.* and *Laurence-Moon s.*

**billowing mitral valve s., billowing posterior leaflet s.**, mitral valve prolapse s.

**Bing-Neel s.**, the central nervous system manifestations of Waldenström's macroglobulinemia; symptoms may include encephalopathy, hemorrhage, stroke, convulsions, delirium, and coma.

**Birt-Hogg-Dubé s.**, an autosomal dominant disorder of proliferation of ectodermal and mesodermal components of the pilar system, occurring as multiple trichodiscomas, acrochordons, and fibrofolliculomas on the head, chest, back, and arms.

**Björnstad's s.**, an autosomal recessive disorder characterized by congenital sensorineural deafness and pili torti.

**Blackfan-Diamond s.**, congenital hypoplastic anemia (def. 1).

**Blatin's s.**, hydatid thrill.

**blind loop s.**, stasis s.

**Bloch-Sulzberger s.**, incontinentia pigmenti.

**Bloom s.**, an autosomal recessive syndrome developing during infancy, consisting of erythema and telangiectasia in a butterfly distribution on the face, photosensitivity, and dwarfism of prenatal onset. Abnormalities in chromosome structure (sister chromatid exchange, q.v.) and in immunoglobulins are present, and there is a high incidence of malignancy, especially leukemia. About one-half of the patients are of Jewish ancestry.

**blue diaper s.**, a defect of tryptophan absorption in which, because of intestinal bacterial action on the tryptophan, the urine contains abnormal indoles, giving it a blue color. It is similar to Hartnup's disease.

**blue rubber bleb nevus s.**, a syndrome of multiple blue rubber bleb nevi associated with hemangiomas of the gastrointestinal tract, which bleed readily and cause chronic iron-deficiency anemia; most cases are sporadic and present in infancy or childhood.

**blue toe s.**, a blue color of the toes, sometimes bilateral, with skin necrosis and ischemic gangrene, resulting from arterial occlusion by emboli, thrombi, or injury.

**body of Luys s.**, hemiballismus.

**Boerhaave's s.**, spontaneous rupture of the esophagus.

**Böök's s.**, PHC s.

**BOR s.**, branchio-oto-renal s.

**Börjeson's s., Börjeson-Forssman-Lehmann s.**, an X-linked syndrome characterized by severe mental retardation, epilepsy, hypogonadism, hypometabolism, marked obesity, swelling of the subcutaneous tissues of the face, and large ears.

**Bouillaud's s.**, pericarditis and endocarditis accompanying rheumatic fever.

**Bourneville-Pringle s.**, tuberous sclerosis.

**Bouveret's s.**, 1. paroxysmal supraventricular tachycardia. 2. obstruction of the gastric outet by a gallstone passed into the duodenal bulb through a cholecystoduodenal or choledochoduodenal fistula.

**bowel bypass s.**, a dermatosis-arthritis syndrome that may occur one to six years after jejunoileal bypass, characterized by rash, malaise, myalgia, polyarthralgia, sterile skin pustules, and a flulike illness; it is probably caused by circulating immune complexes that include bacterial antigens resulting from overgrowth in the bypassed bowel.

**brachial s.**, see under *plexopathy.*

**Brachmann-de Lange s.**, de Lange's s.

**Bradbury-Eggleston s.**, a syndrome of postural hypotension without tachycardia but with visual disturbances, hypohidrosis, impotence, lowered basal metabolic rate, dizziness, syncope, presyncope, and slow unchanging pulse. It occurs predominantly in older males in the early morning hours during the summer and is due to impaired peripheral vasoconstriction; it usually has a progressive course.

**bradycardia-tachycardia s., brady-tachy s.**, a clinical manifestation of the sick sinus syndrome characterized by periods of atrial and ventricular bradycardia alternating with periods of rapid regular or irregular atrial or ventricular tachyarrhythmias.

**branchio-oto-renal s.**, branchial arch anomalies (preauricular pits, branchial fistulas or pits) associated with Mondini's deafness and renal dysplasia, inherited as an autosomal dominant trait with high penetrance and variable expression. Called also *BOR s.*

**Brennemann's s.**, mesenteric and retroperitoneal lymphadenitis as a sequel of throat infections.

**Briquet's s.**, somatization disorder.

**Brissaud-Sicard s.**, spasmodic hemiplegia caused by lesions of the pons.

**Bristowe's s.**, a series of symptoms caused by a tumor of the corpus callosum, including hemiplegia and apraxia.

**brittle bones s.**, osteogenesis imperfecta.

**brittle cornea s.**, an X-linked, recessively inherited syndrome, characterized by brittle cornea, blue sclerae, and red hair.

**Brock's s.**, middle lobe s.

**Brown's vertical retraction s.**, adhesion of the muscles of the eye in the fetus.

**Brown-Séquard's s.**, a syndrome due to damage of one half of the spinal cord, resulting in ipsilateral paralysis and loss of discriminatory and joint sensation, and contralateral loss of pain and temperature sensation. Called also *Brown-Séquard's paralysis* or *sign.*

**Brown-Vialetto-van Laere s.**, an autosomal recessive syndrome consisting of progressive bulbar palsy with any of several cranial nerve disorders, including nerve deafness, facial weakness, dysarthria, and dysphagia.

**Brueghel's s.,** Meige's s. (def. 2).

**Bruns' s.,** intermittent headache, vertigo, vomiting, and visual disturbances on sudden movement of the head, characteristic of cysticercus infection of the fourth ventricle, lesion of the fourth ventricle, or tumors of the midline of the cerebellum and third or lateral ventricles. Called also *Bruns' sign.*

**Brunsting's s.,** a recurrent eruptive syndrome usually affecting middle-aged men, in which grouped, vesicular lesions occur about the head and neck, and result in scarring.

**Brushfield-Wyatt s.,** a congenital syndrome consisting of extensive unilateral nevus flammeus, hemianopia affecting the right or left halves of the visual fields of both eyes, contralateral hemiplegia, cerebral angioma, and mental retardation; it is probably related to the Sturge-Weber syndrome.

**Buckley's s.,** hyperimmunoglobulinemia E s.

**Budd-Chiari s.,** symptomatic obstruction or occlusion of the hepatic veins, causing hepatomegaly, abdominal pain and tenderness, intractable ascites, mild jaundice, and, eventually, portal hypertension and liver failure; the obstruction is caused by thrombi or fibrous obliteration of the veins and has been associated with coagulation disorders, myeloproliferative disorders, invasion of hepatic veins by hepatic, renal, or adrenal carcinoma, and with abdominal trauma. Onset may be acute with death occurring within days in cases of complete occlusion; more often there is a chronic course with survival for months or years. Called also *Chiari's s.* and *endophlebitis hepatica obliterans.* Cf. *veno-occlusive disease of liver.*

**bulbar s.,** any syndrome caused by a lesion in the medulla and its nuclei, with paralysis of the cranial nerves originating there; cf. *progressive bulbar palsy.* Called also *Dejerine's s.*

**Bürger-Grütz s.,** familial hyperlipoproteinemia, type I.

**Burnett's s.,** milk-alkali s.

**burning feet s.,** Gopalan's s.

**Buschke-Ollendorff s.,** dermatofibrosis lenticularis disseminata.

**Bywaters' s.,** crush s.

**Caffey's s., Caffey-Silverman s.,** infantile cortical hyperostosis.

**camptomelic s.,** osteochondrodysplasia associated with flat facies, bowed tibiae with skin dimpling, hypoplastic scapulae, and short vertebrae.

**Canada-Cronkhite s.,** Cronkhite-Canada s.

**Capgras' s.,** a form of delusional misidentification in which the patient believes that other persons in the environment are not their real selves but doubles. Cf. *Frégoli's phenomenon.*

**capillary leak s.,** extravasation of plasma fluid and proteins into the extravascular space, resulting in sometimes fatal hypotension and reduced organ perfusion; an adverse effect of aldesleukin (interleukin-2) therapy.

**Caplan's s.,** pneumoconiosis associated with rheumatoid arthritis. Radiographically, multiple spherical nodular lesions with clearly demarcated borders are found throughout both lungs. Called also *rheumatoid pneumoconiosis.*

**carcinoid s.,** a symptom complex associated with carcinoid tumors and characterized by attacks of severe cyanotic flushing of the skin lasting from minutes to days and by diarrheal watery stools, bronchoconstrictive attacks, sudden drops in blood pressure, edema, and ascites. Symptoms are caused by secretion by the tumor of serotonin, prostaglandins, and other biologically active substances. See also *argentaffinoma s.*

**Carney's s.,** see under *complex.*

**carotid sinus s.,** syncope sometimes associated with convulsive seizures due to overactivity of the carotid sinus reflex (q.v.) when pressure is applied to one or both carotid sinuses. Called also *carotid sinus syncope* and *Charcot-Weiss-Baker s.*

**carpal tunnel s.,** a complex of symptoms resulting from compression of the median nerve in the carpal tunnel, with pain and burning or tingling paresthesias in the fingers and hand, sometimes extending to the elbow.

**Carpenter's s.,** acrocephalopolysyndactyly, type II.

**cat-eye s.,** an association of coloboma of the iris and anal atresia; there may also be many other anomalies, including preauricular skin tags or fistulas, hypertelorism, congenital heart disease, skeletal abnormalities, and renal malformations. It is associated with partial trisomy 22, i.e., the presence of a partial additional copy of chromosome 22.

**cat's cry s.,** cri du chat s.

**cat's eye s.,** cat-eye s.

**cauda equina s.,** 1. dull aching pain of the perineum, bladder, and sacrum, generally radiating in a sciatic fashion, with associated paresthesias and areflexic paralysis, due to compression of the spinal nerve roots. 2. see under *neuritis.*

**caudal dysplasia s., caudal regression s.,** failure of formation of part or all of the coccygeal, sacral, and occasionally lumbar vertebral units and the corresponding segments of the caudal spinal cord, with resulting neurogenic dysfunction of bowel and bladder; called also *sacral agenesis.*

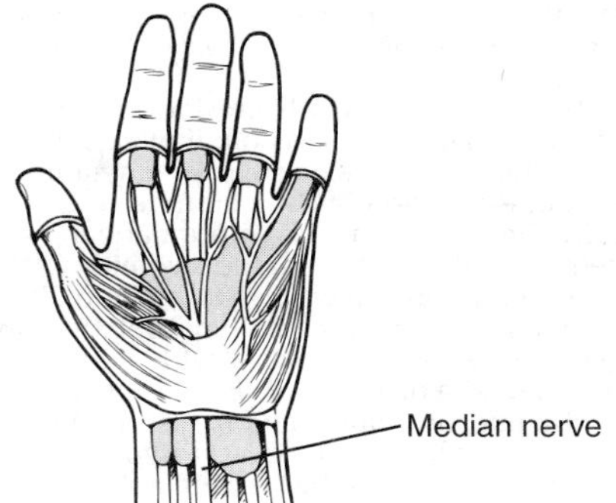


Median nerve entrapped in carpal tunnel.

**cavernous sinus s.,** edema of the conjunctiva, proptosis, edema of upper lid and root of the nose, together with paralysis of the third, fourth, and sixth cranial nerves and the ophthalmic branch of the fifth; it is usually due to thrombosis or tumor of the cavernous sinus. Cf. *Tolosa-Hunt s.* Called also *Foix s.*

**celiac s.,** see under *disease.*

**central alveolar hypoventilation s.,** primary alveolar hypoventilation.

**central cord s.,** syringomyelia.

**central sleep apnea s.,** see under *apnea.*

**centroposterior s.,** syringomyelia.

**cerebellar s.,** see under *ataxia.*

**cerebellopontine angle s.,** a syndrome caused by a tumor of the cerebellopontine angle or an acoustic tumor, characterized by hearing loss, subjective noises, ipsilateral cerebellar ataxia, and eventually ipsilateral impairment of function of the sixth and seventh cranial nerves accompanied by elevated intracranial pressure.

**cerebrocardiac s.,** Krishaber's disease.

**cerebrocostomandibular s.,** an autosomal recessive syndrome of severe micrognathia and costovertebral abnormalities, including small bell-shaped thorax, incompletely ossified aberrant rib structure, and abnormal rib attachment to vertebrae. Also present are palatal defects, glossoptosis, prenatal and postnatal growth deficiencies, and mental retardation, the last perhaps due to the neonatal respiratory distress which is frequently the presenting sign of the disorder.

**cerebrohepatorenal s.,** an autosomal recessive disorder characterized by craniofacial abnormalities, hypotonia, hepatomegaly, polycystic kidneys, jaundice, and death in early infancy, and associated with absence of peroxisomes in the liver and kidneys; called also *Zellweger s.*

**cervical s., cervical disk s.,** a condition caused by irritation or compression of the cervical nerve roots by a protruding disk; symptoms include neck pain radiating into the shoulder, arm, or forearm, paresthesias, and muscle weakness or spasm.

**cervical rib s.,** a thoracic outlet syndrome caused by a cervical rib.

**cervicobrachial s.,** brachial plexopathy.

**Cestan's s., Cestan-Chenais s.,** an association of contralateral hemiplegia, contralateral hemianesthesia, ipsilateral lateropulsion and hemiasynergia, Horner's syndrome, and ipsilateral laryngoplegia, due to scattered lesions of the pyramid, sensory tract, inferior cerebellar peduncle, nucleus ambiguus, and oculopupillary center.

**Cestan-Raymond s.,** Raymond-Cestan s.

**Charcot's s.,** 1. amyotrophic lateral sclerosis. 2. intermittent claudication. 3. intermittent hepatic fever.

**Charcot-Marie s.,** Charcot-Marie-Tooth disease.

**Charcot-Weiss-Baker s.,** carotid sinus s.

**CHARGE s.,** see under *association.*

**Charlin's s.,** pain, iritis, corneitis, rhinorrhea, and tenderness along the nose as a result of neuralgia of the nasociliary nerve. Called also *nasociliary neuralgia.*

**Chauffard's s., Chauffard-Still s.,** Still's disease (polyarthritis with fever, splenomegaly, and enlargement of lymph nodes) in persons infected with bovine or some other type of nonhuman tuberculosis.

**Chédiak-Higashi s.,** a lethal autosomal recessive syndrome associated with oculocutaneous albinism, massive leukocyte inclusions (giant lysosomes), histiocytic infiltration of multiple body organs, development of pancytopenia, hepatosplenomegaly, recurrent or persistent bacterial infections, and a possible predisposition to development of malignant lymphoma. Called also *Béguez César disease* and *Chédiak-Higashi anomaly.*

**Chiari's s.,** Budd-Chiari s.

**Chiari-Arnold s.,** Arnold-Chiari malformation.

**Chiari-Frommel s.,** galactorrhea-amenorrhea syndrome occurring after pregnancy; called also *Frommel-Chiari s., Chiari-Frommel disease,* and *Frommel's disease.*

**chiasma s., chiasmatic s.,** a syndrome indicative of lesion affecting the optic chiasma: impairment of vision, limitations of the field of vision, central scotoma, headache, vertigo, and syncope.

**Chilaiditi s.,** 1. interposition of the colon between the liver and diaphragm. Usually the condition is asymptomatic in adults, but symptoms are evident in children and include vomiting, abdominal pain, anorexia, constipation, aerophagia. Signs include abdominal distention and absence of liver dullness. 2. hepatoptosis (def. 2).

**CHILD s.,** (*c*ongenital *h*emidysplasia with *i*chthyosiform erythroderma and *l*imb *d*efects) a disorder of skin cornification characterized by unilateral erythema and scaling and ipsilateral limb defects, sometimes accompanied by ipsilateral skeletal hypoplasia and brain and visceral defects; it is believed to be an X-linked dominant trait.

**Chinese restaurant s.,** a transient syndrome associated with arterial dilatation, due to ingestion of monosodium glutamate, which is sometimes used liberally in seasoning Chinese food; it is characterized by throbbing of the head, lightheadedness, tightness of the jaw, neck, and shoulders, and backache.

**Chotzen's s.,** an autosomal dominant disorder characterized by acrocephalosyndactyly in which the syndactyly is mild and by hypertelorism, ptosis, and sometimes mental retardation. Called also *acrocephalosyndactyly type III* and *Saethre-Chotzen s.*

**Christian's s.,** Hand-Schüller-Christian disease.

**Christ-Siemens-Touraine s.,** anhidrotic ectodermal dysplasia.

**chronic fatigue s.,** persistent debilitating fatigue of recent onset, with reduction of physical activity to less than half of usual, accompanied by some combination of muscle weakness, sore throat, mild fever, tender lymph nodes, headaches, and depression, with the symptoms not attributable to any other known causes. Its nature is controversial; viral infection (including Epstein-Barr virus and human herpesvirus-6) may be associated with it, but no causal relationship has been demonstrated. A number of names have been used for this syndrome, including *Iceland disease, benign myalgic encephalomyelitis, chronic Epstein-Barr virus infection, chronic mononucleosis,* and *epidemic neuromyasthenia.*

**Churg-Strauss s.,** a form of systemic necrotizing vasculitis in which there is prominent lung involvement with severe asthma, eosinophilia, and granulomatous reactions. If present, cutaneous lesions consist of tender subcutaneous nodules, large ecchymotic plaques, and cutaneous infarcts. Called also *allergic granulomatosis, allergic granulomatous angiitis,* and *Churg-Strauss vasculitis.*

**chylomicronemia s.,** familial hyperchylomicronemia.

**Citelli's s.,** mental dullness, loss of power of concentration, and drowsiness or insomnia, seen in persons with adenoids or sinus infection.

**Clarke-Hadfield s.,** congenital pancreatic disease with infantilism; with enlarged liver, bulky fatty stools, and extensive atrophy of pancreas in an undersized and underweight child.

**Claude's s.,** paralysis of the third (oculomotor) nerve on one side and asynergia on the other side, together with dysarthria; called also *inferior s. of red nucleus* and *rubrospinal cerebellar peduncle s.*

**Claude Bernard–Horner s.,** Horner's s.

**click s., click-murmur s.,** mitral valve prolapse s.

**closed head s.,** the complex of symptoms characteristic of cerebral injury without cranial penetration. See also *concussion* and *postconcussional s.*

**Clouston's s.,** hidrotic ectodermal dysplasia.

**cloverleaf skull s.,** kleeblattschädel s.

**Cockayne's s.,** a hereditary syndrome transmitted as an autosomal recessive trait, consisting of dwarfism with retinal atrophy and deafness, associated with progeria, prognathism, mental retardation, and photosensitivity.

**Coffin-Lowry s.,** a condition with onset in the postnatal period characterized by incapability of speech, severe mental deficiency, and muscle, ligament, and skeletal abnormalities; it is transmitted with X-linked intermediate inheritance.

**Coffin-Siris s.,** hypoplasia or absence of the fifth fingers and toenails associated with growth and mental deficiencies, coarse facies, mild microcephaly, hypotonia, lax joints, mild hirsutism, and occasionally cardiac, vertebral, or gastrointestinal anomalies.

**Cogan's s.,** 1. nonsyphilitic interstitial keratitis with tinnitus and deafness; it usually occurs in children, often associated with polyarteritis nodosa. 2. Cogan's oculomotor apraxia.

**cold agglutinin s.,** the presence of circulating cold agglutinins, usually IgM, which are directed against three types of polysaccharide red cell antigens: *I antigens,* expressed primarily on adult red cells, *i antigens,* expressed primarily on cells of fetuses and infants, and *Pr antigens,* which, unlike I and i antigens, are protease sensitive. The primary clinical manifestations are intravascular hemolysis in exposed extremities and mild hemolytic anemia due to complement fixation, both occurring only upon exposure to cold. There are two major types: *chronic cold agglutinin disease,* a condition seen in the elderly with gradual onset and a chronic course; and *postinfectious cold agglutinin syndrome,* which usually follows *Mycoplasma pneumoniae* infection or infectious mononucleosis and lasts a few months. The syndrome can also develop secondary to malignancy.

**Collet's s., Collet-Sicard s.,** Vernet's syndrome with ipsilateral paralysis of the tongue, due to complete lesion of the ninth, tenth, eleventh, and twelfth cranial nerves. Called also *Sicard's s.*

**compartment s., compartmental s.,** a condition in which increased tissue pressure in a confined anatomical space causes decreased blood flow leading to ischemia and dysfunction of contained myoneural elements, marked by pain, muscle weakness, sensory loss, and palpable tenseness in the involved compartment. Ischemia can lead to necrosis resulting in permanent impairment of function.

**compression s.,** crush s.

**concussion s.,** postconcussional s.

**congenital rubella s.,** transplacental infection of the fetus with rubella, usually in the first trimester of pregnancy, because of maternal infection (which is sometimes subclinical). The newborn infant has developmental abnormalities, which may include cardiac lesions, ocular lesions, deafness, microcephaly, mental retardation, and generalized growth retardation, sometimes associated with acute self-limited conditions such as thrombocytopenic purpura, anemia, hepatitis, encephalitis, and radiolucencies of long bones. Infected infants may shed virus to all contacts for an extended period. Called also *rubella s.*

**congenital tremor s.,** any of several similar congenital neurological diseases of pigs in which piglets have noticeable trembling, often owing to defective myelination of nerves. Mild varieties may clear up within a month but in severe cases the piglets cannot function normally and soon die. One variety is autosomal recessive; another is sex-linked; and others are caused by intrauterine viral infections such as with hog cholera virus. Affected pigs are called *dancing* or *shaker pigs.* Called also *congenital trembles* and *myoclonia congenita.*

**Conn's s.,** primary aldosteronism.

**Conradi's s.,** chondrodysplasia punctata.

**Conradi-Hünermann s.,** an autosomal dominant form of chondrodysplasia punctata, characterized by asymmetric shortening of the extremities and scoliosis; intelligence and life expectancy are normal. The syndrome is also associated with maternal use of warfarin sodium during pregnancy.

**contiguous gene s.,** any syndrome known to be caused by the involvement of contiguous genes on a chromosome, e.g., aniridia–Wilms' tumor association, which may also have genitourinary tract abnormalities, gonadoblastoma, and mental retardation; it is usually caused by chromosome deletions.

**continuous muscle activity s., continuous muscle fiber activity s.,** Isaacs' s.

**Cornelia de Lange's s.,** de Lange's s.

**s. of corpus striatum,** Vogt's s.

**Costen's s.,** a complex of symptoms including partial deafness, stuffiness in the ears, tinnitus, clicking or snapping of the temporomandibular joint, dizziness, headache, and burning pain in the ear, throat, tongue, and nose. Causes proposed include mandibular overclosure, lesions of the temporomandibular joint, and stress. Some researchers question the anatomical and physiological justification for considering this a separate diagnostic entity. Called also *temporomandibular dysfunction s.*

**costoclavicular s.,** a thoracic outlet syndrome caused by compression or friction on nerves and blood vessels between a drooping clavicle and the first rib.

**Cotard's s.,** paranoia with delusions of negation, a suicidal tendency, and sensory disturbances.

**Courvoisier-Terrier s.,** dilatation of the gallbladder, retention jaundice, and discoloration of the feces, indicating obstruction due to a tumor of the ampulla of Vater.

**cracked tooth s.,** a group of symptoms caused by presence of a cracked tooth, including pain on pressure or application of cold, with pulpitis if untreated.

**craniosynostosis–radial aplasia s.,** Baller-Gerold s.

**crazy cow s.,** a type of neurotoxicity seen in cattle in the United States, Brazil, and South Africa after they have eaten any of various plants of the genus *Solanum;* characteristics include cerebellar damage with staggering and incoordination.

**CREST s.,** a form of systemic scleroderma usually less severe than other forms, consisting of *c*alcinosis cutis, *R*aynaud's phenomenon, *e*sophageal dysfunction, *s*clerodactyly, and *t*elangiectasia. When esophageal dysfunction is not prominent, it is known as *CRST s.*

**cricopharyngeal achalasia s.,** Asherson's s.

**cri du chat s.,** a hereditary congenital syndrome characterized by hypertelorism, microcephaly, severe mental deficiency, and a plaintive catlike cry, due to deletion of part of the short arm of chromosome 5. Called also *cat's cry s.*

**Crigler-Najjar s.,** an autosomal recessive form of nonhemolytic jaundice due to the absence of the hepatic enzyme glucuronosyltransferase. It is characterized by the presence in the blood of excessive amounts of unconjugated bilirubin and by kernicterus and severe disorders of the central nervous system. Called also *congenital hyperbilirubinemia* and *congenital nonhemolytic jaundice.*

**s. of crocodile tears,** spontaneous lacrimation occurring parallel with the normal salivation of eating. It follows facial paralysis and seems to be due to inaccurate regrowth of the regenerating nerve fibers into the wrong nerve sheaths, with some of those destined for the salivary glands going to the lacrimal glands.

**Cronkhite-Canada s.,** a rare syndrome of sporadic, widespread intestinal polyps and malabsorption accompanied by ectodermal defects such as alopecia and onychodystrophy; called also *Canada-Cronkhite s.*

**Cross s., Cross-McKusick-Breen s.,** an autosomal recessive syndrome marked by oculocutaneous albinism, microphthalmus, small opaque corneas, oligophrenia with spasticity, high-arched palate, gingival hypertrophy, and scoliosis. Called also *oculocerebral-hypopigmentation s.*

**Crow-Fukase s.,** POEMS s.

**CRST s.,** see *CREST s.*

**crush s.,** the edema, oliguria, and other symptoms of renal failure which follow the crushing of a part, especially a large muscle mass; see *lower nephron nephrosis,* under *nephrosis.*

**Cruveilhier-Baumgarten s.,** cirrhosis of the liver with portal hypertension, associated with congenital patency of the umbilical or paraumbilical veins. It is characterized by hematemesis, ascites, splenomegaly, hypersplenism, esophageal varices, caput medusae, large tortuous veins in the abdominal wall, and a venous hum, often accompanied by a thrill, usually heard over the region of the xiphoid process. Called also *Cruveilhier-Baumgarten cirrhosis.*

**cryptophthalmos s.,** an autosomal recessive abnormality, characterized by absence of the palpebral apertures, disorganization of one or both ocular globes, malformed ears, cleft palate, laryngeal stenosis, syndactyly, meningoencephalocele, imperforate anus, cardiac defects, and maldeveloped kidneys. Called also *Fraser's s.*

**cubital tunnel s.,** a complex of symptoms resulting from injury or compression of the ulnar nerve at the elbow, with pain and numbness along the ulnar aspect of the hand and forearm, and weakness of the hand.

**culture-specific s.,** a form of disturbed behavior highly specific to certain cultural systems and that does not conform to Western nosologic entities; examples are amok, koro, piblokto, and windigo.

**Currarino-Silverman s.,** premature obliteration of the sternal sutures with synostosis as well as a protruding manubrium, causing pectus carinatum; other abnormalities may also be present such as hyperostosis of ribs or hypotrophy of the anterior diaphragm. Called also *Silverman's s.*

**Curschmann-Batten-Steinert s.,** myotonic dystrophy.

**Curtius' s.,** hypertrophy of one side of the entire body or a portion of one side of the body, as of the face; called also *hemihypertrophy.*

**Cushing's s.,** a complex of symptoms caused by hyperadrenocorticism due either to a neoplasm of the adrenal cortex or adenohypophysis, or to excessive intake of glucocorticoids. Symptoms may include adiposity of the face, neck, and trunk; kyphosis from osteoporosis of the spine; hypertension; diabetes mellitus; amenorrhea and hypertrichosis in females; impotence in males; dusky complexion with purple striae; polycythemia; and muscular wasting and weakness. When secondary to excessive secretion of adrenocorticotropic hormone by a pituitary adenoma, it is known as *Cushing's disease.* See also *ectopic ACTH s.* Called also *Cushing's* or *pituitary basophilism.*

**Cushing's s., iatrogenic,** Cushing's syndrome caused by prolonged excessive use of glucocorticoid medications; called also *Cushing's s. medicamentosus.*

**Cushing's s. medicamentosus,** iatrogenic Cushing's s.

**Cyriax's s.,** a syndrome due to slipped rib cartilages pressing on the nerves at the interchondral joint, resulting in pain in the region of the cartilage, radiation of pain to the shoulder and arm, or pain similar to that of angina pectoris.

**Da Costa's s.,** neurocirculatory asthenia.

**Danbolt-Closs s.,** acrodermatitis enteropathica.

**Dandy-Walker s.,** see under *malformation.*

**Danlos' s.,** Ehlers-Danlos s.

**Debré-Sémélaigne s.,** autosomal recessive athyrotic cretinism associated with myotonia and muscular pseudohypertrophy. Called also *Kocher-Debré-Sémélaigne s.*

**de Clérambault s.,** erotomania.

**defibrination s.,** diffuse intravascular coagulation.

**Degos' s.,** malignant atrophic papulosis.

**Dejean's s.,** orbital floor s.

**Dejerine's s.,** 1. symptoms of radiculitis; namely, distribution of the pain, motor, and sensory defects in the region of the radicular or segmental disturbance of the nerve roots rather than along the course of the peripheral nerve. 2. bulbar s. 3. a polyneuropathy resembling tabes dorsalis, secondary to infection by *Corynebacterium diphtheriae* and the resultant lesions of peripheral nerves and of the posterior column of the spinal cord; deep sensibility is depressed but tactile sense is normal. Called also *diphtheritic polyneuropathy.*

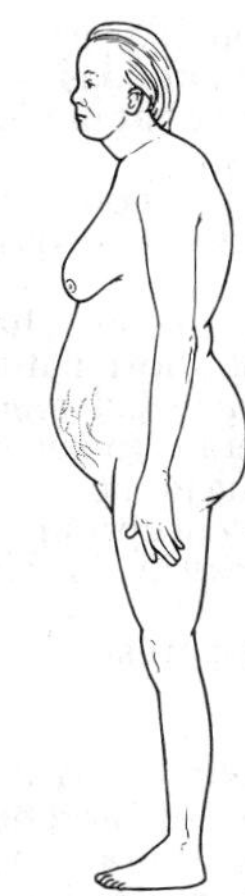

Cushing's syndrome.

**Dejerine-Klumpke s.,** Klumpke's paralysis.

**Dejerine-Roussy s.,** thalamic s.

**Dejerine-Thomas s.,** olivopontocerebellar atrophy.

**de Lange's s.,** a congenital syndrome in which severe mental retardation is associated with many abnormalities, including short stature (Amsterdam dwarf), brachycephaly, low-set ears, webbed neck, carp mouth, depressed bridge of the nose with the end tilted up and forward-directed nostrils, bushy eyebrows meeting at the midline, unruly coarse hair growing low on the forehead and neck, and flat spadelike hands with short tapering fingers. Called also *Brachmann-de Lange s., Cornelia de Lange's s.,* and *typus degenerativus amstelodamensis.*

**del Castillo's s.,** Sertoli-cell–only s.

**dementia s. of depression,** reversible dementia occurring in association with depression in the elderly, the cognitive deficits resolving with treatment of the depression.

**de Morsier's s.,** septo-optic dysplasia.

**dengue shock s.,** see *hemorrhagic dengue,* under *dengue.*

**Dennie-Marfan s.,** spastic paralysis and mental retardation in association with congenital syphilis.

**Denny-Brown's s.,** hereditary sensory radicular neuropathy.

**Denys-Drash s.,** a syndrome of male pseudohermaphroditism, nephropathy leading to renal failure, and, in most cases, Wilms' tumor, caused by a genetic abnormality in the p13 region of chromosome 11.

**depressive s.,** depression, def. 3.

**De Sanctis-Cacchione s.,** a hereditary syndrome, transmitted as an autosomal recessive trait, consisting of xeroderma pigmentosum associated with mental retardation, retarded growth, gonadal hypoplasia, and sometimes neurologic complications and photosensitivity.

**de Toni-Fanconi s.,** see *Fanconi's s.,* def. 2.

**dialysis dysequilibrium s.,** a group of symptoms seen during or after overly rapid hemodialysis or peritoneal dialysis, resulting from an osmotic shift of water into the brain; usually there is headache and less often nausea, muscle cramps, nervous irritability, drowsiness, and convulsions.

**Diamond-Blackfan s.,** congenital hypoplastic anemia (def. 1).

**diarrheogenic s.,** Verner-Morrison s.

**DIDMOAD s.,** [*d*iabetes *i*nsipidus, *d*iabetes *m*ellitus, optic *a*trophy, *d*eafness] Wolfram s.

**diencephalic s.,** failure to thrive, emaciation, and sometimes nevus unius lateralis.

**DiGeorge s.,** a congenital disorder in which defective development of the third and fourth pharyngeal pouches results in hypoplasia or aplasia of the thymus and parathyroid glands, often associated with congenital heart defects, anomalies of the great vessels, esophageal atresia, and abnormalities of facial structures. Depending on the degree of parathyroid and thymic hypoplasia, there is hypocalcemic tetany or seizures due to lack of parathyroid hormone and deficiency of cell-mediated immunity resulting in increased susceptibility to low-grade or opportunistic pathogens, e.g., fungi, viruses, and *Pneumocystis carinii.* Called also *thymic aplasia* or *hypoplasia* and *pharyngeal pouch s.*

**Di Guglielmo's s.,** erythroleukemia.

**disconnection s.,** any neurologic disorder caused by an interruption in impulse transmission along cerebral fiber pathways; one result may be an inability to carry out a desired movement in response to a given sensory input, as in the apraxias.

**disseminated intravascular coagulation s.,** see under *coagulation.*

**Donohue's s.,** leprechaunism.

**DOOR s.,** a rare syndrome of congenital *d*eafness, *o*nycho-*o*steodystrophy, and mental *r*etardation, existing in autosomal dominant and recessive forms.

**Down s.,** a chromosome disorder characterized by a small, anteroposteriorly flattened skull, short, flat-bridge nose, epicanthal fold, short phalanges, widened spaces between the first and second digits of hands and feet, and moderate to severe mental retardation, with Alzheimer's disease developing in the fourth or fifth decade. The chromosomal aberration is trisomy of chromosome 21 associated with late maternal age. Called also *trisomy 21* and *nondisjunction;* formerly called *mongolism.*

**downer cow s.,** parturient paresis in a cow that is intractable to treatment and usually fatal.

**Drash s.,** Denys-Drash s.

**Dresbach's s.,** hereditary eliptocytosis.

**Dressler's s.,** post–myocardial infarction s.

**Duane's s.,** a hereditary congenital syndrome in which the affected eye shows limitation or absence of abduction, restriction of adduction, retraction of the globe on adduction, narrowing of the palpebral fissure on adduction and widening on abduction, and deficient convergence. It is transmitted as an autosomal dominant trait. Called also *retraction s., Stilling's s.,* and *Stilling-Türk-Duane s.*

**Dubin-Johnson s., Dubin-Sprinz s.,** a familial chronic form of nonhemolytic jaundice thought to be due to a defect in the excretion of conjugated bilirubin and certain other organic anions (e.g., sulfobromophthalein) by the liver. It is characterized by the presence of a brown, coarsely granular pigment in the hepatic cells, which is pathognomonic of the condition. Called also *Sprinz-Dubin s.* and *Sprinz-Nelson s.*

**Dubreuil-Chambardel's s.,** dental caries of the incisors, in most instances only the upper ones, usually appearing during adolescence; within a few years the teeth are irreparably damaged. Some authorities do not consider this syndrome a legitimate entity.

**Duchenne's s.,** progressive bulbar palsy.

**Duchenne-Erb s.,** Erb-Duchenne paralysis; see under *paralysis.*

**dumping s.,** a complex reaction thought to be secondary to excessively rapid emptying of the gastric contents into the jejunum, manifested by nausea, weakness, sweating, palpitation, varying degrees of syncope, often a sensation of warmth, and sometimes diarrhea, occurring after ingestion of food by patients who have had partial gastrectomy and gastrojejunostomy. Called also *jejunal s.* and *postgastrectomy s.*

**Duncan's s.,** X-linked lymphoproliferative s.

**Dyke-Davidoff-Masson s.,** a syndrome possibly due to injury to or severe disease affecting one side of the brain during the neonatal period, characterized by mental retardation, asymmetry of the face, and varying degrees of hemiplegia, neurological impairment, and atrophy of the side of the body contralateral to the lesion.

**dyscontrol s.,** a pattern of episodic, abnormal, and often violent and uncontrollable social behavior with little or no provocation; it may result from diseases of the limbic system or the temporal lobe or may accompany abuse of alcohol or some other psychoactive substance. Called also *episodic dyscontrol.*

**dyskinetic cilia s.,** primary ciliary dyskinesia.

**dysmaturity s.,** a syndrome due to placental insufficiency that causes chronic stress and hypoxia, seen in fetuses and newborn infants in post-term pregnancies and characterized by decreased subcutaneous fat, skin desquamation, and long fingernails, often with yellow meconium staining of the nails, skin, and vernix. Called also *dysmaturity, postmaturity s.,* and *placental dysfunction s.*

**dysmnesic s.,** amnestic s.

**dysplasia oculodentodigitalis s.,** oculodentodigital dysplasia.

**dysplastic nevus s.,** the occurrence of dysplastic nevi in persons with or at risk for familial or nonfamilial malignant melanoma.

**Eagle-Barrett s.,** prune-belly s.

**Eaton-Lambert s.,** an autoimmune, myasthenialike syndrome caused by autoantibodies to the voltage-gated calcium channel (anna 1 antibodies) that interfere with the release of acetylcholine at the motor nerve terminal. Weakness usually affects the limbs, but ocular and bulbar muscles are spared; there is reduced muscle action potential on stimulation of its nerve but with repetitive stimulation it becomes augmented. It is often associated with oat-cell carcinoma of the lung. Called also *Lambert-Eaton s., Lambert-Eaton myasthenic s.,* and *myasthenic s.*

**ectopic ACTH s.,** a condition caused by production of adrenocorticotropic hormone by cells outside the pituitary, such as those of carcinoma of the lung; depending on its duration, it may be subtle, resembling true Cushing's disease, but hypokalemic alkalosis and weakness are often prominent.

**ectopic corticotropin-releasing hormone s.,** a disorder clinically indistinguishable from ectopic ACTH syndrome but caused by ectopic secretion of corticotropin-releasing hormone by a variety of tumors, generally bronchial carcinoid tumors.

**ectrodactyly–ectodermal dysplasia–clefting s.,** EEC s.

**Eddowes' s.,** osteogenesis imperfecta, type I.

**Edwards' s.,** trisomy 18 s.

**EEC s.,** a congenital syndrome inherited as an autosomal dominant trait involving both ectodermal and mesodermal tissues, which consists of ectodermal dysplasia associated with hypopigmentation of the skin and hair, scanty hair and eyebrows, absence of lashes, nail dystrophy, hypo- and microdontia, ectrodactyly, and cleft lip and palate. Called also *ectrodactyly–ectodermal dysplasia–clefting s.*

**effort s.,** neurocirculatory asthenia.

**egg drop s.,** a viral disease of ducks and geese, caused by an adenovirus; apparently healthy birds begin laying eggs with thin or soft shells or without shells.

**egg-white s.,** biotin deficiency; see *biotin.*

**Ehlers-Danlos s.,** 1. a group of inherited disorders of the connective tissue, occurring in at least ten types, I to X, based on clinical, genetic, and biochemical evidence, varying in severity from mild to lethal, and transmitted genetically as autosomal recessive, autosomal dominant, or X-linked recessive traits. The major manifestations include hyperextensible skin and joints, easy bruisability, friability of tissues with bleeding and poor wound healing, calcified subcutaneous spheroids, and pseudotumors; variably present in some types are cardiovascular, gastrointestinal, orthopedic, and ocular defects. The biochemical defects are known for several types. *Type IV,* with prominent vascular manifestations, is caused by defects in the structure, synthesis, or secretion of one type of procollagen; *type VI,* with prominent ocular manifestations, is caused by a deficiency of lysyl hydroxylase; *type VII,* with multiple joint dislocations, is called also *arthrochalasis multiplex congenita* and is caused by mutations involving the normal cleavage sites of some procollagen chains; *type IX* is X-linked cutis laxa; and *type X* is due to a defect in fibronectin that interferes with normal platelet aggregation. 2. cutaneous asthenia (def. 1).

**Eisenmenger's s.,** ventricular septal defect with pulmonary hypertension and cyanosis due to right-to-left (reversed) shunt of blood. Sometimes defined as pulmonary hypertension (pulmonary vascular disease) and cyanosis with the shunt being at the atrial, ventricular, or great vessel area.

**Ekbom s.,** restless legs s.

**Ekman's s., Ekman-Lobstein s.,** osteogenesis imperfecta (type I).

**elfin facies s.,** Williams s.

**Ellis-van Creveld s.,** chondroectodermal dysplasia.

**embryonic testicular regression s.,** vanishing testes s.

**EMG s.,** (acronym for *e*xomphalos-*m*acroglossia-*g*igantism) Beckwith-Wiedemann s.

**empty sella s.,** a syndrome diagnosed radiologically in which the diaphragma sellae is vestigial and the enlarged sella turcica forms an extension of the subarachnoid space and is filled with cerebrospinal fluid. The pituitary fossa appears empty, although the pituitary gland is present in a flattened form; pituitary hormone secretion may be normal, deficient, or excessive. Sometimes there is downward herniation of the optic chiasm, which leads to defects in the visual field.

**encephalotrigeminal vascular s.,** Sturge-Weber s.

**eosinophilia-myalgia s.,** a sometimes fatal combined syndrome of eosinophilia and severe generalized myalgia in patients ingesting L-tryptophan, occurring in the absence of infection, neoplasm, or other known causes of eosinophilia; other characteristics may include subjective weakness, fever, arthralgia, shortness of breath, rash, peripheral edema, and pneumonia.

**epiphyseal s.,** precocious development of external genitalia and sexual function, precocious abnormal growth of long bones, appearance of signs of internal hydrocephalus, in the absence of all other motor and sensory symptoms. It has been attributed to pineal body dysfunction and to mechanical effects on the brain caused by tumors of the pineal body. Called also *Pellizzi's s., pineal s.,* and *macrogenitosomia praecox.*

**Epstein's s.,** nephrotic s.

**erythrocyte autosensitization s.,** painful bruising s.

**Escobar s.,** multiple pterygium s.

**euthyroid sick s.,** subnormal levels of triiodothyronine in patients who have systemic illnesses but do not manifest symptoms of hypothyroidism.

**Evans's s.,** acquired hemolytic anemia and thrombocytopenia.

**excited skin s.,** nonspecific cutaneous hyperirritability of the back, sometimes occurring when multiple positive reactions are elicited in patch tests screening a battery of substances. Called also *angry back.*

**exomphalos-macroglossia-gigantism s.,** Beckwith-Wiedemann s.

**extrapyramidal s.,** any of a group of clinical disorders considered to be due to malfunction in the extrapyramidal system and characterized by abnormal involuntary movements; included are parkinsonism, athetosis, and chorea.

**Faber's s.,** hypochromic anemia.

**faciodigitogenital s.,** Aarskog s.

**Fanconi's s.,** 1. a rare recessive disorder with a poor prognosis, characterized by pancytopenia, bone marrow hypoplasia, and patchy brown skin discoloration due to deposition of melanin, as well as multiple congenital anomalies of the musculoskeletal and genitourinary systems. Called also *Fanconi's anemia, pancytopenia,* or *panmyelopathy; congenital hypoplastic anemia; congenital pancytopenia; constitutional infantile panmyelopathy;* and *pancytopenia-dysmelia s.* 2. a general term for a group of diseases marked by dysfunction of the proximal renal tubules, with generalized hyperaminoaciduria, renal glycosuria, hyperphosphaturia, and bicarbonate and water loss; the most common cause is cystinosis (q.v.), but it is also associated with other genetic diseases and occurs in idiopathic and acquired forms. When unassociated with cystinosis, the disorder is also called *de Toni-Fanconi syndrome.*

**Farber s., Farber-Uzman s.,** see under *disease.*

**fat cow s.,** a syndrome seen in overly fat cows just after they have given birth; loss of appetite postpartum leads to mobilization of body fat stores with deposition of fat in the liver and ketosis, sometimes ending in coma and death. Called also *fatty liver disease* and *pregnancy toxemia in cows.*

**Favre-Racouchot s.,** nodular elastosis of Favre and Racouchot.

**feline urological s.,** FUS; dysfunction of the feline lower urinary tract. In male cats there is usually partial or complete obstruction from uroliths or other plugs, and in females there is more often cystitis or urethritis. There may be various causes, including decreased physical activity and excessive dietary magnesium.

**Felty's s.,** a syndrome of splenomegaly with chronic rheumatoid arthritis and leukopenia; there are usually pigmented spots on the skin of the lower extremities, and sometimes there is other evidence of hypersplenism such as anemia or thrombocytopenia.

**feminizing testes s.,** complete androgen resistance; see under *resistance.*

**fertile eunuch s.,** a syndrome of hypogonadotropic hypogonadism, with variable development of secondary sex characters, associated with normal spermatogenesis, normal levels of follicle-stimulating hormone, and variably low levels of luteinizing hormone.

**fetal alcohol s.,** a syndrome of altered prenatal growth and morphogenesis occurring in infants born of women who were chronically alcoholic during pregnancy; it includes maxillary hypoplasia, prominence of the forehead and mandible, short palpebral fissures, microphthalmia, epicanthal folds, severe growth retardation, mental retardation, and microcephaly.

**fetal face s.,** Robinow's s.

**fetal hydantoin s.,** a symptom complex characterized by poor growth and development with craniofacial and skeletal abnormalities, produced by prenatal exposure to hydantoin analogues, including phenytoin.

**Feuerstein-Mims s.,** sebaceous nevus.

**Fèvre-Languepin s.,** popliteal webbing associated with cleft lip and palate, fistula of the lower lip, syndactyly, onychodysplasia, and pes equinovarus. Called also *popliteal pterygium s.*

**FG s.,** an X-linked recessive syndrome of mental retardation, megalencephaly, imperforate anus and other gastrointestinal defects, delayed motor development, congenital hypotonia, characteristic facies and personality, short stature, skeletal anomalies, and congenital cardiac defects.

**Fiessinger-Leroy-Reiter s.,** Reiter's s.

**first arch s.,** anomalies, including macrostomia, hemignathia, and deformities of the external ear, resulting from an inhibitory process occurring toward the seventh week of embryonic life and affecting the facial bones derived from the first pharyngeal (branchial) arch.

**Fisher s.,** 1. a variant of acute idiopathic polyneuritis characterized by areflexia, ataxia, and ophthalmoplegia. Called also *Miller Fisher s.* 2. one-and-a-half s.

**Fitz-Hugh–Curtis s.,** perihepatitis occurring as a complication of gonorrhea or chlamydial infection in women, marked by fever, upper quadrant pain, tenderness and spasm of the abdominal wall, and occasionally by friction rub over the liver.

**floppy infant s.,** a congenital myopathy of infants, characterized clinically by hypotonia and muscle weakness. The pathologic changes in skeletal muscle include numerous eosinophilic intranuclear crystals, characteristic crystal morphology, myofibrillar fragmentation, sarcoplasmic crystals, and expansion of the Z bands.

**floppy valve s.,** mitral valve prolapse s.

**Flynn-Aird s.,** a rare autosomal dominant syndrome with abnormalities of the nervous system and ectodermal structures, including cataracts, retinitis pigmentosa, myopia, dental caries, skin atrophy and ulceration, peripheral neuropathy, ataxia, deafness, and cystic bone changes.

**Foix s.,** cavernous sinus s.

**Foix-Alajouanine s.,** a necrotizing myelopathy characterized by necrosis of the gray matter of the spinal cord, thickening of the walls of the spinal vessels, and abnormal spinal fluid; symptoms include subacute spastic paraplegia of the lower extremities that progresses to flaccid paralysis, often ascending, loss of sphincter control, and progressive sensory loss. Death occurs in one to two years. Called also *subacute necrotic myelitis.*

**folded lung s.,** round atelectasis.

**Forbes-Albright s.,** galactorrhea-amenorrhea syndrome not associated with pregnancy; usually a prolactin-secreting pituitary tumor is present.

**Forsius-Eriksson s.,** an X-linked ocular albinism differing from the Nettleship type in that the males show hypoplastic foveas, axial myopia, and protanomaly and the females show slightly defective color discrimination and latent nystagmus, but no mosaic pigment pattern in the fundus. Called also *Forsius-Eriksson type ocular albinism* and *Åland eye disease.*

**Förster's s., Förster's atonic-astatic s.,** atonic-astatic diplegia.

**Foster Kennedy s.,** Kennedy's s.

**Foville's s.,** a syndrome similar to the Millard-Gubler syndrome, except that, in addition to paralysis of the outward movement of the eye, there is paralysis of conjugate movement.

**fragile X s.,** an X-linked syndrome associated with fragile site on the long arm of the X chromosome at q27.3, associated with mental retardation, enlarged testes, high forehead, and enlarged jaw and ears in most males and mild mental retardation in many heterozygous females. In some families there have been unaffected transmitting males.

**Franceschetti s.,** the complete form of mandibulofacial dysostosis.

**Franceschetti-Jadassohn s.,** an autosomal dominant disorder characterized by the presence of slate-gray to brown reticular pigmentation beginning after infancy without preceding inflammatory changes, and associated with palmoplantar hyperkeratosis, vasomotor changes with hypohidrosis, and yellowing of the dental enamel. Called also *chromatophore nevus of Naegeli, Naegeli syndrome,* and *Naegeli's incontinentia pigmenti.* Cf. *incontinentia pigmenti.*

**François' s.,** oculomandibulofacial s.

**Fraser's s.,** cryptophthalmos s.

**Freeman-Sheldon s.,** craniocarpotarsal dystrophy.

**Frey's s.,** auriculotemporal s.

**Friderichsen-Waterhouse s.,** Waterhouse-Friderichsen s.

**Friedmann's vasomotor s.,** postconcussional s.

**Fröhlich's s.,** adiposogenital dystrophy.

**Froin's s.,** a condition of the lumbar spinal fluid consisting of a transparent clear yellow color (xanthochromia), with the finding of large amounts of protein, rapid coagulation, and the absence of an increased number of cells. It is seen in certain organic nervous diseases in which the lumbar fluid is cut off from communication with the fluid in the ventricles. Called also *loculation s.*

**Frommel-Chiari s.,** Chiari-Frommel s.

**Fuchs' s.,** unilateral heterochromia, fine keratic precipitates, and secondary cataract.

**Fukuhara s.,** MERRF s.

**Fukuyama's s.,** Fukuyama type congenital muscular dystrophy; see under *dystrophy.*

**functional prepubertal castrate s.,** vanishing testes s.

**G s.,** Opitz s.

**Gailliard's s.,** dextrocardia from retraction of lungs and pleura to the right.

**galactorrhea-amenorrhea s.,** amenorrhea and galactorrhea, sometimes associated with increased levels of prolactin; several different types are known. See *Ahumada-del Castillo s., Chiari-Frommel s.,* and *Forbes-Albright s.*

**Ganser s.,** the giving of inappropriate, ridiculous, or approximate answers to questions, sometimes associated with amnesia, disorientation, perceptual disturbances, and conversion symptoms; it is most commonly seen in malingering prisoners feigning psychosis.

**Garcin's s.,** unilateral paralysis of all or most of the cranial nerves due to a tumor at the base of the skull or in the nasopharynx; called also *half base s.*

**Gardner's s.,** familial adenomatous polyposis of the large bowel (with malignant potential), supernumerary teeth, fibrous dysplasia of the skull, osteomas, fibromas, and epithelial cysts.

**Gardner-Diamond s.,** painful bruising s.

**Gasser's s.,** hemolytic uremic s.

**gay bowel s.,** an assortment of sexually transmitted bowel and rectal diseases affecting homosexual males and others who engage in frequent anal intercourse; it is caused by a wide variety of infectious agents.

**Gee-Herter-Heubner s.,** the infantile form of nontropical sprue.

**Gélineau's s.,** narcolepsy.

**gender dysphoria s.,** a group of psychological problems associated with discrepancy between the physical sex assignment and the psychological gender identity.

**general adaptation s.,** a syndrome defined by Hans Selye to include all nonspecific systemic reactions of the body to prolonged exposure to systemic stress; he described three stages in the reacting: the alarm reaction, resistance, and exhaustion.

**genital ulcer s.**, any of the group of diseases causing ulcerations of the genitalia, most commonly syphilis or herpes simplex, but also chancroid, lymphogranuloma venereum, granuloma inguinale, or trauma.

**Gerstmann's s.**, a combination of finger agnosia, right-left disorientation, agraphia, acalculia, and often constructional apraxia; it was formerly attributed to a lesion in the angular gyrus of the dominant hemisphere, but now that etiology is in doubt.

**Gerstmann-Sträussler s., Gerstmann-Sträussler-Scheinker s. (GSS)**, a group of rare prion diseases, of autosomal dominant inheritance but linked to different mutations of the prion protein gene, having the common characteristics of cognitive and motor disturbances and the presence of multicentric amyloid plaques in the brain. In the *ataxic* form, there are progressive cerebellar ataxia and dementia; in the *telencephalic* form, there are dysarthria, dementia, rigidity, tremor, and hyperreflexia; in *GSS with neurofibrillary tangles,* there are progressive short-term memory loss and clumsiness. Death occurs in 1 to 5 years.

**Gianotti-Crosti s.**, a generally benign and self-limited disease of young children representing a primary natural infection with hepatitis B virus, characterized by the appearance of crops of monomorphous, usually nonpruritic, dusky or coppery red, flat-topped, firm papules forming a symmetrical eruption on the face, buttocks, and limbs, including the palms and soles, and associated with malaise, low-grade fever, and few other constitutional symptoms. Called also *acrodermatitis papulosa infantum, infantile papular acrodermatitis,* and *papular acrodermatitis of childhood.*

**giant platelet s.**, Bernard-Soulier s.

**Gilbert s.**, an inborn error of bilirubin metabolism, probably autosomal dominant, a benign elevation of unconjugated bilirubin with no liver damage or hematologic abnormalities. Called also *constitutional hepatic dysfunction, familial cholemia, hyperbilirubinemia I, constitutional hyperbilirubinemia, familial nonhemolytic jaundice,* and *Gilbert cholemia* or *disease.*

**Gilles de la Tourette's s.**, a syndrome comprising both multiple motor and one or more vocal tics, occurring over a period of at least one year, at least intermittently but sometimes as frequently as many times daily. Obsessions, compulsions, hyperactivity, distractibility, and impulsivity are often associated. Onset is in childhood and tics often lessen in severity and frequency and may even remit during adolescence and adulthood. Called also *Gilles de la Tourette's* or *Guinon's disease, maladie des tics,* and *tic de Guinon.*

**Gillespie's s.**, a rare autosomal recessive syndrome consisting of aniridia, cerebellar ataxia, and mental retardation.

**Gitelman's s.**, a syndrome of hypertrophy of juxtaglomerular cells similar to Bartter's syndrome but with hypocalciuria and hypomagnesemia; usually seen in adolescents or adults.

**glioma-polyposis s.**, Turcot's s.

**glucagonoma s.**, the spectrum of symptoms caused by a glucagonoma, associated with high blood levels of glucagon, mild diabetes mellitus, weight loss, anemia, glossitis, stomatitis, angular cheilitis, blepharitis, and necrolytic migrating erythema.

**Goldberg's s.**, galactosialidosis.

**Goldenhar's s.**, oculoauriculovertebral dysplasia.

**Goltz's s., Goltz-Gorlin s.**, focal dermal hypoplasia.

**Good's s.**, immunodeficiency with thymoma.

**Goodman's s.**, acrocephalopolysyndactyly, type IV.

**Goodpasture's s.**, glomerulonephritis associated with pulmonary hemorrhage and circulating antibodies against basement membrane antigens, a condition usually occurring in young men, with rapidly progressing renal failure, hemoptysis, pulmonary infiltrates, and dyspnea. Cf. *anti–glomerular basement membrane antibody disease.*

**Gopalan's s.**, a symptom complex resulting from malnutrition, probably from deficiency of riboflavin or pantothenic acid; it consists of a burning sensation in the extremities, a feeling of "pins and needles" in the distal parts, and hyperhidrosis. Called also *burning feet* and *burning feet s.*

**Gordon's s.**, a type of pseudohypoaldosteronism with hypertension and hyperkalemia but without salt wasting, thought to be due to abnormally increased absorption of chloride by the renal tubules.

**Gorlin's s., Gorlin-Goltz s.**, basal cell nevus s.

**Gougerot-Blum s.**, pigmented purpuric lichenoid dermatitis.

**Gougerot-Carteaud s.**, confluent and reticulated papillomatosis.

**Gougerot-Nulock-Houwer s.**, Sjögren's s.

**Gowers' s.**, 1. vasovagal attack. 2. late distal hereditary myopathy.

**Gradenigo's s.**, paralysis of the abducens nerve and unilateral headache in chronic suppurative otitis media, caused by direct spread of the infection to involve the abducens and trigeminal nerves.

**Graham Little s.**, a syndrome characterized by the presence of cicatricial patches of alopecia of the scalp with prominent follicular plugging and follicular keratoses involving the trunk and extremities, sometimes associated with noncicatricial alopecia of the axillae, pubes, trunk, and extremities.

**gray s.**, a potentially fatal condition seen in neonates, particularly premature infants, due to a reaction to chloramphenicol, characterized by an ashen gray cyanosis, listlessness, weakness, and hypotension.

**gray collie s.**, cyclic neutropenia.

**gray platelet s.**, a rare deficiency of the alpha granules of platelets, resulting in a bleeding disorder that may include ecchymoses, petechiae, and epistaxis from infancy on.

**Greig's s.**, ocular hypertelorism.

**Griscelli s.**, an albinoidism of autosomal recessive inheritance, marked by hypomelanosis, frequent pyogenic infection, hepatosplenomegaly, neutro- and thrombopenia, and possible immunodeficiency. Called also *hypopigmentation-immunodeficiency disease.*

**Grisel's s.**, subluxation of the atlantoaxial joint after an upper respiratory tract infection or an adenoidectomy, usually seen in children.

**Grönblad-Strandberg s.**, angioid streaks in the retina together with pseudoxanthoma elasticum of the skin.

**Gruber's s.**, Meckel's s.

**Guillain-Barré s.**, acute idiopathic polyneuritis.

**Gunn's s.**, unilateral ptosis of the eyelid, with the association of movements of the affected upper eyelid with those of the jaw; called also *Gunn's phenomenon, Marcus Gunn's s.* or *phenomenon,* and *jaw-winking s.* or *phenomenon.*

**gustatory sweating s.**, auriculotemporal s.

**Hadfield-Clarke s.**, Clarke-Hadfield s.

**Hakim's s.**, normal-pressure hydrocephalus.

**half base s.**, Garcin's s.

**Hallermann-Streiff s., Hallermann-Streiff-François s.**, oculomandibulofacial s.

**Hamman's s.**, pneumomediastinum.

**Hamman-Rich s.**, acute interstitial pneumonia.

**hand-arm vibration s.**, Raynaud's phenomenon in people who experience prolonged repetitive hand and arm vibrations.

**hand-foot-and-mouth s.**, see under *disease.*

**hand-foot-uterus s.**, a congenital syndrome consisting of small feet with unusually short great toes, abnormal thumbs, and, in females, duplication of the genital tract.

**Hand-Schüller-Christian s.**, the triad of cranial defects, exophthalmos, and diabetes insipidus sometimes found in multifocal Langerhans cell histiocytosis.

**hand-shoulder s.**, shoulder-hand s.

**Hanhart's s.**, any of several syndromes of variable inheritance, characterized chiefly by severe micrognathia, high nose root, small eyelid fissures, low-set ears, and variable absence of digits or limbs, usually below the elbow or knee.

**Hanot-Chauffard s.**, hypertrophic cirrhosis with pigmentation and diabetes mellitus.

**hantavirus pulmonary s.**, a sometimes fatal febrile illness caused by a hantavirus, characterized by variable respiratory symptoms followed by acute respiratory distress, sometimes progressing to respiratory failure.

**happy puppet s.**, Angelman's s.

**Harada s.**, Vogt-Koyanagi-Harada s.

**HARD s.**, Walker-Warburg s.

**Hare's s.**, Pancoast's s. (def. 1).

**Harris' s.**, hyperinsulinism due to organic endogenous factors, such as insulinoma, manifested by hypoglycemia, weakness, perspiration, jitteriness, tachycardia, mental confusion, and disturbances of vision.

**Hartnup s.**, see under *disease.*

**haw s.**, protrusion of one or both of the nictitating membranes of a dog or cat. Called also *haw.*

**Hay-Wells s.**, an autosomal dominant syndrome of ectodermal dysplasia, cleft lip and palate, and ankyloblepharon filiforme adnatum; it is also characterized by hypodontia, palmar and plantar keratoderma, partial anhidrosis, sparse wiry hair, and sometimes otologic defects. Called also *AEC s.* and *ankyloblepharon–ectodermal dysplasia–clefting s.*

**Hayem-Widal s.**, former name for *hemolytic anemia.*

**heart-hand s.**, Holt-Oram s.

**Hecht s., Hecht-Beals s., Hecht-Beals-Wilson s.**, trismus-pseudocamptodactyly s.

**Heerfordt's s.**, an occasional manifestation of sarcoidosis consisting of enlargement of the parotid and lacrimal glands, anterior uveitis, Bell's palsy, and fever. Called also *Heerfordt's disease* and *uveoparotid fever.*

**Heidenhain's s.**, a rapidly progressive degenerative disease manifested by cortical blindness, presenile dementia, dysarthria, ataxia, athetoid movements, and generalized rigidity.

**HELLP s.**, *h*emolysis, *e*levated *l*iver enzymes, and *l*ow *p*latelet count occurring in association with pre-eclampsia.

**Helweg-Larsen's s.**, an autosomal dominant syndrome consisting of anhidrosis present from birth and labyrinthitis later in life.

**hemangioma-thrombocytopenia s.**, Kasabach-Merritt s.

**hemohistioblastic s.**, reticuloendotheliosis.

**hemolytic uremic s.**, a form of thrombotic microangiopathy with renal failure, hemolytic anemia, and severe thrombocytopenia and purpura, usually seen in children but occurring at any age; some authorities consider it identical to thrombotic thrombocytopenic purpura. Called also *Gasser's s.*

**hemophagocytic s.**, see under *lymphohistiocytosis.*

**hemopleuropneumonic s.**, a syndrome of dyspnea, hemoptysis, tachycardia, fever, pneumonia, and hydrothorax occurring after a puncture wound of the chest.

**Hench-Rosenberg s.**, palindromic rheumatism.

**Henoch-Schönlein s.**, Schönlein-Henoch purpura.

**hepatorenal s.**, functional renal failure, oliguria, and low urinary sodium concentration, without pathological renal changes, associated with cirrhosis and ascites or with obstructive jaundice.

**hereditary benign intraepithelial dyskeratosis s.**, a syndrome characterized by plaques of the bulbar conjunctiva and by oral mucosal thickenings clinically similar to white-folded hypertrophy (white sponge nevus of Cannon); it is inherited as an autosomal dominant trait with a high degree of penetrance.

**Hermansky-Pudlak s.**, an autosomal recessive form of tyrosinase-positive oculocutaneous albinism (ty-pos OCA) with a hemorrhagic diathesis secondary to a platelet defect, and accumulation of a ceroid-like substance in the reticuloendothelial system, oral mucosa, and urine.

**Herrmann's s.**, an autosomal dominant syndrome characterized initially by photomyogenic seizures and progressive deafness, with later development of diabetes mellitus, nephropathy, and mental deterioration progressing to dementia.

**HHH s.**, hyperornithinemia-hyperammonemia-homocitrullinuria s.

**Hick's s.**, hereditary sensory radicular neuropathy.

**Hines-Bannick s.**, intermittent attacks of low temperature and disabling sweating.

**Hinman s.**, a psychogenic disorder seen in children, imitating a neurogenic bladder, consisting of detrusor-sphincter dyssynergia without evidence of any neural lesions. Called also *non-neurogenic neurogenic bladder.*

**Hoffman-Werdnig s.**, Werdnig-Hoffman spinal muscular atrophy.

**holiday heart s.**, paroxysms of arrhythmias, most commonly atrial fibrillation, in patients without overt cardiomyopathy after a weekend bout of alcoholic consumption, especially during the year-end holiday season.

**Holmes-Adie s.**, Adie's s.

**Holt-Oram s.**, autosomal heart disease of varying severity, usually an atrial or ventricular septal defect, associated with skeletal malformation (hypoplastic thumb and short forearm). Called also *heart-hand s.*

**Homén's s.**, postconcussional s.

**honker s.**, a disease of feedlot cattle, of unknown etiology, characterized by edema of the lower trachea with dyspnea and a honking sound during inspiration.

**Horner's s., Horner-Bernard s.**, sinking in of the eyeball, ptosis of the upper eyelid, slight elevation of the lower lid, constriction of the pupil, narrowing of the palpebral fissure, and anhidrosis and flushing of the affected side of the face; caused by a brain stem lesion on the ipsilateral side that interrupts descending sympathetic nerves. See also *Horner's ptosis.* Called also *Bernard's s.* or *Bernard-Horner s.*

**Horton's s.**, 1. cluster headache. 2. giant cell arteritis.

**Howel-Evans' s.**, diffuse palmoplantar keratoderma occurring between the ages of 5 and 15 and associated with the development of esophageal cancer later in life.

**Hughes-Stovin s.**, thrombosis of the pulmonary arteries and peripheral veins, characterized by headache, fever, cough, papilledema, and hemoptysis.

**hungry bone s.**, a condition seen after parathyroidectomy in patients who had had hyperparathyroidism; rapid deposition of calcium in bones leads to hypocalcemia.

**Hunt's s.**, Ramsay Hunt s.

**Hunter's s.**, a mucopolysaccharidosis caused by deficiency of iduronate-2-sulfatase, characterized by excretion of dermatan sulfate and heparan sulfate in the urine, and differing clinically from Hurler's syndrome by (1) X-linked inheritance; (2) slower progression, less severity, and longer survival (thus resembling the Hurler-Scheie syndrome); and (3) absence of corneal clouding. Two clinical forms exist: the severe form has Hurler-Scheie–like symptoms with death before 15, usually from heart disease; the mild form has onset in the first decade, reduced somatic involvement, and near-normal intelligence and lifespan. Called also *mucopolysaccharidosis II.*

**Hurler's s.**, the prototype of the mucopolysaccharidoses, and the gravest of the three allelic disorders of mucopolysaccharidosis I, specifically marked by corneal clouding and death by age 10. It is caused by deficiency of L-iduronidase, and onset is after the first year with progressive physical and mental deterioration. Further symptoms include gargoyle-like facies with hypertelorism, depressed nasal bridge, large tongue, and widely spaced teeth; dwarfism; severe somatic and skeletal changes, including short neck and trunk, scaphocephaly, and kyphosis with gibbus; short broad hands with short fingers; progressive opacities of the cornea; deafness; cardiovascular defects; hepatosplenomegaly; and joint contractures. Death is usually caused by respiratory infection and heart failure. Called also *mucopolysaccharidosis IH.*

**Hurler-Scheie s.**, one of the three allelic disorders of mucopolysaccharidosis I, with clinical features intermediate between the Hurler and the Scheie syndromes, caused by deficiency of L-iduronidase, and specifically characterized by receding chin (micrognathism). Symptoms include mental retardation, dwarfism, dysostosis multiplex, corneal clouding, deafness, hernia, stiff joints (claw hand), and valvular heart disease. Patients survive until their late teens or twenties. Called also *mucopolysaccharidosis I H/S.*

**Hutchinson's s.**, see under *triad.*

**Hutchinson-Gilford s.**, progeria.

**Hutchison s.**, neuroblastoma with metastases to the skull.

**17-hydroxylase deficiency s.**, 17$\alpha$-hydroxylase deficiency; see under *H.*

**hyperabduction s.**, a thoracic outlet syndrome due to compression of the brachial plexus trunk roots and axillary vessels by the pectoralis minor muscle and the coracoid process when the arms are stretched above the head, as during sleep. Called also *Wright's s.*

**hyperactive child s.**, former name for *attention-deficit/hyperactivity disorder.*

**hypercalcemia s.**, milk-alkali s.

**hypereosinophilic s.**, any of several diseases characterized by a massive increase in the number of eosinophils in the blood and bone marrow, with eosinophilic infiltration of other organs. Symptoms vary, depending on the organ involved, and may include pruritic skin ulcers or erythroderma, endomyocarditis, lymph node or spleen enlargement, and ophthalmologic or gastrointestinal complications. Eosinophilic leukemia is a potentially fatal member of the group.

**hyperimmunoglobulinemia E s.**, a primary immunodeficiency disorder characterized by recurrent staphylococcal abscesses of skin, lungs, joints, and other sites, pruritic dermatitis, very high serum IgE levels, normal levels of IgG, IgA, and IgM, blood and sputum eosinophilia, low anamnestic antibody responses to booster immunization, and poor antibody and cell-mediated responses to neoantigens. Called also *Buckley's s.*

**hyperkinetic s.**, former name for *attention-deficit/hyperactivity disorder.*

**hyperkinetic heart s.**, increased cardiac output of unknown cause associated with slightly elevated systolic and pulse pressures, normal mean arterial pressure, and low systemic vascular resistance.

**hyperlucent lung s.**, a syndrome simulating localized emphysema, but due to congenital absence or hypoplasia of pulmonary arteries; there may be lobar or segmental agenesis, as well as accessory lungs, lobes, or segments.

**hyperornithinemia-hyperammonemia-homocitrullinuria s.**, an autosomal recessive syndrome characterized by elevated plasma levels of ornithine, postprandial hyperammonemia and homocitrullinuria, and aversion to protein ingestion. It is believed to result from a defect in the transport of ornithine into mitochondria, which disturbs the cycle of ureagenesis. Called also *HHH s.*

**hypersomnia-bulimia s.**, Kleine-Levin s.

**hypertelorism-hypospadias s.**, Opitz s.

**hyperventilation s.**, a complex of symptoms that accompany hypocapnia caused by hyperventilation, including palpitations, shortness of breath, lightheadedness, profuse perspiration, and tingling sensations in the fingertips, face, or toes; prolonged overbreathing may result in vasomotor collapse and loss of consciousness. Hyperventilation unrecognized by the patient is a common cause of the subjective somatic symptoms associated with chronic anxiety or panic attacks.

**hyperviscosity s.**, any of various syndromes associated with increased viscosity of the blood. One type is due to serum hyperviscosity and is characterized by spontaneous bleeding with neurologic and ocular disorders. Another type is characterized by polycythemia with retarded blood flow, organ congestion, reduced capillary perfusion, and increased cardiac effort. A third group includes conditions in which the deformability of erythrocytes is impaired, such as sickle cell anemia.

**hypoglossia-hypodactyly s.**, a rare syndrome consisting of partial to complete absence of the tongue and of the digits or one or more limbs. Called also *aglossia-adactylia s.*

**hypoplastic left heart s. (HLHS)**, any of a group of congenital anomalies consisting of hypoplasia or atresia of the left ventricle and of the aortic or mitral valve or both and hypoplasia of the ascending aorta; it is characterized by respiratory distress and extreme cyanosis, with cardiac failure and death in early infancy.

**hypothenar hammer s.**, traumatic aneurysm of the ulnar artery at the hypothenar in persons who repeatedly use the hypothenar to push or pound.

**hypotonic s's**, a group of syndromes involving inadequate water excretion in comparison to the amount ingested, so that body fluids become hypotonic and hyponatremic; some are due to excessive water intake as in water intoxication, while others are caused by derangements of the excretory process such as the vasopressin excess in the syndrome of inappropriate diuretic hormone or complications of the nephrotic syndrome, congestive heart failure, or kidney failure.

**idiopathic postprandial s.**, the repeated occurrence of the clinical manifestations of hypoglycemia after meals; a controversial disease entity.

**Imerslund s., Imerslund-Graesbeck s.**, a rare familial form of megaloblastic anemia, usually transmitted as an autosomal recessive trait, characterized by selective intestinal malabsorption of vitamin $B_{12}$ uninfluenced by intrinsic factor, and associated with proteinuria and structural genitourinary tract anomalies.

**immotile cilia s.**, primary ciliary dyskinesia.

**impingement s.**, the progressive pathologic changes resulting from mechanical encroachment of the acromion, coracoacromial ligament, coracoid process, or acromioclavicular joint on the rotator cuff, including reversible edema and hemorrhage, fibrosis, tendinitis, pain, bone spur formation, and tendon rupture.

**s. of inappropriate antidiuretic hormone (SIADH)**, persistent hyponatremia, hypovolemia, and inappropriately elevated urine osmolality, associated with the release of vasopressin in amounts excessive for the state of hydration. Causes include ADH-secreting tumor cells, neoplasms (especially oat cell carcinoma of the lung or pancreatic carcinoma), pulmonary disorders, and central nervous system diseases, including head trauma.

**inferior s. of red nucleus**, Claude's s.

**inhibitory s.**, the manifestations produced by a somatostatinoma, including diabetes mellitus, cholecystolithiasis, steatorrhea, indigestion, hypochlorhydria, and occasionally anemia.

**inspissated bile s.**, biliary obstruction caused by plugging of the outflow tract.

**intrauterine parabiotic s.**, placental transfusion; see under *transfusion.*

**irritable bowel s., irritable colon s.**, a chronic noninflammatory disease characterized by abdominal pain, altered bowel habits consisting of diarrhea or constipation or both, and no detectable pathologic change; a variant form is characterized by painless diarrhea. It is a common disorder with a psychophysiologic basis. Called also *spastic* or *irritable colon.*

**Irukandji s.**, a clinical syndrome observed in Queensland, Australia, due to stinging by the jellyfish *Carukia barnesi;* symptoms include initial neuromuscular paralysis that can be fatal, and in survivors systemic symptoms with pulmonary edema and skin ulcers at the site of infection.

**Isaacs' s., Isaacs-Mertens s.**, progressive muscle stiffness and spasms, with continuous muscle fiber activity similar to that seen with neuromyotonia.

**Ivemark's s.**, congenital splenic agenesis, cardiac defects, and partial situs inversus viscerum; called also *asplenia s.* and *Polhemus-Schafer-Ivemark s.*

**IVIC s.**, a rare autosomal dominant syndrome of internal ophthalmoplegia, hearing impairment, and radial ray defects varying from a long slender thumb to deformity of an entire upper limb, first observed in Venezuela and later in Italy. Called also *oculo-oto-radial s.*

**Jaccoud's s.**, chronic arthritis occurring after rheumatic fever, usually after repeated attacks, and characterized by fibrous changes in the joint capsules and tendons, leading to deformities that may resemble rheumatoid arthritis (especially ulnar deviation of fingers); the joints may be painful and rheumatic nodules are often present, but erosion of bone does not take place. Called also *Jaccoud's arthritis.*

**Jackson's s.**, paralysis of structures innervated by the tenth, eleventh, and twelfth cranial nerves, including the soft palate, larynx, half of the tongue, and the sternomastoid and trapezius muscles. Called also *ambiguo-accessorius-hypoglossal paralysis, Mackenzie's s.,* and *vagoaccessory-hypoglossal s.*

**Jacod's s.**, unilateral blindness and ophthalmoplegia with facial hemiplegia or trigeminal neuralgia as a result of damage to the second, third, fourth, fifth, and sixth cranial nerves, often from a tumor or other lesion just behind the sphenoid bone. Called also *Jacod's triad, Negri-Jacod s.,* and *petrosphenoid s.*

**Jadassohn-Lewandowsky s.**, pachyonychia congenita.

**Jahnke's s.**, a variant of Sturge-Weber syndrome in which glaucoma is absent.

**Janz s.**, juvenile myoclonic epilepsy.

**Jarcho-Levin s.**, an autosomal recessive disorder consisting of multiple vertebral defects, short thorax, rib abnormalities, camptodactyly, and syndactyly; urogenital abnormalities are sometimes present. Death, from respiratory insufficiency, usually occurs in infancy. Called also *spondylothoracic dysplasia.*

**jaw-winking s.**, Gunn's s.

**Jefferson's s.**, cavernous sinus s.

**jejunal s.**, dumping s.

**Jervell and Lange-Nielsen s.**, an autosomal recessive form of the long QT syndrome, characterized by neural deafness and syncope, and sometimes ventricular fibrillation and sudden death. Cf. *Romano-Ward s.*

**Jeune's s.**, asphyxiating thoracic dystrophy.

**Job's s.**, an autosomal recessive disorder of neutrophils, characterized by the presence of abnormal or absent chemotactic responses, which leads to repeated development of cold staphylococcal abscesses and eczema, and by hyperimmunoglobulinemia E. It is usually associated with red hair and fair skin. Most cases reported have been in girls.

**Joubert's s.**, an autosomal recessive syndrome consisting of partial or complete agenesis of the cerebellar vermis, with hypotonia, episodic hyperpnea, mental retardation, and abnormal eye movements; most patients die in infancy.

**jugular foramen s.**, Vernet's s.

**jumping Frenchmen of Maine s.**, a form of jumping disease observed in a group of lumbermen of French-Canadian descent working in a remote area of Maine; affected individuals had exaggerated startle responses, automatic obedience, and often echolalia. It is believed to have represented a form of operant conditioning rather than a true disease.

**juvenile polyposis s.**, juvenile intestinal polyposis.

**Kabuki make-up s.**, a congenital, possibly inherited, syndrome of mental retardation, dwarfism, scoliosis, peculiar facies resembling the makeup of Japanese actors of Kabuki, and frequently cardiovascular abnormalities.

**Kallmann's s.**, hypogonadotropic hypogonadism caused by failure of fetal gonadotropin-releasing hormone neurons to migrate to the thalamus. It is usually associated with anosmia or hyposmia.

**Kanner's s.**, autistic disorder.

**Kartagener's s.**, a hereditary disorder involving a combination of dextrocardia (situs inversus), bronchiectasis, and sinusitis, transmitted as an autosomal recessive trait.

**Kasabach-Merritt s.**, a blood disorder usually occurring in the first few months of life in which severe thrombocytopenia and other evidence of intravascular coagulation are accompanied by rapidly expanding hemangiomas of the trunk, extremities, and abdominal viscera, sometimes associated with bleeding and anemia. Bleeding is thought to be due to trapping and destruction of platelets within the tumor and depletion of circulating clotting factors. Called also *hemangioma-thrombocytopenia s.*

**Kast's s.**, Maffucci's s.

**Kaufman-McKusick s.**, a rare autosomal recessive disorder of hydrometrocolpos accompanied by postaxial polydactyly, congenital cardiac defects, and sometimes subsequent bilateral hydronephrosis. Manifestations in males include hypospadias and prominent scrotal raphe. Called also *McKusick-Kaufman s.*

**Kearns-Sayre s.**, progressive ophthalmoplegia, pigmentary degeneration of the retina, myopathy, ataxia, and cardiac conduction defect; onset is before age 20. Almost all patients have large mitochondrial DNA deletions, and ragged red fibers are seen on muscle biopsy. Called also *ophthalmoplegia plus.*

**Kennedy's s.**, retrobulbar optic neuritis, central scotoma, optic atrophy on the side of the lesion and papilledema on the opposite side, occurring in tumors of the frontal lobe of the brain which press downward.

**keratitis-ichthyosis-deafness s.**, Senter s.

**Key-Gaskell s.**, feline dysautonomia.

**KID s.**, Senter s.

**Kiloh-Nevin s.**, 1. ocular myopathy in patients with ptosis and progressive external ophthalmoplegia. 2. anterior interosseous s.

**Kimmelstiel-Wilson s.**, the nodular type of intercapillary glomerulosclerosis.

**King s.**, a form of malignant hyperthermia (q.v.) in which patients also exhibit characteristic physical abnormalities including short stature, characteristic facies, kyphoscoliosis, pectus carinatum, cryptorchidism, delayed motor development, progressive myopathy, and cardiovascular structural defects.

**kinky-hair s.**, Menkes' s.

**Kinsbourne s.**, myoclonic encephalopathy of childhood; see under *encephalopathy.*

**kleeblattschädel s.**, a congenital disorder, characterized by synostosis of multiple or all cranial sutures, hydrocephalus, and in some cases facial dysostosis and long bone anomalies.

**Klein-Waardenburg s.**, Waardenburg's s. (def. 2).

**Kleine-Levin s.**, episodic periods of excessive sleep and overeating lasting for several weeks, with amnesia for the attacks; it usually occurs in adolescent boys.

**Klinefelter's s.**, a syndrome in males characterized by small testes, hyalinization of seminiferous tubules, azoospermia, variable degrees of masculinization, and increased urinary excretion of gonadotropin; patients tend to be tall, with long legs, and about half have gynecomastia. It is associated typically with an XXY chromosome complement, although variants include XXYY, XXXY, XXXXY, and several mosaic patterns. Called also *seminiferous tubule dysgenesis* and *XXY s.*

**Klippel-Feil s.**, a condition characterized by shortness of the neck resulting from reduction in the number of cervical vertebrae or the fusion of multiple hemivertebrae into one osseous mass; the hairline is low and motion of the neck is limited.

**Klippel-Trénaunay s., Klippel-Trénaunay-Weber s.**, a rare condition usually affecting one extremity, characterized by hypertrophy of the bone and related soft tissues, large cutaneous hemangiomas, persistent nevus flammeus (see *port-wine stain,* under *stain*), and skin varices.

**Klumpke-Dejerine s.**, Klumpke's paralysis.

**Klüver-Bucy s.**, bizarre behavior disturbances seen in monkeys following experimental bilateral temporal lobectomy which destroys important limbic structures; reported in humans after large injuries, usually from trauma, affecting the undersurface of the anterior temporal lobes. It is characterized by a tendency to examine objects orally, depression of drive and emotional reactions, hypermetamorphosis, and lack of sexual inhibitions.

**Kocher-Debré-Sémélaigne s.**, Debré-Sémélaigne s.

**Koerber-Salus-Elschnig s.**, sylvian s.

**König's s.**, constipation alternating with diarrhea and attended with abdominal pain, meteorism, and gurgling sounds in the right iliac fossa.

**Korsakoff's s.**, a syndrome of anterograde and retrograde amnesia with confabulation associated with alcoholic or nonalcoholic polyneuritis described as "cerebropathia psychica toxemica" by Korsakoff; currently used synonymously with the term amnestic syndrome or, more narrowly, to refer to the amnestic component of the Wernicke-Korsakoff syndrome, i.e., an amnestic syndrome resulting from thiamine deficiency. Spelled also *Korsakov's s.* Called also *Korsakoff's psychosis.*

**Kostmann's s.**, infantile genetic agranulocytosis.

**Krause's s.**, a retinal and cerebral dysplasia found in premature infants several months after birth, characterized by malformations of the choroid, retina, and optic nerve, and possible blindness, cataract, coloboma, glaucoma, and microphthalmos. Cerebral symptoms include aplasia, hyperplasia, and hypertrophy of the brain, hydrocephaly, microcephaly, and mental retardation. Called also *encephalo-ophthalmic dysplasia.*

**Kugelberg-Welander s.**, a hereditary form of spinal muscular atrophy, usually transmitted as an autosomal recessive trait, due to lesions of the anterior horns of the spinal cord. Onset is in the first or second decade, principally between two and seventeen years, with atrophy and weakness of the proximal muscles of the lower extremities and pelvic girdle, followed by involvement of the distal muscles and muscular twitchings. Cf. *Werdnig-Hoffmann spinal muscular atrophy.* Called also *juvenile* or *proximal spinal muscular atrophy* and *Wohlfart-Kugelberg-Welander s.*

**Kunkel's s.**, lupoid hepatitis.

**Ladd's s.**, congenital obstruction of the duodenum due to peritoneal bands *(Ladd's bands)* resulting from a malrotated cecum.

**LAMB s.**, a syndrome of familial myxomas with cutaneous, cardiac, and endocrine involvement, manifested as *l*entigines, *a*trial *m*yxoma, and *b*lue nevi. Cf. *NAME s.*

**Lambert-Eaton s., Lambert-Eaton myasthenic s. (LEMS)**, Eaton-Lambert s.

**Landau-Kleffner s.**, an epileptic syndrome of childhood characterized by partial or generalized seizures, psychomotor abnormalities, and aphasia progressing to mutism. The electroencephalogram from bilateral temporal regions is abnormal, with spikes like those of benign rolandic epilepsy. Called also *acquired epileptic aphasia.*

**Landry's s.**, acute idiopathic polyneuritis.

**Langer-Giedion s.**, an inherited disorder characterized by mental retardation, microcephaly, multiple exostosis, characteristic facies with bulbous nose, sparse hair, cone shaped epiphyses, loose redundant skin, joint laxity, and other anomalies.

**Lannois-Gradenigo s.**, Gradenigo's s.

**Laron s.**, an autosomal recessive syndrome of skeletal growth retardation due to impaired inability to synthesize insulin-like growth factor I, usually because of growth hormone receptor defects. Called also *Laron dwarfism.*

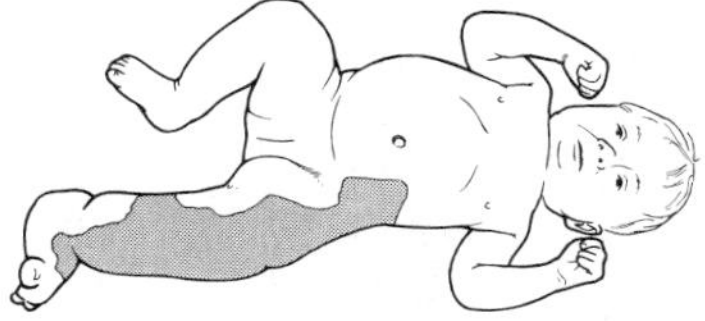

Klippel-Trénaunay-Weber syndrome.

**Larsen's s.**, cleft palate, flattened facies, multiple congenital dislocations, and foot deformities.

**lateral medullary s.**, Wallenberg's s.

**Laubry-Soulle s.**, abnormal localized collections of gas in the colon (splenic flexure) and stomach following acute myocardial infarction.

**Launois' s.**, pituitary gigantism.

**Laurence-Moon s.**, an autosomal recessive disorder characterized by mental retardation, pigmentary retinopathy, hypogonadism, and spastic paraplegia; cf. *Bardet-Biedl s.* and *Biemond s., II.*

**Lawrence-Seip s.**, total lipodystrophy.

**lazy leukocyte s.**, a syndrome of unknown etiology, usually seen in children, marked by recurrent low-grade infections, associated with a defect in neutrophil chemotaxis and deficient random mobility of neutrophils.

**Legg-Calvé-Perthes s.**, osteochondrosis of the capital epiphysis.

**Lemierre s.**, thrombophlebitis of the internal jugular vein with secondary spread of infection, resulting from an acute oropharyngeal infection. Called also *postanginal sepsis.*

**Lemieux-Neemeh s.**, an autosomal dominant syndrome consisting of Charcot-Marie-Tooth disease with progressive deafness.

**Lennox s., Lennox-Gastaut s.**, an atypical form of absence epilepsy characterized by diffuse slow spike waves, often with atonic, tonic, or clonic seizures and mental retardation; there may also be other neurological abnormalities or multiple seizure types. Unlike typical absence epilepsy, it may persist into adulthood. Called also *petit mal variant.*

**Lenz's s.**, a hereditary syndrome, transmitted as an X-linked trait, consisting of microphthalmia or anophthalmos, unilateral or bilateral, and digital anomalies; narrow shoulders, double thumbs, and other skeletal abnormalities; dental, urogenital, and cardiovascular defects may also occur.

**LEOPARD s.**, a hereditary syndrome transmitted as an autosomal dominant trait, consisting of multiple lentigines, asymptomatic cardiac defects, and typical coarse facies; it may also be associated with pulmonary stenosis, sensorineural deafness, skeletal changes, ocular hypertelorism, and abnormalities of the genitalia. Called also *multiple lentigines s.*

**Leredde's s.**, severe dyspnea on exertion, combined with advanced emphysema and recurrent attacks of acute febrile bronchitis; seen in children with congenital syphilis.

**Leriche's s.**, a syndrome caused by obstruction of the terminal aorta, usually occurring in males and characterized by fatigue in the hips, thighs, or calves on exercising, absence of pulsation in the femoral arteries, and impotence, and often pallor and coldness of the lower extremities.

**Lermoyez's s.**, tinnitus and hearing loss preceding an attack of vertigo and then subsiding after the vertigo has become established. Cf. *Meniere's disease.*

**Lesch-Nyhan s.**, a rare X-linked disorder of purine metabolism due to deficient hypoxanthine phosphoribosyltransferase, characterized by physical and mental retardation, compulsive self-mutilation of the fingers and lips by biting, choreoathetosis, spastic cerebral palsy, impaired renal function; and by excessive purine synthesis and consequent hyperuricemia and uricaciduria.

**lethal multiple pterygium s.**, a lethal autosomal recessive disorder characterized by multiple pterygia, lung hypoplasia, flexion contractures of the limbs, characteristic facies, and other abnormalities.

**levator s.**, episodic pain and a sensation of fullness and pressure in the rectum and sacrococcygeal area; attributed to spasm of the levator ani muscle.

**Lévy-Roussy s.**, Roussy-Lévy s.

**Leyden-Möbius s.**, limb-girdle muscular dystrophy; see under *dystrophy.*

**Li-Fraumeni s.**, a familial syndrome of early breast carcinoma associated with soft tissue sarcomas and other tumors.

**Lichtheim's s.**, subacute combined degeneration of spinal cord; see under *degeneration.*

**licking s.**, a form of pica in cattle in which they lick their own or each other's hair and skin, or other surfaces; it is often due to dietary deficiency of copper or sodium.

**Liddle's s.**, a rare autosomal dominant syndrome characterized by hypertension with excessive renal reabsorption of sodium, depletion of potassium, and low activity of renin and aldosterone. Cf. *pseudoprimary aldosteronism.*

**Lightwood's s.**, renal tubular acidosis.

**Lignac's s., Lignac-Fanconi s.**, 1. Fanconi's s. (def. 2). 2. cystinosis.

**linear sebaceous nevus s.**, sebaceous nevus.

**lissencephaly s.**, Miller-Dieker s.

**liver-kidney s.**, hepatorenal s.

**Lobstein's s.**, osteogenesis imperfecta (type I).

**locked-in s.**, quadriplegia and mutism with intact consciousness and the preservation of voluntary vertical eye movements and blinking; usually due to a vascular lesion of the pars ventralis pontis. Called also *coma vigil, de-efferented state,* and *pseudocoma.* Cf. *akinetic mutism.*

**loculation s.,** Froin's s.

**Löffler's s.,** transient infiltrations of the lungs accompanied by cough, fever, dyspnea, and eosinophilia; it may be idiopathic or due to infestation by parasites (particularly *Ascaris lumbricoides*), infection, or drug therapy. See also *Ascaris pneumonitis,* under *pneumonitis.* Called also *Löffler's eosinophilia* or *pneumonia* and *simple pulmonary eosinophilia.*

**Löfgren's s.,** erythema nodosum in conjunction with bilateral adenopathy of hilar lymph nodes, seen as a manifestation of sarcoidosis.

**long QT s.,** prolongation of the Q–T interval combined with torsades de pointes and manifest as several different forms; it may be acquired, usually due to metabolic or cardiac abnormality or to drug administration, or congenital, occurring either with deafness *(Jervell and Lange-Nielsen syndrome)* or without *(Romano-Ward syndrome).* It may lead to serious arrhythmia and sudden cardiac death.

**Looser-Milkman s.,** Milkman's s.

**Lorain-Lévi s.,** hypophysial infantilism.

**Louis-Bar's s.,** ataxia-telangiectasia.

**low cardiac output s.,** see *low-output heart failure,* under *failure.*

**Lowe s., Lowe-Terrey-MacLachlan s.,** oculocerebrorenal s.

**lower radicular s.,** Klumpke's paralysis.

**Lown-Ganong-Levine s.,** a preexcitation syndrome of electrocardiographic abnormality characterized by a short P–R interval with a normal QRS complex, accompanied by atrial tachycardia.

**Lucey-Driscoll s.,** a syndrome of retention jaundice due to defective bilirubin conjugation, occurring in infants; apparently the result of an unidentified factor, presumably a steroid in maternal blood, transmitted to the infant.

**lupus-like s.,** see *systemic lupus erythematosus,* under *lupus.*

**Lutembacher's s.,** atrial septal defect associated with mitral stenosis. Called also *Lutembacher's complex.*

**Lyell's s.,** toxic epidermal necrolysis.

**lymphadenopathy s.,** a condition seen in male homosexuals in the 1980s, characterized by the presence of unexplained lymphadenopathy for 3 or more months involving extrainguinal sites, which on biopsy reveal nonspecific lymphoid hyperplasia; considered by some authorities to be a prodrome of acquired immune deficiency syndrome. See also *AIDS-related complex,* under *complex.*

**lymphoproliferative s's,** see under *disorder.*

**lymphoreticular s's,** see under *disorder.*

**McCune-Albright s.,** Albright's s.

**Mackenzie's s.,** Jackson's s.

**McKusick-Kaufman s.,** Kaufman-McKusick s.

**McLeod s.,** a syndrome seen in some individuals having the McLeod phenotype of blood, characterized by mild hemolytic anemia with acanthocytes, elevated serum creatinine phosphokinase, and sometimes muscle wasting and neurological defects. A few cases have manifested as X-linked types of chronic granulomatous disease.

**Macleod's s.,** Swyer-James s.

**Maffucci's s.,** enchondromatosis associated with multiple cutaneous or visceral hemangiomas. Called also *Kast's s.*

**malabsorption s.,** a group of disorders in which there is subnormal absorption of dietary constituents, and thus excessive loss of nonabsorbed substances in the stool; the malabsorption may be due to an intraluminal (digestive) defect (e.g., pancreatic insufficiency), a mucosal abnormality (celiac disease or disaccharidase deficiency), or a lymphatic obstruction (intestinal lymphangiectasia). Unless there is a specific enzyme or transport defect, steatorrhea is usually present. Deficiency syndromes may result from excessive loss of vitamins, electrolytes, iron, calcium, etc.

**malarial hyperreactive spleen s.,** a syndrome of massive splenomegaly, hepatomegaly, anemia, and elevated serum IgM levels that occurs in some areas where malaria is endemic, such as parts of sub-Saharan Africa and New Guinea. Lymphocytic infiltrates are present in hepatic sinusoids, and the association with chronic malarial infection is suggested by a polyclonal increase in IgM, a very high titer of IgM antibodies to *Plasmodium falciparum,* and often by a therapeutic response to malarial chemoprophylaxis. Called also *tropical splenomegaly* and *tropical splenomegaly s.*

**Mallory-Weiss s.,** hematemesis or melena that follows typically upon many hours or days of severe vomiting and retching, traceable to one or several slitlike lacerations of the gastric mucosa, longitudinally placed at or slightly below the esophagogastric junction.

**manic s.,** mania.

**Marchesani's s.,** Weill-Marchesani s.

**Marchiafava-Micheli s.,** paroxysmal nocturnal hemoglobinuria; see under *hemoglobinuria.*

**Marcus Gunn's s.,** Gunn's s.

**Marfan s.,** one of the manifestations of abnormal fibrillin metabolism, a congenital disorder of connective tissue characterized by abnormal length of the extremities, especially of fingers and toes, subluxation of the lens, cardiovascular abnormalities (commonly dilatation of the ascending aorta), and other deformities. It is an autosomal dominant disorder with variable degree of expression.

**Marie-Bamberger s.,** hypertrophic pulmonary osteoarthropathy.

**Marinesco-Sjögren s.,** a hereditary syndrome transmitted as an autosomal recessive trait, consisting of cerebellar ataxia, mental and somatic growth retardation, congenital cataracts, inability to chew, thin brittle fingernails, and sparse, incompletely keratinized hair.

**Maroteaux-Lamy s.,** a mucopolysaccharidosis caused by deficiency of *N*-acetylgalactosamine-4-sulfatase (arylsulfatase B), and characterized biochemically by the predominance of dermatan sulfate in the urine and the presence of coarse metachromatic granules in the leukocytes, and clinically by Hurler-like signs with normal intelligence. There are three clinical forms: the severe or classic form shows Hurler-like symptoms; the intermediate form has the same phenotype as mucolipidosis III (pseudo-Hurler polydystrophy); the mild form is difficult to distinguish from the Scheie syndrome. Called also *mucopolysaccharidosis VI* and *arylsulfatase B (ARSB) deficiency.*

**Martin-Bell s.,** fragile X s.

**Martorell's s.,** Takayasu's arteritis.

**mastocytosis s.,** an episodic syndrome occurring in certain patients with systemic mastocytosis, usually those with skin lesions, bone lesions, and hepatosplenomegaly, presumably associated with histamine release from degranulation of mast cells, and characterized mainly by intense pruritus, flushing, headache, tachycardia, hypotension, and syncope.

**maternal deprivation s.,** failure to thrive with severe growth retardation, unresponsiveness to the environment, depression, retarded mental and emotional development, and behavioral problems resulting from loss, absence, or neglect of the mother or other primary caregiver.

**Mauriac s.,** dwarfism, hepatomegaly, obesity, and retarded sexual maturation, in association with diabetes mellitus.

**May-White s.,** a rare autosomal dominant syndrome of myoclonus, cerebellar ataxia, and deafness.

**Mayer-Rokitansky-Küster-Hauser s.,** lack of müllerian development, congenital absence of the vagina and a rudimentary uterus (typically bicornuate remnants), with normal uterine tubes, ovaries, and secondary female sex characteristics and normal growth. Called also *Rokitansky-Küster-Hauser s.*

**Meckel's s., Meckel-Gruber s.,** a hereditary syndrome, transmitted as an autosomal recessive trait, most frequently characterized by sloping forehead, posterior meningoencephalocele, polydactyly, and polycystic kidneys, with death occurring in the perinatal period. Called also *Gruber's s.* and *dysencephalia splanchnocystica.*

**meconium aspiration s.,** the respiratory complications resulting from the passage and aspiration of meconium prior to or during delivery. Postterm infants and hypoxic or acidotic fetuses are at higher risk.

**meconium plug s.,** a syndrome of intestinal obstruction caused by unusually thick or hard meconium in which neither enzymatic nor ganglion cell deficiency can be demonstrated.

**median cleft facial s.,** a hereditary form of defective midline development of the head and face, including ocular hypertelorism, occult cleft nose and maxilla, and sometimes mental retardation or other defects. Called also *frontonasal dysplasia.*

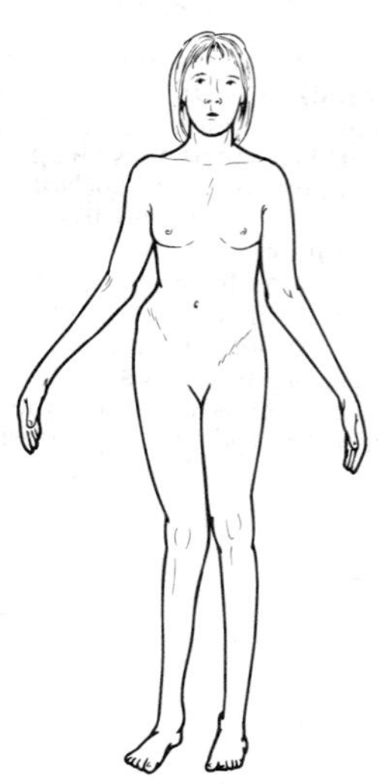

Marfan syndrome.

**megacystis-megaureter s.,** chronic ureteral dilatation (megaureter) associated with hypotonia and dilatation of the bladder (megacystis) and gaping of ureteral orifices, permitting vesicoureteral reflux of urine, and resulting in chronic pyelonephritis.

**megacystis-microcolon–intestinal hypoperistalsis s. (MMIHS),** dilated bladder, microcolon with dilated small intestine, and hypoperistalsis, inherited as an autosomal dominant trait.

**Meige's s.,** 1. Milroy's disease. 2. dystonia of facial and oromandibular muscles with blepharospasm, grimacing mouth movements, and protrusion of the tongue, usually occurring in older women. Called also *Brueghel's s.*

**Meigs' s., Meigs-Salmon s.,** ascites and hydrothorax associated with ovarian fibroma or other pelvic tumor.

**MELAS s.,** *m*itochondrial *e*ncephalopathy, *l*actic *a*cidosis, and *s*troke-like episodes; a familial syndrome, of maternal (mitochondrial) inheritance.

**Melkersson's s., Melkersson-Rosenthal s.,** an autosomal dominant condition usually beginning in childhood or adolescence, characterized chiefly by chronic noninflammatory facial swelling, usually confined to the lips in the form of *granulomatous cheilitis,* with recurrent facial palsy and sometimes fissured tongue. Associated ophthalmic symptoms may include lagophthalmos, blepharochalasis, swollen eyelids, burning sensation of the eyes, corneal opacities, retrobulbar neuritis, and exophthalmos.

**Mendelson's s.,** pulmonary acid aspiration s.

**Mengert's shock s.,** a condition resembling shock that sometimes occurs when pregnant women in the late antepartum period lie in the supine position; it is due to the pressure of the uterus on the vena cava.

**Meniere's s.,** see under *disease.*

**Menkes' s.,** a hereditary abnormality in copper absorption; the resultant copper poisoning causes symptoms such as sparse brittle twisted scalp hair, severe cerebral degeneration, and arterial changes with death in infancy; it is transmitted as an X-linked recessive trait. Called also *kinky-hair s.* and *steely-hair s.*

**Meretoja's s.,** Finnish type familial amyloid polyneuropathy.

**MERRF s.,** *m*yoclonus with *e*pilepsy and with *r*agged *r*ed *f*ibers; a familial syndrome of maternal (mitochondrial) inheritance. Called also *Fukuhara s.*

**metameric s.,** segmentary s.

**methionine malabsorption s.,** an autosomal recessive disorder of methionine absorption in which the urine has a characteristic odor resembling that of the interior of an oasthouse, due to alpha-hydroxybutyric acid formed by bacterial action on the unabsorbed methionine; it is characterized by white hair, mental retardation, convulsions, and attacks of hyperpnea. Called also *oasthouse urine disease* and *Smith-Strang disease.*

**Meyer-Schwickerath and Weyers s.,** oculodentodigital dysplasia.

**middle lobe s.,** lobar atelectasis in the right middle lobe of the lung, with chronic pneumonitis; called also *Brock's s.*

**midsystolic click–late systolic murmur s.,** mitral valve prolapse s.

**Mikulicz's s.,** a chronic bilateral hypertrophy of the lacrimal, parotid, and salivary glands, associated with decreased or absent lacrimation and xerostomia, and often accompanied by chronic lymphocytic infiltration. It may be associated with other diseases, such as Sjögren's syndrome, sarcoidosis, lupus erythematosus, leukemia, lymphoma, and tuberculosis. See also Mikulicz's disease, under *disease.*

**milk-alkali s.,** a syndrome characterized by hypercalcemia without hypercalciuria or hypophosphatemia, with only mild alkalosis, normal serum phosphatase, severe renal insufficiency with hyperazotemia, and calcinosis, attributed to ingestion of milk and absorbable alkali for long periods of time. Called also *Burnett's s.* and *hypercalcemia s.*

**Milkman's s.,** a generalized bone disease marked by multiple transparent stripes of absorption in the long and flat bones; called also *Looser-Milkman s.*

**Millard-Gubler s.,** crossed paralysis, affecting the limbs on one side of the body and the face on the opposite side, together with paralysis of outward movement of the eye; it is due to infarction of the pons, involving the sixth and seventh cranial nerves and the fibers of the corticospinal tract. Called also *Gubler's hemiplegia* or *paralysis* and *Millard-Gubler paralysis.* Cf. *Foville's s.*

**Miller s.,** a syndrome of extensive facial and limb defects, characterized by malar hypoplasia, downslanting palpebral fissures, micrognathia, cleft lip and palate, cup-shaped ears, lower lid ectropion, postaxial limb deficiencies, and syndactyly. Less frequently present are heart defects and hearing loss. The syndrome is probably an autosomal recessive trait. Called also *postaxial acrofacial dysostosis.*

**Miller-Dieker s.,** an autosomal recessive syndrome characterized by lissencephaly, microcephaly, mental retardation, dysmorphic facial appearance, and sometimes polydactyly, cryptorchidism, heart lesions, kidney defects, and defects of the gastrointestinal system. Called also *lissencephaly s.*

**Miller Fisher s.,** 1. Fisher s. (def. 1). 2. one-and-a-half s.

**minimal change nephrotic s.,** minimal change disease.

**Minkowski-Chauffard s.,** hereditary spherocytosis.

**Minot-von Willebrand s.,** von Willebrand's disease.

**mitral valve prolapse s.,** prolapse of the mitral valve, often with regurgitation, associated with myxomatous proliferation of the leaflets of the mitral valve, a common, usually benign, often asymptomatic condition characterized by midsystolic clicks and late systolic murmurs on auscultation. Palpitations and chest discomfort may occur, and in some cases progressive mitral regurgitation necessitates valve replacement. Called also *Barlow's s., click-murmur s., floppy valve s., MVP s.,* and *systolic click–murmur s.*

**Möbius' s.,** agenesis or aplasia of the motor nuclei of the cranial nerves characterized by congenital bilateral facial palsy in various combinations, with unilateral or bilateral paralysis of the abductors of the eye, sometimes associated with involvement of the cranial nerves, particularly the oculomotor, trigeminal, and hypoglossal, and anomalies of the extremities. Called also *nuclear agenesis* or *aplasia, congenital facial diplegia, congenital abducens-facial paralysis,* and *congenital oculofacial paralysis.*

**Mohr s.,** an autosomal recessive disorder characterized by brachydactyly, clinodactyly, polydactyly, syndactyly, and bilateral hallucal polysyndactyly; by cranial, facial, lingual, palatal, and mandibular anomalies; and by episodic neuromuscular disturbances. Called also *orodigitofacial dysostosis, oral-facial-digital s., type II,* and *orofaciodigital s., type II.* See also *oral-facial-digital s., type I.*

**Monakow's s.,** hemiplegia on the side opposite the lesion in occlusion of the anterior choroidal artery, sometimes with hemianesthesia and hemianopia.

**monosomy 9p⁻ s.,** a rare chromosomal disorder in which a piece of the short arm of the ninth chromosome is broken and often lost. Symptoms include mental retardation, a triangular head with forward angulation of the frontal bone, and various other physical deformities.

**Moore's s.,** abdominal epilepsy.

**Morel's s.,** hyperostosis frontalis interna.

**Morgagni-Adams-Stokes s.,** Adams-Stokes s.

**morning glory s.,** a coloboma in which there is a funnel-shaped optic nerve head with a dot of whitish, fluffy material in the center, an elevated ring of pigment around the disk, and vessels radiating from the ring like spokes. Vision is severely affected.

**Morquio's s.,** two biochemically distinct, but clinically nearly indistinguishable, forms of mucopolysaccharidosis characterized by excretion of keratan sulfate in the urine. Clinical features, affecting primarily the skeletal and secondarily the nervous system, include genu valgum, pectus carinatum, progressive platyspondyly, short neck and trunk, normal but broad-mouthed facies with spacing between the teeth, progressive deafness, and very mild corneal clouding. Intelligence is normal. The two enzymatic types are *type A,* caused by *N*-acetylgalactosamine-6-sulfatase deficiency; and *type B,* caused by *β*-galactosidase deficiency. Called also *mucopolysaccharidosis IV.*

**Morris s.,** complete androgen resistance; see under *resistance.*

**Morton's s.,** a congenital insufficiency of the first metatarsal segment of the foot, characterized by metatarsalgia due to shortening or relaxation of the part.

**Morvan's s.,** 1. syringomyelia. 2. a manifestation of syringomyelia in which the subcutaneous tissues of the hands become thickened, edematous, soft, swollen, cyanotic, and cold (see *Marinesco's succulent hand,* under *hand*), associated with analgesic ulceration of the fingertips and paresthesia and atrophy of the hands and forearms.

**Mosse's s.,** polycythemia vera with cirrhosis of the liver.

**Mounier-Kuhn's s.,** tracheobronchomegaly.

**Mount's s., Mount-Reback s.,** a rare autosomal dominant disorder characterized by paroxysmal attacks of choreoathetosis and dystonic movements with Kayser-Fleischer rings on the corneas. It appears in childhood or young adulthood and does not involve a change in consciousness. Called also *paroxysmal* or *familial paroxysmal choreoathetosis.* See also *paroxysmal kinesigenic choreoathetosis.*

**Moynahan s.,** 1. multiple symmetric lentigines, congenital mitral valve stenosis, dwarfism, genital hypoplasia, and mental retardation. Called also *progressive cardiomyopathic lentiginosis.* 2. a familial congenital syndrome consisting of delayed hair growth on the scalp, epilepsy, mental retardation, and unusual electroencephalogram.

**Muckle-Wells s.,** an autosomal dominant syndrome characterized by amyloidosis involving the kidneys and causing nephritis, recurrent urticaria, deafness, and pain in the extremities.

**mucocutaneous lymph node s. (MLNS),** a syndrome of unknown etiology, usually affecting infants and young children, marked by fever, conjunctival injection, reddening of the lips and oral cavity, ulcerative gingivitis, enlarged cervical lymph nodes, and maculoerythematous skin eruption that becomes confluent and bright red in a glove-and-sock distribution; the skin becomes indurated and edematous and desquamates from the fingers and toes. Called also *Kawasaki disease.*

**mucosal neuroma s.,** multiple endocrine neoplasia, Type III.

**Muir-Torre s.,** Torre's s.

**multiple endocrine deficiency s., multiple glandular deficiency s.,**

primary failure of any combination of endocrine glands, including adrenals, thyroid, gonads, parathyroids, and endocrine pancreas, often accompanied by nonendocrine autoimmune abnormalities.

**multiple hamartoma s.,** Cowden disease.

**multiple lentigines s.,** LEOPARD s.

**multiple pterygium s.,** an autosomal recessive syndrome characterized by pterygia of the neck, axillae, and popliteal, antecubital, and intercrural areas, accompanied by hypertelorism, cleft palate, micrognathia, ptosis of eyelids, and short stature. Skeletal abnormalities include camptodactyly, syndactyly, equinovarus, and rocker-bottom feet, as well as vertebral fusion and rib anomalies. Cryptorchidism is present in males and labia majora are absent in females. Called also *Escobar s.* and *pterygium s.*

**Munchausen s.,** a condition characterized by habitual presentation for hospital treatment of an apparent acute physical illness, the patient giving a plausible and dramatic history, all of which is false; it is a subtype of factitious disorder (q.v.).

**Munchausen s. by proxy,** see *factitious disorder by proxy,* under *disorder.*

**MVP s.,** mitral valve prolapse s.

**myasthenic s.,** Eaton-Lambert s.

**myelodysplastic s.,** any of a group of related bone marrow disorders of varying duration preceding the development of overt acute myelogenous leukemia; they are characterized by abnormal hematopoietic stem cells, anemia, neutropenia, and thrombocytopenia. Splenomegaly, hepatomegaly, and lymphadenopathy may not occur until the onset, often explosive, of leukemia. Called also *preleukemia.*

**myelofibrosis-osteosclerosis s.,** agnogenic myeloid metaplasia.

**myeloproliferative s's,** see under *disorder.*

**Naegeli s.,** Franceschetti-Jadassohn s.

**Naffziger's s.,** scalenus s.

**Nager's s., Nager-de Reynier s.,** Nager's acrofacial dysostosis.

**nail-patella s.,** a hereditary syndrome consisting of dystrophy of the nails, absence or hypoplasia of the patella, hypoplasia of the lateral side of the elbow joint, and bilateral iliac horns. Called also *hereditary osteo-onychodysplasia.*

**NAME s.,** a syndrome of familial myxomas with cutaneous, cardiac, and endocrine involvement, manifested as *n*evi, *a*trial *m*yxoma, and neurofibroma *e*phelides. Cf. *LAMB s.*

**neck-tongue s.,** pain in the neck, sometimes followed by numbness of the neck and tongue, on sudden turning of the head; it is thought to be due to compression of C2 nerve roots in the area of the atlantoaxial articulations because the C2 roots contain proprioceptive fibers from the tongue.

**Negri-Jacod s.,** Jacod's s.

**Nélaton's s.,** hereditary sensory radicular neuropathy.

**Nelson's s.,** the development of an ACTH-producing pituitary tumor after bilateral adrenalectomy for Cushing's syndrome; it is characterized by aggressive growth of the tumor and hyperpigmentation of the skin.

**neonatal maladjustment s.,** a disease of newborn foals, caused by perinatal hypoxia and characterized by behavioral disturbances such as inability to nurse, aimless wandering, apparent blindness, and uttering of a barklike sound; it may progress to convulsions, coma, and death. Affected foals are called *barkers, dummies,* or *wanderers.*

**nephrotic s.,** general name for any of a group of diseases involving defective kidney glomeruli, characterized by massive proteinuria and lipiduria with varying degrees of edema, hypoalbuminemia, and hyperlipidemia. See also *nephrosis.*

**nerve compression s.,** entrapment neuropathy.

**Netherton's s.,** a congenital syndrome consisting of lamellar ichthyosis or ichthyosis linearis circumflexa, hair shaft defects, atopic diathesis, and sometimes mental retardation and aminoaciduria. It is believed to be autosomal recessive.

**neurocutaneous s.,** phakomatosis.

**neuroleptic malignant s.,** a rare, sometimes fatal reaction to antipsychotic (neuroleptic) agents, characterized by hyperthermia, rigidity, and coma.

**nevoid basal cell carcinoma s., nevoid basalioma s.,** basal cell nevus s.

**Nezelof s.,** any of a heterogeneous group of immunodeficiency disorders characterized by profoundly deficient cellular immunity and varying degrees of humoral immunodeficiency. Immunoglobulin levels may be normal or increased, but antibody response to immunization may be absent. Patients are highly susceptible to life-threatening infections with low-grade or opportunistic pathogens, such as *Candida albicans, Pneumocystis carinii,* and cytomegalovirus. Both autosomal recessive and X-linked inheritance have been described. Called also *cellular immunodeficiency with immunoglobulins.*

**Noack's s.,** acrocephalopolysyndactyly (type I).

**Nonne-Milroy-Meige s.,** Milroy's disease.

**nonsense s.,** Ganser s.

**nonstaphylococcal scalded skin s.,** toxic epidermal necrolysis.

**Noonan's s.,** the phenotype of Turner's syndrome (webbed neck, ptosis, hypogonadism, congenital heart disease, and short stature) without gonadal dysgenesis; formerly called *male Turner's syndrome* until the female counterpart was identified. Called also *Ullrich-Turner s.*

**Nothnagel's s.,** unilateral oculomotor paralysis combined with cerebellar ataxia, in lesions of the cerebral peduncles.

**Nyssen-van Bogaert s.,** the adult form of metachromatic leukodystrophy.

**OAV s.,** oculoauriculovertebral dysplasia.

**obesity-hypoventilation s.,** a complex of obesity, somnolence, hypoventilation, and erythrocytosis; called also *pickwickian s.*

**obstructive sleep apnea s. (OSAS),** see under *apnea.*

**occipital horn s.,** the X-linked recessive form of cutis laxa.

**oculocerebral-hypopigmentation s.,** Cross s.

**oculocerebrorenal s.,** an X-linked disorder characterized by vitamin D–refractory rickets, hydrophthalmia, congenital glaucoma and cataracts, mental retardation, and tubule reabsorption dysfunction as evidenced by hypophosphatemia, acidosis, and aminoaciduria. Called also *Lowe disease* and *Lowe-Terrey-MacLachlan s.*

**oculodentodigital s., oculodento-osseous s.,** see under *dysplasia.*

**oculomandibulodyscephaly-hypotrichosis s.,** oculomandibulofacial s.

**oculomandibulofacial s.,** a syndrome principally characterized by dyscephaly (usually brachycephaly), parrot nose, mandibular hypoplasia, proportionate nanism, hypotrichosis, bilateral congenital cataracts, and microphthalmia. Called also *Hallermann-Streiff s., Hallermann-Streiff-François s., François' s.,* and *mandibulo-oculofacial dyscephaly.*

**oculo-oto-radial s.,** IVIC s.

**oculopharyngeal s.,** see under *dystrophy.*

**ODD s.,** oculodentodigital dysplasia.

**OFD s.,** oral-facial-digital s.

**Ogilvie's s.,** colonic distention resembling that caused by obstruction, but without evidence of mechanical obstruction; it is usually due to a defect in the sympathetic nerve supply. Called also *false colonic obstruction.*

**Oldfield's s.,** familial polyposis of the colon associated with extensive sebaceous cysts.

**Omenn's s.,** histiocytic medullary reticulosis.

**OMM s.,** ophthalmomandibulomelic dysplasia; see under *dysplasia.*

**one-and-a-half s.,** a disorder of ocular movement caused by a brain stem lesion of one abducens nucleus and the nearby medial longitudinal fasciculus; the ipsilateral eye cannot move beyond the midline horizontally and the contralateral eye abducts on any attempt at conjugate gaze. Called also *Fisher s.* and *Miller Fisher s.*

**Opitz s., Opitz-Frias s.,** an autosomal dominant syndrome consisting of hypertelorism and hernias, and in males hypospadias, cryptorchidism, and bifid scrotum. Cardiac anomalies, laryngotracheal malformations, imperforate anus, renal defects, lung hypoplasia, and downslanted palpebral fissures may also be present. Called also *G s.* and *hypertelorism-hypospadias s.*

**opsoclonus-myoclonus s.,** a syndrome of movements of the eyes (opsoclonus) and trunk (myoclonus), occurring in conjunction with a number of conditions, including viral infections, trauma, drug toxicity, tumors, and hyperosmolar nonketotic coma. It also occurs as a paraneoplastic syndrome; in some women with small cell lung or breast carcinoma, it is associated with an autoantibody (anti-Ri).

**oral-facial-digital (OFD) s., type I,** a male-lethal X-linked dominant disorder characterized by camptodactyly, polydactyly, and syndactyly; by cranial, facial, lingual, and dental anomalies; and by mental retardation, familial trembling, alopecia, and seborrhea of the face and milia. Called also *orodigitofacial dysostosis* and *orofaciodigital s., type I.* See also *Mohr s.*

**oral-facial-digital (OFD) s., type II,** Mohr s.

**oral-facial-digital (OFD) s., type III,** an autosomal recessive disorder characterized by postaxial hexadactyly of the hands and feet, by ocular, lingual, and dental anomalies, and by profound mental retardation. Called also *orodigitofacial dysostosis* and *orofaciodigital s., type III.*

**orbital apex s.,** ophthalmoplegia with impairment of vision that may lead to blindness, swelling of the eyelids, ptosis, hyper- or hypoesthesia of the upper eyelid, one half of the forehead, and cornea, and vasomotor disturbances; it is caused by traumatic, inflammatory, or neoplastic processes involving the sphenoidal fissure and optic canal or the structures they contain.

**orbital floor s.,** exophthalmos, diplopia, and anesthesia in the areas innervated by the trigeminal nerve, occurring with a lesion in the floor of the orbit. Called also *Dejean's s.*

**organic anxiety s.,** a term used in a former system of classification, denoting an organic mental syndrome characterized by prominent, recurrent panic attacks or generalized anxiety caused by a specific organic factor and not associated with delirium. Such disorders are now mainly classified as *substance-induced anxiety disorders* and *anxiety disorders due to a general medical condition.*

**organic brain s.,** organic mental s.

**organic delusional s.,** a term used in a former system of classification, denoting an organic mental syndrome characterized by the presence of delusions caused by a specific organic factor and not associated with delirium. Such disorders are now mainly classified as *substance-induced psychotic disorders* and *psychotic disorders due to a general medical condition.*

**organic dust toxic s.,** pneumonitis, usually hypersensitivity pneumonitis, resulting from an allergic reaction to inhaled organic dust, as in bagassosis and various other conditions.

**organic mental s.,** former term for a constellation of psychological or behavioral signs and symptoms associated with brain dysfunction of unknown or unspecified etiology and grouped according to symptoms (cf. under *disorder*). Designating certain conditions as having an organic basis, possibly implying that others do not, is currently discouraged.

**organic mood s.,** a term used in a former system of classification, denoting an organic mental syndrome characterized by the presence of manic or depressive mood disturbance caused by a specific organic factor and not associated with delirium. Such disorders are now mainly classified as *substance-induced mood disorders* and *mood disorders due to a general medical condition.*

**organic personality s.,** a term used in a former system of classification, denoting an organic mental syndrome characterized by a marked change in behavior or personality, caused by a specific organic factor and not associated with delirium or dementia. The most common causes are space-occupying lesions of the brain, head trauma, and cerebrovascular disease.

**orofaciodigital (OFD) s., type I,** oral-facial-digital s., type I.

**orofaciodigital (OFD) s., type II,** Mohr s.

**orofaciodigital (OFD) s., type III,** oral-facial-digital s., type III.

**Ortner's s.,** laryngeal paralysis associated with heart disease, due to compression of the recurrent laryngeal nerve between the aorta and a dilated pulmonary artery.

**Ostrum-Furst s.,** congenital synostosis of the neck, platybasia, and Sprengel's deformity.

**Othello s.,** delusional belief in the infidelity of the sexual partner, often of sudden onset and usually affecting middle-aged men; it is characterized by repeated accusations, intense searches for evidence, and prolonged interrogation of the partner.

**outlet s.,** thoracic outlet s.

**ovarian hyperstimulation s.,** an iatrogenic condition seen in women undergoing ovulation induction, characterized by mild to severe ovarian enlargement with exudation of fluid and protein, leading to ascites, pleural or pericardial effusion, azotemia, oliguria, and thromboembolism.

**ovarian-remnant s.,** pelvic pain, sometimes cyclic, typically occurring several weeks or months after oophorectomy, usually associated with a pelvic mass, most frequently a corpus luteum cyst, which occasionally leads to unilateral ureteral obstruction. It is due to survival of an ovarian fragment after the operation.

**ovarian vein s.,** obstruction of the ureter due to compression by an enlarged or varicose ovarian vein; typically the vein becomes enlarged during pregnancy, the symptoms being those of obstruction or infection of the upper urinary tract. The right side is usually affected.

**overlap s.,** any of a group of connective tissue disorders that either combine scleroderma with polymyositis or systemic lupus erythematosus or combine systemic lupus erythematosus with rheumatoid arthritis or polymyositis. Cf. *mixed connective tissue disease.*

**overwear s.,** extreme photophobia, pain, and lacrimation associated with contact lenses, particularly non–gas permeable hard lenses, usually caused by wearing them excessively. Prolonged lens-induced corneal hypoxia results in corneal epithelial edema and eventually erosion; it can be a chronic condition or an acute episode that usually occurs several hours after lenses are removed.

**pacemaker s.,** vertigo, syncope, and hypotension, often accompanied by dyspnea, cough, nausea, peripheral edema, and palpitations, induced or exacerbated by abnormalities of the cardiac pacemaker so that it stimulates the ventricle. The symptoms occur because ventricular pacing does not maintain normal atrioventricular synchrony; retrograde ventriculoatrial conduction causes low cardiac output and activates cardiac reflexes that result in increased peripheral vasodilation and hypotension.

**pacemaker twiddler's s.,** twiddler's syndrome in a patient with an artificial cardiac pacemaker.

**Paget-Schroetter s., Paget-von Schroetter s.,** a thoracic outlet syndrome in which a thrombus forms in the axillary vein after strenuous exercise; symptoms include pain, edema, and skin discoloration in the shoulder and upper arm. Called also *effort thrombosis.*

**pain dysfunction s.,** Costen's s.

**painful arc s.,** shoulder pain occurring at a particular portion of the arc described when the arm is abducted from the side to the fully raised position, as in inflammation of the tendons of the supraspinatus muscle.

**painful bruising s.,** a purpuric reaction almost always seen in young to middle-aged women in which spontaneous, chronic recurring painful ecchymoses, single or multiple, occur on the body without antecedent trauma or after insufficient trauma, and may be precipitated by emotional stress. Based on studies that show that certain patients exhibit autoerythrocyte sensitization in which intradermal injection of their own erythrocytes produces a painful ecchymosis, the etiology of the condition has been ascribed by some to an autosensitivity to a component of the erythrocyte membrane; others consider it to be of psychosomatic or factitious origin. Called also *autoerythrocyte sensitization s., erythrocyte autosensitization s.,* and *Gardner-Diamond s.*

**paleostriatal s., pallidal s.,** juvenile paralysis agitans (of Hunt).

**Pancoast's s.,** 1. neuritic pain in the arm, atrophy of the muscles of the arm and hand, and Horner's syndrome, observed with a pulmonary sulcus tumor, due to involvement of the brachial plexus and cervical sympathetic nerves. 2. osteolysis in the posterior part of one or more ribs, sometimes also involving the corresponding vertebra.

**pancreatic cholera s.,** Verner-Morrison s.

**pancreaticohepatic s.,** extensive destruction of pancreatic tissue and fatty metamorphosis of the liver.

**pancytopenia-dysmelia s.,** Fanconi's s. (def. 1).

**Papillon-Lefèvre s.,** an autosomal recessive disorder occurring between the first and fifth years of life, characterized by psoriasiform palmoplantar keratoderma, which may also involve the elbows, knees, tibias, external malleoli, and other areas; ectopic calcifications of the skull; and periodontitis and premature shedding of both the deciduous and permanent teeth.

**paraneoplastic s.,** a symptom-complex arising in a cancer-bearing patient that cannot be explained by local or distant spread of the tumor.

**paratrigeminal s.,** Raeder's paratrigeminal s.

**Parinaud's s.,** paralysis of conjugate upward movement of the eyes without paralysis of convergence, associated with lesions of the midbrain, such as a tumor of the pineal gland.

**Parinaud's oculoglandular s.,** a general term applied to conjunctivitis, most often unilateral, usually of the follicular type, followed by tenderness and enlargement of the preauricular lymph nodes; it is often caused by infection with a leptothrix, or may be associated with other infections, such as cat-scratch fever, lymphogranuloma venereum, and tularemia.

**Parkes Weber s.,** Sturge-Weber s.

**parkinsonian s.,** a form of parkinsonism due to idiopathic degeneration of the corpus striatum or substantia nigra, frequently occurring as a sequel of lethargic encephalitis. Called also *postencephalitic parkinsonism.*

**Parry-Romberg s.,** facial hemiatrophy.

**Patau's s.,** trisomy 13 s.

**Paterson's s., Paterson–Brown Kelly s., Paterson-Kelly s.,** Plummer-Vinson s.

**Pearson's s.,** a rare congenital syndrome of refractory sideroblastic anemia with vacuolization of bone marrow precursors and exocrine pancreatic insufficiency; most affected children die in infancy unless given transfusions.

**Pellegrini-Stieda s.,** calcification of the medial collateral ligament of the knee.

**Pellizzi's s.,** epiphyseal s.

**Pendred's s.,** a hereditary syndrome of congenital bilateral nerve deafness with development in middle childhood of goiter without hypothyroidism; the main biochemical feature is defective thyroxine biosynthesis.

**PEP s.,** [*p*lasma cell dyscrasia, *e*ndocrinopathy, *p*olyneuropathy], POEMS s.

**Pepper s.,** neuroblastoma with metastases to the liver.

**pericolic membrane s.,** symptoms resembling those of chronic appendicitis due to the pressure of pericolic membranes.

**Perlman s.,** a rare, lethal syndrome consisting of renal dysplasia, nephroblastoma, fetal gigantism, and hypertrophy of the islets of Langerhans with hyperinsulinism. It may be transmitted by autosomal recessive inheritance.

**persistent müllerian duct s.,** a hereditary syndrome in males of persistence of müllerian structures in addition to male genital ducts, with undescended testes and bilateral uterine tubes, a uterus, and an upper vagina. There may be cryptorchidism on just one side with a contralateral inguinal hernia that contains a testis, uterus, and uterine tube *(hernia uteri inguinalis).*

**pertussis s.,** 1. pertussis-like s. 2. pertussis.

**pertussis-like s.,** a syndrome clinically indistinguishable from pertussis but in which there is no evidence of infection with *Bordetella pertussis* or *B. parapertussis,* although evidence of other infectious agents, such as adenoviruses types 1, 2, 3, 5, and 6, can be demonstrated. Called also *pertussis s.* Cf. *parapertussis.*

**petrosphenoid s.,** Jacod's s.

**Peutz-Jeghers s.,** an autosomal dominant syndrome, a type of familial adenomatous polyposis characterized by hamartomas of the small intestine and excessive melanin pigmentation of the skin and mucous membranes; gastrointestinal bleeding and intussusception are common complications.

**Pfeiffer's s.**, an autosomal dominant disorder characterized by acrocephalosyndactyly associated with broad short thumbs and big toes. Called also *acrocephalosyndactyly, type V.*

**pharyngeal pouch s.**, DiGeorge s.

**PHC s.**, an autosomal dominant syndrome consisting of premolar aplasia, hyperhidrosis, and premature canities. Called also *Böök's s.*

**Picchini's s.**, inflammation of the three serous membranes connected with the diaphragm, sometimes involving the meninges, synovial sheaths, and tunica vaginalis of the testicle; caused by a trypanosome.

**pickwickian s.**, obesity-hypoventilation s.

**PIE s.** (*p*ulmonary *i*nfiltration with *e*osinophilia), 1. any syndrome characterized by pulmonary infiltrates with eosinophilia, such as Löffler's syndrome or chronic eosinophilic pneumonia. 2. a syndrome of diffuse pulmonary infiltration and peripheral eosinophilia, seen in dogs and sometimes cats; the cause varies but sometimes it may be an allergic reaction. Affected animals are dyspneic with decreased exercise tolerance. Called also *eosinophilic pneumonia.*

**Pierre Robin s.**, an autosomal recessive disorder characterized by brachygnathia and cleft palate, often associated with glossoptosis, backward and upward displacement of the larynx, and angulation of the manubrium sterni; cleft palate makes sucking and swallowing difficult, permitting easy access of fluids into the larynx. It may appear in several syndromes or as an isolated hypoplasia. Called also *Robin's s.* and *Robin's anomalad.*

**pineal s.**, epiphyseal s.

**placental dysfunction s.**, dysmaturity s.

**plica s.**, pain, tenderness, crepitus, and swelling of the knee joint, sometimes accompanied by weakness or locking of the joint, caused by fibrosis and calcification of the synovial plicae, usually the mediopatellar plica.

**Plummer-Vinson s.**, a syndrome usually seen in middle-aged women with hypochromic anemia, chiefly characterized by cracks or fissures at the corners of the mouth, painful tongue with atrophy of filiform and later fungiform papillae, and dysphagia due to esophageal stenosis or webs. Called also *Paterson's s., Paterson-Kelly s., sideropenic dysphagia,* and *Vinson's s.*

**POEMS s.**, a multisystem syndrome combining *p*olyneuropathy *o*rganomegaly, *e*ndocrinopathy, *M* protein, and *s*kin changes. It may be linked to a dysproteinemia such as the presence of unusual monoclonal proteins and light chains. Called also *Crow-Fukase s.* and *PEP s.*

**Poland's s.**, unilateral absence of the sternocostal head of the pectoralis major muscle and ipsilateral syndactyly; called also *Poland's anomaly.*

**Polhemus-Schafer-Ivemark s.**, Ivemark's s.

**polyangiitis overlap s.**, a systemic form of necrotizing vasculitis with clinicopathologic signs overlapping those of polyarteritis nodosa and allergic granulomatous angiitis, but also showing features of hypersensitivity vasculitis. Immunoglobulins are often deposited in involved organs. Called also *overlap vasculitis.*

**polycystic ovary s. (PCOS)**, a clinical symptom complex associated with polycystic ovaries and characterized by oligomenorrhea or amenorrhea, anovulation (hence infertility), and hirsutism. Both hyperestrogenism (from peripheral conversion of androgen) and hyperandrogenism are present. Called also *polycystic ovary disease* and *Stein-Leventhal s.*

**polyglandular autoimmune s's**, a group of syndromes that involve combinations of endocrine and nonendocrine autoimmune diseases. *Type I* (called also *autoimmune polyendocrine-candidiasis s.*), which occurs in infants and children, is a combination of candidiasis, hypoparathyroidism, and adrenal insufficiency; pernicious anemia, vitiligo, gonadal failure, alopecia, insulin-dependent diabetes, or thyroid autoimmune disease may also occur. *Type II* is known as *Schmidt's s.* Called also *polyendocrine* or *polyglandular autoimmune diseases.*

**polysplenia s.**, a congenital syndrome characterized by multiple splenic masses, bilateral left-sidedness, abnormal position and development of visceral organs, complex cardiovascular defects, and abnormal, usually bilobate, lungs. It may be related to Ivemark's syndrome.

**pontine s.**, Raymond-Cestan s.

**popliteal pterygium s.**, 1. popliteal web s. 2. Fèvre-Languepin s.

**popliteal web s.**, a congenital syndrome consisting chiefly of popliteal webs, cleft palate, lower lip pits, and dysplasia of the toenails; a wide variety of other abnormalities may be associated. Called also *popliteal pterygium s.*

**Porak-Durante s.**, osteogenesis imperfecta (type II), recessive form.

**porcine epidemic abortion and respiratory s. (PEARS)**, a disease caused by a virus of the genus *Arterivirus*, affecting pregnant pigs and characterized by fever, anorexia, and respiratory distress followed by unusually high numbers of stillbirths and other piglets born with respiratory distress, weakness, and neurological conditions such as splayleg. Called also *mystery pig disease.*

**porcine stress s.**, sudden death of a pig in response to a stressor such as fighting, transport, or malignant hyperthermia, or as part of a drug reaction. Susceptibility in most cases is inherited as an autosomal recessive gene. Called also *herztod.*

**post–cardiac injury s.**, fever, chest pain, pleuritis, and pericarditis occurring several weeks to months after injury to the heart, including that inflicted by surgery (often called *postpericardiotomy s.*) or myocardial infarction (often called *post–myocardial infarction s.*).

**postcardiotomy s.**, postpericardiotomy s.

**postcardiotomy psychosis s.**, anxiety, confusion, and perceptual disturbances occurring three or more days after open heart surgery.

**postcholecystectomy s.**, the persistence or recurrence of abdominal pain or jaundice following cholecystectomy; it may be due to an incorrect preoperative diagnosis, a retained stone in the common bile duct, or to other physical or psychic abnormalities which are not apparent.

**postcommissurotomy s.**, postpericardiotomy s.

**postconcussion s., postconcussional s.**, physical and personality changes that sometimes occur after concussion of the brain (q.v.); they include amnesia, headache, dizziness, tinnitus, irritability, fatigability, sweating, palpitations of the heart, disordered sleep, and difficulty in concentrating. Called also *traumatic encephalopathy, concussion s., Friedmann's vasomotor s., Homén's s., post-traumatic s.,* and *post-traumatic brain s.* Cf. *boxer's dementia* and *boxer's encephalopathy.*

**posterior column s., posterior cord s.**, sensory deficits and ataxic phenomena derived from a lesion of the posterior columns of the spinal cord.

**posterior inferior cerebellar artery s.**, Wallenberg's s.

**postgastrectomy s.**, dumping s.

**postirradiation s.**, a symptom complex caused by massive irradiation, with hemorrhage, anemia, and malnutrition. See also *acute radiation s.*

**post–lumbar puncture s.**, headache in the erect posture, sometimes with nuchal pain, nausea, vomiting, diaphoresis, and malaise, all relieved by recumbency, occurring several hours after lumbar puncture and lasting a few days; it is due to lowering of intracranial pressure by leakage of cerebrospinal fluid through the needle tract.

**postmaturity s.**, dysmaturity s.

**post–myocardial infarction s.**, pericarditis with fever, leukocytosis, pleurisy, and pneumonia occurring after myocardial infarction; called also *Dressler's s.*

**postperfusion s.**, cytomegalovirus mononucleosis occurring about 3 to 6 weeks after extracorporeal circulation or multiple blood transfusions in open heart or other surgical procedures. Called also *post-transfusion s.* and *post-transfusion mononucleosis.*

**postpericardiotomy s.**, pericardial or pleural reaction occurring more than one week after opening of the pericardium, characterized by fever, chest pain, and signs of pleural and/or pericardial inflammation.

**postphlebitic s.**, the various complications associated with deep vein thrombosis which are caused by greatly increased pressure in the deep and communicating veins, resulting in chronic venous insufficiency, and principally characterized by persistent edema, pain, purpura and increased cutaneous pigmentation, eczematoid dermatitis, pruritus, ulceration, and indurated cellulitis. Called also *post-thrombotic s.*

**postpolio s., postpoliomyelitis s.**, a group of symptoms of unknown etiology seen in patients several years to many years after they have recovered from the major illness of poliomyelitis; it includes new weakness, fatigue, and pain, either generalized or limited to the parts that were affected by the poliomyelitis. Called also *postpoliomyelitis sequela.*

**post-thrombotic s.**, postphlebitic s.

**post-transfusion s.**, postperfusion s.

**post-traumatic s., post-traumatic brain s.**, postconcussional s.

**Potter's s.**, oligohydramnios sequence.

**Prader-Willi s.**, a congenital disorder characterized by obesity, short stature, lack of muscle tone, hypogonadism, and central nervous system dysfunction; there is often a characteristic rounded face with almond-shaped eyes and a low forehead. Mental retardation is common. It can be caused by a deletion on chromosome 15 inherited from the father; the same deletion inherited from the mother causes Angelman's syndrome.

**preexcitation s.**, any syndrome characterized by electrocardiographic evidence of preexcitation, such as Wolff-Parkinson-White syndrome or Lown-Ganong-Levine syndrome; sometimes used as a synonym of the former.

**premenstrual s.**, a syndrome of unknown cause, typically occurring in the period between ovulation and the onset of menstruation, marked by some or all of the following symptoms: feelings of depression, hopelessness, anxiety, or anger, emotional lability, bloating, edema, headache, increased fatigue or lethargy, changes in appetite or cravings for selected foods, breast swelling and tenderness, constipation, and decreased ability to concentrate.

**premotor s.,** the association of spastic hemiplegia with increased reflexes, disturbances of skilled movements, forced grasping, and transient vasomotor disturbance; occurring in very large lesions of the premotor cortex.

**Profichet's s.,** a gradual growth of calcareous nodules in the subcutaneous tissues (skin stones) especially about the larger joints, with a tendency to ulceration or cicatrization and attended by atrophic and nervous symptoms.

**prolonged QT interval s.,** long QT s.

**pronator s., pronator teres s.,** an entrapment neuropathy in which the median nerve or its anterior interosseous branch is compressed by the structures of the cubital fossa or by its passage between the heads of the pronator teres muscle, causing pain in the forearm and weakness or sensory deficits in the radial aspect of the hand.

**Proteus s.,** a rare congenital disorder with highly variable manifestations, including partial gigantism of the hands and feet with hypertrophy of the palms and soles, nevi, hemihypertrophy, subcutaneous tumors, macrocephaly and other skull abnormalities, and abdominal or pelvic lipomatosis. The etiology is unknown, although a genetic origin, possibly of autosomal dominant transmission, has been conjectured.

**prune-belly s.,** a syndrome in which the lower part of the rectus abdominis muscle and the lower and medial parts of the oblique muscles are absent, the bladder and ureters are usually greatly dilated, the kidneys are small and dysplastic, with hydronephrosis, and the testes are undescended. The abdomen is protruding and thin-walled, with wrinkled skin, giving the syndrome its name. Called also *Eagle-Barrett s.*

**pseudo–Cushing's s.,** the presence of clinical or biochemical features of Cushing's syndrome in patients with certain nonendocrine disorders, such as alcoholism or depression.

**pterygium s.,** multiple pterygium s.

**pulmonary acid aspiration s.,** the disorder produced, as a complication of anesthesia, by inhalation of gastric content with a pH of less than 2.5, including bronchoconstriction and destruction of tracheal mucosa, progressing to a syndrome resembling acute respiratory distress syndrome. Called also *Mendelson's s.*

**pulmonary dysmaturity s.,** Wilson-Mikity s.

**pulmonary sling s.,** a constellation of unilateral aeration disturbances caused by a pulmonary artery sling with tracheal stenosis. See also *sling ring complex,* under *complex.*

**Purtilo's s.,** X-linked lymphoproliferative s.

**Putnam-Dana s.,** subacute combined degeneration of spinal cord (see under *degeneration*).

**Rabson-Mendenhall s.,** a rare syndrome seen in children, characterized by a mutation or other defect in an insulin receptor gene, with severe insulin resistance and acanthosis nigricans as well as thick hair, abnormalities of teeth and nails, and hyperplasia of the pineal gland.

**radicular s.,** a syndrome due to lesion of the roots of the spinal nerves, consisting of restricted mobility of the spine and root pain.

**Raeder's s., Raeder's paratrigeminal s.,** unilateral paroxysmal neuralgic pain in the face associated with sympathetic palsy; see also *Horner's s.* Called also *paratrigeminal s.*

**Ramsay Hunt s.,** 1. herpes zoster involving the facial and auditory nerves associated with ipsilateral facial paralysis, usually transitory, and herpetic vesicles of the external ear or tympanic membrane, which also may or may not be associated with tinnitus, vertigo, and hearing disorders. Called also *geniculate neuralgia* or *otalgia, herpes zoster auricularis* or *oticus, otic neuralgia,* and *Hunt's s., disease,* or *neuralgia.* See also *postherpetic neuralgia.* 2. juvenile paralysis agitans (of Hunt). 3. dyssynergia cerebellaris progressiva.

**Raymond-Cestan s.,** a syndrome due to obstruction of twigs of the basilar artery causing lesions of the pontine region; it is characterized by quadriplegia, anesthesia, and nystagmus. Called also *Cestan-Raymond s.* and *pontine s.*

**reactive airways dysfunction s.,** a rare asthmalike disorder consisting of persistent coughing, wheezing, and dyspnea upon only slight irritation, lasting for months after a person has inhaled a high concentration of irritating fumes.

**redundant supraglottic mucosa s.,** redundancy of the aryepiglottic folds, the mucosa overlying the artytenoid cartilages, and the interarytenoid region of the larynx, associated with obstructive sleep apnea, with or without stridor.

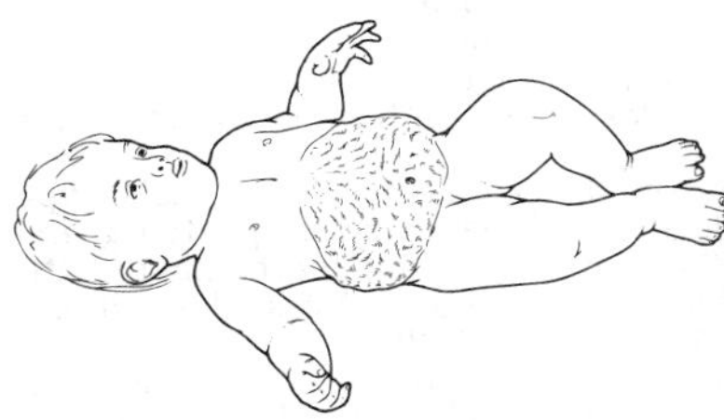

Prune-belly syndrome.

**Reichel's s.,** Henderson-Jones disease.

**Reichmann's s.,** gastrosuccorrhea.

**Reifenstein's s.,** a syndrome of male hypergonadotropic hypogonadism, due to an inherited incomplete androgen resistance (inability to respond to testosterone), with hypospadias, gynecomastia, primary hypogonadism, and postpubertal testicular atrophy and azoospermia.

**Reiter's s.,** a symptom complex consisting of urethritis, conjunctivitis, and arthritis; not all symptoms are present in all patients, and there may also be mucocutaneous manifestations such as keratoderma blennorrhagicum, circinate balanitis, and stomatitis. It usually affects young men and runs a self-limited but relapsing course. Most affected patients have increased levels of the histocompatibility antigen HLA-B27. It may represent an abnormal immune response to infection, perhaps with a hereditary susceptibility. Epidemiologic studies reveal two types: a *venereal* or *postvenereal* type, possibly related to infection with *Chlamydia* or *Ureaplasma;* and a *dysenteric* or *postdysenteric* type, possibly related to *Shigella, Salmonella, Yersinia,* or *Campylobacter fetus* infection. Called also *Fiessinger-Leroy-Reiter s.*

**Rendu-Osler-Weber s.,** hereditary hemorrhagic telangiectasia.

**respiratory distress s.,** see *acute respiratory distress s.* and *respiratory distress s. of the newborn.*

**respiratory distress s. of the newborn,** dyspnea with cyanosis in the newborn, heralded by such prodromal signs as dilatation of the alae nasi, expiratory grunt, and retraction of the suprasternal notch or costal margins, caused by a deficiency in surfactant. It is usually seen in premature infants, children of diabetic mothers, or infants delivered by cesarean section, although sometimes there is no apparent predisposing cause. Some affected infants die of respiratory failure in the first few days of life and at autopsy have eosinophilic hyaline material lining the alveoli, alveolar ducts, and bronchioles. Called also *hyaline membrane disease* and *idiopathic respiratory distress of newborn.*

**restless legs s.,** unpleasant deep discomfort inside the calves when sitting or lying down, especially just before sleep, producing an irresistible urge to move the legs. Called also *restless legs* and *Ekbom s.*

**retraction s.,** Duane's s.

**s. of retroparotid space,** Villaret's s.

**Rett s.** [DSM-IV], a pervasive developmental disorder affecting the gray matter of the brain, occurring exclusively in females and present from birth; it is progressive and is characterized by autistic behavior, ataxia, dementia, seizures, and loss of purposeful use of the hands, with cerebral atrophy, mild hyperammonemia, and decreased levels of biogenic amines. Called also *cerebroatrophic hyperammonemia.*

**Reye's s., Reye-Johnson s.,** a rare, acute, sometimes fatal disease of childhood, characterized by recurrent vomiting and elevated serum transaminase levels, with distinctive changes in the liver and other viscera; an encephalopathic phase may follow with acute brain swelling, disturbances of consciousness, and seizures. It most often occurs as a sequel of chickenpox or a viral upper respiratory infection.

**Rh-null s.,** chronic hemolytic anemia in persons who lack all Rh factors ($Rh_{null}$); it is marked by spherocytosis, stomatocytosis, and increased osmotic fragility.

**Richards-Rundle s.,** a congenital syndrome consisting of ketoaciduria, mental retardation, underdevelopment of secondary sex characteristics, deafness, ataxia, and peripheral muscular wasting which progresses during childhood but eventually becomes static.

**Richner-Hanhart s.,** tyrosinemia, type II.

**Richter's s.,** chronic lymphocytic leukemia with diffuse histiocytic lymphoma.

**Rieger's s.,** Rieger's anomaly accompanied by hypodontia, anal stenosis, hypertelorism, mental deficiency, and agenesis of the facial bones. See also *anterior chamber cleavage s.*

**Riley-Day s.,** familial dysautonomia.

**Riley-Smith s.,** macrocephaly without hydrocephalus, multiple hemangiomas, and pseudopapilledema; presumed to be transmitted as an autosomal dominant trait.

**Roberts' s.,** a hereditary syndrome, transmitted as an autosomal recessive trait, consisting of imperfect development of the long bones of the limbs associated with cleft palate and lip and other anomalies.

**Robin s.,** Pierre Robin s.

**Robinow's s.,** dwarfism associated with increased interorbital distance, malaligned teeth, bulging forehead, depressed nasal bridge, and short limbs. Called also *Robinow dwarfism* and *fetal face s.*

**Rochon-Duvigneaud's s.,** superior orbital fissure s.

**Roger's s.,** a continuous excessive secretion of saliva as the result of cancer in the esophagus, or other esophageal irritation.

**Rokitansky-Küster-Hauser s.,** Mayer-Rokitansky-Küster-Hauser s.

**rolandic vein s.,** hemiplegia resulting from interference with the cerebral venous circulation.

**Rollet's s.,** orbital apex s.

**Romano-Ward s.**, an autosomal dominant form of the long QT syndrome, characterized by syncope and sometimes ventricular fibrillation and sudden death. Cf. *Jervell and Lange-Nielsen s.*

**Rosenberg-Bergstrom s.**, an autosomal recessive syndrome characterized by hyperuricemia, renal insufficiency, ataxia, and deafness, probably due to deficiency of ribose-phosphate pyrophosphokinase.

**Rosenberg-Chutorian s.**, a rare X-linked hereditary syndrome characterized by optic atrophy, progressive neural deafness, and polyneuropathy.

**Rosenthal s.**, hemophilia C.

**Rosenthal-Kloepfer s.**, corneal leukomata, acromegaloid appearance, and cutis verticis gyrata.

**Rosewater's s.**, a mild form of hereditary X-linked hypergonadotropic hypogonadism in males, characterized by sterility and gynecomastia.

**Roth's (Rot's) s., Roth-Bernhardt (Rot-Bernhardt) s.**, meralgia paresthetica.

**Rothmann-Makai s.**, idiopathic circumscribed panniculitis with fat cell necrosis, lipophagic granuloma, and cyst formation; it usually subsides spontaneously.

**Rothmund-Thomson s.**, an autosomal recessive syndrome occurring principally in females, characterized by the presence of reticulated, atrophic, hyperpigmented, telangiectatic cutaneous plaques, often accompanied by juvenile cataracts, saddle nose, congenital bone defects, disturbances in the growth of hair, nails, and teeth, and hypogonadism. Called also *poikiloderma congenitale.* Cf. *Thomson's disease.*

**Rotor's s.**, chronic familial nonhemolytic jaundice differing from Dubin-Johnson syndrome in the lack of liver pigmentation.

**Roussy-Dejerine s.**, thalamic s.

**Roussy-Lévy s.**, a slowly progressive autosomal dominant disorder in which sensory ataxia is associated with areflexia, atrophy of muscles of distal extremities, especially the peroneal muscles, static tremor of the hands, pes cavus or clawfoot, and sometimes kyphoscoliosis. Called also *hereditary areflexic dystasia, Lévy-Roussy s.,* and *Roussy-Lévy hereditary areflexic dystasia.*

**Rovsing's s.**, horseshoe kidney with nausea, abdominal discomfort, and pain on hyperextension.

**rubella s.**, congenital rubella s.

**Rubinstein's s., Rubinstein-Taybi s.**, a congenital condition characterized by mental and motor retardation, broad thumbs and great toes, short stature, characteristic facies, including high-arched palate and straight or beaked nose, various eye abnormalities, pulmonary stenosis, keloid formation in surgical scars, large foramen magnum, and abnormalities of the vertebra and sternum.

**rubrospinal cerebellar peduncle s.**, Claude's s.

**Rud's s.**, congenital syndrome consisting of ichthyosis simplex, mental deficiency, epilepsy, and infantilism.

**rudimentary testis s.**, vanishing testes s.

**Rukavina's s.**, Indiana type familial amyloid polyneuropathy.

**Rundles-Falls s.**, hereditary sideroblastic anemia.

**runting s.**, graft-vs.-host reaction characterized by diarrhea, dermatitis, hepatosplenomegaly, hemolytic anemia, and pancytopenia.

**Russell s., Russell-Silver s.**, Silver-Russell s.

**Rust's s.**, stiff neck, stiff carriage of the head, with the necessity of grasping the head with both hands in lying down or rising up from a horizontal posture, occurring in tuberculosis, cancer, fracture of the spine, rheumatic or arthritic processes, or syphilitic periostitis.

**Ruvalcaba's s.**, brachymetapody, hypogenitalism, and retardation of unknown etiology but present from birth in males; it is characterized by microcephaly, skeletal abnormalities, hypoplastic genitalia, and mental and physical retardation.

**Sabin-Feldman s.**, chorioretinitis and cerebral calcifications, similar to the manifestations of toxoplasmosis, but having all tests for toxoplasmosis negative.

**Saethre-Chotzen s.**, Chotzen's s.

**Sakati-Nyhan s.**, acrocephalopolysyndactyly, type III.

**salt-depletion s., salt-losing s.**, vomiting, dehydration, hypotension, and sudden death due to very large sodium losses from the body (salt wasting). It may be seen in abnormal losses of sodium into the urine (as in congenital adrenal hyperplasia, adrenocortical insufficiency, or one of the forms of salt-losing nephritis) or in large extrarenal sodium losses, usually from the gastrointestinal tract. Called also *salt-depletion* or *salt-losing crisis* and *salt-losing defect.*

**Sandifer's s.**, intermittent torticollis occurring in children as a symptom of reflux esophagitis or hiatal hernia.

**Sanfilippo's s.**, four heterogeneous, biochemically distinct, but clinically indistinguishable forms of mucopolysaccharidosis characterized biochemically by excretion of heparan sulfate in the urine and clinically by severe, rapid mental deterioration and relatively mild somatic symptoms. Onset is from 2 to 6 years of age; the head is large, height normal; Hurler-like features (dysostosis multiplex, hepatomegaly) are mild; hirsutism is generalized; death usually occurs before 20 years of age. The four enzymatic types are *type A,* the most severe, due to deficiency of heparan *N*-sulfatase; *type B,* due to deficiency of α-*N*-acetylglucosaminidase; *type C,* due to deficiency of heparan-α-glucosaminide *N*-acetyltransferase; and *type D,* due to deficiency of *N*-acetylglucosamine-6-sulfatase. Called also *mucopolysaccharidosis III.*

**Santavuori s., Santavuori-Haltia s.**, Haltia-Santovuori disease.

**scalenus s., scalenus anterior s., scalenus anticus s.**, a thoracic outlet syndrome caused by compression of nerves and vessels between a cervical rib and the scalenus anterior muscle; symptoms include pain over the shoulder, often extending down the arm *(brachial plexopathy)* or radiating up the back of the neck. Called also *Naffziger's s.*

**scapulocostal s.**, pain in the superior or posterior aspect of the shoulder girdle, radiating to contiguous regions, as a result of long-standing alteration of the relationship of the scapula and the posterior thoracic wall.

**Schäfer's s.**, pachyonychia congenita associated with retardation of physical and mental development.

**Schanz's s.**, a series of symptoms indicating spinal weakness, consisting of a sense of fatigue, pain on pressure over the spinous processes, pain on lying prone, and indications of spinal curvature.

**Schaumann's s.**, sarcoidosis.

**Scheie's s.**, a relatively mild allelic variant of Hurler's syndrome and the mildest of the three allelic disorders of mucopolysaccharidosis I, characterized by corneal clouding, claw hand, involvement of the aortic valve, somewhat coarse facies with a broad mouth, genu valgum, and pes cavus. Stature, intelligence, and life span are normal; it is caused by a deficiency of L-iduronidase. Called also *mucopolysaccharidosis I S;* formerly called *mucopolysaccharidosis V.*

**Schiff-Sherrington s.**, paraplegia in dogs with rigid extension of the hind limbs, usually associated with acute severe compression of the thoracolumbar spinal cord.

**Schirmer's s.**, a variant of the Sturge-Weber syndrome in which glaucoma occurs early in the course of the disease.

**Schmidt's s.**, 1. [A. Schmidt] paralysis on one side, affecting the vocal cord, the velum palati, the trapezius muscle, and the sternocleidomastoid muscle, due to a lesion of the nucleus ambiguus and nucleus accessorius. Called also *ambiguo-accessorius paralysis* and *vagoaccessory s.* 2. [M. B. Schmidt] hypofunction of more than one endocrine gland, including the thyroid, adrenals, gonads, parathyroids, and endocrine pancreas, in any combination, along with nonendocrine abnormalities of presumed autoimmune origin, such as vitiligo, alopecia, and pernicious anemia; it occurs primarily in adult females. The term was originally applied to primary failure of the adrenal and thyroid glands. Called also *polyglandular autoimmune syndrome, type II.*

**Schönlein-Henoch s.**, see under *purpura.*

**Schüller's s., Schüller-Christian s.**, Hand-Schüller-Christian disease.

**Schultz s.**, agranulocytosis.

**Schwartz-Jampel s., Schwartz-Jampel-Aberfeld s.**, an autosomal recessive disorder characterized by myotonic myopathy, dwarfism, blepharophimosis, joint contractures, and flat facies. Called also *chondrodystrophic myotonia.*

**scimitar s.**, complete or partial venous drainage of the right lung into the inferior vena cava, usually with hypoplasia of the right lung; the anomalous vein has a scimitar shape on a radiograph; see *scimitar sign,* under *sign.*

**sea-blue histiocyte s.**, a rare disorder characterized by the presence of abnormal histiocytes that stain blue with Wright and Giemsa stains *(sea-blue histiocytes)*, accompanied by splenomegaly. Clinically it may range from a benign course with mild purpura secondary to thrombocytopenia, to progressive cirrhosis, hepatic failure, and death. The etiology is unknown, but sometimes it is inherited as an autosomal recessive condition. Called also *sea-blue histiocytosis.*

**Seabright bantam s.**, pseudohypoparathyroidism.

**Seckel's s.**, a syndrome of unknown etiology, characterized by intrauterine growth retardation and postnatal dwarfism with a small head, narrow birdlike face with a beaklike nose, large eyes with an antimongoloid slant, receding mandible, and mild mental retardation. Called also *bird-headed dwarfism, Seckel dwarfism,* and *Virchow-Seckel s.*

**segmentary s.**, a syndrome produced by a lesion of the gray matter of the spinal cord, and marked by weakness and wasting in the affected segment; called also *metameric s.*

**Selye s.**, general adaptation s.

**Senear-Usher s.**, pemphigus erythematosus.

**s. of sensory dissociation with brachial amyotrophy**, see *syringomyelia.*

**Senter s.**, a rare disorder of lamellar ichthyosis, hyperkeratosis, and sensorineural deafness, sometimes with postnatal growth deficiency, variable alopecia, nail dystrophy, tooth malformations, decreased sweating, and inflammatory corneal vascularization. Called also *keratitis-ichthyosis-deafness s.* and *KID s.*

**Sertoli-cell–only s.**, congenital absence of the germinal epithelium of the testes, so that the seminiferous tubules contain only Sertoli cells and the testes are smaller than normal; there is azoospermia with elevated titers of follicle-stimulating hormone and sometimes of luteinizing hormone. Called also *del Castillo's s.*

**serum sickness–like s.**, see *serum sickness*, under *sickness*.

**Sézary s.**, a form of cutaneous T-cell lymphoma manifested by generalized exfoliative erythroderma, intense pruritus, peripheral lymphadenopathy, and abnormal hyperchromatic mononuclear cells in the skin, lymph nodes, and peripheral blood *(Sézary cells)*. Called also *Sézary erythroderma*.

**shaker foal s.**, a type of botulism in young horses, accompanied by flaccid tetraparesis and inability to swallow, so that there is risk of aspiration pneumonia.

**Sheehan's s.**, postpartum pituitary necrosis.

**short-bowel s., short-gut s.**, any of the malabsorption conditions resulting from massive resection of the small bowel, the degree and kind of malabsorption depending on the site and extent of the resection; it is characterized by diarrhea, steatorrhea, and malnutrition.

**shoulder-hand s.**, reflex sympathetic dystrophy limited to the upper extremity; see under *dystrophy*.

**Shprintzen's s.**, velocardiofacial s.

**Shulman's s.**, eosinophilic fasciitis.

**Shwachman s., Shwachman-Diamond s.**, primary pancreatic insufficiency and bone marrow failure, characterized by normal sweat chloride values, pancreatic insufficiency, and neutropenia; it may be associated with dwarfism and metaphyseal dysostosis of the hips.

**Shy-Drager s.**, a progressive disorder of unknown etiology that begins with symptoms of autonomic insufficiency including orthostatic hypotension, impotence in males, constipation, urinary urgency or retention, and anhidrosis; these are followed by signs of generalized neurologic dysfunction such as parkinsonian-like disturbances, cerebellar incoordination, muscle wasting and fasciculations, and coarse tremors of the legs. Called also *chronic, chronic idiopathic,* or *idiopathic orthostatic hypotension*.

**Shy-Magee s.**, central core disease.

**Sicard's s.**, Collet's s.

**sicca s.**, keratoconjunctivitis and xerostomia without connective tissue disease; cf. *Sjögren's s.*

**sick sinus s.**, a syndrome of bradycardia, generally intermittent and sometimes mixed with episodes of atrial tachyarrhythmias (see *bradycardia-tachycardia s.*) or periods of sinus arrest, due to malfunction originating in the supraventricular portion of the cardiac conduction system.

**Silfverskiöld's s.**, a form of eccentro-osteochondrodysplasia in which the skeletal changes are chiefly in the extremities and which is inherited as a dominant character.

**Silver's s., Silver-Russell s.**, a syndrome consisting of low birth weight despite normal length of gestation, short stature, lateral asymmetry, and slight to moderate increase in excretion of gonadotropins, which may be associated with incurved fifth fingers, café-au-lait spots, syndactyly, triangular face, downturned corners of the mouth, and precocious puberty. Called also *Russell s.* or *dwarfism, Russell-Silver s.* or *dwarfism,* and *Silver-Russell dwarfism*.

**Silverman's s.**, Currarino-Silverman s.

**Silvestrini-Corda s.**, a syndrome seen in either men or women with cirrhosis of the liver, consisting of eunuchoid body type, loss of body hair, atrophy of the testes with gynecomastia in males, menstrual disorders such as menorrhagia or amenorrhea in women, sterility, and decreased libido. It results from abnormally high estrogenic activity due to failure of the liver to inactivate the circulating estrogens.

**Simmonds' s.**, see *panhypopituitarism*.

**Sipple's s.**, multiple endocrine neoplasia, type II.

**Sjögren's s.**, a symptom complex of unknown etiology, usually occurring in middle-aged or older women, marked by the triad of keratoconjunctivitis sicca with or without lacrimal gland enlargement, xerostomia with or without salivary gland enlargement, and the presence of a connective tissue disease, usually rheumatoid arthritis but sometimes systemic lupus erythematosus, scleroderma, or polymyositis. An abnormal immune response has been implicated. Called also *Sjögren's disease*. See also *sicca s.*

**Sjögren-Larsson s.**, congenital oligophrenia, ichthyosis, and spastic pyramidal symptoms.

**sleep apnea s.**, sleep apnea.

**sleeper s.**, thromboembolic meningoencephalitis.

**SLE-like s.**, see *systemic lupus erythematosus,* under *lupus*.

**slipping rib s.**, weakness or rupture of the medial fibrous attachments of the eighth, ninth, or tenth ribs, so that their cartilage tip slips upward and impinges on the intercostal nerve, causing chest pain.

**Sluder's s.**, see under *neuralgia*.

**Sly's s.**, a mucopolysaccharidosis caused by deficiency of $\beta$-glucuronidase and characterized biochemically by excretion of dermatan sulfate, heparan sulfate, and chondroitin sulfates A and C in the urine and by granular inclusions in granulocytes. Onset is between 1 and 2 years with mild to moderate Hurler-like features including dysostosis multiplex, pectus carinatum, visceromegaly, cardiac murmurs, short stature, and moderate mental retardation. Milder forms exist. Called also *mucopolysaccharidosis VII*.

**Smith-Lemli-Opitz s.**, a hereditary syndrome, transmitted as an autosomal recessive trait, characterized by multiple congenital anomalies, including microcephaly, mental retardation, hypotonia, incomplete development of male genitalia, short nose with anteverted nostrils, and syndactyly of second and third toes.

**Sneddon's s.**, a rare condition in which cerebral arteriopathy and ischemia are accompanied by diffuse non-inflammatory livedo reticularis.

**SO s.**, orbital apex s.

**social breakdown s.**, deterioration of social and interpersonal skills, work habits, and behavior seen in chronically hospitalized psychiatric patients; due to the effects of long-term institutionalization rather than the primary illness. Symptoms include excessive passivity, assumption of the chronic sick role, withdrawal, and apathy. Such effects are also seen in long-term inmates of prisons or concentration camps.

**Sohval-Soffer s.**, a congenital syndrome consisting of male hypogonadism associated with multiple skeletal abnormalities of the cervical spine and ribs and mental retardation.

**somnolence s.**, a transient condition of drowsiness, lethargy, anorexia, and irritability with electroencephalographic changes, occurring in children after irradiation of the head in the treatment of brain tumors, acute leukemia, or non-Hodgkin's lymphoma.

**Sorsby's s.**, a congenital condition consisting of bilateral macular coloboma associated with apical dystrophy of the hands and feet, usually brachydactyly confined to the distal two phalanges.

**Sotos' s., Sotos' s. of cerebral gigantism,** cerebral gigantism.

**space adaptation s.**, a form of motion sickness occurring in a weightless environment during space flight, with nausea, vomiting, anorexia, headache, malaise, drowsiness, and lethargy. It is probably caused by conflicting signals concerning motion from the otolith (whose proper function depends on the presence of gravity) and the visual system (which affects the autonomic nervous system). Called also *space sickness*.

**Spanish toxic oil s.**, name given to an epidemic of acute pneumonia with pulmonary edema, fever, rash, myalgia, and eosinophilia, sometimes with neuromuscular damage or fatal respiratory failure; it occurred in Spain in 1981 after contaminated cooking oil was sold by traveling salesmen. The toxin has not been identified. Called also *toxic oil s.*

**Spens' s.**, Adams-Stokes s.

**sphenoidal fissure–optic canal s.**, orbital apex s.

**spherophakia-brachymorphia s.**, Weill-Marchesani s.

**splenic flexure s.**, Payr's disease.

**split-brain s.**, an association of symptoms produced by disruption of or interference with the connection between the hemispheres of the brain. See also *split brain,* under *brain*.

**Sprinz-Dubin s., Sprinz-Nelson s.**, Dubin-Johnson s.

**spun glass hair s.**, uncombable hair s.

**Spurway's s.**, osteogenesis imperfecta (type I).

**stagnant loop s.**, stasis s.

**staphylococcal scalded skin s.**, an infectious disease of infants, young children, and occasionally older children and adults occurring following infection with certain strains of *Staphylococcus aureus* (phage group II), which elaborate exfoliatin (q.v.), an epidermolytic erythrogen endotoxin. It causes a clinical spectrum ranging from a localized bulla to widespread fine vesicles and bullae that are easily ruptured, resulting in exfoliation of large sheets of skin, leaving raw, denuded areas that make the skin surface look scalded. Called also *dermatitis exfoliativa neonatorum* and *Ritter's disease*. Cf. *toxic epidermal necrolysis*.

**stasis s.**, overgrowth of bacteria within the small intestine resulting from a variety of conditions causing stasis, particularly disturbances to intestinal motility or decreased acid secretion, but also structural abnormalities such as diverticula, fistulae between the colon and upper bowel, or chronic obstruction; it is characterized by malabsorption of vitamin $B_{12}$, steatorrhea, and anemia. Called also *bacterial overgrowth s., blind loop s.,* and *stagnant loop s.*

**Stauffer s.**, a paraneoplastic syndrome seen in patients with renal cell carcinoma, marked by biochemical hepatic abnormalities without hepatic metastasis of the tumor.

**Steele-Richardson-Olszewski s.**, a progressive neurological disorder, having onset during the sixth decade, characterized by supranuclear ophthalmoplegia, especially paralysis of the downward gaze, pseudobulbar palsy, dysarthria, dystonic rigidity of the neck and trunk, and dementia.

**steely-hair s.**, Menkes' s.

**Stein-Leventhal s.**, polycystic ovary s.

**Steinbrocker's s.**, shoulder-hand s.

**Steiner's s.**, Curtius' s.

**Stevens-Johnson s.**, a sometimes fatal form of erythema multiforme presenting with a flulike prodrome, and characterized by systemic as well as more severe mucocutaneous lesions. The oronasal and anogenital mucous membranes may become involved with a characteristic gray or white pseudomembrane, and hemorrhagic crusts often occur on the lips. Ocular lesions vary, often with injected conjunctivitis, iritis, uveitis, corneal vesicles, erosions, and perforation, which may result in corneal opacities and blindness. Pulmonary, gastrointestinal, cardiac, and renal involvement also occur. Called also *ectodermosis erosiva pluriorificialis, erythema multiforme majus,* and *Johnson-Stevens disease.*

**Stewart-Treves s.,** lymphangiosarcoma which occurs as a late complication of severe lymphedema of the arm following excision of lymph nodes, usually associated with radical mastectomy.

**Stickler's s.,** hereditary progressive arthro-ophthalmopathy.

**stiff heart s.,** any cardiac disease characterized by restrictive hemodynamics; it may result from any pathologic process that renders the myocardial fibers abnormally rigid or that externally applies a constricting pressure and as a consequence impedes flow of blood into the ventricular cavities.

**stiff-man s.,** a condition of unknown etiology characterized by progressive fluctuating rigidity of axial and limb muscles in the absence of signs of cerebral and spinal cord disease but with continuous electromyographic activity.

**Still-Chauffard s.,** Chauffard's s.

**Stilling's s., Stilling-Türk-Duane s.,** Duane's s.

**Stokes' s., Stokes-Adams s.,** Adams-Stokes s.

**Stokvis-Talma s.,** enterogenous cyanosis.

**stomatitis-pneumoenteritis s.,** peste des petits ruminants.

**Strachan's s., Strachan-Scott s.,** a nutritional polyneuropathy of unknown etiology found in impoverished areas of Jamaica and other countries, possibly due to a deficiency in dietary thiamine or riboflavin; characterized by amblyopia, paresthesias, dizziness, glossitis, stomatitis, lesions of the sensory pathways, and various other symptoms.

**straight back s.,** a skeletal deformity characterized by loss of the anterior concavity of the vertebral column in the upper thoracic region, with consequent reduction in the anteroposterior diameter of the thorax and compression of the heart between the dorsal spine and the sternum.

**stroke s.,** a condition with sudden onset caused by acute vascular lesions of the brain, such as infarction from hemorrhage, embolism, or thrombosis, or rupturing aneurysm. It may be marked by any of a variety of symptoms reflecting the focus of infarction or hemorrhage, including hemiparesis, vertigo, numbness, aphasia, and dysarthria; it is often followed by permanent neurologic damage. Called also *cerebrovascular accident* and *stroke.*

**Sturge's s., Sturge-Kalischer-Weber s.,** Sturge-Weber s.

**Sturge-Weber s.,** a congenital syndrome of unknown etiology consisting of a port-wine stain distributed over the trigeminal nerve accompanied by a similar vascular disorder of the underlying meninges and cerebral cortex; it usually occurs unilaterally. Called also *encephalofacial* or *encephalotrigeminal angiomatosis, Sturge's* or *Sturge-Kalischer-Weber s.,* and *Weber's disease.*

**subclavian steal s.,** cerebral or brain stem ischemia resulting from vertebrobasilar insufficiency in cases of subclavian steal.

**sudden infant death s. (SIDS),** the sudden and unexpected death of an apparently healthy infant, typically occurring between the ages of three weeks and five months, and not explained by careful postmortem studies; called also *cot death* and *crib death.*

**sudden unexplained death s.,** death for which no underlying cause can be found of a person 2 years old or older, observed particularly in those of Southeast Asian origin. Abbreviated SUDS.

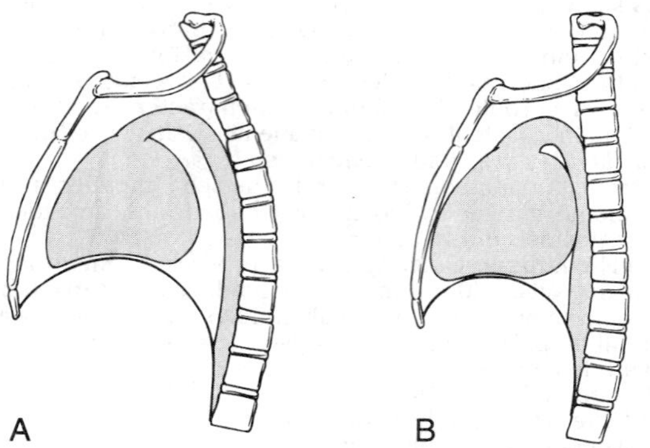


Straight back syndrome. Normal thoracolumbar curvature and anteroposterior chest dimension *(A)* are contrasted with decreased curvature and anteroposterior chest dimension in straight back syndrome *(B).*

**Sudeck-Leriche s.,** post-traumatic osteoporosis associated with vasospasm.

**Sulzberger-Garbe s.,** exudative discoid and lichenoid dermatitis.

**sundown s.,** sundowning.

**superior mesenteric artery s.,** compression of the third, or transverse, portion of the duodenum against the aorta by the superior mesenteric artery, resulting in complete or partial obstruction that may be chronic, intermittent, or acute; symptoms range from mild to severe, including nausea and vomiting, pain, and extreme distention of the stomach and duodenum.

**superior orbital fissure s.,** deep orbital and unilateral frontal headache with progressive sixth, third, and fourth cranial nerve palsies, with oculomotor paralysis, diminution of the field of vision, and other ocular changes; it occurs either as a result of a meningioma of the sphenoid bone that compresses nearby nerves or as an extension of infection from sphenoid sinusitis into the superior orbital fissure. Cf. *Tolosa-Hunt s.*

**superior sulcus tumor s.,** Pancoast's s. (def. 1).

**superior vena cava s.,** a complex of symptoms caused by compression of the superior vena cava, such as by a bronchial tumor or by metastatic mediastinal lymph nodes in lung cancer; characteristics include suffusion and brawny edema of the face, neck, or upper arms; central nervous system disturbances; cyanosis; conjunctival edema; and edema of the trachea and esophagus leading to dyspnea and dysphagia.

**supraspinatus s.,** tenderness over the supraspinatus tendon, a painful arc on movement of the arm, and a reversal of scapulohumeral rhythm.

**supravalvular aortic stenosis s.,** Williams s.

**sweat retention s.,** 1. a dermatologic condition due to occlusion of sweat ducts, which may result in symptoms ranging from pruritus, scratch dermatitis, and miliaria to very persistent inflammatory changes depending upon the extent of the blockage, environmental temperature, and duration of sweating stimulus. 2. tropical anhidrotic asthenia.

**Sweet's s.,** acute febrile neutrophilic dermatosis.

**Swyer s.,** 46,XY gonadal dysgenesis.

**Swyer-James s.,** acquired unilateral emphysema, with severe airway obstruction during expiration, oligemia, and a small hilum; called also *Macleod's s.*

**sylvian s., sylvian aqueduct s.,** impairment of vertical gaze, retraction nystagmus, convergence nystagmus, convergence spasms, and poor or absent reaction of the pupils (which are usually of normal size) to light or near vision. It is caused by a neoplasm, inflammation, or vascular lesion adjacent to the periductal gray matter of the aqueduct of Sylvius. Called also *Koerber-Salus-Elschnig s.* and *retraction nystagmus.*

**syringomyelic s.,** syringomyelia.

**systolic click–murmur s.,** mitral valve prolapse s.

**Takayasu's s.,** see under *arteritis.*

**Tapia's s.,** unilateral paralysis of the tongue and larynx, the soft palate being unaffected. It follows injury to the vagus and hypoglossal nerves, most often from trauma or a tumor. Called also *ambiguohypoglossal paralysis.*

**TAR s.,** thrombocytopenia–absent radius s.

**tarsal tunnel s.,** a complex of symptoms resulting from compression of the posterior tibial nerve or of the plantar nerves in the tarsal tunnel, with pain, numbness, and tingling paresthesia of the sole of the foot.

**Taussig-Bing s.,** a rare congenital malformation of the heart characterized by transposition of the great vessels and a ventricular septal defect straddled by a large pulmonary artery; hemodynamically it is characterized by pulmonary hypertension, pulmonary plethora, cyanosis, and greater $O_2$ saturation of blood in the pulmonary artery than in the aorta.

**tegmental s.,** Benedikt's s.

**temporomandibular dysfunction s., temporomandibular joint s.,** Costen's s.

**Terry's s.,** retinopathy of prematurity.

**Terson's s.,** hemorrhage into the vitreous.

**testicular feminization s.,** complete androgen resistance; see under *resistance.*

**tethered cord s.,** a congenital anomaly resulting from defective closure of the neural tube; the conus medullaris is abnormally low and is tethered by one or more forms of intradural abnormality such as a short, thickened filum terminale, fibrous bands or adhesions, or an intraspinal lipoma.

**thalamic s., thalamic pain s.,** a syndrome caused by a lesion in the thalamus and characterized by contralateral hemianesthesia; some later develop persistent severe pain and choreoathetoid movements on the affected side, mild hemiataxia, and astereognosis. Called also *Dejerine-Roussy s.* and *thalamic hyperesthetic anesthesia.*

**Thévenard's s.,** hereditary sensory radicular neuropathy.

**Thibierge-Weissenbach s.,** calcinosis.

**Thiele s.**, tenderness and pain in the region of the lower portion of the sacrum and coccyx, or in contiguous soft tissues and muscles.

**Thiemann's s.**, see under *disease.*

**thin ewe s.**, chronic caseous lymphadenitis in a ewe, with weight loss and reproductive failure.

**thoracic outlet s.**, any of a variety of neurovascular syndromes resulting from compression of the subclavian artery, the brachial plexus nerve trunks, or less often the axillary vein or subclavian vein, by thoracic outlet abnormalities such as a drooping shoulder girdle, a cervical rib or fibrous band, an abnormal first rib, or occasionally compression of the edge of the scalenus anterior muscle. Continual hyperabduction of the arm may cause another variety *(hyperabduction s.).* Arterial compression leads to ischemia, paresthesias, numbness, and weakness of the affected arm, sometimes with Raynaud's phenomenon of the arm. Nerve compression causes atrophy and weakness of the muscles of the hand and, in advanced cases, of the forearm, with pain and sensory disturbances in the arm. Venous obstruction usually takes the form of the Paget-Schroetter syndrome. Other types include the *cervical rib s., costoclavicular s.,* and *scalenus anticus s.*

**Thorn's s.**, salt-losing nephritis.

**thrombocytopenia–absent radius s.**, an autosomal recessive syndrome consisting of thrombocytopenia associated with absence or hypoplasia of the radius and sometimes congenital heart disease and renal anomalies. Called also *TAR s.*

**thromboembolic s.**, the association between the formation of thrombi in the deep veins of the leg and pulmonary embolism.

**Tietze's s.**, 1. idiopathic painful nonsuppurative swellings of one or more costal cartilages, especially of the second rib; the anterior chest pain may mimic that of coronary artery disease. Called also *costal chondritis.* 2. albinism, except for normal eye pigment, deaf-mutism, and hypoplasia of the eyebrows.

**Tolosa-Hunt s.**, unilateral ophthalmoplegia associated with pain behind the orbit and in the area supplied by the first division of the trigeminal nerve; it is thought to be due to nonspecific inflammation and granulation tissue in the superior orbital fissure or cavernous sinus. Cf. *cavernous sinus s.* and *superior orbital fissure s.*

**Tommaselli's s.**, see under *disease.*

**TORCH s.** (*t*oxoplasmosis, *o*ther agents, *r*ubella, *c*ytomegalovirus, *h*erpes simplex), any of a group of infections seen in neonates due to one of the causative agents having crossed the placental barrier; they all have similar symptoms in babies and may be clinically silent in the mothers. Called also *TORCH infection.*

**Torre's s.**, multiple carcinomas, primarily of the gastrointestinal tract, in association with a large number of sebaceous gland neoplasms.

**Touraine-Solente-Golé s.**, pachydermoperiostosis.

**Tourette's s.**, Gilles de la Tourette's s.

**Townes' s.**, an autosomal dominant syndrome of auricular anomalies, anal defects, limb and digit—particularly thumb—anomalies, and renal deficiencies; it occasionally includes cardiac disease, deafness, or cystic ovary.

**toxic fat s.**, toxicity in 3- to 10-week old chickens that have been fed diets supplemented with fat containing any of several toxins; symptoms are edema of the pericardium and abdomen, waddling gait, and sudden death.

**toxic hypoglycemic s.**, Jamaican vomiting sickness.

**toxic oil s.**, Spanish toxic oil s.

**toxic shock s.**, a severe illness caused by a bacterial infection, characterized by high fever of sudden onset, vomiting, diarrhea, and myalgia, followed by hypotension and, in severe cases, shock. A sunburnlike rash with peeling of the skin, especially of the palms and soles, occurs during the acute phase. It was originally observed almost exclusively in menstruating women using tampons, with the infective agent being *Staphylococcus aureus,* but a nearly identical syndrome has subsequently been seen in males and females of different ages infected with Group A *Streptococcus.*

**translocation Down s.**, Down syndrome in which the excess chromosomal material (the long arm of chromosome 21) is translocated to another acrocentric chromosome (in standard trisomy 21 there is an additional chromosome 21). A carrier of the translocation chromosome has 45 chromosomes including the translocation chromosome and may be at increased risk of having a child with Down syndrome.

**Treacher Collins s.**, the incomplete form of mandibulofacial dysostosis.

**Treacher Collins–Franceschetti s.**, mandibulofacial dysostosis.

**trichorhinophalangeal s.**, an autosomal recessive syndrome consisting of sparse, slowly growing hair, pear-shaped nose with high philtrum, and brachyphalangia with deformity of the fingers and wedge-shaped epiphyses.

**triparanol s.**, alopecia, poliosis, ichthyosis, irreversible cataracts, and impotence, due to the use of triparanol, a drug formerly used to depress the synthesis of cholesterol.

**triple-A s.** [*a*lacrima-*a*chalasia-*a*ddisonian], Allgrove's s.

**trismus-pseudocamptodactyly s.**, a rare autosomal dominant disorder characterized by inability to open the mouth fully, facultative camptodactyly resulting from shortened finger-flexor tendons, and short stature.

**trisomy 8 s.**, a syndrome associated with an extra chromosome 8, usually mosaic (trisomy 8/normal), characterized by mild to severe mental retardation, prominent forehead, deep-set eyes, thick lips, prominent ears, and camptodactyly.

**trisomy 11q s.**, a syndrome resulting from the presence of an extra long arm of chromosome 11; because different segments may be involved, the associated anomalies are highly variable and include preauricular fistulas, hypoplasia of the gallbladder, micropenis, bicornuate uterus, microphthalmos, malformations of the heart, lung, and brain, seizures, and recurrent infection.

**trisomy 13 s.**, a chromosome aberration in which an extra chromosome 13 causes central nervous system defects and mental retardation, together with cleft palate and lip, polydactyly, dermal pattern anomalies, and abnormalities of the heart, viscera, and genitalia. Called also *Patau's s.*

**trisomy 18 s.**, a condition characterized by mental retardation, scaphocephaly or other skull abnormality, micrognathia, blepharoptosis, low-set ears, corneal opacities, deafness, webbed neck, short digits, ventricular septal defects, Meckel's diverticulum, and other deformities. It is due to the presence of an extra chromosome 18. Called also *Edwards' s.* and *trisomy E s.*

**trisomy 21 s.**, Down s.

**trisomy 22 s.**, a syndrome due to an extra chromosome 22, characterized typically by mental and growth retardation, microcephaly, low-set or malformed ears, micrognathia, long philtrum, preauricular skin tag or sinus, and congenital heart disease. In males, there is small penis and/or undescended testes.

**trisomy C s.**, trisomy 8 s.

**trisomy D s.**, trisomy 13 s.

**trisomy E s.**, trisomy 18 s.

**Troisier's s.**, bronzed cachexia occurring in the diabetes associated with hemochromatosis.

**tropical splenomegaly s.**, malarial hyperreactive spleen s.

**Trousseau's s.**, thrombophlebitis migrans occurring primarily as a paraneoplastic syndrome in association with carcinoma of the abdominal viscera, but also with some types of metastatic neoplasms and chemotherapy.

**tumor lysis s.**, severe hyperphosphatemia, hyperkalemia, hyperuricemia, and hypocalcemia occurring after effective induction chemotherapy of rapidly growing malignant neoplasms; thought to be due to release of intracellular products after cell lysis.

**Turcot's s.**, familial adenomatous polyposis of the colon associated with malignant tumors (gliomas) of the central nervous system.

**Turner's s.**, a disorder of gonadal differentiation in patients phenotypically female, marked by short stature, undifferentiated (streak) gonads, and variable abnormalities that may include webbing of the neck, low posterior hair line, cubitus valgus, and cardiac defects; it is typically associated with absence of the second sex chromosome (XO or 45,X), although structural abnormality of one X chromosome or mosaicism (e.g., XX/XX or X/XXX) may also be responsible. Called also *gonadal dysgenesis.*

**Turner's s., male,** Noonan's s.

**twiddler's s.**, dislodgement, breakdown, or other malfunction of an artificial cardiac pacemaker, chemotherapy port, drip infusion valve, or similar implanted diagnostic or therapeutic device as a result of unconscious or habitual manipulation by the patient.

**twin transfusion s., twin-twin transfusion s.**, a syndrome caused by twin-to-twin transfusion (q.v.); the donor twin develops hypovolemia, hypotension, anemia, microcardia, and growth retardation, while the recipient develops hypervolemia, hypertension, polycythemia, cardiomegaly, and congestive heart failure; hydramnios frequently occurs.

**tying-up s.**, azoturia (def. 2).

**Uberreiter's s.**, chronic superficial keratitis.

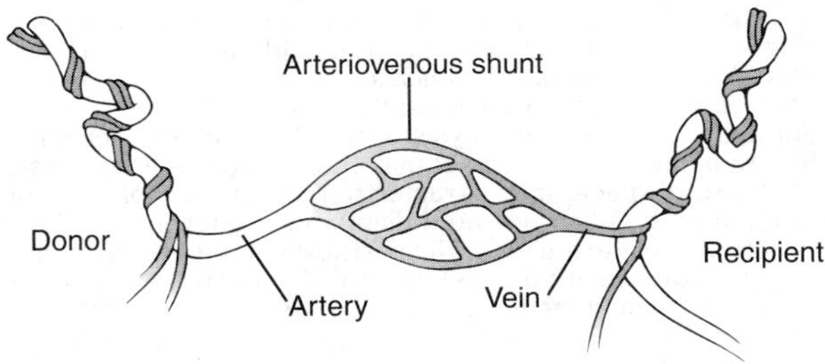


Twin transfusion syndrome characterized by arteriovenous shunt at a shared placental cotyledon in diamniotic monochorionic twins.

**Ullrich-Feichtiger s.,** a condition of micrognathia, hexadactyly, and genital abnormalities, with depressed nose, small eyes, hypertelorism, and protuberant ears, along with other defects.

**Ullrich-Turner s.,** Noonan's s.

**uncombable hair s.,** an abnormality of the hair inherited as an autosomal dominant trait, in which the individual hairs are triangular in cross section, with a longitudinal groove; the hair has a spun-glass appearance and is arranged in bundles that stand out in different directions. Called also *pili canaliculi, pili trianguli et canaliculi,* and *spun glass hair s.*

**unilateral nevoid telangiectasia s.,** generalized essential telangiectasia representing a latent vascular nevus that becomes manifest under the possible influence of estrogens (pregnancy, menarche) or increased venous pressure (liver disease). Called also *unilateral nevoid telangiectasia.*

**Unna-Thost s.,** diffuse palmoplantar keratoderma.

**upper airway resistance s.,** an incomplete form of obstructive sleep apnea in which the upper airway resists air flow and becomes partially obstructed during sleep.

**urethral s.,** suprapubic aching and cramping, urinary frequency, and such bladder complaints as dysuria, urinary tenesmus, and low back pain, without evidence of urinary infection.

**Usher's s.,** an autosomal recessive syndrome in which congenital deafness is accompanied by retinitis pigmentosa, often ending in blindness; sometimes mental retardation and disturbances of gait also occur.

**vagoaccessory s.,** Schmidt's s. (def. 1).

**vagoaccessory-hypoglossal s.,** Jackson's s.

**Vail's s.,** vidian neuralgia.

**Van Allen's s.,** Iowa type familial amyloid polyneuropathy.

**van Bogaert-Nyssen s.,** the adult form of metachromatic leukodystrophy.

**van Buchem's s.,** hyperostosis corticalis generalisata.

**van der Hoeve's s.,** osteogenesis imperfecta (type I).

**Van der Woude's s.,** an autosomal dominant syndrome consisting of cleft lip with or without cleft palate, with cysts of the lower lip.

**vanishing testes s.,** a disorder in males characterized by absence of testes and gonadal tissue (usually unilateral but sometimes bilateral) and a small penis; when it is bilateral the individual will not undergo puberty or adolescent masculinization without testosterone supplements. The testes are thought to have been present in the embryo but to have "vanished" before completion of male sexual differentiation. Called also *embryonic testicular regression s.*

**vanishing twin s.,** the disappearance of one fetus following the sonographic diagnosis of a twin pregnancy, with only one twin eventually being delivered; the vanished twin may be resorbed or incorporated into the placental membrane.

**vascular s.,** any syndrome due to occlusion or stenosis of vessels supplying the nervous system.

**vascular leak s.,** a disorder caused by extravasation of plasma through vessel walls, causing edema in surrounding tissues; the most common cause is a reaction to therapy with interleukin-2.

**VCF s., velocardiofacial s.,** an autosomal dominant syndrome of cardiac defects and characteristic craniofacial abnormalities including cleft palate, jaw abnormalities, and prominent nose; it is often associated with abnormalities of chromosome 22. Learning disabilities occur often; short stature, slender hyperextensible hands and digits, scoliosis, mental retardation, inguinal hernia, auricular abnormalities, and microcephaly occur less frequently. Called also *Shprintzen's s.*

**Verner-Morrison s.,** a rare syndrome of profuse watery diarrhea, hypokalemia, and achlorhydria, usually associated with excess levels of vasoactive intestinal polypeptide resulting from a vipoma in the pancreas; called also *diarrheogenic s., pancreatic cholera, pancreatic cholera s.,* and *WDHA s.*

**Vernet's s.,** paralysis of the ninth, tenth, and eleventh cranial nerves due to a lesion in the region of the jugular foramen, and marked by paralysis of the superior constriction of the pharynx and difficulty in swallowing solids; paralysis of the soft palate and fauces with anesthesia of these parts and of the pharynx, and loss of taste in the posterior third of the tongue; paralysis of the vocal cords and anesthesia of the larynx; and paralysis of the sternocleidomastoid and trapezius muscles. Called also *jugular foramen s.*

**vertebrobasilar s.,** see under *insufficiency.*

**Villaret's s.,** unilateral paralysis of the ninth, tenth, eleventh, and twelfth cranial nerves and sometimes the seventh, due to a lesion in the retroparotid space, and characterized by paralysis of the superior constriction of the pharynx and difficulty in swallowing solids; paralysis of soft palate and fauces with anesthesia of these parts and of the pharynx; loss of taste in the posterior third of the tongue; paralysis of the vocal cords and anesthesia of the larynx; paralysis of the sternocleidomastoid and trapezius; and paralysis of the cervical sympathetic nerves *(Horner's syndrome).* Called also *s. of retroparotid space.*

**Vinson's s.,** Plummer-Vinson s.

**Virchow-Seckel s.,** Seckel's syndrome.

**vitamin E–selenium deficiency s.,** a deficiency disease of pigs whose diet is low in vitamin E and selenium, most commonly rapidly growing, recently weaned piglets. It usually manifests as either hepatosis dietetica or mulberry heart disease, and affected animals may die suddenly during exercise.

**Vogt's s.,** a syndrome associated with birth trauma, characterized by bilateral athetosis, walking difficulties, spasmodic outbursts of laughing or crying, speech disorders, excessive myelination of the nerve fibers of the corpus striatum, giving it a marbled appearance *(status marmoratus),* and sometimes mental deficiency. Called also *s. of corpus striatum.*

**Vogt-Koyanagi s.,** uveomeningitis characterized by exudative iridocyclitis and choroiditis associated with patchy depigmentation of the skin and hair; the lashes and eyebrows also become whitened, and there may also be retinal detachment and associated deafness and tinnitus. Cf. *Vogt-Koyanagi-Harada s.*

**Vogt-Koyanagi-Harada s.,** bilateral uveitis with exudative iridocyclitis, choroiditis, meningism, and temporary or permanent retinal detachment, occurring in association with alopecia, vitiligo, poliosis, loss of visual acuity, headache, vomiting, deafness, and sometimes vertigo or glaucoma. The syndrome may be an inflammatory autoimmune disorder. Called also *Harada s.*

**Vohwinkel's s.,** keratoma hereditarium mutilans.

**Volkmann's s.,** see under *contracture.*

**Waardenburg's s.,** 1. an autosomal dominant disorder characterized by wide bridge of the nose due to lateral displacement of the inner canthi and puncta, pigmentary disturbances, including white forelock, heterochromia iridis, white eyelashes, leukoderma, and sometimes cochlear deafness. 2. an autosomal dominant disorder characterized by acrocephaly, orbital and facial deformities, and brachydactyly with mild soft tissue syndactyly; cleft palate, hydrophthalmos, cardiac malformation, and contractures of the elbows and knees may also be present. Called also *acrocephalosyndactyly type IV* and *Klein-Waardenburg s.*

**WAGR s.,** a syndrome of *W*ilms' tumor, *a*niridia, *g*enitourinary abnormalities or *g*onadoblastoma, and mental *r*etardation, due to a small interstitial deletion of the p13 region of chromosome 11.

**Walker-Warburg s.,** a congenital syndrome, usually fatal before the age of one year, consisting of hydrocephalus, agyria, various ocular anomalies such as retinal dysplasia, corneal opacity, or microphthalmia, and sometimes an encephalocele. Called also *Walker's lissencephaly, HARD s.,* and *Warburg's s.*

**Wallenberg's s.,** a syndrome due usually to occlusion of the vertebral artery, and less often to occlusion of its branch, the posterior inferior cerebellar artery; marked by ipsilateral loss of temperature and pain sensations of the face and contralateral loss of these sensations of the extremities and trunk, ipsilateral ataxia, dysphagia, dysarthria, nystagmus, and Horner's syndrome. Called also *lateral medullary s.* and *posterior inferior cerebellar artery s.*

**Warburg's s.,** Walker-Warburg s.

**Ward-Romano s.,** Romano-Ward s.

**Waterhouse-Friderichsen s.,** the malignant or fulminating form of epidemic cerebrospinal meningitis, marked by sudden onset and short course, fever, coma, and collapse, cyanosis, petechial hemorrhages of the skin and mucous membranes, and bilateral adrenal hemorrhage.

**WDHA s.,** [*w*atery *d*iarrhea, *h*ypokalemia, *a*chlorhydria], Verner-Morrison s.

**WDHH s.,** [*w*atery *d*iarrhea, *h*ypokalemia, *h*ypochlorhydria], Verner-Morrison s.

**Weber's s.,** paralysis of the oculomotor nerve on the same side as the lesion, producing ptosis, strabismus, and loss of light reflex and of accommodation; also spastic hemiplegia on the side opposite the lesion with increased reflexes and loss of superficial reflexes. Called also *alternating oculomotor hemiplegia* and *Weber's paralysis.*

**Weber-Christian s.,** relapsing febrile nodular nonsuppurative panniculitis.

**Weber-Cockayne s.,** localized epidermolysis bullosa simplex.

**Weber-Gubler s., Weber-Leyden s.,** Weber's s.

**Wegener's s.,** see under *granulomatosis.*

**Weil's s.,** a severe form of leptospirosis characterized by jaundice usually with azotemia, hemorrhages, anemia, disturbances of consciousness, and fever. It is usually caused by *Leptospira interrogans* serovar *icterohaemorrhagiae* but may be caused by other serovars. Called also *Fiedler's, Lancereaux-Mathieu,* or *Landouzy's disease, leptospirosis icterohaemorrhagica,* and *infectious, infective, leptospiral,* or *spirochetal jaundice.*

**Weill-Marchesani s.,** a congenital disorder of connective tissue transmitted as an autosomal dominant or recessive trait, characterized by brachycephaly, brachydactyly, short stature with a broad chest and heavy musculature, reduced joint mobility, spherophakia, ectopia lentis, myopia, and glaucoma; called also *dystrophia mesodermalis congenita hyperplastica, Marchesani's s.,* and *spherophakia-brachymorphia s.*

**Weingarten's s.,** tropical eosinophilia.
**Welander's s.,** late distal hereditary myopathy.
**Wells' s.,** cellulitis with erythema, edema, and often blistering of the skin accompanied by eosinophilia, flame figures, and a mild fever; a single episode lasts 2 to 6 weeks and recurrences or exacerbations are common. Called also *eosinophilic cellulitis.*
**Wermer's s.,** multiple endocrine neoplasia, type I.
**Werner's s.,** premature aging in the adult, transmitted as an autosomal recessive trait, and characterized principally by scleroderma-like skin changes, involving especially the extremities, cataracts, subcutaneous calcification, muscular atrophy, a tendency to diabetes mellitus, aged appearance of the face, canities and baldness, and a high incidence of neoplasm. Short stature is common from childhood on; the other features usually develop during adulthood.
**Wernicke's s.,** see under *encephalopathy.*
**Wernicke-Korsakoff s.,** the behavioral disorder caused by thiamine deficiency, most commonly due to chronic alcohol abuse and associated with other nutritional polyneuropathies. *Wernicke's encephalopathy* (confusion, ataxia of gait, nystagmus, and ophthalmoplegia) occurs as an acute attack and is reversible, except for some residual ataxia or nystagmus, by administration of thiamine; *Korsakoff's syndrome* (severe anterograde and retrograde amnesia) may occur in conjunction with Wernicke's encephalopathy or may become apparent later; only about 20 per cent of patients recover completely from the amnesia.
**West's s.,** infantile spasms.
**Weyers' oligodactyly s.,** a congenital syndrome consisting of deficiency of the ulna and ulnar rays, antecubital pterygia, reduced sternal segments, malformations of the kidney and spleen, and cleft lip and palate.
**whiplash shake s.,** a constellation of injuries to the brain and eye that may occur when a child less than 3 years old, usually less than 1 year old, is shaken vigorously while being held by the trunk or limbs with the head unsupported. This causes stretching and tearing of the cerebral vessels and brain substance, commonly leading to subdural hematomas and retinal hemorrhages, and sometimes associated with cerebral contusion. It may result in paralysis, blindness and other visual disturbances, convulsions, and death.
**whistling face s., whistling face–windmill vane hand s.,** craniocarpotarsal dystrophy.
**Widal s.,** former name for *hemolytic anemia.*
**Willebrand's s.,** von Willebrand's disease.
**Williams s., Williams-Beuren s.,** supravalvular aortic stenosis, mental retardation, elfin facies, and transient hypercalcemia in infancy. Called also *elfin facies s.*
**Williams-Campbell s.,** congenital bronchomalacia and bronchiectasis, resulting from absence of annular cartilage distal to the first division of the peripheral bronchi.
**Wilson-Mikity s.,** a rare form of pulmonary insufficiency in low-birth-weight infants, marked by hyperpnea and cyanosis of insidious onset during the first month of life and often resulting in death. Radiographically, there are multiple cystlike foci of hyperaeration throughout the lung with coarse thickening of the interstitial supporting structures. The disorder has been attributed to disparity of maturation of parenchymal elements, especially of alveoli proliferation, and hence has been called *pulmonary dysmaturity.*
**Winter's s.,** a congenital syndrome consisting of renal hypoplasia or aplasia, anomalies of the internal genitalia, especially vaginal atresia, and anomaly of the ossicles of the middle ear.
**Wiskott-Aldrich s.,** an X-linked immunodeficiency syndrome characterized by eczema, thrombocytopenia, and recurrent pyogenic infection. There is an inability to produce antibodies to polysaccharide antigens and increased susceptibility to infection with encapsulated bacteria (*Haemophilus influenzae,* meningococcus, pneumococcus). Typically IgM is low and IgA and IgE are elevated; cutaneous anergy is common. There is also a high incidence of lymphoreticular malignant disease. Called also *Aldrich's s.*
**withdrawal s.,** substance withdrawal.
**wobbler s.,** 1. in large to giant dogs, malformation of the lower cervical vertebrae with compression of the spinal cord so that the animal has ataxia of the hind limbs and a swaying gait; it may progress to paralysis. Called also *wobbles.* 2. in young horses, incoordination of the hind legs with a swaying gait progressing to stumbling, inability to walk, and sometimes paralysis; causes are varied and include stenosis of the spinal canal, malformation of the cervical vertebrae with demyelination, and inflammation of the cord. Called also *equine sensory ataxia* and *wobbles.*
**Wohlfart-Kugelberg-Welander s.,** Kugelberg-Welander s.
**Wolf-Hirschhorn s.,** a syndrome associated with partial deletion of the short arm of chromosome 4, characterized by microcephaly, ocular hypertelorism, epicanthus, cleft palate, micrognathia, low-set ears simplified in form, cryptorchidism, and hypospadias.
**Wolff-Parkinson-White s.,** the association of paroxysmal tachycardia (or atrial fibrillation) and preexcitation, in which the electrocardiogram displays a short P–R interval and a wide QRS complex which characteristically shows an early QRS vector (delta wave); sometimes used synonymously with *preexcitation s.* Called also *WPW s.*
**Wolfram s.,** an autosomal recessive syndrome, first evident in childhood, consisting of diabetes mellitus, diabetes insipidus, optic atrophy, and neural deafness. Called also *DIDMOAD s.*
**Woringer-Kolopp s.,** pagetoid reticulosis.
**WPW s.,** Wolff-Parkinson-White s.
**Wright's s.,** 1. hyperabduction s. 2. a condition marked by multifocal areas of osteitis fibrosa, patchy cutaneous pigmentation, and precocious puberty.
**Wyburn-Mason's s.,** arteriovenous aneurysms on one or both sides of the brain, with ocular anomalies, especially in the retina, facial nevi, and sometimes mental retardation.
**s. X,** a relatively benign syndrome of angina pectoris or angina-like chest pain associated with normal arteriographic appearance of the coronary arteries.
**X-linked lymphoproliferative s.,** an immunodeficiency disorder characterized by defective cellular or humoral immune response to Epstein-Barr virus (EBV). Fulminant infectious mononucleosis, fatal B cell malignancies, or hypogammaglobulinemia can result from EBV infection. Called also *X-linked lymphoproliferative disease* and *Duncan's s.* or *disease.*
**XXY s.,** Klinefelter's s.
**yellow nail s.,** a syndrome associated with lymphedema, especially of the legs, consisting of a yellowish to greenish discoloration of the nails, which may be smooth, thickened, excessively curved on the long axis, and slow growing, and may become loose and be shed.
**Young's s.,** obstructive azoospermia and chronic sinopulmonary infections.
**Zahorsky's s.,** herpangina.
**Zellweger s.,** cerebrohepatorenal s.
**Zieve s.,** hypercholesterolemia, hepatosplenomegaly, fatty infiltration of the liver, hemolytic anemia, and hypertriglyceridemia following the ingestion of large amounts of ethanol.
**Zinsser-Cole-Engman s.,** dyskeratosis congenita.
**Zollinger-Ellison s.,** a triad comprising (1) intractable, sometimes fulminating, and in many ways atypical peptic ulcers; (2) extreme gastric hyperacidity; and (3) gastrin-secreting, non–beta islet cell tumors of the pancreas, which may be single or multiple, small or large, benign or malignant. The gastrinoma sometimes occurs in sites (e.g., the duodenum) other than the pancreas. See also *multiple endocrine neoplasia, type I.*

**syn·drom·ic** (sin-drom′ik) occurring as a syndrome.

**syn·drom·ol·o·gy** (sin″drom-ol′ə-je) the field concerned with the taxonomy, etiology, and patterns of congenital malformations.

**syn·ech·ia** (sĭ-nek′e-ə) pl. *syne′chiae* [Gr. *synecheia* continuity] adhesion of parts, especially adhesion of the iris to the cornea or to the lens.
**annular s.,** adhesion of the whole rim of the iris to the lens.
**anterior s.,** adhesion of the base of the iris to the cornea, producing occlusion of the chamber angle; it may be caused by glaucoma, cataract, or intraocular tumors, or occur after perforation resulting from keratitis, iridocyclitis, trauma, or surgery.
**circular s.,** annular s.
**s. pericar′dii,** concretio cordis.
**posterior s.,** adhesion of the iris to the capsule of the lens or to the surface of the vitreous body, producing an irregularly shaped pupil.
**total anterior s.,** adhesion of the entire surface of the iris to the cornea.
**total posterior s.,** adhesion of the entire surface of the iris to the lens.
**s. vul′vae,** fused vulva: a congenital condition in which the labia minora are sealed in the midline, with only a small opening below the clitoris through which urination and menstruation may occur.

**syn·echo·tome** (sin-ek′o-tōm) a cutting instrument for use in synechotomy.

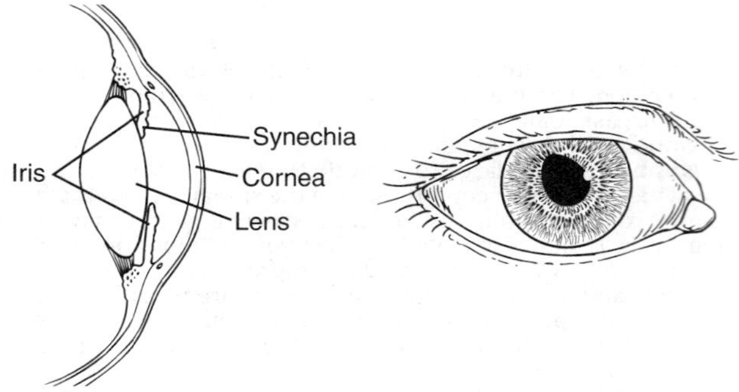


**syn·echot·o·my** (sin″ə-kot′ə-me) [*synechia* + *-tomy*] the operation of cutting a synechia.

**syn·ech·ten·ter·ot·o·my** (sin″ək-ten″tər-ot′ə-me) [Gr. *synechēs* joined together + *entero-* + *-tomy*] division of an intestinal adhesion.

**syn·ecol·o·gy** (sin″ə-kol′ə-je) the study of the environment of organisms in the mass, as distinguished from *autecology.*

**Syn·e·mol** (sin′ə-mol) trademark for a preparation of fluocinolone acetonide.

**syn·en·ceph·a·lo·cele** (sin″ən-sef′ə-lo-sēl″) [*syn-* + *encephalo-* + *-cele*[1]] encephalocele with adhesions to the adjoining parts.

**syn·en·ceph·a·lus** (sin″ən-sef′ə-ləs) a fetus exhibiting synencephaly.

**syn·en·ceph·a·ly** (sin″ən-sef′ə-le) [*syn-* + Gr. *enkephalos* brain] a developmental anomaly in which there are two bodies and one head.

**syn·er·e·sis** (sĭ-ner′ə-sis) [Gr. *synairesis* a taking or drawing together] a drawing together of the particles of the dispersed phase of a gel, with separation of some of the disperse medium and shrinkage of the gel, such as occurs in the clotting of blood.

**syn·er·gen·e·sis** (sin″ər-jen′ə-sis) the doctrine that every cell transmits its protoplasm to every generation of cells derived from it.

**syn·er·get·ic** (sin″ər-jet′ik) synergic.

**syn·er·gia** (sin-er′je-ə) synergy.

**syn·er·gic** (sin-er′jik) acting together or in harmony.

**syn·er·gism** (sin′ər-jizm) synergy.

**syn·er·gist** (sin′ər-jist) 1. a medicine that aids or cooperates with another; an adjuvant. 2. an organ that acts in concert with another. 3. a synergistic muscle.

**syn·er·gis·tic** (sin″ər-jis′tik) 1. acting together. 2. enhancing the effect of another force or agent.

**syn·er·gy** (sin′ər-je) [L. *synergia;* Gr. *syn* together + *ergon* work] 1. correlated action or cooperation on the part of two or more structures or drugs. 2. in neurology, the faculty by which movements are properly grouped for the performance of acts requiring special adjustments.

**syn·es·the·sia** (sin″es-the′zhə) [*syn-* + *esthesia*] 1. a secondary sensation accompanying an actual perception. 2. a dysesthesia in which a stimulus of one sense is perceived as a sensation of a different sense, as when a sound produces a sensation of color. 3. a dysesthesia in which a stimulus to one part of the body is experienced as being at a different location.
**s. al′gica,** synesthesialgia.

**syn·es·the·si·al·gia** (sin″es-the″ze-al′jə) a painful synesthesia.

**syn·e·ze·sis** (sin″ə-ze′sis) synizesis.

**Syn·gam·i·dae** (sin-gam′ĭ-de) a family of nematodes that includes the genera *Cyathostoma, Mammomonogamus,* and *Syngamus.* Many parasitize the respiratory tracts of mammals and birds.

**syn·ga·mous** (sing′gə-məs) [*syn-* + *gam-* + *-ous*] 1. pertaining to or characterized by syngamy. 2. syngonic.

**Syn·ga·mus** (sin′gə-məs) a genus of nematode worms of the family Syngamidae that are parasitic in fowl and other birds.
**S. laryn′geus,** a species that normally infects the upper respiratory tract of ruminants and has occasionally been found in the respiratory tract of humans.
**S. tra′chea,** the gapeworm, a species of parasitic worm found in the trachea in chickens, pheasants, turkeys, and various wild birds, sometimes interfering with respiration and causing gapes (q.v.).

**syn·ga·my** (sing′gə-me) [*syn-* + Gr. *gamos* marriage] 1. sexual reproduction. 2. the union of two gametes in fertilization to form a zygote.

**syn·ge·ne·ic** (sin″jə-ne′ik) [*syn-* + *geno-* + *-ic*] denoting individuals or tissues that have identical genotypes and thus could participate in a syngraft. Cf. *allogeneic* and *xenogeneic.* Called also *isogeneic* and *isogenic.*

**syn·ge·ne·sio·plas·tic** (sin″jə-ne″ze-o-plas′tik) [*syn-* + *genesis* + *plastic*] pertaining to a living related donor; see under *transplantation.*

**syn·ge·ne·sio·trans·plan·ta·tion** (sin″jə-ne″ze-o-trans″plan-ta′shən) living related donor transplantation.

**syn·gen·e·sis** (sin-jen′ə-sis) 1. the origin of an individual from a germ cell derived from both parents, as occurs in nearly all higher animals, and not from just one alone. 2. the state of having descended from a common ancestor.

**syn·gna·thia** (sĭ-na′the-ə) [*syn-* + *gnath-* + *-ia*] a congenital condition characterized by the presence of fibrous bands extending from the maxilla to the mandible.

**syn·gon·ic** (sin-gon′ik) [*syn-* + *gon-*[1] + *-ic*] having the sex of the individual determined at the time the oocyte is fertilized; called also *syngamous.*

**syn·graft** (sin′graft) a graft between genetically identical individuals. Typically, syngrafts are grafts between identical twins, between animals of a single highly inbred strain, or between $F_1$ hybrids produced by crossing inbred strains. Called also *isograft* and *isogeneic, isologous,* or *syngeneic graft.*

**syn·i·ze·sis** (sin″ĭ-ze′sis) [Gr. *synizēsis*] 1. occlusion. 2. a stage in mitosis in which the nuclear chromatin is massed.
**s. pupil′lae,** occlusion of the pupil.

**syn·kary·on** (sin-kar′e-on) [*syn-* + *karyon*] the nucleus produced by the fusion of two pronuclei in karyogamy; the fertilization nucleus.

**Syn·kay·vite** (sin′ka-vīt) trademark for preparations of menadiol sodium diphosphate.

**syn·ki·ne·sia** (sin″ki-ne′zhə) synkinesis.

**syn·ki·ne·sis** (sin″ki-ne′sis) [*syn-* + *-kinesis*] an unintentional movement accompanying a volitional movement, such as the facial contortions accompanying severe exertion. Called also *associated* or *synkinetic movement.*
**imitative s.,** an involuntary movement on the healthy side accompanying an attempt at movement on the paralyzed side.
**mouth-and-hand s.,** Saunders' sign; see under *sign.*
**spasmodic s.,** contralateral associated movement.

**syn·ki·net·ic** (sin″ki-net′ik) pertaining to or of the nature of synkinesis.

**syn·ne·cro·sis** (sin″ə-kro′sis) [*syn-* + *necro-* + *-sis*] a relationship between populations (or individuals) resulting in mutual depression or death.

**syn·ne·ma** (sin-e′mə) a group of erect, sometimes fused conidiophores that produce conidia at or near the apex. Called also *coremium.*

**syn·neu·ro·sis** (sin″u-ro′sis) [Gr. *synneurosis* union by sinews] syndesmosis.

**syn·onych·ia** (sin″o-nik′e-ə) [*syn-* + *onych-* + *-ia*] fusion of the nails of two or more digits in complicated syndactyly.

**syn·oph·rid·ia** (sin″of-rid′e-ə) synophrys.

**syn·oph·rys** (sin-of′ris) [Gr. "with meeting eyebrows"] the condition in which the eyebrows grow together.

**syn·oph·thal·mia** (sin″of-thal′me-ə) [*syn-* + *ophthalm-* + *-ia*] the usual form of cyclopia, in which the two eyes are more or less completely fused into one.

**syn·oph·thal·mus** (sin″of-thal′məs) cyclops.

**Syn·o·phy·late** (sin″o-fi′lāt) trademark for preparations of theophylline sodium glycinate.

**syn·op·to·phore** (sin-op′to-for) [*syn-* + *opto-* + Gr. *phora* movement, range] an instrument for diagnosing strabismus and for treating it by orthoptic methods.

**syn·or·chi·dism** (sin-or′kĭ-diz-əm) synorchism.

**syn·or·chism** (sin′or-kiz-əm) [*syn-* + *orchi-* + *-ism*] fusion of the two testes into one mass, which may be located in the scrotum or in the abdomen.

**syn·os·che·os** (sin-os′ke-os) [*syn-* + Gr. *oscheon* scrotum] adhesion between the penis and scrotum.

**syn·os·te·ol·o·gy** (sin″os-te-ol′ə-je) [*syn-* + *osteo-* + *-logy*] the sum of knowledge regarding the joints and articulations.

**syn·os·te·o·sis** (sin″os-te-o′sis) synostosis.

**syn·os·te·ot·ic** (sin″os-te-ot′ik) pertaining to or marked by synosteosis.

**syn·os·te·ot·o·my** (sin″os-te-ot′ə-me) [*syn-* + *osteo-* + *-tomy*] the dissection of the joints.

**syn·os·to·sis** (sin″os-to′sis) pl. *synosto′ses* [*syn-* + *oste-* + *-osis*] [MeSH: Synostosis] 1. TA alternative for *junctura ossea.* 2. the osseous union of bones that are normally distinct.
**radioulnar s.**, bony fusion of the proximal ends of the radius and ulna.
**sagittal s.**, scaphocephaly.
**tarsal s.**, fusion of various tarsal bones.
**tribasilar s.**, fusion in infancy of the three bones at the base of the skull, producing mental retardation.

**syn·os·tot·ic** (sin″os-tot′ik) synosteotic.

**sy·no·tia** (sĭ-no′she-ə) [*syn-* + *-ot-* + *-ia*] a developmental anomaly characterized by persistence of the ears in their horizontal position inferior to the mandible.

**sy·no·tus** (sĭ-no′təs) [*syn-* + Gr. *ous* ear] a fetus exhibiting synotia.

**syn·o·vec·to·my** (sin″o-vek′tə-me) [*synovi-* + *-ectomy*] excision of a synovial membrane, as of that lining the capsule of the knee joint, performed in treatment of rheumatoid arthritis of the knee, or of the synovial sheath of a tendon.
**radiation s., radioisotope s.**, synoviorthesis.

**sy·no·via** (sĭ-no′ve-ə) [L.; Gr. *syn* with + *ōon* egg] [TA] a transparent alkaline viscid fluid, resembling the white of an egg, secreted by the synovial membrane, and contained in joint cavities, bursae, and tendon sheaths; called also *synovial fluid.*

**sy·no·vi·al** (sĭ-no′ve-əl) [L. *synovialis*] 1. pertaining to a synovium. 2. pertaining to or secreting synovia.

**sy·no·vi·a·lis** (sĭ-no″ve-a′lis) [L.] synovial.

**sy·no·vi·a·lo·ma** (sĭ-no″ve-ə-lo′mə) synovioma.

**sy·no·vi·anal·y·sis** (sĭ-no″ve-ə-nal′ĭ-sis) the laboratory examination of joint fluid (synovia).

**syn·o·vin** (sin′o-vin) the mucin found in synovia.

**synovi(o)-** [L. *synovia,* q.v.] a combining form denoting relationship to the synovia, or to a synovial membrane.

**sy·no·vio·blast** (sĭ-no′ve-o-blast) a fibroblast of synovial membrane.

**sy·no·vio·cyte** (sĭ-no′ve-o-sīt) a cell of the synovial membrane.

**sy·no·vi·o·ma** (sĭ-no″ve-o′mə) [*synovi-* + *-oma*] a tumor of synovial membrane origin.
**benign s.**, giant cell tumor of tendon sheath.
**malignant s.**, synoviosarcoma.

**sy·no·vi·or·the·sis** (sĭ-no″ve-or-the′sis) [*synovi-* + *ortho-* + *-esis*] irradiation of the synovium by intra-articular injection of radiocolloids to destroy inflamed synovial tissue.

**sy·no·vio·sar·co·ma** (sĭ-no″ve-o-sahr-ko′mə) [*synovio-* + *sarcoma*] a malignant neoplasm arising in the synovial membrane of the joints and also in synovial cells of tendons and bursae; called also *malignant synovioma* and *synovial sarcoma.*

**syn·o·vip·a·rous** (sin″o-vip′ə-rəs) [*synovi-* + L. *parere* to produce] producing synovia.

**syno·vi·tis** (sin″o-vi′tis) [MeSH: Synovitis] inflammation of a synovium; it is usually painful, particularly on motion, and is characterized by a fluctuating swelling due to effusion within a synovial sac. Some types are named for accompanying tissue changes, such as *fibrinous, hyperplastic,* or *lipomatous synovitis;* others are named for accompanying disease processes or complications, such as *gonorrheal, metritic, puerperal, rheumatic, scarlatinal, syphilitic,* or *tuberculous synovitis.*
**bursal s.**, bursitis.
**dendritic s.**, that in which villous growths are developed within the synovial sac.
**dry s.**, synovitis with but little effusion.
**fungous s.**, mycotic arthritis.
**infectious s., infectious avian s.**, a disease of young chickens and turkeys caused by infection with *Mycoplasma synoviae*; it ranges from a subclinical respiratory infection to swollen leg joints with lameness and anorexia.
**localized nodular s.**, lesions of the tendon sheaths that give histological evidence of evolution from a number of smaller nodules, or from villous structures.
**pigmented villonodular s.**, synovial proliferation forming brown nodular masses, probably caused by hemangiomas of synovial membrane that become traumatized, resulting in synovial hyperplasia and inflammation; it is characterized by episodic monoarticular pain and swelling, with joint locking and hemorrhagic effusions.
**purulent s.**, that in which there is an effusion of pus in a synovial sac.
**serous s.**, synovitis with copious nonpurulent effusion.
**s. sic′ca**, dry s.
**simple s.**, that in which the effusion is clear or but slightly turbid.
**tendinous s.**, tenosynovitis.
**vaginal s.**, tenosynovitis.
**vibration s.**, synovitis produced by the passage of a missile through the tissues near a joint, but without actually wounding the joint.
**villonodular s.**, proliferation of synovial tissue, especially of the knee joint, composed of synovial villi and fibrous nodules infiltrated by giant cells and by macrophages containing lipids and hemosiderin.

**sy·no·vi·um** (sĭ-no′ve-əm) membrana synovialis capsulae articularis.

**syn·phal·an·gism** (sin-fal′ən-jiz-əm) symphalangia.

**syn·pneu·mon·ic** (sin″noo-mon′ik) occurring in association with pneumonia.

**syn·re·flex·ia** (sin″re-flek′se-ə) the association existing between various reflexes.

**syn·tac·tic** (sin-tak′tik) pertaining to or affecting syntax, or the proper arrangement of words in speech.

**syn·tax·is** (sin-tak′sis) [Gr. "a putting together in order"] articulation, def. 1.

**syn·tec·tic** (sin-tek′tik) pertaining to or characterized by syntexis.

**syn·ten·ic** (sin-ten′ik) pertaining or relating to synteny.

**syn·te·no·sis** (sin″tə-no′sis) [*syn-* + *teno-* + *-osis*] a hinge joint surrounded by tendons.

**syn·te·ny** (sin′tə-ne) [*syn-* + Gr. *tainia* ribbon] the presence together on the same chromosome of two or more gene loci whether or not in such proximity that they may be subject to linkage (q.v., def. 2).

**syn·ter·e·sis** (sin″tər-e′sis) [*syn-* + Gr. *tērein* to watch over] preventive treatment; prophylaxis.

**syn·ter·et·ic** (sin″tər-et′ik) prophylactic.

**syn·tex·is** (sin-tek′sis) [Gr. *syntēxis* colliquation] wasting or emaciation.

**syn·thase** (sin′thās) a term used in the trivial or recommended names of some enzymes, particularly those of the lyase class [EC 4], when the synthetic aspect of the reaction is dominant or emphasized. Cf. *synthetase.*

**syn·the·sis** (sin′thə-sis) [Gr. "a putting together, composition"] 1. the creation of an integrated whole by the combining of simpler parts or entities. 2. the formation of a chemical compound by the union of its elements or from other suitable components. 3. in psychiatry, the integration of the various elements of the personality.
**s. of continuity**, union of the edges of a wound or the ends of a fractured bone.
**morphologic s.**, histogenesis.

**syn·the·size** (sin′thə-sīz) to produce by means of synthesis.

**syn·the·tase** (sin′thə-tās) a term used in the trivial names of most enzymes of the ligase class [EC 6]; formerly part of the recommended name, it is no longer favored because of confusion with the term synthase and because it emphasizes reaction products rather than substrates. Cf. *synthase.*

**syn·thet·ic** (sin-thet′ik) [L. *syntheticus;* Gr. *synthetikos*] 1. pertaining to, of the nature of, or participating in synthesis. 2. produced by synthesis; artificial.

**syn·tho·rax** (sin-thor′aks) thoracopagus.

**Syn·throid** (sin′throid) trademark for a preparation of levothyroxine sodium.

**syn·to·nin** (sin′to-nin) an acid metaprotein which precipitates from a gastric digestion mixture at or near the neutral point.

**syn·to·py** (sin′tə-pe) [*syn-* + Gr. *topos* place] the position of an organ in relation to neighboring organs.

**syn·trip·sis** (sin-trip′sis) [*syn-* + *tripsis*] 1. the comminution or crushing of a bone. 2. comminuted fracture.

**syn·troph·ism** (sin′trōf-iz-əm) [*syn-* + *troph-* + *-ism*] crossfeeding; the stimulation of growth of a cell or organ by a factor released by another cell or organ; especially, growth stimulation of a bacterium resulting from admixture with or nearness of another strain or species, e.g., the growth of *Haemophilus influenzae* as satellite colonies of *Staphylococcus.*

**syn·tropho·blast** (sin-trof′o-blast) syncytiotrophoblast.

**syn·trop·ic** (sin-trop′ik) [*syn-* + *-tropic*] 1. turning or pointing in the same direction, as the ribs or the vertebral spinous processes. 2. denoting the correlation of several factors, as the relation of one disease to the development or incidence of another disease.

**syn·tro·py** (sin′tro-pe) the state of being syntropic.

**syn·u·lo·sis** (sin″u-lo′sis) [Gr. *synoulōsis*] complete cicatrization.

**syn·u·lot·ic** (sin″u-lot′ik) [Gr. *synoulōtikos*] 1. promoting cicatrization. 2. an agent that promotes cicatrization.

**Syn·u·ra** (sin-u′rə) [*syn-* + G. *oura* tail] a genus of free-swimming, colonial, plantlike biflagellate freshwater protozoa (order Chrysomonadida, class Phytomastigophorea), which may impart an unpleasant taste to drinking water.

**syn·xen·ic** (sin-zen′ik) [*syn-* + *xen-* + *-ic*] associated with a known number of microbic species; applied to laboratory animals whose microfauna and microflora are known (gnotobiotes).

**Sy·pha·cia** (si-fa′se-ə) a genus of nematodes of the family Oxyuridae. *S. obveola′ta* is a common intestinal parasite of laboratory rats that has occasionally been reported in human infants.

**syph·i·lid** (sif′ĭ-lid) [MeSH: Syphilis, Cutaneous] one of the skin lesions of secondary syphilis, appearing six weeks to two years after infection in a series of crops lasting a few days to months, and becoming more severe, conspicuous, and persistent, and less widely generalized, in successive outbreaks. Mucous membrane lesions in this stage are typically teeming with *Treponema pallidum* and are clinically the most contagious lesions of the disease. Syphilids may be described by their shape *(annular s., macular s., papular s.)*, location *(palmar s., plantar s.)*, and so on.
**annular s.,** a papular syphilid that is annular and the size of a small coin, usually found on the face, palm, sole, or anogenital area.
**corymbose s.,** a type of papular syphilid characterized by a large central papule surrounded by smaller satellite lesions.
**follicular s.,** lichen syphiliticus.
**lenticular s.,** a type of papular syphilid characterized by small papules resembling lentils, usually on the face or genital region.
**macular s.,** a flat rose-colored spot on the skin, found in groups on various parts of the trunk, one of the earliest signs of secondary syphilis. Called also *syphilitic roseola.*
**maculopapular s.,** a type seen with persistent cases of macular syphilid; the lesions may appear on the face, trunk, palms, or soles, and are darker and more papular than those of macular syphilid.
**palmar s.,** one on the palm, usually pink to brownish in color; it may be either macular or papular.
**papular s.,** one characterized by papules, such as lichen syphiliticus, clovus syphiliticus, or annular, corymbose, or lenticular syphilid.
**plantar s.,** one on the sole, usually pink to brownish in color; it may be either macular or papular.

**syph·i·lide** (sif′ĭ-līd) pl. *syphil′ides* [Fr.] syphilid.

**syph·i·lis** (sif′ĭ-lis) [*Syphilus,* a shepherd infected with the disease in the poem of Fracastorius (1530); the poet may have derived the name from Gr. *syn* together + *philein* to love, or from Gr. *siphlos* crippled, maimed] [MeSH: Syphilis] a subacute to chronic infectious disease caused by the spirochete *Treponema pallidum,* which is usually transmitted by sexual contact or acquired in utero but can be contracted by direct contact with infected tissues and blood or contaminated fomites. Untreated syphilis usually progresses through three clinical stages *(primary, secondary,* and *tertiary s.)*, with a latent period *(latent syphilis)* intervening between the first two and the last. The time of duration of each stage varies, and they are often noticeably shortened in immunocompromised patients. Formerly called *lues* and *pox.* See also *general paresis,* under *paresis,* and *tabes dorsalis.* Cf. *endemic s.*
**cardiovascular s.,** a form of tertiary syphilis in which aortic insufficiency and aortic aneurysm, usually of the ascending aorta, occur as a result of obliterative endarteritis of the vasa vasorum, causing damage to the intima and media of the great vessels, and may result in congestive heart failure. Cf. *syphilitic aortitis.*
**cerebrospinal s.,** Erb's spastic paraplegia.
**congenital s.,** syphilis acquired in utero, and manifested variously by any of several characteristic malformations of the teeth or bones known as stigmata and by active mucocutaneous syphilis at the time of birth or shortly afterward, ocular changes, such as interstitial keratitis, or neurologic changes, such as deafness.
**early s.,** the stage comprising primary, secondary, and early latent syphilis.
**endemic s.,** a chronic, inflammatory, non–sexually transmitted treponemal infection caused by an organism indistinguishable morphologically from *Treponema pallidum, T. pertenue,* and *T. carateum,* mainly affecting children in arid, dry regions, especially of the Middle East, North Africa, and Eastern Mediterranean, and characterized by early mucous patches of the secondary type localized to the oral and faucial mucosa, followed by the appearance of moist papules in the axilla and skin folds, a latent period, and late complications, including osseous and cutaneous gummata. Called also *bejel* and *nonvenereal s.*
**equine s.,** dourine.
**gummatous s.,** late benign s.
**horse s.,** dourine.
**late s.,** tertiary s.
**late benign s.,** a form of tertiary syphilis that responds very rapidly to treatment and is therefore relatively benign, in which the typical lesion is the gumma (q.v.). Called also *gumma* and *gummatous s.*
**latent s.,** a stage after secondary syphilis when an infected patient is free of overt symptoms but has a positive serologic test for syphilis; it may last a short time or many years and may be subdivided into *early latent* and *late latent syphilis,* distinguished by the time since initial infection, degree of infectiousness of the disease, and certain other characteristics.
**latent s., early,** the first period of latent syphilis, when relapses of secondary syphilis are most likely to occur and the patient is considered to be more infectious than at later stages; this usually lasts until one to two years after the initial infection.
**latent s., late,** the later period of latent syphilis, beginning one to two years after the initial infection; relapses of secondary syphilis are rare and patients are resistant to infection. The disease is now usually not infectious, although fetuses in utero may contract congenital syphilis from mothers at this stage.
**meningovascular s.,** see under *neurosyphilis.*
**nonvenereal s.,** endemic s.
**parenchymatous s.,** see under *neurosyphilis.*
**primary s.,** the first stage of syphilis , in which a painless primary lesion *(chancre)* appears at the site of inoculation and is associated with regional adenopathy *(bubo).* Chancres usually appear two to four weeks after infection and heal spontaneously within two weeks. Untreated patients soon develop secondary syphilis.
**rabbit s.,** a venereal disease of rabbits consisting of lesions with scabs around the external genitalia, and sometimes elsewhere on the body, caused by infection with *Treponema paraluiscuniculi;* called also *vent disease.*
**secondary s.,** the second stage of syphilis, usually occurring two to eight weeks after appearance of the primary chancre; characterized chiefly by widespread mucocutaneous lesions (see *syphilid*) and generalized regional lymphadenopathy. It is usually followed by a period of latent syphilis.
**spinal s.,** syphilis primarily affecting the spinal cord; see *tabes dorsalis, meningovascular neurosyphilis,* and *Erb's spastic paraplegia.* Called also *myelosyphilis.*
**tertiary s.,** the third and last stage of syphilis, which may develop soon or many years after the lesions of secondary syphilis have resolved; it is marked by destructive lesions involving many tissues and organs and occurs in three principal forms: *cardiovascular s., late benign syphilis,* and *neurosyphilis.* Called also *late s.*

**syph·i·lit·ic** (sif″ĭ-lit′ik) [L. *syphiliticus*] affected with, caused by, or pertaining to syphilis.

**syph·i·lo·ma** (sif″ĭ-lo′mə) gumma.

**syph·i·lo·pho·bia** (sif″ĭ-lo-fo′be-ə) [*syphilis* + *-phobia*] 1. irrational fear of syphilis. 2. the delusion of being infected with syphilis.

**Syr.** abbreviation for L. *syrupus,* syrup.

**sy·rig·mus** (sĭ-rig′məs) [Gr. *syrigmos* a shrill piping sound] tinnitus.

**syr·ing·ad·e·no·ma** (sə-ring″gad-ə-no′mə) syringocystadenoma.
**s. papilli′ferum,** see under *syringocystadenoma.*

**sy·ringe** (sĭ-rinj′, sir′inj) [L. *syrinxe;* Gr. *syrinx*] [MeSH: Syringes] an instrument for injecting liquids into or withdrawing them from any vessel or cavity.
**air s.,** a small fine-nozzled syringe connected by a hose to the compressed air tank in the dental unit; used to direct a current of air into a tooth cavity during excavation, to remove the small chips detached from the teeth, or to dry the cavity. Called also *chip s.*
**Anel's s.,** a delicate syringe for the treatment of the lacrimal passages.
**chip s.,** air s.
**dental s.,** a small syringe into which is fitted a hermetically sealed cartridge which contains an anesthetic solution; used for intraoral injection anesthesia.
**fountain s.,** an apparatus which injects a liquid by the action of gravity.
**hypodermic s.,** a syringe, usually of small caliber, by means of which drugs in solution or other liquids are injected through a hollow needle of small bore into the subcutaneous tissues.
**Luer's s., Luer-Lok s.,** a glass syringe for intravenous and hypodermic use, with a metallic tip and locking device to hold the needle firmly in place.
**probe s.,** a syringe whose point may be used also as a probe; used mostly in treating the lacrimal passages.
**water s.,** a syringe that is part of the dental unit, designed to permit controlled spraying of water in a desired area.

**syr·in·gec·to·my** (sir″in-jek′tə-me) [*syring-* + *-ectomy*] excision of the walls of a fistula.

**syr·in·gi·tis** (sir″in-ji′tis) inflammation of the auditory tube.

**syring(o)-** [Gr. *syrinx,* gen. *syringos* pipe, tube, fistula] a combining form denoting relationship to a tube or a fistula.

**sy·rin·go·acan·tho·ma** (sə-ring″go-ak″an-tho′mə) [*syringo-* + *acan-*

*thoma*] a rare epithelial neoplasm resembling seborrheic keratosis, characterized by multiple nests of small basaloid cells within the acanthotic epidermis.

**sy·rin·go·ad·e·no·ma** (sĭ-ring′go-ad″ə-no′mə) syringocystadenoma.

**sy·rin·go·bul·bia** (sĭ-ring′go-bul′be-ə) [*syringo-* + *bulbus* + *-ia*] syringomyelia in which the cavity extends to involve the medulla oblongata. Cf. *hydromyelia.*

**sy·rin·go·car·ci·no·ma** (sĭ-ring″go-kahr″sĭ-no′mə) carcinoma of a sweat gland.

**sy·rin·go·cele** (sĭ-ring′go-sēl) myelocele.

**sy·rin·go·coele** (sĭ-ring′go-sēl) [*syringo-* + *-coele*] canalis centralis medullae spinalis.

**sy·rin·go·cys·tad·e·no·ma** (sə-ring″go-sis″tad-ə-no′mə) a benign cystic tumor of the sweat glands.
**s. papilli′ferum,** a hamartoma of an apocrine sweat gland, occurring as a grouping of firm, rose red papules, usually on the scalp but sometimes on the face or trunk or in the genital or inguinal region, and characterized by papillary projections extending into the lumina of dilated cystic sweat glands and ducts.

**sy·rin·go·cys·to·ma** (sə-ring″go-sis-to′mə) [*syringo-* + *cystoma*] syringocystadenoma.

**sy·rin·go·en·ce·pha·lia** (sĭ-ring″go-en″sə-fa′le-ə) [*syringo-* + *enkephal* + *-ia*] the formation of abnormal cavities in the brain substance.

**sy·rin·go·en·ceph·a·lo·my·e·lia** (sĭ-ring″go-ən-sef″ə-lo-mi-e′le-ə) [*syringo-* + *encephal-* + *myel-* + *-ia*] the existence of cavities in the substance of the brain and spinal cord.

**sy·rin·go·hy·dro·my·e·lia** (sə-ring″go-hi″dro-mi-e′le-ə) hydrosyringomyelia.

**sy·rin·goid** (sĭ-ring′goid) [L. *syringoides,* from Gr. *syrinx* pipe + *eidos* form] resembling a pipe or tube; fistulous.

**sy·rin·go·ma** (sir″ing-go′mə) [*syring-* + *-oma*] [MeSH: Syringoma] a benign tumor believed to originate from the ductal portion of the eccrine sweat glands, occurring as multiple small flesh-colored papules on the face, neck, and upper chest, usually in postpubertal women, and characterized by dilated cystic sweat ducts in a fibrous stroma.
**chondroid s.,** a usually benign tumor originating in the sweat glands, occurring as a solitary, firm, deep-seated intradermal or subcutaneous nodule on the head or neck; it is characterized by ductal and cystic glandular proliferation and is believed to be of eccrine origin.

**sy·rin·go·my·e·lia** (sĭ-ring″go-mi-e′le-ə) [*syringo-* + *myel-* + *-ia*] [MeSH: Syringomyelia] a slowly progressive syndrome of cavitation in the central segments of the spinal cord, generally in the cervical region, but sometimes extending up into the medulla oblongata *(syringobulbia)* or down into the thoracic region; it may be of developmental origin, arise secondary to tumor, trauma, infarction, or hemorrhage, or be of unknown cause. It results in neurological deficits, usually segmental muscular weakness and atrophy with a dissociated sensory loss (loss of pain and temperature sensation, with preservation of the sense of touch), and thoracic scoliosis is often present. Sometimes, the use of the term *syringomyelia* is restricted to this condition, with the terms *segmental sensory dissociation with brachial muscular atrophy* and *syndrome of sensory dissociation with brachial amyotrophy* being used for a similar condition that may be associated with other pathological lesions or states. Called also *cavitary myelitis, hydrosyringomyelia, Morvan's syndrome, syringomyelic syndrome,* and *syringomyelus.* See also *Morvan's syndrome* (def. 2).
**post-traumatic s., traumatic s.,** syringomyelia resulting from trauma.

**sy·rin·go·my·elus** (sĭ-ring″go-mi′ə-ləs) syringomyelia.

**Sy·rin·gos·po·ra** (si″ring-gos′pə-rə) former name for *Candida.*

**sy·rin·go·tome** (sĭ-ring′go-tōm) a knife for cutting a fistula.

**sy·rin·got·o·my** (sir″in-got′ə-me) [*syringo-* + *-tomy*] incision of a fistula, particularly an anal fistula.

**syr·inx** (sir′inks) [Gr. "a pipe"] 1. a tube or pipe. 2. a fistula. 3. the lower or posterior part of the trachea of birds in which vocal sounds are produced. 4. an abnormal cavity in the spinal cord in syringomyelia.

**Syr·phi·dae** (sir′phĭ-de) a family of flies, the hover flies, of the order Diptera, including the genera *Eristalis* and *Helophilus.*

**syr·up** (sir′əp) [L. *syrupus,* from Arabic *sharāb*] 1. a concentrated solution of a sugar, such as sucrose, in water or other aqueous liquid, sometimes with some medicinal substance added. 2. [NF] a solution of sucrose in purified water, used as a flavored vehicle in pharmaceutical preparations.
**acacia s.,** a preparation of powdered acacia, sodium benzoate, vanilla tincture, sucrose, and water, used as a flavored vehicle and demulcent for drugs.
**cacao s.,** cocoa s.
**cherry s.,** a mixture of cherry juice, sucrose, alcohol, and purified water, used as a flavored vehicle for drugs.
**citric acid s.,** a preparation of lemon tincture, hydrous citric acid, and purified water, in syrup, used as a flavored vehicle for drugs.
**cocoa s.,** a preparation of cocoa, sucrose, liquid glucose, glycerin, sodium chloride, vanillin, sodium benzoate, and purified water; used as a flavored vehicle for drugs. Called also *cacao s.*
**eriodictyon s., aromatic,** a solution of eriodictyon fluidextract, potassium hydroxide solution, compound cardamom tincture, sassafras oil, lemon oil, clove oil, alcohol, sucrose, and magnesium carbonate, in purified water; used as a vehicle for drugs.
**ipecac s.** [USP], a mixture of ipecac fluidextract, glycerin, and syrup, used as an emetic.
**lactulose s.,** see under *solution.*
**medicated s.,** one to which a medicinal substance has been added.
**orange s.,** a preparation of sweet orange peel tincture, citric acid, talc, and sucrose, in purified water, used as a flavored vehicle for drugs.
**raspberry s.,** a syrup consisting of raspberry juice, sucrose, and alcohol, in purified water, used as a flavored vehicle for drugs.
**simple s.,** one compounded from purified water and sucrose.
**s. of tolu,** tolu balsam s.
**tolu balsam s.,** a mixture of tolu balsam tincture, magnesium carbonate, sucrose, and purified water, used as a flavored vehicle for drugs.
**white pine s., compound,** a solution containing coarsely powdered white pine, wild cherry, aralia, poplar bud, sanguinaria, and sassafras, combined with amaranth solution, chloroform, sucrose, glycerin, alcohol, and water; used as an antitussive and as a vehicle for other drugs.
**white pine s., compound, with codeine,** compound white pine syrup combined with codeine phosphate dissolved in purified water, used as an antitussive.
**wild cherry s.,** a mixture of a percolate of wild cherry, glycerin, sucrose, alcohol, and water; used as a flavored vehicle.
**yerba santa s., aromatic,** eriodictyon s., aromatic.

**sys·sar·co·sic** (sis″ahr-ko′sik) syssarcotic.

**sys·sar·co·sis** (sis″ahr-ko′sis) [*syn-* + *sarc-* + *-osis*] the union or connection of bones by means of muscle, as the connection between the hyoid bone and the mandible, the scapula, and the breast bone.

**sys·sar·cot·ic** (sis″ahr-kot′ik) pertaining to or of the nature of a syssarcosis.

**sys·so·mus** (sĭ-so′məs) [Gr. *syn* with + *sōma* body] conjoined twins with two heads and with the bodies united.

**sys·tal·tic** (sis-tawl′tik) [Gr. *systaltikos* drawing together] alternately contracting and expanding; pulsating.

**sys·tat·ic** (sis-tat′ik) affecting several of the sensory faculties at the same time.

**sys·tem** (sis′təm) [Gr. *systēma* a complex or organized whole] 1. a set or series of interconnected or interdependent parts or entities (objects, organs, or organisms) that function together in a common purpose or produce results impossible of achievement by one of them acting or operating alone. 2. a school or method of practice based on a specific set of principles, as the eclectic or galenic school.

**accessory portal s. of Sappey,** small compensatory blood vessels formed around the liver and gallbladder in cases of cirrhosis of the liver.

**adipose s.,** the fatty tissue of the body, considered collectively.

**AJCC s.,** a method of staging malignant tumors proposed by the American Joint Committee on Cancer, based on TNM staging; it divides cancers into five stages.

**alimentary s.,** the organs concerned with the ingestion, digestion, and absorption of food or nutritional elements; see *apparatus digestorius.*

**anterolateral s.,** lemniscus spinalis.

**APUD s.,** neuroendocrine s.

**arc guidance s.,** an apparatus used in stereotactic surgery consisting of a metal arc-shaped band or bar with degree markings and an attachment for an electrode that is positioned by moving through the arc to aim at a precise location in the brain. Cf. *arc-quadrant.*

**association s.,** the tracts of fibers in the brain by means of which perceptions are associated and thought rendered possible.

**auditory s.,** the series of structures by which sounds are received from the environment and conveyed as signals to the central nervous system; it consists of the outer, middle, and inner ear as well as the tracts in the auditory pathways.

**autonomic nervous s.,** the portion of the nervous system concerned with regulation of the activity of cardiac muscle, smooth muscle, and glands; usually restricted to the two visceral efferent peripheral components, the sympathetic nervous system and the parasympathetic nervous system. Called also *divisio autonomica systematis nervosi peripherici* [TA] and *pars autonomica systematis nervosi peripherici* [TA alternative]. See Plate 48.

**Bethesda S.,** a classification of cervical and vaginal cytology that provides a standardized nomenclature for cytopathologic diagnosis of diseases of the cervix and vagina. it encompasses three elements: comment on the adequacy of the specimen, a general categorization of the specimen, and a descriptive diagnosis.

**biological s.,** a system composed of living material; such systems range from a collection of separate molecules to an assemblage of separate organisms.

**blood group s.,** blood group.

**blood-vascular s.,** the blood vessels of the body; see *circulatory s.*

**brain cooling s.,** thermoregulated equipment for sensing and controlling brain temperature in neurophysiological and neuropsychological applications.

**buffer s.,** see *buffer.*

**cardiovascular s.,** the heart and blood vessels, by which blood is pumped and circulated through the body.

**case s.,** a method of teaching based on the logical analysis of, and deductions formed from, reported cases of disease.

**CD s.** [*c*luster *d*esignation], a system for classifying cell surface markers expressed by lymphocytes based on a computer analysis of monoclonal antibodies against human leukocyte antigens, with antibodies having similar specificity characteristics being grouped together and assigned a number (CD1, CD2, CD3, etc.); these CD numbers are also applied to the specific antigens recognized by the various groups of monoclonal antibodies. See also *CD antigen,* under *antigen.*

**centimeter-gram-second s.,** see *CGS.*

**central nervous s. (CNS),** that portion of the nervous system consisting of the brain and spinal cord. In TA terminology, called *pars centralis systematis nervosi.* See Plates 11 and 12.

**centrencephalic s.,** the system of neurons located in the central core of the upper brain stem from the thalamus down to the medulla oblongata, and connecting the two hemispheres of the brain.

**chemoreceptor s.,** the system of body structures, principally the carotid body, the aortic bodies, and the glomus jugulare, that respond to variations in oxygen tension and carbon dioxide tension of the blood and may play a role in the regulation of respiration.

**chromaffin s.,** the chromaffin cells of the body considered collectively; see under *cell.*

**circulatory s.,** the channels through which the nutrient fluids of the body circulate; often restricted to the vessels conveying blood.

**colloid s., colloidal s.,** see *colloid,* def. 2.

**complement s.,** see *complement.*

**conducting s. of heart, conduction s. of heart,** complexus stimulans cordis.

**coordinate s.,** a method by which a point, a line, a plane, or a geometric solid can be located in space by a set of numbers.

**dentinal s.,** all the tubules radiating from a single pulp cavity.

**dermal s., dermoid s.,** the skin and its appendages, including both the hair and the nails. See *integumentum commune.*

**digestive s.,** the organs associated with the ingestion, digestion, and absorption of food; see *systema digestorium* [TA].

**dioptric s.,** a system of lenses or of different media for refracting light.

**disperse s., dispersion s.,** a colloid system; see *colloid,* def. 2.

**dosimetric s.,** a regular and determinate system of administration of a therapeutic agent.

**ecological s.,** see *ecosystem.*

**endocrine s.,** the system of glands and other structures that elaborate internal secretions (hormones) that are released directly into the circulatory system, and also elaborate paracrine, autocrine, and possibly intracrine regulators that are not released to the blood stream, all of which influence metabolism and other body processes. It includes organs such as the hypothalamus, pituitary, thyroid, parathyroids, adrenal glands, gonads, pancreas, paraganglia, and pineal body; the intestines and the lung also secrete substances that have hormonal functions. See Plate 19.

**endothelial s.,** see *reticuloendothelial s.*

**enteric nervous s.,** the plexus entericus, sometimes considered separately from the autonomic nervous system because it has independent local reflex activity.

**exteroceptive nervous s.,** that portion of the afferent elements of the somatic nervous system which is sensitive to stimuli originating outside the body.

**extracorticospinal s.,** extrapyramidal s.

**extralemniscal s.,** a group of multisynaptic pathways in the spinothalamic tracts, projecting to the intralaminar nuclei of the thalamus.

**extrapyramidal s.,** an imprecise term referring to a functional rather than an anatomical part of the central nervous system that controls motor activities and is not part of the pyramidal tract; it includes the corpus striatum, subthalamic nucleus, substantia nigra, and red nucleus along with their interconnections with the reticular formation, cerebrum, and cerebellum; they control and coordinate especially the postural, static, supporting, and locomotor mechanisms. Called also *extracorticospinal s.* or *tract* and *extrapyramidal tract.*

**Frank lead s.,** in spatial vectorcardiography, the most commonly used corrected system of orthogonal leads, consisting of seven electrodes placed and connected to form leads X, Y, and Z, which describe the transverse, vertical, and sagittal planes, respectively. See also *spatial vectorcardiography,* under *vectorcardiography.*

**genitourinary s.,** urogenital s.

**glandular s.,** the glandular tissue of the body considered collectively.

**glycine cleavage s.,** a group of four mitochondrial enzymes, designated P, H, T, and L, that together catalyze the conversion of glycine to $CO_2$ and a one carbon unit that can be transferred to tetrahydrofolate. Deficiency of one or more of the proteins, an autosomal recessive trait, results in nonketotic hyperglycinemia.

**haversian s.,** a haversian canal and its concentrically arranged lamellae, constituting the basic unit of structure of compact bone; see *osteon.*

**hematopoietic s.,** the tissues concerned in production of the blood, including the bone marrow, liver, lymph nodes, spleen, and thymus. See also *hematopoiesis.*

**heterogeneous s.,** a system or structure made up of mechanically separable parts, as an emulsion.

**hexaxial reference s.,** a series of lines used in electrocardiography to describe the potentials of the heart in the frontal plane by diagram-

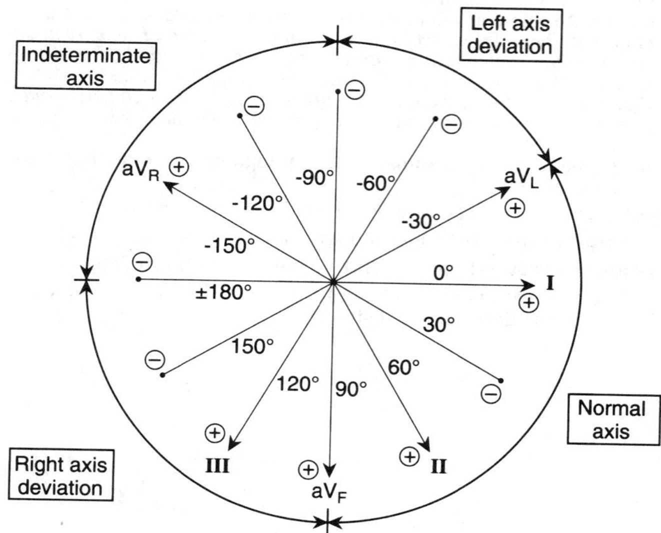


Hexaxial reference system and axes of deviation. The triaxial reference system comprises the vectors I, II, and III (standard dipolar limb leads) only.

# THE AUTONOMIC NERVES

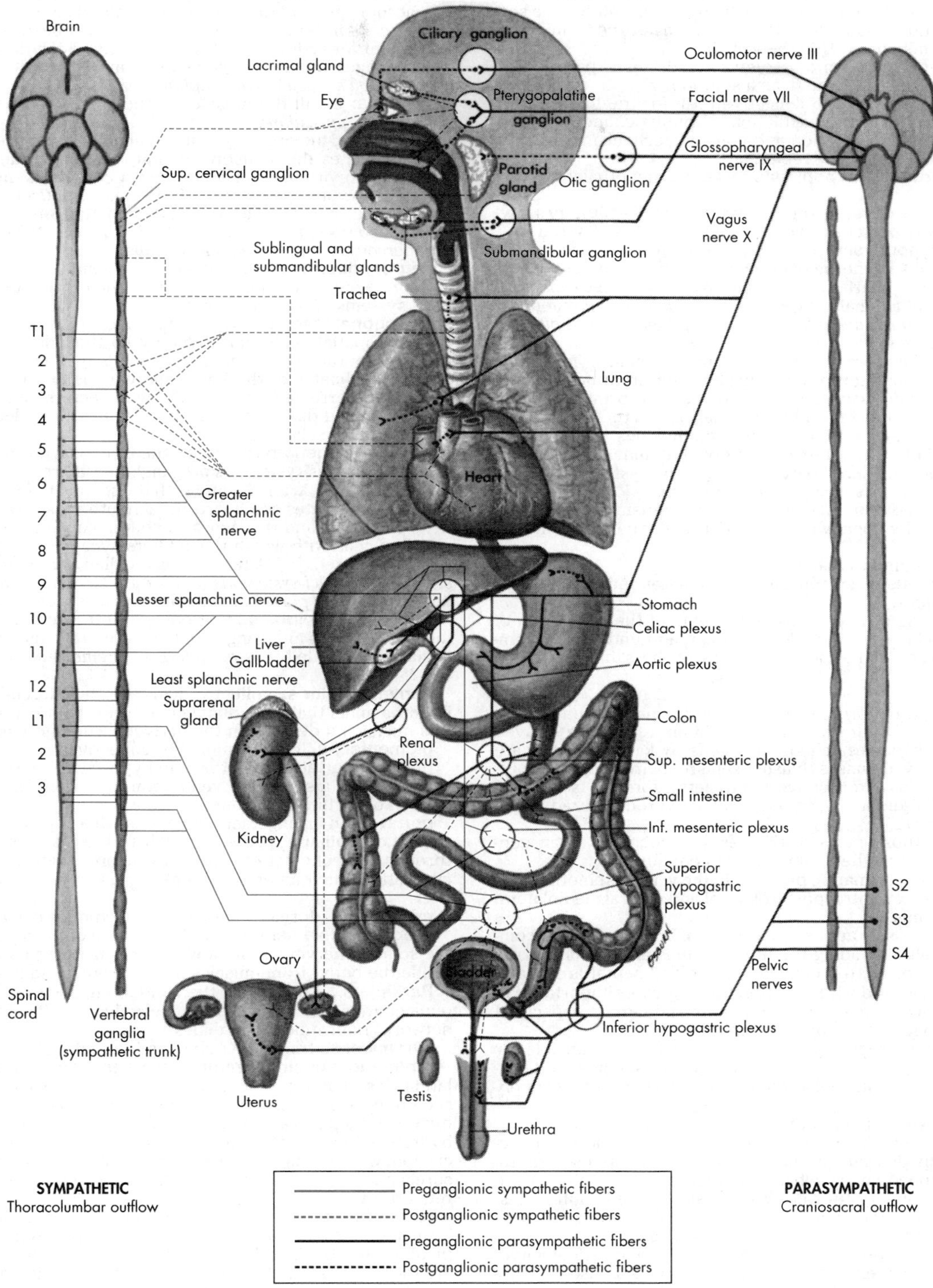


**PLATE 48**—AUTONOMIC NERVOUS SYSTEM

ming vectors that represent the standard bipolar limb leads and the augmented unipolar limb leads. See accompanying illustration.

**His-Purkinje s.**, a portion of the conducting system of the heart (systema conducens cordis), usually referring specifically to the segment beginning with the bundle of His and ending at the terminus of the Purkinje fiber network within the ventricles.

**homogeneous s.**, a system or structure made up of parts which cannot be mechanically separated, as a solution.

**humoral amplification s's**, a collective term for the four enzyme cascades—the complement, coagulation, fibrinolytic, and kinin systems—that serve as amplification and control mechanisms in hemostasis, inflammation, and tissue repair.

**hypophyseoportal s., hypophysioportal s.**, hypothalamo-hypophysial portal s.

**hypothalamic hypophysial portal s., hypothalamic-pituitary s., hypothalamic-pituitary portal s.**, hypothalamo-hypophysial portal s.

**hypothalamo-hypophysial portal s.**, the venules connecting the capillaries (gomitoli) in the median eminence of the hypothalamus with the sinusoidal capillaries of the adenohypophysis. See *venae portales hypophysiales.* Called also *hypophysial portal* or *hypophysioportal circulation, hypothalamic hypophysial portal s., hypothalamic-pituitary s.*, and *pituitary portal s.*

**immune s.**, a complex system of cellular and molecular components having the primary function of distinguishing self from not self and defense against foreign organisms or substances. The primary cellular components are lymphocytes and macrophages, and the primary molecular components are antibodies and lymphokines; granulocytes and the complement system are also involved in immune responses but are not always considered part of the immune system per se.

**International S. of Units**, see *SI unit*, under *unit.*

**interoceptive nervous s.**, that system which transmits afferent impulses from viscera by fibers which run centrally either in autonomic or somatic nerves.

**interstitial s.**, see under *lamella.*

**involuntary nervous s.**, systema nervosum autonomicum.

**kallikrein s.**, kinin s.

**keratinizing s.**, the cells composing the bulk of the epithelium of the epidermis, which are of ectodermal origin and undergo keratinization and form the dead superficial layers of the skin; called also *malpighian s.*

**kinety s.**, kinety.

**kinin s.**, the system of proteins involved in the production and destruction of kinins, e.g., bradykinin and kallidin. Kinins are cleaved from precursor substances called kininogens by kallikreins and are rapidly destroyed by kininases. Plasma kallikrein circulates as a proenzyme (prekallikrein) and is converted to active form by factor XIIa, which cleaves HMW kininogen, an $\alpha_2$-globulin, to produce bradykinin. Called also *kallikrein s.*

**labyrinthine s.**, those parts of the vestibulocochlear organ concerned with hearing and the maintenance of equilibrium.

**lemniscal s.**, an oligosynaptic pathway in the ventral spinothalamic tract, projecting to the ventral posterolateral and ventral mediolateral nuclei of the thalamus.

**limbic s.**, a term loosely applied to a group of brain structures common to all mammals (including the hippocampus and dentate gyrus with their archaeocortex, the cingulate gyrus and septal areas, and the amygdala), associated with olfaction but of greater importance in other activities, such as autonomic functions and certain aspects of emotion and behavior; see also *rhinencephalon.*

**locomotor s.**, the structures in a living organism responsible for locomotion; in humans these consist of the muscles, joints, and ligaments of the lower limbs as well as the arteries and nerves that supply them.

**lymphatic s.**, systema lymphoideum.

**lymphoid s.**, the lymphoid tissue of the body considered collectively; it can be divided into primary (or central) lymphoid tissues, the thymus and bone marrow where lymphocytes differentiate from stem cells, and secondary (or peripheral) tissues, the lymph nodes, spleen, and gut-associated lymphoid tissue (tonsils, Peyer's patches) where lymphocytes take part in immune responses.

**lymphoreticular s.**, the tissues of the lymphoid and reticuloendothelial systems considered together as one system; see also lymphoreticular disorders, under *disorder.*

**macrophage s.**, mononuclear phagocyte s.

**malpighian s.**, keratinizing s.

**masticatory s.**, see under *apparatus.*

**mastigont s.**, an ultrastructural complex characteristic of mastigophorans, comprising all of the organelles associated with the flagella, including basal bodies, axostyle, and Golgi body; it may or may not be associated with a nucleus (see also *karyomastigont* and *akaryomastigont*).

**melanocyte s.**, pigmentary s.

**meter-kilogram-second s.**, see *MKS.*

**metric s.**, a decimal system of weights and measures based on the meter. See also *SI unit*, under *unit*, and see Appendix 3.

**mononuclear phagocyte s. (MPS),** the collection of cells consisting of macrophages and their precursors (blood monocytes and their precursor cells in bone marrow). The term has been proposed as a replacement for reticuloendothelial system, which does not include all macrophages and does include other unrelated cell types. Called also *macrophage s.* See also *macrophage.*

**muscular s.**, all the muscles of the body considered collectively; see *systema musculare.*

**nervous s.**, the organ system which, along with the endocrine system, correlates the adjustments and reactions of an organism to internal and environmental conditions. It comprises the central and peripheral nervous systems: the former is composed of the brain and spinal cord, and the latter includes all the other neural elements. Called also *systema nervosum* [TA]. See also *central nervous s., peripheral nervous s.*, and *autonomic nervous s.*

**neuroendocrine s.**, the APUD cells considered as a system, having endocrine effects on the structures of the central and peripheral nervous systems. Called also *APUD s.*

**orthogonal lead s.**, a system for placing the electrocardiographic leads in spatial vectorcardiography so that ideally the three leads used are mutually perpendicular, each is parallel to one of the rectilinear coordinates of the body, and each is of equal amplitude vectorially. In corrected systems, the lead vectors also retain the same magnitude and direction for all points of cardiac electromotive force generation. See also *Frank lead s.*

**parasympathetic nervous s.**, the craniosacral division of the autonomic nervous system, its preganglionic fibers traveling with cranial nerves III, VII, IX, X, and XI, and with the second to fourth sacral ventral roots; it innervates the heart, the smooth muscle and glands of the head and neck, and the thoracic, abdominal, and pelvic viscera. The ganglion cells with which these fibers synapse are in or near the organs innervated. In TA terminology, called *pars parasympathica divisionis autonomici systematis nervosi.* Called also *craniosacral division* and *craniosacral part of autonomic nervous system.* See Plate 48.

**peripheral nervous s.**, that portion of the nervous system consisting of the nerves and ganglia outside the brain and spinal cord. In TA terminology, called *pars peripherica systematis nervosi.* See Plates 37 to 42.

**periventricular s.**, collective name for the efferent pathways of the hypothalamus that arise mainly in the supraoptic, posterior, and tuberal nuclei and descend in the periventricular gray matter.

**pigmentary s.**, the melanocytes, collectively.

**pituitary portal s.**, hypothalamo-hypophysial portal s.

**plenum s.**, a system of ventilation based on the mechanical propulsion of air into the room.

**portal s.**, an arrangement of vessels whereby blood collected from one set of capillaries passes through a large vessel or vessels and then through a second set of capillaries before it returns to the systemic circulation; such an arrangement occurs in the hypophysis and the liver.

**properdin s.**, former name for the *alternative complement pathway.*

**proprioceptive nervous s.**, that portion of the afferent elements of the somatic nervous system which is sensitive to stimuli originating inside the body (from muscles, bones, joints, and ligaments).

**Purkinje s.**, a portion of the conducting system of the heart (systema conducens cordis), usually referring specifically to the Purkinje network (rami subendocardiales).

**pyramidal s.**, tractus pyramidalis (def. 1).

**renin-angiotensin s., renin-angiotensin-aldosterone s.**, the regulation of sodium balance, fluid volume, and blood pressure by renal secretions: in response to reduced perfusion, renin is secreted, which hydrolyzes a plasma globulin to release angiotensin I, which is rapidly hydrolyzed to angiotensin II; this in turn stimulates aldosterone secretion, which brings about sodium retention, increase in blood pressure, and restoration of renal perfusion, which shuts off the signal for renin release.

**respiratory s.**, the tubular and cavernous organs and structures by means of which pulmonary ventilation and gas exchange between ambient air and the blood are brought about; the chief organs involved are the nose, larynx, trachea, bronchi, bronchioles, and lungs. Called also *respiratory apparatus* or *tract, apparatus respiratorius* [TA] and *systema respiratorium* [TA alternative]. See Plate 49.

**reticular activating s.**, the system of cells of the reticular formation of the medulla oblongata that receive collaterals from the ascending sensory pathways and project to higher centers; they control the overall degree of central nervous system activity, including wakefulness, attentiveness, and sleep; abbreviated RAS.

**reticuloendothelial s. (RES),** a group of cells having the ability to take up and sequester inert particles and vital dyes; it includes macrophages and macrophage precursors; specialized endothelial cells lining the sinusoids of the liver, spleen, and bone marrow; and retic-

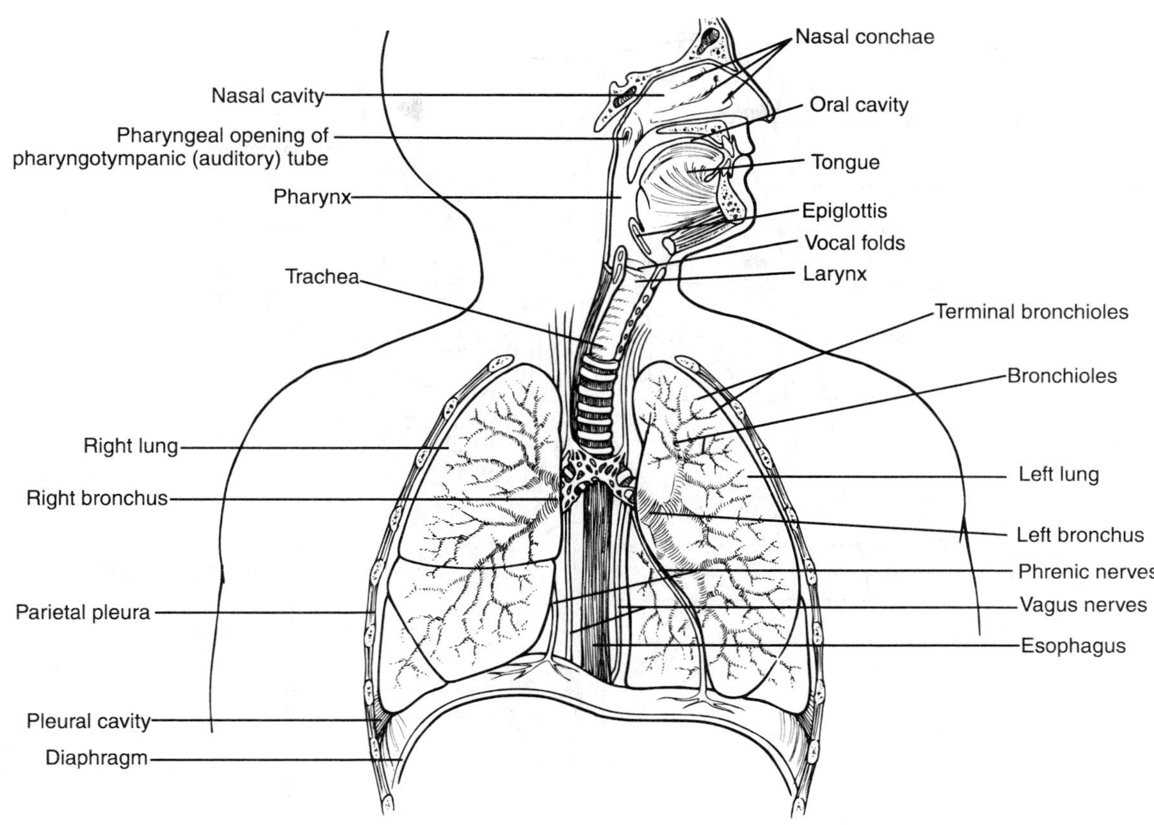


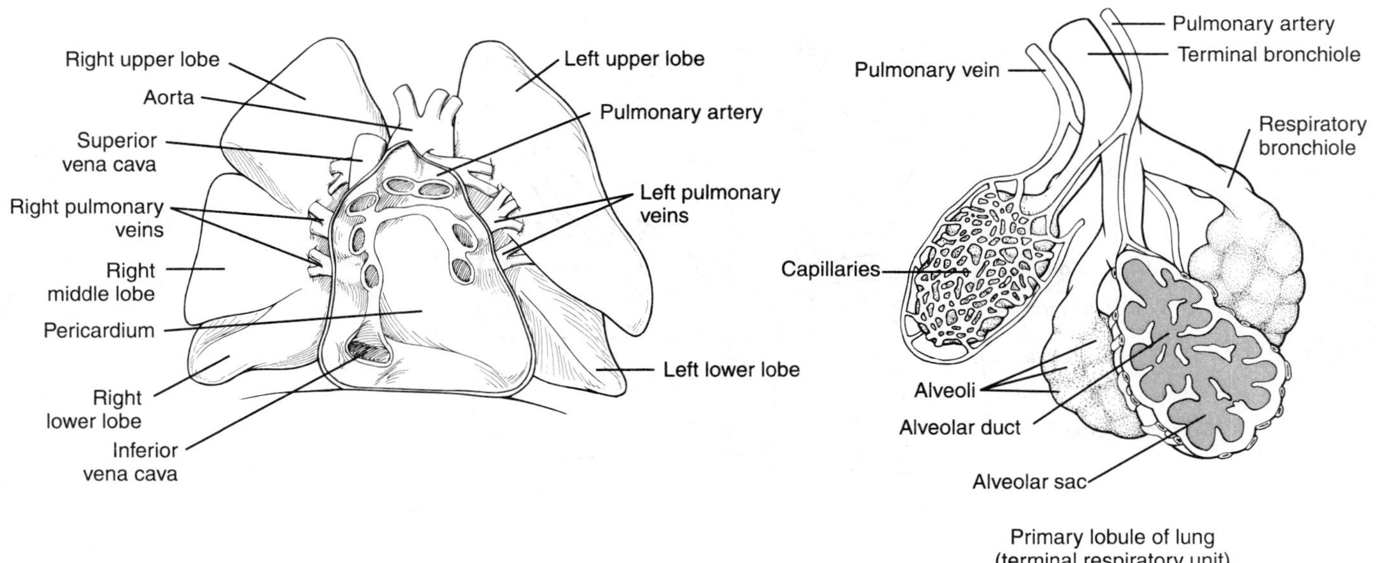


**PLATE 49**—ORGANS OF THE RESPIRATORY SYSTEM

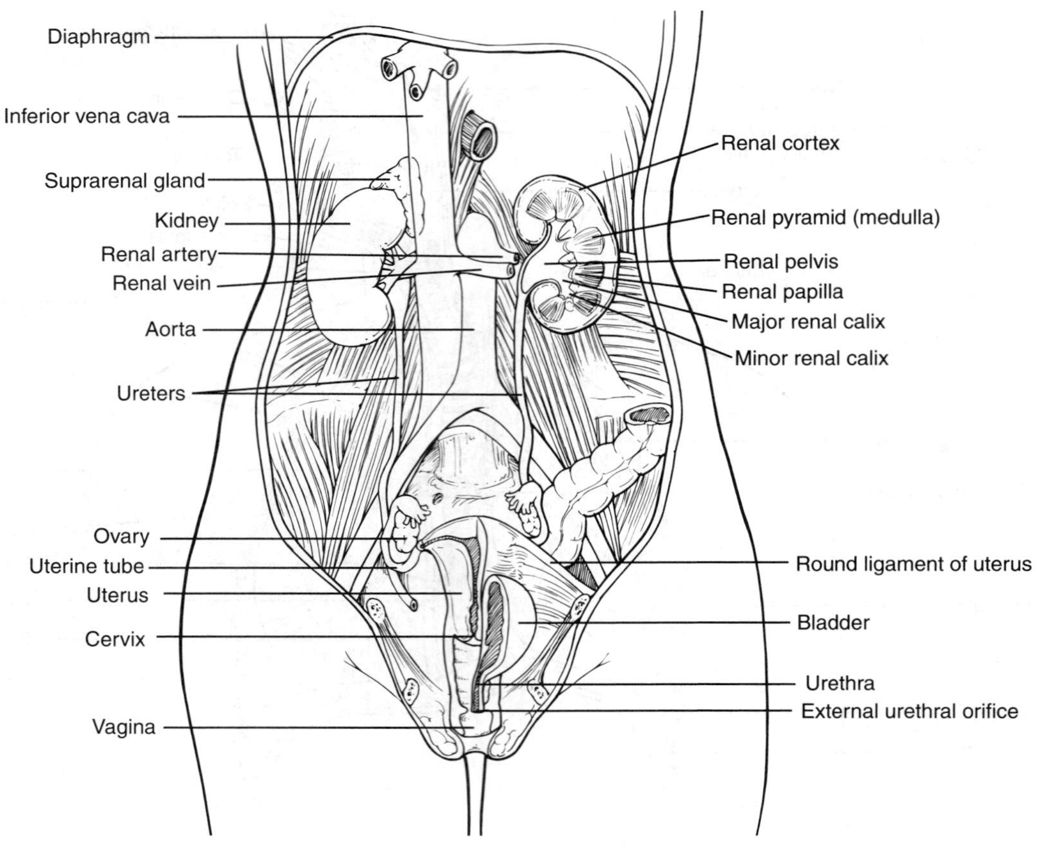


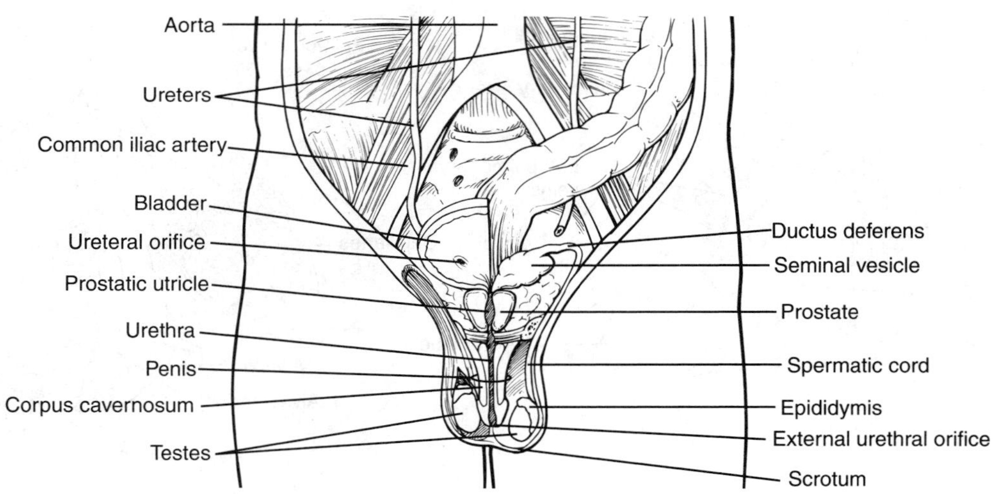


**PLATE 50**—ORGANS OF THE UROGENITAL SYSTEM

ular cells of lymphatic tissue (macrophages) and of bone marrow (fibroblasts). See also *mononuclear phagocyte s.*

**sensory storage s.**, the shortest type of memory, maintaining for less than a second briefly perceived stimuli; see *echoic memory* and *iconic memory,* under *memory.*

**SI s.**, see under *unit.*

**skeletal s.**, systema skeletale.

**somatic nervous s.**, the elements of the nervous system concerned with the transmission of impulses to and from the nonvisceral components of the body, such as the skeletal muscles, bones, joints, ligaments, skin, and eye and ear.

**stereotactic s.**, see under *technique.*

**stomatognathic s.**, the structures of the mouth and jaws, considered collectively, as they subserve the functions of mastication, deglutition, respiration, and speech. See also *masticatory apparatus,* under *apparatus.*

**sympathetic nervous s. (SNS)**, 1. the portion of the autonomic nervous system that receives its fibers of connection with the central nervous system through the thoracolumbar outflow of visceral efferent fibers. These fibers (preganglionic) arise from cells in the thoracic and upper lumbar levels of the spinal cord, leave by way of ventral roots, and, by way of rami communicantes, enter sympathetic trunks, where some synapse with ganglion cells. The fibers (postganglionic) of these ganglion cells return to spinal nerves by way of rami communicantes to supply the blood vessels, smooth muscle, and glands of the trunk and limbs, or go as visceral branches to the blood vessels, smooth muscles, and glands of the head and neck, and the viscera of the thorax, abdomen, and pelvis. Some preganglionic fibers pass through the sympathetic trunks and synapse in the prevertebral ganglia; postganglionic fibers from those ganglia supply adjacent viscera. In TA terminology, called *pars sympathica divisionis autonomici systematis nervosi.* Called also *thoracolumbar division* and *thoracolumbar part of autonomic nervous system.* See Plate 48. 2. former name for the autonomic nervous system.

**T s.**, a system of transverse tubular invaginations *(T,* or *transverse, tubules)* of the sarcolemma, each of which penetrates deep into the muscle fiber. In mammalian skeletal muscle, they are located at the junction of the A band with the I band, and in mammalian cardiac muscle at the level of the Z band; the system plays a role in the excitation and relaxation of muscle and provides an important additional surface for the exchange of metabolites between muscle and the extracellular space. Called also *triad s.* See also *triad of skeletal muscle; terminal cisterns,* under *cistern;* and *T tubule,* under *tubule.*

**triad s.**, T s.

**triaxial reference s.**, a series of lines used in electrocardiography to describe the potentials in the heart by diagramming frontal plane vectors that represent the standard bipolar limb leads; it is a rearrangement of the vectors composing Einthoven's triangle so that they bisect a single central point. See illustration at *hexaxial reference s.*

**UICC s.**, a method of staging malignant tumors proposed by the Union Internationale Contre Cancer, based on TNM staging; it divides cancers into five stages.

**urinary s.**, the organs concerned in secretion of urine; see *organa urinaria* [TA].

**urogenital s.**, the organs concerned in the production and excretion of urine, together with the organs of reproduction. See *apparatus.* See Plate 50.

**vascular s.**, circulatory s.

**vegetative nervous s.**, an old term for the autonomic nervous system (systema nervosum autonomicum [TA]).

**vestibular s.**, the bodily structures connected with receiving and processing sensations of the sense of equilibrium; they include the vestibular labyrinths, the sensory pathways of the vestibular nerves, and the vestibular nuclei.

**visceral nervous s.**, autonomic nervous s.

**visual s.**, the series of structures by which visual sensations are received from the environment and conveyed as signals to the central nervous system; it consists of the photoreceptors in the retina and the afferent fibers in the optic nerve, chiasm, and tract.

**Waring's s.**, see under *method.*

---

**sys·te·ma** (sis-te′mə) [Gr. *systēma* a complex or organized whole] system: a series of interconnected or interdependent organs which together accomplish a specific function.

**s. cardiovascula′re** [TA], the cardiovascular system: the heart and blood vessels; see under *system.*

**s. condu′cens cor′dis,** TA alternative for *complexus stimulans cordis.*

**s. digesto′rium,** the organs associated with the ingestion and digestion of food, including the mouth and associated structures, pharynx, and components of the digestive tube, as well as the associated organs and glands. See also *digestive tract,* under *tract.*

**s. lympha′ticum, s. lymphoi′deum** [TA], lymphatic system: the lymphatic vessels and the lymphoid tissue, considered collectively.

**s. muscula′re** [TA], muscular system: in TA terminology, the nomenclature relating to the muscles and to the bursae and synovial sheaths. Called also *musculi* [TA alternative].

**s. nervo′sum** [TA], the nervous system: the chief organ system that correlates the adjustments and reactions of the organism to internal and environmental conditions; see under *system.*

**s. nervo′sum autono′micum,** divisio autonomica systematis nervosi peripherici. See also *autonomic nervous system,* under *system.*

**s. nervo′sum centra′le,** TA alternative for *pars centralis systematis nervosi.*

**s. nervo′sum periphe′ricum,** TA alternative for *pars peripherica systematis nervosi.*

**s. respirato′rium,** TA alternative for *apparatus respiratorius*; see *respiratory system,* under *system.*

**s. skeleta′le** [TA], skeletal system: the bones *(pars ossea systematis skeletalis)* and cartilages *(pars cartilaginea systematis skeletalis)* of the body.

**s. urogenita′le,** TA alternative for *apparatus urogenitalis;* see *urogenital system,* under *system.*

**s. vaso′rum,** the blood and lymphatic vessels of the body and all their ramifications, considered collectively.

**sys·te·mat·ic** (sis″tə-mat′ik) [Gr. *systēmatikos*] pertaining or according to a system.

**sys·tem·a·ti·za·tion** (sis-tem″ə-tĭ-za′shən) arrangement according to a system. In psychiatry, the arrangement of ideas into a logical sequence, or of delusions into a superficially coherent system.

**sys·te·ma·tol·o·gy** (sis″tə-mə-tol′ə-je) [*system* + *-logy*] the science of classification.

**sys·tème sé·cant** (sis-tem′ sa-kahn′) [Fr. "cutting system"] one of the suture lines seen in ciliate protozoa where fields of kineties from different body areas converge.

**sys·tem·ic** (sis-tem′ik) pertaining to or affecting the body as a whole.

**sys·te·moid** (sis′tə-moid) [*system* + *-oid*] 1. resembling a system. 2. denoting tumors made up of various kinds of tissue.

**sys·to·le** (sis′to-le) [Gr. *systolē* a drawing together, contraction] [MeSH: Systole] the contraction, or period of contraction, of the heart, especially that of the ventricles; sometimes divided into components, as preejection and ejection periods, or isovolumic and ejection.

**aborted s.**, a weak systole, usually premature, not associated with pulsation of a peripheral artery.

**atrial s.**, the contraction of the atria by which blood is propelled from them into the ventricles.

**electromechanical s.**, the interval from the onset of the QRS complex on the electrocardiogram to the aortic component of the second heart sound; it is one of the systolic time intervals (q.v.), encompassing the left ventricular ejection time and the preejection period, and is used to assess left ventricular performance. Symbol $QS_2$.

**extra s.**, extrasystole.

**premature s.**, extrasystole.

**total electromechanical s.**, electromechanical s.

**ventricular s.**, the contraction of the ventricles of the heart by which the blood is forced into the aorta and the pulmonary trunk.

**sys·tol·ic** (sis-tol′ik) 1. pertaining to or produced by systole. 2. occurring during systole.

**sys·trem·ma** (sis-trem′ə) [Gr. "anything twisted up together"] a cramp in the muscles of the calf of the leg.

**Sy·to·bex** (si′to-beks) trademark for preparations of cyanocobalamin.

**sy·zyg·i·al** (sĭ-zij′e-əl) pertaining to syzygy.

**sy·zyg·i·ol·o·gy** (sĭ-zij″e-ol′ə-je) [Gr. *syzygia* yoke + *-logy*] the study of the relationship of the whole as contrasted to that of isolated parts and functions.

**Sy·zy·gi·um** (sĭ-zĭ′je-əm) [Gr. *syzygos* yoked together] a genus of tropical trees of the family Myrtaceae. *S. aroma'ticum* (called also *Eugenia caryophyllus*) is the clove, a species with aromatic flowers that yields the spice clove as well as clove oil.

**sy·zy·gi·um** (sĭ-zĭ'je-əm) syzygy.

**syz·y·gy** (siz'ĭ-je) [Gr. *syzygos* yoked together] the conjunction and fusion of organs without loss of identity.

**Szent-Györ·gyi** (sānt'jor-jĭ) Albert. Hungarian-born American physician and biochemist, 1893–1986; winner of the Nobel prize for medicine or physiology in 1937 for his studies in biological combustion and for his discovery of the catalytic properties of ascorbic acid in the adrenal glands.

# T

**T** symbol for *tesla, tera-, thymine* or *thymidine, thoracic vertebrae* (T1 through T12), *triangulation number,* and *intraocular tension* (see under *pressure*). Normal intraocular tension is indicated by symbol Tn.

**2,4,5-T** a toxic herbicide (2,4,5-trichlorophenoxyacetic acid) that acts as a growth-regulating hormone killing broadleaf plants by overstimulation.

**T-1824** Evans blue.

***T*** symbol for *absolute temperature* and *transmittance.*

**$T_{1/2}$** symbol for *half-life* or *half-time.*

**$T_1$** tricuspid valve closure; see *first heart sound,* under *sound.*

**$T_3$** symbol for *triiodothyronine.*

**$T_4$** symbol for *thyroxine.*

**$T_m$** symbol for *melting temperature* and *tubular maximum* (of the kidneys), a notation used in reporting kidney function studies, with inferior letters representing the substance used in the test, as $T_{m_{PAH}}$ (tubular maximum for para-aminohippuric acid).

**t** in genetics, symbol for *translocation.*

***t*** symbol for *time* and *temperature* (measured on a customary scale). See *t-test* under *tests.*

**$t_{1/2}$** symbol for *half-life* or *half-time.*

**$\theta$** theta, the eighth letter of the Greek alphabet. Symbol for *angle* (def. 2).

**$\tau$** tau, the nineteenth letter of the Greek alphabet. Symbol for *torque* and *mean life.*

**TA** *Terminologia Anatomica*; toxin-antitoxin.

**Ta** symbol for *tantalum.*

**tab•a•co•sis** (tab″ə-ko′sis) a form of pneumoconiosis seen in workers who cut up dried tobacco by hand and inhale tobacco dust.

**tab•a•cum** (tab′ə-kəm) [L., from Amerindian] tobacco.

**tab•a•gism** (tab′ə-jiz-əm) tobacco poisoning.

**tab•a•nid** (tab′ə-nid) any member of the family Tabanidae; called also *gadfly* or *gad fly* and *horse fly.*

**Ta•ba•ni•dae** (tə-ban′ĭ-de) the tabanids or horse flies, a family of insects that bite humans and other animals to get blood. It includes the genera *Chrysops, Chrysozona, Diachlorus, Goniops, Haematopota, Hybomitra, Silvius,* and *Tabanus.* Many species are vectors of disease.

**Ta•ba•nus** (tə-ba′nəs) [L. "gadfly"] a genus of biting, bloodsucking flies of the family Tabanidae; they transmit trypanosomes and anthrax to various animals.
**T. atra′tus,** the common black horsefly of North America.
**T. bovi′nus,** a species that attacks cattle in Asia, Africa, and South America.
**T. ditaenia′tus, T. fascia′tus, T. gra′tus,** the Seroot fly of the Sudan, which is very troublesome to humans and other animals.

**tab•ar•di•llo** (tab″ər-de′yo) [Sp.] murine typhus.

**ta•ba•tière ana•to•mique** (tah-bah″te-ār′ ah-nah-to-mēk′) [Fr. "anatomical snuffbox"] anatomist's snuff-box; see under *box.*

**ta•bel•la** (tə-bel′ə) pl. *tabel′lae* [L.] a medicated tablet or troche.

**tab•er•nan•thine** (tab″ər-nan′thēn) an alkaloid isolated from the root of *Tabernanthe iboga* Baill. (Apocynaceae), which has both analgesic and serotonin antagonist properties. It is isomeric with ibogaine.

**ta•bes** (ta′bēz) [L. "wasting away, decay, melting"] 1. any wasting of the body; progressive atrophy of the body or a part of it. 2. t. dorsalis.
**diabetic t.,** see under *pseudotabes.*
**t. dorsa′lis,** parenchymatous neurosyphilis in which there is slowly progressive degeneration of the posterior columns and posterior roots and ganglia of the spinal cord, occurring 15 to 20 years after the initial infection of syphilis, characterized by lancinating lightning pains, urinary incontinence, ataxia, impaired position and vibratory sense, optic atrophy, hypotonia, hyperreflexia, and trophic joint degeneration (Charcot's joints). Called also *Duchenne's disease, locomotor ataxia, posterior sclerosis* or *posterior spinal sclerosis, tabetic neurosyphilis, tabes,* and *t. spinalis.*
**t. ergo′tica,** a condition resembling tabes dorsalis, due to ergotism.
**Friedreich's t.,** Friedreich's ataxia.
**t. infan′tum,** tabes as seen in infants with congenital syphilis.
**t. mesente′rica, t. mesara′ica,** tuberculosis of the mesenteric glands in children, resulting in digestive derangement and wasting of the body.
**t. spina′lis,** t. dorsalis.

**ta•bes•cent** (tə-bes′ənt) [L. *tabescere* to waste away] wasting away; shriveling.

**ta•bet•ic** (tə-bet′ik) pertaining to or affected with tabes.

**ta•bet•i•form** (tə-bet′ĭ-form) resembling tabes.

**tab•ic** (tab′ik) tabetic.

**tab•id** (tab′id) [L. *tabidus* melting, dissolving] tabetic; wasting away.

**tab•i•fi•ca•tion** (tab″ĭ-fĭ-ka′shən) [L. *tabes* wasting away + *facere* to make] the process of wasting away.

**tab•la•ture** (tab′lə-chər) the separation of the chief cranial bones into inner and outer tables, which are separated by a diploë.

**ta•ble** (ta′bəl) [L. *tabula*] 1. a flat surface or layer. 2. an arrangement of data in rows and columns.
**2 × 2 contingency t.,** a contingency table having two rows and two columns.
**Aub-Dubois t.,** a table of normal basal metabolic rates for persons of various ages.
**cohort life t.,** a table giving the survival data of a cohort of individuals in a clinical study or trial, i.e., the number alive and under observation (not lost to follow-up) at the beginning of each year, the number dying in each year, the number lost to follow-up each year, the conditional probability of survival for each year, and the cumulative probabilities of survival from the beginning of the study to the end of each year.
**contingency t.,** a table used to display statistical data according to two characteristics, each having a number of mutually inclusive categories; categories of one characteristic are listed in rows and categories of the other characteristic are listed in columns. Statistical analysis (often using chi-squared or exact tests) can be readily applied to the rows and columns of the table. The most common is the *2 × 2 contingency t.,* having two rows and two columns. See also *r × c contingency t.*
**external t. of calvaria,** lamina externa calvariae.
**Gaffky t.,** see under *scale.*
**inner t. of frontal bone,** facies interna ossis frontalis.
**inner t. of skull, internal t. of calvaria,** lamina interna calvariae.
**life t.,** any of various tables describing mortality and survival data for groups of individuals at specific times or over defined intervals; tables may summarize combined mortality experience by age over a brief period or may follow a cohort over time *(cohort life t.)* See also *survival curve,* under *curve.*
**Mendeleev's (Mendeléef's, Mendeléeff's) t.,** periodic t.
**outer t. of frontal bone,** facies externa ossis frontalis.
**outer t. of skull,** lamina externa calvariae.
**periodic t.,** an ordering of all the known chemical elements in the form of a chart according to the periodic law, in which corresponding elements from the several periods form groups with similar properties; called also *Mendeleev's t.*
***r* × *c* contingency t.,** a contingency table having more than two categories for at least one of the variables of interest, *r,* standing for the number of rows and *c* standing for the number of columns.
**Reuss' t's,** see under *chart.*
**tilt t.,** a plinth, equipped with a footboard for support, to which a patient can be strapped for rotation to a nearly upright position; used in cases of spinal cord injury and other neurological disorders to enhance blood circulation to the lower limbs, improve posture, and aid in muscle training and sense of balance.
**vitreous t.,** lamina interna calvariae.
**water t.,** the upper surface of the impervious strata on which the ground water lies deep to the surface of the earth.

**ta•ble•spoon** (ta′bəl-spo͞on) a household unit of capacity, approximately equivalent to 4 fluid drams, or 15 milliliters.

**tab•let** (tab′lət) a solid dosage form, of varying weight, size, and shape, which may be molded or compressed, and which contains a medicinal substance in pure or diluted form. Cf. *pill.*
**buccal t.,** a small, flat, oval tablet to be held between the cheek and gum, permitting direct absorption through the oral mucosa of the medicinal substance contained therein.
**dispensing t.,** a compressed or molded tablet containing a large quantity of a drug, used by dispensing pharmacists in compounding prescriptions.
**enteric-coated t.,** one coated with material that delays release of the medication until after it leaves the stomach.
**hypodermic t.,** one containing a medicinal substance to be dissolved in water for hypodermic injection.
**sublingual t.,** a small, flat, oval tablet to be held beneath the tongue, permitting direct absorption of the medicinal substance contained therein.
**t. triturate,** a small, usually cylindrical, molded disk containing a medicinal substance diluted with a mixture of lactose and powdered sucrose, in varying proportions, with a moistening agent.

**ta·boo** (tă-boo′) [Tongan *tabu* forbidden, set apart] [MeSH: Taboo] 1. any of the negative traditions, objects, or behaviors that are generally regarded as harmful to social welfare and are therefore prohibited. Cf. *mores.* 2. excluded from use; prohibited.

**ta·bo·pa·ral·y·sis** (ta″bo-pə-ral′ĭ-sis) taboparesis.

**ta·bo·pa·re·sis** (ta″bo-pə-re′sis) general paresis occurring concomitantly with tabes dorsalis; called also *taboparalysis.*

**ta·bu·la** (tă′bu-lə) gen. and pl. *ta′bulae* [L.] table.
**t. exter′na os′sis cra′nii,** lamina externa calvariae.
**t. inter′na os′sis cra′nii, t. vit′rea,** lamina interna calvariae.

**tab·u·lar** (tab′u-lər) [L. *tabula* a board or table] resembling or shaped like a table.

**ta·bun** (ta′bən) an organophosphorus compound that is a potent cholinesterase inhibitor and is used as a nerve gas; symptoms of poisoning include bronchial constriction, convulsions, and often death. See *organophosphorus compound poisoning,* under *poisoning.*

**TAC** tetracaine, epinephrine, and cocaine; see under *solution.*

**Tac·a·ryl** (tak′ə-ril) trademark for preparations of methdilazine.

**TACE** (tās) trademark for preparations of chlorotrianisene.

**tache** (tahsh) [Fr.] a spot or blemish.
**t. blanche** (blahnsh) [Fr. "white spot"], a white spot on the liver in certain infectious diseases.
**t's bleuâtres** (bloo-ahtr′) [Fr. "bluish spots"], maculae caeruleae.
**t. cérébrale** (sa-ra-brahl′) [Fr. "cerebral spot"], a congested streak produced by drawing the nail across the skin, seen in various nervous or cerebral diseases. Called also *Trousseau's sign* or *spot, meningitic streak* or *stria,* and *t. méningéale.*
**t's laiteuses** (la-tooz′) [Fr. "milky spots"], small spots, of a milky appearance in the omentum, made up of lymphoid cells and macrophages and especially prominent in the rabbit.
**t. méningéale** (ma-nă-zha-ahl′) [Fr. "meningeal spot"], t. cérébrale.
**t. motrice** (mo-trēs′) [Fr. "motor spot"], motor end plate.
**t. noire** (nwahr) [Fr. "black spot"], an ulcer covered with a black adherent crust, a characteristic local reaction occurring at the presumed site of the infective bite in certain tick-borne rickettsioses, such as scrub typhus or boutonneuse fever.
**t. spinale** (spe-nahl′) [Fr. "spinal spot"], a bulla resembling a burn, and due to a spinal cord disease.

**ta·chis·to·scope** (tə-kis′tə-skōp) [Gr. *tachistos* swiftest + *-scope*] a device used in physiological psychology to demonstrate iconic memory; it displays images for controlled times, usually less than one-tenth of a second.

**tach(o)-** [Gr. *tachos* speed] a combining form denoting relationship to speed.

**tacho·gram** (tak′o-gram) [*tacho-* + *-gram*] a graphic record of the movement and velocity of the blood current.

**ta·chog·ra·phy** (tə-kog′rə-fe) [*tacho-* + *-graphy*] the recording of the speed of the blood current.

**tachy-** [Gr. *tachys* swift] a combining form meaning swift or rapid.

**tachy·al·i·men·ta·tion** (tak″e-al″ĭ-mən-ta′shən) [*tachy-* + *alimentation*] hypoglycemia occurring postprandially after gastric resection or gastroenterostomy, due to the accelerated passage of glucose into the small intestine, from which it enters the bloodstream at an increased rate, stimulating the production of insulin by the $\beta$-cells of the pancreas. It is a manifestation of the dumping syndrome.

**tachy·ar·rhyth·mia** (tak″e-ə-rith′me-ə) [*tachy-* + *arrhythmia*] any disturbance of the heart rhythm in which the heart rate is abnormally increased, usually to greater than 100 beats per minute in an adult.

**tachy·aux·e·sis** (tak″e-awk-ze′sis) [*tachy-* + *auxesis*] heterauxesis in which the part grows more rapidly than the whole.

**tachy·car·dia** (tak″ĭ-kahr′de-ə) [*tachy-* + *cardia*] [MeSH: Tachycardia] excessive rapidity in the action of the heart; the term is usually applied to a heart rate above 100 beats per minute in an adult and is often qualified by the locus of origin as well as by whether it is paroxysmal or nonparoxysmal.
**antidromic atrioventricular (AV) reciprocating t.,** a reentrant tachycardia in which the reentrant circuit involves anterograde conduction over the accessory pathway and retrograde conduction over the normal AV node to His bundle pathway. Cf. *orthodromic atrioventricular (AV) reciprocating t.*
**atrial t.,** a rapid cardiac rate, usually between 160 and 190 beats per minute, originating from an atrial locus; it may result from enhanced automaticity or impulse reentry.
**atrioventricular (AV) junctional t., atrioventricular (AV) nodal t.,** junctional t.
**atrioventricular nodal reentrant t.,** that resulting from reentry in or around the atrioventricular node, characterized by a QRS complex of supraventricular origin, sudden onset and termination, and a regular rhythm at a rate of 150 to 250 beats per minute. See also *antidromic atrioventricular (AV) reciprocating t.* and *orthodromic atrioventricular (AV) reciprocating t.*
**atrioventricular reciprocating t. (AVRT),** a reentrant tachycardia in which the reentrant circuit contains both the normal atrioventricular nodal to His bundle pathway and an accessory pathway as integral parts. See *antidromic atrioventricular reciprocating t.* and *orthodromic atrioventricular reciprocating t.*
**chaotic atrial t.,** tachycardia characterized by atrial rates of 100 to 130 beats per minute, markedly variable P wave morphology, and irregular P–P intervals; it occurs predominantly in patients with chronic obstructive pulmonary disease, diabetics, and the elderly, and may lead to atrial fibrillation. Called also *multifocal atrial t.*
**circus movement t.,** reentrant t.
**double t.,** the occurrence of two types of ectopic tachycardia, e.g., nodal and ventricular tachycardia, at the same time.
**ectopic t.,** abnormally rapid heart action in response to impulses arising outside the sinoatrial node.
**endless loop t.,** pacemaker-mediated t.
**junctional t.,** that arising in response to impulses originating in the atrioventricular junction, with a heart rate greater than 75 beats per minute. It may be nonparoxysmal *(nonparoxysmal junctional t.)* or paroxysmal; if the latter, it may be due to reentry (e.g., *atrioventricular nodal reentry t.*) or to enhanced automaticity.
**multifocal atrial t. (MAT),** chaotic atrial t.
**nodal t.,** junctional t.
**nonparoxysmal junctional t.,** a junctional tachycardia of slow onset, with a heart rate of 70 to 130 beats per minute. It is due to enhanced automaticity of the atrioventricular junctional tissue and is often associated with digitalis toxicity, acute myocardial infarction, acute carditis, or surgical trauma.
**orthodromic atrioventricular (AV) reciprocating t.,** a nodal reentrant tachycardia in which the reentrant circuit involves anterograde conduction over the usual AV node to His bundle pathway and retrograde conduction over an accessory pathway. Cf. *antidromic atrioventricular (AV) reciprocating t.*
**orthostatic t.,** disproportionate rapidity of the heart rate on rising from a reclining to a standing position.
**pacemaker-mediated t.,** in patients with dual chamber pacemakers, tachycardia caused by retrograde conduction of ventricular impulses, either premature ventricular complexes or impulses triggered by ventricular pacing which are sensed by the atria and trigger a subsequent ventricular impulse; an endless loop may develop. Called also *endless loop t.*
**paroxysmal t.,** a condition marked by attacks of rapid action of the heart having sudden onset and cessation. It is usually qualified by the locus of impulse origin as either ventricular or supraventricular; some classifications subdivide the latter into atrial and junctional tachycardias.
**paroxysmal supraventricular t. (PSVT),** supraventricular tachycardia occurring in attacks of rapid onset and cessation; it usually is due to a reentrant circuit.
**permanent junctional reciprocating t. (PJRT),** a chronic orthodromic atrioventricular nodal reciprocating tachycardia in which retrograde conduction on a posteroseptal accessory pathway is much slower than anterograde conduction along the normal conduction pathway.
**reciprocating t.,** a tachycardia due to a reentrant mechanism and characterized by a reciprocating rhythm (q.v.).
**reentrant t.,** any tachycardia characterized by a reentrant circuit.
**reflex t.,** rapid action of the heart initiated through a reflex neural arc by an event occurring elsewhere in the body.
**sinus t. (ST),** tachycardia originating in the sinus node; it is normal during exercise or anxiety but is also associated with shock, hypotension, hypoxia, congestive heart failure, fever, and various high output states.
**sinus reentrant t.,** tachycardia arising from a reentrant circuit that encompasses the sinus node.
**supraventricular t. (SVT),** any regular tachycardia in which the point of stimulation is located above the bundle branches, either in the sinus node, atria, or atrioventricular junction; it may also include those arising from large reentrant circuits encompassing both atrial and ventricular sites.
**ventricular t.,** an abnormally rapid ventricular rhythm with aberrant ventricular excitation (wide QRS complexes), usually in excess of 150 per minute, which is generated within the ventricle and is most commonly associated with atrioventricular dissociation. Minor irregularities of rate may also occur. Evidence implicates a reentrant pathway as the usual cause.

**tachy·car·di·ac** (tach″ĭ-kahr′de-ak) 1. pertaining to, characterized by, or causing tachycardia. 2. an agent that acts to accelerate the pulse.

**tachy·car·dic** (tak″ĭ-kahr′dik) having a rapid heart rate.

**tachy·dys·rhyth·mia** (tak″e-dis-rith′me-ə) [*tachy-* + *dysrhythmia*] an abnormal heart rhythm with rate greater than 100 beats per minute in an adult; the term *tachyarrhythmia* is usually used instead.

**tachy·gas·tria** (tak″ĭ-gas′tre-ə) the occurrence of a sequence of electric potentials at abnormally high frequencies in the gastric antrum.

**tachy·gen·e·sis** (tak″ĭ-jen′ə-sis) [*tachy-* + *-genesis*] the acceleration and compression of ancestral stages in embryonic development.

**tachy·ki·nin** (tak″e-ki′nin) any member of the tachykinin family of hormones; see under *family.*

**tachy·lal·ia** (tak″e-la′le-ə) [*tachy-* + *lal-* + *-ia*] logorrhea.

**tachy·lo·gia** (tak″e-lo′jə) [*tachy-* + *log-* + *-ia*] logorrhea.

**ta·chym·e·ter** (tə-kim′ə-tər) [*tachy-* + *-meter*] any instrument for measuring rapidity of motion of any body.

**tachy·pha·gia** (tak″ĭ-fa′je-ə) [*tachy-* + *-phagia*] rapid or hasty eating; seen in some forms of regressed schizophrenia.

**tachy·pha·sia** (tak″e-fa′zhə) [*tachy-* + *-phasia*] logorrhea.

**tachy·phe·mia** (tak″e-fe′me-ə) [*tachy-* + *-phemia*] logorrhea.

**tachy·phra·sia** (tak″e-fra′zhə) logorrhea.

**tachy·phy·lax·is** (tak″e-fə-lak′sis) [*tachy* + *phylaxis*] [MeSH: Tachyphylaxis] 1. rapid immunization against the effect of toxic doses of an extract or serum by previous injection of small doses. 2. rapidly decreasing response to a drug or physiologically active agent after administration of a few doses.

**tach·yp·nea** (tak″ip-ne′ə, tak″e-ne′ə) [*tachy-* + *-pnea*] excessive rapidity of breathing. See also *hyperpnea* and *hyperventilation.*

**tachy·rhyth·mia** (tak″ĭ-rith′me-ə) [*tachy-* + *rhythm* + *-ia*] tachycardia, especially when the mechanism is obscure.

**tach·ys·te·rol** (tak-is′tə-rol) an isomer of ergosterol produced by irradiation.

**tachy·tro·phism** (tak″ĭ-tro′fiz-əm) [*tachy-* + *trophism*] rapid metabolism.

**tachy·zo·ite** (tak″ĭ-zo′īt) [*tachy-* + *zo-* + *-ite*] the crescent or oval, quickly multiplying trophozoite of *Toxoplasma gondii,* found in all tissues except non-nucleated erythrocytes during the acute stage of toxoplasmosis. Called also *endozoite.* Cf. *bradyzoite* and *pseudocyst* (def. 2).

**ta·cla·mine hy·dro·chlo·ride** (tă′klə-mēn) a minor tranquilizer, $C_{21}H_{23}N \cdot HCl$.

**tac·rine** (tak′rēn) [MeSH: Tacrine] a cholinesterase inhibitor used to improve cognitive performance in patients with mild to moderate Alzheimer's disease.

**tac·ro·li·mus** (tak″ro-li′məs) [MeSH: Tacrolimus] a macrolide immunosuppressant derived from *Streptomyces tsukubaensis,* having actions similar to those of cyclosporine; used to prevent rejection of organ transplants, especially liver. Administered orally or intravenously.

**tac·tic** (tak′tik) 1. exhibiting tacticity. 2. pertaining to or characterized by taxis.

**tac·tic·i·ty** (tak-tis′ĭ-te) the condition of having a regular chemical arrangement of the units making up the main chain of a polymer.

**tac·tile** (tak′til) [L. *tactilis*] pertaining to touch.

**tac·tion** (tak′shən) [L. *tactio*] touch.

**tac·tom·e·ter** (tak-tom′ə-tər) [L. *tactus* touch + *-meter*] an instrument for measuring the acuteness of the sense of touch; an esthesiometer.

**tac·tor** (tak′tər) a tactile end-organ.

**tac·tu·al** (tak′choo-əl) [L. *tactus* touch] 1. tactile 2. resulting from touch.

**TAD** a regimen of 6-thioguanine, ara-C (cytarabine), and daunomycin, used in cancer chemotherapy.

**Tae·nia** (te′ne-ə) [L. "a flat band," "bandage," "tape"] [MeSH: Taenia] a genus of large tapeworms of the family Taeniidae.
**T. africa′na,** *T. saginata.*
**T. antarc′tica,** a species from dogs in Antarctic regions.
**T. bala′niceps,** a species from dogs and bobcats in Nevada and New Mexico.
**T. brachyso′ma,** a species that infects dogs in Italy.
**T. brem′neri,** *T. confusa.*
**T. cer′vi,** a species from dogs in Denmark.
**T. confu′sa,** a species found in the Mississippi Valley and in East Africa, believed by some to be a variant of *T. saginata.* Called also *T. bremneri.*
**T. cras′siceps,** a species infecting foxes in Alaska and Canada, found in rodents as an intermediate host.
**T. crassicol′lis,** *T. taeniaeformis.*
**T. cucurbiti′na,** *T. saginata.*
**T. demararien′sis,** *Raillietina demarariensis.*
**T. echinococ′cus,** *Echinococcus granulosus.*
**T. ellip′tica,** *Dipylidium caninum.*
**T. hydati′gena,** a species parasitic in dogs and wild Carnivora; the larval stage (cysticercus) is found in the liver and abdominal cavity of various ruminants and rodents and occasionally in other animals, including humans. Called also *T. marginata.*
**T. krab′bei,** a species that infects the bobcat, dog, and wolf in the northern United States, Canada, Alaska, and Iceland.
**T. madagascarien′sis,** *Raillietina madagascariensis.*
**T. margina′ta,** *T. hydatigena.*
**T. mediocanella′ta,** *T. saginata.*
**T. mul′ticeps,** a species whose adult stage is parasitic in the dog; its larval stage *(Coenurus cerebralis)* infests goats, sheep, and occasionally humans, usually in the central nervous system but sometimes elsewhere, producing coenurosis or gid. Called also *Multiceps multiceps.*
**T. na′na,** *Hymenolepis nana.*
**T. o′vis,** a species parasitic in dogs; found in the musculature of sheep and goats as intermediate hosts.
**T. philippi′na,** *T. saginata.*
**T. pisifor′mis,** a tapeworm commonly found in dogs and also parasitic in cats, foxes, wolves, and other animals; the cysticercus (larval stage) is found in the liver and peritoneal cavity of rabbits.
**T. sagina′ta,** the most common of the large tapeworms infecting humans, a species 4 to 8 meters long, found in the adult form in the human intestine. The cysticerci (larval stage) develop in the muscles and other tissues of cattle and other ruminants. Human infection usually results from eating raw or rare beef. Called also *beef* or *unarmed tapeworm* and *T. africana.*

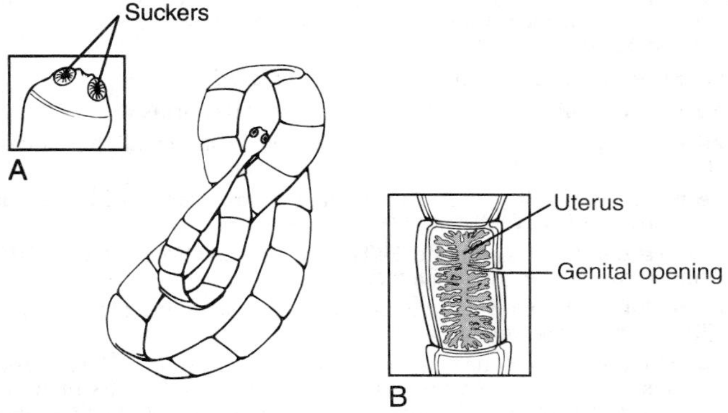

*Taenia saginata* adult. *(A),* Scolex, showing two of the four suckers; *(B),* mature proglottid.

**T. seria′lis,** a species whose adult stage is parasitic in dogs; its larval stage develops in the connective tissues of rabbits, squirrels, other rodents, and occasionally humans. Called also *Multiceps serialis.*
**T. so′lium,** the pork tapeworm, a species 1 to 2 meters long found in the adult form in the human intestine; the cysticerci (larval stage) occur most often in the muscle and various tissues of the pig, but are also found in man, monkeys, camels, sheep, and dogs. It gains access to the human intestine through ingestion of inadequately cooked or measly pork (see *cysticercosis*). It is rare in the United States. Called also *armed* or *measly tapeworm.*
**T. taeniaefor′mis,** a species commonly found in cats, and more rarely in dogs, foxes, and other animals, having rats, mice, and other rodents as intermediate hosts. Called also *T. crassicollis.*

**tae·nia** (te′ne-ə) gen. and pl. *tae′niae* [L. "a flat band," "bandage," "tape"] [MeSH: Taenia] 1. [TA] a flat band or strip of soft tissue; spelled also *tenia.* 2. an individual organism of the genus *Taenia;* called also *tenia.*
**tae′niae acus′ticae,** striae medullares ventriculi quarti.
**t. choroi′dea** [TA], choroid line: the line of attachment of the lateral choroid plexus to the medial wall of the cerebral hemisphere; specifically, the line of attachment of the ependyma of the ventricle to the ependyma of the choroid plexus; called also *t. telae.*
**tae′niae co′li** [TA], three thickened bands, about $\frac{1}{4}$ inch wide and one-sixth shorter than the colon, formed by the longitudinal fibers in the muscular tunic of the large intestine, and extending from the root of the vermiform appendix to the rectum, where the fibers spread out and form a continuous layer encircling the tube; they include the *t. libera, t. mesocolica,* and *t. omentalis.* Called also *taeniae of Valsalva.*
**t. for′nicis** [TA], taenia of fornix: the line of attachment of the choroid plexus of the lateral ventricle to the fornix, including the line of its attachment to the fimbria of the hippocampus.
**t. of fourth ventricle,** t. ventriculi quarti.
**t. li′bera** [TA], the thickened band formed by anterior longitudinal

muscle fibers of the large intestine, almost equidistant from the taenia mesocolica and the taenia omentalis.
**medullary t. of thalamus,** t. thalami.
**t. mesoco'lica** [TA], the thickened band of longitudinal muscle fibers of the large intestine along the site of attachment of the mesocolon.
**t. omenta'lis** [TA], the band of longitudinal muscle fibers of the large intestine along the site of attachment of the greater omentum.
**t. pon'tis,** a bundle of fibers sometimes found on the cerebral peduncle along the rostral border of the pons, running an isolated course to the cerebellum between the superior and middle cerebellar peduncles.
**tae'niae pylo'ri,** ligamenta pylori.
**t. te'lae,** t. choroidea.
**t. termina'lis,** crista terminalis atrii dextri.
**t. tha'lami** [TA], taenia of thalamus: the line of attachment of the ependymal cells of the roof of the third ventricle to the dorsal margin of the thalamus; called also *medullary t. of thalamus* and *t. of third ventricle.*
**t. of third ventricle,** t. thalami.
**t. tu'bae,** a thickened band of peritoneum along the upper border of the uterine tube.
**taeniae of Valsalva,** taeniae coli.
**t. ventri'culi quar'ti,** taenia of fourth ventricle: the line of attachment of the ependymal cells of the choroid plexus to the ependyma along the edge of the caudal part of the fourth ventricle.

**taenia-** [L. *taenia* tape] a combining form denoting relationship to tapeworms or to bands or strips of soft tissue. For words beginning thus, see also those beginning *tenia-.*

**tae•ni•a•cide** (te'ne-ə-sīd") [*taenia-* + *-cide*] 1. destructive to tapeworms. 2. an agent that destroys tapeworms. Called also *teniacide* and *tenicide.*

**tae•niae** (te'ne-e) genitive and plural of *taenia.*

**tae•ni•a•fu•gal** (te"ne-ə-fu'gəl) expelling tapeworms.

**tae•ni•a•fuge** (te'ne-ə-fūj") [*taenia* + *-fuge*] an agent that expels tapeworms. Called also *teniafuge* and *tenifuge.*

**tae•ni•al** (te'ne-əl) 1. of or pertaining to tapeworms of the genus *Taenia.* 2. tenial (def. 1).

**tae•ni•a•sis** (te-ni'ə-sis) [MeSH: Taeniasis] infection with any of the tapeworms of the genus *Taenia.*

**tae•ni•form** (te'nĭ-form) [*taenia* + *form*] resembling the organism *Taenia,* or a tapeworm.

**Tae•ni•i•dae** (te-ni'ĭ-de) a family of medium-sized or large tapeworms of the order Cyclophyllidea, subclass Cestoda, which are parasitic in mammals, including man; medically important genera are *Taenia* and *Echinococcus.*

**tae•ni•o•la** (te-ni'o-lə) [L., dim of *taenia*] a slender bandlike structure.
**t. corporis callosi of Reil,** lamina rostralis.

**tag** (tag) 1. a small appendage, flap, or polyp. 2. label.
**auricular t's,** rudimentary appendages of auricular tissue occurring on the face along the line of union of the first branchial arch.
**cutaneous t.,** acrochordon.
**radioactive t.,** see under *label.*
**skin t.,** acrochordon.

**Tag•a•met** (tag'ə-met) trademark for preparations of cimetidine.

**ta•gli•a•co•tian** (tal-yə-ko'shən) named for Gasparo *Tagliacozzi,* Italian surgeon, 1546–1599.

**tail** (tāl) [L. *cauda;* Gr. *oura*] [MeSH: Tail] 1. any slender appendage; called also *cauda* [TA]. 2. the appendage that extends from the posterior trunk of animals.
**axillary t.,** processus axillaris glandulae mammariae.
**t. of caudate nucleus,** cauda nuclei caudati.
**t. of dentate gyrus,** Giacomini's band.
**t. of epididymis,** cauda epididymidis.
**t. of helix,** cauda helicis.
**occult t.,** supernumerary segments of the coccyx, present in the buttock.
**t. of pancreas,** cauda pancreatis.
**polyadenylate (poly A) t.,** a sequence of about 200 adenylate residues that is added to the 3′ end of many primary mRNA transcripts during post-transcriptional processing in eukaryotes. Its function seems to be protection of the RNA from enzymatic degradation.
**t. of Spence,** the projection of mammary glandular tissue extending into the axillary region, sometimes forming a visible mass which may enlarge premenstrually or during lactation.
**t. of spermatozoon,** the flagellum of a spermatozoon, which contains the axonema; it presents four regions: the *neck, middle piece, principal piece,* and *end piece.*
**t. of spleen,** extremitas anterior splenis.

**tail•gut** (tāl'gut") a prolongation of the hindgut into the tail of the early embryo; it usually undergoes complete obliteration.

**Tail•le•fer's valve** (ti"yə-fāz') [Louis Auguste Horace Sydney Timeléon *Taillefer,* French physician, 1802–1868] see under *valve.*

**tai'pan** (ti-pan') *Oxyuranus scutellatus,* a venomous snake found in northern Australia and New Guinea.

**Ta•ka-di•as•tase** (tah'kah-di"əs-tās) [Jokichi *Takamine,* Japanese chemist in New York, 1854–1922] trademark for an amylolytic enzyme formed by the action of the spores of the fungus *Aspergillus oryzae* on the bran of wheat; used as a digestant.

**Ta•ka•ha•ra's disease** (tah"kah-hah'rahz) [Shigeo *Takahara,* Japanese otolaryngologist, 20th century] acatalasia.

**Ta•ka•ya•su's arteritis (disease, syndrome)** (tah-kah-yah'so͞oz) [Mikito *Takayasu,* Japanese surgeon, 1860–1938] see under *arteritis.*

**Tal.** abbreviation for L. *tal'is,* such a one.

**Ta•la•cen** (tal'ə-sen) trademark for a preparation of pentazocine hydrochloride and acetaminophen.

**tal•al•gia** (tal-al'jə) pain in the heel or ankle.

**tal•amp•i•cil•lin hy•dro•chlo•ride** (tal-amp"ĭ-sil'in) the monohydrochloride salt of the phthalidyl ester of ampicillin, having the actions and uses of ampicillin (q.v.).

**tal•an•tro•pia** (tal"ən-tro'pe-ə) [Gr. *talanton* balance + *trop-* + *-ia*] nystagmus.

**ta•lar** (ta'lər) of or pertaining to the talus.

**tal•bu•tal** (tal'bu-təl) an intermediate-acting barbiturate, used as a sedative and hypnotic, administered orally.

**talc** (talk) [MeSH: Talc] 1. a powdered hydrous form of magnesium silicate, sometimes containing a small proportion of aluminum silicate; solid lumps found in nature are called *soapstone* or *steatite.* Inhalation of the powder can cause talc pneumoconiosis. Called also *French chalk.* 2. [USP] a purified form of talc used as a dusting powder. Called also *purified talc.*

**tal•co•sis** (tal-ko'sis) talc pneumoconiosis.
**pulmonary t.,** talc pneumoconiosis.

**tal•cum** (tal'kəm) [L.] talc.

**ta•li** (ta'li) genitive and plural of *talus.*

**tal•i•a•co•tian** (tal"e-ə-ko'shən) tagliacotian.

**tal•i•ped** (tal'ĭ-ped) 1. clubfooted. 2. a clubfooted person.

**tal•i•pe•dic** (tal"ĭ-pe'dik) clubfooted.

**tal•i•pes** (tal'ĭ-pēz) [L.] a congenital deformity of the foot, which is twisted out of shape or position; called also *clubfoot* and *reel foot.* See also under *pes.*
**t. calcaneoca'vus,** a deformity in which the anterior part of the foot is elevated and the longitudinal arch of the foot is abnormally high.
**t. calcaneoval'gus,** a deformity of the foot in which the heel is

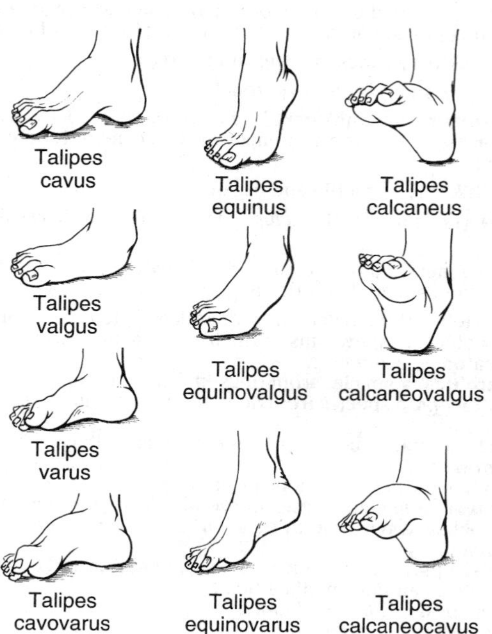

turned outward from the midline of the body and the anterior part of the foot is elevated.
**t. calcaneova'rus,** a deformity of the foot in which the heel is turned toward the midline of the body and the anterior part is elevated.
**t. calca'neus,** a deformity in which the foot is dorsiflexed.
**t. cavoval'gus,** a deformity in which the longitudinal arch of the foot is abnormally high, and the heel is turned outward from the midline of the body.
**t. cavova'rus,** a deformity of the foot in which the longitudinal arch is abnormally high and the heel is turned inward from the midline of the leg.
**t. ca'vus,** exaggerated height of the longitudinal arch of the foot; it may be congenital or secondary to contractures or disturbed balance of the muscles.
**t. equinoval'gus,** a deformity of the foot in which the heel is elevated and turned outward from the midline of the body.
**t. equinova'rus,** a deformity of the foot in which the heel is turned inward from the midline of the leg and the foot is plantar flexed. This is associated with the raising of the inner border of the foot (supination) and displacement of the anterior part of the foot so that it lies medially to the vertical axis of the leg (adduction). With this type of foot the arch is higher (cavus) and the foot is in equinus (plantar flexion). This is a typical clubfoot.
**t. equi'nus,** a deformity in which the foot is plantar flexed, causing the person to walk on the toes without touching the heel.
**t. planoval'gus,** a deformity of the foot in which the heel is turned outward from the midline of the leg and the outer border of the anterior part of the foot is higher than the inner border. This results in a lowering of the longitudinal arch. The condition may be congenital and permanent, or it may be spasmodic as a result of reflex spasm of the muscles controlling the foot.
**t. val'gus,** a deformity of the foot in which the heel is turned outward from the midline of the leg.
**t. va'rus,** a deformity of the foot in which the heel is turned inward from the midline of the leg.

**tal·i·pom·a·nus** (tal″ĭ-pom'ə-nəs) [*talipes* + *manus*] a congenital deformity of the hand; see *clubhand.*

**Tal·ma's disease, operation** (tahl'mahz) [Sape *Talma,* Dutch physician, 1847–1918] see *myotonia tarda,* and see under *operation.*

**ta·lo·cal·ca·ne·al** (ta″lo-kal-ka'ne-əl) pertaining to the talus and calcaneus.

**ta·lo·cal·ca·ne·an** (ta″lo-kal-ka'ne-ən) talocalcaneal.

**ta·lo·cru·ral** (ta″lo-kroo'rəl) [*talus* + *crural*] pertaining to the talus and the bones of the leg.

**ta·lo·fib·u·lar** (ta″lo-fib'u-lər) pertaining to the talus and the fibula.

**tal·on** (tal'on) [L. "bird's claw"] 1. the claw of a bird of prey or other predatory animal. 2. a structure or part resembling such a claw.
**t. noir** (nwahr) [F. "black claw"], black heel.

**ta·lo·na·vic·u·lar** (ta″lo-nə-vik'u-lər) pertaining to the talus and the navicular bone.

**ta·lo·scaph·oid** (ta″lo-skaf'oid) talonavicular.

**ta·lose** (ta'lōs) an aldohexose isomeric with glucose at carbons 2 and 4.

**ta·lo·tib·i·al** (ta″lo-tib'e-əl) pertaining to the talus and the tibia.

**ta·lus** (ta'ləs) pl. *ta'li* [L. "ankle"] [TA] [MeSH: Talus] the highest of the tarsal bones and the one that articulates with the tibia and fibula to form the ankle joint; called also *ankle, ankle bone, astragalus, astragaloid bone,* and *os tarsi tibiale.*

**Tal·win** (tal'win) trademark for preparations of pentazocine lactate.

**Tam·bo·cor** (tam'bo-kor) trademark for a preparation of flecainide acetate.

**tam·bour** (tam-bo͞or') [Fr. "drum"] a drum-shaped appliance used in transmitting movements in a recording instrument. It consists of a cylinder having an elastic membrane stretched over it, from which passes a tube that transmits the changes in air pressure to a recording device.

**Tamm-Hors·fall mucoprotein (protein)** (tam-hors'fal) [Igor *Tamm,* American virologist, born 1922; Frank Lappin *Horsfall,* Jr., American virologist, 1906–1971] see under *mucoprotein.*

**ta·mox·i·fen cit·rate** (tə-mok'sĭ-fən) a nonsteroidal oral antiestrogen, used in the palliative treatment of breast cancer in postmenopausal women and to stimulate ovulation in infertility.

**tam·pan** (tam'pan) 1. *Argas persicus.* 2. *Ornithodoros moubata.*

**tam·pon** (tam'pon) [Fr. "stopper, plug"] [MeSH: Tampons] a pack; a pad or plug made of cotton, sponge, or other material; variously used in surgery to plug the nose, vagina, etc., for the control of hemorrhage or the absorption of secretions.

**tam·pon·ade** (tam″pon-ād') [Fr. *tamponner* to stop up] 1. surgical use of a tampon. 2. pathologic compression of a part.
**balloon t.,** esophagogastric tamponade by means of a device with a triple-lumen tube and two inflatable balloons, the third lumen providing for aspiration of blood clots.
**cardiac t.,** acute compression of the heart caused by increased intrapericardial pressure due to the collection of blood or fluid in the pericardium from rupture of the heart, penetrating trauma, or progressive effusion.
**chronic t.,** chronic compression of the heart caused by chronic pericardial effusion and pericardial thickening.
**esophagogastric t.,** the exertion of direct pressure against bleeding esophageal varices by insertion of a tube with a sausage-shaped balloon in the esophagus and a globular one in the stomach and inflating the balloons.
**heart t.,** cardiac t.
**pericardial t.,** cardiac t.

**tam·pon·age** (tam-po-nahzh') tamponade.

**tam·pon·ing** (tam'pon-ing) tamponade.

**tam·pon·ment** (tam-pon'mənt) the act of plugging with a tampon.

**Ta·mus** (ta'məs) [L.] a genus of plants of the family Dioscoreaceae, having tuberous roots. *T. commu'nis* L. is black bryony, a species native to Europe and Asia whose root is used in homeopathy as a rubefacient and diuretic.

**tan** (tan) 1. to brown or become brown from exposure to sun or to ultraviolet light. 2. the brownish color of the skin acquired by such exposure, resulting from darkening of preformed melanin (Meirowsky phenomenon), accelerated formation of new melanin, and retention of melanin in the epidermis as a result of retardation of keratinization.

**Tan·a·ce·tum** (tan″ə-se'təm) a genus of strongly aromatic, chiefly Old World herbs of the family Compositae.
**T. parthe'nium** [NF], feverfew (q.v.); a species native to southeastern Europe and now widely distributed throughout Europe, North America, and Australia; the dried leaves are used medicinally.

**tan·a·pox** (tan'ə-poks″) [*Tana* River, Kenya] a viral disease occurring in Kenya and Zaire, caused by a poxvirus and characterized by fever and one or two papulovesicular lesions on the extremities.

**Tan·de·a·ril** (tan-de'ə-ril) trademark for a preparation of oxyphenbutazone.

**tan·gen·ti·al·i·ty** (tan-jen″she-al'ĭ-te) a pattern of speech characterized by oblique, digressive, or irrelevant replies to questions; the responses never approach the point of the questions. It differs from *circumstantiality,* in which the responder eventually reaches the point.

**tan·ghin** (tan'gēn) 1. *Tanghinia venenifera.* 2. the poisonous seed of *T. venenifera.*

**Tan·ghin·ia** (tang-gin'e-ə) a genus of trees of the family Apocynaceae. *T. veneni'fera* and other species found in southern Africa and Madagascar have seeds called tanghin that are highly toxic.

**Tan·gier disease** (tan-jēr') [*Tangier* Island, in Chesapeake Bay, where the disease was first discovered] [MeSH: Tangier Disease] see under *disease.*

**tan·gle** (tang'gəl) a knot or snarl.
**neurofibrillary t's,** intracellular knots or clumps of neurofibrils seen in the cerebral cortex in Alzheimer's disease.

**tank** (tank) an artificial receptacle for liquids.
**activated sludge t.,** a tank for the aerobic digestion of sewage.

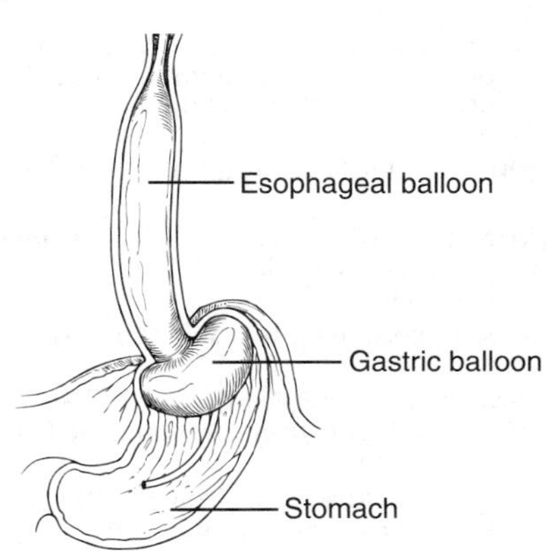


Esophagogastric tamponade.

Screened and sedimented raw sewage, treated with an inoculum of activated sludge (q.v.), flows slowly or intermittently through the tank while being aerated vigorously. The process oxidizes much of the organic material in the sewage, thus reducing the biological oxygen demand.

**digestion t.**, a deep septic tank in which sludge is separated and submitted to anaerobic bacterial action to reduce the mass of material and produce a less offensive product.

**Dortmund t.**, a deep vertical flow settling tank for removing sludge from sewage.

**Emsher t.**, digestion t.

**Hubbard t.**, a tank in which a patient may be immersed for the purpose of permitting him to take underwater exercise.

**Imhoff t.**, digestion t.

**septic t.**, a tank for the receipt of raw sewage, in which putrefaction occurs owing to the presence of anaerobic bacteria, and solid material settles to the bottom.

**settling t.**, a basin in which the rate of flow of the sewage is reduced and the sludge allowed to settle out.

**tan·nase** (tan'ās) an esterase found in various tannin-bearing plants and produced in cultures by *Aspergillus niger* and *Penicillium glaucum*, which catalyzes the hydrolysis of various ester linkages in gallic acid compounds.

**tan·nate** (tan'āt) [L. *tannas*] any salt of tannic acid; all the tannates are astringent.

**tan·nic ac·id** (tan'ik) [USP] [MeSH: Tannic Acid] a tannin obtained from nutgalls and used as an astringent for the mucous membranes of the mouth and throat and as suppositories for the treatment of hemorrhoids; it is no longer used to treat burns because of the possibility of severe liver damage. Called also *gallotannic acid, tannin,* and, erroneously, *digallic acid.*

**tan·nin** (tan'in) tannic acid.

**tan·ta·lum** (tan'tə-ləm) [MeSH: Tantalum] a rare metallic element: symbol, Ta; atomic number, 73; atomic weight, 180.948. It is a noncorrosive and malleable metal which has been used for plates or disks to replace cranial defects, for wire sutures, and for making prosthetic appliances.

**tan·trum** (tan'trəm) a violent display of bad temper.

**tan·y·cyte** (tan'ĭ-sīt) [Gr. *tanyein* to stretch + *-cyte*] a modified ependymal cell of the median eminence, having a body that lies near the third ventricle and sending out processes that extend to the capillary plexus of the portal circulation. Its function is unknown, but it may transport hormones from the cerebrospinal fluid into the portal circulation or from hypothalamic neurons to the cerebrospinal fluid.

**TAO** (ta'o) trademark for preparations of troleandomycin.

**tap** (tap) 1. a quick, light blow. 2. to drain off fluid by paracentesis.

**bloody t.**, a lumbar puncture in which the fluid obtained is bloody or pinkish.

**front t.**, a tap on the muscles of the front of the leg, producing contraction of the muscles of the calf in spinal irritability.

**heel t.**, heel-tap reflex.

**spinal t.**, lumbar puncture.

**Tap·a·zole** (tap'ə-zōl) trademark for a preparation of methimazole.

**tape** (tāp) a long, narrow strip of fabric or other flexible material.

**adhesive t.** [USP], a strip of fabric and/or film evenly coated on one side with a pressure-sensitive, adhesive mixture, the whole having high tensile strength, used for the application of dressings and sometimes to produce immobilization.

**adhesive t., sterile,** adhesive tape, the adhesive surface of which is covered by strips of a protective material of equal width, and which is sterilized after packaging.

**flurandrenolide t.** [USP], flexible polyethylene tape having an adhesive layer impregnated with flurandrenolone; the tape acts as both a vehicle and an occlusive dressing.

**Montgomery's t's**, see under *strap.*

**tap·ei·no·ce·phal·ic** (tap"ĭ-no-sə-fal'ik) characterized by tapeinocephaly.

**tap·ei·no·ceph·a·ly** (tap"ĭ-no-sef'ə-le) [Gr. *tapeinos* low-lying + *-cephaly*] a low form of the skull, which is also flattened at front, having a vertical index below 72.

**ta·pe·tal** (tə-pe'təl) pertaining to a tapetum, especially to the tapetum lucidum.

**ta·pe·to·ret·i·nal** (ta-pe"-to-ret'ĭ-nəl) [*tapetum* + *retinal*] pertaining to the tapetum oculi (*pars pigmentosa retinae* [TA]) and the retina.

**ta·pe·tum** (tə-pe'təm) pl. *tape'ta* [L., from Gr. *tapētion,* dim. of *tapēs* a carpet, rug] 1. a covering structure, or layer of cells. 2. t. corporis callosi.

**t. cellulo'sum,** a type of tapetum lucidum, being the more complex, more cellular type found in all but two species of carnivores and in seals.

**t. choroi'deae,** t. lucidum.

**t. cor'poris callo'si** [TA], a stratum of commissural fibers of the corpus callosum on the superolateral aspect of the occipital horn of the lateral ventricle.

**t. fibro'sum,** a type of tapetum lucidum, being the simpler, fibrous type found in hoofed animals, marsupials, elephants, whales, and a few fish.

**t. lu'cidum,** the iridescent pigment epithelium of the choroid of animals, which gives their eyes the property of shining in the dark; the two primary types are the tapetum cellulosum and the tapetum fibrosum. Called also *t. choroideae.*

**t. ni'grum, t. o'culi,** pars pigmentosa retinae.

**tape·worm** (tāp'wərm) a parasitic intestinal worm having a flattened, bandlike form. Those infecting humans are principally of the genera *Taenia, Diphyllobothrium, Hymenolepis, Echinococcus,* and *Dipylidium.* The eggs are ingested by the intermediate host, whence they make their way into the tissues, where the larval stages are produced (see *hydatid cyst, plerocercoid,* and *cysticercus*). When the flesh of the intermediate host is eaten, the larvae develop within the alimentary canal of the definitive host into adult tapeworms, which consist of an attachment organ, or scolex, an undifferentiated neck, and a strobila made up of a variable number of separate segments, or proglottids, each of which is hermaphroditic and produces eggs. Called also *cestode.*

**African t.**, *Taenia saginata.*

**armed t.**, *Taenia solium.*

**beef t.**, *Taenia saginata.*

**broad t.**, *Diphyllobothrium latum.*

**dog t.**, 1. *Echinococcus granulosus.* 2. *Dipylidium caninum.*

**double-pored dog t.**, *Dipylidium caninum.*

**dwarf t.**, *Hymenolepis nana.*

**fish t.**, *Diphyllobothrium latum.*

**fringed t.**, *Thysanosoma actinioides.*

**heart-headed t.**, *Diphyllobothrium cordatum.*

**hydatid t.**, *Echinococcus granulosus.*

**Madagascar t.**, *Raillietina madagascariensis.*

**Manson's larval t.**, *Diphyllobothrium mansonoides.*

**measly t.**, *Taenia solium.*

**pork t.**, *Taenia solium.*

**rat t.**, *Hymenolepis diminuta.*

**Swiss t.**, *Diphyllobothrium latum.*

**unarmed t.**, *Taenia saginata.*

**taph·e·pho·bia** (taf"ə-fo'be-ə) [Gr. *taphos* grave + *-phobia*] irrational fear of being buried alive.

**Ta·pia's syndrome** (tah'pe-əz) [Antonio García *Tapia,* Spanish otolaryngologist, 1875–1950] see under *syndrome.*

**tap·i·no·ce·phal·ic** (tap"ĭ-no-sə-fal'ik) tapeinocephalic.

**tap·i·no·ceph·a·ly** (tap"ĭ-no-sef'ə-le) tapeinocephaly.

**ta·pi·roid** (ta'pĭ-roid) resembling the snout of a tapir.

**ta·pote·ment** (tah-pōt-maw') [Fr.] a tapping or percussing movement in massage.

**tar** (tahr) a dark brown or black viscid liquid, obtained by roasting the wood of various species of pine, or as a by-product of the destructive distillation of bituminous coal (see *coal t.*). It is a mixture of complex composition, and is the source of organic substances such as cresol, creosol, guaiacol, naphthalene, paraffin, phenol, toluene, and xylene. Once used in chronic bronchitis, diarrhea, and diseases of the urinary organs, it now has only limited use in certain skin diseases, notably psoriasis and chronic eczematous disorders. If it is ingested or its fumes are inhaled, it is toxic and carcinogenic. See also *pitch* and *pitch poisoning.*

**coal t.**, 1. tar obtained as a by-product of the destructive distillation of bituminous coal, used as a raw material for plastics, solvents, waterproofing compounds, sealants, and various other organic chemicals. If it is ingested or its fumes are inhaled it is toxic and carcinogenic; see also *pitch* and *pitch poisoning.* 2. [USP] a preparation of coal tar used as a topical antieczematic and antipsoriatic.

**gas t.**, a coal tar derived from the coal, rosin, petroleum, and other material used in gas works.

**juniper t.** [USP], a volatile thick brown oil with a bitter taste, obtained from the woody portions of *Juniperus oxycedrus,* used as a pharmaceutic necessity and for the topical therapy of dermatoses. Called also *cade oil, Haarlem oil,* and *silver balsam.*

**pine t.**, a viscid, blackish brown liquid obtained by destructive distillation of the wood of various pine trees, used as a local antieczematic and rubefacient; applied topically.

**Tar·ac·tan** (tar-ak'tən) trademark for preparations of chlorprothixene.

**ta·ran·tu·la** (tə-ran'tu-lə) 1. any of numerous large venomous spiders whose bite causes local inflammation and pain. 2. European t.

**American t.,** *Eurypelma hentzii,* a large dark ferocious-looking spider with a poisonous bite.
**black t.,** *Sericopelma communis,* a black venomous species found in Panama.
**European t.,** *Lycosa tarentula,* a large hairy spider whose bite causes pain and was formerly believed to be deadly. Called also *European wolf spider.*

**tar·ba·di·llo** (tahr″bah-de′yo) [Sp.] murine typhus.

**tar·ba·gan** (tahr′bə-gən) *Marmota bobak,* a reddish-brown marmot found on the steppes of Central Asia; it is a natural reservoir of the plague.

**Tar·dieu's spots** (tahr-dyooz′) [Auguste Ambroise *Tardieu,* French physician, 1818–1879] see under *spot.*

**tar·dive** (tahr′div) [Fr. "tardy, late"] marked by lateness, late; said of a disease in which the characteristic lesion is late in appearing.

**tare** (tār) 1. the weight of the vessel in which a substance is weighed. 2. to take the weight of a vessel which is to contain a substance, in order to allow for it when the vessel and the substance are weighed together.

**tar·get** (tahr′gət) 1. an object or area toward which something is directed, such as the metal or plate of an x-ray tube on which the electrons impinge and from which the x-rays are sent out. 2. denoting a cell or organ that is selectively affected by a particular agent, e.g., a hormone or drug.

**tar·get·ing** (tahr′gət-ing) the process of aiming at a specified object or area.
**gene t.,** a process by which precise alterations may be made in the mammalian genome, using the ability of tissue culture cells to induce homologous recombination between introduced DNA molecules and their own genomes.

**Ta·ri·cha** (tə-re′kə) a genus of amphibious newts. *T. toro′sa* contains the poison tarichatoxin (tetrodotoxin) in its body.

**tar·ich·a·tox·in** (tar″ik-ə-tok′sin) a neurotoxin from the newt *(Taricha),* identical with tetrodotoxin (q.v.).

**Ta·rin's (Ta·ri·ni's, Ta·ri·nus′) fascia, fossa,** etc. (tah-raz′, tahre′nēz, tə-ri′nəs) [Pierre *Tarin,* French anatomist, 1725–1761] see *gyrus dentatus* (def. 1), *fossa interpeduncularis, anterior recess of interpeduncular fossa, posterior recess of interpeduncular fossa,* and *velum medullare caudale.*

**Tar·lov's cyst** (tahr′lovz) [Isadore Max *Tarlov,* American surgeon, 1905–1977] perineurial cyst.

**Tar·nier's forceps** (tahr″ne-āz′) [Etienne Stéphane *Tarnier,* French obstetrician, 1828–1897] see under *forceps.*

**tar·sad·e·ni·tis** (tahr″sad-ə-ni′tis) an inflammation of the tarsus of the eyelid and of the meibomian glands.

**tar·sal** (tahr′səl) [L. *tarsalis*] 1. pertaining to the tarsus of an eyelid or to the instep. 2. any of the bones of the tarsus.

**tar·sal·gia** (tahr-sal′jə) pain in the ankle or foot.

**tar·sa·lia** (tahr-sa′le-ə) the bones of the tarsus.

**tar·sa·lis** (tahr-sa′lis) [L.] tarsal.

**tar·sec·to·my** (tahr-sek′tə-me) [*tarso-* + *-ectomy*] 1. excision of the tarsus, or a part of it. 2. excision of a tarsal cartilage.

**tar·sec·to·pia** (tahr″sek-to′pe-ə) [*tarso-* + *ectopia*] dislocation of the tarsus.

**tar·si·tis** (tahr-si′tis) inflammation of the tarsus, or margin of an eyelid; blepharitis.

**tars(o)-** [Gr. *tarsos* a broad flat surface] a combining form denoting relationship to the edge of the eyelid, or to the instep of the foot.

**tar·so·chei·lo·plas·ty** (tahr″so-ki′lo-plas″te) [*tarso-* + *cheilo-* + *-plasty*] a plastic operation upon the edge of the eyelid, as in treatment of trichiasis.

**tar·soc·la·sis** (tahr-sok′lə-sis) [*tarso-* + Gr. *klasis* breaking] the operation of fracturing the tarsus of the foot.

**tar·so·ma·la·cia** (tahr″so-mə-la′shə) [*tarso-* + *malacia*] softening of the tarsus of an eyelid.

**tar·so·meg·a·ly** (tahr″so-meg′ə-le) enlargement of the os calcis.

**tar·so·meta·tar·sal** (tahr″so-met″ə-tahr′səl) pertaining to the tarsus and the metatarsus.

**tar·so·or·bi·tal** (tahr″so-or′bĭ-təl) pertaining to the tarsus of the eyelid and to the orbit.

**tar·so·pha·lan·ge·al** (tahr″so-fə-lan′je-əl) pertaining to the tarsus and the phalanges of the toes.

**tar·so·pla·sia** (tahr″so-pla′zhə) tarsoplasty.

**tar·so·plas·ty** (tahr′so-plas″te) [*tarso-* + *-plasty*] plastic surgery of the tarsus of an eyelid.

**tar·sop·to·sis** (tahr″sop-to′sis) [*tarso-* + *-ptosis*] falling of the tarsus; flatfoot.

**tar·sor·rha·phy** (tahr-sor′ə-fe) [*tarso-* + *-rrhaphy*] suturing together of the upper and lower eyelids in order to shorten or close the palpebral fissure. See also *partial t.* and *total t.* Called also *blepharorrhaphy.*
**external t.,** partial tarsorrhaphy involving the external part of the fissure.
**internal t.,** partial tarsorrhaphy involving the internal part of the fissure.
**median t.,** partial tarsorrhaphy involving the middle part of the fissure.
**partial t.,** tarsorrhaphy that closes only part of a palpebral fissure. See also *external t., median t.,* and *internal t.*
**total t.,** tarsorrhaphy that entirely closes a palpebral fissure.

**tar·so·tar·sal** (tahr″so-tahr′səl) pertaining to the articulation between the two rows of tarsal bones.

**tar·so·tib·i·al** (tahr″so-tib′e-əl) pertaining to the tarsus and the tibia.

**tar·sot·o·my** (tahr-sot′ə-me) [*tarso-* + *-tomy*] the operation of incising the tarsus, or an eyelid; blepharotomy.

**tar·sus** (tahr′səs) [L., from Gr. *tarsos* a frame of wickerwork; any broad flat surface] [MeSH: Tarsus] 1. [TA] the region of the articulation between the foot and the leg; see also *t. osseus.* 2. one of the plates of connective tissue forming the framework of an eyelid; see *t. inferior palpebrae* and *t. superior palpebrae.*
**bony t.,** t. osseus.
**t. infe′rior pal′pebrae** [TA], the firm framework of connective tissue that gives shape to the lower eyelids; see also *palpebral cartilages.*
**t. os′seus** [TA], bony tarsus: the seven bones constituting the articulation between the foot and the leg—the talus, calcaneus, and navicular, in the proximal row; and the cuboid and the lateral, intermediate, and medial cuneiform bones, in the distal row. See also *articulatio talocruralis.*
**t. supe′rior pal′pebrae** [TA], the firm framework of connective tissue that gives shape to the upper eyelids; see also *palpebral cartilages.*

**tar·tar** (tahr′tər) [L. *tartarum;* Gr. *tartaron*] 1. crude potassium bitartrate. 2. dental calculus.
**borated t.,** a white powder prepared by evaporating a solution of 2 parts of sodium borate and 5 parts of potassium bitartrate.
**cream of t.,** potassium bitartrate.

**tar·tar·at·ed** (tahr′tər-āt″əd) charged with tartaric acid.

**tar·tar·ic ac·id** (tahr-tar′ik) 2,3-dihydroxybutanedioic acid; its salts (tartrates) are used in food preparation (cream of tartar) and have been used as cathartics. Tartaric acid has two asymmetric carbon atoms and has three structural isomers: two enantiomers, *d-* and *l-* tartaric acid, and one meso compound, *meso*-tartaric acid, which is a diastereomer of the other two.

**tar·tar·ized** (tahr′tər-īzd) tartarated.

**tar·trate** (tahr′trāt) [L. *tartras*] any salt of tartaric acid.
**acid t.,** a bitartrate; any salt of tartaric acid in which one atom only of hydrogen is replaced by a base.
**ferric ammonium t.,** see under *ammonium.*
**normal t.,** one in which two hydrogen atoms are replaced; various tartrates are employed as remedial agents.

**tar·trat·ed** (tahr′trāt-əd) [L. *tartratus*] containing tartar or tartaric acid.

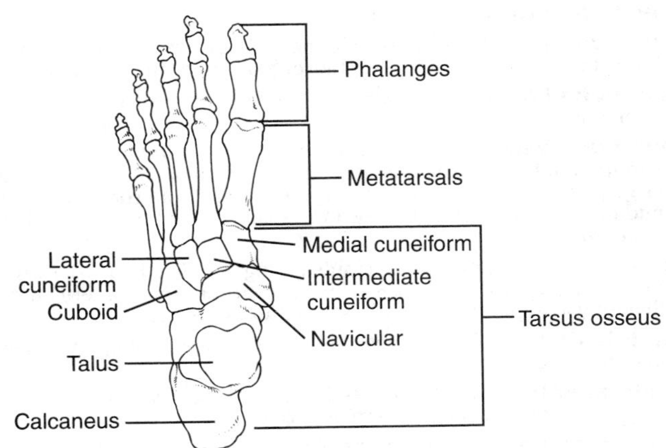


Tarsus osseus (bony tarsus), comprising the seven tarsal bones.

**Ta·rui disease** (tah'roo-e) [Seiichiro *Tarui,* Japanese physician, 20th century] glycogen storage disease (type VII).

**tas·tant** (tās'tənt) any substance, e.g., salt, capable of eliciting gustatory excitation, i.e., stimulating the sense of taste.

**taste** (tāst) [L. *gustus*] [MeSH: Taste] 1. the sense effected by the gustatory receptors in the tongue. Four qualities are distinguished by taste: sweet, sour, salty, and bitter. 2. the act of perceiving by this sense.
**color t.,** a pseudogeusia in which tastes are associated with colors; called also *colored gustation.*
**franklinic t.,** a sour taste produced by stimulating the tongue with static electricity.

**taste·blind·ness** (tāst-blīnd'nəs) inability to taste certain substances, such as phenylthiourea.

**tast·er** (tās'tər) an individual capable of tasting a particular test substance, such as phenylthiourea, used in certain genetic studies.

**TAT** Thematic Apperception Test; toxin-antitoxin.

**Tat·lock·ia mic·da·dei** (tat-lok'e-ə mik-da'de-i) a waterborne legionella-like organism implicated as an etiologic agent of pneumonia, which is probably transmitted by aerosols, direct inoculation into the lung during medical procedures involving the respiratory tract, and aspiration. Called also *Pittsburgh pneumonia agent.*

**tat·too·ing** (tă-too'ing) [MeSH: Tattooing] the insertion of permanent colors in the skin by introducing them through punctures.
**t. of the cornea,** the permanent coloring of the cornea chiefly to conceal leukomatous spots.

**Ta·tum** (ta'təm) Edward Lawrie. American biochemist, 1909–1975; co-winner, with George Wells Beadle and Joshua Lederberg, of the Nobel prize for medicine or physiology in 1958 for proving that genes in bread mold transmit hereditary characteristics by controlling particular chemical reactions.

**Ta·tu·mel·la** (ta″tə-mel'ə) [Harvey *Tatum,* American bacteriologist] a genus of gram-negative, facultatively anaerobic, rod-shaped bacteria of the family Enterobacteriaceae, isolated from human clinical specimens, primarily from the respiratory tract. It is probably an infrequent opportunistic pathogen. The type species is *T. pty'seos.*

**tau** (tou, taw) [T, τ] the nineteenth letter of the Greek alphabet.
**Kendall's t.,** Kendall's rank correlation coefficient.

**tau·rine** (taw'rēn) [MeSH: Taurine] an oxidized sulfur-containing amine occurring conjugated in the bile, usually with cholic acid to form cholyltaurine or with chenodeoxycholic acid to form chenodeoxycholyltaurine; it is also thought to be a central nervous system neurotransmitter or neuromodulator. It is excreted excessively in the urine in hyper-β-alaninemia.

**taur(o)-** [L. *taurus* bull] a combining form denoting relationship to a bull, or to taurine.

**tau·ro·che·no·de·oxy·cho·late** (taw″ro-ke″no-de-ok″se-ko'lāt) chenodeoxycholyltaurine.

**tau·ro·che·no·de·oxy·cho·lic ac·id** (taw″ro-ke″no-de-ok″se-ko'lik) [MeSH: Taurochenodeoxycholic Acid] chenodeoxycholyltaurine.

**tau·ro·cho·lan·er·e·sis** (taw″ro-ko″lən-er'ə-sis) [*taurocholic* acid + Gr. *hairesis* a taking] increase in the output or elimination of cholyltaurine (taurocholic acid) in the bile. Cf. *cholaneresis.*

**tau·ro·cho·lano·poi·e·sis** (taw″ro-ko-lan″o-poi-e'sis) [*taurocholic* acid + *poiesis*] synthesis of cholyltaurine (taurocholic acid) by the liver.

**tau·ro·cho·late** (taw″ro-ko'lāt) cholyltaurine.

**tau·ro·cho·le·mia** (taw″ro-ko-le'me-ə) [*taurocholic* acid + *-emia*] the presence of cholyltaurine (taurocholic acid) in the blood.

**tau·ro·cho·lic ac·id** (taw″ro-ko'lik) [MeSH: Taurocholic Acid] cholyltaurine.

**tau·ro·don·tism** (taw″ro-don'tiz-əm) [*tauro-* + *odont-* + *-ism*] a variation in tooth form characterized by prism-shaped molars with large pulp spaces, resulting from branching of the root only in the middle *(mesotaurodontism),* or in the apical third or not at all *(hypertaurodontism).*

**Taus·sig-Bing syndrome** (tou'sig-bing) [Helen Brooke *Taussig,* American pediatrician, 1898–1986; Richard J. *Bing,* American cardiac physiologist, born 1909] see under *syndrome.*

**taut(o)-** [Gr. *tautos* from *to auto* the same] a combining form meaning the same.

**tau·to·me·ni·al** (taw″to-me'ne-əl) [*tauto-* + Gr. *mēniaia* menses] pertaining to the same menstrual period.

**tau·to·mer** (taw'to-mər) a chemical compound exhibiting, or capable of exhibiting, tautomerism.

**tau·tom·er·al** (taw-tom'ər-əl) [*tauto-* + *mer-*[1] + *-al*[1]] pertaining to the same part, especially sending processes to help in the formation of the white matter in the same side of the spinal cord; said of certain neurons and neuroblasts. See *tautomeral cells,* under *cell.*

**tau·tom·er·ase** (taw-tom'ər-ās) [EC 5.3.2] any member of a sub-subclass of enzymes of the isomerase class that catalyze the interconversion of the keto and enol forms of a substrate. See also *enol.*

**tau·to·mer·ic** (taw″to-mer'ik) exhibiting, or capable of exhibiting, tautomerism.

**tau·tom·er·ism** (taw-tom'ər-iz-əm) [*tauto-* + *mer-*[1] + *-ism*] the relationship that exists between two structural isomers that are in chemical equilibrium and freely change from one form to the other.
**keto-enol t.,** tautomerism between two compounds, one an enol, and the other a ketone, that equilibrate by transfer of a proton. The keto form usually predominates except where the enol form is stabilized by conjugation with other double bonds. See structural formulas at *enol.*

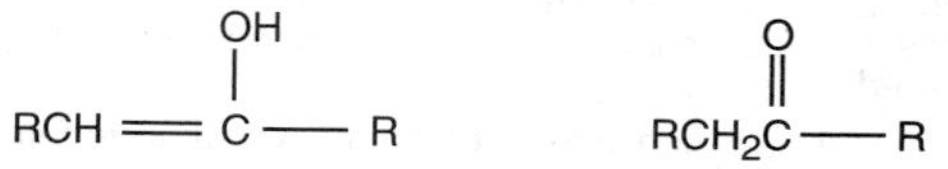

$$RCH{=}C(OH){-}R \qquad\qquad RCH_2C({=}O){-}R$$

Enol form    Keto form

**proton t.,** tautomerism in which an acidic proton is transferred from one position to another in the same molecule, e.g., keto-enol tautomerism. Called also *prototropy.*
**ring-chain t.,** tautomerism involving open-chain and ring forms, as occurs with sugars. See *mutarotation.*

**Tav·ist** (tav'ist) trademark for a preparation of clemastine fumarate.

**Tavist-D** (tav'ist-dee) trademark for a combination preparation of clemastine fumarate and phenylpropanolamine hydrochloride.

**Ta·wa·ra's node** (tah-wah'rahz) [K. Sunao *Tawara,* Japanese pathologist, 1873–1938] nodus atrioventricularis.

**taxa** (tak'sə) plural of *taxon.*

**tax·ane** (tak'sān) any of a group of chemical substances with varying degrees of antitumor activity, acting by promoting and stabilizing the polymerization of microtubules; it includes paclitaxel, docetaxel, and related compounds.

**tax·ine** (tak'sēn) a mixture of alkaloids *(taxine-1* and *taxine-2)* from members of the genus *Taxus,* responsible for their toxicity.

**tax·is** (tak'sis) [Gr. "a drawing up in rank and file"] 1. an orientation movement of a motile organism in response to an external stimulus. Such a response may be either positive (toward) or negative (away from the stimulus). Cf. *tropism.* 2. exertion of force in the manual replacement of a displaced or injured organ or structure, as in the reduction of a fracture or dislocation, or the replacement of a protruded intestine in hernia.

**-taxis** a word termination used to describe an orientation movement of a motile organism in response to a stimulus, affixed to a stem denoting the nature of the stimulus (e.g., chemotaxis, phototaxis).

**Tax·ol** (tak'sol) trademark for a preparation of paclitaxel.

**tax·ol·o·gy** (taks-ol'ə-je) taxonomy.

**tax·on** (tak'son) pl. *tax'a* [Gr. *taxis* a drawing up in rank and file + *on* neuter ending] a particular group (category) into which related organisms are classified; the main categories are (in ascending order): species, genus, family, order, class, phylum, and kingdom.

**taxo·nom·ic** (tak″so-nom'ik) pertaining to taxonomy.

**tax·on·o·mist** (taks-on'ə-mist) a specialist in taxonomy.

**tax·on·o·my** (tak-son'ə-me) [L. *taxinomia;* Gr. *taxis* a drawing up in rank and file + *nomos* law] the orderly classification of organisms into appropriate categories (taxa) on the basis of relationships among them, with the application of suitable and correct names.
**numerical t.,** an arithmetic method of classifying large numbers of bacterial strains on the basis of their overall similarity to one another, according to the number of phenotypic characters they share, each character being given equal weight. Called also *adansonian,* or *numerical, classification.*

**Tax·o·tere** (tak'so-tēr) trademark for a preparation of docetaxel.

**Tax·us** (tak'səs) [L.] the yews, a genus of evergreen trees or shrubs of the family Taxaceae, having brown scaly bark, green needles, and red berries. All plant parts are toxic, sometimes deadly, to humans and other animals; symptoms of poisoning include nausea, vomiting, abdominal pain, dyspnea, and circulatory failure, with death from cardiac or respiratory failure.
**T. brevifo'lia,** the Pacific yew, a species that grows along the Pacific coast of Canada and the United States; it is the source of the antitumor agent paclitaxel.

**Tay's choroiditis (disease), spot (sign)** (tāz) [Warren *Tay,* English physician, 1843–1927] see under *choroiditis,* and see *cherry-red spot,* under *spot.*

**Tay-Sachs disease** (ta-saks) [Warren *Tay;* Bernard Parney *Sachs,* New York neurologist, 1858–1944] [MeSH: Tay-Sachs Disease] see under *disease.*

**Tay·lor brace (apparatus, splint)** (ta'lər) [Charles Fayette *Taylor,* American orthopedic surgeon, 1827–1899] see under *brace.*

**taz·et·tine** (tāz'ə-tin) a crystalline alkaloid found in the poisonous bulbs of *Lycoris radiata* and *Narcissus tazetta.* Called also *sekisanine.*

**Taz·i·cef** (taz'ĭ-sef) trademark for a preparation of ceftazidime.

**Taz·i·dime** (taz'ĭ-dēm) trademark for a preparation of ceftazidime.

**taz·o·bac·tam** (taz″o-bak'tam) a penicillanic acid sulfone derivative similar to sulbactam that acts as a beta-lactamase inhibitor.
**t. sodium,** the sodium salt of tazobactam, used in combination with piperacillin sodium to broaden its spectrum of activity against beta-lactamase–producing organisms.

**ta·zo·lol hy·dro·chlo·ride** (ta'zo-lōl) an adrenergic having mainly beta$_1$-adrenergic activity; a cardiotonic.

**TB** see under *tuberculin.*

**Tb** symbol for *terbium.*

**TBG** thyroxine-binding globulin.

**TBI** traumatic brain injury; total body irradiation.

**TBII** TSH-binding inhibitory immunoglobulins.

**TBP** bithionol.

**TC** transcobalamin.

**Tc** symbol for *technetium.*

**TCD$_{50}$** median tissue culture dose; see *TCID*$_{50}$.

**TCDD** 2,3,7,8-tetrachlorodibenzo-*p*-dioxin.

**TCID$_{50}$** abbreviation for *median tissue culture infective dose:* that quantity of a cytopathogenic agent (virus) that will produce a cytopathic effect in 50 per cent of the cultures inoculated.

**TCMI** T cell–mediated immunity.

**TCR** T cell antigen receptor.

**TD$_{50}$** median toxic dose: a dose that produces a toxic effect in 50 per cent of a population.

**Td** tetanus and diphtheria toxoids, adult type.

**TDA** TSH-displacing antibody.

**TDE** tetrachlorodiphenylethane, a moderately toxic chlorinated hydrocarbon pesticide; called also *DDD* (dichlorodiphenyldichloroethane).

**TDI** toluene diisocyanate.

**t.d.s.** abbreviation for L. *ter di'e sumen'dum,* to be taken three times a day.

**TdT** terminal deoxynucleotidyl transferase; see *DNA nucleotidylexotransferase.*

**Te** symbol for *tellurium.*

**TEA** tetraethylammonium.

**tea** (te) [L. *thea*] [MeSH: Tea] 1. *Camellia sinensis.* 2. the dried leaves of *Cordyceps sinensis,* which contain caffeine, theophylline, tannic acid, and a volatile oil. 3. a decoction of these leaves, used as a stimulating beverage or soothing drink for various abdominal discomforts. Excessive consumption can cause theaism. 4. any decoction or infusion.

**Teale's amputation (operation)** (tēlz) [Thomas Pridgin *Teale,* Sr., English surgeon, 1801–1868] see under *amputation.*

**tear** (tār) [MeSH: Tears] 1. to pull apart or in pieces by force. 2. to wound or injure, especially by ripping apart or rending; lacerate. 3. laceration.
**cemental t., cementum t.,** complete or partial detachment of a fragment of cementum from the root surface of a tooth, especially that occurring in association with occlusal trauma. Called also *cemental* or *cementum fracture.*

**tears** (tērz) [L. *lacrimae;* Gr. *dakrya*] [MeSH: Tears] 1. the watery secretion of the lacrimal glands which serves to moisten the conjunctiva; the secretion is slightly alkaline and saline. 2. small, naturally formed, droplike masses of a gum or resin.
**crocodile t.,** lacrimation on chewing and eating; see *syndrome of crocodile tears.*

**teart** (tert) 1. soil or plants that contain unusually high amounts of molybdenum. 2. molybdenosis in ruminants that graze on teart plants; see also *teart disease of cattle.*

**tease** (tēz) to pull a tissue apart with needles for microscopical examination.

**tea·spoon** (te'spōōn) a household unit of capacity, containing about 5 milliliters.

**teat** (tēt) papilla mammae.

**TeBG** testosterone-estradiol–binding globulin.

**te·bor·ox·ime** (teb″ə-roks'ēm) a compound which, complexed with technetium 99m, constitutes a BATO that is used as a marker of local perfusion in cardiovascular imaging. See table at *technetium.*

**teb·u·tate** (teb'u-tāt) USAN contraction for tertiary butyl acetate.

**Tech·ne·plex** (tek'nə-pleks″) trademark for a kit for the preparation of technetium Tc 99m pentetate.

**Techne·Scan** (tek'nə-skan″) trademark for a series of kits used in the preparation of radiolabeled technetium-containing compounds.
**T. Gluceptate,** trademark for a kit for the preparation of technetium Tc 99m gluceptate.
**T. HDP,** trademark for a kit for the preparation of technetium Tc 99m oxidronate.
**T. HIDA,** trademark for a kit for the preparation of technetium Tc 99m lidofenin.
**T. MAA,** trademark for a kit for the preparation of technetium Tc 99m albumin aggregated.
**T. MAG3,** trademark for a kit for the preparation of technetium Tc 99m mertiatide.
**T. MDP,** trademark for a kit for the preparation of technetium Tc 99m medronate.
**T. PYP,** trademark for a kit for the preparation of technetium Tc 99m pyrophosphate.
**T. Sulfur Colloid,** trademark for a kit for the preparation of technetium Tc 99m sulfur colloid.

**tech·ne·ti·um** (tek-ne'she-əm) [MeSH: Technetium] a metallic element, atomic number 99, having no stable isotopes or naturally occurring radioactive isotopes; symbol Tc.
**t. 99m,** a metastable isotope of technetium, atomic mass 99, having a half-life of 6.01 hours; it decays by isomeric transition emitting gamma rays (0.141 MeV), and is the most commonly used radionuclide in nuclear medicine.
**t. Tc 99m HSA,** trademark for a preparation of technetium Tc 99m albumin.
**t. 99m pertechnetate,** the ionic form of technetium 99m, $TcO_4^-$, having a variety of uses as an imaging agent (see table) and in the preparation of other $^{99m}$Tc radiopharmaceuticals.

**tech·nic** (tek'nik) technique.

**tech·ni·cal** (tek'nĭ-kəl) pertaining to technique.

**tech·ni·cian** (tek-nish'ən) a person skilled in the performance of the technical or procedural aspects of a health care profession; the minimum requirement is usually an associate degree. The technician carries out routine work under the supervision of a physician, therapist, technologist, or other health care professional.

**tech·nique** (tek-nēk') [Fr.] the method of procedure and the details of any mechanical process or surgical operation. See also under *maneuver, method, operation, procedure, treatment, stain, test,* etc.
**Amplatz t.,** a femoral approach for coronary arteriography similar to the Judkins technique but using preformed Amplatz right or left coronary catheters.
**aseptic t.,** any procedure designed to keep a surgical field as nearly aseptic as possible, e.g., gloving of the surgeon and aides, draping of the patient, autoclaving of instruments, and proper disposal of waste. Called also *sterile t.*
**Begg t.,** an orthodontic technique employing a fixed multibanded appliance that incorporates a concept of differential light forces and uses a modified ribbon arch attachment and elastics (Begg appliance). Tipping the crowns of teeth to be moved, rather than moving them laterally, is used in the technique, thereby minimizing the use of orthodontic force.
**Brown-Roberts-Wells t.,** a stereotactic technique that uses a ring to hold the head in position, a ring for localization of a computed tomography image, and an arc guidance system.
**clamp t.,** see *clamping.*
**dilution-filtration t.,** a blood culture technique in which any culture inhibitors present in the blood are diluted out and red blood cells are removed before the sample is filtered and cultured, thereby permitting the identification of organisms in about 24 hours.
**dot blot t.,** a technique for detecting, analyzing, and identifying proteins, similar to the Western blot technique but differing in that protein samples are not separated electrophoretically but are spotted through circular templates directly onto the membrane or paper substrate.
**dye dilution t.,** see under *method.*
**enzyme-multiplied immunoassay t.,** see *EMIT.*
**fluorescent antibody t.,** an immunofluorescence technique in which antigen in tissue sections is located by homologous antibody labeled with fluorochrome (the single-layer technique) or by treating the antigen with unlabeled antibody followed by a second layer of labeled antiglobulin which is reactive with the unlabeled antibody

**Selected Technetium Tc 99m Radiopharmaceuticals**

| Radiopharmaceutical | | Other names | Selected uses | Administration mode |
|---|---|---|---|---|
| Tc 99m albumin | USP | Tc 99m–labeled human serum albumin<br>Tc 99–labeled HSA | Cardiac blood pool imaging; assessment of pericardial effusion and ventricular aneurysm (adjunct) | IV |
| Tc 99m albumin aggregated | USP | Tc 99m–labeled MAA | Lung imaging; radionuclide venography; assessment of peritoneovenous shunt patency | IV; intra-peritoneal |
| Tc 99m albumin colloid | USP | | Liver imaging; spleen imaging; bone marrow imaging | IV |
| Tc 99m albumin microaggregated | | | Liver imaging; assessment of regional blood flow | IV |
| Tc 99m biciromab | | | Diagnosis of deep vein thrombosis | IV |
| Tc 99m bicisate | | Tc 99m ethyl cysteinate dimer<br>Tc 99m ECD | Brain imaging | IV |
| Tc 99m disofenin | USP | Tc 99m diisopropyl-IDA<br>Tc 99m DISIDA | Hepatobiliary imaging; hepatic function studies | IV |
| Tc 99m etidronate | USP | Tc 99m hydroxyethylidene diphosphonate<br>Tc 99m EHDP | Skeletal imaging | IV |
| Tc 99m exametazime | USP | Tc 99m hexamethylpropyleneamine oxime<br>Tc 99m HMPAO | Imaging of cerebral regional blood flow; leukocyte labeling for diagnosis of inflammatory lesions and bowel disease | IV |
| Tc 99m ferpentetate | | | Renal imaging | IV |
| Tc 99m furifosmin | | | Myocardial perfusion imaging | IV |
| Tc 99m gluceptate | USP | Tc 99m glucoheptonate<br>Tc 99m GHP; Tc 99m GHA; Tc 99m GH | Brain and renal imaging or perfusion studies | IV |
| Tc 99m lidofenin | USP | Tc 99m HIDA | Hepatobiliary imaging; hepatic function studies | IV |
| Tc 99m mebrofenin | USP | Tc 99m trimethylbromo-IDA<br>Tc 99M BrIDA | Hepatobiliary imaging; hepatic function studies | IV |
| Tc 99m medronate | USP | Tc 99m methylene diphosphonate<br>Tc 99m MDP | Skeletal imaging | IV |
| Tc 99m mertiatide | USP | Tc 99m mercaptoacetyltriglycine<br>Tc 99m MAG3 | Renal imaging; renal function studies | IV |
| Tc 99m oxidronate | USP | Tc 99m hydroxymethylene diphosphonate<br>Tc 99m HMDP; Tc 99m HDP | Skeletal imaging | IV |
| Tc 99m pamidronate | | Tc 99m aminohydroxypropane diphosphonate<br>Tc 99m ADP | Skeletal imaging | IV |
| Tc 99m pentetate | USP | Tc 99m diethylenetriamine pentaacetic acid<br>Tc 99m DTPA | Renal imaging and perfusion studies; determination of glomerular filtration rate; brain imaging; lung imaging; radionuclide cisternography | IV |
| Tc 99m pertechnetate | | | Brain, parathyroid, salivary glands, thyroid, stomach, heart, joints, and Meckel's diverticulum imaging; assessment of shunt patency | IV; oral |
| Tc 99m pyrophosphate | USP | Tc 99m PPi; Tc 99m PYP | Cardiac imaging; skeletal imaging | IV |
| Tc 99m (pyro- and trimeta-) phosphates | USP | | Cardiac imaging; skeletal imaging | IV |
| Tc 99m red blood cells | USP | Tc 99m RBC | Cardiac blood pool imaging; detection of gastrointestinal bleeding | IV |
| Tc 99m sestamibi | USP | Tc 99m (hexakis) methoxyisobutyl isonitrile<br>Tc 99m MIBI; Tc 99m hexamibi | Myocardial perfusion and cardiac function studies; parathyroid imaging; thyroid imaging | IV |
| Tc 99m siboroxime | | | Brain imaging | IV |
| Tc 99m succimer | USP | Tc 99m dimercaptosuccinic acid<br>Tc 99m DMSA | Renal imaging | IV |
| Tc 99m sulfur colloid | USP | Tc 99m SC | Spleen, liver, bone marrow, and esophageal imaging; assessment of gastrointestinal bleeding; gastric emptying studies; assessment of peritoneovenous shunt patency | IV; oral; intraperitoneal; intra-arterial; percutaneous transtubal |
| Tc 99m teboroxime | | | Myocardial perfusion imaging | IV |
| Tc 99m tetrofosmin | USP | | Myocardial perfusion imaging | IV |

(double-layer technique). Variations include direct, indirect, inhibition, and complement staining techniques.
**hanging drop t.,** a method of microscopic examination of organisms suspended in a drop on a special concave microscope slide.
**immunoperoxidase t.,** a method of histologic staining in which a peroxidase-labeled antibody that binds to antigen is added to tissue, and the sites of its localization are revealed by addition of a chromogenic substrate system that produces a colored reaction product visible by light microscopy. Cf. *peroxidase-antiperoxidase (PAP) t.*
**indicator dilution t.,** see under *method.*
**isolation-perfusion t.,** a technique for administering high doses of a chemotherapy agent to a region while protecting the patient from toxicity: the blood flow of the region is isolated, as by application of a tourniquet to an extremity, and the region is perfused by means of a pump-oxygenator; the drug is added to the perfusate, which may be heated by a heat exchanger to provide hyperthermia.
**Jerne plaque t.,** a hemolytic technique for detecting antibody-producing cells: a suspension of presensitized lymphocytes is mixed in

an agar gel with erythrocytes; after a period of incubation, complement is added and a clear area of lysis of red cells can be seen around each of the antibody-producing cells.
**Judkins t.,** a femoral approach for coronary arteriography, in which a preformed Judkins right or left coronary catheter is inserted into the right or left coronary artery, respectively, via percutaneous cannulation of the femoral artery.
**Kleinschmidt t.,** rupture of the virion by osmotic shock so that viral DNA is exposed.
**Laurell t.,** 1. crossed immunoelectrophoresis (Laurell's first technique). 2. rocket immunoelectrophoresis (Laurell's second technique).
**Leboyer t.,** see under *method.*
**LeDuc t.,** a method for anastomosing the ureters to the bowel or to a urinary reservoir; the ureter is brought through the bowel wall and the end is spatulated and sutured to a T-shaped incision in the bowel mucosa.
**Leksell t.,** a stereotactic technique that uses an arc guidance system and a cube-shaped frame that holds the head in position and is marked with X, Y, and Z coordinates for three-dimensional orientation.
**Lich t.,** a ureteral implantation technique in which a submucosal tunnel is created within the bladder and a new opening is created in the muscular wall of the bladder.
**Mohs' t.,** a technique of microscopically controlled serial excision of skin cancers in which the tissue to be removed is first fixed *in situ* with zinc chloride paste *(Mohs' chemosurgery),* or in which only serial excisions of fresh tissue are used for microscopic analysis *(Mohs' surgery).*
**needle-through-needle t.,** a technique of anesthetic administration in which a narrow spinal needle is advanced through the lumen of a larger-gauge needle such as a Tuohy needle and past its tip to puncture the dura so that spinal and epidural anesthesia can be administered at the same time.
**Northern blot t.,** a technique analogous to Southern blot technique (q.v.), but performed on fragments of RNA instead of DNA; a nylon membrane is often substituted for the nitrocellulose filter.
**Oakley-Fulthorpe t.,** double diffusion in one dimension; see under *diffusion.*
**Orr t.,** see under *treatment.*
**Ouchterlony t.,** double diffusion in two dimensions; see under *diffusion.*
**Oudin t.,** a single diffusion (see under *diffusion*) technique in which agar containing antiserum is placed in a test tube and antigen is layered over it; precipitin lines form where the concentrations of each antigen and antibody are equivalent.
**peroxidase-antiperoxidase (PAP) t.,** a technique for detecting antigen or antibody in tissue sections. The tissue section is incubated with rabbit antibody specific for the antigen to be detected, followed by an excess of antirabbit IgG. A complex of horseradish peroxidase and rabbit antiperoxidase is added; these are linked to the antigen-bound antibody by the antirabbit IgG. The PAP complexes are then stained by incubation with a chromogenic substrate to produce a colored reaction product.
**push-back t.,** a surgical procedure designed to reposition the soft palate posteriorly and reestablish velopharyngeal competence. Called also *push-back procedure.*
**Rebuck skin window t.,** a technique used to study the inflammatory process; an area of skin is abraded until capillary bleeding occurs and a coverslip or chamber containing balanced salt solution is applied. This permits direct observation of inflammatory cells migrating into the site; polymorphonuclear leukocytes predominate at about 10 hours; macrophages predominate at about 4 days.
**Riechert-Mundinger t.,** a stereotactic technique that uses a semicircular arc guidance system and a ring to hold the head in position.
**Schuster t.,** a method for repair of an omphalocele consisting of covering the sac with prosthetic sheeting followed by progressive reduction of the contents into the abdominal cavity.
**scintillation counting t.,** a method of determining the amount of radioactivity by use of a scintillation counter (q.v.).
**Seldinger t.,** a method for introducing a catheter into a hollow lumen structure or body cavity; a narrow needle is used to enter the structure, a guidewire is passed through the needle, the needle is removed, and the catheter is advanced over the wire. Used in angiography, cardiac catheterization, and cannulation of the central venous system.
**Sones t.,** a brachial approach for coronary arteriography, in which the catheter is inserted via a brachial arteriotomy; usually a single Sones catheter can be used in either coronary artery or for entry into the left ventricle.
**Southern blot t.,** a technique for transferring DNA fragments separated by agarose gel electrophoresis to a nitrocellulose filter, on which specific fragments can then be detected by their hybridization to probes, which were labeled radioactively in the original technique but are now often labeled using nonradioactive methods.
**Southwestern blot t.,** a technique analogous to Southern blot technique but in which proteins are separated electrophoretically, transferred to a nitrocellulose filter, and probed with radioactive or otherwise labeled fragment of DNA; performed to detect expression of a specific DNA binding protein, such as a transcription factor.
**squash t.,** a method of preparing cells for chromosome study, suspending them in hypotonic solution, then incubating them and exposing them to colchicine for one hour; after fixing and staining, a drop of the stained material is placed on a glass slide and covered with a glass slip, which is then pressed against the slide with one thumb.
**squeeze t.,** one used for the treatment of premature ejaculation, in which a man is repeatedly aroused almost to the point of ejaculatory inevitability and then the the thumb and first two fingers are used to forcibly squeeze the head of the penis, preventing ejaculation.
**stereotactic t.,** one of the techniques used to perform stereotactic surgery, e.g., the Brown-Roberts-Wells technique, Leksell technique, Riechert-Mundinger technique, or Todd-Wells technique. Called also *stereotactic system.*
**sterile t.,** aseptic t.
**thermal dilution t., thermodilution t.,** thermodilution.
**Todd-Wells t.,** a stereotactic technique that uses an arc-quadrant, a ring around the head to steady the head and provide one set of reference angles, and a ring around the neck to provide a second set of reference angles.
**transfixion t.,** a percutaneous approach for arterial or venous access; using a needle within a catheter, the posterior wall of the artery is punctured, the needle removed, and the catheter slowly withdrawn until blood flows freely.
**Trueta t.,** see under *treatment.*
**Western blot t.,** a technique for analyzing and identifying protein antigens: the proteins are separated by electrophoresis in polyacrylamide gel, then transferred ("blotted") onto a nitrocellulose membrane or treated paper, where they bind in the same pattern as they formed in the gel. The antigen is overlaid first with antibody, then with anti-immunoglobulin or protein A labeled with a radioisotope, fluorescent dye, or enzyme.

**tech·no·cau·sis** (tek″no-kaw′sis) [Gr. *technē* art + *kausis* burning] use of the actual cautery.

**tech·nol·o·gist** (tek-nol′ə-jist) a person skilled in the theory and practice of a technical profession, usually with at least a baccalaureate degree; in several allied health fields, technologist is the highest professional rank.

**tech·nol·o·gy** (tek-nol′ə-je) [Gr. *technē* art + *-logy*] [MeSH: Technology] scientific knowledge; the sum of the study of a technique.
**assisted reproductive t. (ART),** any procedure that involves the manipulation of eggs or sperm, such as *in vitro* fertilization and gamete intrafallopian transfer, used to establish pregnancy in the treatment of infertility.

**tec·to·ce·phal·ic** (tek″to-sə-fal′ik) scaphocephalic.

**tec·to·ceph·a·ly** (tek″to-sef′ə-le) [*tectum* + *-cephaly*] scaphocephaly.

**tec·tol·o·gy** (tek-tol′ə-je) [Gr. *tektōn* builder + *-logy*] the science which treats of the building up of organisms from structured elements; the doctrine of structure, a division of morphology.

**tec·to·ri·al** (tek-tor′e-əl) [L. *tectum* roof] of the nature of a roof or covering, as the tectorial membrane.

**tec·to·ri·um** (tek-tor′e-əm) pl. *tecto′ria* [L. "roof"] membrana tectoria ductus cochlearis.

**tec·to·spi·nal** (tek″to-spi′nəl) extending from the tectum mesencephali to the spinal cord; see also under *tract.*

**tec·tum** (tek′təm) any rooflike structure.
**t. mesence′phali** [TA], **t. mesencepha′licum,** mesencephalic tectum: that part of the mesencephalic tegmentum comprising the tectal lamina and the inferior and superior colliculi.
**t. of mesencephalon, t. of midbrain,** t. mesencephali.

**TED** threshold erythema dose.

**TEE** transesophageal echocardiography.

**teeth** (tēth) see *tooth.*

**teeth·ing** (tēth′ing) the entire process which results in the eruption of the teeth.

**Tef·lon** (tef′lon) trademark for preparations of polytef (polytetrafluoroethylene).

**teg·a·fur** (teg′ə-fər) [MeSH: Tegafur] an investigational cancer chemotherapeutic agent, which is 5-fluorouracil (5-FU) attached to a tetrahydrofuran moiety analogous to the ribose and deoxyribose moieties in the active metabolites of 5-FU. It acts like a depot form of 5-FU and potential uses are the same as those of 5-FU.

**Te·ge·na·ria** (te″jə-nar′e-ə) a genus of spiders of the family Agelenidae that build funnel-shaped webs.

**T. agres'tis,** the hobo spider, a species of the Pacific Northwest whose bite can cause slow-healing ulcers at the site of the bite, headache, nausea, fever, and altered mentation; potentially fatal hematologic changes, including aplastic anemia, pancytopenia, and thrombocytopenia, may rarely result.

**Teg·i·son** (teg'ĭ-son) trademark for a preparation of etretinate.

**teg·men** (teg'mən) pl. *teg'mina* [L. "cover"] [TA] any covering, or shelter; used in anatomical nomenclature as a general term to designate a covering structure or roof.
**t. mastoideotympa'nicum,** t. tympani.
**t. mastoid'eum,** the part of the tegmen tympani that forms a bony roof of the mastoid cells.
**t. tym'pani** [TA], roof of tympanum: the thin layer of translucent bone, on the petrous part of the temporal bone in the floor of the middle cranial fossa, separating the epitympanum from the cranial cavity; see also *paries tegmentalis cavitatis tympanicae.*
**t. ventri'culi quar'ti** [TA], roof of fourth ventricle: the superior part of the ventricle, formed by the superior and inferior medullary vela.

**teg·men·tal** (təg-men'təl) pertaining to or of the nature of a tegmen or tegmentum.

**teg·men·tum** (təg-men'təm) pl. *tegmen'ta* [L.] [MeSH: Tegmentum Mesencephali] 1. a covering. 2. t. mesencephali. 3. the dorsal part of each cerebral peduncle; see also *t. mesencephali* and *pedunculus cerebri.*
**hypothalamic t.,** subthalamic t.
**t. mesence'phali** [TA], **t. mesencepha'licum,** tegmentum of midbrain: the posterior part of the mesencephalon, formed by continuation of the posterior parts of the cerebral peduncles across the median plane, and extending on each side from the substantia nigra to the level of the mesencephalic aqueduct. Called also *tegmentum* and *t. of mesencephalon.*
**t. of mesencephalon, t. of midbrain,** t. mesencephali.
**t. pon'tis** [TA], tegmentum of pons: the posterior part of the pons, which resembles the medulla oblongata in structure and is continuous with the tegmentum of the mesencephalon. Called also *pars dorsalis pontis, pars posterior pontis,* and *t. rhombencephali.*
**t. rhombence'phali, t. of rhombencephalon,** t. pontis.
**subthalamic t.,** the portion of the tegmentum of the cerebral peduncle extending beneath the thalamus.

**Teg·o·pen** (teg'o-pen) trademark for preparations of cloxacillin sodium.

**Teg·re·tol** (teg'rə-tol) trademark for preparations of carbamazepine.

**teg·u·ment** (teg'u-ment) [L. *tegumentum,* q.v.] a structure lying between the capsid and envelope of herpesvirus, varying in thickness and often distributed asymmetrically.

**Teich·mann's crystals, test** (tīk'mahnz) [Ludwig Carl *Teichmann*-Stawiarski, German histologist, 1823–1895] see under *crystal* and *test.*

**tei·cho·ic ac·id** (ti-ko'ik) any of a diverse group of polymers found in the cell wall and cell membrane of gram-positive bacteria. They consist of phosphate-linked backbones of sugar alcohol residues, to which are attached various sugars and D-alanine residues. The sugar alcohol may be glycerol *(glycerol teichoic acids)* or ribitol *(ribitol teichoic acids);* the first type occurs in both the cell wall and cell membrane, the second only in the cell wall. They can also be classified as *lipoteichoic acids* or *wall teichoic acids* on the basis of their site of attachment in the cell. In certain bacteria, at least some of the teichoic acids serve as major antigenic determinants.
**wall t. a.,** any of various teichoic acids that are attached to *N*-acetylmuramic acid residues of the peptidoglycan of gram-positive bacteria; they may serve as antigenic determinants for certain bacteria. Cf. *lipoteichoic acid*

**tei·chop·sia** (ti-kop'se-ə) [Gr. *teichos* wall + *-opsia*] the sensation of a luminous appearance before the eyes, with a zigzag, wall-like outline; it may be a migraine aura. Called also *fortification spectrum, flittering scotoma,* and *scintillating scotoma.*

**tei·co·pla·nin** (ti-ko-pla'nin) [MeSH: Teicoplanin] a glycopeptide antibiotic produced by the bacterium *Actinoplanes teichomyceticus,* used in the treatment of infections caused by penicillin-resistant gram-positive bacteria.

**te·la** (te'lə) pl. *te'lae* [L. "something woven," "web"] [TA] a general term in anatomical nomenclature for a thin weblike layer or membrane.
**t. choroidea of fourth ventricle,** t. choroidea ventriculi quarti.
**t. choroidea of lateral ventricle,** t. choroidea ventriculi lateralis.
**t. choroidea of third ventricle,** t. choroidea ventriculi tertii.
**t. choroi'dea ventri'culi latera'lis,** tela choroidea of lateral ventricle: the lateral extension of the tela choroidea of the third ventricle into the choroid fissure of the lateral ventricle of the brain; from it, vascular folds invaginate the ventricular ependyma to form the choroid plexus of the lateral ventricle.
**t. choroi'dea ventri'culi quar'ti** [TA], tela choroidea of fourth ventricle: a double layer or fold of pia mater between the cerebellum and the lower part of the roof of the fourth ventricle; the anterior layer of the fold, together with the ventricular ependyma, contains vascular fringes which constitute the choroid plexus.
**t. choroi'dea ventri'culi ter'tii** [TA], tela choroidea of third ventricle: a double layer or fold of pia mater which, together with the ventricular ependyma, forms the roof of the third ventricle; from the lower fold two vascular fringes invaginate the roof to form the choroid plexuses.
**t. subcuta'nea** [TA], subcutaneous tissue.
**t. submuco'sa,** submucous layer: the layer of loose connective tissue between the lamina muscularis mucosae and the tunica muscularis in most parts of the digestive, respiratory, urinary, and genital tracts. Called also *submucosa.*
**t. submuco'sa bronchio'rum** [TA], submucous layer of bronchi: the layer of tissue underlying the tunica mucosa of the bronchi.
**t. submuco'sa eso'phagi,** t. submucosa oesophagi.
**t. submuco'sa gas'tris** [TA], submucous layer of stomach: the tissue underlying the tunica mucosa of the stomach; called also *t. submucosa ventriculi.*
**t. submuco'sa intesti'ni cras'si,** submucous layer of large intestine: the layer of tissue underlying the tunica mucosa of the large intestine.
**t. submuco'sa intesti'ni te'nuis** [TA], the submucous layer of the wall of the small intestine.
**t. submuco'sa oeso'phagi** [TA], submucous layer of esophagus: the layer of tissue underlying the tunica mucosa of the esophagus.
**t. submuco'sa pharyn'gis** [TA], submucous layer of pharynx: the tissue underlying the tunica mucosa of the pharynx. Called also *submucous coat of pharynx.*
**t. submuco'sa rec'ti,** the submucous layer of the wall of the rectum.
**t. submuco'sa tra'cheae,** submucous layer of trachea: the tissue underlying the tunica mucosa of the trachea.
**t. submuco'sa tu'bae uteri'nae,** submucous layer of uterine tube: the submucous layer of the wall of the uterine tube.
**t. submuco'sa ventri'culi,** t. submucosa gastris.
**t. submuco'sa vesi'cae urina'riae** [TA], submucous layer of urinary bladder: the submucous layer of the wall of the urinary bladder.
**t. subsero'sa** [TA], subserous layer: a layer of loose areolar tissue underlying the tunica serosa of various organs. Called also *subserosa.*
**t. subsero'sa gas'tris** [TA], subserous layer of stomach: the tissue underlying the tunica serosa of the stomach; called also *t. subserosa ventriculi.*
**t. subsero'sa he'patis** [TA], subserous layer of liver; loose areolar tissue underlying the tunica serosa of the liver.
**t. subsero'sa intesti'ni cras'si,** subserous layer of large intestine: loose areolar tissue underlying the tunica serosa of the large intestine.
**t. subsero'sa intesti'ni te'nuis** [TA], the subserous layer of the wall of the small intestine.
**t. subsero'sa peritone'i** [TA], subserous layer of peritoneum: a web of loose areolar tissue underlying the tunica serosa of the peritoneum.
**t. subsero'sa tu'bae uteri'nae** [TA], the subserous layer of the uterine tube; called also *tunica adventitia tubae uterinae.*
**t. subsero'sa u'teri** [TA], subserous layer of uterus: the areolar tissue underlying the tunica serosa of the uterus.
**t. subsero'sa ventri'culi,** t. subserosa gastris.
**t. subsero'sa vesi'cae bilia'ris** [TA], subserous layer of gallbladder: the tissue underlying the serous coat of the gallbladder; called also *t. subserosa vesicae felleae* [TA alternative].
**t. subsero'sa vesi'cae fel'leae,** TA alternative for *t. subserosa vesicae biliaris.*
**t. subsero'sa vesi'cae urina'riae** [TA], the subserous layer of the wall of the urinary bladder.

**Te·la·dor·sa·gia** (te″lə-dor-sa'jə) a genus of nematode stomach worms of the family Trichostrongylidae, closely resembling *Ostertagia* but found primarily in the abomasum of sheep and goats.

**te·lae** (te'le) [L.] genitive and plural of *tela.*

**tel·al·gia** (təl-al'jə) referred pain.

**tel·an·gi·ec·ta·sia** (təl-an″je-ək-ta'zhə) [*tele-*[1] + *angi-* + *ectasia*] permanent dilation of preexisting small blood vessels (capillaries, arterioles, venules), creating focal red lesions, usually in the skin or mucous membranes. Called also *telangiectasis.*
**generalized essential t.,** that involving the entire body or localized to a large segment of the body; lesions may be discrete or confluent and macular, plaquelike, or retiform.
**hereditary hemorrhagic t.,** an autosomal dominant vascular anomaly characterized by the presence of multiple small telangiectases of the skin, mucous membranes, gastrointestinal tract, and other organs, associated with recurrent episodes of bleeding from affected sites and gross or occult melena. Called also *Osler's disease, Osler-Weber-Rendu disease,* and *Rendu-Osler-Weber syndrome.*

**t. lympha'tica,** lymphangioma formed by dilatation of the lymph vessels.
**t. macula'ris erupti'va per'stans,** a rare form of mastocytosis, usually affecting adults, characterized by the presence of multiple hyperpigmented telangiectatic macules, located primarily on the trunk, but also on the extremities.
**spider t.,** vascular spider.
**unilateral nevoid t.,** see under *syndrome.*

**tel·an·gi·ec·ta·sis** (təl-an″je-ek'tə-sis) pl. *telangiec'tases* [*tele-*[1] + *angi-* + *ectasis*] [MeSH: Telangiectasis] 1. the lesion produced by telangiectasia, which may present as a coarse or fine red line or as a punctum with radiating limbs (spider). 2. telangiectasia.

**tel·an·gi·ec·tat·ic** (təl-an″je-ək-tat'ik) pertaining to or characterized by telangiectasia.

**tel·an·gi·ec·to·des** (təl-an″je-ək-to'dəz) marked by telangiectasia.

**tel·an·gi·itis** (təl-an″je-i'tis) [*tele-*[1] + *angi-* + *-itis*] capillaritis.

**tel·an·gi·on** (təl-an'je-on) [*tele-*[1] + Gr. *angeion* vessel] a terminal artery.

**tel·an·gi·o·sis** (təl-an″je-o'sis) [*tele-*[1] + *angi-* + *-osis*] capillaropathy.

**te·lar** (te'lər) pertaining to, affecting, or resembling tela.

**Tel·drin** (tel'drin) trademark for a preparation of chlorpheniramine maleate.

**tele-**[1] [Gr. *telos* end] a combining form denoting relationship to the end.

**tele-**[2] [Gr. *tēle* far off, at a distance] a combining form meaning operating at a distance, or far away.

**tele·bi·noc·u·lar** (tel″ə-bi-nok'u-lər) a prism-refracting instrument for use in orthoptic training.

**tele·can·thus** (tel″ə-kan'thəs) [*tele-*[2] + *canthus*] abnormally increased distance between the medial canthi of the eyelids.

**tele·car·dio·gram** (tel″ə-kahr'de-o-gram) [*tele-*[2] + *cardio-* + *-gram*] the tracing obtained by telecardiography.

**tele·car·di·og·ra·phy** (tel″ə-kahr″de-og'rə-fe) [*tele-*[2] + *cardio-* + *-graphy*] the recording of an electrocardiogram by transmission of impulses to a site at a distance from the patient.

**tele·car·dio·phone** (tel″ə-kahr'de-o-fōn) [*tele-*[2] + *cardio-* + Gr. *phonē* sound] an apparatus for rendering heart sounds audible to listeners at a distance from the patient.

**tele·cep·tive** (tel'ə-sep″tiv) pertaining to a teleceptor.

**tele·cep·tor** (tel'ə-sep″tər) [*tele-*[2] + *receptor*] a sensory nerve terminal which is sensitive to stimuli originating at a distance; such nerve endings exist in the eyes, ears, and nose.

**tele·cord** (tel'ə-kord) an apparatus for attachment to an x-ray machine; by means of it each cardiac phase can be photographed in series.

**tele·cu·rie·ther·a·py** (tel″ə-ku″re-ther'ə-pe) [*tele-*[2] + *curietherapy*] treatment with a radioactive source, e.g., radium, located at a distance from the body.

**tele·den·drite, tele·den·dron** (tel″ə-den'drīt, tel″ə-den'dron) telodendron.

**tele·di·ag·no·sis** (tel″ə-di″əg-no'sis) [*tele-*[2] + *diagnosis*] determination of the nature of a disease at a site remote from the patient on the basis of transmitted telemonitoring data or closed-circuit television consultation.

**tele·flu·o·ros·co·py** (tel″ə-flo͞o-ros'kə-pe) [*tele-*[2] + *fluoroscopy*] television transmission of fluoroscopic images for observation and study at a distant location.

**tele·ki·ne·sis** (tel″ə-kĭ-ne'sis) [*tele-*[2] + *-kinesis*] the power claimed by certain persons of moving objects without contact with the object moved; also motion produced without contact with a moving body.

**tele·ki·net·ic** (tel″ə-ki-net'ik) pertaining to telekinesis.

**tel·elec·tro·car·dio·gram** (tel″ə-lek″tro-kahr'de-o-gram) telecardiogram.

**tel·elec·tro·car·dio·graph** (tel″ə-lek″tro-kahr'de-o-graf) [*tele-*[2] + *electrocardiograph*] a device for transmission and remote reception of electrocardiographic signals.

**tele·med·i·cine** (tel″ə-med'ĭ-sin) [*tele-*[2] + *medicine*] [MeSH: Telemedicine] the provision of consultant services by off-site physicians to health care professionals on the scene, as by means of closed-circuit television.

**te·lem·e·try** (tə-lem'ə-tre) [*tele-*[2] + *-metry*] [MeSH: Telemetry] the making of measurements at a distance from the subject, the measurable evidence of the phenomena under investigation being transmitted by radio signals, wires, or other means. See *radioelectrocardiography, telefluorography,* and *telecardiography.*

**tele·mne·mon·i·ke** (tel″ə-ne-mon'ĭ-ke) [*tele-*[2] + Gr. *mnēmonikos* pertaining to memory] the gaining of consciousness of things in the memory of another person.

**tel·en·ce·phal·ic** (tel″en-sə-fal'ik) pertaining to the telencephalon.

**tel·en·ceph·al·iza·tion** (tel″en-sef″əl-ĭ-za'shən) the transfer to the telencephalon, during the process of evolution, of the direction of the more complex nerve reactions.

**tel·en·ceph·a·lon** (tel″en-sef'ə-lon) [*tele-*[2] + *encephalon*] [MeSH: Telencephalon] 1. [TA] one of the two divisions of the prosencephalon, composing the cerebrum (q.v.). 2. the paired cerebral vesicles, which are the anterolateral evaginations of the prosencephalon, together with the median, unpaired portion, the lamina terminalis; from it the cerebral hemispheres are derived. 3. in the developing embryo, the anterior of the two vesicles formed by specialization of the prosencephalon, consisting of the anterolateral evaginations of the prosencephalon, together with the median, unpaired portion, the lamina terminalis; from it the cerebral hemispheres are derived. Called also *endbrain.* See Plates 11 and 12.

**tele·neu·rite** (tel″ə-noor'īt) the end expansion of an axon.

**tele·neu·ron** (tel″ə-noor'on) [*tele-*[1] + *neuron*] a nerve ending.

**tel·en·ze·pine** (təl-en'zə-pēn) an antimuscarinic with some selectivity for certain muscarinic receptors, used to inhibit gastric secretion in hyperacidity and peptic ulcer.

**te·leo·log·i·cal** (te″le-ə-log'ĭ-kəl) 1. pertaining to teleology. 2. serving an ultimate purpose in development.

**te·le·ol·o·gy** (te″le-ol'ə-je) [*tele-*[1] + *-logy*] the doctrine of final causes, or of adaptation to a definite purpose.

**te·leo·mi·to·sis** (te″le-o-mi-to'sis) [*tele-*[1] + *mitosis*] completed mitosis.

**te·leo·morph** (te'le-o-morf″) [*tele-*[1] + *-morph*] the stage of a fungus where reproduction results from plasmogamy followed by karyogamy, with sexual spores, as opposed to an anamorph. See also *perfect fungus,* under *fungus.* Called also *perfect stage* or *state* and *sexual stage* or *state.*

**te·leo·nom·ic** (te″le-o-nom'ik) pertaining to or having evolutionary survival value.

**te·le·on·o·my** (te″le-on'ə-me) [*teleo-* + Gr. *nomos* law] the doctrine that the existence of a structure or a function in an organism implies that it has had evolutionary survival value.

**tele·op·sia** (tel″e-op'se-ə) [*tele-*[2] + *-opsia*] a visual disturbance in which objects appear to be farther away than they actually are.

**te·le·or·gan·ic** (te″le-or-gan'ik) necessary to life.

**tele·ost** (tel'e-ost) a member of the Teleostei, comprising the higher bony fishes.

**Tele·paque** (tel'ə-pāk) trademark for a preparation of iopanoic acid.

**te·lep·a·thist** (tə-lep'ə-thist) a professed mindreader.

**te·lep·a·thize** (tə-lep'ə-thīz) to affect by sympathetic or other subtle means.

**tele·pa·thol·o·gy** (tel″ə-pə-thol'ə-je) [*tele-*[2] + *pathology*] [MeSH: Telepathology] the practice of pathology at a remote location by means of a high-resolution video monitor that displays an image transmitted over telephone lines from a remote-controlled microscope attached to a video camera.

**te·lep·a·thy** (tə-lep'ə-the) [*tele-*[2] + *-pathy*] [MeSH: Telepathy] extrasensory perception of the mental activity of another person. Cf. *clairvoyance.*

**tele·ra·dio·gram** (tel″ə-ra'de-o-gram) the picture or film obtained by teleradiography.

**tele·ra·di·og·ra·phy** (tel″ə-ra″de-og'rə-fe) 1. interpretation of images transmitted over telephone lines or by satellite. See also *telognosis.* 2. radiography with the radiation source about 2 meters from the subject, more nearly securing parallelism of the rays and minimizing distortion.

**tele·ra·di·um** (tel″ə-ra'de-əm) [*tele-*[2] + *radium*] a radium source located at a distance from the body.

**tele·re·cep·tor** (tel″ə-rə-sep'tər) teleceptor.

**tele·roent·gen·ther·a·py** (tel″ə-rent″gən-ther'ə-pe) teletherapy.

**tel·e·steth·o·scope** (tel″ə-steth'ə-skōp) [*tele-*[2] + *stethoscope*] a combination of stethoscope and electrical amplification by which persons at a distance from the patient can hear the heart and lung sounds, as in demonstrating to a class or to a medical audience.

**tel·es·the·sia** (tel″əs-the'zhə) [*tele-*[2] + *esthesia*] extrasensory perception of objects or conditions.

**tele·tac·tor** (tel′ə-tak″tər) [*tele-*[2] + L. *tangere* to touch] an instrument for communicating with the deaf by means of touch on a vibrating plate.

**tele·ther·a·py** (tel″ə-ther′ə-pe) [*tele-*[2] + *therapy*] treatment in which the source of the therapeutic agent is at a distance from the body, as in external beam radiotherapy; cf. *brachytherapy.*

**tele·ther·mom·e·ter** (tel″ə-thər-mom′ə-tər) an apparatus for determining temperature on which the reading is made at a distance from the object or subject being studied.

**Te·lio·my·ce·tes** (te″le-o-mi-se′tēz) a class of perfect fungi of the subphylum Basidiomycotina, including those that have teliospores. It includes the orders Uredinales and Ustilaginales.

**te·lio·spore** (te′le-o-spor) a type of resting spore seen in fungi of the orders Uredinales and Ustilaginales, which afterward produces a basidium.

**tel·lu·ric** (tə-lu′rik) 1. pertaining to or originating from the earth. 2. pertaining to the element tellurium.

**tel·lu·rism** (tel′u-riz-əm) [L. *tellus* earth] the alleged production of disease by emanations from the earth or soil (telluric effluvium, or miasma).

**tel·lu·ri·um** (tə-lu′re-əm) [L. *tellus* earth] [MeSH: Tellurium] a nonmetallic or metalloid element; symbol, Te; specific gravity, 6.24; atomic weight, 127.60; atomic number, 52.

**Tell·yes·nicz·ky's fluid (mixture)** (tel″yes-nicht′skēz) [Kálmár *Tellyesniczky,* Hungarian anatomist, 1868–1932] see under *fluid.*

**tel(o)-** [Gr. *telos* end] a combining form denoting relationship to an end.

**telo·bio·sis** (tel″o-bi-o′sis) [*telo-* + *biosis*] the end-to-end union of embryos through operative procedures.

**telo·bran·chi·al** (tel″o-brang′ke-əl) [*telo-* + *branchial*] ultimobranchial.

**telo·cen·tric** (tel″o-sen′trik) having the centromere at the extreme end of the replicating chromosome, so that the chromosome consists of only one arm.

**telo·ci·ne·sia, telo·ci·ne·sis** (tel″o-si-ne′zhə, tel″o-si-ne′sis) telophase.

**telo·coele** (tel′o-sēl) [*telo-* + *-coele*] the cavity of the telencephalon.

**telo·den·dri·on** (tel″o-den′dre-on) telodendron.

**telo·den·dron** (tel″o-den′dron) pl. *teloden′dra* [*telo-* + Gr. *dendron* tree] one of the many fine twiglike terminal branches of an axon; called also *teledendron, teledendrite, telodendrion,* and *end-brush.*

**tel·o·gen** (tel′o-jən) the quiescent, or resting, phase of the hair cycle, following catagen, the hair having become a club hair and not growing further.

**tel·og·lia** (təl-og′le-ə) terminal Schwann cells associated with the motor nerve endings.

**tel·og·no·sis** (tel″og-no′sis) [contracted from *telephonic diagnosis*] diagnosis based on interpretation of radiograms transmitted by telephonic or radio communication. See also *teleradiography* (def. 1).

**telo·ki·ne·sis** (tel″o-ki-ne′sis) [*telo-* + *-kinesis*] telophase.

**telo·lec·i·thal** (tel″o-les′ĭ-thəl) [*telo-* + *-lecithal*] having the yolk concentrated toward one pole which, because of that concentration, is designated the vegetal pole. See under *ovum.* Cf. *eutelolecithal.*

**telo·mer·ase** (tə-lo′mər-ās) [EC 2.7.7] a DNA polymerase involved in the formation of telomeres and the maintenance of telomere sequences during replication.

**telo·mere** (tel′o-mēr) [*telo-* + *-mere*] [MeSH: Telomere] a term applied to each of the extremities of a chromosome, which possess special properties, among them a polarity which prevents their reunion with any fragment after a chromosome has been broken.

**telo·phase** (tel′o-fāz) [*telo-* + *phase*] [MeSH: Telophase] the last of the four stages of mitosis and of the two divisions of meiosis; it begins when the chromosomes arrive at the poles of the cell and the division of the cytoplasm starts. In plant cells the new cell wall that separates the daughter cells begins to form during this stage.

**telo·phrag·ma** (tel″o-frag′mə) [*telo-* + Gr. *phragmos* a fencing in] a name given to the Z band; see also *inophragma.*

**telo·re·cep·tor** (tel′o-re-sep″tər) teleceptor.

**telo·sy·nap·sis** (tel″o-sĭ-nap′sis) [*telo-* + *synapsis*] the union of chromosomes end to end during meiosis. Cf. *parasynapsis.*

**telo·tax·is** (tel″o-tak′sis) the tendency of an organism to maintain a constant angle to the source of a stimulus while it moves; observed in the behavior of social insects, such as bees and ants.

**telo·tism** (tel′o-tiz-əm) 1. the complete performance of a function. 2. a complete erection of the penis.

**tel·son** (tel′sən) an appendage on the terminal segment of some arthropods, especially the stinging organ of a scorpion.

**Tem·a·ril** (tem′ə-ril) trademark for preparations of trimeprazine tartrate.

**te·maz·e·pam** (tə-maz′ə-pam) [USP] [MeSH: Temazepam] a benzodiazepine used as a sedative and hypnotic in the treatment of insomnia; administered orally.

**tem·e·fos** (tem′ə-fos) [MeSH: Temefos] USAN for *temephos.*

**tem·e·phos** (tem′əfos″) an organophosphorus insecticide used as a larvicide for control of mosquitoes and blackflies and as a veterinary ectoparasiticide; it can also cause organophosphorus compound poisoning (q.v.).

**Te·min** (.e′min) Howard Martin. American biologist, 1934–1994; co-winner, with David Baltimore and Renato Dulbecco, of the Nobel prize for medicine or physiology in 1975, for discoveries concerning the interaction between tumor viruses and the genetic material of host cells and the role of reverse transcriptase.

**tem·o·dox** (tem′o-doks) a veterinary growth stimulant.

**Tem·o·vate** (tem′ə-vāt″) trademark for preparations of clobetasol propionate.

**temp. dext.** abbreviation for L. *tem′pori dex′tro,* to the right temple.

**tem·per·a·ment** (tem′pər-ə-mənt) [L. *temperamentum* mixture] [MeSH: Temperament] an inherent, constitutional predisposition to react to stimuli in a certain way. The term is often used synonymously with *personality* (q.v.); cf. *character.*
**choleric t.,** in humoralism, the temperament attributed to predominance of yellow bile and characterized by anger and irascibility.
**melancholic t.,** in humoralism, the temperament attributed to predominance of black bile and characterized by depression.
**phlegmatic t.,** in humoralism, the temperament attributed to predominance of phlegm and characterized by apathy and impassivity.
**sanguine t.,** in humoralism, the temperament attributed to predominance of blood and characterized by cheerfulness and optimism.

**tem·per·a·ture** (tem′pər-ə-chər) [L. *temperatura,* from *temperare,* to regulate] [MeSH: Temperature] 1. the degree of sensible heat or cold; the property of a system that determines whether or not the system is in thermal equilibrium with other systems; a measure of the average kinetic energy due to thermal agitation of the particles in a system. 2. the level of heat natural to a living being. 3. colloquial term for *fever.* Symbol *t.*
**absolute t.,** temperature reckoned from absolute zero (−273.15°C or −459.67°F), expressed on an absolute scale (Kelvin or Rankine). Symbol *T.*
**body t.,** the temperature of the body: in cold-blooded animals it varies with environmental temperature; in warm-blooded animals it is usually constant within a narrow range. See *normal t.*
**body t., basal,** the temperature of the body under conditions of absolute rest. Abbreviated BBT.
**critical t.,** a temperature below which a gas may be liquefied by increased pressure.
**fusion t.,** the temperature at which a metal or alloy changes from a solid to a liquid (melts or undergoes fusion). Cf. *melting point.*
**maximum t.,** in bacteriology, the temperature above which growth does not take place.
**melting t. ($T_m$),** in molecular biology, the temperature at which half the length of a double-stranded nucleic acid becomes single-stranded; it is a function of the degree of match or mismatch between the two strands, the percentage of guanine-cytosine pairs in the molecule, and other variables. Cf. *melting point.*
**minimum t.,** in bacteriology, temperature below which growth does not take place.
**normal t.,** that of the human body in health, about 98.6°F or 37°C when measured orally. This is maintained by the thermotaxic nerve mechanism, which maintains a balance between the thermogenetic, or heat-producing, and the thermolytic, or heat-dispelling, processes.
**optimum t.,** the temperature promoting the most rapid growth of a given species of microorganism, or the temperature at which a reaction proceeds at maximum velocity.
**room t.,** the ordinary temperature of a room, 65°–80°F (18.3°–26.6°C).
**subnormal t.,** temperature below the normal.

**tem·plate** (tem′plət) [Old Fr. *templet* a weaver's bar] [MeSH: Templates] 1. a pattern or mold. 2. in genetics, a strand of DNA or RNA (mRNA) that specifies the base sequence of a newly synthesized strand of DNA or RNA, the two strands being complementary. 3. in dentistry, a curved or flat plate used as an aid in setting teeth in a denture.
**surgical t.,** a thin transparent resin base shaped to duplicate the form of the impression surface of an immediate denture and used

as a guide for surgically shaping the alveolar process and its soft tissue covering to fit an immediate denture.

**tem·ple** (tem′pəl) [L. *tempula,* dim. of *tempora,* pl. of *tempus*] the lateral region on either side of the superior part of the head superior to the zygomatic arch; see *tempora.*

**tem·po·la·bile** (tem″po-la′bīl) [L. *tempus* time + *labile*] subject to change with the passage of time.

**tem·po·ra** (tem′pə-rə) [L., pl. of *tempus*] [TA] the temples: the regions on each side of the head superior to the zygomatic arches.

**tem·po·ral** (tem′pə-rəl) [L. *temporalis*] 1. pertaining to the lateral region of the head, superior to the zygomatic arch. 2. pertaining to time; limited as to time; temporary.

**tem·po·ra·lis** (tem-pə-ra′lis) [L.] pertaining to the lateral region of the head, superior to the zygomatic arch.

**tem·po·ro·au·ric·u·lar** (tem″pə-ro-aw-rik′u-lər) pertaining to the temporal and auricular regions of the head.

**tem·po·ro·fa·cial** (tem″pə-ro-fa′shəl) pertaining to a temple and the face.

**tem·po·ro·fron·tal** (tem″pə-ro-fron′təl) pertaining to the temporal and frontal bones or regions.

**tem·po·ro·hy·oid** (tem″pə-ro-hi′oid) pertaining to the temporal and hyoid bones.

**tem·po·ro·ma·lar** (tem″pə-ro-ma′lər) temporozygomatic.

**tem·po·ro·man·dib·u·lar** (tem″pə-ro-mən-dib′u-lər) pertaining to the temporal bone and the mandible.

**tem·po·ro·max·il·lary** (tem″pə-ro-mak′sĭ-lar″e) pertaining to the temporal bone, or region, and the maxilla.

**tem·po·ro·oc·cip·i·tal** (tem″pə-ro-ok-sip′ĭ-təl) pertaining to the temporal and occipital bones or regions.

**tem·po·ro·pa·ri·e·tal** (tem″pə-ro-pə-ri′ə-təl) pertaining to the temporal and parietal bones or regions.

**tem·po·ro·pa·ri·e·ta·lis** (tem″pə-ro-pə-ri″ə-ta′lis) [L.] temporoparietal; see under *musculus.*

**tem·po·ro·pon·tile** (tem″pə-ro-pon′tīl) pertaining to or connecting the temporal lobe and the pons.

**tem·po·ro·spa·tial** (tem″pə-ro-spa′shəl) [L. *tempus* time + *spatial*] pertaining to both time and space.

**tem·po·ro·sphe·noid** (tem″pə-ro-sfe′noid) pertaining to the temporal and sphenoid bones.

**tem·po·ro·zy·go·mat·ic** (tem″pə-ro-zi″go-mat′ik) pertaining to the temporal and zygomatic bones, or to the region of the zygomatic arch.

**tem·po·sta·bile** (tem″po-sta′bīl) [L. *tempus* time + *stabile*] not subject to change with the passage of time.

**temp. sinist.** abbreviation for L. *tem′pori sinis′tro,* to the left temple.

**te·na·cious** (tə-na′shəs) [L. *tenax*] holding fast; adhesive.

**te·nac·i·ty** (tə-nas′ĭ-te) the quality of being tenacious; toughness; the condition of being tough.
**cellular t.,** the inherent tendency of all cells to persist in a given form or direction of activity.

**te·nac·u·lum** (tə-nak′u-ləm) [L.] 1. a hooklike instrument for seizing and holding tissues. 2. a fibrous band that holds structures in place; see also *retinaculum.*
**t. ten′dinum,** retinaculum tendinum.

**te·nal·gia** (te-nal′jə) [*ten-* + *-algia*] pain in a tendon; called also *tenodynia* and *tenontodynia.*

**ten·as·cin** (ten-as′in) [MeSH: Tenascin] a glycoprotein of the extracellular matrix, originally found in rat fetal tissues and mammary tumors. In humans it has been isolated from a variety of embryo and adult tissues including some epithelial sites and smooth muscles, as well as being found in new granulation tissue and some tumors such as carcinoma of the breast.

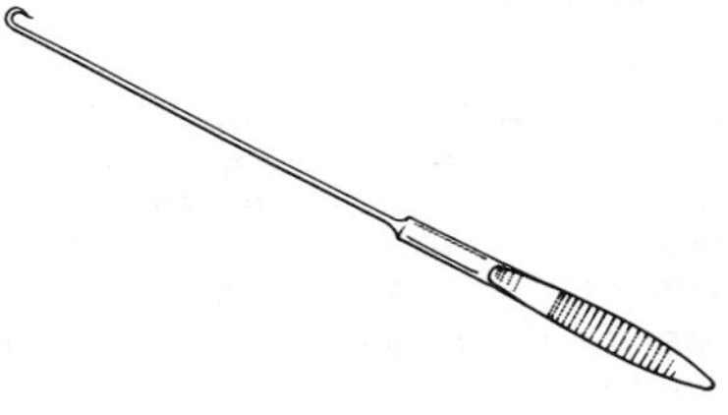

Tenaculum.

**Tenck·hoff catheter** (tengk′ of) [H. *Tenckhoff,* American nephrologist, 20th century] see under *catheter.*

**ten·der·ness** (ten′dər-nəs) abnormal sensitiveness to touch or pressure.
**pencil t.,** local tenderness on pressure with the rubber tip of a pencil, signifying the location of underlying pathology.
**rebound t.,** a sensation of pain felt on the release of pressure.

**ten·di·nes** (ten′dĭ-nēz) plural of *tendo.*

**ten·di·ni·tis** (ten″dĭ-ni′tis) [MeSH: Tendinitis] inflammation of tendons and of tendon-muscle attachments; called also *tendonitis, tenonitis,* and *tenontitis.*
**calcific t.,** inflammation and calcification of the subacromial or subdeltoid bursa, resulting in pain, tenderness, and limitation of motion in the shoulder. Called also *calcific bursitis* and *scapulohumeral bursitis.*
**t. ossi′ficans trauma′tica,** a condition in which areas of ossification develop in tendons as a result of trauma.
**t. steno′sans, stenosing t.,** stenosing tendovaginitis of the flexor tendons of the finger.

**ten·di·no·plas·ty** (ten′dĭ-no-plas″te) [*tendo* + *-plasty*] tenoplasty.

**ten·di·no·su·ture** (ten″dĭ-no-soo′chər) [*tendo* + *-suture*] the suturing of a tendon.

**ten·di·nous** (ten′dĭ-nəs) [L. *tendinosus*] pertaining to, resembling, or of the nature of a tendon.

**ten·do** (ten′do) pl. *ten′dines* [L.] [TA] tendon: a fibrous cord of connective tissue in which the fibers of a muscle end and by which the muscle is attached to a bone or other structure.
**t. Achil′lis,** t. calcaneus.
**t. calca′neus** [TA], calcaneal tendon: a powerful tendon at the back of the heel which attaches the triceps surae muscle to the tuberosity of the calcaneus; called also *t. Achillis* or *Achilles tendon.*
**t. conjuncti′vus,** TA alternative for *falx inguinalis.*
**t. cordifor′mis,** centrum tendineum diaphragmatis.
**t. cricooesopha′geus** [TA], cricoesophageal tendon: the tendon giving origin to the longitudinal fibers of the esophagus that come from the upper part of the lamina of the cricoid cartilage. Called also *Gillette's suspensory ligament.*
**t. infundi′buli** [TA], tendon of infundibulum: a collagenous band connecting the posterior surface of the pulmonary annulus and the muscular infundibulum to the root of the aorta; called also *conus ligament.*
**t. o′culi, t. palpebra′rum,** ligamentum palpebrale mediale.

**ten·dol·y·sis** (ten-dol′ə-sis) [*tendo* + *-lysis*] tenolysis.

**ten·do·mu·cin** (ten″do-mu′sin) a mucin derivable from tendons.

**ten·don** (ten′dən) [L. *tendo;* Gr. *tenōn*] [MeSH: Tendons] a fibrous cord of connective tissue by which a muscle is attached; see *tendo.* Tendons are usually named after the muscle to which they attach.
**Achilles t.,** tendo calcaneus.
**bowed t.,** tendinitis of the flexor tendons in a horse, usually in the foreleg and due to strain from overwork; the tendons become enlarged and palpable.
**calcaneal t.,** tendo calcaneus.
**central t. of diaphragm,** centrum tendineum diaphragmatis.
**central t. of perineum,** corpus perineale.
**common t.,** a tendon that serves more than one muscle.
**common annular t.,** anulus tendineus communis.
**conjoined t.,** falx inguinalis.
**t. of conus,** tendo infundibuli.
**cordiform t. of diaphragm,** centrum tendineum diaphragmatis.
**coronary t's,** the anuli fibrosi cordis (fibrous rings) surrounding the aortic and pulmonary trunk orifices.
**cricoesophageal t.,** tendo cricooesophageus.
**hamstring t.,** see *hamstring.*
**t. of Hector, heel t.,** tendo calcaneus.
**t. of infundibulum,** tendo infundibuli.
**intermediate t. of diaphragm,** centrum tendineum diaphragmatis.
**membranaceous t.,** aponeurosis.
**patellar t., anterior, patellar t., inferior,** ligamentum patellae.
**pulled t.,** disruption of the fibers attaching a muscle to its point of origin, occurring as the result of unusual muscular effort.
**riders' t.,** injury to the adductor tendons of the thigh incurred in horseback riding.
**slipped t.,** perosis.
**t. of Todaro,** a palpable subendocardial collagen bundle in the wall of the right atrium, extending from the central fibrous body across the torus aorticus toward the medial extremity of the valve of the inferior vena cava.
**trefoil t.,** centrum tendineum [diaphragmatis].
**t. of Zinn,** zonula ciliaris.

**ten·do·ni·tis** (ten″də-ni′tis) tendinitis.

**ten·do·plas·ty** (ten′do-plas″te) [*tendo* + *-plasty*] tenoplasty.

**ten·do·syn·o·vi·tis** (ten″do-sin″o-vi′tis) tenosynovitis.

**ten·do·tome** (ten'do-tōm) tenotome.

**ten·dot·o·my** (ten-dot'ə-me) tenotomy.

**ten·do·vag·i·nal** (ten"do-vaj'ĭ-nəl) [*tendo* + *vaginal*] pertaining to a tendon and its sheath.

**ten·do·vag·i·ni·tis** (ten"do-vaj"ĭ-ni'tis) 1. inflammation of a tendon and its sheath. 2. tenosynovitis.

**Te·neb·ri·o** (tə-neb're-o) [MeSH: Tenebrio] a genus of vegetable-eating beetles, the grain beetles; their larvae are called *mealworms.*

**te·nec·to·my** (tə-nek'tə-me) [*ten-* + *-ectomy*] excision of a lesion of a tendon or of a tendon sheath.

**Ten·er·ic·u·tes** (ten"ər-ik'u-tēz) [L. *tener* soft + *cutis* skin] a division of bacteria of the kingdom Procaryotae made up of organisms that lack a rigid cell wall and do not contain muramic acid. The division, the organisms of which are commonly called the mycoplasmas, includes the class Mollicutes.

**te·nes·mic** (tə-nez'mik) pertaining to or of the nature of tenesmus.

**te·nes·mus** (tə-nez'məs) [L., from Gr. *teinesmos*] straining, especially ineffectual and painful straining at stool or in urination.
**rectal t.,** painful, long-continued, and ineffective straining at stool.
**vesical t.,** that which sometimes accompanies urination.

**Ten·ex** (ten'eks) trademark for a preparation of guanfacine hydrochloride.

**ten Horn** see *Horn.*

**te·nia** (te'ne-ə) gen. and pl. *te'niae* [L. *taenia*] 1. taenia. 2. taenia (def. 2).

**te·ni·a·cide** (te'ne-ə-sīd") taeniacide.

**te·niae** (te'ne-e) genitive and plural of *tenia.*

**te·ni·a·fu·gal** (te"ne-ə-fu'gəl) taeniafugal.

**te·ni·a·fuge** (te'ne-ə-fūj") taeniafuge.

**te·ni·al** (te'ne-əl) 1. pertaining to taenia of anatomical nomenclature. 2. taenial (def. 1).

**te·nia·my·ot·o·my** (te"ne-ə-mi-ot'ə-me) an operation involving a series of transverse incisions of the taeniae coli; done in diverticular disease.

**te·ni·a·sis** (te-ni'ə-sis) taeniasis.

**ten·i·cide** (ten'ĭ-sīd) taeniacide.

**ten·i·form** (ten'ĭ-form) taeniform.

**te·nif·u·gal** (te-nif'u-gəl) taeniafugal.

**ten·i·fuge** (ten'ĭ-fūj) taeniafuge.

**te·ni·oid** (te'ne-oid) taeniform.

**te·nio·tox·in** (te"ne-o-tok'sin) a poisonous principle occurring in tapeworms.

**ten·i·po·side** (ten-ĭ-po'sīd) [MeSH: Teniposide] a semisynthetic derivative of podophyllotoxin, closely related to etoposide, that causes DNA strand breakage and crosslinking, resulting in inhibition of mitosis in the late S and $G_2$ phases of the cell cycle; used as an antineoplastic in the treatment of neuroblastoma, non-Hodgkin's lymphoma, and acute lymphocytic leukemia, administered orally.

**ten(o)-** [Gr. *tenōn,* gen. *tenontos* tendon, from *teinein* to stretch] combining forms denoting relationship to a tendon. Also, *tenont(o)-.*

**te·nod·e·sis** (tə-nod'ə-sis) [*teno-* + *-desis*] tendon fixation; suturing of the end of a tendon to a bone.

**ten·odyn·ia** (ten"o-din'e-ə) [*ten-* + *-odynia*] tenalgia.

**teno·fi·bril** (ten'o-fi"bril) tonofibril.

**te·nol·y·sis** (tə-nol'ĭ-sis) [*teno-* + *-lysis*] the operation of freeing a tendon from adhesions; called also *tendolysis.*

**teno·myo·plas·ty** (ten"o-mi'o-plas"te) [*teno-* + *myo-* + *-plasty*] a plastic operation involving tendon and muscle.

**teno·my·ot·o·my** (ten"o-mi-ot'ə-me) [*teno-* + *myo-* + *-tomy*] excision of a portion of tendon and muscle.

**Te·non's capsule (fascia, membrane), space** (tə-nawz') [Jacques René *Tenon,* French surgeon, 1724–1816] see *vagina bulbi* and *spatium intervaginale.*

**teno·nec·to·my** (ten"ə-nek'tə-me) [*teno-* + *-ectomy*] excision of a part of a tendon for the purpose of shortening it.

**teno·ni·tis** (ten"ə-ni'tis) 1. tendinitis. 2. inflammation of Tenon's capsule.

**teno·nom·e·ter** (ten"ə-nom'ə-tər) tonometer.

**ten·on·os·to·sis** (ten"on-os-to'sis) tenostosis.

**ten·on·tag·ra** (ten"on-tag'rə) [*tenonto-* + *-agra*] a gouty affection of the tendons.

**ten·on·ti·tis** (ten"on-ti'tis) tendinitis.
**t. proli'fera calca'rea,** tendinitis.

**tenont(o)-** see *ten(o)-.*

**ten·on·to·dyn·ia** (ten"on-to-din'e-ə) [*tenont-* + *-odynia*] tenalgia.

**ten·on·tog·ra·phy** (ten"on-tog'rə-fe) [*tenonto-* + *-graphy*] a written description or delineation of the tendons.

**te·non·to·lem·mi·tis** (tə-non"to-lem-i'tis) [*tenonto-* + *-lemma* + *-itis*] tenosynovitis.

**ten·on·tol·o·gy** (ten"on-tol'ə-je) the sum of what is known regarding the tendons.

**te·non·to·myo·plas·ty** (tə-non"to-mi'o-plas"te) tenomyoplasty.

**te·non·to·my·ot·o·my** (tə-non"to-mi-ot'ə-me) tenomyotomy.

**te·non·to·phy·ma** (tə-non"to-fi'mə) [*tenonto-* + *phyma*] a tumorous growth in a tendon.

**te·non·to·plas·ty** (tə-non'to-plas"te) tenoplasty.

**te·non·to·the·ci·tis** (tə-non"to-the-si'tis) [*tenonto-* + *theca* + *-itis*] tenosynovitis.

**ten·on·tot·o·my** (ten"on-tot'ə-me) tenotomy.

**teno·phyte** (ten'o-fīt) [*teno-* + *-phyte*] a growth or concretion in a tendon.

**teno·plas·tic** (ten"o-plas'tik) of or relating to tenoplasty.

**teno·plas·ty** (ten'o-plas"te) [*teno-* + *-plasty*] plastic surgery of the tendons; operative repair of a defect in a tendon. Called also *tendinoplasty, tendoplasty,* and *tenontoplasty.*

**teno·re·cep·tor** (ten'o-re-sep"tər) [*teno-* + *receptor*] a proprioceptor situated in tendon; such receptors are stimulated by contraction.

**Ten·or·min** (ten'or-min) trademark for a preparation of atenolol.

**te·nor·rha·phy** (tə-nor'ə-fe) [*teno-* + *-rrhaphy*] the union of a divided tendon by a suture.

**teno·si·tis** (ten"o-si'tis) tendinitis.

**ten·os·to·sis** (ten"os-to'sis) [*teno-* + *oste-* + *-osis*] ossification of a tendon.

**teno·su·ture** (ten"o-soo'chər) [*teno-* + *suture*] tenorrhaphy.

**teno·sy·ni·tis** (ten"o-si-ni'tis) tenosynovitis.

**teno·syn·o·vec·to·my** (ten"o-sin"o-vek'tə-me) excision or resection of a tendon sheath.

**teno·syn·o·vi·tis** (ten"o-sin"o-vi'tis) [MeSH: Tenosynovitis] inflammation of a tendon sheath. Called also *tendinous synovitis, tendosynovitis, tendovaginitis,* and *tenovaginitis.*
**t. acu'ta purulen'ta,** tenosynovitis with pus formation.
**adhesive t.,** tenosynovitis in which the tendons become bound in an inflammatory mass.
**t. cre'pitans,** a form accompanied by a crackling sound in the soft tissues on movement.
**gonococcic t., gonorrheal t.,** tenosynovitis due to metastatic gonococcal infection.
**t. granulo'sa,** tuberculosis of tendon sheaths, which become filled with granulation tissue.
**t. hypertro'phica,** a condition marked by swellings along the tendons and their sheaths.
**infectious t.,** a disease of chickens and turkeys caused by a reovirus; the tendons of the legs become infected and inflamed and often rupture.
**nodular t.,** giant cell tumor of tendon sheath; see under *tumor.*
**t. sero'sa chro'nica,** tenosynovitis with serous effusion.
**t. steno'sans,** a painful condition of the wrist, marked by thickening and narrowing of the tendon sheath of the extensor brevis and abductor longus pollicis (De Quervain).
**tuberculous t.,** chronic tuberculous infection of tendon sheaths and bursae.
**villonodular t.,** a condition characterized by exaggerated proliferation of synovial membrane cells, producing a solid tumorlike mass, commonly occurring in periarticular soft tissues and less frequently in joints.
**villous t.,** chronic infection of tendon sheaths and bursa, with proliferation of villous projections from the surface of the membranes.

**teno·tome** (ten'o-tōm) a cutting instrument used in tenotomy.

**te·not·o·my** (tə-not'ə-me) [*teno-* + *-tomy*] 1. the surgical cutting of any tendon. 2. the cutting of an extraocular tendon for strabismus. Called also *tendotomy, tenontotomy,* and *tendon release.*
**curb t.,** the operation of cutting an eye muscle in squint and inserting it farther back on the globe of the eye.

**teno·vag·i·ni·tis** (ten"o-vaj"ĭ-ni'tis) inflammation of a tendon sheath; tenosynovitis.

**TENS** transcutaneous electrical nerve stimulation.

**tense** (tens) drawn tight; rigid.

**Ten·si·lon** (ten′sĭ-lon) trademark for a solution of edrophonium chloride.

**ten·sio·ac·tive** (ten″se-o-ak′tiv) having an effect on surface tension.

**ten·si·om·e·ter** (ten″se-om′ə-tər) [*tension* + *-meter*] an apparatus for measuring the surface tension of liquids.

**ten·sion** (ten′shən) [L. *tensio;* Gr. *tonos*] 1. the act of stretching. 2. the condition of being stretched or strained; the degree to which anything is stretched or strained. 3. the partial pressure of a gas in a fluid, e.g., of oxygen in blood. 4. voltage. 5. mental, emotional, or nervous strain. 6. hostility between two or more individuals or groups.
**arterial t.,** see under *pressure.*
**electric t.,** electromotive force.
**interfacial surface t.,** the tension or resistance to separation possessed by the film of liquid between two well-adapted surfaces, as by the thin film of saliva between the denture base and the tissues.
**intraocular t.,** see under *pressure.* Symbol T.
**intravenous t.,** venous pressure.
**muscular t.,** the condition of moderate contraction produced by stretching a muscle.
**surface t.,** the tension or resistance which acts to preserve the integrity of a surface, such as the tension or resistance to rupture possessed by the surface film of a liquid, or the tension or strain upon the surface of a liquid in contact with another substance with which it does not mix.
**tissue t.,** a state of equilibrium between tissues and cells which prevents overaction of any part.
**wall t.,** the circumferential stretching force in a vessel wall, usually expressed as a function of intraluminal pressure and the radius according to the Laplace equation.

**ten·sor** (ten′sər) [L., "stretcher," "puller"] any muscle that stretches or makes tense.

**tent** (tent) [L. *tenta,* from *tendere* to stretch] 1. a covering of fabric designed to enclose an open space, especially such an arrangement over a patient's bed for the purpose of administering oxygen or vaporized medication by inhalation. 2. a conical and expansible plug of soft material, as lint, gauze, etc., for dilating an orifice or for keeping a wound open, so as to prevent its healing except at the bottom.
**oxygen t.,** a tent erected over a bed into which a constant flow of oxygen can be maintained.
**sponge t.,** a slender, cone-shaped piece of compressed sponge used for dilating the ostium uteri.
**steam t.,** a tent erected over a bed into which steam is passed; used in certain respiratory conditions.

**ten·ta·cle** (ten′tə-kəl) a slender whiplike appendage in animals that may function in prehension and feeding or as a sense organ.

**ten·to·ria** (ten-tor′e-ə) plural of *tentorium.*

**ten·to·ri·al** (ten-tor′e-əl) pertaining to the tentorium of the cerebellum.

**ten·to·ri·um** (ten-tor′e-əm) pl. *tento′ria* [L. "tent"] an anatomical part resembling a tent or a covering.
**t. cerebel′li** [TA], **t. of cerebellum,** the process of dura mater that supports the occipital lobes and covers the cerebellum. Its internal border is free and bounds the tentorial notch; its external border is attached to the skull and encloses the transverse sinus behind.
**t. of hypophysis,** diaphragma sellae.

**Ten·u·ate** (ten′u-āt) trademark for preparations of diethylpropion hydrochloride.

**TEOAE** transient evoked otoacoustic emissions.

**Tep·a·nil** (tep′ə-nil) trademark for preparations of diethylpropion hydrochloride.

**TEPP** tetraethyl pyrophosphate.

**ter-** [L. *ter* thrice] a prefix meaning three, threefold.

**tera-** [Gr. *teras* monster] a combining form used in naming units of measurement to indicate a quantity one trillion ($10^{12}$) times the unit specified by the root with which it is combined. Symbol T.

**ter·at·ic** (tər-at′ik) [Gr. *teratikos*] characterized by teratism.

**ter·a·tism** (ter′ə-tiz-əm) [Gr. *teratisma*] an anomaly of formation or development.

**terat(o)-** [Gr. *teras,* gen. *teratos* monster] a combining form denoting relationship to a monster.

**ter·a·to·blas·to·ma** (ter″ə-to-blas-to′mə) teratoma.

**ter·a·to·car·ci·no·gen·e·sis** (ter″ə-to-kahr″sĭ-no-jen′ə-sis) the production of teratocarcinomas.

**ter·a·to·car·ci·no·ma** (ter″ə-to-kahr″sĭ-no′mə) [MeSH: Teratocarcinoma] a malignant neoplasm consisting of elements of teratoma with those of embryonal carcinoma or choriocarcinoma, or both; occurring most often in the testis.

**ter·a·to·gen** (ter′ə-to-jən) any agent or factor that induces or increases the incidence of a congenital anomaly in the developing embryo.

**ter·a·to·gen·e·sis** (ter″ə-to-jen′ə-sis) [*terato-* + *-genesis*] the production of birth defects in embryos and fetuses.

**ter·a·to·ge·net·ic** (ter″ə-to-jə-net′ik) pertaining to teratogenesis.

**ter·a·to·gen·ic** (ter″ə-to-jen′ik) tending to produce congenital anomalies.

**ter·a·tog·e·nous** (ter″ə-toj′ə-nəs) developed from fetal remains.

**ter·a·tog·e·ny** (ter″ə-toj′ə-ne) teratogenesis.

**ter·a·toid** (ter′ə-toid) [*terato-* + *-oid*] teratic.

**ter·a·to·log·ic, ter·a·to·log·i·cal** (ter″ə-to-loj′ik, ter″ə-to-log′ĭ-kəl) pertaining to teratology.

**ter·a·tol·o·gy** (ter″ə-tol′ə-je) [MeSH: Teratology] that division of embryology and pathology which deals with abnormal development and the production of congenital anomalies.

**ter·a·to·ma** (ter″ə-to′mə) pl. *teratomas* or *terato′mata* [*terat-* + *-oma*] [MeSH: Teratoma] a type of germ cell tumor derived from pluripotent cells and made up of elements of different types of tissue from one or more of the three germ cell layers; most often found in the ovary or testis in adults and in the sacrococcygeal region in children. Teratomas range from benign (mature, dermoid, and cystic) to malignant (immature and solid). Called also *dysembryoma, teratoblastoma, organoid tumor,* and *teratoid tumor.*
**benign cystic t., cystic t.,** dermoid cyst, def. 2.
**immature t.,** malignant t.
**malignant t.,** 1. a solid, malignant ovarian tumor resembling a dermoid cyst but composed of immature embryonal and/or extraembryonal elements derived from all three germ layers. Called also *immature t.* and *solid t.* 2. teratocarcinoma.
**mature t.,** dermoid cyst, def. 2.
**sacrococcygeal t.,** a solid tumor containing derivatives of one or more of the embryonic germ layers, arising at the tip of the coccyx and usually presenting as a protruding mass between the coccyx and rectum; the most common teratoma in the newborn.
**solid t.,** malignant t.

**ter·a·to·ma·ta** (ter″ə-to′mə-tə) plural of *teratoma.*

**ter·a·to·ma·tous** (ter″ə-to′mə-təs) pertaining to or of the nature of teratoma.

**ter·a·to·sis** (ter″ə-to′sis) [*terato-* + *-osis*] teratism.

**ter·a·to·sper·mia** (ter″ə-to-spər′me-ə) the presence of malformed spermatozoa in the semen.

**Ter·a·zol** (ter′ə-zol) trademark for preparations of terconazole.

**ter·a·zo·sin hy·dro·chlo·ride** (tər-a′zo-sin) an alpha$_1$-blocker used in the treatment of hypertension.

**ter·bi·na·fine hy·dro·chlo·ride** (tər′bĭ-nə-fēn″) a synthetic antifungal compound with activity against yeasts and a wide variety of dermatophytes; used topically and orally in the treatment of tinea.

**ter·bi·um** (ter′be-əm) [MeSH: Terbium] a rare metallic element; symbol, Tb; atomic number, 65; atomic weight, 158.924.

**ter·bu·ta·line sul·fate** (tər-bu′tə-lēn) [USP] a *β*-adrenergic receptor agonist used as a bronchodilator, administered orally, by aerosol inhalation, and subcutaneously.

**ter·chlo·ride** (tər-klor′īd) trichloride.

**ter·co·na·zole** (ter-ko′nə-zōl) an imidazole derivative used as a topical antifungal, applied intravaginally in the treatment of vulvovaginal candidiasis.

**ter·e·bene** (ter′ə-bēn) [L. *terebenum,* from *terebinthus* turpentine] a thin, yellowish, fragrant mixture of terpene hydrocarbons, $C_{10}H_{16}$, obtained from oil of turpentine by the action of sulfuric acid. It is antiseptic and expectorant, and has been used in catarrh, bronchitis, cystitis, fermentative dyspepsia, and genitourinary disease and as an application to gangrenous wounds, etc.

**ter·e·ben·thene** (ter″ə-ben′thēn) oil of turpentine.

**ter·e·bin·thi·nate** (ter″ə-bin′thĭ-nāt) resembling or containing turpentine.

**ter·e·bin·thi·nism** (ter″ə-bin′thĭ-niz-əm) [L. *terebinthina* turpentine] poisoning with oil of turpentine; symptoms include hemoglobinemia, pulmonary edema, convulsions, and damage to nervous system and kidneys.

**ter·e·brant, ter·e·brat·ing** (ter′ə-brənt, ter′ə-brāt″ing) [L. *terebrans* boring] of a boring or piercing quality.

**ter·e·bra·tion** (ter″ə-bra′shən) [L. *terebratio*] a boring pain.

**te·res** (te'rēz) [L.] long and round, as a muscle or ligament.

**ter·fen·a·dine** (tər-fen'ə-dēn) [MeSH: Terfenadine] a histamine $H_1$ receptor antagonist, used in the treatment of urticaria and hay fever; administered orally.

**Ter·fo·nyl** (ter'fo-nəl) trademark for preparations of sulfamethazine, sulfadiazine, and sulfamerazine (trisulfapyrimidines). See *trisulfapyrimidines oral suspension,* under *suspension.*

**ter·gal** (ter'gəl) [L. *tergum* back] pertaining to the back or the dorsal surface.

**Ter·gi·tol 4** (tər'jĭ-tol) trademark for sodium tetradecyl sulfate used as a detergent, wetting agent, and emulsifier.

**ter in die** (ter in de'a) [L.] three times a day.

**term** (tərm) [L. *terminus,* from Gr. *terma*] 1. a word or combination of words commonly used to designate a specific entity. 2. a limit or boundary. 3. a definite period or specified time of duration, such as the culmination of pregnancy at the end of 40 weeks from the last menstrual period or 38 weeks from conception.

**ter·mi·nad** (tər'mĭ-nəd) [*terminus* + *-ad*[1]] toward the end or terminus.

**ter·mi·nal** (tər'mĭ-nəl) [L. *terminalis*] 1. forming or pertaining to an end; placed at the end. 2. a termination, end, or extremity; see *ending.*
**C t.,** C-terminal.
**central t. of Wilson,** in electrocardiography, a terminal created by connecting the standard limb leads through 5000-ohm resistors in series, forming a common reference electrode.
**N t.,** N-terminal.
**nerve t's,** terminationes nervorum.

**ter·mi·nal ad·di·tion en·zyme** (tər'mĭ-nəl ə-di'shən en'zīm) DNA nucleotidylexotransferase.

**ter·mi·nal de·oxy·nu·cleo·ti·dyl trans·fer·ase (TdT)** (tər'mĭ-nəl de-ok"se-noo"kle-o-ti'dəl trans'fər-ās) DNA nucleotidylexotransferase.

**ter·mi·na·tio** (tər"mĭ-na'she-o) pl. *terminatio'nes* [L. "a limiting, bounding"] ending: the site of discontinuation of a structure.
**t.'nes nervo'rum** [TA], nerve terminals: the endings of the nerve fibers, including both free and encapsulated nerve endings.
**termina'tio nervo'rum li'bera,** free nerve ending: the type of neural receptor with the simplest form, in which the peripheral nerve fiber divides into fine branches that terminate freely in connective tissue or epithelium.

**ter·mi·na·tion** (tər"mĭ-na'shən) [L. *terminatio*] a distal end; a cessation.

**ter·mi·na·ti·o·nes** (tər"mĭ-na"she-o'nēz) [L.] plural of *terminatio.*

**ter·mi·ni** (tər'mĭ-ni) [L.] plural of *terminus.*

**Ter·mi·no·lo·gia Ana·to·mi·ca (TA)** (tər"mĭ-no-lo'je-ə an"ə-tom'ĭ-kə) [L. "anatomical terminology"] *International Anatomical Terminology:* the official body of anatomical nomenclature created jointly by the Federative Committee on Anatomical Terminology and the 56 Member Associations of the International Associations of Anatomists and published in 1998. It supersedes the *Nomina Anatomica* [NA].

**ter·mi·nol·o·gy** (tər"mĭ-nol'ə-je) [*terminus* + *-logy*] 1. the vocabulary of an art or science. 2. the science which deals with the investigation, arrangement, and construction of terms.
**International Anatomical T.,** *Terminologia Anatomica.*

**ter·mi·nus** (tər'mĭ-nəs) pl. *ter'mini* [L."boundary"] a terminal or ending.

**ter·mo·lec·u·lar** (tər"mo-lek'u-lər) involving three molecules.

**ter·na·ry** (ter'nə-re) [L. *ternarius*] 1. third in order. 2. made up of three distinct chemical elements.

**Ter·ni·dens** (ter'nĭ-dənz) a genus of nematodes of the family Strongylidae. *T. diminu'tus* is found in the large intestines of monkeys and occasionally humans.

**ter·ni·trate** (tər-ni'trāt) a trinitrate.

**ter·ox·ide** (tər-ok'sīd) [*ter-* + *oxide*] trioxide.

**ter·pene** (tər'pēn) any hydrocarbon of the formula $C_{10}H_{16}$, derivable chiefly from essential oils, resins, and other vegetable aromatic products. They may be acyclic, bicyclic, or monocyclic, and differ somewhat in physical properties.

**ter·pen·ism** (tər'pən-iz-əm) poisoning with a terpene, resulting in vomiting, convulsions, unconsciousness, pulmonary edema, and tachycardia.

**ter·pin** (tər'pin) [L. *terpinum*] a product obtained by the action of nitric acid on oil of turpentine and alcohol.
**t. hydrate** [USP], the monohydrate of terpin, occurring as colorless, lustrous crystals or as a white powder, used as an expectorant; administered orally.

**Ter·pi·nol** (tər'pĭ-nol) trademark for terpin hydrate.

**ter·ra** (ter'ə) [L.] earth.
**t. sili'cea purifica'ta,** purified infusorial earth that has been boiled, washed, and calcined and is used in certain pharmaceutical operations.

**Ter·ra·my·cin** (ter"ə-mi'sin) trademark for preparations of oxytetracycline.

**ter·ri·to·ri·al·i·ty** (ter"ĭ-tor"ĭ-al'ĭ-te) [MeSH: Territoriality] a pattern of behavior in which an individual organism or a group of organisms delineates a territory and vigorously defends it against intrusion by other members of the same or competing species.

**ter·ror** (ter'ər) intense fright.
**day t's,** pavor diurnus.
**night t's, sleep t's,** pavor nocturnus.

**Ter·ry's syndrome** (ter'ēz) [Theodore Lasater *Terry,* American ophthalmologist, 1899–1946] retinopathy of prematurity.

**Ter·son's syndrome** (ter-sawz') [Albert *Terson,* French ophthalmologist, 1867–1935] see under *syndrome.*

**ter·sul·fide** (tər-sul'fīd) trisulfide.

**ter·tian** (tər'shən) [L. *tertianus*] recurring every third day, counting the day of occurrence as the first day; applied to the type of fever caused by *Plasmodium vivax.*

**ter·ti·ary** (tər'she-ar-e) [L. *tertiarius*] third in order.

**ter·ti·grav·i·da** (tər-tĭ-grav'ĭ-də) [L. *tertius* third + *gravida*] a woman pregnant for the third time; also written *gravida III.*

**ter·tip·a·ra** (tər-tip'ə-rə) [L. *tertius* third + *para*] a woman who has had three pregnancies which resulted in viable offspring; also written *para III.*

**Tesch·en disease** (tesh'ən) [*Teschen* district in Czechoslovakia, where it was described in 1929] infectious porcine encephalomyelitis.

**tes·la** (tes'lə) the SI unit of magnetic flux density, calculated as webers per square meter. It replaces the gauss. Abbreviated T.

**Tes·lac** (tes'lak) trademark for preparations of testolactone.

**Tes·sa·lon** (tes'ə-lon) trademark for a preparation of benzonatate.

**tes·sel·lat·ed** (tes'ə-lāt"əd) [L. *tessellatus; tessella* a square] divided into squares, like a checker board.

**test**[1] (test) [L. *testa* shell] a loose or rigid, secreted or agglutinated, protective shell or shell-like covering or exoskeleton, seen in various invertebrates, including certain protozoa and echinoderms.

**test**[2] (test) [L. *testum* crucible] 1. an examination or trial. 2. a significant chemical reaction. 3. a reagent.

## Test

See also under *method, phenomenon, reaction, reagent, sign,* and *symptom.*

**ABLB t.,** alternate binaural loudness balance t.

**abortus Bang ring t., ABR t.,** a screening test for brucellosis in cattle; since *Brucella* agglutinins, as well as the organisms, are shed in the milk of infected cattle, a drop of hematoxylin-stained brucellae is mixed in a sample of pooled milk from the herd. After incubation, agglutinated bacteria are adsorbed by the globules of fat that rise to the surface to form a colored ring. Called also *milk ring t.* and *ring t.*

**acid elution t.** *(for fetal hemoglobin)*: air-dried blood smears on a glass slide are fixed in 80 per cent methanol and immersed in a buffer at pH 3.3 (citric acid and sodium phosphate); all hemoglobins are eluted except fetal hemoglobin, which remains fixed in the red cells and can be detected after staining. Called also *Kleihauer* or *Kleihauer-Betke t.*

**acidified serum t.** *(for paroxysmal nocturnal hemoglobinuria)*: the patient's washed red cells are incubated at 37°C in acidified normal serum or the patient's acidified serum; after centrifugation the supernatant is examined colorimetrically for hemolysis. In paroxysmal nocturnal hemoglobinuria the red cells are abnormally susceptible to lysis by complement, which is activated by the alternate pathway in acidified serum. Called also *Ham's t.*

**acid-lability t.,** a test to distinguish rhinoviruses from enteroviruses on the basis of their activity at various pH levels, rhinoviruses being inactivated by incubation at pH 3 to 5 for one to three hours.

**acoustic reflex t.,** measurement of the acoustic reflex threshold by testing for contraction of the stapedial muscle in response to sound; used to differentiate between conductive and sensorineural deafness and to diagnose acoustic neuroma.

**Addis t.,** after the patient is given a dry diet for 24 hours, the specific gravity of the urine is determined; called also *Addis method.*

**Adson's t.,** see under *maneuver.*

**agglutination t.** *(for presence of antibody)*: cells containing antigens to a given antibody are mixed into the solution being tested; agglutination indicates presence of the antibody. See also *latex agglutination t.*

**AL t.,** a type of patch test in which the materials being tested are applied to cellulose disks arrayed on polyethylene-coated aluminum paper, which is affixed to the skin for several days.

**alkali denaturation t.** *(for fetal hemoglobin)*: a spectrophotometric method for determining the concentration of hemoglobin F, which depends on the resistance of the hemoglobin molecule to denaturation of its globin moiety when exposed to alkali.

**Allen's t.** *(for occlusion of ulnar or radial arteries)*: the patient makes a tight fist so as to express the blood from the skin of the palm and fingers; the examiner digitally compresses either the radial or the ulnar artery. When the patient unclenches the fist, if blood fails to return to the palm and fingers, there is indicated obstruction to blood flow in the artery that has not been compressed.

**Allen-Doisy t.,** a formerly common test for estrogens: the material being tested was injected into spayed laboratory mice and a change from leukocytes to cornified cells in their vaginal secretions was a positive result.

**alpha t.,** a test of intelligence administered by the U.S. Army in World War I to persons who could read.

**alternate binaural loudness balance t.,** ABLB test; comparison of the intensity levels at which a given pure tone sounds equally loud to the normal ear and the ear with hearing loss; done to determine recruitment with unilateral sensorineural loss.

**alternate cover t.,** a test for determining the type of tropia and/or phoria done by alternately covering each eye and noting the movement of the uncovered eye.

**alternate loudness balance t.,** a hearing test done with pure tones that compares the loudness perceived in one ear with that perceived in the other, with the frequency kept constant.

**Ames t.,** a test for mutagenicity of chemical compounds that uses special strains of *Salmonella typhimurium.* The bacteria are incubated on a histidine-deficient medium in the presence of the suspected mutagen and rat liver microsomal cell fraction, which contains mixed-function oxidases known to activate many procarcinogens. Growth of bacterial colonies indicates mutagenicity (reverse mutations restoring the ability to synthesize histidine have occurred). About 90–95 per cent of demonstrated mutagens are also carcinogenic.

**anterior drawer t.,** see *drawer t's.*

**anti-DNA t., anti–double-stranded DNA t.,** an enzyme immunoassay that uses native double-stranded DNA as an antigen to detect and monitor increased serum levels of anti-DNA antibodies, a sign of systemic lupus erythematosus; used in both detection and management of disease.

**antiglobulin t. (AGT),** a test for the presence of nonagglutinating antibodies against red cells that uses antihuman globulin antibody to agglutinate red cells coated with the nonagglutinating antibody. The *direct antiglobulin test* detects antibodies bound to circulating red cells *in vivo.* It is used in the evaluation of autoimmune and drug-induced hemolytic anemia and hemolytic disease of the newborn. The *indirect antiglobulin test* detects serum antibodies that bind to red cells in an *in vitro* incubation step. It is used in typing of erythrocyte antigens and in compatibility testing (cross-match). Called also *Coombs' test.*

**antiglobulin consumption t.,** a test for serum antibodies against cellular antigens. Cells are incubated with the serum sample and then with antiglobulin; any serum antibody that binds to the cells will take up antiglobulin. The amount of antiglobulin consumed is determined by testing the supernatant with antibody-coated red cells; the amount of agglutination is inversely proportional to the antiglobulin consumption.

**Apt t.** *(for differentiating fetal from adult hemoglobin)*: a specimen from an infant's vomitus or stool is mixed with 5 volumes of water and centrifuged so that a clear pink supernatant separates. Sodium hydroxide solution is added to the supernatant; if hemoglobin F (fetal blood) is present, the pink color persists for more than 2 minutes, whereas if hemoglobin A (from swallowed maternal blood) is present, the supernatant turns from pink to yellow within 2 minutes.

**aptitude t's,** tests given to determine aptitude or ability to undertake study or training in a particular field.

**arm ergometry exercise t.,** a variant of the bicycle ergometer stress test in which the patient uses his arms to pedal the bicycle.

**Army General Classification t.,** an intelligence test whose results are used for placement in the military.

**arylsulfatase t.** *(for differentiating species of rapid-growing mycobacteria)*: a sample from a Tween-albumin broth culture of the suspected organism is incubated with tripotassium phenolphthalein disulfate for three days and then alkalinized. Those species producing arylsulfatase *(Mycobacterium fortuitum* and *M. chelonae)* show a pink to red positive reaction; a colorless reaction is negative.

**aspirin tolerance t.,** any of various bleeding time tests in which aspirin is administered and its effect on bleeding time is assessed; aspirin prolongs bleeding time in patients with von Willebrand's disease and certain other platelet disorders.

**association t.,** a test based on associative reaction. It is usually performed by mentioning words to a subject and noting what other words he will give as the ones called up in his mind. The reaction time is also noted.

**atrial pacing stress t.,** a stress test in which temporary immediately reversible atrial pacing is used to stress coronary reserve; used for patients incapable of exercise or in whom an exercise stress test is contraindicated.

**augmented histamine t.** *(of gastric function)*: after a 12-hour fast, the residual gastric contents are aspirated. Basal gastric secretion is then collected for 1 hour in divided 15-minute aliquots. Thirty minutes before completion of collection, a suitable dose of antihistamine is given intramuscularly. At conclusion of basal secretion collection, histamine acid phosphate (0.04 mg per kg of body weight) is given subcutaneously, and gastric contents collected in 15-minute aliquots for 1 hour. Volume, pH, and titratable acidity are measured for each aliquot. When Histalog (1.7 mg per kg of body weight) is used in place of histamine, the antihistamine injection is omitted and 8 (rather than 4) 15-minute aliquots are taken after its injection.

**autohemolysis t.** *(for hereditary spherocytosis)*: a sample of blood is defibrinated and incubated at 37°C for 24 and 48 hours; if hereditary spherocytosis is present, spontaneous hemolysis is increased.

**automated reagin t. (ART),** a modification of the rapid plasma reagin (RPR) test for use with automated analyzers; used in clinical chemistry.

**Ayer's t.** *(for spinal block)*: with a spinal manometer, the pressure in lumbar puncture and that in a cisterna magna puncture should be identical in the normal subject.

**Ayer-Tobey t.,** Tobey-Ayer t.

**Babinski's t.,** see under *sign.*

**Babinski-Weil t.,** the patient, with eyes shut, walks forward and backward ten times. A person with labyrinthine disease deviates from the straight path, bending to one side when walking forward and to the other side when walking backward.

**bacteriolytic t.,** Pfeiffer's phenomenon; see under *phenomenon.*

**Baermann t.** *(for extraction of soil nematodes from earth and detecting larvae of* Strongyloides stercoralis *in feces)*: a specimen of soil or feces is suspended over gauze or wire mesh in a water-filled funnel to which a piece of rubber tubing is attached; larval nematodes migrate from the specimen to the water, and collect in the rubber tubing.

**Bang t.,** abortus Bang ring t.

**Bárány's t.,** caloric t.

**Bárány's pointing t.,** the patient points at a fixed object alternately with the eyes open and closed; a constant error with the eyes closed indicates a brain lesion.

**bar-reading t.,** a test for binocular and stereoscopic vision, which consists of holding a ruler midway between the eyes and the printed page. It is also used as an exercise to develop stereoscopic vision; called also *Welland's t.*

**basophil degranulation t.,** an *in vitro* procedure testing allergic sensitivity to a specific allergen at the cellular level by measuring staining of basophils after exposure to the allergen; a reduction in the number of granulated cells is a positive result.

**Becker's t.** *(for astigmatism)*: the patient looks at a test card containing lines radiating in sets of three and points out which seem blurred.

**Bekhterev's (Bechterew's) t.,** the patient seated in bed is directed to stretch out both legs; in sciatica he cannot do this, but can stretch out each leg in turn.

**Bender Gestalt t., Bender Visual-Motor Gestalt t.,** a psychological test used for evaluating perceptual-motor coordination, for assessing personality dynamics, as a test of organic brain impairment, and for measuring neurological maturation. The subject is asked to make free-hand copies of nine simple geometric designs presented separately on cards or sometimes to reproduce the design from memory.

**Benedict's t.,** 1. *(for glucose in urine)* a test for glucose in the urine using Benedict's reagent. 2. *(for urea)* the urea is hydrolyzed to ammonium carbonate by potassium bisulfate and zinc sulfate made alkaline, and distilled as usual.

**bentonite flocculation t.,** any agglutination test using antigen adsorbed on particles of bentonite; when the antigen is added to serum containing specific antibodies, flocculation occurs.

**benzidine t.** *(for occult blood in urine or feces)*: benzidine, acetic acid, and hydrogen peroxide are added to the specimen; hemoglobin catalyzes the oxidation of benzidine by hydrogen peroxide, giving a blue color. This is the most sensitive screening test for occult blood, but it is seldom used because benzidine is a carcinogen, and its use is restricted.

**Bernstein t.,** esophageal acid infusion t.

**beta t.,** a test of intelligence administered by the U.S. Army in World War I to persons who could not read or did not speak English.

**Bial's t.** *(for pentoses in urine)*: the specimen is heated with a solution of orcinol, hydrochloric acid, and ferric chloride; pentoses are converted to furfural, which reacts with orcinol to form a green product.

**bicycle ergometer exercise t.,** an exercise test in which the patient pedals a stationary bicycle ergometer; the test is usually graded, with incremental or continuous increases in power produced by increases in pedal resistance at a given pedal speed. Cf. *treadmill exercise t.*

**Bielschowsky head-tilting t.,** tilting the head to the right and the left shoulder with the patient looking at a distance fixation device permits distinction between superior rectus paresis and contralateral superior oblique paresis.

**bile solubility t.** *(for differentiation of pneumococci from other streptococci)*: a sample of a broth culture is incubated at pH 7.4 to 7.6 with sodium deoxycholate. A decrease in turbidity (positive test) indicates lysing of the cells. Pneumococci give a positive result, whereas other viridans streptococci give a negative one.

**bilirubin t.,** see specific tests, including *Fouchet's t.* and *Harrison spot t.*

**binaural distorted speech t's,** tests of the capacity of the central nervous system to coordinate two incoming speech patterns, each of which is incomplete.

**Binet's t.,** a method of testing the mental capacity of children and youth by asking a series of questions adapted to, and standardized on, the capacity of normal children at various ages. According to the answers given, the mental age of the subject is ascertained.

**Binet-Simon t.,** Binet's t.

**Bing t.,** a vibrating tuning fork is held to the mastoid process and the auditory meatus is alternately occluded and left open: changes in loudness (positive Bing) are perceived by the normal ear and in sensorineural deafness, but in conduction deafness no difference is perceived (negative Bing).

**biuret t.,** see under *reaction.*

**bleeding time t.,** a test of bleeding time, assessing capillary function and platelet function, such as *Duke's t., Ivy's t.,* or the *template method.*

**Boas' t.,** see under *point.*

**Bodal's t.,** test of color perception by the use of colored blocks.

**bone conduction t's,** tests of bone conduction; see *tuning fork t's.*

**Bozicevich's t.,** a serologic test for the detection of trichinosis.

**breath hydrogen t.,** hydrogen breath t.

**Broadbent's t.** *(for cerebral dominance of language function)*: different numbers (or words) are presented simultaneously to the two ears; right-handed persons tend to report first the words going into the right ear.

**bronchial challenge t.,** see under *challenge.*

**Burchard-Liebermann t.,** Liebermann-Burchard t.

**butyric acid t.,** see *pineapple t.*

**$\chi^2$ t.,** chi-square t.

**California mastitis t. (C.M.T.)** *(for subclinical mastitis in cows)*: equal amounts of milk, bromcresol purple, and an anionic surface-active substance are mixed in four separate cups within a plastic paddle by rapidly rotating the paddle horizontally; a positive reaction is indicated by various degrees of gel formation, according to the degree of abnormality of the milk.

**caloric t.** *(for ocular and vestibular functioning)*: irrigation of the normal ear with warm water produces rotatory nystagmus (*caloric nystagmus*) toward the irrigated side; irrigation with cold water produces similar nystagmus away from that side. Called also *Bárány's t., sign,* or *symptom* and *nystagmus t.*

**CAMP t.** [*C*hristie, *A*tkins, and *M*unch-*P*etersen, discoverers of the phenomenon], *(for the presumptive identification of Group B beta-hemolytic streptococci)*: a culture of streptococcus is streaked on a blood agar plate near a streak of beta-lysin–producing *Staphylococcus aureus.* Group B streptococci produce a substance (CAMP factor) that enlarges the zone of lysis formed by the staphylococcal beta-hemolysin.

**capillary fragility t., capillary resistance t.,** tourniquet t. (def. 1).

**carbohydrate utilization t.,** any of several tests for identification of yeasts and certain other organisms according to a profile of carbohydrate assimilation.

**carbon monoxide t.,** see specific tests, including *Preyer's t., Rubner's t.* (1), *Salkowski's t.* (1), *Wetzel's t., Zaleski's t.*

**Casoni's intradermal t.** *(for hydatid disease)*: injection into the skin of hydatid fluid followed by the immediate or delayed production of a wheal-and-flare reaction denotes hydatid infection; now little used because of its nonspecificity.

**catalase t.** *(for the production of catalase by bacteria)*: a slant culture is treated with hydrogen peroxide. The presence of gas bubbles indicates a positive reaction. Micrococci, staphylococci, most species of *Bacillus,* and anaerobic diphtheroids are catalase-positive; streptococci, pneumococci, and most *Actinomyces* are catalase-negative.

**catoptric t.,** a test for cataract made by observing the reflections from the cornea and from the surfaces of the crystalline lens.

**challenge t.,** challenge (def. 3).

**chemiluminescence t.,** a sensitive test of neutrophil microbicidal function that involves detection of the chemiluminescent energy emitted by unstable and highly reactive oxygen metabolites, e.g., singlet oxygen, produced during the respiratory burst following phagocytosis. It is able to detect heterozygous carriers of chronic granulomatous disease as well as homozygotes and also patients with myeloperoxidase deficiency.

**Chick-Martin t.,** a test for the efficiency of disinfectants in the presence of organic matter; see under *method.*

**Chimani-Moos t.,** a test for detecting simulated deafness.

**chi-square t.,** any statistical hypothesis test that employs the chi-square ($\chi^2$) distribution (q.v.), especially two tests applied to categorical data: the $\chi^2$-test of goodness of fit, which tests whether an observed frequency distribution fits a specified theoretical model, and the $\chi^2$-test of independence or homogeneity, which tests whether two or more series of frequencies (the rows and columns of a contingency table) are independent. In both cases the test statistic is the sum over all categories of the squared difference between the observed and expected frequencies divided by the expected frequency, under the null hypothesis. The sampling distribution of this $\chi^2$-statistic approaches the $\chi^2$-distribution as the sample size increases, under the null hypothesis.

**cholesterol t.,** see specifc tests, including *Liebermann-Burchard t., Salkowski's t.* (2), *Schultze's t.* (2).

**chromatin t.** *(for determination of genetic sex)*: examination of somatic cells for presence of the sex chromatin situated at the periphery of the nucleus in normal females but not in normal males; an index of the presence of XX chromosomal constitution.

**cis-trans t.,** in microbial genetics, a test to determine whether two mutations that have the same phenotypic effect (in a haploid cell or a cell with single phage infection) are located in the same gene (resulting in noncomplementation) or in different genes (resulting in complementation and hence in loss of the mutant defect). The test depends on the independent behavior of two alleles of a gene in a diploid cell or in a cell infected with two phages carrying different alleles.

**citrate t.** *(for differentiation of organisms of the Enterobacter group of bacteria)*: the test organism is grown on a medium containing citrate as its sole carbon source (Simmons citrate agar). The metabolism of citrate (positive reaction) turns the medium from green to blue. The Enterobacteriaceae are mostly positive; *Edwardsiella, Escherichia, Morganella, Shigella,* and *Yersinia* are negative.

**coagulase t.,** a test for coagulase activity in which bacteria are added to citrated or oxalated (human or rabbit) blood plasma; in the presence of coagulase, the plasma gels within three hours. Coagulase activity is also demonstrable by mixing bacteria with blood plasma on a slide; if positive, clumping occurs, with fibrin formation.

**cocaine t.,** after instillation of a cocaine solution in each eye, the pupil of an eye affected by Horner's syndrome remains smaller than that of the normal eye.

**coccidioidin t.,** an intracutaneous test for coccidioidomycosis; see *coccidioidin.*

**Cohn's t.,** a test for color perception by the use of variously colored embroidery patterns.

**colchicine t.,** see *Zeisel's t.*

**cold pressor t.,** immersion of one hand in ice water for several minutes, causing vasoconstriction, tachycardia, and transient hypertension; it is used as an alternative stress test for detection of coronary artery disease in patients incapable of undergoing an exercise stress test and as a test of vasomotor function.

**collateral circulation t.,** see specific tests, including *Korotkoff's t., Pachon's t.,* and *tourniquet t.* (defs. 2 and 3).

**color perception t.,** see specific tests, including *Bodal's t., Cohn's t., Donders' t., Holmgren's t., Ishihara's t., Jenning's t., lantern t., Nagel's t.*

**combined anterior pituitary t.,** a dynamic test of the functioning of the anterior pituitary, such as after surgery or radiation to the gland; four exogenous hypothalamic hormones are administered intravenously (corticotropin-releasing hormone, growth hormone–releasing hormone, luteinizing hormone–releasing hormone, and thyrotropin-releasing hormone) and levels of the corresponding pituitary hormones in the blood are assessed at intervals for about two hours.

**complement fixation t.,** see under *fixation.*

**concentration t.,** 1. *(for renal function)* the patient is placed under conditions which cause the normal person to elaborate urine containing one or more constituents in high concentration and the results are observed to see whether the patient is able to attain this concentration, as in the *urea concentration t.* 2. *(for renal tubular function)* water restriction to measure urine concentration as reflected in specific gravity or osmolality.

**conglutinating complement absorption t. (CCAT),** a test resembling the complement fixation test (see under *fixation*), using as the indicator of antigen-antibody reaction the disappearance of conglutinin (q.v.) activity.

**Congo red t.** *(for amyloidosis)*: Congo red is injected intravenously; if more than 60 per cent of the dye disappears after 1 hour, amyloidosis is indicated.

**conservative t.,** a test having a type I error probability that is at most a stated nominal level.

**contact t's,** patch t.

**contraction stress t. (CST),** the monitoring of the response of the fetal heart rate to uterine contractions by cardiotocography; uterine contractions may be spontaneous or induced by maternal nipple stimulation or by intravenous infusion of oxytocin (oxytocin challenge test). A negative (normal) test consists of three contractions within a 10-minute period with no deceleration of the fetal heart rate; a late deceleration pattern may reflect fetal hypoxia.

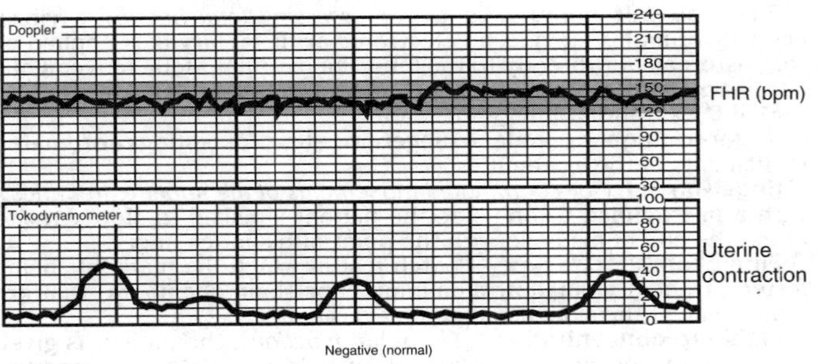


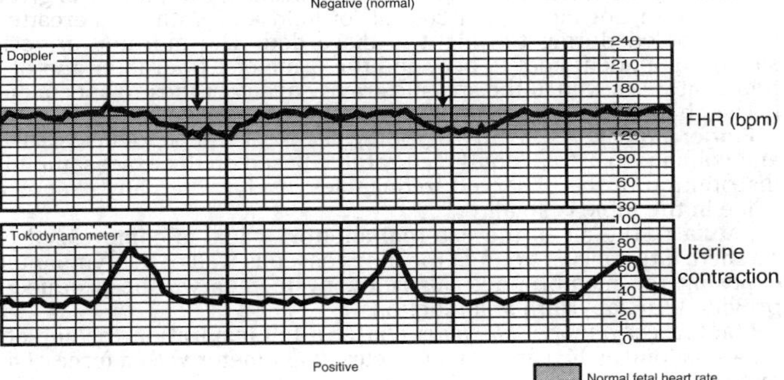


Contraction stress test. The top two tracings show a negative (normal) result, with uterine contractions followed by an unchanged fetal heart rate (FHR); the bottom two tracings show a positive result, with uterine contractions followed by transient decelerations in the fetal heart rate *(arrows).* The shaded strips show the usual range of fetal heart rate.

**Coombs' t.,** antiglobulin t.

**copper t.,** see *Schönbein's t.* (2).

**Corner-Allen t.** *(for progesterone activity)* female rabbits are mated during estrus and the ovaries are removed eighteen hours later; the endometrial changes are measured and compared to those of pregnancy. See also *Corner-Allen unit,* under *unit.*

**cover t.,** see *alternate cover t.* and *cover-uncover t.*

**cover-uncover t.,** a test for determining the type of phoria, by covering one eye and noting its movement as it is uncovered.

**Crafts' t.,** in organic disease of the pyramidal tract, stroking with a blunt point upward over the dorsal surface of the ankle, the leg being extended and the muscles relaxed, produces a dorsal extension of the great toe similar to Babinski's reflex.

**Crampton's t.,** a test for physical resistance and condition based on the difference between the pulse and blood pressure in the recumbent position and in the standing position. A difference of 75 or more indicates good condition; one of 65 or less shows a poor condition.

**creatinine t.,** see specific tests, including *Jaffé's t.* (def. 1), *Kerner's t., Salkowski's t.* (def. 4), *Thudichum's t., von Maschke's t., Weyl's t.* (def. 1). See also *creatinine, methods for,* under *method.*

**Cuignet's t.** *(for simulated unilateral blindness)*: the bar-reading test used to detect simulated unilateral blindness or malingering.

**cycle ergometer t.,** bicycle ergometer exercise t.

**cysteine t.,** see specific tests, including *nitroprusside t.* (1) and *Sullivan's t.*

**cystine t.,** see *Liebig's t.*

**cytosine t.,** see *Wheeler and Johnson's t.*

**dark-adaptation t.** *(for vitamin A deficiency)*: a test based on the fact that with a deficient intake of vitamin A the ability to see a dimly illuminated object in a dark room is diminished.

**darkroom t.,** a test to determine the tendency to develop acute-angle glaucoma: ocular pressure is measured by the applanation tonometer, the subject is placed in a darkroom for one hour, and applanation tonometry is then repeated.

**Davidsohn differential absorption t.,** Paul-Bunnell-Davidsohn t.

**D-dimer t.,** see under *assay.*

**dehydrocholate t.** *(for the speed of blood circulation)*: sodium dehydrocholate solution is injected intravenously; the usual time elapsing until a bitter taste in the mouth occurs is between 10 and 14 seconds.

**Denver Developmental Screening t.,** a test for identification of infants and preschool children with developmental delay.

**deoxyribonuclease t.** *(for the presence of deoxyribonuclease in bacteria)*: a nutrient agar plate containing deoxyribonucleic acid and toluidine blue is inoculated from a young agar slant; after incubation a red zone around the inoculum indicates the presence of deoxyribonuclease. Called also *DNase t.*

**deoxyuridine suppression t.,** a test for folate or cobalamin deficiency, in which lack of 5,10-methylene tetrahydrofolate inhibits incorporation of deoxyuridine into DNA, so that deoxyuridine fails to inhibit incorporation of $^{3}$H-thymidine.

**dexamethasone suppression t., high-dose** *(for Cushing's syndrome)*: urinary levels of cortisol and 17-hydroxycorticosteroid are measured following administration of dexamethasone at 16 times the level used in replacement therapy; cortisol secretion is suppressed in patients with Cushing's syndrome but not in those with ectopic ACTH syndrome or adrenal tumors.

**dexamethasone suppression t., low-dose** *(for Cushing's syndrome)*: urinary levels of cortisol and 17-hydroxycortisone are measured following administration of dexamethasone at three to four times the level used in replacement therapy; cortisol secretion is suppressed in normal patients but not in those with Cushing's syndrome.

**dextrose t.,** glucose t.

**DFA-TP t.,** direct fluorescent antibody–Treponema pallidum t.

**diabetes t.,** a test for diabetes mellitus; see *glucose t.* and *glucose tolerance t.*

**diacetyl t.** *(for urea)*: the solution to be tested is mixed with concentrated hydrochloric acid and diacetyl monoxime; a yellow color develops on boiling if urea is present.

**Dick t.** *(for susceptibility to scarlet fever)*: purified erythrogenic toxin from group A streptococci is injected intradermally; appearance within 24 to 48 hours of a small area of reddening of the skin indicates susceptibility of the subject.

**differential t. for infectious mononucleosis,** a test based on the fact that antisheep agglutinins in infectious mononucleosis are not absorbed by Forssman antigen (whereas those in serum disease and of normal persons are), but are absorbed by beef cells (whereas those in conditions other than infectious mononucleosis may or may not be). See also *Paul-Bunnell-Davidsohn t.*

**diphtheria t.,** see *Schick t.*

**direct fluorescent antibody–*Treponema pallidum* t.,** DFA-TP t.; a serologic test for syphilis using direct immunofluorescence.

**disk diffusion t.** *(for antibiotic sensitivity in bacteria)*: agar plates are inoculated with a standardized suspension of a microorganism. Antibiotic-containing disks are applied to the agar surface. Following overnight incubation, the diameters of the zones of inhibition or clearing surrounding the disks are measured. Zone diameters are interpreted as sensitive (susceptible), indeterminate (or intermediate), or resistant.

**DNase t.,** deoxyribonuclease t.

**Dolman's t.** *(for ocular dominance)*: the patient holds in both hands a card with a hole in it through which to sight at a light.

**Donath-Landsteiner t.** *(for paroxysmal cold hemoglobinuria)*: a test based on the fact that the blood of patients with this disease contains complement-dependent iso- and autohemolysin (Donath-Landsteiner antibody) which unites with red cells only at low temperatures (2° to 10°C), hemolysis occurring only after warming to 37°C.

**Donders' t.,** a color vision test performed by lanterns with sides of colored glass.

**double glucagon t.** *(for deficiency of amylo-1-6-glucosidase)*: glucagon is administered after a 12 hour fast and again shortly after a meal; if the blood sugar fails to rise after the first administration but has a normal rise after the second, the test is positive.

**Draw-a-Person t.,** a commonly used projective test for assessing personality style and psychopathology by interpretation of a drawing of a person done by the subject, based on the assumption that their personality characteristics will be introjected onto the drawing.

**drawer t's** *(for integrity of cruciate ligaments of knee)*: the knee is flexed to a 90° angle; at the femoral-tibial junction, if the tibia can be drawn too far forward there is rupture of the anterior ligaments *(anterior drawer t.)* and if it can be drawn too far back there is rupture of the posterior ligaments *(posterior drawer t.)*. Called also *drawer signs*.

**drinking t.** *(for glaucoma)*: one liter of water is ingested as rapidly as possible into an empty stomach. The intraocular pressure is measured every 15 minutes; a rise of 8 to 15 mm Hg in less than 30 minutes indicates glaucoma. Called also *water provocative t.*

**Duane's t.**, the employment of a candle flame and prisms to measure the degree of ocular heterophoria.

**Dugas' t.**, a test for the existence of dislocation of the shoulder, made by placing the hand of the affected side on the opposite shoulder and bringing the elbow to the side of the chest. If this cannot be accomplished (Dugas' sign), dislocation of the shoulder exists.

**Duke's t.**, a type of bleeding time test in which the incision is made in the earlobe.

**dye exclusion t.**, the determination of cell viability *in vitro*. Following exposure of a cell preparation to trypan blue or eosin, dead cells take up the dye from the medium whereas living cells remain unstained.

**dynamic t.**, one designed to test some physiologic process in the body, such as a challenge, a stimulation test, or a suppression test.

**early pregnancy t.**, a do-it-yourself immunologic test for pregnancy performed in the home as early as one day after menstruation was expected (missed period); a variety of tests exist, all based on an increase in urinary levels of human chorionic gonadotropin after fertilization.

**ECG stress t's**, stress t's.

**Ehrlich's t.**, see *Ehrlich's diazo reaction*, under *reaction*.

**Einhorn string t.**, a test for determining whether the site of bleeding is in the low esophagus, stomach, or duodenum.

**Elek t.**, toxigenicity t.

**Elsberg's t.**, a method of testing the functioning of the sense of smell; variations in function or in rate of fatigue may be used to distinguish between intracerebral and extracerebral tumors or other lesions.

**Ely's t.**, with the patient prone, if flexion of the leg on the thigh causes the buttocks to arch away from the table and the leg to abduct at the hip joint, there is contracture of the lateral fascia of the thigh.

**EP t.**, erythrocyte protoporphyrin t.

**Erhard's t.**, a test for detecting simulated deafness.

**Erichsen t.**, see under *sign*.

**erythrocyte protoporphyrin t.**, EP t.; a screening test for lead toxicity, in which erythrocyte protoporphyrin levels are determined by direct fluorometry of whole blood or fluorescence analysis of whole blood extracts; levels are increased in lead poisoning and iron deficiency.

**esophageal acid infusion t.** *(for diagnosis of gastroesophageal reflux)*: 0.1 N hydrogen chloride infused at a rate of 120 drops per minute produces pain and other symptoms. Called also *Bernstein t.*

**euglobulin lysis t.**, a test that evaluates for hemorrhagic tendencies by measuring time of fibrinolysis, done by determining the time required to dissolve an incubated clot composed of precipitated plasma euglobulin and exogenous thrombin. Lysis in less than 90 minutes indicates abnormally enhanced fibrinolytic activity.

**exact t.**, a statistical test based on the actual probability distribution of the data in the study, rather than on an approximation of it.

**exercise t's, exercise stress t's**, any of various stress tests in which exercise is used in the electrocardiographic assessment of cardiovascular health and function, particularly in the diagnosis of myocardial ischemia. The most widely used forms are the treadmill and bicycle ergometer exercise tests; they are usually graded, consisting of a series of incrementally increasing work loads sustained for defined intervals.

***F*-t.**, a statistical test comparing the means of more than two groups simultaneously by comparing two different measures of variance of the observations. One statistic measures the variations between the means of the groups (the between-groups variation), the other the variations within the groups (the within-group variation). If the two measures of variance yield similar results and their ratio, the F-ratio, approximates 1.0, the null hypothesis that all observations came from the same population cannot be rejected, whereas under the alternative hypothesis, the F-ratio is expected to be larger than 1.0. The test is the first step in the analysis of variance (ANOVA).

**FAB t.**, fluorescent antibody t.

**Farber's t.**, presence of swallowed vernix cells in the meconium of a newborn baby indicates partial intestinal stenosis; their absence indicates intestinal atresia.

**Farr t.**, a radioimmunoassay for measuring absolute amounts of antibody: antibody is reacted with radiolabeled antigen and precipitated with ammonium sulfate; bound antigen or hapten is precipitated while free antigen remains in solution. This test is based on the capacity of antibody to combine with antigen rather than on such secondary properties as precipitation and therefore measures all immunoglobulin classes and subclasses.

**$FE_{Na}$ t.**, excreted fraction of filtered sodium test, a measure of renal tubular reabsorption of sodium, calculated as follows:

$$\frac{(U/P)Na}{(U/P)Cr} \times 100,$$

where U and P represent concentrations of sodium and creatinine in urine and plasma, respectively.

**femoral nerve stretch t.**, *(for lesions of third or fourth lumbar disk)*: passive knee flexion in the prone position causes pain in the back or thighs.

**fermentation t.** *(for glucose and other sugars in urine)*: boil a specimen to destroy bacteria, then add baker's yeast and incubate; perform Benedict's test for reducing sugars on this specimen and an unfermented specimen. Glucose, fructose, and maltose are fermented and give a reaction in the unfermented specimen but not in the fermented specimen.

**fern t.**, see *ferning*.

**ferric chloride t.**, ferric chloride in acidic solution is added to a urine specimen; many substances are oxidized giving colored products. Positive reactions are given by melanin, acetoacetic acid, bilirubin, phenothiazines, salicylates, and the keto acids present in phenylketonuria, alkaptonuria, maple syrup urine disease, and oasthouse urine disease.

**fetal acoustic stimulation t.** *(for assessing fetal health)*: a vibroacoustic stimulus such as an electronic artificial larynx is applied either externally or directly to the fetus and resultant fetal movements, cardioacceleration, and alterations in respiration are evaluated.

**FIGLU excretion t.**, histidine loading t.

**finger-to-finger t.**, similar to finger-nose test, for testing coordinated movements of the extremities.

**finger-nose t.** *(for coordinated movements of the upper extremities)*: with arm extended to one side the patient is asked to slowly try to touch the end of his nose with the point of his index finger.

**Finn chamber t.**, a type of patch test in which the materials being tested are held in shallow aluminum cups (Finn chambers) that are taped against the skin, usually for several days.

**Fishberg concentration t.** *(for renal function)*: the patient is given supper with not more than 200 mL of fluid and nothing thereafter. Urine voided during the night is discarded. The morning urine is saved, the patient kept in bed, and the urine of 1 hour later and of 2 hours later is saved. If the specific gravity of any of these 3 specimens is less than 1.024 there is impairment of renal concentration.

**Fisher exact t.**, a statistical hypothesis test of independence of rows and columns in a 2 × 2 contingency table based on the exact sampling distribution of the observed frequencies, useful when any expected value in the table is small.

**fistula t.**, the air in the external auditory canal is compressed or rarefied: if there is erosion of the inner osseous wall of the tympanum exposing the membranous labyrinth, nystagmus will be produced, provided the labyrinth still functions.

**Flack t.** *(of physical efficiency)*: after a full inspiration the subject blows as long as he can into a mercury manometer with a force of 40 mm mercury.

**flocculation t.**, 1. any of a variety of nonspecific tests of liver function, now obsolete, in which a precipitating reagent is added to serum; positive results generally reflect increased gamma and beta globulins and lipoproteins or decreased albumin. 2. any serologic test in which a flocculent agglomerate is formed; usually the term is applied to a variant form of the precipitin reaction, rarely to agglutination reactions.

**fluorescent antibody t.**, FAB t.; a test for the distribution of cells expressing a specific protein by binding antibody specific for the protein and detecting complexes by fluorescent labeling of the antibody; if it is combined with cell sorting, determinations can be quantitative.

**fluorescent treponemal antibody absorption t.**, FTA-ABS t.; the standard treponemal antigen serologic test for syphilis; patient serum is diluted with an extract of Reiter treponemes to remove nonspecific antibodies, then reacted with the Nichols strain of *Treponema pallidum* fixed to a glass slide; specific antibodies adhering to the treponemes are demonstrated with fluorescein-labeled antihuman globulin. Positive tests are seen in about 85 per cent of cases of primary syphilis, 100 per cent in secondary syphilis, and 98 per cent in late syphilis.

**food challenge t.**, food challenge.

**formaldehyde t.**, see specific tests, including *Jorissen's t.* and *Kentmann's t.*

**Foshay's t.** *(for tularemia)*: a suspension of *Pasteurella tularensis* is injected into the skin; a positive reaction resembles that in a positive tuberculin test.

**Fouchet's t.** *(for bilirubin in urine)*: a few drops of Fouchet's reagent are added to the specimen; a green color is produced if bilirubin is present.

**Fournier t.,** the patient is asked to rise on command from a sitting position; he is asked to rise and walk, then stop quickly on command; he is asked to walk and turn around quickly on command. The ataxic gait is thus brought out.

**Francis' t.,** 1. *(for bile acids in urine)* in a test tube is placed 2 g of glucose in 15 g of sulfuric acid and the urine is placed on top of this; a purple color forms if bile acids are present. 2. an intracutaneous test in pneumonia for ascertaining the body response to the infection and whether the specific antibodies are present after treatment with antipneumococcus serum. The homologous pneumococcus polysaccharide is used in the skin test.

**Fränkel's t.,** examination of the nasal cavity with the patient's head bent down between his knees and rotated so that the side to be examined is turned upward. If pus is seen in the middle meatus, suppuration in some of the anterior accessory sinuses is indicated.

**Friderichsen's t.** *(for vitamin A deficiency)*: determination of the weakest light stimulus which will give rise to an oculomotor reflex. A variation from normal indicates vitamin A deficiency.

**fructosamine t.,** determination of the serum fructosamine level by measurement of the reduction of nitroblue tetrazolium (NBT) to purple under alkaline conditions; it is used as an index of the average glycemic state over the preceding two to three weeks.

**fructose t.,** see *Rubner's t.* (def. 2) and *Selivanoff's t.*

**fructose tolerance t.,** a test of hepatic function based on the power of the liver to absorb and store large quantities of fructose.

**FTA-ABS t.,** fluorescent treponemal antibody absorption t.

**fundus reflex t.,** retinoscopy.

**Funkenstein t.,** an index of central autonomic reactivity, consisting of observing the response in systolic blood pressure after intramuscular injection of 10 mg of acetylcholine.

**Gaenslen's t.,** see under *sign.*

**gastric function t.,** see specific tests, including *augmented histamine t.*

**Gault t.** *(for simulated deafness)*: the patient's good ear is closed and a sound is made near the supposed bad ear; winking on the tested side indicates hearing.

**gaze t.** *(for ocular and vestibular functioning)*: movements of the eye are recorded with the patient gazing straight at an object and at positions off to different sides of it; then with eyes closed for 20 seconds, the patient must perform a small mental exercise. The eyes normally should assume a center gaze while they are closed.

**gel diffusion t.,** see *immunodiffusion.*

**Gerhardt's t.,** 1. *(for acetoacetic acid in the urine)* filter, in order to remove the phosphates, and add a few drops of a solution of ferric chloride, which produces a deep red color, which disappears when sulfuric acid is added. 2. *(for bile pigments in the urine)* shake urine with an equal measure of chloroform and then add iodine tincture and potassium hydroxide to the separated chloroform; a yellow or yellowish brown color is produced (Charles Frédéric Gerhardt).

**germ tube t.** *(for Candida albicans)*: an inoculum of *Candida* is incubated in serum for 2 to 3 hours at 37°C; formation of germ tubes is a positive result.

**Gibbon and Landis t.** *(for peripheral circulation)*: a pair of extremities (the hands, if the feet are to be tested; the feet, if the hands are to be tested) are immersed in a bath of 43°–45°C. If the temperature in the unimmersed extremities rises, the circulation is normal.

**Gies' biuret t.** *(for proteins)*: a form of biuret test employing the following reagent: mix 25 mL of a 3 per cent solution of cupric sulfate and 975 mL of a 10 per cent solution of potassium hydroxide.

**glucagon stimulation t.** *(for deficiency of growth hormone)*: blood samples are taken before and at intervals of 1, 2, 2.5, and 3 hours after subcutaneous or intramuscular injection of glucagon; radioimmunoassay of the serum is then done by enzyme partition.

**glucose t.,** any of various laboratory tests for glucose in the urine; many formerly common ones are no longer used. See *Benedict's t., Rubner's t.,* and *saccharimeter t.*

**glucose tolerance t.,** GTT; a metabolic test of carbohydrate tolerance, measuring active insulin, a hepatic function based on the power of the normal liver to absorb and store large quantities of glucose, and the effectiveness of intestinal absorption of glucose. The most common method is the *oral glucose tolerance test* (q.v.).

**glucose tolerance t., oral,** OGTT; the most common kind of glucose tolerance test. Glucose is ingested into a fasting stomach and measurements of plasma glucose are taken over time; if glucose levels do not return to normal within 2 to 2.5 hours the patient may have impaired glucose tolerance or diabetes mellitus.

**glycosylated hemoglobin t.,** measurement of the percentage of hemoglobin A molecules that have formed a stable keto–amine linkage between the terminal amino acid position of the β-chains and a glucose group; in normal persons this amounts to about 7 per cent of the total, in diabetics about 14.5 per cent. Used in the management of patients with diabetes mellitus.

**glycyltryptophan t.** *(for carcinoma of stomach)*: filtered gastric contents and glycyltryptophan are placed in a test tube and kept at body temperature for 24 hours; if on the addition of a few drops of bromine, a reddish violet color is formed, carcinoma is indicated.

**Gmelin's t.** *(for bile pigments)*: fuming nitric acid is so added to the suspected urine that it forms a layer under it. Near the junction of the two liquids, rings are formed—a green ring above, and under it a blue, violet-red, and reddish yellow. If the green and violet-red rings are absent, the reaction shows the probable presence of lutein.

**Goodenough draw-a-man t., Goodenough draw-a-person t.,** a method of testing the general intelligence of children by asking the subject to draw a picture of a man to the best of his or her ability.

**Goodenough-Harris drawing t.,** a revision of the Goodenough draw-a-man test, in which scoring emphasizes the presence or absence of body and clothing detail rather than artistic skill.

**graded exercise t's (GXT),** see *exercise t's.*

**Graefe's t.** *(for heterophoria)*: on holding a prism of 10 degrees before one eye, base up or down, two images are formed; one of these images is displaced laterally in heterophoria.

**Graham's t.,** the intravenous or oral administration of iodophthalein sodium prior to radiographic examination of the gallbladder.

**Griess t.** *(for nitrites in the saliva)*: mix the saliva with 5 parts of water; add a few drops of dilute solution of sulfuric acid and a few drops of metadiamidobenzene; this produces a strong yellow color if nitrites are present.

**Grigg's t.** *(for proteins)*: metaphosphoric acid precipitates all proteins except the peptones.

**group t.,** a test of intelligence or aptitude given to a number of persons at one time.

**guaiac t.** *(for occult blood)*: glacial acetic acid and a solution of gum guaiac are mixed with the specimen; on addition of hydrogen peroxide, the presence of blood is indicated by a blue tint.

**Guthrie t.** *(for phenylketonuria)*: in the presence of blood containing phenylalanine, β-2-thienylalanine does not inhibit growth of *Bacillus subtilis.*

**Gutzeit's t.** *(for arsenic)*: a paper is moistened with an acidulated silver nitrate solution and exposed to the fumes from the suspected liquid, which is mixed with zinc and dilute sulfuric acid. The formation of a yellow spot on the paper indicates the presence of inorganic arsenic compounds.

**Haagensen t.,** observation of the contour of the breasts when the patient leans forward as a means of detecting malignant changes in the mammae.

**Hallion's t.,** Tuffier's t.

**Ham's t.,** acidified serum t.

**Hamel's t.** *(for slight jaundice)*: a little blood is drawn by puncture from the lobe of the ear into a capillary tube and the tube is allowed to stand for a few hours; the serum which collects in the upper part of the tube will be yellow if jaundice is present.

**Hamilton's t.,** when the shoulder joint is luxated, a rule or straight rod applied to the humerus can be made to touch the outer condyle and the acromion at the same time.

**hapten inhibition t.,** serologic characterization of an antigenic determinant by employing known haptens to mask the antigen binding site of antibody specific for it.

**harmonic acceleration t.** *(for vestibulo-ocular reflex)*: rotation of a patient seated in a chair in complete darkness, with monitoring of eye movements; with normal vestibulo-ocular reflexes the eyes will undergo rotatory nystagmus to the same degree in both eyes in the direction opposite to that of the rotation.

**Harrison spot t.** *(for bilirubin in urine)*: add to 10 mL of urine 5 mL of a 10 per cent solution of barium chloride, mix, and filter. Spread filter paper on dry filter paper. Add one to two drops of Fouchet's reagent (trichloroacetic acid 25 g, water 100 mL, and 10 per cent solution of ferric chloride 10 mL); a positive reaction gives a blue to green color.

**hatching t.,** a test for the detection of live schistosome eggs in urine or feces, dependent upon the eggs hatching to produce miracidia when placed in water; the miracidia are attracted to light and can readily be identified.

**Heaf t.,** Sterneedle tuberculin t.

**heel-knee t.** *(for coordinated movements of the lower extremities)*: the patient, lying on his back, is asked to touch the knee of one leg with the heel of the other and then to pass the heel slowly down the front of the shin to the ankle.

**heel-tap t.,** see under *reflex.*

**hemadsorption t.,** an *in vitro* test for detecting hemagglutinating viruses based on the adherence of red blood cells to cells of the infected tissue in the presence of hemagglutinin.

**hemagglutination inhibition t. (HI, HAI),** 1. a highly sensitive procedure for the measurement of soluble antigens in biologic specimens in which the specimen is first incubated with homologous antibody and then incubated with antigen-coated red cells; the amount of hemagglutination reflects the amount of free antibody present after reaction with the specimen and thus varies inversely with the amount of antigen in the specimen. 2. a procedure for the measurement of serum antibodies directed against a hemagglutinating virus; the highest dilution of serum that completely inhibits hemagglutination by a standardized viral preparation is reported as the hemagglutination titer.

**hemosiderin t.**, see specific tests, including *Perls' t.* and *Rous t.*

**Henshaw t.**, a test to aid in the selection of the appropriate homeopathic remedy in a given case of disease. A visible flocculation zone develops in the patient's blood serum when it is brought into contact with a potentized remedy homeopathically indicated in the case.

**hepatic function t.**, liver function t.

**Hering's t.**, the subject looks with both eyes through a tube blackened within and having a thread running vertically across the farther end, and a small round body is placed either before or behind the thread—if vision is binocular, the subject is able at once to tell whether the ball is nearer to him than the thread or farther off; but if vision is monocular, he cannot tell whether it is nearer or farther than the thread.

**Hess capillary t.**, tourniquet t. (def. 1).

**heterophil antibody t., heterophile antibody t.**, a test for heterophil antibodies associated with infectious mononucleosis; see *horse cell t.*, *Paul-Bunnell t.*, and *Paul-Bunnell-Davidsohn t.*

**Hickey-Hare t.** *(for diabetes insipidus)*: intravenous infusion of hypertonic saline after establishment of water diuresis induces antidiuresis in normal subjects but not in patients with diabetes insipidus.

**Hines and Brown t.**, cold pressor t.

**Histalog t.**, see *augmented histamine t.*

**histamine t.**, 1. one mL of a 0.1 per cent solution of histamine is injected subcutaneously to stimulate gastric secretion; see also *augmented histamine t.* 2. histamine flare t. 3. *(for pheochromocytoma)* following rapid intravenous injection of histamine phosphate administered in a standardized dosage of 0.010 to 0.050 mg of histamine base, normal individuals experience transient headache, flush, and a brief fall in blood pressure, but those with pheochromocytoma, after a fall in blood pressure, experience a marked rise in blood pressure, fear, excitability, etc.

**histamine flare t.** *(for leprosy and postherpetic neuralgia)*: a drop of 1:1000 histamine acid phosphate solution is placed on the skin and a needle puncture is made through it; the test is positive if there is no erythema flare when the puncture is made within the suspected lesion area, or if the flare stops at the border of the lesion when it is made slightly to the outside of it.

**histidine loading t.** *(for folic acid deficiency)*: a loading dose of histidine is given, and the resultant urinary excretion of excess formiminoglutamic acid (FIGLU), secondary to decreased amounts of tetrahydrofolic acid, is measured. Called also *FIGLU excretion t.*

**Hitzig t.** *(for vestibular apparatus)*: the positive electrode of a galvanic current is applied just in front of the ear being examined while the negative electrode is held in the patient's hand, the patient standing with feet together and eyes closed. A current of 5 milliamperes causes a leaning toward the positive pole in normal persons.

**hock t.**, spavin t.

**Hoffmann's t.** *(for tyrosine)*: add mercuric nitrate to the suspected liquid and boil it; then add nitric acid with a little nitrous acid. A red color is produced if tyrosine is present, and a red precipitate is seen.

**Hofmeister's t.**, 1. *(for leucine)* warm the suspected liquid with mercurous nitrate; if leucine is present, metallic mercury is deposited. 2. *(for peptones)* mix phosphotungstic and hydrochloric acids; let the mixture stand twenty-four hours, and filter. With this reagent a solution containing peptones with no albumin will afford a precipitate.

**Hogben t.**, Xenopus t.

**Holmgren's t.**, the use of skeins of colored wool as a test of the perception of colors; a skein is given to the subject of the test, and he is asked to match it out of a set of variously colored skeins.

**Hoppe-Seyler t.**, 1. *(for carbon monoxide in the blood)* add to blood twice its volume of a solution of sodium hydroxide of 1.3 specific gravity: normal blood will form a dingy brown mass with a green shade if spread thin on a white surface; but if carbon monoxide is present, the mass is red, and so is the thin layer. 2. *(for xanthine)* add the substance to be tested to a mixture of chlorinated lime in a porcelain dish; a dark-green ring is formed at first.

**horse cell t.** *(for heterophil antibodies associated with infectious mononucleosis)*: a modification of the Paul-Bunnell-Davidsohn test that uses horse erythrocytes instead of sheep erythrocytes. No centrifugation step is needed and the whole test is performed in minutes. Called also *Monospot t.*

**Hotis t.** *(for mastitis in cows)*: fresh milk containing bromcresol purple is incubated for twenty-four hours; a positive reaction is the formation of yellow flakes on the sides of the test tube.

**Huddleson's t.**, an agglutination test for human brucellosis.

**Huhner t.**, examination of the secretions aspirated from the vaginal fornix and the endocervical canal after coitus, to determine the number and condition of spermatozoa present and the extent to which they have penetrated the cervical mucus.

**hydrochloric acid t.**, see specific tests, including *Leo's t.*, *Mohr's t.*, *Rabuteau's t.* (1,2), *Uffelmann's t.*, *Winckler's t.* (2), and *Witz's t.*

**hydrogen breath t.** *(for deficiency of lactase or other hydrolases, or colonic overgrowth of bacteria)*: a known quantity of carbohydrate is administered and the subject's exhalations are subsequently trapped and measured at timed intervals; patients unable to digest or absorb carbohydrates in the small intestine will have excess carbohydrates in the colon which are broken down there by bacterial fermentation, causing an increase of blood hydrogen and thus of hydrogen exhaled by the lungs.

**hydrogen peroxide t.** *(for blood)*: a 20 per cent solution of hydrogen peroxide is added to the suspected fluid; if blood is present even in minute proportion, bubbles will rise, forming foam on the surface of the fluid.

**hydrostatic t.**, floating of the lungs of a dead infant when placed in water indicates that the child was born alive; called also *Raygat's t.*

**hyperemia t.**, Moschcowitz t.

**hypochlorite-orcinol t.** *(for glycerol)*: to 3 mL of the unknown add 3 drops of N/1 sodium hypochlorite solution and boil one minute to drive off chlorine. Then add an equal volume of strong hydrochloric acid and a little orcinol. Boil, and a violet or greenish blue color indicates glycerol or a sugar, or some substance that can be oxidized to a sugar.

**hypothesis t.**, an abstract procedure for determining whether a set of observations is consistent with a hypothesis under consideration; it is the theoretical basis of most statistical tests. A hypothesis test decides between two hypotheses, one stating that the effect under investigation does not exist (the *null hypothesis*, $H_0$), and the other that some specified effect does exist (the *alternative hypothesis*, $H_a$ or $H_1$), based on the observed value of a test statistic whose sampling distribution is completely determined by $H_0$. When the test statistic falls in a set of values known as the critical region, $H_0$ is rejected. The level of probability of incorrectly rejecting $H_0$ may be set before the data are collected, usually at 0.05 or 0.01; this is called the *significance level* or *α level.* It is now more common to report the smallest $\alpha$ at which the null hypothesis can be rejected; this is called the *significance probability* or P value.

**hypoxanthine t.**, see *Kossel's t.*

**IFA t.**, indirect fluorescent antibody t; see *immunofluorescence.*

**immobilizaton t.**, detection of antibody based on its ability to inhibit the motility of a bacterial cell or protozoon.

**IMViC t.**, [modified acronym from *i*ndole, *m*ethyl red, *V*oges-Proskauer, *c*itrate] a series of metabolic tests used as standard procedure to differentiate genera of the Enterobacteriaceae. See also the individual tests.

**indican t.**, see specific tests, including *Jaffé's t.* (2) and *Weber's t.* (2).

**indirect fluorescent antibody t.**, see *immunofluorescence.*

**indole t.**, see specific tests, including *Nencki's t.*, *nitroso-indole-nitrate t.*, *pine wood t.*, and *Salkowski's t.* (3).

**inhalational challenge t.**, see under *challenge.*

**inkblot t.**, Rorschach t.

**intelligence t.**, a set of problems or tasks posed to assess an individual's innate ability to judge, comprehend, and reason.

**intracutaneous t.**, intradermal t.

**intracutaneous tuberculin t.**, a tuberculin test in which tuberculin is injected below the skin; see specific tests, including *Mantoux t.*, *Sterneedle tuberculin t.*, and *tine t.*

**intradermal t.**, a skin test in which the antigen is injected below the skin. Called also *intracutaneous t.*

**inulin clearance t.**, see under *inulin.*

**iodine t.**, 1. *(for starch)* when a compound solution of iodine is added to starch, and especially to an acid or neutral solution of cooked starch paste, a deep-blue color is produced which disappears on heating and reappears on cooling. Erythrodextrin and glycogen give a red color with iodine. 2. see specific tests, including *Winckler t.* (3).

**Iowa pressure articulation t.**, a test of the ability to produce the consonant sounds in isolated words, particularly the pressure sounds.

**irresistible impulse t.**, see under *impulse.*

**irrigation t.**, the patient is examined with the bladder full. The anterior urethra is washed out with a warm solution of boric acid (3 per cent), the perineum being compressed to prevent the entrance of the fluid into the posterior urethra. When the washings are perfectly clear, the patient voids his urine and any turbidity must come from the posterior urethra.

**Ishihara's t.**, a test for color vision made by the use of a series of pseudoisochromic plates composed of round dots of various sizes and colors.

**isopropanol precipitation t.** *(for unstable hemoglobins)*: a drop of blood is mixed with the nonpolar solvent isopropanol; most unstable hemoglobins precipitate more readily than other hemoglobins. Addition of potassium cyanide reduces false-positive results.

**Ivy's t.**, a bleeding time test in which incisions are made on the forearm, a sphygmomanometer is inflated around the upper arm, and the time until cessation of bleeding is recorded. Called also *Ivy's method.*

**Jacquemin's t.** *(for phenol)*: add to the suspected liquid an equal quantity of aniline and some sodium hypochlorite in solution; a blue color is produced.

**Jadassohn's t.,** irrigation t.

**Jaffe's t.,** 1. *(for creatinine)* to the liquid add trinitrophenol and then make alkaline with sodium hydroxide. A red color indicates presence of creatinine. 2. *(for indican)* to the suspected liquid are added an equal amount of concentrated hydrochloric acid, 1 mL of chloroform, and a few drops of a strong solution of chlorinated soda. The chloroform is colored blue if indican is present.

**Janet's t.** *(for differentiating between functional and organic anesthesia)*: the patient is instructed to say "yes" or "no," according as he does or does not feel the examiner's touch. He may say "no" in functional anesthesia, but he will say nothing in cases of organic anesthesia.

**Javorski's t., Jaworski's t.,** in hourglass stomach a splashing sound will be heard on succussion of the pyloric portion after siphonage.

**Jenning's t.,** a modification of Holmgren's test for color perception. Small patches of colored wool are placed so as to be protected from light and dust. The person to be examined indicates his color selection by pricking the record sheet with a pointed pencil.

**Jones and Cantarow t.,** urea concentration t.

**Jorissen's t.** *(for formaldehyde)*: add 0.5 mL of a 1 per cent solution of phloroglucin in 10 per cent sodium hydroxide to 1 mL of the urine; a bright red color indicates free formaldehyde.

**Kato t.,** a technique for the quantitative estimation of the worm burden of an individual, based on estimation of a standard 50-mg sample of fresh feces cleared with glycerine.

**Kentmann's t.** *(for formaldehyde)*: dissolve in a test tube 0.1 g of morphine in 1 mL of sulfuric acid; add, without mixing, an equal volume of the liquid to be tested; in a short time the latter will take on a reddish violet color if any formaldehyde is present.

**Kerner's t.** *(for creatinine)*: acidify the suspected solution and add phosphomolybdic or phosphotungstic acid in solution; if creatinine is present, it will form a crystalline precipitate.

**kidney function t.,** see specific tests, including *Fishberg concentration t., radioisotope renal excretion t., Rehberg's t., urea concentration t.,* and *D-xylose absorption* or *tolerance t.* Called also *renal function t.*

**Kjeldahl's t.** *(for nitrogen)*, see under *method.*

**Kleihauer t., Kleihauer-Betke t.,** acid elution t.

**Knapp's t.** *(for organic acids in stomach)*: stomach contents are filtered and 1 mL treated with 5 mL of ether; the extract is floated on dilute iron solution in test tubes, and the various colored rings formed will indicate the presence of the various acids.

**Knott t.,** a test for microfilariae or worm larvae in the blood by lysis of the blood in a dilute (2 per cent) formalin solution, centrifugation, and examination of the stained sediment for microfilariae or larvae.

**Kober t.** *(for estrogens)*: when estrogens are treated with a mixture of sulfuric acid and phenolsulfonic acid and then diluted with water, a clear pink color is formed; suitable for qualitative analysis.

**Kolmer t.,** a modification of the Wassermann test, introduced in 1922, or any of its subsequent improvements; these tests used complement fixation rather than flocculation as the indicator reaction and were once the standard confirmatory tests for syphilis; they are now little used.

**Kolmogorov-Smirnov t.,** a statistical test of goodness of fit of a sample to a specified theoretical distribution function, based on the size of the maximum difference between the cumulative distribution functions of the sample and theoretical distributions and using the exact sampling distribution of this difference to determine the significance level. The test can also be used to determine whether two samples are drawn from the same population by examining the maximum difference between the cumulative distribution functions of the two samples.

**Korotkoff's t.** *(for collateral circulation)*: in aneurysm, if the blood pressure in the peripheral circulation remains fairly high while the artery above the aneurysm is compressed, the collateral circulation is good.

**Kossel's t.** *(for hypoxanthine)*: the liquid to be tested is treated with zinc and hydrochloric acid and with sodium hydroxide in excess; if hypoxanthine is present, a ruby-red color is produced.

**Kruskal-Wallis t.,** a nonparametric test for ordinal data, comparing three or more groups simultaneously: all data are ranked numerically and then the rank values are summed and averaged for each group. If the null hypothesis that all groups are drawn from the same population is true, then the mean ranks should be similar across all groups.

**Kuhlmann's t.,** a modification of Binet's test for use in infants.

**Külz's t.** *(for β-hydroxybutyric acid)*: the fermented urine is evaporated to a syrupy consistency, strong sulfuric acid in equal volume is added, and the mixture is distilled. If hydroxybutyric acid is present, α-crotonic acid will be formed, which will crystallize. If, after fermentation, the urine shows dextrorotatory properties, β-hydroxybutyric acid is present.

**Kurzrok-Miller t.,** an *in vitro* test of compatibility of cervical mucus and spermatozoa, involving observation, under the microscope, of the behavior of sperm placed beside a sample of mucus taken from the cervical canal at the time of ovulation.

**Kveim t.** *(for sarcoidosis)*: a skin test using antigen from human sarcoid tissue injected intradermally; any palpable nodule developing at the inoculation site within 6 weeks is biopsied, and histopathologic evidence of epithelioid cell granulomas constitutes a positive reaction. The test is positive in about 60 to 80 per cent of patients.

**Lachman's t.,** an anterior drawer test for cases of severe knee injury, performed at 20 degrees of flexion.

**lactic acid t.,** see specific tests, including *MacLean t.,* and *Uffelmann's t.*

**Lancefield precipitation t.,** a ring precipitation test used to classify and identify streptococci. Group-specific antibody reacts *in vitro* with group-specific polysaccharide to produce a ring of precipitation where the two reagents react at the interface.

**Lang's t.** *(for taurine)*: the solution to be tested is boiled with freshly prepared mercuric oxide; taurine will cause a white precipitate to appear.

**Lange's t.** *(for acetone in urine)*: 15 mL of urine are mixed with 0.5 to 1 mL of acetic acid, and a few drops of a freshly prepared concentrated solution of sodium nitroprusside added. The mixture is overlaid with ammonia. At the point of junction a characteristic violet ring is formed.

**lantern t.,** a test for color blindness made with a set of specially devised lanterns.

**latex agglutination t.** *(for presence of antibody)*: a type of agglutination test in which antigen to a given antibody is adsorbed to latex particles and mixed with a solution to observe for agglutination of the latex. Called also *latex fixation t.*

**latex fixation t.,** latex agglutination t.

**Lee's t.** *(for rennin)*: add 5 drops of gastric juice to 5 mL of milk; coagulation should take place in 20 minutes in the incubator.

**leishmanin t.,** intradermal injection of leishmanin (leishmania promastigote antigens); a positive reaction consists of a palpable nodule developing in 48 to 72 hours and indicates delayed hypersensitivity, but not necessarily immunity, to leishmania organisms. The test is not species-specific. It becomes positive early in the course of cutaneous or mucocutaneous leishmaniasis, particularly the New World forms, except in diffuse cutaneous leishmaniasis; it becomes positive only after recovery from visceral leishmaniasis. Called also *Montenegro t.*

**Leo's t.** *(for free hydrochloric acid)*: calcium carbonate is added to the solution, which is neutralized if the acidity is due to free acid, but not if due to acid salts.

**lepromin t.,** intradermal injection of lepromin (a suspension of heat-killed *Mycobacterium leprae*); a positive reaction consists of a tuberculin-type reaction at 48 to 72 hours *(Fernandez reaction)* or a nodular, occasionally ulcerated, lesion at 3 to 4 weeks *(Mitsuda reaction).* The test is not diagnostic; a large fraction of the normal population exhibits lepromin reactivity owing to sensitivity to cross-reacting antigens. In individuals known to have leprosy, lepromin reactivity is indicative of tuberculoid leprosy or borderline leprosy near the tuberculoid end of the spectrum, whereas lepromin anergy is indicative of lepromatous or near-lepromatous disease.

**Lewis and Pickering t.** *(for peripheral circulation)*: vasodilation of a part is produced by warming it and applying a sphygmomanometer cuff; return of blood to the part is assessed when the cuff is released.

**Lichtheim t.** *(for aphasia)*: if a patient is able to indicate the number of syllables in a word which he cannot utter, it indicates that the cortex is less involved than the association fibers.

**Liebermann-Burchard t.** *(for cholesterol)*: dissolve the sample in chloroform and add acetic anhydride plus concentrated sulfuric acid; cholesterol can be quantitated by the intensity of the resulting blue-green color.

**Liebig's t.** *(for cystine)*: boil the suspected substance with a sodium hydroxide solution and a little lead sulfide; if cystine is present, the lead sulfide will form a black precipitate.

**likelihood ratio t.,** in statistics, a test using the ratio of the maximum value of the likelihood function from one statistical model to that from another model, a smaller ratio indicating a stronger relationship between the variables.

**limulus t.,** an extract of blood cells from the horseshoe crab *(Limulus polyphemus)* is exposed to a blood sample from a patient; if gram-negative endotoxin is present in the sample, it will produce gelation of the extract of blood cells.

**Lindemann's t.** *(for acetoacetic acid in urine)*: to about 10 mL of urine add 5 drops of 30 per cent acetic acid, 5 drops strong iodine solution, and 2 to 3 mL chloroform, and shake. The chloroform does not change color if diacetic acid is present, but becomes reddish violet in its absence. Uric acid also decolorizes iodine, and if much is present, double the amount of strong iodine solution should be used.

**Linder's t.,** see under *sign.*
**lipase t.,** 1. *(for liver function and pancreatic inflammation)* liver or pancreas injury causes a rise in the level of lipase in the blood plasma as measured by the power of the blood to split ethyl butyrate. 2. see specific tests, including *litmus milk t.*
**litmus milk t.** *(for pancreatic lipase)*: add pancreatic lipase to litmus milk, incubate, and note change of color; pancreatic lipase is indicated by a pink coloration.
**liver function t.,** see specific tests, including *fructose tolerance t., lipase t.* (1), *Macdonald's t., phenoltetrachlorophthalein t., Quick's t.* (1), *rose bengal t.*
**log-rank t.,** a statistical test used to test the null hypothesis that two groups have the same distribution of survival by analyzing and comparing the number of observed and expected deaths for each group each time a death occurs in either group.
**Lombard's t.,** a test for simulated deafness using a noise maker.
**Lücke's t.** *(for hippuric acid)*: add boiling hot nitric acid, evaporate, and heat the dry residue; a strong odor of nitrobenzene proves the presence of hippuric acid.
**Lundh t.,** a test for pancreatic function in which the trypsin concentration in duodenal aspirates is measured over several hours following a liquid test meal containing protein, fat, and sugar; a decrease in trypsin concentration indicates abnormally low pancreatic secretion.
**lupus band t.,** an immunofluorescence test to determine the presence and extent of immunoglobulin and complement deposits at the dermal-epidermal junction of skin specimens from patients with systemic lupus erythematosus.
**lymphocyte proliferation t.,** a functional test of the ability of lymphocytes to respond to mitogens, specific antigens, or allogenic cells. Lymphocytes are cultured both with and without the stimulant for several days and then are cultured for several hours with $^3$H-labeled thymidine. The ratio of the thymidine uptake in the stimulated and control cultures is reported as the "stimulation index" (SI) or "stimulation ratio" (SR). The test with allogenic cells, called a mixed lymphocyte culture (MLC), is commonly performed for transplantation tissue typing; all three types of stimulants are used in investigation of immunodeficiency. Commonly used mitogens are phytohemagglutinin (PHA), concanavalin A (ConA), and pokeweed mitogen (PWM); commonly used antigens are PPD (tuberculin), *Candida* antigen, and streptokinase-streptodornase. Called also *blastogenesis assay* and *lymphocyte proliferation assay.*
**Macdonald's t.** *(for liver function)*: inject 2 mg/kg of sodium sulfobromophthalein (Bromsulphalein) and take blood specimens every five minutes for thirty minutes after the injection; of historic interest.
**Machado t., Machado-Guerreiro t.** *(for Chagas' disease)*: a complement-fixation test, using as antigen an extract of the spleen of puppies severely infected with *Trypanosoma cruzi.*
**MacLean t.** *(for lactic acid in gastric juice)*: to 5 mL of gastric juice add 5 drops of the following reagent: ferric chloride, 5 g; concentrated hydrochloric acid, 1.5 mL; saturated solution of mercury bichloride, 100 mL. Lactic acid is indicated by a yellow coloration.
**MacLean-de Wesselow t.,** urea concentration t.
**McMurray's t.** *(for torn meniscus)*: as the patient lies supine with knee fully flexed, the examiner rotates the patient's foot fully outward and the knee is slowly extended; a painful "click" indicates a tear of the medial meniscus of the knee joint. If the click occurs when the foot is rotated inward, the tear is in the lateral meniscus.
**McNemar t.,** a modified chi-squared test performed on data with one degree of freedom to compare findings in a matched analysis or in a before and after study on the same individual.
**MacWilliam's t.** *(for albumin)*: take 20 mL of urine and add 2 drops of a saturated solution of sulfosalicylic acid: if albumin is present, a cloudiness or precipitate will be seen; if other proteolytic digestion products are present, this precipitate will disappear on boiling, but appear again on cooling.
**Magpie's t.** *(for salts of mercury)*: stannous chloride is added to the suspected solution; a white and gray precipitate is formed, consisting of metallic mercury and mild calomel.
**maintenance of wakefulness t.,** MWT; measurement of the length of time for which an individual can remain awake in a dark, quiet room; used as a measure of physiological sleepiness.
**male frog t., male toad t.** *(for pregnancy)*: urine or serum of a woman suspected of being pregnant is injected into the dorsal lymph sac of two male frogs *(Rana pipiens)* or male toads *(Bufo marinus)*. The presence of spermatozoa in the cloacal fluid of both animals is positive; in one animal, inconclusive; in neither animal, negative.
**mallein t.,** see *mallein.*
**Malot's t.,** a test for the quantitative determination of phosphoric acid in urine by the reaction with cochineal and a uranium salt.
**Mann-Whitney t., Mann-Whitney *U* t., Mann-Whitney-Wilcoxon t.,** rank sum t.
**Mantoux t.,** a type of intracutaneous tuberculin test; 0.1 mL of PPD containing 5 TU is administered intradermally, usually to the forearm; the size of the area of any induration on the second or third day, combined with risk factors, is used to determine whether exposure to or infection with *Mycobacterium tuberculosis* or a related organism has occurred.
**manual muscle t.,** a test of muscle function in which the therapist manually puts the patient's body part through a range of motion and records the extent of function and limitations.
**Marlow's t.** *(for heterophoria)*: one eye is occluded by a bandage for some time; after the bandage is removed, measurements for heterophoria are made.
**Master "2-step" exercise t.** *(for coronary insufficiency)*: an early exercise test in which a patient stepped on and off a set of two stairs for a number of trips standardized for age, weight, and sex, with electrocardiograms recorded immediately after test cessation. It has been supplanted by graded exercise tests that can induce higher levels of stress.
**Matas' t.** *(for collateral circulation)*: after hyperemia of the limb has been induced with a tourniquet, the tourniquet is removed and the extent of collateral circulation is determined by compressing the main artery. Called also *tourniquet t.*
**maximal exercise t.,** an exercise test that continues until the maximum capability of the subject to exercise has been reached; the endpoint is usually subjective fatigue, shortness of breath, or chest pain.
**Mayer's t.** *(for alkaloids)*: mercury bichloride, $13\frac{1}{2}$ g, and potassium iodide, 50 g, are dissolved in 1000 mL of water; this is used as a test for alkaloid, with which it gives a white precipitate.
**Mayerhofer's t.,** the reduction of a decinormal solution of potassium permanganate solution by 1 mL of spinal fluid in an acid medium as an index of the amount of protein substance present in the fluid; used as an indication of the existence of tuberculous meningitis.
**Mazzotti t.** *(for onchocerciasis)*: a small dose of diethylcarbamazine is administered orally; the death of microfilariae in the skin causes an intensely pruritic rash within 20 minutes to 24 hours.
**MEGX t.,** monoethylglycinexylidide t.
**Meigs' t.** *(for fat in milk)*: to 10 mL of milk in a special apparatus add 20 mL of water, 20 mL of ethyl ether, and shake. Then add 20 mL of 95 per cent alcohol. Remove the ethereal layer, evaporate, and weigh.
**melanin t.,** see *Thormählen's t.*
**Mendel's t.,** Mantoux t.
**mercury t.,** see specific tests, including *Magpie's t., Reinsch's t.,* and *Vogel and Lee's t.*
**methyl red t.** *(for differentiation of Enterobacteriaceae)*: the organism is inoculated into a buffered glucose-peptone broth containing methyl red. In a positive reaction, the medium remains red after incubation owing to acid metabolic products. Most Enterobacteriaceae are positive; the Klebsielleae are negative and Erwinieae are variable.
**Mett's (Mette's) t.** *(for estimating pepsin)*: tubes (Mett's tubes) of coagulated albumin are introduced into the unknown and into a standard pepsin hydrochloric acid mixture and the amount of digestion occurring in a given time is noted.
**metyrapone t.** *(for Cushing's syndrome)*: plasma 11-deoxycortisol or urinary 17-hydroxycorticosteroids are measured after the administration of metyrapone; levels are increased in patients with Cushing's disease but not in patients with ectopic ACTH syndrome.
**microprecipitation t.,** a precipitin test in which a minute quantity of the serum is employed.
**MIF t.,** migration inhibitory factor t.
**migration inhibitory factor t.,** MIF t.; an *in vitro* test for the production of MIF by lymphocytes in response to specific antigens; used for evaluation of cell-mediated immunity. MIF production is absent in certain immunodeficiency disorders, such as DiGeorge syndrome, Wiskott-Aldrich syndrome, and Hodgkin's disease.
**milk ring t.,** abortus Bang ring t.
**Miller-Kurzrok t.,** a laboratory procedure to test the ability of sperm to penetrate the mucus plug in a woman's cervix.
**40 millimeter t.** *(for athletic efficiency)*: the subject sits with nasal respiration occluded with a clamp, and by expiring through a mouthpiece, sustains a column of mercury at the height of 40 mm as long as he can. The pulse rate is taken meanwhile, every five seconds. In a satisfactory test the pulse rate is unaltered for a minute or more.
**Millon's t.** *(for proteins and nitrogenous compounds)*: a solution is made of 10 g of mercury and 20 g of nitric acid; this is diluted with an equal volume of water and decanted after standing 24 hours. This reagent gives a red color with proteins and other substances, such as tyrosine, phenol, and thymol, which contain the hydroxyphenyl group.
**Mills' t.** *(for tennis elbow)*: with the wrist and fingers fully flexed and the forearm pronated, complete extension of the elbow is painful.
**Mitsuda t.,** lepromin t.
**Mittelmeyer's t.,** the patient tries to march in place with eyes closed; in vestibular disorder he will turn to the side ipsilateral to vestibular loss, or contralateral to vestibular excitation.

**mixed lymphocyte culture t.**, see under *culture*, and see *lymphocyte proliferation t.*

**Mohr's t.** *(for hydrochloric acid in the stomach contents)*: dilute to a light-yellow color a solution of iron acetate, free from alkaline acetates; add a few drops of a solution of potassium thiocyanate, and then the filtered contents of the stomach: if they contain the acid, a red coloring ensues, which is destroyed by sodium acetate.

**Molisch's t.**, 1. *(for glucose in urine)* add 2 mL of urine, 2 drops of a 15 per cent solution of thymol, and an equal volume of strong sulfuric acid; a deep red color results. Called also *Molisch's reaction.* 2. *(for glucose in urine)* to 1 mL of urine add 2 or 3 drops of a 5 per cent solution of α-naphthol in alcohol, then add 2 mL of strong sulfuric acid; a deep violet color is produced, and a violet precipitate follows if water is added. 3. *(for proteins)* the substance is treated with a 15 per cent alcoholic solution of α-naphthol and then with concentrated sulfuric acid; a violet color is formed if proteins are present. Called also *Molisch's reaction;* defs. 2 and 3 called also *alpha-naphthol reaction.*

**Moloney t.** *(for delayed sensitivity to diphtheria toxoid)*: 0.1 mL of 1:10 dilution of fluid toxoid is injected intradermally on the flexor surface of the forearm; the appearance in 12 to 24 hours of an area of redness with induration of more than 12 mm in diameter is a positive reaction.

**monaural loudness balance (MLB) t.**, a test to determine recruitment in bilateral sensorineural deafness; the loudness sensation at impaired frequencies is compared with that at normal frequencies.

**monoethylglycinexylidide t.** *(for liver function)*: MEGX test; the plasma concentration of monoethylglycinexylidide (MEGX) is measured 15 or 30 minutes after the intravenous injection of lidocaine; MEGX levels are reduced in impaired liver function.

**Monospot t.**, horse cell t.

**Montenegro t.**, leishmanin t.

**Morelli's t.** *(to differentiate between an exudate and a transudate)*: add a few drops of the suspected fluid to a saturated solution of mercury bichloride in a test tube; a flaky precipitate indicates a transudate, a clot indicates an exudate.

**Mörner's t.**, 1. *(for tyrosine)* to a small quantity of the crystals in a test tube add a few mL of Mörner's reagent (solution of formaldehyde, 1 mL; distilled water, 45 mL; concentrated sulfuric acid, 55 mL). Heat gently to the boiling point. A green color shows the presence of tyrosine. 2. see *nitroprusside t.* (1).

**Morton's t.**, in metatarsalgia, transverse pressure across the heads of the metatarsals causes a sharp pain, especially between the second and third metatarsals.

**Moschcowitz t.** *(for arteriosclerosis)*: the lower limb is rendered bloodless by means of an Esmarch bandage, which is removed after five minutes; in a normal limb the color returns in a few seconds, but in an arteriosclerotic one color returns more slowly. Called also *hyperemia t.*

**Moynihan's t.** *(for hourglass stomach)*: the two parts of a Seidlitz powder are given separately; in hourglass stomach two separated protrusions on the abdominal wall can be observed; of historic interest.

**multiple-puncture t.**, a skin test in which the material used (e.g., tuberculin) is introduced into the skin by pressure of several needles or pointed tines or prongs. See also *tine t.* and *Sterneedle tuberculin t.*

**multiple sleep latency t.**, MSLT; measurement of the speed at which an individual falls asleep when given multiple opportunities to sleep throughout the day and instructed not to resist doing so; used as a measure of physiological sleepiness.

**mumps skin t.** *(for immunity to mumps)*: an unreliable and little used test consisting of intradermal injection of killed mumps virus, a positive response being development of a tuberculin-type delayed hypersensitivity reaction.

**murexide t.**, Weidel's t. (1).

**Murphy's t.**, the patient sits with his arms folded in front of him; the examiner's thumb is placed under the twelfth rib and short jabbing movements are made. Thus deep-seated tenderness and muscular rigidity are determined. Called also *Murphy's kidney punch.*

**Naffziger's t.** *(for nerve root compression)*: increase or aggravation of pain or sensory disturbance over the distribution of the involved nerve root upon manual compression of the jugular veins bilaterally confirms the presence of an extruded intervertebral disk or other mass.

**Nagel's t.**, a test for color vision in which one half of the field of an anomaloscope is illuminated with standard yellow and the other half is matched to the yellow by the subject who mixes red and green.

**Nagler's t.**, see under *reaction.*

**NBT t.**, nitroblue tetrazolium t.

**Nencki's t.** *(for indole)*: treat the suspected material with nitric acid and a little nitrous acid; a red color follows, and in concentrated solution a red precipitate may appear.

**neostigmine t.** *(for myasthenia gravis)*: used in children, and in adults suspected of having myasthenia gravis but with a negative Tensilon test; neostigmine methylsulfate mixed with atropine sulfate is injected intramuscularly; lessening of myasthenic symptoms is indicative of the disease. Called also *Prostigmine t.*

**Nessler's t.** *(for free ammonia)*, see under *reagent.*

**Neubauer and Fischer's t.**, glycyltryptophan t.

**Neufeld's t.**, see under *reaction.*

**neutralization t.**, a test for the power of an antiserum or other substance to antagonize the pathogenic properties of a microorganism, toxin, virus, bacteriophage, or toxic substance.

**niacin t.** *(for* Mycobacterium tuberculosis*)*: either of two tests to distinguish strains of *M. tuberculosis* by adding aniline, ethanol, and cyanogen bromide to a culture; this will turn human *M. tuberculosis* yellow because of its niacin content.

**Nickerson-Kveim t.**, Kveim t.

**Ninhydrin t.**, triketohydrindene hydrate test.

**nitrate reduction t.** *(for the reduction of nitrate to nitrite by a bacterial culture)*: the organism is cultured in a broth containing nitrate. The medium is tested for nitrite by mixing with solutions containing sulfanilic acid and alpha-naphthylamine in 5 N acetic acid; a red color indicates the presence of nitrite. The test is useful in identifying doubtful strains of Enterobacteriaceae, mycobacteria, and certain aerobic bacteria.

**nitrites t.**, 1. *(for nitrites in saliva)*: to the saliva add 1 or 2 drops of sulfuric acid, a few drops of potassium iodide solution, and some starch paste; a blue color indicates nitrites. 2. a test for the presence of nitrites in any fluid; see specific tests, including *Griess t., nitrate reduction t.,* and *Schaffer's t.*

**nitroblue tetrazolium t. (NBT t.)**, a test of neutrophil microbicidal function; neutrophils are incubated with latex particles and nitroblue tetrazolium (NBT). Normally phagocytosis of the particles is accompanied by reduction of NBT to a blue formazan pigment; absence of NBT reduction indicates a defect in some of the metabolic pathways involved in intracellular microbial killing, as seen in chronic granulomatous disease.

**nitrogen washout t.** *(for functional residual capacity of lungs)*: with the patient inhaling pure oxygen, the concentration of exhaled nitrogen is obtained for each breath until it falls below 1 per cent of the gas being exhaled (usually about seven minutes' time); the total volume of nitrogen that has been exhaled at this point is assumed to be 0.8 of the functional residual capacity.

**nitrogen washout t., single breath**, the patient inhales a vital capacity's volume of pure oxygen and then slowly exhales. The nitrogen concentration of the exhaled gas is measured over the entire breath and a curve is generated; different parts of the curve represent nitrogen concentrations of gas in different components of the vital capacity, and can be analyzed for uniformity of ventilation and determination of anatomic dead space and closing volume. Called also *single breath t.* and *single breath oxygen t.*

**nitroprusside t.**, 1. *(for cysteine)* if a protein containing cysteine is dissolved in water and 2 to 4 drops of a 4 or 5 per cent solution of sodium nitroprusside and then a few drops of ammonia are added, a deep purple-red color appears; called also *Mörner's t.* 2. *(for creatinine)* see *Weyl's t.* (1).

**nitroso-indole-nitrate t.** *(for indole and skatole)*: acidify the unknown with nitric acid and add a few drops of potassium nitrite; a red color or a red precipitate indicates indole, a white turbidity indicates skatole.

**nocturnal penile tumescence t. (NPT t.)**, monitoring of erections occurring during sleep; in the differential diagnosis of psychogenic and organic impotence, the former is generally associated with the presence of normal patterns of nocturnal erection while the latter is not.

**nonparametric t.**, one using nonparametric statistics, such as the rank sum test or signed rank test; nonparametric tests are often less powerful than parametric tests but are valid in cases where parametric tests are not.

**nonstress t. (NST)**, the monitoring of the response of the fetal heart rate to fetal movements by cardiotocography; a reactive (normal) test consists of two or more fetal movements occurring within 20 minutes accompanied by acceleration of the fetal heart rate by at least 15 beats per minute for at least 15 seconds with a long-term variability of at least 10 beats per minute.

**nontreponemal antigen t.**, see *serologic t. for syphilis.*

**Northern blot t.**, see under *technique.*

**NPT t.**, nocturnal penile tumescence t.

**nystagmus t.**, caloric t.

**Oakley-Fulthorpe t.**, see under *technique.*

**Ober's t.**, the patient lies on the side opposite that to be tested, with the underneath hip and knee flexed; with the upper knee flexed to a right angle, the upper hip is flexed to 90 degrees, fully abducted, brought into full hyperextension, and allowed to adduct; the angle that the thigh makes above the horizontal is the degree of abduction contracture.

**occult blood t.**, see specific tests, including *guaiac t.*, and *Hemoccult.*

**one-tailed t.**, a hypothesis test (q.v.) in which the critical region is one tail of the distribution of the test statistic and the null hypothesis is tested against a one-sided alternative that includes deviations from the null hypothesis only in one direction, deviations in the other direction being of no consequence.

**ONPG t.** *(for β-galactosidase in bacteria)*: the organism is grown in a buffered peptone medium containing D-nitrophenyl-β-D-galactopyranoside (ONPG): production of β-galactosidase is indicated by the appearance of a yellow color. Used to differentiate *Salmonella* (positive) from *Arizona* (negative), and *Neisseria lactamicus* (positive) from *N. meningitidis* (negative).

**opticokinetic drum t., optokinetic t., optokinetic drum t.,** a test of vision using a rotating drum or other figure painted with vertical black and white stripes; because the eye involuntarily follows such a figure, it is used in the differential diagnosis of psychogenic blindness, to detect the presence of vision in infants, and is also used in checking the normality of opticokinetic nystagmus.

**orcinol t.** *(for pentose in urine)*, see *Bial's t.*

**organic acid t.,** see *Knapp's t.*

**orientation t.,** see if patient can give correctly the time of day, the day of the week, month, and year, and the place.

**osmotic fragility t.** *(for spherocytosis)*: heparinized or defibrinated blood is placed in tubes of sodium chloride solution (pH 7.4) varying in concentration from 0.85 to 0.00 per cent (w/v); the amount of hemolysis in each tube is determined colorimetrically. Increased fragility indicates spherocytosis.

**Osterberg's t.** *(for β-hydroxybutyric acid)*: to 800 mg of ammonium sulfate add 0.15 mL of concentrated ammonium hydroxide solution, 2 drops of a 5 per cent solution of nitroprusside, and 1 mL of the urine. Dilute to 50 mL and compare with a standard.

**Ouchterlony t.,** double diffusion in two dimensions; see under *diffusion.*

**Oudin t.,** see under *technique.*

**ovarian hyperemia t.** *(for pregnancy)*: the intraperitoneal injection of urine or blood serum of pregnant women into immature female mice produces a reddened appearance of the ovaries.

**oxytocin challenge t. (OCT),** a contraction stress test in which uterine contractions are stimulated by intravenous infusion of oxytocin.

**Pachon's t.** *(for collateral circulation)*: measuring of the blood pressure in cases of aneurysm to determine the state of the collateral circulation.

**Paget's t.,** a solid tumor is most hard in its center, whereas a cyst is least hard in its center.

**pancreatic function t.,** see specific tests, including *litmus milk t., Sahli-Nencki t., secretin t.*

**Pap t., Papanicolaou t.,** an exfoliative cytological staining procedure for the detection and diagnosis of various conditions, particularly malignant and premalignant conditions of the female genital tract (cancer of the vagina, cervix, and endometrium), in which cells which have been desquamated from the genital epithelium are obtained by smears, fixed and stained, and examined under the microscope for evidence of pathologic changes. Each examination should have an individual histological description. The test is also used in detecting human papillomavirus infection, in evaluating endocrine function, and in the diagnosis of malignancies of other organs, as of the respiratory tract and lungs, gastrointestinal tract, urinary tract, and breast. Called also *Pap* or *Papanicolaou smear* and *smear t.* See also *Papanicolaou's stain,* under *stain.*

**parametric t.,** one using parametric statistics, i.e., one that depends upon assumptions about the distribution of the data.

**partial thromboplastin time t.,** see under *time.*

**passive cutaneous anaphylaxis t.,** see *passive cutaneous anaphylaxis,* under *anaphylaxis.*

**passive protection t.,** a test in which antiserum is tested for protective antibody by parenteral inoculation of groups of animals with graded doses in constant volume.

**passive transfer t.,** see *Prausnitz-Küstner reaction,* under *reaction.*

**patch t's,** skin tests, used primarily in the diagnosis of allergies, in which small pieces of gauze or filter paper impregnated with suspected allergens are applied to the skin for fixed time periods; swelling or redness constitutes a positive reaction.

**Patrick's t.,** with the patient supine, the thigh and knee are flexed and the external malleolus is placed over the patella of the opposite leg; the knee is depressed, and if pain is produced thereby arthritis of the hip is indicated. Patrick called this test *fabere sign,* from the initial letters of movements that are necessary to elicit it, namely, flexion, abduction, external rotation, extension.

**Paul-Bunnell t.** *(for heterophil antibodies associated with infectious mononucleosis)*: determination of the highest dilution of the patient's serum capable of agglutinating sheep red blood cells.

**Paul-Bunnell-Davidsohn t.** *(for heterophil antibodies associated with infectious mononucleosis)*: a modification of the Paul-Bunnell test that differentiates among three types of heterophile sheep erythrocyte agglutinins: those associated with infectious mononucleosis, those associated with serum sickness, and natural antibodies against Forssman antigen. The patient's serum is absorbed with guinea pig kidney cells or with beef erythrocytes and centrifuged. Unabsorbed serum has a high heterophile antibody titer in infectious mononucleosis and serum sickness; a low titer is seen in normal individuals. Absorption with guinea pig kidney removes Forssman antibody and serum sickness heterophile antibody. Absorption with beef erythrocytes removes heterophile antibody associated with infectious mononucleosis or serum sickness. Called also *Davidsohn differential absorption t.*

**PCA t.,** see *passive cutaneous anaphylaxis.*

**peptide t.,** see *triketohydrindene hydrate t.*

**peptone t.,** see specific tests, including *Hofmeister's t.* (2) and *triketohydrindene hydrate t.*

**perchlorate discharge t.,** a thyroid function test; one to two hours after administration of radioiodine, perchlorate is administered to block further iodine uptake and flush from the thyroid gland any that has not bound to thyroid proteins. In euthyroid patients only trace amounts will be flushed out; the discharge of significant amounts indicates a defect in thyroid iodine binding.

**performance t.,** an intelligence test in which the subject is required to carry out certain actions rather than to answer questions.

**Peria's t.** *(for tyrosine)*, see *Piria's t.*

**Perls' t.,** a test for hemosiderin made by treating the substance with hydrochloric acid and potassium ferrocyanide; the Prussian blue reaction is produced if hemosiderin is present.

**permanganate t.,** see *Weisz's t.*

**peroxidase t.,** see *Goodpasture's stain,* under *stain.*

**Perthes' t.** *(for collateral circulation in patients with varicose veins)*: a bandage is applied just below the knee and the patient walks around with it on; varicose veins of the leg will become evacuated from continuous compression if there is sufficient collateral circulation in the deep veins. Called also *tourniquet t.*

**phenacetin t.** *(in urine)*: to the urine add a little concentrated hydrochloric acid, a little 1 per cent solution of sodium nitrate, and a little alkaline α-naphthol solution; make alkaline and a red color indicates phenacetin.

**phenol t.,** see specific tests, including *Jacquemin's t.* and *Plugge's t.*

**phenolphthalein t.,** 1. *(for blood)* boil a thin fecal suspension, cool, and add it to half as much reagent (made by dissolving 1 to 2 g of phenolphthalein and 25 g of potassium hydroxide in water). Add 10 g of metallic zinc and heat until decolorized. A pink color indicates the presence of blood. 2. *(in urine)* make the urine alkaline; a red color indicates phenolphthalein.

**phenoltetrachlorophthalein t.** *(for liver function)*: phenoltetrachlorophthalein is injected intravenously, and normally it appears in the feces, being excreted by the liver with the bile, and giving a bright color to the feces. A decrease in the normal excretion of this substance points to liver injury.

**pinch t.** *(for hand dexterity)*: a test measuring any of the various pinches of the hand.

**pineapple t.** *(for butyric acid in stomach)*: a few drops of sulfuric acid and alcohol are added to a dried ether extract of the gastric juice; if butyric acid is present, an odor of pineapple will be given off, caused by the formation of ethylbutyrate.

**pine wood t.** *(for indole)*: a pine splinter moistened with concentrated hydrochloric acid is turned cherry red by a solution of indole.

**Piria's t.** *(for tyrosine)*: moisten the suspected material with strong sulfuric acid and warm it; then dilute and warm it again; neutralize it with barium carbonate, filter, and add ferric chloride in dilute solution: if tyrosine is present, a violet color is seen, which is destroyed by an excess of ferric chloride.

**Pirquet t.,** a formerly much used tuberculin test in which the tuberculin is applied by scarification; called also *Pirquet reaction.*

**pivot shift t.,** see under *phenomenon.*

**P-K t.,** see *Prausnitz-Küstner reaction,* under *reaction.*

**plantar ischemia t.** *(for circulatory disturbances in legs and feet)*: the elevated leg is alternately flexed and extended and the plantar surface of the patient's foot is checked for blanching.

**Plugge's t.** *(for phenol)*: a dilute solution containing phenol becomes red on mixture with a mercuric nitrate solution containing a trace of nitrous acid; mercury is also precipitated and the odor of salicylol is given off.

**pointing t.,** see *Bárány's pointing t.*

**Politzer's t.,** see under *method.*

**porphobilinogen t.,** a test for the presence of porphobilinogen; see *Watson-Schwartz t.*

**Porteus maze t.,** a performance test in which the subject is required to trace with a pencil through printed mazes of increasing difficulty.

**posterior drawer t.,** see *drawer t's.*

**Prausnitz-Küstner t.,** see under *reaction.*

**precipitin t.,** any serologic test based on a precipitin reaction (q.v.).

**pregnancy t.,** see specific tests, including *early pregnancy t., male frog* or *male toad t., ovarian hyperemia t.,* Xenopus *t.*

**Preyer's t.,** a spectroscopic test for carbon monoxide in the blood.

**Proetz t.** *(for acuity of sense of smell)*: use of a series of substances each in 10 different concentrations in a liter of petroleum of specific gravity 0.880, to determine the least concentration at which the substance can be recognized, termed *olfactory coefficient* or *minimal identifiable odor.*

**projective t.**, any of various tests in which an individual interprets ambiguous stimulus situations, e.g., a series of inkblots (Rorschach t.), according to his own unconscious dispositions, thus yielding information about his personality structure, its underlying dynamics, and possible psychopathology.

**Prostigmine t.**, neostigmine t.

**protection t.**, serum neutralization t.

**protein t.**, see specific tests, including *biuret reaction, Gies' biuret t., Grigg's t., Reichl's t., Schulte's t., sulfur t.*, and *triketohydrindene hydrate t.*

**protein-bound iodine t.**, a formerly common thyroid function test in which the amount of iodine firmly bound to protein in the serum was determined by precipitating the proteins, yielding an estimate of serum thyroid hormone concentration. Errors were introduced if iodine compounds from nonthyroid sources were present.

**proteose t.**, proteose does not coagulate on boiling, but gives a ring test with trichloracetic acid.

**prothrombin t.**, a test for prothrombin; see *prothrombin time*, under *time.*

**prothrombin t., one-stage,** prothrombin time; see under *time.*

**prothrombin t., two-stage,** a method of quantitating prothrombin after tissue thromboplastin and excess factor V have converted it to thrombin, by determining the clotting time of a standard fibrinogen solution to which the previously generated thrombin has been added. Called also *two-stage prothrombin time test.*

**prothrombin consumption t.**, a test formerly much used to measure the formation of intrinsic thromboplastin by determining the residual serum prothrombin after the completion of blood coagulation.

**prothrombin-proconvertin t.**, a test formerly used in the control of coumarin-type anticoagulants, employing a saline extract of brain as a thromboplastin and requiring presence of excess blood coagulation factor V.

**prothrombin time t.**, prothrombin time.

**prothrombin time t., one-stage,** prothrombin time; see under *time.*

**prothrombin time t., two-stage,** two-stage prothrombin t.

**provocative t.**, challenge (def. 3).

**psychological t.**, any test to measure a subject's development, achievement, personality, intelligence, thought processes, etc.

**psychomotor t.**, a test that assesses the subject's ability to perceive instructions and perform motor responses, often including measurement of the speed of the reaction.

**pulmonary function t.**, any of numerous tests that measure aspects of the respiratory system in order to assess functional state and presence or nature of any disease process. Factors evaluated include lung mechanics (capacities, flow rates, and volumes), gas exchange, pulmonary blood flow, blood gases, and pH of blood.

**pulp t.**, a diagnostic test to determine tooth pulp vitality or abnormality, usually by means of electric pulp testers or by application of a hot or cold stimulus.

**Queckenstedt's t.**, see under *sign.*

**quellung t.**, see *Neufeld's reaction*, under *reaction.*

**Quick's t.**, 1. *(for liver function)*: a test based on excretion of hippuric acid following the administration of sodium benzoate. 2. prothrombin time; see under *time.*

**Rabuteau's t.**, 1. *(for hydrochloric acid in urine)* add a little indigosulfonic acid to color the urine, and sulfurous acid to decompose what hydrochloric acid may be present; the urine will be decolorized. 2. *(for hydrochloric acid in stomach contents)* 1 g of potassium iodate and 0.5 g of potassium iodide are added to 50 mL of starch mucilage; filtered stomach liquids are added to it; free hydrochloric acid will render the mixture blue.

**radioactive iodine uptake t.**, one of the most common thyroid function tests; a known quantity of radioiodine is administered and 24 hours later the per cent is calculated that has been absorbed by the thyroid gland. Patients who have recently been exposed to iodine compounds, such as in dietary supplements, contrast media, medications, or antiseptics, may not be good candidates for this test.

**radioallergosorbent t. (RAST),** a test used to measure specific IgE antibodies in serum. Allergen extract is coupled to a solid matrix (paper, cellulose particles); this immunosorbent is reacted with serum and washed and then reacted with radiolabeled anti–human IgE antibody and washed. Uptake of the labeled antibody is proportional to the level of specific serum IgE antibodies to the allergen. RAST is used as an alternative to skin tests to determine sensitivity to suspected allergens.

**radioiodine uptake t.**, radioactive iodine uptake t.

**radioimmunosorbent t. (RIST),** a highly sensitive radioimmunoassay for measuring the total IgE antibody concentration in serum; the serum sample is reacted with radiolabeled IgE and anti–human IgE antibody coupled to an insoluble support. The amount of labeled IgE remaining bound to the immunosorbent varies inversely with the amount of (unlabeled) IgE present in the sample.

**radioisotope renal excretion t.** *(for study of renal function)*: radioisotopic material diluted with saline is rapidly injected into a well-hydrated patient; urine collected by an indwelling urethral catheter or a ureteral catheter previously inserted into the kidney is examined at known intervals and the radioactivity of each specimen is determined and recorded.

**Ramon flocculation t.**, to a series of tubes containing a constant amount of toxin, e.g., diphtheria toxin, antitoxin is added in increasing amounts; when a zone of flocculation appears, the tube showing it contains a completely neutralized mixture of toxin and antitoxin. The first tube in which flocculation occurs is taken as the end-point.

**rank sum t.**, a nonparametric statistical test for ordinal data, testing the null hypothesis that two samples are drawn from the same population versus the alternative hypothesis that the two samples are drawn from two populations having probability distributions of the same shape but different locations. It is based on the value of the rank sum statistic, which is calculated as the sum of the ranks of each sample after the observations in both samples are jointly ranked in ascending order; if and only if the null hypothesis is true, the average ranks of the two samples will be similar. Called also *Mann-Whitney* U *t., Mann-Whitney-Wilcoxon t.*, and *Wilcoxon rank sum t.*

**rapid plasma reagin t.**, RPR t.; a flocculation test for syphilis using unheated serum and a modified VDRL antigen containing choline chloride and charcoal particles, enabling macroscopic identification of the flocculation; widely used for screening.

**Raygat's t.**, hydrostatic t.

**Rebuck t.**, Rebuck skin window technique.

**red-glass t.**, a test for ocular deviation using a red glass over the right eye while the patient looks at a light; the position at which the patient sees the red image reveals the affected muscle.

**Rees' t.** *(for albumin)*: small amounts of albumin are precipitated from solution by tannic acid in alcoholic solution.

**Rehberg's t.**, a test of kidney function based on the excretion of creatinine administered 2 g in 500 mL of water.

**Reichl's t.** *(for proteins)*: add 2 or 3 drops of an alcoholic solution of benzaldehyde and a quantity of sulfuric acid previously diluted to twice its volume with water; then add a few drops of ferric sulfate solution. The mixture will take on a deep-blue color if proteins are present.

**Reinsch's t.** *(for heavy metals, including arsenic, mercury, bismuth, antimony, and large amounts of selenium, tellurium, and sulfide)*: insert a strip of clean copper into the suspected acidified liquid or finely ground tissue, and boil; if one or more heavy metals are present, a coating will form on the copper strip.

**renal function t.**, kidney function t.

**resorcinol–hydrochloric acid t.**, Selivanoff's t.

**Reuss' t.** *(for atropine)*: the substance examined is treated with sulfuric acid and oxidizing agents; if atropine is present, an odor of roses and orange-flowers is given off.

**rheumatoid arthritis t.**, see specific tests, such as the *latex agglutination t., Rose-Waaler t.*, and *sheep cell agglutination t.*

**rhubarb t.** *(in urine)*: make the urine alkaline; a red color indicates rhubarb.

**Rideal-Walker t.**, see under *method.*

**RIF t.**, Rubin's t. (def. 2).

**ring t.** *(for antibiotic activity)* the solution is placed in a ring resting on the surface of seeded agar and the size of the surrounding clear area of inhibition indicates the activity.

**Rinne t.**, a hearing test performed, with the opposite ear masked, with tuning forks of 256, 512, and 1024 Hz by alternately placing the stem of the vibrating fork on the mastoid process and $\frac{1}{2}$ inch from the external auditory meatus until it is no longer heard at one of these positions. When air conduction is greater than bone conduction *(positive Rinne test)*, it indicates normal hearing or sensorineural hearing loss. When bone conduction is greater than air conduction *(negative Rinne test)*, it indicates conductive hearing loss.

**Rivalta's t.**, see under *reaction.*

**rollover t.**, a test to assess the risk of preeclampsia in pregnant women. A comparison of blood pressure is made with the woman lying on her left side and on her back; an excessive increase in blood pressure when she rolls to the supine position indicates increased risk of preeclampsia.

**Romberg's t.** *(for differentiating between peripheral and cerebellar ataxia)*: an increase in clumsiness in all movements and in the width and uncertainty of the gait when the patient's eyes are closed indicates peripheral ataxia; no change indicates the cerebellar type. See also *Romberg's sign*, under *sign.*

**Ronchese t.** *(for quantitative determination of ammonia in urine)*: one based on the action of solution of formaldehyde on the ammonia salts. A 10 per cent solution of sodium carbonate is added, a drop at a time, to the urine until the reaction becomes neutral. The solution of formaldehyde (40 per cent) is neutralized with a one-fourth normal soda solution against phenolphthalein until a slight pink tint develops. Then 25 mL of the neutral urine and 10 mL of the neutral solution of formaldehyde are mixed and titrated against decinormal sodium carbonate solution until a deep pink develops. Each mL of the decinormal sodium carbonate solution per 100 mL of urine corresponds to 0.017 g ammonia in 1000 mL of urine.

**Rorschach t.,** a projective test in which the subject is asked to relate his associations to a series of inkblot designs.

**Rose-Waaler t.,** an agglutination test for rheumatoid factor (RF) using tanned sheep red blood cells (SRBC) coated with subagglutinating amounts of rabbit anti-SRBC IgG antibody. These cells agglutinate when exposed to RF (anti-IgG autoantibodies) owing to cross-reaction between human and rabbit IgG.

**rose bengal t.** *(for liver function)*: rose bengal (1 per cent in sodium chloride solution) is injected into the blood stream. Normally it disappears from the blood rapidly; delay in the normal disappearance time points to diminished activity of the liver.

**Rosenbach-Gmelin t.** *(for bile pigment)*: filter the urine through a very small filter, and put a drop of nitric acid with a trace of nitrous acid on the inside of the filter; a pale yellow spot will appear, surrounded with yellowish red, violet, blue, and green rings.

**Rosenthal's t.** *(for blood in urine)*: add potassium hydroxide solution to the urine, remove the precipitate, and dry it; place a small amount on a slide with a crystal of sodium chloride; apply a coverglass and cause a few drops of glacial acetic acid to flow under it; warm the plate. When it is cool, hemin crystals will appear if blood is present.

**Rothera's t.** *(for acetone)*: to 5 mL of urine add a little solid ammonium sulfate and add 2 to 3 drops of a fresh 5 per cent solution of sodium nitroprusside and 1 to 2 mL of ammonium hydroxide; a purple color forms if acetone is present.

**Rous t.** *(for hemosiderin)*: centrifuge the urine; to the sediment add 5 mL of a 2 per cent solution of potassium ferrocyanide and 5 mL of a 1 per cent solution of hydrochloric acid. Hemosiderin granules stain blue.

**Roussin's t.,** microscopic examination of suspected blood stains.

**RPR t.,** rapid plasma reagin t.

**Rubin's t.,** 1. a test for patency of the uterine tubes performed by transuterine insufflation with carbon dioxide. If the tubes are patent the gas enters the peritoneal cavity and may be demonstrated by the fluoroscope or radiograph. This subphrenic pneumoperitoneum may cause pain in one or both shoulders of the patient. If the manometer registers not over 100 mm Hg the tubes are patent; if between 120 and 130, there may be stenosis or stricture, but not complete occlusion; if it rises to 200, the tubes are completely occluded. 2. a test to detect avian leukosis viruses in egg-culture vaccines; if the viruses are present, they induce a cellular resistance to Rous viruses subsequently inoculated (resistance-inducing factor). Called also *RIF t.*

**Rubner's t.,** 1. *(for carbon monoxide in blood)* shake the blood with 4 or 5 volumes of lead acetate in solution: if the blood contains CO, it will retain its bright color; if not, it becomes a chocolate brown. 2. *(for lactose, glucose, maltose, or fructose in urine)* add lead acetate to the urine, boil, and then add an excess of ammonium hydroxide: lactose gives a brick-red color, glucose a coffee-brown color, maltose a light-yellow color, and fructose no color at all.

**ruler t.,** Hamilton's t.

**Rumpel-Leede t.,** see under *phenomenon.*

**Russell's viper venom t.,** Stypven time t.

**Russo's t.,** see under *reaction.*

**Ruttan and Hardisty's t.** *(for blood)*: blood in the presence of a 4 per cent glacial acetic acid solution of orthotoluidine and hydrogen peroxide gives a bluish color.

**Sabin-Feldman dye t.,** a serologic test for the diagnosis of toxoplasmosis, based on the failure of living toxoplasmas, in the presence of specific antibody and accessory factor, to take up methylene blue dye.

**saccharimeter t.,** glucose in solution rotates the plane of polarized light to the right, while fructose turns it to the left.

**saccharin t.** *(for mucociliary clearance)*: the upper respiratory tract is cleaned and small crystals of saccharin are placed on the inferior nasal mucosa. The time is measured until the patient has a sweet taste in the mouth. With normal ciliary transport the time should be 30 minutes or less; a time of more than 1 hour indicates pathology.

**Sahli-Nencki t.** *(for lipolytic activity of the pancreas)*: phenyl salicylate (salol) is administered: it is excreted as salicylic acid when pancreatic activity is normal.

**Sakaguchi t.** *(for arginine)*: a reddish or wine color is produced in the presence of arginine when a tissue section is treated with an alkaline mixture of $\alpha$-naphthol and sodium hypochlorite.

**Salkowski's t.,** 1. *(for carbon monoxide in the blood)* add to the blood 20 volumes of water and sodium hydroxide in solution (specific gravity, 1.34). If CO is present, it becomes cloudy and then red; flakes of red afterward float on the surface. 2. *(for cholesterol)* dissolve the sample in chloroform and add an equal volume of strong sulfuric acid: if cholesterol is present, the solution becomes bluish red, and slowly changes to a violet red, the sulfuric acid becomes red, with a green fluorescence. 3. *(for indole)* to the solution to be tested add a little nitric acid, and drop in slowly a solution of potassium nitrite (2 per cent): a red color shows that indole is present, and a red precipitate is afterward formed. 4. *(for creatinine)* to the yellow solution obtained in Weyl's test add an excess of acetic acid and heat; a green color results, which turns to blue.

**Salkowski-Ludwig t.** *(for uric acid)*: a solution of silver ammonio-nitrate and ammonium and magnesium chlorides precipitates uric acid.

**salol t.,** see *Sahli-Nencki t.*

**Sandrock t.** *(for thrombosis)*: vigorous friction is applied to the part; the degree of hyperemia which follows is an indication of the condition of the circulation.

**scarification t.,** a skin test in which the antigen is introduced by scarification.

**Schaffer's t.** *(for nitrites in urine)*: decolorize 4 mL of urine with animal charcoal and add to it 4 mL of 10 per cent acetic acid and 3 drops of 5 per cent solution of potassium ferrocyanide; an intense yellow color indicates nitrites.

**Schick t.,** intradermal injection of a quantity of diphtheria toxin equal to one-fiftieth of the guinea pig minimal lethal dose in one arm (the test site) and of an equal quantity of heat-inactivated diphtheria toxin in the other arm (the control site). A positive reaction, which consists of an area of redness that appears in 24 to 36 hours at the test site only and persists for 4 to 5 days, leaving an area of brownish pigmentation, indicates a lack of immunity to diphtheria. A pseudoreaction, which consists of an area of redness appearing at both sites and usually disappearing in 48 hours without residual pigmentation, or a negative reaction indicates immunity.

**Schiller's t.** *(for cancer of cervix)*: a test for early squamous cell cancer by treating the tissue with a solution of 1 g of iodine and 2 g of potassium iodide in 300 mL of water: if the cervix is healthy, the surface turns brown; if there is cancer, the treated area turns white or yellow, because cancer cells do not contain glycogen and therefore do not stain with iodine.

**Schilling t.** *(for gastrointestinal absorption of vitamin $B_{12}$)*: a measured amount of radioactively labeled cyanocobalamin is given orally, followed by a parenteral flushing dose of the nonradioactive vitamin, and the percentage of radioactivity is determined in the urine excreted over a 24-hour period. The test is usually performed three times: first with added intrinsic factor, then without it, and then after antibiotic therapy. The results are used in the diagnosis of pernicious anemia and other disorders of vitamin $B_{12}$ metabolism.

**Schirmer's t.** *(for keratoconjunctivitis sicca)*: a test of tear production in which a piece of filter paper is inserted over the conjunctival sac of the lower lid, with the end of the paper hanging down on the outside. The range of normal wetting, determined by measuring the area of moisture on the projecting paper, depends on age, sex, and disease processes.

**Schlichter t.,** serum bactericidal activity t.

**Schönbein's t.,** 1. *(for blood)* blue coloration obtained by adding solution of hydrogen peroxide to tincture of guaiac mixed with suspected blood. 2. *(for copper)* a solution containing a copper salt becomes blue if potassium cyanide and tincture of guaiac are added.

**Schroeder's t.** *(for urea)*: add a crystal of the substance to a solution of bromine in chloroform; the urea will decompose and gas will be formed.

**Schulte's t.** *(for proteins)*: remove all coagulable protein, precipitate with six volumes of absolute alcohol, dissolve the precipitate in water, and apply the biuret test.

**Schultz-Charlton t.,** see under *reaction.*

**Schultze's t.,** 1. *(for cellulose)* iodine is dissolved to saturation in a zinc chloride solution (specific gravity, 1.8), and 6 parts of potassium iodide are added: this reagent colors cellulose blue. 2. *(for cholesterol)* evaporate with nitric acid, using a porcelain dish and water bath; if cholesterol is present, a yellow deposit is formed, which changes to yellowish red when ammonia is added.

**Schumm's t.,** 1. benzidine t. 2. *(for heme in plasma)* a given volume of plasma is covered with a layer of ether; one-tenth the volume of concentrated ammonium sulfide (analar) is then run in with a pipette and subsequently mixed by shaking. A positive reaction is indicated by the appearance of a hemochromogen with a sharply defined $\alpha$ band at 558 nm in a depth up to 4 cm of plasma.

**Schwabach's t.,** a hearing test performed, with the opposite ear masked, with tuning forks of 256, 512, 1024, and 2048 Hz, alternately placing the stem of the vibrating fork on the mastoid process of the patient and that of the examiner (whose hearing should be normal) until it is no longer heard by one of them. The result is expressed as "Schwabach prolonged" if heard longer by the patient (indicative of conduction deafness), as "Schwabach shortened or diminished" if heard longer by the examiner (indicative of sensorineural deafness), and as "Schwabach normal" if heard for the same time by both.

**scratch t.,** a skin test in which the antigen is applied on a superficial scratch.

**screen t.,** 1. alternate cover t. 2. cover-uncover t.

**screening t.,** any test used to eliminate those who are definitely not affected by the disease in question, the remainder (those with positive reactions) being subjected to more refined diagnostic tests.

**secretin t.,** a test for pancreatic function done by examining the pancreatic secretion produced by the intravenous injection of secretin.

**Seidlitz powder t.** *(for diaphragmatic hernia)*: the stomach is distended by the administration of a Seidlitz powder, which will enable radiographic visualization of a herniated stomach loop.

**Selivanoff's (Seliwanow's) t.,** *(for fructose in urine)*: to the urine is added an equal volume of hydrochloric acid containing resorcinol in the following proportion: 5 mg resorcinol, 5 mL water, and 5 mL 25 per cent concentrated hydrochloric acid. Formation of a dark red color after boiling for 10 seconds indicates fructose. Called also *resorcinol–hydrochloric acid t.* and *Selivanoff reaction.*

**sentence completion t.,** a projective test for assessing personality and possible psychopathology, in which the individual is asked to provide endings for unfinished sentences.

**Sereny t.** *(to determine invasiveness of bacteria)*: the organism is inoculated into the eye of a guinea pig; invasiveness is determined by the organism's ability to produce conjunctivitis. The test is used particularly for determining the invasiveness of strains of *Escherichia coli* and *Listeria monocytogenes.*

**serologic t.,** any laboratory test involving serologic reactions (precipitin reaction, agglutination, complement fixation, etc.), especially any such test measuring serum antibody titer.

**serologic t. for syphilis (STS),** any test for serum antibodies indicative of *Treponema pallidum* infection. There are two types: *nontreponemal antigen tests* detect antibodies to substance (reagin) derived from host tissues, now known to consist of the phospholipids cardiolipin and lecithin; they originated with the Wassermann test and are now represented by the VDRL and RPR (rapid plasma reagin) tests. *Treponemal antigen tests* detect specific antitreponemal antibodies; they originated with the TPI (T. pallidum immobilization) test and are now represented by the DFA-TP (direct fluorescent antibody–T. pallidum) test, the FTA-ABS (fluorescent treponemal antibody absorption) test, the MHA-TP (microhemagglutination assay–T. pallidum), and assays using ELISA (enzyme-linked immunosorbent assay) methods. The term "serologic tests for syphilis" is occasionally used with reference only to nontreponemal antigen tests.

**serum bactericidal activity t.,** determination, by serial dilution, of the titer of serum (and antibiotic in serum) that will kill 99.9 per cent of the starting inoculum mixed with the serum sample; used to monitor antibiotic therapy in endocarditis, osteomyelitis, and other serious bacterial infections.

**serum neutralization t.,** a test of the antimicrobial activity of a serum done by inoculating a mixture of the serum and the virus or other microorganism being tested into a susceptible animal; called also *protection t.*

**shadow t.,** retinoscopy.

**sham feeding t.** *(for diagnosis of incomplete vagotomy)*: an appetizing meal is served and chewed but not swallowed, stimulating gastric acid secretion solely by vagal pathways; acid secretion is not stimulated after adequate vagotomy.

**sheep cell agglutination t. (SCAT),** any agglutination test using sheep red blood cells, such as the Rose-Waaler test.

**short increment sensitivity index t.,** see under *index.*

**Sia t.** *(for macroglobulinemia)*: a simple screening test performed by adding a drop of serum to 10 to 100 mL of cold distilled water; a positive reaction is indicated by the formation of a heaving cloud of precipitate at the bottom of the container. It is not diagnostic, because it may be positive in other conditions, as in rheumatoid arthritis.

**sickling t.,** a method for demonstrating hemoglobin S and sickling in erythrocytes, particularly in the heterozygous state, by reducing the environmental oxygen around them. It may be done by simply sealing a drop of blood under a coverslip or may be speeded up by adding 2 per cent sodium metabisulfite or sodium dithionite to the preparation.

**sign t.,** a nonparametric statistical test based on a null hypothesis that by chance the experimental group should outperform the control group for half the outcome variables and vice versa. Results are scored as a series of pluses and minuses awarded to the experimental group depending on its performance relative to that of the control group, a binomial distribution of scores with $p = 0.5$ being expected under the null hypothesis.

**signed rank t.,** a nonparametric statistical test for ordinal data, comparing two populations of data by examining the differences between matched pairs in the two populations. It is based on the signed rank statistic, calculated by arranging all samples in order without regard to which population they are drawn from, identifying pairs, assessing the difference in rankings for the members of each pair, and summing these differences for all pairs. If the null hypothesis is true and there is no difference between the two populations, the median difference in rankings between matched pairs in the population approximates 0. Called also *Wilcoxon's signed rank t.*

**Sims' t.,** a postcoital test for the ability of the spermatozoa to penetrate the cervical mucus.

**single breath t., single breath oxygen t.,** nitrogen washout t., single breath.

**SISI t.,** see *short increment sensitivity index,* under *index.*

**skin t.,** any test in which an antigen is applied to the skin in order to observe the response of the patient, described according to method of application, such as patch tests, scratch tests, and intradermal tests. Skin tests are used to determine prior exposure or immunity to an infectious disease (e.g., tuberculin test), to identify allergens producing allergic reactions, and to assess ability to mount a cellular immune response (using a battery of antigens that give positive tests in most normal individuals).

**skin window t.,** Rebuck skin window technique.

**smear t.,** Papanicolaou t.

**Snellen's t.,** 1. *(for pretended blindness in one eye)* the patient is requested to look at alternate red and green letters; the admittedly sound eye is covered with a red glass and if the green letters are read, evidence of fraud is present. 2. determination of visual acuity by means of Snellen's test types.

**sniff t.,** when a patient sniffs, the paralyzed half of the diaphragm is seen to rise and the intact half to descend, as observed by fluoroscopy.

**Solera's t.** *(for thiocyanates)*: saturate filter paper with 0.5 per cent starch paste containing 1 per cent of iodic acid; dry and preserve as test paper. A piece of this paper moistened with saliva will turn blue if thiocyanate is present.

**solubility t.,** see *bile solubility t.*

**Sonnenschein's t.** *(for strychnine)*: the suspected substance is dissolved in a drop of sulfuric acid, some cerosoceric oxide is added, and stirred with a glass rod; a deep blue color is formed, changing to violet, and finally to cherry red in the presence of strychnine.

**sorting t.,** a type of test for assessing abstract thinking; the patient must arrange objects or cards into groups based on some abstract relationship. Schizophrenics and patients with cortical lesions show impaired performance.

**Southern blot t.,** see under *technique.*

**soybean t.,** urease t. (1).

**spavin t.,** a test for spavin in horses made by holding up the limb with the hock bent sharply; the horse is then started suddenly, and in cases of spavin the first steps are very lame. Called also *hock t.*

**specific gravity t.,** see specific tests, including *Fishberg concentration t.* and *urine concentration t.*

**sphenopalatine t.,** the sphenopalatine ganglion is anesthetized with Novocain in order to determine whether the efferent current which is motivating a symptom is routed through either sphenopalatine ganglion, and if so, whether the left one or the right one.

**STA t., standard tube agglutination t.,** a serologic test for brucellosis, using *Brucella abortus* antigens to detect infections with *B. abortus, B. melitensis,* and *B. suis.*

**Stanford-Binet t.,** a modification of Binet's test, translated, adapted, and standardized on children in the United States.

**starch t.,** see *iodine t.* (1).

**station t.,** Romberg's t.

**Staub-Traugott t.,** see under *effect.*

**Stein's t.,** inability to stand on one foot with the eyes shut; seen in disease of the labyrinth.

**Stenger t.** *(for detecting simulated unilateral hearing loss)*: a signal is presented at an intensity less than the admitted threshold to the affected ear and a less intense signal of the same frequency is presented simultaneously to the unaffected ear. If the subject is feigning a loss of hearing, the signal in the unaffected ear will not be heard.

**Sterneedle tuberculin t.,** a type of intracutaneous tuberculin test; the needle points of the Sterneedle are dipped into 1 to 2 drops of tuberculin P.P.D., then placed on the forearm and made to penetrate the skin, through the P.P.D. solution, to a depth of 1 mm, thus depositing tuberculin in the outer layer of the skin. Palpable, coalescing induration (edema) extending more than 5 mm around the puncture wounds in three to seven days indicates a positive reaction. Called *Heaf t.* in England.

**stimulation t.,** a type of challenge or provocative test used when hypofunction of an endocrine gland is suspected that cannot be detected by other means; either an exogenous releasing hormone or some other substance is administered to stimulate release of the hormone under investigation and levels of it are subsequently measured to assess whether the patient had a normal response.

**Stoll t.,** a technique for the quantitative estimation of the worm burden of an individual based on collection of a 24-hour stool specimen and counting the number of ova present in an aliquot.

**Straus' biological t.** *(for glanders),* see *Straus' reaction,* under *reaction.*

**stress t's,** any of various tests that assess cardiovascular health and function after application of a stress to the heart, usually exercise but sometimes others such as atrial pacing, the cold pressor test, or specific drugs. Subjects are monitored electrocardiographically, symptomatically, by blood pressure and heart rate, and often by recordings of ventilation and tidal volume recordings as well as other applicable noninvasive or invasive methods. See also *exercise t's.*

**strychnine t.**, see specific tests, including *Sonnenschein's t.* and *Wenzell's t.*

**Student's *t*-t.**, *t*-t.

**Stypven time t.**, a prothrombin test similar to the (one-stage) prothrombin time, but performed with Russell's viper venom (Stypven) as the thromboplastic agent; useful in defining deficiencies of blood coagulation factor X. Called also *Russell's viper venom t.* or *time* and *Stypven time.*

**submaximal exercise t.**, an exercise test halted at a predetermined point that is less than the maximal exercise capability of the subject, usually at a particular percentage of the maximal heart rate or after a set time interval.

**sucrose hemolysis t.** *(for paroxysmal nocturnal hemoglobinuria)*: the patient's whole blood is mixed with isotonic sucrose solution, which promotes binding of complement to red cells, then incubated and examined for hemolysis; greater than 10 per cent hemolysis is indicative of paroxysmal nocturnal hemoglobinuria.

**sugar t.**, see *fructose t.* and *glucose t.*

**sulfobromophthalein excretion t.** *(for liver function)*: sulfobromophthalein, a dye that in normal individuals is almost completely cleared from the blood by the liver, is administered intravenously and its rate of disappearance from the blood is determined colorimetrically; of historic interest.

**sulfur t.** *(for protein)*: the suspected liquid is heated with an excess of sodium hydroxide and a small quantity of acetate of lead; if proteins are present, a black precipitate of lead sulfide is formed.

**Sullivan's t.** *(for cysteine)*: to 1 or 2 mL of the unknown solution add 1 to 2 drops of a 0.5 per cent solution of sodium $\beta$-naphthoquinone-4-sulfonate and then 5 mL of a 20 per cent sodium thiosulfate made up in 0.25 normal sodium hydroxide. A brilliant red color indicates a free thiol group, demonstrating cysteine rather than cystine.

**suppression t.**, a type of dynamic test used when hyperfunction of an endocrine gland or presence of a hormone-secreting tumor is suspected; a substance is administered that is normally antagonistic to glandular secretion of a given hormone and hormonal levels are measured to assess whether they drop in the normal fashion.

**susceptibility t.** *(for testing the susceptibility of pathogenic bacteria to antibiotics)*, see *disk diffusion t.*

**swinging flashlight t.**, with the patient's eyes fixed at a distance and a strong light shining before the intact eye, a crisp bilateral contraction of the pupil is noted. On moving the light to the affected eye, both pupils dilate for a short period. Then on return of the light to the intact eye, both pupils contract promptly and remain contracted. Indicative of minimal damage to the optic nerve or retina. See also *Marcus Gunn's pupillary phenomenon,* under *phenomenon.*

**syphilis t.**, see *serologic t. for syphilis.*

***t*-t.**, a statistical hypothesis test based on the *t*-distribution (q.v.) used to test for a difference between the means of two groups. Called also *Student's t-t.*

**taurine t.**, see *Lang's t.*

**Teichmann's t.** *(for blood)*: the suspected liquid is put under a coverglass with a crystal of sodium chloride and a little glacial acetic acid; heat carefully without boiling and then cool. If blood is present, rhombic crystals of hemin will appear.

**Tensilon t.** *(for myasthenia gravis)*: after administration of Tensilon (edrophonium chloride), the patient's eye signs (ptosis and extraocular muscle abnormalities) markedly decrease within two minutes in cases of myasthenia gravis.

**Terman t.**, Stanford-Binet t.

**thalleioquin t.** *(for quinine)*: a neutralized solution of the suspected liquid is treated with chlorine, or bromine water, and then with an excess of ammonia; a green substance, thalleioquin, will be formed.

**thallium stress t.** *(for detection of coronary artery disease)*: stress is placed on the cardiovascular system by exercising the patient on a treadmill or bicycle ergometer and thallous chloride Tl-201 is injected intravenously when stress is maximal, just prior to exercise cessation. Immediate (stress) and delayed (redistribution) images are obtained with a gamma camera (see *thallium-201 myocardial perfusion scintigraphy*); then abnormalities of radionuclide distribution and redistribution are assessed, compared with electrocardiograms obtained during exercise, and used to diagnose areas of ischemia and coronary artery disease. In patients incapable of exercise, stress is induced by injection of dipyridamole or adenosine.

**Thematic Apperception T.**, TAT; a projective test in which the subject tells a story based on each of a series of standard ambiguous pictures, so that his responses reflect a projection of some aspect of his personality and current psychological preoccupations and conflicts.

**thin layer rapid use epicutaneous t.**, TRUE t.

**thiocyanate t.**, see *ferric chloride t.* and *Solera's t.*

**Thomas t.**, with the patient supine, when one leg is flexed so that the knee touches the chest and the lumbar spine is flattened, the angle taken by the other hip is the degree of flexion deformity.

**Thormählen's t.** *(for melanin in urine)*: treat urine with a solution of sodium nitroprusside, potassium hydroxide, and acetic acid; if melanin is present, a deep-blue color will form.

**thromboplastin generation t.**, a test formerly used in the detection of defects in formation of prothrombinase and hence deficiencies of the factors involved.

**Thudichum's t.** *(for creatinine)*: add to the suspected substance a dilute solution of ferric chloride; a dark-red color indicates the presence of creatinine.

**thumbnail t.** *(for fractured patella)*: the examiner's thumbnail is passed over the subcutaneous surface of the patella; a fracture will be felt as a sharp crevice.

**thyroid function t.**, any of various diagnostic procedures measuring the functioning of the thyroid gland, such as the *perchlorate discharge test, protein-bound iodine test, radioactive iodine uptake test, thyroid-stimulating hormone stimulation test, thyroid suppression test, thyrotropin-releasing hormone stimulation test, triiodothyronine resin uptake test,* and measurement of *pertechnetate uptake.*

**thyroid-stimulating hormone stimulation t., thyroid stimulation t.**, a thyroid function test in which thyrotropin (thyroid-stimulating hormone) is administered intramuscularly and the thyroid gland is monitored over time with scintiscanning or radioimmunoassays for a response or areas of decreased responsiveness. The test was formerly also much used for determining whether hypothyroidism was caused by thyroid gland failure or by deficiency in thyrotropin. Called also *TSH stimulation t.*

**thyroid suppression t.**, a thyroid function test; after administration of liothyronine for several days, radioactive iodine uptake is decreased in normal persons but not in those with hyperthyroidism.

**thyrotropin-releasing hormone stimulation t.** *(for pituitary release of thyrotropin)*: a bolus of thyrotropin-releasing hormone is administered and serum concentrations of thyrotropin are assessed at intervals; if serum levels do not increase within 30 to 40 minutes, the pituitary thyrotrophs are dysfunctional. Called also *TRH stimulation t.*

**tine t., tine tuberculin t. (Rosenthal),** a type of intracutaneous tuberculin test; four tines, 2 mm long, attached to a plastic handle, and coated with dip-dried PPD or Old tuberculin (OT) are pressed into the skin of the volar surface of the forearm, where they deposit tuberculin in the outer layer. The skin is checked 48 to 72 hours later for the presence of palpable induration; if the induration around one or more of the puncture wounds is 2 mm or more in diameter or if there is vesiculation, the test is considered positive. If positive, it is usually confirmed with the more specific Mantoux test (q.v.).

**Tizzoni's t.** *(for iron in tissues)*: treat a section of tissue with a 2 per cent solution of potassium ferrocyanide, and then with a 0.5 per cent solution of hydrochloric acid; the tissue will be stained a blue color if iron is present.

**toad t.**, 1. see *male frog* or *male toad t.* 2. see *Xenopus t.*

**Tobey-Ayer t.** *(for sinus thrombosis)*: the jugular vein on the side of the suspected thrombosis is compressed. A rise in spinal fluid pressure should occur; its absence indicates presence of thrombosis. Called also *Ayer-Tobey t.*

**tolbutamide t.** *(for insulinoma)*: one gram of tolbutamide is administered intravenously and plasma levels of glucose and insulin are monitored for 3 hours; prolonged hypoglycemia with hyperinsulinemia indicates presence of an insulinoma.

**tolerance t.**, 1. an exercise test to determine the efficiency of the circulation. 2. a test to determine the body's ability to metabolize a substance or to endure administration of a drug.

**Tollens, Neuberg, and Schwket's t.** *(for uronic acid)*: extract the uronic acid from acidified urine with ether, add water, evaporate the ether, and perform an orcinol test.

**tone decay t.**, an audiometer test in which the patient is asked to raise his hand as long as he hears a continuous tone at his threshold

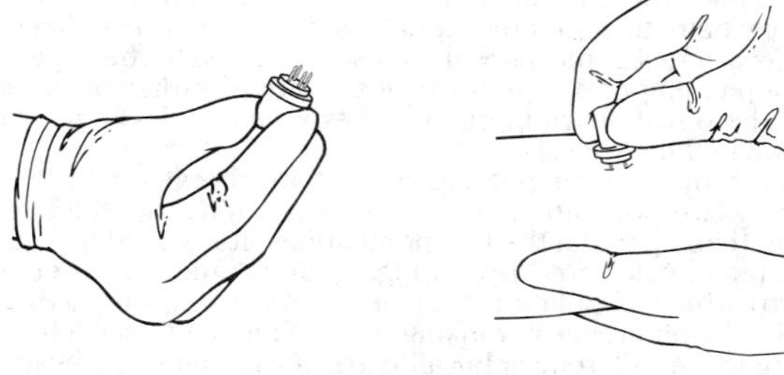

Tine test for tuberculosis.

level and to lower it when it becomes inaudible; whenever he lowers it before 60 seconds, the intensity is raised by 5 decibels and the amount of tone decay from the initial threshold level in decibels is determined.

**tourniquet t.,** 1. *(for capillary fragility)* pressure is applied midway between diastolic and systolic for 5 minutes by a manometer cuff; the cuff is released and petechiae are counted in an area 2.5 cm in diameter, on the inner aspect of the forearm. A number between 10 and 20 is marginal, above 20, abnormal. Called also *capillary fragility t.* and *Hess capillary t.* 2. Matas' t. 3. Perthes' t.

**toxigenicity t.** *(for detection of toxigenic strains of* Corynebacterium diphtheriae*)*: a primary culture is streaked onto a plate of tellurite agar containing a strip of filter paper perfused with diphtheria antitoxin. The exotoxin produced by the bacteria forms a band of precipitation with antitoxin diffusing from the filter paper. Called also *Elek t.*

**Toynbee t.,** performance of the Toynbee maneuver (q.v.) and monitoring of pressure changes in the middle ear. Subsequent middle ear negative pressure or negative pressure followed by ambient pressure usually indicates normal function of the auditory tube.

**TPI t.,** Treponema pallidum immobilization t.

**trapeze t.,** when the patient hangs from a trapeze, a spinal deformity will disappear if the deformity is postural but will remain if it is structural.

**treadmill exercise t. (TET), treadmill stress t. (TMST),** any of various graded exercise tests in which the patient walks on an inclined treadmill, which is generally increased in speed and incline through the test; see also specific test protocols, e.g., *Bruce protocol.* Cf. *bicycle ergometer exercise t.*

**Trendelenburg's t.,** 1. the leg is raised above the level of the heart until the veins are empty, then quickly lowered. If the veins become distended at once, varicosity and incompetence of the valves are indicated. 2. the patient, standing erect with back to the examiner, lifts first one leg and then the other: when weight is supported by the affected limb, the pelvis on the sound side falls instead of rising; seen in disturbances of the gluteus medius mechanism, as in deformity of the femoral neck, dislocated hip joint, and weakness or paralysis of the gluteus medius muscle. Called also *Trendelenburg's sign.*

**treponemal antigen t.,** see *serologic t. for syphilis.*

***Treponema pallidum* complement fixation t's,** nontreponemal antigen serologic tests for syphilis using complement fixation rather than flocculation as the indicator reaction. Once widely used to confirm positive results of flocculation procedures, they have now been replaced by treponemal antigen tests.

***Treponema pallidum* immobilization t.,** TPI t.; the first treponemal antigen serologic test for syphilis, introduced in 1949, now little used; live *Treponema pallidum* is mixed with patient serum and complement and examined microscopically to determine the proportion of treponemes that are immobilized by specific antibodies in the serum.

**TRH t., TRH stimulation t.,** thyrotropin-releasing hormone stimulation t.

**trichophytin t.** *(for Trichophyton infection)*: when filtrates of the fungus are injected into infected persons, a reaction similar to the tuberculin reaction is produced; used to test whether the patient is anergic or can mount a cell-mediated hypersensitivity reaction.

**triiodothyronine resin uptake t.,** a thyroid function test, measuring how many sites on thyroxine-binding globulin are occupied by endogenous triiodothyronine ($T_3$) and how many sites remain available. An excess of radioactive exogenous triiodothyronine is added to the sample, followed by the addition of a resin that also binds $T_3$. A portion of the radioactive $T_3$ binds to sites on TBG not already occupied by endogenous thyroid hormones, and the remainder binds to the resin. The amount of labeled hormones bound to the resin (the triiodothyronine resin uptake) can be subtracted from the total that was added and the remainder is the amount that bound to the unoccupied binding sites on the thyroxine-binding globulin.

**triketohydrindene hydrate t.,** to 25 mL of water add 10 mg of aminoacetic acid. To 1 mL of this solution add a solution of 50 mg of sodium acid in 2 mL of water, then add 0.2 mL of a solution of 5 mg of triketohydrindene hydrate (Ninhydrin) in 1 mL of water. Add the suspected matter and boil for 1–2 minutes. A violet color indicates a free carboxyl and alpha-amino group in proteins, peptones, peptides, or amino acids.

**Trousseau's t.** *(for bile in urine)*: iodine tincture diluted with 10 parts of alcohol is added to urine in a test tube; a green ring is formed where the liquids touch if bilirubin is present.

**TRUE t.,** thin layer rapid use epicutaneous t.; a ready-to-use method for patch testing, consisting of a desiccated mixture of allergen and hydrophilic gel printed on a mylar backing; after application the gel absorbs water from the skin and releases allergen.

**tryptophan load t.** *(for vitamin $B_6$ deficiency)*: a single large dose of tryptophan is administered orally and a 24-hour urine sample is analyzed for xanthurenic acid, and sometimes also kynurenine, hydroxykynurenine, and kynurenic acid. If vitamin $B_6$ deficiency exists, kynureninase activity will be decreased and these metabolites will accumulate in the urine.

**TSH stimulation t.,** thyroid-stimulating hormone stimulation t.

**tuberculin t.,** any of a number of skin tests for tuberculosis using a variety of different types of tuberculin and methods of application. See also *intracutaneous tuberculin t.* and *tine t.*

**tuberculosis t.,** a test for the presence of *Mycobacterium tuberculosis;* see *tuberculin t.* and *niacin t.*

**Tuffier's t.,** in aneurysm, when the main artery and vein of a limb are compressed, swelling of the veins of the hand or foot will occur only if the collateral circulation is free.

**tuning fork t's,** hearing tests using a vibrating tuning fork of known frequency as a source of sound. See *Bing t., Rinne t., Schwabach t.,* and *Weber's t.* (def. 1).

**two step exercise t.,** Master "2-step" exercise t.

**two-tailed t.,** a hypothesis test (q.v.) in which the critical region comprises both tails of the distribution of the test statistic and the null hypothesis is tested against a two-sided alternative that includes deviation from the null hypothesis in both directions.

**tyrosine t.,** see specific tests, including *Hoffmann's t., Mörner's t.* (1), *Piria's t., Udránszky's t.* (2), and *Wurster's t.* (2).

**Tyson's t.** *(for bile acids in urine)*: 180 to 240 mL of urine are evaporated to dryness on the water bath. The residue is extracted with absolute alcohol, and to the extract 12 to 14 volumes of ether are added. The bile acids are precipitated, then are filtered off, dissolved in water, and the aqueous solution decolorized with animal charcoal.

**Tzanck t.,** examination of tissue from the floor of a lesion, in vesicular or bullous diseases, to discover the type of cell present as a means of diagnosing the disease. Multinucleated giant cells are pathognomonic of varicella, herpes simplex, herpes zoster, or pemphigus.

**Udránszky's t.,** 1. *(for bile acids)* take 1 mL of a solution of the suspected substance, add a drop of 0.1 per cent solution of furfurol in water, underlay with strong sulfuric acid, and cool; if bile is present, a bluish-red color is formed. 2. *(for tyrosine)* take 1 mL of the suspected substance in solution, add a drop of 0.5 per cent aqueous solution of furfurol, and underlay with 1 mL of concentrated sulfuric acid; a pink color shows the presence of tyrosine.

**Uffelmann's t.** *(for hydrochloric acid and lactic acid in the gastric contents)*: to a quantity of material taken from the stomach add a few drops of a reagent containing 3 drops of a solution of ferric chloride, 3 drops of a concentrated solution of phenol, and 20 mL of water; hydrochloric acid, if present, decolorizes this solution, while lactic acid turns it yellow.

**Ulrich's t.** *(for albumin)*: the reagent consists of saturated solution of sodium chloride, 98 mL; glacial acetic acid, 2 mL. It must be perfectly clear. Boil a few mL of this fluid in a test tube, and immediately overlay with the urine. Albumin and globulin give a white ring at the zone of contact.

**Ultzmann's t.** *(for bile pigments)*: to 10 mL of the urine to be tested add 3 or 4 mL of a 1:3 solution of potassium hydroxide, and an excess of hydrochloric acid; bile pigments will cause an emerald-green coloration.

**unheated serum reagin t.,** USR t.; a modification of the VDRL test using unheated serum, used primarily for screening.

**uracil t.,** see *Wheeler and Johnson's t.*

**urea t.,** see specific tests, including *Benedict's t.* (def. 2), *diacetyl t., Schroeder's t.,* and *urease t.* (def. 1). See also *urea, methods for,* under *method.*

**urea breath t.** *(for the presence of* Helicobacter pylori *in the stomach):* following the oral administration of urea labeled with $^{13}C$ or $^{14}C$, the carbon dioxide in the patient's breath is analyzed to determine the presence of radiolabeled $CO_2$. If *H. pylori* is present, the action of bacterial urease converts the urea to ammonia and radiolabeled carbon dioxide, which is absorbed into the blood stream and is exhaled by the patient.

**urea concentration t.** *(for renal efficiency)*: a test based on the fact that urea is absorbed rapidly from the stomach into the blood, and is excreted unaltered by the kidneys: 15 g of urea is given with 100 mL of fluid, and the urine which is collected at the end of 2 hours is tested for urea concentration. Called also *MacLean-de Wesselow t.* and *Jones and Cantarow t.*

**urease t.,** 1. a test for urea based on the conversion of urea into ammonium carbonate by the urease of soybean. 2. *(for the production of urease by bacteria)* urease test broth (see under *culture medium*) is prepared in slants. After inoculation of the surface and incubation, urease-positive cultures produce an alkaline reaction (red color) in the medium. *Proteus* cultures show an early urease-positive reaction; other genera may have a delayed response.

**Urecholine supersensitivity t.** *(for neurogenic bladder)*: administer 2.5 mg of Urecholine (bethanechol) subcutaneously; the bladder is neurogenic if it exhibits a rise in intravesical pressure more than 15 cm greater than that of a control.

**uric acid t.,** see specific tests, including *Salkowski-Ludwig t.,* and *Weidel's t.* (def. 1). See also *uric acid, methods for,* under *method.*

**urine concentration t.**, under a controlled diet the specific gravity of the urine should reach 1.18 or more at certain times.

**urochromogen t.**, see *Weisz's t.*

**USR t.**, unheated serum reagin t.

**Valsalva's t.**, Valsalva's maneuver (def. 2).

**van den Bergh's t.**, a test for bilirubin in which diazotized serum or plasma is compared with a standard solution of diazotized bilirubin.

**Van Slyke t.**, 1. *(for amide nitrogen)* nitrous acid acting on amide nitrogen sets free nitrogen gas, which is collected and its volume determined. 2. *(for urea)* treat the sample with urease, pass the ammonia so formed into N/50 normal acid, and titrate the excess of acid.

**VDRL t.** [*V*enereal *D*isease *R*esearch *L*aboratory], the standard nontreponemal antigen serologic test for syphilis, a slide flocculation test using heat-inactivated serum and VDRL antigen, a standardized mixture of cardiolipin, lecithin, and cholesterol. Positive tests are seen in about 70 per cent of cases in primary syphilis, 100 per cent in secondary syphilis, and 70 per cent in tertiary syphilis. There is a 20 to 40 per cent false positive rate.

**ventilation t.**, measurement of the quantity of air expired by a person during a period of exercise. See also *pulmonary function t.*

**Vitali's t.**, 1. *(for alkaloids)* evaporate with fuming nitric acid and add a drop of potassium hydroxide; color reactions will occur. For atropine the color is violet, turning to red. 2. *(for alkaloids)* add sulfuric acid, potassium chlorate, and an alkaline sulfide; various color reactions will follow. 3. *(for bile pigments)* add a few drops of potassium nitrate in solution and dilute sulfuric acid. The color reactions are green, followed by blue or red and yellow. 4. *(for bile pigments)* add quinine bisulfate in solution and follow with diluted ammonia solution, sulfuric acid, a crystal of sugar, and alcohol; a violet color results. 5. *(for thymol)* distill, and pass the vapor through a mixture of chloroform and potassium hydroxide solution; a red color results. 6. *(for pus in the urine)* the urine is acidified with acetic acid and filtered. On the filter paper thus obtained a small quantity of guaiacum is dropped. The paper will turn a dark blue if pus is present.

**vitamin t.**, see specific tests, including *dark-adaptation t., deoxyuridine suppression t., Friderichsen's t., histidine loading t.,* and *Schilling t.*

**Vogel and Lee's t.** *(for mercury)*: add 3 per cent of hydrochloric acid and concentrate the urine to one fifth its original volume. Add a piece of clean copper wire. A silvery film indicates mercury. To confirm, place the wire in a tube with a plug of gold foil and distill the mercury over onto the gold. Sublime a crystal of iodine onto the mercury and form the red iodide of mercury.

**Voges-Proskauer t.** *(for differentiation of Enterobacteriaceae)*: a test for the production of acetylmethylcarbinol from glucose in bacterial cultures. An appropriate culture is treated with a solution of potassium hydroxide and creatine. Development of a red color indicates a positive reaction. *Enterobacter, Klebsiella,* and *Serratia* are V-P positive; *Erwinia, Pectobacterium,* and *Yersinia* are variable; *Escherichia* and other genera of Enterobacteriaceae are V-P negative.

**von Maschke's t.** *(for creatinine)*: to the suspected solution add a few drops of Fehling's solution, after mixing with a cold solution of sodium carbonate; an amorphous, flocculent precipitate proves the presence of creatinine.

**von Pirquet t.**, Pirquet t.

**von Zeynek and Mencki's t.** *(for blood)*: precipitate the urine with acetone, extract the precipitate with acidified acetone, and examine the colored extract under the microscope for small hemin crystals.

**Waaler-Rose t.**, Rose-Waaler t.

**Wada's t.** *(for cerebral dominance of language function)*: amobarbital is injected into an internal carotid artery to produce transient hemiparesis of the contralateral limbs. Injection into the artery of the hemisphere dominant for language produces a transient aphasia, into that of the nondominant hemisphere does not interfere with language function.

**Wagner's t.** *(for occult blood)*, see *benzidine t.*

**Wassermann t.**, the original (1906) nontreponemal antigen serologic test for syphilis.

**water deprivation t.**, a test of the body's ability to concentrate urine when plasma osmolality is artificially increased: without fasting, the patient is deprived of water for at least eight hours. Patient weight and measurements of plasma and urine osmolalities are obtained before the test and each hour after the four-hour point. In a normal individual, the osmolality of the urine should increase to two to four times that of the plasma with eight hours of water deprivation. After eight hours, vasopressin is administered and the patient is allowed to drink as usual; in normal persons this should increase the urine osmolality no more than 9 per cent in the first hour; in those with diabetes insipidus and other abnormalities the osmolality may increase between 10 and 50 per cent.

**water-gurgle t.** *(for stricture of the esophagus)*: the swallowing of water causes a peculiar gurgle heard on auscultation.

**water provocative t.**, drinking t.

**Watson-Schwartz t.**, a simple qualitative procedure for differentiating porphobilinogen from urobilinogen and other Ehrlich reactors, based on the insolubility of porphobilinogen aldehyde in chloroform and butanol; it is useful in diagnosis of acute porphyria.

**Weber's t.**, 1. *(for differentiating between conduction deafness and sensorineural deafness)* the stem of a vibrating tuning fork is placed on the vertex or midline of the forehead; if the sound is heard best in the affected ear, the deafness is probably of the conductive type; if heard best in the normal ear, it is probably of the sensorineural type. (F. E. Weber.) 2. *(for indican)* boil 30 mL of urine with an equal volume of hydrochloric acid containing a little nitric acid; cool it, and shake with ether; if indican is present, the ether will become red or violet and the froth will be blue. (E. H. Weber.) 3. *(for blood)* mix the sample with 30 per cent acetic acid and extract with ether; to the ether extract add an alcoholic solution of guaiac and hydrogen peroxide. A blue color indicates blood. (E. H. Weber.)

**Weidel's t.**, 1. *(for uric acid)* the substance tested is treated with nitric acid, evaporated, and moistened with diluted ammonia solution; if uric acid is present, murexide will be formed, and a purple color is produced. Called also *murexide t.* 2. *(for xanthine)* warm with freshly prepared chlorine water containing a trace of nitric acid until gas ceases to be produced; contact with gaseous ammonia develops a pink or purple color. 3. *(for xanthine bodies)* dissolve in warm chlorine water, evaporate, and treat with diluted ammonia solution; a pink or purple color will form, changing to violet on the addition of sodium or potassium hydroxide solution.

**Weil-Felix t.** *(for diagnosis of typhus and certain other rickettsial diseases)*: the blood serum of a patient with suspected rickettsial disease is tested against certain strains of *Proteus vulgaris* (OX-2, OX-19, OX-K).The agglutination reactions, based on antigens common to both organisms, determine the presence and type of rickettsial infection.

**Weisz's t., Weisz permanganate t.** *(for urochromogen)*: to 2 mL of the urine add 4 mL of distilled water and 3 drops of a 1:1000 solution of potassium permanganate; a canary yellow color indicates urochromogen.

**Welland's t.**, bar-reading t.

**Wenzell's t.** *(for strychnine)*: treat the suspected material with a solution of 1 part of potassium permanganate in 2000 parts of sulfuric acid; strychnine, even in very small proportion, will cause color reactions.

**Wernicke's t.**, see *hemiopic pupillary reaction,* under *reaction.*

**Western blot t.**, see under *technique.*

**Wetzel's t.** *(for carbon monoxide in blood)*: to the blood to be examined add 4 volumes of water and treat with 3 volumes of a 1 per cent tannin solution. If CO is present, the blood becomes carmine red; normal blood slowly assumes a grayish hue.

**Weyl's t.**, 1. *(for creatinine)* to the suspected solution add a little of a dilute solution of sodium nitroprusside, and then carefully put in a few drops of a weak solution of sodium hydroxide; a ruby red color results, changing to blue on warming with acetic acid. 2. *(for nitric acid in the urine)* distill 200 mL of urine with 0.2 part of sulfuric or hydrochloric acid, receiving the distillate in a potassium hydroxide solution. If *m*-phenyldiamine is added, a yellow color will form; if there is added pyrogallic acid in aqueous solution with a little sulfuric acid, the color will be brown; but sulfanilic acid in solution, followed in ten minutes by naphthylamine hydrochlorate, produces a red tint.

**Wheeler and Johnson's t.** *(for uracil and cytosine)*: to the unknown solution add bromine water until the color is permanent, but avoid excess. Then add an excess of barium hydroxide. A purple color indicates one of these substances.

**Widal's t., Widal's serum t.** *(for typhoid fever)*: a test for the presence of agglutinins to O and H antigens of *Salmonella typhi* and *S. paratyphi* in the serum of patients with suspected *Salmonella* infection.

**Wilcoxon rank sum t.**, rank sum t.

**Wilcoxon signed rank t.**, signed rank t.

**Winckler t.**, 1. *(for alkaloids)* a solution of mercury bichloride with an excess of potassium iodide is added; alkaloids will cause a white precipitate. 2. *(for free hydrochloric acid in the gastric juice)* filter the juice into a porcelain cell with a few drops of the 5 per cent alcoholic solution of $\alpha$-naphthol containing 1 per cent or less of glucose. Heat carefully, and a bluish-violet zone will appear, which rapidly grows darker. 3. *(for iodine)* sodium nitrate is mixed with a starch paste; iodine gives a blue color with it.

**Wishart t.** *(for acetonemia)*: a few drops of plasma are placed in a small test tube. Enough dry powdered ammonium sulfate is added to supersaturate, so that at the end of the test there will still be some of the solid sulfate in the bottom of the tube. A couple of drops of a fresh solution of sodium nitroprusside are next added and shaken, and finally 1 or 2 drops of diluted ammonia solution. On shaking, a purple color develops, a little more slowly than in the case of urine. The intensity of the color indicates the degree of acetonemia.

**Witz's t.** *(for hydrochloric acid in the gastric juice)*: a 1:48 aqueous solution of methyl violet causes a violet color, changing to blue and then green.

**Woldman's t.**, a test for gastrointestinal lesion based on the principle that free phenolphthalein may pass through a lesion in the gastrointestinal mucosa and appear in the urine.

**Woodbury's t.** *(for alcohol in the urine)*: to 2 mL of urine 1 mL of sulfuric acid is added, and a crystal of potassium dichromate; a green color will form.

**Wormley's t.,** 1. *(for alkaloids)*: treat the suspected solution with an alcoholic solution of picric acid; a yellow precipitate will be formed. 2. treat the suspected solution with a solution of 1 part of iodine and 2 parts of potassium iodide in 60 parts of water; a colored precipitate will be formed.

**Wurster's t.,** 1. *(for hydrogen peroxide)* test paper is saturated with the solution of tetramethylparaphenylenediamine; hydrogen peroxide turns it to a blue-violet color. 2. *(for tyrosine)* the suspected material is dissolved in boiling water and a little quinone; a ruby-red color will form, changing slowly to brown.

**xanthine t.,** see specific tests, including *Hoppe-Seyler t.* (2) and *Weidel's t.* (2), (3).

***Xenopus* t.** *(for pregnancy)*: a female African clawed toad *(Xenopus laevis)* is injected with 2 mL of urine, or 1 mL of an extract, into the dorsal lymph sac; a deposit of 5–6 or more eggs within four to twelve hours indicates pregnancy.

**D-xylose absorption t., D-xylose tolerance t.** *(for differential diagnosis in malabsorption syndromes)*: after the oral administration of 25 g (sometimes 5 g is used) of D-xylose dissolved in 250 mL of water, followed immediately by an additional 250 mL of water, to a fasting adult, the amount excreted in the urine during a 5-hour period is determined. Since poor renal function may also result in low xylose absorption, blood levels are also determined at two hours. Normally, more than 4.0 g of xylose should be excreted over the 5-hour period; less than this amount suggests intestinal malabsorption. Blood values are normally more than 25 mg xylose per 100 mL of blood.

**Young's t.** *(for cataract)*: on a disk with a varied number of pinholes in different portions, the patient's ability to recognize the number of holes is a test of the integrity of macular function.

***z* t.,** a statistical test using normalized data (*z* values) to compare differences in proportions between sets of data or between individual members of different sets of data.

**Zaleski's t.** *(for carbon monoxide in blood)*: to 2 mL of blood add an equal volume of water and 3 drops of a one-third saturated solution of cupric sulfate: if carbon monoxide is present, the precipitate is brick-red; otherwise it is greenish brown.

**Zeisel's t.** *(for colchicine)*: dissolve in hydrochloric acid, boil with ferric chloride, and shake with chloroform; a brown or dark-red layer will form at the bottom.

---

**tes·ta** (tes'tə) [L. "shell"] test[1].

**Tes·ta·cea** (tes-ta'she-ə) [L. *testa* shell] Arcellinida.

**Tes·ta·ce·a·lo·bo·sia** (tes-ta″se-ə-lo-bo'shə) [Gr. *testa* shell + L. *lobus* lobe] a subclass of ameboid protozoa (class Lobosea, superclass Rhizopoda), characterized by a body enclosed in a test, tectum, or other complex membrane external to the plasma membrane and glycocalyx. It includes two orders: Arcellinida and Trichosida.

**tes·ta·ce·an** (tes-ta'she-ən) 1. any protozoan of the subclass Testacealobosia. 2. pertaining to protozoa of the subclass Testacealobosia.

**tes·ta·ceous** (tes-ta'shəs) [L. *testa* shell] of the nature of shell; having a shell.

**tes·tal·gia** (tes-tal'jə) [*testis* + *-algia*] orchialgia.

**Tes-Tape** (tes'tāp) trademark for a test strip impregnated with glucose oxidase, peroxidase, and *o*-tolidine; used for determining the approximate concentration of glucose in urine.

**test card** (test kahrd) a card printed with various letters or symbols, used in testing vision.

**stigmometric t. c.,** a card with dots and squares arranged in groups, for testing vision (Fridenberg).

**tes·tec·to·my** (təs-tek'tə-me) [*testis* + *-ectomy*] orchiectomy.

**tes·tes** (tes'tēz) [L.] plural of *testis.*

**tes·ti·cle** (tes'tĭ-kəl) [L. *testiculus*] testis.

**tes·ti·cond** (tes'tĭ-kond) [*testis* + L. *condere* to hide] having the testes retained within the abdominal cavity, as occurs normally in many mammals, such as the elephant and armadillo.

**tes·tic·u·lar** (tes-tik'u-lər) pertaining to a testis. Called also *orchic* and *orchidic.*

**tes·tic·u·lo·ma** (tes-tik″u-lo'mə) testicular tumor; see under *tumor.*

**t. ova'rii,** arrhenoblastoma.

**tes·tic·u·lus** (tes-tik'u-ləs) gen. and pl. *testi'culi* [L., dim. of *testis*] testis.

**test·ing** (test'ing) administration of one or more tests.

**reality t.,** objective evaluation of the external world and differentiation between it and the ego or self. Impaired reality testing is seen in psychological defense mechanisms that falsify reality, such as projection and denial, and it is a major criterion for psychosis.

**tes·tis** (tes'tis) pl. *tes'tes* [L.] [TA] [MeSH: Testis] testicle: the male gonad; either of the paired egg-shaped glands normally situated in the scrotum. Each testis is surrounded by an outer mesothelial layer *(tunica vaginalis)* and an inner white capsule *(tunica albuginea),* and is composed of compartments *(lobuli testis)* containing the seminiferous tubules, in which the spermatozoa are produced. Specialized interstitial cells *(Leydig's cells)* secrete testosterone. Called also *orchis* [TA alternative] and *testiculus.*

**Cooper's irritable t.,** a testis affected with neuralgia.

**ectopic t.,** a testis which has become lodged in some abnormal location.

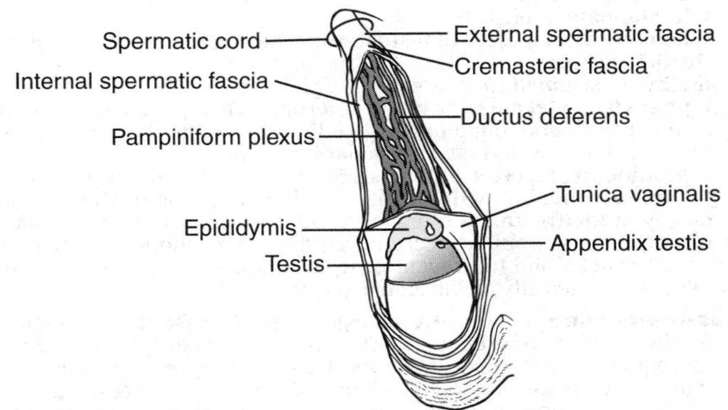


Testis, showing the investing fascial layers.

**inverted t.,** a testis whose position in the scrotum is reversed, the epididymis being attached to the anterior instead of the posterior surface.

**obstructed t.,** a testis whose descent has been prevented by a fascial sheet at the entrance to the scrotum.

**t. re'dux,** retractile t.

**retained t.,** undescended t.

**retractile t.,** a fully descended testis that moves freely between the scrotum and the inguinal canal owing to an exaggerated cremasteric reflex.

**undescended t.,** 1. a testis that has failed to descend into the scrotum and remains in the inguinal canal; see also *cryptorchidism.* Called also *retained t.* 2. cryptorchidism.

**tes·ti·tis** (tes-ti'tis) orchitis.

**test let·ter** (test let'ər) see *test type.*

**test meal** (test mēl) a meal containing material given for the specific purpose of aiding diagnostic examination of the stomach, as by fluoroscopy or by chemical analysis later of the stomach contents. See also *meal.*

**motor t. m.,** a meal or drink containing a radiopaque substance, permitting fluoroscopic observation of its progress through the stomach, pylorus, and other portions of the gastrointestinal tract.

**tes·toid** (tes'toid) an older term applied to testicular hormones and other natural or synthetic androgens.

**tes·to·lac·tone** (tes″to-lak'tōn) [USP] [MeSH: Testolactone] a synthetic antineoplastic agent produced by microbial transformation of progesterone, testosterone, or other steroidal substances, used as adjunctive therapy in the palliative treatment of advanced or disseminated breast cancer in postmenopausal women; administered orally or by intramuscular injection.

**tes·top·a·thy** (təs-top'ə-the) [*testes* + *-pathy*] orchiopathy.

**tes·tos·te·rone** (təs-tos'tə-rōn) [MeSH: Testosterone] 1. the major androgenic hormone produced by the interstitial cells (Leydig's cells) of the testes in response to stimulation by the luteinizing hormone of the adenohypophysis; it regulates gonadotropic secretion and wolffian duct differentiation (formation of the epididymis, vas deferens, and seminal vesicle), and stimulates skeletal muscle. It is also responsible for other male characteristics and spermatogenesis after its conversion to dihydrotestosterone (q.v.) by 5α-reductase in peripheral tissue. In addition, testosterone possesses protein anabolic properties, manifested by retention of nitrogen, calcium, phosphorus, and potassium, and is important in maintaining muscle mass and bone tissue in the adult male. It is also converted by aromatization to estradiol in peripheral tissue. See also *anabolic steroid,* under *steroid.* 2. [USP] the same principle prepared synthetically from cholesterol or isolated from bull testes, used in the form of various esters in treating male hypogonadism, cryptorchidism, and the symptoms of the male climacteric; its derivatives may be used for their anabolic properties. Administered by subcutaneous implantation or intramuscular injection or buccally.
**t. cyclopentylpropionate,** t. cypionate.
**t. cypionate** [USP], an ester of testosterone, having the same actions as the free alcohol but a prolonged duration of effect; used chiefly in the treatment of male hypogonadism, frigidity, and inoperable female breast cancer, to suppress lactation, and as an anabolic agent, administered by intramuscular injection. Called also *t. cyclopentylpropionate.*
**t. enanthate** [USP], an ester of testosterone, having the same actions as the free alcohol but a prolonged duration of effect; used chiefly in the treatment of male hypogonadism, oligospermia, and the symptoms of male climacteric, administered by intramuscular injection. Called also *t. heptanoate.*
**ethinyl t.,** ethisterone.
**t. heptanoate,** t. enanthate.
**t. ketolaurate,** an ester of testosterone, having the same actions as the other esters.
**methyl t.,** see *methyltestosterone.*
**t. phenylacetate,** an ester of testosterone, having the same actions as the free alcohol but a prolonged duration of effect; administered by subcutaneous and intramuscular injection.
**t. propionate,** an ester of testosterone, having the same actions as the free alcohol but with a relatively short duration of effect; used chiefly in the treatment of male hypogonadism, symptoms of male climacteric, postpubertal cryptorchidism, and inoperable female breast cancer, and to prevent postpartum breast engorgement; administered buccally or intramuscularly.

**tes·tos·te·rone 17β-de·hy·dro·gen·ase (NADP⁺)** (tes-tos'tər-ōn de-hi'dro-jən-ās) [EC 1.1.1.64] a microsomal enzyme of the oxidoreductase class that catalyzes the reduction of $\Delta^4$-androstenedione to testosterone using NADPH as an electron donor; it also catalyzes the conversion of estrone to estradiol. Deficiency of the enzyme, an autosomal recessive trait, is called $^{17}\beta$-hydroxysteroid dehydrogenase deficiency. Called also *17β-hydroxysteroid dehydrogenase* and *17-ketosteroid reductase.*

**tes·to·tox·i·co·sis** (tes"to-tok"sĭ-ko'sis) a type of isosexual precocious puberty in males occurring at about age three, caused by excessive amounts of circulating testosterone; it has autosomal dominant inheritance, and patients usually have normal fertility as adults.

**Tes·tryl** (tes'trəl) trademark for a suspension of pure crystalline testosterone.

**test type** (test tīp) printed letters of varying size, used in the testing of visual acuity; see also under *chart.*
**Jaeger's t. t.,** ordinary printer's type of seven different sizes imprinted on a card; used in testing near vision.
**Landolt's t. t.,** see under *ring.*
**Snellen's t. t.,** block letters used in testing visual acuity, so designed that the whole letter subtends, at the appropriate distance, a visual angle usually of 5 minutes, and each component part subtends an angle of 1 minute. See also *Snellen's chart.*

**TET** treadmill exercise test; tubal embryo transfer.

**te·tan·ic** (tə-tan'ik) [Gr. *tetanikos*] 1. pertaining to or of the nature of tetanus. 2. producing tetanus.

**te·tan·i·form** (tə-tan'ĭ-form) [*tetanus* + *form*] like or resembling tetanus or tetany; tetanoid.

**tet·a·nig·e·nous** (tet"ə-nij'ə-nəs) [*tetanus* + *-genous*] producing tetanus or tetanic spasms.

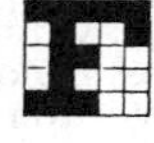 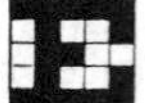

Two of Snellen's test types.

**tet·a·ni·za·tion** (tet"ə-nĭ-za'shən) the act of tetanizing a muscle.

**tet·a·nize** (tet'ə-nīz) to stimulate a muscle at progressively higher frequencies until successive contractions fuse and cannot be distinguished from one another; see *tetanus,* def. 2.

**tet·a·no·can·na·bin** (tet"ə-no-kan'ə-bin) a poisonous principle sometimes found in hemp; it resembles strychnine in its action.

**tet·a·node** (tet'ə-nōd) the unexcited stage occurring between the tetanic contractions in tetanus.

**tet·a·noid** (tet'ə-noid) [*tetanus* + *-oid*] like or resembling tetanus or tetany; tetaniform.

**tet·a·nol·y·sin** (tet"ə-nol'ĭ-sin) [*tetanus* + *lysin*] the hemolytic exotoxin produced by *Clostridium tetani,* the etiologic agent of tetanus; it may or may not contribute to the pathogenicity of the organism. Cf. *tetanospasmin.*

**tet·a·nom·e·ter** (tet"ə-nom'ə-tər) [*tetanus* + *-meter*] an apparatus for measurement and analysis of physiological tetanus.

**tet·a·no·spas·min** (tet"ə-no-spaz'min) [*tetanus* + *spasm-* + *-in* chemical suffix] the neurotoxic component of the exotoxin (tetanus toxin) produced by *Clostridium tetani,* a highly potent protein that binds to gangliosides and blocks the synaptic terminals of the central nervous system, causing the typical muscle spasms of tetanus. It is one of the most powerful poisons known. See also *tetanolysin.*

**tet·a·nus** (tet'ə-nəs) [Gr. *tetanos,* from *teinein* to stretch] [MeSH: Tetanus] 1. an acute, often fatal infectious disease caused by the bacillus *Clostridium tetani,* which produces the neurotoxin tetanospasmin; it usually enters the body through a contaminated puncture wound (such as from a metal nail, wood splinter, or insect bite), although other portals of entry include burns, surgical wounds, cutaneous ulcers, injection sites of drug abusers, the umbilical stump of neonates *(t. neonatorum),* and the postpartum uterus. *Generalized tetanus* is characterized by tetanic muscular contractions and hyperreflexia, resulting in trismus (lockjaw), glottal spasm, generalized muscle spasm, opisthotonos, respiratory spasm, seizures, and paralysis. *Localized tetanus* may be mild, with localized muscular twitching and spasm of muscle groups near the site of injury, or it may progress to the generalized form. 2. physiological tetanus; a state of sustained muscular contraction without periods of relaxation caused by repetitive stimulation of the motor nerve trunk at frequencies so high that individual muscle twitches are fused and cannot be distinguished from one another; called also *tetanic* or *tonic contraction* and *tetanic* or *tonic spasm.*
**cephalic t., cerebral t.,** a rare form of infectious tetanus with an extremely poor prognosis that may occur after an injury to the head or face or in association with otitis media in which *Clostridium tetani* is a constituent of the flora of the middle ear; it is characterized by isolated or combined dysfunction of the cranial nerves, especially the seventh cranial, and may remain localized or progress to generalized tetanus. Called also *cephalotetanus.*
**cryptogenic t.,** tetanus which occurs without any wound or other ascertainable cause.
**neonatal t., t. neonato'rum,** a severe form of infectious tetanus occurring during the first few days of life caused by such factors as unhygienic practice in dressing the umbilical stump or in circumcising male infants and the lack of maternal immunization.
**physiological t.,** tetanus, def. 2.

**tet·a·ny** (tet'ə-ne) [MeSH: Tetany] hyperexcitability of nerves and muscles due to decrease in concentration of extracellular ionized calcium, which may be associated with such conditions as parathyroid hypofunction, vitamin D deficiency, and alkalosis or result from ingestion of alkaline salts; it is characterized by carpopedal spasm, muscular twitching and cramps, laryngospasm with inspiratory stridor, hyperreflexia, and choreiform movements.
**duration t.,** a continuous tetanic contraction in response to a very strong continuous current; it occurs especially in degenerated muscles; abbreviated Dt.
**gastric t.,** a severe form due to disease of the stomach, attended by difficult respiration and painful tonic spasms of the extremities.
**grass t.,** lactation t.
**hyperventilation t.,** tetany produced by forced inspiration and expiration continued for a considerable time.
**hypomagnesemic t.,** 1. lactation t. 2. hypomagnesemia in calves fed only milk (which lacks magnesium); it is often fatal, with symptoms like those of lactation tetany in cows.
**lactation t.,** 1. an often fatal condition seen in cows and sheep in the first few weeks after lactation has begun, when they are turned out into lush pastures, due to deficiency of magnesium in the diet. Symptoms include muscular spasms and convulsions. Called also *grass staggers* and *grass* or *hypomagnesemic t.* 2. puerperal t.
**latent t.,** tetany elicited by the application of electrical and mechanical stimulation.
**neonatal t., t. of newborn,** hypocalcemic tetany occurring in the first few days of life, often marked by irritability, muscular twitch-

ings, jitteriness, tremors, and convulsions, and less frequently by laryngospasm and carpopedal spasm.

**parathyroid t., parathyroprival t.,** tetany due to removal of the parathyroids.

**puerperal t.,** tetany in a nursing mother dog or cat as a result of hypocalcemia; small dogs with large litters are particularly susceptible. Called also *lactation t.* and *eclampsia.*

**transit t., transport t.,** a condition sometimes seen in livestock shipped for long distances, especially well-fed cows and ewes in advanced pregnancy or lactating mares; it may result in paralysis, unconsciousness, and death unless treatment is begun early. The etiology is unknown, but it may be due to acute hypocalcium associated with improper care and feeding. Called also *railroad disease* or *sickness.*

**tet·ar·ta·nope** (tət-ahr'tə-nōp) a person with tetartanopia.

**tet·ar·ta·no·pia** (tet″ər-tə-no'pe-ə) [Gr. *tetartos* fourth + *an-*[1] + *-opia*] 1. quadrantanopia. 2. a rare dichromasy of doubtful existence characterized by retention of the sensory mechanism for two hues only (red and green), and lacking that for blue and yellow, which are replaced in the spectrum by an achromatic (gray) band.

**tet·ar·ta·nop·ic** (tet″ər-tə-nop'ik) pertaining to or characterized by tetartanopia.

**tet·ar·ta·nop·sia** (tet″ər-tə-nop'se-ə) tetartanopia.

**te·tio·thal·ein so·di·um** (te″she-o-thal'ēn) iodophthalein sodium.

**tetra-** [Gr.] a combining form meaning *four.*

**tet·ra·ba·sic** (tet″rə-ba'sik) [*tetra-* + *basic*] containing four atoms of replaceable hydrogen.

**tet·ra·blas·tic** (tet″rə-blas'tik) having four germ layers.

**tet·ra·bo·ric ac·id** (tet″rə-bor'ik) pyroboric acid.

**tet·ra·bra·chi·us** (tet″rə-bra'ke-əs) [*tetra-* + Gr. *brachiōn* arm] conjoined twins having four arms.

**tet·ra·bro·mo·flu·o·res·ce·in** (tet″rə-bro″mo-floo-res'ēn) eosin.

**tet·ra·bro·mo·phe·nol·phthal·ein** (tet″rə-bro″mo-fe″nol-thal'ēn) an indicator which is colorless with acids and violet with alkalis.

**tet·ra·bro·mo·phthal·ein so·di·um** (tet″rə-bro″mo-thal'ēn) the sodium salt of tetrabromophenolphthalein, used for radiologic examination of the gallbladder, in which organ it appears after intravenous injection.

**tet·ra·caine** (tet'rə-kān) [USP] [MeSH: Tetracaine] a local anesthetic applied topically to the eyeball and conjunctiva.

**t. hydrochloride** [USP], the hydrochloride salt of tetracaine, applied topically to the conjunctiva and eyeball, to the mucous membranes of the nose, throat, and respiratory tract, and to the skin to produce surface anesthesia and also used parenterally for spinal, conduction, and infiltration anesthesia. Called also *amethocaine hydrochloride.*

**tet·ra·chi·rus** (tet″rə-ki'rəs) [*tetra-* + Gr. *cheir* hand] a fetus having four hands.

**tet·ra·chlor·eth·ane** (tet″rə-klor-eth'ān) tetrachloroethane.

**tet·ra·chlo·ride** (tet″rə-klor'īd) a compound of a radical with four atoms of chlorine.

**tet·ra·chlor·meth·ane** (tet″rə-klor-meth'ān) carbon tetrachloride, $CCl_4$.

**2,3,7,8-tet·ra·chlo·ro·di·ben·zo-*p*-di·ox·in (TCDD)** (tet″rə-klor″o-di-ben″zo-di-ok'sin) a teratogenic and carcinogenic dioxin that contaminates the herbicide 2,4,5-T.

**tet·ra·chlo·ro·eth·ane** (tet″rə-klor″o-eth'ān) acetylene tetrachloride, formed by the reaction of acetylene and chlorine; an industrial solvent and intermediate in the synthesis of chlorinated hydrocarbons. If ingested it causes a hepatotoxic condition called *tetrachloroethane poisoning* (see under *poisoning*).

**tet·ra·chlo·ro·eth·y·lene** (tet″rə-klor″o-eth'ə-lēn) [MeSH: Tetrachloroethylene] a moderately toxic chlorinated hydrocarbon, formerly used as an anthelmintic but now used only as a dry cleaning solvent and for other industrial uses. Called also *perchloroethylene.*

**tet·ra·chlor·phen·ox·ide** (tet″rə-klor″fən-ok'sīd) a fungicide used for the preservation of lumber; it may cause a dermatitis in workmen.

**tet·ra·chro·mic** (tet″rə-kro'mik) [*tetra-* + *chrom-* + *-ic*] 1. pertaining to or exhibiting four colors. 2. able to distinguish only four of the seven colors of the spectrum according to the Eldridge-Green classification of color blindness.

**tet·rac·id** (tet'ras-id) capable of replacing four atoms of hydrogen in an acid, or having four atoms of hydrogen replaceable by acid radicals.

**tet·ra·co·sa·no·ic ac·id** (tet″rə-ko″sə-no'ik) systematic name for *lignoceric acid*; see also table at *fatty acid.*

**tet·ra·crot·ic** (tet″rə-krot'ik) [*tetra-* + Gr. *krotos* beat] showing four elevations in the sphygmographic tracing of the pulse.

**tet·ra·cyc·lic** (tet″rə-sik'lik) containing four fused rings or closed chains in the molecular structure.

**tet·ra·cy·cline** (tet″rə-si'klēn) [MeSH: Tetracycline] 1. any of a group of biosynthetic antibiotics; some are isolated from certain species of *Streptomyces* and others are produced semisynthetically by catalytic hydrogenation of chlortetracycline or oxytetracycline. The group includes chlortetracycline, oxytetracycline, tetracycline (see def. 2), demeclocycline, rolitetracycline, methacycline, doxycycline, and minocycline. Tetracyclines are effective against a wide variety of organisms, including gram-positive and gram-negative bacteria, rickettsias, mycoplasmas, chlamydias, and certain viruses, protozoa, and actinomycetes. 2. [USP] a semisynthetic antibiotic, having the same wide spectrum of antimicrobial activity as other members of the tetracycline group; used as an antibacterial, antirickettsial, and antiamebic; administered orally.

**t. hydrochloride** [USP], the monohydrochloride salt of tetracycline, having the same actions and uses as the base; administered orally, intramuscularly, or intravenously, or applied topically to the conjunctiva or eyelid.

**t. phosphate complex,** a phosphate complex salt of tetracycline, prepared by the addition of a solution of sodium metaphosphate to a solution of tetracycline or tetracycline hydrochloride; used as an antibacterial, administered orally, intramuscularly, or intravenously.

**Tet·ra·cyn** (tet'rə-sin) trademark for preparations of tetracycline.

**tet·rad** (tet'rad) [Gr. *tetra-* four] a group of four similar or related entities, as (1) any element or radical having a valence, or combining power, of four; (2) a group of four chromosomal elements formed in the pachytene state of the first meiotic prophase; (3) a square of cells produced by the division into two planes of certain cocci *(Sarcina).*

**Fallot's t.,** tetralogy of Fallot.

**narcoleptic t.,** the combination of daytime sleepiness, cataplexy, sleep paralysis, and hypnagogic hallucinations.

**tet·ra·dac·ty·lous** (tet″rə-dak'tə-ləs) pertaining to or characterized by tetradactyly. Called also *quadridigitate.*

**tet·ra·dac·ty·ly** (tet″rə-dak'tə-le) [*tetra-* + Gr. *daktylos* finger] the condition of having four digits on the hand or foot.

**tet·ra·dec·a·no·yl phor·bol ac·e·tate** (tet″rə-dek'ə-no-əl fōr'bol as'ə-tāt) a phorbol ester that is a cancer promoter and is used to produce skin cancer in laboratory animals.

**-tetraene** a suffix denoting a chemical compound in which there are four conjugated double bonds.

**tet·ra·er·y·thrin** (tet″rə-er'ĭ-thrin) crustaceorubin.

**tet·ra·eth·yl·am·mo·ni·um** (tet″rə-eth″əl-ə-mo'ne-əm) the radical $(C_2H_5)_4N$; the bromide and chloride salts are short-acting quaternary ammonium ganglion-blocking agents that have been used in the treatment of acute hypertension, peripheral vascular diseases, and other disorders of the peripheral circulation. They are now seldom employed, having been replaced by more effective drugs. Abbreviated TEA.

**tet·ra·eth·yl py·ro·phos·phate (TEPP)** (tet″rə-eth'il pi″ro-fos'fāt) an organophosphorus agricultural insecticide highly toxic to humans and other animals. See *organophosphorus compound poisoning,* under *poisoning.*

**tet·ra·eth·yl·thi·uram di·sul·fide** (tet″rə-eth″əl-thi'u-ram″) disulfiram.

**tet·ra·fil·con A** (tet″rə-fil'kon) a hydrophilic contact lens material.

**tet·ra·go·num** (tet″rə-go'nəm) [L.; Gr. *tetragōnon*] quadrilateral.

**t. lumba'le,** the quadrangular space bounded by the four lumbar muscles: the serratus posterior inferior superiorly, the internal oblique inferiorly, the erector spinae internally, and the external oblique externally.

**tet·ra·go·nus** (tet″rə-go'nəs) the platysma.

**tet·ra·hy·dric** (tet″rə-hi'drik) containing four atoms of ionizable hydrogen: said of an acid or alcohol.

**tet·ra·hy·dro·bi·op·ter·in** (tet″rə-hi″dro-bi-op'tər-in) a reduced form of dihydrobiopterin that functions as a coenzyme in the reactions hydroxylating phenylalanine, tryptophan, and tyrosine by carrying electrons to oxygen. Defects in the biosynthesis or regeneration of the coenzyme affect all three hydroxylation reactions, interfere with production of the corresponding neurotransmitter precursors, and result in malignant hyperphenylalaninemia.

**tet·ra·hy·dro·can·nab·i·nol** (tet″rə-hi″dro-kə-nab'ĭ-nol) [MeSH: Tetrahydrocannabinol] the active principle of cannabis, occurring in two isomeric forms, both considered psychotomimetically active. Abbreviated THC.

**tet·ra·hy·dro·fo·late (THF)** (tet″rə-hi″dro-fo′lāt) an ester or dissociated form of tetrahydrofolic acid.

**tet·ra·hy·dro·fo·lic ac·id** (tet″rə-hi″dro-fo′lik) a form of folic acid in which the pteridine ring is fully reduced; it is the parent compound of a variety of coenzymes that serve as carriers of one-carbon groups in metabolic reactions. Tetrahydrofolic acid and its derivatives are required for the metabolism of several amino acids, the formation of creatine and choline, the methylation of RNA molecules, the synthesis of purines, and the synthesis of deoxythymidine monophosphate. Abbreviated THF. Called also *tetrahydropteroylglutamic acid.*

**tet·ra·hy·dro·pal·ma·tine** (tet″rə-hi″dro-pal′mə-tin) a crystalline alkaloid, chemically related to berberine, found in corydalis.

**tet·ra·hy·dro·pter·o·yl·glu·ta·mate meth·yl·trans·fer·ase** (tet″rə-hi″dro-ter″o-əl-gloo′tə-māt meth″əl-trans′fər-ās) [MeSH: Tetrahydropteroylglutamate Methyltransferase] 5-methyltetrahydrofolate–homocysteine *S*-methyltransferase.

**tet·ra·hy·dro·pter·o·yl·glu·tam·ic ac·id** (tet″rə-hi″dro-ter″o-əl-gloo-tam′ik) tetrahydrofolic acid.

**tet·ra·hy·droz·o·line hy·dro·chlo·ride** (tet″rə-hi-droz′o-lēn) [USP] an adrenergic, applied topically to the nasal mucosa and to the conjunctiva to produce vasoconstriction.

**Tet·ra·hy·me·na** (tet″rə-hi′mə-nə) [*tetra-* Gr. *hymēn* membrane] [MeSH: Tetrahymena] a genus of ciliate protozoa (suborder Tetrahymenina, order Hymenostomatida) used extensively in physiologic and genetic studies; they have been shown to be capable of parasitic existence when experimentally injected into various hosts. *T limacis* and *T. pyriformis* are representative species.

**Tet·ra·hy·me·ni·na** (tet″rə-hi″mə-ni′nə) [MeSH: Tetrahymenina] a suborder of ciliate protozoa (order Hymenostomatida, subclass Hymenostomatia), characterized by the presence of uniform ciliation, three oral membranelles on the left and an undulating or paroral membrane on the right, and mucocysts. Most are free-living in fresh water, but a few species are symbiotic, mainly in invertebrates. *Tetrahymena* is a representative genus.

**tet·ra·iodo·phe·nol·phthal·ein** (tet″rə-i″o-do-fe″nol-thal′ēn) a dye which after intravenous injection is excreted in the bile in sufficient amount to make possible radiography of the gallbladder.

**tet·ra·iodo·phthal·ein so·di·um** (tet″rə-i″o-do-thal′ēn) iodophthalein sodium.

**tet·ra·iodo·thy·ro·nine** (tet″rə-i″o-do-thi′ro-nēn) thyroxine.

**te·tral·o·gy** (te-tral′ə-je) a combination of four elements or factors, such as four concurrent symptoms or defects.
**t. of Eisenmenger,** Eisenmenger's complex.
**t. of Fallot,** a combination of congenital cardiac defects consisting of pulmonary stenosis, interventricular septal defect, dextroposition of the aorta so that it overrides the interventricular septum and receives venous as well as arterial blood, and right ventricular hypertrophy. See illustration.

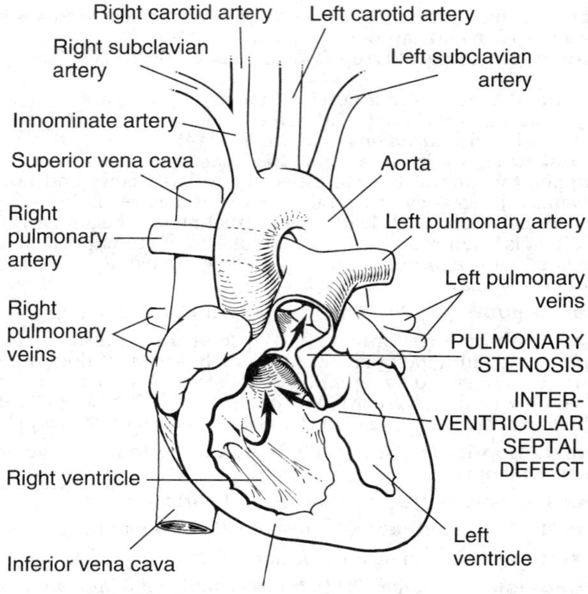

Tetralogy of Fallot.

**tet·ra·mas·ti·gote** (tet″rə-mas′tĭ-gōt) [*tetra-* + *mastigote*] 1. having four flagella. 2. an organism having four flagella.

**tet·ra·ma·zia** (tet″rə-ma′ze-ə) [*tetra-* + *maz-* + *-ia*] the condition of having four mammary glands.

**tet·ra·mer** (tet′rə-mər″) a compound composed of four identical simpler molecules.

**Te·tram·er·es** (tĕ-tram′ər-ēz) a genus of nematodes parasitic in the alimentary tract of chickens and other fowl. *T. america′na* is found in the proventriculus of chickens and other birds; heavy infestations may be fatal to young birds.

**tet·ra·mer·ic** (tet″rə-mer′ik) having four parts.

**tet·ra·meth·yl** (tet″rə-meth′əl) a chemical compound each molecule of which contains four methyl groups.

**tet·ra·meth·yl·am·mo·ni·um hy·drox·ide** (tet″rə-meth″əl-ə-mo′ne-əm hi-drok′sīd) a toxic fraction isolated from the sea anemone, *Actinia equina,* and from the salivary glands of whelks.

**tet·ra·meth·yl·ben·zi·dine** (tet″rə-meth″əl-ben′zĭ-dēn) an analog of benzidine; it acts as a chromogen to detect horseradish peroxidase activity in biochemical assays.

**tet·ra·meth·yl·ene·di·amine** (tet″rə-meth″əl-ēn-di′a-mēn) putrescine.

**tet·ra·meth·yl·pu·tres·cine** (tet″rə-meth″əl-pu-tres′in) an extremely poisonous crystalline base derivable from putrescine; it produces symptoms like those of muscarine poisoning.

**tet·ra·mine** (tet′rə-mēn) tetramethylammonium hydroxide.

**te·tram·i·sole hy·dro·chlo·ride** (tĕ-tram′ĭ-sōl) a veterinary anthelmintic effective against roundworms, hookworms, and strongyloids.

**Te·tram·i·tus mes·ni·li** (tĕ-tram′ĭ-təs məs-ni′le) *Chilomastix mesnili.*

**tet·ra·ni·trol** (tet″rə-ni′trol) erythrityl tetranitrate.

**tet·ran·oph·thal·mos** (tet″ran-of-thal′mos) [*tetra-* + Gr. *ophthalmos* eye] a fetus having four eyes.

**tet·ran·op·sia** (tet″ran-op′se-ə) quadrantanopia.

**Tet·ran·y·chus** (tet-ran′ĭ-kəs) [*tetra-* + Gr. *onyx* nail] a genus of mites. *T. autumna′lis* has been reclassified as *Neotrombicula autumnalis. T. molestis′simus* and *T. tela′rius* (the spider mite) attack humans.

**Tet·ra·odon** (tet″rə-o′don) a genus of poisonous puffer fish of the family Tetraodontidae. Their bodies contain tetrodotoxin, and ingestion without special preparation can cause fatal tetrodotoxism.

**Tet·ra·odon·ti·dae** (tet″rə-o-don′tĭ-de) a family of bony tropical marine fish, including puffers and sunfish; it includes the genera *Fugu, Sphaeroides,* and *Tetraodon.* See also *tetrodotoxin* and *tetrodotoxism.*

**tet·ra·odon·tox·in** (tet″rə-o-don-tok′sin) tetrodotoxin.

**tet·ra·odon·tox·ism** (tet″rə-o-don-tok′siz-əm) tetrodotoxism.

**tet·ra·otus** (tet″rə-o′təs) [Gr. *tetraōtos* four-eared] a fetus with two nearly separate heads, two faces, four eyes, and four ears.

**tet·ra·pa·re·sis** (tet″rə-pə-re′sis) muscular weakness affecting all four extremities.

**tet·ra·pep·tide** (tet″rə-pep′tīd) a peptide which on hydrolysis yields four amino acids.

**tet·ra·ple·gia** (tet″rə-ple′jə) [*tetra-* + *-plegia*] quadriplegia.

**tet·ra·ploid** (tet′rə-ploid) 1. pertaining to or characterized by tetraploidy. 2. an individual or cell having four sets of chromosomes.

**tet·ra·ploi·dy** (tet′rə-ploi-de) the state of having four sets of chromosomes ($4n$).

**tet·ra·pus** (tet′rə-pəs) [*tetra-* + Gr. *pous* foot] a human fetus having four feet.

**tet·ra·pyr·role** (tet′rə-pĭ-rōl″) a compound containing four pyrrole rings, e.g., heme or chlorophyll.

**tet·ra·sac·cha·ride** (tet″rə-sak′ə-rīd) any of a class of carbohydrates composed of four glycosidically linked monosaccharide groups.

**te·tras·ce·lus** (tĕ-tras′ə-ləs) [*tetra-* + Gr. *skelos* leg] a human fetus having four legs.

**tet·ra·som·ic** (tet″rə-som′ik) pertaining to or characterized by tetrasomy.

**tet·ra·so·my** (tet′rə-so″me) [*tetra-* + Gr. *sōma* body] the presence of two additional chromosomes of one type in an otherwise diploid cell ($2n + 2$).

**tet·ra·spore** (tet′rə-spor) in fungi, one of the spores of a four-spored basidium. Cf. *dispore.*

**tet·ras·ter** (tət-ras′tər) [*tetra-* + *aster*] a figure in abnormal mitosis characterized by four centrosomal centers or asters.

**tet·ra·sti·chi·a·sis** (tet″rə-stĭ-ki′ə-sis) [*tetra-* + Gr. *stichos* row + *-iasis*] an extremely rare condition in which there are four rows of eyelashes.

**tet·ra·tom·ic** (tet″rə-tom′ik) 1. consisting of four atoms. 2. having four replaceable atoms.

**Tet·ra·trich·om·o·nas buc·ca·lis** (tet″rə-trik-om′o-nəs bə-ka′lis) *Trichomonas tenax.*

**tet·ra·va·lent** (tət-rə-va′lənt) having a valence of four.

**tet·ro·don·ic ac·id** (tet″ro-don′ik) a poisonous acid from various puffer fish (family *Tetraodontidae*).

**tet·ro·do·tox·in** (tet″ro-do-tok′sin) [MeSH: Tetrodotoxin] a pure, crystalline, highly lethal neurotoxin present in puffer fish of the order Tetraodontidae and in newts of the genus *Taricha* (in which it is called *tarichatoxin*). Ingestion of improperly cooked flesh may result in tetrodotoxism within minutes. Called also *tetraodontoxin.*

**tet·ro·do·tox·ism** (tet″ro-do-tok′siz-əm) [*Tetraodon* + *toxin*] 1. the most severe form of ichthyosarcotoxism, produced by ingestion of puffer fish or other animals containing tetrodotoxin; symptoms include malaise, dizziness, and tingling around the mouth, which may be followed within a short time by ataxia, convulsions, respiratory paralysis, and death. Called also *fugu poisoning* and *puffer* or *puffer fish poisoning.* 2. poisoning from tetrodotoxin after being bitten or stung by an animal such as the blue-ringed octopus. Defs. 1 and 2 called also *tetraodotoxism.*

**tet·ro·fos·min** (tet″ro-foz′min) a phosphine which when labeled with technetium 99m is used in myocardial perfusion imaging; see table at *technetium.*

**tet·ro·nal** (tet′ro-nəl) diethylsulfondiethylmethane, $(C_2H_5)_2 \cdot C \cdot (SO_2C_2H_5)_2$, occurring in the form of colorless scales; it is a hypnotic.

**tet·roph·thal·mos** (tet″rof-thal′mos) [*tetra-* + Gr. *ophthalmos* eye] tetranophthalmos.

**tet·rose** (tet′rōs) a monosaccharide containing four carbon atoms in a molecule.

**tet·ro·tus** (tet-ro′təs) tetraotus.

**te·trox·ide** (tĕ-trok′sīd) a compound of an element or a radical with four oxygen atoms, as osmium tetroxide.

**tet·ru·lose** (tet′roo-lōs) ketotetrose.

**tet·ryl** (tet′rəl) an organic explosive and expellant which may cause an industrial dermatitis.

**tet·ter** (tet′ər) a once popular name for various eczematous skin diseases.
**milky t.,** crusta lactea.

**Teut·le·ben's ligament** (toit′la-benz) [Friedrich Ernst Karl von *Teutleben,* German anatomist, 19th century] see under *ligament.*

**tex·ti·form** (teks′tĭ-form) [L. *textum* any material put together + *form*] formed like a tissue, network, or web.

**tex·to·blas·tic** (teks″to-blas′tik) [L. *textum* any material put together + *blast*[1] + *-ic*] forming adult tissue; regenerative: said of cells.

**tex·tur·al** (teks′chə-rəl) pertaining to the texture, or constitution, of the tissues.

**tex·ture** (teks′chər) [L. *textura*] the structure or organization of a tissue or organ.

**tex·tus** (teks′təs) gen. and pl. *tex′tus* [L., from *texere* to weave] a tissue.

**TF** transfer factor; tuberculin filtrate.

**T-group** [MeSH: Sensitivity Training Groups] training group; see *sensitivity group,* under *group.*

**6-TG** 6-thioguanine.

**TGE** transmissible gastroenteritis.

**TGF** transforming growth factor.

**TGT** thromboplastin generation test.

**Th** symbol for *thorium.*

**Thal procedure** (thal) [Alal P. *Thal,* American surgeon, born 1925] see under *procedure.*

**thal·a·mec·to·my** (thal″ə-mek′tə-me) [*thalamus* + *-tomy*] thalamotomy.

**thal·a·men·ce·phal·ic** (thal″ə-men″sə-fal′ik) pertaining to the thalamencephalon.

**thal·a·men·ceph·a·lon** (thal″ə-mən-sef′ə-lon) the part of the diencephalon that comprises the thalamus, metathalamus, and epithalamus.

**thal·a·mi** (thal′ə-mi) [L.] genitive and plural of *thalamus.*

**tha·lam·ic** (thə-lam′ik) pertaining to the thalamus.

**thal·a·mo·cor·ti·cal** (thal″ə-mo-kor′tĭ-kəl) pertaining to the thalamus and cerebral cortex.

**thal·a·mo·len·tic·u·lar** (thal″ə-mo-lən-tik′u-lər) pertaining to the thalamus and the lenticular nucleus.

**thal·a·mo·mam·mil·lary** (thal″ə-mo-mam′ĭ-lar-e) pertaining to the thalamus and mammillary bodies.

**thal·a·mo·teg·men·tal** (thal″ə-mo-təg-men′təl) pertaining to the thalamus and tegmentum.

**thal·a·mot·o·my** (thal″ə-mot′ə-me) [*thalamus* + Gr. *-otomy*] a stereotaxic surgical technique for the discrete destruction of specific groups of cells within the thalamus; done to relieve pain, to alleviate the tremor and rigidity in paralysis agitans, and as psychosurgery to relieve certain anxiety states, psychoses, and obsessive-compulsive states.
**anterior t.,** production of lesions in the anterior nucleus of the thalamus.
**dorsomedial t.,** production of lesions in the dorsomedial nucleus of the thalamus, a psychosurgical technique for the relief of certain anxiety states, psychoses, and obsessive-compulsive states.

**thal·a·mus** (thal′ə-məs) pl. *thal′ami* [L.; Gr. *thalamos* inner chamber] [TA] [MeSH: Thalamus] a large ovoid mass in the posterior part of the diencephalon forming most of each lateral wall of the third ventricle, composed chiefly of gray substance and associated laminae of white substance. It is divided into anterior, medial, and lateral parts, each part containing groups of nuclei that function as relay centers for sensory impulses and cerebellar and basal ganglia projections to the cerebral cortex. The main groups of thalamic nuclei are the reticular, anterior, median, medial, medullary, intralaminar, ventrolateral, and posterior nuclei. Some authorities consider the subthalamus part of the thalamus and refer to it as the *ventral thalamus,* calling the posterior part the *dorsal thalamus.*

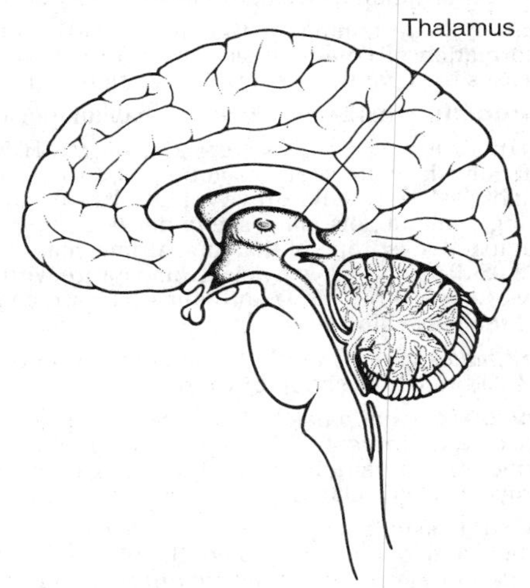


**dorsal t., t. dorsa′lis,** see *thalamus.*
**optic t.,** corpus geniculatum laterale.
**ventral t., t. ventra′lis,** name given to the subthalamus when it is considered part of the thalamus.

**tha·las·sa·ne·mia** (thə-las″ə-ne′me-ə) thalassemia.

**thal·as·se·mia** (thal″ə-se′me-ə) [Gr. *thalassa* sea (because it was observed originally in persons of Mediterranean stock) + *-emia*] [MeSH: Thalassemia] a heterogeneous group of hereditary hemolytic anemias that have in common a decreased rate of synthesis of one or more hemoglobin polypeptide chains and are classified according to the chain involved ($\alpha$, $\beta$, $\delta$); the two major categories are $\alpha$- and $\beta$-thalassemia. Homozygous forms are manifested by profound anemia or death *in utero,* and heterozygous forms by erythrocyte anomalies ranging from mild to severe.
**$\alpha$-t.,** that caused by decreased rate of synthesis of the alpha chains of hemoglobin. The homozygous form is incompatible with life, the stillborn infant displaying severe hydrops fetalis; the heterozygous form may be asymptomatic or marked by mild anemia.
**$\beta$-t.,** that caused by diminished synthesis of beta chains of hemoglobin. The homozygous form is known as *t. major* and the heterozygous form is known as *t. minor.*

**δ-t.,** that involving suppression of the delta chains of hemoglobin; it is usually symptom-free.
**δβ-t.,** a form of heterozygous thalassemia in which synthesis of both delta and beta chains of hemoglobin is decreased; clinically it resembles thalassemia minor.
**hemoglobin C–t.,** see under *disease.*
**hemoglobin E–t.,** see under *disease.*
**hemoglobin S–t.,** sickle cell–thalassemia disease.
**t. interme'dia,** β-thalassemia whose clinical appearance is intermediate between thalassemia major and thalassemia minor.
**t. ma'jor,** the homozygous form of β-thalassemia, a severe condition evident from the neonatal period with complete absence of hemoglobin A; characteristics include hemolytic, hypochromic, microcytic anemia, pronounced hepatosplenomegaly, skeletal deformation, mongoloid facies, and cardiac enlargement. Called also *Cooley's anemia* or *disease.*
**t. mi'nor,** the heterozygous form of β-thalassemia; it is usually asymptomatic, although hemoglobin A synthesis may be retarded and there is sometimes moderate anemia and splenomegaly.
**sickle cell–t.,** see under *disease.*

**tha·las·sin** (thə-las'in) a toxic substance derived from tentacles of the sea anemone, *Anemonia sulcata,* which, when injected into dogs, produces allergic symptoms.

**tha·las·so·ther·a·py** (thə-las″o-ther'ə-pe) [Gr. *thalassa* sea + *therapy*] [MeSH: Thalassotherapy] the treatment of disease by sea bathing, sea voyages, and sea air.

**tha·lid·o·mide** (thə-lid'o-mīd) [MeSH: Thalidomide] a sedative and hypnotic commonly used in Europe in the late 1950's and 1960's. Its use was discontinued because it was discovered to cause serious congenital anomalies in the fetus, notably amelia and phocomelia, when taken by a woman during early pregnancy. It is used investigationally as an immunosuppressant in acute lepra reaction and a number of autoimmune disorders and in the prophylaxis and treatment of graft-versus-host disease.

**Thal·i·tone** (thal'ĭ-tōn) trademark for a preparation of chlorthalidone.

**thal·lei·o·quin** (thə-li'o-kwin) a greenish, resinous substance, produced in a test for quinine; see under *tests.*

**thal·lic** (thal'ik) 1. pertaining to a thallus. 2. said of conidiogenesis in which formation of conidia begins with formation of a septum and progresses to separation of a whole section of the parent cell.

**thal·li·tox·i·co·sis** (thal″ĭ-tok″sĭ-ko'sis) thallium poisoning.

**thal·li·um** (thal'e-əm) [Gr. *thallos* green shoot] [MeSH: Thallium] a heavy, soft, bluish white metal; symbol, Tl; atomic number, 81; atomic weight, 204.37; specific gravity, 11.85. Its salts are active poisons, causing thallium poisoning; see under *poisoning.*
**t. 201,** a radioactive isotope of thallium, atomic mass 201, having a half-life of 3.05 days; it decays by electron capture with emission of gamma rays (0.135, 0.167 MeV) and is used as a diagnostic aid in the form of thallous chloride (q.v.).

**thall(o)-** [Gr. *thallos* green shoot] a combining form denoting a relationship to a branch or shoot, or to thallium.

**Thal·lo·bac·te·ria** (thal″o-bak-tēr'e-ə) [*thallo-* + *bacteria*] a class of bacteria of the Firmicutes, kingdom Procaryotae, made up of gram-positive organisms that show a branching habit. It comprises the actinomycetes and related organisms.

**Thal·loph·y·ta** (thə-lof'ĭ-tə) [*thallo-* + Gr. *phyton* plant] in former classifications, a taxonomic division of the plant kingdom comprising the fungi and algae, i.e., organisms possessing a thallus, and sometimes including bacteria and slime molds.

**thal·lo·phyte** (thal'o-fīt) [*thallo-* + *-phyte*] an individual of the Thallophyta.

**thal·lo·spore** (thal'o-spor) [*thallo-* + *spore*] a thallus modified to serve as an organ of reproduction.

**thal·lo·tox·i·co·sis** (thal″o-tok″sĭ-ko'sis) thallium poisoning.

**thal·lus** (thal'əs) 1. a simple plant body not differentiated into root, stem, and leaf, which is characteristic of mycelial fungi and some algae. 2. the actively growing vegetative organism as distinguished from reproductive or resting portions, as in fungi.

**thal·po·sis** (thal-po'sis) [Gr. *thalpos* warmth] the ability to feel warmth; see *temperature sense,* under *sense.*

**thal·pot·ic** (thal-pot'ik) pertaining to thalposis.

**THAM** tromethamine.

**Tham·nid·ia·ce·ae** (tham-nid″e-a'se-e) a family of perfect fungi of the order Mucorales. Genera *Cokeromyces* and *Thamnidium* contain pathogenic species.

**Tham·nid·i·um** (tham-nid'e-əm) a genus of fungi of the family Thamnidiaceae. Some species contain trichothecenes and can cause alimentary toxic aleukia.

**tham·uria** (tham-u're-ə) [Gr. *thamys* often + *-uria*] pollakiuria.

**thanat(o)-** [Gr. *thanatos* death] a combining form denoting death.

**than·a·to·bi·o·log·ic** (than″ə-to-bi″ə-loj'ik) [*thanato-* + *biologic*] pertaining to death and life.

**than·a·to·gno·mon·ic** (than″ə-to-no-mon'ik) [*thanato-* + Gr. *gnōmonikos* decisive] indicating the approach of death.

**than·a·toid** (than'ə-toid) [*thanato-* + *-oid*] resembling death.

**than·a·tol·o·gy** (than″ə-tol'ə-je) [MeSH: Thanatology] the medicolegal study of death and conditions affecting dead bodies.

**than·a·tom·e·ter** (than″ə-tom'ə-tər) [*thanato-* + *-meter*] a thermometer used to prove the occurrence of death by registering the reduction of the bodily temperature.

**than·a·to·phid·ia** (than″ə-to-fid'e-ə) [*thanato-* + Gr. *ophis* snake] venomous snakes.

**than·a·to·phid·i·al** (than″ə-to-fid'e-əl) pertaining to venomous snakes.

**than·a·to·pho·bia** (than″ə-to-fo'be-ə) [*thanato-* + *-phobia*] irrational fear of death.

**than·a·to·pho·ric** (than″ə-to-for'ik) [*thanato-* + Gr. *pherein* to bear] deadly; lethal.

**than·a·top·sia, than·a·top·sy** (than″ə-top'se-ə, than'ə-top″se) [*thanato-* + Gr. *opsis* view] necropsy.

**than·a·to·sis** (than″ə-to'sis) 1. necrosis. 2. gangrene.

**Thane's method** (thānz) [Sir George Dancer *Thane,* British anatomist, 1850–1930] see under *method.*

**thau·mat·ro·py** (thaw-mat'rə-pe) [Gr. *thauma* wonder + *-tropy*] the transformation of an organ or structure into another organ or structure.

**Thay·sen's disease** (ti'senz) [Thornwald Einar Hess *Thaysen,* Danish physician, 1883–1936] nontropical sprue.

**THC** tetrahydrocannabinol.

**thea·ism** (the'ə-iz-əm) [L. *thea* tea] caffeinism resulting from ingestion of excessive quantities of tea.

**the·ba·ic** (the-ba'ik) [L. *Thebaicus* Theban, named for Thebes, where opium was once prepared] pertaining to or derived from opium.

**the·baine** (the-ba'in) [MeSH: Thebaine] a crystalline, poisonous, and anodyne alkaloid from opium, having properties similar to those of strychnine; called also *dimethyl morphine.*

**the·be·sian** (thə-be'zhən) named for or described by Adam Christian *Thebesius,* German physician, 1686–1732, such as the *thebesian foramina, valve,* or *veins.*

**the·ca** (the'kə) pl. *the'cae* [L.; Gr. *thēkē*] an enclosing case or sheath, as of an ovarian follicle or tendon.
**t. exter'na,** tunica externa thecae folliculi.
**t. of follicle of von Baer,** tunica externa thecae folliculi.
**t. folli'culi,** theca of follicle: an envelope of condensed connective tissue surrounding a vesicular ovarian follicle, comprising an internal vascular layer *(tunica interna)* and an external fibrous layer *(tunica externa).*
**t. inter'na,** tunica interna thecae folliculi.
**t. medulla're spina'lis,** dura mater of the spinal cord.
**t. vertebra'lis,** dura mater of the spinal cord.

**the·cae** (the'se) [L.] genitive and plural of *theca.*

**the·cal** (the'kəl) pertaining to a theca.

**the·ci·tis** (the-si'tis) tenosynovitis.

**the·co·dont** (the'ko-dont) [*theca* + Gr. *odous* tooth] having the teeth inserted in sockets or alveoli.

**the·co·ma** (the-ko'mə) [MeSH: Thecoma] a theca cell tumor.

**the·co·ma·to·sis** (the″ko-mə-to'sis) diffuse hyperplasia of the ovarian stroma.

**the·co·steg·no·sis** (the″ko-stəg-no'sis) [*theca* + *stegnosis*] contraction of a tendon sheath.

**Thee·lin** (the'lin) trademark for preparations of estrone.

**Theile's canal, glands, muscle** (ti'ləz) [Friedrich Wilhelm *Theile,* German anatomist, 1801–1879] see under *gland,* see *musculus transversus perinei superficialis,* and see *sinus transversus pericardii.*

**Thei·ler** (ti'lər) Max. South African–born American physician and microbiologist, 1899–1972; winner of the Nobel prize for medicine or physiology in 1951 for developing a vaccine for yellow fever.

**Thei·ler's disease, virus** (ti'lərz) [Max *Theiler*] see under *disease* and *virus.*

**Thei·le·ria** (thi-lēr-e-ə) [Sir Arnold *Theiler,* Swiss microbiologist, 1867–1936] [MeSH: Theileria] a genus of minute tick-borne protozoa (order Piroplasmida, subclass Piroplasmia) parasitic in the erythrocytes, lymphocytes, and endothelial cells of mammals. Certain species cause economically important diseases in cattle, sheep, and goats. See *theileriasis*.

**T. annula'ta,** a species causing tropical theileriasis in cattle, transmitted by ticks of the genus *Hyalomma*. Called also *T. dispar*.

**T. dis'par,** *T. annulata*.

**T. hir'ci,** a species found in North Africa, the southern part of the former Soviet Union, eastern Europe, India, and Turkey, causing a highly fatal disease in adult sheep and goats; the vector is unknown.

**T. lawren'cei,** the etiologic agent of corridor disease in African cattle, which is antigenically related to and may be a variant of *T. parva*.

**T. mu'tans,** a species parasitic in African cattle and African and Indian water buffaloes, which is usually nonpathogenic or only mildly so but has been known to cause a severe form of theileriasis known as Tzaneen disease.

**T. o'vis,** a species parasitic in sheep and goats in Africa, Europe, the former Soviet Union, India, Sri Lanka, and western Asia, which is nonpathogenic or may cause a mild disease manifested by fever, lymphadenopathy at site of the tick bite, and slight anemia.

**T. par'va,** the etiologic agent of East Coast fever, a highly fatal disease of African cattle, transmitted by ticks of the genera *Rhipicephalus* and *Hyalomma*.

**thei·le·ri·a·sis** (thi″lə-ri'ə-sis) [MeSH: Theileriasis] a group of diseases due to protozoa of the genus *Theileria,* which result in an acute or chronic febrile infection. Called also *theileriosis*.

**bovine t.,** 1. East Coast fever. 2. any of various febrile diseases of cattle caused by species of *Theileria*.

**tropical t.,** an infection in cattle similar to but milder than East Coast fever, caused by *Theileria annulata,* transmitted by *Hyalomma* spp.; it occurs in North Africa, Mediterranean coastal regions, and many parts of Asia, including Turkey, Central Asia, the Middle East, and the Indian subcontinent. Called also *Mediterranean Coast fever,* and *tropical piroplasmosis*.

**thei·le·ri·o·sis** (thi-le″re-o'sis) theileriasis.

**Thei·mich's lip sign** (ti'miks) [Martin *Theimich,* German pediatrician, late 19th century] see under *sign*.

**the·ine** (the'in) caffeine.

**the·in·ism** (the'in-iz-əm) theaism.

**the·lal·gia** (the-lal'jə) [*thel-* + *-algia*] pain in the nipple.

**the·lar·che** (the-lahr'ke) [*thel-* + Gr. *archē* beginning] the beginning of development of the breasts at puberty.

**The·la·zia** (the-la'zhə) a genus of nematodes of the family Thelaziidae. Several species, such as *T. callipae'da* and *T. californien'sis,* are eye worms parasitic in domestic animals.

**the·la·zi·a·sis** (the″lə-zi'ə-sis) infection of the eye with *Thelazia*.

**The·la·zi·i·dae** (the″lə-zi'ĭ-de) a family of nematodes of the superfamily Spiruroidea; some parasitize the eyes of domestic animals. It includes the genus *Thelazia*.

**thele-** [Gr. *thēlē* nipple] a combining form denoting a relationship to the nipple or to a nipplelike structure.

**the·le·plas·ty** (the'le-plas″te) [*thele-* + *-plasty*] a plastic operation upon the nipple.

**the·ler·e·thism** (thə-ler'ə-thiz-əm) [*thele-* + *erethisma* a stirring up] erection or protrusion of the nipple.

**the·lio·lym·pho·cyte** (the″le-o-lim'fo-sīt) intraepithelial lymphocyte; a small lymphocyte found within the epithelium, especially intestinal epithelium.

**the·li·tis** (the-li'tis) [*thel-* + *-itis*] mammillitis.

**the·li·um** (the'le-əm) pl. *the'lia* [L.] 1. a papilla. 2. a nipple.

**thel(o)-** see *thele-*.

**The·lo·ha·nia** (the″lo-ha'ne-ə) a genus of protozoa (suborder Pansporoblastina, order Microsporida) parasitic in the larvae of certain culicine and anopheline mosquitoes and crane flies and in the brains of rodents.

**the·lor·rha·gia** (the″lo-ra'jə) [*thelo-* + *-rrhagia*] hemorrhage from the nipple.

**the·lo·thism, the·lo·tism** (the'lo-thiz-əm, the'lo-tiz-əm) thelerethism.

**thel·y·blast** (thel'ə-blast) [Gr. *thēlys* female + *-blast*] female pronucleus.

**thel·y·blas·tic** (thel″ə-blas'tik) pertaining to or of the nature of a thelyblast (female pronucleus).

**thel·y·gen·ic** (thel″ə-jen'ik) [Gr. *thēlys* female + *-genic*] producing only female offspring.

**thel·y·to·cia** (thel″ə-to'shə) [Gr. *thēlys* female + *toc-* + *-ia*] normal parthenogenesis producing females only.

**the·lyto·cous** (the-lit'ə-kəs) pertaining to or characterized by thelytocia.

**the·lyt·o·ky** (the-lit'ə-ke) thelytocia.

**Them·i·son** (them'ĭ-son) **of Lao·di·cea** [1st century B.C.] a Greek physician who founded the Methodist school of medicine.

**the·nad** (the'nad) toward the thenar eminence or toward the palm.

**the·nal** (the'nəl) pertaining to the palm or thenar.

**the·nar** (the'nər) [Gr.] 1. [TA] the mound on the palm at the base of the thumb; called also *eminentia thenaris* [TA alternative] and *thenar eminence*. 2. pertaining to the palm.

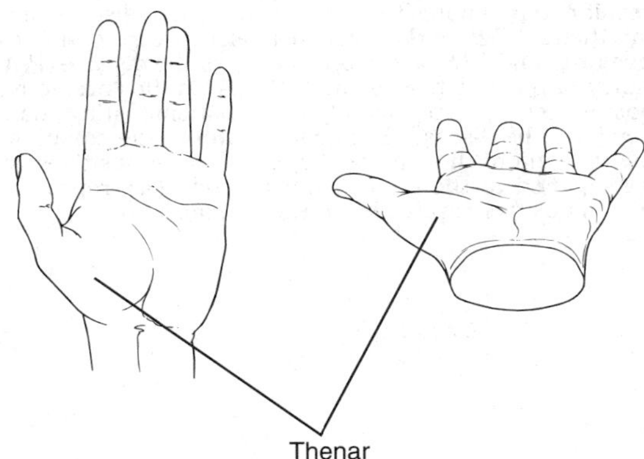


**then·i·um clo·sy·late** (then'e-əm klo'sə-lāt) an anthelmintic formerly widely used to treat hookworm infestations in dogs.

**then·yl·di·amine hy·dro·chlo·ride** (then″əl-di'ə-mēn) an antihistamine used for preoperative sedation, to control postoperative nausea, and to potentiate the action of analgesics.

**Then·y·lene** (then'ə-lēn) trademark for a preparation of methapyrilene.

**then·yl·pyr·amine** (then″əl-pir'ə-mēn) methapyrilene.

**The·o·bal·dia** (the″o-bawl'de-ə) [Frederic Vincent *Theobald,* British zoologist, 1868–1930] *Culiseta*.

**The·o·bro·ma** (the″o-bro'mə) [Gr. *theos* god + *brōma* food] a genus of trees of the family Sterculiaceae, native to tropical parts of the Americas. *T. caca'o* L. is the cacao plant, whose seeds contain the alkaloid theobromine, and yield cacao, cocoa, and cocoa butter.

**the·o·bro·ma** (the″o-bro'mə) cocoa.

**the·o·bro·mine** (the″o-bro'min) [MeSH: Theobromine] one of the methylxanthines, a white crystalline alkaloid found in cocoa or made synthetically from xanthine. It has physiologic properties similar to those of caffeine, and is used as a diuretic, smooth muscle relaxant, myocardial stimulant, and vasodilator. Derivatives such as t. calcium salicylate, t. sodium acetate, t. sodium salicylate, t. sodium formate, and t. salicylate are available for use. Dogs consuming excessive amounts of cocoa sometimes suffer toxic effects from the theobromine, such as vomiting, diarrhea, muscle spasms, and coma.

**The·o·gly·ci·nate** (the″o-gli'sĭ-nāt) trademark for a preparation of theophylline sodium glycinate.

**the·oph·yl·line** (the-of'ə-lin) [USP] [MeSH: Theophylline] a methylxanthine compound occurring in tea leaves and prepared synthetically; theophylline, its salts, and its derivatives act as smooth muscle relaxants, central nervous system and cardiac muscle stimulants, and bronchodilators. Used as a bronchodilator in the prevention and treatment of symptoms of asthma and of reversible bronchospasm associated with chronic bronchitis and emphysema; administered orally and intravenously. Formerly used in the treatment of congestive heart failure and angina pectoris, and as a diuretic, but now replaced by more effective agents.

**t. aminoisobutanol,** ambuphylline.

**t. calcium salicylate,** an equimolar mixture of theophylline calcium and calcium salicylate, having the same actions and uses as the base; administered orally.

**t. cholinate,** oxtriphylline.

**t. sodium,** the sodium salt of theophylline, used in preparations in combination with sodium acetate or sodium glycinate.

**t. sodium glycinate** [USP], an equimolar mixture of theophylline sodium and glycine buffered with an additional mole of glycine and yielding 44.5 to 47.3 per cent anhydrous theophylline, having the same actions and uses as the base; administered orally.

**The·o·rell** (ta-o-rel') Axel Hugo Theodor. Swedish biochemist, born 1903; winner of the Nobel prize in medicine or physiology for 1955, for his discoveries concerning the nature and mode of action of oxidation enzymes.

**the·o·rem** (the'ə-rəm, thēr'əm) [Gr. *theorēma* a principle arrived at by speculation] a proposition capable of demonstration or proof.

**Bayes' t.**, a theorem used to interconvert conditional probabilities:

$$P(B|A) = \frac{P(A|B)\,P(B)}{P(A|B)\,P(B) + P(A|\text{not } B)\,P(\text{not } B)}$$

where $P(A)$ and $P(B)$ are the probabilities of two events, $A$ and $B$, and $P(A|B)$ and $P(B|A)$ are the conditional probabilities of $A$ given $B$ and of $B$ given $A$. For example, if $A$ denotes a positive laboratory test result and $B$ denotes the actual presence of disease in a tested patient, then $P(A|B)$ is the "diagnostic sensitivity" of the test (true positive rate) and $P(B)$ is the prevalence of the disease ($P(A)$ is the frequency of positive test results). $P(B|A)$ is the "predictive value of a positive test," the probability that a patient testing positive will actually have the disease. The denominator of the equation, representing the sum of the true positives and false positives, is sometimes simplified to the equivalent function $P(A)$, representing all those with positive results, both true and false.

**Bernoulli t.**, in an experiment involving probability, the larger the number of trials, the closer the observed probability of an event approaches its theoretical probability.

**central limit t.**, if random samples of size $n$ are taken from a population having a normally distributed variable with mean $\mu$ and standard deviation $\sigma$, the distribution of the sample means is normal, with mean $\mu$ and standard deviation

$$\sigma/\sqrt{n};$$

if the variable in the population is not normally distributed, the sampling distribution of means approximates the normal distribution and the approximation gets better as the sample size increases.

**Gibbs' t.**, substances which lower the surface tension of the pure dispersion medium tend to collect on its surface.

**the·o·ry** (the'ə-re, thēr'e) [Gr. *theōria* speculation as opposed to practice] 1. the doctrine or the principles underlying an art as distinguished from the practice of that particular art. 2. a formulated hypothesis, or, loosely speaking, any hypothesis or opinion not based upon actual knowledge.

## Theory

**acidogenic t.**, a theory of the etiology of dental caries, according to which acids produced by bacteria cause decalcification and softening of the residue.

**aging t. of atherosclerosis, Altmann's t.**, a theory that atherosclerosis is an inevitable consequence of aging and therefore an irreversible process.

**Altmann's t.**, a theory that protoplasm is made up of granular particles (bioblasts) grouped in masses and enclosed in indifferent matter.

**apposition t.**, the theory that tissues grow by the deposit of cells from without.

**Arrhenius' t.**, the theory of electrolytic dissociation, proposed in 1887, which explained the properties of electrolytes based on the presence of free ions in solution and also defined acids and bases as compounds that dissociate to release hydrogen and hydroxide ions, respectively, in solution.

**atomic t.**, the theory that the molecules of a substance are made up of one or more atoms, each representing a definite amount of the element, which amount does not vary in the molecule, whatever combinations the molecule may enter.

**avalanche t.**, the theory that nervous influence increases in force as it descends along an efferent nerve.

**Bolk's retardation t.**, the theory that humans, in their development, are at a stage which, in the higher primates, is still a fetal stage.

**Buergi's t.**, two different substances causing identical therapeutic manifestations when combined are increased in their effects if they possess identical pharmacologic points of attack.

**Cannon's t., Cannon-Bard t.**, emergency t.

**cell t.**, the doctrine that all living matter is composed of cells and that cell activity is the essential process of life.

**cellular immunity t.**, Metchnikoff's cellular immunity t.

**clonal deletion t.**, a theory of immunologic tolerance to self antigens according to which "forbidden clones" of immunocytes, those reactive with self antigens, are eliminated on contact with antigen during fetal life. The terms "clonal abortion," "clonal anergy," "clonal silencing," and "clonal purging" have also been used for this phenomenon. See also *clonal selection t.*

**clonal selection t.**, a modification of the natural selection theory (q.v.): there are in each adult several million clones of antibody-producing cells, each programmed to make antibody of a single specificity and bearing cell-surface receptors capable of reacting with specific antigens; exposure to antigen induces cells of antigen-reactive clones to proliferate and differentiate to produce large quantities of specific antibody. This theory has been found to be essentially correct. See *clonal deletion t.* and *recombinational germline t.*

**closed circulation t.**, one of the theories explaining how the blood in the spleen gets from the arteries to the venous sinuses; it holds that the capillaries empty directly into the venous sinuses. Cf. *open circulation t.* and *closed-open circulation t.* Called also *fast circulation t.*

**closed-open circulation t.**, the theory that both an open and a closed circulation are present in the spleen; e.g., a closed circulation in a contracted spleen may become an open circulation when the organ is distended. Cf. *closed circulation t.* and *open circulation t.*

**Cohnheim's t.**, the theory that tumors develop from embryonic rests which do not participate in the formation of normal surrounding tissue.

**contractile ring t.**, a theory advanced to explain the formation of a furrow in a dividing cell. According to this theory, the gelated ring in the cortex of the dividing cell contracts (cortical gel contraction) like the nonmotile portion of an amoeba, and, therefore, decreases the surface area. Actually, however, before division the surface increases by about 26 per cent.

**convergence-projection t.**, a theory advanced as an explanation for reference of pain, according to which some visceral afferent nerve fibers converge with cutaneous pain afferents to end upon the same neuron at some point in the sensory pathway.

**core conductor t.**, a theory regarding the development of electrotonic potentials and their associated currents along nerve fibers, according to which the nerve fibers are considered to be core conductors, i.e., cylinders of conducting fluid material with a sheath of high electrical resistance, surrounded by a layer of conducting medium.

**darwinian t.**, darwinism.

**dimer t.**, the theory that the tooth organ of primates is composed of two halves, each of which is a representative of an independent tooth in the lower orders of animals.

**dualistic t.**, a variant of the polyphyletic theory that holds that blood cells arise from two distinct types of stem cells, the myeloblasts and lymphoblasts. Cf. *monophyletic t.* and *trialistic t.* Called also *dualism.*

**Ehrlich's t., Ehrlich's side-chain t.**, the first (1896) comprehensive theory of antibody production, which proposed that antibody-producing cells have surface molecules (side chains) that can bind to antigens and that binding to a specific side chain causes the cell to produce more of the same side chain and to release these side chains into the serum as antibodies. Two of Ehrlich's postulates, that antibodies are identical to the antigen receptors and that antigen binding triggers the synthesis of antibody with the same specificity as the receptor, are now known to be essentially correct. Cf. *clonal selection t.*

**electron t.**, all bodies are complex structures composed of small particles called atoms together with still smaller particles called electrons.

**emergency t.**, the theory that the adrenal medulla is stimulated during emotional excitement, pain, and bodily emergencies; see also *alarm reaction,* under *reaction.* Called also *Cannon's t.* and *Cannon-Bard t.*

**encrustation t.**, the theory that fibrinous material derived from the blood is deposited on the inner surface of the intima of vessels and that fatty metamorphosis occurs secondarily in this deposit.

**equilibrium t.**, a theory that the number of breeding species in a biome is a result of the rate of immigration of new species and the rate of extinction.

**expanding surface t.**, a theory of cell division which postulates that a nuclear substance is liberated, probably from chromosomes, which causes expansion of the cellular membrane at the poles; as the polar areas expand, the equator contracts, leading to division.

**fast circulation t.**, closed circulation t.

**frequency t.**, an early theory of hearing, which postulated that the pattern of excitation of auditory nerve fibers was more important in perception of pitch than was the excitation of any of the fibers in any particular area of the cochlear basilar membrane. Called also *Rutherford's t.* Cf. *place t.*

**gate t., gate-control t.,** neural impulses generated by noxious painful stimuli and transmitted to the spinal cord by small-diameter C-fibers and A-delta fibers are blocked at their synapses in the dorsal horn by the simultaneous stimulation of large-diameter myelinated A-fibers, thus inhibiting pain by preventing pain impulses from reaching higher levels of the central nervous system. Called also *gate hypothesis.*

**germ t.,** the doctrine that infectious diseases are of microbic origin.

**germ layer t.,** the theory that the embryo develops three primary germ layers, each of which gives rise to definite organ derivatives.

**gestalt t.,** see *gestaltism.*

**Golgi's t.,** the theory that the neurons communicate by the axons of Golgi's cells and the collaterals of the axons of Deiters' cells.

**Goltz's t.,** the theory that the function of the semicircular canals is to transmit sensations of position, and thus materially aid in the sense of equilibrium.

**Helmholtz t.,** an early theory of sound perception, now disproved; it held that each basilar fiber responded sympathetically to a definite tone and stimulated the hair cells of Corti's organ, causing nerve impulses that were then carried to the brain. Called also *place t.* and *resonance t.*

**Hering's t.,** the doctrine that color sensation depends on decomposition and restitution of the visual substance: disassimilation producing red, yellow, and white, and restitution producing blue, green, and black. Called also *opponent colors t.*

**hit t.,** target t.

**humoral t.,** humoralism.

**incasement t.,** the formerly advocated theory that all animals and plants develop from preexisting germs, and that they encase the germs of all future generations, one within another.

**information t.,** a system for analyzing, chiefly by statistical methods, the characteristics of communicated messages and the systems that encode, transmit, distort, receive, and decode them.

**instructive t.,** template t.

**ionic t.,** a theory that, on going into solution, the molecules of an electrolyte either completely or partially break up or dissociate into two or more portions, these portions being positively and negatively charged electrically, the positively charged portions being different chemically from those negatively charged. When an electric current is passed through the solution of an electrolyte, the positively charged portions are attracted by the negative pole or electrode, and move toward it; the negatively charged portions are attracted by and migrate toward the positive electrode. From this property of moving toward one of the electrodes, these charged molecular fractions of electrolytes are called ions, from the Greek verb meaning "to move."

**Kern plasma relation t.,** the theory that for each cell there exists a definite size relation of nuclear mass to cell mass.

**Ladd-Franklin t.,** a theory of the evolution of color vision: first, light stimulates a substance in the visual cells, producing a sensation of white light; next, molecular changes from the first reaction produce two reactive products, one for each end of the spectrum, for blue and yellow; finally, the reactive product from the yellow becomes two products for red and green. Dichromasies and anomalous trichromasies are considered to be incomplete recapitulations of the evolutionary development.

**Lamarck's t.,** the theory that acquired characteristics may be transmitted.

**Liebig's t.,** the hydrocarbons which oxidize easily are the foods which produce animal heat.

**local circuit t.,** in neurophysiology, the theory that current flows from the unstimulated, positively charged areas of the cell membrane of a neuron to the stimulated, depolarized or negative portion, and that as each new area becomes depolarized or negative, it in turn acts as the sink toward which the current flows from the adjacent area, which results in progressive depolarization, or reversal charge, along the neuron from the point of stimulation; the source of the current is the flow of $Na^+$ into the cell.

**membrane ionic t.,** the theory that the resting potential difference between the inside and outside of the cell is related to (1) the thin, electrically insulating membrane between the cytoplasm and the interstitial conducting medium, which is poorly and variably permeable to diverse ions; (2) the presence of a metabolic cellular pump that promotes the efflux of sodium ions from the cell interior to the outside against its electrochemical gradient and, coupled with this, the influx of potassium ions into the cell against its ionic concentration gradient.

**mendelian t.,** see *Mendel's laws,* under *law.*

**metabolic t. of atherosclerosis,** a theory that atherosclerosis is caused by a disturbance in lipid metabolism, specifically cholesterol metabolism.

**Metchnikoff's (Mechnikov's) cellular immunity t.,** the theory, proposed in the 1880s, that phagocytosis by macrophages and polymorphonuclear leukocytes is the main mechanism of host defense against bacterial infection and that inflammation is the result of the enzymatic digestion process occurring with phagocytosis.

**monophyletic t.,** the theory that all forms of blood cells have their origin in a single type of cell, the blast cell (which develops into a pluripotential stem cell), with the different types of cells arising from there by a process of differentiation. Cf. *dualistic t., polyphyletic t.,* and *trialistic t.* Called also *monophyletism* and *unitarian t.*

**myogenic t.,** the theory that the muscle fibers of the heart possess in themselves the power of originating and maintaining the contraction of the heart.

**natural selection t.,** the first selective theory of antibody formation, according to which about a million different antibody molecules are constantly being produced at low levels; when an antibody combines with a complementary antigen the complex is taken up by antibody-producing cells and the antibody is replicated. This theory explained many features of the immune response but incorrectly located immunologic memory in serum rather than cells. See *clonal selection t.*

**neuron t.,** (Waldeyer, 1891), the theory that the nervous system consists of innumerable neurons in contiguity, but not in continuity. See *neuron.*

**open circulation t.,** one of the theories explaining how the blood in the spleen gets from the arteries to the venous sinuses; it holds that the capillaries open directly into the pulp reticulum, and that the blood gradually filters back into the venous sinuses. Called also *slow circulation t.* Cf. *closed circulation t.* and *closed-open circulation t.*

**open-closed circulation t.,** see *closed-open circulation t.*

**opponent colors t.,** Hering's t.

**overflow t.,** one similar to the underfilling theory (q.v.), but which proposes that the primary event in ascites formation is sodium and water retention with portal hypertension resulting; plasma volume expansion to the point of overflow from the hepatic sinusoids then causes ascites formation.

**overproduction t.,** see *Weigert's law,* under *law.*

**Pasteur's t.,** the theory that the immunity secured by an attack of a disease is caused by the exhaustion of material needed for the growth of the organism of the disease.

**phlogiston t.,** see *phlogiston.*

**pithecoid t.,** the theory that man is descended from apelike ancestors.

**place t.,** an early theory of pitch perception which postulated that excitation of specific areas of the basilar membrane of the cochlea determined the pitch perceived. Cf. *frequency t.*

**Planck's t.,** quantum t.

**polarization-membrane t.,** the theory that living, resting cells are surrounded by a semipermeable membrane lined by a series of electrical doublets, or dipoles, with negative charges on the inner and positive charges on the outer surface. When the membrane is electrically intact, its entire surface is surrounded by doublets, and is said to be polarized.

**polyphyletic t.,** the theory that the various blood cells have their origin from two or more types of stem cells. Cf. *dualistic t., monophyletic t.,* and *trialistic t.* Called also *polyphyletism.*

**P. O. U. t.,** Ishihara's theory of the placenta-ovary-uterus production of internal secretion.

**preformation t.,** the outmoded theory that the individuals of successive generations are contained, completely formed, within the reproductive cell of one of the parents.

**proteolysis-chelation t.,** a theory of the etiology of dental caries, according to which keratolytic microorganisms cause formation of chelates, which in turn cause decalcification.

**proteolytic t.,** a theory of the etiology of dental caries, according to which microorganisms destroy enamel protein.

**quantum t.,** the theory that the radiation and absorption of energy take place in definite quantities called quanta (E) which vary in size and are defined by the equation $E = h\nu$, in which h is Planck's constant and $\nu$ is the frequency of the radiation.

**recapitulation t.,** ontogeny recapitulates phylogeny; that is, an organism in the course of its development goes through the same successive stages as did the species in developing from the lower to the higher forms of animal life. Called also *biogenetic law* and *Haeckel's law.*

**recombinational germline t.,** a theory of the origin of antibody diversity, according to which the DNA coding for a single immunoglobulin chain is assembled by a somatic recombinational event from two genes, one a unique constant region gene and the other one of several million variable region genes. The first theory to propose that two genes might code for a single polypeptide chain, it is now known to be essentially correct, although more than two types of genes are actually involved. Called also *Dreyer and Bennett hypothesis.*

**resonance t.,** 1. Helmholtz t. 2. the theory of specificity which assumes that the surface forces of reacting substances must harmonize.

**Ribbert's t.,** a tumor is formed from the development of cell rests owing to reduced tension in the surrounding tissues.

**Rutherford's t.,** frequency t.

## Theory *Continued*

**Schiefferdecker's symbiosis t.,** the theory that among the tissues of the body there is a sort of symbiosis, so that the products of metabolism in one tissue serve as a stimulus to the activities of other tissues.

**Schön's t.,** the theory (of ocular accommodation) that the ciliary muscle exerts on the lens the same effect as is produced on a rubber ball held in both hands and compressed by the fingers.

**side-chain t.,** Ehrlich's side-chain t.

**single hit t.,** the theory that hemolysis results from a single complement-induced lesion of the erythrocyte surface, rather than that lesions at several sites are necessary.

**sliding filament t.,** 1. a theory which postulates that the thin and thick filaments of a myofibril slide past each other, while maintaining their length, during muscle contraction. 2. a theory that postulates that contraction of cilia involves a sliding of filaments (microtubules) in a manner comparable to the sliding filament mechanism for the contraction of muscle (see def. 1).

**slow circulation t.,** open circulation t.

**spindle elongation t.,** the theory which suggests that the spindle and asters have a decisive role in cell division. The theory is based on the observation that the elongation of the cell at anaphase is accompanied by a shrinkage at the equator. The centers are believed to be pushed apart by the spindle tubules, since the spindles and asters appear to be rigid structures.

**Spitzer's t.,** the formation of the septa in the heart are teleologically conditioned, phylogenetically brought about, and mechanically achieved by the appearance and development of the lungs through phylogeny.

**target t.,** the theory advanced to explain some biological effects of radiation on the basis of ionization occurring in a very small sensitive region within the cell, which postulates that one or more ionizing events, or "hits," within the sensitive volume are necessary to bring about the biological end-effect; called also *hit t.*

**template t.,** a theory of the mechanism of antibody specificity, current during the 1930s and 40s, which proposed that the shape of an antibody molecule is determined as it is synthesized by being molded on an antigen molecule. The antigen thus "instructs" a cell to make specific antibody. Called also *instructive t.*

**thermostat t.,** a theory which suggests that the feeding and satiety centers of the brain, like the thermoregulatory centers, are sensitive to body temperature; a decrease in body temperature activates the feeding center and depresses the satiety center, whereas increased temperature acts on the centers in the opposite way.

**Traube's resonance t.,** resonance t., def. 2.

**trialistic t.,** a variant of the polyphyletic theory that holds that blood cells arise from three distinct types of stem cells, the myeloblasts, lymphoblasts, and monocytes. Cf. *dualistic t.* and *monophyletic t.* Called also *trialism.*

**underfilling t.,** the theory that ascites associated with portal hypertension causes hypovolemia and so both a lowering of portal pressure and retention of sodium and water. The higher sodium concentration causes increases in the plasma volume and portal pressure, and the subsequent formation of ascites renews the cycle. See also *overflow t.*

**undulatory t.,** wave t.

**unitarian t.,** monophyletic t.

**wave t.,** the theory that light, heat, and electricity are transmitted through space in the form of waves.

**Weismann's t.,** see *weismannism.*

**Woods-Fildes t.,** the theory that the antibacterial activity of at least some chemotherapeutic drugs (especially the sulfonamides) is a consequence of a competitive inhibition of essential metabolic reactions of the microorganism.

**Young-Helmholtz t.,** the doctrine that color vision depends on three sets of retinal fibers, corresponding to the colors red, green, and violet.

---

**theo·ther·a·py** (the″o-ther′ə-pe) [Gr. *theos* god + *therapy*] the treatment of disease by prayer and religious exercises.

**Theph·o·rin** (thef′ə-rin) trademark for preparations of phenindamine tartrate.

**theque** (tek) [Fr. a "box or small chest"] a round or oval collection, or nest, of melanin-containing nevus cells occurring at the dermoepidermal junction of the skin or in the dermis proper.

**ther·a·peu·sis** (ther″ə-pu′sis) therapeutics.

**ther·a·peu·tic** (ther″ə-pu′tik) [Gr. *therapeutikos* inclined to serve] [MeSH: Therapeutics] 1. pertaining to therapeutics or to therapy. 2. curative.

**ther·a·peu·tics** (ther″ə-pu′tiks) [MeSH: Therapeutics] 1. the branch of medical science concerned with the treatment of disease. 2. therapy.

**Ther·a·pho·si·dae** (ther″ə-fo′sĭ-de) a family of very large hairy spiders (suborder Orthognatha) found in temperate and tropical areas. *Sericopelma communis* is the only species whose venom has a harmful effect on man, but some are capable of inflicting painful bites. The members of this family are sometimes improperly called tarantulas. See also *bird spider.*

**ther·a·pia** (ther″ə-pi′ə) [L., from Gr.] therapy.

**t. sterili′sans mag′na,** Ehrlich's procedure using a chemical agent that will destroy parasites in the body of a patient without being seriously toxic for the patient.

**ther·a·pist** (ther′ə-pist) [Gr. *therapeutēs* one who attends to the sick] a person skilled in the treatment of disease; often combined with a term indicating the specific type of disorder treated (as *speech t.*) or a particular type of treatment rendered (as *physical t.*).

**physical t.,** a person skilled in the techniques of physical therapy and qualified to administer treatments prescribed by a physician and under his supervision; called also *physiotherapist.*

**respiratory t.,** a person who has graduated from an approved respiratory therapist program or is registered by the National Board for Respiratory Care and is qualified to provide respiratory care under the supervision of a physician.

**speech t.,** a person specially trained to assist patients in overcoming speech and language disorders. Cf. *speech pathologist.*

**ther·a·py** (ther′ə-pe) [Gr. *therapeia* service done to the sick] the treatment of disease; called also *therapeutics.*

---

## Therapy

See also under *treatment.*

**ablation t.,** the destruction of small areas of myocardial tissue, usually by application of electrical or chemical energy, in the treatment of some tachyarrhythmias. See also *electrical* and *chemical ablation,* under *ablation.*

**adjuvant t.,** see under *chemotherapy.*

**aerosol t.,** inhalation therapy using an aerosol.

**anticoagulant t.,** the use of anticoagulants (q.v.) to discourage thrombosis.

**antiplatelet t.,** the use of platelet inhibitors such as aspirin, dipyridamole, sulfinpyrazone, or ticlopidine hydrochloride to inhibit platelet adhesion or aggregation and so prevent thrombosis, alter the course of atherosclerosis, or prolong vascular graft patency.

**autolymphocyte t.,** autopheresis.

**autoserum t.,** treatment of disease by the injection of the patient's own blood serum.

**aversion t., aversive t.,** a form of behavior therapy using aversive conditioning, pairing undesirable behavior or symptoms with unpleasant stimulation in order to reduce or eliminate the behavior or symptoms. The term is sometimes used synonymously with *aversive conditioning.*

**beam t.,** 1. chromotherapy. 2. external beam radiotherapy.

**behavior t.,** a therapeutic approach in which the focus is on the patient's observable behavior, rather than on conflicts and unconscious processes presumed to underlie his maladaptive behavior. This is accomplished through systematic manipulation of the environmental and behavioral variables related to the specific behavior to be modified; operant conditioning, systematic desensitization, token economy, aversive control, flooding, and implosion are examples of techniques that may be used in behavior therapy. Called also *behavior modification* and *conditioning t.*

**behavioral marital t. (BMT),** a form of marital therapy using principles and techniques from behavior therapy; it attempts to alleviate marital distress by increasing positive, pleasant interactions between the members of a couple.

**biological t.,** treatment of disease by the injection of the substances which produce a biological reaction in the organism. The term includes the use of sera, antitoxins, vaccines, and nonspecific proteins.

**buffer t.,** intravenous injection of buffer substances, such as sodium bicarbonate, with the object of lowering the hydrogen ion concentration.

**Chaoul t.,** short source-to-tissue distance, low-voltage x-ray therapy; see also under *tube.*

**client-centered t.,** a form of psychotherapy in which the emphasis is on the patient's self-discovery, interpretation, conflict resolution, and reorganization of values and life approach, which are enabled by the warm, nondirective, unconditionally accepting support of the therapist, who reflects and clarifies the patient's discoveries.

**cognitive t., cognitive behavior t.,** a directive form of psychotherapy based on the theory that emotional problems result from distorted attitudes and ways of thinking that can be corrected. Using techniques drawn in part from behavior therapy, the therapist actively seeks to guide the patient in altering or revising negative or erroneous perceptions and attitudes.

**collapse t.,** a treatment for pulmonary tuberculosis, formerly widely used, in which the diseased lung was collapsed in order to immobilize it and allow it to rest. Common methods were oleothorax, plombage, pneumonolysis, artificial pneumothorax, and thoracoplasty. Pneumonolysis and thoracoplasty are still sometimes done to collapse a lung and allow access during thoracic surgery.

**combined t.,** psychotherapy in which the patient sees the same therapist for both individual and group therapies concurrently. Cf. *conjoint t.*

**combined modality t.,** treatment of cancer using two or more types of therapy, such as radiation therapy, chemotherapy, or surgery in an effort to achieve additive or synergistic effects; see also *chemoradiotherapy.* Called also *multimodality t.*

**compression t.,** treatment of venous insufficiency, varicose veins, or venous ulceration of the lower limbs by having the patient wear compressing garments such as elastic support stockings.

**conditioning t.,** behavior t.

**conjoint t.,** that in which a patient is involved in both group and individual psychotherapy concurrently, seeing separate therapists for each. Cf. *combined t.*

**continuous sleep t.,** treatment of certain mental disorders by inducing prolonged sleep (18 to 20 hours a day for about two weeks) with drugs, usually barbiturates; it is no longer used in the United States.

**convulsive t.,** treatment of mental disorders, primarily depression, by induction of convulsions. The type now almost universally used is electroconvulsive therapy (ECT), in which the convulsions are induced by electric current. In earlier forms, convulsions were induced pharmacologically, at first by pentylenetetrazol and later by flurothyl. Formerly called *shock t.*

**corrective t.,** the planning and administration of progressive physical exercise and activities most effective in improving or maintaining general physical and emotional health, through individual or group participation.

**couples t.,** marital t.

**deep roentgen-ray t.,** orthovoltage radiotherapy.

**deleading t.,** the use of chelating agents in the mobilization and excretion from the body of a heavy metal such as lead or radium.

**diathermic t.,** diathermy.

**diet t.,** treatment of disease by regulation of the diet.

**drug t.,** pharmacotherapy.

**electric convulsive t., electric shock t.,** electroconvulsive t.

**electroconvulsive t. (ECT),** a treatment for mental disorders, primarily depression, in which convulsions and loss of consciousness are induced by application of brief pulses of low-voltage alternating current to the brain via scalp electrodes; a muscle relaxant, generally succinylcholine, is used to prevent injury during the seizure. Awakening usually occurs within 10 to 15 minutes and may be followed by a temporary confusional state; transient memory impairment may be present for weeks to as much as a year after treatment. ECT produces a therapeutic response in a majority of cases of major depression.

**electroshock t. (EST),** electroconvulsive t.

**emotionally focused t.,** a form of marital therapy in which the couple increases intimacy and improves their relationship by each assessing, acknowledging, and expressing their underlying emotions and unmet feelings and needs.

**endocrine t.,** treatment of disease by the use of hormones; called also *hormonal* or *hormone t., endocrinotherapy,* and *hormonotherapy.*

**external beam t.,** see under *radiotherapy.*

**family t.,** *group therapy* of the members of a family, exploring and improving family relationships and processes, understanding and modifying home influences that contribute to mental disorder in one or more family members, and improving communication and collective, constructive methods of problem solving.

**fever t.,** treatment of disease by induction of high body temperature, accomplished by physical means or by injection of fever-producing vaccines.

**fibrinolytic t.,** the use of fibrinolytic agents (prourokinase, streptokinase, t-plasminogen activator, u-plasminogen activator) to lyse thrombi in patients with acute peripheral arterial occlusion, deep venous thrombosis, pulmonary embolism, and acute myocardial infarction. Called also *thrombolytic t.*

**first line t.,** induction t.

**gene t.,** 1. manipulation of the genome of an individual to prevent, mask, or lessen the effects of a genetic disorder. 2. introduction of genetic material into the genome of targeted cells in order to alter cellular metabolism, immune response, or sensitivity to therapeutic agents.

**grid t.,** therapeutic application of ionizing radiations through a metal grid having a pattern of small, evenly spaced perforations.

**group t.,** a form of psychotherapy in which a group of people meet regularly with a group leader, usually a therapist. The group uses therapeutic forces within the group, interactions between members, and the interventions of the trained leader to achieve insight into the cause of problems, provide emotional support, or effect changes in maladaptive behavior, thoughts, or feelings of the individual members. Called also *group psychotherapy.*

**heterovaccine t.,** bacterial vaccine therapy by the use of some infectious agent other than the specific one causing the disease.

**high-voltage roentgen t.,** high-voltage radiotherapy.

**hormonal t., hormone t.,** endocrine t.

**hormone replacement t.,** the administration of sex hormones following menopause or hysterectomy or in amenorrhea; there are a number of indications, including the prevention of postmenopausal osteoporosis and coronary artery disease, and the induction of menses in amenorrhea.

**humidification t.,** inhalation therapy using air supersaturated with moisture in treatment of congestive conditions of the upper and lower respiratory tract.

**immunization t.,** treatment with antiserum and with actively antigenic substances, e.g., vaccines.

**immunosuppressive t.,** treatment with agents, such as x-rays, corticosteroids, and cytotoxic chemicals, which suppress the immune response to antigen(s); it is used in various conditions, including autoimmune disease, allergy, multiple myeloma, and chronic nephritis, and in organ transplantation.

**induction t.,** the first therapeutic measure used to treat a disease, especially when combined modality therapy is planned. Called also *first line t.*

**inhalation t.,** old name for *respiratory care* (def. 3).

**insulin coma t. (ICT),** an older treatment for schizophrenia, not currently used in the United States; sufficient insulin is administered to place the patient in a deep hypoglycemic coma, which is reversed in an hour or less by administration of glucagon, usually for 20 to 60 such treatments.

**intraosseous t.,** the infusion of blood or other solutions into the circulation by injection through the bone marrow.

**intravenous t.,** the introduction of therapeutic liquid agents directly into the venous circulation.

**light t.,** 1. phototherapy (def. 1). 2. photodynamic t.

**locoregional t.,** therapy that affects only a localized area rather than being systemic; said particularly of chemotherapy.

**marital t.,** a type of family therapy aimed at understanding and treating one or both members of a couple in the context of a distressed relationship, but not necessarily addressing the discordant relationship itself. In the past the term has also been used more restrictively as synonymous with marriage therapy (q.v.), but that is increasingly considered a subset of marital therapy. Called also *couples t.*

**marriage t.,** a subset of marital therapy (q.v.) that focuses specifically on the bond of marriage between two people, enhancing and preserving it.

**maintenance t.,** therapy of chronically ill patients that is aimed at keeping the pathology at its present level and preventing exacerbation.

**metatrophic t.**, administration of a diet that acts as an adjunct to the drug taken.
**milieu t.**, treatment, usually in a psychiatric hospital, that emphasizes the provision of an environment and activities appropriate to the patient's emotional and interpersonal needs.
**Morita t.**, a school of psychotherapy originating in Japan, based on the essential elements of conduct in Zen Buddhism. It emphasizes the combating of egocentricity and the correction of alienation from nature.
**multimodality t.**, combined modality t.
**myofunctional t.**, training of the orofacial musculature, including modification of habits, in edentulous conditions, malocclusion, or temporomandibular joint disorders.
**neoadjuvant t.**, in combined modality therapy for cancer, initial use of one modality, such as chemotherapy or radiotherapy, to decrease the tumor burden prior to treatment by another modality, usually surgery. Called also *preoperative t.* and *presurgical t.*
**occupational t.**, the therapeutic use of self-care, work, and play activities to increase function, enhance development, and prevent disability; it may include modification of tasks or the environment to enable the patient to achieve maximum independence and to enhance the quality of the patient's life.
**oral rehydration t. (ORT)**, oral administration of a solution of electrolytes and carbohydrates in the treatment of dehydration.
**orthomolecular t.**, treatment of disease, especially psychiatric disorders, based on the theory that restoration of optimal concentrations of substances normally present in the body, particularly vitamins, will effect a cure.
**oxygen t.**, respiratory care involving inhalation of oxygen.
**photodynamic t.**, intravenous administration of a photosensitizing agent such as hematoporphyrin derivative, which concentrates selectively in metabolically active tumor tissue, followed by exposure of the tumor tissue to red laser light of a specific wavelength, to bring about production of cytotoxic free radicals that selectively destroy the photosensitized tissue. Called also *photochemotherapy, photoradiation, phototherapy, light therapy,* and *light treatment.*
**physical t.**, 1. treatment by physical means. 2. the health profession concerned with the promotion of health, with the prevention of physical disability, with the evaluation and rehabilitation of patients disabled by pain, disease, or injury, and with treatment using physical therapeutic measures as opposed to medical, surgical, or radiologic measures.
**plasma t.**, the therapeutic use of blood plasma.
**play t.**, a method of psychotherapy used in treating children, in which play is used to a considerable extent as the means of communication between the child and therapist, enabling self-expression and the revealing of unconscious material.
**preoperative t.**, neoadjuvant t.
**presurgical t.**, neoadjuvant t.
**primal t.**, psychotherapy in which the patient is encouraged to relive his early traumatic experiences and so relieve the painful emotions with which they are associated.
**protective t.**, prophylaxis.
**pulp canal t.**, root canal t.
**pulse t.**, administration of medication in short intensive courses at regular intervals.
**PUVA t.** [*p*soralen + *u*ltra*v*iolet *A*], a form of photochemotherapy for skin disorders such as psoriasis and vitiligo; oral psoralen administration is followed two hours later by exposure to ultraviolet A.
**radiation t.**, radiotherapy.
**radium t.**, the treatment of disease by means of radium.
**reflex t.**, treatment by producing a reflex action; called also *reflexotherapy.*
**renal replacement t.**, therapy such as hemodialysis or transplantation that takes the place of nonfunctioning kidneys.
**renal replacement t., continuous (CRRT)**, hemodialysis or hemofiltration done 24 hours a day for an extended period, usually in a critically ill patient.
**replacement t.**, 1. treatment to replace deficiencies in body products by administration of natural or synthetic substitutes. Called also *substitution t.* 2. treatment such as hemodialysis or transplantation that replaces or compensates for a nonfunctioning organ.
**respiratory t.**, see under *care.*
**root canal t.**, that aspect of endodontics dealing with the treatment of diseases of the dental pulp, consisting of partial *(pulpotomy)* or complete *(pulpectomy)* extirpation of the diseased pulp, cleaning and sterilization of the empty root canal, enlarging and shaping of the canal to receive sealing material, and obturation of the canal with a nonirritating hermetic sealing agent. Called also *pulp canal t.*
**rotation t.**, in radiotherapy, circular movement of the patient or of the radiation source and beam around a fixed anatomical axis during a treatment exposure; it may entail complete, partial, or skip-field exposure.
**salvage t.**, the use of experimental or strong therapeutic measures in patients whose prognosis is poor after they have failed other therapies.
**serum t.**, see *serotherapy.*
**shock t.**, obsolete term for *convulsive t.*
**short wave t.**, short wave diathermy.
**solar t.**, heliotherapy.
**sparing t.**, treatment directed to the protecting and sparing of an organ by allowing it to rest as much as possible.
**specific t.**, see under *treatment.*
**speech t.**, the use of special techniques for correction of speech and language disorders. Cf. *speech pathology.*
**strategic t.**, a directive form of therapy in which the therapist helps couples or families to change their interactions and behavior by noticing where maladaptive patterns are occurring, then eliminating them by demanding deliberate attempts to behave in ways that, paradoxically, would normally be expected to cause them instead.
**subcoma insulin t.**, intramuscular administration of small doses of insulin to produce mild hypoglycemia, sedation, and weight gain, formerly used to treat schizophrenia and certain other mental disorders.
**substitution t.**, replacement t. (def. 1).
**substitutive t.**, substitutive medication.
**suggestion t.**, a form of psychotherapy characterized by suggestion, reassurance, and sometimes also hypnosis.
**thrombolytic t.**, fibrinolytic t.
**thyroid replacement t., thyroxine replacement t.**, treatment of hypothyroidism by administration of thyroxine, usually in the form of levothyroxine sodium. Called also *thyroidotherapy* and *thyrotherapy.*
**vaccine t.**, active immunization against a disease by the injection of the infectious agents of the disease or their products directly into a patient.
**virus-directed enzyme/prodrug t.**, a method of treating tumors by the introduction of a suicide gene (q.v.) into tumor cells by a viral vector, followed by the administration of a nontoxic prodrug that is converted to a toxic agent, resulting in tumor cell death.

**The•ria** (the're-ə) [Gr. *thērion* beast, animal] in some systems of classification, a subclass of the Mammalia, including the infraclasses Eutheria and Metatheria, the members of which are viviparous.

**the•ri•a•ca** (the-ri'ə-kə) [Gr. *thēriaka* antidotes to the poison of wild animals, from *thērion* wild animal] a mixture of 60 to 70 substances pulverized and made into an electuary with honey, used in the Middle Ages as an antidote to bites by poisonous animals.

**Ther•i•di•i•dae** (ther"ĭ-di'ĭ-de) the comb-footed spiders, a family of small dark spiders of the suborder Labidognatha, whose venomous bite may be fatal to humans. It includes the genus *Latrodectus.*

**the•rio•geno•log•ic** (the"re-o-jen"o-loj'ik) pertaining or relating to theriogenology.

**the•rio•geno•log•i•cal** (the"re-o-jen"o-log'ĭ-kəl) theriogenologic.

**the•rio•gen•ol•o•gist** (the"re-o-jən-ol'ə-jist) one who specializes in theriogenology.

**the•rio•gen•ol•o•gy** (the"re-o-jən-ol'ə-je) [Gr. *thērion* beast + *geno-* + *-logy*] that branch of veterinary medicine dealing with reproduction, including the physiology and pathology of male and female reproductive systems and the clinical practice of veterinary obstetrics, gynecology, and semenology.

**therm** (thərm) [Gr. *thermē* heat] a unit of heat. The word has been used as equivalent to *(a)* large calorie; *(b)* small calorie; *(c)* 1000 large calories; *(d)* 100,000 British thermal units.

**ther•ma•co•gen•e•sis** (thər"mə-ko-jen'ə-sis) [*therm-* + *-genesis*] the production of elevated body temperature by a drug.

**ther•mal** (thər'məl) pertaining to or characterized by heat.

**ther•mal•ge•sia** (thər"məl-je'ze-ə) [*therm-* + *algesia*] a dysesthesia in which the application of heat produces pain; called also *thermoalgesia.* Cf. *thermohyperalgesia.*

**ther•mal•gia** (thər-mal'jə) causalgia.

**therm·an·al·ge·sia** (thərm″an-əl-je′ze-ə) thermoanesthesia.

**therm·an·es·the·sia** (thərm″an-es-the′zhə) thermoanesthesia.

**ther·ma·tol·o·gy** (thər″mə-tol′ə-je) the scientific study of heat as a therapeutic agent.

**ther·mel·om·e·ter** (thər′məl-om′ə-tər) an electric thermometer, used particularly for recording very small temperature variations.

**therm·es·the·sia** (thərm″es-the′zhə) [*therm-* + *esthesia*] temperature sense.

**therm·es·the·si·om·e·ter** (thərm″əs-the″ze-om′ə-tər) [*thermesthesia* + *-meter*] an instrument for measuring sensibility to heat.

**therm·hy·per·es·the·sia** (thərm″hi-pər-es-the′zhə) thermohyperesthesia.

**therm·hy·pes·the·sia** (thərm″hi-pes-the′zhə) thermohypesthesia.

**ther·mic** (thər′mik) of or pertaining to heat.

**ther·mi·on** (thər′me-on) a particle containing an electric charge emitted by an incandescent substance, such as the electrons emitted from the cathode in a Coolidge tube.

**ther·mi·on·ics** (thər″me-on′iks) the science of the phenomena exhibited by thermions.

**ther·mis·tor** (thər-mis′tor) a temperature-sensitive semiconductor whose resistance decreases as the ambient temperature increases; it is used to measure extremely small changes in temperature.

**therm(o)-** [Gr. *thermē* heat] a combining form denoting relationship to heat.

**Ther·mo·ac·ti·no·my·ces** (thər″mo-ak″tĭ-no-mi′sēz) [*thermo-* + Gr. *aktis, aktinos* a ray + *mykēs* fungus] a genus of bacteria of the family Micromonosporaceae, consisting of thermophilic (45° to 60° C) organisms having single spores on the aerial and substrate mycelia. They occur as soil and water saprophytes.
**T. vulga′ris,** a species isolated from soils, manure, and hay; one of the causative organisms of farmer's lung.

**ther·mo·al·ge·sia** (thər″mo-al-je′ze-ə) thermalgesia.

**ther·mo·an·al·ge·sia** (thər″mo-an″əl-je′ze-ə) thermoanesthesia.

**ther·mo·an·es·the·sia** (thər″mo-an″es-the′zhə) [*thermo-* + *anesthesia*] inability to recognize sensations of heat and cold; loss or lack of temperature sense. Called also *thermanalgesia, thermoanalgesia, thermanesthesia,* and *thermal anesthesia.*

**ther·mo·cau·ter·ec·to·my** (thər″mo-kaw″tər-ek′tə-me) [*thermocautery* + *-ectomy*] excision of an organ by thermocautery.

**ther·mo·cau·tery** (thər″mo-kaw′tər-e) cauterization by means of a hot wire or point. See also *electrocautery.*

**ther·mo·chem·is·try** (thər″mo-kem′is-tre) the aspect of physical chemistry dealing with heat changes that accompany chemical reactions.

**ther·mo·chro·ic** (thər″mo-kro′ik) [*thermo-* + Gr. *chroa* color] reflecting some of the heat rays and absorbing or transmitting others.

**ther·mo·chro·ism** (thər″mo-kro′iz-əm) the state or condition of being thermochroic.

**ther·mo·chro·sis** (thər″mo-kro′sis) thermochroism.

**ther·mo·co·ag·u·la·tion** (thər″mo-ko-ag″u-la′shən) coagulation of tissue by the action of high-frequency currents; used in removal of growths and in stereotactic surgery.
**radiofrequency t.,** the use of electromagnetic waves in the radio frequency range to coagulate tissue in stereotactic surgery and rhizotomy.

**ther·mo·cou·ple** (thər′mo-kup″əl) a pair of dissimilar electrical conductors (such as platinum and platinum-rhodium, or copper and constantan), so joined that an electromotive force is developed by the thermoelectric effects when the junctions are at different temperatures; used for measuring temperature differences.

**ther·mo·cur·rent** (thər″mo-kur′ent) a thermoelectric current.

**ther·mo·dif·fu·sion** (thər″mo-dĭ-fu′zhən) diffusion under the influence of a temperature gradient.

**ther·mo·di·lu·tion** (thər″mo-dĭ-loo′shən) [MeSH: Thermodilution] a method of measuring blood flow by injection of a known quantity of a cool or cold indicator, such as a saline solution or distilled water, into the cardiovascular system and measuring with a thermistor the temperature over time at a specific point in the system.

**ther·mo·du·ric** (thər″mo-du′rik) [*thermo-* + L. *durus* enduring] capable of withstanding high temperature.

**ther·mo·dy·nam·ics** (thər″mo-di-nam′iks) [*thermo-* + *dynamics*] [MeSH: Thermodynamics] the branch of science which deals with heat, energy, work, and the interconversion of these, and with related problems. See also under *law.*
**equilibrium t.,** the classic form of thermodynamics, that dealing with the application of the laws of thermodynamics to macroscopic systems in equilibrium states, or undergoing transformations between two equilibrium states.
**laws of t.,** see under *law.*
**nonequilibrium t.,** that dealing with irreversible processes of macroscopic systems and their rates.
**statistical t.,** that correlating the properties of individual atoms and molecules with macroscopic systems.

**ther·mo·elec·tric** (thər″mo-e-lek′trik) pertaining to electricity generated by heat.

**ther·mo·elec·tric·i·ty** (thər″mo-e″lek-tris′ĭ-te) electricity generated by heat.

**ther·mo·es·the·sia** (thər″mo-es-the′zhə) [*thermo-* + *esthesia*] temperature sense.

**ther·mo·es·the·si·om·e·ter** (thər″mo-əs-the″ze-om′ə-tər) thermesthesiometer.

**ther·mo·ex·ci·to·ry** (thər″mo-ək-si′tə-re) exciting or stimulating the production of heat in the body.

**ther·mo·gen·e·sis** (thər″mo-jen′ə-sis) [*thermo-* + *-genesis*] the production of heat, especially within the animal body.
**nonshivering t.,** the production of heat in the animal body without shivering, primarily through the uncoupling of oxidative phosphorylation in brown adipose tissue; it is most important in small mammals with a large surface to mass ratio and in neonates.
**obligatory t.,** the energy required to digest, absorb, and metabolize nutrients; called also *calorigenic effect* and *thermic effect.*
**shivering t.,** the production of heat in the animal body by shivering (q.v.).

**ther·mo·ge·net·ic** (thər″mo-jə-net′ik) 1. pertaining to thermogenesis. 2. thermogenic.

**ther·mo·gen·ic** (thər″mo-jen′ik) producing heat.

**ther·mo·gen·ics** (thər″mo-jen′iks) the science relating to heat production.

**ther·mog·e·nin** (thər-moj′ə-nin) uncoupling protein.

**ther·mog·e·nous** (thər-moj′ə-nəs) pertaining to or caused by heat or elevation of temperature.

**ther·mo·gram** (thər′mo-gram) 1. a graphic record of variations in temperature (heat). 2. the visual record obtained by thermography.

**ther·mo·graph** (thər′mo-graf) 1. an instrument for recording variations in temperature (heat). 2. a thermogram (def. 2). 3. the apparatus or device employed in thermography.
**continuous scan t.,** a thermograph that presents a continuous scan image of the thermal pattern (thermogram) of a patient or object on cathode ray tube.

**ther·mo·graph·ic** (thər″mo-graf′ik) pertaining to a thermogram or to thermography.

**ther·mog·ra·phy** (thər-mog′rə-fe) [*thermo-* + *-graphy*] [MeSH: Thermography] a technique wherein an infrared camera is used to photographically portray the surface temperatures of the body, based on the self-emanating infrared radiation; sometimes employed as a means of diagnosing underlying pathologic processes, such as breast tumors.
**infrared tympanic t.,** determination of body temperature by measuring the infrared radiation emanating from the tympanic membrane, using a probe introduced into the external acoustic meatus.

**ther·mo·gra·vim·e·ter** (thər″mo-grə-vim′ə-tər) an analytical instrument for measuring change in mass of a substance at changing temperature.

**ther·mo·hy·per·al·ge·sia** (thər″mo-hi″pər-al-je′ze-ə) a condition in which the application of moderate heat causes extreme pain.

**ther·mo·hy·per·es·the·sia** (thər″mo-hi″pər-es-the′zhə) a dysesthesia marked by increased sensibility to heat and cold; called also *thermhyperesthesia.*

**ther·mo·hy·pes·the·sia** (thər″mo-hi″pes-the′zhə) [*thermo-* + *hyp-* + *esthesia*] a dysesthesia marked by decreased sensibility to heat and cold; see also *thermoanesthesia.* Called also *thermhypesthesia* and *thermohypoesthesia.*

**ther·mo·hy·po·es·the·sia** (thər″mo-hi″po-əs-the′zhə) thermohypesthesia.

**ther·mo·in·ac·ti·va·tion** (thər″mo-in-ak″tĭ-va′shən) destruction of the power to act by exposure to heat.

**ther·mo·in·hib·i·to·ry** (thər″mo-in-hib′ĭ-tor-e) inhibiting or retarding the production of bodily heat.

**ther·mo·in·te·gra·tor** (thər″mo-in′tə-gra″tor) an apparatus for recording environmental warmth.

**ther·mo·la·bile** (thər″mo-la′bəl) easily altered or decomposed by heat; called also *heat labile.*

**ther·mol·o·gy** (thər-mol′ə-je) [*thermo-* + *-logy*] the science of heat.

**ther·mo·lu·mi·nes·cence** (thər″mo-loo″mĭ-nes′əns) the production of light by a substance when its temperature is increased.

**ther·mol·y·sis** (thər-mol′ĭ-sis) [*thermo-* + *-lysis*] 1. chemical dissociation by means of heat. 2. the dissipation of bodily heat by radiation, evaporation, or some other means.

**ther·mo·lyt·ic** (thər″mo-lit′ik) [*thermo-* + *-lytic*] 1. pertaining to, characterized by, or promoting thermolysis. 2. an agent that promotes thermolysis.

**ther·mo·mas·sage** (thər″mo-mə-sahzh′) massage with heat.

**ther·mo·mas·tog·ra·phy** (thər″mo-mas-tog′rə-fe) the use of thermography in the diagnosis of lesions of the breast.

**ther·mom·e·ter** (thər-mom′ə-tər) [*thermo-* + *-meter*] [MeSH: Thermometers] an instrument for determining temperatures. In principle, it makes use of some substance with a physical property that varies in magnitude with temperature, to determine a value of temperature on some defined scale. See also *scale* and selected subentries thereunder.

**air t.**, one in which the expansible material is air.

**alcohol t.**, a liquid-in-glass thermometer in which alcohol is the liquid used.

**axilla t.**, a surface thermometer to be used in the axilla.

**Beckmann t.**, a thermometer with a large bulb and fine bore stem for measurement of small differences in temperature.

**bimetal t.**, one made of two metals of dissimilar temperature coefficients of expansion so bonded together that a change in temperature causes it to curl.

**Celsius t.**, a thermometer employing the Celsius scale (q.v.).

**centigrade t.**, one having the interval between the two established reference points divided into 100 units; usually specifically denoting a *Celsius t.*

**clinical t.**, one for use in determining temperature of the human body.

**depth t.**, a thermometer whose sensitive element may be introduced into the tissues, for registering the actual temperature of a tissue.

**differential t.**, one for measuring small differences in temperature.

**Fahrenheit t.**, a thermometer employing the Fahrenheit scale (q.v.).

**fever t.**, clinical t.

**gas t.**, one in which the expansible material is a gas, such as air, carbon dioxide, helium, neon, nitrogen, or oxygen.

**half-minute t.**, a clinical thermometer with a short time lag.

**infrared tympanic t.**, a clinical thermometer inserted into the external acoustic meatus to measure body temperature by infrared tympanic thermography.

**kata t.**, see *katathermometer.*

**Kelvin t.**, a thermometer employing the Kelvin scale (q.v.).

**liquid-in-glass t.**, the common type of thermometer, containing a liquid which expands with increase in temperature; most of the liquid is in a bulb, but its free surface is in a capillary tube graduated to indicate the degree of temperature causing expansion to each particular point.

**maximum t.**, one which registers the highest temperature to which it has been exposed.

**mercury t.**, a liquid-in-glass thermometer in which mercury is the liquid used.

**metallic t.**, one in which some solid metal is used as the expansible element.

**metastatic t.**, differential t.

**minimum t.**, one which registers the lowest temperature to which it has been exposed.

**oral t.**, a clinical thermometer which is placed under the tongue, to record the temperature in the mouth; characteristically the bulb containing the mercury is elongated.

**Rankine t.**, a thermometer employing the Rankine scale (q.v.).

**Réaumur t.**, a thermometer employing the Réaumur scale (q.v.).

**recording t.**, a temperature-sensitive instrument by which the temperature to which it has been exposed is continuously recorded on a specially designed chart.

**rectal t.**, a clinical thermometer which is inserted in the rectum, for determining body temperature; characteristically the bulb containing the mercury is pear shaped.

**resistance t.**, a thermometer which uses the electric resistance of metals for determining temperature; it consists of a resistance bulb of platinum or other metal wire, and uses a Wheatstone bridge.

**self-registering t.**, 1. recording t. 2. one that registers the maximum or minimum temperature attained with a single measurement.

**surface t.**, a clinical thermometer for determining the temperature on the surface of the body.

**thermocouple t.**, a combination of a thermocouple with some device for measuring its electromotive force, such as a potentiometer; in use the thermocouple's reference junction is kept at a reference temperature (such as the ice point) and its measuring junction at the temperature being measured.

**tympanic t.**, infrared tympanic t.

**wet-and-dry-bulb t.**, psychrometer.

**ther·mo·met·ric** (thər″mo-met′rik) pertaining to a thermometer or to the measurement of degrees of temperature.

**ther·mom·e·try** (thər-mom′ə-tre) the measurement of temperatures.

**ther·mo·pal·pa·tion** (thər″mo-pal-pa′shən) palpation for the purpose of determining differences of temperature at different portions of the body.

**ther·mo·pen·e·tra·tion** (thər″mo-pen″ə-tra′shən) medical diathermy.

**ther·mo·phile** (thər′mo-fīl) 1. an organism that grows best at elevated temperatures. 2. a bacterium with an optimal growth temperature of 50° to 70° C.

**ther·mo·phil·ic** (thər″mo-fil′ik) [*thermo-* + *-philic*] growing best at or having a fondness for high temperatures. Cf. *mesophilic* and *psychrophilic.*

**ther·mo·phore** (thər′mo-for) [*thermo-* + *-phore*] a device or apparatus for retaining heat; used in therapeutic local application.

**ther·mo·pile** (thər′mo-pīl) [*thermo-* + *pile* (def. 1)] a number of thermocouples in series; used to increase the sensitivity of a temperature-measuring device, or for the direct conversion of heat into electric energy.

**ther·mo·plac·en·tog·ra·phy** (thər″mo-plas″ən-tog′rə-fe) the use of thermography for determining the site of placental attachment.

**ther·mo·plas·tic** (thər″mo-plas′tik) softening under heat and capable of being molded into shape with pressure, then hardening on cooling without undergoing chemical change.

**ther·mo·ple·gia** (thər″mo-ple′jə) [*thermo-* + *-plegia*] heat stroke.

**ther·mo·pre·cip·i·ta·tion** (thər″mo-pre-sip″ĭ-ta′shən) precipitation by heat.

**ther·mo·ra·dio·ther·a·py** (thər″mo-ra″de-o-ther′ə-pe) application of ionizing radiation to an anatomical site whose tissue temperature has been elevated by artificial means on the theory of increasing its radiosensitivity.

**ther·mo·re·cep·tor** (thər″mo-re-sep′tor) [MeSH: Thermoreceptors] a nerve ending, usually in the skin, that is sensitive to a change in temperature; see *cold receptor* and *warmth receptor,* under *receptor.*

**ther·mo·reg·u·la·tion** (thər″mo-reg″u-la′shən) the regulation of heat, such as the body heat of a warm-blooded animal; see also *thermostasis.*

**ther·mo·reg·u·la·tor** (thər″mo-reg′u-la″tor) thermostat.

**ther·mo·re·sis·tance** (thər″mo-re-zis′təns) the quality of being little affected by heat.

**ther·mo·re·sis·tant** (thər″mo-re-zis′tənt) not greatly affected by heat.

**ther·mo·scope** (thər′mo-skōp) [*thermo-* + *-scope*] differential thermometer.

**ther·mo·set** (ther′mo-set″) having undergone thermosetting.

**ther·mo·set·ting** (ther′mo-set″ing) becoming hard or solid when heat is applied and remaining that way upon being recooled; the change is not reversible. Said of resins.

**ther·mo·sta·bile** (thər″mo-sta′bil) unaffected by heat; able to withstand the effects of heat without undergoing change; in immunology, the term usually refers to substances that are not inactivated by heating to 56°C for 30 minutes, which inactivates complement. Called also *heat stable.*

**ther·mo·sta·bil·i·ty** (thər″mo-stə-bil′ĭ-te) the quality of withstanding the effects of heat without undergoing change.

**ther·mo·sta·sis** (thər″mo-sta′sis) [*thermo-* + *stasis*] the maintenance of body temperature in warm-blooded animals.

**ther·mo·stat** (thər′mo-stat) [*thermo-* + *-stat*] a device interposed in a heating system by which the temperature can be automatically maintained between certain levels.

**hypothalamic t.**, the mechanism for control of body temperature, which involves two thermoregulatory centers of the hypothalamus: the preoptic area of the anterior hypothalamus, which senses core temperature and compares it to the set-point, and an area in the posterior hypothalamus that integrates signals from the preoptic area and from cold and warmth receptors in the skin and controls mechanisms of heat dissipation (skin vasodilation, sweating) and production and conservation (skin vasoconstriction, release of epinephrine and thyroid hormones, sympathetic stimulation).

**ther·mo·ste·re·sis** (thər″mo-stə-re′sis) [*thermo-* + Gr. *sterēsis* deprivation] the deprivation of heat.

**ther·mo·stro·muhr** (thər″mo-stro′moor) an instrument for measuring the amount of blood flowing in a blood vessel by noting temperature changes.

**ther·mo·sys·tal·tic** (thər″mo-sis-tawl′tik) [*thermo-* + *systaltic*] contracting under the influence or stimulus of heat; pertaining to thermosystaltism.

**ther·mo·sys·tal·tism** (thər″mo-sis′təl-tiz-əm) [*thermo-* + Gr. *systellein* to contract] muscular contraction in response to temperature changes.

**ther·mo·tac·tic** (thər″mo-tak′tik) pertaining to thermotaxis.

**ther·mo·tax·ic** (thər″mo-tak′sik) thermotactic.

**ther·mo·tax·is** (thər″mo-tak′sis) [*thermo-* + *-taxis*] 1. the normal adjustment of body temperature; see also *thermoregulation.* 2. taxis in response to increased temperature.

**ther·mo·ther·a·py** (thər″mo-ther′ə-pe) [*thermo-* + *therapy*] treatment of disease by the application of heat; usually defined as that which raises body temperature to above 45° C. Cf. *hyperthermia.*

**ther·mot·ics** (thər-mot′iks) the science of heat.

**ther·mo·tol·er·ant** (thər″mo-tol′ər-ənt) enduring heat; said of bacteria whose activity is not checked by high temperature.

**ther·mo·to·nom·e·ter** (thər″mo-to-nom′ə-tər) [*thermo-* + *tono-* + *-meter*] an instrument for measuring the amount of muscular contraction caused by heat.

**ther·mo·trop·ic** (thər″mo-trop′ik) pertaining to or exhibiting thermotropism; called also *caloritropic.*

**ther·mot·ro·pism** (thər-mot′ro-piz-əm) [*thermo-* + *tropism*] tropism of an organism in response to an increase in temperature.

**the·ro·morph** (the′ro-morf) [Gr. *thēr* wild beast + *morph*] a morphologic part of an organism or individual with supernumerary, teratic, or absent parts, giving it a resemblance to a lower animal.

**the·ro·mor·phism** (the″ro-mor′fiz-əm) the abnormal resemblance of some part of the organism to the normal structure of the corresponding part of an animal of lower type.

**Ther·o·my·zon** (ther-o′mī-zon) a genus of leeches of the family Gnathobdellidae; they parasitize the nasal passages and sometimes the conjunctivae of geese.

**the·ront** (the′ront) [Gr. *thēr* wild beast + *on, ontos* being] the free-swimming stage or form in the life cycle of certain ciliate protozoa that arises from a tomite and searches ("hunts") for a new host or food source necessary for the development into the trophont.

**the·sau·ro·cyte** (thə-saw′ro-sīt) an abnormal plasma cell that is distended with homogeneous cytoplasm that stains gray or red, possibly owing to a disturbance in synthesis of immunoglobulin A; it may be related to a flaming plasma cell.

**Thes·sa·lus** (thes′ə-lus) **of Cos** [4th century B.C.] a Greek physician; the son of Hippocrates, whose teachings he followed.

**Thes·sa·lus** (thes′ə-lus) **of Tral·les** [1st century A.D.] a Greek physician of the Methodist school and a pupil of Themison.

**the·ta** (tha′tə) [Θ, θ] the eighth letter of the Greek alphabet.

**Thé·ve·nard's syndrome** (ta-və-nahrz′) [André *Thévenard,* French physician, 20th century] hereditary sensory radicular neuropathy; see under *neuropathy.*

**THF** tetrahydrofolic acid or tetrahydrofolate; see *tetrahydrofolic acid.*

**thi·a·ben·da·zole** (thi″ə-ben′də-zōl) [USP] [MeSH: Thiabendazole] a broad-spectrum benzimidazole anthelmintic with activity against roundworms, pinworms, threadworms, whipworms, and hookworms; used for most types of farm animals in the treatment of enterobiasis, strongyloidiasis, ascariasis, uncinariasis, trichuriasis, and creeping larva migrans.

**thi·ac·et·ar·se·mide so·di·um** (thi-as″ət-ahr′səmīd) [USP] a trivalent arsenical used in veterinary practice for the treatment of dirofilariasis.

**thi·a·di·a·zide, thi·a·di·a·zine** (thi″ə-di′ə-zīd, thi″ə-di′ə-zēn) thiazide.

**thi·am·a·zole** (thi-am′ə-zōl) methimazole.

**thi·a·min** (thi′ə-min) thiamine.

**thi·am·i·nase** (thi-am′ĭ-nās) [EC 3.5.99.2] an enzyme of the hydrolase class that catalyzes the cleavage of thiamine into its component pyrimidine and thiazole moieties, inactivating it. The enzyme is present in intestinal microorganisms. Called also *t. II.*
**t. I,** thiamin pyridinylase.
**t. II,** thiaminase.

**thi·a·mine** (thi′ə-min) [MeSH: Thiamine] vitamin $B_1$, a heat-labile, water-soluble bicyclic compound comprising a substituted pyrimidine linked to a thiazole moiety. It is found particularly in pork, organ meats, legumes, nuts, and whole grain or enriched cereals and breads. The active form is thiamin pyrophosphate (q.v.). Deficiency of the vitamin can result in beri-beri and is a factor in alcoholic neuritis and Wernicke-Korsakoff syndrome. Written also *thiamin.*
**t. hydrochloride** [USP], the monohydrochloride salt of thiamine, administered orally and intramuscularly for the prophylaxis and treatment of thiamine deficiency states.
**t. mononitrate** [USP], the mononitrate salt of thiamine, used in the preparation of various multivitamin dosage forms.
**t. pyrophosphate (TPP),** the active form of thiamine, which serves as a coenzyme in a variety of reactions, particularly those involving oxidative decarboxylation of certain important intermediates in carbohydrate metabolism.

**thi·a·min pyr·i·din·yl·ase** (thi′ə-min pir-ĭ-din′ə-lās) [EC 2.5.1.2] an enzyme of the transferase class that catalyzes the transfer of the pyrimidine moiety of thiamine from the thiazole ring component to pyridine or another base or thiol compound. The reaction inactivates thiamine. The enzyme occurs in the gastrointestinal tract of many fresh water animals. Called also *thiaminase I.*

**thi·am·phen·i·col** (thi-əm-fen′ĭ-kōl) [MeSH: Thiamphenicol] a broad-spectrum antibacterial, effective against a wide range of gram-positive and gram-negative organisms.

**thi·am·y·lal** (thi-am-ĭ-lal) [MeSH: Thiamylal] a very short-acting barbiturate used as an anesthetic.
**t. sodium,** the sodium salt of thiamylal, administered intravenously to produce general anesthesia of brief duration, for induction of anesthesia, to supplement other anesthetics, or to induce hypnosis.

**Thi·a·ra** (thi-ah′rə) a genus of fresh water snails of the family Thiaridae), found mostly in tropical regions of Africa and Asia; formerly called *Melania.* Some species, such as *T. grani′fera* and *T. tubercula ′ta,* act as the main snail hosts of various trematode parasites, including *Paragonimus, Metagonimus,* and *Haplorchis.*

**Thi·ar·i·dae** (thi-ar′ĭ-de) a family of fresh water snails of the subclass Streptoneura, order Mesogastropoda, found in warm regions of Africa, Asia, and various Pacific islands. It includes the genera *Hua* and *Thiara.*

**thi·a·sine** (thi′ə-sin) ergothioneine.

**thi·a·zide** (thi′ə-zīd) any of a group of benzothiadiazenesulfonamide derivatives, typified by chlorothiazide, that act as diuretics by inhibiting the reabsorption of sodium in the proximal renal tubule and stimulating chloride excretion, with resultant increase in excretion of water. They also increase the excretion of potassium, which can cause hypokalemia requiring potassium supplementation, and some increase in bicarbonate excretion. Thiazides are used for the treatment of edema due to congestive heart failure or chronic hepatic or renal disease and, alone or in combination with other drugs, in the treatment of hypertension. Called also *benzothiadiazide, benzothiadiazine, thiadiazide,* and *thiadiazine.*

**-thiazide** a suffix indicating a thiazide diuretic.

**thi·a·zole** (thi′ə-zōl) the chemical ring or any substituted derivative containing such a ring.

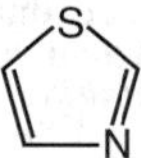


**Thi·bi·erge-Weis·sen·bach syndrome** (te-be-erzh′vīs′ən-bahk) [Georges *Thibierge,* French physician, 1856–1926; Raymond Joseph Emil *Weissenbach,* French physician, 1885–1963] calcinosis.

**thickness** (thik′nəs) a measurement across the smallest dimension of an object.
**triceps skinfold (TSF) t.,** a measurement of subcutaneous fat taken by measuring a fold of skin running parallel to the length of the arm over the triceps muscle midway between the acromion and olecranon; used as a means of estimating percentage of body fat.

**Thiele's syndrome** (thēlz) [George Henry *Thiele,* American proctologist, born 1896] see under *syndrome.*

**Thie·mann's disease** (te′mahnz) [H. *Thiemann,* German physician, early 20th century] see under *disease.*

**thi·emia** (thi-e′me-ə) [*thi-* + *-emia*] an excess of sulfur in the blood.

**thi·en·a·my·cin** (thi-en″ə-mi′sin) an antibacterial produced by *Streptomyces cattleya.*

**Thiersch's graft, operation** (tērsh′əz) [Karl *Thiersch,* German surgeon, 1822–1895] see *Ollier-Thiersch graft,* under *graft,* and see under *operation.*

**thigh** (thi) [MeSH: Thigh] the portion of the lower extremity ex-

tending from the hip above to the knee below; called also *femur*. See also *regio femoris*.
**cricket t.**, rupture of some of the fibers of the rectus femoris, which may occur in playing cricket or football; sometimes the tendon of the quadriceps or that of the patella is also ruptured.
**drivers' t.**, sciatic neuralgia caused by pressure from the use of the accelerator in driving an automobile.
**Heilbronner's t.**, broadening and flattening of the thigh, seen in cases of organic paralysis but not in hysterical paralysis when the patient lies on his back on a hard mattress.

**thig·mes·the·sia** (thig″mes-the′zhə) [*thigm-* + *esthesia*] touch (def. 1).

**thigm(o)-** [Gr. *thigma* touch] a combining form denoting relationship to touch or physical contact.

**thig·mo·tac·tic** (thig″mo-tak′tik) pertaining to, characterized by, or causing thigmotaxis.

**thig·mo·tax·is** (thig″mo-tak′sis) [*thigmo-* + *taxis*] taxis of an organism in response to the stimulus of contact or touch; called also *stereotaxis*.

**thig·mo·trop·ic** (thig″mo-trop′ik) pertaining to or exhibiting thigmotropism; responding to the stimulus of contact or touch; called also *stereotropic*.

**thig·mot·ro·pism** (thig-mot′ro-piz-əm) [*thigmo-* + *tropism*] tropism of an organism elicited by touch or direct contact with a solid or rigid surface; called also *stereotropism*.

**thi·hex·i·nol meth·yl·bro·mide** (thi-hek′sĭ-nōl) an anticholinergic, claimed to inhibit intestinal hypermotility.

**thim·ble** (thim′bəl) 1. coping. 2. see *thimbling*.

**thim·bling** (thim′bling) horizontal cracks or fissures in the hoof of an animal, such as those resulting from laminitis.

**thi·mero·sal** (thi-mer′o-səl) [USP] [MeSH: Thimerosal] an organomercurial antiseptic, which is actively antifungal and bacteriostatic for many nonsporulating bacteria; used as a topical anti-infective and as a preservative in pharmaceutical preparations. Called also *thiomersalate*.

**thi·meth·a·phan cam·phor·sul·fo·nate** (thi-meth′ə-fən kam″for-sul′fo-nāt) trimethaphan camsylate.

**think·ing** (thingk′ing) [MeSH: Thinking] ideational mental activity (in contrast to emotional activity); the flow of ideas, symbols, and associations that brings forth concepts and reasons.
**abstract t.**, that characterized by the ability to appreciate and use metaphors, concepts, and generalizations, to think symbolically, to reason and predict, and to formulate hypotheses and draw conclusions. Cf. *concrete t.*
**autistic t.**, self-absorption; preoccupation with inner thoughts, drives, and idiosyncratic logic; egocentric, subjective thinking lacking objectivity and preferring a narcissistic, inner, private reality to that which is externally validated. Used interchangeably with *dereistic t.*, although differing in emphasis. Called also *autism*.
**concrete t.**, that grounded in the literal, limited in the use or understanding of metaphor or nuance, and representing objects or ideas as specific items rather than as abstractions, generalizations, or totalities. Cf. *abstract t.*
**dereistic t.**, thinking not in accordance with the facts of reality and experience and following illogical, idiosyncratic reasoning. Used interchangeably with *autistic thinking*, although not an exact synonym: dereistic emphasizes disconnection from reality and autistic emphasizes preoccupation with inner experience. Called also *dereism*.
**magical t.**, that characterized by the belief that thinking or wishing something can cause it to occur; it is normal in childhood and dreams but also occurs in schizophrenia and other mental disorders.
**preoperational t.**, a type of thinking usually characteristic of children between the ages of approximately 2 and 7; it is characterized by a capability for symbolic representation but also by egocentricity and by lack of true understanding of relational terms, the principles of conservation, or the ability to arrange series of objects in order.
**primary process t.**, in psychoanalytic theory, the primitive thought processes deriving from the id and marked by illogical form, preverbal content, an emphasis on immediate wish fulfillment, and an equating of thought and action; characteristic of childhood and of dreams.
**secondary process t.**, in psychoanalytic theory, the more sophisticated thought processes, based on logic, obeying the rules of causality, and consistent with external reality; characteristic of mature conscious thought.

**thi(o)-** [Gr. *theion* sulfur] a prefix denoting the presence of sulfur. In systematic chemical nomenclature, it indicates the replacement of oxygen by sulfur as in thiophosphoric acid ($H_3PSO_3$) or ethanethio ($CH_3CH_2SH$).

**thio ac·id** (thi″o) an organic compound produced by replacement of one of the oxygens of the carboxyl group by divalent sulfur.

**thio·al·co·hol** (thi″o-al′kə-hol) mercaptan.

**thio·ar·se·nite** (thi″o-ahr′sə-nīt) any compound of sulfur and arsenic of the type $K_3AsS_3$.

**thio·bar·bi·tal** (thi″o-bahr′bĭ-təl) a salt of thiobarbituric acid, used as a thyroid depressant.

**thio·bar·bit·u·rate** (thi″o-bahr-bit′u-rāt) a salt or derivative of thiobarbituric acid.

**thio·bar·bi·tu·ric ac·id** (thi″o-bahr″bĭ-tu′rik) a condensation of malonic acid and thiourea, differing from barbituric acid only by the presence of a sulfur atom instead of an oxygen atom at the number 2 carbon; it is the parent compound of a class of drugs, thiobarbiturates. Thiobarbiturates and barbiturates are analogous in their effects.

**thio·car·ba·mide** (thi″o-kahr′bə-mīd) thiourea.

**thio·cy·a·nate** (thi″o-si′ə-nāt) the $S{=}C{=}N^-$ anion or a salt or ester containing this ion. Thiocyanate is produced in the metabolism of cysteine and detoxification of cyanide and is excreted in the urine.

**thio·cy·an·ic ac·id** (thi″o-si-an′ik) the molecular species H—S═C═N; aqueous solutions are an equilibrium mixture of thiocyanic and isothiocyanic acid and are very strong acids. Called also *sulfocyanic acid*.

**thio·cy·a·nide** (thi″o-si′ə-nīd) thiocyanate (1).

**thio·di·phen·yl·amine** (thi″o-di-fen″əl-am′in) phenothiazine, def. 1.

**thio·do·ther·a·py** (thi′o-do-ther′ə-pe) [*thio-* + *iodo-* + *therapy*] combined sulfur and iodine therapy.

**thio·es·ter** (thi″o-es′tər) a carboxylic acid and a thiol group in ester linkage, e.g., acetyl coenzyme A.

**thio·ether** (thi″o-e′thər) a sulfur ether; an ether in which sulfur replaces oxygen.

**thio·eth·yl·amine** (thi″o-eth″əl-am′in) an amine, $SH(CH_2)_2NH_2$, formed from cysteine by the loss of $CO_2$.

**thio·fla·vine** (thi″o-fla′vin) [*thio-* + *flavine*] a yellow dye, methyl dehydrothio-*p*-toluidine sulfonate.

**thio·glu·cose** (thi″o-gloo′kōs) a synthetic glucose that contains a sulfhydryl group which replaces the oxygen in the aldehyde group.

**thio·gua·nine** (thi″o-gwah′nēn) [USP] [MeSH: Thioguanine] 6-TG; a purine analogue, closely related to mercaptopurine, which has multiple metabolic effects that lead to blockade of purine nucleotide synthesis and utilization. 6-TG is cell cycle–specific for the S phase and is used for the treatment of acute myelocytic leukemia, administered orally. Called also *6-thioguanine*.

**thio·ki·nase** (thi″o-ki′nās) a term used in the trivial names of some enzymes of the ligase class that catalyze the formation of a thioester by joining a carboxylic acid and coenzyme A, coupled to cleavage of a high-energy phosphate bond.

**thi·ol** (thi′ol) 1. sulfhydryl. 2. any organic compound containing the —SH group; the analogue of an alcohol, which contains the —OH group.

**Thi·o·la** (thi-ol′ə) trademark for a preparation of tiopronin.

**thi·o·lase** (thi′o-lās) an enzyme that cleaves a carbon-carbon bond of a thiol compound to form a thioester. See *acetyl-CoA C-acetyltransferase*, and *acetyl-CoA C-acyltransferase*.

**thi·ol en·do·pep·ti·dase** (thi′ol en″do-pep′tĭ-dās) cysteine endopeptidase.

**thi·ol·his·ti·dine** (thi″ol-his′tĭ-din) the sulfur derivative of histidine occurring in the betaine form as ergothioneine.

**thio·mer·sa·late** (thi″o-mər′sə-lāt) thimerosal.

**thio·ne·ine** (thi″o-ne′in) ergothioneine.

**thi·o·nine** (thi′o-nēn) a dark-green powder, giving a purple color in solution, and used as a metachromatic stain in microscopy. Called also *Lauth's violet*.

**thi·o·nyl** (thi′o-nəl) the radical SO.

**thio·pan·ic ac·id** (thi″o-pan′ik) pantoyltaurine.

**thio·pen·tal so·di·um** (thi″o-pen′təl) [USP] an ultra–short-acting barbiturate, administered intravenously to produce general anesthesia of brief duration, for induction of anesthesia prior to administration of other anesthetics, to supplement regional anesthesia, as an anticonvulsive, and for narcoanalysis in psychiatric disorders.

**thio·pen·tone** (thi″o-pen′tōn) thiopental.

**Thio·plex** (thi′o-pleks″) trademark for a preparation of thiotepa.

**thio·pro·pa·zate hy·dro·chlo·ride** (thi″o-pro′pə-zāt) a phenothiazine tranquilizer, used in the treatment of psychoses and to suppress involuntary muscular activity in Huntington's chorea, administered orally.

**thi·o·rid·a·zine** (thi″o-rid′ə-zēn) [USP] [MeSH: Thioridazine] a phenothiazine compound having antipsychotic and sedative effects, used in the treatment of schizophrenia and acute psychotic episodes, for the relief of anxiety, agitation, and depression in mood disorders, and for the treatment of disruptive behavior disorders in children; administered orally.
**t. hydrochloride** [USP], the monohydrochloride salt of thioridazine, having the same actions and uses as the base; administered orally.

**thio·strep·ton** (thi″o-strep′ton) [USP] [MeSH: Thiostrepton] an antibacterial compound produced by *Streptomyces azureus,* used in topical antibacterial preparations for veterinary use.

**thio·sul·fate** (thi″o-sul′fāt) the $S_2O_3^{2-}$ anion or a salt containing this ion. Thiosulfate is produced in the metabolism of cysteine and excreted in the urine. It has also been used as a tracer for measuring extracellular fluid volume and is a commonly used reducing agent in laboratory chemistry and photography. Called also *hyposulfite.* See also *sodium thiosulfate.*

**thio·sul·fate sul·fur·trans·fer·ase** (thi-o-sul′fāt sul″fər-trans′fər-ās) [EC 2.8.1.1] [MeSH: Thiosulfate Sulfurtransferase] a mitochondrial enzyme of the transferase class that catalyzes the conversion of cyanide to thiocyanate, using thiosulfate as a sulfur donor. The reaction is the major physiologic mechanism for detoxifying cyanide.

**Thio·sul·fil** (thi″o-sul′fil) trademark for preparations of sulfamethizole.

**thio·sul·fur·ic ac·id** (thi″o-səl-fūr′ik) the molecular species $H_2S_2O_3$.

**thio·tepa** (thi″o-tep′ə) [USP] [MeSH: Thiotepa] an alkylating agent that has been used as an antineoplastic in the treatment of carcinoma of the breast, ovary, and bladder, malignant infusions, and lymphomas; now largely supplanted by cyclophosphamide and other nitrogen mustards. Called also *triethylenethiophosphoramide* (TEPA).

**thio·thix·ene** (thi″o-thik′sēn) [USP] [MeSH: Thiothixene] a thioxanthene derivative used for the treatment of symptoms of psychotic disorders; administered orally.
**t. hydrochloride** [USP], the dihydrate dihydrochloride salt of thiothixene, having the same uses as the base; administered orally and intramuscularly.

**thio·ura·cil** (thi″o-u′rə-sil) [MeSH: Thiouracil] thiourea derivative, which affects adversely the synthesis of the thyroid hormones. It has been used as an antithyroid agent in hyperthyroidism, and in angina pectoris and congestive heart failure.

**thio·urea** (thi″o-u-re′-ə) [MeSH: Thiourea] urea in which the oxygen is replaced by sulfur; used as a photographic fixing agent, as an accelerator in vulcanization, and for other purposes. It was formerly used to treat hyperthyroidism but was withdrawn because it is carcinogenic and is a contact allergen. Called also *thiocarbamide.*
**alphanaphthyl t., α-naphthyl t.,** ANTU.

**thio·xan·thene** (thi″o-zan′thēn) 1. a three-ring compound structurally related to phenothiazine but having the nitrogen atom at position 10 replaced by a carbon atom with a double bond. 2. any of a class of structurally related antipsychotic agents derived from thioxanthene, including chlorprothixene, flupenthixol, and thiothixene.

**thio·zine** (thi′o-zin) ergothioneine.

**thi·phen·a·mil hy·dro·chlo·ride** (thi-fen′ə-mil) an anticholinergic, having potent antispasmodic and smooth muscle relaxant properties; used to relieve pain and discomfort due to smooth muscle spasm associated with gastrointestinal disorders, administered orally.

**thi·ram** (thi′ram) [MeSH: Thiram] an antifungal, applied topically and sometimes used to treat seed corn; if animals consume excessive amounts of the corn they may suffer weight loss, dyspnea, lethargy, and convulsions.

**thirst** (thərst) [L. *sitis,* Gr. *dipsa*] [MeSH: Thirst] a sensation, often referred to the mouth and throat, associated with a craving for drink; ordinarily interpreted as a desire for water.
**insensible t.,** subliminal t.
**real t.,** true t.
**subliminal t.,** a sensation of need for water which is insufficient to prompt the ingestion of water but is at times sufficient to maintain drinking once it is initiated.
**true t.,** thirst which is associated with a bodily need for water and is satisfied by the ingestion of water.
**twilight t.,** subliminal t.

**Thi·ry's fistula** (te′rēz) [Ludwig *Thiry,* Austrian physiologist, 1817–1897] see under *fistula.*

**this·tle** (this′əl) any of a number of weedy plants of the family Compositae, having spiny leaves and flower heads surrounded by spiny bracts.
**milk t.,** 1. a tall thistle, *Silybum marianum,* native to southern Europe and naturalized in North America. 2. [NF] the dried ripe fruit of the milk thistle, used for loss of appetite and for supportive treatment in gallbladder and liver disorders.

**thixo·la·bile** (thik″so-la′bil) easily affected by shaking or stirring.

**thix·o·trop·ic** (thik″so-trop′ik) pertaining to or characterized by thixotropy.

**thix·ot·ro·pism** (thik-sot′ro-piz-əm) thixotropy.

**thix·ot·ro·py** (thik-sot′rə-pe) [Gr. *thixis* a touch + *-tropy*] the property, exhibited by certain gels, of becoming fluid when shaken or otherwise agitated and then becoming semisolid again at rest.

**thlip·sen·ceph·a·lus** (thlip″sən-sef′ə-ləs) [Gr. *thlipsis* pressure + *enkephalos* brain] a fetus with a deficient skull; see *craniofenestria* and *craniolacunia.*

**Tho·ma's ampulla, fluid** (to′mahz) [Richard *Thoma,* German histologist, 1847–1923] see under *ampulla* and *fluid.*

**Tho·ma-Zeiss counting chamber (counting cell)** (to′mah-tsīs) [Richard *Thoma;* Carl *Zeiss,* German optician, 1816–1888] see under *chamber.*

**Thom·as** (tom′əs) Edward Donnall. American hematologist, born 1920. Co-winner with Joseph Edward Murray of the Nobel prize for medicine or physiology in 1990 for his pioneering work with bone marrow transplantation.

**Thom·as shunt** (tom′əs) [G.I. *Thomas,* American nephrologist, 20th century] see under *shunt.*

**Tho·mas' sign** (to-mahs′) [André Antoine Henri *Thomas,* French neurologist, 1867–1963] André Thomas sign.

**Thom·as' sign, splint, test** (tom′əs) [Hugh Owen *Thomas,* English orthopedic surgeon, 1834–1891] see under *sign, splint,* and *test.*

**Thomp·son arthroplasty, prosthesis** (tomp′sən) [Frederick Roeck *Thompson,* American orthopedic surgeon, 1907–1983] see under *arthroplasty* and *prosthesis.*

**Thom·sen's disease** (tom′senz) [Asmus Julius Thomas *Thomsen,* Danish physician, 1815–1896] myotonia congenita.

**Thom·son's disease** (tom′sənz) [Mathew Sidney *Thomson,* English dermatologist, 1894–1969] see under *disease.*

**Thom·son scattering** (tom′sən) [Sir Joseph John *Thomson,* English physicist, 1856–1940] see under *scattering.*

**Thom·son's sign** (thom′sənz) [Frederick Holland *Thomson,* British physician, 1867–1938] Pastia's lines.

**thon·zo·ni·um bro·mide** (thon-zo′ne-əm) a cationic detergent used as an additive to ear drops to enhance tissue contact by dispersion and penetration of cellular debris.

**thon·zyl·amine hy·dro·chlo·ride** (thon-zil′ə-mēn) an antihistaminic used for symptomatic relief in hypersensitivity disorders; administered orally, rectally, topically, and intranasally.

**tho·ra·cal** (thor′ə-kəl) thoracic.

**tho·ra·cal·gia** (thor″ə-kal′jə) [*thorac-* + *-algia*] 1. pain in the chest; see also *pleurodynia* and *costalgia.* Called also *pectoralgia, stethalgia,* and *thoracodynia.* 2. pectoralgia (def. 1).

**tho·ra·cec·to·my** (thor″ə-sek′tə-me) [*thorac-* + *-ectomy*] thoracotomy with resection of a portion of a rib.

**tho·ra·cen·te·sis** (thor″ə-sen-te′sis) [*thorac-* + *-centesis*] paracentesis of the parietal cavity for aspiration of fluids; called also *pleuracentesis, pleurocentesis,* and *thoracocentesis.*

**tho·ra·ces** (tho′rə-sēz) plural of *thorax.*

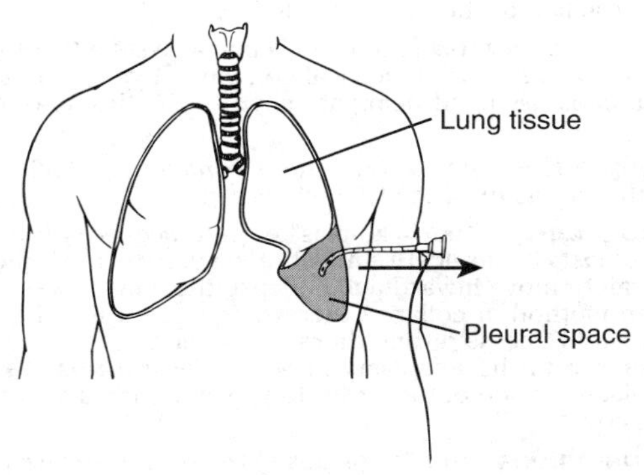


Thoracentesis.

**tho·rac·ic** (thə-ras′ik) [L. *thoracicus;* Gr. *thōrakikos*] pertaining to or affecting the thorax (chest). Called also *pectoral.*

**tho·rac·i·co·ab·dom·i·nal** (thə-ras″ĭ-ko-ab-dom′ĭ-nəl) thoracoabdominal.

**tho·rac·i·co·hu·mer·al** (thə-ras″ĭ-ko-hu′mər-əl) pertaining to the thorax and the humerus.

**tho·raci·spi·nal** (thə-ras″ĭ-spi′nəl) pertaining to the thoracic portion of the spinal column.

**thorac(o)-** [Gr. *thōrax,* gen. *thōrakos* chest] a combining form denoting relationship to the chest.

**tho·ra·co·ab·dom·i·nal** (thor″ə-ko-ab-dom′ĭ-nəl) pertaining to the thorax and the abdomen. Called also *abdominothoracic* and *thoracicoabdominal.*

**tho·ra·co·acro·mi·al** (thor″ə-ko-ə-kro′me-əl) pertaining to the thorax and the acromion.

**tho·ra·co·ce·los·chi·sis** (thor″ə-ko-se-los′kĭ-sis) [*thoraco-* + *celoschisis*] congenital fissure of the thorax and abdomen; cf. *celosomia.* Called also *thoracogastroschisis.*

**tho·ra·co·cen·te·sis** (thor″ə-ko-sən-te′sis) thoracentesis.

**tho·ra·co·cyl·lo·sis** (thor″ə-ko-si-lo′sis) [*thoraco-* + Gr. *kyllōsis* crippling] deformity of the chest.

**tho·ra·co·cyr·to·sis** (thor″ə-ko-sir-to′sis) [*thoraco-* + *cyrtosis*] abnormal curvature of the thorax, or unusual prominence of the chest.

**tho·ra·co·del·phus** (thor″ə-ko-del′fəs) [*thoraco-* + *-adelphus*] conjoined twins with one head, two arms, and four legs, the bodies being joined superior to the umbilicus.

**tho·ra·co·did·y·mus** (thor″ə-ko-did′ĭ-məs) [*thoraco-* + *didymus*] thoracopagus.

**tho·ra·co·dyn·ia** (thor″ə-ko-din′e-ə) [*thorac-* + *-odynia*] 1. thoracalgia (def. 1). 2. pectoralgia (def. 1).

**tho·ra·co·gas·tro·did·y·mus** (thor″ə-ko-gas″tro-did′ĭ-məs) [*thoraco-* + *gastro-* + *didymus*] gastrothoracopagus.

**tho·ra·co·gas·tros·chi·sis** (thor″ə-ko-gas-tros′kĭ-sis) thoracoceloschisis.

**tho·ra·co·graph** (thor′ə-ko-graf) [*thoraco-* + *-graph*] thoracopneumograph.

**tho·ra·co·lap·a·rot·o·my** (thor″ə-ko-lap″ə-rot′ə-me) [*thoraco-* + *laparo-* + *-tomy*] incision through both the thorax and abdomen to gain access to the subphrenic space and adjoining regions.

**tho·ra·co·lum·bar** (thor″ə-ko-lum′bər) pertaining to the thoracic and lumbar parts of the spine.

**tho·ra·col·y·sis** (thor″ə-kol′ĭ-sis) [*thoraco-* + *-lysis*] the freeing of adhesions of the chest wall.

**tho·ra·com·e·lus** (thor″ə-kom′ə-ləs) [*thoraco-* + Gr. *melos* limb] a fetus with a supernumerary limb attached to the thorax.

**tho·ra·com·e·ter** (tho″rə-kom′ə-tər) [*thoraco-* + *-meter*] stethometer.

**tho·ra·com·e·try** (thor″ə-kom′ə-tre) measurement of the thorax.

**tho·ra·co·my·odyn·ia** (thor″ə-ko-mi″o-din′e-ə) [*thoraco-* + *myodynia*] pectoralgia (def. 1).

**tho·ra·co·om·pha·lop·a·gus** (thor″ə-ko-om″fə-lop′ə-gəs) conjoined twins united at the sternum and umbilicus.

**tho·ra·cop·a·gus** (thor″ə-kop′ə-gəs) [*thoraco-* + *-pagus*] conjoined twins united in or near the sternal region, so the two components are face to face. Called also *thoracodidymus.*
**t. epigas′tricus,** asymmetrical conjoined twins in which the parasitic twin is attached to the epigastric region of the larger twin.
**t. parasi′ticus,** asymmetrical conjoined twins in which the parasitic twin is attached to the thorax of the larger twin.

**tho·ra·co·para·ceph·a·lus** (thor″ə-ko-par″ə-sef′ə-ləs) [*thoraco-* + *para-* + *-cephalus*] asymmetrical conjoined twins, a parasitic twin with rudimentary head being attached to the thorax of the larger twin.

**tho·ra·cop·a·thy** (thor″ə-kop′ə-the) [*thoraco-* + *-pathy*] any disorder of the thorax or of the thoracic organs.

**tho·ra·co·plas·ty** (thor′ə-ko-plas″te) [*thoraco-* + *-plasty*] [MeSH: Thoracoplasty] surgical removal of several ribs in order for the chest wall to move inward and collapse the lung; it was formerly a common method of collapse therapy (q.v.) and is still sometimes done to allow access during thoracic surgery.
**costoversion t.,** thoracoplasty in which several ribs are removed and replaced inside out in order to prevent outward movement of the chest wall.

**tho·ra·cos·chi·sis** (thor″ə-kos′kĭ-sis) [*thoraco-* + *-schisis*] congenital fissure of the thorax, which may result in herniation of lung tissue. Called also *schistothorax* and *schizothorax.*

**tho·raco·scope** (thə-rak′o-skōp) an endoscope for examining the pleural cavity; it is inserted into the cavity through a skin incision in an intercostal space.

**tho·ra·cos·co·py** (thor″ə-kəs′kə-pe) [*thoraco-* + *-scopy*] [MeSH: Thoracoscopy] the diagnostic examination of the pleural cavity through an endoscope. Called also *pleuroscopy.*

**tho·ra·co·ste·no·sis** (thor″ə-ko-stə-no′sis) [*thoraco-* + *stenosis*] abnormal contraction of the chest wall.

**tho·ra·cos·to·my** (thor″ə-kos′tə-me) [*thoraco-* + *-stomy*] [MeSH: Thoracostomy] 1. surgical creation of an opening in the wall of the chest for the purpose of drainage. 2. the opening so created.
**tube t.,** thoracostomy with insertion of a chest tube for drainage of air or fluid from the pleural space.

**tho·ra·cot·o·my** (thor″ə-kot′ə-me) [*thoraco-* + *-tomy*] [MeSH: Thoracotomy] surgical incision into the pleural space through the wall of the chest. Called also *pleuracotomy* and *pleurotomy.*

**tho·ra·del·phus** (thor″ə-del′fəs) thoracodelphus.

**tho·rax** (thor′aks) gen. *tho′racis,* pl. *tho′races* [Gr. *thōrax]*] [MeSH: Thorax] 1. [TA] chest: the part of the body between the neck and the thoracic diaphragm, encased by the ribs. 2. cavitas thoracis.
**amazon t.,** a chest with only one mammary gland, or breast.
**barrel-shaped t.,** barrel chest.
**cholesterol t.,** see under *pleurisy.*
**Peyrot's t.,** a chest that is obliquely oval; seen in large pleural effusions.
**pyriform t.,** a pear-shaped thorax, large above, small below.

**Thor·a·zine** (thor′ə-zēn) trademark for preparations of chlorpromazine.

**Tho·rel's bundle** (to′relz) [Christen *Thorel,* German physician, 1868–1935] see under *bundle.*

**tho·ri·um** (thor′e-əm) [*Thor,* a Norse deity] [MeSH: Thorium] a rare, heavy, gray metal, atomic number, 90; atomic weight, 232.038; symbol, Th. The naturally occurring radioactive isotope $^{232}$Th has a half-life of $1.4 \times 10^{10}$ years and is the parent element of a radioactive disintegration series.
**t. dioxide,** a contrast medium formerly used in radiography of the alimentary tract; its use was discontinued after it was linked to hepatic angiosarcoma.
**sodium t. tartrate,** used in radiography, especially of the gastrointestinal tract.

**Thor·mäh·len's test** (tor′ma-lenz) [Johann *Thormählen,* German physician, late 19th century] see under *test.*

**Thorn's syndrome** (thornz) [George Widmer *Thorn,* American physician, born 1906] salt-losing nephritis.

**Thorn·ton's sign** (thorn′tənz) [Knowsley *Thornton,* British physician, 1845–1904] see under *sign.*

**Thorn·waldt** see *Tornwaldt.*

**thor·ough·pin** (thur′o-pin) a distention of the synovial sheath of the flexor perforans tendon of the horse at the hock joint. Called also *knee-gall.*

**thought broad·cast·ing** (thawt brawd′kast-ing) the delusion that one's thoughts are being broadcast to the environment.

**thought in·ser·tion** (thawt in-sər′shən) the delusion that thoughts that are not one's own are being inserted into one's mind.

**thought with·draw·al** (thawt with-draw′əl) the delusion that someone or something is removing thoughts from one's mind.

**Thr** threonine.

**thread** (thred) a long slender structure, such as a continuous filament of some substance used as suture material.
**Simonart's t.,** a band formed by the stretching of adhesions between the amnion and fetus when the amniotic cavity is distended with its fluid; called also *Simonart's band.*

**thread·worm** (thred′wərm) any long slender nematode, such as members of the genera *Capillaria* and *Enterobius.* Called also *hairworm.*

**thre·o·nine** (thre′o-nēn) [MeSH: Threonine] $\alpha$-amino-$\beta$-hydroxybutyric acid, a natural essential amino acid necessary for optimal growth in infants and for nitrogen equilibrium in adults. Symbols Thr and T. See also table at *amino acid.*

**thre·o·nine de·hy·dra·tase** (thre′o-nēn de-hi′drə-tās) [MeSH: Threonine Dehydratase] an enzyme of the lyase class that catalyzes the dehydration and deamination of threonine, an irreversible step in the degradation of this amino acid.

**thre·o·nyl** (thre′o-nəl) the acyl radical of threonine.

**thre·ose** (thre'ōs) an aldotetrose epimeric with erythrose at the 2 carbon.

**thresh·old** (thresh'old) 1. that value at which a stimulus just produces a sensation, is just appreciable, or comes just within the limits of perception; see also *absolute t.* and *differential t.* 2. a hypothetical barrier that stimuli must pass to be detected. 3. that degree of concentration of any of specific substances *(threshold substances)* in the blood plasma above which the substance is excreted by the kidneys and below which it is not excreted. 4. limen. 5. the minimum level of input required to cause some event to occur.
**absolute t.**, the lowest possible limit of stimulation that is capable of producing sensation; called also *stimulus t.*
**achromatic t.**, the least intensity of the spectrum that produces a sensation of color; reduction of intensity below this point produces a sensation of brightness only, without any color distinction.
**anaerobic t.**, the point during exercise at which the ratio of ventilation to oxygen consumption begins to increase as a result of lactic acidosis.
**arousal t.**, the minimal stimulation necessary to awaken a sleeper.
**auditory t.**, the slightest perceptible sound; called also *minimum audible.*
**t. of consciousness**, the lowest limit of sensibility; the point of consciousness at which a stimulus is barely perceived. Called also *minimum sensible.*
**convulsant t.**, the minimum amount of electric current or drug required to produce a convulsion in convulsive therapy.
**differential t.**, the lowest limit of discriminative sensibility; the ratio which the difference of two stimuli must bear to half their sum in order that their difference may be just perceptible.
**displacement t.**, the threshold of perception of a break in the continuity of a contour or of a border; called also *Vernier acuity.*
**double point t.**, the smallest distance apart at which two stimuli of touch are felt as distinct.
**erythema t.**, the size of the radiation dose that is required to cause erythema of the skin.
**flicker fusion t.**, critical fusion frequency.
**insular t.**, limen insulae.
**neuron t.**, that degree of stimulation of a neuron which just suffices to call forth a fruitful excitation (sensation, movement, or the like).
**t. of nose**, limen nasi.
**pacing t.**, the minimal level of electrical stimulation necessary to induce cardiac depolarization consistently.
**relational t.**, the ratio which two stimuli must have to each other in order that the difference between them may be just perceptible.
**renal t.**, that concentration of a substance in plasma at which it begins to be excreted in the urine.
**renal t. for glucose**, the point of sugar (glucose) concentration in the blood (180 mg per mL in the normal) at which the kidney will excrete sugar (glucosuria); called also *transport maximum for glucose.*
**resolution t.**, the least distance that two objects may be apart and still be distinguished as two; called also *minimum separabile.*
**sensing t.**, the minimal level of electrical activity necessary for recognition by the cardiac pacemaker as a signal of depolarization.
**sensitivity t.**, absolute t.
**speech reception t.**, **speech recognition t.**, SRT; the minimum intensity in decibels at which a patient can understand 50 per cent of spoken words; used in tests of speech audiometry.
**stimulus t.**, absolute t.
**swallowing t.**, the minimal stimulation necessary to elicit the reflex action that leads to swallowing.
**t. of visual sensation**, the least possible amount of stimulus that gives rise to the sensation of sight.

**thrill** (thril) a sensation of vibration felt by the examiner on palpation of the body, such as over the heart during loud, harsh cardiac murmurs; cf. *fremitus.*
**aneurysmal t.**, a thrill felt on palpation of an aneurysm.
**aortic t.**, one felt over the aortic orifice in disease of its valves.
**diastolic t.**, a vibratory sensation felt over the precordium during ventricular diastole, as in advanced aortic insufficiency.
**fat t.**, a peculiar thrill sometimes felt in abdominal examinations due to excessive fatness of the parietes.
**hydatid t.**, a tremulous impulse sometimes felt on palpation of the body surface over a hydatid cyst; called also *hydatid fremitus.*
**presystolic t.**, a thrill felt just before the systole by the hand placed over the apex of the heart.
**purring t.**, a thrill of a quality suggesting the purring of a cat.
**systolic t.**, a thrill felt on systole over the precordium, as in aortic stenosis, pulmonary stenosis, and ventricular septal defect.

**thrix** (thriks) [Gr.] hair; see also *pilus* [TA].

**-thrix** word termination denoting relationship to hair.

**throat** (thrōt) 1. pharynx. 2. fauces. 3. the anterior part of the neck.
**sore t.**, see *sore throat,* under S.

**throb** (throb) a pulsating movement or sensation.

**throb·bing** (throb'ing) beating; attended with a rhythmic beating sensation.

**Throck·mor·ton's reflex (sign)** (throk'mor-tənz) [Thomas Bentley *Throckmorton,* American neurologist, 1885–1961] see under *reflex.*

**throe** (thro) a severe pain or paroxysm.

**throm·ba·phe·re·sis** (throm″bə-fə-re'sis) thrombocytapheresis.

**throm·base** (throm'bās) thrombin.

**throm·bas·the·nia** (throm″bəs-the'ne-ə) [*thrombocyte* + *astheneia*] [MeSH: Thrombasthenia] 1. decreased platelet function; called also *thromboasthenia.* 2. Glanzmann's t.
**Glanzmann's t.**, a hereditary platelet abnormality characterized by defective clot retraction, prolonged bleeding time, and related symptoms such as epistaxis and inappropriate bleeding. Clinically there is abnormal glass adhesion and impaired aggregation to ADP, collagen, and thrombin. Most cases are autosomal recessive, but a few are autosomal dominant. Called also *thrombasthenia* and *Glanzmann's disease.*

**throm·bec·to·my** (throm-bek'tə-me) [*thromb-* + *-ectomy*] [MeSH: Thrombectomy] excision of a thrombus from a blood vessel.

**throm·bi** (throm'bi) plural of *thrombus.*

**throm·bin** (throm'bin) [MeSH: Thrombin] 1. the activated form of coagulation factor II (prothrombin); it converts fibrinogen to fibrin. Called also *fibrinogenase* and *thrombase.* 2. [USP] a sterile protein substance *(topical t.)* prepared from prothrombin of bovine origin through interaction with added thromboplastin in the presence of calcium; used therapeutically as a local hemostatic.

**throm·bin·o·gen** (throm-bin'o-jən) [MeSH: Prothrombin] factor II; see under *coagulation factors,* at *factor.*

**thromb(o)-** [Gr. *thrombos* clot] a combining form denoting relationship to a clot, or thrombus.

**throm·bo·ag·glu·ti·nin** (throm″bo-ə-gloo'tĭ-nin) platelet agglutinin.

**throm·bo·an·gi·itis** (throm″bo-an″je-i'tis) [*thrombo-* + *angiitis*] inflammation of a blood vessel (vasculitis) with thrombosis.
**t. obli'terans**, an inflammatory and obliterative disease of the blood vessels of the extremities, primarily the lower extremities, occurring chiefly in young men and leading to ischemia of the tissues and gangrene; called also *Buerger's* or *Winiwarter-Buerger disease.*

**throm·bo·ar·te·ri·tis** (throm″bo-ahr″tər-i'tis) thrombosis occurring in association with inflammation of an artery.
**t. purulen'ta**, purulent softening of an arterial thrombosis, with infiltration of the artery walls.

**throm·bo·as·the·nia** (throm″bo-əs-the'ne-ə) thrombasthenia.

**throm·boc·la·sis** (throm-bok'lə-sis) [*thrombo-* + Gr. *klasis* a breaking] thrombolysis.

**throm·bo·clas·tic** (throm″bo-klas'tik) thrombolytic.

**throm·bo·cyst** (throm'bo-sist) [*thrombo-* + *cyst*] the chronic sac which may form around a thrombus in a hematoma.

**throm·bo·cys·tis** (throm″bo-sis'tis) thrombocyst.

**throm·bo·cy·ta·phe·re·sis** (throm″bo-si″tə-fə-re'sis) [*thrombocyte* + *apheresis*] the selective separation and removal of platelets (thrombocytes) from withdrawn blood, the remainder of the blood then being retransfused into the donor. Called also *plateletpheresis* and *thrombapheresis.*

**throm·bo·cyte** (throm'bo-sīt) [*thrombo-* + *-cyte*] [MeSH: Blood Platelets] platelet.

**throm·bo·cy·the·mia** (throm″bo-si-the'me-ə) [*thrombocyte* + *-emia*] 1. an increase in the number of circulating platelets; called also *thrombocytosis.* 2. essential t.
**essential t.**, **hemorrhagic t.**, a myeloproliferative disorder characterized by a sharp increase in the number of circulating platelets, with repeated spontaneous hemorrhages either externally or into the tissues. Called also *idiopathic* or *primary t.* and *megakaryocytic leukemia.*
**idiopathic t.**, **primary t.**, hemorrhagic t.

**throm·bo·cyt·ic** (throm″bo-sit'ik) 1. pertaining to, characterized by, or of the nature of a platelet (thrombocyte). 2. pertaining to the thrombocytic series.

**throm·bo·cy·tol·y·sis** (throm″bo-si-tol'ĭ-sis) destruction of platelets (thrombocytes).

**throm·bo·cy·to·path·ia** (throm″bo-si″to-path'e-ə) thrombocytopathy.

**throm·bo·cy·to·path·ic** (throm″bo-si″to-path'ik) pertaining to or characterized by thrombocytopathy.

**throm·bo·cy·top·a·thy** (throm″bo-si-top′ə-the) any qualitative disorder of the platelets, due most often to deficiency of platelet factor 3.
**constitutional t.,** thrombasthenia.

**throm·bo·cy·to·pe·nia** (throm″bo-si″to-pe′ne-ə) [*thrombocyte* + *-penia*] [MeSH: Thrombocytopenia] decrease in the number of platelets, such as in thrombocytopenic purpura. See also *pancytopenia.*
**essential t.,** idiopathic thrombocytopenic purpura.
**immune t.,** that associated with the presence of anti-platelet antibodies (IgG).
**infectious cyclic t.,** thrombocytopenia in dogs recurring every one to two weeks, caused by infection with *Ehrlichia platys*; it usually resolves spontaneously in time.
**neonatal t., neonatal alloimmune t.,** immune thrombocytopenia that results when platelets of the fetus express an antigen that is lacking on maternal platelets; fetal platelets enter the maternal circulation and stimulate the production of antibodies, which in turn cross the placenta and destroy fetal platelets.

**throm·bo·cy·to·poi·e·sis** (throm″bo-si″to-poi-e′sis) [*thrombocyte* + *-poiesis*] the production of platelets.

**throm·bo·cy·to·poi·et·ic** (throm″bo-si″to-poi-et′ik) concerned with the formation of platelets.

**throm·bo·cy·to·sis** (throm″bo-si-to′sis) [MeSH: Thrombocytosis] an increase in the number of circulating platelets; called also *thrombocythemia.*
**primary t.,** essential thrombocythemia.
**reactive t., secondary t.,** that occurring in reaction to some other disease process such as an infection, neoplasm, inflammatory process, or rheumatoid process.

**throm·bo·elas·to·gram** (throm″bo-e-las′to-gram) the graphic record of the values determined by thromboelastography.

**throm·bo·elas·to·graph** (throm″bo-e-las′to-graf) an apparatus used in study of the rigidity of blood or plasma during coagulation.

**throm·bo·elas·tog·ra·phy** (throm″bo-e″las-tog′rə-fe) determination of the rigidity of the blood or plasma during coagulation, by use of the thromboelastograph.

**throm·bo·em·bo·lia** (throm″bo-əm-bo′le-ə) thromboembolism.

**throm·bo·em·bo·lism** (throm″bo-em′bo-liz-əm) [MeSH: Thromboembolism] obstruction of a blood vessel with thrombotic material carried by the blood stream from the site of origin to plug another vessel.

**throm·bo·end·ar·ter·ec·to·my** (throm″bo-end″ahr-tər-ek′tə-me) [*thrombo-* + *endarterectomy*] removal of thrombus and atherosclerotic inner lining from an obstructed artery.

**throm·bo·end·ar·ter·itis** (throm″bo-end-ahr″tər-i′tis) inflammation of the innermost coat of an artery, with thrombus formation.

**throm·bo·en·do·car·di·tis** (throm″bo-en″do-kahr-di′tis) [*thrombo-* + *endocarditis*] a term formerly used for nonbacterial thrombotic endocarditis or sometimes incorrectly for nonbacterial verrucous endocarditis.

**throm·bo·gen·e·sis** (throm″bo-jen′ə-sis) the formation of thrombi or blood clots.

**throm·bo·gen·ic** (throm″bo-jen′ik) [*thrombo-* + *-genic*] producing a thrombus or blood clot.

**β-throm·bo·glob·u·lin** (throm″bo-glob′u-lin) a platelet-specific protein released with platelet factor 4 on platelet activation; it mediates several reactions of the inflammatory response, binds and inactivates heparin, and blocks the endothelial cell release of prostacyclin.

**throm·boid** (throm′boid) [Gr. *thromboeidēs*] resembling a thrombus.

**throm·bo·ki·nase** (throm″bo-ki′nās) activated factor X; see under *coagulation factors,* at *factor.*

**throm·bo·ki·ne·sis** (throm″bo-ki-ne′sis) [*thrombo-* + *kinesis*] blood coagulation.

**throm·bo·ki·net·ics** (throm″bo-ki-net′iks) the dynamics of blood coagulation.

**throm·bo·lym·phan·gi·tis** (throm″bo-lim″fan-ji′tis) inflammation of a lymph vessel due to a thrombus.

**Throm·bol·y·sin** (throm-bol′ĭ-sin) trademark for a preparation of fibrinolysin.

**throm·bol·y·sis** (throm-bol′ĭ-sis) [*thrombo-* + *-lysis*] the lysing of thrombi; it involves a complex series of events, of which the most important involves local action of plasmin confined within the substance of the thrombus.
**intracoronary t.,** lysis of clots by thrombolytic agents introduced into the coronary arteries; used in thrombolytic therapy after myocardial infarction.

**throm·boly·so·an·gi·o·plas·ty** (throm-bol″ĭ-so-an′je-o-plas″te) the dissolution of arterial thrombi by intra-arterial infusion of a thrombolytic agent followed by balloon angioplasty.

**throm·bo·lyt·ic** (throm″bo-lit′ik) 1. dissolving or splitting up a thrombus. 2. an agent that so acts. Cf. *antithrombotic.*

**throm·bo·mod·u·lin** (throm″bo-mod′u-lin) [MeSH: Thrombomodulin] an endothelial cell protein that binds protein C and thrombin; the thrombin can then activate bound protein C.

**throm·bon** (throm′bon) [*thrombo-* + Gr. *on* neuter ending] the platelets and their precursors; it is the counterpart of *erythron* and *leukon.*

**throm·bop·a·thy** (throm-bop′ə-the) thrombocytopathy.

**throm·bo·pe·nia** (throm″bo-pe′ne-ə) thrombocytopenia.

**throm·bo·phil·ia** (throm″bo-fil′e-ə) [*thrombo-* + *-philia*] a tendency to the occurrence of thrombosis.

**throm·bo·phle·bi·tis** (throm″bo-flə-bi′tis) [*thrombo-* + *phlebitis*] [MeSH: Thrombophlebitis] inflammation of a vein (phlebitis) associated with thrombus formation (thrombosis).
**iliofemoral t., postpartum,** thrombophlebitis of the iliofemoral vein following childbirth; see also *phlegmasia alba dolens.*
**intracranial t.,** thrombophlebitis in one of the sinuses of the dura mater; see also *sinus thrombosis.*
**t. mi′grans, migratory t.,** a recurring phlebitis usually affecting segments of superficial peripheral veins, and sometimes involving major and visceral veins; it may occur in multiple sites simultaneously or at intervals. Called also *phlebitis migrans.*

**throm·bo·plas·tic** (throm″bo-plas′tik) [*thrombo-* + *-plastic*] causing or accelerating clot formation in the blood.

**throm·bo·plas·tid** (throm″bo-plas′tid) platelet.

**throm·bo·plas·tin** (throm″bo-plas′tin) [MeSH: Thromboplastin] factor III; see under *coagulation factors,* at *factor.*
**tissue t.,** factor III; see under *coagulation factors,* at *factor.* So called because it is released by or derived from extravascular tissues.

**throm·bo·plas·tin·o·gen** (throm″bo-plas-tin′o-jən) [MeSH: Factor VIII] former name for *factor VIII;* see under *coagulation factors,* at *factor.*

**throm·bo·poi·e·sis** (throm″bo-poi-e′sis) 1. thrombogenesis. 2. thrombocytopoiesis.

**throm·bo·poi·et·ic** (throm″bo-poi-et′ik) 1. pertaining to or characterized by thrombopoiesis. 2. thrombogenic.

**throm·bo·poi·e·tin** (throm″bo-poi′ə-tin) [MeSH: Thrombopoietin] a hypothetical substance believed to serve as the humoral regulator of the production of platelets.

**throm·bo·re·sis·tance** (throm″bo-re-zis′təns) resistance by a blood vessel to thrombus formation; see also *anticoagulation.*

**throm·bosed** (throm′bōsd) affected with thrombosis.

**throm·bo·si·nu·si·tis** (throm″bo-si″nu-si′tis) sinus thrombosis.

**throm·bo·sis** (throm-bo′sis) [Gr. *thrombōsis*] [MeSH: Thrombosis] the formation, development, or presence of a thrombus.
**atrophic t.,** marasmic t.
**cardiac t.,** thrombosis in the heart.
**caudal vena caval t.,** thrombosis of the caudal vena cava in cattle, usually because of emboli from a hepatic abscess; it often progresses to embolic pneumonia, which can be fatal.
**cavernous sinus t.,** thrombosis affecting the cavernous sinus.
**cerebral t.,** thrombosis of a cerebral vessel, which may result in cerebral infarction.
**coronary t.,** development of an obstructive thrombus in a coronary artery, usually associated with atherosclerosis and often causing sudden death or a myocardial infarction.
**creeping t.,** thrombosis gradually involving one portion of a vein after another. See also *propagating t.*
**deep venous t.,** DVT; thrombosis of one or more of the deep veins of the lower limb, characterized by swelling, warmth, and erythema, frequently a precursor of a pulmonary embolism.
**dilatation t., dilation t.,** thrombosis due to the slowing of circulation on account of dilation of a vein.
**effort t.,** Paget-Schroetter syndrome.
**infective t.,** thrombosis associated with an infection such as septic phlebitis.
**intracranial t., intracranial sinus t.,** sinus t.
**marantic t., marasmic t.,** thrombosis, usually of one of the sagittal sinuses, occurring in the wasting diseases of infancy and of old age; called also *atrophic t.*
**mesenteric arterial t.,** formation of a clot in an artery or arteriole of the mesentery.
**mesenteric venous t.,** formation of a clot in one of the mesenteric veins, leading to ischemia and infarction of the small bowel or colon.
**placental t.,** 1. a normal formation of thrombi in the placenta. 2. an

abnormal extension of the placental thrombus formation to the veins of the uterus.
**plate t., platelet t.**, the presence or development of a platelet thrombus.
**propagating t.**, progressive clot formation upon an occlusive thrombus, producing an elongated mass sometimes extending into other blood vessels. See also *creeping t.*
**puerperal t.**, coagulation of blood in the veins after childbirth; see also *postpartum iliofemoral thrombophlebitis.*
**sinus t.**, thrombosis of a sinus of the dura mater, usually secondary to head injury or to infection of a nearby structure; called also *intracranial t.* and *intracranial sinus t.*
**traumatic t.**, thrombosis following injury to a part.
**venous t.**, phlebothrombosis.

**throm·bo·spon·din** (throm″bo-spon′din) a 450-kilodalton multifunctional glycoprotein secreted by endothelial cells and by the alpha granules of platelets following activation by thrombin; it interacts with a wide variety of molecules, including heparin, fibrin, fibrinogen, platelet cell membrane receptors, collagen, and fibronectin, and plays a role in platelet aggregation, tumor metastasis, adhesion of *Plasmodium falciparum,* vascular smooth muscle growth, and tissue repair in skeletal muscle following crush injury.

**throm·bos·ta·sis** (throm-bos′tə-sis) stasis of blood in a part, with formation of a thrombus.

**throm·bo·sthe·nin** (throm″bo-sthe′nin) [*thrombo-* + *stheno-* + *-in* chemical suffix] a contractile protein of platelets, active in clot retraction.

**throm·bot·ic** (throm-bot′ik) pertaining to or affected with thrombosis.

**throm·box·ane** (throm-bok′sān) [*thrombocyte* + *oxane* ring] either of two compounds related to prostaglandins and derived from arachidonic acid. *Thromboxane* $A_2$ *(*$TXA_2$*)* is an extremely potent inducer of platelet aggregation and platelet release reactions and is also a vasoconstrictor; it is thus a physiologic antagonist of prostacyclin. It is synthesized by platelets and is very unstable, with a half-life of 30 seconds, undergoing nonenzymatic hydrolysis to *thromboxane* $B_2$ *(*$TXB_2$*),* which is inactive.

**throm·box·ane-A syn·thase** (throm-bok′sān sin′thās) [EC 5.3.99.5] an enzyme of the isomerase class that catalyzes the conversion in platelets of prostaglandin $G_2$ to thromboxane $A_2$, a potent vasoconstrictor and platelet agonist. Deficient enzyme activity, an autosomal dominant trait, causes defects in the release of platelets. See also illustration at *prostaglandin.*

**throm·bus** (throm′bəs) pl. *throm′bi* [Gr. *thrombos* clot] a stationary blood clot along the wall of a blood vessel, frequently causing vascular obstruction. Some authorities differentiate thrombus formation from simple coagulation or clot formation. Cf. *embolus.*

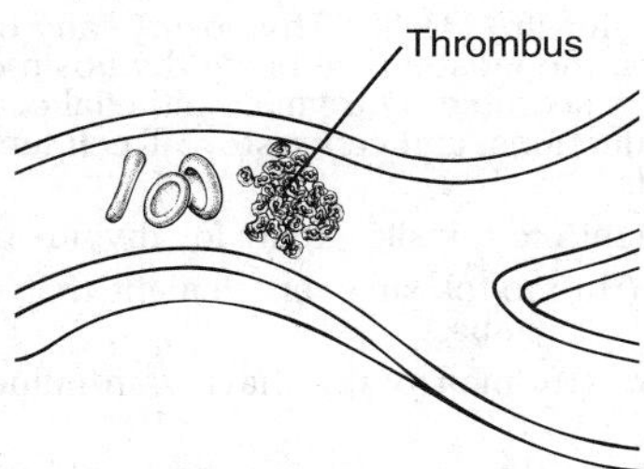


Thrombus obstructing platelet flow near a vascular bifurcation.

**agonal t., agony t.**, see under *clot.*
**annular t.**, one which has an opening through its center, while the circumference is attached to the wall of the vessel.
**antemortem t.**, see under *clot.*
**ball t.**, a roughly spherical, organized thrombus which may obstruct an orifice (usually the mitral valve) intermittently like a ball valve.
**bile t.**, a plug in one of the intrahepatic bile ducts, causing cholestasis.
**blood plate t., blood platelet t.**, platelet t.
**calcified t.**, phlebolith.
**coral t.**, a coral-colored thrombus formed by coagulated fibrin and erythrocytes.
**currant jelly t.**, see under *clot.*
**fibrin t.**, a parietal thrombus composed mainly of fibrin.
**hyaline t.**, a thrombus composed of erythrocytes which have lost their hemoglobin, forming a colorless translucent mass.
**infective t.**, the thrombus seen with infective thrombosis.
**laminated t.**, a thrombus whose substance is in layers, suggesting different periods of formation. Called also *mixed t.* and *stratified t.*
**lateral t.**, parietal t.
**marantic t., marasmic t.**, one associated with severe wasting diseases, often a terminal event; see also under *thrombosis.*
**milk t.**, an accumulation of curdled milk in a lactiferous duct.
**mixed t.**, laminated t.
**mural t.**, a thrombus attached to the wall of the heart adjacent to an area of diseased endocardium, or to the aortic wall overlying an intimal lesion. Cf. *parietal t.*
**obstructive t.**, occlusive t.
**occluding t., occlusive t.**, one that occupies the entire lumen of a vessel and obstructs blood flow. Called also *obstructive t.*
**organized t.**, one which has been invaded by fibroblasts and thereby changed to loose fibrous tissue with varying degrees of vascularity.
**pale t.**, white t.
**parasitic t.**, an accumulation of the pigmented bodies of free malarial parasites and their spores in the capillaries of the brain, causing a condition known as *cerebral malaria.*
**parietal t.**, one attached to the wall of a vessel. Cf. *mural t.* Called also *lateral t.*
**plate t., platelet t.**, one formed by an abnormal accumulation of blood platelets; see also *white t.* (def. 3). Called also *blood plate t.* and *blood platelet t.*
**postmortem t.**, see under *clot.*
**primary t.**, one that remains at its place of origin.
**propagated t.**, one that has grown beyond its original limits.
**red t.**, one with a dark-red color, formed by the coagulation of blood and composed mainly of erythrocytes.
**stratified t.**, laminated t.
**traumatic t.**, the thrombus seen in traumatic thrombosis.
**white t.**, 1. one containing few or no red cells. 2. one composed chiefly of leukocytes. 3. one composed chiefly of platelets and fibrin, usually seen in arterial thrombosis. Called also *pale t.*

**thrush** (thrush) 1. candidiasis of the oral mucosa, usually the buccal mucosa and tongue, and sometimes the palate, gingivae, and floor of the mouth. It is characterized by white plaques of soft curdlike material that may be stripped off, leaving a raw bleeding surface. It usually affects sick or weak infants, individuals in poor health, immunocompromised patients, and less often those who have had treatment with antibiotics. Called also *mycotic stomatitis, acute pseudomembranous candidiasis,* and *oral candidiasis.* 2. an infection of the foot of a horse, with degeneration of the horn and production of a fetid discharge.

**thrust** (thrust) a sudden forceful movement forward.
**paraspinal t.**, the same as spinal thrust, except that the therapist's hands are placed on either side of the spinous processes, the fingers pointing toward the head.
**spinal t.**, with the patient in the prone position on the examining table, the physician stands on the patient's right, facing him, places his right palm over the patient's lumbosacral joint perpendicular to the spinal axis, and using the left hand as reinforcement makes a series of short rapid thrusts downward and toward the head, progressing along each interspace to the midthoracic spine; done for relief of lumbosacral strain.
**tongue t.**, the infantile pattern of the suckle-swallow in which the tongue is placed between the incisor teeth or alveolar ridges during the initial stages of deglutition, resulting sometimes in anterior open bite, deformation of the jaws, and abnormal function.

**thryp·sis** (thrip′sis) [Gr. "a breaking in small pieces"] a comminuted fracture.

**Thu·di·chum's test** (too′de-koomz) [John Lewis William *Thudichum,* German-born physician in England, 1829–1901] see under *test.*

**Thu·ja** (thu′jə) [L.; Gr. *thyia*] a genus of coniferous trees of the family Cupressaceae. *T. occidenta′lis* is the white cedar (also called *arbor vitae*), a species native to eastern North America; its leafy twigs contain the medicinal substance thuja but can be poisonous to humans. Oil from its leaves is used as an expectorant, antirheumatic, and emmenagogue, and externally as a counterirritant and for dermatological diseases. *T. plica′ta* is the western red cedar, which can cause western red cedar asthma in workers with wood products.

**thu·ja** (thu′jə) the fresh tops of *Thuja occidentalis,* a diuretic, antipyretic, sudorific, and emmenagogue used in homeopathic medicine.

**thu·jone** (thu′jōn) an aromatic terpene ketone present in many essential oils and in plants such as species of *Thuja;* it can cause symptoms of neurotoxicity if ingested.

**thu·li·um** (thoo′le-əm) [*Thule,* ancient name of Shetland] [MeSH: Thulium] a very rare metallic element; symbol, Tm; atomic number, 69; atomic weight, 168.934.

**thumb** (thum) [MeSH: Thumb] pollex.
**bifid t.**, a deformed thumb in which the distal phalanx is divided or bifurcated.
**tennis t.**, tendinitis with calcification in the flexor pollicis longus, resulting from repeated friction experienced in playing tennis.

**thumb·print·ing** (thum′print-ing) a radiographic sign appearing as smooth indentations on the barium-filled colon, as though made by depression with the thumb; seen in various disorders of the colon, especially ischemic colitis.

**thump** (thump) 1. to strike or beat with a blunt instrument. 2. the blow so incurred.
**precordial t.,** thumpversion.

**thumps** (thumps) 1. a disease of swine caused by *Ascaris* larvae in the lungs. 2. a kind of singultus, or hiccup, of horses, due to spasm of the diaphragm.

**thump·ver·sion** (thump-vər′zhən) delivery of one or two blows to the chest in initiating cardiopulmonary resuscitation, in order to initiate a pulse or to convert ventricular fibrillation to a normal rhythm.

**thyme** (tīm) [L. *thymus;* from Gr. *thymon*] a plant of the genus *Thymus.*
**creeping t.,** *Thymus serpyllum.*
**garden t.,** *Thymus vulgaris.*
**wild t.,** *Thymus serpyllum.*

**thy·mec·to·mize** (thi-mek′tə-mīz) to remove the thymus gland.

**thy·mec·to·my** (thi-mek′tə-me) [*thym-*[1] + *ectomy*] [MeSH: Thymectomy] surgical removal of the thymus gland.

**thy·mel·co·sis** (thi″məl-ko′sis) [*thym-*[1] + *elcosis*] ulceration of the thymus.

**-thymia** [Gr. *thymos* mind + *-ia*] a word termination denoting a condition of mind.

**thy·mic** (thi′mik) [L. *thymicus*] 1. pertaining to the thymus. 2. contained in or derived from thyme.

**thy·mi·co·lym·phat·ic** (thi″mĭ-ko-lim-fat′ik) pertaining to the thymus and the lymphatic glands.

**thy·mi·dine** (thi′mĭ-dēn) [MeSH: Thymidine] a pyrimidine nucleoside, thymine linked by its N1 nitrogen to the C1 carbon of ribose; symbol T. The term is commonly used as a synonym for deoxythymidine (dT), for it was thought that thymidine-containing ribonucleosides do not exist, which would make the prefix deoxy- unnecessary. However, it is now known that thymine, produced by post-transcriptional methylation of uracil, occurs as a rare base in rRNAs and tRNAs; therefore the term should be restricted to the ribonucleoside and ribonucleotide forms.
**t. monophosphate,** a nucleotide, the 5′-phosphate of thymidine, occurring as a rare base in rRNAs and tRNAs.

**thy·mi·dine ki·nase** (thi′mĭ-dēn ki′nās) [EC 2.7.1.21] [MeSH: Thymidine Kinase] an enzyme of the transferase class that catalyzes the ATP-dependent phosphorylation of thymine deoxyribonucleoside, a reaction of pyrimidine salvage. Because the reaction produces an easily selectable phenotype, the gene and promoter are used extensively in genetic research. Abbreviated TK.

**thy·mi·dyl·ate** (thi″mĭ-dil′āt) 1. deoxythymidylate; see *thymidine.* 2. a dissociated form of thymidylic acid.

**thy·mi·dyl·ate syn·thase** (thi″mĭ-dil′āt sin′thās) [EC 2.1.1.45] an enzyme of the transferase class that catalyzes the transfer of a methyl group from 5,10-methylenetetrahydrofolate to deoxyuridine monophosphate, forming deoxythymidine monophosphate and dihydrofolate in the synthesis of deoxythymidine triphosphate. Improperly called *thymidylate synthetase* in older literature.

**thy·mi·dyl·ic ac·id** (thi″mĭ-dil′ik) 1. deoxythymidylic acid. 2. thymidine monophosphate.

**thy·mi·dyl·yl** (thi″mĭ-dil′əl) 1. deoxythymidylyl. 2. the radical formed by removal of OH from the phosphate group of thymidine monophosphate.

**thy·min** (thi′min) former name for *thymopoietin.*

**thy·mine** (thi′mēn) [MeSH: Thymine] a pyrimidine base, in animal cells usually occurring condensed with deoxyribose to form the nucleoside deoxythymidine, a component of deoxyribonucleic acid. The corresponding ribonucleoside, thymidine, is a rare constituent of ribonucleic acids. See also illustration at *pyrimidine base,* under *base.* Called also *5-methyluracil.*

**thy·mine-ura·cil·uria** (thi″mēn-ūr″ə-sil-u′re-ə) excess of the pyrimidines thymine and uracil in the urine, as occurs in dihydropyrimidine dehydrogenase deficiency.

**thy·min·ic ac·id** (thi-min′ik) an acid formed by the splitting up of deoxyribonucleic acid.

**thym·i·on** (thim′e-on) [Gr.] verruca.

**thy·mi·tis** (thi-mi′tis) inflammation of the thymus.

**thym(o)-**[1] [Gr. *thymos* thymus] a combining form denoting relationship to the thymus gland.

**thym(o)-**[2] [Gr. *thymos* mind, spirit] a combining form denoting relationship to the emotions.

**thy·mo·cyte** (thi′mo-sīt) [*thymo-*[1] + *-cyte*] a lymphocyte found in the thymus; about 10 per cent are mature T cells, and the rest are immature precursors in various stages of maturation. See table accompanying *T lymphocyte,* under *lymphocyte.*

**thy·mo·hy·dro·quin·one** (thi″mo-hi″dro-kwin-ōn′) a compound occurring in the urine after the administration of thymol, and also found in various essential oils.

**thy·mo·ke·sis** (thi″mo-ke′sis) enlargement of the remnant of the thymus that is found in the adult.

**thy·mo·ki·net·ic** (thi″mo-ki-net′ik) tending to stimulate the thymus.

**thy·mol** (thi′mol) [NF] [MeSH: Thymol] a phenol obtained from thyme oil or other volatile oils; used as a stabilizer in pharmaceutical preparations. It has been used for its antiseptic, antibacterial, and antifungal actions, and was formerly used as a vermifuge.
**t. phthalein,** see *thymolphthalein.*

**thy·mo·lep·tic** (thi″mo-lep′tik) [*thymo-*[2] + Gr. *lēpsis* a taking hold] any drug that favorably modifies mood in serious affective disorders such as depression or mania; the main categories of thymoleptics include the tricyclic antidepressants, monoamine oxidase inhibitors, and lithium compounds. Also called *antidepressant.*

**thy·mol·phthal·ein** (thi″mo-thal′ēn) [MeSH: Thymolphthalein] an indicator with a pH range of 9.3 to 10.5, being colorless at 9.3 and blue at 10.5.

**thy·mol·y·sis** (thi-mol′ĭ-sis) [*thymo-*[1] + *lysis*] involution or dissolution of the thymus.

**thy·mo·lyt·ic** (thi″mo-lit′ik) pertaining to, characterized by, or promoting thymolysis.

**thy·mo·ma** (thi-mo′mə) [*thymo-*[1] + *-oma*] [MeSH: Thymoma] a tumor derived from the epithelial or lymphoid elements of the thymus.

**thy·mo·path·ic** (thi″mo-path′ik) pertaining to, characterized by, or causing thymopathy.

**thy·mop·a·thy** (thi-mop′ə-the) any disease of the thymus.

**thy·mo·pen·tin** (thi″mo-pen′tin) [MeSH: Thymopentin] a pentapeptide immunostimulant, corresponding to amino acids 32–36 of thymopoietin; it is effective against certain primary immunodeficiencies, such as DiGeorge syndrome and primary T cell defects.

**thy·mo·poi·e·tin** (thi″mo-poi′ĕ-tin) a 5500-dalton polypeptide hormone secreted by thymic epithelial cells that promotes differentiation of precursor lymphocytes into thymocytes. Formerly called *thymin.*

**thy·mo·priv·ic** (thi″mo-priv′ik) thymoprivous.

**thy·mop·ri·vous** (thi-mop′rĭ-vəs) [*thymo-*[1] + L. *privus* without] pertaining to or caused by removal or atrophy of the thymus.

**thy·mo·sin** (thi′mo-sin) [MeSH: Thymosin] any of several thymic humoral factors, the most active being thymosin $\alpha_1$, a 3100-dalton polypeptide; it is secreted by thymic epithelial cells, maintains immune system functions, and can restore T cell function in thymectomized animals.

**thy·mo·tox·ic** (thi″mo-tok′sik) toxic for thymus tissue.

**thy·mo·tox·in** (thi″mo-tok′sin) an element that exerts a deleterious effect on the thymus.

**thy·mo·troph·ic** (thi″mo-trōf′ik) having an influence on the thymus.

**Thy·mus** (thi′məs) thyme; a genus of herbs of the family Labiatae, native to south central Europe and grown extensively elsewhere. *T. serpyl′lum* is creeping thyme or wild thyme, which contains an oil similar to thyme oil. *T. vulga′ris* L. is garden thyme, a source of thyme oil and thymol.

**thy·mus** (thi′məs) [L., from Gr. *thymos*] [TA] a bilaterally symmetric lymphoid organ consisting of two pyramidal lobes situated in the anterior superior mediastinum. It develops as an outgrowth of the epithelium of the third branchial pouch, which is invaded by lymphoid stem cells that migrate via the blood from the yolk sac and later from the bone marrow. Each lobe is surrounded by a fibrous capsule from which septa penetrate to divide the parenchyma into lobules; each lobule consists of an outer zone, the cortex, relatively rich in lymphocytes (thymocytes), and an inner zone, the medulla, relatively rich in epithelial cells. The thymus is the site of production of T lymphocytes. Precursor cells migrate into the outer cortex, where they actively proliferate. As they mature and acquire T cell surface markers they move through the inner cortex, where approximately 90 per cent die (possibly as part of the acquisition of self-tolerance). The remainder move on to the medulla, become mature T cells, and enter the circulation. T cell maturation is regulated by hormones, including thymopoietin and thymosin, produced by thymic epithelial cells. Congenital athymia or neonatal thymectomy results in complete lack of functional T cells. The thymus reaches its maximal development at about puberty and then

undergoes a gradual process of involution (replacement of parenchyma by fat and fibrous tissue), resulting in a slow decline of immune function throughout adulthood.
**accessory t.,** a separated portion of the thymus gland which may be found occasionally.
**persistent t., t. persis'tens hyperplas'tica,** a thymus which persists into adult life, sometimes even becoming hypertrophied.

**thy·mus-de·pen·dent** (thi″məs-de-pen′dənt) pertaining to T lymphocytes (see under *lymphocyte*). See also under *area.*

**thy·mus·ec·to·my** (thi″məs-ek′tə-me) thymectomy.

**thy·mus-in·de·pen·dent** (thi″məs-in-de-pen′dənt) pertaining to B lymphocytes (see under *lymphocyte*). See also under *area.*

**Thy·rar** (thi′rər) trademark for a preparation of thyroid (def. 3).

**thy·ra·tron** (thi′rə-tron) a form of discharge tube containing mercury vapor and a multiplicity of electrodes, used as an electric valve to rectify alternating current.

**thyre(o)-** for words beginning thus, see those beginning *thyr(o)-*.

**thyr(o)-** [*thyroid,* q.v.] a combining form denoting relationship to the thyroid gland.

**thy·ro·ac·tive** (thi″ro-ak′tiv) 1. thyromimetic. 2. thyrotropic.

**thy·ro·ad·e·ni·tis** (thi″ro-ad″ə-ni′tis) thyroiditis.

**thy·ro·apla·sia** (thi″ro-ə-pla′zhə) [*thyro-* + *aplasia*] defective development of the thyroid gland with hypothyroidism.

**thy·ro·ar·y·te·noid** (thi″ro-ar″ĭ-te′noid) pertaining to the thyroid and arytenoid cartilages.

**thy·ro·cal·ci·to·nin** (thi″ro-kal″sĭ-to′nin) calcitonin.

**thy·ro·car·di·ac** (thi″ro-kahr′de-ak) pertaining to actions of the thyroid hormones on the heart.

**thy·ro·cele** (thi′ro-sēl) [*thyro-* + *-cele*[1]] goiter.

**thy·ro·chon·drot·o·my** (thi″ro-kon-drot′ə-me) [*thyro-* + *chondrotomy*] median laryngotomy.

**thy·ro·col·loid** (thi″ro-kol′oid) thyroid colloid.

**thy·ro·cri·cot·o·my** (thi″ro-kri-kot′ə-me) incision of the cricothyroid membrane.

**thy·ro·epi·glot·tic** (thi″ro-ep″ĭ-glot′ik) pertaining to the thyroid and to the epiglottis.

**thy·ro·fis·sure** (thi″ro-fish′ər) median laryngotomy.

**thy·ro·gen·ic** (thi″ro-jen′ik) thyrogenous.

**thy·rog·e·nous** (thi-roj′ə-nəs) [*thyro-* + *-genous*] originating in the thyroid gland.

**thy·ro·glob·u·lin** (thi-ro-glob′u-lin) [MeSH: Thyroglobulin] 1. an iodine-containing glycoprotein of high molecular weight found in the colloid of thyroid gland follicles; it is made by the follicular cells and secreted into the follicular lumen where it is iodinated, after which its iodinated tyrosyl moieties form the iodothyronines thyroxine and triiodothyronine. Thyroglobulins are then taken up by endocytosis into the follicular cells, where the iodothyronines are liberated by proteolysis, followed by release into the extracellular fluid and thence to the blood stream. 2. a substance obtained by fractionation of thyroid glands from the hog, containing not less than 0.7 per cent of total iodine, formerly used as a powdered oral thyroid supplement in the treatment of hypothyroidism.

**thy·ro·glos·sal** (thi″ro-glos′əl) pertaining to the thyroid gland and the tongue.

**thy·ro·hy·al** (thi″ro-hi′əl) 1. pertaining to the thyroid cartilage and the hyoid bone. 2. cornu majus ossis hyoidei.

**thy·ro·hy·oid** (thi″ro-hi′oid) pertaining to the thyroid gland or cartilage and the hyoid bone.

**thy·roid** (thi′roid) [Gr. *thyreoeidēs,* from *thyreos* oblong shield + *eidos* form] 1. glandula thyroidea. 2. [USP] the cleaned, dried, and powdered thyroid gland, previously deprived of connective tissue and fat, obtained from domesticated food animals; formerly used as a source of thyroid hormones in the treatment of hypothyroidism. 3. pertaining to the thyroid gland *(glandula thyroidea).* 4. scutiform.
**aberrant t's, accessory t's, ectopic t's,** glandulae thyroideae accessoriae.
**intrathoracic t.,** an accessory thyroid gland or thyroid tissue located within the thoracic cavity.
**lingual t.,** an accessory thyroid gland or thyroid tissue located at the base of the tongue, between the foramen cecum and the hyoid bone. It may project into the pharynx, be entirely within the tongue, or be just beneath it; sometimes the normally located thyroid is lacking and this is the only thyroid tissue present.
**retrosternal t., substernal t.,** an accessory thyroid gland or thyroid tissue situated in the thorax behind the sternum.
**suprahyoid t.,** an accessory thyroid gland or thyroid tissue found above the hyoid bone.

**thy·roid·ec·to·mize** (thi″roid-ek′tə-mīz) to remove the thyroid gland or otherwise suppress its function.

**thy·roid·ec·to·my** (thi″roid-ek′tə-me) [*thyroid* + *-ectomy*] [MeSH: Thyroidectomy] 1. surgical removal of the thyroid gland. 2. ablation of thyroid function.
**medical t.,** pharmacologic suppression of thyroid function.

**thy·roid·itis** (thi″roid-i′tis) [MeSH: Thyroiditis] inflammation of the thyroid gland; called also *thyroadenitis.*
**acute pyogenic t., acute suppurative t.,** a rare painful inflammation of the thyroid gland caused by an infectious process such as with *Staphylococcus* or *Streptococcus,* with suppuration and abscess formation, often progressing to the subacute stage. In immunocompromised patients it can be caused by opportunistic pathogens.
**atrophic t.,** a type of autoimmune thyroiditis with atrophy of the follicles and without goiter; called also *atrophic* or *nongoitrous autoimmune t.* and *primary myxedema.*
**autoimmune t.,** 1. any of various types of thyroiditis characterized by the presence of Askanazy cells and autoantibodies that destroy the gland and cause hypothyroidism; they may occur in any age or sex but particularly affect middle-aged to elderly women. A distinction is made between types with goiter *(Hashimoto's disease)* and those without goiter *(atrophic* or *atrophic autoimmune thyroiditis). Riedel's thyroiditis* is a less common type, and *Graves' disease* is a closely related condition. 2. Hashimoto's disease. 3. any of various experimental animal models of thyroiditis.
**autoimmune t., atrophic,** atrophic t.
**autoimmune t., nongoitrous,** atrophic t.
**chronic t., chronic fibrous t.,** Riedel's t.
**chronic lymphadenoid t., chronic lymphocytic t.,** Hashimoto's disease.
**chronic sclerosing t.,** Riedel's t.
**de Quervain's t.,** subacute granulomatous t.
**giant cell t., giant follicular t.,** subacute granulomatous t.
**goitrous t.,** Hashimoto's disease.
**granulomatous t.,** subacute granulomatous t.
**Hashimoto's t.,** see under *disease.*
**invasive t., invasive fibrous t., ligneous t.,** Riedel's t.
**lymphocytic t., lymphoid t.,** Hashimoto's disease.
**painless t.,** painless, self-limited hyperthyroidism with lymphocytic infiltration of the thyroid gland but without the nonthyroidal features of Graves' disease. Called also *silent t.* and *subacute lymphocytic t.*
**postpartum t.,** a type of autoimmune thyroiditis occurring in women after childbirth.
**pseudotuberculous t.,** subacute granulomatous t.
**radiation t.,** thyroiditis during or soon after radioiodine therapy, with painful epithelial swelling and narcosis, edema, and disruption of follicular architecture.
**Riedel's t., sclerosing t.,** a rare chronic type of autoimmune thyroiditis characterized by a proliferating, fibrosing, inflammatory process that involves usually one but sometimes both lobes, with adhesions to the trachea and other adjacent structures. Called also *chronic fibrous t.,invasive* or *invasive fibrous t., ligneous t.* or *struma,* and *Riedel's disease* or *struma.*
**silent t.,** painless t.
**subacute granulomatous t.,** a condition characterized by fever and painful enlargement of the thyroid gland, often following a viral infection, especially of the respiratory tract, with granulomas in the gland consisting of masses of colloid surrounded by giant cells and mononuclear cells, and a moderate amount of fibrosis. Called also *de Quervain's, giant cell, granulomatous,* or *pseudotuberculous t.*
**subacute lymphocytic t.,** painless t.
**woody t.,** Riedel's t.

**thy·roid·iza·tion** (thi″roid-ĭ-za′shən) 1. thyroid replacement therapy. 2. in histopathology, the thyroidlike appearance of a tissue.

**thy·roido·ther·a·py** (thi″roid-o-ther′ə-pe) thyroid replacement therapy.

**thy·roid·ot·o·my** (thi″roid-ot′ə-me) 1. median laryngotomy. 2. thyrotomy.

**thy·roido·tox·in** (thi″roid-o-tok′sin) a toxin specific for thyroid tissue.

**thy·roid per·ox·i·dase** (thi′roid pər-ok′sĭ-dās) iodide peroxidase.

**thy·ro·in·tox·i·ca·tion** (thi″ro-in-tok″sĭ-ka′shən) thyrotoxicosis.

**Thy·ro·lar** (thi′ro-lahr) trademark for a preparation of liotrix.

**thy·ro·lib·er·in** (thi″ro-lib′ər-in) [*thyro*tropin + *-liberin*] thyrotropin-releasing hormone.

**thy·ro·lyt·ic** (thi″ro-lit′ik) [*thyro-* + *-lytic*] destructive to thyroid tissue.

**thy·ro·meg·a·ly** (thi″ro-meg′ə-le) [*thyro-* + *-megaly*] goiter.

**thy·ro·mi·met·ic** (thi″ro-mi-met′ik) producing effects similar to those of thyroid hormones or the thyroid gland.

**thy·ro·nine** (thi′ro-nēn) the *p*-hydroxyphenol ether of tyrosine found in nature as its iodinated derivatives, the iodothyronines.

**thy·ro·para·thy·roid·ec·to·my** (thi″ro-par″ə-thi″roi-dek′tə-me) excision of the thyroid and parathyroids.

**thy·ro·para·thy·ro·priv·ic** (thi″ro-par″ə-thi″ro-priv′ik) lacking thyroid and parathyroid glands or secretions.

**thy·rop·a·thy** (thi-rop′ə-the) [*thyro-* + *-pathy*] any disease of the thyroid gland.

**thy·ro·per·ox·i·dase** (thi″ro-pər-ok′sĭ-dās) iodide peroxidase.

**thy·ro·pri·val** (thi″ro-pri′vəl) [*thyroid* + L. *privus* without] hypothyroid.

**thy·ro·priv·ia** (thi″ro-priv′e-ə) [*thyroid* + L. *privus* without] hypothyroidism.

**thy·ro·priv·ic** (thi″ro-priv′ik) hypothyroid.

**thy·ro·priv·ous** (thi″ro-priv′us) hypothyroid.

**thy·rop·to·sis** (thi″rop-to′sis) [*thyro-* + *ptosis*] downward displacement of the thyroid gland into the thorax.

**thy·ro·ther·a·py** (thi″ro-ther′ə-pe) thyroid replacement therapy.

**thy·ro·tome** (thi′ro-tōm) an instrument for cutting the thyroid cartilage.

**thy·rot·o·my** (thi-rot′ə-me) [*thyro-* + *-tomy*] 1. median laryngotomy. 2. the operation of cutting the thyroid gland. 3. biopsy of the thyroid gland. Called also *thyroidotomy.*

**thy·ro·tox·ic** (thi″ro-tok′sik) 1. pertaining to the effects of thyroid hormone excess. 2. describing a patient suffering from thyrotoxicosis.

**thy·ro·tox·i·co·sis** (thi″ro-tok″sĭ-ko′sis) [MeSH: Thyrotoxicosis] the condition caused by excessive quantities of thyroid hormones (see *hyperthyroidism*); it may be due to overproduction by the thyroid gland as in Graves' disease, overproduction originating outside the thyroid, or loss of storage function and leakage from the gland.

**thy·ro·trope** (thi′ro-trōp) thyrotroph.

**thy·ro·troph** (thi′ro-trōf) a basophil of the adenohypophysis that secretes thyrotropin; called also *beta basophil* and *thyrotrope* or *thyrotropic cell.*

**thy·ro·troph·ic** (thi″ro-trōf′ik) thyrotropic.

**thy·rot·ro·phin** (thi-rot′rə-fin) thyrotropin.

**thy·ro·trop·ic** (thi″ro-trop′ik) having an influence on the thyroid gland.

**thy·rot·ro·pin** (thi-rot′rə-pin) [MeSH: Thyrotropin] a glycoprotein hormone (28,000 daltons) of the adenohypophysis that promotes the growth of, sustains, and stimulates the hormonal secretion of the thyroid gland. Called also *thyroid-stimulating hormone.*

**thy·rox·in** (thi-rok′sin) thyroxine.

**thy·rox·ine ($T_4$)** (thi-rok′sin) [MeSH: Thyroxine] L-3,5,3′,5′-tetraiodothyronine, the major hormone elaborated by the thyroid gland follicular cells, formed from thyroglobulin and transported mainly in the blood serum thyroxine-binding globulin. Its chief function is to increase the rate of cell metabolism. It is also essential for central nervous system maturation and regulates a number of other functions. Thyroxine is deiodinated in peripheral tissues (liver, kidney, and heart) to form triiodothyronine, the active "tissue" form of thyroid hormone, which is much more biologically active. Natural and synthetic preparations are used in the treatment of hypothyroidism. Spelled also *thyroxin.*
**free t.,** the fraction of thyroxine in the serum that is not bound to a binding protein.
**levo t.,** see *levothyroxine sodium.*
**total t., total serum t.,** the total thyroxine in the serum, including both the fraction of free thyroxine and the fraction bound to a binding protein such as thyroxine-binding globulin or transthyretin.

**thy·rox·in·ic** (thi″rok-sin′ik) pertaining to thyroxine.

**Thys·a·no·so·ma** (this″ə-no-so′mə) a genus of cestodes of the family Anoplocephalidae. *T. actinoi′des,* the fringed tapeworm, is found in the bile ducts and small intestines of sheep, cattle, deer, and antelope in the western United States and in Africa.

**Thy·tro·par** (thi′tro-pahr) trademark for a preparation of thyrotropin.

**Ti** symbol for *titanium.*

**TIA** transient ischemic attack.

**ti·ag·a·bine hy·dro·chlo·ride** (ti-ag′ə-bēn) an anticonvulsant agent used as an adjunct to other anticonvulsants in the treatment of partial seizures.

**Ti·a·zac** (ti′ə-zak) trademark for a preparation of diltiazem hydrochloride.

**ti·az·ur·il** (ti-az′ur-il) a coccidiostat for poultry.

**TIBC** total iron-binding capacity.

**tib·ia** (tib′e-ə) [L. "a pipe, flute"] [TA] [MeSH: Tibia] the shin bone: the inner and larger bone of the leg below the knee; it articulates with the femur and head of the fibula above and with the talus below. See plate accompanying *skeleton.*
**saber t., saber-shaped t.,** a tibia curved outward as a result of gummatous periostitis.
**t. val′ga,** a bowing of the leg in which the angulation is away from the midline of the body.
**t. va′ra,** medial angulation of the tibia in the metaphyseal region, due to a growth disturbance of the medial aspect of the proximal tibial epiphysis; there are both infantile and adolescent types. Called also *Blount disease* and *osteochondrosis deformans tibiae.*

**tib·i·ad** (tib′e-ad) toward the tibial aspect.

**tib·i·al** (tib′e-əl) [L. *tibialis*] pertaining to the tibia.

**tib·i·a·le** (tib″e-a′le) a bone on the tibial side of the tarsus of the embryo, partly represented in the adult by the astragalus.
**t. exter′num, t. posti′cum,** a sesamoid bone found in the tendon of the tibialis posterior muscle.

**tib·i·al·gia** (tib″e-al′jə) pain in the tibia (shin).

**tib·i·a·lis** (tib″e-a′lis) [TA] tibial.

**tib·io·cal·ca·ne·an** (tib″e-o-kal-ka′ne-ən) pertaining to the tibia and the calcaneus.

**tib·io·fem·or·al** (tib″e-o-fem′ə-rəl) pertaining to the tibia and the femur.

**tib·io·fib·u·lar** (tib″e-o-fib′u-lər) pertaining to the tibia and the fibula.

**tib·io·na·vic·u·lar** (tib″e-o-nə-vik′u-lər) pertaining to the tibia and the navicular bone.

**tib·io·per·o·ne·al** (tib″e-o-per″o-ne′əl) tibiofibular.

**tib·io·scaph·oid** (tib″e-o-skaf′oid) tibionavicular.

**tib·io·tar·sal** (tib″e-o-tahr′səl) pertaining to the tibia and the tarsus.

**ti·bo·lone** (tĭ′bo-lōn) an anabolic steroid with weak estrogenic, androgenic, and progestogenic properties, used in the treatment of menopausal and postmenopausal symptoms; administered orally.

**ti·bric ac·id** (ti′brik) an antihyperlipidemic with the same uses as clofibrate.

**tic** (tik, Fr. tēk) [Fr.] [MeSH: Tic] an involuntary, compulsive, rapid, repetitive, stereotyped movement or vocalization, experienced as irresistible although it can be suppressed for some length of time; occurrence is exacerbated by stress and diminished during sleep or engrossing activities. Tics may be psychogenic or neurogenic in origin and are subclassified as either simple, such as eye blinking, shoulder shrugging, coughing, grunting, snorting, or barking, or complex, such as facial gestures, grooming motions, coprolalia, echolalia, or echokinesis.
**convulsive t.,** facial spasm.
**diaphragmatic t.,** spasmodic twitching movements of the diaphragm.
**t. douloureux** (doo-loo-roo′), trigeminal neuralgia.

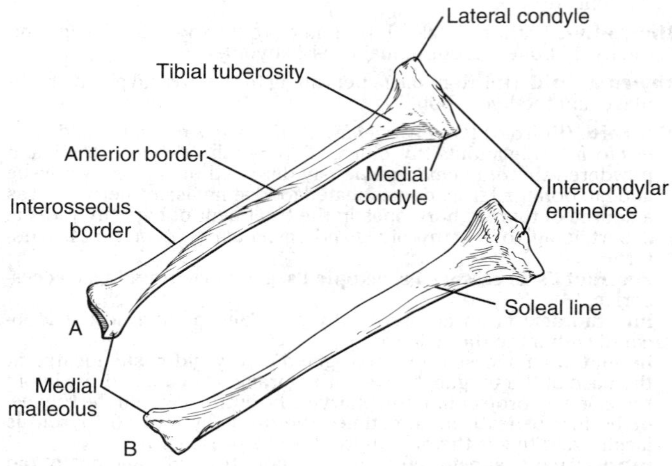

Tibia. Anterior *(A)* and posterior *(B)* views of the right tibia.

**facial t.**, see under *spasm.*
**t. de Guinon,** Gilles de la Tourette's syndrome.
**habit t.**, any tic that is psychogenic in origin.
**local t.**, a tic affecting only a limited locality, as the eye.
**mimic t.**, facial spasm.
**rotatory t.**, see under *spasm.*
**saltatory t.**, see under *spasm.*
**t. de sommeil** (də so-ma'), an involuntary movement of the head during sleep.

**Ti·car** (ti'kər) trademark for a preparation of ticarcillin disodium.

**ti·car·cil·lin** (ti″kahr-sil'in) [MeSH: Ticarcillin] a semisynthetic penicillin bactericidal effective against both gram-negative and gram-positive organisms.
**t. cresyl sodium,** a salt of ticarcillin, $C_{22}H_{21}N_2NaO_6S_2$.
**t. disodium** [USP], the disodium salt of ticarcillin, used in a sterile solution primarily in the treatment of severe systemic infections, septicemia, and infections of the genitourinary tract, the respiratory tract, or the soft tissues due to susceptible strains of *Pseudomonas aeruginosa, Proteus* species, and *Escherichia coli;* administered intramuscularly and intravenously.
**t. monosodium** [USP], the monosodium salt of ticarcillin, having the same actions and uses as the disodium salt.
**t. sodium,** t. disodium.

**tick** (tik) [MeSH: Ticks] a blood-sucking acarid parasite of the suborder Ixodides, superfamily Ixodoidea. The ticks are larger than their relatives, the mites. There are two families: Argasidae (soft ticks) and Ixodidae (hard ticks).
**adobe t.**, *Argas persicus.*
**American dog t.**, *Dermacentor variabilis.*
**bandicoot t.**, *Haemaphysalis humerosa.*
**beady-legged winter horse t.**, *Margaropus winthemi.*
**black-legged t.**, *Ixodes scapularis.*
**black pitted t.**, *Rhipicephalus simus.*
**bont t.**, *Amblyomma hebraeum.*
**British dog t.**, *Ixodes canisuga.*
**brown dog t.**, *Rhipicephalus sanguineus.*
**castor bean t.**, *Ixodes ricinus.*
**cattle t.**, *Boophilus annulatus.*
**Cayenne t.**, *Amblyomma cajennense.*
**eastern deer t.**, see *Ixodes dammini.*
**dog t.**, 1. *Haemaphysalis leachi.* 2. *Dermacentor variabilis.* 3. *Rhipicephalus sanguineus.*
**ear t.**, *Otobius megnini.*
**Gulf Coast t.**, *Amblyomma maculatum.*
**hard t., hard-bodied t.**, ixodid, def. 2.
**Kenya t.**, *Rhipicephalus appendiculatus.*
**Lone Star t.**, *Amblyomma americanum.*
**miana t.**, *Argas persicus.*
**Pacific Coast dog t.**, *Dermacentor occidentalis.*
**pajaroello t.**, *Ornithodoros coriaceus.*
**pigeon t.**, *Argas reflexus.*
**rabbit t.**, *Haemaphysalis leporispalustris.*
**Rocky Mountain wood t.**, *Dermacentor andersoni.*
**russet t.**, *Ixodes pilosus.*
**scrub t.**, *Ixodes holocyclus.*
**seed t.**, the young six-legged larva of a tick: after molting it emerges as an eight-legged nymph.
**sheep t.**, *Melophagus ovinus.*
**soft t., soft-bodied t.**, argasid, def. 2.
**spinous ear t.**, *Otobius megnini.*
**taiga t.**, *Ixodes persulcatus.*
**tampan t.**, 1. *Ornithodoros moubata.* 2. *Argas persicus.*
**winter t.**, *Dermacentor albipictus.*
**wood t.**, *Dermacentor andersoni.*

**tick·ling** (tik'ling) 1. light stimulation of a body surface, such as stroking the skin, causing a tingling sensation. 2. the sensation of being so stimulated, which may cause reflex responses such as involuntary laughter and withdrawal of the body part; called also *gargalesthesia.* Defs. 1 and 2 called also *titillation.*

**tick·over** (tik'o-vər) a continuous, low-level activity needing an additional factor to produce any measurable effect, analogous to the idle of an engine; used in describing regulation of the alternative pathway of complement.

**ti·clo·pi·dine hy·dro·chlo·ride** (ti-klo'pĭ-dēn) a platelet inhibitor used in the treatment of thromboembolic disorders; administered orally.

**tic·po·lon·ga** (tik″po-long'ə) [Sinhalese] Russell's viper.

**t.i.d.** abbreviation for L. *ter in di'e,* three times a day.

**tide** (tīd) a physiological variation or increase of a certain constituent in body fluids.
**acid t.**, temporary increase in the acidity of the urine which sometimes follows fasting.
**alkaline t.**, temporary increase in the alkalinity of the urine during gastric digestion.
**fat t.**, the increase of fat in the lymph and blood following a meal.

**Tie·de·mann's nerve** (te'dĕ-mahnz) [Friedrich *Tiedemann,* German anatomist, 1781–1861] see under *nerve.*

**Tiet·ze's syndrome (disease)** (tēt'səz) [Alexander *Tietze,* German surgeon, 1864–1927] see under *syndrome.*

**Ti·gan** (ti'gən) trademark for preparations of trimethobenzamide hydrochloride.

**tig·lic ac·id** (tig'lik) an unsaturated fatty acid, *trans*-2-methyl-2-butenoic acid, occurring in triglycerides in croton oil.

**tig·li·um** (tig'le-əm) gen. *tig'lii* [L.] *Croton tiglium.*

**ti·groid** (ti'groid) [Gr. *tigroeidēs* tiger-spotted] striped like a tiger, as Nissl bodies or a tigroid fundus oculi.

**ti·grol·y·sis** (ti-grol'ĭ-sis) chromatolysis.

**ti·let·amine hy·dro·chlo·ride** (ti-let'əmēn) [USP] an anesthetic used in veterinary practice in combination with zolazepam hydrochloride.

**Til·ia** (til'e-ə) the lindens or basswoods, a genus of deciduous trees of the family Tiliaceae, native to Europe and eastern North America, which have heart-shaped leaves and fragrant flowers. *T. america'na* is the American linden, whose wood, bark, and flowers are used to make folk remedies for biliary and liver disorders. *T. europae'a* is the European linden.

**Til·laux's disease** (te-yōz') [Paul Jules *Tillaux,* French physician, 1834–1904] see under *disease.*

**Til·le·tia** (tĭ-le'she-ə) a genus of fungi of the family Tilletiaceae, causing smut on cereals. *T. tri'tici* (called also *T. ca'ries*) causes wheat smut.

**Til·le·ti·a·ceae** (tĭ-le″she-a'se-e) a family of fungi of the order Ustilaginales, including the genera *Tilletia* and *Urocystis.*

**til·mi·co·sin** [USP] a macrolide antibiotic used as a veterinary antibacterial.

**til·mus** (til'məs) [Gr. *tilmos* a plucking] floccillation.

**til·or·one** (til'or-ōn) [MeSH: Tilorone] a low-molecular-weight aromatic amine that stimulates the production of interferon in serum.

**til·tom·e·ter** (til-tom'ə-tər) an instrument for measuring the degree of tilting of the operating table in spinal anesthesia and other procedures.

**tim·bre** (tam'bər) [Fr.] a musical quality in a tone or sound.
**t. métallique,** a high-pitched tympanic second sound heard in dilatation of the aorta. When heard in persons under fifty-five years of age it has been considered suggestive of syphilitic aortitis. Called also *Potain's sign* and *bruit de tabourka.*

**time** (tīm) [Gr. *chronos;* L. *tempus*] [MeSH: Time] a measure of duration. Symbol *t.*
**Achilles tendon reflex t.**, assessment of the duration of the triceps surae reflex (Achilles tendon reflex); the phase from the initial tap to half relaxation is prolonged in hypothyroidism, diabetes mellitus, hypothermia, propranolol therapy, local edema, and a few other conditions.
**activated partial thromboplastin t. (APTT; aPTT),** the period required for clot formation in recalcified blood plasma after contact activation and the addition of platelet substitutes (e.g., brain cephalin or similar phospholipids); used to assess the intrinsic and common pathways of coagulation. A prolonged aPTT can indicate a deficiency of a number of factors, including prekallikrein, high-molecular-weight kininogen, factors XII, XI, IX, VIII, X, V, and II, and fibrinogen.
**apex t.**, the interval at which the apex of the summated twitches of a muscle succeeds the second stimulus applied to the same muscle.
**bleeding t.**, the duration of bleeding that follows puncture of the skin; see *bleeding time test,* under *test.*
**chromoscopy t.**, the time elapsing between the intramuscular injection of a dye and its appearance in the gastric secretion.
**circulation t.**, the time required for blood to flow between two designated points, as arm-to-tongue time.
**clot retraction t.**, the time required for 50 per cent of a blood clot to retract from the wall of the vessel containing it; it is prolonged in thrombasthenia and certain other conditions.
**clotting t., coagulation t.**, the time required for blood to clot in a glass tube.
**colonic transit t.**, colonic transit (def. 2).
**conduction t.**, latency (def. 2).
**dead t.**, the amount of time that a system remains unresponsive after the occurrence of some event.
**decimal reduction t.**, the time of heat sterilization required for a 10-fold reduction of viable microorganisms. Symbol D. Called also *D value.*
**dextrinizing t.**, the time required for saliva to convert starch into sugar.
**doubling t.**, generation t., def. 3.

**generation t.**, 1. the period of time between the receipt of an infection by a host and the maximal infectivity of that host. 2. the time elapsing from one generation to the next. 3. the time required for all components of a cell culture to multiply by two. Called also *doubling t.*
**inertia t.**, the time required to overcome the inertia of a muscle after the reception of a stimulus from a nerve.
**isovolumic relaxation t. (IVRT)**, the duration of the period of isovolumic relaxation (see under *period*), normally 50 to 70 msec.
**lead t.**, the interval in the natural history of a disease which can be gained by diagnosing it earlier; the interval between the early and usual times of diagnosis.
**left ventricular ejection t. (LVET)**, the interval from systole to closure of the aortic valve, measured on the carotid pulse tracing from the beginning upstroke to the dicrotic notch; it is one of the systolic time intervals (q.v.) measured to assess left ventricular performance.
**longitudinal relaxation t.**, T1 relaxation t.
**median survival t.**, the length of time at which 50 per cent of the patients have died and 50 per cent still survive.
**one-stage prothrombin t.**, prothrombin t.
**partial thromboplastin t. (PTT)**, a measure of the coagulation factors of the intrinsic pathway of coagulation in plasma; now largely superseded by the test of *activated partial thromboplastin t.*
**prothrombin t. (PT)**, the rate at which prothrombin is converted to thrombin in citrated blood with added calcium; used to assess the extrinsic pathway of coagulation. Results indicate the integrity of the prothrombin complex, i.e., of factors II, V, VII, and X, and the test is often used to monitor administration of coumarin-type anticoagulants. Called also *one-stage prothrombin t.* or *time test* and *Quick's test.*
**reaction t.**, the time elapsing between the application of a stimulus and the resulting reaction.
**recalcification t.**, an insensitive measure of hemostasis, calculating the interval required for clot formation when calcium ion is replaced in anticoagulated platelet-rich plasma.
**relaxation t.**, any of several measures of loss of energy by magnetized materials (particularly hydrogen ions) after a magnetizing current is cut off; in magnetic resonance imaging two particularly useful measures are *T1 relaxation t.* and *T2 relaxation t.* (q.v.).
**reptilase t.**, a test of coagulation time similar to the thrombin time, measuring coagulation time of blood to which reptilase has been added; since reptilase is not affected by the presence of heparin, the test can be used in patients receiving heparin therapy.
**rise t.**, 1. the length of time a waveform takes to rise from 10 per cent to 90 per cent of its peak amplitude. 2. in neurophysiology, the time between the start of a change in potential and when it reaches its positive peak.
**Russell's viper venom t.**, Stypven time test.
**sedimentation t.**, see under *rate.*
**spin-lattice relaxation t.**, T1 relaxation t.
**spin-spin relaxation t.**, T2 relaxation t.
**stimulus-response t.**, reaction t.
**Stypven t.**, see under *test.*
**thermal death t.**, the time required at a given temperature to destroy a population of microorganisms with heat.
**thermal relaxation t.**, T1 relaxation t.
**thrombin t. (TT), thrombin clotting t.**, the time required for plasma fibrinogen to form thrombin: exogenous thrombin is added to citrated plasma and the time to clot formation is measured; it is prolonged with abnormalities of fibrinogen and in the presence of heparin or of fibrin/fibrinogen degradation products.
**transverse relaxation t.**, T2 relaxation t.
**T1 relaxation t.**, a component of relaxation time representing the time required for longitudinal magnetization of a substance to return to equilibrium with its surroundings after administration of a pulse of radiofrequency energy; different substances have different times that are measured in magnetic resonance imaging. Called also *longitudinal relaxation t., spin-lattice relaxation t.,* and *thermal relaxation t.*
**T2 relaxation t.**, a component of relaxation time representing the time required for decay or loss of transverse magnetization after administration of a pulse of radiofrequency energy; different substances have different times that are measured in magnetic resonance imaging. Called also *spin-spin relaxation t.* and *transverse relaxation t.*
**utilization t.**, latency of activation.

**Ti•men•tin** (ti-men'tin) trademark for a combination of ticarcillin disodium and clavulanate potassium.

**tim•er** (tīm'ər) a clock mechanism which may be set to automatically signal the expiration of a given interval of time or to activate or cut off certain other apparatus at the desired time.

**Tim•o•feew's corpuscles** (te-mo-fa'efs) [Dmitri Aleksandrovich *Timofeew,* Russian anatomist, late 19th century] see under *corpuscle.*

**ti•mo•lol mal•e•ate** (ti'mo-lol) a beta-adrenergic blocking agent with antihypertensive and antiarrhythmic properties; it is used topically to lower intraocular pressure in glaucoma, by decreasing the formation of aqueous humor.

**tim•o•thy** (tim'ə-the) *Phleum pratense.*

**tin** (tin) [L. *stannum*] [MeSH: Tin] a white, metallic element, atomic number, 50; atomic weight, 118.69; valence 2 or 4; symbol, Sn. Some of its salts are reagents, others are stains, while some of its compounds, particularly the oxide, have been tried in medicine. Its organic compounds exhibit moderate but variable toxicity.
**t. chloride**, stannous chloride.
**t. oxide**, stannic oxide.

**Tin•ac•tin** (tin-ak'tin) trademark for preparations of tolnaftate.

**Tin•berg•en** (tin'bərg-ən) Nikolaas. Dutch-born British zoologist, born 1907; co-winner, with Karl von Frisch and Konrad Lorenz, of the Nobel prize for medicine or physiology in 1973, for his work on animal behavior.

**tinct.** abbreviation for *tincture,* or *tinctura.*

**tinc•ta•ble** (tink'tə-bəl) stainable or tingible.

**tinc•tion** (tink'shən) [L. *tingere* to dye] 1. the act of staining. 2. the addition of coloring or flavoring agents to a prescription.

**tinc•to•ri•al** (tink-tor'e-əl) pertaining to dyeing or staining.

**tinc•tu•ra** (tink-tu'rə) gen. and pl. *tinctu'rae* [L.] tincture.

**tinc•tur•a•tion** (tink″chər-a'shən) the preparation of a tincture; the treatment of a drug with a menstruum, such as alcohol or ether, for the purpose of preparing a tincture.

**tinc•ture** (tink'chər) [L. *tingere* to wet, to moisten] an alcoholic or hydroalcoholic solution prepared from animal or vegetable drugs or from chemical substances.
**belladonna t.** [USP], an alcoholic preparation of belladonna leaf, used as an anticholinergic for the same purposes as atropine and hyoscyamine.
**benzoin t., compound** [USP], a preparation of benzoin, aloe, storax, and tolu balsam in alcohol, used as a topical protectant.
**cardamom t., compound**, a preparation of powdered cardamom seed, cinnamon, caraway, and cochineal in glycerin and diluted alcohol; used as a flavoring agent.
**ferric citrochloride t.**, a hydroalcoholic solution of ferric chloride and sodium citrate, used as a hematinic.
**green soap t.** [USP], a preparation of green soap, lavender oil, and alcohol used as a skin detergent; called also *medicinal soft soap liniment* and *linimentum saponis mollis.*
**iodine t.** [USP], a preparation of iodine and sodium iodide in diluted alcohol, used as an anti-infective on the skin.
**iodine t., strong**, an alcoholic solution of iodine and potassium iodide, each 100 mL of which contains 6.8–7.5 g of iodine and 4.7–5.5 g of potassium iodide; used as an irritant, antibacterial, and antifungal agent.
**opium t.** [USP], a preparation, obtained by percolation of granulated opium and concentration of the product, used as an antiperistaltic. Called also *deodorized opium t.*
**opium t., camphorated**, paregoric.
**opium t., deodorized**, opium t.
**rhubarb t., aromatic**, a preparation of powdered rhubarb, cinnamon, clove, and myristica in glycerin, alcohol, and water; used as a cathartic.
**sweet orange peel t.**, a preparation produced by the maceration in alcohol of the outer rind of the nonartificially colored fresh ripe fruit of *Citrus sinensis;* used as a flavoring agent.
**thimerosal t.** [USP], a preparation of thimerosal, alcohol, acetone, ethylenediamine solution, and monoethanolamine in water; used as a local anti-infective, applied topically to the skin.
**vanilla t.**, a preparation of vanilla and sucrose in equal parts of diluted alcohol and water; used as a flavor and as an ingredient of acacia syrup.

**Tin•dal** (tin'dəl) trademark for a preparation of acetophenazine maleate.

**tin•ea** (tin'e-ə) [L. "grub," "moth larva," "worm"] [MeSH: Tinea] any of various dermatophytoses of humans, usually designated by a modifying term depending on appearance of lesions, etiologic agent, or site. Popularly called *ringworm.*
**t. amianta'cea, asbestos-like t.**, misnomer for an inflammatory condition of the scalp, not caused by a fungus, characterized by a dense concentration of white to gray scales that extend upward to form an asbestos-like encasement on the hair shafts.
**t. axilla'ris**, misnomer for trichomycosis axillaris, which is not a form of tinea.
**t. bar'bae**, tinea of the bearded area of the face and neck; there are three types: in the *inflammatory type,* usually caused by *Trichophyton mentagrophytes* or *T. verrucosum,* the typical lesions are kerion-like or nodular and may produce crusting; in the *ringworm type,* the

annular lesions resemble those of ringworm of nonhairy skin; and in the *sycosiform type (t. sycosis),* caused by *T. violaceum* or less often *T. rubrum,* the lesions are follicular pustules, each containing a hair that may break off and leave a stub or become epilated. Called also *barber's itch* and *ringworm of the beard.*

**t. ca'pitis,** a type affecting the scalp, caused by species of *Microsporum* and *Trichophyton,* which may occasionally also involve the eyebrows and eyelashes, sometimes occurring in epidemics. Depending upon the etiologic agent, it may vary from a benign scaly noninflammatory subclinical infection to an inflammatory disease marked by scaly, erythematous papular eruptions with loose and broken-off hairs causing areas of alopecia that may become severely inflamed with the formation of deep, ulcerative kerions that often result in keloid formation, scarring, and permanent alopecia. See also *black-dot ringworm* and *gray-patch ringworm,* under *ringworm.* Called also *t. tonsurans* and *ringworm of the scalp.*

**t. cilio'rum,** t. capitis involving the eyelashes.

**t. circina'ta,** t. corporis.

**t. circina'ta tro'pical,** t. imbricata.

**t. cor'poris,** tinea involving glabrous skin areas other than hands and feet, usually caused by *Microsporum canis, Trichophyton rubrum,* or *T. mentagrophytes.* It is typically characterized by one or more well-demarcated erythematous, scaly macules with raised borders and central healing, producing annular outlines. Other types of lesions include vesicular, eczematous, psoriasiform, verrucous, plaquelike, and deep types. Called also *ringworm of the body, t. circinata,* and *t. glabrosa.*

**t. cru'ris,** tinea in the groin or perineal area, sometimes spreading to nearby regions; it is generally seen in males who also have t. pedis, so that the etiologic agent is usually the same for both infections. Characteristics include circumscribed pruritic lesions with raised erythematous margins and thin, dry scaling. Called also *dhobie itch, jock itch, eczema marginatum,* and *ringworm of the groin.*

**t. fa'ciei,** tinea of the nonhairy areas of the face, often with a similar presentation to that of t. corporis. Called also *ringworm of the face.*

**t. favo'sa,** favus.

**t. fla'va,** t. versicolor.

**t. glabro'sa,** t. corporis.

**t. imbrica'ta,** a chronic tropical type of tinea due to *Trichophyton concentricum,* geographically restricted to certain South Pacific islands, Southeast Asia, and Central and South America, seen almost exclusively in those of Indonesian or Polynesian descent; characterized by confluent polycyclic concentric rings of papulosquamous patches of scales frequently covering large areas of the body. Called also *t. circinata tropical, Oriental ringworm, Tokelau ringworm,* and *tokelau.*

**t. ma'nus, t. ma'nuum,** tinea of the interdigital spaces and palmar surfaces of hands; it almost always accompanies t. pedis, so that the etiologic agent is usually the same for both infections. It usually presents as hyperkeratosis of the palm and fingers, usually unilateral, but it may also present as skin exfoliation, circumscribed vesicular patches, discrete, red papulofollicular patches, or red scaly sheets on the dorsum. Called also *ringworm of the hand.*

**t. ni'gra,** a minor fungal infection, caused by *Cladosporium mansoni* or *Exophiala werneckii,* having dark lesions with the appearance of spattered silver nitrate on the skin of the hands or, rarely, on other areas. Called also *cladosporiosis epidermica, keratomycosis nigricans, microsporosis nigra,* and *pityriasis nigra.*

**t. pe'dis,** tinea involving the feet, particularly the interdigital spaces and soles, most often caused by *Trichophyton rubrum, T. mentagrophytes,* or *Epidermophyton floccosum,* and characterized by intensely pruritic lesions varying from mild, chronic, and scaling to acute exfoliative, pustular, and bullous. See also *t. cruris* and *t. manus.* Called also *athlete's foot* and *ringworm of the foot.*

**t. profun'da,** trichophytic granuloma.

**t. syco'sis,** the sycosiform type of tinea barbae.

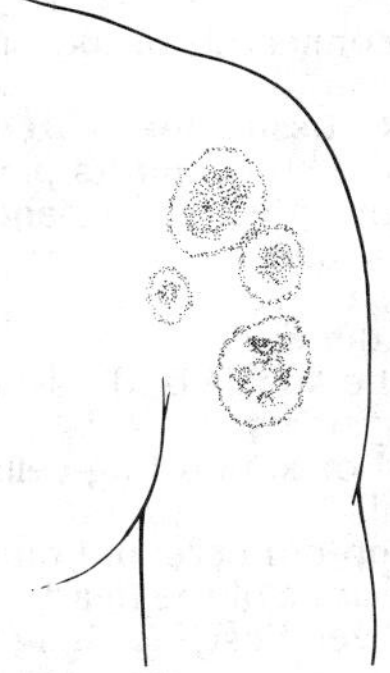

Lesions of tinea corporis on the shoulder.

**t. tonsu'rans,** t. capitis.

**t. un'guium,** tinea involving the nails, usually caused by a combination of bacteria and fungi, particularly species of *Candida;* it usually is seen first as white patches or pits on the nail surface or around its edges, followed by establishment of infection beneath the nail plate. Called also *onychomycosis* or *dermatophytic onychomycosis* and *ringworm of the nail.*

**t. versi'color,** a common chronic, usually symptomless disorder, characterized only by multiple macular patches, of all sizes and shapes, varying from white in pigmented skin to tan or brown in pale skin; usually seen in hot, humid tropical regions, and caused by *Malassezia furfur.* Called also *dermatomycosis furfuracea, liver spots, pityriasis versicolor,* and *t. flava.*

**Ti·nel's sign** (te-nelz') [Jules *Tinel,* French neurologist, 1879–1952] see under *sign.*

**tin·foil** (tin'foil) tin foil.

**tin·gi·bil·i·ty** (tin″jĭ-bil'ĭ-te) the quality of being tingible.

**tin·gi·ble** (tin'jĭ-bəl) [L. *tingere* to stain] susceptible of being tinged or stained.

**ting·ling** (ting'gling) a sensation as of repetitive moving pin pricks, caused by cold or by striking a nerve, or as a result of various diseases of the central or peripheral nervous system.

**distal t. on percussion,** Tinel's sign; see under *sign.*

**ti·nid·a·zole** (ti-nid'ə-zōl) [MeSH: Tinidazole] an antimicrobial having properties and uses similar to those of metronidazole, effective against *Trichomonas vaginalis, Entamoeba histolytica,* and *Giardia intestinalis;* administered orally and intravenously.

**tin·ni·tus** (tin'ĭ-təs, tĭ-ni'təs) [L. "a ringing"] [MeSH: Tinnitus] a noise in the ears, such as ringing, buzzing, roaring, or clicking. It is usually subjective in type (see *subjective t.*). Most classifications stress distinctions between *vibratory* and *nonvibratory* types. Called also *t. aurium.*

**t. au'rium,** tinnitus.

**t. ce'rebri,** tinnitus experienced as being inside the head rather than in an ear.

**clicking t.,** a form of objective tinnitus in which the patient hears a clicking sound; it occurs with serous otitis media.

**Leudet's t.,** a form of objective tinnitus in which the patient hears a crackling sound, produced by involuntary contraction of an internal muscle, coinciding with a tic of fibers of the mandibular division of the trigeminal nerve.

**nonvibratory t.,** tinnitus produced by biochemical changes in the nerve mechanism of hearing. Cf. *vibratory t.*

**objective t.,** a rare type of tinnitus that is audible to others, such as to an examiner with a stethoscope. Cf. *subjective t.*

**pulsatile t.,** vibratory tinnitus in which the sound is rhythmic and synchronous with the heartbeat.

**subjective t.,** the usual type of tinnitus, in which the sound cannot be heard by an examiner or measured by objective instruments. Subtypes include *vibratory* and *nonvibratory t.* Cf. *objective t.*

**vibratory t.,** tinnitus caused by transmission to the cochlea of vibrations from adjacent tissues or organs, most often from blood in vascular malformations. Occasionally the vibrations are loud enough to be heard by an examiner. Cf. *nonvibratory t.*

**tin·tom·e·ter** (tin-tom'ə-tər) [*tint* + *-meter*] an instrument used in determining the relative proportion of coloring matter in a liquid.

**tin·to·met·ric** (tin″to-met'rik) pertaining to tintometry.

**tin·tom·e·try** (tin-tom'ə-tre) the use of the tintometer.

**ti·o·co·na·zole** (ti″o-ko'nə-zōl) an imidazole derivative used as a topical antifungal, applied intravaginally in the treatment of vulvovaginal candidiasis.

**ti·o·pro·nin** (ti-o'pro-nin) a thiol compound that reacts with cystine to form a soluble mixed disulfide, used in the treatment of cystinuria; administered orally.

**tip** (tip) a pointed extremity of a body part; called also *apex.*

**t. of nose,** apex nasi.

**t. of sacral bone,** apex ossis sacri.

**t. of tongue,** apex linguae.

**Woolner's t.,** tuberculum auriculare.

**tip·ping** (tip'ing) 1. a tooth movement in which its vertical position is altered, either spontaneously or as a result of orthodontic therapy. See also *uprighting.* 2. cusp restoration.

**TIPS** transjugular intrahepatic portosystemic shunt.

**ti·queur** (te-kur') [Fr.] a person subject to a tic.

**tir·ing** (tīr'ing) the operation of passing a wire around a fractured patella, like a tire around a wheel; cerclage.

**Ti·se·li·us apparatus** (te-sa'le-əs) [Arne Wilhelm Kaurin *Tiselius,* Swedish biochemist, 1902–1971, winner of the Nobel prize for chemistry in 1948] see under *apparatus.*

**Tis·si·er·el·la** (tis″e-ə-rel′ə) a genus of gram-negative, anaerobic, non–spore-forming, motile rods with peritrichous flagella, containing a single species, *T. praeacuta.*

**T. praeacu′ta,** a bile-sensitive, nonpigmented, nonfermentative or weakly fermentative species isolated from the blood, from gangrenous lesions, and from the intestinal tract of infants and adults; called also *Bacteroides praeacutus.*

**tis·sue** (tish′oo) [Fr. *tissu*] an aggregation of similarly specialized cells united in the performance of a particular function.

## Tissue

**accidental t.,** a tissue growing in or upon a part to which it is foreign; it is either analogous or heterologous.

**adenoid t.,** lymphoid t.

**adipose t.,** fatty tissue; connective tissue made up of fat cells in a meshwork of areolar tissue.

**adipose t., brown,** a thermogenic type of adipose tissue containing a dark pigment. It arises during embryonic life in certain specific areas in many mammals, including humans, and is prominent in newborns. It remains distinct and conspicuous in adults in only certain species, especially those that hibernate. Cf. *white adipose t.* Called also *brown fat.*

**adipose t., white, adipose t., yellow,** the adipose tissue comprising the bulk of the body fat. Cf. *brown adipose t.*

**adrenogenic t.,** fetal zone of adrenal cortex.

**analogous t.,** an accidental tissue similar to one found normally in other parts of the body.

**areolar t., areolar connective t.,** a type of connective tissue made up largely of interlacing fibers. Called also *cribriform t.* and *loose connective t.*

**basement t.,** the substance of a basement membrane.

**bony t.,** bone, whether normal or of a soft tissue, which has become ossified.

**bursa-equivalent t., bursal equivalent t.,** a hypothesized lymphoid tissue in nonavian vertebrates equivalent to the bursa of Fabricius in birds: the site of B lymphocyte maturation. It now appears that B cell maturation occurs primarily in the bone marrow.

**cancellous t.,** the loose spongy tissue of the interior and articular ends of bone.

**cartilaginous t.,** the substance of the cartilages.

**cavernous t.,** erectile t.

**cellular t.,** loose connective tissue with large interspaces.

**chondroid t.,** an embryonic form of cartilage composed of vesicular cells provided with elastic capsules and having collagenous fibers in its interstitial substance.

**chordal t.,** the tissue of the notochord.

**chromaffin t.,** tissue composed largely of chromaffin cells, well supplied with nerves and vessels; it occurs in the adrenal medulla and also forms the paraganglia of the body.

**cicatricial t.,** the dense fibrous tissue forming a scar or cicatrix and derived directly from granulation tissue; called also *scar t.*

**compact t.,** the hard external portion of a bone.

**connective t.,** the tissue that binds together and is the support of the various structures of the body. It is made up of fibroblasts, fibroglia, collagen fibrils, and elastic fibrils, is derived from the mesoderm, and in a broad sense includes the collagenous, elastic, mucous, reticular, osseous, and cartilaginous tissue. Some authorities also include the blood. Cf. *fibroblast.* Connective tissue is classified according to concentration of fibers as loose (areolar) and dense, the latter having more abundant fibers than the former.

**cribriform t.,** areolar t.

**dartoid t.,** that which resembles the dartos in structure.

**dense connective t.,** see *connective t.*

**elastic t., elastic t., yellow,** connective tissue made up of yellow, elastic fibers, frequently massed into sheets.

**endothelial t.,** endothelium.

**episcleral t.,** the loose connective tissue over the sclera, between it and the conjunctiva.

**epithelial t.,** epithelium.

**epivaginal connective t.,** connective tissue surrounding the sheath of the optic nerve.

**erectile t.,** tissue containing large venous spaces with which arteries communicate directly, as in the penis and clitoris. Another type formed of dilated venules occurs in the nasal mucosa. The smooth muscle of the nipples constitutes another erectile organ.

**extracellular t.,** the total of tissues and body fluids outside the cells, including the plasma volume and all plasma components, the extracellular fluid volume and its components, plus the intercellular and extracellular tissue solids, most notably the collagen, cartilage, bone, elastin, and other connective tissues of the body framework and viscera.

**extraperitoneal t.,** fascia extraperitonealis.

**fatty t.,** adipose t.

**fibrohyaline t.,** chondroid t.

**fibrous t.,** the ordinary connective tissue of the body, made up largely of yellow or white fibers.

**fibrous t., white,** that which is composed almost wholly of collagenous fibers.

**Gamgee T.,** trademark for a surgical dressing consisting of a thick layer of absorbent cotton between two layers of absorbent gauze.

**gelatiginous t.,** that which yields gelatin on boiling with water.

**gelatinous t.,** mucous t.

**glandular t.,** an aggregation of epithelial cells that elaborate secretions.

**granulation t.,** the newly formed vascular tissue normally produced in the healing of wounds of soft tissue and ultimately forming the cicatrix; it consists of small, translucent, red, nodular masses or granulations that have a velvety appearance.

**gut-associated lymphoid t. (GALT),** lymphoid tissue associated with the gut, including the tonsils, Peyer's patches, lamina propria of the gastrointestinal tract, and appendix.

**hematopoietic t.,** see under *system.*

**heterologous t.,** tissue unlike any other that is normal to the organism.

**heterotopic t.,** choristoma.

**homologous t.,** tissue identical with another tissue in structural type.

**hyperplastic t.,** 1. tissue affected by hyperplasia. 2. in dentistry, an overgrowth of tissue about the maxilla or mandible that is excessively movable, or more readily displaced than is normal.

**indifferent t.,** undifferentiated embryonic tissue.

**interstitial t.,** stroma.

**junctional t.,** the portion of the conducting system of the heart forming a bridge between the atrium and ventricle of the heart, comprising the atrioventricular node and the bundle of His.

**Kuhnt's intermediary t.,** glial tissue surrounding the optic nerve and separating it from the retina.

**lardaceous t.,** tissue having the appearance of lard as a result of a degenerative process.

**loose connective t.,** areolar t.

**lymphadenoid t.,** tissue resembling that of the lymph nodes, found in the spleen, bone marrow, tonsils, and other organs.

**lymphatic t.,** lymphoid t.

**lymphoid t.,** a latticework of reticular tissue the interspaces of which contain lymphocytes; lymphoid tissue may be diffuse, or densely aggregated as in lymph nodules and nodes. See also *lymphoid system,* under *system.*

**mesenchymal t.,** mesenchyma.

**metanephrogenic t.,** the nephrogenic tissue of the metanephros; it gives rise to the nephrons of the permanent kidney.

**mucosa-associated lymphoid t. (MALT),** a type of specialized lymphoid tissue found in association with certain types of epithelia; it usually has prominent B-cell follicles and sometimes has zones of T cells.

**mucous t.,** a jellylike connective tissue, such as occurs in the umbilical cord.

**muscle t., muscular t.,** tissue specialized for contraction, which produces movement of the body and its parts; it consists of muscle fibers, muscle cells, connective tissue, and extracellular material. Called also *flesh.* See also *muscle.*

**myeloid t.,** medulla ossium rubra.

**nephrogenic t.,** see under *cord.*

**nerve t., nervous t.,** the specialized tissue making up the central and peripheral nervous systems; it consists of neurons with their processes, other specialized or supporting cells such as the neuroglia, and extracellular material.

**nodal t.,** tissue made up of nerve and muscle fibers, such as that composing the sinoatrial node of the heart.

**osseous t.,** the specialized tissue forming the bones.

**osteogenic t.,** that part of the periosteum adjacent to bone and concerned in the formation of osseous tissue; any tissue capable of generating bone.

**osteoid t.,** uncalcified bone tissue.
**parenchymatous t.,** parenchyma.
**protochondral t.,** centers of chondrification.
**reticular t., reticulated t.,** connective tissue consisting of reticular cells and fibers.
**rubber t.,** rubber in sheets for use in surgery.
**scar t.,** cicatricial t.
**sclerous t's,** the cartilaginous, fibrous, and osseous tissues.
**shock t.,** that tissue in the animal body which bears the brunt of the antigen-antibody reaction in anaphylaxis.
**skeletal t.,** the bony, ligamentous, fibrous, and cartilaginous tissue forming the skeleton and its attachments.
**splenic t.,** red pulp; see *pulpa splenica,* under *pulpa.*
**subcutaneous t.,** the layer of loose connective tissue situated just beneath the skin; called also *tela subcutanea* [TA].
**subcutaneous fatty t.,** panniculus adiposus.
**sustentacular t.,** a non-nervous structure of the retina composed of the müllerian fibers of that organ.
**symplastic t.,** symplasm.
**target t.,** 1. tissue, either *in vivo* or *in vitro,* against which humoral or cell-mediated immunity is directed. 2. the tissue that responds specifically to a given hormone.
**tuberculosis granulation t.,** the tissue that forms the characteristic tubercle in tuberculosis, composed of epithelioid cells in concentric masses, lymphocytes, and often Langhans' giant cells.
**vesicular supporting t.,** chondroid t.

---

**tis·sul·ar** (tish'u-lər) pertaining to tissue.

**ti·ta·ni·um** (ti-ta'ne-əm) [L., from Gr. *Titan* a child of Uranus and Gaia] [MeSH: Titanium] a dark gray metallic element of widespread distribution but occurring in small amounts; atomic number, 22; atomic weight, 47.90; symbol, Ti; specific gravity, 4.5; used for fixation of fractures. Titanium and its alloys are the most common metals used in dental implants because of their excellent biocompatibility when in contact with hard or soft tissues and their low corrosion rate due to formation of a stable oxide surface film through passivation.
**t. dioxide,** 1. $TiO_2$, an oxide of titanium used as a white pigment, primarily in paints; workers inhaling excessive amounts of its dust may suffer from titanium dioxide pneumoconiosis. 2. [USP] a purified form of this substance in the form of a white powder, used as a topical protectant against sunburn, in other protectant preparations, in dusting powders, and as a pigment in the manufacture of artificial teeth.

**ti·ter** (ti'tər) [Fr. *titre* standard] the quantity of a substance required to produce a reaction with a given volume of another substance, or the amount of one substance required to correspond with a given amount of another substance.
**agglutination t.,** the highest dilution of a serum which causes clumping of microorganisms or other particulate antigens.
**bacteriophage t.,** the concentration of viable bacteriophage in a given solution.
**whole complement t.,** see *CH50 assay,* under *assay.*

**tit·il·la·tion** (tit"ĭ-la'shən) [L. *titillatio*] tickling (defs. 1 and 2).

**ti·trant** (ti'trənt) the solution of known strength that is added in titration.

**ti·trate** (ti'trāt) to determine by titration.

**ti·tra·tion** (ti-tra'shən) [Fr. *titre* standard] determination of a given component in solution by addition of a liquid reagent of known strength until a given endpoint (e.g., change in color) is reached.
**colorimetric t.,** a method of determining hydrogen ion concentration by adding an indicator to the unknown and then comparing the color with a set of tubes containing this same indicator in solutions of known hydrogen ion concentration.
**complexometric t.,** titration of a substance (e.g., the calcium in clear serum) with a complexing agent (e.g., EDTA); the endpoint of the titration is generally observed as a change in color of the solution.
**coulometric t.,** titration by determining the amount of electricity required to electrochemically generate a titrant which reacts with the substance in question. If the current is kept constant, the amount of electricity (coulombs) used is proportional to the elapsed time.
**Dean and Webb t.,** a test for measuring antibody in which varying dilutions of antigen are mixed with a constant quantity of antiserum; antibody activity is determined by the dilution in which flocculation occurs most rapidly, i.e., the endpoint. In this dilution, antigen and antibody are together at a ratio of optimal proportions.
**formol t.,** see *Sörensen's method,* under *method.*
**potentiometric t.,** a method of determining hydrogen ion concentration by placing a hydrogen electrode in unknown solution and measuring the potential developed as compared with some standard electrode by means of a potentiometer.

**ti·tre** (ti'tər) [Fr.] titer.

**tit·ri·met·ric** (tit"rĭ-met'rik) pertaining to analysis by titration.

**ti·trim·e·try** (ti-trim'ə-tre) [*titration* + *-metry*] [MeSH: Titrimetry] analysis by titration.

**tit·u·bant** (tit'u-bant) pertaining to or characterized by titubation.

**tit·u·ba·tion** (tit"u-ba'shən) [L. *titubatio*] 1. the act of staggering or reeling. 2. a tremor of the head and sometimes trunk, commonly seen in cerebellar disease.
**lingual t.,** 1. stuttering. 2. stammering.

**Tit·y·us** (tit'e-əs) a genus of scorpions found in Central and South America. *T. serrula'tus* is a Brazilian species with a severe, sometimes fatal, sting.

**tix·o·cor·tol piv·a·late** (tic-so'kor-tol) a glucocorticoid with anti-inflammatory action, administered topically in buccal, nasal, throat, or rectal preparations.

**Tiz·zo·ni's test** (te-dzo'nēz) [Guido *Tizzoni,* Italian physician, 1853–1932] see under *test.*

**TK** thymidine kinase.

**TKD** tokodynamometer.

**TKG** tokodynagraph.

**Tl** symbol for *thallium.*

**TLC** total lung capacity; thin-layer chromatography.

**TLI** total lymphoid irradiation.

**TLSO** thoracolumbosacral orthosis.

**TLV** threshold limit value.

**Tm** symbol for *thulium.*

**TMA** trimellitic anhydride.

**TMI** transmandibular implant.

**TMST** treadmill stress test.

**TMV** tobacco mosaic virus.

**Tn** normal intraocular tension; see *intraocular pressure,* under *pressure.*

**TND** transmissible neurodegenerative disease; see *prion disease,* under *disease.*

**TNF** tumor necrosis factor.

**TNM** see under *staging.*

**TNS** transcutaneous nerve stimulation.

**TNT** trinitrotoluene.

**TO** abbreviation for *tinctura opii,* tincture of opium.

**toad** (tōd) any of various tailless leaping amphibians of the order Anura, having rough skin and webbed feet and often used in laboratory experiments. Cf. *frog.* The most common genus is *Bufo.*
**clawed t.,** *Xenopus laevis.*
**fire t.,** *Bombinator igneus.*
**fire-bellied t.,** *Bombina bombina.*

**toad·skin** (tōd'skin) follicular hyperkeratosis.

**toad·stool** (tōd'stōōl) popular name for a poisonous mushroom.

**to·bac·co** (tə-bak'o) [L. *tabacum*] [MeSH: Tobacco] 1. any of various plants of the genus *Nicotiana,* especially *N. tabacum.* 2. the dried and prepared leaves of *N. tabacum*; it contains various alkaloids, the principal one being *nicotine,* has qualities of both a sedative narcotic and an emetic and diuretic, and is also a heart depressant and antispasmodic. See also *tobacco poisoning* and *nicotine poisoning,* under *poisoning.*
**mountain t.,** 1. Arnica. 2. arnica.

**to·bac·co·ism** (tə-bak'o-iz-əm) tobacco poisoning.

**To·bey-Ayer test** (to'be-a'ər) [George L. *Tobey,* Jr., American otolaryngologist, 1881–1947; James Bourne *Ayer,* American neurologist, 1882–1963] see under *test.*

**to·bra·my·cin** (to″brə-mi′sin) [USP] [MeSH: Tobramycin] an aminoglycoside antibiotic, part of the nebramycin complex, effective against a wide range of aerobic gram-negative bacilli and some gram-positive bacteria, having a range of antibacterial activity similar to that of gentamicin; used topically in the treatment of external infections of the eye and its adnexa.
**t. sulfate** [USP], the sulfate salt of tobramycin, used for the treatment of a wide variety of infections caused by susceptible gram-negative organisms; administered intravenously and intramuscularly.

**Tob·rex** (to′breks) trademark for preparations of tobramycin.

**to·cai·nide hy·dro·chlo·ride** (to-ka′nīd) [USP] an oral antiarrhythmic agent, similar to lidocaine in structure and action, used in the treatment of ventricular arrhythmias.

**to·cam·phyl** (to-kam′fəl) a choleretic obtained from turmeric, $C_{19}H_{26}O_4 \cdot C_4H_{11}NO_2$.

**To·clase** (to′klās) trademark for preparations of carbetapentane citrate.

**toc(o)-** [Gr. *tokos* childbirth] a combining form denoting relationship to childbirth, or labor; see also words beginning *tok(o)-.*

**to·co·dy·na·graph** (to″ko-di′nə-graf) tokodynagraph.

**to·co·dy·na·mom·e·ter** (to″ko-di″nə-mom′ə-tər) tokodynamometer.

**to·co·graph** (to′ko-graf) a recording tokodynamometer.

**to·cog·ra·phy** (to-kog′rə-fe) [*toco-* + *-graphy*] the graphic recording of uterine contractions.

**to·col** (to′kol) the basic unit of the tocopherols and tocotrienols, hydroquinone with a saturated polyisoprenoid side chain at the 6 position; it is an antioxidant.

**to·col·y·sis** (to-kol′ĭ-sis) [*toco-* + *lysis*] [MeSH: Tocolysis] inhibition of uterine contractions.

**to·com·e·ter** (to-kom′ə-tər) [*toco-* + *-meter*] tokodynamometer.

**to·coph·er·ol** (to-kof′ər-ol) [*toco-* + Gr. *pherein* to carry + *-ol*] any of a series of structurally similar compounds, methyl-substituted tocols, some of which have biological vitamin E activity.
**α-t., alpha t.,** a doubly methylated tocopherol isomer; it is the most prevalent form of vitamin E occurring in the body and the form administered as a supplement. In nature, it usually occurs with β- and γ-tocopherols. The term is often used synonymously with vitamin E.
**α-t. acetate,** a substituted form of α-tocopherol having the same actions and uses; see also *vitamin E.*
**α-t. acid succinate,** a substituted form of α-tocopherol having the same actions and uses; see also *vitamin E.*

**to·coph·er·yl** (to-kof′ər-əl) the acyl radical of tocopherol.

**to·co·pho·bia** (to″ko-fo′be-ə) [*toco-* + *-phobia*] irrational fear of childbirth.

**to·co·tri·en·ol** (to″ko-tri′ə-nol) any of a series of structurally similar compounds derived from tocol, at least some of which have biological vitamin E activity; they are similar to tocopherols but their isoprenoid side chains are unsaturated.

**To·da·ro's tendon** (to-dah′rōz) [Francesco *Todaro,* Italian physician, 1839–1918] see under *tendon.*

**Todd bodies** (tod) [John Launcelot *Todd,* Canadian physician, 1876–1949] see under *body.*

**Todd's paralysis (palsy), process** (todz) [Robert Bentley *Todd,* British physician, 1809–1860] see under *paralysis,* see *primary biliary cirrhosis,* under *cirrhosis,* and see *fibrae intercrurales.*

**Todd-Wells apparatus, technique** (tod-welz) [Edwin M. *Todd,* American neurosurgeon, 20th century; T.H. *Wells,* Jr., American neurosurgeon, 20th century] see under *apparatus* and *technique.*

**Tod·dal·ia** (to-dal′e-ə) a genus of shrubs of the family Rutaceae. *T. aculea′ta* Pers. is an East Indian species whose root is a stomachic and whose root bark is antimalarial and antipyretic.

**toe** (to) [MeSH: Toes] 1. any of the five digits of the foot. See *hallux, digitus secundus pedis, digitus tertius pedis, digitus quartis pedis,* and *digitus minimus pedis.* 2. the anterior part of a horse's hoof.
**claw t.,** a toe deformity seen in many patients with rheumatoid arthritis, consisting of dorsal subluxation of toes 2 through 5; the metatarsal heads bear weight and become painful during walking so that the patient has a shuffling gait.
**curly t's,** a condition affecting chicks, in which the toes curl underneath the feet, due to a deficiency of riboflavin.
**fifth t.,** digitus minimus pedis.
**first t.,** hallux.

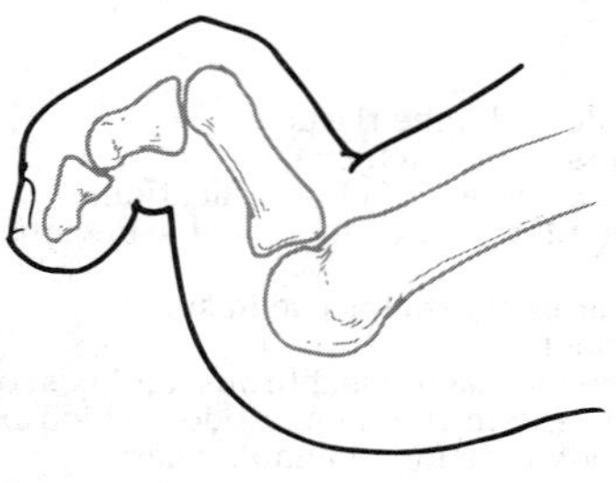

Claw toe.

**fourth t.,** digitus quartus pedis.
**great t.,** hallux.
**hammer t.,** a condition in which the proximal phalanx of a toe—most often that of the second toe—is extended and the second and distal phalanges are flexed, causing a clawlike appearance.
**little t.,** digitus minimum pedis.
**mallet t.,** flexion contracture of the distal interphalangeal joint of any of the lesser toes.
**Morton's t.,** see under *neuralgia.*
**pigeon t.,** a permanent toeing-in position of the feet.
**second t.,** digitus secundus pedis.
**seedy t.,** a disease of horses' hoofs marked by a horny, honeycombed texture between the coffin bone and the wall. Called also *hollow wall* and *dystrophia ungulae.*
**tennis t.,** painful great toe associated with subungual hematoma, which, in the absence of treatment, may lead to subungual abscess; it usually develops after a vigorous tennis game, especially when tennis shoes with protective tips are worn.
**third t.,** digitus tertius pedis.
**webbed t's,** toes abnormally joined by strands of tissue at their base.

**toe·nail** (to′nāl) the nail on any of the digits of the foot. See *unguis* [TA].
**ingrowing t., ingrown t.,** ingrown nail.

**Toep·fer** (terp′fer) see *Töpfer.*

**To·fra·nil** (to-fra′nil) trademark for preparations of imipramine hydrochloride.

**To·fra·nil-PM** (to-fra′nil) trademark for a preparation of imipramine pamoate.

**To·ga·vi·ri·dae** (to″gə-vir′ĭ-de) [MeSH: Togaviridae] the togaviruses: a family of RNA viruses having a spherical virion 60–70 nm in diameter consisting of a lipid-containing envelope, with five peplomers, surrounding an icosahedral nucleocapsid. The genome consists of a single molecule of polyadenylated positive-sense single-stranded RNA (MW $4 \times 10^6$, size 9.7–11.8 kb). Viruses contain three or four major structural proteins and are sensitive to lipid solvents, detergents, and ultraviolet radiation. Replication occurs in the cytoplasm and assembly occurs by budding through the plasma membrane. There are two genera: *Alphavirus* and *Rubivirus.*

**to·ga·vi·rus** (to′gə-vi″rəs) [L. *toga* robe + *virus*] [MeSH: Togaviridae] any virus belonging to the family Togaviridae.

**toi·let** (toi′lət) [Fr. *toilette*] cleansing, as of an accidental wound and the surrounding skin, or of an obstetrical patient after childbirth.

**Toi·son's solution (fluid)** (twah-zawz′) [J. *Toison,* French histologist, 1858–1900] see under *solution.*

**To·ke·lau ringworm** (to-ke-lah′oo) [*Tokelau,* Islands in the South Pacific, part of New Zealand, where the disease is commonly observed] tinea imbricata.

**to·ke·lau** (to-ke-lah′oo) tinea imbricata.

**tok(o)-** [Gr. *tokos* childbirth] for words beginning thus, see also those beginning *toc(o)-.*

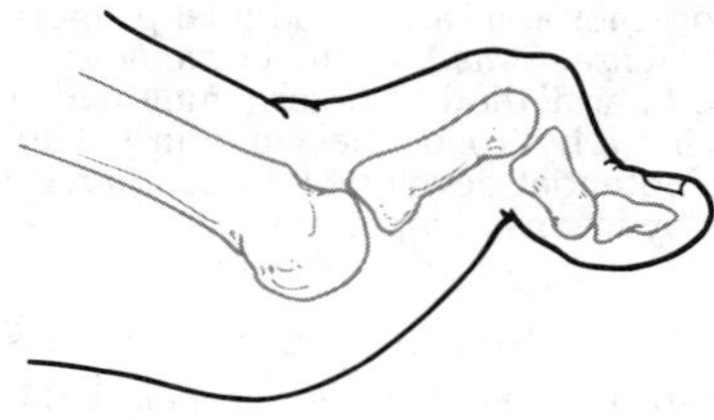

Hammer toe.

**to·ko·dy·na·graph** (to″ko-di′nə-graf) the record obtained with a tokodynamometer. Abbreviated TKG.

**to·ko·dy·na·mom·e·ter** (to″ko-di″nə-mom′ə-tər) [*toko-* + *dynamometer*] an instrument for measuring uterine contractions. Abbreviated TKD.

**to·la·mo·lol** (to-lă′mə-lol) a beta-adrenergic blocking agent which has been used as a coronary vasodilator in the treatment of angina of effort and as a cardiac depressant in the treatment of arrhythmias.

**tol·az·amide** (tol-az′ə-mīd) [USP] [MeSH: Tolazamide] a sulfonylurea compound used as a hypoglycemic in the treatment of type 2 diabetes mellitus; administered orally.

**tol·az·o·line hy·dro·chlo·ride** (tol-az′o-lēn) [USP] an adrenergic blocking agent and peripheral vasodilator used in the treatment of peripheral vascular disorders due to vasospasm, administered orally, and as a vasodilator in pharmacoangiography, administered by intra-arterial infusion.

**tol·bu·ta·mide** (tol-bu′tə-mīd) [USP] [MeSH: Tolbutamide] a sulfonylurea compound used as a hypoglycemic in the treatment of non–insulin-dependent diabetes mellitus; administered orally. It is also used to test for insulinoma in the tolbutamide test (q.v.).
**t. sodium, sterile** [USP], the monosodium salt of tolbutamide, having the same actions as the base; used as a diagnostic test for diabetes mellitus, administered intravenously.

**Toldt's membrane** (tōlts) [Karl *Toldt,* Austrian anatomist, 1840–1920] see under *membrane.*

**Tol·ec·tin** (tol′ek-tin) trademark for a preparation of tolmetin sodium.

**tol·er·ance** (tol′ər-əns) [L. *tolerare* to endure] 1. diminution of response to a stimulus after prolonged exposure. 2. the ability to endure unusually large doses of a poison or toxin. 3. drug t. 4. immunologic t.
**acquired drug t.,** drug t.
**adoptive t.,** immunological tolerance induced by the passive transfer to an irradiated recipient animal of lymphoid cells from a donor rendered tolerant to an antigen.
**alkali t.,** ability of the body to endure the administration of alkalis, measured by the amount of alkali that must be given to cause an alkaline urine; this forms a rough measure of the degree of acidosis.
**crossed t.,** the lessened susceptibility which persons who have acquired a tolerance for one drug or poison may thereafter exhibit toward another drug.
**drug t.,** a decreasing response to repeated constant doses of a drug or the need for increasing doses to maintain a constant response.
**glucose t.,** ability of the body to properly metabolize an administered glucose load; see also *glucose tolerance test,* under *test.*
**glucose t., impaired (IGT),** a term denoting values of fasting plasma glucose or results of an oral glucose tolerance test that are abnormal but not high enough to be diagnostic of diabetes mellitus. Formerly called *chemical, latent, preclinical,* or *subclinical diabetes.*
**high-dose t., high-zone t.,** see *immunologic t.*
**immunologic t.,** an immunologic response consisting of the development of specific nonreactivity of the lymphoid tissues to a given antigen that in other circumstances can induce cell-mediated or humoral immunity; it results from previous contact with the antigen and has no effect on the response to non–cross-reacting antigens. Tolerance is readily induced by administration of antigen to immunologically immature animals (fetuses, neonates). In adults tolerance may be induced by repeated administration of very large doses of antigen *(high-dose* or *high-zone t.),* or of small doses that are below the threshold required for stimulation of an immune response *(low-dose* or *low-zone t.).* Tolerance is most readily induced by soluble antigens administered intravenously; immunosuppression also facilitates the induction of tolerance.
**low-dose t., low-zone t.,** see *immunologic t.*
**self t.,** immunologic unresponsiveness to autoantigens (self antigens), acquired during fetal life by a process of "self recognition." Theories of tolerance induction include deletion of antigen-responsive clones of B cells, antigen-induced inactivation of B or T cells, and induction of antigen-specific T suppressor cells.
**split t.,** 1. following induction of immunologic tolerance to allogeneic cells, tolerance to an antigen or group of antigens on the cell surface occurs, while there is an immune response to other antigens on the cell surface. 2. immunologic tolerance that affects either the humoral immune system or the cell-mediated immune system, but not both simultaneously. Called also *immunodeviation.*
**transplantation t.,** immunologic tolerance of transplanted tissue.

**tol·er·ant** (tol′ər-ənt) able to endure, without effect, the action of any particular drug or other agent; exhibiting tolerance.

**tol·er·a·tion** (tol″ər-a′shən) tolerance.

**tol·ero·gen** (tol′ər-o-jən) an antigen used to introduce tolerance, particularly a form of an antigen (usually a soluble form) that induces tolerance, as distinguished from an immunogen, another form (usually an insoluble form) that induces immunity.

**tol·ero·gen·e·sis** (tol″ər-o-jen′ə-sis) induction of immunologic tolerance.

**tol·er·o·gen·ic** (tol″ər-o-jen′ik) capable of inducing immunologic tolerance.

***o*-to·li·dine** (tol′ĭ-dēn) a compound related to benzidine and formerly used in testing for occult blood; its use is now restricted because it is a carcinogen.

**Tol·in·ase** (tōl′in-ās) trademark for a preparation of tolazamide.

**tol·met·in so·di·um** (tol′met-in) [USP] an anti-inflammatory, analgesic, and antipyretic, used in the treatment of osteoarthritis and rheumatoid arthritis, administered orally.

**tol·naf·tate** (tol-naf′tāt) [USP] [MeSH: Tolnaftate] a synthetic antifungal used topically in the treatment of various forms of tinea of the skin.

**to·lo·ni·um chlo·ride** (to-lo′ne-əm) [MeSH: Tolonium Chloride] an antiheparin compound that has been used in the treatment of idiopathic functional uterine bleeding and menorrhagia, topically to detect and delineate cervical neoplasia, and intravenously to stain the parathyroid glands. Called also *toluidine blue O.*

**To·lo·sa-Hunt syndrome** (to-lo′sah-hunt) [Eduardo S. *Tolosa,* Spanish neurosurgeon, 20th century; William Edward *Hunt,* American neurosurgeon, born 1921] see under *syndrome.*

**tol·u·ene** (tol′u-ēn) [MeSH: Toluene] the hydrocarbon methylbenzene, $C_6H_5 \cdot CH_3$; a colorless liquid derived by the catalytic reforming of petroleum on the fractional distillation of cal-tar light oil. It is an organic solvent used in rubber and plastic cements, paint removers, etc. Poisoning may result from ingesting the solvent or inhaling its concentrated vapors. Called also *toluol* and *methyl benzene.*
**t. diisocyanate (TDI),** a pale yellow liquid with a sharp, pungent odor used in the manufacture of polyurethane foams and elastomers; it is highly toxic and a strong irritant of the skin, eyes, and respiratory system.

**tol·u·i·dine** (tol-u′ĭ-din) a compound homologous with aniline, made by reducing nitrotoluene; used in dyemaking and chemical manufacturing. It has several different isomers, all of which are toxic if inhaled, ingested, or absorbed through the skin. Called also *aminotoluene.*
**t. blue O,** tolonium chloride.
***o*-t.,** the *ortho-* isomer of toluidine, a yellow liquid used in dyemaking and chemical manufacture; it is more carcinogenic than the other isomers. Called also *o-aminotoluene.*

**tol·yl** (tol′əl) the univalent radical, $CH_3 \cdot C_6H_4$, derived from toluene and occurring in three isomeric forms.
**t. hydroxide,** cresol.

**to·mac·u·lous** (to-mak′u-ləs) [L. *tomaculum* sausage] resembling a sausage, usually because of swelling.

**to·ma·tine** (to-ma′tin) [MeSH: Tomatine] an antibiotic substance with antifungal properties, isolated from tomato plants affected with wilt.

**-tome** [Gr. *tomē* a cutting] a word termination signifying *(a)* an instrument for cutting or *(b)* a segment.

**to·men·tum** (to-men′təm) a little-used term for a network of minute blood vessels of the pia mater and the cortex cerebri; called also *tinnitus cerebri.*

**Tomes' layer, process (fiber, fibril)** (tōmz) [Sir John *Tomes,* English anatomist and dentist, 1815–1895] see *process of odontoblast,* and see *granular layer of Tomes,* under *layer.*

**Tomes' process** (tōmz) [Charles Sissmore *Tomes,* English anatomist and dentist, 1846–1928] see under *process* (def. 1).

**to·mite** (to′mīt) [*tom-* + Gr. *mitos* thread] the free-swimming nonfeeding stage or form in the life cycle of certain ciliate protozoa, produced by a tomont and, depending on the species, developing into a phoront, theront, or trophont.

**Tom·ma·sel·li's disease (syndrome)** (tom″ə-sel′ēz) [Salvatore *Tommaselli,* Italian physician, 1834–1906] see under *disease.*

**tom(o)-** [Gr. *tomē* a cutting] a combining form denoting relationship to a cutting, or to a designated layer, as might be achieved by cutting or slicing.

**to·mo·gram** (to′mo-gram) a radiograph of a selected layer of the body made by tomography.

**to·mo·graph** (to′mo-graf) an apparatus for moving an x-ray source in one direction as the film is moved in the opposite direction, thus showing in detail a predetermined plane of tissue while blurring or eliminating detail in other planes.

**to·mog·ra·phy** (to-mog′rə-fe) [*tomo-* + *-graphy*] [MeSH: Tomogra-

phy] the recording of internal body images at a predetermined plane by means of the tomograph; called also *body section radiography.*
**computed t. (CT),** computerized axial t.
**computerized axial t. (CAT),** that in which the emergent x-ray beam is measured by a scintillation counter; the electronic impulses are recorded on a magnetic disk and then are processed by a minicomputer for reconstruction display of the body in cross-section on a cathode ray tube. Called also *computed t.* and *CAT* or *CT scan.*
**electron beam computed t.,** EBCT; ultrafast computed tomography performed using a scanner in which the patient is surrounded by a large circular anode that emits x-rays as the electron beam is guided around it.
**high-resolution computed t. (HRCT),** computed tomography that produces images with a high degree of spatial resolution and anatomic detail using a high-speed scanner, thin slices, and a special algorithm for reconstructing the image.
**hypocycloidal t.,** tomography in which the path of the x-ray source is a hypocycloid, i.e., the path traced by a point on one circle rolling along inside the circumference of another circle.
**positron emission t. (PET),** that accomplished by detection of gamma rays emitted from tissues after administration of a natural biochemical substance (e.g., glucose, fatty acids) into which positron-emitting isotopes have been incorporated. The paths of the gamma rays, which result from collisions of positrons and electrons, are interpreted by a computer, and the resultant tomogram represents local concentrations of the isotope-containing substance.
**single-photon emission computed t. (SPECT),** a type of tomography in which gamma photon–emitting radionuclides are administered to patients and then detected by one or more gamma cameras rotated around the patient. From the series of two-dimensional images produced, a three-dimensional image can be created by computer reconstruction. The technique improves resolution of, and decreases interference by, overlapping organs.
**spiral computed t.,** computed tomography in which the patient is moved through the scanner continuously rather than in increments, so that the path of the beam through the patient is a continuous spiral.
**ultrasonic t.,** the ultrasonographic visualization of a cross-section of a predetermined plane of the body by linear scanning with an ultrasonic probe across the desired site and displaying on a B-scan.

**to·mont** (to'mont) [*tom-* +Gr. *ontos* beings] the nonfeeding, dividing stage or form in the life cycle of certain protozoa that typically encysts and produces tomites by fission.

**-tomy** [Gr. *tomē* a cutting] a word termination signifying the operation of cutting, or incision.

**ton·a·pha·sia** (ton″ə-fa'zhə) [*tono-* + *aphasia*] amusia.

**tone** (tōn) [Gr. *tonos;* L. *tonus*] 1. the normal degree of vigor and tension; in muscle, the resistance to passive elongation or stretch; tonus. 2. a particular quality of sound or of voice. 3. to make permanent, or to change, the color of silver stain by chemical treatment, usually with a heavy metal.
**feeling t.,** the condition or state of mind and feeling which accompanies every thought or act.
**jecoral t.,** the sound produced by percussion over the liver.

**To·ne·ga·wa** (to-na-gah'wah) Susumu. Japanese-born immunologist in United States, born 1939. Winner of the Nobel prize for medicine or physiology in 1987 for his discovery of genetic principles regarding generation of specific antibodies active against any of millions of different disease agents.

**tongs** (tongs) an instrument for grasping and holding, consisting of two arms joined by a hinge or pivot.
**skull t.,** tongs used to exert traction on the skull, as in surgery for fractures of cervical vertebrae; many forms are available, including Crutchfield t., Gardner-Wells t., Barton t., and Vinke t.

**tongue** (tung) [L. *lingua;* Gr. *glōssa*] [MeSH: Tongue] 1. lingua. 2. lingula. 3. any structure or organ having a shape similar to the oral organ of the same name.
**adherent t.,** ankyloglossia.
**amyloid t.,** enlargement of the tongue due to amyloidosis.
**antibiotic t.,** glossitis caused by sensitivity to an antibiotic.
**baked t.,** the dry, brown tongue of typhoid fever.
**bald t.,** Moeller's glossitis.
**beefy t.,** erythematous and/or atrophic glossitis, characterized by red, irregular ulcerations on the dorsal surface of the tongue.
**bifid t.,** a tongue that is divided in its anterior part by a longitudinal fissure; called also *cleft t.*
**black t.,** 1. black hairy t. 2. niacin deficiency in dogs, which is accompanied by severe stomatitis and a dark-colored tongue.
**black hairy t.,** hairy tongue (q.v.) in which the hypertrophied filiform papillae are brown or black. Called also *black t., lingua nigra, melanoglossia, melanotrichia linguae,* and *nigrities linguae.*
**blue t.,** bluetongue.

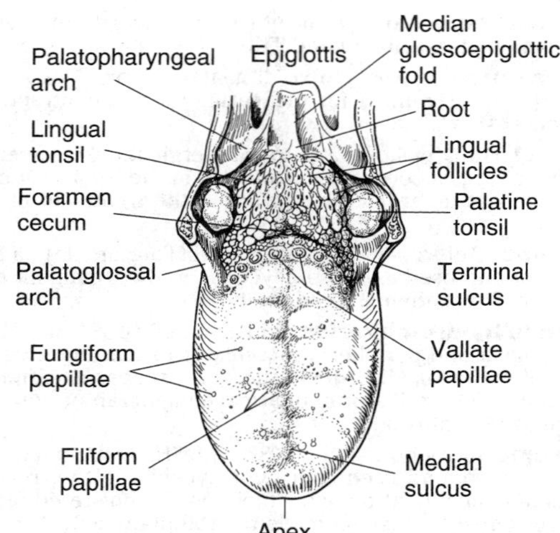

The tongue, showing principal structures.

**burning t.,** glossopyrosis.
**cardinal t.,** a tongue whose surface is denuded of epithelium, giving it a bright red appearance.
**cerebriform t.,** fissured t.
**cleft t.,** bifid t.
**coated t.,** a tongue covered with a whitish or yellowish layer consisting of desquamated epithelium, debris, bacteria, fungi, or other material, which is readily removed by scraping.
**cobble-stone t.,** a condition marked by interstitial glossitis with hypertrophy of the papillae and a verrucous white coating on the tongue, such as seen in riboflavin deficiency.
**crocodile t.,** fissured t.
**dotted t.,** stippled t.
**double t.,** bifid t.
**earthy t.,** a tongue that is coated with a deposit of rough, calcareous matter.
**encrusted t.,** a heavily coated tongue.
**fern leaf t.,** a tongue with a central furrow having lateral branches.
**filmy t.,** one marked with symmetrical whitish patches.
**fissured t.,** a sometimes familial condition characterized by the presence on the dorsal surface of the tongue of numerous furrows, which may radiate outwardly from the median raphe. Called also *cerebriform t., crocodile t., furrowed t., grooved t., plicated t., scrotal t., sulcated t., wrinkled t.,* and *lingua plicata.*
**flat t.,** a condition in which the borders of the tongue cannot be rolled; it is due to paralysis of the transverse lingual muscles occurring as a result of congenital syphilis.
**furred t.,** a tongue with papillae so changed as to give the mucous membrane the appearance of whitish fur.
**furrowed t.,** fissured t.
**geographic t.,** benign migratory glossitis.
**grooved t.,** fissured t.
**hairy t.,** a benign condition characterized by hypertrophy of the filiform papillae, giving the dorsum of the tongue a furry appearance. The color of the elongated papillae varies from yellowish white to brown or black *(black hairy t.),* depending upon staining by substances such as tobacco, foods, or drugs. Called also *glossotrichia* and *trichoglossia.*
**lobulated t.,** a congenital condition marked by a secondary lobe arising from the surface of the tongue.
**magenta t.,** the magenta-colored tongue seen in cases of riboflavin deficiency.
**mappy t.,** benign migratory glossitis.
**parrot t.,** the dry, horny tongue of low fever, which cannot be protruded.
**plicated t.,** fissured t.
**raspberry t.,** the dark red tongue with a glistening smooth surface and prominent filiform papillae seen after desquamation of the white coating characteristic of the early stage of scarlet fever. See also *white strawberry t.* Called also *red strawberry t.*
**Sandwith's bald t.,** an extremely clean tongue sometimes seen in the late stages of pellagra.
**scrotal t.,** fissured t.
**smokers' t.,** oral leukoplakia of the tongue.
**smooth t.,** congenital absence of papillae on the dorsum of the tongue in cattle, with hypersalivation and velvety body hair; called also *epitheliogenesis imperfecta linguae bovis.*
**t. of sphenoid bone,** lingula sphenoidalis.
**split t.,** bifid t.

**stippled t.**, a tongue on which each papilla is covered with a separate white patch of epithelium; called also *dotted t.*
**strawberry t.**, 1. a tongue that is dark red colored and whose surface resembles the surface of a strawberry; seen in conditions such as *Staphylococcus aureus* infection, mucocutaneous lymph node syndrome, and streptococcal pharyngitis. 2. raspberry tongue.
**strawberry t., red,** raspberry t.
**strawberry t., white,** the white-coated tongue with prominent red papillae characteristic of the early stage of scarlet fever; the coating desquamates, leaving a beefy red tongue *(raspberry t.).*
**sulcated t.**, fissured t.
**timber t.**, wooden t.
**white t.**, a condition in which all or part of the papillae and epithelium of the tongue have a dull white color.
**wooden t.**, actinobacillosis of cattle in which hard tumor-like nodules form inside the tongue; called also *timber t.*
**wrinkled t.**, fissured t.

**tongue-tie** (tung'ti) ankyloglossia.

**ton·ic** (ton'ik) [Gr. *tonikos*] 1. producing and restoring the normal tone. 2. characterized by continuous tension. 3. a term formerly used for a class of medicinal preparations believed to have the power of restoring normal tone to tissue.
**bitter t.**, a tonic of bitter taste, used for stimulating the appetite and improving digestion, such as quinine, quassia, and gentian.
**cardiac t.**, one which strengthens the heart's action, such as digitalis, strophanthin, or strychnine.
**digestive t.**, an intestinal or stomachic tonic.
**intestinal t.**, one that improves the tone of the intestinal tract.
**stomachic t.**, one which aids the functions of the stomach; here are classed the alcoholic stimulants, vegetable bitters, hydrochloric and nitrohydrochloric acids.
**vascular t.**, one which increases the tone of the blood vessels; among them are belladonna, digitalis, ergot, and strychnine.

**ton·ic-clon·ic** (ton'ik klon'ik) tonicoclonic.

**to·nic·i·ty** (to-nis'ĭ-te) the state of tissue tone or tension; in body fluid physiology, the effective osmotic pressure equivalent.

**ton·i·co·clon·ic** (ton″ĭ-ko-klon'ik) both tonic and clonic; said of a spasm or seizure consisting of a convulsive twitching of the muscles. Called also *tonic-clonic* and *tonoclonic.*

**ton(o)-** [Gr. *tonos* tension] a combining form denoting relationship to tone or tension.

**Tono·card** (to'no-kahrd) trademark for a preparation of tocainide hydrochloride.

**tono·clon·ic** (ton″o-klon'ik) tonicoclonic.

**tono·fi·bril** (ton'o-fi″bril) a bundle of fine filaments (tonofilaments) in certain cells, especially epithelial cells, the individual strands of which transverse the cytoplasm in all directions and extend into the cell processes to converge and insert on the desmosomes; they are thought to have a supportive or cytoskeletal function and, in keratinizing epithelia, to be the principal precursor of cytokeratin.

**tono·fil·a·ment** (ton″o-fil'ə-mənt) [MeSH: Intermediate Filaments] any of the fine filaments of a tonofibril; because most occur in epithelial cells and are formed of keratin, the term is often used synonymously with *keratin filament.*

**to·no·gram** (to'no-gram) the record produced by tonography.

**to·no·graph** (to'no-graf) [*tono-* + *-graph*] a recording tonometer.

**to·nog·ra·phy** (to-nog'rə-fe) [*tono-* + *-graphy*] the recording of changes in intraocular pressure produced by the constant application of a known weight on the globe of the eye, reflecting the facility of outflow of the aqueous humor from the anterior chamber.
**carotid compression t.**, a test for occlusion of the carotid artery by measuring ocular pressure and pulse before, during, and after the proximal portion of the carotid artery is compressed by the fingers.

**to·nom·e·ter** (to-nom'ə-tər) [*tono-* + *-meter*] 1. an instrument for measuring tension or pressure. 2. specifically, an instrument by which intraocular pressure is measured; called also *ophthalmotonometer.*
**air-puff t.**, an instrument for measuring intraocular pressure; it does not touch the eye, but rather senses deflections of the cornea in reaction to a puff of pressurized air.
**applanation t.**, an instrument that measures intraocular pressure by determination of the force necessary to flatten a corneal surface of constant size.
**electronic t.**, one having an electronic readout.
**Gärtner's t.**, an instrument for measuring blood pressure by means of a compressing ring applied to the finger.
**Goldmann's applanation t.**, an instrument for measuring intraocular pressure which eliminates the effects of scleral resistance.
**impression t., indentation t.**, an instrument that measures direct pressure on the eyeball, such as the Schiøtz, McLean, or MacKay-Marg electronic tonometer.
**MacKay-Marg electronic t.**, an electronic applanation tonometer equipped with a flat plunger which measures intraocular pressure by direct application to the cornea.
**McLean t.**, impression t.
**Recklinghausen's t.**, an instrument for observing oscillatory blood pressure.
**Schiøtz t.**, an instrument that registers intraocular pressure by direct application to the cornea, the reading on the scale being translated into millimeters of mercury by means of a conversion table.

**to·nom·e·try** (to-nom'ə-tre) [*tono-* + *-metry*] [MeSH: Tonometry] 1. the measurement of tension or pressure. 2. ophthalmotonometry.
**digital t.**, estimation of the degree of intraocular pressure by pressure exerted on the eyeball by the finger of the examiner.

**tono·plast** (ton'o-plast) [*tono-* + *-plast*] the limiting membrane of an intracellular vacuole, the vacuole membrane.

**tono·top·ic** (ton″o-top'ik) having a spatial arrangement such that certain tone frequencies are transmitted along a particular portion of the structure, as in the cochlear nuclei.

**tono·top·ic·i·ty** (ton″o-top-is'ĭ-te) the property of being tonotopic.

**ton·sil** (ton'sil) [MeSH: Tonsil] 1. a small rounded mass of tissue, especially lymphoid tissue. Called also *tonsilla.* 2. tonsilla palatina.
**adenoid t.**, tonsilla pharyngea.
**buried t.**, submerged t.
**t. of cerebellum,** tonsilla cerebelli.
**eustachian t.**, tonsilla tubaria.
**faucial t.**, tonsilla palatina.
**Gerlach's t.**, tonsilla tubaria.
**intestinal t.**, see *folliculi lymphatici aggregati.*
**lingual t.**, tonsilla lingualis.
**Luschka's t.**, tonsilla pharyngea.
**palatine t.**, tonsilla palatina.
**pharyngeal t.**, tonsilla pharyngea.
**submerged t.**, a palatine tonsil that is shrunken and atrophied and is partly or entirely hidden by the palatoglossal arch.
**third t.**, tonsilla pharyngea.
**t. of torus tubarius, tubal t.**, tonsilla tubaria.
**tubal t.**, tonsilla tubaria.

**ton·sil·la** (ton-sil'ə) pl. *tonsil'lae* [L.] [TA] tonsil: general anatomical nomenclature for a small rounded mass of tissue, especially lymphoid tissue.
**t. adenoi'dea,** t. pharyngea.
**t. cerebel'li** [TA], tonsilla of cerebellum: a rounded mass forming part of the caudal lobe of the hemisphere of the cerebellum continuous with the uvula of the vermis; called also *ventral paraflocculus* and *paraflocculus ventralis* [TA alternative].
**t. intestina'lis,** see *folliculi lymphatici aggregati.*
**t. lingua'lis** [TA], lingual tonsil: an aggregation of lymph follicles on the floor of the oropharyngeal passageway, at the root of the tongue.
**t. palati'na** [TA], palatine tonsil: either of two small, almond-shaped masses located between the palatoglossal and palatopharyngeal arches, one on either side of the oropharynx, composed mainly of lymphoid tissue, covered with mucous membrane, and containing various crypts and many lymph follicles. Called also *tonsil* and *faucial tonsil.*
**t. pharyn'gea** [TA], pharyngeal tonsil: the diffuse lymphoid tissue and follicles in the roof and posterior wall of the nasopharynx; called also *adenoid tonsil, t. adenoidea,* and *t. pharyngealis.* See also *adenoid* (def. 2).
**t. pharyngea'lis,** t. pharyngea.
**t. tuba'ria** [TA], tubal tonsil: a collection of lymphoid tissue associated with the pharyngeal opening of the auditory tube; called also *eustachian tonsil, Gerlach's tonsil,* and *tonsil of torus tubarius.*

**ton·sil·lar** (ton'sĭ-lər) [L. *tonsillaris*] of or pertaining to a tonsil; called also *amygdaline.*

**ton·sil·lec·to·my** (ton″sĭ-lek'tə-me) [*tonsill-* + *-ectomy*] [MeSH: Tonsillectomy] surgical removal of a tonsil or tonsils.

**ton·sil·lith** (ton'sĭ-lith) tonsillolith.

**ton·sil·lit·ic** (ton″sĭ-lit'ik) pertaining to or affected with tonsillitis.

**ton·sil·li·tis** (ton″sĭ-li'tis) [*tonsill-* + *-itis*] [MeSH: Tonsillitis] inflammation of the tonsils, especially the palatine tonsils.
**acute t.**, tonsillitis of abrupt onset, usually due to infection with a bacteria (commonly a beta-hemolytic streptococcus) or a virus. Characteristics include swelling, chills and fever, headache, and pain in the throat with dysphagia. See also *lacunar t.* and *streptococcal pharyngitis.*
**caseous t.**, lacunar tonsillitis in which the crypts contain caseous material.
**chronic t.**, persistent inflammation of the tonsils resulting from recurrent infections; called also *t. lenta.*
**diphtherial t.**, diphtheria involving the tonsils.
**follicular t.**, lacunar t.

**herpetic t.,** a local manifestation of herpes on the tonsil.
**lacunar t.,** acute tonsillitis affecting the crypts of the tonsils; see also *caseous t.* Called also *follicular t.*
**t. len'ta,** chronic t.
**lingual t.,** inflammation of the lingual tonsils.
**mycotic t.,** tonsillomycosis.
**streptococcal t.,** acute tonsillitis resulting from streptococcal pharyngitis that infects the tonsils.
**Vincent's t.,** acute necrotizing ulcerative gingivitis involving only the tonsils.

**tonsill(o)-** [L. *tonsilla,* q.v.] a combining form denoting relationship to a tonsil or to the tonsils.

**ton·sil·lo·ad·e·noid·ec·to·my** (ton″sĭ-lo-ad″ə-noid-ek'tə-me) adenotonsillectomy.

**ton·sil·lo·lith** (ton-sil'o-lith) [*tonsillo-* + *-lith*] a concretion or calculus in a tonsil. Called also *tonsillar calculus.*

**ton·sil·lo·my·co·sis** (ton-sil″o-mi-ko'sis) a fungal infection of the tonsils. Called also *mycotic tonsillitis.*

**ton·sil·lop·a·thy** (ton″sĭ-lop'ə-the) [*tonsillo-* + *-pathy*] any disease of the tonsil.

**ton·sil·lo·tome** (ton-sil'o-tōm) guillotine.

**ton·sil·lot·o·my** (ton″sĭ-lot'ə-me) [*tonsillo-* + *-tomy*] incision of a tonsil; the surgical removal of a part of a tonsil.

**ton·sil·lo·ty·phoid** (ton″sĭ-lo-ti'foid) pharyngotyphoid.

**ton·so·lith** (ton'so-lith) tonsillolith.

**to·nus** (to'nəs) [L.; Gr. *tonos*] the slight, continuous contraction of muscle, which in skeletal muscles aids in the maintenance of posture and in the return of blood to the heart. See *tone.*

**Tooth's disease (atrophy)** (to͞oths) [Howard Henry *Tooth,* English physician, 1856–1925] Charcot-Marie-Tooth disease.

**tooth** (to͞oth) pl. *teeth* [L. *dens;* Gr. *odous*] [MeSH: Tooth] 1. any of the hard calcified structures set in the alveolar processes of the mandible and maxilla for mastication of food. In humans, there are two sets of teeth (*dentes* [TA]), *deciduous* and *permanent.* Each tooth consists of three parts: the *crown* (see *corona dentis*), the *neck* (see *cervix dentis*), and the *root* (see *radix dentis*). The solid part includes *dentin,* forming most of the tooth and resembling true bone; *enamel,* a very hard inorganic substance, covering the crown; and *cementum,* covering the root. In the center is the soft pulp (see *pulpa dentis*). See also *dentition.* 2. a structure resembling the tooth of an animal.

## Tooth

**abutment t.,** one selected to support a bridge on the basis of the total surface area of a healthy attachment apparatus. See also *abutment,* def. 2.
**accessional teeth,** the molar teeth of the permanent dentition, so called because they do not supplant any deciduous predecessors in the dental arch. Cf. *succedaneous teeth.*
**anatomic teeth,** 1. artificial teeth that duplicate the anatomic forms of natural teeth. 2. teeth that have prominent pointed or rounded cusps on the masticating surfaces and are designed to occlude with the teeth of the opposing denture or natural dentition.
**ankylosed t.,** submerged t.
**anterior teeth,** the incisor and canine teeth, which are in the anterior parts of the dental arches. Called also *labial* or *morsal teeth.*
**artificial t.,** one fabricated for use as a substitute for a natural tooth in a prosthesis, usually made of porcelain or resin. See also *denture.*
**auditory teeth, auditory teeth of Huschke,** dentes acustici.
**t. of axis,** dens axis.
**baby teeth,** deciduous teeth.
**bicuspid t.,** premolar t.
**buccal teeth,** posterior teeth.
**canine t.,** the tooth immediately lateral to the lateral, or second, incisor; it has a long conical crown and the longest, most powerful root of all the teeth. Called also *canine, cuspid, cuspid t.,* and *dens caninus* [TA].
**carnassial t.,** a large molar or premolar of a carnivore, specialized for shearing and tearing.
**cheek teeth,** posterior teeth.
**cog t. of malleus,** spur of malleus.
**conical t.,** peg t.
**connate t.,** geminate t.
**corner t.,** the third incisor on either side of each jaw in the horse. Called also *corner.*
**cross-bite teeth,** artificial posterior teeth designed to permit positioning of the modified buccal cusps of the upper teeth in the fossae of the lower teeth.
**cross-pin teeth,** artificial teeth in which the pins are inserted horizontally.
**cuspid t.,** canine t.
**cuspless t.,** any tooth deprived of a cusp; particularly an artificial tooth designed without cuspal prominences on the occlusal surface.
**deciduous teeth,** the 20 teeth of the first dentition, which are shed and replaced by the permanent teeth. They begin to calcify at about the fourth month of fetal life, and near the end of the sixth month they all have begun to develop. The first incisors appear at about the age of $6\frac{1}{2}$ months; they are followed by the second incisors $\frac{1}{2}$ month later; and, within $1\frac{1}{2}$ months, by the maxillary incisors. The deciduous molars begin eruption a 1 year, and the deciduous canines approximately 4 months later. All the deciduous teeth are expected to erupt by the time the child is $2\frac{1}{2}$ years of age. The deciduous dentition formula (one side) is as follows:

$$I\tfrac{2}{2}\,C\tfrac{1}{1}\,M\tfrac{2}{2} = 10$$

where I = *incisor;* C = *canine;* M = *molar.* Symbol D. Called also *baby, milk, primary,* or *temporary teeth; deciduous, first, primary,* or *temporary dentition;* and *dentes decidui*[TA].

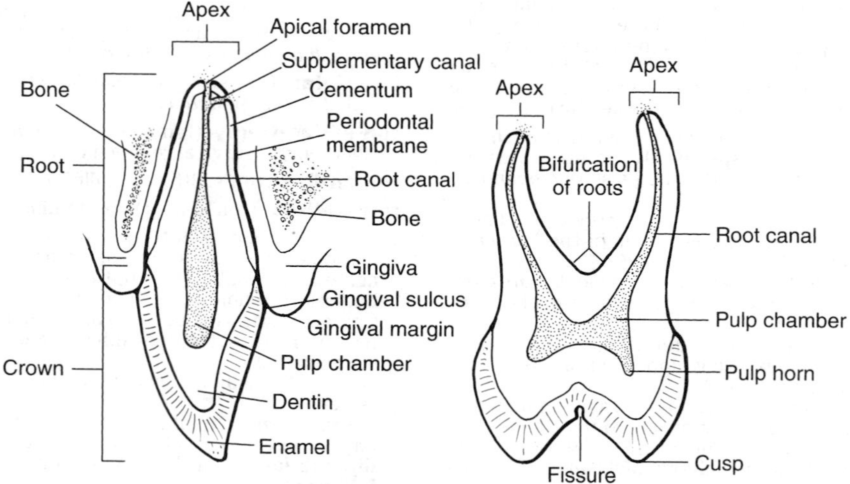


Schematic cross section of an anterior *(left)* and a posterior *(right)* tooth in the maxilla.

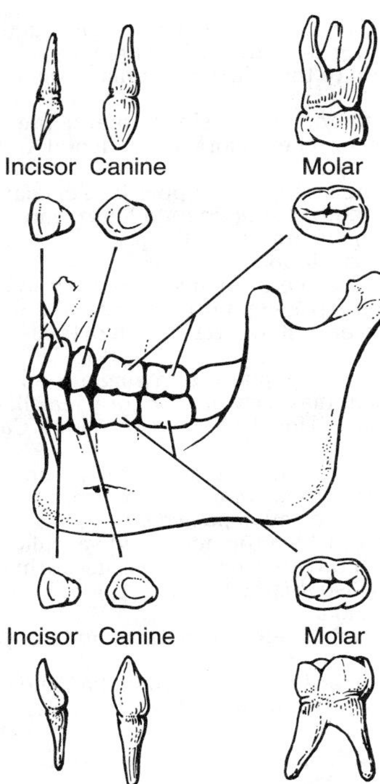


Typical deciduous teeth.

**diatoric teeth,** artificial teeth with holes in their bases into which the denture base material flows and, when processed, attaches the teeth to the base. Called also *pinless teeth.*

**drifting t.,** wandering t.

**embedded t.,** one that is unerupted because of lack of eruptive force.

**t. of epistropheus,** dens axis.

**eye t.,** colloquial term for a canine tooth of the upper jaw.

**Fournier teeth,** Moon's teeth.

**fused teeth,** partial or complete fusion of two or more individual teeth.

**geminate t.,** a tooth with a single root and root canal, but with two completely or incompletely separated crowns, resulting from invagination of a single tooth germ, causing incomplete formation of two teeth. Called also *connate t.*

**Goslee t.,** an interchangeable artificial tooth attached to a metal base.

**hag teeth,** upper medial incisors that are widely separated.

**Horner's teeth,** incisor teeth that are horizontally grooved owing to a deficiency of enamel.

**Hutchinson's teeth,** a tooth abnormality seen in congenital syphilis, in which the permanent incisors have a screwdriver-like shape, sometimes associated with notching of the incisal edges or depressions in the labial surfaces above the cutting edge. Called also *Hutchinson's incisors* and *screwdriver teeth.*

**impacted t.,** one prevented from erupting by a physical barrier. See also *unerupted t.*

**incisor t.,** either of the two most frontal teeth in each jaw, one on either side of the midline; it has a long root and is adapted for cutting. Symbol I. Called also *incisor* and *dens incisivus* [TA].

**labial teeth,** anterior teeth.

**malacotic teeth,** teeth that are soft in structure and are abnormally susceptible to caries.

**malposed t.,** a tooth out of its normal position.

**mandibular teeth,** the teeth of the mandible, or lower jaw.

**maxillary teeth,** the teeth of the maxilla, or upper jaw.

**metal insert t.,** an artificial tooth, usually of acrylic resin, containing an inserted ribbon of metal or a cutting blade in the occlusal surface, with one edge exposed; sometimes used in removable dentures.

**milk t.,** 1. predeciduous t. 2. neonatal t. 3. deciduous t.

**molar t.,** the most posterior teeth on either side in each jaw, totaling 8 in the deciduous dentition (2 on each side, upper and lower), and usually 12 in the permanent dentition (3 on each side, upper and lower). They are the grinding teeth, having large crowns with broad chewing surfaces. The upper molars characteristically have 4 major cusps and three roots. The lower first molars characteristically have 5 cusps, and the remaining lower molars 4 cusps. Normally all lower molars have two roots. The third molars ("wisdom teeth") are often malformed, but when developed normally their crown and root form corresponds in general with neighboring molars in the same jaw. Symbol M. Called also *molars* and *dentes molares* [TA].

**molar t., third,** the tooth most distal to the medial line on either side in each jaw, so called because it is the last of the permanent dentition to erupt, usually at the age of 17 to 21 years. Called also *wisdom t., third molar, dens molaris tertius* [TA], and *dens serotinus* [TA alternative].

**Moon's teeth,** small, domed first molars observed in patients with congenital syphilis.

**morsal teeth** [L. *morsus* a seizing], anterior teeth.

**mottled teeth,** see under *enamel.*

**mulberry t.,** mulberry molar.

**natal t.,** predeciduous t.

**neonatal t.,** one that erupts within the first month of life. Called also *milk t.*

**nonanatomic teeth,** a term applied to artificial teeth the occlusal surfaces of which are especially designed on the basis of engineering concepts, without regard to the features of natural teeth.

**peg t., peg-shaped t.,** one having a conical form, whose sides converge or taper together incisally, instead of being parallel or diverging mesially and distally; a condition frequently observed in the maxillary lateral incisor. Called also *conical t.*

**permanent teeth,** the 32 teeth of the second dentition, which begin to appear in humans at about 6 years of age. The first molars appear first, followed by the mandibular central and lateral incisors, maxillary central incisors, maxillary lateral incisors, mandibular canines, first premolars, second premolars, maxillary canines, second molars, and third molars. They take their position posterior to the deciduous teeth and erupt in succession, whenever the jaws grow sufficiently to accommodate them. Exfoliation of the deciduous teeth is brought about by resorption of their roots, and the succedaneous permanent teeth take their place. The permanent dentition formula (one side) is as follows:

$$I^2_2\,C^1_1\,P^2_2\,M^3_3 = 16$$

where I = *incisor;* C = *canine;* P = *premolar;* M = *molar.* Called also *dentes permanentes* [TA] and *permanent* or *secondary dentition.*

**pink t. of Mummery,** internal tooth resorption (def. 1).

**pinless teeth,** diatoric teeth.

**posterior teeth,** the premolar and molar teeth, which are in the posterior parts of the dental arches. Called also *buccal* or *cheek teeth.*

**predeciduous t.,** any tooth present at birth, which may be normal in all respects or may represent a hornified epithelial rootless structure, found on the gingivae over the crest of the ridge before eruption

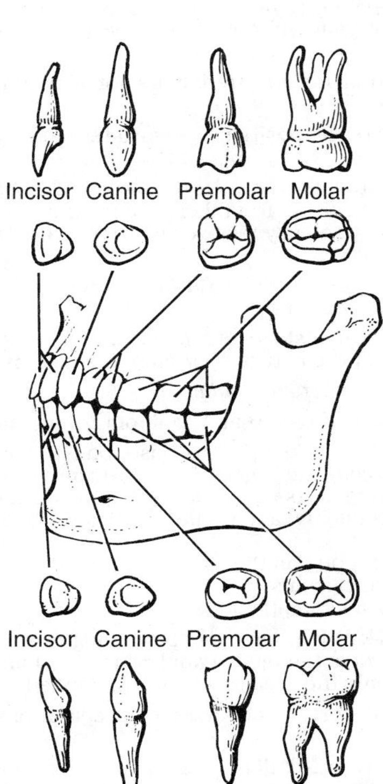


Typical permanent teeth.

of the deciduous teeth. Called also *dentia praecox, milk* or *natal t.,* and *predeciduous dentition.*

**premature teeth,** deciduous teeth that erupt prior to the end of the third month of life, or permanent teeth that erupt prior to the end of the fourth year of life. Called also *dentia praecox* and *precocious* or *premature dentition.* See also *predeciduous teeth.*

**premolar t.,** 1. the permanent teeth between the canines and the molars; there are two on either side in each jaw. The upper premolars are bicuspid and the lower have from one to three cusps. Premolars are succedaneous to the deciduous molar teeth. Symbol P. Called also *dentes premolares* [TA], *premolars, bicuspids,* and *bicuspid teeth.* 2. in animals other than humans, the teeth that succeed the deciduous molars regardless of the number to be succeeded.

**primary teeth,** deciduous teeth.

**pulpless t.,** a tooth from which the pulp has been extirpated.

**rake teeth,** teeth that are widely separated.

**rootless teeth,** dentin dysplasia.

**sclerotic teeth,** teeth that are hard in structure and resistant to caries.

**screwdriver teeth,** Hutchinson's teeth.

**shell t.,** a condition characterized by dysplasia of the dentin, associated with essentially normal enamel, thus resulting in an extremely large pulp chamber and root canal that give the affected tooth the appearance of a shell.

**snaggle t.,** a tooth out of proper line with the others.

**stomach t.,** a canine tooth of the mandible.

**straight-pin teeth,** artificial teeth in which the pins are inserted vertically.

**submerged t.,** a deciduous tooth, usually a second mandibular molar, that has undergone resorption and has become ankylosed to the bone, thus preventing its exfoliation and subsequent replacement by a permanent tooth; it appears to be submerged below the level of occlusion in relation to the adjacent permanent teeth. Called also *ankylosed t.*

**succedaneous teeth, successional teeth,** the permanent teeth that have deciduous predecessors in the dental arch. Cf. *accessional teeth.*

**superior teeth,** the teeth of the upper jaw, or maxilla.

**supernumerary teeth, supplemental teeth,** natural teeth in excess of the number normally present in the jaw.

**temporary teeth,** deciduous teeth.

**tube teeth,** artificial teeth having a vertical, cylindrical aperture from the center of the base up into the body of the tooth, into which a pin may be placed or cast for attachment of the tooth to the denture base.

**Turner's t.,** enamel hypoplasia of a single tooth, most commonly one of the permanent maxillary incisors or a maxillary or mandibular premolar, resulting from local infection or trauma. Called also *Turner's hypoplasia.*

**unerupted t.,** one that failed to erupt; the presence of multiple unerupted permanent teeth is sometimes referred to as *pseudoanodontia.* See also *embedded t.* and *impacted t.*

**vital teeth,** teeth to which the nerve and vascular supply is intact.

**wandering t.,** a tooth that drifts from its normal position in the dental arch. Called also *drifting t.*

**wisdom t.,** third molar t.

**wolf t.,** a vestigial first premolar tooth sometimes present in the jaw of a horse.

**zero degree teeth,** artificial teeth which have no cusp angles in relation to the horizontal on their occlusal surfaces.

---

**tooth·ache** (tōōth'āk) [MeSH: Toothache] pain in a tooth. Called also *dentagra, dentalgia,* and *odontalgia.*

**tooth-borne** (tōōth'born) supported entirely by the teeth; said of a prosthesis or part of a prosthesis entirely supported by the abutment teeth.

**top·ag·no·sia** (top″ag-no'zhə) [*topo-* + *agnosia*] 1. atopognosia. 2. loss of ability to recognize familiar surroundings.

**top·ag·no·sis** (top″ag-no'sis) atopognosia.

**to·pal·gia** (to-pal'jə) [*top-* + *-algia*] pain fixed in one spot, a common feature of pain without organic basis, as seen in conversion disorder.

**To·pa·max** (to'pə-maks) trademark for a preparation of topiramate.

**-tope** [Gr. *topos* place, position] a word termination denoting place or position.

**to·pec·to·my** (to-pek'tə-me) [*top-* + *-ectomy*] ablation of a small and specific area of the frontal cortex, for the treatment of certain forms of epilepsy and psychiatric disorders; called also *corticectomy* and *frontal gyrectomy.*

**top·es·the·sia** (top″es-the'zhə) [*topo-* + *esthesia*] the power of localizing a tactile sensation.

**to·pha·ceous** (to-fa'shəs) [L. *tophaceus: tophus* porous stone] hard or gritty; of the nature of or characterized by tophi.

**to·phi** (to'fi) [L.] plural of *tophus.*

**topho·li·po·ma** (tof″o-lĭ-po'mə) a lipoma containing tophi.

**to·phus** (to'fəs) pl. *to'phi* [L. "porous stone"] a chalky deposit of sodium urate occurring in gout; tophi form most often around joints in cartilage, bone, bursae, and subcutaneous tissue and in the external ear, producing a chronic, foreign-body inflammatory response.

**auricular t.,** a tophus on the ear.

**dental t.,** dental calculus.

**t. syphili'ticus,** a syphilitic node.

**top·i·cal** (top'ĭ-kəl) [Gr. *topikos*] pertaining to a particular surface area, as a topical anti-infective applied to a certain area of the skin and affecting only the area to which it is applied.

**Top·i·cort** (top'ĭ-kort) trademark for preparations of desoximetasone.

**Top·i·cy·cline** (top″ĭ-si'klēn) trademark for a topical preparation of tetracycline hydrochloride; used in treatment of acne.

**Top·i·nard's angle, line** (to″pe-nahrz') [Paul *Topinard,* French physician and anthropologist, 1830–1911] see *ophryospinal angle,* under *angle,* and see under *line.*

**to·pi·ra·mate** (to-pi'rə-māt) a substituted monosaccharide used as an anticonvulsant in the treatment of partial seizures; administered orally.

**top(o)-** [Gr. *topos* place] a combining form meaning place.

**topo·an·es·the·sia** (top″o-an″es-the'zhə) atopognosia.

**topo·chem·is·try** (top″o-kem'is-tre) the chemical composition at specific sites of a structure, as at the surface membrane of a cell.

**top·og·no·sis** (top″og-no'sis) [*topo-* + Gr. *gnōsis* recognition] topesthesia.

**topo·graph·ic** (top″o-graf'ik) describing or pertaining to special regions.

**topo·graph·i·cal** (top″o-graf'ĭ-kəl) pertaining to topography.

**to·pog·ra·phy** (to-pog'rə-fe) [*topo-* + *-graphy*] the description of an anatomical region or of a special part.

**topo·iso·mer** (to″po-i'so-mər) a DNA molecule that differs from another only in linking number, the number of times one strand of the helix wraps around the other in a right hand direction.

**topo·isom·er·ase** (to″po-i-som'ə-rās) an enzyme that interconverts topoisomers of DNA by breaking and rejoining one or more phosphodiester bonds and altering the degree of supercoiling of the DNA.

**type I t.,** DNA topoisomerase.

**type II t.,** DNA topoisomerase (ATP-hydrolyzing).

**topo·log·i·cal** (top-o-loj-ĭ-kəl) pertaining to topology.

**to·pol·o·gy** (tə-pol'ə-je) [*topo-* + *-logy*] 1. the relation between the presenting part of the fetus and the birth canal. 2. regional anatomy. 3. in molecular biology, mathematical description of the tertiary structure of a DNA helix whose ends are not capable of free rotation; it is defined as $L = I \times W$ where $L$ is the linking number, the total number of times one strand winds around the other in a right hand direction, $I$ is the twisting number, the number of helical turns, and $W$ is the writhing number, the number of superhelical turns.

**topo·nym** (top'o-nim) the name of a region as distinguished from an organ.

**to·pon·y·my** (to-pon'ĭ-me) [*topo-* + Gr. *onoma* name] terminology pertaining to the regions of the body.

**To·po·sar** (to'po-sahr) trademark for a preparation of etoposide.

**to·po·te·can hy·dro·chlo·ride** (to″po-te'kan) a cytotoxic inhibitor of DNA topoismerase (type I topoisomerase), which prevents the rejoining of DNA strands following breakage by DNA topoisomerase, leading to double-strand DNA breakage and cell death, used in the treatment of metastatic ovarian carcinoma after failure of first-line or subsequent chemotherapy; administered by intravenous infusion.

**topo·therm·es·the·si·om·e·ter** (top″o-thərm″əs-the-ze-om′ə-tər) [*topo-* + *thermesthesiometer*] an apparatus for measuring the local temperature sense.

**TOPV** poliovirus vaccine live oral trivalent.

**To·ra·dol** (tor′ə-dol) trademark for preparations of ketorolac tromethamine.

**TORCH** toxoplasmosis, other agents, rubella, cytomegalovirus, herpes simplex; see under *syndrome.*

**tor·cu·lar** (tor′ku-lər) [L. "wine-press"] a hollow, or expanded area.
**t. Hero′phili,** confluens sinuum.

**To·rek operation** (to′rek) [Franz J. A. *Torek,* American surgeon, 1861–1938] see under *operation.*

**to·re·mi·fene cit·rate** (tor′ə-mĭ-fēn″) an analogue of tamoxifen that acts as an estrogen antagonist, used in the palliative treatment of metastatic carcinoma of the breast.

**to·ri** (to′ri) [L.] plural of *torus.*

**to·ric** (tor′ik) pertaining to or resembling a torus.

**Tor·kild·sen's shunt (operation)** (tor′kild-senz) [Arne *Torkildsen,* Norwegian neurosurgeon, born 1899] ventriculosternal shunt.

**tor·mi·na** (tor′mĭ-nə) [L.] old name for *colic.*

**tor·mi·nal** (tor′mĭ-nəl) pertaining to or characterized by griping pain, or colic.

**Torn·waldt's (Thorn·waldt's) bursa, bursitis (disease)** (torn′vahlts) [Gustav Ludwig *Tornwaldt* (or *Thornwaldt*), German physician, 1843–1910] see under *abscess* and *bursitis,* and see *bursa pharyngealis.*

**to·rose** (to′rōs) [L. *torosus* muscular, brawny] bulging or knobby; torous.

**to·rous** (to′rəs) torose.

**Tor·o·vi·rus** (tor″o-vi′rəs) [*torus* + *virus* ] [MeSH: Torovirus] the toroviruses; a genus of viruses of the family Coronaviridae having a tubular nucleocapsid that may bend into an open torus; organisms cause gastrointestinal disease. It includes Berne and Breda viruses, as well as human and porcine toroviruses.

**tor·o·vi·rus** (tor′o-vi″rəs) [MeSH: Torovirus] any virus belonging to the genus *Torovirus.*

**tor·pent** (tor′pənt) [L. *torpere* to be sluggish] 1. torpid. 2. an agent that reduces irritation.

**tor·pid** (tor′pid) [L. *torpidus* numb, sluggish] not acting with normal vigor and facility.

**tor·pid·i·ty** (tor-pid′ĭ-te) torpor.

**tor·por** (tor′por) [L.] lack of response to normal or ordinary stimuli.
**t. re′tinae,** a condition in which the retina is excited to action only by stimuli of considerable luminous power.

**torque** (tork) [L. *torquēre* to twist] [MeSH: Torque] 1. a rotatory force causing a part of a structure to twist about an axis. Symbol $\tau$. 2. the rotation of a tooth on its long axis, especially moving the root apex in a buccal or lingual direction through the application of force produced by torsion within the arch wire. See also *torsion.*

**torqu·ing** (tork′ing) the twisting of a tooth into position, as in the correction of malposition.

**torr** (tor) [after Evangelista *Torricelli,* Italian mathematician and physicist, 1608–1647] a unit of pressure equal to exactly $\frac{1}{760}$ atmosphere, equal to one millimeter of mercury (mm Hg) to within one part in 7 million.

**Tor·re's syndrome** (tor′āz) [Douglas Paul *Torre,* American dermatologist, born 1919] see under *syndrome.*

**tor·re·fac·tion** (tor″ə-fak′shən) [L. *torrefactio*] the act of roasting or parching.

**tor·re·fy** (tor′e-fi) [L. *torrefacere*] to parch, roast, or dry by the aid of heat.

**tor·ri·cel·li·an** (tor″e-chel′e-ən) named for Evangelista *Torricelli,* Italian mathematician, 1608–1647; see under *vacuum.*

**tor·sades de pointes** (tor-sahd′ də pwant) [Fr. "fringe of pointed tips"] [MeSH: Torsades de Pointes] an atypical rapid ventricular tachycardia with periodic waxing and waning of amplitude of the QRS complexes on the electrocardiogram as well as rotation of the complexes about the isoelectric line; it may be self-limited or may progress to ventricular fibrillation.

**tor·se·mide** (tor′sə-mīd) a diuretic chemically related to sulfonylurea, used to treat edema in cases of congestive heart failure, hepatic disease, or kidney disease; administered orally or intravenously.

**tor·sion** (tor′shən) [L. *torsio,* from *torquēre* to twist] [MeSH: Torsion] 1. the act or process of twisting; turning or rotating about an axis. 2. a type of mechanical stress, whereby the external forces (load) twist an object about its axis. See also *torque.* 3. in ophthalmology, any rotation of the vertical corneal meridians; such movements are severely limited under normal conditions. See also *extorsion* and *intorsion.* Called also *cyclorotation* and *wheel rotation.*
**abomasal t., t. of the abomasum,** twisting of the abomasum of a cow, often three to six weeks after birth of a calf and after subclinical right displacement of the abomasum (see under *displacement*); symptoms include distention of the abdomen, acute abdominal pain, shock, and (if untreated) circulatory failure and death within 48 hours. Called also *abomasal volvulus.*
**negative t.,** rotation in a counterclockwise direction.
**positive t.,** rotation in a clockwise direction.

**tor·sion·om·e·ter** (tor″shən-om′ə-tər) [*torsion* + *-meter*] an apparatus for estimating the degree of rotation of the spinal column.

**tor·sive** (tor′siv) twisted.

**tor·si·ver·sion** (tor″sĭ-vər′zhən) [L. *torquere* to twist + *version*] the turning or rotation of a tooth on its long axis.

**tor·so** (tor′so) the trunk without the head or limbs.

**tor·ti·col·lar** (tor″tĭ-kol′ər) pertaining to or affected with torticollis.

**tor·ti·col·lis** (tor″tĭ-kol′is) [L. *tortus* twisted + *collum* neck] [MeSH: Torticollis] wryneck; a contracted state of the cervical muscles, producing twisting of the neck and an unnatural position of the head.
**congenital t.,** torticollis due to injury to the sternocleidomastoid muscle on one side at the time of birth and its transformation into a fibrous cord which cannot lengthen with the growing neck.
**dermatogenic t.,** torticollis caused by contraction of the skin of the neck.
**fixed t.,** an unnatural position of the head due to actual and persistent organic muscular shortening.
**hysterical t.,** that of psychogenic origin.
**intermittent t.,** spasmodic t.
**labyrinthine t.,** torticollis due to irritation of the semicircular canals on one side.
**mental t.,** a form of tic, or habit spasm, in which there is spasmodic contraction of the neck muscles, producing deviation of the head. This deviation usually ceases when the patient lies down, or it may be controlled by slight pressure.
**myogenic t.,** a transient condition due to muscular contraction in rheumatism, and to cold.
**neurogenic t.,** spasmodic t.
**ocular t.,** torticollis due to a high degree of astigmatism or to ocular muscle palsy.
**reflex t.,** torticollis caused by inflammation or suppuration in the neck, enlarged cervical lymph nodes, or tumor in the tonsil, neck, or pharynx.
**spasmodic t.,** torticollis due to intermittent dystonia and spasms of neck muscles, particularly the sternocleidomastoid and trapezius muscles. The cause is unknown, although irritation of the accessory nerve has been implicated in some cases. Cf. *retrocollis* and *rotatory spasm.* Called also *intermittent* or *neurogenic t.*
**spurious t.,** twisting or stiffness of the neck due to caries of the cervical vertebrae.
**symptomatic t.,** stiffness of the neck due to spasm of the sternomastoid or adjacent muscles.

**tor·ti·pel·vis** (tor″tĭ-pel′vis) dystonia musculorum deformans.

**tor·tu·ous** (tor′choo-əs) twisted; full of turns and twists.

**To·ru·la** (tə-roo′lə) 1. *Cryptococcus.* 2. a genus of Fungi Imperfecti

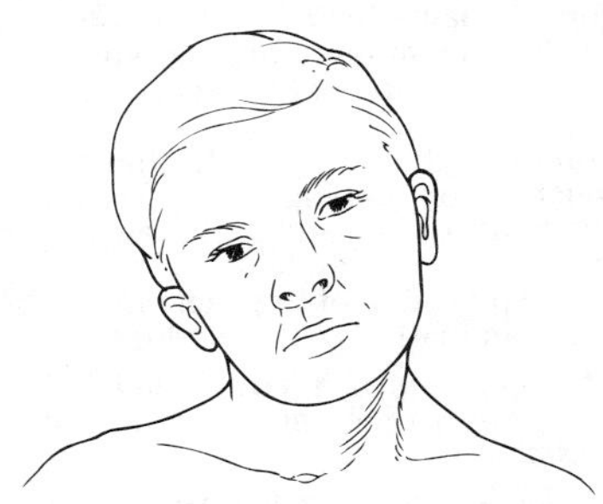

Torticollis.

of the form-class Hyphomycetes, form-family Dematiaceae. *T. jeansel'mei* is a former name for *Exophiala jeanselmei.*

**tor·u·li** (tor'u-li) [L.] plural of *torulus.*

**Tor·u·lop·sis** (tor″u-lop'sis) a genus of Fungi Imperfecti of the family Cryptococcaceae; it is closely related to *Candida* and some authorities have considered it the same genus. Some species are normal inhabitants of the skin, respiratory tract, gastrointestinal tract, and urogenital region but may also cause opportunistic infections.
**T. capsula'tus,** former name for *Histoplasma capsulatum.*
**T. glabra'ta,** a species that is part of the normal flora of the human mouth, gut, and urinary tract but that in weak or immunocompromised patients may cause opportunistic infections such as torulopsosis, meningitis, pneumonia, cystitis, and fungemia. Called also *Candida glabrata.*
**T. neofor'mans,** *Cryptococcus neoformans.*

**tor·u·lop·so·sis** (tor″u-lop'so-sis) infection by *Torulopsis glabrata*; symptoms resemble those of histoplasmosis.

**tor·u·lo·sis** (tor″u-lo'sis) [*Torula* + *-osis*] cryptococcosis.

**tor·u·lus** (tor'u-ləs) pl. *to'ruli* [L., dim. of *torus*] a small elevation or papilla.
**to'ruli tac'tiles** [TA], tactile elevations: the small elevations on the skin of the palm and the sole, richly supplied with sensory nerve endings.

**to·rus** (tor'əs) pl. *to'ri* [L. "a round swelling," "protuberance"] 1. [TA] a general term in anatomical nomenclature for a bulging projection or swelling. 2. the doughnut-shaped geometric figure produced by rotating a circle about an axis that lies in the same plane as the circle but does not cut the circle.
**t. aor'ticus,** a bulge in the anterosuperior part of the right coronary wall, caused by the proximity of the right aortic cusp and sinus.
**t. fronta'lis,** a protuberance in the middle line of the root of the nose, on the external surface of the skull.
**t. levato'rius** [TA], the mucosal fold covering the levator veli palatini muscle in the lateral wall of the nasal part of the pharynx.
**t. mandibula'ris** [TA], mandibular torus: a prominence sometimes seen on the lingual aspect of the mandible at the base of its alveolar part, adjacent to the postcanine teeth.
**t. occipita'lis,** a rounded edge occasionally seen on the occipital bone in the region of the superior nuchal line.
**t. palati'nus** [TA], palatine torus: a bony protuberance sometimes found on the hard palate at the junction of the intermaxillary suture and the transverse palatine suture.
**t. tuba'rius** [TA], tubal prominence: the projecting posterior lip of the pharyngeal opening of the auditory tube. Called also *eustachian cushion* and *tubal protuberance.*
**t. urete'ricus,** plica interureterica.

**to·sy·late** (to'sə-lāt) USAN contraction for *p*-toluenesulfonate.

**To·ta·cil·lin** (to″tə-sil'in) trademark for preparations of ampicillin.

**To·ti's operation** (to'tēz) [Addeo *Toti,* Italian ophthalmologist, early 20th century] dacryocystorhinostomy.

**to·ti·po·ten·cy** (to″tĭ-po'tən-se) [L. *totus* all + *potency*] the ability of a part to develop in any manner, or of a cell to develop into any type of cell.

**to·tip·o·tent** (to-tip'ə-tənt) totipotential.

**to·ti·po·ten·tial** (to″tĭ-po-ten'shəl) [L. *totus* all + *potential*] characterized by ability to develop in any direction; said of cells which can give rise to cells of all orders, i.e., to the complete individual. Cf. *unipotential.*

**to·ti·po·ten·ti·al·i·ty** (to″tĭ-po-ten″she-al'ĭ-te) the ability to differentiate along any line or into any type of cell.

**touch** (tuch) [L. *tactus;* Old Fr. *touchier*] [MeSH: Touch] 1. the sense (actually a group of senses) by which contact with objects gives evidence as to certain of their qualities, as registered by mechanoreceptors in the skin and mucous membranes. Types of touch include light touch, coarse touch, tickling, pressure sense, vibration sense, tissue distortion sense, and pain sense. Called also *tactile sense* and *taction.* 2. palpation or exploration with the finger.
**abdominal t.,** digital palpation of the abdomen.
**double t.,** digital examination of the rectum and vagina at the same time.
**rectal t.,** exploration of the rectum with the finger.
**royal t.,** the touching or tapping of a person with scrofula; once practiced by the kings of England and France as a supposedly curative measure.
**vaginal t.,** digital exploration of the vagina.
**vesical t.,** digital examination of the bladder.

**touch·er·ism** (tuch'ər-iz-əm) a paraphilia in which sexual arousal or orgasm is achieved by touching or fondling or by such fantasies. See also *frotteurism.*

**Tou·raine-So·lente-Go·lé syndrome** (too-ren'so-lahnt'go-la') [Albert *Touraine,* French dermatologist, 1883–1961; G. *Solente,* French physician, 20th century; L. *Golé,* French physician, 20th century] pachydermoperiostosis.

**Tou·rette** see *Gilles de la Tourette.*

**Tour·nay's sign** (tōōr-nāz') [Auguste *Tournay,* French ophthalmologist, 1878–1969] see under *sign.*

**tour·ni·quet** (toor'nĭ-kət) [Fr.] [MeSH: Tourniquets] an instrument for compression of a blood vessel by application around an extremity to control the circulation and prevent the flow of blood to or from the distal area.
**automatic rotating t.,** a system consisting of a motor, air compressor, and four blood pressure cuffs for application to the extremities; the cuffs are inflated and deflated in series and in sequence for treatment of acute pulmonary edema.
**Esmarch's t.,** see under *bandage.*
**garrote t.,** Spanish windlass.
**pneumatic t.,** a narrow rubber bag to be wound around a limb, pressure being applied by pumping air into the inflatable cuff.
**scalp t.,** a tourniquet placed around the scalp with enough pressure to occlude the superficial blood vessels and thereby to lessen the risk of drug-induced alopecia.
**Spanish t., torcular t.,** Spanish windlass.

**Tou·ton giant cell** (toot'on) [Karl *Touton,* German dermatologist, 1858–1934] see under *cell.*

**Towne's projection** (tounz) [Edward Bancroft *Towne,* American physician, 1883–1957] see under *projection.*

**Townes syndrome** (tounz) [Philip Leonard *Townes,* American pediatrician, born 1927] see under *syndrome.*

**Town·send ionization** (toun'zənd) [John *Townsend,* Irish physicist, 1868–1957] see *avalanche ionization,* under *ionization.*

**tox·ane·mia** (tok″sə-ne'me-ə) toxic hemolytic anemia.

**tox·a·phene** (toks'ə-fēn) [MeSH: Toxaphene] a chlorinated hydrocarbon used as an agricultural insecticide; if ingested or absorbed through the skin by a human or other animal, it may cause neurotoxicity such as tremors and potentially fatal convulsions. Called also *camphechlor.*

**Tox·as·ca·ris** (tok-sas'kə-ris) [MeSH: Toxascaris] a genus of parasitic nematodes of the family Ascarididae.
**T. leoni'na,** a species found commonly in large felines such as lions and tigers, and in domestic dogs and cats, especially older ones. Its larvae differ from those of *Toxocara canis* and *T. cati* by not passing through the lungs of the infected animal.

**tox·emia** (tok-se'me-ə) [*tox-* + *-emia*] [MeSH: Toxemia] 1. any condition resulting from the spread of toxins by the bloodstream. 2. any condition resulting from the spread of toxic bacterial products such as endotoxins or exotoxins in the blood.
**eclamptic t., eclamptogenic t.,** eclampsia.
**hydatid t.,** toxemia with urticaria caused by hydatid fluid which has escaped into the peritoneal cavity.
**pregnancy t. in cows,** fat cow syndrome.
**pregnancy t. in ewes,** an acute disorder in ewes caused by ketosis during the last few weeks of pregnancy, especially when they are carrying twins, triplets, or a large single lamb; the usual cause is undernutrition associated with stress. It can lead to impaired nervous function, coma, and death. Called also *twin-lamb disease* and *lambing paralysis.*

**tox·emic** (tok-se'mik) pertaining to or caused by toxemia.

**tox·en·zyme** (toks-en'zīm) any poisonous enzyme.

**toxi-** see *tox(o)-.*

**tox·ic** (tok'sik) [Gr. *toxikon (pharmakon)* poison for arrows, from *toxon* bow] 1. pertaining to, due to, or of the nature of a toxin; called also *poisonous* and *venomous.* 2. manifesting the symptoms of severe infection.

**tox·i·cant** (tok'sĭ-kənt) [L. *toxicans* poisoning] 1. poisonous. 2. a poisonous agent.

**tox·i·ca·tion** (tok″sĭ-ka'shən) poisoning.

**tox·i·ce·mia** (tok″sĭ-se'me-ə) toxemia.

**tox·i·cide** (tok'sĭ-sīd) [*toxi-* + *-cide*] a drug capable of overcoming toxic agents. Cf. *antitoxin.*

**tox·ic·i·ty** (tok-sis'ĭ-te) the quality of being poisonous, especially the degree of virulence of a toxic microbe or of a poison.
**$O_2$ t., oxygen t.,** the effects of hyperoxia due to the breathing of high partial pressures of oxygen for prolonged periods; they include serious, sometimes irreversible, damage to the pulmonary capillary endothelium, followed by cerebral edema and convulsions that can be fatal. Called also *oxygen poisoning.*

**toxic(o)-** a combining form meaning poisonous or denoting relationship to poison. See also *tox(o)-.*

**tox·i·co·den·drol** (tok″sĭ-ko-den'drol) a poisonous, nonvolatile oil found in certain plants of the genus *Rhus (Toxicodendron).*

**Tox·i·co·den·dron** (tok″sĭ-ko-den′dron) [*toxico-* + Gr. *dendron* tree] [MeSH: Toxicodendron] *Rhus.*

**tox·i·co·gen·ic** (tok″sĭ-ko-jen′ik) [*toxico-* + *-genic*] producing or elaborating toxins.

**tox·i·co·he·mia** (tok″sĭ-ko-he′me-ə) toxemia.

**tox·i·coid** (tok′sĭ-koid) resembling a poison.

**tox·i·co·log·ic** (tok″sĭ-ko-loj′ik) pertaining to toxicology.

**tox·i·col·o·gist** (tok″sĭ-kol′ə-jist) an individual who specializes in toxicology.

**tox·i·col·o·gy** (tok″sĭ-kol′ə-je) [MeSH: Toxicology] the sum of what is known regarding poisons; the scientific study of poisons, their actions, their detection, and the treatment of the conditions produced by them.
**developmental t.,** the study of the effects of toxins on embryos in utero. Cf. *teratology.*

**tox·i·cop·a·thy** (tok″sĭ-kop′ə-the) [*toxico-* + *-pathy*] toxicosis.

**tox·i·co·pec·tic** (tok″sĭ-ko-pek′tik) pertaining to, characterized by, or promoting toxicopexis.

**tox·i·co·pex·ic** (tok″sĭ-ko-pek′sik) toxicopectic.

**tox·i·co·pex·is** (tok″sĭ-ko-pek′sis) [*toxico-* + *pexis*] the fixing or neutralizing of a poison in the body.

**tox·i·co·pexy** (tok′sĭ-ko-pek″se) toxicopexis.

**tox·i·co·phid·ia** (tok″sĭ-ko-fid′e-ə) [*toxico-* + Gr. *ophis* snake] venomous snakes.

**tox·i·co·pho·bia** (tok″sĭ-ko-fo′be-ə) [*toxico-* + *-phobia*] irrational fear of being poisoned.

**tox·i·co·sis** (tok″sĭ-ko′sis) [*toxic-* + *-osis*] any disease condition due to poisoning. See also entries under *poisoning.*
**exogenic t.,** poisoning by the ingestion of toxic material, as in the food. See *food poisoning,* under *poisoning.*
**fescue t.,** fescue foot.
**gestational t.,** preeclampsia.
**hemorrhagic capillary t.,** Schönlein-Henoch purpura.
**proteinogenous t.,** an acute and fatal intoxication which appears in white mice which are fed an exclusive diet of various proteins.
**retention t.,** that which is due to the nonexcretion of noxious waste products.
**tick t.,** sweating sickness.

**toxi·cyst** (tok′sĭ-sist) [*toxi-* + *cyst*] one of the numerous toxic subpellicular organelles occurring as slender extrusible tubular structures located apically in certain ciliate protozoa, especially certain of the Kinetofragminophorea, with which the organism penetrates the body of and cytolyzes its prey. Cf. *trichocyst.*

**tox·if·er·ous** (tok-sif′ər-əs) [*toxi-* + *-ferous*] 1. carrying or conveying a poison. 2. toxicogenic.

**tox·i·gen·ic** (tok″sĭ-jen′ik) toxicogenic.

**tox·i·ge·nic·i·ty** (tok″sĭ-jə-nis′ĭ-te) the disease-producing virulence of a parasite which acts by virtue of a soluble toxin.

**tox·ig·nom·ic** (tok″sig-nom′ik) [*toxin* + Gr. *gnōmē* a means of knowing] characteristic of the toxic action of a poison.

**tox·in** (tok′sin) [Gr. *toxikon (pharmakon)* poison for arrows, from *toxon* bow] a poison; frequently used to refer specifically to a protein produced by some higher plants, certain animals, and pathogenic bacteria, which is highly toxic for other living organisms. Such substances are differentiated from the simple chemical poisons and the vegetable alkaloids by their high molecular weight and antigenicity.
**A-B t's,** a class of exotoxins consisting of an active (A) component that crosses the cell membrane and a binding (B) component that binds to cell surface receptors.
***Amanita* t.,** amatoxin.
**animal t.,** zootoxin.
**anthrax t.,** an exotoxin produced by most strains of *Bacillus anthracis* that is immunogenic, produces edema, and is lethal for mice. It consists of three heat-labile, antigenically distinct components: edema factor (EF, factor I), protective antigen (PA, factor II), and lethal factor (LF, factor III).
**bacterial t's,** toxic substances produced by bacteria, including exotoxins, endotoxins, enterotoxins, neurotoxins, and toxic enzymes.
**botulinal t., botulinum t., botulinus t.,** an exotoxin produced by germinating spores and growing cells of *Clostridium botulinum.* The toxin binds to presynaptic terminals of the central nervous system and blocks the release of acetylcholine, leading to paralysis. There are seven immunologically distinct types (A–G). Type A is one of the most powerful poisons known; it is also used therapeutically by injection to inhibit muscular spasm in the treatment of dystonic disorders such as blepharospasm and strabismus and to reduce anal sphincter pressure to promote healing of chronic anal fissure. See also *botulism.*
**cholera t.,** an exotoxin produced by *Vibrio cholerae;* a protein enterotoxin that binds to the membrane of enteric cells and stimulates the adenylcyclase system, causing the hypersecretion of chloride and bicarbonate ions, resulting in increased fluid secretion and the severe diarrhea of cholera.
**clostridial t.,** one elaborated by species of *Clostridium,* including those causing botulism *(botulinus t.),* gas gangrene *(gas gangrene t.),* and tetanus *(tetanus t.).* In addition, *C. difficile* produces an exotoxin causing severe intestinal necrosis. *C. perfringens* produces a number of exotoxins causing gas gangrene, intestinal necrosis, and hemolysis, some with cardiotoxic, deoxyribonuclease, and hyaluronidase activity, and an enterotoxin causing acute food poisoning.
**Dick t.,** streptococcal pyrogenic toxin; used in the Dick test.
**diphtheria t.,** a protein exotoxin produced by virulent (lysogenic) strains of *Corynebacterium diphtheriae* that is primarily responsible for the pathogenesis of diphtheritic infection. It is an enzyme that inhibits protein synthesis by inactivating a factor (EF-2) required for the transfer of polypeptidyl-tRNA from acceptor to donor sites on ribosomes.
**diphtheria t., diagnostic,** diphtheria t. for Schick test.
**diphtheria t., inactivated diagnostic,** Schick test control.
**diphtheria t. for Schick test** [USP], a standardized preparation of diphtheria toxin used in the Schick test (q.v.). Formerly called *diagnostic diphtheria t.*
**dysentery t.,** an exotoxin produced by various species of *Shigella.* That formed by *S. dysenteriae* serotype 1 (Shiga toxin) is a soluble protein with hemorrhagic and paralytic properties. It is a highly potent neurotoxin.
**erythrogenic t.,** streptococcal pyrogenic exotoxin.
**extracellular t.,** a toxin excreted by a bacterial cell; an exotoxin.
**fatigue t.,** kenotoxin.
**fugu t.,** tetrodotoxin.
**fusarial t.,** any mycotoxin produced by molds of the genus *Fusarium.* See also *fusariotoxicosis.*
**gas gangrene t.,** an exotoxin produced by *Clostridium perfringens* and associated with gas gangrene. At least 10 types have been identified. The $\alpha$ toxin is a lethal, necrotizing lecithinase (phospholipase-C) that splits lecithin in cell membranes, is hemolytic, and causes capillary damage. *C. novyi* and *C. septicum* produce similar toxins causing gas gangrene.
**intracellular t.,** a toxin developed and retained within the bacterial cell; an endotoxin.
**plague t.,** a necrotizing exotoxin produced by *Yersinia pestis;* its significance in the pathology of plague is unclear.
**plant t.,** phytotoxin.
**pseudomonal t.,** an exotoxin produced by *Pseudomonas aeruginosa.* It is a protein, lethal for mice and rats and toxic for fibroblast cultures, which inhibits protein synthesis by inactivating elongation factor $EF_2$.
**Shiga t.,** the exotoxin formed by *Shigella dysenteriae* type 1.
**Shiga-like t.,** verocytotoxin.
**soluble t.,** exotoxin.
**staphylococcal t.,** a mixture of exotoxins produced by *Staphylococcus aureus.* There are four chemically and serologically distinct hemolysins ($\alpha$, $\beta$, $\gamma$, and $\delta$) having also dermonecrotic activity ($\alpha$-hemolysin), sphingomyelinase activity ($\beta$-hemolysin), necrotizing activity ($\gamma$-hemolysin), and leukocidin activity ($\delta$-hemolysin). Other toxins produced are leukocytal and exfoliative (causing scalded skin syndrome). Strains of *S. aureus* also produce five serologically distinct enterotoxins: types A and D are major factors in staphylococcal food poisoning.
**streptococcal t.,** a mixture of exotoxins formed by *Streptococcus pyogenes,* including two distinct hemolysins *(streptolysin O* and *streptolysin S),* an erythrogenic toxin (causing scarlet fever rash), and a DPNase that is cardiotoxic.
**T-2 t.,** a trichothecene mycotoxin produced by *Fusarium poae, F. sporotrichioides,* and *F. tricinctum,* which contaminates grain and other foodstuffs, causing fusariotoxicosis with hemorrhaging in livestock and alimentary toxic aleukia in humans.
**tetanus t.,** the potent exotoxin produced by *Clostridium tetani,* consisting of two components, one a neurotoxin *(tetanospasmin)* and the other a hemolysin *(tetanolysin).*
**whooping cough t.,** a dermonecrotic exotoxin produced by *Bordetella pertussis* that appears to be associated with the pathogenicity of the organism in whooping cough.

**tox·in-an·ti·tox·in (TA)** (tok″sin-an′tĭ-tok″sin) a nearly neutral mixture of diphtheria toxin with its antitoxin; formerly used for immunization against diphtheria.

**tox·in·emia** (tok″sĭ-ne′me-ə) [*toxin* + *-emia*] poisoning of the blood.

**tox·in·ol·o·gy** (tok″sin-ol′ə-je) the science dealing with the toxins produced by certain higher plants and animals and by pathogenic bacteria.

**tox·in·o·sis** (tok″sĭ-no′sis) any disease condition due to the presence of a toxin.

**tox·ip·a·thy** (tok-sip'ə-the) toxicosis.

**toxi·pho·bia** (tok"sĭ-fo'be-ə) toxicophobia.

**toxi·res·in** (tok"sĭ-rez'in) a poisonous resinous substance obtainable from digitoxin.

**tox·is·ter·ol** (tok-sis'tər-ol) [*toxi-* + *sterol*] a poisonous isomer of ergosterol, produced by ultraviolet radiation of the latter.

**tox(o)-** [Gr. *toxikon (pharmakon)* poison for arrows, from *toxon* bow] a combining form denoting relationship to a toxin, or poison. Also, *toxi-, toxic(o)-.*

**Tox·o·ca·ra** (tok"so-kar'ə) [MeSH: Toxocara] a genus of nematodes of the family Ascarididae.
**T. ca'nis,** a species parasitic in the intestine of dogs; migrating larvae may cause lesions of the lung, liver, kidney, brain, and eye. In human infections, the larvae do not complete their cycle but cause visceral larva migrans (see under *larva*).
**T. ca'ti,** a species closely related to *T. canis* but commonly found in cats; it has also been reported from humans, both as an accidental intestinal parasite and as causing visceral larva migrans (see under *larva*). Called also *T. mystax.*
**T. mys'tax,** *T. cati.*

**tox·o·car·al** (tok"so-kar'əl) pertaining to or caused by *Toxocara.*

**tox·o·car·i·a·sis** (tok"so-kə-ri'ə-sis) [MeSH: Toxocariasis] infection by roundworms of the genus *Toxocara.*
**human t.,** visceral larva migrans (see under *larva*).

**tox·o·gen** (tok'so-jən) something that produces a poison.

**toxo·glob·u·lin** (tok"so-glob'u-lin) a poisonous globulin.

**tox·oid** (tok'soid) [*toxo-* + *-oid*] a modified or inactivated bacterial exotoxin that has lost toxicity but retains the properties of combining with, or stimulating the formation of, antitoxin.
***Clostridium perfringens*** **t.,** see under *bacterin-toxoid.*
**diphtheria t.,** the formaldehyde-inactivated toxin of *Corynebacterium diphtheriae,* used for immunization against diphtheria; both fluid (diphtheria toxoid [USP]) and adsorbed (on alum, aluminum phosphate, or aluminum hydroxide) (diphtheria toxoid adsorbed [USP]) forms are available. It is generally used in mixtures with tetanus toxoid and pertussis vaccine (DTP) or with tetanus toxoid alone (DT for pediatric use and Td, which contains 5- to 10-fold less diphtheria toxoid, for other use). DTP (adsorbed) is recommended for routine immunization of all children under 6 years of age, except when pertussis vaccine is contraindicated, in which case DT (adsorbed) is used. Td (adsorbed) is used for all others. Official names [USP] are *diphtheria t., diphtheria toxoid adsorbed, diphtheria and tetanus toxoids* (DT), *diphtheria and tetanus toxoids adsorbed, diphtheria and tetanus toxoids and pertussis vaccine* (DTP), *diphtheria and tetanus toxoids and pertussis vaccine adsorbed,* and *tetanus and diphtheria toxoids adsorbed for adult use* (Td).
**tetanus t.,** the formaldehyde-inactivated toxins of *Clostridium tetani,* used for immunization against tetanus; both fluid and adsorbed (on alum, aluminum hydroxide, or aluminum phosphate) forms are available. It is used in mixtures with diphtheria toxoid and pertussis vaccine (DTP, DT, and Td; see under *diphtheria t.*) or by itself (T). DTP (adsorbed) and DT (adsorbed) are used for routine immunization of children under 6 years of age. Td (adsorbed) and T (adsorbed) are used for all others. Official names [USP] are *tetanus t.* (T), *tetanus t. adsorbed, tetanus and diphtheria toxoids adsorbed for adult use* (Td), *diphtheria and tetanus toxoids* (DT), *diphtheria and tetanus toxoids adsorbed, diphtheria and tetanus toxoids and pertussis vaccine* (DTP), and *diphtheria and tetanus toxoids and pertussis vaccine adsorbed.*

**tox·oid-an·ti·tox·oid** (tok"soid-an'tĭ-tok"soid) a toxoid mixed with an equivalent amount of antitoxic serum, the precipitate being suspended in saline.

**toxo·lec·i·thid** (tok"so-les'ĭ-thid) toxolecithin.

**toxo·lec·i·thin** (tok"so-les'ĭ-thin) a lecithin compounded with a toxin, as cobra venom.

**toxo·neme** (tok'so-nēm) rhoptry.

**toxo·no·sis** (tok"so-no'sis) toxicosis.

**toxo·pex·ic** (tok"so-pek'sik) toxicopectic.

**toxo·phil** (tok'so-fil) [*toxo-* + *-phil*] having an affinity for toxins.

**toxo·phil·ic** (tok"so-fil'ik) [*toxo-* + *-philic*] easily susceptible to a poison; having an affinity for toxins (like certain haptophore groups).

**tox·oph·i·lous** (tok-sof'ĭ-ləs) toxophilic.

**toxo·phore** (tok'so-for) [*toxo-* + *-phore*] the group of atoms in the molecule of a toxin that is responsible for the toxic effect.

**tox·oph·o·rous** (tok-sof'ə-rəs) pertaining to the toxophore group of a toxin molecule.

**Toxo·plas·ma** (tok"so-plaz'mə) [*toxo-* + *plasma*] [MeSH: Toxoplasma] a genus of coccidian protozoa (suborder Eimeriina, order Eucoccidiida) comprising intracellular parasites of many organs and tissues of birds and mammals, including humans. See *toxoplasmosis.* The only known complete hosts are cats and other Felidae, in which both asexual and sexual developmental cycles occur in the intestinal epithelium, culminating in the passage of oocysts in the feces. The intestinal stages do not occur in other hosts.
**T. cuni'culi,** *T. gondii.*
**T. gon'dii,** an obligate intracellular species found in a wide range of hosts, including humans and other mammals and birds. The sexual cycle of the organism takes place in the intestinal epithelium of the cat, which is the definitive host. It exists in three forms: tachyzoite, tissue cysts (pseudocysts), and oocysts. Infection (see *toxoplasmosis*) occurs chiefly by ingestion of oocytes shed in cat feces or by ingestion of cysts in raw or uncooked meat.

**tox·o·plas·mo·sis** (tok"so-plaz-mo'sis) [*toxo-* + *plasma* + *-osis*] [MeSH: Toxoplasmosis] infection of humans or other animals by the protozoon *Toxoplasma gondii,* transmitted in oocysts in the feces of cats (the definitive host), usually by contaminated soil, direct exposure to feces, tissue cysts in infected meat, or tachyzoites in blood. Most human infections are asymptomatic, but when symptoms occur they range from a mild disease resembling mononucleosis to a fulminating, disseminated disease (usually in an immunocompromised patient or a fetus infected transplacentally) that can cause extensive damage to the brain, eyes, skeletal and cardiac muscles, liver, and lungs. See also *toxoplasmic meningoencephalitis* and *chorioretinitis.* Chorioretinitis may occur with all forms but is usually a late sequel of the congenital form. In domestic animals toxoplasmosis usually is seen as any of several nonfatal conditions such as a type of infectious abortion in ewes.
**ocular t.,** toxoplasmic chorioretinitis.
**pulmonary t.,** infection of the lungs by *Toxoplasma gondii,* usually seen in immunocompromised patients; symptoms resemble those of interstitial plasma cell pneumonia, with fever, coughing, and dyspnea.

**toxo·pro·tein** (tok"so-pro'tēn) 1. a toxic protein; see *toxin.* 2. a mixture of a toxin and a protein.

**tox·uria** (tok-su're-ə) uremia.

**Toyn·bee's corpuscles, experiment, law, otoscope** (toin'bēz) [Joseph *Toynbee,* English otologist, 1815–1866] see under *maneuver* and *test;* see *corneal corpuscles,* under *corpuscle;* and see *Gull-Toynbee law,* under *law.*

**TPA, t-PA** tissue plasminogen activator.

**TPHA** *Treponema pallidum* hemagglutination assay.

**t-plas·min·o·gen ac·ti·va·tor** (plaz-min'o-jən"ak'tĭ-va-tər) [EC 3.4.21.68] see under *activator.*

**TPN** total parenteral nutrition (see *parenteral hyperalimentation,* under *hyperalimentation*); triphosphopyridine nucleotide.

**TPP** thiamine pyrophosphate.

**TR** tricuspid regurgitation.

**tra·be·cu·la** (trə-bĕ'ku-lə) pl. *trabe'culae* [L., dim. of *trabs*] [TA] a general term in anatomical nomenclature for a supporting or anchoring strand of connective tissue, such as one extending from a capsule into the substance of the enclosed organ.
**arachnoid trabeculae, trabeculae arachnoideae** [TA], delicate fibrous threads connecting the inner surface of the arachnoid to the pia mater.
**trabeculae of bone,** anastomosing bony spicules in cancellous bone which form a meshwork of intercommunicating spaces that are filled with bone marrow.
**trabe'culae car'neae cor'dis** [TA], fleshy trabeculae of heart: irregular bundles and bands of muscle projecting from a great part of the interior of the walls of the ventricles of the heart. They occur as three types: as simple muscular ridges, as bundles attached at both ends but free in the middle, or as papillary muscles (q.v.), projecting from the heart wall and attaching to the chordae tendineae cordis.
**trabe'culae cor'dis,** trabeculae carneae cordis.
**trabe'culae cor'porum cavernoso'rum pe'nis** [TA], trabeculae of corpora cavernosa of penis: numerous bands and cords of fibromuscular tissue traversing the interior of the corpora cavernosa of the penis, attached to the tunica albuginea and to the septum and creating the cavernous spaces that become filled with blood during erection.
**trabe'culae cor'poris spongio'si pe'nis** [TA], trabeculae of corpus spongiosum of penis: numerous bands and cords of fibromuscular tissue traversing the interior of the corpus spongiosum of the penis, creating the cavernous spaces that give the structure its spongy character.
**trabe'culae cra'nii,** a pair of longitudinal cranial bars of cartilage in the embryo, bounding the pituitary space that becomes the sella turcica.

**fleshy trabeculae of heart,** trabeculae carneae cordis.
**trabe′culae lie′nis,** TA alternative for *trabeculae splenicae.*
**trabeculae no′di lympha′tici, trabe′culae no′di lymphoi′dei** [TA], trabeculae of lymph node: strands of dense connective tissue radiating out from the capsule through the interior of the node.
**Rathke's trabeculae,** trabeculae cranii.
**t. septomargina′lis** [TA], septomarginal trabecula: a bundle of muscle at the apical end of the right ventricle of the heart, connecting the base of the anterior papillary muscle to the interventricular septum; it usually contains a branch of the atrioventricular bundle. It has been thought to prevent ventricular overdistention and thus is called also *moderator band.*
**trabe′culae sple′nicae** [TA], trabeculae of spleen: fibrous bands that pass into the spleen from the tunica fibrosa and form the supporting framework of the organ; called also *trabeculae lienis* [TA alternative].

**tra·be·cu·lae** (trah-bek′u-le) [L.] plural of *trabecula.*

**tra·bec·u·lar** (trə-bek′u-lər) pertaining to a trabecula.

**tra·bec·u·lar·ism** (trə-bek′u-lar-iz-əm) trabeculation (def. 2).

**tra·bec·u·late** (trə-bek′u-lāt) [L. *trabecula* a small beam or bar] marked with transverse or radiating bars or trabeculae.

**tra·bec·u·la·tion** (trə-bek″u-la′shən) 1. the formation of trabeculae in a part. 2. the condition of being trabeculated.

**tra·bec·u·lec·to·my** (trə-bek″u-lek′tə-me) [*trabecula* + *-ectomy*] [MeSH: Trabeculectomy] creation of a fistula between the anterior chamber of the eye and the subconjunctival space by surgical removal of a portion of the trabecular meshwork, performed to facilitate drainage of the aqueous humor in glaucoma.

**tra·bec·u·lo·plas·ty** (trə-bek′u-lo-plas″te) plastic surgery of a trabecula.
**laser t.,** an operation for open-angle glaucoma, in which surface burns are placed in the trabecular meshwork of the eye to lower intraocular pressure.

**trace** (trās) 1. a very small amount. 2. a sign of the former presence of something.
**memory t.,** engram (def. 3).

**trac·er** (trās′ər) 1. a dissecting instrument for isolating vessels and nerves. 2. a mechanical device by which the outline of an object or the direction and extent of movement of a part may be graphically recorded; see also *tracing.* 3. a means or agent by which certain substances or structures can be identified or followed, as a radioactive tracer.
**arrow-point t.,** needle-point t.
**needle-point t.,** a mechanical device used in recording jaw movements, in which the tracing is made on a horizontal plate by a weighted or a spring-loaded needle attached to the jaw. Called also *arrow-point t.* and *stylus t.* See also under *tracing.*
**radioactive t.,** a radioactive isotope replacing a stable chemical element in a compound (said to be *radiolabeled*) and so able to be followed or tracked through one or more reactions or systems by means of a radiation detector; used especially for such a compound that is introduced into the body for study of the compound's metabolism, distribution, and passage through the body.
**stylus t.,** needle-point t.

**tra·chea** (tra′ke-ə) pl. *tra′cheae* [L., from Gr. *tracheia artēria*] [MeSH: Trachea] 1. [TA] the cartilaginous and membranous tube descending from the larynx and branching into the right and left main bronchi. It is kept patent by a series of about twenty transverse horseshoe-shaped cartilages. Called also *windpipe.* 2. one of a system of minute tubes ramifying throughout the body of a terrestrial arthropod and delivering air to the tissues; called also *tracheal tubule.* See also *tracheole.*
**scabbard t.,** a trachea which is flattened by approximation of its lateral walls.

**tra·cheae** (tra′ke-e) [L.] plural of *trachea.*

**tra·chea·ec·ta·sy** (tra″ke-ə-ek′tə-se) dilatation of the trachea.

**tra·che·al** (tra′ke-əl) [L. *trachealis*] pertaining to the trachea.

**tra·che·al·gia** (tra″ke-al′jə) [*trache-* + *-algia*] pain in the trachea.

**tra·che·itis** (tra″ke-i′tis) [MeSH: Tracheitis] inflammation of the trachea.
**bacterial t.,** an acute crouplike bacterial infection of the upper airway in children, characterized by coughing and high fever; common causative organisms are *Haemophilus influenzae* type B, *Moraxella catarrhalis, Staphylococcus aureus,* and species of *Streptococcus.* Called also *bacterial, membranous,* and *pseudomembranous croup.*

**tra·che·lec·to·my** (tra″ke-lek′tə-me) cervicectomy.

**tra·che·lism** (tra′kə-liz-əm) [Gr. *trachēlismos*] spasm of the neck muscles; spasmodic retraction of the head in epilepsy.

**tra·che·lis·mus** (tra″kə-liz′məs) trachelism.

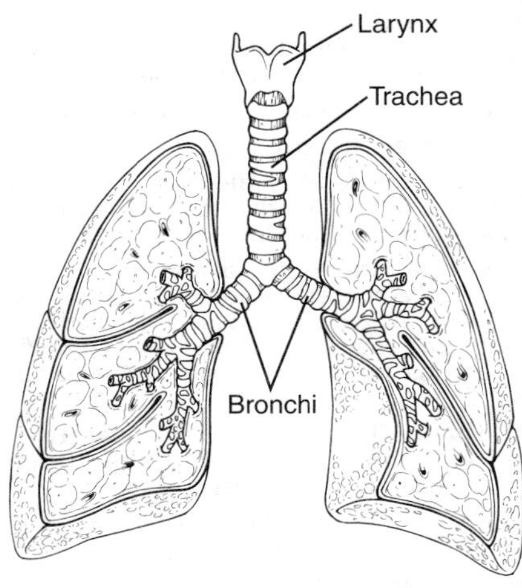


**tra·che·li·tis** (tra″kə-li′tis) cervicitis.

**trachel(o)-** [Gr. *trachēlos* neck] a combining form denoting relationship to the neck or to a necklike structure.

**tra·che·lo·cele** (tra′kə-lo-sēl″) tracheocele.

**tra·che·lo·cyl·lo·sis** (tra″kə-lo-sə-lo′sis) torticollis.

**tra·che·lo·cyr·to·sis** (tra″kə-lo-sir-to′sis) trachelokyphosis.

**tra·che·lo·cys·ti·tis** (tra″kə-lo-sis-ti′tis) [*trachelo-* + *cystitis*] inflammation of the neck of the bladder.

**tra·che·lo·dyn·ia** (tra″kə-lo-din′e-ə) cervicodynia.

**tra·che·lo·ky·pho·sis** (tra″kə-lo-ki-fo′sis) [*trachelo-* + *kyphosis*] abnormal curvature of the cervical portion of the spine.

**tra·che·lol·o·gist** (tra″kə-lol′ə-jist) one skilled in trachelology.

**tra·che·lol·o·gy** (tra″kə-lol′ə-je) [*trachelo-* + *-logy*] the study of the neck and its diseases and injuries.

**tra·che·lo·pexy** (tra′kə-lo-pek″se) [*trachelo-* + *-pexy*] surgical fixation of the neck of the uterus to some other part.

**tra·che·lo·plas·ty** (tra′kə-lo-plas″te) [*trachelo-* + *-plasty*] plastic repair of the cervix uteri.

**tra·che·lor·rha·phy** (tra″kə-lor′ə-fe) [*trachelo-* + *-rrhaphy*] suture of the lacerated cervix uteri.

**tra·che·los·chi·sis** (tra″kə-los′kĭ-sis) [*trachelo-* + *-schisis*] congenital fissure of the neck.

**tra·che·lo·syr·in·gor·rha·phy** (tra″kə-lo-sir″ing-gor′ə-fe) [*trachelo-* + *syringo-* + *-rrhaphy*] trachelorrhaphy for fistula of the vagina.

**tra·che·lot·o·my** (tra″kə-lot′ə-me) [*trachelo-* + *-tomy*] incision of the cervix uteri.

**trache(o)-** [L. *trachea,* q.v.] a combining form denoting relationship to the trachea.

**tra·cheo·aero·cele** (tra″ke-o-ār′o-sēl) [*tracheo-* + *aerocele*] a tracheocele containing air.

**tra·cheo·bron·chi·al** (tra″ke-o-brong′ke-əl) pertaining to the trachea and bronchi. Called also *bronchotracheal.*

**tra·cheo·bron·chi·tis** (tra″ke-o-brong-ki′tis) inflammation of the trachea and bronchi.
**canine infectious t.,** a contagious disease of the respiratory tract, seen in dogs that are confined together in close quarters and spread by aerosol droplets; characteristics include mild cough, laryngitis, and swelling of the air passages. In puppies and weakened animals it may progress to pneumonia. Etiologic agents include *Bordetella bronchiseptica,* adenoviruses, canine parainfluenza virus, and occasionally other bacteria or viruses.

**tra·cheo·bron·cho·meg·a·ly** (tra″ke-o-brong″ko-meg′ə-le) [MeSH: Tracheobronchomegaly] great enlargement of the lumen of the trachea and the larger bronchi, a rare, usually congenital condition. Called also *Mounier-Kuhn syndrome.*

**tra·cheo·bron·chos·co·py** (tra″ke-o-brong-kos′kə-pe) inspection of the interior of the trachea and bronchi.

**tra·cheo·cele** (tra′ke-o-sēl″) [*tracheo-* + *-cele*[2]] hernial protrusion of the tracheal mucous membrane.

**tra·cheo·esoph·a·ge·al** (tra″ke-o-e-sof′ə-je-əl) pertaining to or communicating with both the trachea and esophagus. Called also *esophagotracheal.*

**tra·cheo·fis·tu·li·za·tion** (tra″ke-o-fis″tu-lĭ-za′shən) surgical creation of an opening in the trachea communicating with the cervical skin. See also *tracheostomy* and *tracheotomy.*

**tra·che·o·gen·ic** (tra″ke-o-jen′ik) originating in the trachea.

**tra·cheo·la·ryn·ge·al** (tra″ke-o-lə-rin′je-əl) laryngotracheal.

**tra·che·ole** (tra′ke-ōl) one of the minute, fluid-filled tubules in which the tracheae of a terrestrial arthropod terminate, which contain air cells and permeate all the body tissues.

**tra·cheo·ma·la·cia** (tra″ke-o-mə-la′shə) softening of the tracheal cartilages, often as a congenital condition in infants or in patients of any age after prolonged intubation, and usually accompanied by a barking cough and expiratory stridor or wheezing; nearby organs such as the esophagus or aorta may compress the trachea and cause apnea.

**tra·cheo·path·ia** (tra″ke-o-path′e-ə) tracheopathy.
**t. osteoplas′tica,** a condition marked by the formation of a bony and cartilaginous deposit in the tracheal mucosa.

**tra·che·op·a·thy** (tra″ke-op′ə-the) [*tracheo-* + *-pathy*] disease of the trachea; called also *tracheopathia.*

**tra·cheo·pha·ryn·ge·al** (tra″ke-o-fə-rin′je-əl) pertaining to the trachea and pharynx.

**Tra·che·oph·i·lus** (tra″ke-of′ĭ-ləs) a genus of trematodes. *T. cym′bius* is parasitic in the trachea of ducks in Europe and Asia. *T. cucumeri′nus* is parasitic in the trachea, esophagus, and thoracic cavity of chickens and ducks in Brazil and Madagascar.

**tra·che·oph·o·ny** (tra″ke-of′ə-ne) [*tracheo-* + Gr. *phōnē* voice] a voice sound heard over the trachea.

**tra·cheo·plas·ty** (tra′ke-o-plas″te) [*tracheo-* + *-plasty*] plastic repair of the trachea.

**tra·che·or·rha·gia** (tra″ke-o-ra′jə) [*tracheo-* + *-rrhagia*] hemorrhage from the trachea.

**tra·che·or·rha·phy** (tra″ke-or′ə-fe) [*tracheo-* + *-rrhaphy*] repair of an incised or wounded trachea.

**tra·che·os·chi·sis** (tra″ke-os′kĭ-sis) [*tracheo-* + *-schisis*] fissure of the trachea.

**tra·cheo·scop·ic** (tra″ke-o-skop′ik) pertaining to or of the character of tracheoscopy.

**tra·che·os·co·py** (tra″ke-os′kə-pe) [*tracheo-* + *-scopy*] the inspection of the interior of the trachea.

**tra·cheo·ste·no·sis** (tra″ke-o-stə-no′sis) [*tracheo-* + *stenosis*] contraction or narrowing of the trachea.

**tra·che·os·to·ma** (tra″ke-os′to-mə) [*tracheo-* + *stoma*] an opening into the trachea through the neck. Cf. *tracheostomy,* def. 3.

**tra·che·os·to·mize** (tra″ke-os′tə-mīz) to perform tracheostomy upon.

**tra·che·os·to·my** (tra″ke-os′tə-me) [*tracheo-* + *-stomy*] [MeSH: Tracheostomy] 1. tracheotomy. 2. creation of an opening in the anterior trachea for insertion of a tube to relieve upper airway obstruction and facilitate ventilation. 3. the opening created by either of these processes.

**tra·cheo·tome** (tra′ke-o-tōm) an instrument for use in incising the trachea.

**tra·che·ot·o·mize** (tra″ke-ot′ə-mīz) to perform tracheotomy upon.

**tra·che·ot·o·my** (tra″ke-ot′ə-me) [*tracheo-* + *-tomy*] [MeSH: Tracheotomy] surgical creation of an opening into the trachea through the neck, with the tracheal mucosa being brought into continuity with the skin. Called also *tracheostomy.*
**inferior t.,** one below the isthmus of the thyroid.
**superior t.,** one above the isthmus of the thyroid.

**Tra·chin·i·dae** the weever fishes (q.v.), a family of small stinging bony fishes.

**tra·chi·tis** (trə-ki′tis) tracheitis.

**tra·cho·ma** (trə-ko′mə) pl. *tracho′mata* [Gr. *trachōma* roughness] [MeSH: Trachoma] a chronic infectious disease of the conjunctiva and cornea, producing photophobia, pain, and lacrimation, caused by a strain of *Chlamydia trachomatis.* Clinically, it can be divided into four stages: (1) mild infection with tiny follicles on eyelid conjunctiva and subepithelial infiltration; (2) enlargement of follicles and inflammatory changes forming hard red papillae, usually with vascular invasion of cornea marking the onset of pannus; (3) severe scarring and contraction resulting in symblepharon, entropion, trichiasis, and corneal scarring that may result in blindness; (4) complete arrest with permanent scarring, entropion, and symblepharon. Called also *Arlt's t., Egyptian, granular,* or *trachomatous conjunctivitis, Egyptian* or *granular ophthalmia,* and *granular lids.*
**Arlt's t.,** trachoma.

**tra·cho·ma·ta** (trə-ko′mə-tə) [Gr.] plural of *trachoma.*

**tra·cho·ma·tous** (trə-ko′mə-təs) pertaining to, affected with, or of the nature of trachoma.

**Tra·chyb·del·la** (tra″ke-del′ə) a genus of leeches. *T. bistria′ta* is a species found in Brazil that attacks humans and other animals.

**tra·chy·chro·mat·ic** (tra″ke-kro-mat′ik) [Gr. *trachys* rough + *chromat-* + *-ic*] strongly or deeply staining.

**tra·chy·onych·ia** (trak″e-o-ni′ke-ə) [Gr. *trachys* rough + *onych-* + *-ia*] roughness of nails with brittleness and splitting, often associated with psoriasis, alopecia areata, and lichen planus.

**tra·chy·pho·nia** (tra″kĭ-fo′ne-ə) [Gr. *trachys* rough + *phon-* + *-ia*] hoarseness.

**trac·ing** (trās′ing) 1. a record of movements of the mandible produced by a tracer; the shape of the tracing depends on the relative location of the marking point and the tracing plate, and the apex of a properly made tracing is considered to indicate the most retruded unstrained position of the mandible in relation to the maxilla (centric jaw relation). 2. cephalometric t.
**arrow-point t.,** needle-point t.
**cephalometric t.,** a line drawing of structural outlines of craniofacial landmarks and facial bones made directly from a cephalometric radiogram.
**extraoral t.,** a tracing of mandibular movements made outside the oral cavity.
**Gothic arch t.,** needle-point t.
**intraoral t.,** a tracing of condylar direction made within the oral cavity.
**needle-point t.,** a tracing of the movements of the mandible, resembling an arrowhead or a Gothic arch, made by means of a device attached to the opposing arches, the exact shape depending on the location of the marking point relative to the tracing table; the apex of the tracing is considered as an indication of the centric relation. Called also *arrow point t., Gothic arch t.,* and *stylus t.* See also under *tracer.*
**stylus t.,** needle-point t.

**track** (trak) 1. the path along which something moves, or the mark left by its movement. 2. of pus, to follow the path of least resistance through the tissues, e.g., along an intermuscular septum.
**ionization t.,** see under *path.*

**track·ing** (trak′ing) pursuing or following.
**visual t.,** following an object with one's gaze; it is fundamental to focusing and to the visual aspects of maintaining equilibrium. In brain damaged persons it may be assessed as a test for neurologic status and eye function.

**Tra·cri·um** (tra′cre-um) trademark for a preparation of atracurium besylate.

**tract** (trakt) [L. *tractus*] 1. a region, principally one of some length. 2. a collection or bundle of nerve fibers having the same origin, function, and termination (tractus [TA]); see also under *bundle, fasciculus,* and *lemniscus.* 3. a number of organs, arranged in series, subserving a common function.

## Tract

For descriptions of specific anatomic structures not listed here, see under *tractus,* and see under the entries listed above.

**aerodigestive t., upper,** the respiratory cavities of the head and neck considered together, including the nasal cavity, oral cavity, pharynx, and larynx.
**alimentary t.,** digestive t.
**anterolateral t's,** lemniscus spinalis.
**ascending t.,** any bundle of nerve fibers that conveys impulses toward the brain.
**atriohisian t's,** myocardial fibers that bypass the physiologic delay

of the atrioventricular node and connect the atrium directly to the bundle of His, allowing preexcitation of the ventricle.

**Bekhterev's (Bechterew's) t.,** tractus tegmentalis centralis.

**biliary t.,** the organs, ducts, and other structures that participate in the secretion, storage, and delivery of bile into the duodenum.

**Bruce's t., t. of Bruce and Muir,** fasciculus septomarginalis.

**bulbar t.,** any of the bundles of nerve fibers of the medulla oblongata.

**bulboreticulospinal t.,** tractus bulboreticulospinalis.

**Burdach's t.,** fasciculus cuneatus medullae spinalis.

**central t. of auditory nerve,** a group of fibers that passes from the cochlear nuclei to the superior olive, to the lateral lemniscus on the same and the opposite side and then up through the brachium of the inferior colliculus into the medial geniculate body and from there to the cortex of the transverse temporal gyri.

**cerebellorubral t.,** a group of fibers arising chiefly in the dentate nucleus of the cerebellum and projecting to the opposite red nucleus via the superior cerebellar peduncle; impulses are then relayed to the reticular formation and spinal cord.

**cerebellorubrospinal t.,** a group of fibers that passes from one dentate nucleus of the cerebellum to the contralateral red nucleus, and thence to the spinal cord.

**cerebellospinal t.,** uncinate fasciculus of the cerebellum, from the fastigial nucleus to the cervical cord.

**cerebellotegmental t's of bulb,** fastigiobulbar t's.

**cerebellothalamic t.,** dentatothalamic t.

**comma t. of Schultze,** fasciculus interfascicularis.

**conariohypophyseal t.,** a portion of the cavity of the embryonic brain connecting the pineal body and the pituitary gland.

**corticobulbar t.,** corticonuclear t.

**corticohypothalamic t.,** a diffuse collection of fibers that arise from various parts of the frontal lobe and are distributed directly to the hypothalamus.

**corticonuclear t.,** the nerve fiber tract formed by fibers (corticonuclear fibers) of the pyramidal tract that arise in the cerebral cortex, descend in the internal capsule, and synapse in the various motor nuclei of the mesencephalon, pons, and medulla oblongata. Called also *corticobulbar t.*

**corticopontine t.,** tractus corticopontinus.

**corticorubral t.,** a group of fibers passing from the cerebral cortex to the red nucleus.

**corticospinal t., anterior,** tractus corticospinalis anterior.

**corticospinal t., crossed,** tractus corticospinalis lateralis.

**corticospinal t., direct,** tractus corticospinalis anterior.

**corticospinal t., lateral,** tractus corticospinalis lateralis.

**corticospinal t., ventral,** tractus corticospinalis anterior.

**corticospinal t. of medulla oblongata,** tractus pyramidalis (def. 1).

**corticospinal t's of spinal cord,** the two spinal cord tracts that are continuations of the pyramidal tract of the medulla oblongata; see *tractus corticospinalis lateralis* and *tractus corticospinalis anterior.* Called also *pyramidal t's of spinal cord.*

**corticotectal t., external,** a tract of efferent fibers from visual association areas of the cortex, running transversely into the zonal layer of the superior colliculus.

**corticotectal t., internal,** a tract of efferent fibers from visual association areas of the cortex, running through the intermediate gray and white layers of the superior colliculus and carrying impulses to muscles controlling eye coordination.

**cuneocerebellar t.,** the dorsal external arcuate fibers considered as a unit.

**Deiters' t.,** tractus vestibulospinalis.

**dentatothalamic t.,** a group of fibers arising chiefly in the dentate nucleus of the cerebellum and projecting to the ventral lateral nucleus of the opposite thalamus via the cranial cerebellar peduncle; impulses are then relayed to the frontal lobe. Called also *cerebellothalamic tract.*

**descending t.,** any bundle of nerve fibers that conveys impulses from the brain toward the periphery.

**digestive t.,** the part of the digestive system (q.v.) formed by the esophagus, stomach, and small and large intestines; called also *alimentary canal, alimentary t., canalis alimentarius, digestive canal, digestive tube,* and *tubus digestorius.*

**dorsolateral t.,** tractus posterolateralis.

**extracorticospinal t., extrapyramidal t.,** extrapyramidal system.

**fastigiobulbar t's,** bundles of efferent fibers running from the nucleus fastigii to the medulla oblongata.

**fiber t's of spinal cord,** distinct bundles in the white substance of the spinal cord, made up of fibers which have the same origin, termination, and function.

**Flechsig's t.,** tractus spinocerebellaris posterior.

**flow t. of the heart,** the path of the blood within the chambers of the heart. In the *left flow tract,* blood enters the left atrium through the pulmonary veins, flows through the mitral valve into the left ventricle, and passes through the aortic valve and on into the aorta and systemic circulation. In the *right flow tract,* blood enters the right atrium through the venae cavae, flows through the tricuspid valve into the right ventricle, and passes through the pulmonary valve and on into the pulmonary artery and the pulmonary circulation.

**frontopontine t.,** tractus frontopontinus.

**gastrointestinal t.,** the stomach and intestines in continuity.

**geniculocalcarine t., geniculostriate t.,** radiatio optica.

**genitourinary t.,** apparatus urogenitalis.

**Goll's t.,** fasciculus gracilis medullae spinalis.

**Gowers' t.,** tractus spinocerebellaris anterior.

**habenulointerpeduncular t., habenulopeduncular t.,** tractus habenulointerpeduncularis.

**Helweg's t.,** olivospinal t.

**hypothalamicohypophysial t., hypothalamohypophysial t.,** tractus hypothalamohypophysialis.

**intermediolateral t.,** columna intermediolateralis medullae spinalis.

**internodal t's,** specialized conduction pathways, designated anterior, middle, and posterior, that preferentially transmit the cardiac impulse through the atria; their existence and details remain controversial.

**internuncial t.,** a fiber tract connecting two nuclei or centers.

**intersegmental t. of spinal cord, anterior,** fasciculus proprius anterior medullae spinalis.

**intersegmental t. of spinal cord, dorsal,** fasciculus proprius posterior medullae spinalis.

**intersegmental t. of spinal cord, lateral,** fasciculus proprius lateralis medullae spinalis.

**intersegmental t. of spinal cord, posterior,** fasciculus proprius posterior medullae spinalis.

**intersegmental t. of spinal cord, ventral,** fasciculus proprius anterior medullae spinalis.

**interstitiospinal t.,** tractus interstitiospinalis.

**intestinal t.,** the small and large intestines in continuity.

**Lissauer's t.,** tractus posterolateralis.

**Löwenthal's t.,** tractus tectospinalis.

**Maissiat's t.,** tractus iliotibialis.

**mammillopeduncular t.,** a fiber tract from the mammillary body to nuclei in the interpeduncular fossa.

**mammillotegmental t.,** fasciculus mammillotegmentalis.

**mammillothalamic t.,** fasciculus mammillothalamicus.

**Marchi's t.,** tractus tectospinalis.

**mesencephalic t. of trigeminal nerve,** tractus mesencephalicus nervi trigemini.

**Meynert's t.,** tractus habenulointerpeduncularis.

**Monakow's t.,** tractus rubrospinalis.

**motor t.,** any bundle of nerve fibers conveying motor impulses from the central nervous system to a muscle.

**nigrostriate t.,** a bundle of nerve fibers extending from the substantia nigra to the globus pallidus and putamen in the corpus striatum; injury to it may be a cause of parkinsonism. Its interlacing pattern with fibers of the internal capsule gives it a comblike appearance. Called also *comb bundle.*

**occipitopontile t., occipitopontine t.,** see *occipitopontine fibers,* under *fiber.*

**olfactory t.,** tractus olfactorius.

**olivocerebellar t.,** tractus olivocerebellaris.

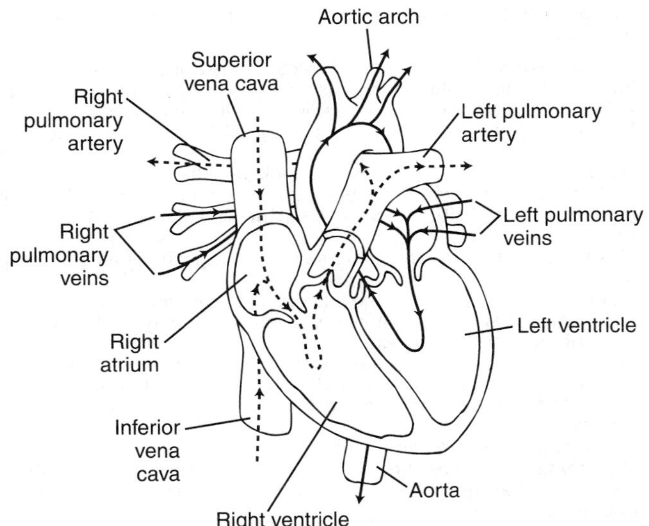


Flow tracts of the heart, left *(solid line)* and right *(dotted line).*

**Tract** *Continued*

**olivocochlear t.,** tractus olivocochlearis.
**olivospinal t.,** a group of nerve fibers in the lateral funiculus, seen as a triangular area in transverse section of the spinal cord; it descends from the olivary nucleus through the medulla oblongata to the upper cervical segments. Called also *Helweg's tract* or *bundle* and *triangular tract.*
**optic t.,** tractus opticus.
**paraventriculohypophysial t.,** tractus paraventriculohypophysialis.
**parietopontine t.,** see *fibrae parietotemporopontinae,* under *fibra.*
**peduncular t., transverse,** a small band of fibers which passes from the brachium of the inferior colliculus to the sulcus medialis cruris cerebri.
**t. of Philippe-Gombault,** Gombault-Philippe triangle.
**pontoreticulospinal t.,** tractus pontoreticulospinalis.
**posterolateral t.,** tractus posterolateralis.
**pyramidal t.,** tractus pyramidalis.
**pyramidal t., anterior,** tractus corticospinalis anterior.
**pyramidal t., crossed,** tractus corticospinalis lateralis.
**pyramidal t., direct,** tractus corticospinalis anterior.
**pyramidal t., lateral,** tractus corticospinalis lateralis.
**pyramidal t., ventral,** tractus corticospinalis anterior.
**pyramidal t. of medulla oblongata,** tractus pyramidalis (def. 1).
**pyramidal t's of spinal cord,** corticospinal t's of spinal cord; see *tractus corticospinalis lateralis* and *tractus corticospinalis anterior.*
**respiratory t.,** see under *system.*
**reticulospinal t., reticulospinal t., anterior,** tractus reticulospinalis anterior.
**reticulospinal t., lateral, reticulospinal t., medullary,** tractus bulboreticulospinalis.
**reticulospinal t., medial,** tractus pontoreticulospinalis.
**reticulospinal t., ventral,** tractus reticulospinalis anterior.
**rubrobulbar t.,** tractus rubrobulbaris.
**rubroreticular t.,** a group of fibers extending from the red nucleus to the reticular formation of the pons and medulla oblongata.
**rubrospinal t.,** tractus rubrospinalis.
**Schultze's t., semilunar t.,** fasciculus interfascicularis.
**Schütz's t.,** fasciculus longitudinalis posterior.
**sensory t.,** any bundle of nerve fibers conveying sensory impulses from a peripheral receptor to the central nervous system.
**septomarginal t.,** fasciculus septomarginalis.
**solitary t. of medulla oblongata,** tractus solitarius medullae oblongatae.
**spinal t. of trigeminal nerve,** tractus spinalis nervi trigemini.
**spinocerebellar t., anterior,** tractus spinocerebellaris anterior.
**spinocerebellar t., direct, spinocerebellar t., dorsal, spinocerebellar t., posterior,** tractus spinocerebellaris posterior.
**spinocerebellar t., ventral,** tractus spinocerebellaris anterior.
**spinocervical t.,** tractus spinocervicalis.
**spinocervicothalamic t.,** a tract ascending uncrossed in the posterior part of the lateral funiculus to the lateral cervical nucleus, which relays to the thalamus by way of the opposite medial lemniscus.
**spinoolivary t.,** tractus spinoolivaris.
**spinoreticular t.,** tractus spinoreticularis.
**spinotectal t.,** tractus spinotectalis.
**spinothalamic t.,** tractus spinothalamicus lateralis.
**spinothalamic t., anterior,** tractus spinothalamicus anterior.
**spinothalamic t., lateral,** tractus spinothalamicus lateralis.
**spinothalamic t., ventral,** tractus spinothalamicus anterior.
**Spitzka's t., Spitzka-Lissauer t.,** tractus posterolateralis.
**strionigral t.,** a bundle of fibers from the corpus striatum to the substantia nigra.
**sulcomarginal t.,** fasciculus sulcomarginalis.
**supraopticohypophysial t.,** tractus supraopticohypophysialis.
**tectobulbar t.,** tractus tectobulbaris.
**tectocerebellar t.,** a bundle of fibers from the tectum of the mesencephalon to the cerebellum.
**tectospinal t.,** tractus tectospinalis.
**tegmental t.,** a tract of fibers in the tegmentum, back of the nucleus posterior corporis trapezoidei, believed to connect the latter with the midbrain.
**tegmental t., central,** tractus tegementalis centralis.
**tegmentospinal t.,** tractus reticulospinalis anterior.
**temporopontine t.,** see *fibrae parietotemporopontinae* and *fibrae temporopontinae,* under *fibra.*
**testobulbar t.,** a bundle of fibers arising mostly in the cranial colliculus; it descends to the lower border of the pons where it ends in the nuclei of the brain stem and in the reticular formation.
**thalamo-olivary t.,** a bundle of fibers descending from the thalamus to the olivary nucleus.
**triangular t.,** olivospinal t.
**triangular t. of Philippe-Gombault,** Gombault-Philippe triangle.
**trigeminothalamic t.,** lemniscus trigeminalis.
**tuberohypophysial t., tuberoinfundibular t.,** a group of nerve fibers arising in the cells of the infundibular nucleus and related nuclei of the intermediate hypothalamic region, believed to provide a neurosecretory pathway associated with the neurocontrol of secretory activity by the anterior lobe of the pituitary gland.
**urinary t.,** the organs and passageways that participate in the excretion of the urine from the kidneys through the bladder and the urinary meatus.
**uveal t.,** tunica vasculosa bulbi.
**ventral amygdalofugal t.,** a diffuse fiber tract connecting the basolateral part of the amygdaloid body with the lateral preoptic and hypothalamic regions. Cf. *stria terminalis.*
**vestibulocerebellar t.,** a group of fibers of the pars vestibularis nervi octavi that extends to the cortex of the cerebellum.
**vestibulospinal t., lateral,** tractus vestibulospinalis lateralis.
**vestibulospinal t., medial,** tractus vestibulospinalis medialis.
**t. of Vicq d'Azyr,** fasciculus mammillothalamicus.

**trac·tel·lum** (trak-tel'əm) pl. *tractel'la* [L.] an anterior locomotive flagellum.

**trac·tion** (trak'shən) [L. *tractio*] [MeSH: Traction] the act of drawing or exerting a pulling force, as along the long axis of a structure.
**axis t.,** traction along an axis, as of the pelvis in obstetrics.
**Bryant's t.,** overhead vertical traction for fracture of the femoral shaft.
**cervical t.,** traction applied to the neck, usually by means of a sling that fits under the chin and behind the occiput; used in the treatment of osteoarthritis, rheumatoid arthritis, and other disorders of the cervical spine.
**elastic t.,** traction by an elastic force or by means of an elastic appliance.
**external t.,** traction applied by means of a fixed anchorage (as by a headgear) outside the oral cavity; used principally in the management of midfacial fractures.
**halo-pelvic t.,** traction applied to the spine by means of two metal hoops, one (the halo) applied to the skull and the other to the pelvis, connected by four extension rods which can be lengthened by turn screws.
**intermaxillary t.,** maxillomandibular t.
**internal t.,** traction applied by using one of the cranial bones above the point of fracture for anchorage; used in the management of facial fractures.
**lumbar t.,** traction applied to the lumbar spine.
**maxillomandibular t.,** traction applied by means of elastic or wire ligatures and interdental wiring and/or splints; called also *intermaxillary t.*
**Russell t.,** traction incorporating a sling beneath the knee that is connected to an overhead pulley.
**skeletal t.,** traction applied directly upon the long bones by means of pins, Kirschner's wire, etc.
**skin t.,** traction on a body part maintained by an apparatus affixed by dressings to the body surface.
**tongue t.,** the pulling forward of the tongue to improve the airway.

**trac·tor** (trak'tər) [L. "drawer"] an instrument for applying traction.
**prostatic t.,** a straight instrument with blades operated by a knob that draws the prostate into view in perineal prostatectomy.
**Syms' t.,** a tube with an inflatable rubber bag at the end; used to bring down a prostate into the perineal incision.
**urethral t.,** a curved instrument with blades operated by a knob that is inserted through the urethra into the bladder in perineal prostatectomy.

**trac·tot·o·my** (trak-tot'ə-me) surgical severing or incising of a nerve tract.
**medullary t.,** interruption of one or more tracts in the medulla oblongata for the relief of pain.
**mesencephalic t.,** mesencephalotomy.
**stereotactic t.,** production of lesions in the fibers of the caudate nucleus; used as a psychosurgical technique to relieve intractable depression, anxiety, or obsessional states.

**trac·tus** (trak′təs) pl. *trac′tus* [L. "track, trail"] 1. a tract; a region, principally one of some length. 2. [TA] a collection or bundle, especially of nerve fibers, having the same origin and termination, and serving the same function. See also under *bundle, fasciculus,* and *lemniscus.*

## Tractus

Descriptions are given on the TA terms, and include anglicized names of specific tracts.

**trac′tus anterolatera′les,** TA alternative for *lemniscus spinalis.*

**t. bulboreticulospina′lis** [TA], bulboreticulospinal tract: a group of reticulospinal nerve fibers in the lateral funiculus of the spinal cord, the axons of which are derived from nerve cells of the medulla oblongata. Called also *lateral reticulospinal tract* and *medullary reticulospinal tract.*

**t. centra′lis thy′mi,** central tract of thymus: the medullary core of the thymus; an irregular fibrous bundle carrying the blood vessels and giving attachment to the lobules of the gland.

**t. corticoponti′nus** [TA], corticopontine tract: the collection of corticopontine fibers (fibrae corticopontinae), arising in various areas of the cerebral cortex, particularly from areas involved in movement, and projecting to the pons.

**t. corticospina′lis ante′rior** [TA], anterior corticospinal tract: a group of nerve fibers in the anterior funiculus of the spinal cord, originating in the cerebral cortex; called also *t. corticospinalis ventralis; t. pyramidalis anterior; direct* or *ventral corticospinal tract;* and *anterior, direct,* or *ventral pyramidal tract.*

**t. corticospina′lis latera′lis** [TA], lateral corticospinal tract: a group of nerve fibers in the lateral funiculus of the spinal cord, originating in the cerebral cortex; called also *crossed corticospinal tract, crossed* or *lateral pyramidal tract,* and *t. pyramidalis lateralis.*

**t. corticospina′lis ventra′lis,** t. corticospinalis anterior.

**t. dorsolatera′lis,** t. posterolateralis.

**t. frontoponti′nus** [TA], frontopontine tract: the collection of nerve fibers that arise in the frontal lobe of the cerebrum, traverse the internal capsule and peduncle, and end in the pontine nuclei.

**t. habenulointerpeduncula′ris** [TA], habenulointerpeduncular tract: a bundle of nerve fibers arising in the habenular nuclei and extending rostroventrally to the interpeduncular nucleus to relay fibers to the reticular formation of the mesencephalon; called also *fasciculus retroflexus* [TA alternative], *habenulopeduncular tract,* and *Meynert's bundle, fasciculus,* or *tract.*

**t. hypothalamohypophysia′lis** [TA], hypothalamicohypophysial tract: the group of nerve fibers making up the efferent pathways of the hypothalamus, arising in the hypothalamic nuclei and ending at various levels in the median eminence, infundibulum, and posterior lobe of the pituitary gland. It contains subgroups of fibers; see *t. paraventriculohypophysialis* and *t. supraopticohypophysialis.* See also *tuberohypophysial tract.*

**t. iliopu′bicus** [TA], iliopubic tract: a thickened band of tissue that strengthens the lower part of the deep inguinal ring and forms the base of the internal spermatic fascia.

**t. iliotibia′lis** [TA], **t. iliotibia′lis [Maissia′ti],** iliotibial tract: a thickened longitudinal band of fascia lata extending from the tensor muscle downward along the lateral side of the thigh to the lateral condyle of the tibia.

**t. interstitiospina′lis** [TA], interstitiospinal tract: a tract of nerve fibers that descends from the interstitial nucleus into the spinal cord as part of the medial longitudinal fasciculus.

**t. mesencepha′licus ner′vi trigemina′lis, t. mesencepha′licus ner′vi trige′mini** [TA], mesencephalic tract of trigeminal nerve: a group of sensory fibers of the entering trigeminal nerve that continues rostrally along the medial aspect of the superior cerebellar peduncle; their cell bodies are located in the nucleus of the mesencephalic tract.

**t. olfacto′rius** [TA], olfactory tract: a narrow triangular band in the olfactory sulcus of the frontal lobe, which arises from the olfactory bulb and extends posteriorly, to end by dividing into medial and lateral olfactory striae, the latter ending in the primary olfactory cortex.

**t. olivocerebella′ris** [TA], olivocerebellar tract: a fiber tract that arises from the olive, crosses to the opposite side to pierce the other olive, and enters the cerebellum through its inferior peduncle.

**t. olivocochlea′ris** [TA], olivocochlear tract: a group of fibers derived from the nucleus of the superior olive that terminates in relation to the hair cells in the spiral organ of the cochlea; called also *olivocochlear fasciculus.*

**t. op′ticus** [TA], optic tract: the tract arising from the optic chiasma, proceeding backward, around the cerebral peduncle, and dividing into a lateral and a medial root; the roots end in the cranial colliculus and lateral geniculate body, respectively.

**t. paraventriculohypophysia′lis** [TA], paraventriculohypophysial tract: the part of the hypothalamicohypophysial tract that arises in the paraventricular nucleus of the hypothalamus; some of the fibers end in the infundibulum and others reach the posterior lobe of the pituitary gland, where their neurosecretory material is stored as oxytocin before being released into the systemic circulation. See also *t. supraopticohypophysialis.*

**t. pontoreticulospina′lis** [TA], pontoreticulospinal tract: a group of reticulospinal nerve fibers in the lateral funiculus of the spinal cord, arising in the pontobulbar region. Called also *medial reticulospinal tract.*

**t. posterolatera′lis** [TA], posterolateral tract: a group of nerve fibers in the lateral funiculus of the spinal cord dorsal to the dorsal column, composed in part of primary pain and temperature fibers which enter the spinal cord, travel the distance of a few segments in the dorsolateral tract, and then synapse in the dorsal column. Called also *dorsolateral fasciculus* or *tract* and *Lissauer's marginal zone.*

**t. pyramida′lis** [TA], 1. pyramidal tract: a term applied to several groups of fibers (corticonuclear, corticospinal, and corticoreticular) arising chiefly in the sensorimotor regions of the cerebral cortex and descending in the internal capsule, cerebral peduncle, and pons to the medulla oblongata, the corticoreticular fibers descending with the corticospinal fibers and synapsing with cells of the reticular formation and the corticonuclear fibers synapsing with motor nuclei throughout the brain stem. Most of the corticospinal fibers cross in the decussation of the pyramids and descend in the spinal cord as the lateral corticospinal tract; most of the uncrossed fibers form the anterior corticospinal tract; both end by synapsing with internuncial and motor neurons. The pyramidal tract is a phylogenetically new tract, most prominent in humans, and provides for direct cortical control and initiation of skilled movements, especially those related to speech and involving the hand and fingers. Called also *corticospinal tract of medulla oblongata, fasciculus pyramidalis medullae oblongatae,* and *pyramidal system.* 2. either of the corticospinal tracts of the spinal cord; see *t. corticospinalis anterior* and *t. corticospinalis lateralis.*

**t. pyramida′lis ante′rior,** t. corticospinalis anterior.

**t. pyramida′lis latera′lis,** t. corticospinalis lateralis.

**t. pyramida′lis ventra′lis,** t. corticospinalis anterior.

**t. reticulospina′lis ante′rior** [TA], **t. reticulospina′lis ante′rior, t. reticulospina′lis ventra′lis,** anterior reticulospinal tract: a group of fibers arising mostly from the reticular formation of the pons and medulla oblongata; chiefly homolateral, the fibers descend in the ventral and lateral funiculi to most levels of the spinal cord; called also *ventral reticulospinal tract* and *tegmentospinal tract.*

**t. rubrobulba′ris** [TA], rubrobulbar tract: a group of nerve fibers arising in the red nucleus and terminating at several different parts of the brain stem including the nucleus of the facial nerve, the motor nucleus of the trigeminal nerve, and the inferior olivary nucleus.

**t. rubrospina′lis** [TA], rubrospinal tract: a group of nerve fibers in the lateral funiculus of the spinal cord, arising in the large cells of the red nucleus of the mesencephalon. Called also *Monakow's bundle, fasciculus,* or *tract.*

**t. solita′rius medul′lae oblonga′tae** [TA], solitary tract of medulla oblongata: a descending tract in the medulla oblongata, ventrolateral to the caudal part of the fourth ventricle, near the dorsal nucleus of the vagus and glossopharyngeal nerves, and comprising primary visceral afferent fibers from the facial, glossopharyngeal, and vagus nerves.

**t. spina′lis ner′vi trigemina′lis, t. spina′lis ner′vi trige′mini** [TA], spinal tract of trigeminal nerve: a descending tract of the trigeminal nerve that extends from the level of entrance of the sensory root of the trigeminal nerves into the pons to the upper cervical segments of the spinal cord. Lying lateral to the nucleus of the spinal tract of the trigeminal nerve, in which its fibers synapse, this tract carries mainly pain and temperature impulses from the face.

**t. spinocerebella′ris ante′rior** [TA], anterior spinocerebellar tract: a group of nerve fibers in the lateral funiculus of the spinal cord, arising mostly in the opposite gray matter and ascending to the cerebellum by way of the anterior part of the lateral funiculus and then the superior cerebellar peduncle; they carry sensory impulses activated by nerve endings in skin, muscles, tendons, and joints. Called also *Gowers' column, fasciculus,* or *tract, ventral spinocerebellar tract,* and *t. spinocerebellaris ventralis.*

**t. spinocerebella′ris dorsa′lis,** t. spinocerebellaris posterior.

**t. spinocerebella′ris poste′rior** [TA], posterior spinocerebellar tract: a group of nerve fibers in the lateral funiculus of the spinal cord, arising chiefly from the columna thoracica and ascending to the cerebellum by way of the posterior part of the lateral funiculus and then the inferior cerebellar peduncle; they carry sensory impulses activated by nerve endings in skin, muscles, tendons, and joints. Called also *direct* or *dorsal spinocerebellar tract* and *t. spinocerebellaris dorsalis.*

**t. spinocerebella′ris ventra′lis,** t. spinocerebellaris anterior.

**t. spinocervica′lis** [TA], spinocervical tract: a somatosensory pathway consisting of fibers that pass out of the posterior spinocerebellar tract, pass through the lateral cervical nucleus, and ascend with the medial lemniscus to the nucleus ventralis posterolateralis of the thalamus.

**t. spinooliva′ris** [TA], spinoolivary tract: an ascending tract of nerve fibers in the lateral funiculus of the spinal cord, arising from the posterior gray columns of the spinal cord and running to the olivary nucleus.

**t. spinoreticula′ris** [TA], spinoreticular tract: an ascending tract of nerve fibers in the lateral funiculus of the spinal cord, passing to the reticular formation of the brain stem.

**t. spinotecta′lis** [TA], spinotectal tract: a group of nerve fibers in the lateral funiculus of the spinal cord, mostly crossed from their origin, which ascend to the superior and inferior colliculi and carry somatic sensory impulses.

**t. spinothala′micus,** t. spinothalamicus lateralis.

**t. spinothala′micus ante′rior** [TA], anterior spinothalamic tract: a group of nerve fibers in the anterior funiculus of the spinal cord, continuous with the spinothalamic tract; they arise in the contralateral gray substance and ascend to the thalamus, joining the medial lemniscus in the brain stem. They carry sensory impulses activated by light touch. Called also *ventral spinothalamic tract* and *t. spinothalamicus ventralis.*

**t. spinothala′micus latera′lis** [TA], lateral spinothalamic tract: a group of nerve fibers in the lateral funiculus of the spinal cord that arise in the opposite gray matter and ascend to the thalamus, running with the lateral lemniscus in the brain stem; they carry sensory impulses activated by pain and temperature.

**t. spinothala′micus ventra′lis,** t. spinothalamicus anterior.

**t. spira′lis foramino′sus** [TA], foraminous spiral tract: a spiral area on the fundus of the internal acoustic meatus, below the crista transversa and in front of the area vestibularis inferior; it corresponds to the base of the cochlea and is perforated with numerous holes for the passage of branches of the vestibulocochlear nerve.

**t. supraopticohypophysia′lis** [TA], supraopticohypophysial tract: the group of fibers of the hypothalamicohypophysial tract arising in the supraoptic nucleus of the thalamus; some of the fibers descend to end in the infundibulum and others reach the posterior lobe of the pituitary gland, where their neurosecretory material is stored as antidiuretic hormone before being released into the systemic circulation. The term has also been used to denote the entire set of fibers of the hypothalamicohypophysial tract entering the infundibulum without regard to point of termination and also to denote the parts of the hypothalamicohypophysial tract that arise in the supraoptic nucleus and the paraventricular nucleus (see *t. paraventriculohypophysialis*).

**t. tectobulba′ris** [TA], tectobulbar tract: a bundle of fibers arising mostly in the superior colliculus; it descends to the lower border of the pons where it ends in the nuclei of the brain stem and in the reticular formation.

**t. tectospina′lis** [TA], tectospinal tract: a group of nerve fibers, chiefly crossed, which arise mostly in the cranial colliculus and descend to the cervical cord, where they lie in the ventral funiculus.

**t. tegmenta′lis centra′lis** [TA], central tegmental tract: a composite nerve tract arising from the midbrain tegmentum, periaqueductal gray matter, and red nucleus; it descends in the tegmentum and reticular formation to end in the inferior olivary complex. The tract includes an ascending component from the reticular formation. Called also *Bekhterev's tract.*

**t. trigeminothala′micus,** TA alternative for *lemniscus trigeminalis.*

**t. vestibulospina′lis latera′lis** [TA], lateral vestibulospinal tract: a group of nerve fibers arising from the lateral vestibular nucleus and descending first ipsilaterally in the periphery of the anterolateral funiculus and then through the medial part of the anterior funiculus at lower levels of the spinal cord, ending ipsilaterally in the medial part of the anterior gray column.

**t. vestibulospina′lis media′lis** [TA], medial vestibulospinal tract: a group of nerve fibers arising mainly from the medial vestibular nucleus and descending via the medial longitudinal fasciculus into the anterior funiculus of the spinal cord, close to the midline; it contains both crossed and uncrossed fibers and projects mainly to the cervical cord segments, ending at the midthoracic cord level.

---

**trag·a·canth** (trag′ə-kanth) [NF] [MeSH: Tragacanth] the dried gummy exudation from *Astragalus gummifer* or other species of *Astragalus;* used as a suspending agent for drugs. Called also *gum tragacanth.*

**tra·gal** (tra′gəl) pertaining to the tragus.

**tra·gi** (tra′ji) [L., pl. of *tragus*] [TA] hair growing on the pinna of the external ear, especially on the cartilaginous projection anterior to the external opening (tragus).

**Tra·gia** (tra′je-ə) a genus of poisonous plants of the family Euphorbiaceae. *T. u′rens* and other species are weeds of the southern United States.

**trag·i·on** (traj′e-on) a cephalometric landmark located at the superior margin of the tragus of the ear.

**trag·o·mas·chal·ia** (trag″o-məs-kal′e-ə) [Gr. *tragos* goat + *maschalē* the armpit] bromidrosis.

**trag·o·pho·nia** (trag″o-fo′ne-ə) egophony.

**tra·goph·o·ny** (trə-gof′ə-ne) [Gr. *tragos* goat + *phōne* voice] egophony.

**trag·o·po·dia** (trag″o-po′de-ə) [Gr. *tragos* goat + *pod-* + *-ia*] genu valgum.

**tra·gus** (tra′gəs) pl. *tra′gi* [L.; Gr. *tragos* goat] [TA] the cartilaginous projection anterior to the external opening of the ear; see also *tragi.*

**train·a·ble** (tra′nə-bəl) capable of being trained; formerly used to describe persons with moderate mental retardation (IQ 35 to 50). See *mental retardation,* under *retardation.*

**train·ing** (trān′ing) a system of instruction or teaching; preparation by instruction and practice.

**assertiveness t.,** a form of behavior therapy in which individuals are taught appropriate interpersonal responses involving direct, forthright expression of their feelings, needs and wishes, both negative and positive.

**bladder t.,** the training of a child or an incontinent adult in habits of urinary continence.

**bowel t.,** the training of a child or an incontinent adult in habits of fecal continence.

**trait** (trāt) 1. any genetically determined characteristic. 2. commonly used in medicine to designate the condition prevailing in the heterozygous state of a recessive disorder, as in sickle cell anemia. 3. a distinctive behavior pattern.

**hemoglobin C t.,** the heterozygous state for hemoglobin C; it is asymptomatic although individuals have increased target cells in the blood. See also *hemoglobin C–thalassemia disease,* under *disease.*

**personality t.,** a consistent pattern of acting, feeling, and thinking that occurs across a variety of situations and endures, and so characterizes a person.

**sickle cell t.,** the condition, usually asymptomatic, caused by heterozygosity for hemoglobin S.

**tra·jec·tor** (trə-jek′tər) an instrument for locating a bullet in a wound.

**Tral** (tral) trademark for preparations of hexocyclium methylsulfate.

**tra·ma·dol hy·dro·chlo·ride** (tram′ə-dol″) an opioid analgesic used for the treatment of moderate to moderately severe pain following surgical procedures and oral surgery; administered orally.

**tra·maz·o·line hy·dro·chlo·ride** (trə-maz′o-lēn) an adrenergic compound used intranasally as a decongestant.

**trance** (trans) a state of altered consciousness characterized by heightened focal awareness and reduced peripheral awareness; a sleeplike state of reduced consciousness and activity.

**hypnotic t.,** the state induced by hypnosis.

**Tran·co·pal** (tran′ko-pəl) trademark for a preparation of chlormezanone.

**Tran·date** (tran′dāt) trademark for a preparation of labetalol hydrochloride.

**tran·ex·am·ic ac·id** (tran-ək-sam′ik) [MeSH: Tranexamic Acid] an antifibrinolytic that acts by competitively inhibiting plasminogen; it is used as a hemostatic in the treatment of severe hemorrhage associated with excessive fibrinolysis.

**tran·qui·liz·er** (trang″kwĭ-līz′ər) [L. *tranquillus* quiet, calm + *-ize* + *-er* agent] a drug with a calming, soothing effect; currently it is usually used to denote a *minor t.*
**major t.,** former name for antipsychotic agent; see *antipsychotic.*
**minor t.,** anxiolytic (def. 2).

***trans*** (tranz) [L., through] 1. in organic chemistry, having certain atoms or radicals on opposite sides. 2. in genetics, denoting two or more loci, particularly pseudoalleles, occurring on opposite chromosomes of a homologous pair. Cf. cis. See also cis-trans *test,* under *test.*

**trans-** a prefix meaning through, across, or beyond.

**trans·ab·dom·i·nal** (trans″ab-dom′ĭ-nəl) through the abdominal wall.

**trans·ac·e·tyl·ase** (trans-ə-set′ə-lās) acetyltransferase.

**trans·ac·e·tyl·a·tion** (trans″ə-set″ə-la′shən) a chemical reaction involving the transfer of an acetyl group. It occurs in many metabolic reactions.

**trans·ac·y·lase** (trans-a′sə-lās) acyltransferase.

**trans·ac·y·la·tion** (trans-a″sə-la′shən) a chemical reaction involving the transfer of the acyl radical between acetic and higher carboxylic acids.

**trans·al·do·lase** (trans-al′do-lās) [EC 2.2.1.2] [MeSH: Transaldolase] an enzyme of the transferase class that catalyzes the transfer of a dihydroxyacetone group from a ketose phosphate to an aldose phosphate in a reaction of the pentose phosphate pathway.

**trans·am·i·din·ase** (trans″ə-mid′in-ās) amidinotransferase.

**trans·am·i·nase** (trans-am′ĭ-nās) [EC 2.6.1] a sub-subclass of enzymes of the transferase class that catalyze the transfer of an amino group from a donor (generally an amino acid) to an acceptor (generally a 2-keto acid). Most are pyridoxal phosphate proteins. Called also *aminotransferase.*

**trans·am·i·na·tion** (trans″am-ĭ-na′shən) the reversible transfer of an amino group from an amino acid to what was originally an $\alpha$-keto acid, forming a new keto acid and a new amino acid, without the appearance of ammonia in the free state.

**trans·an·tral** (trans-an′trəl) performed across or through an antrum, such as brain surgery done through the ethmoid antrum.

**trans·aor·tic** (trans″a-or′tik) performed through the aorta; used especially in reference to surgical procedures on the aortic valve, performed through an incision in the wall of the aorta.

**trans·atri·al** (trans-a′tre-əl) performed through the atrium; used especially in reference to surgical procedures on a cardiac valve, performed through an incision in the wall of the atrium.

**trans·au·di·ent** (trans-aw′de-ənt) permitting passage of the mechanical vibrations perceived as sound.

**trans·ax·i·al** (trans-ak′se-əl) directed at right angles to the long axis of the body or a part.

**trans·ba·sal** (trans-ba′səl) through the base, as a surgical approach through the base of the skull.

**trans·bron·chi·al** (trans-brong′ke-əl) performed through a bronchus.

**trans·ca·lent** (trans-ka′lənt) [*trans-* + L. *calere* to be hot] permitting the passage of radiant heat.

**trans·cal·lo·sal** (trans-kə-lo′səl) performed across or through the corpus callosum.

**trans·cal·var·i·al** (trans″kəl-văr′e-əl) through or across the calvaria.

**trans·can·al** (trans-kə-nal′) done through a canal, such as surgery done through the auditory canals.

**trans·car·bam·o·yl·ase** (trans″kahr-bam′o-ə-lās) carbamoyltransferase.

**trans·car·boxy·lase** (trans″kahr-bok′sə-lās) carboxyltransferase.

**trans·cath·e·ter** (trans-kath′ə-tər) performed through the lumen of a catheter.

**trans·cer·vi·cal** (trans-sər′vĭ-kəl) performed through the cervical opening of the uterus.

**trans·clo·mi·phene** (trans-clo′mĭ-fēn) zuclomiphene.

**trans·co·bal·a·min** (trans″ko-bal′ə-min) any of three plasma glycoproteins, transcobalamin I, II, and III, that bind and transport cobalamin (vitamin $B_{12}$). Abbreviated TC.
**t. I (TCI),** a plasma glycoprotein synthesized by granulocytes; it binds most of the endogenous cobalamin but its function is uncertain. Deficiency of the glycoprotein results in low levels of serum cobalamin but does not cause abnormalities of metabolism. Its concentration is increased in myeloproliferative disorders.
**t. II (TCII),** the plasma glycoprotein that binds vitamin $B_{12}$ absorbed into the blood from the ileum then transports it to the tissues, predominantly the liver, where the complex is absorbed by the cells via receptor-mediated endocytosis. Deficiency of TCII results in failure of immunoglobulin production, megaloblastic anemia, granulocytopenia, thrombocytopenia, and intestinal villous atrophy, all correctable with vitamin $B_{12}$ therapy.
**t. III (TCIII),** a plasma glycoprotein synthesized by granulocytes, differing from TCI only in its carbohydrate content. The serum concentration of TCIII is increased in myeloproliferative disorders, but its function is unknown.

**trans·coch·le·ar** (trnas-kok′le-ər) done through the cochlea, such as removal of a tumor. Cf. *translabyrinthine.*

**trans·con·dy·loid** (trans-kon′də-loid) through the condyles.

**trans·cor·ti·cal** (trans-kor′tĭ-kəl) connecting two different parts of the cerebral cortex; also, dependent on disease of the tracts connecting different parts of the cerebral cortex.

**trans·cor·tin** (trans-kor′tin) [MeSH: Transcortin] an $\alpha$-globulin that specifically and avidly binds and transports in plasma the unconjugated and presumably biologically active cortisol. Called also *corticosteroid-* or *cortisol-binding globulin.*

**trans·cra·ni·al** (trans-kra′ne-əl) performed through the cranium.

**trans·cri·co·thy·roid** (trans-kri″ko-thi′roid) through or across the cricothyroid membrane.

**trans·cript** (trans′kript) a strand of nucleic acid that has been synthesized using another nucleic acid strand as a template.
**primary t.,** the first RNA transcript of a gene, containing introns as well as exons.

**trans·crip·tase** (trans-krip′tās) a general term denoting a DNA-directed RNA polymerase.
**reverse t.,** RNA-directed DNA polymerase.

**trans·crip·tion** (trans-krip′shən) [L. *transcriptio* transfer, copy] the process by which a single-stranded RNA with a base sequence complementary to one strand of a double-stranded DNA is synthesized. The enzymes involved are called DNA-dependent RNA polymerases (see under *polymerase*).

**trans·cu·ta·ne·ous** (trans″ku-ta′ne-əs) transdermal.

**trans·der·mal** (trans-dər′məl) entering through the dermis, or skin, as in administration of a drug applied to the skin in ointment or patch form. Cf. *percutaneous.* Called also *transcutaneous.*

**Trans·derm–Ni·tro** (trans′derm ni′tro) trademark for a preparation of nitroglycerin.

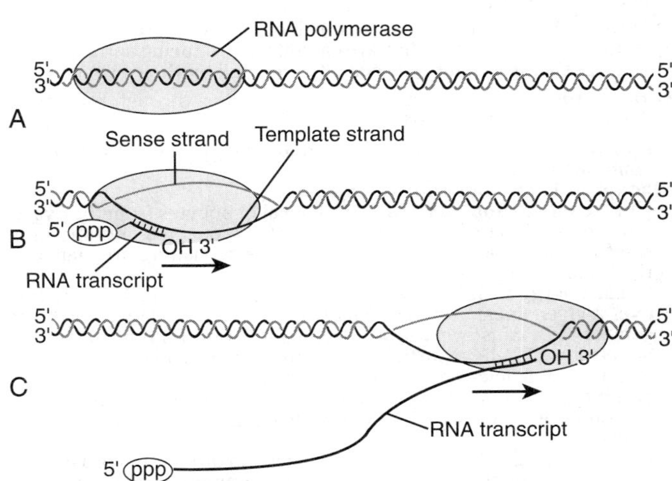


Transcription. Binding of the RNA polymerase at a specific site on DNA to be transcribed *(A)* is followed by unwinding of a region of the DNA helix and initiation of transcription in a 5′ to 3′ direction *(B),* producing an RNA transcript complementary to, and hydrogen bonded with, the template strand of the DNA. The transcript elongates as the polymerase proceeds down the DNA *(C),* helix unwinding before and rewinding after it.

**Trans·derm-Scōp** (trans′dərm-skōp′) trademark for a preparation of scopolamine.

**trans·du·cer** (trans-doo′sər) [MeSH: Transducers] a receptor or artificial device that translates one form of energy to another, such as pressure, temperature, or pulse to an electrical signal.
**neuroendocrine t.,** a neuron having the properties of both nerve and gland, such as a neurohypophysial neuron, that on stimulation secretes a hormone, thereby translating neural information into endocrine information, with consequent inhibition or stimulation of hormonal secretion.
**pressure t.,** an electronic device that converts pressure (such as blood pressure) into electrical signals that can be recorded graphically and monitored.
**ultrasound t.,** a transducer used in ultrasonography, containing a piezoelectric crystal that can translate mechanical energy into electrical signals or electrical signals into mechanical energy.

**trans·du·cin** (trans-doo′sin) [MeSH: Transducin] a G protein of the disk membrane of the retinal rods that interacts with activated rhodopsin and participates in the triggering of a nerve impulse in vision; it stimulates hydrolysis of cyclic guanosine monophosphate, beginning the cascade that closes specific ion channels and generates an action potential.

**trans·duc·tion** (trans-duk′shən) [L. *transducere* to lead across] 1. a method of genetic recombination in bacteria, in which DNA from a lysed bacterium is transferred to another bacterium by bacteriophage, thereby changing the genetic constitution of the second organism. 2. the transforming of one form of energy into another, such as by the sensory mechanisms of the body; see also *sensory t.* and *transducer.*
**sensory t.,** the process by which a sensory receptor converts a stimulus from the environment into an action potential for transmission to the brain. See also *organa sensuum* under *organum.*
**signal t.,** the process by which a cell receives and acts on some external chemical or physical signal, such as a hormone, including receiving the information at specific receptors in the plasma membrane, conveying the signal across the plasma membrane into the cell, and subsequently inducing an intracellular chain of other signalling molecules, thereby stimulating a specific cellular response.
**visual t.,** the transducing of light energy to afferent nerve impulses, such as takes place in the retinal rods and cones.

**trans·du·ral** (trans-doo′rəl) through or across the dura mater.

**tran·sec·tion** (tran-sek′shən) [*trans-* + *section*] a section made across a long axis; a cross section; division by cutting transversely.

**trans·epi·der·mal** (trans″ep-ĭ-dər′məl) occurring through or across the epidermis.

**trans·eth·moi·dal** (trans-eth-moi′dəl) performed across or through the ethmoid bone.

**trans·fau·na·tion** (trans″faw-na′shən) the transfer of animal parasites from one host organism to another.

**trans·fec·tion** (trans-fek′shən) [MeSH: Transfection] the artificial infection of animal or bacterial cells by uptake of nucleic acid isolated from virus or bacteriophage, resulting in the production of mature virus or phage particles.

**trans·fec·to·ma** (trans″fek-to′mə) lymphoid cells transfected with immunoglobulin genes; they are capable of producing antibody molecules separate from the specificity encoded by their own genes.

**trans·fem·o·ral** (trans-fem′ə-rəl) 1. across or through the femur. 2. through the femoral artery.

**trans·fer** (trans′fər) [*trans-* + L. *ferre* to carry] the conveyance of something from one place to another.
**adoptive t.,** see under *immunization.*
**gamete intrafallopian t. (GIFT),** retrieval of oocytes from the ovary, followed by laparoscopic placement of the oocytes and sperm in the fallopian tubes; used as a means of establishing pregnancy in the treatment of infertility.
**linear energy t. (LET),** the energy dissipation of ionizing radiation over a given linear distance. Highly penetrating radiations, such as gamma rays, cause very low ion concentration and thus have a relatively low LET, beta particles and x-rays have an intermediate LET, and alpha particles have a relatively high LET.
**passive t.,** the conferring of immunity to a nonimmune host by injection of antibody or lymphocytes from an immune or sensitized donor.
**tendon t.,** surgical relocation of the insertion of a tendon of a normal muscle to a different site to take over the function of a muscle inactivated by trauma or disease.
**tubal embryo t. (TET),** 1. retrieval of oocytes from the ovary, followed by fertilization and culture of the oocytes in the laboratory and the placement of the resulting embryos in the fallopian tubes by laparoscopy more than 24 hours after oocyte retrieval; used as a means of establishing pregnancy in the treatment of infertility. 2. laparoscopic transfer of cryopreserved embryos to the fallopian tubes.
**zygote intrafallopian t. (ZIFT),** retrieval of oocytes from the ovary, followed by fertilization and culture of the oocytes in the laboratory and the placement of the resulting zygotes in the fallopian tubes by laparoscopy 24 hours after oocyte retrieval; used as a means of establishing pregnancy in the treatment of infertility.

**trans·fer·ase** (trans′fər-ās) [EC 2] a class of enzymes that transfer a chemical group from one compound (the donor) to another compound (the acceptor).

**trans·fer·ence** (trans-fer′əns) in psychotherapy, the unconscious tendency to assign to others in one's present environment feelings and attitudes associated with significant persons in one's early life, especially the patient's transfer to the therapist of feelings and attitudes associated with a parent. The feelings may be affectionate *(positive t.)* or hostile *(negative t.).*
**counter t.,** see *countertransference.*

**trans·fer·rin** (trans-fer′in) [*trans-* + *ferrum* + *-in* chemical suffix] [MeSH: Transferrin] a nonheme serum glycoprotein of molecular weight 79,500, which binds and transports iron; most is produced in the liver. A similar substance called apoferritin is produced in the small intestine. Called also *siderophilin.*

**trans·fix** (trans′fiks) [*trans-* + L. *figere* to fix] to pierce through and through.

**trans·fix·ion** (trans-fik′shən) a cutting through from within outward, as in amputation.

**trans·for·ma·tion** (trans″for-ma′shən) [*trans-* + *formation*] 1. change of form or structure; conversion from one form to another. 2. in oncology, the change that a normal cell undergoes as it becomes malignant. 3. in eukaryotes, the conversion of normal cells to malignant cells in cell culture.
**asbestos t.,** the deposition of extraneous fibers in hyaline cartilage, which gives it a silky, glossy appearance.
**bacterial t.,** the exchange of genetic material between strains of bacteria by the transfer of a fragment of naked DNA from a donor cell to a recipient cell, followed by recombination in the recipient chromosome.
**lymphocyte t.,** the morphologic changes accompanying lymphocyte activation, in which small, resting lymphocytes are transformed into large, active lymphocytes (lymphoblasts).
**nodular t. of the liver,** nodular regenerative hyperplasia.

**trans·fron·tal** (trans-frun′təl) through the frontal bone.

**trans·fu·sion** (trans-fu′zhən) [L. *transfusio*] the introduction of whole blood or blood components directly into the bloodstream. Cf. *infusion.*
**autologous t.,** autotransfusion.
**direct t.,** immediate t.
**exchange t., exsanguination t.,** repetitive withdrawal of small amounts of blood and replacement with donor blood, until a large proportion of the blood volume has been exchanged; used primarily in newborn infants with erythroblastosis fetalis and sometimes in patients with various other blood conditions. Called also *replacement t.* and *substitution t.*
**fetomaternal t.,** transplacental passage of fetal blood into the circulation of the mother; in small amounts it may go unnoticed, but in larger amounts it can cause anemia or edema in the fetus.
**immediate t.,** the transfer of blood from one person to another without use of an intermediate container or anticoagulant. Called also *direct t.*
**indirect t.,** transfer of blood from a donor to a flask or other container, and then to the recipient. Called also *mediate t.*
**intraperitoneal t.,** infusion of blood into the peritoneal cavity; see *intrauterine t.*
**intrauterine t.,** transfusion performed on an unborn infant in utero, often referring to transfusion of Rh-negative blood into the infant's peritoneal cavity in the treatment of erythroblastosis fetalis *in utero.*
**mediate t.,** indirect t.
**placental t.,** return to the newborn, through the umbilical vessels, of some of the blood contained in the fetal placenta.
**replacement t., substitution t.,** exchange t.
**twin-to-twin t.,** an intrauterine abnormality of fetal circulation in monozygotic twins, in which blood is shunted directly from one twin to the other; cf. *placental t.*

**trans·gene** (trans′jēn) [MeSH: Transgenes] a gene that has been spliced into a strand of DNA.

**trans·gen·ic** (trans-jen′ik) [*trans-* + *genic*] pertaining to the experimental splicing of a segment of DNA from one genome onto DNA of a different genome.

**trans·glu·co·syl·ase** (trans″gloo-ko′sə-lās) glucosyltransferase.

**trans·glu·tam·in·ase** (trans″gloo-tam′in-ās) protein-glutamine γ-glutamyltransferase.

**trans·gly·co·si·da·tion** (trans″gli-kōs″ĭ-da′shən) the transfer of a sugar residue from a glycoside to a suitable free hydroxyl group to form a new glycosidic bond, such as is catalyzed by glycosyltransferases.

**trans·gly·co·syl·ase** (trans″gli-ko′sə-lās) glycosyltransferase.

**trans·hi·a·tal** (trans″hi-a′təl) across or through a hiatus.

**trans·hu·mer·al** (trans-hu′mər-əl) across or through the humerus.

**tran·sient** (tran′shent, tran′se-ənt) [L. *transiens* present participle of *transire* to go across] [MeSH: Transients and Migrants] an isolated wave or complex seen on an electroencephalogram.

**trans·il·i·ac** (trans-il′e-ak) across or between the two ilia.

**tran·sil·i·ent** (tran-sil′e-ənt) [*trans-* + L. *salire* to leap] leaping or passing across.

**trans·il·lu·mi·na·tion** (trans″ĭ-loo″mĭ-na′shən) [MeSH: Transillumination] the passage of light through body tissues for the purpose of examination, the object or part under examination being interposed between the observer and the light source; diaphanoscopy.

**trans·in·su·lar** (trans-in′su-lər) across the insula; crossing the insula.

**trans·is·chi·ac** (trans-is′ke-ak) between the two ischia.

**trans·isth·mi·an** (trans-is′me-ən) across an isthmus, especially the isthmus of the gyrus fornicatus.

**trans·is·tor** (tran-zis′tər) [MeSH: Transistors] a small wafer of semiconducting material having three electrodes, called the emitter, base, and collector, which perform functions similar to those of the cathode, grid, and plate of a vacuum tube.

**tran·sit** (tran′sit) passage across or through.
**colonic t.,** 1. passage of feces through the colon. 2. a measure of the time required for feces to pass through the colon; called also *colonic transit time.*

**tran·si·tion** (tran-zĭ′shən) [L. *transitio* crossing over] in molecular genetics, a point mutation in which a purine base replaces a purine base or a pyrimidine base replaces a pyrimidine base. Cf. *transversion.*
**glass t.,** the change in a crystalline polymer or ceramic material from a rubbery or viscous state to a hard, brittle state, usually as a result of a decrease in temperature.
**isobaric t.,** a radioactive decay process in which the daughter and parent are isobars, possessing the same mass number but differing in atomic number. Included are beta decay, positron emission, and electron capture.

**trans·ke·to·lase** (trans-ke′to-lās) [EC 2.2.1.1] [MeSH: Transketolase] an enzyme of the transferase class that catalyzes the transfer to aldose phosphates of glycolaldehyde groups from specific ketose phosphates, reactions that occur in the pentose phosphate pathway. The enzyme contains thiamine pyrophosphate and $Mg^{2+}$ and has displayed reduced thiamine-binding capacity in patients with Wernicke-Korsakoff syndrome.

**trans·lab·y·rin·thine** (trans-lab″ə-rin′thēn) done through the labyrinth, such as otologic surgery. Cf. *transcochlear.*

**trans·lat·er·al** (trans-lat′ər-əl) from side to side; in radiography, referring to the view obtained with the patient supine and the radiation directed horizontally.

**trans·la·tion** (trans-la′shən) [L. *translatio* transfer] in genetics, the process by which polypeptide chains are synthesized, the amino acid sequence being completely determined by the sequence of bases in a messenger RNA (mRNA), which in turn is determined by the sequence of bases in the DNA of the gene from which it was transcribed.
**nick t.,** a process by which radiolabeled nucleotides are incorporated into duplex DNA at single-strand nicks or cleavage points created enzymatically along its two strands.

**trans·lo·case** (trans-lo′kās) 1. transport protein. 2. the prokaryotic elongation factor, involved in protein synthesis.

**trans·lo·ca·tion** (trans″lo-ka′shən) [*trans-* + L. *locus* place] a structural chromosome aberration in which one segment of a chromosome is transferred to a nonhomologous chromosome, the result of breakage of both chromosomes with repair in abnormal arrangement. Called also *interchange.* Abbreviated t. See *insertion,* def. 2, and Plate 1.
**balanced t.,** reciprocal translocation which results in no more or no less than the normal diploid or haploid genetic material. The phenotype is normal, but there will be partial aneuploidy in a percentage of the gametes, with a risk of unbalanced offspring.
**reciprocal t.,** the complete exchange of fragments between two broken nonhomologous chromosomes, one part of one uniting with part of the other, with no fragments left over. Abbreviated rcp. See Plate 1.
**robertsonian t.,** translocation involving two of the acrocentric chromosomes (13, 14, 15, 21, and 22), which fuse at the centromere region and lose their heterochromatic short arms. A carrier of a balanced robertsonian translocation involving chromosome 14 and 21 has a virtually complete chromosomal complement but only 45 chromosomes (including the translocation chromosome), is phenotypically normal, but risks producing offspring with trisomy 21 (translocation Down syndrome). See Plate 1.

**trans·lu·cent** (trans-loo′sənt) [*trans-* + L. *lucens* shining] transmitting light, but diffusing it so that objects beyond are not clearly distinguished.

**trans·me·a·tal** (trans″me-at′əl) through a meatus.

**trans·mem·brane** (trans-mem′brān) extending across a membrane, usually referring to a protein subunit that is exposed on both sides of a cell membrane.

**trans·meta·tar·sal** (trans-met″ə-tahr′səl) across the metatarsal bones.

**trans·meth·y·lase** (trans-meth′ə-lās) methyltransferase.

**trans·meth·y·la·tion** (trans″məth-ə-la′shən) the transfer of a methyl group from one compound to another.

**trans·mi·gra·tion** (trans″mi-gra′shən) 1. a wandering, especially a change of place from one side of the body to the other. 2. diapedesis.
**external t.,** the passage of an ovum from one ovary to the uterine tube of the other side without going through its own oviduct.
**internal t.,** the passage of an ovum from one oviduct to the other by way of the uterus.

**trans·mis·si·ble** (trans-mis′ĭ-bəl) capable of being transmitted from one individual or one species to another.

**trans·mis·sion** (trans-mish′ən) [*trans-* + L. *missio* a sending] 1. a passage or transfer, as of a disease from one individual to another, or of neural impulses from one neuron to another. 2. the communication of inheritable qualities from parent to offspring.
**duplex t.,** the transmission of neural impulses in two directions along a nerve.
**ephaptic t.,** the conduction of a nerve impulse across an ephapse, as opposed to synaptic transmission.
**horizontal t.,** the spread of an infectious agent from one individual to another, usually through contact with bodily excretions or fluids, such as sputum or blood, that contain the agent; cf. *vertical t.*
**neurochemical t.,** transmission of an impulse across a synaptic junction through the medium of a chemical substance (neurotransmitter). Called also *neurohumoral t.*
**neurohumoral t.,** neurochemical t.
**neuromuscular t.,** the chemically mediated transmission of an action potential from nerve to muscle across the myoneural junction.
**synaptic t.,** the communication of a neural impulse from one neuron to another neuron, a muscle fiber, or a gland across a synapse.
**vertical t.,** transmission from one generation to another. The term is restricted by some to genetic transmission and extended by others to include also transmission of infection from one generation to the next, as by milk or through the placenta. Cf. *horizontal heart.*

**trans·mi·tral** (trans-mi′trəl) through the mitral valve.

**trans·mit·tance** (trans-mit′əns) 1. in analytical chemistry, the ratio $I/I_0$ of the light intensity transmitted by the solution under analysis *(I)* to that transmitted by the pure solvent or other reference solution $(I_0)$. 2. in physics, the ratio $I/I_0$ of the radiant energy transmitted by an object divided by the incident radiant energy. Symbol *T.*

**trans·mit·ter** (trans-mit′ər) something that transmits; see also under *substance;* see also *neurotransmitter.*

**trans·mu·ral** (trans-mu′rəl) [*trans-* + *mural*] through the wall of an organ; extending through or affecting the entire thickness of the wall of an organ or cavity.

**trans·mu·ta·tion** (trans″mu-ta′shən) 1. evolutionary change of one species into another. 2. the change of one chemical element into another; nucleonics, the changing of an atomic nucleus to one of a different atomic number by nuclear bombardment, causing rearrangement of the protons and neutrons.

**trans·oc·u·lar** (trans-ok′u-lər) across the eye.

**tran·so·nance** (tran′so-nəns) [*trans-* + L. *sonans* sounding] transmission of a sound originating in one organ through the substance of another organ.

**trans·ovar·i·al** (trans″o-var′e-əl) through the ovary; referring to transmission of pathogens from the maternal organism, by invasion of the ovary and infection of eggs, to individuals of the next generation, as may occur in infections of arthropods, especially mites and ticks.

**trans·ovar·i·an** (trans″o-var′e-ən) transovarial.

**trans·pal·a·tal** (trans-pal′ə-təl) performed through the roof of the mouth, or palate.

**trans·par·ent** (trans-par′ənt) [*trans-* + L. *parere* to appear] permitting the passage of rays of light, so that objects may be seen through the substance.

**trans·pa·ri·e·tal** (trans″pə-ri′ə-təl) [*trans-* + *parietal*] through or across a wall, as through the intact body wall.

**trans·peri·to·ne·al** (trans″per-ĭ-to-ne′əl) through or across the peritoneum.

**trans·phos·phor·y·la·tion** (trans-fos″for-ə-la′shən) the exchange of phosphate groups between organic phosphates, without their going through the stage of inorganic phosphate.

**tran·spi·ra·tion** (tran″spĭ-ra′shən) [*trans-* + L. *spiratio* exhalation] the discharge of air, sweat, or vapor through the skin; insensible perspiration.
**pulmonary t.**, the exhalation of water vapor from the blood circulating through the lungs.

**trans·pla·cen·tal** (trans″plə-sen′təl) through the placenta.

**trans·plant**[1] (trans′plant) 1. an organ or tissue taken from the body for grafting into another area of the same body or into another individual. 2. the process of removing and grafting such an organ or tissue. See also *transplantation.* Called also *graft.*
**Gallie t.**, strips of fascia lata employed as sutures in the repair of hernias.

**trans·plant**[2] (trans-plant′) to transfer tissue from one part to another.

**trans·plan·tar** (trans-plan′tər) [*trans-* + *plantar*] across the sole.

**trans·plan·ta·tion** (trans″plan-ta′shən) [*trans-* + *plantation*] [MeSH: Transplantation] the grafting of tissues taken from the patient's own body or from another; called also *graft, grafting,* and *transplant.*
**allogeneic t.**, transplantation of an allograft; the three types are *cadaveric t., living related donor t.,* and *living unrelated donor t.* Called also *allotransplantation.*
**bone marrow t.**, intravenous infusion of autologous, syngeneic, or allogeneic bone marrow or stem cells (see *peripheral blood progenitor cells,* under *cell*); done to treat malignancies such as leukemia, lymphoma, myeloma, and selected solid tumors, as well as nonmalignant conditions such as aplastic anemia, immunologic deficiencies, inborn errors of metabolism, and the myeloablation resulting from chemotherapy or radiotherapy. Abbreviated *BMT.*
**cadaveric donor t.**, allogeneic transplantation of an organ or tissue from a cadaver.
**heterotopic t.**, transplantation of tissue typical of one area to a different recipient site.
**homotopic t.**, orthotopic t.
**living nonrelated donor t.**, living unrelated donor t.
**living related donor t.**, allogeneic transplantation in which the donor and the recipient have a close biological relationship, such as that of a mother and her child or a brother and sister; called also *syngenesioplastic t.*
**living unrelated donor t.**, allogeneic transplantation in which the donor and the recipient do not have a close biological relationship.
**orthotopic t.**, transplantation of tissue from a donor into its normal anatomical position in the recipient.
**syngeneic t.**, transplantation of a syngraft; called also *isotransplantation.*
**syngenesioplastic t.**, living related donor t.
**tendon t.**, 1. surgical replacement of a damaged segment of tendon by a free tendon graft. 2. tendon transfer.
**tooth t.**, the insertion into a prepared dental alveolus of an autogenous or homologous tooth; it may be a developing tooth germ from the same mouth, a homologous transplant, or a tooth with or without vital pulp, or one having had endodontic treatment, transplanted from one site to another in the same individual or from one individual to another.
**xenogeneic t.**, transplantation of a xenograft; called also *heterotransplantation.*

**trans·pleu·ral** (trans-ploor′əl) through the pleura; by way of the pleural sac.

**trans·port** (trans′port) [L. *transportare* to carry across] the movement of materials in biological systems, particularly into and out of cells and across epithelial layers.
**active t.**, the movement of materials across cell membranes and epithelial layers resulting directly from the expenditure of metabolic energy. Cf. *passive t.*
**bulk t.**, the uptake by or extrusion from a cell of fluid and of particles too large to cross the cell membrane by diffusion or active transport, accomplished by invagination and vacuole formation (uptake) or by evagination (extrusion); it includes endocytosis, phagocytosis, pinocytosis, and exocytosis.
**fast axonal t.**, the rapid bidirectional movement of vesicles containing glycoproteins and neurotransmitters along microtubules between the nerve cell body and the axon terminal.

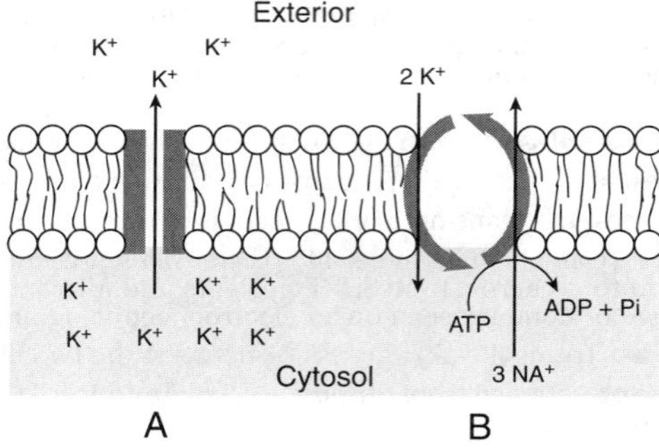


*(A)* Passive transport exemplified by diffusion of potassium ions across the plasma membrane, through specific ion channels, down a concentration gradient; *(B)* active transport exemplified by the cellular sodium pump, which uses ATP hydrolysis to create gradients of sodium and potassium across the plasma membrane.

**oxygen t.**, the carrying of oxygen through the bloodstream bound to hemoglobin (see *oxyhemoglobin*).
**passive t.**, the movement of materials, usually across cell membranes, by processes not requiring expenditure of metabolic energy. Cf. *active t.*
**reverse cholesterol t.**, the process by which high-density lipoproteins (HDL) facilitate the movement of cholesterol from peripheral cells back to the liver for excretion in the bile. Cholesterol released into plasma during cell turnover is adsorbed to HDL where it is esterified by lecithin–cholesterol acyltransferase; most of the cholesteryl esters then are transferred to intermediate- or very-low-density lipoproteins by a specific transfer protein and these lipoproteins are ultimately taken up by the liver.
**slow axonal t.**, the movement of cytoskeletal elements *(component a)* and glycolytic enzymes and actin *(component b)* along an axon away from the nerve cell body, occurring at a rate of 0.2 to 2 mm/day, depending on the species and age of the animal and on the particular nerve. Its function is to renew the cytoskeleton, regulate the axonal caliber, and transport energy-related enzymes.

**trans·port·er** (trans-por′tər) a transport protein; often specifically a transport protein that after binding one to several molecules of substrate, undergoes a conformational change that moves only the substrate across the membrane. Different types facilitate movement with (symport) and against (antiport) concentration gradients.

**trans·po·si·tion** (trans″po-zĭ′shən) [*trans-* + *position*] 1. displacement of a viscus to the opposite side. 2. the operation of carrying a tissue flap from one situation to another without severing its connection entirely until it is united at its new location. 3. the exchange of position of two atoms within a molecule. 4. movement of genetic information from one locus to another, such as via a transposon.
**t. of great vessels**, a congenital cardiovascular malformation in which the aorta arises entirely from the right ventricle and the pulmonary artery from the left ventricle, so that the venous return from the peripheral circulation is recirculated by the right ventricle via the aorta to the systemic circulation without being oxygenated in the lungs. Life then depends on a crossflow of blood between blood in the right heart and that in the left heart, as through a ventricular septal defect or a patent ductus arteriosus. Cyanosis is the chief symptom.
**t. of great vessels, corrected**, a developmental cardiac anomaly characterized by transposition of the great vessels with inversion of the ventricles and atrioventricular valves; termed "corrected" because the inverted ventricles compensate for the transposition, producing a mirror-image blood flow in the heart. Called also *mixed levocardia.*
**t. of great vessels, partial**, Taussig-Bing syndrome.

**trans·po·son** (tranz-po′zon) [MeSH: DNA Insertion Elements] a small mobile genetic (DNA) element that can move around within the genome or to other genomes within the same cell, usually by copying itself to a second site but sometimes by splicing itself out of its original site and inserting in a new location. Complex transposons may carry other genes besides merely those for transposition. Transposons are sometimes called *transposable elements.*

**trans·pu·bic** (trans-pu′bik) performed through the pubic bone after removal of a segment of the bone.

**trans·ra·di·al** (trans-ra′de-əl) 1. through the radial artery. 2. across the radius.

**trans·sa·cral** (tran-sa′krəl) through or across the sacrum.

**trans·sec·tion** (tran-sek′shən) transection.

**trans·seg·men·tal** (trans″səg-men′təl) extending across a segment.

**trans·sep·tal** (tran-sep′təl) through or across a septum.

**trans·sex·u·al** (tran-sek′shoo-əl) 1. a person affected by transsexualism. 2. a person whose external anatomy has been changed to that of the opposite sex.

**trans·sex·u·al·ism** (tran-sek′shoo-əl-iz-əm) [MeSH: Transsexualism] 1. the most severe manifestation of gender identity disorder in adults, being a prolonged, persistent desire to relinquish their primary and secondary sex characteristics and acquire those of the opposite sex; particularly describing those persons who go so far as to live as members of the opposite sex through dress, hormonal treatments, or surgical reassignment. 2. the state of being a transsexual.

**trans·sphe·noi·dal** (trans″sfe-noi′dəl) performed through the sphenoid bone.

**trans·ster·nal** (tran-stər′nəl) through the sternum.

**trans·suc·ci·ny·lase** (trans″sək-sĭ′nə-lās) dihydrolipoamide *S*-succinyltransferase.

**trans·tem·po·ral** (trans-tem′por-əl) 1. crossing the temporal lobe. 2. through the temporal bone, such as otologic surgery.

**trans·tha·lam·ic** (trans″thə-lam′ik) crossing the thalamus.

**trans·tho·rac·ic** (trans″thə-ras′ik) performed through the wall of the thorax, or through the thoracic cavity.

**trans·thy·re·tin** (trans″thi-ret′in) an $\alpha$-globulin secreted by the liver; it forms a complex with retinol binding protein and binds retinol, transporting it to the peripheral tissues. It also acts as a binding protein for thyroxine and triiodothyronine, although those hormones are mainly transported by thyroxine-binding globulin. Called also *prealbumin.*
**amyloid t.,** a mutant form of transthyretin deposited in the tissues in hereditary amyloidosis.

**trans·tra·che·al** (trans-tra′ke-əl) through the wall of the trachea.

**trans·tym·pan·ic** (trans″tim-pan′ik) across the tympanic membrane or the cavity of the middle ear.

**tran·su·date** (trans′u-dāt) [*trans-* + L. *sudare* to sweat] [MeSH: Exudates and Transudates] a fluid substance which has passed through a membrane or been extruded from the blood as a result of hydrodynamic forces. A transudate, in contrast to an exudate, is characterized by high fluidity and a low content of protein, cells, or of solid materials derived from cells.

**tran·su·da·tion** (trans″u-da′shən) 1. the passage of serum or other body fluid through a blood vessel as a result of hydrodynamic forces; it may be the result of inflammation. 2. transudate.

**trans·ura·ni·um** (trans″u-ra′ne-əm) beyond uranium; see *transuranic elements,* under *element.*

**trans·ure·tero·ure·ter·os·to·my** (trans″u-re″tər-o-u-re″tər-os′tə-me) anastomosis of the proximal portion of one ureter to the ureter of the opposite side.

**trans·ure·thral** (trans″u-re′thrəl) performed through the urethra.

**trans·vag·i·nal** (trans-vaj′ĭ-nəl) performed through the vagina.

**trans·va·te·ri·an** (trans″və-tēr′e-ən) through the papilla of Vater.

**trans·vec·tor** (trans-vek′tor) an organism that conveys or transmits a poison which is not generated in its own body but is obtained from another source, such as the mussel, *Mytilus,* which serves as a transvector of paralytic shellfish poison derived from the dinoflagellate *Gonyaulax.*

**trans·ve·nous** (trans-ve′nəs) performed or inserted through a vein.

**trans·ven·tric·u·lar** (trans″vən-trik′u-lər) performed through a ventricle.

**trans·ver·sa·lis** (trans″vər-sa′lis) [*trans-* + L. *vertere, versum* to turn] 1. transverse. 2. [TA] a term designating a structure situated at a right angle to the long axis of the body or of an organ.

**trans·verse** (trans-vərs′) [L. *transversus*] placed crosswise; situated at right angles to the long axis of a part.
**t. abdominal,** see *musculus transversus abdominis,* under *musculus.*

**trans·ver·sec·to·my** (trans″vər-sek′tə-me) [*transverse* + *-ectomy*] surgical removal of the transverse process of a vertebra.

**trans·ver·sion** (trans-vər′zhən) [L. *transvertere* to turn away] 1. displacement of a tooth from its proper numerical position in the jaw. 2. in molecular genetics, a point mutation in which a purine base replaces a pyrimidine base or vice versa. Cf. *transition.*

**trans·ver·so·cos·tal** (trans-vər″so-kos′təl) costotransverse.

**trans·ver·sot·o·my** (trans″vər-sot′ə-me) [*transverse* + *-tomy*] the operation of cutting the transverse process of a vertebra.

**trans·ver·so·ure·thral·is** (trans-vər″so-u″re-thral′is) the transverse fibers of the sphincter urethrae muscle.

**trans·ver·sus** (trans-vər′səs) [L.] [TA] transverse; a general term designating a position at right angles to a long axis.
**t. abdo′minis,** see under *musculus.*
**t. nu′chae,** see under *musculus.*

**trans·ves·i·cal** (trans-ves′ĭ-kəl) through the bladder.

**trans·ves·tism** (trans-ves′tiz-əm) [*trans-* + L. *vestitus* clothed] [MeSH: Transvestism] 1. cross-dressing and otherwise assuming the appearance, manner, or roles traditionally associated with members of the opposite sex. 2. transvestic fetishism.

**trans·ves·tite** (trans-ves′tīt) an individual exhibiting transvestism.

**trans·ves·ti·tism** (trans-ves′tĭ-tiz-əm) transvestism.

**Tran·tas′ dots** (trahn′tahs) [Alexios *Trantas,* Greek ophthalmologist, 1867–1960] see under *dot.*

**Tran·xene** (tran′zēn) trademark for a preparation of clorazepate dipotassium.

**tran·yl·cy·pro·mine sul·fate** (tran″əl-si′pro-mēn) a monoamine oxidase inhibitor with rapid onset of action, used as an antidepressant in patients who have not responded to other antidepressant agents; administered orally.

**tra·pe·zi·al** (trə-pe′ze-əl) pertaining to a trapezium.

**tra·pez·i·form** (trə-pez′ĭ-form) trapezoid (def. 1).

**tra·pe·zio·meta·car·pal** (trə-pe′ze-o-met″ə-kahr′pəl) pertaining to or connecting the trapezium and the metacarpus.

**tra·pe·zi·um** (trə-pe′ze-əm) [L.; Gr. *trapezion*] 1. an irregular four-sided figure. 2. os trapezium.

**trap·e·zoid** (trap′ə-zoid) [L. *trapezoides;* Gr. *trapezoeidēs* table shaped] 1. having the shape of a four-sided plane, with two sides parallel and two diverging. 2. the trapezoid bone (os trapezoideum [TA]).

**Tras·en·tine** (tras′ən-tin) trademark for preparations of adiphenine hydrochloride.

**Tras·y·lol** (tras′ə-lol) trademark for a preparation of aprotinin.

**Trau·be′s sign, semilunar space** (trou′bəz) [Ludwig *Traube,* German physician, 1818–1876] see under *sign* and *space.*

**Traube-Her·ing waves** (trou′bə-her′ing) [Ludwig *Traube;* Edwald *Hering,* German physiologist, 1834–1918] see under *wave.*

**trau·ma** (traw′mə, trow′mə) pl. *traumas* or *trau′mata* [Gr.] 1. injury. 2. psychological or emotional damage.
**birth t.,** 1. an injury to the infant received in or due to the process of being born; called also *birth injury.* 2. in some psychiatric theories, the psychic shock produced in an infant by the experience of being born.
**occlusal t.,** injury to any part of the masticatory system as a result of occlusal dysfunction. See also *traumatic occlusion,* under *occlusion.*
**potential t.,** in dentistry, an alteration in tissue that may occur at any time as a result of an existing dental disharmony.
**psychic t.,** a psychologically upsetting experience that produces an emotional or mental disorder or otherwise has lasting negative effects on a person's thoughts, feelings, or behavior.

**trau·ma·ther·a·py** (traw′mə-ther′ə-pe) [*trauma* + *therapy*] treatment of wounds and injuries.

**trau·mat·ic** (trə-mat′ik) pertaining to, occurring as the result of, or causing trauma.

**trau·ma·tism** (traw′mə-tiz-əm) 1. the physical or psychic state resulting from an injury or wound. Called also *traumatosis.* 2. a wound or injury.

**traumat(o)-** [Gr. *trauma,* gen. *traumatos* wound] a combining form denoting relationship to trauma, or to a wound or injury.

**trau·ma·to·gen·ic** (traw″mə-to-jen′ik) [*traumato-* + *-genic*] 1. caused by or due to a wound or wounds. 2. capable of causing trauma.

**trau·ma·tol·o·gist** (traw″mə-tol′ə-jist) a surgeon experienced in treating accidental injuries.

**trau·ma·tol·o·gy** (traw″mə-tol′ə-je) [*traumato-* + *-logy*] [MeSH: Traumatology] the branch of surgery which deals with wounds and disability from injuries.

**trau·ma·top·a·thy** (traw″mə-top′ə-the) [*traumato-* + *-pathy*] any pathological condition due to wound or injury.

**trau·ma·top·nea** (traw″mə-top′ne-ə) [*traumato-* + *-pnea*] open pneumothorax.

**trau·ma·to·ther·a·py** (traw″mə-to-ther′ə-pe) traumatherapy.

**trau·mat·ro·pism** (trə-mat′ro-piz-əm) [*trauma* + *tropism*] the growth or movement of organisms in relation to injury.

**Traut·mann's triangle** (trout′mahnz) [Moritz Ferdinand *Trautmann,* German surgeon, 1832–1902] see under *triangle.*

**Trav·a·sol** (trav′ə-sol) trademark for a crystalline amino acid solution for intravenous administration, containing a mixture of essential and nonessential amino acids but no peptides.

**tray** (tra) a flat-surfaced utensil for the conveyance of various objects or material.
**acrylic resin t.,** an impression tray made of acrylic resin.
**impression t.,** a horseshoe-shaped receptacle made of metal or other suitable material used to carry the impression material to the mouth, to confine the material in apposition to the surfaces to be recorded, and to control the impression material while it sets to form the impression.

**tra·zo·done hy·dro·chlo·ride** (tra′zo-dōn) [USP] an antidepressant used to treat major depressive episodes with or without prominent anxiety; also used to treat diabetic neuropathy and other types of chronic pain.

**Trea·cher Col·lins syndrome** (tre′chər-kol′inz) [Edward *Treacher Collins,* British surgeon, 1862–1932] see under *syndrome.*

**Trea·cher Col·lins–Fran·ce·schet·ti syndrome** (tre′chər-kol′inz-frahn″cha-sket′e) [E. *Treacher Collins;* Adolphe *Franceschetti,* Swiss ophthalmologist, 1896–1968] mandibulofacial dysostosis; see under *dysostosis.*

**tread** (tred) injury of the coronet of a horse's hoof, such as from being repeatedly struck with the shoe of the opposite side.

**treat·ment** (trēt′mənt) the management and care of a patient for the purpose of combating disease or disorder. See also under *care, maneuver, method, technique, tests,* and *therapy.*
**active t.,** curative t.
**Bouchardat's t.,** treatment of diabetes by use of a diet that excludes substances rich in carbohydrates.
**Brown-Séquard's t.,** organotherapy.
**Carrel's t., Carrel-Dakin t.,** treatment of wounds, based on thorough exposure of the wound, removal of all foreign material and devitalized tissue, meticulous cleansing, and repeated irrigation with a dilute sodium hypochlorite solution. The adjacent skin is protected with petrolatum gauze.
**causal t.,** treatment that is directed against the cause of a disease.
**conservative t.,** treatment designed to avoid radical medical therapeutic measures or operative procedures; often reserved for elderly or debilitated patients.
**curative t.,** treatment designed to cure an existing disease, as opposed to *palliative t.* Called also *active t.*
**drug t.,** pharmacotherapy.
**electroconvulsive t., electroshock t.,** see under *therapy.*
**empiric t.,** treatment by means which experience has proved to be beneficial.
**eventration t.,** application of ionizing radiation to internal anatomical tissues through an open laparotomy wound.
**expectant t.,** treatment designed only to relieve untoward symptoms, leaving the cure mainly to nature.
**fever t.,** pyretotherapy.
**Frenkel's t.,** see under *exercise.*
**Goeckerman t.,** treatment of psoriasis by applying ointments of tar followed by irradiation with ultraviolet B.
**Hartel's t.,** alcoholic injection for trigeminal neuralgia in which the needle is passed through the mouth into the region of the foramen ovale of the sphenoid bone.
**hygienic t.,** that directed to the restoration or maintenance of hygienic conditions.
**Kenny t.,** a treatment formerly used for poliomyelitis consisting of wrapping of the back and limbs in hot cloths, followed, after pain has subsided, by passive exercise and instruction of the patient in exercise of the muscles.
**Klapp's creeping t.,** treatment of scoliosis by having the patient creep about on the floor, with exaggerated movements of the spine.
**Lerich's t.,** *(of strains),* infiltration of the periarticular tissues with a 0.5–2 per cent solution of procaine.
**light t.,** 1. phototherapy (def. 1). 2. photodynamic therapy.
**McPheeters' t.,** treatment of varicose ulcer by bandaging a rubber sponge over the ulcerated area and directing the patient to walk as much as possible; called also *venous heart t.*
**Matas' t.,** treatment of neuralgia by the injection of alcohol under the nerve ganglions at the base of the skull.
**medicinal t.,** pharmacotherapy.
**Orr t.,** treatment of compound fractures and osteomyelitis by débridement of the wound, alignment of fracture, drainage with petrolatum gauze, and immobilization of limb in a plaster cast which is left on until the wound discharge has softened the plaster.
**palliative t.,** treatment designed to relieve pain and distress, but not attempting a cure. See also *curative t.*Called also *supportive t.* and *palliative care.*
**Potter t.,** treatment of intestinal fistulas by administration of tenth normal solution of hydrochloric acid to neutralize the alkalinity of the pancreatic juice, thus preventing tryptic activity.
**preventive t., prophylactic t.,** prophylaxis.
**rational t.,** treatment based upon a knowledge of disease and the action of the remedies employed.
**root canal t.,** see under *therapy.*
**salicyl t.,** treatment of rheumatism with salicylic acid or its derivatives.
**Schlösser's t.,** treatment of trigeminal neuralgia by injections of alcohol into the foramen from which the nerve emerges.
**sewage t.,** the processing of sewage to remove or so alter some of its constituents as to render it less offensive or dangerous and more fit to discharge into a public watercourse.
**shock t.,** obsolete term for *convulsive therapy.*
**slush t.,** the treatment of acne by the application of a mixture of carbon dioxide snow, acetone, and sulfur.
**specific t.,** treatment particularly adapted to a given disease.
**supporting t., supportive t.,** palliative t.
**surgical t.,** therapy using chiefly surgical methods. Cf. *pharmacotherapy* and *physical therapy.*
**symptomatic t.,** expectant t.
**Trueta t.,** immediate treatment of fractures as follows: (1) adopt surgical treatment as soon as possible; (2) thoroughly wash wound and entire limb with water, soap, and a nail brush, shave hair, paint surrounding skin with weak alcoholic solution of iodine, avoiding the wound; (3) débride wound; (4) open neighboring cellular spaces and remove hematomas; (5) remove completely denuded or displaced bone fragments and all foreign matter; (6) reduce fracture; (7) dress wound with sterile gauze and immobilize with plaster, including two adjacent joints if possible; (8) give injection of tetanus antitoxin.
**venous heart t.,** McPheeters' t.

**tree** (tre) 1. a perennial of the plant kingdom characterized by having a main stem or trunk and numerous branches. 2. an anatomical structure with branches resembling a tree. See also *arbor.*
**bronchial t.,** arbor bronchialis.
**decision t.,** a graph resembling a tree in having an increasingly more complex branching structure flowing off an initial stem or point; used in decision analysis (q.v.) to represent choices and outcomes as the results of series of sequential decisions.
**dendritic t.,** the branching arrangement of a dendrite.
**tracheobronchial t.,** the trachea and the bronchial tree considered as a unit.

**tre·foil** (tre′foyl) 1. clover; see *Trifolium.* 2. any of various clover-like plants, such as certain species of *Medicago* and *Lotus.*
**bird's foot t.,** 1. *Lotus americanus.* 2. *Lotus corniculatus.*
**burr t.,** *Medicago polymorpha.*

**α,α-tre·hal·ase** (tre-ha′lās) [EC 3.2.1.28] an enzyme of the hydrolase class that catalyzes the cleavage of the glycosidic bond in trehalose to yield two molecules of glucose. Deficiency of the enzyme, an autosomal recessive disorder, causes trehalose malabsorption, which may be manifested as vomiting and diarrhea after ingestion of large amounts of edible mushrooms.

**tre·ha·lose** (tre-ha′lōs) [MeSH: Trehalose] a disaccharide occurring mainly in insects, algae, and some mushrooms; when hydrolyzed by acids or enzymes it yields glucose.

**Treitz's arch, fascia,** etc. (trīt′səz) [Wenzel *Treitz,* Czech physician, 1819–1872] see under *arch, fascia,* and *hernia,* see *musculus suspensorius duodeni,* and see *recessus duodenalis superior.*

**Trem·a·to·da** (trem″ə-to′də) [Gr. *trēmatōdēs* pierced] [MeSH: Trematoda] the flukes, a class of the phylum Platyhelminthes. Most are parasitic in humans or other animals, infection generally resulting from the ingestion of uncooked or undercooked fish, crustaceans, or vegetation. All flukes require a mollusk as their first intermediate host, in which a complex developmental cycle takes place. The larval stage, which escapes from the mollusk, may then enter a second intermediate host (fish, crustacean, or another mollusk), encyst on vegetation, or penetrate directly into the skin of the definitive host. The important trematodes of humans belong to the genera *Clonorchis, Dicrocoelium, Echinostoma, Fasciola, Fasciolopsis, Gastrodiscoides, Heterophyes, Metagonimus, Opisthorchis, Paragonimus,* and *Schistosoma.*

**trem·a·tode** (trem′ə-tōd) any member of the class Trematoda; called also *fluke.*

**trem·a·to·di·a·sis** (trem″ə-to-di′ə-sis) infection with trematodes; called also *fluke disease.*

**trem·bles** (trem′bəlz) 1. any of various neurological diseases of domestic animals in which tremors are a prominent symptom. 2. poisoning in cattle and sheep that feed on the plants *Eupatorium rugosum* and *Haplopappus heterophyllus,* which contain the toxin tre-

metol; the animal has muscular tremors, becomes weak, and may suddenly stumble and fall. Humans who consume milk, milk products, or flesh from an animal so affected may develop the acute condition called *milk sickness.*
**congenital t.,** congenital tremor syndrome.

**trem•el•loid, tre•mel•lose** (trem'ə-loid, trem'ə-lōs) like jelly.

**trem•e•tol** (trem'ə-tol) a toxin in the white snakeroot, *Eupatorium rugosum,* and the rayless goldenrod, *Haplopappus heterophyllus,* which causes trembles in cattle and sheep and milk sickness in humans. Called also *tremetone.*

**trem•e•tone** (trem'ə-tōn) tremetol.

**Trem•in** (trem'in) trademark for a preparation of trihexyphenidyl hydrochloride.

**tre•mo•gram** (tre'mo-gram) [*tremor* + *-gram*] the tracing or record made by a tremograph; a graphic tracing of a tremor. See *ataxiameter.*

**tre•mo•graph** (tre'mo-graf) [*tremor* + *-graph*] an instrument for recording tremors.

**trem•or** (trem'ər, tre'mər) [L., from *tremere* to shake] [MeSH: Tremor] an involuntary trembling or quivering.
**action t.,** rhythmic, oscillatory, involuntary motion of a part during voluntary movements, as of the outstretched upper limb when writing or lifting a cup. Called also *intention t., kinetic t., postural t.,* and *volitional t.*
**arsenic t.,** a tremor resulting from arsenic poisoning.
**coarse t.,** a tremor in which the vibrations are slow.
**continuous t.,** persistent t.
**darkness t.,** involuntary movements of the eyes, resembling nystagmus, which occur in young animals kept in the dark.
**enhanced physiologic t.,** a tremor that may appear in normal individuals under conditions of stress, such as cold, excitement, hunger, or exercise; it represents an intensification of physiologic tremor to detectable levels.
**epidemic t.,** avian encephalomyelitis.
**essential t.,** a hereditary tremor with onset at varying ages, usually at about 50 years of age, beginning with a fine rapid tremor (as distinct from that of parkinsonism) of the hands, followed by tremor of the arms, tongue, head, legs, and trunk; it is aggravated by emotional factors, is accentuated by volitional movement, and in some cases is temporarily improved by alcohol. Called also *familial t., heredofamilial t.,* and *hereditary essential t.*
**familial t.,** essential t.
**fine t.,** a tremor in which the vibrations are rapid.
**flapping t.,** asterixis.
**hereditary essential t.,** essential t.
**heredofamilial t.,** essential t.
**intention t.,** action t.
**kinetic t.,** action t.
**t. lin'guae,** trembling of the tongue, as seen in alcoholism, typhoid fever, and general paresis.
**t. mercuria'lis,** tremor due to mercury poisoning.
**metallic t.,** a tremor seen in various metallic poisonings.
**orthostatic t.,** a rare tremor of the lower limbs noted when standing but not when walking or sitting.
**parkinsonian t.,** the resting tremor commonly seen with parkinsonism, consisting of slow, regular movements of the hands and sometimes the legs, neck, face, or jaw; it typically stops upon voluntary movement of the part and is intensified by stimuli such as cold, fatigue, and strong emotions.
**passive t.,** resting t.
**persistent t.,** a tremor occurring whether the patient is at rest or in motion.
**physiologic t.,** a rapid tremor of extremely low amplitude found in the limbs and sometimes the neck or face of normal individuals, only subtly detectable on an electromyogram and seldom visible to the naked eye; it may become accentuated and visible under certain conditions. Cf. *enhanced physiologic t.*
**pill-rolling t.,** a parkinsonian tremor of the hand consisting of flexion and extension of the fingers in conjunction with adduction and abduction of the thumb. Called also *pill-rolling.*
**postural t.,** action t.
**purring t.,** a thrill, like the purring of a cat, felt by the hand placed over the heart.
**rest t., resting t.,** a tremor occurring when a limb or other body part is at rest; it may be normal, as in some physiologic tremors, or abnormal, as in parkinsonian tremors. Called also *passive t.*
**senile t.,** a tremor resulting from the infirmities of age.
**static t.,** a tremor occurring on effort to hold one of the limbs in a definite position.
**striocerebellar t.,** a combined form of tremor with both striatal and cerebellar components, usually due to diffuse degeneration of the central nervous system.
**toxic t.,** a tremor seen in states of chronic poisoning.
**trombone t. of tongue,** Magnan's movement.
**volitional t.,** action t.

**trem•or•gram** (trem'ər-gram) tremogram.

**trem•u•lous** (trem'u-ləs) [L. *tremulus*] pertaining to or characterized by tremors.

**Tren•de•len•burg's operation,** etc. (tren'de-lən-bərg) [Friedrich *Trendelenburg,* German surgeon, 1844–1924] see under *operation, position, symptom,* and *test.*

**trend•scrib•er** (trend'skrīb-ər) the apparatus used in trendscription.

**trend•scrip•tion** (trend'skrip-shən) a programmed method of continuous electrocardiographic monitoring, wherein the tracing is condensed on a rotating drum recorder and the program permits selective sampling of rhythm data.

**Tren•tal** (tren'tal) trademark for a preparation of pentoxifylline.

**tre•pan** (trə-pan') [Gr. *trypanon* auger] 1. an obsolete form of the trephine, resembling a carpenter's bit and brace. 2. to trephine.

**trep•a•na•tion** (trep″ə-na'shən) [L. *trepanatio*] trephination.

**tre•pan•ner** (tre-pan'ər) trephiner.

**treph•i•na•tion** (tref″ĭ-na'shən) the operation of trephining.
**corneoscleral t.,** Elliot's operation.
**dental t.,** surgical creation of a fistula by puncturing the soft tissue and cortical bone overlying the root apex to provide drainage. Called also *apicostomy.*

**tre•phine** (trə-fīn', trə-fēn') [L. *trephina*] 1. a saw for removing a disk of bone, chiefly from the skull. 2. an instrument for removing a circular area of cornea, as in corneal transplant operations. 3. to operate upon with the trephine.

**tre•phine•ment** (trĕ-fīn'mənt) the act or process of trephining.

**tre•phin•er** (trĕ-fīn'ər) one who performs the operation of trephining.

**trepho•cyte** (tref'o-sīt) [Gr. *trephein* to feed + *-cyte*] a cell that furnishes nutrition to other cells, as a Sertoli cell.

**trep•i•dant** (trep'ĭ-dənt) tremulous.

**trep•i•da•tion** (trep″ĭ-da'shən) [L. *trepidatio*] 1. tremor. 2. nervous anxiety and fear.

**trepo-** [Gr. *trepein* to turn] a combining form denoting a relationship to a turning movement.

**Trep•o•mo•nas** (trep″o-mo'nəs) [*trepo-* + Gr. *monas* unit, from *monos* single] a genus of flagellate protozoa (suborder Diplomonadina, order Diplomonadida) free-living in fresh water, coprophilic, or parasitic in amphibians, fish, and turtles, and characterized by the presence of one long and three short flagella on each side of the body.

**Trep•o•ne•ma** (trep″o-ne'mə) [*trepo-* + Gr. *nēma* thread] [MeSH: Treponema] a genus of bacteria of the family Spirochaetaceae, consisting of gram-negative, microaerophilic, spiral microorganisms that exhibit motility with a flexing, bending, snapping motion and divide by transverse fission. The outer surfaces have polar flagella (axial filaments) that wind around the organism. They are found in the oral, intestinal, and genital mucosa. Pathogenic species, which cause syphilis, yaws, and pinta, have not been cultured in vitro.
**T. bucca'le,** a species of uncertain status isolated from the human oral cavity. Called also *Borrelia buccalis.*
**T. calligy'rum,** *T. refringens.*
**T. cara'teum,** the causative agent of pinta (carate). Called also *T. herrejoni.*
**T. cuni'culi,** *T. paraluiscuniculi.*
**T. denti'cola,** a nonpathogenic species found in the oral cavity of humans and chimpanzees, usually in calculus occurring at the gingival margin.
**T. genita'lis,** *T. refringens.*
**T. herrejo'ni,** *T. carateum.*
**T. hyodysente'riae,** a species that causes swine dysentery.
**T. macroden'tium,** a nonpathogenic species found in the gingival crevices of humans.
**T. microden'tium,** *T. denticola.*

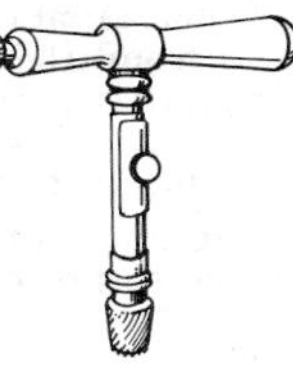

Trephine.

**T. muco'sum,** a species of uncertain status found in the oral cavity of a human with periodontitis.
**T. pal'lidum,** the causative agent of venereal, nonvenereal, and congenital syphilis in humans.
**T. pal'lidum** subsp. **perte'nue,** the causative agent of yaws in humans.
**T. paraluiscuni'culi,** a species causing syphilis in guinea pigs and rabbits; not pathogenic for humans. Called also *T. cuniculi.*
**T. perte'nue,** *T. pallidum* subsp. *pertenue.*
**T. phagede'nis,** a nonpathogenic species found in the genital regions of humans and chimpanzees. Called also *T. reiteri.*
**T. refrin'gens,** a nonpathogenic species that is part of the normal flora of male and female genitalia. Called also *T. calligyrum* and *T. genitalis.*
**T. reite'ri,** *T. phagedenis.*
**T. vincen'tii,** a species isolated from the human oral cavity, especially in acute necrotizing ulcerative gingivitis in association with *Fusobacterium nucleatum.* Called also *Borrelia vincentii* and *spirillum of Vincent.*

**trep·o·ne·ma** (trep″o-ne′mə) [MeSH: Treponema] an organism of the genus *Treponema.* Called also *treponeme.*

**trep·o·ne·mal** (trep″o-ne′məl) of, pertaining to, or caused by treponemas.

**Trep·o·ne·ma·ta·ceae** (trep″o-ne″mə-ta′se-e) in former systems of classification, a family of spirochetes, including the genera *Borrelia, Leptospira,* and *Treponema,* which are now classified in the family Spirochaetaceae.

**trep·o·ne·ma·to·sis** (trep″o-ne-mə-to′sis) an infection with species of *Treponema*; see also *syphilis.* Called also *treponemiasis.*

**trep·o·neme** (trep′o-nēm) treponema.

**trep·o·ne·mi·a·sis** (trep″o-ne-mi′ə-sis) 1. treponematosis. 2. syphilis.

**trep·o·ne·mi·ci·dal** (trep″o-ne″mĭ-si′dəl) destructive to organisms of the genus *Treponema.*

**tre·pop·nea** (tre″pop-ne′ə) [*trepo-* + *-pnea*] dyspnea that is relieved when a person is in a lateral recumbent position.

**trep·pe** (trep′ə) [Ger. "staircase"] the phenomenon of gradual increase in the extent of muscular contraction following rapid repeated stimulation; called also *staircase phenomenon.*

**Tre·sil·i·an's sign** (tre-sil′e-ənz) [Frederick James *Tresilian,* English physician, 1862–1926] see under *sign.*

**Trest** (trest) trademark for a preparation of methixene hydrochloride.

**tret·i·no·in** (tret′ĭ-noin″) [MeSH: Tretinoin] all-*trans*-retinoic acid, applied topically int the treatment of acne vulgaris and as a keratolytic in the treatment of disorders of keratinization, and administered orally as an antineoplastic in the treatment of acute promyelocytic anemia. Called also *retinoic acid* and *vitamin A acid.*

**Treves' fold** (trēvs) [Sir Frederick *Treves,* English surgeon, 1853–1923] see *plica ileocaecalis.*

**Tre·vor's disease** (trev′ərz) [David *Trevor,* British orthopedic surgeon, 1906–1988] dysplasia epiphysealis hemimelica; see under *dysplasia.*

**Trex·an** (trek′san) trademark for a preparation of naltrexone hydrochloride.

**TRH** thyrotropin-releasing hormone.

**tri-** [Gr. *treis;* L. *tres* three] a prefix meaning *three* or *thrice.*

**tri·ac·e·tate** (tri-as′ə-tāt) an acetate which contains three molecules of the acetic acid radical.

**tri·ac·e·tin** (tri-as′ə-tin) [USP] [MeSH: Triacetin] an antifungal agent used topically in the treatment of superficial fungal infections of the skin. Called also *glyceryl triacetate.*

**tri·ace·tyl·ole·an·do·my·cin** (tri-as″ə-təl-o″le-an″do-mi′sin) troleandomycin.

**tri·ac·id** (tri-as′id) a base capable of neutralizing three equivalents of monobasic acid.

**tri·acyl·glyc·er·ol** (tri-a″səl-glis′ər-ol) triglyceride.

**tri·acyl·glyc·er·ol li·pase** (tri-a″səl-glis′ə-rol li′pās) [EC 3.1.1.3] an enzyme of the hydrolase class that catalyzes the cleavage of the two outer fatty acyl groups from triglycerides in the digestion of dietary fats. Individual enzymes are frequently named for the tissues with which they are associated; see entries under *lipase.* The term is sometimes used specifically to denote pancreatic lipase.

**tri·ad** (tri′ad) [L. *trias:* Gr. *trias* group of three] 1. any trivalent element. 2. a group of three entities or objects, as an association of three symptoms.
**acute compression t.,** Beck's t.
**adrenomedullary t.,** the symptoms caused by excessive amounts of adrenomedullary catecholamines: tachycardia, vasoconstriction, and sweating.
**Andersen's t.,** see under *syndrome.*
**Beck's t.,** three symptoms characteristic of cardiac compression: (1) a high venous pressure, (2) a low arterial pressure, and (3) a small quiet heart.
**Bezold's t.,** prolonged bone conduction (negative Rinne test) and lessened perception of low tones, indicating otosclerosis.
**Carney's t.,** see under *complex.*
**Charcot's t.,** 1. nystagmus, intention tremor, and staccato speech, formerly thought to be a sign of multiple sclerosis. 2. the symptom complex of biliary colic, jaundice, and fever and chills characteristic of intermittent cholangitis.
**Currarino's t.,** a complex of congenital anomalies in the anococcygeal region, in various combinations and degrees of seriousness; it consists of scimitar sacrum; presacral anterior meningocele, teratoma, or cyst; and rectal malformations such as stenosis, ectopia, or imperforation.
**Dieulafoy's t.,** hypersensitiveness of the skin, reflex muscular contraction, and tenderness at McBurney's point in appendicitis.
**Grancher's t.,** lessened vesicular quality of breathing, skodaic resonance, and increased vocal fremitus; seen in early pulmonary tuberculosis.
**hepatic t's,** the grouping of the tributaries of the hepatic artery, vein, and bile duct at the angles of the lobules of the liver.
**Hutchinson's t.,** diffuse interstitial keratitis, labyrinthine disease, and Hutchinson teeth, seen in inherited syphilis.
**Jacod's t.,** see under *syndrome.*
**Kartagener's t.,** see under *syndrome.*
**t. of Luciani,** asthenia, atonia, and astasia, the three major symptoms of cerebellar disease.
**Osler's t.,** the telangiectasis, capillary fragility, and hereditary hemorrhagic diathesis seen in hereditary hemorrhagic telangiectasia.
**portal t's,** hepatic t's.
**t. of retinal cone,** the tip of two horizontal cell dendrites and one midget cell dendrite, enclosed in a synaptic invagination of a retinal cone pedicle.
**Saint's t.,** hiatus hernia, colonic diverticula, and cholelithiasis, occurring concomitantly.
**t. of Schultz,** jaundice, gangrenous stomatitis, and leukopenia.
**t. of skeletal muscle,** a pair of terminal cisterns in close apposition to the T tubule, running transversely across a myofibril of skeletal muscle; in mammalian muscle there are two triads to each sarcomere, situated at the A band–I band junction. See also *T system,* under *system* and *T tubule,* under *tubule.*
**Virchow's t.,** three factors predisposing to vascular thrombosis: changes in the vascular wall, changes in the local pattern of blood flow, and changes in the blood constituents.
**Whipple's t.,** three essential clinical features of insulin-producing tumors: (1) spontaneous hypoglycemia with blood sugar levels below 50 mg per 100 mL; (2) central nervous system or vasomotor symptoms; and (3) relief of symptoms by oral or intravenous administration of glucose.

**tri·ad·i·tis** (tri″ad-i′tis) inflammation of a group of three.
**portal t.,** inflammation of the hepatic triads and adjacent connective tissue.

**tri·age** (tre-ahzh′, tre′ahzh) [Fr. "sorting"] [MeSH: Triage] 1. the sorting out and classification of casualties of war or other disaster, to determine priority of need and proper place of treatment. 2. by extension, the sorting and prioritizing of patients for treatment in nonemergency health care settings.

**tri·al** (tri′əl, trīl) a test or experiment.
**Bernoulli t's,** in statistics, a series of independent trials, each having only two mutually exclusive outcomes, commonly called "success" and "failure," so that if the probability of success is $p$ and that of failure is $q$, then $p + q = 1$ and the probability of success remains the same throughout the trials. Cf. *Bernoulli distribution.*
**clinical t.,** an experiment performed on human beings in order to evaluate the comparative efficacy of two or more therapies. The *randomized controlled trial,* which uses an appropriate control group (placebo or sham treatment or the standard well-established therapy) for comparison with the experimental therapy and random allocation of patients to the experimental and control groups, is generally considered to yield the strongest scientific evidence of any well-designed trial. Another element of well-designed trials is called *blinding* (see *single blind, double blind,* and *triple blind*).
**crossover t.,** a multipart clinical trial in which each subject is tested with each (or most) of the treatments being compared in turn, in random order.
**phase I t.,** a clinical trial on normal volunteers, designed to determine the biological activities and range of toxicity or other safety factors of a given therapy.
**phase II t.,** a clinical trial on a small group of patients, designed to determine the effectiveness of the given regimen in treating the disorder in question.
**phase III t.,** a clinical trial using a large sample of patients, designed

to compare the overall course of their disorder under the new treatment with its course untreated and treated with standard therapies previously used; studies are also done on the relative morbidities of the different treatments.

**phase IV t.,** additional studies done after a drug has been approved for distribution or marketing, which could include examination of long-term effects, adverse effects, or specific aspects of a drug's action.

**tri·al·ism** (tri'əl-iz-əm) trialistic theory; see under *theory.*

**tri·al·lyl·am·ine** (tri″ə-ləl-am'in) a volatile, oily, liquid amine, used as an intermediate; it is an irritant and a fire risk.

**tri·am·cin·o·lone** (tri″am-sin'ə-lōn) [USP] [MeSH: Triamcinolone] a synthetic glucocorticoid used in replacement therapy for adrenal insufficiency and as an anti-inflammatory and immunosuppressant in a wide variety of disorders; administered orally.

**t. acetonide** [USP], the acetonide ester of triamcinolone; applied topically to the skin or oral mucosa as an anti-inflammatory, and administered by inhalation for the chronic treatment of bronchial asthma, and by intra-articular, intradermal, intralesional, or intramuscular injection as an anti-inflammatory and immunosuppressant in a wide variety of disorders.

**t. diacetate** [USP], the diacetate ester of triamcinolone, used in replacement therapy for adrenal insufficiency and as an anti-inflammatory and immunosuppressant in a wide variety of disorders; administered orally and by intra-articular, intradermal, intralesional or intramuscular injection.

**t. hexacetonide** [USP], the hexacetonide ester of triamcinolone, used as an anti-inflammatory and immunosuppressant in a wide variety of disorders; administered by intra-articular, intralesional, or sublesional injection.

**tri·am·ine** (tri-am'in) a compound containing three amino (—$NH_2$) groups.

**tri·am·ter·ene** (tri-am'tər-ēn) [USP] [MeSH: Triamterene] a potassium-sparing diuretic that blocks the reabsorption of sodium in the distal convoluted tubules; used for the treatment of edema and hypertension, either alone or in conjunction with a loop or thiazide diuretic; administered orally.

**tri·an·gle** (tri'ang-gəl) [L. *triangulum; tres* three + *angulus* angle] a three-cornered area or figure; called also *trigone* and *trigonum.*

## Triangle

**Alsberg's t.,** an equilateral triangle with its apex upward, formed by a line passing through the long axis of the femur, a second line passing through the long axis of the neck of the femur, and a third line on a plane passing through the base of the head of the femur. The angle at the apex is known as *Alsberg's angle,* or *angle of elevation.*

**anal t.,** regio analis.

**Assézat's t.,** facial t.

**auricular t.,** one bounded by lines drawn from the tip of the auricle and the two ends of its base of insertion.

**t. of auscultation, auscultatory t.,** trigonum auscultationis.

**axillary t.,** the triangular area formed by the inner aspect of the arm, the axilla, and the pectoral region.

**Béclard's t.,** the area lying between the posterior edge of the hyoglossal muscle, the posterior belly of the digastric muscle, and the greater cornu of the hyoid bone.

**Bolton t.,** the triangle formed by drawing a line from the nasion to the sella turcica to the Bolton point.

**Bonwill t.,** one formed by a line connecting the centers of the mandibular condyles and lines connecting either center with the mesial contact area of the mandibular medial incisors, each side being approximately 10 cm long.

**brachial t.,** axillary t.

**Bryant's t.,** iliofemoral t.

**Burger's scalene t.,** a triangle providing a reference frame to represent the quantitative relationships between the electromotive forces of the heart and the extremity leads of the electrocardiograph. As compared to Einthoven's triangle, the lines representing leads I and II are considerably shortened.

**Calot's t.,** the triangle formed by the cystic artery superiorly, the cystic duct inferiorly, and the hepatic duct medially; called also *cystohepatic t.*

**cardiohepatic t.,** the triangular region in the fifth intercostal space of the right side, separating the heart from the superior edge of the liver.

**carotid t.,** trigonum caroticum.

**carotid t., inferior,** trigonum musculare.

**carotid t., superior,** trigonum caroticum.

**cephalic t.,** one on the anteroposterior plane of the skull, between the lines from the occiput to the forehead and to the chin, and a third line extending from the chin to the forehead.

**cervical t.,** trigonum cervicale.

**cervical t., anterior,** regio cervicalis anterior.

**cervical t., posterior,** regio cervicalis lateralis.

**clavipectoral t.,** trigonum clavipectorale.

**Codman's t.,** a triangular area visible radiographically where the periosteum, elevated by a bone tumor, rejoins the cortex of normal bone.

**color t.,** a plane figure with red, green, and blue located at the three apices, and gray at the center, with lines drawn from side to side, as a guide to the color mixing equation needed to produce any intermediate hue.

**crural t.,** the triangular area formed by the inner aspect of the thigh and the lower abdominal, inguinal, and genital regions.

**cystohepatic t.,** Calot's t.

**deltopectoral t.,** trigonum clavipectorale.

**digastric t.,** trigonum submandibulare.

**Einthoven's t.,** an equilateral triangle used as a mathematical model of the standard electrocardiographic limb leads, in which the instantaneous heart vector in the frontal plane may be projected on the sides of the triangle thereby demonstrating that the algebraic sum of the potential differences as recorded in electrocardiographic leads I and III will equal that potential difference recorded in lead II.

**Elant's t.,** a triangular area whose base is the promontory of the sacrum and whose sides are the left and right common iliac arteries.

**t. of elbow,** a triangular area on the front of the elbow, having the brachioradialis muscle on the lateral side and the pronator teres on the medial side, the base being toward the humerus.

**extravesical t.,** Pawlik's t.

**facial t.,** a triangular area whose points are the basion, the alveolar point, and the nasion; called also *Assézat's t.*

**Farabeuf's t.,** a triangular area on the superior part of the neck whose sides are formed by the internal jugular vein and facial vein and whose base is formed by the hypoglossal nerve.

**femoral t.,** 1. trigonum femorale. 2. trigonum femoris.

**fetal t.,** a triangular space made by the side of the fetal trunk, the thigh above, and the arm below.

**frontal t.,** one bounded by the maximum frontal diameter and lines from either end of this diameter to the glabella.

**Garland's t.,** a triangular area of relative resonance in the lower back, close to the spine on the diseased side; seen in pleurisy with effusion.

**Gerhardt's t.,** a triangular area of dullness to percussion above the third left rib, an inconstant sign in patent ductus arteriosus.

**Gombault-Philippe t.,** a triangular field formed in the conus medullaris by the fibers of the septomarginal tract.

**Grocco's t.,** a triangular area of dullness on the back, on the side opposite to that of a pleural effusion. Called also *Grocco's sign* and *paravertebral t.*

**Grynfeltt's t., t. of Grynfeltt and Lesshaft,** Lesshaft's space.

**Henke's t.,** a triangular area between the descending portion of the inguinal fold, the lateral portion of the inguinal fold, and the lateral border of the rectus muscle.

**Hesselbach's t.,** trigonum inguinale.

**hypoglossohyoid t.,** the triangular space in the subhyoid region, bounded superiorly by the hypoglossal nerve, anteriorly by the posterior border of the mylohyoid muscle, and posteriorly and inferiorly by the tendon of the digastric muscle. Called also *Pinaud's t.* and *Pirogoff's t.*

**iliofemoral t.,** a triangular area bounded by Nélaton's line, a line through the anterior superior iliac spine, and one extending from this spine to the great trochanter of the femur.

**infraclavicular t.,** fossa infraclavicularis.

**inguinal t.,** 1. trigonum inguinale. 2. trigonum femorale.

**Jackson's safety t.,** a triangular space bounded above by the lower end of the thyroid cartilage, its apex in the suprasternal notch, and its sides the inner edges of the sternocleidomastoid muscle; so called because it marks the limits of the area through which the trachea may safely be incised in tracheostomy.

**Kanavel's t.,** a triangular area in the middle of the palm beneath which lies the common tendon sheath of the digital flexor tendons.

**Killian's t.,** Killian's dehiscence.

**t. of Koch,** a roughly triangular area on the septal wall of the right atrium, bounded by the base of the septal leaflet of the tricuspid valve, the anteromedial margin of the orifice of the coronary sinus, and the tendon of Todaro; it marks the site of the atrioventricular node.

**Labbé's t.,** one included between a horizontal line along the inferior border of the cartilage of the ninth rib, the line of the false ribs, and the line of the liver, being the area where the stomach lies in contact with the anterior abdominal wall.

**Langenbeck's t.,** one having its apex at the anterior superior spine of the ilium, its base along the anatomical neck of the femur, and its external side by the external face of the great trochanter of the femur.

**Lesser's t.,** one bounded by the hypoglossal nerve superiorly and the two bellies of the digastricus muscle on the other two sides.

**Lesshaft's t.,** see under *space.*

**Lieutaud's t.,** trigonum vesicae.

**Livingston's t.,** an area bounded by lines from the umbilicus to the iliac crest, from the latter to the right pubic spine, and from there to the umbilicus, marking an area hypersensitive to palpation in appendicitis.

**lumbar t., lumbar t., inferior,** trigonum lumbale inferius.

**lumbar t., superior,** trigonum lumbale superius.

**lumbocostoabdominal t.,** a space between the obliquus externus abdominis muscle, the serratus posterior inferior, the erector spinae, and the obliquus internus abdominis.

**Macewen's t.,** foveola suprameatica.

**Malgaigne's t.,** trigonum caroticum.

**mesenteric t.,** a triangular space between the two layers of the mesentery as they diverge to enclose the intestine.

**Minor's t.,** an angular defect posterior to the anus, produced by attachment of the superficial portion of the external sphincter to the coccyx.

**Mohrenheim's t.,** fossa infraclavicularis.

**muscular t.,** trigonum musculare.

**t's of neck,** see *trigonum cervicale.*

**occipital t.,** the area bounded by the sternocleidomastoid muscle anteriorly, the trapezius muscle posteriorly, and the omohyoid muscle inferiorly.

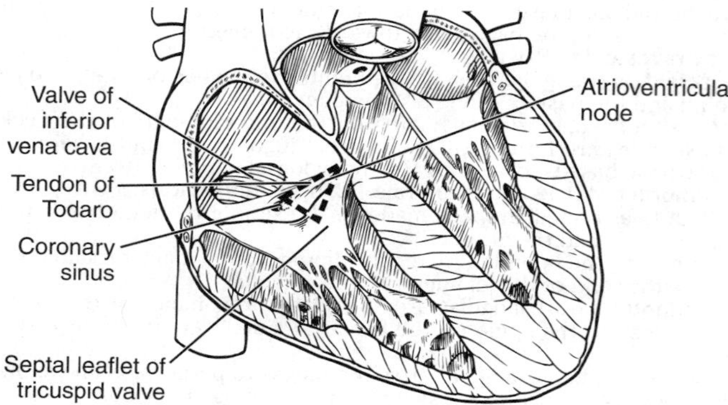


Triangle of Koch, at the apex of which lies the atrioventricular node.

**occipital t., inferior,** a triangular area having a line between the two mastoid processes as its base and the inion as its apex.

**omoclavicular t.,** trigonum omoclaviculare.

**omotracheal t.,** trigonum musculare.

**palatal t.,** one limited by the greatest transverse diameter of the palate and lines from either end of this diameter to the alveolar point.

**paravertebral t.,** Grocco's t.

**Pawlik's t.,** one within the vagina corresponding exactly with the trigonum vesicae, and bounded laterally by Pawlik's folds.

**Petit's t.,** trigonum lumbale inferius.

**Pinaud's t., Pirogoff's t.,** hypoglossohyoid t.

**popliteal t. of femur,** facies poplitea femoris.

**pubourethral t.,** one in the perineum bounded externally by the ischiocavernosus muscle, internally by the bulbocavernosus, and posteriorly by the transversus perinei superficialis.

**Reil's t.,** trigonum lemnisci.

**retromandibular t., retromolar t.,** a triangular shallow fossa on the mandible posterior to the third molar.

**sacral t.,** a shallow triangular depression overlying the sacrum.

**t. of safety,** the fifth or sixth left intercostal space, considered a safe site for pericardial aspiration.

**Scarpa's t.,** trigonum femorale.

**sternocostal t.,** trigonum sternocostale.

**subclavian t.,** trigonum omoclaviculare.

**subinguinal t.,** 1. hiatus saphenus. 2. trigonum femorale.

**submandibular t., submaxillary t.,** trigonum submandibulare.

**submental t.,** trigonum submentale.

**suboccipital t.,** a triangular area lying between the rectus capitis posterior major and the obliquus capitis superior and obliquus capitis inferior muscles.

**supraclavicular t.,** trigonum omoclaviculare.

**suprameatal t.,** foveola suprameatica.

**surgical t.,** any triangular area or region in which certain nerves, vessels, or organs are located; established for reference in surgical operations.

**Trautmann's t.,** a space with its anterior angle at the prominence containing the labyrinth, bounded posteriorly by the transverse sinus and superiorly by the inferior temporal line. When the bone is surgically removed, the superior petrosal sinus will be encountered at the superior posterior angle of this triangle.

**Tweed t.,** a triangle defined by facial and dental landmarks on a lateral cephalometric film, using the Frankfort horizontal plane as a base.

**umbilicomammillary t.,** one having its base formed by the line joining the nipples and its apex at the umbilicus.

**urogenital t.,** 1. diaphragma urogenitale. 2. regio urogenitalis.

**vaginal t.,** Pawlik's t.

**vesical t.,** trigonum vesicae.

**von Weber's t.,** one on the sole of the foot formed by lines connecting the head of the first metatarsal, the head of the fifth metatarsal, and the center of the undersurface of the heel.

**Ward's t.,** the space formed by the angle of the trabeculae in the neck of the femur; a vulnerable point for fracture.

**Wernicke's t.,** the area within the posterior limb on the internal capsule in which the optic radiation, having just left the lateral geniculate body, comes into close proximity to the auditory and somesthetic radiations.

**tri·an·gu·lar** (tri-ang′gu-lər) [L. *triangularis*] having three angles or corners.

**tri·an·gu·la·ris** (tri-ang″gu-lar′is) [L.] triangular.

**tri·an·te·bra·chia** (tri″an-te-bra′ke-ə) [*tri-* + *antebrachium* + *-ia*] a developmental anomaly characterized by tripling of the forearm.

**Tri·at·o·ma** (tri-at′o-mə) [MeSH: Triatoma] a genus of cone-nose bugs of the family Reduviidae; many species are important vectors of *Trypanosoma cruzi,* the etiologic agent of Chagas' disease. These include *T. dimidia′ta, T. genicula′ta,* and *T. mexica′na* in Mexico and Central America; *T. gerstacek′eri, T. protrac′ta,* and *T. sanguisu′ga* in the southern United States; *T. recu′va* and *T. rubi′da* in Arizona; and *T. infes′tans* (the unchuca or great black bug), *T. nigrova′rius, T. sor′dida,* and *T. vit′ticeps* in South America. Several of the species in the Uni

**T. megis′ta,** former name for *Panstrongylus megistus.*

**tri·atom·ic** (tri″ə-tom′ik) made up of three atoms.

**tri·a·zene** (tri′ə-zēn) 1. the chemical species HN=N—$NH_2$. 2. a group of cytotoxic alkylating agents containing this moiety, typified by dacarbazine.

**tri·a·zo·lam** (tri-a′zə-lam) [USP] [MeSH: Triazolam] a benzodiazepine used as a sedative and hypnotic in the treatment of insomnia; administered orally.

**tri·a·zole** (tri′əzōl, tri-a′zōl) 1. a five-membered ring containing two carbon and three nitrogen atoms. 2. any of a class of compounds containing this ring.

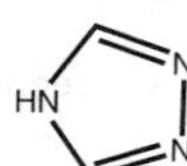


**trib·a·dism** (trib′ə-diz-əm) [Gr. *tribein* to rub] 1. lesbianism; usually used to denote that in which heterosexual intercourse is simulated; sometimes used to refer to the use of an artificial penis. 2. mutual friction of the genitals between women.

**tri·ba·sic** (tri-ba′sik) [*tri-* + *basic*] having three replaceable hydrogen atoms.

**tribe** (trīb) a taxonomic category subordinate to a family (or subfamily) and superior to a genus (or subtribe).

**tri·ben·o·side** (tri-ben′o-sīd) a sclerosing agent which has been used in inflammatory and varicose disorders of the veins.

**Tri·bo·li·um** (tri-bo′le-əm) [MeSH: Tribolium] a genus of small beetles that live in and are very destructive to flour and other cereal products. The two most common species, *T. confu′sum* and *T. casta′neum,* are reddish brown in color and 3.5 mm in length.

**tri·bol·o·gy** (trĭ-bol′ə-je) [Gr. *tribē* a rubbing + *-logy*] the study of the lubrication, friction, and wear of the joints.

**tri·bo·lu·mi·nes·cence** (tri″bo-loo″mĭ-nes′əns) [Gr. *tribein* to rub + *luminescence*] luminescence produced by mechanical energy, as by the grinding, rubbing, or breaking of certain crystals.

**tri·bra·chia** (tri-bra′ke-ə) [*tri-* + *brachia*] a developmental anomaly characterized by tripling of an arm.

**tri·bra·chi·us** (tri-bra′ke-əs) 1. a fetus exhibiting tribrachia. 2. conjoined twins having only three arms.

**tri·brom·sa·lan** (tri-brom′sə-lən) a bromsalan disinfectant with antibacterial and antifungal activities, used mainly in medicated soaps.

**trib·u·lo·sis** (trib″u-lo′sis) poisoning in sheep in South Africa caused by eating wilted plants of the species *Tribulus terrestris;* symptoms include hepatic injury, photosensitization, and encephalopathy.

**tri·bu·tyl cit·rate** (tri-bu′til) [NF] the ester of *n*-butyl alcohol and citric acid, used as a plasticizer in pharmaceutical preparations.

**Trib·u·lus** (trib′u-ləs) a genus of tropical and subtropical herbs. *T. terres′tris* is the puncture vine, which causes tribulosis in sheep in Australia and South Africa.

**Trib·u·ron** (trib′u-ron) trademark for preparations of triclobisonium chloride.

**tri·bu·tyr·in** (tri-bu′tər-in) the triglyceride formed from butyric acid and occurring in butter; it is a liquid fat with an acrid taste. Called also *butyrin.*

**TRIC** (trik) acronym for *tr*achoma *i*nclusion *c*onjunctivitis (group of organisms); see *Chlamydia trachomatis.*

**tri·cal·cic** (tri-kal′sik) containing three atoms of calcium.

**tri·cel·lu·lar** (tri-sel′u-lər) three celled.

**tri·ceph·a·lus** (tri-sef′ə-ləs) [*tri-* + *-cephalus*] a fetus having three heads.

**tri·ceps** (tri′seps) [L., from *tri-* + *caput* head] having three heads, as a triceps muscle.
**t. su′rae,** see under *musculus.*

**tri·chei·ria** (tri-ki′re-ə) [*tri-* + *cheir-* + *-ia*] a developmental anomaly characterized by tripling of a hand.

**trich·es·the·sia** (trik″əs-the′zhə) trichoesthesia.

**tri·chi·a·sis** (trĭ-ki′ə-sis) [Gr.] 1. a condition of ingrowing hairs about an orifice, or of ingrowing eyelashes. 2. the appearance of hairlike filaments in the urine.

**trich·i·lem·mo·ma** (trik″ĭ-ləm-o′mə) a benign neoplasm of the lower outer root sheath of the hair.

**Tri·chi·na** (trĭ-ki′nə) *Trichinella.*

**tri·chi·na** (trĭ-ki′nə) pl. *trichi′nae.* An individual organism of the genus *Trichinella.*

**Trich·i·nel·la** (trik″ĭ-nel′ə) [Gr. *trichinos* of hair] [MeSH: Trichinella] a genus of nematode parasites of the family Trichinellidae, superfamily Trichuroidea.
**T. nati′va,** a species that infects the human intestine in arctic and subarctic areas.
**T. nelso′ni,** a species that infects the human intestine in hot regions, especially in Africa.
**T. spira′lis,** a small parasitic nematode, 1.5 mm long, the usual etiologic agent of trichinosis; it is found coiled in a cyst in the muscles of bears, rats, pigs, and humans. When infected meat is eaten without proper cooking the cyst dissolves and the parasite matures and deposits its larvae in the deep mucosa; from there they enter the lymphatics, are carried to all parts of the body, and again encyst. An extract of *Trichinella* larvae is used in an intradermal skin test for trichinosis. Called also *pork worm.*

**Trich·i·nel·li·dae** a family of nematodes of the superfamily Trichuroidea; it contains the genus *Trichinella.*

**trich·i·nel·li·a·sis** (trik″ĭ-nə-li′ə-sis) trichinosis.

**trich·i·nel·lo·sis** (trik″ĭ-nə-lo′sis) trichinosis.

**trich·i·ni·a·sis** (trik″ĭ-ni′ə-sis) trichinosis.

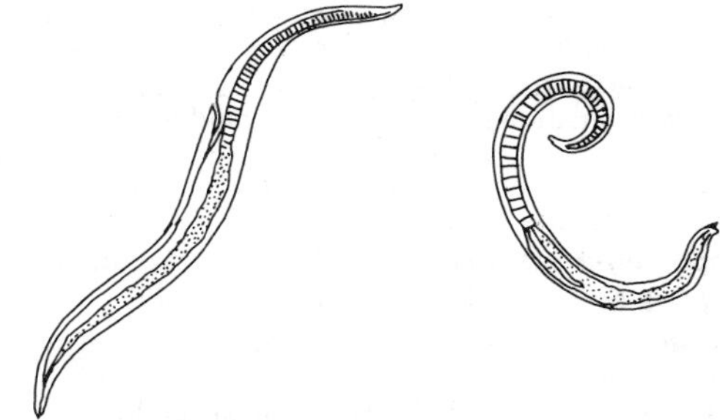

*Trichinella spiralis,* female *(left)* and male *(right).*

**trich·i·nif·er·ous** (trik″ĭ-nif′ər-əs) [*trichina* + *-ferous*] containing trichinae.

**trich·i·ni·za·tion** (trik″ĭ-nĭ-za′shən) trichinosis.

**trich·i·no·sis** (trik″ĭ-no′sis) [MeSH: Trichinosis] a disease due to infection with *Trichinella spiralis,* seen following the eating of undercooked contaminated meat; early symptoms are diarrhea, nausea, colic, and fever, followed later by stiffness, pain, muscle swelling, fever, eosinophilia, circumorbital edema, splinter hemorrhages, sweating, and insomnia.

**trich·i·nous** (trik′ĭ-nəs) affected with or containing trichinae.

**trich·i·on** (trik′e-on) pl. *trich′ia* [Gr.] an anthropometric landmark, the point at which the midsagittal plane of the head intersects the hairline.

**tri·chite** (tri′kīt) [Gr. *thrix* hair] 1. trichocyst. 2. nematodesma. 3. a hollow, rodlike, subpellicular component of the skeleton of oligotrich ciliates.

**tri·chlor·fon** (tri-klor′fon) [USP] [MeSH: Trichlorfon] an organophosphorous insecticide having potent anticholinesterase activity; especially effective against *Schistosoma haematobium.* Administered topically as an ectoparasiticide in humans, and sometimes orally as an anthelmintic; used more commonly in veterinary medicine as an oral anthelmintic. Overdosage can cause organophosphorus compound poisoning (q.v.). Called also *metrifonate* and *trichlorphon.*

**tri·chlo·ride** (tri-klor′īd) any combination of three atoms of chlorine with one of another element.

**tri·chlor·me·thi·a·zide** (tri-klor″mə-thi′ə-zīd) [USP] [MeSH: Trichlormethiazide] a thiazide diuretic used in the treatment of hypertension and edema; administered orally.

**tri·chlo·ro·ac·et·al·de·hyde** (tri-klor″o-as″ət-al′də-hīd) chloral.

**tri·chlo·ro·ace·tic ac·id** (tri-klor″o-ə-se′tik) [USP] [MeSH: Trichloroacetic Acid] a strong acid used as a protein precipitant in clinical chemistry and also as a caustic for removing warts.

**tri·chlo·ro·eth·y·lene** (tri-klor″o-eth′ə-lēn) [MeSH: Trichloroethylene] a toxic liquid widely used as an industrial solvent; formerly used as an inhalation anesthetic.

**tri·chlo·ro·meth·yl·chlo·ro·for·mate** (tri-klor″o-meth″əl-klor″o-for′māt) a chlorine-containing gas which is irritating to lung tissue.

**tri·chlo·ro·mono·flu·o·ro·meth·ane** (tri-klor″o-mon″o-floor′o-meth′ān) [NF] chemical name: trichlorofluoromethane. A clear, colorless gas having a faint, ethereal odor, $CCl_3F$, used as an aerosol propellant.

**tri·chlo·ro·phe·nol** (tri″klor-o-fe′nol) a disinfectant and external antiseptic.

**2,4,5-tri·chlo·ro·phen·oxy·ace·tic ac·id** (tri-klor″o-fən-ok″se-ə-se′tik) [MeSH: 2,4,5-Trichlorophenoxyacetic Acid] 2,4,5-T.

**tri·chlo·ro·tri·vi·nyl·ar·sine** (tri-klor″o-tri-vi″nəl-ahr′sin) a sternutatory war gas.

**tri·chlor·phon** (tri-klor′fon) trichlorfon.

**trich(o)-** [Gr. *thrix,* gen. *trichos,* hair] a prefix denoting relationship to hair.

**tricho·ad·e·no·ma** (trik″o-ad″ə-no′mə) [*tricho-* + *adenoma*] a benign follicular tumor occurring on the face or trunk, with histologic features midway between those of trichofolliculoma and trichoepithelioma, with large cystic spaces lined by squamous epithelium and squamous cells.

**tricho·bac·te·ria** (trik″o-bak-tēr′e-ə) [*tricho-* + *bacteria*] 1. a group of bacteria including those forms which possess flagella. 2. the filamentous or threadlike bacteria.

**tricho·be·zoar** (trik″o-be′zor) [*tricho-* + *bezoar*] [MeSH: Bezoars] a concretion within the stomach or intestines formed of hairs; called also *hairball* or *hair ball.*

**Tricho·bil·har·zia** (trik″o-bil-hahr′ze-ə) a genus of flukes of the family Schistosomatidae. *T. ocella′ta* is found in the portal veins of ducks.

**tricho·car·dia** (trik″o-kahr′de-ə) [*tricho-* + Gr. *kardia* heart] shaggy pericardium.

**tricho·ceph·a·li·a·sis** (trik″o-sef″ə-li′ə-sis) trichuriasis.

**tricho·ceph·a·lo·sis** (trik″o-sef″ə-lo′sis) trichuriasis.

**Tricho·ceph·a·lus** (trik″o-sef′ə-ləs) [*tricho-* + *-cephalus*] former name for *Trichuris.*

**tricho·cla·sia** (trik″o-kla′zhə) trichorrhexis nodosa.

**trich·oc·la·sis** (trik-ok′lə-sis) [*tricho-* + Gr. *klasis* fracture] trichorrhexis nodosa.

**Trich·o·co·ma·ceae** (trik″o-ko-ma′se-e) [Gr. *trichokomos* hairdresser] a family of fungi of the order Eurotiales, containing the perfect (sexual) stage of certain species of *Aspergillus, Paecilomyces,* and *Penicillium.* Medically important genera include *Emericella* and *Eurotium.*

**tricho·cyst** (trik′o-sist) [*tricho-* + *-cyst*] one of the extrusible and explosive, nontoxic, spindle-shaped subpellicular organelles occurring in many protozoa, which can discharge long, striated, fibrous shafts. Its true function is unknown, but it may serve to anchor the organism during feeding, serve an offensive or defensive function, or serve in prey capture. Called also *trichite.*

**Tricho·dec·tes** (trik″o-dek′tēz) [*tricho-* + Gr. *dēktēs* biter] a genus of parasitic biting lice (order Mallophaga). *T. ca′nis* infests dogs and is an intermediate host for the tapeworm *Dipylidium caninum. T. la′tus* also infests dogs. *T. sphaeroce′phalus* infests the wool of sheep in Europe and North America. *T. e′qui, T. herm′si,* and *T. pilo′sus* have been reclassified into the genus *Damalinia.*

**Tricho·der·ma** (trik-o-dər′mə) [*tricho* + *derma* skin] [MeSH: Trichoderma] a genus of soil-inhabiting Fungi Imperfecti of the form-class Hyphomycetes, form-family Moniliaceae; some species contain trichothecenes and cause alimentary toxic aleukia. Its perfect (sexual) stage when found is in the genera *Hypocrea* and *Pododerma.*

**tricho·dis·co·ma** (trik″o-dis-ko′mə) [*tricho-* + *disc-* + *-oma*] a hamartoma of the mesodermal portion of the hair disk, usually occurring as multiple small papules that histologically resemble acrochordons; they may occur in association with fibrofolliculomas and acrochordons as the autosomal dominant Birt-Hogg-Dubé syndrome.

**tricho·epi·the·li·o·ma** (trik″o-ep″ĭ-the-le-o′mə) [*tricho-* + *epithelioma*] a benign skin tumor originating in the hair matrix, generally occurring on the face and characterized histologically by strands of basal cells surrounded by fibrocellular stroma. It usually occurs in young women as an autosomal dominant disorder, characterized by multiple smooth, flesh-colored, cystic and solid nodules or papules *(multiple trichoepithelioma),* but it may occur as a nonhereditary solitary lesion, usually in young adult women *(solitary trichoepithelioma).*
**desmoplastic t.,** a benign, solitary, whitish, hard nodule with a central nonulcerated depression, usually occurring on the face in young to middle-aged women and characterized by strands of basaloid cells and epidermal cysts infiltrating fibrotic stroma. Called also *sclerosing epithelial hamartoma.*
**t. papillo′sum mul′tiplex,** multiple t.; see *trichoepithelioma.*

**tricho·es·the·sia** (trik″o-əs-the′zhə) [*tricho-* + *esthesia*] the perception that one of the hairs of the skin has been touched, caused by stimulation of a hair follicle receptor.

**tricho·es·the·si·om·e·ter** (trik″o-əs-the″ze-om′ə-tər) [*tricho-* + *esthesio-* + *-meter*] an electric apparatus for measuring the hair sensibility, or the sensitiveness of the scalp by means of the hairs.

**tricho·fol·lic·u·lo·ma** (trik″o-fə-lik″u-lo′mə) [*tricho-* + *folliculus* + *-oma*] a benign usually solitary dome-shaped nodular lesion with a central pore that frequently contains a woolly hair-like tuft; it usually occurs on the head or neck, is derived from a hair follicle, and is characterized histologically by a central keratinous cystic cavity into which numerous abortive hair follicles radiate.

**tricho·glos·sia** (trik″o-glos′e-ə) [*tricho-* + *gloss-* + *-ia*] hairy tongue.

**tricho·graph·ism** (tri-kog′rə-fiz-əm) pilomotor reflex.

**tricho·hy·a·lin** (trik″o-hi′ə-lin) [*tricho-* + *hyalin*] a keratohyaline-like substance occurring in granules in the cytoplasm of the cells of Huxley's layer of a hair follicle.

**trich·oid** (trik′oid) [*tricho-* + *-oid*] like or resembling a hair, or the hair.

**tricho·lem·mo·ma** (trik″o-lem-o′mə) trichilemmoma.

**tricho·leu·ko·cyte** (trik″o-loo′ko-sīt) hairy cell.

**tricho·lith** (trik′o-lith) [*tricho-* + *-lith*] a hairy concretion.

**trich·ol·o·gy** (trĭ-kol′ə-je) the study of hair, or the sum of what is known about the hair.

**tri·cho·ma** (trĭ-ko′mə) entropion.

**tri·chom·a·tous** (trĭ-kom′ə-təs) affected with, of the nature of, or pertaining to trichoma (entropion).

**tri·chome** (tri′kōm) [Gr. *trichōma* a growth of hair, hair generally] 1. a filamentous or hairlike structure. 2. a colony of filamentous blue-green algae in which the member cells grow end-to-end to form a chain-like structure.

**tricho·meg·a·ly** (trik″o-meg′ə-le) [*tricho-* + *-megaly*] a congenital syndrome consisting of excessive growth of the eyelashes and brow hair associated with dwarfism, mental retardation, and pigmentary degeneration of the retina.

**tricho·mo·na·ci·dal** (trik″o-mo″nə-si′dəl) destructive to trichomonads.

**tricho·mo·na·cide** (trik″o-mo′nə-sīd) an agent destructive to trichomonads.

**tricho·mo·nad** (trik″o-mo′nad, trik″o-mon′ad) [*tricho-* + *monad*] any protozoan of the order Trichomonadida.

**Tricho·mo·nad·i·da** (trik″o-mo-nad′e-də) [MeSH: Trichomonadida] an order of chiefly parasitic protozoa (superorder Parabasalidea, class Zoomastigophora), typically characterized by the presence of karyomastigonts with four to six flagella, one of which is recurrent or free or has a proximal segment or the entire length adherent to the body surface; an undulating membrane (if present) associated with adherent segments of recurrent flagellum; and a pelta and noncontractile axostyle in each mastigont. Representative genera include *Dientamoeba, Histomonas, Monocercomonas,* and *Trichomonas.*

**tricho·mo·nal** (trik″o-mo′nəl) pertaining to or caused by trichomonads.

**Tricho·mo·nas** (trik″o-mo′nəs) [*tricho-* + Gr. *monas* unit, from *monas* single] [MeSH: Trichomonas] a genus of parasitic flagellated protozoa of the order Trichomonadida, class Zoomastigophorea, found in the intestinal and genitourinary tracts of various invertebrates and vertebrates, including humans, and characterized by the presence of a pelta, an axostyle, an undulating membrane, and three to five anterior flagella. In some systems of classification, those with three flagella have been assigned to genus *Tritrichomonas,* and those with five to genus *Pentatrichomonas.*
**T. bucca′lis,** *T. tenax.*
**T. foe′tus,** a species with three anterior flagella, found in the genital tract of cattle; it causes a contagious venereal disease (bovine trichomoniasis) transmitted from bulls to cows by coitus or by artificial insemination, and characterized by early abortion, pyometra, and sterility.
**T. galli′nae,** a species with four anterior flagella found in the upper digestive tract and associated structures and in other organs, especially the liver, of domestic pigeons and various other birds, in which it causes a form of avian trichomoniasis. Infection varies from mild to a rapidly fatal disease manifested by caseous accumulations and necrosis in involved tissues and severe weight loss.
**T. gallina′rum,** a species with four anterior flagella found in the lower digestive tract of chickens, turkeys, and other domestic birds in which it sometimes causes a fatal form of avian trichomoniasis. Infection is manifested by lesions of the cecum and liver, diarrhea, and loss of appetite and weight.
**T. ho′minis,** a species with five flagella that is one of the most common enteric flagellates seen in humans, in whom it may be present in large numbers but is generally considered to be nonpathogenic. Called also *T. intestinalis.*
**T. te′nax,** a commensal species with four anterior flagella found in the mouth of primates, including humans, where it is most often seen in the tartar around teeth, cavities of carious teeth, pockets associated with periodontal disease, and tonsillar crypts. Called also *T. buccalis.*
**T. vagina′lis,** a species with four flagella found in the vagina and male genital tract, the cause of trichomoniasis vaginalis.

**tricho·mo·ni·a·sis** (trik″o-mo-ni′ə-sis) infection with *Trichomonas.*
**avian t.,** trichomoniasis in birds and poultry, especially pigeons, caused by *Trichomonas gallinae* and *T. gallinarum,* and marked by necrotic lesions of the upper digestive tract.
**bovine t.,** venereal trichomoniasis in cattle, caused by *Trichomonas foetus* and marked by abortion and pyometra.
**t. vagina′lis,** human trichomoniasis caused by *Trichomonas vaginalis,* seen in both females and males; it is usually transmitted by coitus and is sometimes asymptomatic. The symptomatic condition in females may take the form of a severe vaginitis associated with discharge, burning, pruritus, and chafing; in males it may produce urethritis, enlargement of the prostate, and epididymitis.

**Trich·o·my·ce·tes** (trik″o-mi-se′tēs) [*tricho-* + Gr. *mykēs* fungus]

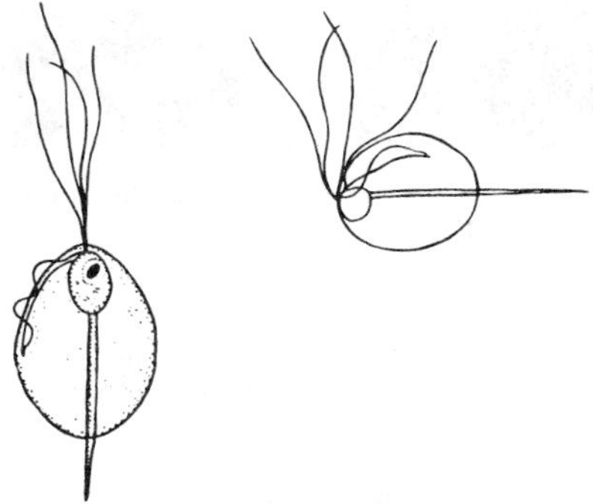

*Trichomonas vaginalis.*

a class of perfect fungi of the phylum Zygomycota, most of whose members are found as parasites in the digestive tract or on the external cuticle of living arthropods.

**tricho·my·co·sis** (trik″o-mi-ko′sis) [*tricho-* + *mycosis* ] 1. t. axillaris. 2. any disease of the hair due to infection by a fungus.
**t. axilla′ris,** a superficial infection of the axillary or pubic hair in which yellow, black, or red nodular concretions form around the hair shaft; it is caused by *Corynebacterium tenuis,* a nocardia-like microorganism of uncertain affiliation that was formerly thought to be a fungus.
**t. nodo′sa, t. nodula′ris,** piedra.

**trich·on** (trik′on) trichophytin.

**tricho·no·do·sis** (trik″o-no-do′sis) [*tricho-* + L. *nodus* knot + *-osis*] a rare condition characterized by apparent or actual knotting of the hair, thought to be the result of inability of new hairs to grow freely from their follicles, because of toughness of the surrounding tissues.

**tricho·path·ic** (trik″o-path′ik) pertaining to disease of the hair.

**trich·op·a·thy** (trĭ-kop′ə-the) [*tricho-* + *-pathy*] disease of the hair.

**tricho·pha·gia** (trik″o-fa′jə) [*tricho-* + *-phagia*] the practice or habit of eating hair.

**trich·oph·a·gy** (trĭ-kof′ə-je) trichophagia.

**tricho·phyt·ic** (trik″o-fit′ik) pertaining to trichophytosis.

**tri·choph·y·tid** (trĭ-kof′ĭ-tid) [*Trichophyton* + *-id*] a dermatophytid associated with trichophytosis; applied especially to allergic manifestations of any ringworm infection.

**tri·choph·y·tin** (trĭ-kof′ĭ-tin) [MeSH: Trichophytin] the soluble broth culture products of various species of *Trichophyton;* used in the trichophytin test.

**tricho·phy·to·be·zoar** (trik″o-fi″to-be′zor) [*tricho-* + *phyto-* + *bezoar*] a bezoar composed of animal hair and vegetable fibers.

**Tri·choph·y·ton** (tri-kof′ĭ-ton) [*tricho-* + Gr. *phyton* plant] [MeSH: Trichophyton] a genus of Fungi Imperfecti of the form-class Hyphomycetes, form-family Moniliaceae, consisting of flat, branched filaments. Many species are dermatophytes and attack the skin, nails, and hair, and most are either of the large-spored ectothrix or endothrix type. As the perfect (sexual) stages are identified they are classified in the genus *Arthroderma.*
**T. concen′tricum,** an anthropophilic species that is the usual cause of tinea imbricata.
**T. equi′num,** a zoophilic species that causes ringworm in horses.
**T. ferrugi′neum,** *Microsporum ferrugineum.*
**T. galli′nae,** a zoophilic species that is a large-spored ectothrix and causes favus in fowls. Called also *Microsporum gallinae.*
**T. mentagrophy′tes,** a small-spored ectothrix species that causes ringworm (tinea) of various types in farm animals and humans. It has perfect (sexual) stages in genus *Arthroderma.*
**T. ru′brum,** an anthropophilic species that commonly causes various types of ringworm (tinea).
**T. schoenlei′nii,** an anthropophilic species that causes favus.
**T. si′mii,** a geophilic species found in India that causes ringworm in monkeys and chickens and tinea corporis in humans. Its perfect (sexual) stage is *Arthroderma simii.*
**T. tonsu′rans,** an anthropophilic species that is an endothrix and causes tinea capitis and tinea corporis; it occurs throughout the world but is particularly prevalent in the Americas.
**T. verruco′sum,** a species that causes ringworm (tinea) in farm animals and humans.
**T. viola′ceum,** an anthropophilic species that is an endothrix and usually causes tinea capitis but sometimes also causes tinea corporis and tinea unguium.

**tricho·phy·to·sis** (trik″o-fi-to′sis) a fungal infection caused by species of *Trichophyton*; see also *favus.*

**Tri·chop·tera** (tri-kop′tər-ə) [*tricho-* + Gr. *pteron* wing] an order of flies, the caddis flies. The hair and scales from the wings may produce allergic symptoms in susceptible persons.

**trich·op·ti·lo·sis** (trik″o-tĭ-lo′sis) [*tricho-* + Gr. *ptilon* feather + *-osis*] the condition in which the hairs are split and feather-like.

**trich·or·rhex·is** (trik″o-rek′sis) [*tricho-* + *-rrhexis*] a condition in which the hairs break.
**t. nodo′sa,** a condition characterized by what look like white nodes on the hairs but are actually sites where the cortex of the shaft has fractured and split into strands. The most common type affects the proximal hair shafts, so that hairs grow a few centimeters and break off; it may be either idiopathic and congenital or acquired, usually in persons with tightly curled hair who repeatedly straighten their hair. Called also *bamboo hair, clastothrix, trichoclasia,* and *trichoclasis.*

**trich·os·chi·sis** (trik-os′kĭ-sis) [*tricho-* + *-schisis*] splitting of the hairs.

**tri·chos·co·py** (trĭ-kos′kə-pe) [*tricho-* + *-scopy*] examination of the hair.

**tricho·sid·er·in** (trik″o-sid′ər-in) [*tricho-* + Gr. *sidēros* iron] an iron-containing brown pigment found in normal human red hair.

**tri·cho·sis** (tri-ko′sis) [Gr. *trichōsis*] any disease or abnormal growth of the hair.
**t. carun′culae,** abnormal development of the hair on the lacrimal caruncle.

**Tricho·so·ma** (trik″o-so′mə) [*tricho-* + Gr. *sōma* body] *Capillaria.*
**T. contor′tum,** *Capillaria contorta.*

**Tricho·so·moi·des** (trik″o-so-moi′dēz) a genus of nematodes of the family Trichuridae. *T. crassicau′da* is parasitic in rats; the male is much smaller than the female and lives inside the uterus.

**Tri·chos·po·ron** (tri-kos′pə-ron) [*tricho-* + Gr. *sporos* seed] [MeSH: Trichosporon] a genus of Fungi Imperfecti of the form-family Cryptococcaceae, closely related to *Geotrichum.* Called also *Trichosporum. T. beige′lii* (also called *T. cuta′neum* and *T. gigan′teum*) is a normal inhabitant of the human skin, respiratory tract, and digestive tract but sometimes causes white piedra (q.v.) or a potentially fatal opportunistic infection. *T. capita′tum* is a former name for *Blastischizomyces capitatus. T. pedrosia′num* is a former name for *Fonsecaea pedrosoi.*

**tri·chos·po·ro·no·sis** (tri-kos″pə-rə-no′sis) infection by species of *Trichosporon;* the term is usually limited to opportunistic infections and does not include white piedra. Called also *trichosporosis.*

**tricho·spo·ro·sis** (trik″o-spə-ro′sis) 1. trichosporonosis. 2. white piedra.

**Tri·chos·po·rum** (tri-kos′pə-rəm) *Trichosporon.*

**tri·chos·ta·sis spin·u·lo·sa** (trĭ-kos′tə-sis spin″u-lo′sə) [*tricho-* + *stasis* + L. *spinulosus* thorny] a condition in which the hair follicles contain a dark, horny, comedo-like keratin plug, which contains a bundle of villus hair.

**Tricho·sto·mat·i·da** (trik″o-sto-mat′ĭ-də) [*tricho-* + Gr. *stoma* mouth] [MeSH: Trichostomatida] an order of ciliate protozoa (subclass Vestibuliferia, class Kinetofragminophorea), many of which are endocommensals in vertebrates; most have uniform somatic ciliature, sometimes asymmetrical, and no buccal ciliature in the oral region is present. It comprises two suborders: Trichostomatina and Blepharocorynthina.

**Tricho·sto·ma·ti·na** (trik″o-sto″mə-ti′nə) [MeSH: Trichostomatina] a suborder of ciliate protozoa (order Trichostomatida, subclass Vestibuliferia) in which the somatic ciliature is not reduced. *Balantidium* and *Isotricha* are representative genera.

**tricho·stron·gy·li·a·sis** (trik″o-stron″jə-li′ə-sis) infection of humans or other animals by nematodes of the genus *Trichostrongylus;* it is usually asymptomatic, but diarrhea may occur. Called also *trichostrongylosis.*

**Tricho·stron·gyl·i·dae** (trik″o-stron-jil′ĭ-de) a family of nematodes that includes many parasites of humans, domestic animals, and ruminants. Genera of medical or veterinary interest include *Cooperia, Dictyocaulus, Hyostrongylus, Mecistocirrus, Nematodirus, Nippostrongylus, Ostertagia, Teladorsagia,* and *Trichostrongylus.*

**tricho·stron·gy·lo·sis** (trik″o-stron″jə-lo′sis) [MeSH: Trichostrongylosis] trichostrongyliasis.

**Tricho·stron·gy·lus** (trik″o-stron′jə-ləs) [MeSH: Trichostrongylus] a genus of nematodes of the family Trichostrongylidae, comprising some species formerly included in the genus *Strongylus.* Adult worms are small and embed their heads in the mucosa of the small intestine of humans and other mammals; their eggs are often mistaken for those of the hookworm. See *trichostrongyliasis.*
**T. caprico′la,** a species commonly found in ruminants.
**T. colubrifor′mis,** a species frequently present in sheep and goats

and occasionally in humans; called also *Strongylus subtilis* and *T. instabilis.*
**T. insta'bilis,** *T. colubriformis.*
**T. orienta'lis,** a species found in humans and sheep in Asia.
**T. probolu'rus,** a species found in sheep, mountain goats, dromedaries, gazelles, and occasionally humans in Europe, Africa, and North America.
**T. vitri'nus,** a species found in sheep, goats, dromedaries, and occasionally humans.

**tri·choth·e·cene** (tri-koth'ə-sēn) any of a group of mycotoxins found contaminating grain and other foods; those from species of *Fusarium* cause fusariotoxicosis and those from species of *Stachybotrys* cause stachybotryotoxicosis. The group includes deoxynivalenol, diacetoxyscirpenol, roridins, satratoxins, T-2 toxin, and verrucarins.

**Tricho·the·ci·um** (trik″o-the'se-əm) [*tricho-* + Gr. *thēkē* case] a genus of Fungi Imperfecti of the form-class Hyphomycetes, form-family Moniliaceae. Certain species contain trichothecenes and occasionally cause alimentary toxic aleukia. *T. ro'seum* causes pinkrot on apples and lumber and is occasionally recovered from human otitis externa and mycotic keratitis.

**tricho·thio·dys·tro·phy** (trik″o-thi″o-dis'trə-fe) a hair abnormality, probably congenital, in which hair is sparse and brittle, has an unusually low sulfur content, and has a banded appearance under polarized light; often accompanied by short stature and varying degrees of mental retardation.

**tricho·til·lo·ma·nia** (trik″o-til″o-ma'ne-ə) [*tricho-* + Gr. *tillein* to pull + *-mania*] [MeSH: Trichotillomania] [DSM-IV] compulsive pulling out of one's hair, associated with tension or an irresistible urge before pulling and followed by pleasure or relief.

**tri·chot·o·mous** (tri-kot'ə-məs) [Gr. *tricha* three-fold + *tom-* + *-ous*] divided into three parts.

**tri·cho·tox·in** (tri″ko-tok'sin) an antibody that has a toxic action on epithelial cells.

**tri·chro·ic** (tri-kro'ik) pertaining to or characterized by trichroism.

**tri·chro·ism** (tri'kro-iz-əm) [*tri-* + Gr. *chroa* color] the exhibition of three different colors in three different aspects.

**tri·chro·ma·sy** (tri-kro'mə-se) [*tri-* + Gr. *chrōma* color] 1. ability to distinguish the three primary colors, red, yellow, and blue and mixtures thereof. 2. normal color vision.
**anomalous t.,** defective color vision in which the patient has all three cone pigments, one of which is deficient or anomalous, but not absent. There are three types of anomalous trichromasy—protanomaly, deuteranomaly, and tritanomaly, and they may be: (1) *acquired,* resulting from a retinal, cerebral, systemic, or toxic disorder; or (2) *congenital* and inherited as an X-linked recessive trait. Called also *anomalous trichromatism.*

**tri·chro·mat** (tri'kro-mat) a person with trichromasy.

**tri·chro·mat·ic** (tri″kro-mat'ik) trichromic.

**tri·chro·ma·tism** (tri-kro'mə-tiz-əm) trichroism.
**anomalous t.,** anomalous trichromasy.

**tri·chro·ma·top·sia** (tri″kro-mə-top'se-ə) trichromasy.

**tri·chro·mic** (tri-kro'mik) [*tri-* + *chrom-* + *-ic*] 1. pertaining to or exhibiting three colors. 2. able to distinguish the three primary colors (red, blue, green); having normal color vision.

**trich·ter·brust** (trich'ter-broost) [Ger.] pectus excavatum.

**trich·u·ri·a·sis** (trik″u-ri'ə-sis) [MeSH: Trichuriasis] infection with nematodes of the genus *Trichuris.*
**canine t.,** infection of the cecum of a dog with *Trichuris vulpis*; mild cases may be asymptomatic but severe cases may be characterized by bloody diarrhea.

**Trich·u·ri·dae** a family of nematodes of the superfamily Trichuroidea. It includes the genera *Capillaria, Trichosomoides,* and *Trichuris.*

**Trich·u·ris** (trik-u'ris) [*tricho-* + Gr. *oura* a tail] [MeSH: Trichuris] the whipworms, a genus of nematodes of the family Trichuridae; several species parasitize the intestines of dogs, cats, or other mammals. *T. trichiu'ra* parasitizes humans. *T. vul'pis* causes canine trichuriasis. Formerly called *Trichocephalus.*
**T. trichiu'ra,** the species that principally infects humans. It is about 5 cm long, with the front part of its body (the esophageal zone) thin like a hair. It inhabits the large intestine and may cause diarrhea, vomiting, and rectal prolapse in heavily infected children, although it usually produces no symptoms. Also known as *whipworm.*

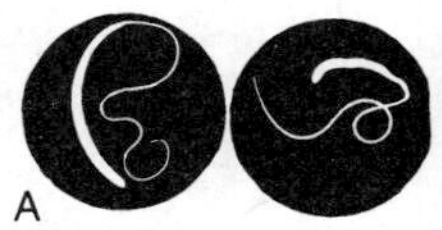

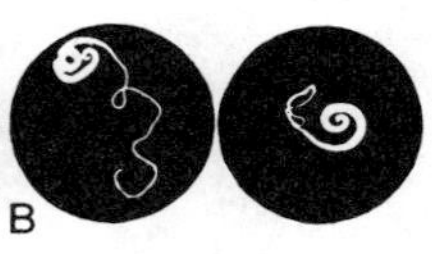


*Trichuris trichiura: (A)* females, *(B)* males. The posterior portion of the male is usually coiled as shown in *(B).*

**Trich·u·roi·dea** (trik″u-roi'de-ə) [MeSH: Trichuroidea] a superfamily of aphasmid nematodes including the families *Trichinellidae,* and *Trichuridae.*

**tri·cip·i·tal** (tri-sip'ĭ-təl) [L. *tricipitis*] 1. pertaining to the triceps muscle. 2. having three heads.

**tri·clo·bi·so·ni·um chlo·ride** (tri″klo-bĭ-so'ne-əm) a quaternary ammonium compound used as a local anti-infective, primarily in the treatment of vulvitis, vaginitis, and other gynecological conditions due to *Trichomonas vaginalis, Candida albicans,* and *Haemophilus vaginalis* or to staphylococci and streptococci, administered intravaginally.

**tri·clo·car·ban** (tri″klo-kahr'ban) a disinfectant, effective against gram-positive bacteria and to a lesser extent against gram-negative bacteria and against fungi; used in the preparation of soaps and other cleansing products and dermatological compositions to control skin infections.

**tri·clo·fen·ol pi·per·a·zine** (tri-klo'fən-ol) 2,4,5-trichlorophenol compound with piperazine (2:1); an anthelmintic effective against roundworms and hookworms.

**tri·clo·fos so·di·um** (tri'klo-fōs) an oral hypnotic and sedative used especially to induce sleep in the treatment of insomnia. It may also be used as premedication for sleep induction in electroencephalography.

**Tri·clos** (tri'klōs) trademark for a preparation of triclofos sodium.

**tri·clo·san** (tri-klo'san) [USP] [MeSH: Triclosan] an antibacterial effective against gram-positive and most gram-negative organisms and exhibiting slight activity against yeasts and fungi; used as a detergent in surgical scrubs, soaps, and deodorants.

**Tri·co·fu·ron** (tri″ko-fu'ron) trademark for preparations of furazolidone.

**Tri·co·loid** (tri'ko-loid) trademark for a preparation of tricyclamol chloride.

**tri·corn** (tri'korn) [*tri-* + *cornu*] a lateral ventricle of the brain.

**tri·cor·nute** (tri-kor'nūt) [*tri-* + L. *cornutus* horned] having three horns, cornua, or processes.

**tri·cre·sol** (tri-kre'sol) cresol.

**tri·crot·ic** (tri-krot'ik) [Gr. *trikrotos* rowed with a triple stroke; triple beating] pertaining to or characterized by tricrotism. See also *anatricrotic* and *catatricrotic.*

**tri·cro·tism** (tri'kro-tiz-əm) presence of a tricrotic pulse.

**tri·cus·pid** (tri-kus'pid) [*tri-* + *cuspid*] 1. having three points or cusps. 2. pertaining to the tricuspid valve of the heart.

**tri·cy·cla·mol chlo·ride** (tri-si'klə-mol) a quaternary ammonium anticholinergic derived from procyclidine which inhibits gastrointestinal hypermotility and reduces secretion of gastric juices; it has been used in the treatment of peptic ulcer and as a gastrointestinal antispasmodic.

**tri·cyc·lic** (tri-sik'lik) containing three fused rings or closed chains in the molecular structure; see also under *antidepressant.*

**Trid.** abbreviation for L. *trid'uum,* three days.

**tri·dac·ty·lism** (tri-dak'tə-liz-əm) [*tri-* + *dactyl-* + *-ism*] the condition of having three digits on the hands or feet.

**tri·dac·ty·lous** (tri-dak'tə-ləs) pertaining to or characterized by tridactylism.

**tri·dent** (tri'dent) tridentate.

**tri·den·tate** (tri-den'tāt) three-pronged.

**tri·der·mal** (tri-der'məl) pertaining to or possessing all three germ cell layers.

**tri·der·mic** (tri-dər'mik) [*tri-* + *dermic*] derived from the ectoderm, endoderm, and mesoderm.

**tri·der·mo·gen·e·sis** (tri″dər-mo-jen'ə-sis) [*tri-* + *dermo-* + *-genesis*] the formation of the three germ layers and, by extension, the stage in embryonic development during which it occurs.

**tri·der·mo·ma** (tri″dər-mo'mə) [*tri-* + *derm-* + *-oma*] a teratoma containing representatives of all three germ layers.

**Tri·des·i·lon** (tri-des'ĭ-lon) trademark for preparations of desonide.

**tri·di·hex·eth·yl chlo·ride** (tri″di-hək-seth'əl) quaternary ammonium anticholinergic which inhibits gastrointestinal hypermotility and spasms and reduces secretion of gastric juices; used as adjunctive therapy in the treatment of peptic ulcer and in the irritable bowel syndrome, administered orally and parenterally.

**tri·en·ceph·a·lus** (tri″ən-sef′ə-ləs) [*tri-* + Gr. *enkephalos* brain] a fetus having no organs of sight, hearing, or smell. Cf. *triocephalus.*

**-triene** a chemical suffix indicating the presence of three double bonds.

**tri·es·ter** (tri′es-tər) a compound containing three ester groups.

**tri·eth·a·nol·amine** (tri″eth-ə-nol′ə-mēn) former name for *trolamine.*

**tri·eth·yl·amine** (tri″eth-əl-am′in) a liquid ptomaine with a fishy, ammoniacal smell, occurring during putrefaction, especially in fish; it is also synthesized for use in a variety of industrial processes. It is an irritant to tissue and is toxic by inhalation and ingestion.

**tri·eth·yl cit·rate** (tri-eth′il) [NF] the ethyl ester of citric acid, used as a plasticizer in pharmaceutical preparations.

**tri·eth·yl·ene·thio·phos·pho·ra·mide** (tri-eth″ə-lēn-thi″o-fos-for′ə-mīd) thiotepa.

**tri·fa·cial** (tri-fa′shəl) [L. *trifacialis*] designating the fifth cranial nerve (nervus trigeminus [TA]).

**tri·fid** (tri′fid) [L. *trifidus,* from *tres* three + *findere* to split] split into three parts.

**tri·flu·o·per·a·zine hy·dro·chlo·ride** (tri-floo-o-per′ə-zēn) [USP] a phenothiazine antipsychotic agent, used in the treatment of symptoms of psychotic disorders and for the short-term relief of anxiety; administered orally and intramuscularly.

**tri·flu·per·i·dol** (tri-floo-per′ĭ-dol) [MeSH: Trifluperidol] a butyrophenone used in the treatment of mania and schizophrenia; administered orally.

**tri·flu·pro·ma·zine** (tri″floo-pro′mə-zēn) [USP] [MeSH: Triflupromazine] an antipsychotic agent, occurring as a viscous amber-colored oily liquid that crystallizes on long standing to large irregular crystals; administered orally.
**t. hydrochloride** [USP], the monohydrochloride salt of triflupromazine, having the same uses as the base; administered orally and intramuscularly.

**tri·flur·i·dine** (tri-floor′ĭ-dēn) [USP] [MeSH: Trifluridine] an antiviral compound that interferes with viral DNA synthesis, used in the treatment of keratitis and keratoconjunctivitis caused by human herpesviruses 1 and 2.

**tri·flu·tate** (tri′floo-tāt″) USAN contraction for trifluoroacetate.

**tri·fo·li·o·sis** (tri″fo-le-o′sis) a disease usually seen in horses, marked by photosensitization and irritation of the oral mucous membranes, sometimes with liver damage; attributed to the eating of *Trifolium hybridum* (hybrid clover) and related plants.

**Tri·fo·li·um** (tri-fo′le-əm) the clovers, a genus of herbs commonly fed to livestock. *T. hy′bridum,* the hybrid clover, can cause trifoliosis. *T. re′pens,* the white clover, contains cyanogenetic compounds and can cause cyanide poisoning.

**tri·fur·ca·tion** (tri″fər-ka′shən) [*tri-* + *furcation*] 1. division into three branches or parts, such as with blood vessels, or teeth that have three roots. 2. the site of such division.

**tri·gas·tric** (tri-gas′trik) [*tri-* + Gr. *gastēr* belly] having three bellies; said of a muscle.

**tri·gem·i·nal** (tri-jem′ĭ-nəl) [*tri-* + L. *geminus* twin] 1. triple. 2. pertaining to the fifth cranial nerve (nervus trigeminus [TA]).

**tri·gem·i·nus** (tri-jem′ĭ-nəs) [L.] triple; see *nervus trigeminus.*

**tri·gem·i·ny** (tri-jem′ĭ-ne) [*tri-* + L. *geminus* twin] 1. occurrence in threes. 2. the occurrence of a trigeminal pulse.
**ventricular t.,** an arrhythmia consisting of the repetitive sequence of one ventricular premature complex followed by two normal beats.

**Tri·glo·chin** (tri-glo′kin) arrow grass, a genus of grasses (family Gramineae), some species of which have pollen that can cause hay fever.

**tri·glyc·er·ide** (tri-glis′ər-īd) a compound consisting of three molecules of fatty acid esterified to glycerol; it is a neutral fat synthesized from carbohydrates for storage in animal adipose cells. On enzymatic hydrolysis, it releases free fatty acids in the blood.

**tri·glyc·er·ide lip·ase** (tri-glis′ə-rīd li′pās) triacylglycerol lipase.

**tri·go·ceph·a·lus** (tri″go-sef′ə-ləs) trigonocephalus.

**tri·go·na** (tri-go′nə) [L.] plural of *trigonum.*

**tri·go·nal** (tri′go-nəl) triangular; pertaining to a trigone.

**tri·gone** (tri′gōn) 1. triangle. 2. the first three cusps of an upper molar tooth; see *hypocone, paracone,* and *protocone.*
**t. of bladder,** trigonum vesicae.
**carotid t.,** trigonum caroticum.
**cerebral t.,** fornix (def. 2).
**collateral t. of fourth ventricle,** trigonum nervi vagi.
**collateral t. of lateral ventricle,** trigonum collaterale ventriculi lateralis.
**fibrous t. of heart, left,** trigonum fibrosum sinistrum cordis.
**fibrous t. of heart, right,** trigonum fibrosum dextrum cordis.
**t. of habenula, habenular t.,** trigonum habenulare.
**Henke's t.,** see under *triangle.*
**hypoglossal t., t. of hypoglossal nerve,** trigonum nervi hypoglossi.
**iliopectineal t.,** fossa iliopectinea.
**interpeduncular t.,** fossa interpeduncularis.
**t. of lateral lemniscus,** trigonum lemnisci lateralis.
**olfactory t.,** trigonum olfactorium.
**omoclavicular t.,** trigonum omoclaviculare.
**Pawlik's t.,** see under *triangle.*
**pontocerebellar t.,** trigonum pontocerebellare.
**t. of Reil,** trigonum lemnisci.
**retromolar t.,** see under *triangle.*
**urogenital t.,** diaphragma urogenitale.
**vagal t., t. of vagus nerve,** trigonum nervi vagi.
**vesical t.,** trigonum vesicae.

**tri·go·nec·to·my** (tri″go-nek′to-me) [*trigone* + *-ectomy*] excision of the base of the bladder (trigonum vesicae).

**Tri·go·nel·la** (tri-gə-nel′ə) a genus of leguminous plants. *T. foenumgrae′cum* L. is fenugreek, a species found in Southern Europe, North Africa, and India whose seeds are the medicinal substance fenugreek; if eaten in large quantities it is toxic to livestock.

**trig·o·nel·line** (trig″o-nel′in) an alkaloid found in fenugreek, cannabis, strophanthus, and various other plants, in sea urchins and jellyfish, and also in the urine after administration of nicotinic acid. It is a betaine of methyl nicotinic acid.

**tri·gon·id** (tri-gon′id) the first three cusps of a lower molar tooth. See *hypoconid, paraconid,* and *protoconid.*

**trig·o·ni·tis** (trig″o-ni′tis) [*trigone* + *-itis*] inflammation or localized hyperemia of the trigone of the bladder.

**trig·o·no·ce·pha·lia** (trig″o-no-sə-fa′le-ə) trigonocephaly.

**trig·o·no·ce·phal·ic** (trig″o-no-sə-fal′ik) pertaining to or characterized by trigonocephaly.

**trig·o·no·ceph·a·lus** (trig″o-no-sef′ə-ləs) an individual exhibiting trigonocephaly.

**trig·o·no·ceph·a·ly** (trig″o-no-sef′ə-le) [Gr. *trigonos* triangular + *-cephaly*] a deformity of the head characterized by sharp angulation ventrad of the squamous portion of the frontal bones at the site of the suture between them.

**tri·go·num** (tri-go′nəm) pl. *trigo′na* [L.; Gr. *trigōnon* triangle] [TA] triangle.
**t. auscultatio′nis** [TA], triangle of auscultation: the area limited by the lower edge of the trapezius muscle, the latissimus dorsi, and the medial margin of the scapula.
**t. caro′ticum** [TA], carotid triangle: the triangular region bounded by the posterior belly of the digastric muscle and the stylohyoid, the sternocleidomastoid muscle, and the superior belly of the omohyoid; called also *fossa carotica* and *superior carotid triangle.*

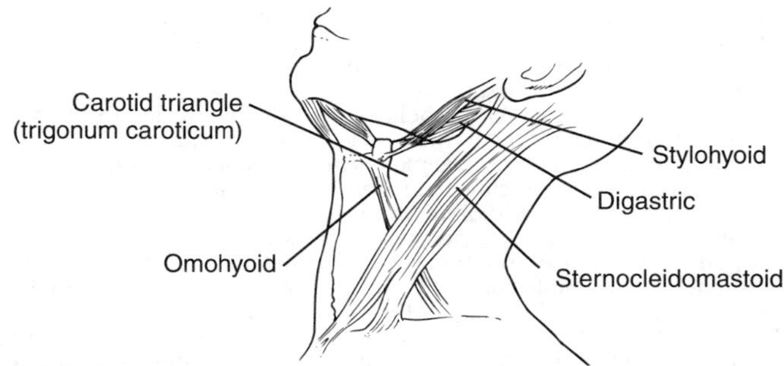


**t. cervica′le,** cervical triangle: any of the triangles of the neck; see *t. caroticum, t. musculare, t. omoclaviculare, t. submandibulare,* and *t. submentale.*
**t. cervica′le ante′rius,** TA alternative for *regio cervicalis anterior.*
**t. cervica′le poste′rius,** TA alternative for *regio cervicalis lateralis.*
**t. clavipectora′le** [TA], clavipectoral triangle: the triangular region separating the upper border of the pectoralis minor muscle from the clavicle, which contains the clavipectoral fascia. Called also *t. deltopectorale* [TA alternative] and *deltopectoral triangle.*
**t. collatera′le ventri′culi latera′lis** [TA], collateral trigone of lateral ventricle: the triangular area in the floor of the lateral ventricle between the diverging temporal and occipital horns.
**t. col′li ante′rius,** TA alternative for *regio cervicalis anterior.*
**t. col′li latera′le,** TA alternative for *regio cervicalis lateralis.*
**t. coracoacromia′le,** a triangle bounded by the coracoid process, the apex of the acromion, and the concave border of the clavicle.

**t. deltoideopectora'le,** fossa infraclavicularis.
**t. deltopectora'le,** TA alternative for *t. clavipectorale.*
**t. femora'le** [TA], femoral triangle: a triangular subfascial area bounded superiorly by the inguinal ligament, laterally by the medial border of the sartorius muscle, and medially by the medial border of the adductor longus muscle; called also *Scarpa's triangle.*
**t. fe'moris** [TA], femoral triangle: the surface area of the thigh overlying the trigonum femorale.
**t. fibro'sum dex'trum cor'dis** [TA], right fibrous trigone of heart: a thickened, irregularly triangular portion of the fibrous skeleton of the base of the heart, located between the right and left atrioventricular fibrous rings, posterior to the aortic orifice. Called also *central fibrous body of heart.*
**t. fibro'sum sinis'trum cor'dis** [TA], left fibrous trigone of heart: a thickened and irregularly triangular portion of the fibrous skeleton of the base of the heart, located between the left atrioventricular fibrous ring and the left posterior margin of the aortic fibrous ring.
**t. habe'nulae, t. habenula're** [TA], habenular trigone: the small, depressed triangular area on the dorsomedial aspect of the posterior part of the thalamus which contains the habenular nuclei and marks the habenular commissure.
**t. hypoglossa'le,** TA alternative for *t. nervi hypoglossi.*
**t. inguina'le** [TA], inguinal triangle: the triangular area on the anteroinferior abdominal wall bounded by the rectus abdominis muscle, the inguinal ligament, and the inferior epigastric vessels: the site in which a direct inguinal hernia begins.
**t. lemnis'ci latera'lis** [TA], trigone of lateral lemniscus: a small, more or less distinct triangular area lateral to the isthmus and the inferior colliculus, superior to the superior cerebellar peduncle and the lateral lemniscus, posteromedially by the brachium of the inferior colliculus, and anterolaterally by the lateral sulcus of the mesencephalon.
**t. lumba'le infe'rius** [TA], inferior lumbar triangle: a small triangular interval between the inferolateral margin of the latissimus dorsi muscle and the external oblique muscle of the abdomen, just superior to the ilium; called also *trigonum lumbare, lumbar triangle,* and *Petit's triangle.*
**t. lumba'le supe'rius** [TA], superior lumbar triangle: an inconstant triangle or rhombus bounded by the twelfth rib and the serratus posterior inferior, erector spinae, and internal oblique muscles, and overlapped by the latissimus dorsi and the external oblique, with the thoracolumbar fascia as its floor. When present it is sometimes a site through which abscesses point or hernias occur.
**t. lumba're, t. lumba're [Peti'ti],** trigonum lumbale inferius.
**t. lumbocosta'le** [TA], a triangular opening of variable size between the lateral lumbocostal arch and the pars costalis diaphragmatis.
**t. muscula're** [TA], muscular triangle: the part of the trigonum caroticum medial to the omohyoid muscle; called also *t. omotracheale* [TA alternative], *inferior carotid triangle,* and *omotracheal triangle.*
**t. ner'vi hypoglos'si** [TA], trigone of hypoglossal nerve: the tapering lower end of the medial eminence of the rhomboid fossa just superficial to the position of the hypoglossal nucleus. Called also *hypoglossal trigone.*
**t. ner'vi va'gi** [TA], trigone of vagus nerve: an area in the floor of the fourth ventricle immediately lateral to the trigonum nervi hypoglossi; beneath it lies the dorsal nucleus of the vagus nerve. Called also *t. vagale* [TA alternative] and *vagal trigone.*
**t. olfacto'rium** [TA], olfactory trigone: the area of the anterior perforated substance between the diverging lateral and medial olfactory striae, and bounded posteriorly by the diagonal band.
**t. omoclavicula're** [TA], omoclavicular triangle: a deep region of the neck, corresponding to the fossa supraclavicularis major on the surface, in which the brachial plexus may be palpated, and by downward pressure the subclavian artery can be compressed against the first rib; called also *subclavian triangle.*
**t. omotrachea'le,** TA alternative for *t. musculare.*
**t. pontocerebella're,** pontocerebellar triangle: the angular depression between the inferior border of the pons, the interior cerebellar peduncle, and the flocculus of the cerebellum.
**t. sternocosta'le** [TA], sternocostal triangle: a triangular opening between the pars costalis and the pars sternalis diaphragmatis; beyond this point the internal thoracic vessels become the superior epigastric vessels. Called also *Larrey's cleft.*
**t. submandibula're** [TA], submandibular triangle: the triangular region of the neck bounded by the mandible, the stylohyoid muscle and posterior belly of the digastric muscle, and the anterior belly of the digastric muscle.
**t. submenta'le** [TA], submental triangle: a triangle bounded on either side by the anterior belly of the digastric muscle and below by the hyoid bone.
**t. urogenita'le,** diaphragma urogenitale.
**t. vaga'le,** TA alternative for *t. nervi vagi.*
**t. vesi'cae** [TA], **t. vesi'cae [Lieutau'di],** trigone of bladder: a smooth triangular portion of the mucous membrane at the base of the bladder; it is bounded behind by the interureteric fold and ends in front in the uvula of the bladder.

**tri·hex·o·syl·cer·a·mide** (tri-hek″so-səl-ser′ə-mīd) ceramide trihexoside.

**tri·hex·y·phen·i·dyl hy·dro·chlo·ride** (tri-hek″sĭ-fen′ĭ-dəl) [USP] an anticholinergic, occurring as a white or slightly off-white crystalline powder, having atropine-like actions; used as an oral antiparkinsonian agent.

**tri·hy·brid** (tri-hi′brid) [*tri-* + *hybrid*] a hybrid offspring of parents differing in three mendelian characters.

**tri·hy·drate** (tri-hi′drāt) trihydroxide; a compound containing three hydroxyl groups.

**tri·hy·dric** (tri-hi′drik) containing three hydrogen atoms that are replaceable by bases.

**tri·hy·drol** (tri-hi′drol) the associated water or ice molecule, $(H_2O)_3$.

**tri·hy·drox·ide** (tri″hi-drok′sīd) trihydrate.

**tri·hy·droxy** (tri″hi-drok′se) a term denoting a compound containing three molecules of the hydroxy (OH) radical; used also as a prefix (trihydroxy-) to denote such a compound.

**tri·hy·droxy·es·trin** (tri″hi-drok″se-es′trin) estriol.

**tri·in·i·od·y·mus** (tri″in-e-od′ĭ-məs) [*tri-* + *inio-* + *-didymus*] a fetus with a single body and three heads united posteriorly.

**tri·io·dide** (tri-i′o-dīd) a compound containing three atoms of iodine to one of another element.

**tri·io·do·eth·i·on·ic ac·id** (tri-i″o-do-eth″e-on′ik) iophenoxic acid.

**tri·io·do·meth·ane** (tri-i″o-do-meth′ān) iodoform.

**tri·io·do·thy·ro·nine ($T_3$)** (tri-i″o-do-thi′ro-nēn) [MeSH: Triiodothyronine] 3,5,3′-triiodothyronine, an iodine-containing thyroid hormone secreted in smaller amounts than thyroxine; most circulating triiodothyronine is produced by the deiodination of thyroxine in the peripheral tissues, chiefly the liver. It has several times the biological activity of thyroxine and is the "tissue-active" form of thyroid hormone.
**free t.,** the fraction of triiodothyronine in the serum that is not bound to a binding protein.
**reverse t. ($rT_3$),** 3,3′,5′-triiodothyronine, a thyroxine derivative that has little if any biologic activity; it is produced in increased amounts in hypothyroidism, hyperthyroidism, and the euthyroid sick syndrome, as well as during febrile illness or carbohydrate deprivation.
**total t., total serum t.,** the total triiodothyronine in the serum, including both the fraction of free triiodothyronine and the fraction bound to a binding protein such as thyroxine-binding globulin or transthyretin.

**tri·ke·to·hy·drin·dene hy·drate** (tri-ke″to-hi-drin′dēn) chemical name: 1,2,3-indantrione monohydrate. A compound, $C_9H_4O_3 \cdot H_2O$, occurring as white to brownish white crystals or crystalline powder, used as a reagent. See under *tests.*

**tri·ke·to·pu·rine** (tri″ke-to-pu′rin) uric acid.

**tri·labe** (tri′lāb) [*tri-* + Gr. *labē* a handle] a three-pronged instrument for taking calculi from the bladder.

**Tri·la·fon** (tri′lə-fon) trademark for preparations of perphenazine.

**tri·lam·i·nar** (tri-lam′ĭ-nər) consisting of three layers.

**tri·lat·er·al** (tri-lat′ər-əl) [*tri-* + *lateral*] having three sides; see *triangle.*

**tri·lau·rin** (tri-law′rin) the triglyceride formed from lauric acid residues, forming the principal constituent of coconut oil, and found in bayberry oil and palm nut oil.

**tri·lin·o·le·in** (tri″lin-o′le-in) an unsaturated triglyceride formed from linoleic acid, found in drying oils such as linseed or sunflower oil.

**Tril·i·sate** (tril′ĭ-sāt) trademark for choline magnesium trisalicylate.

**tri·lo·bate** (tri-lo′bāt) [*tri-* + *lobate*] having three lobes.

**tri·lobed** (tri′lōbd) trilobate.

**tri·loc·u·lar** (tri-lok′u-lər) [*tri-* + *locular*] having three compartments or cells.

**tril·o·gy** (tril′ə-je) a combination of three elements, such as three concurrent defects or symptoms.
**t. of Fallot,** a term sometimes applied to the combination of pulmonic stenosis, atrial septal defect, and right ventricular hypertrophy.

**tri·lo·stane** (tri′lo-stān) an adrenocortical suppressant used experimentally to inhibit aldosterone synthesis and raise potassium levels in patients with adrenal hyperfunction and in hypertensive patients undergoing diuretic therapy.

**tri·mas·ti·gote** (tri-mas′tĭ-gōt) 1. having three flagella. 2. a cell having three flagella.

**tri·me·dox·ime** (tri″mə-dok′sēm) [MeSH: Trimedoxime] a cholinesterase reactivator used for treatment of organophosphate poisoning. Available as *trimedoxime bromide.*

**tri·men·su·al** (tri-men′su-əl) occurring every three months.

**tri·mep·ra·zine tar·trate** (tri-mep′rə-zēn) [USP] a phenothiazine derivative having mild central nervous system depressant, moderate antiemetic and anticonvulsant properties, and powerful antihistaminic actions; used as an antipruritic, administered orally.

**tri·mer** (tri′mər) 1. a compound formed by combination of three identical simpler molecules. 2. a capsomer having three structural units.

**tri·mer·cu·ric** (tri″mər-ku′rik) containing three atoms of bivalent mercury.

**Trim·e·re·su·rus** (trim″ə-re-su′rəs) [MeSH: Trimeresurus] a genus of venomous pit vipers of the family Crotalidae, found in East and Southeast Asia and nearby islands; they are usually green with a prehensile tail. *T. flavovi′ridis* and *T. mucrosqua′matus* are both known as *habu.* See table at *snake.*

**tri·mer·ic** (tri′mər-ik) exhibiting the characteristics of a trimer.

**tri·mes·ter** (tri-mes′tər) a period of three months.

**tri·meth·a·di·one** (tri″meth-ə-di′ōn) [MeSH: Trimethadione] an anticonvulsant with analgesic properties, used for the control of petit mal seizures, administered orally. In veterinary medicine, used as an anticonvulsant and analgesic for cats. Called also *troxidone.*

**tri·meth·a·phan cam·sy·late** (tri-meth′ə-fən) a short-acting ganglionic blocking agent with direct vasodilator action, used as an antihypertensive to produce controlled hypotension during surgery and for the emergency treatment of hypertensive crises and pulmonary edema due to hypertension, administered by intravenous infusion. Called also *t. camphorsulfonate.*

**tri·meth·i·din·i·um meth·o·sul·fate** (tri-meth″ĭ-din′e-əm) a quaternary ammonium ganglion blocking agent, used as an oral antihypertensive in the treatment of moderate to severe hypertension in certain patients.

**tri·meth·o·ben·za·mide hy·dro·chlo·ride** (tri-meth″o-ben′zə-mīd) [USP] an antiemetic, administered orally, intramuscularly, or rectally.

**tri·meth·o·prim** (tri-meth′o-prim) [USP] [MeSH: Trimethoprim] an antibacterial closely related to the antimalarial pyrimethamine; administered orally, in combination with a sulfonamide because the two drugs markedly potentiate each other, in the treatment of urinary tract infections due to *Escherichia coli, Klebsiella-Enterobacter* group, *Proteus vulgaris, P. mirabilis,* and *P. morganii,* and in *Pneumocystis carinii* pneumonitis in children with reduced host defenses. In certain countries, it is used alone as an antimalarial.
**t. sulfate** [USP], the sulfate salt of trimethoprim, having the same actions and uses as the base.

**tri·meth·y·lene** (tri-meth′ə-lēn) cyclopropane.

**tri·meth·yl·xan·thine** (tri-meth″əl-zan′thin) caffeine.

**tri·me·trex·ate** (tri″mə-trek′sāt) [MeSH: Trimetrexate] a folic acid antagonist structurally related to methotrexate, used investigationally as an antineoplastic; also used in combination with leukovorin to treat *Pneumocystis carinii* pneumonia in acquired immune deficiency syndrome.

**tri·mip·ra·mine** (tri-mip′rə-mēn) [MeSH: Trimipramine] a tricyclic antidepressant of the dibenzazepine class.
**t. maleate,** the maleate salt of trimipramine, used particularly in the treatment of endogenous depression; used also in the treatment of peptic ulcer. Administered orally.

**tri·mor·phous** (tri-mor′fəs) [*tri-* + *morph-* + *-ous*] existing in three different forms.

**Tri·mox** (tri′moks) trademark for preparations of amoxicillin.

**tri·neg·a·tive** (tri-neg′ə-tiv) having three negative valences or charges.

**tri·ni·trate** (tri-ni′trāt) a nitrate which contains three radicals of nitric acid, as glycerol trinitrate.

**tri·ni·trin** (tri-ni′trin) nitroglycerin.

**tri·ni·tro·cel·lu·lose** (tri″ni-tro-sel′u-lōs) pyroxylin.

**tri·ni·tro·glyc·er·in** (tri-ni″tro-glis′ər-in) nitroglycerin.

**tri·ni·tro·glyc·er·ol** (tri-ni″tro-glis′ər-ol) nitroglycerin.

**tri·ni·tro·phe·nol** (tri″ni-tro-fe′nol) a yellow crystalline substance used as a dye and a tissue fixative; its toxic effects are similar to those of dinitrophenol. It can be detonated by percussion or heating above 300°C. Called also *picric acid.*

**tri·ni·tro·tol·u·ene** (tri″ni-tro-tol′u-ēn) [MeSH: Trinitrotoluene] a high explosive obtained by nitrating toluene; called also TNT.

**tri·no·mi·al** (tri-no′me-əl) [*tri-* + L. *nomen* name] composed of three names or terms.

**tri·nu·cle·ate** (tri-noo′kle-āt) having three nuclei.

**tri·nu·cleo·tide** (tri-noo′kle-o-tīd) a polymer made up of three mononucleotides.

**trio·ceph·a·lus** (tri″o-sef′ə-ləs) [*tri-* + *-cephalus*] a fetus in which the structures of the mouth, nose, and eyes are absent and the head is a shapeless mass. Cf. *triencephalus.*

**Trio·don·toph·o·rus** (tri″o-don-tof′ə-rəs) a genus of nematodes of the family Strongylidae. *T. tenuicol′lis* is found in ulcers in the colons of horses.

**tri·o·ki·nase** (tri″o-ki′nās) [EC 2.7.1.28] an enzyme of the transferase class that catalyzes the phosphorylation of glyceraldehyde to form glyceraldehyde 3-phosphate. The reaction occurs in the liver and is part of the series funneling fructose into the Embden-Meyerhof pathway. Called also *triose kinase.*

**tri·o·le·in** (tri-o′lēn) [MeSH: Triolein] olein.

**tri·oph·thal·mos** (tri″of-thal′mos) [*tri-* + Gr. *ophthalmos* eye] a double-faced fetus with three eyes.

**tri·o·pod·y·mus** (tri″o-pod′ĭ-məs) [*tri-* + Gr. *ops* face + *-didymus*] triprosopus.

**tri·or·chid** (tri-or′kid) [*tri-* + Gr. *orchis* testis] an individual with three testes.

**tri·or·chi·dism** (tri-or′ki-diz-əm) the condition of having three testes.

**tri·or·chis** (tri-or′kis) triorchid.

**tri·or·chism** (tri-or′kiz-əm) triorchidism.

**tri·ose** (tri′ōs) a monosaccharide containing three atoms of carbon in the molecule.
**t. phosphate,** a phosphorylated triose, particularly glyceraldehyde 3-phosphate and dihydroxyacetone phosphate, two important intermediates in glycolysis, alcoholic fermentation, and gluconeogenesis. Called also *phosphotriose.*

**tri·ose ki·nase** (tri′ōs ki′nās) triokinase.

**tri·ose·phos·phate de·hy·dro·gen·ase** (tri′ōs fos′fāt de-hi′dro-jən-ās) glyceraldehyde-3-phosphate dehydrogenase.

**tri·ose·phos·phate isom·er·ase** (tri′ōs fos′fāt i-som′ər-ās) [EC 5.3.1.1] an enzyme of the isomerase class that catalyzes the reversible interconversion of glyceraldehyde 3-phosphate and dihydroxyacetone phosphate in the Embden-Meyerhof pathway (see illustration at *pathway*). Deficiency of the enzyme, an autosomal recessive trait, causes hemolytic anemia, neuromuscular dysfunction, and susceptibility to infection.

**tri·otus** (tri-o′təs) [*tri-* + Gr. *ous* ear] an individual with a supernumerary ear.

**tri·ox·ide** (tri-ok′sīd) a compound containing three atoms of oxygen to one of another element.

**tri·ox·sa·len** (tri-ok′sə-lən) [USP] [MeSH: Trioxsalen] a synthetic psoralen used orally in conjunction with exposure to ultraviolet light to facilitate repigmentation in vitiligo, and also as a suntan accelerator and sun protectant.

**tri·oxy·pu·rine** (tri″ok-se-pu′rin) uric acid.

**tri·pal·mi·tin** (tri-pal′mĭ-tin) palmitin.

**trip·a·ra** (trip′ə-rə) [*tri-* + *para*] tertipara.

**tri·par·tite** (tri-pahr′tīt) having three parts.

**Tri·pe·dia** (tri-pe′de-ə) trademark for a preparation of diphtheria and tetanus toxoids and acellular pertussis vaccine.

**tri·pe·len·na·mine** (tri″pə-len′ə-min) [MeSH: Tripelennamine] a histamine antagonist.
**t. citrate,** the citrate salt of tripelennamine, used as antihistaminic in the symptomatic treatment of allergic disorders, administered orally.
**t. hydrochloride** [USP], the monohydrochloride salt of tripelennamine, having the same appearance, actions, and uses as the citrate salt; administered orally, parenterally, and topically.

**tri·pep·tide** (tri-pep′tid) a peptide which on hydrolysis yields three amino acids.

**tri·pep·ti·dyl-pep·ti·dase** (tri-pep″tĭ-dəl-pep′tĭ-dās) [EC 3.4.14] any member of a sub-subclass of enzymes of the hydrolase class that catalyze the cleavage of a tripeptide residue from a free N-terminal end of a peptide or polypeptide.

**tri·pha·lan·ge·al** (tri″fə-lan′je-əl) pertaining to or characterized by triphalangia.

**tri·pha·lan·gia** (tri″fə-lan′jə) triphalangism.

**tri·phal·an·gism** (tri-fal′ən-jiz-əm) the presence of three phalanges in the longitudinal axis of a digit normally composed of only two.

**tri·pha·sic** (tri-fa′zik) [*tri-* + Gr. *phasis* phase] triply varied or triply phasic; used in describing the electromotive actions of muscles. Cf. *diphasic* and *monophasic.*

**Tri·pha·sil** (tri-fa′zil) trademark for preparations of a combination of levonorgestrel and ethinyl estradiol.

**tri·phen·yl·eth·y·lene** (tri-fen″əl-eth′ə-lēn) a synthetic estrogen, not related to naturally occurring estrogens with the phenanthrene nucleus.

**tri·phen·yl·meth·ane** (tri-fen″əl-meth′ān) a substance from coal tar, the basis of various dyes and stains, including aurin, rosaniline, basic fuchsin, and gentian violet.

**tri·phos·phate** (tri-fos′fāt) a salt containing three phosphate radicals.

**tri·phos·pho·pyr·i·dine nu·cle·o·tide** (tri-fos″fo-pir′ĭ-dēn noo′kle-o-tid″) former name for *nicotinamide adenine dinucleotide phosphate (NADP).* Abbreviated TPN.

**Tri·pier's amputation** (tre″pe-āz′) [Léon *Tripier,* French surgeon, 1842–1891] see under *amputation.*

**trip·le-an·gle** (trip′əl-ang″gəl) having three angles; a dental instrument having three angulations in the shank connecting the handle, or shaft, with the working portion of the instrument, known as the blade, or nib. Cf. *binangle, monangle,* and *quadrangle* (def. 2).

**trip·le blind** (trip′əl blīnd) pertaining to a clinical trial or other experiment in which neither the subject nor the person administering treatment nor the person evaluating the response to treatment knows which treatment any particular subject is receiving.The term *triple mask* is sometimes preferred to avoid confusion associated with the use of the term "blind."

**trip·le mask** (trip′əl mask) triple blind.

**tri·ple·gia** (tri-ple′jə) [*tri-* + *-plegia*] paralysis of three of the extremities.

**trip·let** (trip′lət) [MeSH: Triplets] 1. one of three individuals having coextensive gestation periods and produced at the same birth. 2. a combination of three objects or entities occurring or acting together, as three lenses constituting a microscope eyepiece or objective. 3. codon. 4. a triple discharge.

**tri·plex** (tri′pleks) [Gr. *triploos* triple] triple or three-fold.

**trip·lo·blas·tic** (trip″lo-blas′tik) [Gr. *triploos* triple + *blast-* + *-ic*] having three germ layers or blastodermic membranes; said of an embryo.

**trip·loid** (trip′loid) 1. pertaining to or characterized by triploidy. 2. an individual or cell having three sets of chromosomes.

**trip·loi·dy** (trip′loi-de) the presence in humans of 69 chromosomes, or three full sets, a frequent finding in abortuses.

**trip·lo·ko·ria** (trip″lo-kor′e-ə) [Gr. *triploos* triple + *cor-* + *-ia*] the presence of three pupils in one eye.

**trip·lo·pia** (trip-lo′pe-ə) [Gr. *triploos* triple + *-opia*] the perception of three images of a single object; triple vision.

**tri·pod** (tri′pod) [*tri-* + Gr. *pous* foot] anything having three feet or supports.
**Haller's t.,** truncus coeliacus.
**t. of life, vital t.,** the brain, heart, and lungs regarded as the triple support of life.

**tri·po·dia** (tri-po′de-ə) [*tri-* + *pod-* + *-ia*] tripodial symmelia.

**tri·po·di·al** (tri-po′de-əl) having three feet; see *symmelia.*

**tri·pod·ing** (tri′pod-ing) the use of three points of support, as adopted by paralyzed patients when changing from a sitting or standing position. See also *tripod position,* under *position.*

**trip·o·li** (trip′o-le) [*Tripoli,* Libya] a granulated porous siliceous rock originally mined in North Africa and presently produced from silica; used as a dental polishing agent.

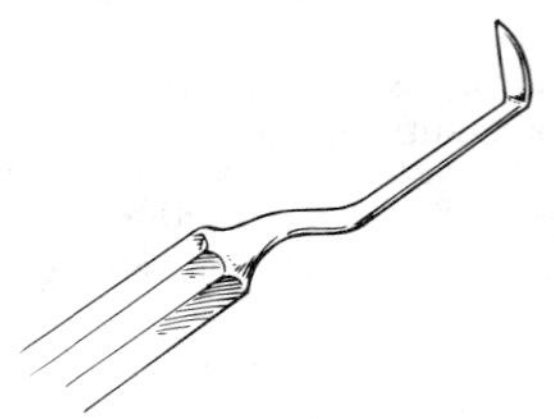

Triple-angle.

**tri·pos·i·tive** (tri-pos′ĭ-tiv) having three positive valences or charges.

**tri·pro·li·dine hy·dro·chlo·ride** (tri-pro′lĭ-dēn) [USP] an antihistaminic used in the treatment of various allergic conditions and their manifestations, administered orally.

**tri·pro·so·pus** (tri″pro-so′pəs) [*tri-* + Gr. *prosōpon* face] a fetus having a triple face.

**trip·sis** (trip′sis) [Gr. *tripsis* rubbing] 1. a trituration; the process of trituration. 2. massage.

**-tripsy** [Gr. *tripsis* a rubbing, friction] a word termination designating a surgical procedure in which a structure is intentionally crushed.

**trip·to·ko·ria** (trip″to-kor′e-ə) triplokoria.

**trip·to·rel·in** (trip″tə-rel′in) [MeSH: Triptorelin] a synthetic analogue of gonadorelin used as an antineoplastic in the palliative treatment of advanced ovarian carcinoma and in the treatment of prostatic carcinoma.

**tri·pus** (tri′pəs) [*tri-* + *pous* foot] 1. a tripod. 2. conjoined twins with tripodial symmelia.

**tri·que·trous** (tri-kwe′trəs) [L. *triquetrus*] triangular; three cornered.

**tri·que·trum** (tri-kwe′trəm) [L.] three cornered; see *os triquetrum.*

**tri·ra·di·al** (tri-ra′de-əl) triradiate.

**tri·ra·di·ate** (tri-ra′de-āt) [*tri-* + L. *radiatus* rayed] having three rays; radiating in three directions; triradial.

**tri·ra·di·a·tion** (tri″ra-de-a′shən) radiation in three directions.

**TRIS** tris(hydroxymethyl)aminomethane; see *tromethamine.*

**tris** (tris) 1. tromethamine. 2. tris(2,3-dibromopropyl) phosphate.

**tri·sac·cha·ride** (tri-sak′ə-rīd) any of a class of carbohydrates composed of three glycosidically linked monosaccharide groups.

**tris·(2,3-di·bro·mo·pro·pyl) phos·phate** (tris″di-bro″mo-pro′pəl fos′fāt) a yellow liquid flame retardant, formerly used in children's clothing but now restricted in use because it is carcinogenic. Called also *tris.*

**Tri·se·tum** (tri-se′tum) a genus of grasses found in pastures. *T. flaves′cens* is yellow or golden oat grass, a European variety that causes enzootic calcinosis in ruminants.

**tri·seg·men·tec·to·my** resection of the liver in which three segments are removed.
**left t.,** that in which the left lobe and anterior segment of the right lobe are removed.
**right t.,** that in which the right lobe and medial segment of the left lobe are removed.

**tris·(hy·droxy·meth·yl)·am·i·no·meth·ane** (tris″hi-drok″se-meth″əl-ə-me″no-meth′ān) tromethamine.

**tris·mic** (triz′mik) of the nature of or pertaining to trismus.

**tris·mus** (triz′məs) [Gr. *trismos* grating, grinding] [MeSH: Trismus] motor disturbance of the trigeminal nerve, especially spasm of the masticatory muscles, with difficulty in opening the mouth; a characteristic early symptom of tetanus. Called also *lockjaw.*

**tri·so·di·um phos·pho·no·for·mate** (tri-so′de-əm fos″fon-o-for′māt) foscarnet sodium.

**tri·so·mia** (tri-so′me-ə) trisomy.

**tri·so·mic** (tri-so′mik) pertaining to or characterized by trisomy.

**tri·so·my** (tri′so-me) [*tri* + Gr. *sōma* body] [MeSH: Trisomy] the presence of an extra chromosome of one type in an otherwise diploid cell (2n +1). See various types of trisomy syndromes under *syndrome.*

**Tri·sor·a·len** (tri-sor′ə-lən) trademark for a preparation of trioxsalen.

**tri·splanch·nic** (tri-splangk′nik) [*tri-* + *splanchnic*] pertaining to or supplying the three great body cavities and their viscera.

**tri·ste·a·rin** (tri-ste′ə-rin) the saturated triglyceride formed from stearic acid; it occurs mainly in harder fats such as tallow and cacao butter and can be prepared by hydrogenation of oils. Called also *stearin.*

**tri·stich·ia** (tri-stik′e-ə) [Gr. *treis* three + *stichos* row] the existence of three rows of eyelashes.

**tri·sub·sti·tut·ed** (tri-sub′stĭ-to͞ot″əd) having three molecules or atoms replaced by three other molecules or atoms.

**tri·sul·cate** (tri-sul′kāt) having three furrows.

**tri·sul·fa·py·rim·i·dines** (tri-sul″fə-pi-rim′ĭ-dēnz) preparations containing a mixture of the sulfonamides sulfadiazine, sulfamerazine, and sulfamethazine.

**tri·sul·fate** (tri-sul′fāt) a binary compound containing three sulfate ($SO_4$) groups in the molecule.

**tri·sul·fide** (tri-sul′fīd) a sulfur compound containing three atoms of sulfur to one of the base.

**Trit.** abbreviation for L. *tri′tura,* triturate.

**tri·tan** (tri′tən) 1. pertaining to tritanomaly or tritanopia. 2. a person with tritanomaly or tritanopia.

**tri·ta·nom·al** (tri″tə-nom′əl) a person with tritanomaly.

**tri·ta·nom·a·lous** (tri″tə-nom′ə-ləs) pertaining to or characterized by tritanomaly.

**tri·ta·nom·a·ly** (tri″tə-nom′ə-le) [Gr. *tritos* third + *anomaly*] a very rare anomalous trichromasy in which the third, blue-sensitive, cones have decreased sensitivity; therefore a greater than normal proportion of blue light to green light is required to match a blue-green stimulus. Tritanomaly is an X-linked trait and occurs in about 0.0001 per cent of white males; it is therefore of little clinical importance.

**tri·ta·nope** (tri′tə-nōp″) an individual exhibiting tritanopia.

**tri·ta·no·pia** (tri″tə-no′pe-ə) [Gr. *tritos* third + *an-*[1] + *-opia*] a rare dichromasy characterized by retention of the sensory mechanism for two hues only (red and green) of the normal 4-primary quota, and lacking blue and yellow, with loss of luminance and shift of brightness and hue curves toward the long-wave end of the spectrum. Often associated with drug administration, retinal detachment, or diseases of the nervous system.

**tri·ta·nop·ic** (tri″tə-nop′ik) pertaining to or characterized by tritanopia.

**tri·ta·nop·sia** (tri″tə-nop′se-ə) tritanopia.

**tri·ter·pene** (tri-tər′pēn) any of a class of compounds biosynthesized from or comprising six isoprene, and thus three terpene, units; most are tetra- or pentacyclic steroids.

**tri·ti·ceous** (tri-tish′əs) [L. *triticeus*] resembling a grain of wheat.

**tri·tic·e·um** (tri-tis′e-əm) [L.] cartilago triticea.

**Trit·i·ra·chi·um** (trit″ĭ-ra′ke-əm) a genus of Fungi Imperfecti of the form-class Hyphomycetes. *T. ory′zae* has been isolated from human infections such as corneal ulcers.

**trit·i·um** (trit′e-əm) [Gr. *tritos* third] [MeSH: Tritium] the mass three isotope of hydrogen, $^3$H, a radioactive gas with a half-life of 12.33 years and emitting beta particles (0.0186 MeV); it has been used as tracer in metabolic studies. Cf. *deuterium* and *protium.*

**Tri·tricho·mo·nas** (tri″trik-o-mo′nas, tri″trik-o-mon′as) [*tri-* + *tricho-* + Gr. *monas* unit, from *monos* single] [MeSH: Tritrichomonas] in some systems of classification, a genus established to include the species of *Trichomonas* having three anterior flagella, i.e., *T. foetus.*

**trit·ur·ate** (trich′ūr-āt) 1. to rub to a powder. 2. to create a homogeneous whole by mixing; see trituration (def. 3). 3. a triturated substance.

**trit·ur·a·tion** (trich″ūr-a′shən) [L. *tritura* the treading out of corn] 1. the reduction of solid bodies to a powder by continuous rubbing. 2. a triturated drug, especially one rubbed up with lactose. 3. the creation of a homogeneous whole by mixing, as the combining of particles of an alloy with mercury to form dental amalgam; called also *amalgamation.*

**trit·ur·a·tor** (trich′ūr-a″tər) an apparatus in which substances can be continuously rubbed, as in the process of amalgamating an alloy with mercury. Called also *amalgamator.*

**tri·va·lence** (tri-va′ləns) the condition or quality of being trivalent.

**tri·va·lent** (tri-va′lənt) [*tri-* + L. *valens* powerful] having a valence of three.

**tri·valve** (tri′valv) having three valves or three blades, as a speculum.

**tri·zo·nal** (tri-zo′nəl) arranged in three zones.

**tRNA** transfer RNA; see under *RNA.*

**Tro·bi·cin** (tro-bi′sin) trademark for a preparation of spectinomycin hydrochloride.

**tro·car** (tro′kahr) [Fr. *trois quarts* three quarters] a sharp-pointed instrument equipped with a cannula, used to puncture the wall of a body cavity and withdraw fluid.

**troch.** trochiscus.

**tro·chan·ter** (tro-kan′tər) [L.; Gr. *trochantēr*] either of the two processes below the neck of the femur.
**greater t.,** t. major.
**lesser t.,** t. minor.
**t. ma′jor** [TA], greater trochanter: a broad, flat process at the upper end of the lateral surface of the femur, to which several muscles are attached.
**t. mi′nor** [TA], lesser trochanter: a short conical process projecting medially from the lower part of the posterior border of the base of the neck of the femur.
**rudimentary t.,** t. tertius.
**small t.,** t. minor.
**t. ter′tius** [TA], third trochanter: a term applied to the gluteal tuberosity of the femur when it is unusually prominent.

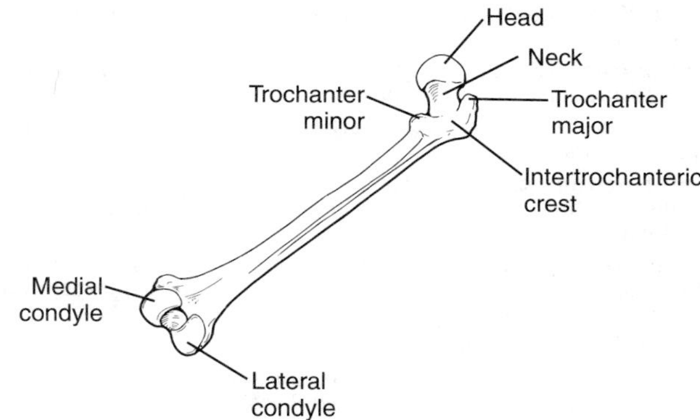

Posterior aspect of right femur, showing the greater and lesser trochanters.

**tro·chan·ter·i·an** (tro″kən-ter′e-ən) trochanteric.

**tro·chan·ter·ic** (tro″kən-ter′ik) pertaining to a trochanter.

**tro·chan·ter·plas·ty** (tro-kan′tər-plas″te) surgical excision of a ridge of bone to form a new femoral neck.

**tro·chan·tin** (tro-kan′tin) trochanter minor.

**tro·chan·tin·i·an** (tro″kən-tin′e-ən) pertaining to the lesser trochanter.

**tro·che** (tro′ke) [Gr. *trochos* a round cake] a small circular or oblong tablet usually for solution in the mouth, especially for medication of the throat, consisting of an active ingredient incorporated in a mass made up of sugar and mucilage or fruit base, and air dried. Called also *lozenge, morsulus, rotula,* and *trochiscus.*

**tro·chis·cus** (tro-kis′kəs) pl. *trochis′chi* [L., from Gr. *trochiskos,* dim. of *trochos,* a small wheel or disk] a medicated tablet; a troche.

**troch·i·ter** (trok′ĭ-tər) 1. trochanter major. 2. tuberculum majus humeri.

**troch·i·te·ri·an** (trok″ĭ-tēr′e-ən) pertaining to the trochiter.

**troch·lea** (trok′le-ə) pl. *troch′leae* [L.; Gr. *trochilia* pulley] [TA] a general term in anatomical nomenclature for a pulley-shaped part or structure.
**t. fibula′ris calca′nei,** a small eminence on the lateral surface of the calcaneus, separating the tendons of the peroneus brevis and longus muscles; called also *processus trochlearis calcanei* and *t. peronealis calcanei* [TA alternative].
**t. hu′meri** [TA], trochlea of humerus: the pulleylike medial portion of the distal end of the humerus for articulation with the semilunar notch of the ulna; called also *trochlear eminence.*
**t. muscula′ris** [TA], muscular trochlea: an anatomical part that serves to change the direction of pull of a tendon; it may be fibrous or bony.
**t. mus′culi obli′qui superio′ris bul′bi** [TA], **t. mus′culi obli′qui superio′ris o′culi,** trochlea of superior oblique muscle: the fibrocartilaginous pulley near the internal angular process of the frontal bone, through which the tendon of the superior oblique muscle of the eyeball passes.
**peroneal t. of calcaneus,** t. fibularis calcanei.
**t. peronea′lis calca′nei** [TA], TA alternative for *t. fibularis calcanei.*
**t. phalan′gis ma′nus** [TA], trochlea of phalanx of hand: the pulleylike concavity of the head of a proximal or middle phalanx, to which the base of the articulating phalanx is adapted.
**t. phalan′gis pe′dis** [TA], trochlea of phalanx of foot: the pulleylike concavity of the head of a proximal or middle phalanx (except in the big toe, which has only two phalanges), to which the base of the articulating phalanx is adapted.
**t. of superior oblique muscle,** t. musculi obliqui superioris bulbi.
**t. ta′li** [TA], trochlea of talus: the surface of the talus for articulation with the tibia and fibula.

**troch·le·ar** (trok′le-ər) [L. *trochlearis*] 1. of the nature of or resembling a pulley. 2. pertaining to a trochlea.

**troch·le·ar·i·form** (trok″le-ar′ĭ-form) pulley-shaped.

**troch·le·a·ris** (trok″le-ar′is) [L.] trochlear.

**tro·cho·ce·pha·lia** (tro″ko-sə-fa′le-ə) trochocephaly.

**tro·cho·ceph·a·ly** (tro″ko-sef′ə-le) [Gr. *trochos* wheel + *-cephaly*] a rounded appearance of the head caused by synostosis of the frontal and parietal bones.

**tro·choid** (tro'koid) [Gr. *trochos* wheel + *-oid*] resembling a pivot or a pulley.

**tro·choi·des** (tro-koi'dēz) [Gr. *trochoeidēs,* from *trochos* wheel + *eidos* form] articulatio trochoidea.

**Tro·ci·nate** (tro'sĭ-nāt) trademark for a preparation of thiphenamil hydrochloride.

**tro·gli·ta·zone** (tro"glĭ-ta'zōn) an antihyperglycemic that lowers insulin resistance, used in the treatment of type 2 diabetes mellitus; administered orally.

**Trog·lo·stron·gy·lus** (trog"lo-stron'jĭ-lus) a genus of nematodes of the family Crenosomatidae. Some species infect the respiratory tract or lungs of cats.

**Trog·lo·tre·ma** (trog"lo-tre'mə) Nanophyetus.

**Trog·lo·tre·ma·ti·dae** (trog"lo-tre-mot'ĭ-dae) a family of trematodes that includes the genera *Nanophyetus* and *Paragonimus.*

**Troi·sier's node (ganglion, sign), syndrome** (trwah-ze-āz') [Charles Emile *Troisier,* French physician, 1844–1919] see under *syndrome* and see *signal node,* under *node.*

**tro·la·mine** (tro'lə-mēn) [NF] 1. a mixture of alkanolamines, consisting largely of triethanolamine and containing some di- and monoethanolamine; used as an alkalizing agent in pharmaceutical preparations. Called also *triethanolamine.* 2. USAN contraction for triethanolamine.
**t. salicylate** [USP], a mixture of trolamine and salicylic acid in propylene glycol having analgesic and anesthetic properties and also acting as a sunscreen that absorbs ultraviolet light in the UVA range; used topically as an analgesic and as a sunscreen.

**tro·land** (tro'lənd) [for Leonard Thompson *Troland,* American psychologist and physicist, 1889–1932] the retinal illuminance produced by the image of an object the luminance of which is 1 lumen per square meter for an area of the entrance pupil of 1 square millimeter.

**Tro·lard's plexus (net), vein** (tro-lahrz') [Paulin *Trolard,* French anatomist, 1842–1910] see *plexus venosus canalis hypoglossi* and *vena anastomotica inferior.*

**tro·le·an·do·my·cin** (tro"le-an-do-mi'sin) [USP] [MeSH: Troleandomycin] a macrolide antibiotic, the synthetically prepared triacetyl ester of oleandomycin, to which it is converted in the body, used in the treatment of pneumococcal pneumonia and Group A $\beta$-hemolytic streptococcal infections resistant to other systemic antibiotics; administered orally.

**trol·ni·trate phos·phate** (trol-ni'trāt) an organic nitrate having vasodilating actions; used to reduce the frequency and severity of anginal attacks, administered orally.

**Tröltsch's corpuscles, recesses (spaces)** (trerl'chez) [Anton Friedrich von *Tröltsch,* German otologist, 1829–1890] see under *corpuscle,* and see *recessus membranae tympani anterior* and *recessus membranae tympani posterior.*

**Trom·bic·u·la** (trom-bik'u-lə) a genus of mites of the family Trombiculidae; it is further divided into the subgenera *Eutrombicula* and *Leptotrombidium.* Their larvae, called *chiggers,* cause an irritating dermatitis in many vertebrates, including humans; some species spread scrub typhus in Asia and the Pacific.
**T. akamu'shi,** the kedani mite, whose larvae (chiggers) transmit *Rickettsia tsutsugamushi,* the etiologic agent of scrub typhus; it is the chief vector in Japan. Called also *Microtrombidium akamushi.*
**T. alfreddugè'si,** *Eutrombicula alfreddugèsi.*
**T. autumna'lis,** *Neotrombicula autumnalis.*
**T. delien'sis,** a species whose larvae transmit *Rickettsia tsutsugamushi,* the etiologic agent of scrub typhus; it is believed to be the chief vector outside of Japan.
**T. flet'cheri,** a carrier of *Rickettsia tsutsugamushi,* the causative agent of scrub typhus.
**T. holoseri'ceum,** *Neotrombicula autumnalis.*
**T. interme'dia,** a carrier of *Rickettsia tsutsugamushi,* the causative agent of scrub typhus.
**T. ir'ritans,** *Eutrombicula alfreddugèsi.*
**T. mus'cae domes'ticae,** a red acarid parasite on the housefly.
**T. musca'rum,** *T. muscae domesticae.*
**T. pal'lida,** a carrier of *Rickettsia tsutsugamushi,* the causative agent of scrub typhus.
**T. scutella'ris,** a carrier of *Rickettsia tsutsugamushi,* the causative agent of scrub typhus.
**T. splen'dens,** *Eutrombicula splendens.*
**T. tsalsahua'tl,** *Eutrombicula alfreddugèsi.*

**trom·bic·u·li·a·sis** (trom-bik"u-li'ə-sis) [MeSH: Trombiculiasis] infestation with mites of the family Trombiculidae; it usually occurs in the form of dermatitis when the larval forms (see *chigger*) attach to the skin of a human, other mammal, or bird. Called also *trombiculidiasis, trombidiiasis,* and *trombidiosis.*

**trom·bic·u·lid** a mite of the family Trombiculidae; called also *chigger mite.*

**Trom·bic·u·li·dae** (trom-bik'u-lĭ"de) a family of mites found in many parts of the world; their larvae are parasitic on vertebrates. Genera of medical and significance include *Trombicula* and *Neotrombicula.*

**trom·bic·u·li·di·a·sis** (trom-bik"u-lĭ-di'ə-sis) trombiculiasis.

**trom·bid·i·i·a·sis** (trom-bid"e-i'ə-sis) trombiculiasis.

**trom·bid·i·o·sis** (trom-bid"e-o'sis) trombiculiasis.

**Trom·bid·i·um** (trom-bid'e-əm) a name formerly given a genus of mites, now included in the genus *Trombicula.*

**tro·meth·amine** (tro-meth'ə-mēn) [USP] [MeSH: Tromethamine] an amine base used intravenously as an alkalizer for the correction of metabolic acidosis. Called also *THAM, TRIS* and *tris(hydroxymethyl)aminomethane.*

**tromo·pho·nia** (trom"o-fo'ne-ə) a form of dysphonia characterized by a tremulous voice.

**Tron·o·thane** (tron'o-thān) trademark for preparations of pramoxine hydrochloride.

**tro·pate** (tro'pāt) a salt of tropic acid.

**troph·ec·to·derm** (trof-ek'to-dərm) [*tropho-* + *ectoderm*] the outer layer of cells of the early blastocyst; the earliest trophoblast.

**troph·ede·ma** (trof"ə-de'mə) [*tropho-* + *edema*] a disease marked by permanent edema of the feet or legs.
**congenital t., hereditary t.,** Milroy's disease.

**Tro·phe·ry·ma** (tro-fer'ĭ-mə) [*troph-* + Gr. *eryma* defense] a genus of aerobic, gram-positive actinomycetes not closely related to any known genus.
**T. whippe'lii,** a species that is the cause of Whipple's disease.

**troph·ic** (trof'ik) [Gr. *trophikos*] nutritional.

**-trophic** [Gr. *trophikos* nourishing] word termination denoting relationship to nutrition.

**tro·phic·i·ty** (tro-fis'ĭ-te) a trophic function or relation.

**-trophin** see *-tropin.*

**troph·ism** (trof'iz-əm) direct trophic influence.

**troph(o)-** [Gr. *trophē* nutrition] a combining form denoting relationship to food or nourishment.

**tropho·blast** (trof'o-blast) [*tropho-* + *-blast*] [MeSH: Trophoblast] a layer of extraembryonic ectodermal tissue on the outside of the blastocyst. It attaches the blastocyst to the endometrium of the uterine wall and supplies nutrition to the embryo. From it are derived the chorion and amnion. The inner cellular layer of the trophoblast covering a chorionic villus is called *cytotrophoblast* and its outer syncytial layer *syncytiotrophoblast.* The mesoblast, once thought to be trophoblastic, is now traced in primates to the caudal end of the primitive streak.

**tropho·blas·tic** (trof"o-blas'tik) pertaining to the trophoblast.

**tropho·cyte** (trof'o-sīt) a lower type of cell which furnishes nourishment to a higher type of cell of a tissue. Cf. *trophospongium* (def. 1).

**tropho·derm** (trof'o-dərm) [*tropho-* + *-derm*] trophoblast.

**tropho·der·ma·to·neu·ro·sis** (trof"o-der"mə-to-noo͝-ro'sis) acrodynia.

**tropho·dy·nam·ics** (trof"o-di-nam'iks) the study of the forces engaged in nutrition.

**tropho·ede·ma** (trof"o-ə-de'mə) trophedema.

**tropho·lec·i·thal** (trof"o-les'ĭ-thəl) pertaining to the tropholecithus.

**tropho·lec·i·thus** (trof"o-les'ĭ-thəs) [*tropho-* + Gr. *lekithos* yolk] the food yolk of a meroblastic egg.

**tro·phol·o·gy** (tro-fol'ə-je) nutriology.

**tropho·neu·ro·sis** (trof"o-noo͝-ro'sis) any functional disease due to the failure of nutrition in part because of defective nerve supply.
**facial t.,** facial hemiatrophy.
**lingual t.,** progressive lingual hemiatrophy.
**t. of Romberg,** facial hemiatrophy.

**tropho·neu·rot·ic** (trof"o-noo͝-rot'ik) pertaining to or of the nature of a trophoneurosis.

**troph·o·no·sis** (trof"o-no'sis) [*tropho-* + *nos-* + *-sis*] any disease or disorder due to nutritional causes.

**tro·phont** (tro'font) [*troph-* + Gr. *on, ontos* being] the active, motile, feeding stage or form in the life cycle of certain ciliate protozoa, especially that produced by a tomite and developing into a theront. Cf. *trophozoite.*

**tropho·nu·cle·us** (trof″o-noo′kle-əs) macronucleus.

**tropho·path·ia** (trof″o-path′e-ə) trophopathy.

**tro·phop·a·thy** (tro-fop′ə-the) [*tropho-* + *-pathy*] any derangement of nutrition.

**tropho·plast** (trof′o-plast) [*tropho-* + *-plast*] a granular protoplasmic body; a plastid.

**tropho·spon·gia** (trof″o-spon′je-ə) plural of *trophospongium.*

**tropho·spon·gi·um** (trof″o-spon′je-əm) pl. *trophospon′gia* [*tropho-* + Gr. *spongion* sponge] 1. a canalicular network in the cytoplasm of certain cells which was once believed to be instrumental in the circulation of nutritive material. 2. (pl.) the vascular endometrium between the myometrium and the trophoblast.

**tropho·tax·is** (tro″fo-tak′sis) [*tropho-* + *taxis*] chemotaxis of an organism in response to nutritive material.

**tropho·ther·a·py** (tro″fo-ther′ə-pe) diet therapy.

**tropho·tro·pism** (tro″fo-tro′piz-əm) [*tropho-* + *tropism*] chemotropism of an organism in response to nutritive material.

**tropho·zo·ite** (trof″o-zo′īt) [*tropho-* + Gr. *zōon* animal] the active, motile, feeding stage of a protozoan organism, as contrasted with the nonmotile encysted stage. In the malarial parasite, it is the stage between the merozoite and the mature schizont. Trophozoites of *Toxoplasma gondii* (tachyzoites) are found in the tissues during the acute stage of toxoplasmosis. Cf. *trophont.*

**-trophy** [Gr. *trophē* nutrition] a word termination denoting food or nutrition.

**tro·pia** (tro′pe-ə) [Gr. *tropē* a turning] a manifest deviation of an eye from the normal position when both eyes are open and uncovered; strabismus, or squint. See *cyclotropia, esotropia, exotropia, hypertropia,* and *hypotropia.*

**-tropic** [Gr. *tropikos* turning] a word termination denoting turning toward, changing, or tending to turn or change; see *tropism.*

**tro·pic ac·id** (tro′pik) 2-phenyl-3-hydroxypropanoic acid, a constituent of atropine and scopolamine.

**trop·i·cal** (trop′ĭ-kəl) [Gr. *tropikos* turning] pertaining to the regions of the earth bounded by the parallels of latitude 23° 27′ north and south of the equator.

**tro·pic·a·mide** (tro-pik′ə-mīd) [USP] [MeSH: Tropicamide] an anticholinergic applied topically to the conjunctiva to produce mydriasis and cycloplegia.

**trop·i·dine** (trop′ĭ-din) an oily, liquid base with an odor like that of coniine, formed by the dehydration of tropine.

**-tropin** [Gr. *tropos* a turning] a word termination denoting an affinity for the structure or thing indicated by the stem to which it is affixed, as gonadotropin. Also, *-trophin.*

**tro·pine** (tro′pin) a crystalline alkaloid with a smell like tobacco, derivable from atropine and from various plants.

**tro·pism** (tro′piz-əm) [Gr. *tropē* a turn, turning] [MeSH: Tropism] the turning, bending, movement, or growth of an organism or part of an organism in response to an external stimulus. Such response may be either positive (toward) or negative (away from the stimulus). By extension, used as a word termination affixed to a stem denoting the nature of the stimulus (phototropism) or the material or entity for which an organism or substance shows a special affinity (neurotropism), usually applied to nonmotile organisms. Cf. *taxis,* def. 1.

**trop(o)-** [Gr. *tropos* a turn, turning] a combining form denoting a turn, reaction, or change.

**tro·po·chrome** (tro′po-krōm″) [*tropo-* + *-chrome*] refusing to stain with mucin stains after formol-bichromate fixation, as applied to certain serous cells of the salivary glands. Cf. *homeochrome.*

**tro·po·col·la·gen** (tro″po-kol′ə-jən) [*tropo-* + *collagen*] [MeSH: Tropocollagen] the basic structural unit of collagen; a helical structure consisting of three polypeptide chains, each chain composed of about a thousand amino acids, coiled around each other to form a spiral and stabilized by inter- and intrachain covalent bonds. It is rich in glycine, which occurs nearly one residue out of three, as well as proline, hydroxyproline, and hydroxylysine, the last two rarely occurring in other proteins.

**tro·po·elas·tin** (tro″po-e-las′tin) [MeSH: Tropoelastin] the precursor of elastin.

**tro·pom·e·ter** (tro-pom′ə-tər) [*tropo-* + *-meter*] an instrument for measuring the twist or torsion of a long bone.

**tro·po·my·o·sin** (tro″po-mi′o-sin) [MeSH: Tropomyosin] muscle protein of the I band that inhibits contraction unless its position is modified by troponin so that the myosin molecules can make contact with the actin molecules. See Plate 35.

**t. A,** paramyosin.

**tro·po·nin** (tro′po-nin) [MeSH: Troponin] a complex of globular muscle proteins of the I band that inhibits contraction by blocking the interaction of actin and myosin; when combined with $Ca^{2+}$, it so modifies the position of the tropomyosin molecules that interaction takes place. See Plate 35.

**-tropy** [Gr. *tropos* a turn, turning] a word termination denoting a turn, turning, or change in response to a stimulus.

**trough** (trof) a shallow longitudinal depression or channel.

**synaptic t.,** an invagination of the membrane of a striated muscle fiber, surrounding a motor end plate at a neuromuscular junction. Called also *synaptic cleft* and *primary synaptic cleft.*

**Trous·seau's phenomenon, sign, spot, twitching** (troo-sōz′) [Armand *Trousseau,* French physician, 1801–1867] see under *phenomenon, sign,* and *twitching,* and see *tache cérébrale.*

**tro·va·flox·a·cin mes·y·late** (tro″və-flok′sə-sin) an antibacterial related to the fluoroquinolones, effective against a broad spectrum of gram-positive and gram-negative organisms, used in the treatment of infections caused by susceptible organisms; administered orally.

**Tro·van** (tro′van) trademark for preparations of alatrofloxacin mesylate and trovafloxacin mesylate.

**trox·i·done** (trok′sĭ-dōn) trimethadione.

**troy** (troi) a system of weights commonly used in England and the United States for expressing quantities of gold and silver; for equivalents see *tables of weights and measures.*

**Trp** tryptophan.

**TRU** turbidity reducing unit.

**Tru·e·ta treatment (method, technique)** (troo-a′tah) [José *Trueta,* Spanish surgeon in England, 1897–1977] see under *treatment.*

**trun·cal** (trung′kəl) pertaining to the trunk.

**trun·cate** (trung′kāt) [L. *truncatus*] having the end cut squarely off.

**trun·cus** (trung′kəs) pl. *trun′ci* [L. "trunk"] [TA] 1. a general term in anatomical nomenclature for a major, undivided, and usually short portion of a nerve, blood vessel, lymphatic vessel, or duct. 2. the main part of the body, to which the head and limbs are attached.

**t. arterio′sus,** an arterial trunk, especially the artery connected with the embryonic heart, which gives off the aortic arches and develops into the aortic and pulmonary arteries.

**t. arteriosus, persistent,** a congenital anomaly, characterized by a single arterial trunk arising from the heart, receiving blood from both ventricles and supplying blood to the coronary, pulmonary, and systemic circulations; sometimes classified according to the arrangement of the arteries supplying the lungs.

**t. brachiocepha′licus** [TA], brachiocephalic trunk: the first branch of the arch of the aorta, which behind the right sternoclavicular joint divides into the right common carotid and right subclavian arteries, with distribution to the right side of the head and neck and to the right arm; the lowest thyroid artery may arise from this trunk. Called also *brachiocephalic artery* and *innominate artery.*

**t. bronchomediastina′lis** [TA], bronchomediastinal trunk: either of the two lymphatic vessels, right and left, draining the pulmonary, bronchopulmonary, tracheobronchial, tracheal, and parasternal lymph nodes: that on the right side into the right lymphatic duct or subclavian vein, and that on the left into the thoracic duct or the subclavian vein.

**t. coeli′acus** [TA], celiac trunk: the arterial trunk that arises from the abdominal aorta, gives off the left gastric, common hepatic, and splenic arteries, and supplies the esophagus, stomach, duodenum, spleen, pancreas, liver, and gallbladder.

**t. cor′poris callo′si** [TA], trunk of corpus callosum: the main central portion of the corpus callosum as distinguished from the rostrum and the splenium.

**t. costocervica′lis** [TA], costocervical trunk: an artery that arises from the back of the subclavian artery, arches backward, and at the neck of the first rib divides into the deep cervical and highest intercostal arteries, thus supplying blood to the structures of the first two intercostal spaces, the vertebral column, the muscles of the back, and the deep neck muscles.

**t. ence′phali** [TA], **t. encepha′licus,** encephalic trunk: the stemlike portion of the brain connecting the cerebral hemispheres with the spinal cord and comprising the pons, medulla oblongata, and mesencephalon; the diencephalon is considered part of the truncus encephalicus by some. Called also *brain stem.*

**t. fasci′culi atrioventricula′ris,** trunk of atrioventricular bundle: the undivided portion of the atrioventricular bundle, from its origin at the atrioventricular node to the point of division into the right and left bundle branches at the superior end of the muscular part of the interventricular septum. It contains the penetrating portion of the bundle, a short segment of multiple small fascicles that penetrate the fibrous tissue of the atrioventricular septum.

**t. infe′rior plex′us brachia′lis** [TA], inferior trunk of brachial plexus: the trunk of the brachial plexus that is formed by the anterior branches of the eighth cervical and first thoracic nerves; medial pectoral nerves may arise from it. Its anterior division becomes the medial cord of the plexus, and its posterior division helps form the posterior cord; *modality,* general sensory and motor. Called also *lower trunk of brachial plexus.*

**trun′ci intestina′les** [TA], intestinal trunks: short lymphatic vessels which leave the gastrointestinal tract and participate in formation of the thoracic duct.

**t. jugula′ris** [TA], jugular trunk: either of the two vessels, right and left, draining the deep cervical lymph nodes: on the right side, into the right lymphatic duct or subclavian vein, and on the left side, into the thoracic duct or subclavian vein.

**t. linguofacia′lis** [TA], linguofacial trunk: the common trunk by which the facial and lingual arteries often arise from the external carotid artery.

**t. lumba′lis** [TA], **t. lumba′ris,** lumbar trunk: either of the two lymphatic vessels, right and left, draining lymph upward from the lumbar lymph nodes and helping form the thoracic duct.

**t. lumbosacra′lis** [TA], lumbosacral trunk: a trunk formed by union of the lower division of the anterior branch of the fourth lumbar nerve with the anterior branch of the fifth lumbar nerve; it descends to the sacral plexus.

**trun′ci lympha′tici,** lymphatic trunks: the lymphatic vessels (right or left lumbar, intestinal, right or left bronchomediastinal, right or left subclavian, and right or left jugular trunks) that drain lymph from various regions of the body into the right lymphatic or thoracic duct.

**t. me′dius plex′us brachia′lis** [TA], middle trunk of brachial plexus: the trunk of the brachial plexus that is formed by the anterior branch of the seventh cervical nerve. Its anterior division, from which lateral pectoral nerves may arise, helps form the lateral cord of the plexus, and its posterior division helps form the posterior cord; *modality,* general sensory and motor.

**t. ner′vi accesso′rii** [TA], trunk of accessory nerve: the nerve trunk formed by the cranial and spinal roots of the accessory nerve, which separates into an internal and external terminal branch. See also *nervus accessorius.*

**t. ner′vi spina′lis** [TA], trunk of spinal nerve: the usually very short nerve trunk formed by the ventral and dorsal roots of a spinal nerve.

**trun′ci plex′us brachia′lis** [TA], trunks of brachial plexus: the three trunks (superior, middle, and inferior) of the brachial plexus, arising from the anterior branches of the lower four cervical nerves and the first thoracic nerve near the lateral border of the scalenus anterior muscle; they continue laterally and downward, above and behind the subclavian artery, and near the clavicle each splits into an anterior and a posterior division. The anterior divisions of the superior and medial trunks unite to form the lateral fasciculus and that of the inferior trunk forms the medial fasciculus of the plexus; and the posterior divisions of the three trunks form the posterior fasciculus of the plexus.

**t. pulmona′lis** [TA], pulmonary trunk: the vessel arising from the conus arteriosus of the right ventricle, extending upward obliquely to divide into the right and left pulmonary arteries beneath the arch of the aorta, and conveying unaerated blood toward the lungs. Called also *arteria pulmonalis* or *pulmonary artery.*

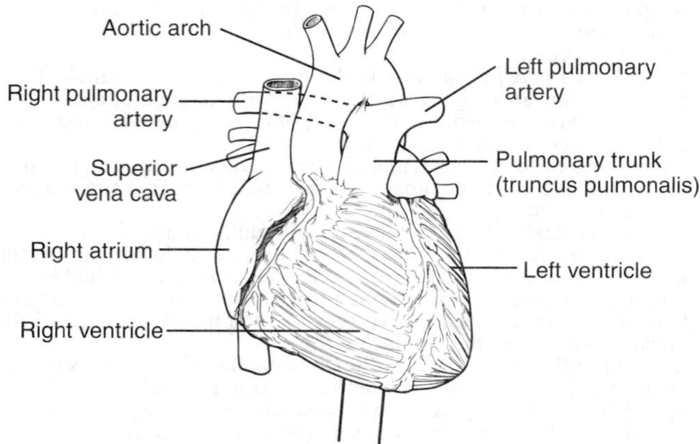


**t. subcla′vius** [TA], subclavian trunk: either of two lymphatic vessels, right and left, draining the axillary lymph nodes; that on the right into the right lymphatic duct or subclavian vein, that on the left into the thoracic duct or the subclavian vein.

**t. supe′rior plex′us brachia′lis** [TA], superior trunk of brachial plexus: the trunk of the brachial plexus that is formed by the anterior branches of the fifth and sixth cervical nerves. Its anterior division helps form the lateral cord of the plexus, its posterior division helps form the posterior cord, and it gives rise directly to the suprascapular and subclavian nerves; *modality,* general sensory and motor. Called also *upper trunk of brachial plexus.*

**t. sympathe′ticus, t. sympa′thicus** [TA], sympathetic trunk: two long nerve strands, one on each side of the vertebral column, extending from the base of the skull to the coccyx. Interconnected by nerve strands, each has cervical, thoracic, lumbar, and sacral sympathetic ganglia. These receive preganglionic fibers from thoracic and upper lumbar anterior roots by way of rami communicantes, send postganglionic fibers to anterior roots by rami communicantes, and give branches to prevertebral plexuses and adjacent viscera and blood vessels.

**t. thyrocervica′lis** [TA], thyrocervical trunk: a short artery that arises from the convex side of the subclavian artery just medial to the anterior scalene muscle and at once divides into the inferior thyroid, transverse cervical, and suprascapular arteries, supplying thyroid, neck, and scapular regions.

**t. vaga′lis ante′rior** [TA], anterior vagal trunk: a nerve trunk (or trunks) formed by fibers from both left and right vagus nerves, collected from the anterior part of the esophageal plexus; it descends through the esophageal opening of the diaphragm to supply branches to the anterior surface of the stomach.

**t. vaga′lis poste′rior** [TA], posterior vagal trunk: a nerve trunk or trunks formed by fibers from both left and right vagus nerves, collected from the posterior part of the esophageal plexus; it descends through the esophageal opening of the diaphragm to supply branches to the posterior surface of the stomach.

**trunk** (trungk) [L. *truncus* the stem or trunk of a tree] 1. the main part of the body, to which head and limbs are attached. 2. a major, undivided and usually short, portion of a nerve or of a blood or lymphatic vessel, or other duct. For entries not found here, see under *truncus.*

**t. of accessory nerve,** truncus nervi accessorii.
**t. of atrioventricular bundle,** truncus fasciculi atrioventricularis.
**t's of brachial plexus,** trunci plexus brachialis.
**bronchomediastinal t.,** truncus bronchomediastinalis.
**t. of bundle of His,** truncus fasciculi atrioventricularis.
**celiac t.,** truncus coeliacus.
**t. of corpus callosum,** truncus corporis callosi.
**encephalic t.,** truncus encephali.
**inferior t. of brachial plexus,** truncus inferior plexus brachialis.
**intestinal t's,** trunci intestinales.
**jugular t.,** truncus jugularis.
**lower t. of brachial plexus,** truncus inferior plexus brachialis.
**lumbar t.,** truncus lumbalis.
**lumbosacral t.,** truncus lumbosacralis.
**lymphatic t's,** trunci lymphatici.
**middle t. of brachial plexus,** truncus medius plexus brachialis.
**pulmonary t.,** truncus pulmonalis.
**t. of spinal nerve,** truncus nervi spinalis.
**subclavian t.,** truncus subclavius.
**superior t. of brachial plexus,** truncus superior plexus brachialis.
**sympathetic t.,** truncus sympathicus.
**upper t. of brachial plexus,** truncus superior plexus brachialis.
**vagal t., anterior,** truncus vagalis anterior.
**vagal t., posterior,** truncus vagalis posterior.

**Tru·sopt** (troo′sopt) trademark for a preparation of dorzolamide hydrochloride.

**truss** (trus) an elastic, canvas, or metallic device for retaining a hernia reduced within the abdominal cavity.

**nasal t.,** a trusslike support for fractured nasal bones.

**try-in** (tri′in) a preliminary insertion of a dental prosthesis or orthodontic appliance to determine its fit and suitability.

**try·pan·id** (tri′pan-id) trypanosomid.

**try·pano·ci·dal** (tri-pan″o-si′dəl) trypanosomicidal.

**try·pano·cide** (tri-pan′o-sīd) trypanosomicide.

**try·pan·ol·y·sis** (tri″pan-ol′ĭ-sis) the destruction of trypanosomes.

**try·pano·lyt·ic** (tri″pan-o-lit′ik) destructive to trypanosomes.

**Try·pano·so·ma** (tri-pan″o-so′mə) [Gr. *trypanon* borer +*sōma* body] [MeSH: Trypanosoma] a genus of protozoa (suborder Trypanosomatina, order Kinetoplastida) comprising hemoflagellates parasitic in invertebrates and vertebrates, including humans; several species are pathogenic. Their life cycle involves amastigote, promastigote, epimastigote, and trypomastigote stages; the first three stages are found in the vector (usually a bloodsucking invertebrate) and the last in the vertebrate (definitive) host. In some systems of classification, trypanosomes are categorized in two groups according to where they develop in the digestive system of the vector: *salivaria,* including the subgenera *Duttonella, Nannomonas,* and *Trypanozoon;* and *stercoraria,* including the subgenera *Megatrypanum, Herpetosoma,* and *Schizotrypanum.* Another system classifies them into four groups based on biological similarities: (1) *lewisi group,* including *T. lewisi, T. duttoni, T. theileri, T. cruzi, T. nabiasi, T. melophagium,* and *T. rangeli;* (2) *vivax group,* including *T. vivax* and *T. uniforme;* (3) *congolense group,* including *T. congolense, T. dimorphon,* and *T. simiae;* and (4) *brucei group,* including *T. brucei, T. gambiense, T. rhodesiense, T. evansi, T. equinum,* and *T. epiperdum.*

**T. bru'cei,** a salivarian species widely distributed in Africa where it is transmitted by the bites of tsetse flies from a reservoir in wild animals, in which it causes a mild infection, to domestic animals, especially cattle, in which it causes a severe, often fatal disease (see *nagana*). Some systems of classification consider *T. brucei* to consist of three morphologically indistinguishable subspecies or varieties: *T. brucei brucei,* which causes trypanosomiasis in animals; *T. brucei gambiense,* the etiologic agent of Gambian trypanosomiasis; and *T. brucei rhodesiense,* the cause of Rhodesian trypanosomiasis. Other authorities prefer to grant specific status to *T. gambiense* and *T. rhodesiense* because of their biologic and epidemiologic differences.

**T. bru'cei bru'cei,** a subspecies of *T. brucei* that infects mammals, but not humans, being transmitted from a reservoir in wild animals, in which it causes a relatively mild infection, to various domestic animals, especially cattle, in which it causes a severe, often fatal, disease (see *nagana*). Called also *T. brucei.*

**T. bru'cei gambien'se,** a polymorphic subspecies of *T. brucei* causing the chronic or Gambian form of trypanosomiasis in West and Central Africa, transmitted by the bite of infected tsetse flies, chiefly *Glossina palpalis, G. tachinoides,* and *G. fuscipes,* with humans being the only important reservoir. Called also *T. gambiense, T. hominis,* and *T. ugandense.*

**T. bru'cei rhodesien'se,** a polymorphic subspecies of *T. brucei* causing acute or Rhodesian trypanosomiasis throughout East Africa, transmitted by the bite of infected tsetse flies, chiefly *Glossina morsitans, G. pallidipes,* and *G. swynnertoni.* Although many animals can become infected, the most important reservoirs are the antelopes (particularly the bushbuck and hartebeest); domestic animals, particularly cattle, may also serve as reservoirs. Transmission to humans is usually via these animals, although intrahuman cycles of infection are possible. Called also *T. rhodesiense.*

**T. congolen'se,** a tsetse fly–transmitted salivarian species found in Central Africa that is a cause of nagana in domestic animals, which is especially severe in cattle. Called also *T. nanum.*

**T. cru'zi,** a stercorarian species commonly infecting many wild and domestic animals throughout North, Central, and South America, with armadillos, cats, dogs, bats, rodents, and other mammals serving as reservoir hosts, and usually transmitted by reduviid bugs of the genera *Panstrongylus, Triatoma,* and *Rhodnius.* It is the etiologic agent of Chagas' disease in humans. Called also *T. triatomae* and *Schizotympanum cruzi.*

**T. dimor'phon,** a tsetse fly–transmitted salivarian species widely distributed in Central Africa, which was formerly thought to be identical with *T. congolense* but has been shown to be a distinct species. It is found in horses, pigs, goats, sheep, cattle, and dogs, in the latter three of which it has been shown to be more pathogenic than *T. congolense.*

**T. equi'num,** a salivarian species transmitted mechanically primarily by tabanid flies and causing mal de caderas in horses in Central and South America. Except for the absence of a kinetoplast it is identical with *T. evansi.*

**T. equiper'dum,** a salivarian species structurally indistinguishable from *T. evansi* that causes the venereal disease dourine in horses in Africa, Asia, and certain regions of Europe and North and South America. Called also *T. rougeti.*

**T. evan'si,** a salivarian species transmitted mechanically usually by tabanid flies in the Far and Middle East, in North Africa outside of tsetse fly–inhabiting areas, and in certain parts of Central and South America where the vampire bat is also a vector. *T. evansi* causes surra, which is an economically important disease in domestic animals such as camels, equines, cattle, elephants, and dogs. Called also *T. hippicum.*

**T. gambien'se,** a polymorphic salivarian species causing the chronic or Gambian form of trypanosomiasis in West and Central Africa, transmitted by the bites of infected tsetse flies, chiefly *Glossina palpalis, G. tachinoides,* and *G. fuscipes,* with humans being the only important reservoir. Called also *T. hominis* and *T. ugandense.* See also *T. brucei.*

**T. hip'picum,** *T. evansi.*

**T. ho'minis,** *T. brucei gambiense.*

**T. lew'isi,** a stercorarian species commonly found in the blood of rats worldwide, usually nonpathogenic in adults but causing lethal infection in sucklings, and transmitted by the rat flea, *Nosopsyllus fasciatus.* The species is much used in laboratory research.

**T. melopha'gium,** a nonpathogenic stercorarian species commonly found in sheep worldwide and transmitted by the sheep kid, *Melophagus ovinus.*

**T. na'num,** *T. congolense.*

**T. neoto'mae,** a species found in wood rats in California, possibly identical with *T. cruzi.*

**T. range'li,** a nonpathogenic, stercorarian species infecting humans and various animals, especially cats and dogs, primarily in Venezuela, Brazil, Colombia, Costa Rica, El Salvador, Guatemala, and Panama, and usually transmitted by reduviid flies of the genus *Rhodnius.*

**T. rhodesien'se,** *T. brucei rhodesiense.*

**T. rotato'rium,** the type species of the genus, and found in the blood of several species of frogs.

**T. rouge'ti,** *T. equiperdum.*

**T. si'miae,** a salivarian species found especially in East Africa and eastern Zaire, first reported from the monkey although its natural reservoir is the warthog, and usually transmitted by tsetse flies (*Glossina* spp.) but sometimes also by bloodsucking flies. It causes nagana in various domestic animals, being highly pathogenic for camels (causing death in several days), mildly pathogenic for goats, and apparently nonpathogenic for cattle, horses, and dogs.

**T. su'is,** a species that causes nagana in pigs.

**T. thei'leri,** a large stercorarian species found in the blood of cattle worldwide, transmitted by tabanid flies, and usually nonpathogenic although under stressful conditions it may be associated with illness and perhaps death.

**T. theodo'ri,** a nonpathogenic, stercorarian species similar to (and perhaps the same as) *T. melophagium* that is found in goats and has the hippoboscid *Lipoptena caprina* as an intermediate host.

**T. tria'tomae,** *T. cruzi.*

**T. uganden'se,** *T. brucei gambiense.*

**T. unifor'me,** a tsetse fly–transmitted salivarian species similar to but smaller than *T. vivax* that is a cause of nagana in cattle, goats, sheep, and antelopes in Zaire.

**T. vi'vax,** a tsetse fly–transmitted salivarian species found in many animals, including cattle, sheep, goats, camels, horses, antelopes, and giraffes in Africa, Central and South America, the West Indies, and Mauritius. It is a cause of nagana, the severity of which depends on the species affected, being fatal in certain types of cattle in certain areas.

**try·pano·so·mal** (tri-pan″o-so′məl) 1. pertaining to or caused by trypanosomes. 2. see *trypomastigote.*

**try·pano·so·ma·tid** (tri-pan″o-so′mə-tid) 1. any protozoan of the suborder Trypanosomatina. 2. pertaining to or caused by a protozoan of the suborder Trypanosomatina.

**Try·pano·so·ma·ti·na** (tri-pan″o-so″mə-ti′nə) [MeSH: Trypanosomatina] a suborder of parasitic protozoa (order Kinetoplastida, class Zoomastigophorea) comprising the hemoflagellates, which are found in the hosts' blood, lymph, and tissues, and are characterized by a leaflike or rounded body with one nucleus, one flagellum that is free or attached to the body by an undulating membrane, and a relatively small compact kinetoplast. All trypanosomatids have morphologically distinct stages in their life cycles during which the organisms of one genus may pass through forms characteristic of other genera of the suborder. These forms include: amastigote, choanomastigote, epimastigote, opisthomastigote, promastigote, and trypomastigote. Not all species pass through all of the stages, but all have at least two such forms during their development. Representative genera include *Blastocrithidia, Crithidia, Leishmania, Leptomonas,* and *Trypanosoma.*

**try·pano·so·ma·to·trop·ic** (tri-pan″o-so″mə-to-trop′ik) having a selective affinity for trypanosomes.

**try·pano·some** (tri-pan′o-sōm) 1. any protozoan of the genus *Trypanosoma* or of the suborder Trypanosomatina. 2. denoting a morphologic stage in the development of certain trypanosomatid protozoa; see *trypomastigote.*

**try·pano·so·mi·a·sis** (tri-pan″o-so-mi′ə-sis) [MeSH: Trypanosomiasis] infection with protozoa of the genus *Trypanosoma.* Trypanosomal infections of humans include the Gambian and Rhodesian forms of African trypanosomiasis, and Chagas' disease. When it affects domestic animals, trypanosomiasis is usually called *nagana.* Other trypanosomal syndromes seen in animals include dourine, mal de caderas, and surra.

**African t.,** human trypanosomiasis endemic in tsetse fly–infested areas of tropical Africa. The early stage is manifested by hemolymphatic involvement with intermittent fever, anemia, rash, and transitory, localized edema. Later, invasion of the central nervous system occurs, with resultant meningoencephalitis, leading to extreme mental and physical lethargy, tremors, convulsions, and eventually coma and death. The disease occurs in two forms: *Gambian* (chronic) and *Rhodesian* (acute). Called also *African sleeping sickness.*

**American t.,** Chagas' disease.

**East African t.,** Rhodesian t.

**Gambian t.,** the usually chronic and less severe form of African trypanosomiasis, occurring in Central and West Africa, caused by

*Trypanosoma brucei gambiense,* and transmitted by the bites of infected tsetse flies, chiefly *Glossina palpalis, G. tachinoides,* and *G. fuscipes.* This form differs from Rhodesian trypanosomiasis in that the duration of the chronic disease is several months to years and central nervous system involvement usually occurs later in its course. Called also *Gambian sleeping sickness* and *West African t.*
**Rhodesian t.,** the usually acute, more severe, often fatal form of African trypanosomiasis, occurring in East Africa, caused by *Trypanosoma brucei rhodesiense,* transmitted by the bites of infected tsetse flies, chiefly *Glossina pallidipes, G. morsitans,* and *G. swynnertoni.* This form differs from Gambian trypanosomiasis in that the acute form has a duration of 3 to 9 months and central nervous system involvement occurs earlier in its course. Called also *East African t.* and *Rhodesian sleeping sickness.*
**South American t.,** Chagas' disease.
**West African t.,** Gambian t.

**try·pano·so·mi·ci·dal** (tri-pan″o-so″mĭ-si′dəl) destructive to trypanosomes.

**try·pano·so·mi·cide** (tri-pan″o-so′mĭ-sīd) [*trypanosome* + *-cide*] 1. destructive to trypanosomes. 2. a substance which destroys trypanosomes.

**try·pano·so·mid** (tri-pan′o-so-mid) a skin eruption occurring in trypanosomiasis; called also *trypanid.*

**Try·pano·zo·on** (tri-pan″o-zo′ən) [Gr. *trypanon* borer + *zoon* animal] in some systems of classification, a subgenus of salivarian trypanosomes, including *Trypanosoma brucei, T. rhodesiense, T. gambiense, T. evansi, T. equinum,* and *T. equiperdum.*

**try·par·o·san** (tri-par′o-san) a preparation formed by introducing a halogen radical (e.g., chlorine) into the parafuchsin molecule; used by injection in trypanosomiasis.

**tryp·ar·sa·mide** (trip-ahr′sə-mīd) an antitrypanosomal agent formerly used in the treatment of late-stage Gambian trypanosomiasis; because of increased resistance, it has been replaced by melarsoprol.

**try·pe·sis** (tri-pe′sis) [Gr. *trypēsis*] trephination.

**try·po·mas·ti·gote** (tri″po-mas′tĭ-gōt) [Gr. *trypanon* borer + *mastigote*] any of the bodies representing the morphologic (trypanosomal) stage in the life cycle of certain trypanosomatid protozoa, resembling the typical adult form of members of the genus *Trypanosoma,* in which the slender elongate cell has a kinetoplast and basal body located at the posterior end and a flagellum running anteriorly along an undulating membrane to become a free-flowing structure. Cf. *amastigote, choanomastigote, epimastigote, opisthomastigote,* and *promastigote.*

**try·po·nar·syl** (tri″po-nahr′səl) tryparsamide.

**try·po·tan** (tri′po-tan) tryparsamide.

**tryp·sin** (trip′sin) [EC 3.4.21.4] [MeSH: Trypsin] a serine endopeptidase that catalyzes the cleavage of peptide bonds on the carboxyl side of either arginine or lysine. It is secreted by the pancreas as the proenzyme trypsinogen and converted to the active form in the small intestine by enteropeptidase; the active enzyme catalyzes the cleavage and activation of additional trypsinogen and other pancreatic proenzymes important to protein digestion.
**crystallized t.** [USP], a purified, crystallized preparation from an extract of the pancreas of the ox, *Bos taurus;* used topically for its proteolytic effect in the débridement of necrotic wounds and ulcers, abscesses, fistulas, and sinuses, and in the treatment of empyema.

**tryp·sin·o·gen** (trip-sin′o-jən) [MeSH: Trypsinogen] the inactive proenzyme of trypsin secreted by the pancreas, activated in the duodenum via cleavage by enteropeptidase.

**tryp·ta·mine** (trip′tə-mēn) a chemical product of the decarboxylation of tryptophan effecting vasoconstriction by causing the release of norepinephrine at postganglionic nerve endings; it is a precursor of many natural and synthetic compounds, including psychoactive ones such as diethyltryptamine and dimethyltryptamine.

**Tryp·tar** (trip′tahr) trademark for a preparation of crystallized trypsin.

**tryp·tic** (trip″tik) relating to or produced as a result of digestion by trypsin.

**tryp·tone** (trip′tōn) a peptone produced by proteolytic digestion with trypsin.

**tryp·to·phan** (trip′to-fan) [MeSH: Tryptophan] an essential amino acid, α-amino-3-indolepropionic acid, existing in proteins, from which it is set free by tryptic digestion; necessary for optimal growth in infants and for nitrogen equilibrium in human adults. It is a precursor of serotonin. Adequate levels of tryptophan in the diet may compensate for deficiencies of niacin and thus mitigate pellagra. Before the name tryptophan was accepted, *proteinochromagen* was also suggested, both names being derived from the color produced in tests. Symbols Trp and W. See table at *amino acid.*

**tryp·to·phan 2,3-di·oxy·gen·ase** (trip′to-fan di-ok′sə-jən-ās) [EC 1.13.11.11] an enzyme of the oxidoreductase class that catalyzes the first step in tryptophan catabolism, the oxidation of tryptophan to formylkynurenine. The enzyme is a heme protein.

**tryp·to·phan 5-mono·oxy·ge·nase** (trip′to-fan mon″o-ok′sə-jən-ās) [EC 1.14.16.4] a monooxygenase that activates molecular oxygen to catalyze the hydroxylation of tryptophan to hydroxytryptophan, a precursor of serotonin; it requires the cofactor tetrahydrobiopterin. The enzyme occurs in the central nervous system and is inactivated in malignant hyperphenylalaninemia.

**tryp·to·phan hy·droxy·lase** (trip′to-fan hi-drok′sə-lās) [MeSH: Tryptophan Hydroxylase] tryptophan 5-monooxygenase.

**tryp·to·phan pyr·ro·lase** (trip′to-fan pə-rōl′ās) tryptophan 2,3-dioxygenase.

**tryp·to·phan·uria** (trip″to-fə-nu′re-ə) the presence of excessive amounts of tryptophan in the urine; the symptoms resemble those of pellagra.

**tryp·to·phyl** (trip′to-fəl) the acyl radical of tryptophan.

**TS** test solution; tricuspid stenosis.

**TSA** tumor-specific antigen.

**TSE** transmissible spongiform encephalopathy.

**tset·se** (tset′se) an African fly of the genus *Glossina.*

**TSF** triceps skinfold; see under *thickness.*

**TSH** thyroid-stimulating hormone; see *thyrotropin.*

**TSTA** tumor-specific transplantation antigen.

**Tsu·ga** (tsoo′gə) the hemlocks, a genus of coniferous trees of the family Pinaceae. *T. canaden′sis* L. Carr. is the eastern hemlock, a source of Canada pitch, of the volatile oil of hemlock, and of an astringent extract.

**TT** thrombin time.

**TU** tuberculin unit.

**Tu·a·mine** (too′ə-min) trademark for preparations of tuaminoheptane.

**tu·am·i·no·hep·tane** (too″ə-me″no-hep′tān) an adrenergic administered by inhalation to produce vasoconstriction of the nasal mucosa for relief of congestion.
**t. sulfate,** the sulfate of tuaminoheptane, having the same actions and uses as the base; applied topically to the nasal mucosa.

**tu·ba** (too′bə) pl. *tu′bae* [L. "trumpet"] [TA] tube: a general term in anatomical nomenclature for an elongated hollow cylindrical organ.
**t. acus′tica,** t. auditiva.
**t. auditi′va** [TA], auditory tube: a channel about 3.6 cm long, lined with mucous membrane, that establishes communication between the tympanic cavity and the nasopharynx and serves to adjust the pressure of gas in the cavity to the external pressure, as well as for mucociliary clearance of the middle ear. It comprises a pars ossea, located in the temporal bone, and a pars cartilaginea, ending in the nasopharynx. Called also *t. acustica, t. auditoria* [TA alternative], *eustachian canal* or *tube, otopharyngeal tube,* and *pharyngotympanic tube.*
**t. audito′ria,** TA alternative for *t. auditiva.*
**t. uteri′na** [TA], **t. uteri′na [fallo′pii],** uterine tube: a long slender

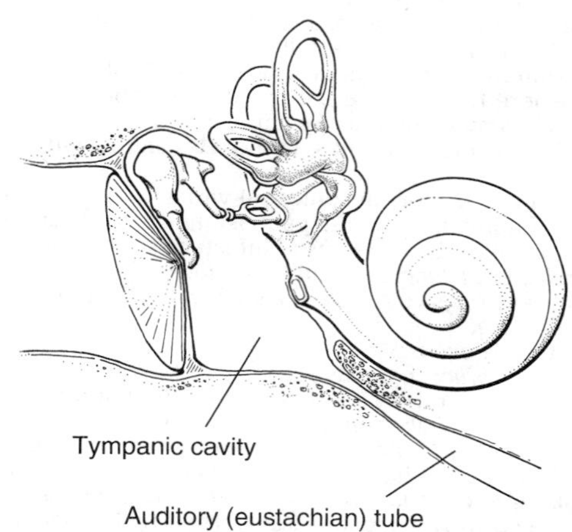

tube that extends from the upper lateral cornu of the uterus to the region of the ovary of the same side; it is attached to the broad ligament by the mesosalpinx, and consists of an ampulla, an infundibulum, an isthmus, two ostia, and a pars uterina. Called also *fallopian tube* and *salpinx* [TA alternative].

**Tu·ba·dil** (too'bə-dil) trademark for a preparation of tubocurarine chloride.

**tu·bae** (too'be) plural of *tuba.*

**tu·bal** (too'bəl) pertaining to or occurring in a tube, as a tubal pregnancy.

**Tu·ba·rine** (too'bə-rin) trademark for a preparation of tubocurarine chloride.

**tu·ba·tor·sion** (too″bə-tor'shən) torsion or twisting of the uterine tube.

**tube** (to͞ob) [L. *tubus*] an elongated hollow cylindrical organ or instrument.

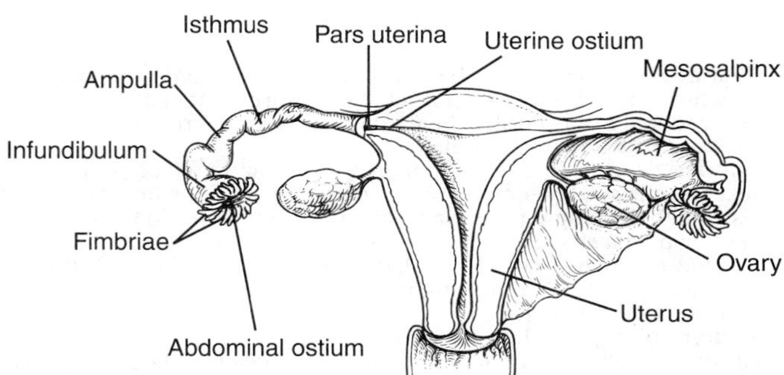


Tuba uterina (uterine, or fallopian, tube), divisible into the infundibulum and fimbriae, ampulla, isthmus, and pars uterina.

## Tube

**Abbott-Miller t.,** Miller-Abbott t.

**Abbott-Rawson t.,** a double barreled tube through which fluid may be both injected and aspirated; it may be used for lavage or decompression of the stomach.

**air t.,** 1. airway. 2. any tubular passage of the respiratory system; see *trachea, bronchus,* and *bronchiolus.*

**auditory t.,** tuba auditiva.

**Bouchut's t's,** a set of tubes for use in the intubation of the larynx.

**Bowman's t's,** tubes formed artificially between the lamellae of the cornea in the process of injection; called also *corneal t's.*

**buccal t.,** see *end t.*

**Cantor t.,** a mercury-weighted tube for intestinal intubation.

**Carlens' t.,** an early type of endobronchial tube equipped with a small hook to hold the tube in position at the tracheal bifurcation; used for ventilation of the left lung.

**cathode-ray t.,** a vacuum tube in which the cathode rays are accelerated as a beam to form luminous spots on a fluorescent screen.

**Celestin's t.,** a plastic tube used to keep the esophagus open in inoperable esophageal carcinoma.

**cerebromedullary t.,** neural t.

**Chaoul t.,** a low voltage x-ray tube so designed as to permit the anode to be located at 2 cm. from the body, thus permitting intense but very superficial tissue penetration of the ionizing radiation beam.

**collecting t's,** tubulus renalis colligens.

**Coolidge t.,** a vacuum tube for the generation of x-rays in which the cathode consists of a spiral filament of incandescent tungsten and the anode (the target) of massive tungsten.

**corneal t's,** Bowman's t's.

**Craigie's t.,** a tube apparatus used for separating motile from nonmotile bacteria; it consists of a length of glass tubing with slanted bottom inserted into a larger tube of semisolid culture medium with the top of the smaller tube protruding above the medium. The medium is inoculated by stab inside the smaller tube. Organisms isolated from the medium outside the tubing are motile; nonmotile types remain inside.

**digestive t.,** see under *tract.*

**discharge t.,** a vessel of insulating material (usually glass) provided with metal electrodes which is exhausted to a low gas pressure and permits the passage of electricity through the residual gas when a moderately high voltage is applied to the electrodes.

**drainage t.,** a tube used in surgery to facilitate the escape of fluids.

**Durham's t.,** 1. [Arthur Edward *Durham*] a jointed tracheostomy tube. 2. [Herbert Edward *Durham*] a small inverted test tube used in determining bacterial gas production.

**empyema t.,** a tube for draining an empyema from the thoracic cavity.

**end t.,** an orthodontic attachment on the buccal surface of a terminal banded molar; often referred to as *buccal t.* when using an edgewise arch mechanism.

**endobronchial t.,** a double-lumen tube inserted into the bronchus of one lung and permitting the complete deflation of the other lung; used in anesthesia and thoracic surgery.

**endotracheal t.,** a tube inserted into the trachea through the mouth, the nose, or a tracheostomy for administration of anesthesia, maintenance of an airway, aspiration of secretions, ventilation of the lungs, or prevention of entrance of foreign material into the tracheobronchial tree. Called also *tracheal t.*

**esophageal t.,** stomach t.

**eustachian t.,** tuba auditiva.

**Ewald t.,** a tube of large bore used to evacuate the stomach.

**fallopian t.,** tuba uterina.

**feeding t.,** a tube for introducing fluids of high caloric value into the stomach.

**fermentation t.,** a U-shaped tube with one arm closed for determining gas production by bacteria.

**Ferrein's t's,** the convoluted uriniferous tubules.

**fusion t's,** heteroscope.

**germ t.,** the short tube formed by a germinating hypha, conidium, or yeast cell.

**Harris t.,** a single-lumen tube with a mercury weight, used as a diagnostic aid in the study of the small intestine; similar to the Miller-Abbott tube.

**horizontal t.,** a metal tube attachment placed in a horizontal position on the buccal surface of each anchor molar.

**hot-cathode t.,** a vacuum tube in which the cathode is electrically heated to incandescence and in which the stream of electrons depends on the temperature of the cathode.

**Kobelt's t's,** the remains of the tubules of the mesonephros in the paroöphoron.

**Levin t.,** a type of nasogastric tube.

**medullary t.,** neural t.

**Mett's (Mette's) t's,** small glass tubes filled with coagulated egg white for testing peptic activity; see also under *test.*

**Miescher's t.,** sarcocyst.

**Miller-Abbott t.,** a double-channel intestinal tube with an inflatable balloon at its distal end, for use in the treatment of obstruction of the small intestine; occasionally useful also as a diagnostic aid.

**nasogastric t.,** a tube of soft rubber or plastic inserted through a nostril and into the stomach, for instilling liquid foods or other substances, or for withdrawing gastric contents.

**nasotracheal t.,** an endotracheal tube that passes through the nose.

**nephrostomy t.,** a tube inserted through the abdominal wall into the pelvis of the kidney, for direct drainage of the urine.

**neural t.,** the neuroepithelial tube developed from the neural plate and forming the central nervous system of the embryo; called also *medullary t.* and *cerebromedullary t.*

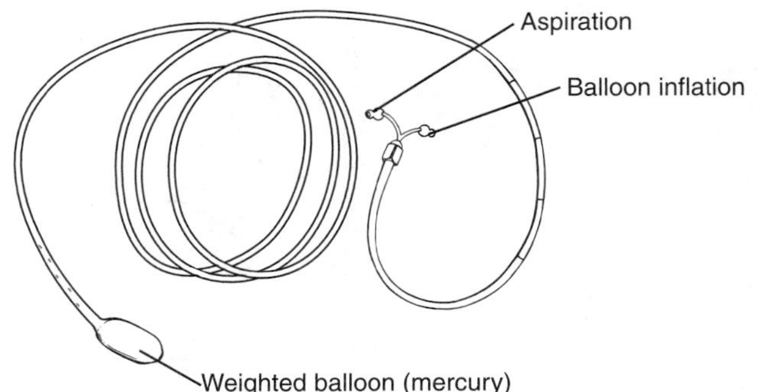


Miller-Abbott tube; the balloon is weighted with mercury after placement into the stomach, to aid its passage into the intestine.

**Olshevsky t.,** an x-ray tube constructed to use only the stronger rays which pass through the target and armoring the rest of the tube.
**orotracheal t.,** an endotracheal tube that passes through the mouth.
**otopharyngeal t.,** tuba auditiva.
**ovarian t's,** groups of cells that grow down and are cut off from the thickened surface layer of the ovary; they surround the primordial sex cells, which develop into primary oocytes, each with a follicular layer. Called also *Pflüger's t's.*
**Paul-Mixter t.,** a large-calibered, flanged drainage tube of glass used for temporary intestinal decompression.
**Pflüger's t's,** ovarian t's.
**pharyngotympanic t.,** tuba auditiva.
**photomultiplier t.,** a vacuum tube that converts electromagnetic radiation signals into electrical pulses, consisting of a light-sensitive surface that emits electrons when light is incident on it, the electrons then passing through successive stages with electron multiplication at each stage.
**polar t.,** a hollow, extensible, filamentous tubular organelle found coiled in the spore of microsporidan protozoa, through which the sarcoplasm is injected into the host's tissues. Called also *polar injecting filament.*
**pus t.,** pyosalpinx.
**Rainey's t.,** sarcocyst.
**Robertshaw t.,** an endobronchial tube that has various improvements over the Carlens tube such as lack of the positioning hook and availability for ventilation of either lung.
**Roida's t.,** a tube designed for the separation of motile from nonmotile bacteria; the motile organisms make their way through sand, glass-wool, and other obstructions.
**roll t.,** see *roll-tube culture,* under *culture.*
**Ruysch's t.,** a very small tubular opening on the nasal septum, just anterior and inferior to the nasopalatine foramen: it is a relic of the fetal Jacobson's organ.
**Ryle's t.,** a thin rubber tube with an olive-shaped end used in giving a test meal.
**Schachowa's spiral t's,** the tubuli renales.
**Sengstaken-Blakemore t.,** a multilumen tube used for the tamponade of bleeding esophageal varices: one lumen leads to a balloon which is inflated in the stomach, to retain the instrument in place, and to compress the vessels around the cardia; another leads to a long narrow balloon by which pressure is exerted against the varices in the wall of the esophagus; and a third provides for aspirating contents of the stomach.
**Shiner's t.,** a flexible plastic radiopaque tube for obtaining biopsy material from the jejunum under fluoroscopic control; the jejunal mucosa is drawn by suction into a small aperture in the knife cylinder head at the end of the tube, and a portion is excised.
**sputum t.,** a graduated capillary tube for containing sputum to be rotated in the centrifuge.
**stomach t.,** a tube for feeding or for irrigation of the stomach; the most common kind is the nasogastric tube. Called also *esophageal t.*
**T t.,** a self-retaining drainage tube in the shape of a T.
**tampon t.,** a piece of stout rubber tubing wound with iodoform gauze, used in plugging the rectum to control oozing and at the same time to allow the escape of gas.
**test t.,** a tube of thin glass closed at one end, used for various procedures in chemistry and for the growth of bacterial or viral cultures.
**thoracostomy t.,** a tube inserted through an opening in the chest wall, for application of suction to the pleural cavity; used to drain fluid or blood or to reexpand the lung in pneumothorax.
**tracheal t.,** endotracheal t.

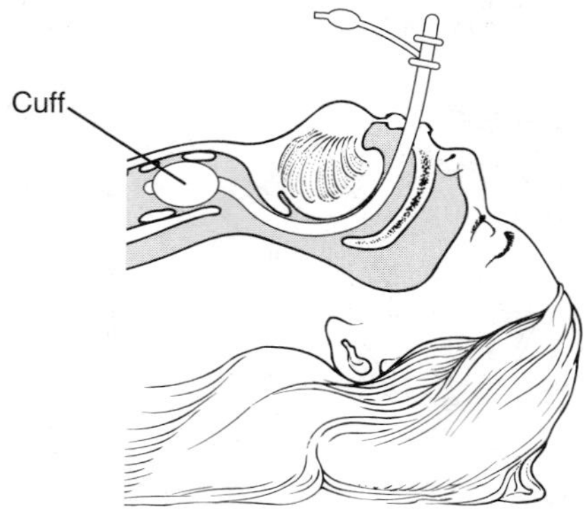


Orotracheal tube.

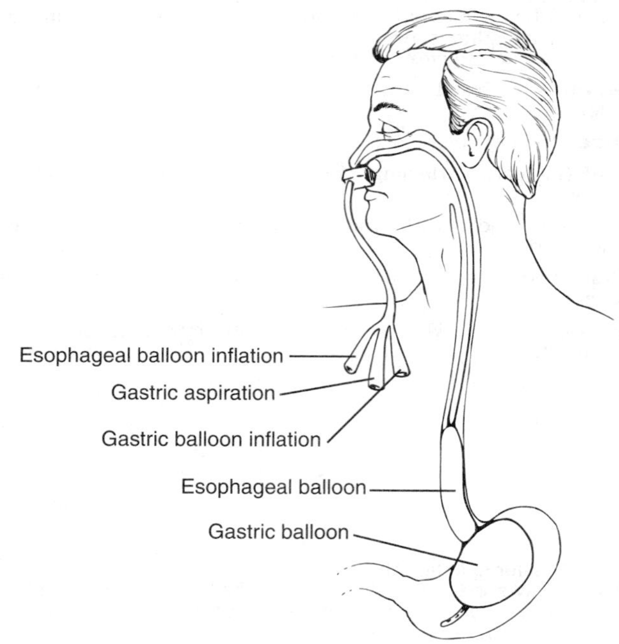


Sengstaken-Blakemore tube for esophagogastric tamponade.

**tracheostomy t.,** a curved endotracheal tube inserted into the trachea through the opening made in tracheostomy.
**tympanostomy t.,** ventilation t.
**uterine t.,** tuba uterina.
**vacuum t.,** a glass tube from which the air has been exhausted to a high degree of vacuum.
**valve t.,** a vacuum tube used to rectify an alternating current.
**Veillon t.,** a piece of glass tubing with a rubber cork at one end and a plug of cotton at the other, used in bacterial culture work.
**ventilation t.,** a tube inserted after myringotomy in chronic cases of middle ear effusion, such as in secretory or mucoid otitis media; it provides ventilation and drainage for the middle ear during healing. Called also *tympanostomy t.*
**vertical t.,** an orthodontic attachment usually placed on the lingual surface of the anchor band to allow for the insertion of the lingual arch wire.
**Wangensteen t.,** a small nasogastric tube connected with a special suction apparatus to maintain gastric and duodenal decompression; called also *Wangensteen's apparatus.*
**Westergren t.,** a straight glass pipette 30 cm long and 2.5 mm in internal diameter, marked in millimeters from 0 to 200 and used in the Westergren method of determining the erythrocyte sedimentation rate.
**Wintrobe hematocrit t.,** a thick-walled glass tube with a uniform internal bore, a flat bottom, and millimeter calibrations from 0 to 105; used in the Wintrobe method of calculating hematocrit.
**x-ray t.,** a glass vacuum bulb containing two electrodes. Electrons are obtained either from gas in the tube or from a heated cathode. When suitable potential is applied, electrons travel at high velocity from cathode to anode, where they are suddenly arrested, giving rise to x-rays.

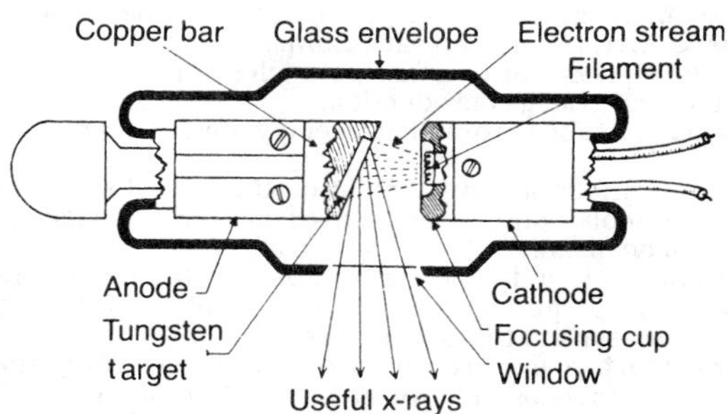


Standard stationary anode x-ray tube; diagram in longitudinal section.

**tu·bec·to·my** (too-bek'to-me) salpingectomy.

**tu·ber** (too'bər) pl. *tubers* or *tu'bera* [L.] 1. [TA] a general term in anatomical nomenclature for a swelling or protuberance. Called also *tuberosity.* 2. the essential lesion of tuberous sclerosis, presenting as a pale, firm, nodular phakomalike glial hamartomatous brain lesion that sometimes becomes calcified, which develops predominantly in the cerebral hemispheres, cerebellum, medulla, and spinal cord.

**t. calca'nei** [TA], tuberosity of calcaneus: the posteroinferior projection of the calcaneus that forms the heel.

**t. cine'reum** [TA], 1. gray tubercle: a layer of gray matter which is part of the hypothalamus; forming a part of the floor of the third ventricle, it lies in front of and between the corpora mammillaria and merges anteriorly into the infundibulum; called also *tuberculum cinereum.* 2. tuberculum trigeminale.

**t. coch'leae,** promontorium tympani.

**eustachian t.,** an eminence on the medial wall of the tympanum, below the vestibular window.

**external t. of Henle,** tuberculum mentale mandibulae.

**t. fronta'le** [TA], frontal tuber: one of the slight rounded prominences on the frontal bone on either side superior to the eyes, forming the most prominent portions of the forehead; called also *eminentia frontalis* [TA alternative] and *frontal eminence.*

**iliopubic t.,** eminentia iliopubica.

**t. ischia'dicum** [TA], **t. ischia'le,** tuberosity of ischium: a large elongated mass on the inferior part of the posterior margin of the body of the ischium, to which several muscles are attached. Called also *ischial tuberosity.*

**t. maxil'lae** [TA], **t. maxilla're, maxillary t.,** tuberosity of maxilla: a rounded eminence at the posteroinferior angle of the infratemporal surface of the maxilla; called also *maxillary eminence* or *tuberosity* and *eminentia maxillae* [TA alternative].

**mental t.,** tuberculum mentale mandibulae.

**omental t. of body of pancreas,** t. omentale corporis pancreatis.

**omental t. of liver,** t. omentale hepatis.

**t. omenta'le cor'poris pancre'atis** [TA], omental eminence of body of pancreas: a rounded prominence chiefly on the anterior surface of the neck of the pancreas.

**t. omenta'le he'patis** [TA], omental tuber of liver: the rounded prominence on the posteroinferior surface of the left lobe of the liver, just cranial to the lesser curvature of the stomach.

**papillary t. of liver,** processus papillaris hepatis.

**t. parieta'le** [TA], parietal tuber: the somewhat laterally bulging prominence just superior to the superior temporal line on the external surface of the parietal bone. Called also *eminentia parietalis* [TA alternative] and *parietal eminence.*

**t. ra'dii, t. of radius,** tuberositas radii.

**sciatic t.,** t. ischiadicum.

**t. ver'mis** [TA], tuber of vermis: the part of the vermis of the cerebellum between the folium vermis and the pyramids.

**t. zygoma'ticum,** tuberculum articulare ossis temporalis.

**tu·be·ra** (too'bə-rə) [L.] plural of *tuber.*

**tu·ber·cle** (too'bər-kəl) 1. the characteristic lesion of tuberculosis, a small round gray translucent granulomatous lesion, usually with central caseation; it is made up of modified macrophages resembling epithelial cells *(epithelioid cells),* surrounded by a rim of mononuclear cells, principally lymphocytes, and sometimes a center of giant multinucleate cells *(Langhans' giant cells).* Called also *gray t.* 2. a nodule, or small eminence, such as a rough, rounded eminence on a bone; called also *tuberculum.* See also *tuber, tuberositas,* and *tuberosity.* 3. dental t.

## Tubercle

For descriptions of specific anatomic structures not found here, see under *tuberculum* or under one of the other entries referred to in definition 2.

**acoustic t.,** auditory t.

**adductor t. of femur,** tuberculum adductorium femoris.

**anatomical t.,** tuberculosis verrucosa cutis.

**t. of anterior scalene muscle,** tuberculum musculi scaleni anterioris.

**articular t. of temporal bone,** tuberculum articulare ossis temporalis.

**t. of atlas, anterior,** tuberculum anterius atlantis.

**t. of atlas, posterior,** tuberculum posterius atlantis.

**auditory t.,** an eminence in the lateral recess of the fourth ventricle, formed by an extension of the vestibular area and the underlying dorsal nucleus and the cochlear part of the vestibulocochlear nerve; called also *acoustic t.*

**auricular t.,** tuberculum auriculare.

**Babès' t's,** see under *nodule.*

**brachial t. of humerus,** processus supracondylaris humeri.

**calcaneal t.,** tuberculum calcanei.

**Carabelli t.,** see under *cusp.*

**carotid t.,** tuberculum caroticum.

**caseous t.,** a tubercle having a central necrotic yellowish mass of cheesy material, such as occurs in tuberculosis.

**caudal t. of liver,** processus caudatus hepatis.

**cervical t's,** two small eminences on the femur, a *superior* one on the upper and anterior part of the neck at its junction with the greater trochanter, and an *inferior* one at the junction with the lesser trochanter.

**t. of cervical vertebrae, anterior,** tuberculum anterius vertebrarum cervicalium.

**t. of cervical vertebrae, posterior,** tuberculum posterius vertebrarum cervicalium.

**Chassaignac's t.,** tuberculum caroticum.

**condyloid t.,** an eminence on the condylar process of the mandible for attachment of the lateral ligament of the temporomandibular articulation.

**conglomerate t.,** a mass made up of an aggregation of many smaller tubercles or nodules.

**conoid t.,** tuberculum conoideum.

**corniculate t.,** tuberculum corniculatum.

**cuneate t., t. of cuneate nucleus,** tuberculum cuneatum.

**cuneiform t.,** tuberculum cuneiforme.

**Darwin's t., darwinian t.,** tuberculum auriculare.

**deltoid t.,** 1. a prominence on the clavicle for attachment of the deltoid muscle. 2. tuberositas deltoidea humeri.

**dental t.,** 1. tuberculum dentis. 2. cuspis dentis.

**dorsal t. of radius,** tuberculum dorsale radii.

**epiglottic t.,** tuberculum epiglotticum.

**Farre's t's,** masses beneath the capsule of the liver, felt on palpation in some cases of hepatocellular carcinoma.

**fibrous t.,** a tubercle that has undergone chronic inflammatory scarring.

**t. of fibula, posterior,** apex capitis fibulae.

**genial t.,** tuberculum mentale mandibulae.

**genital t.,** an eminence ventral to the cloaca in the early embryo, which is the primordium of the penis or the clitoris.

**Ghon t.,** see under *focus.*

**gracile t.,** tuberculum gracile.

**gray t.,** 1. tubercle (def. 1). 2. tuberculum trigeminale. 3. tuber cinereum.

**greater t. of calcaneus,** processus medialis tuberis calcanei.

**t. of greater multangular bone,** tuberculum ossis trapezii.

**hard t.,** a noncaseating tubercle, the characteristic lesion of sarcoidosis, composed of discrete aggregations of large, pale-staining, epithelioid cells intermingled with histiocytes, lymphocytes, and Langhans' giant cells, sometimes surrounded by a narrow band of lymphocytes; when necrosis is present, it is minimal. Similar lesions may be seen in association with foreign bodies in the tissues and in such conditions as tuberculoid leprosy, tuberculosis, cutaneous leishmaniasis, and deep fungal infections.

**t. of humerus,** capitulum humeri.

**t. of humerus, anterior, of Meckel,** tuberculum majus humeri.

**t. of humerus, anterior, of Weber,** tuberculum minus humeri.

**t. of humerus, external,** tuberculum majus humeri.

**t. of humerus, greater,** tuberculum majus humeri.

**t. of humerus, internal,** tuberculum minus humeri.

**t. of humerus, lesser,** tuberculum minus humeri.

**t. of humerus, posterior,** tuberculum majus humeri.

**iliac t.,** tuberculum iliacum.

**iliopectineal t., iliopubic t.,** eminentia iliopubica.

**inferior t. of Humphrey,** processus accessorius.

**infraglenoid t.,** tuberculum infraglenoidale.

**intercolumnar t.,** organum subfornicale.

**intercondylar t.,** eminentia intercondylaris.

**intercondylar t., lateral,** tuberculum intercondylare laterale.

**intercondylar t., medial,** tuberculum intercondylare mediale.

**intervenous t.,** tuberculum intervenosum.

**jugular t. of occipital bone,** tuberculum jugulare ossis occipitalis.
**labial t.,** tuberculum labii superioris.
**lacrimal t.,** papilla lacrimalis.
**lateral orbital t., lateral palpebral t.,** Whitnall's t.
**lateral t. of posterior process of talus,** tuberculum laterale processus posterioris tali.
**lesser t. of calcaneus,** processus lateralis tuberis calcanei.
**Lisfranc's t.,** tuberculum musculi scaleni anterioris.
**Lister's t.,** tuberculum dorsale radii.
**Lower's t.,** tuberculum intervenosum.
**Luschka's t.,** carina urethralis vaginae.
**mammillary t.,** processus mammillaris.
**mammillary t. of hypothalamus,** corpus mammillare.
**marginal t. of zygomatic bone,** tuberculum marginale ossis zygomatici.
**medial t. of posterior process of talus,** tuberculum mediale processus posterioris tali.
**mental t.,** tuberculum mentale mandibulae.
**mental t., external,** protuberantia mentalis.
**mental t. of mandible,** tuberculum mentale mandibulae.
**miliary t.,** one of the minute tubercles formed in organs in miliary tuberculosis.
**Montgomery's t's,** greatly enlarged Morgagni's tubercles observed on the surface of the areola of the mammary gland during pregnancy.
**Morgagni's t.,** 1. bulbus olfactorius. 2. one of the small nodules on the surface of the areola of the mammary gland produced by the superficially situated large sebaceous glands.
**Müller's t.,** a protrusion into the urogenital sinus caused by the caudally-growing paramesonephric ducts.
**muscular t. of atlas,** tuberculum anterius atlantis.
**t. of navicular bone,** tuberculum ossis scaphoidei.
**nuchal t.,** the prominence formed by the spinous process of the seventh cervical vertebra.
**t. of nucleus cuneatus,** tuberculum cuneatum.
**t. of nucleus gracilis,** tuberculum gracile.
**obturator t., anterior,** tuberculum obturatorium anterius.
**obturator t., posterior,** tuberculum obturatorium posterius.
**papillary t.,** processus papillaris hepatis.
**pharyngeal t.,** tuberculum pharyngeum.
**plantar t.,** tuberositas ossis metatarsalis primi.
**postglenoid t.,** a small conical tubercle projecting inferiorly from the zygomatic process of the temporal bone between the mandibular fossa and the external auditory meatus.
**pterygoid t.,** tuberositas pterygoidea mandibulae.
**pubic t. of pubic bone,** tuberculum pubicum ossis pubis.
**quadrate t. of femur,** tuberculum quadratum femoris.
**rabic t's,** Babès' nodes.
**t. of rib,** tuberculum costae.
**t. of Rolando,** tuberculum trigeminale.
**t. of root of zygoma,** tuberculum articulare ossis temporalis.
**t. of Santorini,** tuberculum corniculatum.
**scalene t.,** tuberculum musculi scaleni anterioris.
**t. of scaphoid bone,** tuberculum ossis scaphoidei.
**t. of sella turcica,** tuberculum sellae turcicae.
**superior t. of Henle,** tuberculum obturatorium posterius.
**superior t. of Humphrey,** processus mammillaris.
**supraglenoid t.,** tuberculum supraglenoidale.
**supratragic t.,** tuberculum supratragicum.
**thalamic t., anterior,** tuberculum anterius thalami.
**thalamic t., posterior,** pulvinar.
**thyroid t., inferior,** tuberculum thyroideum inferius.
**thyroid t., superior,** tuberculum thyroideum superius.
**t. of tibia,** eminentia intercondylaris.
**transverse t. of fourth tarsal bone,** tuberositas ossis cuboidei.
**t. of trapezium,** tuberculum ossis trapezii.
**trigeminal t.,** tuberculum trigeminale.
**trochlear t.,** spina trochlearis.
**t. of ulna,** tuberositas ulnae.
**t. of upper lip,** tuberculum labii superioris.
**t's of vertebra,** three elevations *(superior, inferior,* and *external)* upon the transverse process of the last thoracic vertebra, and represented on the lumbar vertebrae by more or less rudimentary structures.
**Whitnall's t.,** a small eminence on the internal aspect of the middle of the orbital surface of the zygomatic bone; called also *lateral orbital* or *palpebral t.*
**Wrisberg's t.,** tuberculum cuneiforme.
**zygomatic t., t. of zygomatic arch,** tuberculum articulare ossis temporalis.

**tu·ber·cu·la** (too-ber'ku-lə) [L.] plural of *tuberculum.*

**tu·ber·cu·lar** (too-ber'ku-lər) 1. pertaining to or resembling tubercles. 2. tuberculous.

**Tu·ber·cu·lar·i·a·ceae** (too-ber"ku-lar"ĭ-a'se-e) in some systems of classification, a form-family of Fungi Imperfecti of the form-order Moniliales; it includes the genus *Fusarium.*

**tu·ber·cu·late** (too-ber'ku-lāt") having tubercles; tuberculated.

**tu·ber·cu·lat·ed** (too-ber'ku-lāt"əd) tuberculate.

**tu·ber·cu·la·tion** (too-bər"ku-la'shən) the development of tubercles; becoming affected with tubercles.

**tu·ber·cu·lid** (too-ber'ku-lid) recurrent eruptions of the skin usually characterized by spontaneous involution. Some believe tuberculids to occur as local hyperergic reactions to mycobacteria or their antigens that are spread hematogenously to the skin from foci of active tuberculosis, while others believe that the lesions are unrelated to tuberculosis. Considered to comprise erythema induratum, lichen scrofulosorum, and papulonecrotic tuberculid, and sometimes lupus miliaris disseminatus faciei.
**micronodular t.,** granulomatous rosacea.
**papulonecrotic t.,** a grouped symmetric eruption of symptomless papules appearing in successive crops and healing spontaneously with superficially depressed scars, which occur chiefly on the extensor surface of the extremities in infants, children, and young adults. Called also *acne scrofulosorum* and *papulonecrotic tuberculosis.*
**rosacea-like t.,** granulomatous rosacea.

**tu·ber·cu·lin** (too-ber'ku-lin) [USP] [MeSH: Tuberculin] a sterile solution containing growth products of the tubercle bacillus *(Mycobacterium tuberculosis* or *M. bovis)* used in skin tests for tuberculosis (see *tuberculin test,* under *test*); also a commonly used antigen in laboratory immunology. Tuberculin was introduced in 1890 by Koch as a cure for tuberculosis, but proved to be an ineffective and dangerous treatment. Although many different tuberculin preparations have been devised, all are now obsolete except Old tuberculin (OT) and purified protein derivative (PPD) tuberculin. Dosages are expressed in tuberculin units (TU), which measure biologic activity as compared with a standard tuberculin preparation. Three dosages are used: first strength tuberculin (1 TU), used for young children or persons in whom extreme hypersensitivity is expected, intermediate strength tuberculin (5 TU), the standard test dose, and second strength tuberculin (250 TU), used for retests.
**Koch's t.,** Old t.
**Old t. (OT),** a heat-concentrated filtrate of tubercle bacillus culture grown on a special medium, used for tuberculin tests. Called also *Koch's t.*
**PPD t., purified protein derivative t.,** a soluble purified protein fraction precipitated by trichloracetic acid from filtrate of tubercle bacillus culture grown on a special medium, used for tuberculin tests.
**Seibert's t.,** purified protein derivative t.

**tu·ber·cu·li·tis** (too"bər-ku-li'tis) [*tubercle* + *-itis*] inflammation of or near a tubercle.

**tu·ber·cu·li·za·tion** (too-ber"ku-lĭ-za'shən) the formation of or conversion into tubercles.

**tu·ber·cu·lo·cele** (too-ber'ku-lo-sēl") [*tubercle* + *-cele*[1]] tuberculous disease of the testis.

**tu·ber·cu·lo·ci·dal** (too-ber"ku-lo-si'dəl) lethal to *Mycobacterium tuberculosis.*

**tu·ber·cu·lo·der·ma** (too-ber"ku-lo-der'mə) [*tuberculo-* + *derma*] 1. any tuberculous condition or disease of the skin. 2. a tuberculous lesion of the skin.

**tu·ber·cu·loid** (too-ber'ku-loid) 1. resembling a tubercle. 2. resembling tuberculosis.

**tu·ber·cu·lo·ma** (too-ber"ku-lo'mə) [MeSH: Tuberculoma] a tumor-like mass resulting from the aggregation or enlargement of caseous tubercles.
**t. en plaque,** a flat plaque on the surface of the frontoparietal cortex in tuberculous meningitis, producing the symptoms of brain tumor.

**tu·ber·cu·lo·sil·i·co·sis** (too-ber″ku-lo-sil″ĭ-ko′sis) silicotuberculosis.

**tu·ber·cu·lo·sis** (too-ber″ku-lo′sis) [MeSH: Tuberculosis] 1. any of the infectious diseases of humans or other animals caused by species of *Mycobacterium* and characterized by the formation of tubercles and caseous necrosis in the tissues. The usual causative species are *M. tuberculosis* and *M. bovis.* Tuberculosis varies widely in its manifestations and has a tendency to great chronicity. Any organ may be affected, although in humans the lung is the major seat of the disease (see *pulmonary t.*) and is the usual portal of entry into the body. See also *nontuberculous mycobacteria,* under *mycobacterium.* 2. pulmonary t.
**adult t.,** former name for *postprimary t.*
**aerogenic t.,** inhalation t.
**anthracotic t.,** tuberculosis associated with anthracosis.
**atypical t.,** mycobacteriosis.
**avian t.,** a variety of tuberculosis affecting various birds, including chickens and ducks, caused by *Mycobacterium avium,* and characterized by tubercles consisting principally of epithelioid cells. It may be communicated to other animals and humans.
**basal t.,** pulmonary tuberculosis situated in the lower part of the affected lung.
**t. of bones and joints,** tuberculosis involving the bones and joints, producing strumous arthritis, or white swelling, and cold abscess.
**bovine t.,** tuberculosis in cattle caused by infection with *Mycobacterium bovis;* it is transmissible to humans and other animals. Characteristics include tubercles or nodular lesions in lymph nodes and various organs, such as the udder, kidneys, uterus, and meninges.
**cerebral t.,** tuberculous meningitis.
**cestodic t.,** a disease simulating tuberculosis, but due to excessive infestation with cestode parasites.
**chicken t.,** avian tuberculosis occurring in chickens.
**childhood t.,** former name for *primary t.*
**t. colliquati′va, t. colliquati′va cu′tis,** 1. scrofuloderma. 2. tuberculous gumma.
**t. cu′tis,** tuberculosis of the skin, occurring as a result of exogenous (e.g., autoinoculation) or endogenous (e.g., by extension of an existing infection) infection or by lymphatic or hematogenous spread of infection, presenting in a large variety of clinical expressions, including lupus vulgaris, tuberculosis verrucosa cutis, scrofuloderma, tuberculous chancre, and papulonecrotic tuberculid.
**t. cu′tis indurati′va,** erythema induratum.
**t. cu′tis lichenoi′des,** lichen scrofulosorum.
**t. cu′tis milia′ris dissemina′ta,** t. miliaris disseminata.
**t. cu′tis orificia′lis,** tuberculous infection of the mucosal orifices and adjacent skin (nose, mouth and tongue, anus, vulva, penis), usually either by direct hematogenous or lymphatic extension of infection from an internal organ or by inoculation; characteristics include nodules that break down to form painful, shallow oval ulcers with undermined bluish edges. It generally occurs as a manifestation of advanced systemic disease in middle-aged and elderly males. Called also *orificial t.* and *t. ulcerosa.*
**disseminated t.,** 1. hematogenous or lymphohematogenous spread of tubercle bacilli from a primary focus of infection; its incidence is increased among immunocompromised patients. 2. miliary t.
**exudative t.,** the simplest form of pulmonary tuberculosis, frequently the earliest reaction to infection, in which the alveolar spaces and the smaller bronchi become filled with a cellular exudate consisting mainly of large mononuclear cells. See also *tuberculous pneumonia.*
**fowl t.,** avian tuberculosis occurring in fowl.
**genital t.,** tuberculosis of the genital tract, e.g., tuberculous endometritis.
**genitourinary t.,** tuberculosis involving the genitourinary tract, often the result of hemic dissemination of pulmonary tuberculosis.
**hematogenous t.,** infection with *Mycobacterium tuberculosis* carried through the bloodstream to other organs from the primary site of infection.
**hilus t.,** pulmonary tuberculosis involving the hilus of the lung.
**t. indurati′va,** erythema induratum.
**inhalation t.,** tuberculosis caused by aspiration of the tubercle bacilli into the lungs.
**t. of intestines,** a form that involves the intestines, with diarrhea, formation of spreading ulcers (especially of the lymphoid tissue), and sometimes eventual cicatricial stricture.
**laryngeal t., t. of larynx,** tuberculosis involving the larynx, producing ulceration of the vocal cords and elsewhere on the mucosa, and commonly attended by hoarseness, cough, pain on swallowing, and hemoptysis.
**t. lichenoi′des,** lichen scrofulosorum.
**t. of lungs,** pulmonary t.
**t. milia′ris dissemina′ta,** a severe form of acute miliary tuberculosis involving the skin, seen especially in children, occurring as a generalized cutaneous eruption of brownish, acuminate papules that become necrotic, and may form minute circular ulcers with red borders and pale granulating bases covered by a seropurulent exudate. It may occur in immunocompromised patients, or following an exanthematous disease or some other type of serious infection. Called also *t. cutis miliaris disseminata.*
**miliary t.,** a type that varies from a chronic, slowly progressive debilitating infection to an acute fulminating disease; it is caused by hematogenous or lymphohematogenous dissemination of infected caseous material into the bloodstream and seeding of many organs with millet seed–like tubercles. See also *t. miliaris disseminata.* Called also *disseminated t.*
**open t.,** 1. tuberculosis in which there are lesions from which the tubercle bacilli are being discharged out of the body. 2. pulmonary tuberculosis with cavitation.
**oral t.,** a rare condition usually occurring as a bloodborne complication of pulmonary tuberculosis, most often involving the gingivae and tongue, and characterized by the presence of small, crateriform, painless ulcers that bleed readily and are surrounded by edema or reddish nodules. See also *tuberculous gingivitis,* under *gingivitis.*
**orificial t.,** t. cutis orificialis.
**papulonecrotic t.,** see under *tuberculid.*
**postprimary t.,** pulmonary tuberculosis that is typical of a fresh infection but in which the person has actually had an earlier, probably subclinical, attack; it is distinguished by caseation and cavitation with healing that results in fibrosis. Called also *reactivation t., secondary t.,* and formerly *adult t.*
**primary t.,** pulmonary tuberculosis when a person is first infected; it is often asymptomatic, with simply a positive result on a tuberculin test. In children there may be exudation (see *exudative t.*), with the primary complex consisting of a parenchymal pulmonary lesion and a corresponding lymph node focus. Formerly called *childhood t.*
**primary inoculation t.,** the cutaneous reaction at the site of inoculation of tubercle bacilli in individuals with no previous exposure to *Mycobacterium tuberculosis,* associated with prominent involvement of regional lymph nodes, and manifested by a chancriform (tuberculous chancre, the most common manifestation), impetiginous, or ecthymatous lesion. Called also *primary inoculation complex* and *primary tuberculous complex.*
**productive t.,** pulmonary tuberculosis in which a new type of tissue appears at the site of infection (tuberculosis granulation tissue, consisting of epithelioid cells in concentric masses, lymphocytes, and often Langhans' giant cells).
**pulmonary t.,** infection of the lungs by *Mycobacterium tuberculosis.* The usual course of untreated disease is tuberculous pneumonia, formation of tuberculous granulation tissue, caseous necrosis, calcification, and cavity formation. It may spread to other lung segments via the bronchi, or to other organs via the blood or lymph vessels. Symptoms may include weight loss, lassitude and fatigue, night sweats, and wasting, with purulent sputum, hemoptysis, and chest pain. See also *primary t.* and *postprimary t.* Called also *t. of lungs.*
**reactivation t.,** postprimary t.
**reinfection t.,** a new infection with tuberculosis in a patient who was previously infected and cured.
**secondary t.,** postprimary t.
**t. of serous membranes,** tuberculosis involving the pleura, peritoneum, pericardium, and cerebral meninges, producing inflammation of those structures.
**t. of skin,** t. cutis.
**spinal t., t. of spine,** osteitis or caries of the vertebrae, usually occurring as a complication of tuberculosis of the lungs; it is marked by stiffness of the vertebral column, pain on motion, tenderness on pressure, prominence of certain of the vertebral spines, and occasionally abdominal pain, abscess formation, and paralysis. Called also *David's disease, Pott's disease, spondylitis tuberculosa,* and *tuberculous spondylitis.*
**surgical t.,** tuberculosis that can be treated by surgical means.
**tracheobronchial t.,** productive tuberculous involvement of the bronchi, characterized by wheezing, mucosal redness and edema, granulation tissue, and sometimes ulceration and bronchial stricture due to cicatrization.
**t. ulcero′sa,** t. cutis orificialis.
**t. verruco′sa cu′tis,** a tuberculous warty granulomatous lesion acquired accidentally by inoculation, from an infected source, of an individual having a certain degree of immunity or tuberculin sensitivity owing to previous infection or contact with *Mycobacterium* spp., and occurring often as a result of occupational inoculation (e.g., in pathologists, surgeons, postmortem attendants, or farmers) or as a consequence of autoinoculation or of superinfection from contact with tuberculous sputum. Called also *anatomical tubercle* or *wart, necrogenic, postmortem, prosector's,* or *tuberculous wart, verruca necrogenica,* and *warty t.*
**warty t.,** t. verrucosa cutis.

**tu·ber·cu·lo·stat·ic** (too-ber″ku-lo-stat′ik) inhibiting the growth of *Mycobacterium tuberculosis.*

**tu·ber·cu·lot·ic** (too-ber″ku-lot′ik) tuberculous.

**tu·ber·cu·lous** (too-ber′ku-ləs) 1. pertaining to or affected with tuberculosis: caused by *Mycobacterium tuberculosis.* Called also *tubercular* and *tuberculotic.*

**tu·ber·cu·lum** (too-ber'ku-ləm) pl. *tuber'cula* [L., dim. of *tuber*] [TA] a general term in anatomical nomenclature for a tubercle, nodule, or small eminence. See also *tubercle, tuber, tuberositas,* and *tuberosity.*

## Tuberculum

Descriptions of tubercles are given on TA terms, and include anglicized names of specific tubercles.

**t. adducto'rium fe'moris** [TA], adductor tubercle of femur: a small projection from the upper part of the medial epicondyle of the femur, to which the tendon of the adductor magnus muscle is attached.

**t. ante'rius atlan'tis** [TA], anterior tubercle of atlas: the conical eminence on the front of the anterior arch of the atlas.

**t. ante'rius tha'lami** [TA], anterior thalamic tubercle: a distinct enlargement on the dorsal surface of the most rostral part of the thalamus; it contains the anterior nuclear group.

**t. ante'rius ver'tebrae cervica'lis** [TA], anterior tubercle of cervical vertebra: a tubercle on the anterior part of the extremity of each transverse process, lying lateral to the posterior tubercle and at a slightly higher level in all except the sixth vertebra, to which are attached the scalenus anterior, longus capitis, and longus colli muscles.

**t. arthri'ticum,** a gouty concretion in a joint.

**t. articula're os'sis tempora'lis** [TA], articular tubercle of temporal bone: an enlargement of the inferior border of the zygomatic process of the temporal bone, forming the anterior boundary of the mandibular fossa and marking the termination of the anterior root of the zygomatic arch; it gives attachment to the lateral ligament of the temporomandibular articulation. Called also *tubercle of root of zygoma.*

**t. auri'culae, t. auricula're** [TA], auricular tubercle: a small projection sometimes found on the edge of the helix, and conjectured by some to be a relic of a simian ancestry. Called also *darwinian apex* or *tubercle* and *Darwin's tubercle.* Cf. *apex auriculare.*

**t. calca'nei** [TA], calcaneal tubercle: the eminence, often double, on the inferior surface of the calcaneus at the anterior extremity of the rough area for the attachment of the long plantar ligament.

**t. caro'ticum** [TA], carotid tubercle: the large anterior tubercle of the transverse process of the sixth cervical vertebra, which lies lateral to and at a slightly higher level than the posterior tubercle. Called also *Chassaignac's tubercle.*

**t. cine'reum,** 1. t. trigeminale. 2. tuber cinereum.

**t. conoi'deum** [TA], conoid tubercle: a prominent elevation on the inferior aspect of the lateral part of the clavicle, to which the conoid part of the coracoclavicular ligament is attached.

**t. cornicula'tum** [TA], **t. cornicula'tum [Santori'ni],** corniculate tubercle: a rounded eminence near the posterior end of the aryepiglottic fold, posterior to the cuneiform tubercle, corresponding to the corniculate cartilage. Called also *tubercle of Santorini.*

**t. coro'nae,** t. dentis.

**t. cos'tae** [TA], tubercle of rib: a small eminence on the posterior surface of a rib where the neck and body join; it protrudes inferiorly and posteriorly, and bears on its medial part a surface that articulates with the transverse process of the corresponding vertebra.

**t. cunea'tum** [TA], cuneate tubercle: an enlargement of the fasciculus cuneatus in the medulla oblongata, just lateral to the tuberculum gracile, produced by the underlying nucleus cuneatus.

**t. cuneifor'me** [TA], **t. cuneifor'me [Wrisber'gi],** cuneiform tubercle: a rounded eminence in the posterior portion of the aryepiglottic fold, anterior to the corniculate tubercle, corresponding to the cuneiform cartilage; called also *Wrisberg's tubercle.*

**t. denta'le, t. den'tis** [TA], dental tubercle: a small elevation of indiscriminate size on some portion of the crown of a tooth, produced by extra formation of enamel; called also *t. coronae.* See also *cuspis dentis.*

**t. doloro'sum,** a painful nodule or tubercle, such as one situated in the subcutaneous tissue near a joint, produced by enlargement of the end of a sensory nerve.

**t. dorsa'le ra'dii** [TA], dorsal tubercle of radius: an easily palpable prominence on the distal dorsal aspect of the radius; it is grooved by the tendon of the extensor pollicis longus muscle. Called also *Lister's tubercle.*

**t. epiglot'ticum** [TA], epiglottic tubercle: a posterior projection on the inferior part of the posterior surface of the epiglottic cartilage. Called also *cushion of epiglottis.*

**t. genia'le,** t. mentale mandibulae.

**t. gra'cile** [TA], gracile tubercle: an enlargement of the nucleus gracilis in the medulla oblongata, forming the lower lateral border of the posterior part of the fourth ventricle, produced by the underlying nucleus gracilis.

**t. ilia'cum** [TA], iliac tubercle: a prominence on the iliac crest about 5 cm behind the anterior superior iliac spine.

**t. im'par,** a small tubercle in the midline on the floor of the pharynx of the embryo, between the ends of the first and second pharyngeal arches (mandibular and hyoid arches), which is a primordium of the tongue. It forms no recognizable part of the adult tongue. Called also *median tongue bud.*

**t. infraglenoida'le** [TA], infraglenoid tubercle: a roughened area, just below the glenoid cavity of the scapula, that gives origin to the long head of the triceps muscle; called also *tuberositas infraglenoidalis* or *infraglenoid tuberosity.*

**t. intercondyla're latera'le** [TA], lateral intercondylar tubercle: a lateral spur projecting upward from the intercondylar eminence at the proximal end of the tibia; called also *t. intercondyloideum laterale.*

**t. intercondyla're media'le** [TA], medial intercondylar tubercle: a medial spur projecting upward from the intercondylar eminence at the proximal end of the tibia; called also *t. intercondyloideum mediale.*

**t. intercondyloi'deum,** eminentia intercondylaris.

**t. intercondyloi'deum latera'le,** t. intercondylare laterale.

**t. intercondyloi'deum media'le,** t. intercondylare mediale.

**t. interveno'sum** [TA], intervenous tubercle: a more or less distinct ridge across the inner surface of the right atrium between the openings of the venae cavae. Called also *Lower's tubercle.*

**t. jugula're os'sis occipita'lis** [TA], jugular tubercle of occipital bone: a smooth eminence overlying the hypoglossal canal on the superior surface of the lateral part of the occipital bone.

**t. la'bii superio'ris** [TA], tubercle of upper lip: the central prominence of the superior border between the skin and the mucous membrane of the upper lip, marking the distal termination of the philtrum. Called also *procheilon* and *labial tubercle.*

**t. latera'le proces'sus posterio'ris ta'li** [TA], the lateral tubercle of the posterior process of the talus.

**t. ma'jus hu'meri** [TA], greater tubercle of humerus: a large flattened prominence at the upper end of the lateral surface of the humerus, just lateral to the highest part of the anatomical neck, giving attachment to the infraspinatus, the supraspinatus, and the teres minor muscles.

**t. margina'le os'sis zygoma'tici** [TA], marginal tubercle of zygomatic bone: a process on the superior part of the temporal border of the zygomatic bone to which a strong slip of the temporal fascia is attached; called also *marginal process of zygomatic bone.*

**t. media'le proces'sus posterio'ris ta'li** [TA], the medial tubercle of the posterior process of the talus.

**t. menta'le mandi'bulae** [TA], mental tubercle of mandible: a more or less distinct prominence on the inferior border of either side of the mental protuberance of the mandible. Called also *genial* or *mental tubercle* and *t. geniale.*

**t. mi'nus hu'meri** [TA], lesser tubercle of humerus: a distinct prominence at the proximal end of the anterior surface of the humerus, just lateral to the anatomical neck; it gives insertion to the subscapular muscle.

**t. mus'culi scale'ni anterio'ris** [TA], tubercle of anterior scalene muscle: the tubercle on the cranial surface of the first rib for the insertion of the anterior scalene muscle; called also *t. scaleni* [*Lisfranci*].

**t. obturato'rium ante'rius** [TA], anterior obturator tubercle: a small spur sometimes present on the margin of the obturator foramen, projecting from the superior ramus of the pubis.

**t. obturato'rium poste'rius** [TA], posterior obturator tubercle: a small protuberance often present on the margin of the obturator foramen, projecting from the free edge of the acetabular fossa near the junction of the pubis and ischium.

**t. os'sis multan'guli majo'ris,** t. ossis trapezii.

**t. os'sis navicula'ris,** t. ossis scaphoidei.

**t. os'sis scaphoi'dei** [TA], tubercle of scaphoid bone: a projection on the volar surface of the scaphoid bone of the wrist, giving attachment to the transverse carpal ligament; called also *t. ossis navicularis.*

**t. os'sis trape'zii** [TA], tubercle of trapezium: a prominent ridge on the volar surface of the trapezium bone, forming the lateral margin of the groove that transmits the tendon of the flexor carpi radialis muscle; called also *t. ossis multanguli majoris.*

**t. pharyn'geum** [TA], pharyngeal tubercle: a midline eminence on the inferior surface of the basilar part of the occipital bone, for attachment of the pharynx (superior constrictor and pharyngeal raphe).

**t. poste'rius atlan'tis** [TA], posterior tubercle of atlas: a variable prominence on the posterior surface of the posterior arch of the atlas, which represents a spinous process and gives attachment to the rectus capitis posterior minor muscle.

**t. poste'rius ver'tebrae cervica'lis** [TA], posterior tubercle of cervical vertebra: a tubercle on the posterior part of the extremity of each transverse process of a cervical vertebra, lying lateral to the anterior tubercle and at a slightly lower level in all except the sixth vertebra, to which are attached the splenius, longissimus and iliocostalis cervicis, levator scapulae, and scalenus posterior and medius muscles.

**t. pu'bicum os'sis pu'bis** [TA], pubic tubercle of pubic bone: a prominent tubercle situated at the lateral end of the pubic crest and at the medial end of the superior border of the superior ramus of the pubic bone; it is the anterior medial terminal of the obturator crest and of the pecten of the pubic bone.

**t. quadra'tum fe'moris** [TA], quadrate tubercle of femur: an elevation just above the intertrochanteric crest that gives attachment to the quadratus femoris muscle.

**t. scale'ni [Lisfran'ci],** t. musculi scaleni anterioris.

**t. sel'lae tur'cicae** [TA], tubercle of sella turcica: a transverse ridge on the superior surface of the body of the sphenoid bone; it is anterior to the sella turcica, posterior to the sulcus chiasmatis, and between the anterior clinoid processes.

**t. sep'ti,** a tubercle or prominence on the superior anterior part of the nasal septum.

**t. supraglenoida'le** [TA], supraglenoid tubercle: a raised roughened area, just superior to the glenoid cavity of the scapula, that gives attachment to the long head of the biceps muscle of the arm; called also *tuberositas supraglenoidalis scapulae.*

**t. supratra'gicum** [TA], supratragic tubercle: a small tubercle sometimes seen on the pinna just superior to the tragus.

**t. thyroi'deum infe'rius** [TA], inferior thyroid tubercle: a more or less distinct tubercle at the inferior end of the oblique line of the thyroid cartilage.

**t. thyroi'deum supe'rius** [TA], superior thyroid tubercle: a more or less distinct tubercle at the superior extremity of the oblique line of the thyroid cartilage.

**t. trigemina'le** [TA], trigeminal tubercle: an elevation in the caudal part of the posterior surface of the medulla oblongata located between the fasciculus cuneatus and the roots of the accessory nerve, produced by the descending spinal tract of the trigeminal nerve and the caudal (inferior) cerebellar peduncle. Called also *t. cinereum, gray tubercle, tubercle of Rolando,* and *tuber cinereum.*

**tu·ber·o·sis** (too″bər-o'sis) a condition characterized by the development of nodules.

**tu·be·ros·i·tas** (too″bə-ros'ĭ-təs) pl. *tuberosita'tes* [L.] [TA] tuberosity: a general term in anatomical nomenclature for an elevation or protuberance. See also *tuber, tubercle,* and *tuberculum.*

**t. coracoi'dea,** coracoid tuberosity.

**t. cos'tae II,** t. musculi serrati anterioris.

**t. costa'lis clavi'culae,** impressio ligamenti costoclavicularis.

**t. deltoi'dea hu'meri** [TA], deltoid tuberosity of humerus: a rough, triangular elevation, about the middle of the anterolateral border of the shaft of the humerus, for attachment of the deltoid muscle.

**t. fe'moris exter'na,** epicondylus lateralis femoris.

**t. fe'moris inter'na,** epicondylus medialis femoris.

**t. glu'tea fe'moris** [TA], gluteal tuberosity of femur: an elevation on the upper part of the shaft of the femur for attachment of the gluteus maximus muscle.

**t. ili'aca** [TA], iliac tuberosity: a roughened area on the sacropelvic surface of the ilium, between the iliac crest and the auricular surface, for the attachment of muscles and ligaments.

**t. infraglenoida'lis,** tuberculum infraglenoidale.

**t. ligamen'ti coracoclavicula'ris** [TA], a protuberance on the inferior surface of the acromial extremity of the clavicle, giving attachment to the coracoclavicular ligament and including the surface for the acromial joint.

**t. massete'rica** [TA], masseteric tuberosity: an elongated, raised and roughened area on the lateral side of the angle of the mandible, for the insertion of tendinous bundles of the masseter muscles.

**t. mus'culi serra'ti anterio'ris** [TA], tuberosity for serratus anterior muscle: a roughened, raised area on the second rib that gives attachment to a slip of the anterior serratus muscle; called also *t. costae II.*

**t. os'sis cuboi'dei** [TA], tuberosity of cuboid bone: a transverse ridge on the lower surface of the cuboid bone over which the tendon of the peroneus longus muscle plays.

**t. os'sis metatarsa'lis pri'mi** [TA], tuberosity of first metatarsal bone: a blunt process projecting downward and laterally from the lower surface of the base of the first metatarsal bone, to which the tendon of the peroneus longus muscle is attached.

**t. os'sis metatarsa'lis quin'ti** [TA], tuberosity of fifth metatarsal bone: a large conical protuberance projecting backward and laterally from the base of the fifth metatarsal bone, to which the tendon of the peroneus brevis muscle is attached.

**t. os'sis navicula'ris** [TA], tuberosity of navicular bone: a rough protuberance on the navicular bone of the foot, projecting downward and medially, and giving attachment to the tendon of the posterior tibial muscle.

**t. os'sis sa'cri** [TA], sacral tuberosity: a roughened area on the pars lateralis of the sacrum, on the dorsal surface between the lateral sacral crest and the auricular surface, which gives attachment to the sacroiliac ligaments. Called also *t. sacralis.*

**t. patella'ris,** t. tibiae.

**t. phalan'gis dista'lis ma'nus** [TA], distal tuberosity of fingers: a roughened, raised bony mass on the palmar surface of the tip of a distal phalanx of the hand; called also *t. unguicularis manus.*

**t. phalan'gis dista'lis pe'dis** [TA], distal tuberosity of toes: a roughened, raised bony mass on the plantar surface of the tip of a distal phalanx of the foot; called also *t. unguicularis pedis.*

**t. pronato'ria** [TA], pronator tuberosity: the apex of the lateral curve of the radius, where there is a roughened ridge for the insertion of the pronator teres muscle.

**t. pterygoi'dea mandi'bulae** [TA], pterygoid tuberosity of mandible: a roughened area on the inner side of the angle of the mandible for the insertion of the internal pterygoid muscle; called also *pterygoid tubercle.*

**t. ra'dii** [TA], radial tuberosity: the tuberosity on the anterior inner surface of the neck of the radius, for the insertion of the tendon of the biceps muscle.

**t. sacra'lis,** t. ossis sacri.

**t. supraglenoida'lis sca'pulae,** tuberculum supraglenoidale.

**t. ti'biae** [TA], tuberosity of tibia: a longitudinally elongated, raised and roughened area on the anterior crest of the tibia, located just distal to the intercondylar eminence, and giving attachment to the patellar ligament.

**t. ti'biae exter'na,** condylus lateralis tibiae.

**t. ti'biae inter'na,** condylus medialis tibiae.

**t. ul'nae** [TA], tuberosity of ulna: a large roughened area on the volar surface of the ulna, located just distal to the coronoid process, and giving attachment to the brachialis muscle.

**t. unguicula'ris ma'nus,** t. phalangis distalis manus.

**t. unguicula'ris pe'dis,** t. phalangis distalis pedis.

**tu·be·ros·i·ta·tes** (too″bər-os'ĭ-tah'tēs) [L.] plural of *tuberositas.*

**tu·be·ros·i·ty** (too″bə-ros'ĭ-te) an elevation or protuberance; called also *tuber* and *tuberositas.*

**t. for anterior serratus muscle,** tuberositas musculi serrati anterioris.

**bicipital t.,** tuberositas radii.

**t. of calcaneus,** tuber calcanei.

**t. of clavicle,** impressio ligamenti costoclavicularis.

**coracoid t.,** the tuberculum conoideum and linea trapezoidea considered as a unit.

**costal t. of clavicle,** impressio ligamenti costoclavicularis.

**t. of cuboid bone,** tuberositas ossis cuboidei.

**deltoid t. of humerus,** tuberositas deltoidea humeri.

**distal t. of fingers,** tuberositas phalangis distalis manus.

**distal t. of toes,** tuberositas phalangis distalis pedis.

**t. of femur, external,** epicondylus lateralis femoris.

**t. of femur, internal,** epicondylus medialis femoris.

**t. of femur, lateral,** epicondylus lateralis femoris.

**t. of femur, medial,** epicondylus medialis femoris.

**t. of fifth metatarsal,** tuberositas metatarsalis quinti.

**t. of first carpal bone,** tuberculum ossis scaphoidei.

**t. of first metatarsal,** tuberositas metatarsalis primi.

**t. of fourth tarsal bone,** tuberositas ossis cuboidei.

**gluteal t. of femur,** tuberositas glutea femoris.

**greater t. of humerus,** tuberculum majus humeri.

**t. of greater multangular bone,** tuberculum ossis trapezii.

**t's of humerus,** the three elevations on the humerus; see *tuberculum*

*majus humeri, tuberculum minus humeri,* and *tuberositas deltoidea humeri.*
**iliac t.,** tuberositas iliaca.
**infraglenoid t.,** tuberculum infraglenoidale.
**ischial t., t. of ischium,** tuber ischiadicum.
**lesser t. of humerus,** tuberculum minus humeri.
**malar t.,** the lateral prominence of the zygomatic bone.
**masseteric t.,** tuberositas masseterica.
**t. of maxilla, maxillary t.,** tuber maxillae.
**t. of navicular bone,** tuberositas ossis navicularis.
**patellar t.,** tuberositas tibiae.
**pronator t.,** tuberositas pronatoria.
**pterygoid t. of mandible,** tuberositas pterygoidea mandibulae.
**t. of pubic bone,** tuberculum pubicum ossis pubis.
**pyramidal t. of palatine bone,** processus pyramidalis ossis palatini.
**radial t., t of radius,** tuberositas radii.
**sacral t.,** tuberositas sacralis.
**t. of scaphoid bone,** 1. tuberculum ossis scaphoidei. 2. tuberositas ossis navicularis.
**scapular t. of Henle,** processus coracoideus scapulae.
**t. of second rib, t. for serratus anterior muscle,** tuberositas musculi serrati anterioris.
**supraglenoid t.,** tuberculum supraglenoidale.
**t. of tibia,** tuberositas tibiae.
**t. of tibia, external,** condylus lateralis tibiae.
**t. of tibia, internal,** condylus medialis tibiae.
**t. of trapezium,** tuberculum ossis trapezii.
**t. of ulna,** tuberositas ulnae.
**ungual t., unguicular t.,** see *tuberositas phalangis distalis manus* and *tuberositas phalangis distalis pedis.*

**tu·ber·ous** (too′bər-əs) covered with tubers; called also *tubiferous.*

**tu·bi** (too′bi) [L.] genitive and plural of *tubus.*

**Tu·bif·era** (too-bif′ər-ə) *Eristalis.*

**tu·bif·er·ous** (too-bif′ər-əs) tuberous.

**tubo-** [L. *tubus* pipe, tube] a combining form denoting relationship to a tube.

**tu·bo·ab·dom·i·nal** (too″bo-ab-dom′ĭ-nəl) pertaining to the oviduct and the abdomen.

**tu·bo·ad·nexo·pexy** (too″bo-ad-nek′so-pek″se) the operation of suturing the uterine adnexa in a fixed position.

**tu·bo·cu·ra·rine** (too″bo-ku-rah′rin) [MeSH: Tubocurarine] an alkaloid isolated from the bark and stems of *Chondodendron tomentosum* R. & P. (Menispermaceae); it is the active principle of curare (q.v.).
**t. chloride** [USP], a neuromuscular blocking agent administered intravenously to relax skeletal muscles in surgery, tetanus, and shock therapy, and may be used for diagnosis of myasthenia gravis in certain cases.
**dimethyl t. iodide,** metocurine iodide.

**tu·bo·lig·a·men·tous** (too″bo-lig″ə-men′təs) pertaining to a uterine tube and a broad ligament.

**tu·bo·ovar·i·an** (too″bo-o-var′e-ən) of or pertaining to a uterine tube and ovary. Called also *ovariotubal.*

**tu·bo·ovar·i·ot·o·my** (too″bo-o-var″e-ot′ə-me) salpingo-oophorectomy.

**tu·bo·ova·ri·tis** (too″bo-o″və-ri′tis) salpingo-oophoritis.

**tu·bo·peri·to·ne·al** (too″bo-per″ĭ-to-ne′əl) pertaining to a uterine tube and the peritoneum.

**tu·bo·plas·ty** (too′bo-plas″te) plastic repair of a tube, such as the uterine tube or the auditory tube; see also *salpingoplasty.*
**eustachian t.,** plastic repair of the eustachian tube.
**transcervical balloon t.,** recanalization of an obstructed fallopian tube by inflation of a balloon catheter introduced through the cervix under fluoroscopic guidance.

**tu·bor·rhea** (too″bo-re′ə) [*tubo-* + *-rrhea*] a fluid discharge from the auditory tube.

**tu·bo·tor·sion** (too″bo-tor′shən) a twisting of a tube, especially of the auditory tube.

**tu·bo·tym·pa·nal** (too″bo-tim′pə-nəl) tubotympanic.

**tu·bo·tym·pan·ic** (too″bo-tim-pan′ik) pertaining to the auditory tube and tympanic cavity.

**tu·bo·tym·pa·num** (too″bo-tim′pə-nəm) the auditory tube and tympanic cavity considered together.

**tu·bo·uter·ine** (too″bo-u′tər-īn) pertaining to a uterine tube and the uterus.

**tu·bo·vag·i·nal** (too″bo-vaj′ĭ-nəl) pertaining to a uterine tube and the vagina.

**tu·bu·lar** (too′bu-lər) [L. *tubularis*] shaped like a tube; of or pertaining to a tubule.

**tu·bule** (too′būl) a small tube; called also *tubulus.*
**Albarrán's t's,** small branching tubules in the cervical part of the prostate gland.
**arcuate renal t.,** tubulus renalis arcuatus.
**attenuated t.,** thin tubule.
**Bellini's t.,** ductus papillaris.
**biliferous t.,** any small channel conveying bile.
**caroticotympanic t's,** canaliculi caroticotympanici.
**collecting t.,** a channel through which fluids pass from the secreting cells; see *tubulus renalis colligens,* under *tubulus.*
**connecting t.,** tubulus renalis arcuatus.
**convoluted t.,** a channel that follows a tortuous course; see *tubulus contortus distalis, tubulus contortus proximalis,* and *tubuli seminiferi contorti,* under *tubulus.*
**convoluted t., distal,** tubulus contortus distalis.
**convoluted t., proximal,** tubulus contortus proximalis.
**cortical collecting t.,** the more proximal parts of the renal tubule, which lie within the cortex.
**dental t's, dentinal t's,** canaliculi dentales.
**discharging t's,** channels by which a fluid is discharged from the substance of the gland or organ in which it is secreted, such as tubuli renales recti.
**Ferrein's t's,** the portions of the renal tubules making up the pars radiata of the lobules of the renal cortex.
**galactophorous t's,** ductus lactiferi.
**Henle's t.,** ansa nephroni.
**junctional t.,** tubulus renalis arcuatus.
**Kobelt's t's,** 1. the outer series of tubules in the epoophoron. 2. a similar series of tubules in the paradidymis of the male.
**lactiferous t's,** ductus lactiferi.
**malpighian t.,** one of the tubular or hairlike excretory organs arising from the midgut-hindgut junction of many arthropods; two to several hundred such tubules may be present.
**medullary collecting t.,** the distal part of the renal tubule, including the loop of Henle, lying within the medulla.
**mesonephric t's,** the tubules constituting the mesonephros, or temporary kidney of amniotes.
**metanephric t's,** the tubules comprising the permanent kidney of amniotes.
**Miescher's t.,** sarcocyst.
**paraurethral t's,** ductus paraurethrales.
**pronephric t's,** the tubules constituting the primordial kidney of vertebrates; they are rudimentary in amniotes.
**Rainey's t.,** sarcocyst.
**renal t's,** tubuli renales.
**renal collecting t.,** tubulus renalis colligens.
**segmental t's,** the tubules of the mesonephros.
**seminiferous t's,** channels in the testis in which the spermatozoa develop and through which they leave the gland; see *tubuli seminiferi contorti* and *tubuli seminiferi recti.*
**seminiferous t's, convoluted,** tubuli seminiferi contorti.
**seminiferous t's, straight,** tubuli seminiferi recti.
**Skene's t's,** ductus para-urethrales urethrae femininae.
**spiral t.,** convoluted t.
**straight t.,** a channel that follows a comparatively straight course; see *tubulus rectus distalis, tubulus rectus proximalis,* and *tubuli seminiferi recti,* under *tubulus.*
**straight t., distal,** tubulus rectus distalis.
**straight t., proximal,** tubulus rectus proximalis.
**straight collecting t.,** tubulus colligens rectus.
**subtracheal t.,** ductus thyroglossalis.
**T t's,** the transverse intracellular tubules invaginating from the cell membrane and surrounding the myofibrils of the T system of skeletal and cardiac muscle, serving as a pathway for the spread of electrical excitation within a muscle cell, enabling the nearly simultaneous activation of all myofibrils; in skeletal muscle, a T tubule is the intermediate element of a triad of tubular structures, the other elements being a pair of terminal cisterns. See also *T system,* under *system, terminal cistern,* under *cistern,* and *triad of skeletal muscle.*
**thin t.,** part of the renal tubule where the walls are especially thin, extending from the proximal straight tubule to the distal straight tubule; this concept is now considered outdated. Called also *tubulus attenuatus.*
**tracheal t.,** trachea (def. 2).
**transverse t.,** T t.
**uriniferous t., uriniparous t.,** tubulus renalis.
**vertical t's,** the inner set of tubules in the epoophoron.

**tu·bu·li** (too′bu-li) [L.] plural of *tubulus.*

**tu·bu·lin** (too′bu-lin) [MeSH: Tubulin] the constituent protein of microtubules; thought to be involved in phagocyte motility.

**tu·bu·li·tis** (too″bu-li′tis) inflammation of a renal tubule.

**Tu·bu·li·na** (too″bu-li′nə) [L. *tubulus,* dim. of *tubus* tube] [MeSH: Tubulina] a suborder of ameboid protozoa (order Amoebida, subclass Gymnamoebia) having a branched or unbranched cylindrical body. Representative genera include *Amoeba* and *Entamoeba.*

**tu·bu·li·za·tion** (too″bu-lĭ-za′shən) a method of treating injured nerves by isolating the nerve stump in an absorbable cylinder, which serves as a guide for new growth.

**tu·bu·lo·ac·i·nar** (too″bu-lo-as′ĭ-nər) composed of tubular acini, as a tubuloacinar gland.

**tu·bu·lo·cyst** (too′bu-lo-sist) any cystic dilatation of a vestigial canal or functionless duct.

**tu·bu·lo·in·ter·sti·tial** (too″bu-lo-in″tər-stĭ′shəl) pertaining to the renal tubules and interstitial tissues.

**tu·bu·lop·a·thy** (too″bu-lop′ə-the) any disease of the kidney tubules.

**tu·bu·lo·rac·e·mose** (too″bu-lo-ras′ə-mōs) both tubular and racemose.

**tu·bu·lor·rhex·is** (too″bu-lo-rek′sis) [*tubule* + *-rrhexis*] disruption of continuity of kidney tubules, the basement membrane being suddenly interrupted, or disintegrated into fibrils.

**tu·bu·lo·sac·cu·lar** (too″bu-lo-sak′u-lər) both tubular and saccular.

**tu·bu·lous** (too′bu-ləs) containing tubules.

**tu·bu·lo·ves·icle** (too″bu-lo-ves′ĭ-kəl) a membranous inclusion of nonsecreting parietal cell cytoplasm that contains the hydrogen ion pump. Upon stimulation of acid secretion, the tubulovesicles coalesce to form canaliculi with elongated microvilli, which have the greater surface area conducive to rapid secretion.

**tu·bu·lo·ve·sic·u·lar** (too″bu-lo-və-sik′u-lər) composed of small tubes and sacs; used particularly to describe cytoplasmic membranes of the resting state parietal cell.

**tu·bu·lus** (too′bu-ləs) pl. *tu′buli* [L., dim. of *tubus*] [TA] a general term in anatomical nomenclature for such a tubule or small tube.
**t. attenua′tus,** thin tubule.
**t. bili′ferus,** a channel for conveying bile; see *ductus cysticus.*
**t. col′ligens rec′tus,** straight collecting tubule: the lower straight part of the renal collecting tubule, extending from the arcuate renal tubule to the papillary duct.
**t. contor′tus dista′lis,** distal convoluted tubule: a distal, convoluted part of the ascending limb of the renal tubule, extending from the distal straight tubule to the junctional (connecting) tubule.
**t. contor′tus proxima′lis,** proximal convoluted tubule: the most proximal part of the renal tubule, extending from the glomerular capsule to the proximal straight tubule.
**t. rec′tus dista′lis,** distal straight tubule: part of the renal tubule primarily on the ascending limb, extending from the thin tubule to the distal convoluted tubule. Called also *thick ascending limb.*
**t. rec′tus proxima′lis,** proximal straight tubule: part of the descending limb of the renal tubule, extending from the proximal convoluted tubule to the thin tubule. Called also *pars recta tubuli renalis.*
**t. rena′lis,** renal tubule: one of the minute, reabsorptive, secretory, and collecting canals, made up of basement membrane lined with epithelium, that form the substance of the kidneys. See also *nephron.* See Plate 22.
**t. rena′lis arcua′tus,** arcuate renal tubule: a short, curved part of the distal end of the renal tubule, extending from the distal convoluted tubule to the straight collecting tubule. Called also *connecting tubule* or *junctional tubule.*
**t. rena′lis col′ligens,** renal collecting tubule: the arcuate renal tubule, straight collecting tubule, and papillary duct considered together. Called also *collecting duct.*
**tu′buli semini′feri contor′ti** [TA], convoluted seminiferous tubules: the numerous delicate, contorted canals within each lobule of the testis; its epithelial lining contains Sertoli's cells and germ cells.

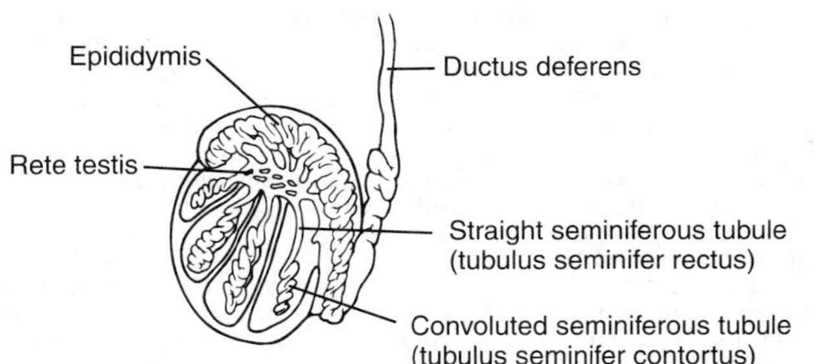


**tu′buli semini′feri rec′ti** [TA], straight seminiferous tubules: the straight terminal portion of the seminiferous tubules; they join to form the rete testis.

**tu·bus** (too′bəs) gen. and pl. *tu′bi* [L.] tube; used as a general term in anatomical nomenclature.
**t. digesto′rius,** digestive tract.

**Tuerck** see *Türck.*

**Tuf·fier's test** (too-fe-āz′) [Marin Théodore *Tuffier,* French surgeon, 1857–1929] see under *test.*

**tuft** (tuft) a small clump or cluster.
**enamel t's,** bunches of tuftlike structures extending from the dentinoenamel junction through about one third of the thickness of the enamel, representing defects in mineralization; confined to the innermost 20–30 per cent of the enamel.
**hair t's,** groups of several hairs from one follicle, consisting of one main hair and some secondary hairs.
**synovial t's,** villi synoviales.

**tuft·sin** (tuft′sin) [*Tufts* University + *-in*] [MeSH: Tuftsin] a tetrapeptide (Thr-Lys-Pro-Arg) cleaved from IgG that stimulates phagocytosis by neutrophils. It is produced primarily in the spleen; hereditary tuftsin deficiency and tuftsin deficiency following splenectomy result in increased susceptibility to certain infections.

**tug·ging** (tug′ing) a pulling sensation.
**tracheal t.,** a pulling sensation in the trachea, due to aneurysm of the arch of the aorta; it is most apparent when the head is extended and a finger is placed on the thyroid cartilage. Called also *Oliver's* or *Porter's sign.*

**tu·la·re·mia** (too″lə-re′me-ə) [*Tulare* County, California, where it was first described] [MeSH: Tularemia] an infectious, plaguelike, zoonotic disease caused by infection with the bacillus *Francisella tularensis.* It is found primarily in rodents but also affects humans and many other animals; rabbits, squirrels, and muskrats are the primary source of infection. It is transmitted by the bites of deer flies, fleas, and ticks; by contact with contaminated animals or their products; by inhalation of aerosolized *F. tularensis;* and by ingestion of contaminated food or water. In addition to a marked reaction at the portal of entry of the pathogen, which has led to classification of the various forms of tularemia, most cases are characterized by abrupt onset of fever, chills, weakness, headache, backache, and malaise. Called also *deer fly fever, Francis' disease, Pahvant Valley fever* or *plague, rabbit fever,* and in Japan *Ohara's disease.*
**gastrointestinal t.,** a rare form of tularemia due to ingestion of large numbers of *Francisella tularensis,* characterized by cramping abdominal pain, acute watery diarrhea, fever, and, infrequently, superficial ulcerations of the colon resulting in bloody diarrhea or acute hemorrhage with minimal diarrhea.
**glandular t.,** tularemia identical to the oculoglandular type except that there is no visible primary lesion.
**oculoglandular t.,** a form of tularemia in which the primary site of entry of *Francisella tularensis* is the conjunctival sac, characterized by conjunctivitis, itching, lacrimation, pain, granulomatous corneal lesions that if untreated may result in perforation of the cornea and optic atrophy, and enlargement of preauricular lymph nodes.
**oropharyngeal t.,** typhoidal tularemia, usually seen in children, associated with ulcerative pharyngitis with pustular lesions on the tonsils, with or without membrane formation, cervical lymph node involvement resembling the bull neck of diphtheria, and dysphagia.
**pulmonary t., pulmonic t.,** tularemia with lung involvement, caused by lymphohematogenous spread of a primary infection or by inhalation of aerosolized *Francisella tularensis,* and characterized by nonproductive cough, headache, fever, malaise, substernal pain, and bloody, mucoid sputum. Called also *tularemic pneumonia.*
**typhoidal t.,** the most serious form of tularemia, which may be caused by swallowing an inoculum of the pathogen or by inhaling the organisms while chewing contaminated food, characterized by abdominal pain, high fever, and other symptoms similar to those of typhoid; oropharyngeal involvement and pneumonia and pleural effusion may be associated in many cases.
**ulceroglandular t.,** the most common form of human tularemia, beginning as a painful, swollen, erythematous papule at the point of inoculation with *Francisella tularensis* that becomes pustular and then ruptures to form a shallow ulcer; mild, generalized lymphadenopathy, hepatosplenomegaly, and pneumonia may be associated.

**tulle gras** (tool-grah′) [Fr. "fatty tulle"] a close-meshed net cut into squares and impregnated with soft paraffin, Peruvian balsam, and vegetable oil; used in treating raw surfaces.

**Tul·lio's phenomenon** (too′le-ōz) [Pietro *Tullio,* Italian physician, 20th century] see under *phenomenon.*

**Tul·pi·us' valve** (tul′pe-əs) [Nicolas *Tulpius* (Nikolaas *Tulp*), Dutch physician, 1593–1674] valva ileocecalis.

**tu·me·fa·cient** (too″mə-fa′shənt) [L. *tumefaciens*] tending to cause or causing a swelling.

**tu·me·fac·tion** (too″mə-fak′shən) [L. *tumefactio*] swelling (def. 1).

**tu·men·tia** (too-men′shə) [L.] swelling (def. 1).

**tu·mes·cence** (too-mes′əns) swelling (def. 1).
**nocturnal penile t.**, tumescence or erection of the penis when sleeping at night; it may be assessed in an impotent individual to determine whether the impotence is psychogenic or organic.

**tu·meur** (too-moor′) [Fr.] tumor.
**t. perlée** (per-la′) [Fr. "pearly tumor"], cholesteatoma.
**t. pileuse** (pe-looz′) [Fr. "hairy tumor"], trichobezoar.

**tu·mid** (too′mid) [L. *tumidus*] swollen or edematous.

**tu·mor** (too′mər) [L., from *tumere* to swell] [MeSH: Neoplasms] 1. swelling, one of the cardinal signs of inflammation; morbid enlargement. 2. a new growth of tissue in which the multiplication of cells is uncontrolled and progressive; called also *neoplasm*.

## Tumor

See also under specific types of tumors, e.g., *angioma, sarcoma*.

**Abrikosov's (Abrikossoff's) t.**, granular cell t.
**acinar cell t., acinic cell t.**, see under *carcinoma*.
**acoustic nerve t.**, acoustic neuroma.
**acute splenic t.**, a swelling resulting from acute splenitis.
**adenoid t.**, adenoma.
**adenomatoid t.**, a small, circumscribed, benign tumor of the genital tract (the epididymis, tunic of testis, uterine corpus, or uterine tube), composed of small glandlike spaces lined by flattened or cuboidal mesothelium-like cells.
**adenomatoid odontogenic t.**, a benign odontogenic tumor characterized by ductlike or glandlike arrangements of columnar epithelial cells; it usually occurs in the anterior jaw region in children and young adults. Formerly called *adenoameloblastoma*.
**adipose t.**, lipoma.
**adrenal rest t.**, 1. a rare neoplasm of the testis of young boys, consisting of adrenal tissue; it may be secondary to hyperplasia of an adrenal gland. 2. lipoid cell t. of ovary.
**aldosterone-producing t., aldosterone-secreting t.**, aldosteronoma.
**alveolar cell t.**, bronchioloalveolar carcinoma.
**ameloblastic adenomatoid t.**, adenomatoid odontogenic t.
**aniline t.**, see under *carcinoma*.
**Askin's t.**, a malignant small-cell tumor of soft tissue in the thoracopulmonary region in children, one of the peripheral neuroectodermal tumors.
**benign t.**, one that lacks the properties of invasion and metastasis and that is usually surrounded by a fibrous capsule; its cells also show a lesser degree of anaplasia than those of malignant tumors. Called also *innocent t.*
**benign epithelial odontogenic t.**, squamous odontogenic t.
**Brenner t.**, a rare, usually benign, tumor of the ovary whose structure consists of groups of epithelial cells lying in a fibrous connecting tissue stroma. When small the tumor may be solid, resembling fibroma; when large it may resemble a cystadenoma with nodular masses of the tumor (Brenner nodules) in the cyst wall. Called by Brenner *oophoroma folliculare*.
**bronchial carcinoid t.**, carcinoid t. of bronchus.
**Brooke's t.**, multiple trichoepithelioma; see *trichoepithelioma*.
**brown t.**, a giant-cell granuloma produced in and replacing bone, occurring in osteitis fibrosa cystica and due to hyperparathyroidism.
**Burkitt's t.**, see under *lymphoma*.
**Buschke-Löwenstein t.**, a destructive tumor clinically resembling squamous cell carcinoma but microscopically representing a form of condyloma acuminatum, usually occurring on the uncircumcised penis, but also seen elsewhere in the anogenital area such as about the anus and vulva. It presents as a large verrucous to fungating, cauliflower-like mass that erodes the involved skin and progresses to penetrate and destroy the deeper tissues. Called also *giant condyloma* and *verrucous carcinoma*.
**calcifying epithelial odontogenic t.**, a rare benign odontogenic neoplasm of the jaw, particularly the mandible, believed to arise from the epithelial elements of the enamel organ. It is slow growing but potentially invasive and is characterized histologically by sheets of polyhedral epithelial cells with occasional Liesegang rings. Called also *Pindborg t.*
**carcinoid t.**, carcinoid.
**carcinoid t. of bronchus**, a highly vascular tumor of the bronchus similar to carcinoid (argentaffinoma) of the gastrointestinal tract; it may be invasive and malignant. Called also *argentaffinoma of bronchus, bronchial carcinoid, bronchial carcinoid t.*, and *carcinoid adenoma of bronchus*.
**carcinoma ex mixed t.**, carcinoma ex pleomorphic adenoma.
**carotid body t.**, a chemodectoma of the carotid body; a benign, encapsulated, firm round mass at the bifurcation of the common carotid artery, with nests of large polyhedral cells in alveolar or organoid arrangement; usually asymptomatic, but sometimes causing dizziness and nausea or vomiting. Called also *potato t.*
**cartilaginous t.**, a chondroma or an enchondroma.
**cavernous t.**, see under *hemangioma*.
**cellular t.**, a tumor made up chiefly of cells in a homogeneous stroma.
**chromaffin cell t.**, pheochromocytoma.
**Codman's t.**, chondroblastoma.
**collision t.**, an area of mixing of malignant cells from two distinct tumors (such as a carcinoma and a sarcoma) that have developed separately but near each other.
**colloid t.**, myxoma.
**connective-tissue t.**, any tumor developed from some structure of the connective tissue, such as a lipoma, fibroma, glioma, chondroma, or sarcoma.
**craniopharyngeal duct t.**, craniopharyngioma.
**cystic t.**, a tumor that contains cysts; specific types often have the prefixes *cyst-* or *cysto-*, such as *cystadenoma, cystocarcinoma,* and *cystosarcoma*. Called also *cystoma*.
**dermal duct t.**, a small, intradermal, papular, eccrine lesion occurring on the head and neck in older adults.
**dermoid t.**, dermoid cyst (def. 2).
**desmoid t.**, a fibromatous tumor arising in the musculoaponeurotic tissue, usually of the abdominal wall, and often closely resembling fibrosarcoma; desmoid tumors are not encapsulated, are locally invasive, and rarely metastasize.
**diarrheogenic t.**, vipoma.
**dumbbell t.**, hourglass t.
**embryonal t., embryoplastic t.**, embryoma.
**endodermal sinus t.**, yolk sac t.
**epidermoid t.**, see under *cyst*.
**erectile t.**, cavernous hemangioma.
**Ewing's t.**, see under *sarcoma*.
**false t.**, pseudotumor.
**fatty t.**, lipoma.
**fecal t.**, stercoroma.
**feminizing t.**, a functional tumor that produces feminization in boys and men or precocious sexual development in girls; common types are germinomas, tumors of the anterior pituitary, and tumors of the adrenal cortex. Cf. *virilizing t.*
**fibrocellular t.**, fibroma.
**fibrohistiocytic t.**, a tumor containing cells resembling fibroblasts and cells resembling histiocytes in varying proportions; often used to denote the most general meaning of benign or malignant fibrous histiocytoma.
**fibroid t.**, 1. fibroma. 2. leiomyoma.
**fibroplastic t.**, 1. fibroma. 2. fibrosarcoma.
**t. of follicular infundibulum**, a smooth papular lesion of the hair follicle occurring on the face and neck of older patients, characterized by plate-like proliferation of squamous cells that are connected at many points to the lower surface of the epidermis.
**functional t., functioning t.**, a hormone-secreting tumor in an endocrine gland; cf. *endocrine-active adenoma*.
**gelatinous t.**, myxoma.
**germ cell t.**, any of a group of tumors arising from primitive germ cells, usually of the testis or ovum; they range from benign to highly malignant. Types include germinoma, yolk sac or endodermal sinus tumor, teratoma, embryonal carcinoma, polyembryoma, gonadoblastoma, and some types of choriocarcinoma; many tumors are mixtures of types.
**giant cell t.**, a benign or malignant tumor containing giant cells; see under *carcinoma, granuloma,* and *sarcoma*.
**giant cell t., familial bilateral**, cherubism.
**giant cell t. of bone**, a bone tumor composed of cellular spindle cell stroma containing scattered multinucleated giant cells resembling osteoclasts; symptoms may include local pain and tenderness, functional disability, and, occasionally, pathologic fractures. The tumors remain benign or progress to frankly malignant lesions. See also *giant cell sarcoma*, under *sarcoma*. Called also *osteoclastoma*.
**giant cell t. of tendon sheath**, a benign tumor-like lesion of tendon sheath origin forming a small, yellow, discrete nodule, most commonly of the wrist and fingers, or ankle and toes; the tissue is laden with lipophages and contains multinucleated giant cells. It is sometimes

considered a variant or subtype of benign fibrous histiocytoma (q.v). Called also *benign synovioma* and *nodular tenosynovitis.*

**glomus t.,** 1. a benign but painful tumor involving a glomeriform arteriovenous anastomosis (glomus body), which may be found anywhere in the skin, most often on the distal part of a finger or toe, especially beneath the nail. It may also occur in the stomach or nasal cavity. Called also *glomangioma.* 2. chemodectoma.

**glomus jugulare t.,** a chemodectoma involving the tympanic body (glomus jugulare). It may cause symptoms in the ear (see *glomus tympanicum t.*) or in the mouth (hoarseness, dysphagia, aspiration, or tongue atrophy).

**glomus tympanicum t.,** a type of glomus jugulare tumor involving the glomus tympanicum adjacent to the promontory of the tympanic cavity. When large, the tumor may fill the tympanic cavity, causing tinnitus and conductive hearing loss.

**glomus vagale t.,** a chemodectoma of a glomus vagale. Those along the auricular branch of the nerve often cause vocal cord paralysis with subsequent tinnitus and deafness.

**gonadal stromal t.,** androblastoma (def. 1).

**granular cell t.,** a relatively common, usually benign neoplasm whose cells have a granular appearance under light microscopy; found throughout the body, but most commonly in the oral cavity, especially the tongue, and sometimes occurring as multiple tumors. Its histogenesis is uncertain but a Schwann cell derivation is favored. Originally named *granular cell myoblastoma* because of postulated muscle cell origin, which has now been disproven. Called also *Abrikosov's t.* and *granular cell schwannoma.* See also *congenital epulis,* under *epulis.*

**granulation t.,** a granuloma.

**granulosa t., granulosa cell t.,** an ovarian tumor originating in the cells of the primordial membrana granulosa; it may be associated with excessive production of estrin, inducing endometrial hyperplasia with menorrhagia. See also *granulosa-theca cell t.* and *granulosa cell carcinoma.*

**granulosa-theca cell t.,** an ovarian tumor predominantly composed of either granulosa cells (follicular cells) or theca cells, and often associated with excessive production of estrogen, with hyperplasia and carcinoma of the endometrium. When luteinized, i.e., having cells resembling those of the corpus luteum, it is known as luteoma.

**Grawitz's t.,** renal cell carcinoma.

**Gubler's t.,** a tumor on the back of the wrist, with paralysis of the extensors of the hand, in cases of lead poisoning.

**gummy t.,** gumma.

**heterologous t.,** one made up of tissue which differs from that in which it grows.

**heterotypic t.,** heterologous t.

**hilar cell t., hilum cell t.,** a rare benign neoplasm of the hilum of the ovary, histologically resembling Leydig cell tumor of the testis; it may cause virilization. Called also *Leydig cell t.*

**histioid t.,** one which is formed of a single tissue resembling that of the surrounding parts.

**homoiotypic t., homologous t.,** a tumor which resembles the surrounding parts in its structure.

**hourglass t.,** a spinal tumor made up of intradural and extradural masses joined by a narrow pedicle passing through an enlarged intervertebral foramen.

**Hürthle cell t.,** a new growth of the thyroid gland composed wholly or predominantly of large cells *(Hürthle* or *Askanazy cells)* that have abundant granular, eosinophilic cytoplasm. Such tumors are usually benign (Hürthle cell adenoma) but on occasion may be locally invasive or may metastasize (Hürthle cell carcinoma or malignant Hürthle cell tumor). Called also *oxyphil cell t.*

**innocent t.,** benign t.

**interstitial cell t.,** Leydig cell t. (def. 1).

**islet cell t.,** a tumor of the islets of Langerhans; many secrete excessive amounts of hormones. Types include *gastrinoma, glucagonoma, insulinoma, somatostatinoma,* and *VIPoma.* Called also *nesidioblastoma.*

**ivory-like t.,** osteoma durum.

**Jensen's t.,** see under *sarcoma.*

**juxtaglomerular t., juxtaglomerular cell t.,** a rare benign tumor of renal juxtaglomerular cells in young men, causing hyperreninemia. Called also *hemangiopericytoma of kidney.*

**Klatskin's t.,** hilar cholangiocarcinoma.

**Koenen's t.,** periungual fibroma.

**Krukenberg's t.,** a special type of carcinoma of the ovary, usually metastatic from cancer of the gastrointestinal tract, especially of the stomach. It is characterized by areas of mucoid degeneration and the presence of signet-ring–like cells. Called also *carcinoma mucocellulare.*

**Leydig cell t.,** 1. the most common nongerminal tumor of the testis, derived from the Leydig cells of the testis; such tumors are rarely malignant; called also *interstitial cell t.* 2. hilar cell t.

**t. lie'nis,** enlargement of the spleen less in degree than splenomegaly.

**Lindau's t.,** hemangioblastoma.

**lipoid cell t. of ovary,** a rare, usually benign, ovarian tumor composed of eosinophilic cells or cells with lipoid vacuoles, arising from ovarian cells or embryonic rest cells of the adrenals; it causes masculinization. Called also *adrenal rest t.*

**luteinized granulosa-theca cell t.,** luteoma.

**malignant t.,** one that has the properties of invasion and metastasis and that shows a greater degree of anaplasia than do benign tumors.

**march t.,** syndesmitis metatarsea.

**margaroid t.,** a cholesteatoma.

**mast cell t.,** mastocytoma.

**melanotic neuroectodermal t.,** a benign, rapidly growing, deeply pigmented tumor of the jaw and occasionally of other sites, consisting of an infiltrating mass of cells arranged in an alveolar pattern, and occurring almost exclusively in infants. Its source of origin is in dispute, the various theories giving rise to its several names. Called also *melanoameloblastoma, melanotic ameloblastoma, pigmented ameloblastoma, melanotic progonoma,* and *retinal anlage t.*

**Merkel cell t.,** see under *carcinoma.*

**mesodermal mixed t.,** müllerian mixed t.

**mixed t.,** a tumor composed of more than one type of neoplastic tissue, particularly a benign or malignant mixed tumor of the salivary glands.

**mixed t., benign,** pleomorphic adenoma.

**mixed t., malignant,** a type of malignant pleomorphic adenoma usually occurring in the salivary glands of older adults in one of two forms: in the first both epithelial and mesenchymal components are malignant and may metastasize *(carcinosarcoma)* and in the second a histologically benign appearance persists in both the primary tumor and metastatic foci. The term is sometimes used synonymously with *carcinoma ex pleomorphic adenoma* or with the more general term *malignant pleomorphic adenoma.*

**mixed t. of skin,** chondroid syringoma.

**mucoepidermoid t.,** see under *carcinoma.*

**mucous t.,** myxoma.

**müllerian mixed t.,** a malignant mixed tumor of the uterus containing both endometrial adenocarcinoma and sarcomatous cells that may be of either uterine or extrauterine origin.

**muscular t.,** myoma.

**Nélaton's t.,** a dermoid tumor of the wall of the abdomen.

**nerve sheath t.,** a tumor of the sheaf of a nerve, such as an acoustic nerve tumor or a schwannoma; called also *sheaf t.*

**neuroectodermal t. of infancy,** melanotic neuroectodermal t.

**neuroendocrine t., neuroendocrine cell t.,** any of a diverse group of tumors containing neurosecretory cells that cause endocrine dysfunction; most are carcinoids or carcinomas. They occur most often in the gastrointestinal tract, in bronchial and tracheal mucous membranes, and in teratoid ovarian tumors.

**neuroepithelial t.,** any of several closely related types of highly malignant tumors that develop from elements derived from the neural crest and are seen mainly in children. They may be found outside the central nervous system but resemble central nervous system tumors. Included are ependymoblastoma, medulloblastoma, medulloepithelioma, neuroblastoma, pinealoblastoma, and spongioblastoma. They compose the majority of the proposed new category, the *primitive neuroectodermal tumors.*

**nonfunctional t., nonfunctioning t.,** a tumor located in an endocrine gland but not secreting hormones; cf. *endocrine-inactive adenoma.*

**odontogenic t.,** a lesion derived from epithelial or mesenchymal elements, or both, that are associated with the development of the teeth; it occurs in the mandible or maxilla, or occasionally the gingiva.

**organoid t.,** teratoma.

**oxyphil cell t.,** 1. oncocytoma. 2. Hürthle cell t.

**Pancoast's t.,** pulmonary sulcus t.

**papillary t.,** papilloma.

**papillary cystic t. of pancreas,** a rare, low-grade tumor of endothelial origin, predominantly affecting young women beginning in adolescence, consisting of a well-circumcribed mass containing both solid and cystic elements; tumor cells are small, polygonal, and eosinophilic and form solid sheets or papillary projections.

**pearl t., pearly t.,** cholesteatoma.

**Pepper t.,** see under *syndrome.*

**peripheral neuroectodermal t.,** a primitive neuroectodermal tumor occurring outside of the central nervous system in a site such as an extremity, the pelvis, or the chest wall; seen most often in adolescents and young adults, frequently with widespread metastases.

**phyllodes t.,** a large fibroadenoma in the breast, with an unusually cellular, sarcoma-like stroma; it is locally aggressive and sometimes metastasizes. Called also *cystosarcoma phyllodes* and *giant fibroadenoma of the breast.*

**Pindborg t.,** calcifying epithelial odontogenic t.

**plasma cell t.,** 1. plasma cell dyscrasia. 2. solitary myeloma.

**potato t.,** carotid body t.

**Pott's puffy t.**, a circumscribed area of edema surrounding lesions of osteomyelitis of the skull.
**pregnancy t.**, tumorous gingivitis histologically and clinically identical to angiogranuloma or to pyogenic granuloma seen in pregnant women, especially after the third trimester, and occurring as a result of minor trauma or irritation probably intensified by the endocrine alteration during pregnancy. It may or may not regress after delivery. Identical lesions are also seen in men and in nonpregnant women.
**premalignant fibroepithelial t.**, premalignant fibroepithelioma.
**primitive neuroectodermal t. (PNET)**, proposed name for a heterogeneous group of neoplasms thought to derive from undifferentiated neuroglial cells of the neural crest. Some occur in the brain and some (the *peripheral neuroectodermal tumors*) in sites such as the extremities, the pelvis, or the chest wall. The classification also includes the neuroepithelial tumors of childhood.
**primitive neuroepithelial t.**, neuroepithelial t.
**prolactin-secreting t.**, prolactinoma.
**proliferating trichilemmal t.**, a large, solitary, multilobulated lesion of the hair follicle occurring on the scalp, usually in middle-aged or older women; it is composed of large follicular sheath cells with glycogen-rich cytoplasms and is often confused with squamous cell carcinoma.
**pulmonary sulcus t.**, one at the apex of the lung, extending outward to destroy the ribs and vertebrae and invading the brachial plexus; see also *Pancoast's syndrome* (def. 1), under *syndrome.* Called also *Pancoast's t.* and *superior sulcus t.*
**Rathke's t., Rathke's pouch t.**, craniopharyngioma.
**Recklinghausen's t.**, an adenomatoid tumor of the posterior uterine wall or of the wall of an oviduct.
**recurring digital fibrous t's of childhood**, infantile digital fibromatosis.
**Regaud's t.**, lymphoepithelioma.
**renomedullary interstitial cell t.**, small, round, grayish white, benign nodules consisting of medullary interstitial cells and spindle cells, found occasionally in the renal medulla at autopsy.
**retinal anlage t.**, melanotic neuroectodermal t.
**rhabdoid t. of the kidney**, a malignant kidney tumor similar to Wilms' tumor but with a poorer prognosis; it has large cells with large nuclei and eosinophilic fibrils in the cytoplasm. It often metastasizes to the brain.
**sand t.**, psammoma.
**Schmincke's t.**, lymphoepithelioma.
**Schwann cell t.**, schwannoma.
**Sertoli cell t.**, androblastoma (def. 1).
**Sertoli-Leydig cell t.**, androblastoma (def. 2).
**sex cord–stromal t's**, stromal t's.
**sheath t.**, nerve sheath t.
**solid-cystic t. of pancreas, solid pseudopapillary t. of pancreas**, papillary cystic t. of pancreas.
**solitary fibrous t.**, a usually benign, localized tumor of mesenchymal origin with a wide range of histologic growth patterns, arising most often in the pleura but also occurring in the mediastinum, upper respiratory tract, head and neck, and abdomen. Called also *localized fibrous mesothelioma.*
**squamous odontogenic t.**, a benign odontogenic epithelial neoplasm occurring in the mandible or maxilla and believed to derive from transformation of the rests of Malassez; it is characterized by islands of mature squamous epithelium surrounded by flattened or cuboidal cells.
**stercoral t.**, stercoroma.
**stromal t's**, a diverse group of tumors derived from the ovarian stroma; many of them secrete sex hormones. Included are granulosa-theca cell tumor, hilar cell tumor, lipoid cell tumor, arrhenoblastoma, and gynandroblastoma. Called also *sex cord–stromal t's.*
**superior sulcus t.**, pulmonary sulcus t.
**teratoid t.**, teratoma.
**testicular t.**, general term for any tumor of the testes; in adults these are nearly always malignant germinomas, whereas in children many are yolk sac tumors or benign varieties such as teratomas, Leydig cell tumors or androblastomas. Called also *orchidoncus, orchioncus,* and *testiculoma.*
**theca cell t.**, a fibroid-like tumor of the ovary containing yellow areas of lipoid material derived from theca cells. It may be associated with excessive production of estrogen and have a tendency to cystic degeneration. The tumor is rarely composed entirely of theca cells; commonly both theca and follicular cells (granulosa cells) are found. Called also *thecoma* and *fibroma thecocellulare xanthomatodes.* See also *granulosa-theca cell t.*
**thyrotrope t., thyrotroph t.**, see under *adenoma.*
**tomato t.**, cylindroma, def. 1, particularly a large lesion. Cf. *turban t.*
**transmissible venereal t., canine**, a venereal tumor found on the external genitalia of male or female dogs, usually wartlike or pedunculated and varying in size from less than 1 cm to 10 cm. Ulceration and hemorrhaging sometimes occur. Called also *canine venereal granuloma.*
**tridermic t.**, tridermoma.
**Triton t.**, a malignant schwannoma, associated with neurofibromatosis 1, with rhabdomyoblastic differentiation.
**turban t.**, a term used to describe the gross appearance of multiple cylindromas of the scalp. See *cylindroma,* def. 1.
**vascular t.**, 1. angioma. 2. any tumor with a copious blood supply.
**villous t.**, papilloma.
**virilizing t.**, a functional tumor that produces virilization in girls and women or precocious sexual development in boys; common types are germinomas, tumors of the anterior pituitary, and tumors of the adrenal cortex. Cf. *feminizing t.*
**Warthin's t.**, adenolymphoma.
**white t.**, chronic tuberculous arthritis.
**Wilms' t.**, a rapidly developing malignant mixed tumor of the kidneys, made up of embryonal elements; it usually affects children before the fifth year, but may occur in the fetus and rarely in later life. Called also *embryonal adenomyosarcoma,* or *adenosarcoma, embryonal carcinosarcoma,* or *nephroma,* and *nephroblastoma.*
**yolk sac t.**, a malignant germ cell tumor of children that represents a proliferation of both yolk sac endoderm and extraembryonic mesenchyme. It is characterized by a labyrinthine glandular pattern with a papillary projection into a sinuslike space; frequently there are hyaline bodies and Schiller-Duval bodies. It produces α-fetoprotein and most often occurs in the testes, but is also seen in the ovaries and some extragonadal sites. Called also *adenocarcinoma of infantile testis, infantile embryonal carcinoma, juvenile embryonal carcinoma, yolk sac carcinoma, orchioblastoma,* and *endodermal sinus t.*

**tu·mor·af·fin** (too″mər-af′in) [*tumor* + L. *affinis* related] oncotropic.

**tu·mor·ec·to·my** (too-mər-ek′tə-me) [*tumor* + *-ectomy*] an imprecise term usually used to denote either debulking or removal of most or all of a primary tumor, particularly of the breast, with only minimal removal of surrounding tissue.

**tu·mor·i·ci·dal** (too″mər-ĭ-si′dal) oncolytic.

**tu·mor·i·gen·e·sis** (too″mər-ĭ-jen′ə-sis) the production of tumors. Called also *oncogenesis.*

**tu·mor·i·gen·ic** (too″mər-ĭ-jen′ik) giving rise to either benign or malignant tumors; said especially of a cell or group of cells capable of producing a tumor. Cf. *oncogenic.*

**tu·mor·let** (too′mər-lət) a type of tiny, often microscopic, benign neoplasm occurring singly or multiply in bronchial and bronchiolar mucosa of middle-aged to elderly people; it often occurs in areas of scarring or chronic irritation and is asymptomatic.

**tu·mor·ous** (too′mər-əs) neoplastic (def. 1).

**tu·mul·tus** (too-mul′təs) [L.] excessive organic action or motility.

**Tun·ga** (tung′gə) a genus of fleas of the family Hectopsyllidae. *T. pe′netrans* is the chigoe (q.v.).

**tun·gi·a·sis** (təng-gi′ə-sis) infestation of the skin with the chigoe *(Tunga penetrans).*

**tung·sten** (tung′stən) [Swed. "heavy stone"] [MeSH: Tungsten] the chemical element of atomic number 74, symbol W, and atomic weight 183.85; used in electric light filaments and in steel alloys to secure hardness.
**t. carbide**, WC, an extremely hard material used for dental drills and burs. Inhalation of its fine dust during manufacturing can cause hard metal disease (see under *disease*).

**tu·nic** (too′nik) 1. tunica. 2. coat (def. 2).
**Bichat's t.**, tunica intima vasorum.
**Brücke's t.**, tunica nervea of Brücke.
**fibrous t. of eyeball**, tunica fibrosa bulbi.
**fibrous t. of liver**, tunica fibrosa hepatis.
**internal t. of eyeball**, tunica interna bulbi.
**pharyngeal t., pharyngobasilar t.**, fascia pharyngobasilaris.
**Ruysch's t.**, see under *membrane.*

**sensory t. of eyeball,** tunica interna bulbi.
**t's of spermatic cord,** tunicae funiculi spermatici.
**vascular t. of eyeball,** tunica vasculosa bulbi.

**tu·ni·ca** (too'nĭ-kə) pl. *tu'nicae* [L.] [TA] a general term in anatomical nomenclature for a membrane or other structure covering or lining a body part or organ. Called also *coat* and *tunic.*

## Tunica

Descriptions of coats are given on TA terms, and include anglicized names of specific coats.

**t. abdomina'lis,** the aponeurosis of the abdominal muscles in certain quadrupeds, as the horse.
**t. adna'ta o'culi,** tunica conjunctiva; sometimes applied specifically to the tunica conjunctiva bulbaris.
**t. adna'ta tes'tis,** lamina parietalis tunicae vaginalis propriae testis.
**t. adventi'tia** [TA], adventitial or adventitious coat: the outer coat of various tubular structures, made up of connective tissue and elastic fibers.
**t. adventi'tia duc'tus deferen'tis** [TA], the adventitious coat of the ductus deferens.
**t. adventi'tia eso'phagi,** t. adventitia oesophagi.
**t. adventi'tia glan'dulae semina'lis,** TA alternative for *t. adventitia glandulae vesiculosae.*
**t. adventi'tia glan'dulae vesiculo'sae** [TA], the adventitious coat of a seminal gland (seminal vesicle); called also *t. adventitia glandulae seminalis* and *t. adventitia vesiculae seminalis* [TA alternatives].
**t. adventi'tia oeso'phagi** [TA], the adventitious coat of the esophagus.
**t. adventi'tia tu'bae uteri'nae,** tela subserosa tubae uterinae.
**t. adventi'tia ure'teris** [TA], the adventitious coat of the ureter.
**t. adventi'tia vaso'rum,** t. externa vasorum.
**t. adventi'tia vesi'culae semina'lis,** TA alternative for *t. adventitia glandulae vesiculosae.*
**t. albugi'nea** [TA], white coat: a dense, white, fibrous sheath enclosing a part or organ.
**t. albugi'nea cor'poris spongio'si** [TA], the dense, white, fibroelastic sheath that encloses the corpus spongiosum of the penis.
**t. albugi'nea corpo'rum cavernoso'rum** [TA], the dense, white, fibroelastic sheath that encloses the corpora cavernosa penis. Its superficial, longitudinal fibers form a tunic surrounding both corpora, and the deep circularly coursing fibers surround them separately, uniting medially to form the septum of the penis.
**t. albugi'nea ova'rii** [TA], the layer of dense connective tissue beneath the germinal epithelium of the ovary.
**t. albugi'nea tes'tis** [TA], the dense, white, inelastic tissue immediately covering the testis, beneath the visceral layer of the tunica vaginalis.
**t. conjuncti'va** [TA], conjunctiva: the thin, transparent mucous membrane lining the eyelids and covering the front surface of the eyeball, consisting of the *t. conjunctiva bulbaris* and the *t. conjunctiva palpebralis.*
**t. conjuncti'va bulba'ris, t. conjuncti'va bul'bi** [TA], bulbar conjunctiva: the portion of the tunica conjunctiva covering the cornea and front part of the sclera, appearing white because of the sclera behind it.
**t. conjuncti'va palpebra'lis, t. conjuncti'va palpebra'rum** [TA], palpebral conjunctiva: the portion of the tunica conjunctiva lining the eyelids, appearing red because of its great vascularity.
**t. dar'tos,** 1. [TA] the thin layer of subcutaneous tissue underlying the skin of the scrotum, consisting mainly of nonstriated muscle fibers (*musculus dartos,* which is sometimes used to refer to the entire tunica dartos). Called also *dartos* and *dartos muscle.* 2. musculus dartos.
**t. deci'dua,** decidua.
**t. elas'tica,** the tunica media vasorum of a large (elastic) artery.
**t. exter'na the'cae folli'culi,** external coat of theca folliculi: the outer, fibrous layer of the theca folliculi.
**t. exter'na vaso'rum** [TA], external coat of vessels: the outer, fibroelastic coat of the blood vessels; called also *adventitia* and *t. adventitia vasorum.*
**t. fibro'sa** [TA], fibrous tunic or coat: an enveloping fibrous membrane.
**t. fibro'sa bul'bi** [TA], fibrous tunic of eyeball: the outer of the three tunics of the eye, comprising the cornea and the sclera; called also *t. fibrosa oculi.*
**t. fibro'sa he'patis** [TA], fibrous tunic of liver: the fibroelastic layer that surrounds the liver beneath the peritoneum; it is continuous at the hepatic portal with the perivascular fibrous capsule.
**t. fibro'sa lie'nis,** TA alternative for *capsula splenis.*
**t. fibro'sa o'culi,** t. fibrosa bulbi.
**t. fibro'sa re'nis,** capsula fibrosa renis.
**t. fibro'sa sple'nis,** TA alternative for *capsula splenis.*

**tu'nicae funi'culi sperma'tici,** tunics of spermatic cord: the coverings of the spermatic cord, comprising the external spermatic fascia, the cremasteric muscle and fascia, the internal spermatic fascia, and the tunica vaginalis testis.
**t. inter'na bul'bi** [TA], internal tunic of eye: the innermost of the three tunics of the eye; it is nervous and sensory and consists primarily of the retina and its blood vessels. Called also *t. sensoria bulbi.* See *retina.*
**t. inter'na the'cae folli'culi,** internal coat of theca folliculi: the inner, vascular layer of secretory cells of the theca folliculi; called also *theca interna* and *internal coat of capsule of graafian follicle.*
**t. in'tima vaso'rum** [TA], the inner coat of the blood vessels, made up of endothelial cells surrounded by longitudinal elastic fibers and connective tissue. Called also *intima* and *Bichat's tunic.*
**t. me'dia vaso'rum** [TA], the middle coat of the blood vessels, made up of transverse elastic and muscle fibers.
**t. muco'sa** [TA], mucous tunic or coat: the mucous lining of various tubular structures, comprising the epithelium, basement membrane, lamina propria mucosae, and lamina muscularis mucosae. Called also *mucous membrane* and *mucosa.*
**t. muco'sa bronchio'rum** [TA], mucous coat of bronchi: the mucous membrane lining the bronchi.
**t. muco'sa cavita'tis tympa'nicae** [TA], mucous coat of tympanic cavity: the mucous membrane covering the walls and much of the contents of the tympanic cavity; called also *t. mucosa tympanica.*
**t. muco'sa duc'tus deferen'tis** [TA], the mucous coat of the ductus deferens.
**t. muco'sa eso'phagi,** t. mucosa oesophagi.
**t. muco'sa gas'tris** [TA], the mucous coat of the stomach.
**t. muco'sa glan'dulae semina'lis,** TA alternative for *t. mucosa glandulae vesiculosae.*
**t. muco'sa glan'dulae vesiculo'sae** [TA], the mucous coat of the seminal gland (seminal vesicle); called also *t. mucosa glandulae seminalis* and *t. mucosa vesiculae seminalis* [TA alternatives].
**t. muco'sa intesti'ni cras'si** [TA], the mucous coat of the large intestine.
**t. muco'sa intesti'ni rec'ti,** t. mucosa recti.
**t. muco'sa intesti'ni ten'uis** [TA], the mucous coat of the small intestine.
**t. muco'sa laryn'gis** [TA], the mucous coat of the larynx.
**t. muco'sa lin'guae** [TA], the mucous membrane covering the tongue.
**t. muco'sa na'si** [TA], the mucous membrane lining the nasal cavity; called also *schneiderian membrane.* See also *pars olfactoria cavitatis nasi* and *pars respiratoria cavitatis nasi.*
**t. muco'sa oeso'phagi** [TA], the mucous coat of the esophagus.
**t. muco'sa o'ris** [TA], the tunica mucosa of the mouth.
**t. muco'sa pharyn'gis** [TA], the mucous coat of the pharynx.
**t. muco'sa rec'ti,** the mucous coat of the rectum; called also *t. mucosa intestini recti.*

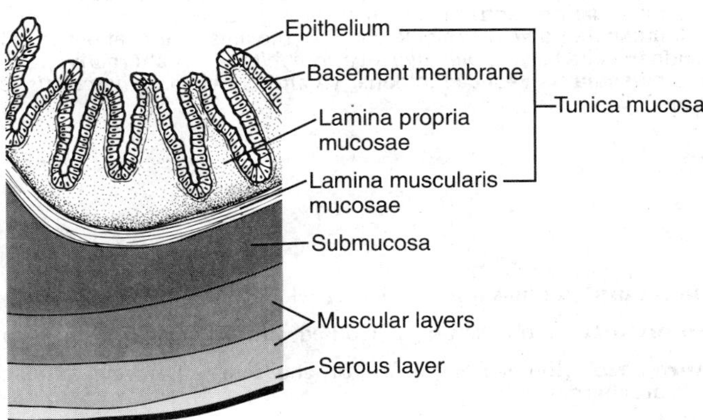


.Tunica mucosa lining the walls of the small intestine.

**t. muco'sa tra'cheae** [TA], the mucous coat of the trachea.
**t. muco'sa tu'bae auditi'vae** [TA], the mucous membrane lining the auditory tube; called also *t. mucosa tubae auditoriae* [TA alternative].
**t. muco'sa tu'bae audito'riae,** TA alternative for *t. mucosa tubae auditivae.*
**t. muco'sa tu'bae uteri'nae** [TA], mucous coat of uterine tube: the mucous membrane lining the uterine tube, arranged in longitudinal rugae or folds, and continuous with the mucous lining of the uterus. Called also *endosalpinx.*
**t. muco'sa tympa'nica,** t. mucosa cavitatis tympanicae.
**t. muco'sa ure'teris** [TA], the mucous coat of the ureter.
**t. muco'sa ure'thrae femini'nae** [TA], **t. muco'sa ure'thrae mulie'bris,** the mucous coat of the female urethra.
**t. muco'sa u'teri** [TA], the inner mucous membrane of the uterus, the thickness and structure of which vary with the phase of the menstrual cycle. It is functionally divisible into three layers: the stratum basale, stratum spongiosum, and stratum compactum; the latter two layers together form the *stratum functionale*. Called also *endometrium* [TA alternative].
**t. muco'sa vagi'nae** [TA], the mucous coat of the vagina.
**t. muco'sa ventri'culi,** t. mucosa gastris.
**t. muco'sa vesi'cae bilia'ris** [TA], the mucous coat of the gallbladder; called also *t. mucosa vesicae felleae* [TA alternative].
**t. muco'sa vesi'cae fel'leae,** TA alternative for *t. mucosa vesicae biliaris.*
**t. muco'sa vesi'cae urina'riae** [TA], the mucous coat of the urinary bladder.
**t. muco'sa vesi'culae semina'lis,** TA alternative for *t. mucosa glandulae vesiculosae.*
**t. muscula'ris** [TA], muscular tunic or coat: the muscular coat or layer surrounding the tela submucosa in most portions of the digestive, respiratory, urinary, and genital tracts.
**t. muscula'ris bronchio'rum,** the muscular coat of the bronchi.
**t. muscula'ris co'li** [TA], the muscular coat of the colon, consisting of layers of longitudinally and circularly coursing fibers.
**t. muscula'ris duc'tus deferen'tis** [TA], the muscular coat of the ductus deferens.
**t. muscula'ris eso'phagi,** t. muscularis oesophagi.
**t. muscula'ris gas'tris** [TA], the muscular coat of the stomach, composed of longitudinal, circular, and oblique fibers.
**t. muscula'ris glan'dulae semina'lis,** TA alternative for *t. muscularis glandulae vesiculosae.*
**t. muscula'ris glan'dulae vesiculo'sae** [TA], the muscular coat of the seminal gland (seminal vesicle); called also *t. muscularis glandulae seminalis* and *t. muscularis vesiculae seminalis* [TA alternatives].
**t. muscula'ris intesti'ni te'nuis** [TA], the muscular coat of the small intestine, consisting of an inner circular and an outer longitudinal layer.
**t. muscula'ris oeso'phagi** [TA], the muscular coat of the esophagus.
**t. muscula'ris pharyn'gis,** TA alternative for *musculi pharyngis.*
**t. muscula'ris rec'ti** [TA], the muscular coat of the rectum, consisting of an outer longitudinal and an inner circular layer.
**t. muscula'ris tra'cheae,** the muscular coat of the trachea.
**t. muscula'ris tu'bae uteri'nae** [TA], the muscular coat of the uterine tube.
**t. muscula'ris ure'teris** [TA], the muscular coat of the ureter.
**t. muscula'ris ure'thrae femini'nae** [TA], **t. muscula'ris ure'thrae mulie'bris,** the muscular coat of the female urethra.
**t. muscula'ris u'teri** [TA], the smooth muscle coat of the uterus, which forms the mass of the organ; called also *myometrium* [TA alternative] and *mesometrium.*
**t. muscula'ris vagi'nae** [TA], the muscular coat of the vagina.
**t. muscula'ris ventri'culi,** t. muscularis gastris.
**t. muscula'ris vesi'cae bilia'ris** [TA], the muscular coat of the gallbladder; called also *t. muscularis vesicae felleae* [TA alternative].
**t. muscula'ris vesi'cae fel'leae,** TA alternative for *t. muscularis vesicae biliaris.*
**t. muscula'ris vesi'cae urina'riae** [TA], the smooth muscle coat of the urinary bladder.
**t. muscula'ris vesi'culae semina'lis,** TA alternative for *t. muscularis glandulae vesiculosae.*
**t. nervea of Brücke,** the cerebral layer of the retina, exclusive of the rod and cone layer with its fibers and nuclei.
**t. pro'pria,** tunic proper: a general term in anatomical nomenclature for the actual coat or layer of a part, as distinguished from an investing membrane.
**t. pro'pria co'rii,** stratum reticulare dermidis.
**t. pro'pria tu'buli tes'tis,** the proper coat of the seminiferous tubules.
**t. ruyschia'na,** Ruysch's membrane.
**t. senso'ria bul'bi,** t. interna bulbi.
**t. sero'sa** [TA], serous tunic: the membrane lining the external walls of the body cavities and reflected over the surfaces of protruding organs; it consists of mesothelium lying upon a connective tissue layer, and it secretes a watery exudate; called also *serosa, serous coat,* and *serous membrane.*
**t. sero'sa gas'tris** [TA], the serous coat of the stomach.
**t. sero'sa he'patis** [TA], the serous coat of the liver.
**t. sero'sa intesti'ni cras'si** [TA], the serous coat of the large intestine.
**t. sero'sa intesti'ni te'nuis** [TA], the serous coat of the small intestine.
**t. sero'sa lie'nis,** TA alternative for *t. serosa splenis.*
**t. sero'sa peritone'i** [TA], the serous coat of the peritoneum.
**t. sero'sa sple'nis** [TA], the serous coat of the spleen; called also *t. serosa lienis* [TA alternative].
**t. sero'sa tes'tis,** serous layer of tunica vaginalis of testis: the inner part of the tunica vaginalis of the testis, firmly attached to the testis and epididymis.
**t. sero'sa tu'bae uteri'nae** [TA], the serous coat of the uterine tube.
**t. sero'sa u'teri** [TA], the serous coat of the uterus; called also *perimetrium* [TA alternative].
**t. sero'sa ventri'culi,** t. serosa gastris.
**t. sero'sa vesi'cae bilia'ris** [TA], the serous coat of the gallbladder; called also *t. serosa vesicae felleae* [TA alternative].
**t. sero'sa vesi'cae fel'leae,** TA alternative for *t. serosa vesicae biliaris.*
**t. sero'sa vesi'cae urina'riae** [TA], the serous coat of the urinary bladder.
**t. spongio'sa ure'thrae femini'nae** [TA], a thin layer of spongiose erectile tissue located just beneath the mucous coat of the female urethra, which contains a plexus of large veins.
**t. spongio'sa vagi'nae** [TA], a thin layer of spongiose erectile tissue located between the muscular and mucous coats of the vagina, which contains a large plexus of blood vessels.
**t. submuco'sa ure'thrae femini'nae,** the submucous coat of the female urethra.
**tu'nicae tes'tis,** the coverings of the testis; see *tunicae funiculi spermatici.*
**t. u'vea,** t. vasculosa bulbi.
**t. vagina'lis tes'tis** [TA], the serous membrane covering the front and sides of the testis and epididymis, composed of a visceral layer *(lamina visceralis)* and a parietal layer *(lamina parietalis).*
**t. vasculo'sa,** a vascular coat, or a layer well supplied with blood vessels.
**t. vasculo'sa bul'bi** [TA], vascular tunic of eye: the middle, pigmented, vascular coat of the eye, comprising the choroid, the ciliary body, and the iris; called also *uvea* and *uveal tract.*
**t. vasculo'sa len'tis,** the vascular envelope which encloses and nourishes the developing lens of the fetus; it consists of the *pupillary membrane* in the region of the pupil, the *capsulopupillary membrane* around the edge of the lens, and the *capsular membrane* at the back of the lens. It normally degenerates during the late fetal period when the hyaloid artery degenerates.
**t. vasculo'sa o'culi,** t. vasculosa bulbi.

**tu•ni•cary** (too″nĭ-kar′e) tunicate (def. 1).

**Tu•ni•ca•ta** (too″nĭ-ka′tə) [L. "clothed with a tunic"] Urochordata.

**tu•ni•cate** (too′nĭ-kāt) [MeSH: Urochordata] 1. having a tunic. 2. urochordate.

**tu•ni•cin** (too′nĭ-sin) a substance resembling cellulose occurring in the body covering of some of the lowest vertebrates, such as the tunicates or ascidians; animal cellulose.

**tun•nel** (tun′əl) a passageway through a solid body, completely enclosed except for the open ends, permitting entrance and exit. Cf. *canal.*
**aortico–left ventricular t.,** a congenital communication between the ascending aorta just above the coronary arteries, and the left ventricle.
**carpal t.,** canalis carpi.
**cervical t's,** small tubular canals which are extensions of the clefts in the uterine endocervical mucosa.

**Corti's t.,** inner t.
**cubital t.,** the opening between the two heads of the flexor carpi ulnaris muscle through which the ulnar nerve enters the forearm.
**flexor t.,** carpal t.
**inner t.,** a canal extending the length of the cochlea, formed by the pillar cells of the organ of Corti; called also *cuniculus internus, canal of Corti, Corti's t., arcuate zone, zona arcuata,* and *zona tecta.*
**outer t.,** a fluid-filled space in the organ of Corti between the outermost hair cells and Hensen's cells; called also *Nuel's space* and *cuniculus externus.*
**tarsal t.,** the osseofibrous passage for the posterior tibial vessels, tibial nerve, and flexor tendons, formed by the flexor retinaculum and tarsal bones.

**tu·ra·nose** (tōōr'ə-nōs) a reducing disaccharide composed of fructose and glucose; it is isomeric with sucrose and is part of the trisaccharide melezitose.

**tur·ban** (tur'bən) [Turkish *tülbend* gauze] a headdress made of a long strip of material wound around the head.
**ice t.,** a soft head wrapping filled with ice, used to promote scalp hypothermia and prevent alopecia during chemotherapy.

**Tur·ba·trix** (tər-ba'triks) a genus of nematodes.
**T. ace'ti,** a minute nematode found in vinegar and sometimes occurring in the urine of patients who have used vinegar douches. It may also occur in sour paste and fermenting vegetable substances. Formerly called *Anguillula aceti.*

**tur·bid** (tur'bid) [L. *turba* a tumult] cloudy; showing turbidity.

**tur·bi·dim·e·ter** (tur"bĭ-dim'ə-tər) an instrument that measures the turbidity of a solution by measuring the loss of intensity of a beam of light as it passes through the solution. Cf. *nephelometer.*

**tur·bid·i·met·ric** (tur"bid-ĭ-met'rik) performed by the turbidimeter.

**tur·bi·dim·e·try** (tur"bĭ- dim'ə-tre) measurement of the turbidity of a fluid.

**tur·bid·i·ty** (tur-bid'ĭ-te) cloudiness of a solution caused by the scattering of light by colloidal particles or by suspended precipitate or sediment.

**tur·bi·nal** (tur'bĭ-nəl) [L. *turbinalis,* from *turbo* a child's top] turbinate.

**tur·bi·nate** (tur'bĭ-nāt) [L. *turbineus*] [MeSH: Turbinates] 1. shaped like a top. 2. any of the nasal conchae; see terms beginning *concha nasalis.* Called also *turbinal.*
**inferior t.,** concha nasalis inferior.
**middle t.,** concha nasalis media.
**sphenoid t.,** concha sphenoidalis.
**superior t.,** concha nasalis superior.
**supreme t.,** concha nasalis suprema.

**tur·bi·nat·ed** (tur'bĭ-nāt"əd) shaped like a top.

**tur·bi·nec·to·my** (tur"bĭ-nek'tə-me) [*turbinate* + *-ectomy*] the surgical removal of a nasal concha (turbinate bone).

**tur·bino·tome** (tur-bin'ə-tōm) an instrument used for removal or cutting of a nasal concha (turbinate bone). Called also *conchotome.*

**tur·bi·not·o·my** (tur"bĭ-not'ə-me) [*turbinate* + *-tomy*] the surgical cutting of a nasal concha (turbinate bone). Called also *conchotomy.*

**Tur·bo·hal·er** (tər'bo-hāl"ər) trademark for a type of dry powder inhaler that can deliver multiple doses of medication.

**TURBT** transurethral resection of bladder tumor.

**Türck's bundle, column,** etc. (tērks) [Ludwig *Türck,* Austrian neurologist and laryngologist, 1810–1868] see under *degeneration* and see *tractus corticospinalis anterior* and *fibrae parietotemporopontinae.*

**Turck's zone** (turks) [Fenton Benedict *Turck,* New York physician, 1857–1932] see *zona transformans.*

**Tur·cot's syndrome** (tēr-kōz') [Jacques *Turcot,* Canadian physician, born 1914] see under *syndrome.*

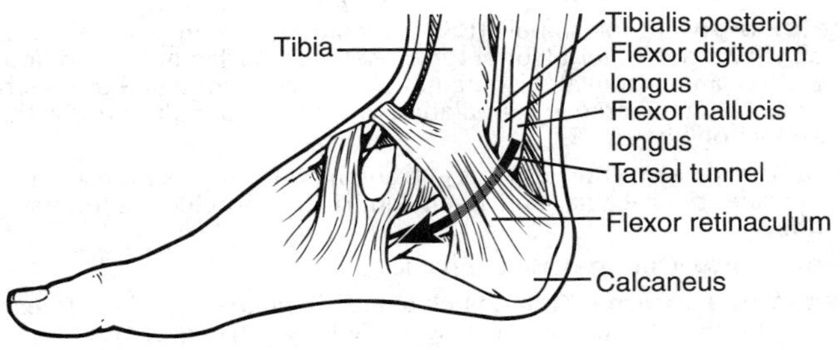


Tarsal tunnel.

**tur·ges·cence** (tər-jes'əns) [L. *turgescens* swelling] swelling (def. 1).

**tur·ges·cent** (tər-jes'ənt) [L. *turgescens*] 1. swollen. 2. beginning to swell.

**tur·gid** (tur'jid) [L. *turgidus*] swollen and congested.

**tur·gid·iza·tion** (tur"jid-ĭ-za'shən) the creation of turgor in a tissue by the injection of fluid.

**tur·gom·e·ter** (tər-gom'ə-tər) [*turgor* + *-meter*] an instrument for measuring the amount of turgescence.

**tur·gor** (tur'gər) [L.] the condition of being turgid; normal or other fullness. See also *swelling* (def. 1).
**t. vita'lis,** the normal consistency of living tissue.

**tu·ris·ta** (too-rēs'tah) [Sp.] Mexican name for traveler's diarrhea.

**Türk's cell (irritation leukocyte)** (tērks) [Willhelm *Türk,* Austrian physician, 1871–1916] see under *cell.*

**tur·mer·ic** (tur'mər-ik) 1. *Curcuma longa.* 2. the rhizome of *C. longa,* which contains curcumin, an orange-yellow coloring principle, and several aromatic principles that give it a pepper-like and bitter taste; used as a coloring agent, chemical indicator, and condiment (as curry powder).

**turm·schä·del** (toorm'sha-dəl) [Ger.] a developmental anomaly in which the skull is high and rounded, due to early synostosis of the three major sutures of the skull.

**Tur·ner's sign** (tur'nərz) [George Grey *Turner,* English surgeon, 1877–1951] see under *sign.*

**Tur·ner's sulcus** (tur'nərz) [Sir William *Turner,* English anatomist, 1832–1916] sulcus intraparietalis.

**Tur·ner's syndrome** (tur'nərz) [Henry Hubert *Turner,* American endocrinologist, 1892–1970] [MeSH: Turner's Syndrome] see under *syndrome.*

**Tur·ner tooth (hypoplasia)** (tur'nər) [Joseph George *Turner,* British dentist, died 1955] see under *tooth.*

**tur·nera** (tur'nər-ə) damiana.

**turn·over** (turn'o-vər) 1. the movement of something into, through, and out of a place. 2. the rate at which something is depleted and replaced.
**erythrocyte iron t. (EIT),** the rate at which iron moves from the bone marrow into circulating red cells, calculated as: plasma iron turnover (PIT) × red cell utilization (RCU). Called also *red blood cell iron t.*
**plasma iron t. (PIT),** the rate at which iron leaves the blood plasma for bone marrow or other tissues, expressed in mg/day; calculated as: (plasma iron concentration) × (plasma volume) × 0.693 ÷ (plasma iron clearance half-time).
**red blood cell iron t. (RBC IT),** erythrocyte iron t.

**turn·sick** (tərn'sik) gid.

**turn·sick·ness** (tərn'sik-nəs) gid.

**TURP** transurethral resection of the prostate.

**tur·pen·tine** (tur'pən-tīn) [L. *terebinthina*] [MeSH: Turpentine] the concrete oleoresin obtained from *Pinus palustris* and other species of *Prunus.* It contains a volatile oil, turpentine oil (q.v.). to which its properties are due, and in which form it is generally used.

**tur·ri·ceph·a·ly** (tur"ĭ-sef'ə-le) oxycephaly.

**tu·run·da** (tu-run'də) [L.] 1. tent (def. 2). 2. a suppository.

**Tu·ryn's sign** (too'rinz) [Felix *Turyn,* Polish physician, born 1899] see under *sign.*

**tus.** abbreviation for L. *tus'sis,* a cough.

**tus·sal** (tus'əl) [L. *tussis* cough] tussive.

**tus·sic·u·la** (tə-sik'u-lə) [L., dim. of *tussis* cough] a slight cough.

**tus·sic·u·lar** (tə-sik'u-lər) [L. *tussicula*] tussive.

**tus·sic·u·la·tion** (tə-sik"u-la'shən) hacking cough.

**tus·si·gen·ic** (tus"ĭ-jen'ik) [*tussis* + *-genic*] causing cough.

**tus·sis** (tus'is) [L.] cough.

**tus·sive** (tus'iv) pertaining to or due to a cough; called also *bechic, tussal,* and *tussicular.*

**tu·ta·men** (tu-ta'mən) pl. *tuta'mina* [L.] a protective covering or structure.
**tuta'mina o'culi,** organa oculi accessoria.

**Tut·tle's proctoscope** (tut'əlz) [James Percival *Tuttle,* American surgeon, 1857–1912] see under *proctoscope.*

**Tween** (twēn) trademark for preparations of polysorbates, used with a numerical suffix; e.g., *Tween 80* is a trademark for polysorbate 80.

**twig** in anatomy, a final ramification, as of branches of nerves or blood vessels.

**twin** (twin) [MeSH: Twins] one of two offspring produced in the same pregnancy and developed from one ovum (monozygotic) or from two ova (dizygotic) fertilized at the same time.
**acardiac t.**, acardius.
**allantoidoangiopagous t's,** twins joined by the vessels of the umbilical cord only; called also *omphaloangiopagous t's.*
**binovular t's,** dizygotic t's.
**conjoined t's,** monozygotic twins ranging from two well-developed individuals joined by a superficial connection of varying extent, usually in the frontal, transverse, or sagittal body plane *(symmetrical* or *equal conjoined t's),* to those in which only a small part of the body is duplicated or one small and incompletely developed parasitic twin is attached to a much larger and more fully developed twin *(asymmetrical* or *unequal t's).* Called also *Siamese t's.*
**conjoined t's, asymmetrical,** see *conjoined t's.*
**conjoined t's, equal,** see *conjoined t's.*
**conjoined t's, symmetrical,** see *conjoined t's.*
**conjoined t's, unequal,** see *conjoined t's.*
**diamnionic t's, diamniotic t's,** twins developing within separate amniotic cavities; such twins may be monochorionic or dichorionic.
**dichorial t's, dichorionic t's,** twins having distinct chorions; this includes monozygotic twins separated within 72 hours of fertilization and all dizygotic twins.
**dissimilar t's, dizygotic t's,** two offspring developed from two zygotes that resulted from fertilization of two ova fertilized at the same time; they may be of the same or different sex, and they have different genomes. Called also *binovular, false, fraternal, heterologous, hetero-ovular, two-egg,* and *unlike t's.*
**enzygotic t's,** monozygotic t's.
**false t's, fraternal t's,** dizygotic t's.
**heterologous t's, hetero-ovular t's,** dizygotic t's.
**identical t's,** monozygotic t's.
**impacted t's,** twins so situated during delivery that the pressure of one against the other prevents simultaneous engagement of both.
**membranous t.,** fetus papyraceus.
**monoamnionic t's, monoamniotic t's,** twins developing within a single amniotic cavity; they are always monozygotic and monochorionic.

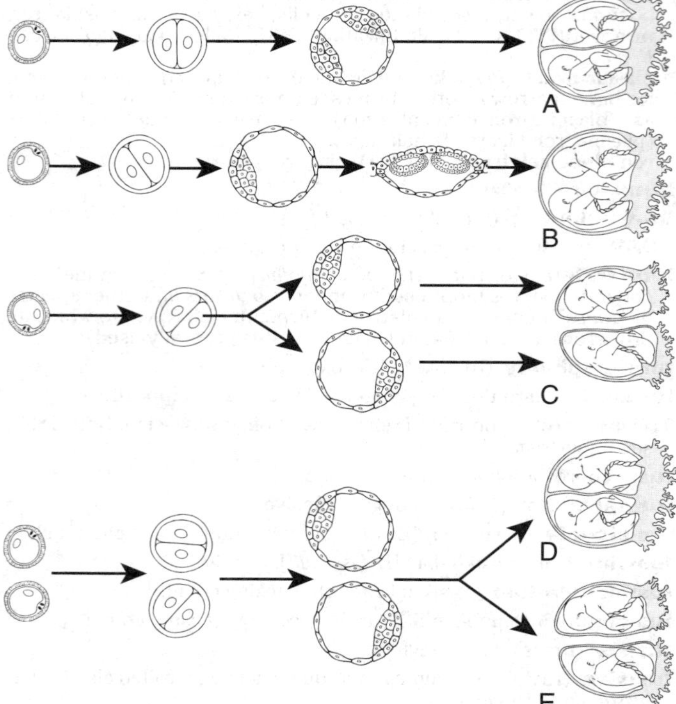

Twins. *(A),* The most common type of monozygotic twinning, with division of the inner cell mass of the blastocyst resulting in separate amnions but a single chorion and placenta; *(B),* a rare form of monozygotic twinning, with complete division of the embryonic disk resulting in two embryos in a single amniotic sac with a single placenta and chorionic sac; *(C),* monozygotic twinning with division occurring between the two-cell and morula stages to produce identical blastocysts, resulting in separate amniotic and chorionic sacs and either separate *(shown)* or fused placentas; *(D,E),* dizygotic twinning, with *(D)* or without *(E)* fusion of the placenta and chorion.

**monochorial t's, monochorionic t's,** twins developing with a single chorion; such twins are always monozygotic and may be monoamnionic or diamnionic.
**mono-ovular t's, monovular t's,** monozygotic t's.
**monozygotic t's,** two offspring developed from one zygote that divided into two embryos at an early stage (usually during the first eight days); the twins therefore have identical genomes. Called also *enzygotic, identical, mono-ovular, monovular, similar, true,* and *uniovular t's.*
**omphaloangiopagous t's,** allantoidoangiopagous t's.
**one-egg t's,** monozygotic t's.
**Siamese t's,** conjoined t's.
**similar t's, true t's,** monozygotic t's.
**two-egg t's,** dizygotic t's.
**uniovular t's,** monozygotic t's.
**unlike t's,** dizygotic t's.

**twinge** (twinj) a short, sharp pain.

**twin·ning** (twin'ing) 1. the simultaneous production of two (or more) offspring. 2. the production of symmetrical structures or parts by division.
**experimental t.,** embryonic duplication produced by purposeful external intervention.
**spontaneous t.,** embryonic duplication without external intervention, as occurs in nature.

**twin·ship** (twin'ship) the state of being a twin.

**Twis·ton** (twis'ton) trademark for preparations of rotoxamine tartrate.

**twitch** (twich) 1. a brief contractile response of a skeletal muscle elicited by a single maximal volley of impulses in the motor neurons supplying it. 2. a noose passed around the lip or ear and through a perforation in a board, used for restraining a horse during minor surgery.
**fast t.,** see *muscle fibers,* under *fiber.*
**slow t.,** see *muscle fibers,* under *fiber.*

**twitch·ing** (twich'ing) the occurrence of a single contraction or a series of contractions of a muscle; see *twitch.*
**fascicular t.,** repetitive brief contraction of large groups of bundles of muscle fibers.
**fibrillar t.,** repetitive brief contraction of single bundles of muscle fibers.
**Trousseau's t.,** repetitive brief contraction involving muscles of the face.

**Twort-d'He·relle phenomenon** (twort-dĕ-rel') [Frederick William *Twort,* English bacteriologist, 1877–1950; Félix Hubert *d'Herelle,* Canadian bacteriologist in France, 1873–1949] see under *phenomenon.*

**TWZ** triangular working zone; see *Kambin's triangular working zone,* under *zone.*

**$TXA_2$, $TXB_2$** thromboxanes $A_2$ and $B_2$; see *thromboxane.*

**ty·ba·mate** (ti'bə-māt) a minor tranquilizer, occurring as a clear viscous liquid; administered orally.

**ty·ing up** (ti'ing up) azoturia (def. 2).

**ty·lec·to·my** (ti-lek'tə-me) [Gr. *tylos* knot + *-ectomy*] lumpectomy.

**Ty·le·nol** (ti'lə-nol) trademark for preparations of acetaminophen.

**tyl·i·on** (til'e-on) [Gr. *tyleion* cushion] the point on the anterior edge of the optic groove in the median line.

**ty·lo·ma** (ti-lo'mə) [Gr. *tylōma*] callus.

**ty·lo·sin** (ti'lo-sin) [USP] a macrolide antibiotic, similar to erythromycin, used in veterinary practice.

**ty·lo·sis** (ti-lo'sis) [Gr. *tylōs* a knob or callus] formation of a callus.
**t. cilia'ris,** thickening of the eyelids due to long-term ulcerative blepharitis.
**t. palma'ris et planta'ris,** palmoplantar keratoderma.

**ty·lot·ic** (ti-lot'ik) pertaining to or affected with tylosis.

**Ty·lox** (ti'loks) trademark for a combination preparation of oxycodone hydrochloride and acetaminophen.

**ty·lox·a·pol** (ti-lok'sə-pol) [USP] a nonionic liquid polymer of the alkyl aryl polyether alcohol type; used as a surfactant to aid liquefaction and removal of mucopurulent bronchopulmonary secretions, administered by inhalation through a nebulizer or with a stream of oxygen.

**Tym·pa·ge·sic** (tim"pə-je'zik) trademark for a preparation of antipyrine, benzocaine, and phenylephrine hydrochloride otic solution.

**tym·pa·nal** (tim'pə-nəl) tympanic (def. 1).

**tym·pa·nec·to·my** (tim"pə-nek'tə-me) [*tympan-* + *-ectomy*] excision of the tympanic membrane. Called also *myringectomy.*

**tym·pan·ia** (tim-pan'e-ə) tympanites.

**tym·pan·ic** (tim-pan'ik) [L. *tympanicus*] 1. of or pertaining to the tympanic cavity or the tympanic membrane. 2. bell-like or resonant; called also *tympanitic.*

**tym·pa·nic·i·ty** (tim"pə-nis'ĭ-te) a tympanic quality.

**tym·pa·nism** (tim'pə-niz-əm) [Gr. *tympanon* drum] tympanites.

**tym·pa·ni·tes** (tim"pə-ni'tēz) [Gr. *tympanitēs,* from *tympanon* drum] distention of the abdomen, due to the presence of gas or air in the intestine or in the peritoneal cavity, as in peritonitis and typhoid fever.
**uterine t.,** physometra.

**tym·pa·nit·ic** (tim"pə-nit'ik) 1. pertaining to or affected with tympanites. 2. tympanic (def. 2).

**tympan(o)-** [Gr. *tympanon* drum] a combining form denoting relationship to the tympanic cavity or to the tympanic membrane.

**tym·pa·no·cen·te·sis** (tim"pə-no-sən-te'sis) surgical puncture of the membrana tympani for removal of fluid from the middle ear. Cf. *myringotomy.*

**tym·pa·no·eu·sta·chi·an** (tim"pə-no-u-sta'ke-ən) pertaining to the tympanic cavity and auditory tube.

**tym·pa·no·gen·ic** (tim"pə-no-jen'ik) [*tympano-* + *-genic*] arising from the tympanic cavity.

**tym·pa·no·gram** (tim-pan'o-gram") [*tympano-* + *-gram*] a graphic representation of the relative compliance and impedance of the tympanic membrane and ossicles of the middle ear obtained by tympanometry.

**tym·pa·no·hy·al** (tim"pə-no-hi'əl) 1. pertaining to the tympanic cavity and the hyoid arch. 2. a small bone or cartilage at the base of the styloid process of the temporal bone; in early life it becomes a part of the temporal bone.

**tym·pa·no·lab·y·rin·tho·pexy** (tim"pə-no-lab"ĭ-rin'tho-pek"se) Sourdille's operation of uniting a neotympanic system to a labyrinthine fistula for the cure of progressive hearing loss from otosclerosis; of historical interest.

**tym·pa·no·mal·le·al** (tim"pə-no-mal'e-əl) pertaining to the tympanic membrane and the malleus.

**tym·pa·no·mas·toid·ec·to·my** (tim"pə-no-mas"toid-ek'tə-me) mastoidectomy with tympanectomy.
**canal wall down t.,** open-cavity t.
**canal wall up t.,** closed-cavity t.
**closed-cavity t.,** tympanomastoidectomy with tympanoplasty and maintenance of an intact posterior wall of the ear canal. Called also *closed-cavity mastoidectomy, canal wall up t.* or *mastoidectomy,* and *intact canal wall t.* or *mastoidectomy.* Cf. *open-cavity t.*
**intact canal wall t.,** closed-cavity t.
**open-cavity t.,** tympanomastoidectomy with removal of the posterior wall of the ear canal, such as radical mastoidectomy and modified radical mastoidectomy. Called also *open-cavity mastoidectomy,* and *canal wall down t.* or *mastoidectomy.* Cf. *closed-cavity t.*

**tym·pa·no·mas·toid·itis** (tim"pə-no-mas"toi-di'tis) inflammation of the tympanic cavity and the pneumatic cells of the mastoid process.

**tym·pa·no·me·a·tal** (tim"pə-no-me-a'təl) pertaining to the tympanum and the external acoustic meatus.

**tym·pa·no·met·ric** (tim"pə-no-met'rik) pertaining to tympanometry.

**tym·pa·nom·e·try** (tim"pə-nom'ə-tre) indirect measurement of the compliance (mobility) and impedance of the tympanic membrane and ossicles of the middle ear; it is done by subjecting the external acoustic meatus to positive, normal, and negative air pressure and monitoring the resultant sound energy flow.

**tym·pa·no·plas·tic** (tim"pə-no-plas'tik) relating to tympanoplasty.

**tym·pa·no·plas·ty** (tim"pə-no-plas'te) [*tympano-* + *-plasty*] [MeSH: Tympanoplasty] surgical reconstruction of the hearing mechanism of the middle ear, with restoration of the drum membrane to protect the round window from sound pressure, and establishment of ossicular continuity between the tympanic membrane and the oval window. See also *myringoplasty.*

**tym·pa·no·scle·ro·sis** (tim"pə-no-sklə-ro'sis) the presence of masses of hard, dense connective tissue around the auditory ossicles.

**tym·pa·no·scle·rot·ic** (tim"pə-no-sklə-rot'ik) characterized by or pertaining to tympanosclerosis.

**tym·pa·no·squa·mo·sal** (tim"pə-no-skwah-mo'səl) pertaining to the pars tympanica and pars squamosa of the temporal bone.

**tym·pa·no·sta·pe·di·al** (tim"pə-no-stə-pe'de-əl) pertaining to the tympanic cavity and the stapes.

**tym·pa·nos·to·my** (tim"pə-nos'tə-me) myringotomy.

**tym·pa·no·tem·po·ral** (tim"pə-no-tem'pə-rəl) pertaining to the tympanic cavity and the region over the temporal bone or region.

**tym·pa·not·o·my** (tim"pə-not'ə-me) [*tympano-* + *-tomy*] 1. tympanocentesis. 2. myringotomy.
**facial recess t.,** posterior t.
**posterior t.,** tympanotomy with exenteration of the air cells posterior to the facial recess. Called also *facial recess t.*

**tym·pa·nous** (tim'pə-nəs) pertaining to or marked by tympanites; distended with gas.

**tym·pa·num** (tim'pə-nəm) [L., from Gr. *tympanon* drum] 1. membrana tympani. 2. cavitas tympani.

**tym·pa·ny** (tim'pə-ne) [Gr. *tympanias*] 1. tympanites. 2. a tympanic, or bell-like, percussion note.
**bell t.,** a modified tympanitic note heard on percussion of the chest in some cases of pneumothorax.
**ruminal t.,** a kind of indigestion in cattle and sheep, marked by an abnormal collection of gas in the rumen; the usual cause is a diet too high in carbohydrates. As gas volume increases, the rumen presses against adjacent organs; it may occlude the vena cava and cause circulatory problems or press against the diaphragm and lungs and cause death from asphyxia. Called also *bloat.*
**ruminal t., primary,** ruminal tympany caused by eating too much wet or frothy legume, particularly alfalfa or clover, which forms a stable foam in the rumen. Called also *frothy bloat.*
**ruminal t., secondary,** ruminal tympany caused by an esophageal obstruction that prevents eructation; called also *free gas bloat.*
**Skoda's t., skodaic t.,** skodaic resonance.
**t. of the stomach,** bloat, def. 1.

**Tyn·dall cone, effect (phenomenon), light** (tin'dəl) [John *Tyndall,* British physicist, 1820–1893] see under *cone, effect,* and *light.*

**tyn·dal·li·za·tion** (tin"dəl-ĭ-za'shən) [John *Tyndall*] fractional sterilization.

**type** (tīp) [Gr. *typos* mark] something with particular characteristics, such as a person, substance, or case of a disease. Cf. *constitution* and *diathesis.*
**asthenic t.,** a constitutional type marked by a slender body, long neck, long, flat chest and abdomen, and poor muscular development.
**athletic t.,** a constitutional type marked by broad shoulders, deep chest, flat abdomen, thick neck, and good muscular development.
**blood t.,** blood group; see under *B.*
**body t.,** constitutional t.
**buffalo t.,** see under *type.*
**constitutional t.,** a constellation of traits related to body build.
**dysplastic t.,** any constitutional type that differs from the asthenic, the athletic, and the pyknic types.
**mating t.,** in ciliate protozoa, certain bacteria, and certain fungi, the equivalent of a sex; as many as eight sexes are present in some species of protozoa.
**personality t.,** any of various categories of both normal and abnormal personality variants; usually they derive from a theory-based topology, such as introvert/extrovert or oral/anal/phallic.
**phage t.,** an intraspecies type of bacterium demonstrated by phage typing (see under *typing*); called also *phagotype.*
**pyknic t.,** a constitutional type marked by a rounded body, large chest, thick shoulders, broad head, and short neck.
**sympatheticotonic t.,** a type of physical constitution characterized by sympathicotonia.
**test t.,** see *test type.*
**wild t.,** in genetics, the standard phenotype for any experimental organism; also a gene that determines a standard phenotypic trait.

**typh·lec·ta·sis** (tif-lek'tə-sis) [*typhlo-* + *ectasis*] distention of the cecum.

**typh·lec·to·my** (tif-lek'tə-me) cecectomy.

**typh·li·tis** (tif-li'tis) cecitis.

**typhl(o)-**[1] [Gr. *typhlos* blind] a combining form denoting relationship to blindness.

**typhl(o)-**[2] [Gr. *typhlon* cecum, from *typhlos* blind] a combining form denoting relationship to the cecum.

**Typh·lo·coe·lum** (tif"lo-se'ləm) old name for a genus of trematodes, now classified as part of *Tracheophilus.*

**typh·lo·dic·li·di·tis** (tif"lo-dik"lĭ-di'tis) [*typhlo-*[2] + Gr. *diklis* door + *-itis*] inflammation of the ileocecal valve.

**typh·lol·o·gy** (tif-lol'ə-je) [*typhlo-*[1] + *-logy*] the study of blindness.

**typh·lo·pexy** (tif'lo-pek"se) [*typhlo-*[2] + *-pexy*] operative suspension and fixation of the cecum.

**typh·lo·sis** (tif-lo'sis) [Gr. *typhlōsis* a making blind] blindness.

**typh·los·to·my** (tif-los'tə-me) [*typhlo*[2] + *-stomy*] cecostomy.

**typh·lot·o·my** (tif-lot'ə-me) [*typhlo*[2] + *-tomy*] cecotomy.

**ty·pho·bac·ter·in** (ti″fo-bak′tər-in) typhoid vaccine.

**ty·phoid** (ti′foid) [Gr. *typhōdes* like smoke; delirious] [MeSH: Typhoid] 1. typhus-like. 2. see under *fever.* 3. typhoidal.
**fowl t.,** an acute infectious disease of fowl caused by *Salmonella enteritidis,* serotype *gallinarum,* marked by drowsiness, anorexia, extreme weakness, and usually diarrhea, finally ending in death in four days to two weeks after onset. Called also *Klein's disease.*
**provocation t.,** the systemic reaction to the endotoxin of killed typhoid bacilli in typhoid vaccine.

**ty·phoid·al** (ti-foid′əl) pertaining or relating to or resembling typhoid fever; typhoid. See also *enteric fever,* under *fever.*

**ty·phous** (ti′fəs) pertaining to or resembling typhus.

**ty·phus** (ti′fəs) [Gr. *typhos* stupor arising from fever] a group of acute, arthropod-borne infections caused by rickettsiae that are closely related clinically and pathologically but differ in signs and symptoms and severity; all are characterized by severe headache, chills, high fever, stupor, and a macular, maculopapular, petechial, or papulovesicular eruption. The three entities making up the group are *epidemic t.,* its recrudescent form *(Brill-Zinsser disease),* and *murine t.* Called also *typhus fever.* In English-speaking countries, often used alone to refer to epidemic typhus, whereas in several European languages it refers to typhoid fever.
**Australian tick t.,** Queensland tick t.
**canine t.,** Stuttgart disease.
**cat flea t.,** a flea-borne form of typhus clinically similar to murine typhus, caused by *Rickettsia felis* and transmitted by the cat flea *(Ctenocephalides felis).*
**classic t.,** epidemic t.
**endemic t.,** murine t.
**epidemic t.,** the classic, louse-borne form of typhus, caused by *Rickettsia prowazekii,* which is transmitted from person to person by the human body louse, *Pediculus humanus corporis,* although the organism can also grow in the head louse, *P. humanus capitis.* Characteristics include abrupt onset, chills, fever, malaise, headache that progresses in severity, backache, and myalgia; an eruption that may be macular, maculopapular, or petechial and spreads from the trunk to cover the entire body except for the face, palms, and soles; and central nervous system involvement that progresses from dullness to stupor and sometimes coma and death. Recrudescences occur (see *Brill-Zinsser disease,* under *disease*). Epidemic typhus has been known by various names, including *camp, jail, prison, ship,* and *war fever, European t.,* and *exanthematous t.*
**European t.,** epidemic t.
**exanthematic t. of São Paulo,** Rocky Mountain spotted fever.
**t. exanthematique, exanthematous t.,** epidemic t.
**flea-borne t.,** murine t.
**flying squirrel t., flying squirrel–associated t.,** an acute infectious disease occurring in the southeastern United States, particularly during the winter months, caused by *Rickettsia prowazekii,* which is transmitted to humans by the fleas and lice of the flying squirrel; it is clinically similar to epidemic typhus but has a lower mortality rate.
**Gubler-Robin t.,** the renal form of typhus.
**Indian tick t.,** boutonneuse fever.
**Kenya tick t.,** boutonneuse fever.
**latent t.,** Brill-Zinsser disease.
**louse-borne t.,** epidemic t.
**Manchurian t.,** murine t.
**Mexican t.,** murine t.
**mite-borne t.,** scrub t.
**Moscow t.,** murine t.
**murine t.,** an acute, flea-borne endemic infectious disease clinically similar to but milder than epidemic typhus; caused by *Rickettsia typhi,* which is transmitted from rats to humans chiefly by the rat flea, *Xenopsylla cheopis.* Infections identical or nearly identical to murine typhus have been known by various names, including *Congo red fever, Manchurian, Mexican,* or *Moscow t.,* and *tabardillo* or *tarbadillo.* See also *Toulon t.* and *urban t.*
**North Asian tick t.,** Siberian tick t.
**North Queensland tick t.,** Queensland tick t.
**Queensland tick t.,** an acute, febrile, exanthematous disease marked by a primary lesion (tache noire), caused by *Rickettsia australis,* and transmitted by the Australian ticks *Ixodes holocyclus* and *I. tasmani.* Called also *Australian* and *North Queensland tick t.*
**recrudescent t.,** Brill-Zinsser disease.
**São Paulo t.,** Rocky Mountain spotted fever.
**scrub t.,** an acute typhuslike infectious disease caused by *Rickettsia tsutsugamushi,* transmitted by the bite of infected larval trombiculid mites (chiggers), occurring chiefly in Asia and the southern and western Pacific, and characterized chiefly by the formation of a pathognomonic primary cutaneous lesion or eschar at the site of inoculation (tache noire) accompanied by regional lymphadenopathy, fever, and a maculopapular rash. It has many synonyms and local names, including *akamushi, shimamushi, island,* or *tsutsugamushi disease; inundation, island, Japanese flood, Japanese river, Kedani, Mossman,* or *tsutsugamushi fever;* and *mite-borne* or *tropical t.*
**shop t.,** urban t.
**Siberian tick t.,** a relatively mild, acutely febrile, spotted fever, characterized by headache, malaise, conjunctival injection, a maculopapular rash, and a primary ulcerative lesion at the site of the tick bite; it occurs in north, central, and east Asia. The causative agent is *Rickettsia sibirica,* which is transmitted by ticks of the genera *Dermacentor* and *Haemaphysalis.* Called also *North Asian tick t.*
**tick t., tick-borne t.,** Rocky Mountain spotted fever; also, any tick-borne infectious disease (see *tick fever,* under *fever*).
**Toulon t.,** a mild form of murine typhus occurring in the Mediterranean region.
**tropical t.,** scrub t.
**urban t.,** a mild form of murine typhus observed in indoor workers in Malaysia and the Mediterranean region; called also *shop t.*

**typ·i·cal** (tip′ĭ-kəl) [Gr. *typikos*] presenting the distinctive features of any type.

**typ·ing** (tīp′ing) determination of the type category to which an individual, object, or other entity belongs; e.g., bacteria, blood cells, cell cultures, or tissues.
**t. of blood,** classification of the blood with reference to various erythrocytic membrane antigens. See *blood group.*
**HLA t.,** determination of the HLA antigens possessed by an individual. Class I antigens (HLA-A, -B, and -C) are detected by lymphocyte microcytotoxicity assay using standard typing sera. Class II antigens are detected by one-way mixed lymphocyte reactions (MLR) using panels of homozygous typing cells (HTC); they may also be identified by primed lymphocyte typing (PLT). DR Class II antigens are also detected by lymphocyte microtoxicity assay using B-lymphocytes and anti-DR antibody types. HLA typing is used to identify compatible donors and recipients for transplantation or platelet or granulocyte transfusion, to establish associations of HLA antigens with diseases, and in paternity testing.
**phage t.,** characterization of bacteria, extending to strain differences, by demonstration of susceptibility to one or more (a spectrum) races of bacteriophage; widely applied to staphylococci, typhoid bacilli, etc., for epidemiological purposes.
**primed lymphocyte t. (PLT),** a technique used for typing of Class II HLA antigens: unknown cells are exposed to a panel of lymphocytes primed against specific HLA antigens by prior coculture with stimulator cells that matched the primed cells at all but one HLA locus; when restimulated by the same HLA antigen the primed cells give a secondary proliferative response, which shows that the unknown cells bear the same antigen as the stimulator cells.
**tissue t.,** HLA t.

**ty·po·dont** (ti′po-dont) an artificial model that contains artificial teeth or natural teeth that are used for teaching exercises.

**ty·pol·o·gy** (ti-pol′ə-je) the study of types; the science of classifying, as bacteria according to type.

**ty·po·scope** (ti′po-skōp) [Gr. *typos* type + *-scope*] an instrument to aid amblyopia and help cataract patients in reading.

**ty·pus** (ti′pəs) [L.] type.
**t. degenerati′vus amstelodamen′sis,** de Lange's syndrome.

**Tyr** tyrosine.

**ty·ra·mine** (ti′rə-mēn) [MeSH: Tyramine] a decarboxylation product of tyrosine, which may be converted to cresol and phenol; closely related structurally to epinephrine and norepinephrine, it has a similar but weaker action. It is found in decayed animal tissue, ripe cheese, and ergot.

**ty·re·sin** (ti-re′sin) a principle derivable from the venom of serpents and from the juice of mushrooms; it was thought to be an antidote for snake poisoning.

**tyr(o)-** [Gr. *tyros* cheese] a combining form denoting relationship to cheese.

**ty·ro·ci·din** (ti″ro-si′din) tyrocidine.

**ty·ro·ci·dine** (ti″ro-si′din) [MeSH: Tyrocidine] a crystalline polypeptide antibiotic substance which is the major component of tyrothricin, the lesser component being gramicidin.

**Ty·rode's solution** (ti′rōdz) [Maurice Vejux *Tyrode,* American pharmacologist, 1878–1930] see under *solution.*

**ty·rog·e·nous** (ti-roj′ə-nəs) [*tyro-* + *-genous*] originating in cheese.

**Ty·rog·ly·phus** (ti-rog′lĭ-fəs) [*tyro-* + Gr. *glyphein* to carve] *Tyrophagus.*
**T. si′ro,** *Acarus siro.*

**ty·roid** (ti′roid) [*tyro-* + *-oid*] caseous; resembling cheese.

**ty·ro·ma·to·sis** (ti″ro-mə-to′sis) a condition characterized by caseous degeneration.

**ty·ro·pa·no·ate so·di·um** (ti″ro-pə-no′āt) a diagnostic radiopaque medium for use in cholecystography.

**Ty·roph·a·gus** (ti-rof′ə-gəs) the meal mites, a genus of pale, soft-bodied mites of the family Acaridae; called also *Tyroglyphus.*
**T. castella′ni,** the copra mite, the species that causes copra itch.
**T. fari′nae,** the flour mite, found in flour mills and granaries.
**T. lon′gior,** the cheese mite, which has been reported from both the urinary and digestive tracts and may be found in feces.
**T. si′ro,** *Acarus siro.*

**ty·ros·amine** (ti-rōs′ə-mēn) tyramine.

**ty·ro·sin·ase** (ti-ro′sin-ās) a monophenol monooxygenase (q.v.); it can also act as a catechol oxidase (q.v.). Absence of enzyme activity, an autosomal recessive trait, leads to tyrosinase-negative oculocutaneous albinism.

**ty·ro·sine** (ti′ro-sēn) [MeSH: Tyrosine] a crystallizable, nonessential amino acid, *β-p*-hydroxyphenylalanine, found in most proteins and synthesized metabolically from phenylalanine; it is a precursor of thyroid hormones, catecholamines, and melanin. Symbols Tyr and Y. See also table at *amino acid.*

**ty·ro·sine ami·no·trans·fer·ase** (ti′ro-sēn ə-me″no-trans′fər-ās) tyrosine transaminase.

**ty·ro·sine hy·droxy·lase** (ti′ro-sēn hi-drok′sə-lās) tyrosine 3-monooxygenase.

**ty·ro·sine ki·nase** (ti′ro-sēn ki′nās) protein-tyrosine kinase.

**ty·ro·sin·e·mia** (ti″ro-sĭ-ne′me-ə) an aminoacidopathy of tyrosine metabolism characterized by hypertyrosinemia, tyrosinuria, and urinary excretion of related metabolites such as *p*-hydroxyphenylpyruvic acid. Several forms exist: *type I, type II, neonatal t.* (q.v.), and *hawkinsinuria* (q.v.). *Type I* is due to deficiency of fumarylacetoacetase, an autosomal recessive trait. It is characterized by accumulation of succinylacetoacetate and succinylacetone, leading to secondary deficiencies in porphobilinogen synthase and other enzymes and subsequent hepatorenal damage. Its *acute* form shows onset soon after birth, with cabbagelike odor and death from liver failure in infancy; its *chronic* form is characterized by chronic liver disease, renal tubular dysfunction, hypophosphatemic rickets, and death in childhood. *Type II* is an oculocutaneous syndrome due to deficiency of hepatic tyrosine transaminase, an autosomal recessive trait, and is clinically marked by the crystallization of the accumulated tyrosine in the epidermis as palmoplantar hyperkeratoses and in the corneas as herpetiform ulcers and frequently by mental retardation; it is called also *Richner-Hanhart syndrome.* See also *hyperphenylalaninemia.*
**hepatorenal t.,** t., type I.
**hereditary t.,** t., type I.
**neonatal t.,** an asymptomatic, transitory, neonatal disorder of uncertain etiology, characterized by increased serum tyrosine and phenylalanine and urinary tyrosine and related metabolites. It may result in mild mental retardation.

**ty·ro·sine 3-mono·oxy·ge·nase** (ti′ro-sēn mon″o-ok′sə-jən-ās) [EC 1.14.16.2] [MeSH: Tyrosine 3-Monooxygenase] a monooxygenase that activates molecular oxygen to catalyze the hydroxylation of tyrosine to dopa; it requires the cofactor tetrahydrobiopterin. The enzyme occurs in the brain and is inactivated in malignant hyperphenylalaninemia.

**ty·ro·sine trans·am·i·nase** (ti′ro-sēn trans-am′ĭ-nās) [EC 2.6.1.5] [MeSH: Tyrosine Transaminase] an enzyme of the transferase class that catalyzes the transamination of tyrosine to form the keto acid *p*-hydroxyphenylpyruvate as the first step in the catabolism of tyrosine. Deficiency of the enzyme, an autosomal recessive trait, causes tyrosinemia, type II.

**ty·ro·sin·o·sis** (ti″ro-sĭ-no′sis) older term for tyrosinemia, used particularly for tyrosinemia, type I.

**ty·ro·sin·uria** (ti″ro-sĭ-nu′re-ə) the presence of tyrosine in urine, as in tyrosinemia.

**ty·ro·sis** (ti-ro′sis) caseation, def. 2.

**ty·ro·syl** (ti′ro-səl) the acyl radical of tyrosine.

**ty·ro·syl·uria** (ti″ro-səl-u′re-ə) the increased urinary excretion of para-hydroxyphenyl compounds derived from tyrosine, as in tyrosinemia.

**ty·ro·thri·cin** (ti″ro-thri′sin) [MeSH: Tyrothricin] an antibiotic substance isolated from the soil bacillus *Bacillus brevis,* occurring as a white, grayish white, or brownish white powder, consisting principally of two polypeptides, the major one being tyrocidine and the other gramicidin. It is effective against many gram-positive bacteria, and is applied topically in pyodermic, ocular, and other localized infections due to susceptible organisms.

**Tyr·rell's fascia, hook** (tir′əlz) [Frederick *Tyrrell,* English anatomist, 1793–1843] see *septum rectovesicale,* and see under *hook.*

**Ty·son's crypts (glands)** (ti′sənz) [Edward *Tyson,* English physician and anatomist, 1650–1708] glandulae preputiales.

**ty·so·ni·an** (ti-so′ne-ən) named for Edward *Tyson.*

**ty·so·ni·tis** (ti″sə-ni′tis) inflammation of Tyson's glands.

**ty·vel·ose** (ti′vəl-ōs) an unusual sugar found in the lipopolysaccharides of certain serotypes of *Salmonella.* It is the determinant of somatic (O) antigen factor 9 of group D salmonellae.

**Ty·zine** (ti′zēn) trademark for preparations of tetrahydrozoline hydrochloride.

**Tyz·ze·ria** (ti-zēr′e-ə) a genus of coccidian protozoa (suborder Eimeriina, order Eucoccidiida), characterized by the presence of oocysts containing eight naked sporozoites. *T. pernicio′sa* is highly pathogenic for domestic ducklings, being parasitic in the small intestine, especially in the upper half.

**Tzanck cell, test** (tsahngk) [Arnault *Tzanck,* Russian dermatologist in Paris, 1886–1954] see under *cell* and *test.*

**Tza·neen disease** (tsah-nēn′) [*Tzaneen,* South Africa, where the disease was first reported] see under *disease.*

**tzet·ze** (tset′se) tsetse.

# U

**U** symbol for *uranium, uracil* or *uridine, international unit of enzyme activity,* and *unit.*

**u** symbol for *atomic mass unit.*

**uar·thri·tis** (u″ahr-thri′tis) gouty arthritis.

**uber·ous** (u′bər-əs) prolific.

**uber·ty** (u′bər-te) [L. *ubertas* fruitfulness] fertility.

**ubiq·ui·nol** (u-bik′wĭ-nol) the reduced form of a ubiquinone.

**ubi·qui·nol–cy·to·chrome-*c* re·duc·tase** (u-bik′wĭ-nol si′to-krōm rĕ-duk′tās) [EC 1.10.2.2] an enzyme complex of the inner mitochondrial membrane that catalyzes the transfer of electrons from ubiquinol to cytochrome *c,* oxidizing the former and reducing the latter in a reaction of the electron transport chain (q.v.). The enzyme contains cytochromes *b* and $c_1$ and iron-sulfur prosthetic groups and is associated with proton translocation and the resultant synthesis of ATP. Called also *ubiquinol dehydrogenase.*

**ubiq·ui·nol de·hy·dro·gen·ase** (u-bik′wĭ-nol de-hi′dro-jən-ās) ubiquinol–cytochrome-*c* reductase.

**ubiq·ui·none** (u-bik′wĭ-nōn) [MeSH: Ubiquinone] a quinone derivative with a variable length side chain of isoprene units; in mammals it usually contains ten such units. It occurs in the lipid core of inner mitochondrial membranes and functions in the electron transport chain (q.v.), acting as a point of entry for electrons from FAD and transferring them to ubiquinol–cytochrome-*c* reductase. Abbreviated Q or $Q_{10}$. Formerly called *coenzyme Q.*

**ud·der** (ud′ər) the mammary organ of cattle and certain other mammals; within the large baglike envelope are two or more glands, each having a teat.

**UDP** uridine diphosphate.

**UDP-*N*-ac·e·tyl·ga·lac·to·sa·mine** (as″ə-tēl-gal″ak-tōs′ə-mēn) a nucleotide derivative of *N*-acetylgalactosamine; it donates acetylgalactosamine groups in the synthesis of glycosaminoglycans.

**UDP-*N*-ac·e·tyl·glu·co·sa·mine** (as″ə-tēl″gloo-kōs′ə-mēn) a nucleotide derivative of *N*-acetylglucosamine; it donates acetylglucosamine groups in the synthesis of glycosaminoglycans and is the parent compound for other hexosamines.

**UDP-*N*-ac·e·tyl·glu·co·sa·mine 4-epim·er·ase** (as″ə-tēl″gloo-kōs′ə-mēn ə-pim′ə-rās) [EC 5.1.3.7] an enzyme of the isomerase class that catalyzes the interconversion of the epimers UDP-*N*-acetylglucosamine and UDP-*N*-acetylgalactosamine.

**UDP-*N*-ac·e·tyl·glu·co·sa·mine–ly·so·so·mal-en·zyme *N*-ac·e·tyl·glu·co·sa·mine·phos·pho·trans·fer·ase** (as″ə-tēl″gloo-kōs′ə-mēn li″so-so′məl en′zīm as″ə-tēl″gloo-kōs″ə-mēn-fos″fo-trans′fər-ās) [EC 2.7.8.17] an enzyme of the transferase class that catalyzes a step in the synthesis of the mannose 6-phosphate recognition markers necessary on most lysosomal enzymes for internalization of the enzymes into lysosomes. Deficiency of the enzyme, an autosomal recessive trait, causes mucolipidosis types II and III. Called also N-*acetylglucosaminylphosphotransferase.*

**UDP-*N*-ac·e·tyl·glu·co·sa·mine py·ro·phos·phor·y·lase** (as″ə-tēl″gloo-kōs′ə-mēn pi″ro-fos-for′ə-lās) [EC 2.7.7.23] an enzyme of the transferase class that catalyzes the attachment of a UMP group from UTP to *N*-acetylglucosamine 1-phosphate, forming UDP-*N*-acetylglucosamine.

**UDP·ga·lac·tose** (gə-lak′tōs) a nucleotide derivative of galactose; it donates galactosyl groups in the synthesis of lactose, polysaccharides, and glycosaminoglycans and is an intermediate in the metabolism of galactose.

**UDP·ga·lac·tose 4-epim·er·ase** (gə-lak′tōs ə-pim′ər-ās) UDPglucose 4-epimerase.

**UDP·glu·cose** (gloo′kōs) a nucleotide derivative of glucose; it donates glucosyl groups in the synthesis of glycogen and other polysaccharides. It is the parent compound from which the other UDPhexoses are synthesized.

**UDP·glu·cose 6-de·hy·dro·gen·ase** (gloo′kōs de-hi′dro-jən-ās) [EC 1.1.1.22] an enzyme of the oxidoreductase class that catalyzes the oxidation of UDPglucose to UDPglucuronate, using $NAD^+$ as an electron acceptor.

**UDP·glu·cose 4-epim·er·ase** (gloo′kōs ə-pim′ər-ās) [EC 5.1.3.2] an enzyme of the isomerase class that catalyzes the interconversion of UDPgalactose and UDPglucose in the metabolism of galactose, requiring $NAD^+$ as a cofactor. Deficiency of the enzyme in erythrocytes, an autosomal recessive trait, causes accumulation in red cells of galactose 1-phosphate. Called also *UDPgalactose 4-epimerase.*

**UDP·glu·cose–hex·ose-1-phos·phate uri·dyl·yl·trans·fer·ase** (gloo″kōs hek″sōs fos′fāt u-rĭ-dil-″əl-trans′fər-ās) [EC 2.7.7.12] an enzyme of the transferase class that catalyzes the exchange of galactose 1-phosphate for the glucose 1-phosphate moiety of UDPglucose, forming UDPgalactose and glucose 1-phosphate. The reaction is the second step in the utilization of galactose as a fuel. Lack of enzyme activity, an autosomal recessive trait, causes galactosemia. Called also *galactose 1-phosphate uridyltransferase, hexose 1-phosphate uridylyltransferase,* and *uridyl transferase.*

**UDP·glu·cose py·ro·phos·pho·ry·lase** (gloo′kōs pi″ro-fos-for′ə-lās) UTP–glucose-1-phosphate uridylyltransferase.

**UDP·glu·cu·ro·nate** (gloo-ku′ro-nāt) a nucleotide derivative of glucuronate; it donates glucuronate groups for the synthesis of glucuronides, polysaccharides, and glycosaminoglycans, as well as for the reduction and solubilization of bilirubin and the detoxification of foreign phenols and amines in the liver.

**UDP·glu·cu·ro·nate–bil·i·ru·bin - glu·cu·ro·no·syl·trans·fer·ase** (gloo-ku′ro-nāt bil″ĭ-roo′bin gloo″ku-ron″ə-səl-trans′-fər-ās) former nomenclature for an enzyme that is now described formally by general classification as a glucuronosyltransferase.

**UDP·glu·cu·ro·nate de·car·boxy·lase** (gloo″ku-ro′nāt de-kahr-bok′sə-lās) [EC 4.1.1.35] an enzyme of the lyase class that catalyzes the decarboxylation of UDPglucuronate to form UDPxylose.

**UDP·hex·ose** a nucleotide consisting of hexose linked to the terminal phosphoryl group of uridine diphosphate (q.v.). The UDPhexoses act as activated intermediates in the syntheses of polysaccharides, glycosaminoglycans, and glycolipids.

**UDP·id·uron·ate** (īd″u-ron′āt) a nucleotide derivative of iduronate, synthesized from UDPglucuronate; it donates iduronate groups in proteoglycan synthesis.

**UDP·xy·lose** (zi′lōs) a nucleotide derivative of xylose, synthesized from UDPglucuronate; it donates xylose groups in the synthesis of proteoglycans.

**Udrán·szky's test** (oo-drahn′skēz) [László *Udránszky,* Hungarian physiologist, 1862–1914] see under *test.*

**Uf·fel·mann's test** (oof′el-mahnz) [Julius August Christian *Uffelmann,* German physician, 1837–1894] see under *test.*

**Uhl's anomaly** (yo͞olz) [Henry Stephen Magraw *Uhl,* American physician, born 1921] see under *anomaly.*

**UK** urokinase.

**ulag·an·ac·te·sis** (u-lag″an-ak-te′sis) [*ul-*[2] + *aganaktēsis* irritation] irritation or itching of the gingiva.

**ulal·gia** (u-lal′jə) [*ul-*[2] + *-algia*] gingivalgia.

**ulat·ro·phy** (u-lat′ro-fe) [*ul-*[2] + *atrophy*] atrophy of the gingiva associated with its recession and exposure of the root portion of the tooth.

**afunctional u.,** ulatrophy occurring in congenital malocclusion.

**atrophic u.,** ischemic u.

**calcic u.,** ulatrophy that is caused by the presence of salivary concretions.

**ischemic u.,** ulatrophy due to deficient blood supply. Called also *atrophic u.*

**traumatic u.,** ulatrophy due to gingival trauma.

**ul·cer** (ul′sər) [L. *ulcus;* Gr. *helkōsis*] [MeSH: Ulcer] a local defect, or excavation, of the surface of an organ or tissue, which is produced by the sloughing of inflammatory necrotic tissue.

**Aden u.,** Old World cutaneous leishmaniasis.
**amebic u.,** the ulcerous lesion of amebiasis cutis.
**amputating u.,** ulceration which encircles a part and destroys the tissues to the bone.
**anastomotic u.,** ulcer at the anastomotic site occurring as a complication after gastroenterostomy performed for duodenal ulcer.
**aphthous u.,** the ulcerative lesion of recurrent aphthous stomatitis.
**atheromatous u.,** a loss of intima over an atheroma, often causing thrombus formation.
**atonic u.,** a chronic ulcer with unhealthy granulations.
**Barrett's u.,** chronic peptic ulcer of the esophagus, usually associated with heterotopic gastric mucosa and stricture formation; it is usually a late complication of reflux esophagitis.
**burrowing phagedenic u.,** 1. progressive synergistic gangrene. 2. Meleney's u. (def. 1).
**Buruli u.,** a cutaneous infection caused by *Mycobacterium ulcerans,* manifested by a small, firm, painless, movable subcutaneous nodule that enlarges and becomes fluctuant and ulcerates, leaving an undermined edge. It occurs principally in Uganda and Zaire but has also been seen elsewhere in Central Africa, in Southeast Asia, in Australia, and sometimes in Central and South America.
**catarrhal corneal u.,** an ulcer near the corneal limbus seen in catarrhal conjunctivitis.
**chancroid u.,** chancroid.
**chicle u., chiclero u.,** an endemic, zoonotic form of New World cutaneous leishmaniasis, found mainly in forest workers in the Yucatan and adjacent areas of Mexico, Belize, and Guatemala. It is caused by *Leishmania mexicana mexicana,* transmitted by *Lutzomyia olmeca,* and characterized by one or a few lesions that are usually self-limited and heal within 6 months, except when the pinna of the ear is involved, in which case over a period of many years the chronic lesion invades and slowly destroys the cartilage of the ear.
**chrome u.,** an ulcer produced by chromium or its salts; seen in tanners and others working in chromium. Called also *tanner's u.*
**concealed u.,** destructive inflammation affecting some internal tissue.
**corneal u.,** ulcerative keratitis.
**Cruveilhier's u.,** gastric u.
**Cushing's u.,** a peptic ulcer associated with manifest or occult lesions of the central nervous system.
**Cushing-Rokitansky u's,** Rokitansky-Cushing u.
**decubital u., decubitus u.,** an ulceration caused by prolonged pressure in a patient allowed to lie too still in bed for a long period of time; called also *decubitus, bed sore,* and *pressure u.* or *sore.*
**dendriform u., dendritic u.,** ulcer of the cornea branching in various directions, usually caused by herpes simplex infection.
**diabetic u.,** an ulcer, usually of the lower extremity, associated with diabetes mellitus. Cf. *diabetic gangrene.*
**Dieulafoy's u.,** Dieulafoy's vascular malformation.
**diphtheritic u.,** one whose surface is partly or entirely covered by a gray membrane, as in cutaneous diphtheria.
**duodenal u.,** a peptic ulcer in the duodenum.
**elusive u.,** Hunner's u.
**eosinophilic u.,** a type of rodent ulcer in cats, usually on the upper lip near a canine tooth and seldom pruritic or painful; it is part of the eosinophilic granuloma complex and may progress to a more serious lesion.
**Fenwick-Hunner u.,** Hunner's u.
**fistulous u.,** the ulcerated superficial end of a fistula.
**flask u.,** an ulcer of the intestine in amebic dysentery.
**follicular u.,** a small ulcer on the mucous membrane having its origin in a lymph follicle.
**gastric u.,** a peptic ulcer of the gastric mucosa.
**giant peptic u.,** a rare type of large peptic ulcer with characteristic clinical and radiological manifestations.
**girdle u.,** a tuberculous ulcer that spreads along the wall of the intestine in an encircling manner.
**gouty u.,** a superficial ulcer occurring over a gouty joint.
**gummatous u.,** a broken-down superficial gumma.
**Hunner's u.,** a lesion occurring in chronic interstitial cystitis, involving all the layers of the bladder wall, and appearing as a small brownish red patch on the mucosa; it tends to heal superficially and is notoriously difficult to detect.
**hypertensive ischemic u.,** a manifestation of infarction of the skin due to arteriolar occlusion as part of a longstanding vascular disease, seen especially in women in late middle age, and presenting as a red painful plaque on the leg or ankle that later breaks down into a superficial ulcer surrounded by a zone of purpuric erythema.
**hypopyon u.,** a corneal ulcer accompanied by hypopyon.
**Jacob's u.,** rodent ulcer, especially that of an eyelid.
**jejunal u.,** an ulcer of the jejunum; one developing after gastroenterostomy is called *secondary jejunal u.*
**kissing u's,** ulcers on directly opposing surfaces of the stomach, as on opposite sides of the lesser curvature.
**Kocher's dilatation u.,** ulceration occurring in a greatly distended intestine or in the course of ileus.
**Lipschütz u.,** ulcus vulvae acutum.
**lupoid u.,** a skin ulcer that simulates or resembles lupus.
**Mann-Williamson u.,** a progressive peptic ulcer produced in experimental animals by means of a gastric resection or gastroenterostomy.
**marginal u.,** a gastric ulcer in the jejunal mucosa near the site of a gastrojejunal anastomosis; called also *stoma u.*
**Marjolin's u.,** an ulcer seated upon an old cicatrix; it may degenerate into a squamous cell carcinoma with a propensity for metastasis.
**Meleney's u., Meleney's chronic undermining u.,** 1. a variety of progressive synergistic gangrene associated with the formation of burrowing cutaneous fissures and sinus tracts that open at distant sites. Called also *burrowing phagedenic u.* and *undermining burrowing u.* 2. progressive synergistic gangrene.
**Mooren's u.,** chronic serpiginous ulceration, usually bilateral, of the marginal cornea, seen in elderly individuals; it is of unknown etiology.
**neurogenic u., neurotrophic u.,** an ulcer resulting from separation of tissue from its nerve supply, as in sensory neuropathy.
**penetrating u.,** an ulcerative lesion which involves also the wall or substance of an adjacent organ.
**penetrating u. of foot,** plantar u.
**peptic u.,** an ulceration of the mucous membrane of the esophagus, stomach, or duodenum, caused by the action of the acid gastric juice.
**perambulating u.,** phagedenic u. (def. 1).
**perforating u.,** an ulcer which involves the entire thickness of an organ, as the foot, or the wall of the stomach or intestine, creating an opening on both surfaces.
**phagedenic u.,** 1. any of a group of conditions due to secondary bacterial invasion of a preexisting cutaneous lesion or the intact skin of a person with impaired resistance as a result of a systemic disease; it is characterized by necrotic ulceration associated with prominent tissue destruction. The group includes desert sore, Meleney's ulcer, and tropical phagedenic ulcer. Called also *perambulating u.* and *sloughing u.* 2. tropical phagedenic u.
**plantar u.,** a deep neurotrophic ulcer of the sole of the foot, resulting from repeated injury because of lack of sensation in the part; seen with diseases such as diabetes mellitus and leprosy. Called also *penetrating u. of foot* and *mal perforant du pied.*
**pneumococcus u.,** ulcus serpens corneae.
**pressure u.,** decubitus u.
**pudendal u.,** granuloma inguinale.
**ring u.,** fusion of foci of ulceration in the cornea to form a peripheral ring of ulceration.
**rodent u.,** ulcerating basal cell carcinoma of the skin.
**Rokitansky-Cushing u's,** an occasional ulcerative accompaniment of severe lesions of the central nervous system, affecting the lower third of the esophagus, the fundus of the stomach, or the duodenum.
**round u.,** gastric u.
**Saemisch's u.,** ulcus serpens corneae.
**sea anemone u.,** an intestinal ulcer in amebiasis, with a deep crater and partly necrotic undermined edges which are raised above the level of the surrounding mucosa.
**secondary jejunal u.,** see *jejunal u.*
**serpiginous corneal u.,** ulcus serpens corneae.
**simple u.,** a mild form of ulcer which is neither of septic origin nor the expression of a general disease.
**sloughing u.,** phagedenic u. (def. 1).
**soft u.,** chancroid.
**stasis u.,** ulceration on the ankle due to venous insufficiency and venous stasis.
**stercoraceous u., stercoral u.,** an ulcer caused by the pressure of impacted feces; also a fistulous ulcer through which fecal matter escapes.
**stoma u., stomal u.,** marginal u.
**stress u.,** a peptic ulcer, usually gastric, resulting from stress; possible predisposing factors include changes in the microcirculation of the gastric mucosa, increased permeability of the gastric mucosa barrier to $H^+$, and impaired cell proliferation.
**sublingual u.,** an ulcer on the frenum of the tongue.
**submucous u.,** Hunner's u.; so called because of the tendency of the lesion to heal superficially.
**symptomatic u.,** an ulcer that indicates some general disease.
**tanner's u.,** chrome u.
**trophic u.,** an ulcer due to imperfect nutrition of the part.
**trophoneurotic u.,** neurotrophic u.
**tropical u.,** 1. a lesion of cutaneous leishmaniasis. 2. tropical phagedenic u.
**tropical phagedenic u.,** a chronic, painful phagedenic ulcer usually occurring on the lower extremities of malnourished children in the tropics; the etiology is unknown but spirochetes, fusiform bacilli, and other bacteria are often present in the developing lesion, and protein and vitamin deficiency with lowered resistance to infection may play a role in the etiology. Called also *phagedenic u.* and *tropical u.,* and

also known by various native names and by names having only geographical significance.
**undermining burrowing u.,** 1. progressive synergistic gangrene. 2. Meleney's u. (def. 1).
**varicose u.,** one that is due to varicose veins, such as a stasis ulcer.
**venereal u.,** a nonspecific term referring to the formation of ulcers resembling chancre or chancroid around the external genitalia, both sexually transmitted and of other types.

**ul·cera** (ul'sər-ə) [L.] plural of *ulcus*.

**ul·cer·ate** (ul'sər-āt) [L. *ulcerare, ulceratus*] to become affected with ulceration.

**ul·cer·a·tion** (ul″sər-a'shən) [L. *ulceratio*] 1. the formation or development of an ulcer. 2. an ulcer.

**ul·cer·a·tive** (ul'sər-a″tiv) pertaining to or characterized by ulceration.

**ul·cero·gan·gre·nous** (ul″sər-o-gang'rə-nəs) characterized by both ulceration and gangrene; pertaining to a gangrenous ulcer.

**ul·cer·o·gen·ic** (ul″sər-o-jen'ik) causing ulceration; leading to the production of ulcers.

**ul·cero·gran·u·lo·ma** (ul″sər-o-gran″u-lo'mə) a granuloma developing on an ulcer.

**ul·cero·mem·bra·nous** (ul″sər-o-mem'brə-nəs) characterized by ulceration and by a membranous exudation.

**ul·cer·ous** (ul'sər-əs) [L. *ulcerosus*] 1. of the nature of an ulcer. 2. affected with ulceration.

**ul·cus** (ul'kəs) pl. *ul'cera* [L.] ulcer.
**u. am'bulans,** phagedenic ulcer.
**u. interdigita'le,** keratolysis of the horny layer of the skin between the toes, a disease similar to cracked heel.
**u. pe'netrans,** one that penetrates not into the peritoneal cavity but into an abutting organ.
**u. ser'pens cor'neae,** an ulcer of the cornea; a creeping central suppurative ulcer of the cornea due usually to pneumococcus. Called also *pneumococcus ulcer, Saemisch's ulcer,* and *serpiginous corneal ulcer.*
**u. sim'plex vesi'cae,** Hunner's ulcer.
**u. ventri'culi,** gastric ulcer.
**u. vul'vae acu'tum,** a nonvenereal, usually shallow lesion of the vulva, often associated with a febrile illness; its etiology is uncertain. Called also *Lipschütz's disease* and *Lipschütz ulcer.*

**ule-** see *ul(o)-*.

**ulec·to·my** (u-lek'tə-me) 1. [*ul-*[1] + *ectomy*] excision of scar tissue. 2. [*ul-*[2] + *ectomy*] gingivectomy.

**ule·gy·ria** (u″le-ji're-ə) [*ule-* + *gyr-* + *-ia*] a condition in which the cerebral gyri are narrow and distorted by scars, resulting from lesions existing in fetal life or early infancy.

**uler·y·the·ma** (u″lər-ĭ-the'mə) [*ul-*[1] + *erythēma* redness] an erythematous disease of the skin characterized by the formation of cicatrices and by atrophy.
**u. ophryo'genes,** keratosis pilaris affecting the follicles of the eyebrow hairs of young men, associated with erythema, and leading to scarring and atrophy; it is transmitted as an autosomal dominant trait.

**ulig·i·nous** (u-lij'ĭ-nəs) [L. *uliginosus* moist] muddy or slimy.

**uli·tis** (u-li'tis) gingivitis.

**Ull·mann's line** (ool'mahnz) [Emerich *Ullmann,* Hungarian surgeon, 1861–1937] see under *line.*

**Ull·rich-Feich·ti·ger syndrome** (ool'rik-fīk'tĭ-gər) [Otto *Ullrich,* German pediatrician, 1894–1957; H. *Feichtiger,* German physician, 20th century] see under *syndrome.*

**Ull·rich-Tur·ner syndrome** (o͞ol'rik-tər'nər) [O. *Ullrich;* Henry Hubert *Turner,* American endocrinologist, 1892–1970] Noonan's syndrome.

**Ul·mus** (ul'məs) [L. "elm"] the elms, a genus of trees of the family Ulmaceae. *U. ru'bra* Muhlenberg (*U. ful'va* Micheaux) is the slippery elm, source of slippery elm bark (see under *bark*).

**ul·na** (ul'nə) pl. *ul'nae* [L. "the arm"] [TA] [MeSH: Ulna] the inner and larger bone of the forearm, on the side opposite that of the thumb; it articulates with the humerus and with the head of the radius at its proximal end, and with the radius and bones of the carpus at the distal end. See Plate 45.

**ul·nad** (ul'nad) toward the ulna.

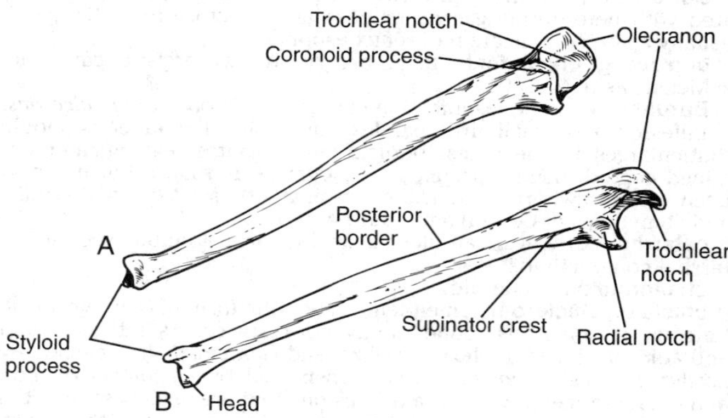

Ulna, anterior *(A)* and lateral *(B)* aspects.

**ul·nar** (ul'nər) [L. *ulnaris*] pertaining to the ulna or to the ulnar (medial) aspect of the arm as compared with the radial (lateral) aspect.

**ul·na·re** (əl-na're) [L.] os triquetrum.

**ul·na·ris** (əl-na'ris) [L., from *ulna,* q.v.] [TA] ulnar; a general term denoting relationship to the ulna or to the ulnar aspect of the forearm.

**ul·nen** (ul'nən) pertaining to the ulna alone.

**ul·no·car·pal** (ul″no-kahr'pəl) pertaining to the ulna and carpus.

**ul·no·ra·di·al** (ul″no-ra'de-əl) pertaining to the ulna and radius.

**ul(o)-**[1] [Gr. *oulē* scar] a combining form denoting relationship to a scar, or cicatrix. Also, *ule-*.

**ul(o)-**[2] [Gr. *oulon* gum] a combining form denoting relationship to the gingivae.

**ulo·glos·si·tis** (u″lo-glos-i'tis) [*ulo-*[2] + *glossitis*] gingivoglossitis.

**ulor·rha·gia** (u″lo-ra'jə) [*ulo-*[2] + *-rhagia*] hemorrhage from the gingivae.

**-ulose** a suffix indicating that the substance is a ketose.

**ulot·o·my** (u-lot'ə-me) 1. [*ulo-*[1] + *-tomy*] the cutting or division of scar tissue. 2. [*ulo-*[2] + *-tomy*] incision of the gingivae.

**ulo·trip·sis** (u″lo-trip'sis) [*ulo-*[2] + *tripsis*] revitalization of the gingivae by massage.

**ul·ti·mate** (ul'tĭ-mət) [L. *ultimus* last] the last or farthest; final or most remote.

**Ul·tane** (ul'tān) trademark for a preparation of sevoflurane.

**ul·ti·mi·ster·nal** (ul″tĭ-mĭ-stər'nəl) pertaining to the xiphoid process.

**ul·ti·mo·bran·chi·al** (ul″tĭ-mo-brang'ke-əl) [L. *ultimus* last + *branchial*] pertaining to or derived from the fifth pharyngeal pouch.

**ul·ti·mum mo·ri·ens** (ul'tĭ-məm mo're-ənz) [L. "last to die"] the right atrium; said to be the last part of the body to cease moving in death.

**Ul·ti·va** (ul-te'vah) trademark for a preparation of remifentanil hydrochloride.

**ult. praes.** abbreviation for L. *ul'timum praescriptus,* last prescribed.

**ultra-** [L. "beyond"] a prefix denoting excess, or beyond.

**ul·tra·brachy·ce·phal·ic** (ul″trə-brak″e-sə-fal'ik) [*ultra-* + *brachy-* + *cephal-* + *-ic*] pertaining to or characterized by an extremely broad, short skull, with a cephalic index of more than 90.0.

**ul·tra·cen·trif·u·ga·tion** (ul″trə-sən-trif″u-ga'shən) [MeSH: Ultracentrifugation] subjection to the action of an ultracentrifuge.

**ul·tra·cen·tri·fuge** (ul″trə-sen'trĭ-fūj) a centrifuge with an exceedingly high rate of rotation which will separate and sediment the molecules of a substance.

**ul·tra·di·an** (əl-trə'de-ən) [*ultra-* + L. *dies* day] pertaining to the rhythmic repetition of certain phenomena in living organisms occurring in cycles of greater frequency than circadian, that is, more frequently than once a day. Cf. *circadian* and *infradian.*

**ul·tra·dol·i·cho·ce·phal·ic** (ul″trə-dol″ĭ-ko-sə-fal'ik) [*ultra-* + *dolichocephalic*] pertaining to or characterized by an extremely long, narrow head, with a cephalic index of not more than 64.9.

**ul·tra·fil·ter** (ul″trə-fil'tər) an apparatus for performing ultrafiltration through a semipermeable membrane.

**ul·tra·fil·trate** (ul″trə-fil'trāt) the liquid that has passed through an ultrafilter.

**ul·tra·fil·tra·tion** (ul″trə-fil-tra'shən) [MeSH: Ultrafiltration] filtration through filters with minute pores, thus allowing the separation of extremely minute particles. It occurs naturally, as in the filtration of plasma at the capillary membrane, and is also performed clinically and in the laboratory, such as in hemodialysis, where it involves the bulk movement of solute and solvent across the membrane down pressure gradients and is usually performed under pressure to accelerate the process.

**Ul·tram** (ul'tram) trademark for a preparation of tramadol hydrochloride.

**ul·tra·mi·cro·chem·is·try** (ul″trə-mi″kro-kem'is-tre) the chemical study of materials in extremely minute quantities.

**ul·tra·mi·cro·pi·pet** (ul″trə-mi″kro-pi-pet′) a pipet designed to handle extremely small quantities of liquid (less than 0.005 mL).

**ul·tra·mi·cro·scope** (ul″trə-mi'kro-skōp) a special darkfield microscope for the examination of particles of colloidal size. See *darkfield illumination,* under *illumination,* and *darkfield microscope,* under *microscope.*

**ul·tra·mi·cro·scop·ic** (ul″trə-mi″kro-skop'ik) 1. pertaining to the ultramicroscope. 2. too small to be seen with an ordinary microscope.

**ul·tra·mi·cros·co·py** (ul″trə-mi-kros'kə-pe) the employment of the ultramicroscope.

**ul·tra·mi·cro·tome** (ul″trə-mi'kro-tōm) an instrument for making very thin tissue sections for electron microscopy.

**ul·tra·phago·cy·to·sis** (ul″trə-fag″o-si-to'sis) ingestion of particles of submicroscopic dimensions.

**ul·tra·pro·phy·lax·is** (ul″trə-pro″fə-lak'sis) prophylaxis directed toward the prevention of diseased or abnormal children by regulation of the marriage of the unfit.

**ul·tra·son·ic** (ul″trə-son'ik) [*ultra-* + L. *sonus* sound] [MeSH: Ultrasonics] pertaining to mechanical radiant energy having a frequency beyond the upper limit of perception by the human ear, that is, beyond about 20,000 Hz (20 KHz); called also *supersonic.* See also *ultrasonics.*

**ul·tra·son·ics** (ul″trə-son'iks) [MeSH: Ultrasonics] the study and use of ultrasonic waves; these could include any frequencies above 20 kHz, but the term is usually restricted to those above 500 kHz. Such waves are injurious to living tissue because of their thermal effects, but controlled doses may be used therapeutically to break down pathologic tissue or diagnostically in ultrasonography.

**ul·tra·sono·gram** (ul″trə-son'o-gram) the record obtained by ultrasonography.

**ul·tra·sono·graph·ic** (ul″trə-son″o-graf'ik) pertaining to or accomplished by ultrasonography; called also *sonographic.*

**ul·tra·so·nog·ra·phy** (ul″trə-sə-nog'rə-fe) [MeSH: Ultrasonography] the visualization of deep structures of the body by recording the reflections of (echoes of) pulses of ultrasonic waves directed into the tissues. Diagnostic ultrasonography, as in echocardiography and echoencephalography, utilizes a frequency range of 1 million to 10 million hertz (cycles per second), or 1 to 10 MHz. Such sound waves are transmissible only in liquids and solids. See also *scan* (def. 2). Called also *echography* and *sonography.*
**Doppler u.,** that in which the shifts in frequency between emitted ultrasonic waves and their echoes are used to measure the velocities of moving objects, based on the principle of the Doppler effect. The waves may be continuous or pulsed; the technique is frequently used to examine cardiovascular blood flow (Doppler echocardiography). See also *pulsed wave Doppler u., continuous wave Doppler u.,* and *color flow Doppler imaging,* under *imaging.*
**duplex u.,** a type that combines real-time with Doppler ultrasonography.
**Doppler u., continuous wave,** Doppler ultrasonography using two transducers, with one continually transmitting and the other continually recording the ultrasonic waves. It is used to record signals with very high velocities, such as occur in severely stenotic valves, but cannot provide spatial resolution of the signals. Cf. *pulsed wave Doppler u.*
**Doppler u., pulsed wave,** Doppler ultrasonography in which a single transducer alternately transmits and records ultrasonic waves. It can be used to determine the site of signal origin precisely but cannot record signals with high velocities. Cf. *continuous wave Doppler u.*
**endorectal u.,** endosonography of the rectum with a transducer on a rigid rectal probe, used particularly in the staging of rectal cancer.
**endoscopic u.,** endosonography of the esophagus, stomach, or duodenum to provide views of the mediastinum or abdominal organs.
**gray-scale u.,** a B-scan technique in which a television video-scan converter amplifies and processes echoes according to their strength into a visual display ranging from white for the strongest echoes to varying shades of gray.
**intravascular u.,** visualization of the interior of blood vessels by ultrasound; the transducer is mounted on the end of a catheter that is introduced percutaneously.
**real-time u.,** a series of ultrasound images produced in rapid succession so that the video display shows motion of an organ or part.

**ul·tra·so·nom·e·try** (ul″trə-sə-nom'ə-tre) the measurement of certain physical properties of biologic fluids by means of ultrasound.

**ul·tra·sound** (ul'trə-sound) 1. mechanical radiant energy (see *sound*) with a frequency greater than 20,000 hertz (cycles per second); see *ultrasonics.* 2. ultrasonography.

**ul·tra·struc·ture** (ul'trə-struk″chər) the arrangement of the smallest elements making up a body; the structure beyond the resolution power of the light microscope, i.e., the structure visible only under the ultramicroscope and electron microscope. Called also *fine structure.*

**Ultra·Tag RBC** (ul'trə-tag″) trademark for a kit for the preparation of technetium Tc 99m red blood cells.

**Ul·tra·tard** (ul'trə-tahrd) trademark for preparations of extended insulin zinc suspension.

**ul·tra·vi·o·let** (ul″trə-vi'ə-lət) beyond the violet end of the spectrum; said of electromagnetic rays or radiation between the violet rays and the x-rays, that is, with wavelengths between 200 and 400 nm. These rays have powerful actinic and chemical properties, inducing sunburn and tanning of the skin and producing ergocalciferol (vitamin $D_2$) by their action on ergosterol in the skin.
**u. A (UVA),** ultraviolet radiation with wavelengths between 320 and 400 nm, comprising over 99 per cent of ultraviolet radiation reaching the surface of the earth. UVA enhances the harmful effects of ultraviolet B radiation and is also responsible for some photosensitivity reactions; it is used therapeutically in the treatment of a variety of skin disorders.
**u. B (UVB),** ultraviolet radiation with wavelengths between 290 and 320 nm, comprising less than 1 per cent of the ultraviolet radiation reaching the earth's surface. UVB causes sunburn and a number of damaging photochemical changes within cells, including damage to DNA, leading to premature aging of the skin, premalignant and malignant changes, and a variety of photosensitivity reactions; it is also used therapeutically in the treatment of skin disorders.
**u. C (UVC),** ultraviolet radiation with wavelengths between 200 and 290 nm; all UVC radiation is filtered out by the ozone layer so that none reaches the earth's surface. UVC is germicidal and is also used in ultraviolet phototherapy.
**far u.,** ultraviolet radiation of shortest wavelength, between 200 and 300 nm.
**near u.,** that portion of the ultraviolet near the visible spectrum, that is, with wavelengths between 300 and 400 nm.

**ul·tra·vis·i·ble** (ul″trə-viz'ĭ-bəl) ultramicroscopic.

**Ul·tra·vist** (ul'trə-vist″) trademark for a preparation of iopromide.

**ul·tro·mo·tiv·i·ty** (ul″tro-mo-tiv'ĭ-te) ability to move spontaneously.

**Ultz·mann's test** (ooltz'mahnz) [Robert *Ultzmann,* German urologist, 1842–1889] see under *test.*

**um·bau·zo·nen** (um″bou-zo'nen) [Ger., "rebuilding zones"] Looser's transformation zones; see under *zone.*

**um·bel** (um'bəl) [L. *umbella* parasol] a more or less flat-topped cluster of small flowers whose stalks arise from a common small area at the top of the main stem; it is characteristic of the family Umbelliferae.

**Um·bel·li·fe·rae** (um″bə-lif'ĭ-re) the parsley family, a large family of plants with fragrant leaves and flower clusters arranged in umbels; many species are used as foods and spices in the human diet. Important genera include *Anethum, Carum, Cicuta, Conium, Coriandrum, Daucus, Foeniculum,* and *Pimpinella.*

**um·bel·lif·er·ous** (um″bə-lif'ər-us) 1. pertaining to or characteristic of the family Umbelliferae. 2. bearing umbels.

**um·bel·lif·er·one** (um″bə-lif′ər-ōn) a substance present in many plants, particularly those of the family Umbelliferae; used to absorb ultraviolet rays in sunscreen creams and lotions.

**um·ber** (um′bər) a natural earth containing chiefly manganese, iron oxide, and silica; used as a pigment.

**um·bil·i·cal** (əm-bil′ĭ-kəl) [L. *umbilicalis*] pertaining to the umbilicus.

**um·bil·i·cate** (əm-bil′ĭ-kāt) [L. *umbilicatus*] shaped like or resembling the umbilicus.

**um·bil·i·cat·ed** (əm-bil′ĭ-kāt″əd) marked by depressed areas resembling the umbilicus.

**um·bil·i·ca·tion** (əm-bil″ĭ-ka′shən) a pit or depression resembling the umbilicus.

**um·bil·i·cus** (əm-bil′ĭ-kəs) [L.] [MeSH: Umbilicus] 1. the navel: the cicatrix marking the site of attachment of the umbilical cord in the fetus. Called also *omphalus.* 2. [TA] the region of the abdomen surrounding the umbilicus; called also *regio umbilicalis* [TA alternative] and *umbilical region.*
**amniotic u.,** the oval aperture formed by converging amnion folds.
**decidual u.,** a small cicatricial mark over the human blastocyst shortly after its migration through the uterine epithelium into the stroma, marking the place of the closure of the decidua capsularis.

**um·bo** (um′bo) gen. *umbo′nis,* pl. *umbo′nes* [L. "a boss"] a round projection; the projecting center of any rounded surface.
**u. membra′nae tym′pani, u. membra′nae tympa′nicae** [TA], umbo of tympanic membrane: the slight projection at the center of the outer surface of the tympanic membrane, corresponding to the point of attachment of the tip of the manubrium of the malleus. Called also *spatula mallei.*

**um·bo·nate** (um′bo-nāt) [L. *umbo* a knob] knoblike; buttonlike; having a buttonlike, raised center.

**um·bo·nes** (əm-bo′nēz) [L.] plural of *umbo.*

**um·bra** (um′brə) [L. "shadow"] 1. the area of a shadow where there is no illumination; Cf. *penumbra.* 2. in radiography, the area of sharp contrast.

**um·bras·co·py** (əm-bras′kə-pe) retinoscopy.

**UMP** uridine monophosphate.

**UMP syn·thase** (sin′thās) the combined activities of the enzymes orotate phosphoribosyltransferase and orotidine-5′-phosphate decarboxylase, which together catalyze the last steps in pyrimidine nucleotide biosynthesis.

**UMP syn·thase de·fi·cien·cy** oroticaciduria, type I.

**Un·a·syn** (u′nə-sin) trademark for a preparation of ampicillin sodium and sulbactam sodium.

**un·azo·tized** (ən-a′zo-tīzd) containing no nitrogen.

**un·bal·ance** (ən-bal′əns) lack or loss of normal balance.

**un·cal** (ung′kəl) of or pertaining to the uncus.

**Un·ca·ria** (ən-kar′e-ə) [L.] a genus of shrubs of the family Rubiaceae, native to Asia. The twigs and bark of *U. gam′bier* [Hunter] Roxb. (called also *U. gam′bir*) are used medicinally and called gambir.

**un·car·thro·sis** (ung″kahr-thro′sis) bone disease involving the uncinate processes of vertebrae.

**un·ci** (un′si) [L.] genitive and plural of *uncus.*

**un·cia** (un′se-ə) pl. *un′ciae* [L.] 1. ounce. 2. inch.

**un·ci·form** (un′sĭ-form) [*uncus* (def. 1) + *form*] uncinate.

**un·ci·for·me** (un″sĭ-for′me) [L.] unciform.

**un·ci·nal** (un′sĭ-nəl) uncinate.

**Un·ci·na·ria** (un″sĭ-nar′e-ə) [L. *uncus* hook] a genus of nematode hookworms of the family Ancylostomatidae.
**U. america′na,** *Necator americanus.*
**U. duodena′lis,** *Ancylostoma duodenale.*
**U. stenoce′phala,** a hookworm commonly causing hookworm disease in dogs; also parasitic in foxes, cats, and other carnivores.

**un·cin·a·ri·a·sis** (un″sin-ə-ri′ə-sis) hookworm disease in a carnivore caused by infection with worms of the genus *Uncinaria.*

**un·cin·a·ri·at·ic** (un″sin-a″re-at′ik) pertaining to or exhibiting uncinariasis.

**un·ci·nate** (un′sĭ-nāt) 1. shaped like a hook; cf. *hamate.* Called also *uncinal.* 2. pertaining to or affecting the uncinate gyrus.

**un·ci·na·tum** (un″sĭ-na′təm) [L.] uncinate.

**un·ci·pres·sure** (un′sĭ-presh″ər) [*uncus* (def. 1) + *pressure*] pressure with a hook to control hemorrhage.

**un·com·ple·ment·ed** (ən-kom′plə-ment″əd) not joined with complement, and therefore not active.

**un·con·scious** (ən-kon′shəs) 1. insensible; incapable of responding to sensory stimuli and of having subjective experiences; see also *coma* and *consciousness.* 2. the part of the mind that is not readily accessible to conscious awareness by ordinary means but whose existence may be manifested in symptom formation, in dreams, or under the influence of drugs; it is one of the systems of Freud's topographic model of the mind. Cf. *conscious* and *preconscious.*
**collective u.,** in jungian psychology, the elements of the unconscious that are theoretically common to all mankind.

**un·co·os·si·fied** (un″ko-os′ĭ-fīd) not united into one bone.

**un·cot·o·my** (əng-kot′ə-me) [*uncus* (def. 2) + *-tomy*] the production of a circumscribed lesion in the uncus in the treatment of psychotic states.

**un·co·ver·te·bral** (ung″ko-ver′tə-brəl) pertaining to or affecting the uncinate processes of a vertebra.

**unc·tion** (ungk′shən) [L. *unctio*] 1. an ointment. 2. the application of an ointment or salve; inunction.

**unc·tu·ous** (ungk′choo-əs) greasy or oily; oleaginous.

**un·cus** (ung′kəs) [L. "hook"] 1. any hook-shaped structure. 2. [TA] the medially curved anterior end of the parahippocampal gyrus; called also *u. gyri fornicati, u. gyri hippocampi,* and *u. gyri parahippocampalis.*
**u. cor′poris ver′tebrae cervica′lis** [TA], uncus of body of cervical vertebra: a hooklike projection found on each side of the superior surface of the third to seventh cervical vertebral bodies. This is a frequent site of formation of spurs (osteophytes), leading to spondylosis uncovertebralis. Callec also *uncinate process of cervical vertebra.*
**u. gy′ri fornica′ti, u. gy′ri hippocam′pi, u. gy′ri parahippocampa′lis,** uncus (def. 2).
**u. of hamate bone,** hamulus ossis hamati.

**un·dec·e·no·ic ac·id** (ən-des″ə-no′ik) systematic name for undecylenic acid.

**un·dec·yl·en·ic ac·id** (un″des-əl-en′ik) [USP] a fungicide (against *Epidermophyton, Trichophyton,* and *Microsporum* spp.) applied topically either alone or with zinc undecylenate.

**un·der·bite** (un′dər-bīt) popular name for *retrognathia.*

**un·der·cut** (un′dər-kət) 1. that portion of a tooth which lies between the survey line (height of contour) and the gingivae. 2. the contour of a cross-section of a residual ridge or dental arch which would prevent the insertion of a denture. 3. the contour of flasking stone which interlocks in such a way as to prevent the separation of the parts. 4. a depressed or intaglio irregularity in the wall of a prepared tooth that prevents the ready withdrawal and seating of a wax pattern and the metal alloy casting.

**un·der·horn** (un′dər-horn) cornu temporale ventriculi lateralis.

**un·der·nu·tri·tion** (un″dər-noo-trish′ən) malnutrition due to inadequate food supply or to inability to metabolize or use necessary food elements.

**un·der·sens·ing** (un′dər-sens″ing) missed sensing of cardiac electrical signals by an artificial cardiac pacemaker, resulting in too frequent or irregular delivery of stimuli; causes include head dislodgment, malfunctioning of the pulse generator, fibrosis, infarct, and drugs.

**un·der·stain** (un′dər-stān) to stain less deeply than usual.

**un·der·toe** (un′dər-to) hallux valgus in which the great toe is displaced under the others.

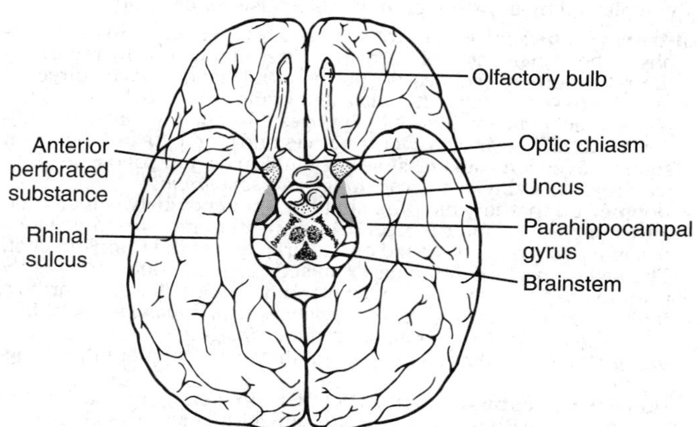


Uncus shown on the inferior (ventral) surface of the cerebral hemispheres, the cerebellum and most of the brainstem removed.

**Un·der·wood's disease** (un'dər-woodz) [Michael *Underwood,* English obstetrician and pediatrician, 1737–1820] sclerema.

**un·dif·fer·en·ti·at·ed** (ən-dif″ər-en'she-āt-əd) without identifiable pattern, usually referring to the cellular arrangement of neoplastic tissue; anaplastic.

**un·dif·fer·en·ti·a·tion** (un″dif-ər-en″she-a'shən) anaplasia.

**un·dine** (ən-dēn', un'din) [L. *unda* wave, water] a small glass flask for irrigating the eye.

**un·din·ism** (un'din-iz-əm) [*Undine* a water nymph, from L. *unda* wave] the association of sexual ideas with water, including urine and urination.

**Un·dritz anomaly** (oon'drits) [E. *Undritz,* Swiss physician, 20th century] hereditary hypersegmentation of neutrophils; see under *hypersegmentation.*

**un·du·lant** (un'jə-lənt) [L. *unda* wave] characterized by wavelike fluctuations; see also under *fever.*

**un·du·late** (un'jə-lət) [L. *undulatus,* from *unda* wave] having a wavy, curved border; said of a colony of microorganisms.

**un·du·la·tion** (un″jə-la'shən) [L. *undulatio*] a wavelike motion in any medium; see also *pulsation.*
**respiratory u.,** the variation of the blood pressure curve due to respiration.

**ung.** abbreviation for L. *unguen'tum,* ointment.

**un·gual** (ung'gwəl) [L. *unguis* nail] pertaining to the nails.

**un·guent** (ung'gwənt) [L. *unguentum*] an ointment, salve, or cerate.

**un·guen·tum** (əng-gwen'təm) gen. *unguen'ti,* pl. *unguen'ta* [L.] ointment.

**un·gues** (ung'gwēz) [L.] plural of *unguis.*

**un·guic·u·late** (əng-gwik'u-lāt) 1. provided with claws or nails. 2. resembling a claw.

**un·guic·u·lus** (əng-gwik'u-ləs) [L., dim. of *unguis*] claw.

**un·guis** (ung'gwis) pl. *un'gues* [L.] 1. [TA] nail: the horny cutaneous plate on the dorsal surface of the distal end of the terminal phalanx of a finger or toe, made up of flattened epithelial scales developed from the stratum lucidum of the skin. See illustration at *nail.* 2. a collection of pus in the cornea; an onyx. 3. a nail-like part or structure.
**u. incarna'tus,** ingrown nail; see under *nail.*
**u. ventri'culi latera'lis ce'rebri,** calcar avis.

**un·gu·la** (ung'gu-lə) [L. "hoof," "claw," "talon"] hoof.

**un·gu·late** (ung'gu-lāt) [L. *ungula* hoof] a hoofed mammal. Formerly all classified into one order, they are now divided into the orders Artiodactyla and Perissodactyla.

**un·gu·li·grade** (ung'gu-lĭ-grād″) [*ungula* + L. *gradi* to walk] characterized by standing or walking on hooves (the tips of the toes); applied to certain quadrupeds known as *ungulates,* including horses, cattle, pigs, sheep, and deer. Cf. *digitigrade* and *plantigrade.*

**uni-** [L. *unus* one] a prefix meaning one.

**uni·ar·tic·u·lar** (u″ne-ahr-tik'u-lər) [*uni-* + *articular*] pertaining to a single joint.

**uni·au·ral** (u″ne-aw'rəl) monaural.

**uni·ax·i·al** (u″ne-ak'se-əl) [*uni-* + *axial*] 1. having but one axis; said of a joint. 2. developing in an axial direction only, as a uniaxial organism.

**uni·ba·sal** (u″nĭ-ba'səl) [*uni-* + *basal*] having only one base.

**uni·cam·er·al** (u″nĭ-kam'ər-əl) [*uni-* + *camera* + *-al*[1]] having only one cavity or compartment.

**uni·cel·lu·lar** (u″nĭ-sel'u-lər) [*uni-* + *cellular*] made up of but a single cell, as the bacteria.

**uni·cen·tral** (u″nĭ-sen'trəl) [*uni-* + *central*] pertaining to or having a single center.

**uni·cen·tric** (u″nĭ-sen'trik) unicentral.

**uni·ceps** (u″nĭ-seps) [*uni-* + L. *caput* head] having one head or origin; said of a muscle.

**uni·col·lis** (u″nĭ-kol'is) [L., from *uni-* + L. *collum* neck] having a single cervix; see *uterus unicornis unicollis,* under *uterus.*

**uni·cor·nous** (u″nĭ-kor'nəs) [L. *unicornis*] having only one horn or cornu.

**uni·cus·pid** (u″nĭ-kus'pid) a tooth with only one cusp.

**uni·cus·pi·date** (u″nĭ-kus'pĭ-dāt) having only one cusp.

**uni·di·rec·tion·al** (u″nĭ-di-rek'shən-əl) flowing in only one direction.

**uni·flag·el·late** (u″nĭ-flaj'ə-lāt) having one flagellum.

**uni·fo·cal** (u″nĭ-fo'kəl) arising from or pertaining to a single focus.

**uni·fo·rate** (u″nĭ-for'āt) [*uni-* + L. *foratus* pierced] having only one opening.

**uni·gem·i·nal** (u″nĭ-jem'ĭ-nəl) [*uni-* + *geminus*] pertaining to or affecting one twin of a pair.

**uni·ger·mi·nal** (u″nĭ-jər'mĭ-nəl) 1. pertaining to a single germ or ovum. 2. monozygotic.

**uni·glan·du·lar** (u″nĭ-glan'du-lər) pertaining to or affecting only one gland.

**uni·grav·i·da** (u″nĭ-grav'ĭ-də) primigravida.

**uni·lam·i·nar** (u″nĭ-lam'ĭ-nər) having only one layer or lamina.

**uni·lat·er·al** (u″nĭ-lat'ər-əl) [*uni-* + *lateral*] affecting but one side.

**uni·lo·bar** (u″nĭ-lo'bər) having only one lobe; consisting of a single lobe.

**uni·loc·u·lar** (u″nĭ-lok'u-lər) [*uni-* + *locular*] having but one loculus or compartment.

**uni·mo·dal** (u″nĭ-mo'dəl) having only one mode.

**uni·ne·phrec·to·my** (u″nĭ-nə-frek'tə-me) [*uni-* + *nephrectomy*] surgical removal of a single kidney.

**uni·nu·cle·ar** (u″nĭ-noo'kle-ər) pertaining to a single nucleus; mononuclear.

**uni·nu·cle·at·ed** (u″nĭ-noo'kle-āt″əd) having but one nucleus; mononuclear; mononucleate.

**uni·oc·u·lar** (u″ne-ok'u-lər) pertaining to or affecting only one eye.

**un·ion** (ūn'yən) [L. *unio*] the process of healing; the renewal of continuity in a broken bone or between the edges of a wound. See *healing.*
**faulty u.,** an ununited fracture.
**primary u.,** healing by first intention.
**radioulnar u., middle,** syndesmosis radioulnaris.
**vicious u.,** union of the ends of a fractured bone so as to produce deformity.

**uni·ov·u·lar** (u″ne-ov'u-lər) [*uni-* + *ovular*] monozygotic; monovular.

**unip·a·ra** (u-nip'ə-rə) primipara.

**uni·pa·ren·tal** (u″nĭ-pə-ren'təl) pertaining to one of the parents only.

**unip·a·rous** (u-nip'ə-rəs) [*uni-* + L. *parere* to bring forth, produce] 1. producing only one ovum or offspring at one time. 2. primiparous.

**Uni·pen** (u'nĭ-pen) trademark for preparations of nafcillin sodium.

**uni·po·lar** (u″nĭ-po'lər) [*uni-* + *polar*] 1. having but a single pole or process, as a nerve cell. 2. pertaining to mood disorders in which only depressive episodes occur.

**uni·po·ten·cy** (u″nĭ-po'tən-se) [*uni-* + *potency* (def. 3)] the ability of a part to develop in one manner only, or of a cell to develop into only one type of cell.

**uni·po·tent** (u-nip'ə-tənt) unipotential.

**uni·po·ten·tial** (u″nĭ-po-ten'shəl) [*uni-* + *potential*] capable in one way only; said of cells which have had their fates determined and can give rise to cells of one order only. Cf. *totipotential.*

**un·ir·ri·ta·ble** (un-ir'ĭ-tə-bəl) not irritable; not capable of being stimulated.

**uni·sep·tate** (u″ne-sep'tāt) having only one septum.

**uni·sex·u·al** (u″nĭ-sek'shoo-əl) [*uni-* + *sexual* (def. 1)] of only one sex; having the sexual organs of one sex only.

**unit** (u'nit) [L. *unus* one] 1. a single thing. 2. a quantity assumed as a standard of measurement. Symbol U.

**Allen-Doisy u.**, in the Allen-Doisy test, the least amount of estrogen that causes cornification of vaginal epithelium in a spayed laboratory mouse. Called also *mouse u.*

**amboceptor u.**, in complement fixation tests, the smallest amount of anti-RBC antibody (amboceptor) that produces complete red cell lysis in the presence of an excess of complement.

**Angström u.**, angstrom.

**Ansbacher u.**, a unit of vitamin K dosage.

**antigen u.**, in complement fixation tests, the smallest amount of antigen that will fix one unit of complement.

**antitoxic u.**, a unit for expressing the strength of an antitoxin. The unit of diphtheria antitoxin is approximately the amount that will preserve the life of a guinea pig weighing 250 g for at least four days after it is injected subcutaneously with a mixture of 100 times the minimum lethal dose of diphtheria toxin. The unit of tetanus antitoxin is approximately ten times the amount that will preserve the life of a guinea pig weighing 350 g for at least 96 hours after injection of a mixture with 100 times minimum lethal dose of tetanus toxin. The U.S. Public Health Service unit for scarlet fever antitoxin neutralizes 50 skin test doses of scarlet fever toxin.

**atomic mass u.**, the unit mass equal to $\frac{1}{12}$ the mass of the nuclide of carbon-12, equivalent to $1.657 \times 10^{-24}$ gm; abbreviated amu. Symbol u. Called also *atomic weight u.* and *dalton.*

**atomic weight u.**, atomic mass u.

**Behnken's u.**, a unit of x-ray exposure, being that quantity which, when applied in 1 cc of air at 18°C and 760 mm Hg of pressure, engenders sufficient electric conductivity to equal one electrostatic unit, as measured by the saturation current. Symbol R.

**Bethesda u.**, a measure of the level of inhibitor to coagulation factor VIII; equal to the amount of inhibitor in patient plasma that will inactivate 50 per cent of factor VIII in an equal volume of normal plasma following a 2-hour incubation period.

**Bodansky u.**, the quantity of alkaline phosphatase that liberates 1 mg of phosphate ion from glycerol 2-phosphate in 1 hour at 37°C and under other standardized conditions.

**British thermal u.**, the amount of heat necessary to raise the temperature of one pound of water one degree Fahrenheit, usually from 39°F to 40°F; abbreviated BTU.

**burst-forming u.–erythroid (BFU-E)**, the earliest erythrocyte precursor in the erythrocytic series, detectable mainly in vitro and having a high requirement for erythropoietin; it gets its name from the fact that its growth is composed of subcolonies resembling bursts. It is followed by the colony-forming unit–erythroid.

**CGS u.**, any unit in the centimeter-gram-second system.

**CH50 u.**, the amount of complement that will lyse 50 per cent of a standard preparation of sheep red blood cells coated with antisheep erythrocyte antibody.

**colony-forming u. (CFU)**, 1. any of several hematopoietic stem cells identified by their ability to give rise to monoclonal colonies in the spleen when transplanted into isogeneic, lethally irradiated mice. 2. in microbiology, estimation of the number of bacteria or yeasts by counting the colonies on a solid medium, with one bacterium being considered equal to one colony; some colonies develop from two or more organisms attached to or lying close to each other when inoculated.

**colony-forming u.–culture (CFU-C)**, colony-forming u.–granulocyte-macrophage.

**colony-forming u.–erythroid (CFU-E)**, an erythrocyte precursor in the erythrocyte series that follows the burst-forming unit–erythroid and precedes the proerythroblast; detectable mainly in vitro.

**colony-forming u.–granulocyte-macrophage (CFU-GM)**, a precursor cell in the granulocytic series that can grow into a myeloblast in the presence of appropriate stimulators in vitro. Called also *colony forming u.–culture.*

**colony-forming u.–spleen (CFU-S)**, a name for the hematopoietic stem cell, based on the fact that in mice whose marrow has been ablated by irradiation this cell gives rise to colonies of marrow cells in the spleen.

**complement u.**, in complement fixation tests, the smallest amount of complement or serum that will produce complete hemolysis of sensitized red cells. Called also *hemolytic u.*

**Corner-Allen u.**, a unit of activity of progestational agents; see also *Corner-Allen test,* under *test.*

**coronary care u.**, a specially designed and equipped hospital area containing a small number of private rooms, with all facilities necessary for constant observation and possible emergency treatment of patients with severe heart disease.

**dental u.**, 1. a single tooth and its adnexa, considered as a unit in the physiology of mastication. 2. a mobile or fixed article of dental equipment, which may be combined with a chair, consisting of items and attachments needed for dental examination and operations, and housing the electrical, mechanical, and plumbing facilities needed to operate the equipment and fixtures of the unit.

**electromagnetic u's**, that system of units based on the fundamental definition of a unit magnetic pole as one which will repel an exactly similar pole with a force of one dyne when the poles are 1 cm apart.

**electrostatic u's**, that system of units based on the fundamental definition of a unit charge as one which will repel an equal and like charge with a force of one dyne when the two charges are 1 cm apart in a vacuum. Abbreviated ESE (Ger., *elektrostatische Einheit*) and *esu.*

**enzyme u.**, see *international u. of enzyme activity.*

**Felton's u.**, a mouse protective unit of antipneumococcic serum; it is that quantity of antibody capable of protecting a white Swiss mouse against one million fatal doses of a standard pneumococcus culture of the corresponding type. Frequently, it is considered to be the equivalent of the National Institutes of Health control serum (P-11).

**French u.**, a linear unit for diameter size in the French scale, equivalent to 0.33 mm.

**Hampson u.**, a unit of x-ray exposure; it is one quarter of the erythema dose.

**hemolytic u.**, complement u.

**hemorrhagin u.**, the amount of snake venom necessary to produce hemorrhagins in the vascular network of a three-day-old chick embryo.

**Hounsfield u.**, a unit of x-ray attenuation used for CT scans, each pixel being assigned a value on a scale on which air is −1000, water is 0, and compact bone is +1000. Symbol H.

**intensive care u.**, a hospital unit in which are concentrated special equipment and skilled personnel for the care of seriously ill patients requiring immediate and continuous attention; abbreviated ICU.

**International u. (IU)**, a unit of biological material, as of enzymes, hormones, vitamins, etc., established by the International Conference for the Unification of Formulas.

**international u. of enzyme activity**, that amount of an enzyme that will catalyze the transformation of 1 micromole of substrate per minute under standard conditions of temperature, optimal pH, and optimal substrate concentration. Symbol U.

**international insulin u.**, one twenty-second of a milligram (.045 mg) of the pure crystalline product of insulin, now adopted as the standard.

**international u. of penicillin**, the specific penicillin activity contained in 0.6 microgram of the international standard sodium salt of penicillin G.

**international u. of vitamin A**, an older unit of vitamin A activity, equal to the activity of 0.3 microgram retinol or 0.6 microgram β-carotene; because the provitamin A carotenoids are absorbed less efficiently than is retinol, the source must be specified. Although largely supplanted by retinol equivalent (q.v.), the unit is still used in labeling. When the source is retinol, the unit is officially *vitamin A u.*

**international u. of vitamin D**, the specific biological activity of 0.025 microgram of cholecalciferol.

**international u. of vitamin E**, the specific biological activity of 0.671 milligram of *d*-alpha-tocopherol or 1.0 milligram of *dl*-alpha-tocopherol acetate. See also *alpha-tocopherol equivalent.*

**Karmen u.**, the amount of transaminase that under specified conditions will cause a change of 0.001 in the absorbance of NADH when measured at 340 nm in a 1 cm light path.

**Kienböck u.**, a unit of x-ray exposure equal to 0.1 erythema dose; symbol X.

**King u., King-Armstrong u.**, the amount of phosphatase that liberates 1 mg of phenol from an excess of disodium phenylphosphate under defined conditions; alkaline phosphatase can be measured under alkaline conditions and acid phosphatase under acidic conditions.

**Lf u.**, see under *dose.*

**map u.**, centimorgan.

**motor u.**, the unit of motor activity formed by a motor nerve cell and its many innervated muscle fibers.

**mouse u.**, Allen-Doisy u.

**Noon pollen u.**, the activity present in the saline extract from one millionth of a grain of pollen.

**u. of oxytocin**, a USP unit expressing the uterus-stimulating activity of preparations of synthetic oxytocin; one unit is approximately equivalent to the strength of 2 μg of pure hormone.

**pepsin u.**, a unit for measuring the proportion of pepsin in the gastric juice.

**peripheral resistance u. (PRU)**, a conventional unit of vascular resistance equal to the resistance that produces a pressure difference of 1 mm Hg, corresponding to a blood flow of 1 mL/sec.

**pilosebaceous u.**, the hair follicle and the associated apocrine gland.

**plaque-forming u.**, an estimate of the titer of a bacteriophage solution, determined by mixing the bacteriophage with a solution of susceptible bacteria, plating, incubating, and counting the number of plaques present on the bacterial lawn, with each plaque representing a viable bacteriophage.

**quantum u.**, see *Planck's constant,* under *constant.*

**SI u.**, any of the units of the Système International d'Unités, or International System of Units, adopted in 1960 at the Eleventh General Conference of Weights and Measures. SI units are based on the metric

## **Unit** *Continued*

system and many are derived from natural constants. For units and for multiples and submultiples of these units formed by the use of prefixes, see Appendices 2 and 3.

**Somogyi u.,** that amount of amylase that will liberate reducing equivalents equal to 1 mg of glucose per 30 minutes under defined conditions.

**sudanophobic u.,** the smallest amount of adrenocorticotropic hormone that will cause the disappearance of the sudanophobic zone of the adrenal cortex in at least two of three hypophysectomized rats when they are injected morning and evening on eight consecutive days.

**Svedberg u.,** a unit equal to $10^{-13}$ second used for expressing sedimentation coefficients (q.v.) of macromolecules. Symbol S.

**Svedberg flotation u.,** a unit equal to $10^{-13}$ second used for expressing negative sedimentation coefficients of macromolecules that float rather than sink in a centrifuge, e.g., lipoproteins. Symbol $S_f$.

**terminal respiratory u.,** the part of the lung distal to a single terminal bronchiole; it is the anatomical and functional unit of the lung and consists of a respiratory bronchiole, two or more alveolar ducts, and alveoli. Called also *primary lobule of lung, pulmonary acinus,* and *transitional and respiratory zone.* See Plate 49.

**toxic u., toxin u.,** the smallest dose of toxin which will kill a guinea pig weighing about 250 g in three to four days.

**tuberculin u. (TU),** an arbitrary unit of tuberculin dosage defined by comparison of clinical response with a standard preparation of PPD tuberculin.

**turbidity reducing u. (TRU),** the amount of hyaluronidase which is just sufficient to reduce the turbidity produced by 0.2 mg of hyaluronate to that produced by 0.1 mg after addition of acidified horse serum.

**USP u.,** one used in the United States Pharmacopeia in expressing the potency of antibiotic, pharmacodynamic, and endocrine preparations, as well as most of the sera, toxins, vaccines, and related products, corresponding to units established internationally, by the Food and Drug Administration, or by the National Institutes of Health.

**vitamin A u.** [USP], the specific biological activity of 0.3 mg of the all-*trans* isomer of retinol. See also *international u. of vitamin A* and *retinol equivalent.*

**vitamin D u.,** see *international u. of vitamin D.*

**Wood's u.,** peripheral resistance u.

**x-ray u.,** Kienböck u.

---

**unit·age** (u′nit-əj) a statement of the unit quantity in any system of measurement.

**uni·tary** (u′nĭ-tar″e) [L. *unitas* oneness] composed of or pertaining to a single unit.

**Unit·ed States Phar·ma·co·peia** see *USP.*

**Uni·ten·sen** (u″nĭ-ten′sən) trademark for a preparation of cryptenamine acetates or cryptenamine tannates.

**uni·ter·mi·nal** (u″nĭ-tər′mĭ-nəl) 1. monopolar. 2. a monopolar apparatus.

**unit·less** (u′nit-ləs) lacking units.

**Uni·tu·ni·ca·tae** (u″ne-too″nĭ-ka′te) in fungal taxonomy, a series of the subphylum Ascomycotina, consisting of those having a unitunicate ascus. It is usually subdivided into operculate and inoperculate groups according to whether or not the ascus has an operculum (small cap that pops open for ejection of spores).

**uni·va·lence** (u″nĭ-va′ləns) the state or condition of being univalent.

**uni·va·lent** (u″nĭ-va′lənt) monovalent.

**uni·var·iate** (u″nĭ-văr′e-ət) pertaining to only one variable.

**Uni·vasc** (u′nĭ-vask″) trademark for a preparation of moexipril hydrochloride.

**uni·vi·tel·line** (u″nĭ-vi-tel′in) pertaining to or derived from a single ovum.

**un·med·ul·lat·ed** (ən-med′u-lāt″əd) unmyelinated.

**un·my·eli·nat·ed** (ən-mi′ə-lĭ-nāt″əd) not possessing a myelin sheath; said of a nerve fiber. Called also *nonmedullated, nonmyelinated,* and *unmedullated.*

**Un·na's paste boot, alkaline methylene blue** (oon′ahz) [Paul Gerson *Unna,* German dermatologist, 1850–1929] see under *boot,* and *Table of Stains.*

**Un·na-Pap·pen·heim stain** (oon′ah-pahp′en-hīm) [Paul Gerson *Unna;* Artur *Pappenheim,* German physician, 1870–1916] see under *stain.*

**Un·na-Thost disease, syndrome** (oon′ah-tost) [P.G. *Unna;* Arthur *Thost,* German physician, late 19th century] diffuse palmoplantar keratoderma.

**un·or·ga·nized** (ən-or′gən-īzd) not developed into an organic structure; not having organs.

**un·phys·i·o·log·ic** (un″fiz-e-o-loj′ik) not physiologic in character.

**un·rest** (ən-rest′) a state of uneasiness or restlessness.

**peristaltic u.,** a state of disturbed peristalsis of the stomach or intestine.

**un·sat·u·rat·ed** (ən-sach′ə-rāt″əd) not saturated; applied to a chemical compound in which two or more atoms are united by double or triple bonds, which contain multiple pairs of shared electrons. Such compounds may still add atoms or groups to the unsaturated bonding atoms up to a limit of bonding power, or saturation. Most commonly refers to carbon-carbon bonds, as in unsaturated fatty acids. Also applied to a solution in which more solute may still be dissolved under stated conditions.

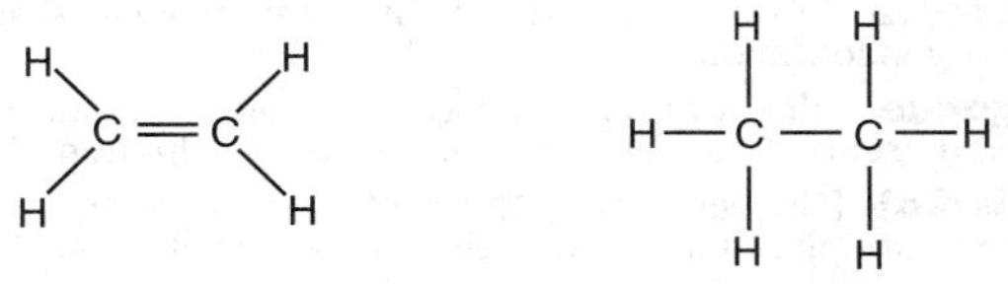

A Ethylene B Ethane

Unsaturated *(A)* and saturated *(B)* two-carbon hydrocarbons.

**Un·schuld's sign** (oon′shooldz) [Paul *Unschuld,* German internist, 1835–c. 1905] see under *sign.*

**un·sex** (ən-seks′) castrate.

**un·sharp·ness** (un-shahrp′nes) in radiology, the measure or degree to which sharp boundaries of an object or person being imaged are blurred in that image.

**un·spe·cif·ic mono·oxy·ge·nase** (un″spə-sif′ik mon″o-ok′sə-jən-ās) [EC 1.14.14.1] a broadly specific monooxygenase for which the hydrogen donor is a reduced flavoprotein; it contains cytochrome P-450 as its oxygen activator. It acts on a wide range of substrates, including xenobiotics, steroids, fatty acids, vitamins, and prostaglandins.

**un·stri·at·ed** (ən-stri′āt-əd) having no striations or striae; see under *muscle.*

**un·thrif·ti·ness** (un-thrif′te-nes) failure of a young animal to grow or gain weight at a normal rate in spite of an adequate diet and lack of overt illness. Called also *ill thrift.*

**Un·ver·richt's disease (syndrome)** (oon′fer-ikts) [Heinrich *Unverricht,* German physician, 1853–1912] myoclonus epilepsy.

**Un·ver·richt-Lund·borg disease** (oon′fer-ikt-loond′borg) [H. *Unverricht;* Herman Bernhard *Lundborg,* Swedish physician, 1868–1943] Baltic myoclonic epilepsy.

**un·voiced** (un-voist′) voiceless.

**u-plas·min·o·gen ac·ti·va·tor** (plaz-min′ə-jən″ ak′tĭ-va-tər) [EC 3.4.21.74] see under *activator.*

**up-reg·u·la·tion** (up reg-u-la′shən) an increase in the number of receptors for a chemical or drug on cell surfaces in a given area so that the cells are more reactive to the effects of the agent. See also *down-regulation.*

**UPPP** uvulopalatopharyngoplasty.

**up·right·ing** (up′rīt-ing) tipping inclined teeth to a more vertical axial inclination. See also *tipping,* def. 1.

**up·si·loid** (up′sĭ-loid) [Gr. *upsilon* + *-oid*] shaped like the Greek upsilon (υ or Υ); see *hyoid* (def. 1) and *hypsiloid.*

**up·si·lon** (up′si-lon) [Υ, υ] the twentieth letter of the Greek alphabet.

**up·stream** (up′strēm) in molecular biology, a term used to denote a region of nucleic acid to the 5′ side of a gene or region of interest.

**up·take** (up′tāk) absorption and incorporation of a substance by living tissue.
**pertechnetate u.,** a thyroid function test in which, along with radioiodine, radioactive technetium is administered in the form of the pertechnetate ion (technetium 99m pertechnetate) to measure early uptake and trapping of the ion by the thyroid gland.
**radioactive iodine u. (RAIU), radioiodine u.,** uptake of radioiodine from the blood by the thyroid gland; see under *test.*
**triiodothyronine resin u.,** the uptake of radioactive triiodothyronine at binding sites on resin, contrasted to uptake at sites on thyroxine-binding globulin in the triiodothyronine resin uptake test (see under *test*).

**ura·chal** (u′rə-kəl) pertaining to the urachus.

**ura·cho·ves·i·cal** (u″rə-ko-ves′ĭ-kəl) pertaining to the urachus and the urinary bladder.

**ura·chus** (u′rə-kəs) [Gr. *ourachos*] [MeSH: Urachus] the derivative of the allantoic stalk in the fetus that connects the urinary bladder with the umbilicus; it persists throughout life as a fibrous cord, the *median umbilical ligament,* into which a patent canal may extend for part of the distance to the umbilicus.

**ura·cil** (ūr′ə-sil) [MeSH: Uracil] a pyrimidine base, in animal cells usually occurring condensed with ribose to form the ribonucleoside uridine, a component of ribonucleic acid and of free nucleotides with functions in metabolism. The corresponding deoxyribonucleoside, deoxyuridine, is a component of free nucleotides involved in pyrimidine biosynthesis. See also illustration at *pyrimidine base,* under *base.* Symbol U.

**ura·cra·sia** (u″rə-kra′zhə) [*ur-* + *a-*[1] + *-crasia*] a disordered state of the urine.

**ura·cra·tia** (u″rə-kra′shə) [*ur-* + Gr. *akrateia* lack of self control] urinary incontinence.

**ura·gogue** (u′rə-gog) [*ur-* + *agogue*] 1. increasing urinary volume flow; diuretic. 2. an agent that increases production of urine.

**uranisc(o)-** [Gr. *ouraniskos,* the roof of the mouth] a combining form denoting relationship to the palate; see also *uran(o)-.*

**ura·nis·co·chas·ma** (u″rə-nis″ko-kaz′mə) [*uranisco-* + Gr. *chasma* cleft] cleft palate.

**ura·nis·co·la·lia** (u″rə-nis″ko-la′le-ə) [*uranisco-* + *lal-* + *-ia*] cleft palate speech.

**ura·nis·co·plas·ty** (u″rə-nis′ko-plas″te) palatoplasty.

**ura·nis·cor·rha·phy** (u″rə-nis-kor′ə-fe) [*uranisco-* + *-rrhaphy*] palatorrhaphy.

**ura·nis·cus** (u″rə-nis′kəs) [Gr. *ouraniskos,* dim. of *ouranos*] the palate.

**ura·ni·um** (u-ra′ne-əm) [L. *Uranus* a planet] [MeSH: Uranium] a hard and heavy radioactive metallic element; symbol, U; atomic number, 92; atomic weight, 238.03; specific gravity, 18.68. Naturally occurring uranium is composed of three isotopes of mass numbers 234, 235, and 238. Uranium 235 separated from U 238 undergoes fission with slow neutrons, giving up neutrons which can join the nucleus of U 238 to form neptunium, which in turn decays by beta particle emission to form plutonium. Cf. *neptunium* and *plutonium.*

**uran(o)-** [Gr. *ouranos* the vault of heaven or of a ceiling, the roof of the mouth or palate] a combining form denoting relationship to the palate.

**ura·no·plas·ty** (u′rə-no-plas′te) palatoplasty.

**ura·no·ple·gia** (u″rə-no-ple′jə) palatoplegia.

**ura·nor·rha·phy** (u″rə-nor′ə-fe) palatorrhaphy.

**ura·nos·chi·sis** (u″rə-nos′kĭ-sis) cleft palate.

**ura·nos·chism** (u″rə-nos′kiz-əm) cleft palate.

**ura·no·staph·y·lo·plas·ty** (u″rə-no-staf′ə-lo-plas″te) an operation for repairing a defect of both the soft and hard palate. See also *palatoplasty.*

**ura·no·staph·y·lor·rha·phy** (u″rə-no-staf″ə-lor′ə-fe) [*urano-* + *staphylo-* + *-rrhaphy*] suture of both the soft and hard palate. See also *palatorrhaphy.*

**ura·no·staph·y·los·chi·sis** (u″rə-no-staf″ə-los′kĭ-sis) cleft palate involving both the soft palate and the hard palate.

**Ura·no·tae·nia** (u″rə-no-te′ne-ə) a genus of culicine mosquitoes. *U. sappari′nus* is found in the eastern United States.

**ura·nyl** (u′rə-nəl) the $UO_2^{2+}$ ion.

**ura·pos·te·ma** (u″rə-pos-te′mə) [*ur-* + Gr. *apostēma* abscess] an abscess which contains urine.

**urar·thri·tis** (u″rahr-thri′tis) gouty arthritis.

**urate** (ūr′āt) any salt or anion of uric acid (q.v.).

**ura·te·mia** (u″rə-te′me-ə) the presence of urates in the blood.

**urate ox·i·dase** (ūr′āt ok′sĭ-dās) [EC 1.7.3.3] [MeSH: Urate Oxidase] an enzyme of the oxidoreductase class that catalyzes the oxidation of uric acid to allantoin with liberation of $CO_2$ and $H_2O_2$. It is a copper enzyme, found in most mammals but not in primates; it is frequently used in clinical assays of uric acid concentrations. Called also *uricase.*

**urat·ic** (u-rat′ik) pertaining to urates or to gout.

**ura·to·his·tech·ia** (u″rə-to-his-tek′e-ə) [*urate* + *hist-* + *echein* to hold] the presence of an excessive amount of urate, urea, or uric acid in a tissue.

**ura·to·ma** (u″rə-to′mə) a tophus or concretion made up of urates.

**ura·to·sis** (u″rə-to′sis) the deposition of crystalline urates in the tissues.

**ura·tu·ria** (u″rə-tu′re-ə) the presence of an excess of urates in the urine; lithuria.

**Ur·bach-Wiethe disease** (ur′bak-vēt′ĕ) [Erich *Urbach,* American dermatologist, 1893–1946; Camillo *Wiethe,* Austrian otologist, 1888–1949] lipoid proteinosis.

**ur·ce·i·form** (ər-se′ĭ-form) [L. *urceus* pitcher + *form*] pitcher-shaped.

**ur·ce·o·late** (ər-se′ə-lāt) urceiform.

**urea** (u-re′ə) [USP] [MeSH: Urea] 1. a compound, $CO(NH_2)_2$, formed in the liver via the urea cycle (q.v.) from ammonia produced by the deamination of amino acids and later excreted by the kidney; it is the principal end product of protein catabolism and constitutes about one half of the total urinary solids. Elevation of the blood levels of urea and other nitrogenous compounds (azotemia) occurs with decreased glomerular filtration rate due to inadequate renal perfusion, acute or chronic renal disease, or urinary tract obstruction (see *uremia*). Called also *carbamide.* 2. [USP] a preparation of urea administered intravenously as an osmotic diuretic to reduce intracranial or intraocular pressure and in topical preparations to moisten and soften rough dry skin. Urea is a common feed additive for ruminants because it enhances protein synthesis from dietary roughage and stimulates multiplication of microorganisms that digest cellulose.
**u. nitrogen,** the urea concentration of blood or serum stated in terms of nitrogen content; converted to urea concentration by multiplying by 60/28 or 2.14. The serum or plasma urea nitrogen is traditionally referred to as *blood urea nitrogen (BUN).*

**urea·ge·net·ic** (u-re″ə-jə-net′ik) [*urea* + Gr. *gennan* to produce] forming or producing urea.

**ure·al** (u′re-əl) pertaining to urea.

**ure·am·e·try** (u″re-am′ə-tre) the measurement of the urea present in the urine.

**Urea·phil** (u-re′ə-fil) trademark for a preparation of urea.

**Urea·plas·ma** (u-re″ə-plaz′mə) [*urea* + Gr. *plasma* anything formed or molded] [MeSH: Ureaplasma] a genus of bacteria of the family Mycoplasmataceae, made up of pleomorphic, gram-negative organisms that lack a cell wall and that hydrolyze urea. Called also *T-mycoplasma* and *T-strain mycoplasma* (T for *tiny*).

**urea·poi·e·sis** (u-re″ə-poi-e′sis) [*urea* + *-poiesis*] the formation of urea.

**ure·ase** (u′re-ās) [EC 3.5.1.5] [MeSH: Urease] an enzyme of the hydrolase class that catalyzes the hydrolysis of urea to $CO_2$ and ammonia; it is a nickel protein found in microorganisms and plants that is frequently used in clinical assays of plasma urea concentrations.

**urec·chy·sis** (u-rek′ĭ-sis) [*uro-* + Gr. *ekchysis* a pouring out] the effusion of urine into the cellular tissue.

**Urech·i·tes** (u-rek′ĭ-tēz) a genus of plants of the family Apocyanaceae, native to tropical parts of the Americas. *U. lu′tea* is a Cuban plant that causes fatal heart failure in cattle. *U. suberec′ta* is the Savannah flower, whose leaves are poisonous and antipyretic.

**urech·i·tin** (u-rek′ĭ-tin) a poisonous glycoside from *Urechites suberecta.*

**urech·i·tox·in** (u-rek″ĭ-tok′sin) a poisonous glycoside from *Urechites suberecta.*

**Ure·cho·line** (u″re-ko′lin) trademark for preparations of bethanechol chloride.

**ure·de·ma** (u″rə-de′mə) [*uro-* + *edema*] a puffy condition of the tissues caused by infiltration of extravasated urine.

**Ure·di·na·les** (u″rə-dĭ-na′lēz) the rusts, an order of perfect fungi of the class Teliomycetes; they cause damage to numerous different economically important food plants.

**ure·ide** (u′re-id) a compound of urea and an acid or aldehyde.

Those from one molecule of urea, as alloxan, are monoureides; those derived from two, as uric acid, are diureides.

**urel·co·sis** (u″rəl-ko′sis) [*uro-* + *elcosis*] 1. ulceration of the urinary passages. 2. an ulcer due to derangement of the urinary apparatus.

**ure·mia** (u-re′me-ə) [*ur-* + *-emia*] [MeSH: Uremia] 1. an excess in the blood of urea, creatinine, and other nitrogenous end products of protein and amino acid metabolism; more correctly referred to as *azotemia.* 2. in current usage the entire constellation of signs and symptoms of chronic renal failure, including nausea, vomiting, anorexia, a metallic taste in the mouth, a characteristic odor of the breath, pruritus, urea frost on the skin, neuromuscular disorders, pain and twitching in the muscles, hypertension, edema, mental confusion, and acid-base and electrolyte imbalances.

**ure·mic** (u-re′mik) pertaining to or characterized by uremia.

**ure·mi·gen·ic** (u-re″mĭ-jen′ik) 1. caused by or due to uremia. 2. causing uremia.

**ure(o)-** [*urea,* q.v.] for words beginning thus, see also those beginning *urea-*.

**ure·ol·y·sis** (u″re-ol′ĭ-sis) [*ureo-* + *-lysis*] the decomposition of urea to carbon dioxide and ammonia.

**ureo·lyt·ic** (u″re-o-lit′ik) pertaining to, characterized by, or promoting ureolysis.

**ure·om·e·try** (u″re-om′ə-tre) ureametry.

**ureo·tel·ic** (u″re-o-tel′ik) [*ureo-* + *tel-* + *-ic*] having urea as the chief excretory product of nitrogen metabolism.

**ure·si·es·the·sis** (u-re″se-əs-the′sis) [*uresis* + *esthesis*] the normal impulse to pass the urine.

**ure·sis** (u-re′sis) [Gr. *ourēsis*] urination.

**-uresis** a word termination denoting excretion in the urine of the substance indicated by the stem to which it is affixed, as chloruresis, cupruresis, or saluresis.

**ure·tal** (u-re′təl) ureteral.

**ure·ter** (u-re′tər) [Gr. *ourētēr*] [TA] [MeSH: Ureter] the fibromuscular tube which conveys the urine from the kidney to the bladder. It begins with the pelvis of the kidney, a funnel-like dilatation, and empties into the base of the bladder, being 16 to 18 inches long. It is divided into a pars abdominalis and a pars pelvina. See Plate 50.
**circumcaval u.,** postcaval u.
**ectopic u.,** a ureter which opens elsewhere than in the bladder wall, usually arising from the upper segment of a double kidney, and, in the female, opening in the vestibule, terminal urethra, vagina, cervix, or uterine cavity; in the male it invariably enters the genital or urinary tract above the level of the external sphincter.
**postcaval u.,** a congenital anomaly in which the right ureter passes behind the inferior vena cava and curves round this vessel to regain its anterior position as it descends to the bladder; called also *circumcaval u.* and *retrocaval u.*
**retrocaval u.,** postcaval u.
**retroiliac u.,** a congenital anomaly in which a ureter passes behind the iliac artery.

**ure·ter·al** (u-re′tər-əl) pertaining to or used upon the ureter.

**ure·ter·al·gia** (u″re-tər-al′jə) pain in the ureter; neuralgia of the ureter.

**ure·ter·ec·ta·sia** (u-re″tər-ək-ta′zhə) ureterectasis.

**ure·ter·ec·ta·sis** (u-re″tər-ek′tə-sis) [*ureter* + *ectasis*] distention of the ureter.

**ure·ter·ec·to·my** (u″re-tər-ek′tə-me) [*ureter* + *-ectomy*] the surgical removal of a ureter or of a part of it.

**ure·ter·ic** (u″rə-ter′ik) ureteral.

**ure·ter·itis** (u″re-tər-i′tis) inflammation of a ureter.
**u. cys′tica,** ureteritis characterized by the formation of multiple submucosal cysts.
**u. glandula′ris,** ureteritis characterized by the conversion of transitional mucosal into cylindrical epithelium, with formation of glandular acini.

**ureter(o)-** [*ureter,* q.v.] a combining form denoting relationship to the ureter.

**ure·tero·cele** (u-re′tər-o-sēl″) [*uretero-* + *-cele*[1]] [MeSH: Ureterocele] sacculation of the terminal portion of the ureter into the bladder, as a result of stenosis of the ureteral meatus. See illustration.
**ectopic u.,** one which is located distal to the trigone of the bladder and which may extend into the urethra.

**ure·tero·ce·lec·to·my** (u-re″tər-o-se-lek′tə-me) excision of a ureterocele.

**ure·tero·cer·vi·cal** (u-re″tər-o-ser′vĭ-kəl) pertaining to a ureter and to the cervix uteri.

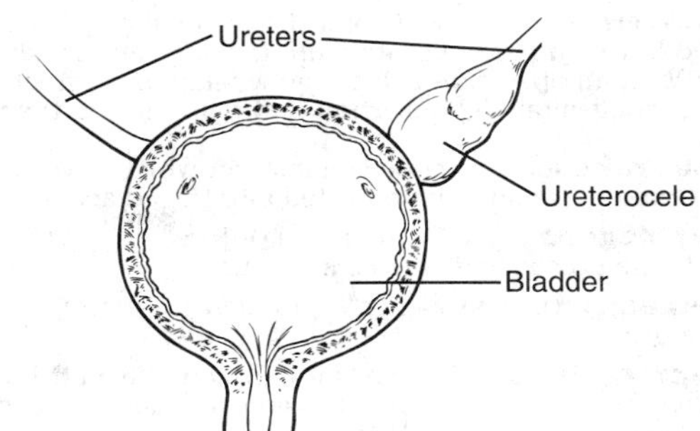


**ure·tero·co·los·to·my** (u-re″tər-o-ko-los′tə-me) [*uretero-* + *colostomy*] anastomosis of a ureter to the colon.

**ure·tero·cu·ta·ne·os·to·my** (u-re″tər-o-ku-ta″ne-os′tə-me) surgical creation of a ureteral opening on the skin, permitting drainage of urine directly to the exterior of the body.

**ure·tero·cys·ta·nas·to·mo·sis** (u-re″tər-o-sis″tə-nas″tə-mo′sis) ureteroneocystostomy.

**ure·tero·cys·to·ne·os·to·my** (u-re″tər-o-sis″to-ne-os′tə-me) [*uretero-* + *cysto-* + *neo-* + *-stomy*] ureteroneocystostomy.

**ure·tero·cys·to·scope** (u-re″tər-o-sis′to-skōp) [*uretero-* + *cystoscope*] a cystoscope designed for catheterizing the ureters.

**ure·tero·cys·tos·to·my** (u-re″tər-o-sis-tos′tə-me) [*uretero-* + *cystostomy*] ureteroneocystostomy.

**ure·tero·du·o·de·nal** (u-re″tər-o-doo″o-de′nəl) pertaining to or communicating with a ureter and the duodenum, as a ureteroduodenal fistula.

**ure·tero·en·ter·ic** (u-re″tər-o-ən-ter′ik) pertaining to or connecting the ureter and the intestine.

**ure·tero·en·tero·anas·to·mo·sis** (u-re″tər-o-en″tər-o-ə-nas″tə-mo′sis) ureteroenterostomy.

**ure·tero·en·ter·os·to·my** (u-re″tər-o-en″tər-os′tə-me) [*uretero-* + *enterostomy*] surgical creation of an opening between a ureter and the intestine.

**ure·tero·gram** (u-re′tər-o-gram) a radiograph of the ureter.

**ure·ter·og·ra·phy** (u-re″tər-og′rə-fe) [*uretero-* + *-graphy*] radiography of the ureter after injection of an opaque medium into the ureter.

**ure·tero·il·e·os·to·my** (u-re″tər-o-il″e-os′tə-me) anastomosis of the ureters to an isolated loop of the ileum, drained through a stoma on the abdominal wall. See also *ileal conduit,* under *conduit.*

**ure·tero·in·tes·ti·nal** (u-re″tər-o-in-tes′tĭ-nəl) pertaining to or connecting the ureter and intestine.

**ure·tero·lith** (u-re′tər-o-lith) [*uretero-* + *-lith*] a calculus lodged or formed in a ureter.

**ure·tero·li·thi·a·sis** (u-re″tər-o-lĭ-thi′ə-sis) the formation of a calculus in the ureter.

**ure·tero·li·thot·o·my** (u-re″tər-o-lĭ-thot′ə-me) [*uretero-* + *litho-* + *-tomy*] the removal of a calculus from the ureter by incision.

**ure·ter·ol·y·sis** (u-re″tər-ol′ĭ-sis) [*uretero-* + *-lysis*] 1. rupture of the ureter. 2. paralysis of the ureter. 3. the operation of freeing the ureter from adhesions.

**ure·tero·me·a·tot·o·my** (u-re″tər-o-me″ə-tot′ə-me) incision of the opening of the ureter in the bladder wall.

**ure·tero·neo·cys·tos·to·my** (u-re″tər-o-ne″o-sis-tos′tə-me) [*uretero-* + *neo-* + *cystostomy*] surgical transplantation of the ureter to a different site in the bladder. Called also *ureterocystostomy* and *ureterocystoneostomy.*

**ure·tero·neo·py·elos·to·my** (u-re″tər-o-ne″o-pi″ə-los′tə-me) [*uretero-* + *neo-* + *pyelostomy*] ureteropyeloneostomy.

**ure·tero·ne·phrec·to·my** (u-re″tər-o-nə-frek′tə-me) [*uretero-* + *nephr-* + *-ectomy*] extirpation of a kidney and its ureter.

**ure·ter·op·a·thy** (u-re″tər-op′ə-the) [*uretero-* + *-pathy*] any disease of the ureter.

**ure·tero·pel·vic** (u-re″tər-o-pel′vik) pertaining to or affecting the ureter and the renal pelvis.

**ure·tero·pel·vio·ne·os·to·my** (u-re″tər-o-pel″ve-o-ne-os′tə-me) ureteropyeloneostomy.

**ure·tero·pel·vio·plas·ty** (u-re″tər-o-pel′ve-o-plas″te) surgical reconstruction of the junction of the ureter and renal pelvis.

**Culp-DeWeerd u.**, ureteropelvioplasty in which a spiral pelvic flap is turned down and incorporated into the adjacent ureter.
**Foley Y-V u.**, an operation using a pelvic flap for correction of obstructive, congenital high insertion of the ureter into the renal pelvis.
**Scardino-Prince u.**, ureteropelvioplasty in which a vertical pelvic flap is turned down and incorporated into the adjacent ureter.

**ure·tero·phleg·ma** (u-re″tər-o-fleg′mə) [*uretero-* + Gr. *phlegma* phlegm] the presence of mucus in the ureter.

**ure·tero·plas·ty** (u-re′tər-o-plas″te) [*uretero-* + *-plasty*] plastic surgery of a ureter.

**ure·tero·proc·tos·to·my** (u-re″tər-o-prok-tos′tə-me) [*uretero-* + *proctostomy*] surgical creation of an anastomosis between a ureter and the lower rectum. Called also *ureterorectostomy.*

**ure·tero·py·eli·tis** (u-re″tər-o-pi-ə-li′tis) [*uretero-* + *pyelitis*] inflammation of a ureter and of the pelvis of a kidney.

**ure·tero·py·elog·ra·phy** (u-re″tər-o-pi-ə-log′rə-fe) radiography of the ureter and pelvis of the kidney. Called also *pelviureteroradiography.*

**ure·tero·py·elo·ne·os·to·my** (u-re″tər-o-pi″ə-lo-ne-os′tə-me) [*uretero-* + *pyelo-* + *neo-* + *-stomy*] surgical formation of a new passage from the pelvis of a kidney to the ureter. Called also *ureteroneopyelostomy, ureteropelvioneostomy, ureteropyelonephrostomy,* and *pelvioneostomy.*

**ure·tero·py·elo·ne·phri·tis** (u-re″tər-o-pi″ə-lo-nə-fri′tis) [*uretero-* + *pyelo-* + *nephritis*] inflammation of the ureter and the pelvis of the kidney.

**ure·tero·py·elo·ne·phros·to·my** (u-re″tər-o-pi″ə-lo-nə-fros′tə-me) ureteropyeloneostomy.

**ure·tero·py·elo·plas·ty** (u-re″tər-o-pi′ə-lo-plas″te) any plastic operation on the ureter and renal pelvis. Called also *pyeloureteroplasty.*

**ure·tero·py·elos·to·my** (u-re″tər-o-pi″ə-los′tə-me) ureteropyeloneostomy.

**ure·tero·py·o·sis** (u-re″tər-o-pi-o′sis) [*uretero-* + *pyo-* + *-osis*] suppurative inflammation of the ureter.

**ure·tero·rec·tal** (u-re″tər-o-rek′təl) pertaining to or communicating with a ureter and the rectum, as a ureterorectal fistula.

**ure·tero·rec·to·ne·os·to·my** (u-re″tər-o-rek″to-ne-os′tə-me) ureteroproctostomy.

**ure·tero·rec·tos·to·my** (u-re″tər-o-rək-tos′tə-me) ureteroproctostomy.

**ure·tero·re·no·scope** (u-re″tər-o-re′no-skōp) a fiberoptic endoscope used in ureterorenoscopy.

**ure·tero·re·nos·co·py** (u-re″tər-o-re-nos′kə-pe) visual inspection of the interior of the ureter and kidney by means of a fiberoptic endoscope for such purposes as biopsy, removal or crushing of stones, etc.

**ure·ter·or·rha·gia** (u-re″tər-o-ra′jə) [*uretero-* + *-rrhagia*] a discharge of blood from the ureter.

**ure·ter·or·rha·phy** (u-re″tər-or′ə-fe) [*uretero-* + *-rrhaphy*] suture of a ureter.

**ure·tero·scope** (u-re′tər-o-skōp″) a fiberoptic endoscope used in ureteroscopy.

**ure·ter·os·copy** (u-re″tər-os′kə-pe) [MeSH: Ureteroscopy] examination of the ureter by means of a fiberoptic endoscope.

**ure·tero·sig·moi·dos·to·my** (u-re″tər-o-sig″moi-dos′tə-me) the operation of implanting the ureter into the sigmoid colon.

**ure·tero·steg·no·sis** (u-re″tər-o-stəg-no′sis) [*uretero-* + *stegnosis*] ureterostenosis.

**ure·tero·ste·no·ma** (u-re″tər-o-stə-no′mə) [*uretero-* + Gr. *stenōma* stricture] ureterostenosis.

**ure·tero·ste·no·sis** (u-re″tər-o-stə-no′sis) [*uretero-* + *stenosis*] stricture of the ureter.

**ure·ter·os·to·ma** (u″re-tər-os′to-mə) [*uretero-* + *stoma*] 1. the vesical orifice of the ureter (ostium ureteris [TA]). 2. a ureteral fistula.

**ure·ter·os·to·my** (u″re-tər-os′tə-me) [*uretero-* + *-stomy*] [MeSH: Ureterostomy] surgical formation of a fistula through which a ureter may discharge its contents.
**cutaneous u.**, the operation of bringing the ureter to the skin through an incision in the iliac region; ureterocutaneostomy.

**ure·ter·ot·o·my** (u″re-tər-ot′ə-me) [*uretero-* + *-tomy*] surgical incision of a ureter.

**ure·tero·tri·go·no·en·ter·os·to·my** (u-re″tər-o-tri-go″no-en″tər-os′tə-me) implantation into the intestine of the ureter with the part of the bladder wall surrounding its termination.

**ure·tero·tri·go·no·sig·moi·dos·to·my** (u-re″tər-o-tri-go″no-sig″moi-dos′tə-me) implantation of the ureter with part of the bladder wall into the sigmoid colon.

**ure·tero·ure·ter·al** (u-re″tər-o-u-re′tər-əl) connecting two parts of the ureter.

**ure·tero·ure·ter·os·to·my** (u-re″tər-o-u-re″tər-os′tə-me) end-to-end anastomosis of the two portions of a transected ureter; see also *transureteroureterostomy.*

**ure·tero·uter·ine** (u-re″tər-o-u′tər-in) pertaining to or communicating with a ureter and the uterus.

**ure·tero·vag·i·nal** (u-re″tər-o-vaj′ĭ-nəl) pertaining to or communicating with a ureter and the vagina.

**ure·tero·ves·i·cal** (u-re″tər-o-ves′ĭ-kəl) pertaining to a ureter and the bladder.

**ure·tero·ves·i·co·plas·ty** (u-re″tər-o-ves′ĭ-ko-plas″te) plastic repair of the ureterovesical junction for correction of ureterovesical reflux or obstruction.

**ure·tero·ves·i·cos·to·my** (u-re″tər-o-ves″ĭ-kos′tə-me) the operation of reimplanting the ureter at a different site in the bladder wall.

**ure·thra** (u-re′thrə) [Gr. *ourēthra*] [MeSH: Urethra] the membranous canal conveying urine from the bladder to the exterior of the body. See Plate 50.
**anterior u.**, the portion of the male urethra extending from the bulb to the meatus on the summit of the glans penis, tunneling the corpus spongiosum; it consists of three parts: the bulbous, the pendulous, and the most distal, glandular part.
**double u.**, congenital complete or partial reduplication of the urethra; the urethral openings may be side by side or one above the other.
**u. femini′na** [TA], female urethra: a canal about 3.7 cm. long, extending from the neck of the bladder, running above the anterior vaginal wall and piercing the urogenital diaphragm, to reach the urinary meatus; called also *u. muliebris.*
**u. masculi′na** [TA], male urethra: a canal extending from the neck of the bladder to the urinary meatus, measuring about 20 cm. in length, and presenting a double curve when the penis is flaccid; it is divided into a *pars spongiosa, pars intermedia,* and *pars prostatica.* Called also *u. virilis.*
**membranous u.**, pars intermedia urethrae masculinae.
**u. mulie′bris**, u. feminina.
**posterior u.**, the portion of the male urethra extending from the bladder to the bulb, and consisting of the membranous and prostatic parts.
**prostatic u.**, pars prostatica urethrae masculinae.
**spongiose u., spongy u.**, pars spongiosa urethrae masculinae.
**u. viri′lis**, u. masculina.

**ure·thral** (u-re′thrəl) pertaining to the urethra.

**ure·thral·gia** (u″re-thral′jə) pain in the urethra; called also *urethrodynia.*

**ure·thra·scope** (u-re′thrə-skōp) urethroscope.

**ure·thra·tre·sia** (u-re″thrə-tre′zhə) imperforation of the urethra. Called also *atreturethria.*

**ure·threc·to·my** (u″rə-threk′tə-me) [*urethr-* + *-ectomy*] the surgical removal of the urethra or a part of it.

**ure·threm·phrax·is** (u″rə-thrəm-frak′sis) [*urethr-* + *emphraxis*] obstruction of the urethra.

**ureth·reu·ryn·ter** (u-rēth″roo-rin′tər) [*urethra* + Gr. *eurynein* to make wide] an instrument for dilating the urethra.

**ure·thrism** (u′rə-thriz-əm) [L. *urethrismus*] irritability or chronic spasm of the urethra.

**ure·thri·tis** (u″rə-thri′tis) [MeSH: Urethritis] inflammation of the urethra.
**u. cys′tica**, inflammation of the urethra, with the formation of multiple submucosal cysts.
**u. glandula′ris**, inflammation of the urethra, with conversion of transitional mucosal into cylindrical epithelium, with formation of glandular acini.
**gonococcal u., gonorrheal u.**, gonorrhea in the male.
**gouty u.**, urethritis due to gout.
**u. granulo′sa**, urethritis in which the anterior urethra is filled with granulations.
**nongonococcal u., nonspecific u.**, urethritis without evidence of gonococcal infection, as, for example, that caused by *Chlamydia trachomatis;* called also *simple u.*
**u. orifi′cii exter′ni**, inflammation and ulceration of the external urethral meatus.
**u. petri′ficans**, urethritis with the formation of calcareous matter in the urethral wall.
**prophylactic u.**, a mild urethritis that sometimes follows irrigations used to prevent venereal infections.
**simple u.**, nongonococcal u.

**specific u.**, that due to infection with the gonococcus.
**u. vene'rea,** gonorrhea.

**urethr(o)-** [*urethra,* q.v.] a combining form denoting relationship to the urethra.

**ure•thro•blen•nor•rhea** (u-re″thro-blen″o-re′ə) a purulent discharge from the urethra.

**ure•thro•bul•bar** (u-re″thro-bul′bər) pertaining to the urethra and the bulbus penis.

**ure•thro•cele** (u-re′thro-sēl) [*urethro-* + *-cele*[1]] 1. prolapse of the female urethra through the meatus urinarius. 2. a diverticulum of the urethral walls encroaching upon the vaginal canal.

**ure•thro•cys•ti•tis** (u-re″thro-sis-ti′tis) inflammation of the urethra and bladder; called also *cystourethritis.*

**ure•thro•cys•to•gram** (u-re″thro-sis′to-gram) a radiograph of the urethra and bladder.

**ure•thro•cys•tog•ra•phy** (u-re″thro-sis-tog′rə-fe) [*urethro-* + *cysto-* + *-graphy*] radiography of the urethra and bladder after the injection of a contrast medium.

**ure•thro•cys•to•pexy** (u-re″thro-sis′to-pek″se) [*urethro-* + *cysto-* + *-pexy*] surgical fixation of the urethrovesical junction, and the area of the bladder just above it, to the back of the pubic bones, for relief of stress incontinence.

**ure•thro•dyn•ia** (u-re″thro-din′e-ə) [*urethro-* + *-odynia*] urethralgia.

**ure•thro•graph** (u-re′thro-graf) an instrument for recording graphically the caliber of the urethra.

**ure•throg•ra•phy** (u″rə-throg′rə-fe) radiography of the urethra after the injection of an opaque medium.

**ure•throm•e•ter** (u″rə-throm′ə-tər) [*urethro-* + *-meter*] an instrument for measuring the urethra.

**ure•throm•e•try** (u″rə-throm′ə-tre) 1. determination of the resistance of various segments of the urethra to retrograde flow of fluid. 2. measurement of the urethra.

**ure•thro•pe•nile** (u-re″thro-pe′nīl) pertaining to the urethra and the penis.

**ure•thro•peri•ne•al** (u-re″thro-per″ĭ-ne′əl) pertaining to or communicating with the urethra and the perineum.

**ure•thro•peri•neo•scro•tal** (u-re″thro-per″ĭ-ne″o-skro′təl) pertaining to the urethra, perineum, and scrotum.

**ure•thro•pexy** (u-re′thro-pek″se) [*urethro-* + *-pexy*] surgical fixation of the urethra to the overlying symphysis pubis and fascia of the rectus abdominis muscle, in correction of stress incontinence in the female.

**ure•thro•phrax•is** (u-re″thro-frak′sis) [*urethro-* + Gr. *phrassein* to stop up] urethremphraxis.

**ure•thro•phy•ma** (u-re″thro-fi′mə) [*urethro-* + *phyma*] a tumor or growth in the urethra.

**ure•thro•plas•ty** (u-re′thro-plas″te) [*urethro-* + *-plasty*] plastic surgery of the urethra.

**ure•thro•pros•tat•ic** (u-re″thro-pros-tat′ik) pertaining to the urethra and the prostate.

**ure•thro•rec•tal** (u-re″thro-rek′təl) pertaining to or communicating with the urethra and the rectum.

**ure•thror•rha•gia** (u-re″thro-ra′je-ə) [*urethro-* + *-rrhagia*] a flow of blood from the urethra.

**ure•thror•rha•phy** (u″rə-thror′ə-fe) [*urethro-* + *-rrhaphy*] suture of the urethra.

**ure•thror•rhea** (u-re″thro-re′ə) [*urethro-* + *-rrhea*] an abnormal discharge from the urethra.

**ure•thro•scope** (u-re′thro-skōp) [*urethro-* + *-scope*] an instrument for viewing the interior of the urethra.

**ure•thro•scop•ic** (u-re″thro-skop′ik) pertaining to the urethroscope or urethroscopy.

**ure•thros•co•py** (u″rə-thros′kə-pe) [*urethro-* + *-scopy*] visual inspection of the interior of the urethra.

**ure•thro•scro•tal** (u-re″thro-skro′təl) pertaining to or communicating with the urethra and scrotum, as a urethroscrotal fistula.

**ure•thro•spasm** (u-re′thro-spaz-əm) [*urethro-* + *spasm*] spasm of the muscular tissue of the urethra.

**ure•thro•stax•is** (u-re″thro-stak′sis) [*urethro-* + *staxis*] oozing of blood from the urethra.

**ure•thro•ste•no•sis** (u-re″thro-stə-no′sis) [*urethro-* + *stenosis*] stricture or stenosis of the urethra.

**ure•thros•to•my** (u″rə-thros′tə-me) [*urethro-* + *-stomy*] surgical formation of a permanent opening of the urethra at the perineal surface.

**ure•thro•tome** (u-re′thro-tōm) an instrument for cutting a urethral stricture.
**Maisonneuve's u.**, a urethrotome in which the knife is concealed until it reaches the stricture.

**ure•throt•o•my** (u″rə-throt′ə-me) [*urethro-* + *-tomy*] incision of the urethra for relief of stricture.
**external u.**, incision of the urethra through the perineum.
**internal u.**, incision of the urethra from within, either blindly or with an instrument that permits direct visualization.

**ure•thro•tri•go•ni•tis** (u-re″thro-tri″go-ni′tis) inflammation of the urethra and trigone of the bladder.

**ure•thro•vag•i•nal** (u-re″thro-vaj′ĭ-nəl) pertaining to or communicating with the urethra and the vagina.

**ure•thro•ves•i•cal** (u-re″thro-ves′ĭ-kəl) vesicourethral.

**uret•ic** (u-ret′ik) [L. *ureticus;* Gr. *ourētikos*] 1. pertaining to the urine. 2. diuretic.

**Urex** (u′reks) trademark for a preparation of methenamine hippurate.

**ur•gen•cy** (ur′jən-se) the sudden compelling urge to urinate.

**Ur•gin•ea** (ər-jin′e-ə) [L.] a genus of plants of the family Liliaceae. *U. mari'tima* (L.) Baker, a white Mediterranean species, and *U. in'dica* Kunth., an Indian species, are varieties of squill.

**ur•hid•ro•sis** (ūr″hid-ro′sis) [*ur-* + *hidro-* + *-sis*] the presence in the sweat of urinous materials, such as uric acid, urea, etc. Called also *uridrosis.*
**u. crystal'lina,** a form in which crystals of uric acid are deposited upon the skin. Called also *urea frost.*

**-uria** [Gr. *ouron* urine + *-ia*] a word termination denoting a characteristic or constituent of the urine, indicated by the stem to which it is affixed, as oliguria, proteinuria.

**uri•an** (u′re-an) urochrome.

**uric** (u′rik) [Gr. *ourikos*] urinary. See also *uric acid.*

**uric ac•id** (u′rik) [MeSH: Uric Acid] the end-product of purine catabolism in primates. Urate is very insoluble in water, and disorders of purine metabolism produce gout, in which deposition of sodium urate crystals (tophi) in the joints and skin is followed by a foreign-body inflammatory response. Called also *lithic acid.*

**uric•ac•i•de•mia** (u″rik-as″ĭ-de′me-ə) hyperuricemia.

**uric•ac•i•du•ria** (u″rik-as″ĭ-du′re-ə) hyperuricuria.

**uri•case** (u′rĭ-kās) urate oxidase.

**uri•ce•mia** (u″rĭ-se′me-ə) hyperuricemia.

**uric(o)-** [Gr. *ouron* urine] of or pertaining to the urine or to uric acid.

**uri•co•cho•lia** (u″rĭ-ko-ko′le-ə) [*urico-* + *chol-* + *-ia*] the presence of uric acid in the bile.

**uri•col•y•sis** (u″rĭ-kol′ĭ-sis) [*urico-* + *-lysis*] the cleavage of uric acid or of urates.

**uri•co•lyt•ic** (u″rĭ-ko-lit′ik) pertaining to, characterized by, or promoting uricolysis.

**uri•com•e•ter** (u″rĭ-kom′ə-tər) [*urico-* + *-meter*] an instrument for measuring the amount of uric acid in the urine.
**Ruhemann's u.**, one based on the principle that uric acid will absorb iodine.

**uri•co•poi•e•sis** (u″rĭ-ko-poi-e′sis) the formation of uric acid.

**uri•co•su•ria** (u″rĭ-ko-su′re-ə) hyperuricuria.

**uri•co•su•ric** (u″rĭ-ko-su′rik) 1. pertaining to, characterized by, or promoting uricosuria. 2. an agent that promotes uricosuria.

**uri•co•tel•ic** (u″rĭ-ko-tel′ik) [*urico-* + *tel-* + *-ic*] having uric acid as the chief excretory product of nitrogen metabolism, as in reptiles and birds.

**uri•co•tel•ism** (u″rĭ-ko-tel′iz-əm) the excretion of uric acid as the end product of nitrogen metabolism, as in reptiles and birds.

**Uri•cult** (u′rĭ-kəlt) trademark for a bacterial culture device, consisting of a glass slide in a sterile plastic container. On one face of the slide a 13 sq cm area is coated with MacConkey's medium; on the other a similar area is coated with nutrient agar. The slide is dipped into freshly voided urine, removed, and replaced in the container, where growth takes place.

**uri•dine** (ūr′ĭ-dēn) [MeSH: Uridine] a pyrimidine nucleoside, uracil linked by its N1 nitrogen to the C1 carbon of ribose. It is a component of ribonucleic acid, and its nucleotides participate in the biosynthesis of polysaccharides and some polysaccharide-containing compounds. Symbol U.
**u. diphosphate (UDP),** a nucleotide, the 5′-pyrophosphate of uridine, which serves as a carrier for hexoses, hexosamines, and hexuronic acids in the synthesis of glycogen, glycoproteins, and gly-

cosaminoglycans. UDPglucose and UDP-*N*-acetylglucosamine are the parent compounds from which are synthesized the other UDP-linked hexoses, hexosamines, and hexuronic acids. See also specific UDP-linked compounds (e.g., UDPgalactose).

**u. monophosphate (UMP),** a nucleotide, the 5′-phosphate of uridine; it is a component of ribonucleic acid. Called also *uridylic acid.*

**u. triphosphate (UTP),** a nucleotide, the 5′-triphosphate of uridine; it is an activated precursor in the synthesis of ribonucleic acid and of UDP-linked hexoses involved in glycogen and glycoprotein metabolism.

**uri·dro·sis** (u″rĭ-dro′sis) urhidrosis.

**uri·dyl·ate** (ur″ĭ-dil′āt) a dissociated form of uridylic acid.

**uri·dyl·ic ac·id** (ur″ĭ-dil′ik) phosphorylated uridine, uridine monophosphate unless otherwise specified.

**uri·dyl trans·fer·ase** (u′ri-dəl trans′fər-ās) UDPglucose–hexose-1-phosphate uridylyltransferase.

**uri·dyl·yl** (ur′ĭ-dil′əl) the radical formed by removal of OH from the phosphate group of uridine monophosphate.

**uri·es·the·sis** (u″re-es′thə-sis) uresiesthesis.

**urin·a·ble** (u′rin-ə-bəl) capable of being excreted in the urine.

**urin·ac·cel·er·a·tor** (u″rin-ək-sel′ər-a″tor) musculus bulbospongiosus.

**urin·ac·i·dom·e·ter** (u″rin-as″ĭ-dom′ə-tər) an instrument for estimating the pH of urine.

**uri·nae·mia** (u″rĭ-ne′me-ə) uremia.

**uri·nal** (u′rĭ-nəl) [L. *urinalis* urinary] a vessel or other receptacle for urine.

**uri·nal·y·sis** (u″rĭ-nal′ĭ-sis) [MeSH: Urinalysis] physical, chemical, or microscopic analysis or examination of urine.

**uri·nary** (u′rĭ-nar″e) pertaining to the urine; containing or secreting urine.

**uri·nate** (u′rĭ-nāt) to void or discharge urine.

**uri·na·tion** (u″rĭ-na′shən) [MeSH: Urination] the discharge or passage of urine. Called also *micturition* and *uresis.*

**precipitant u.,** urgency.

**stuttering u.,** an intermittent flow of urine, due to vesical spasm. Called also *urinary stuttering.*

**uri·na·tive** (u′rĭ-na″tiv) diuretic.

**urine** (u′rin) [L. *urina;* Gr. *ouron*] [MeSH: Urine] the fluid excreted by the kidneys, passed through the ureters, stored in the bladder, and discharged through the urethra; its constituents and volume vary widely from day to day in order to maintain normal fluid and electrolyte homeostasis.

**black u.,** urine colored black by melanin (melanuria), or by derivatives of homogentisic acid (ochronosis).

**chylous u.,** chyluria.

**cloudy u.,** urine having a cloudy appearance, usually due to phosphaturia or uraturia, but sometimes caused by pyuria; called also *nebulous u.*

**crude u.,** light-colored, watery urine, which deposits little sediment.

**diabetic u.,** that which contains an excess of glucose.

**dyspeptic u.,** the urine in dyspepsia, frequently containing calcium oxalate crystals.

**febrile u.,** strong, odorous, high-colored, concentrated urine, such as is secreted in fever.

**gouty u.,** scanty, high-colored urine containing large quantities of urates.

**milky u.,** urine having a milky appearance, which may be due to chyluria or pyuria.

**nebulous u.,** cloudy u.

**residual u.,** the urine that remains in the bladder after urination in disease of the bladder and hypertrophy of the prostate.

**uri·ne·mia** (u″rĭ-ne′me-ə) [*urin-* + *-emia*] uremia.

**urin·i·dro·sis** (u″rin-ĭ-dro′sis) urhidrosis.

**uri·nif·er·ous** (u″rĭ-nif′ər-əs) [*urine* + *-ferous*] transporting or conveying the urine.

**uri·nif·ic** (u″rĭ-nif′ik) uriniparous.

**uri·nip·a·rous** (u″rĭ-nip′ə-rəs) [*urine* + L. *parere* to produce] producing or elaborating urine.

**urin(o)-** [L. *urina,* q.v.] a combining form denoting relationship to urine; see also *ur(o)-.*

**uri·no·cry·os·co·py** (u-ri″no-kri-os′kə-pe) cryoscopy of the urine.

**uri·no·gen·i·tal** (u″rĭ-no-jen′ĭ-təl) genitourinary.

**uri·nog·e·nous** (u″rĭ-noj′ə-nəs) urogenous (def. 2).

**uri·no·glu·co·som·e·ter** (u″rĭ-no-gloo″ko-som′ə-tər) an instrument for measuring the glucose in the urine.

**uri·nol·o·gist** (u″rĭ-nol′ə-jist) urologist.

**uri·nol·o·gy** (u″rĭ-nol′ə-je) urology.

**uri·no·ma** (u″rĭ-no′mə) [*urine* + *-oma*] a collection of urine encapsulated by fibrous tissue, resulting from leakage of urine from a tear in the ureter or renal pelvis or calices while the ureter is obstructed; it may be a result of external trauma or a postoperative complication. Called also *pararenal pseudocyst.*

**uri·nom·e·ter** (u″rĭ-nom′ə-tər) [*urino-* + *-meter*] an instrument for determining the specific gravity of the urine.

**uri·nom·e·try** (u″rĭ-nom′ə-tre) the ascertainment of the specific gravity of the urine.

**uri·noph·i·lous** (u″rĭ-nof′ĭ-ləs) [*urino-* + Gr. *philein* to love] having an affinity for urine, as a microorganism that grows best in urine.

**uri·nos·co·py** (u″rĭ-nos′kə-pe) uroscopy.

**uri·no·sex·u·al** (u″rĭ-no-sek′shoo-əl) genitourinary.

**uri·no·tho·rax** (u″rĭ-no-tho′raks) hydrothorax in which the fluid is urine, secondary to an obstruction in the renal pelvis or urinary tract.

**uri·nous** (u′rĭ-nəs) urinary.

**uri·po·sia** (u″rĭ-po′ze-ə) [*urine* + *-posia*] the drinking of urine.

**urish·i·ol** (u-rish′e-ol) an extremely allergenically active mixture of catechol derivatives forming the major constituent of the irritant resin of poison ivy and other members of Anacardiaceae.

**Uri·spas** (u′rĭ-spaz) trademark for a preparation of flavoxate hydrochloride.

**Uri·tone** (u′rĭ-tōn) trademark for preparations of methenamine.

**ur(o)-** [Gr. *ouron* urine] a combining form denoting relationship to urine, the urinary tract, or urination. Also, *uron(o)-.*

**uro·ac·i·dim·e·ter** (u″ro-as″ĭ-dim′ə-tər) an instrument for measuring the acidity of the urine.

**uro·am·mo·ni·ac** (u″ro-ə-mo′ne-ak) containing uric acid and ammonia.

**uro·an·the·lone** (u″ro-an′thə-lōn) former name for *human epidermal growth factor.*

**uro·az·o·tom·e·ter** (u″ro-az″o-tom′ə-tər) an apparatus for measuring the nitrogenous matter of the urine.

**uro·ben·zo·ic ac·id** (u″ro-ben-zo′ik) hippuric acid.

**uro·bi·lin** (u″ro-bi′lin) [*uro-* + *bilin*] [MeSH: Urobilin] an amorphous, brownish pigment, an oxidized form of urobilinogen, found in the feces and sometimes in urine left standing in the air.

**uro·bil·in·emia** (u″ro-bil″ĭ-ne′me-ə) [*urobilin* + *-emia*] the presence of urobilin in the blood.

**uro·bi·lino·gen** (u″ro-bĭ-lin′o-jən) [*urobilin* + *-gen*] [MeSH: Urobilinogen] a colorless compound formed in the intestines by the reduction of bilirubin. Some is excreted in the feces, where by oxidation it becomes urobilin, and some is reabsorbed and re-excreted either in the bile as bilirubin or at times in the urine, where it may be later oxidized to urobilin.

**uro·bi·lino·gen·emia** (u″ro-bĭ-lin″o-jə-ne′me-ə) the presence of urobilinogen in the blood.

**uro·bi·lino·gen·uria** (u″ro-bĭ-lin″o-jə-nu′re-ə) the presence of urobilinogen in the urine.

**uro·bil·i·noid** (u″ro-bil′ĭ-noid) resembling urobilin.

**uro·bil·i·noi·den** (u″ro-bil″ĭ-noi′dən) a reduction product of hematin, resembling urobilin, sometimes found in the urine.

**uro·bil·in·uria** (u″ro-bil″ĭ-nu′re-ə) [*urobilin* + *-uria*] the presence of an excess of urobilin in the urine, as in cirrhosis of the liver.

**uro·can·ase** (u″ro-kan′ās) urocanate hydratase.

**uro·can·ase de·fi·cien·cy** an inherited disorder of histidine catabolism caused by deficiency of urocanate hydratase; it is characterized by excess urinary excretion of urocanic acid and growth retardation and may also be associated with mental retardation.

**uro·can·ate** (u″ro-kan′at) the anionic form of urocanic acid.

**uro·can·ate hy·dra·tase** (u″ro-kan′āt hy′drə-tās) [EC 4.2.1.49] [MeSH: Urocanate Hydratase] an enzyme of the lyase class that catalyzes the reduction of urocanate to formiminoglutamate, a step in the catabolism of histidine. Deficiency of the enzyme, presumed to be an autosomal recessive trait, causes urocanase deficiency. Called also *urocanase.*

**uro·can·ic ac·id** (u″ro-kan′ik) [MeSH: Urocanic Acid] a product of the direct deamination of histidine, one of the pathways of histidine catabolism; it is accumulated and excreted in the urine in urocanase deficiency.

**uro·cele** (u'ro-sēl) [*uro-* + *-cele*[1]] distention of the scrotum with extravasated urine.

**uroch·er·as** (u-rok'ər-əs) [*uro-* + Gr. *cheras* gravel] uropsammus.

**uro·che·zia** (u″ro-ke'ze-ə) [*uro-* + Gr. *chezein* to defecate + *-ia*] the discharge of urine in the feces.

**Uro·chor·da·ta** (u″ro-kor-da'tə) [Gr. *oura* tail + L. *chorda* string] [MeSH: Urochordata] a subphylum of chordates intermediate between the invertebrates and true vertebrates, including the sea squirts and their allies, the members of which have a saclike body and a leathery tunic; the notochord is present only during the larval stage. Called also *Tunicata.*

**uro·chor·date** (u-ro-kor'dāt) [MeSH: Urochordata] any member of the Urochordata; called also *tunicate.*

**uro·chrome** (u'ro-krōm) [*uro-* + *-chrome*] a yellow, amorphous pigment of the urine, which gives the urine its yellow color.

**uro·chro·mo·gen** (u″ro-kro'mo-jən) a low oxidation product found in the urine, which on further oxidation becomes urochrome.

**uro·ci·net·ic** (u″ro-si-net'ik) urokinetic.

**uro·clep·sia** (u″ro-klep'se-ə) [*uro-* + Gr. *kleptein* to steal] the unconscious escape of urine.

**uro·cris·ia** (u″ro-kriz'e-ə) [*uro-* + Gr. *krinein* to judge] diagnosis by observing or examining the urine. Cf. *uromancy.*

**uro·cri·te·ri·on** (u″ro-kri-tēr'e-on) [*uro-* + *criterion*] an indication of disease observed in examination of the urine.

**Uro·cys·tis** (u″ro-sis'tis) a genus of fungi of the family Tilletiaceae. *U. tri'tici* causes flag smut on wheat in Australia and southern and eastern Asia.

**uro·cys·ti·tis** (u″ro-sis-ti'tis) cystitis.

**uro·di·al·y·sis** (u″ro-di-al'ĭ-sis) [*uro-* + *dialysis*] partial or complete suppression of the urine.

**uro·dy·nam·ic** (u″ro-di-nam'ik) [MeSH: Urodynamics] pertaining to the flow and motion of liquids in the urinary tract.

**uro·dy·nam·ics** (u″ro-di-nam'iks) [MeSH: Urodynamics] the dynamics of the propulsion and flow of urine in the urinary tract.

**uro·dyn·ia** (u″ro-din'e-ə) [*ur-* + *-odynia*] pain accompanying urination.

**uro·ede·ma** (u″ro-ə-de'mə) edema due to infiltration of urine.

**uro·en·ter·one** (u″ro-en'tər-ōn) former name for *human epidermal growth factor.*

**uro·er·y·thrin** (u″ro-er'ĭ-thrin) [*uro-* + Gr. *erythros* red] a dark reddish coloring matter found in the urine; it gives the red color seen in deposits of urates. Called also *purpurin.*

**uro·fla·vin** (u″ro-fla'vin) a fluorescent compound closely related to riboflavin, excreted in the urine.

**uro·flo·me·ter, uro·flow·me·ter** (u″ro-flo'me-tər) a device for the continuous recording of urine flow in milliliters per second, consisting of a cylinder placed on a transducer that weighs the urine entering the cylinder and records it on a time scale.

**uro·fol·li·tro·pin** (u″ro-fol'e-tro″pin) a preparation of gonadotropins from the urine of postmenopausal women, used to induce ovulation; administered by injection.

**uro·fus·cin** (u″ro-fus'in) [*uro-* + *fuscin*] a pigment of the urine which is the precursor of hematoporphyrin.

**uro·fus·co·hem·a·tin** (u″ro-fus″ko-hem'ə-tin) a red-brown pigment in the urine in certain diseases.

**uro·gas·ter** (u″ro-gas'tər) [*uro-* + Gr. *gastēr* stomach] the urinary intestine; a part of the allantoic cavity of the embryo.

**uro·gas·trone** (u″ro-gas'trōn) human epidermal growth factor.

**uro·gen·i·tal** (u″ro-jen'ĭ-təl) genitourinary.

**urog·e·nous** (u-roj'ə-nəs) [*uro-* + *-genous*] 1. producing urine. 2. produced from or in the urine. Called also *urinogenous.*

**Uro·gra·fin** (ūr-o-graf'in) trademark for a contrast medium containing diatrizoate meglumine and diatrizoate sodium.

**uro·gram** (u'ro-gram) a radiograph of part of the urinary tract.

**urog·ra·phy** (u-rog'rə-fe) [MeSH: Urography] radiography of a part of the urinary tract which has been rendered opaque by some opaque medium.
**ascending u.,** retrograde u.
**cystoscopic u.,** retrograde u.
**descending u., excretion u., excretory u., intravenous u.,** radiographic examination of the urinary tract after the intravenous injection of an opaque medium that is rapidly excreted in the urine.
**oral u.,** urography in which the opaque medium is given by the mouth.
**retrograde u.,** urography in which the contrast medium is injected into the bladder through the urethra.

**uro·gra·vim·e·ter** (u″ro-grə-vim'ə-tər) [*uro-* + *gravimeter*] urinometer.

**uro·hem·a·tin** (u″ro-hem'ə-tin) the coloring matter or pigments of the urine; regarded as identical with heme.

**uro·hem·a·to·ne·phro·sis** (u″ro-hem″ə-to-nə-fro'sis) distention of the kidney with urine and blood.

**uro·hem·a·to·por·phy·rin** (u″ro-hem″ə-to-por'fĭ-rin) hematoporphyrin derived from the urine.

**uro·ki·nase (UK)** (u″ro-ki'nās) [MeSH: Urokinase] u-plasminogen activator.

**uro·ki·net·ic** (u″ro-kĭ-net'ik) [*uro-* + *kinetic*] caused by a reflex from the urinary organs; said of a form of dyspepsia.

**uro·ky·mog·ra·phy** (u″ro-ki-mog'rə-fe) kymography applied to study of the urogenital system.

**uro·lag·nia** (u″ro-lag'ne-ə) [*uro-* + Gr. *lagneia* lust] sexual excitement associated with the sight or thought of urine or urination. Cf. *urophilia.*

**uro·lith** (u'ro-lith) [*uro-* + *-lith*] urinary calculus.

**uro·li·thi·a·sis** (u″ro-lĭ-thi'ə-sis) 1. the formation of urinary calculi (see under *calculus*). 2. the diseased condition associated with the presence of urinary calculi.
**feline u.,** urolithiasis in cats, usually males; it is one type of feline urological syndrome.

**uro·lith·ic** (u″ro-lith'ik) pertaining to urinary calculi.

**uro·li·thol·o·gy** (u″ro-lĭ-thol'ə-je) the sum of knowledge regarding urinary calculi.

**uro·log·ic, uro·log·i·cal** (u″ro-loj'ik, u″ro-loj'ĭ-kəl) pertaining to urology.

**urol·o·gist** (u-rol'ə-jist) a physician who specializes in urology.

**urol·o·gy** (u-rol'ə-je) [MeSH: Urology] the medical specialty concerned with the urinary tract in both male and female, and with the genital organs in the male.

**uro·man·cy** (u'ro-man″se) [*uro-* + Gr. *manteia* a divination] prognosis based on examination of urine. Cf. *urocrisia.*

**uro·mel·a·nin** (u″ro-mel'ə-nin) [*uro-* + *melanin*] a black pigment sometimes found in urine; it results from the decomposition of urochrome.

**urom·e·lus** (u-rom'ə-ləs) [Gr. *oura* tail + *melos* limb] sympus monopus.

**urom·e·ter** (u-rom'ə-tər) [*uro-* + *-meter*] urinometer.

**uro·met·ric** (u″ro-met'rik) pertaining to urometry.

**urom·e·try** (u-rom'ə-tre) the measurement and recording of pressure changes caused by contraction of the ureter during ureteral peristalsis.

**uro·mod·u·lin** (u″ro-mod'u-lin) Tamm-Horsfall mucoprotein.

**uro·nate** (u'ro-nāt) a salt, anion, or ester of a uronic acid.

**uron·cus** (u-rong'kəs) [*uro-* + Gr. *onkos* mass] a swelling containing urine.

**uro·ne·phro·sis** (u″ro-nə-fro'sis) abnormal distention of the pelvis and tubules of the kidney with urine.

**ur·on·ic ac·id** (ūr-on'ik) a carboxylic acid produced by oxidation of the terminal —$CH_2OH$ group in a sugar farthest from the carbonyl group to a carboxyl (=COOH) group, e.g., glucuronic acid.

**uron(o)-** see *ur(o)-.*

**uro·nol·o·gy** (u″ro-nol'ə-je) urology.

**uron·on·com·e·try** (u″ron-on-kom'ə-tre) [*urono-* + *onco-*[1] + *-metry*] the measurement of the quantity of urine excreted in twenty-four hours.

**uro·patho·gen** (u″ro-path'o-jən) a microorganism which causes diseases of the urinary tract.

**urop·a·thy** (u-rop'ə-the) [*uro-* + *-pathy*] any disease or other pathologic change in the urinary tract. Called also *urosis.*
**obstructive u.,** any pathologic change in the urinary tract due to obstruction.

**uro·pe·nia** (u″ro-pe'ne-ə) [*uro-* + *-penia*] deficiency of urine or urinary secretion.

**uro·pep·sin·o·gen** (u″ro-pep-sin'o-jən) pepsinogen occurring in the urine.

**uro·phan·ic** (u″ro-fan'ik) [*uro-* + Gr. *phainein* to show] appearing in the urine.

**uro·phe·in** (u″ro-fe′in) [*uro-* + Gr. *phaios* gray] an odoriferous gray pigment of the urine.

**uro·phil·ia** (u″ro-fil′e-ə) [*uro-* + *-philia*] a paraphilia in which sexual arousal or activity is linked to urine. Cf. *urolagnia.*

**uro·phos·phom·e·ter** (u″ro-fos-fom′ə-tər) an instrument for measuring the quantity of phosphorus in the urine.

**uro·pit·tin** (u″ro-pit′in) [*uro-* + Gr. *pitta* pitch] a resinous product of the decomposition of urochrome.

**uro·pla·nia** (u″ro-pla′ne-ə) [*uro-* + Gr. *planē* wandering + *-ia*] the presence of urine in, or its discharge from, organs not of the urogenital tract.

**uro·pod** (u′ro-pod) [Gr. *oura* tail + *pous,* gen. *podos* foot] the cytoplasmic footlike process that trails behind locomoting leukocytes; the term is used particularly of lymphocytes, in which the trailing process and large nucleus produce a characteristic "hand mirror" shape. The uropod serves as a point of attachment to the substrate and may also be involved in cell-cell interactions.

**uro·poi·e·sis** (u″ro-poi-e′sis) [*uro-* + *-poiesis*] the production of the urine.

**uro·poi·et·ic** (u″ro-poi-et′ik) pertaining to or concerned in the production of the urine.

**uro·por·phyr·ia** (u″ro-por-fir′e-ə) porphyria in which there is excessive excretion of uroporphyrin.
**erythropoietic u.,** congenital erythropoietic porphyria.

**uro·por·phy·rin** (u″ro-por′fə-rin) the porphyrin (q.v.) produced by oxidation of the methylene bridges in uroporphyrinogen. Excessive amounts of uroporphyrin I are excreted in congenital erythropoietic porphyria, and both types I and III are excreted in porphyria cutanea tarda. See *uroporphyrinogen.*

**uro·por·phy·rin·o·gen** (u″ro-por″fə-rin′ə-jən) a porphyrinogen (q.v.) in which each pyrrole ring has one acetate side chain and one propionate side chain; it is formed by condensation of four molecules of porphobilinogen. Four isomers are possible but only two exist naturally, types I and III; the latter is a functional intermediate in heme biosynthesis while the former is produced in an abortive side reaction.

**uro·por·phy·rin·o·gen III co·syn·thase** (u″ro-por″fə-rin′ə-jən ko-sin′thās) uroporphyrinogen-III synthase.

**uro·por·phy·rin·o·gen de·car·boxy·lase** (u″ro-por″fə-rin′ə-jən de-kahr-bok′sə-lās) [EC 4.1.1.37] [MeSH: Uroporphyrinogen Decarboxylase] an enzyme of the lyase class that catalyzes the decarboxylation of uroporphyrinogen III to coproporphyrinogen III in the biosynthesis of heme. Decreased enzyme activity is associated with porphyria cutanea tarda and the variant hepatoerythropoietic porphyria.

**uro·por·phy·rin·o·gen I syn·thase** (u″ro-por″fə-rin′ə-jən sin′thās) hydroxymethylbilane synthase.

**uro·por·phy·rin·o·gen-III syn·thase** (u″ro-por″fə-rin′ə-jən sin′thās) [EC 4.2.1.75] an enzyme of the lyase class that acts concertedly with hydroxymethylbilane synthase to convert porphobilinogen to uroporphyrinogen III in the biosynthesis of porphyrins and heme. Deficiency of the enzyme, an autosomal recessive trait, causes congenital erythropoietic porphyria. Called also *uroporphyrinogen III cosynthase.*

**uro·pro·tec·tion** (u″ro-pro-tek′shən) protection of the urinary tract, especially against urotoxic substances.

**uro·pro·tec·tive** (u″ro-pro-tek′tiv) providing uroprotection.

**uro·psam·mus** (u″ro-sam′əs) [*uro-* + *psammous*] sediment or gravel in the urine.

**urop·ter·in** (u-rop′tər-in) a pigment, identical with xanthopterin, isolated from human urine; see *pterin.*

**uro·pyo·ne·phro·sis** (u″ro-pi″o-nə-fro′sis) the presence of urine and pus in the pelvis of the kidney.

**uro·pyo·ure·ter** (u″ro-pi″o-u-re′tər) [*uro-* + *pyo-* + *ureter*] a collection of urine and pus in the ureter.

**uro·ra·di·ol·o·gy** (u″ro-ra″de-ol′ə-je) radiology of the urinary tract.

**uro·rhyth·mog·ra·phy** (u″ro-rith-mog′rə-fe) [*uro-* + *rhythm* + *-graphy*] graphic registration of the ejaculation of the urine from the ureteral orifices.

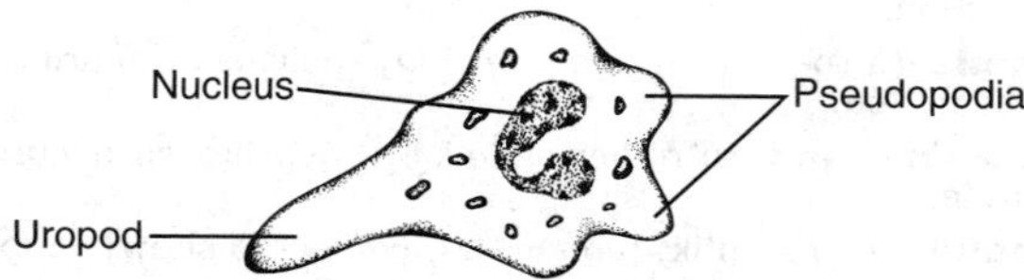

Uropod trailing behind a leukocyte locomoting on a flat surface.

**uro·ro·se·in** (u″ro-ro′ze-in) urorrhodin.

**uro·ro·se·in·o·gen** (u″ro-ro″se-in′ə-jən) urorrhodinogen.

**uror·rho·din** (u″ro-ro′din) a rose-colored pigment found in the urine in typhoid fever, nephritis, pulmonary tuberculosis, and other diseases. See under *tests.*

**uror·rho·din·o·gen** (u″ro-ro-din′ə-jən) a chromogen in the urine which, on decomposition, yields urorrhodin.

**uro·ru·bin** (u″ro-roo′bin) [*uro-* + *rubin*] a red pigment derivable from the urine by the action of hydrochloric acid.

**uro·ru·bin·o·gen** (u″ro-roo-bin′ə-jən) a chromogen from which urorubin is derived.

**uro·sac·cha·rom·e·try** (u″ro-sak″ə-rom′ə-tre) the measurement or estimation of sugar in the urine.

**uro·sa·cin** (u-ro′sa-sin) urorrhodin.

**uros·cheo·cele** (u-ros′ke-o-sēl″) [*uro-* + *oscheocele*] urocele.

**uros·che·sis** (u-ros′kə-sis) [*uro-* + Gr. *schesis* holding] retention of urine.

**uro·scop·ic** (u″ro-skop′ik) pertaining to uroscopy.

**uros·co·py** (u-ros′kə-pe) [*uro-* + *-scopy*] diagnostic examination of the urine.

**uro·se·mi·ol·o·gy** (u″ro-se″me-ol′ə-je) diagnostic study of the urine.

**uro·sep·sis** (u″ro-sep′sis) [*uro-* + *sepsis*] a syndrome characterized by fever, chills, hypotension, and occasionally altered mental status, resulting from invasion from the urinary tract to the bloodstream by microorganisms or their products.

**uro·sep·tic** (u″ro-sep′tik) pertaining to or marked by urosepsis.

**uro·sis** (u-ro′sis) uropathy.

**uro·spec·trin** (u″ro-spek′trin) [*uro-* + L. *spectrum* image] one of the pigments of normal urine; a substance obtainable from certain specimens of urine, allied to hematoporphyrin.

**uro·stal·ag·mom·e·try** (u″ro-stal″əg-mom′ə-tre) the use of the stalagmometer in the study of the urine.

**uro·ste·a·lith** (u″ro-ste′ə-lith) [*uro-* + *stear-* + *-lith*] a fatty constituent of certain urinary calculi; a urinary calculus having fatty constituents.

**uro·the·li·al** (u″ro-the′le-əl) pertaining to the urothelium.

**uro·the·li·um** (u″ro-the′le-əm) [*uro-* + *thelium*] [MeSH: Urothelium] a layer of transitional epithelium in the wall of the bladder, ureter, and renal pelvis, external to the lamina propria.

**uro·tox·ia** (u″ro-tok′se-ə) [*uro-* + *tox-* + *-ia*] 1. the toxicity of the urine. 2. the toxic substances of the urine.

**uro·tox·ic** (u″ro-tok′sik) pertaining to the toxic materials of the urine.

**uro·tox·ic·i·ty** (u″ro-tok-sis′ĭ-te) the toxic quality of the urine.

**uro·tox·in** (u″ro-tok′sin) the toxic or poisonous constituents of the urine.

**uro·toxy** (u′ro-tok″se) urotoxia.

**Urot·ro·pin** (u-rot′ro-pin) trademark for a preparation of methenamine.

**uro·ure·ter** (u″ro-u-re′tər) distention of the ureter with urine.

**urox·in** (u-rok′sin) alloxantin.

**ur·rho·din** (u-ro′din) urorrhodin.

**ur·so·de·oxy·cho·late** (ur″so-de-ok″se-ko′lāt) a salt, ester, or anionic form of ursodeoxycholic acid.

**ur·so·de·oxy·cho·lic ac·id** (ur″so-de-ok″se-ko′lik) [MeSH: Ursodeoxycholic Acid] a secondary bile acid formed in the intestine from chenodeoxycholic acid; it is choleretic and decreases the concentration of cholesterol in the bile. The pharmaceutical preparation is called *ursodiol.*

**ur·so·de·oxy·cho·lyl·gly·cine** (ur″so-de-ok″se-ko″ləl-gli′sēn) a bile salt, the glycine conjugate of ursodeoxycholic acid.

**ur·so·de·oxy·cho·lyl·tau·rine** (ur″so-de-ok″se-ko″ləl-taw′rēn) a bile salt, the taurine conjugate of ursodeoxycholic acid.

**ur·so·di·ol** (ur″so-di′ol) [USP] ursodeoxycholic acid used as an anticholelithic to dissolve radiolucent, noncalcified gallstones; administered orally.

**Ur·ti·ca** (ər-ti′kə) [L.] the nettles, a genus of plants of the family Urticaceae that are covered with stinging hairs and secrete a poisonous fluid. *U. dio′ica* is a type of stinging nettle that grows in temperate regions and is stimulating, diuretic, and hemostatic.

**ur·ti·cant** (ur'tĭ-kənt) causing an itching or stinging sensation, or creating a wheal, or both.

**ur·ti·ca·ria** (ur"tĭ-kar'e-ə) [*Urtica* + *-ia*] [MeSH: Urticaria] a vascular reaction in the upper dermis, usually transient, consisting of localized edema caused by dilatation and increased capillary permeability, with development of wheals. Many different stimuli may induce it, and it may be classified as either immune-mediated, complement-mediated (involving either immunologic or nonimmunologic mechanisms), urticariogenic material–induced, physical agent–induced, stress-induced, or idiopathic. Urticaria may be either acute or chronic; the former evolves over a few days to weeks and the latter is continuous or persists episodically for six weeks or more. *Angioedema* is the same physiological response in the deep dermis or subcutaneous or submucosal tissues. Called also *hives.*
**acute u.,** see *urticaria.*
**aquagenic u.,** contact urticaria that may be due to a combination of water and sweat or sebum, regardless of the temperature, which produces urticariogenic substances, and characterized by the development of small perifollicular wheals with surrounding erythema.
**u. bullo'sa, bullous u.,** that in which bullae are superimposed on the characteristic wheals.
**cholinergic u.,** that characterized by the presence of distinctive punctate wheals surrounded by areas of erythema, thought to be a nonimmunologic hypersensitivity reaction in which acetylcholine released from parasympathetic or motor nerve terminals induces release of mediators from mast cells, and evoked by conditions of exertion, stress, or increased environmental heat. Cf. *heat u.*
**chronic u.,** see *urticaria.*
**cold u.,** urticaria precipitated by cold air, water, or objects, occurring in two forms: In the autosomal dominant form, which is associated with fever, arthralgias, and leukocytosis, the lesions present as erythematous, burning papules and macules. The more common acquired form is usually idiopathic and self-limited.
**colonic u.,** the lifting up of the mucosal surface of the colon owing to edema, resulting in a characteristic mosaic pattern on radiology.
**contact u.,** a localized or generalized, transient wheal-and-flare response elicited by exposure to rapidly absorbable urticariogenic agents.
**giant u.,** angioedema.
**heat u.,** localized or generalized urticaria produced by application of heat to the skin or by exposure to high environmental temperature, sometimes associated with cramps, weakness, flushing, salivation, and collapse, which is probably mediated by acetylcholine. Cf. *cholinergic u.*
**light u.,** solar u.
**u. medicamento'sa,** a drug eruption manifested by the development of wheals.
**u. multifor'mis endem'ica,** harara.
**papular u.,** a persistent cutaneous eruption representing a hypersensitivity reaction to insect bites (e.g., mites, fleas, bedbugs, gnats, mosquitoes, animal lice), seen primarily in atopic children, and characterized by crops of small urticarial papules and wheals and transitional forms of these lesions, which may become secondarily infected or lichenified owing to rubbing and excoriation. Called also *lichen urticatus* and *strophulus.*
**u. pigmento'sa,** the most common form of mastocytosis, occurring primarily in children, typically characterized by multiple persistent small, reddish brown, hyperpigmented, pruritic macules and papules, located most commonly on the trunk but also seen on the extremities, head, and neck, which tend to urticate upon mild mechanical trauma or chemical irritation (Darier's sign). See also *mastocytoma.*
**pressure u.,** urticaria of unknown cause occurring hours after local pressure on the skin, most often seen on the feet after walking and on the buttocks after sitting, and associated with pain.
**solar u., u. sola'ris,** rapidly developing urticaria occurring on brief exposure to sunlight. Called also *light u.*

**ur·ti·car·i·al** (ur"tĭ-kar'e-əl) pertaining to, characterized by, or of the nature of urticaria. Called also *urticarious.*

**ur·ti·car·i·o·gen·ic** (ur"tĭ-kar"e-o-jen'ik) causing urticaria.

**ur·ti·car·i·ous** (ur"tĭ-kar'e-əs) urticarial.

**ur·ti·cate** (ur'tĭ-kāt) 1. marked by the presence of wheals. 2. to produce urtication.

**ur·ti·ca·tion** (ur"tĭ-ka'shən) [L. *urtica* a stinging nettle] 1. the development or formation of urticaria. 2. a burning sensation as of stinging with nettles.

**uru·shi·ol** (u-roo'she-ol) the chief constituent of the irritant oil of poison ivy, poison oak, and related plants; it consists of a mixture of several oleoresins.

**US** ultrasound.

**USAN** (u'san) acronym for *United States Adopted Names,* a nonproprietary designation for any compound used as a drug, established by negotiation between the manufacturer of the compound and a nomenclature committee known as the USAN Council, which is sponsored jointly by the American Medical Association, the American Pharmaceutical Association, and The United States Pharmacopeial Convention. A liaison representative of the United States Food and Drug Administration sits on the USAN Council. The term is currently limited to names adopted by the Council since June, 1961. These names will appear as the monograph titles in the official compendia, USP and NF, when and if the respective drugs are admitted to either compendium.

**USDA** United States Department of Agriculture.

**Ush·er's syndrome** (ush'ərz) [Charles Howard *Usher,* British ophthalmologist, 1865–1942] see under *syndrome.*

**Us·nea** (us'ne-ə) a genus of lichens of the family Usneaceae. *U. barba'ta* (L.) Wigg. is a species that grows on forest trees and contains usnic acid; it is used as a homeopathic preparation and as a dressing for wounds.

**us·ne·in** (us'ne-in) usnic acid.

**us·nic ac·id** (us'nik) an antibacterial compound occurring in the lichen *Usnea barbata.*

**USP** the United States Pharmacopeia, a legally recognized compendium of standards for drugs, published by The United States Pharmacopeial Convention, Inc., and revised periodically. It includes also assays and tests for the determination of strength, quality, and purity.

**USPHS** United States Public Health Service.

**Us·ti·lag·i·na·ceae** (us"tĭ-laj"ĭ-na'se-e) a family of smuts, fungi of the order Ustilaginales. It includes the genus *Ustilago.*

**Us·ti·lag·i·na·les** (us"tĭ-laj"ĭ-na'lēz) [MeSH: Ustilaginales] the smuts, an order of perfect fungi of the class Teliomycetes, characterized by lack of a basidiocarp; it includes the families Ustilaginaceae and Tilletiaceae.

**us·ti·lag·i·nism** (us"tĭ-laj'ĭ-niz-əm) a condition resembling ergotism, seen in humans and other animals after eating corn contaminated with *Ustilago maydis* or *U. zeae.*

**Us·ti·la·go** (us"tĭ-la'go) [L.] [MeSH: Ustilago] a genus of smuts, fungi of the family Ustilaginaceae that are parasitic on plants. *U. may'dis* and *U. ze'ae* cause corn smut, and the ingestion of contaminated seeds causes ustilaginism.

**us·tion** (us'chən) [L. *ustio*] burning with the actual cautery.

**us·tu·la·tion** (us"tu-la'shən) [L. *ustulare* to scorch] the drying of a moist drug by heat.

**uta** (oo'tah) [from Peruvian Indian name for the disease] a form of New World cutaneous leishmaniasis occurring in the Peruvian Andes, caused by *Leishmania viannia peruviana,* which is found only at 900 to 3000 meters, probably transmitted by *Lutzomyia verrucarum* and *L. peruensis,* and characterized by the presence of a single or a few ulcer-like, self-limited lesions.

**Ut dict.** abbreviation for L. *ut dic'tum,* as directed.

**Utend.** abbreviation for L. *uten'dus,* to be used.

**uter·al·gia** (u"tər-al'jə) hysteralgia.

**uteri** (u'tər-i) [L.] genitive and plural of *uterus.*

**uter·ine** (u'tər-in) [L. *uterinus*] of or pertaining to the uterus.

**uter(o)-** [L. *uterus,* q.v.] a combining form denoting relationship to the uterus. See also words beginning with *hyster(o)- and metr(o)-.*

**utero·ab·dom·i·nal** (u"tər-o-ab-dom'ĭ-nəl) pertaining to the uterus and the abdomen.

**utero·cer·vi·cal** (u"tər-o-ser'vĭ-kəl) pertaining to the uterus and the cervix uteri.

**uter·odyn·ia** (u"tər-o-din'e-ə) hysteralgia.

**utero·fix·a·tion** (u"tər-o-fik-sa'shən) hysteropexy.

**uter·o·gen·ic** (u"tər-o-jen'ik) formed in the uterus.

**utero·ges·ta·tion** (u"tər-o-jəs-ta'shən) [*utero-* + *gestation*] 1. uterine pregnancy; any pregnancy which is not extrauterine. 2. the full period of time of normal pregnancy.

**utero·glob·u·lin** (u"tər-o-glob'u-lin) blastokinin.

**uter·og·ra·phy** (u"tər-og'rə-fe) hysterography.

**utero·lith** (u'tər-o-lith") [*utero-* + *-lith*] a hysterolith.

**uter·om·e·ter** (u"tər-om'ə-tər) an instrument for measuring the uterus.

**uter·om·e·try** (u"tər-om'ə-tre) measurement of the uterus.

**utero-ovar·i·an** (u"tər-o-o-var'e-ən) pertaining to the uterus and ovary.

**utero·pexy** (u'tər-o-pek"se) hysteropexy.

**utero·pla·cen·tal** (u″tər-o-plə-sen′təl) pertaining to the uterus and the placenta.

**utero·plas·ty** (u′tər-o-plas″te) any plastic operation on the uterus.

**utero·rec·tal** (u″tər-o-rek′təl) pertaining to the uterus and rectum, or communicating with the uterine cavity and rectum, as a utero-rectal fistula.

**utero·sa·cral** (u″tər-o-sa′krəl) pertaining to the uterus and the sacrum.

**utero·sal·pin·gog·ra·phy** (u″tər-o-sal″ping-gog′rə-fe) hysterosalpingography.

**utero·scle·ro·sis** (u″tər-o-sklə-ro′sis) sclerosis of the uterus.

**utero·scope** (u′tər-o-skōp″) [*utero-* + *-scope*] hysteroscope.

**utero·ther·mom·e·try** (u″tər-o-thər-mom′ə-tre) the measurement of the temperature in the uterus.

**uter·ot·o·my** (u″tər-ot′ə-me) hysterotomy.

**utero·ton·ic** (u″tər-o-ton′ik) 1. giving muscular tone to the uterus. 2. an agent that increases the tonus of the uterine muscle.

**utero·trop·ic** (u″tər-o-trop′ik) having a special affinity for or exerting its principal influence upon the uterus.

**utero·tu·bal** (u″tər-o-too′bəl) pertaining to the uterus and the oviducts.

**utero·tu·bog·ra·phy** (u″tər-o-too-bog′rə-fe) hysterosalpingography.

**uter·o·vag·i·nal** (u″tər-o-vaj′ĭ-nəl) pertaining to the uterus and the vagina.

**utero·ven·tral** (u″tər-o-ven′trəl) pertaining to the uterus and the cavity of the abdomen.

**uter·o·ves·i·cal** (u″tər-o-ves′ĭ-kəl) pertaining to the uterus and the bladder.

**uter·us** (u′tər-əs) pl. *u′teri* [L.; Gr. *hystera*] [TA] [MeSH: Uterus] the hollow muscular organ in female mammals in which the fertilized ovum normally becomes embedded and in which the developing embryo and fetus is nourished. In the nongravid human, it is a pear-shaped structure, about 3 inches in length, consisting of a fundus body, isthmus, and cervix. Its cavity opens into the vagina below, and into the uterine tube on either side at the cornu. It is supported by direct attachment to the vagina and by indirect attachment to various other nearby pelvic structures. Called also *metra.*
**u. arcua′tus,** a uterus with a depressed fundus.
**u. bicamera′tus vetula′rum,** a uterus in which the cervical orifices are closed by adhesions, resulting in distention of the cervix and corpus uteri.
**u. bicor′nis,** a uterus which has two horns, or cornua.
**u. bicor′nis bicol′lis,** a uterus with two horns and two cervices.
**u. bicor′nis unicol′lis,** a uterus with two horns and a single cervix.
**u. bi′foris,** a uterus in which the external os is divided by a septum.
**u. bilocula′ris,** a uterus whose cavity is divided into two parts by a septum; called also *bipartite* or *septate u.*
**bipartite u., u. biparti′tus,** u. bilocularis.
**cochleate u.,** a small adult uterus with a conical cervix and body which is small, globular, and acutely flexed.
**u. cordifor′mis,** a heart-shaped uterus.
**Couvelaire u.,** see *uteroplacental apoplexy,* under *apoplexy.*
**u. didel′phys,** the existence of two distinct uteri in the same individual; called also *didelphia* and *u. duplex.*
**duplex u., u. du′plex,** 1. u. didelphys. 2. a double uterus, as occurs normally in marsupial mammals.
**fetal u.,** a uterus in which the cervical canal is longer than the cavity of the corpus.
**gravid u.,** the pregnant uterus.
**u. incudifor′mis,** a uterus bicornis which is broad between the two horns.

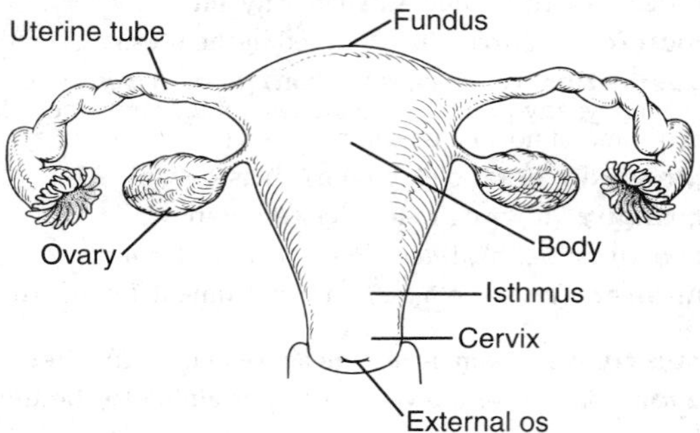

Uterus, comprising the fundus, body, isthmus, and cervix.

**infantile u.,** pubescent u.
**u. masculi′nus,** utriculus prostaticus.
**u. parvicol′lis,** a uterus in which the cervical portion is very small, but the corpus is of normal size.
**u. planifunda′lis,** u. incudiformis.
**pubescent u.,** one which is adult in type but is undeveloped; called also *infantile u.*
**ribbon u.,** an aplastic uterus found as a transverse ribbon of fibromuscular tissue between the blind ends of the uterine tubes and the bladder.
**u. rudimenta′rius,** a hypoplastic uterus measuring 1 to 3 cm. in length; affected women are amenorrheic and sterile.
**saddle-shaped u.,** u. arcuatus.
**septate u., u. sep′tus,** u. bilocularis.
**u. simplex,** one that is single throughout its length, as in the human.
**u. subsep′tus,** u. bicornis.
**u. triangula′ris,** u. incudiformis.
**u. unicor′nis,** one with only one cornu, one lateral half being undeveloped or imperfectly developed.

**Uti·bid** (u′tĭ-bid) trademark for a preparation of oxolinic acid.

**Uti·cort** (u′tĭ-kort″) trademark for preparations of betamethasone benzoate.

**util·iza·tion** (u″til-ĭ-za′shən) the use of something.
**red cell u. (RCU),** the fraction of iron leaving the blood plasma that is incorporated in circulating red blood cells; iron-59 bound to the patient's own transferrin is administered, and the red cell utilization is calculated as: (radioactive iron/mL blood at 10–14 days) ÷ (extrapolated radioactive iron/mL blood at time zero) × 100 per cent.

**UTP** uridine triphosphate.

**UTP–glu·cose-1-phos·phate uri·dyl·yl·trans·fer·ase** (gloo′kōs fos′fāt u″rĭ-del′əl-trans′fər-ās) [EC 2.7.7.9] an enzyme of the transferase class that catalyzes the reaction UTP + glucose 1-phosphate = pyrophosphate + UDPglucose, a reaction in the glycogen storage mechanism. Called also *UDPglucose pyrophosphorylase.*

**UTP–hex·ose-1-phos·phate uri·dyl·yl·trans·fer·ase** (hek′sōs fos′fāt u″rĭ-dil″əl-trans′fər-ās) [EC 2.7.7.10] an enzyme of the transferase class that catalyzes the transfer of galactose 1-phosphate to UTP to form UDPgalactose. The reaction is an alternative minor pathway for producing UDPgalactose for galactose utilization (cf. *UDPglucose–hexose-1-phosphate uridylyltransferase*). The enzyme is present in the liver of adults, but is lacking in infants. Called also *galactose 1-phosphate uridylyltransferase.*

**utri·cle** (u′trĭ-kəl) [L. *utriculus*] 1. any small sac. 2. utriculus (def. 2).
**prostatic u., urethral u.,** utriculus prostaticus.

**utric·u·lar** (u-trik′u-lər) 1. pertaining to a utricle. 2. resembling a bladder.

**utric·u·li** (u-trik′u-li) [L.] genitive and plural of *utriculus.*

**utric·u·li·tis** (u-trik″u-li′tis) 1. inflammation of the prostatic utricle. 2. inflammation of the utricle of the ear.

**utric·u·lo·sac·cu·lar** (u-trik″u-lo-sak′u-lər) pertaining to the utricle and saccule of the labyrinth.

**utric·u·lus** (u-trik′u-ləs) pl. *utric′uli* [L., dim. of *uter*] 1. a small sac. 2. [TA] utricle: the larger of the two divisions of the membranous labyrinth, located in the posterosuperior region of the vestibule. It is the major organ of the vestibular system, which gives information about position and movements of the head. Called also *u. vestibuli.*
**u. masculi′nus,** u. prostaticus.
**u. prosta′ticus** [TA], prostatic utricle: the remains of the lower part of the paramesonephric duct in the male; it is a small blind pouch arising in the prostatic substance and opening onto the seminal colliculus.
**u. vesti′buli,** utriculus (def. 2).

**utri·form** (u′trĭ-form) having the shape of a bottle.

**UVA** ultraviolet A.

**uva** (u′və) pl. *u′vae* [L. "grape"] 1. the raisin; the dried fruit of *Vitis vinifera.* 2. any of various other fruits resembling that of *V. vinifera.*
**u. ur′si** [L. "bear's grapes"] 1. *Arctostaphylos uva-ursi.* 2. the leaves of *A. uva-ursi,* used medicinally as an astringent, diuretic tea.

**Uval** (u′val) trademark for preparations of sulisobenzone.

**UVB** ultraviolet B.

**UVC** ultraviolet C.

**uvea** (u′ve-ə) [MeSH: Uvea] tunica vasculosa bulbi.

**uve·al** (u′ve-əl) pertaining to the uvea.

**uve·it·ic** (u″ve-it′ik) pertaining to uveitis.

**uve·itis** (u″ve-i′tis) [*uvea* + *-itis*] [MeSH: Uveitis] an inflammation of part or all of the uvea, commonly involving the other tunics of the eye (sclera, cornea, and retina).

**anterior u.**, uveitis involving the structures of the iris and/or ciliary body, including iritis, cyclitis, and iridocyclitis.
**equine recurrent u.**, periodic ophthalmia.
**Förster's u.**, syphilitic involvement of the entire uvea.
**granulomatous u.**, uveitis of any part of the uveal tract but particularly the posterior portion, characterized by nodular collections of epithelioid cells and giant cells surrounded by lymphocytes.
**heterochromic u.**, see under *iridocyclitis.*
**lens-induced u.**, three disorders—phacoantigenic uveitis, phacotoxic uveitis, and phacolytic glaucoma—of greater or lesser severity caused by autoimmune response to lens protein leaking through the capsule. The leakage may be from hypermature cataract, capsular rupture, extracapsular lens extraction, or other trauma.
**nongranulomatous u.**, inflammation of the anterior portion of the uveal tract (iris and ciliary body).
**phacoantigenic u.**, one of the lens-induced uveitides, it is a severe anterior uveitis, similar to sympathetic ophthalmia, observed weeks or even months after extracapsular lens surgery or other trauma to the capsule. Called also *phacoanaphylactic endophthalmitis.*
**phacotoxic u.**, an extremely rare lens-induced uveitis that is a low-grade reaction to lens protein, and not a separate disease entity.
**posterior u.**, uveitis involving the posterior segment of the eye, including choroiditis and chorioretinitis.
**sympathetic u.**, see under *ophthalmia.*
**toxoplasmic u.**, chorioretinitis as a complication of toxoplasmosis.
**tuberculous u.**, granulomatous uveitis due to infection with the tubercle bacillus, usually a severe caseating granulomatous chorioretinitis.

**uveo·me·nin·gi·tis** (u′ve-o-men″in-ji′tis) a disorder characterized by lesions of the uvea accompanied by meningeal inflammation.

**uveo·pa·rot·id** (u″ve-o-pə-rot′id) affecting the uvea and the parotid gland; see under *fever.*

**uveo·scle·ri·tis** (u″ve-o-sklə-ri′tis) scleritis resulting from an extension of the inflammation from the uvea to the sclera.

**uvi·form** (u′vĭ-form) [*uva* + *form*] having the form of a grape.

**uvu·la** (u′vu-lə) pl. *u′vulae* [L. "little grape"] [MeSH: Uvula] 1. [TA] a general term in anatomical terminology for a pendent, fleshy mass. 2. u. palatina.
**bifid u.**, bifurcation of the uvula, considered an incomplete form of cleft palate. Called also *cleft, forked,* or *split u., u. fissa,* and *staphyloschisis.*
**u. of bladder**, u. vesicae.
**u. cerebel′li, u. of cerebellum**, u. vermis.
**cleft u.**, bifid u.
**u. fis′sa, forked u.**, bifid u.
**Lieutaud's u.**, u. vesicae.

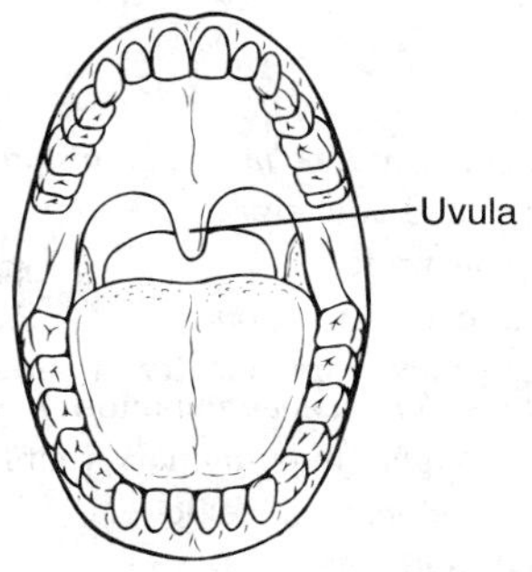


**u. palati′na** [TA], palatine uvula: the small, fleshy mass hanging from the soft palate above the root of the tongue, composed of the levator and tensor palati muscles and the muscle of the uvula, connective tissue, and mucous membrane.
**split u.**, bifid u.
**u. ver′mis** [TA], uvula of vermis: the part of the vermis of the cerebellum between the pyramis and the nodulus; called also *u. of cerebellum.*
**u. vesi′cae** [TA], uvula of bladder: a rounded elevation at the neck of the bladder, formed by convergence of many fibers of the trigonal muscle as they pass through the encircling musculus sphincter vesicae to terminate in the urethra.

**uvu·lar** (u′vu-lər) pertaining to the uvula; called also *staphyline.*

**uvu·la·ris** (u″vu-lar′is) [L., from *uvula*] uvular.

**uvu·lec·to·my** (u″vu-lek′tə-me) [*uvula* + *-ectomy*] excision of the uvula.

**uvu·li·tis** (u″vu-li′tis) [*uvula* + *-itis*] inflammation of the uvula; staphylitis.

**uvu·lo·pal·a·to·phar·yn·go·plas·ty (UPPP)** (u″vu-lo-pal″ə-to″fəring′go-plas″te) palatopharyngoplasty.

**uvu·lo·pal·a·to·plas·ty** (u″vu-lo-pal′ə-to-plas″te) palatopharyngoplasty.

**uvu·lop·to·sis** (u″vu-lop-to′sis) [*uvula* + *ptosis*] elongation or relaxation of the palate; called also *staphyloptosis.*

**uvu·lo·tome** (u′vu-lo-tōm) an instrument for cutting the uvula; called also *staphylotome.*

**uvu·lot·o·my** (u″vu-lot′ə-me) [*uvula* + *-tomy*] surgical removal of all or part of the uvula; cf. *uvulectomy.* Called also *staphylotomy.*

# V

**V** symbol for *vanadium, volt, volume,* and *vision.*

***V*** symbol for *voltage* and *volume.*

**$V_H$** see *variable region,* under *region.*

**$V_L$** see *variable region,* under *region.*

***$V_{max}$*** symbol for the maximum velocity of an enzyme-catalyzed reaction; see *Michaelis-Menten equation* under *equation.*

**$V_T$** symbol for *tidal volume* (in pulmonary ventilation).

**v** abbreviation for L. *ve'na,* vein; velocity.

***v*** symbol for *velocity* and *voltage.*

**VA** visual acuity; Veterans Administration (now the Department of Veterans Affairs [DVA]).

**VAC** a regimen of vincristine, dactinomycin, and cyclophosphamide, used in cancer chemotherapy.

**vac·cen·ic ac·id** (vak-sen'ik) a monounsaturated fatty acid isomeric with oleic and elaidic acids; it occurs naturally in both *cis* and *trans* configurations, the former in bacteria and the latter in beef fat and butterfat. See table accompanying *fatty acid.*

**vac·ci·na** (vak-si'nə) vaccinia.

**vac·ci·nal** (vak'sĭ-nəl) [L. *vaccinus*] 1. pertaining to vaccinia, to vaccine, or to vaccination. 2. having protective qualities when used by way of inoculation.

**vac·ci·nate** (vak'sĭ-nāt) to inoculate with vaccine for the purpose of producing immunity.

**vac·ci·na·tion** (vak″sĭ-na'shən) [L. *vacca* cow] [MeSH: Vaccination] the introduction of vaccine into the body for the purpose of inducing immunity. Coined originally to apply to the injection of smallpox vaccine, the term has come to mean any immunizing procedure in which vaccine is injected.

**vac·ci·na·tor** (vak'sĭ-na″tər) 1. one who vaccinates. 2. an instrument for use in vaccination.

**vac·cine** (vak-sēn') [L. *vaccinus* pertaining to cows, from *vacca* cow (so named from the use of cowpox virus inoculation for immunization against smallpox)] a suspension of attenuated or killed microorganisms (bacteria, viruses, or rickettsiae), or of antigenic proteins derived from them, administered for the prevention, amelioration, or treatment of infectious diseases.

## Vaccine

**acellular v.,** a cell-free vaccine prepared from purified antigenic components of pathogenic microorganisms, thus carrying less risk of adverse reactions than whole-cell preparations.

**anthrax v.,** a cell-free protein extract of cultures of *Bacillus anthracis,* used for immunization of persons with occupational exposure to anthrax, e.g., workers with imported animal hides or hair.

**anthrax spore v.,** a live vaccine consisting of *Bacillus anthracis* spores in saponified diluent, used for vaccination of domestic farm animals against anthrax.

**attenuated v.,** a vaccine prepared from live microorganisms or viruses cultured under adverse conditions leading to loss of their virulence but retention of their ability to induce protective immunity.

**autogenous v.,** a vaccine prepared from microorganisms which have been freshly isolated from the lesion of the patient who is to be treated with it.

**avian encephalomyelitis v.,** a live virus vaccine of chick embryo origin, used for immunization of layer or breeder replacement pullets against avian encephalomyelitis.

**bacterial v.,** a preparation of killed or attenuated bacteria used as an active immunizing agent; many are used in veterinary medicine. Called also *bacterin.*

**BCG v.** [USP] [bacille Calmette-Guérin], a vaccine made from the Calmette-Guérin strain of *Mycobacterium bovis,* which was made avirulent by culture by Calmette and Guérin for many years on a medium enriched in beef bile; it is administered by intradermal injection or scarification to tuberculin-negative individuals for prevention of tuberculosis. It is used for routine vaccination of children only in regions where there is a high incidence of tuberculosis. In the United States it is recommended only for immunization of high-risk individuals. BCG vaccine is also used in cancer immunotherapy, particularly in malignant melanoma; it is thought to act as a nonspecific stimulator of cell-mediated immunity.

**bluetongue v.,** a live virus vaccine of bovine tissue culture origin, used for prevention of bluetongue in sheep.

**bovine rhinotracheitis v.,** a modified live virus vaccine of tissue culture origin used for immunization of healthy cattle against infectious bovine rhinotracheitis.

**bovine virus diarrhea v.,** a modified live virus vaccine of tissue culture origin, used for immunization of cattle against bovine virus diarrhea.

**bronchitis v.,** a live virus vaccine of chick embryo origin prepared from the Massachusetts or Connecticut variant strains of bronchitis virus, used for prevention of infectious bronchitis in chickens and other birds.

***Brucella abortus* v.,** a live virus vaccine of *Brucella abortus* strain 19, used for immunization of healthy calves against brucellosis.

**bursal disease v.,** a modified live virus of chick embryo origin, used for immunization of chicks against infectious bursal disease.

**Calmette's v.,** BCG v.

**canine distemper v.,** a modified live virus vaccine consisting of an attenuated strain of canine distemper virus propagated in tissue culture, used for immunization of dogs against canine distemper.

**cholera v.** [USP], a killed bacteria vaccine containing equal portions of the Inaba and Ogawa strains of *Vibrio cholerae,* used for immunization against cholera. It enhances protection in adults for about six months, but does not reduce fecal shedding of bacteria or reduce disease transmission.

**coccidiosis v.,** live sporulated oocysts of chicken origin, used to introduce subclinical coccidial infection in chickens in order to establish immunity against clinical infections.

**distemper v.–mink,** a modified live virus vaccine of chick embryo tissue culture origin, used for prevention of canine distemper in mink.

**duck embryo v.,** vaccine prepared from embryonate duck eggs infected with inactivated fixed virus.

**duck virus enteritis v.,** a modified live virus vaccine of chick embryo origin, used for prevention of duck virus enteritis.

**duck virus hepatitis v.,** a modified live virus vaccine of chick embryo origin, used for prevention of duck virus hepatitis.

**encephalomyelitis v.,** a bivalent killed virus vaccine of chicken tissue culture origin, used for immunization of horses against Eastern and Western equine encephalomyelitis.

**equine influenza v.,** a bivalent killed virus vaccine of chick embryo origin, used for immunization of horses against equine influenza due to influenza virus A equine strains 1 and 2.

**equine rhinopneumonitis v.,** an attenuated live virus vaccine of tissue culture origin or a killed virus vaccine, used for immunization of horses against equine viral rhinopneumonitis due to equine herpesvirus type 1.

***Erysipelothrix rhusiopathiae* v.,** an avirulent live culture of *Erysipelothrix rhusiopathiae,* used for prevention of erysipelas in swine.

**feline panleukopenia v.,** a modified live virus vaccine or killed virus vaccine of tissue culture origin, used for immunization of cats against feline panleukopenia.

**feline pneumonitis v.,** a modified live vaccine of chick embryo origin, used for immunization of cats against *Chlamydia psittaci.*

**feline rhinotracheitis v.,** a modified live virus vaccine of tissue culture origin, used for immunization of cats against feline rhinotracheitis.

**fowl laryngotracheitis v.,** a modified live virus vaccine of chick embryo origin, used for prevention of laryngotracheitis in chickens.

**fowlpox v.,** a modified live virus vaccine of chicken embryo or tissue culture origin, used to immunize chickens and turkeys against fowlpox.

***Haemophilus influenzae* b conjugate v. (HbCV),** a preparation of *Haemophilus influenzae* type b capsular polysaccharide covalently bound to diphtheria toxoid; it stimulates both B- and T-lymphocyte responses and is much more immunogenic than the polysaccharide vaccine. Used as an immunizing agent in children between the ages of 18 months and 5 years who belong to certain high-risk groups.

***Haemophilus influenzae* b polysaccharide v. (HbPV),** a sterile preparation of highly purified capsular polysaccharide derived from *Haemophilus influenzae* type b, which stimulates an immune response in B lymphocytes only; used as an immunizing agent in children between the ages of 18 months and 5 years who belong to certain high-risk groups.

**hepatitis B v.**, formalin-treated hepatitis B surface antigen isolated from plasma of human carriers of hepatitis B, used for immunization of persons at high risk, e.g., medical and dental personnel, immunocompromised patients and patients requiring hemodialysis or frequent transfusions, residents and staff of closed institutions, contacts of carriers, and male homosexuals.

**hepatitis B v. (recombinant)**, a noninfectious viral vaccine derived by recombination from hepatitis B surface antigen and cloned in yeast cells.

**heterologous v.**, a vaccine that confers protective immunity against a pathogen not present in the vaccine, because it contains microorganisms that possess cross-reacting antigens which they share in common with that pathogen. For example, vaccinia virus protects against smallpox. Called also *heterotypic v.*

**heterotypic v.**, heterologous v.

**human diploid cell v. (HDCV)**, rabies v.

**influenza virus v.** [USP], a killed virus vaccine; both whole virion and subvirion vaccines are available. The composition of the vaccine is changed each year in response to antigenic shifts and changes in prevalence of influenza virus strains; the vaccine is usually bivalent or trivalent, containing one or two influenza virus A strains and one influenza virus B strain. Annual immunization before November is recommended for high-risk individuals (persons over 65 years of age and persons with chronic disease).

**Japanese encephalitis virus v.**, a formaldehyde-inactivated vaccine prepared from infected mouse brains, used for immunization against Japanese encephalitis; recommended for persons staying a month or more in endemic or epidemic regions of Asia and for laboratory workers who may be exposed to Japanese encephalitis virus.

**live v.**, a vaccine prepared from live microorganisms or viruses that have been attenuated but that retain their immunogenic properties.

**Lyme disease v. (recombinant OspA)**, a preparation of outer surface protein A (OspA), a cell surface lipoprotein of *Borrelia burgdorferi*, produced by recombinant technology; used for active immunization against Lyme disease in persons between 15 and 70 years of age.

**Marek's disease v.**, a live virus vaccine of tissue culture origin, used for immunization of 1-day-old chicks against Marek's disease, prepared from one or more of the three serotypes of Marek's disease virus.

**measles v.**, a modified live virus vaccine of canine tissue culture origin, used to induce resistance to canine distemper in 3- to 6-week-old puppies in which response to canine distemper vaccine would be neutralized because of interference by maternal antibody.

**measles, mumps, and rubella virus v. live** [USP], a combination of live attenuated measles virus, live mumps virus, and live attenuated rubella virus, used for simultaneous immunization against measles, mumps, and rubella.

**measles and mumps virus v. live** [USP], a combination of live attenuated measles virus and live mumps virus, used for simultaneous immunization against measles and mumps.

**measles and rubella virus v. live** [USP], a combination of live attenuated measles virus and live attenuated rubella virus, used for simultaneous immunization against measles and rubella.

**measles virus v. live** [USP], a live attenuated virus vaccine of chick embryo origin, used for routine immunization of children and for immunization of adolescents and adults who have not had measles or been immunized with live measles vaccine and have no serum antibodies against measles. Children are usually immunized with measles-mumps-rubella (MMR) combination vaccine.

**meningococcal polysaccharide v.**, a preparation of the capsular polysaccharide antigen of *Neisseria meningitidis*, types A, C, Y, or W-135; monovalent group A [USP] or C [USP], bivalent group A and C [USP], and quadrivalent vaccines are available. The vaccine is administered to persons over 2 years of age at risk in event of an epidemic of meningococcal disease caused by these serotypes and routinely only to military recruits.

**mink enteritis v.**, a killed virus vaccine of feline tissue culture origin, used for immunization of mink against mink viral enteritis.

**mixed v.**, polyvalent v.

**mumps virus v. live** [USP], a live attenuated virus vaccine of chick embryo origin, used for routine immunization of children and for immunization of adolescents and adults who have not had mumps or been immunized with live mumps vaccine. Children are usually immunized with measles-mumps-rubella (MMR) combination vaccine.

**Newcastle disease v.**, live virus vaccine or chemically inactivated, adsorbed killed virus vaccine, both of chick embryo origin, used for immunization of chickens against Newcastle disease, the live vaccine for mass immunization in drinking water, aerosol spray, or eye drops, the killed vaccine for immunization by injection.

**ovine ecthyma v.**, a live virus vaccine of ovine origin, used for immunization of sheep and goats against contagious ecthyma (orf).

***Pasteurella multocida* v.**, a live bacterial vaccine, used for prevention of pasteurellosis in turkeys due to *Pasteurella multocida*, types 3 and 4.

**pertussis v.**, a suspension of killed *Bordetella pertussis* organisms, used for immunization against pertussis (whooping cough); both fluid and adsorbed (on alum, aluminum hydroxide, or aluminum phosphate) forms are available. It is generally used in a mixture with diphtheria and tetanus toxoids (DTP). Routine pertussis immunization is recommended for all children under 6, except when a specific contraindication exists. Official names [USP] are *pertussis v., pertussis vaccine adsorbed, diphtheria* and *tetanus toxoids and pertussis vaccine* (DTP), and *diphtheria and tetanus toxoids and pertussis vaccine adsorbed.*

**pertussis v., acellular**, a vaccine for immunization against pertussis prepared from the purified antigenic components of *Bordetella pertussis;* it causes fewer adverse reactions than the whole-cell vaccine and, like the whole-cell vaccine, is generally used in a mixture with diphtheria and tetanus toxoids (DTP). In the United States, it is licensed for use only in children at least 15 months of age.

**pigeonpox v.**, a live virus vaccine of chick embryo origin, used for prevention of fowlpox in chickens and turkeys.

**plague v.** [USP], a suspension of killed *Yersinia pestis* bacilli, used for immunization of persons having occupational or avocational exposure to wild rodents in plague enzootic areas.

**pneumococcal polysaccharide v.**, a 23-valent vaccine containing capsular polysaccharide of *Streptococcus pneumoniae* types 1–5, 8, 9, 12, 14, 17, 19, 20, 22, 23, 26, 34, 43, 51, 54, 56, 57, 68, and 70, which are responsible for about 90 per cent of pneumococcal disease in the United States; used for immunization of persons over 2 years of age having chronic cardiac, pulmonary, hepatic, or renal disease, diabetes mellitus, sickle cell anemia, or anatomic or functional asplenia, and persons in nursing homes or other institutions where there is high risk of pneumococcal disease.

**poliomyelitis v.**, poliovirus v. inactivated.

**poliovirus v. inactivated (IPV)** [USP], a suspension of formalin-inactivated poliovirus, types I, II, and III, grown in monkey kidney cell tissue culture, used in the United States only for immunization of immunologically deficient patients and for primary immunization of unimmunized adults at risk. Called also *Salk v.* and (formerly) *poliomyelitis v.*

**poliovirus v. live oral (OPV)** [USP], **poliovirus v. live oral trivalent (TOPV)**, a live vaccine containing attenuated poliovirus, types I, II, and III, grown in monkey kidney cell tissue culture, used for routine immunization of children against polio. OPV induces long-lasting intestinal and humoral immunity; IPV (killed vaccine) induces only humoral immunity. OPV should not be administered to immunocompromised individuals or their household contacts. Called also *Sabin v.*

**polyvalent v.**, a vaccine prepared from cultures or antigens of more than one strain or species.

**pseudorabies v.**, any of several vaccines used for immunization of swine against pseudorabies. Four types are used: one using an attenuated virus, one with an inactivated virus, one with a thymidine kinase–deficient virus, and a subunit vaccine.

**purified chick embryo cell v. (PCEC)**, a lyophilized vaccine used for pre- and post-exposure rabies prophylaxis, prepared from rabies virus grown in primary cultures of chicken fibroblasts and inactivated with β-propiolactone; administered intramuscularly.

**rabies v.** [USP], an inactivated virus vaccine, used for preexposure immunization to persons at high risk of exposure, e.g., veterinarians, and in conjunction with rabies immune globulin, for postexposure prophylaxis. The official preparation is *human diploid cell v.* (HDCV) produced from rabies virus grown in cultures of human diploid embryo lung cells and inactivated with propiolactone; it has a much lower incidence of adverse reactions than the previously used *duck embryo v.* (DEV).

**rabies v. adsorbed (RVA)**, a rabies vaccine for pre- and postexposure rabies prophylaxis in humans, administered intramuscularly. It is prepared from rabies virus grown in cultures of fetal rhesus lung; the virus is inactivated by β-propiolactone and concentrated by adsorption to aluminum phosphate.

**reo-corona viral calf diarrhea v.**, a modified live virus vaccine of bovine tissue culture origin, used for immunization of newborn calves against enteric disease caused by reoviruses and coronaviruses.

**replicative v.**, any vaccine containing organisms that are able to reproduce, including live and attenuated viruses and bacteria.

**Rocky Mountain spotted fever v.**, a killed rickettsia vaccine produced from *Rickettsia rickettsii* grown in yolk sacs of embryonated chicken eggs; it had limited effectiveness and is no longer available. A new chick embryo cell culture vaccine is under investigation.

**rotavirus v. live oral**, a live virus vaccine produced from a mixture of four rotavirus types grown in fetal rhesus diploid cells; used to immunize infants against rotaviral gastroenteritis.

**rubella and mumps virus v. live** [USP], a combination of live attenuated rubella virus and live mumps virus, used for simultaneous immunization against rubella and mumps.

**rubella virus v. live** [USP], a live attenuated virus vaccine of duck embryo or human diploid cell tissue culture origin, used for routine immunization of children and for immunization of nonpregnant adolescent and adult females of childbearing age who are unimmunized and do not have serum antibodies to rubella. Children are usually immunized with measles-mumps-rubella (MMR) combination vaccine.
**Sabin v.**, poliovirus v. live oral.
**Salk v.**, poliovirus v. inactivated.
**smallpox v.** [USP], a live vaccina virus vaccine of calf lymph or chick embryo origin, used for immunization against smallpox. Now recommended only for laboratory workers exposed to smallpox virus; certain countries continue to vaccinate those in the military forces. Complications that result from smallpox vaccination include vaccinia, secondary bacterial infections, and encephalomyelitis.
**split-virus v.**, subunit v.
**streptococcus group E v.**, an oral modified live virus vaccine of Lancefield group E streptococcus, used for prevention of streptococcal lymphadenitis (jowl or cervical abscesses) in swine.
**subunit v.**, a vaccine produced from specific protein subunits of a virus and thus having less risk of adverse reactions than live or killed whole virus vaccines, e.g., hepatitis B vaccine and some influenza vaccines. Called also *split-virus v.,* and *subvirion v.*
**subvirion v.**, subunit v.
**tenosynovitis v.**, a modified live virus vaccine of chick embryo origin, administered to broiler-breeder replacement chickens for prevention of infectious tenosynovitis.
**transmissible gastroenteritis v.**, a modified live virus vaccine of porcine tissue culture origin, used for prevention of transmissible gastroenteritis in swine.
**tuberculosis v.**, BCG v.
**typhoid v.** [USP], a killed bacteria vaccine, either acetone-dried or phenol-inactivated, used for immunization against typhoid fever. It confers about 70 per cent protection, which can be overcome by a large challenge. Immunization is recommended only for exposure due to travel, epidemic, or household contact with a carrier.
**typhoid Vi polysaccharide v.**, a sterile solution of the cell surface Vi polysaccharide extracted from the strain *Salmonella typhi* Ty2, used for immunization against typhoid fever in persons at risk for exposure to *S. typhi* due to travel or household contact; administered intramuscularly.
**typhus v.**, a formalin-inactivated vaccine of chick embryo origin, used for immunization against epidemic *(Rickettsia prowazeki)* typhus. Efficacy of this vaccine has not been established and it is no longer available in the United States. A live vaccine containing the attenuated Madrid E strain of *R. prowazeki* is protective but can cause mild symptomatic infection; it also is not generally available.
**yellow fever v.**, a live attenuated virus vaccine of chick embryo origin, used for prevention of yellow fever; recommended for immunization of persons residing or traveling in endemic areas of Africa and South America.

---

**vac·cin·ia** (vak-sin'e-ə) [L., from *vacca* cow] [MeSH: Vaccinia] the cutaneous and sometimes systemic reactions associated with vaccination with smallpox vaccine. Cf. *cowpox* and *paravaccinia.*
**fetal v.**, vaccinia of the fetus due to bloodborne dissemination of vaccinia virus in the pregnant woman after primary smallpox vaccination; it is frequently lethal to the fetus.
**v. gangreno'sa**, progressive v.
**generalized v.**, a usually self-limited generalized skin eruption resembling smallpox, sometimes occurring after primary smallpox vaccination, caused by transient viremia with localization of the virus in the skin.
**progressive v.**, a rare but often fatal complication of smallpox vaccination in those with deficient immune mechanisms or receiving immunosuppressive therapy, characterized by tissue necrosis that spreads from the inoculation site, which may result in metastatic vaccinial lesions in the skin, bones, and viscera. Called also *v. gangrenosa.*

**vac·cin·i·al** (vak-sin'e-əl) pertaining to or characteristic of vaccinia.

**vac·cin·i·form** (vak-sin'ĭ-form) resembling vaccinia.

**vac·cino·gen** (vak-sin'o-jən) a source from which vaccine is derived.

**vac·ci·nog·e·nous** (vak″sĭ-noj'ə-nəs) producing vaccine.

**vac·cino·style** (vak-sin'o-stīl) a small lance used in vaccination.

**vac·ci·no·ther·a·py** (vak″sĭ-no-ther'ə-pe) therapeutic use of vaccines.

**VACTERL** an acronym for *v*ertebral, *a*nal, *c*ardiac, *t*racheal, *e*sophageal, *r*enal, and *l*imb; used to designate a pattern of congenital anomalies sometimes seen in infants whose mothers had taken progestogen-estrogen birth control pills.

**vac·u·o·lar** (vak″u-o'lər) pertaining to a vacuole; characterized by the presence of vacuoles.

**vac·u·o·late** (vak'u-o-lāt″) to form small spaces, or vacuoles.

**vac·u·o·lat·ed** (vak'u-o-lāt″əd) pertaining to or characterized by vacuoles.

**vac·u·o·la·tion** (vak″u-o-la'shən) the process of forming vacuoles; the condition of being vacuolated.

**vac·u·ole** (vak'u-ōl) [L. *vacuus* empty + *-ole* diminutive ending] [MeSH: Vacuoles] any small space or cavity formed in the protoplasm of a cell.
**autophagic v.**, autophagosome.
**condensing v's**, membrane-bound spherical vacuoles in the Golgi complex of secretory cells, which contain secretory product in varying degrees of condensation and which mature, pass to the cell surface as secretory granules or droplets, and discharge their contents.
**contractile v.**, an osmoregulatory organelle of protozoa and sponges that alternately fills with water extracted from the adjacent cytoplasm and then ejects the water to the outside; thus it acts as a pumping mechanism to remove excess water from the cell. Called also *water expulsion vesicle.*
**digestive v.**, secondary lysosome.
**food v.**, a fluid-containing intracytoplasmic space in which food material is suspended; it occurs in holozoic protozoa.
**heterophagic v.**, heterophagosome.
**plasmocrine v.**, a small cavity containing crystalloids in a secretory cell.
**rhagiocrine v.**, a small cavity containing colloids in a secretory cell.
**water v.**, a small drop of water within the protoplasm of a cell.

**vac·u·o·li·za·tion** (vak″u-o-lĭ-za'shən) vacuolation.

**vac·u·ome** (vak'u-ōm) the system of vacuoles in a cell which stain with neutral red.

**vac·u·um** (vak'ūm) [L.] [MeSH: Vacuum] a space devoid of air or of other gas; a space from which the air has been exhausted.
**high v.**, a vacuum in which the attenuation is extreme.
**torricellian v.**, the vacuum in a barometric tube.

**VAD** ventricular assist device.

**va·dum** (va'dəm) [L. "a shallow"] an occasional elevation from the bottom of a cerebral sulcus, rendering the sulcus more or less shallow.

**va·gal** (va'gəl) pertaining to the vagus nerve.

**va·gec·to·my** (va-jek'tə-me) surgical vagotomy.

**va·gi** (va'ji) [L.] genitive and plural of *vagus.*

**va·gi·na** (və-ji'nə) pl. *vagi'nae* [L.] [TA] [MeSH: Vagina] 1. sheath: general anatomical nomenclature for a tubular enveloping structure. 2. the genital canal in the female, extending from the vulva to the cervix uteri, which receives the penis in copulation.
**v. bul'bi** [TA], sheath of eyeball: connective tissue that forms the capsule enclosing the posterior part of the eyeball, extending anteriorly to the conjunctival fornix, and continuous with the muscular fascia of the eye; called also *bulbar fascia, capsula bulbi, fascia bulbi [Tenoni], bulbar sheath,* and *Bonnet's, ocular,* or *Tenon's capsule.*
**v. caro'tica fas'ciae cervica'lis** [TA], carotid sheath of cervical fascia: the portion of the cervical fascia that encloses the carotid vessels and vagus nerve.
**v. commu'nis musculo'rum flexo'rum** [TA], the common synovial sheath for the flexor tendons as they pass through osteofibrous canals of the fingers; called also *v. synovialis communis musculorum flexorum.*
**v. commu'nis ten'dinum musculo'rum fibula'rium** [TA], common sheath of tendons of fibular muscles: the double tendon sheath for the long and short fibular muscles; called also *v. communis tendinum musculorum peroneorum* [TA alternative], *v. synovialis musculorum fibularium communis,* and *v. synovialis musculorum peroneorum communis.*

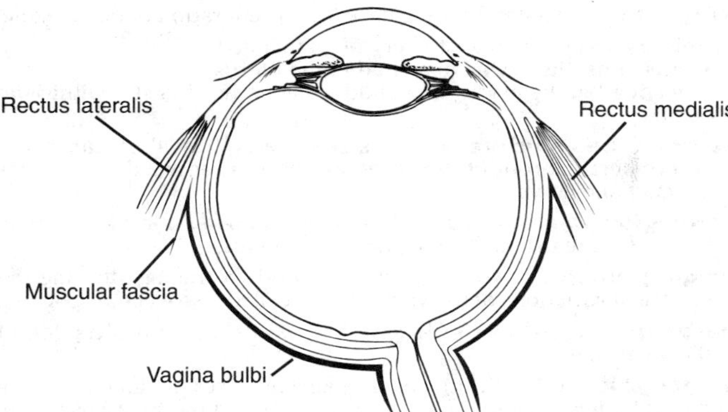


Section through the eyeball, showing the vagina bulbi continuous with the muscular fascia.

**v. commu'nis ten'dinum musculo'rum peroneo'rum,** TA alternative for *v. communis tendinum musculorum fibularium.*
**v. exter'na ner'vi op'tici** [TA], external sheath of optic nerve: the thick outer sheath of the optic nerve, continuous with the dura mater and connecting it with the sclera; called also *fibrous* or *outer sheath of optic nerve* and *dural sheath.*
**v. fe'moris,** fascia lata.
**v. fibro'sa,** TA alternative for *stratum fibrosum vaginae tendinis.*
**vagi'nae fibro'sae digito'rum ma'nus** [TA], fibrous sheaths of fingers: strong fibrous, semicylindrical sheaths investing the grooved palmar surface of the proximal and middle phalanges of the fingers; called also *ligamenta vaginalia digitorum manus.*
**vagi'nae fibro'sae digito'rum pe'dis** [TA], fibrous sheaths of toes: more or less complete fascial sheaths surrounding the phalanges of the toes, for attachment of the tendons and their synovial membranes; called also *ligamenta vaginalia digitorum pedis.*
**v. fibro'sa ten'dinis,** stratum fibrosum vaginae tendinis.
**v. inter'na ner'vi op'tici** [TA], internal sheath of optic nerve: the inner sheath of the optic nerve, continuous with the pia mater and arachnoidea mater; called also *inner sheath of optic nerve.* See also *arachnoid sheath* and *pial sheath,* under *sheath.*
**v. masculi'na,** utriculus prostaticus.
**vagi'na muco'sa,** v. synovialis.
**v. muco'sa ten'dinis,** v. synovialis tendinis.
**v. mus'culi rec'ti abdo'minis** [TA], sheath of rectus abdominis muscle: a sheath formed by the aponeuroses of other abdominal muscles, within which the rectus abdominis can move. Called also *rectus sheath.*
**vagi'nae ner'vi op'tici,** sheaths of optic nerve; see also *v. externa nervi optici* and *v. interna nervi optici.*
**v. o'culi,** v. bulbi.
**v. planta'ris ten'dinis mus'culi fibula'ris lon'gi** [TA], the tendon sheath of the peroneus longus muscle, beginning in the peroneal groove of the cuboid bone.
**v. planta'ris ten'dinis mus'culi pero'nei lon'gi,** TA alternative for *v. plantaris tendinis musculi fibularis longi.*
**v. proces'sus styloi'dei** [TA], sheath of styloid process: a ridge on the inferior surface of the temporal bone, partly enclosing the base of the styloid process.
**v. synovia'lis** [TA], synovial sheath: a double-layered, fluid-filled sheath such as the type usually found surrounding tendons running in osseofibrous tunnels.
**v. synovia'lis commu'nis musculo'rum flexo'rum,** v. communis musculorum flexorum.
**vagi'nae synovia'les digito'rum ma'nus** [TA], the synovial sheaths of the tendons of the fingers.
**vagi'nae synovia'les digito'rum pe'dis** [TA], the synovial sheaths of the tendons of the toes.
**v. synovia'lis intertubercula'ris** [TA], intertubercular synovial sheath: the synovial membrane that surrounds the long head of the biceps brachii muscle as it passes through the intertubercular sulcus; called also *synovial sheath of intertubercular groove.*
**v. synovia'lis musculo'rum fibula'rium commu'nis,** v. communis tendinum musculorum fibularium.
**v. synovia'lis mus'culi obli'qui superio'ris,** v. tendinis musculi obliqui superioris.
**v. synovia'lis musculo'rum peroneo'rum commu'nis,** v. communis tendinum musculorum fibularium.
**v. synovia'lis ten'dinis,** 1. synovial sheath of tendon: a double-layered, fibrous sheath usually found surrounding a tendon running in an osteofibrous canal, with synovial fluid present between the layers. Called also *v. mucosa tendinis.* 2. TA alternative for stratum synoviale vaginae tendinis.
**vagi'nae synovia'les ten'dinum digito'rum ma'nus,** vaginae tendinum digitorum manus.
**vagi'nae synovia'les ten'dinum digito'rum pe'dis,** vaginae tendinum digitorum pedis.
**v. synovia'lis ten'dinis mus'culi flexo'ris car'pi radia'lis,** v. tendinis musculi flexoris carpi radialis.
**v. synovia'lis ten'dinis mus'culi flexo'ris hal'lucis lon'gi,** v. tendinis musculi flexoris hallucis longi.
**v. synovia'lis ten'dinis mus'culi tibia'lis posterio'ris,** v. tendinis musculi tibialis posterioris.
**v. ten'dinis** [TA], tendon sheath: a sheath of tissue that covers a tendon; it has both fibrous and synovial layers (*stratum fibrosum vaginae tendinis* and *stratum synoviale vaginae tendinis*). Called also *epitendineum.*
**vagi'nae ten'dinum digito'rum ma'nus,** the tendon sheaths of the long and short flexors of the fingers; called also *vaginae synoviales tendinum digitorum manus.*
**vagi'nae ten'dinum digito'rum pe'dis** [TA], the synovial sheaths of the tendons of the toes; called also *vaginae synoviales tendinum digitorum pedis.*
**v. ten'dinum musculo'rum abducto'ris lon'gi et extenso'ris pol'licis bre'vis** [TA], the tendon sheath of the long abductor and short extensor muscles of the thumb.
**v. ten'dinum musculo'rum extenso'rum car'pi radia'lium** [TA], the tendon sheath of the short and long extensor carpi radialis muscles.
**v. ten'dinis mus'culi extenso'ris car'pi ulna'ris** [TA], the tendon sheath of the extensor carpi ulnaris muscle.
**v. ten'dinum musculo'rum extenso'ris digito'rum commu'nis et extenso'ris in'dicis,** v. tendinum musculorum extensoris digitorum et extensoris indicis.
**v. ten'dinum musculo'rum extenso'ris digito'rum et extenso'ris in'dicis** [TA], the tendon sheath of the extensor digitorum and extensor indicis muscles.
**v. ten'dinis mus'culi extenso'ris dig'iti min'mimi** [TA], the tendon sheath of the extensor digiti minimi muscle.
**vagi'nae ten'dinum mus'culi extenso'ris digito'rum lon'gi pe'dis** [TA], the tendon sheaths of the extensor digitorum longus muscle, running from the cruciate ligament to the intermediate cuneiform bone.
**v. ten'dinis mus'culi extenso'ris hal'lucis lon'gi** [TA], the tendon sheath of the extensor hallucis longus muscle, extending from the cruciate ligament to the dorsal fascia of the foot.
**v. ten'dinis mus'culi extenso'ris pol'licis lon'gi** [TA], the sheath of the extensor pollicis longus tendon.
**v. ten'dinis mus'culi flexo'ris car'pi radia'lis** [TA], the tendon sheath of the flexor carpi radialis muscle.
**vagi'nae ten'dinum mus'culi flexo'ris digito'rum lon'gi pe'dis** [TA], the tendon sheaths of the flexor digitorum longus muscle, extending from the medial malleolus to below the navicular bone.
**v. ten'dinis mus'culi flexo'ris hal'lucis lon'gi** [TA], the tendon sheath of the flexor hallucis longus muscle, extending from the medial malleolus to where it crosses the tendon of the flexor digitorum longus; called also *v. synovialis tendinis musculi flexoris hallucis longi.*
**v. ten'dinis mus'culi flexo'ris pol'licis lon'gi** [TA], the tendon sheath for the long flexor muscle of the thumb in the wrist and palm.
**v. ten'dinis mus'culi obli'qui superio'ris** [TA], the synovial sheath of the superior oblique muscle, particularly where its tendon passes through the trochlea; called also *synovial bursa of trochlea, trochlear synovial bursa,* and *v. synovialis musculi obliqui superioris.*
**v. ten'dinis mus'culi tibia'lis anterio'ris** [TA], the tendon sheath of the tibialis anterior muscle, extending from the transverse crural ligament to the talonavicular joint.
**v. ten'dinis mus'culi tibia'lis posterio'ris** [TA], the tendon sheath of the tibialis posterior muscle, beginning at the medial malleolus and extending into the foot; called also *v. synovialis tendinis musculi tibialis posterioris.*
**v. vaso'rum,** a fibrous sheath that encloses any of various arteries, sometimes along with their veins and nerves.

**va·gi·nae** (və-ji'ne) genitive and plural of *vagina.*

**vag·i·nal** (vaj'ĭ-nəl) 1. of the nature of a sheath; ensheathing. 2. pertaining to the vagina. 3. pertaining to the tunica vaginalis testis.

**vag·i·na·lec·to·my** (vaj"ĭ-nə-lek'tə-me) vaginectomy.

**vag·i·na·li·tis** (vaj"ĭ-nə-li'tis) periorchitis.
**plastic v.,** pachyvaginalitis.

**vag·i·na·pexy** (vaj"ĭ-nə-pek'se) vaginofixation.

**vag·i·nate** (vaj'ĭ-nāt) [L. *vaginatus* sheathed] provided with a sheath.

**vag·i·nec·to·my** (vaj"ĭ-nek'tə-me) excision of the vagina.

**vag·i·ni·peri·ne·ot·o·my** (vaj"ĭ-nĭ-per"ĭ-ne-ot'ə-me) paravaginal incision.

**vag·i·nis·mus** (vaj″ĭ-niz′məs) [L.] painful spasm of the vagina due to involuntary contraction of the vaginal musculature, usually severe enough to prevent intercourse; the cause may be organic or psychogenic.

**vag·i·ni·tis** (vaj″ĭ-ni′tis) [MeSH: Vaginitis] 1. inflammation of the vagina; it is marked by pain and by a purulent discharge. Called also *colpitis.* 2. inflammation of a sheath.
**v. adhaesi′va, adhesive v.,** atrophic vaginitis with ulceration and exfoliation of the mucosa resulting in adhesions of the membranes; opposite surfaces may adhere to each other, causing obliteration of the vaginal canal. Called also *senile v.*
**atrophic v.,** vaginitis occurring in postmenopausal women, associated with estrogen deficiency. The two most common types are *senile vulvovaginitis* and *adhesive vaginitis.*
***Candida* v., candidal v.,** vaginitis caused by infection with *Candida* species and characterized by a thick creamy discharge, pruritus, and erythema. Called also *vaginal candidiasis.*
**desquamative inflammatory v.,** vaginitis of unknown etiology, resembling atrophic vaginitis clinically and microscopically, but occurring in the absence of estrogen deficiency, and characterized chiefly by recrudescent reddened superficial ulcerations.
**diphtheritic v.,** diphtheritic inflammation of the vagina.
**v. emphysemato′sa, emphysematous v.,** inflammation of the vagina and adjacent cervix, characterized by numerous, asymptomatic, gas-filled cystlike lesions; the gas filling the lesions has been shown to have a carbon dioxide content.
**granular v.,** vaginitis in cows with small nodules on the vulvar mucosa, apparently a nonspecific response of lymphatic tissue to irritation.
**senile v.,** see *atrophic v.*
**v. tes′tis,** perididymitis.
**trichomonas v.,** vaginitis produced by *Trichomonas.*

**vag·i·no·ab·dom·i·nal** (vaj″ĭ-no-ab-dom′ĭ-nəl) pertaining to the vagina and the abdomen.

**vag·i·no·cele** (vaj′ĭ-no-sēl″) [*vagina* + *-cele*[1]] 1. vaginal hernia. 2. prolapse or falling of the vagina; called also *colpoptosis.*

**vag·i·no·cu·ta·ne·ous** (vaj″ĭ-no-ku-ta′ne-əs) pertaining to the vagina and skin, or communicating with the vagina and the cutaneous surface of the body, as a vaginocutaneous fistula.

**vag·in·odyn·ia** (vaj″ĭ-no-din′e-ə) [*vagina* + *-odynia*] pain in the vagina; colpodynia.

**vag·i·no·fix·a·tion** (vaj″ĭ-no-fik-sa′shən) colpopexy.

**vag·i·no·gram** (vaj′ĭno-gram) a radiograph of the vagina.

**vag·i·nog·ra·phy** (vaj″ĭ-nog′rə-fe) radiography of the vagina.

**vag·i·no·la·bi·al** (vaj″ĭ-no-la′be-əl) pertaining to the vagina and the labia.

**vag·i·nom·e·ter** (vaj″ĭ-nom′ə-tər) [*vagina* + *-meter*] an instrument for measuring the length and diameter of the vagina.

**vag·i·no·my·co·sis** (vaj″ĭ-no-mi-ko′sis) [*vagina* + *mycosis*] fungal disease of the vagina; see also Candida vaginitis.

**vag·i·nop·a·thy** (vaj″ĭ-nop′ə-the) [*vagina* + *-pathy*] any disease of the vagina.

**vag·i·no·per·i·ne·al** (vaj″ĭ-no-per″ĭ-ne′əl) pertaining to the vagina and perineum.

**vag·i·no·peri·neo·plas·ty** (vaj″ĭ-no-per″ĭ-ne′o-plas″te) [*vagino-* + *perineoplasty*] plastic surgery of the vagina and perineum.

**vag·i·no·peri·ne·or·rha·phy** (vaj″ĭ-no-per″ĭ-ne-or′ə-fe) suture repair of the vagina and perineum.

**vag·i·no·peri·ne·ot·o·my** (vaj′ĭ-no-per″ĭ-ne-ot′ə-me) paravaginal incision.

**vag·i·no·peri·to·ne·al** (vaj″ĭ-no-per″ĭ-to-ne′əl) pertaining to the vagina and peritoneum.

**vag·i·no·pexy** (vaj″ĭ-no-pek′se) [*vagina* + *-pexy*] colpopexy.

**vag·i·no·plas·ty** (vaj″ĭ-no-plas′te) [*vagina* + *-plasty*] plastic surgery of the vagina; called also *colpoplasty.*

**vag·i·no·scope** (vaj′ĭ-no-skōp) [*vagina* + *-scope*] a vaginal speculum; called also *colposcope.*

**vag·i·nos·co·py** (vaj″ĭ-nos′kə-pe) [*vagina* + *-scopy*] inspection of the vagina; colposcopy.

**vag·i·no·sis** (vaj″ĭ-no′sis) a disease of the vagina.
**bacterial v.,** a type of vaginitis frequently associated with positive cultures for *Gardnerella vaginalis* or *mobiluncus,* characterized by increased malodorous gray vaginal discharge that cannot be attributed to other cause.

**vag·i·not·o·my** (vaj″ĭ-not′ə-me) [*vagina* + *-tomy*] colpotomy.

**vag·i·no·ves·i·cal** (vaj″ĭ-no-ves′ĭ-kəl) pertaining to the vagina and bladder.

**vag·i·no·vul·var** (vaj″ĭ-no-vul′vər) vulvovaginal.

**Va·gi·stat** (vaj′ĭ-stat″) trademark for a preparation of tioconazole.

**va·gi·tus** (və-ji′təs) [L.] the cry of an infant.
**v. uteri′nus,** the crying of a child in the uterus.
**v. vagina′lis,** the crying of a child while its head is still within the vagina.

**va·go·ac·ces·so·ri·us** (va″go-ak″sĕ-sor′e-əs) [L.] the vagus nerve and the cranial root of the accessory nerves regarded as together forming one nerve.

**va·go·glos·so·pha·ryn·ge·al** (va″go-glos″o-fə-rin′je-əl) pertaining to the vagus and glossopharyngeal nerves.

**va·go·gram** (va′go-gram) [*vagus* + *-gram*] a tracing showing the electrical variations of the vagus nerve; called also *electrovagogram.*

**va·gol·y·sis** (va-gol′ĭ-sis) [*vagus* + *-lysis*] surgical destruction of the vagus nerve.

**va·go·lyt·ic** (va″go-lit′ik) having an effect resembling that produced by interruption of impulses transmitted by the vagus nerve; parasympatholytic.

**va·go·mi·met·ic** (va″go-mĭ-met′ik) having an effect which resembles that produced by vagal stimulation.

**va·go·splanch·nic** (va″go-splank′nik) vagosympathetic.

**va·go·sym·pa·thet·ic** (va″go-sim″pə-thet′ik) pertaining to both the vagus and sympathetic innervation.

**va·got·o·my** (va-got′ə-me) [*vagus* + *-tomy*] [MeSH: Vagotomy] interruption of the impulses carried by the vagus nerve or nerves.
**bilateral v.,** transection of the right and left vagus nerves.
**highly selective v.,** division of only those vagal fibers supplying the acid-secreting glands of the stomach, with preservation of those supplying the antrum as well as the hepatic and celiac branches.
**medical v.,** interruption of the impulses carried by the vagus nerve by administration of suitable drugs; vagus block.
**parietal cell v.,** selective severing of the vagus nerve fibers supplying the proximal two-thirds (parietal area) of the stomach; done for duodenal ulcer.
**posterior truncal v.,** a variation of the highly selective vagotomy in which the posterior vagal trunk is surgically cut for treatment of severe intractable gastric ulcers.
**selective v.,** division of the vagal fibers to the stomach with preservation of the hepatic and celiac branches.
**truncal v.,** surgical division of the two main trunks of the abdominal vagus nerve as they emerge through the esophageal hiatus.

**va·go·to·nia** (va″go-to′ne-ə) [*vagus* + *ton-* + *-ia*] hyperexcitability of the vagus nerve, particularly with respect to its parasympathetic effects on body organs; this results in vasomotor instability, constipation, sweating, and involuntary motor spasms with pain. Called also *parasympathicotonia, sympathetic imbalance,* and *vagotony.* Cf. sympatheticotonia.

**va·go·ton·ic** (va″go-ton′ik) pertaining to or characterized by vagotonia.

**va·got·o·ny** (va-got′ə-ne) vagotonia.

**va·go·trop·ic** (va″go-trop′ik) having an effect on the vagus nerve; see also *vagotropism.*

**va·got·ro·pism** (va-got′rə-piz-əm) [*vagus* + *tropism*] affinity of a drug or poison for the vagus nerve.

**va·go·va·gal** (va″go-va′gəl) arising as a result of afferent and efferent impulses which are both mediated through the vagus nerve.

**va·grant** (va′grənt) [L. *vagrans,* from *vagare* to wander] wandering; moving from one place to another.

**va·gus** (va′gəs) pl. *va′gi* [L. "wandering"] designating the tenth cranial nerve; see *nervus vagus.*

**Vahl·kamp·fia** (vahl-kamp′fe-ah) a genus of freshwater or parasitic ameboid protozoa (suborder Schizopyrenida, subclass Gymnamoeba), characterized by the presence of one broad pseudopodium.

**Vail's neuralgia (syndrome)** (vālz) [Harris Holmes *Vail,* American otorhinolaryngologist, 1892–1939] vidian neuralgia.

**Val** valine.

**val·a·cy·clo·vir hy·dro·chlo·ride** (val″a-si′klo-vir) the hydrochloride salt of the L-valyl ester of acyclovir, used as an antiviral agent in the treatment of herpes zoster in immunocompetent adults; administered orally. Following absorption, valacyclovir is converted by intestinal and hepatic metabolism to the active drug acyclovir.

**va·lence** (va′lens) [L. *valēre* to be strong] 1. a positive number that represents the combining power of an element in a chemical compound, i.e., the number of bonds each atom of that element makes with other atoms. In this most general sense "valence" has been superseded by the concept "oxidation number." However, "valence" is still used to indicate *(a)* the number of covalent bonds formed by an atom in a covalent compound or *(b)* the charge on a monatomic or polyatomic molecule. 2. in immunology, the number of antigen binding sites possessed by an antibody molecule, two per immunoglobulin monomer, or the number of antigenic determinants possessed by an antigen, usually a large number.

**va·len·cy** (va'lən-se) [L. *valentia*] 1. strength; ability. 2. valence.

**Val·en·tin's corpuscles, ganglion (pseudoganglion), nerve** (val'ən-tinz) [Gabriel Gustav *Valentin,* German physiologist, 1810–1883] see under *corpuscle* and *nerve,* and see *intumescentia tympanica.*

**Val·en·tine's position** (val'ən-tīnz) [Ferdinand C. *Valentine,* American surgeon, 1851–1909] see under *position.*

**val·er·ate** (val'ər-āt) a salt or ester of valeric acid.

**va·le·ri·an** (və-lēr'e-ən) [L. *valeriana*] [NF] [MeSH: Valerian] any plant of the genus *Valeriana.* The dried roots and rhizome of *V. officinalis* L. (Valerianaceae) of Europe are antispasmodic and sedative and are used for nervousness and insomnia.
**Greek v.,** the European plant *Polemonium caeruleum* L. (Polemoniaceae), or Jacob's ladder, used as a topical application to ulcers.

**va·le·ric ac·id** (və-lēr'ik) a monobasic organic acid derived from valerian, used as an intermediate in pharmaceutical manufacture.

**val·eth·a·mate bro·mide** (vəl-eth'ə-māt) a quaternary ammonium anticholinergic, used as an antispasmodic in the treatment of hypermotility and spasm of the gastrointestinal, genitourinary, and biliary tracts, administered orally, intramuscularly, or intravenously.

**val·e·tu·di·nar·i·an** (val″ə-too″dĭ-nar'ne-ən) [L. *valetudinarius* sickly] an invalid; a feeble person.

**val·e·tu·di·nar·i·an·ism** (val″ə-too″dĭ-nar'e-ən-iz-əm) an infirm or feeble habit of body.

**val·gus** (val'gəs) [L.] bent outward, twisted; denoting a deformity in which the angulation of the part is away from the midline of the body, as in *talipes valgus.* The term valgus is an adjective and should be used only in connection with the noun it describes, as talipes valgus, genu valgum, coxa valga. The meanings of *valgus* and *varus* are often reversed, so that genu valgum is knock-knee, not bowleg. Cf. *varus.*

**val·i·da·tion** (val″ĭ-da'shən) confirmation or corroboration; the declaration of validity.
**consensual v.,** the confirmation of reality by comparison of one's own perceptions and concerns with those of others, including the recognition and modification of distortions.

**va·lid·i·ty** (və-lid'ĭ-te) the extent to which a measurement, test, or study measures what it purports to measure.
**construct v.,** the degree to which an instrument measures the characteristic being investigated; the extent to which the conceptual definition matches the operational definition.
**content v.,** verification that the method of measurement actually measures what it is expected to measure, covering all areas under investigation reasonably and thoroughly.
**criterion v.,** verification that the instrument correlates with external criteria of the phenomenon under study, either concurrently or predictively.
**external v.,** the extent to which study results can be generalized beyond the sample used in the study.
**face v.,** a type of content validity, determining the suitability of a given instrument as a source of data on the subject under investigation, using common-sense criteria.
**internal v.,** the extent to which the effects detected in a study are truly caused by the treatment or exposure in the study sample, rather than being due to other biasing effects of extraneous variables.

**val·ine** (va'lēn, val'ēn) [MeSH: Valine] an essential amino acid, α-aminoisovaleric acid, produced by the digestion or hydrolytic decomposition of proteins; it is essential for optimal growth in infants and for nitrogen equilibrium in human adults. Symbols Val and V. See also table at *amino acid.*

**val·in·emia** (val″in-e'me-ə) hypervalinemia.

**val·ine trans·am·i·nase** (va'lēn trans-am'ĭ-nās) a branched-chain-amino-acid transaminase acting on valine.

**Val·i·sone** (val'ĭ-sōn) trademark for preparations of betamethasone valerate.

**Val·i·um** (val'e-əm) trademark for preparations of diazepam.

**val·late** (val'āt) [L. *vallatus* walled] having a wall or rim; cup-shaped.

**val·lec·u·la** (və-lek'u-lə) pl. *vallec'ulae* [dim. of L. *valles* a hollow] [TA] 1. a general term in anatomical nomenclature for a depression or furrow. 2. v. epiglottica.
**v. cerebel'li** [TA], vallecula of cerebellum: the longitudinal hollow on the inferior surface of the cerebellum, between the hemispheres, in which the medulla oblongata rests.
**v. epiglot'tica** [TA], epiglottic vallecula: a depression between the lateral and median glossoepiglottic folds on each side.
**v. ova'ta,** fossa vesicae biliaris.
**v. for petrosal ganglion,** fossula petrosa.
**v. syl'vii,** fossa lateralis cerebralis.
**v. un'guis,** sulcus matricis unguis.

**val·lec·u·lar** (və-lek'u-lər) pertaining to or affecting a vallecula.

**Val·les·tril** (və-les'tril) trademark for a preparation of methallenestril.

**val·lic·e·po·bu·fa·gin** (və-lis″ə-po-bu'fə-jin) a cardiac poison from the skin glands of the toad, *Bufo valliceps.*

**val·lum** (val'əm) [L. "rampart"] a wall.
**v. un'guis** [TA], nail wall: the fold of skin overlapping the sides and the proximal end of a nail.

**Val·mid** (val'mid) trademark for a preparation of ethinamate.

**Val·nac** (val'nak) trademark for preparations of betamethasone valerate.

**val·one** (val'ōn) an indanedione anticoagulant compound used as an insecticide and rodenticide; it can cause fatal anticoagulant rodenticide poisoning (q.v.) in many mammalian species.

**Val·pin** (val'pin) trademark for preparations of anisotropine methylbromide.

**val·pro·ate so·di·um** (val-pro'āt) the sodium salt of valproic acid, having the same uses as the parent compound.

**val·pro·ic ac·id** (val-pro'ik) [USP] [MeSH: Valproic Acid] a simple eight-carbon branched-chain fatty acid used in the treatment of epileptic seizures, particularly absence seizures; administered orally.

**Val·sal·va's ligaments, maneuver,** etc. (vahl-sahl'vəz) [Antonio Maria *Valsalva,* Italian anatomist, 1666–1723] see under *maneuver,* and see *sinus aortae.*

**val·sar·tan** (val-sahr'tan) an angiotensin II blocker used as an antihypertensive; administered orally.

**Val·trex** (val'treks) trademark for a preparation of valacyclovir hydrochloride.

**val·ue** (val'u) 1. a measure of worth or efficiency. 2. a quantitative measurement of the activity, concentration, or some other quality of a substance; see *normal v's.*
**acetyl v.,** see under *number.*
**acid v.,** see under *number.*
**buffer v.,** a numerical expression of the degree of change in pH of a solution in response to the addition of acid or alkali.
**D v.,** decimal reduction time. See under *time.*
**expected v.,** in statistics, the value of an estimate that is the mean of its sampling distribution.
**fuel v.,** the potential heat energy of a food.
**Hehner's v.,** see under *number.*
**liminal v.,** that intensity of a stimulus which produces a just noticeable impression.
**negative predictive v.,** see *predictive v.*
**normal v's,** see *reference v's.*
***P* v., *p* v.,** the probability of obtaining by chance a result at least as extreme as that observed, even when the null hypothesis is true and no real difference exists; when $P \leq 0.05$ the sample results are usually deemed significant at a statistically important level and the null hypothesis rejected. See also *Type I error;* under *error.*
**positive predictive v.,** see *predictive v.*
**predictive v.,** the conditional probability that a clinical test result correctly identifies a patient as having or not having a disease, i.e., the predictive value of a positive test *(positive predictive v.)* is the probability that a person with a positive test is a true positive (i.e., does have the disease) and the predictive value of a negative test *(negative predictive v.)* is the probability that a person with a negative test does not have the disease. Cf. *sensitivity* and *specificity.* The predictive value of a screening test is determined by the sensitivity and specificity of the test, and by the prevalence of the condition for which the test is used.
**reference v's,** a set of values of a quantity measured in the clinical laboratory that characterize a specified population in a defined state of health. The values obtained from a statistical sample are used to establish a *reference interval* that covers 95 per cent of the values of the healthy general population or of specific subpopulations differing in age and sex. These concepts were originally and are still widely referred to as "normal values" and the "normal range," but the use of these terms is now discouraged because of their implication that values falling outside of the reference interval are "abnormal" or "unhealthy," which has led to much confusion. It must be remembered that, by definition, 5 per cent of healthy individuals fall outside of the reference interval.
**saponification v.,** see under *number.*
**threshold v.,** liminal v.
**threshold limit v. (TLV),** a value assigned to an industrial chemical by the American Conference of Governmental Hygienists, repre-

senting the maximum concentration to which most workers can be repeatedly exposed without adverse health effects.
**valence v.,** the number obtained by multiplying the lowering of the freezing point in degrees by the amount of urine in milliliters.
***z* v.,** a normalized value created from a member of a set of data by expressing it in terms of standard deviations from the mean, using the equation

$$z = \frac{x - \bar{x}}{\sigma}$$

where $x$ is an item of data, $\bar{x}$ is the mean of the data, and $\sigma$ is the standard deviation. The mean and standard deviation of the set of such $z$ values are 0 and 1, respectively.

**val·va** (val'və) pl. *val'vae* [sing. of L. *valvae* folding doors] [TA] valve: a membranous fold in a canal or passage, which prevents the
**v. aor'tae** [TA], aortic valve: a valve composed of three semilunar cusps or segments (semilunar cusps of aortic valve), guarding the aortic orifice in the left ventricle of the heart; it prevents backflow into the left ventricle.
**v. atrioventricula'ris dex'tra** [TA], right atrioventricular valve: the valve between the right atrium and right ventricle of the heart; it usually has three cusps (anterior, posterior, and septal), but additional small cusps may be present. Called also *v. tricuspidalis* [TA alternative] and *tricuspid valve.*
**v. atrioventricula'ris sinis'tra** [TA], left atrioventricular valve: the valve between the left atrium and left ventricle of the heart; it usually has two cusps (anterior and posterior), but additional small cusps may be present. Called also *v. mitralis* [TA alternative] and *mitral valve.*
**v. ilea'lis,** 1. v. ileocaecalis. 2. papilla ilealis.
**v. ileocaeca'lis,** ileocecal valve: a so-called valve formed by the flaps or lips, one above and one below, of the ileocecal opening. In the cadaver the flaps project into the lumen of the large intestine as thickened folds, but in the living individual the ileum forms a conical or papillary projection, the *papilla ilealis.* Called also *ileocolic valve, v. ilealis,* and *valvula ileocolica.*
**v. mitra'lis,** TA alternative for *v. atrioventricularis sinistra.*
**v. pulmona'ria,** v. trunci pulmonalis.
**v. tricuspida'lis,** TA alternative for *v. atrioventricularis dextra.*
**v. trun'ci pulmona'lis** [TA], valve of pulmonary trunk: a valve composed of three semilunar cusps or segments (semilunar cusps of pulmonary valve), guarding the pulmonary orifice in the right ventricle of the heart; it prevents backflow of blood into the right ventricle. Called also *pulmonary* or *pulmonic valve* and *v. pulmonaria.*

**val·val** (val'vəl) pertaining to a valve; valvar.

**val·var** (val'vər) valval.

**val·vate** (val'vāt) pertaining to or having valves.

**valve** (valv) a membranous fold in a canal or passage, which prevents the reflux of the contents passing through it; see also *valve* and *valvula.*
**anal v's,** valvulae anales.
**v. of aorta, aortic v.,** valva aortae.
**aortic v., bicuspid,** a congenital anomaly of the aortic valve, caused by incomplete separation of two of the three cusps; it is generally asymptomatic early in life but is predisposed to calcification and stenosis later on.

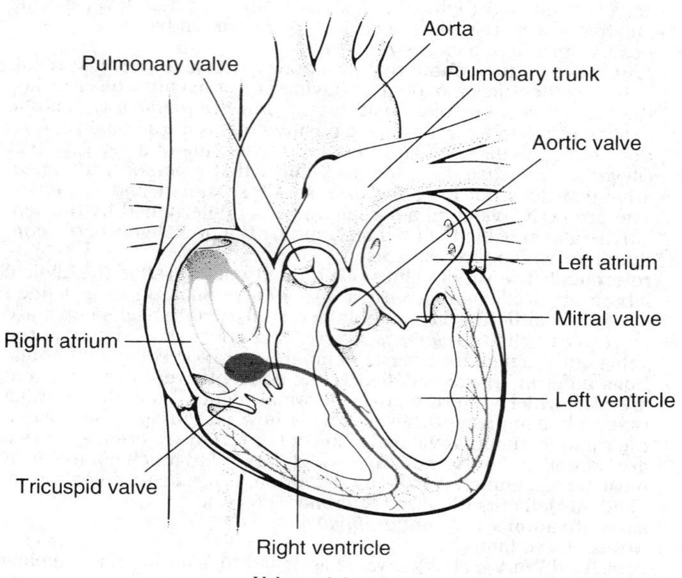

Valves of the heart.

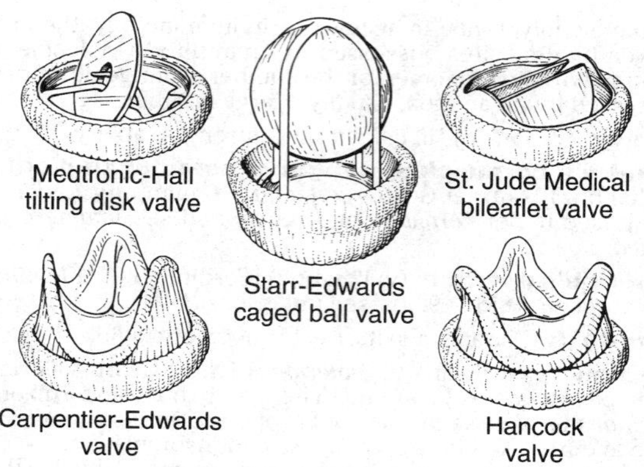

Artificial cardiac valves.

**atrioventricular v., left,** valva atrioventricularis sinistra.
**atrioventricular v., right,** valva atrioventricularis dextra.
**Ball's v's,** valvulae anales.
**Bauhin's v.,** valva ileocaecalis.
**Béraud's v.,** a fold of mucous membrane sometimes found at the junction of the lacrimal sac and the nasolacrimal duct; called also *Krause's v.*
**Bianchi's v.,** plica lacrimalis.
**bileaflet v.,** a type of artificial cardiac valve consisting of a sewing ring surrounding a circular valve seat, to which are attached two semicircular occluding disks that swing open and closed to regulate blood flow.
**bioprosthetic v.,** an artificial cardiac valve composed of biological tissue, sterilized and mounted on a plastic or metallic supporting structure; it is inaudible and does not require anticoagulation; a common type is the porcine valve. Called also *tissue v.*
**Björk-Shiley v.,** a tilting-disk valve consisting of a cobalt alloy cage, a Teflon fabric–covered sewing ring, and a disk made of pyrolytic carbon that opens to an angle of 60 degrees.
**Bochdalek's v.,** a fold within the lacrimal duct near the punctum lacrimale.
**caged-ball v.,** a type of artificial cardiac valve consisting of a sewing ring to which is attached a cage made of curved struts; a ball within the cage floats freely, allowing passage of blood or occluding the orifice to prevent reflux.
**cardiac v's,** valves that control the flow of blood through and from the heart; they are the atrioventricular, aortic, and pulmonary trunk valves.
**cardiac v., artificial,** a substitute, mechanical or composed of tissue, for a cardiac valve. See illustration. Called also *heart valve prosthesis.*
**Carpentier-Edwards v.,** a porcine valve mounted on an Elgiloy alloy stent with a Teflon cloth–covered sewing ring. See illustration.
**caval v.,** valvula venae cavae inferioris.
**Cooley-Cutter v.,** a caged-ball valve consisting of an open cage with four metal struts forming foot-like projections into the orifice, a cloth-covered sewing ring, and a disk-shaped or biconical poppet.
**coronary v., v. of coronary sinus,** valvula sinus coronarii.
**eustachian v.,** valvula venae cavae inferioris.
**fallopian v.,** valva ileocaecalis.
**femoral v.,** one of the valves of the femoral vein; there are usually four or five.
**flail mitral v.,** a mitral valve having a cusp that has lost its normal support (as in ruptured chordae tendineae) and flutters in the blood stream.
**Foltz's v.,** a fold of membrane at the lacrimal canaliculus.
**v. of foramen ovale,** valvula foraminis ovalis.
**Gerlach's v.,** valvula processus vermiformis.
**Guérin's v.,** valvula fossae navicularis.
**Hancock v.,** a porcine valve mounted on a semiflexible stent made of a Stellite ring and flexible struts of polypropylene. See illustration.
**Hasner's v.,** plica lacrimalis.
**heart v's,** cardiac v's.
**Heister's v.,** plica spiralis.
**Hoboken's v's,** foldlike thickenings of the vessels of the umbilical cord, especially the arteries, which protrude into the lumen of the vessels.
**homograft v.,** a transplanted cardiac valve obtained from a human donor and antibiotic-sterilized or cryopreserved, then sewn into the native anulus.
**Houston's v's,** plicae transversae recti.
**Huschke's v.,** plica lacrimalis.

**hymenal v. of male urethra,** valvula fossae navicularis.
**ileocecal v., ileocolic v.,** valva ileocaecalis.
**v. of inferior vena cava,** valvula venae cavae inferioris.
**Ionescu-Shiley v.,** a type of artificial cardiac valve consisting of glutaraldehyde-fixed bovine pericardium constructed as a three-cusp valve mounted on a Dacron-covered titanium frame.
**Kerckring's (Kerkring's) v's,** plicae circulares.
**Kohlrausch's v's,** plicae transversae recti.
**Krause's v.,** Béraud's v.
**Lillehei-Kaster v.,** a tilting-disk valve consisting of a titanium valve housing, Teflon sewing ring, and flat, free-floating, pivoting pyrolytic carbon disk that opens to 80 degrees.
**lymphatic v.,** valvula lymphaticum.
**v. of Macalister,** valva ileocaecalis.
**Medtronic-Hall v.,** a tilting-disk valve comprising a titanium valve housing an S-shaped disk guide strut, a Teflon cloth sewing ring, and a centrally perforated pyrolytic carbon–coated graphite disk that opens to an angle of 75 degrees. See illustration.
**Mercier's v.,** plica interureterica.
**mitral v.,** valva atrioventricularis sinistra.
**mitral v., floppy,** mitral valve prolapse.
**Morgagni's v's,** valvulae anales.
**nasal v.,** limen nasi.
**v. of navicular fossa,** valvula fossae navicularis.
**O'Beirne's v.,** see under *sphincter.*
**Omnicarbon v.,** a tilting-disk valve similar to the Omniscience valve but entirely coated with pyrolytic carbon, including the sewing ring.
**Omniscience v.,** a modification of the Lillehei-Kaster tilting-disk valve, having a curvilinear pyrolytic carbon disk suspended in a one piece titanium frame with fin-like projections and a Teflon sewing ring.
**porcine v.,** a type of artificial cardiac valve made from a pig aortic valve cured in glutaraldehyde and mounted on a supporting structure.
**pulmonary v., v. of pulmonary trunk,** valva trunci pulmonalis.
**pulmonic v.,** valva trunci pulmonalis.
**pyloric v.,** valvula pylori.
**Rosenmüller's v.,** plica lacrimalis.
**St. Jude Medical v.,** a bileaflet valve with a Dacron sewing ring and pyrolytic carbon leaflets and housing, the leaflets opening to 85 degrees. See also illustration.
**semilunar v.,** a valve having semilunar cusps, i.e., the aortic valve and the pulmonary valve. The term is sometimes used to designate the semilunar cusps composing these valves; see entries beginning *valvula semilunaris.*
**semilunar v's of colon,** plicae semilunares coli.
**semilunar v's of Morgagni,** sinus anales.
**sigmoid v's of colon,** plicae semilunares coli.
**Smeloff-Cutter v.,** a caged-ball valve with two open titanium cages, one on each side of the valve ring, a barium-impregnated silicone rubber ball, and a Teflon sewing ring.
**spiral v. of cystic duct, spiral v. of Heister,** plica spiralis.
**Starr-Edwards v.,** a caged-ball heart valve prosthesis consisting of a Stellite retaining cage containing a Silastic ball and a Teflon and polypropylene cloth–covered sewing ring. See illustration.
**v. of Sylvius,** valvula venae cavae inferioris.
**Taillefer's v.,** a fold of the mucous membrane of the nasolacrimal duct near the middle of its course.
**Tarinus' v.,** velum medullare inferius.
**thebesian v.,** valvula sinus coronarii.
**tilting-disk v.,** a type of artificial cardiac valve consisting of a sewing ring and a valve housing containing a suspended disk that swings between closed and open positions.
**tissue v.,** bioprosthetic v.
**tricuspid v.,** valva atrioventricularis dextra.
**v. of Tulpius,** valva ileocaecalis.
**ureteral v.,** a congenital transverse fold across the lumen of the ureter, composed of redundant mucosa prominent by circular muscle fibers; it usually disappears in time but may rarely cause urinary obstruction. Pathological valves or kinks also occur.
**urethral v., anterior,** a rare type of obstructing fold in the distal part of the male urethra, usually a type of diverticulum in the corpus spongiosum.
**urethral v., posterior,** any of various types of congenital folds across the proximal part of the male urethra near the seminal colliculus, which cause obstruction.
**v. of Varolius,** valva ileocaecalis.
**v. of veins, venous v.,** valvula venosa.
**v. of vermiform appendix,** valvula processus vermiformis.
**v. of Vieussens, Willis' v.,** velum medullare rostralis.

**valved** (valvd) having valves; opening by valves.

**val•vi•form** (val'vĭ-form) shaped like a valve.

**val•vo•tome** (val'vo-tōm) a surgical instrument for incising a valve.

**val•vot•o•my** (val-vot'ə-me) [*valve* + *-tomy*] incision of a valve. Called also *valvulotomy.*
**mitral v.,** dilation of the left atrioventricular (mitral) valve, the commissures being split with or without the aid of a knife or a mechanical dilator.
**pulmonary v.,** incision of the pulmonary valve to correct valvular stenosis.
**transventricular closed v.,** correction of pulmonary valvular stenosis by passage of a valvotome through the wall of the right ventricle into the pulmonary artery to open the valve; called also *Brock's operation.*

**val•vu•la** (val'vu-lə) pl. *val'vulae* [L., dim of *valva*] [TA] valvule: a small valve; formerly used in official nomenclature to designate any valve, but now restricted to certain small valves in the body and cusps of heart valves.
**val'vulae ana'les** [TA], anal valves: archlike folds of mucous membrane connecting the caudal ends of the anal columns.
**val'vulae conniven'tes,** [L. "closing valves"], plicae circulares.
**v. corona'ria dex'tra val'vae aor'tae,** TA alternative for *v. semilunaris dextra valvae aortae.*
**v. corona'ria sinis'tra val'vae aor'tae,** TA alternative for *valvula semilunaris sinistra valvae aortae.*
**v. fora'minis ova'lis** [TA], 1. valve of foramen ovale: in the adult, a crescentic ridge on the left side of the interatrial septum, representing the edge of what was the septum primum before fusion of the septum; called also *falx septi.* 2. a fold in the left atrium of the fetal heart, derived from the embryonic septum primum.
**v. fos'sae navicula'ris** [TA], valve of navicular fossa: a fold of mucous membrane occasionally occurring in the roof of the fossa navicularis of the urethra.
**v. ileoco'lica,** valva ileocaecalis.
**v. lympha'ticum** [TA], lymphatic valve: any of the usually doubled cusps in the collecting lymphatic vessels, serving to ensure flow in only one direction.
**v. non corona'ria val'vae aor'tae,** TA alternative for *v. semilunaris posterior valvae aortae.*
**v. proces'sus vermifor'mis,** an inconstant fold of mucous membrane at the opening into the cecum of the canal of the vermiform appendix.
**v. pylo'ri,** pyloric valve: a prominent circular fold of mucous membrane at the pyloric orifice of the stomach.
**v. semiluna'ris,** semilunar cusp.
**v. semiluna'ris ante'rior val'vae trun'ci pulmona'lis** [TA], the anterior cusp of the valve of the pulmonary trunk.
**v. semiluna'ris dex'tra val'vae aor'tae** [TA], the right cusp of the aortic valve; called also *v. coronaria dextra valvae aortae* [TA alternative].
**v. semiluna'ris dex'tra val'vae trun'ci pulmona'lis** [TA], the right cusp of the valve of the pulmonary trunk.
**v. semiluna'ris poste'rior val'vae aor'tae** [TA], the posterior cusp of the aortic valve; called also *v. non coronaria valvae aortae* [TA alternative].
**v. semiluna'ris sinis'tra val'vae aor'tae** [TA], the left cusp of the aortic valve; called also *v. coronaria sinistra valvae aortae* [TA alternative].
**v. semiluna'ris sinis'tra val'vae trun'ci pulmona'lis** [TA], the left cusp of the valve of the pulmonary trunk.
**v. si'nus corona'rii** [TA], valve of coronary sinus: a fold of endocardium along the right and inferior margins of the opening of the coronary sinus into the right atrium of the heart; it covers the lower part of the sinus and prevents regurgitation into the sinus during atrial contractions.
**v. spira'lis [Heis'teri],** plica spiralis.
**v. ve'nae ca'vae inferio'ris** [TA], valve of inferior vena cava: the variably sized crescentic fold of endocardial tissue, enclosing a few muscle fibers, that is attached to the anterior margin of the opening of the inferior vena cava into the right atrium of the heart. Rudimentary in the adult, in the fetus it directs blood flow from the inferior vena cava into the left atrium via the foramen ovale. Called also *caval* or *eustachian valve* and *valve of Sylvius.*
**v. veno'sa** [TA], venous valve: any of the small cusps or folds found in the tunica intima of many veins, serving to prevent backflow of blood.
**v. vesti'buli,** either of the two thin folds bordering the opening of the sinus reuniens into the right atrium of the embryonic heart; they develop into the valves of the inferior vena cava and coronary sinus.

**val•vu•lae** (val'vu-le) [L.] genitive and plural of *valvula.*

**val•vu•lar** (val'vu-lər) pertaining to, affecting, or of the nature of a valve.

**val•vule** (val'vūl) [L. *valvula,* q.v.] a small valve; see *valvula.*

**val•vu•li•tis** (val"vu-li'tis) inflammation of a valve or valvula, especially a valve of the heart.
**rheumatic v.,** that due to rheumatic fever, characterized by numerous small, translucent vegetations, composed of fibrin and platelets, located on the edges of the valve cusps along the lines of closure. The mitral valve is most frequently involved. It is sometimes incorrectly called *rheumatic endocarditis* (q.v.).

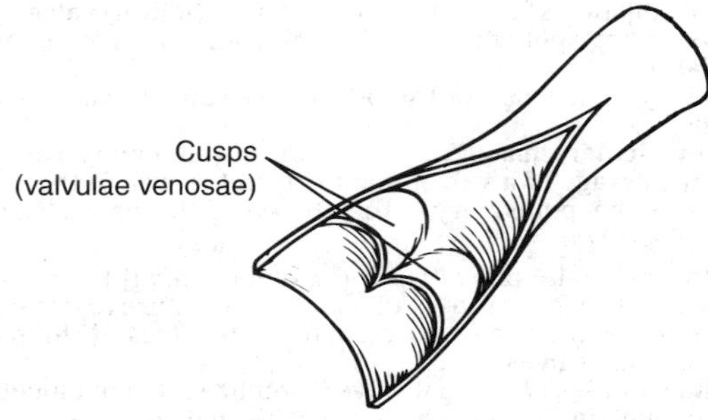

Vein laid open to show the valvulae venosae.

**val·vu·lo·plas·ty** (val'vu-lo-plas″te) plastic repair of a cardiac or venous valve.
**balloon v.,** dilation of a stenotic cardiac valve by means of a balloon-tipped catheter that is introduced into the valve and inflated.
**internal v.,** repair of a venous valve through a venotomy incision, using sutures to shorten the floppy cusps.

**val·vu·lo·tome** (val'vu-lo-tōm″) valvotome.

**val·vu·lot·o·my** (val″vu-lot'ə-me) valvotomy.

**val·yl** (val'əl, va'ləl) the acyl radical of valine.

**VAMP** a regimen of vincristine, methotrexate, 6-mercaptopurine, and prednisone, used in cancer chemotherapy.

**vam·pire** (vam'pīr) vampire bat.

**van·a·date** (van'ə-dāt) any salt of vanadic acid; the salts have various industrial applications and many are toxic.

**va·nad·ic ac·id** (və-nad'ik) an inorganic acid produced by dissolving vanadium pentoxide in water; there are various degrees of hydration, $HVO_3$, $H_3VO_4$, $H_4V_2O_7$, etc., seen in salts (vanadates).

**va·na·di·um** (və-na'de-əm) [*Vanadis,* a Norse deity] [MeSH: Vanadium] a rare, gray, metallic element; symbol, V; atomic number, 23; atomic weight, 50.942. Its salts have been used in treating various diseases. See also *vanadiumism.*
**v. pentoxide,** a yellow to brown oxide of vanadium, used to add color and ultraviolet blocking to glass and as a component of photographic developers; its fumes can cause vanadiumism and vanadium bronchitis.

**va·na·di·um·ism** (və-na'de-əm-iz-əm) a chronic intoxication caused by absorption of vanadium compounds, usually via the lungs; symptoms include irritation of the respiratory tract *(vanadium bronchitis),* pneumonitis, conjunctivitis, and anemia.

**Van Al·len type familial amyloid polyneuropathy (syndrome)** (van-al'ən) [Maurice Wright *Van Allen,* American physician, born 1918] Iowa type familial amyloid polyneuropathy; see under *polyneuropathy.*

**van Bo·gaert's encephalitis, sclerosing leukoencephalitis** (vahn-bo'gārts) [Ludo *van Bogaert,* Belgian neuropathologist, born 1897] subacute sclerosing panencephalitis.

**van Bo·gaert-Nys·sen syndrome** (vahn-bo'gārt-ni'sen) [L. *van Bogaert;* René *Nyssen,* Belgian neurologist, 20th century] metachromatic leukodystrophy (adult form); see under *leukodystrophy.*

**van Bo·gaert-Nys·sen-Peif·fer syndrome** (vahn-bo'gārt-ni'sen-pi'fer) [L. *van Bogaert;* R. *Nyssen;* Jürgen *Peiffer,* German physician, born 1922] metachromatic leukodystrophy (adult form); see under *leukodystrophy.*

**van Bu·chem's syndrome** (vahn-boo'kemz) [Francis Steven Peter *van Buchem,* Dutch physician, born 1897] hyperostosis corticalis generalisata; see under *hyperostosis.*

**van Bu·ren's disease** (van-bu'rənz) [William Holme *van Buren,* American surgeon, 1819–1883] see *Peyronie's disease,* under *disease.*

**Van·ce·nase** (van'sə-nāz″) trademark for a preparation of beclomethasone dipropionate.

**Van·cer·il** (van'sər-il″) trademark for a preparation of beclomethasone dipropionate.

**Van·co·cin** (van'ko-sin) trademark for a preparation of vancomycin hydrochloride.

**van·co·my·cin hy·dro·chlo·ride** (van″ko-mi'sin) [USP] an antibiotic produced by the soil bacillus *Streptomyces orientalis,* which is highly effective against cocci, especially staphylococci, and other gram-positive bacteria, occurring as a tan to brown, free-flowing powder; used in the treatment of severe staphylococcal infections resistant to other antibiotics, administered intravenously or by intravenous infusion.

**Van de Graaff machine** (van də grahf) [Robert Jemison *Van de Graaff,* American physicist, 1901–1967] see under *machine.*

**van den Bergh's disease, test** (vahn dən bərgz') [A. A. Hymans *van den Bergh,* Dutch physician, 1869–1943] see under *disease* and *test.*

**van der Hoeve's syndrome** (vahn dār hoo'vəz) [Jan *van der Hoeve,* Dutch ophthalmologist, 1878–1952] osteogenesis imperfecta (type I).

**van der Kolk's law** (vahn dār kolks) [Jacob Ludwig Conrad Schroeder *van der Kolk,* Dutch physiologist, 1797–1862] Schroeder van der Kolk's law; see under *law.*

**van der Vel·den's test** (vahn dār vel'denz) [Reinhardt *van der Velden,* German physician, 1851–1903] Maly's test.

**van der Waals forces** (vahn dər vahlz') [Johannes Diderik *van der Waals,* Dutch physicist, 1837–1923] see under *force.*

**Van der Woude's syndrome** (van der wo'dəz) [Anne *Van der Woude,* American physician, 20th century] see under *syndrome.*

**Vane** (vān) John Robert. British pharmacologist, born 1927; co-winner, with Sune Bergström and Bengt Ingemar Samuelsson, of the Nobel prize for medicine or physiology in 1982 for their discovery of prostaglandins and related substances.

**van Ge·huch·ten's method** (vahn ga-hook'tenz) [Arthur *van Gehuchten,* Belgian anatomist, 1861–1914] see under *method.*

**van Gie·son's stain** (van ge'sonz) [Ira *van Gieson,* American neuropathologist, 1865–1913] see under *Stains and Staining Methods.*

**Van·gue·ria** (van-ger'e-ə) a genus of shrubs of the family Rubiaceae. *V. pygmo'ra* is a shrub of southern Africa that is poisonous to sheep and cattle, causing gousiekte.

**van Hook's operation** (van hooks') [Weller *van Hook,* American surgeon, 1862–1933] ureteroureterostomy.

**van Hoorne's canal** (vahn hornz') [Jan *van Hoorne,* Dutch anatomist, 1621–1670] the thoracic duct (ductus thoracicus [TA]).

**Va·nil·la** (və-nil'ə) [L.] a genus of climbing plants of the family Orchidaceae, native to hot climates. *V. planifo'lia* Andr. is Mexican or Bourbon vanilla and *V. tahiten'sis* Moor. is Tahitian vanilla; both have fruits called vanilla beans, which are sources of the flavoring vanilla.

**va·nil·la** (və-nil'ə) [Sp. *vainilla* little sheath] 1. any plant of the genus *Vanilla.* 2. the fruit of *Vanilla planifolia* or *V. tahitensis,* an elongated pod that is the source of the flavoring called vanilla. Called also *vanilla bean.* 3. a preparation of the cured unripe fruit of *V. planifolia* or *V. tahitensis,* used in medicine as a flavoring agent, usually in the form of vanilla tincture (see under *tincture*).
**Bourbon v., Mexican v.,** *Vanilla planifolia.*
**Tahitian v.,** *Vanilla tahitensis.*

**va·nil·lal** (və-nil'əl) ethyl vanillin.

**va·nil·lic ac·id** (və-nil'ik) [MeSH: Vanillic Acid] 4-hydroxy-3-methoxybenzoic acid, obtained by oxidation of vanillin.
**v. a. diethylamide,** ethamivan.

**va·nil·lin** (və-nil'in, van'ĭ-lin) [NF] a constituent of vanilla and other plants, which also may be prepared synthetically; used as a flavor in pharmaceutical preparations.
**ethyl v.** [NF], fine white or slightly yellowish crystals, used as a flavor in pharmaceutical preparations.

**va·nil·lism** (və-nil'iz-əm) symptoms of dermatitis, coryza, and malaise seen in those handling raw vanilla, caused by the mite *Acarus siro.*

**va·nil·lyl·man·del·ic ac·id** (və-nil'əl-mən-del'ik) [MeSH: Vanilmandelic Acid] the primary end-product of catecholamine metabolism excreted in the urine; urinary levels are used in screening patients for pheochromocytoma. Abbreviated VMA.

**va·nil·man·del·ic ac·id** (van″əl-man-del'ik) [MeSH: Vanilmandelic Acid] vanillylmandelic acid.

**Van·sil** (van'sil) trademark for a preparation of oxamniquine.

**Van Slyke's formula, test (method)** (van slīks') [Donald Dexter *Van Slyke,* American biochemist, 1883–1971] see under *formula* and *test.*

**van't Hoff's law, rule** (vahnt hofs') [Jacobus Hendricus *van't Hoff,* Dutch chemist, 1852–1911; winner of the Nobel prize for chemistry in 1901] see under *law* and *rule.*

**Van·tin** (van'tin) trademark for preparations of cefpodoxime proxetil.

**Van·zet·ti's sign** (vahn-tset'ēz) [Tito *Vanzetti,* Italian surgeon, 1809–1888] see under *sign.*

**va·por** (va′por) pl. *vapo′res, vapors* [L.] 1. an atmospheric dispersion of a substance that in its normal state is a liquid or solid. 2. steam, gas, or an exhalation.

**va·por·iza·tion** (va″pər-ĭ-za′shən) 1. the conversion of a solid or liquid into a vapor without chemical change. See also *nebulization.* 2. distillation.

**va·por·ize** (va′pər-īz) to convert into vapor or to be transformed into vapor.

**va·por·iz·er** (va″por-īz′ər) [MeSH: Nebulizers and Vaporizers] a device for producing an aerosol or mist, as from a solution containing a medication to ease breathing. Cf. *nebulizer.*

**va·pors** (va′porz) obsolete term for *hypochondriasis* or *hysteria.*

**Va·quez's disease** (vah-kāz′) [Louis Henri *Vaquez,* French physician, 1860–1936] polycythemia vera.

**var.** variety.

**var·i·a·bil·i·ty** (var″e-ə-bil′ĭ-te) the state of being variable.

**var·i·a·ble** (var′e-ə-bəl) [L. *variare* to change] 1. changing from time to time. 2. in mathematics, a symbol that represents an arbitrary number or an arbitrary element of a set.
**categorical v.,** one of the variables that are not continuous but instead put data into categories.
**confounding v.,** confounder.
**continuous v.,** a variable that can assume the complete continuum of values (a theoretically infinite variety) through its distribution; cf. *discrete v.*
**dependent v.,** in a mathematical equation or relationship between two or more variables, a variable whose value depends on those of others; e.g., in the formula $x = 3y + z^2$, $x$ is the dependent variable.
**discrete v.,** an experimental variable that can assume only certain specific values in its distribution; the possible list of values is finite and often countable; cf. *continuous v.*
**independent v.,** in a mathematical equation or relationship between two or more variables, any variable whose value determines that of others; e.g., in the formula $x = 3y + z^2$, $y$ and $z$ are the independent variables.
**outcome v.,** one that measures consequences or results; it may be primary, ancillary, or incidental to a particular study.
**random v.,** an outcome of a random process that has a numerical value.

**var·i·ance** (var′e-əns) in statistics, a measure of the variation shown by a set of observations: the average of the squared deviations from the mean; it is the square of the standard deviation (q.v.). Symbol $\sigma^2$.

**var·i·ant** (var′e-ənt) 1. something that differs in some characteristic from the class to which it belongs, as a variant of a disease, trait, species, etc. 2. exhibiting such variation.
**L-phase v.,** a variant phase of certain bacteria, induced by osmotic shock, temperature shock, or the presence of antibiotics, and consisting of a spherical or ellipsoidal body without a rigid cell wall. The cells are capable of growth and multiplication; they may be stable or may revert to a normal bacterial cell. Called also *L-form.*
**migraine v.,** migraine associated with non-neurologic symptoms, such as occurs in ophthalmic migraine, basilar migraine, or abdominal migraine.
**petit mal v.,** Lennox-Gastaut syndrome.

**var·i·ate** (var′e-āt) a variable or random variable.

**var·i·a·tion** (var″e-a′shən) in genetics, deviation in characters in an individual from those typical of the group to which it belongs; also, deviation in characters of the offspring from those of its parents.
**allotypic v.,** the antigenic differences that characterize immunoglobulin allotypes.
**antigenic v.,** 1. a mechanism whereby parasites, such as trypanosomes, plasmodia, and *Borrelia,* are enabled to escape immune surveillance of a host by modifying or completely altering their surface antigens. 2. a phenomenon occurring in the influenza virus, in which the virus spontaneously exhibits both slow antigenic drift and sharp antigenic changes at intervals.
**contingent negative v. (CNV),** a small negative potential recorded on an electroencephalogram over the front central scalp of some subjects who perform tasks requiring close attention or who have just received a warning stimulus. Called also *E wave* and *expectancy wave.*
**continuous v.,** phenotypic differences so numerous and minute that the values selected for observation form a continuous spectrum, and no one phenotype or group of phenotypes predominates.
**discontinuous v.,** phenotypic differences that are marked, do not grade into one another, and form two or more separate, discontinuous classes.
**idiotypic v.,** the antigenic differences that characterize the different amino acid sequences and structures of immunoglobulin variable regions (idiotypes) and corresponding differences in antigen specificity.
**impressed v.,** differences among individuals or groups arising from a particular environmental, nongenetic stimulus.
**inborn v.,** one which arises from changes in the germ cells and not from the somatic cells.
**isotypic v.,** the antigenic differences that characterize the immunoglobulin classes and subclasses (isotypes).
**meristic v.,** variation in the number of parts in the offspring.
**microbial v.,** the range of characteristics within a species used in identification and differentiation.
**phenotypic v.,** the total range of variation, of whatever cause, observed in one character.
**quasicontinuous v.,** variation in which the underlying distribution of variability is continuous but a threshold effect makes it appear discontinuous.
**saltatory v.,** halmatogenesis.
**smooth-rough v., S-R v.,** a genetic mutation or an adaptation seen in bacteria, most often evidenced by a change in the surface of colonies from smooth (S, glossy) to rough (R, dull). The change correlates with pathogenicity, S strains being generally more virulent and R strains less so. The cells in S colonies have polysaccharide capsules and are more antigenically complete; R cells contain little or no capsule. The term may also refer to changes in other cell structures such as flagella and somatic antigens, as well as susceptibility to bacteriophage. Variations are often reversible and tend to result in mixed types on repeated subculture. See also *bacterial dissociation,* under *dissociation.*

**var·i·ca·tion** (var″ĭ-ka′shən) 1. the formation of a varix. 2. varicosity (def. 1).

**var·i·ce·al** (var″ĭ-se′əl) varicose.

**var·i·cel·la** (var″ĭ-sel′ə) [L.] chickenpox.
**v. gangreno′sa,** a rare form of chickenpox in which the eruption leads to a gangrenous ulceration, occurring mainly in children with leukemia, immunodeficiency, or some other severe underlying disease.

**Var·i·cel·lo·vi·rus** (var″ĭ-sel′o-vi″rəs) [*varicella* + *virus*] varicella and pseudorabies-like viruses; a genus of viruses of the subfamily Alphaherpesvirinae (family Herpesviridae) that infect both humans and animals, including human herpesvirus 3 and, tentatively, pseudorabies virus, bovine herpesvirus 1, and equid herpesviruses 1 and 4.

**var·i·cel·li·form** (var″ĭ-sel′ĭ-form) resembling chickenpox (varicella); called also *varicelloid.*

**var·i·cel·loid** (var″ĭ-sel′oid) varicelliform.

**var·i·ces** (vār′ĭ-sēz) [L.] plural of *varix.*

**var·ic·i·form** (var-is′ĭ-form) 1. varicoid. 2. varicose.

**varic(o)-** [L. *varix* a varicose vein] a combining form denoting relationship to a varix, or meaning twisted and swollen.

**var·i·co·bleph·a·ron** (var″ĭ-ko-blef′ə-ron) [*varico-* + Gr. *blepharon* eyelid] a varicose swelling of the eyelid.

**var·i·co·cele** (var′ĭ-ko-sēl″) [*varico-* + *-cele*[1]] [MeSH: Varicocele] a varicose condition of the veins of the pampiniform plexus, forming a swelling that feels like a "bag of worms," appearing bluish through the skin of the scrotum, and accompanied by a constant pulling, dragging, or dull pain in the scrotum.
**ovarian v., pelvic v.,** a varicose condition of the veins of the broad ligament.
**utero-ovarian v.,** a varicose condition of the veins of the pampiniform plexus of the female.

**var·i·co·ce·lec·to·my** (var″ĭ-ko-sə-lek′tə-me) [*varicocele* + *-ectomy*] ligation and excision of the enlarged veins for varicocele.

**var·i·cog·ra·phy** (var″ĭ-kog′rə-fe) [*varico-* + *-graphy*] radiographic visualization of varicose veins.

**var·i·coid** (var′ĭ-koid) [*varico-* + *-oid*] resembling a varix; called also *variciform.*

**var·i·cole** (var′ĭ-kōl) varicocele.

**var·i·com·pha·lus** (var″ĭ-kom′fə-ləs) [*varico-* + *omphalus*] a varicose tumor at the umbilicus.

**var·i·co·phle·bi·tis** (var″ĭ-ko-flə-bi′tis) varicose veins with inflammation.

**var·i·cose** (var′ĭ-kōs) [L. *varicosus*] pertaining to a varix; unnaturally and permanently distended. Called also *variceal* and *variciform.*

**var·i·co·sis** (var″ĭ-ko′sis) [L.] varicosity (def. 1).

**var·i·cos·i·ty** (var″ĭ-kos′ĭ-te) 1. a varicose condition; the state of being varicose. Called also *varication, varicosis,* and *phlebectasia.* 2. varix. 3. varicose vein.

**var•i•cot•o•my** (var″ĭ-kot′ə-me) [*varico-* + *-tomy*] incision into a varix or a varicose vein.

**va•ric•u•la** (və-rik′u-lə) [L.] a varix of the conjunctiva.

**Var•i•dase** (var′ĭ-dās) trademark for preparations of streptokinase-streptodornase.

**va•ri•e•ty** (və-ri′ə-te) in taxonomy, a subcategory of a species.

**va•ri•o•la** (və-ri′o-lə) [L.] smallpox.

**v. capri′na,** goatpox.

**v. haemorha′gica,** hemorrhagic smallpox.

**v. ma′jor,** the classic severe form of smallpox (q.v.); its mortality rate is 20 to 50 per cent. Cf. *v. minor.*

**v. mi′nor,** a mild form of smallpox (q.v.), found only in certain regions, such as South America and West Africa; it has a much lower mortality rate (1 to 2 per cent) than variola major. It has many synonyms and local names, including *alastrim, cottonpox, Cuban itch, milkpox,* and *whitepox.*

**v. ovi′na,** sheep-pox.

**v. si′ne eruptio′ne,** modified smallpox in which no rash is present.

**va•ri•o•lar** (və-ri′o-lər) pertaining to smallpox; variolic.

**Va•ri•o•la•ria ama•ra** (va″re-o-lar′e-ə ə-ma′rə) a febrifugal and anthelmintic lichen of the Old World, which is a source of litmus.

**va•ri•o•late** (var′e-o-lāt) 1. having the nature or appearance of smallpox. 2. to inoculate with smallpox virus.

**va•ri•o•la•tion** (var″e-o-la′shən) deliberate inoculation with the virus of unmodified smallpox to produce immunity to the naturally occurring disease. As practiced in the Orient in ancient times, the dried crusts of smallpox lesions were applied to the skin or nasal mucous membranes, or were ingested. The method employed in Europe in the eighteenth century consisted in subcutaneous injection of material from the lesions. Variolation is now used only experimentally in animals.

**var•i•ol•ic** (var″e-ol′ik) variolar.

**va•ri•ol•i•form** (var″e-o′lĭ-form) resembling smallpox.

**va•ri•o•li•za•tion** (var″e-o-lĭ-za′shən) variolation.

**va•ri•o•loid** (və-ri′o-loid″) 1. modified smallpox. 2. resembling smallpox; varioliform.

**va•ri•o•lous** (və-ri′o-ləs) pertaining to or of the nature of smallpox.

**va•ris•tor** (və-ris′tər) a voltage-variable resistor; a resistor, usually a semiconductor, designed to change its resistance with the voltage applied across it.

**va•rix** (var′iks) pl. *va′rices* [L.] an enlarged and tortuous vein, artery, or lymphatic vessel.

**anastomotic v.,** aneurysmal v. (def. 2).

**aneurysmal v., aneurysmoid v.,** 1. a markedly dilated tortuous vessel. 2. a form of arteriovenous aneurysm in which the blood flows directly into a neighboring vein without the intervention of a connecting sac; called also *anastomotic v.* and *Pott's aneurysm.*

**arterial v.,** a racemose aneurysm or varicose artery.

**cirsoid v.,** racemose aneurysm.

**esophageal v.,** varicosities of the branches of the azygos vein which anastomose with tributaries of the portal vein in the lower esophagus, occurring in patients with portal hypertension.

**lymph v., v. lympha′ticus,** a soft, lobulated swelling of a lymph node, resulting from obstruction and dilatation of the lymphatic vessels.

**Var•mus** (vahr′məs) Harold Eliot. American microbiologist, born 1939. Co-winner with John Michael Bishop of the Nobel prize for medicine or physiology in 1989 for their discovery that oncogenes of animal tumor viruses are derived from proto-oncogenes.

**var•nish** (vahr′nish) 1. a solution of resin or of natural gum, such as copal or rosin, in a suitable solvent, such as acetone, ether, or chloroform, which is capable of hardening into a thin film. 2. cavity v.

**cavity v.,** a cavity lining agent consisting of a solution of one or more natural or synthetic resins, gums, and rosin in an organic solvent such as chloroform, ethanol, acetone, or benzene; applied to the floor and walls of the prepared cavity.

**va•ro•li•an** (və-ro′le-ən) 1. described by or named for Costanzo *Varolius.* 2. pertaining to the pons.

**Va•ro•li•us′ bridge, valve** (və-ro′le-əs) [Costanzo *Varolius (Varoli, Varolio),* Italian anatomist, 1543–1575] see *pons* (def. 2) and *valva ileocaecalis.*

**va•rus** (var′əs) [L. "knock-kneed"] bent inward; denoting a deformity in which the angulation of the part is toward the midline of the body, as talipes varus. The term varus is an adjective and should be used only in connection with the noun it describes, as talipes varus, genu varum, coxa vara. The meanings of *varus* and *valgus* are often reversed, so that genu varum is bowleg, not knock-knee. Cf. *valgus.*

**vas** (vas) pl. *va′sa* [L.] [TA] vessel: a general term in anatomical nomenclature for a canal for carrying fluid, especially those carrying blood, lymph, or spermatozoa.

**v. aber′rans,** 1. ductulus aberrans superior 2. any anomalous or unusual vessel.

**v. aber′rans of Roth,** see *ductuli aberrantes.*

**va′sa aberran′tis he′patis,** numerous vessels found in the inconstant fibrous appendix and in the capsule of the liver.

**va′sa afferen′tia,** vessels that convey fluid to a structure or part.

**v. af′ferens glome′ruli,** arteriola glomerularis afferens.

**va′sa afferen′tia lymphoglan′dulae,** vasa afferentia nodi lymphatici.

**va′sa afferen′tia no′di lympha′tici,** afferent vessels of lymph node: lymphatic vessels that carry lymph to a lymph node, entering through the capsule.

**v. anastomo′ticum** [TA], anastomotic vessel: a vessel that serves to interconnect other vessels; such communications are present in the palm of the hand, sole of the foot, base of the brain, and other regions.

**va′sa au′ris inter′nae,** vasa sanguinea auris internae.

**va′sa bre′via,** arteriae gastricae breves.

**v. capilla′re** [TA], capillary.

**v. collatera′le** [TA], collateral vessel: a vessel that parallels another vessel, nerve, or other structure.

**v. de′ferens,** ductus deferens.

**va′sa efferen′tia,** efferent vessels: vessels that convey fluid away from a structure or part; see *vasa efferentia nodi lymphatici* and *ductuli efferentes testis.*

**v. ef′ferens glome′ruli,** arteriola glomerularis efferens.

**va′sa efferen′tia lymphoglan′dulae,** vasa efferentia nodi lymphatici.

**va′sa efferen′tia no′di lympha′tici,** efferent vessels of lymph node: lymphatic vessels that carry lymph away from a lymph node, emerging at the hilus.

**v. epididy′midis,** ductus epididymidis.

**va′sa lympha′tica** [TA], lymphatic vessels: collectively, the lymphocapillary vessels, collecting vessels, and trunks which collect lymph from the tissues and through which the lymph passes to reach the bloodstream.

**v. lympha′ticum profun′dum** [TA], deep lymphatic vessel: any lymphatic vessel that drains lymph from deep body structures; deep lymphatic vessels accompany the deeply placed blood vessels.

**v. lympha′ticum superficia′le** [TA], superficial lymphatic vessel: any lymphatic vessel located under the skin and superficial fascia, in the submucous areolar tissue of the digestive, respiratory, and genitourinary tracts, and in the subserous tissue of the walls of the abdomen and thorax.

**v. lymphocapilla′re** [TA], lymphocapillary vessel: one of the minute vessels of the lymphatic system, having a caliber greater than a blood capillary; they form closed networks (sing. *rete lymphocapillare*) by which they communicate freely with one another.

**va′sa nervo′rum** [TA], blood vessels supplying the nerves.

**va′sa prae′via,** presentation, in front of the fetal head during labor, of the blood vessels of the umbilical cord where they enter the placenta.

**v. pro′minens duc′tus cochlea′ris** [TA], a small vessel often seen deep to the spiral prominence in the cochlear duct.

**vasa propria of Jungbluth,** vessels situated beneath the amnion of the early embryo.

**va′sa rec′ta re′nis,** TA alternative for *arteriolae rectae renis.*

**va′sa sangui′nea au′ris inter′nae** [TA], the blood vessels of the inner ear; called also *vasa auris internae.*

**va′sa sangui′nea re′tinae** [TA], the blood vessels of the retina, including all the arterioles, derived from the central artery of the retina, and the venules, which return blood to the central vein.

**v. sinusoi′deum** [TA], sinusoid: a form of terminal blood channel consisting of a large, irregular anastomosing vessel, having a lining of reticuloendothelium but little or no adventitia; sinusoids are found in the liver, adrenals, heart, parathyroid, carotid gland, spleen, hemolymph glands, and pancreas. Those in the anterior pituitary gland, adrenal cortex, and islets of Langerhans have a continuous basal lamina and a thin endothelium penetrated by pores closed by thin diaphragms *(fenestrated sinusoids);* in many mammals the endothelial cells lining those of the liver meet and overlap in some areas, while there are gaps between the cells in other areas *(discontinuous sinusoids).* Called also *sinusoidal capillary.*

**v. spira′le** [TA], a prominent vessel in the basilar membrane near the osseous spiral lamina.

**va′sa vaso′rum** [TA], the small nutrient arteries and the veins in the walls of the larger blood vessels.

**va′sa vortico′sa,** venae vorticosae.

**va•sa** (va′sə) [L.] plural of *vas.*

**Vas•al** (vas′əl) trademark for a preparation of papaverine hydrochloride.

**va•sal** (va′səl) 1. pertaining to a vas. 2. vascular.

**va•sal•gia** (və-sal′jə) angialgia.

**va•sa•li•um** (və-sa′le-əm) true vascular tissue, such as is found in closed or vascular organs.

**Vas•co•ray** (vas′ko-ra) trademark for a preparation of iothalamate meglumine and iothalamate sodium.

**vas•cu•lar** (vas′ku-lər) 1. pertaining to vessels, particularly blood vessels; called also *vasal.* 2. having a copious blood supply.

**vas•cu•lar•i•ty** (vas″ku-lar′ĭ-te) the condition of being vascular.

**vas•cu•lar•iza•tion** (vas″ku-lər-ĭ-za′shən) 1. the process of becoming vascular. 2. angiogenesis. 3. the surgically induced development of vessels in a tissue.

**vas•cu•lar•ize** (vas′ku-lər-īz) to supply with vessels.

**vas•cu•la•ture** (vas′ku-lə-chər) 1. circulatory system. 2. any specific part of the circulatory system.

**vas•cu•lit•ic** (vas″ku-lit′ik) pertaining to vasculitis.

**vas•cu•li•tis** (vas″ku-li′tis) [*vasculum* + *-itis*] [MeSH: Vasculitis] inflammation of a blood or lymph vessel; see *arteritis, lymphangitis,* and *phlebitis.* Called also *angiitis.*
**allergic v.,** hypersensitivity v.
**Churg-Strauss v.,** see under *syndrome.*
**consecutive v.,** vasculitis caused by extension of the inflammation from the neighboring tissues.
**granulomatous v. of central nervous system, granulomatous cerebral v.,** isolated v. of central nervous system.
**hypersensitivity v.,** a group of systemic necrotizing vasculitides thought to represent hypersensitivity to an antigenic stimulus, such as a drug, infectious agent, or exogenous or endogenous protein; all disorders in this group involve the small vessels. Types include varieties of Schönlein-Henoch purpura and serum sickness, as well as urticarial v. Called also *allergic* or *leukocytoclastic v.* and *hypersensitivity* or *leukocytoclastic angiitis.*
**hypocomplementemic v.,** hypersensitivity vasculitis accompanied by hypocomplementemia.
**isolated v. of central nervous system,** an idiopathic vasculitis affecting small and medium-sized intracranial vessels, marked by headache, progressive intellectual deterioration, and recurrent cerebral infarcts; some show segmental markings of small arteries on an angiogram, and some have evidence of pleocytosis and elevated protein in the cerebrospinal fluid. Called also *granulomatous v. of central nervous system, granulomatous cerebral v.,* and *isolated angiitis of central nervous system.*
**leukocytoclastic v.,** hypersensitivity v.
**livedo v.,** segmented hyalinizing v.
**necrotizing v.,** see *systemic necrotizing v.*
**nodular v.,** a chronic vasculitis of the lower legs, usually seen in young or middle-aged women, with an unknown etiology; characteristics include painful, reddish blue nodular lesions that may ulcerate, leaving scars, or resorb, leaving atrophic depressions. In the late stages, the subcutaneous fat is replaced by fibrosis and atrophy. See also *erythema induratum.*
**overlap v.,** polyangiitis overlap syndrome.
**pulmonary v.,** any of numerous inflammatory conditions of the walls of the pulmonary vessels; the most common ones are allergic granulomatous angiitis and Wegener's granulomatosis.
**rheumatoid v.,** systemic vasculitis associated with rheumatoid arthritis, affecting small and medium-sized vessels, and generally occurring in patients with long-standing disease, rheumatoid nodules, and a high titer of rheumatoid factor.
**segmented hyalinizing v.,** a chronic relapsing vasculitis of the lower legs, usually affecting middle-aged persons; lesions are nodular or purpuric at the onset and later become superficially ulcerated, resulting in scars; histologically, endothelial proliferations, hyaline degeneration, and thrombosis are seen in the mid and lower dermis. Called also *livedo v.*
**systemic v., systemic necrotizing v.,** any of a group of disorders characterized by inflammation and necrosis of blood vessels, occurring in a broad spectrum of cutaneous and systemic disorders. It includes Churg-Strauss syndrome, polyarteritis nodosa, polyangiitis overlap syndrome, the various kinds of hypersensitivity vasculitis, and other conditions. Called also *necrotizing v.* or *angiitis.*
**urticarial v.,** a type of hypersensitivity vasculitis in which urticaria lasts more than 24 hours, often with systemic symptoms such as arthralgias, arthritis, nephritis, and abdominal pain; many patients also have hypocomplementemia *(hypocomplementemic vasculitis).* The condition may be idiopathic or secondary to a disorder such as systemic lupus erythematosus or Sjögren's syndrome.

**vas•cu•lo•gen•e•sis** (vas″ku-lo-jen′ə-sis) [*vasculum* + *-genesis*] angiogenesis.

**vas•cu•lo•gen•ic** (vas″ku-lo-jen′ik) angiogenic (def. 1).

**vas•cu•lo•lym•phat•ic** (vas″ku-lo-lim-fat′ik) pertaining to blood or lymph vessels.

**vas•cu•lo•mo•tor** (vas″ku-lo-mo′tor) vasomotor.

**vas•cu•lop•a•thy** (vas″ku-lop′ə-the) any disorder of blood vessels.

**vas•cu•lo•tox•ic** (vas″ku-lo-tok′sik) pertaining to or characterized by a deleterious or toxic effect on the vessels of the body.

**vas•cu•lum** (vas′ku-ləm) [L., dim. of *vas*] a small vessel.
**v. aber′rans,** vas aberrans.

**va•sec•to•mized** (və-sek′tə-mīzd) having undergone removal of the ductus deferentes (vasa deferentia) by surgical means.

**va•sec•to•my** (və-sek′tə-me) [*vas* + *-ectomy*] [MeSH: Vasectomy] surgical removal of the ductus (vas) deferens, or of a portion of it; done to induce infertility or in association with prostatectomy. Called also *vasoresection* and *vasosection.*
**cross-over v.,** vasectomy in which the right and the left vas deferens are transected, the lower portion of each (the portions still attached to the epididymis) then being tied together. The technique prevents recanalization while allowing surgical reconstruction.

**Va•se•ret•ic** (vas-ə-ret′ik) trademark for a preparation of enalapril maleate and hydrochlorothiazide.

**vas•i•fac•tive** (vas″ĭ-fak′tiv) [*vas* + L. *facere* to make] angiogenic (def. 1).

**vas•i•form** (vas′ĭ-form) [*vas* + *form*] having the appearance of a vessel.

**va•si•tis** (və-si′tis) deferentitis.

**vas(o)-** [L. *vas,* q.v.] a combining form denoting relationship to a vessel or to a duct.

**vaso•ac•tive** (vas″o-, va″zo-ak′tiv) said of a chemical that exerts an effect upon the caliber of blood vessels.

**vaso•con•stric•tion** (vas″o-, va″zo-kən-strik′shən) [MeSH: Vasoconstriction] the diminution of the caliber of vessels, especially constriction of arterioles leading to decreased blood flow to a part.

**vaso•con•stric•tive** (vas″o-, va″zo-kən-strik′tiv) pertaining to, characterized by, or producing vasoconstriction.

**vaso•con•stric•tor** (vas″o-, va″zo-kən-strik′tər) 1. causing constriction of the blood vessels. 2. a motor nerve or chemical compound that causes constriction of the blood vessels.

**vaso•de•pres•sion** (vas″o, va″zo-de-presh′ən) decrease in vascular resistance with hypotension.

**vaso•de•pres•sor** (vas″o-, va″zo-de-pres′ər) 1. having the effect of lowering the blood pressure through reduction in peripheral resistance. 2. an agent that causes vasodepression.

**Va•so•di•lan** (va″zo-di′lan) trademark for preparations of isoxsuprine hydrochloride.

**vaso•di•la•ta•tion** (vas″o-, va″zo-dĭ-lə-ta′shən) vasodilation.

**vaso•di•la•tion** (vas″o-, va″zo-di-la′shən) [MeSH: Vasodilation] dilation of a vessel, especially dilation of arterioles leading to increased blood flow to a part; extreme, abnormal vasodilation is called *angiectasis.* Called also *vasodilatation.*
**reflex v.,** vasodilation occurring as a reflex response to stimuli applied elsewhere, or subsequent to an initial vasoconstrictive response.

**vaso•di•la•tive** (vas″o-, va″zo-di-la′tiv) pertaining to, characterized by, or producing vasodilatation.

**vaso•di•la•tor** (vas″o-, va″zo-di′la-tər) 1. causing dilation of the blood vessels. 2. a motor nerve or chemical compound that causes dilation of the blood vessels.

**vaso•epi•did•y•mog•ra•phy** (vas″o-, va″zo-ep″ĭ-did″ĭ-mog′rə-fe) radiography of the vas deferens and epididymis after injection of a contrast medium.

**vaso•epi•did•y•mos•to•my** (vas″o-, va″zo-ep″ĭ-did-ĭ-mos′tə-me) operative formation of a communication between the ductus (vas) deferens and the epididymis.

**vaso•fac•tive** (vas″o-, va″zo-fak′tiv) angiogenic (def. 1).

**vaso•for•ma•tive** (vas″o-, va″zo-for′mə-tiv) angiogenic (def. 1).

**vaso•gan•gli•on** (vas″o-, va″zo-gang′gle-on) any vascular ganglion or rete.

**va•sog•ra•phy** (va-zog′rə-fe) [*vaso-* + *-graphy*] angiography.

**vaso•hy•per•ton•ic** (vas″o-, va″zo-hi″pər-ton′ik) vasoconstrictor (def. 1).

**vaso•hy•po•ton•ic** (vas″o-, va″zo-hi″po-ton′ik) vasodilator (def. 1).

**vaso•in•ert** (vas″o-, va″zo-in-ərt′) exerting no effect on the caliber of blood vessels.

**vaso•in•hib•i•tor** (vas″o-, va″zo-in-hib′ĭ-tər) an agent that inhibits the action of the vasomotor nerves.

**va·so·in·hib·i·to·ry** (vas″o-, va″zo-in-hib′ĭ-tor-e) hindering the action of the vasomotor nerves.

**va·so·li·ga·tion** (vas″o-, va″zo-lĭ-ga′shən) ligation of the ductus (vas) deferens.

**va·so·mo·tion** (vas″o-, va″zo-mo′shən) [*vaso-* + *motion*] change in the caliber of a vessel, especially of a blood vessel.

**va·so·mo·tor** (vas″o-, va″zo-mo′tər) [*vaso-* + *motor*] affecting the caliber of a vessel, especially of a blood vessel. Cf. *vasoactive.*

**va·so·mo·tor·ic·i·ty** (vas″o-, va″zo-mo-tər-is′ĭ-te) the power of producing change in the caliber of blood vessels.

**va·so·neu·rop·a·thy** (vas″o-, va″zo-noo-rop′ə-the) a combined vascular and neurologic defect, the lesions being caused by simultaneous action of both the vascular and the nervous systems, or by the interaction of the two systems. See also *angiopathic neuropathy* and *angioneuropathy* (def. 2).

**va·so·neu·ro·sis** (vas″o-, va″zo-noo-ro′sis) angioneuropathy.

**va·so·or·chid·os·to·my** (vas″o-, va″zo-or″kid-os′tə-me) the operation of suturing tubules of the epididymis to the ductus (vas) deferens.

**va·so·pa·re·sis** (vas″o-, va″zo-pə-re′sis) [*vaso-* + *paresis*] partial vasomotor paralysis (q.v.); called also *angioparesis.*

**va·so·per·me·a·bil·i·ty** (vas″o-, va″zo-pər″me-ə-bil′ĭ-te) the permeability of a blood vessel; the extent to which a blood vessel is permeable.

**va·so·pres·sin** (vas″o-, va″zo-pres′in) 1. one of two nonapeptide hormones (the other being oxytocin) that are formed by neuronal cells of hypothalamic nuclei and stored in the neurohypophysis. It stimulates contraction of muscles of capillaries and arterioles, raising blood pressure; promotes contraction of the intestinal musculature, increasing peristalsis; exerts contractile influence on the uterus; and has a specific effect on the epithelial cells of renal collecting tubules, augmenting resorption of water independently of solutes to cause concentration of urine and dilution of blood serum. Its rate of secretion is regulated chiefly by the osmolarity of the plasma. 2. [USP] a pharmaceutical preparation of the same principle, prepared from the neurohypophyses of domesticated food animals or produced synthetically; used mainly as an antidiuretic in treatment of diabetes insipidus, administered intranasally or by injection. It is also used to induce vasoconstriction to treat hemorrhage or administered intramuscularly as a test of hypothalamo-neurohypophysial-renal function in distinguishing central from nephrogenic diabetes insipidus. Called also *antidiuretic hormone.*
**arginine v. (AVP),** vasopressin containing arginine, as that from humans and most other mammals; for medicinal uses, see *vasopressin* (def. 2). Called also *argipressin.*
**lysine v.,** the antidiuretic hormone of the pig family, differing from arginine vasopressin in having lysine instead of arginine at position 8. Both natural and synthetic preparations are used as antidiuretics and vasoconstrictors to treat central diabetes insipidus when desmopressin acetate is too potent; administered by intranasal spray. Called also *lypressin.*
**v. tannate,** the water-insoluble tannate salt of vasopressin, having the same actions and uses as the base; administered intramuscularly in an oil suspension.

**va·so·pres·sor** (vas″o-, va″zo-pres′ər) 1. stimulating contraction of the muscular tissue of the capillaries and arteries. 2. an agent that stimulates contraction of the muscular tissue of the capillaries and arteries.

**va·so·punc·ture** (vas″o-, va″zo-punk′chər) puncture of the ductus (vas) deferens.

**va·so·re·flex** (vas″o-, va″zo-re′fleks) a reflex involving a blood vessel.

**va·so·re·lax·a·tion** (vas″o-, va″zo-re-lak-sa′shən) decrease of vascular pressure.

**va·so·re·sec·tion** (vas″o-, va″zo-re-sek′shən) vasectomy.

**vas·or·rha·phy** (vas-or′ə-fe) suture of the ductus (vas) deferens.

**va·so·sec·tion** (vas″o-, va″zo-sek′shən) [*vaso-* + *section*] 1. the severing of a vessel or vessels. 2. vasectomy.

**va·so·sen·so·ry** (vas″o-, va″zo-sen′sər-e) supplying sensory filaments to the vessels.

**va·so·spasm** (vas′o-, va′zo-spaz-əm) spasm of the blood vessels, resulting in vasoconstriction. Called also *angiospasm.*

**va·so·spas·mo·lyt·ic** (vas″o-, va″zo-spaz″mo-lit′ik) arresting spasm of the vessels.

**va·so·spas·tic** (vas″o-, va″zo-spas′tik) producing or affected by vasospasm.

**va·so·stim·u·lant** (vas″o-, va″zo-stim′u-lənt) vasotonic.

**va·sos·to·my** (vas-os′, va-zos′tə-me) [*vas* deferens + *-stomy*] the operation of forming an opening into the ductus (vas) deferens.

**Va·so·tec** (vas′o-tek) trademark for a preparation of enalapril maleate.

**va·so·to·cin** (vas″o-, va″zo-to′sin) [MeSH: Vasotocin] a nonapeptide hormone having some properties similar to those of vasopressin and oxytocin, made in the supraoptico-neurohypophysial unit of birds, reptiles, amphibians, and fishes. It is found in the pituitary gland and hypothalamus of the human fetus but amounts in humans after birth are minute to indetectable.

**va·sot·o·my** (va-zot′ə-me) [*vaso-* + *-tomy*] incision into or cutting of the ductus (vas) deferens.

**va·so·to·nia** (vas″o-, va″zo-to′ne-ə) [*vaso-* + *ton-* + *-ia*] tone or tension of the vessels; called also *angiotonia.*

**va·so·ton·ic** (vas″o-, va″zo-ton′ik) pertaining to, characterized by, or promoting vasotonia. Called also *angiotonic* and *vasostimulant.*

**va·so·tribe** (vas″o-, va′zo-trīb) angiotribe.

**va·so·trip·sy** (vas″o-, va″zo-trip′se) angiotripsy.

**va·so·troph·ic** (vas″o-, va″zo-trof′ik) [*vaso-* + *-trophic*] pertaining to the nutrition of blood vessels.

**va·so·trop·ic** (vas″o-, va″zo-trop′ik) tending to act on blood vessels.

**va·so·va·gal** (vas″o-, va″zo-va′gəl) vascular and vagal; see *vasovagal attack,* under *attack.*

**va·so·va·sos·to·my** (vas″o-, va″zo-va-zos′tə-me) [MeSH: Vasovasostomy] anastomosis of the ends of the severed ductus (vas) deferens; done to restore fertility in vasectomized males.

**va·so·ve·sic·u·lec·to·my** (vas″o-, va″zo-və-sik″u-lek′tə-me) excision of the ductus (vas) deferens and seminal vesicles.

**va·so·ve·sic·u·li·tis** (vas″o-, va″zo-və-sik″u-li′tis) inflammation of the ductus deferentes (vasa deferentia) and seminal vesicles.

**Vas·ox·yl** (va-zok′səl) trademark for preparations of methoxamine hydrochloride.

**vas·tus** (vas′təs) [L.] great or vast; description of muscles, as musculus vastus lateralis.

**VATER** acronym for *v*ertebral defects, imperforate *a*nus, *t*racheoesophageal fistula, and *r*adial and *r*enal dysplasia; see under *complex.*

**Va·ter's ampulla, corpuscles,** etc. (fah′terz) [Abraham *Vater,* German anatomist, 1684–1751] see under *fold* and see *ampulla hepatopancreatica, corpusculum lamellosum, ductus thyroglossalis,* and *papilla duodeni major.*

**Va·ter-Pa·ci·ni corpuscles** (fah′ter-pa-che′ne) [Abraham *Vater;* Filippo *Pacini,* Italian anatomist, 1812–1883] corpusculum lamellosum.

**vault** (vawlt) 1. any arched or domelike structure. See also *fornix.* 2. the longest palatal border obtainable through a coronal section of the maxilla. 3. a cavity or a prepared area within a bone for an implant.
**cranial v.,** calvaria.

**VC** vital capacity.

**VCG** vectorcardiogram.

**V-Cil·lin** (ve-sil′in) trademark for preparations of penicillin V.

**VCU** voiding cystourethrography.

**VCUG** voiding cystourethrogram.

**VD** venereal disease; see also *sexually transmitted disease,* under *disease.*

**VDEL** Venereal Disease Experimental Laboratory.

**VDH** valvular disease of the heart.

**VDRL** Venereal Disease Research Laboratories; see also under *antigen* and *test.*

**vec·tion** (vek′shən) [L. *vectio* a carrying] the carrying of disease germs from an infected person to a well person. It is *circumferential, indirect,* or *mediate* when pathogens are carried by an intermediate host; *direct, immediate,* and *radial* when transferred directly from one person to another.

**vec·tor** (vek′tər) [L. "one who carries," from *vehere* to carry] 1. a carrier, especially the animal (usually an arthropod) that transfers an infective agent from one host to another. 2. a plasmid or viral chromosome into whose genome a fragment of foreign DNA is inserted, used to introduce the foreign DNA into a host cell in the cloning of DNA. 3. a quantity possessing magnitude and direction and commonly represented by a straight line resembling an arrow: the length of the line denotes magnitude and the arrowhead and the position of the line with respect to an axis of reference denote

direction. 4. in mathematics, an ordered set of values. For example, the vector $x$ denotes the ordered set $(x_1, x_2, \ldots. x_n)$.
**biological v.,** an animal vector in whose body the pathogenic organism develops and multiplies before being transmitted to the next host.
**cloning v.,** a plasmid or viral chromosome so constructed that it will accept insertion of a foreign DNA fragment while retaining the ability to replicate.
**mechanical v.,** an animal vector not essential to the life cycle of the parasite.
**recombinant v.,** a vector into which a foreign DNA fragment has been inserted.
**shuttle v.,** in molecular biology, a plasmid capable of replicating in both bacteria and mammalian cells; used for mutation and transfer of specific segments of DNA among various hosts.
**spatial v.,** one representing a three-dimensional force; see *vectorcardiography*.

**vec·tor-borne** (vek'tər-born") spread or transmitted from one host to another by a vector, as an infectious disease.

**vec·tor·car·dio·gram (VCG)** (vek"tər-kahr'de-o-gram") the record, usually a photograph, of the loop formed on the oscilloscope in vectorcardiography, the inscribed loop representing the ends of the instantaneous vectors.

**vec·tor·car·dio·graph** (vek"tər-kahr'de-o-graf) the instrument used in vectorcardiography.

**vec·tor·car·di·og·ra·phy** (vek"tər-kahr"de-og'rə-fe) [MeSH: Vectorcardiography] the registration, usually by formation of a loop display on an oscilloscope, of the direction and magnitude (vector) of the moment-to-moment electromotive forces of the heart during one complete cycle, as transmitted by electrocardiographic leads.
**spatial v.,** that in which the potential vectors of cardiac excitation are projected upon three mutually perpendicular coordinates, usually designated X, Y, and Z, where X is the transverse (right or left), Y the vertical (up or down), and Z the sagittal (anterior or posterior). See also *orthogonal lead system*, under *system*.

**vec·to·ri·al** (vek-tor'e-əl) pertaining to a vector.

**Vec·trin** (vek'trin) trademark for preparations of minocycline hydrochloride.

**vec·u·ro·ni·um bro·mide** (vek"u-ro'ne-əm) [MeSH: Vecuronium Bromide] a nondepolarizing neuromuscular blocking agent, used as an adjunct to general anesthesia to induce relaxation of skeletal muscle and to facilitate endotracheal intubation and mechanical ventilation; administered intravenously.

**VEE** Venezuelan equine encephalomyelitis.

**Vee·tids** (ve'tidz) trademark for a preparation of penicillin V potassium.

**veg·an** (vej'ən, ve'gən) an extreme vegetarian who excludes all food of animal origin from the diet.

**veg·a·nism** (vej'ə-niz-əm) strict limitation to a vegetable diet, with exclusion of all food of animal origin.

**veg·e·ta·ble** (vej'ə-tə-bəl) [L. *vegetabilis* quickening] [MeSH: Vegetables] 1. pertaining to or derived from plants. 2. any plant or species of plant, especially one cultivated as a source of food.

**veg·e·tal** (vej'ə-təl) 1. pertaining to plants or to a plant. 2. vegetative.

**veg·e·tal·i·ty** (vej"ə-tal'ĭ-te) the aggregate of phenomena that are common to plants.

**veg·e·tar·i·an** (vej"ə-tər'e-ən) one who practices vegetarianism.

**veg·e·tar·i·an·ism** (vej"ə-tər'e-ə-niz"əm) [MeSH: Vegetarianism] restriction of the diet to disallow some or all foods of animal origin, consuming mainly or wholly foods of plant origin. See also *lacto-vegetarianism, ovolactovegetarianism, ovovegetarianism,* and *veganism*.

**veg·e·ta·tion** (vej"ə-ta'shən) [L. *vegetatio*] any plantlike fungoid neoplasm or growth; a luxuriant fungus-like growth of pathologic tissue.
**bacterial v's,** irregular excrescences on the cardiac valves or endocardium that are formed by bacteria.
**dendritic v.,** 1. the shaggy appearance of a villous cancer. 2. the arachnoidal tufts and villous neoplasms on the pleura and other serous membranes.
**marantic v's,** small, sterile, verrucous, fibrinous excrescences occurring in the left-side heart valves in nonbacterial thrombotic (marantic) endocarditis.
**verrucous v's,** small irregular fibrinous excrescences usually occurring along the line of closure of the cardiac valve cusps, sometimes extending into the mural endocardium or chordae tendineae, and rarely also present on the left ventricular papillary muscles.

**veg·e·ta·tive** (vej'ə-ta"tiv) 1. concerned with growth and with nutrition. 2. functioning involuntarily or unconsciously, as the vegetative nervous system; see under *system*. 3. resting; denoting the portion of a cell cycle during which the cell is not involved in replication. 4. of, pertaining to, or characteristic of plants. 5. of or pertaining to asexual reproduction, as by budding or fission.

**veg·e·to·an·i·mal** (vej"ə-to-an'ĭ-məl) common to plants and animals.

**ve·hi·cle** (ve'ĭ-kəl) [L. *vehiculum*] excipient.

**veil** (vāl) 1. a covering structure; see *velum*. 2. caul.
**Fick's v.,** see under *phenomenon*.
**Jackson's v.,** see under *membrane*.
**Sattler's v.,** Fick's phenomenon.

**Veil·lon tube** (va-yaw') [Adrien *Veillon,* Paris bacteriologist, 1864–1931] see under *tube*.

**Veil·lon·el·la** (va"on-el'ə) [Adrien *Veillon*] [MeSH: Veillonella] a genus of bacteria of the family Veillonellaceae made up of small, gram-negative, anaerobic cocci occurring in pairs or short chains. They are found as nonpathogenic parasites in the mouth and intestines of humans and animals. The type species is *V. par'vula*.

**Veil·lon·el·la·ceae** (va"on-əl-a'se-e) [MeSH: Veillonellaceae] a family of gram-negative, anaerobic, coccoid bacteria occurring in pairs and short chains. They are asporogenous nonmotile organisms found in the alimentary tract of humans, ruminants, rodents, and pigs. The family includes the genera *Acidaminococcus, Megasphaera,* and *Veillonella;* only *Veillonella* is of medical importance.

**vein** (vān) [L. *vena*] [MeSH: Veins] a vessel through which blood passes from various organs or parts back to the heart; all veins except the pulmonary veins carry blood low in oxygen. Like arteries, veins have three coats, an *inner, middle,* and *outer,* but the coats are not so thick, and they collapse when the vessel is cut. Many veins have *valves* formed of reduplications of their lining membrane, which prevent the backward flow of blood away from the heart. Called also *vena* [TA].

## Vein

For descriptions of specific veins, see under *vena*.

**accompanying v.,** vena comitans.
**accompanying v. of hypoglossal nerve,** vena comitans nervi hypoglossi.
**afferent v's,** veins that carry blood to an organ.
**allantoic v's,** paired vessels that accompany the allantois, growing out from the primitive hindgut and entering the connecting stalk of the early embryo; they fuse later into one vessel, the umbilical vein.
**anastomotic v., inferior,** vena anastomotica inferior.
**anastomotic v., superior,** vena anastomotica superior.
**angular v.,** vena angularis.
**antebrachial v., median,** vena mediana antebrachii.
**anterior v's of heart,** venae ventriculi dextri anteriores.
**anterior v's of right ventricle,** venae ventriculi dextri anteriores.
**appendicular v.,** vena appendicularis.
**v. of aqueduct of cochlea,** vena aqueductus cochleae.
**v. of aqueduct of vestibule,** vena aqueductus vestibuli.
**aqueous v's,** microscopic, blood vessel–like pathways on the surface of the eye, containing aqueous humor or diluted blood and connecting the sinus venosus sclerae (Schlemm's canal) with conjunctival or subconjunctival veins.
**arciform v's, arcuate v's of kidney,** venae arcuatae renis.
**arterial v.,** truncus pulmonalis.
**articular v's,** venae articulares.
**atrial v's of heart, left,** venae atriales sinistrae.
**atrial v's of heart, right,** venae atriales dextrae.
**atrioventricular v's of heart,** venae atrioventriculares cordis.
**auditory v's, internal,** venae labyrinthi.
**auricular v's, anterior,** venae auriculares anteriores.
**auricular v., posterior,** vena auricularis posterior.
**axillary v.,** vena axillaris.

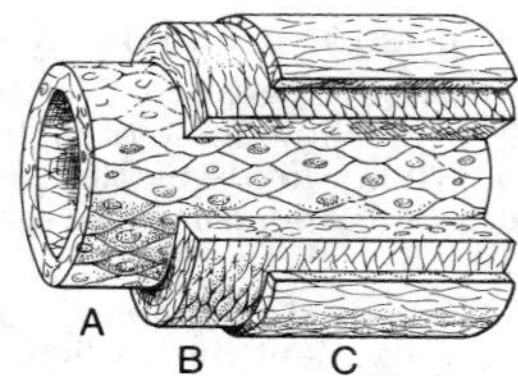


The three coats of a vein: *(A)*, tunica intima (endothelium); *(B)*, tunica media; *(C)*, tunica externa.

**azygos v.,** vena azygos.
**azygos v., left,** vena hemiazygos.
**basal v.,** 1. vena basalis. 2. see *vena basalis communis, vena basalis inferior,* and *vena basalis superior.*
**basal v., anterior,** vena basalis anterior.
**basal v., common,** vena basalis communis.
**basal v., inferior,** vena basalis inferior.
**basal v., superior,** vena basalis superior.
**basilic v.,** vena basilica.
**basilic v., intermediate,** vena intermedia basilica.
**basivertebral v's,** venae basivertebrales.
**brachial v's,** venae brachiales.
**brachiocephalic v.,** vena brachiocephalica.
**Breschet's v's,** venae diploicae.
**bronchial v's,** venae bronchiales.
**Browning's v.,** vena anastomotica inferior.
**v. of bulb of penis,** vena bulbi penis.
**v. of bulb of vestibule,** vena bulbi vestibuli.
**Burow's v.,** an inconstant vessel formed by the two inferior epigastric veins and a branch from the bladder; it joins the portal vein.
**v. of canaliculus of cochlea,** vena aqueductus cochleae.
**cardiac v's,** venae cordis.
**cardiac v's, anterior,** venae ventriculi dextri anteriores.
**cardiac v., great,** vena cardiaca magna.
**cardiac v., middle,** vena cardiaca media.
**cardiac v., small,** vena cardiaca parva.
**cardiac v's, smallest,** venae cardiacae minimae.
**cardinal v's,** embryonic vessels that include the precardinal, postcardinal, and common cardinal veins.
**cardinal v's, anterior,** precardinal v's.
**cardinal v's, common,** two short venous trunks in the embryo that open into the primordial atrium of the heart; the right one combines with the anterior cardinal vein to become the superior vena cava; called also *ducts* or *sinuses of Cuvier.*
**cardinal v's, posterior,** postcardinal v's.
**v's of caudate nucleus,** venae nuclei caudati.
**cavernous v's of penis,** venae cavernosae penis.
**central v.,** a vein that occupies the axis of an organ.
**central v's of hepatic lobules, central v's of liver,** venae centrales hepatis.
**central v. of retina,** vena centralis retinae.
**central v. of suprarenal gland,** vena centralis glandulae suprarenalis.
**cephalic v.,** vena cephalica.
**cephalic v., accessory,** vena cephalica accessoria.
**cephalic v., median,** vena intermedia cephalica.
**cerebellar v's,** venae cerebelli.
**cerebellar v's, inferior,** see *venae cerebelli.*
**cerebellar v's, superior,** see *venae cerebelli.*
**cerebral v's,** venae encephali.
**cerebral v's, anterior,** venae anteriores cerebri.
**cerebral v's, deep,** venae profundae cerebri.
**cerebral v., deep middle,** vena media profunda cerebri.
**cerebral v., great,** vena magna cerebri.
**cerebral v's, inferior,** venae inferiores cerebri.
**cerebral v's, internal,** venae internae cerebri.
**cerebral v's, superficial,** venae superficiales cerebri.
**cerebral v's, superficial middle,** vena media superficialis cerebri.
**cerebral v's, superior,** venae superiores cerebri.
**cervical v., deep,** vena cervicalis profunda.
**cervical v's, transverse,** venae transversae cervicis.
**choroid v., inferior,** vena choroidea inferior.
**choroid v., superior,** vena choroidea superior.
**ciliary v's,** venae ciliares.
**ciliary v's, anterior,** see *venae ciliares.*
**ciliary v's, posterior,** 1. see *venae ciliares.* 2. venae vorticosae.
**circumflex femoral v's, lateral,** venae circumflexae femoris laterales.
**circumflex femoral v's, medial,** venae circumflexae femoris mediales.
**circumflex iliac v., deep,** vena circumflexa ilium profunda.
**circumflex iliac v., superficial,** vena circumflexa ilium superficialis.
**v. of cochlear canaliculus,** vena aqueductus cochleae.
**colic v., intermediate,** vena colica media.
**colic v., left,** vena colica sinistra.
**colic v., middle,** vena colica media.
**colic v., right,** vena colica dextra.
**communicating v's,** 1. venae perforantes. 2. perforating v's (def. 2).
**conjunctival v's,** venae conjunctivales.
**coronary v., left,** vena coronaria sinistra.
**coronary v., right,** vena coronaria dextra.
**v. of corpus callosum, dorsal,** vena dorsalis corporis callosi.
**v. of corpus callosum, posterior,** vena posterior corporis callosi.
**costoaxillary v's,** venae costoaxillares.
**cubital v., median,** vena mediana cubiti.
**cutaneous v.,** vena cutanea.
**cystic v.,** vena cystica.
**deep v.,** vena profunda.
**deep v's of clitoris,** venae profundae clitoridis.
**deep v's of lower limb,** venae profundae membri inferioris.
**deep v's of penis,** venae profundae penis.
**deep v. of thigh,** vena profunda femoris.
**deep v. of tongue,** vena profunda linguae.
**deep v's of upper limb,** venae profundae membri superioris.
**digital v's, palmar,** venae digitales palmares.
**digital v's, plantar,** venae digitales plantares.
**digital v's of foot, common,** venae digitales communes pedis.
**digital v's of foot, dorsal,** venae digitales dorsales pedis.
**diploic v's,** venae diploicae.
**diploic v., anterior temporal,** vena diploica temporalis anterior.
**diploic v., frontal,** vena diploica frontalis.
**diploic v., occipital,** vena diploica occipitalis.
**diploic v., posterior temporal,** vena diploica temporalis posterior.
**dorsal v. of clitoris, deep,** vena dorsalis profunda clitoridis.
**dorsal v's of clitoris, superficial,** venae dorsales superficiales clitoridis.
**dorsal v. of penis, deep,** vena dorsalis profunda penis.
**dorsal v's of penis, superficial,** venae dorsales superficiales penis.
**dorsal v's of tongue,** venae dorsales linguae.
**emissary v.,** vena emissaria.
**emissary v., condylar,** vena emissaria condylaris.
**emissary v., mastoid,** vena emissaria mastoidea.
**emissary v., occipital,** vena emissaria occipitalis.
**emissary v., parietal,** vena emissaria parietalis.
**v's of encephalic trunk,** venae trunci encephalici.
**epigastric v., inferior,** vena epigastrica inferior.
**epigastric v., superficial,** vena epigastrica superficialis.
**epigastric v's, superior,** venae epigastricae superiores.
**epiploic v., left,** vena gastroomentalis sinistra.
**epiploic v., right,** vena gastroomentalis dextra.
**episcleral v's,** venae episclerales.
**esophageal v's,** venae oesophageales.
**ethmoidal v's,** venae ethmoidales.
**facial v.,** vena facialis.
**facial v., anterior,** see *vena facialis.*
**facial v., common,** see *vena facialis.*
**facial v., deep,** vena profunda faciei.
**facial v., posterior,** vena retromandibularis.
**facial v., transverse,** vena transversa faciei.
**femoral v.,** vena femoralis.
**femoral v., deep,** vena profunda femoris.
**femoropopliteal v.,** vena femoropoplitea.
**fibular v's,** venae fibulares.
**frontal v's,** 1. venae frontales. 2. venae supratrochleares.
**Galen's v.,** 1. either of the internal cerebral veins; see *venae internae cerebri.* 2. vena magna cerebri.
**gastric v., left,** vena gastrica sinistra.
**gastric v., right,** vena gastrica dextra.
**gastric v's, short,** venae gastricae breves.
**gastroepiploic v., left,** vena gastroomentalis sinistra.
**gastroepiploic v., right,** vena gastroomentalis dextra.
**gastroomental v., left,** vena gastroomentalis sinistra.
**gastroomental v., right,** vena gastroomentalis dextra.
**genicular v's,** venae geniculares.
**gluteal v's, inferior,** venae gluteae inferiores.
**gluteal v's, superior,** venae gluteae superiores.
**gonadal v's,** the left and right ovarian veins and left and right testicular veins considered as a group.
**hemiazygos v.,** vena hemiazygos.
**hemiazygos v., accessory,** vena hemiazygos accessoria.
**hepatic v's,** venae hepaticae.
**hepatic v's, intermediate,** venae hepaticae intermediae.
**hepatic v's, middle,** venae hepaticae intermediae.
**hypophyseoportal v's,** venae portales hypophysiales.

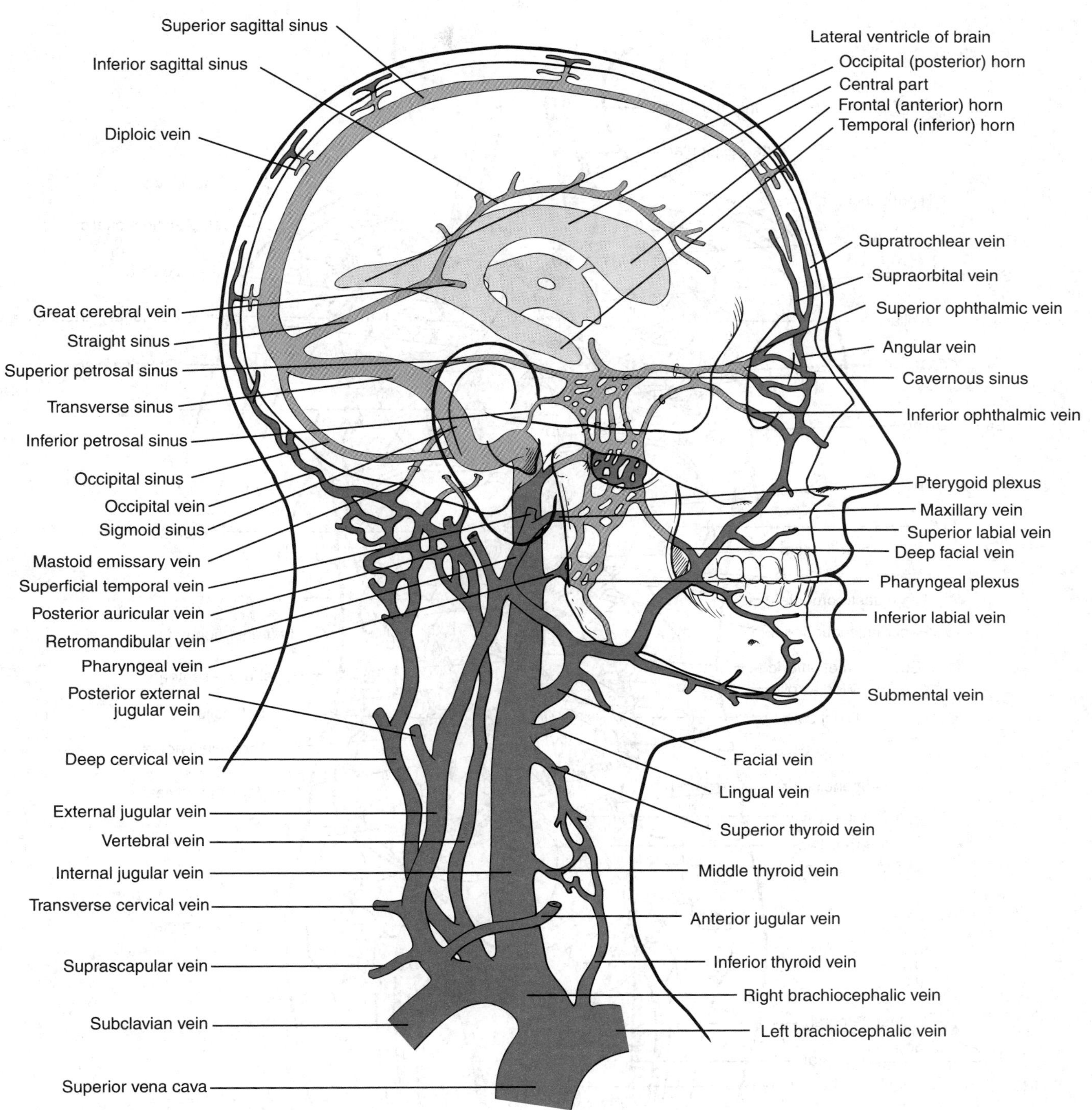


**PLATE 51**—VEINS OF THE HEAD AND NECK

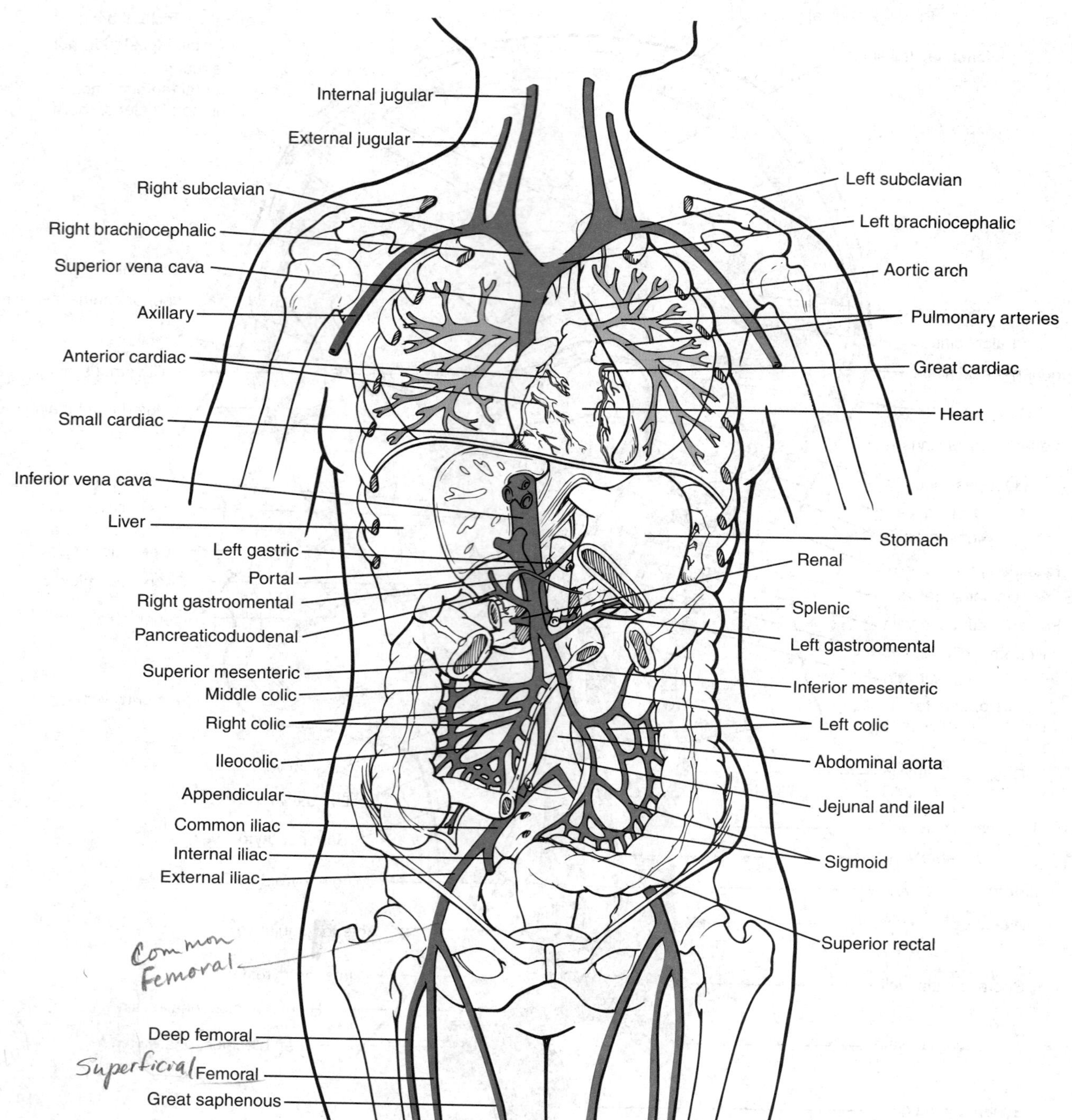


**PLATE 52**—PRINCIPAL VEINS OF THE BODY

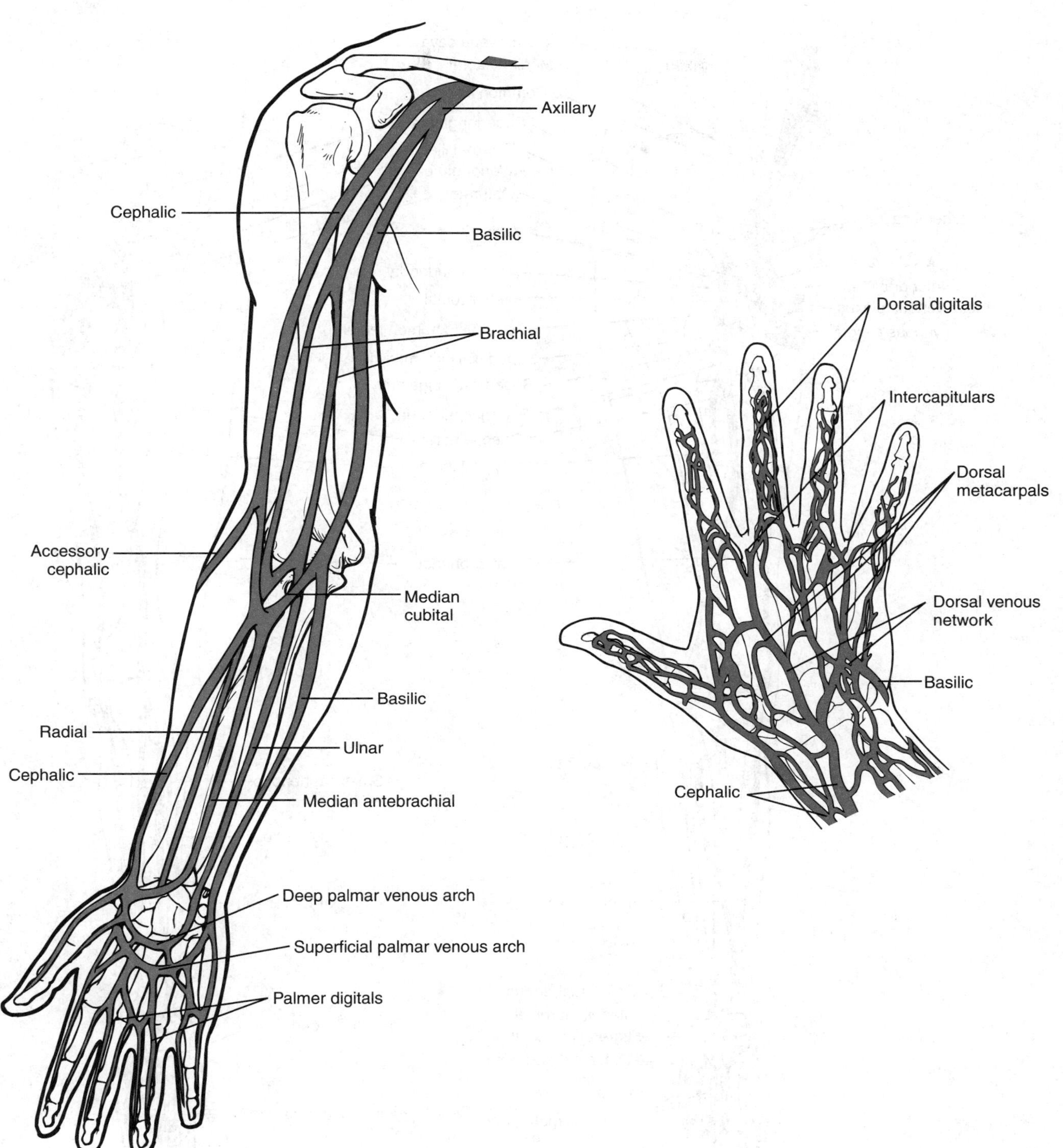


**PLATE 53—**SUPERFICIAL VEINS OF THE UPPER LIMB

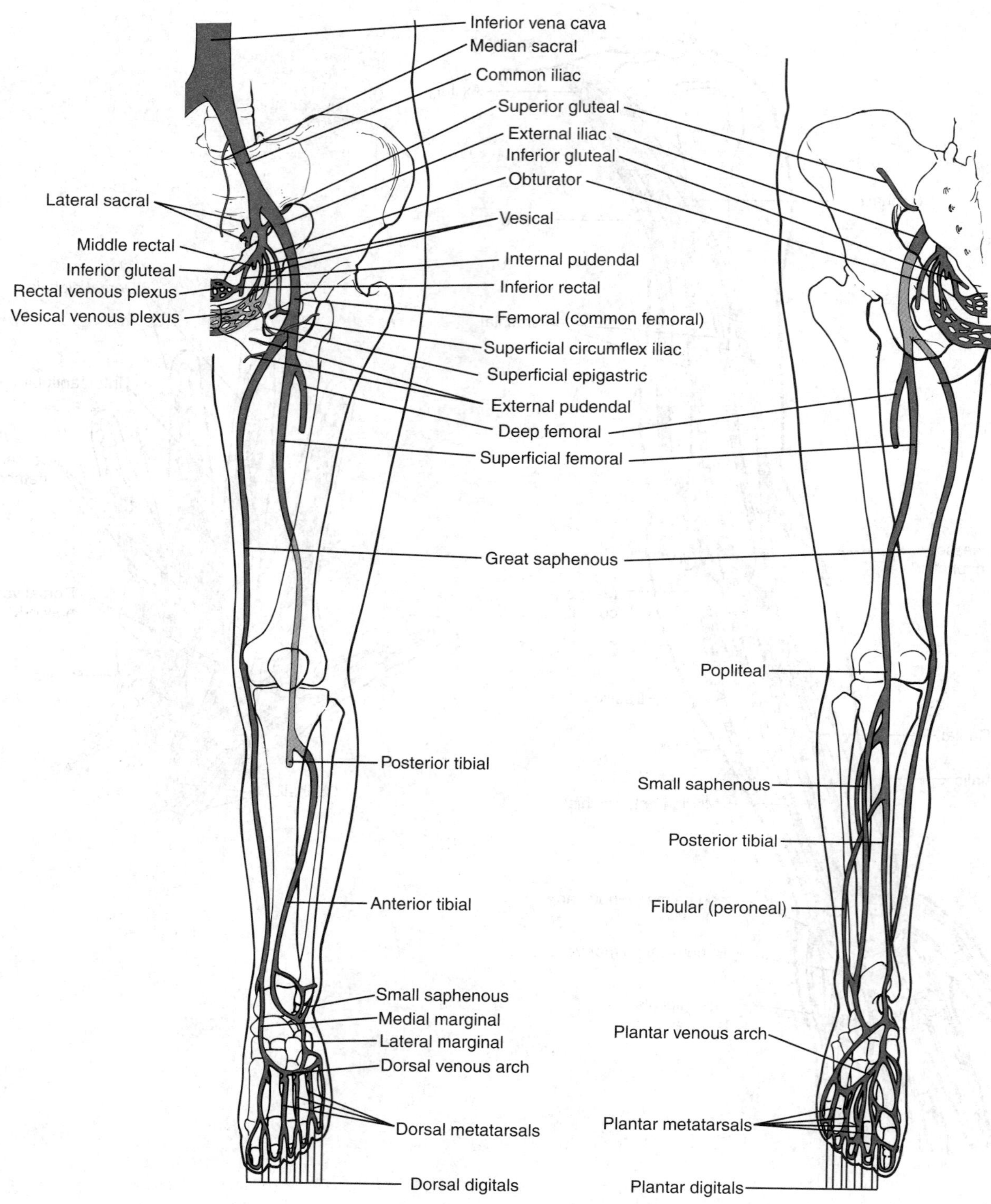


**PLATE 54—**SUPERFICIAL VEINS OF THE LOWER LIMB

**ileal v's,** venae ileales.
**ileocolic v.,** vena ileocolica.
**iliac v., common,** vena iliaca communis.
**iliac v., external,** vena iliaca externa.
**iliac v., internal,** vena iliaca interna.
**iliolumbar v.,** vena iliolumbalis.
**inferior v's of cerebellum,** venae inferiores cerebelli.
**infralobar v.,** pars infralobaris rami posterior.
**infrasegmental v.,** pars intersegmentalis.
**innominate v.,** vena brachiocephalica.
**insular v's,** venae insulares.
**intercapitular v's of foot,** venae intercapitulares pedis.
**intercapitular v's of hand,** venae intercapitulares manus.
**intercostal v's, anterior,** venae intercostales anteriores.
**intercostal v., highest,** vena intercostalis suprema.
**intercostal v., left superior,** vena intercostalis superior sinistra.
**intercostal v's, posterior,** venae intercostales posteriores.
**intercostal v., right superior,** vena intercostalis superior dextra.
**interlobar v's of kidney,** venae interlobares renis.
**interlobular v's of kidney,** venae interlobulares renis.
**interlobular v's of liver,** venae interlobulares hepatis.
**interosseous v's, anterior,** venae interosseae anteriores.
**interosseous v's, posterior,** venae interosseae posteriores.
**intersegmental v.,** 1. pars intersegmentalis. 2. pars infralobaris rami posterior.
**interventricular v., anterior,** vena interventricularis anterior.
**interventricular v., posterior,** vena cardiaca media.
**intervertebral v.,** vena intervertebralis.
**jejunal v's,** venae jejunales.
**jugular v., anterior,** vena jugularis anterior.
**jugular v., external,** vena jugularis externa.
**jugular v., internal,** vena jugularis interna.
**v's of kidney,** venae renales.
**Kohlrausch v's,** superficial veins passing from the under surface of the penis to the dorsal vein.
**Krukenberg's v's,** venae centrales hepatis.
**Kuhnt's postcentral v.,** a vein branching from the vena centralis retina, extending posteriorly from the center of the optic nerve, and draining into the canalis opticus.
**Labbé's v.,** vena anastomotica inferior.
**labial v's, anterior,** venae labiales anteriores.
**labial v's, inferior,** venae labiales inferiores.
**labial v's, posterior,** venae labiales posteriores.
**labial v., superior,** vena labialis superior.
**v's of labyrinth, labyrinthine v's,** venae labyrinthi.
**lacrimal v.,** vena lacrimalis.
**laryngeal v., inferior,** vena laryngea inferior.
**laryngeal v., superior,** vena laryngea superior.
**lateral direct v's,** venae directae laterales.
**v. of lateral recess of fourth ventricle,** vena recessus lateralis ventriculi quarti.
**v. of lateral ventricle, lateral,** vena lateralis ventriculi lateralis.
**v. of lateral ventricle, medial,** vena medialis ventriculi lateralis.
**lingual v.,** vena lingualis.
**lingual v., deep,** vena profunda linguae.
**lingual v's, dorsal,** venae dorsales linguae.
**lobar v., middle,** vena lobi medii pulmonis dextri.
**v's of lower limb,** venae membri inferioris.
**lumbar v's,** venae lumbales.
**lumbar v., ascending,** vena lumbalis ascendens.
**mammary v's, external,** venae costoaxillares.
**mammary v's, internal,** venae thoracicae internae.
**marginal v., lateral,** vena marginalis lateralis.
**marginal v., left,** a vein ascending along the left margin of the heart that drains the left ventricle and empties into the great cardiac vein.
**marginal v., medial,** vena marginalis medialis.
**marginal v., right,** vena marginalis dextra.
**v. of Marshall, Marshall's oblique v.,** vena obliqua atrii sinistri.
**masseteric v's,** venae massetericae.
**maxillary v's,** venae maxillares.
**Mayo's v.,** vena prepylorica.
**median v. of elbow,** vena mediana cubiti.
**median v. of forearm,** vena mediana antebrachii.
**median v. of neck,** vena mediana colli.
**mediastinal v's,** venae mediastinales.
**v's of medulla oblongata,** venae medullae oblongatae.
**meningeal v's,** venae meningeae.
**meningeal v's, middle,** venae meningeae mediae.
**mesencephalic v's,** venae trunci encephalici.
**mesenteric v., inferior,** vena mesenterica inferior.
**mesenteric v., superior,** vena mesenterica superior.
**metacarpal v's, dorsal,** venae metacarpales dorsales.
**metacarpal v's, palmar,** venae metacarpales palmares.
**metatarsal v's, dorsal,** venae metatarsales dorsales.
**metatarsal v's, plantar,** venae metatarsales plantares.
**musculophrenic v's,** venae musculophrenicae.
**nasal v's, external,** venae nasales externae.
**nasofrontal v.,** vena nasofrontalis.
**oblique v. of left atrium,** vena obliqua atrii sinistri.
**obturator v's,** venae obturatoriae.
**obturator v., accessory,** ramus pubicus venae epigastricae inferioris.
**occipital v.,** 1. vena occipitalis. 2. (pl.) venae occipitales.
**v. of olfactory gyrus,** vena gyri olfactorii.
**omphalomesenteric v's,** vitelline v's.
**ophthalmic v., inferior,** vena ophthalmica inferior.
**ophthalmic v., superior,** vena ophthalmica superior.
**ophthalmomeningeal v.,** vena ophthalmomeningea.
**v's of orbit,** venae orbitae.
**ovarian v., left,** vena ovarica sinistra.
**ovarian v., right,** vena ovarica dextra.
**palatine v., palatine v., external,** vena palatina externa.
**palpebral v's,** venae palpebrales.
**palpebral v's, inferior,** venae palpebrales inferiores.
**palpebral v's, superior,** venae palpebrales superiores.
**pancreatic v's,** venae pancreaticae.
**pancreaticoduodenal v's,** venae pancreaticoduodenales.
**paraumbilical v's,** venae paraumbilicales.
**parietal v's,** venae parietales.
**parietal v. of Santorini,** vena emissaria parietalis.
**parotid v's,** venae parotideae.
**parotid v's, anterior,** rami parotidei venae facialis.
**parotid v's, posterior,** venae parotideae.
**parumbilical v's,** venae para-umbilicales.
**peduncular v's,** venae pedunculares.
**perforating v's,** 1. venae perforantes. 2. an inconstant group of veins seen as tributaries of the great saphenous vein, anastomosing between it and other veins of the lower leg.
**pericardiac v's,** venae pericardiacae.
**pericardiacophrenic v's,** venae pericardiacophrenicae.
**pericardial v's,** venae pericardiacae.
**peroneal v's,** venae fibulares.
**petrosal v.,** vena petrosa.
**pharyngeal v's,** venae pharyngeae.
**phrenic v's, inferior,** venae phrenicae inferiores.
**phrenic v's, superior,** venae phrenicae superiores.
**v's of pons,** venae pontis.
**pontomesencephalic v., anterior,** vena pontomesencephalica anterior.
**popliteal v.,** vena poplitea.
**portal v., portal v., hepatic,** vena portae hepatis.
**portal v's of hypophysis,** venae portales hypophysiales.
**portal v. of liver,** vena portae hepatis.
**postcardinal v's,** paired vessels in the embryo caudal to the heart; called also *posterior cardinal v's.*
**posterior v. of left ventricle,** vena ventriculi sinistri posterior.
**precardinal v's,** paired venous trunks in the embryo cranial to the heart; called also *anterior cardinal v's.*
**precentral v. of cerebellum,** vena precentralis cerebelli.
**prefrontal v's,** venae prefrontales.
**prepyloric v.,** vena prepylorica.
**primary head v's,** vessels alongside the embryonic brain that continue into the precardinal veins.
**v. of pterygoid canal,** vena canalis pterygoidei.
**pudendal v's, external,** venae pudendae externae.
**pudendal v., internal,** vena pudenda interna.
**pulmonary v's,** venae pulmonales.
**pulmonary v., left inferior,** vena pulmonalis sinistra inferior.
**pulmonary v., left superior,** vena pulmonalis sinistra superior.
**pulmonary v., right inferior,** vena pulmonalis dextra inferior.
**pulmonary v., right superior,** vena pulmonalis dextra superior.
**pulp v's,** vessels draining the splenic sinuses.
**pyloric v.,** vena gastrica dextra.
**radial v's,** venae radiales.
**ranine v.,** vena sublingualis.
**rectal v's, inferior,** venae rectales inferiores.
**rectal v's, middle,** venae rectales mediae.
**rectal v., superior,** vena rectalis superior.
**renal v's,** venae renales.
**retromandibular v.,** vena retromandibularis.
**Retzius' v's,** inconstant venous anastomoses that connect veins from the walls of the intestine to the tributaries of the inferior vena cava rather than to the superior mesenteric vein.
**revehent v's,** venae revehentes.
**Rosenthal's v.,** vena basalis.
**sacral v's, lateral,** venae sacrales laterales.
**sacral v., median, sacral v., middle,** vena sacralis mediana.
**saphenous v., accessory,** vena saphena accessoria.

**saphenous v., great,** vena saphena magna.
**saphenous v., small,** vena saphena parva.
**v's of Sappey,** venae paraumbilicales.
**scleral v's,** venae sclerales.
**scrotal v's, anterior,** venae scrotales anteriores.
**scrotal v's, posterior,** venae scrotales posteriores.
**segmental v., apicoposterior,** vena apicoposterior lobi superioris pulmonis sinistri.
**segmental v., inferior lingular,** pars inferior venae lingularis.
**segmental v., superior lingular,** pars superior venae lingularis.
**segmental v. of left lung, anterior,** vena anterior lobi superioris pulmonis sinistri.
**segmental v. of left lung, superior,** vena superior lobi inferioris pulmonis sinistri.
**segmental v. of right lung, anterior,** vena anterior lobi superioris pulmonis dextri.
**segmental v. of right lung, apical,** vena apicalis lobi superioris pulmonis dextri.
**segmental v. of right lung, lateral,** pars lateralis venae lobi medii.
**segmental v. of right lung, medial,** pars medialis venae lobi medii.
**segmental v. of right lung, posterior,** vena posterior lobi superioris pulmonis dextri.
**segmental v. of right lung, superior,** vena superior lobi inferioris pulmonis dextri.
**v. of septum pellucidum, anterior,** vena anterior septi pellucidi.
**v. of septum pellucidum, posterior,** vena posterior septi pellucidi.
**sigmoid v's,** venae sigmoideae.
**small v. of heart,** vena cardiaca parva.
**spermatic v.,** either of the testicular veins; see *vena testicularis dextra* and *vena testicularis sinistra.*
**spinal v's, anterior,** venae spinales anteriores.
**spinal v's, posterior,** venae spinales posteriores.
**spiral v. of modiolus,** vena spiralis modioli.
**splenic v.,** vena splenica.
**stellate v's of kidney,** venae stellatae renis.
**Stensen's v's,** venae vorticosae.
**sternocleidomastoid v.,** vena sternocleidomastoidea.
**striate v's,** venae thalamostriatae inferiores.
**stylomastoid v.,** vena stylomastoidea.
**subcardinal v's,** paired vessels in the embryo, replacing the postcardinal veins and persisting to some degree as definitive vessels.
**subclavian v.,** vena subclavia.
**subcostal v.,** vena subcostalis.
**subcutaneous v's of abdomen,** venae subcutaneae abdominis.
**sublingual v.,** vena sublingualis.
**sublobular v's,** tributaries of the hepatic veins that receive the central veins of hepatic lobules.
**submental v.,** vena submentalis.
**superficial v.,** vena superficialis.
**superficial v's of lower limb,** venae superficiales membri inferioris.
**superficial v's of upper limb,** venae superficiales membri superioris.
**superior v's of cerebellum,** venae superiores cerebelli.
**supracardinal v's,** paired vessels in the embryo, developing later than the subcardinal veins and persisting chiefly as the inferior segment of the inferior vena cava.
**supraorbital v.,** vena supraorbitalis.
**suprarenal v., left,** vena suprarenalis sinistra.
**suprarenal v., right,** vena suprarenalis dextra.
**suprascapular v.,** vena suprascapularis.
**supratrochlear v's,** venae supratrochleares.
**sural v's,** venae surales.
**sylvian v's, v's of sylvian fossa,** see *vena media superficialis cerebri.*
**temporal v's, deep,** venae temporales profundae.
**temporal v., middle,** vena temporalis media.
**temporal v's, superficial,** venae temporales superficiales.
**temporomandibular articular v's,** venae articulares.
**terminal v.,** vena thalamostriata superior.
**testicular v., left,** vena testicularis sinistra.
**testicular v., right,** vena testicularis dextra.
**thalamostriate v's, inferior,** venae thalamostriatae inferiores.
**thalamostriate v., superior,** vena thalamostriata superior.
**thebesian v's, v's of Thebesius,** venae cardiacae minimae.
**thoracic v's, internal,** venae thoracicae internae.
**thoracic v., lateral,** vena thoracica lateralis.
**thoracoacromial v.,** vena thoracoacromialis.
**thoracoepigastric v's,** venae thoracoepigastricae.
**thymic v's,** venae thymicae.
**thyroid v., inferior,** vena thyroidea inferioris.
**thyroid v's, middle,** venae thyroideae mediae.
**thyroid v., superior,** vena thyroidea superior.
**tibial v's, anterior,** venae tibiales anteriores.
**tibial v's, posterior,** venae tibiales posteriores.
**trabecular v's,** vessels coursing in splenic trabeculae, formed by tributary pulp veins.
**tracheal v's,** venae tracheales.
**transverse v. of face,** vena transversa faciei.
**transverse v's of neck,** venae transversae cervicis.
**transverse v. of scapula,** vena suprascapularis.
**Trolard's v.,** vena anastomotica superior.
**tympanic v's,** venae tympanicae.
**ulnar v's,** venae ulnares.
**umbilical v.,** vena umbilicalis.
**umbilical v., left,** vena umbilicalis sinistra.
**v. of uncus,** vena uncalis.
**v's of upper limb,** venae membri superioris.
**uterine v's,** venae uterinae.
**varicose v.,** a dilated tortuous vein, usually in the subcutaneous tissues of the leg, often associated with incompetency of the venous valves.
**ventricular v's of heart,** venae ventriculares cordis.
**ventricular v., inferior,** vena ventricularis inferior.
**v. of vermis, inferior,** vena inferior vermis.
**v. of vermis, superior,** vena superior vermis.
**vertebral v.,** vena vertebralis.
**vertebral v., accessory,** vena vertebralis accessoria.
**vertebral v., anterior,** vena vertebralis anterior.
**vertebral v's, superficial,** the veins of the external vertebral plexuses; see *plexus venosus vertebralis externus anterior* and *posterior.* Called also *external v's of vertebral column.*
**v's of vertebral column,** venae columnae vertebralis.
**v's of vertebral column, external,** superficial vertebral v's.
**vesalian v.,** an emissary vein connecting the cavernous sinus with the pterygoid venous plexus, sometimes passing through an opening in the great wing of the sphenoid bone.
**vesical v's,** venae vesicales.
**vestibular v's,** venae vestibulares.
**vidian v.,** vena canalis pterygoidei.
**v's of Vieussens,** venae ventriculi dextri anteriores.
**vitelline v's,** veins that return the blood from the yolk sac to the primordial heart of the early embryo. Called also *omphalomesenteric v's.*
**vorticose v's,** venae vorticosae.

---

**Vel blood group** (vel) [from part of the name of the propositus first described in 1952] see under *blood group.*

**ve·la** (ve'lə) [L.] plural of *velum.*

**Vel·a·cy·cline** (vel"ə-si'klēn) trademark for preparations of rolitetracycline.

**ve·la·men** (ve-la'mən) pl. *vela'mina* [L. "a covering"] a membrane, velum, meninx, or tegument.

**vel·a·men·ta** (vel"ə-men'tə) [L.] plural of *velamentum.*

**vel·a·men·tous** (vel"ə-men'təs) [L. *velamen* veil] membranous and pendent; like a veil.

**vel·a·men·tum** (vel"ə-men'təm) pl. *velamen'ta* [L.] any covering, velum, or envelope.
**velamen'ta ce'rebri,** the meninges.

**ve·lar** (ve'lər) 1. pertaining to a velum, especially to the velum palatinum (palatum molle). 2. said of consonantal speech sounds produced with the tongue near the soft palate, such as *g* and *k.*

**Vel·ban** (vel'ban) trademark for a preparation of vinblastine sulfate.

**vel·i·form** (vel'ĭ-form) velamentous.

**Vel·la's fistula** (va'lahz) [Luigi *Vella,* Italian physiologist, 1825–1886] see under *fistula.*

**vel·lo·sine** (və-lo'sin) a poisonous alkaloid from the bark of *Geissosperum laeve* and *G. vellosii.*

**vel·lus** (vel'əs) [L. "fleece"] 1. the fine hair which succeeds the lanugo over most of the body. 2. a structure resembling this fine hair.
**v. oli'vae,** a narrow band of tangential fibers surrounding the olive.

**ve·lo·cim·e·try** (ve″lo-sim′ə-tre) measurement of speed, such as speed of flow. See also *flowmeter.*
**laser-Doppler v.**, measurement of the flow of red cells in a microcirculatory bed by means of laser light delivered to and detected from the region of interest by fiberoptic probes.

**ve·loc·i·ty** (və-los′ĭ-te) [L. *velox* swift] the rate of movement of a body in a given direction. Symbol *v.*
**nerve conduction v.**, the speed, in meters per second, at which an impulse moves along the largest fibers of a peripheral nerve.
**thrombotic threshold v.**, TTV; the minimum velocity of blood flow through a vascular graft or prosthesis below which thrombogenicity would begin along the intimal surface; variables affecting it include lumen diameter and type of material the graft or prosthesis is made of.

**ve·lo·no·ski·as·co·py** (ve″lo-no-ski-as′kə-pe) belonoskiascopy.

**ve·lo·pha·ryn·ge·al** (ve″lo-fə-rin′je-əl) pertaining to the soft palate (velum palatinum) and pharynx.

**Vel·o·sef** (vel′o-sef) trademark for preparations of cephradine.

**Ve·lo·su·lin** (ve-lo′soo-lin) trademark for preparations of insulin injection (regular insulin).

**Vel·peau's bandage, canal, deformity, hernia** (vel-pōz′) [Alfred Armand Louis Marie *Velpeau,* French surgeon, 1795–1867] see under *bandage* and *hernia,* see *canalis inguinalis,* and see *silver fork fracture,* under *fracture.*

**ve·lum** (ve′ləm) pl. *ve′la* [L.] [TA] a general term in anatomical nomenclature for a veil or veillike structure.
**artificial v.**, an artificial palate (q.v.) for the soft palate.
**v. interpo′situm ce′rebri,** tela choroidea ventriculi tertii.
**v. medulla′re ante′rius,** v. medullare superius.
**v. medulla′re cauda′le,** v. medullare inferius.
**v. medulla′re infe′rius** [TA], **v. medulla′re poste′rius,** inferior medullary velum: either of two thin layers of white substance symmetrically located on the sides of the nodule of the vermis; their internal surface forms the lower wall of the lateroposterior recess of the fourth ventricle. On the sides the velum is continuous with the pedunculus flocculi and the taenia, and anteriorly it is fused with the choroid plexus. Called also *caudal* or *posterior medullary v.*
**v. medulla′re rostra′lis, v. medulla′re supe′rius** [TA], superior medullary velum: a thin layer of white substance forming the roof of the superior part of the fourth ventricle, and extending from the tectal lamina in front to the fastigium behind, and between the superior cerebellar peduncles; called also *anterior* or *rostral medullary v.*
**medullary v., anterior,** v. medullare superius.
**medullary v., caudal, medullary v., inferior, medullary v., posterior,** v. medullare inferius.
**medullary v., rostral, medullary v., superior,** v. medullare superius.
**v. pala′ti,** palatum molle.
**v. palati′num,** TA alternative for *palatum molle.*
**v. of Tarinus,** v. medullare inferius.
**v. transver′sum,** a transverse fold of the tela choroidea marking the boundary between the diencephalon and the telencephalon in the embryonic brain.

**ve·na** (ve′nə) pl. *ve′nae* [L.] [TA] vein.

## Vena

Descriptions of veins are given on TA terms, and include anglicized names of specific veins.

**v. adrena′lis dex′tra,** v. suprarenalis dextra.

**ve′nae advehen′tes,** channels in the early embryo that convey blood to the sinusoids of the liver and later join to form the portal vein.

**v. anastomo′tica infe′rior** [TA], inferior anastomotic vein: a vein that interconnects the superficial middle cerebral vein and the transverse sinus. Called also *Browning's vein.*

**v. anastomo′tica supe′rior** [TA], superior anastomotic vein: a vein that interconnects the superficial middle cerebral vein and the superior sagittal sinus. Called also *Trolard's vein.*

**v. angula′ris** [TA], angular vein: a short vein between the eye and the root of the nose; it is formed by union of the supratrochlear and supraorbital veins and continues inferiorly as the facial vein.

**ve′nae anterio′res ce′rebri** [TA], anterior cerebral veins: veins that accompany the anterior cerebral artery and join the basal vein; called also *venae cerebri anteriores.*

**v. ante′rior lo′bi supe′rioris pulmo′nis dex′tri** [TA], anterior vein of superior lobe of right lung: a branch that drains the anterior segment of the right upper lobe and empties into the right superior pulmonary vein; called also *ramus anterior venae pulmonalis dextrae superioris* [TA alternative] and *anterior segmental vein of right lung.*

**v. ante′rior lo′bi supe′rioris pulmo′nis sinis′tri** [TA], 1. anterior branch of left superior pulmonary vein: a venous branch that drains the anterior segment of the left lung and empties into the left superior pulmonary vein. Called also *anterior segmental vein of left lung.* 2. anterior vein of superior lobe of left lung: a branch that drains the anterior segment of the left upper lobe and empties into the left superior pulmonary vein; called also *ramus anterior venae pulmonalis sinistrae superioris* [TA alternative] and *anterior segmental vein of left lung.*

**v. ante′rior sep′ti pellu′cidi** [TA], anterior vein of septum pellucidum: a vein that drains the anterior septum pellucidum into the superior thalamostriate vein; called also *v. septi pellucidi anterior.*

**v. apica′lis lo′bi superio′ris pulmo′nis dex′tri** [TA], apical artery of superior lobe of right lung: a branch that drains the apical segment of the right upper lobe; called also *ramus apicalis venae pulmonalis dextrae superioris* [TA alternative] and *apical segmental vein of right lung.*

**v. apicoposte′rior lo′bi superio′ris pulmo′nis sinis′tri** [TA], apicoposterior vein of superior lobe of left lung: a venous branch that drains the apicoposterior segment of the left lung and empties into the left superior pulmonary vein. Called also *ramus apicoposterior venae pulmonalis dextrae superioris* [TA alternative] and *apicoposterior segmental vein.*

**v. appendicula′ris** [TA], appendicular vein: the vena comitans of the appendicular artery; it unites with the anterior and posterior cecal veins to form the ileocolic vein.

**v. aqueduc′tus coch′leae** [TA], vein of aqueduct of cochlea: a vein along the aqueduct of the cochlea that empties into the superior bulb of the internal jugular vein; called also *vein of cochlear canaliculus* and *v. canaliculi cochleae.*

**v. aqueduc′tus vesti′buli** [TA], vein of aqueduct of vestibule: a small vein from the internal ear that passes through the aqueduct of the vestibule and empties into the superior petrosal sinus.

**ve′nae arcifor′mes re′nis,** venae arcuatae renis.

**ve′nae arcua′tae re′nis** [TA], arcuate veins of kidney: a series of complete arches across the bases of the pyramids of the kidneys; they are formed by union of the interlobular veins and the venulae rectae and drain into the interlobar veins. Called also *venae arciformes renis.*

**ve′nae articula′res** [TA], articular veins: small vessels that drain the plexus around the temporomandibular articulation into the retromandibular vein; called also *temporomandibular articular veins.*

**ve′nae atria′les dex′trae** [TA], right atrial veins: the veins of the right atrium of the heart.

**ve′nae atria′les sinis′trae** [TA], left atrial veins: the veins of the left atrium of the heart.

**ve′nae atrioventricula′res cor′dis** [TA], atrioventricular veins of heart: the veins that supply the atria and ventricles of the heart.

**ve′nae auditi′vae inter′nae,** venae labyrinthi.

**ve′nae auricula′res anterio′res** [TA], anterior auricular veins: branches from the anterior part of the pinna that enter the superficial temporal vein.

**v. auricula′ris poste′rior** [TA], posterior auricular vein: a vein that begins in a plexus on the side of the head, passes down behind the pinna, and joins with the retromandibular vein to form the external jugular vein.

**v. axilla′ris** [TA], axillary vein; the venous trunk of the upper member; it begins at the lower border of the teres major muscle by junction of the basilic and brachial veins, and at the lateral border of the first rib is continuous with the subclavian vein.

**v. a′zygos** [TA], azygos vein: an intercepting trunk for the right intercostal veins as well as a connecting branch between the superior and inferior venae cavae: it arises from the ascending lumbar vein, passes up in the posterior mediastinum to the level of the fourth thoracic vertebra, where it arches over the root of the right lung *(arcus venae azygou),* and empties into the superior vena cava.

**v. basa′lis** [TA], basal vein: a vein that arises at the anterior perforated substance, passes backward and around the cerebral peduncle, and empties into the internal cerebral vein; called also *Rosenthal's vein.*

**v. basa′lis ante′rior** [TA], anterior basal vein: a venous branch draining the anterior basal segment of either lung and emptying into the common basal vein. Called also *ramus basalis anterior venae basalis communis* [TA alternative].

**v. basa'lis commu'nis** [TA], common basal vein: either of two veins, one draining the lower lobe of each lung and draining into the corresponding inferior pulmonary vein; both are formed by the union of superior and inferior basal veins.

**v. basa'lis infe'rior** [TA], inferior basal vein: either of two veins, each draining the inferior segments of an inferior lobe of the corresponding lung and draining into a common basal vein.

**v. basa'lis supe'rior** [TA], superior basal vein: either of two veins, each draining the apical segment of an inferior lobe of the corresponding lung and draining into a common basal vein.

**v. basi'lica** [TA], basilic vein: the superficial vein that arises from the ulnar side of the dorsal rete of the hand, passes up the forearm, and joins with the brachial veins to form the axillary vein.

**ve'nae basivertebra'les** [TA], basivertebral veins: venous sinuses in the cancellous tissue of the bodies of the vertebrae, which communicate with the plexus of veins on the anterior surface of the vertebrae and with the anterior internal vertebral plexus.

**ve'nae brachia'les** [TA], brachial veins: the venae comitantes of the brachial artery, which join with the basilic vein to form the axillary vein.

**v. brachiocepha'lica** [TA], brachiocephalic vein: either of the two veins that drain blood from the head, neck, and upper extremities, and unite to form the superior vena cava. Each is formed at the root of the neck by union of the ipsilateral internal jugular and subclavian veins. The right vein *(v. brachiocephalica dextra)* passes almost vertically downward in front of the brachiocephalic artery, and the left vein *(v. brachiocephalica sinistra)* passes from left to right behind the upper part of the sternum. Each vein receives the vertebral, deep cervical, deep thyroid, and internal thoracic veins. The left vein also receives intercostal, thymic, tracheal, esophageal, phrenic, mediastinal, and pericardiac branches, as well as the thoracic duct; and the right vein receives the right lymphatic duct. Called also *innominate vein.*

**ve'nae bronchia'les** [TA], bronchial veins: vessels that drain blood from the larger subdivisions of the bronchi; on the left they drain into the azygos vein and on the right they drain into the hemiazygos vein or superior intercostal vein.

**ve'nae bronchia'les anterio'res,** see *venae bronchiales.*

**ve'nae bronchia'les posterio'res,** see *venae bronchiales.*

**v. bul'bi pe'nis** [TA], vein of bulb of penis: a vein draining blood from the bulb of the penis into the internal pudendal vein.

**v. bul'bi vesti'buli** [TA], vein of bulb of vestibule: a vein draining blood from the bulb of the vestibule of the vagina into the internal pudendal vein.

**v. canali'culi coch'leae,** v. aqueductus cochleae.

**v. cana'lis pterygoi'dei** [TA], vein of pterygoid canal: one of the veins that pass through the pterygoid canal and empty into the pterygoid plexus; called also *vidian vein.*

**ve'nae cardi'acae anterio'res,** venae ventriculi dextri anteriores.

**v. cardi'aca mag'na** [TA], great cardiac vein: a vein that collects blood from the anterior surface of the ventricles, follows the anterior longitudinal sulcus, and empties into the coronary sinus; called also *v. cordis magna* [TA alternative]. See also *v. coronaria sinistra* and *v. interventricularis anterior.*

**v. cardi'aca me'dia** [TA], middle cardiac vein: a vein that collects blood from the diaphragmatic surface of the ventricles, follows the posterior longitudinal sulcus, and empties into the coronary sinus; called also *v. cordis media* [TA alternative]. See *v. coronaria dextra* and *v. interventricularis posterior.*

**ve'nae cardi'acae mi'nimae** [TA], smallest cardiac veins: numerous small veins arising in the muscular walls and draining independently into the cavities of the heart, and most readily seen in the atria; called also *thebesian veins* and *venae cordis minimae* [TA alternative].

**v. cardi'aca par'va** [TA], small cardiac vein: a vein that collects blood from both parts of the right heart, follows the coronary sulcus to the left, and opens into the coronary sinus; called also *v. cordis parva* [TA alternative].

**ve'nae ca'vae,** the vena cava inferior and vena cava superior considered together.

**v. ca'va infe'rior** [TA], inferior vena cava: the venous trunk for the lower extremities and for the pelvic and abdominal viscera; it begins at the level of the fifth lumbar vertebra by union of the common iliac veins, passes upward on the right of the aorta, and empties into the right atrium of the heart.

**v. ca'va supe'rior** [TA], superior vena cava: the venous trunk draining blood from the head, neck, upper extremities, and chest; it begins by union of the two brachiocephalic veins, passes directly downward, and empties into the right atrium of the heart.

**ve'nae caverno'sae pe'nis** [TA], cavernous veins of penis: veins that return the blood from the corpora cavernosa to the deep veins and the dorsal vein of the penis.

**v. centra'lis glan'dulae suprarena'lis** [TA], central vein of suprarenal gland: the large single vein into which the various veins within the substance of the gland empty, and which continues at the hilum as the suprarenal vein.

**ve'nae centra'les he'patis** [TA], central veins of liver: veins in the middle of the hepatic lobules, draining into the hepatic vein. Called also *central veins of hepatic lobules* and *Krukenberg's veins.*

**v. centra'lis re'tinae** [TA], central vein of retina: the vein that is formed by union of the retinal veins; it passes out of the eyeball in the optic nerve to empty into the superior ophthalmic vein.

**v. cepha'lica** [TA], cephalic vein: the superficial vein that arises from the radial side of the dorsal rete of the hand, and winds anteriorly to pass along the anterior border of the brachioradialis muscle; above the elbow it ascends along the lateral border of the biceps muscle and the pectoral border of the deltoid muscle, and opens into the axillary vein.

**v. cepha'lica accesso'ria** [TA], accessory cephalic vein: a vein arising from the dorsal rete of the hand, passing up the forearm to join the cephalic vein just above the elbow.

**ve'nae cerebel'li** [TA], cerebellar veins: the veins on the surface of the cerebellum; see *venae inferiores cerebelli* and *venae superiores cerebelli.*

**ve'nae ce'rebri,** venae encephali.

**ve'nae ce'rebri ante'riores,** venae anteriores cerebri.

**ve'nae ce'rebri inferio'res,** venae inferiores cerebri.

**ve'nae ce'rebri inter'nae,** venae internae cerebri.

**v. ce'rebri mag'na,** v. magna cerebri.

**ve'nae ce'rebri profun'dae,** venae profundae cerebri.

**ve'nae ce'rebri superficia'les,** venae superficiales cerebri.

**ve'nae ce'rebri superio'res,** venae superiores cerebri.

**v. cervica'lis profun'da** [TA], deep cervical vein: a vein that arises from a plexus in the suboccipital triangle, follows the deep cervical artery down the neck, and empties into the vertebral or the brachiocephalic vein.

**v. choroi'dea infe'rior** [TA], inferior choroid vein: a vein that drains the inferior choroid plexus into the basal vein.

**ve'nae choroi'deae o'culi,** venae vorticosae.

**v. choroi'dea supe'rior** [TA], superior choroid vein: the vein that runs along the whole length of the choroid plexus, draining it and the hippocampus, fornix, and corpus callosum; it unites with the superior thalamostriate vein to form the internal cerebral vein.

**ve'nae cilia'res** [TA], ciliary veins: veins that arise inside the eyeball by branches from the ciliary muscle and drain into the superior ophthalmic vein. The *anterior ciliary veins* follow the anterior ciliary arteries, and receive branches from the sinus venosus, sclerae, the episcleral veins, and the tunica conjunctiva bulbi. The *posterior ciliary veins* follow the posterior ciliary arteries and empty also into the inferior ophthalmic vein.

**ve'nae circumflex'ae fe'moris latera'les** [TA], lateral circumflex femoral veins: venae comitantes of the lateral circumflex femoral artery, emptying into the femoral or the deep femoral vein; called also *venae circumflexae laterales femoris.*

**ve'nae circumflex'ae fe'moris media'les,** medial circumflex femoral veins: venae comitantes of the medial circumflex femoral artery, emptying into the femoral or the deep femoral vein; called also *venae circumflexae mediales femoris.*

**v. circumflex'a ili'aca profun'da,** v. circumflexa ilium profunda.

**v. circumflex'a ili'aca superficia'lis** [TA], v. circumflexa ilium superficialis.

**v. circumflex'a i'lium profun'da** [TA], deep circumflex iliac vein: a common trunk formed from the venae comitantes of the homonymous artery and emptying into the external iliac vein. Called also *v. circumflexa iliaca profunda.*

**v. circumflex'a i'lium superficia'lis,** superficial circumflex iliac vein: a vein that follows the homonymous artery and empties into the great saphenous vein. Called also *v. circumflexa iliaca superficialis.*

**ve'nae circumflex'ae latera'les fe'moris,** venae circumflexae femoris laterales.

**ve'nae circumflex'ae media'les fe'moris** [TA], venae circumflexae femoris mediales.

**v. circumflex'a superficia'lis i'lium,** v. circumflexa ilium superficialis.

**v. co'lica dex'tra** [TA], right colic vein: a vein that follows the distribution of the right colic artery and empties into the superior mesenteric vein.

**v. co'lica interme'dia,** v. colica media.

**v. co'lica me'dia** [TA], middle colic vein: a vein that follows the distribution of the middle colic artery and empties into the superior mesenteric vein; called also *intermediate colic vein* and *v. colica intermedia.*

**v. co'lica sinis'tra** [TA], left colic vein: a vein that follows the left colic artery and opens into the inferior mesenteric vein.

**ve'nae colum'nae vertebra'lis** [TA], veins of the vertebral column: a plexiform venous network extending the entire length of the vertebral column, outside or inside the vertebral canal; the anterior and posterior external and anterior and posterior internal groups freely anastomose and end in the intervertebral veins. See terms beginning *plexus venosus vertebralis.*

**v. co'mitans** [TA], accompanying vein: a vein, usually occurring in a pair (venae comitantes), that closely accompanies its homonymous artery and is found especially in the extremities.

**v. co'mitans ner'vi hypoglos'si** [TA], accompanying vein of hypoglossal nerve: a vessel, formed by union of the vena profunda linguae and the vena sublingualis, that accompanies the hypoglossal nerve; it empties into the facial, lingual, or internal jugular vein.

**ve'nae conjunctiva'les** [TA], conjunctival veins: small veins that drain blood from the conjunctiva to the superior ophthalmic vein.

**ve'nae cor'dis** [TA], cardiac veins: the veins of the heart, which drain blood from the various tissues making up the organ.

**ve'nae cor'dis anterio'res,** venae ventriculi dextri anteriores.

**v. cor'dis mag'na,** TA alternative for *v. cardiaca magna.*

**v. cor'dis me'dia,** TA alternative for *v. cardiaca media.*

**ve'nae cor'dis mi'nimae,** TA alternative for *venae cardiacae minimae.*

**v. cor'dis par'va,** TA alternative for *v. cardiaca parva.*

**v. corona'ria dex'tra,** right coronary vein: the portion of the middle cardiac vein that receives blood from the posterior interventricular vein and empties into the coronary sinus.

**v. corona'ria sinis'tra,** left coronary vein: the portion of the great cardiac vein lying in the coronary sulcus; it receives blood from the anterior interventricular vein and empties into the coronary sinus.

**ve'nae costoaxilla'res,** costoaxillary veins: veins that arise from the areolar venous plexus, anastomose with the upper six or seven posterior intercostal veins, and empty into the axillary vein. Called also *external mammary veins.*

**v. cuta'nea** [TA], cutaneous vein: one of the small veins that begin in the papillae of the skin, form subpapillary plexuses, and open into the subcutaneous veins.

**v. cys'tica** [TA], cystic vein: a small vein that returns the blood from the gallbladder to the right branch of the portal vein, within the substance of the liver.

**ve'nae digita'les commu'nes pe'dis,** common digital veins of foot: short veins formed by union of the dorsal digital and the intercapitular veins of the foot.

**ve'nae digita'les dorsa'les pe'dis** [TA], dorsal digital veins of foot: the veins on the dorsal surfaces of the toes that unite in pairs around each cleft to form the dorsal metatarsal veins; called also *venae digitales pedis dorsales.*

**ve'nae digita'les palma'res** [TA], palmar digital veins: the venae comitantes of the proper and common palmar digital arteries, which join the superficial palmar venous arch.

**ve'nae digita'les pe'dis dorsa'les,** venae digitales dorsales pedis.

**ve'nae digita'les planta'res** [TA], plantar digital veins: veins from the plantar surfaces of the toes which unite at the clefts to form the plantar metatarsal veins of the foot.

**ve'nae diplo'icae** [TA], diploic veins: veins of the skull, including the frontal, occipital, anterior temporal, and posterior temporal diploic veins, which form sinuses in the cancellous tissue between the laminae of the cranial bones. They send branches to the external and the internal lamina, the periosteum, and the dura mater, and empty in part inside and in part outside the skull.

**v. diplo'ica fronta'lis** [TA], frontal diploic vein: a vein that drains the frontal bone, emptying externally into the supraorbital vein or internally into the superior sagittal sinus.

**v. diplo'ica occipita'lis** [TA], occipital diploic vein: the largest of the diploic veins, which drains blood from the occipital bone and empties into the occipital vein or the transverse sinus.

**v. diplo'ica tempora'lis ante'rior** [TA], anterior temporal diploic vein: a vein that drains the lateral portion of the frontal and the anterior part of the parietal bone, opening internally into the sphenoparietal sinus and externally into a deep temporal vein.

**v. diplo'ica tempora'lis poste'rior** [TA], posterior temporal diploic vein: a vein that drains the parietal bone and empties into the transverse sinus.

**ve'nae direc'tae latera'les** [TA], lateral direct veins: veins of the lateral ventricle, draining into the great cerebral vein.

**v. dorsa'lis clito'ridis profun'da,** v. dorsalis profunda clitoridis.

**ve'nae dorsa'les clito'ridis superficia'les,** venae dorsales superficiales clitoridis.

**v. dorsa'lis cor'poris callo'si** [TA], dorsal vein of corpus callosum: a vein that drains the superior surface of the corpus callosum into the great cerebral vein.

**ve'nae dorsa'les lin'guae** [TA], dorsal lingual veins: veins that unite with a small vena comitans of the lingual artery and join the main lingual trunk.

**v. dorsa'lis pe'nis profun'da,** v. dorsalis profunda penis.

**ve'nae dorsa'les pe'nis superficia'les,** venae dorsales superficiales penis.

**v. dorsa'lis profun'da clito'ridis** [TA], deep dorsal vein of clitoris: a vein that follows the course of its homonymous artery and opens into the vesical plexus; called also *v. dorsalis clitoridis profunda.*

**v. dorsa'lis profun'da pe'nis** [TA], deep dorsal vein of penis: a vein lying subfascially in the midline of the penis between the dorsal arteries; it begins in small veins around the corona glandis, is joined by the deep veins of the penis as it passes proximally, and passes between the arcuate pubic and transverse perineal ligaments where it divides into a left and right vein to join the prostatic plexus. Called also *v. dorsalis penis profunda.*

**ve'nae dorsa'les superficia'les clito'ridis** [TA], superficial dorsal veins of clitoris: veins that collect blood subcutaneously from the clitoris and drain into the external pudendal vein; called also *venae dorsales clitoridis superficiales.*

**ve'nae dorsa'les superficia'les pe'nis** [TA], superficial dorsal veins of penis: veins that collect blood subcutaneously from the penis and drain into the external pudendal vein; called also *venae dorsales penis superficiales.*

**v. emissa'ria** [TA], emissary vein: one of the small, valveless veins that pass through foramina of the skull, connecting the dural venous sinuses with scalp veins or with deep veins below the base of the skull. Called also *emissarium* and *emissary.*

**v. emissa'ria condyla'ris** [TA], **v. emissa'ria condyloi'dea,** condylar emissary vein: a small vein running through the condylar canal of the skull, connecting the sigmoid sinus with the vertebral or the internal jugular vein; called also *emissarium condyloideum.*

**v. emissa'ria mastoi'dea** [TA], mastoid emissary vein: a small vein passing through the mastoid foramen of the skull and connecting the sigmoid sinus with the occipital or the posterior auricular vein; called also *emissarium mastoideum.*

**v. emissa'ria occipita'lis** [TA], occipital emissary vein: an occasional small vein running through a minute foramen in the occipital protuberance of the skull and connecting the confluence of the sinuses with the occipital vein; called also *emissarium occipitale.*

**v. emissa'ria parieta'lis** [TA], parietal emissary vein: a small vein passing through the parietal foramen of the skull and connecting the superior sagittal sinus with the superficial temporal veins; called also *emissarium parietale.*

**ve'nae ence'phali** [TA], cerebral veins: veins that drain the surfaces or inner regions of the cerebral hemispheres; they are divided into superficial and deep groups (see *venae superficiales cerebri* and *venae profundae cerebri*). Called also *venae cerebri.*

**v. epigas'trica infe'rior** [TA], inferior epigastric vein: a vein that accompanies the inferior epigastric artery and opens into the external iliac vein.

**v. epigas'trica superficia'lis** [TA], superficial epigastric vein: a vein that follows its homonymous artery and opens into the great saphenous or the femoral vein.

**ve'nae epigas'tricae superio'res** [TA], superior epigastric veins: the venae comitantes of the superior epigastric artery, which open into the internal thoracic vein.

**v. epiplo'ica dex'tra,** v. gastroomentalis dextra.

**v. epiplo'ica sinis'tra,** v. gastroomentalis sinistra.

**ve'nae episclera'les** [TA], episcleral veins: the veins that ring the cornea and drain into the vorticose and ciliary veins.

**ve'nae esopha'geae, ve'nae esophagea'les,** venae oesophageales.

**ve'nae ethmoida'les** [TA], ethmoidal veins: veins that follow the anterior and posterior ethmoidal arteries, emerge from the ethmoidal foramina, and empty into the superior ophthalmic vein.

**v. ethmoida'lis ante'rior,** see *venae ethmoidales.*

**v. ethmoida'lis poste'rior,** see *venae ethmoidales.*

**v. facia'lis** [TA], facial vein: the vein that begins at the medial angle of the eye as the angular vein, descends behind the facial artery, and usually ends in the internal jugular vein; formerly called the *anterior facial vein* or *vena facialis anterior,* this vessel sometimes joins the retromandibular vein to form a common trunk previously known as the *common facial vein* or *vena facialis communis.*

**v. facia'lis ante'rior,** see *v. facialis.*

**v. facia'lis commu'nis,** see *v. facialis.*

**v. facia'lis poste'rior,** v. retromandibularis.

**v. facie'i profun'da,** v. profunda faciei.

**v. femora'lis** [TA], femoral vein: a vein that lies in the proximal two-thirds of the thigh; it is a direct continuation of the popliteal vein, follows the course of the femoral artery, and at the inguinal ligament becomes the external iliac vein. NOTE: Vascular surgeons refer to the portion of the femoral vein proximal to the branching of the deep femoral vein as the *common femoral vein,* and to its continuation distal to the branching as the *superficial femoral vein.*

**v. femoropopli'tea,** femoropopliteal vein: an inconstant superficial descending vein draining the lower and back part of the thigh and opening into the small saphenous vein just before it perforates the deep fascia.

**ve'nae fibula'res** [TA], fibular veins: the venae comitantes of the fibular artery, emptying into the posterior tibial vein; called also *venae peroneae* [TA alternative] and *peroneal veins.*

**ve'nae fronta'les** [TA], frontal veins: a group of superior cerebral veins, superficial cerebral veins that drain the cortex of the frontal lobe.

**ve'nae gas'tricae bre'ves** [TA], short gastric veins: small vessels draining the left portion of the greater curvature of the stomach and emptying into the splenic vein.

**v. gas'trica dex'tra** [TA], right gastric vein: the vena comitans of the right gastric artery, emptying into the portal vein.

**v. gas'trica sinis'tra** [TA], left gastric vein: the vena comitans of the left gastric artery, emptying into the portal vein.

**v. gastroepiplo'ica dex'tra,** TA alternative for *v. gastroomentalis dextra.*

**v. gastroepiplo'ica sinis'tra,** TA alternative for *v. gastroomentalis sinistra.*

**v. gastroomenta'lis dex'tra** [TA], right gastroomental vein: a vein that follows the distribution of its homonymous artery and empties into the superior mesenteric vein; called also *right epiploic vein, right gastroepiploic vein, epiploica dextra,* and *v. gastroepiploica dextra* [TA alternative].

**v. gastroomenta'lis sinis'tra** [TA], left gastroomental vein: a vein that follows the distribution of its homonymous artery and empties into the splenic vein; called also *left epiploic vein, left gastroepiploic vein, v. epiploica sinistra,* and *v. gastroepiploica sinistra* [TA alternative].

**ve'nae genicula'res** [TA], **ve'nae ge'nus,** genicular veins: veins accompanying the genicular arteries and draining into the popliteal vein.

**ve'nae glu'teae inferio'res** [TA], inferior gluteal veins: venae comitantes of the inferior gluteal artery; they drain the subcutaneous tissue of the back of the thigh and the muscles of the buttock, unite into a single vein after passing through the greater sciatic foramen, and empty into the internal iliac vein.

**ve'nae glu'teae superio'res** [TA], superior gluteal veins: venae comitantes of the superior gluteal artery; they drain the muscles of the buttock, pass through the greater sciatic foramen, and empty into the internal iliac vein.

**v. gy'ri olfacto'rii** [TA], vein of olfactory gyrus: a vein that drains the olfactory gyrus into the basal vein.

**v. hemia'zygos** [TA], hemiazygos vein: an intercepting trunk for the lower left posterior intercostal veins; it arises from the ascending lumbar vein, passes up on the left side of the vertebrae to the eighth thoracic vertebra, where it may receive the accessory branch, and crosses over the vertebral column to open into the azygos vein.

**v. hemia'zygos accesso'ria** [TA], accessory hemiazygos vein: the descending intercepting trunk for the upper, often the fourth through the eighth, left posterior intercostal veins. It lies on the left side and at the eighth thoracic vertebra joins the hemiazygos vein or crosses to the right side to join the azygos vein directly; above, it may communicate with the left superior intercostal vein.

**ve'nae hepa'ticae** [TA], hepatic veins: several veins that receive blood from the central veins of the liver. The upper group usually consists of two or three large veins, and the lower group consists of six to twenty small veins; all form successively larger vessels *(right, left,* and *middle hepatic veins)* that ultimately open into the inferior vena cava on the posterior aspect of the liver.

**ve'nae hepa'ticae dex'trae** [TA], right hepatic veins: the larger veins that drain the right side of the liver and ultimately empty into the inferior vena cava.

**ve'nae hepa'ticae interme'diae** [TA], intermediate hepatic veins: the larger veins that drain the middle part of the liver and ultimately empty into the inferior vena cava. Called also *middle hepatic veins* and *venae hepaticae mediae.*

**ve'nae hepa'ticae me'diae,** venae hepaticae intermediae.

**ve'nae hepa'ticae sinis'trae** [TA], left hepatic veins: the larger veins that drain the left side of the liver and ultimately empty into the inferior vena cava.

**ve'nae ilea'les** [TA], ileal veins: veins draining blood from the ileum into the superior mesenteric vein.

**v. ileoco'lica** [TA], ileocolic vein: a vein that follows the distribution of its homonymous artery and empties into the vena mesenterica superior.

**v. ili'aca commu'nis** [TA], common iliac vein: a vein that arises at the sacroiliac articulation by union of the external iliac and the internal iliac veins, and passes upward to the right side of the fifth lumbar vertebra where the two unite to form the inferior vena cava.

**v. ili'aca exter'na** [TA], external iliac vein: the continuation of the femoral vein from the inguinal ligament to the sacroiliac articulation, where it joins with the internal iliac vein to form the common iliac vein.

**v. ili'aca inter'na** [TA], internal iliac vein: a short trunk formed by union of parietal branches; it extends from the greater sciatic notch to the brim of the pelvis, where it joins the external iliac vein to form the common iliac vein.

**v. iliolumba'lis** [TA], iliolumbar vein: a vein that follows the distribution of the iliolumbar artery and opens into the internal iliac or the common iliac vein, or it may divide to end in both.

**ve'nae inferio'res cerebel'li** [TA], inferior veins of cerebellum: veins that drain the inferior surface of the cerebellum and empty into the transverse, sigmoid, inferior petrosal, and occipital sinuses.

**ve'nae inferio'res ce'rebri** [TA], inferior cerebral veins: rather large superficial cerebral veins that ramify on the base and the inferolateral surface of the brain: those on the inferior surface of the frontal lobe drain into the inferior sagittal sinus and the cavernous sinus; those on the temporal lobe, into the superior petrosal sinus and the transverse sinus; those on the occipital lobe into the straight sinus. Called also *venae cerebri inferiores.*

**v. infe'rior ver'mis** [TA], inferior vein of vermis: a vein that drains the inferior surface of the cerebellum; it runs backward on the inferior vermis to empty into the straight sinus or one of the sigmoid sinuses; called also *v. vermis inferior.*

**ve'nae insula'res** [TA], insular veins: veins that drain the insula and join the deep middle cerebral vein.

**ve'nae intercapita'les,** venae intercapitulares manus.

**ve'nae intercapita'les ma'nus,** venae intercapitulares manus.

**ve'nae intercapitula'res ma'nus** [TA], intercapitular veins of hand: veins at the clefts of the finger which pass between the heads of the metacarpal bones and establish communication between the dorsal and the palmar venous system of the hand; called also *venae intercapitales manus.*

**ve'nae intercapitula'res pe'dis** [TA], intercapitular veins of foot: veins at the clefts of the toes which pass between the heads of the metatarsal bones and establish communication between the dorsal and the plantar venous system.

**ve'nae intercosta'les anterio'res** [TA], anterior intercostal veins: the twelve paired venae comitantes of the anterior thoracic arteries, which drain into the internal thoracic veins.

**ve'nae intercosta'les posterio'res** [TA], posterior intercostal veins: the veins that accompany the corresponding intercostal arteries and drain the intercostal spaces posteriorly; the first ends in the brachiocephalic or the vertebral vein, the second and third join the superior intercostal vein, and the fourth to eleventh join the azygos vein on the right and the hemiazygos veins on the left.

**v. intercosta'lis supe'rior dex'tra** [TA], right superior intercostal vein: a common trunk formed by union of the second, third, and sometimes fourth posterior intercostal veins, which drains into the azygos vein.

**v. intercosta'lis supe'rior sinis'tra** [TA], left superior intercostal vein: the common trunk formed by union of the second, third, and sometimes fourth posterior intercostal veins, which crosses the arch of the aorta and joins the left brachiocephalic vein.

**v. intercosta'lis supre'ma** [TA], highest intercostal vein: the first posterior intercostal vein of either side, which passes over the apex of the lung and ends in the brachiocephalic, vertebral, or superior intercostal vein.

**ve'nae interloba'res re'nis** [TA], interlobar veins of kidney: veins that drain the venous arcades of the kidney, pass down between the pyramids, and unite to form the renal vein.

**ve'nae interlobula'res he'patis** [TA], interlobular veins of liver: the veins that arise as tributaries of the portal vein between the hepatic lobules.

**ve'nae interlobula'res re'nis** [TA], interlobular veins of kidney: veins that collect blood from the capillary network of the cortex and empty into the venous arcades of the kidney.

**v. interme'dia antebra'chii,** v. mediana antebrachii.

**v. interme'dia basi'lica,** median basilic vein: a vein sometimes present as the medial branch, ending in the basilic vein, of a bifurcation of the median antebrachial vein; called also *v. mediana basilica.*

**v. interme'dia cepha'lica,** median cephalic vein: a vein sometimes present as the lateral branch, ending in the cephalic vein, formed by bifurcation of the median antebrachial vein; called also *v. mediana cephalica.*

**v. interme'dia cu'biti,** v. mediana cubiti.

**ve'nae inter'nae ce'rebri** [TA], internal cerebral veins: two veins that arise at the interventricular foramen by the union on the thalamostriate and the choroid veins; they pass backward through the tela choroidea, collecting blood from the basal nuclei, and unite at the splenium of the corpus callosum to form the great cerebral vein. Called also *venae cerebri internae.*

**ve'nae interos'seae anterio'res** [TA], anterior interosseous veins: the veins accompanying the anterior interosseous artery, which join the ulnar veins near the elbow.

**ve'nae interos'seae posterio'res** [TA], posterior interosseous veins: the veins accompanying the posterior interosseous artery, which join the ulnar veins near the elbow.

**v. interventricula'ris ante'rior** [TA], anterior interventricular vein: the portion of the great cardiac vein ascending in the anterior interventricular sulcus and emptying into the left coronary vein.

**v. interventricula'ris poste'rior,** TA alternative for *v. cardiaca media.*

**v. intervertebra'lis** [TA], intervertebral vein: any one of the veins that drain the vertebral plexuses, passing out through the intervertebral foramina and emptying into the regional veins: in the neck, into the vertebral; in the thorax, the intercostal; in the abdomen, the lumbar; and in the pelvis, the lateral sacral veins.

**ve'nae jejuna'les** [TA], jejunal veins: veins draining blood from the jejunum into the superior mesenteric vein.

**v. jugula'ris ante'rior** [TA], anterior jugular vein: a vein that arises under the chin, passes down the neck, and opens into the external jugular or the subclavian vein or into the jugular venous arch.

**v. jugula'ris exter'na** [TA], external jugular vein: the vein that begins in the parotid gland behind the angle of the jaw by union of the retromandibular and the posterior auricular vein, passes down the neck, and opens into the subclavian, the internal jugular, or the brachiocephalic vein.

**v. jugula'ris inter'na** [TA], internal jugular vein: the vein that begins as the superior bulb in the jugular fossa, draining much of the head and neck; it descends with first the internal carotid and then the common carotid artery in the neck, and joins with the subclavian vein to form the brachiocephalic vein.

**ve'nae labia'les anterio'res** [TA], anterior labial veins: veins that collect blood from the anterior aspect of the labia and drain into the external pudendal vein; they are homologues of the anterior scrotal veins in the male.

**ve'nae labia'les inferio'res** [TA], inferior labial veins: veins that drain the region of the lower lip into the facial vein.

**ve'nae labia'les posterio'res** [TA], posterior labial veins: small branches from the labia which open into the vesical venous plexus; they are homologues of the posterior scrotal veins in the male.

**v. labia'lis supe'rior** [TA], superior labial vein: the vein that drains blood from the region of the upper lip into the facial vein.

**ve'nae labyrin'thi** [TA], **ve'nae labyrinthi'nae,** veins of labyrinth: several small veins that pass through the internal acoustic meatus from the cochlea into the inferior petrosal or the transverse sinus; called also *internal auditory veins* and *labyrinthine veins.*

**v. lacrima'lis** [TA], lacrimal vein: the vein that drains blood from the lacrimal gland into the superior ophthalmic vein.

**v. laryn'gea infe'rior** [TA], inferior laryngeal vein: a vein draining blood from the larynx into the inferior thyroid vein.

**v. laryn'gea supe'rior** [TA], superior laryngeal vein: a vein that drains blood from the larynx into the superior thyroid vein.

**v. latera'lis ventri'culi latera'lis** [TA], lateral vein of lateral ventricle: a vein passing through the lateral wall of the lateral ventricle to drain the temporal and parietal lobes into the superior thalamostriate vein.

**v. liena'lis,** TA alternative for *v. splenica.*

**v. lingua'lis** [TA], lingual vein: the deep vein that follows the distribution of the lingual artery and empties into the internal jugular vein.

**v. lingula'ris** [TA], lingular vein: a venous branch that drains the lingular segments of the superior lobe of the left lung, emptying into the left superior pulmonary vein and formed by the union of superior and inferior parts. Called also *ramus lingularis venae pulmonalis sinistrae superioris* [TA alternative].

**v. lo'bi me'dii pulmo'nis dex'tri** [TA], middle lobar vein of right lung: a branch that drains the middle lobe of the right lung, emptying into the right superior pulmonary vein and formed by the union of lateral and medial parts. Called also *ramus lobi medii venae pulmonalis dextrae superior* [TA alternative].

**ve'nae lumba'les** [TA], lumbar veins: the veins, four or five on each side, that accompany the corresponding lumbar arteries and drain the posterior wall of the abdomen, vertebral canal, spinal cord, and meninges; the first four usually end in the inferior vena cava, although the first may end in the ascending lumbar vein; the fifth is a tributary of the iliolumbar or of the common iliac vein; and all are generally united by the ascending iliac vein.

**v. lumba'lis ascen'dens** [TA], ascending lumbar vein: an ascending intercepting vein for the lumbar veins of either side; it begins in the lateral sacral veins and passes up the spine to the first lumbar vertebra, where by union with the subcostal vein it becomes on the right side the azygos vein, and on the left side, the hemiazygos vein.

**v. mag'na ce'rebri** [TA], great cerebral vein: a short median trunk formed by union of the two internal cerebral veins, which curves around the splenium of the corpus callosum and empties into, or is continued as, the straight sinus; called also *v. cerebri magna.*

**v. margina'lis dex'tra** [TA], right marginal vein: a vein ascending along the right margin of the heart, draining adjacent parts of the right ventricle and opening into the right atrium or anterior cardiac veins.

**v. margina'lis latera'lis** [TA], lateral marginal vein: a vein running along the lateral side of the foot, returning blood from the dorsal venous arch, dorsal venous network, and superficial veins of the sole and draining into the small saphenous vein.

**v. margina'lis media'lis** [TA], medial marginal vein: a vein running along the medial side of the dorsum of the foot, returning blood from the dorsal venous arch, the dorsal venous network, and superficial veins of the sole and draining into the great saphenous vein.

**ve'nae massete'ricae,** masseteric veins: veins from the masseter muscle that empty into the facial vein.

**ve'nae maxilla'res** [TA], maxillary veins: veins from the pterygoid plexus, usually forming a single short trunk, passing back and uniting with the superficial temporal vein in the parotid gland to form the retromandibular vein.

**v. me'dia profun'da ce'rebri** [TA], deep middle cerebral vein: the vein that accompanies the middle cerebral artery in the floor of the lateral sulcus, and joins the basal vein.

**v. me'dia superficia'lis ce'rebri** [TA], superficial middle cerebral vein: either of the two veins, one in each hemisphere, that drain the lateral surface of the cerebrum, follow the lateral cerebral fissure, and empty into the cavernous sinus; they are fed by the inferior and superior anastomotic veins. Called also *sylvian vein and vein of sylvian fossa.*

**v. media'lis ventri'culi latera'lis** [TA], medial vein of lateral ventricle: a vein passing through the medial wall of the lateral ventricle to drain the parietal and occipital lobes into the internal cerebral or great cerebral vein.

**v. media'na antebra'chii** [TA], median antebrachial vein: a vein that arises from a palmar venous plexus and passes up the forearm between the cephalic and the basilic veins to the elbow, where it either joins one of these, bifurcates to join both, or joins the median cubital vein; called also *median vein of forearm* and *v. intermedia antebrachii.*

**v. media'na basi'lica,** v. intermedia basilica.

**v. media'na cepha'lica,** v. intermedia cephalica.

**v. media'na col'li,** median vein of neck: a vein sometimes formed when the anterior jugular veins unite as they pass down the neck.

**v. media'na cu'biti** [TA], median cubital vein: the large connecting branch that arises from the cephalic vein below the elbow and passes obliquely upward over the cubital fossa to join the basilic vein; called also *median vein of elbow* and *v. intermedia cubiti.*

**ve'nae mediastina'les** [TA], mediastinal veins: numerous small branches that drain blood from the anterior mediastinum into the brachiocephalic vein, azygos vein, or the superior vena cava.

**ve'nae medul'lae oblonga'tae** [TA], veins of medulla oblongata: the veins that drain the medulla oblongata, which empty into the veins of the spinal cord, the adjacent dural venous sinuses, or along the last four cranial nerves to the inferior petrosal sinus or superior bulb of the jugular vein.

**ve'nae mem'bri inferio'ris** [TA], veins of lower limb: veins that drain the thigh, leg, and foot, divided into *superficial veins* (those in the superficial fascia) and *deep veins* (those that accompany arteries). See also *venae profundae membri inferioris* and *venae superficiales membri inferioris.*

**ve'nae mem'bri superio'ris** [TA], veins of upper limb: veins that drain the arm, forearm, and hand, divided into *superficial veins* (those in the superficial fascia) and *deep veins* (those that accompany arteries); there are frequent anastomoses between the two groups. See also *venae profundae membri superioris* and *venae superficiales membri superioris.*

**ve'nae menin'geae** [TA], meningeal veins: the venae comitantes of the meningeal arteries, which drain the dura mater, communicate with the lateral lacunae, and empty into the regional sinuses and veins.

**ve'nae menin'geae me'diae** [TA], middle meningeal veins: the venae comitantes of the middle meningeal artery, which end in the pterygoid venous plexus.

**ve'nae mesencepha'licae,** venae trunci encephalici.

**v. mesente'rica infe'rior** [TA], inferior mesenteric vein: a vein that follows the distribution of its homonymous artery and empties into the splenic vein.

**v. mesente'rica supe'rior** [TA], superior mesenteric vein: a vein that follows the distribution of its homonymous artery and joins with the splenic vein to form the hepatic portal vein.

**ve'nae metacarpa'les dorsa'les** [TA], dorsal metacarpal veins: veins that arise from the union of dorsal veins of adjacent fingers and pass proximally to join in forming the dorsal venous rete of the hand; called also *venae metacarpeae dorsales.*

**ve'nae metacarpa'les palma'res** [TA], palmar metacarpal veins: the venae comitantes of the palmar metacarpal arteries, which open into the deep palmar venous arch; called also *venae metacarpeae palmares.*

**ve'nae metacar'peae dorsa'les,** venae metacarpales dorsales.

**ve'nae metacar'peae palma'res,** venae metacarpales palmares.

**ve'nae metatarsa'les dorsa'les** [TA], dorsal metatarsal veins: veins that are formed by the dorsal digital veins of the toes at the clefts of the toes, joining the dorsal venous arch; called also *venae metatarseae dorsales.*

**ve'nae metatarsa'les planta'res** [TA], plantar metatarsal veins: deep veins of the foot that arise from the plantar digital veins at the clefts of the toes and pass back to open into the plantar venous arch; called also *venae metatarseae plantares.*

**ve'nae metatar'seae dorsa'les,** venae metatarsales dorsales.

**ve'nae metatar'seae planta'res,** venae metatarsales plantares.

**ve'nae musculophre'nicae** [TA], musculophrenic veins: the venae comitantes of the musculophrenic artery, draining blood from parts of the diaphragm and from the wall of the thorax and abdomen.

**ve'nae nasa'les exter'nae** [TA], external nasal veins: small ascending branches from the nose that open into the angular and facial veins.

**v. nasofronta'lis** [TA], nasofrontal vein: a vein that begins at the supraorbital vein, enters the orbit, and joins the superior ophthalmic vein.

**ve'nae nu'clei cauda'ti** [TA], the veins of the caudate nucleus, located within the corpus striatum.

**v. obli'qua a'trii sinis'tri** [TA], oblique vein of left atrium: a small vein from the left atrium that opens into the coronary sinus. Called also *vein of Marshall* and *Marshall's oblique vein.*

**ve'nae obturato'riae** [TA], obturator veins: veins that drain the hip joint and the regional muscles, enter the pelvis through the obturator canal, and empty into the internal iliac or the inferior epigastric vein, or both.

**ve'nae occipita'les** [TA], occipital veins: a group of superior cerebral veins, superficial cerebral veins that drain the cortex of the occipital lobe.

**v. occipita'lis** [TA], occipital vein: a vein in the scalp that follows the distribution of the occipital artery and opens under the trapezius muscle into the suboccipital venous plexus; it may continue with the occipital artery and end in the internal jugular vein.

**ve'nae oesophagea'les** [TA], esophageal veins: small veins that drain blood from the esophagus into the hemiazygos and azygos veins, or into the left brachiocephalic vein; called also *venae esophageae* and *venae esophageales.*

**v. ophthal'mica infe'rior** [TA], inferior ophthalmic vein: a vein formed by confluence of muscular and ciliary branches, and running backward either to join the superior ophthalmic vein or to open directly into the cavernous sinus; it sends a communicating branch through the inferior orbital fissure to join the pterygoid venous plexus.

**v. ophthal'mica supe'rior** [TA], superior ophthalmic vein: the vein that begins at the medial angle of the eyelid, where it communicates with the frontal, supraorbital, and angular veins; it follows the distribution of the ophthalmic artery, and may be joined by the inferior ophthalmic vein at the superior orbital fissure before opening into the cavernous sinus.

**v. ophthalmomenin'gea,** ophthalmomeningeal vein: a small inferior meningeal vein that opens usually into the superior ophthalmic vein, or occasionally into the superior petrosal sinus.

**ve'nae or'bitae** [TA], veins of orbit: the veins that drain the orbit and its structures, including the superior ophthalmic vein and its tributaries and the inferior ophthalmic vein.

**v. ova'rica dex'tra** [TA], right ovarian vein: a vein that drains the pampiniform plexus of the broad ligament on the right into the inferior vena cava.

**v. ova'rica sinis'tra** [TA], left ovarian vein: a vein that drains the pampiniform plexus of the broad ligament on the left into the left renal vein.

**v. palati'na,** v. palatina externa.

**v. palati'na exter'na** [TA], external palatine vein: the vein that drains blood from the tonsils and the soft palate into the facial vein; called also *v. palatina.*

**ve'nae palpebra'les** [TA], palpebral veins: small branches from the eyelids that open into the superior ophthalmic vein.

**ve'nae palpebra'les inferio'res** [TA], inferior palpebral veins: branches that drain the blood from the lower eyelid into the facial vein.

**ve'nae palpebra'les superio'res** [TA], superior palpebral veins: branches that drain the blood from the upper eyelid to the angular vein.

**ve'nae pancrea'ticae** [TA], pancreatic veins: numerous branches from the pancreas which open into the splenic and the superior mesenteric veins.

**ve'nae pancreaticoduodena'les** [TA], pancreaticoduodenal veins: four veins that drain blood from the pancreas and duodenum, closely following the homonymous arteries. A superior and an inferior vein originate from both an anterior and a posterior venous arcade. The anterior superior vein joins the right gastroomental vein; the posterior superior vein joins the portal vein. The anterior and posterior inferior veins join, sometimes as one trunk and other times joining the uppermost jejunal vein or the superior mesenteric vein.

**ve'nae paraumbilica'les** [TA], paraumbilical veins: veins that communicate with the portal vein and anastomose with the superior and inferior epigastric and the superior vesical veins in the region of the umbilicus. They form a part of the collateral circulation of the portal vein in the event of hepatic obstruction. Called also *parumbilical veins* and *veins of Sappey.*

**ve'nae parieta'les** [TA], parietal veins: a group of superior cerebral veins, superficial cerebral veins that drain the cortex of the parietal lobe.

**ve'nae paroti'deae** [TA], parotid veins: small veins from the parotid gland that open into the superficial temporal vein; called also *posterior parotid veins.*

**ve'nae pectora'les** [TA], pectoral veins: collective term for branches of the subclavian vein that drain the pectoral region.

**ve'nae peduncula'res** [TA], peduncular veins: veins that drain the cerebral peduncle into the basal vein.

**ve'nae perforan'tes** [TA], perforating veins: veins that accompany the perforating arteries and connect superficial and deep veins, establishing an anastomosis between the deep femoral vein and the popliteal vein below and the inferior gluteal vein above. Called also *communicating veins.*

**ve'nae pericardi'acae** [TA], pericardial veins: numerous small branches that drain blood from the pericardium into the brachiocephalic, inferior thyroid and azygos veins, and the superior vena cava; called also *venae pericardiales* and *pericardiac veins.*

**ve'nae pericardiacophre'nicae** [TA], pericardiacophrenic veins: small veins that drain blood from the pericardium and diaphragm into the left brachiocephalic vein.

**ve'nae pericardia'les,** venae pericardiacae.

**ve'nae perone'ae,** TA alternative for *venae fibulares.*

**v. petro'sa** [TA], petrosal vein: a short trunk arising from the union of four or five cerebellar and pontine veins opposite the middle cerebellar peduncle and terminating in the superior petrosal sinus.

**ve'nae pharyn'geae** [TA], **ve'nae pharyngea'les,** pharyngeal veins: veins that drain the pharyngeal plexus and empty into the internal jugular vein.

**ve'nae phre'nicae inferio'res** [TA], inferior phrenic veins: veins that follow the homonymous arteries, the one on the right entering the inferior vena cava, and the one on the left entering the left suprarenal or renal vein or the inferior vena cava.

**ve'nae phre'nicae superio'res** [TA], superior phrenic veins: small veins on the superior surface of the diaphragm that drain into the azygos and hemiazygos veins.

**ve'nae pon'tis** [TA], veins of pons: the veins that drain the pons, which empty into the basal vein, cerebellar veins, petrosal or venous sinuses, or venous plexus of the foramen ovale.

**v. pontomesencepha'lica ante'rior** [TA], anterior pontomesencephalic vein: a vein lying on the superior and anterior aspects of the pons in the midline of the interpeduncular fossa, communicating superiorly with the basal vein and inferiorly with the petrosal vein.

**v. popli'tea** [TA], popliteal vein: a vein following the popliteal artery, and formed by union of the venae comitantes of the anterior and posterior tibial arteries; at the adductor hiatus it becomes continuous with the femoral vein.

**v. por'tae he'patis** [TA], **v. porta'lis he'patis,** portal vein of liver: a short thick trunk formed by union of the superior mesenteric and the splenic veins behind the neck of the pancreas; it passes upward to the right end of the porta hepatis, where it divides into successively smaller branches, following the branches of the hepatic artery, until it forms a capillary-like system of sinusoids that permeates the entire substance of the liver. Called also *hepatic portal vein* and *portal vein.*

**ve'nae porta'les hypophysia'les** [TA], hypophyseoportal veins: a system of venules connecting capillaries in the hypothalamus with sinusoidal capillaries in the anterior lobe of the hypophysis. Called also *portal veins of hypophysis.*

**v. poste'rior cor'poris callo'si** [TA], posterior vein of corpus callosum: a vein that drains the posterior surface of the corpus callosum into the great cerebral vein.

**v. poste'rior lo'bi superio'ris pulmo'nis dex'tri** [TA], posterior branch of right superior pulmonary vein: a branch that drains the posterior segment of the right upper lobe; called also *ramus posterior venae pulmonalis dextrae superioris* [TA alternative] and *posterior segmental vein of right lung.*

**v. poste'rior sep'ti pellu'cidi** [TA], posterior vein of septum pellucidum: a vein that drains the posterior septum pellucidum into the superior thalamostriate vein; called also *v. septi pellucidi posterior.*

**v. poste'rior ventri'culi sinis'tri cor'dis,** v. ventriculi sinistri posterior cordis.

**v. precentra'lis cerebel'li** [TA], precentral vein of cerebellum: a vein arising in the precentral cerebellar fissure and passing anterior and superior to the culmen, terminating in the great cerebral vein.

**ve'nae prefronta'les** [TA], prefrontal veins: a group of superior cerebral veins, superficial cerebral veins that drain the prefrontal area of the cerebral cortex.

**v. prepylo'rica** [TA], prepyloric vein: a vein that accompanies the prepyloric artery, passing upward over the anterior surface of the junction between the pylorus and the duodenum and emptying into the right gastric vein. Called also *Mayo's vein.*

**v. profun'da** [TA], deep vein: any deeply situated vein.

**ve'nae profun'dae ce'rebri** [TA], deep cerebral veins: the veins that drain the inner regions of the cerebral hemispheres, consisting of the basal veins, the great cerebral veins, the veins of the encephalic trunk, and their tributaries. Called also *venae cerebri profundae.*

**ve'nae profun'dae clito'ridis** [TA], deep veins of clitoris: small veins of the clitoris that drain into the vesical venous plexus.

**v. profun'da facia'lis,** TA alternative for *v. profunda faciei.*

**v. profun'da facie'i** [TA], deep facial vein: a vein draining from the pterygoid plexus to the facial vein; called also *v. faciei profunda* and *v. profunda facialis* [TA alternative].

**v. profun'da fe'moris** [TA], deep femoral vein: a vein that follows the distribution of the deep femoral artery and opens into the femoral vein.

**v. profun'da lin'guae** [TA], deep lingual vein: a vein that drains blood from the deep aspect of the tongue and joins the sublingual vein to form the vena comitans of the hypoglossal nerve.

**ve'nae profun'dae mem'bri inferio'ris** [TA], deep veins of lower limb: veins that drain the lower limb, found accompanying homonymous arteries, and anastomosing freely with the superficial veins; the principal deep veins are the femoral and popliteal veins.

**ve'nae profun'dae mem'bri superio'ris** [TA], deep veins of upper limb: veins that drain the upper limb, found accompanying homonymous arteries, and anastomosing freely with the superficial veins; they include the brachial, ulnar, and radial veins, and their tributaries, all of which ultimately drain into the axillary vein.

**ve'nae profun'dae pe'nis** [TA], deep veins of penis: veins that follow the distribution of the homonymous artery and empty into the dorsal vein of the penis.

**ve'nae puden'dae exter'nae** [TA], external pudendal veins: veins that follow the distribution of the external pudendal artery and open into the great saphenous vein.

**v. puden'da inter'na** [TA], internal pudendal vein: a vein that follows the course of the internal pudendal artery, and drains into the internal iliac vein.

**ve'nae pulmona'les** [TA], pulmonary veins: the four veins, right and left superior and right and left inferior, that return aerated blood from the lungs to the left atrium of the heart. See also *segmenta bronchopulmonalia.*

**v. pulmona'lis dex'tra infe'rior** [TA], right inferior pulmonary vein: the vein that returns blood from the lower lobe of the right lung (from the superior [apical] branch and from the common, superior, and inferior basal veins) to the left atrium of the heart; called also *v. pulmonalis inferior dextra.*

**v. pulmona'lis dex'tra supe'rior** [TA], right superior pulmonary vein: the vein that returns blood from the upper and middle lobes of the right lung (from the superior [apical], anterior, and posterior branches and the middle lobar branch) to the left atrium of the heart; called also *v. pulmonalis superior dextra.*

**v. pulmona'lis infe'rior dex'tra,** v. pulmonalis dextra inferior.

**v. pulmona'lis infe'rior sinis'tra,** v. pulmonalis sinistra inferior.

**v. pulmona'lis sinis'tra infe'rior** [TA], left inferior pulmonary vein: the vein that returns blood from the lower lobe of the left lung (from the superior apical branch and the common basal vein) to the left atrium of the heart; called also *v. pulmonalis inferior sinistra.*

**v. pulmona'lis sinis'tra supe'rior** [TA], left superior pulmonary vein: the vein that returns blood from the upper lobe of the left lung (from the apicoposterior, anterior, and lingular branches) to the left atrium of the heart; called also *v. pulmonalis superior sinistra.*

**v. pulmona'lis supe'rior dex'tra,** v. pulmonalis dextra superior.

**v. pulmona'lis supe'rior sinis'tra,** v. pulmonalis sinistra superior.

**ve'nae radia'les** [TA], radial veins: the venae comitantes of the radial artery, which open into the brachial veins.

**v. reces'sus latera'lis ventri'culi quar'ti** [TA], vein of lateral recess of fourth ventricle: a small vein arising in the tonsil of the cerebellum, passing the lateral recess of the fourth ventricle, and terminating in the petrosal vein.

**ve'nae recta'les inferio'res** [TA], inferior rectal veins: veins that drain the rectal plexus into the internal pudendal vein.

**ve'nae recta'les me'diae** [TA], middle rectal veins: veins that drain the rectal plexus and empty into the internal iliac and superior rectal veins.

**v. recta'lis supe'rior** [TA], superior rectal vein: the vein that drains the upper part of the rectal plexus into the inferior mesenteric vein and thus establishes connection between the portal system and the systemic circulation.

**ve'nae rena'les** [TA], **ve'nae re'nis,** renal veins: the veins within the kidney, including the interlobular, arcuate, and interlobular veins, the venulae stellatae, and the venulae rectae.

**v. retromandibula'ris** [TA], retromandibular vein: the vein that is formed in the upper part of the parotid gland behind the neck of the mandible by union of the maxillary and superficial temporal veins; it passes downward through the gland, communicates with the facial vein, and emerging from the gland joins with the posterior auricular vein to form the external jugular vein. Called also *v. facialis posterior.*

**ve'nae revehen'tes,** revehent veins: channels in the early embryo that convey blood from the sinusoids of the liver to the sinus venosus and later become the hepatic veins.

**ve'nae sacra'les latera'les** [TA], lateral sacral veins: veins that follow the homonymous arteries, help to form the lateral sacral plexus, and empty into the internal iliac vein or the superior gluteal veins.

**v. sacra'lis me'dia,** v. sacralis mediana.

**v. sacra'lis media'na** [TA], median sacral vein: a vein that follows the middle sacral artery and opens into the common iliac vein; called also *v. sacralis media* and *middle sacral vein.*

**v. saphe'na accesso'ria** [TA], accessory saphenous vein: a vein that, when present, drains the medial and posterior superficial parts of the thigh and opens into the great saphenous vein.

**v. saphe'na mag'na** [TA], great saphenous vein: the longest vein in the body, extending from the dorsum of the foot to just below the inguinal ligament, where it opens into the femoral vein.

**v. saphe'na par'va** [TA], small saphenous vein: the vein that continues the marginal vein from behind the malleolus and passes up the back of the leg to the knee joint, where it opens into the popliteal vein.

**v. scapula'ris dorsa'lis** [TA], dorsal scapular vein: a branch occasionally seen contributing to the subclavian vein.

**ve'nae sclera'les** [TA], scleral veins: tributaries of the anterior ciliary veins that drain the sclera.

**ve'nae scrota'les anterio'res** [TA], anterior scrotal veins: veins that collect blood from the anterior aspect of the scrotum and drain into the external pudendal vein.

**ve'nae scrota'les posterio'res** [TA], posterior scrotal veins: small branches from the scrotum that open into the vesical venous plexus.

**v. sep'ti pellu'cidi ante'rior,** v. anterior septi pellucidi.

**v. sep'ti pellu'cidi poste'rior,** v. posterior septi pellucidi.

**ve'nae sigmoi'deae** [TA], sigmoid veins: veins from the sigmoid colon that empty into the inferior mesenteric vein.

**ve'nae spina'les anterio'res** [TA], anterior spinal veins: a group of longitudinal veins forming a plexus on the dorsal surface of the spinal cord, comprising a median vein lying anterior to the anterior median fissure and two anterolateral veins lying slightly posterior to the ventral nerve roots; they drain the anterior spinal cord. See also *plexus venosus vertebralis externus anterior* and *plexus venosus vertebralis internus anterior.*

**ve'nae spina'les posterio'res** [TA], posterior spinal veins: a group of longitudinal, usually discontinuous, veins forming a plexus on the posterior surface of the spinal cord, comprising a median vein lying behind the posterior median septum and two posterolateral veins lying posterior to the dorsal nerve roots; they drain the posterior spinal cord. See also *plexus venosus vertebralis externus posterior* and *plexus venosus vertebralis internus posterior.*

**v. spira'lis modi'oli,** spiral vein of modiolus: a small vein in the spiral modiolus, a tributary of the labyrinthine veins.

**v. sple'nica** [TA], splenic vein: the vein formed by union of several branches at the hilum of the spleen, passing from left to right to the neck of the pancreas, where it joins the superior mesenteric vein to form the portal vein; called also *v. lienalis* [TA alternative].

**ve'nae stella'tae re'nis** [TA], stellate veins of kidney: veins on the surface of the kidney that collect blood from the superficial parts of the cortex and empty into the interlobular veins; called also *Verheyen's stars* or *stellulae.*

**v. sternocleidomastoi'dea** [TA], sternocleidomastoid vein: a vein that follows the course of the homonymous artery and opens into the internal jugular vein.

**ve'nae stria'tae,** venae thalamostriatae inferiores.

**v. stylomastoi'dea** [TA], stylomastoid vein: a vein following the stylomastoid artery and emptying into the retromandibular vein.

**v. subcla'via** [TA], subclavian vein: the vein that continues the axillary as the main venous stem of the upper member, follows the subclavian artery, and joins with the internal jugular vein to form the brachiocephalic vein.

**v. subcosta'lis** [TA], subcostal vein: the vena comitans of the subcostal artery on the left or right side; it joins the ascending lumbar vein to form the azygos vein on the right or the hemiazygos vein on the left.

**ve'nae subcuta'neae abdo'minis** [TA], subcutaneous veins of abdomen: the superficial veins of the abdominal wall.

**v. sublingua'lis** [TA], sublingual vein: a vein that follows the sublingual artery and opens into the lingual vein.

**v. submenta'lis** [TA], submental vein: a vein that follows the submental artery and opens into the facial vein.

**v. superficia'lis** [TA], superficial vein: any superficially situated vein.

**ve'nae superficia'les ce'rebri** [TA], superficial cerebral veins: the veins that drain the surfaces of the cerebral hemispheres, comprising the superior, inferior, and middle superficial cerebral veins and their tributaries; called also *venae cerebri superficiales.*

**ve'nae superficia'les mem'bri inferio'ris** [TA], superficial veins of lower limb: veins that drain the lower limb, found immediately beneath the skin, and anastomosing freely with the deep veins; the principal superficial veins are the great and small saphenous veins.

**ve'nae superficia'les mem'bri superio'ris** [TA], superficial veins of upper limb: veins that drain the upper limb, found immediately beneath the skin, and anastomosing freely with the deep veins; they include the cephalic, basilic, and median cubital and antebrachial veins, and their tributaries, all of which ultimately drain into the axillary vein.

**superior v. cava, persistent left,** a developmental anomaly in which the left superior vena cava persists into postnatal life, usually draining into the left atrium; it is due to failure of the upper part of the left anterior cardinal vein to become obliterated. It may be an isolated anomaly or accompany other cardiovascular defects, such as tetralogy of Fallot.

**ve'nae superio'res cerebel'li** [TA], superior veins of cerebellum: veins that drain the superior surfaces of the cerebellar hemisphere and empty into the straight sinus and the great cerebral vein or into the transverse and superior petrosal sinuses.

**ve'nae superio'res ce'rebri** [TA], superior cerebral veins: the 8 to 12 superficial cerebral veins (prefrontal, frontal, parietal, and occipital) that drain the superior, lateral, and medial surfaces of the cerebrum toward the longitudinal cerebral fissure, where they open into the superior sagittal sinus; called also *venae cerebri superiores.*

**v. supe'rior lo'bi inferio'ris pulmo'nis dex'tri** [TA], superior vein of inferior lobe of right lung: a venous branch that drains the superior segment of the inferior lobe of the right lung and empties into the right inferior pulmonary vein. Called also *ramus superior venae pulmonalis dextrae inferioris* [TA alternative] and *superior segmental vein of right lung.*

**v. supe'rior lo'bi inferio'ris pulmo'nis sinis'tri** [TA], superior vein of inferior lobe of left lung: a venous branch that drains the superior segment of the inferior lobe of the left lung and empties into the left inferior pulmonary vein. Called also *ramus superior venae pulmonalis sinistrae inferioris* [TA alternative] and *superior segmental vein of left lung.*

**v. supe'rior ver'mis** [TA], superior vein of vermis: a vein that drains the superior surface of the cerebellum; it runs forward and medially across the superior vermis to empty into the straight sinus or the great cerebral vein; called also *v. vermis superior.*

**v. supraorbita'lis** [TA], supraorbital vein: the vein that passes down the forehead lateral to the supratrochlear vein, joining it at the root of the nose to form the angular vein.

**v. suprarena'lis dex'tra** [TA], right suprarenal vein: a vein that drains the right suprarenal gland into the inferior vena cava; called also *v. adrenalis dextra.*

**v. suprarena'lis sinis'tra** [TA], left suprarenal vein: the vein that returns blood from the left suprarenal gland to the left renal vein.

**v. suprascapula'ris** [TA], suprascapular vein: the vein that accompanies the homonymous artery (sometimes as two veins that unite), opening usually into the external jugular, or occasionally into the subclavian vein; called also *transverse vein of scapula.*

**ve'nae supratrochlea'res** [TA], supratrochlear veins: two veins, each beginning in a venous plexus high up on the forehead and descending to the root of the nose, where it joins with the supraorbital to form the angular vein. Called also *frontal veins.*

**ve'nae sura'les** [TA], sural veins: veins that ascend with the sural arteries and drain blood from the calf into the popliteal vein.

**v. tempora'lis me'dia** [TA], middle temporal vein: the vein that arises in the substance of the temporal muscle and passes down under the fascia to the zygoma, where it breaks through to join the superficial temporal vein.

**ve'nae tempora'les profun'dae** [TA], deep temporal veins: veins that drain the deep portions of the temporal muscle and empty into the pterygoid plexus.

**ve'nae tempora'les superficia'les** [TA], superficial temporal veins: veins that drain the lateral part of the scalp in the frontal and parietal regions, the tributaries forming a single superficial temporal vein in front of the ear, just above the zygoma. This descending vein receives the middle temporal and transverse facial veins and, entering the parotid gland, unites with the maxillary vein deep to the neck of the mandible to form the retromandibular vein.

**v. termina'lis,** TA alternative for *v. thalamostriata superior.*

**v. testicula'ris dex'tra** [TA], right testicular vein: a vein that drains the right pampiniform plexus into the inferior vena cava.

**v. testicula'ris sinis'tra** [TA], left testicular vein: a vein that drains the left pampiniform plexus into the left renal vein.

**ve'nae thalamostria'tae inferio'res** [TA], inferior thalamostriate veins: veins that pass through the anterior perforate substance and join the deep middle cerebral and anterior cerebral veins to form the basal vein; called also *striate veins* and *venae striatae.*

**v. thalamostria'ta supe'rior** [TA], superior thalamostriate vein: a vein that collects blood from the corpus striatum and thalamus, and joins with the choroid vein to form the internal cerebral vein; called also *terminal vein* and *v. terminalis* [TA alternative].

**v. thoraca'lis latera'lis,** v. thoracica lateralis.

**ve'nae thora'cicae inter'nae** [TA], internal thoracic veins: two veins formed by junction of the venae comitantes of the internal thoracic artery of either side; each continues along the artery to open into the brachiocephalic vein. Called also *internal mammary veins.*

**v. thora'cica latera'lis** [TA], lateral thoracic vein: a large vein accompanying the lateral thoracic artery and draining into the axillary vein; called also *v. thoracalis lateralis.*

**v. thoracoacromia'lis** [TA], thoracoacromial vein: the vein that follows the homonymous artery and opens into the subclavian vein.

**ve'nae thoracoepigas'tricae** [TA], thoracoepigastric veins: long, longitudinal, superficial veins in the anterolateral subcutaneous tissue of the torso, which empty superiorly into the lateral thoracic and inferiorly into the femoral vein.

**ve'nae thy'micae** [TA], thymic veins: small branches from the thymus gland that open into the left brachiocephalic vein.

**v. thyroi'dea i'ma,** an occasional vein formed by high junction of the right and left inferior thyroid veins, and usually emptying into the left brachiocephalic vein.

**v. thyroi'dea inferio'ris** [TA], inferior thyroid vein: either of two veins, left and right, that drain the thyroid plexus into the left and right brachiocephalic veins; occasionally they may unite into a common trunk to empty, usually, into the left brachiocephalic vein.

**ve'nae thyroi'deae me'diae** [TA], middle thyroid veins: veins that drain blood from the thyroid gland into the internal jugular vein.

**v. thyroi'dea supe'rior** [TA], superior thyroid vein: a vein arising from the upper part of the thyroid gland on either side, opening into the internal jugular vein, occasionally in common with the facial vein.

**ve'nae tibia'les anterio'res** [TA], anterior tibial veins: venae comitantes of the anterior tibial artery, which unite with the posterior tibial veins to form the popliteal vein.

**ve'nae tibia'les posterio'res** [TA], posterior tibial veins: venae comitantes of the posterior tibial artery, which unite with the anterior tibial veins to form the popliteal vein.

**ve'nae trachea'les** [TA], tracheal veins: small branches that drain blood from the trachea into the brachiocephalic vein.

**ve'nae transver'sae cer'vicis** [TA], **ve'nae transver'sae col'li,** transverse cervical veins: veins that follow the transverse artery of the neck and open into the subclavian vein.

**v. transver'sa facia'lis,** TA alternative for *v. transversa faciei.*

**v. transver'sa facie'i** [TA], transverse facial vein: a vein that passes backward with the transverse facial artery just below the zygomatic arch to join the retromandibular vein; called also *v. transversa facialis* [TA alternative].

**v. transver'sa sca'pulae,** v. suprascapularis.

**ve'nae trun'ci encepha'lici** [TA], veins of encephalic trunk: the veins that drain the brain stem and empty into the basal or great cerebral vein; see *v. pontomesencephalica anterior, venae pontis, venae medullae oblongatae,* and *v. recessus lateralis ventriculi quarti.* Called also *venae mesencephalicae.*

**ve'nae tympa'nicae** [TA], tympanic veins: small veins from the tympanic cavity that pass through the petrotympanic fissure, open into the plexus around the temporomandibular articulation, and finally drain into the retromandibular vein.

**ve'nae ulna'res** [TA], ulnar veins: the venae comitantes of the ulnar artery, which unite with the radial veins at the elbow to form the brachial veins.

**v. umbilica'lis** [TA], umbilical vein: the vein formed by fusion of the atrophied right umbilical vein with the left umbilical vein, which carries all the blood from the placenta to the ductus venosus.

**v. umbilica'lis sinis'tra,** left umbilical vein: former official anatomical nomenclature for the left of the two veins that carry blood from the chorion to the sinus venosus and heart in the early embryo; they later fuse to form the vena umbilicalis.

**v. unca'lis** [TA], vein of uncus: a vein that drains the uncus into the ipsilateral inferior cerebral vein.

**ve'nae uteri'nae** [TA], uterine veins: veins that drain the uterine plexus into the internal iliac veins.

**ve'nae vaso'rum,** small veins that return blood from the tissues making up the walls of the blood vessels themselves.

**ve'nae ventricula'res cor'dis** [TA], the veins of the ventricles of the heart.

**v. ventricula'ris infe'rior** [TA], inferior ventricular vein: a vein that drains the temporal lobe into the basal vein.

**ve'nae ventri'culi dex'tri anterio'res** [TA], anterior veins of right ventricle: small veins that drain blood from the ventral aspect of the right ventricle and empty into the right atrium. Called also *venae cardiacae anteriores, venae cordis anteriores, anterior cardiac veins,* and *anterior veins of heart.*

**v. ventri'culi sinis'tri poste'rior** [TA], posterior vein of left ventricle: the vein that drains blood from the posterior surface of the left ventricle into the coronary sinus. Called also *v. posterior ventriculi sinistri cordis.*

**v. ver'mis infe'rior,** v. inferior vermis.

**v. ver'mis supe'rior,** v. superior vermis.

**v. vertebra'lis** [TA], vertebral vein: a vein that arises from the suboccipital venous plexus, passes with the vertebral artery through the foramina of the transverse processes of the upper six cervical vertebrae, and opens into the brachiocephalic vein.

**v. vertebra'lis accesso'ria** [TA], accessory vertebral vein: a vein that sometimes arises from a plexus formed around the vertebral artery by the vertebral vein, descends with the vertebral vein, and emerges through the transverse foramen of the seventh cervical vertebra to empty into the brachiocephalic vein.

**v. vertebra'lis ante'rior** [TA], anterior vertebral vein: a small vein accompanying the ascending cervical artery; it arises in a venous plexus adjacent to the more cranial cervical transverse processes, and descends to end in the vertebral vein.

**ve'nae vesica'les** [TA], vesical veins: veins passing from the vesical plexus to the internal iliac vein.

**ve'nae vestibula'res** [TA], vestibular veins: branches draining blood from the vestibule into the labyrinthine veins.

**ve'nae vortico'sae** [TA], vorticose veins: four veins that pierce the sclera and carry blood from the choroid to the superior ophthalmic vein; called also *posterior ciliary veins* and *venae choroideae oculi.*

**ve•na•ca•val** (ve'nə ka'vəl) caval.

**ve•na ca•val** caval.

**ve•na•ca•vo•gram** (ve″nə-ka'vo-gram) the film obtained by venacavography.

**ve•na•ca•vog•ra•phy** (ve″nə-ka-vog'rə-fe) radiography of a vena cava, usually of the inferior vena cava.

**ve•nae** (ve'ne) [L.] genitive and plural of *vena.*

**Ve•na med•i•nen•sis** (ve'nə med″ĭ-nen'sis) former name for *Dracunculus medinensis.*

**ve•na•tion** (ve-na'shən) [L. *vena,* q.v.] the manner of distribution of the veins of a part.

**ve•nec•ta•sia** (ve″nək-ta'zhə) a varicosity of a vein.

**ve•nec•to•my** (ve-nek'tə-me) phlebectomy.

**ve•neer** (və-nēr') a thin layer of tooth-colored material, usually porcelain, some other ceramic, or acrylic resin, attached to the surface by direct fusion, cementation, or mechanical retention in the construction of crowns or pontics, or cemented directly to the prepared surface of a tooth to modify its shape or color.
**full v.,** full crown.

**ven•e•na•tion** (ven″ə-na'shən) [L. *venenum* poison] poisoning; a condition of being poisoned.

**ven•e•nif•er•ous** (ven″ə-nif'ər-əs) [L. *venenum* poison + *-ferous*] carrying poison.

**ven•e•nif•ic** (ven″ə-nif'ik) [L. *venenum* poison + *facere* to make] forming poison.

**ven•e•no•sal•i•vary** (ven'ə-no-sal'ĭ-var-e) venomosalivary.

**ven•e•nos•i•ty** (ven″ə-nos'ĭ-te) toxicity.

**ven•e•nous** (ven'ə-nəs) [L. *venenosus*] venomous.

**vene•punc•ture** (ven'ə-punk″chər) phlebotomy (def. 2).

**ve•ne•re•al** (və-nēr'e-əl) [L. *venereus*] pertaining or related to or transmitted by sexual contact; see *sexually transmitted disease,* under *disease.*

**ve•ne•re•ol•o•gist** (və-nēr″e-ol'ə-jist) a specialist in venereology.

**ve•ne•re•ol•o•gy** (və-nēr″e-ol'ə-je) [MeSH: Venereology] the branch of medicine that deals with sexually transmitted diseases.

**vene•sec•tion** (ven″ə-sek'shən) [*vena* + *section*] phlebotomy.

**vene•su•ture** (ven″ə-soo'chər) phleborrhaphy.

**veni•punc•ture** (ven'ĭ-punk″chər) phlebotomy (def. 2).

**veni•sec•tion** (ven″ĭ-sek'shən) phlebotomy.

**veni•su•ture** (ven″ĭ-soo'chər) phleborrhaphy.

**ven•la•fax•ine hy•dro•chlo•ride** (ven″lə-fak'sēn) an inhibitor of serotonin and norepinephrine reuptake, unrelated chemically to any other antidepressants, that potentiates neurotransmitter activity in the central nervous system, used as an antidepressant; administered orally.

**ven(o)-** [L. *vena,* q.v.] a combining form denoting relationship to a vein. See also words beginning *phleb(o)-.*

**ve•no•at•ri•al** (ve″no-a'tre-əl) pertaining to the vena cava and the right atrium.

**ve•noc•ly•sis** (ve-nok'lĭ-sis) [*veno-* + *clysis*] phleboclysis.

**ve•no•fi•bro•sis** (ve″no-fi-bro'sis) phlebosclerosis.

**Ve•no•glob•u•lin-I** (ve″no-glob'u-lin) trademark for a preparation of immune globulin.

**ve•no•gram** (ve'no-gram) 1. phlebogram. 2. a venous-pulse tracing.

**ve•nog•ra•phy** (ve-nog'rə-fe) phlebography (def. 1).
**intraosseous v.,** radiography of the veins after injection of the contrast medium into bone marrow at an appropriate site, such as the iliac crest, ischium, pubic bones, greater trochanter, spinous processes of the vertebrae, or sternum.
**portal v.,** portography.
**splenic v.,** splenic portography.

**ven•om** (ven'um) [L. *venenum* poison] [MeSH: Venoms] a poison, especially one secreted by an animal such as a snake or arthropod.
**Russell's viper v.,** the venom of Russell's viper, *Vipera russelli,* which acts in vitro as an intrinsic thromboplastin and is useful in defining deficiencies of coagulation factor X.
**snake v.,** the poisonous secretion of snakes, containing hemotoxins, hemagglutinins, neurotoxins, leukotoxins, or endotheliotoxins. The venoms of various species have been used as hemostatics. See also *antivenomous serum,* under *serum.*
**spider v.,** the venom of a spider such as *Atrax, Ctenus, Latrodectus,* or *Lycosa.*

**ven•o•mo•sal•i•vary** (ven″ə-mo-sal'ĭ-var″e) secreting a poisonous saliva.

**ve•no•mo•tor** (ve″no-mo'tor) pertaining to or producing constriction or dilatation of the veins.

**ven•o•mous** (ven'ə-məs) secreting venom; see *toxic,* def. 1.

**ve•no•oc•clu•sive** (ve″no-ə-kloo'siv) pertaining to or characterized by obstruction of the veins.

**ve•no•peri•to•ne•os•to•my** (ve″no-per″ĭ-to″ne-os'tə-me) [*veno-* + *peritoneostomy*] anastomosis of the saphenous vein with the peritoneum for permanent drainage of the peritoneal cavity in ascites.

**ve•no•pres•sor** (ve-no-pres″ər) 1. pertaining to venous blood pressure. 2. an agent that causes venous constriction.

**ve•nor•rha•phy** (ve-nor'ə-fe) [*veno-* + *-rrhaphy*] phleborrhaphy.

**ve•no•scle•ro•sis** (ve″no-sklə-ro'sis) phlebosclerosis.

**ve•nose** (ve'nōs) provided with veins.

**ve•no•si•nal** (ve″no-si'nəl) pertaining to the venae cavae and the right atrium of the heart.

**ve•nos•i•ty** (ve-nos'ĭ-te) 1. the condition of being venous. 2. excess of venous blood in a part. 3. a plentiful supply of veins.

**ve•no•sta•sis** (ve″no-sta'sis) [*veno-* + *-stasis*] venous stasis.

**ve•not•o•my** (ve-not'ə-me) phlebotomy.

**ve•nous** (ve'nəs) [L. *venosus*] of or pertaining to the veins.

**ve•no•ve•nos•to•my** (ve″no-ve-nos'tə-me) phlebophlebostomy.

**ve•no•ve•nous** (ve″no-ve'nəs) beginning at a vein and ending at a vein, such as a tube for access in hemodialysis or hemofiltration.

**vent** (vent) [Fr. *fente* slit] 1. any opening or outlet; especially the anus. 2. an opening that discharges pus. 3. cloacal aperture.

**Ven•taire** (ven'tār) trademark for a preparation of protokylol hydrochloride.

**ven•ter** (ven'tər) pl. *ven'tres* [L. "belly"] 1. any belly-shaped part. 2. [TA] belly: a general term for a fleshy contractile part of a muscle. 3. abdomen. 4. any hollowed part or cavity.
**v. ante'rior mus'culi digas'trici** [TA], anterior belly of digastric muscle: the shorter belly of the digastric muscle, arising from the digastric fossa on the mandible and extending posteriorly to join the posterior belly through an intermediate tendon attached to the hyoid bone.

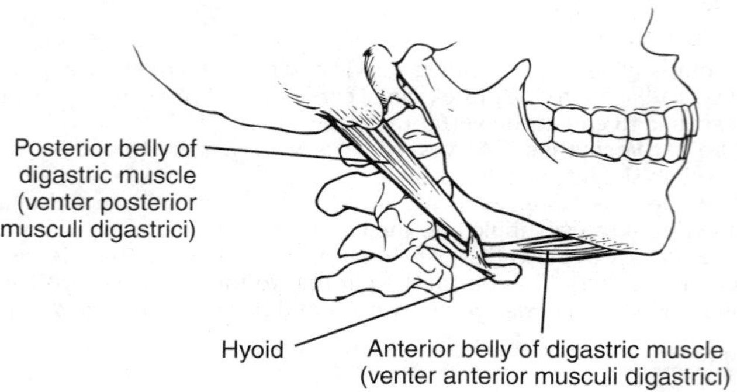


**v. fronta′lis mus′culi occipitofronta′lis** [TA], frontal belly of occipitofrontal muscle: a part that originates from the galea aponeurotica and inserts into the skin of the eyebrows and the root of the nose. Called also *musculus frontalis.*
**v. i′lii,** the free (pelvic) portion of the sacropelvic surface of the ilium.
**v. infe′rior mus′culi omohyoi′dei** [TA], inferior belly of omohyoid muscle: a narrow band that attaches to the superior margin of the scapula.
**v. occipita′lis mus′culi occipitofronta′lis** [TA], occipital belly of occipitofrontal muscle: a part that originates from the highest nuchal line of the occipital bone and inserts into the galea aponeurotica; called also *musculus occipitalis.*
**v. poste′rior mus′culi digas′trici** [TA], posterior belly of digastric muscle: the longer belly of the digastric muscle, arising from the mastoid notch of the temporal bone and extending anteriorly to join the anterior belly through an intermediate tendon attached to the hyoid bone.
**v. propen′dens,** pendulous abdomen.
**v. sca′pulae,** fossa subscapularis.
**v. supe′rior mus′culi omohyoi′dei** [TA], superior belly of omohyoid muscle: a part that ascends and attaches to the hyoid bone.

**ven·ti·la·tion** (ven″tĭ-la′shən) [L. *ventilare* to fan, from *ventus* wind] [MeSH: Ventilation] 1. circulation, replacement, or purification of air or other gas in a defined or enclosed space. 2. in respiratory physiology, the process of exchange of air between the lungs and the environment, including *inspiration* and *expiration.* See also *alveolar v.* and *pulmonary v.* Called also *breathing, pneusis,* and *respiration.* 3. in psychiatry, verbalization of one's problems, emotions, or feelings.
**alveolar v.,** a fraction of the pulmonary ventilation, being the amount of air that reaches the alveoli and is available for gas exchange with the blood.
**artificial v.,** see under *respiration.*
**assist/control mode v.,** positive pressure ventilation in the assist-control mode (see under *mode*); if the spontaneous ventilation rate falls below a preset level, the ventilator enters the control mode.
**assisted v.,** artificial respiration.
**assist mode v.,** positive pressure ventilation in which the ventilator is in assist mode (see under *mode*); cf. *control mode v.* and *assist/control mode v.*
**collateral v.,** the entrance of air into alveoli through pulmonary alveolar pores and other pathways so that a lobule may remain aerated even though its bronchiole is obstructed. Called also *collateral respiration.*
**continuous positive pressure v.,** control mode ventilation using continuous positive airway pressure.
**controlled v., controlled mechanical v.,** control mode v.
**control mode v.,** positive pressure ventilation in which the ventilator is in control mode, with its cycle entirely controlled by the apparatus and not influenced by the patient's efforts at spontaneous ventilation. Called also *controlled* or *controlled mechanical v.*
**downward v.,** ventilation of a building or room in which the outlets have places lower than those of the inlets.
**exhausting v.,** ventilation of a building or room by means of an exhaust fan or some other process that withdraws the foul air.
**expired air v.,** an artificial respiration technique in which ventilation is supplied by blowing into the patient's nose or throat, or into a laryngectomy site, an airway, or a special mask made for the purpose.
**high-frequency v.,** mechanical ventilation in which small tidal volumes are delivered at a high respiration rate; it may either be positive pressure ventilation or be delivered in the form of frequent jets of air.
**intermittent mandatory v.,** IMV; a type of control mode ventilation in which the patient breathes spontaneously while the ventilator delivers a positive-pressure breath at preset intervals. Cf. *intermittent positive-pressure breathing.*
**intermittent mandatory v., synchronized,** SIMV; positive pressure ventilation in which the patient breathes spontaneously while the ventilator delivers a positive-pressure breath at intervals that are predetermined but synchronized with the patient's breathing.
**intermittent positive pressure v.,** see under *breathing.*
**inverse ratio v.,** a type of assisted ventilation in which inspiratory time is artificially increased until it is longer than expiratory time; believed to improve distribution of ventilation at lower airway-inflating pressures and to decrease intrapulmonary shunting. Used for patients with acute lung injury or acute respiratory distress syndrome that is refractory to other methods.
**mandatory minute v.,** a type of intermittent positive pressure ventilation designed to maintain a constant minute ventilation.
**maximal voluntary v., maximum voluntary v.,** MVV; the greatest volume of gas that can be breathed per minute by voluntary effort. Called also *maximal breathing capacity.*
**mechanical v.,** ventilation accomplished by extrinsic means, usually distinguished as either *negative pressure v.* or *positive pressure v.* Cf. *spontaneous v.*
**minute v.,** the total volume of gas in liters expelled from the lungs per minute. See also *minute volume,* under *volume.* Called also *total v.*
**natural v.,** ventilation of a building or room done without the aid of any special appliance.
**negative pressure v.,** a type of mechanical ventilation in which negative pressure is generated on the outside of the patient's chest and transmitted to the interior of the thorax in order to expand the lungs and allow air to flow in; used primarily with patients having extreme weakness or paralysis of the chest muscles. See also *negative pressure ventilator,* under *ventilator.*
**plenum v.,** ventilation of an entire building by fan blowers.
**positive pressure v.,** any of numerous types of mechanical ventilation in which gas is delivered into the airways and lungs under positive pressure, producing positive airway pressure during inspiration; it may be done via either an endotracheal tube or a nasal mask.
**pressure control v.,** positive pressure ventilation in which breaths are augmented by air at a fixed rate and amount of pressure, with tidal volume not being fixed; used particularly for patients with acute respiratory distress syndrome.
**pressure support v.,** positive pressure ventilation in which the patient breathes spontaneously and breathing is augmented with air at a preset amount of pressure, with tidal volume not being fixed.
**proportional assist v.,** positive pressure ventilation in which the ventilator can sense the patient's level of inspiratory flow and deliver pressure support to achieve a given tidal volume.
**pulmonary v.,** a measure of the rate of ventilation, referring to the total exchange of air between the lungs and the ambient air, usually in liters per minute.
**spontaneous v.,** term used to denote breathing accomplished naturally, without any artificial aids, as opposed to mechanical ventilation and other forms of artificial respiration.
**total v.,** minute v.
**upward v.,** ventilation of a building or room in which air is introduced below the place of its withdrawal.
**vacuum v.,** ventilation of a room or building by the forced extraction of air.

**ven·ti·la·tor** (ven″tĭ-la′tor) [MeSH: Ventilators, Mechanical] 1. an apparatus designed to qualify the air that passes through it. 2. an apparatus used in artificial respiration, usually in mechanical ventilation (see under *ventilation*). Called also *inhaler* and *respirator.*
**cuirass v.,** a type of negative pressure ventilator in which a cuirass-like apparatus either completely surrounds the trunk or is applied only to the front of the chest and abdomen, and allows intermittent negative pressure by evacuation of air to force the chest to expand. Called also *cuirass respirator.*
**negative pressure v.,** a type of ventilator that uses negative pressure ventilation (q.v.) for patients having extreme weakness or paralysis of the chest muscles; the most common types are the Drinker respirator and the cuirass ventilator.
**tank v.,** Drinker respirator.

**ven·ti·la·to·ry** (ven′tĭ-lə-tor″e) pertaining to ventilation.

**Ven·to·lin** (ven′tə-lin) trademark for preparations of albuterol.

**ven·trad** (ven′trad) [*ventr-* + *-ad*[1]] toward the abdomen, a venter, or a ventral aspect.

**ven·tral** (ven′trəl) [L. *ventralis*] 1. pertaining to the abdomen or to any venter. 2. denoting a position more toward the belly surface than some other object of reference; a synonym of *anterior* in human anatomy and of *inferior* in quadruped anatomy.

**ven·tra·lis** (vən-tra′lis) [TA] ventral.

**ven·tral·ward** (ven′trəl-wərd) ventrad.

**ventri-** see *ventr(o)-.*

**ven·tri·cle** (ven′trĭ-kəl) ventriculus (def. 2).
**v. of Arantius,** the fossa rhomboidea, especially its lower end.
**auxiliary v.,** an implanted pumping mechanism designed to assist

the left ventricle of the heart in maintaining normal output, rate, and blood pressure; called also *booster heart.*
**v's of the brain,** the cavities within the brain which are filled with cerebrospinal fluid, including the two lateral, the third, and, linked by the aqueduct, the fourth ventricles. They are lined by ependyma which, in certain regions, is invaginated by vascular fringes of pia mater to form the choroid plexuses. The cavum septi pellucidi, to which the term ventricle is sometimes applied, is not a true ventricle.
**double-inlet v.,** a congenital anomaly in which both atrioventricular valves or a single common atrioventricular valve open into a single ventricle, which usually resembles the left ventricle morphologically *(double inlet left v.)* but may resemble the right *(double inlet right v.)* or neither or both ventricles.
**double-outlet left v.,** a rare anomaly in which both great arteries arise from the left ventricle; it is often associated with a hypoplastic right ventricle, ventricular septal defect, valvular or subvalvular pulmonic stenosis, and a variety of associated malformations.
**double-outlet right v.,** incomplete transposition of the great vessels in which both the aorta and the pulmonary artery arise from the right ventricle, associated with a ventricular septal defect. The defect may be remote from or close to either or both semilunar valves; it may be related to the aorta *(subaortic),* to the pulmonary trunk *(subpulmonic),* to both vessels *(doubly committed),* or to neither *(uncommitted);* and it may be associated with pulmonary stenosis.
**Duncan's v., fifth v.,** cavum septi pellucidi.
**first v. of cerebrum,** ventriculus lateralis cerebri.
**fourth v. of cerebrum,** ventriculus quartus cerebri.
**Galen's v.,** ventriculus laryngis.
**v. of heart,** ventriculus cordis.
**v. of larynx,** ventriculus laryngis.
**lateral v. of cerebrum,** ventriculus lateralis cerebri.
**left v. of heart,** ventriculus sinister cordis.
**Morgagni's v.,** ventriculus laryngis.
**pineal v.,** recessus pinealis.
**right v. of heart,** ventriculus dexter cordis.
**second v. of cerebrum,** ventriculus lateralis cerebri.
**single v.,** cor triloculare biatriatum.
**sixth v.,** Verga's v.
**v. of Sylvius,** cavum septi pellucidi.
**terminal v. of spinal cord,** ventriculus terminalis medullae spinalis.
**third v. of cerebrum,** ventriculus tertius cerebri.
**Verga's v.,** an occasional space (not a true ventricle) between the corpus callosum and the fornix; called also *cavum vergae, cavum psalterii,* and *sixth v.*
**Vieussens' v.,** cavum septi pellucidi.

**ven·tri·cose** (ven'trĭ-kōs) having an expansion or belly on one side.

**ven·tric·u·lar** (ven-trik'u-lər) pertaining to a ventricle.

**ven·tric·u·li** (ven-trik'u-li) [L.] genitive and plural of *ventriculus.*

**ven·tric·u·li·tis** (ven-trik"u-li'tis) inflammation of a ventricle, especially of a ventricle of the brain.

**ventricul(o)-** [L. *ventriculus,* dim. of *venter* belly] a combining form denoting relationship to a ventricle, of the heart or brain.

**ven·tric·u·lo·atri·os·to·my** (ven-trik"u-lo-a"tre-os'tə-me) ventriculoatrial shunt.

**ven·tric·u·lo·cis·ter·nos·to·my** (ven-trik"u-lo-sis"tər-nos'to-me) ventriculocisternal shunt.

**ven·tric·u·lo·en·ceph·a·li·tis** (ven-trik"u-lo-en-sef"ə-li'tis) [*ventriculo-* + *encephalitis*] ventriculitis accompanied by encephalitis.
**cytomegalovirus v.,** a late-appearing type of cytomegalovirus encephalitis seen in immunocompromised patients, characterized by high protein levels and pleocytosis of the cerebrospinal fluid, encephalitis, cranial nerve deficits, ventriculomegaly with necrotizing ventriculitis, and sometimes ascending muscle weakness with nystagmus.

**ven·tric·u·lo·gram** (ven-trik'u-lo-gram) a radiograph of the cerebral ventricles or of the ventricles of the heart.

**ven·tric·u·log·ra·phy** (ven-trik"u-log'rə-fe) [*ventriculo-* + *-graphy*] 1. radiography of the head following removal of cerebrospinal fluid from the cerebral ventricles and its replacement by air or other contrast medium. 2. radiography of a ventricle of the heart after injection of a contrast medium.
**first pass v.,** see under *angiocardiography.*
**gated blood pool v.,** equilibrium radionuclide angiocardiography.
**left v.,** cineangiography of the heart after insertion of a catheter into the left ventricle, usually retrograde across the aortic valve, and injection of iodinated contrast material; used to assess various ventricular function parameters and to detect regurgitation through the atrioventricular valves.
**radionuclide v.,** see under *angiocardiography.*

**ven·tric·u·lo·meg·a·ly** (ven-trik"u-lo-meg'ə-le) [*ventriculo-* + *-megaly*] gross enlargement of a ventricle of the brain, as by hydrocephalus.

**ven·tric·u·lom·e·try** (ven-trik"u-lom'ə-tre) [*ventriculo-* + *-metry*] the measurement of the intraventricular (intracranial) pressure.

**ven·tric·u·lo·my·ot·o·my** (ven-trik"u-lo-mi-ot'ə-me) incision of the muscular wall of the heart.

**ven·tric·u·lo·punc·ture** (ven-trik'u-lo-pungk"chər) ventricular puncture.

**ven·tric·u·lo·scope** (ven-trik'u-lo-skōp) an endoscope for examining the cerebral ventricles and for cauterizing the choroid plexus.

**ven·tric·u·los·co·py** (ven-trik"u-los'kə-pe) [*ventriculo-* + *-scopy*] direct examination of the cerebral ventricles by means of an endoscope or cystoscope.

**ven·tric·u·los·ti·um** (ven-trik"u-los'te-əm) [*ventriculo-* + *ostium*] an artificial opening created between one of the cerebral ventricles and the external surface of the brain; see also *shunt.*

**ven·tric·u·los·to·my** (ven-trik"u-los'tə-me) [*ventriculo-* + *-stomy*] [MeSH: Ventriculostomy] the operation of establishing a free communication or shunt between the floor of the third ventricle and the underlying cisterna interpeduncularis; for the treatment of hydrocephalus.

**ven·tric·u·lo·sub·arach·noid** (ven-trik"u-lo-sub"ə-rak'noid) pertaining to the cerebral ventricles and the subarachnoid spaces.

**ven·tric·u·lot·o·my** (ven-trik"u-lot'ə-me) [*ventriculo-* + *-tomy*] incision of a ventricle of the brain or heart.
**partial encircling endocardial v.,** the encompassing and isolation of visible areas of endocardial fibrosis in the left ventricle by an incision extending part way through the endocardium; done to relieve ventricular tachycardia in patients with ischemic heart disease.

**ven·tric·u·lo·ve·nos·to·my** (ven-trik"u-lo-ve-nos'tə-me) ventriculovenous shunt.

**ven·tric·u·lus** (ven-trik'u-ləs) pl. *ventri'culi* [L., dim. of *venter* belly] 1. gaster. 2. [TA] ventricle: a small, normal cavity in an organ such as the heart or brain. 3. the midgut of an invertebrate.

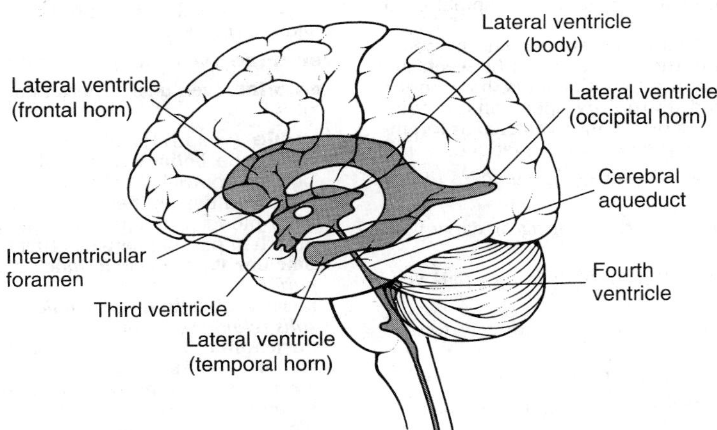


Ventricles of the brain.

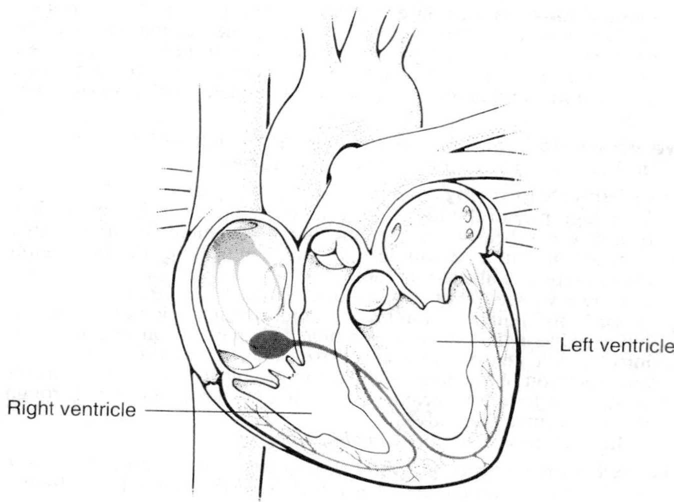


Ventricles of the heart.

**v. cor'dis dex'ter/sinis'ter** [TA], right/left ventricle of heart: the pair of cavities, with thick muscular walls, that make up the bulk of the heart. See *v. dexter cordis* and *v. sinister cordis.*
**v. dex'ter ce'rebri,** the ventriculus lateralis cerebri of the right cerebral hemisphere.
**v. dex'ter cor'dis** [TA], right ventricle of heart: the cavity of the heart that propels the blood through the pulmonary trunk and arteries into the lungs. See Plate 20.
**v. laryn'gis** [TA], **v. laryn'gis [Morgag'nii],** ventricle of larynx: a lateral evagination of mucous membrane between the vocal and vestibular folds, reaching nearly to the angle of the thyroid cartilage.
**v. latera'lis ce'rebri** [TA], lateral ventricle of cerebrum: the cavity in each cerebral hemisphere, derived (developed) from the cavity of the embryonic neural tube; it consists of a pars centralis and three horns—frontal (anterior), temporal (inferior), and occipital (occipital) in the frontal, temporal, and occipital lobes, respectively. They are separated from each other by the septum pellucidum, and each communicates with the third ventricle by an interventricular foramen (the foramen of Monro), through which also the choroid plexuses of the lateral ventricles become continuous with that of the third ventricle. Cerebrospinal fluid formed in the lateral ventricle flows into the third ventricle through the interventricular foramina.
**v. quar'tus ce'rebri** [TA], fourth ventricle of cerebrum: an irregularly shaped cavity in the rhombencephalon, between the medulla oblongata, the pons, and the isthmus in front, and the cerebellum behind; it is continuous with the central canal of the cord below and with the cerebral aqueduct above, and through its lateral and median apertures it communicates with the subarachnoid space.
**v. sinis'ter ce'rebri,** the ventriculus lateralis cerebri of the left cerebral hemisphere.
**v. sinis'ter cor'dis** [TA], left ventricle of heart: the cavity of the heart that propels the blood out through the aorta into the systemic arteries. See Plate 20.
**v. termina'lis medul'lae spina'lis** [TA], terminal ventricle of spinal cord: a saclike expansion of the central canal of the spinal cord within the conus medullaris.
**v. ter'tius ce'rebri** [TA], third ventricle of cerebrum: a narrow cleft below the corpus callosum, within the diencephalon between the two thalami. Its floor is formed by the hypothalamus, its anterior wall by the lamina terminalis, and its roof by ependyma. It communicates with the lateral ventricles by the interventricular foramina, and with the fourth ventricle by the cerebral aqueduct.

**ven·tri·cum·bent** (ven″trĭ-kum'bənt) [*ventri-* + L. *cumbere* to lie] lying upon the belly; prone.

**ven·tri·duct** (ven'trĭ-dukt) [*ventri-* + *duct*] to bring or carry ventrad.

**ven·tri·duc·tion** (ven″trĭ-duk'shən) the act of drawing a part ventrad.

**ven·tri·flex·ion** (ven″trĭ-flek'shən) [*ventri-* + *flexion*] flexion toward the belly or ventral surface.

**ven·tri·me·sal** (ven″trĭ-me'səl) pertaining to the ventrimeson.

**ven·trim·e·son** (vən-trim'ə-son) [*ventri-* + *meson*] the middle line on the ventral surface.

**ventr(o)-** [L. *venter* belly or abdomen] combining forms denoting relationship to the belly, or to the front (anterior) aspect of the body. Also, *ventri-*.

**ven·tro·cys·tor·rha·phy** (ven″tro-sis-tor'ə-fe) the stitching of a cyst, or of the bladder, to the abdominal wall.

**ven·tro·dor·sad** (ven″tro-dor'sad) from the ventral toward the dorsal aspect.

**ven·tro·dor·sal** (ven″tro-dor'səl) pertaining to the ventral and dorsal surfaces.

**ven·tro·fix·a·tion** (ven″tro-fik-sa'shən) [*ventro-* + *fixation*] the operation of suspending the retroplaced uterus to the abdominal wall. Cf. *hysteropexy.*

**ven·tro·hys·tero·pexy** (ven″tro-his'tər-o-pek″se) ventrofixation of the uterus.

**ven·tro·in·gui·nal** (ven″tro-ing'gwĭ-nəl) pertaining to the abdomen and the inguinal region.

**ven·tro·lat·er·al** (ven″tro-lat'ər-əl) both ventral and lateral.

**ven·tro·me·di·an** (ven″tro-me'de-ən) both ventral and median.

**ven·tro·pos·te·ri·or** (ven″tro-pos-tēr'e-or) both ventral and posterior.

**ven·trop·to·sia** (ven″trop-to'se-ə) [*ventro-* + *ptosis* + *-ia*] gastroptosis.

**ven·trop·to·sis** (ven″trop-to'sis) gastroptosis.

**ven·tros·co·py** (ven-tros'kə-pe) [*ventro-* + *-scopy*] peritoneoscopy.

**ven·trose** (ven'trōs) [L. *ventrosus*] having a bellylike expansion.

**ven·tro·sus·pen·sion** (ven″tro-səs-pen'shən) ventrofixation.

**ven·trot·o·my** (ven-trot'ə-me) [*ventro-* + *-tomy*] celiotomy.

**Ven·tu·ri mask** (ven-too're) [Giovanni Battista *Venturi,* Italian physicist, 1746–1822] see under *mask.*

**ven·tu·rim·e·ter** (ven″tu-rim'ə-tər) [G. B. *Venturi* + *-meter*] an instrument for measuring the flow of liquids, as of the blood in vessels, by relating difference of pressures between a constricted and a nonconstricted portion of a tube through which fluid is flowing.

**ven·u·la** (ven'u-lə) pl. *ven'ulae* [L., dim. of *vena*] [TA] venule: any of the small vessels that collect blood from the capillary plexuses and join to form veins.
**v. macula'ris infe'rior** [TA], inferior macular venule: the inferior venule draining blood from the macula retinae.
**v. macula'ris me'dia** [TA], medial macular venule: a small branch draining blood from the central region of the retina to the central retinal vein; called also *v. retinae medialis.*
**v. macula'ris supe'rior** [TA], superior macular venule: the superior venule draining blood from the macula retinae.
**v. nasa'lis re'tinae infe'rior** [TA], inferior nasal venule of retina: a small vein returning blood from the inferior nasal region of the retina to the central vein.
**v. nasa'lis re'tinae supe'rior** [TA], superior nasal venule of retina: a small vein returning blood from the superior nasal region of the retina to the central vein.
**ve'nulae rec'tae re'nis** [TA], straight venules of kidney: venules that drain the papillary part of the kidney and empty into the arcuate veins.
**v. re'tinae media'lis,** v. macularis media.
**ve'nulae stella'tae re'nis,** venae stellatae renis.
**v. tempora'lis re'tinae infe'rior** [TA], inferior temporal venule of retina: a small vein returning blood from the inferior temporal region of the retina to the central vein.
**v. tempora'lis re'tinae supe'rior** [TA], superior temporal venule of retina: a small vein returning blood from the superior temporal region of the retina to the central vein.

**ven·u·lae** (ven'u-le) [L.] genitive and plural of *venula.*

**ven·u·lar** (ven'u-lər) pertaining to, composed of, or affecting venules.

**ven·ule** (ven'ūl) [MeSH: Venules] venula.
**high endothelial v's,** specialized postcapillary venules with tall cuboidal endothelial cells, found in lymph nodes and gut-associated lymphoid tissue; they are the sites where lymphocytes recirculate from blood to lymph, binding specifically to the endothelial cells and then passing between them. Called also *postcapillary v's.*
**macular v.,** see *venula macularis inferior* and *venula macularis superior.*
**nasal v. of retina,** see *venula nasalis retinae inferior* and *venula nasalis retinae superior.*
**postcapillary v.,** 1. venous capillary. 2. (pl.) high endothelial v's.
**stellate v's of kidney,** venae stellatae renis.
**straight v's of kidney,** venulae rectae renis.
**temporal v. of retina,** see *venula temporalis retinae inferior* and *venula temporalis retinae superior.*

**ven·u·li·tis** (ven″u-li'tis) inflammation of the venules.

**cutaneous necrotizing v.,** a necrotizing vasculitis affecting the venules of the skin, usually of the extremities, caused by deposition of circulating immune complexes and associated with infection, chronic disease, or drug administration; some cases are idiopathic. Manifestations are variable, the most common being palpable purpura; angioedema, urticaria, and deposition of fibrinoid material and cellular infiltrates also occur.

**VEP** visual evoked potential.

**Ve·Pe·sid** (ve'pe-sid) trademark for a preparation of etoposide.

**Ver·a·cil·lin** (ver"ə-sil'in) trademark for a preparation of dicloxacillin sodium.

**Ver·al·ba** (ver-al'bə) trademark for a mixture of protoveratrines A and B.

**ver·ap·a·mil hy·dro·chlo·ride** (vər-ap'ə-mil) a calcium channel blocker that dilates coronary arteries and decreases myocardial oxygen demand, used in the treatment and prophylaxis of angina and in the intravenous therapy of supraventricular tachyarrhythmias.

**Ve·ra·trum** (ve-ra'trəm) [L.] [MeSH: Veratrum] a genus of plants of the genus Liliaceae. Some species contain antihypertensive alkaloids that are used medicinally; most are poisonous to humans and livestock.
**V. al'bum,** the European or white hellebore, a poisonous variety that is a source of the protoveratrines.
**V. califor'nicum,** skunk cabbage, a variety found in the western United States that contains teratogenic alkaloids, causing cyclopia and other conditions in fetal sheep when their mothers eat the plant.
**V. viri'de,** Aiton, the American or green hellebore, a poisonous variety that is a source of alkavervir and cryptenamine.

**ver·bal** (vər'bəl) [L. *verbum*] consisting of words; pertaining to words or speech.

**Ver·be·na** (vər-be'nə) a genus of herbs of the family Verbenaceae, mostly native to the Americas. *V. triphyl'la* L. is the source of verbenone.

**ver·be·none** (vər-be'nōn) a terpene ketone from *Verbena triphylla,* an American herb.

**ver·big·er·a·tion** (vər-bij"ər-a'shən) [L. *verbigerare* to chatter] stereotyped and meaningless repetition of words and phrases; seen in some cases of schizophrenia. See also *logorrhea* and *perseveration.* Called also *cataphasia.*

**ver·bo·ma·nia** (vər"bo-ma'ne-ə) [L. *verbum* word + *-mania*] logorrhea.

**Ver·cyte** (ver'sīt) trademark for a preparation of pipobroman.

**ver·do·he·mo·glo·bin** (ver"do-he"mo-glo"bin) choleglobin.

**ver·do·per·ox·i·dase** (ver"do-pər-ok'sĭ-dās) myeloperoxidase.

**Ver·ess needle** (və-res') [J. *Veress,* German surgeon, 20th century] see under *needle.*

**Ver·ga's lacrimal groove, ventricle** (ver'gahz) [Andrea *Verga,* Italian neurologist, 1811–1895] see under *groove* and *ventricle.*

**verge** (vərj) a circumference, or ring.
**anal v.,** the external or distal boundary of the anal canal; the line where the walls of the anus come in contact during the normal state of apposition.

**ver·gence** (vər'jəns) [L. *vergere* to bend] 1. the amount of convergence or divergence of a pencil of rays entering or leaving a lens or mirror, expressed as the reciprocal of the distance from the lens or mirror to the focus of the rays. For rays through a principal focus, the vergence is equal to the focal power of the lens or mirror. See *convergence* (def. 2) and *divergence* (def. 1). 2. a disjunctive reciprocal rotation of both eyes around their horizontal, vertical, or anteroposterior axes such that the axes of fixation are not parallel. The kind of vergence is indicated by a prefix. See *convergence* (def. 3), *divergence* (def. 2), *infravergence, supravergence, cyclovergence,* and see *duction* and *version* (def. 5).

**ver·gen·cy** (vər'jən-se) vergence.

**Ver·hey·en's stars** (ver-hi'enz) [Philippe *Verheyen,* Flemish anatomist, 1648–1710] venae stellatae renis.

**Ver·hoeff's stain** (ver'hefz) [Frederick Herman *Verhoeff,* American ophthalmologist, 1874–1968] see under *stain.*

**Ver·i·loid** (ver'ĭ-loid) trademark for a preparation of alkavervir.

**ver·mes** (vər'mēz) [L.] plural of *vermis.*

**ver·me·toid** (vər'mə-toid) 1. vermiform. 2. vermicular.

**ver·mi·an** (vər'me-ən) pertaining to the vermis cerebelli.

**Ver·mi·cel·la** (vər"mĭ-sel'ə) [L.] a genus of mildly venomous Australian serpents.

**ver·mi·ci·dal** (vər"mĭ-si'dəl) anthelmintic (def. 1).

**ver·mi·cide** (vər'mĭ-sīd) [*vermis* + *-cide*] anthelmintic (def. 2).

**ver·mic·u·lar** (vər-mik'u-lər) [L. *vermicularis*] wormlike in shape or appearance. Called also *helminthoid, vermiculose,* and *vermiculous.*

**ver·mic·u·la·tion** (vər-mik"u-la'shən) [L. *vermiculatio,* from *vermis* worm] peristaltic or wormlike movements, as of the intestine; peristalsis.

**ver·mi·cule** (vər'mĭ-kūl) a wormlike structure; see also *ookinete.*

**ver·mic·u·lose** (vər-mik'u-lōs) vermicular.

**ver·mic·u·lous** (vər-mik'u-ləs) 1. vermicular. 2. infected with worms.

**ver·mi·form** (vər'mĭ-form) [L. *vermiformis,* from *vermis* worm + *forma* shape] shaped like a worm.

**ver·mif·u·gal** (vər-mif'u-gəl) [*vermis* + *-fugal*] anthelmintic, def. 1.

**ver·mi·fuge** (vər'mĭ-fūj) anthelmintic (def. 2).

**ver·mil·ion·ec·to·my** (vər-mil"yon-ek'tə-me) excision of the vermilion border of the lip, the surgically created defect being resurfaced by advancement of the undermined labial mucosa.

**ver·min** (vər'min) [L. *vermis* worm] an external animal parasite; animal ectoparasites collectively.

**ver·mi·nal** (vər'mĭ-nəl) verminous.

**ver·mi·na·tion** (vər"mĭ-na'shən) [L. *verminatio*] 1. infection with worms; called also *helminthiasis.* 2. infestation with vermin. Defs. 1 and 2 called also *verminosis.*

**ver·mi·no·sis** (vər"mĭ-no'sis) vermination.

**ver·mi·not·ic** (vər"mĭ-not'ik) 1. pertaining to or caused by infection with worms. 2. pertaining to or caused by infestation with vermin. See also *vermination.*

**ver·mi·nous** (vər'mĭ-nəs) [L. *verminosus*] 1. pertaining to, due to, or abounding in worms. 2. pertaining to, due to, or abounding in vermin. Called also *verminal.*

**ver·mis** (vər'mis) [L.] 1. worm (def. 1). 2. a wormlike structure. 3. v. cerebelli.
**v. cerebel'li** [TA], vermis of cerebellum: the narrow median part of the cerebellum, between the two lateral hemispheres; the *cranial* or *superior* portion extends from the lingula to the folium vermis, and the *inferior* or *caudal* portion from the tuber vermis to the nodulus. See also *cerebellum.*

**ver·mix** (vər'miks) appendix vermiformis.

**ver·mog·ra·phy** (vər-mog'rə-fe) radiography of the vermiform appendix.

**Ver·mox** (vər'moks) trademark for preparations of mebendazole.

**ver·nal** (vər'nəl) [L. *vernalis* of the spring] pertaining to or occurring in the spring.

**Ver·ner-Mor·ri·son syndrome** (vər'nər-mor'ĭ-sən) [John Victor *Verner,* American physician, born 1927; Ashton Byrom *Morrison,* American physician, born 1922] see under *syndrome.*

**Ver·net's syndrome** (ver-nāz') [Maurice *Vernet,* French neurologist, 20th century] see under *syndrome.*

**Ver·neuil's canals, disease, neuroma** (ver-nwēz') [Aristide Auguste Stanislaus *Verneuil,* French surgeon, 1823–1895] see under *canal* and *disease,* and see *plexiform neurofibroma* under *neurofibroma.*

**Ver·ni·er acu·i·ty** (vār-nya') [Pierre *Vernier,* French physicist, 1580–1637] see *displacement threshold,* under *threshold.*

**ver·ni·er** (vər'ne-ər) [Pierre *Vernier*] a finely graduated scale accessory to a more coarsely graduated one for measuring fractions of the divisions of the latter.

**ver·nix** (vər'niks) [L. "sandarac" (resin), from Gr. *Berenikē* (now *Benghazi*) where first made] varnish.
**v. caseo'sa,** ["cheesy varnish"], an unctuous substance composed of sebum and desquamated epithelial cells, which covers the skin of the fetus.

**Ver·no·nia** (vər-no'ne-ə) a genus of mostly tropical herbs and shrubs of the family Compositae. *V. anthelmin'tica* Willd. is an Indian species used as an anthelmintic, abortifacient, and treatment for skin diseases.

**Ver·o·cay bodies** (ver'o-ka) [José *Verocay,* Czechoslovakian pathologist, 1876–1927] see under *body.*

**ver·o·cy·to·tox·in** (ver"o-si"to-tok'sin) either of two toxins closely related to the Shiga toxin, found in *Shigella dysenteriae* type I and some strains of *Escherichia coli;* they cause one type of hemolytic uremic syndrome. Humans are infected by ingesting undercooked meat, unpasteurized milk, and foods contaminated with cattle feces. Called also *Shiga-like toxin.*

**Ve·ron·i·cel·la** (və-ron"ĭ-sel'ə) a genus of slugs of the family Veronicellidae, order Pulmonata. *V. leydi'gi* and other species are intermediate hosts of *Angiostrongylus cantonensis* on various islands in the Pacific.

**ver·o·tox·in** (ver″o-tok'sin) [*Vero* cells, q.v.] either of two enterotoxins, designated I and II, elaborated by certain enterohemorrhagic serotypes of *Escherichia coli*; both are cytotoxic to intestinal villi and colonic epithelial cells and v. I is also cytotoxic to vascular endothelial cells. They are similar to toxins of *Shigella dysenteriae* and have been implicated in at least some cases of hemorrhagic colitis and enterocolitis.

**ver·ru·ca** (və-roo'kə) gen. and pl. *verru'cae* [L.] 1. a lobulated hyperplastic epidermal lesion with a horny surface caused by a human papillomavirus, transmitted by contact or autoinoculation, and usually occurring on the dorsa of the fingers and hands. Called also *wart* and *verruga*. 2. any of various nonviral epidermal proliferations resembling this lesion.
**v. acumina'ta,** condyloma acuminatum.
**v. digita'ta,** a wart with finger-like excrescences growing from its surface.
**v. filifor'mis,** a wart with soft, thin, threadlike projections on its surface.
**v. necroge'nica,** tuberculosis verrucosa cutis.
**v. perua'na, v. peruvia'na,** verruga peruana.
**v. pla'na, v. pla'na juveni'lis,** a small, smooth, usually skin-colored or light brown, slightly raised wart sometimes occurring in great numbers on the face, neck, back of the hands, wrists, and knees; seen most frequently in children but also in adults. Called also *flat, fugitive, juvenile,* and *plane wart.* See also *epidermodysplasia verruciformis.*
**v. planta'ris,** plantar wart: a viral epidermal tumor on the sole.
**v. seborrhe'ica,** seborrheic keratosis.
**v. vulga'ris,** verruca, def. 1.

**ver·ru·cae** (və-roo'se) [L.] genitive and plural of *verruca.*

**ver·ru·ca·rin** (və-roo'kə-rin) any of several trichothecene mycotoxins found in species of *Stachybotrys,* especially *S. alternans,* causing stachybotryotoxicosis.

**ver·ru·ci·form** (və-roo'sĭ-form) [*verruca* + *form*] resembling or shaped like a verruca, or wart.

**ver·ru·cose** (ver'oo-kōs) [L. *verrucosus*] verrucous.

**ver·ru·co·sis** (ver″oo-ko'sis) a condition marked by the presence of multiple warts, or verrucae.

**ver·ru·cous** (ver'oo-kəs) rough; warty.

**ver·ru·ga** (və-roo'gə) [Sp.] verruca.
**v. perua'na,** the second or chronic stage of bartonellosis; called also *verruca peruana* or *peruviana, hemorrhagic pian,* and *Peruvian wart.*

**Ver·sa·pen** (vər'sə-pən) trademark for preparations of hetacillin.

**Versed** (ver-sed') trademark for a preparation of midazolam.

**ver·si·co·lor** (vər″si-kol'or) [L. *vertere* to turn + *color*] variegated; changing color.

**ver·sion** (vər'zhən) [L. *versio,* turning] 1. the act or process of turning something or of changing direction. 2. the situation of an organ or part in relation to an established normal position. 3. in gynecology, the tilting of the uterus; cf. *flexion* (def. 2). 4. in obstetrics, the manual conversion of or changing of the polarity of the fetus with reference to the mother; cf. *presentation.* 5. in ophthalmology, the conjugate rotation of both eyes in the same direction. See *infraversion* and *sursumversion,* and see *duction* and *vergence* (def. 2).
**abdominal v.,** external v.
**bimanual v.,** version done by combined external and internal manipulation, the cervix being open enough to admit the hand; called also *combined v.*
**bipolar v.,** version done by purely external manipulation or by combined internal and external manipulation.
**Braxton Hicks v.,** internal podalic version performed through a partially but not completely dilated cervix; used on a nonviable fetus.
**cephalic v.,** version in which the fetal head is brought down into the maternal pelvis.
**combined v.,** bimanual v.
**Denman's spontaneous v.,** see under *evolution.*
**external v.,** manipulation of the fetal body applied through the abdominal wall of the mother.
**Hicks v.,** Braxton Hicks v.
**internal v.,** turning of the fetus effected by the hand or fingers inserted through the dilated cervix.
**pelvic v.,** version done by manipulating the buttocks of the fetus.
**podalic v.,** version in which one or both legs of the fetus are brought down into the maternal pelvis.
**Potter v.,** podalic version in head presentation when the cervix is fully effaced and dilated.
**spontaneous v.,** conversion of an abnormal position of the fetus into a normal or relatively normal one, occurring without the aid of manipulation.
**Wigand's v.,** external conversion of a transverse lie into a cephalic presentation, accomplished by pushing the fetal head down with one hand and its buttocks up with the other; called also *Wigand's maneuver.*

**ver·te·bra** (vər'tə-brə) gen. and pl. *ver'tebrae* [L.] [TA] any of the thirty-three bones of the spinal column (columna vertebralis), comprising the seven *cervical,* twelve *thoracic,* five *lumbar,* five *sacral,* and four *coccygeal* vertebrae.
**abdominal vertebrae,** vertebrae lumbales.
**basilar v.,** the lowest or last of the lumbar vertebrae.
**caudal vertebrae, caudate vertebrae,** 1. vertebrae coccygeae. 2. the vertebrae in the tail of an animal.
**cervical vertebrae, ver'tebrae cervica'les** [TA], the upper seven vertebrae, constituting the skeleton of the neck. Symbols C1 through C7.
**ver'tebrae coccy'geae, coccygeal vertebrae,** TA alternative for *os coccygis.*
**ver'tebrae col'li,** vertebrae cervicales.
**cranial vertebrae,** the segments of the skull and facial bones, by some regarded as modified vertebrae.
**v. denta'ta,** the second cervical vertebra (*axis* [TA]).
**dorsal vertebrae,** vertebrae thoracicae.
**false vertebrae,** the vertebrae that become fused, i.e., the sacral and coccygeal vertebrae.
**ver'tebrae lumba'les** [TA], **lumbar vertebrae,** the five vertebrae between the thoracic vertebrae and the sacrum. Symbols L1 through L5.
**v. mag'na,** os sacrum.
**odontoid v.,** the second cervical vertebra (*axis* [TA]).
**v. pla'na,** a condition of spondylitis in which the body of the vertebra is reduced to a sclerotic disk; often due to eosinophilic granuloma.
**v. pro'minens** [TA], prominent vertebra: the seventh cervical vertebra, so called because of the length of its spinous process, although it is only the spine that is prominent. (NOTE: the spinous process of the first thoracic vertebra is often more prominent.)
**sacral vertebrae, ver'tebrae sacra'les** [TA], TA alternative for *os sacrum*
**sternal v.,** sternebra.
**terminal v., great,** os sacrum.
**ver'tebrae thoraca'les, ver'tebrae thora'cicae** [TA], thoracic vertebrae: the vertebrae, usually twelve in number, situated between the cervical and the lumbar vertebrae, giving attachment to the ribs and forming part of the posterior wall of the thorax. Symbols T1 through T12.
**true vertebrae,** the vertebrae that normally remain unfused throughout life, i.e., the cervical, thoracic, and lumbar vertebrae.

**ver·te·brae** (vər'tə-bre) [L.] genitive and plural of *vertebra.*

**ver·te·bral** (vər'tə-brəl) [L. *vertebralis*] of or pertaining to a vertebra.

**ver·te·brar·te·ri·al** (ver″tə-brahr-tēr'e-əl) vertebroarterial.

**Ver·te·bra·ta** (vər″tə-bra'tə) a subphylum of the Chordata comprising all animals that have a vertebral column, including mammals, birds, reptiles, amphibians, and fishes.

**ver·te·brate** (vər'tə-brāt) [L. *vertebratus*] [MeSH: Vertebrates] 1. having a vertebral column. 2. any member of the subphylum Vertebrata.

**ver·te·brate col·la·gen·ase** (vər'tə-brāt kol'ə-jen-ās) see under *collagenase.*

**ver·te·brat·ed** (vər'tə-brāt'əd) made up of joints resembling the vertebrae.

**ver·te·brec·to·my** (ver″tə-brek'tə-me) [*vertebr-* + *-ectomy*] excision of a vertebra.

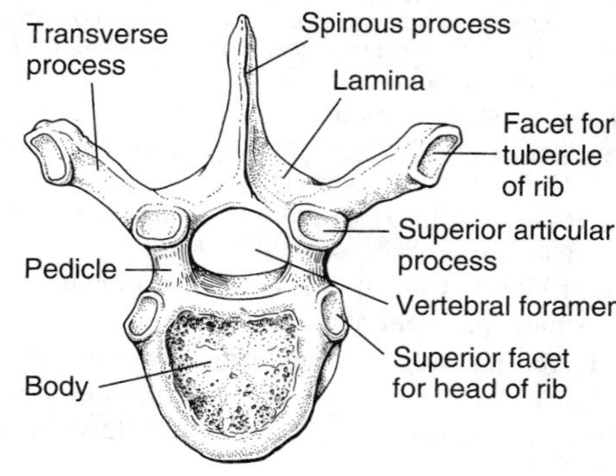


Typical (sixth) thoracic vertebra viewed from above.

**vertebr(o)-** [L. *vertebra,* q.v.] a combining form denoting relationship to a vertebra, or to the vertebral column.

**ver·te·bro·ar·te·ri·al** (vər″tə-bro-ahr-tēr′e-əl) 1. pertaining to vertebrae and arteries. 2. pertaining to the vertebral artery. Called also *vertebrarterial.*

**ver·te·bro·bas·i·lar** (vər″tə-bro-bas′ĭ-lər) pertaining to or involving the vertebral and basilar arteries.

**ver·te·bro·chon·dral** (vər″tə-bro-kon′drəl) pertaining to a vertebra and a costal cartilage.

**ver·te·bro·cos·tal** (vər″tə-bro-kos′təl) [*vertebro-* + *costal*] pertaining to a vertebra and a rib.

**ver·te·bro·did·y·mus** (vər″tə-bro-did′ĭ-məs) [*vertebro-* + *-didymus*] conjoined twins united in the region of the vertebral column.

**ver·te·brod·y·mus** (vər″tə-brod′ĭ-məs) vertebrodidymus.

**ver·te·bro·fem·or·al** (vər″tə-bro-fem′or-əl) relating to the vertebrae and the femur.

**ver·te·bro·gen·ic** (vər″tə-bro-jen′ik) arising in a vertebra or in the vertebral column.

**ver·te·bro·il·i·ac** (vər″tə-bro-il′e-ak) pertaining to the vertebrae and the ilium.

**ver·te·bro·mam·ma·ry** (vər″tə-bro-mam′ə-re) pertaining to or extending between the vertebral column and the pectoral region.

**ver·te·bro·sa·cral** (vər″tə-bro-sa′krəl) pertaining to the vertebrae and the sacrum.

**ver·te·bro·ster·nal** (vər″tə-bro-stər′nəl) pertaining to the vertebrae and the sternum.

**ver·tex** (vər′təks) pl. *ver′tices* [L.] [TA] 1. a general term in anatomical nomenclature for a summit or top. 2. the top or crown of the head; called also *v. cranii.*
**v. of bony cranium,** the highest point or crown of the skull; generally located on the sagittal suture, usually near the midpoint. Called also *v. cranii ossei.*
**v. cor′neae** [TA], vertex of cornea: the central, thinner portion of the cornea.
**v. cra′nii,** vertex (def. 2).
**v. cra′nii os′sei,** v. of bony cranium.

**ver·ti·cal** (vər′tĭ-kəl) 1. perpendicular to the plane of the horizon; see also *verticalis.* 2. relating to the vertex. 3. spreading from one generation to another; see under *transmission.*

**ver·ti·ca·lis** (vər″tĭ-ka′lis) [L.] 1. vertical (def. 1). 2. [TA] a general term used in reference to structures with the body in the anatomical, that is, upright, position.

**ver·tic·il·late** (vər-tis′ĭ-lāt) [L. *vertex* a whorl] arranged in the form of a whorl.

**Ver·ti·cil·li·um** (vər″tĭ-sil′e-əm) a genus of Fungi Imperfecti of the form-class Hyphomycetes, form-family Moniliaceae. Some species cause apple wilt, and some contain trichothecenes and can cause alimentary toxic aleukia. A species called *V. gra′phii,* isolated from otitis externa and mycotic keratitis, may actually be a species of *Trichosporon.*

**ver·ti·co·men·tal** (vər″tĭ-ko-men′təl) pertaining to the vertex and the chin.

**ver·tig·i·nous** (vər-tij′ĭ-nəs) [L. *vertiginosus*] pertaining to or affected with vertigo.

**ver·ti·go** (vər′tĭ-go) [L. *vertigo*] [MeSH: Vertigo] an illusory sense that either the environment or one's own body is revolving; it may result from diseases of the inner ear or may be due to disturbances of the vestibular centers or pathways in the central nervous system. The term is sometimes erroneously used to mean any form of dizziness. Cf. *dysequilibrium.*
**alternobaric v.,** a transient vertigo sometimes affecting those such as caisson workers and members of airplane crews who are subjected to large, rapid variations in barometric pressure; see also *barotrauma.* Called also *pressure v.*
**angiopathic v.,** vertigo due to arteriosclerosis of cerebral vessels, particularly the vertebral or basilar arteries; called also *arteriosclerotic v.*
**apoplectic v.,** scotodinia.
**arteriosclerotic v.,** angiopathic v.
**benign paroxysmal v. of childhood,** a form of paroxysmal vertigo occurring in young children otherwise in good health; sudden attacks are accompanied by pallor, sweating, and immobility and less often by vomiting and nystagmus.
**benign paroxysmal positional v., benign paroxysmal postural v.,** recurrent positional vertigo and nystagmus occurring when the head is placed in certain positions such as with one ear down, and relieved by returning to an upright position. It is usually due to otolithiasis that causes exaggerated movement of the endolymph, rather than to a central nervous system lesion.
**benign positional v., benign postural v.,** benign paroxysmal positional v.
**central v.,** vertigo due to disease of the central nervous system. See also *cerebral v.*
**cerebral v.,** vertigo resulting from a brain lesion, such as a cerebellar infarct. Called also *organic v.*
**cervical v.,** vertigo after injury to the neck such as whiplash.
**disabling positional v.,** constant positional vertigo or dysequilibrium and nausea in the upright position, without hearing disturbance or loss of vestibular function.
**encephalic v.,** a sensation of movement of tissues within the skull, as of the brain turning over and over.
**endemic paralytic v.,** vestibular neuronitis.
**epidemic v.,** vestibular neuronitis.
**epileptic v.,** vertigo that accompanies epilepsy, usually as part of an aura. See also *vertiginous epilepsy.*
**essential v.,** vertigo whose cause is unknown.
**gastric v.,** a form associated with disease or disorder of the stomach.
**height v.,** dizziness (not a true vertigo) felt on looking down from a high location.
**horizontal v.,** positional vertigo experienced when a person lies down.
**labyrinthine v.,** Meniere's disease.
**laryngeal v.,** tussive syncope.
**lateral v.,** vertigo caused by rapidly passing a row of similar objects, such as a fence or a series of pillars.
**mechanical v.,** vertigo due to long-continued turning or vibration of the body, as in motion sickness.
**nocturnal v.,** a sensation of falling occurring as the subject is going to sleep.
**objective v.,** a form in which the objects seen by the patient seem to be moving around him, in contrast to *subjective vertigo.*
**ocular v.,** a form due to eye disease, especially to paralysis of or lack of balance in the eye muscles.
**organic v.,** cerebral v.
**paralytic v.,** vestibular neuronitis.
**paralyzing v.,** vertigo so severe that the patient is afraid to move.
**paroxysmal v.,** vertigo occurring in sudden, brief attacks; see *benign paroxysmal positional v.* and *benign paroxysmal v. of childhood.*
**peripheral v.,** vestibular v.
**pilot's v.,** spatial disorientation.
**positional v.,** vertigo associated with a specific position of the head in space or changes in the position of the head in space. See also *benign paroxysmal positional v., disabling positional v., horizontal v,* and *vertical v.* Called also *postural v.*
**posttraumatic v.,** vertigo following some injury, such as fracture of the temporal bone, whiplash (see *cervical v.*), or lesions of the cerebral cortex or cerebellum.
**postural v.,** positional v.
**pressure v.,** alternobaric v.
**primary v.,** vestibular v.
**recurrent aural v.,** Meniere's disease.
**residual v.,** 1. vertigo in the aftermath of some disease process. 2. vertigo associated with motion, resulting from hypofunction or absence of vestibular sensory or neural elements; see also *positional v.*
**riders' v.,** motion sickness.
**rotary v., rotatory v.,** subjective v.
**stomachal v.,** gastric v.
**v. ab sto′macho lae′so,** gastric v.
**subjective v.,** that in which the patient has a sensation of turning round and round, in contrast to *objective vertigo.* Called also *rotatory v.* and *systematic v.*
**systematic v.,** subjective v.
**tenebric v.,** scotodinia.
**toxic v.,** vertigo as a result of ototoxicity; see also *acute serous labyrinthitis.*
**vertical v.,** 1. height v. 2. positional vertigo experienced when a person is in an upright position.
**vestibular v.,** vertigo due to disturbances of the vestibular system; cf. *Meniere's disease.* Called also *peripheral v.* and *primary v.*

**ver·tig·ra·phy** (vər-tig′rə-fe) [*vertigo* + *-graphy*] tomography.

**ve·ru·mon·ta·ni·tis** (ver″u-mon″tə-ni′tis) colliculitis.

**ve·ru·mon·ta·num** (ver″u-mon-ta′nəm) [L. "mountain ridge"] colliculus seminalis.

**ve·sa·li·an** (və-sa′le-ən) named in honor of Andreas *Vesalius,* as the vesalian bone (os vesalianum) or vein.

**ve·sa·li·a·num** (və-sa″le-a′nəm) [Andreas *Vesalius*] a name applied to several sesamoid bones: one on the outer border of the foot between the cuboid and fifth metatarsal bone, and one (sometimes more) in the tendon of origin of the gastrocnemius muscle.

**Ve·sa·li·us** (və-sa′le-əs) Andreas (1514–1564). A Flemish physician and professor of anatomy of Padua, where in 1543 he produced his

*De humani corporis fabrica libri septem* (Seven Books on the Structure of the Human Body) and founded the modern science of anatomy. Following Galen's exhortations to dissect and observe, Vesalius dissected and observed and overthrew Galen's anatomy (which was founded on nonhuman dissection). Vesalius standardized anatomical nomenclature and made important contributions in osteology and myology; in cardiology he rejected Galen's doctrine of the pervious septum. The riot of criticism for the old orthodoxy and against Vesalius drove him from Padua to Spain, where he became physician to Emperor Charles V.

**Ve•sa•li•us' foramen, ligament** (ve-sa'le-əs) [A. *Vesalius*] see *foramen venosum,* under *foramen,* and *ligamentum inguinale.*

**Vesic.** abbreviation for L. *vesic'ula, vesicato'rium,* a blister.

**ve•si•ca** (və-si'kə) gen. and pl. *vesi'cae* [L.] [TA] bladder: a general term in anatomical nomenclature for a membranous sac or receptacle for a secretion.
**v. bilia'ris** [TA], gallbladder: the pear-shaped reservoir for the bile on the posteroinferior surface of the liver between the right and quadrate lobes; from its neck, the cystic duct projects to join the common bile duct. Called also *cholecyst, cystis fellea* and *v. fellea* [TA alternative].
**v. fel'lea,** TA alternative for *v. biliaris.*
**v. prosta'tica,** utriculus prostaticus.
**v. urina'ria** [TA], urinary bladder: the musculomembranous sac, situated in the anterior part of the pelvic cavity, that serves as a reservoir for urine; it receives the excretory products of the kidneys through the ureters, and expels them through the urethra. Called also *bladder.*

**ve•si•cae** (və-si'se) [L.] genitive and plural of *vesica.*

**ves•i•cal** (ves'ĭ-kəl) pertaining to the urinary bladder.

**ves•i•cant** (ves'ĭ-kənt) [L. *vesica* blister] 1. causing blisters; blistering. 2. a blistering drug or agent.

**ves•i•ca•tion** (ves″ĭ-ka'shən) 1. the process of blistering. 2. a blistered spot or surface.

**ves•i•ca•to•ry** (ves″ĭ-kə-tor'e) [L. *vesicare* to blister] vesicant.

**ves•i•cle** (ves'ĭ-kəl) [L. *vesicula,* dim. of *vesica* bladder] 1. a small bladder or sac containing liquid; see also *vesicula.* 2. a small circumscribed epidermal elevation, usually containing a clear fluid. Cf. *bulla.* 3. the swollen end of a conidiophore from which sterigmata are produced.
**acoustic v.,** otic v.
**acrosomal v.,** a membrane-bounded vacuolelike structure containing the enlarging acrosomal granule, which undergoes collapse and spreads over the upper two thirds of the head (acrosome) of a spermatozoon to form a head cap.
**allantoic v.,** see under *diverticulum.*
**amniocardiac v's,** fissures in the mesoderm of the early embryo representing the paired primordia of the pericardial sac and the heart.
**archoplasmic v.,** a sac developed from the attraction sphere of a spermatid and growing into the sheath of the tail of the spermatozoon.
**auditory v.,** otic v.
**blastodermic v.,** blastocyst.
**brain v's,** the five divisions of the closed neural tube in the developing embryo, including, in craniocaudal sequence, the telencephalon, diencephalon, mesencephalon, metencephalon, and myelencephalon.
**brain v's, primary,** the three earliest subdivisions of the embryonic neural tube, including the prosencephalon, mesencephalon, and rhombencephalon.
**brain v's, secondary,** the five brain vesicles formed by specialization of the prosencephalon (telencephalon and diencephalon), mesencephalon, and rhombencephalon (metencephalon and myelencephalon) in later embryonic development.
**cephalic v's, cerebral v's,** brain v's.
**cervical v.,** a temporary sac in the cervical region of the embryo formed by the closing off of the cervical sinus.
**chorionic v.,** the chorion of a mammal.
**concentrating v's,** condensing vacuoles.
**encephalic v's,** brain v's.
**germinal v.,** the fluid-filled nucleus of an oocyte toward the end of prophase of its meiotic division.
**graafian v's,** folliculi ovarici vesiculosi.
**intermediate v's,** transfer v's.
**lens v.,** a vesicle formed from the lens pit of the embryo; it later develops into the crystalline lens.
**matrix v's,** small membrane-limited structures at sites of calcification of the cartilage matrix.
**ocular v.,** vesicula ophthalmica.
**olfactory v.,** 1. the vesicle in the embryo which later develops into the olfactory bulb and tract. 2. a bulbous expansion at the distal end of an olfactory cell, from which the olfactory hairs project.
**ophthalmic v., optic v.,** vesicula ophthalmica.
**otic v.,** a detached ovoid sac formed by closure of the otic pit in embryonic development of the external ear; called also *acoustic* or *auditory v.*
**phagocytotic v.,** phagosome.
**pinocytotic v.,** pinosome.
**pituitary v.,** Rathke's pouch.
**plasmalemmal v.,** caveola.
**prostatic v.,** utriculus prostaticus.
**Purkinje v.,** germinal v.
**secretory v's,** condensing vacuoles.
**seminal v.,** glandula vesiculosa.
**sense v.,** the vesicular primordium of a sense organ in the embryo.
**spermatic v., false,** utriculus prostaticus.
**synaptic v's,** small membrane-bound structures behind a presynaptic membrane, containing neurotransmitters; when depolarization occurs they fuse with the presynaptic membrane and release the neurotransmitter into the synaptic cleft.
**transfer v's, transitional v's, transport v's,** small vesicles formed by budding off of the granular endoplasmic reticulum, in which secretory material is transferred to the Golgi complex, where it is concentrated in condensing vacuoles (q.v.). Called also *intermediate v's.*
**umbilical v.,** the pear-shaped expansion of the yolk sac growing out into the cavity of the chorion at the end of the fourth week of development, and joined to the midgut of the embryo by the yolk stalk.
**water expulsion v.,** contractile vacuole.

**vesic(o)-** [L. *vesica* bladder] a combining form denoting relationship to the bladder, or to a blister.

**ves•i•co•ab•dom•i•nal** (ves″ĭ-ko-ab-dom'ĭ-nəl) abdominocystic.

**ves•i•co•cav•er•nous** (ves″ĭ-ko-kav'ər-nəs) both vesicular and cavernous.

**ves•i•co•cele** (ves'ĭ-ko-sēl″) [*vesico-* + *-cele*[1]] hernial protrusion of the bladder.

**ves•i•co•cer•vi•cal** (ves″ĭ-ko-sər'vĭ-kəl) [*vesico-* + *cervical*] pertaining to the urinary bladder and the cervix uteri, or communicating with the bladder and the cervical canal, as a vesicocervical fistula. Called also *cervicovesical.*

**ves•i•coc•ly•sis** (ves″ĭ-kok'lĭ-sis) [*vesico-* + *clysis*] the injection of a fluid into the urinary bladder.

**ves•i•co•col•ic** (ves″ĭ-ko-kol'ik) vesicocolonic.

**ves•i•co•co•lon•ic** (ves″ĭ-ko-ko-lon'ik) pertaining to or communicating with the urinary bladder and colon, as a vesicocolonic fistula. Called also *colovesical* and *vesicocolic.*

**ves•i•co•en•ter•ic** (ves″ĭ-ko-en-ter'ik) vesicointestinal.

**ves•i•co•fix•a•tion** (ves″ĭ-ko-fik-sa'shən) the surgical fixation of the urinary bladder; cystopexy.

**ves•i•co•in•tes•ti•nal** (ves″ĭ-ko-in-tes'tĭ-nəl) pertaining to or communicating with the urinary bladder and intestine, as a vesicointestinal fistula. Called also *enterovesical* and *vesicoenteric.*

**ves•i•co•per•i•ne•al** (ves″ĭ-ko-per″ĭ-ne'əl) pertaining to or communicating with the urinary bladder and perineum, as a vesicoperineal fistula.

**ves•i•co•pros•tat•ic** (ves″ĭ-ko-pros-tat'ik) pertaining to the urinary bladder and the prostate.

**ves•i•co•pu•bic** (ves″ĭ-ko-pu'bik) pertaining to the urinary bladder and the pubic region. Called also *pubovesical.*

**ves•i•co•pus•tule** (ves″ĭ-ko-pus'tūl) a vesicle which is developing into a pustule by entry of leukocytes into its contents.

**ves•i•co•rec•tal** (ves″ĭ-ko-rek'təl) pertaining to the urinary bladder and the rectum.

**ves•i•co•re•nal** (ves″ĭ-ko-re'nəl) pertaining to the urinary bladder and the kidney.

**ves•i•co•sig•moid** (ves″ĭ-ko-sig'moid) pertaining to the urinary bladder and sigmoid flexure.

**ves•i•co•sig•moid•os•to•my** (ves″ĭ-ko-sig″moi-dos'tə-me) [*vesico-*

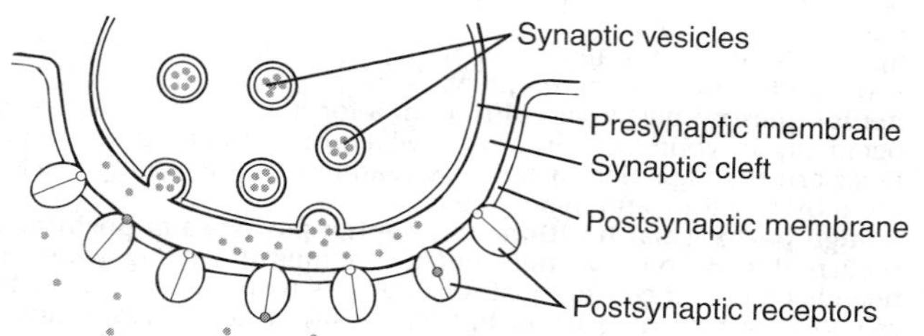


Diagram of synaptic vesicles in a synapse.

+ *sigmoidostomy*] surgical creation of an opening between the urinary bladder and the sigmoid colon.

**ves·i·co·spi·nal** (ves″ĭ-ko-spi′nəl) pertaining to the urinary bladder and the spinal cord.

**ves·i·cos·to·my** (ves″ĭ-kos′tə-me) cystostomy.
**cutaneous v.,** surgical anastomosis of the bladder mucosa to an opening in the skin below the umbilicus, creating a stoma for bladder drainage; done in infants as a temporary alternative to suprapubic cystostomy.

**ves·i·cot·o·my** (ves″ĭ-kot′ə-me) cystotomy.

**ves·i·co·um·bil·i·cal** (ves″ĭ-ko-əm-bil′ĭ-kəl) pertaining to the urinary bladder and the umbilicus.

**ves·i·co·ura·chal** (ves″ĭ-ko-u′rə-kəl) pertaining to the urinary bladder and the urachus.

**ves·i·co·ure·ter·al** (ves″ĭ-ko-u-re′ter-al) vesicoureteric.

**ves·i·co·ure·ter·ic** (ves″ĭ-ko-u-re′ter-ik) pertaining to or communicating with the urinary bladder and the ureter.

**ves·i·co·ure·thral** (ves″ĭ-ko-u-re′thrəl) pertaining to or communicating with the urinary bladder and the urethra.

**ves·i·co·uter·ine** (ves″ĭ-ko-u′tər-in) pertaining to or communicating with the urinary bladder and the uterus.

**ves·i·co·utero·vag·i·nal** (ves″ĭ-ko-u″tər-o-vaj′ĭ-nəl) pertaining to or communicating with the urinary bladder, uterus, and vagina.

**ves·i·co·vag·i·nal** (ves″ĭ-ko-vaj′ĭ-nəl) pertaining to or communicating with the urinary bladder and vagina.

**ves·i·co·vag·i·no·rec·tal** (ves″ĭ-ko-vaj″ĭ-no-rek′təl) pertaining to or communicating with the urinary bladder, vagina, and rectum.

**ve·sic·u·la** (və-sik′u-lə) pl. *vesic′ulae* [L., dim. of *vesica*] vesicle: general anatomical nomenclature for a small bladder or sac containing liquid.
**v. bi′lis, v. fel′lea,** vesica biliaris.
**v. germinati′va,** germinal vesicle.
**vesi′culae graafia′nae,** folliculi ovarici vesiculosi.
**vesi′culae nabo′thi,** Naboth's follicles.
**v. ophthal′mica,** optic vesicle: an evagination developing on either side of the forebrain of the early embryo, from which the percipient parts of the eye are formed.
**v. prosta′tica,** utriculus prostaticus.
**v. semina′lis,** TA alternative for *glandula vesiculosa.*
**v. sero′sa,** chorion.

**ve·sic·u·lae** (və-sik′u-le) [L.] genitive and plural of *vesicula.*

**ve·sic·u·lar** (və-sik′u-lər) composed of or relating to vesicles.

**ve·sic·u·lat·ed** (və-sik′u-lāt″əd) having vesicles.

**ve·sic·u·la·tion** (və-sik″u-la′shən) the presence or formation of vesicles.

**ve·sic·u·lec·to·my** (və-sik″u-lek′tə-me) [*vesicle* + *-ectomy*] excision of a vesicle, especially the seminal vesicle.

**ve·sic·u·li·form** (və-sik′u-lĭ-form″) [*vesicle* + *form*] shaped like a vesicle.

**ve·sic·u·li·tis** (və-sik″u-li′tis) inflammation of a vesicle, especially of a seminal vesicle.

**ve·sic·u·lo·bron·chi·al** (və-sik″u-lo-brong′ke-əl) said of breath sounds having characteristics of both vesicular and bronchial sounds.

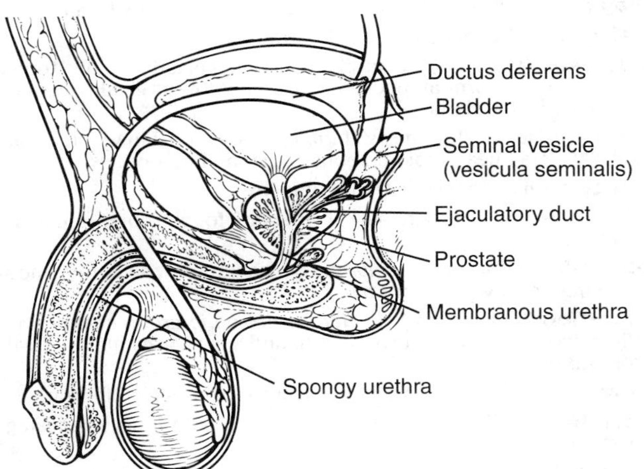


Vesicula seminalis (seminal vesicle) in a median sagittal section of the male urogenital organs.

**ve·sic·u·lo·cav·er·nous** (və-sik″u-lo-kav′ər-nəs) having both vesicular and cavernous qualities, such as abnormal respiration.

**ve·sic·u·lo·gram** (və-sik′u-lo-gram″) a radiograph of the seminal vesicles.

**ve·sic·u·log·ra·phy** (və-sik″u-log′rə-fe) radiography of the seminal vesicles.

**ve·sic·u·lo·pap·u·lar** (və-sik″u-lo-pap′u-lər) pertaining to or characterized by vesicles and papules.

**ve·sic·u·lo·pus·tu·lar** (və-sik″u-lo-pus′tu-lər) consisting of or pertaining to vesicles and pustules.

**ve·sic·u·lot·o·my** (və-sik″u-lot′ə-me) [*vesicle* + *-tomy*] incision of a vesicle, especially the seminal vesicle.

**ve·sic·u·lo·tu·bu·lar** (və-sik″u-lo-too′bu-lər) having both a vesicular and a tubular quality; said of auscultatory sounds.

**ve·sic·u·lo·tym·pan·ic** (və-sik″u-lo-tim-pan′ik) vesiculotympanitic.

**ve·sic·u·lo·tym·pa·nit·ic** (və-sik″u-lo-tim-pə-nit′ik) having both a vesicular and tympanitic quality; said of auscultatory sounds or resonance. Called also *vesiculotympanic.*

**Ves·ic·u·lo·vi·rus** (və-sik′u-lo-vi″rəs) [L. *vesicula* vesicle + *virus*] [MeSH: Vesiculovirus] vesicular stomatitis-like viruses: a genus of viruses of the family Rhabdoviridae that includes viruses that cause vesicular stomatitis in swine, cattle, and horses and related viruses that infect man and other animals. Mosquitoes, sandflies, and ticks are vectors, and some viral species have been isolated only from arthropods.

**Ves·pa** (ves′pə) a genus of wasps and hornets of the family Vespidae; several species live in Europe or North America and have painful stings.

**ves·per·al** (ves′pər-əl) [L. *vespera* evening] pertaining to or occurring in the evening.

**Ves·pi·dae** (ves′pĭ-de) the social wasps, a family of flying insects of the order Hymenoptera that have a long thin body and delicate wings; many species can sting. Members of this family live in complicated social units with castes. Genera include *Polistes, Vespa,* and *Vespula.*

**Ves·prin** (ves′prin) trademark for preparations of triflupromazine.

**Ves·pu·la** (ves′pu-lə) a genus of wasps and hornets of the family Vespidae; several species are common in North America and have painful stings.

**ves·sel** (ves′əl) any channel for carrying a fluid, such as the blood or lymph; see also *vas.*
**absorbent v.,** vas lymphaticum.
**afferent v. of glomerulus,** arteriola glomerularis afferens.
**afferent v's of lymph node,** vasa afferentia nodi lymphatici.
**anastomotic v.,** vas anastomoticum.
**arterioluminal v's,** small branches of coronary arterioles that lie near the endocardium, and after a short course open directly into the lumen of the heart.
**arteriosinusoidal v's,** small branches of coronary arterioles that soon break up into sinusoids that lie between bundles or individual muscle fibers of the heart.
**bile v's,** ductuli biliferi.
**blood v.,** any of the vessels conveying the blood; an artery, arteriole, capillary, venule, or vein.
**chyliferous v.,** lacteal, def. 2.
**collateral v.,** 1. vas collaterale. 2. a vessel important in establishing and maintaining collateral circulation (q.v.).
**efferent v. of glomerulus,** arteriola glomerularis efferens.
**efferent v's of lymph node,** vasa efferentia nodi lymphatici.
**great v's,** the large vessels entering the heart, including the aorta, the pulmonary arteries and veins, and the venae cavae.
**hemorrhoidal v's,** veins of the rectum which have become dilated and swollen; see *hemorrhoid.*
**Jungbluth's v's,** vasa propria of Jungbluth.
**lacteal v.,** lacteal, def. 2.
**lymphatic v's,** vasa lymphatica.
**lymphatic v., deep,** vas lymphaticum profundum.
**lymphatic v., superficial,** vas lymphaticum superficiale.
**lymphocapillary v.,** vas lymphocapillare.
**nutrient v's,** vessels that supply nutritive elements to special tissues, such as arteries entering the substance of bone, or supplying walls of the blood vessels themselves. See also *arteria nutricia.*
**sinusoidal v.,** vas sinusoideum.

**ves·tib·u·la** (ves-tib′u-lə) [L.] plural of *vestibulum.*

**ves·tib·u·lar** (ves-tib′u-lər) [L. *vestibularis*] 1. pertaining to or toward a vestibule. 2. in dental anatomy, used to refer to the tooth surface directed toward the vestibule of the mouth; see *facies vestibularis dentis.*

**ves·ti·bule** (ves′tĭ-būl) [MeSH: Vestibule] a space or cavity at the entrance to a canal; called also *vestibulum* [TA].
**v. of aorta,** a space within the left ventricle at the root of the aorta.
**buccal v.,** that portion of the vestibule of the mouth that lies between the cheeks and the teeth and gingivae or residual alveolar ridges.
**v. of ear,** vestibulum auris.
**labial v.,** that portion of the vestibule of the mouth that lies between the lips and the teeth and gingivae, or residual alveolar ridges.
**v. of larynx,** vestibulum laryngis.
**v. of mouth,** vestibulum oris.
**nasal v., v. of nose,** vestibulum nasi.
**v. of omental bursa,** vestibulum bursae omentalis.
**Sibson's v.,** v. of aorta.
**v. of vagina, v. of vulva,** vestibulum vaginae.

**Ves·ti·bu·li·fer·ia** (vəs-ti″bu-lĭ-fer′e-ə) [*vestibule* + Gr. *phōros* bearing] a subclass of free-living or parasitic (especially in the digestive tract of vertebrates and invertebrates) ciliate protozoa (class Kinetofragminophorea, phylum Ciliophora), characterized by the presence of a cytosome within a groove (vestibulum) bearing distinct ciliature at or near the apical end of the body and a cytopharynx. It comprises three orders: Trichostomatida, Entodiniomorphida, and Colpodida.

**ves·tib·u·li·tis** (ves-tib″u-li′tis) inflammation of the vulvar vestibule and the periglandular and subepithelial stroma; it results in a burning sensation and dyspareunia.

**ves·tib·u·lo·cer·e·bel·lum** (vəs-tib″u-lo-ser″ə-bel′əm) [*vestibular system* + *cerebellum*] [TA] the portion of the cerebellum serving as the primary site of termination of the vestibular afferents, roughly corresponding to the flocculonodular lobe; therefore, the term is sometimes equated with archicerebellum, which is the anatomical division of the cerebellum comprising the flocculonodular lobe. Cf. *spinocerebellum* and *pontocerebellum.*

**ves·tib·u·lo·coch·le·ar** (ves-tib″u-lo-kok′le-ər) pertaining to the vestibule of the ear and the cochlea.

**ves·tib·u·lo·gen·ic** (vəs-tib″u-lo-jen′ik) arising in a vestibule, as that of the ear.

**ves·tib·u·lo·oc·u·lar** (vəs-tib″u-lo-ok′u-lər) pertaining to the vestibular and oculomotor nerves; or to the maintenance of visual stability during head movements.

**ves·tib·u·lo·plas·ty** (vəs-tib′u-lo-plas″te) [MeSH: Vestibuloplasty] the surgical modification of the gingival–mucous membrane relationships in the vestibule of the mouth, including deepening of the vestibular trough, repositioning of the frenum or muscle attachments, and broadening of the zone of attached gingiva, after periodontal treatment.

**ves·tib·u·lot·o·my** (vəs-tib″u-lot′ə-me) [*vestibule* + *-tomy*] surgical opening of the vestibule of the inner ear.

**ves·tib·u·lo·ure·thral** (vəs-tib″u-lo-u-re′thrəl) pertaining to the vestibulum vaginae and to the urethra.

**ves·tib·u·lum** (vəs-tib′u-ləm) pl. *vestib′ula* [L.] 1. [TA] vestibule: a general term in anatomical nomenclature for a space or cavity at the entrance to a canal. 2. a depression, invagination, chamber, or cavity in the body of an organism that gives access to another such space, e.g., as the preoral chamber of certain ciliate protozoa.
**v. au′ris** [TA], vestibule of ear: an oval cavity in the middle of the bony labyrinth, communicating anteriorly with the cochlea and posteriorly with the semicircular canals, and containing perilymph surrounding the sacculus and utriculus.
**v. bur′sae omenta′lis** [TA], vestibule of omental bursa: that part of the omental bursa dorsal to the lesser omentum and adjacent to the epiploic foramen.
**v. glot′tidis,** v. laryngis.
**v. laryn′gis** [TA], vestibule of larynx: the portion of the laryngeal cavity above the vestibular folds.
**v. nasa′le, v. na′si** [TA], vestibule of nose: the anterior part of the nasal cavity situated just inferior to the nares and limited posteriorly by the limen nasi. It is lined with stratified squamous epithelium and contains hairs (vibrissae) and sebaceous glands. Called also *nasal vestibule.*
**v. o′ris** [TA], vestibule of mouth: the portion of the oral cavity bounded on one side by the teeth and gingivae, or the residual alveolar ridges, and on the other side by the lips *(labial vestibule)* and cheeks *(buccal vestibule)*; called also *cavitas oris externa, cavum oris externum,* and *external oral cavity.*
**v. vagi′nae** [TA], vestibule of vagina: the space between the labia minora into which the urethra and vagina open.

**ves·tige** (ves′tij) the remnant of a structure which functioned in a previous stage of species or individual development; called also *vestigium.*

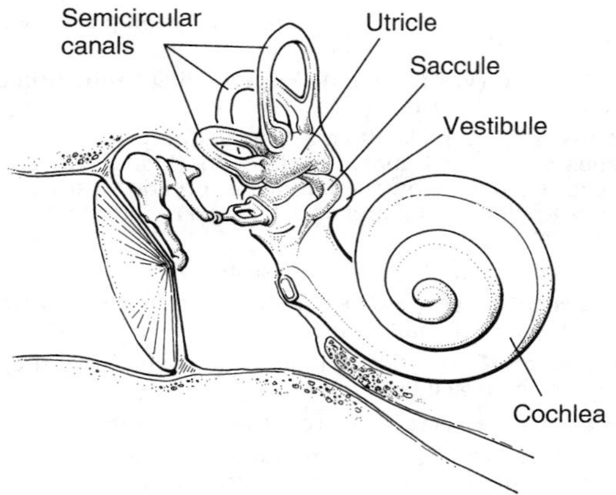


Vestibule of the ear.

**coccygeal v.,** the remnant of the caudal end of the neural tube.
**v. of vaginal process,** vestigium processus vaginalis.

**ves·tig·ia** (vəs-tij′e-ə) [L.] plural of *vestigium.*

**ves·tig·i·al** (vəs-tij′e-əl) of the nature of a vestige, trace, or relic; rudimentary.

**ves·ti·gi·um** (vəs-tĭ′je-əm) pl. *vesti′gia* [L. "a trace"] [TA] vestige: a general term in anatomical nomenclature for the degenerating remains of any structure which served as a functioning entity in the embryo or fetus.
**v. proces′sus vagina′lis** [TA], vestige of vaginal process: a band of connective tissue in the spermatic cord which is that vestige of the processus vaginalis; called also *rudimentum processus vaginalis.*

**ve·su·vine** (ve-su′vēn) Bismark brown R.

**vetch** (vech) 1. any plant of the genus *Vicia.* 2. any of several plants of the genus *Lathyrus.*

**vet·er·i·nar·i·an** (vet″ər-ĭ-nar′e-ən) [MeSH: Veterinarians] a doctor of veterinary medicine, trained and authorized to practice veterinary medicine and surgery.

**vet·er·i·nary** (vet′ər-ĭ-nar″e) [L. *veterinarius*] pertaining to the diseases and other disorders of domestic animals.

**Vex·ol** (vek′sol) trademark for a preparation of rimexolone.

**VF** vocal fremitus.

**vf** visual field.

**VFib** ventricular fibrillation.

**VFl** ventricular flutter.

**VHDL** very-high-density lipoprotein.

**vi·a·bil·i·ty** (vi″ə-bil′ĭ-te) ability to live after birth.

**vi·a·ble** (vi′ə-bəl) capable of living; especially said of a fetus that has reached such a stage of development that it can live outside of the uterus. This usually connotes a fetus that weighs at least 500 gm and has reached a gestational age of 20 weeks (22 weeks after fertilization).

**Vi·ag·ra** (vi-ag′rə) trademark for a preparation of *sildenafil citrate.*

**vi·al** (vi′əl) [Gr. *phialē*] a small bottle.

**vi·be·sate** (vi′bə-sāt) a modified polyvinyl plastic applied topically as a spray, to form an occlusive dressing for surgical wounds and other surface lesions.

**vi·bex** (vi′beks) pl. *vi′bices* [L. *vibix* mark of a blow] 1. a line or streak. 2. a linear subcutaneous effusion of blood.

**vi·bi·ces** (vĭ-bi′sēz) [L.] plural of *vibex.*

**Vi·bra·my·cin** (vi-brə-mi′sin) trademark for a preparation of doxycycline.

**vi·bra·tile** (vi′brə-til) [L. *vibratilis*] having an oscillatory motion; swaying or moving to and fro.

**vi·bra·tion** (vi-bra′shən) [L. *vibratio,* from *vibrare* to shake] [MeSH: Vibration] 1. a rapid movement to and fro; cf. *oscillation.* 2. vibratory massage.

**vi·bra·tor** (vi′bra-tər) an instrument for producing vibrations.

**vi·bra·to·ry** (vi′brə-tor″e) [L. *vibratorius*] vibrating or causing vibration.

**Vi·bra·zole** (vi′brə-zōl) trademark for a preparation of ribavirin.

**Vib·rio** (vib′re-o) [L. *vibrare* to move rapidly, vibrate] [MeSH: Vibrio] a genus of gram-negative, facultatively anaerobic, straight or

curved, rod-shaped bacteria of the family Vibrionaceae; they are actively motile and have one or more polar flagella. Some species (the *cholera vibrios*) cause cholera; others (the *noncholera vibrios*) cause milder forms of diarrhea in humans; and others infect only animals other than humans.
**V. alginoly'ticus,** a halophilic species found in seawater and seafoods that is sometimes associated with diarrhea, septicemias, and wound infections.
**V. anguilla'rum,** the etiologic agent of an epidemic disease of carp and other fish. Called also *V. piscium.*
**V. cho'lerae,** the etiologic agent of human Asiatic cholera, found in the intestinal tract of normal and diseased humans and animals and in water. The species is divided into four biotypes. Six serogroups are based on somatic (O) antigens. Pathogenic, virulent strains produce a potent enterotoxin and agglutinate specific polyvalent 01 antiserum. Serotypes that are not agglutinated by 01 antiserum generally cause a milder diarrheal disease. Called also *V. comma.*
**V. cho'lerae** biotype **alben'sis,** a strain that may be luminescent, isolated from fresh water and from human feces and bile specimens, which does not agglutinate 01 serum and is not pathogenic. Called also *V. phosphorescens.*
**V. cho'lerae** biotype **cho'lerae,** a pathogenic strain producing epidemic and pandemic cholera. It belongs to serogroup 0:1.
**V. cho'lerae** biotype **el'tor,** a pathogenic strain first isolated in Egypt in 1960; it is the cause of the present pandemic of cholera. It belongs to serogroup 0:1. Called also *El Tor vibrio* and *V. eltor.*
**V. cho'lerae** biotype **pro'teus,** *V. metschnikovii.*
**V. co'li,** *Campylobacter jejuni.*
**V. com'ma,** *V. cholerae.*
**V. dam'sela,** a halophilic species isolated from human clinical specimens. It is oxidase positive and sucrose and lactose negative.
**V. danu'bicus,** a type of noncholera vibrio; see under *vibrio.*
**V. el'tor,** *V. cholerae* biotype *eltor.*
**V. fe'tus,** *Campylobacter fetus.*
**V. fluvia'lis,** a halophilic species isolated from human clinical specimens. It is oxidase and sucrose positive and lactose negative.
**V. ghin'da,** a type of noncholera vibrio; see under *vibrio.*
**V. har'veyi,** a luminescent species found in sea water and on the surface of dead marine animals. The organisms were formerly classified as a separate genus, *Lucibacterium.*
**V. hol'lisae,** a halophilic species isolated from human clinical specimens. It is oxidase positive and sucrose and lactose negative.
**V. jeju'ni,** *Campylobacter jejuni.*
**V. massau'ah,** a type of noncholera vibrio; see under *vibrio.*
**V. metschniko'vii,** a halophilic species found in rivers and sewage and in the intestinal tract or feces of humans and other animals, especially birds. It is pathogenic for humans and guinea pigs, producing gastroenteritis. Called also *V. cholerae* biotype *proteus* and *V. proteus.* See also *fowl septicemia,* under *septicemia.*
**V. mi'micus,** a halophilic species isolated from human clinical specimens.
**V. parahaemoly'ticus,** a halophilic species that is a major cause of gastroenteritis due to the consumption of raw or improperly cooked fish or seafood, especially in Japan.
**V. phosphores'cens,** *V. cholerae* biotype *albensis.*
**V. pis'cium,** *V. anguillarum.*
**V. pro'teus,** *V. metschnikovii.*
**V. sep'ticus,** *Clostridium septicum.*
**V. succino'genes,** *Wolinella succinogenes.*
**V. vulni'ficus,** a halophilic species whose strains are similar to *V. parahaemolyticus* and *V. alginolyticus* but differ in that they can ferment lactose. Infection by eating raw seafood causes septicemia and cellulitis, and may be especially severe or even fatal in those with preexisting hepatic disease. Wound infection may occur following exposure to sea water or from injury when handling crabs.

**vib·rio** (vib're-o) pl. *vib'rios* or *vibrio'nes* [MeSH: Vibrio] an organism of the genus *Vibrio.*
**Celebes v.,** *Vibrio cholerae,* biotype *eltor.*
**cholera v.,** *Vibrio cholerae.*
**El Tor v.,** *Vibrio cholerae* biotype *eltor.*
**v. group EF-6, v. group F,** a group of vibrios isolated from individuals with diarrheal disease.
**NAG v's, nonagglutinating v's,** nonpathogenic paracholera vibrios, unrelated to the cholera vibrio O antigenic group.
**noncholera v's (NCVs),** a group of microorganisms similar to *Vibrio cholerae,* but differing from it immunologically; they have variable pathogenic properties. Many have been isolated from water or from the feces of persons with mild diarrhea and have been named for the place of their discovery, as *V. danu'bicus, V. ghin'da,* and *V. massau'ah.* Called also *paracholera v's.*
**paracholera v's,** noncholera v's.

**vib·rio·ci·dal** (vib″re-o-si'dəl) destructive to organisms of the genus *Vibrio,* especially *V. cholerae.*

**Vib·rio·na·ceae** (vib″re-o-na'se-e) [MeSH: Vibrionaceae] a family of gram-negative, facultatively anaerobic, motile, straight or curved, rod-shaped bacteria. It contains the genera *Aeromonas, Photobacterium, Plesiomonas,* and *Vibrio.*

**vib·ri·o·nes** (vib″re-o'nēz) plural of *vibrio.*

**vib·ri·o·sis** (vib″re-o'sis) infection with bacteria of the genus *Vibrio.*
**bovine genital v.,** see under *campylobacteriosis.*
**ovine genital v.,** see under *campylobacteriosis.*

**vi·bris·sa** (vi-bris'ə) [L.] singular of *vibrissae.*

**vi·bris·sae** (vi-bris'e) sing. *vibris'sa* [L. pl. of *vibrissa*] [MeSH: Vibrissae] 1. [TA] the hairs growing in the vestibular region of the nasal cavity. 2. long coarse hairs growing around the nose (muzzle) of an animal, as of the dog or cat.

**vi·bro·acous·tic** (vi″bro-ə-kōōs'tik) 1. containing both vibratory and acoustic elements. 2. referring to sound associated with tactile vibration as well as, or instead of, auditory stimuli.

**Vi·bur·num** (vi-bur'nəm) [L.] a genus of trees and shrubs of the family Caprifoliaceae. *V. o'pulus* is the cranberry bush or tree, whose dried bark is medicinal; see *cramp bark,* under *bark. V. prunifo'lium* L. is the black haw, whose root and stem have bark that has been used as a uterine sedative.

**vi·car·i·ous** (vi-kar'e-əs) [L. *vicarius*] acting in the place of another or of something else; occurring at an abnormal site.

**Vic·ia** (vish'e-ə) the vetches, a genus of climbing plants of the family Leguminosae.
**V. fa'ba, V. fa'va,** a species whose beans or pollen contain a component that causes favism (q.v.) in susceptible individuals; called also *fava, fava bean,* and *broad bean.*
**V. sati'va,** a common species of vetch that contains cyanogenetic compounds and also causes photosensitization and liver damage in livestock.

**vi·cine** (vi'sin) a pyrimidine-based glycoside occurring in species of *Vicia*; in fava beans it is cleaved by an endogenous $\beta$-glucosidase to form the toxic compound divicine.

**Vi·co·pro·fin** (vi-ko-pro'fin) trademark for a preparation of hydrocodone bitartrate plus ibuprofen.

**Vicq d'Azyr's band,** etc. (vēk dah-zērz') [Félix *Vicq d'Azyr,* French anatomist, 1748–1794] see *fasciculus mammillothalamicus, foramen caecum medullae oblongatae,* and see *Kaes-Bekhterev layer,* under *layer.*

**Vi·cryl** (vi'krəl) trademark for polyglactin 910.

**vi·dar·a·bine** (vi-dar'ə-bēn) [MeSH: Vidarabine] a purine analogue that inhibits DNA synthesis; used in a sterile solution as a topical antiviral agent in the treatment of herpes simplex keratitis and intravenously in the treatment of herpes simplex encephalitis. Called also *adenine arabinoside* or *ara-A.*

**vid·eo·den·si·tom·e·try** (vĭ'de-o-den″sĭ-tom'ə-tre) densitometry using a video camera to record the images to be analyzed.

**vid·eo·flu·o·ros·co·py** (vid″e-o-flōō-ros'kə-pe) the recording on videotape of the images appearing on a fluoroscopic screen.

**vid·e·og·no·sis** (vid″e-og-no'sis) [*video-,* from L. *videre* to see + *diagnosis*] diagnosis based on the interpretation of radiographs transmitted by television techniques to a radiologic center.

**vid·eo·lap·a·ros·co·py** (vid″e-o-lap″ə-ros'kə-pe) laparoscopic surgery aided by a video camera.

**vid·eo·la·ser·os·co·py** (vid″e-o-la-zər-os'kə-pe) [*video-* + *laser* + *-scopy*] a modification of laser laparoscopy in which the inside of the cavity is visualized through a video camera that projects an enlarged image onto a video monitor.

**vid·eo·mi·cros·co·py** (vid″e-o-mi-kros'kə-pe) television microscopy.

**Vi·dex** (vi'deks) trademark for a preparation of didanosine.

**vid·i·an artery, canal, nerve, veins** (vid'e-ən) [Guido Guidi (L. *Vidius*), Italian anatomist, 1500–1569] see *arteria canalis pterygoidei, canalis pterygoideus, nervus canalis pterygoidei, nervus petrosus profundus,* and *venae canalis pterygoidei.*

**Vieus·sens' ansa,** etc. (vyōō-sahz') [Raymond de *Vieussens,* French anatomist, 1641–1715] see *ansa subclavia, cavum septi pellucidi, foramina venarum minimarum atrii dextri, limbus fossae ovalis,* and *venae ventriculi dextri anteriores.*

**view** (vu) projection (def. 5).

**VIG** vaccinia immune globulin.

**vi·ga·ba·trin** (vi-ga'bə-trin) an antiepileptic also used to control tardive dyskinesias; administered orally.

**vig·il·am·bu·lism** (vij″il-am'bu-liz-əm) an ambulatory automatism resembling somnambulism but occurring in the waking state.

**vig·i·lance** (vij'ĭ-ləns) [L. *vigilantia*] alert watchfulness, particularly with regard to danger or other changes in the environment; attentiveness; readiness to respond to stimuli.

**vi·gin·ti·nor·mal** (vi-jin″tĭ-nor′məl) [L. *viginti* twenty + *normal*] having one twentieth the strength of normal, as a solution.

**Vig·nal's cells** (vēn-yahlz′) [Guillaume *Vignal,* French physiologist, 1852–1893] see under *cell.*

**vig·or** (vig′ər) [L. *vigere* to flourish] a combination of attributes of living organisms which expresses itself in rapid growth, high fertility and fecundity, large size, and long life.
**hybrid v.,** heterosis.

**Vil·lar·et's syndrome** (ve-yahr-āz′) [Maurice *Villaret,* French neurologist, 1877–1946] see under *syndrome.*

**vil·li** (vil′i) [L.] genitive and plural of *villus.*

**vil·lif·er·ous** (vĭ-lif′ər-əs) having or bearing villi.

**vil·li·ki·nin** (vil″ĭ-ki′nin) [*villi* + Gr. *kinein* to move] a hormone hypothesized to exist in the duodenum, stimulating villus movement and being released by action of hydrochloric acid on the mucous membrane.

**vil·lin** (vil′in) an intracellular protein found in the intestinal epithelium and elsewhere; it severs microfilaments at high calcium concentrations and blocks their growth at low calcium concentrations.

**vil·li·tis** (vĭ-li′tis) [*villi* + *-itis*] 1. *villositis.* 2. inflammation of the villous tissue of the coronet and of the plantar substance of a horse's foot.

**vil·lo·ma** (vĭ-lo′mə) [*villus* + *-oma*] papilloma.

**vil·lo·nod·u·lar** (vil″o-nod′u-lər) characterized by villous and nodular thickening; said of a proliferative disorder of the synovial tissue.

**vil·lose** (vil′ōs) [L. *villosus*] shaggy with soft hairs; covered with villi.

**vil·lo·si·tis** (vil″o-si′tis) a bacterial disease characterized by alterations in the villi of the placenta. Called also *villitis.*

**vil·los·i·ty** (vĭ-los′ĭ-te) 1. the condition of being covered with villi. 2. a villus.

**vil·lous** (vil′əs) villose.

**vil·lus** (vil′əs) pl. *vil′li* [L. "tuft of hair"] 1. a small protrusion resembling a tuft of hair. 2. [TA] a general term in anatomical nomenclature for a small vascular process or protrusion, especially such a protrusion from the free surface of a membrane.
**amniotic v.,** one of the irregular, flat, opaque areas of imperfect skin on the amnion near the distal end of the umbilical cord.
**anchoring v.,** a chorionic villus that attaches to the decidua basalis.
**arachnoid villi,** 1. granulationes arachnoideae. 2. numerous microscopic projections of the arachnoid into some of the venous sinuses, which are thought by some to enlarge in man with advancing age to become the granulationes arachnoideae (q.v.).
**branch v.,** a branch of a tertiary (stem) villus through which the main transport of substances between the mother and fetus occurs.
**chorionic v.,** one of the threadlike projections growing in tufts on the external surface of the chorion; see *primary, secondary,* and *tertiary v.*
**villi of choroid plexus,** tiny hairlike processes of varying sizes along the edges of the choroid plexus, containing blood vessels; their exact function is unknown.
**free v.,** a chorionic villus that projects into the intervillous space.
**vil′li intestina′les** [TA], intestinal villi: the multitudinous threadlike projections that cover the surface of the mucosa of the small intestine and serve as the sites of absorption (by active transport and diffusion) of fluids and nutrients.

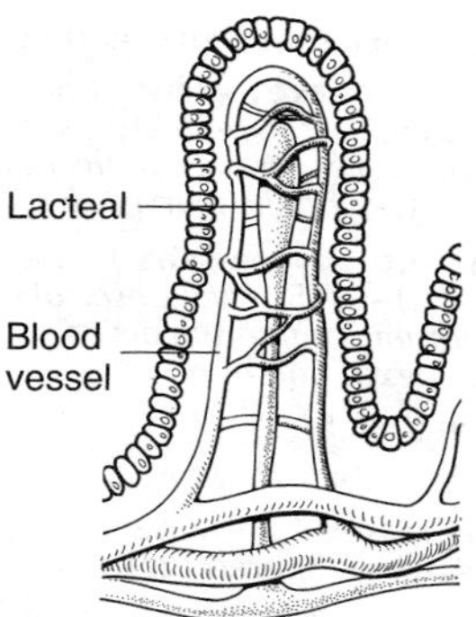

Intestinal villus.

**lingual villi,** papillae filiformes.
**vil′li pleura′les,** pleural villi: the shaggy appendages on the surface of the pleura near the costomediastinal sinus.
**primary v.,** one of the earliest chorionic villi, composed of trophoblast only.
**secondary v.,** an intermediate stage of chorionic villi, having a core of connective tissue (mesoblast) covered with trophoblast.
**villi of small intestine,** villi intestinales.
**stem v.,** tertiary v.
**vil′li synovia′les** [TA], synovial villi: slender projections of the synovial membrane from its free inner surface into the joint cavity.
**tertiary v.,** one of the definitive type of chorionic villi, having trophoblastic cover, connective tissue (mesoblastic) core, and blood vessels. Called also *stem v.*

**vil·lus·ec·to·my** (vil″əs-ek′tə-me) synovectomy; excision of a synovial villus.

**vi·men·tin** (vĭ-men′tin) [MeSH: Vimentin] a protein that forms the vimentin filaments (q.v.); it is used as an immunohistochemical marker for cells derived from the embryonic mesenchyme.

**vin·bar·bi·tal** (vin-bahr′bĭ-təl) an intermediate-acting barbiturate that has been used as a hypnotic and sedative, administered orally.
**sodium v.,** the sodium salt of vinbarbital, having the same actions and uses as the base; administered orally and parenterally.

**vin·blas·tine sul·fate** (vin-blas′tēn) [USP] the sulfate salt of a vinca alkaloid, used as an antineoplastic in the palliative treatment of lymphomas, including generalized Hodgkin's disease, lymphosarcoma, reticulum-cell sarcoma, and advanced mycosis fungoides, as well as of neuroblastoma, Letterer-Siwe disease, choriocarcinoma resistant to other agents, breast carcinoma resistant to other agents, and embryonal carcinoma of the testis. Administered intravenously.

**Vin·ca** (vin′kə) [L. pervinca *periwinkle*] a genus of woody herbs of the family Apocynaceae, including periwinkles. *V. mi′nor* L. is the common, or lesser, periwinkle. *V. ro′sea* L. is the Madagascar periwinkle, source of the vinca alkaloids (see under *alkaloid*).

**vin·ca** (ving′kə) any plant of the genus *Vinca.*

**vin·ca·mine** (vin′kə-mēn) [MeSH: Vincamine] a major alkaloid obtained from *Vinca minor,* used to help improve intellectual capacity in patients with cerebrovascular disorders.

**Vin·cent's angina, gingivitis,** etc. (vă-sahz′) [Henri *Vincent,* French physician, 1862–1950] see under *angina* and *tonsillitis,* and see *acute necrotizing gingivitis,* under *gingivitis,* and *Treponema vincenti.*

**vin·cris·tine sul·fate** (vin-kris′tēn) [USP] the sulfate salt of a vinca alkaloid, used as an antineoplastic agent, primarily as a component of combination chemotherapy regimens for Hodgkin's disease, acute lymphocytic leukemia, and non-Hodgkin's lymphomas, as well as in the treatment of Wilms' tumor, neuroblastoma, breast carcinoma, rhabdomyosarcoma and other sarcomas, and certain brain tumors. Administered intravenously.

**vin·cu·lin** (vin′ku-lin) [MeSH: Vinculin] a protein found in muscle, fibroblasts, and epithelial cells that binds actin and appears to mediate attachment of actin filaments to integral proteins of the plasma membrane. See also *α-actinin.*

**vin·cu·lum** (ving′ku-ləm) pl. *vin′cula* [L.] [TA] a general term in anatomical nomenclature for a band or bandlike structure.
**v. bre′ve digito′rum ma′nus** [TA], either of two fan-shaped expansions near the ends of the flexor tendons of a finger, one connecting the superficial tendon to the proximal interphalangeal joint and the other connecting the deep tendon to the intermediate interphalangeal joint.
**v. lin′guae,** frenulum linguae.
**vin′cula lin′gulae cerebel′li,** lateral prolongations of the lingula of the cerebellum.
**v. lon′gum digito′rum ma′nus** [TA], either of two independent pairs of slender bands in each finger, one connecting the deep flexor tendon to the superficial tendon after the latter becomes subjacent, and the other connecting the superficial tendon to the proximal phalanx.
**vin′cula ten′dinum digito′rum ma′nus** [TA], vincula of tendons of fingers: small vascular bands that connect the tendons of the flexor digitorum profundus and flexor digitorum superficialis muscles to the phalanges and interphalangeal articulations of the hand. The tendon blood supply is also carried in them. See *v. breve digitorum manus* and *v. longum digitorum manus.*
**vin′cula ten′dinum digito′rum pe′dis** [TA], vincula of tendons of toes: bands connecting the tendons of the flexor digitorum longus and flexor digitorum brevis muscles to the phalanges and interphalangeal articulations of the foot. They are similar to the vincula found in the hand.
**vincula of tendons of fingers,** vincula tendinum digitorum manus.
**vincula of tendons of toes,** vincula tendinum digitorum pedis.

**vin·de·sine sul·fate** (vin'də-sēn) a synthetic vinca alkaloid derived from vinblastine sulfate, used as an antineoplastic in the treatment of acute lymphocytic leukemia; administered intravenously.

**Vine·berg operation** (vīn'bərg) [Arthur M. *Vineberg,* Canadian surgeon, born 1903] see under *operation.*

**vin·e·gar** (vin'ə-gər) [Fr. *vinaigre* sour wine] 1. a weak and impure dilution of acetic acid; especially a sour liquid consisting chiefly of acetic acid, formed by the fermentation of cider, wine, etc., or by the distillation of wood. 2. a medicinal solution of a drug in dilute acetic acid.

**vin·e·ga·roon** (vin"ə-gə-ro͞on') *Mastigoproctus giganteus,* a species of whip scorpion so called because it produces an irritating excretion with an odor resembling that of vinegar.

**vi·no·rel·bine tar·trate** (vī-nor'el-bēn) a semisynthetic derivative of vinblastine, used in the treatment of non–small cell lung carcinoma; administered intravenously.

**Vin·son's syndrome** (vin'sənz) [Porter Paisley *Vinson,* American surgeon, 1890–1959] Plummer-Vinson syndrome; see under *syndrome.*

**vi·nyl** (vi'nəl) the univalent group $CH_2{=}CH{-}$.
**v. acetate,** a vinyl group to which the monovalent radical $CH_3COO{-}$ is attached, the monomer which polymerizes to polyvinyl acetate.
**v. benzene,** styrene.
**v. chloride,** a vinyl group to which an atom of chlorine is attached, the monomer which polymerizes to polyvinyl chloride, used in organic synthesis and in the plastics industry; it is toxic and carcinogenic. Called also *chloroethylene.* See also *vinyl chloride disease,* under *disease.*
**v. cyanide,** acrylonitrile.

**Vi·o·cin** (vi'o-sin) trademark for a preparation of viomycin sulfate.

**Vi·o·form** (vi'o-form) trademark for preparations of iodochlorhydroxyquin.

**Vi·o·kase** (vi'o-kās) trademark for a preparation of pancreatin.

**vi·o·la·ce·in** (vi"o-la'se-in) a violet pigment with antibiotic properties produced by species of *Chromobacter.* It is soluble in ethanol but not in water or chloroform.

**vi·o·la·ceous** (vi"o-la'shəs) having a violet color, usually describing a discoloration of the skin.

**vi·o·les·cent** (vi"o-les'ənt) somewhat violet in color.

**vi·o·let** (vi'o-lət) 1. the hue seen in the most refracted end of the spectrum. 2. a violet-colored dye.
**ammonium oxalate crystal v.,** a type of Gram stain prepared by mixing 2 gm of crystal violet (90 per cent dye content) and 20 mL of ethyl alcohol (95 per cent) with 0.8 gm of ammonium oxalate and 80 mL of distilled water.
**v. 7 B or C,** gentian v.; see under *G.*
**cresyl v. acetate,** a basic violet dye used as a stain for the central nervous system.
**cresyl v., cresylecht v.,** a dye used in pathologic staining.
**crystal v.,** gentian v.; see under *G.*
**v. G,** gentian v.; see under *G.*
**gentian v.,** see under *G.*
**hexamethyl v.,** gentian v.; see under *G.*
**Hofmann's v., iodine v.,** dahlia.
**iris v.,** amethyst v.
**Lauth's v.,** thionine.
**methyl v.,** gentian v.; see under *G.*
**methylene v.,** one of the constituents of polychrome methylene blue.
**neutral v.,** a dye that resembles neutral red, but is more violet in color.
**Paris v., pentamethyl v.,** gentian v.; see under *G.*

**vi·o·my·cin sul·fate** (vi'o-mi"sin) the sulfate salt of an antibacterial antibiotic produced by *Streptomyces puniceus, S. floridae,* and *Actinomyces vinaceus,* or by other means; used as a tuberculostatic, administered intramuscularly.

**vi·os·ter·ol** (vi-os'tər-ol) ergocalciferol.

**VIP** vasoactive intestinal polypeptide.

**vi·per** (vi'pər) 1. any member of the families Viperidae and Crotalidae. 2. any venomous snake. See table at *snake.*
**European v.,** *Vipera berus,* a venomous snake native to Europe, North Africa, and the Middle East; it may be either red, brown, or gray with dark markings, or completely black. Called also *adder.*
**carpet v.,** saw-scaled v.
**Gaboon v.,** *Bitis gabonica,* a deadly, brightly marked, viperine snake found in tropical West Africa.
**horned v.,** *Cerastes cerastes,* a venomous species found in the Sahara Desert and from Lebanon south to the Arabian peninsula.
**nose-horned v.,** sand v.
**Old World v.,** true v.
**palm v.,** any of various small, greenish, arboreal pit vipers of the genera *Bothrops* and *Trimeresurus,* which have prehensile tails that enable them to move from tree to tree.
**pit v.,** crotalid (def. 1).
**pit v., Malayan,** *Calloselasma rhodostoma.*
**rhinoceros v.,** *Bitis nasicornis,* a venomous, brightly colored, viperine snake found in tropical Africa, characterized by the presence of a pair of hornlike growths on its snout.
**Russell's v.,** *Vipera russelli,* an extremely venomous, brightly colored, viperine snake of southeastern Asia and Indonesia. Called also *daboia* and *ticpolonga.*
**sand v.,** *Vipera ammodytes,* a venomous snake found in southern Europe and Turkey that has a hornlike protuberance on its snout for burrowing; called also *nose-horned v.*
**saw-scaled v.,** either of two venomous snakes, *Echis carinatus* and *E. coloratus*; called also *carpet v.*
**true v.,** any of the snakes of the family Viperidae.

**Vi·pera** (vi'pər-ə) a genus of venomous snakes of the family Viperidae. *V. ammody'tes* is the sand viper; *V. be'rus* is the adder or European viper; and *V. rus'selli* is Russell's viper.

**vi·per·id** (vi'pər-id) viperine.

**Vi·per·i·dae** (vi-per'ĭ-de) [MeSH: Viperidae] a family of venomous snakes, the true or Old World vipers, characterized by front, movable, hollow fangs. It includes the genera *Bitis, Cerastes, Echis,* and *Vipera.* Cf. *Crotalidae.* See table at *snake.*

**vi·per·ine** (vi'pər-in, vi'pər-īn) 1. of or pertaining to the family Viperidae. 2. true viper.

**VIP·oma** (vĭ-po'mə) [*v*asoactive *i*ntestinal *p*olypeptide + *-oma*] an endocrine tumor, usually a type of islet cell tumor, that produces excessive vasoactive intestinal polypeptide, causing severe diarrhea and other symptoms of the Verner-Morrison syndrome. Called also *diarrheogenic tumor.* Written also *vipoma.*

**Vira-A** (vi'rə-a) trademark for a preparation of vidarabine.

**Vi·ra·cept** (vi'rə-sept) trademark for a preparation of nelfinavir mesylate.

**vi·ra·gin·i·ty** (vi"rə-jin'ĭ-te) [L. *virago* a manlike woman] the adoption by a woman of traditionally qualities and behaviors usually considered masculine.

**vi·ral** (vi'rəl) pertaining to, caused by, or of the nature of virus.

**Vi·ra·mune** trademark for a preparation of nevirapine.

**Vir·chow** (fēr'ko) Rudolf Ludwig Karl (1821–1902). German writer and editor, politician and statesman, anthropologist, ethnologist, archaeologist, and pathologist; Virchow's *Cellularpathologie* (1858) finally overthrew humoralism and marked the beginning of modern pathology. Virchow made valuable contributions to anatomy, parasitology, the history of medicine, public health, histology, and anatomic pathology. He regarded the body as a cell-state in which every cell is a citizen, and disease as a civil war brought about by external forces among the cells; he thought all cells arose from other cells (implicitly rejecting spontaneous generation), and that cell theory applied to diseased tissue. Virchow opposed Pasteur's theory of germs, Darwin's of natural selection and evolution, and Semmelweiss's washing of hands to prevent puerperal fever.

**Vir·chow's angle,** etc. (fēr'kōz) [R.L.K. *Virchow*] see under *angle, cell, corpuscle, crystal, granulation, line,* and *node.*

**Vir·chow-Rob·in spaces** (fēr'ko ro-bă') [R.L.K. *Virchow;* Charles Philippe *Robin,* French anatomist, 1821–1885] see under *space.*

**Vir·chow-Seck·el syndrome** (fēr'ko sek'əl) [R. L. K. *Virchow;* Helmut Paul George *Seckel,* American physician, 1900–1960] Seckel's syndrome; see under *syndrome.*

**vi·re·mia** (vi-re'me-ə) [MeSH: Viremia] the presence of viruses in the blood, usually characterized by malaise, fever, and aching of the back and extremities.

**vir·gin** (vir'jin) [L. *virgo*] 1. a person who has not had sexual intercourse. 2. a laboratory animal that has been kept free from sexual intercourse.

**vir·gin·al** (vir'jĭ-nəl) pertaining to a virgin or to virginity.

**vir·gin·ia·my·cin** (vir-jin'yə-mi'sin) [MeSH: Virginiamycin] an antibiotic produced by *Streptomyces virginiae* or by other means, consisting chiefly of two components, virginiamycin $M_1$ (factor $M_1$) and virginiamycin $S_1$ (factor S); administered as a feed additive to pigs as a growth stimulant and to combat infections, especially those with gram-positive cocci.

**vir·gin·i·ty** (vir-jin'ĭ-te) [L. *virginitas*] the condition of being a virgin.

**vi·ri·ci·dal** (vi"rĭ-si'dəl) virucidal.

**vi·ri·cide** (vi'rĭ-sīd) virucide.

**vi·rid·in** (vi-rid′in) an antifungal antibiotic isolated from *Gliocladium virens.*

**vir·i·do·bu·fa·gin** (vir″ĭ-do-bu′fə-jin) a cardiac poison from the skin glands of the toad *Bufo viridis.*

**vir·ile** (vir′il) [L. *virilis*] 1. masculine. 2. specifically, having male copulative power.

**vir·i·les·cence** (vir″ĭ-les′əns) masculinization.

**vir·i·lism** (vir′ĭ-liz-əm) [MeSH: Virilism] 1. masculinity 2. masculinization.

**adrenal v.,** that due to inappropriate adrenal cortical androgen production, particularly noticeable in a girl, woman, or prepubertal boy.

**vi·ril·i·ty** (vĭ″-ril′ĭ-te) [L. *virilitas,* from *vir* man] masculinity.

**vir·il·iza·tion** (vir″il-ĭ-za′shən) masculinization.

**vir·i·liz·ing** (vir′ĭ-līz″ing) masculinizing.

**vi·ri·on** (vi′re-on) [MeSH: Virion] the complete viral particle, found extracellularly and capable of surviving in crystalline form and infecting a living cell; it comprises the nucleoid (genetic material) and the capsid. Called also *viral particle.*

**vi·ro·gene** (vi′ro-jēn) [*virus* + *gene*] in theoretical genetics, an RNA tumor virus assembled by the normal genetic complement of a cell.

**vi·ro·ge·net·ic** (vi″ro-jə-net′ik) having a viral origin; caused by a virus.

**vi·roid** (vi′roid) [MeSH: Viroids] any of a class of infectious agents consisting of a small strand of RNA not associated with any protein. The RNA does not code for proteins and is not translated; it is replicated by host cell enzymes. Viroids are known to cause several plant diseases.

**vi·ro·lac·tia** (vi″ro-lak′shə) secretion of viruses in the milk.

**vi·rol·o·gist** (vi-rol′ə-jist) a microbiologist specializing in virology.

**vi·rol·o·gy** (vi-rol′ə-je) [MeSH: Virology] that branch of microbiology which is concerned with viruses and viral diseases.

**vi·ro·mi·cro·some** (vi″ro-mi′kro-sōm) a name sometimes applied to an incomplete virus particle released by premature disruption of the host cell.

**vi·ro·pex·is** (vi″ro-pek′sis) [*virus* + *pexis*] the fixation of virus to the membrane of an animal cell and its subsequent engulfment by the cell.

**vi·ro·plasm** (vi′ro-plaz-əm) plaques of very fine granular substance that appear in cells before virions are observed and which correspond to the DNA material, as in poxvirus infections.

**vi·ro·sis** (vi-ro′sis) pl. *viro′ses..* A disease caused by a virus.

**vi·ro·stat·ic** (vi″ro-stat′ik) 1. inhibiting the replication of viruses. 2. an agent that inhibits the replication of viruses.

**vi·ru·ci·dal** (vi″rə-si′dəl) capable of neutralizing or destroying a virus.

**vi·ru·cide** (vi′rə-sīd) an agent that neutralizes or destroys a virus.

**vir·u·lence** (vir′u-ləns) [L. *virulen′tia,* from *virus* poison] [MeSH: Virulence] the degree of pathogenicity of a microorganism as indicated by the severity of the disease produced and its ability to invade the tissues of a host. It is measured experimentally by the median lethal dose ($LD_{50}$) or median infective dose ($ID_{50}$). By extension, the competence of any infectious agent to produce pathologic effects.

**vir·u·lent** (vir′u-lənt) [L. *virulentus,* from *virus* poison] pertaining to or characterized by virulence; exceedingly pathogenic, noxious, or deleterious.

**vir·u·lic·i·dal** (vir″u-lis′ĭ-dəl) destructive of virulence; capable of destroying the deleterious potency of a virus or other noxious agent.

**vir·u·lif·er·ous** (vir″u-lif′ər-əs) [*virus* + *-ferous*] conveying or producing a virus or other noxious agent.

**vir·uria** (vīr-oo′re-ə) the presence of viruses in the urine.

**vi·rus** (vi′rəs) [L.] [MeSH: Viruses] one of a group of minute infectious agents, with certain exceptions (e.g., poxviruses) not resolved in the light microscope, and characterized by a lack of independent metabolism and by the ability to replicate only within living host cells. Like living organisms, they are able to reproduce with genetic continuity and the possibility of mutation. They range from 200–300 nm to 15 nm in size and are morphologically heterogeneous, occurring as rod-shaped, spherical, or polyhedral, and tadpole-shaped forms; masses of the spherical or polyhedral forms may be made up of orderly arrays, to give a crystalline structure. The individual particle, or virion, consists of nucleic acid (the nucleoid), DNA or RNA (but not both) and a protein shell, or capsid, which contains and protects the nucleic acid and which may be multilayered. Viruses are customarily separated into three subgroups on the basis of host specificity, namely bacterial viruses, animal viruses, and plant viruses. They are also classified as to their origin (e.g., reoviruses), mode of transmission (arboviruses, tickborne viruses), or the manifestations they produce (polioviruses, polyomaviruses, poxviruses). They are sometimes named for the geographical location in which they were first isolated (e.g., coxsackievirus).

## Virus

Many of the names listed below are names of virus species; species names in viral taxonomy do not use Latin binomial nomenclature and are neither capitalized (unless the species name includes a proper name) nor italicized.

**Absettarov v.,** a strain of Central European encephalitis virus belonging to the Far Eastern subgroup of the tick-borne encephalitis viruses, which causes disease in Central Europe, Scandinavia, and the western part of the former Soviet Union.

**acute laryngotracheobronchitis v.,** human parainfluenza viruses 1 and 2.

**adeno-associated v. (AAV),** Dependovirus.

**African horse sickness v.,** a virus of the genus *Orbivirus* that is the etiologic agent of African horse sickness.

**African swine fever v.,** a double-stranded DNA virus that is the etiological agent of African swine fever; it was formerly classified as a member of the Iridoviridae but is now assigned to the genus African swine fever–like viruses, which belongs to no family and of which it is the only member.

**Akabane v.,** a bunyavirus that causes arthrogryposis and other congenital deformities in fetal cattle and sheep in utero when the mothers become infected; it is spread between animals by biting insects.

**Aleutian mink disease v.,** a virus of the genus *Parvovirus* that is the etiologic agent of Aleutian mink disease.

**animal v's,** viruses that produce diseases of man and other animals.

**Argentine hemorrhagic fever v.,** Junin v.

**attenuated v.,** one whose pathogenicity has been reduced by serial animal passage or by other means.

**Australian X disease v.,** Murray Valley encephalitis v.

**avian infectious bronchitis v.,** a virus of the genus *Coronavirus* that is the etiologic agent of infectious avian bronchitis.

**avian influenza v.,** a subspecies of influenza A virus, influenza virus A avian, that causes avian influenza (fowl plague).

**avian leukosis v's,** any of a complex of type C oncoviruses, classified in ten subgroups (A–J), causing erythroblastosis, granulomatosis, lymphomatosis, and myelocytomatosis. Subgroups A–E and J infect chickens; Subgroups F–I infect other birds. See *avian leukosis,* under *leukosis.*

**B v.,** herpesvirus B.

**B19 v.,** a species belonging to the genus *Erythrovirus* that binds to the erythrocyte P blood group antigen and is the cause of erythema infectiosum. In patients with hemolytic anemia or sickle cell disease it causes aplastic crisis; it can also cause acute arthritis. Fetal infection can cause hydrops fetalis, fetal death, and spontaneous abortion. Persistent infection in immunocompromised patients can lead to chronic bone marrow failure. Called also *human parvovirus B19.*

**bacterial v.,** a virus capable of producing transmissible lysis of bacteria; the virus particle attaches to the bacterial cell wall and viral nucleoprotein enters the cell, resulting in the synthesis of virus and its liberation on physical disruption of the cell. Bacterial viruses are usually specific for bacterial species, but they may be strain-specific or may infect more than one species of bacteria. Called also *bacteriophage* or *phage.* See *Twort-d'Herelle phenomenon,* under *phenomenon.*

**Belgrade v.,** see *Dobrava-Belgrade v.*

**Berne v.,** a virus of the genus *Torovirus* associated with diarrhea in horses.

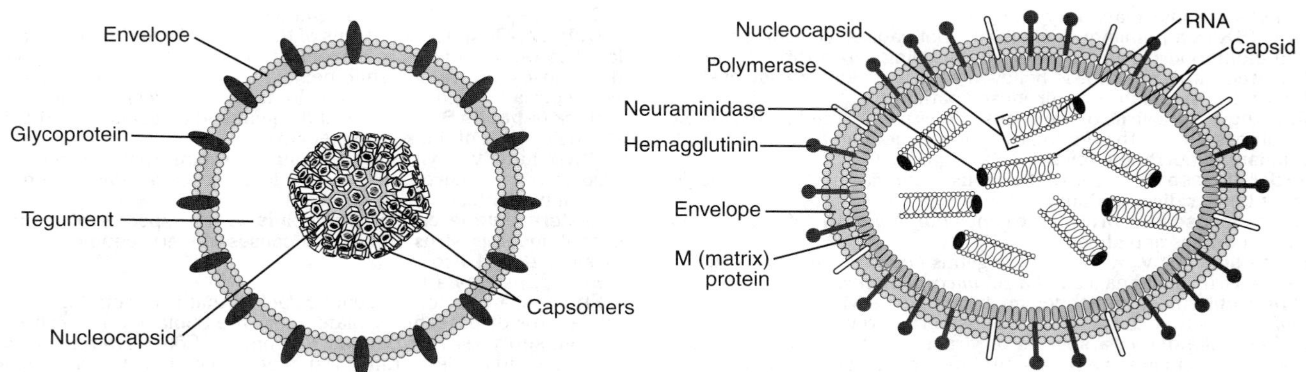


Herpes simplex virus. The nucleocapsid comprises a capsid shell surrounding a linear double-stranded DNA and toroidal core protein.

Influenza virus. The nucleocapsids, helical assemblies of single-stranded RNA and nucleoprotein capsids, are twisted on themselves to form tightly coiled helical superstructures (not shown)

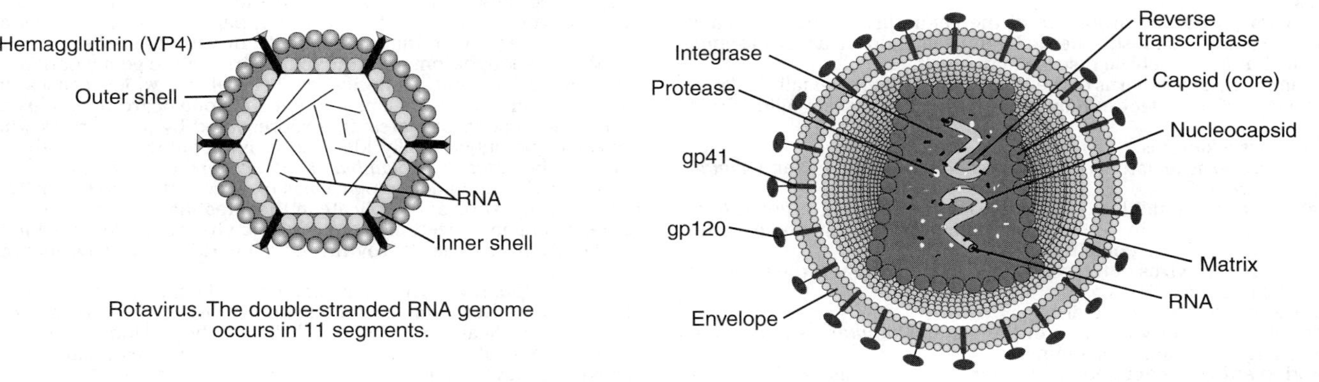


Rotavirus. The double-stranded RNA genome occurs in 11 segments.

Human immunodeficiency virus (HIV). Within the core capsid, the diploid, single-stranded, positive-sense RNA is complexed to nucleoprotein.

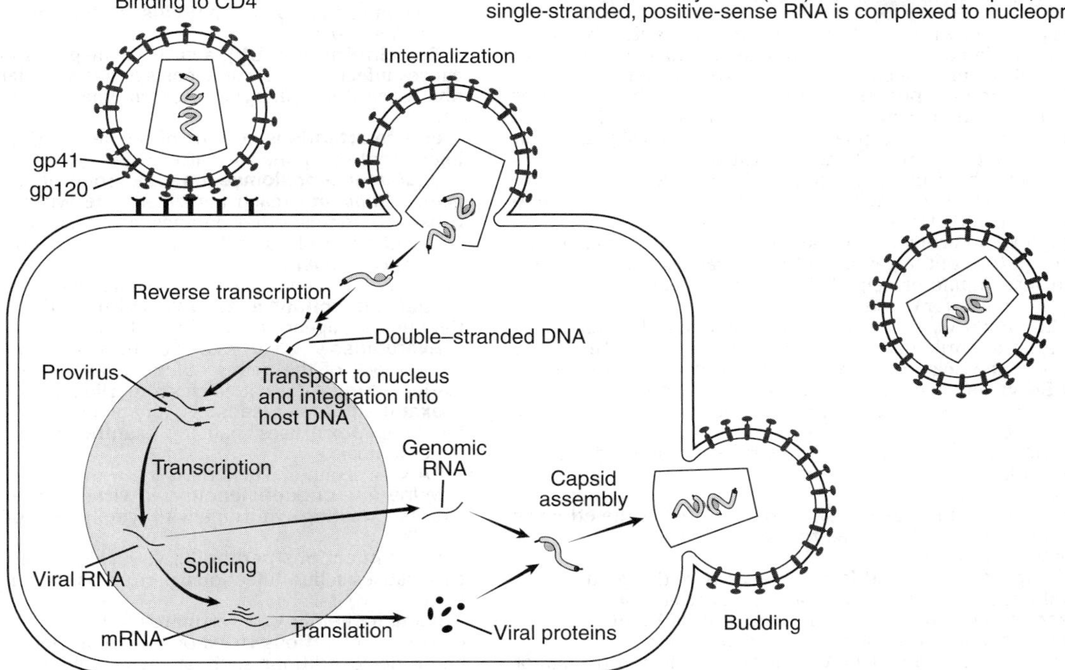


Life cycle of the human immunodeficiency virus. The extracellular envelope protein gp120 binds to CD4 on the surface of T lymphocytes or mononuclear phagocytes, while the transmembrane protein gp41 mediates the fusion of the viral envelope with the cell membrane. (gp=glycoprotein)

**PLATE 55—**STRUCTURE OF VARIOUS VIRUSES AND LIFE CYCLE OF HUMAN IMMUNODEFICIENCY VIRUS

**Bittner v.,** mouse mammary tumor v.

**BK v. (BKV),** a human polyomavirus that causes widespread infection in childhood (80 per cent of adults being seropositive) and remains latent in the host; it is believed to cause hemorrhagic cystitis and nephritis in immunocompromised patients.

**bluetongue v.,** a virus of the genus *Orbivirus,* separable into at least 24 serotypes, that is the etiologic agent of bluetongue.

**Bolivian hemorrhagic fever v.,** Machupo v.

**border disease v.,** a virus of the genus *Pestivirus* that is the etiologic agent of border disease (hairy shaker disease).

**Borna disease v.,** a virus of the genus *Bornavirus* that causes Borna disease in horses and sheep.

**bovine diarrhea v.,** a virus of the genus *Pestivirus* that is the agent of bovine virus diarrhea; called also *mucosal disease v.*

**bovine ephemeral fever v.,** an insect-borne virus of the genus *Ephemerovirus* that causes bovine ephemeral fever.

**bovine leukemia v.,** a species of viruses of the genus BLV-HTLV retroviruses that causes a persistent infection in cattle that is usually asymptomatic but may result in enzootic bovine leukosis.

**bovine papillomatosis v.,** bovine papillomavirus.

**bovine papular stomatitis v.,** a virus of the genus *Parapoxvirus* that is the etiologic agent of bovine papular stomatitis.

**bovine respiratory syncytial v.,** see *respiratory syncytial v's.*

**Breda v.,** a virus of the genus *Torovirus* associated with diarrhea in calves.

**Bunyamwera v.,** an arbovirus of the genus *Bunyavirus,* originally isolated from *Aedes* mosquitoes in Uganda; infection is usually asymptomatic, but a mild febrile disease may result.

**Bwamba v.,** an arbovirus of the genus *Bunyavirus,* originally isolated in Uganda but prevalent in much of Africa, that causes a mild febrile disease.

**C v.,** coxsackievirus.

**CA v.,** croup-associated v.; see *human parainfluenza v. 1* and *human parainfluenza v. 2.*

**California encephalitis v.,** a mosquito-borne virus of the genus *Bunyavirus* occurring in the western United States and Canada; it is the cause of California encephalitis.

**camelpox v.,** a virus of the genus *Orthopoxvirus* that is the etiologic agent of camelpox.

**cancer-inducing v.,** oncovirus.

**canine distemper v.,** a virus of the genus *Morbillivirus* that is the etiologic agent of canine distemper.

**caprine arthritis-encephalitis v.,** a virus of the genus *Lentivirus* that in young goats causes acute encephalitis and in older goats causes chronic arthritis, sometimes with mastitis, pneumonia, or glomerulonephritis.

**Catu v.,** a species of viruses of the genus *Bunyavirus* closely related to Guama virus, isolated from a Brazilian patient with a febrile illness.

**CELO v.** [*c*hicken-*e*mbyro-*l*ethal *o*rphan], fowl adenovirus.

**Central European encephalitis v.,** a species of tick-borne viruses in the genus *Flavivirus* that includes the members of the European subgroup of tick-borne encephalitis viruses (Hanzalova, Hypr, Kumlinge, and Neudoerfl viruses) and Absettarov virus.

**Chagres v.,** an arbovirus of the genus *Phlebovirus,* causing fever associated with malaise, headache, and pains of localized and generalized distribution, in Panama.

**chikungunya v.,** an arbovirus of the genus *Alphavirus* transmitted chiefly by mosquitoes of the genus *Aedes* that causes chikungunya, a dengue-like disease found principally in Southeast Asia and Africa.

**Coe v.,** former name for *coxsackievirus A21.*

**Colorado tick fever v.,** a virus of the family Reoviridae that is the etiologic agent of a febrile disease occurring in regions of the Rocky Mountains where the tick vector *Dermacentor andersoni* is prevalent.

**Columbia SK v.,** an encephalomyocarditis virus originally isolated in 1940 from a monkey which had previously been inoculated with the Yale SK strain of poliovirus.

**common cold v's,** viruses such as rhinoviruses considered to cause the common cold.

**coryza v.,** rhinovirus.

**cowpox v.,** a virus of the genus *Orthopoxvirus* that is the etiologic agent of cowpox; it is closely related to vaccinia virus.

**Coxsackie v.,** coxsackievirus.

**Crimean-Congo hemorrhagic fever v.,** a virus of the genus *Nairovirus,* the etiologic agent of Crimean-Congo hemorrhagic fever.

**croup-associated v.,** human parainfluenza viruses 1 and 2.

**cytomegalic inclusion disease v.,** see *cytomegalovirus.*

**defective v.,** one that cannot be completely replicated or cannot form a protein coat; in some cases replication can proceed if missing gene functions are supplied by other (helper) viruses; see *helper v.*

**dengue v.,** a species of the genus *Flavivirus* existing as four antigenically related but distinct types (designated 1, 2, 3, and 4) that causes classic dengue and hemorrhagic dengue.

**DNA v.,** a virus whose genome consists of DNA; called also *deoxyribovirus.*

**Dobrava v.,** see *Dobrava-Belgrade v.*

**Dobrava-Belgrade v.,** a virus of the genus *Hantavirus,* originally isolated as Dobrava virus in Slovenia and Belgrade virus in Yugoslavia, that causes severe epidemic hemorrhagic fever in the Balkans. The reservoir is the yellow-necked field mouse, *Apodemus flavicollis.*

**duck hepatitis B v.,** a virus of the genus *Avihepadnavirus* that is the etiologic agent of duck virus hepatitis.

**Duvenhage v.,** a virus of the genus *Lyssavirus* that is widely distributed in bats in Europe and Africa and causes a rabies-like disease; fatal human infection has occurred.

**eastern equine encephalomyelitis v.,** the species of equine encephalomyelitis virus (q.v.) that causes eastern equine encephalomyelitis. Called also *EEE v.*

**EB v.,** Epstein-Barr v.

**Ebola v.,** a virus of the genus *Filovirus* that is the etiologic agent of Ebola virus disease, first isolated near the Ebola River in Zaire; there are four subtypes: Zaire, Sudan, Reston, and Côte d'Ivoire. The natural reservoir and mode of transmission of primary infection are unknown, but secondary infection is by direct contact with infected blood and other body secretions and by airborne particles.

**ectromelia v.,** a virus of the genus *Orthopoxvirus* that is the etiologic agent of infectious ectromelia in mice.

**EEE v.,** eastern equine encephalomyelitis v.; see *equine encephalomyelitis v.*

**egg drop syndrome 1976 v.,** an adenovirus (duck adenovirus 1), first recognized in 1976, that causes apparently healthy ducks and geese to lay eggs with thin or soft shells or without shells.

**EMC v., encephalomyocarditis v.,** a virus of the genus *Cardiovirus* found in Africa, South America, and elsewhere, which causes mild aseptic meningitis in humans and encephalomyocarditis in pigs and certain nonhuman primates; it is represented by four strains which appear to be substantially identical in immunological and other respects. It includes the *Columbia SK, Mengo,* and *MM viruses.*

**enteric v's,** an epidemiologic class of viruses that are normally acquired by ingestion and replicate in the intestinal tract, causing local rather than generalized infection. Enteric viruses are included in the families Adenoviridae, Astroviridae, Caliciviridae, Coronaviridae, and Reoviridae.

**enteric orphan v's,** viruses isolated from the intestinal tract of man and various other animals, called orphan viruses because they are often not specifically associated with illness; they include such viruses isolated from cattle (ecboviruses), dogs (ecdoviruses), man (echoviruses), monkeys (ecmoviruses), and swine (ecsoviruses).

**enveloped v.,** a virus having an outer lipoprotein bilayer acquired by budding through the host cell membrane.

**epidemic keratoconjunctivitis v.,** human adenovirus type 8; see *Mastadenovirus.*

**Epstein-Barr v. (EBV),** a virus of the genus *Lymphocryptovirus* that causes infectious mononucleosis and is associated with Burkitt's lymphoma and nasopharyngeal carcinoma. Called also *human herpesvirus 4.*

**equine arteritis v.,** a virus of the genus *Arterivirus* that is the etiologic agent of equine viral arteritis.

**equine encephalomyelitis v.,** a group of arbovirus species of the genus *Alphavirus,* each named for the type of encephalomyelitis it causes in horses, other equines, and humans; they have a reservoir of infection in birds and transmission by mosquitoes. Included are *eastern equine encephalomyelitis virus, western equine encephalomyelitis virus,* and *Venezuelan equine encephalomyelitis virus.*

**equine infectious anemia v.,** a virus of the genus *Lentivirus* that is the etiologic agent of equine infectious anemia.

**Everglades v.,** an arbovirus of the genus *Alphavirus,* transmitted by mosquitoes of the genus *Culex,* isolated from rodents in the Everglades National Park; it causes a febrile illness in humans.

**exanthematous disease v.,** any of a group of dermotropic viruses, including poxviruses, causing exanthematous disease in man and lower animals.

**FA v.,** a strain of Theiler's v.

**feline immunodeficiency v.,** a virus of the genus *Lentivirus* that causes a wasting syndrome with lymphadenopathy and lymphopenia in cats.

**feline infectious peritonitis v.,** a species of the genus *Coronavirus* that causes feline infectious peritonitis in domestic cats and other felines.

**feline leukemia v.,** a retrovirus found in domestic cats, which can cause any of various types of contagious leukemias and lymphomas and other conditions such as anemia, glomerulonephritis, spontaneous abortion, and immunosuppression. See also *feline leukemia,* under *leukemia.*

**feline panleukopenia v.,** a virus of the genus *Parvovirus* that causes panleukopenia in cats and infections in other animals; it is antigenically closely related to canine parvovirus and mink enteritis virus. See also *feline parvovirus.*

**feline rhinotracheitis v.,** felid herpesvirus 1.

**v. fixé, fixed v.**, rabies virus whose virulence and incubation period have been stabilized by serial passage and remain fixed during further transmission; used for inoculating animals from which rabies vaccine is prepared. Cf. *street v.*

**foamy v's**, *Spumavirus.*

**fowlpox v.**, a virus of the genus *Avipoxvirus* that is the etiologic agent of fowlpox.

**Friend v., Friend murine leukemia v.**, a mammalian type C retrovirus causing erythroleukemia in mice.

**Germisten v.**, an arbovirus of the genus *Bunyavirus* that causes a mild febrile disease in South Africa.

**goatpox v.**, a virus of the genus *Capripoxvirus* that is the etiologic agent of goatpox.

**Graffi v.**, a strain of murine leukemia virus which causes chloroma in mice.

**Gross v.**, a strain of murine leukemia virus that induces lymphomas in mice.

**Guama v.**, a virus of the genus *Bunyavirus* isolated in the region of Belem, Brazil, from foresters suffering from hyperthermia, headache, muscular and articular pains, and occasionally nausea and vertigo.

**Guanarito v.**, a virus of the Tacaribe complex, first isolated from patients in Guanare, Portuguesa state, Venezuela, that is the etiologic agent of Venezuelan hemorrhagic fever.

**Guaroa v.**, an arbovirus of the genus *Bunyavirus* isolated in Colombia from the blood of patients with a febrile disease.

**Hantaan v.**, a virus of the genus *Hantavirus* that causes severe epidemic hemorrhagic fever in Asia. The reservoir is mice of the genus *Apodemus.*

**Hanzalova v.**, a strain of Central European encephalitis virus, antigenically very similar or identical to Hypr virus, first isolated in the Czech Republic.

**helper v.**, a virus (e.g., the Rous-associated virus) that aids the development of a defective virus by supplying or restoring the activity of a viral gene or enabling a defective virus (e.g., the Rous sarcoma virus) to form a protein coat.

**hemadsorption v., type 1 (HA1)**, former name for *human parainfluenza virus 3.*

**hemadsorption v., type 2 (HA2)**, former name for *human parainfluenza virus 1.*

**hemagglutinating encephalomyelitis v. of pigs**, porcine hemagglutinating encephalomyelitis v.

**hepatitis A v. (HAV)**, a virus of the genus *Hepatovirus,* the etiologic agent of hepatitis A.

**hepatitis B v. (HBV)**, a virus of the genus *Orthohepadnavirus* that is the etiologic agent of hepatitis B.

**hepatitis C v.**, a species of the genus *Hepacivirus,* the etiologic agent of hepatitis C.

**hepatitis C–like v's**, *Hepacivirus.*

**hepatitis D v. (HDV)**, a satellite virus of the genus *Deltavirus,* the etiologic agent of hepatitis D. The presence of hepatitis B virus to provide helper functions is required, and the viral envelope is composed of hepatitis B surface antigen. Called also *hepatitis delta v.*

**hepatitis delta v.**, hepatitis D v.

**hepatitis E v.**, a virus of the genus *Calicivirus*, the enterically transmitted etiologic agent of hepatitis E, consisting of a spherical virion 27–34 nm in diameter with a positive-sense single-stranded RNA genome.

**hepatitis G v. (HGV)**, a parenterally transmitted flavivirus originally isolated from a patient with chronic hepatitis and considered to be identical to hepatitis GB virus-C; most infections are benign, and the role of HGV in the etiology of liver disease is uncertain.

**hepatitis GB v. (HBGV)**, a group of viruses isolated from a patient with hepatitis and classified as HGBV-A, HGBV-B, and HGBV-C; HGBV-C belongs to the same species as hepatitis G virus. The name is derived from the patient's initials (G.B.).

**herpangina v.**, any of several virus types of the coxsackievirus A group, causing a febrile disease, usually of children, characterized by small herpes-like lesions on the soft palate or in the faucial area.

**herpes v.**, see *herpesvirus.*

**herpes simplex v. (HSV)**, see human herpesvirus 1 and human herpesvirus 2, under *herpesvirus.*

**hog cholera v.**, a virus of the genus *Pestivirus* that is the etiologic agent of hog cholera.

**human immunodeficiency v. (HIV)**, a virus of the genus *Lentivirus,* separable into two serotypes (HIV-1 and HIV-2), that is the etiologic agent of acquired immunodeficiency syndrome (AIDS). HIV-1, which comprises at least three subgroups (M, N, and O), is of worldwide distribution, while HIV-2 is largely confined to West Africa; transmission and manifestations are very similar. HIV-1 was formerly called *human T-cell lymphotropic v. type III (HTLV-III)* and *lymphadenopathy-associated v. (LAV).* See Plate 55.

**human parainfluenza v. 1**, a virus of the genus *Paramyxovirus* that causes croup in young children and mild upper respiratory infections in older children and adults. Called also *acute laryngotracheobronchitis v., CA v.,* and *croup-associated v.*

**human parainfluenza v. 2**, a virus of the genus *Rubulavirus* that causes croup in young children. Called also *acute laryngotracheobronchitis v., CA v.,* and *croup-associated v.*

**human parainfluenza v. 3**, a virus of the genus *Paramyxovirus* that causes croup and lower respiratory tract infections in young children.

**human parainfluenza v. 4**, a virus of the genus *Rubulavirus* that causes upper respiratory infections, chiefly in young children.

**human respiratory syncytial v.**, see *respiratory syncytial v's.*

**human T-cell leukemia v.**, synonym for *human T-lymphotropic v.*; see there for entries for specific strains.

**human T-cell lymphotropic v. type I (HTLV-I)**, human T-lymphotropic virus 1.

**human T-cell lymphotropic v. type II (HTLV-II)**, human T-lymphotropic virus 2.

**human T-cell lymphotropic v. type III (HTLV-III)**, former name for *human immunodeficiency v. 1.*

**human T-lymphotropic v. 1 (HTLV-1)**, a species in the genus BLV-HTLV retroviruses, of worldwide distribution, having an affinity for helper/inducer T lymphocytes; it causes chronic infection and is associated with adult T-cell leukemia/lymphoma and chronic progressive myelopathy. Called also *human T-cell leukemia v. type I* and *human T-cell lymphotrophic virus type I.*

**human T-lymphotropic v. 2 (HTLV-2)**, a species in the genus BLV-HTLV retroviruses having extensive serologic cross-reactivity with HTLV-1, isolated from an atypical T-cell variant of hairy cell leukemia and from patients with other hematologic disorders; no clear association with disease has been established. Called also *human T-cell leukemia v. type II* and *human T-cell lymphotropic v. type II.*

**Hypr v.**, a strain of Central European encephalitis virus, antigenically very similar or identical to Hanzalova virus, that infects many mammalian species and is a frequent cause of human infection in Central Europe and Scandinavia.

**igbo-ora v.**, an arbovirus of the genus *Alphavirus,* closely related to chikungunya virus and o'nyong-nyong virus, that has been associated with a dengue-like disease in Nigeria, the Central African Republic, and the Ivory Coast.

**Ilheus v.**, an arbovirus of the genus *Flavivirus,* first isolated from species of *Aedes* and *Psorophora* in Brazil; also found in Panama, where birds may be hosts. It is related to St. Louis encephalitis virus, Japanese B encephalitis virus, and West Nile virus.

**infectious bovine rhinotracheitis v.**, bovine herpesvirus 1.

**infectious bursal disease v.**, a virus of the genus *Avibirnavirus* that is the etiologic agent of infectious bursal disease in chickens.

**infectious ectromelia v.**, a virus of the genus *Orthopoxvirus* that is the etiologic agent of infectious ectromelia in mice.

**infectious laryngotracheitis v.**, gallid herpesvirus 1.

**infectious pancreatic necrosis v.**, a virus of the genus *Aquabirnavirus* that is the etiologic agent of infectious pancreatic necrosis in fish.

**infectious porcine encephalomyelitis v.**, porcine enterovirus.

**influenza v.**, any of a group of orthomyxoviruses that cause influenza, including at least three serotypes: *Influenzavirus A, Influenzavirus B,* and *Influenzavirus C.* Antigenic variants are classified on the basis of their surface antigens (hemagglutinin and neuraminidase) as H1N1, H2N2, etc. Serotype A viruses are subject to major antigenic changes (antigenic shifts) as well as minor gradual antigenic changes (antigenic drift) and cause the major pandemics. Serotype B viruses appear to undergo only antigenic drift and cause more localized epidemics. Serotype C viruses appear to be antigenically stable and cause only sporadic disease. See Plate 55.

**influenza A v., influenza B v., influenza C v.**, species in the genera *Influenzavirus A, Influenzavirus B,* and *Influenzavirus C;* see *influenza v.*

**insect v's**, viruses capable of causing disease in insects.

**iridescent v.**, iridovirus.

**Jamestown Canyon v.**, a virus of the genus *Bunyavirus,* serologically related to California encephalitis virus, that occasionally causes encephalitis.

**Japanese encephalitis v.**, a mosquito-borne virus of the genus *Flavivirus,* antigenically related to St. Louis encephalitis virus, that is the etiologic agent of Japanese encephalitis.

**JC v. (JCV)**, a human polyomavirus that causes widespread infection in childhood (80 per cent of adults being seropositive) and remains latent in the host; it is the cause of progressive multifocal leukoencephalopathy.

**Junin v.**, an arenavirus of the Tacaribe complex that is the etiologic agent of Argentine hemorrhagic fever, transmitted by contact with infected rodents, especially of the genus *Calomys.* Called also *Argentine hemorrhagic fever v.*

**K v.**, a nononcogenic virus of the genus *Polyomavirus* that produces fatal pneumonia on inoculation into newborn mice.

**Kemerovo v.,** a tickborne virus of the genus *Orbivirus* that causes a benign febrile disease in western Siberia and Egypt.

**Korean hemorrhagic fever v.,** Hantaan v.

**Kumba v.,** a strain of Semliki Forest virus isolated from mosquitoes in the Kumba region of Cameroon.

**Kumlinge v.,** a strain of Central European encephalitis virus that causes a febrile illness accompanied by encephalitis in Finland.

**Kunjin v.,** a mosquito-borne virus of the genus *Flavivirus,* antigenically related to Japanese encephalitis virus, that causes febrile disease and encephalitis in Australia and the Malay Archipelago.

**Kyasanur Forest disease v.,** a virus of the genus *Flavivirus* transmitted by ticks of the genus *Haemaphysalis,* especially *H. spinigera,* first isolated in an epidemic of hemorrhagic fever among forest workers and monkeys in the Kyasanur Forest in Mysore State, India; it is antigenically related to the Omsk hemorrhagic fever virus.

**La Crosse v.,** a virus of the California serogroup of the genus *Bunyavirus,* the etiologic agent of La Crosse encephalitis.

**Lansing v.,** the prototype strain of poliovirus type 2.

**Lassa v.,** an arenavirus of the LCMV-LASV complex, existing in several serologically distinct strains and distributed throughout West and Central Africa. It causes an inapparent infection in the multimammate mouse; human infection (Lassa fever) results from contact with mouse urine.

**latent v.,** masked v.

**LCM v.,** lymphocytic choriomeningitis v.

**Leon v.,** the prototype strain of *poliovirus type 3.*

**louping ill v.,** a virus of the genus *Flavivirus* transmitted by the tick *Ixodes ricinus;* it causes louping ill of sheep, and is transmissible to humans, in whom it may cause meningitis and encephalitis.

**lumpy skin disease v.,** a virus of the genus *Capripoxvirus* that is the etiologic agent of lumpy skin disease in African cattle.

**lymphadenopathy-associated v. (LAV),** human immunodeficiency v. I.

**lymphocystis v's,** *Lymphocystivirus.*

**lymphocyte-associated v.,** any virus of the subfamily Gammaherpesvirinae, members of which are specific for either B- or T-lymphocytes; infection is often arrested at a prelytic or lytic stage without production of infectious virions. Latent virus may frequently be demonstrated in lymphoid tissue. Host range is very narrow.

**lymphocytic choriomeningitis v.,** a virus of the genus the LCMV-LASV complex that is the etiologic agent of lymphocytic choriomeningitis. Called also *LCM v.*

**lytic v.,** one that is replicated in the host cell and causes death and lysis of the cell.

**M-25 v.,** a virus with the properties of a myxovirus, although antigenically unrelated; isolated from a person with upper respiratory illness.

**Machupo v.,** an arenavirus of the Tacaribe complex that is the etiologic agent of Bolivian hemorrhagic fever, transmitted by contact with infected rodents of the species *Calomys callosus.* Called also *Bolivian hemorrhagic fever v.*

**maedi/visna v.,** a virus of the genus *Lentivirus* that is the etiologic agent of ovine progressive pneumonia (maedi-visna).

**Makonde v.,** Uganda S v.

**mammary tumor v.,** mouse mammary tumor v.

**Marburg v.,** a virus of the genus *Filovirus* that is the etiologic agent of Marburg virus disease, transmitted by direct physical contact with African green monkeys or their organs or with an infected person.

**Marek's disease v.,** a group of serologically related viruses in the family *Herpesviridae,* comprising three serotypes: *type 1,* which contains all pathogenic strains, *type 2,* which contains nonpathogenic strains infecting chickens, and *type 3,* which contains nonpathogenic strains infecting turkeys. See also *gallid herpesvirus 2* and *gallid herpesvirus 3,* under *herpesvirus.*

**masked v.,** a virus which ordinarily occurs in a noninfective state and is demonstrable by indirect methods which activate it, as by blind passage in experimental animals.

**Mayaro v.,** an arbovirus of the genus *Alphavirus,* originally isolated in Mayaro County, Trinidad, that causes a dengue-like illness in Central and South America; transmission is by mosquitoes of the genus *Haemagogus.*

**measles v.,** a virus of the genus *Morbillivirus* that is the etiologic agent of measles.

**measles-like v's,** *Morbillivirus.*

**Mengo v.,** an encephalomyocarditis virus isolated in 1948 in Uganda from a monkey with encephalomyelitis, and later from mosquitoes and a mongoose in the same area; identified also as the cause of an epizootic disease of swine in Panama.

**milker's node v.,** pseudocowpox v.

**mink enteritis v.,** a virus of the genus *Parvovirus* that is the etiologic agent of mink viral enteritis; it is sometimes considered to be a species-specific variant of feline parvovirus.

**MM v.,** an encephalomyocarditis virus originally isolated in 1943 from the brain of a hamster that was previously inoculated with material from a human case of paralytic disease.

**molluscum contagiosum v.,** the single species of the genus *Molluscipoxvirus,* the etiologic agent of molluscum contagiosum.

**Moloney v.,** a strain of murine leukemia virus which causes lymphoid leukemia in mice.

**monkeypox v.,** a virus of the genus *Orthopoxvirus* that produces a mild, epidemic exanthematous disease in monkeys and a smallpox-like disease in humans.

**mouse mammary tumor v.,** the sole member of the mammalian type B retroviruses, which induces mammary adenocarcinoma in certain strains of mice, usually transmitted from mother to offspring through the milk; viral expression and carcinogenesis are influenced by estrogen stimulation. Called also *Bittner v.*

**mucosal disease v.,** bovine diarrhea v.

**mumps v.,** a virus of the genus *Rubulavirus* that causes mumps and, in some cases, tenderness and swelling of the testes, pancreas, ovaries, or other organs.

**murine leukemia v.,** a species in the genus mammalian type C retroviruses, comprising a number of strains that can be grouped by their envelope antigens or by the antigens induced on the surface of the infected cell. It causes leukemia and solid tumors in rats, mice, hamsters, and other animals; the genus includes the Gross, Rauscher, Friend, Moloney, and Graffi viruses.

**Murray Valley encephalitis v.,** a mosquito-borne virus of the genus *Flavivirus,* antigenically related to Japanese encephalitis virus, that is the etiologic agent of Murray Valley encephalitis.

**myxoma v.,** a virus of the genus *Leporipoxvirus* that is the etiologic agent of infectious myxomatosis in rabbits.

**Nairobi sheep disease v.,** a tick-borne virus of the genus *Nairovirus* that is the etiologic agent of Nairobi sheep disease.

**naked v.,** a virus lacking an outer lipoprotein bilayer.

**Nakiwogo v.,** Semunya v.

**Negishi v.,** a tick-borne virus of the genus *Flavivirus* isolated from cases of fatal encephalitis in Japan.

**Neudoerfl v.,** a strain of Central European encephalitis virus.

**neurotropic v.,** one that has a predilection for and causes infection in nervous tissues, e.g., the rabies virus.

**newborn pneumonitis v.,** human parainfluenza v. 1.

**Newcastle disease v.,** a virus of the genus *Rubulavirus* that is the etiologic agent of Newcastle disease in birds; human infection is mild and characterized by conjunctivitis and brief generalized symptoms. Called also *avian paramyxovirus 1.*

**non-A, non B-hepatitis v.,** a hepatitis virus other than hepatitis A virus or hepatitis B virus, usually referring to hepatitis C virus.

**nonenveloped v.,** naked v.

**non-oncogenic v.,** a virus that does not induce cell transformation or malignancy.

**Norwalk v.,** a human calicivirus that is a common cause of epidemics of acute gastroenteritis, with diarrhea and vomiting lasting 24 to 48 hours.

**Omsk hemorrhagic fever v.,** a virus of the genus *Flavivirus* transmitted by ticks of the genera *Dermacentor* and *Ixodes,* isolated from patients with hemorrhagic fever in a forested region of Siberia.

**oncogenic v's,** an epidemiologic class of viruses that are acquired by close contact (including sexual contact) or injection and cause usually persistent infection; they may induce cell transformation and malignancy. Oncogenic viruses are included in the families Adenoviridae, Hepadnaviridae, Herpesviridae, Papovaviridae, and Retroviridae.

**o'nyong-nyong v.,** an arbovirus of the genus *Alphavirus,* closely related to chikungunya virus, that causes o'nyong-nyong, a dengue-like disease, in Uganda, Kenya, Tanzania, Malawi, and Senegal; it is transmitted by anopheline mosquitoes.

**orf v.,** a virus of the genus *Parapoxvirus* that is the etiologic agent of contagious ecthyma (orf).

**Oropouche v.,** a member of the Simbu serogroup of the genus *Bunyavirus* that causes illness in Brazil; infection may be severe and is characterized by fever, chills, malaise, headache, myalgia, and arthralgia, sometimes with nausea and vomiting, and occasionally with central nervous system involvement.

**orphan v's,** viruses which when isolated originally in tissue culture showed no specific association with disease, such as the enteric orphan viruses; some have since been found to occur in association with human disease.

**Orungo v.,** a mosquito-borne virus of the genus *Orbivirus* that causes a febrile illness in Nigeria and Uganda.

**papilloma v.,** papillomavirus.

**pappataci fever v.,** *Phlebovirus.*

**parainfluenza v.,** a group of viruses of the family Paramyxoviridae that cause upper respiratory tract disease in humans and other animals. Species that infect humans are classified in two genera: *Paramyxovirus* (human parainfluenza viruses 1 and 3) and *Rubulavirus* (human parainfluenza viruses 2 and 4). Also included here are simian parainfluenza viruses and Sendai virus.

**paravaccinia v.**, pseudocowpox v.
**peste-des-petits-ruminants v.**, a virus of the genus *Morbillivirus* that is the etiologic agent of peste des petits ruminants.
**pharyngoconjunctival fever v.**, human adenovirus type 3; see *Mastadenovirus.*
**Pichinde v.**, a virus of the Tacaribe complex infecting rodents in Colombia, and isolated from human subclinical infections.
**Piry v.**, a virus of the genus *Vesiculovirus,* related to vesicular stomatitis virus, isolated from an opossum in Brazil; laboratory infections have occurred, marked by fever, myalgia, and abdominal tenderness.
**plant v's,** viruses that replicate in and may produce diseases of higher plants.
**poliomyelitis v.**, see *poliovirus.*
**polyoma v.**, polyomavirus.
**Pongola v.**, a mosquito-borne virus of the Bwamba serogroup of the genus *Bunyavirus,* occurring in central and southern Africa. Natural hosts are donkeys, horses, and monkeys; human infection is asymptomatic.
**porcine hemagglutinating encephalomyelitis v.**, a virus of the genus *Coronavirus* that causes vomiting and wasting disease (q.v.) in piglets.
**porcine transmissible gastroenteritis v.**, a virus of the genus *Coronavirus* that is the etiologic agent of transmissible gastroenteritis of swine.
**Powassan v.**, a tickborne virus of the genus *Flavivirus* that causes encephalitis in the eastern United States and Canada.
**pox v.**, see *poxvirus.*
**pseudocowpox v.**, a virus of the genus *Parapoxvirus* that produces nodular lesions similar to those of cowpox and orf on the udders and teats of milk cows and the oral mucosa of suckling calves (paravaccinia), which can be transmitted to humans during milking. Called also *milker's node v.* and *paravaccinia v.*
**pseudorabies v.**, a virus of the genus *Varicellovirus* that is the etiologic agent of pseudorabies. Called also *suid herpesvirus 1.*
**Puumala v.**, a virus of the genus *Hantavirus* that causes nephropathia epidemica in Scandinavia, Russia, and several other European countries; the natural host is the bank vole, *Clethrionomys glareolus.*
**Quaranfil v.**, an arbovirus found in Egypt, where it was isolated from the blood of children with febrile disease, from the blood of young egrets, and from ticks *(Argas arboreus* and *A. hermanni).* It is ether-sensitive and presumed to contain RNA.
**rabbit fibroma v.**, a virus of the genus *Leporipoxvirus* that is the etiologic agent of rabbit fibroma.
**rabbit hemorrhagic disease v.**, a virus of the genus *Calicivirus* that is the etiologic agent of rabbit hemorrhagic disease.
**rabies v.**, a virus of the genus *Lyssavirus* that is the etiologic agent of rabies.
**rabies-like v's,** *Lyssavirus.*
**Rauscher v.**, a strain of murine leukemia virus that causes lymphoid leukemia in mice.
**respiratory v's,** an epidemiologic class of viruses that are acquired by inhalation of fomites and replicate in the respiratory tract, causing local rather than generalized infection. Respiratory viruses are included in the families Adenoviridae, Coronaviridae, Orthomyxoviridae, Paramyxoviridae, and Picornaviridae.
**respiratory syncytial v's (RSV),** viruses belonging to the genus *Pneumovirus,* isolated originally from chimpanzees with coryza. In humans, they cause respiratory disease that is particularly severe in infants, in whom it causes bronchiolitis (q.v.) and sometimes pneumonia. Other viruses (bovine respiratory syncytial virus) cause respiratory disease in cattle. In tissue RSV causes syncytium formation. RSV is separable into two groups (A and B) on the basis of the antigenic structure of the G protein and into subgroups within the two groups.
**Rift Valley fever v.**, a virus of the genus *Phlebovirus,* which is the etiologic agent of Rift Valley fever in domestic animals and humans, first seen in the Rift Valley of Kenya, but now widespread in southern and eastern Africa to Egypt; transmitted by mosquitoes of the genera *Aedes, Culex,* and *Erethmapodites* or by contact with tissues and secretions of infected animals.
**rinderpest v.**, a virus of the genus *Morbillivirus* that is the etiologic agent of cattle plague (rinderpest).
**Rio Bravo v.**, a virus of the genus *Flavivirus,* isolated from bats in Mexico and the southwestern United States, that has caused orchitis in laboratory workers. No arthropod vector is known.
**RNA v.**, a virus whose genome consists of RNA; called also *ribovirus.*
**Rocio v.**, a mosquito-borne virus of the genus *Flavivirus* occurring in Brazil that causes a sometimes fatal encephalitis.
**Ross River v.**, an arbovirus of the genus *Alphavirus* that is the etiologic agent of epidemic polyarthritis.
**Rous-associated v. (RAV),** a helper virus in whose presence a defective Rous sarcoma virus is able to form a protein coat.
**Rous sarcoma v. (RSV),** a usually defective avian leukosis virus producing fibrosarcoma in fowl, especially chickens; some strains have been shown to produce tumors in other animals. See *Rous sarcoma,* under *sarcoma.*
**RS v.**, respiratory syncytial v.
**rubella v.**, the sole species of the genus *Rubivirus,* the etiologic agent of rubella.
**Russian spring-summer encephalitis v.**, a tick-borne virus of the genus *Flavivirus* that causes spring-summer encephalitis in the former Soviet Union and Central Europe.
**SA v.**, a parainfluenza virus isolated from the hamster brain following inoculation with a chick embryo allantoic culture of nasal washings from a person with acute upper respiratory infection; identical to simian virus SV5.
**Sabia v.**, a species isolated from a fatal case of hemorrhagic fever in São Paulo, Brazil, and tentatively assigned to the genus *Arenavirus;* the reservoir is unknown but assumed to be a rodent.
**St. Louis encephalitis v.**, a virus of the genus *Flavivirus,* antigenically related to Japanese encephalitis virus, that is the etiologic agent of St. Louis encephalitis; transmitted by mosquitoes.
**salivary gland v.**, cytomegalovirus.
**sandfly fever v's,** *Phlebovirus.*
**sandfly fever-Naples v.**, a virus of the Naples serogroup of the genus *Phlebovirus,* an etiologic agent of phlebotomus fever.
**sandfly fever-Sicilian v.**, a virus of the Sicilian serogroup of the genus *Phlebovirus,* an etiologic agent of phlebotomus fever.
**satellite v.**, a strain of virus unable to replicate except in the presence of helper virus; considered to be deficient in coding for capsid formation.
**Schwartz leukemia v.**, a virus that causes lymphoid leukemia in Swiss mice.
**Semliki Forest v.**, a species of viruses of the genus *Alphavirus,* originally isolated from *Aedes* mosquitoes in Western Uganda; it is widespread in Africa, where it appears to be non-pathogenic, although infections of laboratory workers have occurred.
**Semunya v.**, an arbovirus isolated from East African patients with an acute febrile syndrome; called also *Nakiwogo v.*
**Sendai v.**, a virus of the genus *Paramyxovirus* that causes latent infection in laboratory mice and asymptomatic infection in other animals, used experimentally as a model for paramyxoviruses in molecular studies and to induce syncytium formation in tissue culture.
**Seoul v.**, a virus of the genus *Hantavirus* that causes mild to moderately severe epidemic hemorrhagic fever. *Rattus rattus* and *Rattus norvegicus* are the natural hosts.
**Sepik v.**, a mosquito-borne virus, tentatively assigned to the genus *Flavivirus,* that causes febrile disease in New Guinea.
**sheeppox v.**, a virus of the genus *Capripoxvirus* that is the etiologic agent of sheep-pox.
**sigma v.**, a congenitally transmitted genus of rhabdoviruses that induces carbon dioxide sensitivity in *Drosophila melanogaster* and other fruit flies.
**Simbu v.**, a virus of the genus *Bunyavirus* isolated from a species of mosquitoes *(Aedes circumluteolis)* in Africa; serologically related species infect humans and other animals.
**simian v's,** viruses that have been recovered from monkeys; they belong to many different groups, including adenoviruses, enteroviruses, herpesviruses, and reoviruses.
**simian v. 40 (SV40),** a polyomavirus isolated from *Rhesus* monkey kidney tissue, which produces transformation in human and newborn hamster kidney cell cultures and tumors on inoculation into newborn hamsters. It has caused progressive multifocal leukoencephalopathy in humans.
**simian immunodeficiency v. (SIV),** a virus of the genus *Lentivirus,* closely related to human immunodeficiency virus, that causes inapparent infection in African green monkeys and a disease resembling acquired immunodeficiency syndrome in macaques.
**Sindbis v.**, a virus of the genus *Alphavirus,* transmitted by *Culex* mosquitoes, that causes Sindbis fever in southern and eastern Africa, Egypt, Israel, India, the Philippines, and eastern Australia.
**slow v.**, any virus causing a disease characterized by a very long preclinical course and very gradual progression once the symptoms appear.
**Spondweni v.**, a mosquito-borne virus of the genus *Flavivirus* that causes a febrile illness with hepatitis in South Africa, Nigeria, Mozambique, and Cameroon.
**street v.**, virulent rabies virus from a naturally infected animal, as opposed to a laboratory-adapted strain of the virus. Cf. *fixed v.*
**swine infertility and respiratory syndrome v.**, a virus of the genus *Arterivirus* that is the etiologic agent of porcine epidemic abortion and respiratory syndrome.
**swine influenza v.**, a type A influenza virus that causes swine influenza; in rare cases, direct transmission to humans has caused sometimes fatal infection.
**swinepox v.**, the sole species of the genus *Suipoxvirus,* the etiologic agent of swinepox.
**Tacaribe v.**, a virus of the genus *Arenavirus,* isolated from bats in

**Selected Tick-Borne Encephalitis Viruses**

| European Subtypes | Far Eastern Subtypes |
|---|---|
| Hanzalova virus | Absettarov virus |
| Hypr virus | Kyasanur forest disease virus |
| Kumlinge virus | Louping ill virus |
| Neudoerfl virus | Negishi virus |
| | Omsk hemorrhagic fever virus |
| | Powassan virus |
| | Russian spring-summer encephalitis virus |

Trinidad, which is immunologically related to the Junin and Machupo viruses.

**Tahyna v.**, a virus belonging to the California serogroup of the genus *Bunyavirus* that causes a febrile illness in Russia and Central Europe.

**Tamiami v.**, a virus of the Tacaribe complex, originally isolated from bats in Trinidad, that has been serologically linked to human infection.

**tanapox v.**, a virus of the genus *Yatapoxvirus* that is the etiologic agent of tanapox.

**temperate v.**, see under *bacteriophage.*

**Teschen v.**, porcine enterovirus.

**Theiler's v., Theiler's murine encephalomyelitis v.**, a species of the genus *Cardiovirus* that is the etiologic agent of Theiler's disease in mice; called also *murine poliovirus.*

**Thogoto v.**, a species of tick-borne orthomyxoviruses that infect humans, cattle, and sheep in Africa. Human infection results in sometimes severe encephalitis and optic neuritis.

**Thogoto-like v's**, a genus of tick-borne viruses of the family Orthomyxoviridae that cause infection in vertebrates in Africa, Europe, and Asia.

**tick-borne v's**, viruses that are transmitted by ticks.

**tick-borne encephalitis v's**, a serogroup of the genus *Flavivirus,* consisting of viruses that are transmitted by ticks and cause encephalitis in humans and animals that ranges in severity from subclinical to fatal. It comprises European and Far Eastern subtypes. See accompanying table.

**Toscana v.**, a virus of the Naples serogroup of the genus *Phlebovirus,* an etiologic agent of phlebotomus fever.

**tumor v.**, oncovirus.

**U v.**, echovirus 11; isolated from children with subglottic laryngitis, it causes respiratory and gastrointestinal disease and rashes. Called also *Uppsala v.*

**Uganda S v.**, an arbovirus of the genus *Flavivirus,* first isolated from species of *Aedes* in Bwamba county in Uganda. It causes mild febrile disease in certain areas in Africa, especially in Nigeria.

**Uppsala v.**, U v.

**Uukuniemi v.**, the type species of the Uukuniemi group of the genus *Phlebovirus* (q.v.).

**vaccinia v.**, an virus of the genus *Orthopoxvirus* that does not occur in nature, being propagated only in the laboratory for use as an active vaccine against smallpox. The present virus is derived from the original one used by Jenner, obtained from the lesions of cowpox, but the origin of the original virus remains unclear. Some believe that vaccinia virus is a derivative of the immunologically similar but antigenically different viruses of cowpox and variola (smallpox), while others think that it may be a recombinant of these viruses.

**varicella-zoster v.**, human herpesvirus 3.

**variola v.**, the virtually extinct virus, belonging to the genus *Orthopoxvirus,* that is the etiologic agent of smallpox. No natural infection has occurred since 1977, and no reservoir of the virus now exists.

**VEE v., Venezuelan equine encephalomyelitis v.**, the species of the genus *Alphavirus* that causes Venezuelan equine encephalomyelitis.

**vesicular exanthema of swine v.**, a virus of the genus *Calicivirus* having at least 13 serotypes, designated A–M, which is the etiologic agent of vesicular exanthema in swine.

**vesicular stomatitis v.**, any of several antigenically distinct species of the genus *Vesiculovirus* (vesicular stomatitis Alagoas, vesicular stomatitis Indiana, and vesicular stomatitis New Jersey viruses) that cause vesicular stomatitis in swine, cattle, and horses.

**vesicular stomatitis–like v's**, *Vesiculovirus.*

**WEE v.**, western equine encephalomyelitis v.

**Wesselsbron v.**, a mosquito-borne virus of the genus *Flavivirus* that is the etiologic agent of Wesselsbron disease in sheep and cattle and a mild febrile illness in humans.

**western equine encephalomyelitis (WEE) v.**, a species of the genus *Alphavirus* that causes western equine encephalomyelitis.

**West Nile v.**, a virus of the genus *Flavivirus,* antigenically closely related to Murray Valley virus, St. Louis encephalitis virus, and Japanese encephalitis virus, that causes West Nile encephalitis; it is transmitted by *Culex* mosquitoes, with wild birds serving as the reservoir and occurs widely in Africa, Europe, the Middle East, and Asia, and has recently been reported in the United States.

**Wyeomyia v.**, a virus belonging to the Bunyamwera serogroup of the genus *Bunyavirus,* originally isolated from the mosquito *Wyeomyia melanocephala* and occurring in Central and South America and Trinidad, that causes a febrile illness.

**Yaba monkey tumor v.**, a virus of the genus *Yatapoxvirus* that is the etiologic agent of yabapox.

**Yale SK v.**, a strain of poliovirus.

**yellow fever v.**, a mosquito-borne species of the genus *Flavivirus* that causes yellow fever in Central and South America and Africa.

**Zika v.**, a mosquito-borne virus of the genus *Flavivirus,* occurring in Central Africa, that causes a febrile illness with rash.

**vi·rus·emia** (vi″rəs-e′me-ə) viremia.

**viru·stat·ic** (vir″u-stat′ik) [*virus* + *-static*] inhibiting the replication of viruses.

**vis·ce·ra** (vis′ər-ə) [L.] [MeSH: Viscera] plural of *viscus.*

**vis·cer·ad** (vis′ər-ad) toward the viscera.

**vis·cer·al** (vis′ər-əl) [L. *visceralis,* from *viscus* a viscus] pertaining to a viscus.

**vis·cer·al·gia** (vis″ər-al′jə) [*viscer-* + *-algia*] pain in the viscera or in any bodily organ.

**vis·cer·al·ism** (vis′ər-əl-iz-əm) the opinion that the viscera are the principal seats of disease.

**vis·ceri·mo·tor** (vis″ər-ĭ-mo′tər) visceromotor.

**viscer(o)-** [L. *viscus,* gen. *visceris*] a combining form denoting relationship to the organs (viscera) of the body.

**vis·cero·cra·ni·um** (vis″ər-o-kra′ne-əm) [*viscero-* + *cranium*] [TA] that part of the skull that is derived from the branchial (or pharyngeal) arches and comprises the bones of the face; cf. *neurocranium.* Called also *splanchnocranium.*

**cartilaginous v.**, that part of the viscerocranium formed by endochondral ossification of the pharyngeal (branchial) arch cartilages. It includes the malleus, incus, stapes, styloid process of temporal bone, hyoid bone, and laryngeal cartilages other than the epiglottis.

**membranous v.**, that part of the viscerocranium formed by intramembranous ossification in the first pharyngeal (branchial) arch. It includes the maxilla, mandible, nasal bone, and zygomatic arch.

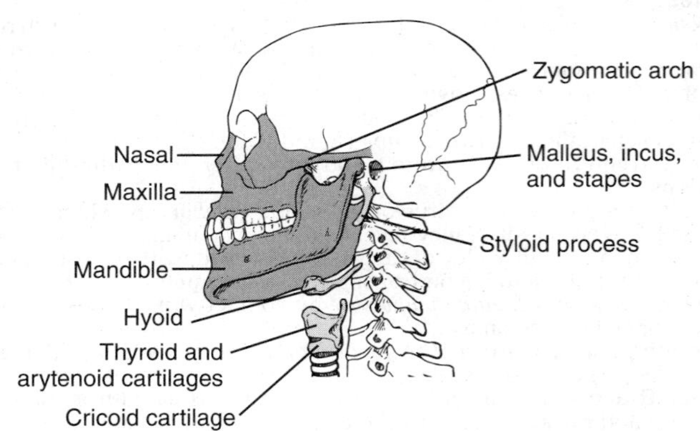


Viscerocranium, comprising the membranous viscerocranium *(dark shading)* and cartilaginous viscerocranium *(light shading).*

**vis·cer·og·ra·phy** (vis″ər-og′rə-fe) radiography of the viscera.

**vis·cero·in·hib·i·to·ry** (vis″ər-o-in-hib′ĭ-tor-e) inhibiting the essential movements of any viscus or organ.

**vis·cero·meg·a·ly** (vis″ər-o-meg′ə-le) [*viscero-* + *-megaly*] enlargement of the viscera; called also *organomegaly* and *splanchnomegaly.*

**vis·cero·mo·tor** (vis″ər-o-mo′tər) [*viscero-* + *motor*] conveying or concerned with motor impulses to the viscera.

**vis·cero·pa·ri·e·tal** (vis″ər-o-pə-ri′ə-təl) pertaining to the viscera and the abdominal wall.

**vis·cero·peri·to·ne·al** (vis″ər-o-per″ĭ-to-ne′əl) pertaining to the viscera and the peritoneum.

**vis·cero·pleu·ral** (vis″ər-o-ploor′əl) pertaining to both the viscera and the pleura.

**vis·cero·sen·so·ry** (vis″ər-o-sen′sə-re) pertaining to sensation in the viscera.

**vis·cero·skel·e·tal** (vis″ər-o-skel′ə-təl) pertaining to the visceral skeleton.

**vis·cero·so·mat·ic** (vis″ər-o-so-mat′ik) pertaining to the viscera and body.

**vis·cero·tome** (vis′ər-o-tōm) 1. an instrument designed for obtaining specimens of liver tissue from cadavers by simple puncture. 2. an area on an abdominal viscus which is supplied with afferent nerve fibers by a single posterior root.

**vis·cer·ot·o·my** (vis″ər-ot′ə-me) [*viscero-* + *-tomy*] incision of an organ, especially postmortem excision of a portion of the liver.

**vis·cero·to·nia** (vis″ər-o-to′ne-ə) [*viscero-* + *ton-* + *-ia*] a temperament type characterized by love of physical comfort, sociability, tolerance for others, and extroversion; the behavioral counterpart of endomorphy.

**vis·cero·troph·ic** (vis″ər-o-trof′ik) trophic and dependent upon the viscera.

**vis·cer·o·trop·ic** (vis″ər-o-trop′ik) [*viscero-* + *-tropic*] primarily acting on the viscera; having a predilection for the abdominal or thoracic viscera.

**vis·cid** (vis′id) [L. *viscidus*] glutinous or sticky.

**vis·cid·i·ty** (vĭ-sid′ĭ-te) the quality of being viscid.

**vis·co·elas·tic** (vis″ko-e-las′tik) both viscous and elastic; said of viscous substances used to restore or maintain the shape of the eye, especially the anterior chamber, during cataract surgery or other procedures performed on the anterior chamber.

**vis·co·gel** (vis′ko-jel) a gel which on melting gives a sol of high viscosity.

**vis·com·e·ter** (vis-kom′ə-tər) viscosimeter.

**vis·com·e·try** (vis-kom′ə-tre) viscosimetry.

**vis·cose** (vis′kōs) 1. viscous. 2. a form of cellulose acetate, used in dialysis membranes and other products.

**vis·co·sim·e·ter** (vis″ko-sim′ə-tər) an apparatus used in determination of the viscosity of a substance. Called also *viscometer.*
**Ostwald v.**, one which measures relative viscosity by comparing the time required for the meniscus of the solution under study to fall a fixed distance in a capillary tube with the time required for the same movement by a meniscus of a liquid of known viscosity.
**Stormer v.**, an apparatus for determining viscosity by measurement of the time required, under controlled conditions, for a definite number of revolutions of a rotating cylinder immersed in the substance to be tested.

**vis·co·sim·e·try** (vis″ko-sim′ə-tre) the measurement of the viscosity of a substance. Called also *viscometry.*

**vis·cos·i·ty** (vis-kos′ĭ-te) [MeSH: Viscosity] resistance to flow; a physical property of a substance that depends on the friction of its component molecules as they slide past one another.
**absolute v.**, the frictional resistance generated in a fluid when two parallel planes are flowing at different velocities, defined as the frictional force per unit area times the separation of the planes divided by the relative velocity of the planes; measured in poises. Called also *dynamic v.* Symbol $\eta$.
**dynamic v.**, absolute v.
**kinematic v.**, absolute viscosity divided by the density of the fluid; measured in stokes as the time for an exact quantity of liquid to flow by gravity through a capillary tube. Symbol $\nu$.

**vis·cous** (vis′kəs) [L. *viscosus*] sticky or gummy; characterized by a high degree of viscosity.

**Vis·cum** (vis′kəm) [MeSH: Viscum] a genus of parasitic plants of the family Loranthaceae, native to Europe and Asia. *V. al′bum* is European mistletoe, whose berries were formerly used as an oxytocic, emmenagogue, cardiac stimulant, and vasodilator.

**vis·cus** (vis′kəs) pl. *vis′cera* [L.] any large interior organ in any one of the three great cavities of the body, especially in the abdomen; see Plate 56.

**vis·ile** (viz′īl) pertaining to vision; understanding or recalling most readily what has been seen. Cf. *audile.*

**Vi·sine** (vi-zēn′) trademark for a preparation of tetrahydrozoline hydrochloride.

**vi·sion** (vizh′ən) [L. *visio,* from *vidēre* to see] [MeSH: Vision] 1. the special sense by which objects in the external environment are perceived by means of light they give off or reflect, which stimulates the photoreceptors in the retina; called also *sight.* 2. the act of seeing. 3. an apparition; a subjective sensation of vision not elicited by actual visual stimuli. 4. visual acuity; symbol V.
**achromatic v.**, monochromatism.
**binocular v.**, the use of both eyes together without diplopia.
**central v.**, that which is elicited by stimuli impinging directly on the macula retinae.
**chromatic v.**, color v.
**color v.**, 1. perception of the different colors making up the spectrum of visible light; it is mediated by the cones of the retina. 2. chromatopsia.
**day v.**, visual perception in the daylight, or under conditions of bright illumination; see also *light adaptation.*
**dichromatic v.**, dichromasy.
**direct v.**, central v.
**double v.**, diplopia.
**facial v.**, the ability, formerly thought to be possessed by some blind people, to judge distance, direction, etc., of objects in one's environment by sensation felt in the skin of the face.
**foveal v.**, central v.
**gun-barrel v.**, tunnel v.
**halo v.**, perception of a colored halo about a light source, one of the symptoms of glaucoma, punctate cataract, and sometimes conjunctivitis.
**haploscopic v.**, stereoscopic v.
**indirect v.**, peripheral v.
**low v.**, impairment of vision such that there is significant visual handicap but also significant usable residual vision; such impairment may involve visual acuity, visual fields, or ocular motility.
**monocular v.**, vision with one eye.
**multiple v.**, polyopia.
**night v.**, visual perception in the darkness of night, or under conditions of reduced illumination; see also *dark adaptation.*
**v. null, v. obscure,** the existence of scotomas in the field of vision of which the patient is not aware.
**oscillating v.**, oscillopsia.
**peripheral v.**, that which is elicited by stimuli falling on areas of the retina distant from the macula.
**photopic v.**, day v.
**Pick's v.**, a visual condition in which objects lose their normal horizontal-vertical alignment and converge toward or diverge from one another.
**pseudoscopic v.**, the reverse of stereoscopic vision, an illusion produced by reversing the pictures in a stereoscope, with apparent reversal of concavity and convexity, near and far, etc.
**rainbow v.**, halo v.
**rod v.**, vision in which the cones of the retina play little or no part, as in night vision.
**scotopic v.**, night v.
**solid v., stereoscopic v.**, perception of the relief of objects or of their depth; vision in which objects are perceived as having three dimensions, and not merely as two-dimensional pictures.
**triple v.**, triplopia.
**tubular v.**, tunnel v.
**tunnel v.**, 1. that in which the visual field is severely constricted. When due to organic causes such as glaucoma or retinitis pigmentosa the field expands as it is tested at increasing distances; when due to functional disorders such as conversion disorder or malingering it remains constant or contracts at increasing distances. 2. in psychiatry, restriction of psychological or emotional perception to a limited range.
**twilight v.**, night v.
**yellow v.**, xanthopsia.

**Vis·i·paque** (viz′ĭ-pāk) trademark for a preparation of iodixanol.

**Vis·ken** (vis′ken) trademark for a preparation of pindolol.

**vis·na** (vis′nə) [Icelandic "wasting"] [MeSH: Visna] the meningoencephalitic form of ovine progressive pneumonia.

**Vis·ta·ril** (vis′tə-ril) trademark for preparations of hydroxyzine.

**Vis·tide** (vis′tīd) trademark for a preparation of cidofovir.

**vis·u·al** (vizh′oo-əl) [L. *visualis,* from *videre* to see] pertaining to vision or sight.

**vis·u·al·iza·tion** (vizh″oo-əl-ĭ-za′shən) the act of viewing, or of achieving a complete visual impression of an object, as by radiography.
**double contrast v.**, see *mucosal relief radiography,* under *radiography.*

**vis·u·al·ize** (vizh′oo-əl-īz) to achieve a complete view of; to become visible.

**vis·u·al·spa·tial** (vizh′oo-əl spa′shəl) visuospatial.

**vis·uo·au·di·to·ry** (vizh″oo-o-aw′dĭ-tor″e) simultaneously stimu-

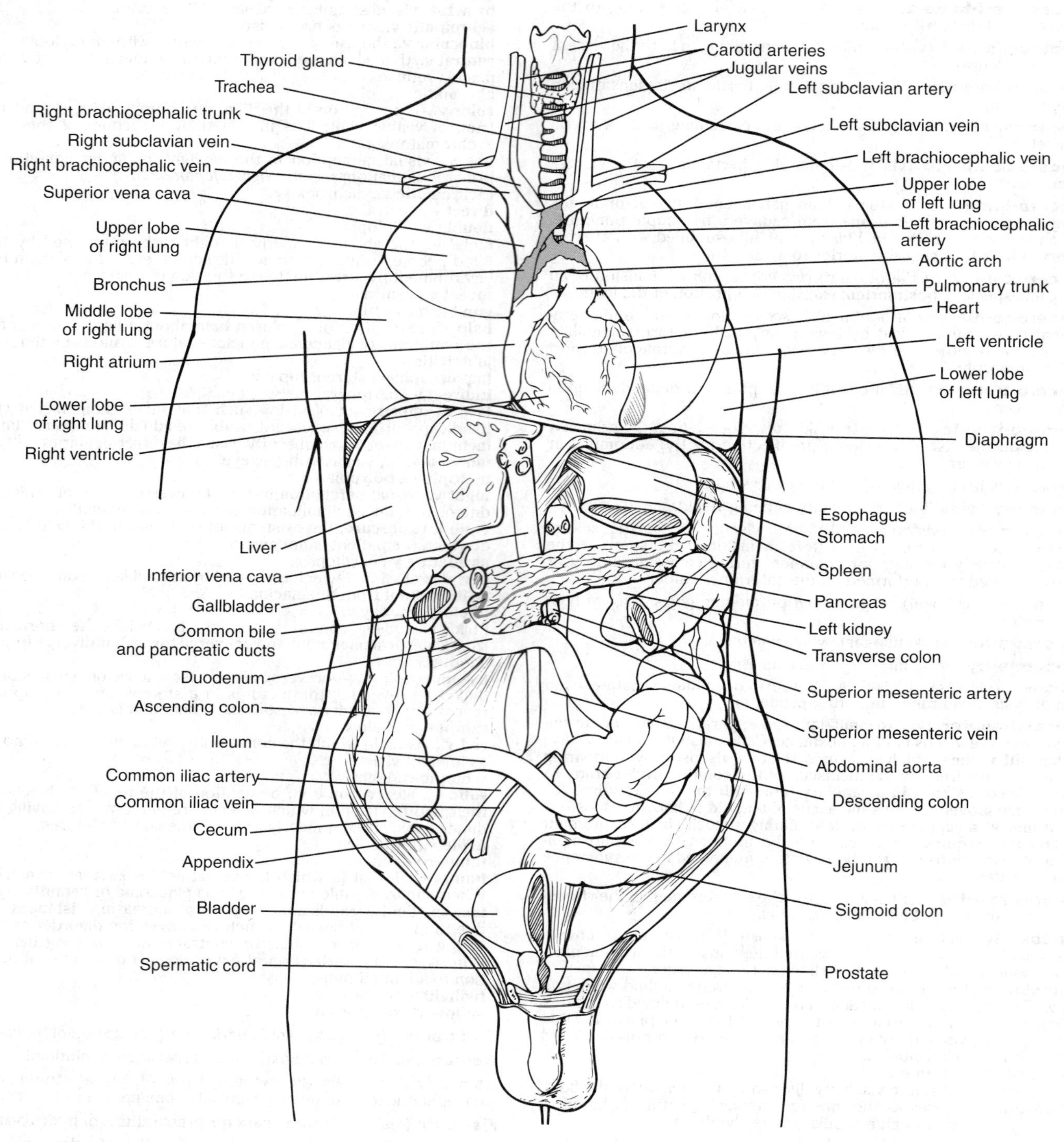


**PLATE 56**—THORACIC AND ABDOMINAL VISCERA

lating, or pertaining to simultaneous stimulation of, the senses of both hearing and sight.

**visu·og·no·sis** (vizh″oo-og-no′sis) [L. *visus* sight + Gr. *gnōsis* knowledge] the recognition and interpretation of visual impressions.

**vis·uo·mo·tor** (vizh″oo-o-mo′tər) pertaining to connections between visual and motor processes, such as the use of visual cues to maintain coordinated movements.

**vis·uo·psy·chic** (vizh″oo-o-si′kik) visual and psychic; a term applied to that area of the cerebral cortex concerned in the judgment of visual sensations.

**vis·uo·sen·so·ry** (vizh″oo-o-sen′sə-re) pertaining to the perception of stimuli giving rise to visual impressions.

**vis·uo·spa·tial** (vizh″oo-o-spa′shəl) pertaining to the ability to understand visual representations and their spatial relationships; called also *visual-spatial.* Cf. *visual-spatial agnosia.*

**vi·tag·o·nist** (vi-tag′ə-nist) a vitamin antagonist; a substance that produces deficiency of a given vitamin.

**vi·tal** (vi′təl) [L. *vitalis,* from *vita* life] necessary to or pertaining to life.

**Vi·ta·li's test** (ve-tah′lēz) [Dioscoride *Vitali,* Italian physician, 1832–1917] see under *test.*

**vi·ta·lism** (vi′tə-liz-əm) [L. *vita* life] [MeSH: Vitalism] the theory, opposed to mechanism (def. 3), that biological activities are due to a vital force or principle distinct from physical and chemical forces.

**Vi·tal·li·um** (vi-tal′e-əm) [MeSH: Vitallium] trademark for a cobalt-chromium alloy used in dentures and in surgical appliances, prostheses, and instruments.

**vi·ta·mer** (vi′tə-mər) any of a number of compounds that possess a given vitamin activity, i.e., that act to overcome a given vitamin deficiency in one or another organism, plant or animal. Thus, there are biotin vitamers, niacin vitamers, thiamine vitamers, pyridoxin vitamers, A vitamers, D vitamers, K vitamers, etc.

**vi·ta·min** (vi′tə-min) [L. *vita* life + *amine*] a general term for a number of unrelated organic substances that occur in many foods in small amounts and that are necessary in trace amounts for the normal metabolic functioning of the body. They may be water-soluble or fat-soluble.
**v. A,** 1. retinol or any of several related fat-soluble compounds having similar biological activity; the vitamin acts in numerous capacities, particularly in the functioning of the retina, the growth and differentiation of epithelial tissue, the growth of bone, reproduction, and the immune response. Deficiency of vitamin A causes skin disorders such as xeroderma and follicular hyperkeratosis, increased susceptibility to infection, nyctalopia, xerophthalmia and other eye disorders, anorexia, and sterility. As vitamin A, it is mostly found in liver, particularly of fish, egg yolks, and the fat component of dairy products; its other major dietary source is the provitamin A carotenoids of plants. 2. [USP] a preparation of retinol or esters of retinol formed from edible fatty acids, usually acetic and palmitic acids, used in the prophylaxis and treatment of vitamin A deficiency. Vitamin A is toxic when taken in excess; see *hypervitaminosis A.* The term vitamin A is sometimes used to refer specifically to retinol.
**v. $A_1$,** retinol.
**v. $A_2$,** dehydroretinol.
**v. B,** a member of the vitamin B complex.
**v. $B_1$,** thiamine.
**v. $B_2$,** riboflavin.
**v. $B_6$,** water-soluble substances (including pyridoxine, pyridoxal, and pyridoxamine) found in most foods, especially meats, liver, vegetables, whole grain cereals, and egg yolk, and concerned in the metabolism of amino acids, in the degradation of tryptophan, and in the breakdown of glycogen to glucose-1-phosphate.
**v. $B_{12}$,** cyanocobalamin (q.v.) by chemical definition, but generally any substituted cobalamin (def. 2) derivative with similar biological activity; it is a water-soluble hematopoietic vitamin occurring in meats and animal products. To be absorbed by the intestine, it must combine with intrinsic factor, and its metabolism is interconnected with that of folic acid. The vitamin is necessary for the growth and replication of all body cells and the functioning of the nervous system, being required for purine and pyrimidine (and hence DNA, protein, and nucleoprotein) synthesis, methylation reactions, hematopoiesis, and myelin synthesis; at least some of these effects are mediated through its role in folic acid metabolism. Deficiency of the vitamin causes pernicious anemia and other forms of megaloblastic anemia, and neurologic lesions. See also *adenosylcobalamin, cobalamin, hydroxocobalamin,* and *methylcobalamin.*
**v. $B_{12a}$,** hydroxocobalamin.
**v. B complex,** a group of water-soluble substances including thiamine, riboflavin, niacin (nicotinic acid), niacinamide (nicotinamide), the vitamin $B_6$ group (including pyridoxine, pyridoxal, pyridoxamine), biotin, pantothenic acid, folic acid, possibly para-aminobenzoic acid, inositol, vitamin $B_{12}$, and possibly choline. Niacin and niacinamide are also known, together, as the *pellagra-preventing factor, P.-P. factor,* or *antipellagra factor.*
**v. C,** ascorbic acid.
**v. D,** either of two fat-soluble compounds with antirachitic activity, or both collectively: cholecalciferol (q.v.), which is synthesized in the skin and is considered a hormone, and ergocalciferol (q.v.), which is the form generally used as a dietary supplement. Dietary sources include some fish liver oils, egg yolks, and fortified dairy products. Deficiency of vitamin D can result in rickets in children and osteomalacia in adults, while ingestion of excess levels can lead to hypercalcemia, mobilization of calcium from bone, and renal dysfunction. References to metabolites of vitamin D may denote those of cholecalciferol, of ergocalciferol, or of both collectively.
**v. $D_2$,** ergocalciferol.
**v. $D_3$,** cholecalciferol.
**v. E,** 1. any of a group of at least eight related compounds with similar biological antioxidant activity, particularly $\alpha$-tocopherol but also including other isomers of tocopherol and the related compound tocotrienol. It occurs naturally in wheat germ oil, cereal germs, egg yolk, liver, green plants, milk fat, and vegetable oils and is also prepared synthetically. In various species, it is important for normal reproduction, muscle development, and resistance of erythrocytes to hemolysis, but deficiency in human children and adults is rare except in severe cases of malabsorption. The term is sometimes used synonymously with $\alpha$-tocopherol. 2. [USP] an official preparation containing 96 to 102 per cent of the *d-* or *dl* -isomers of $\alpha$-tocopherol, $\alpha$-tocopheryl acid succinate, or $\alpha$-tocopheryl acetate; used as dietary supplement for neonates, particularly if they are premature or have steatorrhea.
**fat-soluble v's,** those (vitamins A, D, E, and K) that are soluble in fat solvents and are absorbed along with dietary fats; they are not normally excreted in the urine and tend to be stored in the body in moderate amounts.
**v. K,** any of a group of structurally similar fat-soluble compounds that promote blood clotting by increasing hepatic biosynthesis of prothrombin and other coagulation factors, activating these factors by $\gamma$-carboxylation of glutamic acid moieties in inactive precursor proteins. Two forms exist naturally, phytonadione (vitamin $K_1$) and menaquinone (vitamin $K_2$), as well as one synthetic provitamin form, menadione (vitamin $K_3$). The best sources are green leafy vegetables, liver, cheese, butter, and egg yolk, and as menaquinone it is synthesized by the intestinal flora. Deficiency, usually seen only in neonates, in disorders of absorption, or during antibiotic therapy, is characterized by hemorrhage.
**v. $K_1$,** phytonadione.
**v. $K_2$,** menaquinone.
**v. $K_3$,** menadione.
**water-soluble v's,** all the vitamins soluble in water (i.e., all but vitamins A, D, E, and K); they are excreted in the urine and are not stored in the body in appreciable quantities.

**vi·ta·min A ac·id** (vi′tə-min) tretinoin.

**vi·tan·i·tion** (vi″tə-nĭ′shən) hypovitaminosis.

**vi·tel·la·ri·um** (vi″tə-lar′e-əm) an accessory genital gland found in flukes and tapeworms which secretes the yolk and shell for the fertilized egg; called also *vitelline gland.*

**vit·el·lary** (vit′ə-lar″e) vitelline.

**vi·tel·li·cle** (vi-tel′ĭ-kəl) [L. *vitellus* yolk] yolk sac.

**vi·tel·lin** (vi-tel′in) [L. *vitellus* yolk] a phosphoprotein found in the yolk of eggs.

**vi·tel·line** (vi-tel′in) [L. *vitellus* yolk] resembling or pertaining to a yolk.

**vi·tel·lo·gen·e·sis** (vi″təl-o-jen′ə-sis) [MeSH: Vitellogenesis] production of yolk.

**vi·tel·lo·lu·te·in** (vi″təl-o-loo′tēn) [*vitellus* + *lutein*] a yellow pigment obtainable from lutein.

**vi·tel·lo·ru·bin** (vi″təl-o-roo′bin) [*vitellus* + *ruber*] 1. a reddish pigment obtainable from lutein. 2. crustaceorubin.

**vi·tel·lose** (vi-tel′ōs) a form of proteose derived from vitellin.

**vi·tel·lus** (vi-tel′əs) [L.] yolk (def. 1).

**vi·ti·a·tin** (vi-ti′ə-tin) a compound sometimes occurring in the urine along with creatine and creatinine; it is a homologue of choline.

**vi·ti·a·tion** (vish″e-a′shən) [L. *vitiatio*] impairment of efficiency; the perversion of any process so as to render it faulty or ineffective.

**vit·i·lig·i·nes** (vit″ĭ-lij′ĭ-nēz) [pl. of *vitiligo*] depigmented areas of the skin, as those occurring in vitiligo, or the whitened lines of striae atrophicae.

**vit·i·lig·i·nous** (vit″ĭ-lij′ĭ-nəs) relating to or affected with vitiligo.

**vit·i·li·go** (vit″ĭ-li′go) [L.] [MeSH: Vitiligo] a chronic anomaly of the skin, usually progressive, consisting of depigmented white patches that may be surrounded by a hyperpigmented border; there is an

autosomal dominant predisposition to the condition, and the etiology is thought to be an autoimmune mechanism. Cf. *leukoderma* and *piebaldism*.
**v. i'ridis,** depigmentation of the iris.

**Vi·tis** (vi'tis) [L.] a genus of plants of the family Vitaceae, including grapes. *V. vini'fera* L. is the species most widely cultivated as fruit and wine grapes for human consumption.

**vit·i·um** (vish'e-əm) pl. *vi'tia* [L.] fault, defect.
**v. conformatio'nis,** a defect in shape; a malformation.
**v. pri'mae formatio'nis,** a developmental anomaly.

**vit. ov. sol.** abbreviation for L. *vitel'lo o'vi solu'tus,* dissolved in yolk of egg.

**Vit·ra·sert** (vit'rə-sərt) trademark for a preparation of ganciclovir.

**vi·trec·to·my** (vĭ-trek'tə-me) [*vitreum* + *-ectomy*] [MeSH: Vitrectomy] surgical extraction usually via the pars plana of the contents of the vitreous chamber of the eye.

**vit·re·i·tis** (vit″re-i'tis) hyalitis.

**vit·reo·cap·su·li·tis** (vit″re-o-kap″su-li'tis) [*vitreous* + *capsulitis*] inflammation of the capsule enclosing the vitreous; hyalitis.

**vit·reo·ret·i·nal** (vit″re-o-ret'ĭ-nəl) of or pertaining to the vitreous and retina.

**vit·re·ous** (vit're-əs) glasslike or hyaline; often used alone to designate the vitreous body of the eye (corpus vitreum [TA]).
**detached v.,** vitreous separated from its attachments, especially from the retina.
**primary v.,** the earliest vitreous in the embryo, formed from a mass of ectodermal and mesodermal fibrils and vascularized by the proliferating hyaloid system. It ceases to be formed when the hyaline capsule of the lens is formed, and is then enveloped by secondary vitreous.
**primary persistent hyperplastic v.,** a congenital anomaly, usually unilateral, due to persistence of embryonic remnants of the fibromuscular tunic of the eye and part of the hyaloid vascular system. Clinically, there is a white pupil, elongated ciliary processes, and often microphthalmia; the lens, although clear initially, may become completely opaque.
**secondary v.,** embryonic vitreous composed of densely packed fine fibrils formed around the primary vitreous by the inner layer of the optic cup.
**tertiary v.,** embryonic zonular fibers derived from the primary vitreous and the basement membrane of the nonpigmented epithelium of the ciliary body; the fibers eventually attach to the lens capsule, giving rise to the zonule of Zinn.

**vit·re·um** (vit're-əm) corpus vitreum.

**vit·ri·fi·ca·tion** (vit″rĭ-fĭ-ka'shən) [L. *vitrum* glass] the forming of a supercooled liquid such as glass.

**vit·ri·ol** (vit're-ol) [L. *vitriolum*] any crystalline sulfate.
**blue v.,** the pentahydrate form of cupric sulfate.

**vit·ri·tis** (vĭ-tri'tis) hyalitis.

**vit·ro·nec·tin** (vit″ro-nek'tin) [MeSH: Vitronectin] a multifunctional adhesive glycoprotein occurring in serum and various tissues and having binding sites for integrins, collagen, heparin, complement components and perforin. Its functions include regulation of the coagulation, fibrinolytic, and complement cascades, and it plays a role in hemostasis, wound healing, tissue remodeling, and cancer. It binds plasminogen activator inhibitor (PAI-1); mediates the inflammatory and repair reactions occurring at sites of tissue injury; and promotes adhesion, spreading, and migration of cells. It has been shown to be identical to *S protein,* which was identified as an inhibitor of complement activation, binding the membrane attack complex and preventing its insertion into the membrane.

**Vi·vac·til** (vi-vak'til) trademark for a preparation of protriptyline hydrochloride.

**vivi-** [L. *vivus* alive] a combining form meaning alive or denoting relationship to life.

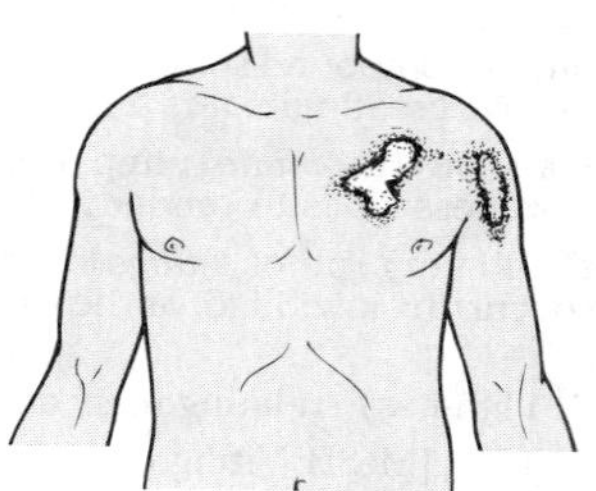

Vitiligo.

**vivi·di·al·y·sis** (viv″ĭ-di-al'ĭ-sis) removal by dialysis through a living membrane (the peritoneum). Cf. *peritoneal lavage,* under *lavage.*

**vivi·dif·fu·sion** (viv″ĭ-dĭ-fu'zhən) removal of diffusible substances from the circulating blood of living subjects by dialysis, performed by the continuous passage of the blood from an artery through a system of tubes made of celloidin immersed in saline solution, and its return to a vein, thus yielding by dialysis certain of its constituents to the fluid surrounding the tubes.

**vivi·par·i·ty** (viv″ĭ-par'ĭ-te) the quality of being viviparous.

**vi·vip·a·rous** (vi-vip'ə-rəs) [*vivi-* + L. *parere* to bring forth, produce] bearing living young which derive nutrition directly from the maternal organism.

**Vi·vip·a·rus** (vi-vip'ə-rəs) a genus of fresh water snails of the family Viviparidae, order Mesogastropoda. *V. java'nicus* is a second intermediate host of the fluke *Echinostoma ilocanum* in Indonesia.

**vivi·pa·tion** (viv″ĭ-pa'shən) the form of reproduction in which the embryo develops within and derives nutrition directly from the maternal organism.

**vivi·sec·tion** (viv″ĭ-sek'shən) [MeSH: Vivisection] the performance of surgical procedures upon living animals for purposes of research.

**vivi·sec·tion·ist** (viv″ĭ-sek'shən-ist) one who practices or defends vivisection.

**VLA** very late activation (antigen); see $\beta_1$ *integrin,* under *integrin.*

**Vla·di·mir·off's operation** (vlah″dĭ-mēr'ofs) [Alexander A. *Vladimiroff,* Russian surgeon, 1837–1903] see *Mikulicz's operation,* def. 3, under *operation.*

**Vla·di·mir·off-Mik·u·licz amputation** (vlah″dĭ-mēr'of-me-koo'lich) [Alexander A. *Vladimiroff;* Johann von *Mikulicz*-Radecki, Polish surgeon in Germany, 1850–1905] see under *amputation.*

**VLBW** very low birth weight; see under *infant.*

**VLCD** very low calorie diet.

**VLDL** very-low-density lipoprotein.
**$\beta$-VLDL, beta VLDL,** a mixture of lipoproteins with diffuse electrophoretic mobility approximately that of $\beta$-lipoproteins but having lower density; they are remnants derived from mutant chylomicrons and very-low-density lipoproteins that cannot be metabolized completely and therefore accumulate in plasma. Called also *floating beta lipoproteins.* See also *familial dysbetalipoproteinemia.*
**pre-$\beta$-VLDL,** very-low-density lipoprotein; the term is used to emphasize its normal electrophoretic mobility.

**VM-26** teniposide.

**VMA** vanillylmandelic acid.

**VMD** Doctor of Veterinary Medicine [L. Veterinariae Medicinae Doctor].

**vo·cal** (vo'kəl) [L. *vocalis,* from *vox* voice] pertaining to the voice.

**Vo·ges-Pros·kau·er test (reaction)** (fo'ges-pros'kou-er) [Daniel Wilhelm Otto *Voges,* German physician, early 20th century; Bernhard *Proskauer,* German hygienist, 1851–1915] see under *test.*

**Vogt's angle** (fōkts) [Karl *Vogt,* German naturalist and physiologist, 1817–1895] see under *angle.*

**Vogt's point** (fōkts) [Paul Frederick Emmanuel *Vogt,* German surgeon, 1844–1885] see under *point.*

**Vogt's syndrome** (fōkts) [Cécile *Vogt,* French physician in Germany, 1875–1962, and Oskar *Vogt,* German neurologist, 1870–1959] see under *syndrome.*

**Vogt-Hue·ter point** (fōkt-he'ter) [P. F. E. *Vogt;* Karl *Hueter,* German surgeon, 1838–1882] see Vogt's *point,* under *point.*

**Vogt-Ko·ya·na·gi syndrome** (fōgt-ko-yah-nah'ge) [Alfred *Vogt,* Swiss ophthalmologist, 1879–1943; Yoshizo *Koyanagi,* Japanese ophthalmologist, 1880–1954] see under *syndrome.*

**Vogt-Ko·ya·na·gi-Ha·ra·da syndrome** (fōkt-ko-yah-nah'ge-hah-rah'dah) [Alfred *Vogt; Y. Koyanagi; Einosuke Harada,* Japanese surgeon, 1892–1947] Harada syndrome.

**Vogt-Spiel·mey·er disease** (fōgt-shpēl'mi-er) [Heinrich *Vogt,* German physician, 20th century; Walter *Spielmeyer,* German physician, 1879–1935] see under *disease.*

**Voh·win·kel's syndrome** (fo-ving'kelz) [Karl Hermann *Vohwinkel,* German dermatologist, 20th century] keratoma hereditarium mutilans.

**voice** (vois) [L. *vox* voice] [MeSH: Voice] a sound produced by the larynx and modified by the vocal cords and other structures in the pharynx and oral cavity.
**amphoric v.,** cavernous v.
**cavernous v.,** a type of pectoriloquy consisting of hollow voice sounds heard over a lung cavity when the patient speaks. Called also *amphoric v., amphoriloquy,* and *amphorophony.*

**double v.,** diphonia.
**eunuchoid v.,** a high falsetto voice in a man, resembling that of a eunuch or a woman.
**whispered v.,** see under *pectoriloquy.*

**voiced** (voist) said of speech sounds produced with vibration of the vocal cords, such as *b, d,* or *z.* Called also *sonant* and *sonorant.*

**voice·less** (vois'ləs) said of speech sounds produced without vibration of the vocal cords, such as *p, t,* or *s.* Called also *surd* and *unvoiced.*

**void** (void) excrete.

**Voigt's lines** (foits) [Christian August *Voigt,* Austrian anatomist, 1809–1890] see under *line.*

**Voille·mi·er's point** (vwahl"me-āz') [Léon Clémont *Voillemier,* French urologist, 1809–1878] see under *point.*

**Voit's nucleus** (foits) [Karl von *Voit,* German physiologist, 1831–1908] see under *nucleus.*

**voix** (vwah) [Fr.] voice.
**v. de Polichinelle** (də po-le-she-nel'), [Fr. "Punch's voice"], egophony.

**vo·la** (vo'lə) gen. and pl. *vo'lae* [L.] 1. a concave or hollow surface. 2. TA alternative for *palma.*

**vo·lar** (vo'lər) [L. *volaris*] pertaining to the palm or sole; see *palmar* and *plantar.*

**vo·lar·dor·sal** (vo"lər-dor'səl) from the volar to the dorsal surface.

**vo·la·ris** (vo-lar'is) [L., from *vola* (q.v.)] volar; TA alternative for *palmaris.*

**vol·a·tile** (vol'ə-til) [L. *volatilis,* from *volare* to fly] tending to evaporate rapidly; readily vaporizable at low temperature.

**vol·a·til·iza·tion** (vol"ə-til"ī-za'shən) [MeSH: Volatilization] the conversion into vapor or gas without chemical change.

**vol·a·til·ize** (vol'ə-til-īz) to convert into vapor.

**vol·a·til·iz·er** (vol'ə-til-īz"ər) an apparatus for producing volatilization.

**vole** (vōl) [MeSH: Microtinae] any of various small rodents of the genera *Clethrionomys* and *Microtus,* found in northern Europe, Asia, and North America; some serve as reservoirs for disease.
**bank v.,** *Clethrionomys glareolus.*
**field v.,** either *Microtus agrestis* or *M. montebelli,* species found in northern Europe and North America and presumed to be the host of *Leptospira interrogans* serovar *hebdomadis,* an etiologic agent of nanukayami.

**vo·li·tion** (vo-lish'ən) [L. *velle* to will] [MeSH: Volition] the act or power of willing.

**vo·li·tion·al** (vo-lish'ən-əl) pertaining to the will.

**Volk·mann's canal, membrane** (fōk'mahnz) [Alfred Wilhelm *Volkmann,* German physiologist, 1800–1877] see under *canal* and *membrane.*

**Volk·mann's contracture (ischemic paralysis, syndrome),** etc. (fōk'mahnz) [Richard von *Volkmann,* German surgeon, 1830–1889] see under *contracture, disease, paralysis,* and *spoon.*

**vol·ley** (vol'e) [Fr. *volée* flight] a number of simultaneous muscle twitches or nerve impulses all caused by the same stimulus.
**antidromic v.,** a volley of nerve impulses that travel in a direction opposite to normal, usually under experimental stimulation.

**vol·sel·la** (vol-sel'ə) [L.] vulsella.

**volt** (vōlt) [Alessandro *Volta,* Italian physiologist and physicist, 1745–1827] the SI unit of electric potential or electromotive force equal to one joule per coulomb or one ampere-ohm. Symbol V.
**electron v. (eV, ev),** the energy acquired by an electron accelerated through a potential difference of one volt, equal to $1.6022 \times 10^{-19}$ joule. Larger units, used for specifying rest masses and kinetic energies of particles, are obtained by attaching SI prefixes, giving *kilo electron volt* (keV = $10^3$ eV), *mega electron volt* (MeV = $10^6$ eV), and *giga electron volt* (GeV = $10^9$ eV).

**vol·tage** (vōl'təj) electromotive force measured in volts. Symbol *V* or *v.*

**vol·ta·ic** (vol-ta'ik) galvanic (def. 2).

**vol·tam·me·ter** (vōl-tam'ə-tər) an instrument for measuring both volts and amperes.

**volt·am·pere** (vōlt-am'pēr) the product of multiplying a volt by a milliampere.

**Vol·ta·ren** (vōl'tə-ren) trademark for a preparation of diclofenac sodium.

**volt·me·ter** (vōlt'me-tər) an instrument for measuring electromotive force in volts.

**Vol·to·li·ni's disease, sign** (vol"to-le'nēz) [Friedrich Edward Rudolf *Voltolini,* German otorhinolaryngologist, 1819–1889] see under *disease.*

**vol·ume** (vol'ūm) the measure of the quantity or capacity of a substance. Symbol V or *V.*
**atomic v.,** the value obtained by dividing the atomic weight of an element by its specific gravity in the solid condition.
**blood v.,** the plasma volume added to the red cell volume.
**circulation v., v. of circulation,** the amount of blood pumped through the lungs and out to all the organs of the body by the heart, expressed in liters of blood flow per minute.
**closing v. (CV),** the difference between the closing capacity and the residual volume; the volume of gas still in the lungs in excess of the residual volume when dependent small airways are assumed to have closed. Seen in the test results (such as with the single breath nitrogen washout test) near the end of the vital capacity period as a sharp rise in nitrogen concentration, indicating that most gas at this point is coming from the upper lung areas. It has sometimes been analyzed for indications of early lung disease.
**v. of distribution,** a dilution method for determining the volume of fluids, e.g., plasma, in a body fluid compartment. A solute (e.g., inulin) is injected into the compartment and, after it is equally distributed, a sample is taken. Then the quantity of solute removed (as by metabolism, excretion, etc.) is subtracted from the quantity administered, and the result is divided by the concentration per milliliter in the sample.
**end-diastolic v. (EDV),** the volume of blood in each ventricle at the end of diastole, usually about 120–130 mL but sometimes reaching 200–250 mL in the normal heart; it is a measure of preload (q.v.) and is the sum of the stroke volume plus end-systolic volume.
**end-systolic v. (ESV),** the volume of blood remaining in each ventricle at the end of systole, usually about 50–60 mL but sometimes as little as 10–30 mL in the normal heart; it is the difference between the end-diastolic volume and the stroke volume and is determined by the contractility of the ventricles and the state of the venous system.
**expiratory reserve v.,** ERV: the maximal amount of gas that can be expired from the resting end-expiratory level. See illustration at *capacity.*
**forced expiratory v.,** the fraction of the forced vital capacity that is exhaled in a specific number of seconds; abbreviated FEV, with a subscript telling how many seconds the measurement lasted. See also *forced expiratory flow,* under *flow.*
**functional venous v.,** the increase in volume of blood in veins of the legs, measured in milliliters, when a patient who has been supine with legs elevated changes to a standing position.
**inspiratory reserve v.,** the maximal amount of gas that can be inspired from the end-inspiratory position. Abbreviated IRV.
**mean corpuscular v. (MCV),** the average volume of erythrocytes, conventionally expressed in cubic micrometers or femtoliters per red cell, obtained by multiplying the hematocrit (in L/L) by 1000 and dividing by the red cell count (in millions per $\mu$L): MCV = Hct/RBC. Automated electronic blood cell counters generally obtain the MCV directly from the average pulse height of the voltage pulses produced during the red cell count. These instruments obtain the hematocrit indirectly from the equation Hct = MCV × RBC.
**minute v.,** the quantity of gas expelled from the lungs per minute; tidal volume multiplied by respiratory rate. Abbreviated MV.
**packed-cell v. (PCV), v. of packed red cells (VPRC),** hematocrit.
**plasma v.,** the total volume of blood plasma, i.e., the extracellular fluid volume of the vascular space, measured by tracer dilution using $^{125}$I- or $^{131}$I-labeled albumin or T-1824 Evans blue dye as the tracer.
**red cell v.,** the total volume of red cells in the body measured by isotopic dilution methods, usually with $^{51}$Cr-labeled autologous red cells.
**residual v.,** RV; the amount of gas remaining in the lung at the end of a maximal expiration. See illustration at *capacity.*
**stroke v.,** the amount of blood ejected from a ventricle at each beat of the heart, equal to the difference between the end-diastolic volume and the end-systolic volume.
**tidal v.,** $V_T$; the amount of gas that is either inspired or expired during one respiratory cycle. See *ventilation* (def. 2) and see illustration at *capacity.* Called also *tidal air.*

**vol·u·men·om·e·ter** (vol"u-mən-om'ə-tər) volumometer.

**vol·u·met·ric** (vol"u-met'rik) [*volume* + *metric*] pertaining to or accomplished by measurement in volumes.

**vol·u·mette** (vol"u-met') an instrument for delivering repeatedly quantities of fluid in accurate predetermined amounts.

**vol·u·mom·e·ter** (vol"u-mom'ə-tər) [*volume* + *-meter*] an instrument for measuring volume or changes in volume.

**vol·un·tary** (vol'ən-tar"e) [L. *voluntas* will] accomplished in accordance with the will.

**vo·lun·to·mo·to·ry** (vo"lən-to-mo'tə-re) [L. *voluntas* will + *motor*] subject to voluntary motor influence.

**vo·lute** (vo-lūt′) rolled up.

**vo·lu·tin** (vo-lu′tin) a complex molecule containing large amounts of orthophosphate polymers, nucleoprotein, and lipid, occurring as cytoplasmic granular inclusions (granules) in certain bacteria, yeasts, yeastlike fungi, and protozoa, and serving as an intracellular phosphate reserve. Because volutin granules stain red with blue basic dyes they are sometimes called *metachromatic granules.*

**vol·u·trau·ma** (vol′u-traw″mə) damage to the lung caused by overdistension by a mechanical ventilator set for an excessively high tidal volume.

**vol·vu·late** (vol′vu-lāt) [L. *volvere* to twist round] to twist or form a knot; see also *volvulus.*

**vol·vu·lo·sis** (vol″vu-lo′sis) onchocerciasis.

**vol·vu·lus** (vol′vu-ləs) [L. *volvere* to twist round] intestinal obstruction due to a knotting and twisting of the bowel.
**abomasal v.,** see under *torsion.*
**gastric dilatation-v.,** excessive dilatation of the stomach of a dog, usually seen in large deep-chested breeds and often resulting from swallowed air; if untreated, the dilatation often progresses to fatal volvulus.
**v. neonato′rum,** volvulus occurring in the newborn.

**vo·mer** (vo′mər) [L. "plowshare"] [TA] the unpaired flat bone that forms the inferior and posterior part of the nasal septum.

**vo·mer·ine** (vo′mər-in) of or pertaining to the vomer.

**vo·mero·bas·i·lar** (vo″mər-o-bas′ĭ-lər) pertaining to the vomer and to the basilar portion of the cranium.

**vo·mero·na·sal** (vo″mər-o-na′səl) pertaining to the vomer and the nasal bone.

**vom·it** (vom′it) [L. *vomitare*] 1. to cast up from the stomach by the mouth. 2. matter cast up from the stomach; vomited matter.
**Barcoo v.,** vomiting and nausea, with bulimia, occurring in southern Australia.
**bilious v.,** vomited matter stained with bile.
**black v.,** vomit discolored black in yellow fever and other conditions in which blood collects in the stomach.
**coffee-ground v.,** vomit containing dark altered blood mixed with stomach contents; see *black v.*

**vom·it·ing** (vom′it-ing) [MeSH: Vomiting] forcible expulsion of stomach contents through the mouth; called also *emesis* and *regurgitation.*
**cerebral v.,** spontaneous vomiting without nausea, frequently due to stimulation of the vomiting center in the brain.
**cyclic v.,** vomiting recurring at irregular intervals, especially in children; called also *periodic v.* and *recurrent v.*
**dry v.,** nausea with attempts at vomiting, but with the ejection of nothing but gas.
**fecal v.,** stercoraceous v.
**hysterical v.,** vomiting accompanying an attack of hysteria.
**periodic v.,** cyclic v.
**pernicious v.,** vomiting in pregnancy, so severe as to threaten the life of the mother.
**v. of pregnancy,** vomiting occurring in pregnancy, especially the early morning vomiting common in that condition.
**projectile v.,** vomiting in which the vomitus is ejected with force.
**psychogenic v.,** that due to emotional anxiety or other psychological factors.
**recurrent v.,** cyclic v.
**stercoraceous v.,** the vomiting of fecal matter; it is seen in intestinal obstruction, appendicitis, etc., when bacterial overgrowth in the upper intestine has modified the intestinal contents.

**vom·i·tive** (vom′ĭ-tiv) emetic.

**vom·i·to·ry** (vom′ĭ-tor″e) an emetic.

**vom·i·tox·in** (vom″ĭ-tok′sin) deoxynivalenol.

**vom·it·u·ri·tion** (vom″it-u-rish′ən) repeated ineffectual attempts at vomiting.

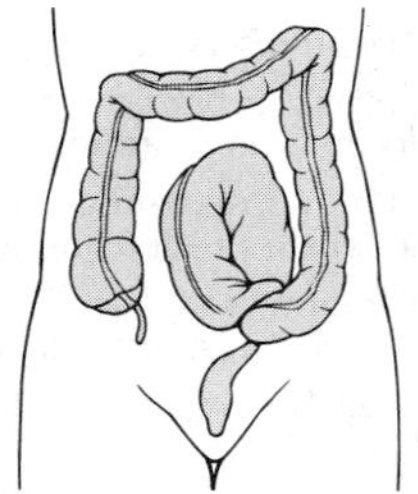

Volvulus.

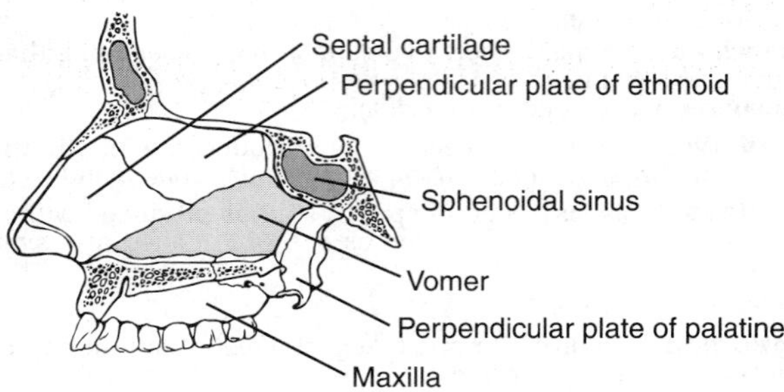


Vomer, in a median section of the anterior portion of the skull.

**vom·i·tus** (vom′ĭ-təs) [L.] 1. vomiting. 2. matter vomited.
**v. cruen′tus,** bloody vomit.
**v. matuti′nus,** the morning vomiting of chronic gastritis.

**von Arlt** see *Arlt.*

**von Behr·ing** see *Behring.*

**von Be·zold** see *Bezold.*

**v-*onc*** [*v*iral *onc*ogene] a nucleic acid sequence in a virus responsible for the oncogenicity of the virus; it is derived from the cellular proto-oncogene and acquired from the host by recombination. Cf. *c*-onc. See also table of oncogenes at *oncogene.*

**von Econ·o·mo** see *Economo.*

**von Frisch** see *Frisch.*

**von Gier·ke** see *Gierke.*

**von Grae·fe** see *Graefe.*

**von Hal·ler** see *Haller.*

**von Han·se·mann cells** (fōn hahn′sə-mahnz) [David Paul von *Hansemann,* German pathologist, 1858–1920] see under *cell.*

**von Hip·pel** see *Hippel.*

**von Lan·gen·beck** see *Langenbeck.*

**von Ley·den** see *Leyden.*

**von Mi·ku·licz** see *Mikulicz.*

**von Mo·na·kow** see *Monakow.*

**von Pir·quet** see *Pirquet.*

**von Reck·ling·hau·sen** see *Recklinghausen.*

**Von·trol** (von′trōl) trademark for preparations of diphenidol.

**von Tröltsch** see Tröltsch.

**von Wil·le·brand** see *Willebrand.*

**von Zen·ker** see *Zenker.*

**von Zum·busch** see *Zumbusch.*

**Vor·a·nil** (vor′ə-nil) trademark for a preparation of clortermine hydrochloride.

**vor·bei·re·den** (for′bi-ra-dən) the giving of approximate or otherwise ridiculous answers or talking past the point, as occurs in Ganser syndrome and other mental disorders but which also may occur in tired or stressed but otherwise mentally healthy individuals.

**vor·tex** (vor′teks) pl. *vor′tices* [L. "whirl"] 1. a whorled arrangement. 2. [TA] a general term in anatomical nomenclature for a structure having a whorled arrangement, design, or pattern.
**v. coccy′geus,** coccygeal vortex: a spiral arrangement of hairs over the region of the coccyx.
**v. cor′dis** [TA], vortex of heart: the whorled arrangement of muscle fibers at the apex in the left ventricle of the heart, through which the more superficial fibers pass to the interior of the left ventricle toward the base.
**Fleischer's v.,** a rare congenital opacity characterized by ochre-colored whorls which radiate from the center of the cornea at the level of Bowman's membrane; called also *cornea verticillata.*
**v. len′tis,** a spiral figure on the surface of the lens of the eye produced by the concentric arrangement of the fibers composing it; called also *nuclear arc* or *zone.*
**vor′tices pilo′rum** [TA], hair whorls: whorled patterns of hair growth on the body, as that on the crown of the head.

**vor·ti·ces** (vor′tĭ-sēz) [L.] plural of *vortex.*

**v. o. s.** abbreviation for L. *vitel′lo o′vi solu′tus,* dissolved in yolk of egg.

**Vos·si·us' ring** (fos′e-əs) [Adolf *Vossius,* German ophthalmologist, 1855–1925] see under *ring.*

**vox** (voks) gen. *vo′cis,* pl. *vo′ces* [L.] voice.

**v. chole'rica,** the faint, sometimes inaudible, high-pitched voice of patients with severe cholera.

**vox·el** (vok'sel) [*volume element*, by analogy with *pixel*] each defined volume unit of an element being scanned in computerized axial tomography. Cf. *pixel.*

**vo·yeur** (voi-yoor') a person who practices voyeurism.

**vo·yeur·ism** (voi'yər-iz-əm) [MeSH: Voyeurism] [DSM-IV] a paraphilia characterized by recurrent, intense sexual urges or arousal involving real or fantasized observation of unsuspecting people who are naked, disrobing, or engaging in sexual activity.

**VP** variegate porphyria.

**VP-16** etoposide.

**VPB** ventricular premature beat; see *ventricular premature complex,* under *complex.*

**VPC** ventricular premature complex.

**VPD** ventricular premature depolarization; see *ventricular premature complex,* under *complex.*

**VPRC** volume of packed red cells.

**VR** vocal resonance.

**Vro·lik's disease** (vro'liks) [Willem *Vrolik,* Dutch anatomist, 1801–1863] osteogenesis imperfecta (type II), recessive form; see under *osteogenesis.*

**VS** volumetric solution.

**VSG** variable surface glycoprotein.

**VT** ventricular tachycardia.

**vu·er·om·e·ter** (vu″ər-om'ə-tər) [Fr. *vue* sight + *-meter*] an instrument for measuring the interpupillary distance.

**vul·ca·nize** (vul'kə-nīz) to subject raw rubber, in the presence of sulfur, to heat and high steam pressure, producing a flexible or hard rubber.

**vul·ga·ris** (vəl-ga'ris) [L.] ordinary; common. See *acne vulgaris, lupus vulgaris,* etc.

**vul·ner·a·bil·i·ty** (vul″nər-ə-bil'ĭ-te) susceptibility to injury or to contagion.

**vul·ner·ant** (vul'nər-ənt) 1. inflicting injury or causing a wound. 2. an agent that causes injury.

**vul·ner·ary** (vul'nər-ar″e) [L. *vulnerarius,* from *vulnus* wound] 1. pertaining to wounds or the healing of wounds. 2. an agent that promotes the healing of wounds.

**vul·ner·ate** (vul'nər-āt) [L. *vulnerare*] to wound.

**vul·nus** (vul'nəs) pl. *vul'nera* [L.] wound.

**Vul·pi·an's atrophy** (vūl-pyahz') [Edme Felix Alfred *Vulpian,* French physician, 1826–1887] see under *atrophy.*

**vul·sel·la** (vəl-sel'ə) [L.] a forceps with clawlike hooks at the extremity of each blade.

**vul·sel·lum** (vəl-sel'əm) [L.] vulsella.

**vul·va** (vəl'və) [L.] [MeSH: Vulva] the region of the external genital organs of the female, including the labia majora, labia minora, mons pubis, clitoris, bulb of the vestibule, vestibule of the vagina, greater and lesser vestibular glands, and vaginal orifice. See *pudendum femininum* [TA].
**fused v.,** synechia vulvae.

**vul·val, vul·var** (vul'vəl, vul'vər) pertaining to the vulva.

**vul·vec·to·my** (vəl-vek'tə-me) excision of the vulva.

**vul·vis·mus** (vəl-viz'məs) vaginismus.

**vul·vi·tis** (vəl-vi'tis) [*vulva* + *-itis*] [MeSH: Vulvitis] inflammation of the vulva.
**atrophic v.,** lichen sclerosus in females; see under *lichen.*
**diabetic v.,** vulvitis occurring in diabetes.
**eczematiform v.,** vulvitis marked by the formation of vesicular pustules.
**erosive v.,** a condition due to mixed microbial infection in which gangrenous ulcerations similar to the lesions seen in noma of the oral tissues affect one labium majus and then the other. Called also *noma vulvae* and *phlegmonous v.*
**leukoplakic v.,** lichen sclerosus in females.
**phlegmonous v.,** erosive v.
**plasma cell v., v. plasmocellula'ris,** the counterpart of balanitis circumscripta plasmacellularis in women, in which the vulva has a lacquer-like appearance; erosions, punctate hemorrhage, synechiae, and a slate- to ochre-colored pigmentation may supervene.
**pseudoleukoplakic v.,** lichen sclerosus in females.
**ulcerative v.,** a form with ulceration, pain, and lymphangitis.

**vul·vo·cru·ral** (vul″vo-kroo'rəl) pertaining to the vulva and the thigh.

**vul·vop·a·thy** (vəl-vop'ə-the) [*vulva* + *-pathy*] any disease of the vulva.

**vul·vo·rec·tal** (vul″vo-rek'təl) pertaining to or communicating with the vulva and rectum, as a vulvorectal fistula.

**vul·vo·uter·ine** (vul″vo-u'tər-in) pertaining to the vulva and uterus.

**vul·vo·vag·i·nal** (vul″vo-vaj'ĭ-nəl) pertaining to the vulva and vagina.

**vul·vo·vag·i·ni·tis** (vul″vo-vaj″ĭ-ni'tis) [MeSH: Vulvovaginitis] inflammation of the vulva and vagina, or of the vulvovaginal glands.
***Candida* v.,** a common form caused by infection with species of *Candida;* it is usually asymptomatic but may be characterized by pruritus, white discharge, vulvar erythema and swelling, and dyspareunia. See also *Candida vaginitis,* under *vaginitis.* Called also *vulvovaginal candidiasis.*
**infectious pustular v.,** a venereal infection of cows, caused by bovine herpesvirus I and characterized by inflammation, necrosis, and pustule formation of varying degree in the vulva and vagina. It is the female counterpart of infectious pustular balanoposthitis.
**senile v.,** atrophic vaginitis in which there is intense itching around the vagina, almost complete lack of vaginal secretions, and tissue atrophy.

**Vu·mon** (voo'mon) trademark for a preparation of teniposide.

**vv.** abbreviation for L. *ve'nae* (veins).

**v/v** volume (of solute) per volume (of solvent).

**VW** vessel wall.

**VX** an organophosphorus compound that is a potent cholinesterase inhibitor and is used as a nerve gas; symptoms of poisoning include bronchial constriction, convulsions, and often death. See *organophosphorus compound poisoning,* under *poisoning.*

**vWF** von Willebrand's factor.

**V-Y plas·ty** V-Y procedure.

**VZIG** varicella-zoster immune globulin.

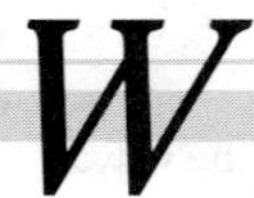

**W** symbol for *tungsten* [Ger. *Wolfram*] and *watt.*

***W*** symbol for *work.*

**Waar·den·burg's syndrome** (vahr'den-bərgz) [Petrus Johannes *Waardenburg,* Dutch ophthalmologist, 1886–1979] [MeSH: Waardenburg's Syndrome] see under *syndrome.*

**Wach·en·dorf's membrane** (vahk'en-dorfs) [Eberhard Jacob *Wachendorf,* Dutch physician, 1703–1758] see under *membrane.*

**Wa·da's test** (wah'dəz) [Juhn Atsushi *Wada,* Japanese-born Canadian neurosurgeon, born 1924] see under *test.*

**Wag·staffe's fracture** (wag'stafs) [William Warwick *Wagstaffe,* English surgeon, 1843–1910] see under *fracture.*

**WAIS** Wechsler Adult Intelligence Scale.

**waist** (wāst) the portion of the body between the thorax and the hips.

**wake·ful·ness** (wāk'fəl-nəs) [MeSH: Wakefulness] 1. a condition of alertness or watchfulness. 2. a state marked by indisposition to sleep; sleeplessness; see also *consciousness.*

**Waks·man** (waks'mən) Selman Abraham. Russian-born American microbiologist, 1888–1973; winner of the Nobel prize for medicine or physiology in 1952 for his discovery of streptomycin and its effectiveness against tuberculosis.

**Wald** (wahld) George. American biologist, born 1906; co-winner, with Ragnar Arthur Granit and Haldan Keffer Hartline, of the Nobel prize for medicine or physiology in 1967 for discoveries regarding the molecular basis of visual excitation.

**Wal·den·ström's disease** (vahl'den-strermz) [Johan Henning *Waldenström,* Swedish orthopedic surgeon, 1877–1972] see *osteochondrosis.*

**Wal·den·ström's macroglobulinemia** (vahl'den-strermz) [Jan Gosta *Waldenström,* Swedish physician, 1906–1996] see under *macroglobulinemia.*

**Wal·dey·er's fluid,** etc. (vahl'di-erz) [Heinrich Wilhelm Gottfried von *Waldeyer,* German anatomist, 1836–1921] see under *fluid, fossa, gland, layer,* and *ring.*

**walk** (wawk) 1. to move on foot. 2. gait.

**walk·er** (wawk'ər) [MeSH: Walkers] an enclosing framework made of lightweight metal tubing, sometimes with wheels, for patients who need more support for walking than that given by a cane or a crutch.

**Walk·er's lissencephaly** (waw'kərz) [Arthur Earl *Walker,* American surgeon, born 1907] Walker-Warburg syndrome.

**Walk·er-War·burg syndrome** (waw'kər-vahr'boorg) [A.E. *Walker;* Mette *Warburg,* Danish ophthalmologist, 20th century] see under *syndrome.*

**walk·ing** (wawk'ing) [MeSH: Walking] 1. progressing on foot; called also *ambulation.* 2. gait.
**chromosome w.,** in molecular genetics, the sequential isolation of clones carrying overlapping DNA sequences so that the isolation "walks" along part of a chromosome.
**heel w.,** a gait marked by walking on the heels to avoid the pain of pressure upon the hyperalgesic soles of the feet in cases of peripheral neuritis.
**sleep w.,** somnambulism.

**wall** (wawl) 1. the limiting structure of a space, hollow organ, or definitive mass of material. See also *paries.* 2. the rigid external surface of a horse's hoof.
**anterior w. of stomach,** paries anterior gastris.
**anterior w. of tympanic cavity,** paries caroticus cavitatis tympani.
**anterior w. of vagina,** paries anterior vaginae.
**axial w.,** a cavity wall approximating the pulp tissue, parallel with the long axis of the tooth.
**carotid w. of tympanic cavity,** paries caroticus cavitatis tympani.
**cavity w.,** the walls of a prepared cavity, named according to the surface of a tooth toward which they are placed, extracoronal walls being named after surfaces that have been reduced, and intracoronal ones after surfaces from which they derive.
**cell w.,** a rigid structure that lies just outside of and is joined to the plasma membrane of plant cells and most prokaryotic cells; it protects the cell and maintains its shape.
**chest w.,** the bony and muscular structures that form the outer framework of the thorax and move during breathing.
**external w. of cochlear duct,** paries externus ductus cochlearis.
**gastric w., anterior,** paries anterior gastris.
**gastric w., posterior,** paries posterior gastris.
**germ w.,** a ringlike thickening around the blastoderm of the bird, consisting of the advancing boundary zone at its margin.
**gingival w.,** a peripheral cavity wall near the apical end of the crown of the tooth.
**hollow w.,** seedy toe.
**inferior w. of orbit,** paries inferior orbitae.
**jugular w. of tympanic cavity,** paries jugularis cavitatis tympani.
**labyrinthic w. of tympanic cavity,** paries labyrinthicus cavitatis tympani.
**lateral w. of nasal cavity,** the lateral surface of the cavity, containing the nasal conchae and meatus.
**lateral w. of orbit,** paries lateralis orbitae.
**lateral w. of tympanic cavity,** paries membranaceus cavitatis tympani.
**mastoid w. of tympanic cavity,** paries mastoideus cavitatis tympani.
**medial w. of nasal cavity,** septum nasi.
**medial w. of orbit,** paries medialis orbitae.
**medial w. of tympanic cavity,** paries labyrinthicus cavitatis tympani.
**membranous w. of trachea,** paries membranaceus tracheae.
**membranous w. of tympanic cavity,** paries membranaceus cavitatis tympani.
**nail w.,** vallum unguis.
**parietal w.,** somatopleure.
**party w.,** a bony septum in the nose.
**periotic w.,** the wall of the otic vesicle.
**posterior w. of stomach,** paries posterior gastris.
**posterior w. of tympanic cavity,** paries mastoideus cavitatis tympani.
**posterior w. of vagina,** paries posterior vaginae.
**pulpal w.,** the cavity wall on the occlusal surface that covers the pulp in a plane at right angles to the long axis of the tooth.
**splanchnic w.,** splanchnopleure.
**subpulpal w.,** the floor of a prepared cavity formed when the pulp is removed and the cavity is extended to include the pulp chamber.
**superior w. of orbit,** paries superior orbitae.
**tegmental w. of tympanic cavity,** paries tegmentalis cavitatis tympani.
**tympanic w. of cochlear duct,** paries tympanicus ductus cochlearis.
**vestibular w. of cochlear duct,** paries vestibularis ductus cochlearis.

**Wal·len·berg's syndrome** (vahl'en-bergz) [Adolf *Wallenberg,* German physician, 1862–1949] [MeSH: Wallenberg's Syndrome] see under *syndrome.*

**wal·le·ri·an degeneration** (wahl-e're-ən) [Augustus Volney *Waller,* English physiologist, 1816–1870] [MeSH: Wallerian Degeneration] see under *degeneration.*

**wall·eye** (wawl'i) 1. leukoma of the cornea. 2. exotropia.

**Wal·thard's islets (cell nests, cell rests, inclusions)** (vahl'tahrdz) [Max *Walthard,* Swiss gynecologist, 1867–1933] see under *islet.*

**Wal·ther's ducts, oblique ligament** (vahl'terz) [August Friedrich *Walther,* German anatomist, 1688–1746] see *ductus sublinguales minores* and *ligamentum talofibulare posterius.*

**wan·der·er** (wahn'dər-ər) a foal with neonatal maladjustment syndrome.

**wan·der·ing** (wahn'dər-ing) 1. moving about freely, as a wandering cell. 2. abnormally movable; too loosely attached.
**pathologic tooth w.,** see under *migration.*

**Wan·gen·steen drainage, tube (apparatus, suction)** (wang'gən-stēn) [Owen Harding *Wangensteen,* American surgeon, 1898–1981] see under *drainage* and *tube.*

**Wang·i·el·la** (wang″e-el'ə) *Exophiala.*

**war·bles** (wor'bəlz) 1. larvae of the flies *Hypoderma bovis* and *H. lineatum.* 2. cysts containing these larvae, especially on the backs of cattle near the spinal canal. 3. infection of cattle by these larvae, seen around the world in the Northern Hemisphere. Symptoms include damage to the hide, periesophagitis, sometimes anaphylaxis, and, if the larvae invade the nervous system, partial paralysis; serious cases may prove fatal. Called also *ox w.*
**ox w.,** warbles.

**War·burg's syndrome** (vahr'bərgz) [Mette *Warburg,* Danish ophthalmologist, 20th century] Walker-Warburg syndrome.

**Ward-Ro·ma·no syndrome** (word-ro-mah'no) [O.C. *Ward,* Irish physician, 20th century; C. *Romano,* Italian physician, born 1923] Romano-Ward syndrome.

**ward** (wawrd) a large room in a hospital for the accommodation of several patients.

**war·fa·rin** (wor'fər-in) [named for *Wisconsin Alumni Research Foun-*

*dation*] [MeSH: Warfarin] a synthetic coumarin anticoagulant; it is also used as a rodenticide, causing fatal hemorrhaging in any mammal that consumes a sufficient dose.
**w. potassium,** the potassium salt of warfarin, having anticoagulant actions and uses similar to those of the sodium salt; administered orally.
**w. sodium** [USP], the sodium salt of warfarin, the anticoagulant action of which is of intermediate duration and cumulative; administered orally, intravenously, or intramuscularly. It is also used as a rodenticide.

**War·ing's method (system)** (war'ings) [George Edwin *Waring,* Jr., American sanitary engineer, 1833–1898] see under *method.*

**War·ren's incision** (wor'ənz) [John Collins *Warren,* American surgeon, 1778–1856] see under *incision.*

**War·ren shunt** (wor'en) [W. Dean *Warren,* American surgeon, 1924–1989] see under *shunt.*

**wart** (wort) [L. *verruca*] [MeSH: Warts] verruca.
**acuminate w.,** condyloma acuminatum.
**anatomical w.,** tuberculosis verrucosa cutis.
**cattle w.,** one of the lesions of bovine papillomatosis.
**common w.,** verruca (def. 1).
**digitate w.,** verruca digitata.
**filiform w.,** verruca filiformis.
**flat w.,** verruca plana.
**fugitive w.,** verruca plana.
**genital w.,** condyloma acuminatum.
**Hassall-Henle w's,** hyaline excrescences in the periphery of Descemet's membrane (lamina limitans posterior corneae) occurring with advancing age.
**juvenile w.,** verruca plana.
**moist w.,** condyloma latum.
**mosaic w.,** an irregularly shaped lesion on the sole of the foot, with a granular surface, formed by an aggregation of contiguous plantar warts.

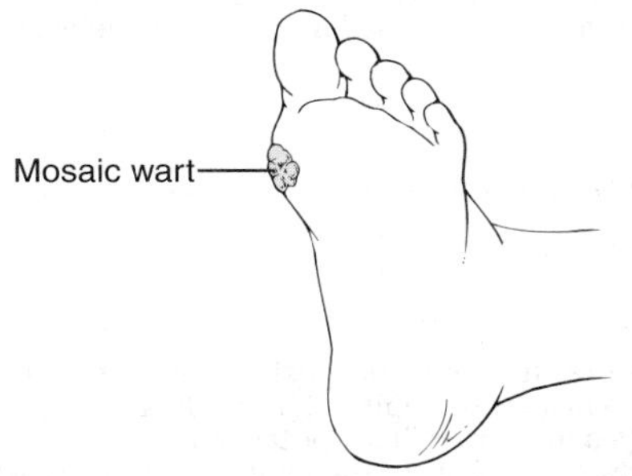


**necrogenic w.,** tuberculosis verrucosa cutis.
**Peruvian w.,** verruga peruana.
**pitch w's,** precancerous, keratotic, epidermal tumors occurring in individuals who work in gas, tar, pitch, or various oils derived from coal.
**plane w.,** verruca plana.
**plantar w.,** verruca plantaris.
**pointed w.,** condyloma acuminatum.
**postmortem w., prosector's w.,** tuberculosis verrucosa cutis.
**seborrheic w.,** seborrheic keratosis.
**seed w.,** verruca or common wart; so called because of the minute black specks or "seeds" within it, which are actually thrombosed elongated capillary loops extending up into the substance of the wart.
**soot w.,** a sign of chimney sweeps' cancer, which occurs beneath the wart.
**telangiectatic w.,** a misnomer for the verrucous papule of angiokeratoma.
**tuberculous w.,** tuberculosis verrucosa cutis.
**venereal w.,** condyloma acuminatum.

**War·ten·berg's disease, sign** (wor'tən-bərgz) [Robert *Wartenberg,* American neurologist, 1887–1956] see *cheiralgia paresthetica* and see under *sign.*

**War·thin's tumor** (wor'thinz) [Aldred Scott *Warthin,* American pathologist, 1866–1931] see *papillary adenocystoma lymphadenomatosum,* under *adenocystoma.*

**War·thin-Fin·kel·dey cell** (wor'thin fing'kəl-da) [Aldred Scott *Warthin,* American pathologist, 1866–1931; Wilhelm *Finkeldey,* German pathologist, 20th century] see under *cell.*

**wash** (wahsh) a solution used for cleansing or bathing a part; see *irrigation* and *lavage.*
**eye w.,** collyrium.
**mouth w.,** see *mouthwash.*

**wash·out** (wahsh'owt) a cleansing or sweeping clean.
**nitrogen w.,** see under *test.*

**wasp** (wahsp) [L. *vespa*] [MeSH: Wasps] 1. a general term for almost any member of the families Vespidae and Sphecidae, flying hymenopteran insects with long thin bodies, many of which have painful stings. Some live in complicated social colonies and others live in solitary social settings. Cf. *hornet* and *yellowjacket.* 2. any of various other animals thought to resemble these insects.
**sea w.,** any of various venomous stinging cubomedusan jellyfish; species dangerous to humans include *Chironex fleckeri* and *Chiropsalmus quadrigatus.*

**was·ser·hel·le** (vahs'ər-hel″ĕ) [Ger. "water-clear"] see *water-clear cell,* under *cell.*

**Was·ser·mann test** (vahs'er-mahn) [August Paul von *Wassermann,* German bacteriologist, 1866–1925] see under *test.*

**Was·ser·mann-fast** (vahs'er-mahn-fast) showing a persistent positive reaction to the Wassermann test despite antisyphilitic treatment.

**waste** (wāst) 1. gradual loss, decay, or diminution of bulk. 2. useless and effete material, unfit for further use within the organism. 3. to pine away or dwindle.

**wast·ing** (wāst'ing) 1. gradual loss or decay; emaciation. See also *wasting disease,* under *disease.* 2. excessive depletion.
**salt w.,** inappropriate sodium excretion in the urine (natriuresis) with hyponatremia and hyperkalemia; see also *salt-losing syndrome,* under *syndrome.*

**wa·ter** (waw'tər, wah'tər) [MeSH: Water] 1. a tasteless, odorless, colorless liquid, $(H_2O)_n$, used as the standard of specific gravity and of specific heat. It freezes at 32°F (0°C) and boils at 212°F (100°C). It is present in all organic tissues and in many other substances and is the most universal of the solvents. 2. aromatic w. 3. purified w.
**ammonia w.,** dilute ammonia solution.
**ammonia w., stronger,** strong ammonia solution.
**aromatic w.,** a solution, usually saturated, of a volatile oil or other aromatic or volatile substance in purified water, prepared by distillation or solution; called also *aqua aromatica.*
**bound w.,** water in the tissues of the body bound to macromolecules or organelles.
**capillary w.,** the water contained in the soil above the water table of the ground water.
**chlorine w.,** a saturated solution of chlorine in water.
**cinnamon w.,** a clear, saturated solution of cinnamon oil in purified water, used as a flavored vehicle in pharmaceutical preparations; called also *aqua cinnamomi.*
**w. of combustion,** metabolic w.
**w. of crystallization,** that which is chemically combined in many salts; it forms a structural part of the crystal but can be removed by heating.
**distilled w.,** water which has been purified by distillation; called also *aqua destillata.*
**egg w.,** 1. water that has bathed eggs of various invertebrates and acquired one or another substance detectable by a physiological reaction; e.g., oyster egg water may stimulate spawning of male oysters. 2. water containing fertilizin exuded from the ripe eggs of sea urchins and other aquatic animals, by which the spermatozoa are agglutinated.
**free w.,** that portion of the water in body tissues which is not bound by macromolecules or organelles.
**ground w.,** the water which lies in the depth of soils, being carried along underground over impervious strata.
**hamamelis w.,** witch hazel (def. 2).
**hard w.,** water that contains salts of calcium or magnesium, which resist the action of soap, so that it does not readily form lather.
**heavy w.,** a compound analogous to water but containing deuterium, the mass two isotope of hydrogen, the formula being $D_2O$ or $^2H_2O$. It differs from ordinary water in having a higher freezing point (3.8°C) and boiling point (101.4°C), and in the fact that it is incapable of supporting life. It is the stable isotope used as a moderator in nuclear reactors. Called also *deuterium oxide.*
**w. for injection** [USP], water for parenteral use, prepared by distillation, and meeting certain standards as to sterility and clarity.
**w. for injection, sterile bacteriostatic** [USP], sterile water for injection, containing one or more suitable antimicrobial agents.
**w. for injection, sterile** [USP], water for injection that has been sterilized and suitably packaged.
**lime w.,** calcium hydroxide topical solution.
**metabolic w.,** water in the body derived from metabolism of a food element such as starch, glucose, or fat; called also *w. of combustion.*
**mineral w.,** water containing mineral salts in solution in sufficient quantity to give it special properties and taste.
**w. O 15** [USP], water in which a portion of the molecules are labeled with $^{15}O$; used for positron emission tomography in the diagnosis of vascular disorders.
**orange flower w.,** a saturated solution of the odoriferous principles

of the flowers of *Citrus aurantium;* used as a vehicle, flavor, and perfume in pharmaceutical preparations.
**peppermint w.** [NF], a clear, saturated solution of peppermint oil in purified water, used as a vehicle in pharmaceutical preparations. Called also *aqua menthae piperitae.*
**potable w.,** water that is suitable for drinking purposes.
**purified w.** [USP], water obtained by distillation or deionization, used for pharmaceutical or other purposes requiring mineral-free water.
**purified w., sterile** [USP], purified water that has been sterilized and suitably packaged, and containing no antimicrobial agents.
**rose w.,** a solution prepared by diluting stronger rose water with an equal volume of purified water; used as a perfuming agent in pharmaceutical preparations.
**rose w., stronger** [NF], a saturated solution of the odoriferous principles of the flowers of *Rosa centifolia* Linné, used as a perfuming agent in pharmaceutical preparations; called also *aqua rosae fortior.*
**saline w.,** water which contains neutral salts.
**soft w.,** water that contains little or no mineral matter.

**wa·ter-borne** (waw′tər-born″) conveyed or spread by water, as an infectious disease; see under *infection.*

**wa·ter brash** (waw′tər brash″) heartburn with regurgitation of sour fluid or almost tasteless saliva into the mouth.

**Wa·ter·house-Fri·der·ich·sen syndrome** (waw′tər-hous-frid″ər-ik′sen) [Rupert *Waterhouse,* British physician, 1873–1958; Carl *Friderichsen,* Danish pediatrician, 20th century] [MeSH: Waterhouse-Friderichsen Syndrome] see under *syndrome.*

**wa·ter-jet** (waw′tər-jet″) see under *dissector.*

**Wa·ters' position, projection** (waw′tərz) [Charles Alexander *Waters,* American radiologist, 1888–1961] see under *projection.*

**wa·ters** (waw′tərz) a popular name for the amniotic fluid.

**wa·ter·shed** (waw′tər-shed) 1. a ridge that directs drainage toward either side. 2. an area where the peripheries of two vascular beds meet, particularly in the brain; small anastomoses link the adjoining beds. See also *watershed area,* under *area.*
**abdominal w's,** the ridges formed in the supine position by the forward projection of the lumbar vertebrae and the projecting brim of the pelvis, causing free effusions to gravitate into the lumbar fossae and pelvis.

**Wa·ter·ston operation (anastomosis, shunt)** (waw′tər-stən) [David J. *Waterson,* British thoracic and pediatric surgeon, b. 1910] see under *operation.*

**Wat·kins' operation** (waht′kinz) [Thomas James *Watkins,* American gynecologist, 1863–1925] see under *operation.*

**Wat·son** (waht′sən) James Dewey. American biochemist, born 1928; co-winner, with Maurice Hugh Frederick Wilkins and Francis Harry Compton Crick, of the Nobel prize for medicine or physiology in 1962 for the discovery of the molecular structure of nuclear acids and its significance for information transfer in living material.

**Wat·son-Schwartz test** (waht′sən-shworts) [Cecil James *Watson,* American physician, born 1901; Samuel *Schwartz,* American physician, 1916–1983] see under *test.*

**Wat·so·ni·us** (waht-so′ne-əs) [Malcolm *Watson,* British physician, 1873–1955] a genus of pear-shaped trematodes of the family Paramphistomatidae. *W. watso′ni* (formerly called *Amphistoma watsoni*) is a cause of paramphistomiasis in humans and monkeys in Africa.

**watt** (waht) [after James *Watt,* 1736–1819] a unit of electric power, being the work done at the rate of 1 joule per second. It is equivalent to a current of 1 ampere under a pressure of 1 volt. Symbol W.

**watt·age** (waht′əj) the power output or consumption of an electrical device; expressed in watts.

**watt-hour** (waht′our) a unit of electrical work or energy, equal to the wattage multiplied by the time in hours.

**watt·me·ter** (waht′me-tər) an instrument for measuring electric activity in watts.

**wave** (wāv) a uniformly advancing disturbance in which the parts moved undergo a double oscillation; any wavelike pattern.

## Wave

**A w.,** 1. a compound muscle action potential evoked by a submaximal stimulus to the motor nerve of a muscle, occurring because of an axon reflex and due to axonal branching; it has an amplitude similar to that of the F wave but a shorter more constant latency. Called also *axon w.* 2. in an intracardiac electrogram, the complex waveform due to depolarization of the atria, usually specifically the lower atrial septum in the His bundle electrogram. See also illustration at *electrogram.*
**a w.,** 1. in a tracing of the venous pulse, a positive deflection representing contraction of the right atrium, occurring just prior to the carotid arterial pulse and first heart sound. See also illustration at *pulse.* 2. in the electroretinogram, the small negative deflection occurring after stimulus presentation, related to the photoreceptor processes of the rods and cones. 3. in the apexcardiogram, a small positive deflection in late diastole, coinciding with the third heart sound; it represents the passage of blood into the left ventricle as a result of atrial systole.
**alpha w's,** brain waves in the electroencephalogram which have a frequency of 8 to 13 per second; they are typical of the normal person awake and in a quiet resting state and occur principally in the occipital region.
**anacrotic w.,** the wave on a tracing of an anacrotic pulse.
**anadicrotic w.,** the wave on a tracing of an anadicrotic pulse.
**atrial pressure w's,** the three elevations commonly seen on the graphic representation of the cardiac cycle, known as the *a wave, c wave,* and *v wave.* See illustration at *cycle.*
**axon w.,** A w. (def. 1).
**b w.,** in the electroretinogram, a high-amplitude, positive deflection occurring immediately after the a wave and representing complex activity of the retinal bipolar layer.
**beta w's,** brain waves in the electroencephalogram, which have a frequency of 18 to 30 per second; they are typical during periods of intense activity of the nervous system and occur principally in the parietal and frontal regions.
**brain w's,** the fluctuations of electrical potential in the brain, as recorded by electroencephalography. See *alpha, beta, delta,* and *theta w's.*
**c w.,** 1. in a tracing of the venous pulse, a small positive deflection representing the bulging back toward the atria of the tricuspid valve at the onset of ventricular contraction. See also illustration at *pulse.* 2. in the electroretinogram, the positive deflection representing the response of the pigmented epithelium of the retina to photoreceptor-induced changes in extracellular potassium.
**cannon a w's,** in tracings of the jugular venous pulse, abnormal tall a waves seen in rhythm disturbances in which the atrium contracts against a closed tricuspid valve. See also *giant a w's.*
**catacrotic w.,** the wave of a tracing of a catacrotic pulse.
**catadicrotic w.,** the wave of a tracing of a catadicrotic pulse.
**contraction w.,** the wave of progression of the contraction in a muscle from the point of stimulation; also the graphic representation of a contracting muscle.
**d w.,** in the electroretinogram, a small positive deflection produced by cone receptors in the latent period after stimulus termination.
**delta w.,** a small hump occurring on the upstroke of the QRS complex in electrocardiography; it is characteristic of preexcitation.
**delta w's,** waves in the electroencephalogram which have a frequency below 3.5 per second; they are typical in deep sleep, in infancy, and in serious brain disorders.
**dicrotic w.,** the second portion of the arterial pulse or arterial pressure recording after the dicrotic notch, attributed to the reflected impulse of closure of the aortic valves. Called also *recoil w.*
**E w.,** contingent negative variation.
**electroencephalographic w's,** see *brain w's.*
**electromagnetic w's,** the spectrum of waves propagated through space or matter by the oscillation of an electric field and a magnetic field at right angles to one another; the waves travel perpendicularly to both the electric and magnetic fields, having a velocity in a vacuum of $3 \times 10^8$ m/s. They include, in order of decreasing wavelength, radio waves; microwaves; infrared, visible, and ultraviolet light; x-rays; gamma rays; and cosmic rays.
**excitation w.,** an electric wave flowing from a muscle just previous to its contraction.
**expectancy w.,** contingent negative variation.
**F w's,** 1. rapid sawtooth-edged atrial waves without isoelectric intervals between them, seen in the electrocardiogram in atrial flutter. Written also *f w's.* Called also *flutter w's.* 2. compound muscle action potentials with a smaller amplitude and a longer latency than the corresponding M waves; caused by antidromic activation of the motor neuron. 3. f w's, def. 1.

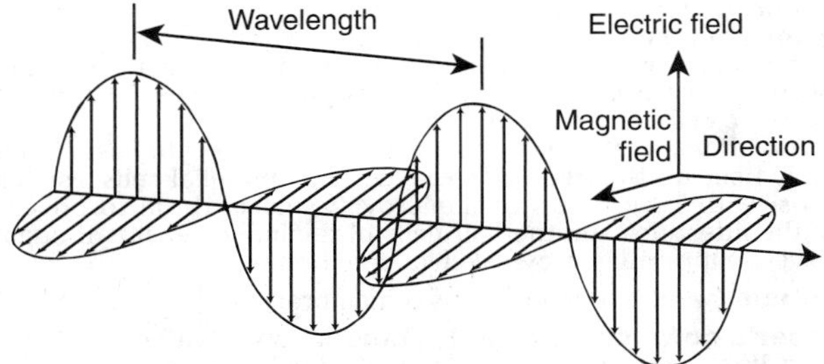


Diagrammatic representation of electromagnetic waves.

**f w's,** 1. small, irregular, rapid deflections in the electrocardiogram in atrial fibrillation. Written also *F w's.* Called also *fibrillary w's.* 2. F w's, def. 1.
**fibrillary w's,** f w's, def. 1.
**flutter w's,** F w's, def. 1.
**giant a w's,** abnormally tall a waves in tracings of the jugular venous pulse; they occur when either inflow resistance to or outflow resistance from the right ventricle is increased or when atrial contractions occur out of phase, during the period the tricuspid valve is closed (cannon a waves).
**H w.,** 1. a compound muscle action potential of consistently longer latency and smaller amplitude than the corresponding M wave; evoked primarily from extensor muscles, usually in the calf, and thought to be due to a spinal reflex (the H-reflex). It is evoked only by submaximal stimulation and disappears when the stimulation increases to the supramaximal level. 2. His bundle deflection.
**J w.,** a deflection occurring in the electrocardiogram between the QRS complex and the onset of the ST segment; it occurs prominently in hypothermia and in hypercalcemia.
**lambda w's,** electropositive sharp waves of medium amplitude sometimes seen on an electroencephalogram of the occipital region during concentration on a visual stimulus or during saccadic eye movements.
**Liesegang's w's,** see under *phenomenon.*
**light w's,** the electromagnetic waves that produce sensations in the retina; see *light.*
**longitudinal w.,** one in which the oscillatory motion is parallel to the direction of propagation of the wave.
**M w.,** a compound muscle action potential evoked from a muscle by a single electric stimulus to its motor nerve; the waveform is usually biphasic and relatively similar on repeated stimulations.
**Mayer w's,** regular variations in blood pressure over intervals longer than those of Traube-Hering waves, associated with pathologic mechanisms such as abnormal oscillations in the baroreceptor system or activation of vasopressor reflexes.
**Osborne w.,** J w.
**P w.,** in the electrocardiogram, the initial deflection of the cardiac cycle, representing excitation of the atria. See illustration at *electrocardiogram.*
**papillary w., percussion w.,** the chief ascending portion of a sphygmographic tracing.
**positive sharp w.,** a short burst of biphasic electrical activity recorded from a muscle fiber, usually evoked by stimulation or injury by electrode insertion or other electrode movement; spontaneous occurrence of such waves at other times may be a sign of a myopathic disorder or a denervated muscle.
**pulse w.,** the elevation of the pulse felt by the finger or shown graphically in a recording of pulse or pressure.
**Q w.,** in the QRS complex, the initial downward (negative) deflection, related to the initial phase of depolarization (excitation) of the ventricular myocardium and the depolarization of the interventricular septum; see also illustration at *electrocardiogram.*
**R w.,** the initial upward deflection of the QRS complex, following the Q wave in the normal electrocardiogram and representing early depolarization of the ventricles; see also illustration at *electrocardiogram.*
**$R_1$ w.,** the earlier of the two blink responses.
**$R_2$ w.,** the later of the two blink responses.
**radio w's,** electromagnetic radiation of wavelength between $10^{-1}$ and $10^6$ cm and frequency of about $10^{11}$ to $10^4$ hertz.
**random w's,** brain waves showing irregular changes in potential and no fixed frequency.
**rapid filling w.,** in the apexcardiogram, the steep positive deflection following the O point, or mitral valve opening, representing the period of rapid blood flow into the left ventricle. Its transition to the slow filling wave is marked by the third heart sound.
**recoil w.,** dicrotic w.
**S w.,** a downward deflection of the QRS complex following the R wave in the normal electrocardiogram and representing late depolarization of the ventricles; see also illustration at *electrocardiogram.*
**sharp w.,** a wave on an electroencephalogram that has a sharp peak but is longer in duration than a spike.
**short w.,** a wave having a wavelength of 60 meters or less.
**sine w.,** the waveform of an alternating current characterized by a rise from zero to maximum positive potential, descending back through zero to its maximum negative value, and then rising back to zero. Called also *sinusoidal w.* and *sinusoidal waveform.*
**sinusoidal w.,** sine w.
**slow filling w.,** in the apexcardiogram, the shallow-sloped positive deflection following the rapid filling wave; it represents continued, but slowed, blood flow into the left ventricle.
**sonic w's,** audible sound waves.
**sound w's,** longitudinal waves of mechanical energy that transmit the vibrations interpreted as sound.
**stimulus w.,** excitation w.
**T w.,** the deflection of the normal electrocardiogram following the QRS complex; it represents repolarization, or recovery, of the ventricles. See also illustration at *electrocardiogram.*
**Ta w.,** a small asymmetric wave, of opposite polarity to the P wave, representing atrial repolarization; together with the P wave it defines atrial electrical systole. In most electrocardiograms, it is obscured by the QRS complex.
**theta w's,** brain waves in the electroencephalogram which have a frequency of 4 to 7 per second; they occur mainly in children but also in adults during periods of emotional stress.
**tidal w.,** the sphygmographic wave after the percussion wave; the second elevation of the sphygmographic tracing between the percussion and dicrotic waves.
**transverse w.,** one in which the oscillatory motion is perpendicular to the direction of propagation of the wave.
**Traube-Hering w's,** rhythmical rises and falls in the arterial pressure, attributed to rhythmical activity of the vasoconstrictor center.
**tricrotic w.,** a third wave in the sphygmographic curve in addition to the tidal and dicrotic waves, occurring during systole.
**U w.,** in the electrocardiogram, a small positive deflection usually immediately following the T wave but often poorly separated from it and so concealed; it is postulated to represent repolarization of the Purkinje fibers or a mechanical event such as ventricular relaxation. It is not invariably present and is most often seen in tachyarrhythmias and electrolyte disturbances. See also illustration at *electrocardiogram.*
**ultrashort w.,** an electromagnetic wave of wavelength of less than 10 meters; called also *microwave.*
**ultrasonic w's,** waves similar to sonic waves but of such high frequency (20,000 hertz or higher) that the human ear does not perceive them as sound; see *ultrasonics.*
**v w.,** in a tracing of the venous pulse, a positive deflection representing the filling of the right atrium against the closed tricuspid valve during ventricular contraction. See also illustration at *pulse.*
**x w.,** in a tracing of the venous pulse, a negative deflection representing relaxation of the atria. See also illustration at *pulse.*
**y w.,** in a tracing of the venous pulse, a negative deflection representing emptying of the right atrium upon right ventricular relaxation and opening of the tricuspid valve. See also illustration at *pulse.*

**wave·form** (wāv′fōrm) the shape of a wave on a graph; sometimes used as a synonym for *wave.*
**sinusoidal w.,** sine wave.

**wave·length** (wāv′length) the distance between the top of one wave and the identical phase of the succeeding one. Symbol λ.
**effective w., equivalent w.,** in radiology, the wavelength of monochromatic x-rays which would undergo the same percentage attenuation in a specified absorber as the heterogeneous beam under consideration.
**minimum w.,** the shortest wavelength in an x-ray spectrum.

**wax** (waks) [L. *cera*] a low-melting, high-molecular-weight, organic mixture or compound, similar to fats and oils but lacking glycerides; it may be deposited by insects, obtained from plants, or prepared synthetically. Most waxes are esters of fatty acids and alcohols, with some hydrocarbons. The wax of pharmacy is principally *yellow w.* and its bleached form is *white w.*
**baseplate w.**, a dental wax containing about 75 per cent paraffin or ceresin with additions of beeswax and other waxes and resins; used chiefly to establish the initial arch form in making trial plates for the construction of complete dentures. Called also *try-in w.*
**blockout w.**, a dental wax used as a blockout (q.v.) material to eliminate undercuts on master casts prior to duplication.
**bone w.**, a waxy substance used for packing small bone cavities, as in bones of the skull, and for controlling bleeding from them.
**boxing w.**, a dental wax used for boxing (q.v.) impressions in the fabrication of restorations and appliances.
**candelilla w.**, a wax from the candelilla plant, *Euphorbia antisyphilitica,* used as a substitute for beeswax.
**carding w.**, dental wax used as a base for mounting artificial teeth, organized by standard sizes, shades, and so forth.
**carnauba w.** [NF], a wax obtained from the leaves of the palm *Copernicia cerifera,* used as a tablet coating agent.
**casting w.**, a mixture of several dental waxes; used for making patterns to determine the shape of the metallic framework and other parts of removable partial dentures.
**cetyl esters w.** [NF], a mixture consisting primarily of esters of saturated fatty alcohols and saturated fatty acids; used as a stiffening agent in pharmaceutical preparations. Called also *synthetic spermaceti.*
**dental w.**, a mixture of two or more natural and synthetic waxes, resins, coloring agents, and other additives; used for pattern making for casting purposes and in the construction of nonmetallic denture bases, for registering jaw relations, and as aids in laboratory work.
**dental inlay casting w.**, a wax used to make a pattern for an inlay (wax pattern), usually containing paraffin, carnauba, ceresin, and candelilla waxes, beeswax, and gum dammar; synthetic waxes are sometimes used to replace the carnauba wax. Called also *inlay casting w.* and *inlay pattern w.*
**ear w.**, cerumen.
**emulsifying w.** [NF], a waxy solid prepared from cetostearyl alcohol, containing a polyoxyethylene derivative of a fatty acid ester of sorbitan; used as an emulsifying and stiffening agent in pharmaceutical preparations.
**grave w.**, adipocere.
**Horsley's w.**, a bone wax composed of wax, petrolatum, and phenol.
**inlay casting w., inlay pattern w.**, dental inlay casting w.
**palm w.**, carnauba w.
**paraffin w.**, paraffin, def. 1.
**set-up w.**, a dental wax used in laboratories to align artificial teeth in dentures.
**try-in w.**, baseplate w.
**tubercle bacillus w.**, a high-molecular-weight phosphatidic glycolipid extracted from the cell walls of *Mycobacterium tuberculosis,* made up of arabinoglycans and mycolic and muramic acids. It is used as an adjuvant to enhance the immunogenicity of tuberculin preparations.
**utility w.**, a soft, pliable, adhesive dental wax used for various purposes in the laboratory, such as to give the desired contour to a perforated tray to be used with hydrocolloids.
**vegetable w.**, a waxy substance, resembling beeswax, derived from various vegetable sources.
**white w.** [NF], the bleached, purified wax from the honeycomb of the bee, *Apis mellifera,* used as an ingredient in several ointments.
**yellow w.** [NF], the purified wax from the honeycomb of the bee *Apis mellifera;* used as a stiffening agent in pharmaceutical preparations and as an ingredient of yellow ointment. It was formerly used internally, in the treatment of diarrhea. Called also *beeswax* and *cera flava.*

**wax·ing** (wak'sing) the contouring of a wax pattern or the wax base of a trial denture into the desired shape. Called also *waxing up.*

**wax·ing up** (wak'sing up) waxing.

**Wb** weber.

**WBC** white blood cell; white blood [cell] count (see *blood count,* under *count*).

**wean** (wēn) to discontinue the breast feeding of an infant, with substitution of other feeding habits.

**wean·ling** (wēn'ling) 1. recently weaned. 2. a recently weaned human infant or other animal.

**web** (web) a tissue or membrane.
**antral w.**, see under *membrane.*
**esophageal w.**, a fibrous, weblike, circumferential fold of the mucous membrane of the esophagus.
**laryngeal w.**, a common congenital malformation of the larynx that may be thin and translucent or thicker and more fibrotic; it is spread between the vocal folds near the anterior commissure and may cause hoarseness, aphonia, and other symptoms. See also *laryngeal atresia,* under *atresia.*
**pyloric w.**, see under *membrane.*
**subsynaptic w.**, a system of filaments or fine canaliculi which have been observed to penetrate at a varying distance into the postsynaptic cell.
**terminal w.**, a feltwork of fine filaments in the cytoplasm immediately beneath the free surface of certain epithelial cells, especially those with a brush border of microvilli, such as the absorptive cells of the intestines and the hair cells of the inner ear; it is thought to have a supportive or cytoskeletal function.

**webbed** (webd) connected by a membrane.

**We·ber's corpuscle (organ), glands, zone** (va'berz) [Moritz Ignatz *Weber,* German anatomist, 1795–1875] see under *gland,* and see *utriculus prostaticus* and *zona orbicularis articulationis coxae.*

**Web·er's disease** (va'bərz) [Frederick Parkes *Weber,* English physician, 1863–1962] Sturge-Weber syndrome.

**We·ber's paradox, test** (va'berz) [Ernest Heinrich *Weber,* German anatomist and physiologist, 1795–1878] see under *paradox* and see *Weber's test* (def. 2 and 3).

**Web·er's syndrome (paralysis, sign)** (web'ərz) [Sir Hermann David *Weber,* English physician, 1823–1918] see under *syndrome.*

**We·ber's test** (va'berz) [Friedrich Eugen *Weber,* German otologist, 1832–1891] see *Weber's test* (def. 1).

**Web·er-Chris·tian disease, panniculitis, syndrome** (va'bər-kris'chən) [F.P. *Weber;* Henry Asbury *Christian,* American physician, 1876–1951] relapsing febrile nodular nonsuppurative panniculitis.

**Web·er-Cock·ayne syndrome** (va'bər-kok-ān') [F.P. *Weber;* Edward Alfred *Cockayne,* English physician, 1880–1956] localized epidermolysis bullosa simplex.

**Web·er-Gub·ler syndrome** (web'ər- go͞ob'lər) [Sir H.D. *Weber;* Adolphe Marie *Gubler,* French physician, 1821–1879] Weber's syndrome.

**We·ber-Ley·den syndrome** (web'ər-li'dən) [Sir H.D. *Weber;* Ernst Victor von *Leyden,* German physician, 1832–1910] Weber's syndrome.

**web·er** (web'ər) a unit of magnetic flux which, linking a circuit of one turn, produces in it an electromotive force of one volt as it is reduced to zero at a uniform rate in one second. In SI, it replaces the maxwell. Abbreviated Wb.

**Web·ster's operation** (web'stərz) [John Clarence *Webster,* American gynecologist, 1863–1950] see under *operation.*

**Wechs·ler Adult Intelligence Scale, Intelligence Scale for Children** (weks'lər) [David *Wechsler,* Romanian-born American psychologist, 1896–1981] see under *scale.*

**wed·dell·ite** (wed'ə-līt) [*Weddell* Sea in the Antarctic, where minute quantities were first found] a dihydrate of calcium oxalate, seen in urinary calculi.

**We·den·sky facilitation, inhibition, phenomenon** (və-den'ske) [Nikolai Yevgenyevich *Wedensky,* Russian neurologist, 1852–1922] see under *facilitation, inhibition,* and *phenomenon.*

**wedge** (wej) [A.S. *wecg*] 1. a piece of material thick at one end and tapering to a thin edge at the other end. 2. to force something into a space of limited size; see under *pressure.*
**step w.**, penetrometer; a block of an absorber, usually aluminum, machined in steps of increasing thickness, used to measure the penetrability of x-rays.

**WEE** western equine encephalomyelitis.

**Weeks' bacillus** (wēks) [John Elmer *Weeks,* New York ophthalmologist, 1853–1949] *Haemophilus aegyptius.*

**weep** (wēp) 1. to shed tears. Called also *cry.* 2. to ooze serum.

**wee·ver fish** (we'vər fish) a fish of the family Trachinidae; most species are small in size and are found in the eastern Atlantic or the Mediterranean. They have 5 to 8 dorsal venomous spines; stings cause severe pain in humans and other animals.

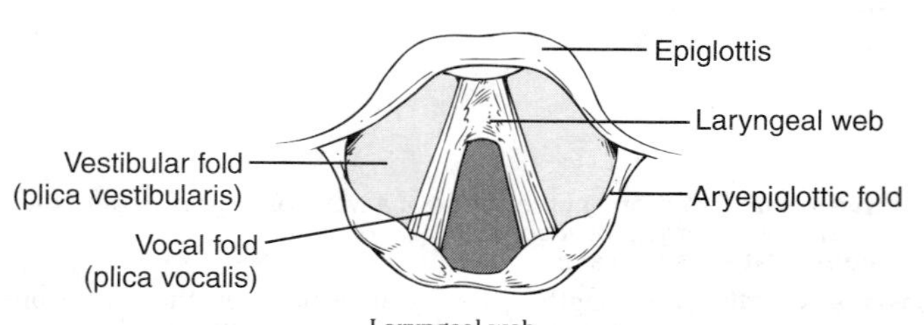


Laryngeal web.

**wee·vil** (we'vəl) any of various beetles, some of which are highly destructive to plants and food.
**wheat w.,** *Sitophilus granarius.*

**We·ge·ner's granulomatosis** (veg'ĕ-nerz) [Friedrich *Wegener,* German pathologist, born 1907] see under *granulomatosis.*

**Weg·ner's disease, sign** (veg'nerz) [Friedrich Rudolf Georg *Wegner,* German pathologist, 1843–1917] see under *disease* and *sign.*

**Wei·bel-Pa·lade bodies** (vi'bəl pah-lād') [Ewald R. *Weibel,* Swiss physician, 20th century; George E. *Palade,* Romanian-born American cytologist, born 1912] see under *body.*

**Wei·del's test** (vi'delz) [Hugo *Weidel,* Austrian chemist, 1849–1899] see under *test.*

**Wei·gert's law, stain (method)** (vi'gerts) [Karl *Weigert,* German pathologist, 1845–1904] see under *law,* and see *stain.*

**weight** (wāt) 1. heaviness; the degree to which a body is drawn toward the earth by gravity. See tables of weights and measures (Appendix 11). 2. in statistics, the process of assigning greater importance to some observations than to others, or a mathematical factor used to apply such a process.
**apothecaries' w.,** a system of weights used in compounding prescriptions based on the grain (equivalent 64.8 mg). Its units are the scruple (20 grains), dram (3 scruples), ounce (8 drams), and pound (12 ounces).
**atomic w.,** the sum of the masses of the constituents of an atom, either that of a single isotope or that obtained using weighted averages of the masses of the natural isotopes. It can be expressed in atomic mass units (or daltons), in SI units (i.e., kilograms), or as a dimensionless ratio derived by comparing the mass to the mass of the $^{12}$C isotope of carbon, which is defined as exactly 12.000. Abbreviated at wt. Called also *atomic mass.*
**avoirdupois w.,** the system of weight commonly used for ordinary commodities in English-speaking countries; its units are the dram (27.344 grains), ounce (16 drams), and pound (16 ounces).
**combining w.,** equivalent w.
**equivalent w.,** the amount of a substance that combines with or displaces 8.0 g of oxygen (or 1.008 g of hydrogen), usually expressed in grams; for acid/base reactions, one equivalent donates or receives a mole of protons, and the equivalent weight is the ratio of the molecular weight to the number of protons involved in the reaction. For redox reactions, one equivalent donates or receives a mole of electrons, and the equivalent weight is the ratio of the molecular weight to the number of electrons involved in the reaction.
**gram molecular w.,** the molecular weight of a substance expressed in grams; one gram molecular weight of any molecular substance contains one mole of the molecules. Cf. *mole*[1].
**molecular w.,** the weight of a molecule of a substance as compared with that of an atom of carbon 12; it is equal to the sum of the atomic weights of its constituent atoms and is dimensionless (cf. *molecular mass* and *molar mass*). Abbreviated Mol wt or MW. Although widely used, the term is not technically correct; relative molecular mass ($M_r$) is preferable.

**Weil's basal layer (zone)** (vīlz) [Ludwig A. *Weil,* German dentist, 1849–1895] see under *layer.*

**Weil's stain** (wīlz) [Arthur *Weil,* American neuropathologist, 1887–1969] see under *Stains and Staining Methods.*

**Weil's syndrome (disease)** (vīlz) [Adolf *Weil,* German physician, 1848–1916] see under *syndrome.*

**Weil-Fe·lix test (reaction)** (vīl-fa'liks) [Edmund *Weil,* Austrian physician in Czechoslovakia, 1880–1922; Arthur *Felix,* Polish-born bacteriologist in England, 1887–1956] see under *test.*

**Weill's sign** (vīlz) [Edmond *Weill,* French pediatrician, 1858–1924] see under *sign.*

**Weill-Mar·che·sa·ni syndrome** (vīl-mahr-kə-sah'ne) [Georges *Weill,* French ophthalmologist, 1866–1952; Oswald *Marchesani,* German ophthalmologist, 1900–1952] see under *syndrome.*

**Wein·gar·ten's syndrome** (wīn'gahr-tənz) [R.J. *Weingarten,* American physician, 20th century] tropical eosinophilia; see under *eosinophilia.*

**Weir Mitch·ell** (wēr-mich'əl) see *Mitchell.*

**Weis·bach's angle** (vīs'bahks) [Albin *Weisbach,* Austrian anthropologist, 1837–1914] see under *angle.*

**Weis·mann's theory** (vīs'mahnz) [August Friedrich Leopold *Weismann,* German biologist, 1834–1914] weismannism.

**weis·mann·ism** (wīs'man-iz-əm) [August *Weismann*] the doctrine of the noninheritance of acquired characters.

**Weiss' reflex** (vīs) [Leopold *Weiss,* German oculist, 1848–1901] see under *reflex.*

**Weit·brecht's cartilage, cord (ligament),** etc. (vīt'brekts) [Josias *Weitbrecht,* German anatomist in Russia, 1702–1747] see *chorda obliqua membranae interosseae antebrachii* and *discus articularis articulationis acromioclavicularis,* and see under *foramen* and *retinaculum.*

**We·lan·der's distal myopathy (myopathy, syndrome)** (va'lahn-dərz) [Lisa *Welander,* Swedish neurologist, born 1909] late distal hereditary myopathy.

**Welch's bacillus** (welch'əz) [William Henry *Welch,* American pathologist, 1850–1934] *Clostridium perfringens.*

**Welck·er's angle** (vel'kerz) [Hermann *Welcker,* Austrian physician, 1822–1897] see *angulus sphenoidalis ossis parietalis.*

**Well·bu·trin** (wel-bu'trin) trademark for a preparation of bupropion hydrochloride.

**Wel·ler** (wel'ər) Thomas Huckle. American physician and parasitologist, born 1915; co-winner, with John Franklin Enders and Frederick Chapman Robbins, of the Nobel prize for medicine or physiology in 1954 for the discovery that viruses (specifically, poliomyelitis viruses) can be grown in tissue culture and thereby isolated and studied, making possible the production of vaccines.

**Wells's syndrome** (welz) [G.C. *Wells,* British dermatologist, 20th century] see under *syndrome.*

**welt** (welt) wheal.

**wen** (wen) 1. epidermal cyst. 2. pilar cyst.

**Wen·cke·bach's period, phenomenon** (veng'kə-bahks) [Karel Frederik *Wenckebach,* Dutch internist in Austria, 1864–1940] see under *period* and *phenomenon.*

**Wen·zell's test** (wen'zəlz) [William Theodore *Wenzell,* American physician, 1829–1913] see under *test.*

**Werd·nig-Hoff·mann spinal muscular atrophy (disease)** (verd'nig-hof'mahn) [Guido *Werdnig,* Austrian neurologist, 1844–1919; Johann *Hoffmann,* German neurologist, 1857–1919] see under *atrophy.*

**Werl·hof's disease** (verl'hofs) [Paul Gottlieb *Werlhof,* German physician, 1699–1767] idiopathic thrombocytopenic purpura.

**Wer·mer's syndrome** (wər'mərz) [Paul *Wermer,* American internist, 1898–1975] multiple endocrine neoplasia, type I; see under *neoplasia.*

**Wer·ner's syndrome** (ver'nerz) [C. W. Otto *Werner,* German physician, 1879–1936] [MeSH: Werner's Syndrome] see under *syndrome.*

**Wer·ner-His disease** (ver'ner-his') [Heinrich *Werner,* German physician, 1874–1947; Wilhelm *His,* Jr., German physician, 1863–1934] trench fever.

**Wer·ner Schultz disease** (ver'ner-shooltz) [*Werner Schultz,* German internist, 1878–1947] agranulocytosis.

**Wer·ni·cke's encephalopathy (disease, syndrome),** etc. (ver'nĭ-kəz) [Karl *Wernicke,* German neurologist, 1848–1905] see under *area, encephalopathy,* and *triangle;* see *receptive aphasia,* under *aphasia;* and see *hemiopic pupillary reaction,* under *reaction.*

**Wer·ni·cke-Kor·sa·koff syndrome** (ver'nĭ-kə-kor'sə-kof) [Karl *Wernicke;* Sergei Sergeivich *Korsakoff,* Russian neurologist, 1854–1900] see under *syndrome.*

**Wer·ni·cke-Mann hemiplegia** (ver'nĭ-kə-mahn) [Karl *Wernicke;* Ludwig *Mann,* German neurologist, 1866–1936] see under *hemiplegia.*

**Wert·heim's operation** (vert'hīmz) [Ernst *Wertheim,* German gynecologist, 1864–1920] see under *operation.*

**West's syndrome** (wests) [Charles *West,* British physician, 1816–1898] infantile spasms.

**West·berg's space** (vest'bergz) [Friedrich *Westberg,* German physician, late 19th century] see under *space.*

**Wes·ter·gren method, tube** (ves'ter-gren) [Alf *Westergren,* Swedish physician, born 1891] see under *method* and *tube.*

**Wes·ter·mark's sign** (ves'ter-mahrks) [Neil *Westermark,* German radiologist, born 1904] see under *sign.*

**Wes·tern blot technique (blot analysis, blot hybridization, blot test)** (wes'tərn) [facetious coinage by analogy with *Southern blot technique*] see under *technique.*

**West Nile encephalitis (fever), virus** (west nīl) [*West Nile* River valley and region in northern Uganda, where the disease was first observed in 1937] see under *encephalitis* and *virus.*

**West·phal's nucleus, sign (phenomenon)** (vest'fahlz) [Carl Friedrich Otto *Westphal,* German neurologist, 1833–1890] see under *sign,* and see *nucleus nervi accessorius.*

**West·phal's phenomenon, pupillary reflex** (vest'fahlz) [Alexander Karl Otto *Westphal,* German neurologist, 1863–1941] orbicularis pupillary reflex.

**West·phal-Piltz phenomenon, reflex** (vest'fahl-pilts) [A. K. O.

*Westphal;* Jan *Piltz,* Austrian neurologist, 1870–1930] orbicularis pupillary reflex.

**West·phal-Strüm·pell disease, pseudosclerosis** (vest′fahl-strēm′pel) [C. F. O. *Westphal;* Ernst Adolf Gustav Gottfried von *Strümpell,* German physician, 1853–1925] Wilson's disease; see under *disease.*

**wet-nurse** (wet′nərs) see under *nurse.*

**wet·pox** (wet′poks) a form of fowlpox, with lesions occurring in the mouth and surrounding region, frequently causing death by suffocation.

**Wet·zel's grid** (wet′səlz) [Norman Carl *Wetzel,* American pediatrician, 1897–1984] see under *grid.*

**Wet·zel's test** (vet′selz) [Georg *Wetzel,* German anatomist, 1871–1951] see under *test.*

**We·ver-Bray phenomenon** (we′vər bra) [Ernest Glen *Wever,* American psychologist, born 1902; Charles William *Bray,* American otologist, born 1904] cochlear microphonic.

**Wey·ers' oligodactyly syndrome** (vi′ərz) [Helmut *Weyers,* German pediatrician, 20th century] see under *syndrome.*

**Weyl's test** (vīlz) [Theodor *Weyl,* German chemist 1851–1913] see under *test.*

**Whar·ton's duct, jelly (gelatin)** (hwawr′tənz) [Thomas *Wharton,* English physician and anatomist, 1614–1673] see *ductus submandibularis,* and see under *jelly.*

**wheal** (hwēl, wēl) a smooth, slightly elevated area on the body surface, which is redder or paler than the surrounding skin; it is often accompanied by severe itching and is usually evanescent, changing its size or shape or disappearing within a few hours. It is the typical lesion of urticaria, the dermal evidence of allergy, and in sensitive persons may be provoked by mechanical irritation of the skin. Called also *hive* and *welt.*

**wheel** (hwēl) [A.S. *hwēol*] 1. a circular frame or disk designed to revolve around a central axis. 2. any of various round, engine-driven cutting or polishing dental instruments that may be of uniform thickness or knife-edge.
**rag w.,** a dental disk made up of several layers of cloth stitched together and wetted down with pumice; used to polish dentures. Called also *cloth disk.*

**wheeze** (hwēz) 1. a continuous sound (q.v.) consisting of a whistling noise with a high pitch, thought to be generated by gas flowing through narrowed airways. Called also *sibilant* or *whistling rhonchus.* 2. to breathe making such a high-pitched sound.
**asthmatoid w.,** a sound similar to the wheezing of an asthmatic, heard in cases of foreign body in the trachea or bronchus.

**whelk** (hwelk) any of various large ocean-dwelling snails with pointed spiral shells. Some are edible, but others are poisonous; see under *poison* and *poisoning.*

**whelp** (hwelp) 1. to give birth to; said of the female dog. 2. an unweaned puppy.

**whe·well·ite** (hwu′wə-līt) [William *Whewell,* English philosopher, 1794–1866] a monohydrate of calcium oxalate, seen in urinary calculi.

**whey** (hwa) the thin serum of milk remaining after the casein and fat have been removed; it contains proteins and the bulk of the lactose and water-soluble vitamins and minerals. The whey proteins, chiefly lactalbumins and lactoglobulins, constitute the majority of the protein content of human milk.

**WHHL** Watanabe heritable hyperlipidemic; see under *rabbit.*

**whip** (hwip) 1. to move suddenly and quickly. 2. a sudden, quick, thrashing movement.
**catheter w.,** excessive mobility of the tip of an intracardiac catheter due to cardiac contraction, causing pressure measurements to be alternately artificially elevated and reduced.

**whip·lash** (hwip′lash) see under *injury.*

**Whip·ple** (hwip′əl) George Hoyt. American pathologist, 1878–1976; co-winner, with George R. Minot and William P. Murphy, of the Nobel prize for medicine or physiology in 1934 for their research into the therapeutic value of liver in cases of pernicious anemia and in the regeneration of hemoglobin.

**Whip·ple's disease** (hwip′əlz) [George Hoyt *Whipple*] [MeSH: Whipple's Disease] see *intestinal lipodystrophy,* under *lipodystrophy.*

**Whip·ple procedure (operation), triad** (hwip′əl) [Allen O. *Whipple,* American surgeon, 1881–1963] see under *procedure* and *triad.*

**whip·worm** (hwip′werm) any member of the genus *Trichuris.*

**whis·per** (hwis′pər) a soft, low, sibilant breathing sound produced by the unvoiced passage of the breath through the glottis. Cf. *hypophonia.*

**White** (hwīt) Charles. English surgeon and obstetrician, 1728–1813, whose *Treatise on the Management of Pregnant and Lying-in Women* (1773) antedated the work of Semmelweis in its appeal for surgical cleanliness to combat puerperal fever.

**White's operation** (hwīts) [J. William *White,* American surgeon, 1850–1916] see under *operation.*

**white** (hwīt) [A.S. *hwīt*] reflecting all the rays of the spectrum; the opposite of black.
**visual w.,** exhausted or decolorized rhodopsin; called also *leukopsin.*

**White·head's operation** (hwīt′hedz) [Walter *Whitehead,* English surgeon, 1840–1913] see under *operation.*

**white·head** (hwīt′hed) 1. milium. 2. closed comedo.

**white·leg** (hwīt′leg) phlegmasia alba dolens.

**white·pox** (hwīt′poks) variola minor.

**Whit·field's ointment** (hwit′fēldz) [Arthur *Whitfield,* British dermatologist, 1868–1947] benzoic and salicylic acids ointment.

**whit·lock·ite** (hwit′lə-kīt) [Herbert P. *Whitlock,* American mineralogist, 1868–1948] a type of tribasic calcium phosphate found in urinary calculi.

**whit·low** (hwit′lo) a felon.
**herpetic w.,** a primary herpes simplex infection of the terminal segment of a finger, usually occurring in persons exposed to infected oral or respiratory secretions (such as dentists, physicians, nurses). It begins with intense itching and pain, followed by the formation of deep coalescing vesicles. The process is associated with much tissue destruction and may be accompanied by systemic symptoms. A similar lesion may occur as a result of nail biting during the course of primary herpetic gingivostomatitis. Called also *herpetic paronychia.*
**melanotic w.,** subungual melanoma.
**thecal w.,** suppurative tenosynovitis of the terminal phalanx of a finger.

**Whit·man's operation** (hwit′mənz) [Royal *Whitman,* American orthopedic surgeon, 1857–1946] see under *operation.*

**Whit·more's disease (fever)** (hwit′morz) [Major Alfred *Whitmore,* English surgeon in India, 1876–1946] see *melioidosis.*

**Whit·nall's tubercle** (hwit′nalz) [Samuel Ernest *Whitnall,* English anatomist, 1876–1950] see under *tubercle.*

**WHO** World Health Organization.

**whoop** (hōōp) the sonorous and convulsive inspiration of pertussis (whooping cough).

**whoop·ing cough** (hōōp′ing kawf) [MeSH: Whooping Cough] pertussis.

**whorl** (hwerl) a spiral turn or twist, such as one of the turns of the cochlea of the inner ear, the arrangement of muscle fibers in the heart *(vortex),* or a spiral arrangement of the ridges apparent in a fingerprint.
**bone w.,** an enostosis.

**Whytt's disease** (hwits) [Robert *Whytt,* Scottish physician, 1714–1766] see under *disease.*

**Wick·ers·hei·mer's fluid (medium)** (vik′ərz-hi″mərz) [J. *Wickersheimer,* German anatomist, 1832–1896] see under *fluid.*

**Wick·ham's striae** (wik′amz) [Louis-Frédéric *Wickham,* French dermatologist, 1861–1913] see under *stria.*

**Wi·dal's syndrome, test (reaction, serum test)** (ve-dahlz′) [Georges Fernand Isidore *Widal,* French physician, 1862–1929] see *hemolytic anemia,* under *anemia,* and see under *test.*

**Wi·do·witz's sign** (vid′o-vit-səz) [Jannak *Widowitz,* Polish physician, 20th century] see under *sign.*

**width** (width) the extent of something from side to side.
**window w.,** the energy range of gamma radiation that, once detected, will be accepted by the detection system; determined by the upper and lower window settings of the pulse height analyzer.

**Wie·sel** (ve′zel) Torsten Nils. Swedish physician residing in the United States, born 1924; co-winner, with David Hunter Hubel and Roger Wolcott Sperry, of the Nobel prize for medicine or physiology in 1981 for their research on information processing in the visual system.

**Wi·gand's version (maneuver)** (ve′gahnts) [Justus Heinrich *Wigand,* German gynecologist, 1766–1817] see under *version.*

**Wig·gers di·a·gram** (wig′ərz) [Carl John *Wiggers,* American surgeon, 1883–1963] see under *diagram.*

**Wil·cox·on rank sum test, signed rank test** (wil-kok′sonz) [Frank *Wilcoxon,* American chemist and statistician, 1892–1962] see *rank sum test* and *signed rank test,* under *test.*

**wild** (wīld) 1. raised in a natural environment and not in captivity or a laboratory. 2. referring to a genetic strain used as a standard, usually presumed to be the type found in nature; see *wild type,* under *type,* and *wild-type strain,* under *strain.*

**Wil·der's sign** (wīl'dərz) [William Hamlin *Wilder,* American ophthalmologist, 1860–1935] see under *sign.*

**Wil·der·muth's ear** (vil'der-moots) [Hermann A. *Wildermuth,* German neurologist, 1852–1907] see under *ear.*

**Wil·kins** (wil'kinz) Maurice Hugh Frederick. British biochemist, born 1916; co-winner, with Francis Harry Compton Crick and James Dewey Watson, of the Nobel prize for medicine or physiology in 1962 for the discovery of the molecular structure of nuclear acids and its significance for information transfer in living material.

**Wil·lett forceps (clamp)** (wil'ət) [John Abernethy *Willett,* English obstetrician, 1872–1932] see under *forceps.*

**Wil·lia** (wil'e-ə) former name for *Hansenula.*

**Wil·liams' exercises (flexion exercises)** (wil'yəmz) [P.C. *Williams,* physician, 20th century] see under *exercise.*

**Wil·liams syndrome** (wil'yəmz) [J.C.P. *Williams,* New Zealand cardiologist, 20th century] [MeSH: Williams Syndrome] see under *syndrome.*

**Wil·liams-Beu·ren syndrome** (wil'yəmz-bu'rən) [J.C.P. *Williams,* Alois J. *Beurer,* 20th century] see under *syndrome.*

**Wil·liams-Camp·bell syndrome** (wil'yəmz-kam'bəl) [Howard *Williams,* Australian physician, 20th century; Peter E. *Campbell,* Australian physician, 20th century] see under *syndrome.*

**Wil·liam·son's sign** (wil'yəm-sənz) [Oliver K. *Williamson,* English physician, 1866–1941] see under *sign.*

**Wil·lis' antrum,** etc. (wil'is) [Thomas *Willis,* English anatomist and physician, 1621–1675] see *antrum pyloricum, circulus arteriosus cerebri,* and *nervus accessorius,* and see under *cord* and *paracusis.*

**Wilms' tumor** (vilmz) [Max *Wilms,* German surgeon, 1867–1918] see under *tumor.*

**Wil·son's disease (degeneration, syndrome)** (wil'sənz) [Samuel Alexander Kinnier *Wilson,* English neurologist, 1877–1937] see under *disease.*

**Wil·son's muscle** (wil'sənz) [James *Wilson,* English surgeon, 1765–1821] musculus sphincter urethrae.

**Wil·son-Mik·i·ty syndrome** (wil'sən mik'ə-te) [Miriam Geisendorfer *Wilson,* American pediatrician, born 1922; Victor G. *Mikity,* American radiologist, born 1919] see under *syndrome.*

**Wim·ber·ger's sign** (vim'ber-gerz) [Heinrich *Wimberger,* German radiologist, 20th century] see under *sign.*

**Wims·hurst machine** (wimz'hərst) [James *Wimshurst,* English engineer, 1832–1903] see under *machine.*

**Win·ckel's disease** (ving'kelz) [Franz Karl Ludwig Wilhelm von *Winckel,* German gynecologist, 1837–1911] see under *disease.*

**wind·burn** (wind'bərn) chapping of the skin caused by excessive exposure to wind.

**wind·chill** (wind'chil) loss of heat from bodies subjected to wind.

**wind·gall** (wind'gawl) distention of the joint capsule or of a tendon sheath in the region of the fetlock of a horse, caused by a collection of synovial fluid; it is unsightly but usually does not interfere with functioning. Also written *wind gall.* Called also *windpuff.*

**win·di·go** (win'dĭ-go) [Ojibwa a cannibalistic monster of the mythology of Eskimos and certain Native Americans] a culture-specific syndrome characterized by delusions of being possessed by the windigo, with fears of becoming cannibalistic and agitated depression. Called also *witigo.*

**wind·lass** (wind'ləs) an apparatus for lifting or hauling, consisting of a bar that can be turned to reel in a cable attached to a load.
**Spanish w.,** an improvised tourniquet consisting of a handkerchief tied around a body part and twisted by a stick passed under it.

**win·dow** (win'do) [L. *fenestra*] 1. a circumscribed opening in a surface; called also *fenestra.* 2. the upper and lower voltage limits that determine which pulses a pulse height analyzer will accept and pass on.
**aortic w.,** a region below the aortic arch and above the pulmonary artery that contains mediastinal lymph nodes, visible on a radiograph.
**aorticopulmonary w.,** aortic septal defect.
**w. of cochlea, cochlear w.,** fenestra cochleae.
**nasoantral w.,** a surgically created opening between the maxillary sinus and the nasal cavity; see *nasoantrostomy.*
**oval w.,** fenestra vestibuli.
**round w.,** fenestra cochleae.
**skin w.,** see *Rebuck skin window technique,* under *technique.*
**therapeutic w.,** the range between the minimum and maximum doses of an agent. See also *therapeutic index,* under *index.*
**vestibular w., w. of vestibule,** fenestra vestibuli.

**wind·pipe** (wind'pīp) the trachea.

**wind·puff** (wind'pəf) windgall.

**wind·suck·ing** (wind'sək-ing) cribbing.

**wing** (wing) [L. *ala*] [MeSH: Wing] 1. either of the paired anterior appendages of birds, which are modified for flight. 2. a structure or part resembling the wing of a bird; called also *ala.*
**w. of central lobule,** ala lobuli centralis.
**great w. of sphenoid bone, greater w. of sphenoid bone,** ala major ossis sphenoidalis.
**w. of ilium,** ala ossis ilii.
**w. of Ingrassia,** ala minor ossis sphenoidalis.
**lateral w. of sacrum,** pars lateralis ossis sacri.
**lesser w. of sphenoid bone,** ala minor ossis sphenoidalis.
**major w. of sphenoid bone,** ala major ossis sphenoidalis.
**minor w. of sphenoid bone,** ala minor ossis sphenoidalis.
**w. of nose,** ala nasi.
**orbital w. of sphenoid bone, small w. of sphenoid bone,** ala minor ossis sphenoidalis.
**w's of sphenoid bone,** the laterally projecting processes of the sphenoid bone; see *ala major ossis sphenoidalis major ossis sphenoidalis* and *ala minor ossis sphenoidalis.*
**temporal w. of sphenoid bone,** ala major ossis sphenoidalis.
**w. of vomer,** ala vomeris.

**Win·Gel** (win'jəl) trademark for a preparation of alumina and magnesia.

**Win·i·war·ter-Buer·ger disease** (vin'ĭ-vahr″ter-bēr'gər) [Felix von *Winiwarter,* German physician, 1848–1917; Leo *Buerger,* American physician, 1879–1943] thromboangiitis obliterans.

**wink·ing** (wingk'ing) [A.S. *wincian*] quick closing and opening of the eyelids, particularly of only one eye.
**jaw w.,** Gunn's syndrome.

**Wink·ler's disease** (vink'lerz) [Max *Winkler,* Swiss physician, 1875–1952] chondrodermatitis nodularis chronica helicis.

**Wins·low's foramen,** etc. (winz'lōz) [Jacob Benignus *Winslow,* Danish anatomist in Paris, 1669–1760] see under *foramen, ligament,* and *star.*

**Win·strol** (win'strol) trademark for a preparation of stanozolol.

**Win·ter's syndrome** (win'tərz) [Jeremy Stephen Drummond *Winter,* Canadian physician, born 1937] see under *syndrome.*

**win·ter·ber·ry** (win'tər-ber″e) *Ilex verticillata.*

**Win·ter·bot·tom's sign** (win'tər-bot″əmz) [Thomas Masterman *Winterbottom,* English physician, 1765–1859] see under *sign.*

**win·ter·green** (win'tər-grēn) *Gaultheria procumbens.*

**Win·ter·nitz's sound** (vin'ter-nits″əz) [Wilhelm *Winternitz,* German physician in Austria, 1835–1917] see under *sound.*

**Win·trobe hematocrit tube, method** (win'trōb) [Maxwell Myer *Wintrobe,* American hematologist, 1901–1986] see under *tube* and *method.*

**wire** (wīr) 1. a long, slender, flexible structure of metal, used in surgery and dentistry. 2. to insert wires into a body structure, as into a broken bone to immobilize the fragments, or into an aneurysm to promote the formation of clots.
**arch w.,** a wire attached to molar bands or an orthodontic appliance and applied around the dental arch to control and force tooth movement in orthodontic therapy. Called also *orthodontic w.*
**arch w., ideal,** the configuration of an arch wire that conforms as closely as possible to the desired ultimate shape of the arch for a particular individual.
**Kirschner w.,** a steel wire for skeletal fixation of fractured bones and for obtaining skeletal traction in fractures; it is inserted through the soft tissues and the bone.
**ligature w.,** a soft, thin wire used to tie an arch wire to band attachments or brackets in an orthodontic appliance.
**orthodontic w.,** arch w.
**separating w.,** a brass wire threaded between two teeth having tight contact in an effort to wedge them slightly apart before fitting a band in the application of an orthodontic appliance.
**twin w.,** see under *appliance.*

**wire·worm** (wīr'werm) *Haemonchus contortus.*

**wir·ing** (wīr'ing) the fixing into position by means of wire, as of segments of fractured bone.
**circumferential w.,** a technique for fixation of mandibular fractures in which wires are passed around a section of bone with the ends exiting into the oral cavity and then around a fixed intraoral splint.
**continuous loop w.,** wiring of the teeth for the reduction and fixation of fractures, by using a single length of wire to form wire loops on both the maxillary and mandibular teeth, over which intermaxillary elastics can be placed; called also *Stout w.*
**craniofacial suspension w.,** wiring of noncontiguous areas of bone

(piriform aperture, zygomatic arch, zygomatic process of the frontal bone) for the support of fractured jaw segments.
**Gilmer w.**, a method of intermaxillary fixation in which single opposing teeth are wired circumferentially and the wires twisted together.
**Ivy loop w.**, wiring of adjacent teeth in groups of two to provide an attachment for intermaxillary elastics.
**perialveolar w.**, the fixing of a splint to the maxillary arch by passing a wire through the alveolar process from the buccal plate to the palate.
**piriform aperture w.**, wiring through the nasal bones at the piriform aperture for the stabilization of fractures of the jaws.
**Stout w.**, continuous loop w.

**Wir·sung's canal, duct** (vēr'soongz) [Johann Georg *Wirsung,* German physician in Italy, 1600–1643] ductus pancreaticus.

**WISC** Wechsler Intelligence Scale for Children.

**Wis·kott-Al·drich syndrome** (vis'kot-awl'drik) [Alfred *Wiskott,* German pediatrician, 1898–1978; Robert Anderson *Aldrich,* American pediatrician, born 1917] [MeSH: Wiskott-Aldrich Syndrome] see under *syndrome.*

**witch ha·zel** (wich' ha'zəl) 1. *Hamamelis virginiana.* 2. [USP] a clear, colorless distillate prepared from recently cut, partially dried twigs of *H. virginiana* macerated in water, used topically as a mild astringent. Called also *hamamelis water.*

**with·draw·al** (with-draw'əl) 1. a pathological retreat from interpersonal contact and social involvement, as may occur in schizophrenia, depression, or schizoid, avoidant, or schizotypal personality disorders. 2. substance w.
**substance w.** [DSM-IV], a substance-specific mental disorder that follows the cessation of use or reduction in intake of a psychoactive substance that had been regularly used to induce a state of intoxication. DSM-IV includes specific withdrawal syndromes for alcohol; amphetamines or similarly acting sympathomimetics; cocaine; nicotine; opioids; and sedatives, hypnotics, or anxiolytics. Called also *withdrawal, withdrawal symptoms* or *syndrome,* and *abstinence symptoms* or *syndrome.*

**with·ers** (with'ərz) the top of the shoulders of the horse.
**fistulous w.**, distention and rupture of the bursa in the withers region of horses, with suppuration; it is caused by a dual infection with *Brucella* species and *Actinomyces* species and is virtually identical to poll evil.

**wi·ti·go** (wĭ-ti'go) windigo.

**wit·kop** (wit'kop) [Afrikaans "whitehead"] a South African term for *favus.*

**Wit·zel gastrostomy (operation)** (vit'səl) [Friedrich Oskar *Witzel,* German surgeon, 1856–1925] see under *gastrostomy.*

**wit·zel·sucht** (vit'sel-zo͞okt) [Ger.] a mental condition characteristic of frontal lobe lesions and marked by the making of poor jokes and puns and the telling of pointless stories, at which the patient himself is intensely amused.

**WMA** World Medical Association.

**wob·ble** (wob'əl) to move unsteadily or unsurely back and forth or from side to side. See under *hypothesis.*

**wob·bles** (wob'əlz) wobbler syndrome, defs. 1 and 2.

**Wohl·fart-Ku·gel·berg-We·lan·der syndrome** (vōl'fahrt-koo'gəl-bārg-va'lahn-dər) [Karl Gunnar Vilhelm *Wohlfart,* Swedish neurologist, 1910–1961; Eric Klas Henrik *Kugelberg,* Swedish neurologist, born 1913; Lisa *Welander,* Swedish neurologist, born 1909] Kugelberg-Welander syndrome.

**Wohl·fahr·tia** (vōl-fahr'te-ə) [Peter *Wohlfahrt,* German medical writer, 1675–1726] a genus of flesh flies of the family Sarcophagidae, the cause of myiasis in humans and other animals. *W. magni'fica* is found in Russia and the Middle East and causes wound myiasis. *W. opa'ca* and *W. vi'gil* are found in North America and cause cutaneous myiasis.

**Wold·man's test** (wōld'mənz) [Edward Elbert *Woldman,* American physician, 20th century] see under *test.*

**Wolf-Hirsch·horn syndrome** (volf-hərsh'horn) [Ulrich *Wolf,* German physician, born 1933; Kurt *Hirschhorn,* American physician, born 1926] see under *syndrome.*

**Wolfe's graft** (woolfs) [John Reissberg *Wolfe,* Scottish ophthalmologist, 1824–1904] Krause-Wolfe graft.

**Wolfe-Krause graft** (woolf-krou'zə) [J. R. *Wolfe;* Fedor *Krause,* German surgeon, 1857–1937] Krause-Wolfe graft.

**Wolff's duct** (volfs) [Kaspar Friedrich *Wolff,* German anatomist and physiologist, 1733–1794] see *ductus mesonephricus.*

**Wolff's law** (volfs) [Julius *Wolff,* German anatomist, 1836–1902] see under *law.*

**Wolff-Chai·koff effect** (woolf cha'kof) [J. *Wolff,* American physiologist, 20th century; Israel Lyon *Chaikoff,* British-born American physiologist, born 1902] see under *effect.*

**Wolff-Par·kin·son-White syndrome** (woolf-pahr'kin-sən-hwīt) [Louis *Wolff,* American cardiologist, born 1898; Sir John *Parkinson,* English physician, 1885–1976; Paul Dudley *White,* American cardiologist, 1886–1973] [MeSH: Wolff-Parkinson-White Syndrome] see under *syndrome.*

**wolf·fi·an** (wool'fe-ən) described by Kaspar Friedrich *Wolff,* as wolffian body (mesonephros), cyst, duct (ductus mesonephricus), and ridge (mesonephric ridge).

**Wölf·ler's glands** (verlf'lerz) [Anton *Wölfler,* Austrian surgeon, 1850–1917] glandulae thyroideae accessoriae.

**Wölf·ler's operation** (verlf'lerz) [A. *Wölfler*] see under *operation.*

**Wol·fram syndrome** (wool'frəm) [D.J. *Wolfram,* American physician, 20th century] [MeSH: Wolfram Syndrome] see under *syndrome.*

**wol·fram** (wool'fram) tungsten.

**Wolf·ring's glands** (volf'ringz) [Emilij Franzevic von *Wolfring,* Polish ophthalmologist, 1832–1906] see under *gland.*

**wolfs·bane** (woolfs'bān) 1. *Arnica.* 2. arnica. 3. *Aconitum napellus.* 4. aconite.

**Wo·li·nel·la** (wo″lĭ-nel'ə) [M.J. *Wolin,* American bacteriologist] [MeSH: Wolinella] a genus of gram-negative, anaerobic, helical, curved or straight, rod-shaped bacteria of the family Bacteroidaceae, motile with a polar flagellum, found in cattle and the human oral cavity.
**W. rec'ta,** *Campylobacter rectus.*
**W. succino'genes,** a species found in the bovine rumen. Called also *Vibrio succinogenes.*

**Woll·as·ton's doublet** (wool'əs-tənz) [William Hyde *Wollaston,* English physician, 1766–1828] see under *doublet.*

**Wol·man disease** (wol'mən) [Moshe *Wolman,* Israeli neuropathologist, born 1914] [MeSH: Wolman Disease] see under *disease.*

**Wo·mack procedure** (wo'mak) see under *procedure.*

**womb** (wo͞om) the uterus.

**Wood's light (filter, glass)** (woodz) [Robert Williams *Wood,* American physicist, 1868–1955] see under *light.*

**Wood's sign** (woodz) [Horatio Charles *Wood,* American physician and pharmacologist, 1874–1958] see under *sign.*

**wood·chuck** (wood'chuk) [MeSH: Marmota] *Marmota monax,* a large, fat, brown rodent of northeastern North America, sometimes a natural reservoir of the plague. Called also *groundhog.*

**wool** (wool) [L. *lana*] [MeSH: Wool] 1. the hair of sheep. Called also *lana.* 2. by extension, any material existing as fine threads.
**lumpy w.**, dermatophilosis in sheep.

**Wool·ner's tip** (wool'nərz) [Thomas *Woolner,* English sculptor and poet, 1825–1892] tuberculum auriculare.

**word sal·ad** (wərd sal'əd) a meaningless mixture of words and phrases characteristic of advanced schizophrenia; called also *schizophasia.*

**Wo·rin·ger-Ko·lopp disease (syndrome)** (vo″rin-zhār'ko-lop') [Frédéric *Woringer,* French dermatologist, 1903–1964; P. *Kolopp,* French dermatologist, 20th century] pagetoid reticulosis; see under *reticulosis.*

**work** (wərk) in physics, the force applied to an object times the distance traveled in the direction of the force. Symbol *W.* The SI unit of work is the joule.

**work-up** (werk'əp) the procedures done to arrive at a diagnosis, including history taking, laboratory tests, x-rays, and so on.

**World Health Or·ga·ni·za·tion (WHO)** [MeSH: World Health Organization] an agency of the United Nations, devoted to attainment of the highest level of health by all peoples of the world; the permanent secretariat is located in Geneva, Switzerland.

**worm** (werm) [L. *vermis*] 1. any of the soft-bodied, naked, elongated invertebrates of the phyla Platyhelminthes, Annelida, Acanthocephala, and Aschelminthes. See also *helminth.* Called also *vermis.* 2. vermis, def. 2.
**barber's pole w.**, *Haemonchus contortus.*
**bilharzia w.**, *Schistosoma.*
**bladder w.**, 1. cysticercus. 2. coenurus.
**case w.**, *Echinococcus.*
**cayor w.**, the larva of *Cordylobia anthropophaga.*
**dragon w.**, *Dracunculus medinensis.*
**eel w.**, nematode.
**eye w.**, any of various parasitic nematodes that infest the conjunc-

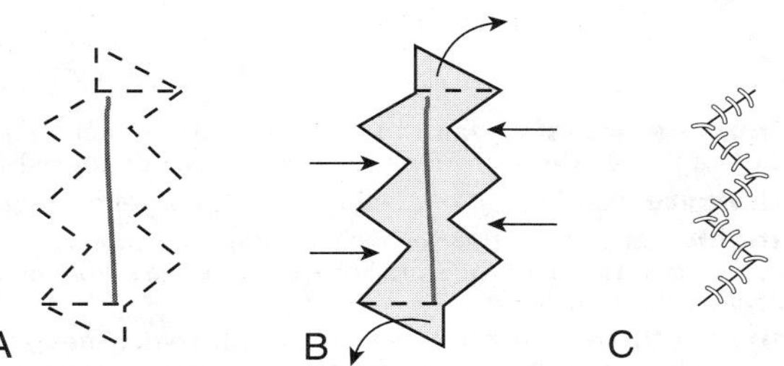

W-plasty. *(A)*, lines of excision; *(B)*, removal of triangular end flaps and apposition of segments; *(C)*, after suturing.

tivae and conjunctival glands or sacs of humans or other animals; see *Loa loa, Onchocerca,* and *Thelazia.*
**flat w.,** platyhelminth.
**fleece w.,** wool maggot.
**giant kidney w.,** *Dioctophyma renale.*
**guinea w.,** *Dracunculus medinensis.*
**heart w.,** *Dirofilaria immitis.*
**horsehair w.,** *Gordius.*
**kidney w.,** *Dioctophyma renale.*
**lung w.,** see *lungworm.*
**maw w.,** *Ascaris.*
**meal w.,** mealworm.
**Medina w.,** *Dracunculus medinensis.*
**nodular w.,** any nematode of the genus *Oesophagostomum.*
**palisade w.,** *Strongylus equinus.*
**pork w.,** *Trichinella spiralis.*
**round w.,** nematode.
**scour w.,** a parasitic worm that causes diarrhea (scours) in ruminants, such as a nematode of one of the genera *Cooperia, Nematodirus, Ostertagia,* or *Trichostrongylus.*
**screw w.,** see *screwworm.*
**serpent w.,** *Dracunculus medinensis.*
**spinyheaded w.,** acanthocephalan.
**stomach w.,** any parasitic worm that lives in the stomach of an animal, such as species of *Haemonchus, Ostertagia,* and *Teladorsagia.*
**thorny-headed w.,** acanthocephalan.
**tongue w.,** pentastome.
**trichina w.,** *Trichinella.*
**wire w.,** *Haemonchus contortus.*

**Worm·ley's test** (worm'lēz) [Theodore George *Wormley,* American chemist, 1826–1897] see under *test.*

**worm·seed** (werm'sēd) 1. *Artemisia maritima.* 2. santonica (def. 2). 3. *Chenopodium maritima.*

**worm·wood** (werm'wood) 1. *Artemisia absinthium.* 2. absinthium (def. 2).

**Woulfe's bottle** (woolfs) [Peter *Woulfe,* English chemist, 1727–1803] see under *bottle.*

**wound** (wo͞ond) [L. *vulnus*] [MeSH: Wounds and Injuries] an injury or damage, usually restricted to those caused by physical means with disruption of normal continuity of structures. Called also *injury* and *trauma.*
**aseptic w.,** one which is not infected with pathogens.
**blowing w.,** open pneumothorax.
**contused w.,** nonpenetrating w.
**incised w.,** one made by a cutting instrument.
**lacerated w.,** laceration.
**nonpenetrating w.,** one in which there is no disruption of the skin but there is injury to underlying structures. See also *contusion.*
**open w.,** one that communicates with the atmosphere by direct exposure.
**penetrating w.,** one caused by a sharp, usually slender object, such as a nail or ice pick, which passes through the skin into the underlying tissues. Called also *puncture w.*
**perforating w.,** a penetrating wound which extends into a viscus or bodily cavity.
**puncture w.,** penetrating w.
**septic w.,** one that is infected with pathogens.
**seton w.,** one which enters and exits on the same side of the injured part.
**subcutaneous w.,** one which involves only the skin and subcutaneous tissue.
**sucking w.,** a penetrating wound of the chest through which air is drawn in and out. See also *open pneumothorax.*
**tangential w.,** an oblique glancing wound which results in one edge being undercut.

**W-plas·ty** a technique in plastic surgery used mainly in the repair of straight scars that require the redistribution of tension. It consists of excising a series of consecutive small triangular areas of tissue on each side of the wound or scar and imbricating the resultant triangular flaps.

**wrapping** (rap'ing) the act or process of putting a cover around a thing.
**fundic w.,** fundoplication.

**Wright blood group** [from the name of the English propositus family first reported on in 1953] see under *blood group.*

**Wright's stain** (rītz) [James Homer *Wright,* American pathologist, 1869–1928] see under *Stains and Staining Methods.*

**Wright's syndrome** (rītz) [Irving Sherwood *Wright,* American physician, born 1901] see under *syndrome.*

**Wris·berg's cartilage,** etc. (ris'bərgz) [Heinrich August *Wrisberg,* German anatomist, 1739–1808] see *cartilago cuneiformis, ganglia cardiaca, ligamentum meniscofemorale posterius, nervus intermedius, nervus cutaneus brachii medialis,* and *tuberculum cuneiforme.*

**wrist** (rist) [MeSH: Wrist] 1. carpus, defs. 1 and 3. 2. articulatio radiocarpalis.
**SLAC w.,** a wrist affected by scapholunate advanced collapse (SLAC).
**tennis w.,** tenovaginitis of the tendons of the wrist in tennis players.

**wrist·drop** (rist'drop) a condition resulting from paralysis of the extensor muscles of the hand and fingers. Called also *carpoptosis* and *drop hand.*

**writ·ing** (rīt'ing) [MeSH: Writing] the inscription of letters or other symbols, and of words, phrases, and sentences, so that they may be perceived by the eyes or, by the blind, through the fingertips.
**mirror w.,** writing in which the right and left relationships of letters and words are reversed, as if seen in a mirror.

**wry·neck** (ri'neck) torticollis.

**wt** weight.

**Wu·cher·e·ria** (voo″ker-e're-ə) [Otto *Wucherer,* German physician in Brazil, 1820–1873] [MeSH: Wuchereria] a genus of nematodes of the superfamily Filarioidea that affect mainly humans in various countries of warmer regions of the world.
**W. bancrof'ti,** a white threadlike worm which causes elephantiasis, lymphangitis, and chyluria by interfering with the lymphatic circulation. The immature forms, or microfilariae *(microfilaria bancrofti),* are found in the circulating blood, especially at night, and are carried by *Culex* and other mosquitoes. In the Pacific form of *W. bancrofti,* sometimes called *W. bancrofti* var. *pacifica,* the microfilariae do not show the nocturnal periodicity seen elsewhere.
**W. ma'layi,** *Brugia malayi.*

**wu·cher·e·ri·a·sis** (voo-ker″e-ri'ə-sis) infection with trematodes of the genus *Wuchereria.*

**Wun·der·lich's curve** (voon'der-liks) [Carl Reinhold August *Wunderlich,* German physician, 1815–1877] see under *curve.*

**Wur·ster's test** (voor'sterz) [Casimir *Wurster,* German physiologist, 1856–1913] see under *test.*

**w/v** weight (of solute) per volume (of solvent).

**Wy·a·mine** (wi'ə-min) trademark for preparations of mephentermine sulfate.

**Wy·burn-Ma·son's syndrome** (wi'bərn-ma'sənz) [Roger *Wyburn-Mason,* British physician, 20th century] see under *syndrome.*

**Wy·cil·lin** (wi-sil'lin) trademark for preparations of penicillin G procaine.

**Wy·dase** (wi'dās) trademark for preparations of hyaluronidase for injection.

**Wye·o·my·ia** (we″o-mi'yə) a genus of mosquitoes of the subfamily Culicinae, native to Central and South America, the vector of the Wyeomyia virus.

**Wy·mox** (wi'moks) trademark for preparations of amoxicillin.

**Wynn method** (win) [Sidney Keith *Wynn,* American plastic surgeon, born 1917] see under *method.*

**Wy·ten·sin** (wi-ten'sin) trademark for a preparation of guanabenz acetate.

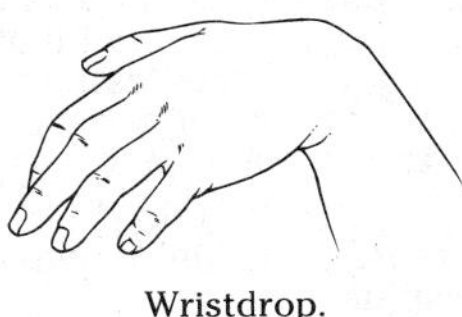
Wristdrop.

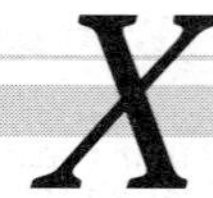

**X** symbol for *Kienbock unit* and *xanthine* or *xanthosine.*

**$\bar{X}$** symbol for *sample mean.*

***X*** symbol for *reactance.*

***x*** symbol for *abscissa.*

*ξ* xi, the fourteenth letter of the Greek alphabet.

**Xal·a·tan** (zal'ə-tan) trademark for a preparation of latanoprost.

**Xan·ax** (zan'aks) trademark for a preparation of alprazolam.

**xan·chro·mat·ic** (zan"kro-mat'ik) xanthochromic.

**xan·thel·as·ma** (zan"thəl-az'mə) [*xanth-* + Gr. *elasma* plate] planar xanthoma involving the eyelid(s). Called also *xanthoma palpebrarum.*

**xan·thel·as·ma·to·sis** (xan"thəl-az"mə-to'sis) xanthomatosis.

**xan·them·a·tin** (zan-them'ə-tin) a yellow substance derivable from hematin by the action of nitric acid.

**xan·thene** (zan'thēn) the compound $(C_6H_4)_2(O)CH_2$, or dibenzpyran, from which the xanthene dyes and indicators are derived.

**xan·thic** (zan'thik) 1. yellow. 2. pertaining to xanthine.

**xan·thin** (zan'thin) any of the yellow pigments obtained from yellow flowers and other plants, probably consisting of oxygen-containing carotenoids.

**xan·thine** (zan'thēn) [Gr. *xanthos* yellow: named from the yellow color of its nitrate] a purine base found in most body tissues and fluids, certain plants, and some urinary calculi. It is an intermediate in the degradation of adenosine monophosphate to uric acid, being formed by oxidation of hypoxanthine. Methylated xanthines (see *methylxanthine*) are used medicinally. Xanthine also occurs complexed with ribose as xanthose. Abbreviated X.

**xan·thine de·hy·dro·gen·ase** (zan'thēn de-hi'dro-jən-ās) [EC 1.1.1.204] [MeSH: Xanthine Dehydrogenase] an enzyme of the oxidoreductase class that catalyzes the hydroxylation of xanthine or hypoxanthine to urate, using $NAD^+$ as an electron acceptor. The enzyme is a molybdoflavoprotein with a bound FAD and two iron-sulfur centers. Under certain conditions the enzyme is converted to a form that can reduce molecular oxygen and is called xanthine oxidase. Deficiency of enzyme activity, due to isolated defect in the enzyme or to molybdenum cofactor deficiency (q.v.), results in xanthinuria and deposition of xanthine calculi.

**xan·thine ox·i·dase** (zan'thēn ok'sĭ-dās) [EC 1.1.3.22] [MeSH: Xanthine Oxidase] an enzyme of the oxidoreductase class that catalyzes the oxidation of hypoxanthine to xanthine and of xanthine to uric acid, the final steps in the degradation of purines. It is an iron-molybdenum flavoprotein containing FAD. Deficiency of the enzyme, an autosomal recessive trait, causes xanthinuria.

**xan·thin·uria** (zan"thin-u're-ə) 1. a rare autosomal recessive hereditary disorder of purine metabolism due to deficiency of the enzyme xanthine oxidase, which results in excessive urinary secretion of xanthine and hypoxanthine, in place of uric acid, and may lead to the formation of xanthine calculi in the urinary tract. 2. excretion of xanthine in the urine.

**xan·thin·uric** (zan"thin-u'-rik) pertaining to or resulting from xanthinuria.

**xan·thism** (zan'thiz-əm) [Gr. *xanthos* auburn] an autosomal recessive form of oculocutaneous albinism occurring in blacks and characterized by a red to reddish brown coloration of the skin and hair and reddish brown, slightly translucent irides; photophobia and nystagmus are mild and visual acuity is normal or nearly normal. Called also *red* or *rufous albinism.*

**Xan·thi·um** (zan'the-um) the cockleburrs, a genus of composite plants. In several species, the small new shoots that appear after rainstorms are poisonous, causing hepatic necrosis and fatal encephalopathy in livestock.

**xan·thi·uria** (zan"the-u're-ə) xanthinuria.

**xanth(o)-** [Gr. *xanthos* yellow] a combining form meaning yellow.

**xan·tho·chro·mat·ic** (zan"tho-kro-mat'ik) xanthochromic.

**xan·tho·chro·mia** (zan"tho-kro'me-ə) [*xantho-* + *chrom-* + *-ia*] any yellowish discoloration, as of the skin or of the spinal fluid.
**x. stria'ta palma'ris,** planar xanthoma involving the volar creases of the palms and finger joints, manifested by yellowish brown discoloration of the creases of the palmar aspect of the hands, which is assumed by some to gradually progress to xanthoma striatum palmare.

**xan·tho·chro·mic** (zan"tho-kro'mik) having a yellow discoloration; said of cerebrospinal fluid.

**xan·tho·cy·a·nop·sia** (zan"tho-si"ə-nop'se-ə) [*xantho-* + *cyano-* + *-opsia*] ability to discern yellow and blue tints, but not red or green.

**xan·tho·cyte** (zan'tho-sīt) a cell that contains yellow pigment.

**xan·tho·der·ma** (zan"tho-der'mə) [*xantho-* + *derma*] any yellowish discoloration of the skin. For example, see *carotenemia, jaundice,* and *xanthochromia.*

**xan·tho·eryth·ro·der·mia** (zan"tho-ə-rith"ro-der'me-ə) a yellowish red discoloration of the skin.
**x. per'stans,** small plaque parapsoriasis.

**xan·tho·gran·u·lo·ma** (zan"tho-gran"u-lo'mə) [*xanthoma* + *granuloma*] a tumor having the histologic characteristics of both granuloma and xanthoma.
**juvenile x.,** a benign, self-limited disorder of infants and children, usually present at birth, manifested by the development of single or multiple papules or nodules, which may be yellow, pink, orange, or reddish brown in color, found typically on the scalp, face, proximal extremities, or trunk; involvement of mucous membranes, viscera, eye, and other organs may also occur. Mature lesions are characterized histologically by a dermal infiltrate of lipid-laden histiocytes, admixed inflammatory cells, and Touton giant cells. Most lesions regress spontaneously during the first few years of life. It is sometimes considered a variant or subtype of benign fibrous histiocytoma (q.v.). Formerly called *nevoxanthoendothelioma.*

**xan·tho·ky·an·o·py** (zan"tho-ki-an'ə-pe) xanthocyanopsia.

**xan·tho·ma** (zan-tho'mə) [*xanth-* + *-oma*] a tumor composed of lipid-laden foam cells, which are histiocytes containing cytoplasmic lipid material. See also *xanthomatosis.*
**craniohypophyseal x.,** deposits of cholesterol esters in bones around the hypophysis in Hand-Schüller-Christian disease.
**diabetic x., x. diabetico'rum,** eruptive x.
**disseminated x., x. dissemina'tum,** a rare form of normolipoproteinemic xanthomatosis manifested by the development of reddish yellow to brown papules and nodules that may coalesce to form furrowed plaques and have a predilection for flexural creases, mucous membranes of the mouth and respiratory tract, cornea, sclera, and central nervous system, including the pituitary gland, the involvement of which often produces diabetes insipidus. Called also *x. multiplex.*
**eruptive x., x. erupti'vum,** crops of small yellowish orange or yellow papules surrounded by an erythematous halo, occurring suddenly, usually on the buttocks, posterior thighs, knees, and elbows; the papules may be intensely pruritic and may ulcerate. It is caused by high concentrations of plasma triglycerides, such as with uncontrolled diabetes mellitus, and it usually disappears when the underlying condition is corrected. See also *tuberoeruptive x.* Called also *diabetic x.*
**fibrous x.,** benign fibrous histiocytoma.
**x. mul'tiplex,** disseminated x.
**x. palpebra'rum,** xanthelasma.
**planar x., plane x., x. pla'num,** a form manifested as soft yellowish, tannish, or dark red flat macules or slightly raised plaques, sometimes having a white central area, which may be localized or generalized, often occurring in association with other types of xanthomas and certain types of hyperlipoproteinemia, and may be associated with lymphoma and multiple myeloma.
**x. stria'tum palma're,** planar xanthoma involving the creases of the palms and volar finger joints, manifested by linear, slightly elevated papules in the palmar creases, especially of the fingers; assumed by some authorities to be a gradual transition from xanthochromia striata palmaris.
**x. tendino'sum, tendinous x.,** a form manifested by the presence of freely movable papules or nodules in the tendons, ligaments, fascia, and periosteum, especially on the dorsum of the hands, fingers, elbows, knees, and heels, which occurs in association with certain types of hyperlipoproteinemia, tuberous xanthoma, xanthelasma, and cerebrotendinous xanthomatosis.
**tuberoeruptive x.,** a form in which lesions of eruptive xanthoma develop in association with already existing tuberous xanthoma and have a tendency to coalesce; this usually occurs in combination with hyperlipoproteinemia type III.
**x. tubero'sum, x. tubero'sum mul'tiplex, tuberous x.,** development of groups of large, flat or elevated, yellow to orange, indurated nodules on the extensor surfaces and areas subjected to trauma, particularly on the elbows and knees; lesions tend to coalesce. Seen associated with such conditions as hyperlipoproteinemias, biliary cirrhosis, and myxedema. See also *tuberoeruptive x.*
**verruciform x.,** an uncommon solitary xanthoma of the oral mucosa; it is covered with a rough parakeratinized layer and usually occurs on the lower alveolar ridge.

**xan·tho·ma·to·sis** (zan"tho-mə-to'sis) [MeSH: Xanthomatosis] a

condition characterized by the presence of xanthomas. Called also *xanthelasmatosis.* See also *xanthoma.*
**biliary hypercholesterolemic x.,** widespread xanthomatosis resulting from hypercholesterolemia due to biliary tract obstruction.
**x. bul'bi,** fatty degeneration of the cornea.
**cerebrotendinous x.,** a lipid storage disease, inherited as an autosomal recessive trait, characterized by xanthomas of the tendons, the white matter of the brain, and the lungs and by spasticity, ataxia, pyramidal paresis, mental retardation, dementia, early cataracts, and atherosclerosis. It is associated with elevated plasma and tissue levels of cholestanol and defective bile synthesis, with the deposition of cholestanol in the central nervous system and in the myelin of peripheral nerves. The lesions contain cholesterol and dehydrocholesterol.
**chronic idiopathic x.,** Hand-Schüller-Christian disease.
**x. cor'neae,** dystrophia adiposa corneae.
**x. generalisa'ta os'sium,** Hand-Schüller-Christian disease
**x. i'ridis,** the formation of yellow patches in the discolored iris of an eye blinded as the result of protracted iritis or glaucoma.
**primary familial x., Wolman x.,** Wolman's disease.

**xan·tho·ma·tous** (zan-tho'mə-təs) pertaining to or of the nature of xanthoma.

**Xan·tho·mo·nas** (zan"tho-mo'nəs) [Gr. *xanthos* yellow + Gr. *monas* unit, from *monos* single] [MeSH: Xanthomonas] a genus of gram-negative, aerobic, rod-shaped bacteria of the family Pseudomonadaceae. The organisms produce a yellow pigment; most species are plant pathogens. *X. campes'tris* is used in the production of xanthan gum.
**X. maltophi'lia,** a widespread species that is occasionally an opportunistic pathogen, found in infections of the upper respiratory tract, wounds, blood, and urine. Called also *Pseudomonas maltophilia.*

**xan·thone** (zan'thōn) xanthene ketone, a derivative of xanthine.

**xan·tho·phore** (zan'tho-for) [*xantho-* + *-phore*] a chromatophore of cold-blooded animals containing granules of yellow-red pigment.

**xan·tho·phyll** (zan'tho-fil) [*xantho-* + Gr. *phyllon* leaf] [MeSH: Xanthophyll] a yellow coloring matter of plants, one of a group of oxygenated carotenoids occurring along with carotene in green leaves, grass, egg yolks, human plasma, and other organic matter.

**xan·tho·pia** (zan-tho'pe-ə) xanthopsia.

**xan·tho·pro·te·ic ac·id** (zan"tho-pro-te'ik) the product of treating protein with nitric acid.

**xan·tho·pro·tein** (zan"tho-pro'tēn) an orange pigment produced by heating proteins with nitric acid.

**xan·thop·sia** (zan-thop'se-ə) [*xantho-* + *-opsia*] a form of chromatopsia in which objects appear yellow.

**xan·thop·ter·in** (zan-thop'tər-in) [*xantho-* + *pterin*] [MeSH: Xanthopterin] a yellow pigment from the integument of wasps and hornets and from butterfly wings, which has some hematopoietic activity in anemic animals. It is an inhibitor of xanthine oxidase. See *pterin.*

**xan·tho·sar·co·ma** (zan"tho-sahr-ko'mə) a tumor in the inflammatory subtype of malignant fibrous histiocytoma.

**xan·tho·sine** (zan'tho-sēn) a pyrimidine nucleoside; xanthine linked by its N1 nitrogen to the C1 carbon of ribose. Symbol X.
**x. monophosphate (XMP),** a nucleotide, the 5′-phosphate of xanthosine, that is an intermediate in the synthesis of guanosine monophosphate (GMP).

**xan·tho·sis** (zan-tho'sis) a yellowish discoloration; degeneration with yellowish pigmentation.

**xan·thous** (zan'thəs) yellow or yellowish.

**xanth·u·ren·ic ac·id** (zanth"u-ren'ik) a bicyclic aromatic compound formed as a minor catabolite of tryptophan and present in increased amounts in the urine in vitamin $B_6$ deficiency and some disorders of tryptophan catabolism.

**xan·thu·ria** (zan-thu're-ə) xanthinuria.

**xan·thyl** (zan'thəl) the monovalent radical of xanthene.

**xan·thyl·ic ac·id** (zan-thil'ik) phosphorylated xanthine, usually xanthosine monophosphate.

**X-bite** crossbite.

**Xe** symbol for *xenon.*

**xe·nia** (ze'ne-ə) [Gr. "a friendly relation between two foreigners"] the appearance in the endosperm (seed) resulting from cross-pollination of dominant characters inherited from the male (pollen) plant.

**Xen·i·cal** (zen'ĭ-cal) trademark for a preparation of orlistat.

**xen(o)-** [Gr. *xenos* strange, foreign] a combining form meaning strange, or denoting relationship to foreign material.

**xeno·an·ti·gen** (zen"o-an'tĭ-jən) an antigen occurring in organisms of more than one species, e.g., the A and B antigens of the ABO blood group.

**xeno·bi·ot·ic** (zen"o-bi-ot'ik) a chemical foreign to the biologic system.

**xeno·cy·to·phil·ic** (zen"o-si"to-fil'ik) [*xeno-* + *cyto-* + *-philic*] having an affinity for cells derived from a different species.

**xeno·di·ag·no·sis** (zen"o-di"əg-no'sis) [*xeno-* + *diagnosis*] a method of animal inoculation using laboratory-bred bugs and animals in the diagnosis of certain parasitic infections when it is not possible to demonstrate the infecting organism in blood films. Originally used in the diagnosis of *Trypanosoma cruzi* (Chagas' disease), the method is also used in *Trichinella spiralis* infections. In the original method, bugs are fed or offered the patient's blood through a membrane, and the feces or intestinal contents are examined later for the presence of the organisms. For the diagnosis of trichinosis, muscle tissue from patients is fed to laboratory rats to detect larvae of the parasite.

**xeno·di·ag·nos·tic** (zen"o-di"əg-nos'tik) pertaining to xenodiagnosis.

**xeno·ge·ne·ic** (zen"o-jə-ne'ik) [*xeno-* + *gennan* to produce] in transplantation biology, denoting individuals from different species or tissues transplanted between species; called also *heterogenic* and *heterologous.* See *xenograft* and *xenogeneic transplantation.*

**xeno·gen·e·sis** (zen"o-jen'ə-sis) 1. heterogenesis (def 1). 2. the hypothetical production of offspring unlike either parent.

**xen·og·e·nous** (zen-oj'ə-nəs) [*xeno-* + *-genous*] caused by a foreign body, or originating outside the organism.

**xeno·graft** (zen'o-graft) a graft of tissue transplanted between animals of different species. Called also *heterograft, heterologous graft,* and *heteroplastic graft.*
**Carpentier-Edwards porcine x.,** see under *valve.*
**concordant x.,** a graft between members of closely related species, in which the recipient lacks natural antibodies specific for the transplanted tissue.
**discordant x.,** a graft between members of divergent species, in which the recipient has natural antibodies specific for the transplanted tissue.
**Hancock porcine x.,** see under *valve.*
**Ionescu-Shiley pericardial x.,** see under *valve.*

**xen·ol·o·gy** (ze-nol'ə-je) the science of the relations of parasites to their hosts.

**xeno·me·nia** (xen"o-me'ne-ə) [*xeno-* + *men-* + *-ia*] vicarious menstruation.

**xe·non** (ze'non) [Gr. *xenos* stranger] [MeSH: Xenon] a chemically unreactive gaseous element found in the atmosphere; atomic number, 54; atomic weight, 131.30; symbol, Xe.
**x. Xe 127** [USP], a radioactive isotope of xenon, atomic mass 127, having a half-life of 36.41 days and decaying by electron capture with emission of gamma rays (0.172, 0.203 MeV); administered by inhalation as a gas for assessment of respiratory perfusion and in lung imaging.
**x. Xe 133** [USP], a radioisotope of xenon, atomic mass 133, having a half-life of 5.25 days and emitting beta particles (0.346 MeV) and gamma rays (0.081 MeV); used for assessment of respiratory perfusion and in cerebral blood flow studies, administered by inhalation as a gas or intra-arterially or intramuscularly as a gas in solution.

**xeno·para·site** (zen"o-par'ə-sīt) an organism not usually parasitic on the host but which becomes so because of a weakened condition of the host.

**xeno·pho·bia** (zen"o-fo'be-ə) [*xeno-* + *-phobia*] irrational fear of strangers.

**xeno·pho·nia** (zen"o-fo'ne-ə) [*xeno-* + *phon-* + *-ia*] an abnormal alteration of the accent and intonation of a person's speech.

**xen·oph·thal·mia** (zen"of-thal'me-ə) [*xen-* + *ophthalmia*] ophthalmia caused by a foreign body in the eye.

**Xen·op·syl·la** (zen"op-sil'ə) [*xeno-* + Gr. *psylla* flea] a genus of fleas, many of which transmit disease-producing microorganisms.
**X. as'tia,** a rat flea of parts of Sri Lanka and India that has been implicated in the transmission of plague.
**X. brasilien'sis,** a rat flea of Africa, Brazil, and India, a transmitter of plague.
**X. cheo'pis,** a rat flea of worldwide distribution which transmits plague and murine typhus; called also *Pulex cheopis* and *Asiatic rat flea.*
**X. hawaiien'sis,** *X. vexabilis.*
**X. vexa'bilis,** a species infesting field rats in Hawaii; called also *X. hawaiiensis.*

**Xeno·pus** (zen'o-pəs) [MeSH: Xenopus] a genus of frogs and toads that have large clawed hindlimbs and weak forelimbs. *X. lae'vis* is the clawed frog or clawed toad, an African species used in the *Xenopus* test (see under *test*).

**xeno·trop·ic** (zen"o-trop'ik) [*xeno-* + *-tropic*] pertaining to a virus that is found benignly in cells of one animal species but will replicate into complete virus particles only when it infects cells of a different species. Cf. *ecotropic*.

**xen·yl** (zen'əl) the univalent chemical group $C_6H_5{\cdot}C_6H_4$—.

**xen·yl·amine** (zə-nil'ə-mēn) *p*-aminobiphenyl.

**xer(o)-** [Gr. *xēros* dry] a combining form meaning dry, or denoting relationship to dryness.

**xe·ro·col·lyr·i·um** (zēr"o-ko-lir'e-əm) [*xero-* + *collyrium*] a dry collyrium; an eye salve.

**xe·ro·cyte** (ze'ro-sīt) an erythrocyte that is dehydrated and has decreased cations due to abnormal permeability of the membrane that allows leakage of potassium ions and water out of the cell. See also *xerocytosis*.

**xe·ro·cy·to·sis** (ze"ro-si-to'sis) presence of xerocytes in the blood.
**hereditary x.,** a hereditary type of hemolytic anemia characterized by xerocytes, sometimes containing phosphatidylcholine.

**xe·ro·der·ma** (zēr"o-der'mə) [*xero-* + *derma*] a mild form of ichthyosis, marked by a dry, rough, discolored state of the skin, with the formation of a scaly desquamation.
**x. pigmento'sum,** a rare pigmentary and atrophic autosomal recessive disease affecting all races, in which there is extreme cutaneous photosensitivity to ultraviolet light, as a result of a deficient enzyme in the excisional repair of ultraviolet-damaged DNA. It begins in childhood with the early development of senile changes in sun-exposed skin, including excessive freckling, telangiectases, keratoses, papillomas, and malignancies, and of severe ophthalmologic abnormalities, including photophobia, lacrimation, keratitis, opacities, and tumors of the lid and cornea. Mental retardation, areflexia, and other neurological disorders may be associated. Subtypes of the disorder have been identified based on the capacity for excisional DNA repair. See also *pigmented xerodermoid*, under *xerodermoid*.

**xe·ro·der·mat·ic** (zēr"o-dər-mat'ik) pertaining to or of the nature of xeroderma.

**xe·ro·der·mia** (zēr"o-der'me-ə) xeroderma.

**xe·ro·der·moid** (zēr"o-der'moid) [*xeroderma* + *-oid*] resembling xeroderma.
**pigmented x.,** a condition considered to be a variant of xeroderma pigmentosum in which there is no defect in the excisional repair of ultraviolet-damaged DNA; it is characterized by a late onset, associated with prolonged exposure to the sun, with freckling appearing in the second decade and no skin cancers until age 40.

**xe·ro·gel** (zēr'o-jəl) a gel containing little liquid. Cf. *lyogel*.

**xe·rog·ra·phy** (ze-rog'rə-fe) xeroradiography.

**xe·ro·ma** (zēr-o'mə) an abnormally dry condition of the conjunctiva; xerophthalmia.

**xe·ro·mam·mog·ra·phy** (zēr"o-mə-mog'rə-fe) [MeSH: Xeromammography] xeroradiography of the breast.

**xe·ro·me·nia** (zēr"o-me'ne-ə) [*xero-* + *men-* + *-ia*] a condition in which the bodily symptoms of menstruation occur without any bloody flow.

**xe·ro·myc·te·ria** (zēr"o-mik-tēr'e-ə) [*xero-* + Gr. *myktēr* nose] dryness of the nasal mucous membrane.

**xe·roph·thal·mia** (zēr"of-thal'me-ə) [*xero-* + *ophthalmia*] [MeSH: Xerophthalmia] dryness of the conjunctiva and cornea due to vitamin A deficiency. The condition begins with night blindness and conjunctival xerosis and progresses to corneal xerosis and, in the late stages, to keratomalacia.

**xe·roph·thal·mus** (zēr"of-thal'məs) xerophthalmia.

**xe·ro·ra·di·og·ra·phy** (zēr"o-ra"de-og'rə-fe) [MeSH: Xeroradiography] a dry, totally photoelectric process for recording x-ray images, using metal plates coated with a semiconductor, such as selenium.

**xe·ro·si·a·log·ra·phy** (zēr"o-si"ə-log'rə-fe) sialography in which the images are recorded by xeroradiography.

**xe·ro·sis** (zēr-o'sis) [Gr. *xērosis*] abnormal dryness, as of the eye, skin, or mouth.
**x. conjuncti'vae, conjunctival x.,** dryness of the conjunctiva. When associated with Bitot's spots, it is due to vitamin A deficiency and may progress to xerophthalmia and keratomalacia.
**x. cor'neae, corneal x.,** dryness of the cornea, giving it a hazy or milky appearance; see *xerophthalmia*.
**x. cu'tis,** xerotic eczema.
**x. generalisa'ta,** dryness of the skin, with pruritus and branny scaling, seen in patients with acquired immunodeficiency syndrome.
**x. parenchymato'sa,** xerophthalmia due to trachoma.
**x. superficia'lis,** xerophthalmia due to abnormal exposure of the eyeball to the air.

**xe·ro·sto·mia** (zēr"o-sto'me-ə) [*xero-* + *stom-* + *-ia*] [MeSH: Xerostomia] dryness of the mouth from salivary gland dysfunction, as in Sjögren's syndrome.

**xe·rot·ic** (zēr-ot'ik) characterized by xerosis or dryness.

**xe·ro·to·mog·ra·phy** (zēr"o-tə-mog'rə-fe) tomography in which the images are recorded by xeroradiography.

**xe·ro·trip·sis** (zēr"o-trip'sis) [*xero-* + *tripsis*] dry friction.

**X-His di·pep·ti·dase** (di-pep'tĭ-dās) [EC 3.4.13.3] an enzyme of the hydrolase class that catalyzes the cleavage of the dipeptide carnosine into component amino acids *β*-alanine and histidine; it also acts on some other aminoacyl-L-histidine dipeptides. The tissue isozyme requires zinc ions and does not hydrolyze anserine or homocarnosine; the serum isozyme requires cadmium and does hydrolyze anserine and homocarnosine. Deficiency of the serum isozyme causes serum carnosinase deficiency. Called also *carnosinase* and *aminoacyl-histidine dipeptidase*. See also *homocarnosinase*.

**xi** (zi, kse) [Ξ, ξ] the fourteenth letter of the Greek alphabet.

**xip·amide** (zip'ə-mīd) [MeSH: Xipamide] a diuretic and antihypertensive with actions and uses similar to those of the thiazide diuretics; administered orally.

**xiphi-** see *xiph(o)-*.

**xiphi·ster·nal** (zif"ĭ-stər'nəl) pertaining to the xiphisternum.

**xiphi·ster·num** (zif"ĭ-stər'nəm) [*xiphi-* + *sternum*] processus xiphoideus.

**xiph(o)-** [Gr. *xiphos* sword] a combining form denoting relationship to the xiphoid process. Also, *xiphi-*.

**xipho·cos·tal** (zif"o-kos'təl) [*xipho-* + *costal*] pertaining to the xiphoid process and the ribs.

**xipho·did·y·mus** (zif"o-did'ĭ-məs) [*xipho-* + *-didymus*] xiphopagus.

**xi·phod·y·mus** (zĭ-fod'ĭ-məs) xiphopagus.

**xiph·odyn·ia** (zif"o-din'e-ə) [*xipho-* + *-odynia*] pain in the xiphoid process.

**xiph·oid** (zif'oid, zi'foid) [Gr. *xiphoeidēdes* sword-shaped, from *xiphos* sword + *eidos* form] 1. shaped like a sword; ensiform. 2. pertaining to the processus xiphoideus. 3. processus xiphoideus.

**xiph·oi·di·tis** (zif"oi-di'tis) inflammation of the xiphoid process.

**xi·pho·om·pha·lo·is·chi·op·a·gus** (zi"fo-om"fə-lo-is"ke-op'ə-gəs) [*xipho-* + *omphalo-* + *ischio-* + *-pagus*] conjoined twins united from the level of the xiphoid process to the ischia.

**xi·phop·a·gus** (zĭ-fop'ə-gəs) [*xipho-* + *-pagus*] symmetrical conjoined twins fused in the region of the xiphoid process.

**X-linked** (eks'linkt) see under *gene*.

**XMP** xanthosine monophosphate.

**XO** an unapproved but widely used symbol to indicate the presence of only one sex chromosome, the other X or the Y chromosome being absent.

**XOAN** X-linked (Nettleship) ocular albinism.

**X-Prep** (eks'prep) trademark for a preparation of senna.

**X-Pro di·pep·ti·dase** (di-pep'tĭ-dās") [EC 3.4.13.9] a dipeptidase that catalyzes the cleavage of a C-terminal proline or another imino acid from imidodipeptides, an important step in intestinal absorption of the imino acid portion of dipeptides. Reduced enzyme activity, an autosomal recessive trait, causes prolidase deficiency. Called also *prolidase* and *proline dipeptidase*.

**x-ray** (eks'ra) [MeSH: X-Rays] see under *ray*.

**XU** excretory urography.

**xy·lan** (zi'lan) any of a group of pentosans composed of xylose residues; they are major structural constituents of wood, straw, and bran.

**xy·la·zine hy·dro·chlo·ride** (zi'lə-zēn) [USP] a veterinary analgesic, sedative, and muscle relaxant, used in most domestic animals except pigs.

**xy·lene** (zi'lēn) [Gr. *xylon* wood] 1. any of three isomeric hydrocarbons, $C_6H_4(CH_3)_2$, from methyl alcohol or coal tar; usually qualified by the substituent positions. Called also *dimethylbenzene*. 2. a mixture of all three isomers, with uses including solvent and clarifier for microscopy, protective coating, and in various syntheses.

**xy·li·dine** (zi'lĭ-din) a compound, dimethylaniline $(CH_3)_2C_6H_3{\cdot}NH_2$, used as a dyestuff intermediate and for blending gasoline.

**xy·li·tol** (zi'lĭ-tol) [NF] [MeSH: Xylitol] a five-carbon sugar alcohol derived from xylose by reduction of the carbonyl group; it is as sweet as sucrose and is used as a noncariogenic sweetener and also as a sugar substitute in diabetic diets.

**xy·li·tol de·hy·dro·gen·ase** (zi′lĭ-tol de-hi′dro-jən-ās) L-xylulose reductase.

**xyl(o)-** [Gr. *xylon* wood] a combining form denoting relationship to wood.

**Xy·lo·caine** (zi′lo-kān) trademark for preparations of lidocaine.

**Xy·lo·hy·pha** (zi″lo-hi′fə) a genus of Fungi Imperfecti of the form-class Hyphomycetes, form-family Dematiaceae. *X. nigres′cens* is a species commonly found on trees. *X. bantia′na* has been renamed *Cladosporium bantianum.*

**xy·lol** (zi′lol) xylene.

**xy·lo·met·a·zo·line hy·dro·chlo·ride** (zi″lo-met″ə-zo′lēn) [USP] an adrenergic used topically as a vasoconstrictor to reduce swelling and congestion of the nasal mucosa.

**xy·lo·py·ra·nose** (zi″lo-pi′rə-nōs) xylose in the cyclic pyranose form.

**Xy·lor·rhi·za** (zi″lə-ri′zə) a genus of plants of the family Compositae; all species preferentially seek seleniferous soil and may be high in selenium, causing selenium poisoning in livestock.

**xy·lose** (zi′lōs) [MeSH: Xylose] 1. an aldopentose epimeric with ribose at the 3 carbon and occurring in pyranose form; it is found in plants in the form of xylans. 2. [USP] an official preparation of xylose, used as a diagnostic aid in the determination of intestinal function.

**xy·lo·side** (zi-lo-sīd) a glycoside of xylose.

**xy·lu·lose** (zi′lu-lōs) [MeSH: Xylulose] a ketopentose epimeric with ribulose at the 3 carbon, occurring naturally as both the D- and L-isomers. The latter is excreted in the urine in essential pentosuria; the former, phosphorylated at the 5 carbon *(D-xylulose 5-phosphate),* is an intermediate in the pentose phosphate pathway.

**L-xy·lu·lose re·duc·tase** (zi′lu-lōs re-duk′tās) [EC 1.1.1.10] an enzyme of the oxidoreductase class that catalyzes the reduction of xylulose to xylitol, using NADPH as an electron donor. Deficiency of the enzyme, an autosomal recessive trait, leads to essential pentosuria.

**L-xy·lu·los·u·ria** (zi″lu-lo-su′re-ə) essential pentosuria.

**xy·lyl** (zi′ləl) the hydrocarbon radical $CH_3C_6H_4CH_2$—.

**xyph·oid** (zif′oid, zi′foid) sword-shaped; xiphoid.

**xys·ma** (zis′mə) [Gr. "that which is scraped or shaved off"] material such as bits of membrane that is seen in the stools of diarrhea.

**xys·ter** (zis′tər) [Gr. *xystēr* scraper] rasp (def. 1).

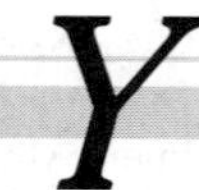

**Y** symbol for *yttrium.*

***y*** symbol for *ordinate.*

**Υ** the Greek capital letter upsilon.

***υ*** upsilon, the twentieth letter of the Greek alphabet.

**yab·a·pox** (yab'ə-poks") [*Yaba,* Nigeria, where the disease was first recognized in a rhesus monkey colony] a viral disease caused by the Yaba monkey tumor virus that causes subcutaneous tumorlike growths in African monkeys, especially cynomolgus monkeys; accidental human infection has occurred, characterized by localized skin nodules that resolve spontaneously.

**Yal·ow** (yal'o) Rosalyn Sussman. American medical physicist, born 1921; co-winner, with Roger Charles Louis Guillemin and Andrew Victor Schally, of the Nobel prize for medicine or physiology in 1977 for her work in endocrinology and the development of the radioimmunoassay technique.

**Yat·a·pox·vi·rus** (yat'ə-poks-vi"rəs) [*ya*bapox + *ta*napox + *virus*] [MeSH: Yatapoxvirus] a genus of viruses of the subfamily Chordopoxvirinae (family Poxviridae) comprising tanapox virus and Yaba monkey tumor virus.

**yaw** (yaw) a lesion of yaws (q.v.).
**guinea corn y.,** a lesion of yaws that resembles a grain of corn (maize).
**mother y.,** the initial cutaneous lesion of yaws; called also *frambesioma* and *framboesioma.*
**ringworm y.,** a circular or ring-shaped lesion of yaws.

**yawn·ing** (yawn'ing) [MeSH: Yawning] a deep, involuntary inspiration with the mouth open, often accompanied by the act of stretching. Cf. *pandiculation.* Called also *hiation* and *oscitation.*

**yaws** (yawz) [from Caribbean Indian name for the disease] [MeSH: Yaws] an endemic, infectious, tropical disease caused by *Treponema pertenue,* usually affecting persons under age 15, and spread by direct contact with skin lesions or contaminated fomites. The spirochete initially appears at the site of inoculation and then enters the body through abraded or otherwise compromised skin; then a painless papule appears and grows into a papilloma (mother yaw); when that heals, it leaves a scar, followed by crops of generalized secondary granulomatous papules that may relapse repeatedly. Late manifestations include destructive and deforming lesions of the skin, bones, and joints. Called also *frambesia, frambesia tropica, framboesia, granuloma tropicum, polypapilloma tropicum,* and *thymiosis.*
**crab y.,** yaws characterized by hyperkeratosis with fissuring and ulceration of the soles of the feet, and less commonly involving the palms of the hands.
**forest y.,** pian bois.

**Yb** symbol for *ytterbium.*

**yd** yard.

**yeast** (yēst) an imprecise term used to refer to a member of one of the two largest groupings of fungi (the other being *molds*); yeasts are single-celled, usually rounded fungi that produce by budding (blastospore formation). Some transform to a mycelial (mold) stage under certain environmental conditions, while others always remain single-celled. Many of the perfect yeasts are classified in the order Endomycetales, and many imperfect ones are classified in the form-family Moniliaceae. A few yeasts are pathogenic for humans.
**bakers' y., brewers' y.,** *Saccharomyces cerevisiae.*
**dried y.,** the dry cells of any suitable strain of *Saccharomyces cerevisiae,* usually a by-product of the brewing industry; used as a natural source of protein and B-complex vitamins.
**imperfect y.,** one whose perfect (sexual) stage is unknown; such yeasts are classified in the subphylum Deuteromycotina.
**perfect y.,** one whose perfect (sexual) stage is known; such yeasts are classified in the subphyla Ascomycotina and Basidiomycotina, or the phylum Zygomycota.

**yel·low** (yel'o) 1. one of the primary colors of wavelength of 571.5 to 578.5 millimicrons. 2. a dye or stain that produces a yellow color.
**acid y.,** fast y.
**alizarin y.,** an indicator used in the determination of hydrogen ion concentration with a pH range of 10.1–12.1.
**brilliant y.,** an indicator used in determining hydrogen ion concentration, with a pH range of 6–8.
**butter y.,** *p*-dimethylaminoazobenzene.
**corallin y.,** yellow corallin.
**fast y.,** a yellow, acid azo dye, used in staining bone.
**imperial y.,** aurantia.
**Manchester y., Martius y.,** a poisonous, yellow, azo dye used as a stain and in the preparation of light filters.
**metanil y., metaniline y. (extra),** an indicator used in the determination of hydrogen ion concentration, with a pH range of 1.2–2.3.
**methyl y.,** *p*-dimethylaminoazobenzene.
**naphthol y.,** Manchester y.
**Philadelphia y.,** phosphine, def. 3.

**yel·low·jack·et** (yel'o-jak"ət) any of various wasps that have dark bodies with yellow or brown markings.

**yel·lows** (yel'ōz) 1. a form of canine leptospirosis resembling the human condition Weil's syndrome, caused by *Leptospira interrogans*; formerly believed to be caused specifically by the serovar *L. icterohaemorrhagiae.* 2. hepatogenous photosensitization seen in sheep and goats in Scotland in the summertime, usually after ingestion of *Narthecium ossifragum* (the bog asphodel).

**yer·ba san·ta** (yer'bə sahn'tə) [Sp. "sacred herb"] *Eriodictyon californicum.*

**Yer·kes discrimination box** (yər'kēz) [Robert M. *Yerkes,* American psychobiologist, 1876–1956] see under *box.*

**Yer·sin·ia** (yər-sin'e-ə) [Alexandre J.E. *Yersin,* Swiss bacteriologist in Paris, 1863–1943] [MeSH: Yersinia] a genus of gram-negative, facultatively anaerobic, rod-shaped to ovoid bacteria of the family Enterobacteriaceae. It contains the organism responsible for bubonic plague (see *Y. pestis*) and other species that cause gastroenteritis and mesenteric lymphadenitis. Numerous serotypes based on the presence of an O antigen have been described.
**Y. enterocoli'tica,** a ubiquitous species isolated from mammals, birds, and frogs, and from material contaminated by feces; it is transmitted by infected food and water and by person-to-person contact and causes yersiniosis in humans.
**Y. frederikse'nii,** an opportunistic pathogen, a species that resembles *Y. enterocolitica* except that it ferments L-rhamnose.
**Y. interme'dia,** an opportunistic pathogen, a species that resembles *Y. enterocolitica* except that it ferments L-rhamnose, raffinose, and melibiose.
**Y. kristense'nii,** an opportunistic pathogen, a species that resembles *Y. enterocolitica* except that it does not ferment sucrose.
**Y. pes'tis,** the etiologic agent of bubonic and pneumonic plague in humans and rats, ground squirrels, and other rodents, transmitted from rat to rat and from rat to human by the rat flea, and from human to human by the human body louse; pathogenic for mice, guinea pigs, and rabbits. Formerly called *Bacterium pestis* and *Pasteurella pestis.*
**Y. pseudotuberculo'sis,** a species found in the intestinal tract of birds, rodents, and other animals. It is pathogenic, causing mesenteric lymphadenitis in humans and pseudotuberculosis in guinea pigs, white rats, rabbits, and occasionally other animals. Human infection occurs from contact with infected food or animals. Formerly called *Pasteurella pseudotuberculosis.*
**Y. ruc'keri,** a species that resembles *Y. enterocolitica* except that it does not ferment cellobiose. It is found in fresh waters and can cause red mouth disease in fish.

**yer·sin·ia** (yər-sin'e-ə) [MeSH: Yersinia] a bacterium of the genus *Yersinia.*

**Yer·sin·i·eae** (yər-sin'e-e) in some systems of classification, a tribe of gram-negative, facultatively anaerobic, rod-shaped bacteria of the family Enterobacteriaceae, consisting of the single genus *Yersinia.*

**yer·sin·i·o·sis** (yər-sin"e-o'sis) 1. infection with bacteria of the genus *Yersinia.* 2. specifically, infection with *Yersinia enterocolitica*; symptoms include acute gastroenteritis and mesenteric lymphadenitis in children and arthritis, septicemia, and erythema nodosum in adults. 3. pseudotuberculosis caused by *Yersinia pseudotuberculosis,* seen in guinea pigs, white rats, rabbits, and birds.

**yew** (yu) any of the evergreens of the genus *Taxus.*
**Pacific y.,** *Taxus brevifolia.*

**-yl** [Gr. *hylē* matter, substance] a chemical suffix signifying a radical, particularly a univalent hydrocarbon radical.

**-ylene** a suffix used in chemistry to denote a bivalent hydrocarbon radical.

**Yo·dox·in** (yo-dok'sin) trademark for preparations of iodoquinol.

**yo·him·bine** (yo-him'bēn) [MeSH: Yohimbine] an alkaloid from *Corynanthe johimbe* K. Schum. (Rubiaceae) and from *Rauwolfia serpentina* L. Benth. (Apocynaceae). It possesses adrenergic blocking properties and is used in arteriosclerosis and angina pectoris, and formerly as a local anesthetic and mydriatic and for its purported aphrodisiac properties.

**yoke** (yōk) 1. a connecting structure. 2. jugum.
**alveolar y's of mandible,** juga alveolaria mandibulae.
**alveolar y's of maxilla,** juga alveolaria maxillae.
**sphenoidal y.,** jugum sphenoidale.

**yolk** (yōk) [L. *vitellus*] 1. the stored nutrient of an egg or ovum. 2. crude wool fat or suint.
**accessory y.,** the part of the yolk that serves for the nutrition of the formative portion.
**egg y.,** the yellow portion of the egg of a bird.
**formative y.,** that part of the ovum from which the embryo is developed, as in birds.
**nutritive y.,** accessory y.

**Yo·me·san** (yo'me-sən) trademark for preparations of niclosamide.

**Young's operation** (yungz) [Hugh Hampton *Young,* American urologist, 1870–1945] see under *operation.*

**Young's rule** (yungz) [Thomas *Young,* English physician, physicist, and philologist, 1773–1829, the "father of physiologic optics"] see under *rule.*

**Young-Helm·holtz theory** (yung helm'hōlts) [Thomas *Young;* Herman Ludwig Ferdinand von *Helmholtz,* German physiologist, 1821–1894] see under *theory.*

**yper·ite** (i'pər-īt) dichlorodiethyl sulfide.

**yp·sil·i·form** (ip-sil'ĭ-form) upsiloid.

**yp·si·loid** (ip'sĭ-loid) upsiloid.

**yt·ter·bi·um** (ĭ-tər'be-əm) [from *Ytterby,* in Sweden] [MeSH: Ytterbium] a very rare metal; symbol, Yb; atomic number, 70; atomic weight, 173.04.

**yt·tri·um** (ĭ'tre-əm) [from *Ytterby,* in Sweden] [MeSH: Yttrium] a very rare metal, allied to cerium; symbol Y; atomic number, 39; atomic weight, 88.905.
**y. 90,** a radioactive isotope of yttrium, atomic mass 90, having a half-life of 64.1 hours and emitting beta particles (2.288 MeV); it localizes predominantly to bone, and also liver, and has been used in radiation synovectomy and, linked to antibody, in radioimmunotherapy.

# Z

**Z** symbol for *atomic number* and *impedance*.

**Z-** [Ger. *zusammen* together] a stereodescriptor used to specify the absolute configuration of compounds having double bonds. See *E-*.

*ζ* zeta, the sixth letter of the Greek alphabet.

**Zac·tane** (zak'tān) trademark for a preparation of ethoheptazine citrate.

**za·fir·lu·kast** (zə-fir'loo-kast) an antiasthmatic agent that acts as a leukotriene receptor antagonist; administered orally.

**Za·gam** (za'gam) trademark for a preparation of sparfloxacin.

**Zahn's infarct, lines (ribs)** (tsahnz) [Friedrich Wilhelm *Zahn*, German-born pathologist in Switzerland, 1845–1904] see under *infarct* and *line*.

**Za·hor·sky's disease** (zə-hor'skēz) [John *Zahorsky*, Hungarian-born American physician, 1871–1963] see *exanthema subitum* and *herpangina*.

**zal·ci·ta·bine** (zal-si'tə-bēn) [USP] [MeSH: Zalcitabine] 2′3′-dideoxycytidine, an analogue of 2′-deoxycytidine; an antiretroviral agent that is converted intracellularly into the active metabolite dideoxycytidine 5′-triphosphate that inhibits the action of reverse transcriptase; used in combination with zidovudine for the treatment of advanced HIV-1 infection, administered orally. Formerly called *dideoxycytidine (ddC)*.

**Za·mia** (za'me-ə) a genus of zamia palms whose leaves and seeds contain macrozamin and other toxic glycosides and cause hepatotoxicity, spinal cord degeneration, and cancer in humans and other animals. See also *zamia staggers*, under *staggers*.

**za·mia** (za'me-ə) 1. a poisonous cycad palm of genus *Zamia, Macrozamia*, or related genera; these trees contain toxic glycosides such as macrozamin. 2. misnomer for any cycad. See also *zamia staggers*, under *staggers*.

**Zang's space** (tsahngz) [Christoph Bonifacius *Zang*, German-born surgeon in Austria, 1772–1835] fossa supraclavicularis minor.

**Zan·o·sar** (zan'o-sər) trademark for preparations of streptozocin.

**Zan·tac** (zan'tak) trademark for a preparation of ranitidine hydrochloride.

**Zap·pert's chamber** (tsah'perts) [Julius *Zappert*, Czechoslovakian physician in Austria, 1867–1942] see under *chamber*.

**Za·ron·tin** (zə-ron'tin) trademark for a preparation of ethosuximide.

**Za·rox·o·lyn** (zə-rok'so-lin) trademark for a preparation of metolazone.

**Z-DNA** see under *DNA*.

**Zea** (ze'ə) [Gr. *zeia* single-grained wheat; maize] a genus of large grasses (family Gramineae), originally native to the Americas. *Z. mays* is maize or corn, a tall cereal plant that produces seeds or kernels on large ears. See also *corn oil*, under *oil*.

**zea·ral·e·nol** (zə-ral'ə-nol) zeranol.

**zea·ral·e·none** (zə-ral'ə-nōn) [MeSH: Zearalenone] an estrogenic mycotoxin produced by the fungus *Fusarium graminearum*; animals eating contaminated grain or flour products may develop fertility problems or vulvovaginitis. See also *zeranol*.

**zed·o·ary** (zed'o-ar″e) [L. *zedoaria*] the rhizome of *Curcuma zedoaria*, a plant of India, which resembles ginger; used medicinally as an aromatic stimulant and carminative.

**Zee·man effect** (tsa'mahn) [Pieter *Zeeman*, Dutch physicist, 1865–1943] see under *effect*.

**zein** (ze'in) [MeSH: Zein] a protein of the prolamin group, molecular weight about 40,000, found in corn; it does not contain tryptophan or lysine.

**zei·o·sis** (zi-o'sis) [Gr. *zein* to boil, seethe + *-osis*] bubbling or blebbing activity, giving the appearance of boiling in slow motion, observed at the periphery of cells cultured in artificial media.

**Zeis' glands** (tsīs) [Eduard *Zeis*, German ophthalmologist, 1807–1868] see under *gland*.

**zei·si·an stye** (zi'se-ən) [Eduard *Zeis*] see under *stye*.

**ze·ism** (ze'iz-əm) [L. *zea* maize, corn] any condition attributed to excessive use of maize in the diet, principally pellagra.

**ze·is·mus** (ze-is'məs) zeism.

**zeit·ge·ber** (zīt'ga-ber) [Ger. "time giver"] any of a number of periodic natural fluctuations, such as the cycle of light and darkness, that act as signals to control circadian rhythms.

**Zell·weg·er syndrome** (zel'weg-ər) [Hans Ulrich *Zellweger*, American pediatrician, born 1909] [MeSH: Zellweger Syndrome] cerebrohepatorenal syndrome; see under *syndrome*.

**Zem·u·ron** (zem'u-ron) trademark for a preparation of rocuronium bromide.

**Zen·a·pax** (zen'ə-paks) trademark for a preparation of daclizumab.

**Zen·ker's degeneration (necrosis), diverticulum** (tseng'kerz) [Friedrich Albert von *Zenker*, German pathologist, 1825–1898] see under *degeneration* and *diverticulum*.

**Zen·ker's fixative (fluid, solution)** (tseng'kerz) [Konrad *Zenker*, German histologist, died 1894] see under *fixative*.

**zen·ker·ism** (zeng'kər-iz-əm) [F. A. von *Zenker*] Zenker's degeneration; see under *degeneration*.

**zen·ker·ize** (zeng'kər-īz) [K. *Zenker*] to treat with Zenker's fixative.

**ze·o·lite** (ze'o-lit) any of a group of hydrated aluminum silicate minerals; some have ion-exchange properties and others are used as absorbents or filters. See also *erionite*.

**zeo·scope** (ze'o-skōp) [Gr. *zein* to boil, seethe + *-scope*] an apparatus for determining the alcoholic strength of a liquid by means of its boiling point.

**Zeph·i·ran Chloride** (zef'ĭ-rən) trademark for preparations of benzalkonium chloride.

**ze·ra·nol** (zer'ə-nol) [MeSH: Zeranol] a reduction product of zearalenone; an anabolic-estrogenic agent that has been used for estrogen replacement in humans but is used primarily in veterinary medicine as a growth stimulant. Called also *zearalenol*.

**ze·ro** (ze'ro) [Ital. "naught"] the point on a thermometer scale at which the graduation begins; the ice point on the Celsius and Réaumur scales and 32° below the ice point on the Fahrenheit.
**absolute z.**, the lowest possible temperature, designated as 0 on the Kelvin or Rankine scale; by definition this is equivalent to −273.15°C or −459.67°F.
**limes z.**, limes nul dose.
**physiologic z.**, the temperature at which a thermal stimulus ceases to cause a sensation.

**Zes·to·ret·ic** (zes″tə-ret'ik) trademark for a preparation of lisinopril and hydrochlorothiazide.

**Zes·tril** (zes'tril) trademark for a preparation of lisinopril.

**ze·ta** (za'tə) [Z, *ζ*] the sixth letter of the Greek alphabet.

**ze·ta·crit** (za'tə-krit) the packed-cell volume produced by the zeta sedimentation ratio procedure (see under *ratio*).

**Ze·ta·fuge** (za'tə-fūj) trademark for a specially designed centrifuge used in determination of the zeta sedimentation ratio.

**Ze·tar** (ze'tahr) trademark for a preparation of coal tar.

**zeu·go·po·di·um** (zoo″go-po'de-əm) zygopodium (see *limb*).

**zi·do·vu·dine** (zi-do'vu-dēn) [USP] [MeSH: Zidovudine] a synthetic thymidine analog that inhibits replication of some retroviruses, including the human immunodeficiency virus; used in the management of acquired immunodeficiency syndrome and advanced AIDS-related complex. Formerly called *azidothymidine*.

**Zie·gler's operation** (zēg'lərz) [Samuel Louis *Ziegler*, American ophthalmologist, 1861–1926] see under *operation*.

**Zie·hen-Op·pen·heim disease** (tse'hen-op'en-hīm) [Georg Theodor *Ziehen*, German neurologist, 1862–1950; Herman *Oppenheim*, German neurologist, 1858–1919] dystonia musculorum deformans.

**Ziehl-Neel·sen stain (method)** (tsēl-nāl'sen) [Franz *Ziehl*, German bacteriologist, 1857–1926; Friedrich Karl Adolf *Neelsen*, German pathologist, 1854–1894] see under *Stain*.

**Zielke in·stru·men·ta·tion** (tsēl'kə) [K. *Zielke*, German orthopedic surgeon, 20th century] see under *instrumentation*.

**Ziems·sen's motor point** (tsēm'senz) [Hugo Wilhelm von *Ziemssen*, German physician, 1829–1902] see under *point*.

**Zieve syndrome** (zēv) [Leslie *Zieve*, American physician, born 1915] see under *syndrome*.

**ZIFT** zygote intrafallopian transfer.

**zig·zag·plas·ty** (zig'zag-plas″te) the surgical technique of minimizing the visual impact of a long linear scar by breaking it up into short irregular segments at right or acute angles to each another.

**zimb** (zim) a fly of the genus *Pangonia*.

**Zim·mer·lin's atrophy** (tsĭ'mer-linz) [Franz *Zimmerlin*, Swiss physician, 1858–1932] see under *atrophy*.

**Zim·mer·mann's arch** (tsĭ'mer-mahnz) [Karl Wilhelm *Zimmermann*, German histologist, 1861–1935] see under *arch*.

**Zin·a·cef** (zin′ə-sef) trademark for a preparation of cefuroxime sodium.

**zinc** (zingk) [L. *zincum*] [MeSH: Zinc] a blue-white metal, many of whose salts are used in medicine; symbol, Zn; atomic number, 30; atomic weight, 65.37. Zinc is necessary in trace amounts in the body, and hence in the diet; it forms an essential part of many enzymes (e.g., carbonic anhydrase, important in carbon dioxide metabolism) and plays an important role in protein synthesis and in cell division. Deficiency in zinc is associated with anemia, short stature, hypogonadism, impaired wound healing, and geophagia. Zinc salts are often poisonous when inhaled or absorbed by the system, producing zinc poisoning (q.v.).
**z. acetate** [USP], a salt produced by the reaction of zinc oxide with acetic acid, used as a pharmaceutic necessity for zinc-eugenol cement and as an astringent, styptic, and formerly as an emetic.
**z. carbonate** [USP], a zinc salt used as a topical antiseptic and astringent. It may be used in the preparation of calamine (calamine [USP] contains zinc oxide).
**z. chloride,** 1. a compound, $ZnCl_2$, with a variety of industrial uses; if its fumes are inhaled they can cause zinc poisoning (q.v.). 2. [USP] a preparation used as a nutritional supplement in total parenteral nutrition. Zinc chloride is also used topically as an astringent and desensitizer for dentin.
**z. gluconate** [USP], a zinc salt used as a dietary supplement; administered orally.
**z. hydroxide,** a white powder, $Zn(OH)_2$, an ingredient of medicinal zinc peroxide.
**z. oxide,** 1. a compound, ZnO, used in welding; inhalation of its fumes can cause zinc poisoning (q.v.). 2. [USP] a powdered form of this compound, used topically as an astringent and protectant in various cutaneous conditions and as an ingredient in calamine. It is also found in several dental cements. Called also *white z.*
**z. peroxide,** a white to yellowish white odorless powder used in pharmaceuticals.
**z. peroxide, medicinal,** a mixture of zinc peroxide, zinc carbonate, and zinc hydroxide, used topically in a 40 per cent solution as a local anti-infective and oxidant. It is also used as an astringent and deodorant.
**z. phosphide,** the phosphide salt of zinc, a rodenticide that is toxic to most mammalian species, including humans; it causes vomiting, convulsions, and dyspnea from pulmonary edema.
**z. pyrithione,** a compound used as an antibacterial, topical antifungal, and antiseborrheic.
**z. salicylate,** a salt which has been used as an antiseptic and astringent.
**z. stearate** [USP], a compound of zinc with variable proportions of stearic acid and palmitic acid, used as a dusting powder.
**z. sulfate** [USP], the heptahydrate zinc salt of sulfuric acid, used as an astringent for the mucous membranes, especially for those of the eye, and considered specific for conjunctivitis due to *Haemophilus duplex.* It has also been used in various dermatological preparations and internally as an antiemetic, especially in the treatment of poisoning.
**z. undecylenate** [USP], see *undecylenic acid.*
**white z.,** z. oxide.

**zinc·al·ism** (zingk′əl-iz-əm) zinc poisoning; see under *poisoning.*

**zin·cif·er·ous** (zing-kif′ər-əs) containing zinc.

**zin·coid** (zing′koid) [*zinc* + *-oid*] pertaining to or resembling zinc.

**Zin·e·card** (zin′ə-kahrd) trademark for a preparation of dexrazoxane.

**Zin·gi·ber** (zin′jĭ-bər) a genus of leafy herbs of the family Zingiberaceae, native to southern Asia and southern Pacific islands. *Z. officina′le* is ginger, whose rhizome is ground into the spice also called ginger.

**Zink·er·na·gel** (tsing′kər-nah″gəl) Rolf M. Swiss immunologist, born 1944. Co-winner, with Peter C. Doherty, of the Nobel prize for medicine or physiology in 1996 for their discovery about how the immune system detects virus-infected cells.

**Zinn's artery,** etc. (tsinz) [Johann Gottfried *Zinn,* German anatomist, 1727–1759] see *anulus tendineus communis, arteria centralis retinae, circulus vasculosus nervi optici, fibrae zonulares,* and *zonula ciliaris;* and see under *cap.*

**Zins·ser-Cole-Eng·man syndrome** (tsin′ser-kōl-eng′mən) [Ferdinand *Zinsser,* German dermatologist, 1865–1952; Harold Newton *Cole,* American dermatologist, 1884–1966; Martin Feeney *Engman,* American dermatologist, 1869–1953] dyskeratosis congenita.

**zip·per** (zip′ər) a fastener made of two rows of protruding teeth which may be made to interdigitate, linking the rows.
**leucine z.,** a stretch of amino acids consisting of four to seven leucine residues, each separated by six amino acids, occurring adjacent to a highly basic stretch of amino acids in some DNA-binding proteins. The configuration of the region is a helix, arranged such that leucine residues from two separate helices can interdigitate or interact to form dimers; the basic regions are arranged so as to recognize and bind specific DNA sequences.

**zir·co·ni·um** (zir-ko′ne-əm) [MeSH: Zirconium] a rather rare metallic element; symbol Zr; atomic number, 40; atomic weight, 91.22; chiefly obtained from a mineral called zircon.

**Zith·ro·max** trademark for preparations of azithromycin.

**Zn** symbol for zinc.

**zo·ac·an·tho·sis** (zo″ak-ən-tho′sis) any dermatitis caused by the retention of animal structures, such as bristles, stings, or hairs.

**zo·an·throp·ic** (zo″ən-throp′ik) pertaining to or characterized by zoanthropy.

**zo·an·thro·py** (zo-an′thro-pe) [*zo-* + Gr. *anthrōpos* man] the delusion that one has become an animal.

**Zo·cor** (zo′kor) trademark for a preparation of simvastatin.

**Zo·fran** (zo′fran) trademark for a preparation of ondansetron hydrochloride.

**zo·ic** (zo′ik) [Gr. *zōikos* of or proper to animals] pertaining to or characterized by animal life.

**Zo·la·dex** (zo′lə-deks) trademark for a preparation of goserelin acetate.

**zo·la·ze·pam hy·dro·chlo·ride** (zo′la-zə-pam) [USP] a sedative-hypnotic compound used in veterinary practice in combination with tiletamine hydrochloride.

**Zol·lin·ger-El·li·son syndrome** (zol′in-jər-el′ĭ-son) [Robert Milton *Zollinger,* American surgeon, 1903–1992; Edwin H. *Ellison,* American surgeon, 1918–1970] [MeSH: Zollinger-Ellison Syndrome] see under *syndrome.*

**Zöll·ner's lines (figures)** (tserl′nerz) [Johann Karl Friedrich *Zöllner,* German physicist, 1834–1882] see under *line.*

**zol·mi·trip·tan** (zōl″mĭ-trip′tan) an antimigraine agent used to relieve acute migraine headaches, with or without aura; administered orally.

**Zo·loft** (zo′loft) trademark for a preparation of sertraline hydrochloride.

**zol·pi·dem tar·trate** (zōl-pi′dem) a non-benzodiazepine sedative-hypnotic administered orally.

**Zo·mig** (zo′mig) trademark for a preparation of zolmitriptan.

**zo·na** (zo′nə) gen. and pl. *zo′nae* [L. "a girdle"] 1. a zone: an encircling region or area. 2. herpes zoster. 3. [TA] a general term for an area with a specific boundary or characteristics.
**z. arcua′ta,** inner tunnel.
**z. cartilagi′nea,** limbus spiralis.
**z. cilia′ris,** ciliary zone.
**z. denticula′ta,** denticulate zone: the inner zone of the lamina basilaris ductus cochlearis with the limbus of the osseous spiral lamina.
**z. derma′tica,** an elevation of thick skin around the protruding mass in spina bifida.
**z. epitheliosero′sa,** an area of membranous tissue inside the zona dermatica.
**z. fascicula′ta,** fascicular zone: the thick middle layer of the adrenal cortex; it is the major source of glucocorticoids.
**z. glomerulo′sa,** glomerular zone: the thin outer layer of the adrenal cortex, contiguous with the capsule; it is the source of aldosterone.
**z. granulo′sa,** the peripheral stratified cuboidal epithelium of the ovarian follicle.
**z. hemorrhoida′lis,** hemorrhoidal zone: that part of the anal canal extending from the anal valves to the anus and containing the rectal venous plexus.
**z. incer′ta** [TA], a narrow layer of gray matter extending throughout most of the diencephalon, ventral to and separated from the thalamus by the thalamic fasciculus and laterally continuous with the reticular nucleus of the thalamus. See also *fields of Forel,* under *field.*
**z. ophthal′mica,** herpes zoster ophthalmicus.
**z. orbicula′ris articulatio′nis cox′ae** [TA], orbicular zone of hip joint: circular fibers of the articular capsule of the hip joint which form a ring around the neck of the femur; they are especially prominent at the inferior and posterior part of the capsule.
**z. pectina′ta,** pectinate zone: the outer part of the lamina basilaris ductus cochlearis running from the rods of Corti to the spiral ligament.
**z. pellu′cida,** 1. pellucid zone: a thick, transparent, noncellular layer or envelope of uniform thickness surrounding an oocyte; called also *oolemma.* Under the light microscope, it appears as a radially striated layer, which can be seen to be microvillous under the electron microscope, and is therefore called *z. radiata, zona striata,* or *striated membrane.* 2. area pellucida.
**z. perfora′ta,** the inner portion of the lamina basilaris ductus cochlearis.
**z. radia′ta,** see *z. pellucida,* def. 1.
**z. reticula′ris,** reticular zone: the inner layer of the adrenal cortex,

consisting of cells arranged as clearly anastomosing cords, and abutting the medulla.

**z. rolan'dica,** primary somatomotor area.

**z. stria'ta,** see *z. pellucida,* def. 1.

**z. tec'ta,** inner tunnel.

**z. transfor'mans,** transformation zone: the connective tissue layer of the intestinal wall where bacteria penetrating from the intestine are destroyed; called also *Turck's zone.*

**z. vasculo'sa,** vascular zone: a region in the supramastoid fossa containing many foramina for the passage of blood vessels.

**z. We'beri,** z. orbicularis articulationis coxae.

**zo·nae** (zo'ne) [L.] genitive and plural of *zona.*

**zo·nal** (zo'nəl) [L. *zona'lis*] of the nature of a zone.

**Zon·a·lon** (zon'əlon) trademark for a preparation of doxepin hydrochloride.

**zo·na·ry** (zo'nə-re) zonal.

**zone** (zōn) [Gr. *zōnē* a belt, girdle] a region or area, especially one with specific characteristics or boundary; called also *zona.*

## Zone

**abdominal z's,** regiones abdominales.

**active z.,** a site in a presynaptic membrane that is especially adapted for the release of synaptic vesicles.

**adoral z. of membranelles,** an area of serially arranged membranelles (three or more) along the left side of the oral area, typically in a buccal cavity or peristome, in ciliate protozoa.

**androgenic z.,** fetal z. of adrenal cortex.

**anelectrotonic z.,** polar z.

**z. of antibody excess,** prozone.

**z. of antigen excess,** in a precipitin reaction, the region of relatively high antigen concentration, in which soluble complexes are formed and the reaction is inhibited. Called also *postzone.*

**apical z.,** a narrow area along the mucous membrane over the apexes of the roots of the teeth.

**arcuate z.,** inner tunnel.

**biokinetic z.,** the range of temperatures within which the living cell carries on its life activities, lying approximately between 10° and 45°C.

**border z.,** a zone at the boundary of two contiguous structures, as that where the trophoblast and the endometrium meet.

**cervical z.,** that third of the coronal zone which is nearest the cervix of the tooth, marked by the cementoenamel junction of crown and root.

**chemoreceptor trigger z.,** part of the area postrema in the fourth ventricle that mediates physiological reactions to various chemicals and drugs and plays an indirect role in stimulation of vomiting. It mediates some impulses that in turn stimulate the vomiting center in the medulla.

**ciliary z.,** the outer of the two regions into which the anterior surface of the iris is divided by the collarette. Cf. *pupillary z.*

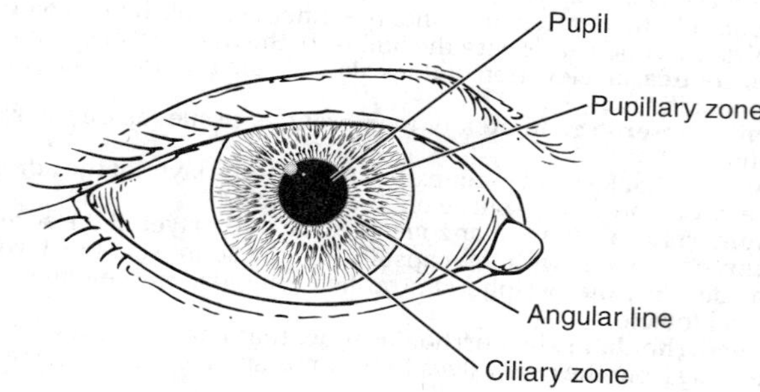


**comfort z.,** an environmental temperature between 13° and 21°C (55° to 70°F) with a humidity of 30 to 55 per cent.

**contact area z.,** the zone which includes the contact area of adjoining teeth; usually it is in the middle third of the coronal zone between the occlusal and the cervical zones.

**cornuradicular z.,** the outer part of the fasciculus cuneatus medullae spinalis.

**coronal z.,** the entire enamel area of the tooth crown above the cementoenamel junction, the demarcation between crown and root. The coronal zone is subdivided horizontally into three areas; the occlusal zone, the contact area zone, and the cervical zone. These divisions are also spoken of as the occlusal third, the middle third, and the cervical third.

**Cozzolino's z.,** fissula ante fenestram.

**definitive z. of adrenal cortex,** the smaller outer zone of the primordial adrenal cortex and that of the fetus and newborn, which develops into the zona fasciculata and zona glomerulosa. See also *fetal z. of adrenal cortex.*

**denticulate z.,** zona denticulata.

**dentofacial z.,** the entire lower part of the face; the region of the face overlying the teeth and the alveolar processes of the jaws.

**z's of discontinuity,** zones of varying optic density, seen with the slit lamp, in the lens of the eye; these zones are formed at particular periods in the prenatal development of the lens.

**dolorogenic z.,** a trigger zone to which stimulation produces pain or an attack of neuralgia.

**dorsal z. of His,** the smaller upper thickening of the dorsal portion of the embryonic spinal cord projecting into the central canal.

**entry z.,** the area where the dorsal roots enter the spinal cord on the brain stem.

**ependymal z.,** see under *layer.*

**epigastric z.,** epigastrium.

**epileptogenic z.,** see under *focus.*

**z. of equivalence,** z. of optimal proportions.

**erogenous z., erotogenic z.,** in psychoanalytic theory, an area of the body through which the libido expresses itself and which is therefore susceptible to erotic excitation upon stimulation; the primary sites are the oral, anal, and genital regions, but the other body orifices, breasts, and skin are also included.

**z. of exclusion,** the area of the cytoplasm devoid of all cytoplasmic components except the Golgi complex.

**extravisual z's,** those dioptric surfaces and media outside the visual zone that are practically incapable of accurately focusing light.

**fascicular z.,** zona fasciculata.

**fetal z. of adrenal cortex,** the inner zone of the primordial adrenal cortex and that of the fetus and newborn, which begins to involute shortly after birth; see also *definitive z. of adrenal cortex.* Called also *fetal adrenal cortex* and *provisional cortex.*

**Flechsig's primordial z's,** the cortex of the ascending frontal gyrus and the ascending parietal gyrus of the brain.

**glomerular z.,** zona glomerulosa.

**Golgi z.,** the intracellular zone close to the nucleus and containing the Golgi complex; in most secretory cells, it is between the nucleus and the apical surface through which expulsion of the secretion occurs.

**grenz z.,** a narrow layer in the upper dermis just below the epidermis, made up of densely packed collagen fibrils that are not infiltrated in the same way other layers of the dermis are.

**Head's z's,** areas of cutaneous sensitiveness associated with diseases of the viscera; called also *z's of hyperalgesia.*

**hemorrhoidal z.,** zona hemorrhoidalis.

**His' z's,** four thickenings which run the entire length of the embryonic spinal cord.

**z's of hyperalgesia,** Head's z's.

**hyperesthetic z.,** a region of the body surface marked by abnormal sensibility.

**hypogastric z.,** hypogastrium.

**inner z. of renal medulla,** the part of the medulla farthest in from the cortex, containing ascending and descending limbs of the thin tubule as well as the inner part of the medullary collecting duct.

**intermediate z. of spinal cord,** columna intermedia medullae spinalis.

**interpalpebral z.,** the part of the cornea not covered by the eyelids when the eye is open.

**juxtanuclear z.,** that part of the cytoplasm immediately adjoining the nucleus of a cell.

**Kambin's triangular working z.,** a triangular space free of significant vascular and neural structures that allows safe access to a lumbar disk in microdiskectomy; it is bounded anteriorly by the spinal nerve, inferiorly by the upper rim of the next lower vertebral plate, and posteriorly by the lateral edge of the superior articular process.

**keratogenous z.,** the zone immediately above the dome of the dermal papilla, in which the cellular components of a hair follicle undergo keratinization and form the hair shaft.

**language z.,** see under *area.*

**lateral z. of hypothalamus,** a longitudinal division of the hypothalamus, containing part of the preoptic nuclei as well as the supraoptic and tuberal nuclei and the nuclei of the mammillary body.

**Lissauer's marginal z.,** tractus posterolateralis.
**Looser's transformation z's,** dark lines seen on radiographs of bones, thought to represent pathological healing phases of fatigue fractures occurring in certain bone diseases.
**mantle z.,** see under *layer.*
**marginal z.,** 1. border z. 2. see under *layer.*
**medial z. of hypothalamus,** a longitudinal division of the hypothalamus, containing part of the preoptic nuclei as well as the anterior, dorsomedial, and ventromedial hypothalamic nuclei.
**motor z.,** see under *area.*
**nephrogenic z.,** the subcapsular layer of the kidney.
**neutral z.,** the potential space between the lips and cheeks on one side and the tongue on the other, natural or artificial teeth in this zone being subject to equal and opposite forces from the surrounding musculature.
**neutral z. of His,** a thickening of the dorsal portion of the embryonic spinal cord projecting into the central canal.
**Nitabuch z.,** see under *layer.*
**nuclear z.,** vortex lentis.
**occlusal z.,** that third of the coronal zone of the teeth which is nearest the occlusal plane.
**z. of optimal proportions,** in a precipitin reaction, the region of maximal precipitation, the antigen and antibody combining to form a cross-linked lattice. Called also *z. of equivalence.*
**orbicular z. of hip joint,** zona orbicularis articulationis coxae.
**outer z. of renal medulla,** the part of the medulla nearest to the cortex; containing the medullary part of the distal straight tubule as well as the outer part of the medullary collecting duct. It is subdivided into the *inner stripe* and the *outer stripe.*
**z. of oval nuclei,** a narrow band of sustentacular cells with oval nuclei in the olfactory mucosa.
**z. of partial preservation,** in spinal cord injury, a region where there may be only partial damage to nerves, including one to three spinal segments below the level of the injury.
**pectinate z.,** zona pectinata.
**pellucid z.,** zona pellucida.
**peripolar z.,** the region surrounding a polar zone.
**periventricular z.,** a longitudinal division of the hypothalamus, containing part of the preoptic nuclei as well as the periventricular, infundibular, and posterior nuclei.
**placental z.,** the area of the uterus to which the placenta is attached.
**polar z.,** the region immediately around an electrode applied to the body.
**pupillary z.,** the inner of the two regions into which the anterior surface of the iris is divided by the collarette. Cf. *ciliary z.*
**reticular z.,** zona reticularis.
**Rolando's z.,** primary somatomotor area.
**root z.,** entry z.
**z. of round nuclei,** a broad band of olfactory cells with round nuclei in the olfactory mucosa.
**rugae z.,** see under *area.*
**z's of Schreger,** see under *line.*
**segmental z.,** a zone of undifferentiated mesoderm between somites already formed and the primitive node, from which additional somites will be produced.
**sudanophobic z.,** a broad zone of cells that appears in the adrenal cortex of rats following hypophysectomy and does not stain with Sudan; see also *sudanophobic unit,* under *unit.*
**tendinous z's of heart,** see anulus fibrosus dexter/sinister cordis.
**thymus-dependent z.,** see under *area.*
**thymus-independent z.,** see under *area.*
**transformation z.,** zona transformans.
**transition z., transitional z.,** any anatomical region that marks the point at which the constituents of a structure change from one type to another; for example, the circle in the equator of the ocular lens in which epithelial fibers are developed into lens fibers, or the zone *(anocutaneous line)* that marks the junction of stratified squamous epithelium with columnar epithelium.
**transitional and respiratory z.,** terminal respiratory unit.
**triangular working z. (TWZ),** Kambin's triangular working z.
**trigger z.,** an area to which stimulation may cause physiological or pathological changes. See also *dolorogenic z.* and *trigger point.*
**Turck's z.,** zona transformans.
**umbau z's,** Looser's transformation z's.
**vascular z.,** zona vasculosa.
**visual z.,** those dioptric surfaces and media around an optic axis in which there is practically no aberration of light rays.
**Weber's z.,** zona orbicularis articulationis coxae.
**Weil's basal z.,** see under *layer.*
**Wernicke's z.,** see under *area.*
**Westphal's z.,** a zone of the posterior gray column of the spinal cord in the lumbar region; it is said to contain the exodic fibers concerned in the patellar reflex.
**X z.,** fetal z. of adrenal cortex.
**z. of Zinn,** zonula ciliaris.

**zo·nes·the·sia** (zo″nəs-the′zhə) [*zone* + *-esthesia*] a dysesthesia consisting of a sensation of constriction, as by a girdle. Called also *cincture sensation, girdle sensation,* and *strangalesthesia.*

**zo·nif·u·gal** (zo-nif′ə-gəl) [*zona* + *-fugal*[1]] passing outward from any area or region.

**zon·ing** (zōn′ing) the occurrence of a stronger fixation of complement in a lesser amount of suspected serum.

**zo·nip·e·tal** (zo-nip′ə-təl) [*zona* + *-petal*] passing from outside into any area or region.

**zo·no·skel·e·ton** (zo″no-skel′ə-ton) see *limb.*

**zo·nu·la** (zō′nu-lə) gen. and pl. *zo′nulae* [L., dim. of *zona*] a small zone, or zonule.
**z. adhe′rens,** an intermediate junction occurring between columnar epithelial cells, where it forms a complete band around the cell surface, just deep to the zonula occludens. The plasma membranes are separated by 15–30 nm and linked by and to actin filaments of the terminal web. Called also *belt desmosome.*
**z. cilia′ris** [TA], **z. cilia′ris [Zin′nii],** ciliary zonule: a system of fibers extending between the ciliary body and the equator of the lens, holding the lens in place; called also *Zinn's membrane* and *tendon* or *zonule of Zinn.*
**z. occlu′dens,** a type of tight junction (q.v.) occurring just below the apical surface in columnar epithelial cells; it extends completely around the cell perimeter above the zonula adherens and partially or wholly eliminates intercellular exchange. Called also *tight junction.*

**zo·nu·lae** (zo′nu-le) [L.] genitive and plural of *zonula.*

**zo·nu·lar** (zo′nu-lər) pertaining to a zonule.

**zo·nule** (zo′nūl) a small zone; called also *zonula.*
**ciliary z.,** zonula ciliaris.
**lens z.,** zonula ciliaris.

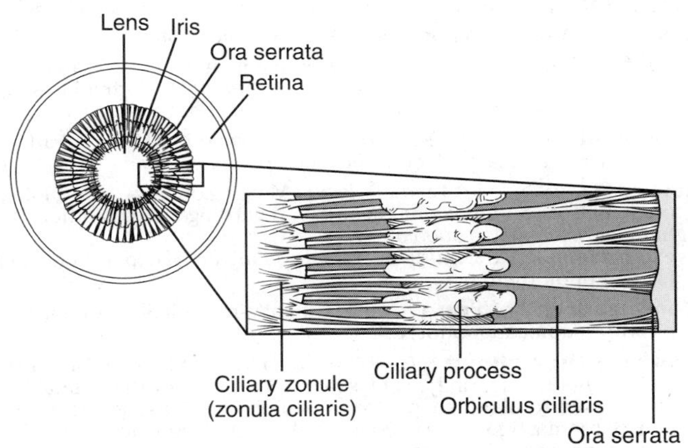


Zonula ciliaris (ciliary zonule), the system of suspensory ligaments holding the lens in position.

**z. of Zinn,** zonula ciliaris.

**zo·nu·li·tis** (zo″nu-li′tis) inflammation of the zonula ciliaris.

**zo·nu·lol·y·sis** (zo″nu-lol′ĭ-sis) [*zonule* + *lysis*] dissolution of the zonula ciliaris in surgery by means of enzymes such as chymotrypsin.

**zon·u·lot·o·my** (zon″u-lot′o-me) [*zonule* + *-tomy*] incision of the zonula ciliaris.

**zo·nu·ly·sis** (zon″u-li′sis) zonulolysis.

**zo(o)-** [Gr. *zōon* animal] a combining form denoting relationship to an animal.

**zoo·ag·glu·ti·nin** (zo″o-ə-gloo′tĭ-nin) a substance in animal poisons having the power of agglutinating red blood cells.

**zoo·bi·ol·o·gy** (zo″o-bi-ol′ə-je) [*zoo-* + *bio-* + *-logy*] zoology.

**zoo·bio·tism** (zo″o-bi′o-tiz-əm) biotics.

**zoo·blast** (zo′o-blast) [*zoo-* + *-blast*] an animal cell.

**zoo·chem·i·cal** (zo″o-kem′ĭ-kəl) pertaining to zoochemistry.

**zoo·chem·is·try** (zo″o-kem′is-tre) the study of the chemical reactions occurring in animal tissues.

**zoo·der·mic** (zo″o-dər′mik) [*zoo-* + *derm-* + *-ic*] performed with the skin of an animal; said of skin grafting in which the grafts are from the skin of an animal.

**zoo·de·tri·tus** (zo″o-de-tri′təs) biodetritus produced by the disintegration and decomposition of animal organisms. Cf. *phytodetritus.*

**zoo·dy·nam·ic** (zo″o-di-nam′ik) pertaining to zoodynamics (animal physiology).

**zoo·dy·nam·ics** (zo″o-di-nam′iks) [*zoo-* + *dynamics*] animal physiology.

**zoo·eras·tia** (zo″o-e-ras′te-ə) [*zoo-* + Gr. *erastēs* lover] bestiality.

**zoo·flag·el·late** (zo″o-flaj′ə-lāt) [*zoo-* + *-flagellate*] an animal-like flagellate protozoan of the class Zoomastigophorea. Cf. *phytoflagellate.*

**zoo·gen·e·sis** (zo″o-jen′ə-sis) zoogeny.

**zo·og·e·nous** (zo-oj′ə-nəs) 1. acquired from animals. 2. viviparous.

**zo·og·e·ny** (zo-oj′ə-ne) [*zoo-* + *-geny*] the development and evolution of animals.

**zoo·ge·og·ra·phy** (zo″o-je-og′rə-fe) the study of the distribution of animal life on the earth.

**zoo·glea** (zo″o-gle′ə) pl. *zoogle′ae* [*zoo-* + Gr. *gloios* gum] any microorganism of the genus *Zoogloea.*

**zoo·gle·al** (zo″o-gle′əl) pertaining to or characterized by the presence of zoogleae.

**Zoo·gloea** (zo″o-gle′ə) [MeSH: Zoogloea] a genus of gram-negative, aerobic, rod-shaped bacteria of the family Pseudomonadaceae, occurring in a gelatinous macroscopic flocculant mass and found in water and sewage.

**zo·o·gloea** (zo″o-gle′ə) [MeSH: Zoogloea] zooglea.

**zo·og·o·nous** (zo-og′ə-nəs) viviparous.

**zo·og·o·ny** (zo-og′ə-ne) [*zoo-* + Gr. *gonē* offspring] viviparity.

**zoo·graft·ing** (zo′o-graft″ing) xenografting of tissue from a different species into a human.

**zo·og·ra·phy** (zo-og′rə-fe) [*zoo-* + *-graphy*] a treatise on animals.

**zoo·hor·mone** (zo″o-hor′mōn) an animal hormone.

**zo·oid** (zo′oid) [*zoo-* + *-oid*] 1. resembling an animal. 2. an object or form which resembles an animal. 3. one of the individuals in a united colony of animals. See *blastozooid* and *oozooid.*

**zoo·lag·nia** (zo″o-lag′ne-ə) [*zoo-* + Gr. *lagneia* lust] sexual attraction toward animals. Cf. *bestiality* and *zoophilia.*

**zo·ol·o·gy** (zo-ol′ə-je) [*zoo-* + *-logy*] [MeSH: Zoology] the biology of animals; the sum of what is known regarding animals other than humans. Called also *zoobiology.*
**experimental z.,** the study of animals by means of experiments performed upon them.

**Zoo·mas·ti·goph·o·ra** (zo″o-mas″tĭ-gof′ə-rə) [MeSH: Zoomastigophora] Zoomastigophorea.

**Zoo·mas·ti·go·pho·rea** (zo″o-mas″tĭ-gə-for′e-ə) [*zoo-* + Gr. *mastix* whip + *phōros* bearing] a class comprising all of the animal-like, as opposed to plantlike, protozoa (subphylum Mastigophora, phylum Sarcomastigophora), collectively called zooflagellates. Zoomastigophoreans lack chromatophores and are heterotrophic, and most are either commensal or parasitic. They have one to many flagella and some are capable of ameboid movement with or without flagella. It comprises one superorder, Parabasilidea, and six orders: Choanoflagellida, Kinetoplastida, Proteromonadina, Retortamonadida, Diplomonadida, and Oxymonadida. Cf. *Phytomastigophorea.*

**zoo·mas·ti·go·pho·re·an** (zo″o-mas″tĭ-gə-for′e-ən) a protozoan of the class Zoomastigophorea.

**Zoon's erythroplasia** (zōnz) [Johannes Jacobus *Zoon,* Dutch dermatologist, born 1902] balanitis circumscripta plasmacellularis.

**zo·on·er·y·thrin** (zo″on-er′ĭ-thrin) [*zoo-* + Gr. *erythros* red] crustaceorubin.

**zoo·nite** (zo′o-nīt) a cerebrospinal metamere.

**zo·on·o·my** (zo-on′ə-me) [*zoo-* + Gr. *nomos* law] zoology.

**zoo·no·sis** (zo″o-no′sis, zo-on′ə-sis) pl. *zoono′ses* [*zoo-* + *nos-* + *-is*] a disease of animals that may be transmitted to humans under natural conditions, such as brucellosis or rabies.

**zoo·no·sol·o·gy** (zo″o-no-sol′ə-je) [*zoo-* + *noso-* + *-logy*] the classification of diseases of animals. Cf. *zoopathology.*

**zoo·not·ic** (zo″o-not′ik) transmissible from animals to humans under natural conditions; pertaining to or constituting a zoonosis.

**Zoo·pa·ga·les** (zo″ə-pə-ga′lēz) an order of perfect fungi of the phylum Zygomycota, class Zygomycetes, many of which are saprobes; it includes the genus *Piptocephalis,* which can infect humans.

**zoo·para·site** (zo″o-par′ə-sīt) animal parasite.

**zoo·para·sit·ic** (zo″o-par″ə-sit′ik) pertaining to or produced by zooparasites.

**zoo·pa·thol·o·gy** (zo″o-pə-thol′ə-je) animal pathology; the study of the diseases of animals. Cf. *veterinary medicine.*

**zo·op·er·al** (zo-op′ər-əl) pertaining to zoopery.

**zo·op·ery** (zo-op′ər-e) [*zoo-* + Gr. *peiran* to experiment] the performing of experiments on animals.

**zo·oph·a·gous** (zo-of′ə-gəs) [*zoo-* + *phag-* + *-ous*] carnivorous.

**zoo·phile** (zo′o-fīl) [*zoo-* + *-phile*] 1. zoophilic. 2. an antivivisectionist.

**zoo·phil·ia** (zo″o-fil′e-ə) abnormal fondness for animals; in particular, a paraphilia in which intercourse or other sexual activity with animals is the preferred method of achieving sexual excitement.

**zoo·phil·ic** (zo″o-fil′ik) preferring other animals to human beings, such as certain mosquitoes and dermatophytes. Cf. *anthropophilic* and *anthropozoophilic.*

**zoo·phil·ism** (zo-of′ĭ-liz-əm) 1. fondness for animals; antivivisection. 2. the state of being zoophilic.
**erotic z.,** sexual pleasure experienced in the fondling of animals.

**zo·oph·i·lous** (zo-of′ĭ-ləs) zoophilic.

**zoo·pho·bia** (zo″o-fo′be-ə) [*zoo-* + *-phobia*] irrational fear of animals.

**zoo·phys·i·ol·o·gy** (zo″o-fiz″e-ol′ə-je) animal physiology.

**zoo·phyte** (zo′o-fīt) [*zoo-* + *-phyte*] [MeSH: Bryozoa] any plantlike animal, such as a sponge or hydroid.

**zoo·plank·ton** (zo″o-plangk′ton) [*zoo-* + *plankton*] [MeSH: Zooplankton] the minute animal organisms which, with those of the vegetable kingdom (phytoplankton), make up the plankton of natural waters.

**zoo·plas·ty** (zo′o-plast″te) [*zoo-* + *-plasty*] zoografting.

**zoo·pre·cip·i·tin** (zo″o-pre-sip′ĭ-tin) a precipitin obtained by injections of protein substances of animal origin.

**zoo·pro·phy·lax·is** (zo″o-pro″fĭ-lak′sis) 1. prophylaxis applied to animals; veterinary prophylaxis. Cf. *veterinary medicine.* 2. the prevention or amelioration of disease (e.g., smallpox) in humans as a result of previous exposure to heterologous infection of animal origin (e.g., cowpox). 3. protection of humans from bites of mosquitoes by providing cattle or other animals for the mosquitoes to feed on.

**zo·op·sia** (zo-op′se-ə) [*zoo-* + *-opsia*] a hallucination in which the patient thinks he sees animals.

**zoo·psy·chol·o·gy** (zo″o-si-kol′ə-je) animal psychology.

**zoo·sa·dism** (zo″o-sa′diz-əm) sadism directed toward animals.

**zo·o·sis** (zo-o′sis) [*zoo-* + *-osis*] any disease due to animal agents.

**zoo·sperm** (zo′o-spərm) [*zoo-* + *sperm*] spermatozoon.

**zoo·sper·mia** (zo″o-spər′me-ə) the presence of live spermatozoa in the ejaculated semen.

**zoo·spo·ran·gi·um** (zo″o-spə-ran′je-əm) pl. *zoosporan′gia* [*zoo-* + *sporangium*] the case within which zoospores are developed.

**zoo·spore** (zo′o-spor) [*zoo-* + *spore*] a motile spore, such as an asexual flagellate of certain algae and lower fungi, or a minute sexual or asexual flagellate or ameboid spore produced by certain protozoa; it forms within a case called a zoosporangium. Called also *flagellospore.*

**zoo·ste·roid** (zo″o-ste′roid) any steroid of animal origin.

**zoo·ste·rol** (zo″o-ste′rol) any sterol of animal origin.

**zoo·tech·nics** (zo″o-tek′niks) the raising, breeding, and handling of animals in domestication or captivity. Called also *zootechny.*

**zoo·tech·ny** (zo″o-tek′ne) [*zoo-* + Gr. *technē* art] zootechnics.

**zo·ot·ic** (zo-ot′ik) pertaining to animals other than humans.

**zo·ot·o·mist** (zo-ot′ə-mist) a comparative anatomist.

**zoo·tox·in** (zo″o-tok′sin) [*zoo-* + *toxin*] a toxic substance of animal origin, such as the venoms of snakes, spiders, and scorpions.

**zoo·troph·ic** (zo″o-trof′ik) [*zoo-* + *-trophic*] pertaining to the nutrition of animals.

**zoo·tropho·tox·ism** (zo″o-trof″o-tok′siz-əm) [*zoo-* + *tropho-* + *tox-* + *-ism*] poisoning with animal foods.

**Zop·fi·us** (zop′fe-əs) in former systems of classification, a genus of bacteria made up of organisms now classified as *Kurthia.*

**zor·ba·my·cin** (zor-bə-mi′sin) an antibacterial antibiotic derived from a variant of *Streptomyces bikiniensis.*

**zo·ru·bi·cin hy·dro·chlo·ride** (zo-roo′bĭ-sin) an antineoplastic, $C_{34}H_{35}N_3O_{10}$·HCl.

**zos·ter** (zos′tər) [Gr. *zōstēr* a girdle] herpes zoster.
**z. si′ne eruptio′ne, z. si′ne her′pete,** pain typical of herpes zoster in an appropriate sensory area but not followed by the development of characteristic lesions.
**ophthalmic z.,** herpes zoster ophthalmicus.

**zos·ter·i·form** (zos-ter′ĭ-form) zosteroid.

**zos·ter·oid** (zos′tər-oid) resembling herpes zoster.

**Zos·trix** (zos′triks) trademark for a preparation of capsaicin.

**Zo·syn** (zo′zin) trademark for a combination preparation of piperacillin sodium and tazobactam sodium.

**Zo·vir·ax** (zo-vi′raks) trademark for preparations of acyclovir.

**Z-plas·ty** (ze-plas′te) a plastic operation for the relaxation of contractures, in which a Z-shaped incision is made, the middle bar of the Z being over the contracted scar, and the triangular flaps rotated so that their apices cross the line of contracture.

**Zr** symbol for *zirconium.*

**ZSR** zeta sedimentation ratio.

**Zu·ber·el·la** (zoo″bər-el′ə) in former systems of classification, a genus of bacteria made up of organisms now classified in the genera *Bacteroides* and *Fusobacterium.*

**zuck·er·guss·darm** (tsook′er-goos″dahrm) [Ger. "sugar-icing intestine"] peritonitis chronica fibrosa encapsulans.

**zuck·er·guss·le·ber** (tsook′er-goos″la-ber) [Ger. "sugar-icing liver"] perihepatitis chronica hyperplastica.

**Zuck·er·kan·dl's bodies (organs), convolution, dehiscences** (tsook′er-kahn″dəlz) [Emil *Zuckerkandl,* Hungarian-born anatomist in Germany and Austria, 1849–1910] see *corpora para-aortica,* under *corpus,* see *gyrus paraterminalis,* and see under *dehiscence.*

**zu·clo·mi·phene** (zoo-klo′mĭ-fēn) the *trans*-isomer of the gonad-stimulating principle clomiphene citrate (q.v.); called also *trans-clomiphene.* Cf. *enclomiphene.*

**Zum·busch's psoriasis** (tsoom′boosh-əz) [Leo von *Zumbusch,* German dermatologist, 1874–1940] generalized pustular psoriasis.

**zwit·ter·ion** (tsvit′er-i″on) a dipolar ion, i.e., an ion that has both positive and negative regions of charge; amino acids, for example, occur as zwitterions in neutral solution, and the pH value at which the zwitterion state is at a maximum is the isoelectric point.

**Zy·ban** (zi′ban) trademark for a preparation of bupropion hydrochloride.

**zy·gal** (zi′gəl) [*zyg-* + *-al*[1]] shaped like a yoke.

**zy·ga·po·phys·e·al** (zi″gə-po-fiz′e-əl) pertaining to an articular process of a vertebra (zygapophysis).

**zy·ga·poph·y·sis** (zi″gə-pof′ĭ-sis) pl. *zygapoph′yses* [*zyg-* + *apophysis*] an articular process of a vertebra.

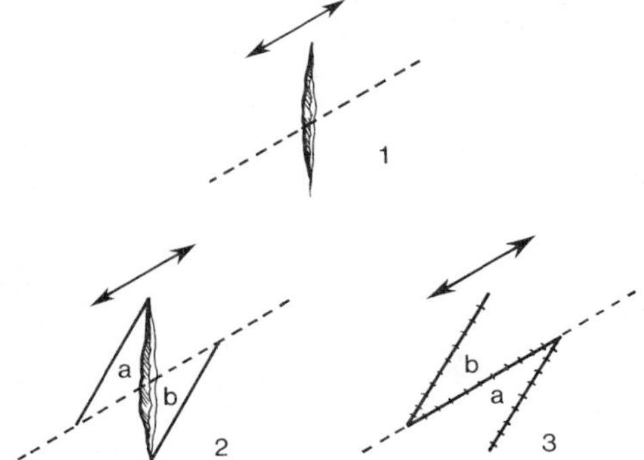


Z-plasty, showing the direction of relaxed skin tension lines *(arrow),* desired position of final scar *(dotted line),* and the two flaps to be juxtaposed *(a, b).*

**z. inferior,** TA alternative for *processus articularis inferior vertebrae.*
**z. superior,** TA alternative for *processus articularis superior vertebrae.*

**zyg·ia** (zij′e-ə) plural of *zygion.*

**zyg·i·on** (zij′e-on) pl. *zyg′ia* [Gr.] a craniometric and cephalometric landmark, being the most laterally situated point on either zygomatic arch.

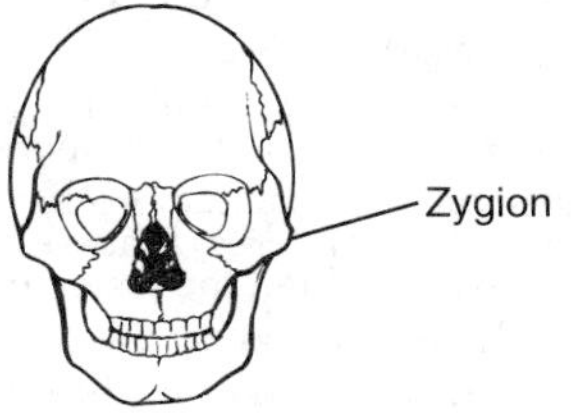


**zyg(o)-** [Gr. *zygon* yoke] a combining form meaning yoked or joined, or denoting relationship to a junction.

**Zy·go·co·ty·le lu·na·tum** (zi″go-ko′tĭ-le loo-na′təm) a trematode parasitic in the intestine of a variety of hosts, including rats, cattle, and ducks in North America.

**zy·go·dac·ty·ly** (zi″go-dak′tə-le) [*zygo-* + Gr. *daktylos* finger] a term sometimes used to designate simple syndactyly, as distinguished from syndactyly in which there is bony fusion between the phalanges of the digits involved; usually occurring in the hand between the third and fourth digits and in the foot between the fourth and fifth.

**zy·go·ma** (zi-go′mə) [Gr. *zygōma* bolt or bar] [MeSH: Zygoma] 1. processus zygomaticus ossis temporalis. 2. arcus zygomaticus. 3. a term sometimes applied to the os zygomaticum.

**zy·go·mat·ic** (zi″go-mat′ik) 1. see *os zygomaticum* (zygomatic bone). 2. connecting with or in the region of the os zygomaticum.

**zy·go·mat·i·co·fa·cial** (zi″go-mat″ĭ-ko-fa′shəl) pertaining to the zygomatic arch, process, or bone and the face.

**zy·go·mat·i·co·fron·tal** (zi″go-mat″ĭ-ko-frun′təl) pertaining to the zygomatic arch, process, or bone and the frontal bone.

**zy·go·mat·i·co·max·il·lary** (zi″go-mat″ĭ-ko-mak′sĭ-lar″e) pertaining to the zygomatic arch, process, or bone and the maxilla.

**zy·go·mat·i·co·or·bi·tal** (zi″go-mat″ĭ-ko-or′bĭ-təl) pertaining to the zygomatic arch, process, or bone and the orbit.

**zy·go·mat·i·co·sphe·noid** (zi″go-mat″ĭ-ko-sfe′noid) pertaining to the zygomatic arch, process, or bone and the sphenoid bone.

**zy·go·mat·i·co·tem·po·ral** (zi″go-mat″ĭ-ko-tem′pər-əl) pertaining to the zygomatic arch, process, or bone and the temporal bone.

**zy·go·max·il·la·re** (zi″go-mak′sĭ-lar″e) [L.] a craniometric point at the inferior end of the zygomatic suture.

**zy·go·max·il·lary** (zi″go-mak′sĭ-lar″e) zygomaticomaxillary.

**Zy·go·my·ce·tes** (zi″go-mi-se′tēz) [*zygo-* + Gr. *mykēs* fungus] a class of saprobic and parasitic fungi of the phylum Zygomycota, having a mycelial thallus, coenocytic hyphae, and chitinous cell walls; sexual reproduction is by means of zygospores. Pathogenic organisms are included in the orders Entomophthorales, Mucorales, and Zoopagales.

**zy·go·my·co·sis** (zi″go-mi-ko′sis) 1. mucormycosis. 2. any fungal infection with members of the class Zygomycetes, including entomophthoromycosis and mucormycosis.
**rhinocerebral z.,** zygomycosis that has spread from the paranasal sinuses to the brain; see *rhinocerebral mucormycosis* and *entomophthoromycosis conidiobolae.*
**rhinofacial z.,** rhinoentomophthoromycosis.
**subcutaneous z.,** entomophthoromycosis basidiobolae.

**Zy·go·my·co·ta** (zi″go-mi-ko′tə) a phylum of perfect fungi consisting of soil saprobes and invertebrate parasites; it includes the classes Zygomycetes and Trichomycetes. Organisms may cause human or animal infection in debilitated or highly stressed individuals. In some systems of classification, it is considered a subphylum, Zygomycotina, and placed under the phylum Eumycota.

**Zy·go·my·co·ti·na** (zi″go-mi″ko-ti′nə) [MeSH: Zygomycotina] name given to Zygomycota when it is seen as a subphylum under Eumycota.

**zy·gon** (zi′gon) [Gr. "bar" or "yoke"] the bar or stem connecting the two branches of a zygal fissure.

**zy·go·phore** (zi′go-for) a specialized branch of a hypha containing isogametes (zygospheres) that unite to form a zygospore.

**zy·go·po·di·um** (zi″go-po′de-əm) see *limb.*

**zy·go·sis** (zi-go′sis) [Gr. *zygōsis* a balancing] conjugation; the sexual union of two unicellular organisms.

**zy·gos·i·ty** (zi-gos′ĭ-te) [*zygon* + *-ity* state or condition] the condition relating to conjugation, or to the zygote, as *(a)* the state of a cell or individual in regard to the alleles determining a specific character, whether identical (homozygosity) or different (heterozygosity); or *(b),* in the case of twins, whether developing from one zygote (monozygosity) or two (dizygosity). Often used as a word termination affixed to a root descriptive of the condition.

**zy·go·sperm** (zi′go-spərm) zygospore.

**zy·go·sphere** (zi′go-sfēr) a gamete arising from a zygophore which unites with another to form a zygospore.

**zy·go·spore** (zi′go-spor) a sexual spore formed by the conjugation of two isogametes (zygospheres) that are morphologically identical, or in the Zygomycetes, from the fusion of like gametangia.

**zy·go·style** (zi′go-stīl) the last coccygeal vertebra.

**zy·gote** (zi′gōt) [Gr. *zygōtos* yoked together] [MeSH: Zygote] the fertilized ovum; the cell resulting from union of a male and a female gamete (sperm and ovum). More precisely, the cell after synapsis at the completion of fertilization until first cleavage. Also, used loosely to refer to the fertilized ovum and early derivatives for an indefinite period. Cf. *conceptus.*

**zy·go·tene** (zi′go-tēn) [Gr. *zygōtos* yoked together] the synaptic stage of the first meiotic prophase in which the two leptotene chromosomes undergo pairing by the formation of synaptonemal complexes to form a bivalent structure. See also *diplotene, leptotene,* and *pachytene.* Called also *amphitene.*

**zy·got·ic** (zi-got′ik) pertaining to a zygote.

**Zy·lo·prim** (zi′lo-prim) trademark for a preparation of allopurinol.

**zym(o)-** [Gr. *zymē* leaven] a combining form denoting relationship to an enzyme, or to fermentation.

**zy·mo·chem·is·try** (zi″mo-kem′is-tre) the chemistry of fermentation.

**zy·mo·gen** (zi′mo-jən) a proenzyme, particularly of a proteolytic enzyme.

**zy·mo·gen·ic** (zi″mo-jen′ik) pertaining to a zymogen (proenzyme) or to its transformation into an active enzyme form.

**zy·mog·e·nous** (zi-moj′ə-nəs) zymogenic.

**Zy·mo·mo·nas** (zi″mo-mo′nəs) [*zyme* + Gr. *monas* unit, from *monos* single] [MeSH: Zymomonas] a genus of facultatively anaerobic, gram-negative, rod-shaped bacteria that are motile with polar flagella, occurring as a spoiler in beer and cider, as fermenting agents in plant saps, and present on bees, and in ripening honey. The type species is *Z. mo′bilis.*

**zy·mo·san** (zi′mo-sən) [MeSH: Zymosan] a mixture of polysaccharides, proteins, and ash, of variable concentration, derived from the cell walls, or the entire cell, of yeast, commonly *Saccharomyces cerevisiae.* It is anticomplementary, absorbing the C3 component of complement, and is used in assaying properdin.

**zy·mos·ter·ol** (zi-mos′tər-ol) a mycosterol occurring in yeast as an intermediate in the synthesis of cholesterol.

**Zyr·tec** (zir′tek) trademark for a preparation of cetirizine hydrochloride.

**Zz.** abbreviation for L. *zin′giber,* ginger.

# APPENDICES

# APPENDIX 1

## Selected Abbreviations Used in Medicine

| Abbreviation | Meaning |
|---|---|
| **A** | accommodation |
| | adenine |
| | adenosine |
| | alveolar gas (as subscript) |
| | ampere |
| | anode |
| | anterior |
| **AI** | first auditory area |
| **AII** | second auditory area |
| ***A*** | absorbance |
| | activity |
| | admittance |
| | area |
| | mass number |
| **$A_2$** | aortic second sound |
| **Å** | angstrom |
| **a** | accommodation |
| | arterial blood (as subscript) |
| **a.** | L. arteria (artery) |
| ***a*** | specific absorptivity |
| | acceleration |
| | activity |
| **$\alpha$** | the $\alpha$ chain of hemoglobin |
| | Bunsen coefficient |
| | the heavy chain of IgA |
| **AA** | achievement age |
| | Alcoholics Anonymous |
| | amino acid |
| **aa.** | L. arteriae (arteries) |
| **AAV** | adeno-associated virus |
| **Ab** | abbreviation for antibody |
| **ABC** | aspiration biopsy cytology |
| **ABE** | acute bacterial endocarditis |
| **ABG** | arterial blood gases |
| **ABP** | arterial blood pressure |
| **abst** | abstract |
| **abstr** | abstract |
| **AC** | air conduction |
| | alternating current |
| | aortic closure |
| | anodal closure |
| | axiocervical |
| | acromioclavicular |
| **ACAT** | acyl CoA: cholesterol acyltransferase |
| **Acc** | accommodation |
| **ACCl** | anodal closure clonus |
| **ACD** | acid citrate dextrose |
| **ACE** | angiotensin converting enzyme |
| | adrenocortical extract |
| **ACG** | angiocardiography |
| **AcG** | accelerator globulin |
| **ACh** | acetylcholine |
| **AChE** | acetylcholinesterase |
| **ACP** | acid phosphatase |
| **ACTH** | adrenocorticotropic hormone |
| **AD** | alcohol dehydrogenase |
| | anodal duration |
| **A.D.** | L. auris dextra (right ear) |
| **ADA** | adenosine deaminase |
| **ADCC** | antibody-dependent cell-mediated cytotoxicity |
| **ADL** | activities of daily living |
| **ADH** | alcohol dehydrogenase |
| | antidiuretic hormone |
| **ADP** | adenosine diphosphate |
| **AEP** | auditory evoked potential |
| **AF** | atrial fibrillation |
| **AFib** | atrial fibrillation |
| **AFl** | atrial flutter |
| **AFO** | ankle-foot orthosis |
| **AFP** | alpha-fetoprotein |
| **AFX** | atypical fibroxanthoma |
| **AG** | atrial gallop |
| **Ag** | antigen |
| **AGEPC** | acetyl glyceryl ether phosphoryl choline |
| **AGT** | antiglobulin test |
| **AGTH** | adrenoglomerulotropin |
| **AGV** | aniline gentian violet |
| **ah** | hyperopic astigmatism |
| **AHF** | antihemophilic factor (blood coagulation Factor VIII) |
| **AHG** | antihemophilic globulin (blood coagulation Factor VIII) |
| **AI** | anaphylatoxin inhibitor |
| | aortic incompetence |
| | aortic insufficiency |
| | apical impulse |
| | artificial insemination |
| **AICD** | automatic implantable cardioverter-defibrillator |
| **AID** | donor insemination |
| **AIDS** | acquired immunodeficiency syndrome |
| **AIH** | homologous insemination |
| **AIHA** | autoimmune hemolytic anemia |
| **AILD** | angioimmunoblastic lymphadenopathy with dysproteinemia |
| **ALA** | $\alpha$-aminolevulinic acid |
| **Ala** | alanine |
| **ALARA** | as low as reasonably achievable (exposure dose of radiation) |
| **ALAT** | alanine aminotransferase |
| **ALG** | antilymphocyte globulin |
| **ALL** | acute lymphoblastic anemia |
| **ALP** | alkaline phosphatase |
| **ALS** | amyotrophic lateral sclerosis |
| | antilymphocyte serum |
| **Am** | americium |
| **am** | myopic astigmatism |
| | meterangle |
| | ametropia |
| **Amh** | mixed astigmatism with myopia predominating over hyperopia |
| **AMI** | acute myocardial infarction |
| **AMP** | adenosine monophosphate |
| **3′5′-AMP** | cyclic adenosine monophosphate |
| | cyclic AMP |
| **AML** | acute myelogenous leukemia |
| **amp** | ampere |
| **amu** | atomic mass unit |
| **An** | anode |
| | anodal |
| **ANA** | antinuclear antibodies |
| **anat.** | anatomy |
| | anatomical |
| **ANF** | antinuclear factor |
| **ANOVA** | analysis of variance |
| **ANS** | anterior nasal spine |
| | autonomic nervous system |
| **ant.** | anterior |
| **ANUG** | acute necrotizing ulcerative gingivitis |
| **AO** | anodal opening |
| | opening of the atrioventricular valves |
| **AOS** | anodal opening sound |
| **AP** | action potential |
| | angina pectoris |
| | anterior pituitary |
| | anteroposterior |
| | arterial pressure |

| Abbreviation | Meaning |
|---|---|
| **APB** | atrial premature beat |
| **APC** | atrial premature complex |
| **APD** | atrial premature depolarization |
| **APE** | anterior pituitary extract |
| **APTT, aPTT** | activated partial thromboplastin time |
| **AQ** | achievement quotient |
| **AR** | alarm reaction |
| | aortic regurgitation |
| | artificial respiration |
| **ARC** | anomalous retinal correspondence |
| | AIDS-related complex |
| **ARD** | acute respiratory disease |
| **ARDS** | acute respiratory distress syndrome |
| | adult respiratory distress syndrome |
| **Arg** | arginine |
| **AROA** | autosomal recessive ocular albinism |
| **ART** | assisted reproductive technology |
| | automated reagin test |
| **AS** | aortic stenosis |
| | arteriosclerosis |
| **A.S.** | L. auris sinistra (left ear) |
| **As** | astigmatism |
| **ASA** | acetylsalicylic acid |
| | argininosuccinic acid |
| **ASAT** | aspartate aminotransferase |
| **ASCVD** | arteriosclerotic cardiovascular disease |
| **ASH** | asymmetrical septal hypertrophy |
| **ASHD** | arteriosclerotic heart disease |
| **ASL** | antistreptolysin |
| **Asn** | asparagine |
| **ASO** | arteriosclerosis obliterans |
| **Asp** | aspartic acid |
| **ASS** | anterior superior spine |
| **AST** | aspartate transaminase |
| **Ast** | astigmatism |
| **Asth** | asthenopia |
| **AT** | atrial tachycardia |
| **ATA** | alimentary toxic aleukia |
| **ATCC** | American Type Culture Collection |
| **ATG** | antithymocyte globulin |
| **ATL** | adult T-cell leukemialymphoma |
| **atm** | atmosphere |
| **ATN** | tyrosinase-negative oculocutaneous albinism |
| **ATP** | adenosine triphosphate |
| **ATPase** | adenosinetriphosphatase |
| **ATS** | antitetanic serum |
| **at vol** | atomic volume |
| **At wt** | atomic weight |
| **Au** | gold (L. aurum) |
| | Australian antigen |
| **AUL** | acute undifferentiated leukemia |
| **AV, A-V** | atrioventricular |
| | arteriovenous |
| **AVN** | atrioventricular node |
| **AVP** | arginine vasopressin |
| **AVRT** | atrioventricular reciprocating tachycardia |
| **awu** | atomic weight unit |
| **ax.** | axis |
| **AZQ** | diaziquone |
| **B** | bel |
| | boron |
| ***B*** | magnetic flux density |
| **b** | born |
| | base (nucleic acids) |
| **$\beta$** | the $\beta$ chain of hemoglobin |
| **BAEP** | brainstem auditory evoked potential |
| **BAL** | dimercaprol |
| **BBB** | blood-brain barrier |
| | bundle branch block |
| **BBBB** | bilateral bundle branch block |
| **BBT** | basal body temperature |
| **BC** | bone conduction |
| **BCAA** | branched chain amino acid |
| **BCDF** | B cell differentiation factors |

| Abbreviation | Meaning |
|---|---|
| **BCF** | basophil chemotactic factor |
| **BCG** | bacille Calmette-Guérin |
| | bicolor guaiac test |
| **BCGF** | B cell growth factors |
| **BEI** | butanol-extractable iodine |
| **BF** | blastogenic factor |
| **BFP** | biologic false-positive |
| **BHA** | butylated hydroxyanisole |
| **BHT** | butylated hydroxytoluene |
| **bid** | twice a day (L. bis in die) |
| **BKV** | BK virus |
| **BMI** | body mass index |
| **BMR** | basal metabolic rate |
| **BMT** | behavioral marital therapy |
| | bone marrow transplantation |
| **BOOP** | bronchiolitis obliterans with organizing pneumonia |
| **BP** | blood pressure |
| | British Pharmacopoeia |
| **bp** | base pair |
| | boiling point |
| **B Ph** | British Pharmacopoeia |
| **BPIG** | bacterial polysaccharide immune globulin |
| **Bq** | becquerel |
| **BRM** | biological response modified |
| **BS** | blood sugar |
| | breath sounds |
| **BSA** | body surface area |
| **BSP** | Bromsulphalein |
| **BSS** | Bernard-Soulier syndrome |
| **BTU** | British thermal unit |
| **BUDR** | 5-bromodeoxyuridine |
| **BUN** | blood urea nitrogen |
| **BVAD** | biventricular assist device |
| **C** | canine (tooth) |
| | carbon |
| | cathode |
| | cathodal |
| | cervical vertebrae (C1–C7) |
| | clonus |
| | closure |
| | color sense |
| | complement (C1 through C9) |
| | compliance (subscripts denote the structure, e.g., $C_L$, lung compliance) |
| | contraction |
| | coulomb |
| | cylinder |
| | cylindrical lens |
| | cytidine |
| | cytosine |
| ***C*** | capacitance |
| | clearance (subscripts denote the substance, e.g., $C_I$ or $C_{In}$ (inulin clearance) |
| | heat capacity |
| **°C** | degree Celsius |
| **c** | contact |
| ***c*** | molar concentration |
| | specific heat capacity |
| | velocity of light in a vacuum |
| **CA** | cardiac arrest |
| | coronary artery |
| | chronological age |
| | croup-associated (virus) |
| **CABG** | coronary artery bypass graft |
| **CAD** | coronary artery disease |
| **cal** | calorie |
| **CALLA** | common acute lymphoblastic leukemia antigen |
| **CAM** | cell adhesion molecules |
| **cAMP** | cyclic adenosine monophosphate |
| **CAPD** | continuous ambulatory peritoneal dialysis |
| **CAT** | computerized axial tomography |
| **CAVB** | complete atrioventricular block |
| **cbc** | complete blood count |

| Abbreviation | Meaning |
|---|---|
| **CBF** | cerebral blood flow |
| **CBG** | corticosteroid-binding globulin |
| **Cbl** | cobalamin |
| **CBS** | chronic brain syndrome |
| **CC** | chief complaint |
| **CCA** | congenital contractural arachnodactyly |
| **CCAT** | conglutinating complement absorption test |
| **CCF** | crystal-induced chemotactic factor |
| **CCK** | cholecystokinin |
| **CCNU** | lomustine |
| **CCU** | critical care unit |
| **CD** | cadaveric donor |
| | L. conjugata diagonalis (diagonal conjugate diameter of the pelvic inlet) |
| | curative dose |
| | cluster designation (for antigens) |
| **cd** | candela |
| **CDC** | Centers for Disease Control and Prevention |
| **cdf** | cumulative distribution function |
| **cDNA** | complementary DNA |
| | copy DNA |
| **CDP** | cytidine diphosphate |
| **CEA** | carcinoembryonic antigen |
| **CEP** | congenital erythropoietic porphyria |
| **ces** | central excitatory state |
| **CESD** | cholesteryl ester storage disease |
| **CF** | carbolfuchsin |
| | cardiac failure |
| | Christmas factor |
| | citrovorum factor |
| **cff** | critical fusion frequency |
| **CFT** | complement-fixation test |
| **CFU** | colony-forming unit |
| **CGD** | chronic granulomatous disease |
| **cGMP** | cyclic guanosine monophosphate |
| **cGy** | centrigray |
| **CH** | crown-heel (length of fetus) |
| **CHD** | congenital heart disease |
| | coronary heart disease |
| **ChE** | cholinesterase |
| **CHF** | congestive heart failure |
| **CHO** | Chinese hamster ovary (cell) |
| **CI** | color index |
| | Colour Index |
| **Ci** | curie |
| **CIE** | counterimmunoelectrophoresis |
| **Ci-hr** | curie-hour |
| **CIN** | cervical intraepithelial neoplasia |
| **CK** | creatine kinase |
| **CLIP** | corticotropin-like intermediate lobe peptide |
| **CMAP** | compound muscle action potential |
| **CMD** | cerebromacular degeneration |
| **CMHC** | community mental health center |
| **CMI** | cell-mediated immunity |
| **CML** | cell-mediated lympholysis |
| **CMP** | cytidine monophosphate |
| **CMR** | cerebral metabolic rate |
| **CMV** | cytomegalovirus |
| **CN-Cbl** | cyanocobalamin |
| **CNS** | central nervous system |
| **CNV** | contingent negative variation |
| **CO** | cardiac output |
| **Co** | cobalt |
| **CoA** | coenzyme A |
| **CoA-SH** | coenzyme A |
| **COC** | calcifying odontogenic cyst |
| **COLD** | chronic obstructive lung disease |
| **ConA** | concanavalin A |
| **COPD** | chronic obstructive pulmonary disease |
| **cp** | centipoise |
| **CPAP** | continuous positive airway pressure |
| **CPC** | clinicopathological conference |

| Abbreviation | Meaning |
|---|---|
| **CPD** | citrate phosphate dextrose |
| **CPDA-1** | citrate phosphate dextrose adenine |
| **CPDD** | calcium pyrophosphate deposition disease |
| **CPI** | congenital palatopharyngeal incompetency |
| **CPK** | creatine phosphokinase |
| **CPS** | carbamoyl phosphate synthetase |
| **CPR** | cardiopulmonary resuscitation |
| **CPSII** | carbamoyl phosphate synthetase II |
| **CR** | conditioned response |
| | complement receptor |
| | crown-rump (length of fetus) |
| **CREG** | cross-reactive group (of HLA antigens) |
| **CRH** | corticotropin-releasing hormone |
| **CRL** | crown-rump length (of fetus) |
| **CRM** | cross-reacting material |
| **cRNA** | complementary RNA |
| **CRP** | C-reactive protein |
| **CRRT** | continuous renal replacement therapy |
| **CRS** | Chinese restaurant syndrome |
| **CS** | cesarean section |
| | conditioned stimulus |
| | coronary sinus |
| **CSF** | cerebrospinal fluid |
| | colony-stimulating factor |
| **CSF-1** | macrophage colony–stimulating factor |
| **CSII** | continuous subcutaneous insulin infusion |
| **CSM** | cerebrospinal meningitis |
| **CST** | contraction stress test |
| **CT** | computed tomography |
| **CTBA** | cetrimonium bromide |
| **CTL** | cytotoxic lymphocytes |
| **CTP** | cytidine triphosphate |
| **CV** | cardiovascular |
| | closing volume |
| | coefficient of variation |
| **CVA** | cardiovascular accident |
| | cerebrovascular accident |
| | costovertebral angle |
| **CVID** | common variable immunodeficiency |
| **CVP** | central venous pressure |
| **CVS** | cardiovascular system |
| | chorionic villus sampling |
| **CX** | circumflex artery |
| **Cx** | cervix |
| | convex |
| **Cy** | cyanogen |
| **CYC** | cyclophosphamide |
| **cyl** | cylinder |
| | cylindrical lens |
| **Cys** | cysteine |
| **Cys-Cys** | cystine |
| **D** | dalton |
| | deciduous (teeth) |
| | decimal reduction timedeuterium |
| | died |
| | diffusing capacity |
| | diopter |
| | distal |
| | dorsal vertebrae (D1–D12) |
| | dose |
| | dwarf (colony) |
| $\mathbf{D_L}$ | diffusing capacity of the lung |
| **d** | day |
| | deoxyribose |
| $\delta$ | the $\delta$ chain of hemoglobin |
| | the heavy chain of IgD |
| **DA** | developmental age |
| | diphenylchlorarsine |
| **Da** | dalton |
| **DAC** | decitabine |
| **DAD** | delayed afterdepolarization |
| **DADDS** | diacetyl diaminodiphenylsulfone |
| **dADP** | deoxyadenosine diphosphate |

| Abbreviation | Meaning |
|---|---|
| **DAF** | decay accelerating factor |
| **dAMP** | deoxyadenosine monophosphate |
| **D and C** | dilation and curettage |
| **dATP** | deoxyadenosine triphosphate |
| **dB, db** | decibel |
| **DBA** | dibenzanthracene |
| **DC** | direct current |
| **D & C** | dilation and curettage |
| **dC** | deoxycytidine |
| **DCA** | desoxycorticosterone acetate |
| **DCc** | double concave |
| **dCDP** | deoxycytidine diphosphate |
| **DCF** | direct centrifugal flotation |
| **DCI** | dichloroisoproterenol |
| **DCIS** | ductal carcinoma in situ |
| **dCMP** | deoxycytidine monophosphate |
| **dCTP** | deoxycytidine triphosphate |
| **DCx** | double convex |
| **DDS** | diaminodiphenylsulfone (dapsone) |
| **Deg** | degeneration |
| | degree |
| **DES** | diethylstilbestrol |
| **DET** | diethyltryptamine |
| **DEV** | duck embryo rabies vaccine |
| **DFP** | diisopropyl flurophosphate |
| **dG** | deoxyguanosine |
| **dGDP** | deoxyguanosine diphosphate |
| **dGMP** | deoxyguanosine monophosphate |
| **dGTP** | deoxyguanosine triphosphate |
| **DH** | delayed hypersensitivity |
| **DHA** | docosahexaenoic acid |
| **DHEA** | dehydroepiandrosterone |
| **DHF** | dihydrofolate |
| | dihydrofolic acid |
| **DHT** | dihydrotestosterone |
| **DIC** | disseminated intravascular coagulation |
| **DLE** | discoid lupus erythematosus |
| **DM** | diabetes mellitus |
| **DMAPN** | dimethylaminopropionitrile |
| **DMBA** | 7,12-dimethylbenz[a]anthracene |
| **DMFO** | eflornithine |
| **DMPE** | 3,4-dimethoxyphenylethylamine |
| **DMSA** | succimer |
| **DMSO** | dimethyl sulfoxide |
| **DMT** | dimethyltryptamine |
| **DN** | dibucaine number |
| **DNA** | deoxyribonucleic acid |
| **DNase** | deoxyribonuclease |
| **DNB** | dinitrobenzene |
| **DNCB** | dinitrochlorobenzene |
| **DNFB** | dinitrofluorobenzene |
| **DNOC** | dinitro-*o*-cresol |
| **DNR** | do not resuscitate |
| **DOA** | dead on arrival |
| **DOC** | 11-deoxycorticosterone |
| **DOM** | 2,5-dimethoxy-4-methylamphetamine |
| **DPN** | diphosphopyridine nucleotide |
| **DPT** | diphtheria-pertussis-tetanus (vaccine) |
| **DR** | reaction of degeneration |
| **DRG** | diagnosis-related group |
| **dsDNA** | double-stranded DNA |
| **dsRNA** | double-stranded RNA |
| **Dt** | duration tetany |
| **dT** | deoxythymidine |
| **DTaP** | diphtheria and tetanus toxoids and acellular pertussis vaccine |
| **dTDP** | deoxythymidine diphosphate |
| **DTH** | delayed-type hypersensitivity |
| **DTIC, Dtic** | dacarbazine |
| **dTMP** | deoxythymidine monophosphate |
| **DTPA** | pentetic acid |
| **dTTP** | deoxythymidine triphosphate |
| **dU** | deoxyuridine |
| **dUMP** | deoxyuridine monophosphate |
| **dUTP** | deoxyuridine triphosphate |

| Abbreviation | Meaning |
|---|---|
| **DVT** | deep venous thrombosis |
| **Dy** | dysprosium |
| **dyn** | dyne |
| **E** | emmetropia |
| | enzyme |
| $E_1$ | estrone |
| $E_2$ | estradiol |
| $E_3$ | estriol |
| $E_4$ | estetrol |
| $E^\circ$ | standard reduction potential |
| $e^-$ | electron |
| $e^+$ | positron |
| $e$ | elementary unit |
| $\eta$ | absolute viscosity |
| **EAC** | erythrocyte antibody and complement |
| **EACA** | epsilon-aminocaproic acid |
| **EAD** | early afterdepolarization |
| **EAE** | experimental allergic encephalomyelitis |
| **EAP** | epiallopregnanolone |
| **EB** | elementary body |
| **EBCT** | electron beam computed tomography |
| **EBV** | Epstein-Barr virus |
| **EC** | Enzyme Commission |
| **ECF** | eosinophil chemotactic factor |
| | extended care facility |
| | extracellular fluid |
| **ECF-A** | eosinophil chemotactic factor of anaphylaxis |
| **ECG** | electrocardiogram |
| **ECI** | electrocerebral inactivity |
| **ECM** | extracellular matrix |
| **ECMO** | extracorporeal membrane oxygenation |
| **ECS** | electrocerebral silence |
| **ECT** | electroconvulsive therapy |
| **ED** | effective dose |
| | erythema dose |
| **EDR** | effective direct radiation |
| | electrodermal response |
| **EDRF** | endothelium-derived relaxing factor |
| **EDTA** | ethylenediaminetetraacetic acid |
| **EDV** | end-diastolic volume |
| **EEE** | eastern equine encephalomyelitis |
| **EEG** | electroencephalogram |
| **EENT** | eye-ear-nose-throat |
| **EERP** | extended endocardial resection procedure |
| **EFA** | essential fatty acids |
| **EGD** | esophagogastroduodenoscopy |
| **EGF** | epidermal growth factor |
| **EGTA** | egtazic acid |
| **EHBF** | estimated hepatic blood flow |
| **EI** | erythema infectiosum |
| **EIA** | enzyme immunoassay |
| **EIT** | erythrocyte iron turnover |
| **EKG** | electrocardiogram |
| **EKY** | electrokymogram |
| **Em** | emmetropia |
| **EMC** | encephalomyocarditis (virus) |
| **EMF** | electromotive force |
| **EMG** | electromyogram |
| **ENA** | extractable nuclear antigens |
| **ENG** | electronystagmography |
| **ENT** | ear, nose, and throat |
| **EOG** | electro-olfactogram |
| **EP** | evoked potential |
| **EPP** | erythrohepatic protoporphyria |
| | erythropoietic protoporphyria |
| **EPR** | electrophrenic respiration |
| **EPSP** | excitatory postsynaptic potential |
| **ER** | endoplasmic reticulum |
| | estrogen receptor |
| **ERBF** | effective renal blood flow |
| **ERCP** | endoscopic retrograde cholangiopancreatography |
| **ERG** | electroretinogram |
| **ERP** | endocardial resection procedure |

| Abbreviation | Meaning |
|---|---|
| **ERPF** | effective renal plasma flow |
| **ERV** | expiratory reserve volume |
| **ESF** | erythropoietic stimulating factor |
| **ESP** | extrasensory perception |
| **ESR** | erythrocyte sedimentation rate |
| **ESRD** | end-stage renal disease |
| **EST** | electric shock therapy |
| | electroshock therapy |
| **esu** | electrostatic unit |
| **ESV** | end-systolic volume |
| **Et** | ethyl group |
| **ETF** | electron transfer flavoprotein |
| **ET-NANB** | enterically transmitted non-A, non-B hepatitis |
| **eV, ev** | electron volt |
| **ext** | extract |
| **F** | farad |
| | fertility |
| | fluorine |
| | formula |
| | French (scale) |
| | visual field |
| **°F** | degree Fahrenheit |
| ***F*** | faraday |
| | force |
| | gilbert |
| $\mathbf{F_1}$ | first filial generation |
| $\mathbf{F_2}$ | second filial generation |
| **f** | focal length |
| ***f*** | frequency |
| **FA** | fatty acid |
| | fluorescent antibody |
| **FACS** | fluorescence-activated cell sorter |
| **FAD** | flavin adenine dinucleotide |
| **fasc.** | L. fasciculus (bundle) |
| **fCi** | femtocurie |
| **FDP** | fibrin degradation products |
| | fibrinogen degradation products |
| **F-dUMP** | 5-fluorodeoxyuridine monophosphate |
| **FEF** | forced expiratory flow |
| **FEP** | free erythrocyte protoporphyrin |
| **FES** | functional electrical stimulation |
| **FEV** | forced expiratory volume |
| **FFA** | free fatty acids |
| **FFT** | flicker fusion threshold |
| **FIA** | fluoroimmunoassay |
| **FIGLU** | formiminoglutamic acid |
| **FITC** | fluorescein isothiocyanate |
| **fld** | fluid |
| **fl dr** | fluid dram |
| **fl oz** | fluidounce |
| **FMN** | flavin mononucleotide (riboflavin 5′-phosphate) |
| **FNH** | focal nodular hyperplasia |
| **FNTC** | fine needle transhepatic cholangiography |
| **FPG** | fasting plasma glucose |
| **FRC** | functional residual capacity |
| **FSF** | fibrin-stabilizing factor |
| **FSG, FSGS** | focal segmental glomerulosclerosis |
| **FSH** | follicle-stimulating hormone |
| **FSH/LH-RH** | follicle-stimulating hormone and luteinizing hormone releasing hormone |
| **FSH-RH** | follicle-stimulating hormone releasing hormone |
| **5-FU** | 5-fluorouracil |
| **FUDR, FUdR** | 5-fluorouracil deoxyribonucleoside |
| **FUO** | fever of undetermined origin |
| **FVC** | forced vital capacity |
| **G** | gauss |
| | gravida |
| | guanine |
| | guanosine |
| ***G*** | conductance |
| | G force |
| | Gibbs free energy |
| | gravitational constant |
| **g** | gram |
| ***g*** | standard gravity |
| $\gamma$ | the $\gamma$ chains of fetal hemoglobin |
| | the heavy chain of IgG |
| **GABA** | $\gamma$-aminobutyric acid |
| **GAD** | generalized anxiety disorder |
| **GAG** | glycosaminoglycan |
| **GalNAc** | *N*-acetylgalactosamine |
| **GALT** | gut-associated lymphoid tissue |
| **GAPD** | glyceraldehyde-3-phosphate dehydrogenase |
| **GBM** | glomerular basement membrane |
| **GC** | gas chromatography |
| **G-CSF** | granulocyte colony–stimulating factor |
| **GDP** | guanosine diphosphate |
| **GFAP** | glial fibrillary acidic protein |
| **GFR** | glomerular filtration rate |
| **GGT** | $\gamma$-glutamyltransferase |
| **GH** | growth hormone |
| **GH-RH** | growth hormone releasing hormone |
| **GI** | gastrointestinal |
| **GIP** | gastric inhibitory polypeptide |
| **gl.** | L. glandula (gland) |
| **GLC** | gas-liquid chromatography |
| **GlcNAc** | *N*-acetylglucosamine |
| **GLI** | glucagon-like immunoreactivity |
| **Glu** | glutamic acid |
| **Gly** | glycine |
| **GM-CSF** | granulocyte-macrophage colony–stimulating factor |
| **GMP** | guanosine monophosphate |
| **3′,5′-GMP** | cyclic guanosine monophosphate |
| **Gn-RH** | gonadotropin-releasing hormone |
| **GP** | general practitioner |
| | general paresis |
| **G6PD** | glucose-6-phosphate dehydrogenase |
| **GPI** | general paralysis of the insane |
| **GPT** | glutamic-pyruvic transaminase |
| **gr** | grain |
| **GRH** | growth hormone releasing hormone |
| **GSC** | gas-solid chromatography |
| **GSH** | reduced glutathione |
| **GSS** | Gerstmann-Sträussler-Scheinker syndrome |
| **GSSG** | oxidized glutathione |
| **GTH** | gonadotropic hormone |
| **GTN** | gestational trophoblastic neoplasia |
| **GTP** | guanosine triphosphate |
| **GTT** | glucose tolerance test |
| **GU** | genitourinary |
| **GVH** | graft-versus-host (disease or reaction) |
| **GXT** | graded exercise test |
| **Gy** | gray |
| **H** | henry |
| | Holzknecht unit |
| | horizontal |
| | Hounsfield unit |
| | hydrogen |
| | hypermetropia |
| | hyperopia |
| ***H*** | enthalpy |
| | magnetic field strength |
| $H_0$ | null hypothesis |
| $H_1$ | alternate hypothesis |
| $H_a$ | alternative hypothesis |
| **h** | hour |
| ***h*** | Planck's constant |
| | height |
| **HA** | hemadsorbent |
| **HAA** | hepatitis-associated antigen |
| **HAI** | hemagglutination inhibition |
| **H and E** | hematoxylin and eosin |
| **HANE** | hereditary angioneurotic edema |
| **HAT** | hypoxanthine-aminopterin-thymidine (medium) |
| **HAV** | hepatitis A virus |

| Abbreviation | Meaning |
|---|---|
| **HB** | hepatitis B |
| **HBc** | hepatitis B core (antigen) |
| **HBe** | hepatitis B e (antigen) |
| **HBs** | hepatitis B surface (antigen) |
| **Hb** | hemoglobin |
| **HBcAg** | hepatitis B core antigen |
| **HbCV** | *Haemophilus influenzae* b conjugate vaccine |
| **HBE** | His bundle electrogram |
| **HBeAg** | hepatitis B e antigen |
| **HBsAg** | hepatitis B surface antigen |
| **$HbO_2$** | oxyhemoglobin |
| **HbPV** | *Haemophilus influenzae* b polysaccharide vaccine |
| **HBV** | hepatitis B virus |
| **HC** | hospital corps |
| **HCG, hCG** | human chorionic gonadotropin |
| **HCM** | hypertrophic cardiomyopathy |
| **HCP** | hereditary coproporphyria |
| **HCT** | hematocrit |
| **HCV** | hepatitis C virus |
| **HDCV** | human diploid cell rabies vaccine |
| **HDL** | high-density lipoprotein |
| **$HDL_1$** | Lp(a) lipoprotein |
| **HDN** | hemolytic disease of the newborn |
| **HDV** | hepatitis D virus |
| **H & E** | hematoxylin and eosin |
| **hEGF** | human epidermal growth factor |
| **HEK** | human embryo kidney (cell culture) |
| **HEL** | human embryo lung (cell culture) |
| **HEP** | hepatoerythropoietic porphyria |
| **HETE** | hydroxyeicosatetaraenoic acid |
| **HF** | Hageman factor (coagulation Factor XII)<br>high frequency |
| **Hgb** | hemoglobin |
| **HGBV** | hepatitis GB virus |
| **HGE** | human granulocytic ehrlichiosis |
| **HGF** | hyperglycemic-glycogenolytic factor (glucagon) |
| **HGG** | human gamma globulin |
| **HGH, hGH** | human growth hormone |
| **hGHr** | growth hormone recombinant |
| **HGPRT** | hypoxanthine-guanine phosphoribosyltransferase |
| **HGV** | hepatitis G virus |
| **HHT** | hydroxyheptadecatrienoic acid |
| **HI** | hemagglutination inhibition |
| **5-HIAA** | 5-hydroxyindoleacetic acid |
| **HIDA** | hepatobiliary iminodiacetic acid |
| **His** | histidine |
| **HIV** | human immunodeficiency virus |
| **HKAFO** | hip-knee-ankle-foot orthosis |
| **Hl** | latent hyperopia |
| **HLHS** | hypoplastic left heart syndrome |
| **Hm** | manifest hyperopia |
| **HMM** | hexamethylmelamine |
| **HMO** | health maintenance organization |
| **HMSN** | hereditary motor and sensory neuropathy |
| **HMW-NCF** | high-molecular-weight neutrophil chemotactic factor |
| **HMWK** | high-molecular-weight kininogen |
| **hnRNA** | heterogeneous nuclear RNA |
| **HOCM** | hypertrophic obstructive cardiomyopathy |
| **HOP** | high oxygen pressure |
| **HP** | house physician |
| **Hp** | haptoglobin |
| **HPETE** | hydroperoxyeicosatetraenoic acid |
| **HPF** | high-power field |
| **HPL, hPL** | human placental lactogen |
| **HPLC** | high-performance liquid chromatography |
| **HPRT** | hypoxanthine phosphoribosyltransferase |
| **HPV** | human papillomavirus |
| **HRA** | high right atrium |
| **HRCT** | high-resolution computed tomography |
| **HRF** | histamine releasing factor |
| **HRIG** | human rabies immune globulin |
| **HRP** | horseradish peroxidase |
| **HS** | house surgeon |
| **HSA** | human serum albumin |
| **HSAN** | hereditary sensory and autonomic neuropathy |
| **HSF** | hydrazine-sensitive factor |
| **HSR** | homogeneously staining regions |
| **HSV** | herpes simplex virus |
| **5-HT** | 5-hydroxytryptamine (serotonin) |
| **Ht** | total hyperopia |
| **HTACS** | human thyroid adenylate cyclase stimulators |
| **HTC** | homozygous typing cells |
| **HTLV** | human T-cell leukemia/lymphoma virus |
| **HuIFN** | human interferon |
| **HVA** | homovanillic acid |
| **HVL** | half-value layer |
| **Hz** | hertz |
| **I** | incisor<br>inosine<br>iodine |
| ***I*** | electric current<br>intensity (of radiant energy)<br>ionic strength |
| **IAB** | intra-aortic balloon |
| **IABP** | intra-aortic balloon pump |
| **IAHA** | immune adherence hemagglutination assay |
| **IB** | inclusion body |
| **IBC** | iron-binding capacity |
| **IBF** | immunoglobulin-binding factor |
| **IC** | inspiratory capacity<br>irritable colon |
| **ICAM-1** | intercellular adhesion molecule 1 |
| **ICAM-2** | intercellular adhesion molecule 2 |
| **ICD** | International Classification of Diseases<br>intrauterine contraceptive device |
| **ICP** | intracranial pressure |
| **ICSH** | interstitial cell–stimulating hormone |
| **ICSI** | intracytoplasmic sperm injection |
| **ICT** | insulin coma therapy |
| **ICU** | intensive care unit |
| **ID** | inside diameter<br>intradermal |
| **$ID_{50}$** | median infective dose |
| **IDA** | iminodiacetic acid |
| **IDD** | insulin-dependent diabetes |
| **IDL** | intermediate-density lipoprotein |
| **IDU** | idoxuridine |
| **IEP** | immunoelectrophoresis |
| **IF** | intrinsic factor |
| **IFA** | immunofluorescence assay |
| **IFN** | interferon |
| **Ig** | immunoglobulin |
| **IGF** | insulin-like growth factor |
| **IGT** | impaired glucose tolerance |
| **IH** | infectious hepatitis |
| **IHD** | ischemic heart disease |
| **IL** | interleukin |
| **Ile** | isoleucine |
| **IM** | intramuscularly |
| **$ImD_{50}$** | median immunizing dose |
| **IMPA** | incisal mandibular plane angle |
| **IMV** | intermittent mandatory ventilation |
| **$InsP_3$** | inositol 1,4,5-triphosphate |
| **IOP** | intraocular pressure |
| **IP** | intraperitoneally<br>isoelectric point |
| **$IP_3$** | inositol 1,4,5-triphosphate |
| **IPD** | intermittent peritoneal dialysis |
| **IPPB** | intermittent positive pressure breathing |
| **IPSP** | inhibitory postsynaptic potential |

| Abbreviation | Meaning |
|---|---|
| **IPV** | poliovirus vaccine inactivated |
| **IQ** | intelligence quotient |
| **IRC** | inspiratory reserve capacity |
| **IRMA** | immunoradiometric assay |
| **IRV** | inspiratory reserve volume |
| **IS** | intercostal space |
| **ISA** | intrinsic sympathomimetic activity |
| **ITP** | idiopathic thrombocytopenic purpura |
| **IU** | immunizing unit |
| | international unit |
| **IUD** | intrauterine contraceptive device |
| **IUGR** | intrauterine growth retardation |
| **IV** | intravenously |
| **IVC** | inferior vena cava |
| **IVF** | in vitro fertilization |
| **IVP** | intravenous pyelogram |
| | intravenous pyelography |
| **IVRT** | isovolumic relaxation time |
| **IVS** | interventricular septum |
| **J** | joule |
| **JCV** | JC virus |
| **K** | potassium (L. kalium) |
| | kelvin |
| $K$ | equilibrium constant |
| $K_a$ | acid dissociation constant |
| $K_b$ | base dissociation constant |
| $K_d$ | dissociation constant |
| $K_{eq}$ | equilibrium constant |
| $K_M$, $K_m$ | Michaelis constant |
| $K_p$ | solubility product constant |
| $K_W$ | ion product of water |
| $k$ | Boltzmann's constant |
| | rate constant |
| $\kappa$ | one of the two types of immunoglobulin light chains |
| **KAF** | conglutinogen activating factor (factor I) |
| **KAFO** | knee-ankle-foot orthosis |
| **kb** | kilobase (1000 base pairs) |
| **kbp** | kilobase pairs |
| **kcal** | kilocalorie |
| **kCi** | kilocurie |
| **kg** | kilogram |
| **kHz** | kilohertz |
| **kj** | knee jerk |
| ***K*m** | Michaelis constant |
| **KP** | keratitic precipitates |
| **KUB** | kidney, ureter, and bladder |
| **kV** | kilovolt |
| **kVp** | kilovolts peak |
| **kW** | kilowatt |
| **kW-hr** | kilowatt-hour |
| **L** | lambert |
| | left |
| | light chain |
| | liter |
| | lumbar vertebra (L1–L5) |
| | lung |
| $L$ | self-inductance |
| | luminance |
| $L_0$ | limes null |
| $L+$, $L_+$ | limes tod |
| **l.** | L. ligamentum (ligament) |
| **L0** | limes null |
| **L & A** | light and accommodation (reaction of pupils) |
| **LAD** | left anterior descending (coronary artery) |
| | left axis deviation |
| **LAE** | left atrial enlargement |
| **LAH** | left anterior hemiblock |
| **LAO** | left anterior oblique |
| **LAP** | leukocyte adhesion protein |
| | leukocyte alkaline phosphate |
| **LATS** | long-acting thyroid stimulator |
| **LATS-p** | LATS protector |

| Abbreviation | Meaning |
|---|---|
| **LAV** | lymphadenopathy-associated virus |
| **LBBB** | left bundle branch block |
| **LBP** | low back pain |
| **LBW** | low birth weight |
| **LCA** | left coronary artery |
| | leukocyte common antigen |
| **LCAT** | lecithin-cholesterol acyltransferase |
| **LCIS** | lobular carcinoma in situ |
| **LD** | lethal dose |
| | light difference |
| $LD_{50}$ | median lethal dose |
| **LDH** | lactate dehydrogenase |
| **LDL** | low-density lipoproteins |
| **LE** | left eye |
| | lupus erythematosus |
| **LEMS** | Lambert-Eaton myasthenic syndrome |
| **les** | local excitatory state |
| **LET** | linear energy transfer |
| **Leu** | leucine |
| **Lf** | limit of flocculation |
| **LFA-1** | leukocyte function–associated antigen 1 |
| **LFA-2** | leukocyte function–associated antigen 2 |
| **LFA-3** | leukocyte function–associated antigen 3 |
| **LH** | luteinizing hormone |
| **LH-RH** | luteinizing hormone–releasing hormone |
| **LIA** | leukemia-associated inhibitory activity |
| **LIF** | left iliac fossa |
| | leukocyte inhibitory factor |
| **lig.** | L. ligamentum (ligament) |
| **ligg.** | L. ligamenta (ligaments) |
| **LLL** | left lower lobe (of the lung) |
| **LM** | light minimum |
| | linguomesial |
| **LMF** | lymphocyte mitogenic factor |
| **LMP** | last menstrual period |
| | latent membrane protein |
| **LNPF** | lymph node permeability factor |
| **LOAEL** | lowest observed adverse effect level |
| **LOEL** | lowest observed effect level |
| **LPF** | low-power field |
| **LPH** | lipotropic hormone |
| | left posterior hemiblock |
| **LPN** | licensed practical nurse |
| **LPS** | lipopolysaccharide |
| **LPV** | lymphotropic papovavirus |
| **LRF** | luteinizing hormone releasing factor |
| **LSD** | lysergic acid diethylamide |
| **LSO** | lumbosacral orthosis |
| **LT** | lymphotoxin |
| **LTF** | lymphocyte transforming factor |
| **LTH** | luteotropic hormone |
| **LTR** | long terminal repeat |
| **LUL** | left upper lobe (of lungs) |
| **LVAD** | left ventricular assist device |
| **LVEDP** | left ventricular end-diastolic pressure |
| **LVEDV** | left ventricular end-diastolic volume |
| **LVET** | left ventricular ejection time |
| **LVH** | left ventricular hypertrophy |
| **LVN** | licensed vocational nurse |
| **Lys** | lysine |
| **M** | molar |
| | morgan |
| | mucoid |
| | myopia |
| $M$ | molar |
| | molar mass |
| | mutual inductance |
| $M_1$ | mitral valve closure |
| $M_r$ | relative molecular mass |
| **m** | median |
| | meter |
| **m.** | L. musculus (muscle) |
| $m$ | mass |
| | molal |

| Abbreviation | Meaning |
|---|---|
| **$\mu$** | electrophoretic mobility |
| | the heavy chain of IgM |
| | linear attenuation coefficient |
| | micron |
| | population mean |
| **MA** | mental age |
| | meter angle |
| **$\mu$A** | microampere |
| **mA** | milliampere |
| **MAA** | macroaggregated albumin |
| **MAC** | membrane attack complex |
| | minimal alveolar concentration |
| **MAC INH** | membrane attack complex inhibitor |
| **MADD** | multiple acyl CoA dehydrogenation deficiency |
| **MAF** | macrophage activating factor |
| **MALT** | mucosa-associated lymphoid tissue |
| **MAO** | monoamine oxidase |
| **MAOI** | monoamine oxidase inhibitor |
| **MAP** | mean arterial pressure |
| **masc** | mass concentration |
| **MAST** | military or medical anti-shock trousers |
| **MAT** | multifocal atrial tachycardia |
| **MBP** | major basic protein |
| | myelin basic protein |
| **MCA** | 3-methylcholanthrene |
| **MCD** | mean of consecutive differences |
| **MCF** | macrophage chemotactic factor |
| **MCH** | mean corpuscular hemoglobin |
| **MCHC** | mean corpuscular hemoglobin concentration |
| **mCi-hr** | millicurie-hour |
| **MCP** | membrane cofactor protein |
| **M-CSF** | macrophage colony–stimulating factor |
| **MCT** | mean circulation time |
| **MCV** | mean corpuscular volume |
| **MDA** | methylenedioxyamphetamine |
| **MDF** | myocardial depressant factor |
| **MDP** | methylene diphosphonate |
| **MDS** | myelodysplasia |
| **Me** | methyl |
| **MeCbl** | methylcobalamin |
| **MED** | minimal effective dose |
| | minimal erythema dose |
| **MEGX** | monoethylglycinexylidide |
| **MEN** | multiple endocrine neoplasia |
| **MEP** | maximum expiratory pressure |
| **mEq, meq** | milliequivalent |
| **Met** | methionine |
| **mg** | milligram |
| **$\mu$g** | microgram |
| **MHA-TP** | microhemagglutination assay–*Treponema pallidum* |
| **MHC** | major histocompatibility complex |
| **MHD** | minimum hemolytic dose |
| **MI** | myocardial infarction |
| **MIBG** | metaiodobenzylguanidine |
| **MID** | minimum infective dose |
| **MIF** | migration inhibiting factor |
| **MIO** | minimal identifiable odor |
| **MIP** | maximum inspiratory pressure |
| **MIRL** | membrane inhibitor of reactive lysis |
| **MIT** | monoiodotyrosine |
| **MK** | monkey lung (cell culture) |
| **mL** | milliliter |
| **$\mu$L** | microliter |
| **MLBW** | moderately low birth weight |
| **MLC** | mixed lymphocyte culture |
| **MLD** | median lethal dose |
| | minimum lethal dose |
| **MLNS** | mucocutaneous lymph node syndrome |
| **MLR** | mixed lymphocyte reaction |
| **MM** | mucous membranes |
| **mM** | millimolar |

| Abbreviation | Meaning |
|---|---|
| **mm** | millimeter |
| **$\mu$m** | micromolar |
| **MMIHS** | megacystis-microcolon–intestinal hypoperistalsis syndrome |
| **MMR** | measles-mumps-rubella (vaccine) |
| **MODY** | maturity-onset diabetes of youth |
| **molc** | molar concentration |
| **Mol wt** | molecular weight |
| **mOsm** | milliosmol |
| **MOTT** | mycobacteria other than tubercle bacilli |
| **6-MP** | 6-mercaptopurine |
| **mp** | melting point |
| **MPD** | maximum permissible dose |
| **MPO** | myeloperoxidase |
| **MPS** | mononuclear phagocyte system |
| | mucopolysaccharidosis |
| **MR** | mitral regurgitation |
| **MRA** | magnetic resonance angiography |
| **MRD** | minimum reacting dose |
| **MRDM** | malnutrition-related diabetes mellitus |
| **mrem** | millirem |
| **MRI** | magnetic resonance imaging |
| **mRNA** | messenger RNA |
| **MS** | multiple sclerosis |
| **MSH** | melanocyte-stimulating hormone |
| **MSL** | midsternal line |
| **MSUD** | maple syrup urine disease |
| **MSLT** | multiple sleep latency test |
| **MT** | L. membrana tympani (tympanic membrane) |
| **MTD** | maximum tolerated dose |
| **mtDNA** | mitochondrial DNA |
| **MTU** | methylthiouracil |
| **MTX** | methotrexate |
| **MUAP** | motor unit action potential |
| **MUGA** | multiple gated acquisition (scan) |
| **MUP** | motor unit potential |
| **MVP** | mitral valve prolapse |
| **MW** | molecular weight |
| **My** | myopia |
| **N** | newton |
| | nitrogen |
| ***N*** | normal (solution) |
| | neutron number |
| | number |
| | population size |
| **$N_A$** | Avogadro's number |
| **n** | refractive index |
| | neutron |
| **n.** | L. nervus (nerve) |
| ***n*** | (haploid) chromosome number |
| | refractive index |
| | sample size |
| **$n_D$** | refractive index |
| **$\nu$** | degrees of freedom |
| | frequency |
| | neutrino |
| | kinematic viscosity |
| **NA** | Nomina Anatomica |
| | numerical aperture |
| **NAD** | nicotinamide-adenine dinucleotide |
| | no appreciable disease |
| **$NAD^+$** | the oxidized form of NAD |
| **NADH** | the reduced form of NAD |
| **NADP** | nicotinamide-adenine dinucleotide phosphate |
| **$NADP^+$** | the oxidized form of NADP |
| **NADPH** | the reduced form of NADP |
| **NAN** | *N*-acetylneuraminic acid |
| **NANBH** | non-A, non-B hepatitis |
| **NAP** | nasion, point A, pogonion |
| **NASH** | nonalcoholic steatohepatitis |
| **NBT** | nitroblue tetrazolium |
| **NBTE** | nonbacterial thrombotic endocarditis |

| Abbreviation | Meaning |
|---|---|
| **NCF** | neutrophil chemotactic factor |
| **NCV** | nerve conduction velocity |
| **nDNA** | nuclear DNA |
| **NDV** | Newcastle disease virus |
| **Nd:YAG** | neodymium:yttrium-aluminum-garnet (laser) |
| **NED** | no evidence of disease |
| **NEFA** | nonesterified fatty acids |
| **ng** | nanogram |
| **NGF** | nerve growth factor |
| **NIDD** | non–insulin-dependent diabetes |
| **nm** | nanometer |
| **NMN** | nicotinamide mononucleotide |
| **NMR** | nuclear magnetic resonance |
| **NMS** | neuroleptic malignant syndrome |
| **nn.** | L. nervi (nerves) |
| **NOAEL** | no observed adverse effect level |
| **NOEL** | no observed effect level |
| **NPN** | nonprotein nitrogen |
| **NPO** | L. nil per os (nothing by mouth) |
| **NRC** | normal retinal correspondence |
| **NREM** | non-rapid eye movement |
| **NSAIA** | nonsteroidal anti-inflammatory analgesic |
| **NSAID** | nonsteroidal anti-inflammatory drug |
| **NSCLC** | non–small cell lung carcinoma |
| **NSR** | normal sinus rhythm |
| **NST** | nonstress test |
| **NTP** | normal temperature and pressure |
| **nU** | nanounit |
| **NUG** | necrotizing ulcerative gingivitis |
| **nvCJD** | new variant Creutzfeldt-Jakob disease |
| **NYD** | not yet diagnosed |
| **O** | oxygen |
| **O.** | oculus |
| **Ω** | ohm |
| **OA** | ocular albinism |
| **OAE** | otoacoustic emissions |
| **OAF** | osteoclast activating factor |
| **OAT** | ornithine aminotransferase |
| **OB** | obstetrics |
| **OCA** | oculocutaneous albinism |
| **OCD** | obsessive-compulsive disorder |
| **OCT** | ornithine carbamoyltransferase |
| | oxytocin challenge test |
| **OD** | L. oculus dexter (right eye) |
| | optical density |
| | outside diameter |
| | overdose |
| **ODC** | orotidine 5-phosphate decarboxylase |
| **OFD** | oral-facial-digital (syndrome) |
| **OGTT** | oral glucose tolerance test |
| **OH-Cbl** | hydroxocobalamin |
| **17-OHCS** | 17-hydroxycorticosteroid |
| **OI** | osteogenesis imperfecta |
| **OIC** | osteogenesis imperfecta congenita |
| **OIH** | orthoiodohippurate |
| **OL** | L. oculus laevus (left eye) |
| **OMPA** | octamethyl pyrophosphoramide |
| **OPRT** | orotate phosphoribosyltransferase |
| **OPV** | poliovirus vaccine live oral |
| **OR** | operating room |
| **Orn** | ornithine |
| **ORS** | oral rehydration salts |
| **ORT** | oral rehydration therapy |
| **OS** | L. oculus sinister (left eye) |
| **OSAS** | obstructive sleep apnea syndrome |
| **OT** | old term (anatomy) |
| | Old tuberculin |
| **OTC** | ornithine transcarbamoylase |
| | over the counter |
| **OTD** | organ tolerance dose |
| **OVD** | occlusal vertical dimension |
| **P** | para |
| | phosphate group |

| Abbreviation | Meaning |
|---|---|
| | phosphorus |
| | poise |
| | posterior |
| | premolar |
| | pupil |
| ***P*** | power |
| | pressure |
| | probability |
| $\mathbf{P_1}$ | parental generation |
| $\mathbf{P_2}$ | pulmonic second sound |
| $\mathbf{P_i}$ | orthophosphate |
| **p** | proton |
| | short arm of a chromosome |
| **PA** | posteroanterior |
| | physician assistant |
| **Pa** | protactinium |
| | pascal |
| **PAB, PABA** | para-aminobenzoic acid |
| **PAF** | platelet activating factor |
| **PAGE** | polyacrylamide gel electrophoresis |
| **PAH, PAHA** | para-aminohippuric acid |
| **PAI** | plasminogen activator inhibitor |
| **PALS** | periarterial lymphoid sheath |
| **PAN** | polyarteritis nodosa |
| **PAP** | peroxidase-antiperoxidase |
| **PAS** | para-aminosalicylic acid |
| **PASG** | pneumatic antishock garment |
| **PAT** | paroxysmal atrial tachycardia |
| **PAWP** | pulmonary artery wedge pressure |
| **PBG** | porphobilinogen |
| **PBI** | protein-bound iodine |
| **PBPC** | peripheral blood progenitor cells |
| **PC** | phosphocreatine choline |
| **PCA** | passive cutaneous anaphylaxis |
| **PCB** | polychlorinated biphenyl |
| **PCE** | pseudocholinesterase |
| **PCEC** | purified chick embryo cell vaccine |
| **PCG** | phonocardiogram |
| **pCi** | picocurie |
| **PCOS** | polycystic ovary syndrome |
| **PCP** | phencyclidine hydrochloride |
| | *Pneumocystis carinii* pneumonia |
| **PCR** | polymerase chain reaction |
| **PCV** | packed cell volume |
| **PCWP** | pulmonary capillary wedge pressure |
| **PD** | interpupillary distance |
| | peritoneal dialysis |
| | prism diopter |
| **PDA** | patent ductus arteriosus |
| | posterior descending (coronary) artery |
| **PE** | phosphatidylethanolamine |
| **PEEP** | positive end-expiratory pressure |
| **PEFR** | peak expiratory flow rate |
| **PEG** | pneumoencephalography |
| | polyethylene glycol |
| **PEM** | protein-energy malnutrition |
| **PEN** | pharmacy equivalent name |
| **PEP** | phosphoenolpyruvate |
| **PET** | positron emission tomography |
| **PG** | prostaglandin |
| **pg** | picogram |
| **Ph** | Pharmacopeia |
| **PHA** | phytohemagglutinin |
| **phar, pharm** | pharmacy |
| | pharmaceutical |
| | pharmacopeia |
| **PhB** | British Pharmacopoeia |
| **Phe** | phenylalanine |
| **PHPPA** | *p*-hydroxyphenylpyruvic acid |
| **PI** | phosphatidylinositol |
| **PID** | pelvic inflammatory disease |
| **PIE** | pulmonary interstitial emphysema |
| **PIF** | prolactin inhibiting factor |
| | proliferation inhibitory factor |

| Abbreviation | Meaning |
|---|---|
| **PIP** | phosphatidylinositol 4-phosphate |
| **$PIP_2$** | phosphatidylinositol 4,5-biphosphate |
| **PIT** | plasma iron turnover |
| **PJRT** | permanent junctional reciprocating tachycardia |
| **PJT** | paroxysmal junctional tachycardia |
| **PK** | pyruvate kinase |
| **PKU** | phenylketonuria |
| **PLED** | periodic lateralized epileptiform discharge |
| **PLP** | proteolipid protein |
| **PLT** | primed lymphocyte typing |
| | psittacosis-lymphogranuloma venereum-trachoma (group of organisms) |
| **PMB** | polymorphonuclear basophil leukocytes |
| **PME** | polymorphonuclear eosinophil leukocytes |
| **PMI** | point of maximal impulse |
| **PMM** | pentamethylmelamine |
| **PMMA** | polymethyl methacrylate |
| **PMN** | polymorphonuclear neutrophil leukocytes |
| **PMR** | proportionate mortality ratio |
| **PMSG** | pregnant mare serum gonadotropin |
| **PNET** | peripheral neuroectodermal tumor |
| **PNH** | paroxysmal nocturnal hemoglobinuria |
| **PO** | L. per os (by mouth, orally) |
| **POA** | pancreatic oncofetal antigen |
| **poly A** | polyadenylate |
| | polyadenylic acid |
| **POR** | problem-oriented record |
| **pot AGT** | potential abnormality of glucose tolerance |
| **PP** | L. punctum proximum (near point of accommodation) |
| **$PP_i$** | pyrophosphate |
| **PPD** | purified protein derivative (tuberculin) |
| **PPLO** | pleuropneumonia-like organisms |
| **ppm** | parts per million |
| **Ppt** | precipitate |
| | prepared |
| **PR** | prosthion |
| | pulmonic regurgitation |
| **PR** | L. punctum remotum (far point of accommodation) |
| **Pr** | presbyopia |
| | prism |
| **PRA** | panel-reactive antibody |
| **prev AGT** | previous abnormality of glucose tolerance |
| **PRF** | prolactin releasing factor |
| **PRL, Prl** | prolactin |
| **prn** | L. pro re nata (according as circumstances may require) |
| **Pro** | proline |
| **pro-UK** | prourokinase |
| **PrP** | prion protein |
| **PRPP** | phosphoribosylpyrophosphate |
| **PRU** | peripheral resistance unit |
| **PS** | phosphatidylserine |
| | pulmonary stenosis |
| **PSA** | prostate-specific antigen |
| **PSM** | presystolic murmur |
| **PSMA** | prostate-specific membrane antigen |
| **PSP** | phenolsulfonphthalein |
| **PSVT** | paroxysmal supraventricular tachycardia |
| **PT** | prothrombin time |
| **PTA** | plasma thromboplastin antecedent (blood coagulation Factor XI) |
| **PTC** | plasma thromboplastin component (blood coagulation Factor IX) |
| | phenylthiocarbamide |
| **PTEN** | pentaerythritol tetranitrate |
| **PTFE** | polytetrafluoroethylene (polytef) |
| **PTH** | parathyroid hormone |
| **PTT** | partial thromboplastin time |
| **PUO** | pyrexia of unknown origin |
| **PUVA** | psoralen plus ultraviolet A |
| **PVC** | polyvinyl chloride |
| | postvoiding cystogram |
| | premature ventricular contraction |
| | pulmonary venous congestion |
| **PVP** | polyvinylpyrrolidone |
| **PVP-I** | povidone-iodine |
| **PWM** | pokeweed mitogen |
| **PZI** | protamine zinc insulin |
| **Q** | ubiquinone |
| ***Q*** | electric charge |
| | heat |
| | reaction quotient |
| **$Q_{10}$** | temperature coefficient |
| | ubiquinone |
| **$\dot{Q}$** | rate of blood flow |
| **q** | long arm of a chromosome |
| ***q*** | electric charge |
| | ubiquinone |
| **qid** | four times a day (L. quater in die) |
| **$QS_2$** | electromechanical systole |
| **R** | Behnken's unit |
| | organic radical |
| | Rankine scale |
| | rate |
| | Réaumur scale |
| | respiratory exchange ratio |
| | resistance |
| | respiration |
| | rhythm |
| | right |
| | roentgen |
| | rough (colony) |
| ***R*** | resistance |
| | gas constant |
| **℞** | L. recipe (take) |
| **$R_A$, $R_{AW}$** | airway resistance |
| **$R_e$** | Reynold's number |
| **r** | drug resistance |
| | ring chromosome |
| ***r*** | correlation coefficient |
| | distance radius |
| | drug resistance |
| **$r_s$** | Spearman's rank correlation coefficient |
| **$\rho$** | correlation coefficient |
| | electric charge density |
| | mass density |
| **RAD** | right axis deviation |
| **rad** | radian |
| | radiation absorbed dose |
| **rad.** | L. radix (root) |
| **RAE** | right atrial enlargement |
| **RAO** | right anterior oblique |
| **RAST** | radioallergosorbent test |
| **RBBB** | right bundle branch block |
| **RBC** | red blood cell |
| | red blood (cell) count |
| **RBC IT** | red blood cell iron turnover |
| **RBE** | relative biological effectiveness |
| **RBP** | retinol binding protein |
| **RCA** | right coronary artery |
| **rcp** | reciprocal translocation |
| **RCU** | red cell utilization |
| **RD** | reaction of degeneration |
| **rd** | rutherford |
| **RDE** | receptor-destroying enzyme |
| **RE** | retinol equivalent |
| | right eye |
| **REG** | radioencephalogram |
| **REM** | rapid eye movements |
| **RES** | reticuloendothelial system |
| **RF** | rheumatoid factor |
| **RFLP** | restriction fragment length polymorphism |
| **Rh** | rhodium |
| **r-HuEPO** | recombinant human erythropoietin |
| **RID** | radial immunodiffusion |
| **RIF** | right iliac fossa |
| **RIND** | reversible ischemic neurologic deficit |

| Abbreviation | Meaning |
|---|---|
| **RIST** | radioimmunosorbent test |
| **RLF** | retrolental fibroplasia |
| **RLL** | right lower lobe |
| **RML** | right middle lobe |
| **RNA** | ribonucleic acid |
| **RNP** | ribonucleoprotein |
| **RPF** | renal plasma flow |
| **RPS** | renal pressor substance |
| **RQ** | respiratory quotient |
| **rRNA** | ribosomal RNA |
| **RSV** | Rous sarcoma virus |
| **RTF** | resistance transfer factor |
| **RU** | rat unit |
| **RUL** | right upper lobe |
| **RV** | residual volume |
| **RVA** | rabies vaccine adsorbed |
| **RVAD** | right ventricular assist device |
| **RVH** | right ventricular hypertrophy |
| **S** | sacral vertebrae (S1–S5) |
| | siemens |
| | smooth (colony) |
| | spherical lens |
| | substrate |
| | sulfur |
| | Svedberg unit |
| ***S*** | entropy |
| **$S_1$** | first heart sound |
| **$S_2$** | second heart sound |
| **$S_3$** | third heart sound |
| **$S_4$** | fourth heart sound |
| **s** | second |
| **s.** | L. sinister (left) |
| **$\bar{s}$** | L. sine (without) |
| ***s*** | sample standard deviation |
| **$s^{-}$** | reciprocal second |
| **$\sigma$** | standard deviation |
| **SA** | sinoatrial |
| **SB** | sinus bradycardia |
| **SBE** | subacute bacterial endocarditis |
| **SC** | secretory component |
| **SC** | closure of the semilunar valves |
| **SCAT** | sheep cell agglutination test |
| **SCID** | severe combined immunodeficiency |
| **scu-PA** | single chain urokinase-type plasminogen activator |
| **SD** | skin dose |
| | standard deviation |
| **SDE** | specific dynamic effect |
| **SDS** | sodium dodecyl sulfate |
| **SDS-PAGE** | SDS–polyacrylamide gel electrophoresis |
| **SE** | standard error |
| | sphenoethmoidal suture |
| **SED** | skin erythema dose |
| **SEP** | somatosensory evoked potential |
| **Ser** | serine |
| **SFEMG** | single fiber electromyography |
| **SGOT** | serum glutamic-oxaloacetic transaminase |
| **SGPT** | serum glutamate pyruvate transaminase |
| **SH** | serum hepatitis |
| **SHML** | sinus histiocytosis with massive lymphadenopathy (Rosai-Dorfman disease) |
| **SI** | stimulation index |
| | Système International d'Unités (International System of Units) |
| **SIADH** | syndrome of inappropriate antidiuretic hormone |
| **sid** | once a day (L. semel in die) |
| **SIDS** | sudden infant death syndrome |
| **SIMV** | synchronized intermittent mandatory ventilation |
| **SISI** | short increment sensitivity index |
| **SLE** | systemic lupus erythematosus |
| **SMAF** | specific macrophage arming factor |
| **SMC** | selenomethylnorcholesterol |

| Abbreviation | Meaning |
|---|---|
| **SMON** | subacute myelo-opticoneuropathy |
| **SMR** | standard mortality (or morbidity) ratio |
| **SNAP** | sensory nerve action potential |
| **snRNA** | small nuclear RNA |
| **snRNP** | small nuclear ribonucleoprotein |
| **SNS** | sympathetic nervous system |
| **SO** | spheno-occipital (synchondrosis) |
| **SOB** | shortness of breath |
| **Sol** | solution |
| **SOMI** | sternal-occipital-mandibular immobilizer |
| **SPCA** | serum prothrombin conversion accelerator (blood coagulation factor VII) |
| **SPECT** | single photon emission computed tomography |
| **sp gr** | specific gravity |
| **sph** | spherical or spherical lens |
| **SQ** | subcutaneous |
| **SR** | stimulation ratio |
| **sr** | steradian |
| **SRBC** | sheep red blood cell |
| **SRF** | skin reactive factor |
| **SRH** | somatotropin-releasing hormone |
| **sRNA** | soluble ribonucleic acid |
| **SRS-A** | slow-reacting substance of anaphylaxis |
| **SS** | somatostatin |
| **SSD** | source-skin distance |
| **ssDNA** | single-stranded DNA |
| **SSPE** | subacute sclerosing panencephalitis |
| **ssRNA** | single-stranded RNA |
| **SSS** | sick sinus syndrome |
| | specific soluble substance |
| **ST** | sinus tachycardia |
| **STD** | sexually transmitted disease |
| **STI** | systolic time intervals |
| **STP** | standard temperature and pressure (0° C and 760 mm Hg) |
| **STS** | serologic test for syphilis |
| **SUDS** | sudden unexplained death syndrome |
| **SV** | simian virus |
| | sinus venosus |
| | stroke volume |
| **Sv** | sievert |
| **SVC** | superior vena cava |
| **T** | intraocular tension |
| | tesla |
| | thoracic vertebrae (T1–T12) |
| | thymine |
| | thymidine |
| | transmittance |
| **$T_{\frac{1}{2}}$** | half-life |
| | half-time |
| **$T_1$** | tricuspid valve closure |
| **$T_3$** | triiodothyronine |
| **$T_4$** | thyroxine |
| **$T_m$** | melting temperature |
| | tubular maximum |
| **t** | translocation |
| ***t*** | temperature |
| | time |
| **$t_{\frac{1}{2}}$** | half-life |
| | half-time |
| **$\theta$** | angle |
| **$\tau$** | mean life |
| | torque |
| **TA** | Terminologia Anatomica |
| | toxin-antitoxin |
| **TAC** | tetracaine, epinephrine, and cocaine |
| **TAT** | thematic apperception test |
| | toxin-antitoxin |
| **TBG** | thyroxine-binding globulin |
| **TBII** | TSH-binding inhibitory immunoglobulins |
| **TC** | transcobalamin |
| **$TCD_{50}$** | median tissue culture dose |
| **$TCID_{50}$** | median tissue culture infective dose |
| **TCMI** | T cell–mediated immunity |

| Abbreviation | Meaning |
|---|---|
| **TCR** | T cell antigen receptor |
| **Td** | tetanus and diphtheria toxoids, adult type |
| **$TD_{50}$** | median toxic dose |
| **TDA** | TSH-displacing antibody |
| **TDI** | toluene diisocyanate |
| **TdT** | terminal deoxynucleotidyl transferase |
| **TEA** | tetraethylammonium |
| **TeBG** | testosterone-estradiol–binding globulin |
| **TED** | threshold erythema dose |
| **TEE** | transesophageal echocardiography |
| **TENS** | transcutaneous electrical nerve stimulation |
| **TET** | treadmill exercise test |
| **TF** | transfer factor |
| **TGF** | transforming growth factor |
| **TGT** | thromboplastin generation test |
| **THC** | tetrahydrocannabinol |
| **Thr** | threonine |
| **TIA** | transient ischemic attack |
| **tid** | three times a day (L. ter in die) |
| **TK** | thymidine kinase |
| **TKD** | tokodynamometer |
| **TKG** | tokodynagraph |
| **TLC** | thin-layer chromatography |
| | total lung capacity |
| **TLSO** | thoracolumbosacral orthosis |
| **TLV** | threshold limit value |
| **TMA** | trimellitic anhydride |
| **TMI** | transmandibular implant |
| **TMST** | treadmill stress test |
| **TMV** | tobacco mosaic virus |
| **TND** | transmissible neurodegenerative disease |
| **TNF** | tumor necrosis factor |
| **TNS** | transcutaneous nerve stimulation |
| **TNT** | trinitrotoluene |
| **TOPV** | poliovirus vaccine live oral trivalent |
| **t-PA, TPA** | tissue plasminogen activator |
| **TPHA** | *Treponema pallidum* hemagglutination assay |
| **TPN** | total parenteral nutrition |
| **TR** | tricuspid regurgitation |
| **TRH** | thyrotropin-releasing hormone |
| **tRNA** | transfer RNA |
| **Trp** | tryptophan |
| **TRU** | turbidity reducing unit |
| **TS** | test solution |
| **TSA** | tumor-specific antigen |
| **TSF** | triceps skinfold |
| **TSH** | thyroid-stimulating hormone |
| **TSTA** | tumor-specific transplantation antigen |
| **TT** | thrombin time |
| **TU** | tuberculin unit |
| **TURP** | transurethral prostatic resection |
| **TWZ** | triangular working zone |
| **$TXA_2$, $TXB_2$** | thromboxanes $A_2$ and $B_2$ |
| **Tyr** | tyrosine |
| **U** | international unit of enzyme activity |
| | unit |
| | uracil |
| | uranium |
| | uridine |
| **u** | atomic mass unit |
| **UDP** | uridine diphosphate |
| **UK** | urokinase |
| **UMP** | uridine monophosphate |
| **US** | ultrasound |
| **UTP** | uridine triphosphate |
| **UVA** | ultraviolet A |
| **UVB** | ultraviolet B |
| **UVC** | ultraviolet C |
| **V** | vanadium |
| | volt |
| ***V*** | voltage |
| | volume |
| **$V_{max}$** | maximum velocity of an enzyme-catalyzed reaction |
| **$V_T$** | tidal volume |
| **v.** | L. vena (vein) |
| ***v*** | velocity |
| | voltage |
| **VA** | visual acuity |
| **VAD** | ventricular assist device |
| **Val** | valine |
| **var.** | variety |
| **VC** | vital capacity |
| **VCG** | vectorcardiogram |
| **VD** | venereal disease |
| **VDH** | valvular disease of the heart |
| **VEE** | Venezuelan equine encephalomyelitis |
| **VEP** | visual evoked potential |
| **VF** | vocal fremitus |
| **vf** | visual field |
| **VFib** | ventricular fibrillation |
| **VFl** | ventricular flutter |
| **VIG** | vaccinia immune globulin |
| **VIP** | vasoactive intestinal polypeptide |
| **VLA** | very late activation (antigen) |
| **VLBW** | very low birth weight |
| **VLDL** | very low-density lipoprotein |
| **VMA** | vanillylmandelic acid |
| **VPB** | ventricular premature beat |
| **VPC** | ventricular premature complex |
| **VPD** | ventricular premature depolarization |
| **VPRC** | volume of packed red cells |
| **VR** | vocal resonance |
| **VS** | volumetric solution |
| **VSG** | variable surface glycoprotein |
| **VT** | ventricular tachycardia |
| **vv.** | L. venae (veins) |
| **v/v** | volume (of solute) per volume (of solvent) |
| **VW** | vessel wall |
| **vWF** | von Willebrand's factor |
| **VZIG** | varicella-zoster immune globulin |
| **W** | tungsten (Ger. Wolfram) |
| | watt |
| ***W*** | work |
| **Wb** | weber |
| **WBC** | white blood cell |
| | white blood (cell) count |
| **WEE** | western equine encephalomyelitis |
| **wt** | weight |
| **w/v** | weight (of solute) per volume (of solvent) |
| **X** | Kienbock's unit |
| | xanthine |
| | xanthosine |
| **$\overline{X}$** | sample mean |
| ***X*** | reactance |
| ***x*** | abscissa |
| **XMP** | xanthosine monophosphate |
| **XOAN** | X-linked (Nettleship) ocular albinism |
| **Y** | yttrium |
| ***y*** | ordinate |
| ***Z*** | atomic number and impedance |
| **ZSR** | zeta sedimentation rate |

APPENDIX 2

# Anatomy: Arteries

**Arteries**

| Common Name* | TA Equivalent† | Origin* | Branches* | Distribution |
|---|---|---|---|---|
| accompanying a. of sciatic nerve. *See* sciatic a. | | | | |
| acromiothoracic a. *See* thoracoacromial a. | | | | |
| a's of Adamkiewicz | rami spinales arteriae vertebralis | transverse part of vertebral a. | | spinal cord, meninges, vertebral bodies, intervertebral disks |
| alveolar a's, anterior superior | aa. alveolares superiores anteriores | infraorbital a. | dental branches | incisor and canine regions of upper jaw, maxillary sinus |
| alveolar a., inferior | a. alveolaris inferior | maxillary a. | dental, peridental, mental mylohyoid branches | lower jaw, lower lip, chin |
| alveolar a., posterior superior | a. alveolaris superior posterior | maxillary a. | dental and peridental branches | molar and premolar regions of upper jaw, maxillary sinus, buccinator muscle |
| angular a. | a. angularis | facial a. | | lacrimal sac, lower eyelid, nose |
| aorta | aorta | left ventricle | | |
| abdominal aorta | pars abdominalis aortae | lower portion of descending aorta, from aortic hiatus of diaphragm to bifurcation into common iliac a's | inferior phrenic, lumbar, median sacral, superior and inferior mesenteric, middle suprarenal, renal, and testicular or ovarian a's, celiac trunk | |
| arch of aorta | arcus aortae | continuation of ascending aorta | brachiocephalic trunk, left common carotid and left subclavian a's; continues as descending (thoracic) aorta | |
| ascending aorta | pars ascendens aortae | proximal portion of aorta, arising from left ventricle | right and left coronary a's; continues as arch of aorta | |
| descending aorta. *See* thoracic aorta; abdominal aorta | pars descendens aortae | continuation of aorta from arch of aorta to division into common iliac arteries | | |
| thoracic aorta | pars thoracica aortae | proximal portion of descending aorta, continuing from arch of aorta to aortic hiatus of diaphragm | bronchial, esophageal, pericardiac, and mediastinal branches, superior phrenic a's, posterior intercostal a's [III–XI], subcostal a's, continues as abdominal aorta | |
| appendicular a. | a. appendicularis | ileocolic a. | | vermiform appendix |
| arcuate a. of foot | a. arcuata pedis | dorsalis pedis a. | deep plantar branch, dorsal metatarsal a's | foot, toes |
| arcuate a's of kidney | aa. arcuatae renis | interlobar a. | interlobar a's, straight arterioles of kidney | parenchyma of kidney |
| auditory a., internal. *See* a. of labyrinth | | | | |
| auricular a., deep | a. auricularis profunda | maxillary a. | | skin of auditory canal, tympanic membrane, temporomandibular joint |
| auricular a., posterior | a. auricularis posterior | external carotid a. | auricular and occipital branches, stylomastoid a. | middle ear, mastoid cells, auricle, parotid gland, digastric and other muscles |

* a. = artery; a's = (pl.) arteries.
† a. = [L.] arteria; aa. = [L. (pl.)] arteriae; r. = [L.] ramus (branch); rr. = [L.] rami (branches).

**Arteries** *Continued*

| Common Name | TA Equivalent | Origin | Branches | Distribution |
|---|---|---|---|---|
| axillary a. | a. axillaris | continuation of subclavian a. | subscapular branches, superior thoracic, thoracoacromial, lateral thoracic, subscapular, and anterior and posterior circumflex humeral a's | upper limb, axilla, chest, shoulder |
| basilar a. | a. basilaris | from junction of right and left vertebral a's | pontine branches, anterior inferior cerebellar, labyrinthine, superior cerebellar, posterior cerebral a's | brain stem, internal ear, cerebellum, posterior cerebrum |
| brachial a. | a. brachialis | continuation of axillary a. | superficial and deep brachial, nutrient of humerus, superior and inferior ulnar collateral, radial, ulnar a's | shoulder, arm, forearm, hand |
| brachial a., deep | a. profunda brachii | brachial a. | nutrient to humerus, deltoid branch, middle and radial collateral a's | humerus, muscles and skin of arm |
| brachial a., superficial | a. brachialis superficialis | variant brachial a., taking a more superficial course than usual | see *brachial a.* | see *brachial a.* |
| brachiocephalic trunk | truncus brachiocephalicus | arch of aorta | right common carotid, right subclavian a's | right side of head and neck, right arm |
| buccal a. | a. buccalis | maxillary a. | | buccinator muscle, oral mucous membrane |
| a. of bulb of penis | a. bulbi penis | internal pudendal a. | | bulbourethral gland, bulb of penis |
| a. of bulb of urethra. *See* a. of bulb of penis | | | | |
| a. of bulb of vestibule | a. bulbi vestibuli | internal pudendal a. | | bulb of vestibule of vagina, Bartholin glands |
| callosomarginal a. | a. callosomarginalis | anterior cerebral a. | anteromedial frontal, mediomedial frontal, posteromedial frontal, cingular branches | medial and upper lateral surfaces of cerebral hemisphere |
| capsular a's | rr. capsulares arteriae renalis | renal a. | | renal capsule |
| caroticotympanic a's | aa. caroticotympanicae | internal carotid a. | | tympanic cavity |
| carotid a., common | a. carotis communis | brachiocephalic trunk (right), arch of aorta (left) | external and internal carotid a's | see *carotid a., external* and *carotid a., internal* |
| carotid a., external | a. carotis externa | common carotid a. | superior thyroid, ascending pharyngeal, lingual, facial, sternocleidomastoid, occipital, posterior auricular, superficial temporal, maxillary a's | neck, face, skull |
| carotid a., internal | a. carotis interna | common carotid a. | caroticotympanic, ophthalmic, posterior communicating, anterior choroid, anterior cerebral, middle cerebral a's | middle ear, brain, hypophysis, orbit, choroid plexus |
| caudal a. *See* sacral a., median | | | | |
| cecal a., anterior | a. caecalis anterior | ileocolic a. | | cecum |
| cecal a., inferior | a. caecalis inferior | ileocolic a. | | cecum |
| celiac trunk | truncus celiacus | abdominal aorta | left gastric, common hepatic, splenic a's | esophagus, stomach, duodenum, spleen, pancreas, liver, gallbladder |
| central a's, anterolateral | aa. anterolaterales | middle cerebral a. | medial and lateral branches | anterior lenticular and caudate nuclei and internal capsule of brain |
| central a's, anteromedial | aa. centrales anteromediales | anterior cerebral a. | | anterior and medial corpus striatum |
| central a's, posterolateral | aa. centrales posterolaterales | posterior cerebral a. | | cerebral peduncle, posterior thalamus, colliculi, pineal and medial geniculate bodies |

**Arteries** *Continued*

| Common Name | TA Equivalent | Origin | Branches | Distribution |
|---|---|---|---|---|
| central a's, posteromedial | aa. centrales posteromediales | posterior cerebral a. | | anterior thalamus, lateral wall of third ventricle, globus pallidus |
| central a., long | | anterior cerebral a. | | |
| central a. of retina | a. centralis retinae | ophthalmic a. | | retina |
| central a., short | | anterior cerebral a. | | |
| cerebellar a., anterior, inferior | a. inferior anterior cerebelli | basilar a. | posterior, spinal (usually), and labyrinthine (usually) a's | lower anterior cerebellum, lower and lateral parts of pons, (sometimes) upper part of medulla oblongata |
| cerebellar a., posterior inferior | a. inferior posterior cerebelli | vertebral a. | | lower part of cerebellum, medulla, choroid plexus of fourth ventricle |
| cerebellar a., superior | a. superior cerebelli | basilar a. | | upper part of cerebellum, midbrain, pineal body, choroid plexus of third ventricle |
| cerebral a's | aa. cerebri | internal carotid a., basilar a. | | cerebral hemispheres |
| cerebral a., anterior | a. cerebri anterior | internal carotid a. | *precommunical part:* anteromedial central, long and short central, anterior communicating a's; *postcommunical part:* medial frontobasal, callosomarginal, paracentral, precuneal, parietooccipital a's | orbital, frontal, and parietal cortex, corpus callosum, diencephalon, corpus striatum, internal capsule, choroid plexus of lateral ventricle |
| cerebral a., middle | a. cerebri media | internal carotid a. | *sphenoidal part:* anterolateral central a; *insular part:* insular lateral frontobasilar, temporal a's; *terminal* or *cortical part:* a's of sulcus, parietal a's, a. of angular gyri | orbital, frontal, parietal, and temporal cortex, corpus striatum, internal capsule |
| cerebral a., posterior | a. cerebri posterior | terminal bifurcation of basilar a. | *precommunical part:* posteromedial central a's; *postcommunical part:* posterolateral central a's, medial and lateral posterior choroidal, peduncular branches; *terminal* or *cortical part:* lateral and medial occipital a's | occipital and temporal lobes, basal ganglia, choroid plexus of lateral ventricle, thalamus, midbrain |
| cervical a., ascending | a. cervicalis ascendens | inferior thyroid a. | | muscles of neck, vertebrae, vertebral canal |
| cervical a., deep | a. cervicalis profunda | costocervical trunk | | deep neck muscles |
| cervical a., transverse | a. transversa cervicis | subclavian a. | deep and superficial branches | root of neck, muscles of scapula interior of brain, including choroid plexus of lateral ventricle and adjacent parts |
| ciliary a's, anterior | aa. ciliares anteriores | ophthalmic and lacrimal a's | episcleral and anterior conjunctival a's | iris, conjunctiva |
| ciliary a's, posterior, long | aa. ciliares posteriores longae | ophthalmic a. | | iris, ciliary processes |
| ciliary a's, posterior, short | aa. ciliares posteriores breves | ophthalmic a. | | choroid coat of eye |
| circumflex a. | ramus circumflexus arteriae coronariae sinistrae | left coronary a. | atrial, atrial anastomotic, atrioventricular, intermediate atrial, left marginal, and left posterior ventricular branches | left ventricle, left atrium |
| circumflex femoral a., lateral | a. circumflexa femoris lateralis | deep femoral a. | ascending, descending, and transverse branches | hip joint, thigh muscles |
| circumflex femoral a., medial | a. circumflexa femoris medialis | deep femoral a. | acetabular, ascending, deep, and transverse branches | hip joint, thigh muscles |

**Arteries** *Continued*

| Common Name | TA Equivalent | Origin | Branches | Distribution |
|---|---|---|---|---|
| circumflex humeral a., anterior | a. circumflexa humeri anterior | axillary a. | | shoulder joint and head of humerus, long tendon of biceps, tendon of greater pectoral muscle |
| circumflex humeral a., posterior | a. circumflexa humeri posterior | axillary a. | | deltoid, shoulder joint, teres minor and triceps muscles |
| circumflex iliac a., deep | a. circumflexa ilium profunda | external iliac a. | ascending branches | iliac region, abdominal wall, groin |
| circumflex iliac a., superficial | a. circumflexa ilium superficialis | femoral a. | | groin, abdominal wall |
| circumflex a. of scapula | a. circumflexa scapulae | subscapular a. | | inferolateral muscles of scapula |
| coccygeal a. *See* sacral a., median | | | | |
| colic a., left | a. colica sinistra | inferior mesenteric a. | | descending colon |
| colic a., middle | a. colica media | superior mesenteric a. | | transverse colon |
| colic a., right | a. colica dextra | superior mesenteric a. | | ascending colon |
| colic a., right, inferior. *See* ileocolic a. | | | | |
| colic a., superior accessory. *See* colic a., middle | | | | |
| collateral a., inferior ulnar | a. collateralis ulnaris inferior | brachial a. | | arm muscles at back of elbow |
| collateral a., middle | a. collateralis media | deep brachial a. | | triceps muscle, elbow joint |
| collateral a., radial | a. collateralis radialis | deep brachial a. | | brachioradial and brachial muscles |
| collateral a., superior ulnar | a. collateralis ulnaris superior | brachial a. | | elbow joint, triceps muscle |
| communicating a., anterior | a. communicans anterior | precommunical part of anterior cerebral a. | | interconnects anterior cerebral a's |
| communicating a., posterior | a. communicans posterior | interconnects internal carotid and posterior cerebral a's | branches to optic chiasm, oculomotor nerve, thalamus, hypothalamus, and tail of caudate nucleus | |
| conjunctival a's, anterior | aa. conjunctivales anteriores | anterior ciliary a's | | conjunctiva |
| conjunctival a's, posterior | aa. conjunctivales posteriores | medial palpebral a. | | lacrimal caruncle, conjunctiva |
| coronary a., left anterior descending | ramus interventricularis anterior arteriae coronariae sinistrae | left coronary a. | conus a., lateral and interventricular septal branches | ventricles, interventricular septum |
| coronary a., posterior descending | ramus interventricularis posterior arteriae coronariae dextrae | right coronary a. | interventricular septal | diaphragmatic surface of ventricles, part of interventricular septum |
| coronary a. of heart, left | a. coronaria sinistra | left aortic sinus | anterior interventricular and circumflex branches | left ventricle, left atrium |
| coronary a. of heart, right | a. coronaria dextra | right aortic sinus | conus a., atrial, atrioventricular node, intermediate atrial, posterior interventricular, right marginal, and sinoatrial node branches | right ventricle, right atrium |
| coronary a. of stomach, left | a. gastrica sinistra | celiac a. | esophageal | esophagus, lesser curvature of stomach |
| coronary a. of stomach, right | a. gastrica dextra | common hepatic a. | | |
| costocervical trunk | truncus costocervicalis | subclavian a. | deep cervical and highest intercostal a's | deep neck muscles, first two intercostal spaces, vertebral column, back muscles |
| cremasteric a. | a. cremasterica | inferior epigastric a. | | cremaster muscle, coverings of spermatic cord |
| cystic a. | a. cystica | right branch of hepatic a., proper | | gallbladder |
| deep brachial a. *See* brachial a., deep | | | | |

**Arteries** *Continued*

| Common Name | TA Equivalent | Origin | Branches | Distribution |
|---|---|---|---|---|
| deep a. of clitoris | a. profunda clitoridis | internal pudendal a. | | clitoris |
| deep femoral a. *See* femoral a., deep | | | | |
| deep lingual a. *See* profunda linguae a. | | | | |
| deep a. of penis | a. profunda penis | internal pudendal a. | | corpus cavernosum penis |
| deferential a. *See* a. of ductus deferens | | | | |
| deltoid a. | ramus deltoideus arteriae profundae brachii | deep brachial a. | | brachialis and deltoid muscles |
| | ramus deltoideus arteriae thoracoacromialis | thoracoacromial a. | | deltoid and pectoralis major muscles |
| dental a's. *See* alveolar a's | | | | |
| diaphragmatic a's. *See* phrenic a's | | | | |
| digital a's, collateral. *See* digital a's, palmar, proper | | | | |
| digital a's of foot, common. *See* metatarsal a's, plantar | | | | |
| digital a's of foot, dorsal | aa. digitales dorsales pedis | dorsal metatarsal a's | | dorsum of toes |
| digital a's of hand, dorsal | aa. digitales dorsales manus | dorsal metacarpal a's | | dorsum of fingers |
| digital a's, palmar, common | aa. digitales palmares communes | superficial palmar arch | proper palmar digit a's | fingers |
| digital a's, palmar, proper | aa. digitales palmares propriae | common palmar digital a's | | fingers |
| digital a's, plantar, common | aa. digitales plantares communes | plantar metatarsal a's | proper plantar digital a's | toes |
| digital a's, plantar, proper | aa. digitales plantares propriae | common plantar digital a's | | toes |
| dorsal a. of clitoris | a. dorsalis clitoridis | internal pudendal a. | | clitoris |
| dorsal a. of foot. *See* dorsalis pedis a. | | | | |
| dorsal a. of nose | a. dorsalis nasi | ophthalmic a. | lacrimal branch | dorsum of nose |
| dorsal a. of penis | a. dorsalis penis | internal pudendal a. | | glans, corona, and prepuce of penis |
| dorsalis pedis a. | a. dorsalis pedis | continuation of anterior tibial a. | lateral and medial tarsal, arcuate, and deep plantar a's | foot, toes |
| a. of ductus deferens | a. ductus deferentis | umbilical a. | ureteral artery | ureter, ductus deferens, seminal vesicles, testes |
| duodenal a's. *See* pancreaticoduodenal a's, inferior | | | | |
| epigastric a., external. *See* circumflex iliac a., deep | | | | |
| epigastric a., inferior | a. epigastrica inferior | external iliac a. | pubic branch, cremasteric a., a. of round ligament of uterus | abdominal wall |
| epigastric a., superficial | a. epigastrica superficialis | femoral a. | | abdominal wall, groin |
| epigastric a., superior | a. epigastrica superior | internal thoracic a. | | abdominal wall, diaphragm |
| episcleral a's | aa. episclerales | anterior ciliary a. | | iris, ciliary processes |
| ethmoidal a., anterior | a. ethmoidalis anterior | ophthalmic a. | anterior meningeal, anterior septal, anterior lateral nasal branches | dura mater, nose, frontal sinus, anterior ethmoidal cells |
| ethmoidal a., posterior | a. ethmoidalis posterior | ophthalmic a. | | conjunctival ethmoidal cells, dura mater, nose |
| facial a. | a. facialis | external carotid a. | ascending palatine, submental, inferior and superior labial, septal, lateral nasal, and angular a's; tonsillar and glandular branches | face, tonsil, palate, submandibular gland |
| facial a., deep. *See* maxillary a. | | | | |
| facial a., transverse | a. transversa faciei | superficial temporal a. | | parotid region |
| fallopian a. *See* uterine a. | | | | |

**Arteries** Continued

| Common Name | TA Equivalent | Origin | Branches | Distribution |
|---|---|---|---|---|
| femoral a. | a. femoralis | continuation of external iliac a. | superficial epigastric, superficial circumflex iliac, external pudendal, profunda femoris, and descending genicular a's | lower abdominal wall, external genitalia, lower limb |
| femoral a., deep | a. profunda femoris | femoral a. | medial and lateral circumflex femoral a's, perforating a's | thigh muscles, hip joint, gluteal muscle, femur |
| fibular a. *See* peroneal a. | | | | |
| frontal a. *See* supratrochlear a. | | | | |
| frontobasal a., lateral | a. frontobasalis lateralis | middle cerebral a. | | cortex of frontal lobe |
| frontobasal a., medial | a. frontobasalis medialis | anterior cerebral a. | | cortex of frontal lobe |
| funicular a. *See* testicular a. | | | | |
| gastric a., left | a. gastrica sinistra | celiac trunk | esophageal branches | esophagus, lesser curvature of stomach |
| gastric a., posterior | a. gastrica posterior | splenic a. | | posterior gastric wall |
| gastric a., right | a. gastrica dextra | common hepatic a. | | lesser curvature of stomach |
| gastric a's, short | aa. gastricae breves | splenic a. | | upper part of stomach |
| gastroduodenal a. | a. gastroduodenalis | common hepatic a. | superior pancreaticoduodenal and right gastroepiploic a's | stomach, duodenum, pancreas, greater omentum |
| gastroepiploic a., left. *See* gastro-omental a., left | | | | |
| gastroepiploic a., right. *See* gastro-omental a., right | | | | |
| gastro-omental a., left | a. gastroomentalis sinistra | splenic a. | gastric and omental branches | stomach and greater omentum |
| gastro-omental a., right | a. gastroomentalis dextra | gastroduodenal a. | gastric and omental branches | stomach and greater omentum |
| genicular a., descending | a. descendens genus | femoral a. | saphenous, articular branches | knee joint, upper and medial part of leg |
| genicular a., lateral inferior | a. inferior lateralis genus | popliteal a. | | knee joint |
| genicular a., lateral superior | a. superior lateralis genus | popliteal a. | | knee joint, femur, patella, contiguous muscles |
| genicular a., medial inferior | a. inferior medialis genus | popliteal a. | | knee joint |
| genicular a., medial superior | a. superior medialis genus | popliteal a. | | knee joint, femur, patella, contiguous muscles |
| genicular a., middle | a. media genus | popliteal a. | | knee joint, cruciate ligaments, patellar synovial and alar folds |
| gluteal a., inferior | a. glutea inferior | internal iliac a. | sciatic a. | buttock, back of thigh |
| gluteal a., superior | a. glutea superior | internal iliac a. | superficial and deep branches | buttocks |
| helicine a's | aa. helicinae penis | deep and dorsal a's of penis | superficial and deep branches | erectile tissue of penis |
| hemorrhoidal a's. *See* rectal a's | | | | |
| hepatic a., common | a. hepatica communis | celiac trunk | right gastric, gastroduodenal, proper hepatic a's | stomach, pancreas, duodenum, liver, gallbladder, greater omentum |
| hepatic a., proper | a. hepatica propria | common hepatic a. | right and left branches | liver, gallbladder |
| hyaloid a. | a. hyaloidea | fetal ophthalmic a. | | fetal lens (usually not present after birth) |
| hypogastric a. *See* iliac a., internal | | | | |
| hypophyseal a., inferior | a. hypophysialis inferior | internal carotid a. | | pituitary gland |
| hypophyseal a., superior | a. hypophysialis superior | internal carotid a. | | pituitary gland |
| iliac a., common | a. iliaca communis | abdominal aorta | internal and external iliac a's | pelvis, abdominal wall, lower limb |
| iliac a., external | a. iliaca externa | common iliac a. | inferior epigastric, deep circumflex iliac a's | abdominal wall, external genitalia, lower limb |

**Arteries** *Continued*

| Common Name | TA Equivalent | Origin | Branches | Distribution |
|---|---|---|---|---|
| iliac a., internal | a. iliaca interna | continuation of common iliac a. | iliolumbar, obturator, superior and inferior gluteal, umbilical, inferior vesical, uterine, middle rectal, and internal pudendal a's | wall and viscera of pelvis, buttock, reproductive organs, medial aspect of thigh |
| ileal a's | aa. ileales | superior mesenteric a. | | ileum |
| ileocolic a. | a. ileocolica | superior mesenteric a. | anterior and posterior cecal and appendicular a's, colic (ascending) and ileal branches | ileum, cecum, vermiform appendix, ascending colon |
| iliolumbar a. | a. iliolumbalis | internal iliac a. | iliac and lumbar branches, lateral sacral a's | pelvic muscles and bones, fifth lumbar vertebra, sacrum |
| infraorbital a. | a. infraorbitalis | maxillary a. | anterior superior alveolar a's | maxilla, maxillary sinus, upper teeth, lower eyelid, cheek, nose |
| innominate a. *See* brachiocephalic trunk | | | | |
| insular a's | aa. insulares | insular part of cerebral a. | | cortex of insula |
| intercostal a., highest | a. intercostalis suprema | costocervical trunk | posterior intercostal a's I and II | upper thoracic wall |
| intercostal a's, posterior, I and II | aa. intercostales posteriores I et II | highest intercostal a. | dorsal and spinal branches | upper thoracic wall |
| intercostal a's, posterior, III–XI | aa. intercostales posteriores III–XI | thoracic aorta | dorsal, spinal, lateral and medial cutaneous collateral, and lateral mammary branches | thoracic wall |
| interlobar a's of kidney | aa. interlobares renis | lower branches of segmental a's | arcuate a's | parenchyma of kidney |
| interlobular a's of kidney | aa. interlobulares renis | arcuate a's of kidney | | renal glomeruli |
| interlobular a's of liver | aa. interlobulares hepatis | right or left branch of proper hepatic a. | between lobules of liver | |
| interosseous a., anterior | a. interossea anterior | posterior or common interosseous a. | median a. | deep parts of front of forearm |
| interosseous a., common | a. interossea communis | ulnar a. | anterior and posterior interosseous a's | antecubital fossa |
| interosseous a., posterior | a. interossea posterior | common interosseous a. | recurrent interosseous a. | deep parts of back of forearm |
| interosseous a., recurrent | a. interossea recurrens | posterior or common interosseous a. | | back of elbow joint |
| intestinal a's | | vessels arising from superior mesenteric a. and supplying intestines; they include pancreaticoduodenal, jejunal, ileal, ileocolic, and colic a's | | |
| jejunal a's | aa. jejunales | superior mesenteric a. | | jejunum |
| labial a., inferior | a. labialis inferior | facial a. | | lower lip |
| labial a., superior | a. labialis superior | facial a. | septal and alar branches | upper lip and nose |
| a. of labyrinth | a. labyrinthi | basilar or anterior inferior cerebellar a. | vestibular and cochlear branches | internal ear |
| lacrimal a. | a. lacrimalis | ophthalmic a. | lateral palpebral a. | lacrimal gland, eyelids, conjunctiva |
| laryngeal a., inferior | a. laryngea inferior | inferior thyroid a. | | larynx, trachea, esophagus |
| laryngeal a., superior | a. laryngea superior | superior thyroid a. | | larynx |
| lingual a. | a. lingualis | external carotid a. | suprahyoid, sublingual, dorsal lingual, profunda linguae branches | tongue, sublingual gland, tonsil, epiglottis |
| lingual a., deep. *See* profunda linguae a. | | | | |
| lumbar a's | aa. lumbales | abdominal aorta | dorsal and spinal branches | posterior abdominal wall, renal capsule |
| lumbar a., lowest | aa. lumbales imae | median sacral a. | | sacrum, greatest gluteal muscle |
| mammary a., external. *See* thoracic a., lateral | | | | |
| mammary a., internal. *See* thoracic a., internal | | | | |
| mandibular a. *See* alveolar a., inferior | | | | |
| marginal a. of colon | a. marginalis coli | branches from superior and inferior mesenteric a's | runs along inner perimeter of large intestine from ileocolic junction to rectum and gives off straight arteries that supply intestinal wall | |

**Arteries** *Continued*

| Common Name | TA Equivalent | Origin | Branches | Distribution |
|---|---|---|---|---|
| marginal a. of Drummond. *See* marginal a. of colon. | | | | |
| masseteric a. | a. masseterica | maxillary a. | | masseter muscle |
| maxillary a. | a. maxillaris | external carotid a. | pterygoid branches; deep auricular, anterior tympanic, inferior alveolar, middle meningeal, masseteric, deep temporal, buccal, posterior superior alveolar, infra-orbital, descending palatine, and sphenopalatine a's, and a. of pterygoid canal | both jaws, teeth, muscles of mastication, ear, meninges, nose, paranasal sinuses, palate |
| maxillary a., external. *See* facial a. | | | | |
| maxillary a., internal. *See* maxillary a. | | | | |
| median a. | a. comitans nervi mediani | anterior interosseous a. | | median nerve, muscles of front of forearm |
| meningeal a., middle | a. meningea media | maxillary a. | frontal, parietal, lacrimal, anastomotic, accessory meningeal, and petrous branches, and superior tympanic a. | cranial bones, dura mater |
| meningeal a., posterior | a. meningea posterior | ascending pharyngeal a. | | bones and dura mater of posterior cranial fossa |
| mesencephalic a's | aa. mesencephalicae | basilar a. | | cerebral peduncle |
| mesenteric a., inferior | a. mesenterica inferior | abdominal aorta | left colic, sigmoid, and superior rectal a's | descending colon, rectum |
| mesenteric a., superior | a. mesenterica superior | abdominal aorta | inferior pancreaticoduodenal, jejunal, ileal, ileocolic, right and middle colic a's | small intestine, proximal half of colon |
| metacarpal a's, dorsal | aa. metacarpales dorsales | dorsal carpal rete and radial a. | dorsal digital a's | dorsum of fingers |
| metacarpal a's, palmar | aa. metacarpales palmares | deep palmar arch | | deep parts of metacarpus |
| metatarsal a's, dorsal | aa. metatarsales dorsales | arcuate a. of foot | dorsal digital a's | dorsum of foot, including toes |
| metatarsal a's, plantar | aa. metatarsales plantares | plantar arch | perforating branches, common and proper plantar digital a's | plantar surface of toes |
| musculophrenic a. | a. musculophrenica | internal thoracic a. | | diaphragm, abdominal and thoracic walls |
| nasal a's, posterior lateral | aa. nasales posteriores laterales | sphenopalatine a. | | frontal, maxillary, and sphenoidal sinuses |
| nutrient a's of femur | aa. nutriciae femoris | third perforating a. | | femur |
| nutrient a's of fibula | aa. nutriciae fibulae | fibular a. | | fibula |
| nutrient a's of humerus | aa. nutriciae humeri | brachial and deep brachial a's | | humerus |
| nutrient a's of tibia | aa. nutriciae tibiae | posterior tibial a. | | tibia |
| obturator a. | a. obturatoria | internal iliac a. | pubic, acetabular, anterior and posterior branches | pelvic muscles, hip joint |
| obturator a., accessory | a. obturatoria accessoria | variant obturator a., arising from inferior epigastric instead of internal iliac a. | | |
| occipital a. | a. occipitalis | external carotid a. | auricular, meningeal, mastoid, descending, occipital, and sternocleidomastoid branches | muscles of neck and scalp, meninges, mastoid cells |
| occipital a., lateral | a. occipitalis lateralis | posterior cerebral a. | anterior temporal, middle intermediate temporal, and posterior temporal branches | anterior, medial, intermediate, and posterior parts of temporal lobe |
| occipital a., middle | a. occipitalis medialis | posterior cerebral a. | dorsal corpus callosum, parietal, parieto-occipital, calcarine, occipital, occipitotemporal branches | dorsum of corpus callosum, precuneus, cuneus, lingual gyrus, posterior part of lateral surface of occipital lobe |

**Arteries** *Continued*

| Common Name | TA Equivalent | Origin | Branches | Distribution |
|---|---|---|---|---|
| ophthalmic a. | a. ophthalmica | internal carotid a. | lacrimal and supraorbital a's, central a. of retina, ciliary, posterior and anterior ethmoidal, palpebral, supratrochlear, and dorsal nasal a's | eye, orbit, adjacent facial structures |
| ovarian a. | a. ovarica | abdominal aorta | ureteral and tubal branches | ureter, ovary, uterine tube |
| palatine a., ascending | a. palatina ascendens | facial a. | | soft palate, wall of pharynx, tonsil, auditory tube |
| palatine a., descending | a. palatina descendens | maxillary a. | greater and lesser palatine a's | soft and hard palates, tonsil |
| palatine a., greater | a. palatina major | descending palatine a. | | hard palate |
| palatine a's, lesser | aa. palatinae minores | descending palatine a. | | soft palate, tonsil |
| palpebral a's, lateral | aa. palpebrales laterales | lacrimal a. | | eyelids, conjunctiva |
| palpebral a's, medial | aa. palpebrales mediales | ophthalmic a. | posterior conjunctival a's | eyelids |
| pancreaticoduodenal a., anterior superior | a. pancreaticoduodenalis superior anterior | gastroduodenal a. | pancreatic and duodenal branches | pancreas, duodenum |
| pancreaticoduodenal a's, inferior | a. pancreaticoduodenalis inferior | superior mesenteric a. | anterior and posterior branches | pancreas, duodenum |
| pancreaticoduodenal a., posterior superior | a. pancreaticoduodenalis superior posterior | gastroduodenal a. | pancreatic and duodenal branches | pancreas, duodenum |
| paracentral a's | rr. paracentrales | pericallosal | | cerebral cortex and medial central sulcus |
| parietal a., anterior | a. parietalis anterior | middle cerebral a. | | anterior parietal lobe |
| parietal a., posterior | a. parietalis posterior | middle cerebral a. | | posterior temporal lobe |
| parieto-occipital a's | rr. parietooccipitales | pericallosal | | parietal lobe and sometimes occipital lobe |
| perforating a's | aa. perforantes | deep femoral a. | nutrient a's | adductor, hamstring, and gluteal muscles, femur |
| pericardiacophrenic a. | a. pericardiacophrenica | internal thoracic a. | | pericardium, diaphragm, pleura |
| perineal a. | a. perinealis | internal pudendal a. | | perineum, skin of external genitalia |
| peroneal a. | a. fibularis | posterior tibial a. | perforating, communicating, calcaneal, and lateral and medial malleolar branches, calcaneal rete | lateral side and back of ankle, deep calf muscles |
| pharyngeal a., ascending | a. pharyngea ascendens | external carotid a. | posterior meningeal, pharyngeal, inferior tympanic branches | pharynx, soft palate, ear, meninges |
| phrenic a's, great. *See* phrenic a's, inferior | | | | |
| phrenic a., inferior | a. phrenica inferior | abdominal aorta | superior suprarenal a's | diaphragm, suprarenal gland |
| phrenic a's, superior | aa. phrenicae superiores | thoracic aorta | | upper surface of vertebral portion of diaphragm |
| plantar a., lateral | a. plantaris lateralis | posterior tibial a. | plantar arch, plantar metatarsal a's | sole of foot, toes |
| plantar a., medial | a. plantaris medialis | posterior tibial a. | deep and superficial branches | sole of foot, toes |
| pontine a's | aa. pontis | basilar a. | | pons and adjacent areas of the brain |
| popliteal a. | a. poplitea | continuation of femoral a. | lateral and medial superior genicular, middle genicular, sural, lateral and medial inferior genicular, anterior and posterior tibial a's; articular rete of knee, patellar rete | knee and calf |
| precuneal a's | rr. precuneales | pericallosal a. | | inferior precuneus |
| prepancreatic a. | a. prepancreatica | splenic a., anterior superior pancreaticoduodenal a. | | between the neck and uncinate process of pancreas |
| princeps pollicis a. | a. princeps pollicis | radial a. | radialis indicis a. | sides and palmar aspect of thumb |
| principal a. of thumb. *See* princeps pollicis a. | | | | |
| profunda linguae a. | a. profunda linguae | lingual a. | | tongue |

**Arteries** *Continued*

| Common Name | TA Equivalent | Origin | Branches | Distribution |
|---|---|---|---|---|
| a. of pterygoid canal | a. canalis pterygoidei | maxillary a. | pterygoid | roof of pharynx, auditory tube |
| pudendal a's, external | aa. pudendae externae | femoral a. | anterior scrotal or anterior labial branches, inguinal branches | external genitalia, upper medial thigh |
| pudendal a., internal | a. pudenda interna | internal iliac a. | posterior scrotal or posterior labial branches, inferior rectal, perineal, urethral a's, a. of bulb of penis or vestibule, deep a. and dorsal a. of penis or clitoris | external genitalia, anal canal, perineum |
| pulmonary a., left | a. pulmonalis sinistra | pulmonary trunk | numerous branches named according to segments of lung to which they distribute unaerated blood | left lung |
| pulmonary a., right | a. pulmonalis dextra | pulmonary trunk | numerous branches named according to segments of lung to which they distribute unaerated blood | right lung |
| pulmonary trunk | truncus pulmonalis | right ventricle | right and left pulmonary a's | conveys unaerated blood toward lungs |
| radial a. | a. radial | brachial a. | palmar carpal, superficial palmar and dorsal carpal branches; recurrent radial a., princeps pollicis a., deep palmar arch | forearm, wrist, hand |
| radial a., collateral. *See* collateral a., radial | | | | |
| radial a. of index finger. *See* radialis indicis a. | | | | |
| radialis indicis a. | a. radialis indicis | princeps pollicis a. | | index finger |
| radiate a's of kidney. *See* interlobular a's of kidney | | | | |
| ranine a. *See* profunda linguae a. | | | | |
| rectal a., inferior | a. rectalis inferior | internal pudendal a. | | rectum, anal canal |
| rectal a., middle | a. rectalis media | internal iliac a. | | rectum, prostate, seminal vesicles, vagina |
| rectal a., superior | a. rectalis superior | inferior mesenteric a. | | rectum |
| recurrent a., radial | a. recurrens radialis | radial a. | | brachioradial and brachial muscles, elbow region |
| recurrent a., tibial, anterior | a. recurrens tibialis anterior | anterior tibial a. | | anterior tibial muscle and long extensor muscle of toes; knee joint, contiguous fascia and skin |
| recurrent a., tibial, posterior | a. recurrens tibialis posterior | anterior tibial a. | | knee |
| recurrent a., ulnar | a. recurrens ulnaris | ulnar a. | anterior and posterior branches | elbow region |
| renal a. | a. renalis | abdominal aorta | ureteral branches, inferior suprarenal a. | kidney, suprarenal gland, ureter |
| renal a's. *See* arcuate, interlobar, *and* interlobular a's of kidney, *and* straight arterioles of kidney | | | | |
| a. of round ligament of uterus | a. ligamenti teretis uteri | inferior epigastric a. | | round ligament of uterus |
| sacral a's, lateral | aa. sacrales laterales | iliolumbar a. | spinal branches | structures about coccyx and sacrum |
| sacral a., median | a. sacralis mediana | central continuation of abdominal aorta, beyond origin of common iliac a's | lowest lumbar a. | sacrum, coccyx, rectum |
| scapular a., dorsal | a. dorsalis scapulae | subclavian (deep) branch of transverse cervical a. | | rhomboid, latissimus dorsi, trapezius muscles |

**Arteries** *Continued*

| Common Name | TA Equivalent | Origin | Branches | Distribution |
|---|---|---|---|---|
| scapular a., transverse. *See* suprascapular a. | | | | |
| sciatic a. | a. comitans nervi ischiadici | inferior gluteal a. | | accompanies sciatic nerve |
| septal a's, anterior | rami interventriculares septales rami interventricularis anterioris arteriae coronariae sinistrae | left coronary a. | | anterior interventricular septum |
| septal a's, posterior | rami interventriculares septales rami interventricularis posterioris arteriae coronariae dextrae | right coronary a. | | posterior interventricular septum |
| sigmoid a's | aa. sigmoideae | inferior mesenteric a. | | sigmoid colon |
| spermatic a., external. *See* cremasteric a. | | | | |
| sphenopalatine a. | a. sphenopalatina | maxillary a. | posterior lateral nasal a. and posterior septal branches | structures adjoining nasal cavity, nasopharynx |
| spinal a., anterior | a. spinalis anterior | vertebral a. | | spinal cord |
| spinal a., posterior | a. spinalis posterior | vertebral a. | | spinal cord |
| splenic a. | a. splenica | celiac trunk | pancreatic and splenic branches, prepancreatic, left gastroepiploic, short gastric a's | spleen, pancreas, stomach, greater omentum |
| straight arterioles of kidney | arteriolae rectae renis | arcuate a's of kidney | | renal pyramids |
| stylomastoid a. | a. stylomastoidea | posterior auricular a. | mastoid and stapedial branches, posterior tympanica | middle ear walls, mastoid cells, stapedius |
| subclavian a. | a. subclavia | brachiocephalic trunk (right), arch of aorta (left) | vertebral, internal thoracic a's, thyrocervical and costocervical trunks | neck, thoracic wall, spinal cord, brain, meninges, upper limb |
| subcostal a. | a. subcostalis | thoracic aorta | dorsal and spinal branches | upper posterior abdominal wall |
| sublingual a. | a. sublingualis | lingual a. | | sublingual gland |
| submental a. | a. submentalis | facial a. | | tissue under chin |
| subscapular a. | a. subscapularis | axillary a. | thoracodorsal and circumflex scapular a's | scapular and shoulder region |
| a. of central sulcus | a. sulci centralis | middle cerebral a. | | cortex on either side of central sulcus |
| a. of postcentral sulcus | a. sulci postcentralis | middle cerebral a. | | cortex on either side of postcentral sulcus |
| a. of precentral sulcus | a. sulci precentralis | middle cerebral a. | | cortex on either side of precentral sulcus |
| supraduodenal a. | a. supraduodenalis | gastroduodenal a. | duodenal branch | superior part of duodenum |
| supraorbital a. | a. supraorbitalis | ophthalmic a. | superficial, deep, diploic branches | forehead, superior muscles of orbit, upper eyelid, frontal sinus |
| suprarenal a., inferior | a. suprarenalis inferior | renal a. | | suprarenal gland |
| suprarenal a., middle | a. suprarenalis media | abdominal aorta | | suprarenal gland |
| suprarenal a's, superior | aa. suprarenales superiores | inferior phrenic a. | | suprarenal gland |
| suprascapular a. | a. suprascapularis | thyrocervical trunk | acromial branch | clavicular, deltoid, and scapular regions |
| supratrochlear a. | a. supratrochlearis | ophthalmic a. | | anterior scalp |
| sural a's | aa. surales | popliteal a. | | popliteal space, calf |
| sylvian a. *See* cerebral a., middle | | | | |
| tarsal a., lateral | a. tarsalis lateralis | dorsalis pedis a. | | tarsus |
| tarsal a's, medial | aa. tarsales mediales | dorsalis pedis a. | | side of foot |
| temporal a., anterior | a. temporalis anterior | middle cerebral a. | | cortex of anterior temporal lobe |
| temporal a., anterior deep | a. temporalis profunda anterior | maxillary a. | to zygomatic bone and greater wing of sphenoid bone | temporal muscle |
| temporal a., middle | a. temporalis media | 1. superficial temporal a.<br>2. middle cerebral a. | | 1. temporal region<br>2. cortex of temporal lobe |
| temporal a., posterior | a. temporalis posterior | middle cerebral a. | | cortex of posterior temporal lobe |

**Arteries** Continued

| Common Name | TA Equivalent | Origin | Branches | Distribution |
|---|---|---|---|---|
| temporal a., posterior deep | a. temporalis profunda posterior | maxillary a. | | temporal muscle |
| temporal a., superficial | a. temporalis superficialis | external carotid a. | parotid, auricular, and occipital branches; transverse facial, zygomaticoorbital, middle temporal a's | parotid and temporal regions |
| testicular a. | a. testicularis | abdominal aorta | ureteral and epididymal branches | ureter, epididymis, testis |
| thoracic a., internal | a. thoracica interna | subclavian a. | mediastinal, thymic, bronchial, tracheal, sternal, perforating, medial mammary, lateral costal and anterior intercostal branches; pericardiacophrenic, musculophrenic, superior epigastric a's | anterior thoracic wall, mediastinal structures, diaphragm |
| thoracic a., lateral | a. thoracica lateralis | axillary a. | mammary branches | pectoral muscles, mammary gland |
| thoracic a., superior | a. thoracica superior | axillary a. | | axillary aspects of chest wall |
| thoracoacromial a. | a. thoracoacromialis | axillary a. | clavicular, pectoral, deltoid, and acromial branches | deltoid, clavicular, thoracic regions |
| thoracodorsal a. | a. thoracodorsalis | subscapular a. | | subscapular and teres major and minor muscles |
| thyrocervical trunk | truncus thyrocervicalis | subclavian a. | inferior thyroid, suprascapular and transverse cervical a's | deep neck, including thyroid gland, scapular region |
| thyroid a., inferior | a. thyroidea inferior | thyrocervical trunk | pharyngeal, esophageal, tracheal branches; inferior laryngeal, ascending cervical a's | thyroid gland and adjacent structures |
| thyroid a., lowest. *See* thyroidea ima a. | | | | |
| thyroid a., superior | a. thyroidea superior | external carotid a. | hyoid, sternocleidomastoid, superior laryngeal, cricothyroid, muscular, and glandular branches | thyroid gland and adjacent structures |
| thyroidea ima a. | a. thyroidea ima | arch of aorta, brachiocephalic trunk or right common carotid a. | | thyroid gland |
| tibial a., anterior | a. tibialis anterior | popliteal a. | posterior and anterior tibial recurrent a's, lateral and medial anterior malleolar a's, lateral and medial malleolar retes | leg, ankle, foot |
| tibial a., posterior | a. tibialis posterior | popliteal a. | fibular circumflex branch; peroneal, medial plantar, lateral plantar a's | leg, foot |
| transverse a. of face. *See* facial a., transverse | | | | |
| transverse a. of neck. *See* cervical a., transverse | | | | |
| transverse a. of scapula. *See* suprascapular a. | | | | |
| tympanic a., anterior | a. tympanica anterior | maxillary a. | | tympanic cavity |
| tympanic a., inferior | a. tympanica inferior | ascending pharyngeal a. | | tympanic cavity |
| tympanic a., posterior | a. tympanica posterior | stylomastoid a. | | tympanic cavity |
| tympanic a., superior | a. tympanica superior | middle meningeal a. | | tympanic cavity |
| ulnar a. | a. ulnaris | brachial a. | palmar carpal, dorsal carpal, and deep palmar branches; ulnar recurrent and common interosseous a's; superficial palmar arch | forearm, wrist, hand |
| ulnar a., collateral. *See* collateral a., inferior ulnar, *and* collateral a., superior ulnar | | | | |

**Arteries** *Continued*

| Common Name | TA Equivalent | Origin | Branches | Distribution |
|---|---|---|---|---|
| umbilical a. | a. umbilicalis | internal iliac a. | a. of ductus deferens, superior vesical a's | ductus deferens, seminal vesicles, testes, urinary bladder, ureter |
| urethral a. | a. urethralis | internal pudendal a. | | urethra |
| uterine a. | a. uterina | internal iliac a. | ovarian and tubal branches; vaginal a. | uterus, vagina, round ligament of uterus, uterine tube, ovary |
| vaginal a. | a. vaginalis | uterine a. | | vagina, fundus of bladder |
| vertebral a. | a. vertebralis | subclavian a. | *transverse part:* spinal and muscular branches; *intracranial part:* anterior spinal a., and posterior inferior cerebellar a. and its branches | muscles of neck, vertebrae, spinal cord, cerebellum, interior of cerebrum |
| vesical a., inferior | a. vesicalis inferior | internal iliac a. | prostatic | bladder, prostate, seminal vesicles, lower ureter |
| vesical a's, superior | aa. vesicales superiores | umbilical a. | | bladder, urachus, ureter |
| zygomatico-orbital a. | a. zygomatico-orbitalis | superficial temporal a. | | lateral side of orbit |

# Appendix 3

## Anatomy: Bones, Listed by Regions of the Body

| Region | Name | Total Number | Region | Name | Total Number |
|---|---|---|---|---|---|
| *Axial skeleton* | | | *Upper limb (×2)* | | 64 |
| | Skull | 21 | Shoulder | scapula | |
| | (eight paired—16) | | | clavicle | |
| | inferior nasal concha | | Upper arm | humerus | |
| | lacrimal | | Lower arm | radius | |
| | maxilla | | | ulna | |
| | nasal | | Wrist | carpal (8) | |
| | palatine | | | (capitate) | |
| | parietal | | | (hamate) | |
| | temporal | | | (lunate) | |
| | zygomatic | | | (pisiform) | |
| | (five unpaired—5) | | | (scaphoid) | |
| | ethmoid | | | (trapezium) | |
| | frontal | | | (trapezoid) | |
| | occipital | | | (triquetral) | |
| | sphenoid | | Hand | Metacarpal (5) | |
| | vomer | | Fingers | Phalanges (14) | |
| | Ossicles of each ear | 6 | *Lower limb (×2)* | | 62 |
| | incus | | Pelvis | Hip bone (1) | |
| | malleus | | | (ilium) | |
| | stapes | | | (ischium) | |
| | Lower jaw | | | (pubis) | |
| | mandible | 1 | Thigh | femur | |
| | Neck | | Knee | patella | |
| | hyoid | 1 | Leg | tibia | |
| | Vertebral column | 26 | | fibula | |
| | cervical vertebrae (7) | | Ankle | tarsal (7) | |
| | (atlas) | | | (calcaneus) | |
| | (axis) | | | (cuboid) | |
| | thoracic vertebrae (12) | | | (cuneiform, medial) | |
| | lumbar vertebrae (5) | | | (cuneiform, intermediate) | |
| | sacrum (5 fused) | | | (cuneiform, lateral) | |
| | coccyx (4–5 fused) | | | (navicular) | |
| | Chest | | | (talus) | |
| | sternum | 1 | Foot | Metatarsal (5) | |
| | ribs (12 pairs) | 24 | Toes | Phalanges (14) | |

# APPENDIX 4

## Anatomy: Bones

### Bones

| Common Name* | TA Equivalent† | Region | Description | Articulations |
|---|---|---|---|---|
| astragalus. *See* talus | | | | |
| atlas | atlas | neck | first cervical vertebra, ring of bone supporting the skull | with occipital b. and axis |
| axis | axis | neck | second cervical vertebra, with thick process (odontoid process) around which first cervical vertebra pivots | with atlas above and third cervical vertebra below |
| calcaneus | calcaneus | foot | the "heel bone," of irregular cuboidal shape, largest of the tarsal bones | with talus and cuboid b. |
| capitate b. | o. capitatum | wrist | with second, third, and fourth metacarpal b's, and hamate, lunate, trapezoid, and scaphoid b's | |
| carpal b's | oss. carpi | wrist | see *capitate, hamate, lunate, pisiform b's, scaphoid, trapezium, trapezoid,* and *triquetral b's* | |
| clavicle | clavicula | shoulder | elongated slender, curved bone (collar bone) lying horizontally at root of neck, in upper part of thorax | with sternum and ipsilateral scapula and cartilage of first rib |
| coccyx | o. coccygis | lower back | triangular bone formed usually by fusion of last 4 (sometimes 3 or 5) (coccygeal) vertebrae | with sacrum |
| concha, inferior nasal | concha nasalis inferior | skull | thin, rough plate of bone attached by one edge to side of each nasal cavity, the free edge curling downward | with ethmoid and ipsilateral lacrimal and palatine b's and maxilla |
| cuboid b. | o. cuboideum | foot | pyramidal bone, on lateral side of foot, in front of calcaneus | with calcaneus, lateral cuneiform b., fourth and fifth metatarsal b's, occasionally with navicular b. |
| cuneiform b., intermediate | o. cuneiforme intermedium | foot | smallest of 3 cuneiform b's, located between medial and lateral cuneiform b's | with navicular, medial and lateral cuneiform b's, and second metatarsal b. |
| cuneiform b., lateral | o. cuneiforme laterale | foot | wedge-shaped bone at lateral side of foot, intermediate in size between medial and intermediate cuneiform b's | with cuboid, navicular, intermediate cuneiform b's and second, third, and fourth metatarsal b's |
| cuneiform b., medial | o. cuneiforme mediale | foot | largest of 3 cuneiform b's, at medial side of foot | with navicular, intermediate cuneiform, and first and second metatarsal b's |
| epistropheus. *See* axis | | | | |
| ethmoid b. | o. ethmoidale | skull | unpaired bone in front of sphenoid b. and below frontal b., forming part of nasal septum and superior and medial conchae of nose | with sphenoid and frontal b's, vomer, and both lacrimal, nasal, and palatine b's, maxillae, and inferior nasal conchae |
| fabella | | knee | sesamoid b. in lateral head of gastrocnemius muscle | with femur |
| femur | femur | thigh | longest, strongest, heaviest bone of the body (thigh b.) | proximally with hip b., distally with patella and tibia |
| fibula | fibula | leg | lateral and smaller of 2 bones of leg | proximally with tibia, distally with tibia and talus |
| frontal b. | o. frontale | skull | unpaired bone constituting anterior part of skull | with ethmoid and sphenoid b's, and both parietal, nasal, lacrimal, and zygomatic b's, and maxillae |
| hamate b. | o. hamatum | wrist | most medial of 4 bones of distal row of carpal b's | with fourth and fifth metacarpal b's and lunate, capitate, and triquetral b's |

* b. = bone; b's = (pl.) bones.
† o. = os; oss. = (L. pl.) ossa.

**Bones** *Continued*

| Common Name | TA Equivalent | Region | Description | Articulations |
|---|---|---|---|---|
| hip b. | o. coxae | pelvis and hip | broadest bone of skeleton, composed originally of 3 bones which become fused together in acetabulum: *ilium,* broad, flaring, uppermost portion; *ischium,* thick three-sided part behind and below acetabulum and behind obturator foramen; *pubis,* consisting of body (expanded anterior portion), inferior ramus (extending backward and fusing with ramus of ischium), and superior ramus (extending from body to acetabulum) | with femur, anteriorly with its fellow (at symphysis pubis), posteriorly with sacrum |
| humerus | humerus | arm | long bone of upper arm | proximally with scapula, distally with radius and ulna |
| hyoid b. | o. hyoideum | neck | U-shaped bone at root of tongue, between mandible and larynx | none; attached by ligaments and muscles to skull and larynx |
| ilium | o. ilium | pelvis | see *hip b.* | |
| incus | incus | ear | middle ossicle of chain in the middle ear, so named because of its resemblance to an anvil | with malleus and stapes |
| innominate b. *See* hip b. | | | | |
| ischium | o. ischii | pelvis | see *hip b.* | |
| lacrimal b. | o. lacrimale | skull | thin, uneven scale of bone near rim of medial wall of each orbit | with ethmoid and frontal b's, and ipsilateral inferior nasal concha and maxilla |
| lunate b. | o. lunatum | wrist | second from thumb side of 4 bones of proximal row of carpus | with radius, and capitate, hamate, scaphoid, and triquetral b's |
| malleus | malleus | ear | most lateral ossicle of chain in middle ear, so named because of its resemblance to a hammer | with incus; fibrous attachment to tympanic membrane |
| mandible | mandibula | lower jaw | horseshoe-shaped bone carrying lower teeth | with temporal b's |
| maxilla | maxilla | skull (upper jaw) | paired bone, below orbit and at either side of nasal cavity, carrying upper teeth | with ethmoid and frontal b's, vomer, fellow maxilla, and ipsilateral inferior nasal concha and lacrimal, nasal, palatine, and zygomatic b's |
| maxilla, inferior. *See* mandible | | | | |
| maxilla, superior. *See* maxilla | | | | |
| metacarpal b's | oss. metacarpi | hand | five miniature long bones of hand proper, slightly concave on palmar surface | first—trapezium and proximal phalanx of thumb; second—third metacarpal b., trapezium, trapezoid, capitate, and proximal phalanx of index finger (second digit); third—second and fourth metacarpal b's, capitate and proximal phalanx of middle finger (third digit); fourth—third and fifth metacarpal b's, capitate, hamate, and proximal phalanx of ring finger (fourth digit); fifth—fourth metacarpal b., hamate b., and proximal phalanx of little finger (fifth digit) |
| metatarsal b's | oss. metatarsi | foot | five miniature long bones of foot, concave on plantar and slightly convex on dorsal surface | first—medial cuneiform b., proximal phalanx of great toe, and occasionally with second metatarsal b.; second—medial, intermediate, and lateral cuneiform b's, third and occasionally with first metatarsal b., and proximal phalanx of second toe; third—lateral cuneiform b., second and fourth metatarsal b's and proximal phalanx of third toe; fourth—lateral cuneiform b., cuboid b., third and fifth metatarsal b's and proximal phalanx of fourth toe; fifth—cuboid b., fourth metatarsal b., and proximal phalanx of fifth toe |
| multiangulum majus. *See* trapezium; trapezoid b. | | | | |
| nasal b. | o. nasale | skull | paired bone, the two uniting in median plane to form bridge of nose | with frontal and ethmoid b's, fellow of opposite side, and ipsilateral maxilla |

**Bones** *Continued*

| Common Name | TA Equivalent | Region | Description | Articulations |
|---|---|---|---|---|
| navicular b. | o. naviculare | foot | bone at medial side of tarsus, between talus and cuneiform b's | with talus and 3 cuneiform b's, occasionally with cuboid b. |
| occipital b. | o. occipitale | skull | unpaired bone constituting back and part of base of skull | with sphenoid b. and atlas and both parietal and temporal b's |
| os magnum. *See* capitate b. | | | | |
| palatine b. | o. palatinum | skull | paired bone, the two forming posterior portions of bony palate | with ethmoid and sphenoid b's, vomer, fellow of opposite side, and ipsilateral inferior nasal concha and maxilla |
| parietal b. | o. parietale | skull | paired bone between frontal and occipital b's, forming superior and lateral parts of skull | with frontal, occipital, sphenoid, fellow parietal, and ipsilateral temporal b's |
| patella | patella | knee | small, irregularly rectangular compressed (sesamoid) bone over anterior aspect of knee (kneecap) | with femur |
| phalanges (proximal, middle, and distal phalanges) | oss. digitorum (phalanx proximalis, phalanx media, and phalanx distalis) | fingers and toes | miniature long bones, two only in thumb and great toe, three in each of other fingers and toes | proximal phalanx of each digit with corresponding metacarpal or metatarsal b., and phalanx distal to it; other phalanges with phalanges proximal and distal (if any) to them |
| pisiform b. | o. pisiforme | wrist | medial and palmar of 4 bones of proximal row of carpal b's | with triquetral b. |
| pubic b. | o. pubis | pelvis | see *hip b.* | |
| radius | radius | forearm | lateral and shorter of 2 bones of forearm | proximally with humerus and ulna; distally with ulna and lunate and scaphoid b's |
| ribs | costae | chest | 12 pairs of thin, narrow, curved long bones, forming posterior and lateral walls of chest | all posteriorly with thoracic vertebrae; upper 7 pairs (true ribs) with sternum; lower 5 pairs (false ribs), by costal cartilages, with rib above or (lowest 2—floating ribs) unattached anteriorly |
| sacrum | o. sacrum | lower back | wedge-shaped bone formed usually by fusion of 5 vertebrae below lumbar vertebrae, constituting posterior wall of pelvis | with fifth lumbar vertebra above, coccyx below, and with ilium at each side |
| scaphoid | o. scaphoideum | wrist | most lateral of 4 bones of proximal row of carpal b's | with radius, trapezium, and trapezoid, capitate and lunate b's |
| scapula | scapula | shoulder | wide, thin, triangular bone (shoulder blade) opposite second to seventh ribs in upper part of back | with ipsilateral clavicle and humerus |
| sesamoid b's | oss. sesamoidea | chiefly hands and feet | small, flat, round bones related to joints between phalanges or between digits and metacarpal or metatarsal b's; include also 2 at knee (fabella and patella) | |
| sphenoid b. | o. sphenoidale | base of skull | unpaired, irregularly shaped bone, constituting part of sides and base of skull and part of lateral wall or orbit | with frontal, occipital, and ethmoid b's, vomer, and both parietal, temporal, palatine, and zygomatic b's |
| stapes | stapes | ear | most medial ossicle of chain in middle ear, so named because of its resemblance to a stirrup | with incus; ligamentous attachment to fenestra vestibuli |
| sternum | sternum | chest | elongated flat bone, forming anterior wall of chest, consisting of 3 segments: *manubrium* (topmost segment), *body* (in youth composed of 4 separate segments joined by cartilage), and *xiphoid process* (lowermost segment) | with both clavicles and upper 7 pairs of ribs |
| talus | talus | ankle | the "ankle bone," second largest of tarsal b's | with tibia, fibula, calcaneus, and navicular b. |
| tarsal b's | oss. tarsi | ankle and foot | see *calcaneus, cuboid, intermediate, lateral,* and *medial cuneiform b's, navicular b.,* and *talus* | |
| temporal b. | o. temporale | skull | irregularly shaped bone, one on either side, forming part of side and base of skull, and containing middle and inner ear | with occipital, sphenoid, mandible, and ipsilateral parietal and zygomatic b's |
| tibia | tibia | leg | medial and larger of 2 bones of lower leg (shin b.) | proximally with femur and fibula, distally with talus and fibula |
| trapezium | o. trapezium | wrist | most lateral of 4 bones of distal row of carpal b's | with first and second metacarpal b's and trapezoid and scaphoid b's |

**Bones** *Continued*

| Common Name | TA Equivalent | Region | Description | Articulations |
|---|---|---|---|---|
| trapezoid b. | o. trapezoideum | wrist | second from thumb side of 4 bones of distal row of carpal b's | with second metacarpal b. and capitate, trapezium, and scaphoid b's |
| triquetral b. | o. triquetrum | wrist | third from thumb side of 4 bones of proximal row of carpal b's | with hamate, lunate, and pisiform b's and articular disk |
| turbinate b., inferior. *See* concha, inferior nasal | | | | |
| ulna | ulna | forearm | medial and longer of 2 bones of forearm | proximally with humerus and radius, distally with radius and articular disk |
| vertebrae (cervical, thoracic [dorsal], lumbar, sacral, and coccygeal) | vertebrae (vertebrae cervicales, vertebrae thoracicae, vertebrae lumbales, vertebrae sacrales, vertebrae coccygeae) | back | separate segments of vertebral column; about 33 in the child; uppermost 24 remain separate as true, movable vertebrae; the next 5 fuse to form the sacrum; the lowermost 3–5 fuse to form the coccyx | except first cervical (atlas) and fifth lumbar, each vertebra articulates with adjoining vertebrae above and below; the first cervical articulates with the occipital b. and second cervical vertebra (axis); the fifth lumbar with the fourth lumbar vertebra and sacrum; the thoracic vertebrae articulate also with the heads of the ribs |
| vomer | vomer | skull | thin bone forming posterior and posteroinferior part of nasal septum | with ethmoid and sphenoid b's and both maxillae and palatine b's |
| zygomatic b. | o. zygomaticum | skull | bone forming hard part of cheek and lower, lateral portion of rim of each orbit | with frontal and sphenoid b's and ipsilateral maxilla and temporal b. |

# Anatomy: Muscles

**Muscles**

| Common Name* | TA Term† | Origin* | Insertion* | Innervation | Action |
|---|---|---|---|---|---|
| abductor m. of great toe | m. abductor hallucis | medial tubercle of calcaneus, plantar fascia | medial site of base of proximal phalanx of great toe | medial plantar | abducts, flexes great toe |
| abductor m. of little finger | m. abductor digiti minimi manus | pisiform bone, tendon of ulnar flexor m. of wrist | medial side of base of proximal phalanx of little finger | ulnar | abducts little finger |
| abductor m. of little toe | m. abductor digiti minimi pedis | medial and lateral tubercle of calcaneus, plantar fascia | lateral side of base of proximal phalanx of little toe | lateral plantar | abducts little toe |
| abductor m. of thumb, long | m. abductor pollicis longus | posterior surfaces of radius and ulna | lateral side of bone of first metacarpal bone and trapezium | posterior interosseous | abducts, extends thumb |
| abductor m. of thumb, short | m. abductor pollicis brevis | tubercles of scaphoid and trapezium, flexor retinaculum of hand | lateral side of base of proximal phalanx of thumb | median | abducts thumb |
| adductor m., great | m. adductor magnus | *deep part*—inferior ramus of pubis, ramus of ischium; *superficial part*—ischial tuberosity | *deep part*—linea aspera of femur; *superficial part*—adductor tubercle of femur | *deep part*—obturator; *superficial part*—sciatic | *deep part*—adducts thigh; *superficial part*—extends thigh |
| adductor m. of great toe | m. adductor hallucis | *oblique head*—long plantar ligament; *transverse head*—plantar ligaments | lateral side of proximal phalanx of great toe | lateral plantar | flexes, adducts great toe |
| adductor m., long | m. adductor longus | body of pubis | linea aspera of femur | obturator | adducts, rotates, flexes thigh |
| adductor m., short | m. adductor brevis | body and inferior ramus of pubis | upper part of linea aspera of femur | obturator | adducts, rotates, flexes thigh |
| adductor m., smallest | m. adductor minimus | a name given to the anterior portion of the great adductor m. | ischium, body, and ramus of pubis | obturator, sciatic | adducts thigh |
| adductor m. of thumb | m. adductor pollicis | *oblique head*—second metacarpal, capitate, and trapezoid; *transverse head*—front of third metacarpal | medial side of base of proximal phalanx of thumb | ulnar | adducts, opposes thumb |
| anconeus m. | m. anconeus | back of lateral epicondyle of humerus | olecranon and posterior surface of ulna | radial | extends forearm |
| antitragus m. | m. antitragicus | outer part of antitragus | caudate process of helix and anthelix | temporal, posterior auricular branches of facial | |
| arrector m. of hair | m. arrector pili | dermis | hair follicle | sympathetic | elevate hairs of skin |
| articular m. of elbow | m. articularis cubiti | a name applied to a few fibers of the deep surface of the triceps m. of arm that insert into the posterior ligament and synovial membrane of the elbow joint | | | |
| articular m. of knee | m. articularis genus | front of lower part of femur | upper part of capsule of knee joint | femoral | raises capsule of knee joint |
| aryepiglottic m. | pars aryepiglottica musculi arytenoidei obliqui | a name applied to inconstant fibers of oblique arytenoid m., from apex of arytenoid cartilage to lateral margin of epiglottis | | | |
| arytenoid m., oblique | m. arytenoideus obliquus | muscular process of arytenoid cartilage | apex of opposite arytenoid cartilage | recurrent laryngeal | closes inlet of larynx |
| arytenoid m., transverse | m. arytenoideus transversus | medial surface of arytenoid cartilage | medial surface of opposite arytenoid cartilage | recurrent laryngeal | approximates arytenoid cartilage |

* m. = muscle; m's = (pl.) muscles
† m. = [L.] musculus; mm. = ([L.] pl.) musculi

**Muscles** *Continued*

| Common Name | TA Term | Origin | Insertion | Innervation | Action |
|---|---|---|---|---|---|
| auricular m., anterior | m. auricularis anterior | superficial temporal fascia | cartilage of ear | facial | draws auricle forward |
| auricular m., oblique | m. obliquus auriculae | cranial surface of concha | cranial surface of auricle above concha | posterior auricular, temporal | |
| auricular m., posterior | m. auricularis posterior | mastoid process | cartilage of ear | facial | draws auricle backward |
| auricular m., superior | m. auricularis superior | galea aponeurotica | cartilage of ear | facial | raises auricle |
| biceps m. of arm | m. biceps branchii | *long head*—supraglenoid tubercle of scapula; *short head*—apex of coracoid process | tuberosity of radius, antebrachial fascia, ulna | musculocutaneous | flexes, supinates forearm |
| biceps m. of thigh | m. biceps femoris | *long head*—ischial tuberosity; *short head*—linea aspera of femur | head of fibula, lateral condyle of tibia | *long head*—tibial; *short head*—peroneal, popliteal | flexor, rotates leg laterally, extends thigh |
| brachial m. | m. brachialis | anterior aspect of humerus | coronoid process of ulna | musculocutaneous, radial | flexes forearm |
| brachioradial m. | m. brachioradialis | lateral supracondylar ridge of humerus | lateral surface of lower end of radius | radial | flexes forearm |
| bronchoesophageal m. | m. bronchooesophageus | a name applied to muscle fibers arising from wall of left bronchus, reinforcing musculature of esophagus | | | |
| buccinator m. | m. buccinator | buccinator ridge of mandible, alveolar processes of maxilla, pterygomandibular ligament | orbicular m. of mouth at angle of mouth | buccal branch of facial | compresses cheek and retracts angle of mouth |
| bulbocavernous m. | m. bulbocavernosus, m. bulbospongiosus | tendinous center of perineum, median, raphe of bulb | fascia of penis or clitoris | pudendal | constricts urethra in male, vagina in female |
| canine m. *See* levator m. of angle of mouth | | | | | |
| ceratocricoid m. | m. ceratocricoideus | a name applied to muscle fibers from cricoid cartilage to inferior horn of thyroid cartilage | | | |
| chin m. | m. mentalis | incisive fossa of mandible | skin of chin | facial | wrinkles skin of chin |
| chondroglossus m. | m. chondroglossus | lesser horn and body of hyoid bone | substance of tongue | hypoglossal | depresses, retracts tongue |
| ciliary m. | m. ciliaris | *longitudinal division* (Brücke's m's)—junction of cornea and sclera; *circular division* (Müller's m.)—sphincter of ciliary body | outer layer of choroid and ciliary processes | short ciliary | makes lens more convex in visual accommodation |
| coccygeus m. | m. coccygeus | ischial spine | lateral border of lower part of sacrum, coccyx | third and fourth sacral | supports and raises coccyx |
| constrictor m. of pharynx, inferior | m. constrictor pharyngis inferior | undersurfaces of cricoid and thyroid cartilages | median raphe of posterior wall of pharynx | glossopharyngeal, pharyngeal plexus, external branch of superior laryngeal and recurrent laryngeal | constricts pharynx |
| constrictor m. of pharynx, middle | m. constrictor pharyngis medius | horns of hyoid bone, stylohyoid ligament | median raphe of posterior wall of pharynx | pharyngeal plexus of vagus, glossopharyngeal | constricts pharynx |
| constrictor m. of pharynx, superior | m. constrictor pharyngis superior | pterygoid plate, pterygomandibular raphe, mylohyoid ridge of mandible, mucous membrane of floor of mouth | median raphe of posterior wall of pharynx | pharyngeal plexus of vagus | constricts pharynx |
| coracobrachial m. | m. coracobrachialis | coracoid process of scapula | medial surface of shaft of humerus | musculocutaneous | flexes, adducts arm |
| corrugator m., superciliary | m. corrugator supercilii | medial end of superciliary arch | skin of eyebrow | facial | draws eyebrow downward and medially |

**Muscles** *Continued*

| Common Name | TA Term | Origin | Insertion | Innervation | Action |
|---|---|---|---|---|---|
| cremaster m. | m. cremaster | inferior margin of internal oblique m. of abdomen | pubic tubercle | genital branch of genitofemoral | elevates testis |
| cricoarytenoid m., lateral | m. cricoarytenoideus lateralis | lateral surface of cricoid cartilage | muscular process of arytenoid cartilage | recurrent laryngeal | approximates vocal folds |
| cricoarytenoid m., posterior | m. cricoarytenoideus posterior | back of lamina of cricoid cartilage | muscular process of arytenoid cartilage | recurrent laryngeal | separates vocal folds |
| cricothyroid m. | m. cricothyroideus | front and side of cricoid cartilage | lamina and inferior horn of thyroid cartilage | external branch of superior laryngeal | tenses vocal folds |
| deltoid m. | m. deltoideus | clavicle, acromion, spine of scapula | deltoid tuberosity of humerus | axillary | abducts, flexes, or extends arm |
| depressor m. of angle of mouth | m. depressor anguli oris | lateral border of mandible | angle of mouth | facial | pulls down angle of mouth |
| depressor m. of lower lip | m. depressor labii inferioris | anterior surface of lower border of mandible | orbicular m. of mouth and skin of lower lip | facial | depresses lower lip |
| depressor m. of septum of nose | m. depressor septi nasi | incisive fossa of maxilla | ala and septum of nose | facial | constricts nostril and depresses ala |
| depressor m., superciliary | m. depressor supercilii | a name applied to a few fibers of orbital part of orbicular m. of eye that are inserted into the eyebrow, which they depress | | | |
| detrusor m. of bladder | m. detrusor vesicae | bundles of smooth muscle fibers forming the muscular coat of the urinary bladder, which are arranged in a longitudinal and a circular layer and on contraction serve to expel urine | | | |
| detrusor urinae. *See* detrusor m. of bladder. | | | | | |
| diaphragm | diaphragma | back of xiphoid process, inner surfaces of lower 6 costal cartilages and lower 4 ribs, medial and lateral arcuate ligaments, bodies of upper lumbar vertebrae | central tendon of diaphragm | phrenic | increases volume of thorax in inspiration |
| digastric m. | m. digastricus | *anterior belly*—digastric fossa on lower border of mandible near symphysis; *posterior belly*—mastoid notch of temporal bone | intermediate tendon on hyoid bone | *anterior belly*—mylohyoid branch of inferior alveolar; *posterior belly*—digastric branch of facial | elevates hyoid bone, lowers jaw |
| dilator m. of pupil | m. dilatator pupillae | a name applied to fibers extending radially from sphincter of pupil to ciliary margin | | sympathetic | dilates iris |
| epicranial m. | m. epicranius | a name applied to muscular covering of scalp, including occipitofrontal and temporoparietal m's and galea aponeurotica | | | |
| erector m. of spine | m. erector spinae | a name applied to fibers of the more superficial of deep muscles of back, originating from sacrum, spines of lumbar and eleventh and twelfth thoracic vertebrae, and iliac crest, which split and insert as iliocostal, longissimus, and spinal m's | | | |
| extensor m. of fingers | m. extensor digitorum | lateral epicondyle of humerus | extensor expansion of 4 medial fingers | posterior interosseous | extends wrist joint and phalanges |
| extensor m. of great toe, long | m. extensor hallucis longus | front of fibula, interosseous membrane | base of distal phalanx of great toe | deep peroneal | extends great toe, dorsiflexes ankle joint |
| extensor m. of great toe, short | m. extensor hallucis brevis | a name applied to portion of short extensor m. of toes that goes to great toe | | | |
| extensor m. of index finger | m. extensor indicis | posterior surface of ulna, interosseous membrane | extensor expansion of index finger | posterior interosseous | extends index finger |
| extensor m. of little finger | m. extensor digiti minimi | lateral epicondyle of humerus | extensor aponeurosis of little finger | deep branch of radial | extends little finger |
| extensor m. of thumb, long | m. extensor pollicis longus | posterior surface of ulna and interosseous membrane | back of distal phalanx of thumb | posterior interosseous | extends, adducts thumb |
| extensor m. of thumb, short | m. extensor pollicis brevis | posterior surface of radius | back of proximal phalanx of thumb | posterior interosseous | extends thumb |

**Muscles** *Continued*

| Common Name | TA Term | Origin | Insertion | Innervation | Action |
|---|---|---|---|---|---|
| extensor m. of toes, long | m. extensor digitorum longus | anterior surface of fibula, lateral condyle of tibia, interosseous membrane | extensor expansion of 4 lateral toes | deep peroneal | extends toes |
| extensor m. of toes, short | m. extensor digitorum brevis | upper surface of calcaneus | extensor tendons of first, second, third, fourth toes | deep peroneal | extends toes |
| extensor m. of wrist, radial, long | m. extensor carpi radialis longus | lateral supracondylar ridge of humerus | back of base of second metacarpal bone | radial | extends, abducts wrist joint |
| extensor m. of wrist, radial, short | m. extensor carpi radialis brevis | lateral epicondyle of humerus | back of bases of second and third metacarpal bones | radial or its deep branch | extends, abducts wrist joint |
| extensor m. of wrist, ulnar | m. extensor carpi ulnaris | *humeral head*—lateral epicondyle of humerus; *ulnar head*—posterior border of ulna | base of fifth metacarpal bone | deep branch of radial | extends, abducts wrist joint |
| fibular m. *See* peroneal m. | | | | | |
| flexor m. of fingers, deep | m. flexor digitorum profundus | shaft of ulna, coronoid process, interosseous membrane | bases of distal phalanges of 4 medial fingers | anterior interosseous, ulnar | flexes distal phalanges |
| flexor m. of fingers, superficial | m. flexor digitorum superficialis | *humeroulnar head*—medial epicondyle of humerus, coronoid process of ulna; *radial head*—anterior border of radius | sides of middle phalanges of 4 medial fingers | median | flexes middle phalanges |
| flexor m. of great toe, long | m. flexor hallucis longus | posterior surface of fibula | base of distal phalanx of great toe | tibial | flexes great toe |
| flexor m. of great toe, short | m. flexor hallucis brevis | undersurface of cuboid, lateral cuneiform | both sides of base of proximal phalanx of great toe | medial plantar | flexes great toe |
| flexor m. of little finger, short | m. flexor digiti minimi brevis manus | hook of hamate bone, transverse carpal ligament | medial side of proximal phalanx of little finger | ulnar | flexes little finger |
| flexor m. of little toe, short | m. flexor digiti minimi brevis pedis | sheath of long peroneal muscle | lateral surface of base of proximal phalanx of little toe | lateral plantar | flexes little toe |
| flexor m. of thumb, long | m. flexor pollicis longus | anterior surface of radius, medial epicondyle of humerus, coronoid process of ulna | base of distal phalanx of thumb | anterior interosseous | flexes thumb |
| flexor m. of thumb, short | m. flexor pollicis brevis | tubercle of trapezium, flexor retinaculum | lateral side of base of proximal phalanx of thumb | median, ulnar | flexes, adducts thumb |
| flexor m. of toes, long | m. flexor digitorum longus pedis | posterior surface of shaft of tibia | distal phalanges of 4 lateral toes | tibial | flexes toes, extends foot |
| flexor m. of toes, short | m. flexor digitorum brevis pedis | medial tuberosity of calcaneus, plantar fascia | middle phalanges of 4 lateral toes | medial plantar | flexes toes |
| flexor m. of wrist, radial | m. flexor carpi radialis | medial epicondyle of humerus | bases of second and third metacarpal bones | median | flexes, abducts wrist joint |
| flexor m. of wrist, ulnar | m. flexor carpi ulnaris | *humeral head*—medial epicondyle of humerus; *ulnar head*—olecranon and posterior border of ulna | pisiform bone, hook of hamate bone, base of fifth metacarpal bone | ulnar | flexes, adducts wrist joint |
| gastrocnemius m. | m. gastrocnemius | *medial head*—popliteal surface of femur, upper part of medial condyle, capsule of knee; *lateral head*—lateral condyle, capsule of knee | aponeurosis unites with tendon of soleus to form Achilles tendon | tibial | plantar flexes foot, flexes knee joint |
| gemellus m., inferior | m. gemellus inferior | tuberosity of ischium | internal obturator tendon | nerve to quadrate m. of thigh | rotates thigh laterally |
| gemellus m., superior | m. gemellus superior | spine of ischium | internal obturator tendon | nerve to internal obturator | rotates thigh laterally |
| genioglossus m. | m. genioglossus | superior genial tubercle | hyoid bone, undersurface of tongue | hypoglossal | protrudes, depresses tongue |

**Muscles** *Continued*

| Common Name | TA Term | Origin | Insertion | Innervation | Action |
|---|---|---|---|---|---|
| geniohyoid m. | m. geniohyoideus | inferior genial tubercle | body of hyoid bone | a branch of first cervical nerve through hypoglossal | draws hyoid bone forward |
| glossopalatine m. *See* palatoglossus m. | | | | | |
| gluteus maximus m. (gluteal m., greatest) | m. gluteus maximus | dorsal aspect of ilium, dorsal surfaces of sacrum, coccyx, sacrotuberous ligament | iliotibial tract of fascia lata, gluteal tuberosity of femur | inferior gluteal | extends, abducts, rotates thigh laterally |
| gluteus medius m. (gluteal m., middle) | m. gluteus medius | dorsal aspect of ilium between anterior and posterior gluteal lines | greater trochanter of femur | superior gluteal | abducts, rotates thigh medially |
| gluteus minimus m. (gluteal m., least) | m. gluteus minimus | dorsal aspect of ilium between anterior and posterior gluteal lines | greater trochanter of femur | superior gluteal | abducts, rotates thigh medially |
| gracilis m. | m. gracilis | body and inferior ramus of pubis | medial surface of shaft of tibia | obturator | adducts thigh, flexes knee joint |
| m. of helix, greater | m. helicis major | spine of helix | anterior border of helix | auriculotemporal, posterior auricular | tenses skin of acoustic meatus |
| m. of helix, smaller | m. helicis minor | anterior rim of helix | concha | temporal, posterior auricular | |
| hyoglossus m. | m. hyoglossus | body and greater horn of hyoid bone | side of tongue | hypoglossal | depresses, retracts tongue |
| iliac m. | m. iliacus | iliac fossa, ala of sacrum | greater psoas tendon, lesser trochanter of femur | femoral | flexes thigh, trunk on limb |
| iliococcygeus m. | m. iliococcygeus | a name applied to posterior portion of levator ani m., including fibers originating as far forward as obturator canal, and inserting on side of coccyx and in anococcygeal ligaments | | | |
| iliocostal m. | m. iliocostalis | a name applied to lateral division of erector m. of spine | | | |
| iliocostal m. of loins | m. iliocostalis lumborum | iliac crest | angles of lower 6 or 7 ribs | thoracic and lumbar | extends lumbar spine |
| iliocostal m. of neck | m. iliocostalis cervicis | angles of third, fourth, fifth, and sixth ribs | transverse processes of lower fourth, fifth, and sixth cervical vertebrae | cervical | extends cervical spine |
| iliocostal m. of thorax | m. iliocostalis thoracis | upper borders of angles of 6 lower ribs | angles of upper ribs and transverse process of seventh cervical vertebra | thoracic | keeps thoracic spine erect |
| iliopsoas m. | m. iliopsoas | a name applied collectively to iliac and greater psoas m's | | | |
| incisive m's of inferior lip | | incisive fossae of mandible | angle of mouth | facial | make vestibule of mouth shallow |
| incisive m's of superior lip | | incisive fossae of maxilla | angle of mouth | facial | make vestibule of mouth shallow |
| infraspinous m. | m. infraspinatus | infraspinous fossa of scapula | greater tubercle of humerus | suprascapular | rotates arm laterally |
| intercostal m's, external | mm. intercostales externi | inferior border of rib | superior border of rib below | intercostal | elevate ribs in inspiration |
| intercostal m's, innermost | mm. intercostales intimi | a name applied to the layer of muscle fibers separated from the internal intercostal m's by the intercostal nerves and vessels | | | |
| intercostal m's, internal | mm. intercostales interni | inferior border of rib and costal cartilage | superior border of rib and costal cartilage below | intercostal | act on ribs in expiration |
| interosseous m's of foot, dorsal | mm. interossei dorsales pedis | sides of adjacent metatarsal bones | base of proximal phalanges of second, third, and fourth toes | lateral plantar | flex, abduct toes |
| interosseous m's of hand, dorsal | mm. interossei dorsales manus | each by two heads from adjacent sides of metacarpal bones | extensor tendons of second, third, and fourth fingers | ulnar | abduct, flex proximal, extend middle and distal phalanges |

**Muscles** *Continued*

| Common Name | TA Term | Origin | Insertion | Innervation | Action |
|---|---|---|---|---|---|
| interosseous m's, palmar | mm. interossei palmares | sides of first, second, fourth, and fifth metacarpal bones | extensor tendons of first, second, fourth, and fifth fingers | ulnar | adduct, flex proximal, extend middle and distal phalanges |
| interosseous m's, plantar | mm. interossei plantares | medial side of third, fourth, and fifth metatarsal bones | medial side of base of proximal phalanges of third, fourth, and fifth toes | lateral plantar | flex, abduct toes |
| interspinal m's | mm. interspinales | a name applied to short bands of muscle fibers extending on each side between spinous processes of contiguous vertebrae | | spinal | extend vertebral column |
| interspinal m's of loins | mm. interspinales lumborum | extend between contiguous lumbar vertebrae | | spinal | extend vertebral column |
| interspinal m's of head | mm. interspinales cervicis | extend between contiguous cervical vertebrae | | spinal | extend vertebral column |
| interspinal m's of thorax | mm. interspinales thoracis | extend between contiguous thoracic vertebrae | | spinal | extend vertebral column |
| intertransverse m's | mm. intertransversarii | a name applied to small muscles passing between transverse processes of adjacent vertebrae | | spinal | bend vertebral column laterally |
| ischiocavernous m. | m. ischiocavernosus | ramus of ischium | crus of penis or clitoris | perineal branches of pudendal | maintains erection of penis or clitoris |
| latissimus dorsi m. | m. latissimus dorsi | spines of lower thoracic vertebrae, spines of lumbar and sacral vertebrae through attachment to thoracolumbar fascia, iliac crest, lower ribs, inferior angle of scapula | floor or intertubercular groove of humerus | thoracodorsal | adducts, extends, rotates humerus medially |
| levator m. of angle of mouth | m. levator anguli oris | canine fossa of maxilla | orbicular m. of mouth, skin at angle of mouth | facial | raises angle of mouth |
| levator ani m. | m. levator ani | a name applied collectively to important muscular components of pelvic diaphragm, arising mainly from back of body of pubis and running backward toward coccyx; includes pubococcygeus (levator m. of prostate in male and pubovaginal in female), puborectal, and iliococcygeus m's | | third and fourth sacral | helps support pelvic viscera and resist increases in intra-abdominal pressure |
| levator m. of palatine velum | m. levator veli palatini | apex of pars petrosa of temporal bone and cartilage of auditory tube | aponeurosis of soft palate | pharyngeal plexus | raises and draws back soft palate |
| levator m. of prostate | m. levator prostatae | a name applied to part of anterior portion of pubococcygeus m., which in male is inserted into prostate and tendinous center of perineum | | sacral, pudendal | supports, compresses prostate, helps control micturition |
| levator m's of ribs | mm. levatores costarum | transverse processes of seventh cervical and first 11 thoracic vertebrae | medial to angle of rib below | intercostal | aid elevation of ribs in respiration |
| levator m. of scapula | m. levator scapulae | transverse processes of 4 upper cervical vertebrae | vertebral border of scapula | third and fourth cervical | raises scapula |
| levator m. of thyroid gland | m. levator glandulae thyroideae | isthmus or pyramidal lobule of thyroid gland | body of hyoid bone | external branch of superior laryngeal | |
| levator m. of upper eyelid | m. levator palpebrae superioris | sphenoid bone above optic foramen | skin and tarsal plate of upper eyelid | oculomotor | raises upper eyelid |
| levator m. of upper lip | m. levator labii superioris | lower margin of orbit | musculature of upper lip | facial | raises upper lip |
| levator m. of upper lip and ala of nose | m. levator labii superioris alaeque nasi | frontal process of maxilla | skin and cartilage of ala of nose, upper lip | infraorbital branch of facial | raises upper lip, dilates nostril |
| long m. of head | m. longus capitis | transverse processes of third to sixth cervical vertebrae | basilar portion of occipital bone | cervical | flexes head |

**Muscles** *Continued*

| Common Name | TA Term | Origin | Insertion | Innervation | Action |
|---|---|---|---|---|---|
| long m. of neck | m. longus cervicis | *superior oblique portion*—transverse processes of third to fifth cervical vertebrae; *inferior oblique portion*—bodies of first to third thoracic vertebrae; *vertical portion*—bodies of 3 upper thoracic and 3 lower cervical vertebrae | *superior oblique portion*—tubercle of anterior arch of atlas; *inferior oblique portion*—transverse processes of fifth and sixth cervical vertebrae; *vertical portion*—bodies of second to fourth cervical vertebrae | anterior cervical | flexes, supports cervical vertebrae |
| longissimus m. of head | m. longissimus capitis | transverse processes of 4 or 5 upper thoracic vertebrae, articular processes of 3 or 4 lower cervical vertebrae | mastoid process of temporal bone | cervical | draws head backward, rotates head |
| longissimus m. of neck | m. longissimus cervicis | transverse processes of 4 or 5 upper thoracic vertebrae | transverse processes of second or third to sixth cervical vertebrae | lower cervical and upper thoracic | extends cervical vertebrae |
| longissimus m. of thorax | m. longissimus thoracis | transverse and articular processes of lumbar vertebrae and thoracolumbar fascia | transverse processes of all thoracic vertebrae, 9 or 10 lower ribs | lumbar and thoracic | extends thoracic vertebrae |
| longitudinal m. of tongue, inferior | m. longitudinalis inferior linguae | undersurface of tongue at base | tip of tongue | hypoglossal | changes shape of tongue in mastication and deglutition |
| longitudinal m. of tongue, superior | m. longitudinalis superior linguae | submucosa and septum of tongue | margins of tongue | hypoglossal | changes shape of tongue in mastication and deglutition |
| lumbrical m's of foot | mm. lumbricales pedis | tendons of long flexor m's of toes | medial side of base of proximal phalanges of 4 lateral toes | medial and lateral plantar | flex metatarsophalangeal joints, extend distal phalanges |
| lumbrical m's of hand | mm. lumbricales manus | tendons of deep flexor m's of fingers | extensor tendons of 4 lateral fingers | median, ulnar | flex metacarpophalangeal joints, extend middle and distal phalanges |
| masseter m. | m. masseter | *superficial part*—zygomatic process of maxilla, lower border of zygomatic arch; *deep part*—lower border and medial surface of zygomatic arch | *superficial part*—angle and ramus of mandible; *deep part*—upper half of ramus and lateral surface of coronoid process of mandible | masseteric, from mandibular division of trigeminal | raises mandible, closes jaws |
| multifidus m's | mm. multifidi | sacrum, sacroiliac ligament, mamillary processes of lumbar, transverse processes of thoracic, and articular processes of cervical vertebrae | spines of contiguous vertebrae above | spinal | extend, rotate vertebral column |
| mylohyoid m. | m. mylohyoideus | mylohyoid line of mandible | body of hyoid bone, median raphe | mylohyoid branch of inferior alveolar | elevates hyoid bone, supports floor of mouth |
| nasal m. | m. nasalis | maxilla | *alar part*—ala of nose; *transverse part*—by aponeurotic expansion with fellow of opposite side | facial | *alar part*—aids in widening nostril; *transverse part*—depresses cartilage of nose |
| oblique m. of abdomen, external | m. obliquus externus abdominus | lower 8 ribs at costal cartilages | crest of ilium, linea alba through rectus sheath | lower thoracic | flexes, rotates vertebral column, compresses abdominal viscera |

**Muscles** *Continued*

| Common Name | TA Term | Origin | Insertion | Innervation | Action |
|---|---|---|---|---|---|
| oblique m. of abdomen, internal | m. obliquus internus abdominis | thoracolumbar fascia, iliac crest, iliac fascia, inguinal fascia | lower 3 or 4 costal cartilages, linea alba, conjoined tendon to pubis | lower thoracic | flexes, rotates vertebral column, compresses abdominal viscera |
| oblique m. of eyeball, inferior | m. obliquus inferior bulbi | orbital surface of maxilla | sclera | oculomotor | abducts, rotates eyeball upward and outward |
| oblique m. of eyeball, superior | m. obliquus superior bulbi | lesser wing of sphenoid above optic foramen | sclera | trochlear | abducts, rotates eyeball downward and outward |
| oblique m. of head, inferior | m. obliquus capitis inferior | spinous process of axis | transverse process of atlas | spinal | rotates atlas and head |
| oblique m. of head, superior | m. obliquus capitis superior | transverse process of atlas | occipital bone | spinal | extends and moves head laterally |
| obturator m., external | m. obturatorius externus | pubis, ischium, external surface of obturator membrane | trochanteric fossa of femur | obturator | rotates thigh laterally |
| obturator m., internal | m. obturatorius internus | pelvic surface of hip bone and obturator membrane, margin of obturator foramen | greater trochanter of femur | fifth lumbar, first and second sacral | rotates thigh laterally |
| occipitofrontal m. | m. occipitofrontalis | *frontal belly*—galea aponeurotica; *occipital belly*—highest nuchal line of occipital bone | *frontal belly*—skin of eyebrow, root of nose; *occipital belly*—galea aponeurotica | *frontal belly*—temporal branch of facial; *occipital belly*—posterior auricular branch of facial | *frontal belly*—raises eyebrow; *occipital belly*—draws scalp backward |
| omohyoid m. | m. omohyoideus | superior border of scapula | body of hyoid bone | upper cervical through ansa cervicalis | depresses hyoid bone |
| opposing m. of little finger | m. opponens digiti minimi manus | hook of hamate bone | front of fifth metacarpal | eighth cervical through ulnar | abducts, flexes, rotates fifth metacarpal |
| opposing m. of thumb | m. opponens pollicis | tubercle of trapezium, flexor retinaculum | lateral side of first metacarpal | sixth and seventh metacarpal through median | flexes, opposes thumb |
| orbicular m. of eye | m. orbicularis oculi | *orbital part*—medial margin of orbit, including frontal process of maxilla; *palpebral part*—medial palpebral ligament; *lacrimal part*—posterior lacrimal crest | *orbital part*—near origin after encircling orbit; *palpebral part*—orbital tubercle of zygomatic bone; *lacrimal part*—lateral palpebral raphe | facial | closes eyelids, wrinkles forehead, compresses lacrimal sac |
| orbicular m. of mouth | m. orbicularis oris | a name applied to complicated sphincter muscle of mouth, comprising 2 parts: *labial part*—consisting of fibers restricted to lips; *marginal part*—consisting of fibers blending with those of adjacent muscles | | facial | closes, protrudes lips |
| orbital m. | m. orbitalis | bridges inferior orbital fissure | fascia of inferior orbital fissure | sympathetic fibers | protrudes eye |
| palatoglossus m. | m. palatoglossus | undersurface of soft palate | side of tongue | pharyngeal plexus | elevates tongue, constricts fauces |
| palatopharyngeal m. | m. palatopharyngeus | posterior border of bony palate, palatine, aponeurosis | posterior border of thyroid cartilage, side of pharynx and esophagus | pharyngeal plexus | constricts pharynx, aids swallowing |
| palmar m., long | m. palmaris longus | medial epicondyle of humerus | flexor retinaculum, palmar aponeurosis | median | tenses palmar aponeurosis |
| palmar m., short | m. palmaris brevis | palmar aponeurosis | skin of medial border of hand | ulnar | assists in deepening hollow of palm |
| papillary m's | mm. papillares cordis | a name applied to conical muscular projections from walls of cardiac ventricles, attached to cusps of atrioventricular valves by chordae tendineae | | | steady and strengthen atrioventricular valves and prevent eversion of their cusps |
| pectinate m's | mm. pectinati atrii | a name applied to small ridges of muscular fibers projecting from inner walls of auricles of heart, and extending in right atrium from auricle to crista terminalis | | | |
| pectineal m. | m. pectineus | pectineal line of pubis | pectineal line of femur | femoral, obturator | flexes, adducts thigh |

**Muscles** *Continued*

| Common Name | TA Term | Origin | Insertion | Innervation | Action |
|---|---|---|---|---|---|
| pectoral m., greater | m. pectoralis major | clavicle, sternum, 6 upper costal cartilages, aponeurosis of external oblique m. of abdomen | crest of greater tubercle of humerus | lateral and medial pectoral | adducts, flexes, rotates arm medially |
| pectoral m., smaller | m. pectoralis minor | second, third, fourth, and fifth ribs | coracoid process of scapula | medial and lateral pectoral | draws shoulder forward and downward, raises third, fourth, and fifth ribs in forced inspiration |
| peroneal m., long | m. peroneus longus | lateral condyle of tibia, head of fibula, lateral surface of fibula | medial cuneiform, first metatarsal | superficial peroneal | plantar flexes, everts, abducts foot |
| peroneal m., short | m. peroneus brevis | lateral surface of fibula | tuberosity of fifth metatarsal | superficial peroneal | everts, abducts, plantar flexes foot |
| peroneal m., third | m. peroneus tertius | anterior surface of fibula, interosseous membrane | fascia or base of fifth (or fourth) metatarsal | deep peroneal | everts, dorsiflexes foot |
| piriform m. | m. piriformis | ilium, second to fourth sacral vertebrae | greater trochanter of femur | first and second sacral | rotates thigh laterally |
| plantar m. | m. plantaris | popliteal surface of femur | Achilles tendon or back of calcaneus | tibial | plantar flexes foot, flexes leg |
| platysma | platysma | a name applied to a platelike muscle originating from the fascia of cervical region and inserting on mandible and skin around mouth | | cervical branch of facial | wrinkles skin of neck, depresses jaw |
| pleuroesophageal m. | m. pleuroesophageus | a name applied to a bundle of smooth muscle fibers, usually connecting esophagus with left mediastinal pleura | | | |
| popliteal m. | m. popliteus | lateral condyle of femur, lateral meniscus | posterior surface of tibia | tibial | flexes leg, rotates leg medially |
| procerus m. | m. procerus | fascia over nasal bones | skin of forehead | facial | draws medial angle of eyebrows down |
| pronator m., quadrate | m. pronator quadratus | anterior surface and border of distal third or fourth of shaft of ulna | anterior surface and border of distal fourth of shaft of radius | anterior interosseous | pronates forearm |
| pronator m., round | m. pronator teres | *humeral head*—medial epicondyle of humerus; *ulnar head*—coronoid process of ulna | lateral surface of radius | median | pronates and flexes forearm |
| psoas m., greater | m. psoas major | lumbar vertebrae | lesser trochanter of femur | second and third lumbar | flexes thigh or trunk |
| psoas m., smaller | m. psoas minor | last thoracic and first lumbar vertebrae | arcuate line of hip bone | first lumbar | assists greater psoas m. |
| pterygoid m., lateral (external) | m. pterygoideus lateralis | *upper head*—infratemporal surface of greater wing of sphenoid, infratemporal crest; *lower head*—lateral surface of lateral pterygoid plate | neck of mandible, capsule of temporomandibular joint | mandibular | protrudes mandible, opens jaws, moves mandible from side to side |
| pterygoid m., medial (internal) | m. pterygoideus medialis | medial surface of lateral pterygoid plate, tuber of maxilla | medial surface of ramus and angle of mandible | mandibular | closes jaws |
| pubococcygeus m. | m. pubococcygeus | a name applied to anterior portion of levator ani m., originating in front of obturator canal and inserting in anococcygeal ligament and side of coccyx | | third and fourth sacral | helps support pelvic viscera and resist increases in intra-abdominal pressure |
| puboprostatic m. | m. puboprostaticus | a name applied to smooth muscle fibers contained within medial puboprostatic ligament, which pass from prostate anteriorly to pubis | | | |
| puborectal m. | m. puborectalis | a name applied to portion of levator ani m., with a more lateral origin from pubic bone, and continuous posteriorly with corresponding muscle of opposite side | | third and fourth sacral | helps support pelvic viscera and resist increases in intra-abdominal pressure |
| pubovaginal m. | m. pubovaginalis | a name applied to part of anterior portion of pubococcygeus m., which is inserted into urethra and vagina | | sacral and pudendal | helps control micturition |

**Muscles** *Continued*

| Common Name | TA Term | Origin | Insertion | Innervation | Action |
|---|---|---|---|---|---|
| pubovesical m. | m. pubovesicalis | a name applied to smooth muscle fibers extending from neck of urinary bladder to pubis | | | |
| pyloric sphincter m. | m. sphincter pyloricus | a thickening of the circular muscle of the stomach around its opening into the duodenum | | | |
| pyramidal m. | m. pyramidalis | body of pubis | linea alba | last thoracic | tenses abdominal wall |
| pyramidal m. of auricle | m. pyramidalis auriculae | a name applied to inconstant prolongation of fibers of m. of tragus to spine of helix | | | |
| quadrate m. of loins | m. quadratus lumborum | iliac crest, thoracolumbar fascia | twelfth rib transverse processes of lumbar vertebrae | first and second lumbar, twelfth thoracic | flexes trunk laterally |
| quadrate m. of lower lip. *See* depressor m. of lower lip | | | | | |
| quadrate m. of sole | m. quadratus plantae | calcaneus, plantar fascia | tendons of long flexor m. of toes | lateral plantar | aids in flexing toes |
| quadrate m. of thigh | m. quadratus femoris | tuberosity of ischium | intertrochanteric crest and quadrate tubercle of femur | fourth and fifth lumbar, first sacral | adducts, rotates thigh laterally |
| quadrate m. of upper lip. *See* levator m. of upper lip | | | | | |
| quadriceps m. of thigh | m. quadriceps femoris | a name applied collectively to rectus m. of thigh and intermediate, lateral, and medial vastus m's, inserting by a common tendon that surrounds patella and ends on tuberosity of tibia | | femoral | extends leg upon thigh |
| rectococcygeus m. | m. rectococcygeus | a name applied to smooth muscle fibers originating on anterior surface of second and third coccygeal vertebrae and inserting on posterior surface of rectum | | autonomic | retracts, elevates rectum |
| recto-urethral m. | m. rectourethralis | a name applied to band of smooth muscle fibers in male, extending from perineal flexure of rectum to membranous part of urethra | | | |
| recto-uterine m. | m. rectouterinus | a name applied to band of fibers in female, running between cervix uteri and rectum, in rectouterine fold | | | |
| rectovesical m. | m. rectovesicalis | a name applied to band of fibers in male, connecting longitudinal musculature of rectum with external muscular coat of bladder | | | |
| rectus m. of abdomen | m. rectus abdominis | pubic crest and symphysis | xiphoid process, fifth, sixth, and seventh costal cartilages | lower thoracic | flexes lumbar vertebrae, supports abdomen |
| rectus m. of eyeball, inferior | m. rectus inferior bulbi | common tendinous ring | underside of sclera | oculomotor | adducts, rotates eyeball downward and medially |
| rectus m. of eyeball, lateral | m. rectus lateralis bulbi | common tendinous ring | lateral side of sclera | abducens | abducts eyeball |
| rectus m. of eyeball, medial | m. rectus medialis bulbi | common tendinous ring | medial side of sclera | oculomotor | adducts eyeball |
| rectus m. of eyeball, superior | m. rectus superior bulbi | common tendinous ring | upper side of sclera | oculomotor | adducts, rotates eyeball upward and medially |
| rectus m. of head, anterior | m. rectus capitis anterior | lateral mass of atlas | basilar part of occipital bone | first and second cervical | flexes, supports head |
| rectus m. of head, lateral | m. rectus capitis lateralis | transverse process of atlas | jugular process of occipital bone | first and second cervical | flexes, supports head |
| rectus m. of head, posterior, greater | m. rectus capitis posterior major | spinous process of axis | occipital bone | suboccipital, greater occipital | extends head |
| rectus m. of head, posterior, smaller | m. rectus capitis posterior minor | posterior tubercle of atlas | occipital bone | suboccipital, greater occipital | extends head |
| rectus m. of thigh | m. rectus femoris | anterior inferior iliac spine, rim of acetabulum | base of patella, tuberosity of tibia | femoral | extends leg, flexes thigh |
| rhomboid m., greater | m. rhomboideus major | spinous processes of second, third, fourth, and fifth thoracic vertebrae | vertebral margin of scapula | dorsal scapular | retracts and fixes scapula |

**Muscles** *Continued*

| Common Name | TA Term | Origin | Insertion | Innervation | Action |
|---|---|---|---|---|---|
| rhomboid m., smaller | m. rhomboideus minor | spinous processes of seventh cervical and first thoracic vertebrae, lower part of nuchal ligament | vertebral margin of scapula at root of spine | dorsal scapular | retracts and fixes scapula |
| risorius m. | m. risorius | fascia over masseter | skin at angle of mouth | buccal branch of facial | draws angle of mouth laterally |
| rotator m's | mm. rotatores | a name applied to a series of small muscles deep in groove between spinous and transverse processes of vertebrae | | spinal | extend and rotate vertebral column toward opposite side |
| sacrococcygeal m., dorsal (posterior) | | a name applied to muscular slip passing from dorsal surface of sacrum to coccyx | | | |
| sacrococcygeal m., ventral (anterior) | | a name applied to musculotendinous slip passing from lower sacral vertebrae to coccyx | | | |
| sacrospinal m. *See* erector m. of spine | | | | | |
| salpingopharyngeal m. | m. salpingopharyngeus | cartilage of auditory tube | posterior part of palatopharyngeus | pharyngeal plexus | raises pharynx |
| sartorius m. | m. sartorius | anterior superior iliac spine | upper part of medial surface of tibia | femoral | flexes thigh and leg |
| scalene m., anterior | m. scalenus anterior | transverse processes of third to sixth cervical vertebrae | scalene tubercle of first rib | second to seventh cervical | raises first rib, flexes cervical vertebrae laterally |
| scalene m., middle | m. scalenus medius | transverse processes of first to seventh cervical vertebrae | upper surface of first rib | second to seventh cervical | raises first rib, flexes cervical vertebrae laterally |
| scalene m. of pleura. *See* scalene m., smallest | | | | | |
| scalene m., posterior | m. scalenus posterior | transverse processes of fourth to sixth cervical vertebrae | second rib | second to seventh cervical | raises first and second ribs, flexes cervical vertebrae laterally |
| scalene m., smallest | m. scalenus minimus | a name applied to muscular band occasionally found between anterior and middle scalene m's | | | |
| semimembranous m. | m. semimembranosus | tuberosity of ischium | lateral condyle of femur, medial condyle and border of tibia | sciatic | flexes leg, extends thigh |
| semispinal m. of head | m. semispinalis capitis | transverse processes of upper thoracic and lower cervical vertebrae | occipital bone | suboccipital, greater occipital, branches of cervical | extends head |
| semispinal m. of neck | m. semispinalis cervicis | transverse processes of upper thoracic vertebrae | spinous processes of second to fifth (or fourth) cervical vertebrae | branches of cervical | extends, rotates vertebral column |
| semispinal m. of thorax | m. semispinalis thoracis | transverse processes of lower thoracic vertebrae | spinous processes of lower cervical and upper thoracic vertebrae | spinal | extends, rotates vertebral column |
| semitendinous m. | m. semitendinosus | tuberosity of ischium | upper part of medial surface of tibia | sciatic | flexes and rotates leg medially, extends thigh |
| serratus m., anterior | m. serratus anterior | 8 upper ribs | vertebral border of scapula | long thoracic | draws scapula forward, rotates scapula to raise shoulder in abduction of arm |
| serratus m., posterior, inferior | m. serratus posterior inferior | spines of lower thoracic and upper lumbar vertebrae | 4 lower ribs | ninth to twelfth (or eleventh) thoracic | lowers ribs in expiration |
| serratus m., posterior, superior | m. serratus posterior superior | nuchal ligament, spinous processes of upper thoracic vertebrae | second, third, fourth, and fifth ribs | upper 4 thoracic | raises ribs in inspiration |
| soleus m. | m. soleus | fibula, tendinous arch, tibia | calcaneus by Achilles tendon | tibial | plantar flexes foot |
| sphincter m. of anus, external | m. sphincter ani externus | tip of coccyx, anococcygeal ligament | tendinous center of perineum | inferior rectal, perineal branch of fourth sacral | closes anus |

**Muscles** *Continued*

| Common Name | TA Term | Origin | Insertion | Innervation | Action |
|---|---|---|---|---|---|
| sphincter m. of anus, internal | m. sphincter ani internus | a name applied to a thickening of circular layer of muscular tunic at caudal end of rectum | | | |
| sphincter m. of bile duct | m. sphincter ductus biliaris | a name applied to annular sheath of muscle fibers investing bile duct within wall of duodenum | | | |
| sphincter m. of hepatopancreatic ampulla | m. sphincter ampullae hepatopancreaticae | a name applied to annular band of muscle fibers investing hepatopancreatic ampulla | | | |
| sphincter m. of pupil | m. sphincter pupillae | a name applied to circular fibers of iris | | parasympathetic through ciliary | constricts pupil |
| sphincter m. of pylorus | m. sphincter pyloricus | a name applied to a thickening of circular muscle of stomach around its opening into duodenum pylorus | | | |
| sphincter m. of urethra, external | m. sphincter urethrae externus | inferior ramus of pubis | median raphe behind and in front of urethra | perineal | compresses membranous urethra |
| sphincter m. of urethra, internal | m. sphincter urethrae internus | a name applied to circular layer of fibers surrounding internal urethral orifice | | vesical | closes internal orifice of urethra |
| spinal m. of head | m. spinalis capitis | spinous processes of upper thoracic and lower cervical vertebrae | occipital bone | spinal | extends head |
| spinal m. of neck | m. spinalis cervicis | spinous process of seventh cervical vertebra, nuchal ligament | spinous processes of axis | branches of cervical | extends vertebral column |
| spinal m. of thorax | m. spinalis thoracis | spinous processes of upper lumbar and lower thoracic vertebrae | spinous processes of upper thoracic vertebrae | branches of spinal | extends vertebral column |
| splenius m. of head | m. splenius capitis | lower half of nuchal ligament, spinous processes of seventh cervical and upper thoracic vertebrae | mastoid part of temporal bone, occipital bone | cervical | extends, rotates head |
| splenius m. of neck | m. splenius cervicis | spinous process of upper thoracic vertebrae | transverse processes of upper cervical vertebrae | cervical | extends, rotates head and neck |
| stapedius m. | m. stapedius | interior of pyramidal eminence of tympanic cavity | neck of stapes | facial | dampens movement of stapes |
| sternal m. | m. sternalis | a name applied to muscular band occasionally found parallel to sternum on sternocostal head of greater pectoral m. | | | |
| sternocleidomastoid m. | m. sternocleidomastoideus | *sternal head*—manubrium; *clavicular head*—medial third of clavicle | mastoid process, superior nuchal line of occipital bone | accessory, cervical plexus | flexes vertebral column, rotates head to opposite side |
| sternocostal m. *See* transverse m. of thorax | | | | | |
| sternohyoid m. | m. sternohyoideus | manubrium sterni and/or clavicle | body of hyoid bone | ansa cervicalis | depresses hyoid bone and larynx |
| sternothyroid m. | m. sternothyroideus | manubrium sterni | lamina of thyroid cartilage | ansa cervicalis | depresses thyroid cartilage |
| styloglossus m. | m. styloglossus | styloid process | margin of tongue | hypoglossal | raises, retracts tongue |
| stylohyoid m. | m. stylohyoideus | styloid process | body of hyoid bone | facial | draws hyoid bone and tongue upward and backward |
| stylopharyngeus m. | m. stylopharyngeus | styloid process | thyroid cartilage, side of pharynx | glossopharyngeal, pharyngeal plexus | raises, dilates pharynx |
| subclavius m. | m. subclavius | first rib and its cartilage | lower surface of clavicle | nerve to subclavius | depresses lateral end of clavicle |
| subcostal m's | mm. subcostales | lower border of ribs | upper border of second or third rib below | intercostal | raise ribs in inspiration |
| subscapular m. | m. subscapularis | subscapular fossa of scapula | lesser tubercle of humerus | subscapular | rotates arm medially |

**Muscles** *Continued*

| Common Name | TA Term | Origin | Insertion | Innervation | Action |
|---|---|---|---|---|---|
| supinator m. | m. supinator | lateral epicondyle of humerus, ligaments of elbow | radius | deep branch of radial | supinates forearm |
| supraspinous m. | m. supraspinatus | supraspinous fossa of scapula | greater tubercle of humerus | suprascapular | abducts arm |
| suspensory m. of duodenum | m. suspensorius duodeni | a name applied to flat band of smooth muscle fibers originating from left crus of diaphragm and inserting continuous with muscular coat of duodenum at its junction with jejunum | | | |
| tarsal m., inferior | m. tarsalis inferior | inferior rectus m. of eyeball | tarsal plate of lower eyelid | sympathetic | widens palpebral fissure |
| tarsal m., superior | m. tarsalis superior | levator m. of upper eyelid | tarsal plate of upper eyelid | sympathetic | widens palpebral fissure |
| temporal m. | m. temporalis | temporal fossa and fascia | coronoid process of mandible | mandibular | closes jaws |
| temporoparietal m. | m. temporoparietalis | temporal fascia above ear | galea aponeurotica | temporal branches of facial | tightens scalp |
| tensor m. of fascia lata | m. tensor fasciae latae | iliac crest | iliotibial tract of fascia lata | superior gluteal | flexes, rotates thigh medially |
| tensor m. of palatine velum | m. tensor veli palatine | scaphoid fossa and spine of sphenoid | aponeurosis of soft palate, wall of auditory tube | mandibular | tenses soft palate, opens auditory tube |
| tensor m. of tympanum | m. tensor tympani | cartilaginous portion of auditory tube | handle of malleus | mandibular | tenses tympanic membrane |
| teres major m. | m. teres major | inferior angle of scapula | crest of lesser tubercle of humerus | lower subscapular | adducts, extends, and rotates arm medially |
| teres minor m. | m. teres minor | lateral margin of scapula | greater tubercle of humerus | axillary | rotates arm laterally |
| m. of terminal notch | m. incisurae terminalis | a name applied to inconstant slips of fibers continuing forward from m. of tragus to bridge notch of cartilaginous part of meatus | | | |
| thyroarytenoid m. | m. thyroarytenoideus | medial surface of lamina of thyroid cartilage | muscular process of arytenoid cartilage | recurrent laryngeal | relaxes, shortens vocal folds |
| thyroepiglottic m. | pars thyroepiglottica musculi thyroarytenoidei | lamina of thyroid cartilage | epiglottis | recurrent laryngeal | closes inlet to larynx |
| thyrohyoid m. | m. thyrohyoideus | lamina of thyroid cartilage | greater horn of hyoid bone | ansa cervicalis | raises and changes form of larynx |
| tibial m., anterior | m. tibialis anterior | lateral condyle and surface of tibia, interosseous membrane | medial cuneiform, base of first metatarsal | deep peroneal | dorsiflexes, inverts foot |
| tibial m., posterior | m. tibialis posterior | tibia, fibula, interosseous membrane | bases of second to fourth metatarsal bones and tarsal bones, except talus | tibial | plantar flexes, inverts foot |
| tracheal m. | m. trachealis | a name applied to transverse smooth muscle fibers filling gap at back of each cartilage of trachea | | autonomic | lessens caliber of trachea |
| m. of tragus | m. tragicus | a name applied to short, flattened vertical band on lateral surface of tragus, innervated by auriculotemporal and posterior auricular nerves | | | |
| transverse m. of abdomen | m. transversus abdominis | lower 6 costal cartilages, thoracolumbar fascia, iliac crest | linea alba through rectus sheath, conjoined tendon to pubis | lower thoracic | compresses abdominal viscera |
| transverse m. of auricle | m. transversus auriculae | cranial surface of auricle | circumference of auricle | posterior auricular branch of facial | retracts helix |
| transverse m. of chin | m. transversus menti | a name applied to superficial fibers of depressor m. of angle of mouth which turn medially and cross to opposite side | | | |
| transverse m. of nape | m. transversus nuchae | a name applied to small muscle often present, passing from occipital protuberance to posterior auricular m.; it may be either superficial or deep to trapezius | | | |
| transverse m. of perineum, deep | m. transversus perinei profundus | ramus of ischium | tendinous center of perineum | perineal | fixes tendinous center of perineum |
| transverse m. of perineum, superficial | m. transversus perinei superficialis | ramus of ischium | tendinous center of perineum | perineal | fixes tendinous center of perineum |

**Muscles** *Continued*

| Common Name | TA Term | Origin | Insertion | Innervation | Action |
|---|---|---|---|---|---|
| transverse m. of thorax | m. transversus thoracis | posterior surface of body of sternum and of xiphoid process | second to sixth costal cartilages | intercostal | perhaps narrows chest |
| transverse m. of tongue | m. transversus linguae | median septum of tongue | dorsum and margins of tongue | hypoglossal | changes shape of tongue in mastication and swallowing |
| transversospinal m's | mm. transversospinales | a name applied collectively to semispinal, multifidus, and rotator m's | | | |
| trapezius m. | m. trapezius | occipital bone, nuchal ligament, spinous processes of seventh cervical and all thoracic vertebrae | clavicle, acromion, spine of scapula | accessory, cervical plexus | elevates shoulder, rotates scapula to raise shoulder in abduction of arm, draws scapula backward |
| triangular m. *See* depressor m. of angle of mouth | | | | | |
| triceps m. of arm (triceps brachii m.) | m. triceps brachii | *long head*—infraglenoid tubercle of scapula; *lateral head*—posterior surface of humerus; *medial head*—posterior surface of humerus below groove for radial nerve | olecranon of ulna | radial | extends forearm; *long head* adducts, extends arm |
| triceps m. of calf (triceps surae m.) | m. triceps surae | a name applied collectively to gastrocnemius and soleus m's | | | |
| m. of uvula | m. uvulae | posterior nasal spine of palatine bone and aponeurosis of soft palate | uvula | pharyngeal plexus | raises uvula |
| vastus m., intermediate | m. vastus intermedius | anterior and lateral surfaces of femur | patella, common tendon of quadriceps m. of thigh | femoral | extends leg |
| vastus m., lateral | m. vastus lateralis | lateral aspects of femur | patella, common tendon of quadriceps m. of thigh | femoral | extends leg |
| vastus m., medial | m. vastus medialis | medial aspect of femur | patella, common tendon of quadriceps m. of thigh | femoral | extends leg |
| vertical m. of tongue | m. verticalis linguae | dorsal fascia of tongue | sides and base of tongue | hypoglossal | changes shape of tongue in mastication and deglutition |
| vocal m. | m. vocalis | angle between laminae of thyroid cartilage | vocal process of arytenoid cartilage | recurrent laryngeal | causes local variations in tension of vocal fold |
| zygomatic m., greater | m. zygomaticus major | zygomatic bone | angle of mouth | facial | draws angle of mouth upward and backward |
| zygomatic m., smaller | m. zygomaticus minor | zygomatic bone | orbicular m. of mouth, levator m. of upper lip | facial | draws upper lip upward and laterally |

# APPENDIX 6

## Anatomy: Nerves

**Nerves**

| Common Name* [Modality] | TA Term† | Origin* | Branches* | Distribution* |
|---|---|---|---|---|
| abducent n. (6th cranial) [motor] | n. abducens | a nucleus in the pons, beneath floor of fourth ventricle | | lateral rectus muscle of eyeball |
| accessory n. (11th cranial) [parasympathetic, motor] | n. accessorius | by cranial roots from side of medulla oblongata, and by spinal roots of spinal cord | | internal branch to vagus, thereby to palate, pharynx, larynx, and thoracic viscera; external to sternocleidomastoid and trapezius muscles |
| acoustic n. *See* vestibulocochlear n. | | | | |
| alveolar n., inferior [motor, general sensory] | n. alveolaris inferior | mandibular n. | inferior dental, mental, and inferior gingival nerves; mylohyoid n. | teeth and gums of lower jaw, skin of chin and lower lip, mylohyoid muscle and anterior belly of digastric muscle |
| alveolar n's, superior | nn. alveolares superiores | superior alveolar branches (anterior, middle, and posterior) that arise from infraorbital and maxillary n's, innervating teeth of upper jaw and maxillary sinus, and forming superior dental plexus | | |
| ampullary n., anterior | n. ampullaris anterior | branch of vestibular part of eighth cranial (vestibulocochlear) n. that innervates ampulla of anterior semicircular duct, ending around hair cells of ampullary crest | | |
| ampullary n., inferior. *See* ampullary n., posterior | | | | |
| ampullary n., lateral | n. ampullaris lateralis | branch of vestibular n. that innervates ampulla of lateral semicircular duct, ending around hair cells of ampullary crest | | |
| ampullary n., posterior | n. ampullaris posterior | branch of vestibular part of eighth cranial (vestibulocochlear) n. that innervates ampulla of posterior semicircular duct, ending around hair cells of ampullary crest | | |
| ampullary n., superior. *See* ampullary n., anterior | | | | |
| anal n's, inferior. *See* rectal n's, inferior | | | | |
| anococcygeal n. [general sensory] | n. anococcygeus | coccygeal plexus | | sacrococcygeal joint, coccyx, skin over coccyx |
| auditory n. *See* vestibulocochlear n. | | | | |
| auricular n's, anterior [general sensory] | nn. auriculares anteriores | auriculotemporal n. | | skin of anterosuperior part of external ear |
| auricular n., great [general sensory] | n. auricularis magnus | cervical; plexus—C2–C3 | anterior and posterior branches | skin over parotid gland and mastoid process, and both surfaces of auricle |
| auricular n., posterior [motor, general sensory] | n. auricularis posterior | facial n. | occipital branch | posterior auricular and occipitofrontal muscles, skin of external acoustic meatus |
| auriculotemporal n. [general sensory] | n. auriculotemporalis | by two roots from mandibular n. | anterior auricular n., n. of external acoustic meatus, parotid branches, branch to tympanic membrane, branch communicating with facial n.; terminal branches superficial temporal to scalp | parotid gland, scalp in temporal region, tympanic membrane. *See also* auricular n., anterior *and* n. of external acoustic meatus |

* n = nerve; n's = (pl.) nervus.
† n. = [L.] nervus; nn = ([L.] pl.) nervi.

**Nerves** *Continued*

| Common Name [Modality] | TA Term | Origin | Branches | Distribution |
|---|---|---|---|---|
| axillary n. [motor, general sensory] | n. axillaris | posterior cord of brachial plexus—C5–C6 | lateral superior brachial cutaneous n., muscular branches | deltoid and teres minor muscles, skin over back of arm |
| buccal n. [general sensory] | n. buccalis | mandibular n. | | skin and mucous membrane of cheeks, gums, and perhaps first two molars and the premolars |
| cardiac n., cervical, inferior [sympathetic (accelerator), visceral afferent (chiefly pain)] | n. cardiacus cervicalis inferior | cervicothoracic ganglion | | heart via cardiac plexus |
| cardiac n., cervical, middle [sympathetic (accelerator), visceral afferent (chiefly pain)] | n. cardiacus cervicalis medius | middle cervical ganglion | | heart |
| cardiac n., cervical, superior [sympathetic (accelerator)] | n. cardiacus cervicalis superior | superior cervical ganglion | | heart |
| cardiac n., inferior. *See* cardiac n., cervical, inferior | | | | |
| cardiac n., middle, *See* cardiac n., cervical, middle | | | | |
| cardiac n., superior. *See* cardiac n., cervical, superior | | | | |
| cardiac n's, thoracic [sympathetic (accelerator), visceral afferent (chiefly pain)] | rami cardiaci thoracici | ganglia T2–T4 or T5 of sympathetic trunk | together with tympanic n. forms tympanic plexus | heart |
| caroticotympanic n's [sympathetic] | nn. caroticotympanici | internal carotid plexus | help form tympanic plexus | tympanic region, parotid gland |
| caroticotympanic n's, inferior and superior [sympathetic] | nn. caroticotympanici | internal carotid plexus | with tympanic n. form tympanic plexus | tympanic region, parotid gland |
| carotid n's, external [sympathetic] | nn. carotici externi | superior cervical ganglion | | cranial blood vessels and glands via external carotid plexus |
| carotid n., internal [sympathetic] | n. caroticus internus | superior cervical ganglion | | cranial blood vessels and glands via internal carotid plexus |
| cavernous n's of clitoris [parasympathetic, sympathetic, visceral afferent] | nn. cavernosi clitoridis | uterovaginal plexus | | erectile tissue of clitoris |
| cavernous n's of penis [sympathetic, parasympathetic, visceral afferent] | nn. cavernosi penis | prostatic plexus | | erectile tissue of penis |
| cerebral n's. *See* cranial n's | | | | |
| cervical n's | nn. cervicales | the 8 pairs of n's that arise from cervical segments of spinal cord and, except last pair, leave vertebral column above correspondingly numbered vertebra; the ventral branches of upper 4, on either side, unite to form cervical plexus; those of lower 4, together with ventral branch of first thoracic n., form most of brachial plexus | | |
| cervical n., transverse [general sensory] | n. transversus cervicalis | cervical plexus—C2–C3 | superior and inferior branches | skin on side and front of neck |
| ciliary n's, long [sympathetic, general sensory] | nn. ciliares longi | nasociliary n., from ophthalmic n. | | dilator muscle of pupil, uvea, cornea |
| ciliary n's, short [parasympathetic, sympathetic, general sensory] | nn. ciliares breves | ciliary ganglion | | smooth muscles and tunics of eye |
| clunial n's, inferior [general sensory] | nn. clunium inferiores | posterior femoral cutaneous n. | | skin of lower part of buttock |
| clunial n's, middle [general sensory] | nn. clunium medii | plexus formed by lateral branches of dorsal branches of first 4 sacral nerves behind sacrum and coccyx | | ligaments of sacrum and skin over posterior part of buttock |

**Nerves** *Continued*

| Common Name [Modality] | TA Term | Origin | Branches | Distribution |
|---|---|---|---|---|
| clunial n's, superior [general sensory] | nn. clunium superiores | lateral branches of dorsal branch of upper lumbar n's | | skin of upper part of buttock |
| coccygeal n. | n. coccygeus | one of the pair of nerves arising from coccygeal segment of spinal cord | | |
| cochlear n. | n. cochlearis | the part of the vestibulocochlear n. concerned with hearing, consisting of fibers that arise from the bipolar cells in the spiral ganglion and have their receptors in the spiral organ of the cochlea | | |
| cranial n's | nn. craniales | the 12 pairs of n's connected with brain, including olfactory (I), optic (II), oculomotor (III), trochlear (IV), trigeminal (V), abducens (VI), facial (VII), vestibulocochlear (VIII), glossopharyngeal (IX), vagus (X), accessory (XI), and hypoglossal (XII) nerves | | |
| cubital n. *See* ulnar n. | | | | |
| cutaneous n. of arm, lateral, inferior [general sensory] | n. cutaneus brachii lateralis inferior | radial n. | | skin of lateral surface of lower arm |
| cutaneous n. of arm, lateral, superior [general sensory] | n. cutaneus brachii lateralis superior | axillary n. | | skin of back of arm |
| cutaneous n. of arm, medial [general sensory] | n. cutaneus brachii medialis | medial cord of brachial plexus (T1) | | skin on medial and posterior aspects of arm |
| cutaneous n. of arm, posterior [general sensory] | n. cutaneus brachii posterior | radial n. in axilla | | skin on back of arm |
| cutaneous n. of calf, lateral [general sensory] | n. cutaneus surae lateralis | common fibular n. | | skin of lateral side of back of leg, rarely may continue as sural n. |
| cutaneous n. of calf, medial [general sensory] | n. cutaneus surae medialis | tibial n.; usually joins fibular communicating branch of common fibular n. to form sural n. | | may continue as sural n. |
| cutaneous n., dorsal, intermediate [general sensory] | n. cutaneus dorsalis intermedius | superficial fibular n. | dorsal digital n's of foot | skin of front of lower third of leg and dorsum of foot; ankle; skin and joints of adjacent sides of third and fourth, and of fourth and fifth toes |
| cutaneous n., dorsal, lateral [general sensory] | n. cutaneus dorsalis lateralis | continuation of sural n. | | skin and joints of lateral side of foot and fifth toe |
| cutaneous n. dorsal, medial [general sensory] | n. cutaneus dorsalis medialis | superficial fibular n. | | skin and joints of medial side of foot and big toe; adjacent sides of second and third toes |
| cutaneous n. of forearm, lateral [general sensory] | n. cutaneus antebrachii lateralis | continuation of musculocutaneous n. | | skin over radial side of forearm; sometimes an area of skin of back of hand |
| cutaneous n. of forearm, medial [general sensory] | n. cutaneus antebrachii medialis | medial cord of brachial plexus (C8, T1) | anterior and ulnar | skin of front, medial, and posteromedial aspects of forearm |
| cutaneous n. of forearm, posterior [general sensory] | n. cutaneus antebrachii posterior | radial n. | | skin of dorsal aspect of forearm |
| cutaneous n. of neck, anterior. *See* cutaneous n. of neck, transverse | | | | |
| cutaneous n. of neck, transverse [general sensory] | n. transversus cervicalis | cervical plexus—C2–C3 | superior and inferior rami | skin on side and front of neck |
| cutaneous n. of thigh, lateral [general sensory] | n. cutaneus femoris lateralis | lumbar plexus—L2–L3 | | skin of lateral aspect and front of thigh |
| cutaneous n. of thigh, posterior [general sensory] | n. cutaneus femoralis posterior | sacral plexus—S1–S3 | inferior clunial n's, perineal branches | skin of buttock, external genitalia, back of thigh and calf |
| digital n's, dorsal, radial. *See* digital n's of radial n., dorsal | | | | |
| digital n's, dorsal, ulnar. *See* digital n's of ulnar n., dorsal | | | | |

**Nerves** *Continued*

| Common Name [Modality] | TA Term | Origin | Branches | Distribution |
|---|---|---|---|---|
| digital n's of foot, dorsal [general sensory] | nn. digitales dorsales pedis | intermediate dorsal cutaneous n. | | skin and joint of adjacent sides of third and fourth, and of fourth and fifth toes |
| digital n's of lateral plantar n., plantar, common [general sensory] | nn. digitales plantares communes nervi plantaris lateralis | superficial branch of lateral plantar n. | medial n. gives rise to 2 proper plantar digital n's | lateral one to short flexor muscle of little toe, skin and joints of lateral side of sole and little toe; medial one to adjacent sides of fourth and fifth toes |
| digital n's of lateral plantar n., plantar, proper [motor general sensory] | nn. digitales plantares proprii nervi plantaris lateralis | common plantar digital n's | | short flexor muscle of little toe, skin and joints of lateral side of sole and little toe, and adjacent surfaces of fourth and fifth toes |
| digital n's of medial plantar n., plantar, common [motor, general sensory] | nn. digitales plantares communes nervi plantaris medialis | medial plantar n. | muscular and proper plantar digital n's | flexor hallucis brevis muscle and first lumbrical muscles, skin and joints of medial side of foot and first toe, and adjacent sides of first and second, second and third, and third and fourth toes |
| digital n's of medial plantar n., plantar, proper [general sensory] | nn. digitales plantares proprii nervi plantaris medialis | common plantar digital n's | | skin and joints of first toe, and adjacent sides of first and second, second and third, and third and fourth toes; the nerves extend to the dorsum to supply nail beds and tips of toes |
| digital n's of median n., palmar, common [motor, general sensory] | nn. digitales palmares communes nervi mediani | lateral and medial divisions of median n. | proper palmar digital n's | thumb, index, middle, and ring fingers, and first two lumbrical muscles |
| digital n's of median n., palmar, proper [motor, general sensory] | nn. digitales palmares proprii nervi mediani | common palmar digital n's | | first two lumbrical muscles, skin and joints of both sides and palmar aspect of thumb, index, and middle fingers, radial side of ring finger, back of distal aspect of these digits |
| digital n's of radial n., dorsal [general sensory] | nn. digitales dorsales nervi radialis | superficial branch of radial n. | | skin and joints of back of thumb, index finger, and part of middle finger, as far distally as digital phalanx |
| digital n's of ulnar n., dorsal [general sensory] | nn. digitales dorsales nervi ulnaris | dorsal branch of ulnar n. | | skin and joints of medial side of little finger, dorsal aspects of adjacent sides of little and ring fingers and of ring and middle fingers |
| digital n's of ulnar n., palmar, common [general sensory] | nn. digitales palmares communes nervi ulnaris | superficial branch of ulnar n. | proper palmar digital n's | little and ring fingers |
| digital n's of ulnar n., palmar, proper [general sensory] | nn. digitales palmares proprii nervi ulnaris | the lateral of the two common palmar digital n's from superficial branch of ulnar n. | | skin and joints of adjacent sides of fourth and fifth fingers |
| dorsal n. of clitoris [general sensory, motor] | n. dorsalis clitoridis | pudendal n. | | deep transverse muscle of perineum, sphincter muscle of urethra, corpus cavernosum of clitoris, and skin, prepuce, and glans of clitoris |
| dorsal n. of penis [general sensory, motor] | n. dorsalis penis | pudendal n. | | deep transverse muscle of perineum, sphincter muscle of urethra, corpus cavernosum of penis, and skin, prepuce, and glans of penis |

**Nerves** *Continued*

| Common Name [Modality] | TA Term | Origin | Branches | Distribution |
|---|---|---|---|---|
| dorsal scapular n. [motor] | n. dorsalis scapulae | brachial plexus—ventral branch of C5 | | rhomboid muscles and occasionally the levator muscle of scapula |
| ethmoidal n., anterior [general sensory] | n. ethmoidalis anterior | continuation of nasociliary n., from ophthalmic n. | internal, external, lateral, and medial nasal branches | mucosa of upper and anterior nasal septum, lateral wall of nasal cavity, skin of lower bridge and tip of nose |
| ethmoidal n., posterior [general sensory] | n. ethmoidalis posterior | nasociliary n., from ophthalmic n. | | mucosa of posterior ethmoid cells and of sphenoidal sinus |
| n. of external acoustic meatus [general sensory] | n. meatus acustici externi | auriculotemporal n. | | skin lining external acoustic meatus, and tympanic membrane |
| facial n. (7th cranial) [motor, parasympathetic, general sensory, special sensory]. *See also* intermediate n. | n. facialis | inferior border of pons, between olive and inferior cerebellar peduncle | stapedius n.; posterior auricular n.; parotid plexus; digastric, temporal, zygomatic, buccal, lingual, marginal mandibular, and cervical branches, and communicating branch with tympanic plexus | various structures of face, head, and neck (see also individual branches in this table) |
| femoral n. [general sensory, motor] | n. femoralis | lumbar plexus—L2–L4; descending behind inguinal ligament to femoral triangle | saphenous n., muscular and anterior cutaneous branches | skin of thigh and leg, muscles of front of thigh, and hip and knee joints (see also individual branches in this table) |
| fibular n., common [general sensory, motor] | n. fibularis communis | sciatic n. in lower part of thigh | supplies short head of biceps femoris muscle; gives off lateral sural cutaneous n. and communicating branch as it descends in popliteal fossa, supplies knee and superior tibiofibular joints and tibialis anterior muscle; divides into superficial and deep fibular n's | |
| fibular n., deep [general sensory, motor] | n. fibularis profundus | common fibular n. | winds around neck of fibula and descends on the interosseous membrane to front of ankle; muscular branches given off to tibialis anterior, extensor hallucis, extensor digitorum longus, and third peroneal muscles, and a twig to ankle joint; a lateral terminal division supplies extensor brevis muscle and tarsal joints; medial terminal division, or digital branch, divides into dorsal digital n's for skin and joints of adjacent sides of first and second toes | |
| fibular n., superficial common [general sensory, motor] | n. fibularis superficialis | common fibular n. | descends in front of fibula, supplies peroneus longus and brevis muscles and, in the lower part of the leg, divides into the muscular rami, medial and intermediate dorsal cutaneous n's | |
| frontal n. [general sensory] | n. frontalis | ophthalmic division of trigeminal n.; enters orbit through superior orbital fissure | supraorbital and supratrochlear n's | chiefly to forehead and scalp (see individual branches listed in this table) |
| genitofemoral n. [general sensory, motor] | n. genitofemoralis | lumbar plexus—L1–L2 | genital and femoral branches | cremaster muscle, skin of scrotum or labium majus and of adjacent area of thigh and femoral triangle |
| glossopharyngeal n. (9th cranial) [motor, parasympathetic, general sensory, special sensory, visceral sensory] | n. glossopharyngeus | several rootlets from lateral side of upper medulla oblongata, between olive and inferior cerebellar peduncle | tympanic n., pharyngeal, stylopharyngeal, tonsillar, and lingual branches, branch to carotid sinus, communicating branch with auricular branch of vagus n. | has two enlargements (superior and inferior ganglia) and supplies tongue, pharynx, and parotid nerve (see also individual branches in this table) |
| gluteal n., inferior [motor] | n. gluteus inferior | sacral plexus—L5–S2 | | gluteus maximus muscle |
| gluteal n., superior [motor, general sensory] | n. gluteus superior | sacral plexus—L4–S1 | | gluteus medius and minimus muscles, tensor fasciae latae, and hip joint |
| hemorrhoidal n's, inferior. *See* rectal n's, inferior | | | | |
| hypogastric n. | n. hypogastricus | a nerve trunk situated on either side (right and left), interconnecting superior and inferior hypogastric plexuses | | |

**Nerves** Continued

| Common Name [Modality] | TA Term | Origin | Branches | Distribution |
|---|---|---|---|---|
| hypoglossal n. (12th cranial) [motor] | n. hypoglossus | several rootlets in anterolateral sulcus between olive and pyramid of medulla oblongata; passes through hypoglossal canal to tongue | lingual branches | styloglossus, hyoglossus, and genioglossus muscles, intrinsic muscles of tongue |
| iliohypogastric n. [motor, general sensory] | n. iliohypogastricus | lumbar plexus—L1 (sometimes T12) | lateral and anterior cutaneous branches | skin above pubis and over lateral side of buttock, and occasionally pyramidal muscle |
| ilioinguinal n. [general sensory] | n. ilioinguinalis | lumbar plexus—L1 (sometimes T12); accompanies spermatic cord through inguinal canal | anterior scrotal or labial branches | skin of scrotum or labia majora, and adjacent part of thigh |
| infraoccipital n. *See* suboccipital n. | | | | |
| infraorbital n. [general sensory] | n. infraorbitalis | continuation of maxillary n., entering orbit through inferior orbital fissure, occupying in succession infraorbital groove, canal, and foramen | middle and anterior superior alveolar, inferior palpebral, internal and external nasal, and superior labial branches | incisor, cuspid, and premolar teeth of upper jaw, skin and conjunctiva of lower eyelid, mobile septum and skin of side of nose, mucous membrane of mouth, skin of upper lip |
| infratrochlear n. [general sensory] | n. infratrochlearis | nasociliary n., from ophthalmic n. | palpebral branches | skin of root and upper bridge of nose and lower eyelid, conjunctiva, lacrimal duct |
| intercostobrachial n's [general sensory] | nn. intercostobrachiales | second and third intercostal n's | | skin on back and medial aspect of arm |
| intermediate n. [parasympathetic, special sensory] | n. intermedius | smaller root of facial n., between main root and vestibulocochlear n. | greater petrosal n., chorda tympani | lacrimal, nasal, palatine, submandibular, and sublingual glands, and anterior two thirds of tongue |
| intermediofacial n. *See* facial n. and intermediate n. | | | | |
| interosseous n. of forearm, anterior [motor, general sensory] | n. interosseous antebrachii anterior | median n. | | flexor pollicis longus, flexor digitorum profundus, and pronator quadratus muscles, wrist and intercarpal joints |
| interosseous n. of forearm, posterior [motor, general sensory] | n. interosseus antebrachii posterior | continuation of deep branch of radial n. | | long abductor muscle of thumb, extensor muscles of thumb and index finger, and wrist and intercarpal joints |
| interosseous n. of leg [general sensory] | interosseus cruris | tibial n. | | interosseous membrane and tibiofemoral syndesmosis |
| ischiadic n. *See* sciatic n. | | | | |
| jugular n. | n. jugularis | a branch of the superior cervical which communicates with glossopharyngeal and vagus n's | | |
| labial n's, anterior [general sensory] | nn. labiales anteriores | ilioinguinal n. | | skin of anterior labial region of labia majora and adjacent part of thigh |
| labial n's, posterior [general sensory] | nn. labiales posteriores | pudendal n. | | labium majus |
| lacrimal n. [general sensory] | n. lacrimalis | ophthalmic division of trigeminal n. entering orbit through superior orbital fissure | | lacrimal gland, conjunctiva, lateral commissure of eye, skin of upper eyelid |
| laryngeal n., external [motor] | ramus externus nervi laryngei superioris | superior laryngeal n. | | cricothyroid, inferior constrictor of pharynx |
| laryngeal n., inferior [motor] | | recurrent laryngeal n., especially the terminal portion | | intrinsic muscles of larynx, except cricothyroid communicates with internal laryngeal n. |
| laryngeal n., internal [general sensory] | ramus internus nervi laryngealis superioris | superior laryngeal n. | | mucosa of epiglottis, base of tongue, and larynx |

**Nerves** *Continued*

| Common Name [Modality] | TA Term | Origin | Branches | Distribution |
|---|---|---|---|---|
| laryngeal n., recurrent [parasympathetic, visceral afferent, motor] | n. laryngealis recurrens | vagus n. (chiefly the cranial part of the accessory n.) | inferior laryngeal n., tracheal, esophageal, and inferior cardiac branches | tracheal mucosa, esophagus, cardiac plexus (see also individual branches in this table) |
| laryngeal n., superior [motor, general sensory, visceral afferent, parasympathetic] | n. laryngealis superior | inferior ganglion of vagus n. | external, internal, and communicating branches | cricothyroid muscle and inferior constrictor muscle of pharynx, mucous membrane of back of tongue and larynx |
| lingual n. [general sensory] | n. lingualis | mandibular n., descending to tongue, first medial to mandible and then under cover of mucosa of mouth | sublingual n., lingual branch, branch to isthmus of fauces, branch communicating with hypoglossal n. and chorda tympani | anterior two thirds of tongue, adjacent areas of mouth, gums, isthmus of fauces |
| lumbar n's | nn. lumbales | the 5 pairs of n's that arise from lumbar segments of spinal cord, each pair leaving vertebral column below correspondingly numbered vertebrae; ventral branches of these nerves participate in formation of lumbosacral plexus | | |
| mandibular n. (third division of trigeminal n.) [general sensory, motor] | n. mandibularis | trigeminal ganglion | meningeal branch, masseteric, deep temporal, lateral and medial pterygoid, buccal, auriculotemporal, lingual and inferior alveolar n's | extensive distribution to muscles of mastication, skin of face, mucous membrane of mouth, and teeth (see also individual branches in this table) |
| masseteric n. [motor, general sensory] | n. massetericus | mandibular division of trigeminal n. | | masseter muscle, temporomandibular joint |
| maxillary n. (second division of trigeminal n.) [general sensory] | n. maxillaris | trigeminal ganglion | meningeal branch, zygomatic n., posterior superior alveolar branches, infraorbital n., pterygopalatine n's, and indirectly branches of pterygopalatine ganglion | extensive distribution to skin of face and scalp, mucous membrane of maxillary sinus and nasal cavity, and teeth |
| median n. [general sensory] | n. medianus | lateral and medial cords of brachial plexus—C6–T1 | anterior interosseous n. of forearm, common palmar digital n's, and muscular and palmar branches, and a communicating branch with ulnar n. | ultimately, skin on front of lateral part of hand, most of flexor muscles of front of forearm, most of short muscles of thumb, elbow joint, and many joints of hand |
| mental n. [general sensory] | n. mentalis | inferior alveolar n. | mental, gingival, and inferior labial branches | skin of chin, lower lip |
| musculocutaneous n. [general sensory, motor] | n. musculocutaneus | lateral cord of brachial plexus—C5–C7 | lateral cutaneous n. of forearm, muscular branches | coracobrachial, biceps, brachial muscles, elbow joint, skin of radial side of forearm |
| musculocutaneous n. of foot. *See* fibular n., superficial | | | | |
| musculocutaneous n. of leg. *See* fibular n., deep | | | | |
| mylohyoid n. [motor] | n. mylohyoideus | inferior alveolar n. | | mylohyoid muscle, anterior belly of digastric muscle |
| nasociliary n. [general sensory] | n. nasociliaris | ophthalmic division of trigeminal nerve | long ciliary, posterior ethmoidal, anterior ethmoidal, and infratrochlear n's and a communicating branch to ciliary ganglion | (see individual branches in this table) |
| nasopalatine n. [parasympathetic, general sensory] | n. nasopalatinus | pterygopalatine ganglion | | mucosa and glands of most of nasal septum and anterior part of hard palate |
| obturator n. [general sensory, motor] | n. obturatorius | lumbar plexus—L3–L4 | anterior, posterior, and muscular branches | gracilis and adductor muscles, skin of medial part of thigh, and hip joints |
| obturator n., accessory [general sensory, motor] | n. obturatorius accessorius | ventral branches of ventral rami of L3–L4 | | pectineus muscle, hip joint, obturator nerve |
| obturator n., internal [general sensory, motor] | n. musculi obturatorii interni | ventral branches of ventral rami of L5, S1–S2 | | posterior gemellus superior, obturator internus muscle |

**Nerves** *Continued*

| Common Name [Modality] | TA Term | Origin | Branches | Distribution |
|---|---|---|---|---|
| occipital n., greater [general sensory, motor] | n. occipitalis major | medial branch of dorsal branch of C2 | | semispinal muscle of head and skin of head as far forward as vertex |
| occipital n., lesser [general sensory] | n. occipitalis minor | superficial cervical plexus—C2–C3 | | ascends behind auricle and supplies some of the skin of side of head and on cranial surface of auricle |
| occipital n., third [general sensory] | n. occipitalis tertius | medial branch of dorsal branch of C3 | | skin of upper part of back of neck and head |
| oculomotor n. (3rd cranial) [motor, parasympathetic] | n. oculomotorius | brain stem, emerging medial to cerebral peduncles, running forward in the cavernous sinus | superior and inferior branches | entering orbit through superior orbital fissure, the branches supply levator muscle of upper lid, all extrinsic muscles except lateral rectus and superior oblique, and carry parasympathetic fibers from ciliary muscle to sphincter of pupil |
| olfactory n. (1st cranial) [special sensory] | nn. olfactorius | the nerve of smell, consisting of about 20 bundles arising in the olfactory epithelium and passing through the cribriform plate of ethmoid bone to olfactory bulb | | |
| ophthalmic n. (first division of trigeminal n.) [general sensory] | n. ophthalmicus | trigeminal ganglion | tentorial branches, frontal, lacrimal, nasociliary n's | eyeball and conjunctiva, lacrimal sac and gland, nasal mucosa and frontal sinus, external nose, eyelid, forehead, and scalp (see also individual branches in this table) |
| optic n. (2nd cranial) [special sensory] | n. opticus | the nerve of sight, consisting chiefly of axons and central processes of cells of the ganglionic layer of retina leaving the orbit through the optic canal, joining the optic chiasm (the medial ones crossing over to opposite side), and continuing as the optic tract | | |
| palatine n., anterior. *See* palatine n., greater | | | | |
| palatine n., greater [parasympathetic, sympathetic, general sensory] | n. palatinus major | pterygopalatine ganglion | posterior inferior [lateral] nasal branches | emerges through greater palatine foramen and supplies palate |
| palatine n's, lesser [parasympathetic, sympathetic, general sensory] | nn. palatini minores | pterygopalatine ganglion | | emerge through lesser palatine foramen and supply soft palate and tonsil |
| perineal n's [motor, general sensory] | nn. perineales | pudendal n. in pudendal canal | muscular branches and posterior scrotal or labial nerves | muscular branches supply bulbospongiosus, ischiocavernosus, superficial transverse perinei muscles and bulb of penis and, in part, sphincter ani externi and levator ani; the scrotal (labial) n's supply the scrotum or labium majus |
| peroneal n's. *See* entries under fibular n. | | | | |
| petrosal n., deep [sympathetic] | n. petrosus profundus | internal carotid plexus | | joins greater petrosal n. to form n. of pterygoid canal, and supplies lacrimal, nasal, and palatine glands via pterygopalatine ganglion and its branches |
| petrosal n., greater [parasympathetic, general sensory] | n. petrosus major | intermediate n. via geniculate ganglion | | running forward from geniculate ganglion, joins deep petrosal n. of pterygoid canal, and reaches lacrimal, nasal, and palatine glands and nasopharynx via pterygopalatine ganglion and its branches |

**Nerves** *Continued*

| Common Name [Modality] | TA Term | Origin | Branches | Distribution |
|---|---|---|---|---|
| petrosal n., lesser [parasympathetic] | n. petrosus minor | tympanic plexus | | parotid gland via otic ganglion and auriculotemporal n. |
| phrenic n. [motor, general sensory] | n. phrenicus | cervical plexus—C4–C5 | pericardial and phrenicoabdominal branches | pleura, pericardium, diaphragm, peritoneum, sympathetic plexuses |
| phrenic n's, accessory | nn. phrenici accessorii | inconstant contribution of fifth cervical n. to phrenic n.; when present, they run a separate course to root of neck or into thorax before joining phrenic n. | | |
| piriform n. [general sensory, motor] | n. musculi piriformis | dorsal branches of ventral rami of S1–S2 | | anterior piriform muscle |
| plantar n., lateral [general sensory, motor] | n. plantaris lateralis | smaller of terminal branches of tibial n. | muscular, superficial, and deep branches | lying between first and second layers of muscles of sole, supplies quadratus plantae, abductor digiti minimi, flexor digiti minimi brevis, adductor hallucis, interossei, and second, third, and fourth lumbrical muscles, and gives off cutaneous and articular twigs to lateral side of sole and fourth and fifth toes (see also individual branches in this table) |
| plantar n., medial [general sensory, motor] | n. plantaris medialis | larger of terminal branches of tibial n. | common plantar digital n's and muscular branches | abductor hallucis, flexor digitorum brevis, flexor hallucis brevis, and first lumbrical muscles and cutaneous and articular twigs to medial side of sole and first to fourth toes (see also individual branches in this table) |
| pneumogastric n. *See* vagus n. | | | | |
| popliteal n., external. *See* fibular n., common | | | | |
| popliteal n., lateral. *See* fibular n., common | | | | |
| pterygoid n., lateral [motor] | n. pterygoideus lateralis | mandibular n. | | lateral pterygoid, tensor tympani, and tensor veli palatini muscles |
| pterygoid n., medial [motor] | n. pterygoideus medialis | mandibular n. | | medial pterygoid muscle |
| n. of pterygoid canal [parasympathetic, sympathetic] | n. canalis pterygoidei | union of deep and greater petrosal n's | | pterygopalatine ganglion and branches |
| pterygopalatine n's [general sensory] | | two nerves connecting maxillary n. to pterygopalatine ganglion; they are the sensory roots of the ganglion | | |
| pudendal n. [general sensory, motor, parasympathetic] | n. pudendus | sacral plexus—S2–S4 | enters pudendal canal, gives off inferior rectal n., then divides into perineal n. and dorsal n. of penis (clitoris) | muscles, skin, and erectile tissue of perineum (see also individual branches in this table) |
| n. of quadrate muscle of thigh [sensory, motor] | n. musculi quadrati femoris | ventral branches of ventral rami of L4–L5 | | gemellus inferior, anterior quadratus femoris muscle, hip joint |
| radial n. [general sensory, motor] | n. radialis | posterior cord of brachial plexus—C6–C8, and sometimes C5 and T1 | posterior cutaneous and inferior lateral cutaneous n's of arm, posterior cutaneous n. of forearm, muscular, deep, and superficial branches | descending in back of arm and forearm, ultimately distributed to skin on back of forearm, arm, and hand, extensor muscles on back of arm and forearm, and elbow joint and many joints of hand |
| rectal n's, inferior [general sensory, motor] | nn. rectales inferiores | pudendal n., or independently from sacral plexus | | sphincter ani externus muscle, skin around anus, lining of anal canal up to pectinate line |
| recurrent n. *See* laryngeal n., recurrent | | | | |

**Nerves** *Continued*

| Common Name [Modality] | TA Term | Origin | Branches | Distribution |
|---|---|---|---|---|
| saccular n. | n. saccularis | the branch of vestibular part of eighth cranial (vestibulocochlear) nerve that innervates macula of saccule | | |
| sacral n's | nn. sacrales | the 5 pairs of n's that arise from sacral segments of spinal cord; the ventral branches of first 4 pairs participate in formation of sacral plexus | | |
| saphenous n. [general sensory] | n. saphenus | termination of femoral n. | infrapatellar and medial crural cutaneous | knee joint, subsartorial and patellar plexuses, skin on medial side of leg and foot |
| sciatic n. [general sensory, motor] | n. ischiadicus | sacral plexus—L4–S3; leaves pelvis through greater sciatic foramen | divides into common peroneal and tibial n's, usually in lower third of thigh | (see individual branches in this table) |
| scrotal n's, anterior [general sensory] | nn. scrotales anteriores | ilioinguinal n. | | skin of anterior scrotal region |
| scrotal n's, posterior [general sensory] | nn. scrotales posteriores | perineal n's | | skin of scrotum |
| sphenopalatine n's. *See* pterygopalatine n's. | | | | |
| spinal n's | nn. spinales | the 31 pairs of n's that arise from spinal cord, and pass between the vertebrae, including 8 cervical, 12 thoracic, 5 lumbar, 5 sacral, and 1 coccygeal | | |
| splanchnic n., greater [preganglionic sympathetic, visceral afferent] | n. splanchnicus major | thoracic sympathetic trunk and thoracic ganglia T5–T10 of sympathetic trunk | | descending through diaphragm or its aortic opening, ends in celiac ganglia and plexuses, with a splanchnic ganglion commonly near the diaphragm |
| splanchnic n., lesser [preganglionic sympathetic, visceral afferent] | n. splanchnicus minor | thoracic ganglia T9, T10 or sympathetic trunk | renal branch | pierces diaphragm, joins aorticorenal ganglion and celiac plexus, and communicates with renal and superior mesenteric plexuses |
| splanchnic n., lowest [sympathetic, visceral afferent] | n. splanchnicus imus | last ganglion of sympathetic trunk or lesser thoracic n. | | aorticorenal ganglion and adjacent plexus |
| splanchnic n's, lumbar [preganglionic sympathetic, visceral afferent] | nn. splanchnici lumbales | lumbar ganglia or sympathetic trunk | | upper nerves join celiac and adjacent plexuses, middle ones go to mesenteric and adjacent plexuses, lower ones descend to superior hypogastric plexus |
| splanchnic n's, pelvic [preganglionic sympathetic, visceral afferent] | nn. splanchnici pelvici | sacral plexus—S3–S4 | | leaving sacral plexus, they enter inferior hypogastric plexus and supply pelvic organs |
| splanchnic n's, sacral [preganglionic sympathetic, visceral afferent] | nn. splanchnici sacrales | sacral part of sympathetic trunk | | pelvic organs and blood vessels via inferior hypogastric plexus |
| stapedius n. [motor] | n. stapedius | facial n. | | stapedius muscle |
| subclavian n. [motor, general sensory] | n. subclavius | upper trunk of brachial plexus—C5 | | subclavius muscle, sternoclavicular joint |
| subcostal n. [general sensory, motor] | n. subcostalis | ventral branch of T12 | | skin of lower abdomen and lateral side of gluteal region, parts of transverse, oblique, and rectus muscles, and usually pyramidal muscle, and adjacent peritoneum |
| sublingual n. [parasympathetic, general sensory] | n. sublingualis | lingual n. | | sublingual gland and overlying mucous membrane |
| suboccipital n. [motor] | n. suboccipitalis | dorsal branch of C1 | | emerges above posterior arch of atlas, supplies muscles of suboccipital triangle and semispinal muscle of head |

**Nerves** *Continued*

| Common Name [Modality] | TA Term | Origin | Branches | Distribution |
|---|---|---|---|---|
| subscapular n's [motor] | nn. subscapulares | posterior cord of brachial plexus—C5 | | usually two or more nerves, upper and lower, supplying subscapular and teres major muscles |
| supraclavicular n's, anterior. *See* supraclavicular n's, medial | | | | |
| supraclavicular n's, intermediate [general sensory] | nn. supraclaviculares intermedii | cervical plexus—C3–C4 | | descend in posterior triangle, cross clavicle, supplying skin over pectoral and deltoid regions |
| supraclavicular n's, lateral [general sensory] | nn. supraclaviculares laterales | cervical plexus—C3–C4 | | descend in posterior triangle, cross clavicle, supplying skin of superior and posterior aspects of shoulder |
| supraclavicular n's, medial [general sensory] | nn. supraclaviculares mediales | cervical plexus—C3–C4 | | descend in posterior triangle, cross clavicle, supplying skin of medial infraclavicular region |
| supraclavicular n's, middle. *See* supraclavicular n's, intermediate | | | | |
| supraclavicular n's, posterior. *See* supraclavicular n's, lateral | | | | |
| supraorbital n. [general sensory] | n. supraorbitalis | continuation of frontal n., from ophthalmic n. | lateral and medial branches | leaves orbit through supraorbital notch or foramen, supplying skin of upper eyelid, forehead, anterior part of scalp (to vertex), mucosa of frontal sinus |
| suprascapular n. [motor, general sensory] | n. suprascapularis | brachial plexus—C5–C6 | | descends through suprascapular and spinoglenoid notches, supplying acromioclavicular and shoulder joints, and supraspinous and infraspinous muscles |
| supratrochlear n. [general sensory] | n. supratrochlearis | frontal n., from ophthalmic n. | | leaves orbit at end of supraorbital margin, supplying forehead and upper eyelid |
| sural n. [general sensory] | n. suralis | medial sural n. and communicating branch of common peroneal n. | lateral dorsal cutaneous n. and lateral calcaneal branches | skin on back of leg, and skin and joints on lateral side of foot and heel |
| temporal n's, deep [motor] | nn. temporales profundi | mandibular n. | | temporal muscles |
| n. of tensor tympani muscle [motor] | n. musculi tensoris tympani | mandibular n. via n. to medial pterygoid muscle and otic ganglion | | tensor muscle of tympanum |
| n. of tensor veli palatini muscle [motor] | n. musculi tensoris veli palatini | mandibular n. via n. to medial pterygoid muscle and otic ganglion | | tensor muscle of palatine velum |
| tentorial n. [general sensory] | ramus tentorius nervi ophthalmici | ophthalmic n. | | dura mater of tentorium cerebelli |
| thoracic n's | nn. thoracici | the 12 pairs of spinal n's that arise from thoracic segments of spinal cord, each pair leaving vertebral column below correspondingly numbered vertebra | | body wall of thorax and upper part of abdomen |
| thoracic n., long [motor] | n. thoracicus longus | brachial plexus—ventral branches of C5–C7 | | descends behind brachial plexus to anterior serratus muscle |
| thoracic splanchnic n., greater. *See* splanchnic n., greater | | | | |
| thoracic splanchnic n., lesser. *See* splanchnic n., lesser | | | | |
| thoracic splanchnic n., lowest. *See* splanchnic n., lowest | | | | |
| thoracodorsal n. [motor] | n. thoracodorsalis | posterior cord of brachial plexus—C7–C8 | | latissimus dorsi muscle |

**Nerves** *Continued*

| Common Name [Modality] | TA Term | Origin | Branches | Distribution |
|---|---|---|---|---|
| tibial n. [general sensory, motor] | n. tibialis | sciatic n. in lower thigh | interosseous n. of leg, medial cutaneous n. of calf, sural and medial and lateral plantar n's, and muscular and medial calcaneal branches | while still incorporated in sciatic n., supplies semimembranous and semitendinous muscles, long head of biceps, and adductor magnus muscle; supplies knee joint as it descends in popliteal fossa; continuing into leg, supplies muscles and skin of calf, sole, and toes (see also individual branches in this table) |
| trigeminal n. (5th cranial) [general sensory, motor] | n. trigeminus | emerges from lateral surface of pons as a motor and a sensory root, the latter expanding into trigeminal ganglion, from which the 3 divisions of nerve arise (see mandibular n., maxillary n., and ophthalmic n.) | | face, teeth, mouth, nasal cavity, muscles of mastication |
| trochlear n. (4th cranial) [motor] | n. trochlearis | fibers of each nerve (one on either side) decussate across median plane, and emerge from back of brain stem below corresponding inferior colliculus | | runs forward in lateral wall of cavernous sinus, traverses superior orbital fissure, supplying superior oblique muscle of eyeball |
| tympanic n. [general sensory, parasympathetic] | n. tympanicus | inferior ganglion of glossopharyngeal n. | helps form tympanic plexus | mucous membrane of tympanic cavity, mastoid air cells, auditory tube, and, via lesser petrosal n. and otic ganglion, parotid gland |
| ulnar n. [general sensory, motor] | n. ulnaris | medial and lateral cords of brachial plexus—C7–T1 | muscular, dorsal, palmar, superficial, and deep branches | ultimately to skin on front and medial part of hand, some flexor muscles on front of forearm, many short muscles of hand, elbow joint, many joints of hand |
| utricular n. | n. utricularis | the branch of vestibular n. that innervates macula of utricle | | |
| utriculoampullary n. | n. utriculoampullaris | a n. that arises by peripheral division of vestibular n., and supplies utricle and ampullae of semicircular ducts | | |
| vaginal n's [sympathetic, parasympathetic] | nn. vaginales | uterovaginal plexus | | vagina |
| vagus n. (10th cranial) [parasympathetic, visceral afferent, motor, general sensory] | n. vagus | by numerous rootlets from lateral side of medulla oblongata in groove between olive and inferior cerebellar peduncle | superior and recurrent laryngeal n's, meningeal, auricular, pharyngeal, cardiac, bronchial, gastric, hepatic, celiac, and renal branches, pharyngeal, pulmonary, and esophageal plexuses, and anterior and posterior trunks | descending through jugular foramen, presents as a superior and inferior ganglion, continues through neck and thorax into abdomen, supplying sensory fibers to ear, tongue, pharynx, and larynx, motor fibers to pharynx, larynx, esophagus, and parasympathetic and visceral fibers to thoracic and abdominal viscera (see also individual branches in this table) |
| vertebral n. [sympathetic] | n. vertebralis | cervicothoracic and vertebral | | ascends with vertebral artery and gives fibers to spinal meninges, cervical n's, and posterior cranial fossa |
| vestibular n. | n. vestibularis | the posterior part of the vestibulocochlear n., concerned with equilibration, consisting of fibers arising from bipolar cells in vestibular ganglion; divides peripherally into rostral and caudal parts, with receptors in the ampullae of the semicircular canals, the ventricle, and the saccule | | |

**Nerves** *Continued*

| Common Name [Modality] | TA Term | Origin | Branches | Distribution |
|---|---|---|---|---|
| vestibulocochlear n. (8th cranial) | n. vestibulocochlearis | emerges from brain between pons and medulla oblongata, at cerebellopontine angle and behind facial n.; divides near lateral end of internal acoustic meatus into two functionally distinct and incompletely united components, the vestibular n. and the cochlear n. and is connected with brain by corresponding roots (vestibular and cochlear roots) | | |
| vidian n. *See* n. of pterygoid canal | | | | |
| vidian n., deep. *See* petrosal n., deep | | | | |
| zygomatic n. [general sensory] | n. zygomaticus | maxillary n., entering orbit through inferior orbital fissure | zygomaticofacial and zygomaticotemporal branches | communicates with lacrimal nerve, supplying skin of temple and adjacent part of face |

# Anatomy: Veins

**Veins**

| Common Name* | TA Term† | Region* | Receives Blood From* | Drains Into* |
|---|---|---|---|---|
| accompanying v. of hypoglossal nerve | v. comitans nervi hypoglossi | accompanies hypoglossal nerve | formed by union of profunda linguae v. and sublingual v. | facial, lingual, or internal jugular |
| adrenal v's. *See* suprarenal v., left and right. | | | | |
| anastomotic v., inferior | v. anastomotica inferior | interconnects superficial middle cerebral v. and transverse sinus | | |
| anastomotic v., superior | v. anastomotica superior | interconnects superficial middle cerebral v. and superior sagittal sinus | | |
| angular v. | v. angularis | between eye and root of nose | formed by union of supratrochlear v. and supraorbital v. | continues inferiorly as facial v. |
| antebrachial v., median | v. mediana antebrachii | forearm between cephalic v. and basilic v. | a palmar venous plexus | cephalic v. and/or basilic v., or median cubital v. |
| anterior v's of right ventricle | vv. ventriculi dextri anteriores | ventral surface of right ventricle | | right atrium |
| appendicular v. | v. appendicularis | accompanies appendicular artery | | joins anterior and posterior cecal v's to form ileocolic v. |
| v. of aqueduct of cochlea | v. aqueductus cochleae | along aqueduct of cochlea | cochlea | superior bulb of internal jugular v. |
| v. of aqueduct of vestibule | v. aqueductus vestibuli | passes through aqueduct of vestibule | internal ear | superior petrosal sinus |
| arcuate v's of kidney | vv. arcuatae renis | a series of complete arches across the bases of the renal pyramids, formed for union of interlobular v's and straight venules of kidney | | interlobar v's |
| articular v's | vv. articulares | | plexus around temporomandibular joint | retromandibular v. |
| auditory v's, internal. *See* labyrinthine v's | | | | |
| auricular v's, anterior | vv. auriculares anteriores | anterior part of auricle | | superficial temporal v. |
| auricular v., posterior | v. auricularis posterior | passes down behind auricle | a plexus on side of head | joins retromandibular v. to form external jugular v. |
| axillary v. | v. axillaris | the upper limb | formed at lower border of teres major muscle by junction of basilic v. and brachial v. | at lateral border of first rib is continuous with subclavian v. |
| azygos v. | v. azygos | intercepting trunk for right intercostal v's as well as connecting branch between superior and inferior venae cavae; it ascends in front of and on right side of vertebrae | ascending lumbar v. | superior vena cava |
| azygos v., left. *See* hemiazygos v. | | | | |
| azygos v., lesser superior. *See* hemiazygos v., accessory | | | | |
| basal v. | v. basalis | passes from anterior perforated substance backward and around cerebral peduncle | anterior perforated substance | internal cerebral v. |
| basilic v. | v. basilica | forearm, superficially | ulnar side of dorsal rete of hand | joins brachial v's to form axillary v. |
| basilic v., median | | sometimes present as medial branch of a bifurcation of median antebrachial v. | | basilic v. |

*v. = vein; v's = (pl.) veins.
†v. = vena; vv. = [L.(pl.)] venae.

**Veins** *Continued*

| Common Name | TA Term | Region | Receives Blood From | Drains Into |
|---|---|---|---|---|
| basivertebral v's | vv. basivertebrales | venous sinuses in cancellous tissue of bodies of vertebrae, which communicate with venous plexus on anterior surface of vertebrae and with external and internal vertebral plexuses | | |
| brachial v's | vv. brachiales | accompany brachial artery | | joins basilic v. to form axillary v. |
| brachiocephalic v's | vv. brachiocephalicae | thorax | head, neck, and upper limbs; formed at root of neck by union of ipsilateral internal jugular and subclavian v's | unite to form superior vena cava |
| bronchial v's | vv. bronchiales | | larger subdivisions of bronchi | azygos v. on left; hemiazygos or superior intercostal v. on right |
| v. of bulb of penis | v. bulbi penis | | bulb of penis | internal pudendal v. |
| v. of bulb of vestibule | v. bulbi vestibuli | | bulb of vestibule of vagina | internal pudendal v. |
| cardiac v's, anterior | vv. ventriculi dextri anteriores | | anterior wall of right ventricle | right atrium of heart, or lesser cardiac v. |
| cardiac v., great | | | anterior surface of ventricles | coronary sinus |
| cardiac v., middle | | | diaphragmatic surface of ventricles | coronary sinus |
| cardiac v., small | v. cardiaca parva | | right atrium and ventricle | coronary sinus |
| cardiac v's, smallest | vv. cardiacae minimae | numerous small veins arising in myocardium, draining independently into cavities of heart and most readily seen in the atria | | |
| carotid v., external. *See* retromandibular v. | | | | |
| cavernous v's of penis | vv. cavernosae penis | | corpora cavernosa | deep v's and dorsal v. of penis |
| central v's of liver | vv. centrales hepatis | in middle of hepatic lobules | liver substance | hepatic v. |
| central v. of retina | v. centralis retinae | eyeball | retinal v's | superior ophthalmic v. |
| central v. of suprarenal gland | v. centralis glandulae suprarenalis | the large single vein into which the various veins within the substance of the gland empty, and which continues at the hilum as the suprarenal v. | | |
| cephalic v. | v. cephalica | winds anteriorly to pass along anterior border of brachioradial muscle; above elbow, ascends along lateral border of biceps of deltoid muscle | radial side of dorsal rete of hand | axillary v. |
| cephalic v., accessory | v. cephalica accessoria | forearm | dorsal rete of hand | joins cephalic v. just above elbow |
| cephalic v's, median | | sometimes present as lateral branch formed by bifurcation of median antebrachial v. | | cephalic v. |
| cerebellar v's, inferior | vv. inferiores cerebelli | | inferior surface of cerebellum | transverse, sigmoid, and inferior petrosal sinuses, or occipital sinus |
| cerebellar v's, superior | vv. superiores cerebelli | | superior surface of cerebellum | straight sinus and great cerebral v., or transverse and superior petrosal sinuses |
| cerebral v's, anterior | vv. anteriores cerebri | accompany anterior cerebral artery | | basal v. |
| cerebral v., great | v. magna cerebri | curves around splenium of corpus callosum | formed by union of the 2 internal cerebral veins | continues as or drains into straight sinus |
| cerebral v's, inferior | vv. inferiores cerebri | veins that ramify on base and inferolateral surface of brain, those on inferior surface of frontal lobe draining into inferior sagittal sinus and cavernous sinus; those on temporal lobe into superior petrosal sinus and transverse sinus; and those on occipital lobe into straight sinus | | |
| cerebral v's, internal (2) | vv. internae cerebri | pass backward from interventricular foramen through tela choroidea | formed by union of thalamostriate v. and choroid v.; collect blood from basal ganglia | unite at splenium or corpus callosum to form great cerebral v. |
| cerebral v., middle, deep | v. media profunda cerebri | accompanies middle cerebral artery in floor of lateral sulcus | | basal v. |

**Veins** *Continued*

| Common Name | TA Term | Region | Receives Blood From | Drains Into |
|---|---|---|---|---|
| cerebral v., middle, superficial | v. media superficialis cerebri | follows lateral cerebral fissure | lateral surface of cerebrum | cavernous sinus |
| cerebral v's, superior | vv. superiores cerebri | about 12 veins draining superolateral and medial surfaces of cerebrum toward longitudinal fissure | | superior sagittal sinus |
| cervical v., deep | v. cervicalis profunda | accompanies deep cervical artery down neck | a plexus in suboccipital triangle | vertebral v. or brachiocephalic v. |
| cervical v's, transverse | vv. transversae cervicis | accompany transverse cervical artery | | subclavian v. |
| choroid v., inferior | v. choroidea inferior | | inferior choroid plexus | basal v. |
| choroid v., superior | v. choroidea superior | runs whole length of choroid plexus | choroid plexus, hippocampus, fornix, corpus callosum | joins superior thalamostriate v. to form internal cerebral v. |
| ciliary v's | vv. ciliares | anterior vessels follow anterior ciliary arteries; posterior follow posterior ciliary arteries | arise in eyeball by branches from ciliary muscle; anterior ciliary v's also receive branches from sinus venosus, sclerae, episcleral v's, and conjunctiva of eyeball | superior ophthalmic v.; posterior ciliary v's empty also into inferior ophthalmic v. |
| circumflex femoral v's, lateral | vv. circumflexae femoris laterales | accompany lateral circumflex femoral artery | | femoral v. or profunda femoris v. |
| circumflex femoral v's, medial | vv. circumflexae femoris mediales | accompany medial circumflex femoral artery | | femoral v. or profunda femoris v. |
| circumflex iliac v., deep | v. circumflexa ilium profunda | a common trunk formed by veins accompanying deep circumflex iliac artery | | external iliac v. |
| circumflex iliac v., superficial | v. circumflexa ilium superficialis | accompanies superficial circumflex iliac artery | | great saphenous v. |
| v. of cochlear canal. *See* v. of aqueduct of cochlea. | | | | |
| colic v., left | v. colica sinistra | accompanies left colic artery | | inferior mesenteric v. |
| colic v., middle | v. colica media | accompanies middle colic artery | | superior mesenteric v. |
| colic v., right | v. colica dextra | acompanies right colic artery | | superior mesenteric v. |
| conjunctival v's | vv. conjunctivales | | conjunctiva | superior ophthalmic v. |
| coronary v., left | | the portion of the great cardiac v. lying in the coronary sulcus | anterior interventricular v. | coronary sinus |
| coronary v., right | | | posterior interventricular v. | coronary sinus |
| v. of corpus callosum, posterior | v. posterior corporis callosi | | posterior surface of corpus callosum | great cerebral v. |
| cubital v., median | v. mediana cubiti | the large connecting branch passing obliquely upward across cubital fossa | cephalic v, below | basilic v. |
| cutaneous v. | v. cutanea | one of the small veins that begin in papillae of skin, form subpapillary plexuses, and open into the subcutaneous veins | | |
| cystic v. | v. cystica | within substance of liver | gallbladder | right branch of portal v. |
| deep v's of clitoris | vv. profundae clitoridis | | clitoris | vesical venous plexus |
| deep v's of penis | vv. profundae penis | accompany deep artery of penis | penis | dorsal v. of penis |
| digital v's of foot, dorsal | vv. digitales dorsales pedis | dorsal surfaces of toes | | unite at clefts to form dorsal metatarsal v's |
| digital v's, palmar | vv. digitales palmares | accompany proper and common palmar digital arteries | | superficial palmar venous arch |
| digital v's, plantar | vv. digitales plantares | plantar surfaces of toes | | unite at clefts to form plantar metatarsal v's |
| diploic v., frontal | v. diploica frontalis | | frontal bone | supraorbital v. externally, or superior sagittal sinus internally |
| diploic v., occipital | v. diploica occipitalis | | occipital bone | occipital v. or transverse sinus |
| diploic v., temporal, anterior | v. diploica temporalis anterior | | lateral portion of frontal bone, anterior part of parietal bone | sphenoparietal sinus internally, or a deep temporal v. externally |
| diploic v., temporal, posterior | v. diploica temporalis posterior | | parietal bone | transverse sinus |
| direct v's, lateral | vv. directae laterales | | lateral ventricle | great cerebral v. |

**Veins** *Continued*

| Common Name | TA Term | Region | Receives Blood From | Drains Into |
|---|---|---|---|---|
| dorsal v. of clitoris, deep | v. dorsalis profunda clitoridis | accompanies dorsal artery of clitoris | | vesical plexus |
| dorsal v's of clitoris, superficial | vv. dorsales superficiales clitoridis | | clitoris, subcutaneously | external pudendal v. |
| dorsal v. of corpus callosum | v. dorsalis corporis callosi | | superior surface of corpus callosum | great cerebral vein |
| dorsal v. of penis, deep | v. dorsalis profunda penis | the single median vein lying subfascially in penis between the dorsal arteries; it begins in small veins around corona of glans, is joined by deep veins of penis as it passes proximally, and passes between arcuate pubic and transverse perineal ligaments, where it divides into a left and a right vein to join prostatic plexus | | |
| dorsal v's of penis, superficial | vv. dorsales superficiales penis | | penis, subcutaneously | external pudendal v. |
| dorsal v's, of tongue. *See* lingual v's, dorsal. | vv. dorsales linguae | | | |
| emissary v. | vv. emissaria | foramina of skull | dural venous sinuses | scalp vv., deep vv. below base of skull |
| emissary v., condylar | v. emissaria condyloidea | a small vein running through condylar canal of skull connecting sigmoid sinus with vertebral v. or internal jugular v. | | |
| emissary v., mastoid | v. emissaria mastoidea | a small vein passing through mastoid foramen of skull, connecting sigmoid sinus with occipital v. or posterior auricular v. | | |
| emissary v., occipital | v. emissaria occipitalis | an occasional small vein running through a minute foramen in occipital protuberance of skull, connecting confluence of sinuses with occipital v. | | |
| emissary v., parietal | v. emissaria parietalis | a small vein passing through parietal foramen of skull, connecting superior sagittal sinus with superficial temporal v's | | |
| epigastric v., inferior | v. epigastrica inferior | accompanies inferior epigastric artery | | external iliac v. |
| epigastric v., superficial | v. epigastrica superficialis | accompanies superficial epigastric artery | | great saphenous v. or femoral v. |
| epigastric v's, superior | vv. epigastricae superiores | accompany superior epigastric artery | | internal thoracic v. |
| episcleral v's | vv. episclerales | around cornea | | vorticose v's and ciliary v's |
| esophageal v's | vv. oesophageales | | esophagus | hemiazygos v. and azygos v., or left brachiocephalic v. |
| ethmoidal v's | vv. ethmoidales | accompany anterior and posterior ethmoidal arteries and emerge from ethmoidal foramina | | superior ophthalmic v. |
| facial v. | v. facialis | the vein beginning at medial angle of eye as angular v., descending behind facial artery, and usually ending in internal jugular v.; sometimes joins retromandibular v. to form a common trunk | | |
| facial v., deep | v. profunda faciei | | pterygoid plexus | facial v. |
| facial v., posterior. *See* retromandibular v. | | | | |
| facial v., transverse | v. transversa faciei | passes backward with transverse facial artery just below zygomatic arch | | retromandibular v. |
| femoral v. | v. femoralis | follows course of femoral artery in proximal two thirds of thigh | continuation of popliteal v. | at inguinal ligament becomes external iliac v. |
| femoral v., deep | v. profunda femoris | accompanies deep femoral artery | | femoral v. |
| fibular v's. *See* peroneal v's. | | | | |
| frontal v's | vv. frontales | superficial superior cerebral veins that drain the frontal cortex | | |
| gastric v., left | v. gastrica sinistra | accompanies left gastric artery | | portal v. |
| gastric v., right | v. gastrica dextra | accompanies right gastric artery | | portal v. |
| gastric v's, short | vv. gastricae breves | | left portion of greater curvature of stomach | splenic v. |
| gastroepiploic v., left. *See* gastroomental v., left. | | | | |

**Veins** *Continued*

| Common Name | TA Term | Region | Receives Blood From | Drains Into |
|---|---|---|---|---|
| gastroepiploic v., right. *See* gastroomental v., right. | | | | |
| gastroomental v., left | v. gastroomentalis sinistra | accompanies left gastroomental artery | | splenic v. |
| gastroomental v., right | v. gastroomentalis dextra | accompanies right gastroomental artery | | superior mesenteric v. |
| genicular v's | vv. geniculares | accompany genicular arteries | | popliteal v. |
| gluteal v's, inferior | vv. gluteae inferiores | accompany inferior gluteal artery; unite into a single vessel after passing through greater sciatic foramen | subcutaneous tissue of back of thigh, muscles of buttock | internal iliac v. |
| gluteal v's, superior | vv. gluteae superiores | accompany superior gluteal artery and pass through greater sciatic foramen | muscles of buttock | internal iliac v. |
| hemiazygos v. | v. hemiazygos | an intercepting trunk for lower left posterior intercostal v's; ascends on left side of vertebrae to eighth thoracic vertebra, where it may receive accessory branch, and crosses vertebral column | ascending lumbar v. | azygos v. |
| hemiazygos v., accessory | v. hemiazygos accessoria | the descending intercepting trunk for upper, often fourth through eighth, left posterior intercostal v's; it lies on left side and at eighth thoracic vertebra joins hemiazygos v. or crosses to right side to join azygos v. directly; above, it may communicate with left superior intercostal v. | | |
| hemorrhoidal v's. *See* entries under rectal v's | | | | |
| hepatic v's | vv. hepaticae | 2 or 3 large veins in an upper group and 6 to 20 small veins in a lower group, forming successively larger vessels | central v's of liver | interior vena cava on posterior aspect of liver |
| hypogastric v. *See* iliac v., internal. | | | | |
| ileal v's | vv. ileales | | ileum | superior mesenteric v. |
| ileocolic v. | v. ileocolica | accompanies ileocolic artery | | superior mesenteric v. |
| iliac v., common | v. iliaca communis | ascends to right side of fifth lumbar vertebra | arises at sacroiliac joint by union of external and internal iliac v's | unites with fellow of opposite side to form inferior vena cava |
| iliac v., external | v. iliaca externa | extends from inguinal ligament to sacroiliac joint | continuation of femoral v. | joins internal iliac v. to form common iliac v. |
| iliac v., internal | v. iliaca interna | extends from greater sciatic notch to brim of pelvis | formed by union of parietal branches | joins external iliac v. to form common iliac v. |
| iliolumbar v. | v. iliolumbalis | accompanies iliolumbar artery | | internal iliac v. and/or common iliac v. |
| innominate v's. *See* brachiocephalic v's. | | | | |
| insular v's | vv. insulares | | insula | deep middle cerebral v. |
| intercapital v's | vv. intercapitulares manus | veins at clefts of fingers that pass between heads of metacarpal bones and establish communication between dorsal and palmar venous systems of hand | | |
| intercostal v's, anterior (12 pairs) | vv. intercostales anteriores | accompany anterior thoracic arteries | | internal thoracic v's |
| intercostal v., highest | v. intercostalis suprema | first posterior intercostal vein of either side, which passes over apex of lung | | brachiocephalic, vertebral, or superior intercostal v. |
| intercostal v's, posterior | vv. intercostales posteriores | accompany posterior intercostal arteries | intercostal spaces | azygos v. on right; hemiazygos or accessory hemiazygos v. on left |

**Veins** *Continued*

| Common Name | TA Term | Region | Receives Blood From | Drains Into |
|---|---|---|---|---|
| intercostal v., superior, left | v. intercostalis superior sinistra | crosses arch of aorta | formed by union of second, third, and sometimes fourth posterior intercostal v's | left brachiocephalic v. |
| intercostal v., superior, right | v. intercostalis superior dextra | | formed by union of second, third, and sometimes fourth posterior intercostal v's | azygos v. |
| interlobar v's of kidney | vv. interlobares renis | pass down between renal pyramids | venous arcades of kidney | unite to form renal v. |
| interlobular v's of kidney | vv. interlobulares renis | | capillary network of renal cortex | venous arcades of kidney |
| interlobular v's of liver | vv. interlobulares hepatis | arise between hepatic lobules | liver | portal v. |
| interosseous v's, anterior | vv. interosseae anteriores | accompany anterior interosseous artery | | ulnar vv. |
| interosseous v's, posterior | vv. interosseae posteriores | accompany posterior interosseous artery | | ulnar vv. |
| interosseous v's of foot, dorsal. *See* metatarsal v's, dorsal. | | | | |
| interventricular v., anterior | v. interventricularis anterior | the portion of the great cardiac v. ascending in the anterior interventricular sulcus | | left coronary v. |
| interventricular v., posterior | v. interventricularis posterior | the portion of the middle cardiac v. ascending in the posterior interventricular sulcus | | right coronary v. |
| intervertebral v. | v. intervertebralis | vertebral column | vertebral venous plexuses | in neck, vertebral v.; in thorax, intercostal v's; in abdomen, lumbar v's; in pelvis, lateral sacral v's |
| jejunal v's | vv. jejunales | | jejunum | superior mesenteric v. |
| jugular v., anterior | v. jugularis anterior | arises under chin and passes down neck | | external jugular v. or subclavian v., or jugular venous arch |
| jugular v., external | v. jugularis externa | begins in parotid gland behind angle of jaw and passes down neck | formed by union of retromandibular v. and posterior auricular v. | subclavian v., internal jugular v., or brachiocephalic v. |
| jugular v., internal | v. jugularis interna | from jugular fossa, descends in neck with internal carotid artery and then with common carotid artery | begins as superior bulb, draining much of head and neck | joins subclavian v. to form brachiocephalic v. |
| labial v's, anterior | vv. labiales anteriores | | anterior aspect of labia in female | external pudendal v. |
| labial v's, inferior | vv. labiales inferiores | | region of lower lip | facial v. |
| labial v's, posterior | vv. labiales posteriores | | labia in female | vesical venous plexus |
| labial v., superior | v. labialis superior | | region of upper lip | facial v. |
| labyrinthine v's | vv. labyrinthi | pass through internal acoustic meatus | cochlea | inferior petrosal sinus or transverse sinus |
| lacrimal v. | v. lacrimalis | | lacrimal gland | superior ophthalmic v. |
| laryngeal v., inferior | v. laryngea inferior | | larynx | inferior thyroid v. |
| laryngeal v., superior | v. laryngea superior | | larynx | superior thyroid v. |
| v. of lateral ventricle, lateral | v. lateralis ventriculi lateralis | passes through lateral wall of lateral ventricle | temporal and parietal lobes | superior thalamostriate v. |
| v. of lateral ventricle, medial | v. medialis ventriculi lateralis | passes through medial wall of lateral ventricle | parietal and occipital lobes | internal cerebral or great cerebral v. |
| lingual v. | v. lingualis | a deep vein, following distribution of lingual artery | | internal jugular v. |
| lingual v., deep | v. profunda linguae | | deep aspect of tongue | joins sublingual v. to form accompanying v. of hypoglossal nerve |
| lingual v's, dorsal | vv. dorsales linguae | veins that unite with a small vein accompanying lingual artery and join main lingual trunk | | |
| lumbar v's | vv. lumbales | four or five v's on each side accompanying corresponding lumbar arteries and draining posterior wall of abdomen, vertebral canal, spinal cord, and meninges; first four usually end in inferior vena cava, although first may end in ascending lumbar v.; fifth is generally a tributary of common iliac v. | | |

**Veins** *Continued*

| Common Name | TA Term | Region | Receives Blood From | Drains Into |
|---|---|---|---|---|
| lumbar v., ascending | v. lumbalis ascendens | an ascending intercepting vein for lumbar v's on either side; it begins in lateral sacral region and ascends to first lumbar vertebra, where by union with subcostal v. it becomes on right side the azygos v. and on left the hemiazygos v. | | |
| marginal v., right | v. marginalis dextra | ascends along right margin of heart | right ventricle | right atrium, anterior cardiac v's |
| maxillary v's | vv. maxillares | usually form a single short trunk with pterygoid plexus | | join superficial temporal v. in parotid gland to form retromandibular v. |
| mediastinal v's | vv. mediastinales | | anterior mediastinum | brachiocephalic v., azygos v., or superior vena cava |
| v's of medulla oblongata | vv. medullae oblongatae | | medulla oblongata | v's of spinal cord, dural venous sinuses, inferior petrosal sinus, superior bulb of jugular v. |
| meningeal v's | vv. meningeae | accompany meningeal arteries | dura mater (also communicate with lateral lacunae) | regional sinuses and veins |
| meningeal v's, middle | vv. meningeae mediae | accompany middle meningeal artery | | pterygoid venous plexus |
| mesenteric v., inferior | v. mesenterica inferior | follows distribution of inferior mesenteric artery | | splenic v. |
| mesenteric v., superior | v. mesenterica superior | follows distribution of superior mesenteric artery | | joins splenic v. to form portal v. |
| metacarpal v's, dorsal | vv. metacarpales dorsales | veins arising from union of dorsal veins of adjacent fingers and passing proximally to join in forming dorsal venous network of hand | | |
| metacarpal v's, palmar | vv. metacarpales palmares | accompany palmar metacarpal arteries | | deep palmar venous arch |
| metatarsal v's, dorsal | vv. metatarsales dorsales | | arise from dorsal digital v's of toes at clefts of toes | dorsal venous arch |
| metatarsal v's, plantar | vv. metatarsales plantares | deep veins of foot | arise from plantar digital v's at clefts of toes | plantar venous arch |
| musculophrenic v's | vv. musculophrenicae | accompany musculophrenic artery | parts of diaphragm and wall of thorax and abdomen | internal thoracic v's |
| nasal v's, external | vv. nasales externae | small ascending branches from nose | | angular v., facial v. |
| nasofrontal v. | v. nasofrontalis | | supraorbital v. | superior ophthalmic v. |
| oblique v. of left atrium | v. obliqua atrii sinistri | left atrium of heart | | coronary sinus |
| obturator v's | vv. obturatoriae | enter pelvis through obturator canal | hip joint and regional muscles | internal iliac v. and/or inferior epigastric v. |
| occipital v. | v. occipitalis | scalp; follows distribution of occipital artery | | opens under trapezius muscle into suboccipital venous plexus, or accompanies occipital artery to end in internal jugular v. |
| ophthalmic v., inferior | v. ophthalmica inferior | a vein formed by confluence of muscular and ciliary branches, and running backward either to join superior ophthalmic v. or to open directly into cavernous sinus; it sends a communicating branch through inferior orbital fissure to join pterygoid venous plexus | | |
| ophthalmic v., superior | v. ophthalmica superior | a vein beginning at medial angle of eye, where it communicates with frontal, supraorbital, and angular v's; it follows distribution of ophthalmic artery, and may be joined by inferior ophthalmic v. at superior orbital fissure before opening into cavernous sinus | | |
| ovarian v., left | v. ovarica sinistra | | pampiniform plexus of broad ligament on left | left renal v. |
| ovarian v., right | v. ovarica dextra | | | inferior vena cava |
| palatine v., external | v. palatina externa | | tonsils and soft palate | facial v. |
| palpebral v's | vv. palpebrales | small branches from eyelids | | superior ophthalmic v. |
| palpebral v's, inferior | vv. palpebrales inferiores | | lower eyelid | facial v. |
| palpebral v's, superior | vv. palpebrales superiores | | upper eyelid | angular v. |
| pancreatic v's | vv. pancreaticae | | pancreas | splenic v., superior mesenteric v. |

**Veins** *Continued*

| Common Name | TA Term | Region | Receives Blood From | Drains Into |
|---|---|---|---|---|
| pancreaticoduodenal v's | vv. pancreaticoduodenales | 4 veins that drain blood from pancreas and duodenum, closely following pancreaticoduodenal arteries, a superior and an inferior vein originating from an anterior and a posterior venous arcade; anterior superior v. joins right gastroepiploic v., and posterior superior v. joins portal v.; anterior and posterior inferior v's join, sometimes as one trunk, uppermost jejunal v. or superior mesenteric v. | | |
| paraumbilical v's | vv. paraumbilicales | veins that communicate with portal v. above and descend to anterior abdominal wall to anastomose with superior and inferior epigastric and superior vesical v's in region of umbilicus; they form a significant part of collateral circulation of portal v. in event of hepatic obstruction | | |
| parotid v's | vv. parotideae | | parotid gland | superficial temporal v. |
| perforating v's | vv. perforantes | empty into deep femoral v. and establish anastomosis between deep femoral v. and popliteal v. (below) and inferior gluteal v. (above) | | |
| pericardiac v's | vv. pericardiacae | | pericardium | brachiocephalic, inferior thyroid, and azygos v's, superior vena cava |
| pericardiacophrenic v's | vv. pericardiacophrenicae | | pericardium and diaphragm | left brachiocephalic v. |
| peroneal v's | vv. fibulares | accompany peroneal artery | | posterior tibial v. |
| pharyngeal v's | vv. pharyngeae | | pharyngeal plexus | internal jugular v. |
| phrenic v's, inferior | vv. phrenicae inferiores | accompany inferior phrenic arteries | | on right, enters inferior vena cava; on left, enters left suprarenal or renal v., or inferior vena cava |
| v's of pons | vv. pontis | | pons | basal v., cerebellar v's, petrosal or venous sinuses, or venous plexus of foramen ovale |
| popliteal v. | v. poplitea | follows popliteal artery | formed by union of anterior and posterior tibial v's | at adductor hiatus becomes femoral v. |
| portal v. | v. portae hepatis | a short, thick trunk formed by union of superior mesenteric and splenic v's behind neck of pancreas; it ascends to right end of porta hepatis, where it divides into successively smaller branches, following branches of hepatic artery, until it forms a capillary-like system of sinusoids that permeates entire substance of liver | | |
| posterior v's. of left ventricle | vv. ventriculi sinistri posteriores | | posterior surface of left ventricle | coronary sinus |
| prepyloric v. | v. prepylorica | accompanies prepyloric artery, passing upward over anterior surface of junction between pylorus and duodenum | | right gastric v. |
| profunda femoris v. *See* femoral v., deep. | | | | |
| profunda linguae v. *See* lingual v., deep. | | | | |
| v. of pterygoid canal | v. canalis pterygoidei | passes through pterygoid canal | | pterygoid plexus |
| pudendal v's, external | vv. pudendae externae | follow distribution of external pudendal artery | | great saphenous v. |
| pudendal v., internal | v. pudenda interna | follows course of internal pudendal artery | | internal iliac v. |
| pulmonary v., inferior, left | v. pulmonalis sinistra inferior | | lower lobe of left lung | left atrium of heart |
| pulmonary v., inferior, right | v. pulmonalis dextra inferior | | lower lobe of right lung | left atrium of heart |
| pulmonary v., superior, left | v. pulmonalis sinistra superior | | upper lobe of left lung | left atrium of heart |
| pulmonary v., superior, right | v. pulmonalis dextra superior | | upper and middle lobes of right lung | left atrium of heart |
| pyloric v. *See* gastric v., right. | | | | |
| radial v's | vv. radiales | accompany radial artery | | brachial v's |

**Veins** *Continued*

| Common Name | TA Term | Region | Receives Blood From | Drains Into |
|---|---|---|---|---|
| ranine v. *See* sublingual v. | | | | |
| rectal v's, inferior | vv., rectales inferiores | | rectal plexus | internal pudendal v. |
| rectal v's, middle | vv. rectales mediae | | rectal plexus | internal iliac and superior rectal v's |
| rectal v., superior | v. rectalis superior | establishes connection between portal and systemic systems | upper part of rectal plexus | inferior mesenteric v. |
| retromandibular v. | v. retromandibularis | the vein formed in upper part of parotid gland behind neck of mandible by union of maxillary and superficial temporal v's; it passes downward through the gland, communicates with facial v. and, emerging from the gland, joins with posterior auricular v. to form external jugular v. | | |
| sacral v's, lateral | vv. sacrales laterales | follow lateral sacral arteries | | help form lateral sacral plexus; empty into internal iliac v. or superior gluteal v's |
| sacral v., median | v. sacralis mediana | follows median sacral artery | | common iliac v. |
| saphenous v., accessory | v. saphena accessoria | | when present, medial and posterior superficial parts of thigh | great saphenous v. |
| saphenous v., great | v. saphena magna | extends from dorsum of foot to just below inguinal ligament | | femoral v. |
| saphenous v., small | v. saphena parva | from behind ankle passes up back of leg to knee | | popliteal v. |
| scleral v's | vv. sclerales | | sclera | anterior ciliary v's |
| scrotal v's, anterior | vv. scrotales anteriores | | anterior aspect of scrotum | external pudendal v. |
| scrotal v's, posterior | vv. scrotales posteriores | scrotum | | vesical venous plexus |
| v. of septum pellucidum, anterior | v. anterior septi pellucidi | | anterior septum pellucidum | superior thalamostriate v. |
| v. of septum pellucidum, posterior | v. posterior septi pellucidi | | septum pellucidum | superior thalamostriate v. |
| sigmoid v's | vv. sigmoideae | | sigmoid colon | inferior mesenteric v. |
| spinal v's, anterior and posterior | vv. spinales anteriores<br>vv. spinales posteriores | anastomosing networks of small veins that drain blood from spinal cord and its pia mater into internal vertebral venous plexuses | | |
| spiral v. of modiolus | | modiolus | | labyrinthine v's |
| splenic v. | v. splenica | passes from left to right of neck of pancreas | formed by union of several branches at hilus of spleen | joins superior mesenteric v. to form portal v. |
| stellate v's of kidney | venulae stellatae renis | | superficial parts of renal cortex | interlobular v's of kidney |
| sternocleidomastoid v. | v. sternocleidomastidea | follows course of sternocleidomastoid artery | | internal jugular v. |
| stylomastoid v. | v. stylomastoidea | follows stylomastoid artery | | retromandibular v. |
| subclavian v. | v. subclavia | follows subclavian artery | continues axillary v. as main venous channel of upper limb | joins internal jugular v. to form brachiocephalic v. |
| subcostal v. | v. subcostalis | accompanies subcostal artery | | joins ascending lumbar v. to form azygos v. on right<br>hemiazygos v. on left |
| subcutaneous v's of abdomen | vv. subcutaneae abdominis | superficial layers of abdominal wall | | |
| sublingual v. | v. sublingualis | follows sublingual artery | | lingual v. |
| submental v. | v. submentalis | follows submental artery | | facial v. |
| supraorbital v. | v. supraorbitalis | passes down forehead lateral to supratrochlear v. | | joins supratrochlear v. at root of nose to form angular v. |
| suprarenal v., left | v. suprarenalis sinistra | | left suprarenal gland | left renal v. |
| suprarenal v., right | v. suprarenalis dextra | | right suprarenal gland | inferior vena cava |
| suprascapular v. | v. suprascapularis | accompanies suprascapular artery (sometimes as 2 veins that unite) | | usually into external jugular v., occasionally into subclavian v. |
| supratrochlear v's (2) | vv. supratrochleares | | venous plexuses high up on forehead | joins supraorbital v. at root of nose to form angular v. |
| sural v's | vv. surales | accompany sural arteries | calf | popliteal v. |
| temporal v's, deep | vv. temporales profundae | | deep portions of temporal muscle | pterygoid plexus |

**Veins** *Continued*

| Common Name | TA Term | Region | Receives Blood From | Drains Into |
|---|---|---|---|---|
| temporal v., middle | v. temporalis media | descends deep to fascia to zygoma | arises in substance of temporal muscle | joins superficial temporal v. |
| temporal v's, superficial | vv. temporales superficiales | veins that drain lateral part of scalp in frontal and parietal regions, the branches forming a single superficial temporal v. in front of ear, just above zygoma; this descending vein receives middle temporal and transverse facial v's and, entering parotid gland, unites with maxillary v. deep to neck of mandible to form retromandibular v. | | |
| testicular v., left | v. testicularis sinistra | | left pampiniform plexus | left renal v. |
| testicular v., right | v. testicularis dextra | | right pampiniform plexus | inferior vena cava |
| thalamostriate v's, inferior | vv. thalamostriatae inferiores | | anterior perforated substance of brain | join deep middle cerebral and anterior cerebral v's to form basal v. |
| thalamostriate v., superior | v. thalamostriata superior | | corpus striatum and thalamus | joins choroid v. to form internal cerebral v. |
| thoracic v's, internal | vv. thoracicae internae | 2 veins formed by junction of the veins accompanying internal thoracic artery of either side; each continues along the artery to open into brachiocephalic v. | | |
| thoracic v., lateral | v. thoracica lateralis | accompanies lateral thoracic artery | | axillary v. |
| thoracoacromial v. | v. thoracoacromialis | follows thoracoacromial artery | | subclavian v. |
| thoracoepigastric v's | vv. thoracoepigastricae | long, longitudinal, superficial veins in anterolateral subcutaneous tissue of trunk | | superiorly into lateral thoracic v.; inferiorly into femoral v. |
| thymic v's | vv. thymicae | | thymus | left brachiocephalic v. |
| thyroid v's., inferior | vv. thyroideae inferiores | two veins, left and right, that drain thyroid plexus into left and right brachiocephalic v's; occasionally they may unite into a common trunk to empty, usually into left brachiocephalic v. | | |
| thyroid v's, middle | vv. thyroideae mediae | | thyroid gland | internal jugular v. |
| thyroid v., superior | v. thyroidea superior | arises from side of upper part of thyroid gland | thyroid gland | internal jugular v., occasionally in common with facial v. |
| tibial v's, anterior | vv. tibiales anteriores | accompany anterior tibial artery | | join posterior tibial v's to form popliteal v. |
| tibial v's, posterior | vv. tibiales posteriores | accompany posterior tibial artery | | join anterior tibial v's to form popliteal v. |
| tracheal v's | vv. tracheales | | trachea | brachiocephalic v. |
| tympanic v's | vv. tympanicae | small veins from middle ear that pass through petrotympanic fissure and open into the plexus around temporomandibular joint | | retromandibular v. |
| ulnar v's | vv. ulnares | accompany ulnar artery | | join radial v's at elbow to form brachial v's |
| umbilical v. | v. umbilicalis | in the early embryo, either of the paired veins that carry blood from chorion to sinus venosus and heart; they later fuse and become left umbilical v. of fetus. | | |
| umbilical v. of fetus, left | | the vein formed by fusion of atrophied right umbilical v. with the left umbilical v., which carries all the blood from placenta to ductus venosus | | |
| v. of uncus | v. uncalis | | uncus | ipsilateral inferior cerebral v. |
| uterine v's | vv. uterinae | | uterine plexus | internal iliac v's |
| vena cava, inferior | vena cava inferior | the venous trunk for the lower limbs and for pelvic and abdominal viscera; it begins at level of fifth lumbar vertebra by union of common iliac v's and ascends on right of aorta | | right atrium of heart |
| vena cava, superior | vena cava superior | the venous trunk draining blood from head, neck, upper limbs, and thorax; it begins by union of 2 brachiocephalic v's and passes directly downward | | right atrium of heart |
| ventricular v., inferior | v. ventricularis inferior | | temporal lobe | basal v. |
| vertebral v., anterior | v. vertebralis anterior | accompanies ascending cervical artery | | vertebral vein |
| v. of vermis, inferior | v. inferior vermis | | inferior surface of cerebellum | straight sinus or one of the sigmoid sinuses |
| v's of Vieussens | vv. cardiacae anteriores | ascend through right part of atrioventricular sulcus | anterior wall of right ventricle | right atrium, lesser cardiac v. |

# APPENDIX 8

## Phobias

| Fear of: | Phobia |
|---|---|
| air | aerophobia |
| amphibians | herpetophobia |
| animals | zoophobia |
| bacilli | bacillophobia |
| bad men | scelerophobia |
| barren space | cenophobia, kenophobia |
| bearing a deformed child | teratophobia |
| beating | mastigophobia, rhabdophobia |
| bees | apiphobia, melissophobia |
| being alone | autophobia, eremophobia, monophobia |
| being beaten | mastigophobia, rhabdophobia |
| being buried alive | taphephobia |
| being enclosed | claustrophobia, clithrophobia |
| being laughed at | catagelophobia, katagelophobia |
| being locked in | clithrophobia |
| being looked at | scopophobia, scoptophobia |
| being scratched | amychophobia |
| being touched | aphephobia, haphephobia, haptephobia |
| being unclean | automysophobia |
| being unclothed | gymnophobia, nudophobia |
| birds | ornithophobia |
| blood | hematophobia, hemophobia |
| blushing | ereuthophobia, erythrophobia |
| body defect, imaginary | dysmorphophobia |
| brain disease | meningitophobia |
| bridge, crossing | gephyrophobia |
| building, being inside | domatophobia |
| burglars | scelerophobia |
| burial alive | taphephobia |
| cancer | cancerophobia, cancerphobia, carcinomatophobia, carcinophobia |
| cats | ailurophobia, galeophobia, gatophobia |
| change | kainophobia, kainotophobia, neophobia |
| childbirth | maieusiophobia, tocophobia |
| children | pedophobia |
| choking | anginophobia, pnigophobia |
| climbing | climacophobia |
| coitus | coitophobia |
| cold | cheimaphobia, cryophobia, psychropophobia |
| colors | chromatophobia, chromophobia |
| comets | cometophobia |
| confinement | claustrophobia |
| contamination | coprophobia, molysmophobia, mysophobia, scatophobia |
| corpses | necrophobia |
| crossing a bridge or river | gephyrophobia |
| crossing a street | dromophobia |
| crowds | demophobia, ochlophobia |
| dampness | hygrophobia |
| darkness | achluphobia, noctiphobia, nyctophobia, scotophobia |
| dawn | eosophobia |
| daylight | phengophobia |
| dead bodies | necrophobia |
| death | necrophobia, thanatophobia |
| defecation | coprophobia |
| deformed child, bearing | teratophobia |
| deformity | dysmorphophobia |
| demons | demonophobia |
| dental operations | odontophobia |
| depths | bathophobia |
| devils or the devil | demonophobia, satanophobia |

| Fear of: | Phobia |
|---|---|
| dirt | coprophobia, mysophobia, rhypophobia, rupophobia |
| dirtiness, personal | automysophobia |
| disease | nosophobia, pathophobia |
| disease, specific | monopathophobia |
| disorder | ataxiophobia, ataxophobia |
| dogs | cynophobia |
| dolls | pediophobia |
| drafts | aerophobia, anemophobia |
| drugs | pharmacophobia |
| dust | amathophobia |
| eating | cibophobia, phagophobia, sitophobia |
| electricity | electrophobia |
| emptiness | cenophobia, kenophobia |
| enclosed spaces | claustrophobia |
| endlessness | apeirophobia |
| error | hamartophobia |
| everything | panophobia, panphobia, pantophobia |
| excrement | coprophobia, scatophobia |
| eyes | ommatophobia |
| failure | kakorrhaphiophobia |
| fatigue | kopophobia |
| fearing or fears | phobophobia |
| feathers | pteronophobia |
| feces | coprophobia |
| female genitals | eurotophobia |
| fever | febriphobia, pyrexiophobia |
| filth | mysophobia, rhypophobia, rupophobia |
| filth, personal | automysophobia |
| fire | pyrophobia |
| fish | icthyophobia |
| flogging | mastigophobia, rhabdophobia |
| floods | antlophobia |
| flutes | aulophobia |
| flying | aviophobia |
| fog | homichlophobia |
| food | cibophobia, phagophobia, sitophobia |
| forests | hylophobia |
| fresh air | aerophobia |
| frogs | batrachophobia |
| functioning | ergasiophobia |
| fur | doraphobia |
| germs | microbiophobia, microphobia |
| ghosts | phasmophobia, demonophobia |
| girls | parthenophobia |
| glare | photaugiaphobia |
| glass | crystallophobia, hyalophobia |
| God | theophobia |
| gravity | barophobia |
| hair | trichopathophobia, trichophobia |
| heart disease | cardiophobia |
| heat | thermophobia |
| heaven | siderophobia, uranophobia |
| heights | acrophobia, hyposophobia |
| hell | hadephobia, stygiophobia |
| hereditary disease or heredity | patroiophobia, patriophobia |
| high objects | batophobia |
| home, returning to | nostophobia |
| horses | equinophobia, hippophobia |
| houses | domatophobia, oikophobia |
| human society | anthropophobia |
| humiliation | catagelophobia, katagelophobia |
| ideas | ideophobia |
| infinity | apeirophobia |

| Fear of: | Phobia |
|---|---|
| inherited disease | patroiophobia, patriophobia |
| injury | traumatophobia |
| innovation | neophobia |
| insanity | lyssophobia, maniaphobia |
| insects | acarophobia, entomophobia |
| instrument of punishment | rhabdophobia |
| jealousy | zelophobia |
| justice | dikephobia |
| knives | aichmophobia |
| large objects | megalophobia |
| left or objects to the left | levophobia |
| light | photophobia |
| lightning | astraphobia, astrapophobia, keraunophobia |
| loneliness | eremophobia, monophobia |
| love | erotophobia |
| machinery | mechanophobia |
| malignancy | cancerophobia, cancerphobia, carcinomatophobia, carcinophobia |
| many things | polyphobia |
| marriage | gamophobia |
| medicines | pharmacophobia |
| men | androphobia |
| messiness | ataxiophobia, ataxophobia |
| metals | metallophobia |
| meteors | meteorophobia |
| mice | musophobia |
| microorganisms | microbiophobia, microphobia |
| mind | psychophobia |
| minute objects | acarophobia, microbiophobia, microphobia |
| mirrors | eisoptrophobia, spectrophobia |
| missiles | ballistophobia |
| mites | acarophobia |
| moisture | hygrophobia |
| money | chrematophobia |
| motion | kinesophobia |
| movement | ergasiophobia |
| myths | mythophobia |
| naked body or nakedness | gymnophobia, nudophobia |
| names or naming or being named | onomatophobia |
| needles | belonephobia |
| neglecting duty | paralipophobia |
| new things | kainophobia, kainotophobia, neophobia |
| night | achluphobia, noctiphobia, nyctophobia |
| northern lights | auroraphobia |
| novelty | kainophobia, kainotophobia, neophobia |
| nudity | gymnophobia, nudophobia |
| ocean | nautophobia, thalassophobia |
| odor, personal | automysophobia, bromidrosiphobia |
| odors | olfactophobia, osmophobia, osphresiophobia |
| one's own voice | phonophobia |
| oneself | autophobia, monophobia |
| open spaces | agoraphobia, agyiophobia |
| overwork | ponophobia |
| pain | algophobia, odynophobia |
| parasites | acarophobia, parasitophobia |
| passing high objects | batophobia |
| people | anthropophobia |
| personal odor or uncleanliness | automysophobia, bromidrosiphobia |
| phobia, development of | phobophobia |
| pins | belonephobia |
| places | topophobia |
| pleasure | hedonophobia |
| points or pointed objects | aichmophobia |
| poison | iophobia, toxiphobia, toxicophobia |
| poverty | peniaphobia |

| Fear of: | Phobia |
|---|---|
| precipices | cremnophobia |
| public places | agoraphobia, agyiophobia |
| punishment | poinephobia |
| rabies | cynophobia, lyssophobia |
| radiation | radiophobia |
| railroads | siderodromophobia |
| rain or rainstorms | ombrophobia |
| rectal excreta | coprophobia, scatophobia |
| rectum | proctophobia |
| red | erythrophobia |
| reptiles | herpetophobia |
| responsibility | hypengyophobia |
| ridicule | catagelophobia, katagelophobia |
| right or objects to the right | dextrophobia |
| rivers | potamophobia |
| rivers, crossing | gephyrophobia |
| robbers | harpaxophobia |
| rod | mastigophobia, rhabdophobia |
| ruin | atephobia |
| sacred objects | hierophobia |
| scabies | scabiophobia |
| scratch, receiving | amychophobia |
| sea | nautophobia, thalassophobia |
| self | autophobia |
| semen | spermatophobia |
| sex | genophobia |
| sexual intercourse | coitophobia, cypridophobia, cypriophobia |
| sexual love | erotophobia |
| sharp objects | aichmophobia, belonephobia |
| ships | nautophobia |
| shock | hormephobia |
| sickness | nosophobia, pathophobia |
| sin or sinning | enosiophobia, hamartophobia, peccatiphobia |
| sitting | thaasophobia |
| sitting down, the act | cathisophobia, kathisophobia |
| skin, animal | doraphobia |
| skin disease | dermatosiophobia |
| skin lesion | dermatophobia |
| sleep | hypnophobia |
| small objects or animals | microbiophobia, microphobia |
| smelling bad | automysophobia, bromidrosiphobia |
| smothering | pnigerophobia |
| snakes | ophidiophobia |
| snow | chionophobia |
| solitude | autophobia, eremophobia, monophobia |
| sounds | acousticophobia, phonophobia |
| sourness | acerophobia |
| speaking | glossophobia, laliophobia, lalophobia |
| speaking aloud | phonophobia |
| specific disease | monopathophobia |
| specific word | onomatophobia |
| spiders | arachnephobia, arachnophobia |
| spirits | demonophobia |
| stairs | climacophobia |
| standing up | stasiphobia |
| standing up and walking | stasibasiphobia |
| stars | siderophobia |
| stating untruths | mythophobia |
| stealing | kleptophobia |
| stories | mythophobia |
| strangers | xenophobia |
| street, crossing | dromophobia |
| streets | agoraphobia, agyiophobia |
| string | linonophobia |
| sunlight | heliophobia |
| symbolism | symbolophobia |
| syphilis | syphilophobia |
| talking | laliophobia, lalophobia |
| tapeworms | taeniophobia |
| taste or tasting | geumaphobia |

| Fear of: | Phobia |
|---|---|
| teeth | odontophobia |
| thinking | phronemophobia, psychophobia |
| thirteen | triskaidekaphobia |
| thunder | astraphobia, astrapophobia, brontophobia, keraunophobia, tonitrophobia |
| time | chronophobia |
| touching | aphephobia, haphephobia, haptephobia |
| trains | siderodromophobia |
| travel | hodophobia, dromophobia |
| trembling | tremophobia |
| trichinosis | trichinophobia |
| tuberculosis | phthisiophobia, tuberculophobia |
| uncleanliness, self | automysophobia |
| untruths | mythophobia |

| Fear of: | Phobia |
|---|---|
| vaccination | vaccinophobia |
| vehicles | amaxophobia |
| venereal disease | cypridophobia, cypriphobia |
| voices | phonophobia |
| voids | cenophobia, kenophobia |
| vomiting | emetophobia |
| walking | basiphobia |
| water | aquaphobia, hydrophobia, nautophobia |
| weakness | asthenophobia |
| wind | anemophobia |
| wind instruments | aulophobia |
| women | gynephobia, gynophobia |
| word, specific | onomatophobia |
| work | ergasiophobia, ponophobia |
| writing | graphophobia |
| x-rays | radiophobia |

# *Appendix* 9

## Celsius and Fahrenheit Temperature Equivalents

**Celsius—Fahrenheit**

| °C | °F | °C | °F | °C | °F |
|---|---|---|---|---|---|
| −40 | −40.0 | 9 | 48.2 | 58 | 136.4 |
| −39 | −38.2 | 10 | 50.0 | 59 | 138.2 |
| −38 | −36.4 | 11 | 51.8 | 60 | 140.0 |
| −37 | −34.6 | 12 | 53.6 | 61 | 141.8 |
| −36 | −32.8 | 13 | 55.4 | 62 | 143.6 |
| −35 | −31.0 | 14 | 57.2 | 63 | 145.4 |
| −34 | −29.2 | 15 | 59.0 | 64 | 147.2 |
| −33 | −27.4 | 16 | 60.8 | 65 | 149.0 |
| −32 | −25.6 | 17 | 62.6 | 66 | 150.8 |
| −31 | −23.8 | 18 | 64.4 | 67 | 152.6 |
| −30 | −22.0 | 19 | 66.2 | 68 | 154.4 |
| −29 | −20.2 | 20 | 68.0 | 69 | 156.2 |
| −28 | −18.4 | 21 | 69.8 | 70 | 158.0 |
| −27 | −16.6 | 22 | 71.6 | 71 | 159.8 |
| −26 | −14.8 | 23 | 73.4 | 72 | 161.6 |
| −25 | −13.0 | 24 | 75.2 | 73 | 163.4 |
| −24 | −11.2 | 25 | 77.0 | 74 | 165.2 |
| −23 | −9.4 | 26 | 78.8 | 75 | 167.0 |
| −22 | −7.6 | 27 | 80.6 | 76 | 168.8 |
| −21 | −5.8 | 28 | 82.4 | 77 | 170.6 |
| −20 | −4.0 | 29 | 84.2 | 78 | 172.4 |
| −19 | −2.2 | 30 | 86.0 | 79 | 174.2 |
| −18 | −0.4 | 31 | 87.8 | 80 | 176.0 |
| −17 | +1.4 | 32 | 89.6 | 81 | 177.8 |
| −16 | 3.2 | 33 | 91.4 | 82 | 179.6 |
| −15 | 5.0 | 34 | 93.2 | 83 | 181.4 |
| −14 | 6.8 | 35 | 95.0 | 84 | 183.2 |
| −13 | 8.6 | 36 | 96.8 | 85 | 185.0 |
| −12 | 10.4 | 37 | 98.6 | 86 | 186.8 |
| −11 | 12.2 | 38 | 100.4 | 87 | 188.6 |
| −10 | 14.0 | 39 | 102.2 | 88 | 190.4 |
| −9 | 15.8 | 40 | 104.0 | 89 | 192.2 |
| −8 | 17.6 | 41 | 105.8 | 90 | 194.0 |
| −7 | 19.4 | 42 | 107.6 | 91 | 195.8 |
| −6 | 21.2 | 43 | 109.4 | 92 | 197.6 |
| −5 | 23.0 | 44 | 111.2 | 93 | 199.4 |
| −4 | 24.8 | 45 | 113.0 | 94 | 201.2 |
| −3 | 26.6 | 46 | 114.8 | 95 | 203.0 |
| −2 | 28.4 | 47 | 116.6 | 96 | 204.8 |
| −1 | 30.2 | 48 | 118.4 | 97 | 206.6 |
| 0 | 32.0 | 49 | 120.2 | 98 | 208.4 |
| +1 | 33.8 | 50 | 122.0 | 99 | 210.2 |
| 2 | 35.6 | 51 | 123.8 | 100 | 212.0 |
| 3 | 37.4 | 52 | 125.6 | 101 | 213.8 |
| 4 | 39.2 | 53 | 127.4 | 102 | 215.6 |
| 5 | 41.0 | 54 | 129.2 | 103 | 217.4 |
| 6 | 42.8 | 55 | 131.0 | 104 | 219.2 |
| 7 | 44.6 | 56 | 132.8 | 105 | 221.0 |
| 8 | 46.4 | 57 | 134.6 | 106 | 222.8 |

**Fahrenheit—Celsius**

| °F | °C | °F | °C | °F | °C |
|---|---|---|---|---|---|
| −40 | −40.0 | 55 | 12.7 | 146 | 63.3 |
| −39 | −39.4 | 60 | 15.5 | 147 | 63.8 |
| −38 | −38.9 | 65 | 18.3 | 148 | 64.4 |
| −37 | −38.3 | 70 | 21.1 | 149 | 65.0 |
| −36 | −37.8 | 75 | 23.8 | 150 | 65.5 |
| −35 | −37.2 | 80 | 26.6 | 151 | 66.1 |
| −34 | −36.7 | 85 | 29.4 | 152 | 66.6 |
| −33 | −36.1 | 86 | 30.0 | 153 | 67.2 |
| −32 | −35.6 | 87 | 30.5 | 154 | 67.7 |
| −31 | −35.0 | 88 | 31.0 | 155 | 68.3 |
| −30 | −34.4 | 89 | 31.6 | 156 | 68.8 |
| −29 | −33.9 | 90 | 32.2 | 157 | 69.4 |
| −28 | −33.3 | 91 | 32.7 | 158 | 70.0 |
| −27 | −32.8 | 92 | 33.3 | 159 | 70.5 |
| −26 | −32.2 | 93 | 33.8 | 160 | 71.1 |
| −25 | −31.7 | 94 | 34.4 | 161 | 71.6 |
| −24 | −31.1 | 95 | 35.0 | 162 | 72.2 |
| −23 | −30.6 | 96 | 35.5 | 163 | 72.7 |
| −22 | −30.0 | 97 | 36.1 | 164 | 73.3 |
| −21 | −29.4 | 98 | 36.6 | 165 | 73.8 |
| −20 | −28.9 | 98.6 | 37.0 | 166 | 74.4 |
| −19 | −28.3 | 99 | 37.2 | 167 | 75.0 |
| −18 | −27.8 | 100 | 37.7 | 168 | 75.5 |
| −17 | −27.2 | 101 | 38.3 | 169 | 76.1 |
| −16 | −26.7 | 102 | 38.8 | 170 | 76.6 |
| −15 | −26.1 | 103 | 39.4 | 171 | 77.2 |
| −14 | −25.6 | 104 | 40.0 | 172 | 77.7 |
| −13 | −25.0 | 105 | 40.5 | 173 | 78.3 |
| −12 | −24.4 | 106 | 41.1 | 174 | 78.8 |
| −11 | −23.9 | 107 | 41.6 | 175 | 79.4 |
| −10 | −23.3 | 108 | 42.2 | 176 | 80.0 |
| −9 | −22.8 | 109 | 42.7 | 177 | 80.5 |
| −8 | −22.2 | 110 | 43.3 | 178 | 81.1 |
| −7 | −21.7 | 111 | 43.8 | 179 | 81.6 |
| −6 | −21.1 | 112 | 44.4 | 180 | 82.2 |
| −5 | −20.6 | 113 | 45.0 | 181 | 82.7 |
| −4 | −20.0 | 114 | 45.5 | 182 | 83.3 |
| −3 | −19.4 | 115 | 46.1 | 183 | 83.8 |
| −2 | −18.9 | 116 | 46.6 | 184 | 84.4 |
| −1 | −18.3 | 117 | 47.2 | 185 | 85.0 |
| 0 | −17.8 | 118 | 47.7 | 186 | 85.5 |
| +1 | −17.2 | 119 | 48.3 | 187 | 86.1 |
| 5 | −15.0 | 120 | 48.8 | 188 | 86.6 |
| 10 | −12.2 | 121 | 49.4 | 189 | 87.2 |
| 15 | −9.4 | 122 | 50.0 | 190 | 87.7 |
| 20 | −6.6 | 123 | 50.5 | 191 | 88.3 |
| 25 | −3.8 | 124 | 51.1 | 192 | 88.8 |
| 30 | −1.1 | 125 | 51.6 | 193 | 89.4 |
| 31 | −0.5 | 126 | 52.2 | 194 | 90.0 |
| 32 | 0 | 127 | 52.7 | 195 | 90.5 |
| 33 | +0.5 | 128 | 53.3 | 196 | 91.1 |
| 34 | 1.1 | 129 | 53.8 | 197 | 91.6 |
| 35 | 1.6 | 130 | 54.4 | 198 | 92.2 |
| 36 | 2.2 | 131 | 55.0 | 199 | 92.7 |
| 37 | 2.7 | 132 | 55.5 | 200 | 93.3 |
| 38 | 3.3 | 133 | 56.1 | 201 | 93.8 |
| 39 | 3.8 | 134 | 56.6 | 202 | 94.4 |
| 40 | 4.4 | 135 | 57.2 | 203 | 95.0 |
| 41 | 5.0 | 136 | 57.7 | 204 | 95.5 |
| 42 | 5.5 | 137 | 58.3 | 205 | 96.1 |
| 43 | 6.1 | 138 | 58.8 | 206 | 96.6 |
| 44 | 6.6 | 139 | 59.4 | 207 | 97.2 |
| 45 | 7.2 | 140 | 60.0 | 208 | 97.7 |
| 46 | 7.7 | 141 | 60.5 | 209 | 98.3 |
| 47 | 8.3 | 142 | 61.1 | 210 | 98.8 |
| 48 | 8.8 | 143 | 61.6 | 211 | 99.4 |
| 49 | 9.4 | 144 | 62.2 | 212 | 100.0 |
| 50 | 10.0 | 145 | 62.7 | 213 | 100.5 |

# Multiples and Submultiples of the Metric System

| Multiples and Submultiples | | Prefix | Symbol |
|---|---|---|---|
| 1,000,000,000,000 | ($10^{12}$) | tera- | T |
| 1,000,000,000 | ($10^{9}$) | giga- | G |
| 1,000,000 | ($10^{6}$) | mega- | M |
| 1,000 | ($10^{3}$) | kilo- | k |
| 100 | ($10^{2}$) | hecto- | h |
| 10 | (10) | deka- | da |
| 0.1 | ($10^{-1}$) | deci- | d |
| 0.01 | ($10^{-2}$) | centi- | c |
| 0.001 | ($10^{-3}$) | milli- | m |
| 0.000 001 | ($10^{-6}$) | micro- | $\mu$ |
| 0.000 000 001 | ($10^{-9}$) | nano- | n |
| 0.000 000 000 001 | ($10^{-12}$) | pico- | p |
| 0.000 000 000 000 001 | ($10^{-15}$) | femto- | f |
| 0.000 000 000 000 000 001 | ($10^{-18}$) | atto- | a |

# Appendix 11

## Tables of Weight and Measures

### Measures of Mass

#### Avoirdupois Weight

| Grains | Drams | Ounces | Pounds | Metric Equivalents (grams) |
|---|---|---|---|---|
| 1 | 0.0366 | 0.0023 | 0.00014 | 0.0647989 |
| 27.34 | 1 | 0.0625 | 0.0039 | 1.772 |
| 437.5 | 16 | 1 | 0.0625 | 28.350 |
| 7000 | 256 | 16 | 1 | 453.5924277 |

#### Apothecaries' Weight

| Grains | Scruples (℈) | Drams (ʒ) | Ounces (℥) | Pounds (℔) | Metric Equivalents (grams) |
|---|---|---|---|---|---|
| 1 | 0.05 | 0.0167 | 0.0021 | 0.00017 | 0.0647989 |
| 20 | 1 | 0.333 | 0.042 | 0.0035 | 1.296 |
| 60 | 3 | 1 | 0.125 | 0.0104 | 3.888 |
| 480 | 24 | 8 | 1 | 0.0833 | 31.103 |
| 5760 | 288 | 96 | 12 | 1 | 373.24177 |

#### Metric Weight

| Microgram | Milligram | Centigram | Decigram | Gram | Decagram | Hectogram | Kilogram | Metric Ton | Equivalents | |
|---|---|---|---|---|---|---|---|---|---|---|
| | | | | | | | | | *Avoirdupois* | *Apothecaries'* |
| 1 | — | — | — | — | — | — | — | — | 0.000015 gr | |
| $10^3$ | 1 | — | — | — | — | — | — | — | 0.015432 gr | |
| $10^4$ | 10 | 1 | — | — | — | — | — | — | 0.154323 gr | |
| $10^5$ | 100 | 10 | 1 | — | — | — | — | — | 1.543235 gr | |
| $10^6$ | 1000 | 100 | 10 | 1 | — | — | — | — | 15.432356 gr | |
| $10^7$ | $10^4$ | 1000 | 100 | 10 | 1 | — | — | — | 5.6438 dr | 7.7162 scr |
| $10^8$ | $10^5$ | $10^4$ | 1000 | 100 | 10 | 1 | — | — | 3.527 oz | 3.215 oz |
| $10^9$ | $10^6$ | $10^5$ | $10^4$ | 1000 | 100 | 10 | 1 | — | 2.2046 lb | 2.6792 lb |
| $10^{12}$ | $10^9$ | $10^8$ | $10^7$ | $10^6$ | $10^5$ | $10^4$ | 1000 | 1 | 2204.6223 lb | 2679.2285 lb |

#### Troy Weight

| Grains | Pennyweights | Ounces | Pounds | Metric Equivalents (grams) |
|---|---|---|---|---|
| 1 | 0.042 | 0.002 | 0.00017 | 1.0647989 |
| 24 | 1 | 0.05 | 0.0042 | 1.555 |
| 480 | 20 | 1 | 0.083 | 31.103 |
| 5760 | 240 | 12 | 1 | 373.24177 |

## Measures of Capacity

### Apothecaries' (Wine) Measure

| Minims | Fluid Drams | Fluid Ounces | Gills | Pints | Quarts | Gallons | Cubic Inches | Equivalents | |
|---|---|---|---|---|---|---|---|---|---|
| | | | | | | | | *Milliliters* | *Cubic Centimeters* |
| 1 | 0.0166 | 0.002 | 0.0005 | 0.00013 | — | — | 0.00376 | 0.06161 | 0.06161 |
| 60 | 1 | 0.125 | 0.0312 | 0.0078 | 0.0039 | — | 0.22558 | 3.6967 | 3.6967 |
| 480 | 8 | 1 | 0.25 | 0.0625 | 0.0312 | 0.0078 | 1.80468 | 29.5737 | 29.5737 |
| 1920 | 32 | 4 | 1 | 0.25 | 0.125 | 0.0312 | 7.21875 | 118.2948 | 118.2948 |
| 7680 | 128 | 16 | 4 | 1 | 0.5 | 0.125 | 28.875 | 473.179 | 473.179 |
| 15360 | 256 | 32 | 8 | 2 | 1 | 0.25 | 57.75 | 946.358 | 946.358 |
| 61440 | 1024 | 128 | 32 | 8 | 4 | 1 | 231 | 3785.434 | 3785.434 |

### Metric Measure

| Microliter | Milliliter | Centiliter | Deciliter | Liter | Dekaliter | Hectoliter | Kiloliter | Megaliter | Equivalents (Apothecaries' Fluid) |
|---|---|---|---|---|---|---|---|---|---|
| 1 | — | — | — | — | — | — | — | — | 0.01623108 min |
| $10^3$ | 1 | — | — | — | — | — | — | — | 16.23 min |
| $10^4$ | 10 | 1 | — | — | — | — | — | — | 2.7 fl dr |
| $10^5$ | 100 | 10 | 1 | — | — | — | — | — | 3.38 fl oz |
| $10^6$ | $10^3$ | 100 | 10 | 1 | — | — | — | — | 2.11 pts* |
| $10^7$ | $10^4$ | $10^3$ | 100 | 10 | 1 | — | — | — | 2.64 gal |
| $10^8$ | $10^5$ | $10^4$ | $10^3$ | 100 | 10 | 1 | — | — | 26.418 gals |
| $10^9$ | $10^6$ | $10^5$ | $10^4$ | $10^3$ | 100 | 10 | 1 | — | 264.18 gals |
| $10^{12}$ | $10^9$ | $10^8$ | $10^7$ | $10^6$ | $10^5$ | $10^4$ | $10^3$ | 1 | 26418 gals |

*1 liter = 2.113363738 pints (Apothecaries')

## Measures of Length

### Metric Measure

| Micrometer | Millimeter | Centimeter | Decimeter | Meter | Dekameter | Hectometer | Kilometer | Megameter | Equivalents |
|---|---|---|---|---|---|---|---|---|---|
| 1 | 0.001 | $10^{-4}$ | — | — | — | — | — | — | 0.000039 inch |
| $10^3$ | 1 | $10^{-1}$ | — | — | — | — | — | — | 0.03937 inch |
| $10^4$ | 10 | 1 | — | — | — | — | — | — | 0.3937 inch |
| $10^5$ | 100 | 10 | 1 | — | — | — | — | — | 3.937 inches |
| $10^6$ | 1000 | 100 | 10 | 1 | — | — | — | — | 39.37 inches |
| $10^7$ | $10^4$ | 1000 | 100 | 10 | 1 | — | — | — | 10.9361 yards |
| $10^8$ | $10^5$ | $10^4$ | 1000 | 100 | 10 | 1 | — | — | 109.3612 yards |
| $10^9$ | $10^6$ | $10^5$ | $10^4$ | 1000 | 100 | 10 | 1 | — | 1093.6121 yards |
| $10^{10}$ | $10^7$ | $10^6$ | $10^5$ | $10^4$ | 1000 | 100 | 10 | — | 6.2137 miles |
| $10^{12}$ | $10^9$ | $10^8$ | $10^7$ | $10^6$ | $10^5$ | $10^4$ | 1000 | 1 | 621.370 miles |

# Conversion Tables

**Avoirdupois—Metric Weight**

| Ounces | Grams | Ounces | Grams | Pounds | Grams | Kilograms |
|---|---|---|---|---|---|---|
| 1/16 | 1.772 | 7 | 198.447 | 1 (16 oz) | 453.59 | |
| 1/8 | 3.544 | 8 | 226.796 | 2 | 907.18 | |
| 1/4 | 7.088 | 9 | 255.146 | 3 | 1360.78 | 1.36 |
| 1/2 | 14.175 | 10 | 283.495 | 4 | 1814.37 | 1.81 |
| 1 | 28.350 | 11 | 311.845 | 5 | 2267.96 | 2.27 |
| 2 | 56.699 | 12 | 340.194 | 6 | 2721.55 | 2.72 |
| 3 | 85.049 | 13 | 368.544 | 7 | 3175.15 | 3.18 |
| 4 | 113.398 | 14 | 396.893 | 8 | 3628.74 | 3.63 |
| 5 | 141.748 | 15 | 425.243 | 9 | 4082.33 | 4.08 |
| 6 | 170.097 | 16 (1 lb) | 453.59 | 10 | 4535.92 | 4.54 |

**Metric—Avoirdupois Weight**

| Grams | Ounces | Grams | Ounces | Grams | Pounds |
|---|---|---|---|---|---|
| 0.001 (1 mg) | 0.000035274 | 1 | 0.035274 | 1000 (1 kg) | 2.2046 |

**Apothecaries'—Metric Weight**

| Grains | Grams |
|---|---|
| 1/150 | 0.0004 |
| 1/120 | 0.0005 |
| 1/100 | 0.0006 |
| 1/90 | 0.0007 |
| 1/80 | 0.0008 |
| 1/64 | 0.001 |
| 1/60 | 0.0011 |
| 1/50 | 0.0013 |
| 1/48 | 0.0014 |
| 1/40 | 0.0016 |
| 1/36 | 0.0018 |
| 1/32 | 0.002 |
| 1/30 | 0.0022 |
| 1/25 | 0.0026 |
| 1/20 | 0.003 |
| 1/16 | 0.004 |
| 1/12 | 0.005 |
| 1/10 | 0.006 |
| 1/9 | 0.007 |
| 1/8 | 0.008 |
| 1/7 | 0.009 |
| 1/6 | 0.01 |
| 1/5 | 0.013 |
| 1/4 | 0.016 |
| 1/3 | 0.02 |

| Grains | Grams |
|---|---|
| 2/5 | 0.03 |
| 1/2 | 0.032 |
| 3/5 | 0.04 |
| 2/3 | 0.043 |
| 3/4 | 0.05 |
| 7/8 | 0.057 |
| 1 | 0.065 |
| 1 1/2 | 0.097 (0.1) |
| 2 | 0.12 |
| 3 | 0.20 |
| 4 | 0.24 |
| 5 | 0.30 |
| 6 | 0.40 |
| 7 | 0.45 |
| 8 | 0.50 |
| 9 | 0.60 |
| 10 | 0.65 |
| 15 | 1.00 |
| 20 (1 ℈) | 1.30 |
| 30 | 2.00 |

| Scruples | Grams |
|---|---|
| 1 | 1.296 (1.3) |
| 2 | 2.592 (2.6) |
| 3 (1 ʒ) | 3.888 (3.9) |

| Drams | Grams |
|---|---|
| 1 | 3.888 |
| 2 | 7.776 |
| 3 | 11.664 |
| 4 | 15.552 |
| 5 | 19.440 |
| 6 | 23.328 |
| 7 | 27.216 |
| 8 (1 ℥) | 31.103 |

| Ounces | Grams |
|---|---|
| 1 | 31.103 |
| 2 | 62.207 |
| 3 | 93.310 |
| 4 | 124.414 |
| 5 | 155.517 |
| 6 | 186.621 |
| 7 | 217.724 |
| 8 | 248.828 |
| 9 | 279.931 |
| 10 | 311.035 |
| 11 | 342.138 |
| 12 (1 ℔) | 373.242 |

**Metric—Apothecaries' Weight**

| Milligrams | Grains | Grams | Grains | Grams | Equivalents |
|---|---|---|---|---|---|
| 1 | 0.015432 | 0.1 | 1.5432 | 10 | 2.572 drams |
| 2 | 0.030864 | 0.2 | 3.0864 | 15 | 3.858 " |
| 3 | 0.046296 | 0.3 | 4.6296 | 20 | 5.144 " |
| 4 | 0.061728 | 0.4 | 6.1728 | 25 | 6.430 " |
| 5 | 0.077160 | 0.5 | 7.7160 | 30 | 7.716 " |
| 6 | 0.092592 | 0.6 | 9.2592 | 40 | 1.286 oz |
| 7 | 0.108024 | 0.7 | 10.8024 | 45 | 1.447 " |
| 8 | 0.123456 | 0.8 | 12.3456 | 50 | 1.607 " |
| 9 | 0.138888 | 0.9 | 13.8888 | 100 | 3.215 " |
| 10 | 0.154320 | 1.0 | 15.4320 | 200 | 6.430 " |
| 15 | 0.231480 | 1.5 | 23.1480 | 300 | 9.644 " |
| 20 | 0.308640 | 2.0 | 30.8640 | 400 | 12.859 " |
| 25 | 0.385800 | 2.5 | 38.5800 | 500 | 1.34 lb |
| 30 | 0.462960 | 3.0 | 46.2960 | 600 | 1.61 " |
| 35 | 0.540120 | 3.5 | 54.0120 | 700 | 1.88 " |
| 40 | 0.617280 | 4.0 | 61.728 | 800 | 2.14 " |
| 45 | 0.694440 | 4.5 | 69.444 | 900 | 2.41 " |
| 50 | 0.771600 | 5.0 | 77.162 | 1000 | 2.68 " |
| 100 | 1.543240 | 10.0 | 154.324 | | |

**Apothecaries'—Metric Liquid Measure**

| Minims | Milliliters | Fluid Drams | Milliliters | Fluid Ounces | Milliliters |
|---|---|---|---|---|---|
| 1 | 0.06 | 1 | 3.70 | 1 | 29.57 |
| 2 | 0.12 | 2 | 7.39 | 2 | 59.15 |
| 3 | 0.19 | 3 | 11.09 | 3 | 88.72 |
| 4 | 0.25 | 4 | 14.79 | 4 | 118.29 |
| 5 | 0.31 | 5 | 18.48 | 5 | 147.87 |
| 10 | 0.62 | 6 | 22.18 | 6 | 177.44 |
| 15 | 0.92 | 7 | 25.88 | 7 | 207.01 |
| 20 | 1.23 | 8 (1 fl oz) | 29.57 | 8 | 236.58 |
| 25 | 1.54 | | | 9 | 266.16 |
| 30 | 1.85 | | | 10 | 295.73 |
| 35 | 2.16 | | | 11 | 325.30 |
| 40 | 2.46 | | | 12 | 354.88 |
| 45 | 2.77 | | | 13 | 384.45 |
| 50 | 3.08 | | | 14 | 414.02 |
| 55 | 3.39 | | | 15 | 443.59 |
| 60 (1 fl dr) | 3.70 | | | 16 (1 pt) | 473.17 |
| | | | | 32 (1 qt) | 946.33 |
| | | | | 128 (1 gal) | 3785.32 |

**Metric—Apothecaries' Liquid Measure**

| Milliliters | Minims | Milliliters | Fluid Drams | Milliliters | Fluid Ounces |
|---|---|---|---|---|---|
| 1 | 16.231 | 5 | 1.35 | 30 | 1.01 |
| 2 | 32.5 | 10 | 2.71 | 40 | 1.35 |
| 3 | 48.7 | 15 | 4.06 | 50 | 1.69 |
| 4 | 64.9 | 20 | 5.4 | 500 | 16.91 |
| 5 | 81.1 | 25 | 6.76 | 1000 (1 L) | 33.815 |
| | | 30 | 7.1 | | |

**U.S.—Metric Length**

| Inches | Millimeters | Centimeters | Meters |
|---|---|---|---|
| 1/25 | 1.00 | 0.1 | 0.001 |
| 1/8 | 3.18 | 0.318 | 0.00318 |
| 1/4 | 6.35 | 0.635 | 0.00635 |
| 1/2 | 12.70 | 1.27 | 0.00127 |
| 1 | 25.40 | 2.54 | 0.0254 |
| 12 (1 foot) | 304.80 | 30.48 | 0.3048 |

# APPENDIX 13

## Reference Values for the Interpretation of Laboratory Tests*

**Reference Intervals for Hematology**

| Test | Conventional Units | SI Units |
|---|---|---|
| Acid hemolysis (Ham test) | No hemolysis | No hemolysis |
| Alkaline phosphatase, leukocyte | Total score 14–100 | Total score 14–100 |
| Cell counts | | |
| Erythrocytes | | |
| Males | 4.6–6.2 million/$mm^3$ | 4.6–6.2 × $10^{12}$/L |
| Females | 4.2–5.4 million/$mm^3$ | 4.2–5.4 × $10^{12}$/L |
| Children (varies with age) | 4.5–5.1 million/$mm^3$ | 4.5–5.1 × $10^{12}$/L |
| Leukocytes, total | 4500–11,000/$mm^3$ | 4.5–11.0 × $10^9$/L |
| Leukocytes, differential counts† | | |
| Myelocytes | 0% | 0/L |
| Band neutrophils | 3–5% | 150–400 × $10^6$/L |
| Segmented neutrophils | 54–62% | 3000–5800 × $10^6$/L |
| Lymphocytes | 25–33% | 1500–3000 × $10^6$/L |
| Monocytes | 3–7% | 300–500 × $10^6$/L |
| Eosinophils | 1–3% | 50–250 × $10^6$/L |
| Basophils | 0–1% | 15–50 × $10^6$/L |
| Platelets | 150,000–400,000/$mm^3$ | 150–400 × $10^9$/L |
| Reticulocytes | 25,000–75,000/$mm^3$ (0.5–1.5% of erythrocytes) | 25–75 × $10^9$/L |
| Coagulation tests | | |
| Bleeding time (template) | 2.75–8.0 min | 2.75–8.0 min |
| Coagulation time (glass tube) | 5–15 min | 5–15 min |
| D-Dimer | <0.5 μg/mL | <0.5 mg/L |
| Factor VIII and other coagulation factors | 50–150% of normal | 0.5–1.5 of normal |
| Fibrin split products (Thrombo-Wellco test) | <10 μg/mL | <10 mg/L |
| Fibrinogen | 200–400 mg/dL | 2.0–4.0 g/L |
| Partial thromboplastin time, activated (aPTT) | 20–35 s | 20–35 s |
| Prothrombin time (PT) | 12.0–14.0 s | 12.0–14.0 s |
| Coombs' test | | |
| Direct | Negative | Negative |
| Indirect | Negative | Negative |
| Corpuscular values of erythrocytes | | |
| Mean corpuscular hemoglobin (MCH) | 26–34 pg/cell | 26–34 pg/cell |
| Mean corpuscular volume (MCV) | 80–96 $\mu m^3$ | 80–96 fL |
| Mean corpuscular hemoglobin concentration (MCHC) | 32–36 g/dL | 320–360 g/L |
| Haptoglobin | 20–165 mg/dL | 0.20–1.65 g/L |
| Hematocrit | | |
| Males | 40–54 mL/dL | 0.40–0.54 |
| Females | 37–47 mL/dL | 0.37–0.47 |
| Newborns | 49–54 mL/dL | 0.49–0.54 |
| Children (varies with age) | 35–49 mL/dL | 0.35–0.49 |
| Hemoglobin | | |
| Males | 13.0–18.0 g/dL | 8.1–11.2 mmol/L |
| Females | 12.0–16.0 g/dL | 7.4–9.9 mmol/L |
| Newborns | 16.5–19.5 g/dL | 10.2–12.1 mmol/L |
| Children (varies with age) | 11.2–16.5 g/dL | 7.0–10.2 mmol/L |
| Hemoglobin, fetal | <1.0% of total | <0.01 of total |
| Hemoglobin $A_{1c}$ | 3–5% of total | 0.03–0.05 of total |
| Hemoglobin $A_2$ | 1.5–3.0% of total | 0.015–0.03 of total |
| Hemoglobin, plasma | 0.0–5.0 mg/dL | 0.0–3.2 μmol/L |
| Methemoglobin | 30–130 mg/dL | 19–80 μmol/L |
| Sedimentation rate (ESR) | | |
| Wintrobe: Males | 0–5 mm/h | 0–5 mm/h |
| Females | 0–15 mm/h | 0–15 mm/h |
| Westergren: Males | 0–15 mm/h | 0–15 mm/h |
| Females | 0–20 mm/h | 0–20 mm/h |

*From William Z. Borer, Reference Values for the Interpretation of Laboratory Tests. *In* Robert E. Rakel (ed.): Conn's Current Therapy 2000. Philadelphia, W.B. Saunders Company, 2000.

†Conventional units are percentages; SI units are absolute counts.

**Reference Intervals* for Clinical Chemistry (Blood, Serum, and Plasma)**

| Analyte | Conventional Units | SI Units |
|---|---|---|
| Acetoacetate plus acetone | | |
| Qualitative | Negative | Negative |
| Quantitative | 0.3–2.0 mg/dL | 30–200 μmol/L |
| Acid phosphatase, serum (thymolphthalein monophosphate substrate) | 0.1–0.6 U/L | 0.1–0.6 U/L |
| ACTH (see Corticotropin) | | |
| Alanine aminotransferase (ALT) serum (SGPT) | 1–45 U/L | 1–45 U/L |
| Albumin, serum | 3.3–5.2 g/dL | 33–52 g/L |
| Aldolase, serum | 0.0–7.0 U/L | 0.0–7.0 U/L |
| Aldosterone, plasma | | |
| Standing | 5–30 ng/dL | 140–830 pmol/L |
| Recumbent | 3–10 ng/dL | 80–275 pmol/L |
| Alkaline phosphatase (ALP), serum | | |
| Adult | 35–150 U/L | 35–150 U/L |
| Adolescent | 100–500 U/L | 100–500 U/L |
| Child | 100–350 U/L | 100–350 U/L |
| Ammonia nitrogen, plasma | 10–50 μmol/L | 10–50 μmol/L |
| Amylase, serum | 25–125 U/L | 25–125 U/L |
| Anion gap, serum, calculated | 8–16 mEq/L | 8–16 mmol/L |
| Ascorbic acid, blood | 0.4–1.5 mg/dL | 23–85 μmol/L |
| Aspartate aminotransferase (AST) serum (SGOT) | 1–36 U/L | 1–36 U/L |
| Base excess, arterial blood, calculated | 0 ± 2 mEq/L | 0 ± 2 mmol/L |
| Bicarbonate | | |
| Venous plasma | 23–29 mEq/L | 23–29 mmol/L |
| Arterial blood | 21–27 mEq/L | 21–27 mmol/L |
| Bile acids, serum | 0.3–3.0 mg/dL | 0.8–7.6 μmol/L |
| Bilirubin, serum | | |
| Conjugated | 0.1–0.4 mg/dL | 1.7–6.8 μmol/L |
| Total | 0.3–1.1 mg/dL | 5.1–19.0 μmol/L |
| Calcium, serum | 8.4–10.6 mg/dL | 2.10–2.65 mmol/L |
| Calcium, ionized, serum | 4.25–5.25 mg/dL | 1.05–1.30 mmol/L |
| Carbon dioxide, total, serum or plasma | 24–31 mEq/L | 24–31 mmol/L |
| Carbon dioxide tension ($P_{CO_2}$), blood | 35–45 mm Hg | 35–45 mm Hg |
| β-carotene, serum | 60–260 μg/dL | 1.1–8.6 μmol/L |
| Ceruloplasmin, serum | 23–44 mg/dL | 230–440 mg/L |
| Chloride, serum or plasma | 96–106 mEq/L | 96–106 mmol/L |
| Cholesterol, serum or ethylenediaminetetraacetic acid (EDTA) plasma | | |
| Desirable range | <200 mg/dL | <5.20 mmol/L |
| Low-density lipoprotein (LDL) cholesterol | 60–180 mg/dL | 1.55–4.65 mmol/L |
| High-density lipoprotein (HDL) cholesterol | 30–80 mg/dL | 0.80–2.05 mmol/L |
| Copper | 70–140 μg/dL | 11–22 μmol/L |
| Corticotropin (ACTH), plasma, 8 AM | 10–80 pg/mL | 2–18 pmol/L |
| Cortisol, plasma | | |
| 8 AM | 6–23 μg/dL | 170–630 nmol/L |
| 4 PM | 3–15 μg/dL | 80–410 nmol/L |
| 10 PM | <50% of 8 AM value | <50% of 8 AM value |
| Creatine, serum | | |
| Males | 0.2–0.5 mg/dL | 15–40 μmol/L |
| Females | 0.3–0.9 mg/dL | 25–70 μmol/L |
| Creatine kinase (CK), serum | | |
| Males | 55–170 U/L | 55–170 U/L |
| Females | 30–135 U/L | 30–135 U/L |
| Creatine kinase MB isoenzyme, serum | <5% of total CK activity<br><5.0 ng/mL by immunoassay | <5% of total CK activity<br><5.0 ng/mL by immunoassay |
| Creatinine, serum | 0.6–1.2 mg/dL | 50–110 μmol/L |
| Estradiol-17β, adult | | |
| Males | 10–65 pg/mL | 35–240 pmol/L |
| Females | | |
| Follicular | 30–100 pg/mL | 110–370 pmol/L |
| Ovulatory | 200–400 pg/mL | 730–1470 pmol/L |
| Luteal | 50–140 pg/mL | 180–510 pmol/L |
| Ferritin, serum | 20–200 ng/mL | 20–200 μg/L |
| Fibrinogen, plasma | 200–400 mg/dL | 2.0–4.0 g/L |
| Folate, serum | 3–18 ng/mL | 6.8–41 nmol/L |
| Erythrocytes | 145–540 ng/mL | 330–1220 nmol/L |
| Follicle-stimulating hormone (FSH), plasma | | |
| Males | 4–25 mU/mL | 4–25 U/L |
| Females, premenopausal | 4–30 mU/mL | 4–30 U/L |
| Females, postmenopausal | 40–250 mU/mL | 40–250 U/L |
| Gamma-glutamyltransferase (GGT), serum | 5–40 U/L | 5–40 U/L |
| Gastrin, fasting, serum | 0–100 pg/mL | 0–100 mg/L |
| Glucose, fasting, plasma or serum | 70–115 mg/dL | 3.9–6.4 nmol/L |
| Growth hormone (hGH), plasma, adult, fasting | 0–6 ng/mL | 0–6 μg/L |
| Haptoglobin, serum | 20–165 mg/dL | 0.20–1.65 gm/L |

**Reference Intervals* for Clinical Chemistry (Blood, Serum, and Plasma)** *Continued*

| Analyte | Conventional Units | SI Units |
|---|---|---|
| Immunoglobulins, serum (see table of Reference Intervals for Tests of Immunologic Function) | | |
| Iron, serum | 75–175 μg/dL | 13–31 μmol/L |
| Iron binding capacity, serum | | |
| Total | 250–410 μg/dL | 45–73 μmol/L |
| Saturation | 20–55% | 0.20–0.55 |
| Lactate | | |
| Venous whole blood | 5.0–20.0 mg/dL | 0.6–2.2 mmol/L |
| Arterial whole blood | 5.0–15.0 mg/dL | 0.6–1.7 mmol/L |
| Lactate dehydrogenase (LD), serum | 110–220 U/L | 110–220 U/L |
| Lipase, serum | 10–140 U/L | 10–140 U/L |
| Lutropin (LH), serum | | |
| Males | 1–9 U/L | 1–9 U/L |
| Females | | |
| Follicular phase | 2–10 U/L | 2–10 U/L |
| Midcycle peak | 15–65 U/L | 15–65 U/L |
| Luteal phase | 1–12 U/L | 1–12 U/L |
| Postmenopausal | 12–65 U/L | 12–65 U/L |
| Magnesium, serum | 1.3–2.1 mg/dL | 0.65–1.05 mmol/L |
| Osmolality | 275–295 mOsm/kg water | 275–295 mOsm/kg water |
| Oxygen, blood, arterial, room air | | |
| Partial pressure ($Pao_2$) | 80–100 mm Hg | 80–100 mm Hg |
| Saturation ($Sao_2$) | 95–98% | 95–98% |
| pH, arterial blood | 7.35–7.45 | 7.35–7.45 |
| Phosphate, inorganic, serum | | |
| Adult | 3.0–4.5 mg/dL | 1.0–1.5 mmol/L |
| Child | 4.0–7.0 mg/dL | 1.3–2.3 mmol/L |
| Potassium | | |
| Serum | 3.5–5.0 mEq/L | 3.5–5.0 mmol/L |
| Plasma | 3.5–4.5 mEq/L | 3.5–4.5 mmol/L |
| Progesterone, serum, adult | | |
| Males | 0.0–0.4 ng/mL | 0.0–1.3 mmol/L |
| Females | | |
| Follicular phase | 0.1–1.5 ng/mL | 0.3–4.8 mmol/L |
| Luteal phase | 2.5–28.0 ng/mL | 8.0–89.0 mmol/L |
| Prolactin, serum | | |
| Males | 1.0–15.0 ng/mL | 1.0–15.0 μg/L |
| Females | 1.0–20.0 ng/mL | 1.0–20.0 μg/L |
| Protein, serum, electrophoresis | | |
| Total | 6.0–8.0 g/dL | 60–80 g/L |
| Albumin | 3.5–5.5 g/dL | 35–55 g/L |
| Globulins | | |
| $Alpha_1$ | 0.2–0.4 g/dL | 2.0–4.0 g/L |
| $Alpha_2$ | 0.5–0.9 g/dL | 5.0–9.0 g/L |
| Beta | 0.6–1.1 g/dL | 6.0–11.0 g/L |
| Gamma | 0.7–1.7 g/dL | 7.0–17.0 g/L |
| Pyruvate, blood | 0.3–0.9 mg/dL | 0.03–0.10 mmol/L |
| Rheumatoid factor | 0.0–30.0 IU/mL | 0.0–30.0 kIU/L |
| Sodium, serum or plasma | 135–145 mEq/L | 135–145 mmol/L |
| Testosterone, plasma | | |
| Males, adult | 300–1200 ng/dL | 10.4–41.6 nmol/L |
| Females, adult | 20–75 ng/dL | 0.7–2.6 nmol/L |
| Pregnant females | 40–200 ng/dL | 1.4–6.9 nmol/L |
| Thyroglobulin | 3–42 ng/mL | 3–42 μg/L |
| Thyrotropin (hTSH), serum | 0.4–4.8 μIU/mL | 0.4–4.8 mIU/L |
| Thyrotropin-releasing hormone (TRH) | 5–60 pg/mL | 5–60 ng/L |
| Thyroxine ($FT_4$), free, serum | 0.9–2.1 ng/dL | 12–27 pmol/L |
| Thyroxine ($T_4$), serum | 4.5–12.0 μg/dL | 58–154 nmol/L |
| Thyroxine-binding globulin (TBG) | 15.0–34.0 μg/mL | 15.0–34.0 mg/L |
| Transferrin | 250–430 mg/dL | 2.5–4.3 g/L |
| Triglycerides, serum, 12-h fast | 40–150 mg/dL | 0.4–1.5 g/L |
| Triiodothyronine ($T_3$), serum | 70–190 ng/dL | 1.1–2.9 nmol/L |
| Triiodothyronine uptake, resin ($T_3RU$) | 25–38% | 0.25–0.38 |
| Urate | | |
| Males | 2.5–8.0 mg/dL | 150–480 μmol/L |
| Females | 2.2–7.0 mg/dL | 130–420 μmol/L |
| Urea, serum or plasma | 24–49 mg/dL | 4.0–8.2 nmol/L |
| Urea nitrogen, serum or plasma | 11–23 mg/dL | 8.0–16.4 nmol/L |
| Viscosity, serum | 1.4–1.8 × water | 1.4–1.8 × water |
| Vitamin A, serum | 20–80 μg/dL | 0.70–2.80 μmol/L |
| Vitamin $B_{12}$, serum | 180–900 pg/mL | 133–664 pmol/L |

*Reference values may vary, depending on the method and sample source used.

**Reference Intervals for Therapeutic Drug Monitoring (Serum)**

| Analyte | Therapeutic Range | Toxic Concentrations | Proprietary Name(s) |
|---|---|---|---|
| *Analgesics* | | | |
| Acetaminophen | 10–20 μg/mL | >250 μg/mL | Tylenol<br>Datril |
| Salicylate | 100–250 μg/mL | >300 μg/mL | Aspirin<br>Bufferin |
| *Antibiotics* | | | |
| Amikacin | 25–30 μg/mL | Peak >35 μg/mL<br>Trough >10 μg/mL | Amikin |
| Gentamicin | 5–10 μg/mL | Peak >10 μg/mL<br>Trough >2 μg/mL | Garamycin |
| Tobramycin | 5–10 μg/mL | Peak >10 μg/mL<br>Trough >2 μg/mL | Nebcin |
| Vancomycin | 5–35 μg/mL | Peak >40 μg/mL<br>Trough >10 μg/mL | Vancocin |
| *Anticonvulsants* | | | |
| Carbamazepine | 5–12 μg/mL | >15 μg/mL | Tegretol |
| Ethosuximide | 40–100 μg/mL | >150 μg/mL | Zarontin |
| Phenobarbital | 15–40 μg/mL | 40–100 ng/mL (varies widely) | Luminal |
| Phenytoin | 10–20 μg/mL | >20 μg/mL | Dilantin |
| Primidone | 5–12 μg/mL | >15 μg/mL | Mysoline |
| Valproic acid | 50–100 μg/mL | >100 μg/mL | Depakene |
| *Antineoplastics and Immunosuppressives* | | | |
| Cyclosporine | 50–400 ng/mL | >400 ng/mL | Sandimmune |
| Methotrexate, high dose, 48-h | Variable | >1 μmol/L 48 h after dose | |
| Tacrolimus (FK-506), whole blood | 3–10 μg/L | >15 μg/L | Prograf |
| *Bronchodilators and Respiratory Stimulants* | | | |
| Caffeine | 3–15 ng/mL | >30 ng/mL | |
| Theophylline (aminophylline) | 10–20 μg/mL | >20 μg/mL | Elixophyllin<br>Quibron |
| *Cardiovascular Drugs* | | | |
| Amiodarone<br>(obtain specimen more than 8 h after last dose) | 1.0–2.0 μg/mL | >2.0 μg/mL | Cordarone |
| Digitoxin<br>(obtain specimen 12–24 h after last dose) | 15–25 ng/mL | >35 ng/mL | Crystodigin |
| Digoxin<br>(obtain specimen more than 6 h after last dose) | 0.8–2.0 ng/mL | >2.4 ng/mL | Lanoxin |
| Disopyramide | 2–5 μg/mL | >7 μg/mL | Norpace |
| Flecainide | 0.2–1.0 ng/mL | >1 ng/mL | Tambocor |
| Lidocaine | 1.5–5.0 μg/mL | >6 μg/mL | Xylocaine |
| Mexiletine | 0.7–2.0 ng/mL | >2 ng/mL | Mexitil |
| Procainamide | 4–10 μg/mL | >12 μg/mL | Pronestyl |
| Procainamide plus *N*-acetyl-*p*-aminophenol (NAPA) | 8–30 μg/mL | >30 μg/mL | |
| Propranolol | 50–100 ng/mL | Variable | Inderal |
| Quinidine | 2–5 μg/mL | >6 μg/mL | Cardioquin<br>Quinaglute |
| Tocainide | 4–10 ng/mL | >10 ng/mL | Tonocard |
| *Psychopharmacologic Drugs* | | | |
| Amitriptyline | 120–150 ng/mL | >500 ng/mL | Elavil<br>Triavil |
| Bupropion | 25–100 ng/mL | Not applicable | Wellbutrin |
| Desipramine | 150–300 ng/mL | >500 ng/mL | Norpramin |
| Imipramine | 125–250 ng/mL | >400 ng/mL | Tofranil |
| Lithium<br>(obtain specimen 12 h after last dose) | 0.6–1.5 mEq/L | >1.5 mEq/L | Lithobid |
| Nortriptyline | 50–150 ng/mL | >500 ng/mL | Aventyl<br>Pamelor |

**Reference Intervals* for Clinical Chemistry (Urine)**

| Analyte | Conventional Units | SI Units |
|---|---|---|
| Acetone and acetoacetate, qualitative | Negative | Negative |
| Albumin | | |
| Qualitative | Negative | Negative |
| Quantitative | 10–100 mg/24 h | 0.15–1.5 μmol/d |
| Aldosterone | 3–20 μg/24 h | 8.3–55 nmol/d |
| δ-Aminolevulinic acid (δ-ALA) | 1.3–7.0 mg/24 h | 10–53 μmol/d |
| Amylase | <17 U/h | <17 U/h |
| Amylase/creatinine clearance ratio | 0.01–0.04 | 0.01–0.04 |
| Bilirubin, qualitative | Negative | Negative |
| Calcium (regular diet) | <250 mg/24 h | <6.3 nmol/d |

**Reference Intervals* for Clinical Chemistry (Urine)** *Continued*

| Analyte | Conventional Units | SI Units |
|---|---|---|
| Catecholamines | | |
| Epinephrine | <10 µg/24 h | <55 nmol/d |
| Norepinephrine | <100 µg/24 h | <590 nmol/d |
| Total free catecholamines | 4–126 µg/24 h | 24–745 nmol/d |
| Total metanephrines | 0.1–1.6 mg/24 h | 0.5–8.1 µmol/d |
| Chloride (varies with intake) | 110–250 mEq/24 h | 110–250 mmol/d |
| Copper | 0–50 µg/24 h | 0.0–0.80 µmol/d |
| Cortisol, free | 10–100 µg/24 h | 27.6–276 nmol/d |
| Creatine | | |
| Males | 0–40 mg/24 h | 0.0–0.30 mmol/d |
| Females | 0–80 mg/24 h | 0.0–0.60 mmol/d |
| Creatinine | 15–25 mg/kg/24 h | 0.13–0.22 mmol/kg/d |
| Creatinine clearance (endogenous) | | |
| Males | 110–150 mL/min/1.73 $m^2$ | 110–150 mL/min/1.73 $m^2$ |
| Females | 105–132 mL/min/1.73 $m^2$ | 105–132 mL/min/1.73 $m^2$ |
| Cystine or cysteine | Negative | Negative |
| Dehydroepiandrosterone | | |
| Males | 0.2–2.0 mg/24 h | 0.7–6.9 µmol/d |
| Females | 0.2–1.8 mg/24 h | 0.7–6.2 µmol/d |
| Estrogens, total | | |
| Males | 4–25 µg/24 h | 14–90 nmol/d |
| Females | 5–100 µg/24 h | 18–360 nmol/d |
| Glucose (as reducing substance) | <250 mg/24 h | <250 mg/d |
| Hemoglobin and myoglobin, qualitative | Negative | Negative |
| Homogentisic acid, qualitative | Negative | Negative |
| 17-Ketogenic steroids | | |
| Males | 5–23 mg/24 h | 17–80 µmol/d |
| Females | 3–15 mg/24 h | 10–52 µmol/d |
| 17-Hydroxycorticosteroids | | |
| Males | 3–9 mg/24 h | 8.3–25 µmol/d |
| Females | 2–8 mg/24 h | 5.5–22 µmol/d |
| 5-Hydroxyindoleacetic acid | | |
| Qualitative | Negative | Negative |
| Quantitative | 2–6 mg/24 h | 10–31 µmol/d |
| 17-Ketosteroids | | |
| Males | 8–22 mg/24 h | 28–76 µmol/d |
| Females | 6–15 mg/24 h | 21–52 µmol/d |
| Magnesium | 6–10 mEq/24 h | 3–5 mmol/d |
| Metanephrines | 0.05–1.2 ng/mg creatinine | 0.03–0.70 mmol/mmol creatinine |
| Osmolality | 38–1400 mOsm/kg water | 38–1400 mOsm/kg water |
| pH | 4.6–8.0 | 4.6–8.0 |
| Phenylpyruvic acid, qualitative | Negative | Negative |
| Phosphate | 0.4–1.3 g/24 h | 13–42 mmol/d |
| Porphobilinogen | | |
| Qualitative | Negative | Negative |
| Quantitative | <2 mg/24 h | <9 µmol/d |
| Porphyrins | | |
| Coproporphyrin | 50–250 µg/24 h | 77–380 nmol/d |
| Uroporphyrin | 10–30 µg/24 h | 12–36 nmol/d |
| Potassium | 25–125 mEq/24 h | 25–125 mmol/d |
| Pregnanediol | | |
| Males | 0.0–1.9 mg/24 h | 0.0–6.0 µmol/d |
| Females | | |
| Proliferative phase | 0.0–2.6 mg/24 h | 0.0–8.0 µmol/d |
| Luteal phase | 2.6–10.6 mg/24 h | 8–33 µmol/d |
| Postmenopausal | 0.2–1.0 mg/24 h | 0.6–3.1 µmol/d |
| Pregnanetriol | 0.0–2.5 mg/24 h | 0.0–7.4 µmol/d |
| Protein, total | | |
| Qualitative | Negative | Negative |
| Quantitative | 10–150 mg/24 h | 10–150 mg/d |
| Protein/creatinine ratio | <0.2 | <0.2 |
| Sodium (regular diet) | 60–260 mEq/24 h | 60–260 mmol/d |
| Specific gravity | | |
| Random specimen | 1.003–1.030 | 1.003–1.030 |
| 24-hour collection | 1.015–1.025 | 1.015–1.025 |
| Urate (regular diet) | 250–750 mg/24 h | 1.5–4.4 mmol/d |
| Urobilinogen | 0.5–4.0 mg/24 h | 0.6–6.8 µmol/d |
| Vanillylmandelic acid (VMA) | 1.0–8.0 mg/24 h | 5–40 µmol/d |

*Values may vary depending on the method used.

**Reference Intervals for Toxic Substances**

| Analyte | Conventional Units | SI Units |
|---|---|---|
| Arsenic, urine | <130 μg/24 h | <1.7 μmol/d |
| Bromides, serum, inorganic | <100 mg/dL | <10 mmol/L |
| Toxic symptoms | 140–1000 mg/dL | 14–100 mmol/L |
| Carboxyhemoglobin, blood: | Saturation | |
| Urban environment | <5% | <0.05 |
| Smokers | <12% | <0.12 |
| Symptoms | | |
| Headache | >15% | >0.15 |
| Nausea and vomiting | >25% | >0.25 |
| Potentially lethal | >50% | >0.50 |
| Ethanol, blood | <0.05 mg/dL<br><0.005% | <1.0 mmol/L |
| Intoxication | >100 mg/dL<br>>0.1% | >22 mmol/L |
| Marked intoxication | 300–400 mg/dL<br>0.3–0.4% | 65–87 mmol/L |
| Alcoholic stupor | 400–500 mg/dL<br>0.4–0.5% | 87–109 mmol/L |
| Coma | >500 mg/dL<br>>0.5% | >109 mmol/L |
| Lead, blood | | |
| Adults | <25 μg/dL | <1.2 μmol/L |
| Children | <15 μg/dL | <0.7 μmol/L |
| Lead, urine | <80 μg/24 h | <0.4 μmol/d |
| Mercury, urine | <30 μg/24 h | <150 nmol/d |

**Reference Intervals for Tests Performed on Cerebrospinal Fluid**

| Test | Conventional Units | SI Units |
|---|---|---|
| Cells | <5/$mm^3$, all mononuclear | <5 × $10^6$/L, all mononuclear |
| Protein electrophoresis | Albumin predominant | Albumin predominant |
| Glucose | 50–75 mg/dL (20 mg/dL less than in serum) | 2.8–4.2 mmol/L (1.1 mmol less than in serum) |
| IgG | | |
| Children under 14 | <8% of total protein | <0.08 of total protein |
| Adults | <14% of total protein | <0.14 of total protein |
| IgG index* $\left(\frac{\text{CSF/serum IgG ratio}}{\text{CSF/serum albumin ratio}}\right)$ | 0.3–0.6 | 0.3–0.6 |
| Oligoclonal banding on electrophoresis | Absent | Absent |
| Pressure, opening | 70–180 mm $H_2O$ | 70–180 mm $H_2O$ |
| Protein, total | 15–45 mg/dL | 150–450 mg/L |

**Abbreviation:* CSF = cerebrospinal fluid.

**Reference Intervals for Tests of Gastrointestinal Function**

| Test | Conventional Units |
|---|---|
| Bentiromide test | 6-h urinary arylamine excretion greater than 57% excludes pancreatic insufficiency |
| β-Carotene, serum | 60–260 ng/dL |
| Fecal fat estimation | |
| Qualitative | No fat globules seen by high-power microscope |
| Quantitative | <6 g/24 h (>95% coefficient of fat absorption) |
| Gastric acid output | |
| Basal | |
| Males | 0.0–10.5 mmol/h |
| Females | 0.0–5.6 mmol/h |
| Maximum (after histamine or pentagastrin) | |
| Males | 9.0–48.0 mmol/h |
| Females | 6.0–31.0 mmol/h |
| Ratio: basal maximum | |
| Males | 0.0–0.31 |
| Females | 0.0–0.29 |
| Secretin test, pancreatic fluid | |
| Volume | >1.8 mL/kg/h |
| Bicarbonate | >80 mEq/L |
| D-Xylose absorption test, urine | >20% of ingested dose excreted in 5 h |

**Reference Intervals for Tests of Immunologic Function**

| Test | Conventional Units | SI Units |
|---|---|---|
| Complement, Serum | | |
| C3 | 85–175 mg/dL | 0.85–1.75 gm/L |
| C4 | 15–45 mg/dL | 150–450 mg/L |
| Total hemolytic ($CH_{50}$) | 150–250 U/mL | 150–250 U/mL |
| Immunoglobulins, Serum, Adult | | |
| IgG | 640–1350 mg/dL | 6.4–13.5 g/L |
| IgA | 70–310 mg/dL | 0.70–3.1 g/L |
| IgM | 90–350 mg/dL | 0.90–3.5 g/L |
| IgD | 0.0–6.0 mg/dL | 0.0–60 mg/L |
| IgE | 0.0–430 ng/dL | 0.0–430 μg/L |

**Lymphocyte Subsets, Whole Blood, Heparinized**

| Antigen(s) Expressed | Cell Type | Percentage | Absolute Cell Count |
|---|---|---|---|
| CD3 | Total T cells | 56–77% | 860–1880 |
| CD19 | Total B cells | 7–17% | 140–370 |
| CD3 and CD4 | Helper-induced cells | 32–54% | 550–1190 |
| CD3 and CD8 | Suppressor-cytotoxic cells | 24–37% | 430–1060 |
| CD3 and DR | Activated T cells | 5–14% | 70–310 |
| CD2 | E rosette T cells | 73–87% | 1040–2160 |
| CD16 and CD56 | Natural killer (NK) cells | 8–22% | 130–500 |
| Helper/suppressor ratio: 0.8–1.8 | | | |

**Reference Values for Semen Analysis**

| Test | Conventional Units | SI Units |
|---|---|---|
| Volume | 2–5 mL | 2–5 mL |
| Liquefaction | Complete in 15 min | Complete in 15 min |
| pH | 7.2–8.0 | 7.2–8.0 |
| Leukocytes | Occasional or absent | Occasional or absent |
| Spermatozoa | | |
| Count | $60–150 \times 10^6$/mL | $60–150 \times 10^6$/mL |
| Motility | >80% motile | >0.80 motile |
| Morphology | 80–90% normal forms | >0.80–0.90 normal forms |
| Fructose | >150 mg/dL | >8.33 mmol/L |

# Credits

## Plates

Plate 13 *(bottom)* King, BG, and Showers, MJ: Human Anatomy and Physiology. 6th ed. Philadelphia, WB Saunders Company, 1969.

## Illustrations and Tables

Page 279 Bargmann, W: Histologie und Mikronscopische Anatomie des Menschen. Stuttgart. Georg Thieme Verlag, 1977.

351 Courtesy of RG Worton. *In* Thompson, MW: Genetics in Medicine. 4th ed. Philadelphia, WB Saunders Company, 1986.

638 Chou, T-C: Electrocardiography in Clinical Practice. 3rd ed. Philadelphia, WB Saunders Company, 1991.

1302 Bernstein, AD, et al: The NASPE/BPEG Generic Pacemaker Code for Antibradyarrhythmia and Adaptive-Rate Pacing and Antitachyarrhythmia Devices. PACE10:794, 1987.

Page 1493 Bennett, JC, Plum, F, eds.: Cecil Textbook of Medicine, 20th ed. Philadelphia, WB Saunders Company, 1996.

1875 Markell, EK, John, DT, Krotoski, WA: Markell and Voge's Medical Parasitology. 8th ed. Philadelphia, WB Saunders Company, 1999.

1876 Henry, JB: Clinical Diagnosis and Management by Laboratory Methods. 19th ed. Philadelphia, WB Saunders Company, 1996.

1888 Meschan, I: Synopsis of Radiologic Anatomy with Computed Tomography. Revised Reprint. Philadelphia, WB Saunders Company, 1980.

## Color Insert

Hematopoiesis
Carr, JH, Rodak, BF: Clinical Hematology Atlas. Philadelphia, WB Saunders Company, 1999.

Erythrocyte Abnormalities
Carr, JH, Rodak, BF: Clinical Hematology Atlas, Philadelphia, WB Saunders Company, 1999.

Stains
Bibbo, M, ed.: Comprehensive Cytopathology, 2nd ed. Philadelphia, WB Saunders Company, 1997 (I-A, I-D, I-E, II).
Henry, JB, ed.: Clinical Diagnosis and Management by Laboratory Methods. 19th ed. Philadelphia, WB Saunders Company, 1996 (I-C, I-F).

Kumar, V, Cotran, RS, Robbins, SL: Basic Pathology, 6th ed. WB Saunders Company, 1997 (IB).

Infectious Disease
Cotran, RS, Kumar, V, Collins, T, eds.: Robbins Pathologic Basis of Disease, 6th ed. Philadelphia, WB Saunders Company, 1999 (I-A through C, I-E, II-A, II-B through E).
Goldman L, and Bennett JC, eds.: Cecil Textbook of Medicine, 21st ed. Philadelphia, WB Saunders Company, 2000 (I-D, II-F).

Skin Lesions
Goldman L, and Bennett JC, eds.: Cecil Textbook of Medicine, 21st ed. Philadelphia, WB Saunders Company, 2000 (I and II).